WITHDRAWN

SINGLE USER SOFTWARE & LICENCE AGREEMENT

PLEASE READ THE FOLLOWING AGREEMENT CAREFULLY BEFORE USING THIS PRODUCT. THIS PRODUCT IS LICENSED UNDER THE TERMS CONTAINED IN THIS LICENCE AGREEMENT ('Agreement'). BY USING THIS PRODUCT, YOU, AN INDIVIDUAL OR ENTITY INCLUDING EMPLOYEES, AGENTS AND REPRESENTATIVES ('You' or 'Your'), ACKNOWLEDGE THAT YOU HAVE READ THIS AGREEMENT, THAT YOU UNDERSTAND IT, AND THAT YOU AGREE TO BE BOUND BY THE TERMS AND CONDITIONS OF THIS AGREEMENT. ELSEVIER LIMITED ('Elsevier') EXPRESSLY DOES NOT AGREE TO LICENSE THIS PRODUCT TO YOU UNLESS YOU ASSENT TO THIS AGREEMENT. IF YOU DO NOT AGREE WITH ANY OF THE FOLLOWING TERMS, YOU MAY, WITHIN THIRTY (30) DAYS AFTER YOUR RECEIPT OF THIS PRODUCT RETURN THE UNUSED PRODUCT AND ALL ACCOMPANYING DOCUMENTATION TO ELSEVIER FOR A FULL REFUND.

DEFINITIONS As used in this Agreement, these terms shall have the following meanings:

'Proprietary Material' means the valuable and proprietary information content of this Product including without limitation all indexes and graphic materials and software used to access, index, search and retrieve the information content from this Product developed or licensed by Elsevier and/or its affiliates, suppliers and licensors.

'Product' means the copy of the Proprietary Material and any other material delivered on CD-ROM and any other human-readable or machine-readable materials enclosed with this Agreement, including without limitation documentation relating to the same.

OWNERSHIP This Product has been supplied by and is proprietary to Elsevier and/or its affiliates, suppliers and licensors. The copyright in the Product belongs to Elsevier and/or its affiliates, suppliers and licensors and is protected by the copyright, trademark, trade secret and other intellectual property laws of the United Kingdom and international treaty provisions, including without limitation the Universal Copyright Convention and the Berne Copyright Convention. You have no ownership rights in this Product. Except as expressly set forth herein, no part of this Product, including without limitation the Proprietary Material, may be modified, copied or distributed in hardcopy or machine-readable form without prior written consent from Elsevier. All rights not expressly granted to You herein are expressly reserved. Any other use of this Product by any person or entity is strictly prohibited and a violation of this Agreement.

SCOPE OF RIGHTS LICENSED (PERMITTED USES) Elsevier is granting to You a limited, non-exclusive, non-transferable licence to use this Product in accordance with the terms of this Agreement. You may use or provide access to this Product on a single computer or terminal physically located at Your premises and in a secure network or move this Product to and use it on another single computer or terminal at the same location for personal use only, but under no circumstances may You use or provide access to any part or parts of this Product on more than one computer or terminal simultaneously.

You shall not (a) copy, download, or otherwise reproduce the Product or any part(s) thereof in any medium, including, without limitation, online transmissions, local area networks, wide area networks, intranets, extranets and the Internet, or in any way, in whole or in part, except for printing out or downloading nonsubstantial portions of the text and images in the Product for Your own personal use; (b) alter, modify, or adapt the Product or any part(s) thereof, including but not limited to decompiling, disassembling, reverse engineering, or creating derivative works, without the prior written approval of Elsevier; (c) sell, license or otherwise distribute to third parties the Product or any part(s) thereof; or (d) alter, remove, obscure or obstruct the display of any copyright, trademark or other proprietary notice on or in the Product or on any printout or download of portions of the Proprietary Materials.

RESTRICTIONS ON TRANSFER This Licence is personal to You, and neither Your rights hereunder nor the tangible embodiments of this Product, including without limitation the Proprietary Material, may be sold, assigned, transferred or sublicensed to any other person, including without limitation by operation of law, without the prior written consent of Elsevier. Any purported sale, assignment, transfer or sublicense without the prior written consent of Elsevier will be void and will automatically terminate the Licence granted hereunder.

TERM This Agreement will remain in effect until terminated pursuant to the terms of this Agreement. You may terminate this Agreement at any time by removing from Your system and destroying the Product and any copies of the Proprietary Material. Unauthorized copying of the Product, including without limitation, the Proprietary Material and documentation, or otherwise failing to comply with the terms and conditions of this Agreement shall result in automatic termination of this licence and will make available to Elsevier legal remedies. Upon termination of this Agreement, the licence granted herein will terminate and You must immediately destroy the Product and all copies of the Product and of the Proprietary Material, together with any and all accompanying documentation. All provisions relating to proprietary rights shall survive termination of this Agreement.

LIMITED WARRANTY AND LIMITATION OF LIABILITY Elsevier warrants that the software embodied in this Product will perform in substantial compliance with the documentation supplied in this Product, unless the performance problems are the result of hardware failure or improper use. If You report a significant defect in performance in writing to Elsevier within ninety (90) calendar days of your having purchased the Product, and Elsevier is not able to correct same within sixty (60) days after its receipt of Your notification, You may return this Product, including all copies and documentation, to Elsevier and Elsevier will refund Your money. In order to apply for a refund on your purchased Product, please contact the return address on the invoice to obtain the refund request form ('Refund Request Form'), and either fax or mail your signed request and your proof of purchase to the address indicated on the Refund Request Form. Incomplete forms will not be processed. Defined terms in the Refund Request Form shall have the same meaning as in this Agreement.

YOU UNDERSTAND THAT, EXCEPT FOR THE LIMITED WARRANTY RECITED ABOVE, ELSEVIER, ITS AFFILIATES, LICENSORS, THIRD PARTY SUPPLIERS AND AGENTS (TOGETHER 'THE SUPPLIERS') MAKE NO REPRESENTATIONS OR WARRANTIES, WITH RESPECT TO THE PRODUCT, INCLUDING, WITHOUT LIMITATION THE PROPRIETARY MATERIAL. ALL OTHER REPRESENTATIONS, WARRANTIES, CONDITIONS OR OTHER TERMS, WHETHER EXPRESS OR IMPLIED BY STATUTE OR COMMON LAW, ARE HEREBY EXCLUDED TO THE FULLEST EXTENT PERMITTED BY LAW.

IN PARTICULAR BUT WITHOUT LIMITATION TO THE FOREGOING NONE OF THE SUPPLIERS MAKE ANY REPRESENTATIONS OR WARRANTIES (WHETHER EXPRESS OR IMPLIED) REGARDING THE PERFORMANCE OF YOUR PAD, NETWORK OR COMPUTER SYSTEM WHEN USED IN CONJUNCTION WITH THE PRODUCT, NOR THAT THE PRODUCT WILL MEET YOUR REQUIREMENTS OR THAT ITS OPERATION WILL BE UNINTERRUPTED OR ERROR-FREE.

EXCEPT IN RESPECT OF DEATH OR PERSONAL INJURY CAUSED BY THE SUPPLIERS' NEGLIGENCE AND TO THE FULLEST EXTENT PERMITTED BY LAW, IN NO EVENT (AND REGARDLESS OF WHETHER SUCH DAMAGES ARE FORESEEABLE AND OF WHETHER SUCH LIABILITY IS BASED IN TORT, CONTRACT OR OTHERWISE) WILL ANY OF THE SUPPLIERS BE LIABLE TO YOU FOR ANY DAMAGES (INCLUDING, WITHOUT LIMITATION, ANY LOST PROFITS, LOST SAVINGS OR OTHER SPECIAL, INDIRECT, INCIDENTAL OR CONSEQUENTIAL DAMAGES ARISING OUT OF OR RESULTING FROM: (I) YOUR USE OF, OR INABILITY TO USE, THE PRODUCT; (II) DATA LOSS OR CORRUPTION; AND/OR (III) ERRORS OR OMISSIONS IN THE PROPRIETARY MATERIAL.

IF THE FOREGOING LIMITATION IS HELD TO BE UNENFORCEABLE, OUR MAXIMUM LIABILITY TO YOU IN RESPECT THEREOF SHALL NOT EXCEED THE AMOUNT OF THE LICENCE FEE PAID BY YOU FOR THE PRODUCT. THE REMEDIES AVAILABLE TO YOU AGAINST ELSEVIER AND THE LICENSORS OF MATERIALS INCLUDED IN THE PRODUCT ARE EXCLUSIVE.

If the information provided in the Product contains medical or health sciences information, it is intended for professional use within the medical field. Information about medical treatment or drug dosages is intended strictly for professional use, and because of rapid advances in the medical sciences, independent verification of diagnosis and drug dosages should be made.

The provisions of this Agreement shall be severable, and in the event that any provision of this Agreement is found to be legally unenforceable, such unenforceability shall not prevent the enforcement or any other provision of this Agreement.

GOVERNING LAW This Agreement shall be governed by the laws of England and Wales. In any dispute arising out of this Agreement, you and Elsevier each consent to the exclusive personal jurisdiction and venue in the courts of England and Wales.

GRAY'S Anatomy

The Anatomical Basis of Clinical Practice

THIRTY-NINTH EDITION

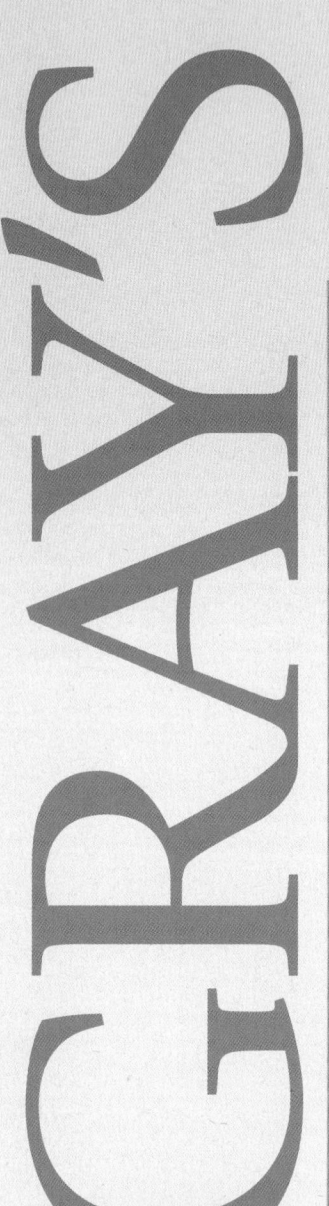

GRAY'S Anatomy

The Anatomical Basis of Clinical Practice

EDITOR-IN-CHIEF

Susan Standring PhD DSc

Professor of Experimental Neurobiology and Head, Division of Anatomy, Cell and Human Biology,
Guy's, King's and St Thomas' School of Biomedical Sciences, King's College London, London, UK

LEAD EDITORS

Harold Ellis CBE MCh FRCS

Emeritus Professor of Surgery of the former Westminster Hospital Medical School,
Clinical Anatomist, Division of Anatomy, Cell and Human Biology,
Guy's, King's and St Thomas' School of Biomedical Sciences, King's College London, London, UK

Jeremiah C Healy MA MB BChir MRCP FRCR

Consultant Radiologist, Chelsea and Westminster Hospital, London, UK

David Johnson MA BM BCh DM FRCS(Eng)

Specialist Registrar in Plastic and Reconstructive Surgery,
Department of Plastic and Reconstructive Surgery, Radcliffe Infirmary, Oxford, UK

Andrew Williams MB BS FRCS FRCS(Orth)

Consultant Orthopaedic Surgeon, Trauma and Orthopaedics Department,
Chelsea and Westminster Hospital, London, UK

THEME EDITORS

Patricia Collins PhD

Associate Professor of Anatomy, Anglo-European College of Chiropractic, Bournemouth, UK

Caroline Wigley BSc PhD

Honorary University Teaching Fellow, The Peninsula Medical School, Exeter, UK

THIRTY-NINTH EDITION

EDITORS

Barry KB Berkovitz BDS FDSRCS(Eng) MSc PhD
(Chapters 25, 27, 29–33, 35, 36, 38 & 41)
Reader, Division of Anatomy, Cell and Human Biology,
Guy's, King's and St Thomas' School of Biomedical Sciences,
King's College London, London, UK

Neil R Borley FRCS FRCS(Ed) MS
(Chapters 66–89 & 108)
Consultant Colorectal Surgeon,
Department of Gastrointestinal Surgery,
Cheltenham General Hospital,
Gloucestershire Hospitals NHS Trust, Cheltenham, UK

Alan R Crossman BSc PhD DSc
(Chapters 12, 13, 15–19 & 21–24)
Professor of Anatomy,
The University of Manchester, Manchester, UK

Mark S Davies MB BS FRCS FRCS(Orth)
(Chapter 115)
Consultant Orthopaedic Surgeon,
Guy's and St Thomas' Hospitals,
and The London Foot and Ankle Centre,
The Hospital of St John and St Elizabeth, London, UK

MJ Turlough FitzGerald MD, PhD, DSc, MRIA
(Chapter 20)
Emeritus Professor of Anatomy,
National University of Ireland, Galway, Ireland

Jonathan Glass MB BS FRCS(Urol)
(Chapters 91–101)
Consultant Urologist,
Guy's and St Thomas' Hospitals, London, UK

Carole M Hackney PhD
(Chapter 39)
Professor of Auditory Neuroscience,
MacKay Institute of Communication and Neuroscience,
School of Life Sciences, Keele University, Keele, UK

Thomas Ind MD MRCOG
(Chapters 102–107)
Consultant Gynaecological Surgeon,
Royal Marsden and St George's Hospitals, London, UK

Anthony R Mundy MS FRCP FRCS
(Chapters 91–101 & 108)
Professor of Urology,
Institute of Urology and Nephrology, London, UK

Richard LM Newell BSc MB BS FRCS
(Chapters 44–46 & 110–114)
Clinical Anatomist, Cardiff School of Biosciences,
Cardiff University, Wales, and Honorary Consultant Orthopaedic Surgeon,
Royal Devon and Exeter Healthcare NHS Trust,
Exeter, UK

The late Gordon L Ruskell PhD
(Chapter 42)
Emeritus Professor, Department of Optometry and Visual Science,
City University, London, UK

Pallav Shah MD FRCP
(Chapters 56–60 & 62–64)
Consultant Physician,
Royal Brompton Hospital, London, and
Department of Respiratory Medicine,
Chelsea and Westminster Hospital,
London, UK

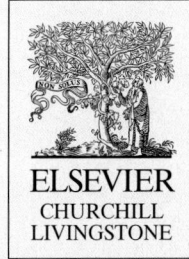

ELSEVIER
CHURCHILL
LIVINGSTONE

EDINBURGH • LONDON • NEW YORK • OXFORD • PHILADELPHIA • ST LOUIS • SYDNEY • TORONTO • 2005

ELSEVIER
CHURCHILL LIVINGSTONE

© Elsevier Ltd 2005

No part of this publication may be reproduced, stored in a retrieval system, or transmitted in any form or by any means, electronic, mechanical, photocopying, recording or otherwise, without either the prior permission of the publishers or a licence permitting restricted copying in the United Kingdom issued by the Copyright Licensing Agency, 90 Tottenham Court Road, London W1T 4LP. Permissions may be sought directly from Elsevier's Health Sciences Rights Department in Philadelphia, USA: phone: (+1) 215 238 7869, fax: (+1) 215 238 2239, e-mail: healthpermissions@elsevier.com. You may also complete your request on-line via the Elsevier homepage (http://www.elsevier.com), by selecting 'Customer Support' and then 'Obtaining Permissions'.

First edition JW Parker & Son 1858
Second edition 1860
Third to eleventh editions, Longman, Green & Co. 1864–1887
Twenty-fifth edition Longman, Green & Co. 1932
Twenty-sixth edition Longman, Green & Co. 1935
Twenty-seventh edition Longman, Green and Co. 1938
Twenty-eighth edition Longman, Green & Co. 1942
Twenty-ninth edition Longman, Green & Co. 1947
Thirtieth edition Longman, Green & Co. 1949
Thirty-first edition Longman, Green & Co. 1954
Thirty-second (centenary) edition Longman, Green & Co. 1958
Thirty-third edition Longman 1964
Thirty-fourth edition Longman 1967
Thirty-fifth edition Longman 1973
Thirty-sixth edition Churchill Livingstone 1980
Thirty-seventh edition Churchill Livingstone 1989
Thirty-eighth edition Churchill Livingstone 1999
Thirty-ninth edition Elsevier Limited 2005
Reprinted 2005

ISBN:
Main Edition 0 443 07168 3
International Student Edition 0 443 07169 1
edition™ 0 443 06676 0
edition™ online access only 0 443 06675 2

British Library Cataloguing in Publication Data
A catalogue record for this book is available from the British Library

Library of Congress Cataloging in Publication Data
A catalog record for this book is available from the Library of Congress

For Elsevier

Commissioning Editors: Inta Ozols, Richard Furn
Senior Project Development Manager: Alison Whitehouse
Project Development Managers: Martin Mellor, with Jim Killgore and Gus Gomes
Head of Project Management: Colin Arthur
Project Manager: Lesley W Small
Illustration Manager: Bruce Hogarth
Illustrators (39th edition): Robert Britton, Graeme Chambers, Michael Courtney, Peter Cox, Ethan Danielson, Brian Evans, Sandie Hill, Bruce Hogarth, Gillian Lee, Gillian Oliver, Richard Tibbitts (Antbits), Philip Wilson
Illustrators (recent editions): Andrew Bezear, Marks Creative, Patrick Elliot, Jenny Halstead, Dr AA van Horssen, Peter Jack, Peter Lamb, Paul Richardson, Lesley J Skeates, Denise Smith
Photographers: Sarah-Jane Smith (38th and 39th editions), Kevin Fitzpatrick (38th edition)
Designers: Sarah Russell, Keith Kail
Copyeditors: Carolyn Holleyman, with Lewis Derrick, Sue Lowry and Ruth Swan
Proofreaders: Isobel Black, Christian Simpson, Ian Ross
Index: Merrall-Ross International Ltd

The publisher's policy is to use **paper manufactured from sustainable forests**

Printed in Spain

Preface

When I was a student at Guy's Hospital Medical School, London, in the mid sixties, anatomy was regarded as one of the cornerstones of basic medical science. I remember using the 33rd edition of *Gray's Anatomy*, not as a course book, but as a source of additional information and detailed illustration: it became an old friend. I still have my copy and often refer to it – indeed it was used when preparing some of the illustrations in this new edition.

Almost four decades later, anatomy occupies a less prominent place within an overcrowded undergraduate medical curriculum. Paradoxically, over the same period, the need for detailed anatomical knowledge at the postgraduate level has increased dramatically, fuelled particularly by developments in imaging and computer-assisted three-dimensional reconstruction (both macro- and microscopically); anaesthetics; endoscopic surgery, and the miniaturization of instruments. Anatomists and clinicians have learned to look with a fresh eye at familiar structures revealed in new ways, e.g. the arthroscopic appearance of joint cavities; high-resolution CT images of the petrous bone; images of the coronary circulation during MRI-guided cardiovascular catheter-based interventions; radionuclide imaging of the thyroid gland.

As I write this, I have opened in front of me on my desk an English translation of Wilhelm Braune's *Atlas of Topographical Anatomy*, which was published by J and A Churchill in 1877: it contains detailed woodcuts of plane sections of frozen bodies, and displays a level of detail comparable with that seen in the best modern atlases of sectional anatomy. The following passage from the translator's preface to Braune's Atlas (published in Liepsig [sic] in 1874) speaks about the fundamental place of anatomy in medicine. *'By means of the sections found in this Atlas the exact position and relations of the structures which must be divided or avoided in the course of an operation are indicated: and the track of a bullet or puncture wound suggested. At the same time they afford an absolutely correct representation of the intimate relations of the viscera of the thorax and abdomen.'* For clinicians who work at the cutting edge (quite literally) of medicine, the message has not changed over the intervening years – anatomical knowledge remains an essential item in their armamentarium.

The 39th edition of *Gray's Anatomy* is radically different from earlier editions because the body is described in regions rather than in systems. In an ideal world, an anatomical reference book should contain both systematic and regional anatomy. In the real world, the editorial team for the 39th edition decided that a book which would be of the greatest benefit to practising clinicians should mirror their daily practice and describe anatomy in the way in which they use it, i.e. regionally. Talking to colleagues around the world, this view has been the one that we have heard most frequently. We have responded to these comments by updating and clarifying the text, and have also paid particular attention to issues of navigability and clinical relevance.

The members of the editorial team who have worked with me in preparing the 39th edition brought a wide range of experience as academic anatomists and clinicians: I am indebted to them all for their dedication and enthusiasm. The Lead Editors – Harold Ellis, Jeremiah Healy, David Johnson and Andrew Williams – have been responsible with me for overseeing the revision of specific parts of the book, initially by drawing together relevant material from the various sections of the 38th edition, and subsequently by guiding and advising the Editors of the sections and chapters. They also helped me to take strategic decisions about the overall content and organization of the 39th edition. Thus, for example, we have included descriptions of the blood supply to the skin and muscles, on the grounds that they have surgical relevance when raising flaps for reconstructive surgery, and we have made extensive use of new imaging modalities. The Theme Editors, Caroline Wigley and Pat Collins, worked closely with all members of the editorial team to update microstructure and embryology respectively throughout the book.

The work of drilling down into the existing text, updating it and setting it in a clinical context, was undertaken by the Editors of the sections and chapters, a group of clinicians and anatomists (sometimes both) with a wealth of experience of teaching applied anatomy and neuroanatomy to medical and dental undergraduates and postgraduates. Editors and Specialist Contributors have provided new insights into topics such as the anatomy of the pelvic floor, inner ear, peritoneum, preimplantation embryology, assisted fertilization, spread of infection via fascial planes in the head and neck, smooth and cardiac muscle, wrist kinematics and kinetics, and the temporomandibular joint. Neuroanatomy has been comprehensively revised and now focuses on the human nervous system. The manuscript has been submitted to rigorous scrutiny by Specialist Reviewers (who commented on specific chapters), and by General Reviewers (who were able to comment on the text at first proof stage): their comments have been incorporated into the text. I am grateful to them all for their encouragement and suggestions.

As far as possible, the orientation of diagrams and photographs throughout the book has been standardized to show the left side of the body, irrespective of whether a lateral or medial view is presented; transverse sections are viewed from below to facilitate comparison with clinical images. Clinicopathological examples have been selected where the pathology is either a direct result of, or a consequence of, the anatomy, or where the anatomical features are instrumental in the diagnosis/treatment/management of the condition. Wherever possible, the new photomicrographs illustrate human histology and embryology. I recognize that re-orientating a great many of the illustrations from previous editions has created an enormous amount of work for the artwork staff, who were asked to reposition thousands of leader lines and their associated names. I am very grateful to Dr Michael Hutchinson for checking the accuracy of these changes. However, I have no doubt that eagle-eyed readers will alert me to any errors that may have slipped undetected through several iterations of proof reading of both text and figures.

The Lead Editorial team took the view that *Gray's Anatomy* is not, and should not attempt to be, a source book for molecular biology, pathology, neuroscience, physiology or operative procedures. Moreover, space considerations mean that it is not an appropriate vehicle in which to rehearse experimental data, and preclude the level of descriptive detail that is found in highly specialized dedicated texts. Mindful of these caveats, reference lists have been provided at the end of all but a few very short chapters to guide further reading: the references have been annotated when the content of the paper or book is not evident from its title. A list of general texts and references covering material presented in more than one chapter, e.g. the distribution of angiosomes, or other basic medical sciences, is included on page xv.

I offer my thanks to the production team at Elsevier, initially under the leadership of Richard Furn (1999–2002) and latterly of Inta Ozols (2003–2004), for their guidance, professionalism, good humour and unfailing support. In what has truly been a team effort, it is difficult to single out individuals for especial mention.

I would like to place on record my heartfelt thanks to Alison Whitehouse, Colin Arthur, Martin Mellor and Lesley Small, for being at the end of a phone or e-mail whenever I needed advice. I am grateful to Guy Standring, my long-suffering husband, for his patience and tolerance throughout the last four years.

Susan Standring
August 2004

Specialist contributors and reviewers

SPECIALIST CONTRIBUTORS

Dr Leila Abbas
Whitfield Laboratory, Centre for Developmental Genetics,
Department of Biomedical Science, University of Sheffield,
Sheffield, UK

Dr Martin E Atkinson
Senior Lecturer, Department of Biomedical Science,
University of Sheffield, Sheffield, UK

Professor Clive Bartram
Consultant Radiologist, St Mark's Hospital,
Harrow, and Honorary Professor of Gastrointestinal Radiology,
Faculty of Medicine, Imperial College, London, UK

Dr Gina Brown
Consultant Radiologist and Honorary Senior Lecturer,
The Royal Marsden Hospital NHS Trust, Surrey, UK

Professor Helen M Cox
Professor of Pharmacology, Centre for Neuroscience Research,
Guy's, King's and St Thomas' School of Biomedical Sciences,
King's College London, London, UK

Dr Wolfgang Hamann
Senior Lecturer in Pain Management,
Guy's, King's and St Thomas' School of Biomedical Sciences,
Pain Management Centre, St Thomas' Hospital, London, UK

Mr Simon A Hickey
Consultant ENT Surgeon, ENT Department,
Torbay Hospital, Devon, UK

Professor John D Langdon
Department of Maxillofacial Surgery,
Guy's, King's and St Thomas' Dental Institute,
King's College Hospital, London, UK

Miss Vivien C Lees
Consultant Plastic and Hand Surgeon,
Department of Plastic Surgery, Wythenshawe Hospital,
Manchester, UK

Dr Daniel E Lieberman
Professor of Anthropology, Peabody Museum,
Harvard University, Cambridge, USA

Professor Vishy Mahadevan
The Royal College of Surgeons of England, London, UK

Professor BJ Moxham
Professor of Anatomy and Deputy Director (Head of Teaching) in
Biosciences, Cardiff School of Biosciences, Cardiff University,
Cardiff, UK

Professor Jeff Osborn
Professor Emeritus, Faculty of Dentistry, University of Alberta,
Alberta, Canada

Dr Ruth Richardson
Research Associate, Centre for Medical Humanities,
University College London, and The Wellcome Trust Centre for
The History of Medicine at University College London, London, UK

Mr Gregory P Sadler
Consultant Endocrine Surgeon, John Radcliffe Hospital, Oxford, UK

Dr Allan Thexton
[Formerly] Division of Physiology,
Guy's, King's and St Thomas' School of Biomedical Sciences,
King's College London, London, UK

Mr Giles Toogood
Consultant Hepatobiliary Surgeon,
St James's University Hospital, Leeds, UK

CRITICAL REVIEWERS

Dr Michael A Adams
Senior Research Fellow, Department of Anatomy,
University of Bristol, Bristol, UK

Professor Tipu Aziz
Consultant Neurosurgeon, Radcliffe Infirmary, Oxford,
and Charing Cross Hospital, London, UK

Mr John Bidmead
Consultant Urogynaecologist, King's College Hospital, London, UK

Professor Peter Braude
Head of Department of Women's Health,
Guy's, King's and St Thomas' School of Medicine,
St Thomas' Hospital, London, UK

Dr Robert Brooks
Lecturer, Division of Anatomy, Cell and Human Biology,
Guy's, King's and St Thomas' School of Biomedical Sciences,
London, UK

Dr Paul Cartwright
Consultant Anaesthetist, Derby City Hospital, Derby, UK

Dr Fred Cody
Senior Lecturer, The University of Manchester, Manchester, UK

Mr Steven A Corbett
Consultant Orthopaedic Surgeon,
Guy's and St Thomas' Hospitals NHS Trust, London, UK

Mr Michael Dilkes
Consultant Ear, Nose and Throat Surgeon, and Honorary Senior
Lecturer, St Bartholomew's Hospital, London, UK

Dr Michael A Gatzoulis
Consultant Cardiologist, Director, Adult Congenital Heart Unit,
Royal Brompton Hospital, London, UK

Professor Paul Griffiths
Professor of Radiology, University of Sheffield,
Royal Hallamshire Hospital, Sheffield, UK

Dr Mike Hall
Consultant Neonatologist, and Honorary Senior Clinical Lecturer in
Child Health, Princess Anne Hospital, Southampton, UK

Dr Michael Hutchinson
Clinical Anatomist, Division of Anatomy, Cell and Human Biology,
Guy's, King's and St Thomas' School of Biomedical Sciences,
King's College London, London, UK

Professor Alan Jackson
Professor of Neuroradiology,
Department of Imaging Science and Biomedical Engineering,
The University of Manchester, Manchester, UK

Dr Mark Johnson
Senior Lecturer, Obstetrics and Gynaecology,
Chelsea and Westminster Hospital, Imperial College School of
Medicine at Chelsea and Westminster Hospital, London, UK

Dr Jonathan C Kentish
Reader in Pharmacology,
Centre for Cardiovascular Biology and Medicine,
King's College London, The Rayne Institute,
St Thomas's Hospital, London, UK

Professor Birgit Lane
Cox Professor of Anatomy and Cell Biology,
Cancer Research UK Cell Structure Research Group,
Division of Cell and Developmental Biology,
University of Dundee School of Life Sciences, Dundee, UK

Professor Andres Lozano
Professor and R R Tasker Chair in Neurosurgery,
Division of Neurosurgery, Toronto Western Hospital,
University of Toronto, Toronto, Canada

Dr Alison McGregor
Senior Lecturer in Biodynamics, Division of Surgery,
Anaesthetics and Intensive Care, Faculty of Medicine,
Imperial College, Charing Cross Hospital, London, UK

Professor Peter Morgan
Professor of Oral Pathology and Honorary Consultant,
Guy's, King's and St Thomas' Hospitals Dental Institute, London, UK

Professor David Neary
Professor of Neurology, Department of Neurology,
Hope Hospital, Salford, UK

Professor John Pepper
Professor of Cardiac Surgery, Imperial College School of Medicine,
London, and Consultant Surgeon, Department of Surgery,
Royal Brompton Hospital, London, UK

Dr Susan Pickering
Senior Lecturer, Women's Services, King's College London,
Division of Women's Health, Guy's and St Thomas' Hospitals,
London, UK

Professor Mary Ritter
Director, Graduate School of Life Sciences and Medicine,
Department of Immunology, Division of Medicine,
Imperial College, London, UK

Dr Anthea Rowlerson
Lecturer in Physiology, Guy's, King's and St Thomas' School of
Biomedical Sciences, London, UK

Professor Jeremy PT Ward
Professor of Respiratory Cell Physiology,
Department of Asthma, Allergy and Respiratory Science,
King's College London, London, UK

Mr David Woods
Consultant Orthopaedic Surgeon, Great Western Hospital,
Swindon, UK

Professor Stuart Stanton
Emeritus Professor, St George's Hospital Medical School,
London, UK

GENERAL REVIEWERS

Riaz Agha
Guy's, King's and St Thomas' School of Biomedical Sciences,
King's College London, London, UK

Professor Kirby I Bland
Professor and Chairman, Department of Surgery,
Deputy Director of the Comprehensive Cancer Center,
University of Alabama at Birmingham, Birmingham, USA

Professor John D Corson
Professor of Vascular Surgery,
University of Iowa Health Care, Iowa City, USA

Professor Charles Cummings
Andelot Professor, Otolaryngology–Head and Neck Surgery,
The Johns Hopkins Hospital, Baltimore, USA

Professor Daniel J Deziel
Senior Attending Surgeon at Rush–Presbyterian–St. Luke's Medical
Center, Professor of Surgery at Rush Medical College,
Chicago, USA

Mr David Evans
Consultant Hand Surgeon and Director,
The Hand Clinic, Windsor, and Honorary Consultant Hand Surgeon,
The Royal National Orthopaedic Hospital, London, UK

Professor Mark K Ferguson
Professor of Surgery, University of Chicago, Chicago, USA

Professor Lee A Fleisher
Professor and Chair of Anesthesia, Professor of Medicine,
University of Pennsylvania School of Medicine, Philadelphia, USA

Professor Thomas R Gest
Associate Professor of Anatomy,
Director of the Anatomical Donations Program,
University of Michigan Medical School, Office of Medical Education,
Ann Arbor, USA

Dr Duaine Haines
Chairman and Professor of Anatomy,
University of Mississippi Medical Center, Jackson, USA

Dr Rajeev M Joshi
Professor of Surgery, LTM Medical College, Mumbai, India

Dr John Paul Judson
Associate Dean (VMU) and Associate Professor of Human Biology,
Cells and Molecules, International Medical University,
Kuala Lumpur, Malaysia

Professor Subramaniam Krishnan
Head of Department of Anatomy, Faculty of Medicine,
University of Malaya, Kuala Lumpur, Malaysia

Professor Ling Eng Ang
Head of Department of Anatomy, National University of Singapore,
Singapore

Professor Nancy M Major
Associate Professor of Radiology,
Duke University Medical Center, Durham, USA

Professor Suleman Merchant
Head, Department of Radiology and Imaging,
LTM Medical College and General Hospital, Mumbai, India

Professor Gillian Morriss-Kay
Department of Human Anatomy and Genetics,
University of Oxford, Oxford, UK

Dr Ian Parkin
Clinical Anatomist, Department of Anatomy,
Cambridge University, Cambridge, UK

Professor Thomas H Quinn
Professor of Anatomy, Creighton University School of Medicine,
Omaha, USA

Dr Lakshmi Selvaratnam
Department of Anatomy, Faculty of Medicine,
University of Malaya, Kuala Lumpur, Malaysia

Professor Roger Soames
Associate Professor and Head of Anatomy,
School of Biomedical Sciences, James Cook University,
Townsville, Australia

Dr Anil H Walji
Professor and Director, Division of Anatomy,
Professor of Radiology and Diagnostic Imaging,
Faculty of Medicine and Dentistry, University of Alberta,
Edmonton, Canada

Acknowledgements

We are indebted to Dr Michael Hutchinson for checking the labelling and placement of labels in anatomical illustrations across the book.

NEW PHOTOGRAPHY COMMISSIONED FOR THIS EDITION

We thank Sarah-Jane Smith for the following photos

Microstructure: 3.4, 3.10, 3.15, 3.17, 3.19, 5.2, 5.4A–F, 5.6, 5.8, 5.12, 5.13, 5.14, 5.18, 6.6, 6.15, 6.17, 6.19A, 6.20, 6.28, 6.29, 6.37, 6.42, 6.48, 7.15, 7.17, 8.4, 8.8, 8.11, 8.13, 8.14, 8.16, 8.17, 9.1, 9.2, 9.3, 17.1, 21.14, 21.15, 31.31, 33.40, 33.41, 58.3, 71.16A, 71.17, 72.1, 75.3, 75.4, 85.16, 86.5, 88.6, 88.7, 89.4, 89.6, 96.3, 104.6.

Osteology: 45.11, 45.17, 45.18, 45.19, 45.21, 45.22, 45.23, 45.24, 45.26, 45.31, 45.32, 45.33A, 45.34, 49.1A,B, 49.3, 49.4, 49.5, 49.6, 49.8A,B, 49.9A,B, 49.10A,B, 49.11, 52.5, 52.6, 52.7, 52.8, 52.12, 57.4A,B, 57.7, 57.8, 57.9A,B, 57.10A,B, 57.11A,B, 111.4A,B, 111.5A,B, 111.6, 111.15A,B, 111.16A,B, 111.17, 111.18, 111.19, 113.5, 113.6, 113.13, 114.1A,B, 114.2A,B, 114.5.

Surface anatomy: 25.1, 25.2, 25.3, 25.4, 25.5, 25.6, 25.7, 25.8, 44.1, 44.2, 44.3, 48.14, 48.15, 48.16A–C, 48.17, 56.3, 110.12, 110.13, 110.14, 110.15, 110.16, 110.17, 110.18, 110.19, 110.20, 110.21, 110.22, 110.24, 110.25, 110.26, 110.27.

Diagrammatic overlays for figures: 25.1, 25.2, 25.3, 25.4, 25.5, 25.6, 25.7, 25.8, 110.12, 110.13, 110.14, 110.15, 110.16, 110.17, 110.18, 110.20, 110.21, 110.22, 110.24.

PREVIOUSLY PUBLISHED ILLUSTRATIONS

Within individual figure captions, we have acknowledged all figures kindly loaned from other sources. However, we would particularly like to thank the following authors who have generously loaned so many figures from other books published by Elsevier:

Microstructure:
Kerr JB 1999 Atlas of Functional Histology. London: Mosby.
Figures 3.8, 3.9, 3.14, 4.23, 6.11, 7.5, 7.18, 7.21, 33.12B, 58.2B, 59.23, 71.18, 72.5, 85.14, 85.15, 87.7, 88.5, 91.17, 97.5A, 102.8, 103.5.

Kierszenbaum AL 2002 Histology and Cell Biology: An Introduction to Pathology. St Louis: Mosby.
Figures 3.6, 3.11, 4.16, 6.25, 8.3, 8.5, 32.5, 33.42, 59.17, 62.2, 62.3, 71.15, 96.4A,B, 97.7, 104.5.

Stevens A, Lowe JS 1996 Human Histology, 2nd edn. London: Mosby.
Figures 2.9, 2.17, 4.17, 31.30, 32.6, 62.5, 91.22, 92.4, 102.6, 102.9.

Young B, Heath JW 2000 Wheater's Functional Histology: A Text and Colour Atlas, 4th edn. Edinburgh: Churchill Livingstone
Figures 2.4, 2.5B, 2.12, 2.15, 2.16A,B, 2.18B, 2.24, 3.2, 3.3, 3.13, 3.16, 4.1, 4.10B,C, 5.11, 5.17, 6.41, 7.10, 7.20, 33.10, 33.11, 35.7A, 42.15, 58.5, 62.7, 62.8, 62.9, 72.3, 85.18, 91.19, 91.20, 97.4, 102.10.

Head and neck:
Berkovitz BKB, Holland GR, Moxham BJ 2002 Oral Anatomy, Embryology and Histology, 3rd edn. Edinburgh: Mosby.
Figures 33.2, 33.12A, 33.18B–E, 33.25, 33.26, 33.28, 33.29, 33.30, 33.32, 33.34, 34.10D, 35.12, Table 33.1.

Berkovitz BKB, Moxham BJ 1994 Color Atlas of the Skull. London: Mosby-Wolfe.
Figures 27.1, 27.3, 27.4, 27.5, 27.7, 27.8, 27.9, 27.10, 27.11, 27.13, 27.14, 27.16, 27.17, 27.19, 27.20, 27.21, 27.22, 27.23, 27.24, 27.25, 27.27, 27.28, 32.1, 32.2, 33.16.

Surface anatomy:
Lumley JSP 2002 Surface Anatomy: the Anatomical Basis of Clinical Examination, 2nd edn. Edinburgh: Churchill Livingstone.
Figures 27.2, 27.6, 41.15, 41.16, 48.13A,B, 48.18B, 56.1, 56.2, 56.4, 66.1, 66.2, 66.3, 66.4, 110.23.

Diagrammatic overlays for figures 25.1, 25.2, 25.3, 25.4, 25.5, 25.6, 25.7, 25.8, 110.12, 110.13, 110.14, 110.15, 110.16, 110.17, 110.18, 110.20, 110.21, 110.22, 110.24.

NEW ILLUSTRATIONS COMMISSIONED FOR THIS EDITION

We thank the illustrators for their valuable contribution to the new edition

Antbits: 1.1, 16.3, 16.11, 19.16, 19.18, 41.13, 59.1. All of surface anatomy and bones overlays.

Robert Britton: 2.1, 2.3, 2.5A, 2.6, 2.11, 2.18A, 2.22, 2.23, 3.1, 3.12, 4.11, 4.12, 4.27, 6.39, 7.3, 8.5, 8.12, 8.20, 8.22, 12.40, 21.3, 30.8, 30.11, 33.39, 39.22, 42.17, 42.19, 42.23, 59.18, 62.1, 62.6, 65.5, 71.14, 85.17, 87.6, 87.8, 102.5, 105.8, 110.29, 110.30, 110.31.

Graeme Chambers: 53.32.

Michael Courtney: 17.6, 17.7, 17.13, 17.15, 17.16, 45.50, 45.51, 45.52, 45.53, 45.55, 45.56, 45.57, 48.5, 49.16, 49.18, 49.21, 49.23, 49.24, 50.1, 50.2, 50.3, 50.4, 51.1, 51.9, 51.11, 51.12, 52.1, 52.2, 52.3, 52.9, 52.15, 52.16, 52.17, 52.18, 52.19, 52.20, 52.21, 52.22, 52.23, 53.2, 53.3, 53.4, 53.12, 53.34, 53.36, 53.37, 53.38, 53.40, 53.42, 53.43, 53.51, 53.52, 53.53, 53.55, 53.56, 53.58, 53.59, 63.5, 63.13, 64.3, 113.19, 115.1, 115.7, 115.17, 115.37, 115.42.

Peter Cox: 13.3, 13.15, 15.6, 15.10, 15.12, 16.2, 23.4, 23.5, 23.9, 23.12, 23.15, 23.16, 24.4, 24.5.

Ethan Danielson: 4.19, 6.49, 10.22, 10.23, 10.24, 11.1, 11.4, 11.5, 11.6B, 12.2, 14.5, 14.15, 14.26, 14.27, 14.28, 15.3, 18.10, 18.11, 18.12, 19.1, 19.17, 20.4, 20.6, 20.7, 20.8, 20.9, 20.10, 20.11, 20.12, 20.13, 20.14, 20.15, 22.30, 23.14, 26.6, 29.10, 31.18, 34.5, 34.8, 38.11, 45.1, 45.2, 45.5, 46.12, 47.6, 47.8, 47.9, 47.10, 48.1, 48.4, 49.27, 49.29, 54.2, 54.3, 57.1, 57.2, 61.3, 65.1, 72.4, 85.3, 89.5, 90.3, 90.5, 90.6, 91.12, 91.15, 97.6, 105.3, 109.1, 109.2, 109.3, 109.4, 109.5, 109.6, 109.7, 109.11, 109.12, 109.13, 109.14, 109.15, 109.16, 109.18, 109.19, 109.20, 110.4, 110.5, 110.9.

Brian Evans: 15.1, 15.3, 29.3, 29.15, 31.1, 31.4, 31.9, 31.26, 33.7, 41.4, 41.6, 76.1, 76.10, 76.11, 76.14, 76.16, 76.17, 82.1, 82.2, 83.8, 83.9, 108.2, 108.3, 108.9, 108.11, 108.12.

Sandie Hill: 35.2, 35.11A, 36.1, 36.2, 36.3, 36.4, 36.6, 36.7, 36.8, 36.9, 36.10, 36.11, 36.13, 36.14, 36.15, 67.4, 67.5B, 67.6B, 67.12, 67.13, 67.15, 67.16, 71.2, 71.11A,B, 73.1, 84.1, 84.3, 84.5B, 84.6A, 84.7, 85.1, 85.2, 85.3, 85.5, 85.12, 86.1, 87.2, 87.3, 87.4, 87.8.

Bruce Hogarth: 8.28, 16.5, 16.6, 16.9, 18.23, 19.13, 19.14, 19.23, 22.1, 22.3, 22.6, 29.2, 44.4, 45.3, 45.4, 48.6, 48.8, 53.34, 71.1, 71.3, 71.5, 71.8, 71.10, 71.12, 110.3, 110.28.

Gillian Lee: 6.33, 6.34, 6.35, 6.36, 31.2, 31.16, 32.3, 32.8, 33.43, 41.3, 41.22, 60.17, 63.1, 63.11, 63.34C, 69.2, 69.7, 92.2.

Gillian Oliver: 71.4.

Philip Wilson: 30.10, 44.6, 44.8, 45.5, 45.6, 45.10, 45.13, 45.14, 45.38, 45.41, 45.43, 45.44, 46.8, 46.11, 46.13, 49.9, 57.21, 58.4, 67.7, 68.1, 68.3, 68.4, 68.8, 68.12, 68.15, 76.15, 80.1, 92.3, 111.21.

COVER ILLUSTRATION

An oblique paracoronal shaded volume-rendition slab image of the head and neck superimposed on a photograph of a young male subject, posterior view. The image was derived from a coronally acquired T1-weighted volumetric magnetic resonance dataset: it was produced using a Voxar 3D workstation (Voxar Ltd, Edinburgh, Scotland).

Image supplied by Dr RJS Chinn, Consultant Radiologist, Chelsea and Westminster Hospital, London, UK.

Contents

Bibliography of selected titles

The following references contain information relevant to numerous chapters in this edition. They are therefore cited here rather than at the end of individual chapters.

TERMINOLOGY

Federative Committee on Anatomical Terminology 1998 Terminologia Anatomica. International Anatomical Nomenclature. Stuttgart: Thieme.

Dorland, 2003, Dorland's Illustrated Medical Dictionary, 30th edn. Philadelphia: W B Saunders.

BASIC SCIENCES

Abrahams PH, Marks SC Jr, Hutchings R 2002 McMinn's Colour Atlas of Human Anatomy, 5th edn. London: Churchill Livingstone.

Alberts B, Johnson A, Lewis J, Raff M, Roberts K, Walter P 2002 Molecular Biology of the Cell, 4th edn. New York: Garland Science Publishing.

Berkovitz BKB, Kirsh C, Moxham BJ, Alusi G, Cheeseman T 2002 Interactive Head and Neck. London: Primal Pictures.

Boron W, Boulpaep E 2002 Medical Physiology. Philadelphia: W B Saunders.

Crossman AR, Neary D 2000 Neuroanatomy, 2nd edn. Edinburgh: Churchill Livingstone.

Fitzgerald MJT, Folan-Curran J 2001 Clinical Neuroanatomy and Related Science, 4th edn. Edinburgh: Churchill Livingstone.

Guyton AC, Hall JE 1996 Human Physiology and Mechanisms of Disease, 6th edn. Philadelphia: W B Saunders.

Kerr JB 1999 Atlas of Functional Histology. London: Mosby.

Kierszenbaum AL 2002 Histology and Cell Biology: An Introduction to Pathology. St Louis: Mosby.

Moore KL, Persaud TVN 2003 Before We Are Born: Essentials of Embryology and Birth Defects, 6th edn. Philadelphia: W B Saunders.

Pollard TD, Earnshaw WC 2002 Cell Biology. Philadelphia: W B Saunders.

Roitt I, Brostoff J, Male D 2001 Immunology, 6th edn. London: Mosby.

Salmon M 1994 Anatomic Studies: Book 1 Arteries of the Muscles of the Extremities and the Trunk, Book 2 Arterial Anastomotic Pathways of the Extremities. Ed. by Taylor G, Razaboni RM. St Louis: Quality Medical Publishing Inc.

Stevens A, Lowe JS 1996 Human Histology, 2nd edn. London: Mosby.

Young B, Heath JW 2000 Wheater's Functional Histology: A Text and Colour Atlas. Edinburgh: Churchill Livingstone.

IMAGING AND RADIOLOGY/RADIOLOGICAL ANATOMY

Butler P, Mitchell AWM, Ellis H 1999 Applied Radiological Anatomy. New York: Cambridge University Press.

Ellis H, Dixon A, Logan BM 1999 Human Sectional Anatomy: Atlas of Body Sections, CT and MRI Images, 2nd edn. Oxford: Oxford University Press.

Haaga JR, Lanzieri CF, Gilkeson RC 2002 CT and MR Imaging of the Whole Body, 4th edn. St Louis: Mosby.

Lasjaunias P, Berenstein A, ter Brugge K 2001 Surgical Neuroangiography, vol 1. Clinical Vascular Anatomy and Variations, 2nd edn. Berlin, New York: Springer.

Meyers MA 1994 Dynamic Radiology of the Abdomen: Normal and Pathologic Anatomy, 4th edn. New York: Springer.

Pomeranz SJ 1992 MRI Total Body Atlas. Cincinnati: MRI-EFI Publications.

Sutton D 2002 Textbook of Radiology and Imaging, 7th edn. Edinburgh: Churchill Livingstone.

Weir J, Abrahams PH 2003 Imaging Atlas of Human Anatomy, 3rd edn. London: Mosby.

Wicke L 1998 Atlas of Radiologic Anatomy, 6th edn. Baltimore: Williams and Wilkins.

Whaites E 2002 Essential of Dental Radiography and Radiology, 3rd edn. Edinburgh: Churchill Livingstone.

CLINICAL

Birch R, Bonney G, Wynn Parry CB 1998 Surgical Disorders of the Peripheral Nerves. Edinburgh: Churchill Livingstone.

Bogduk N 1997 Clinical Anatomy of the Lumbar Spine and Sacrum, 3rd edn. Edinburgh: Churchill Livingstone.

Borges AF 1984 Relaxed skin tension lines (RSTL) versus other skin lines. Plast Reconstr Surg 73: 144–50.

Burnand K, Young A, Rowlands B, Scholefield J 2004 The New Aird's Companion in Surgical Studies, 3rd edn. Edinburgh: Churchill Livingstone.

Canale ST 2003 Campbell's Operative Orthopaedics, 10th edn. Philadelphia: Mosby.

Cormack GC, Lamberty BGH 1994 The Arterial Anatomy of Skin Flaps. Edinburgh: Churchill Livingstone.

Dyck PJ, Thomas PK 2004 Peripheral Neuropathy, 4th edn. Philadelphia: W B Saunders.

Ellis H 2002 Clinical Anatomy: A Revision and Applied Anatomy for Clinical Students, 10th edn. Maldem MA: Blackwell Scientific Publications.

Ellis H, Feldman S, Harrop-Griffiths W 2003 Anatomy for Anaesthetists, 8th edn. Oxford: Blackwell Science.

Rosai J 2004 Rosai and Ackerman's Surgical Pathology, 2-volume set with CD-ROM, 9th edn. London: Mosby

Shah J 2003 Head and Neck Surgery and Oncology, 3rd edn. Edinburgh; New York: Mosby

Taylor GI, Palmer JH, McManamy D 1987 The vascular territories of the body (angiosomes): experimental study and their clinical applications. In McCarthy JG, 1990, Plastic Surgery, vol I General Principles. Philadelphia: W B Saunders.

Zancolli E A, Cozzi E P 1992 Atlas of Surgical Anatomy of the Hand, Edinburgh: Churchill Livingstone.

CLINICAL EXAMINATION

Aids to the Examination of the Peripheral Nervous System, 4th Edition. London: W B Saunders, 2000.

Lumley JSP 2002 Surface Anatomy: The Anatomical Basis of Clinical Examination, 3rd edn. Edinburgh: Churchill Livingstone.

All references from the 38th edition are available on the website which accompanies the e-dition of Gray's Anatomy - ISBN 0443066760 for the book and website package, and ISBN 0443066752 for online access only.

A historical introduction to *Gray's Anatomy*

The shortcomings of existing anatomical textbooks probably impressed themselves upon Henry Gray when he was still a student at St George's Hospital Medical School, near London's Hyde Park Corner, in the mid 1840s. He began thinking about creating a new anatomy textbook a decade later, while war was being fought in the Crimea. New legislation was being planned which would establish the General Medical Council (1858) to regulate professional education and standards.

Gray was now 28 years old, and a teacher himself at St George's. Although little is known about his personal life, we do know he was very able and highly ambitious, already a Fellow of the Royal Society, and of the Royal College of Surgeons. His was a glittering career thus far, achieved while he served and taught on the hospital wards and in the dissecting room (Anon 1908).

Gray shared the idea for the new book with a gifted artistic colleague on the teaching staff at St George's, Dr Henry Vandyke Carter, in November 1855. Neither was interested in producing a pretty book, or an expensive one. Their purpose was to supply an affordable, accurate teaching aid for students like their own, who might soon be required to operate on soldiers injured at Sebastopol or on some other battlefield. The book they planned together was a practical one, designed to encourage youngsters to study anatomy, help them pass exams, and assist them as budding surgeons.

Now, at the turn of the twenty-first century, in this 39th edition of *Gray's Anatomy*, we can look back over nearly 150 years of continuous publication to consider the long-term value of their efforts, to discern how the book they created triumphed over its competitors and survived pre-eminent.

Gray and Carter belonged to a generation of anatomists ready to infuse the study of human anatomy with a new, and respectable, scientificity. Disreputable aspects of the profession's history, acquired during the days of bodysnatching, were assiduously being forgotten. The Anatomy Act of 1832 had legalized the requisition of unclaimed bodies from workhouse and hospital mortuaries, and the study of anatomy (now with its own Inspectorate) was rising in respectability in Britain. The private anatomy schools which had flourished in the Regency period had finally closed their doors, and the major teaching hospitals were erecting new purpose-built dissection rooms (Richardson 2000).

The best-known student works when Gray and Carter had qualified were probably Erasmus Wilson's *Anatomist's Vade Mecum*, and *Elements of Anatomy* by Jones Quain. Both works were small – pocket-sized – but Quain was a 'triple-decker' in three volumes. Both were good books in their way, but their small pages of dense type, and even smaller illustrations, were somewhat daunting, seeming to demand much nose-to-the-grindstone effort from the reader.

The planned new textbook's dimensions and character were serious matters. Pocket manuals were commercially successful because they appealed to students by offering much knowledge in a small compass. But pocket-sized books had button-sized illustrations. Knox's *Manual of Human Anatomy*, for example, was only six inches by four (17 × 10 cm) and few of its illustrations occupied more than a third of a page. Gray and Carter must have discussed this between themselves, and with Gray's publisher JW Parker & Son, before the decision was finalized.

The two men were earnestly engaged for the following 18 months in the work which would form the basis of the book. All the dissections were undertaken jointly: Gray wrote the text, and Carter prepared the illustrations. Their working days were long, all the hours of daylight, eight or nine hours at a stretch – right through 1856. We can infer from the warmth of Gray's appreciation of Carter in his published acknowledgements that their collaboration was a happy one.

The Author gratefully acknowledges the great services he has derived in the execution of this work, from the assistance of his friend, Dr HV Carter, late Demonstrator of Anatomy at St George's Hospital. All the drawings from which the engravings were made, were executed by him. (Gray 1858)

With all the dissections done, and Carter's inscribed blocks at the engravers, Gray took six months' leave from his teaching at St George's to see the book through the press. Carter sat the examination for medical officers in the East India Company, and sailed for India in the spring of 1858, when the book was still in its proof stages. Gray was assisted in the checking of the galley proofs by an older colleague, Timothy Holmes, whose association with the book would later prove vital to its survival.

THE FIRST EDITION

The book Gray and Carter created, *Anatomy: Descriptive and Surgical*, appeared in August 1858, to immediate acclaim. Reviews in the *Lancet* and *British Medical Journal* were highly complimentary, and students flocked to buy.

It is not difficult to understand why it was a runaway success. *Gray's Anatomy* knocked its competitors into a cocked hat. The book holds well in the hand, it feels substantial, it contains everything required. It was smaller and more slender than the doorstopper with which modern readers are familiar. To contemporaries it was small enough to be portable, but large enough for decent illustrations: 'octavo' – nine-and-a-half inches by six (24 × 15 cm) – about two-thirds of modern A4 size. Its medium size, single volume format was far removed from Quain's book, yet double the size of Knox's *Manual*.

Simply organized and well designed, the book explains itself confidently and well: the clarity and authority of the prose is manifest. But what made it unique for its day was the outstanding size and quality of the illustrations. Gray thanked the wood engravers Butterworth and Heath for the 'great care and fidelity' they had displayed in the engravings, but it was really to Carter that the book owed its extraordinary success.

The beauty of Carter's illustrations resides in their diagrammatic clarity, quite atypical for their time. Contemporary anatomical images were usually *proxy labelled*: dotted with tiny numbers or letters, or bristling with a sheaf of numbered arrows, referring to a key situated elsewhere. Proxy labels require the reader's eye to move to and fro: from the structure to the proxy label to the legend and back again. Carter's illustrations, by contrast, unify name and structure, enabling the eye to assimilate both at a glance. The volume made human anatomy look new, exciting, accessible, and do-able.

The spine of the first edition read:

GRAY

ANATOMY

CARTER

with both surnames in equal sized type. Carter was given equal credit with Gray on the book's title page for undertaking all the dissections on which the book was based, and sole credit for all the illustrations.

Gray was paid £150 for every thousand copies sold, but Carter received no royalty payments, only a one-off fee at publication, which may have allowed him to purchase the long-desired microscope he took with him to India.

The first edition print-run of 2000 copies sold out swiftly. An edition was published in the United States in 1859, and Gray must have been deeply gratified to have to revise and pilot an enlarged new English edition through the press in 1860, though he was surely saddened and worried by the death of John Parker junior, aged 40, that same year. The second edition came out in December and it, too, sold well.

The following summer, in June 1861, at the height of his powers and full of promise, Henry Gray died suddenly at the age of only 34. Gray had contracted smallpox while nursing his little nephew Charles, and although he had been vaccinated in infancy the disease became confluent, and Gray died within days.

THE BOOK SURVIVES

Anatomy: Descriptive and Surgical could have died too. With Carter in India, the death of Gray, so swiftly after the younger Parker, might have spelled catastrophe. Certainly at St George's there was a sense of calamity. The grand old medical man Sir Benjamin Brodie – Sergeant-Surgeon to the Queen, and a great supporter of Gray – to whom *Anatomy* had been dedicated, cried forlornly: 'Who is there to take his place?' (Anon 1908).

But old JW Parker ensured the survival of the book by inviting Timothy Holmes, the doctor who had helped proof-read the first edition, and who had filled Gray's shoes at the medical school, to serve as editor for the next edition. Other long-running anatomy works remained in print in a similar way: Quain, for example, was co-edited by other hands (Quain 1856).

Holmes (1825–1907) was another gifted St George's man. A scholarship boy who won an exhibition to Cambridge, where his brilliance was recognized, Holmes had been a Fellow of the Royal College of Surgeons at the age of 28. John Parker junior had commissioned Holmes to edit *A System of Surgery* (1860–1864), an important essay series by distinguished surgeons on subjects of their own choosing. Many of Holmes's authors remain important figures even today: John Simon, James Paget, Henry Gray, Ernest Hart, Jonathan Hutchinson, Brown Séquard, and Joseph Lister. Holmes lost an eye in an operative accident, and had a gruff manner which terrified students, yet he published a lament for young Parker which reveals him capable of deep feeling (Holmes 1860).

John Parker senior's heart, however, was no longer in publishing. His son's death had diminished his interest in the future. The business, with all its stocks and copyrights, was sold to Messrs Longman. Parker retired to the village of Farnham, where he later died.

With Holmes as editor, and Longmans as publisher, the immediate future of Gray's *Anatomy* was assured. The third edition appeared in 1864 with relatively few changes, Gray's estate receiving the balance of his royalty after Holmes was paid £100 for his work.

THE MISSING OBITUARY

Why no obituary appeared for Gray in *Gray's Anatomy* is curious. Gray had referred to Holmes as his 'friend' in the preface to the first edition, yet it would also be true to say that they were rivals. Both had just applied for a post at St George's, for Assistant Surgeon. Had Gray lived, it is thought that Holmes may not have been appointed, despite his seniority in age (Gray 1858).

Later commentators have promulgated the mistaken idea that Holmes's 'proof-reading' included improving Gray's writing style, which is probably a reflection of Holmes's own self-regard. There can be no doubt that as editor of seven editions of *Gray's Anatomy*, Holmes added new material, and had to correct and compress passages, but Gray's original writing style was lucid, in this as in other works.

It may be that Gray's glittering career or perhaps the patronage which unquestionably advanced it created jealousies among his colleagues; or that there was something in Gray's manner which precluded affection, or which created resentments among clever social inferiors like Carter and Holmes. Whatever the explanation, no reference to Gray's life or death appeared in *Gray's Anatomy* until the twentieth century (20th edition 1918).

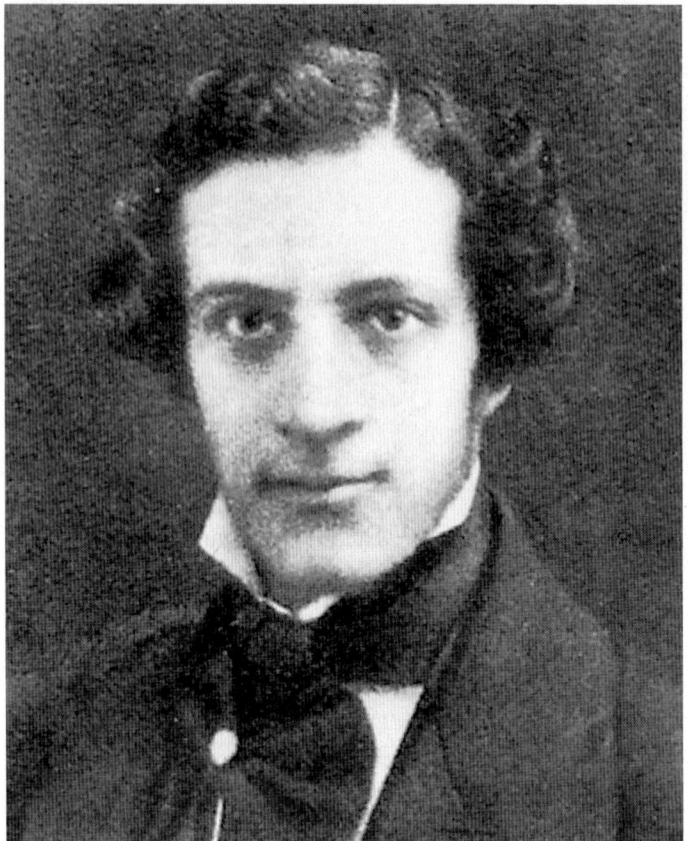

Fig. 1 Henry Gray (1827–1861).

A SUCCESSION OF EDITORS

Holmes expanded areas of the book which Gray himself had developed in the second edition (1860), notably in 'general' anatomy (histology) and 'development' (embryology). In Holmes's era the volume grew from 788 pages in 1864 to 960 in 1880 (9th edition), with the histological section paginated separately in roman numerals at the front of the book. Extra illustrations were added, mainly from other published sources.

The connections with Gray, Carter and with St George's were maintained with the appointment of the next editor, T Pickering Pick, who had been a student at St George's in Gray's and Carter's time. From 1883 (10th edition) onwards, Pick kept up with current research, rewrote and integrated the histology and embryology into the volume, dropped Holmes from the title page, removed Gray's preface to the first edition, and added emboldened subheadings which certainly improved the appearance and accessibility of the text. Pick said he had 'tried to keep before himself the fact that the work is intended for students of anatomy rather than for the Scientific Anatomist' (13th edition 1893).

Pick also introduced colour printing (11th edition 1887) and experimented with the addition of illustrations using the new printing method of half-tone dots: for colour (which worked) and for new black-and-white illustrations (which did not). Half-tone shades of grey compared poorly with Carter's wood engravings, still sharp and clear by comparison.

What Henry Carter made of these changes is a rich topic for speculation. He returned to England in 1888, having retired from the Indian Medical Service full of honours – Deputy Surgeon General, and in 1890 was made Honorary Surgeon to Queen Victoria. Carter died in Scarborough in 1897, aged 65. Like Gray, he received no obituary in the book.

When Pick was joined on the title page by Robert Howden (a professional anatomist from the University of Durham) in 1901 (15th edition), the volume was still easily recognizable as the book Gray and Carter had created. Although many of Carter's illustrations had been revised or replaced, many still remained. Sadly, an entire section (embryology) was again separately paginated, as its revision

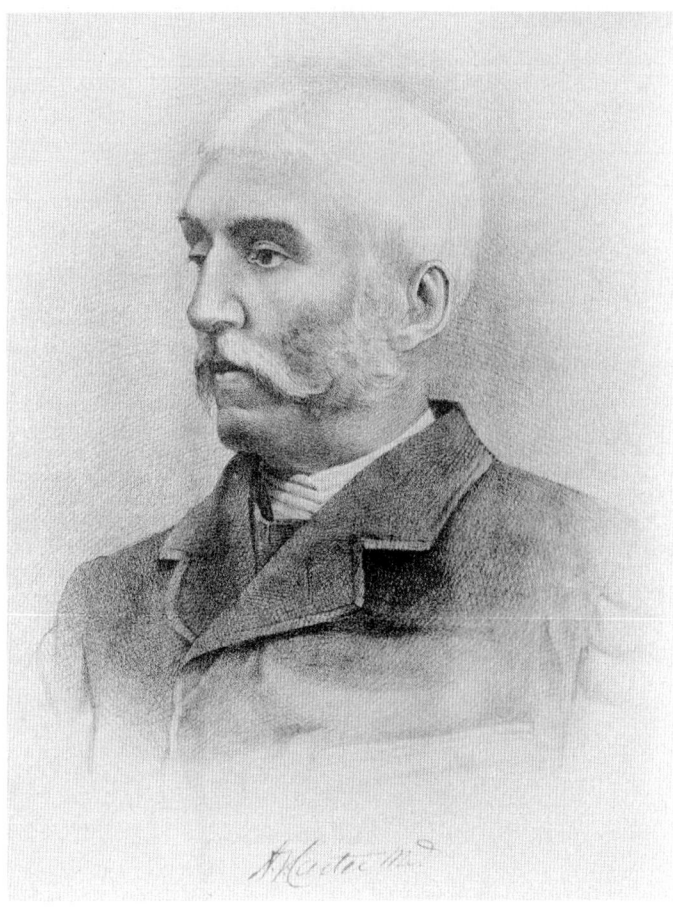

Fig. 2 Henry Vandyke Carter (1831–1897). Carter was appointed Honorary Surgeon to the Queen in 1890.

had taken longer than anticipated. *Gray's Anatomy* had grown, seemingly inexorably, and was now quite thick and heavy, 1244 pages weighing 5 lb 8 oz (2.5 kg). Both co-editors, and perhaps also its publisher, were dissatisfied with it.

KEY EDITION: 1905

Serious decisions were taken in advance of the next edition, which turned out to be Pick's last with Howden. Published 50 years after Gray had first suggested the idea to Carter, the 1905 (16th) edition was a landmark edition.

The period 1880–1930 was a difficult time for anatomical illustration, because the new techniques of photolitho and half-tone were not as yet perfected, and in any case could not provide the bold simplicity of line required for a book like *Gray's* which depended so heavily on clear illustration. Recognizing the inferiority of half-tone illustrations to Carter's wood-engraved originals, Pick and Howden courageously decided to jettison them altogether. Most of the book's new illustrations and even some older ones, were newly commissioned wood engravings or line drawings, intended 'to harmonise with Carter's original figures', and they did successfully emulate Carter's verve. Having fewer pages and lighter paper, the 1905 (16th edition) weighed less than its predecessor, at 4 lb 11 oz (2.1 kg). Typographically, the new edition was superb.

Howden took over as sole editor in 1909 (17th edition) and immediately stamped his personality on *Gray's*. He excised 'Surgical' from the title, changing it to *Anatomy Descriptive and Applied*, and removed Carter's name altogether. He also instigated the beginnings of an editorial board of experts for *Gray's*, by adding to the title page: 'Notes on Applied Anatomy' by AJ Jex-Blake, and W Fedde Fedden, both St George's men. For the first time, the number of illustrations exceeded one thousand. Howden was responsible for the significant innovation of a short historical note on Henry Gray himself, nearly 60 years after his death, which included a portrait photograph (20th edition 1918).

THE NOMENCLATURE CONTROVERSY

Howden's era, and that of his successor TB Johnston (of Guy's) was overshadowed by international controversy concerning anatomical terminology. European anatomists were endeavouring to standardize anatomical terms, often using Latinate constructions, a move resisted in Britain and the United States. *Gray's* became mired in these debates for over twenty years. The endeavour to be fair to all sides by using multiple terms doubtless generated much confusion amongst students, until a working compromise was arrived at, in 1955 (32nd edition 1958).

Johnston oversaw the second retitling of the book (27th edition 1938): it was now, officially, *Gray's Anatomy*, finally ending the fiction that it had ever been known as anything else. *Gray's* suffered from paper shortages and printing difficulties in World War II, but successive editions nevertheless continued to grow in size and weight, while illustrations were replaced and added as the text was revised. Between Howden's first sole effort (17th edition 1909) and Johnston's last edition (32nd edition 1958) *Gray's* expanded by over 300 pages from 1296 to 1604 pages, and almost 300 additional illustrations brought the total to over 1300. Johnston also introduced X-ray plates (1938) and in 1958 (32nd edition) electron micrographs by AS Fitton-Jackson, one of the first occasions on which a woman was credited for a contribution to *Gray's*. Johnston felt compelled to mention that she was 'a blood relative of Henry Gray himself', perhaps by way of mitigation.

AFTER WORLD WAR II

The editions of *Gray's* issued in the decades immediately following World War II give the impression of intellectual stagnation. Steady expansion continued in an almost formulaic fashion, with the insertion of additional detail.

The central historical importance of innovation in the success of *Gray's* seems to have been lost sight of by its publishers and editors – Johnston (24th to 32nd editions 1930–1958); James Whillis (co-editor with Johnston 1938–1954), DV Davies (32nd to 34th editions 1958–1967) and F Davies (co-editor with DV Davies: 32nd to 33rd editions 1958–1964). *Gray's* had become so pre-eminent that perhaps complacency crept in, or editors were too daunted or too busy to confront the 'massive undertaking' of a root and branch revision (Tansey 1995). The unexpected deaths of three major figures associated with *Gray's* in this era, James Whillis, Francis Davies, and David Vaughan Davies – all of whom had been groomed to take the editorial reins – may have contributed to retard the process. The work became somewhat dull.

KEY EDITION: 1973

DV Davies had recognized the need for modernization, but his unexpected death left the work to other hands. Peter Williams, who had been involved as an indexer for *Gray's* for several years, and Roger Warwick (both Professors of Anatomy at Guy's) regarded it as an honour to fulfil Davies' intentions.

Their 35th edition of 1973 was a significant departure from tradition. Over 780 pages (of 1471) were newly written, almost a third of the illustrations were newly commissioned, and the illustration captions were freshly written throughout. With a complete resetting of the text in larger double column pages, a new index, and the innovation of a bibliography, this edition of *Gray's* looked and felt quite unlike its 1967 (34th edition) predecessor, and much more like its modern incarnation.

This 1973 edition departed from earlier volumes in other significant ways. The editors made explicit their intention to try to counter the impetus towards specialization and compartmentalization in twentieth century medicine by embracing and attempting to reintegrate the complexity of the available knowledge. Warwick and Williams openly renounced the pose of omniscience adopted by many textbooks, believing it important to accept and mention areas of ignorance or uncertainty. They shared with the reader the difficulty of keeping abreast in the sea of research, and accepted with a refreshing humility the impossibility of fulfilling their own ambitious programme.

Warwick and Williams's 1973 edition had much in common with Gray and Carter's first edition. It was bold and innovative, respectful of its heritage while also striking out into new territory. It was visually attractive and visually informative. It embodied a sense of a treasury of information laid out for the reader (preface to 35th edition 1973). It was published simultaneously in the United States (the American *Gray's* had developed a distinct character of its own in the interval; Tansey 1995), and sold extremely well there.

The influence of Warwick and Williams's edition was forceful and long-lasting, and set a new pattern for the following quarter century. As has transpired several times before, wittingly or unwittingly a new editor was being prepared for the future: Dr Susan Standring, who created the bibliography for the 1973 edition of *Gray's*, went on to serve on the editorial board and is now the Editor in Chief of the current edition (39th edition 2005).

THE DOCTOR'S BIBLE

Neither Gray nor Carter, young men who – by their committed hard work between 1855 and 1858 – created the original edition of *Gray's Anatomy*, would have conceived that years after their deaths their book would not only be a household name but regarded as a work of such pre-eminent importance that a novelist half a world away would rank it as cardinal – alongside the Bible and Shakespeare – to a doctor's education (Lewis 1925). With this fine new edition, their book goes marching on.

Ruth Richardson MA DPhil FR Hist Soc
Research Associate, Centre for Medical Humanities,
University College of London, and The Wellcome
Trust for The History of Medicine at
University College London, London, UK

REFERENCES

Anon 1908 Henry Gray. St George's Hospital Gazette 16(4): 49–54.

Gray H 1858 Anatomy: Descriptive and Surgical. London: JW Parker & Son: preface.

Holmes T (ed) 1860 A System of Surgery. London: JW Parker & Son: I, preface.

Lewis S 1925 Arrowsmith. New York: Harcourt Brace: 4.

Quain J 1856 Elements of Anatomy. Sharpey W, Ellis GV (eds). London, Walton & Maberly.

Richardson R 2000 Death, Dissection and the Destitute. Chicago: Chicago University Press: 193–249, 287, 357.

Tansey EM 1995 A Brief History of Gray's Anatomy. In: Gray's Anatomy, 38th edn. London: Churchill Livingstone: xvii–xx.

ACKNOWLEDGEMENTS

For their assistance while I was undertaking the research for this essay, I should like to thank the librarians and archivists at the British Library, Society of Apothecaries, London School of Hygiene & Tropical Medicine, Royal College of Surgeons, Royal Society of Medicine, St Bride Printing Library, St George's Hospital Tooting, Scarborough City Museum & Art Gallery, University of Reading, Wellcome Institute Library, Westminster City Archives and Windsor Castle; and the following individuals: Anne Bayliss, David Buchanan, Dee Cook, Chris Hamlin, Victoria Killick, Sarah Potts, Mark Smalley, Nallini Thevakarrunai. Above all, my thanks to Brian Hurwitz, who has read and advised on the evolving text.

INTRODUCTION AND SYSTEMIC OVERVIEW

Editors:

Susan Standring *(Lead Editor)*
Caroline Wigley *(Microstructure)*
Patricia Collins *(Embryology, Growth and Development)*
Andrew Williams *(Biomechanics)*

Critical reviewers:

Peter Braude *(chapter 10)*, **Robert Brooks** *(2 & 3)*, **Fred Cody** *(4 & 6)*, **Mike Hall** *(11)*, **Jonathan C Kentish** *(7)*, **Birgit Lane** *(2 & 8)*, **Susan Pickering** *(10)*, **Mary Ritter** *(5)*, **Anthea Rowlerson** *(4 & 6)*, **Jeremy PT Ward** *(7)*

Anatomical nomenclature

Anatomy is the study of the structure of the body, from the submicroscopic to the macroscopic. It is conventionally divided into topographical or gross anatomy (including surface, endoscopic and radiological anatomy), histology, embryology and neuroanatomy.

Anatomical language is one of the fundamental languages of medicine. The unambiguous description of thousands of structures is impossible without an extensive and often highly specialized vocabulary. Ideally, these terms, which are often derived from Latin or Greek, should be used to the exclusion of any other, throughout the world. In reality, many terms are vernacularized. The *Terminologia Anatomica*, drawn up by the Federative Committee on Anatomical Terminology (FCAT) in 1998, has served as our guide in preparing the 39th Edition of *Gray's Anatomy*. Where we have anglicized some of the Latin terms, we have given the official form, at least once, in parentheses. We have also included eponyms, since these are often used, possibly more so by clinicians than anatomists. Indeed, certain eponyms are so firmly entrenched in the language of the clinician that to avoid them could lead to confusion: the eponymous term is often the only way to describe a particular structure, because there is no simple alternative anatomical term.

PLANES, DIRECTIONS AND RELATIONSHIPS

To avoid ambiguity, all anatomical descriptions assume that the body is in the conventional 'anatomical position', i.e. standing erect and facing forwards, upper limbs by the side with the palms facing forwards, and lower limbs together with the feet facing forwards (**Fig. 1.1**). Descriptions are based on four imaginary planes, median, sagittal, coronal and horizontal, applied to a body in the anatomical position. The median plane passes longitudinally through the body and divides it into right and left halves. The sagittal plane is parallel to the median plane. The coronal plane is orthogonal to the median plane and divides the body into anterior (front) and posterior (back). The horizontal (transverse) plane is orthogonal to both median and sagittal planes. Radiologists refer to transverse planes as (trans)axial. Convention dictates that axial anatomy is viewed as though looking from the feet towards the head.

Structures nearer the head are superior; cranial may be used when talking about the head. Structures closer to the feet are inferior; caudal is frequently used in embryology to refer to the tail end of the embryo. Medial and lateral indicate closeness to the midline, medial being nearer to the midline than lateral. External (outer) and internal (inner) refer to the distance from the centre of an organ or cavity, e.g. the layers of the body wall. Various degrees of obliquity are acknowledged using compound terms, e.g. posterolateral. When referring to structures in the trunk and upper limb we have used freely the synonyms anterior, ventral, flexor, palmar, volar, and posterior, dorsal and extensor. We recognize that these synonyms are not always satisfactory, e.g. the extensor aspect of the leg is anterior with respect to the knee and ankle joints, and superior in the foot and digits; the plantar (flexor) aspect of the foot is inferior. Dorsal (dorsum) and ventral are terms used particularly by embryologists and neuroanatomists: they therefore feature most often in Sections 1 and 2. Distal and proximal are used to describe structures in the limbs, taking the datum point as the attachment of the limb to the trunk, such that a proximal structure is closer to the attachment of the limb than a distal structure; they are also used in describing branching structures, e.g. bronchi. Superficial and deep are used to describe the relationships between adjacent structures. Ipsilateral refers to the same side (of the body, organ or structure), bilateral to both sides, and contralateral to the opposite side.

MOVEMENTS

Movements at joints, e.g. flexion, extension, adduction and abduction, and the many possible combinations of these 'pure' movements, are described in Chapter 6. Specialized movements, such as those that occur at the elbow, wrist, ankle and temporomandibular joints, are described in the appropriate chapters.

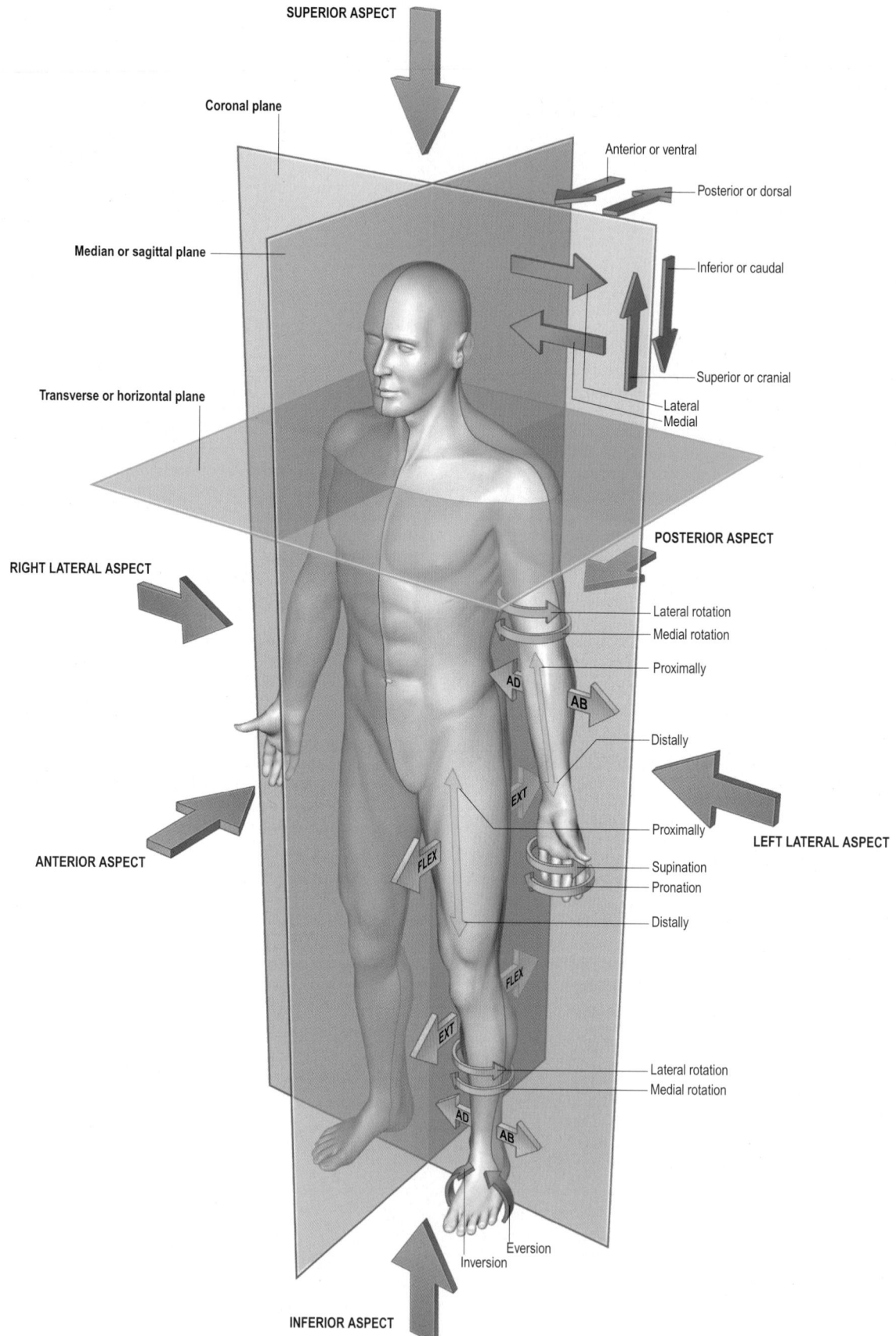

Fig. 1.1 The terminology widely used in descriptive anatomy. Abbreviations shown on arrows: AD, adduction; AB, abduction; FLEX, flexion (of the thigh at the hip joint); EXT, extension (of the leg at the knee joint).

Basic structure and function of cells

CELL STRUCTURE

GENERAL CHARACTERISTICS OF CELLS

Most cells lie within the size range 5–50 μm in diameter: e.g. resting lymphocytes are c.6 μm across, red blood cells c.7.5 μm and columnar epithelial cells are c.20 μm tall and 10 μm wide. Some cells are much larger than this: e.g. megakaryocytes of the bone marrow are more than 200 μm in diameter. Large neurones and skeletal muscle cells have relatively enormous volumes because of their extended shapes, some of the former being over 1 metre in length. Cell size is limited by rates of diffusion, either that of material entering or leaving cells, or of diffusion within them. Diffusion can be much accelerated by processes of active transport across membranes and also directed by transport mechanisms within the cell.

Motility is a characteristic of most cells, in the form of movements of cytoplasm or specific organelles from one part of the cell to another. It also includes: the extension of parts of the cell surface such as pseudopodia, membrane ruffles, filopodia and microvilli; locomotion of entire cells as in the amoeboid migration of tissue macrophages; the beating of flagella or cilia to move the cell (e.g. in spermatozoa) or fluids overlying it (e.g. in respiratory epithelium); cell division and muscle contraction. Cell movements are also involved in the uptake of materials from their environment (endocytosis, phagocytosis) and the passage of large molecular complexes out of cells (exocytosis, secretion).

The shapes of cells vary widely depending on their interactions with each other, their extracellular environment and internal structures. Their surfaces are often highly folded when absorptive or transport functions take place across their boundaries. According to the location of absorptive or transport functions, apical microvilli or basolateral infoldings create a large surface area for transport or diffusion.

Cells rarely operate independently of each other and commonly form aggregates by adhesion, often assisted by specialized intercellular junctions. They may also communicate with each other either by releasing and detecting molecular signals that diffuse across intercellular spaces, or more rapidly by membrane contact, which often involves small, transient, transmembrane channels. Cohesive groups of cells constitute tissues and more complex assemblies of tissues form functional systems or organs.

CELLULAR ORGANIZATION

Cytoplasm is contained within a limiting plasma membrane. All cells except mature red blood cells also contain a nucleus that is surrounded by a nuclear membrane (**Figs 2.1, 2.2**). The nucleus includes the genome of the cell contained within the chromosomes, and the nucleolus. The cytoplasm contains several systems of organelles. These include a series of membrane-bound structures that form separate compartments within the cytoplasm, such as rough and smooth endoplasmic reticulum, Golgi apparatus, lysosomes, peroxisomes, mitochondria and vesicles for transport, secretion and storage of cellular components. There are also structures that lie free in the non-membranous, cytosolic compartment. They include ribosomes and several filamentous protein structures known collectively as the cytoskeleton. The cytoskeleton determines general cell shape and supports specialized extensions of the cell surface (microvilli, cilia, flagella). It is involved in the assembly of new filamentous organelles (e.g. centrioles) and controls internal movements of the cytoplasm and cytoplasmic vesicles. The cytosol contains many soluble proteins, ions and metabolites.

Cell domains

In polarized cells, particularly in epithelia, the cell is generally subdivided into domains that reflect the polarization of activities within

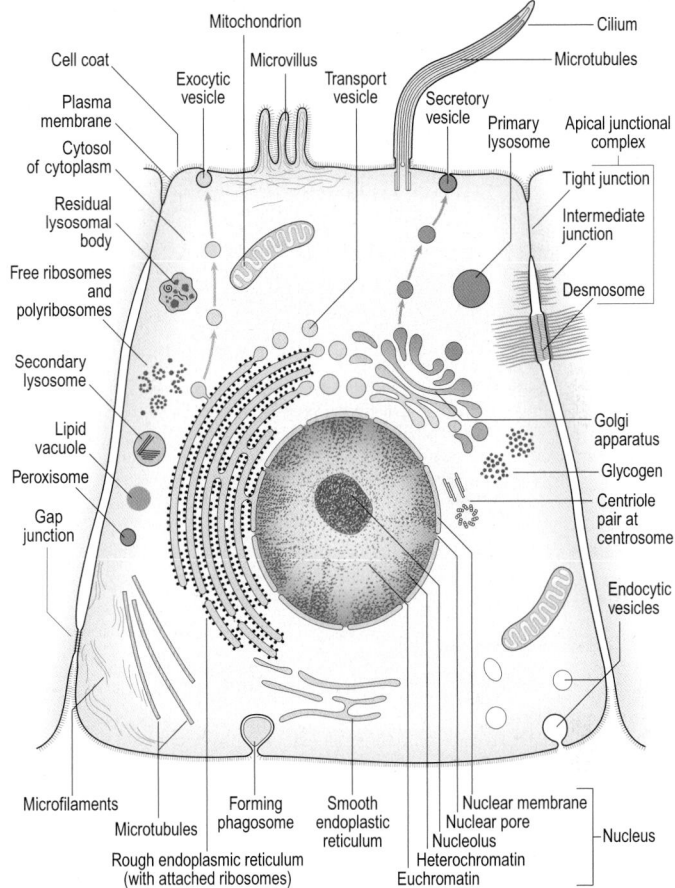

Fig. 2.1 The main structural components and internal organization of a generalized cell.

the cell. The free surface, e.g. that facing the intestinal lumen or airway, is the apical surface, and its adjacent cytoplasm is the apical cell domain. This is where the cell interfaces with a specific body compartment (or, in the case of the epidermis, with the outside world). The apical surface is specialized to act as a barrier, restricting access of substances from this compartment to the rest of the body. Specific components are selectively absorbed from, or added to, the external compartment by the active processes, respectively, of active transport and endocytosis inwardly or exocytosis and secretion outwardly.

The surface of the cell opposite to the apical surface is the basal surface, with its associated basal cell domain. In a single-layered epithelium, this surface is apposed to the basal lamina. The remaining surfaces are known as the lateral cell surfaces. In many instances the lateral and basal surfaces perform similar functions and the cellular domain is termed the basolateral domain. Cells actively transport substances, such as digested nutrients from the intestinal lumen or endocrine secretions, across their basal (or basolateral) surfaces into the subjacent connective tissue matrix and the blood capillaries within it. Dissolved non-polar gases (oxygen and carbon dioxide) diffuse freely between the cell and the bloodstream across the basolateral surface.

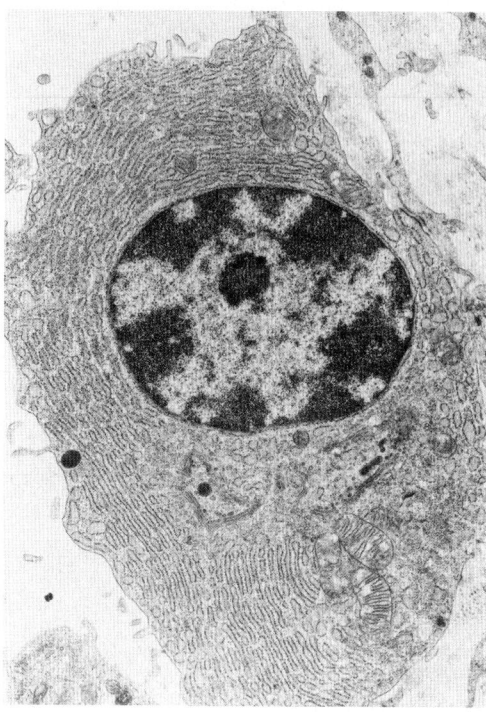

Fig. 2.2 A protein-synthesizing cell (immunoglobulin-secreting plasma cell) in connective tissue. The main ultrastructural features are a nucleus surrounded by a nuclear envelope and containing peripheral heterochromatin, central euchromatin and a nucleolus; and cytoplasm containing rough endoplasmic reticulum, mitochondria, Golgi apparatus, transport vesicles and small lysosomes.

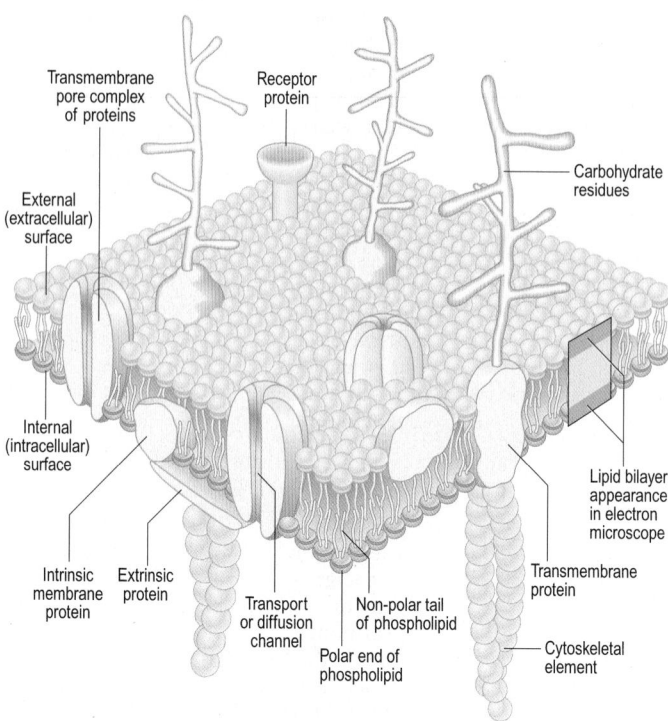

Fig. 2.3 The molecular organization of the plasma membrane, according to the fluid mosaic model of membrane structure. Intrinsic or integral membrane proteins include diffusion or transport channel complexes, receptor proteins and adhesion molecules. These may span the thickness of the membrane (transmembrane proteins) and can have both extracellular and cytoplasmic domains. Transmembrane proteins have hydrophobic zones, which cross the phospholipid bilayer and allow the protein to 'float' in the plane of the membrane. Some proteins are restricted in their freedom of movement where their cytoplasmic domains are tethered to the cytoskeleton.

Plasma membrane

Cells are bounded by a distinct plasma membrane, which shares features with the system of internal membranes that compartmentalize the cytoplasm and surround the nucleus. They are all composed of lipids (mainly phospholipids, cholesterol and glycolipids) and proteins, in approximately equal ratios. Plasma membrane lipids form a layer two molecules thick, the lipid bilayer. The hydrophobic ends of each lipid molecule face the interior of the membrane and the hydrophilic ends face outwards. Most proteins are embedded within, or float in, the lipid bilayer as a fluid mosaic. Some proteins, because of extensive hydrophobic regions of their polypeptide chains, span the entire width of the membrane (transmembrane proteins), whereas others are only superficially attached to the bilayer by lipid groups. Both are integral (intrinsic) membrane proteins, as distinct from peripheral (extrinsic) membrane proteins, which are membrane-bound only through their association with other proteins. Carbohydrates in the form of oligosaccharides and polysaccharides are bound either to proteins (glycoproteins) or to lipids (glycolipids), and project mainly into the extracellular domain.

Combinations of biochemical, biophysical and biological techniques have revealed that lipids are not homogenously distributed in membranes, but that some are organized into microdomains in the bilayer, called 'detergent-resistant membranes' or lipid 'rafts', rich in sphingomyelin and cholesterol (Morris et al 2003). The ability of select subsets of proteins to partition into different lipid microdomains has profound effects on their function, e.g. in T-cell receptor and neurotrophin signalling. The highly organized environment of the domains provides a signalling, trafficking and membrane fusion environment very different from that found in the disorganized fluid mosaic membrane.

In the electron microscope, membranes fixed and contrasted by heavy metals such as osmium appear in section as two densely stained layers separated by an electron-translucent zone – the classic unit membrane (Figs 2.3, 2.4). The total thickness is c.5 nm. Freeze-fracture cleavage planes usually pass along the midline of each membrane, where the hydrophobic tails of phospholipids meet. This technique has also demonstrated intramembranous particles embedded in the lipid bilayer; these are in the 5–15 nm range and in most cases represent large

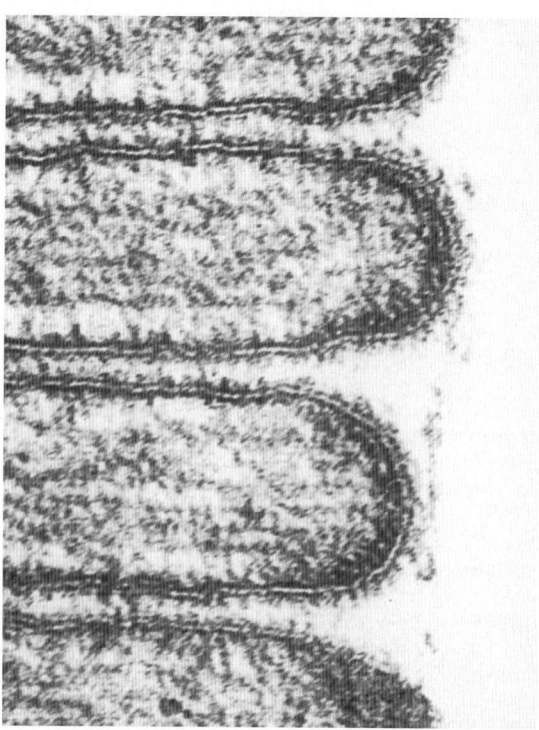

Fig. 2.4 The plasma membrane covering microvilli on absorptive epithelial cells in the small intestine. The lipid bilayer is clearly seen at this high magnification, as is the cell coat or glycocalyx projecting into extracellular space (the gut lumen, right) as an outer fuzzy layer. (By permission from Young B, Heath JW 2000 Wheater's Functional Histology. Edinburgh: Churchill Livingstone.)

transmembrane protein molecules or complexes of molecules. Intramembranous particles are distributed asymmetrically between the two half-membranes, usually adhering more to one face than to the other. In plasma membranes, the inner or protoplasmic (cytoplasmic) half-membrane carries most particles, seen on its surface facing the exterior (the P face). Where they have been identified, particles usually represent channels for the transmembrane passage of ions or molecules.

Biophysical measurements show the lipid bilayer to be highly fluid, allowing diffusion in the plane of the membrane. Thus proteins are able to move freely in such planes unless anchored from within the cell. Membranes in general, and the plasma membrane in particular, form boundaries selectively limiting diffusion and creating physiologically distinct compartments. Lipid bilayers are impermeable to hydrophilic solutes and ions and so membranes actively control the passage of ions and small organic molecules such as nutrients, through the activity of membrane transport proteins. However, lipid-soluble substances can pass directly through the membrane so that, for example, steroid hormones enter the cytoplasm freely. Their receptor proteins are either cytosolic or nuclear, rather than being located on the cell surface.

Plasma membranes are able to generate electrochemical gradients and potential differences by selective ion transport, and actively take up or export small molecules by energy dependent processes. They also provide surfaces for the attachment of enzymes, sites for the receptors of external signals, including hormones and other ligands, and sites for the recognition and attachment of other cells. Internally, plasma membranes can act as points of attachment for intracellular structures, in particular those concerned with motility and other cytoskeletal functions. Cell membranes are synthesized by the rough endoplasmic reticulum in conjunction with the Golgi apparatus.

THE CELL COAT (GLYCOCALYX)

The plasma membrane differs structurally from internal membranes in that it possesses an external, diffuse, carbohydrate-rich coat, the cell coat or glycocalyx. The cell coat forms an integral part of the plasma membrane, projecting as a diffusely filamentous layer 2–20 nm or more from the lipoprotein surface (**Fig. 2.4**). The overall thickness of the plasma membrane is therefore variable, but is typically 8–10 nm. The cell coat is composed of the carbohydrate portions of glycoproteins and glycolipids embedded in the plasma membrane (**Fig. 2.3**).

The precise composition of the glycocalyx varies with cell type: many tissue and cell type-specific antigens are located in the coat, including the major histocompatibility antigen systems and, in the case of erythrocytes, blood group antigens. It also contains adhesion molecules, which enable cells to adhere selectively to other cells or to the extracellular matrix. They have important roles in maintaining the integrity of tissues and in a wide range of dynamic cellular processes, e.g. the formation of intercommunicating neural networks in the developing nervous system and the extravasation of leukocytes. Cells tend to repel each other because of the predominance of negatively charged carbohydrates at cell surfaces. There is consequently a distance of at least 20 nm between the plasma membranes of adjacent cells, other than at specialized junctions.

CELL SURFACE CONTACTS

The plasma membrane is the surface which establishes contact with other cells and with structural components of extracellular matrices. These contacts may have a predominantly adhesive role, or initiate instructive signals within and between cells, or both; they frequently affect the behaviour of cells. Structurally, there are two main classes of contact, both associated with cell adhesion molecules. One class is associated with specializations at discrete regions of the cell surface that are ultrastructurally distinct. These are described on page 7. The second, general, class of adhesive contact has no obvious associated ultrastructural features.

GENERAL ADHESIVE CONTACTS

One class of transmembrane or membrane-anchored glycoproteins that project externally from the plasma membrane, and which form adhesive contacts, are the cell adhesion molecules. There are a number of molecular subgroups, which are broadly divisible on the basis of their calcium dependence.

Calcium-dependent adhesion molecules

Cadherins, selectins and integrins are calcium-dependent adhesion molecules. Cadherins are transmembrane proteins, with five heavily glycosylated external domains. They are responsible for strong general intercellular adhesion, as well as being components of some specialized adhesive contacts, and are attached by linker proteins (catenins) at their cytoplasmic ends to underlying cytoskeletal fibres (either actin or intermediate filaments). Different cell types possess different members of the cadherin family, e.g. N-cadherins in nervous tissue, E-cadherins in epithelia, and P-cadherins in the placenta. These molecules bind to those of the same type in other cells (homophilic binding), so that cells of the same class adhere to each other preferentially, forming tissue aggregates or layers, as in epithelia.

Selectins are found on leukocytes, platelets and vascular endothelial cells. They are transmembrane lectin glycoproteins that can bind with low affinity to the carbohydrate groups on other cell surfaces to permit movement between the two, e.g. the rolling adhesion of leukocytes on the walls of blood vessels (p. 146). They function cooperatively in sequence with integrins, which strengthen the selectin adhesion.

Integrins are glycoproteins that typically mediate adhesion between cells and extracellular matrix components such as fibronectin, collagen, laminin. They integrate interactions between the matrix and the cell cytoskeleton to which they are linked, and so facilitate cell migration within the matrix. An integrin molecule is formed of two subunits (α and β), each of which has several subtypes. Combinations of alternative subunits provide more than 20 integrin heterodimers, each one directed to a particular extracellular molecule, although there is considerable overlap in specificity. Some integrins depend for their binding on magnesium, rather than calcium.

Calcium-independent adhesion molecules

The best known calcium-independent adhesion molecules are glycoproteins that have external domains related to immunoglobulin molecules. Most are transmembrane proteins. Some are entirely external, either attached to the plasma membrane by a glycosylphosphatidylinositol anchor, or secreted as soluble components of the extracellular matrix. Different types are expressed in different tissues. Neural cell adhesion molecules are found on a number of cell types, but are expressed widely by neural cells. Intercellular adhesion molecules are expressed on vascular endothelial cells. Cell adhesion molecule binding is predominantly homophilic, although some, e.g. intercellular adhesion molecules, use a heterophilic mechanism and can bind to integrins.

For further information on all aspects of cell adhesion molecules and intercellular contacts, see Alberts et al (2002).

SPECIALIZED ADHESIVE CONTACTS

Specialized adhesive contacts, some of which mediate activities other than simple mechanical cohesion, are localized regions of the cell surface with particular ultrastructural characteristics. Three major classes exist: occluding, adhesive and communicating junctions (**Fig. 2.5**).

Occluding junctions (tight junctions, zonula occludens)

Occluding junctions create diffusion barriers in continuous layers of cells, including epithelia, mesothelia and endothelia, and prevent the passage of materials across the cellular layer through intercellular spaces. They form a continuous belt (zonula) around the cell perimeter, near the apical surface in cuboidal or columnar epithelial cells. At a tight junction, the membranes of the adjacent cells come into contact, so that the gap between them is obliterated. Freeze-fracture electron microscopy shows that the contacts between the membranes lie along branching and anastomosing ridges formed by the incorporation of chains of intramembranous protein particles on the P face of the lipid bilayer (**Fig. 2.5C**).

This arrangement ensures that substances can only pass through the layer of cells by diffusion or transport through their apical membranes and cytoplasm. The cells thus selectively modify the environment on either side of the layer. Occluding junctions also create regional differences in the plasma membranes of the cells in which they are found. For example, in epithelia, the composition of the apical plasma membrane differs from that of the basolateral regions, and this allows these regions to engage in functions such as directional transport of ions and uptake of macromolecules. Because tight junctions have high concentrations of fixed transmembrane proteins, they act as barriers to lateral diffusion of lipid and protein within membranes. The integrity of tight junctions

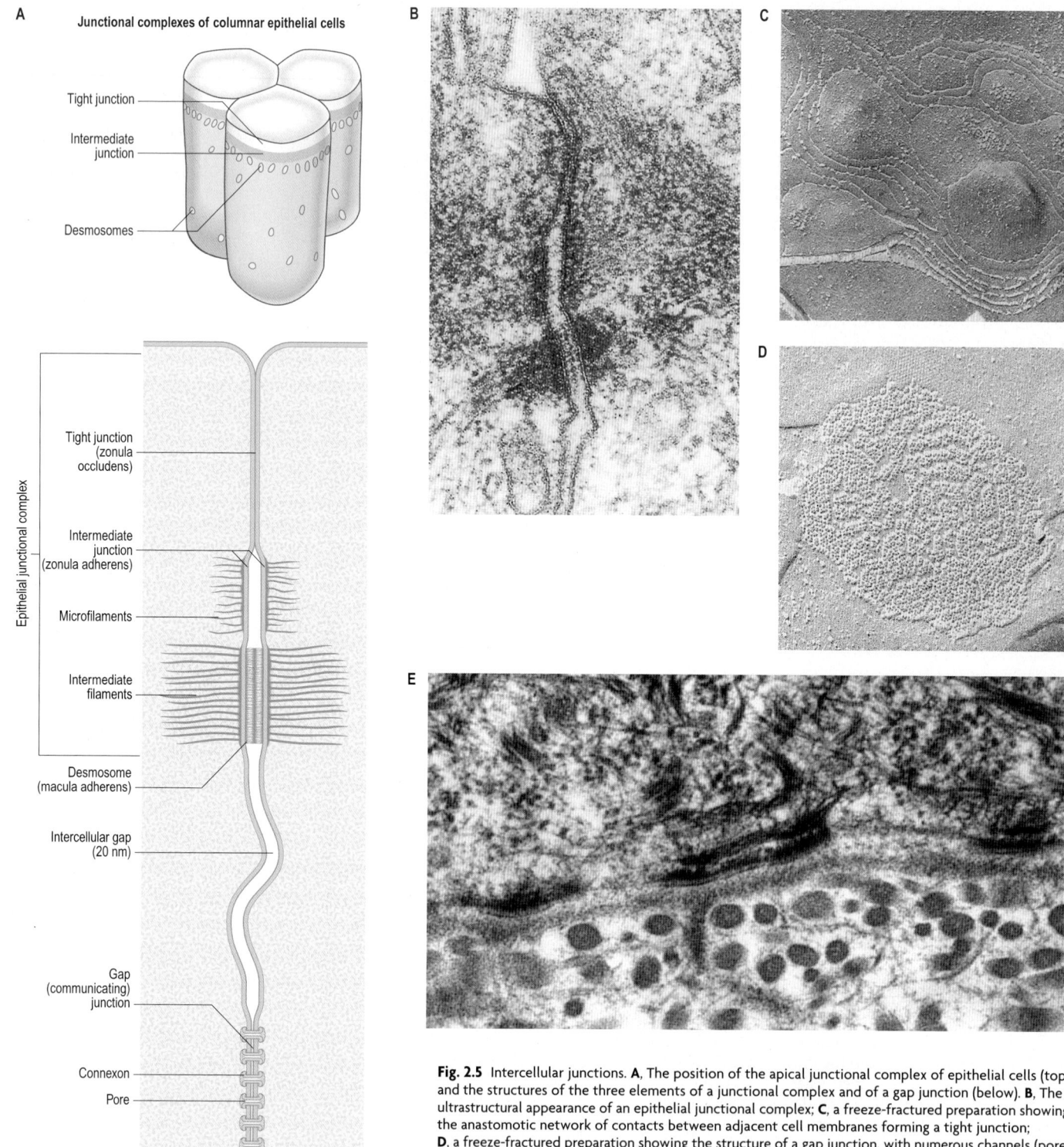

A

Junctional complexes of columnar epithelial cells

Tight junction

Intermediate junction

Desmosomes

Epithelial junctional complex

Tight junction (zonula occludens)

Intermediate junction (zonula adherens)

Microfilaments

Intermediate filaments

Desmosome (macula adherens)

Intercellular gap (20 nm)

Gap (communicating) junction

Connexon

Pore

B

C

D

E

Fig. 2.5 Intercellular junctions. **A**, The position of the apical junctional complex of epithelial cells (top) and the structures of the three elements of a junctional complex and of a gap junction (below). **B**, The ultrastructural appearance of an epithelial junctional complex; **C**, a freeze-fractured preparation showing the anastomotic network of contacts between adjacent cell membranes forming a tight junction; **D**, a freeze-fractured preparation showing the structure of a gap junction, with numerous channels (pores within connexons) clustered to form a plaque-like junctional region between adjacent plasma membranes; **E**, hemidesmosomes in the basal layer of the epidermis, contacting the underlying basal lamina. Dermal collagen fibrils are sectioned transversely below. (**B**, by permission from Young B, Heath JW 2000 Wheater's Functional Histology. Edinburgh: Churchill Livingstone; **C**, by kind permission from Dr Andrew Kent, King's College London; **D**, by kind permission from Professor Dieter Hülser, University of Stuttgart; **E**, by permission from the Company of Biologists Ltd, Cambridge, UK, and Frye M, Gardner C, Li ER, Arnold I, Watt FM 2003 Evidence that Myc activation depletes the epidermal stem cell compartment by modulating adhesive interactions with the local microenvironment. Development 130: 2793–2808.)

is calcium-dependent. Cells can transiently alter the permeability of their tight junctions to increase passive paracellular transport in some circumstances.

Adhesive junctions

Adhesive junctions include intercellular and cell–extracellular matrix contacts, where cells adhere strongly to each other or to adjacent matrix components. Intercellular contacts can be subdivided according to the extent and location of the contact. They all display a high concentration of cell adhesion molecules, which externally bind adjacent cells, and internally link to the cytoskeleton via intermediary proteins.

Zonula adherens (intermediate junction)

A zonula adherens is a continuous, belt-like zone of adhesion around the apical perimeters of epithelial, mesothelial and endothelial cells, parallel and just basal to the tight junction in epithelia. High concentrations of cadherins occur in this zone; their cytoplasmic ends are anchored via the proteins vinculin and α-actinin to a layer of actin microfilaments. These junctions help to reinforce the intercellular attachment of the tight junction and prevent its mechanical disruption. The gap between cell surfaces is c.20 nm. Usually, no electron-dense material is observed within this intercellular space.

Fascia adherens

A fascia adherens is similar to a zonula adherens, but is more limited in extent and forms a strip or patch of adhesion, e.g. between smooth muscle cells, in the intercalated discs of cardiac muscle cells (p. 152) and between glial cells and neurones. The junctions involve cadherins attached indirectly to actin filaments on the inner side of the membrane.

Desmosomes (macula adherens)

Desmosomes are limited, plaque-like areas of particularly strong intercellular contact. They can be located anywhere on the cell surface. In epithelial cells, there may be a circumferential row of desmosomes parallel to the tight and intermediate junctional zones, an arrangement that forms the third, most basally situated, component of the epithelial apical junctional complex (**Fig. 2.5A,B** and p. 29). The intercellular gap is c.25 nm, is filled with electron-dense filamentous material running transversely across it and is also marked by a series of densely staining bands running parallel to the cell surfaces. Adhesion is mediated by calcium-dependent cadherins, desmoglein and desmocollin. Within the cells on either side, a cytoplasmic density underlies the plasma membrane and includes the anchor proteins desmoplakin and plakoglobin, into which the ends of intermediate filaments are inserted. The type of intermediate filament depends on cell type, e.g. cytokeratins are found in epithelia and desmin filaments in cardiac muscle cells. Desmosomes form strong anchorage points, likened to spot-welds, between cells subject to mechanical stress, e.g. in the spinous layer of the epidermis, where they are extremely numerous and large (p. 157).

Hemidesmosomes

Hemidesmosomes are best known as anchoring junctions between the bases of epithelial cells and the basal lamina. Ultrastructurally, they resemble a single-sided desmosome, anchored on one side to the plasma membrane, and on the other to the basal lamina and adjacent collagen fibrils (**Fig. 2.5E**). On the cytoplasmic side of the membrane there is a dense coat into which cytokeratin filaments are inserted. Hemidesmosomes use integrins as their adhesion molecules, whereas desmosomes use cadherins.

Less highly structured attachments with a similar arrangement exist between many other cell types and their surrounding matrix, e.g. between smooth muscle cells and their matrix fibrils, and between the ends of skeletal muscle cells and tendon fibres. The smaller, punctate adhesions resemble focal adhesion plaques.

Focal adhesion plaques

Focal adhesion plaques are regions of local attachment between cells and the extracellular matrix. They are typically situated at or near the ends of actin filament bundles (stress fibres), which are anchored through intermediary proteins to the cytoplasmic domains of integrins. In turn, these are attached at their external ends to collagen or other filamentous structures in the extracellular matrix. They are usually short-lived: their formation and subsequent disruption are part of the motile behaviour of migratory cells.

Gap junctions (communicating junctions)

Gap junctions resemble tight junctions in transverse section, but the two apposed lipid bilayers are separated by an apparent gap of 3 nm which is bridged by numerous transmembrane channels (connexons). Connexons are formed by a ring of six connexin proteins in each membrane. Their external surfaces meet those of the adjacent cell in the middle. A minute central pore links one cell to the next (**Fig. 2.5A**). These channels may exist in small numbers, and this makes them difficult to detect structurally. However, they lower the transcellular electrical resistance and so can be detected by microelectrodes. Larger assemblies of many thousands of channels are often packed in hexagonal arrays (**Fig. 2.5D**). Such junctions form limited attachment plaques rather than continuous zones, and so allow free passage of substances within the adjacent intercellular space, unlike tight junctions. They occur in numerous tissues including the liver, epidermis, pancreatic islet cells, connective tissues, cardiac muscle and smooth muscle, and are also common in embryonic tissues. In the central nervous system, they are found in the ependyma and between neuroglial cells, and they form electrical synapses between some types of neurone, although this is rare in humans.

Although gap junctions form diffusion channels between cells, the size of their apertures limits diffusion to small molecules and ions (up to a molecular weight of about 1000 kDa). Thus they admit sodium, potassium and calcium ions, various second messenger components, and a number of metabolites, but they exclude messenger RNA and other macromolecules. In some excitable tissues (e.g. cardiac and smooth muscle), one cell can activate another electrically by current flow through gap junctions. Communicating junctions probably permit metabolic cooperation between groups of adjacent cells; the significance of this activity in embryogenesis, normal tissue function, homeostasis and repair is only beginning to be understood.

Other types of junction

Chemical synapses and neuromuscular junctions are specialized areas of intercellular adhesion where neurotransmitters secreted from a neuronal terminal gain access to specialized receptor molecules on a recipient cell surface. They are described on pages 44 and 64, respectively.

CELL SIGNALLING

Cellular systems in the body communicate with each other to coordinate and integrate their functions. This occurs through a variety of processes known collectively as cell signalling, in which a signalling molecule produced by one cell is detected by another, almost always by means of a specific receptor protein molecule. The recipient cell transduces the signal, which it most usually detects at the plasma membrane, into intracellular chemical messages that change cell behaviour.

The signal may act over a long distance, as in endocrine signalling through the release of hormones into the bloodstream or neuronal synaptic signalling via electrical impulse transmission along axons (p. 44) and subsequent release of chemical transmitters of the signal at synapses (p. 44) or neuromuscular junctions (p. 64). A specialized variation of endocrine signalling (neurocrine signalling) occurs when neurones or paraneurones (e.g. chromaffin cells of the suprarenal medulla) secrete a hormone into the bloodstream.

Alternatively, signalling may occur at short range through a paracrine mechanism, in which cells of one type release molecules into the interstitial fluid of the local environment, to be detected by nearby cells of a different type that express the specific receptor protein. Cells may generate and respond to the same signal. This is autocrine signalling, a phenomenon that reinforces the coordinated activities of a group of like cells, which respond together to a high concentration of a local signalling molecule. The most extreme form of short-distance signalling is contact-dependent signalling, where one cell responds to transmembrane proteins of an adjacent cell that bind to surface receptors in the responding cell membrane. This type of signalling is important during development and in immune responses.

These different types of signalling mechanism are illustrated in **Fig. 2.6**. For further reading, see Alberts et al (2002) and Pollard and Earnshaw (2002).

SIGNALLING MOLECULES AND THEIR RECEPTORS

The majority of signalling molecules (ligands) are hydrophilic. They cannot cross the plasma membrane of a recipient cell to effect changes intracellularly unless they first bind to a plasma membrane receptor protein. Ligands are mainly proteins, polypeptides or highly charged biogenic amines. They include: classic peptide hormones of the endocrine system (Ch. 9); cytokines, which are mainly of haemopoietic cell origin and involved in inflammatory responses and tissue remodelling, e.g. the interferons, interleukins, tumour necrosis factor, leukaemia inhibitory factor; polypeptide growth factors, e.g. the epidermal growth factor superfamily, nerve growth factor, platelet-derived growth factor, the fibroblast growth factor family, transforming growth factor beta and the insulin-like growth factors. Polypeptide growth factors are multifunctional molecules with more widespread actions and cellular sources than their names suggest. They and their receptors are commonly mutated or aberrantly expressed in certain cancers. The cancer-causing gene variant is termed a transforming oncogene and the normal (wild-type) version of the gene is a cellular oncogene or proto-oncogene. The activated receptor acts as a transducer to generate intracellular signals, which are either small diffusible second

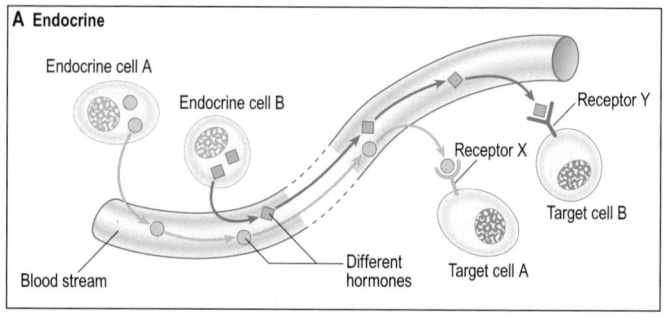

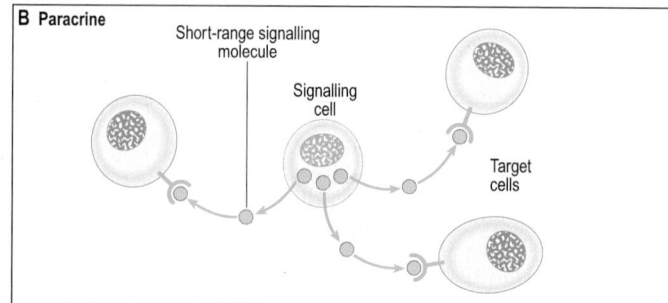

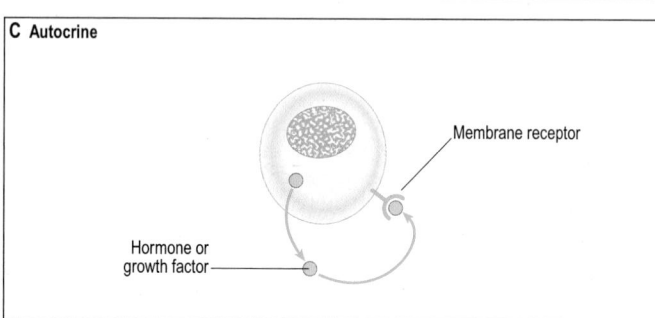

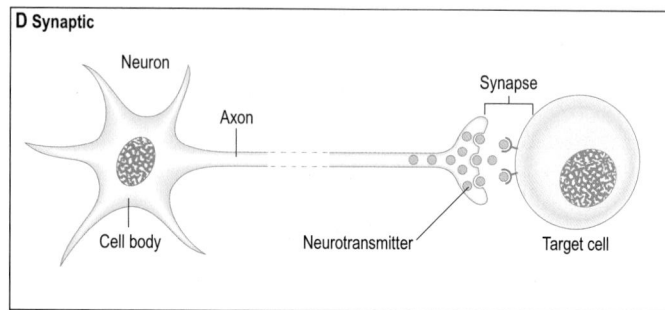

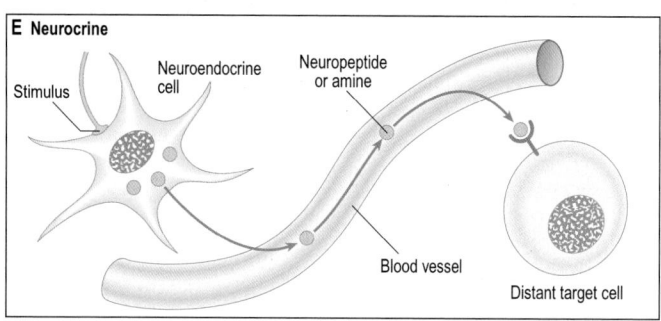

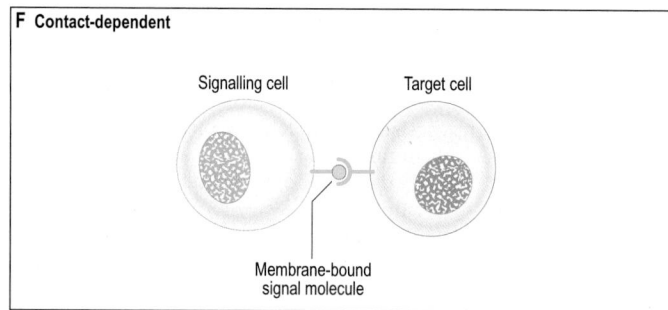

Fig. 2.6 The different modes of cell–cell signalling.

messengers (e.g. calcium, cyclic adenosine monophosphate or the plasma membrane lipid-soluble diacylglycerol), or larger protein complexes that amplify and relay the signal to target control systems. For further reading on growth factors and other signalling molecules, see Epstein (2003).

Some signals are hydrophobic and able to cross the plasma membrane freely. Classic examples are the steroid hormones, thyroid hormones, retinoids and vitamin D. Steroids, for instance, enter cells non-selectively, but elicit a specific response only in those target cells which express specific cytoplasmic or nuclear receptors. Light stimuli also cross the plasma membranes of photoreceptor cells and interact intracellularly, at least in rod cells, with membrane-bound photosensitive receptor proteins. Hydrophobic ligands are transported in the bloodstream or interstitial fluids, generally bound to carrier proteins, and they often have a longer half-life and longer-lasting effects on their targets than do water-soluble ligands.

A separate group of signalling molecules that are able to cross the plasma membrane freely is typified by the gas, nitric oxide. The principal target of short-range nitric oxide signalling is smooth muscle, which relaxes in response. Nitric oxide is released from vascular endothelium as a result of the action of autonomic nerves that supply the vessel wall. It causes local relaxation of smooth muscle and dilation of vessels. In the penis, this mechanism is responsible for penile erection. Nitric oxide is unusual among signalling molecules in having no specific receptor protein; instead, it acts directly on intracellular enzymes of the response pathway.

Receptor proteins

There are c.20 different families of receptor proteins, each with several isoforms responding to different ligands. The great majority of these receptors are transmembrane proteins. Members of each family share structural features that indicate either shared ligand-binding characteristics in the extracellular domain or shared signal transduction

properties in the cytoplasmic domain, or both. There is little relationship either between the nature of a ligand and the family of receptor proteins to which it binds and activates, or the signal transduction strategies by which an intracellular response is achieved. The same ligand may activate fundamentally different types of receptor in different cell types.

Cell surface receptor proteins are generally grouped according to their linkage to one of three intracellular systems: ion channel-linked receptors; G-protein-coupled receptors; receptors that link to enzyme systems. Other receptors do not fit neatly into any of these categories. All the known G-protein-coupled receptors belong to a structural group of proteins that pass through the membrane seven times in a series of serpentine loops. These receptors are thus known as seven-pass transmembrane receptors or, because the transmembrane regions are formed from α-helical domains, as seven-helix receptors. The most well-known of this large group of phylogenetically ancient receptors are the odorant-binding proteins of the olfactory system, the light-sensitive receptor protein, rhodopsin, and many of the receptors for clinically useful drugs. A comprehensive list of receptor proteins, their activating ligands and examples of the resultant biological function, is given in Pollard and Earnshaw (2002).

TRANSPORT ACROSS CELL MEMBRANES

Lipid bilayers are increasingly impermeable to molecules as they increase in size or hydrophilicity. Transport mechanisms are therefore required to carry essential polar molecules, including ions, nutrients, nucleotides and metabolites of various kinds, across the plasma membrane and into or out of membrane-bound intracellular compartments. Transport is facilitated by a variety of membrane transport proteins, each with specificity for a particular class of molecule, e.g. sugars. Transport proteins fall mainly into two major classes, channel proteins and carrier proteins.

Channel proteins form aqueous pores in the membrane, which open and close under the regulation of intracellular signals, e.g. G-proteins, to allow the flux of solutes (usually inorganic ions) of specific size and charge. Transport through ion channels is always passive and ion flow through an open channel depends only on the ion concentration gradient and its electronic charge, and the potential difference across the membrane. These factors combine to produce an electrochemical gradient, which governs ion flux. Channel proteins are utilized most effectively by the excitable plasma membranes of nerve cells, where the resting membrane potential can change transiently from about −70 mV (negative inside the cell) to +50 mV (positive inside the cell) when stimulated by a neurotransmitter (as a result of the opening and subsequent closure of channels selectively permeable to sodium and potassium).

Carrier proteins bind their specific solutes, such as amino-acids, and transport them across the membrane through a series of conformational changes. This latter process is slower than ion transport through membrane channels. Transport by carrier proteins can occur either passively by simple diffusion, or actively against the electrochemical gradient of the solute. Active transport must therefore be coupled to a source of energy, such as ATP generation, or energy released by the coordinate movement of an ion down its electrochemical gradient. Linked transport can be in the same direction as the solute, in which case the carrier protein is described as a symporter, or in the opposite direction, when the carrier acts as an antiporter.

TRANSLOCATION OF PROTEINS ACROSS INTRACELLULAR MEMBRANES

Proteins are generally synthesized on ribosomes in the cytosol or on the rough endoplasmic reticulum. A few are made on mitochondrial ribosomes. Once synthesized, many proteins remain in the cytosol, where they carry out their functions. Others, such as integral membrane proteins or proteins for secretion, are translocated across intracellular membranes for post-translational modification and targeting to their destinations. This is achieved by the signal sequence, an addressing system contained within the protein sequence of amino-acids, which is recognized by receptors or translocators in the appropriate membrane. Proteins are thus sorted by their signal sequence (or set of sequences that become spatially grouped as a signal patch when the protein folds into its tertiary configuration), so that they are recognized by and enter the correct intracellular membrane compartment.

EXOCYTOSIS AND ENDOCYTOSIS

Secreted proteins, lipids, mucins, small molecules such as amines and other cellular products destined for export from the cell are transported to the plasma membrane in small vesicles released from the *trans* face of the Golgi apparatus. This pathway is either constitutive, in which transport and secretion occur more or less continuously, or it is regulated by external signals, as in the control of salivary secretion by autonomic neural stimulation. In regulated secretion, the secretory product is stored temporarily in membrane-bound secretory granules or vesicles. Exocytosis is achieved by fusion of the secretory vesicular membrane with the plasma membrane and release of the vesicle contents into the extracellular domain.

In polarized cells, e.g. most epithelia, exocytosis occurs at the apical plasma membrane and the cells secrete into a duct lumen or onto a free surface such as the lining of the stomach. In hepatocytes, bile is secreted across a very small area of plasma membrane forming the wall of the bile canaliculus (p. 1222). This region is defined as the apical plasma membrane, and is the site of exocrine secretion (p. 34), whereas secretion of hepatocyte plasma proteins into the bloodstream is targeted to the basolateral surfaces facing the sinusoids. Packaging of different secretory products into appropriate vesicles takes place in the *trans*-Golgi network. Delivery of secretory vesicles to their correct plasma membrane domains is achieved by sorting sequences in the cytoplasmic tails of vesicular membrane proteins.

There are other mechanisms in which initial delivery of secretory products is less selective, but is followed by selective retention (or degradation) or reprocessing and redistribution by endosomes. Ultimately, secretory vesicles undergo docking, priming (to prepare the vesicle for a regulatory signal, where secretion is regulation-dependent) and fusion with the plasma membrane to release their contents. The

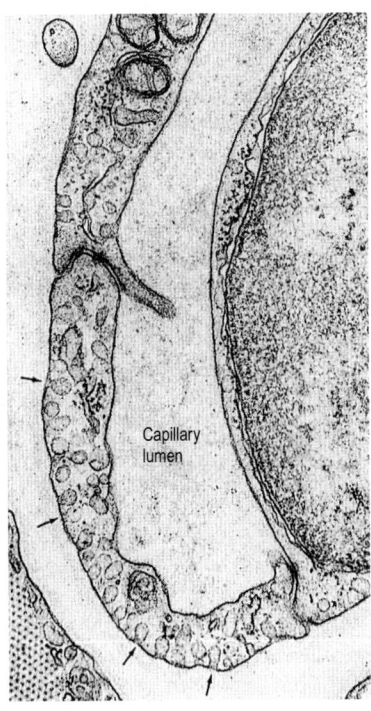

Fig. 2.7 Transcytotic vesicles (arrows) shuttle in both directions between blood plasma and extracellular fluid, across the cytoplasm of these endothelial cells in the wall of a capillary.

Capillary lumen

process of exocytosis also delivers integral membrane components to the cell surface in the normal turnover and recycling of the plasma membrane. However, excess plasma membrane generated by vesicle fusion during exocytosis is rapidly removed by concurrent endocytosis.

The process of endocytosis involves the internalization of vesicles derived from the plasma membrane. The vesicles may contain: engulfed fluids and solutes from the extracellular interstitial fluid (pinocytosis); larger macromolecules, often bound to surface receptors (receptor-mediated endocytosis); particulate matter, including microorganisms or cellular debris (phagocytosis). Pinocytosis generally involves small fluid-filled vesicles and is a marked property of capillary endothelium, e.g. where vesicles containing nutrients and oxygen dissolved in blood plasma are transported from the vascular lumen to the endothelial basal plasma membrane (**Fig. 2.7**). Interstitial fluid containing dissolved carbon dioxide is also taken up by pinocytosis for simultaneous transportation across the endothelial cell wall in the opposite direction, for release into the bloodstream by exocytosis. This shuttling of pinocytotic vesicles is also termed transcytosis. Larger volumes of fluid are engulfed by dendritic cells, e.g. in the process of sampling interstitial fluids by macropinocytosis in immune surveillance for antigens (p. 81). Interstitial fluid is inevitably taken up during receptor-mediated endocytosis when ligands are internalized.

Receptor-mediated endocytosis, also known as clathrin-dependent endocytosis, is initiated at specialized regions of the plasma membrane known as clathrin-coated pits. Clathrin is a protein that cross-links adjacent adaptor protein (adaptin) complexes to form a basket-like structure, bending the membrane inwards into a hemisphere. Much, but not all, fluid-phase pinocytosis also utilizes clathrin-coated pits. Ligands such as the iron-transporting protein, transferrin, and the cholesterol-transporting low-density lipoprotein bind to their receptors, which cluster in clathrin-coated pits through an interaction with adaptins. The pits then invaginate and pinch off from the plasma membrane, internalizing both receptor and ligand. The processing of endocytic vesicles and their contents is described on page 14. For further details of the molecular mechanisms of endocytosis, see Alberts et al (2002) or Pollard and Earnshaw (2002).

PHAGOCYTOSIS

Phagocytosis is a property of many cell types, but is most efficient in cells specialized for this activity. The professional phagocytes of the body belong to the monocyte lineage of haemopoietic cells, in particular the tissue macrophages (p. 80). Other effective phagocytes are neutrophil granulocytes and most dendritic cells (p. 81), which are also of haemopoietic origin. Phagocytosis plays an important part in the immune defence system of the body, in which the amoeboid process of ingestion of organisms for nutrition has evolved into a mechanism for the clearance of microorganisms invading the body. Macrophages also ingest particulate material including inorganic matter, such as inhaled dust particles, in addition to debris from dead cells and protein aggregates such as immune complexes in the blood, airways, interstitial spaces and connective tissue matrices.

Phagocytosis is a triggered process, initiated when a phagocytic cell binds to a particle or organism, often through a process of molecular recognition. Typically, a pathogenic microorganism may first be coated by antibodies, which are bound in turn by receptors for the Fc portion of the antibody molecule expressed by macrophages and neutrophils; in this way the microorganism is attached to the cell. This triggers the production of large pseudopodia, which engulf the organism and internalize it, as their pseudopod tips fuse together. The process appears to depend on actin–myosin-based cellular motility and, unlike receptor-mediated endocytosis, it is energy dependent. Phagosomes thus formed are as large as the body they engulf and can be a considerable proportion of the volume of the phagocytic cell. Inside the cell, the phagosome fuses with lysosomes, which degrade its contents.

Cytoplasm

ENDOPLASMIC RETICULUM

Endoplasmic reticulum is a system of interconnecting membrane-lined channels within the cytoplasm (Fig. 2.8). These channels take various forms, including cisternae (flattened sacs), tubules and vesicles. The membranes divide the cytoplasm into two major compartments. The intramembranous compartment includes the space where secretory products are stored or transported to the Golgi complex and cell exterior. The extramembranous cytosol is made up of the colloidal proteins such as enzymes, carbohydrates and small protein molecules, together with ribosomes and ribonucleic acids, and elements of the cytoskeleton.

Structurally, the channel system can be divided into rough or granular endoplasmic reticulum, which has ribosomes attached to its outer cytosolic surface, and smooth or agranular endoplasmic reticulum, which lacks ribosomes.

ROUGH ENDOPLASMIC RETICULUM

The rough endoplasmic reticulum, studded with ribosomes, is a site of protein synthesis (Fig. 2.8A). Most proteins pass through its membranes and accumulate within its cisternae, although some integral membrane proteins, e.g. plasma membrane receptors, are inserted into the rough endoplasmic reticulum membrane, where they remain. After passage from the rough endoplasmic reticulum, proteins remain in membrane-bound cytoplasmic organelles such as lysosomes, become incorporated into new plasma membrane, or are secreted by the cell. Some carbohydrates are also synthesized by enzymes within the cavities of the rough endoplasmic reticulum and may be attached to newly formed protein (glycosylation). Vesicles are budded off from the rough endoplasmic reticulum for transport to the Golgi as part of the protein-targeting mechanism of the cell.

SMOOTH ENDOPLASMIC RETICULUM

The smooth endoplasmic reticulum (Fig. 2.8B) is associated with carbohydrate metabolism and many other metabolic processes, including detoxification and synthesis of lipids, cholesterol and other steroids. The membranes of the smooth endoplasmic reticulum serve as surfaces for the attachment of many enzyme systems, e.g. the enzyme cytochrome P450, which is involved in important detoxification mechanisms and is thus accessible to its substrates, which are generally lipophilic. They also cooperate with the rough endoplasmic reticulum and the Golgi apparatus to synthesize new membranes; the protein, carbohydrate and lipid components are added in different structural compartments. Highly specialized types of endoplasmic reticulum are present in some cells. For example, in skeletal muscle cells, the smooth endoplasmic reticulum (sarcoplasmic reticulum) stores calcium ions, which are released into the cytosol to initiate contraction after stimulation initiated by a motor neurone at the neuromuscular junction (p. 64).

RIBOSOMES

Ribosomes are macromolecular machines that catalyse the synthesis of proteins from amino-acids. They are granules c.15 nm in diameter, composed of ribosomal RNA (rRNA) molecules assembled into two unequal subunits. A large number of proteins, mostly small and basic, are applied mainly to the surfaces of the subunit cores of RNA. The subunits can be separated by their sedimentation coefficients (S) in an ultracentrifuge, into larger 60S and smaller 40S components. These are associated with 73 different proteins (40 in the large subunit and 33 in the small), which have structural and enzymatic functions. Three small, highly convoluted rRNA strands (28S, 5.8S and 5S) make up the large subunit, and one strand (18S) is in the small subunit. Their synthesis and assembly into subunits takes place in the nucleolus, and includes association with ribosomal proteins translocated from their site of synthesis in the cytoplasm. The individual subunits are then transported into the cytoplasm, where they remain separate from each other when not actively synthesizing proteins.

A typical cell contains millions of ribosomes. They may be solitary, relatively inactive structures, or may form groups (polyribosomes or polysomes) attached to messenger RNA (mRNA), which they translate during protein synthesis (Fig. 2.9). Polysomes may be attached to the membranes of the rough endoplasmic reticulum or may lie free in the cytosol, where they synthesize proteins for use outside the system of membrane compartments, including enzymes of the cytosol and cytoskeletal proteins. Some of the cytosolic products include proteins that can be inserted directly into (or through) membranes of selected organelles, such as mitochondria and peroxisomes.

In a mature polysome, all the attachment sites of the mRNA are occupied as ribosomes move along it, synthesizing protein according to its nucleic acid sequence. Consequently, the number of ribosomes in a polysome indicates the length of the mRNA molecule and hence the size of the protein being made. The two subunits have separate roles in protein synthesis. The 40S subunit is the site of attachment and translation of mRNA. The 60S subunit is responsible for the release of the new protein and, where appropriate, attachment to the endoplasmic

A
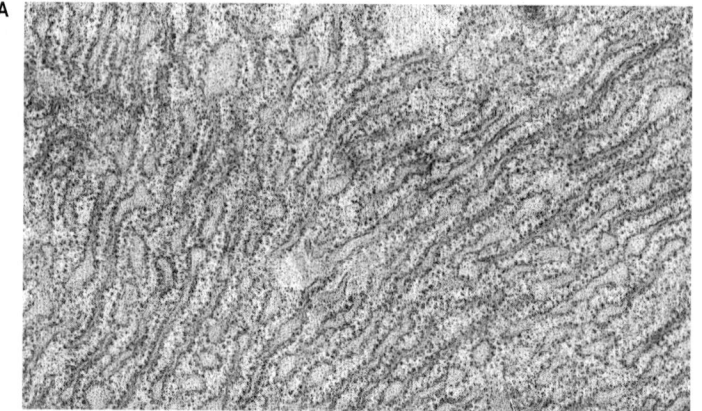

B
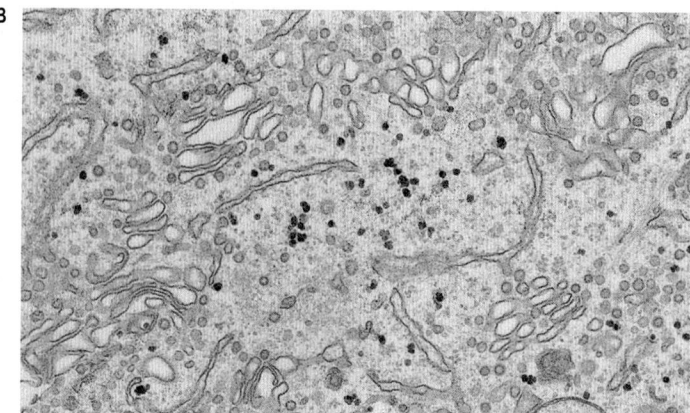

Fig. 2.8 The endoplasmic reticulum. **A**, Rough endoplasmic reticulum with attached ribosomes; **B**, smooth endoplasmic reticulum with associated vesicles. The dense particles are glycogen granules. (By kind permission from Rose Watson, Cancer Research UK.)

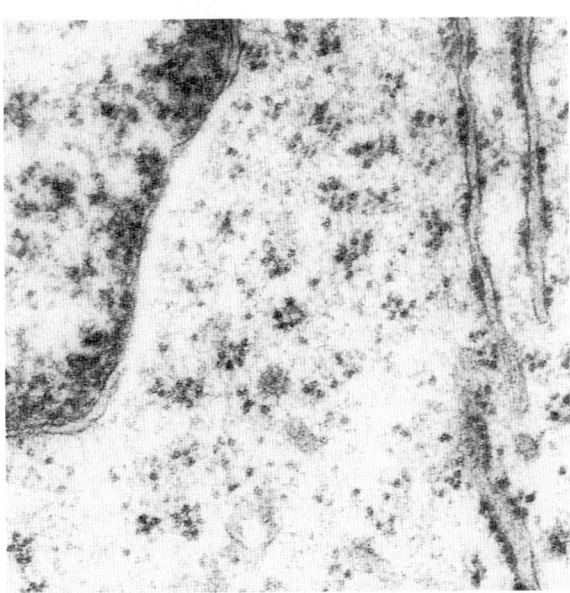

Fig. 2.9 Ribosomes, distributed either singly, clustered as polyribosomes (polysomes), or attached to the rough endoplasmic reticulum (right). (By permission from Stevens A, Lowe JS 1996 Human Histology, 2nd edn. London: Mosby.)

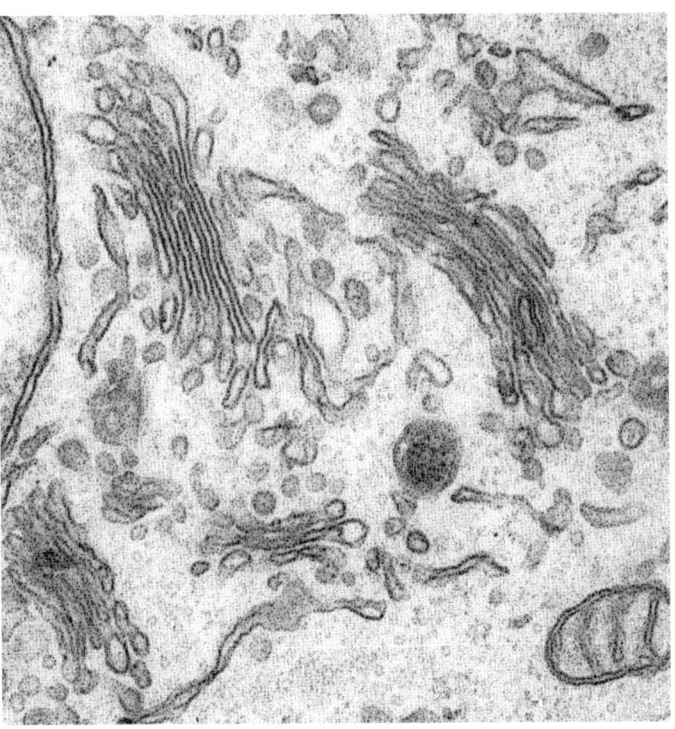

Fig. 2.10 Golgi apparatus in a fibroblast. Several Golgi stacks are present, each with convex *cis*- and concave *trans*-Golgi surfaces, and associated transport vesicles. The edge of the nucleus appears on the left. (By kind permission from Rose Watson, Cancer Research UK.)

reticulum via an intermediate docking protein that directs the newly synthesized protein through the membrane into the cisternal space.

GOLGI APPARATUS (GOLGI COMPLEX) (Figs 2.10, 2.11)

The Golgi apparatus is a distinct cytoplasmic region near the nucleus, and is particularly prominent in secretory cells when stained with silver or other metallic salts. The Golgi apparatus forms part of the pathway by which proteins synthesized in the rough endoplasmic reticulum undergo post-translational modification and are targeted to the cell surface for secretion or for storage in membranous vesicles. Ultra-

structurally, the Golgi apparatus is a membranous organelle consisting of a stack of several flattened membranous cisternae, together with clusters of vesicles surrounding its surfaces. Seen in vertical section, it is often cup-shaped. Small transport vesicles from the rough endoplasmic reticulum, generated by a process of budding and pinching off, are

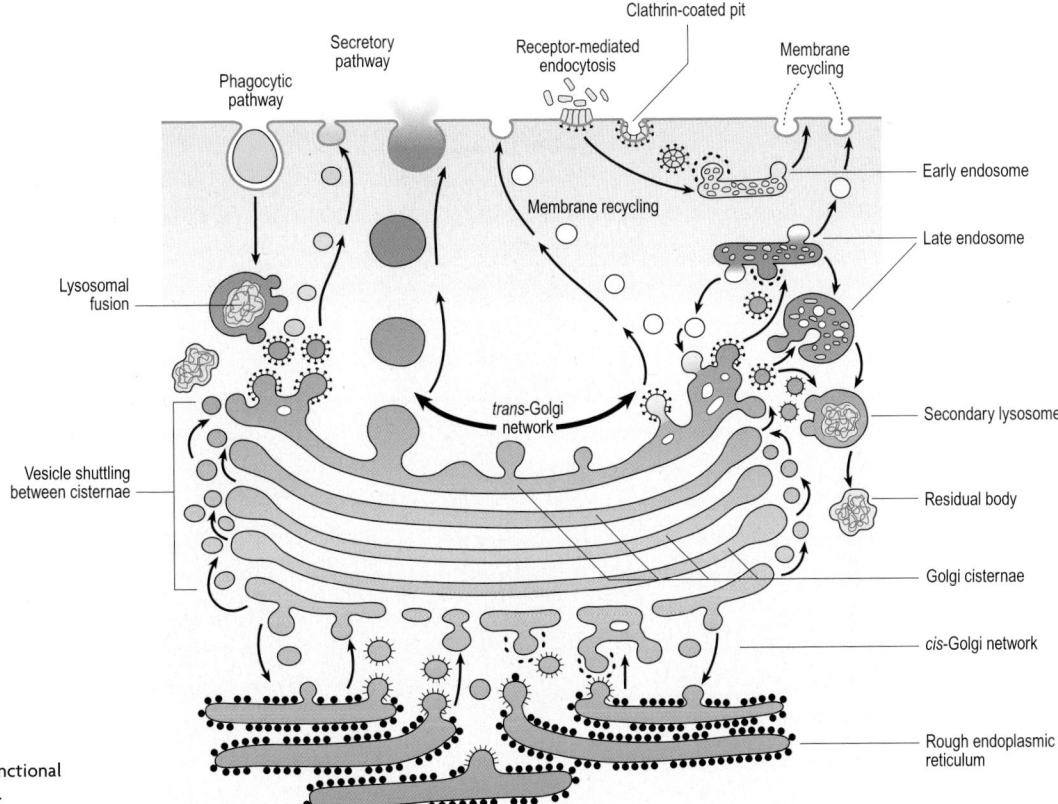

Fig. 2.11 The Golgi apparatus and its functional relationships with associated structures.

received at one face of the Golgi stack, the convex *cis*-face (entry or forming surface). Here, they deliver their contents to the first cisterna in the series by membrane fusion. From the edges of this cisterna, the protein is transported to the next cisterna by vesicular budding and then fusion, and this process is repeated until the final cisterna at the concave *trans* face (exit or condensing surface) is reached. Here, larger vesicles are formed for delivery to other parts of the cell.

In addition to these cisternae, there are other membranous structures that form an integral part of the Golgi apparatus, termed the *cis*-Golgi and *trans*-Golgi networks. The *cis*-Golgi network is a region of complex membranous channels interposed between the rough endoplasmic reticulum and the Golgi *cis* face (Golgi–rough endoplasmic reticulum complex), which receives and transmits vesicles in both directions. Its function is to select appropriate proteins synthesized on the rough endoplasmic reticulum for delivery by vesicles to the Golgi stack, while inappropriate proteins are shuttled back to the rough endoplasmic reticulum.

The *trans*-Golgi network, at the other side of the Golgi stack, is also a region of interconnected membrane channels engaged in protein sorting. Here, modified proteins processed in the Golgi cisternae are packaged selectively into vesicles and dispatched to different parts of the cell. The packaging depends on the detection, by the *trans*-Golgi network, of particular amino-acid signal sequences, leading to their enclosure in membranes of appropriate composition that will further modify their contents, e.g. by extracting water to concentrate them or by pumping in protons to acidify their contents. The membranes contain specific signal proteins, which may allocate them to microtubule-based transport pathways and allow them to dock with appropriate targets elsewhere in the cell, e.g. the plasma membrane in the case of secretory vesicles. Vesicle formation and budding at the *trans*-Golgi network involves the addition of clathrin on their external surface, to form coated pits.

Within the Golgi stack proper, proteins undergo a series of sequential chemical modifications that started in the rough endoplasmic reticulum. These include: changes in glycosyl groups, e.g. removal of mannose, addition of *N*-acetyl glucosamine and sialic acid; sulphation of attached glycosaminoglycans; protein phosphorylation. Lipids formed in the endoplasmic reticulum are also routed for incorporation into vesicles.

The role of the Golgi apparatus in the synthesis of primary lysosomes is a major activity in cells with abundant lysosomes, such as those with phagocytic roles. In glandular cells with an apical secretory zone, the Golgi apparatus lies between the secretory surface and the nucleus. In fibroblasts, there are two or more groups of Golgi stacks; up to 50 groups are found in liver cells. The Golgi apparatus is often closely associated with the centrosome (a region of the cell containing a centriole pair and related microtubules), reflecting a link with the microtubule-mediated vesicle transport system.

ENDOSOMES, LYSOSOMES AND PEROXISOMES

The endosome system of vesicles originates in small endocytic vesicles or larger phagosomes taken up by the cell from the exterior. The system is linked functionally to a second series of membranous structures, the lysosomes. Lysosomes contain acid hydrolases, which process or degrade exogenous materials (heterophagy), and intracellular organelles that are exhausted, damaged or no longer required (autophagy). There is a continual exchange of vesicles between this system and the Golgi–rough endoplasmic reticulum complex, so that the endosomal/lysosomal system is provided with hydrolytic enzymes and the Golgi receives depleted vesicles for recharging. Once internalized, endocytic vesicles shed their coat of adaptin and clathrin, and fuse with a tubular cisterna termed an early endosome, where the receptor molecules release their bound ligands. Membrane and receptors from the early endosomes can be recycled to the cell surface as exocytic vesicles.

LATE ENDOSOMES

After a brief period in the early endosomes, materials can be passed on to late endosomes, which are a more deeply placed set of tubules, vesicles or cisternae. Late endosomes receive lysosomal enzymes via vesicles (small lysosomes) transported from the Golgi apparatus. The pH of late endosomes is low (about 5.0) and this activates lysosomal acid hydrolases to degrade the endosomal contents. The products of hydrolysis are either passed through the membrane into the cytosol, or may be retained in the endosome. Late endosomes may grow considerably in size by vesicle fusion to form multivesicular bodies (**Fig. 2.12**), and the enzyme concentration may increase greatly to form the large, dense classic lysosomes described by de Duve. However, such large organelles do not appear in all cells, perhaps because late endosomes often deal very rapidly with endocytosed material.

LYSOSOMES

Lysosomes are dense, spheroidal, membrane-bound bodies 80–800 nm in diameter (**Fig. 2.12**), often with complex inclusions of material undergoing hydrolysis (secondary lysosomes). They contain acid hydrolases able to degrade a wide variety of substances. To date, more than 40 lysosomal enzymes have been described, including proteases, lipases, carbohydrases, esterases and nucleases. The enzymes are heavily glycosylated, and are maintained at a low pH by proton pumps in the lysosomal membranes.

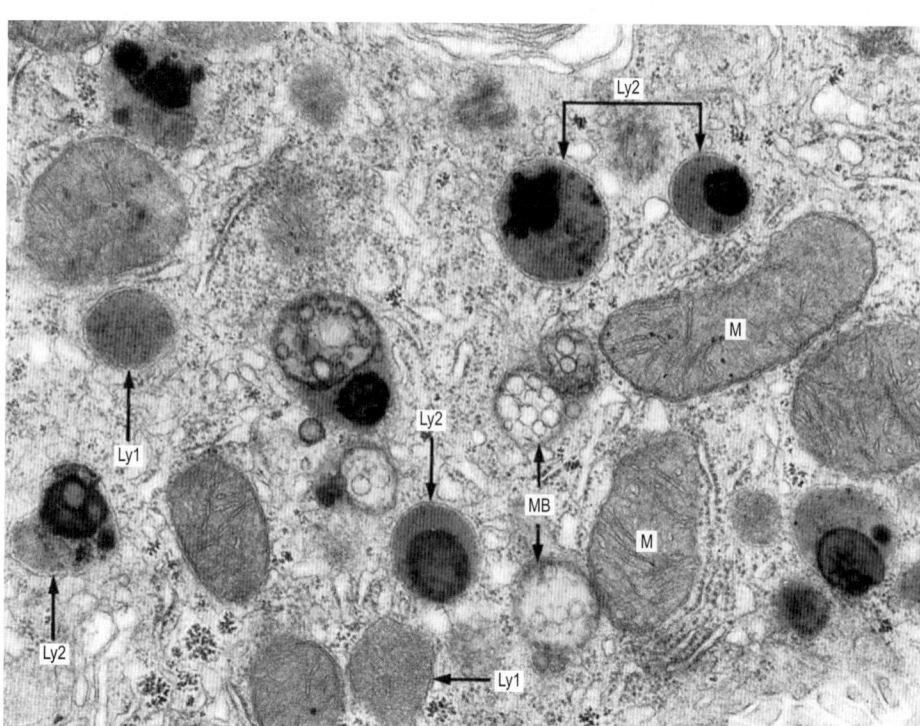

Fig. 2.12 The typical features of primary and secondary lysosomes in the cytoplasm of a liver cell. Primary lysosomes (Ly1) are homogeneous membrane-bound bodies, whereas secondary lysosomes (Ly2) are typically variable in density and content, and often difficult to distinguish from later-stage residual bodies. Note their size relative to mitochondria (M). A number of late endosomes (multivesicular bodies, MB) are also shown. (By permission from Young B, Heath JW 2000 Wheater's Functional Histology. Edinburgh: Churchill Livingstone.)

Lysosomes are numerous in actively phagocytic cells, e.g. macrophages and neutrophil granulocytes, in which lysosomes are responsible for destroying phagocytosed bacteria. In these cells, the phagosome containing the bacterium may fuse with several lysosomes. Lysosomes are also frequent in cells with a high turnover of organelles, e.g. exocrine gland cells and neurones. Effete organelles are targeted for demolition by a process that is not fully understood, but which results in engulfment of areas of cytoplasm, including entire organelles, in a membranous cisterna. The structure then fuses with lysosomes and the contents are rapidly degraded.

Material that has been hydrolysed within late endosomes and lysosomes may be completely degraded to soluble products, e.g. aminoacids, which are recycled through metabolic pathways. However degradation is usually incomplete, and some debris remains. A debris-laden vesicle is called a residual body, and may be passed to the cell surface, where it is ejected by exocytosis; alternatively, it may persist inside the cell as an inert residual body. Considerable numbers of residual bodies can accumulate in long-lived cells, often fusing to form larger dense vacuoles with complex lamellar inclusions. As their contents are often darkly pigmented, this may change the colour of the tissue, e.g. in neurones the end-product of lysosomal digestion, lipofuscin (neuromelanin or senility pigment), gives ageing brains a brownish-yellow colouration.

Lysosomal enzymes may also be secreted – often as part of a process to alter the extracellular matrix, as in osteoclast erosion of bone (p. 92). Abnormal release of enzymes can cause tissue damage, as in certain types of arthritis. Some drugs, e.g. cortisone, can stabilize lysosomal membranes and may therefore inhibit many lysosomal activities, including the secretion of enzymes, and their fusion with phagocytic vesicles.

Lysosomal storage diseases

If any of the lysosomal enzymes are defective because of gene mutations, the materials that they normally degrade will accumulate within late endosomes and lysosomes. Many such lysosomal storage diseases are known, e.g. Tay–Sachs disease, in which a faulty gangliosidase leads to the accumulation of glycolipid in neurones, causing death during childhood. In Hurler's syndrome, failure to metabolize certain glycosaminoglycans causes the accumulation of large amounts of matrix within connective tissue, which distorts growth of many parts of the body.

PEROXISOMES

Peroxisomes are membrane-bound vacuoles c.0.5–0.15 μm across, present in all nucleated cell types. They often contain dense cores or crystalline interiors composed mainly of high concentrations of the enzyme urate oxidase. Large (0.5 μm) peroxisomes are particularly numerous in hepatocytes and kidney tubule cells. Peroxisomes are important in the oxidative detoxification of various substances taken into or produced within cells, including ethanol and formaldehyde. Oxidation is carried out by a number of enzymes, including D-aminoacid oxidase and urate oxidase, which generate hydrogen peroxide as a source of molecular oxygen. Excess amounts of hydrogen peroxide are broken down by the enzyme, catalase. Peroxisomes also oxidize fatty acid chains by β-oxidation.

The formation of peroxisomes is unusual in that they appear to be derived by the growth and fission of previously existing peroxisomes. Their internal proteins are passed from the cytosol directly through channels in their membranes, rather than by packaging from the rough endoplasmic reticulum and Golgi apparatus. These features are also found in mitochondria, although peroxisomal proteins are coded for entirely in the nucleus. A genetic abnormality in the translocation of proteins into peroxisomes, leading to peroxisomal enzyme deficiencies, is seen in Zellweger syndrome, caused by a gene mutation in an integral membrane protein (peroxisome assembly factor-1). In homozygotes, this is usually fatal shortly after birth.

MITOCHONDRIA

The mitochondrion is a membrane-bound organelle (**Fig. 2.13**). It is the principal source of chemical energy in most cells. Mitochondria are the site of the citric acid (Kreb's, tricarboxylic acid) cycle and the electron transport (cytochrome) pathway by which complex organic molecules are finally oxidized to carbon dioxide and water. This process provides the energy to drive the production of ATP from ADP and inorganic

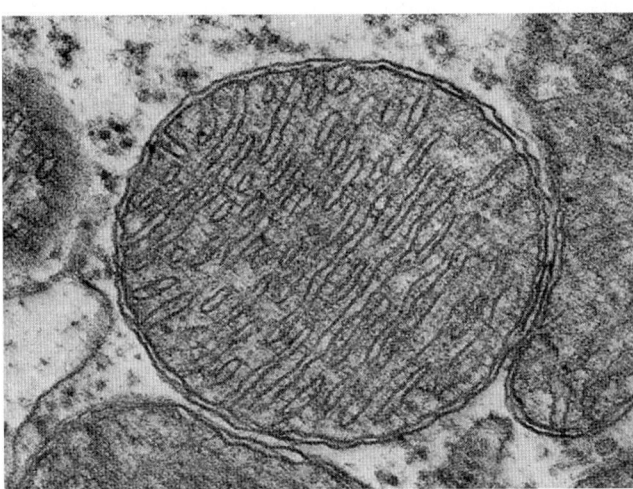

Fig. 2.13 A mitochondrion. The folded cristae project into the matrix from the inner mitochondrial membrane.

phosphate (oxidative phosphorylation). The various enzymes of the citric acid cycle are located in the mitochondrial matrix, whereas those of the cytochrome system and oxidative phosphorylation are localized chiefly in the inner mitochondrial membrane.

The numbers of mitochondria in a particular cell reflect its general energy requirements; e.g. in hepatocytes there may be as many as 2000, whereas in resting lymphocytes there are usually very few. Mature erythrocytes lack mitochondria altogether. Cells with few mitochondria generally rely largely on glycolysis for their energy supplies. These include some very active cells, e.g. fast twitch skeletal muscle fibres, which are able to work rapidly, but for only a limited duration. Mitochondria appear in the light microscope as long thin threads, or alternatively as spherical or ellipsoid bodies in the cytoplasm of most cells, particularly those with a high metabolic rate, e.g. secretory cells in exocrine glands. In living cells, mitochondria constantly change shape and intracellular position; they multiply by growth and fission and may undergo fusion.

In the electron microscope, mitochondria usually appear as elliptical bodies 0.5–2.0 μm long. Each mitochondrion is lined by an outer and an inner unit membrane, separated by a variable gap termed the intermembrane space. The lumen is surrounded by the inner membrane and contains the mitochondrial matrix. The outer membrane is smooth and sometimes attached to other organelles, particularly microtubules. The inner membrane is deeply folded to form incomplete transverse or longitudinal tubular invaginations, cristae, which create a relatively large surface area of membrane. Mitochondrial shape, and the shape and organization of the cristae, vary with the cell type. Cristae are most numerous and complex in cells with a high metabolic rate, e.g. cardiac muscle cells. The permeabilities of the two mitochondrial membranes differ considerably: the outer membrane is freely permeable to many substances because of the presence of large non-specific channels formed by proteins (porins), whereas the inner membrane is permeable to only a narrow range of molecules. The presence of cardiolipin, a phospholipid, in the inner membrane may contribute to this relative impermeability.

The mitochondrial matrix is an aqueous environment. It contains a variety of enzymes, and strands of mitochondrial DNA with the capacity for transcription and translation of a unique set of mitochondrial genes (mitochondrial mRNAs and transfer RNAs, mitochondrial ribosomes with rRNAs). The DNA forms a closed loop, c.5 μm across; several identical copies are present in each mitochondrion. The ratio between its bases differs from that of nuclear DNA, and the RNA sequences also differ in the precise genetic code used in protein synthesis. At least 13 respiratory chain enzymes of the matrix and inner membrane are encoded by the small number of genes along the mitochondrial DNA. The great majority of mitochondrial proteins are encoded by nuclear genes and made in the cytosol, then inserted through special channels in the mitochondrial membranes to reach their destinations. Their membrane lipids are synthesized in the endoplasmic reticulum.

Mitochondrial ribosomes are smaller and quite distinct from those of the rest of the cell. Mitochondrial ribosomes and nucleic acids resemble those of bacteria. This similarity underpins the theory that mitochondrial ancestors were oxygen-utilizing bacteria that existed in a symbiotic relationship with eukaryotic cells unable to metabolize the oxygen produced by early plants. As mitochondria are formed only from previously existing ones, it follows that all mitochondria in the body are descended from those in the cytoplasm of the fertilized ovum. It has also been shown that mitochondria are of maternal origin because the mitochondria of the sperm are not generally incorporated into the ovum at fertilization. Thus mitochondria (and mitochondrial genetic variations and mutations) are passed only through the female line.

Mitochondria are distributed within a cell according to regional energy requirements, e.g. near the bases of cilia in ciliated epithelia, in the basal domain of the cells of proximal convoluted tubules in the renal cortex (where considerable active transport occurs) and around the proximal end of the flagellum in spermatozoa. They may be involved with tissue-specific metabolic reactions, e.g. various urea-forming enzymes in liver cell mitochondria. Moreover, a number of genetic diseases of mitochondria affect particular tissues exclusively, e.g. mitochondrial myopathies (skeletal muscle) and mitochondrial neuropathies (nervous tissue). For further information see Graff et al (2002).

CYTOSOLIC ORGANELLES

The aqueous cytosol surrounds the membranous organelles described above. It also contains various non-membranous organelles, including free ribosomes, a system of filamentous proteins known as the cytoskeleton, and other inclusions, such as storage granules (e.g. glycogen) and lipid vacuoles.

LIPID VACUOLES

Lipid vacuoles are spherical bodies of various sizes found within many cells, but are especially prominent in the adipocytes (lipocytes) of adipose connective tissue. They do not belong to the Golgi-related vacuolar system of the cell. They are not membrane bound, but are droplets of lipid suspended in the cytosol. In cells specialized for lipid storage the vacuoles reach 80 μm or more in diameter.

Lipid vacuoles are often surrounded by cytoskeletal filaments that help to stabilize them within cells and to prevent their fusion with the membranes of other organelles, including the plasma membrane. They function as stores of chemical energy, thermal insulators and mechanical shock absorbers in adipocytes. In many cells, they may represent end-products of other metabolic pathways, e.g. in steroid-synthesizing cells, where they are a prominent feature of the cytoplasm. They may also be secreted, as in the alveolar epithelium of the lactating breast.

CYTOSKELETON

The cytoskeleton is a system of filamentous intracellular proteins of different shapes and sizes that form a complex, often interconnected, network throughout the cytoplasm. It provides mechanical support, maintains cell shape and rigidity, and enables cells to adopt highly asymmetric or irregular profiles, e.g. in neurones. The cytoskeleton plays an important part in establishing structural polarity and different functional domains within a cell. It also provides mechanical support for projections from the cell surface such as microvilli and cilia, and anchors them into the cytoplasm.

The cytoskeleton restricts specific organelles to particular cellular locations, e.g. the Golgi apparatus is near the nucleus and endoplasmic reticulum, and mitochondria are near sites of energy requirement. Most specifically, the cytoskeleton is concerned with motility, either within the cell (e.g. shuttling vesicles and macromolecules between cytoplasmic sites, or the movement of chromosomes during mitosis), or of the entire cell (e.g. in embryonic morphogenesis or the chemotactic migration of leukocytes). One of the most highly developed and specialized functions of the cytoskeleton is seen in the contractility of muscle cells.

The catalogue of cytoskeletal structural proteins is extensive and still increasing. The major filamentous structures found in non-muscle cells are microfilaments (actin), microtubules (tubulin), and intermediate filaments (varieties of cell specific intermediate filament proteins). Other important components are generally smaller proteins that bind to the principal filamentous types to link them together or to generate

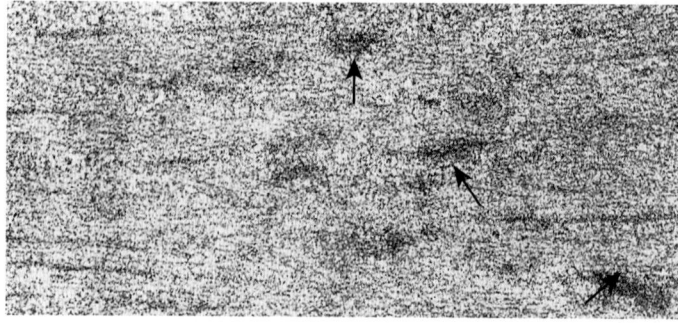

Fig. 2.14 Actin microfilaments present at high density in the cytoplasm of a smooth muscle cell. Cytoplasmic dense bodies (arrows) are points of attachment for the actin filaments.

movement. These include actin-binding proteins such as myosin, which in some cells can assemble into thick filaments, and microtubule-associated proteins.

Actin filaments (microfilaments)

Actin filaments are well-defined, fine filaments with a width of 6–8 nm (**Fig. 2.14**), and a solid cross-section. Within most cell types, actin constitutes the most abundant protein and in some motile cells its concentration may exceed 200 μM (10 mg protein per ml cytoplasm). The filaments are formed by the ATP-dependent polymerization of actin monomer into a characteristic linear form in which the subunits are arranged in a single tight helix with a distance of 13 subunits between turns. The polymerized form is termed F-actin (fibrillar actin) and the unpolymerized form is G-actin (globular actin), with a molecular mass of 43 kDa. Each monomer has an asymmetric structure. When monomers polymerize, they confer a defined polarity on the filament: the plus end favours monomer addition, and the minus end favours monomer dissociation. Myosins bind to filamentous actin at an angle to give the appearance of a series of arrowheads pointing towards the minus end of the filament, and the barbs point towards the plus end. There is a dynamic equilibrium between G-actin and F-actin: in most cells c.50% of the actin is estimated to be in the polymerized state.

Actin-binding proteins

A wide variety of actin-binding proteins exist that are capable of modulating the form of actin within the cell. These interactions are fundamental to the organization of cytoplasm and to cell shape. Actin-binding proteins can be divided into bundling proteins, gel-forming proteins and filament severing proteins.

Bundling proteins tie actin filaments together in longitudinal arrays to form cables or core structures. The bundles may be closely spaced, e.g. in microvilli, microspikes and filopodia, where parallel filaments are tied tightly together to form stiff bundles orientated in the same direction. Proteins with this function include fimbrin and villin (also classified as a severing protein). Other actin-bundling proteins form rather looser bundles of filaments that run anti-parallel to each other with respect to their plus and minus ends. They include α-actinin and myosin II, which can form cross-links with ATP-dependent motor activity, and cause adjacent actin filaments to slide on each other, and either change the shape of cells or (if the actin bundles are anchored into the cell membrane at both ends), maintain a degree of active rigidity.

Gel-forming proteins, such as filamin, interconnect adjacent actin filaments to produce loose filamentous meshworks (gels) composed of randomly orientated F-actin. These networks are frequently found in the outer cortical regions of cells, e.g. fibroblasts. They form a semi-rigid zone from which most other organelles are excluded. Severing proteins, such as gelsolin and severin, bind to F-actin filaments and sever them, which produces profound changes within the actin cytoskeleton and in its coupling to the cell surface.

Other classes of actin-binding proteins link the actin cytoskeleton to the plasma membrane either directly or indirectly through a variety of membrane-associated proteins. The latter may also create links via trans-membrane proteins to the extracellular matrix. Best known of these is the family of spectrin-like molecules, which can bind to actin and also to each other and various membrane-associated proteins to create supportive networks beneath the plasma membrane. Spectrin is found in erythrocytes, and closely related molecules are present in many other cells; for instance, fodrin is found in nerve cells, and dystrophin occurs in muscle cells, linking the contractile apparatus with the extracellular matrix via integral membrane proteins. Proteins such as ankyrin (which also binds actin directly), vinculin, talin, zyxin and paxillin connect actin-binding proteins to integral plasma membrane proteins such as integrins (directly or indirectly), and thence to focal adhesions. Myosin I and other unconventional myosins connect actin filaments to membranous structures, including the plasma membrane and transport vesicle membranes. Tropomyosin, an important regulatory protein of muscle fibres, is also present in non-muscle cells, where its function may be primarily to stabilize actin filaments against depolymerization. For further reading see Pollard and Earnshaw (2002).

Myosins – the motor proteins

The myosin family of microfilaments is often classified within a distinct category of motor proteins. Myosin proteins have a globular head region consisting of a heavy and a light chain. The heavy chain bears an α-helical tail of varying length. The head has an ATPase activity and can bind to and move along actin filaments – the basis for myosin function as a motor protein. The best-known class is myosin II, which occurs in muscle and in many non-muscle cells. Its molecules have two heads and two tails, intertwined to form a long rod. The rods can bind to each other to form long, thick filaments, as seen in striated and smooth muscle fibres, myoepithelial cells and myofibroblasts. Myosin II molecules can also assemble into smaller groups, especially dimers, which can cross-link individual actin microfilaments in stress fibres and other F-actin arrays. The ATP-dependent sliding of myosin on actin forms the basis for muscle contraction and the extension of microfilament bundles, as seen in cellular motility or in the contraction of the ring of actin and myosin around the cleavage furrow of dividing cells. There are a number of known subtypes of myosin II: they assemble in different ways and have different dynamic properties. In skeletal muscle the myosin molecules form filaments c.15 nm thick, reversing their direction of assembly at the midpoint, which is bare of head regions, to produce a symmetric arrangement of subunits. In smooth muscle the molecules form thicker, flattened ribbons and are orientated in different directions on either face of the ribbon. These arrangements have important consequences for the contractile force characteristics of the different types of muscle cell.

Related molecules are known as unconventional myosins. They include the myosin I subfamily of single-headed molecules with tails of varying length. These molecules are associated with membranes to which their tails can attach, and are implicated in the movements of membranes on actin filaments. So, for example, vesicles track along F-actin in a similar manner to kinesin and dynein-related movements along microtubules. Other functions of myosin I are the movements of membranes in endocytosis, microspike formation in neuronal growth cones, actin–actin sliding and attachment of actin to membranes, e.g. of microvilli. Other myosins have been isolated; the significance of their diversity is not fully understood.

Other thin filaments

A heterogeneous group of filamentous structures with diameters of 2–4 nm occur in various cells. The two most widely studied forms, titin and nebulin, constitute c.13% of the total protein of skeletal muscle. They are amongst the largest known molecules, and have subunit weights of around 10^6; native molecules are c.1 μm in length. Their elastic properties are important for the effective functioning of muscle, and possibly for other cells.

Intermediate filaments

Intermediate filaments are c.10 nm thick and formed by a heterogeneous group of filamentous proteins. They are found in different cell types and are often present in large numbers, either where structural strength is needed (**Fig. 2.15**), or to provide scaffolding for the attachment of other structures. Intermediate filaments of different molecular classes are characteristic of particular tissues or states of maturity. They are therefore important indicators of the origins of cells or levels of differentiation, and are of considerable value in histopathology.

Of the different classes of intermediate filaments, keratin (cytokeratin) proteins are found in epithelia, where keratin filaments are always composed of equal ratios of types I (acidic) and II (basic to neutral) keratins.

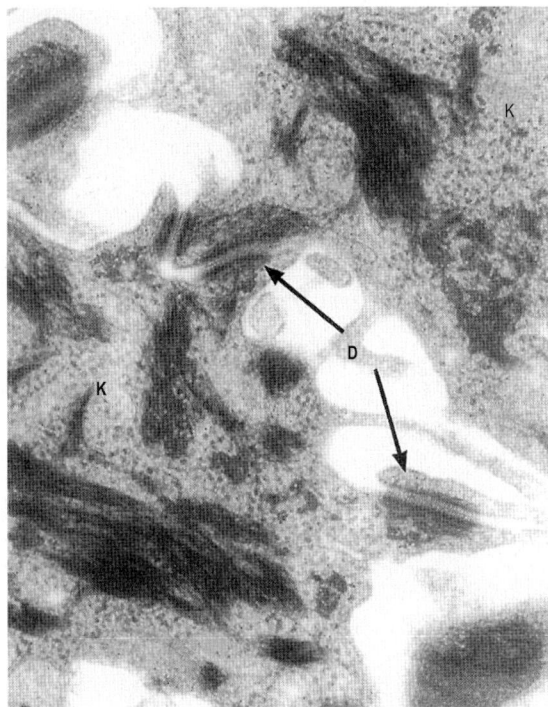

Fig. 2.15 Keratin filaments (tonofilaments) in two adjacent keratinocytes (K) of the epidermis. Keratin filaments also insert into the desmosome contacts (D) between cells. (By permission from Young B, Heath JW 2000 Wheater's Functional Histology. Edinburgh: Churchill Livingstone.)

About 20 types of each of the acidic and basic/neutral keratin proteins are known. Within the epidermis, expression of keratin heterodimer combinations changes as keratinocytes mature during their transition from basal to superficial layers. Genetic abnormalities of keratins are known to affect the mechanical stability of epithelia. For example, the disease epidermolysis bullosa simplex causes lysis of epidermal basal cells and blistering of the skin after mechanical trauma. It is caused by defects in genes encoding keratins 5 and 14, which produce cytoskeletal instability and thus cellular fragility in the basal cells. When keratins 1 and 10 are affected, cells in the spinous layer of the epidermis lyse, and this produces the intraepidermal blistering of epidermolytic hyperkeratosis. For a recent review, see Porter and Lane (2003).

Vimentins occur in mesenchyme-derived cells of connective tissue, desmins in muscle cells, glial fibrillary acidic protein in glial cells, and peripherin in peripheral axons. Neurofilaments are a major cytoskeletal element in neurones, particularly in axons (**Fig. 2.16**), where they are the dominant protein. They are heteropolymers of low, medium and high molecular weight neurofilament proteins; the low molecular weight form is always present in combination with either the medium- or the high-molecular weight neurofilament. Abnormal accumulations of neurofilaments (neurofibrillary tangles) are characteristic features of a number of neuropathological conditions.

Other intermediate filament proteins include nestin, a molecule resembling neurofilament protein which forms intermediate filaments in neurectodermal stem cells in particular. Nuclear lamins form intermediate filaments that line the inner surface of the nuclear envelope of all nucleated cells. They provide a mechanical framework for the nucleus and act as attachment sites for chromosomes. They are unusual in that they form a square lattice of regularly spaced crossing filaments rather than bundles, reflecting their unusual molecular composition.

The exact manner in which intermediate filament proteins polymerize to form linear filaments is much more complex than that of tubulin or actin, and has not been fully determined. The individual intermediate filament proteins are chains with a middle α-helical region flanked on either side by non-helical domains. The proteins associate as coiled coil dimers that form short rods c.48 nm long. These assemble in pairs in a staggered antiparallel formation to form soluble tetramers, eight of which pack together laterally and twist into the rope-like 10 nm intermediate filament. The 32 α-helices in parallel give the filaments their

17

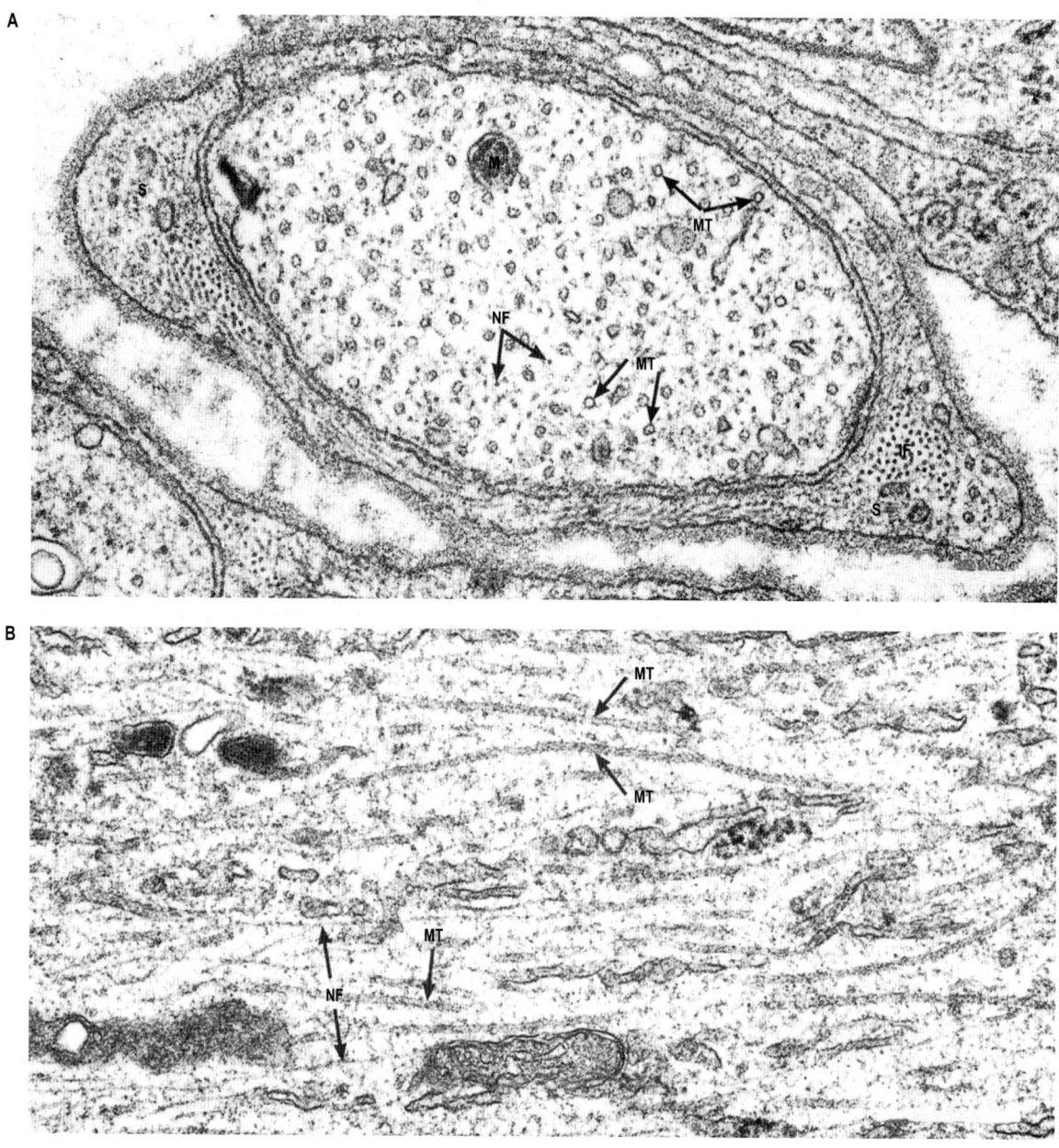

Fig. 2.16 Microtubules (MT) in axons in peripheral nerve. **A,** In transverse section, microtubules appear as hollow spherical structures. The axon is ensheathed by a Schwann cell (S) and its associated basal lamina. **B,** In longitudinal section, microtubules appear as straight, unbranched tubes. Neurofilaments (intermediate filaments of neurones; NF) appear in transverse section as solid punctate structures, smaller than microtubules. (By permission from Young B, Heath JW 2000 Wheater's Functional Histology. Edinburgh: Churchill Livingstone.)

tensile strength. However, unlike actin and myosin, the antiparallel arrangement of the dimers produces a filamentous protein with no intrinsic polarity. The non-coiled regions of the subunits project outwards as side arms that can link intermediate filaments into bundles or attach them to other structures. The existence of different combinations of subunit proteins within one filament is the basis of their functional diversity. In the living cell they have been shown to be quite dynamic structures, possibly as a result of reversible phosphorylation.

Microtubules

Microtubules are polymers of tubulin with the form of hollow, relatively rigid cylinders, c.25 nm in diameter and of varying length (up to 70 μm in spermatozoan flagella) (**Fig. 2.16**). They are present in most cell types, and are particularly abundant in neurones, leukocytes, blood platelets and the mitotic spindles of dividing cells. They also form part of the structure of cilia, flagella and centrioles.

There are two major classes of tubulin: α- and β-tubulins. Before microtubule assembly, tubulins are associated as dimers with a combined molecular mass of 100 kDa (50 kDa each). Each protein subunit is c.5 nm across and arranged along the long axis in straight rows of alternating α– and β-tubulins, forming protofilaments. About 13 protofilaments (the number varies between 11 and 16), associate in a ring to form the wall of a hollow cylindrical microtubule. Each longitudinal row is slightly out of alignment with its neighbour, so that a spiral pattern of alternating α and β subunits appears when the microtubule is viewed from the side. There is a dynamic equilibrium between the dimers and assembled microtubules: dimeric asymmetry creates polarity (α-tubulins are all orientated towards the minus end, β-tubulins towards the plus end). Tubulin is added preferentially to the plus end; the minus end is relatively slow growing. When tubulin is added at one end while being removed at the other (treadmilling), the microtubule gradually shifts its position longitudinally. Polymerization requires phosphorylation of tubulins by guanosine triphosphate, and either a nucleation site (e.g. the end of a pre-existing microtubule), or a microtubule-organizing centre (e.g. those surrounding, and including, centrioles), around which spindle microtubules polymerize during cell division and from which cilia can grow.

Various drugs (e.g. colcemid, vinblastine, griseofulvin, nocodazole) cause microtubule depolymerization by binding the soluble tubulin dimers and so shifting the equilibrium towards the unpolymerized state. Microtubule demolition causes a wide variety of effects, including the inhibition of cell division by disruption of the mitotic spindle. Conversely, the drug taxol stabilizes microtubules and promotes abnormal microtubule assembly which causes a peripheral neuropathy.

Different microtubules possess varying degrees of stability, e.g. microtubules in cilia are generally unaffected by many drugs that cause microtubular demolition. There are also differences between tissues, e.g. neurones have a special tubulin subclass. Tubulins associated with microtubule organizing centres include γ-tubulin.

Microtubule-associated proteins

Various small proteins that can bind to assembled tubulins may be concerned with structural properties or associated with motility. Structural microtubule-associated proteins (MAPs) form cross-bridges between adjacent microtubules or between microtubules and other structures such as intermediate filaments, mitochondria and the plasma membrane. Microtubule-associated proteins found in neurones include: MAPs 1A and 1B, which are present in neuronal dendrites and axons; MAPs 2A and 2B, found chiefly in dendrites; and tau, found only in axons. MAP 4 is the major microtubule-associated protein in many other cell types. Structural microtubule-associated proteins are implicated in microtubule formation, maintenance and demolition, and are therefore of considerable significance in cell morphogenesis, mitotic division, and the maintenance and modulation of cell shape. Motility-associated microtubule-associated proteins are found in situations in which movement occurs over the surfaces of microtubules, e.g. the transport of cytoplasmic vesicles, bending of cilia and flagella, and some movements of mitotic spindles. They include a large family of motor proteins, the best known of which are the dyneins and kinesins. Another protein, dynamin, is involved in endocytosis. The kinetochore proteins assemble at the centromere during mitosis and meiosis. They attach to spindle microtubules; some of the kinetochore proteins are responsible for chromosomal movements in mitotic and meiotic anaphase.

All of these microtubule-associated proteins bind to microtubules and actively slide along their surfaces. Kinesins and dyneins can simultaneously attach to membranes such as transport vesicles and convey them along microtubules for considerable distances, thus enabling selective targeting of materials within the cell. Such movements occur in both directions along microtubules. Kinesin-dependent motion is mostly towards the plus ends of microtubules, e.g. from the cell body towards the axon terminals in neurones, and away from the centrosome in other cells. Conversely, dynein-related movements are in the opposite direction, i.e. to the minus ends of microtubules. Dyneins also form the arms of peripheral microtubules in cilia and flagella, where they make dynamic cross-bridges to adjacent microtubule pairs. The resulting shearing forces cause the axonemal array of microtubules to bend, generating ciliary and flagellar beating movements. A number of related motor proteins can also interact with microtubules, e.g. kinesin-related proteins cross-link mitotic spindle microtubules to push the two centriolar poles apart during mitotic prophase.

Centrioles, centrosomes and basal bodies

Centrioles are microtubular cylinders c.0.2 μm in diameter and 0.4 μm long (**Fig. 2.17**). They are formed by a ring of nine microtubule triplets linked by a number of other proteins. At least two centrioles occur in all cells that are capable of mitotic division. They usually lie close together, at right angles or, most usually, at an oblique angle to each other (an arrangement often termed a diplosome), within the centrosome, a densely filamentous region of cytoplasm at the centre of the cell. The centrosome is the major microtubule-organizing centre of the cell; it is the site at which new microtubules are formed and the mitotic spindle is generated during cell division. Before cell division, a new centriole forms at right angles to each one of the existing centrosomal pair; the resulting new pairs are passed on to the daughter cells. The proximity of the centrosome to the Golgi apparatus provides a means of targeting Golgi vesicular products to different parts of the cell.

The microtubule-organizing centre contains complexes of γ-tubulin that bind the minus ends of microtubules. Basal bodies are microtubule-organizing centres that are closely related to centrioles, and are believed to be derived from them. They are located at the bases of cilia and flagella, which they anchor to the cell surface. The outer microtubule doublets of cilia and flagella originate from two of the microtubules in each triplet of the basal body.

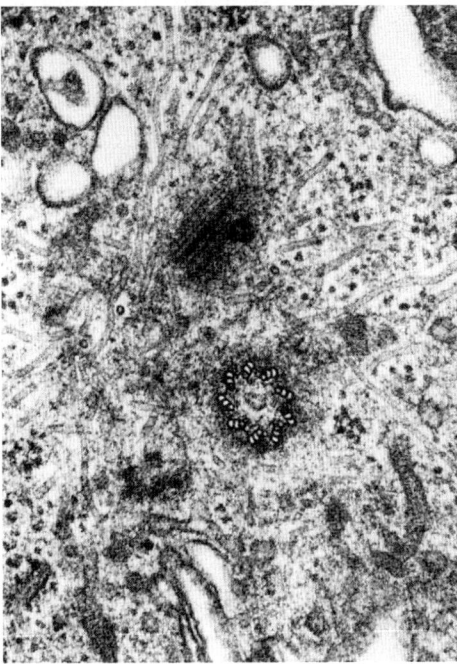

Fig. 2.17 In electron microscopic preparations, one centriole is usually visible in cross-section, revealing the circular arrangement of tubules, while its partner is cut either longitudinally or slightly obliquely (above). (By permission from Stevens A, Lowe JS 1996 Human Histology, 2nd edn. London: Mosby.)

CELL SURFACE PROJECTIONS

The surfaces of many different types of cell are specialized to form structures that project from the surface. These projections may permit movement of the cell itself (flagella), or of fluids across the apical cell surface (cilia), or increase the surface area available for absorption (microvilli). Infoldings of the basolateral plasma membrane also increase the area for transport across this surface of the cell.

CILIA AND FLAGELLA

Cilia and flagella are motile, hair-like projections of the cell surface which create currents in the surrounding fluid, movements of the cell to which they are attached, or both. Cilia occur on many internal surfaces of the body, in particular: the epithelia of most of the respiratory tract; parts of the male (p. 1307) and female (p. 1329) reproductive tracts; the ependyma that line the central canal of the spinal cord and ventricles of the brain (p. 53). They also occur at the endings of olfactory receptors and vestibular hair cells, and, in modified form, as portions of the rods and cones of the retina (p. 710). A single cell may bear many cilia, e.g. in bronchial epithelium, or only one or two. Each male gamete possesses a single flagellum c.70 μm long.

A cilium or flagellum consists of a shaft (c.0.25 μm diameter) constituting most of its length, a tapering tip and a basal body at its base, which lies within the surface cytoplasm of the cell (**Fig. 2.18**). Other than at its base, the entire structure is covered by plasma membrane. The core of the cilium is the axoneme, a cylinder of nine microtubule doublets that surrounds a central pair of single microtubules.

Several filamentous structures are associated with the microtubules in the shaft, e.g. radial spokes extend inwards from the outer microtubules towards the central pair. The outer doublet microtubules bear two rows of tangential dynein arms attached to the A subfibre of the doublet, which point towards the B subfibre of the adjacent doublet. Adjacent doublets are also linked by thin filaments. Other filaments partially encircle the central pair of microtubules, which are also united by ladder-like spokes. The '9 + 2' pattern of microtubules imparts a plane of symmetry that passes perpendicular to a line joining the central pair and corresponds to the direction of bending.

Movements of cilia and flagella are broadly similar. Flagella move by rapid undulation, which passes from the attached to the free end. In human spermatozoa there is an additional helical component to this motion. In cilia, the beating is planar, but asymmetric. In the effective stroke, the cilium remains stiff except at the base, where it bends to

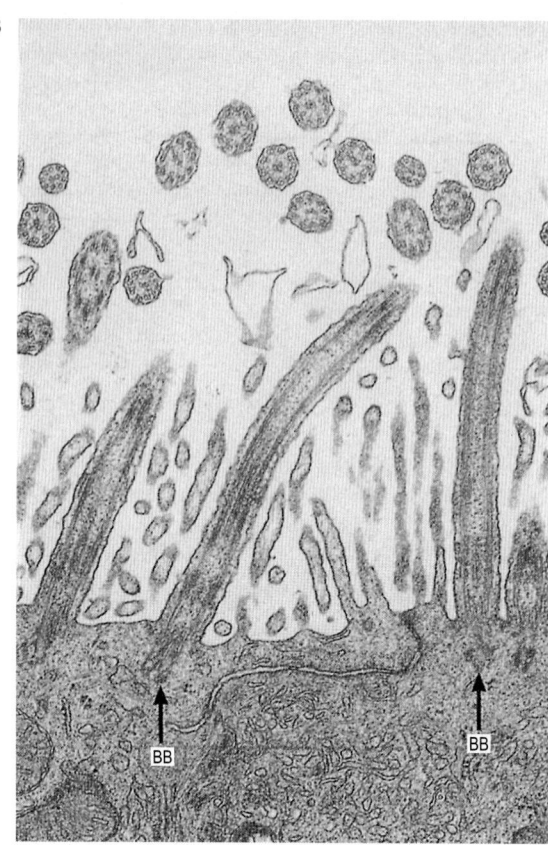

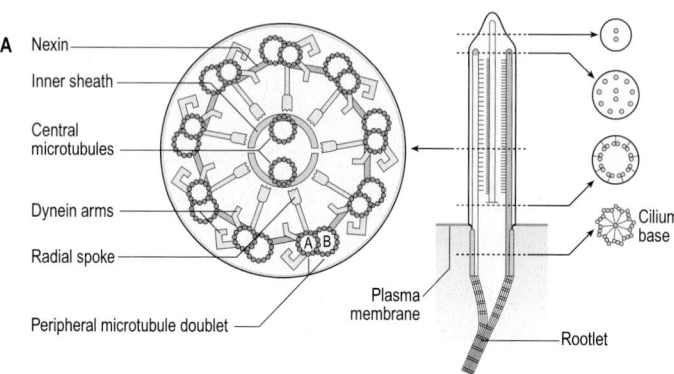

Fig. 2.18 **A**, Structure of a cilium shown in (left) transverse and (right) longitudinal section. **B**, Apical region of respiratory epithelial cells, showing the proximal parts of three cilia sectioned longitudinally, anchored into the cytoplasm by basal bodies (BB). Other cilia project out of the plane of section and are cut transversely, showing the '9 + 2' arrangement of microtubules. (**A**, redrawn by permission from Sleigh MA 1977 The nature and action of respiratory tract cilia. In: Brain JD, Proctor DF, Reid LM (eds) Respiratory Defense Mechanisms. Part 1. New York: Dekker; pp247–288. **B**, by permission from Young B, Heath JW 2000 Wheater's Functional Histology. Edinburgh: Churchill Livingstone.)

produce an oar-like stroke. The recovery stroke follows, during which the bend passes from base to tip, returning the cilium to its initial position for the next cycle. The activity of groups of cilia is usually coordinated so that the bending of one is rapidly followed by the bending of the next and so on, resulting in long travelling waves of metachronal synchrony. These pass over the tissue surface in the same direction as the effective stroke.

When a cilium bends, the microtubules do not change in length, but slide on one another. The dynein arms of peripheral doublets slant towards the base of the cilium from their attached ends. Dynein has an ATPase activity, which is stimulated by magnesium ions, and causes mutual sliding of adjacent doublets by initially attaching sideways to the next pair, then swinging upwards towards the tip of the cilium. There is a group of genetic diseases in which cilia beat either ineffectively or not at all, e.g. Kartagener's immotile cilium syndrome. Affected cilia exhibit various ultrastructural defects in their internal structure, such as a lack of dynein arms or missing spokes. Patients with this syndrome suffer various respiratory problems caused by the accumulation of particles in the lungs; males are typically sterile because of the loss of sperm motility, and c.50% have an alimentary tract that is a mirror image of the usual pattern (situs inversus) – i.e. it rotates in the opposite direction during early development (p. 1257).

MICROVILLI

Microvilli are finger-like cell surface extensions usually c.0.1 μm in diameter and up to 2 μm long (**Fig. 2.19**). When arranged in a regular parallel series, they constitute a striated border, as typified by the absorptive surfaces of the epithelial enterocytes of the small intestine. When they are less regular, as in the gallbladder epithelium and proximal kidney tubules, the term brush border is used.

Microvilli are covered by plasma membrane, and supported internally by closely packed bundles of actin microfilaments linked by cross-bridges of the actin-bundling proteins, villin and fimbrin. Other bridges composed of myosin I and calmodulin connect the microfilaments to the plasma membrane. The microfilament bundles of microvilli are embedded in the apical cytoplasm amongst a meshwork of transversely running microfilaments linked by spectrin to form the terminal web (**Fig. 2.19**). The web is anchored laterally to the zonula adherens.

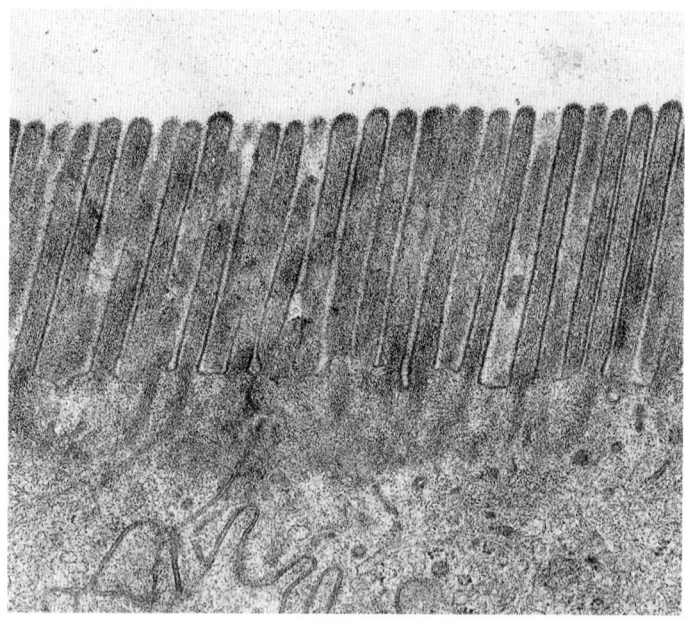

Fig. 2.19 Microvilli sectioned longitudinally in the striated border of two adjacent intestinal absorptive cells with interlocking lateral plasma membranes (below, centre). Actin filaments fill the cores of the microvilli and insert into a terminal web of actin filaments in the apical cytoplasm.

Myosin is also found in the terminal web, where it is believed to bind to the actin and so stiffen this part of the cell. At the apex of each microvillus, the free ends of microfilaments are inserted into a dense mass that includes the protein, α-actinin.

Microvilli greatly increase the area of cell surface (up to 40 times), particularly at sites of active absorption. In the small intestine, they have a very thick cell coat or glycocalyx, which reflects the presence of integral membrane glycoproteins, including enzymes concerned with digestion and absorption. Irregular microvilli, filopodia, are also found on the surfaces of many types of cell, particularly of free macrophages and fibroblasts, where they may be associated with phagocytosis and cell motility.

Long, regular microvilli are called stereocilia, an early misnomer, as they are not motile and lack microtubules. They are found on cochlear and vestibular receptor cells (p. 663), where they act as sensory transducers, and also in the absorptive epithelium of the epididymis (p. 1307).

Nucleus

The nucleus (Figs 2.1, 2.2) is generally the largest intracellular structure and is usually spherical or ellipsoid in shape, with a diameter of 3–10 μm. Histological stains used to identify nuclei in tissue sections mainly detect the acidic molecules of deoxyribonucleic acid (DNA), which are largely confined to the nucleus.

NUCLEAR MEMBRANE

The nucleus is surrounded by two layers of membrane, each of which is a lipid bilayer, and which together form the nuclear membrane or envelope. The outer membrane layer and the lumen between the two layers are continuous with the rough endoplasmic reticulum. Like the rough endoplasmic reticulum, the outer membrane of the nuclear envelope is studded with ribosomes that are active in protein synthesis; the newly synthesized proteins pass into the perinuclear space between the two membrane layers.

Intermediate filaments are associated with both the inner (nuclear) and outer (cytoplasmic) surfaces of the nuclear membrane. Within the nucleus they form a dense shell beneath the membrane, the nuclear lamina, consisting of specialized nuclear intermediate filaments called nuclear lamins. These cross each other at right angles to create a meshwork that covers the interior surface of the nuclear membrane. In so doing, they reinforce the nuclear membrane mechanically, determine the shape of the nucleus and anchor the ends of chromosomes. Condensed chromatin (heterochromatin) also tends to aggregate near the nuclear membrane during interphase. At the end of mitotic and meiotic prophase (p. 23), the lamin filaments disassemble, causing the nuclear membranes to vesiculate. At the end of anaphase, the lamins reattach to the chromosomes and create a new nuclear compartment around which the nuclear membranes reform. A network of filamentous proteins, the nuclear matrix, is also present throughout the nucleus. It is associated with newly replicated DNA and with genes that are being actively transcribed, and incorporates enzymes of the replication machinery.

The transport of molecules between the nucleus and the cytoplasm is achieved by specialized nuclear pore structures that perforate the nuclear membrane (Fig. 2.20). They act as highly selective directional molecular filters, permitting proteins such as histones and gene regulatory proteins (which are synthesized in the cytoplasm but function in the nucleus) to enter the nucleus, and molecules that are synthesized in the nucleus but destined for the cytoplasm (e.g. ribosomal subunits, transfer RNAs and messenger RNAs), to leave the nucleus.

Ultrastructurally, nuclear pores appear as disc-like structures with an outer diameter of c.130 nm and an inner pore with an effective diameter for free diffusion of 9 nm (Fig. 2.20B). The nuclear membrane of an active cell is bridged by up to 4000 such pores. The nuclear pore complex has an octagonal symmetry and is formed by an assembly of more than 50 proteins, the nucleoporins. The inner and outer nuclear membranes fuse around the pore complex (Fig. 2.20A). Transfer of lipids and proteins between the two is prevented, possibly by the luminal subunits of the pore. Nuclear pores are freely permeable to small molecules, ions and proteins up to about 17 kDa. Proteins of up to 60 kDa seem to be able to equilibrate slowly between the nucleus and cytoplasm through the pore, but larger proteins are normally excluded. However, certain proteins are selectively transported into the nucleus and some of these, such as the DNA polymerases, are very large. Proteins that are selectively transported into the nucleus possess a nuclear localization signal within their amino-acid sequence. This is recognized by cytoplasmic proteins that facilitate the docking of the proteins to be transported with the cytoplasmic surface of the pore. Subsequent translocation into the nucleus is energy dependent and requires the hydrolysis of GTP. The nuclear pore can open to a maximum of c.25 nm to permit the entry or exit of large, actively transported molecules. Steroid hormone receptors, which are gene regulatory proteins, associate with the cytoskeleton until they bind their ligands, when they dissociate from the cytoskeleton and are transported into the nucleus. Transport also occurs from the nucleus to the cytoplasm, e.g. RNAs synthesized in the nucleus are transported through nuclear pores into the cytoplasm.

CHROMATIN

DNA is organized within the nucleus in a DNA–protein complex known as chromatin. The protein constituents of chromatin are the histones and the non-histone proteins. Non-histone proteins are an extremely heterogeneous group that includes DNA and RNA polymerases and gene regulatory proteins. Histones are the most abundant group of proteins in chromatin, primarily responsible for the packaging of chromosomal DNA into its primary level of organization, the nucleosome. There are

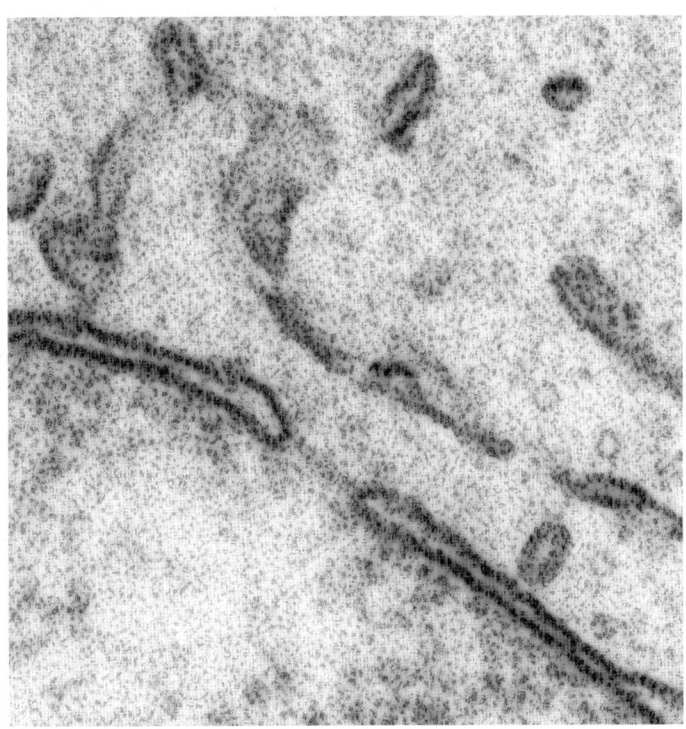

A

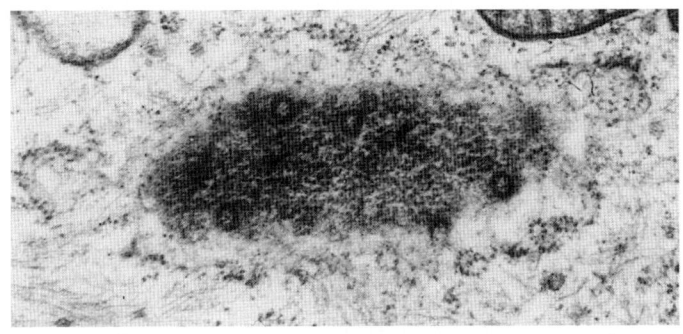

B

Fig. 2.20 A, Nuclear envelope with a nuclear pore (centre field) in transverse section, showing the continuity between the inner and outer phospholipid layers of the envelope on either side of the pore. The fine 'membrane' spanning the pore is formed by proteins of the pore complex. **B,** Nuclear pores seen 'en face' in a tangential section through the nuclear membrane. (**A,** by kind permission from Rose Watson, Cancer Research UK.)

five histone proteins: H1, H2A, H2B, H3 and H4; the last four combine in equal ratios to form a compact octameric nucleosome core. The DNA molecule (one per chromosome) winds 1.65 times around each nucleosome core, taking up 146 nucleotide pairs. This packaging organizes the DNA into a chromatin fibre 11 nm in diameter, and imparts to this form of chromatin the electron microscopic appearance of beads on a string, in which each bead is separated by a variable length of DNA, c.50 nucleotide pairs long. The nucleosome core region and one of the linker regions constitute the nucleosome proper, which is thus c.200 nucleotide pairs in length. However, chromatin rarely exists in this simple form and is usually packaged further into a 30 nm thick fibre, involving a single H1 histone per nucleosome, which interacts with both DNA and protein to impose a higher order of nucleosome packing. Usually, 30 nm fibres are further folded into loop-like domains, but individual loops are believed to decondense and extend during active transcription. In a typical interphase nucleus, euchromatin (nuclear regions that appear pale in appropriately stained tissue sections, or relatively electron-lucent in electron micrographs; **Fig. 2.2**) is likely to consist mainly of 30 nm fibres and loops, and contains the transcriptionally active genes. Transcriptionally active cells, such as most neurones, have nuclei that are predominantly euchromatic and often described as 'open face' nuclei.

Heterochromatin (nuclear regions that appear dark in appropriately stained tissue sections or electron-dense in electron micrographs) is characteristically located mainly around the periphery of the nucleus, except over the nuclear pores, and around the nucleolus (**Fig. 2.2**). It is a highly compacted form of chromatin, containing additional proteins; its higher order packaging is poorly understood. Heterochromatin includes non-coding regions of DNA, such as centromeric and telomeric regions, which are known as constitutive heterochromatin. DNA that is inactivated (becoming resistant to transcription) in some cells as they differentiate during development or cell maturation contributes to heterochromatin, and is known as facultative heterochromatin. The inactive X chromosome in females is an example of facultative heterochromatin and can be identified in the light microscope as the deeply staining Barr body (drumstick chromosome) that projects from the nuclear periphery.

In transcriptionally inactive cells, chromatin is predominantly in the condensed, heterochromatic state, and may comprise as much as 90% of the total. Examples of such cells are mature neutrophil leukocytes (in which the condensation of chromatin induces the formation of a multilobed, densely staining nucleus), and the highly condensed nuclei of orthochromatic erythroblasts (late-stage erythrocyte precursors). In most mature cells, a mixture of the two occurs, indicating that only a proportion of the DNA is being transcribed. A particular instance of this is seen in the mature B lymphocyte (plasma cell), in which much of the chromatin is in the condensed condition and is arranged in regular masses around the perimeter of the nucleus, producing the so-called 'clock-face' nucleus (**Fig. 2.2**). Although this cell is actively transcribing, much of its protein synthesis is of a single immunoglobulin type, and consequently much of its genome is in an inactive state.

During mitosis, the chromatin is further condensed to form the much shortened chromosomes characteristic of metaphase. This shortening is achieved through further levels of close packing of the chromatin, and is an energy dependent process involving proteins known as condensins. Progressive folding of the chromosomal DNA by interactions with specific proteins can reduce c.5 cm of chromosomal DNA by 10,000 fold, to a length of c.5 μm in the mitotic chromosome.

CHROMOSOMES AND KARYOTYPES

The nuclear DNA of eukaryotic cells is organized into linear units called chromosomes. The DNA in a normal human diploid cell contains 6×10^9 nucleotide pairs organized in the form of 46 chromosomes (44 autosomes and 2 sex chromosomes). The largest human chromosome (number 1) contains c.2.5×10^8 nucleotide pairs, and the smallest (the Y chromosome) c.5×10^7 nucleotide pairs.

Each chromosomal DNA molecule contains a number of specialized nucleotide sequences that are associated with its maintenance. One is the centromere. During mitosis, a disc-shaped structure composed of a complex array of proteins, the kinetochore, associates with the centromeric region of DNA in order to attach it to the microtubular spindle. Another sequence, the telomere, defines the end of each chromosomal DNA molecule. Telomeres consist of tandem repeats of

a short sequence enriched in guanosine nucleotides. They are not replicated by the same DNA polymerase as the rest of the chromosome, but by a specific enzyme called telomerase. The number of tandem repeats of the telomeric DNA sequence varies. It appears to shorten with successive cell divisions, because telomerase activity reduces or is absent in differentiated cells with a finite lifespan. It is believed that this mechanism regulates cell senescence and protects against proliferative disorders, including cancer.

CLASSIFICATION OF HUMAN CHROMOSOMES

A number of genetic abnormalities can be directly related to the chromosomal pattern. The characterization or karyotyping of chromosome number and structure is therefore of considerable diagnostic importance. The identifying features of individual chromosomes are most easily seen during metaphase, although prophase chromosomes can be used for more detailed analyses.

Lymphocytes separated from blood samples, or cells taken from other tissues, are used as a source of chromosomes. Diagnosis of fetal chromosome patterns is generally carried out on samples of amniotic fluid containing fetal cells aspirated from the uterus by amniocentesis, or on a small piece of chorionic villus tissue removed from the placenta. Whatever their origin, the cells are cultured *in vitro* and stimulated to divide by treatment with agents that stimulate cell division. Mitosis is interrupted at metaphase with spindle inhibitors. The chromosomes are dispersed by first causing the cells to swell in a hypotonic solution, then the cells are gently fixed and mechanically ruptured on a slide to spread the chromosomes. They are subsequently stained in various ways to allow the identification of individual chromosomes by size, shape and distribution of stain (**Fig. 2.21**). General techniques show the obvious landmarks, e.g. lengths of arms and positions of constrictions. Banding techniques demonstrate differential staining patterns, characteristic for each chromosome type. Fluorescence staining with quinacrine mustard and related compounds produces Q bands, and Giemsa staining (after treatment that partially denatures the chromatin) gives G bands (**Fig. 2.21A**). Other less widely used methods include: reverse-Giemsa staining, in which the light and dark areas are reversed (R bands); the staining of constitutive heterochromatin with silver salts (C-banding); T-banding to stain the ends (telomeres) of chromosomes. Collectively, these methods permit the classification of chromosomes into numbered autosomal pairs in order of decreasing size, from 1 to 22 plus the sex chromosomes.

A summary of the major classes of chromosomes is given below:

Group	Features
1–3 (A)	Large metacentric chromosomes
4–5 (B)	Large submetacentric chromosomes
6–12 + X (C)	Metacentrics of medium size
13–15 (D)	Medium-sized acrocentrics with satellites
16–18 (E)	Shorter metacentrics (16) or submetacentrics (17,18)
19–20 (F)	Shortest metacentrics
21–22 + Y (G)	Short acrocentrics; 21, 22 with satellites, Y without

Methodological advances in banding techniques improved the recognition of abnormal chromosome patterns. The use of *in-situ* hybridization with fluorescent DNA probes specific for each chromosome (**Fig. 2.21B**) permits the identification of even very small abnormalities.

NUCLEOLUS

Nucleoli are a prominent feature of an interphase nucleus (**Fig. 2.2**). They are the site of most of the synthesis of rRNA and assembly of ribosome subunits. Ultrastructurally, the nucleolus appears as a pale fibrillar region (non-transcribed DNA), containing dense fibrillar cores (sites of rRNA gene transcription) and granular regions (sites of ribosome subunit assembly) within a diffuse nucleolar matrix. Five pairs of chromosomes carry rRNA genes organized in clusters of tandemly repeated units on each chromosome. Each rRNA unit is transcribed individually and encodes the 28S, 18S and 5.8S rRNA molecules. During mitosis the nucleolus breaks down. It reforms after telophase, in a process initiated by the onset of transcription in nucleolar organizing centres on each chromosome. The 28S, 18S and 5.8S rRNA molecules are assembled into their ribosomal subunits in the granular region of the nucleolus together with the 5S rRNA, which is not synthesized in the nucleolus.

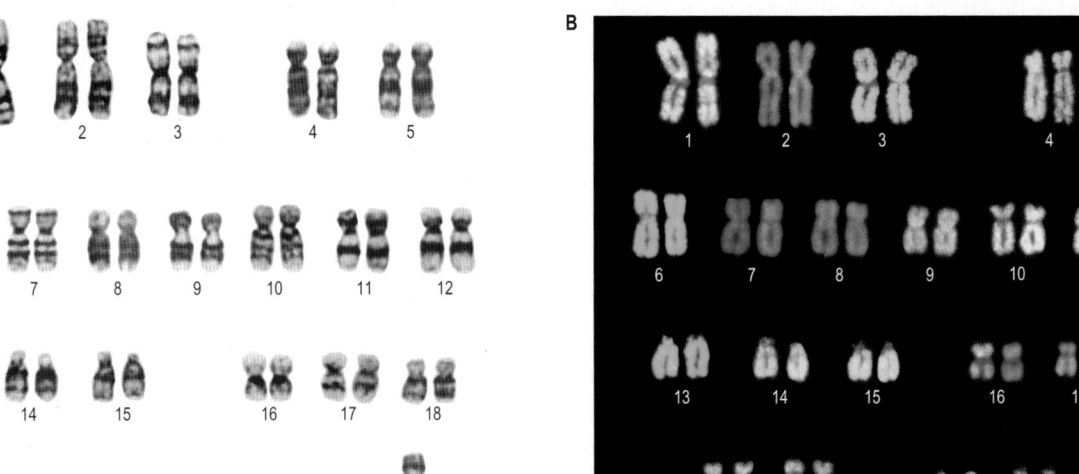

Fig. 2.21 Chromosomes from normal males, arranged as karyotypes. **A**, G-banded preparation; **B**, preparation stained by multiplex fluorescence *in-situ* hybridization to identify each chromosome. (By kind permission from Dr Denise Sheer, Cancer Research UK.)

The newly formed ribosomal subunits are then translocated to the cytoplasm through the nuclear pores.

CELL DIVISION AND THE CELL CYCLE

During prenatal development, most cells undergo repeated division as the body grows in size and complexity. As cells mature, they differentiate structurally and functionally. Some cells, such as neurones, lose the ability to divide. Others may persist throughout the lifetime of the individual as replication-competent stem cells, e.g. cells in the haemopoietic tissue of bone marrow. Many stem cells divide infrequently, but give rise to daughter cells that undergo repeated cycles of mitotic division as transit (or transient) amplifying cells. Their divisions may occur in rapid succession, as in cell lineages with a short lifespan and similarly fast turnover and replacement time. Transit amplifying cells are all destined to differentiate and ultimately to die and be replaced, unlike the population of parental stem cells, which self-renews.

Patterns and rates of cell division within tissues vary considerably. In many epithelia, such as the crypts between intestinal villi, the replacement of damaged or effete cells by division of stem cells can be rapid. Rates of cell division may also vary according to demand, as occurs in the healing of wounded skin, in which cell proliferation increases to a peak and then returns to the normal replacement level. The rate of cell division is tightly coupled to the demand for growth and replacement. Where this coupling is faulty, tissues either fail to grow or replace their cells, or they can overgrow, producing neoplasms.

The cell cycle is the period of time between the birth of a cell and its own division to produce two daughter cells. It lasts a minimum of 12 hours, but in most adult tissues is considerably longer, and is divided into four distinct phases, which are known as G_1, S, G_2 and M. The combination of G_1, S and G_2 phases is known as interphase. M is the mitotic phase. G_1 is the period when cells respond to growth factors directing the cell to initiate another cycle; once made, this decision is irreversible. It is also the phase in which most of the molecular machinery required to complete another cell cycle is generated. Cells that retain the capacity for proliferation, but which are no longer dividing, have entered a phase called G_0 and are described as quiescent. Growth factors can stimulate quiescent cells to leave G_0 and re-enter the cell cycle, whereas the proteins encoded by certain tumour suppressor genes (e.g. the gene mutated in retinoblastoma, *Rb*) block the cycle in G_1. DNA replication occurs during S phase, at the end of which the DNA content of the cell has doubled. During G_2, the cell prepares for division; this period ends with the breakdown of the nuclear membrane and the onset of chromosome condensation. The times taken for S, G_2 and M are similar for most cell types, and occupy c.6–8, 2–4 and 1–2 hours respectively. In contrast, the duration of G_1 shows considerable variation, sometimes ranging from less than 2 hours in rapidly dividing cells, to more than 100 hours within the same tissue.

The regulation of the transitions between the cell cycle phases is now becoming understood at the molecular level. At the G_1–S and G_2–M transitions, members of a family of proteins called cyclins attain their maximum abundance in the cell. The G_1 cyclins progressively accumulate during G_1. The M phase cyclins accumulate during late S phase and throughout G_2. High concentrations of cyclin proteins activate a family of cyclin-dependent protein kinase enzymes (CDKs), which are present in constant concentrations during the cell cycle, although their state of activation varies. The activation of different cyclin–CDK complexes regulates the G_1–S and G_2–M transitions. The activities of these enzymes and their cyclin activators are themselves subject to complex regulation, beyond the scope of this text.

There are important checkpoints in the cell cycle at which progress will be arrested if, for instance, DNA replication or mitotic spindle assembly and chromosome attachment are incomplete. Negative regulation systems also operate to delay cell cycle progression when DNA has been damaged by radiation or chemical mutagens. Cells with checkpoint defects, such as loss of the protein p53 which is a major negative control element in the division cycle of all cells, are commonly associated with the development of malignancy. Cells lacking one of the critical checkpoint functions are then able to progress through the cycle carrying defects, which increases the probability that further abnormalities will accumulate in their progeny. The p53 gene is an example of a tumour suppressor gene. For further reading on cell cycle regulation, see Alberts et al (2002).

Mitosis and meiosis (Figs 2.22, 2.23)

Mitosis occurs in most somatic cells. It results in the distribution of identical copies of the parent cell genome to the two daughter cells. In meiosis, the divisions immediately before the final production of gametes halve the number of chromosomes to the haploid number, so that at fertilization the diploid number is restored. Moreover, meiosis includes a phase in which exchange of genetic material occurs between homologous chromosomes. This allows a reassortment of genes to take place, which means that the daughter cells differ from the parental cell in both their precise genetic sequence and their haploid state. Mitosis and meiosis are alike in many respects, and differ principally in chromosomal behaviour during the early stages of cell division. In meiosis, two divisions occur in quick succession. Meiosis I is unlike mitosis, whereas meiosis II is more like mitosis.

MITOSIS

New DNA is synthesized during the S phase of the cell cycle interphase. This means that the amount of DNA in diploid cells has doubled to the tetraploid value by the onset of mitosis, although the chromosome number is still diploid. During mitosis, this amount is halved between

23

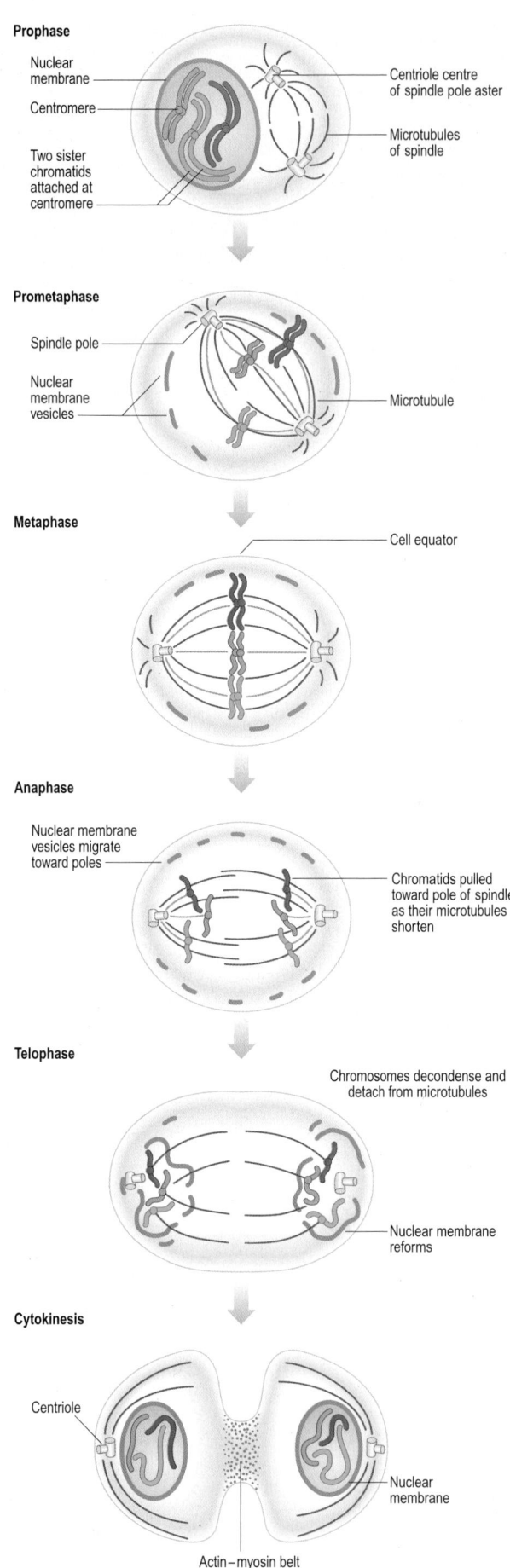

Prophase

Nuclear membrane

Centromere

Two sister chromatids attached at centromere

Centriole centre of spindle pole aster

Microtubules of spindle

Prometaphase

Spindle pole

Nuclear membrane vesicles

Microtubule

Metaphase

Cell equator

Anaphase

Nuclear membrane vesicles migrate toward poles

Chromatids pulled toward pole of spindle as their microtubules shorten

Telophase

Chromosomes decondense and detach from microtubules

Nuclear membrane reforms

Cytokinesis

Centriole

Nuclear membrane

Actin–myosin belt at cleavage furrow

Fig. 2.22 The stages in mitosis, including the appearance and distribution of the chromosomes.

the two daughter cells, so that DNA quantity and chromosome number are diploid in both cells. The nuclear changes that achieve this distribution are conventionally divided into four phases called prophase, metaphase, anaphase and telophase (**Figs 2.22, 2.24**).

PROPHASE

During prophase, the strands of chromatin, which are highly extended during interphase, shorten, thicken and resolve themselves into recognizable chromosomes. Each chromosome is made up of duplicate chromatids joined at their centromeres. Outside the nucleus, the two centriole pairs begin to separate, and move towards opposite poles of the cell. Parallel microtubules are assembled between them to create the mitotic spindle, and others radiate to form the asters, which come to lie at the spindle poles. As prophase proceeds, the nucleoli disappear, and the nuclear membrane suddenly disintegrates into small vesicles to release the chromosomes, an event that marks the end of prophase.

PROMETAPHASE–METAPHASE

As the nuclear membrane disappears, the spindle microtubules extend into the central region of the cell, attaching to the chromosomes which move towards the equator of the spindle (prometaphase). This plane is called the metaphase or equatorial plate. The chromosomes, attached at their centromeres, appear to be arranged in a ring when viewed from either pole of the cell, or to lie linearly across this plane when viewed from above. Cytoplasmic movements during late metaphase effect the approximately equal distribution of mitochondria and other organelles around the cell periphery.

ANAPHASE

The centromere in metaphase is a double structure (one per sister chromatid). During anaphase its halves separate, each carrying an attached chromatid. Each original chromosome appears therefore to split lengthwise into two new chromosomes, which move apart, one towards each pole. At the end of anaphase the chromosomes are grouped at either end of the cell, and both clusters are diploid in number. An infolding of the cell equator begins, and deepens during telophase as the cleavage furrow.

TELOPHASE

During telophase the chromosomes decondense. Each nuclear membrane forms, beginning as membranous vesicles at the ends of the chromosomes, and the nucleoli appear. At the same time, cytoplasmic division, which usually begins in early anaphase, continues until the new cells separate, each with its derived nucleus. The spindle remnant now disintegrates. While the cleavage furrow is active, a peripheral band or belt of actin and myosin appears in the constricting zone: contraction of this band is responsible for furrow formation.

Failure of disjunction of chromatids, so that paired chromatids pass to the same pole, may sometimes occur. Of the two new cells, one will have more, and the other fewer, chromosomes than the diploid number. Exposure to ionizing radiation promotes non-disjunction and may, by chromosomal damage, inhibit mitosis altogether. A typical symptom of radiation exposure is the failure of rapidly dividing epithelia to replace lost cells, with consequent ulceration of the skin and mucous membranes. Mitosis can also be disrupted by chemical agents, particularly colchicine and its derivatives. These compounds inhibit or reverse spindle microtubule formation, so that mitosis is arrested in metaphase. This underpins the rationale for many types of cytotoxic drugs used in cancer therapy.

MEIOSIS

There are two cell divisions during meiosis. Details of this process differ at a cellular level for male and female lineages.

MEIOSIS I

Prophase I

Prophase I is a long and complex phase that differs considerably from mitotic prophase and is customarily divided into five substages, called leptotene, zygotene, pachytene, diplotene and diakinesis.

Leptotene stage – Chromosomes appear as individual threads that are attached at one end to the nuclear membrane. They show characteristic

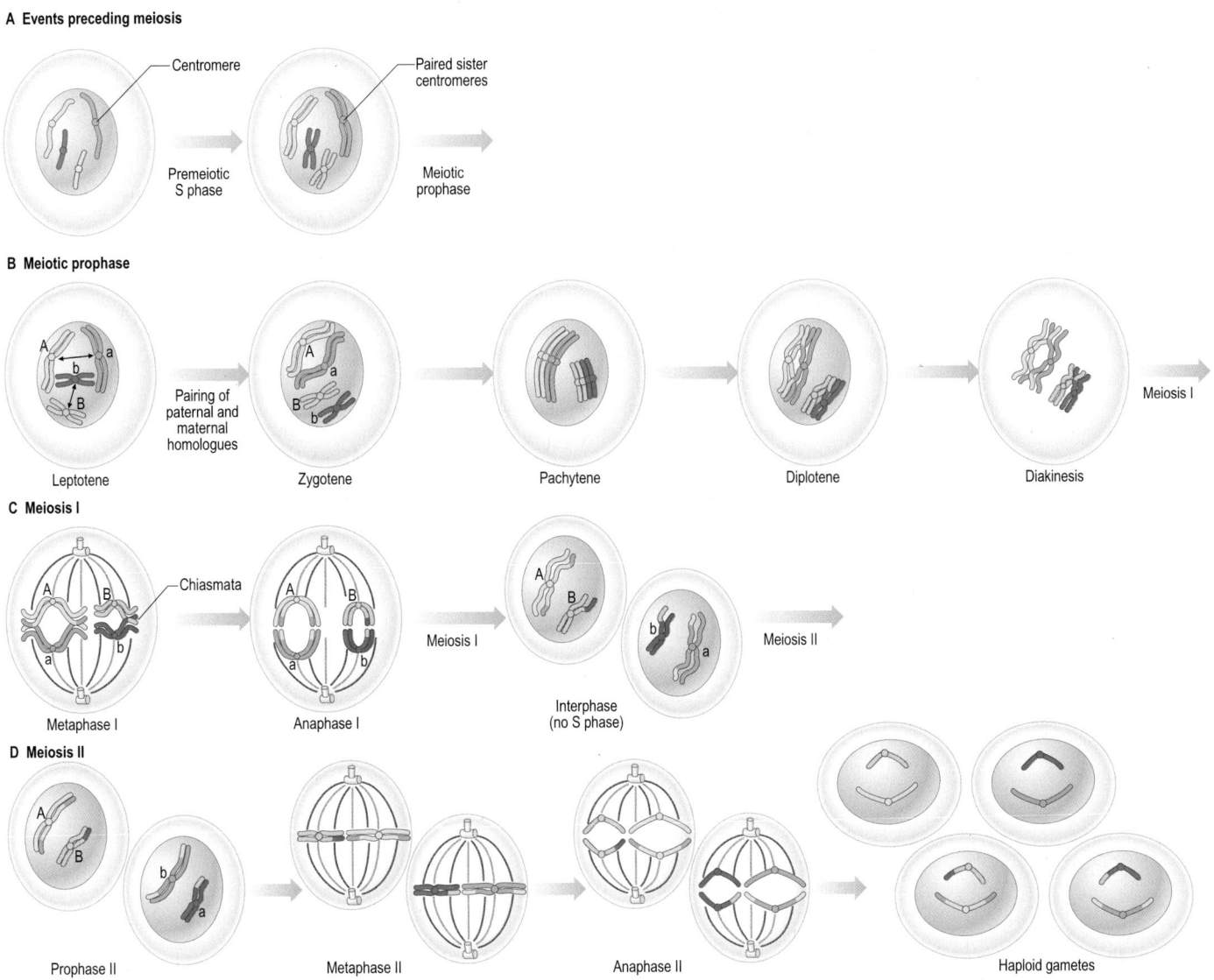

Fig. 2.23 The stages in meiosis, depicted by two pairs of maternal and paternal homologues (dark and pale colours). DNA and chromosome complement changes and exchange of genetic information between homologues are indicated.

beading throughout their length. Their DNA has been replicated in the preceding S phase.

Zygotene stage – Chromosomes lie together side by side in homologous pairs, a process which may be initiated during the previous mitotic division. The homologous chromosomes pair point for point progressively, beginning at their attachment to the nuclear membrane, so that corresponding regions lie in contact. This process is known as synapsis, conjugation or pairing, and each pair is now a bivalent. In the case of the unequal X and Y sex chromosomes, only limited pairing segments are homologous and these pair end to end. Homologous chromosomes are held together by a highly structured fibrillar band, the synaptonemal complex.

Pachytene stage – As shortening and thickening of each chromosome progress, its two chromatids, which are joined at the centromere, become visible. Each bivalent pair therefore consists of four chromatids, forming a tetrad. Two chromatids, one from each bivalent chromosome, partially coil round each other, and during this stage, exchange of DNA (crossing over or decussation) occurs by breaking and rejoining of strands.

Diplotene stage – Homologous pairs, now much shortened, separate except where crossing over has occurred (chiasmata). At least one chiasma forms between each homologous pair and up to five have been observed. In the ovaries, primary oocytes become diplotene by the fifth

month *in utero* and each remains at this stage until the period before ovulation (up to 50 years).

Diakinesis – The chromosomes, still as bivalents, become even shorter and thicker. They subsequently disperse, as bivalents, to lie against the nuclear membrane.

During prophase, the nucleoli disappear and the spindle and asters form as they do in mitosis. At the end of prophase the nuclear membrane disappears and bivalent chromosomes move towards the equatorial plate (prometaphase).

Metaphase I

Metaphase I resembles mitotic metaphase, except that the bodies attaching to the spindle microtubules are bivalents, not single chromosomes. These become arranged so that the homologous pairs lie parallel to the equatorial plate, with one on either side.

Anaphase and telophase I

Chiasmata finally disappear. Anaphase and telophase I also occur as in mitosis, except that in anaphase the centromeres do not split. Instead of paired chromatids separating to move towards the poles, entire homologous chromosomes (made up of two joined chromatids) move to opposite poles. As positioning of bivalent pairs is random, assortment of maternal and paternal chromosomes in each telophase nucleus is also random.

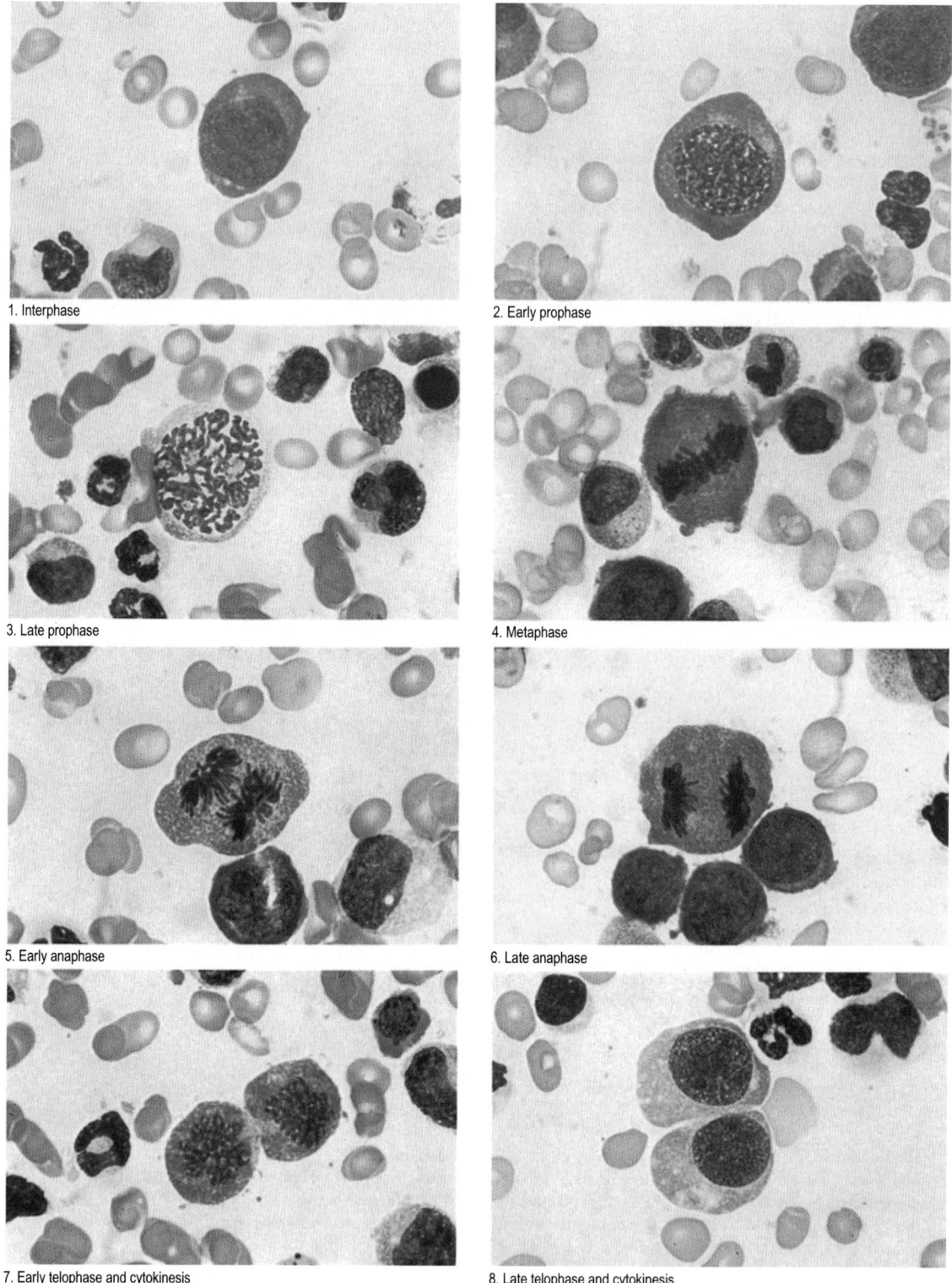

1. Interphase

2. Early prophase

3. Late prophase

4. Metaphase

5. Early anaphase

6. Late anaphase

7. Early telophase and cytokinesis

8. Late telophase and cytokinesis

Fig. 2.24 Stages in mitosis, seen in immature blood cells in a smear preparation of human bone marrow. (By permission from Young B, Heath JW 2000 Wheater's Functional Histology. Edinburgh: Churchill Livingstone.)

During meiosis I, cytoplasmic division occurs as it does in mitosis, to produce two new cells.

MEIOSIS II
Meiosis II commences after only a short interval during which no DNA synthesis occurs. This second division is more like mitosis, in that chromatids separate during anaphase, but, unlike mitosis, the separating chromatids are genetically different. Cytoplasmic division also occurs and thus, in the male, four haploid cells result from meiosis I and II.

CELL DIFFERENTIATION

As the embryo develops, its cells pass through a series of changes in gene expression, reflected in alterations of cell structure and behaviour. They begin to diversify, separating first into two main tissue arrangements, epithelium and embryonic mesenchyme, then into more restricted subtypes of tissue, until finally they mature into cells of their particular adult lineage. In this process, and in the maturation of functioning cells of the different lineages from their stem cells, there is a sequential pattern of gene expression that changes and limits the cell to a particular specialized range of activities. Such changes involve alterations in cell structure and biochemical characteristics, particularly in the types of proteins that are synthesized. At the genetic level, differentiation is based on a change in the pattern of repression and activation of the DNA sequences encoding proteins specific to that stage of development.

A cell may be committed to a particular differentiated fate without manifesting its commitment until later. Once switched in this way, cells are not usually able to revert to an earlier stage of differentiation, so that an irreversible repression of some gene sequences must have occurred. Differentiation signals include interactions between cells that are mediated by diffusible signalling molecules elaborated by one cell and detected by another, and by contact-mediated signalling (such as Delta-Notch signalling). The latter is particularly important in establishing boundaries between different cell populations in development.

Differentiation may also depend in some instances on a temporal sequence such as the number of previous cell divisions. In mature tissues in which cell turnover occurs, similar mechanisms appear to ensure the final differentiation to a functional end cell. This may be linked to the presence of a physiological stimulus, e.g. B lymphocytes respond to exposure to an antigen by differentiating into plasma cells that secrete a neutralizing antibody. In other cases, particularly where a cell is part of a highly organized tissue system, more subtle mechanisms exists to ensure a balance between cell proliferation, differentiation and programmed cell death (apoptosis) (p. 203).

APOPTOSIS

Cells die as a result of either tissue injury (necrosis) or the internal activation of a 'suicide' programme (apoptosis). Apoptosis (programmed cell death, regulated cell suicide) is a central mechanism controlling multicellular development. During morphogenesis, apoptosis mediates activities such as the separation of the developing digits, and has an important role in regulating the number of neurones in the nervous system (the majority of neurones die during development). Apoptosis also ensures that inappropriate or inefficient cells of the acquired immune system are eliminated.

The morphological changes exhibited by necrotic cells are very different from those seen in apoptotic cells. Necrotic cells swell and subsequently rupture; the resulting debris may induce an inflammatory response. Apoptotic cells shrink, their nuclei and chromosomes fragment, forming apoptotic bodies, and their plasma membranes undergo conformational changes that act as a signal to local phagocytes. The dead cells are removed rapidly, and as their intracellular contents are not released into the extracellular environment, inflammatory reactions are avoided.

Apoptosis and cell proliferation are intimately coupled: several cell cycle regulators can influence both cell division and apoptosis. The signals that trigger apoptosis include withdrawal of survival factors or exposure to inappropriate proliferative stimuli. The current model of the intracellular pathway(s) that lead to apoptosis implicates permeabilization of the mitochondrial membrane, the release of cytochrome c (from the space between the inner and outer mitochondrial membranes) into the cytosol, and subsequent activation of a family of cysteine proteases known as caspases. Caspases are the intracellular mediators of apoptosis: when activated, they initiate a cascade of degradative processes targeting, in particular, proteins of the nuclear lamina and cytoskeleton.

Subversion of the apoptotic response is a key characteristic of many cancer cells. Thus the tumour suppressor gene *p53* (which functions in cell-cycle control, regulation of apoptosis and the maintenance of genetic stability), is mutated in about 50% of all human cancers. For further details, see Alberts et al (2002).

REFERENCES

Alberts B, Johnson A, Lewis J, Raff M, Roberts K, Walter P 2002 Molecular Biology of the Cell, 4th edn. New York: Garland Press.

Epstein RJ 2003. Human Molecular Biology. An Introduction to the Molecular Basis of Health and Disease. Cambridge: Cambridge University Press.
Reviews signalling molecules and their receptors in the context of human disease.

Graff C, Bui T-H, Larsson N-G 2002. Mitochondrial diseases. Best Pract Res Clin Obstet Gynaecol 16: 715–28.
Reviews clinical conditions related to the inheritance of maternal mitochondrial gene mutations.

Morris R, Cox H, Mombelli E, Quinn P 2004. Rafts, little caves and large potholes: how lipid structure interacts with membrane proteins to create functionally diverse membrane environments. In: Quinn PJ (ed) Membrane Dynamics and Domains. London: Kluwer Academic/Plenum Publishers: (in press).
Reviews how lipids partition proteins into different environments within membranes, and the benefits that accrue to the proteins as a result.

Pollard TD, Earnshaw WC 2002. Cell Biology. Philadelphia: Saunders.
Reviews cytoskeletal and motor proteins.

Porter RM, Lane EB 2003. Phenotypes, genotypes and their contribution to understanding keratin function. Trends Genet 19: 278–85.
Reviews the largest family of intermediate filament proteins, providing evidence for the functional roles of this diverse group, and addresses inherited tissue fragility disorders resulting from keratin gene mutations.

Integrating cells into tissues

Although some cells in the body are essentially migratory, most exist as cellular aggregates in which individual cells carry out similar or closely related functions in a coordinated manner. These aggregates are termed tissues, and can be classified into a fairly small number of broad categories on the basis of their structure, function and molecular properties. On the basis of their structure, most tissues are divided into four major types: epithelia, connective or supporting tissue, muscle and nervous tissue. Epithelia are continuous layers of cells with little intercellular space, which cover or line surfaces, or have been so derived. In connective tissues, the cells are embedded in an intercellular matrix which, typically, forms a substantial and important component of the tissue. Muscle consists largely of specialized contractile cells. Nervous tissue consists of cells specialized for conducting and transmitting electrical and chemical signals and the cells that support this activity.

There is molecular evidence that this structure-based scheme of classification has validity. Thus the intermediate filament proteins (p. 17) characteristic of all epithelia are keratins; those of connective tissue are vimentins; those of muscle are desmins; and those of nervous tissue are neurofilament and glial fibrillary acidic proteins. However, cells such as myofibroblasts, neuroepithelial sensory receptors and ependymal cells of the central nervous system have features of more than one tissue type. Despite its anomalies, the scheme is useful for descriptive purposes and widely used, and will be adopted here.

In this section, two of the major tissue categories, epithelia and general connective and supporting tissues, will be described. Specialized skeletal connective tissues, i.e. cartilage and bone, together with skeletal muscle, are described in detail in Chapter 6 as part of the musculoskeletal system overview. Smooth muscle and cardiac muscle are described in Chapter 7. Nervous system tissues are described in Chapter 4. Specialized defensive cells, which also form a migrant population within the general connective tissues, are considered in more detail in Chapter 5, with blood, lymphoid tissues and haemopoiesis.

EPITHELIA

The term epithelium is applied to the layer or layers of cells that cover the body surfaces or line the body cavities that open on to it. Developmentally, epithelia are derived from all three layers of the early embryo (p. 206). The ectoderm gives rise to the epidermis, glandular tissue of the breast, cornea and the junctional zones of the buccal cavity and anal canal. The endoderm forms the epithelial lining of the alimentary canal and its glands, most of the respiratory tract and the distal parts of the urogenital tract. Mesodermal derivatives include the epithelia of the kidney, the suprarenal (adrenal) cortex and endocrine cells of the ovary and testis. These endocrine cells are atypical epithelia in that they differentiate from embryonic mesenchyme (p. 207) and, in common with endocrine cells in general, they lack a free surface that communicates with the exterior. This atypical category also includes endothelia that line blood vessels and lymphatics (p. 146), and the epithelium-like cell layers of mesodermal (and mesenchymal) origin that line internal cavities of the body and are usually classified separately as mesothelia (p. 41): they line the pericardial, pleural and peritoneal cavities.

Epithelia function generally as selective barriers that facilitate, or inhibit, the passage of substances across the surfaces they cover. In addition, they may: protect underlying tissues against dehydration, chemical or mechanical damage; synthesize and secrete products into the spaces that they line; function as sensory surfaces. In this respect, many features of nervous tissue can be regarded as those of a modified epithelium and the two tissue types share an origin (p. 207) in embryonic ectoderm.

Epithelia (**Fig. 3.1**) are predominantly cellular and the little extracellular material they possess is limited to the basal lamina. Intercellular junctions, which are usually numerous, maintain the mechanical cohesiveness of the epithelial sheet and contribute to its barrier functions. A series of three intercellular junctions forms a typical epithelial junctional complex: in sequence from the apical surface, this consists of a tight junctional zone, an adherent (intermediate) junctional zone and a region of discrete desmosome junctions (p. 7). Epithelial cell shape is most usually polygonal and partly determined by cytoplasmic features such as secretory granules. The basal surface of an epithelium lies in contact with a thin layer of filamentous protein and proteoglycan termed the basal lamina, which is synthesized predominantly by the epithelial cells. The basal lamina is described in the section on extracellular matrix (p. 38).

Epithelia can usually regenerate when injured. Indeed, many epithelia continuously replace their cells to offset cell loss caused by mechanical abrasion. Blood vessels do not penetrate typical epithelia and so cells receive their nutrition by diffusion from capillaries of neighbouring connective tissues. This arrangement limits the maximum thickness of living epithelial cell layers. Epithelia, together with their supporting connective tissue, can often be removed surgically as one layer, which is collectively known as a membrane. Where the surface of a membrane is moistened by mucous glands it is called a mucous membrane or mucosa (p. 41), whereas a similar layer of connective tissue covered by mesothelium is called a serous membrane or serosa (p. 41).

Classification

Epithelia can be classified as unilaminar (single-layered, simple), in which a single layer of cells rests on a basal lamina, or multilaminar, in which the layer is more than one cell thick. The latter includes: stratified squamous epithelia, in which superficial cells are constantly replaced from the basal layers; urothelium (transitional epithelium), which serves special functions in the urinary tract; and other multilaminar epithelia which, like urothelium, are replaced only very slowly under normal conditions. Seminiferous epithelium is a specialized multilaminar tissue found only in the testis.

UNILAMINAR (SIMPLE) EPITHELIA

Unilaminar epithelia are further classified according to the shape of their cells, into squamous, cuboidal, columnar and pseudostratified types. Cell shape is largely related to cell volume. Where little cytoplasm is present, there are generally few organelles and therefore low metabolic activity and cells are squamous or low cuboidal. Highly active cells, e.g. secretory epithelia, contain abundant mitochondria and endoplasmic reticulum and are typically tall cuboidal or columnar. Unilaminar epithelia can also be subdivided into those which have special functions, such as those with cilia, numerous microvilli, secretory vacuoles (in mucous and serous glandular cells), or sensory features. Myoepithelial cells, which are contractile, are found as isolated cells associated with glandular structures, e.g. salivary and mammary glands.

SQUAMOUS EPITHELIUM

Simple squamous epithelium is composed of flattened, tightly apposed, polygonal cells (squames). This type of epithelium is described as tessellated when the cells have complex, interlocking borders rather than straight boundaries. The cytoplasm may in places be only 0.1 μm thick and the nucleus usually bulges into the overlying space (**Fig. 3.2**). These cells line the alveoli of the lungs and form the outer capsular wall

29

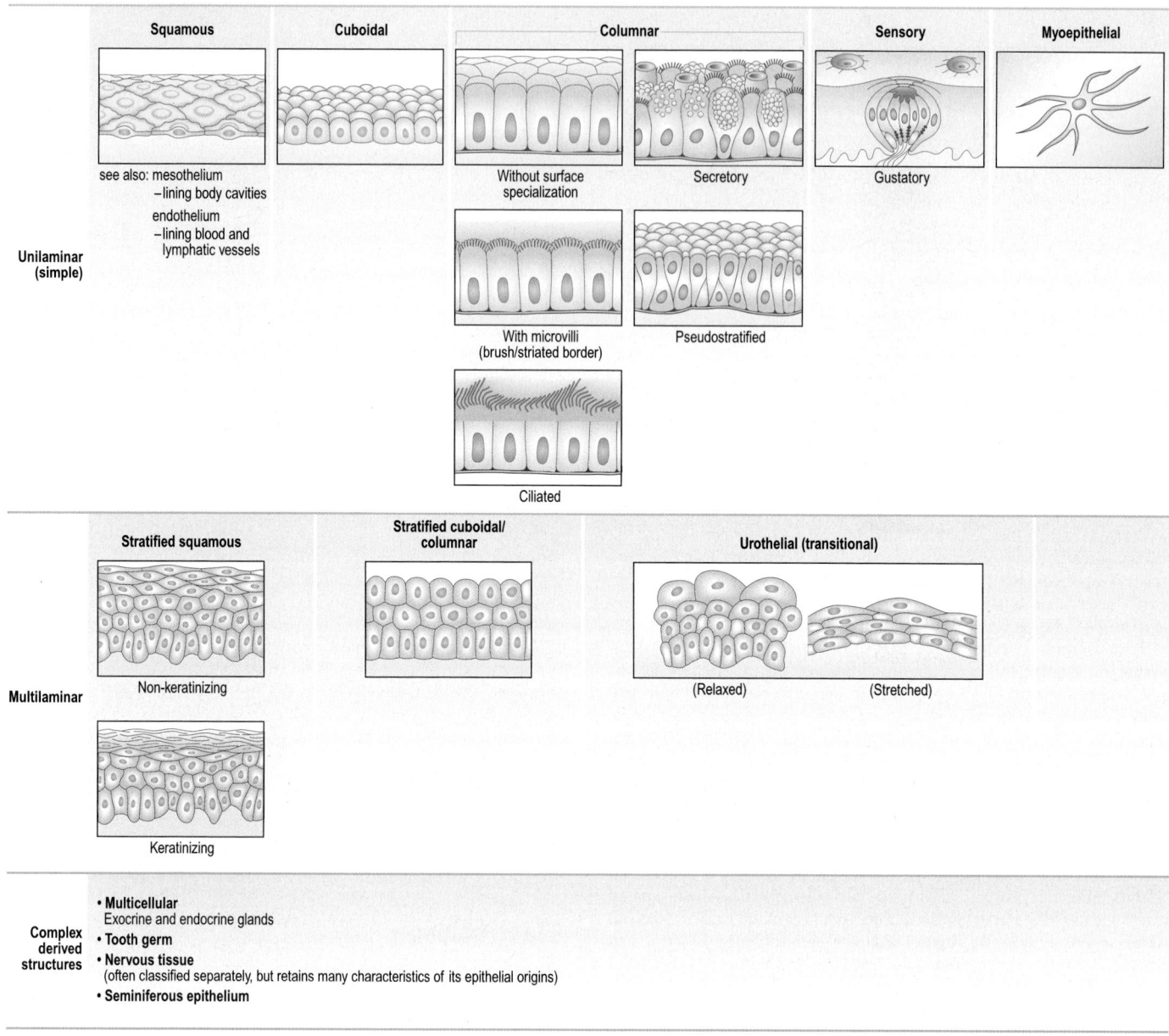

Squamous

see also: mesothelium
– lining body cavities
endothelium
– lining blood and
lymphatic vessels

Cuboidal

Columnar

Without surface
specialization

With microvilli
(brush/striated border)

Secretory

Pseudostratified

Ciliated

Sensory

Gustatory

Myoepithelial

**Unilaminar
(simple)**

Multilaminar

Stratified squamous

Non-keratinizing

Keratinizing

**Stratified cuboidal/
columnar**

Urothelial (transitional)

(Relaxed)   (Stretched)

**Complex
derived
structures**

• **Multicellular**
  Exocrine and endocrine glands
• **Tooth germ**
• **Nervous tissue**
  (often classified separately, but retains many characteristics of its epithelial origins)
• **Seminiferous epithelium**

Fig. 3.1 Classification of epithelial tissues and cells.

of renal corpuscles, the thin segments of the renal tubules and various parts of the inner ear. Because it is so thin, simple squamous epithelium allows rapid diffusion of gases and water; it may also engage in active transport, as indicated by the presence of numerous endocytic vesicles in these cells. Tight junctions between adjacent cells ensure that materials pass primarily through cells, rather than between them.

CUBOIDAL AND COLUMNAR EPITHELIA

Cuboidal and columnar epithelia consist of regular rows of cylindrical cells (**Figs 3.3, 3.4**). Cuboidal cells are approximately square in vertical section, whereas columnar cells are taller than their diameter, and both are polygonal when sectioned horizontally. Commonly, microvilli are found on their free surfaces, which considerably increases the absorptive area, e.g. in the epithelia of the small intestine (columnar cells with a striated border of very regular microvilli), the gallbladder (columnar cells with a brush border) and proximal and distal convoluted tubules of the kidney (large cuboidal to low columnar cells with brush borders).

Ciliated columnar epithelium lines: most of the respiratory tract (except for the lower pharynx and vocal folds) where it is pseudo-stratified (**Fig. 3.5**) as far as the terminal bronchioles; some of the tympanic cavity and auditory tube; the uterine tube; the efferent ductules of the testis. Mucous glands also line much of the respiratory

tract and cilia sweep a layer of mucus and trapped dust particles etc., from the lung towards the pharynx in the mucociliary rejection current, which clears the respiratory passages of inhaled particles. Cilia in the uterine tube assist the passage of oocytes and fertilized ova to the uterus (p. 1329).

Some columnar cells are glandular, and their apical domains (p. 5) contain mucus- or protein-filled (zymogen) vesicles, e.g. mucin-secreting and chief cells of the gastric epithelium. Where mucous cells lie among non-secretory cells, e.g. in the intestinal epithelium, their apical cytoplasm and its secretory contents often expand to produce a characteristic cell shape, and they are known as goblet cells (**Fig. 3.5**). For further details of glandular tissue, see page 34 and for the characteristics of mucus, see page 41.

PSEUDOSTRATIFIED EPITHELIUM

Pseudostratified epithelium is a single-layered (simple) columnar epithelium in which nuclei lie at different levels in a vertical section (**Figs 3.5, 3.6**). All cells are in contact with the basal lamina throughout their lifespan, but not all cells extend through the entire thickness of the epithelium. Some constitute an immature basal cell layer of smaller cells, which are often mitotic and able to replace damaged mature cells. Migrating lymphocytes and mast cells within columnar epithelia may also give a pseudostratified appearance because their nuclei are found

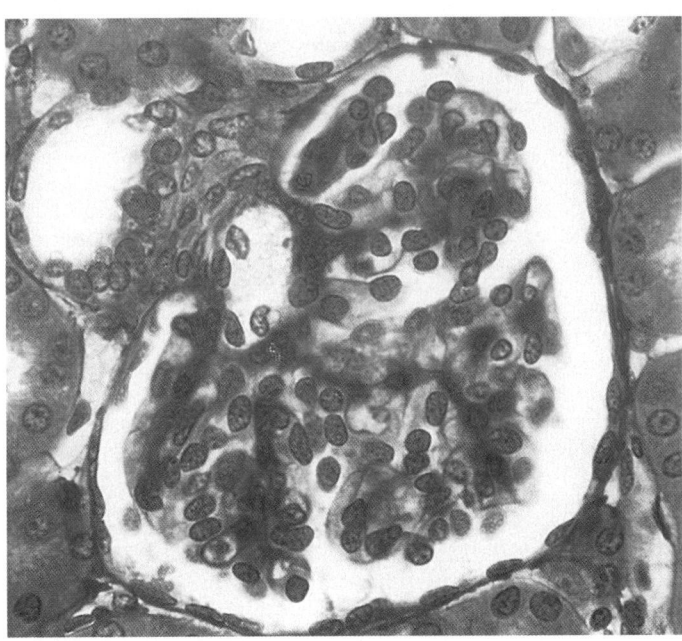

Fig. 3.2 Simple squamous epithelium lining the outer parietal layer of Bowman's capsule in the renal corpuscle. Oval nuclei project into the urinary space, covered by a highly attenuated cytoplasm. The underlying basement membrane is stained blue in this azan preparation. (By permission from Young B, Heath JW 2000 Wheater's Functional Histology. Edinburgh: Churchill Livingstone.)

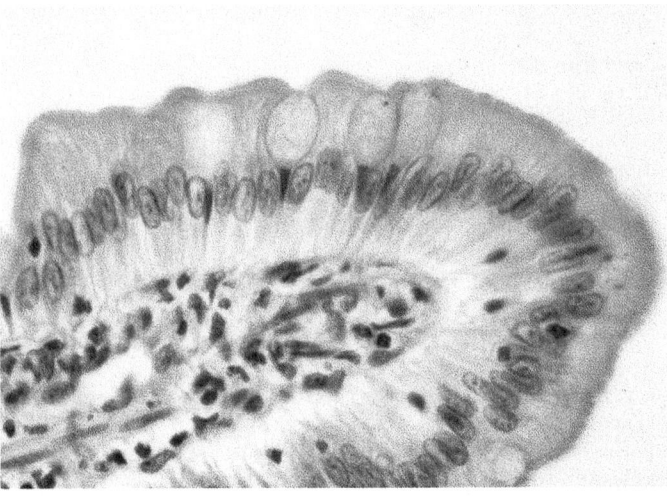

Fig. 3.4 Simple columnar epithelium covering the tip (right) of a villus in the small intestine. Tall, columnar absorptive cells bear a striated border of microvilli, just visible as a deeper-stained apical fringe. A few interspersed goblet cells are present, with pale apical secretory granules and dark, elongated nuclei. (Photograph by Sarah-Jane Smith.)

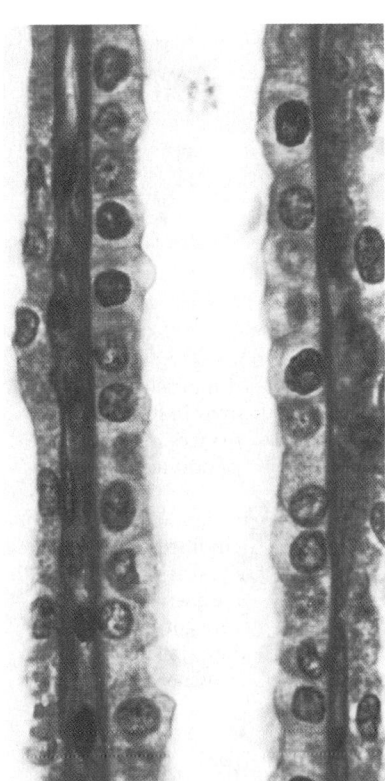

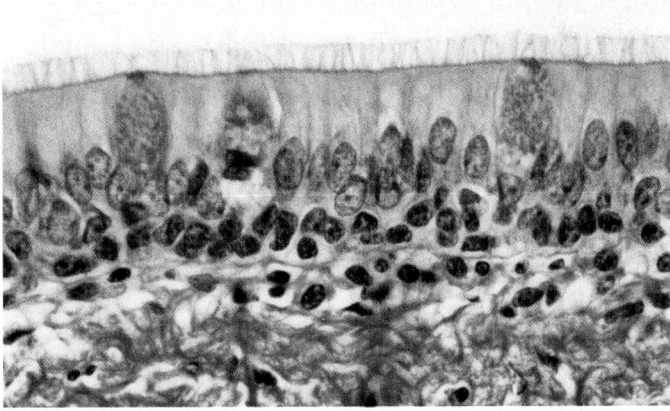

Fig. 3.5 Ciliated columnar epithelium lining a bronchus in the respiratory tract, stained with alcian blue to show the goblet cells with blue-stained mucinogen granules in their apical cytoplasm.

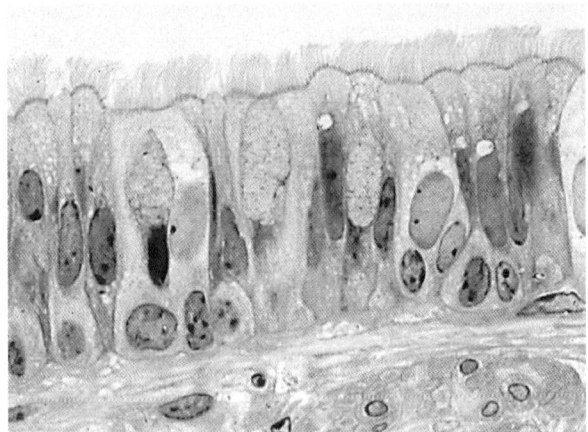

Fig. 3.3 Simple cuboidal epithelium lining a collecting tubule in the renal medulla. Azan preparation; the basement membrane is stained blue. (By permission from Young B, Heath JW 2000 Wheater's Functional Histology. Edinburgh: Churchill Livingstone.)

Fig. 3.6 Pseudostratified columnar epithelium, with ciliated cells, goblet cells with their apical cytoplasm distended by mucinogen granules, and basal cells. This type of epithelium is found almost exclusively in the larger airways of the respiratory system and is thus also known as respiratory epithelium. (By permission from Kierszenbaum AL 2002 Histology and Cell Biology. St Louis: Mosby.)

at different depths. Much of the ciliated lining of the respiratory tract is of the pseudostratified type, and so is the sensory epithelium of the olfactory area.

SENSORY EPITHELIA

Sensory epithelia are found in special sense organs of the olfactory, gustatory and vestibulocochlear receptor systems. All of these contain sensory cells surrounded by supportive, non-receptor cells. Olfactory receptors are modified neurones, and their axons pass directly to the brain, but the other types are specialized epithelial cells that synapse with terminals of afferent (and sometimes efferent) nerve fibres.

MYOEPITHELIAL CELLS

Myoepithelial cells, which are also sometimes termed basket cells, are fusiform or stellate in shape (**Fig. 3.7**), contain actin and myosin filaments, and contract when stimulated by nervous or endocrine signals. They surround the secretory portions and ducts of some glands, e.g. mammary, lacrimal, salivary and sweat glands, and lie between the basal lamina and the glandular or ductal epithelium. Their contraction assists the initial flow of secretion into larger conduits. Myoepithelial cells are ultrastructurally similar to smooth muscle cells in the arrangement of their actin and myosin, but differ from them because they originate from embryonic ectoderm or endoderm. They can be identified immunohistochemically on the basis of the co-localization of myofilament proteins (which signify their contractile function), and keratin intermediate filaments (which accords with their epithelial lineage).

MULTILAMINAR (STRATIFIED) EPITHELIA

Multilaminar epithelia are found at surfaces subjected to mechanical damage or other potentially harmful conditions. They can be divided into those which continue to replace their surface cells from deeper layers, designated stratified squamous epithelia, and others in which replacement is extremely slow except after injury.

STRATIFIED SQUAMOUS EPITHELIA

Stratified squamous epithelia are multilayered tissues in which the formation, maturation and loss of cells is continuous, although the rates of these processes can change, e.g. after injury. New cells are formed in the most basal layers by the mitotic division (p. 23) of stem cells and transit (or transient) amplifying cells. The daughter cells move more superficially, changing gradually from a cuboidal shape to a more flattened form and are eventually shed from the surface as a highly flattened squame. Typically, the cells are held together by numerous desmosomes to form strong, contiguous cellular sheets that provide protection to the underlying tissues against mechanical, microbial and chemical damage. Stratified squamous epithelia may be broadly subdivided into keratinized and non-keratinized types.

Keratinized epithelium

Keratinized epithelium (**Fig. 3.8**) is found at surfaces that are subject to drying or mechanical stresses, or are exposed to high levels of abrasion. These include the entire epidermis and the mucocutaneous junctions of the lips, nostrils, distal anal canal, outer surface of the tympanic membrane and parts of the oral lining (gingivae, hard palate and filiform papillae on the anterior part of the dorsal surface of the tongue). Their cells, keratinocytes, are described in more detail on page 158. A distinguishing feature of keratinized epithelia is that cells of the superficial layer, the stratum corneum, are anucleate, dead, flattened squames that eventually flake off from the surface. In addition, the tough keratin intermediate filaments become firmly embedded in a matrix protein. This unusual combination of strongly coherent layers of living cells and more superficial strata made of plates of inert, mechanically robust protein complexes, interleaved with water-resistant lipid, makes this type of epithelium an efficient barrier against different types of injury and water loss.

Non-keratinized epithelium

Non-keratinized epithelium is present at surfaces that are subject to abrasion but protected from drying (**Fig. 3.9**). These include: the buccal cavity (except for the areas noted above); oropharynx and laryngopharynx; oesophagus; part of the anal canal; vagina; distal uterine cervix; distal urethra; conjunctiva and cornea; inner surfaces of the eyelids; the vestibule of the nasal cavities. Cells go through the same transitions in general shape as are seen in the keratinized type, but they do not fill completely with keratin or secrete glycolipid, and they retain their nuclei until they desquamate at the surface. In sites where considerable abrasion occurs, e.g. parts of the buccal cavity, the epithelium is thicker and its most superficial cells may partly keratinize, so that it is referred to as parakeratinized, in contrast to the orthokeratinized state of fully keratinized epithelium. Diets deficient in vitamin A may induce keratinization of such epithelia, and excessive doses may lead to its transformation into mucus-secreting epithelium.

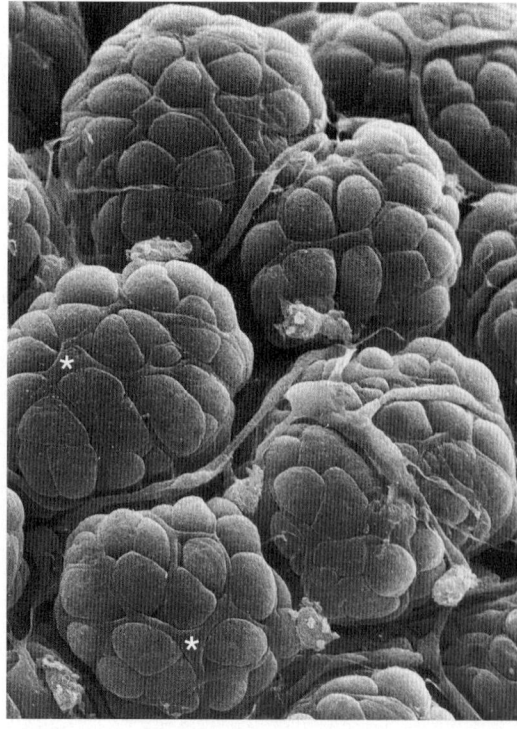

Fig. 3.7 Stellate myoepithelial cells wrapped around secretory acini in the lactating mammary gland, seen in the scanning electron microscope after enzymatic removal of extracellular matrix. Rodent tissue. (Reproduced from Cell Tissue Res 209: 1–10. A scanning electron microscope study of myoepithelial cells in exocrine glands. Nagato T et al, 1980 © Springer-Verlag.)

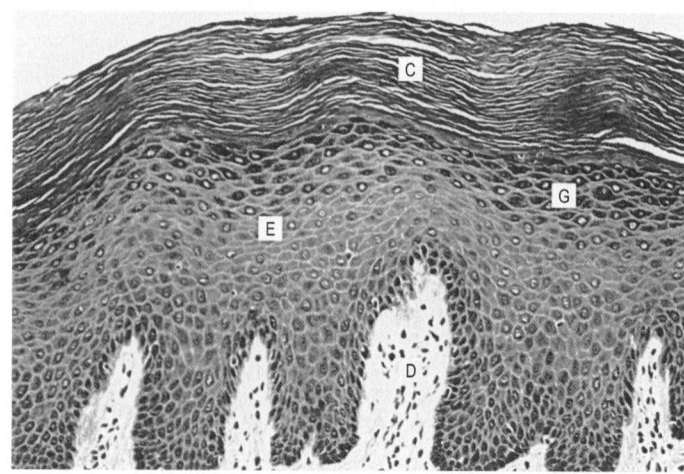

Fig. 3.8 Keratinized stratified squamous epithelium from the epidermis (E) of the lateral surface of a toe, showing thick skin with a prominent cornified layer (C) of dead keratinized squames. The granular layer (G) is prominent in thick skin. (By permission from Dr JB Kerr, Monash University, from Kerr JB 1999 Atlas of Functional Histology. London: Mosby.)

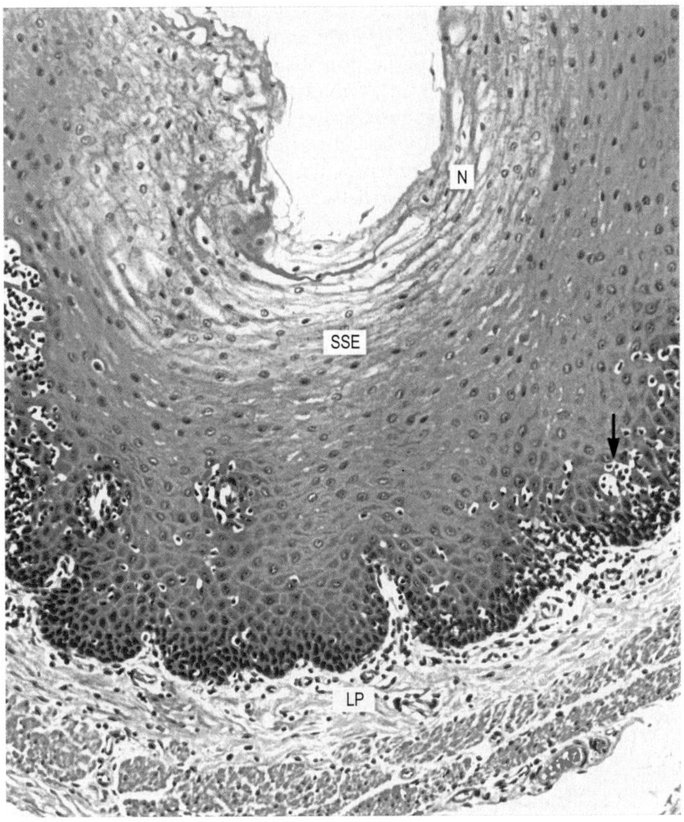

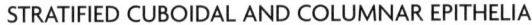

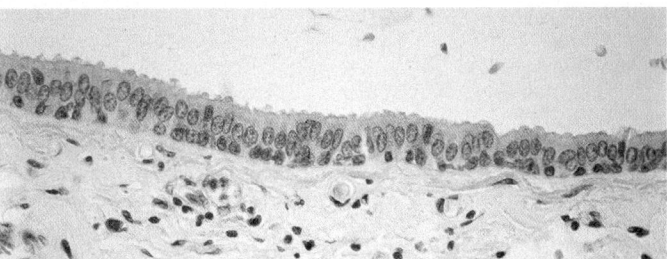

Fig. 3.10 Stratified cuboidal epithelium lining a large interlobular collecting duct of the parotid salivary gland. (Photograph by Sarah-Jane Smith.)

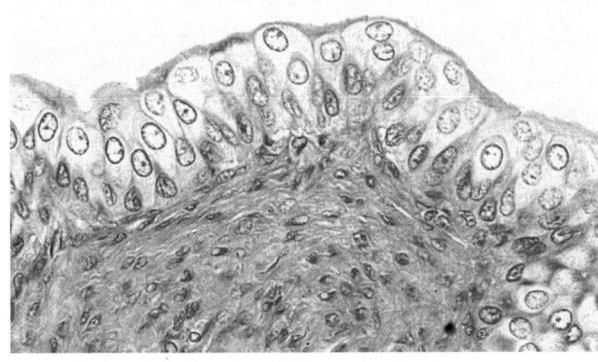

Fig. 3.11 Urothelium (transitional epithelium) lining the urinary bladder. The most superficial cells have a thickened plasma membrane as a result of the presence of intramembranous plaques, which give an eosinophilic appearance to the luminal surface. (By permission from Kierszenbaum AL 2002 Histology and Cell Biology. St Louis: Mosby.)

Fig. 3.9 The luminal surface of the oesophagus is nonkeratinized, stratified squamous epithelium (SSE), similar to much of the epithelial lining of the oral cavity. The most superficial layers of stratum corneum are only several cells thick, and the nuclei (N) are retained with little or no transformation into plaques of keratin. Individual lymphocytes are noted in the epithelium (arrow) and at intervals in the subjacent lamina propria (LP). (By permission from Dr JB Kerr, Monash University, from Kerr JB 1999 Atlas of Functional Histology. London: Mosby.)

STRATIFIED CUBOIDAL AND COLUMNAR EPITHELIA

Two or more layers of cuboidal or low columnar cells (**Fig. 3.10**) are typical of the walls of the larger ducts of some exocrine glands, e.g. the pancreas, salivary glands and the ducts of sweat glands and they presumably provide more strength than a single layer. Parts of the male urethra are also lined by stratified columnar epithelium. The layers are not continually replaced by basal mitoses and there is no progression of form from base to surface, but they can repair themselves if damaged.

UROTHELIUM (URINARY OR TRANSITIONAL EPITHELIUM)

Urothelium (**Fig. 3.11**) is a specialized epithelium that lines much of the urinary tract and prevents its rather toxic contents from damaging surrounding structures. It extends from the ends of the collecting ducts of the kidneys, through the ureters (p. 1277) and bladder (p. 1292), to the proximal portion of the urethra. In males it covers the urethra as far as the ejaculatory ducts, then becomes intermittent and is finally replaced by stratified columnar epithelium in the membranous urethra. In females it extends as far as the urogenital membrane. During development, part of it is derived from mesoderm and part from ectoderm and endoderm.

The epithelium appears to be four to six cells thick, and lines organs that undergo considerable distension and contraction. It can therefore stretch greatly without losing its integrity. In stretching, the cells become flattened, without altering their positions relative to each other, as they are firmly connected by numerous desmosomes. However, the urothelium appears to be reduced to two to three cells thick. The epithelium is called transitional because of the apparent transition between a stratified cuboidal epithelium and a stratified squamous epithelium, which occurs as it is stretched to accommodate urine, particularly in the bladder. The basal cells are basophilic, with many ribosomes, and are cuboidal, uninucleate (diploid) when relaxed. More apically, they form large binucleate, or, more often, polyploid

uninucleate cells. The surface cells are largest and may even be octaploid: in the relaxed state, they typically bulge into the lumen as dome-shaped cells with a thickened, eosinophilic glycocalyx or cell coat (p. 6). Their luminal surfaces are covered by a specialized plasma membrane in which plaques of intramembranous glycoprotein particles are embedded. These plaques stiffen the membrane. When the epithelium is in the relaxed state, and the surface area of the cells is reduced, the plaques are partially internalized by the hinge-like action of the more flexible interplaque membrane regions. They re-emerge onto the surface when it is stretched.

Normally, cell turnover is very slow; cell division is infrequent and is restricted to the basal layer. However, when damaged, the epithelium regenerates quite rapidly.

SEMINIFEROUS EPITHELIUM

Seminiferous epithelium is a highly specialized, complex stratified epithelium. It consists of a heterogeneous population of cells that form the lineage of the spermatozoa (spermatogonia, spermatocytes, spermatids), together with supporting cells (Sertoli cells). It is described in detail in Chapter 97 (p. 1307).

GLANDS

One of the features of many epithelia is their ability to alter the environment facing their free surfaces by the directed transport of ions, water or macromolecules. This is particularly well demonstrated in glandular tissue, in which the metabolism and structural organization of the cells is specialized for the synthesis and secretion of macromolecules, usually from the apical surface. Such cells may exist in isolation amongst other non-secretory cells of an epithelium, e.g. goblet cells in the absorptive lining of the small intestine, or may form highly coherent sheets of epithelium with a common secretory function, e.g. the mucous lining of the stomach and, in a highly invaginated structure, the complex salivary glands.

Glands may be subdivided into exocrine glands and endocrine glands. Exocrine glands secrete, often via a duct, onto surfaces that are continuous with the exterior of the body, including the alimentary tract, respiratory system, urinary and genital ducts and their derivatives, and the skin. Endocrine glands are ductless and secrete hormones directly into the circulatory system, which then conveys them throughout the body to affect the activities of other cells (p. 179).

Paracrine glandular cells are similar to endocrine cells, but their secretions diffuse locally to cellular targets in the immediate vicinity. In addition to strictly epithelial glands, some tissues derived from the nervous system, including the suprarenal medulla (p. 1247) and neurohypophysis (p. 380), are neurosecretory. Modes of signalling by secretory cells are illustrated in **Fig. 2.6**.

Exocrine glands

TYPES OF SECRETORY PROCESSES (Fig. 3.12)

The mechanism of secretion varies considerably. If the secretions are initially packaged into vesicles, these are conveyed to the cell surface (p. 11), where they are discharged in a number of different ways. In merocrine secretion, which is by far the most common mechanism, vesicle membranes fuse with the plasma membrane to release their contents to the exterior. Specialized transmembrane molecules in the secretory vacuole wall recognize marker proteins on the cytoplasmic side of the plasma membrane and bind to them. This initiates interactions with other proteins that cause the fusion of the two membranes and the consequent release of the vesicle contents. The stimulus for secretion varies with the type of cell, but often appears to involve a rise in intracellular calcium. Glands such as the simple sweat glands of the skin, where ions and water are actively transported from plasma, were once classified as eccrine glands. They are now known to synthesize and secrete small amounts of protein by a merocrine mechanism, and are thus reclassified as merocrine glands.

In apocrine glands, some of the apical cytoplasm is pinched off with the contained secretions, which are stored in the cell as membrane-free droplets. The best understood example of this is the secretion of milk fat by mammary gland cells (p. 972), in which a small amount of cytoplasm is incorporated into the plasma membrane-bound lipid globule as it is released from the cell. Larger amounts of cytoplasm are included in secretions by specialized apocrine sweat glands in the axilla and genitoanal regions of the body. In some tissues there is a combination of different types of secretion, e.g. mammary gland cells secrete milk fat by apocrine secretion and milk protein, casein, by merocrine secretion.

In holocrine glands, e.g. sebaceous glands in the skin, the cells first fill with secretory products (lipid droplets or sebum, in this instance) and then the entire cell disintegrates to liberate the accumulated mass of secretion into the duct or hair follicle.

STRUCTURAL AND FUNCTIONAL CLASSIFICATION

Exocrine glands are either unicellular or multicellular. The latter may be in the form of simple sheets of secretory cells, e.g. at the surface of the stomach, or may be structurally more complex and invaginated to a variable degree. Such glands (**Fig. 3.12**) may be single units or their connection to the surface may be branched. Simple unbranched tubular glands exist in the walls of many of the hollow viscera, e.g. the small intestine and uterus, whereas some single glands have expanded, flasklike ends (acini or alveoli). Such glands may consist entirely of secretory cells, or may have a blind-ending secretory portion that leads through a non-secretory duct to the surface, in which case the ducts may modify the secretions as they pass along them.

Glands with ducts may be branched (compound), and sometimes form elaborate ductal trees. Such glands generally have acinar or alveolar secretory lobules, as in the exocrine pancreas, but the secretory units may alternatively be tubular or mixed tubulo-acinar. More than one type of secretory cell may occur within a particular secretory unit, or individual units may be specialized to just one type of secretion (e.g. serous acini of salivary glands).

Exocrine glands are also classified by their secretory products. Secretory cells in mucus-secreting or mucous glands have frothy cyto-

plasm and basal, flattened nuclei. They stain deeply with metachromatic stains and periodic acid-Schiff (PAS) methods that detect carbohydrate residues. However, in general (i.e. non-specific) histological preparations they are weakly stained because much of their content of water-rich mucin is extracted by the processing procedures. Secretory cells in serous glands have centrally placed nuclei and eosinophilic secretory storage granules in their cytoplasm. They secrete mainly glycoproteins (including lysozyme and digestive enzymes).

Some glands are almost entirely mucous (e.g. the sublingual salivary gland), whereas others are mainly serous (e.g. the parotid salivary gland). The submandibular gland is mixed, in that some lobules are predominantly mucous and others serous. In some regions, mucous acini share a lumen with clusters of serous cells (seen in routine preparations as serous demilunes). Although this simple approach to classification is useful for general descriptive purposes, the diversity of molecules synthesized and secreted by glands is such that complex mixtures often exist within the same cell.

Endocrine glands

Endocrine glands secrete directly into the circulation. Their cells are grouped around beds of capillaries or sinusoids (p. 143) which typically are lined by fenestrated endothelia to allow the rapid passage of macromolecules through their walls. Endocrine cells may be arranged in clusters around vascular networks, in cords between parallel vascular channels or as hollow structures (follicles) surrounding their stored secretions. Isolated endocrine cells also exist scattered amongst other tissues as part of the dispersed neuroendocrine system (p. 180), e.g. throughout the alimentary and respiratory tracts.

Control of glandular secretion

Glandular activity may be controlled directly by autonomic secretomotor fibres, which may either form synapses on the bases of gland cells (e.g. in the suprarenal medulla) or release neuromediators in the vicinity of the glands, to reach them by diffusion. Alternatively, the autonomic nervous system may act indirectly on gland cells, e.g. via histamine released neurogenically from another cell, as occurs in the gastric lining. Paracrine activities of neuroendocrine cells are important in the alimentary and bronchial glands. Circulating hormones from the adenohypophysis stimulate synthesis and secretion by target cells in many endocrine glands. Such signals, mostly detected by receptors at the cell surface and mediated by second messenger systems, may increase the synthetic activity of gland cells, and may cause them to discharge their secretions by exocytosis. Secretions already released into ducts are expressed rapidly from certain glands by the contraction of associated myoepithelial cells that enclose the secretory units and smaller ducts. These may be under direct neural control, as in the salivary glands, or they may respond to circulating hormones, e.g. cells in the mammary gland respond to the concentration of circulating oxytocin.

BASEMENT MEMBRANE AND BASAL LAMINA

There is a narrow layer of extracellular matrix (p. 38), which stains strongly for carbohydrates at the interface between connective and other tissues, e.g. between epithelia and their supporting connective tissues. In early histological texts this layer was termed the basement membrane. As almost all of its components are synthesized by the epithelium or other tissue (e.g. muscle), rather than the adjacent connective tissue, it will be discussed here.

Electron microscopy revealed that the basement membrane is composed of two distinct components. A thin, finely fibrillar layer, the basal lamina, is associated closely with the cell surface (**Fig. 3.13**). A variable reticular lamina of larger fibrils and glycosaminoglycans of the extracellular matrix underlies this layer and is continuous with the connective tissue proper, although it is much reduced or largely absent in some tissues, e.g. surrounding muscle fibres, Schwann cells and capillary endothelia. In other tissues, the basal lamina separates two layers of cells and there are no intervening typical connective tissue elements. This occurs in the thick basal lamina of the renal glomerular filter (p. 1277), the basal lamina of the thin portions of the lung interalveolar septa across which gases exchange between blood and air

Mechanism of secretion

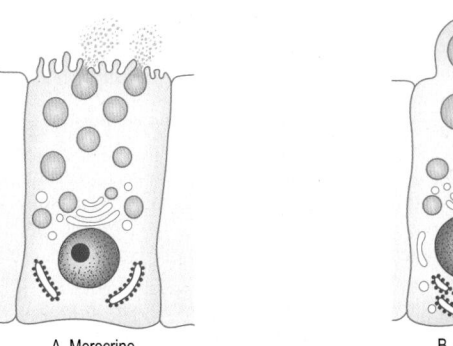

A. Merocrine   B. Apocrine   C. Holocrine

Arrangement of cells and structural classification of glands

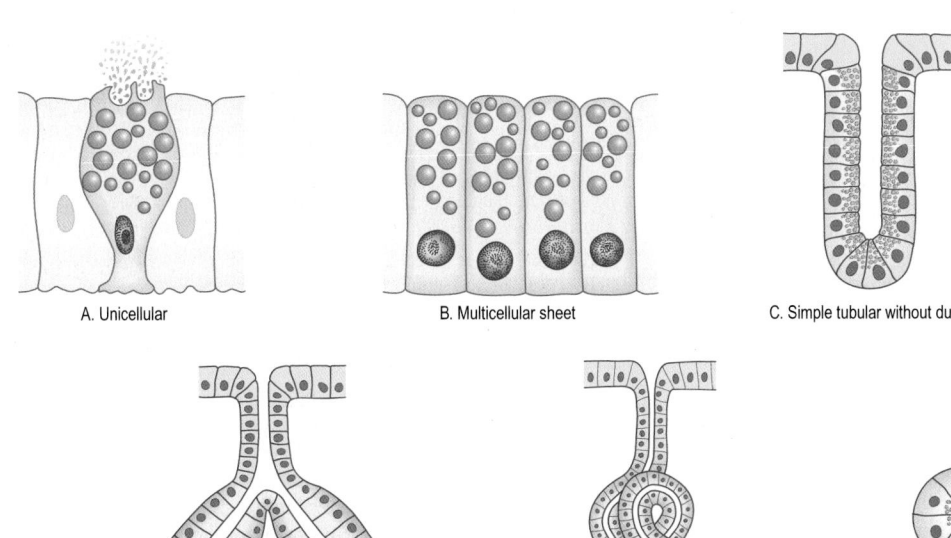

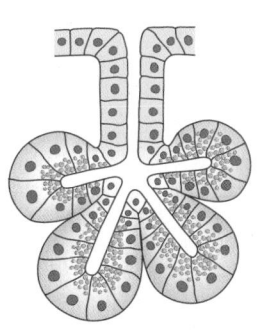

A. Unicellular   B. Multicellular sheet   C. Simple tubular without duct   D. Simple tubular with duct

E. Simple branched tubular   F. Simple coiled tubular   G. Simple acinar or alveolar

Branching pattern of complex glands

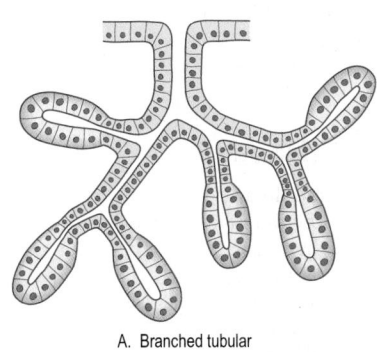
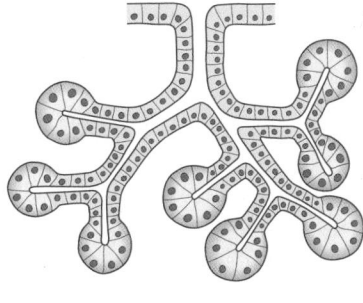
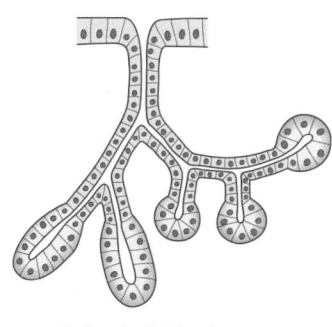

A. Branched tubular   B. Branched acinar/alveolar   C. Branched tubulo-acinar

Fig. 3.12 Classification of the different types of epithelial gland.

p. 1060), and the anterior limiting (Descemet's) lamina in the cornea (p. 703).

The basal lamina is usually c.80 nm thick, varying between 40 and 120 nm, and consists of a sheet-like fibrillar layer, the lamina densa (20–50 nm wide), separated from the plasma membrane of the cell it supports by a narrow electron-lucent zone, the lamina lucida. The lamina lucida is absent from tissues prepared by rapid freezing and so may be an artefact. In many tissues this zone is crossed by integral plasma membrane proteins, e.g. keratinocyte hemidesmosomes are anchored into the lamina densa in the basal lamina of the epidermis. The basal lamina is a delicate felt-like network composed largely of two glyco-protein polymers, laminin and type IV collagen, which self-assemble into two-dimensional sheets interwoven with each other. Early embryonic basal lamina is formed only of the laminin polymer. Two other

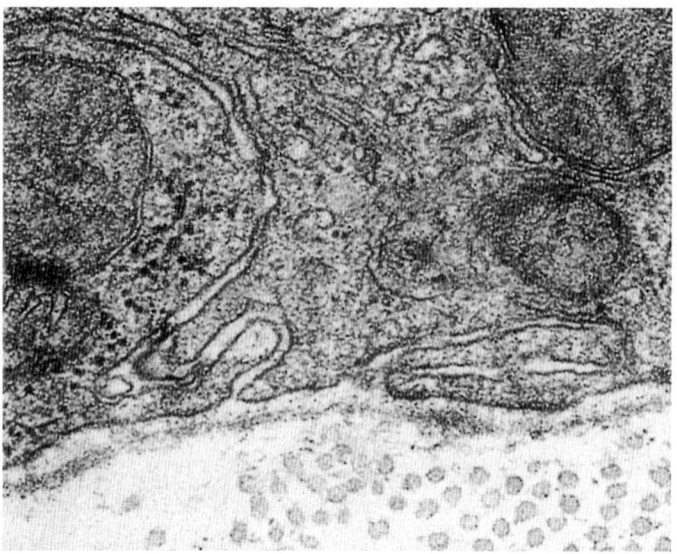

Fig. 3.13 The basal lamina, underlying an epithelium (top). The finely fibrillar dense layer corresponds to the lamina densa and spherical collagen fibrils sectioned transversely lie in the subjacent connective tissue. These contribute to the appearance of the basement membrane in light microscope preparations stained for carbohydrate-rich structures. (By permission from Young B, Heath JW 2000 Wheater's Functional Histology. Edinburgh: Churchill Livingstone.)

molecules cross-link and stabilize the network: entactin (nidogen) and perlecan (a large heparan sulphate proteoglycan).

Although all basal laminae have a similar form, their thickness and precise molecular composition vary between tissues and even within a tissue, e.g. between the crypts and villi of the small intestine. The isoforms of laminin and collagen type IV differ in various tissues, thus Schwann cells and muscle cells express laminin-2 (merosin) rather than the prototypical laminin-1. Laminin-5, although not itself a basal lamina component, is found in the hemidesmosomes of the basal epidermis and links the basal lamina with epidermal transmembrane proteins, $\alpha_6\beta_4$ integrin and collagen type XVII (formerly known as bullous pemphigoid antigen, the target of the autoimmune blistering skin disease, bullous pemphigoid). The particular isoform of collagen type IV in the basal lamina of different tissues is reflected in tissue-specific disease patterns. Mutations in a collagen expressed by muscle and kidney glomeruli cause Allport syndrome, a form of renal failure. Renal failure also occurs in Goodpasture syndrome, in which renal basal lamina collagen is targeted by autoantibodies.

In Descemet's membrane in the cornea, collagen type VIII replaces collagen type IV in the much thickened endothelial basal lamina. The basal lamina of the neuromuscular junction (p. 64) contains agrin, a heparan sulphate proteoglycan, which plays a part in the clustering of muscle acetylcholine receptors in the plasma membrane at these junctions.

RETICULAR LAMINA

The reticular lamina consists of a dense extracellular matrix that contains collagen. In skin, it contains fibrils of type VII collagen (anchoring fibrils), which bind the lamina densa to the adjacent connective tissue. The high concentration of proteoglycans in the reticular lamina is responsible for the positive reaction of the entire basement membrane to stains for carbohydrates, seen in sections prepared for light microscopy.

Functions of basal lamina

Basal laminae perform a number of important roles. They form selectively permeable barriers between adjacent tissues, e.g. in the glomerular filter of the kidney; they anchor epithelial and connective tissues and so stabilize and orient the tissue layers; they may exert instructive effects on adjacent tissues, and so determine their polarity, rate of cell division, cell survival, etc. In addition, they may act as pathways for the migration and pathfinding of growing cell processes, both in development and

in tissue repair, e.g. in guiding the outgrowth of axons and the re-establishment of neuromuscular junctions during regeneration after injury in the peripheral nervous system. Changes in basal lamina thickness are often associated with pathological conditions, e.g. the thickening of the glomerular membrane in glomerulonephritis and diabetes.

CONNECTIVE AND SUPPORTING TISSUES

The connective tissues are defined as those composed predominantly of intercellular material, the extracellular matrix, which is secreted mainly by the connective tissue cells. The cells are therefore usually widely separated by their matrix, which is composed of fibrous proteins and a relatively amorphous ground substance. Many of the special properties of connective tissues are determined by the composition of the matrix, and their classification is also largely based on its characteristics. In some types of connective tissue, the cellular component eventually dominates the tissue, even though the tissue originally has a high matrix:cell ratio, e.g. adipose tissue. Connective tissues are derived from embryonic mesoderm or, in the head region, largely from neural crest.

Connective tissues have several essential roles in the body. These may be subdivided into structural roles, which largely reflect the special mechanical properties of the extracellular matrix components, and defensive roles, in which the cellular component has the dominant role. Connective tissues often also play important trophic and morphogenetic parts in organizing and influencing the growth and differentiation of surrounding tissues, e.g. in the development of glands from an epithelial surface.

Structural connective tissues are divided into ordinary (or general) types, which are widely distributed, and special skeletal types, i.e. cartilage and bone, which are described in Chapter 6. A third type, haemolymphoid tissues, consists of peripheral blood cells, lymphoid tissues and their precursors; these tissues are described in Chapter 5. They are often grouped with other types of connective tissue, because of their similar mesenchymal origins and because the various defensive cells of the blood also form part of a typical connective tissue cell population. They reach connective tissues via the blood circulation and migrate into them through the endothelial walls of vessels.

Cells of general connective tissues

Cells of general connective tissue can be separated into the resident cell population (fibroblasts, adipocytes, mesenchymal stem cells, etc.) and a population of migrant cells with various defensive functions (macrophages, lymphocytes, mast cells, neutrophils and eosinophils), which may change in number and moderate their activities according to demand. Embryologically, fibroblasts and adipocytes arise from mesenchymal stem cells, some of which may remain in the tissues to provide a source of replacement cells postnatally. As noted above, the cells of haemopoietic origin migrate into the tissue from bone marrow and lymphoid tissue.

RESIDENT CELLS

FIBROBLASTS

Fibroblasts are usually the most numerous resident cells. They are flattened and irregular in outline, with extended processes, and in profile they appear fusiform or spindle-shaped (**Figs 3.14, 3.16**). Fibroblasts synthesize most of the extracellular matrix of connective tissue; accordingly they have all the features typical of cells active in the synthesis and secretion of proteins. Their nuclei are relatively large and euchromatic and possess prominent nucleoli. In young, highly active cells, the cytoplasm is abundant and basophilic (reflecting the high concentration of rough endoplasmic reticulum), mitochondria are abundant and several sets of Golgi apparatus are present. In old and relatively inactive fibroblasts (often termed fibrocytes) the cytoplasmic volume is reduced, the endoplasmic reticulum is sparse and the nucleus is flattened and heterochromatic.

Fibroblasts are usually adherent to the fibres of the matrix (collagen and elastin), which they lay down. In some highly cellular structures, e.g. liver, kidney and spleen, and in most lymphoid tissue, fibroblasts and delicate collagenous fibres (type III collagen; reticular fibres) form fibrocellular networks which are often called reticular tissue. The fibroblasts may then be termed reticular cells.

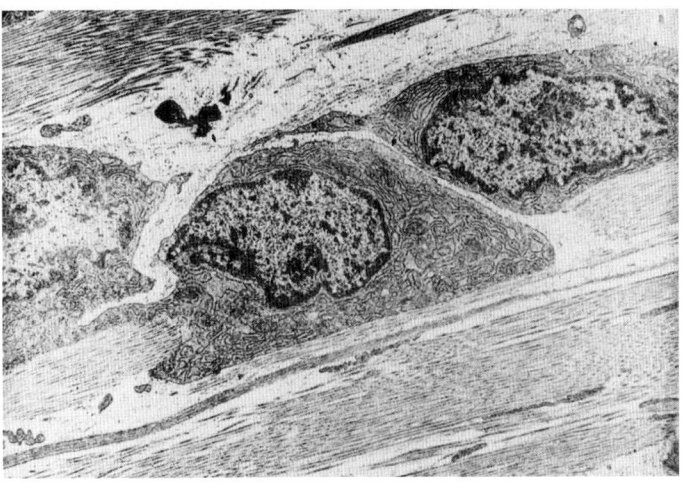

Fig. 3.14 Fibroblasts in connective tissue, surrounded by bundles of finely banded collagen fibrils which they secrete. (From Dr B Oakes, Anatomy and Cell Biology, Monash University, and by permission from Kerr JB 1999 Atlas of Functional Histology. London: Mosby.)

Fibroblasts are particularly active during wound repair, when they proliferate and lay down a fibrous matrix that becomes invaded by numerous blood vessels (granulation tissue). Contraction of wounds is at least in part caused by the shortening of specialized contractile fibroblasts (myofibroblasts) that arise in such areas. Fibroblast activity is influenced by various factors such as steroid hormone concentrations, dietary content and prevalent mechanical stresses. In vitamin C deficiency, there is an impairment of collagen formation.

ADIPOCYTES (LIPOCYTES, FAT CELLS)

Adipocytes occur singly or in groups in many, but not all, connective tissues. They are numerous in adipose tissue (**Fig. 3.15**). Individually, the cells are oval or spherical in shape, but when packed together they are polygonal. They vary in diameter, averaging c.50 μm. Each cell consists of a peripheral rim of cytoplasm, in which the nucleus is embedded, surrounding a single large central globule of fat, which consists of glycerol esters of oleic, palmitic and stearic acids. There is a small accumulation of cytoplasm around the nucleus, which is oval in shape and compressed against the cell membrane by the lipid droplet, as is the Golgi complex. Many cytoskeletal filaments, some endoplasmic reticulum and a few mitochondria lie around the lipid droplet, which is in direct contact with the surrounding cytoplasm and not enclosed within a membrane. In sections of tissue not specially treated to preserve lipids, the lipid droplet is usually dissolved out by the solvents used in routine preparations, so that only the nucleus and the peripheral rim of cytoplasm surrounding a central empty space remain.

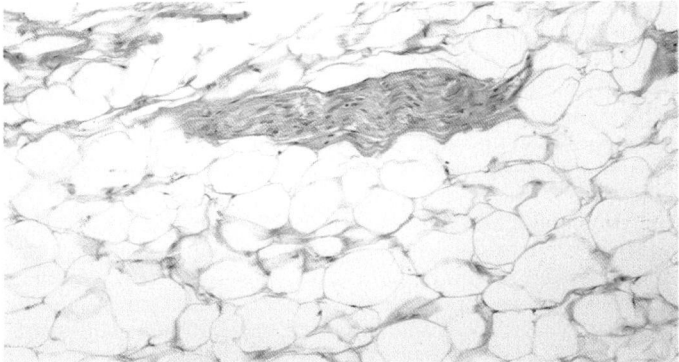

Fig. 3.15 Adipose tissue in the fibrous pericardium of the heart. Adipocytes are distended polygonal cells filled with lipid, which is extracted by the tissue processing. This leaves only the plasma membranes with scant cytoplasm and nuclei, occasionally visible compressed against the cell periphery. An autonomic nerve fibre is shown sectioned longitudinally on its course through the adipose tissue. (Photograph by Sarah-Jane Smith.)

In neonates, a special form of adipose tissue known as brown fat is present in the interscapular region and may be more widespread. Brown fat is characterized by the presence of a large cell type in which the fat is present as several separate droplets and not as a single globule, and the mitochondria have unusually large and numerous cristae. These deposits of fat are concerned with heat production, mediated by mitochondria.

The mobilization of fat is under nervous or hormonal control: noradrenaline (norepinephrine) released at sympathetic nerve endings in adipose tissue is particularly important in this respect.

MESENCHYMAL STEM CELLS

Mesenchymal stem cells are normally inconspicuous cells in connective tissues. They are derived from embryonic mesenchyme (p. 207) and are able to differentiate into the mature cells of connective tissue during normal growth and development, in the turnover of cells throughout life and, most conspicuously, in the repair of damaged tissues in wound healing. There is evidence that, even in mature tissues, mesenchymal stem cells remain pluripotent and able to give rise to all the resident cells of connective tissues in response to local signals and cues.

MIGRANT CELLS

MACROPHAGES

Macrophages are typically numerous in connective tissues, where they are either attached to matrix fibres or are motile and migratory. They are relatively large cells, c.15–20 μm in diameter, with indented and relatively heterochromatic nuclei and a prominent nucleolus. Their cytoplasm is slightly basophilic, contains many lysosomes (p. 14) and typically has a foamy appearance under the light microscope. Macrophages are important phagocytes, and form part of the mononuclear phagocyte system (p. 80). They can engulf and digest particulate organic materials, such as bacteria, and are also able to clear dead or damaged cells from a tissue. They are also the source of a number of secreted cytokines that have profound effects on many other cell types. Macrophages are able to proliferate in connective tissues to a limited extent, but are derived primarily from haemopoietic stem cells (p. 80) in the bone marrow, which circulate in the blood as monocytes before migrating through vessel walls into connective tissues.

Many properties of macrophages in general connective tissue (**Fig. 3.16**) are similar to those of related cells in other sites. These include: circulating monocytes, from which they are derived; alveolar macrophages in the lungs; phagocytic cells in the lymph nodes, spleen and bone marrow; Kupffer cells of the liver sinusoids; microglial cells of the central nervous system.

LYMPHOCYTES

Lymphocytes are typically present in small numbers (**Fig. 3.16**), and are numerous in general connective tissue only in pathological states, when they migrate in from adjacent lymphoid tissue or from the circulation. The majority are small cells (6–8 μm) with highly heterochromatic nuclei, but they enlarge when stimulated. Two major functional classes exist, termed B and T lymphocytes (p. 80). B lymphocytes originate in the bone marrow, then migrate to various lymphoid tissues, where they proliferate. When antigenically stimulated, they undergo further mitotic divisions, then enlarge as they mature, commonly in general connective tissues, to form plasma cells that synthesize and secrete antibodies (immunoglobulins). Mature plasma cells are rounded or ovoid, up to 15 μm across, and have an extensive rough endoplasmic reticulum. Their nuclei are spherical and have a characteristic 'clock-face' configuration of heterochromatin that is regularly distributed in peripheral clumps. The prominent Golgi complex is visible with a light microscope as a pale region to one side of the nucleus and the remaining cytoplasm is deeply basophilic because of the abundant endoplasmic reticulum. Mature plasma cells do not divide.

T lymphocytes originate from precursors in bone marrow haemopoietic tissue, but later migrate to the thymus, where they develop T cell identity, before passing into the peripheral lymphoid system where they continue to multiply. When antigenically stimulated, T cells enlarge and their cytoplasm becomes filled with free polysome clusters. The functions of T lymphocytes are numerous: different subsets recognize and destroy virus-infected cells, tissue and organ grafts, or interact with B lymphocytes and several other defensive cell types (p. 73).

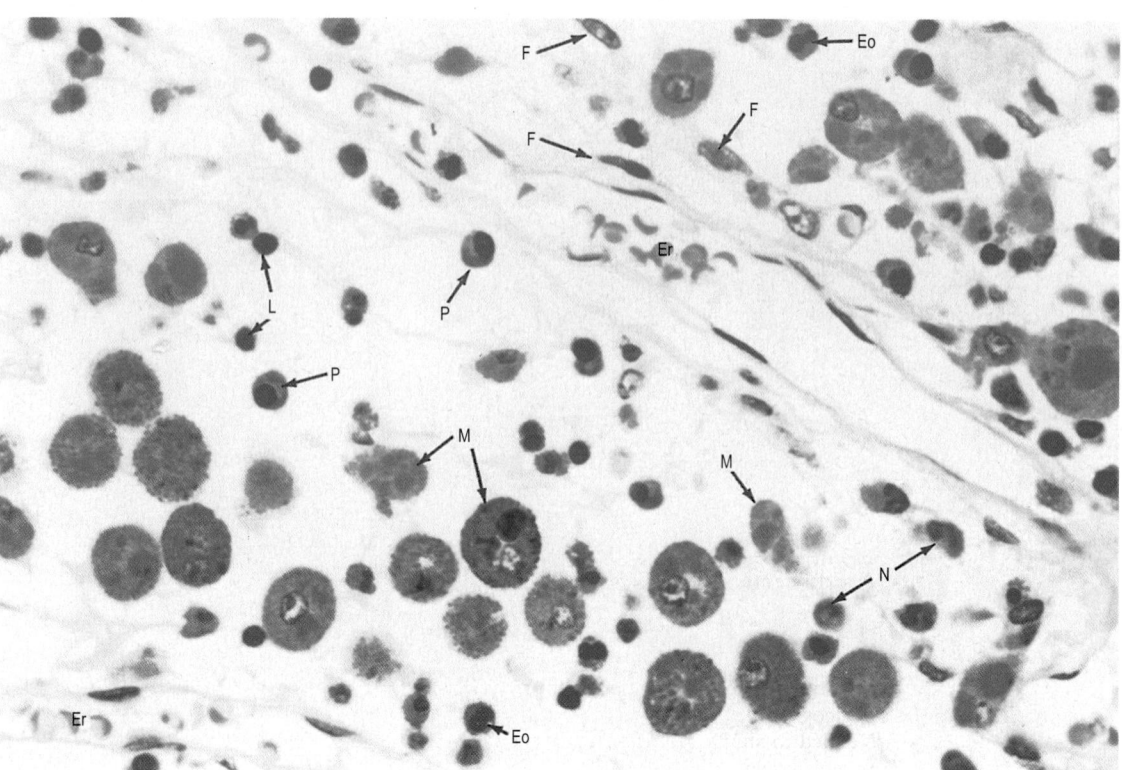

Fig. 3.16 Macrophages (M) in loose connective tissue. Their actively phagocytic properties are indicated by the brown material visible in their cytoplasm; these are residual bodies from engulfed particles. Other leukocytes are shown, including lymphocytes (L), eosinophils (Eo), neutrophils (N) and plasma cells (P). Elongated nuclei of fibroblasts (F) and erythrocytes (Er) in small vessels are also visible. (By permission from Young B, Heath JW 2000 Wheater's Functional Histology. Edinburgh: Churchill Livingstone.)

MAST CELLS

Mast cells are important defensive cells which occur particularly in loose connective tissues and often in the fibrous capsules of certain organs such as the liver. They are characteristically numerous around blood vessels and nerves. Mast cells are round or oval, c.12 μm in diameter, with many filopodia extending from the cell surface. The nucleus is centrally placed and relatively small, and is surrounded by large numbers of prominent vesicles and a well developed Golgi apparatus, but scant endoplasmic reticulum. The vesicles have a high content of glycosaminoglycans and show a strongly positive reaction with the periodic acid-Schiff stain for carbohydrates. The membrane-bounded vesicles vary in size and shape (mean diameter c.0.5 μm) and have a rather heterogeneous content of dense, lipid-containing material, which may be finely granular, lamellar or in the form of membranous whorls.

The major granule components, many of them associated with inflammation, are the proteoglycan heparin, histamine, tryptase, superoxide dismutase, aryl sulphatase, β-hexosaminidase and various other enzymes, together with chemotactic factors for neutrophil and eosinophil granulocytes. Mast cells may be disrupted to release some or all of their contents, either by direct mechanical or chemical trauma, or after contact with particular antigens to which the body has previously been exposed. The consequences of granule release include alteration of capillary permeability, smooth muscle contraction, and activation and attraction to the locality of various other defensive cells. Responses to mast cell degranulation may be localized, e.g. urticaria, or there may occasionally be a generalized response to the release of large amounts of histamine into the circulation (anaphylactic shock). Mast cells closely resemble basophil granulocytes of the general circulation but are now known to be derived from a separate lineage precursor. It is believed that they are generated in the bone marrow and circulate to the tissues as basophil-like cells, migrating through the capillary and venule walls to their final destination.

GRANULOCYTES (POLYMORPHONUCLEAR LEUKOCYTES)

Neutrophil and eosinophil granulocytes are immigrant cells from the circulation. Relatively infrequent in normal connective tissues, their numbers may increase dramatically in infected tissues, where they are important components of cellular defence. Neutrophils are highly phagocytic, especially towards bacteria. The functions of eosinophils are less well understood. These cells are described further in Chapter 5.

Cells of specialized connective tissues

Skeletal tissues, namely cartilage and bone, are generally classified with the connective tissues, but their structure and functions are highly specialized; they are described in Chapter 6. As with the general connective tissues, these specialized types are characterized by their extracellular matrix, which forms the major component of the tissues and is responsible for their properties. The resident cells are different from those in general connective tissues. Cartilage is populated by chondroblasts, which synthesize the matrix, and by mature chondrocytes. Bone matrix is elaborated by osteoblasts. Their mature progeny, osteocytes, are embedded within the matrix, which they help to mineralize, turn over and maintain. A third cell type, the osteoclasts, have a different lineage origin and are derived from haemopoietic tissue; they are responsible for bone degradation and remodelling in collaboration with osteoblasts.

Extracellular matrix

The term extracellular matrix is applied collectively to the extracellular components of connective and supporting tissues. Essentially it consists of a system of insoluble protein fibres, adhesive glycoproteins and soluble complexes composed of carbohydrate polymers linked to protein molecules (proteoglycans and glycosaminoglycans), which bind water. The extracellular matrix distributes the mechanical stresses on tissues and also provides the structural environment of the cells embedded in it, forming a framework to which they adhere and on which they can move. With the exception of bone matrix, it provides a highly hydrated medium, through which metabolites, gases and nutrients can diffuse freely between cells and the blood vessels traversing it or, in the case of cartilage, passing nearby. There are many complex interactions between connective tissue cells and the extracellular matrix. The cells continually synthesize, secrete, modify and degrade extracellular matrix components, and themselves respond to contact with the matrix in the regulation of cell metabolism, proliferation and motility.

The insoluble fibres are mainly of two types of structural protein: members of the collagen family, and elastin (**Fig. 3.17**). The interfibrillar matrix (ground substance) includes a number of adhesive glycoproteins that perform a variety of functions in connective tissues, including cell–matrix adhesion and matrix–cell signalling. These glycoproteins include fibronectin, laminin, tenascin and vitronectin, in addition to a number of other less well characterized proteins. The glycosaminoglycans

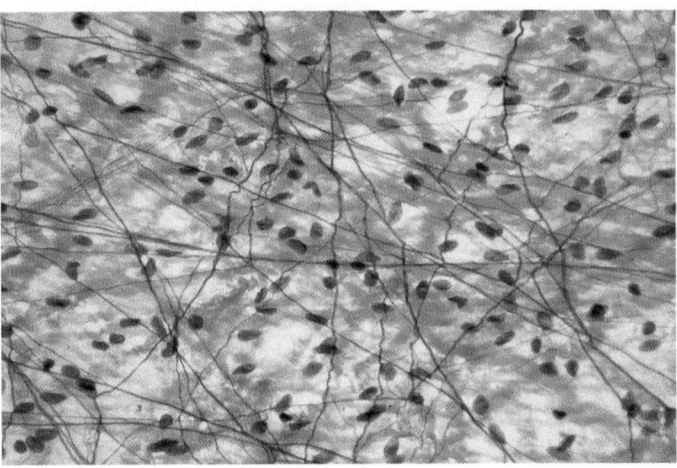

Fig. 3.17 Elastic fibres, seen as fine, dark, relatively straight fibres in a whole-mount preparation of mesentery, stained for elastin. The wavy pink bands are collagen bundles and oval grey nuclei are mainly of fibroblasts. (Photograph by Sarah-Jane Smith.)

of the interfibrillar matrix are, with one notable exception, post-translationally modified proteoglycan molecules in which long poly-saccharide side chains are added to short core proteins during transit through the secretory pathway between the rough endoplasmic reticulum and the *trans*-Golgi network. The exception, the polymeric disaccharide, hyaluronan, has no protein core and is synthesized entirely by cell surface enzymes. For further reading on extracellular matrix molecules, see Pollard and Earnshaw (2002).

Functional attributes of connective tissues vary and depend on the abundance of its different components. Collagen fibres resist tension, whereas elastin provides a measure of resilience to deformation by stretching. The highly hydrated, soluble polymers of the interfibrillar material (proteoglycans and glycosaminoglycans, mainly hyaluronan) generally form a stiff gel resisting compressive forces. Thus tissues that are specialized to resist tensile forces (e.g. tendons) are rich in collagen fibrils, tissues that accommodate changes in shape and volume (e.g. mesenteries) are rich in elastic fibres and those that absorb compressive forces (e.g. cartilages) are rich in glycosaminoglycans and proteoglycans. In bone, mineral crystals take the place of most of the soluble polymers, and endow the tissue with incompressible rigidity.

FIBRILLAR MATRIX: COLLAGENS

Collagens make up a very large proportion (c.30%) of all the proteins of the body. They consist of a wide range of related molecules that have various roles in the organization and properties of connective (and some other) tissues. The first collagen to be characterized was type I, the most abundant of all the collagens and a constituent of the dermis, fasciae, bone, tendon, ligaments, blood vessels and the sclera of the eyeball. The characteristic collagen of cartilage and the vitreous body of the eye, with a slightly different chemical composition, is type II, whereas type III is present in several tissues, including the dermis and blood vessels, and type IV is in basal lamina. The other types are widely distributed in various tissues. Five of the collagens, types I, II, III, V and XI, form fibrils; types IV, VIII and X form sheets or meshworks; types VI, VII, IX, XII, XIV and XVIII have an anchoring or linking role; types XIII and XVII are transmembrane proteins.

Biochemically, all collagens have a number of features in common. Unlike most other proteins, they contain high levels of hydroxyproline and all are composed of three polypeptides that form triple helices and are substantially modified post-translationally. After secretion, individual molecules are further cross-linked to form stable polymers. Functionally, collagens are structural proteins with considerable mechanical strength. Just a few of their distinguishing structural features are described below. For further reading on the molecular structure and functions of the collagens, see Pollard and Earnshaw (2002).

Type I collagen

Type I collagen is very widely distributed. It forms inextensible fibrils in which collagen molecules (triple helices) are aligned side by side in a staggered fashion, with three-quarters of the length of each molecule in contact with neighbouring molecules. The fibril has well-marked bands of charged and uncharged amino-acids arranged across it (these stain with heavy metals in a banding pattern that repeats every 65 nm in longitudinal sections viewed in the electron microscope (**Fig. 3.14**).

Fibril diameters vary between tissues and with age. Developing tissues often have thinner fibrils than mature tissues. Corneal stroma fibrils are of uniform and thin diameter, whereas tendon fibrils may be up to 20 times thicker and quite variable. Tissues in which the fibrils are subject to high tensile loading tend to have thicker fibrils. Thick fibrils are composites of uniform thin fibrils with a diameter of 8–12 nm. The fibrils themselves are relatively flexible, but when mineralized (as in bone) or surrounded by high concentrations of proteoglycan (as in cartilage), the resulting fibre-reinforced composite materials are rigid.

Fresh type I collagen fibres are white and glistening. They form bundles of various sizes that are generally visible at the light microscope level. The component fibres may leave one bundle and interweave with others. In many situations, collagen fibrils are laid down in precise geo-metrical patterns, in which successive layers alternate in direction, e.g. corneal stroma, where the high degree of order is essential for trans-parency. Tendons, aponeuroses and ligaments are also highly ordered tissues.

Types II, III, V and XI collagens

Types II, III, V and XI collagens can also aggregate to form linear fibrils. Type II collagen occurs in extremely thin (10 nm) short fibrils in the vitreous humour and in very thick fibrils in ageing human cartilage. The amino-acid sequence and banding pattern are very similar to those of type I collagen, as are the post-translational modifications of the triple helical protein molecule. The fine fibrils in the vitreous may fuse into thicker aggregates in older tissue.

Type III collagen is very widely distributed, particularly in young and repairing tissues. It usually co-localizes with type I collagen, and covalent links between Type I and Type III collagen have been demonstrated. In skin, many fibrils are probably composites of Types I and III collagens.

Reticular fibres

Fine branching and anastomosing reticular fibres form the supporting mesh framework of many glands, the kidney and lymphoreticular tissue (lymph nodes, spleen, etc.). Classically, these fibres stained intensely with silver salts, although they are poorly stained using conventional histological techniques. They associate with basal laminae and are often found in the neighbourhood of collagen fibre bundles. Reticular fibres are formed principally of type III collagen.

Elastin

Elastin is a 70 kDa protein, rich in the hydrophobic amino-acids valine and alanine. Elastic fibrils, which also contain fibrillin, are highly cross-linked via two elastin-specific amino-acids, desmosine and iso-desmosine, which are formed extracellularly from lysine residues. They are less widely distributed than collagen, yellowish in colour, typically cross-linked and are usually thinner (10–20 nm) than collagen fibrils. They can be thick, e.g. in the ligamenta flava and ligamentum nuchae. Unlike collagen type I, they show no banding pattern in the electron microscope. They stain poorly with routine histological stains, but are stained with orcein-containing preparations. They sometimes appear as sheets, as in the fenestrated elastic lamellae of the aortic wall. Elastin-rich structures stretch easily with almost perfect recoil, although they tend to calcify with age and lose elasticity. Elastin is highly resistant to attack by acid and alkali, even at high temperatures.

INTERFIBRILLAR MATRIX: GLYCOSAMINOGLYCANS

The structural soluble polymers characteristic of the extracellular matrix are the acidic glycosaminoglycans, which are unbranched chains of repeating disaccharide units, each unit carrying one or more negatively charged groups (carboxylate or sulphate esters, or both). The anionic charge is balanced by cations (Na^+, K^+, etc.) in the interstitial fluid. Their polyanionic character endows the glycosaminoglycans with high osmotic activity, which helps keep the fibrils apart, confers stiffness on the porous gel that they collectively create and gives the tissue a varying degree of basophilia. Glycosaminoglycans are named according to the tissues in which they were first found, e.g. hyaluronan (vitreous body), chondroitins (cartilage), dermatan (skin), keratan (cornea), heparan (liver). This terminology is no longer relevant, as most glycosaminoglycans are very widely distributed, whereas, conversely, some corneas contain little or no keratan sulphate. Of the glycosaminoglycans, all except hyaluronan have short protein cores and are highly variable in their carbohydrate side chain structure.

Hyaluronan

Hyaluronan was formerly called hyaluronic acid (or hyaluronate, as only the salt exists at physiological pH). It is a very large, highly hydrated molecule (25,000 kDa). Hyaluronan is found in all extracellular matrices and in most tissues and is a prominent component of embryonic and developing tissues.

Hyaluronan is important in the aggregation of proteoglycans and link proteins that possess specific hyaluronan binding sites (e.g. laminin). Indeed, the very large aggregates that are formed may be the essential compression-resisting units in cartilage. Hyaluronan also forms very viscous solutions, which are probably the major lubricants in synovial joints. Because of its ability to bind water, it is often present in semi-rigid structures (e.g. vitreous humour in the eye), where it co-operates with sparse but regular meshworks of thin collagen fibrils.

Proteoglycans

Proteoglycans have been classified according to the size of their protein core: their nomenclature is under review. The same core protein can bear different glycosaminoglycan side chains in different tissues. The functions of many proteoglycans are poorly understood. Some of the better known proteoglycans are: aggrecan in cartilage; perlecan in basal laminae; decorin associated with fibroblasts in collagen fibril assembly; syndecan in embryonic tissues.

Adhesive glycoproteins

These proteins include molecules that mediate adhesion between cells and the extracellular matrix, often in association with collagens, proteoglycans or other matrix components. All of them are glycosylated and they are, therefore, glycoproteins. General connective tissue contains the well known families of fibronectins (and osteonectin in bone), laminins and tenascins; there is a rapidly growing list of other glycoproteins associated with extracellular adhesion (Pollard & Earnshaw 2002). They possess binding sites for other extracellular matrix molecules and for cell adhesion molecules (p. 7), especially the integrins; in this way they enable cells selectively to adhere to appropriate matrix structures (e.g. the basal lamina). They also function as signalling molecules, which are detected by cell surface receptors and initiate changes within the cytoplasm (e.g. to promote the formation of hemidesmosomes or other areas of strong adhesion; reorganize the cytoskeleton; promote or inhibit locomotion and cell division).

Fibronectin – Fibronectin is a large glycoprotein consisting of a dimer joined by disulphide links. Each subunit is composed of a string of large repetitive domains linked by flexible regions. Fibronectin subunits have binding sites for collagen, heparin and cell surface receptors, especially integrins, and so can promote adhesion between all these elements. In connective tissues, the molecules are able to bind to cell surfaces in an orderly fashion, to form short fibronectin filaments. The liver secretes a related protein, plasma fibronectin, into the circulation. The selective adhesion of different cell types to the matrix during development and in postnatal life is mediated by numerous isoforms of fibronectin generated by alternative splicing. Isoforms found in embryonic tissues are also expressed during wound repair, when they facilitate tissue proliferation and cell movements; the adult form is re-expressed once repair is complete.

Laminin – Laminin is a large (850 kDa) flexible molecule composed of three polypeptide chains (designated α, β, and γ). There are many isoforms of the different chains, and at least 18 types of laminin. The prototypical molecule has a cruciform shape, in which the terminal two-thirds are wound round each other to form the stem of a cross, and the shorter free ends form the upright and transverse members. Laminin bears binding sites for other extracellular matrix molecules such as heparan sulphate, type IV collagen and entactin and also for laminin receptor molecules situated in cell plasma membranes. Laminin molecules can assemble themselves into flat regular meshworks, e.g. in the basal lamina.

Tenascin – Tenascin is large glycoprotein composed of six subunits that are joined at one end to form a structure that resembles the spokes of a wheel. There is a family of tenascin molecules, generated by alternative splicing of the tenascin gene. Tenascin is abundant in embryonic tissues, but its distribution is restricted in the adult. It appears to be important in guiding cell migration and axonal growth in early development: it may either promote or inhibit these activities depending on the cell type and tenascin isoform.

Classification of connective tissues

Connective and supporting tissues differ considerably in appearance, consistency and composition in different regions. These differences reflect local functional requirements and are related to the predominance of the cell types, the concentration, arrangement and types of fibre and the characteristics of the interfibrillar matrix. On these bases, general connective tissues can be classified into irregular and regular types, according to the degree of orientation of their fibrous components.

IRREGULAR CONNECTIVE TISSUES

Irregular connective tissues can be further subdivided into loose, dense and adipose connective tissue.

LOOSE (AREOLAR) CONNECTIVE TISSUE

Loose connective tissue is the most generalized form (**Fig. 3.18**) and is extensively distributed. Its chief function is to bind structures together, while still allowing a considerable amount of movement to take place. It constitutes the submucosa in the digestive tract and other viscera lined by mucosae, and the subcutaneous tissue in regions where this is devoid of fat (e.g. eyelids, penis, scrotum and labia), and it surrounds muscles, vessels and nerves, connecting them with surrounding structures. It is present in the interior of organs, where it binds together the lobes and lobules of glands, forms the supporting layer (lamina propria) of mucosal epithelia and vascular endothelia, and lies within and between fascicles of muscle and nerve fibres.

Loose connective tissue consists of a meshwork of thin collagen and elastin fibres interlacing in all directions to give a measure of both elasticity and tensile strength. The large meshes contain the soft, semi-fluid interfibrillar matrix or ground substance, and different connective tissue cells, which are scattered along the fibres or in the meshes. It also contains adipocytes, usually in small groups, and particularly around blood vessels.

A variant of loose connective tissue occurs in the choroid and the sclera of the eye, where large numbers of pigment cells (melanocytes) are also present.

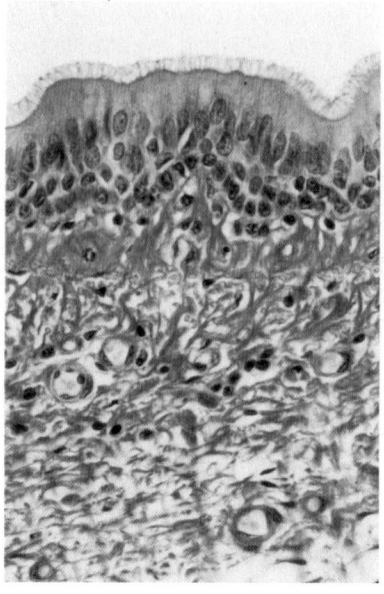

Fig. 3.18 General connective tissue supporting a respiratory epithelium, with fibroblasts and other cells of connective tissue, bundles of collagen (red) and small blood vessels.

DENSE IRREGULAR CONNECTIVE TISSUE

Dense irregular connective tissue is found in regions that are under considerable mechanical stress and where protection is given to ensheathed organs. The matrix is relatively acellular and contains a high proportion of collagen fibres organized into thick bundles interweaving in three dimensions and imparting considerable strength. There are few active fibroblasts, which are usually flattened with heterochromatic nuclei. Dense irregular connective tissue occurs in: the reticular layer of the dermis; the connective tissue sheaths of muscle and nerves and the adventitia of large blood vessels; the capsules of various glands and organs (e.g. testis, sclera of the eye, periostea and perichondria).

ADIPOSE TISSUE

A few adipocytes occur in loose connective tissue in most parts of the body. However, they constitute the principal component of adipose tissue, where they are embedded in a vascular loose connective tissue, usually divided into lobules by stronger fibrous septa carrying the larger blood vessels (**Fig. 3.15**). Adipose tissue only occurs in certain regions. In particular it is found in: subcutaneous tissue; the mesenteries and omenta; the female breast; bone marrow; as retro-orbital fat behind the eyeball; around the kidneys; deep to the plantar skin of the foot; as localized pads in the synovial membrane of many joints. Its distribution in subcutaneous tissue shows characteristic age and sex differences. Fat deposits serve as energy stores, sources of metabolic lipids, thermal insulation (subcutaneous fat) and mechanical shock-absorbers (e.g. soles of the feet, palms of the hands, gluteal region and synovial membranes).

REGULAR CONNECTIVE TISSUES (Fig. 3.19)

Regular connective tissues include highly fibrous tissues in which fibres are regularly orientated, either to form sheets such as fasciae and aponeuroses, or as thicker bundles such as ligaments or tendons. The direction of the fibres within these structures is related to the stresses which they undergo, moreover, fibrous bundles display considerable interweaving, even within tendons, which increases their structural stability and resilience.

The fibroblasts that secrete the fibres may eventually become trapped within the fibrous structure, where they become compressed, relatively inactive cells with stellate profiles and small heterochromatic nuclei. Fibroblasts on the external surface may be active in continued fibre formation and they constitute a pool of cells available for repair of injured tissue.

Although regular connective tissue is predominantly collagenous, some ligaments contain significant amounts of elastin, e.g. the ligamenta flava of the vertebral laminae and the vocal folds. The collagen fibres may form precise geometrical patterns, as in the cornea (p. 702).

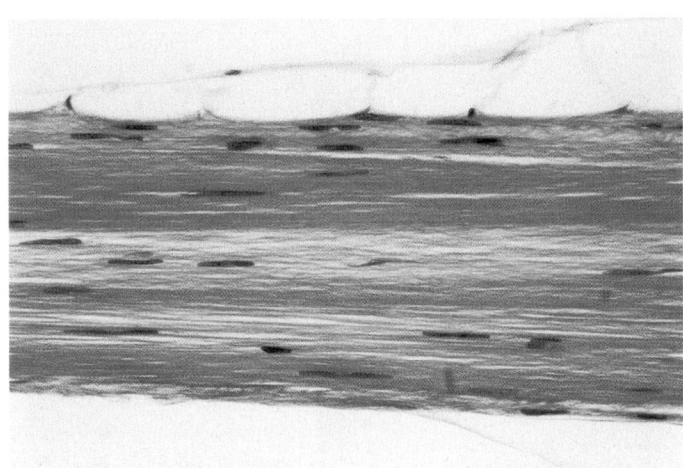

Fig. 3.19 Dense regular connective tissue in a tendon. Thick parallel bundles of type 1 collagen (pink) give tendon its white colour in life. The elongated nuclei of fibroblasts are visible between collagen bundles. (Photograph by Sarah-Jane Smith.)

MUCOID TISSUE

Mucoid tissue is a fetal or embryonic type of connective tissue, found chiefly as a stage in the development of connective tissue from mesenchyme. It exists in Wharton's jelly, which forms the bulk of the umbilical cord, and consists substantially of extracellular matrix, largely made up of hydrated mucoid material and a fine meshwork of collagen fibres, in which nucleated, fibroblast-like cells with branching process are found. Fibres are usually rare in typical mucoid tissue, although the full-term umbilical cord contains perivascular collagen fibres. Postnatally, mucoid tissue is seen in the pulp of a developing tooth, the vitreous body of the eye (a persistent form of mucoid tissue that contains few fibres or cells) and the nucleus pulposus of the intervertebral disc.

MUCOSA (MUCOUS MEMBRANE)

A mucosa or mucous membrane lines many internal hollow organs of which the inner surfaces are moistened by mucus, such as the intestines, conducting portions of the airway, and the genital and urinary tracts. The mucosa proper consists of an epithelial lining, which may have mucosal glands opening on to its surface, the underlying loose connective tissue, the lamina propria, and a thin layer of smooth muscle, the muscularis mucosae. This last layer is either absent from some mucosae, or is replaced by a layer of elastic fibres. The term mucous membrane reflects the fact that these tissues can all be peeled away as a sheet or membrane from underlying structures; the plane of separation occurs along the muscularis mucosae.

Submucosa is a layer of supporting connective tissue, which usually lies below the muscularis mucosae. It may contain mucous or seromucous submucosal glands, which convey their secretions through ducts to the mucosal surface. Most mucosae are also supported by one or more layers of smooth muscle, the muscularis externa. Contraction of this muscle may constrict the mucosal lumen (e.g. in the airway) or, where there are two or more muscle layers orientated in opposing directions (e.g. in the intestines), cause peristaltic movement of the viscus and the contents of its lumen. The outer surface of the muscle may be covered by a serosa or, where the structure is retroperitoneal or passes through the pelvic floor, by a connective tissue adventitia.

MUCUS

Mucus is a viscous suspension of complex glycoproteins (mucins) of various kinds, and is secreted by scattered individual epithelial (goblet) cells, a secretory surface epithelium (e.g. the stomach) or mucous and sero-mucous glands. The precise composition of the mucus varies with the tissue and secretory cells that produce it. All mucins consist of filamentous core proteins to which are attached carbohydrate chains, usually branched; salivary mucus contains nearly 600 chains. Carbohydrate residues include glucose, fucose, galactose and N-acetylglucosamine (sialic acid). The terminals of some carbohydrate chains are identical with the blood group antigens of the ABO group in the majority of the population (secretors, bearing the secretor gene S^e), and can be detected in salivary mucus by means of appropriate clinical tests. The long polymeric carbohydrate chains bind water and protect surfaces against drying; they also provide good lubricating properties. In concentrated form, mucins form viscous layers that protect the underlying tissues against damage.

Synthesis of mucus starts in the rough endoplasmic reticulum. It is then passed to the Golgi complex, where it is conjugated with sulphated carbohydrates to form the glycoprotein, mucinogen, and this is exported in small dense vesicles, which swell as they approach the cell surface, with which they fuse before releasing their contents.

SEROSA (SEROUS MEMBRANE)

Serosa consists of a single layer of squamous mesothelial cells supported by an underlying layer of loose connective tissue that contains numerous blood and lymphatic vessels. Serosal cells are derived from embryonic mesenchyme and so share a common lineage with connective tissue cells. However, structurally they resemble squamous epithelia and they express keratin intermediate filaments. Serosa lines the pleural, pericardial and peritoneal cavities, covers the external surfaces of organs lying within those cavities and, in the abdomen, the mesenteries that envelop them. A potential space, filled with a small amount of protein-containing serous fluid (largely an exudate of interstitial fluid), exists between the outer parietal and the inner visceral layer of the serosa.

FASCIA

Fascia is a term applied to masses of connective tissue large enough to be visible to the unaided eye. Its structure is highly variable but, in general, collagen fibres in fascia tend to be interwoven and seldom show the compact, parallel orientation seen in tendons and aponeuroses.

Fascia that is organized into condensations on the surfaces of muscles and other tissues is termed investing fascia, but this may not be its sole function. Between muscles that move extensively, it takes the form of loose areolar connective tissue and provides a degree of mechanical isolation. It constitutes the loose packing of connective tissue around peripheral nerves, blood and lymph vessels as they pass between other structures and often links them together as neurovascular bundles. It forms a dense connective tissue layer investing some large vessels, e.g. the common carotid and femoral arteries, and its presence here may be functionally significant, aiding venous return by approximating large veins to pulsating arteries.

SUPERFICIAL FASCIA
Superficial fascia is a layer of loose connective tissue of variable thickness that merges with the deep aspect of the dermis. It is often adipose, particularly between muscle and skin. It allows increased mobility of skin, and the adipose component contributes to thermal insulation and constitutes a store of energy for metabolic use. Subcutaneous nerves, vessels and lymphatics travel in the superficial fascia; their main trunks lie in its deepest layer, where adipose tissue is sparse. In the head and neck, superficial fascia also contains a group of striated muscles (collectively termed the muscles of facial expression), which are a remnant of more extensive sheets of skin-associated musculature found in other mammals.

The quantity and distribution of subcutaneous fat differs in the sexes. It is generally more abundant and widely distributed in females. In males, it diminishes from the trunk to the extremities; this distribution becomes more obvious in middle age, when the total amount increases in both sexes. There is an association with climate (rather than race), and superficial fat is more abundant in colder geographical regions. Superficial fascia is most distinct on the lower anterior abdominal wall, where it contains much elastic tissue and appears many-layered as it passes through the inguinal regions into the thighs. It is well differentiated in the limbs and the perineum, but is thin where it passes over the dorsal aspects of the hands and feet, the sides of the neck and face, around the anus and over the penis and scrotum, and is almost absent from the external ears. Superficial fascia is particularly dense in the scalp, palms and soles, where it is permeated by numerous strong connective tissue bands that bind the superficial fascia and skin to underlying structures.

DEEP FASCIA
Deep fascia is also composed mainly of collagenous fibres, but these are compacted and in many cases arranged so regularly that the deep fascia may be indistinguishable from aponeurotic tissue. In limbs, where deep fascia is well developed, the collagen fibres are longitudinal or transverse, and condense into tough, inelastic sheaths around the musculature.

REFERENCES

Pollard TD, Earnshaw WC 2002 Cell Biology. Philadelphia: Saunders.
A cell biology text with extensive coverage of extracellular matrix components.

Nervous system

The nervous system has two major divisions, the central nervous system (CNS) and the peripheral nervous system (PNS). The CNS consists of the brain and spinal cord and contains the majority of neuronal cell bodies. The PNS includes all nervous tissue outside the central nervous system and is subdivided into the cranial and spinal nerves, autonomic nervous system (ANS) (including the enteric nervous system of the gut wall, ENS) and special senses (taste, olfaction, vision, hearing and balance). It is composed mainly of the axons of sensory and motor neurones which pass between the CNS and the body. However, the ENS contains as many intrinsic neurones in its ganglia as the entire spinal cord, is not connected directly to the CNS, and may be considered separately as a third division of the nervous system.

The CNS is derived from the neural tube (p. 207). The cell bodies of neurones are often grouped together in areas termed nuclei, or they may form more extensive layers or masses of cells collectively called grey matter. Neuronal dendrites and synaptic activity are mostly confined to areas of grey matter, and they form part of its meshwork of neuronal and glial processes which is collectively termed the neuropil (**Fig. 4.1**). Their axons pass into bundles of nerve fibres which tend to be grouped separately to form tracts. In the spinal cord, cerebellum, cerebral cortices (Chs 20, 22) and some other areas, concentrations of tracts constitute the white matter, so called because the axons are often ensheathed in myelin which is white when fresh (**Figs 18.1, 18.4**).

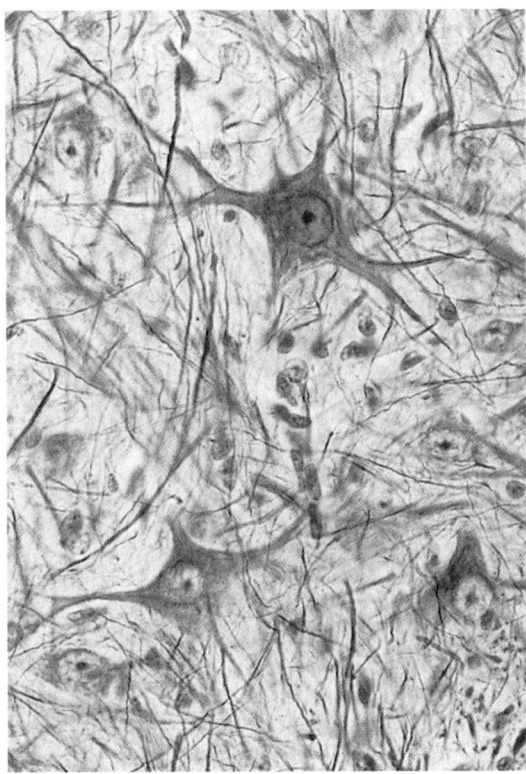

Fig. 4.1 Neuronal somata, dendrites and axons in the CNS neuropil; their cytoskeleton has been stained using a gold method. The toluidine blue counterstaining reveals the nuclei of surrounding glial cells. (By permission from Young B, Heath JW 2000 Wheater's Functional Histology. Edinburgh: Churchill Livingstone.)

The PNS is composed of the axons of motor neurones situated inside the CNS, and the cell bodies of sensory neurones (grouped together as ganglia) and their processes. Sensory cells in dorsal root ganglia give off both centrally and peripherally directed processes: there are no synapses on their cell bodies. Ganglionic neurones of the ANS receive synaptic contacts from various sources. Neuronal cell bodies in peripheral ganglia are all derived embryologically from cells which migrate from the neural crest (p. 207).

When the neural tube is formed during prenatal development its walls thicken greatly but do not completely obliterate the cavity within. The latter remains in the spinal cord as the narrow central canal, and in the brain it becomes greatly expanded to form a series of interconnected cavities called the ventricular system. In the fore- and hindbrains, parts of the neural tube roof do not generate nerve cells but become thin folded sheets of secretory tissue which are invaded by blood vessels and are called the choroid plexuses. The plexuses secrete cerebrospinal fluid which fills the ventricles and subarachnoid spaces (p. 282), and penetrates the intercellular spaces of the brain and spinal cord to create their interstitial fluid. The CNS has a rich blood supply, which is essential to sustain its high metabolic rate. The blood–brain barrier places considerable restrictions on the substances which can diffuse from the bloodstream into the nervous tissue.

Neurones encode information, conduct it over considerable distances, and then transmit it to other neurones or to various non-neural cells. The movement of this information within the nervous system depends on the rapid conduction of transient electrical impulses along neuronal plasma membranes. Transmission to other cells is mediated by secretion of neurotransmitters at special junctions either with other neurones (synapses), or with cells outside the nervous system, e.g. muscle cells (neuromuscular junctions), gland cells, adipose tissue, etc. and this causes changes in their behaviour.

The nervous system contains large populations of non-neuronal cells, neuroglia or glia, which, whilst not electrically active in the same way, are responsible for creating and maintaining an appropriate environment in which neurones can operate efficiently. In the CNS, glia outnumber neurones by 10–50 times and consist of microglia and macroglia. Macroglia are further subdivided into three main types, oligodendrocytes, astrocytes and ependymal cells. The principal glial cell of the PNS is the Schwann cell. Satellite cells surround each neuronal soma in ganglia.

NEURONES

Most of the neurones in the CNS are either clustered into nuclei, columns or layers, or dispersed within grey matter. Neurones of the PNS are confined to ganglia. Irrespective of location, neurones share many general features, which are discussed here in the context of central neurones. Special characteristics of ganglionic neurones and their adjacent tissues are discussed on page 58.

Neurones exhibit great variability in their size (cell bodies range from 5 to 100 μm diameter) and shapes. Their surface areas are extensive because most neurones display numerous narrow branched cell processes. They usually have a rounded or polygonal cell body (perikaryon or soma). This is a central mass of cytoplasm which encloses a nucleus and gives off long, branched extensions, with which most intercellular contacts are made. Typically, one of these processes, the axon, is much longer than the others, the dendrites (**Fig. 4.2**). Dendrites conduct electrical impulses towards a soma whereas axons conduct impulses away from it.

43

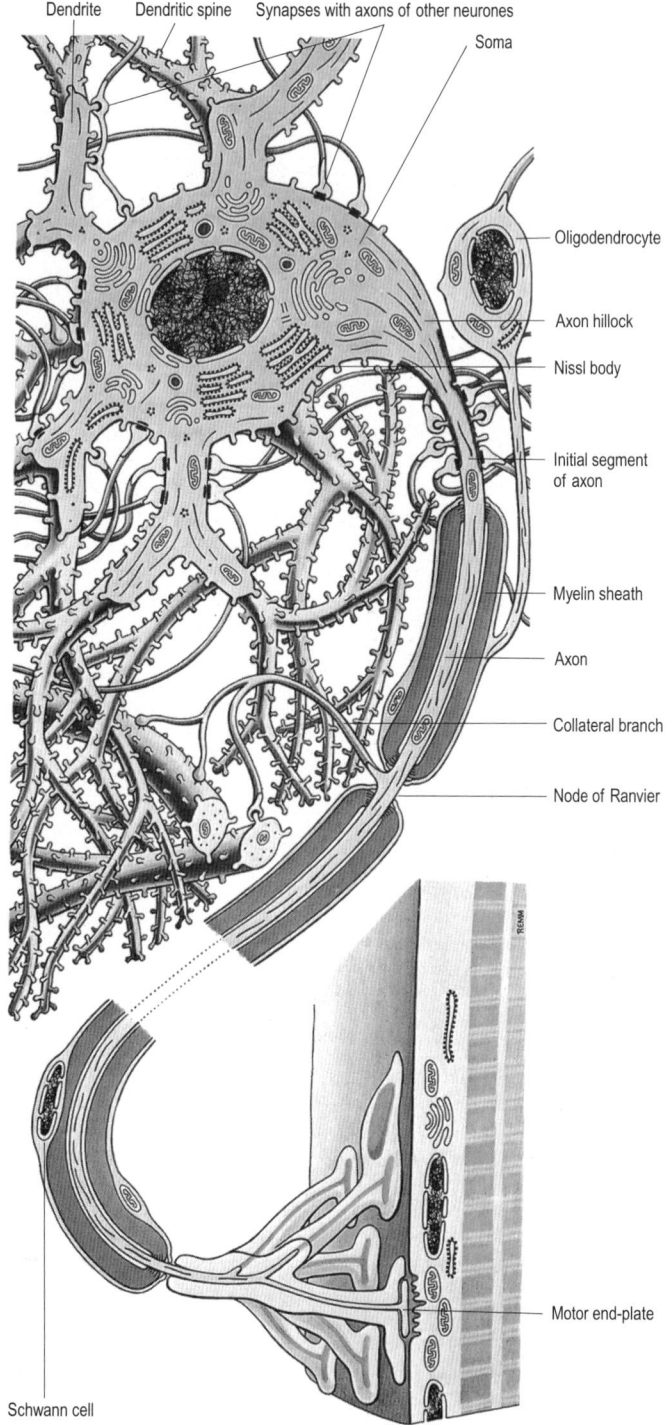

Fig. 4.2 A typical neurone (here, a motor neurone), showing the soma, part of the dendritic tree with dendritic spines and synaptic contacts, and an axon myelinated by oligodendrocytes and (in the PNS) by Schwann cells and ending at a neuromuscular junction.

Neurones can be classified according to the number and arrangement of their processes. Multipolar neurones (Figs 4.3, 22.9) are common: they have an extensive dendritic tree which arises from either a single primary dendrite or directly from the soma, and a single axon. Bipolar neurones, which typify neurones of the special sensory systems, e.g. retina (p. 712), have only a single dendrite which emerges from the soma opposite the axonal pole. Unipolar neurones which transmit general sensation, e.g. dorsal root ganglion neurones, have a single short process which bifurcates into peripheral and central processes (p. 58), an arrangement which arises by the fusion of the proximal axonal and dendritic processes of a bipolar neurone during development.

Neurones are postmitotic cells and, with few exceptions, they are not replaced when lost.

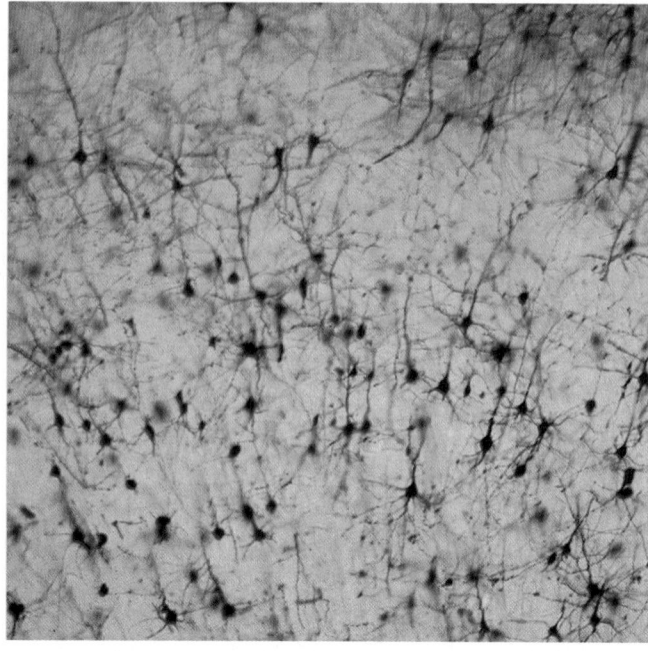

Fig. 4.3 Section through the cerebral cortex (mouse) stained by the Golgi method which demonstrates only a small proportion of the total neuronal population. (Specimen prepared by Martin Sadler, Division of Anatomy and Cell Biology, GKT School of Medicine, London.)

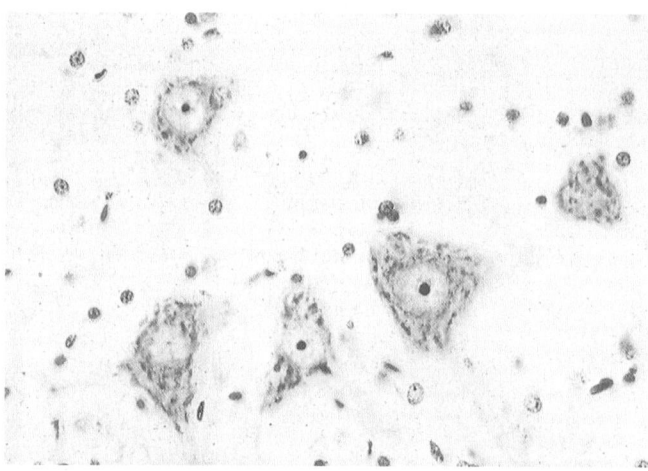

Fig. 4.4 Large multipolar neuronal perikarya in the magnocellular part of the feline red nucleus, showing prominent Nissl granules, bases of dendrites and axon hillocks. The nuclei are euchromatic and vesicular, with prominent nucleoli. The small nuclei scattered in the surrounding neuropil are characteristic of the various categories of neuroglial cell. (Photograph by Kevin Fitzpatrick on behalf of GKT School of Medicine, London.)

SOMA

The plasma membrane of the soma is unmyelinated and contacted by inhibitory and excitatory axosomatic synapses (p. 44): very occasionally, somasomatic and dendrosomatic contacts may be made. The non-synaptic surface is covered by either astrocytic or satellite oligodendrocyte processes.

The cytoplasm of a typical soma (Fig. 4.2) is rich in rough and smooth endoplasmic reticulum and free polyribosomes, which reveals a high level of protein synthetic activity. Free polyribosomes often congregate in large groups associated with the rough endoplasmic reticulum. These aggregates of RNA-rich structures are visible by light microscopy as basophilic Nissl (chromatin) bodies or granules (Fig. 4.4). They are more obvious in large, highly active cells, such as spinal motor neurones, which contain large stacks of rough endoplasmic reticulum and polyribosome aggregates. Maintenance and turnover of cytoplasmic and membranous components are necessary in all cells:

the huge total volume of cytoplasm within the soma and processes of many neurones requires a considerable commitment of protein synthetic machinery. Neurones synthesize other proteins (enzyme systems, etc.) which are involved in the production of neurotransmitters and in the reception and transduction of incoming stimuli. Various transmembrane channel proteins and enzymes are located at the surfaces of neurones where they are associated with ion transport. The apparatus for protein synthesis (including RNA and ribosomes) occupies the soma and dendrites, but is usually absent from axons.

The nucleus is characteristically large, round and euchromatic, with one or more prominent nucleoli, as is typical of all cells engaged in substantial levels of protein synthesis. The cytoplasm contains many mitochondria and moderate numbers of lysosomes. Golgi complexes are typically seen close to the nucleus, near the bases of the main dendrites and opposite the axon hillock.

The neuronal cytoskeleton is a prominent feature of its cytoplasm, and it gives shape, strength and rigidity to the dendrites and axons. Neurofilaments (the intermediate filaments of neurones) and micro-tubules are abundant: they occur in the soma and extend along den-drites and axons, in proportions which vary with the type of neurone and cell process. Bundles of neurofilaments constitute neurofibrils which can be seen by light microscopy in silver stained sections. Neurofilaments are heteropolymers of proteins assembled from three polypeptide subunits, NF-L (68 kDa), NF-M (160 kDa) and NF-H (200 kDa). NF-M and NF-H have long C-terminal domains which project as side arms from the assembled neurofilament and bind to neighbouring filaments. They can be heavily phosphorylated, particularly in the highly stable neurofilaments of mature axons, and are thought to give axons their tensile strength. Some axons are almost filled by neurofilaments. Dendrites usually have more microtubules than axons.

Microtubules are important in axonal transport. Centrioles persist in mature postmitotic neurones, where they are concerned with the generation of microtubules rather than cell division. Centrioles are associated with cilia on the surfaces of developing neuroblasts. Their significance, other than at some sensory endings (e.g. the olfactory mucosa, p. 568), is not known.

Pigment granules appear in certain regions, e.g. neurones of the substantia nigra contain neuromelanin, probably a waste product of catecholamine synthesis (p. 344). In the locus coeruleus a similar pigment, rich in copper, gives a bluish colour to the neurones. Some neurones are unusually rich in certain metals, which may form a component of enzyme systems, e.g. zinc in the hippocampus and iron in the oculomotor nucleus. Ageing neurones especially in spinal ganglia accumulate granules of lipofuscin (senility pigment). They represent residual bodies, which are lysosomes packed with partially degraded lipoprotein material (corpora amylaceae).

DENDRITES

Dendrites are highly branched, usually short processes which project from the soma (**Fig. 4.2**). The branching patterns of many dendritic arrays are probably established by random adhesive interactions between dendritic growth cones and afferent axons which occur during development. There is an overproduction of dendrites in early develop-ment, which is pruned in response to functional demand as the indi-vidual matures and information is processed through the dendritic tree. There is evidence that dendritic trees may be plastic structures through-out adult life, expanding and contracting as the traffic of synaptic activity varies through afferent axodendritic contacts (for review see Berry 1991). Groups of neurones with similar functions have a similar stereotypic tree structure (**Fig. 4.5**), suggesting that the branching patterns of dendrites are important determinants of the integration of afferent inputs which converge on the tree.

Dendrites differ from axons in many respects. They represent the afferent rather than the efferent system of the neurone, and receive both excitatory and inhibitory axodendritic contacts. They may also make dendrodendritic and dendrosomatic connections (see **Fig. 4.8**), some of which are reciprocal. Synapses occur either on small projections called dendritic spines or on the smooth dendritic surface. Dendrites contain ribosomes, smooth endoplasmic reticulum, microtubules, neurofilaments, actin filaments and Golgi complexes. The neuro-filament proteins of dendrites are poorly phosphorylated. Dendrite microtubules express the microtubule-associated protein (MAP-2) almost exclusively in comparison with axons.

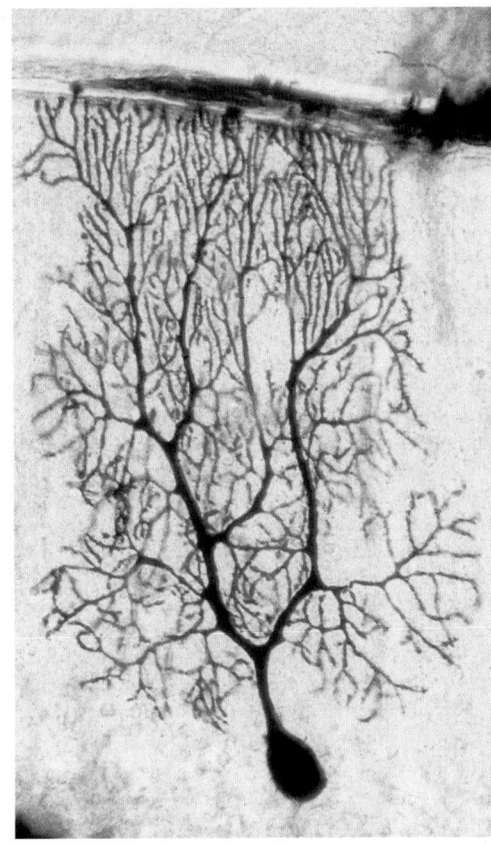

Fig. 4.5 Purkinje neurone from the cerebellum of a rat stained by the Golgi–Cox method, showing the extensive two-dimensional array of dendrites. (Provided by Martin Sadler and M Berry, Division of Anatomy and Cell Biology, GKT School of Medicine, London.)

Dendritic spine shapes range from simple protrusions to structures with a slender stalk and expanded distal end. Most spines are not more than 2 μm long, and have one or more terminal expansions, but they can also be short and stubby, branched or bulbous. Free ribosomes and polyribosomes are concentrated at the base of the spine. Ribosomal accumulations near synaptic sites provide a mechanism for activity-dependent synaptic plasticity through the local regulation of protein synthesis.

AXONS

The axon originates either from the soma or from the proximal segment of a dendrite, at a specialized region, the axon hillock (**Fig. 4.2**), which is free of Nissl granules. Action potentials are initiated here. The axonal plasma membrane (axolemma) is undercoated at the hillock by a concentration of cytoskeletal molecules, including spectrin and actin fibrils, which are thought to be important in anchoring numerous voltage sensitive channels to the membrane. The axon hillock is unmyelinated and often participates in inhibitory axo-axonal synapses. This region of the axon is unique because it contains ribosomal aggregates immediately below the postsynaptic membrane.

When present, myelin begins at the distal end of the axon hillock. Myelin thickness and internodal segment lengths are positively correlated with axon diameter. In the PNS unmyelinated axons are embedded in Schwann cell cytoplasm, in the CNS they lie free in the neuropil. Nodes of Ranvier are specialized constricted regions of myelin-free axolemma where action potentials are generated and where an axon may branch. The density of sodium channels in the axolemma is highest at nodes of Ranvier, and very low along internodal mem-branes. In contrast, sodium channels are spread more evenly within the axolemma of unmyelinated axons. Fast potassium channels are also present in the paranodal regions of myelinated axons. Fine processes of glial cytoplasm (astrocyte in the CNS, Schwann cell in the PNS) surround the nodal axolemma. The terminals of an axon are unmyelinated. They expand into presynaptic boutons which may form connections with axons, dendrites, neuronal somata or, in the periphery, muscle fibres, glands and lymphoid tissue. They may themselves be contacted by other axons, forming axoaxonal presynaptic inhibitory circuits. Further details of neuronal microcircuitry are given in Kandel & Schwartz (2000).

Axons contain microtubules, neurofilaments, mitochondria, membrane vesicles, cisternae, and lysosomes: they do not usually contain ribosomes or Golgi complexes, except at the axon hillock. However, ribosomes are found in the neurosecretory fibres of hypothalamo-hypophyseal neurones which contain the mRNA of neuropeptides. Organelles are differentially distributed along axons, e.g. there is a greater density of mitochondria and membrane vesicles in the axon hillock, at nodes, and in presynaptic endings. Axonal microtubules are interconnected by cross-linking microtubule-associated proteins (MAPs) of which tau is the most abundant. Microtubules have an intrinsic polarity (p. 18): in axons all microtubules are uniformly orientated with their rapidly growing ends directed away from the soma towards the axon terminal. Neurofilament proteins ranging from high to low molecular weights are highly phosphorylated in mature axons, whereas growing and regenerating axons express a calmodulin-binding membrane-associated phosphoprotein, growth-associated protein-43 (GAP-43), as well as poorly phosphorylated neurofilaments.

Axons respond differently to injury, depending on whether the damage occurs in the CNS or PNS. The glial microenvironment of a damaged central axon does not facilitate regrowth, and reconnection with original synaptic targets does not normally occur. In the PNS, the glial microenvironment is capable of facilitating axonal regrowth, however the functional outcome of clinical repair of a large mixed peripheral nerve, especially if the injury occurs some distance from the target organ, or produces a long defect in the damaged nerve, is frequently unsatisfactory.

Axoplasmic flow

Neuronal organelles and cytoplasm are in continual motion. Bidirectional streaming of vesicles along axons results in a net transport of materials from the soma to the terminals, with more limited movement in the opposite direction. Two major types of transport occur, one slow, and one relatively fast. Slow axonal transport is a bulk flow of axoplasm only in the anterograde direction, carrying cytoskeletal proteins and soluble, non-membrane bound proteins at a rate of c.0.1–3 mm a day. In contrast, fast axonal transport carries vesicular material at c.200 mm a day in the retrograde direction and c.40 mm per day anterogradely.

Rapid flow depends on microtubules. Vesicles with side projections line up along microtubules and are transported along them by their side-arms. Two microtubule-based motor proteins with ATPase activity are involved in fast transport. Kinesin family proteins are responsible for the fast component of anterograde transport, and cytoplasmic dynein is responsible for retrograde transport. Fast anterograde transport carries vesicles, including synaptic vesicles containing neurotransmitters, from the soma to the axon terminals. Retrograde axonal transport accounts for the flow of mitochondria, endosomes and lysosomal autophagic vacuoles from the axonal terminals into the soma. Retrograde transport mediates the movement of neurotrophic viruses, e.g. herpes zoster, rabies and polio, from peripheral terminals, and their subsequent concentration in the neuronal soma.

SYNAPSES

Transmission of impulses across specialized junctions (synapses) between two neurones is largely chemical. It depends on the release of neurotransmitters from the presynaptic side: this causes a change in the electrical state of the postsynaptic neuronal membrane, resulting in either its depolarization or hyperpolarization.

The patterns of axonal termination vary considerably. A single axon may synapse with one neurone, e.g. climbing fibres ending on cerebellar Purkinje neurones, or more often with many, e.g. cerebellar parallel fibres, which provide an extreme example of this phenomenon (p. 357). In synaptic glomeruli, e.g. in the olfactory bulb, and synaptic cartridges, groups of synapses between two or many neurones form interactive units encapsulated by neuroglia (Fig. 4.6).

Electrical synapses (direct communication via gap junctions) are rare in the human CNS and are confined largely to groups of neurones with tightly coupled activity, e.g. the inspiratory centre in the medulla. They will not be discussed further here.

Classification of chemical synapses

Chemical synapses have an asymmetric structural organization (see Figs 4.7, 4.8) in keeping with the unidirectional nature of their transmission. Typical chemical synapses share a number of important features. They all display an area of presynaptic membrane apposed to a corresponding postsynaptic membrane: the two are separated by a narrow (20–30 nm) gap, the synaptic cleft. Synaptic vesicles containing neurotransmitter lie on the presynaptic side, clustered near an area of dense material on the cytoplasmic aspect of the presynaptic membrane. A corresponding region of submembrane density is present on the postsynaptic side. Together these define the active zone, the area of the synapse where neurotransmission takes place.

Chemical synapses can be classified according to a number of different parameters, including the neuronal regions forming the synapse; their ultrastructural characteristics; the chemical nature of their neurotransmitter(s); their effects on the electrical state of the postsynaptic neurone. The following classification is limited to associations between neurones. Neuromuscular junctions share many (though not all) of these parameters, and are often referred to as peripheral synapses. They are described separately on page 64.

Synapses can occur between almost any surface regions of the participating neurones. The most common type occurs between an axon and either a dendrite or a soma, when the axon is expanded as a small bulb or bouton (Figs 4.7, 4.8). This may be a terminal of an axonal branch (terminal bouton) or one of a row of bead-like endings, when the axon makes contact at several points, often with more than one neurone (bouton de passage). Boutons may synapse with dendrites, including dendritic spines or the flat surface of a dendritic shaft; a soma, usually

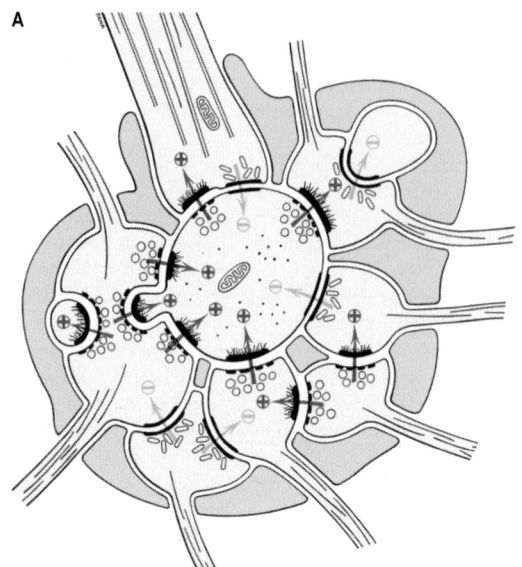

A

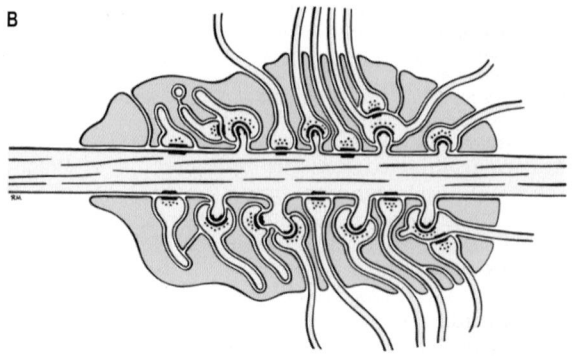

B

Fig. 4.6 The arrangement of complex synaptic units. **A**, Synaptic glomerulus with excitatory ('+') and inhibitory ('–') synapses grouped around a central dendritic terminal expansion. The directions of transmission are shown by the arrows. **B**, Synaptic cartridge with a group of synapses surrounding a dendritic segment. Each complex unit is enclosed within a glial capsule (green).

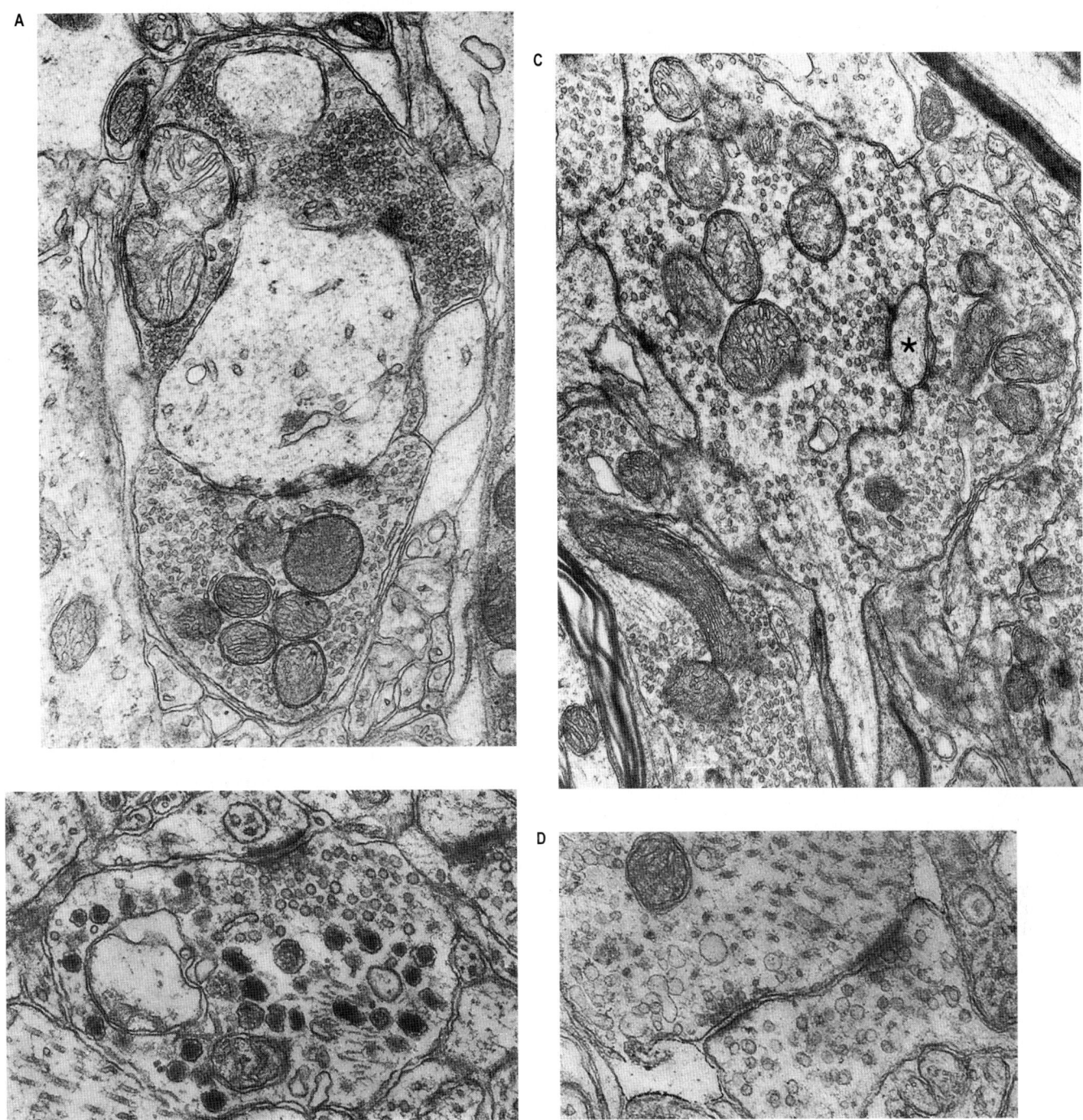

Fig. 4.7 Electron micrographs demonstrating various types of synapse. **A**, A pale cross-section of a dendrite upon which two synaptic boutons end. The upper bouton contains round vesicles, and the lower bouton contains flattened vesicles of the small type. A number of pre- and postsynaptic thickenings mark the specialized zones of contact. **B**, A type I synapse containing both small, round, clear vesicles and also large dense-cored vesicles of the neurosecretory type. **C**, A large terminal bouton of an optic nerve afferent fibre, which is making contact with a number of postsynaptic processes, in the dorsal lateral geniculate nucleus of the rat. One of the postsynaptic processes (*) also receives a synaptic contact from a bouton containing flattened vesicles (right). **D**, Reciprocal synapses between two neuronal processes in the olfactory bulb. (**A**, **B**, **D** and **E**, provided by AR Lieberman, Department of Anatomy, University College, London.)

on its flat surface, but occasionally on spines; the axon hillock; the terminal boutons of other axons.

The connection is classified according to the direction of transmission, with the incoming terminal region named first. Most common are axodendritic synapses, although axosomatic connections are frequent. All other possible combinations are found, but they are less common, i.e. axoaxonic, dendroaxonic, dendrodendritic, somatodendritic or somatosomatic. Axodendritic and axosomatic synapses occur in all regions of the CNS and in autonomic ganglia including those of the ENS. The other types appear restricted to regions of complex interaction between larger sensory neurones and microneurones, e.g. in the thalamus.

Ultrastructurally, synaptic vesicles may be internally clear or dense, and of different size (loosely categorized as small or large) and shape (round, flat or pleomorphic, i.e. irregularly shaped). The submembranous densities may be thicker on the postsynaptic than on the presynaptic side (asymmetric synapses), or equivalent in thickness (symmetrical synapses). Synaptic ribbons are found at sites of neurotransmission in the retina and inner ear. They have a distinctive morphology, in that the synaptic vesicles are grouped around a ribbon- or rod-like density orientated perpendicular to the cell membrane (**Fig. 4.8**).

Synaptic boutons make obvious close contacts with postsynaptic structures, but many other terminals lack specialized contact zones. Areas of transmitter release occur in the varicosities of unmyelinated

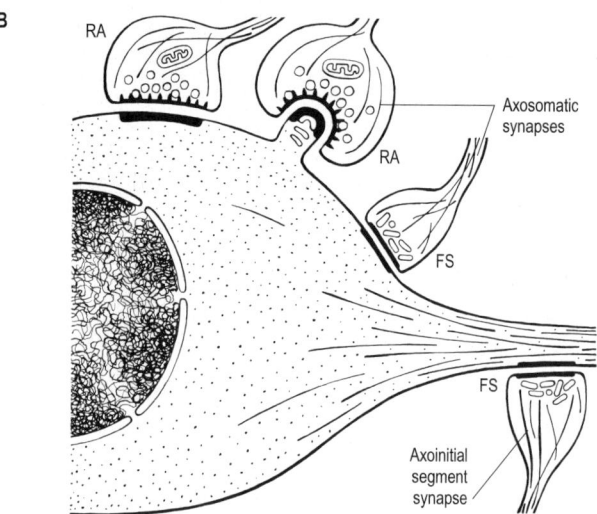

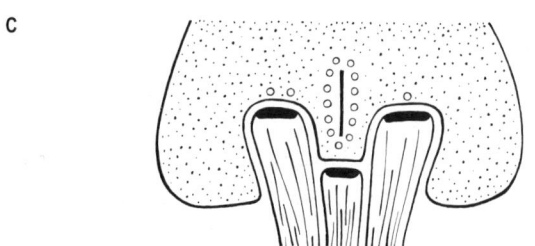

Fig. 4.8 The structural arrangements of different types of synaptic contact. **A**, The gap junction (B) and the desmosome (E) are without synaptic significance. Excitatory synaptic boutons are shown (C, G) containing small spherical translucent vesicles. D: a bouton with dense-cored, catecholamine-containing vesicles; F: an inhibitory synapse containing small flattened vesicles; H: a reciprocal synaptic structure between two dendritic profiles, inhibitory towards dendrite A and excitatory in the opposite direction; I: an inhibitory synapse containing large flattened vesicles. J and K: two serial synapses; J is excitatory to the dendrite; K is inhibitory to J; L: a neurosecretory ending adjacent to a vascular channel (M), surrounded by a fenestrated endothelium. All the boutons in this diagram are of the terminal type, except G which is a bouton de passage. **B**, Axosomatic and axoinitial segment synapses: RA, asymmetrical synapses with rounded vesicles; FS, symmetrical synapses with flattened vesicles. **C**, Ribbon synapse: triad at base of retinal rod.

axons, where effects are sometimes diffuse, e.g. the aminergic pathways of the basal ganglia (p. 428) and in autonomic fibres in the periphery (p. 65). In some instances, such axons may ramify widely throughout extensive areas of the brain and affect the behaviour of very large populations of neurones, e.g. the diffuse cholinergic innervation of the cerebral cortices. Pathological degeneration of these pathways can therefore cause widespread disturbances in neural function.

Neurones express a variety of neurotransmitters, either as one class of neurotransmitter per cell or more often as several. Good correlations exist between some types of transmitter and specialized structural features of synapses. In general, asymmetric synapses with relatively small spherical vesicles are associated with acetylcholine (ACh), glutamate, serotonin (5-hydroxytryptamine, 5-HT), and some amines; those with dense-core vesicles include many peptidergic synapses and other amines (e.g. noradrenaline (norepinephrine), adrenaline (epinephrine), dopamine). Symmetrical synapses with flattened or pleomorphic vesicles have been shown to contain either γ-aminobutyric acid (GABA) or glycine.

Neurosecretory endings found in various parts of the brain and in neuroendocrine glands have many features in common with presynaptic boutons. They all contain peptides or glycoproteins within dense-core vesicles of characteristic size and appearance, which are often ellipsoidal or irregular in shape, and are relatively large, e.g. oxytocin and vasopressin vesicles in the neurohypophysis may be up to 200 nm across.

Synapses may cause depolarization or hyperpolarization of the postsynaptic membrane, depending on the neurotransmitter released and the classes of receptor molecule in the postsynaptic membrane. Depolarization of the postsynaptic membrane results in excitation of the postsynaptic neurone, whereas hyperpolarization has the effect of transiently inhibiting electrical activity. Subtle variations in these responses may also occur at synapses where mixtures of neuromediators are present and their effects are integrated.

Type I and II synapses

There are two broad categories of synapse: type I synapses, in which the subsynaptic zone of dense cytoplasm is thicker than on the presynaptic side, and type II synapses, in which the two zones are more symmetrical but thinner. Other differences include the widths of the synaptic clefts, which are c.30 nm in type I and c.20 nm in type II synapses, and their vesicle content. Type I boutons contain a predominance of small spherical vesicles c.50 nm in diameter, and type II boutons contain a variety of flat forms. The general principle found to apply in broad outline throughout the CNS classifies type I synapses as excitatory and type II as inhibitory. In a few instances types I and II synapses are found in close proximity, orientated in opposite directions across the synaptic cleft (a reciprocal synapse).

Mechanisms of synaptic activity

Synaptic activation begins with arrival of one or more action potentials at the presynaptic bouton, which causes the opening of voltage-sensitive calcium channels in the presynaptic membrane. The response time in typical fast-acting synapses is then very rapid; classic neurotransmitter (e.g. ACh) is released in less than a millisecond, which is faster than the activation time of a classic second messenger system on the presynaptic side. The influx of calcium activates Ca^{2+}-dependent protein kinases. This uncouples synaptic vesicles from a spectrin-actin meshwork within the presynaptic ending, to which they are bound via synapsins I and II. The vesicles dock with the presynaptic membrane, through processes not yet fully understood, and their membranes fuse to open a pore through which neurotransmitter diffuses into the synaptic cleft.

Once the vesicle has discharged its contents, its membrane is incorporated into the presynaptic plasma membrane and is then more slowly recycled back into the bouton by endocytosis around the edges of the active site. The time between endocytosis and re-release may be c.30 seconds; newly recycled vesicles compete randomly with previously stored vesicles for the next cycle of neurotransmitter release. The fusion of vesicles with the presynaptic membrane is responsible for the observed quantal behaviour of neurotransmitter release, both during neural activation and spontaneously, in the slightly leaky resting condition.

Postsynaptic events vary greatly, depending on the receptor molecules and their related molecular complexes. Receptors are generally classed as either ionotropic or metabotropic. Ionotropic receptors function as ion channels, so that conformational changes induced in the receptor protein when it binds the neurotransmitter cause the opening of an ion channel within the same protein assembly, thus causing a voltage change within the postsynaptic cell. Examples are the nicotinic ACh receptor and the N-methyl-D-aspartate (NMDA) glutamate receptor. Alternatively, the receptor and ion channel may be separate molecules, coupled by G-proteins, some via a complex cascade of chemical interactions (a second messenger system), e.g. the adenylate cyclase pathway (p. 9). Postsynaptic effects are generally rapid and short-lived, because the transmitter is quickly inactivated either by an extracellular enzyme (e.g. acetylcholinesterase, AChE), or by uptake by neuroglial cells. Examples of such metabotropic receptors are the muscarinic Ach receptor and 5-HT receptor.

Neurohormones

Neurohormones are included in the range of transmitter activities. They are synthesized in neurones and released into the blood circulation by exocytosis at synaptic terminal-like structures. As with classic endocrine gland hormones (Ch. 9, they may act at great distances from their site of secretion. Neurones secrete into the cerebrospinal fluid or local interstitial fluid to affect other cells, either diffusely or at a distance. To encompass this wide range of phenomena the general term neuromediation has been used, and the chemicals involved are called neuromediators.

Neuromodulators – Some neuromediators do not appear to affect the postsynaptic membrane directly, but they can affect its responses to other neuromediators, either enhancing their activity (increasing the immediate response in size, or causing a prolongation), or perhaps limiting or inhibiting their action. These substances are called neuromodulators. A single synaptic terminal may contain one or more neuromodulators in addition to a neurotransmitter, usually (though not always) in separate vesicles. Neuropeptides (see below and p. 180) are nearly all neuromodulators, at least in some of their actions. They are stored within dense granular synaptic vesicles of various sizes and appearances.

Development and plasticity of synapses

Embryonic synapses first appear as inconspicuous dense zones flanking synaptic clefts. Immature synapses often appear after birth, suggesting that they may be labile, and are reinforced if transmission is functionally effective, or withdrawn if redundant. This is implicit in some theories of memory, which postulate that synapses are modifiable by frequency of use, to establish preferential conduction pathways. Evidence from hippocampal neurones suggests that even brief synaptic activity can increase the strength and sensitivity of the synapse for some hours or longer (long-term potentiation, LTP). During early postnatal life, the normal developmental increase in numbers and sizes of synapses and dendritic spines depends on the degree of neural activity and is impaired in areas of damage or functional deprivation.

Neurotransmitters

Until recently the molecules known to be involved in chemical synapses were limited to a fairly small group of classic neurotransmitters, e.g. ACh, noradrenaline, adrenaline, dopamine and histamine, all of which had well-defined rapid effects on other neurones, muscle cells or glands. However, many synaptic interactions cannot be explained on the basis of classic neurotransmitters, and it now appears that other substances, particularly some amino acids such as glutamate, glycine, aspartate, GABA and the monoamine, serotonin, also function as transmitters. Substances first identified as hypophyseal hormones or as part of the dispersed neuroendocrine system of the alimentary tract, can be detected widely throughout the CNS and PNS, often associated with functionally integrated systems. Many of these are peptides: more than 50 (together with other candidates), function mainly as neuromodulators and influence the activities of classic transmitters.

Acetylcholine

Acetylcholine (ACh) is perhaps the most extensively studied neurotransmitter of the classic type. Its precursor, choline, is synthesized in the neuronal soma and transported to the axon terminals where it is acetylated by the enzyme choline acetyl transferase (ChAT), and stored in clear spherical vesicles c.50 nm in diameter. ACh is synthesized by motor neurones and released at all their motor terminals on skeletal muscle and at synapses in parasympathetic and sympathetic ganglia.

Many parasympathetic, and some sympathetic, ganglionic neurones are also cholinergic.

In some sites ACh is also associated with the degradative extracellular enzyme acetyl cholinesterase (AChE), e.g. at neuromuscular junctions. The effects of ACh on nicotinic receptors (i.e. those in which nicotine is an agonist) are rapid and excitatory. In the peripheral ANS, the slower, more sustained excitatory effects of cholinergic autonomic endings are mediated by muscarinic receptors via a second messenger system.

Monoamines

Monoamines include the catecholamines (noradrenaline, adrenaline and dopamine), the indoleamine serotonin (5-hydroxytryptamine, 5-HT) and histamine. Neurones which synthesize the monoamines include sympathetic ganglia and their homologues, the chromaffin cells of the suprarenal medulla (pp. 180, 1247) and paraganglia (p. 181). Within the CNS, their somata lie chiefly in the brainstem, although their axons spread and ramify widely into all parts of the nervous system. Monoaminergic cells are also present in the retina (p. 710).

Noradrenaline is the chief transmitter present in sympathetic ganglionic neurones with endings in various tissues, notably smooth muscle and glands, and in other sites including adipose and haemopoietic tissues, and the corneal epithelium. It is also found at widely distributed synaptic endings within the CNS, many of them terminals of neuronal somata situated in the locus coeruleus in the medullary floor. The actions of noradrenaline depend on its site of action, and vary with the type of postsynaptic receptor. In some cases, e.g. the neurones of the submucosal plexus of the intestine and of the locus coeruleus, it is strongly inhibitory via actions on the α_2-adrenergic receptor, whereas the β-receptors, e.g. of vascular smooth muscle, mediate depolarization and therefore vasoconstriction. Adrenaline is present in central and peripheral nervous pathways and occurs with noradrenaline in the suprarenal medulla. Both of these monoamines are found in dense-cored synaptic vesicles c.50 nm diameter.

Dopamine is a neuromediator of considerable clinical importance, present mainly in the CNS, where it is found in neurones with cell bodies in the telencephalon, diencephalon and mesencephalon. A major dopaminergic neuronal population in the midbrain constitutes the substantia nigra, so called because its cells contain neuromelanin, a black granular byproduct of dopamine synthesis. Dopaminergic endings are particularly numerous in the corpus striatum, limbic system and cerebral cortex. Pathological reduction in dopaminergic activity has widespread effects on motor control, affective behaviour and other neural activities, as seen in Parkinson's syndrome. Structurally, dopaminergic synapses contain numerous dense-cored vesicles resembling those of noradrenaline.

Serotonin and histamine are found in neurones mainly in the CNS. Serotonin is synthesized chiefly in small median neuronal clusters of the brainstem, mainly in the raphe nuclei, whose axons spread and branch extensively throughout the entire brain and spinal cord. Synaptic terminals contain rounded, clear vesicles c.50 nm diameter and are of the asymmetrical type. Histaminergic neurones appear to be relatively sparse, and are restricted largely to the hypothalamus.

Amino acids

The best understood amino acid is GABA, which is a major inhibitory transmitter released at the terminals of local circuit neurones within the brainstem and spinal cord (e.g. the recurrent inhibitory Renshaw loop; p. 307), cerebellum (as the main transmitter of Purkinje neurones) and elsewhere. It is stored in flattened or pleomorphic vesicles within symmetrical synapses: it may be inhibitory to the postsynaptic neurone, or it may mediate either presynaptic inhibition or facilitation, depending on the synaptic arrangement.

Glutamate and aspartate are major excitatory transmitters present widely within the CNS, including the major projection pathways from the cortex to the thalamus, tectum, substantia nigra and pontine nuclei. They are found in the central terminals of the auditory and trigeminal nerves, and glutamate is present in the terminals of parallel fibres ending on Purkinje cells in the cerebellum. Structurally, they are associated with asymmetrical synapses containing small (c.30 nm) round, clear synaptic vesicles.

Glycine is a well-established inhibitory transmitter of the CNS, particularly the lower brainstem and spinal cord, where it is mainly found in local circuit neurones.

Nitric oxide

Nitric oxide (NO) is of considerable importance at autonomic and enteric synapses, where it mediates smooth muscle relaxation. NO has been implicated in the mechanism of long-term potentiation. The gas is able to diffuse freely through cell membranes, and so is not under such tight quantal control as vesicle-mediated neurotransmission.

Neuropeptides

Many neuropeptides coexist with other neuromediators in the same synaptic terminals. As many as three peptides often share a particular ending with a well-established neurotransmitter, in some cases within the same synaptic vesicles. Some peptides occur both in the CNS and PNS, particularly in the ganglion cells and peripheral terminals of the ANS, whilst others are entirely restricted to the CNS. Only a few examples are given here.

Most of the neuropeptides are classified according to the site where they were first discovered; for example, the gastrointestinal peptides were initially found in the gut wall, and a group first associated with the pituitary gland includes releasing hormones, adenohypophyseal and neurohypophyseal hormones. Some of these peptides are closely related to each other in their chemistry, because they are derived from the same gene products (e.g. the pro-opiomelanocortin group), which are cleaved to produce smaller peptides.

Substance P (SP) was the first of the peptides to be characterized as a gastrointestinal neuromediator. It consists of 11 amino acid residues and is a major neuromediator in the brain and spinal cord. It occurs in c.20% of dorsal root and trigeminal ganglion cells, in particular in small nociceptive neurones. It is also present in some fibres of the facial, glossopharyngeal and vagal nerves. Within the CNS, SP is present in several apparently unrelated major pathways. It is contained within large granular synaptic vesicles. Its known action is prolonged post-synaptic excitation.

Vasoactive intestinal polypeptide (VIP), another gastrointestinal peptide, is widely present in the CNS, where it is probably an excitatory neurotransmitter or neuromodulator. Its distribution includes distinctive bipolar neurones of the cerebral cortex, small dorsal root ganglion cells, particularly of the sacral region, the median eminence of the hypothalamus, where it may be involved in endocrine regulation, intramural ganglion cells of the gut wall and sympathetic ganglia.

Somatostatin (ST, somatotropin release inhibiting factor) has a broad distribution within the nervous system, and may be a central neurotransmitter or neuromodulator. It occurs in small dorsal root ganglion cells.

β-Endorphin, leu- and metenkephalins and the dynorphins belong to a group of peptides (naturally occurring opiates) which have aroused much interest because of their analgesic properties. They bind to opiate receptors in the brain where, in general, their action seems to be inhibitory. The enkephalins have been localized in many areas of the brain, particularly the septal nuclei, amygdaloid complex, basal ganglia and hypothalamus, from which it has been inferred that they are important mediators in the limbic system and in the control of endocrine function. They have been implicated strongly in the central control of pain pathways, because they are found in the periaqueductal grey matter of the midbrain, a number of reticular raphe nuclei, the spinal nucleus of the trigeminal nerve and the substantia gelatinosa of the spinal cord. The enkephalinergic pathways exert an important presynaptic inhibitory action on nociceptive afferents in the spinal cord and brainstem. Like many other neuromediators, the enkephalins also occur widely in other parts of the brain in lower concentrations.

CENTRAL GLIA

Glial (neuroglial) cells vary considerably in type and number in different regions of the CNS. There are two major groups which are classified according to origin. Macroglia arise within the neural plate, in parallel with neurones, and constitute the great majority of glial cells. Microglia are smaller cells, generally considered to be monocytic in origin, and are derived from haemopoietic tissue (**Fig. 4.9**).

ASTROCYTES

Astrocytes are star-shaped glia whose processes ramify through the entire central neuropil (**Fig. 4.9**). Their processes are functionally coupled at gap junctions and form an interconnected network which ensheathes all neurones, except at synapses and along the myelinated segments of axons. Astrocyte processes terminate as end-feet at the basal lamina of blood vessels and where they form the glia limitans (glial limiting membrane) at the pial surface (p. 284). Ultrastructurally, astrocytes

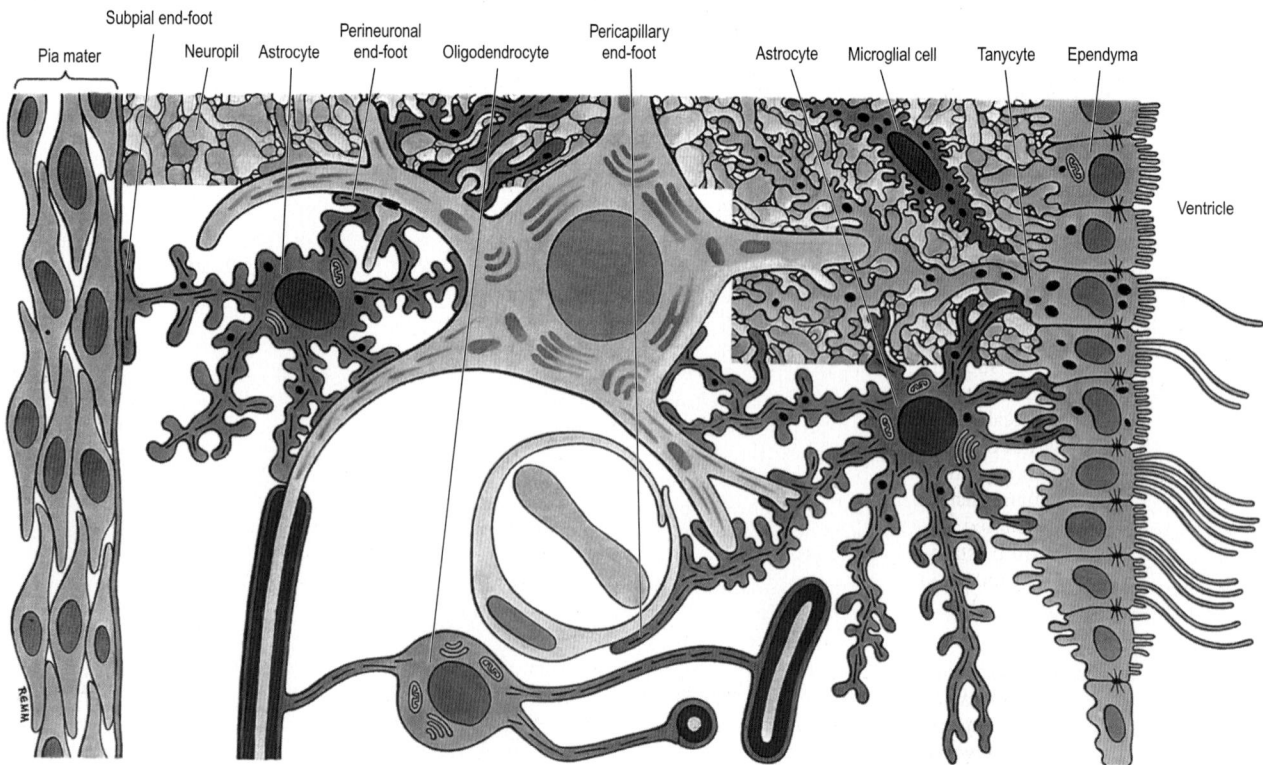

Fig. 4.9 The different types of non-neuronal cell in the CNS and their structural organization and interrelationships with each other and with neurones.

typically have a pale nucleus with a narrow rim of heterochromatin, although this is variable. They have a pale cytoplasm containing glycogen, lysosomes, Golgi complexes and bundles of glial intermediate filaments within their processes (these last are found particularly in fibrous astrocytes, which occur predominantly in white matter). Glial intermediate filaments are formed from glial fibrillary acidic protein (GFAP): its presence can be used clinically to identify tumour cells of glial origin. A second morphological type of astrocyte, the protoplasmic astrocyte, is found mainly in grey matter. The significance of these subtypes is unclear: there are few known functional differences between fibrous and protoplasmic astrocytes.

Astrocytes are thought to provide a network of communication in the brain via interconnecting low resistance gap junctional complexes (p. 7). They signal to each other using intracellular calcium wave propagation, triggered by synaptically released glutamate. Functionally, this may coordinate astrocyte activities, e.g. ion (particularly potassium) buffering; neurotransmitter uptake and metabolism (e.g. of excess glutamate, which is excitotoxic); membrane transport; the secretion of peptides, amino acids, trophic factors etc., essential for efficient neuronal activity.

Injury to the CNS induces astrogliosis, which is seen as a local increase in the number and size of cells expressing GFAP and in the extent of their meshwork of processes which form a glial scar. It is thought that the local glial scar environment, which may include oligodendrocytes and myelin debris, inhibits regeneration of CNS axons and/or fails to provide the necessary stimuli for axonal regrowth.

Pituicytes are glial cells found in the neural parts of the pituitary gland, the infundibulum and neurohypophysis. They resemble astrocytes, but their processes end mostly on endothelial cells in the neurohypophysis and tuber cinereum.

Blood–brain barrier

Proteins circulating in the blood enter most tissues of the body except those of the brain, spinal cord or peripheral nerves. This concept of a blood–brain barrier (and blood–nerve barrier) covers many substances, some of which are actively transported across the blood–brain barrier, whereas others are actively excluded. The blood–brain barrier is located at the capillary endothelium within the brain. It depends upon the presence of tight junctions between endothelial cells and a relative lack of transcytotic vesicular transport (pp. 11, 146). The tightness of the barrier depends upon the close apposition of astrocytes to blood capillaries (**Figs 4.10C, 4.11**).

The blood–brain barrier develops during embryonic life but may not be fully completed by birth. Moreover, there are certain areas of the adult brain in which the endothelial cells do not have tight junctions and a free exchange of molecules occurs between blood and adjacent brain. Most of these areas are situated close to the ventricles and are known as circumventricular organs (p. 53). Otherwise unrestricted diffusion through the blood–brain barrier is only possible for substances which can cross biological membranes because of their lipophilic character. Lipophilic molecules may be actively re-exported by the brain endothelium.

Breakdown of the blood–brain barrier occurs following brain damage caused by ischaemia or infection, and this permits an influx of fluid, ions, protein and other substances into the brain. It is also associated with primary and metastatic cerebral tumours. CT and MRI scans can demonstrate such breakdown of the blood–brain barrier clinically. A similar breakdown of the blood–brain barrier may be seen at postmortem in patients who are jaundiced. Normally brain, spinal cord and peripheral nerves remain unstained by the bile, except for the choroid plexus, which is often stained a deep yellow. However, areas of recent infarction (1–3 days), will be stained by bile pigment as a result of localized breakdown of the blood–brain barrier.

OLIGODENDROCYTES

Oligodendrocytes myelinate CNS axons and are most commonly seen as intrafascicular cells in myelinated tracts (**Figs 4.12, 4.13**). They usually have round nuclei and their cytoplasm contains numerous mitochondria, microtubules and glycogen. They display a spectrum of morphological variation, from large euchromatic nuclei and pale cytoplasm, to heterochromatic nuclei and dense cytoplasm. Oligodendrocytes may enclose up to 50 axons in separate myelin sheaths: the largest calibre axons are usually ensheathed on a 1:1 basis. Some oligo-

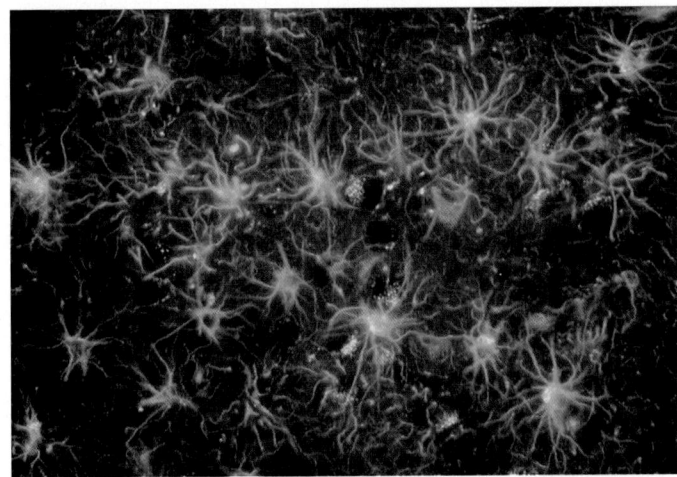

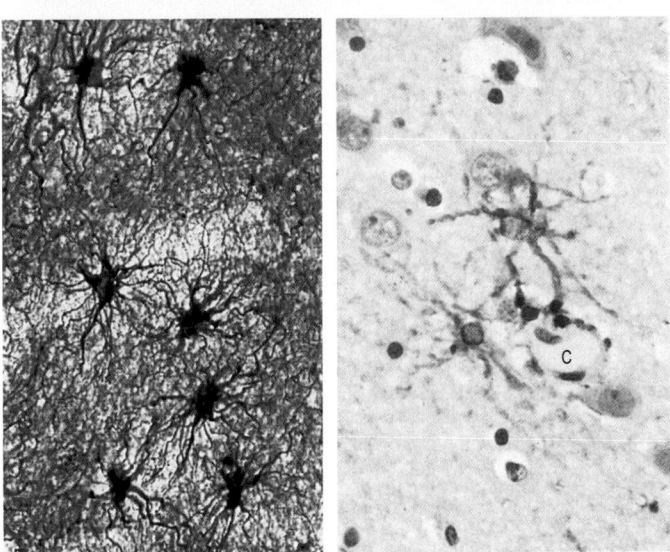

Fig. 4.10 Astrocytes. **A**, Immunofluorescent technique, human cerebral cortex, showing astrocytes immunopositive for glial fibrillary acidic protein (GFAP). **B**, Classic heavy metal impregnation technique (Cajal method). **C**, Immunoperoxidase technique, GFAP. Note perivascular end-feet embracing the capillary, C. (**A**, preparation by Jonathan Carlisle, Division of Anatomy and Cell Biology, GKT School of Medicine, London.) (**B** and **C**, by permission from Young B, Heath JW 2000 Wheater's Functional Histology. Edinburgh: Churchill Livingstone.)

dendrocytes are not associated with axons, and are either precursor cells or perineuronal (satellite) oligodendrocytes whose processes ramify around neuronal somata.

Within tracts, interfascicular oligodendrocytes are arranged in long rows in which single astrocytes intervene at regular intervals. Groups of oligodendrocytes myelinate the surrounding axons: their processes are radially aligned to the axis of each row. Myelinated tracts therefore consist of cables of axons, which are predominantly myelinated by a row of oligodendrocytes running down the axis of each cable.

Oligodendrocytes originate from the ventricular neurectoderm and the subependymal layer in the fetus (p. 262), and continue to be generated from the subependymal plate postnatally. Stem cells migrate and seed into white and grey matter to form a pool of adult progenitor cells which may later differentiate to replenish lost oligodendrocytes, and possibly remyelinate pathologically demyelinated regions.

Nodes of Ranvier and incisures of Schmidt–Lanterman

The territory ensheathed by an oligodendrocyte process defines an internode, the interval between internodes is called a node of Ranvier and the territory immediately adjacent to the nodal gap is a paranode, where loops of oligodendrocyte cytoplasm abut the axolemma. Nodal axolemma is contacted by the end-feet of perinodal cells which have been shown in animal studies to have a presumptive adult oligodendrocyte progenitor phenotype: their function is unknown (Butt &

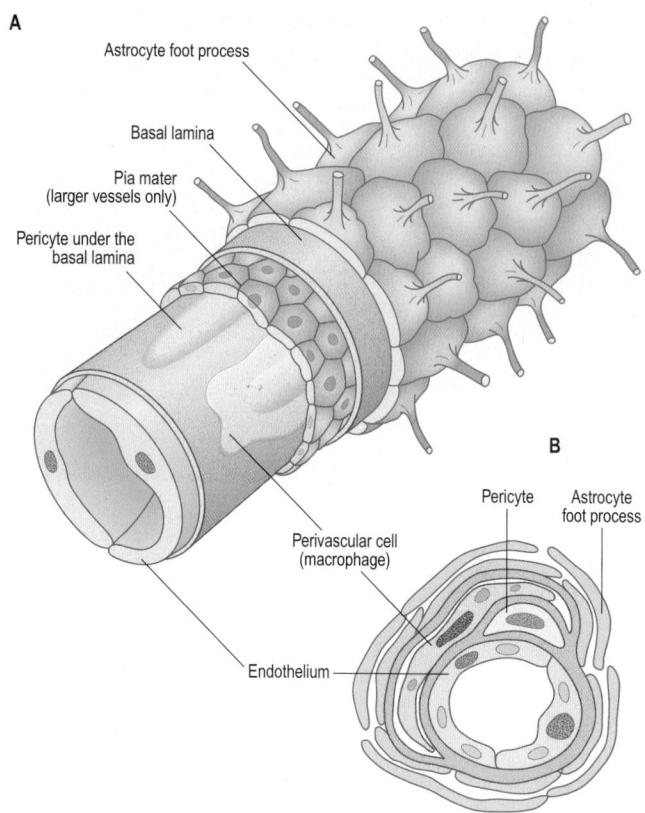

Fig. 4.11 The relationship between the glia limitans, perivascular cells and blood vessels within the brain, in longitudinal and transverse section. A sheath of astrocytic end-feet wraps around the vessel and, in vessels larger than capillaries, its investment of pial meninges. Vascular endothelial cells are joined by tight junctions and supported by pericytes; perivascular macrophages lie outside the endothelial basal lamina.

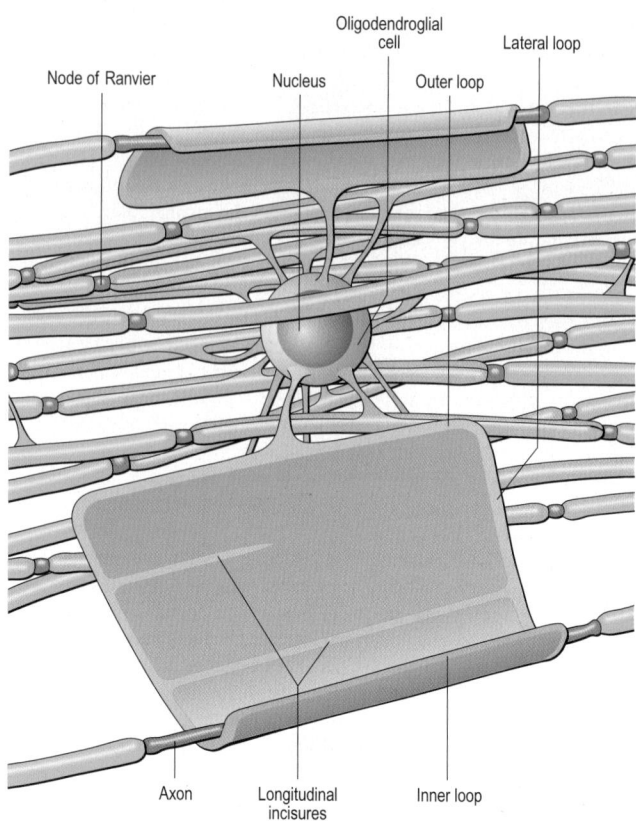

Fig. 4.12 The ensheathment of a number of axons by the processes of an oligodendrocyte. The oligodendrocyte soma is shown in the centre and its myelin sheaths are unfolded to varying degrees to show their extensive surface area. (Modified from Morell and Norton 1980 by Raine 1984, by permission.)

Berry 2000). Schmidt–Lanterman incisures are helical decompactions of internodal myelin where the major dense line of the myelin sheath splits to enclose a spiral of oligodendrocyte cytoplasm. Their function is unknown: their structure suggests that they may play a role in the transport of molecules across the myelin sheath.

MYELIN AND MYELINATION

Myelin is secreted by oligodendrocytes (CNS) and Schwann cells (PNS). A single oligodendrocyte may ensheathe up to 50 separate axons, depending upon calibre, whereas myelinating Schwann cells ensheathe axons on a 1:1 basis.

In general, myelin is laid down around axons above 2 μm diameter. However, the critical minimal axon diameter for myelination is smaller and more variable in the CNS than in the PNS and is c.0.2 μm (compared with 1–2 μm in the PNS). Since there is considerable overlap between the size of the smallest myelinated and the largest unmyelinated axons, axonal calibre is unlikely to be the only factor in determining myelination. Additionally, the first axons to become ensheathed ultimately reach larger diameters than later ones. There is a reasonable linear relationship between axon diameter and internodal length and myelin sheath thickness. As the sheath thickens from a few lamellae to up to 200, the axon may also grow from 1 to 15 μm in diameter. Internodal lengths increase about tenfold during the same time.

It is not known how myelin is formed in either PNS or CNS. The ultrastructural appearance of myelin (**Fig. 4.14**) is usually explained in terms of the spiral wrapping of a flat glial process around an axon, and the subsequent extrusion of cytoplasm from the sheath at all points other than incisures and paranodes (p. 56). In this way, the compacted external surfaces of the plasma membrane of the ensheathing glial cell are thought to produce the minor dense lines, and the compacted inner

cytoplasmic surfaces, the major dense lines, of the mature myelin sheath (**Fig. 4.15**). These correspond to the intraperiod and period lines respectively defined in X-ray studies of myelin. The inner and outer zones of occlusion of the spiral process are continuous with the minor dense line and are called the inner and outer mesaxons.

There are significant differences between central and peripheral myelin, reflecting the fact that oligodendrocytes and Schwann cells express different proteins during myelinogenesis. The basic dimensions of the myelin membrane are different. CNS myelin has a period repeat thickness of 15.7 nm whereas PNS myelin has a period to period line thickness of 18.5 nm. The major dense line space is c.1.7 nm in CNS myelin, compared with 2.5 nm in PNS myelin.

Myelin membrane contains protein, lipid and water, which forms at least 20% of the wet weight. It is a relatively lipid-rich membrane and contains 70–80% lipid. All classes of lipid have been found: the precise lipid composition of PNS and CNS myelin is different. The major lipid species are cholesterol (the commonest single molecule), phospholipids and glycosphingolipids. Minor lipid species include galactosylglycerides, phosphoinositides and gangliosides. The major glycolipids are galacto-cerebroside and its sulphate ester, sulphatide: these lipids are not unique to myelin, but they are present in characteristically high concentrations. CNS and PNS myelin also contain low concentrations of acidic glycolipids, which constitute important antigens in some inflammatory demyelinating states. Gangliosides, which are glycosphingolipids characterized by the presence of sialic acid (N-acetylneuraminic acid), account for less than 1% of the lipid.

A relatively small number of protein species account for the majority of myelin protein. Some of these proteins are common to both PNS and CNS myelin, but others are different. Proteolipid protein (PLP) and its splice variant DM20 are found only in CNS myelin, whereas myelin basic protein (MBP) and myelin associated glycoprotein (MAG) occur in both. MAG is a member of the immunoglobulin supergene family, and is localized specifically at those regions of the myelin segment where compaction starts, namely, the mesaxons and inner periaxonal

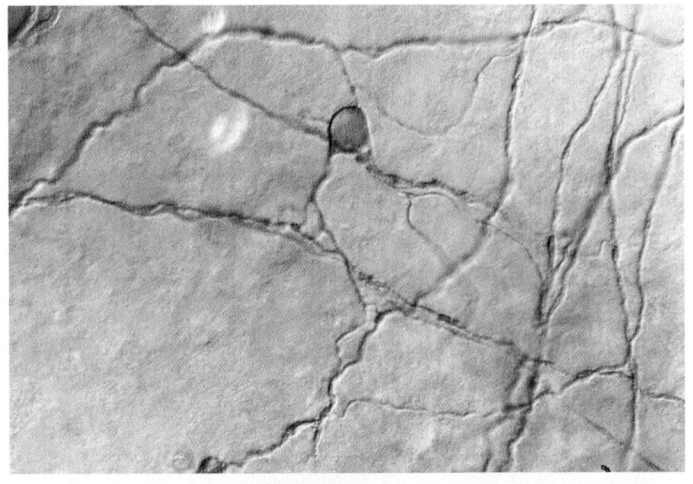

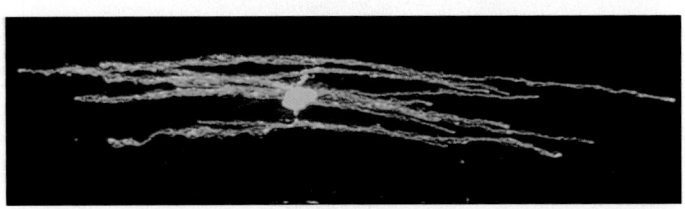

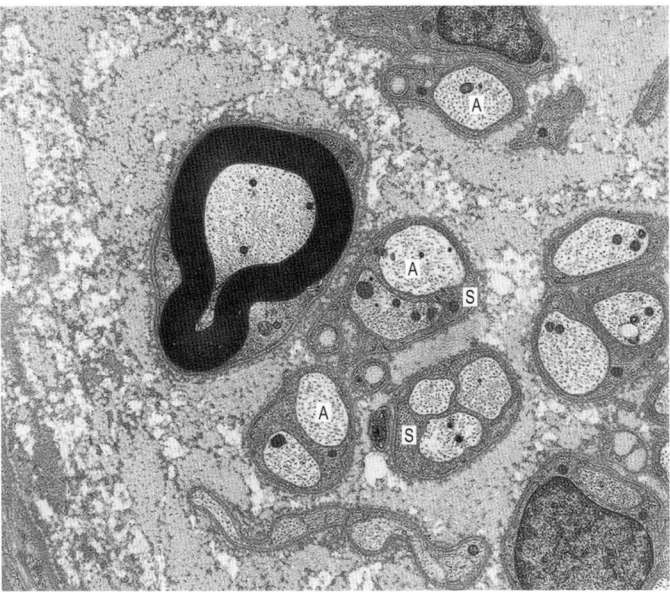

Fig. 4.14 Transverse section of sciatic nerve showing a myelinated axon and several non-myelinated axons (A), ensheathed by Schwann cells (S). (Provided by Professor Susan Standring, GKT School of Medicine, London.)

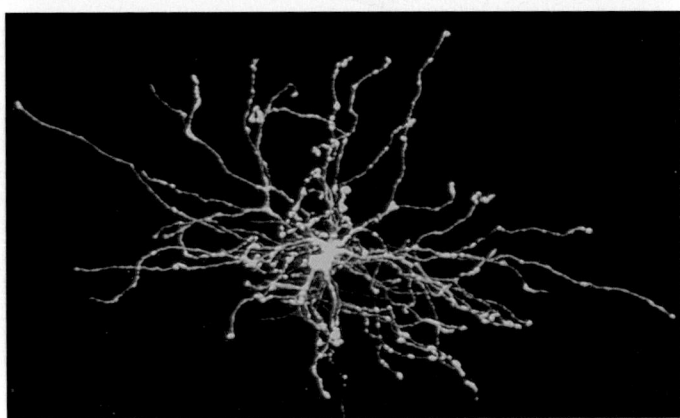

Fig. 4.13 A, An oligodendrocyte enwrapping several axons with myelin, demonstrated in a whole-mounted rat anterior medullary velum, immunolabelled with antibody to an oligodendrocyte membrane antigen. **B, C,** Confocal micrographs of a mature myelin forming oligodendrocyte (B) and astrocyte (C) iontophoretically filled in the adult rat optic nerve with an immunofluorescent dye by intracellular microinjection. (**A,** provided by Fiona Ruge; **B** and **C,** prepared by Dr A Butt and Kate Colquhoun, Division of Physiology, GKT School of Medicine, London. Photograph by Sarah-Jane Smith using the pseudocolour technique, Division of Anatomy and Cell Biology, GKT School of Medicine, London.)

membranes, paranodal loops and incisures, in both CNS and PNS sheaths. It is thought to have a functional role in membrane adhesion.

In the developing CNS, axonal outgrowth precedes the migration of oligodendrocyte precursors, and oligodendrocytes associate with and myelinate axons after their phase of elongation: oligodendrocyte myelin gene expression is not dependent on axon-association. In marked contrast, Schwann cells in the developing PNS are associated with axons during the entire phase of outgrowth from CNS to target organ.

Myelination does not occur simultaneously in all parts of the body in late fetal and early postnatal development. White matter tracts and nerves in the periphery have their own specific temporal patterns, which relate to their degree of functional maturity.

Mutations of the major myelin structural proteins have now been recognized in a number of inherited human neurological diseases. As would be expected, these mutations produce defects in myelination, and in the stability of nodal and paranodal architecture, which are consistent with the suggested functional roles of the relevant proteins in maintaining the integrity of the myelin sheath. The molecular organization of myelinated axons is described in Scherer & Arroyo (2002).

EPENDYMA

Ependymal cells line the ventricles and central canal of the spinal cord (**Fig. 4.16**). They form a single-layered epithelium which varies from squamous to columnar in form. At the ventricular surface, cells are joined by gap junctions and occasional desmosomes. Their apical surfaces have numerous microvilli and cilia, which contribute to the flow of cerebrospinal fluid (p. 292). There is considerable regional variation in the ependymal lining of the ventricles, but four major types have been described. These are general ependyma which overlies grey matter; general ependyma which overlies white matter; specialized areas of ependyma in the third and fourth ventricles; choroidal epithelium.

The ependymal cells overlying areas of grey matter are cuboidal; each cell bears c.20 central apical cilia, surrounded by short microvilli. The cells are joined by gap junctions and desmosomes and do not have a basal lamina. Beneath them there may be a subependymal zone, from two to three cells deep, which consists of cells which generally resemble ependymal cells. The capillaries beneath them have no fenestrations and few transcytotic vesicles, which is typical of the CNS. Where the ependyma overlies myelinated tracts of white matter, the cells are much flatter and few are ciliated. There are gap junctions and desmosomes between cells, but their lateral margins interdigitate, unlike those overlying grey matter. No subependymal zone is present.

Specialized areas of ependymal cells are found in four areas around the margins of the third ventricle which are called the circumventricular organs. These are the lining of the median eminence of the hypothalamus; the subcommissural organ; the subfornical organ and the vascular organ of the lamina terminalis (p. 375). The area postrema, at the inferoposterior limit of the fourth ventricle, has a similar structure. In all of these sites the ependymal cells are only rarely ciliated and their ventricular surfaces bear many microvilli and apical blebs. They have numerous mitochondria, well-formed Golgi complexes and a rather flattened basal nucleus. They are joined laterally by tight junctions which form a barrier to the passage of materials across the ependyma, and desmosomes. Many of the cells are tanycytes (ependymal astrocytes) and have basal processes which project into the perivascular space surrounding the underlying capillaries. Significantly these capillaries are fenestrated and therefore do not form a blood–brain barrier. It is believed that neuropeptides can pass from nervous tissue into the cerebrospinal fluid (CSF) by active transport through the ependymal cells in these specialized areas, and in this way access a wide population of neurones via the permeable ependymal lining of the rest of the ventricle.

The ependyma is highly modified where it lies adjacent to the vascular layer of the choroid plexuses (p. 292).

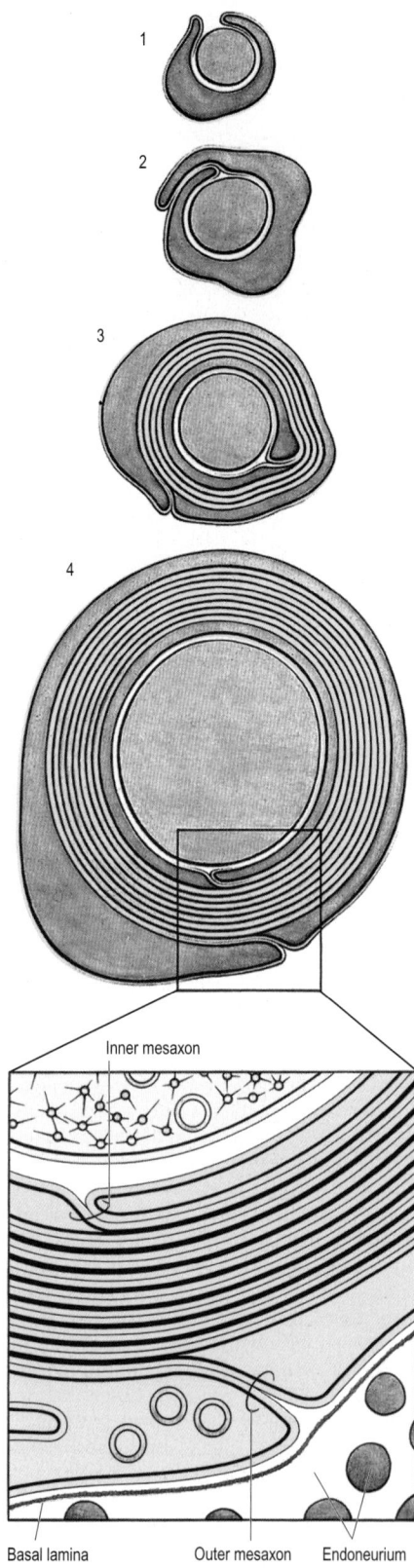

Fig. 4.15 Stages in myelination of a peripheral axon.

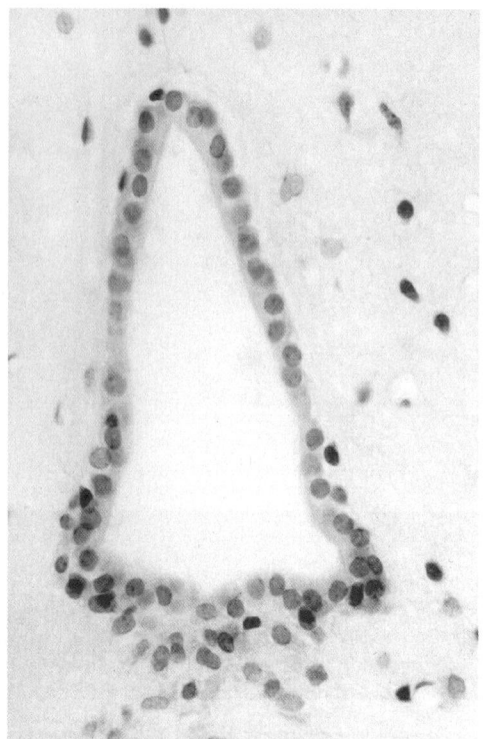

Fig. 4.16 Ciliated cuboidal ependymal cells lining the central canal of the spinal cord. Similar cells line most of the ventricular system of the brain. (By permission from Kierszenbaum AL 2002 Histology and Cell Biology. St Louis: Mosby, and by kind permission from Dr Wan-hua Amy Yu.)

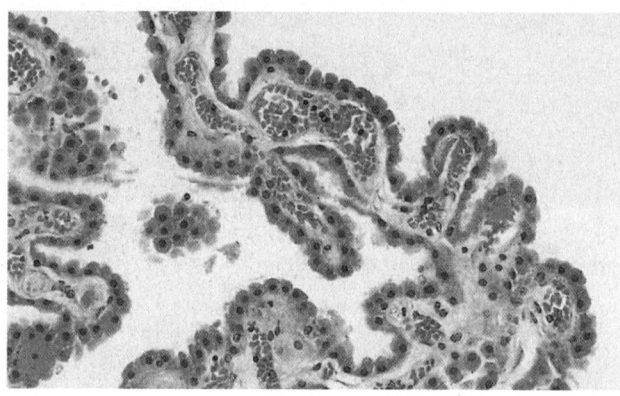

Fig. 4.17 Choroid plexus within a ventricle. Frond-like projections of vascular stroma derived from the pial meninges are covered with a low columnar epithelium which secretes cerebrospinal fluid. (By permission from Stevens A, Lowe JS 1996 Human Histology, 2nd edn. London: Mosby.)

Choroid plexus

The ependymal cells in the choroid plexuses resemble those of the circumventricular organs, except that they do not have basal processes, but form a cuboidal epithelium which rests on a basal lamina adjacent to the enclosed fold of pia mater (p. 284) and its capillaries (**Figs 4.17, 4.18**). Capillaries of the choroid plexuses are lined by a fenestrated endothelium. Cells have numerous long microvilli with only a few cilia interspersed between them. They also have many mitochondria, large Golgi complexes and basal nuclei, which is consistent with their secretory activity: they produce most components of the CSF. They are linked by tight junctions which form a transepithelial barrier (a component of the blood–CSF barrier), and by desmosomes. Their lateral margins are highly folded.

The choroid plexus has a villous structure where the stroma is composed of pial meningeal cells, and contains fine bundles of collagen and blood vessels. During fetal life, erythropoiesis occurs in the stroma, which is then occupied by bone marrow-like cells. In adult life the stroma contains phagocytic cells, and these, together with the cells of the choroid plexus epithelium, phagocytose particles and proteins from the ventricular lumen.

Age-related changes occur in the choroid plexus which can be detected on imaging the brain. Calcification of the choroid plexus can be detected by X-ray or CT scan in 0.5% of individuals in the first decade of life and in 86% in the eighth decade. There is a sharp rise in the incidence of calcification, from 35% of CT scans in the fifth decade, to 75% in the sixth decade. The visible calcification is usually restricted

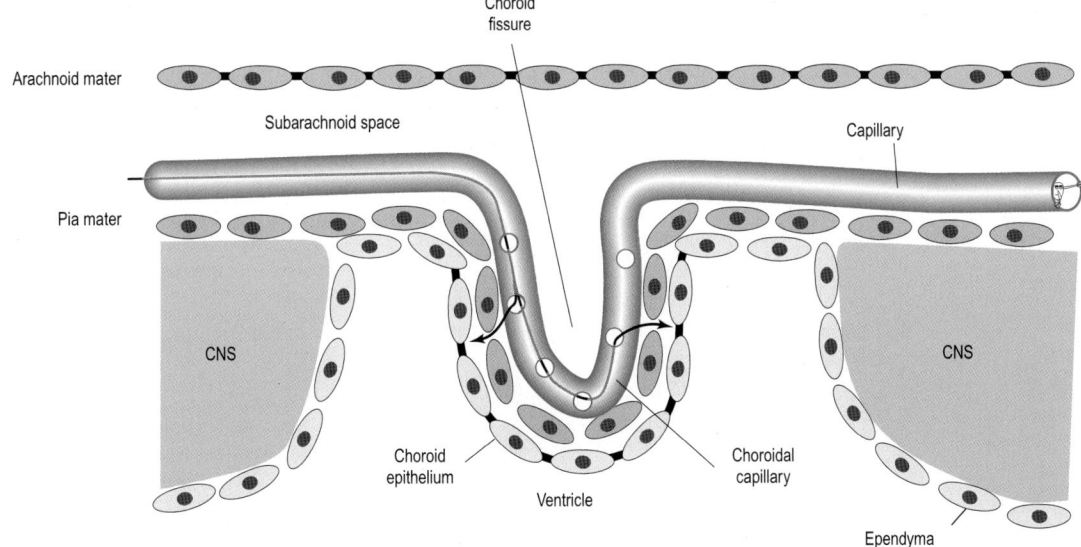

Fig. 4.18 Schematic representation of the arrangement of tissues forming the choroid plexus. (By permission from Nolte J 2002 The Human Brain, 5th edn. London: Mosby.)

to the glomus region of the choroid plexus, i.e. the vascular bulge in the choroid plexus as it curves to follow the anterior wall of the lateral ventricle into the temporal horn (p. 287).

MICROGLIA

Microglia are small dendritic cells found throughout the CNS (**Fig. 4.19**) including the retina (p. 712). Evidence largely supports the view that they are derived from fetal monocytes, or their precursors, which invade the developing nervous system. An alternative hypothesis holds that microglia share a lineage with ependymal cells and are thus neural tube derivatives. According to the monocyte theory, haematogenous cells pass through the walls of neural blood vessels and invade CNS tissue prenatally as amoeboid cells. Later they lose their motility and transform into typical microglia, bearing branched processes which ramify in non-overlapping territories within the brain. All microglial domains, defined by their dendritic fields, are equivalent in size, and form a regular mosaic throughout the brain. The expression of microglia-specific antigens changes with age: many are downregulated as microglia attain the mature dendritic form.

Microglia have elongated nuclei with peripheral heterochromatin. The scant cytoplasm is pale staining, and contains granules, scattered cisternae of rough endoplasmic reticulum and Golgi complexes at both poles. Two or three primary processes stem from opposite poles of the cell body and branch repeatedly to form short terminal processes. The function of microglia in the normal brain is obscure. Like astrocytes, microglia are activated by traumatic and ischaemic injury. In many diseases including Parkinson's disease, Alzheimer's disease, multiple sclerosis, acquired immunodeficiency syndrome (AIDS), amyotrophic lateral sclerosis (motor neurone disease) and paraneoplastic encephalitis, they become phagocytic and are actively involved in synaptic stripping and clearance of neuronal debris. Some transform into amoeboid, motile cells.

ENTRY OF INFLAMMATORY CELLS INTO THE BRAIN

Although the CNS has long been considered to be an immunologically privileged site, lymphocyte surveillance of the brain may be a normal, low-grade activity, which is enhanced in disease. Lymphocytes are able to enter the brain in response to virus infections and as part of the auto-immune response in multiple sclerosis. Activated, but not resting, lymphocytes pass through the endothelium of small venules, a process that requires the expression of recognition and adhesion molecules, which are induced following cytokine activation. They subsequently migrate into the brain parenchyma. Within the CNS, microglia and astrocytes can be induced by T-cell cytokines to act as efficient antigen-presenting cells. Lymphocytes probably drain along lymphatic pathways to regional cervical lymph nodes.

Polymorphonuclear leukocyte entry into the CNS is less common than lymphocyte entry, but is seen in the early stages of infarction and autoimmune disease and, in particular, in pyogenic infections. These cells probably enter the nervous system following expression of adhesion molecules on endothelium and pass through the endothelial layer. In the later stages of inflammation, monocytes may follow similar pathways.

Within the subarachnoid space, polymorphonuclear leukocytes and lymphocytes pass through the endothelium of large veins into the CSF during the inflammatory phase of meningitis.

PERIPHERAL NERVES

Afferent nerve fibres connect peripheral receptors to the CNS: their neuronal somata are located either in special sense organs (e.g. the olfactory epithelium) or in the sensory ganglia of craniospinal nerves. Efferent nerve fibres connect the CNS to the effector cells and tissues: they are the peripheral axons of neurones with somata in the central grey matter.

Peripheral nerve fibres are grouped in widely variable numbers into bundles (fasciculi). The size, number and pattern of fasciculi (**Fig. 4.20**) vary in different nerves and at different levels along their paths. Their number increases and their size decreases some distance proximal to a point of branching. Where nerves are subjected to pressure, e.g. deep to a retinaculum, fasciculi are increased in number but reduced in size, and the amount of associated connective tissue and degree of vascularity

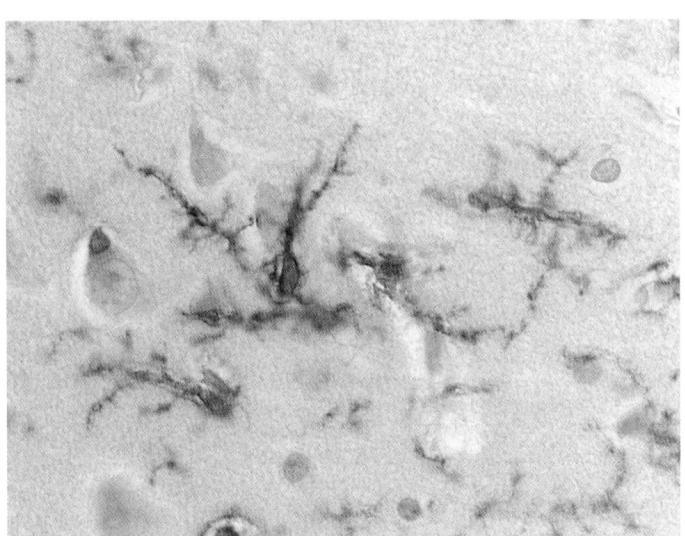

Fig. 4.19 Micrograph showing activated microglial cells in the central nervous system, in a biopsy from a patient with Rasmussen's encephalitis, visualized using MHC class II antigen immunohistochemistry. (By kind permission from Dr Norman Gregson, Division of Neurology, GKT School of Medicine, London.)

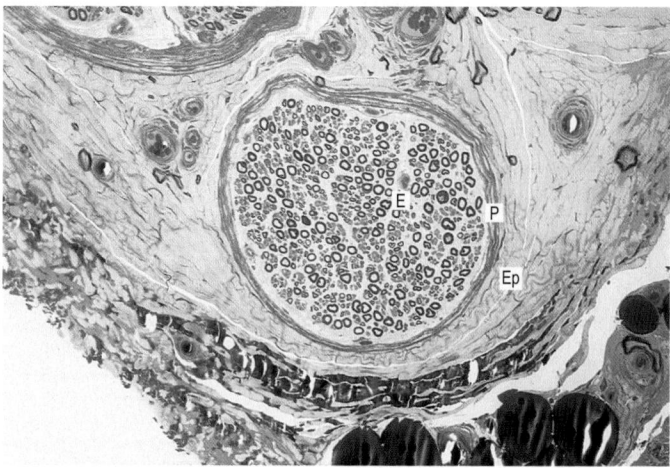

Fig. 4.20 Transverse section through a peripheral nerve, showing the arrangement of its connective tissue sheaths. Individual axons, myelinated and unmyelinated, are arranged in a small fascicle bounded by a perineurium. Abbreviations: P, perineurium; Ep, epineurium; E, endoneurium. (Provided by Professor Susan Standring, GKT School of Medicine, London.)

also increase. At these points, nerves may occasionally show a pink, fusiform dilatation, sometimes termed a pseudoganglion or gangliform enlargement.

PERIPHERAL NERVE FIBRES

The classification of peripheral nerve fibres is based on various parameters such as conduction velocity, function and fibre diameter. Of two classifications in common use, the first divides fibres into three major classes, designated A, B and C, corresponding to peaks in the distribution of their conduction velocities. In man, group A fibres are subdivided into α, δ and γ subgroups: B group fibres are preganglionic autonomic efferents, and C fibres are unmyelinated. Fibre diameter and conduction velocity are proportional in most fibres. Group Aα fibres are the largest and conduct most rapidly, and C fibres are the smallest and slowest.

The largest afferent axons (Aα fibres) innervate encapsulated cutaneous, joint and muscle receptors, and some large alimentary enteroceptors. Aδ fibres innervate thermoreceptors and nociceptors, including those in dental pulp, skin and connective tissue. C fibres have thermoreceptive, nociceptive and interoceptive functions. The largest somatic efferent fibres (Aα) are up to 20 μm in diameter. They innervate extrafusal muscle fibres exclusively and conduct at a maximum of 120 m/s. Fibres to fast twitch muscles are larger than those to slow twitch muscle. Aβ fibres are restricted to collaterals of Aα fibres, and form plaque endings on some intrafusal muscle fibres. Aγ fibres are exclusively fusimotor to plate and trail endings on intrafusal muscle fibres. C fibres are postganglionic sympathetic and parasympathetic axons. This scheme can be applied to all fibres of spinal and cranial nerves except perhaps those of the olfactory nerve, whose fibres form a uniquely small and slow group.

A different classification, used for afferent fibres of somatic muscles, divides myelinated fibres into groups I, II and III. Group I fibres are large (12–22 μm), and include primary sensory fibres of muscle spindles (Group Ia) and smaller fibres of Golgi tendon organs (Group Ib). Group II fibres are the secondary sensory terminals of muscle spindles, with diameters of 6–12 μm. Group III fibres, 1–6 μm in diameter, have free sensory endings in the connective tissue sheaths around and within muscles, and are believed to be nociceptive, relaying pressure pain in externally stimulated muscles. Paciniform (encapsulated) endings of muscle sheaths may also contribute fibres to this class. Group IV fibres are unmyelinated, with diameters below 1.5 μm: they include free endings in muscles, and are primarily nociceptive.

CONNECTIVE TISSUE SHEATHS

Nerve trunks, whether uni- or multifascicular, are surrounded by an epineurium. Individual fasciculi are enclosed by a multilayered perineurium, which in turn surrounds the endoneurium or intrafascicular connective tissue (**Fig. 4.20**).

Epineurium

Epineurium is a condensation of loose (areolar) connective tissue, and is derived from mesoderm. As a general rule, the more fasciculi present in a peripheral nerve, the thicker the epineurium. Epineurium contains fibroblasts, collagen (types I and III), and variable amounts of fat, and it cushions the nerve it surrounds. Loss of this protective layer may be associated with pressure palsies seen in wasted, bedridden patients. The epineurium also contains lymphatics (which probably pass to regional lymph nodes) and blood vessels, the vasa nervorum, which pass across the perineurium to communicate with a network of fine vessels within the endoneurium.

Perineurium

Perineurium extends from the CNS–PNS transition zone to the periphery, where it is continuous with the capsules of muscle spindles and encapsulated sensory endings. At unencapsulated endings and neuromuscular junctions the perineurium ends openly. It consists of alternating layers of flattened polygonal cells which are thought to be derived from fibroblasts, and collagen. It can often contain 15–20 layers of such cells, each layer enclosed by a basal lamina up to 0.5 μm thick. Cells within each layer interdigitate along extensive tight junctions and their cytoplasm contains numerous pinocytotic vesicles and often, bundles of microfilaments. These features indicate that the perineurium functions as a metabolically active diffusion barrier, and together with the blood–nerve barrier (p. 58), probably plays an essential role in maintaining the osmotic milieu and fluid pressure within the endoneurium.

Endoneurium

Strictly speaking, the term endoneurium is restricted to interfascicular connective tissue excluding the perineurial partitions within fascicles. Endoneurium consists of a fibrous matrix composed predominantly of type I collagen fibres, which are mainly organized in fine bundles lying parallel to the long axis of the nerve, and condensed around individual Schwann cell-axon units and endoneurial vessels. The fibrous and cellular components of the endoneurium are bathed in endoneurial fluid at a slightly higher pressure than that outside in the surrounding epineurium. The major cellular constituents of the endoneurium are Schwann cells, associated with axons, and endothelial cells. Schwann cell-axon units and endothelial cells are enclosed within individual basal laminae. Other cells which are always present within the endoneurium are fibroblasts (constituting c.4% of the total endoneurial cell population), resident macrophages and mast cells.

Endoneurial arterioles have a poorly developed smooth muscle layer, and do not autoregulate well. In sharp contrast, epineurial and perineurial vessels have a dense perivascular plexus of peptidergic, serotoninergic and adrenergic nerves.

SCHWANN CELLS

Schwann cells are the major glial type in the PNS. *In vitro* they are fusiform in appearance. Both *in vitro* and *in vivo* they ensheathe peripheral axons, and myelinate those greater than 2 μm diameter. In a mature peripheral nerve fibre, they are distributed along the axons in longitudinal chains. The precise geometry of their association depends on whether the axon is myelinated or unmyelinated. In myelinated axons the territory of a Schwann cell defines an internode.

The molecular phenotype of mature myelin-forming Schwann cells is different from that of the mature non-myelinating Schwann cell. Adult myelin-forming Schwann cells are characterized by the presence of several myelin proteins, some, but not all, of which are shared with oligodendrocytes and central myelin. In contrast, expression of the low affinity neurotrophin receptor (p75[NTR]) and GFAP intermediate filament protein (which differs from the CNS form in its post-translational modification), characterize adult non-myelin forming Schwann cells.

Schwann cells arise during development from multipotent cells of the very early migrating neural crest (p. 244) which also give rise to peripheral neurones. Axon-associated signals are critical in controlling the proliferation of developing Schwann cells and their precursors. Neurones may also regulate the developmentally programmed death of Schwann cell precursors, as a mechanism for matching numbers of axons and glia within each peripheral nerve bundle. Neuronal signals appear to control the production of basal laminae by Schwann cells; the induction and maintenance of myelination; and, in the mature nerve, Schwann cell survival (few Schwann cells persist in chronically denervated nerves). Schwann cell signals may influence axonal calibre, and they are of crucial importance in the repair of damaged peripheral nerves. The acute Schwann cell response to axonal injury and degeneration involves mitotic division and the elaboration of signals which promote the regrowth of axons.

Unmyelinated axons

Unmyelinated axons are commonly <1.0 μm in diameter, although some may be 1.5 μm or even 2 μm in diameter. Groups of up to 10 small axons (0.15–2.0 μm in diameter), are enclosed within a chain of overlapping Schwann cells and surrounded by a basal lamina. Within each Schwann cell, individual axons are usually sequestered from their neighbours by delicate processes of cytoplasm (**Fig. 4.14**). Axons move between Schwann cell chains as they pass proximodistally along a nerve fasciculus. It seems likely, on the basis of quantitative studies in subhuman primates, that axons from adjacent cord segments may share Schwann cell columns: this phenomenon may play a role in the evolution of neuropathic pain after nerve injury. In the absence of a myelin sheath and nodes of Ranvier, conduction along unmyelinated axons is not saltatory but electrotonic: the passage of impulses is therefore relatively slow (c.0.5–4.0 m/s).

Myelinated axons

Myelinated axons (**Fig. 4.14**) have a 1:1 relationship with their ensheathing Schwann cells. The territory of an individual Schwann cell defines an internode (**Fig. 4.21**): internodal length varies directly with the diameter of the fibre, from 150 to 1500 μm. The interval between two internodes is a node of Ranvier. In the PNS, the myelin sheaths on either side of a node terminate in asymmetrically swollen paranodal bulbs. Schwann cell cytoplasm only forms a continuous layer in the perinuclear (mid-internodal) and paranodal regions. Between these sites, internodal Schwann cytoplasm forms a delicate network over the inner (abaxonal) surface of the myelin sheath. The outer (adaxonal)

layer of Schwann cell cytoplasm is frequently discontinuous, and axons are surrounded by a narrow periaxonal space (15–20 nm) which, although nominally part of the extracellular space, is functionally isolated from it at the paranodes. For further details, see Scherer & Arroyo (2002).

Nodes of Ranvier (Fig. 4.21)

PNS nodes of Ranvier are typically c.0.8–1.1 μm in length. The calibre of the nodal axon is characteristically reduced relative to that of the internodal axon: this is most marked in the largest calibre axons. Nodes are filled with an amorphous gap substance and processes of Schwann cell cytoplasm, and are surrounded by a continuous basal lamina elaborated by the ensheathing Schwann cells. In large calibre axons the surfaces of the paranodal bulbs and of the underlying axon are fluted as they approach the nodes. The grooves in the external surface of the myelin sheath that are produced by fluting are filled by Schwann cell cytoplasm characterized by large numbers of mitochondria. In smaller fibres this arrangement is less obvious, although the paranodal cytoplasm usually contains mitochondria. Fine processes arise from the paranodal collar of Schwann cell cytoplasm and extend into the nodal gap substance where they interdigitate with their counterparts from the adjacent Schwann cell. In small calibre axons the processes contact the nodal axolemma. In large calibre axons, where the processes are more numerous, they form regular hexagonal arrays which fill the nodal gap. Expanded terminal loops of paranodal Schwann cell cytoplasm either abut the paranodal axolemma directly or, in the case of the largest calibre myelinated axons, abut each other to form stacks with a typical 'ear of wheat' configuration.

Schmidt–Lanterman incisures

Schmidt–Lanterman incisures are helical decompactions of internodal myelin. The major dense line of the myelin sheath is split to enclose a continuous spiral band of granular cytoplasm which passes between

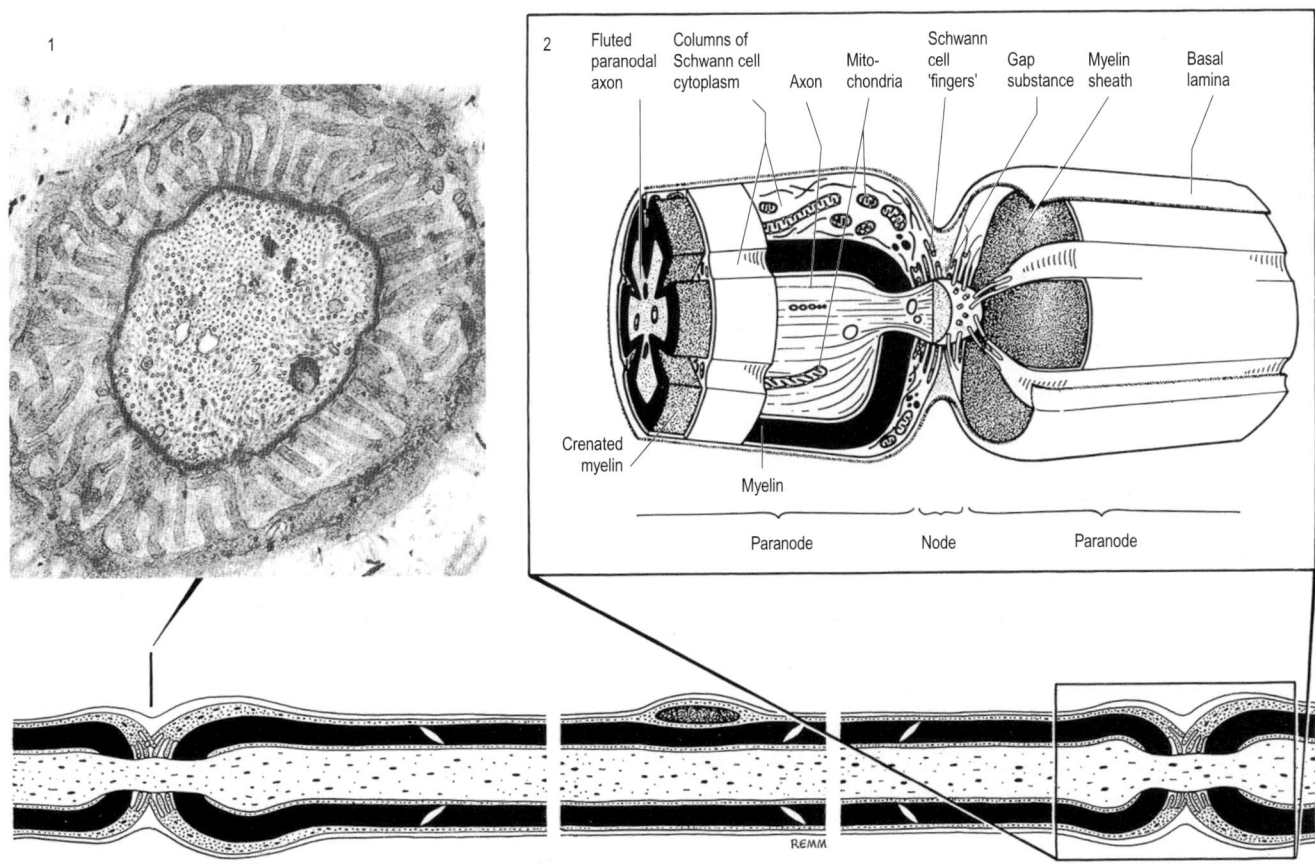

Fig. 4.21 General plan of a myelinated nerve fibre in longitudinal section including one complete internodal segment and two adjacent paranodal bulbs, used as a key for the more detailed microarchitecture of specific subregions. **1**: transverse section through the centre of a node of Ranvier, with numerous finger-like processes of adjacent Schwann cells converging towards the nodal axolemma. Many microtubules and neurofilaments are visible within the axoplasm. **2**: The arrangement of the axon, myelin sheath and Schwann cell cytoplasm at the node of Ranvier and in the paranodal bulbs. (**1**, provided by Professor Susan Standring, GKT School of Medicine, London; **2** provided by PL Williams and DN Landon.)

the abaxonal and adaxonal layers of Schwann cell cytoplasm. The minor dense line of the incisural myelin sheath separates to create a long channel which connects the periaxonal space with the extracellular fluid in the endoneurium. The function of incisures is not known: their structure suggests that they may participate in transport of molecules across the myelin sheath.

SATELLITE CELLS

Many non-neuronal cells of the nervous system have been called satellite cells. The list includes small round extracapsular cells in peripheral ganglia, ganglionic capsular cells and Schwann cells. The term is sometimes used to describe all non-neuronal cells, both central and peripheral, which are closely associated with neuronal somata. The name is also given to precursor cells associated with striated muscle fibres (p. 114). Within the nervous system, the term is most commonly reserved for the flat, epithelioid satellite cells (ganglionic glial cells, capsular cells) (see **Fig. 4.22**), which surround the neuronal somata of peripheral ganglia. The cytoplasm of capsular cells resembles that of Schwann cells and their deep surfaces interdigitate with reciprocal infoldings in the membranes of the enclosed neurones. The capsular layer is continuous with similar cells which enclose the initial part of the dendroaxonal process in unipolar sensory neurones of the dorsal spinal roots, and subsequently with the Schwann cells surrounding their peripheral and central processes.

Enteric glia

Autonomic nerves of the ENS (Ch. 70) have more in common with central tracts than with other peripheral nerves. Enteric nerves do not have the collagenous coats of other peripheral nerves, and they lack an endoneurium. The enteric ganglionic neurones are supported by glia which closely resemble astrocytes and contain more glial fibrillary acidic protein (GFAP) than non-myelinating Schwann cells. The enteric glia also differ from Schwann cells in that they do not produce a surrounding basal lamina.

Olfactory ensheathing glia

Olfactory ensheathing glia resemble Schwann cells in many respects but share a common origin with olfactory receptor neurones in the olfactory placode (p. 245). They ensheathe olfactory sensory axons in a manner which is reminiscent of developing peripheral nerves, because they surround, but do not segregate, bundles of up to 50 fine unmyelinated fibres to form c.20 fila olfactoria. Olfactory ensheathing glia accompany olfactory axons from the lamina propria of the olfactory epithelium to their synaptic contacts in the glomeruli of the olfactory bulbs. This unusual arrangement is quite unlike that seen at the CNS–PNS transition zone elsewhere in the nervous system, where there is an obvious boundary between the territories of peripheral and central glia.

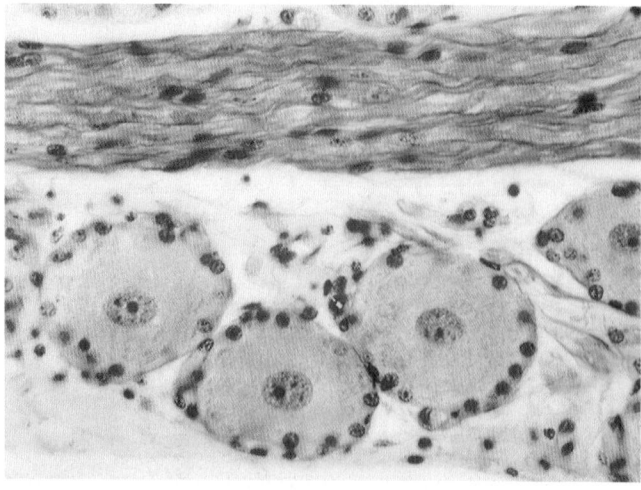

Fig. 4.22 A typical field in a dorsal root ganglion. Note the characteristic juxtaposition of large ovoid neuronal somata and the fascicles of myelinated and non-myelinated axons (top). Note also the nuclei of the capsular (satellite) cells which surround each neuronal soma. Grübler's stain. (By permission from Dr JB Kerr, Monash University, from Kerr JB 1999 Atlas of Functional Histology. London: Mosby.)

Ensheathing glia, and the end-feet of astrocytes which lie between olfactory axon bundles, both contribute to the glia limitans at the pial surface of the olfactory bulbs. Ensheathing glia have a malleable phenotype, indeed there may be more than one subtype. Some express GFAP as fine cytoplasmic filaments, and some express the low affinity neurotrophin receptor.

BLOOD SUPPLY OF PERIPHERAL NERVES

The blood vessels supplying a nerve end in a capillary plexus which pierces the perineurium. Its branches run parallel with the fibres, connected by short transverse vessels, forming narrow, oblong meshes similar to those found in muscle. The blood supply of peripheral nerves is unusual. Endoneurial capillaries have atypically large diameters and intercapillary distances are greater than in many other tissues. Peripheral nerves have two separate, functionally independent vascular systems: an extrinsic system (regional nutritive vessels and epineurial vessels) and an intrinsic system (longitudinally running microvessels in the endoneurium). Anastomoses between the two systems produce considerable overlap between the territories of the segmental arteries. This unique pattern of vessels, together with a high basal nerve blood flow relative to metabolic requirements, confer a high degree of resistance to ischaemia on peripheral nerves.

Blood–nerve barrier

Just as the neuropil within the central nervous system is protected by a blood–brain barrier, the endoneurial contents of peripheral nerve fibres are protected by a blood–nerve barrier and by the cells of the perineurium. The blood–nerve barrier operates at the level of the endoneurial capillary walls. The endothelial cells are joined by tight junctions, are non-fenestrated and surrounded by continuous basal laminae. The barrier is much less efficient in dorsal root and autonomic ganglia and in the distal parts of peripheral nerves.

GANGLIA

Ganglia are aggregations of neuronal somata. They occur in the dorsal roots of spinal nerves; in the sensory roots of the trigeminal, facial, glossopharyngeal, vagal and vestibulocochlear cranial nerves; in autonomic nerves and the enteric nervous system. They vary in form and size. Each ganglion is enclosed within a capsule of fibrous connective tissue and contains neuronal somata and neuronal processes. Some ganglia, particularly in the ANS, contain fibres whose cell bodies lie elsewhere in the nervous system and which pass through or terminate within them.

SENSORY GANGLIA

The sensory ganglia of dorsal spinal roots (**Fig. 4.22**) and the ganglia of the trigeminal, facial, glossopharyngeal and vagal cranial nerves are enclosed in periganglionic connective tissue, which resembles the perineurium. Ganglionic neurones are unipolar. They have spherical or oval somata of varying size, which are aggregated in groups between fasciculi of myelinated and unmyelinated nerve fibres. For each neurone, the single axodendritic process bifurcates into central and peripheral processes: in myelinated fibres the junction occurs at a node of Ranvier. The peripheral process reaches a sensory ending and, since it conducts impulses towards the soma, strictly speaking it functions as an elongated dendrite. However, since it has the typical structural and other functional properties of a peripheral axon, it is conventionally described as an axon.

Each soma has a capsule of satellite glial cells. Outside this lie the axodendritic process and its peripheral and central divisions which are ensheathed by Schwann cells. The cells lie within a delicate vascular connective tissue which is continuous with the endoneurium of the nerve root.

Sensory ganglionic neurones are not entirely confined to discrete craniospinal ganglia: they often occupy heterotopic positions, either singly or in small groups, distal or proximal to their ganglia.

Herpes zoster – Primary infection with the varicella zoster virus causes chickenpox. Following recovery, the virus remains dormant within dorsal root ganglia. Reactivation of the virus leads to shingles, which involves the dermatome supplied by the sensory nerve affected (p. 175). Severe pain and a rash similar to chickenpox, often confined to one of the divisions of the trigeminal nerve, or to a spinal nerve dermatome, are diagnostic. Herpes zoster involving the geniculate ganglion results in a lower motor neurone facial paralysis, known as Ramsay Hunt syndrome. Occasionally, if the vestibulocochlear nerve is involved, there is vertigo, tinnitus and some deafness.

AUTONOMIC GANGLIA

Neurones in autonomic ganglia are multipolar, and have dendritic trees on which preganglionic autonomic motor fibres synapse. They are surrounded by a mixed neuropil of afferent and efferent fibres, dendrites, synapses and non-neural cells. Autonomic ganglia are largely relay stations. A small fraction of their fibres traverse one or more ganglia without synapsing: some are efferent fibres en route to another ganglion, and some are afferents from the viscera and glands. There is considerable variation in the ratio between pre- and postganglionic fibres. Preganglionic sympathetic axons may synapse with many postganglionic neurones for the wide dissemination and perhaps amplification of sympathetic activity, a feature not found to the same degree in parasympathetic ganglia. Dissemination may also be achieved by connections with ganglionic interneurones or by the diffusion within the ganglion of transmitter substances either produced locally (paracrine effect) or elsewhere (endocrine effect).

Most neurones of autonomic ganglia have somata ranging from 25–50 μm; a less frequent type is smaller, 15–20 μm, and often clustered in groups. Dendritic fields of these multipolar neurones are complex and dendritic glomeruli have been observed in many ganglia. Clusters of small granular adrenergic vesicles occupy the soma and dendrites, probably representing the storage of catecholamines. Ganglionic neurones receive many axodendritic synapses from preganglionic nerve fibres; axosomatic synapses are less numerous. Postganglionic fibres commonly arise from the initial stem of a large dendrite and produce few or no collateral processes.

ENTERIC GANGLIA

The enteric nervous system is composed of ganglionic neurones and associated nerves (**Fig. 4.23**) serving different functions, including regulation of gut motility and mucosal transport. Extrinsic autonomic fibres supply the gut wall and, together with intrinsic enteric ganglionic

neurones, and the endocrine and cardiovascular systems, they integrate the activities of the digestive system either as a result of interaction with enteric neurones (e.g. via vagal fibres), or the direct regulation of the local blood flow (via postganglionic sympathetic fibres).

Enteric ganglionic neurones are predominantly peptidergic or monoaminergic and can be classified accordingly. Other neurones express nitric oxide synthase and release NO. There are regional differences in the numbers of ganglia and the classes of neurone they contain. For example, myenteric plexus ganglia are less frequent in oesophageal smooth muscle (1.5 per cm) than in the small and large intestines (c.10 per cm length of bowel). Oesophageal enteric neurones all coexpress vasoactive polypeptide (VIP) and neuropeptide Y (NPY), whereas gastrin- and somatostatin-containing fibres are rare. In contrast, gastrin and somatostatin-containing neurones are abundant in the small and large intestines, and although both types are present, very few VIP neurones coexpress NPY.

Correlations can be made between some phenotypic classes of enteric neurone and their functional properties, although much remains undetermined. Cholinergic neurones are excitatory, cause muscular contraction and mainly project orally. NO-releasing neurones are generally larger and project for longer distances, mainly anally. They are inhibitory neurones, some of which also express VIP, and they promote muscular relaxation.

SENSORY ENDINGS (Fig. 4.24)

GENERAL FEATURES OF SENSORY RECEPTORS

There are three major forms of sensory receptor.

A neuroepithelial receptor is a neurone with a soma situated near a sensory surface and an axon which conveys sensory signals into the CNS to synapse on second order neurones. This is an evolutionarily primitive arrangement, and the only example in man is the sensory neurone of the olfactory epithelium.

An epithelial receptor is a cell which is modified from a non-nervous sensory epithelium and innervated by a primary sensory neurone, whose soma lies near the CNS. Examples are epidermal Merkel cells, auditory receptors and taste buds. Activity in this type of receptor elicits the passage of excitation from the receptor by neurotransmission across a synaptic gap. In taste receptors, individual cells are constantly being renewed from the surrounding epithelium. In many ways visual receptors in the retina (p. 710) are similar in their form and relations. These cells are derived from the ventricular lining of the fetal brain and are not replaced.

A neuronal receptor is a primary sensory neurone which has a soma in a craniospinal ganglion and a peripheral axon, the end of which is a sensory terminal. All cutaneous sensors (with the exception of Merkel cells) and proprioceptors are of this type: their sensory terminals may be encapsulated or linked to special mesodermal or ectodermal structures to form a part of the sensory apparatus. The extraneural cells are not necessarily excitable, but create the environment for the excitation of the neuronal process.

The receptor stimulus is transduced into a graded change of electrical potential at the receptor surface (receptor potential), which initiates an all-or-none action potential transmitted to the CNS. This may occur in the receptor, where this is a neurone, or partly in the receptor and partly in the neurone innervating it, in the case of epithelial receptors.

Transduction varies with the modality of stimulus, usually causing depolarization of the receptor membrane (or, in the retina, hyperpolarization). In mechanoreceptors it may involve the deformation of membrane structure, which results in strain- or voltage-sensitive transducing protein molecules opening ion channels. In chemoreceptors, receptor action may resemble that for ACh at neuromuscular junctions. Visual receptors share similarities with chemoreceptors: light causes changes in receptor proteins, which activate G proteins, resulting in the release of second messengers, and this affects membrane permeability.

The quantitative responses of sensory endings to stimuli vary greatly and increase the flexibility of functional design of sensory systems. Although increased excitation with the increasing stimulus level is a common pattern ('on' response), some receptors respond to decreased stimulation ('off' response). Even unstimulated receptors show varying degrees of spontaneous background activity against which an increase or decrease in activity occurs with changing levels of stimulus. In all receptors studied, when stimulation is maintained at a steady level,

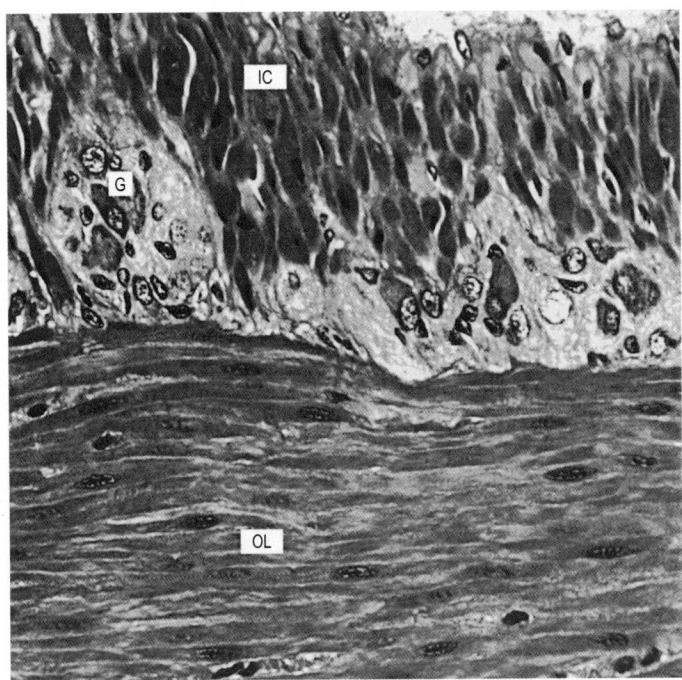

Fig. 4.23 The myenteric plexus of ganglia (G) and fibres which lies between the inner circular (IC) and outer longitudinal (OL) smooth muscle layers of the gut wall.

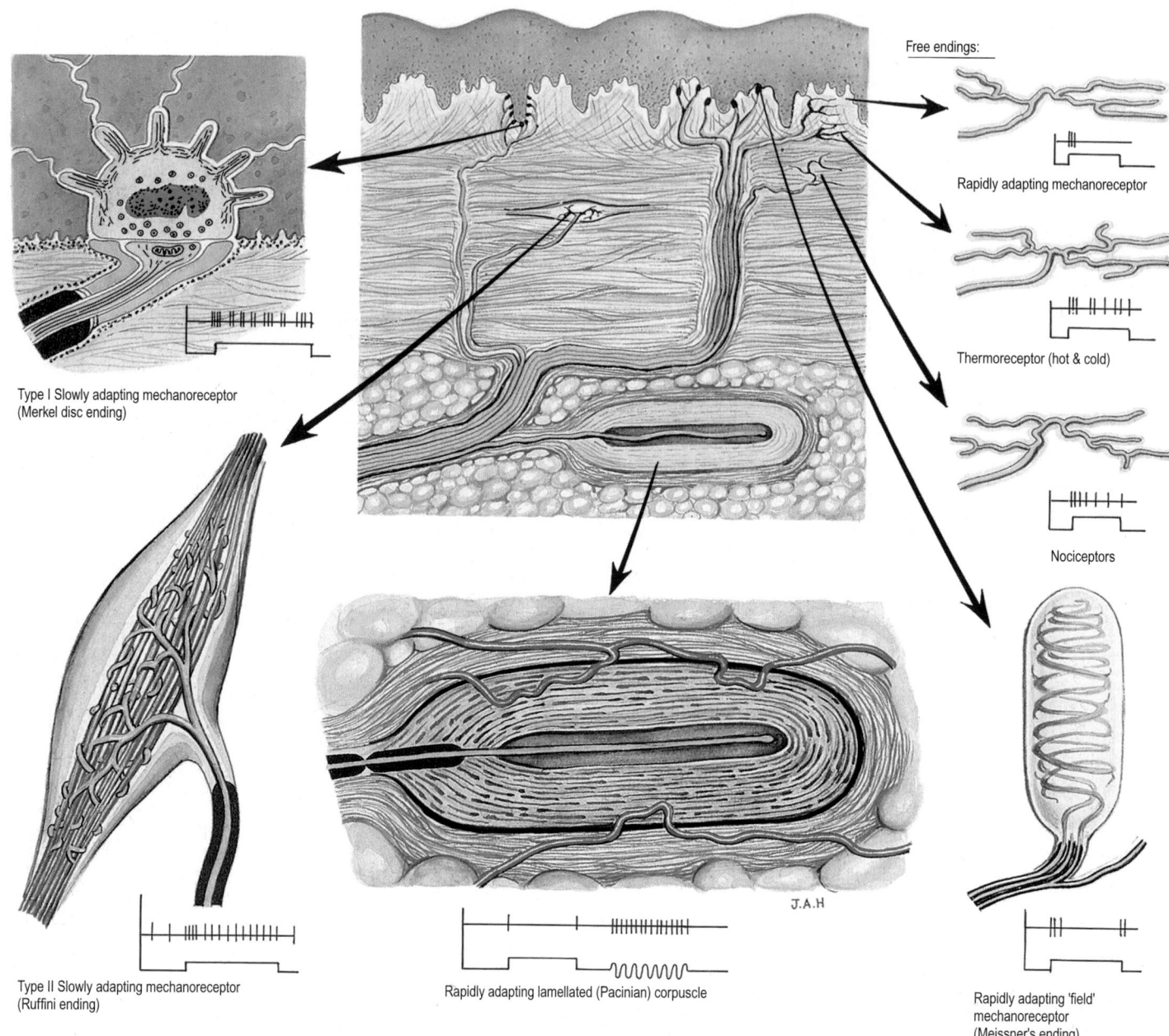

Type I Slowly adapting mechanoreceptor
(Merkel disc ending)

Free endings:

Rapidly adapting mechanoreceptor

Thermoreceptor (hot & cold)

Nociceptors

Type II Slowly adapting mechanoreceptor
(Ruffini ending)

Rapidly adapting lamellated (Pacinian) corpuscle

Rapidly adapting 'field'
mechanoreceptor
(Meissner's ending)

J.A.H

Fig. 4.24 Some major types of sensory ending of general afferent fibres (omitting neuromuscular, neurotendinous and hair-related types).

there is an initial burst (the dynamic phase) followed by a gradual adaptation to steady level (the static phase). Though all receptors show these two phases, one or other may predominate, providing a distinction between rapidly adapting endings which accurately record the rate of stimulus onset, and slowly adapting endings which signal the constant amplitude of a stimulus, e.g. position sense. Dynamic and static phases are reflected in the amplitude and duration of the receptor potential and also in the frequency of action potentials in the sensory fibres. The stimulus strength necessary to elicit a response in a receptor, i.e. its threshold level, varies greatly between receptors, and provides an extra level of information about stimulus strength.

For further information on sensory receptors, see Nolte (2002).

FUNCTIONAL CLASSIFICATION OF RECEPTORS

Receptors may be classified in several ways. They may be classified by the modalities to which they are sensitive, such as mechanoreceptors (which are responsive to deformation, e.g. touch, pressure, sound waves, etc.), chemoreceptors, photoreceptors and thermoreceptors. Some receptors respond selectively to more than one modality (polymodal receptors): they usually have high thresholds and respond to damaging stimuli associated with irritation or pain (nociceptors).

Another widely used classification divides receptors on the basis of their distribution in the body into exteroceptors, proprioceptors and interoceptors. Exteroceptors and proprioceptors are receptors of somatic afferent components of the nervous system, while interoceptors are receptors of the visceral afferent pathways.

Exteroceptors respond to external stimuli and are found at, or close to, body surfaces. They can be subdivided into the general or cutaneous sense organs and special sensory organs. General sensory receptors include free and encapsulated terminals in skin and near hairs. Special sensory organs are the olfactory, visual, acoustic, vestibular and taste receptors.

Proprioceptors respond to stimuli to deeper tissues, especially of the locomotor system, and are concerned with detecting movement, mechanical stresses and position. They include Golgi tendon organs, neuromuscular spindles, Pacinian corpuscles, other endings in joints, and vestibular receptors. Proprioceptors are stimulated by the contraction of muscles, movements of joints and changes in the position of the body. They are essential for the coordination of muscles, the grading of muscular contraction, and the maintenance of equilibrium.

Interoceptors are found in the walls of the viscera, glands and vessels, where their terminations include free nerve endings, encapsulated terminals and endings associated with specialized epithelial cells. Nerve terminals are found in the layers of visceral walls and the adventitia of blood vessels (p. 148), but the detailed structure and function of many of these endings is not well-established. Encapsulated (lamellated) endings occur in the heart, adventitia, and mesenteries. Free terminal arborizations occur in the endocardium, loose connective tissue, the endomysium of all muscles and connective tissue generally.

Visceral nerve terminals are not usually responsive to stimuli which act on exteroceptors, and do not respond to localized mechanical and thermal stimuli. Tension produced by excessive muscular contraction or by visceral distension often causes pain, particularly in pathological states, which is frequently poorly localized and of a deep-seated nature. Visceral pain is often referred to the corresponding dermatome (see **Fig. 8.28**).

Interoceptors include vascular chemoreceptors such as the carotid body, and baroceptors which are concerned with the regulation of blood flow and pressure and in the control of respiration. Irritant receptors respond polymodally to noxious chemicals or damaging mechanical stimuli and are widely distributed in the epithelia of the alimentary and respiratory tracts: they may initiate protective reflexes.

FREE NERVE ENDINGS

Sensory endings that branch to form plexuses (**Fig. 4.24**) occur in many sites. They occur in all connective tissues, including those of the dermis, fasciae, capsules of organs, ligaments, tendons, adventitia of blood vessels, meninges, articular capsules, periosteum, perichondrium, Haversian systems in bone, parietal peritoneum, walls of viscera and the endomysium of all types of muscle. They also innervate the epithelium of the skin, cornea, buccal cavity, and alimentary and respiratory tracts and their glands. Within epithelia they lack Schwann cell ensheathment and are enveloped instead by epithelial cells. Afferent fibres from free terminals may be myelinated or unmyelinated but are always of small diameter and low conduction velocity. When afferent axons are myelinated, their terminal arborizations are not. These terminals serve several sensory modalities. In the dermis, they may be responsive to moderate cold or heat (thermoreceptors); light mechanical touch (mechanoreceptors); damaging heat, cold or deformation (unimodal nociceptors); damaging stimuli of several kinds (polymodal nociceptors). Similar fibres in deeper tissues may also signal extreme conditions, and these are experienced, as with all nociceptors, as pain. Free endings in the cornea, dentine and periosteum may be exclusively nociceptive.

Special types of free ending are associated with epidermal structures in the skin. They include terminals associated with hair follicles (peritrichial receptors) which branch from myelinated fibres in the deep dermal cutaneous plexus: the number, size and form of the endings are related to the size and type of hair follicle innervated. These endings respond mainly to movement when hair is deformed and belong to the rapidly adapting mechanoreceptor group.

Merkel tactile endings lie at the base of the epidermis or around the apical ends of some hair follicles and are innervated by large myelinated axons. The axon expands into a disc which is applied closely to the base of the Merkel cell in the basal layer of the epidermis. Merkel cells, which are believed to be derived from the neural crest, contain many large (50–100 nm) dense-cored vesicles, presumably containing transmitters, which are concentrated near the junction with the axon. Merkel endings are slow-adapting mechanoreceptors and are responsive to sustained pressure and sensitive to the edges of applied objects.

ENCAPSULATED ENDINGS

Encapsulated endings are a major group of special endings, although they exhibit considerable variety in their size, shape and distribution. They all share a common feature, which is that the axon terminal is encapsulated by non-excitable cells. This category of ending includes lamellated corpuscles of various kinds (e.g. Meissner's, Pacinian), Golgi tendon organs, neuromuscular spindles and Ruffini endings (**Fig. 4.24**).

Meissner's corpuscles

Meissner's corpuscles are found in the dermal papillae (p. 162) of all parts of the hand and foot, the front of the forearm, the lips, palpebral conjunctiva and mucous membrane of the apical part of the tongue. They are most concentrated in thick hairless skin, especially of the finger pads, where there may be up to 24 corpuscles per cm^2 in young adults. Mature corpuscles are cylindrical in shape, c.80 μm long and

30 μm across, with their long axes perpendicular to the skin surface. Each corpuscle has a connective tissue capsule and central core (**Fig. 4.25**). Meissner's corpuscles are rapidly adapting mechanoreceptors, sensitive to shape and textural changes in exploratory and discriminatory touch: their acute sensitivity provides the neural basis for reading Braille text.

Pacinian corpuscles

Pacinian corpuscles are situated subcutaneously in the palmar and plantar aspects of the hand and foot and their digits; the external genitalia; arm; neck; nipple; periostea; interosseous membranes; near the joints, and in the mesentries. They are oval, spherical or irregularly coiled and are up to 2 mm in length and 100–500 μm or more across: the larger ones are visible to the naked eye. Each corpuscle has a capsule, an intermediate growth zone and a central core which contains an axon terminal. The capsule is formed by c.30 concentrically arranged lamellae of flat cells c.0.2 μm thick (**Fig. 4.26**). Adjacent cells overlap

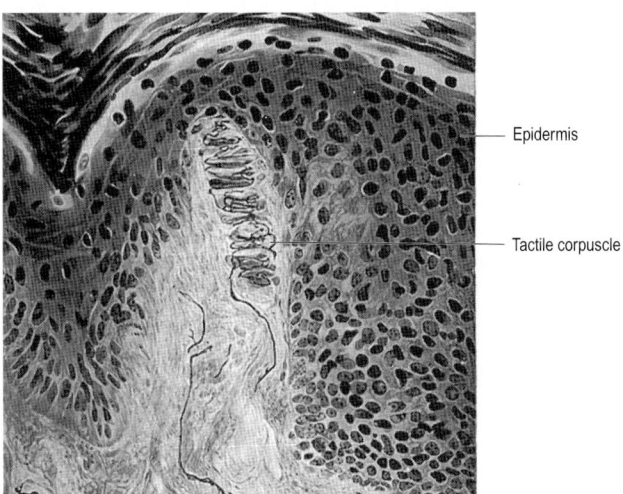

Epidermis

Tactile corpuscle

Fig. 4.25 A tactile Meissner's corpuscle in a dermal papilla in the skin, demonstrated using the Gros–Bielschowsky technique. (Provided by N Cauna, University of Pittsburgh.)

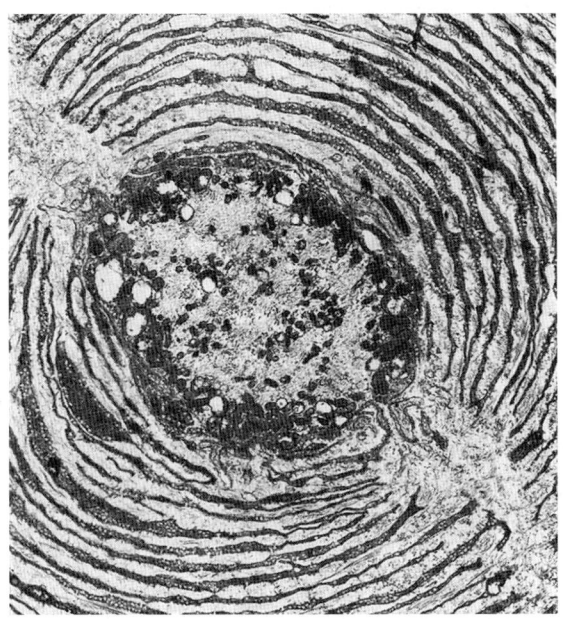

Fig. 4.26 A Pacinian corpuscle in transverse section, showing the central core region and lamellar cells surrounding the axon. Note the presence of large intercellular spaces between the lamellar cells and the numerous mitochondria in the axon (Rhesus monkey finger). (Material provided by W Hamann, Department of Anaesthetics, Guy's Hospital Medical School, London.)

and successive lamellae are separated by an amorphous proteoglycan matrix which contains circularly orientated collagen fibres, closely applied to the surfaces of the lamellar cells. The amount of collagen increases with age. The intermediate zone is cellular and its cells become incorporated into the capsule or core, so that it is not clearly defined in mature corpuscles. The core consists of c.60 bilateral, compacted lamellae, which lie on both sides of a central nerve terminal.

Each corpuscle is supplied by a myelinated axon, which loses its myelin sheath and, at its junction with the core, its ensheathing Schwann cell. The naked axon runs through the central axis of the core and ends in a slightly expanded bulb. It is in contact with the innermost core lamellae, is transversely oval and sends short projections of unknown function into clefts in the lamellae. It contains numerous large mitochondria, and minute vesicles, c.5 nm in diameter, which aggregate opposite the clefts. The cells of the capsule and core lamellae are thought to be specialized fibroblasts but some may be Schwann cells. Elastic fibrous tissue forms an overall external capsule to the corpuscle. Pacinian corpuscles are supplied by capillaries which accompany the axon as it enters the capsule.

Pacinian corpuscles act as very rapidly adapting mechanoreceptors. They respond only to sudden disturbances and are especially sensitive to vibration. The rapidity may be partly due to the lamellated capsule acting as a high pass frequency filter, damping slow distortions by fluid movement between lamellar cells. Groups of corpuscles respond to pressure changes, e.g. on grasping or releasing an object.

Ruffini endings

Ruffini endings are slowly adapting mechanoreceptors. They are found in the dermis of thin, hairy skin, where they function as dermal stretch receptors and are responsive to maintained stresses in dermal collagen. They consist of highly branched, unmyelinated endings of myelinated afferents. They ramify between bundles of collagen fibres within a spindle-shaped structure which is enclosed partly by a fibrocellular sheath derived from the perineurium of the nerve. They appear electrophysiologically similar to Golgi tendon organs, which they resemble, although they are less organized structurally. Similar structures appear in joint capsules.

Golgi tendon organs

Golgi tendon organs are mainly found near musculotendinous junctions (Fig. 4.27), where more than 50 may occur at any one site. Each terminal is related closely to a group of muscle fibres (up to 20) as they insert into the tendon. Golgi tendon endings are c.500 µm long and 100 µm in diameter, and consist of small bundles of tendon fibres enclosed in a delicate capsule. The collagen bundles (intrafusal fasciculi) are less compact than elsewhere in the tendon, the collagen fibres are smaller and the fibroblasts larger and more numerous. One or more thickly myelinated axons enter the capsule and divide. Their branches, which may lose their Schwann cell sheaths, terminate in leaf-like enlargements containing vesicles and mitochondria, which wrap around the tendon. A basal lamina or process of Schwann cell cytoplasm separates the nerve terminals from the collagen bundles which make up the tendon. The endings are activated by passive stretch of the tendon, but are much more sensitive to active contraction of the muscle. They are

important in providing proprioceptive information complementing that from neuromuscular spindles. Their responses are slowly adapting and they signal maintained tension.

NEUROMUSCULAR SPINDLES

Neuromuscular spindles are essential for the control of muscle contraction. Each spindle contains a few small, specialized intrafusal muscle fibres (p. 116), innervated by both sensory and motor nerve fibres (Figs 4.28, 4.29). The whole is surrounded equatorially by a fusiform spindle capsule of connective tissue, consisting of an outer perineurial-like sheath of flattened fibroblasts and collagen and an inner sheath which forms delicate tubes around individual intrafusal fibres. A gelatinous fluid rich in glycosaminoglycans fills the space between the two sheaths.

There are usually 5–14 intrafusal fibres (the number varies between muscles) and two major types of fibre, nuclear bag and nuclear chain fibres, which are distinguished by the arrangement of nuclei in their sarcoplasm. In the former, the equatorial cluster of nuclei makes the fibre bulge slightly, whereas in the latter the nuclei form a single axial row. Nuclear bag fibres are greater in diameter than chain fibres and extend beyond the surrounding capsule to the endomysium of nearby extrafusal muscle fibres. Nuclear chain fibres are attached at their poles to the capsule or to the sheaths of nuclear bag fibres.

The intrafusal fibres resemble typical skeletal muscle fibres, except that the zone of myofibrils is thin around the nuclei. One subtype of nuclear bag fibre (dynamic bag 1) generally lacks M lines, possesses little sarcoplasmic reticulum and has an abundance of mitochondria and oxidative enzymes, but little glycogen. A second subtype of bag fibre (static bag 2) has distinct M lines and abundant glycogen. Nuclear chain fibres have marked M lines, sarcoplasmic reticulum and T-tubules, and abundant glycogen, but few mitochondria. These variations reflect, as they do in muscle generally, the contractile properties of different intrafusal fibres (Boyd 1985).

The sensory innervation of muscle spindles is of two types, both of which are the unmyelinated terminations of large myelinated axons. Primary (anulospiral) endings are equatorially placed and form spirals around the nucleated parts of intrafusal fibres. They are the endings of large sensory fibres (Group Ia afferents), each of which sends branches to a number of intrafusal muscle fibres. Each terminal lies in a deep sarcolemmal groove in the spindle plasma membrane beneath its basal lamina. Secondary (flowerspray) endings, which may be spray-shaped or anular, are largely confined to nuclear chain fibres, and are the branched terminals of somewhat thinner myelinated (Group II) afferents. They are varicose and spread in a narrow band on both sides of the primary endings. They lie close to the sarcolemma, though not in grooves. In essence primary endings are rapidly adapting, while secondary endings have a regular, slowly adapting, response to static stretch.

There are three types of motor endings in muscle spindles. Two are from fine, myelinated, fusimotor (γ) efferents and one is from myelinated (β) efferent collaterals of extrafusal slow twitch muscle fibres. The fusimotor efferents terminate nearer the equatorial region where their terminals either resemble the motor end-plates of extrafusal fibres (plate endings) or are more diffuse (trail endings). Stimulation of

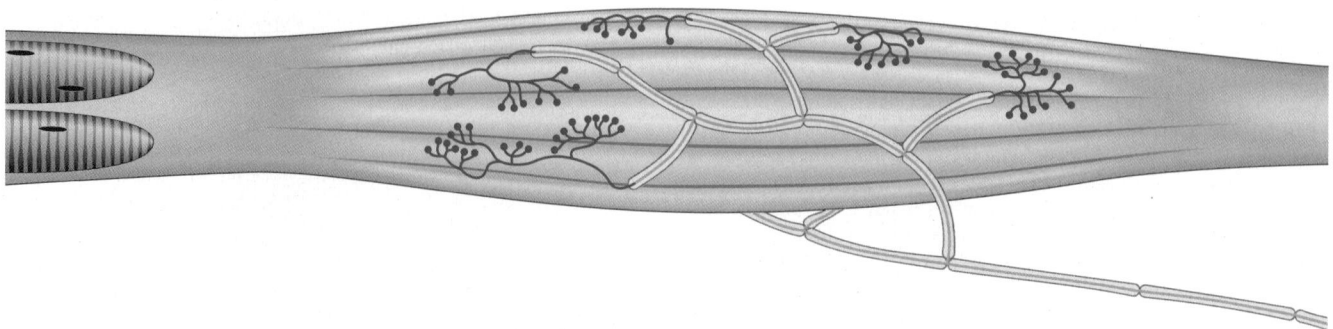

Fig. 4.27 The structure and innervation of a Golgi tendon organ. For clarity the perineurium and endoneurium have been omitted to show the distribution of nerve fibres ramifying between the collagen fibre bundles of the tendon.

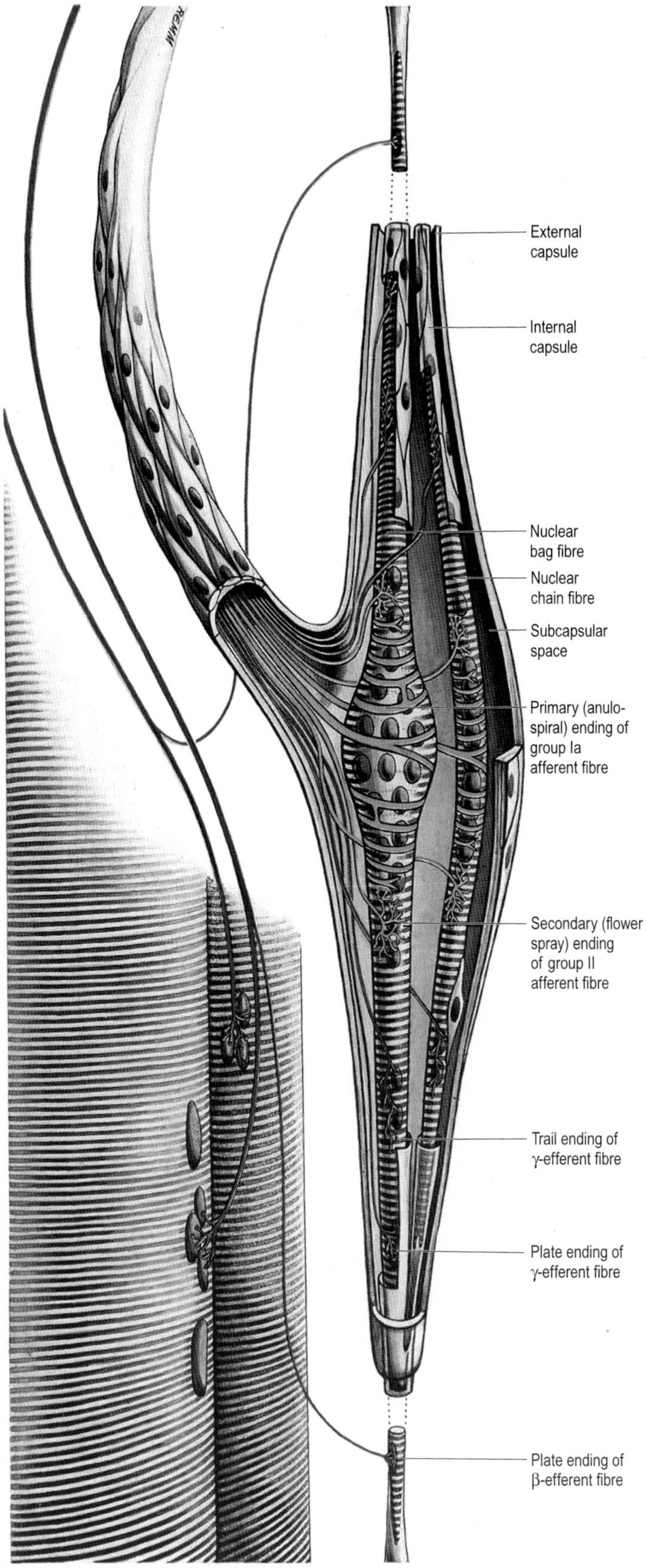
External capsule
Internal capsule
Nuclear bag fibre
Nuclear chain fibre
Subcapsular space
Primary (anulo-spiral) ending of group Ia afferent fibre
Secondary (flower spray) ending of group II afferent fibre
Trail ending of γ-efferent fibre
Plate ending of γ-efferent fibre
Plate ending of β-efferent fibre

Fig. 4.28 Schematic three-dimensional representation of a neuromuscular spindle, showing nuclear bag and nuclear chain fibres; these are innervated by the sensory anulospiral and 'flower spray' terminals (blue) and by the γ and β fusimotor terminals (red). See also **Fig. 4.29**.

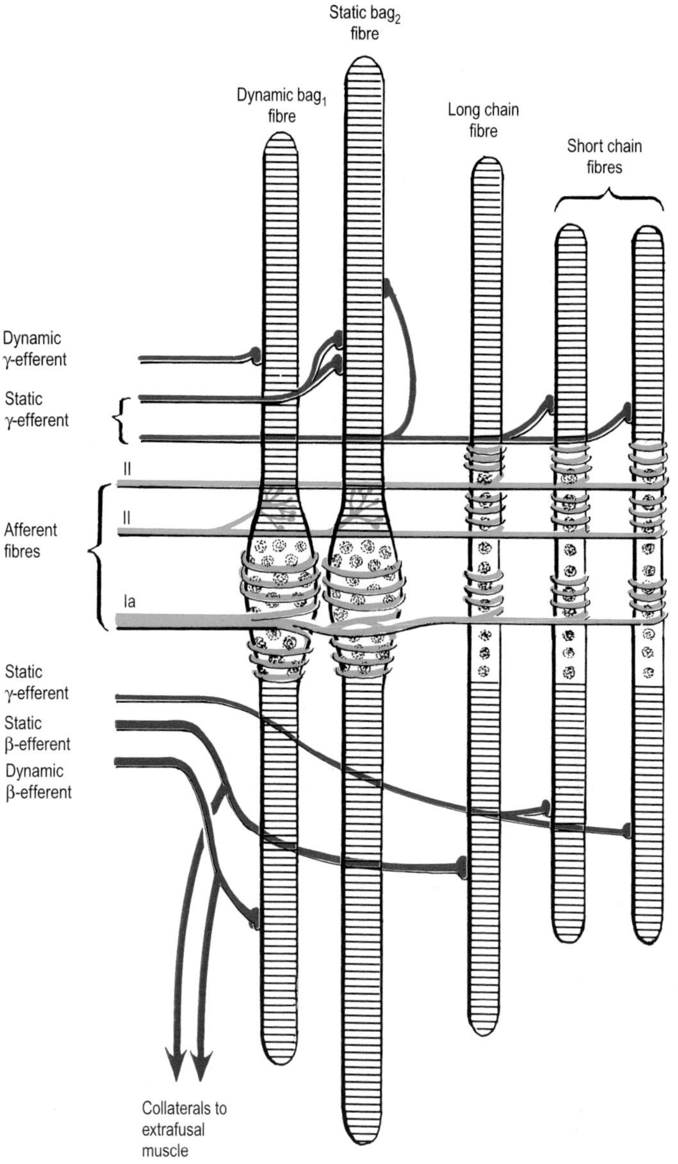
Static bag$_2$ fibre
Dynamic bag$_1$ fibre
Long chain fibre
Short chain fibres
Dynamic γ-efferent
Static γ-efferent
II
Afferent fibres
II
Ia
Static γ-efferent
Static β-efferent
Dynamic β-efferent
Collaterals to extrafusal muscle

Fig. 4.29 Schematic three-dimensional representation of nuclear bag and nuclear chain fibres in a neuromuscular spindle. Dynamic β- and γ-efferents innervate dynamic bag 1 intrafusal fibres, whereas static β- and γ-efferents innervate static bag 2 and nuclear chain intrafusal fibres.

the fusimotor and β efferents causes contraction of the intrafusal fibres and activation of their sensory endings.

Muscle spindles signal: the length of extrafusal muscle both at rest and throughout contraction and relaxation; the velocity of their contraction; changes in velocity. These modalities may be related to the different behaviours of the three major types of intrafusal fibre and their sensory terminals. The sensory endings of one type of nuclear bag fibre (dynamic bag 1) are particularly concerned with signalling rapid changes in length occurring during movement, whilst those of the second bag fibre type (static bag 2), are less responsive to movement. The afferents from chain fibres have relatively slowly adapting responses at all times. These elements can therefore detect complex changes in the state of the extrafusal muscle surrounding spindles and can signal fluctuations in length, tension, velocity of length change and acceleration. Moreover, they are under complex central control: efferent (fusimotor) nerve fibres, by regulating the strength of contraction, can adjust the length of the intrafusal fibres and thereby the responsiveness of spindle sensory endings. In summary, the organization of spindles allows them to actively monitor muscle conditions in order to compare intended and actual movements, and provide a detailed input to spinal, cerebellar, extrapyramidal and cortical centres about the state of the locomotor apparatus.

JOINT RECEPTORS

The arrays of receptors situated in and near articular capsules provide information on the position, movements and stresses acting on joints. Structural and functional studies have demonstrated at least four types of joint receptor: their proportions and distribution vary with site. Three are encapsulated endings, the fourth a free terminal arborization.

Type I endings are capsulated corpuscles of the slowly adapting mechanoreceptor (Ruffini) type, situated in the superficial layers of fibrous joint capsules in small clusters and supplied by myelinated afferent axons. Being slowly adapting, they provide awareness of joint position and movement, and respond to patterns of stress in articular capsules. They are particularly common in joints where static positional sense is necessary for the control of posture (e.g. hip, knee).

Type II endings are lamellated receptors, and resemble small versions of the large Pacinian corpuscles found in general connective tissue. They occur in small groups throughout joint capsules, particularly in the deeper layers and other articular structures (e.g. the fat pad of the temporomandibular joint). They are rapidly adapting, low-threshold mechanoreceptors, sensitive to movement and pressure changes, and they respond to joint movement and transient stresses in the joint capsule. They are supplied by myelinated afferent axons, but are probably not involved in the conscious awareness of joint sensation.

Type III endings are identical to Golgi tendon organs in structure and function: they occur in articular ligaments, but not in joint capsules. They are high-threshold, slowly adapting receptors and apparently serve, at least in part, to prevent excessive stresses at joints by reflex inhibition of the adjacent muscles. They are innervated by large myelinated afferent axons.

Type IV endings are free terminals of myelinated and unmyelinated axons. They ramify in articular capsules, the adjacent fat pads and around the blood vessels of the synovial layer. They are high-threshold, slowly adapting receptors and are thought to respond to excessive movements, providing a basis for articular pain.

NEUROMUSCULAR JUNCTIONS

SKELETAL MUSCLE

The most intensively studied effector endings are those which innervate muscle, particularly skeletal muscle. All neuromuscular (myoneural) junctions are axon terminals of somatic motor neurones. They are specialized for the release of neurotransmitter onto the sarcolemma of skeletal muscle fibres, causing a change in their electrical state which leads to contraction. Each axon branches near its terminal and subsequently innervates from several to hundreds of muscle fibres, depending on the precision of motor control required. The detailed structure of a motor terminal varies with the type of muscle innervated. Two major endings are recognized, those typical of extrafusal muscle fibres, and endings on the intrafusal fibres of neuromuscular spindles. In the former, each axonal terminal usually ends midway along a muscle fibre in a discoidal motor end-plate (**Figs 4.30, 4.31, 4.32**). This type usually initiates action potentials which are rapidly conducted to all parts of the muscle fibre. In the latter, the axon has numerous subsidiary branches which form a cluster of small expansions extending along the muscle fibre. In the absence of propagated muscle excitation, these excite the fibre at several points. Both types are associated with a specialized receptive region of the muscle fibre, the sole plate, where a number of muscle cell nuclei are grouped within the granular sarcoplasm.

The sole plate contains numerous mitochondria, endoplasmic reticulum and Golgi complexes (**Figs 4.31, 4.32**). The neuronal terminal branches are plugged into shallow grooves in the surface of the sole plate (primary clefts), from where numerous pleats extend for a short distance into the underlying sarcoplasm (secondary clefts). The axon terminal contains mitochondria and many clear 60 nm spherical vesicles similar to those in presynaptic boutons, clustered over the zone of membrane apposition. The motor terminal is ensheathed by Schwann cells whose cytoplasmic projections extend into the synaptic cleft. The plasma membranes of the nerve terminal and the muscle cell are separated by a 30–50 nm gap, with a basal lamina interposed. The basal lamina follows the surface folding of the sole plate membrane into the secondary clefts. It contains specialized components including specific isoforms of type IV collagen and laminin and the heparan sulphate proteoglycan, agrin. Endings of fast and slow twitch muscle fibres (p. 122) differ in detail: the sarcolemmal grooves are deeper, and the presynaptic vesicles more numerous, in the fast fibres.

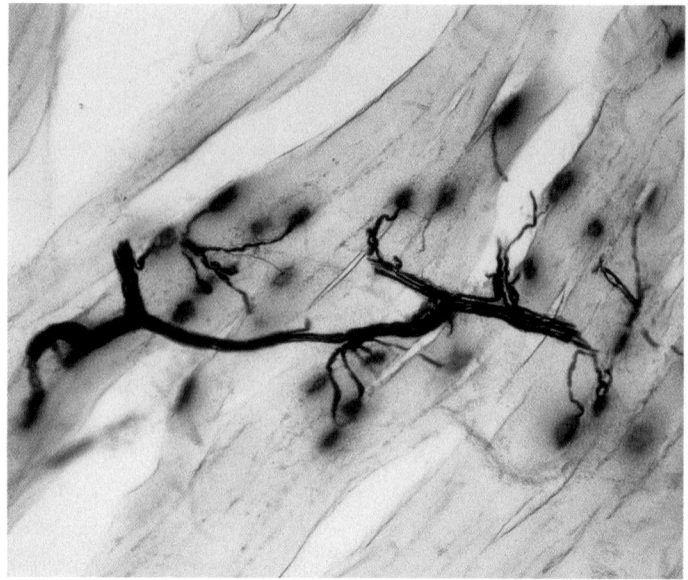

Fig. 4.30 A neuromuscular junction in a whole-mount preparation of teased skeletal muscle fibres (pale, faintly striated, diagonally orientated structures). The terminal part of the axon (silver-stained, brown) branches to form motor end-plates on adjacent muscle fibres. The sole plate recesses in the sarcolemma, into which the motor end-plates fit, are demonstrated by the presence of acetylcholinesterase (shown by enzyme histochemistry, blue). (By kind permission from Dr Norman Gregson, Division of Neurology, GKT School of Medicine, London; photograph by Sarah-Jane Smith.)

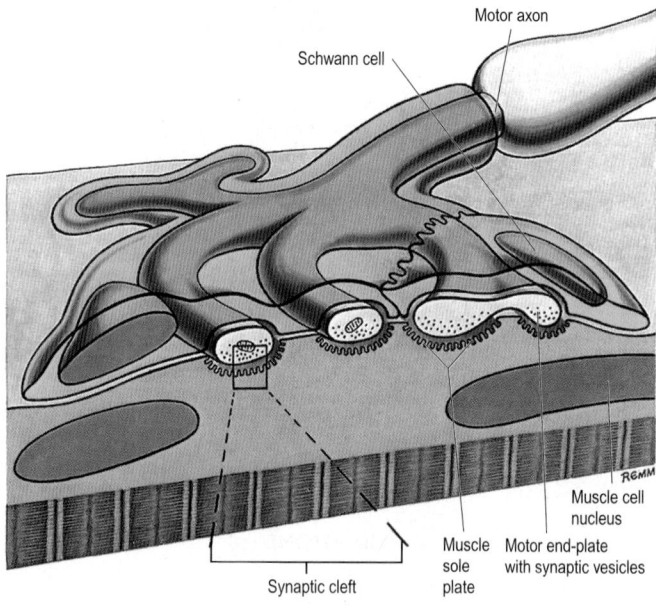

Fig. 4.31 A neuromuscular junction. Note the axonal motor end-plate and the deeply infolded sarcolemma.

Junctions with skeletal muscle are cholinergic, and the release of ACh changes the ionic permeability of the muscle fibre. Clustering of ACh receptors at the neuromuscular junction depends in part on the presence of agrin, synthesized by the motor neurone. Agrin affects muscle cytoskeletal attachments to the ACh receptor cytoplasmic domain, and prevents their lateral diffusion out of the junction. When the depolarization of the sarcolemma reaches a particular threshold, it initiates an all-or-none action potential in the sarcolemma, which is then propagated rapidly over the whole cell surface and also deep within the fibre via the invaginations (T-tubules) of the sarcolemma (p. 114), causing contraction. The amount of ACh released by the arrival of a single nerve impulse is sufficient to trigger an action

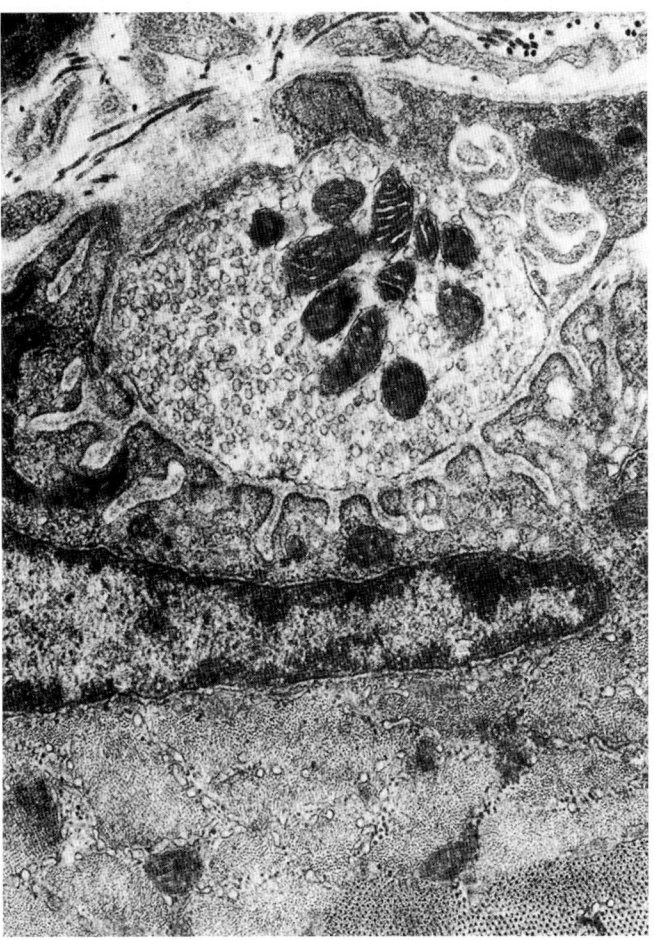

Fig. 4.32 A neuromuscular junction in skeletal muscle. The expanded motor end-plate of the axon is filled with vesicles containing synaptic transmitter (ACh) (above) and the deep infoldings of the sarcolemmal sole plate (below) form subsynaptic gutters. (By kind permission from DN Landon, Institute of Neurology, University College London.)

potential. However, because ACh is very rapidly hydrolysed by the enzyme acetylcholinesterase (AChE) present at the sarcolemmal surface of the sole plate, a single nerve impulse only gives rise to one muscle action potential, i.e. there is a one-to-one relationship between neural and muscle action potentials. Thus the contraction of a muscle fibre is controlled by the firing frequency of its motor neurone.

Neuromuscular junctions are partially blocked by high concentrations of lactic acid, as in some types of muscle fatigue.

AUTONOMIC MOTOR TERMINATIONS

Autonomic neuromuscular junctions differ in several important ways from the skeletal neuromuscular junction and from synapses in the CNS and PNS. There is no fixed junction with well defined pre- and postjunctional specializations. Unmyelinated, highly branched, post-ganglionic autonomic axons become beaded or varicose as they reach the effector smooth muscle. These varicosities are not static but are able to move along axons. They are packed with mitochondria and vesicles containing neurotransmitters which are released from the varicosities during conduction of an impulse along the axon. The distance (cleft) between the varicosity and smooth muscle membrane varies consider-ably depending on the tissue, from 20 nm in densely innervated struc-tures such as the vas deferens to 1–2 μm in large elastic arteries. Unlike skeletal muscle, the effector tissue is a muscle bundle rather than a single cell. Gap junctions between individual smooth muscle cells are low resistance pathways, which allow electronic coupling and the spread of activity within the effector bundle: they vary in size from punctate junctions to junctional areas of more than 1 μm in diameter.

Adrenergic sympathetic postganglionic terminals contain dense-cored vesicles. Cholinergic terminals, which are typical of all parasympathetic and some sympathetic endings, contain clear spherical vesicles like those

in motor end-plates of skeletal muscle. A third category of autonomic neurones has non-adrenergic, non-cholinergic endings, which contain a wide variety of chemicals with transmitter properties. Conjugated purine (ATP, a nucleoside), is probably the neurotransmitter at these terminals, which are thus classed as purinergic. Typically, their axons contain large, 80–200 nm, dense opaque vesicles, congregated in varicosities at intervals along axons. They are formed in many sites, including the external muscle layers and sphincters of the alimentary tract, lungs, vascular walls, urogenital tract and CNS. In the intestinal wall, neuronal somata lie in the myenteric plexus, and their axons spread caudally for a few millimetres, mainly to innervate circular muscle. Purinergic neurones are under cholinergic control from pre-ganglionic sympathetic neurones. Their endings mainly hyperpolarize smooth muscle cells, causing relaxation, e.g. preceding peristaltic waves, opening sphincters and, probably, causing reflex distension in gastric filling.

Autonomic efferents also innervate glands, myoepithelial cells, adipose and lymphoid tissue.

CNS–PNS TRANSITION ZONE

The transition between CNS and PNS usually occurs some distance from the point at which nerve roots emerge from the brain or the spinal cord. The segment of root which contains components of both CNS and PNS tissue is called the CNS–PNS transition zone (TZ). All axons in the PNS, other than postganglionic autonomic neurones, cross such a transition zone. Macroscopically, as a nerve root is traced towards the spinal cord or the brain, it splits into several thinner rootlets which may, in turn, subdivide into minirootlets. The transition zone is located within either rootlet or minirootlet (**Fig. 4.33**). The arrangement of roots and rootlets varies according to whether the root trunk is ventral, dorsal or cranial. Thus, in dorsal roots, the main root trunk separates into a fan of rootlets and minirootlets which enter the spinal cord in sequence along the dorsolateral sulcus. In certain cranial nerves the minirootlets come together central to the transition zone and enter the brain as a stump of white matter.

Microscopically, the transition zone is characterized by an axial CNS compartment surrounded by a PNS compartment. The zone lies more peripherally in sensory than in motor nerves, but in both, the apex of the transition zone is described as a glial dome, whose convex surface is directed distally. The centre of the dome consists of fibres with a typical CNS organization, surrounded by an outer mantle of astrocytes (corresponding to the glia limitans). From this mantle, numerous glial processes project into the endoneurial compartment of the peripheral nerve where they interdigitate with its Schwann cells. The astrocytes form a loose reticulum through which axons pass. Peripheral myelinated axons usually cross the zone at a node of Ranvier, which is here termed a PNS–CNS compound node.

A cell type, the boundary cap cell, has been described recently in avian and mammalian species which transiently occupies the presumptive dorsal root transition zone of the embryonic spinal cord. Boundary cap cells are derived from the neural crest and are thought to prevent cell mixing at this interface and to help dorsal root ganglion afferents navigate their path to targets in the spinal cord. Further details are given in Golding & Cohen (1997).

CONDUCTION OF THE NERVOUS IMPULSE
(Fig. 4.34)

All cells generate a steady electrochemical potential across their plasma membranes (a membrane potential) because of the different ionic concentrations inside and outside the cell. Neurones use minute fluctu-ations in this potential to receive, conduct, and transmit information across their surfaces.

The membrane potential of a neurone, known as the resting potential, is similar to that of non-excitable cells. In most neurones it is c.80 mV, inside being negative. The entry into neurones of sodium or, in some sites, calcium, ions causes depolarization of the cell, while an increased chloride influx or an increased potassium efflux results in hyper-polarization. Plasma membrane permeability to these ions is altered by the opening or closing of ion-specific transmembrane channels, triggered by chemical or electrical stimuli. Chemically triggered ionic fluxes occur

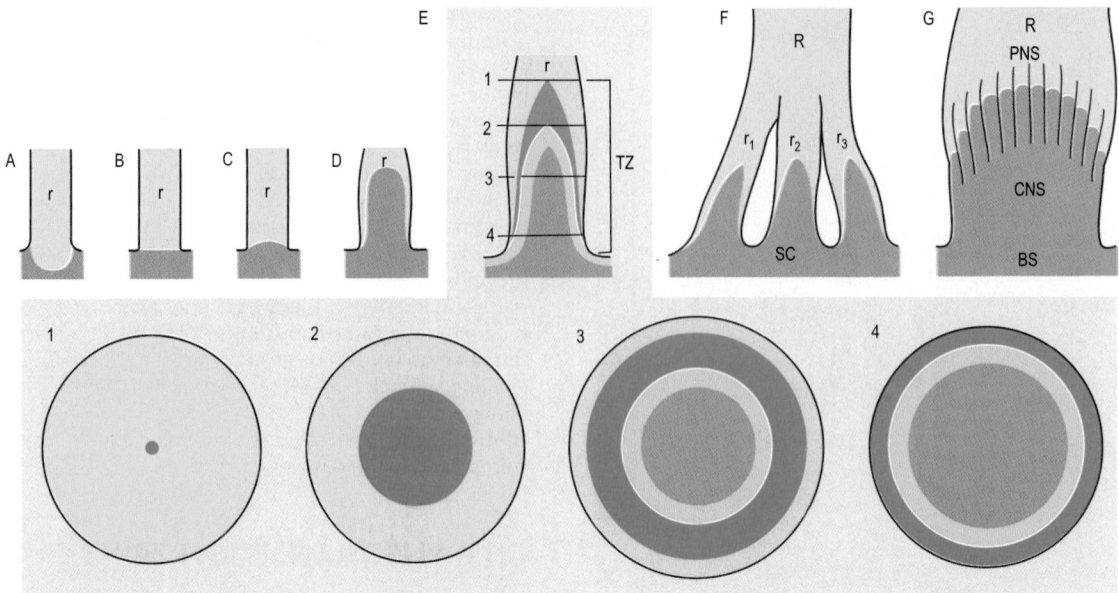

Fig. 4.33 Schematic representation of the nerve root–spinal cord junction. **A–E**, Different CNS–PNS borderline arrangements. **A**, Concave borderline (white line) and inverted transitional zone (TZ). **B**, Flat borderline situated at the level of the rootlet (r)–spinal cord junction. **C** and **D**, Convex, dome-shaped borderline; the CNS expansion into the rootlet is moderate in C and extensive in D. Brown denotes CNS tissue. The glial fringe is not shown. **E**, Pointed borderline. The extent of the TZ is indicated. The cross-sectional appearance at four different TZ levels (A, B, C, and D) and the distribution of the different TZ are shown in the lower part of the illustration. Yellow, endoneurial zone; dark green, glial fringe; light green, mantle zone; brown, core zone. **F**, Root–spinal cord junction. The root (R) splits into rootlets (r), each with its own TZ and attaching separately to the spinal cord (SC). **G**, Arrangement noted in several cranial nerve roots (e.g. vestibulocochlear nerve). The PNS component of the root separates into a bundle of closely packed minirootlets, each equipped with a TZ. The minirootlets reunite centrally. BS, brain stem. (By permission from Dyck PJ et al 1993 Peripheral Neuropathy, 3rd edn. Philadelphia: WB Saunders.)

at synapses, and may be either direct, where the chemical agent (neurotransmitter) binds to the channel itself to cause it to open, or indirect, where the neurotransmitter is bound by a transmembrane receptor molecule which is not itself a channel, but which activates a complex second messenger system within the cell to open separate transmembrane channels. Electrically induced changes in membrane potential depend on the presence of voltage-sensitive ion channels which, when the transmembrane potential reaches a critical level, open to allow the influx or efflux of specific ions. In all cases, the channels remain open only transiently, and the numbers which open and close determine the total flux of ions across the membrane.

The types and concentrations of transmembrane channels and related proteins, and therefore the electrical activity of the membranes, vary in different parts of the cell. Dendrites and neuronal somata depend mainly on neurotransmitter action and show graded potentials, whereas axons have voltage-gated channels which give rise to action potentials.

In graded potentials, a flow of current from or into adjacent areas of the cell occurs when a synapse is activated, and this contributes to the total degree of polarization of the membrane covering the cell body. However, the influence of an individual synapse on neighbouring regions decreases with distance so that, for instance, synapses on the distal tips of dendrites may, on their own, have relatively little effect. The electrical state of a neurone therefore depends on many factors, including the numbers and positions of thousands of excitatory and inhibitory synapses, their degree of activation, and the branching pattern of the dendritic tree and geometry of the cell body. The target of these integrated factors is a small part of the neurone surface, the axon hillock (p. 44), where voltage sensitive channels are concentrated (unlike the dendrites or soma). The axon hillock is the site where action potentials are generated prior to their conduction along the axon.

ACTION POTENTIAL

The action potential is a brief complete reversal of polarity, which propagates itself along membranes. It depends on an initial influx of

sodium ions which causes a reversal of polarity to about 40 mV (positive inside), followed by a rapid return to the resting potential as potassium ions flow out (the detailed mechanism differs somewhat between CNS and PNS). The whole process is completed in c.5 m/s. For a particular neurone, the size and duration of action potentials are always the same (described as all or none), no matter how much a stimulus may exceed the threshold value.

Once initiated, an action potential spreads rapidly and at constant velocity because it triggers the opening of neighbouring voltage-gated channels of the same sort. The velocity of conduction, ranging from 4–120 m/s, depends on a number of factors related to the way in which the current spreads, e.g. axonal cross-sectional area, membrane capacitance (influenced by the presence of myelin), and the numbers and positioning of ion channels. At the end of an action potential, there is an irreducible delay, the refractory period, during which another action potential cannot be triggered. This determines the maximum frequency at which action potentials can be conducted along a nerve fibre: its value differs in different neurones and affects the amount of information which can be carried by an individual fibre.

Myelinated fibres are electrically insulated along most of their lengths, except at nodes of Ranvier. Voltage-gated sodium channels are clustered at nodes, and the nodal membrane is the only place where an action potential can be propagated down the axon. The action potential thus jumps from node to node across internodal distances of 0.2–2.0 mm, depending on the axon diameter, a process known as saltatory conduction. This greatly speeds the rate of conduction. In demyelinating diseases, such as multiple sclerosis, the speed and the security of conduction are severely compromised.

Axonal conduction is naturally unidirectional, from dendrites and soma to axon terminals. When an action potential reaches the axonal terminals, it causes depolarization of the presynaptic membrane and as a result, quanta of neurotransmitter (which correspond to the content of individual vesicles) are released to change the degree of excitation of the next neurone, muscle fibre or glandular cell. For further information, see Kandel & Schwartz (2000).

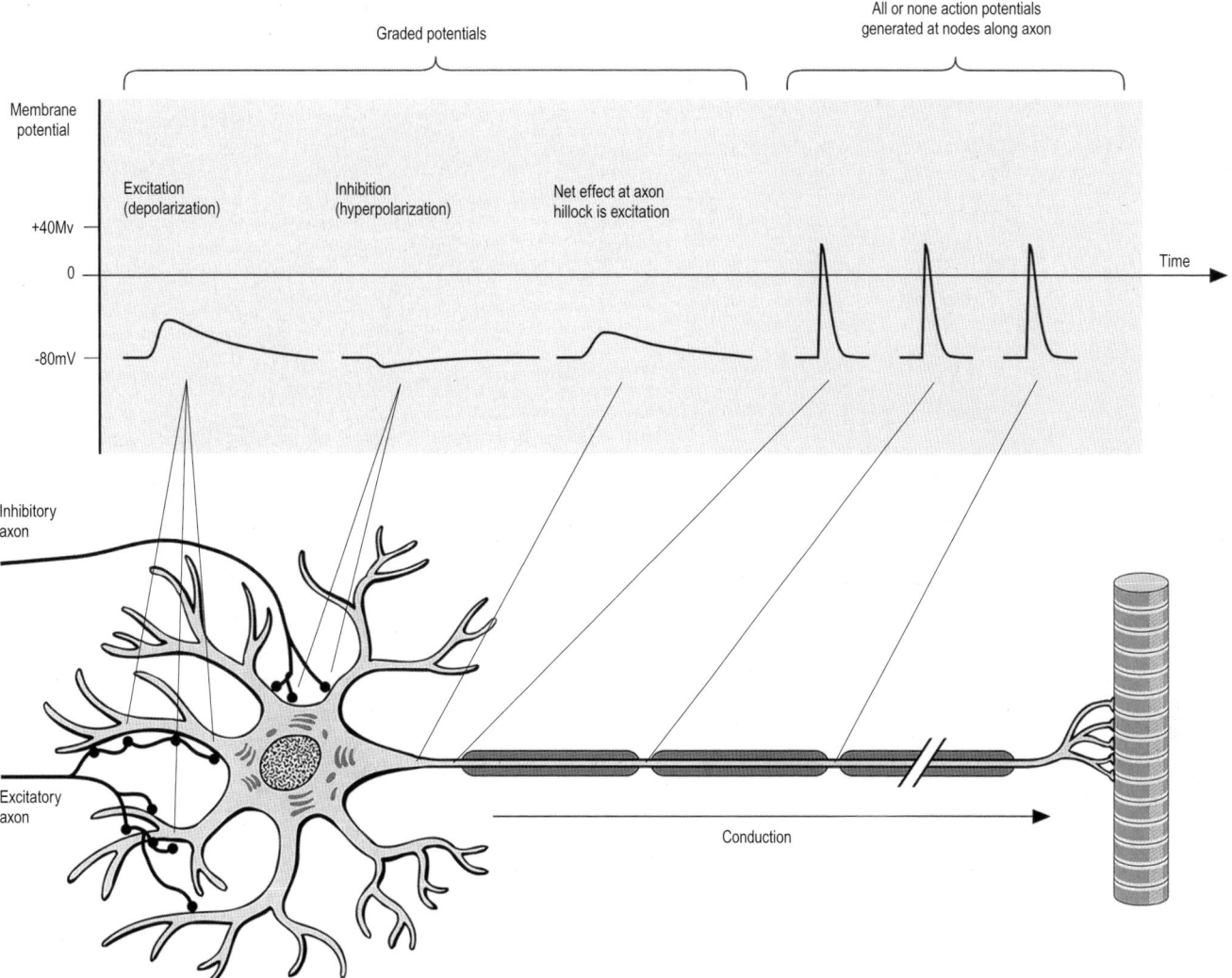

Fig. 4.34 The types of change in electrical potential that can be recorded across the cell membrane of a motor neurone at the points indicated by the arrows. Excitatory and inhibitory synapses on the surfaces of the dendrites and soma cause local graded changes of potential which summate at the axon hillock and may initiate a series of all-or-none action potentials, which in turn are conducted along the axon to the effector terminals.

REFERENCES

Boyd IA 1985 Muscle spindles and stretch reflexes. In: Swash M, Kennard C (eds) Scientific Basis of Clinical Neurology. Edinburgh: Churchill Livingstone: pp. 74–97.
A detailed account of the functional aspects of neuromuscular spindles.

Butt AM, Berry M 2000 Oligodendrocytes and the control of myelination in vivo: new insights from the rat anterior medullary velum. J Neurosci Res 59; 477–88.
Describes the characteristics of a glial cell which contacts nodes of Ranvier in the central nervous system.

Golding J, Cohen J 1997 Border controls at the mammalian spinal cord: late-surviving neural crest boundary cap cells at dorsal root entry sites may regulate sensory afferent ingrowth and entry zone morphogenesis. Mol Cell Neurosci 9: 381–96.
Describes the characteristics of a novel type of cell concerned with establishing the boundary between central and peripheral nervous systems during embryogenesis.

Kandel ER, Schwartz JH 2000 Principles of Neural Science, 4th edn. New York: McGraw-Hill.

Scherer SS, Arroyo EJ 2002 Recent progress on the molecular organization of myelinated axons. J Peripheral Nervous System 7: 1–12.
Review of the molecular architecture of myelinated peripheral axons and their myelin sheaths.

Blood, lymphoid tissues and haemopoiesis

Blood cells are formed postnatally in the bone marrow. Haemopoiesis produces red cells (erythrocytes), and a wide variety of defensive cells (white blood cells, leukocytes) (p. 77). The latter include neutrophil, eosinophil and basophil granulocytes, B lymphocytes and monocytes. T lymphocytes develop in the thymus from bone marrow-derived progenitors. Platelets are produced in the bone marrow as cellular fragments of megakaryocytes. Only erythrocytes and platelets are generally confined to the blood vascular system, whereas all leukocytes can leave the circulation and enter extravascular tissues. The numbers of cells doing so increases greatly in local infections and diseases.

The lymphoid tissues are the thymus, lymph nodes, spleen and the lymphoid nodules associated mainly with the alimentary and respiratory tracts. Lymphocytes populate lymphoid tissues and are concerned with various types of immune defence. Lymphoid tissue also contains supportive stromal cells which are non-haemopoietic in origin (e.g. thymic epithelium), non-haemopoietic follicular dendritic cells of lymph node and splenic follicles, interdigitating dendritic cells, and macrophages of the mononuclear phagocyte system. Dendritic cells and macrophages, derived from blood monocytes, are found additionally in most tissues and organs where they function as immunostimulatory antigen-presenting cells (APCs).

CELLS OF PERIPHERAL BLOOD

Blood

Blood is an opaque fluid with a viscosity greater than that of water (mean relative viscosity 4.75 at 18°C), and a specific gravity of c.1.06 at 15°C. It is bright red when oxygenated, in the systemic arteries, and dark red to purple when deoxygenated, in systemic veins. Blood is a mixture of a clear liquid, plasma, and cellular elements, and consequently the hydrodynamic flow of blood in vessels behaves in a complex, non-Newtonian manner.

PLASMA

Plasma is a clear, yellowish fluid which contains many substances in solution or suspension: low molecular weight solutes give a mean freezing-point depression of c.0.54°C. Plasma contains high concentrations of sodium and chloride ions, potassium, calcium, magnesium, phosphate, bicarbonate, traces of many other ions, glucose, amino acids, vitamins. The colloids include high molecular weight plasma proteins, e.g. clotting factors, particularly prothrombin; immunoglobulins and complement proteins involved in immunological defence; glycoproteins, lipoproteins, polypeptide and steroid hormones and globulins for the transport of hormones and iron. Since most of the metabolic activities of the body are reflected in the plasma composition, its routine chemical analysis is of great diagnostic importance.

The precipitation of the protein fibrin from plasma to form a clot (**Fig. 5.1**) is initiated by the release of specific materials from damaged cells and blood platelets in the presence of calcium ions. If blood or plasma samples are allowed to stand, they will separate into a clot and a clear yellowish fluid, the serum. Clot formation is prevented by removal of calcium ions, e.g. by addition of citrate, oxalate or various organic calcium chelators (EDTA, EGTA) to the sample. Heparin is also widely used as an anticlotting agent, because it interferes with another part of the complex series of chemical interactions which lead to fibrin clot formation.

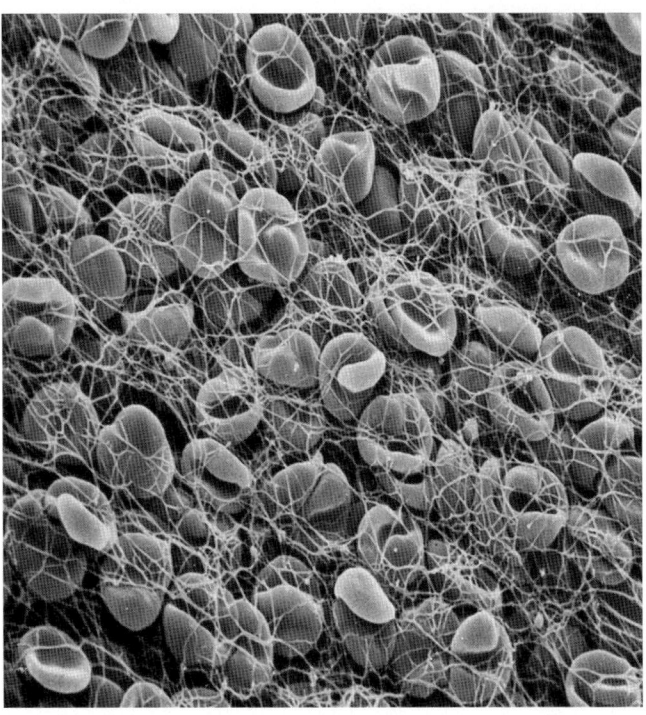

Fig. 5.1 Erythrocytes enmeshed in filaments of fibrin in a clot. (By kind permission from Michael Crowder.)

Erythrocytes (Figs 5.1, 5.2, 5.3)

Erythrocytes (red blood cells, red blood corpuscles) account for the largest proportion of blood cells (99% of the total number), with normal values of $4.1–6.0 \times 10^6/\mu l$ in adult males and $3.9–5.5 \times 10^6/\mu l$ in adult females. Each cell is a biconcave disc with a mean diameter in dried smear preparations of 7.1 μm; in fresh preparations the mean diameter is 7.8 μm, decreasing slightly with age. Mature erythrocytes lack nuclei. They are pale red by transmitted light, with paler centres because of their biconcave shape. The properties of their cell coat cause them to adhere to one another by their rims to form loose piles of cells (rouleaux). In normal blood, a few cells assume a shrunken star-like, crenated form: this shape can be reproduced by placing normal biconcave erythrocytes in a hypertonic solution, which causes osmotic shrinkage. In hypotonic solutions erythrocytes take up water and become spherical; they may eventually lyse to release their haemoglobin (haemolysis), leaving red cell ghosts.

Erythrocytes have a limiting plasma membrane which encloses mainly a single protein, haemoglobin, as a 33% solution. The plasma membrane of erythrocytes is c.60% lipid and glycolipid, and 40% protein and glycoprotein. More than 15 classes of protein are present, including two major types. Glycophorins A and B (each with a molecular mass of c.50 kDa) span the membrane, and their negatively charged carbohydrate chains project from the outer surface of the cell. Their sialic acid groups confer most of the fixed charge on the cell surface. A second transmembrane macromolecule, band 3 protein, forms an important anion channel, exchanging bicarbonate for chloride ions

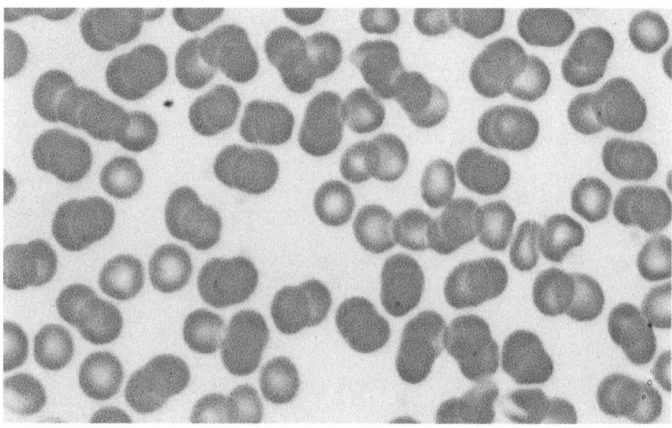

Fig. 5.2 Erythrocytes in peripheral blood. The pale centre visible in some cells reflects the reduced thickness of the biconcave disc in this region. Groups of cells adhere to each other in loose piles (rouleaux). (Photograph by Sarah-Jane Smith.)

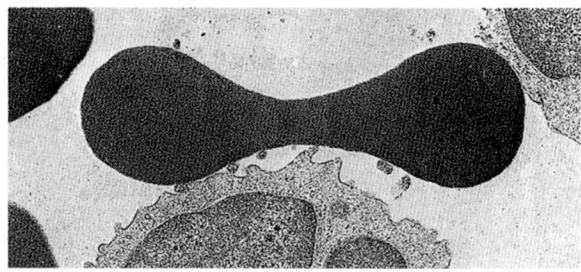

Fig. 5.3 An erythrocyte. Note the biconcave profile and dense homogeneous contents.

across the membrane and allowing the release of CO_2 in the lung. The ABO blood group antigens are all membrane glycolipids.

The shape of the erythrocyte is largely determined by the filamentous protein dimer, spectrin, a name which reflects its original isolation from red cell ghosts. Spectrin dimers associate as tetramers through their head regions, and are attached to the cytoplasmic domain of band 3 protein via ankyrin. Other proteins, including tropomyosin, short actin filaments and band 4.1 protein, form junctional complexes which link spectrin to glycophorin transmembrane proteins, forming a stabilizing cytoskeletal network. This gives the membrane great flexibility: red cells are deformable but regain their biconcave shape and dimensions after passing through the smallest capillaries, which are c.4 μm in diameter. Erythrocyte membrane flexibility also contributes to the normally low viscosity of blood. Defects in the cytoskeleton occur in autosomal dominant disorders (elliptocytosis and spherocytosis) which result in abnormalities of red cell shape, membrane fragility and premature destruction of erythrocytes in the spleen (p. 1242).

Fetal erythrocytes up to the fourth month of gestation differ markedly from those of adults, in that they are larger, are nucleated and contain a different type of haemoglobin (HbF). After this time they are progressively replaced by the adult type of cell.

HAEMOGLOBIN

Haemoglobin (Hb) is a globular protein with a molecular mass of 67 kDa. It consists of globulin molecules bound to haem, an iron-containing porphyrin group. The oxygen-binding power of haemoglobin is provided by the iron atoms of the haem groups, and these are maintained in the ferrous (Fe^{++}) state by the presence of glutathione within the erythrocyte. The haemoglobin molecule is a tetramer, made up of four subunits, each a coiled polypeptide chain holding a single haem group. In normal blood, five types of polypeptide chain can occur, namely, α, β and two β-like polypeptides, γ and δ. A third, β-like η chain is restricted to early fetal development. Each haemoglobin molecule

contains two α-chains and two others, so that several combinations, and hence a number of different types of haemoglobin molecule, are possible. For example, haemoglobin A (HbA), which is the major adult class, contains 2α- and 2β-chains; a variant, HbA_2 accounts for only c.2% of adult haemoglobin. Haemoglobin F (HbF), found in fetal and early postnatal life, consists of 2α- and 2γ-chains. Adult red cells normally contain less than 1% of HbF.

In the pathological genetic condition thalassaemia, only one type of chain is expressed normally, the mutant chain being absent or present at much reduced levels. Thus, a molecule may contain 4 α-chains (β-thalassaemia) or, more commonly, 4 β-chains (α-thalassaemia) where individuals affected carry haemoglobin H (HbH). In haemoglobin S (HbS) of sickle-cell disease, a point mutation in the β-chain gene (valine substituted for glutamine) causes a major alteration in the behaviour of the red cell and its oxygen-carrying capacity.

LIFE SPAN

Erythrocytes last between 100 and 120 days before being destroyed. As erythrocytes age they become increasingly fragile, and their surface charges decrease as their content of negatively charged membrane glycoproteins diminishes. The lipid content of their membranes also reduces. Aged erythrocytes are eventually ingested by the macrophages of the spleen and liver sinusoids, usually without prior lysis, and are hydrolysed in phagocytic vacuoles where the haemoglobin is split into its globulin and porphyrin moieties. Globulin is further degraded to amino acids which pass into the general amino acid pool. Iron is removed from the porphyrin and used either directly in the synthesis of new haemoglobin in the bone marrow, or stored in the liver as ferritin or haemosiderin. The remainder of the haem group is converted in the liver to bilirubin and excreted in the bile.

The recognition of effete erythrocytes by macrophages appears to depend in part on the exposure of normally inaccessible parts of membrane proteins, enabling autoantibodies to these erythrocyte senescence antigens to bind to them and flag them for macrophage removal. Red cells are destroyed at the rate of c.5×10^{11} cells a day and are normally replaced from the bone marrow at the same rate.

BLOOD GROUPS

Over 300 red cell antigens are recognizable with specific antisera. They can interact with naturally occurring antibodies in the plasma of recipients of an unmatched transfusion, causing agglutination and lysis of the erythrocytes. Erythrocytes of a single individual can carry several different types of antigen, each type belonging to an antigenic system in which a number of alternative antigens are possible in different persons. So far 19 major groups have been identified. They vary in their distribution frequencies between different populations, and include the ABO, Rhesus, MNS, Lutheran, Kell, Lewis, Duffy, Kidd, Diego, Cartwright, Colton, Sid, Scianna, Yt, Auberger, Ii, Xg, Indian and Dombrock systems. Clinically, the ABO and Rhesus groups are of most importance.

In the ABO system, two allelic genes are inherited in simple Mendelian fashion. Thus the genome may be homozygous and carry the AA complement, the blood group being A, or the BB complement which gives blood group B, or it may carry neither (OO), producing blood group O. In the heterozygous condition the following combinations can occur: AB (blood group AB), AO (blood group A) and BO (blood group B).

Individuals with group AB blood lack antibodies to both A and B antigens, and so can be transfused with blood of any group: they are termed universal recipients. Conversely, those with group O, universal donors, can give blood to any recipient, since anti-A and anti-B antibodies in the donated blood are diluted to insignificant levels. Normally, however, blood is only transfused between persons with precisely corresponding groups, because anomalous antibodies of the ABO system are occasionally found in blood and may cause agglutination or lysis. The anti-ABO agglutinins, unlike those of the Rhesus system, belong to the immunoglobulin M (IgM) class and do not cross the placenta during pregnancy.

The Rhesus antigen system is determined by three sets of alleles, namely Cc, Dd and Ee: the most important clinically is Dd. Inheritance of the Rh factor also obeys simple Mendelian laws and it is therefore possible for a Rhesus-negative mother to bear a Rhesus-positive child.

Fetal Rh antigens can, under these circumstances, stimulate the production of anti-Rh antibodies by the mother: since these belong to the immunoglobulin G (IgG) class of antibodies they are able to cross the placental barrier (generally in the last trimester) and cause agglutination of fetal erythrocytes. In the first such pregnancy little damage usually occurs, but in subsequent Rh-positive pregnancies massive destruction of fetal red cells (haemolytic disease of the newborn) may result, causing fetal or neonatal death. Sensitization of the maternal immune system can also result from abortion or miscarriage, or even occasionally amniocentesis, which may introduce fetal antigens into the maternal circulation. Treatment is by exchange transfusion of the neonate or, prophylactically, by giving Rh-immune (anti-D) serum to the mother after the first Rh-positive pregnancy, which destroys the fetal Rh antigen in her circulation before sensitization can occur.

Leukocytes also bear highly polymorphic antigens encoded by allelic gene variants. These belong to the group of major histocompatibility complex (MHC) antigens, also termed human leukocyte antigens (HLA) in man. They play important roles in cell–cell interactions in the immune system, particularly in the presentation of antigens by antigen presenting cells to T lymphocytes.

Leukocytes (Fig. 5.4)

Leukocytes (white blood cells or white corpuscles) belong to at least five different categories, and are distinguishable by their size, nuclear shape and cytoplasmic inclusions. In practice, leukocytes are often divided into two main groups, namely those with prominent stainable cytoplasmic granules, the granulocytes, and those without.

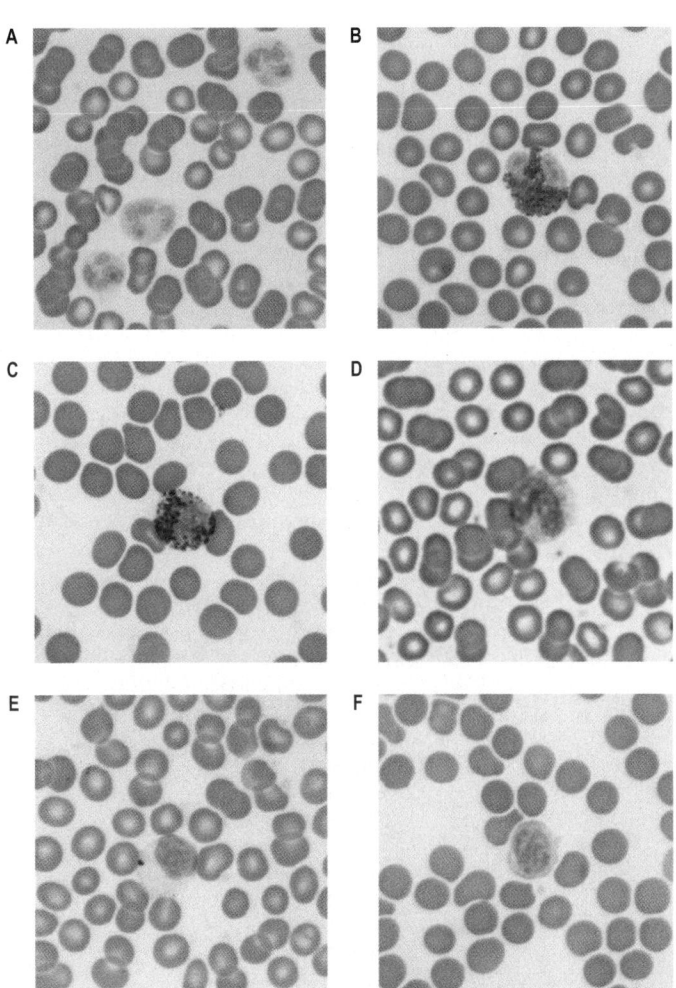

Fig. 5.4 Leukocytes in peripheral blood. **A**, neutrophil granulocytes; **B**, eosinophil granulocyte; **C**, basophil granulocyte; **D**, monocyte; **E**, small lymphocyte; **F**, medium lymphocyte. (Photographs by Sarah-Jane Smith.)

GRANULOCYTES

This group consists of eosinophil granulocytes, with granules which bind acidic dyes such as eosin; basophil granulocytes, with granules which bind basic dyes strongly; and neutrophil granulocytes, with granules which stain only weakly with either type of dye. Granulocytes all possess irregular or multilobed nuclei and belong to the myeloid series of blood cells (p. 78).

NEUTROPHIL GRANULOCYTES (Fig. 5.4A)

Neutrophil granulocytes (neutrophils), are also referred to as polymorphonuclear leukocytes (polymorphs) because of their segmented nuclei. They form the largest proportion of the white blood cells (40–75% in adults, with a normal count of 2500–7500/μl) and have a diameter of 12–14 μm. In the living state the cells may be spherical in the circulation, but they can flatten and become actively motile within the extracellular matrix of connective tissues.

The numerous cytoplasmic granules are heterogeneous in size, shape and content, but all are membrane-bound and contain hydrolytic and other enzymes. Two major categories can be distinguished according to their developmental origin and contents. Non-specific or primary (azurophilic) granules are formed early in neutrophil maturation. They are relatively large (0.5 μm) spheroidal lysosomes containing myeloperoxidase, acid phosphatase, elastase and several other enzymes. Specific or secondary granules are formed later, and occur in a wide range of shapes including spheres, ellipsoids and rods. These contain strong bacteriocidal components including alkaline phosphatase, lactoferrin and collagenase, none of which are found in primary granules. Conversely, secondary granules lack peroxidase and acid phosphatase. Some enzymes, e.g. lysozyme, are present in both types of granule.

In mature neutrophils the nucleus is characteristically multilobed with up to six (usually three or four) segments joined by narrow nuclear strands: this is known as the segmented stage. Less mature cells have fewer lobes. The earliest to be released under normal conditions are juveniles (band or stab cells) in which the nucleus is an unsegmented crescent or band. In certain clinical conditions, even earlier stages in neutrophil formation, when cells display indented or rounded nuclei (metamyelocytes or myelocytes) may be released from the bone marrow. In mature cells the edges of the nuclear lobes are often irregular. In females c.3% of the nuclei of neutrophils show a conspicuous 'drumstick' formation which represents the sex chromatin of the inactive X chromosome (Barr body). Neutrophil cytoplasm contains few mitochondria but abundant cytoskeletal elements, including actin filaments, microtubules and their associated proteins, all characteristic of highly motile cells.

Neutrophils are important in the defence of the body against microorganisms. They can phagocytose microbes and small particles in the circulation and, after extravasation, they carry out similar activities in other tissues. They function effectively in relatively anaerobic conditions, relying largely on glycolytic metabolism, and they fulfil an important role in the acute inflammatory phase of tissue injury, responding to chemotoxins released by damaged tissue. Phagocytosis of cellular debris or invading microorganisms is followed by fusion of the phagocytic vacuole, first with specific granules, whose pH is reduced to 5.0 by active transport of protons, then with non-specific (primary) granules, which complete the process of bacterial killing and digestion. Actively phagocytic neutrophils are able to reduce oxygen enzymatically to form superoxide radicals and hydrogen peroxide, which enhance bacterial destruction.

Phagocytosis is greatly facilitated by circulating antibodies, secreted by plasma cells, to molecules such as bacterial antigens which the body has previously encountered. Antibodies coat the antigenic target and bind the plasma complement protein, C1, to their non-variable Fc regions. This activates the complement cascade, which involves some 20 plasma proteins synthesized mainly in the liver, and completes the process of opsonization. The complement cascade involves the sequential cleavage of the complement proteins into a large fragment, which generally binds to the antigenic surface, and a small bioactive fragment which is released. The final step is the recognition of complement by receptors on the surfaces of neutrophils (and macrophages), which promotes phagocytosis of the organism. Organisms which do not become opsonized may escape phagocytosis and are thus potential pathogens.

Neutrophils are short-lived; they spend some 6–7 hours circulating in the blood and a few days in connective tissues. The number of circulating neutrophils varies, and often rises during episodes of acute bacterial infection. They die after carrying out their phagocytic role: dead neutrophils, bacteria, tissue debris (including tissue damaged by neutrophil enzymes and toxins) and interstitial fluid form the characteristic, greenish-yellow pus of infected tissue. The colour is derived from the natural colour of neutrophil myeloperoxidase.

Granules may also be inappropriately released from neutrophils. Their enzymes are implicated in various pathological conditions, e.g. rheumatoid arthritis, where tissue destruction and chronic inflammation occur.

EOSINOPHIL GRANULOCYTES (Fig. 5.4B)

Eosinophil granulocytes (eosinophils) are similar in size (12–15 μm), shape and motile capacity to neutrophils, but are present only in small numbers in normal blood (100–400/μl). The nucleus has two prominent lobes connected by a thin strand. Their cytoplasmic specific granules are uniformly large (0.5 μm) and give the living cell a slightly yellowish colour. The cytoplasm is packed with granules which are spherical or ellipsoid and membrane-bound. The core of each granule is composed of a lattice of major basic protein, which is responsible for its strong eosinophilic staining properties. The surrounding matrix contains several lysosomal enzymes including acid phosphatase, ribonuclease, phospholipase and a myeloperoxidase unique to eosinophils.

Like other leukocytes, eosinophils are motile. When suitably stimulated, they are able to pass into the extravascular tissues from the circulation. They are typical minor constituents of the dermis, and of the connective tissue components of the bronchial tree, alimentary tract, uterus and vagina. The total lifespan of these cells is a few days, of which some 10 hours is spent in the circulation, and the remainder in the extravascular tissues.

Eosinophil numbers rise (eosinophilia) in worm infestations and also in certain allergic disorders, and it is thought that they evolved as a primary defence against parasitic attack. They have surface receptors for IgE which bind to IgE-antigen complexes, triggering phagocytosis and release of granule contents. However, they are only weakly phagocytic and their most important function is the destruction of parasites too large to phagocytose. This anti-parasitic effect is mediated via toxic molecules released from their granules (e.g. eosinophil cationic protein and major basic protein).They also release histaminase, which limits the inflammatory consequences of mast cell degranulation. High local concentrations of eosinophils, e.g. in bronchial asthma and in cutaneous contact sensitivity and allergic eczema, can cause tissue destruction as a consequence of the release of molecules such as collagenase from their granules.

BASOPHIL GRANULOCYTES (Fig. 5.4C)

Slightly smaller than other granulocytes, basophil granulocytes are 10–14 μm in diameter, and form only 0.5–1% of the total leukocyte population of normal blood, with a count of 25–200/μl. Their distinguishing feature is the presence of large, conspicuous basophilic granules. The nucleus is somewhat irregular or bilobed, and is usually obscured in stained blood smears by the similar colour of the basophilic granules. The granules are membrane-bound vesicles which display a variety of crystalline, lamellar and granular inclusions. They contain heparin, histamine and several other inflammatory agents, and closely resemble those of tissue mast cells (p. 38). Both basophils and mast cells have membrane receptors for IgE and respond to antibody-coated antigen, which triggers their degranulation. This produces vasodilation, chemotactic stimuli for other granulocytes, and the symptoms of immediate hypersensitivity, e.g. in allergic rhinitis (hay fever). Despite these similarities, basophils and mast cells develop as separate lineages from the haemopoietic stem cell in the bone marrow.

MONONUCLEAR LEUKOCYTES

MONOCYTES (Fig. 5.4D)

Monocytes are the largest of the leukocytes (15–20 μm in diameter), but they form only a small proportion of the total population (2–8% with a count of 100–700/μl of blood). The nucleus, which is euchromatic, is relatively large and irregular, often with a characteristic indentation on one side. The cytoplasm is pale-staining, particulate and typically vacuolated. Near the nuclear indentation it contains a prominent Golgi

complex and vesicles. Monocytes are actively phagocytic cells, and contain numerous lysosomes. Phagocytosis is triggered by recognition of opsonized material, as described for neutrophils. Monocytes are highly motile, and possess a well-developed cytoskeleton.

Monocytes express Class II MHC antigens and share other similarities to tissue macrophages and dendritic cells. Most monocytes are thought to be in transit via the bloodstream from the bone marrow to the peripheral tissues where they give rise to macrophages and dendritic cells. Like other leukocytes, they pass into extravascular sites through the walls of capillaries and venules.

LYMPHOCYTES (Fig. 5.4E,F, and see Figs 5.5, 5.7)

Lymphocytes are the second most numerous type of leukocyte in adulthood, forming 20–30% of the total population (1500–2700/μl of blood). In young children they are the most numerous blood leukocyte. Most circulating lymphocytes are small, 6–8 μm in diameter; a few are medium-sized and have an increased cytoplasmic volume, often in response to antigenic stimulation. Occasionally, cells up to 16 μm are seen in peripheral blood. Lymphocytes, like other leukocytes, are found in extravascular tissues, however, they are the only white blood cells which return to the circulation. The life span of lymphocytes ranges from a few days (short-lived) to many years (long-lived). Long-lived lymphocytes play a significant role in the maintenance of immunological memory.

Blood lymphocytes are a heterogeneous collection mainly of B and T cells and consist of different subsets and different stages of activity and maturity. About 85% of all circulating lymphocytes in normal blood are T cells. Included with the lymphocytes, but probably a separate lineage subset, are the natural killer (NK) cells. These are also known as 'null' cells, because they lack the antigens which characterize B and T lymphocytes. NK cells most closely resemble large T cells morphologically.

Small lymphocytes (both B and T cells) contain a rounded, densely staining nucleus which is surrounded by a very narrow rim of cytoplasm, barely visible in the light microscope. In the electron microscope (Fig. 5.5), few cytoplasmic organelles can be seen apart from a small number of mitochondria, single ribosomes, sparse profiles of endoplasmic reticulum and occasional lysosomes: these features indicate a low metabolic rate and a quiescent phenotype. However, these cells become motile when they contact solid surfaces, and can pass between endothelial cells to exit from, or re-enter, the vascular system. They migrate extensively within various tissues, including epithelia (Fig. 5.6).

Larger lymphocytes include both B and T cell classes and also NK cells. This group contains cells which are functionally activated or proliferating after stimulation, e.g. by the presence of antigen. They contain a nucleus, which is at least in part euchromatic, and a basophilic cytoplasm, which may appear granular, and numerous polyribosome clusters, consistent with active protein synthesis. The ultrastructural appearance of these cells varies according to their class and is described below.

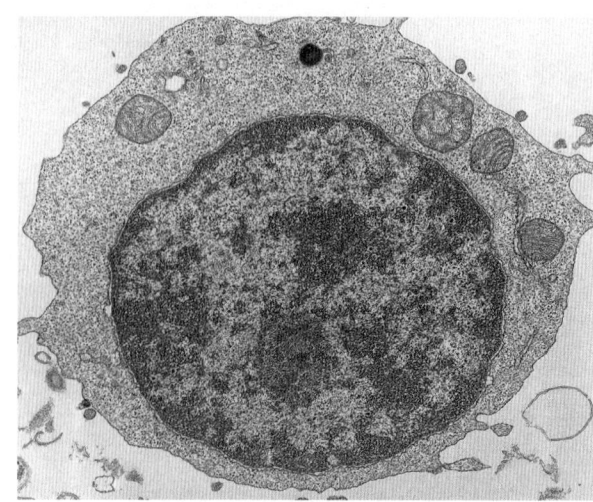

Fig. 5.5 A small relatively quiescent (resting) lymphocyte in peripheral blood. This cell measures c.6 μm in diameter and contains scant cytoplasm and few organelles.

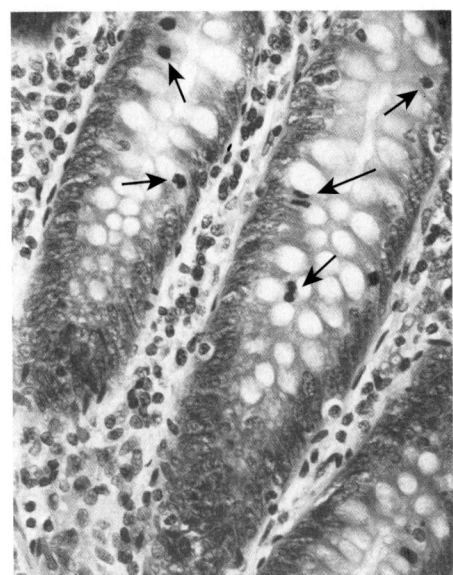

Fig. 5.6 Tubular glands in the appendix, showing proliferating intraepithelial lymphocytes (arrowed). A lymphocyte in anaphase is indicated (longer arrow). (Photograph by Sarah-Jane Smith.)

B cells

B cells and the plasma cells that develop from them synthesize and secrete antibodies which can specifically recognize and neutralize foreign (non-self) macromolecules (antigens), and can prime various non-lymphocytic cells (e.g. neutrophils, macrophages and dendritic cells) to phagocytose pathogens. B cells differentiate from haemopoietic stem cells in the bone marrow. After deletion of autoreactive cells, the selected B lymphocytes then leave the bone marrow and migrate to peripheral lymphoid sites (e.g. lymph nodes). Here, following stimulation by antigen, they undergo further proliferation and selection, forming germinal centres in the lymphoid tissues. Following this, some B cells mature into large basophilic (RNA-rich) plasma cells, either within or outside the lymphoid tissues. Plasma cells produce antibodies in their extensive rough endoplasmic reticulum (**Fig. 5.7**) and secrete them into the adjacent tissues. Other germinal centre B cells develop into long-lived memory cells capable of responding to their specific antigens not only with a more rapid and higher antibody output, but also with an increased antibody affinity compared with the primary response.

Antibodies are immunoglobulins, grouped into five classes according to their heavy polypeptide chain. Immunoglobulin G (IgG) forms the bulk of circulating antibodies. Immunoglobulin M (IgM) is normally synthesized early in immune responses. Immunoglobulin A (IgA) is present in breast milk, tears, saliva and other secretions of the alimentary tract, coupled to a secretory piece (a 70 kDa protein) which is synthesized by the epithelial cells and protects the immunoglobulin from proteolytic degradation. Immunoglobulin E (IgE) is a cytophilic antibody found on the surfaces of mast cells, eosinophils and blood basophils. Immunoglobulin D (IgD) is found together with IgM as a major membrane-bound immunoglobulin on mature immunocompetent naïve (prior to antigen exposure) B cells, acting as the cellular receptor for antigen.

When circulating antibodies bind to antigens they form immune complexes. If present in abnormal quantities, these may cause pathological damage to the vascular system and other tissues, either by interfering mechanically with permeability of the basal lamina (e.g. some types of glomerulonephritis), or by causing local activation of the complement system which generates inflammatory mediators (e.g. C5a), attacks cell membranes and causes vascular disease. In pregnancy, some maternal IgG is transferred across the placenta, and confers passive immunity on the fetus. In the case of Rhesus factor incompatibility, this brings about the destruction of Rhesus-positive fetal erythrocytes and subsequent fetal anaemia and death if it is not treated. Maternal milk contains secretory immunoglobulins (IgA) which help to combat bacterial and viral organisms in the alimentary tract of the baby during the first few weeks of postnatal life.

T cells

There are a number of sub-sets of T (thymus-derived) lymphocytes, which are all progeny of haemopoietic stem cells in the bone marrow. They require the thymus for their development and maturation before leaving to populate the peripheral, secondary, lymphoid organs (p. 981). T cells undertake a wide variety of cell-mediated defensive functions which are not directly dependent on antibody activity, and which constitute the basis of cellular immunity. T cell responses focus on the destruction of cellular targets such as virus-infected cells, certain bacterial infections, fungi, some protozoal infections, neoplastic cells and the cells of grafts from other individuals (allografts) when the tissue antigens of the donor and recipient are not sufficiently similar. Targets may be killed directly by cytotoxic T cells, or indirectly by accessory cells (e.g. macrophages) which have been recruited and activated by cytokine-secreting helper T cells. A third group, regulatory T cells, may be distinct or a subset of helper T cells, and appear to regulate or limit immune responses.

Functional groups of T cells are classified according to the molecules they express on their surfaces. The majority of cytokine-secreting helper T cells express CD4, while cytotoxic T cells are characterized by CD8. Regulatory T cells coexpress CD4 and CD25. The CD (cluster of differentiation) prefix provides a standard nomenclature for these molecules. More than 150 CD antigens have now been identified: their range of functions includes cell–cell interactions, cell adhesion, interaction with soluble ligands and signalling. Further details of the classification are beyond the scope of this publication and are given in Roitt et al (2001).

Structurally, T lymphocytes present different appearances depending on their type and state of activity. When resting, they are typical small lymphocytes and are morphologically indistinguishable from B lymphocytes. When stimulated, they become large (up to 15 μm), moderately basophilic cells, with a partially euchromatic nucleus and numerous free ribosomes, rough and smooth endoplasmic reticulum, a Golgi complex and a few mitochondria, in their cytoplasm. Cytotoxic T cells contain dense lysosome-like vacuoles which function in cytotoxic killing.

Cytotoxic T cells

Cytotoxic T lymphocytes are responsible for the direct cytotoxic killing of target cells (e.g. virus-infected cells): the requirement for direct cell–cell contact ensures the specificity of the response. Recognition of antigen, presented as a peptide fragment on MHC class I molecules, triggers the calcium-dependent release of lytic granules by the T cell. These lysosome-like granules contain perforin which forms a pore in the target cell membrane. They also contain several different serine protease enzymes (granzymes) which enter the target cell via the perforin pore and induce the programmed cell death (apoptosis; p. 27) of the target. These apoptotic cells are recognized and rapidly ingested and destroyed by phagocytes such as macrophages. The mechanism of apoptotic cell uptake does not activate the phagocyte for antigen presentation, and so the process is immunologically silent.

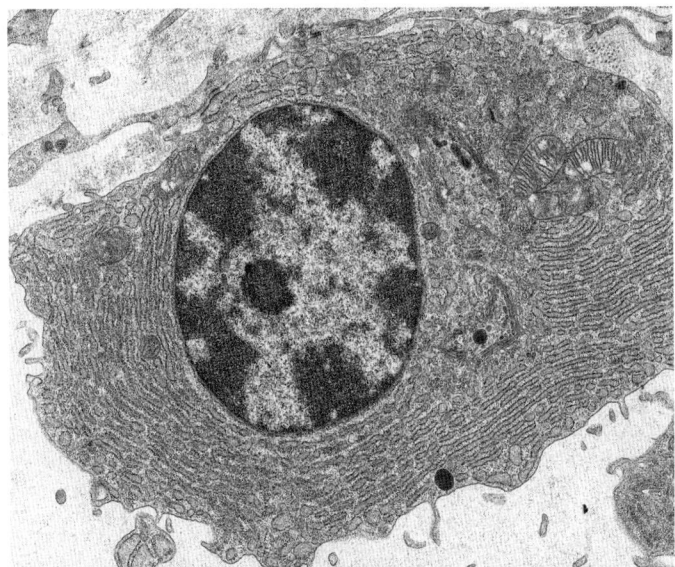

Fig. 5.7 A mature B lymphocyte (plasma cell) in loose connective tissue. The abundant rough endoplasmic reticulum is characteristic of cells synthesizing secretory proteins (in this case, immunoglobulin).

Helper T cells

Helper T cells are characterized by the secretion of cytokines. Two major populations have been identified according to the range of cytokines produced. Th1 helper T cells typically secrete interleukin (IL)-2, tumour necrosis factor (TNF) alpha and interferon gamma, while Th2 cells produce cytokines such as IL-4, IL-5 and IL-13. These two CD4-expressing populations are termed 'helper' T cells because one aspect of their function is to stimulate the proliferation and maturation of B lymphocytes and cytotoxic T lymphocytes (mediated via cytokines such as IL-4, IL-2 and interferon gamma), thus enabling and enhancing the immune responses mediated by these cells.

However, helper T cells are also important in directing the destruction of pathogens by recruiting accessory cells (e.g. macrophages, neutrophils, eosinophils) to the site of infection and by activating their effector functions. This process is tightly coordinated. For example, Th1 helper T cells secrete cytokines that not only attract and activate macrophages but also provide help for B cells and guide their immunoglobulin production to the subclasses that fix complement. Thus these antibodies opsonize the pathogen target which can then be recognized, ingested and destroyed by the macrophage accessory cells that bear receptors for complement and the Fc region of IgG. These Th1 cells are sometimes referred to as delayed type hypersensitivity T cells. In contrast, Th2 cells secrete cytokines that induce the development and activation of eosinophils, and also induce B cells to switch their immunoglobulins to non-complement fixing classes (e.g. IgE). Pathogens such as parasitic worms can then be coated with IgE antibody and hence recognized and destroyed by the effector functions of the eosinophil accessory cells which bear receptors for the Fc region of IgE.

If helper T cell activities are non-functional, a state of immunodeficiency results. This means that potentially pathogenic organisms, which are normally kept in check by the immune system, may proliferate and cause overt pathology, e.g. acquired immune deficiency syndrome (AIDS), where a virus (HIV I) specifically infects and kills (predominantly) helper T cells, but also a variety of antigen-presenting cells.

Regulatory T cells

A third population of T cells, 'regulatory' or 'T reg' T cells has recently been identified. These CD4, CD25-expressing cells have an immunomodulatory function and can dampen the effector functions of both cytotoxic and helper T cells. Regulatory T cells are produced in the thymus and are likely to be an important additional mechanism for maintaining self-tolerance. T reg function is antigen-specific and depends upon direct cell–cell contact with the target cell. The cytokine transforming growth factor (TGF) beta plays a role in mediating their function. Similar regulatory T cells can be induced in the periphery and may be important in the induction of oral tolerance to ingested antigens.

Natural killer (NK) cells

Natural killer (NK) cells have functional similarities to cytotoxic T cells. However they lack other typical lymphocyte features, and do not express antigen-specific receptors. They normally form only a small percentage of all lymphocyte-like cells and are usually included in the large granular lymphocyte category. When mature, NK cells have a mildly basophilic cytoplasm and a partially euchromatic nucleus. Ultrastructurally, their cytoplasm contains ribosomes, rough endoplasmic reticulum and dense, membrane-bound vesicles 200–500 nm in diameter with crystalline cores. These contain the protein perforin (cytolysin), capable of inserting holes in the plasma membranes of target cells, and granzymes (serine proteases) that trigger subsequent target cell death by apoptosis. NK cells are activated to kill target cells by a number of factors, including antibody-coated virus-infected cells (antibody-dependent cell-mediated cytotoxicity, ADCC), and the loss of MHC class I antigens on abnormal cells, e.g. tumour cells, which leads to loss of signalling via the NK cell inhibitory receptors that recognize MHC class I. They represent a relatively non-specific means of attacking virus-infected cells and some tumour cells.

PLATELETS (Fig. 5.8)

Blood platelets, also known as thrombocytes, are relatively small (2–4 μm across) irregular or oval discs present in large numbers (200,000–400,000/μl) in blood. In freshly harvested blood samples they readily adhere to each other and to all available surfaces, unless

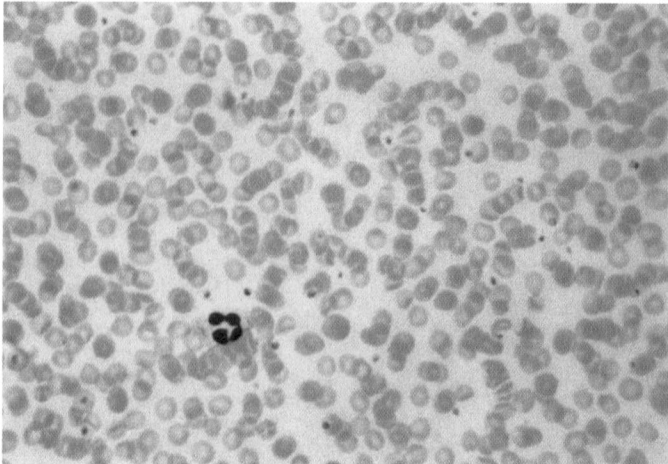

Fig. 5.8 Platelets in peripheral blood, seen as small particles staining more deeply than the surrounding erythrocytes. A neutrophil granulocyte is shown in the lower left side of the field. (Photograph by Sarah-Jane Smith.)

the blood is treated with citrate or other substances which reduce the availability of calcium ions. Platelets are anucleate cell fragments, derived from megakaryocytes in the bone marrow. They are surrounded by a plasma membrane with a thick glycoprotein coat, which is responsible for their adhesive properties. A band of c.10 microtubules lies around the perimeter of the platelet beneath the plasma membrane: the microtubules are associated with actin filaments, myosin and other proteins related to cell contraction. The cytoplasm also contains mitochondria, glycogen, a few profiles of smooth endoplasmic reticulum, tubular invaginations of the plasma membrane, and three major types of membrane-bound vesicle, designated alpha, delta and lambda granules.

Alpha granules are the largest, and have diameters of up to 500 nm. They contain platelet-derived growth factor (PDGF), fibrinogen and other substances. Delta granules are smaller (up to 300 nm), and contain 5-hydroxytryptamine (serotonin) which has been endocytosed from the blood plasma. Lambda granules are the smallest (up to 250 nm) and contain lysosomal enzymes.

Platelets play an important role in haemostasis. When a blood vessel is damaged, platelets become activated, evert their membrane invaginations to form pseudopodia and aggregate at the site of injury, plugging the wound. They adhere to each other (agglutination), and to other tissues. Adhesion is a function of the thick platelet coat and is promoted by the release of ADP and calcium ions from the platelets in response to vessel injury. The contents of released alpha granules, together with factors released from the damaged tissues, initiate a complex sequence of chemical reactions in the blood plasma, which leads to the precipitation of insoluble fibrin filaments in a three-dimensional meshwork, the fibrin clot (**Fig. 5.1**). More platelets attach to the clot, inserting extensions of their surfaces (filopodia) deep into the spaces between the fibrin filaments, to which they adhere strongly. The platelets then contract (clot retraction) by actin–myosin interactions within their cytoplasm, and this concentrates the fibrin clot and pulls the walls of the blood vessel together, which limits any further leakage of blood. After repair of the vessel wall, which may be promoted by the mitogenic activity of PDGF, the clot is dissolved by enzymes such as plasmin. Plasmin is formed by plasminogen activators in the plasma, probably assisted by lysosomal enzymes derived from the lambda granules of platelets. Platelets circulate for c.10 days before they are removed, mainly by splenic macrophages.

LYMPHOID TISSUES

Lymphocytes are located in many sites in the body, most obviously at strategic sites which are liable to infection, e.g. the oropharynx. The main areas of lymphocyte concentration are classified as primary or secondary lymphoid organs, according to whether they are involved in *de novo* lymphocyte generation (primary lymphoid organs, bone marrow and thymus) or the site of mature lymphocyte activation and initiation of an immune response (secondary lymphoid organs; e.g. lymph nodes, spleen).

All lymphocytes arise from pluripotent haemopoietic stem cells in the bone marrow. The B lymphocyte lineage develops through a series of differentiation stages within the bone marrow. The newly formed B cells then leave through the circulation and migrate to peripheral sites. In contrast, T lymphocyte development requires the thymus; the bone marrow-derived stem cells must therefore migrate via the blood circulation to the thymus (p. 981). After their differentiation and maturation into immunocompetent T cells which have survived thymic selection processes (1–3%), they re-enter the circulation and are transported to peripheral sites where they join the pool of naïve lymphocytes which recirculate through the secondary lymphoid organs via blood and lymphatic circulation systems. As recirculating cells, their major function is immune surveillance. Their activation and subsequent proliferation and functional maturation is under the control of antigen-presenting cells.

The secondary or peripheral lymphoid organs are the specialized sites where B and T lymphocytes and antigen presenting cells come together to initiate immune responses to foreign antigens. These secondary tissues include lymph nodes, spleen, and lymphoid tissue associated with epithelial surfaces (mucosa-associated lymphoid tissue, MALT), e.g. the palatine and nasopharyngeal tonsils, Peyer's patches in the small intestine, lymphoid nodules in the respiratory and urinogenital systems, the skin and conjunctiva of the eye. The microstructure of lymph nodes and of general MALT are described below. Details of all other lymphoid tissues and organs are included in the descriptions of the appropriate regional anatomy.

Lymphocytes enter secondary lymphoid tissues from the blood, usually by migration through the walls of capillaries or venules (high endothelial venules, HEV) and leave by the lymphatic system. In the spleen, lymphocyte entry and exit is via the marginal zone and venous drainage respectively. Antigen presenting cells (dendritic cells) enter via the lymphatics, bringing with them antigen from peripheral infected sites. In all the secondary tissues there are specific areas where either B or T cells are concentrated. After activation, functionally competent lymphocytes migrate to other sites in the body, where they combat the original infection.

Lymph nodes (Figs 5.9, 5.10, 5.11, 5.12)

Lymph nodes are encapsulated centres of antigen presentation and lymphocyte activation, differentiation and proliferation. They generate mature, antigen-primed, B and T cells, and filter particles, including microbes, from the lymph by the action of numerous phagocytic macrophages. A normal young adult body contains up to 450 lymph nodes,

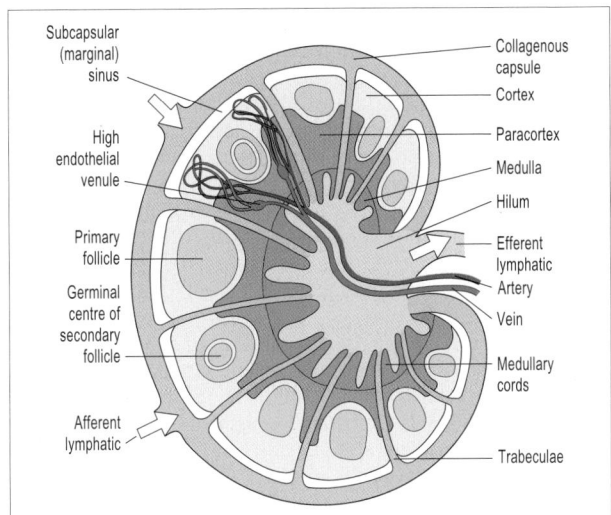

Fig. 5.9 Structure of a lymph node. (By permission from Roitt I, Brostoff J, Male D 2001 Immunology, 6th edn. London: Mosby.)

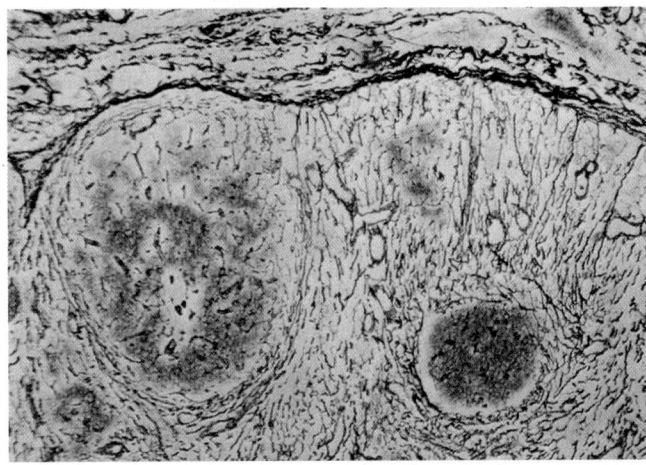

Fig. 5.10 A lymph node stained for reticulin (collagen type III). Note the heavy concentration of fibres in the capsule (top) and trabeculae. A fine network permeates the rest of the node, with a concentric distribution surrounding the cortical lymphatic follicles.

of which 60–70 are found in the head and neck, c.100 in the thorax and c.250 in the abdomen and pelvis. Lymph nodes are particularly numerous in the neck, mediastinum, posterior abdominal wall, abdominal mesenteries, pelvis and proximal regions of the limbs. By far the greatest number lie close to the viscera, especially in the mesenteries.

MICROSTRUCTURE

Lymph nodes are small, oval or kidney-shaped bodies, 0.1–2.5 cm long, lying along the course of the lymphatic vessels. Each usually has a slight indentation on one side, the hilum, through which blood vessels enter and leave and the efferent lymphatic vessel leaves. Several afferent lymphatic vessels enter the capsule around the periphery. Lymph nodes have a highly cellular cortex and a medulla (**Fig. 5.9**) which contains a network of minute lymphatic channels (sinuses) through which lymph from the afferent lymphatics is filtered, to be collected at the hilum by the efferent lymphatic. The cortex is absent at the hilum, where the medulla reaches the surface.

The capsule is composed mainly of collagen fibres, elastin fibres (especially in the deeper layers), and a few fibroblasts. From the capsule, trabeculae of dense connective tissue extend radially into the interior of the node. They are continuous with a network of fine type III collagen (reticulin) (**Fig. 5.10**) which supports the lymphoid tissue. At the hilum, dense fibrous tissue may extend into the medulla, surrounding the efferent lymphatic vessel.

The fine reticulin bundles branch and interconnect to form a very dense network in the cortex: there are fewer fibres in the germinal centres of follicles. They provide attachment for various cells, mostly dendritic cells, macrophages and lymphocytes. Reticulin and the associated proteoglycan matrix are produced by fibroblasts, a few of which are associated with the fibre network.

LYMPHATIC AND VASCULAR SUPPLY

Lymph nodes are permeated by channels through which lymph percolates after its entry from the afferent vessels. Macrophages line the channels or migrate along the reticulin which crosses them, and so lymph is exposed to their phagocytic activities, as well as to B and T lymphocytes which lie within the various regions of a node. Afferent lymphatic vessels enter at many points on the periphery, branch to form a dense intracapsular plexus, and then open into the subcapsular sinus, a cavity which is peripheral to the whole cortex except at the hilum (**Fig. 5.9**). Numerous radial cortical sinuses lead from the subcapsular sinus to the medulla, where they coalesce as larger medullary sinuses. The latter become confluent at the hilum with the efferent vessel which drains the node. All of these spaces are lined by a continuous endothelium.

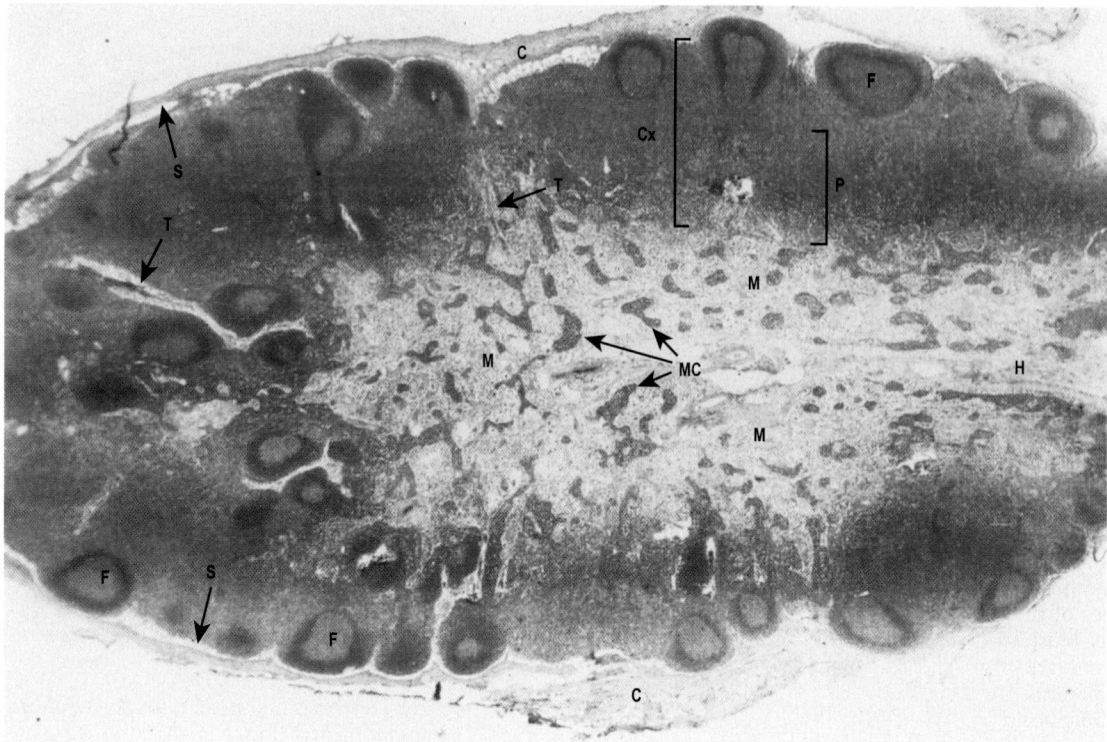

Fig. 5.11 A lymph node surrounded by an outer capsule (C). Beneath the capsule is the subcapsular sinus (S) which receives lymph via afferent lymphatic vessels. The outer cortex (Cx) is subdivided into peripheral follicles (F), many of which have a pale germinal centre, and an inner paracortex (P). The innermost medulla (M) is less densely cellular and thus pale-staining between the medullary cords (MC); it carries blood vessels, which enter and leave at the hilum (H), where the efferent lymphatic vessel also drains the node. (By permission from Young B, Heath JW 2000 Wheater's Functional Histology. Edinburgh: Churchill Livingstone.)

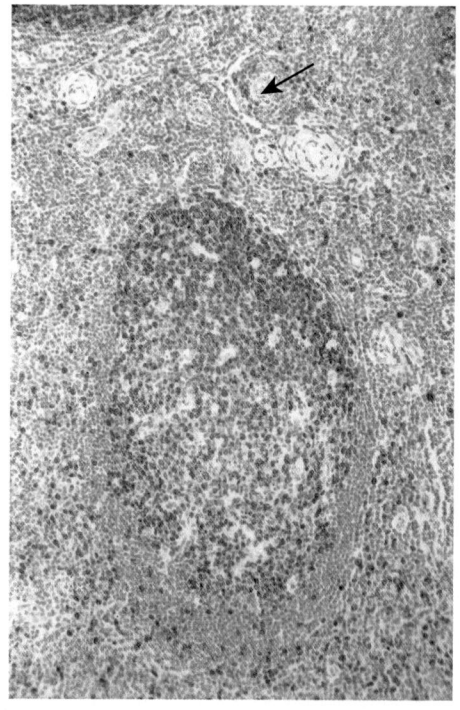

Fig. 5.12 A germinal centre in a lymphoid follicle in the tonsil, immunolabelled to demonstrate B cell-specific antigens (brown coloration); B cells are also found scattered in the surrounding mantle zone and subcapsular tissue (below) but there are few in the paracortex (above), which is mainly populated by T cells. Note the high endothelial venules (arrow) in the paracortex. (Photograph by Sarah-Jane Smith.)

CELLS AND CELLULAR ZONES OF LYMPH NODES

Although most of the cells in a lymph node are B and T lymphocytes, their distribution is not homogeneous. In the cortex, cells are densely packed and in the outer cortical area they form lymphoid follicles or nodules (**Fig. 5.11**), which are populated mainly by B cells and specialized follicular dendritic cells (FDC). The number, degree of isolation and staining characteristics of follicles vary according to their state of antigenic stimulation. A primary follicle is uniformly populated by small, quiescent lymphocytes, whereas a secondary follicle has a germinal centre which is composed mainly of antigen-stimulated B cells which are larger, less deeply staining and more rapidly dividing than those at its periphery. The follicular dendritic cells in the germinal centres display whole unprocessed antigen which is important in selecting B cells with the highest affinity, and is characteristic of the secondary immune response. After numerous mitotic divisions the selected B cells give rise to small lymphocytes, some of which become memory B cells and leave the lymph node to join the recirculating pool. Others leave to mature as antibody-secreting plasma cells either in the lymph node medulla or in peripheral tissues.

The mantle zones of cortical follicles are otherwise populated by cells similar to those of primary follicles, mainly quiescent B cells with condensed heterochromatic nuclei and little cytoplasm (hence the deeply basophilic staining of this region). They also contain a few helper T cells, follicular dendritic cells and macrophages.

The deep cortex or paracortex lies between the cortical follicles and the medulla, and is populated mainly by T cells, which are not organized into follicles. Both CD4 and CD8 T cell subsets are present. The paracortex also contains interdigitating dendritic cells. These dendritic cells include Langerhans cells from the skin and other squamous epithelia which have migrated as veiled cells via the afferent lymphatics into the draining lymph nodes. Their role is to present processed antigen to T cells. The region expands greatly in T cell-dominated immune responses, when its cells are stimulated to proliferate and disperse to peripheral sites. Macrophages, particularly in the cortical follicles and germinal centres, phagocytose apoptotic lymphocytes which have responded inadequately or inappropriately to antigenic stimulation and consequently macrophage cytoplasm becomes filled with engulfed lipid and nuclear debris.

In the medulla, lymphocytes are much less densely packed, forming irregular branching medullary cords between which the reticulin network is easily seen. Other cells include macrophages, which are

Arteries and veins serving lymph nodes pass through the hilum, giving off straight branches which traverse the medulla, and sending out minor branches as they do so. In the cortex, arteries form dense arcades of arterioles and capillaries in numerous anastomosing loops, eventually returning to highly branched venules and veins. Capillaries are especially profuse around the follicles, which contain fewer vessels. Postcapillary high endothelial venules (HEV) are abundant in the paracortical zones. They form an important site of blood-borne lymphocyte extravasation into lymphoid tissue, apparently by migration through labile endothelial tight junctions. The density of the capillary beds increases greatly when lymphocytes multiply in response to antigenic stimulation. Veins leave a node through its principal trabeculae and capsule, and drain them and the surrounding connective tissue.

more numerous in the medulla than in the cortex, plasma cells and a few granulocytes.

Mucosa-associated lymphoid tissue (MALT)

Large amounts of unencapsulated lymphoid tissue exist in the walls of the alimentary, respiratory, reproductive and urinary tracts, and in the skin: they are collectively termed mucosa-associated lymphoid tissue (MALT). Some authorities distinguish between lymphoid tissues associated with different organ systems of the body. Although there may be functional differences between them related to the different antigenic challenges encountered, this is not evident in their microstructure. Anatomically, the main subclasses are gut-associated lymphoid tissue (GALT) and bronchus-associated lymphoid tissue (BALT).

Throughout the body, MALT includes an extremely large population of lymphocytes, principally because of the size of the alimentary tract. The lymphoid cells are located in the lamina propria and in the submucosa as discrete follicles or nodules (p. 41). More scattered cells, derived from these follicles, are found throughout the lamina propria and in the base of the epithelium (**Figs 5.6, 5.13**). MALT includes macroscopically visible lymphoid masses, notably the peripharyngeal lymphoid ring of tonsillar tissue (palatine, nasopharyngeal, tubal and lingual), and the Peyer's patches of the small intestine (Chapter 72), which are described elsewhere. Most MALT consists of microscopic aggregates of lymphoid tissue, and lacks a fibrous capsule. Lymphocyte populations are supported mechanically by a fine network of fine type III collagen (reticulin) fibres and associated fibroblasts, as they are in lymph nodes.

In common with lymph nodes, MALT provides centres for the activation and proliferation of B and T lymphocytes in its follicles and parafollicular zones, respectively. The function of cells in these zones, including antigen presenting cells (follicular dendritic cells and interdigitating dendritic cells) and macrophages as well as T and B cells, is similar to that found in lymph nodes. The close proximity of lymphocytes within the MALT to an epithelial surface facilitates their access to pathogens. The lymphocyte population in MALT is not fixed: lymphocytes migrate into MALT through its high endothelial venules and leave mainly via its efferent lymphatics, which drain interstitial fluid as lymph. MALT lacks afferent lymphatic vessels. Migration from MALT follows a different route from the major peripheral route of recirculation. After antigen activation, lymphocytes travel via the regional lymph nodes and are dispersed along all mucosal surfaces so that pathogen entry at a single site in the MALT leads to protective T and B cell immunity which is disseminated throughout the mucosal system.

FOLLICLE-ASSOCIATED EPITHELIUM

The epithelium covering mucosa-associated lymphoid tissue, which varies in type according to its location, is unusual in possessing cells which are involved in sampling antigens and passing them to the underlying tissues. The main function of B lymphocytes in MALT is to produce IgA for secretion into the lumen of the tracts which they line. They are exposed to antigens present in the lumen because the epithelium samples and transfers these antigens to antigen-presenting cells in the underlying lymphoid tissue. Appropriate clones of T and B cells are then activated and amplified prior to their exit via the lymphatics. In the small and large intestine these specialized epithelial cells have characteristic short microvilli on their luminal surface and are known as microfold (M) cells (Ch. 72). In the palatine tonsils they include modified stratified squamous reticulated epithelial cells (see **Fig. 35.7B**).

Thus, many of the lymphocytes migrating between cells in the basal regions of epithelia (**Fig. 5.6**) are effector cytotoxic and helper T cells that have already been selected in lymphoid nodules and are engaged in immune responses. Similar cells, and activated IgA-producing B cells and plasma cells, are also scattered throughout the entire mucosal lamina propria.

HAEMOPOIESIS

Postnatally, blood cells are formed primarily in the bone marrow. Other tissues, particularly the spleen and liver, may develop haemopoietic activity once more, if production from the marrow is inadequate.

Bone marrow (Fig. 5.14)

Bone marrow is a soft pulpy tissue which is found in the marrow cavities of all bones and even in the larger Haversian canals of lamellar bone (p. 88). It differs in composition in different bones and at different ages and occurs in two forms, yellow and red marrow. In old age the marrow of the cranial bones undergoes degeneration and is then termed gelatinous marrow.

YELLOW MARROW

Yellow marrow consists of a framework of connective tissue which supports numerous blood vessels and cells, most of which are adipocytes. A small population of typical red marrow cells persists and may be reactivated when the demand for blood cells becomes sufficiently great.

RED MARROW

Red marrow is found throughout the skeleton in the fetus and during the first years of life. After about the fifth year the red marrow, which represents actively haemopoietic tissue, is gradually replaced in the long bones by yellow marrow. The replacement starts earlier, and is generally more advanced, in the more distal bones. By 20–25 years of age, red marrow persists only in the vertebrae, sternum, ribs, clavicles, scapulae, pelvis, cranial bones and in the proximal ends of the femur and humerus.

Red bone marrow consists of a network of loose connective tissue, the stroma, which supports clusters of haemopoietic cells (haemopoietic

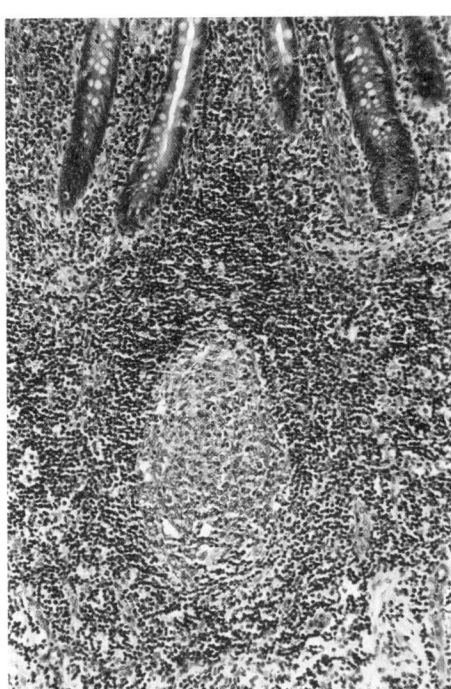

Fig. 5.13 Germinal centre in a follicle of mucosa-associated lymphoid tissue (MALT) in the mucosa and submucosa of the appendix. The bases of tubular glands of the mucosal epithelium are seen in the upper field. (Photograph by Sarah-Jane Smith.)

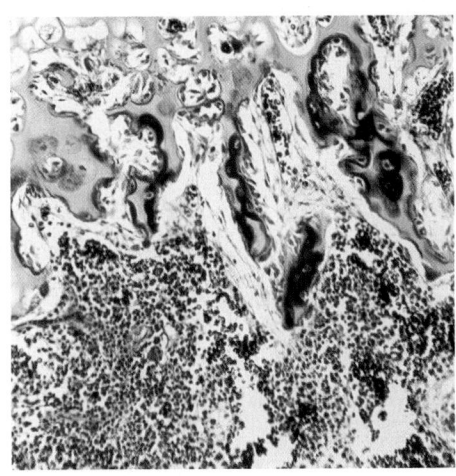

Fig. 5.14 Haemopoietic tissue in the marrow cavity of a foetal long bone undergoing endochondral ossification (top). Islands of densely-packed nucleated haemopoietic cells of different lineages are separated by large vascular sinusoids (bottom centre and right) which are filled with mature red blood cells in the general circulation. (Photograph by Sarah-Jane Smith.)

cords or islands) and a rich vascular supply in which large, thin-walled sinusoids are the main feature (**Fig. 5.14**). The vascular supply is derived from the nutrient artery to the bone, which ramifies in the bone marrow, and terminates in thin-walled arterioles from which the sinusoids arise. These, in turn, drain into disproportionately large veins. Lymphatic vessels are absent from bone marrow. The stroma contains a variable amount of fat, depending on age, site and the haematological status of the body, and small patches of lymphoid tissue are also present. Marrow thus consists of vascular and extravascular compartments, both enclosed within a bony framework from which they are separated by a thin layer of endosteal cells (p. 93).

Stroma

Stroma is composed of a delicate network of fine type III collagen (reticulin) fibres secreted by highly branched, specialized fibroblast-like cells (reticular cells) derived from embryonic mesenchyme. When haemopoiesis stops, as occurs in most limb bones in adult life, these cells (or closely related cells) become distended with lipid droplets, and fill the marrow with yellow fatty tissue (yellow marrow). If there is a later demand for haemopoiesis, the stellate stromal cells reappear. The stroma also contains numerous macrophages attached to extracellular matrix fibres. These cells actively phagocytose cellular debris created by haemopoietic development, especially the extruded nuclei of erythroblasts, remnants of megakaryocytes and cells which have failed the B lymphocyte selection process. Stromal cells play a major role in the control of haemopoietic cell differentiation, proliferation and maturation.

Marrow sinusoids are lined by a single layer of endothelial cells, supported by reticulin on their basal surfaces. Although the endothelial cells are interconnected by tight junctions, their cytoplasm is extremely thin in places, and the underlying basal lamina is discontinuous. The passage of newly formed blood cells from the haemopoietic compartment into the bloodstream appears to occur through an interactive process with the endothelium, producing temporary apertures (large fenestrae) in their attenuated cytoplasm.

Haemopoietic tissue

Cords and islands of haematogenous cells consist of clusters of immature blood cells in various stages of development; several different cell lineages are typically represented in each focal group. One or more macrophages lie at the core of each such group of cells. These macrophages engage in phagocytic functions, are important in transferring iron to developing erythroblasts for haemoglobin synthesis, and may play a role, with other stromal cells, in regulating the rate of cell proliferation and maturation of the neighbouring haemopoietic cells.

Cell lineages (Figs 5.15, 5.16)
HAEMOPOIETIC STEM CELLS

Within the adult marrow there is a very small number (c.0.05% of haemopoietic cells) of self-renewing, pluripotent stem cells which are capable of giving rise to all blood cell types, including lymphocytes. Although they cannot be identified morphologically in the marrow, they can be recognized in aspirates by the expression of specific cell surface marker proteins (e.g. CD34).

Progressively more lineage-restricted committed progenitor cells develop from these ancestors to produce the various cell types found in peripheral blood. The committed progenitor cells are often termed colony-forming units (CFU) of the lineage(s), e.g. CFU-GM cells give rise, after proliferation, to neutrophil granulocytes, monocytes and certain dendritic cells, whereas CFU-E produce only erythrocytes (**Figs 5.15, 5.16**). Each cell type undergoes a period of maturation in the marrow, often accompanied by several structural changes, before release into the general circulation. In some lineages, e.g. the erythroid series, the final stages of maturation take place in the circulation, whereas in the monocytic lineage, they occur after the cells have left the circulation and entered peripheral tissues where they differentiate into macrophages and some dendritic cells.

To generate a complete set of blood cells from a single pluripotent cell may take some months. The later progenitor cells form mature cells

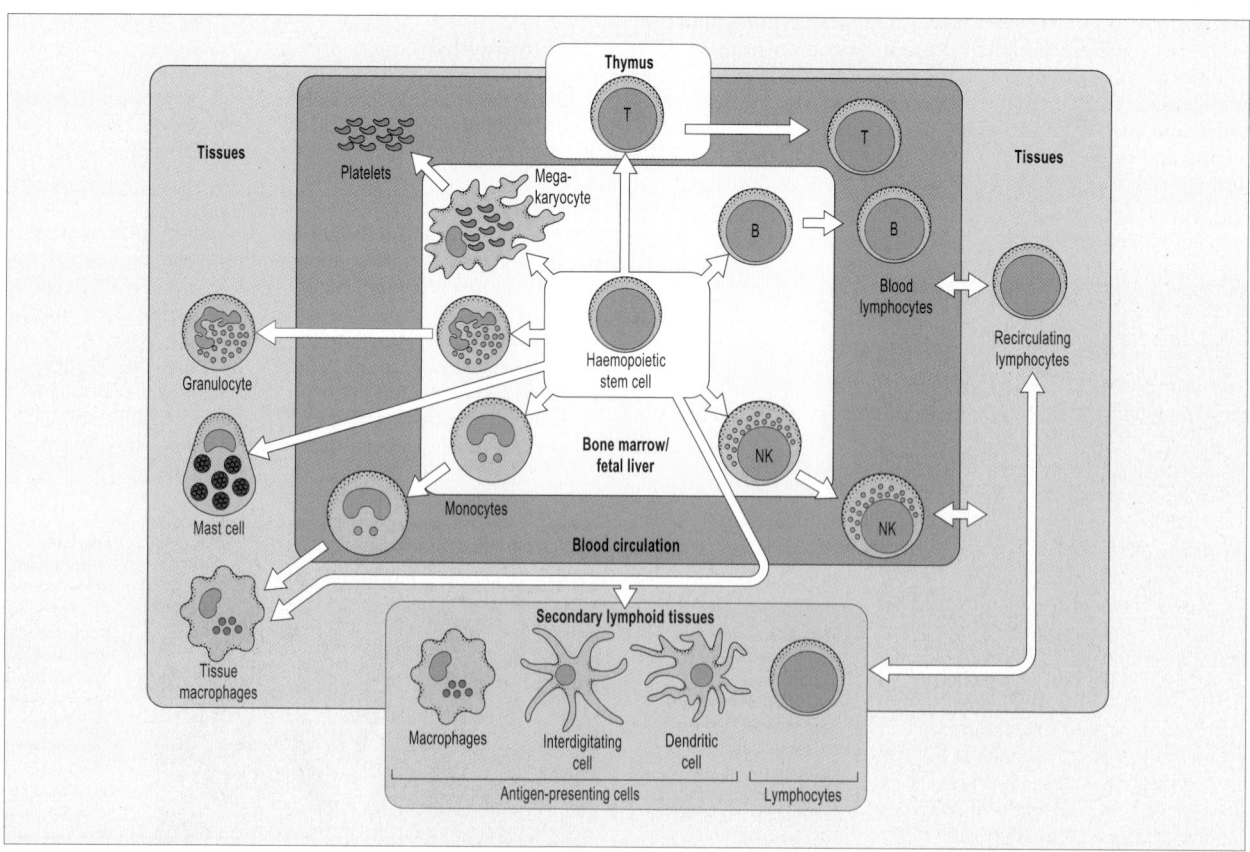

Fig. 5.15 Developmental origins of cells of the immune system. All the cells shown originate from haemopoietic stem cells and are released into the blood circulation, through which certain cells reach peripheral tissues. (By permission from Roitt I, Brostoff J, Male D 2001 Immunology, 6th edn. London: Mosby.)

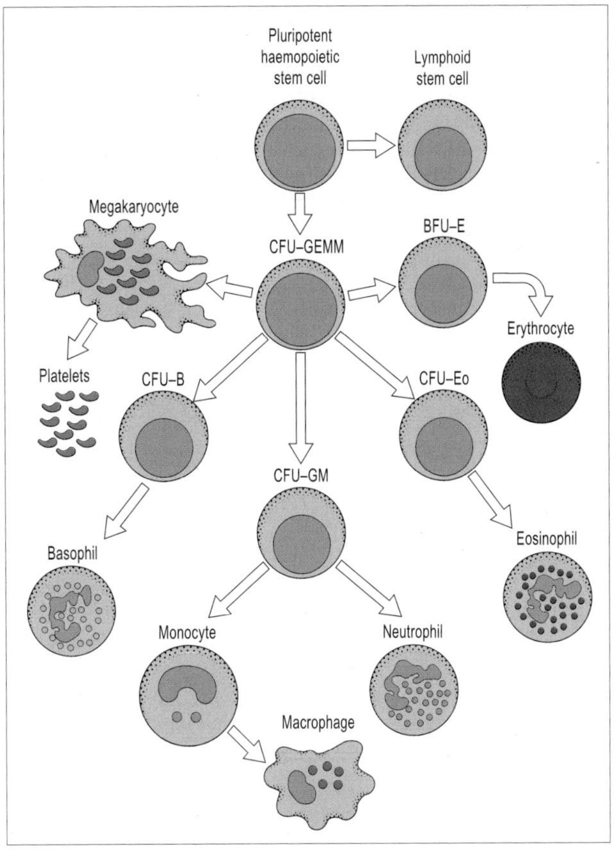

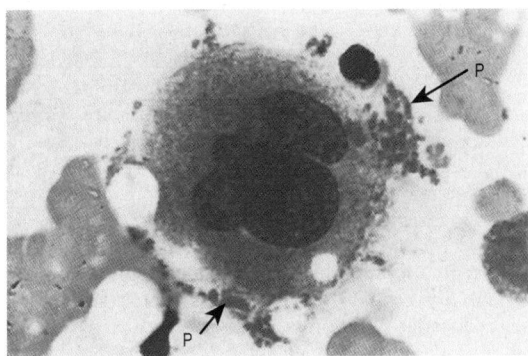

Fig. 5.16 Development of granulocytes and monocytes. Haemopoietic stem cells give rise to colony-forming units (CFUs). CFU-GEMMs have the potential to give rise to all blood cells except lymphocytes. These are granulocytes (G), erythrocytes (E), monocytes (M) and megakaryocytes (M), which each develop in response to specific cytokines and hormones. Intermediate CFUs or, for erythrocytes, burst-forming units (BFUs), are shown. (By permission from Roitt I, Brostoff J, Male D 2001 Immunology, 6th edn. London: Mosby.)

of their particular lineages more quickly. However, because they are not self-renewing, grafts of these later cells eventually fail because the cells they produce all ultimately die. This is of considerable importance in bone marrow replacement therapy. The presence of pluripotent stem cells in the donor marrow is essential for success: only c.5% of the normal number are needed to repopulate the marrow. Following replacement therapy, T lymphocytes reconstitute more slowly than the other haemopoietic lineages, reflecting the progressive reduction in size of the thymus with age (chronic involution).

ERYTHROCYTES

Erythrocytes and granulocytes belong to the myeloid lineage. The earliest identifiable erythroid stem cells are capable of rapid bursts of cell division to form numerous daughter cells; they have thus been named burst-forming units of the erythroid line (BFU-E). They give rise to the CFU-E, which, with their immediate progeny, are sensitive to the hormone erythropoietin. This hormone, produced in the kidney, induces further differentiation along the erythroid line.

The first readily identifiable cell of the erythroid series is the pro-erythroblast, a large (c.20 μm) cell with a large euchromatic nucleus and moderately basophilic cytoplasm. It also responds to erythropoietin. The proerythroblast contains small amounts of ferritin and bears some of the protein spectrin on its plasma membrane (p. 69). Proerythroblasts proliferate to produce smaller (12–16 μm) basophilic erythroblasts, rich in ribosomes, in which haemoglobin-RNA synthesis begins. The cytoplasm becomes partially, and then uniformly, eosinophilic (the polychromatic erythroblast and orthochromatic erythroblast respectively). These cells are only 8–10 μm in diameter and contain very little cytoplasmic RNA. The nucleus becomes intensely pyknotic and is finally extruded from the cell, leaving an anucleate reticulocyte, which enters a sinusoid. Its reticular staining pattern, visible using special stains,

results from residual cytoplasmic RNA which is lost within c.24 hours of entering the peripheral blood circulation. Reticulocyte numbers in peripheral blood are therefore a good indicator of the rate of red cell production. The whole process of erythropoiesis takes 5–9 days.

GRANULOCYTES

Granulocyte formation involves major changes in nuclear morphology and cytoplasmic contents which are best known for the neutrophil. Initially, myeloid stem cells transform into large (10–20 μm) myeloblasts which are similar in general size and appearance to proerythroblasts. These proliferative cells have large euchromatic nuclei and lack cytoplasmic granules. They differentiate into slightly larger promyelocytes, in which the first group of specific proteins is synthesized in the rough endoplasmic reticulum and Golgi apparatus. The proteins are stored in large (0.3 μm) primary (non-specific) granules, which are large lysosomes containing acid phosphatase. Smaller secondary (specific) granules are formed in the smaller myelocyte, which is the last proliferative stage. The nucleus is typically flattened or slightly indented on one side in myelocytes.

In the next, metamyelocyte, stage, the cell size (10–15 μm) decreases, the nucleus becomes heterochromatic and horse-shoe shaped, and protein synthesis almost stops. As the neutrophil is released, the nucleus becomes first heavily indented (the juvenile stab or band form), and subsequently segmented into up to six lobes, characteristic of the mature neutrophil. The whole process takes c.7 days to complete, of which c.3 days are spent proliferating, and 4 days maturing. Neutrophils may then be stored in the marrow for a further 4 days, depending on demand, before their final release into the circulation.

Eosinophils and basophils pass through a similar sequence but their nuclei do not become as irregular as that of the neutrophil. It is thought that these cells each arise from distinct colony-forming units, which are separate from the CFU-GM.

PLATELETS

Platelets arise in a unique manner by the shedding of thousands of cytoplasmic fragments from the tips of processes of megakaryocytes in the bone marrow (**Fig. 5.17**). The first detectable cell of this line is the highly basophilic megakaryoblast (15–50 μm), followed by a pro-megakaryocyte stage (20–80 μm), in which synthesis of granules begins. Finally, the fully differentiated megakaryocyte, a giant cell (35–160 μm) with a large, dense, polyploid, multilobed nucleus, appears. Once differentiation is initiated from the CFU-Meg, DNA replicates without cytoplasmic division (endoreduplication) and the chromosomes are retained within a single polyploid nucleus which may contain 8n, 16n or 32n chromosomes.

The cytoplasm contains fine basophilic granules and becomes partitioned into proplatelets by invaginations of the plasma membrane. These are seen ultrastructurally as a network of tubular profiles which coalesce to form cytoplasmic islands c.3–4 μm in diameter. Individual platelets are shed into the circulation from a long, narrow process of

Fig. 5.17 Megakaryocytes in an aspirate of bone marrow (Giemsa-stained). Note the enormous cell size compared with the clustered erythrocytes (orange), the multilobed nucleus and irregular cytoplasmic outline. P, platelets. (By permission from Young B, Heath JW 2000 Wheater's Functional Histology. Edinburgh: Churchill Livingstone.)

megakaryocyte cytoplasm which is protruded through an aperture in the sinusoidal endothelium.

MONOCYTES

Monocytes are formed in the bone marrow. Monocytes and neutrophils appear to be closely related cells: together with some of the antigen-presenting dendritic cells, they arise from a shared progenitor, the colony-forming unit for granulocytes and macrophages (CFU-GM). Different colony-stimulating factors (CSF) act on the common progenitor to direct its subsequent differentiation pathway. Monocyte progenitors pass through a proliferative monoblast stage (14 μm) and then form differentiating promonocytes, which are slightly smaller cells in which production of small lysosomes begins. After further divisions, monocytes (up to 20 μm) are released into the general circulation. Most migrate into perivascular and extravascular sites, which they then populate as macrophages, while others may give rise to dendritic cells.

LYMPHOCYTES

Lymphocytes are a heterogeneous group of cells (p. 72) which may share a common ancestral lymphoid stem cell, distinct from the myeloid stem cell which gives rise to all of the cell types described above. The first identifiable progenitor cell is the lymphoblast, which divides several times to form prolymphocytes: both cells are characterized by a high nuclear to cytoplasmic ratio. B cells undergo differentiation to their specific lineage subset entirely within the bone marrow and migrate to peripheral or secondary lymphoid tissues as naïve B cells, ready to respond to antigen. However, T cells require the specialized thymic microenvironment for their development. Progenitor cells migrate to the thymus (p. 981) during fetal and early postnatal life, and at lower levels throughout life. In the thymus they undergo a process of differentiation and selection as T cells, before populating secondary lymphoid tissues.

B CELL DEVELOPMENT

B cells start their development in the subosteal region of the bone marrow, moving centripetally as differentiation progresses. Their development entails the rearrangement of immunoglobulin genes to create a unique receptor for antigen on each B cell, and the progressive expression of cell surface and intracellular molecules required for mature B lymphocyte function. Autoreactive cells which meet their self-antigen within the bone marrow are eliminated. Overall c.25% of B cells successfully complete these developmental and selection processes, and those that fail die by apoptosis and are removed by macrophages. Bone marrow stromal cells (fibroblasts, fat cells and macrophages) express cell surface molecules and secreted cytokines which control B lymphocyte development. The mature naïve B lymphocytes leave via the central sinuses. They express antigen receptors (immunoglobulin) of IgM and IgD classes. Class switching to IgG, A and E occurs in the periphery in response to antigen activation.

T CELL (THYMOCYTE) DEVELOPMENT

T cells develop within the thymus from blood-borne bone marrow-derived progenitors. These cells enter the thymus via high endothelial venules at the corticomedullary junction. They first migrate to the outer (subcapsular) region of the thymus and then, as in the bone marrow, move progressively inwards as development continues. T cell development involves gene rearrangements in the T cell receptor (TcR) loci to create unique receptors for antigen on each cell, together with the progressive expression of molecules required for mature T cell function. Selection of the receptor repertoire is more stringent for T cells than for B cells because of the way in which mature T cells 'see' cell-bound antigens presented in conjunction with specific proteins of the major histocompatibility complex (MHC) expressed on the surfaces of antigen-presenting cells. Thus selection must ensure the survival of those T cells which can respond only to foreign antigens (i.e. are self-tolerant), bound to their own (self) class of MHC molecule. Cells which fail to bind to self MHC molecules or which bind to self-antigens are eliminated by apoptotic cell death. It is estimated that up to 95% of T cell progenitors undergo apoptosis in this way. Those which express appropriate molecules and have effective, MHC-restricted binding properties, survive to become mature, naïve T cells which leave the thymus and populate the periphery.

Thymic stromal cells play a crucial role in T cell development and selection (p. 981). Thymic epithelial cells in the cortex express both MHC class I and II molecules and are unique in their ability to select T cells which recognize self MHC (positive selection). Deletion of self-antigen reactive cells (negative selection) is mainly controlled by thymic dendritic cells located at the corticomedullary junction and in the medulla, although the epithelium can also perform this function. Apoptotic thymocytes are removed by thymic macrophages. The role of the thymic epithelium in thymocyte differentiation is complex and involves cell–cell contact as well as the secretion of soluble mediators such as cytokines, chemokines, neuroactive peptides (e.g. somatostatin) and thymic hormones (e.g. thymulin). Thymic fibroblasts and the extracellular matrix also play a role.

MACROPHAGES AND DENDRITIC CELLS

Macrophages and dendritic cells are important accessory cells in immune defence. Dendritic cells (e.g. Langerhans cells of the skin) are the professional antigen-presenting cells (APC) of the immune system, taking up foreign material by endocytosis and macropinocytosis, and they are uniquely capable of efficiently activating naïve as well as mature T lymphocytes. Macrophages are able to process and present antigen to lymphocytes, but are less effective than dendritic cells. In addition macrophages play an important role in the effector arm of the immune response, clearing the infectious agent by phagocytosis. Thus, monocytes and macrophages ingest particulate material, including potential pathogens, and they kill organisms intracellularly, like neutrophils. The third major cell type involved in antigen presentation and T cell activation is the B lymphocyte. Follicular dendritic cells of lymph nodes, MALT and the spleen form a distinct group which, although not classic APCs, participate as accessory cells of the immune system by presenting non-processed antigen to B lymphocytes.

APCs endocytose antigen, digest it intracellularly, mostly to peptide fragments, and present the fragments on their surfaces, in conjunction with MHC class II molecules. Some endocytosed material is presented on Class I molecules, which are expressed by all nucleated cells. Class II molecules are normally found only on APC, although there is evidence that certain other cells can express class II molecules in pathological situations.

Recognition of foreign antigen is controlled by a variety of APC cell surface receptors. In addition to Fc and complement receptors which mediate uptake of opsonized material, pathogen-derived molecules are directly recognized via pattern recognition receptors (PRR) such as Toll-like receptors (TLR) and scavenger receptors.

Macrophages

The mononuclear phagocyte system consists of the blood monocytes, from which the other types are derived, and various tissue macrophages, some of which have tissue-specific names. Certain dendritic cells are sometimes included in the mononuclear phagocyte system; however, although they share a common lineage ancestor, they appear to form a discrete branch of the family tree. Most monocytes and macrophages express class II MHC molecules (e.g. HLA-DR).

Macrophages are very variable in size (generally 15–25 μm) and are found in many tissues of the body. They are migrant cells in all general connective tissues, the alveolar macrophages in the lung (**Fig. 5.18**; Chapter 62), Kupffer cells in liver sinusoids (p. 1222), in bone marrow (p. 77) and in all lymphoid tissues (p. 74). Macrophages often aggregate in subserous connective tissue of the pleura and peritoneum, where they are visible as milky spots near small lymphatic trunks. They cluster around the terminations of small (penicillar) arterioles in the spleen and, are distributed more diffusely, throughout the splenic cords (p. 1242).

Osteoclasts (up to 100 μm) in bone (p. 92) are closely related to macrophages. However they are syncytial cells derived from the fusion of up to 30 progenitor monocytes in bone tissue, where they differentiate further (p. 92). Microglia of the central nervous system (CNS) are thought to be monocytic in origin: they migrate into the CNS during its development (p. 55). They differ from macrophages in that normally they are quiescent cells in which MHC class II expression is down-regulated, and they display little phagocytic activity.

Macrophages vary in structure depending on their location in the body. All have a moderately basophilic cytoplasm containing some

(activated macrophages) by cytokines, e.g. interferon (IFN)-γ, which are secreted by other cells of the immune system, especially T lymphocytes.

Close antibody-mediated binding may initiate the release of lysosomal enzymes onto the surfaces of the cellular targets to which the macrophages bind. This process of antibody-dependent cell-mediated cytotoxicity (ADCC), is also used by other cells, including NK cells, neutrophils and eosinophils, particularly if the targets are too large to be phagocytosed (e.g. nematode worm parasites).

SECRETORY ACTIVITIES

Activated macrophages can synthesize and secrete various bioactive substances, e.g. IL-1, which stimulate the proliferation and maturation of other lymphocytes, greatly amplifying the reaction of the immune system to foreign antigens. They also synthesize tumour necrosis factor (TNF)-α, which is able to kill small numbers of neoplastic cells. TNF-α depresses the anabolic activities of many cells in the body, and may be a major factor mediating cachexia (wasting) which typically accompanies more advanced cancers. Other macrophage products include plasminogen activator, which promotes clot removal; various lysosomal enzymes; several complement and clotting factors; and lysozyme (an antibacterial protein). In pathogenesis, these substances may be released inappropriately and damage healthy tissues, e.g. in rheumatoid arthritis and various other inflammatory conditions.

Dendritic cells (Fig. 5.19)

There are two distinct groups of dendritic cells, myeloid and lymphoid. The groups are morphologically similar but have different developmental origins and functions. They are derived from haemopoietic stem cells, and a major subset are of myeloid lineage, closely related to monocytes and responsive to bacterial antigens. The other group may share lineage with the lymphocytic line and respond primarily to viral antigens.

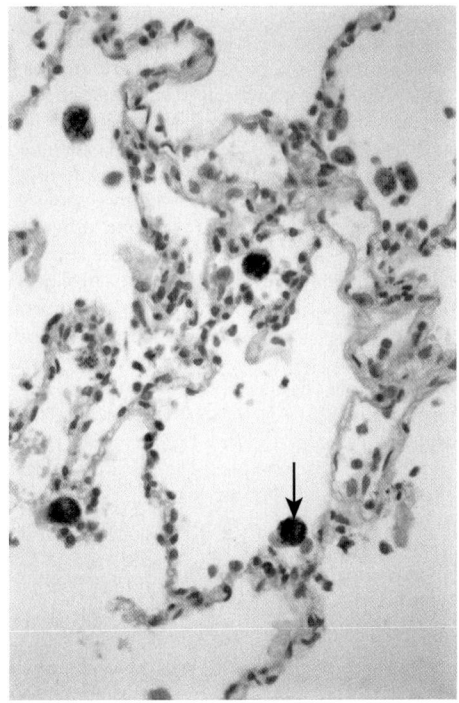

Fig. 5.18 Alveolar macrophages (dust cells, arrow) with ingested carbon particles, in a section through pulmonary alveoli. (Photograph by Sarah-Jane Smith.)

rough and smooth endoplasmic reticulum, an active Golgi complex and a large, euchromatic and somewhat irregular nucleus. These features are consistent with an active metabolism: synthesis of lysosomal enzymes continues in mature cells. All macrophages have irregular surfaces studded with filopodia and they contain varying numbers of endocytic vesicles, larger vacuoles and lysosomes. Some macrophages are highly motile, whereas others tend to remain attached and sedentary, e.g. in hepatic and lymphoid sinuses. Within connective tissues, macrophages may fuse to form large syncytia (giant cells) around particles which are too large to be phagocytosed, or when stimulated by the presence of infectious organisms, e.g. tubercle bacilli.

When blood-borne monocytes enter the tissues through the endothelial walls of capillaries and venules, they can undergo a limited number of rounds of mitosis as tissue macrophages before they die and are replaced from the bone marrow, typically after several weeks. There is some evidence that alveolar macrophages of the lung are able to undergo many more mitoses than other macrophages.

PHAGOCYTOSIS

The uptake of particulate material and microorganisms is carried out by macrophages in many tissues and organs. When present in general connective tissue, they ingest and kill invading microorganisms and remove debris produced as a consequence of tissue damage. They engulf apoptotic cells in all situations. In the lung, alveolar macrophages constantly patrol the respiratory surfaces, to which they migrate from pulmonary connective tissue. They engulf inhaled particles including bacteria, surfactant and debris and many enter the sputum (hence their alternative names, dust cells or, in cardiac disease, heart failure cells, which are full of extravasated erythrocytes). They perform similar scavenger functions in the pleural and peritoneal cavities. In lymph nodes, macrophages line the walls of sinuses and remove particulate matter from lymph as it percolates through them. In the spleen and liver, macrophages are involved in particle removal and in the detection and destruction of aged or damaged erythrocytes. They begin the degradation of haemoglobin for recycling iron and amino acids.

Macrophages bear surface receptors for the Fc portions of antibodies and for the C3 component of complement. Phagocytic activity is greatly increased when the target has been coated in antibody (opsonized) or complement, or both. Once phagocytosis has occurred, the vacuole bearing the ingested particle fuses with endosomal vesicles which contain a wide range of lysosomal enzymes, including many hydrolases, and oxidative systems capable of rapid bacteriocidal action. These activities are much enhanced when macrophages are stimulated

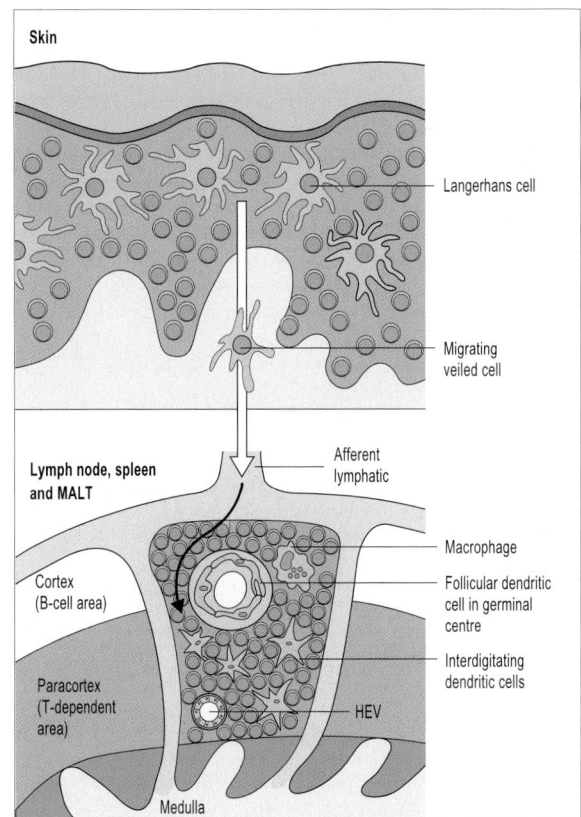

Fig. 5.19 Dendritic cells in the skin and lymphoid tissues. In the skin, these are known as Langerhans cells. They migrate (as veiled cells) with processed antigen to the paracortex of draining lymph nodes, where, as interdigitating dendritic cells, they make contact with and present antigen to T cells. Follicular dendritic cells in germinal centres of lymph nodes expose B cells to antigen. (By permission from Roitt I, Brostoff J, Male D 2001 Immunology, 6th edn. London: Mosby.)

The myeloid dendritic cells are professional antigen-presenting cells (APC), which are able to process and present antigen to T lymphocytes, including naïve T cells. They are present as immature dendritic cells in the epidermis of the skin and other stratified squamous epithelia, e.g. the oral mucosa (Langerhans cells), and in the dermis and most other tissues (interstitial dendritic cells), where they are concerned with immune surveillance. Immature dendritic cells have an antigen-capturing function. They express pattern recognition receptors (e.g. Toll-like receptors) on their surface. Binding of bacterial molecules (e.g. carbohydrate or DNA) to these receptors stimulates the dendritic cells to migrate via the lymphatics to nearby secondary lymphoid tissues where they mature and acquire an antigen-presenting function. Mature dendritic cells are known as veiled cells when in the afferent lymphatics and the subcapsular sinuses of lymph nodes (p. 75), and as inter-digitating dendritic cells once they are within the lymphoid tissue proper. Their function within the secondary lymphoid tissue is to present their processed antigen to T lymphocytes, and thus to initiate and stimulate the immune response.

LANGERHANS CELLS

Langhans cells are one of the most well-studied type of immature dendritic cell. They are present throughout the epidermis, but are most clearly identifiable in the stratum spinosum (p. 157). They have an irregular nucleus and a clear cytoplasm, and contain characteristic elongated membranous vesicles (Birbeck granules). Langerhans cells endocytose and process antigens, undergoing a process of maturation from antigen-capturing to antigen-presenting cells which express high levels of MHC class I and II molecules, co-stimulatory proteins and adhesion molecules. They migrate to lymph nodes to activate T lymphocytes.

INTERDIGITATING DENDRITIC CELLS

Immature dendritic cells are found all over the body and function in antigen-processing and immune surveillance. Mature dendritic cells are present in T cell-rich areas of secondary lymphoid tissue (paracortical areas of lymph nodes, interfollicular areas of MALT, periarteriolar sheaths of splenic white pulp), where they are frequently referred to as interdigitating dendritic cells. Within the secondary lymphoid tissues, they are involved in the presentation of antigen to T lymphocytes in the context of either MHC class I (CD8 T cells) or MHC class II (CD4 T cells). Binding is accompanied by co-stimulatory protein recognition by T cell surface molecules, and by adhesive interactions between the two cell types. Appropriate T cells are thus activated to proliferate and are primed for carrying out their immunological functions. Only T cells which possess receptors corresponding to the specific antigen presented to them in combination with MHC class I or II molecules can be triggered in this way. These processes are known as class I and class II MHC restriction, respectively. Naïve T cells can only respond to antigen presented by dendritic cells. Once primed, T cells can be stimulated by any APC, including macrophages. Mature dendritic cells not only present antigen to activate T lymphocytes, but also secrete cytokines which direct the nature of the T cell response (e.g. Th1 versus Th2).

FOLLICULAR DENDRITIC CELLS (Fig. 5.20)

Follicular dendritic cells, FDCs, are a non-migratory population of cells found in the follicles of secondary lymphoid tissues, where they attract and interact with B cells. Unlike other dendritic cells, FDCs are not haemopoietic in origin, but are probably derived from the stromal cells of lymphoid tissues. They are unable to endocytose and process antigen, and they lack MHC class II molecules. However, Fc receptors and complement receptors CD21 and CD35 on FDCs allow the cells to bind immune complexes (iccosomes) to their surface for subsequent presentation, as unprocessed antigen, to germinal centre B cells. Complex interactions between B cells, CD4 helper T cells and FDCs in the germinal centres are important in the selection of high affinity B cells and their maturation to either plasma cells or memory B lymphocytes.

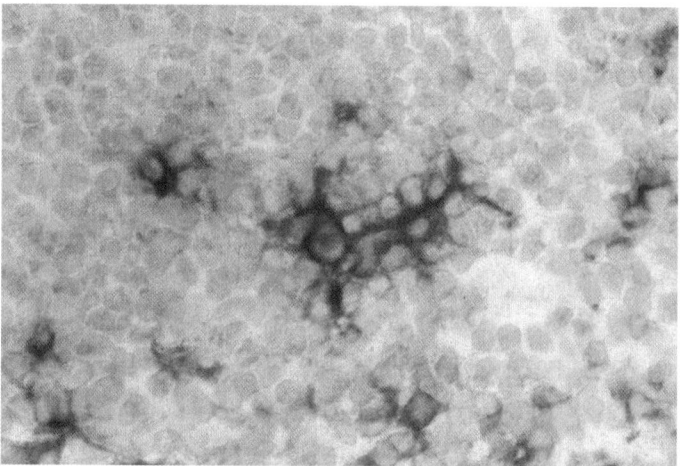

Fig. 5.20 Follicular dendritic cells in a germinal centre of the palatine tonsil (immunoperoxidase labelled). (By kind permission from Dr Marta Perry, UMDS, London.)

REFERENCES

Janeway C, Walport M, Travers P 2004 Immunobiology: the Immune System in Health and Disease, 5th edn. New York: Garland Publishing.
Emphasizes the unifying principles of structure and function of the immune system in health and disease.

Liu Y-J 2001 Dendritic cell subsets and lineages, and their functions in innate and adaptive immunity. Cell 106: 259–62.
Review of current research and a re-evaluation of the lineage of and functional relationships between different dendritic cell types.

Roitt I, Brostoff J, Male D 2001 Immunology, 6th edn. London: Mosby.
Sets out the scientific principles of clinical immunology, integrated with histology, pathology and clinical examples.

Functional anatomy of the musculoskeletal system

The skeletal system consists of the specialized supporting connective tissues of the bony skeleton and associated tissues of joints, including cartilage. Cartilage is the fetal precursor tissue in the development of many bones; it also supports non-skeletal structures, as in the ear, larynx and tracheobronchial tree. Bone provides a rigid framework which protects and supports most of the soft tissues of the body and acts as a system of struts and levers which, through the action of attached skeletal muscles, permits movement of the body. Bones of the skeleton are connected with each other at joints which, according to their structure, allow varying degrees of movement. Some joints are stabilized by fibrous tissue connections between the articulating surfaces, while others are stabilized by tough but flexible ligaments. Skeletal muscles are attached to bone by strong flexible, but inextensible, tendons which insert into bone tissue. The entire assembly forms the musculoskeletal system; all its cells are related members of the connective tissue family (p. 36) and are derived from mesenchymal stem cells.

CARTILAGE

During early fetal life the human skeleton is mostly cartilaginous, but is subsequently largely replaced by bone. In adults, cartilage persists at the surfaces of synovial joints, in the walls of the larynx and epiglottis, trachea, bronchi, nose and external ears. Developmental replacement by bone is a complex process: cells in cartilaginous growth plates – which lie between ossifying epiphyses and the diaphyses of long bones (and elsewhere) – continue to proliferate, increasing the length of the bones concerned until they eventually ossify, when growth ceases.

Microstructure of cartilage

Cartilage is a type of load-bearing connective tissue. It has a low metabolic rate and its vascular supply is confined to its surface or to large cartilage canals. It has a capacity for continued and often rapid interstitial and appositional growth, and a high resistance to tension, compression and shearing, with some resilience and elasticity. Cartilage is covered by a fibrous perichondrium except at its junctions with bone and at synovial surfaces, which are lubricated by a secreted nutrient synovial fluid.

The cells of cartilage are chondroblasts and chondrocytes. Like connective tissues generally, the extracellular matrix is a dominant component and gives the tissue its distinguishing characteristics. The extracellular matrix of cartilage varies in appearance, composition and in the nature of its fibres in the different types of cartilage, namely, hyaline cartilage, white fibrocartilage and yellow elastic cartilage. A densely cellular cartilage, with thin septa of matrix between its cells, is typical of early embryonic cartilage. Hyaline cartilage is the prototypical form but it varies more in composition and properties according to age and location, than either elastic or fibrocartilage. Hyaline cartilage may become calcified as part of the normal process of bone development, or as an age-related, degenerative change.

Cartilage cells occupy small lacunae in the matrix which they secrete. Young cells (chondroblasts) are smaller, often flat and irregular in contour, and bear many surface processes, which fit into complementary recesses in the matrix. Newly generated chondroblasts often retain intercellular contacts, including gap junctions. These are lost when daughter cells are separated by the synthesis of new matrix. As cartilage cells mature, they lose the ability to divide and become metabolically less active. Some authors reserve the name chondrocytes for such cells, but this term is commonly employed, as it is here, to denote all cartilage cells. Mature chondrocytes enlarge with age and become more rounded. The ultrastructure of chondrocytes is typical of cells which are active in making and secreting proteins. The nucleus is round or oval, euchromatic and possesses one or more nucleoli. The cytoplasm is filled with rough endoplasmic reticulum, transport vesicles and Golgi complexes, and contains many mitochondria and frequent lysosomes, together with numerous glycogen granules, intermediate filaments (vimentin) and pigment granules. When these cells mature to the relatively inactive chondrocyte stage, the nucleus becomes heterochromatic, the nucleolus smaller, and the protein synthetic machinery much reduced: the cells may also accumulate large lipid droplets.

Cartilage is often described as totally avascular. Most cartilage cells are usually distant from exchange vessels, which are mostly perichondrial, and so nutrient substances and metabolites diffuse along concentration gradients across the matrix between the perichondrial capillary network and chondrocytes. This limitation is reflected in the fact that most living cartilage tissue is restricted to a few millimetres in thickness. Cartilage cells situated further than this from a nutrient vessel do not survive, and their surrounding matrix typically becomes calcified. In the larger cartilages and during the rapid growth of some fetal cartilages, vascular cartilage canals penetrate the tissue at intervals, providing an additional source of nutrients. In some cases these canals are temporary structures, but others persist throughout life.

EXTRACELLULAR MATRIX

The extracellular matrix is composed of collagen and, in some cases, elastic fibres, embedded in a highly hydrated but stiff ground substance (Fig. 6.1). The components are unique to cartilage, and endow it with unusual mechanical properties. The ground substance is a firm gel, rich in carbohydrates and therefore predominantly acidic. The chemistry of the ground substance is complex. It consists mainly of water and dissolved salts, held in a meshwork of long interwoven proteoglycan molecules together with various other minor constituents, mainly proteins or glycoproteins.

COLLAGEN

Collagen forms up to 50% of the dry weight of cartilage. It is chemically distinct from that of most other tissues, and is classed as type II collagen. This variety is only found elsewhere in the notochord, the nucleus pulposus of the intervertebral disc, the vitreous body of the eye, and in the primary corneal stroma. Its tropocollagen subunits are composed of triple helices of identical polypeptides (three α-1 chains). Collagen in the outer layers of the perichondrium and much of the collagen in white fibrocartilage is the general connective tissue type I.

The majority of the collagen fibres of cartilage are relatively short and thin (mainly 10–20 nm diameter), with a characteristic cross-banding (65 nm periodicity). They are interwoven to create a three-dimensional meshwork linked by lateral projections of the proteoglycans associated with their surfaces. Proteoglycans and other organic molecules link collagen fibres with the interfibrillar ground substance and with cartilage cells. The amount, size and orientation of collagen fibres vary in different types of cartilage, and with maturity and position within the cartilage mass. In articular cartilage, collagen fibres close to the surfaces of cells are particularly narrow (4–6 nm diameter) and resemble fibres of type II collagen in non-cartilaginous tissue, i.e. the vitreous body of the eye. Cartilage contains minor quantities of other classes unique to cartilage, including types IX, X and XI.

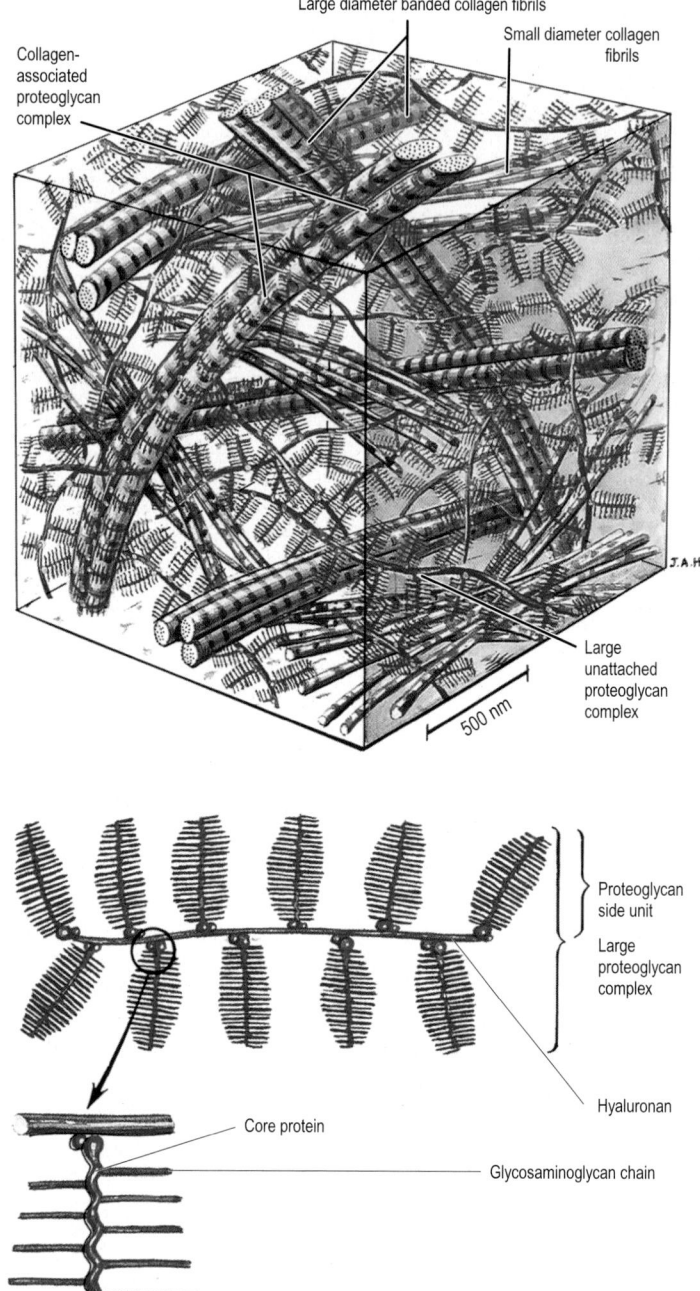

Fig. 6.1 Fine structural organization of hyaline cartilage matrix. Depicted are large proteoglycan complexes and type II collagen fibres of the coarse cross-banded and the narrow varieties. Proteoglycan complexes bind to the surface of these fibres and link them together. Detail shows the arrangement of glycosaminoglycans and core protein.

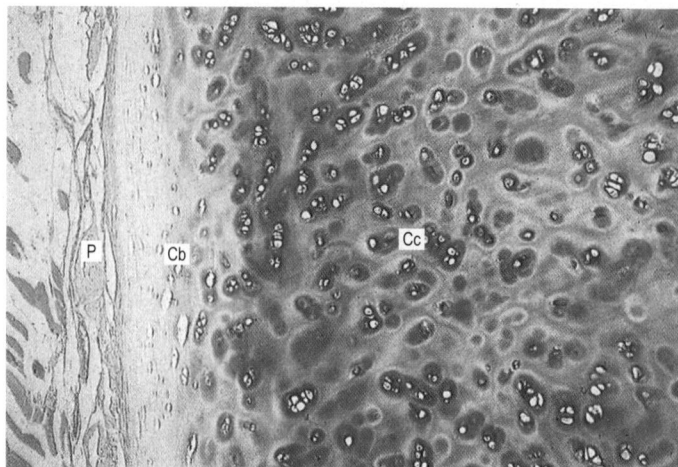

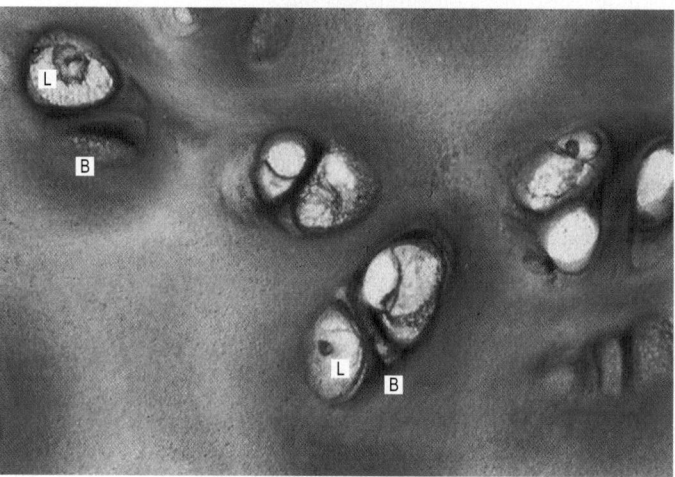

Fig. 6.2 Sections through hyaline cartilage of human rib. **A**, Low-power view, showing perichondrium (P, left), chondroblasts (Cb) embedded in pale-staining matrix and mature chondrocytes (Cc) embedded in the basophilic matrix (centre and right). **B**, Higher magnification, showing groups of chondrocytes within lacunae (L) (shrinkage artifacts seen in light microscopic preparations following dehydration of the water-rich matrix). Note the basophilic zones (B) (rich in acidic proteoglycans) around the cell clusters.

PROTEOGLYCANS AND GLYCOSAMINOGLYCANS (GAGS)

Proteoglycans are similar in general outline to those of general connective tissue, although with features peculiar to cartilage. Chondroitin sulphate and keratan sulphate play important roles in the water retention properties of cartilage.

SYNTHESIS OF MATRIX

Chondrocytes synthesize and secrete all of the major components of the matrix. Collagen is synthesized within the rough endoplasmic reticulum in the same way as in fibroblasts, except that type II rather than type I procollagen chains are made. These assemble into triple helices and some carbohydrate is added at this stage. After transport to the Golgi apparatus, where further glycosylation occurs, they are secreted as procollagen molecules into the extracellular space. Here, terminal registration peptides are cleaved from their ends, so forming tropo-collagen molecules, and final assembly into collagen fibres takes place. Core proteins of the proteoglycan complexes are also synthesized in the rough endoplasmic reticulum and addition of GAG chains begins. The process is completed in the Golgi complex. Hyaluronan, which lacks a protein core, is synthesized by enzymes on the surface of the chondrocyte; it is not modified post-synthetically, and is extruded directly into the matrix without passing through the endoplasmic reticulum.

HYALINE CARTILAGE (Figs 6.2, 6.3)

Hyaline cartilage has a homogeneous glassy, bluish opalescent appearance. It has a firm consistency and some elasticity. Costal, nasal, some laryngeal, tracheobronchial, all temporary and most articular, cartilages are hyaline. The arytenoid cartilage changes from hyaline at its base, to elastic cartilage at its apex. Size, shape and arrangement of cells, fibres and proteoglycan composition vary at different sites and with age. The chondrocytes are flat near the perichondrium and rounded or angular deeper in the tissue. They are often in grouped in pairs, sometimes more, forming cell nests (isogenous cell groups) which are the offspring of a common parent chondroblast: apposing cells have a straight outline. The matrix is typically basophilic and metachromatic, particularly in the lacunar capsule, where recently formed, territorial matrix borders the lacuna of a chondrocyte. The pale-staining interterritorial matrix between cell nests is older synthetically. Fine collagen fibres are arranged

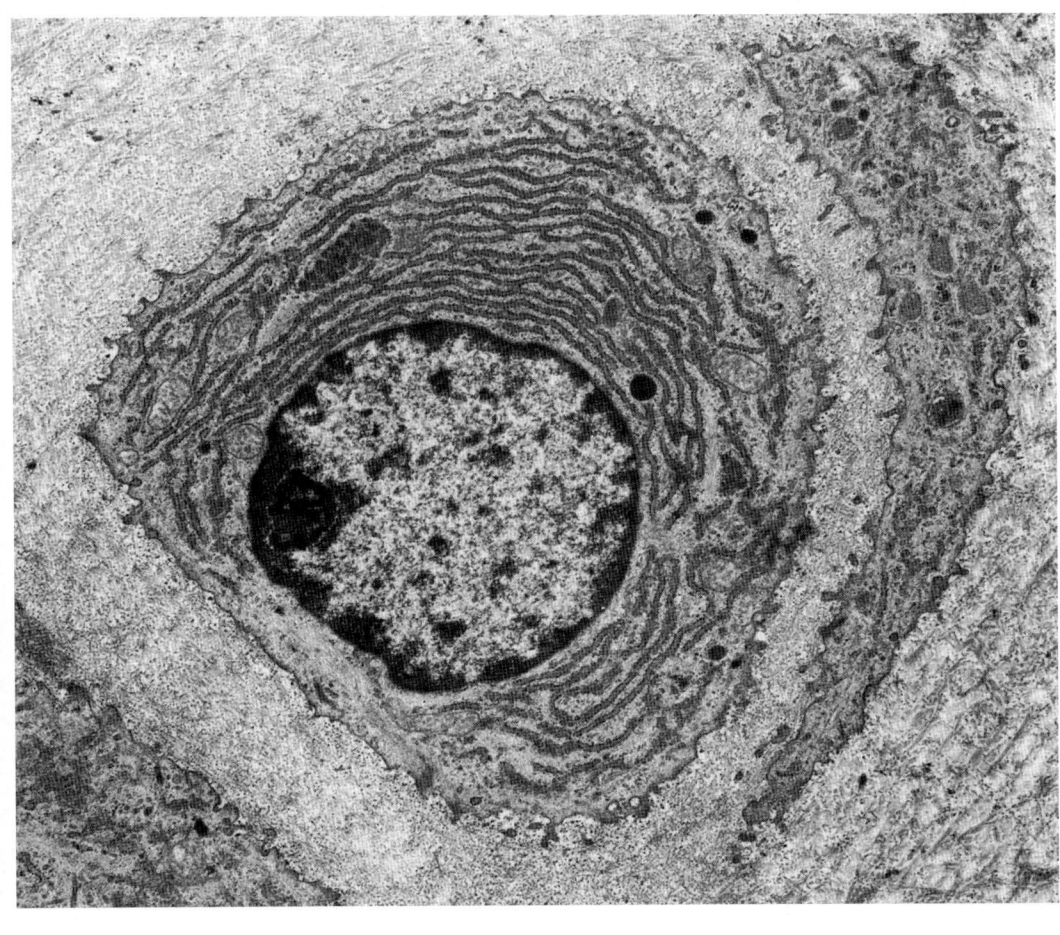

Fig. 6.3 Electron micrograph of chondroblasts in rabbit femoral condylar cartilage. The central cell has an active euchromatic nucleus with a prominent nucleolus, and its cytoplasm contains concentric cisternae of rough endoplasmic reticulum, scattered mitochondria, lysosomes and glycogen aggregates. The plasma membrane bears numerous short filopodia which project into the surrounding matrix. The latter shows a delicate feltwork of collagen fibrils within finely granular interfibrillary material. No pericellular lacuna is present; the matrix separates the central chondroblast from the cytoplasm of two adjacent chondroblasts (left, and crescentic profile). (Preparation by Susan Smith, Department of Anatomy, GKT School of Medicine, London.)

in a basket-like network, but are often absent from a narrow zone immediately surrounding the lacuna. An isogenous cell group, together with the enclosing pericellular matrix, is sometimes referred to as a chondron.

After adolescence, hyaline cartilages are prone to calcification, especially in costal and laryngeal sites. In costal cartilage, the matrix tends to fibrous striation, especially in old age when cellularity diminishes. The xiphoid process and the cartilages of the nose, larynx and trachea (except the elastic cartilaginous epiglottis and corniculate cartilages) resemble costal cartilage in microstructure. The regenerative capacity of hyaline cartilage is poor.

ARTICULAR HYALINE CARTILAGE

Articular hyaline cartilage covers articular surfaces (**Fig. 6.4**) in synovial joints. It provides an extremely smooth, resistant surface bathed by synovial fluid, which allows almost frictionless movement. Its elasticity, together with that of other articular structures, dissipates stresses, and gives the whole articulation some flexibility, particularly near extremes of movement. Articular cartilage is particularly effective as a shock-absorber, and resists the large compressive forces generated by weight transmission, especially during movement.

Articular cartilage does not ossify. It varies from 1 to 7 mm in thickness and is moulded to the shape of the underlying bone, indeed it often accentuates and modifies the surface geometry of the bone. It is thickest centrally on convex osseous surfaces, and the reverse is true of concave surfaces. Its thickness decreases from maturity to old age. The surface of articular cartilage lacks a perichondrium; synovial membrane overlaps and then merges into its structure circumferentially (p. 110, **Fig. 6.37**).

Adult articular cartilage shows a structural zonation with increasing depth from the surface. The arrangement of collagen fibres has been variously described as plexiform, helical, or in the form of serial arcades which radiate from the deepest zone to the surface, where they follow a short tangential course before returning radially. If the surface of an articular cartilage is pierced by a needle, a longitudinal split-line remains after withdrawal. For any given joint, the patterns of split-lines are constant and distinctive and follow the predominant directions of collagen bundles in tangential zones of cartilage. These patterns may

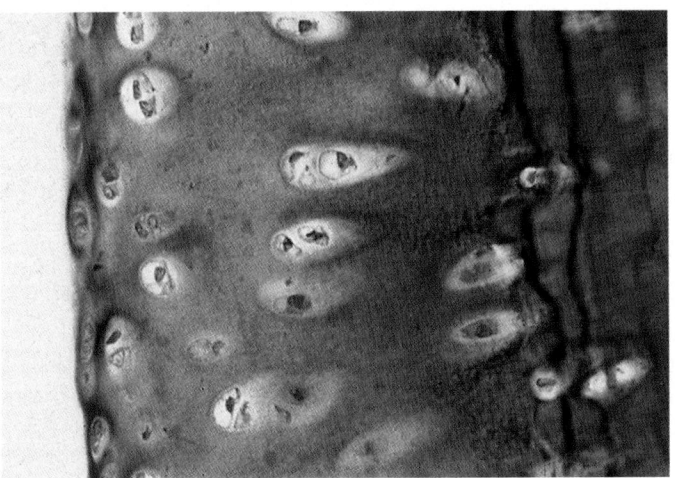

Fig. 6.4 Articular cartilage stained with silver, showing the cellular arrangement of the different layers. Note the absence of a periosteum, the superficial flattened cells of the articular surface (left), the more rounded chondrocytes of deeper layers, the lines of calcification in the deepest layer (right) and the lamellar bone adjacent to the cartilage (far right). Interphalangeal joint (rhesus monkey).

reveal tension trajectories set up in surrounding cartilage during joint movement.

Zone 1 is the superficial or tangential layer. The free articular surface is a thin, cell-free layer, 3 μm thick, which contains fine collagen type II fibrils covered superficially by a protein coating. The cells are small, oval or elongated. They are flat and parallel to the surface, relatively inactive, and surrounded by fine tangential fibres. The collagen fibres deeper within this zone are regularly tangential, their diameters and density increase with depth. Zone 2 is the transitional or intermediate layer. The cells are larger, rounder, and are either single or in isogenous groups.

Most are typical active chondrocytes, surrounded by oblique collagen fibres. Deeper still, in the radiate layer (zone 3), cells are large, round and often disposed in vertical columns, with intervening radial collagen fibres. As elsewhere, the cells, either singly or in groups, are encapsulated in pericellular matrix which has fine fibrils and contains fibronectin and types II, IX and XI collagen. The deepest layer or calcified layer (zone 4) lies adjacent to the subchondral bone (hypochondral osseous lamina) of the epiphysis. The adjacent surfaces show reciprocal fine ridges, grooves and interdigitations, which, with the confluence of their fibrous arrays, resist shearing stresses produced by postural changes and muscle action. The junction between zones 3 and 4 is called the tidemark. With age, articular cartilage thins and degenerates by advancement of the tidemark zone, and the replacement of calcified cartilage by bone.

Concentrations of GAGs vary according to site and, in particular, with age. The proportion of keratan sulphate increases linearly with depth, mainly in the older matrix between cell nests, whereas chondroitin sulphates are concentrated around lacunae. The turnover rates of GAGs in cartilage are faster than those of collagen, and the smaller, more soluble GAGs turn over fastest. Turnover decreases with age and distance from the cells. The proteoglycan turnover time is estimated at nearly 5 years for adult human articular cartilage.

The sequence of structural features outlined above is also typical of cartilaginous growth plates (p. 101). It follows radial epiphyseal growth by the extension of endochondral ossification into overlying calcified cartilage. This ceases in maturity, but the zones persist throughout life. The same terminal mechanism also occurs in bones which lack epiphyses.

Cells of articular cartilage divide by mitosis, but mitoses are few except in young bones. Superficial cells are lost progressively from normal young joint surfaces, and they are replaced by cells from deeper layers. Degenerating cells may occur in any of the four zones. This probably accounts for the progressive reduction in cellularity of cartilage with advancing age, particularly in superficial layers.

Articular cartilages derive nutrients by diffusion from vessels of the synovial membrane, synovial fluid and hypochondral vessels of an adjacent medullary cavity, some capillaries from which penetrate and occasionally traverse the calcified cartilage. The contributions from these sources are uncertain and may change with age. Small molecules freely traverse articular cartilage, with diffusion coefficients about half those in aqueous solution. Larger molecules have diffusion coefficients inversely related to their molecular size. The permeability of cartilage to large molecules is greatly affected by variations in its GAG, and hence water, content, e.g. a three-fold increase multiplies the diffusion coefficient a hundred-fold.

FIBROCARTILAGE

Fibrocartilage is dense, fasciculated, opaque white fibrous tissue. It contains fibroblasts and small interfascicular groups of chondrocytes. The cells are ovoid and surrounded by concentrically striated matrix (**Fig. 6.5**). When present in quantity, as in intervertebral discs, fibrocartilage has great tensile strength and appreciable elasticity. In lesser amounts, as in articular discs, glenoid and acetabular labra, the cartilaginous lining of bony grooves for tendons and some articular cartilages, it provides strength, elasticity and resistance to repeated pressure and friction. It is resistant to degenerative change.

Fibrocartilage is unlike other types of cartilage in containing a considerable amount of type I (general connective tissue) collagen which is synthesized by the fibroblasts in its matrix. It is perhaps best regarded as a mingling of the two types of tissue, e.g. where a ligament or tendinous tissue inserts into hyaline cartilage, rather than as a separate type of cartilage. However, fibrocartilage in joints often lacks type II collagen altogether, and so possibly represents a distinct class of connective tissue.

The articular surfaces of bones which ossify in mesenchyme (e.g. squamous temporal, mandible and clavicle) are covered by white fibrocartilage. The deep layers, adjacent to hypochondral bone, resemble calcified regions of the radial zone of hyaline articular cartilage. The superficial zone contains dense parallel bundles of thick collagen fibres, interspersed with typical dense connective tissue fibroblasts and little ground substance. Fibre bundles in adjacent layers alternate in direction, as they do in the cornea. A transitional zone of irregular bundles of coarse collagen and active fibroblasts separates the superficial and deep layers. The fibroblasts are probably involved in elaboration of proteoglycans and collagen, and may also constitute a germinal zone

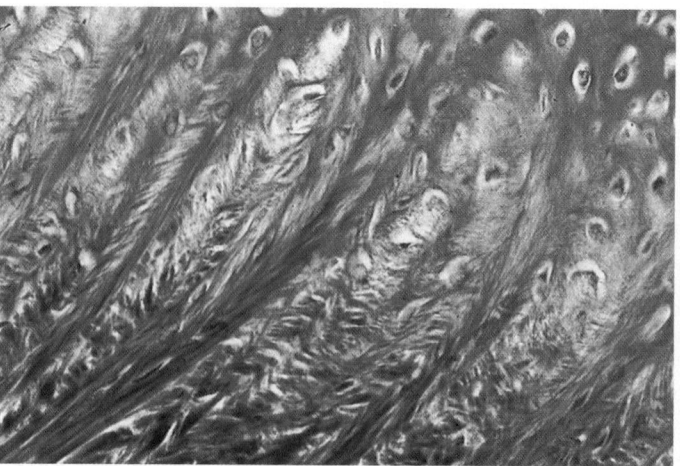

Fig. 6.5 White fibrocartilage in a late fetal intervertebral disc. Chondroblasts lie between coarse collagen type I fibres (blue) derived from the annulus fibrosus. Mallory's triple stain.

for deeper cartilage. Fibre diameters and types may differ at different sites according to the functional load.

ELASTIC CARTILAGE

Elastic cartilage (**Fig. 6.6**) occurs in the external ear, corniculate cartilages, epiglottis and apices of the arytenoids. It contains typical chondrocytes, but its matrix is pervaded by yellow elastic fibres, except around lacunae (where it resembles typical hyaline matrix with fine type II collagen fibrils). Its elastic fibres are irregularly contoured and show no periodic banding. Most sites in which elastic cartilage occurs have vibrational functions, such as laryngeal sound wave production, or the collection and transmission of sound waves in the ear. Elastic cartilage is resistant to degeneration; it can regenerate to a limited degree following traumatic injury, e.g. the distorted repair of a 'cauliflower ear'.

Development and growth of cartilage

Cartilage is usually formed in embryonic mesenchyme. Mesenchymal cells proliferate and become tightly packed: the shape of their condensation foreshadows that of subsequent cartilage. The cells become rounded, with prominent round or oval nuclei and a low cytoplasm: nucleus ratio. Gap junctions are present between the cells. Each cell

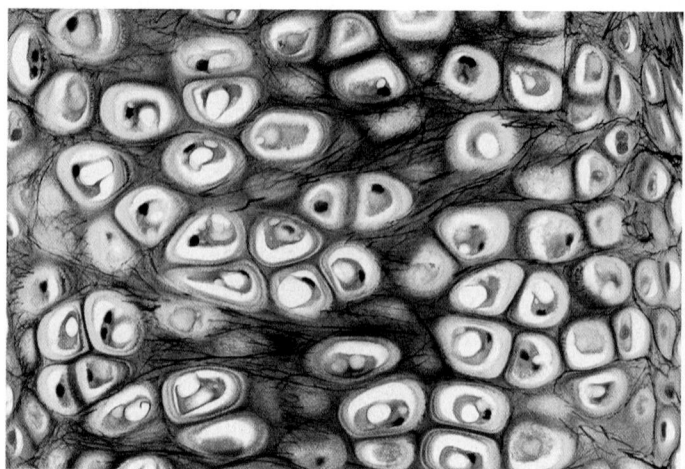

Fig. 6.6 Elastic cartilage, stained with Gomori's elastin stain to demonstrate elastin fibres (blue-black). Chondroblasts and larger chondrocytes are embedded in the matrix, which also contains collagen type II fibres. (Photograph by Sarah-Jane Smith.)

secretes a surrounding basophilic halo of matrix, composed of a delicate network of fine type II collagen filaments, type IX collagen and cartilage proteoglycan core protein, i.e. they differentiate into chondroblasts (**Figs 6.7**, **6.8**). In some sites, continued secretion of matrix further separates the cells, and produces typical hyaline cartilage. Elsewhere, many cells become fibroblasts, and collagen synthesis predominates; chondroblastic activity appears only in isolated groups or rows of cells which become surrounded by dense bundles of collagen fibres to form white fibrocartilage. In yet other sites, the matrix of early cellular cartilage is permeated first by anastomosing oxytalan fibres, and later by elastin fibres. In all cases, developing cartilage is surrounded by condensed mesenchyme which differentiates into a bilaminar perichondrium. The cells of the outer layer become fibroblasts and secrete a dense collagenous matrix lined externally by vascular mesenchyme. The cells of the inner layer contain differentiated, but mainly resting, chondroblasts or prechondroblasts.

Cartilage grows by interstitial and appositional mechanisms. Interstitial growth is the result of continued mitosis of early chondroblasts throughout the tissue mass. When a chondroblast divides, its descendants temporarily occupy the same lacuna. They are soon separated by a thin septum of secreted matrix, which thickens and further separates the daughter cells. Continuing division produces isogenous groups. Interstitial growth is obvious only in young cartilage, where plasticity of the matrix permits continued expansion. Appositional growth is the result of continued proliferation of cells of the internal, chondrogenic layer of the perichondrium. Newly formed chondroblasts secrete matrix around themselves, creating superficial lacunae beneath the perichondrium. This continuing process adds additional surface, while the entrapped cells participate in interstitial growth. Apposition is thought to be most prevalent in mature cartilages, but interstitial growth must persist for long periods in epiphyseal cartilages. Relatively little is known about the factors which determine the overall shape of a cartilage.

BONE

Bone, and the struts and levers which it forms, is exquisitely adapted to resist stress with suitable resilience, support the body and provide leverage for movement. It is a highly vascular mineralized connective tissue, consisting of cells and an intercellular matrix in which the great majority of its cells are embedded. The matrix is composed in part (c.40% dry weight in mature bone) of organic materials, which are mainly collagen fibres, and the rest consists of inorganic salts rich in calcium and phosphate.

Macroscopic anatomy of bone

Macroscopically, living bone is white, and it has either a dense texture like ivory (compact bone), or it is honeycombed by large cavities (cancellous, trabecular, or spongy bone), where the bony element is reduced to a latticework of bars and plates (trabeculae) (**Figs 6.9**, **6.10**, **6.11**). Compact bone is usually limited to the cortices of mature bones (cortical bone) and is of great importance in providing their strength. Its thickness and architecture vary for different bones, according to their overall shape, position and functional roles. The cortex plus the hollow medullary canal of long bones allows combination of strength with low weight. Cancellous bone is usually internal; it gives additional strength to cortices and supports the bone marrow. Bone forms a reservoir of metabolic calcium (99% of body calcium is in the bony skeleton) and phosphate: the content is under hormonal and cytokine control. In cancellous bone this property may be enhanced by its large surface area and its proximity to blood vessels and sources of cytokines in the bone marrow.

The proportions of compact to cancellous bone vary greatly. In the shaft (diaphysis) of a long bone, a thick cylinder of compact bone presents only a few trabeculae and spicules on its inner surface. It encloses a large central medullary or marrow cavity, which communicates freely with the intratrabecular spaces of the expanded bone ends. In other bones, especially flat ones such as the ribs, the interior is uniformly cancellous, and compact bone forms the surface. These cavities are filled with marrow, either red haemopoietic or yellow adipose, according to age and site. In some bones of the skull, notably the mastoid process of the temporal bone, and sinuses of the maxilla and ethmoid, many of the internal cavities are filled with air (pneumatized).

Bones vary not only in their primary shape but also in lesser surface details, or secondary markings which appear mainly in postnatal life. Most bones display features such as elevations and depressions, smooth areas and rough ridges. For example, bones display articular surfaces at synovial joints with their neighbours; if small, these are termed facets or foveae. Knuckle-shaped surfaces are condyles, and a trochlea is grooved like a pulley. Adapted in shape to the movement of particular joints, such surfaces are smooth, and in life are covered by articular cartilage which forms the articular surfaces of synovial joints. The texture of these osseous surfaces is partly due to the fact that they lack the vascular foramina typical of most other bone surfaces.

Large tendons (e.g. adductor magnus, subscapularis) are attached to facets which lack the regular contours of articular surfaces, but which resemble them in texture, because they are poorly vascularized. These tendon facets are sometimes depressed, alternatively they may surmount large elevations, e.g. the humeral tubercles.

Depressions (fossae) and elevations vary in size and shape and interrupt otherwise featureless osseous surfaces. Some articular surfaces are fossae (e.g. the temporomandibular joint); lengthy depressions are

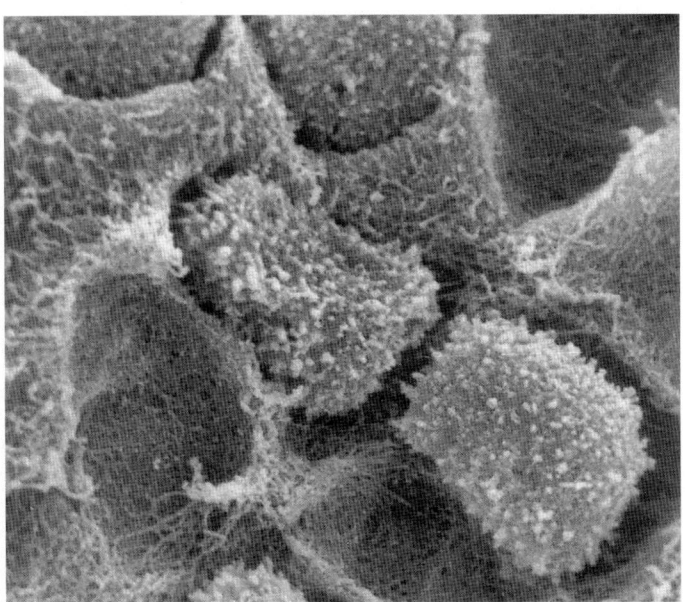

Fig. 6.7 Chondrocytes in phalangeal cartilage. Note that the cells have many short microvilli. 17-day mouse embryo.

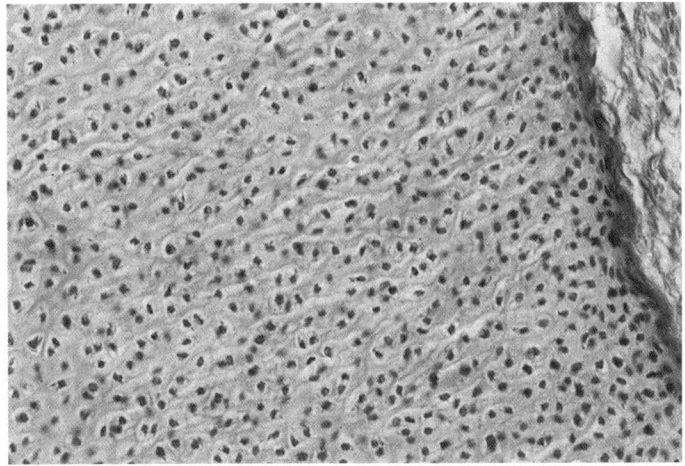

Fig. 6.8 Highly cellular fetal cartilage, human phalanx. The cells are small and almost uniform in distribution. Mallory's triple stain.

A

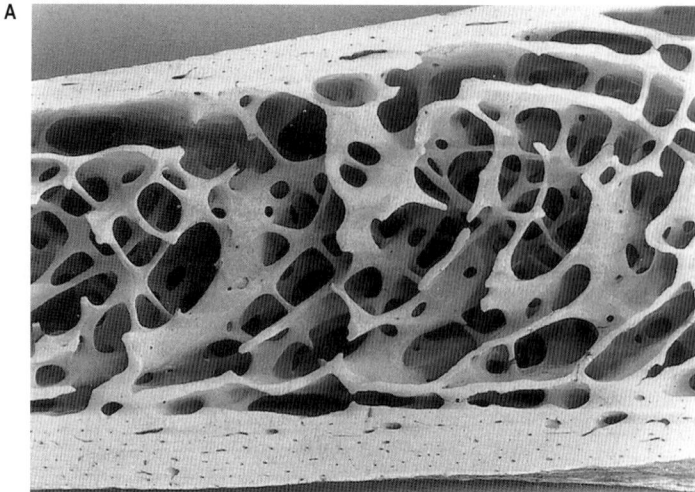

B

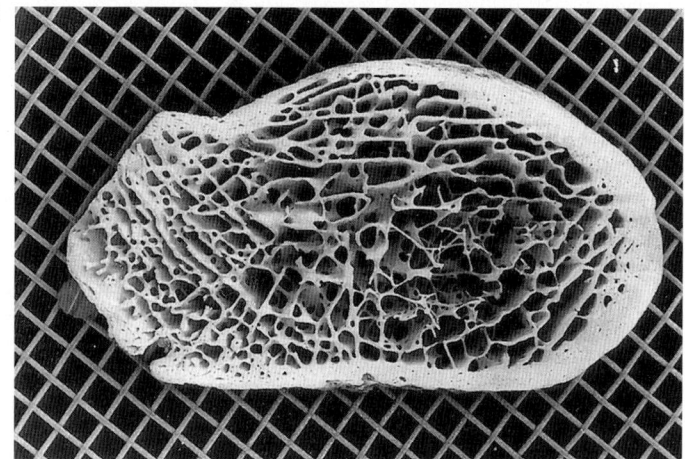

Fig. 6.9 A, Vertical section 2 cm below the anterosuperior border of the iliac crest (to the right of the field view as oriented; female, 42 years). The cancellous bone consists of intersecting curved plates and struts. Osteonal (Haversian) canals can just be seen in the two cortices at this magnification. **B**, Transverse section, femoral neck (male, 45 years) viewed from the distolateral aspect towards the femoral head, showing the predominant pattern of curved intersecting plates in the cancellous bone.

grooves or sulci (e.g. humeral bicipital sulcus); a notch is an incisura, and an actual gap is a hiatus. A large projection is termed a process or, if elongated and slender or pointed, a spine. A curved process is a hamulus or cornu (e.g. sphenoidal pterygoid hamuli and hyoid cornua). A rounded projection is a tuberosity or tubercle, occasionally a trochanter. Long elevations are crests, or lines, if less developed; crests are wider and present boundary edges or lips. An epicondyle is a projection close to a condyle and is usually an attachment for the collateral ligaments of the adjacent joint or common myotendinous attachments for superficial muscle groups. The terms protuberance, prominence, eminence and torus are less often applied to certain bony projections. The expanded proximal ends of many long bones are often termed the 'head' or caput (e.g. humerus, femur, radius). A hole in bone is a foramen; foramina are known as canals when lengthy. Large holes may be called apertures or, if covered largely by connective tissue, fenestrae. Clefts in or between bones are fissures. A lamina is a thin plate; larger laminae may be called squamae (e.g. the temporal squama).

Large areas on many bones are featureless and often smoother than articular surfaces, from which they differ because they are pierced by many visible vascular foramina. This texture occurs where muscle is directly attached to bone, and small blood vessels pass through the foramina from bone to muscle, and perhaps vice versa. Areas covered only by periosteum are similar, but vessels are less numerous.

Tendons are usually attached at roughened bone surfaces. Wherever any aggregation of collagen in a muscle reaches bone, surface irregularities correspond in form and extent to the pattern of such 'tendinous

fibres'. Such markings are almost always elevated above the general surface, as if ossification advanced into the collagen bundles from periosteal bone. How such secondary markings are induced is uncertain but they may result from the continued incorporation of new collagen fibres into the bone, perhaps necessary for minor functional adjustment. Evidence suggests that their prominence may be related to the power of the muscles involved and they increase with advancing years, as if the pull of muscles and ligaments exercised a cumulative effect over a limited area. Surface markings delineate the shape of attached connective tissue structures, whether these are an obvious tendon, intramuscular tendon or septum, aponeurosis, or tendinous fibres mediating what is otherwise a direct muscular attachment. These markings may be facets, ridges, nodules, rough areas or complex mixtures: they afford accurate indications of the junctions of bone with muscles, tendons, ligaments or articular capsules.

When a muscle is apparently attached directly to bone, its fibres do not themselves adhere directly to periosteum or bone. The route of transmission of tension from contracting muscle to bone is through the connective tissue which encapsulates (as the epimysium) and pervades all muscles (as the perimysium and endomysium). These two forms of attachment of muscles, at the extremes of a range of admixtures, differ in the density of collagen fibres between muscle and bone. Where collagen is visibly concentrated, markings appear on the bone surface. In contrast, the multitude of microscopic connective tissue ties of direct attachment, necessarily over a larger area, do not visibly mark the bone and so it appears smooth to unaided vision and touch.

Microstructure of bone

Bone contains an extracellular mineralized matrix and a number of different cell types, including osteoblasts, osteocytes and osteoclasts, the cells of its vascular and nervous supply, and components of the periosteum, endosteum and marrow. These components will be described in detail below, first individually and then in terms of their overall organization.

BONE MATRIX

Bone matrix is the extracellular mineralized material of bone and, like general connective tissues, consists of a ground substance in which numerous collagen fibres are embedded, usually ordered in bone in parallel arrays (**Fig. 6.12**). In mature bone, the matrix is moderately hydrated, and 10–20% of its mass is water. Of its dry weight, 60–70% is made up of inorganic, mineral salts (mainly microcrystalline calcium and phosphate hydroxides, hydroxyapatite), 30–40% is collagen and the remainder (c.5%) is non-collagenous protein and carbohydrate, mainly conjugated as glycoproteins. The proportions of these various components vary with age, location and metabolic status. In the early stages of bone formation, before mineralization, the matrix is termed osteoid. In adult bones the amount of osteoid is very small, reflecting local remodelling of the bone in which mineralization follows the deposition of the organic matrix. In certain disease states where mineralization is defective, notably rickets, the amounts of osteoid are greatly increased.

COLLAGEN

Collagen in bone closely resembles that of many other connective tissues, and is mainly type I, with trace amounts of type V which is thought to regulate fibrillogenesis. However, unlike collagen in general connective tissue, its molecular structure is more strongly covalently cross-linked internally, and the transverse spacings within its fibrils are somewhat larger. The cross-links make it stronger and chemically more inert, and the internal gaps provide the space for deposition of minerals. Up to two-thirds of the mineral content of bone is thought to be located within collagen fibrils. Crystal formation is probably initiated in the hole zones, which are gaps between the ends of tropocollagen subunits.

Collagen contributes greatly to the mechanical strength of bone tissue, although its precise role in bone mechanics is not understood in detail. As well as contributing to the tensile, compressive and shearing strengths of bone, the small degree of elasticity shown by collagen imparts a measure of resilience to the tissue, and helps to resist fracture when bone is mechanically loaded.

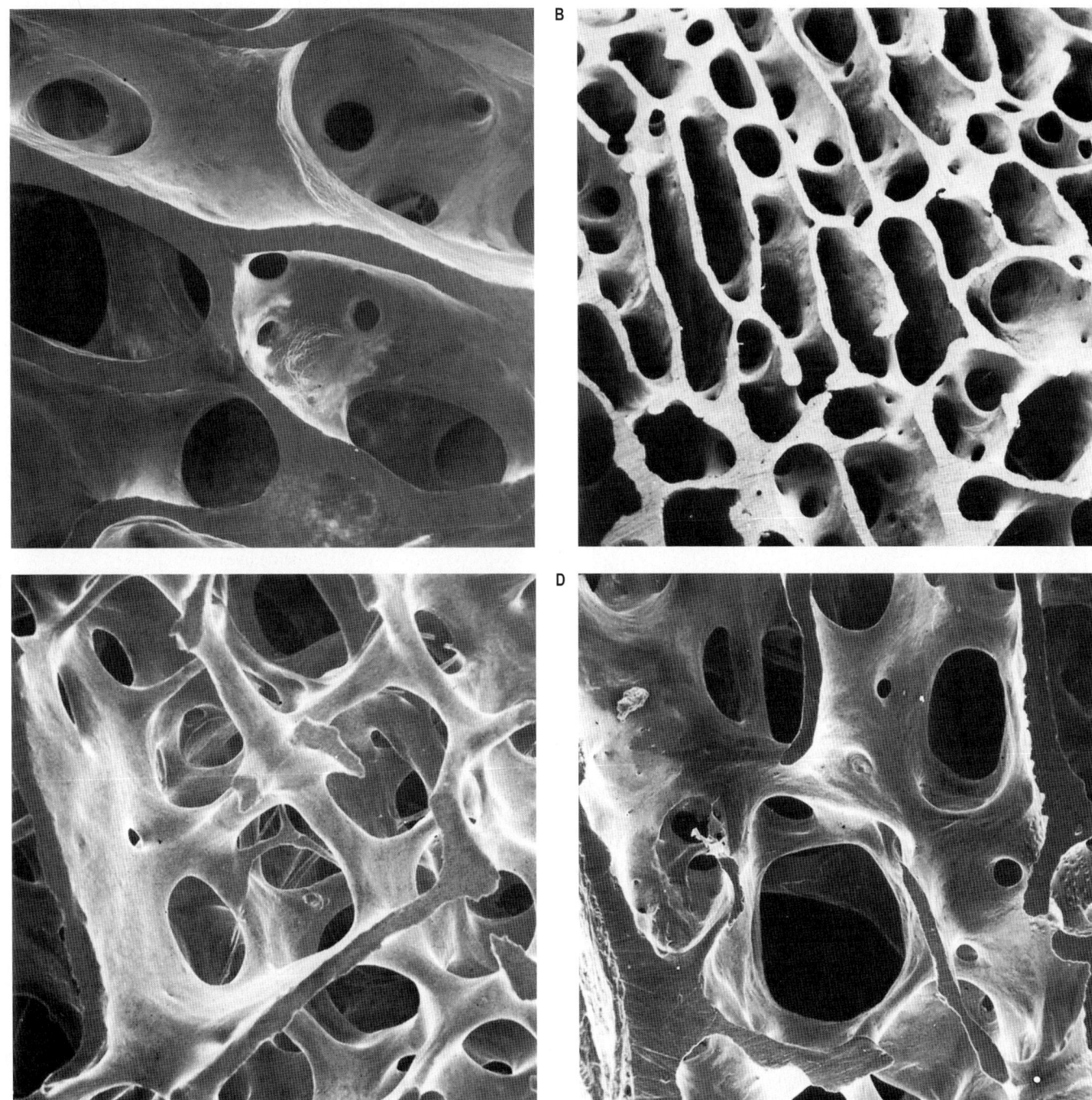

Fig. 6.10 Trabecular bone at different sites in the proximal part of the same human femur. All fields are at the same scale. **A**, Subcapital part of the neck; **B** and **C**, Greater trochanter; **D**, Rim of the articular surface of the head. Note the wide variation in thickness, orientation and spacing of the trabeculae. (Original photographs from Whitehouse WJ, Dyson ED 1974 Scanning electron microscope studies of trabecular bone in the proximal end of the human femur. J Anat 118: 417–414, by permission from Blackwell Publishing.)

Collagen fibres are synthesized by osteoblasts, polymerize from tropocollagen extracellularly and become progressively more cross-linked as they mature. In primary bone, collagen fibres form a complex interwoven meshwork (non-lamellar woven or bundle bone (**Fig. 6.13**)), which in most sites is almost entirely replaced by regular laminar arrays of nearly parallel collagen fibres (lamellar bone). Partially mineralized collagen networks can be seen within osteoid on the outer and internal surfaces of bone, and in the endosteal linings of vascular canals. Collagen fibres from the periosteum are incorporated in cortical bone (extrinsic fibres), and anchor this fibrocellular layer at its surface (**Fig. 6.12**). Terminal collagen fibres of tendons and ligaments are incorporated deep into the matrix of cortical bone. They may be interrupted by new osteons during cortical drift (modelling) and turnover (remodelling), and remain as islands of interstitial lamellae or even trabeculae.

NON-COLLAGENOUS ORGANIC COMPONENTS

Small amounts of various complex macromolecules are attached to collagen fibres and surrounding bone crystals. Osteonectin is a phosphorylated glycoprotein secreted by osteoblasts. It binds to collagen and hydroxyapatite and may play a role in initiating hydroxyapatite crystallization. Osteocalcin is a glycoprotein synthesized by osteoblasts which binds hydroxyapatite and calcium, and is used as a marker of new bone formation. The bone proteoglycans biglycan and decorin may bind transforming growth factor-β (TGF-β). Bone sialoproteins, osteopontin and thrombospondin, mediate osteoclast adhesion to bone surfaces via binding to osteoclast integrins.

Bone matrix also contains many growth factors, proteases and protease inhibitors which are secreted by osteoblasts, often in a latent form. TGF-β, secreted by osteoclasts as well as osteoblasts, is activated in the acid conditions of the ruffled border zone of the osteoclast, and

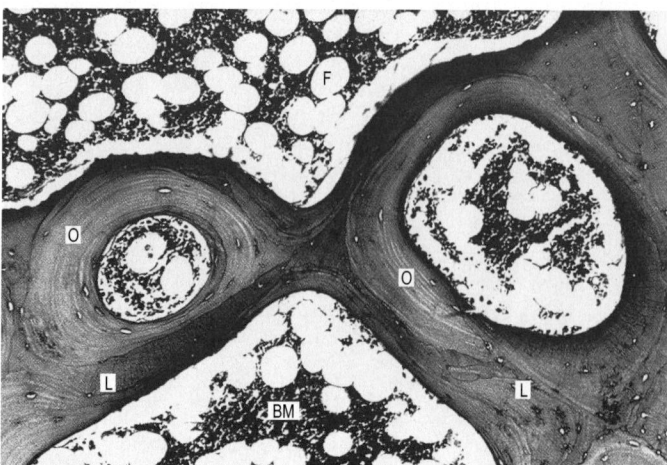

Fig. 6.11 Cancellous (spongy) bone, containing a mixture of lamellar bone (L) and concentric lamellae resembling osteons (O). Fat cells (F) are prevalent amongst islands of haemopoietic bone marrow (BM). (By permission from Dr JB Kerr, Monash University, from Kerr JB 1999 Atlas of Functional Histology. London: Mosby.)

may be a coupling factor for stimulating new bone formation at resorption sites.

BONE MINERALS

Bone minerals are the inorganic constituents of the bone matrix. They confer the hardness and much of the rigidity of bone, and are the main reason that bone is easily seen on radiographs (bone has to be 50% mineralized to be visible on X-ray). The mineral substances of bone are mostly acid-soluble. If they are removed, using calcium chelators such as citrates or ethylene diamine tetraacetic acid (EDTA), the bone retains its shape but becomes highly flexible.

The mineral portion of mature bones is composed largely of crystals made of a substance generally referred to as hydroxyapatite (but with an important carbonate content, and a lower Ca/P ratio than pure hydroxyapatite ($Ca_{10}(PO_4)_6(OH)_2$), together with a small amount of calcium phosphate. Bone crystals are small but have a large surface area. They take the form of thin plates or leaf-like structures and range in size up to 150 nm long × 80 nm wide × 5 nm thick, although most are half that size. They are often packed quite closely together, with their long axes nearly parallel to the collagen fibril axes. The narrow gaps between the crystals contain associated water and organic macromolecules.

The major ions which make up the mineral part of bone include calcium, phosphate, hydroxyl and carbonate. Less numerous ions are citrate, magnesium, sodium, potassium, fluoride, chloride, iron, zinc, copper, aluminium, lead, strontium, silicon and boron, many of which are present only in trace quantities. Fluoride ions can substitute for hydroxyl ions, and carbonate can substitute for either hydroxyl or phosphate groups. Group IIA cations, e.g. radium, strontium and lead, all readily substitute for calcium and are therefore known as bone-seeking cations. Since they can be either radioactive or chemically toxic, their presence in bone, where they may be close to haemopoietic bone marrow, may cause illness and characteristic appearances on X-rays.

The concentration of mineral in young osteons is low but increases with age: it is highest in the older, more peripheral lamellae. In established, highly mineralized osteons, mineral distribution is uniform. Mineralization reaches 70–80% in c.3 weeks. Immature woven bone mineralizes faster and can be identified from adjacent lamellar bone by its higher degree of mineralization. Osteons may show one or more highly mineralized arrest lines within their walls.

OSTEOBLASTS (Fig. 6.14)

Osteoblasts are derived from osteoprogenitor ('stem') cells of mesenchymal origin, which are present in the bone marrow and other connective tissues. They proliferate and differentiate into osteoblasts prior to bone formation. Osteoblasts are basophilic, roughly cuboidal mononuclear cells c.15–30 μm across. Ultrastructurally, they have features typical of protein-secreting cells. They are found on the forming surfaces

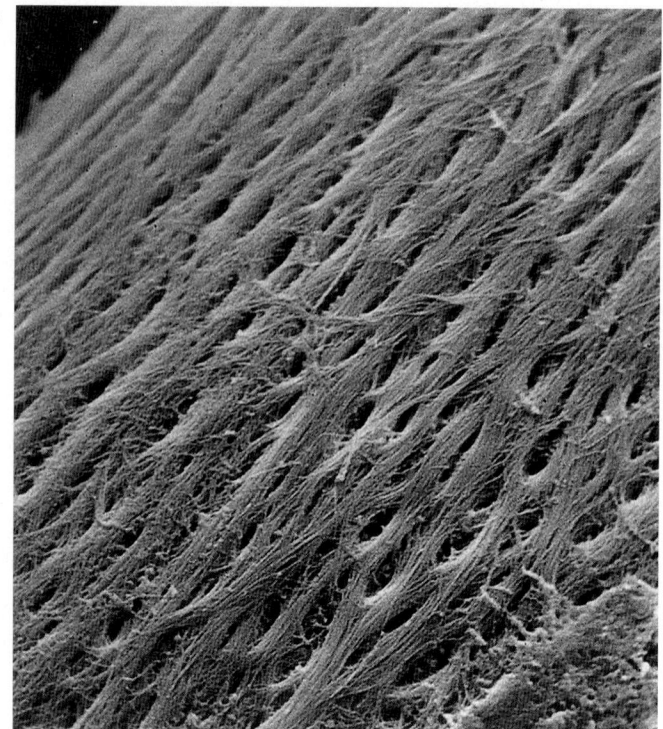

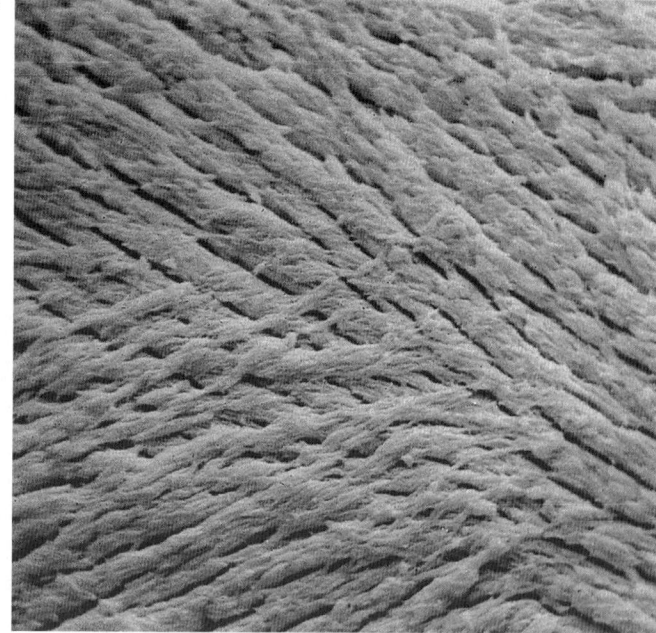

Fig. 6.12 Scanning electron micrographs of collagen fibres on the surface of human trabecular bone. **A**, Note branching fibres (female, 2 months, sixth rib). **B**, Tapering collagen fibres border a new patch of lamellar bone and lie across those of the underlying layer (male, 35 years, fourth lumbar vertebra).

of growing or remodelling bone, where they constitute a covering monolayer. In relatively quiescent adult bones they appear to be present mostly on endosteal rather than periosteal surfaces, but they also occur deep within compact bone where osteons are being remodelled. They are responsible for the synthesis, deposition and mineralization of the bone matrix, which they secrete. Once embedded in the matrix, they change into osteocytes.

Osteoblasts contain prominent bundles of actin, myosin and other cytoskeletal proteins which are associated with the maintenance of cell shape, attachment and motility. Their plasma membranes display many extensions, some of which contact neighbouring osteoblasts and embedded osteocytes at intercellular gap junctions. This arrangement facilitates coordination of the activities of groups of cells, e.g. in the formation of large domains of parallel collagen fibres.

A major activity of osteoblasts is the synthesis and secretion of organic matrix, i.e. type I collagen; small amounts of type V collagen; and various other macromolecules. Collagen synthesis occurs in the rough endoplasmic reticulum and Golgi apparatus. Type I collagen is secreted as monomers which assemble into the triple helical procollagen extracellularly. Other glycoprotein products include osteocalcin (required for bone mineralization); osteonectin (which binds strongly to mineral and collagen and may also be a cell adhesion factor); osteopontin; RANKL (the cell surface ligand for RANK, an osteoclast progenitor receptor protein); osteoprotegerin; and some proteoglycans, latent proteases and growth factors, including bone morphogenetic proteins (BMPs).

Prior to its mineralization the organic matrix is called osteoid. Osteoblasts play a significant role in the mineralization of osteoid. Extracellular fluid is supersaturated with respect to the basic calcium phosphates, yet mineralization is not a widespread phenomenon. The conditions in osteoid matrix favour crystallization. Alkaline phosphatase activity at osteoblast cell surfaces raises local concentrations of calcium and phosphate. Some enzyme is shed and reaches the blood circulation where it can be detected in conditions of rapid bone formation or turnover. Osteoblasts secrete osteocalcin which binds calcium weakly, but at levels sufficient to concentrate the ion locally. They also release matrix vesicles which bud off from their plasma membranes into newly formed osteoid. The vesicles contain alkaline phosphatase (which can cleave phosphate ions from various molecules to elevate concentrations locally), and pyrophosphatase (which degrades inhibitory pyrophosphate in the extracellular fluid). The vesicles are membrane-bound spheres 0.1–0.2 µm in diameter, with an electron-dense core. They appear to be the sites of earliest crystal formation in newly forming bone (**Fig. 6.26**).

Osteoblasts probably play an indirect role in the hormonal regulation of bone resorption, since they express receptors for parathyroid hormone (PTH), 1,25-dihydroxy vitamin D3 and other promoters of bone resorption. During bone deposition, osteoblasts inhibit the extent of osteoclast activity via RANKL binding to RANK on immature osteoclasts. In the presence of PTH, osteoblasts secrete osteoprotegerin, a soluble ligand with higher affinity for RANK, displacing the inhibitory contact-mediated signal, RANKL. Immature osteoclasts then mature into bone resorbing cells which remove osseous tissue. (For further details, consult Kierszenbaum 2002; see Bibliography of selected titles for publication details.)

Bone-lining cells are flattened epithelioid cells found on the surfaces of adult bone not undergoing active deposition or resorption, and are generally considered to be quiescent osteoblasts or osteoprogenitor cells. They form the outer boundary of the marrow tissue on the endosteal surface of marrow cavities; are present on the periosteal surface; and line the system of vascular canals within osteons.

OSTEOCYTES (Fig. 6.15)

Osteocytes constitute the major cell type of mature bone, and are scattered within its matrix, interconnected by numerous dendritic processes to form a complex cellular network. They are derived from osteoblasts and are enclosed within their matrix but, unlike chondrocytes, have ceased formation of new matrix and do not divide. They retain contacts with each other and with cells at the surfaces of bone (osteoblasts and bone-lining cells) throughout their lifespan.

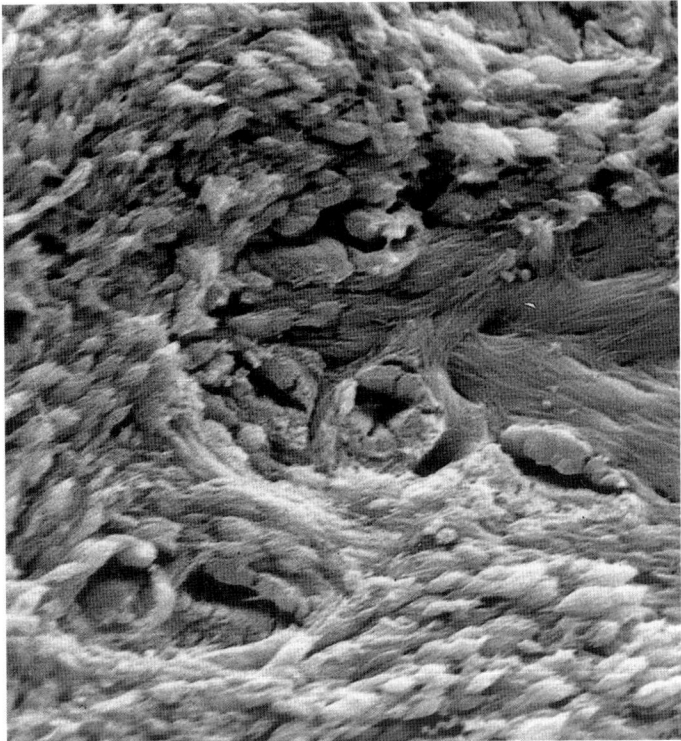

Fig. 6.13 Scanning electron micrograph of human bundle bone lining the socket of an upper first molar: unmineralized osteoid and periodontal ligament have been removed to reveal the interface with mineralized tissue. The mineralized segments of the intrinsic fibres lie in the plane of the surface, and the ends of extrinsic fibres have unmineralized cores. The back wall of an osteocyte lacuna (centre right) accommodates several extrinsic fibres; it is well mineralized and shows canalicular openings.

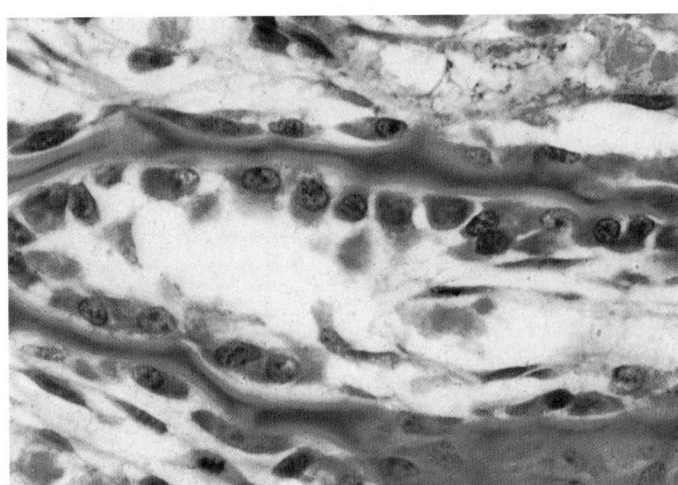

Fig. 6.14 Section through the metaphysis of a fetal bone showing developing spicules of early bone. Each spicule contains a deeply stained basophilic core of calcified cartilage, which is covered on both aspects by a lightly stained eosinophilic layer of young bone along which are ranged rows of active osteoblasts.

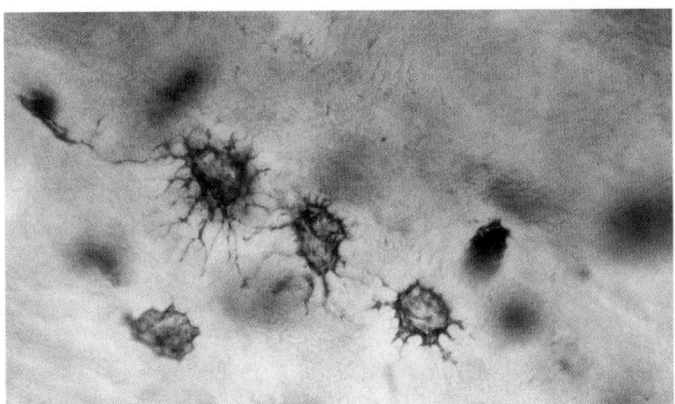

Fig. 6.15 Osteocyte lacunae shown at high magnification in a dry ground section of lamellar bone. The territories of three osteocytes are shown. Their branching dendrites contact those of neighbouring cells via the canaliculi seen here within the bone matrix. Several other osteocyte lacunae are present, out of the focal plane in this section, and tangential to the osteon axis. (Photograph by Sarah-Jane Smith.)

Mature, relatively inactive, osteocytes possess an ellipsoid cell body with the longest axis (c.25 μm) parallel to the surrounding bony lamella. The rather narrow rim of cytoplasm is faintly basophilic, contains relatively few organelles and surrounds an oval nucleus. Osteocytes in woven bone are larger and more irregular in shape (**Fig. 6.16**).

Numerous fine dendritic processes emerge from the cell body of each osteocyte and branch a number of times. They contain bundles of microfilaments and some smooth endoplasmic reticulum. At their distal tips they contact the processes of adjacent cells (i.e. other osteocytes and, at surfaces, osteoblasts and bone-lining cells), with which they form communicating gap junctions: they are thus in electrical and metabolic continuity.

Bone matrix surrounds the cell bodies and processes. There appears to be a variable space between each osteocyte and its enclosing wall which contains extracellular fluid. Each cell body lies in a lacuna from which extend many narrow, branched channels (canaliculi) c.0.5–0.25 μm wide, containing the dendritic processes of the osteocytes. In this way the bony matrix is penetrated extensively by minute channels which provide a route for the diffusion of nutrients, gases and waste products between its osteocytes and the blood vessels. Canaliculi do not usually extend through and beyond the reversal line surrounding an osteon and so do not communicate with neighbouring systems. The walls of lacunae may be lined with a variable (0.2–2 μm) layer of unmineralized organic matrix.

In well-vascularized bone, osteocytes are long-lived cells which actively maintain the bone matrix. The average lifespan of an osteocyte varies with the metabolic activity of the bone and the likelihood that it will be remodelled, but is measured in years. Old osteocytes may retract their processes from the canaliculi and, when dead, their lacunae and canaliculi may become plugged with cell debris and minerals, which hinders diffusion through the bone. Dead osteocytes occur commonly in interstitial bone and the inner regions of trabecular bone which escape surface remodelling, and become particularly noticeable by the

second and third decades. Bones which experience little turnover, e.g. ear ossicles, are most likely to contain aged osteocytes and low osteocyte viability.

Osteocytes play an essential role in the maintenance of bone: their death leads to the resorption of the matrix by osteoclast activity. They remain responsive to parathyroid hormone and $1,25(OH)_2$ vitamin D3, and it is possible that they are involved in mineral exchange at adjacent bone surfaces. Osteocytes themselves are often mineralized.

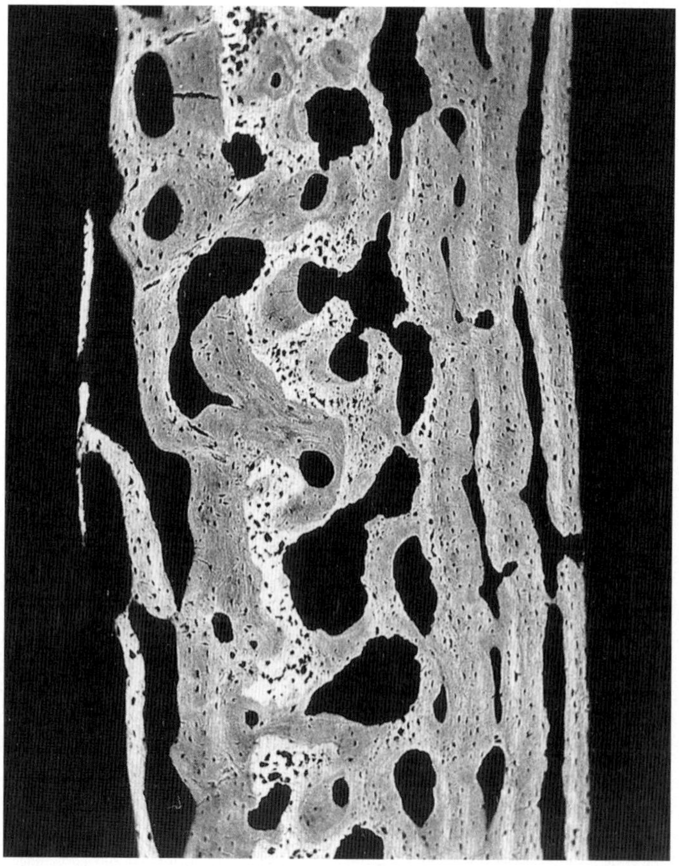

OSTEOCLASTS (Fig. 6.17)

Functionally, osteoclasts are responsible for the local removal of bone during bone growth and subsequent remodelling of osteons and surface bone. They are large (40 μm or more) polymorphic cells with a variable number (up to 15–20) of oval, closely packed nuclei, and lie in close contact with the bone surface in pits termed resorption bays (Howship's lacunae).

Osteoclasts contain numerous mitochondria and vacuoles, many of which are acid phosphatase-containing lysosomes. The rough endoplasmic reticulum is relatively sparse for the size of cell, but the Golgi complex is extensive. The cytoplasm also contains numerous coated transport vesicles and vacuoles, and microtubule arrays. The latter are involved in the transport of vesicles between the Golgi stacks and the ruffled membrane, the highly infolded cell surface which contains the sites of local bone resorption. There is a well-defined zone of actin filaments around the perimeter of the ruffled membrane.

Osteoclasts cause demineralization by proton release, which creates an acidic local environment, and organic matrix destruction by releasing lysosomal (cathepsin K) and non-lysosomal (e.g. collagenase) enzymes. Factors stimulating osteoclasts to resorb bone include osteoblast-derived signals; cytokines from other cells, e.g. macrophages and lymphocytes; blood-borne factors, e.g. parathyroid hormone and $1,25(OH)_2$ vitamin D3 (calcitriol).

Osteoclasts arise by fusion of monocytes derived from the bone marrow or other haemopoietic tissue. They probably share a common precursor with macrophages within the granulocyte–macrophage lineage (p. 78), but it is thought that they subsequently form a distinct class of cells.

OSTEONS AND REMODELLING

The mechanical properties of bone are dependent on the general composition of its matrix: the manner in which the different components are arranged is important in determining its strength and resilience. There are two quite distinct types of organization: woven and lamellar bone.

In woven, or bundle, bone, the collagen fibres and bone crystals are irregularly arranged. The diameters of the fibres vary, so that fine and

Fig. 6.16 Human parietal bone (male neonate) showing primary osteonal bone (grey) and woven bone (white containing many connecting osteocyte lacunae, black). Internal resorption of the bone has produced large irregular dark spaces (trabecularization).

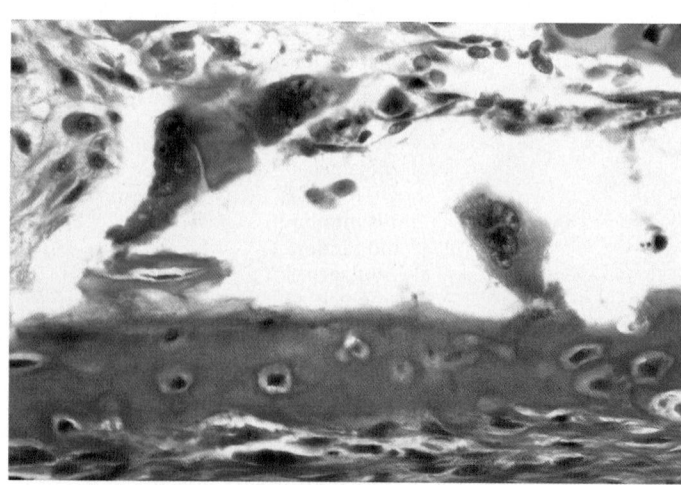

Fig. 6.17 Osteoclasts in a Heidenhain's azan-stained preparation of developing bone (solid blue matrix). Three large multinucleate osteoclasts are seen, contacting a free flat surface of woven bone (below) and a residual spicule of trabecular bone (above, left). (Photograph by Sarah-Jane Smith.)

coarse fibres intermingle, producing the appearance of the warp and weft of a woven fabric. Woven bone is typical of young fetal bones, but is also seen in adults during excessively rapid bone remodelling and repair of fractures. It is formed by highly active osteoblasts during development, and is stimulated in the adult by fracture, growth factors, or prostaglandin E_2.

Lamellar bone (**Figs 6.18, 6.19**) makes up almost all of the adult osseous skeleton. The precise arrangement of lamellae varies from site to site, particularly between compact cortical bone and the trabecular bone within. In many bones a few lamellae form continuous circumferential layers at the outer (periosteal) and inner (endosteal) surfaces. However, by far the greatest proportion are arranged in concentric cylinders around neurovascular channels (Haversian canals), forming the basic units of bone tissue, the Haversian systems or osteons. Osteons usually lie parallel to each other (**Fig. 6.20**) and, in elongated bones such as those of the appendicular skeleton, with the long axis of the bone. They may also spiral, branch or intercommunicate: some end blindly.

It has been estimated that there are c.21 million osteons in the adult skeleton. In transverse section they are round or ellipsoidal, varying from c.100 to 400 μm in diameter. There are c.30 lamellae, each c.3 μm thick, in medium-sized osteons. Each osteon is permeated with the canaliculi of its resident osteocytes, and these form pathways for diffusion of nutrients, gases, etc. between the vascular system and the osteocytes. The maximum diameter of an osteon ensures that no osteocyte is more than c.200 μm from a blood vessel, a distance which may be a limiting factor in cellular survival. The fragmentary remains of osteons and the circumferential lamellae of older bone, which have been partially eroded before the new osteons were formed, lie in the spaces between osteons and constitute the interstitial lamellae.

The central Haversian canals of osteons vary in size, with a mean diameter of 50 μm; those near the marrow cavity are somewhat larger. Each canal contains one or two capillaries lined by fenestrated endothelium and surrounded by a basal lamina which also encloses typical pericytes. They usually contain a few unmyelinated and occasional myelinated axons. The bony surfaces of osteonic canals are perforated by the openings of osteocyte canaliculi and are lined by collagen fibres.

Haversian canals communicate directly or indirectly with the marrow cavity via vascular channels, Volkmann's canals, which run obliquely or perpendicular to the direction of the osteons (**Fig. 6.20**). The majority of these channels appear to anastomose, but there are also a few large vascular connections with the periosteum and endosteum.

Osteons are distinguished from their neighbours by a cement line which contains little or no collagen, and is strongly basophilic because it has a high content of glycoproteins and proteoglycans. It marks the limit of bone erosion prior to the formation of an osteon, and is therefore also known as a reversal line. Similar basophilic lines also occur in the absence of erosion, where bony growth has been interrupted and then resumed, and are called resting lines. Canaliculi occasionally pass through cement lines, and so provide a route for exchange between interstitial bone lamellae and vascular channels within osteons.

Each lamella consists of a sheet of mineralized matrix containing collagen fibres of similar orientation locally, which run in branching bundles c.2–3 μm thick, and often extend the full width of a lamella. This interconnecting, three-dimensional construction increases the strength of the bone. The orientation of the collagen fibres and associated mineral crystals differs in adjacent lamellae: the difference varies between 0° and 90°, and is clearly shown by polarized light microscopy. A less perfect packing of collagen fibrils into bundles occurs at the borders of lamellae, where intermediate and random orientations predominate.

The main direction of the collagen fibres within osteons of long bone shafts varies between sites which are subjected predominantly to tension, where the fibres are more longitudinal, and those subjected mostly to compression, where the fibres are more oblique. At any site in a diaphysis, the peripheral lamellae of osteons contain more transverse fibres.

TRABECULAR BONE (Figs 6.9, 6.21)

The organization of trabecular bone is basically lamellar, and takes the form of branching and anastomosing curved plates, tubes and bars of various widths and lengths which bound marrow cavities (p. 77) and are lined by endosteal tissue. Their thickness ranges from c.50 to 400 μm. In general, bone lamellae are oriented parallel with the adjacent bone surface, and the arrangement of cells and matrix is similar to that found in circumferential and osteonic bone. Thick trabeculae and regions

close to compact bone may contain small osteons, but blood vessels do not otherwise lie within the bony tissue, and osteocytes therefore rely on canalicular diffusion from adjacent medullary vessels. In young bone, calcified cartilage may occur in the cores of trabeculae, but this is generally replaced by bone during subsequent remodelling.

REMODELLING

Remodelling of the interior of bone depends upon the balance of removal and deposition of bone, i.e. on the balanced activities of osteoclasts and osteoblasts. Osteoclasts first excavate a cylindrical tunnel by concerted action. A 'cutting cone' is formed by groups of osteoclasts moving at c. 50 μm/day, followed by osteoblasts which fill in the space so created. The osteoblasts deposit new osteoid matrix concentrically around a centrally ingrowing blood vessel, starting at the peripheral surface of the tunnel. This forms a 'closing cone' with c.4000 osteoblasts/mm^2. Deposition of successive, concentric lamellae follows, as cohorts of osteoblasts become embedded in the matrix they secrete, and are succeeded by new osteoblasts which line the free surface thus created, and secrete the next layer. In this way the walls of resorption cavities are lined with new lamellar matrix, and the vascular channels are progressively narrowed (**Fig. 6.22**). The pattern and extent of remodelling is dictated by the mechanical loads applied to the bone (Wolff's Law; Wolff 1892).

A hypermineralized basophilic cement line marks a site of reversal from resorption to deposition. Formation of osteons does not end with growth but continues variably throughout life. Remnants of circumferential lamellae and aged osteons form interstitial lamellae between osteons which are formed later (**Figs 6.18, 6.19A**).

It has been estimated that c.10% of the adult bony skeleton turns over each year by the process of remodelling. The degree of remodelling varies with age; the number of osteons and osteon fragments have therefore been used in attempts to estimate the age of skeletal material at death.

Bone growth is appositional. New layers are added only to preexisting surfaces and, unlike chondrocytes, osteocytes enclosed in lacunae do not divide or secrete new matrix. The rigidity of mineralized bone matrix prevents internal expansion, which means that interstitial growth, which is characteristic of most tissues, is absent in bone.

PERIOSTEUM, ENDOSTEUM AND BONE MARROW

The outer surface of bone is covered by a condensed, fibrocollagenous layer, the periosteum, and the inner surface is lined by a thinner, more cellular, endosteum. Osteoprogenitor cells, osteoblasts, osteoclasts and other cells important in the turnover and homeostasis of bone tissue lie in these layers.

The periosteal layer is tethered to the underlying bone by extrinsic collagen fibres, Sharpey's fibres, which penetrate deep into the outer cortical bone tissue. It is absent from articular surfaces, and from the points of insertion of tendons and ligaments. The periosteum is highly active during fetal development, when it generates osteoblasts for the appositional growth of bone. These cells form a layer, two to three cells deep, between the fibrous periosteum and new woven bone matrix. Osteoprogenitor cells within the mature periosteum are indistinguishable morphologically from fibroblasts. Periosteum is important in the repair of fractures: where it is absent, e.g. within the joint capsule of the femoral neck, fractures are slow to heal.

In resting adult bone, quiescent osteoblasts and osteoprogenitor cells are present chiefly on the endosteal surfaces, which act as the principal reservoir of new bone-forming cells for remodelling or repair. The endosteum provides a surface of c.7.5 m^2, thought to be important in calcium homeostasis. It is formed by flattened osteoblast precursor cells and reticular (type III collagen) fibres, and lines all the internal cavities of bone, including the Haversian canals. It overlies the endosteal circumferential lamellae, and encloses the medullary cavity.

Neurovascular supply of bone
VASCULAR SUPPLY AND LYMPHATIC DRAINAGE

The osseous circulation supplies bone tissue, marrow, perichondrium, epiphyseal cartilages in young bones, and, in part, articular cartilages. The vascular supply of a long bone depends on several points of inflow, which feed complex and regionally variable sinusoidal networks within

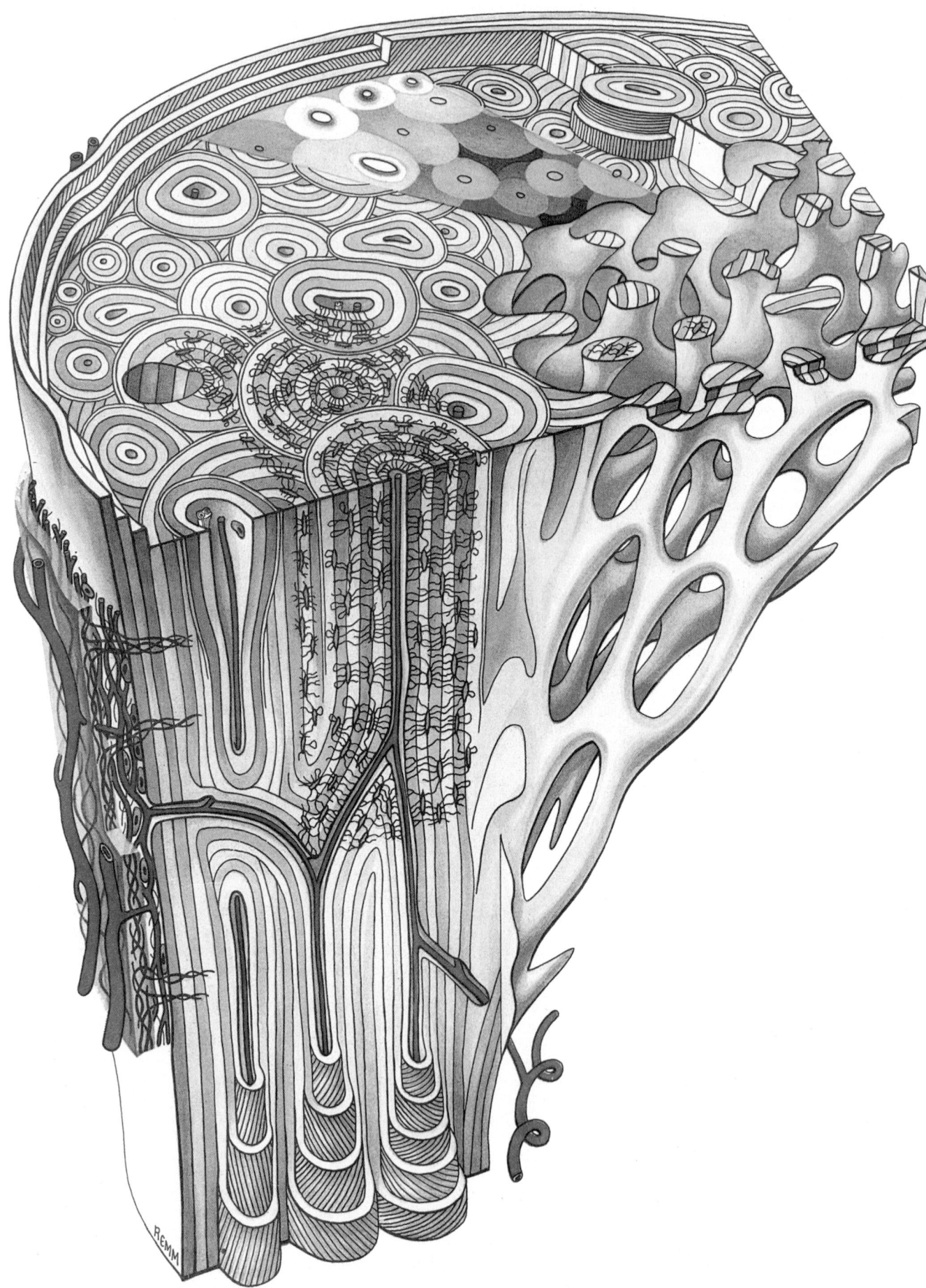

Fig. 6.18 Main features of the microstructure of mature lamellar bone. Areas of compact and trabecular (cancellous) bone are included. The central grey area in the transverse section simulates a microradiograph, the densities reflecting variations in mineralization. Note the general construction of the osteons, distribution of the osteocyte lacunae; Haversian canals and their contents; resorption spaces; and the different views of the structural basis of bone lamellation.

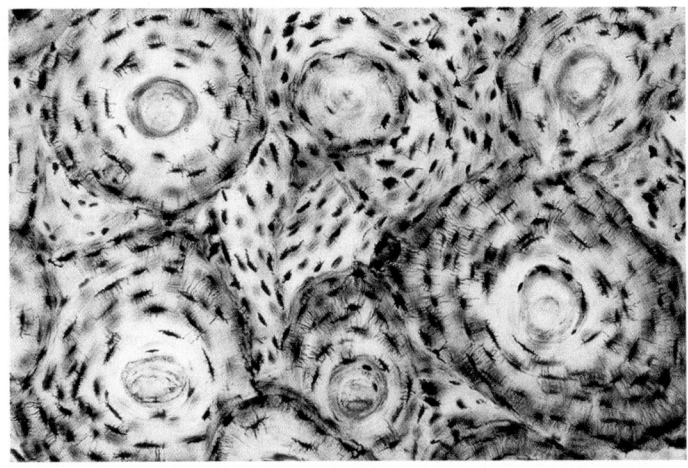

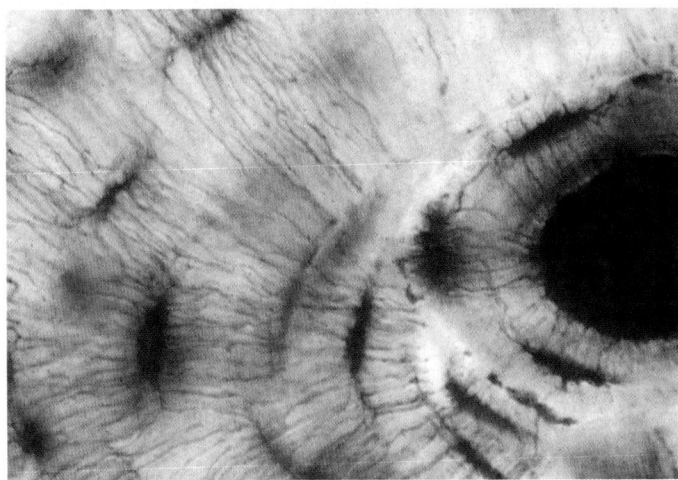

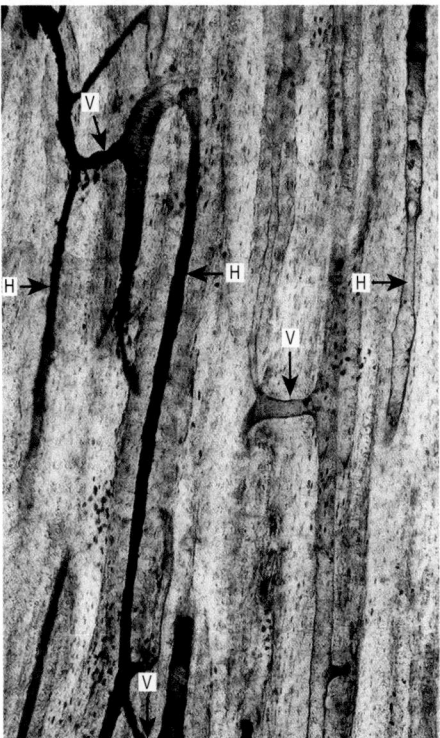

Fig. 6.20 Osteons in a dry ground longitudinal section of bone. The central Haversian canals (H: tubular structures, mainly dark) show transverse nutrient (Volkmann's) canals (V) which form bridges between adjacent osteons and their blood vessels. (Photograph by Sarah-Jane Smith.)

Fig. 6.19 A, Osteons in a dry ground transverse section of bone. Concentric lamellae surround the central Haversian canal of each complete osteon; they contain the dark lacunae of osteocytes and the canaliculi which are occupied in life by their dendrites. These canaliculi interconnect with canaliculi of osteocytes in adjacent lamellae. Incomplete (interstitial) lamellae (e.g. centre field) are the remnants of osteons remodelled by osteoclast erosion.
B, High-power view of osteocytes within lamellae; a Haversian canal is seen on the right. (**A**, photograph by Sarah-Jane Smith.)

it. These drain to venous channels which leave through all surfaces not covered by articular cartilage. The flow of blood through cortical bone in the shafts of long bones is mainly centrifugal (**Fig. 6.23**). These vascular patterns are summarized in **Fig. 6.24**.

One or two main diaphyseal nutrient arteries enter the shaft obliquely through nutrient foramina leading into nutrient canals. Their sites of entry and angulation are almost constant and characteristically directed away from the dominant growing epiphysis. A study of metacarpal and metatarsal bones showed that, apart from a few with double or no foramina, over 90% had a single nutrient foramen in the middle third of the shaft. Nutrient arteries do not branch in their canals, but divide into ascending and descending branches in the medullary cavity. These approach the epiphyses, dividing repeatedly into smaller helical branches close to the endosteal surface. These endosteal vessels are vulnerable during operations which involve passing metal implants into the medullary canal, e.g. intramedullary nailing for fractures. Near the epiphyses they are joined by terminal branches of numerous metaphyseal and epiphyseal arteries. The former are direct branches of neighbouring systemic vessels, the latter come from periarticular vascular arcades formed on non-articular bone surfaces. Numerous vascular foramina penetrate bones near their ends, often at fairly specific sites; some are occupied by arteries, but most contain thin-walled veins. Within bone, the arteries are unusual in consisting of endothelium with only a thin layer of supportive connective tissue. The epiphyseal and metaphyseal arterial supply is richer than the diaphyseal supply.

Medullary arteries of the shaft give off centripetal branches to a hexagonal mesh of medullary sinusoids which drain into a wide, thin-walled central venous sinus. They also possess cortical branches which pass through endosteal canals to feed fenestrated capillaries in Haversian systems. The central sinus drains veins which retrace the paths of nutrient arteries, sometimes piercing the shaft elsewhere as independent emissary veins. Cortical capillaries follow the pattern of Haversian canals, and are mainly longitudinal with oblique connections via Volkmann's canals (**Fig. 6.20**). At bone surfaces, cortical capillaries make capillary and venous connections with periosteal plexuses (**Fig. 6.24**). The latter are formed by arteries from neighbouring muscles which contribute vascular arcades with longitudinal links to the fibrous periosteum. From this external plexus a capillary network permeates the deeper, osteogenic periosteum. At muscular attachments, periosteal and muscular plexuses are confluent and the cortical capillaries then drain into interfascicular venules.

In addition to the centrifugal supply of cortical bone, there is an appreciable centripetal arterial flow to outer cortical zones from periosteal vessels. The large nutrient arteries of epiphyses form many intraosseous anastomoses, their branches passing towards the articular surfaces within the trabecular spaces of the bone. Near the articular cartilages these form serial anastomotic arcades (e.g. three or four in the femoral head), which give off end-arterial loops. These often pierce the thin hypochondral compact bone to enter, and sometimes traverse, the calcified zone of articular cartilage, before returning to the epiphyseal venous sinusoids.

In immature long bones the supply is similar, but the epiphysis is a discrete vascular zone. Epiphyseal and metaphyseal arteries enter on both sides of the growth cartilage; there are few, if any, anastomoses between them. Growth cartilages probably receive a supply from both sources, and from an anastomotic collar in the adjoining periosteum. Occasionally, cartilage canals are incorporated into a growth plate. Metaphyseal bone is nourished by terminal branches of metaphyseal arteries and by primary nutrient arteries of the shaft which form terminal blind-ended sprouts or sinusoidal loops in the zone of advancing ossification. Young periosteum is more vascular; its vessels communicate more freely with those of the shaft than their adult counterparts, and they have more metaphyseal branches.

Large irregular bones, e.g. the scapula and innominate, receive a periosteal supply. In addition, they often have large nutrient arteries which penetrate directly into their cancellous bone: the two systems anastomose freely. Short bones receive numerous fine vessels which

95

A

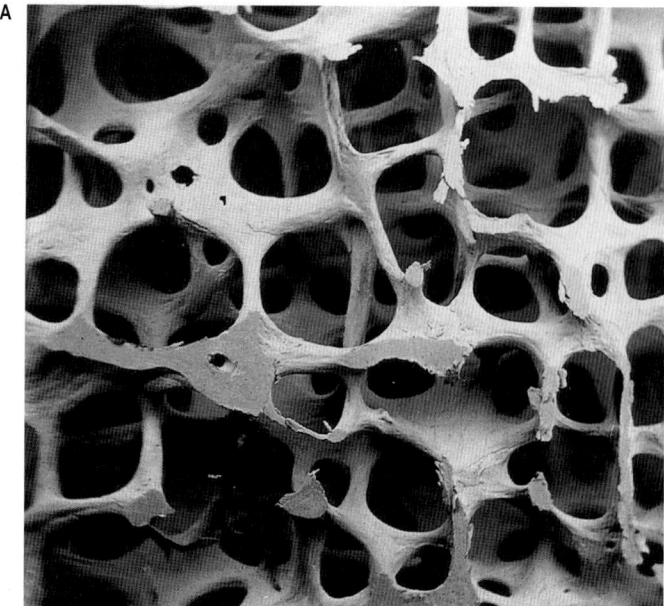

B

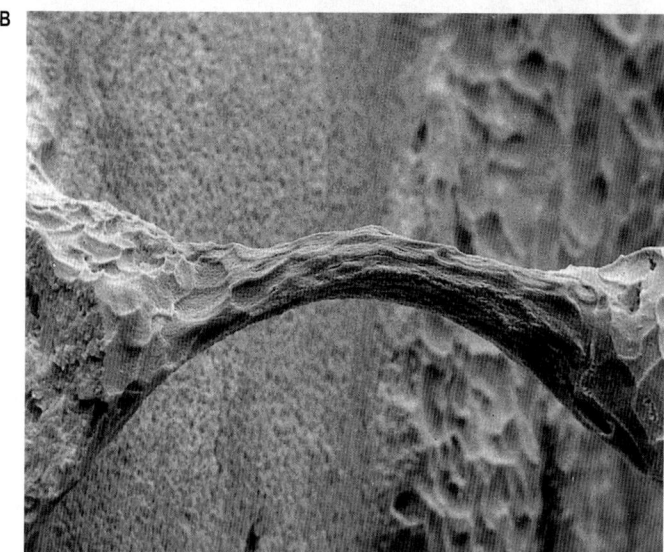

Fig. 6.21 **A**, Vertical section of cancellous bone, second lumbar vertebra (female, 42 years); **B**, Endosteal surface, sixth rib (female, 3.5 months), showing extensive resorption of a trabecular (foreground) and of the endosteal surface (right background). Scanning electron micrographs of inorganic preparations.

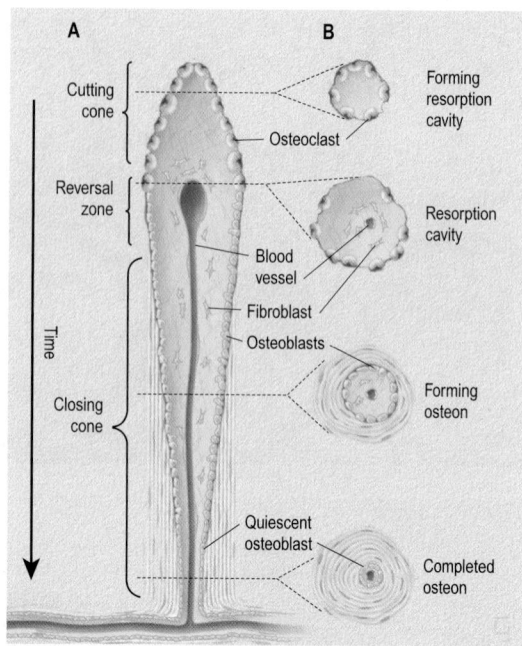

Fig. 6.22 Bone remodelling. Longitudinal and cross-sections of a time line illustrating the formation of an osteon. Osteoclasts cut a cylindrical channel through bone. Osteoblasts follow, laying down bone on the surface of the channel until matrix surrounds the central blood vessel of the newly formed osteon (closing cone of a new osteon). (By permission from Pollard T, Earnshaw W 2002 Cell Biology. Philadelphia: Saunders, and redrawn by permission from Parfitt AM 1976 The action of parathyroid hormone on bone. Metabolism 25: 809–844.)

supply their compact and cancellous bone and medullary cavities from the periosteum covering non-articular surfaces. Arteries enter vertebrae close to the bases of their transverse processes. Each vertebral medullary cavity drains to two large basivertebral veins which converge to a foramen on the posterior surface of the vertebral body. Flatter cranial bones are supplied by numerous periosteal or mucoperiosteal vessels. Large thin-walled veins run tortuously in cancellous bone. Lymphatic vessels accompany periosteal plexuses but have not been convincingly demonstrated in bone.

INNERVATION

Nerves are most numerous in the articular extremities of long bones, vertebrae and larger flat bones, and in periosteum. Fine myelinated and unmyelinated axons accompany nutrient vessels into bone and marrow and lie in the perivascular spaces of Haversian canals. Bone has a complex autonomic and sensory innervation, and bone cells have receptors for several neuropeptides which are found in the nerves which supply bone, e.g. neuropeptide Y, calcitonin gene-related peptide, vasoactive intestinal peptide and substance P.

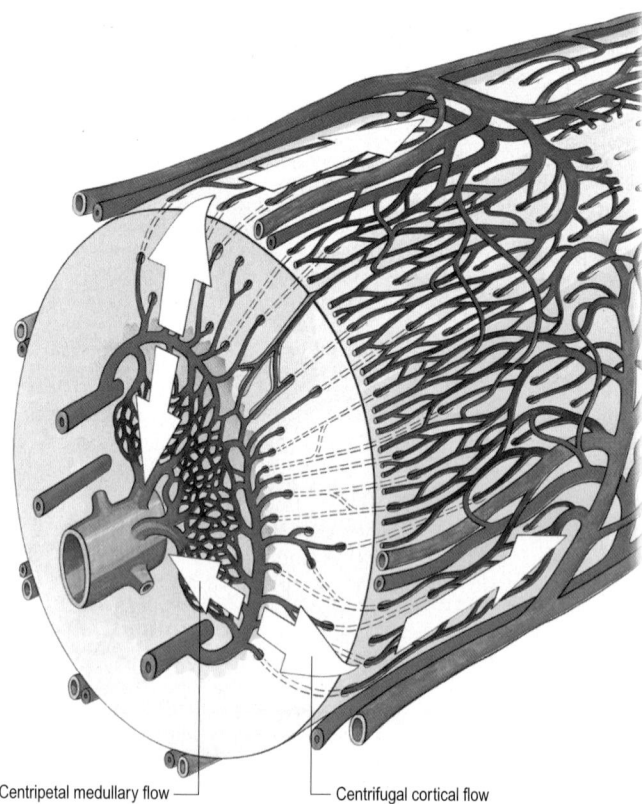

Fig. 6.23 Part of the diaphysis of a typical long bone, showing the organization of the blood vessels. The marrow cavity contains a large central venous sinus, a dense network of medullary sinusoids, and longitudinal medullary arteries and their circumferential rami. Longitudinally oblique transcortical capillaries emerge through minute 'cornet-shaped' foramina to become confluent with the periosteal capillaries and venules. Not to scale. The obliquity of the cortical capillaries is emphasized for clarity. (Constructed with the collaboration of the late Professor Murray Brookes, Department of Anatomy, GKT School of Medicine, London.)

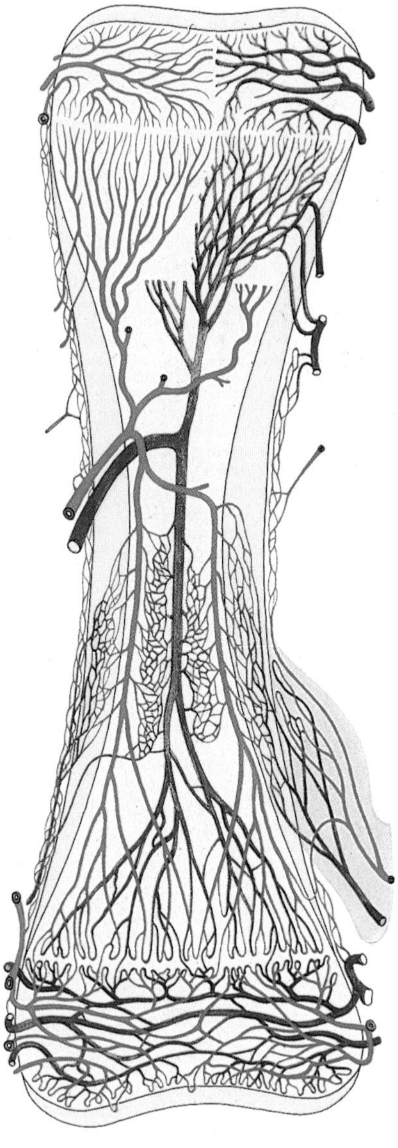

Fig. 6.24 The main features of the blood supply of a long bone. Note the contrasting supplies of the diaphysis, metaphysis and epiphysis, and their connections with periosteal, endosteal, muscular and periarticular vessels. (Constructed with the collaboration of the late Professor Murray Brookes, Department of Anatomy, GKT School of Medicine, London.)

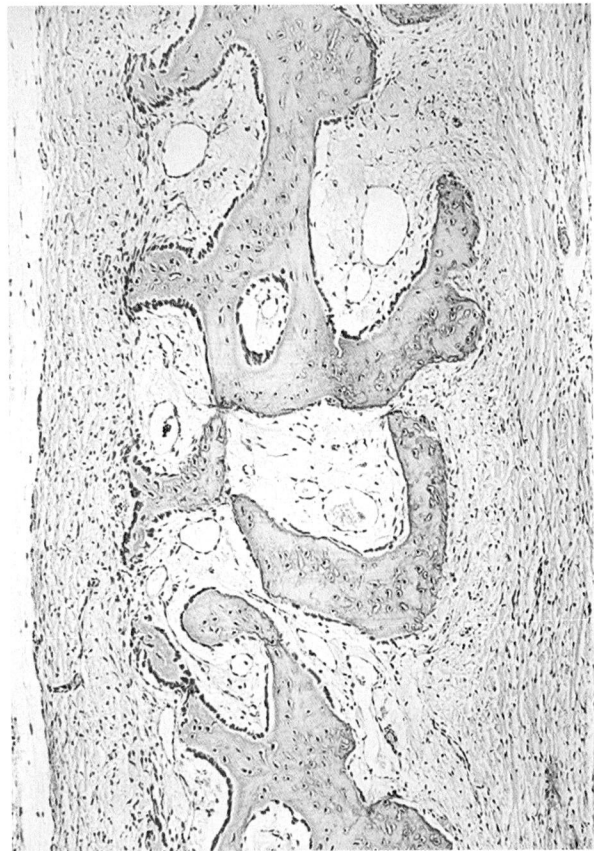

Fig. 6.25 Bone formation by intramembranous ossification. Focal deposition of osteoid follows osteoblastic differentiation within condensations of mesenchyme. Islands of bone (solid pink matrix, enclosing osteocytes) enlarge, fuse and are remodelled by osteoclasts to form mature lamellar bone. (By permission from Kierszenbaum AL 2002 Histology and Cell Biology. St Louis: Mosby.)

Development and growth of bone

Most bones are formed by a process of endochondral ossification, in which preformed cartilage templates (models) define their initial shapes and positions, and the cartilage is replaced by bone in an ordered sequence. Bones such as those in the cranial vault are laid down within a fibrocellular membrane, by a process known as intramembranous ossification.

INTRAMEMBRANOUS OSSIFICATION

Intramembranous ossification is the direct formation of bone (membrane bone) within highly vascular sheets or 'membranes' of condensed primitive mesenchyme (Fig. 6.25). At centres of ossification, mesenchymal stem cells differentiate into osteoprogenitor cells which proliferate around the branches of a capillary network, forming incomplete layers of osteoblasts in contact with the primitive bone matrix. The cells are polarized because they secrete a fine mesh of collagen fibres and ground substance, osteoid, from the surface which faces away from the blood vessels. The earliest crystals appear in association with extracellular matrix vesicles produced by the osteoblasts; crystal formation subsequently extends into collagen fibrils in the surrounding matrix, producing an early labyrinth of woven bone, the primary

spongiosa (Fig. 6.26). As layers of calcifying matrix are added to these early trabeculae, the osteoblasts enclosed by matrix come to lie within primitive lacunae. New osteocytes retain intercellular contact by means of their surface processes (dendrites) and, as these elongate, matrix condenses around them to form canaliculi.

As matrix secretion, calcification and enclosure of osteoblasts proceed, the trabeculae thicken and the intervening vascular spaces become narrower. Where bone remains trabecular, the process slows and the spaces between trabeculae become occupied by haemopoietic tissue. Where compact bone is forming, trabeculae continue to thicken and vascular spaces continue to narrow. Meanwhile the collagen fibres of the matrix, secreted on the walls of the narrowing spaces between trabeculae, become organized as parallel, longitudinal or spiral bundles, and the cells they enclose occupy concentric sequential rows. These irregular, interconnected masses of compact bone each has a central canal, and may be called primary osteons (primary Haversian systems). They are later eroded, together with the intervening woven bone, and replaced by generations of mature (secondary) osteons.

While these changes occur, mesenchyme condenses on the outer surface to form a fibrovascular periosteum. Bone is laid down increasingly by new osteoblasts which differentiate from osteoprogenitor cells in the deeper layers of the periosteum. Modelling of the growing bone is achieved by varying rates of resorption and deposition at different sites.

ENDOCHONDRAL OSSIFICATION (Figs 6.27, 6.28)

The hyaline cartilage model which forms during embryogenesis is a miniature template of the bone (cartilage bone) that will subsequently develop. It becomes surrounded by a condensed, vascular mesenchyme or perichondrium, which resembles the mesenchymal 'membrane' in which intramembranous ossification occurs. Its deeper layers contain osteoprogenitor cells.

The first appearance of a centre of primary ossification occurs when chondroblasts deep in the centre of the primitive shaft (Figs 6.27B,

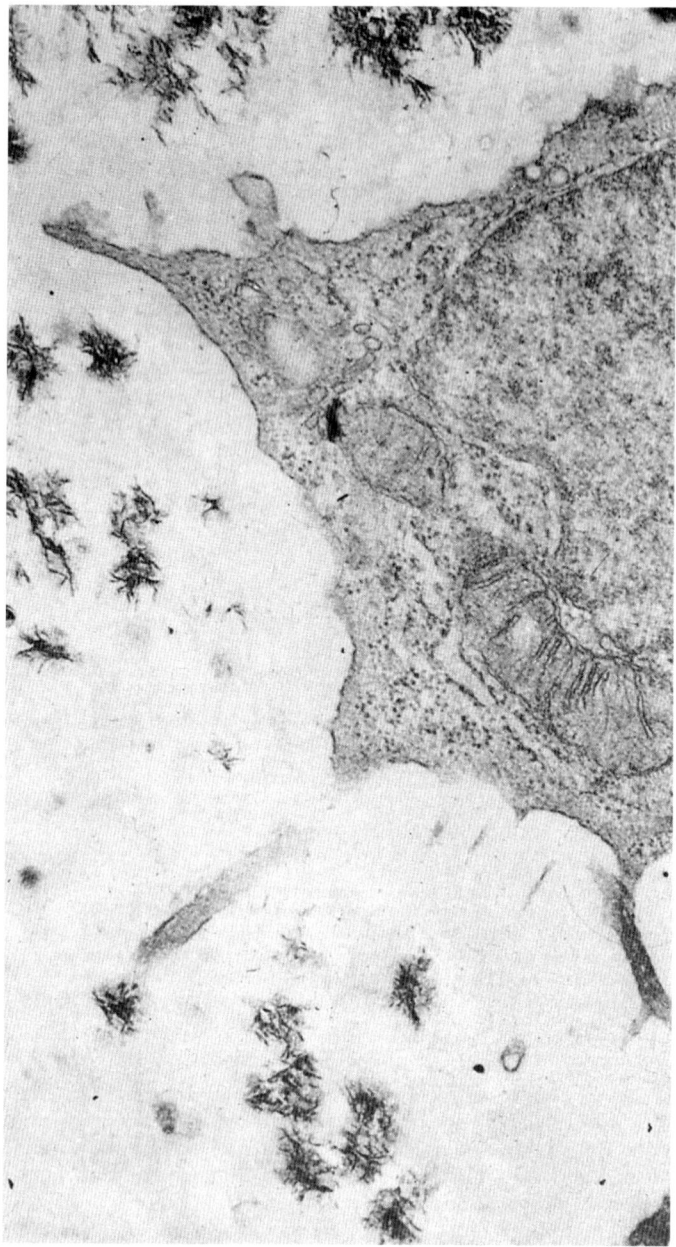

A

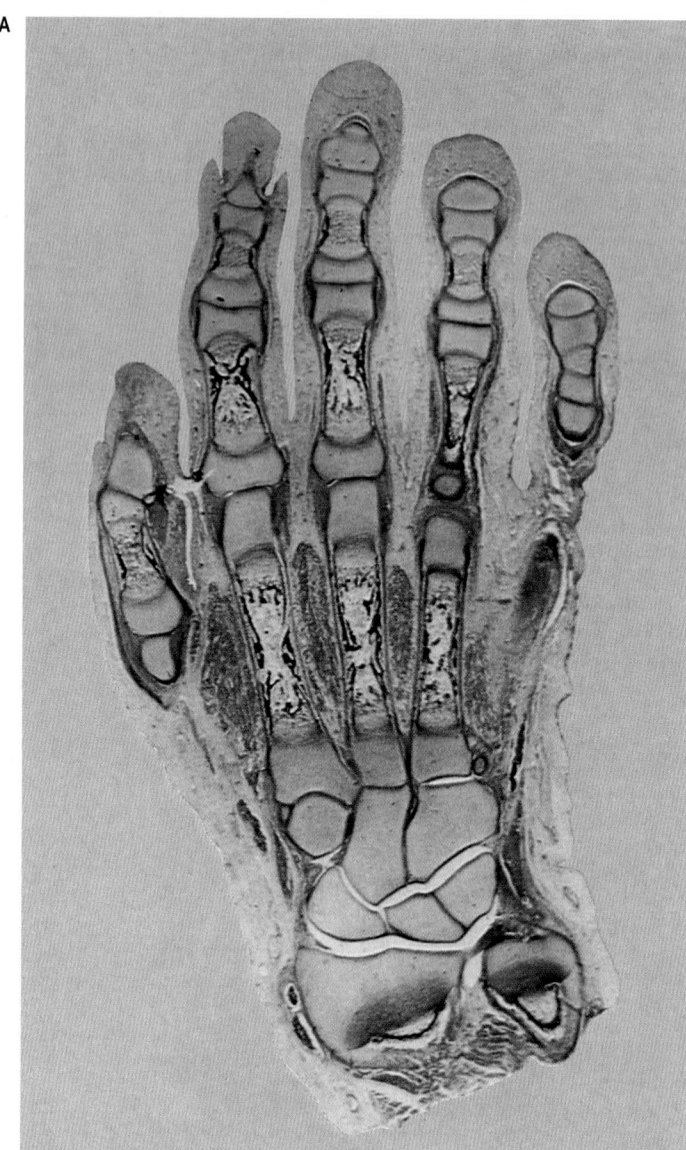

Fig. 6.26 Part of a young osteocyte. Its surface bears long filopodia which project into the surrounding extracellular matrix. The latter contains clusters of electron-dense matrix vesicles: these provide the initial nucleation sites for the formation of hydroxyapatite crystallites in the early mineralization of bone. The specimen is a cultured cell, growing from the subperiosteal ossifying front of the tibia of a chick.

B

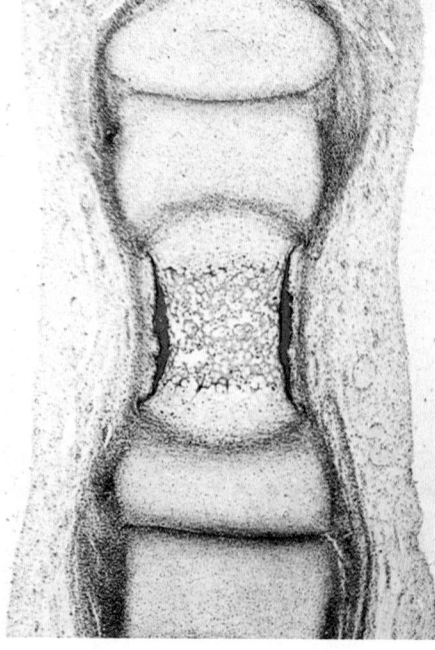

Fig. 6.27 A, Section of a fetal hand showing cartilaginous models of the carpal bones, and the primary ossification centres, which display varying stages of maturity, in the metacarpals and phalanges. Note that none of the carpal elements shows any evidence of ossification. **B**, Higher power view of an early primary ossification centre. The cartilage cells in the shaft have hypertrophied and this region is surrounded by a delicate tube or collar of subperiosteal bone (red). (Photographs by Kevin Fitzpatrick on behalf of GKT School of Medicine, London.)

6.29) enlarge greatly, and their cytoplasm becomes vacuolated and accumulates glycogen. Their intervening matrix is compressed into thin, often perforated, septa. The cells degenerate and may die, leaving enlarged and sometimes confluent lacunae (primary areolae) whose thin walls become calcified during the final stages. Type X collagen is produced in the hypertrophic zone of cartilage. Matrix vesicles originating from chondrocytes in the proliferation zone are most evident in the inter-columnar regions, where they appear to initiate crystal formation. At the same time, cells in the deep layer of perichondrium around the centre of the cartilage model differentiate into osteoblasts and form a peripheral layer of bone. Initially, this periosteal collar, formed by intra-membranous ossification within the perichondrium, is a thin-walled tube which encloses the central shaft (**Figs 6.27B, 6.29**). As it increases in diameter it also extends towards both ends of the shaft.

The periosteal collar which overlies the calcified cartilaginous walls of degenerate chondrocyte lacunae is invaded from the deep layers of the periosteum (formerly perichondrium) by osteogenic buds. These

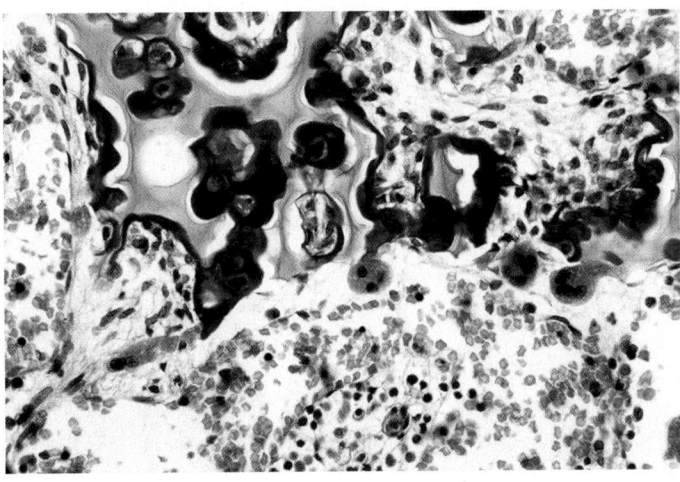

Fig. 6.28 Endochondral ossification in fetal bone. Spicules of cartilage remnant (pale blue) serve as surfaces for the deposition of osteoid (dark blue), shown in the upper half of the field. Mineralized, woven bone is stained red. Three large multinucleate osteoclasts are seen centre right, further eroding cartilage and remodelling the developing bone. Blood sinusoids and haemopoietic tissue (below) fill the spaces between areas of ossification. Heidenhain's azan trichrome preparation. (Photograph by Sarah-Jane Smith.)

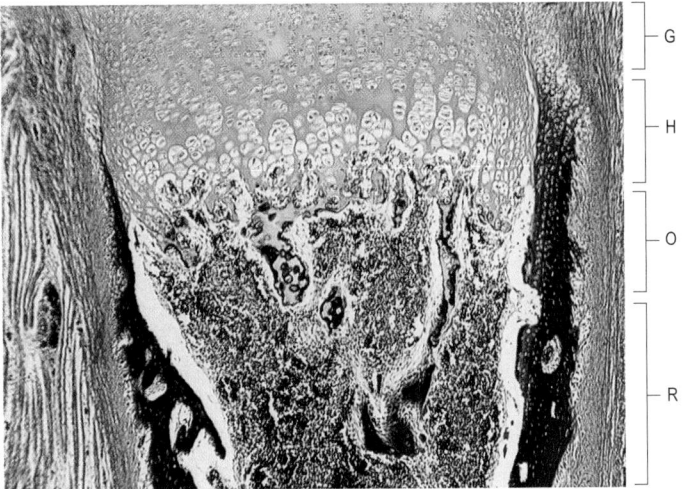

Fig. 6.29 The sequence of cellular events in endochondral ossification. This low magnification micrograph shows the primary ossification centre in a fetal bone. *See* **Fig. 6.30** for further details. G, growth zone; H, hypertrophic zone; O, ossification zone; R, remodelling zone. (Photograph by Sarah-Jane Smith.)

are blind-ended capillary sprouts and are accompanied by osteo-progenitor cells and osteoclasts. The latter excavate newly formed bone to reach adjacent calcified cartilage where they continue to erode the walls of primary chondrocyte lacunae. This process leads to their fusion into larger and irregular communicating spaces, secondary areolae, which fill with embryonic medullary tissue (vascular mesenchyme, osteoblasts and osteoclasts, haemopoietic and marrow stromal cells, etc.). Osteoblasts attach themselves to the delicate residual walls of calcified cartilage and lay down osteoid which rapidly becomes confluent, forming a continuous lining of bone. Further layers of bone are added, enclosing young osteocytes in lacunae, and narrowing the perivascular spaces. Bone deposition on the more central calcified cartilage ceases as the formation of subperiosteal bone continues.

Osteoclastic erosion of the early bone spicules then creates a primitive medullary cavity in which only a few trabeculae, composed of bone with central cores of calcified cartilage, remain to support the developing marrow tissues. These trabeculae soon become remodelled and replaced by more mature bone or by marrow. Meanwhile new,

adjacent, cartilaginous regions undergo similar changes. Since these are most advanced centrally, and the epiphyses remain cartilaginous, the intermediate zones exhibit a temporospatial sequence of changes when viewed in longitudinal section (**Fig. 6.30F**). This region of dynamic change from cartilage to bone persists until longitudinal growth of the bone ceases.

Expansion of the cartilaginous extremity (usually an epiphysis) keeps pace with the growth of the rest of the bone both by appositional and interstitial growth. The growth zone expands in all dimensions. Growth in thickness of a developing long bone is caused by occasional transverse mitoses in its chondrocytes, and by appositional growth as a result of matrix deposition by cells from the perichondrial collar or ring at this level. The future growth plate therefore expands in concert with the shaft and adjacent future epiphysis. A zone of relatively quiescent chondrocytes (the resting zone) lies on the side of the plate closest to the epiphysis. An actively mitotic zone of cells faces towards the shaft of the bone: the more frequent divisions in the long axis of the bone soon create numerous longitudinal columns (palisades) of disc-shaped chondrocytes, each in a flattened lacuna (**Fig. 6.30A–G**). Proliferation and column formation occurs in this region, the zone of cartilage growth (the proliferative zone), and its continued longitudinal interstitial expansion provides the basic mode of elongation of a bone.

The columns of cells show increasing maturity towards the centre of the shaft. Their chondrocytes increase in size and accumulate glycogen. In the hypertrophic zone, energy metabolism is depressed at the level of the mineralizing front (**Fig. 6.31**). The lacunae are now separated by transverse and longitudinal walls. The longitudinal walls are impregnated with apatite crystals (the zone of calcified cartilage). The calcified partitions enter the zone of bone formation and are invaded by vascular mesenchyme, which contains osteoblasts, osteoclasts, etc. The partitions, especially the transverse ones, are then partly eroded; osteoid deposition, bone formation and osteocyte enclosure occur on the surfaces of the longitudinal walls. Lysis of calcified partitions has been ascribed to osteoclast (chondroclast) action, aided by cells associated with the terminal buds of vascular sinusoids which occupy, and come into close contact with, each incomplete columnar trabecular framework.

Continuing cell division in the growth zone adds to the epiphyseal ends of cell columns, and the bone grows in length as this sequence of changes proceeds away from the diaphyseal centre. The bone also grows in diameter as further subperiosteal bone deposition occurs near the epiphyses, and its medullary cavity enlarges transversely and longitudinally. Internal erosion and remodelling of the newly formed bone tissue continues.

Growth continues in this way for many months or years in different bones but eventually one or more secondary centres of ossification usually appear in the cartilaginous extremities. These epiphyseal centres (or ends of bones which lack epiphyses) do not at first display cell columns. Instead, isogenous cell groups hypertrophy, with matrix calcification, and are then invaded by osteogenic vascular mesenchyme, sometimes from cartilage canals. Bone is formed on calcified cartilage, as described above. As an epiphysis enlarges, its cartilaginous periphery also forms a zone of proliferation in which cell columns are organized radially; hypertrophy, calcification, erosion and ossification occur at increasing depths from the surface. The early osseous epiphysis is thus surrounded by a superficial growth cartilage, and the growth plate adjacent to the metaphysis soon becomes the most active region.

As a bone reaches maturity, epiphyseal and metaphyseal ossification processes gradually encroach upon the growth plate from either side: they eventually meet when bony fusion of the epiphysis occurs and longitudinal growth of the bone ceases. The events which take place during fusion are broadly as follows. As growth ceases, the cartilaginous plate becomes quiescent and gradually thins: proliferation, palisading and hypertrophy of chondrocytes stop, and the cells form short, irregular conical masses. Patchy calcification is accompanied by resorption of calcified cartilage and some of the adjacent metaphyseal bone, forming resorption channels which are invaded by vascular mesenchyme. Some endothelial sprouts pierce the thin plate of cartilage, and the metaphyseal and epiphyseal vessels unite. Ossification around these vessels spreads into the intervening zones and results in fusion of epiphysis and metaphysis.

This bone is visible in radiographs as a radio-dense epiphyseal line (a term which is also used to describe the level of the perichondrial collar or ring around the growth cartilage of immature bones, or the

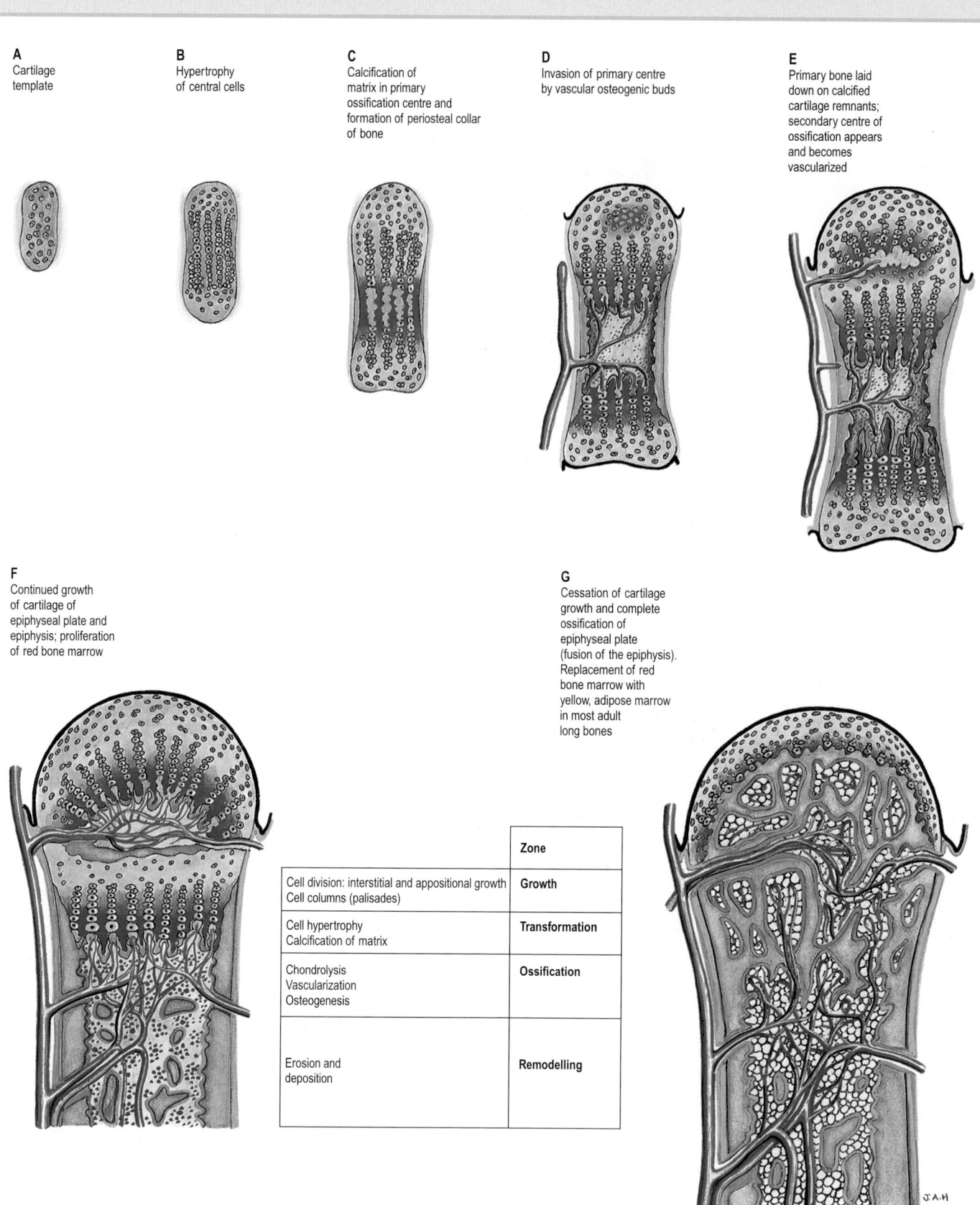

A
Cartilage
template

B
Hypertrophy
of central cells

C
Calcification of
matrix in primary
ossification centre and
formation of periosteal collar
of bone

D
Invasion of primary centre
by vascular osteogenic buds

E
Primary bone laid
down on calcified
cartilage remnants;
secondary centre of
ossification appears
and becomes
vascularized

F
Continued growth
of cartilage of
epiphyseal plate and
epiphysis; proliferation
of red bone marrow

G
Cessation of cartilage
growth and complete
ossification of
epiphyseal plate
(fusion of the epiphysis).
Replacement of red
bone marrow with
yellow, adipose marrow
in most adult
long bones

	Zone
Cell division: interstitial and appositional growth Cell columns (palisades)	Growth
Cell hypertrophy Calcification of matrix	Transformation
Chondrolysis Vascularization Osteogenesis	Ossification
Erosion and deposition	Remodelling

Fig. 6.30 A–G, The stages of endochondral ossification in a long bone.

surface junction between epiphysis and metaphysis in a mature bone). In smaller epiphyses, which unite earlier, there is usually one initial eccentric area of fusion, and thinning of the residual cartilaginous plate. The original sites of fusion are subsequently resorbed and replaced by new bone. Medullary tissue extends into the whole cartilaginous plate until union is complete and no epiphyseal 'scar' persists. In larger epiphyses, which unite later, similar processes also involve multiple

perforations in growth plates, and islands of epiphyseal bone often persist as epiphyseal scars. Calcified cartilage coated by bone forms the epiphyseal scar, and is also found below articular cartilage. It has been called metaplastic bone, a term also applied to attachments of tendons, ligaments and other dense connective tissues.

The cartilaginous surfaces of epiphyses forming synovial joints remain unossified, but the typical sequence of cartilaginous zones in

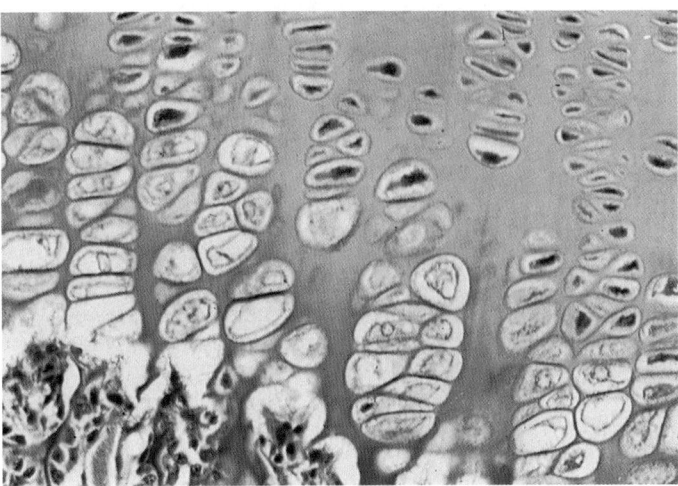

Fig. 6.31 Section showing the hypertrophy and palisading of cartilage cells as the ossifying front of an early primary centre of ossification is approached (below). Lacunae are enlarged, and matrix partitions are reduced in width and exhibit increased staining density (eosinophilia) following calcification.

them persists throughout life. A similar developmental sequence occurs at synchondroses, except that the proliferative rates of chondrocytes and the replacement of cartilage by bone are similar, although not identical, at each side of the synchondrosis.

POSTNATAL GROWTH AND MAINTENANCE

Changes in general shape, modelling, occur in all growing bones; the process has been studied mainly in cranial and long bones with expanded extremities. A bone such as the parietal thickens and expands during growth, but decreases in curvature. Accretion continues at its edges by proliferation of osteoprogenitor cells at sutures. Periosteal bone is mainly added externally and eroded internally, but not at uniform rates or at all times. The rate of formation increases with radial distance from the centre of ossification (the future parietal eminence), and formation may also occur endocranially as well as ectocranially, changing the curvature of the bone. As the skull bones thicken and grow at the sutures, the relative positions of original centres of ossification change in three dimensions, the vault of the skull expanding with growth of the brain. The development of diploë (trabeculae of spongy bone) and marrow space internally produces outer and inner cortical plates.

Long bones elongate mainly by extension of endochondral ossification into calcified zones of adjacent growth cartilages, which are continually replaced by the longitudinal interstitial growth of their proliferative zones, with minor additions by radial epiphyseal growth. Simultaneously, diametric increases of growth cartilages and shafts occur by continuing subperiosteal deposition and endosteal erosion. However, in many bones growth is at different rates, or even reversed, at different places. A bone which is initially tubular may thus become triangular in section, e.g. the tibia. Similarly, the waisted contours of metaphyses are preserved by differential rates of periosteal erosion and endosteal deposition, as metaphyseal bone becomes diaphyseal in position. The junction between a field of resorption and one of deposition on the surface of a bone during its growth is called a surface reversal line. The relative position of such a line may remain stable over long periods of cortical drift.

Lamellar bone forms at variable rates which reflect the slow turnover of osteons throughout adult life. Each Haversian system resorption canal (cutting cone) of c.2 mm long takes 1–3 months to form, and a new infilling osteon (closing cone) forms in a similar period (**Fig. 6.22**). Internal remodelling continuously supplies young osteons with labile calcium reserves, and provides a malleable osseous architecture responsive to altering patterns of stress. The remodelling unit in cancellous bone, equivalent to the secondary osteon of compact bone, is the bone structural unit. This has an average thickness of 40–70 μm and length of c.100 μm, but may be more extensive and irregular in shape.

The morphogenetic control of shape is not clear, but is thought largely to involve responses to strain. Bone resorption typically occurs when gravitational or other mechanical stresses are reduced, as in bed rest, or in the zero gravity conditions in space. Likewise bone subjected to constant pressure tends to resorb. This underpins much orthodontic treatment, since teeth can be made to migrate slowly through alveolar bone by the application of steady lateral or medial pressure. Conversely, with constant tension, bone is deposited, e.g. the bones in the racket arm of tennis players are more robust than in the contralateral limb.

The normal development and maintenance of bone requires adequate intake and absorption of calcium, phosphorus, vitamins A, C and D, and a balance between growth hormone, thyroid hormones, oestrogens and androgens. Various other factors, including different prostaglandins and glucocorticoids, may also play important roles in the maintenance and turnover of osseous tissue. Prolonged deficiency of calcium causes loss of bone mineral via a loss of bone tissue (osteoporosis) and consequent bone fragility. Vitamin D influences intestinal transport of calcium and phosphate, and therefore affects circulatory calcium levels. Prolonged deficiency (with or without low intake) leads, in adults, to bones which contain regions of deformable, uncalcified osteoid (osteomalacia). Similar deficiencies, during growth, lead to severe disturbance of growth cartilages and ossification, e.g. reductions of regular columnar organization in growth plates, and failure of cartilage calcification (although chondrocytes proliferate). Growth plates also become thicker and less regular than normal (classic rickets or juvenile osteomalacia). In rickets, the uncalcified or poorly calcified cartilage trabeculae are only partially eroded: osteoblasts secrete layers of osteoid, but these fail to ossify in the metaphyseal region, and ultimately gravity deforms these softened bones.

Vitamin C is essential for the adequate synthesis of collagen and matrix proteoglycans in connective tissues. When vitamin C is deficient, growth plates become thin, ossification almost stops, and metaphyseal trabeculae and cortical bone are reduced in thickness. This causes fragility and delayed healing of fractures. Vitamin A is necessary for normal growth, and for a correct balance of deposition and removal of bone. Deficiency retards growth as a result of the failure of internal erosion and remodelling, particularly in the cranial base. Foramina are narrowed, sometimes causing pressure atrophy of contained nerves, and the cranial cavity and spinal canal may fail to expand with the central nervous system, which impairs nervous function. Conversely, excess vitamin A stimulates vascular erosion of growth cartilages, which become thin or totally lost, and longitudinal growth ceases. Retinoic acid, a vitamin A derivative, is involved in pattern formation in limb buds, and in the differentiation of osteoblasts.

Balanced endocrine functions are also essential to normal bone maturation, and disturbances in this balance may have profound effects. In addition to its role in calcium metabolism, parathyroid hormone in excess (primary hyperparathyroidism) stimulates unchecked osteoclastic erosion of bone, particularly subperiosteally and later endosteally (osteitis fibrosa cystica).

Growth hormone (GH; somatotropin) is required for normal interstitial proliferation in growth cartilages, and hence increase in stature. Termination of normal growth is imperfectly understood, but may involve a fall in hormone production or in the sensitivity of chondroblasts to insulin-like growth factors regulated by GH. Reduction of GH production in the young leads to quiescence and thinning of growth plates and hence pituitary dwarfism. Conversely, continued hypersecretion in the immature leads to gigantism, and in the adult results in thickening of bones by subperiosteal deposition; the mandible, hands and feet are the most affected, a condition known as acromegaly.

While continued longitudinal growth of bones depends on adequate levels of GH, effective remodelling to a mature shape also requires the action of the thyroid hormones. Growth and skeletal maturity are also closely related to endocrine activities of the ovaries, testes and suprarenal cortices. High oestrogen levels increase deposition of endosteal and trabecular bone; conversely, osteoporosis in postmenopausal women reflects reduced ovarian function. Fluctuations in the rate of growth and the timing of skeletal maturation are a function of circulating levels of suprarenal and testicular androgens. In hypogonadism, maturation (marked by growth plate fusion) is late and the limbs therefore elongate excessively; conversely, in hypergonadism, premature fusion of the epiphyses results in diminished stature.

GROWTH OF INDIVIDUAL BONES

Ossification centres appear over a long period during bone growth, many in embryonic life (**Fig. 11.6A**), some in prenatal life, and others well into the postnatal growing period. Initially microscopic, the ossification centres soon become macroscopic and their growth can then be followed by radiological and other scanning techniques.

Many bones, including carpal, tarsal, lacrimal, nasal, and zygomatic bones, inferior nasal conchae and auditory ossicles, ossify from a single centre. Even in this limited group, centres appear between the eighth intrauterine week and the tenth year, a wide sequence for studying growth or estimating age. However, most bones ossify from several centres, one of which appears in late embryonic or early fetal life (seventh week to fourth month), in the centre of the future bone. Ossification progresses from the centres towards the ends, which are still cartilaginous at birth (**Fig. 6.32**). These terminal regions ossify from separate centres, sometimes multiple, which appear between birth and the late teens, and so they are secondary to the earlier primary centre from which much of the bone ossifies. This is the pattern in long bones, as well as in some shorter elements such as the metacarpals and metatarsals, and in the ribs and clavicles.

At birth a bone such as the tibia is typically ossified throughout its diaphysis by a primary centre which appears in the seventh intrauterine week, whereas its cartilaginous epiphyses ossify from secondary centres. As the epiphyses enlarge almost all the cartilage is replaced by bone, except for a specialized layer of articular hyaline cartilage which persists at the joint surface, and a thicker zone between the diaphysis and epiphysis. Persistence of this epiphyseal plate or disc (growth plate or growth cartilage) allows increase in bone length until the usual dimensions are reached, by which time the epiphyseal plate has ossified. The bone has then reached maturity. Coalescence of the epiphysis and diaphysis is fusion, the amalgamation of separate osseous units into one.

Many bones, e.g. long bones, have epiphyses at both ends. Metacarpals, metatarsals, phalanges, clavicles and ribs have only one epiphysis, although the costal cartilages may represent epiphyses which are normally devoid of ossification centres. Epiphyseal ossification is sometimes more complex; e.g. the proximal end of the humerus, which is wholly cartilaginous at birth, develops three centres during childhood, and these coalesce into a single mass before they fuse with the diaphysis. Only one of these centres forms an articular surface, the others form the greater and lesser tubercles which give muscular attachments. Similar composite epiphyses occur at the distal end of the humerus and in the femur and ribs and vertebrae.

Many cranial bones ossify from multiple centres. The sphenoid, temporal and occipital bones are almost certainly composites of multiple elements in their evolutionary history. Some show evidence of fusion between membrane and cartilage bones which unite during growth to form a complex whole.

Disparate rates of ossification occur at different sites and do not appear to be related to bone size. If the growth rate was uniform, ossification centres would appear in a strict descending order of bone size. However, the appearance of primary centres for bones of such different sizes as the phalanges and femora are separated by, at most, a week of embryonic life. Those for carpal and tarsal bones show some correlation between size and order of ossification, from largest (calcaneus in the fifth fetal month) to smallest (pisiform in the ninth to twelfth postnatal year). In individual bones, succession of centres is related to the volume of bone which each produces. The largest epiphyses, e.g. the adjacent ends of the femur and tibia, are the earliest to begin to ossify (immediately before or after birth, which are points of forensic interest).

At epiphyseal plates, the rate of growth is initially equal at both ends of bones which possess two epiphyses. However, experimental observations in other species have revealed that one generally grows faster than the other after birth. Since the faster-growing end also usually fuses later with the diaphysis, its contribution to length is greater. Though faster rate has not been measured directly in human bones, later fusion has been documented radiologically.

The more active end of a long limb bone is often termed the growing end, but this is a misnomer. The rate of increase of stature, which is rapid in infancy and again at puberty, demonstrates that rates of growth at epiphyses vary. The spurt at puberty, or slightly before, decreases as epiphyses fuse in post-adolescent years, and has been the subject of much study.

Growth cartilages do not grow uniformly at all points, which presumably accounts for changes such as the alteration in angle between the humeral shaft and its neck. The junctions between epiphysis and diaphysis at growth plates are not uniformly flat on either surface. Osseous surfaces usually become reciprocally curved by differential growth, and the epiphysis forms a shallow cup over the convex end of the shaft, with cartilage intervening. This arrangement may resist shearing forces at this relatively weak region. Reciprocity of bone surfaces is augmented by small nodules and ridges, as can be seen when the surfaces are stripped of cartilage. These adaptations emphasize the formation of many immature bones from several elements which are held together by epiphyseal cartilages. Most human bones exhibit these complex junctions, at which bone is bonded to bone through cartilage, not only through the active years of childhood, but also through the even more vigorous years of adolescence.

Forces at growth cartilages are largely compressive, but with an element of shear. Interference with epiphyseal growth may occur as a result of violence, but disturbance by constitutional disease, such as fevers, is more frequent, and produces changes in trabecular patterns of bone, which are visible radiographically as dense transverse lines of arrested growth (Harris' lines). Several such lines may appear in the limb bones of children afflicted by successive illnesses.

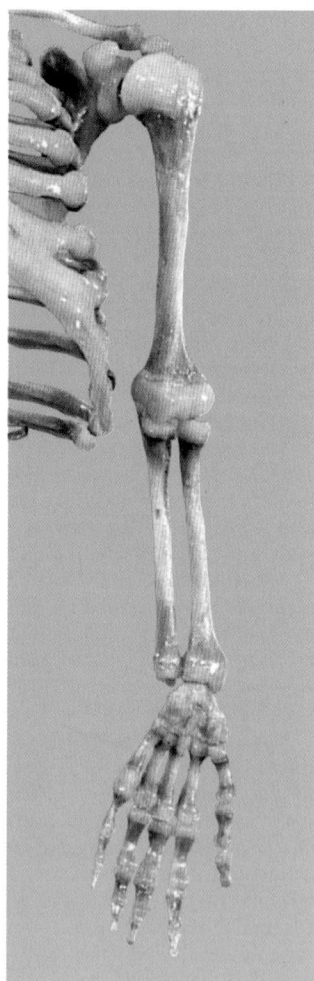

A B

Fig. 6.32 **A**, Radiograph of a neonatal arm. Ossification from primary centres is well advanced in all of the limb bones except the carpals, which are still wholly cartilaginous. The gaps by which individual elements appear to be separated are filled by radiolucent hyaline cartilage, in which epiphyseal or carpal ossification will subsequently occur. Note the flaring contours, narrow midshaft and relatively expanded metaphyses of the long bones, and the proportions of the limb segments, in particular the relatively large hand, which are characteristic of this age. **B**, The bones and cartilages of a neonatal left arm. Compare the radiolucent areas in the radiograph (A) with the preserved cartilaginous epiphyses and carpal elements in this specimen. (**B**, provided by the Department of Nuclear Medicine, GKT School of Medicine; photograph by Kevin Fitzpatrick and Sarah-Jane Smith on behalf of GKT School of Medicine, London.)

Variation in skeletal development occurs between individuals, sexes and possibly also races. However, the sequence of events shows little variation; it is their timing which varies. Females antedate males in all groups studied, and differences, which are perhaps insignificant before birth, increase thereafter, rising to two years or so in the later epiphyseal fusions of adolescence.

JOINTS

The bones of the skeleton are joined by a variety of structural arrangements collectively termed joints (arthroses). Joints allow differential growth, the transmission of forces (compressive, shear and torsion), and movement (from consolidation and complete rigidity at one extreme, to relatively free but controlled movement at the other). They may be classified in a number of ways.

The specialized connective tissues forming joints may remain solid, often changing character with time, or they may develop a narrow but extensive, enclosed, fluid-containing cavity. Solid (non-synovial) joints are called synarthroses and are commonly grouped into fibrous joints and cartilaginous joints, according to the principal type of intervening connective tissue. Synovial joints are called diarthroses: with few exceptions (the temporomandibular joint and those involving the clavicle, which have intervening fibrocartilaginous discs), they occur between the ends or other defined surfaces of endochondral bones.

Fibrous joints

In most instances fibrous joints consist mainly of collagenous junctions between bones. In a minority of situations fibroelastic tissue predominates. Three main groups of fibrous articulation are generally recognized, namely, sutures, gomphoses and syndesmoses (**Figs 6.33, 6.34**).

SUTURE

Sutures are limited to the skull (Chapter 27). They occur wherever margins or broader surfaces of bones are separated only by connective tissue, the sutural ligament or membrane, which is a surviving, unossified part of the mesenchymal sheets in which membrane bones develop. Sutural ligaments display regions of differentiation which are involved in growth and the binding of apposed bone surfaces. On its sutural aspect each bone is covered by a layer of osteogenic cells, the cambial layer, which is itself overlaid by a capsular lamella of fibrous tissue. Collectively these correspond to, and are continuous with, the periosteum at the margins of the sutural surfaces, both inside and outside the skull. Between these two layers of sutural periosteum there is a central stratum of loose fibrous connective tissue which varies in width according to age and the interval between the bones involved. It contains thin-walled blood vessels; the veins communicate with diploic vessels, intracranial venous sinuses and external veins in the scalp. The

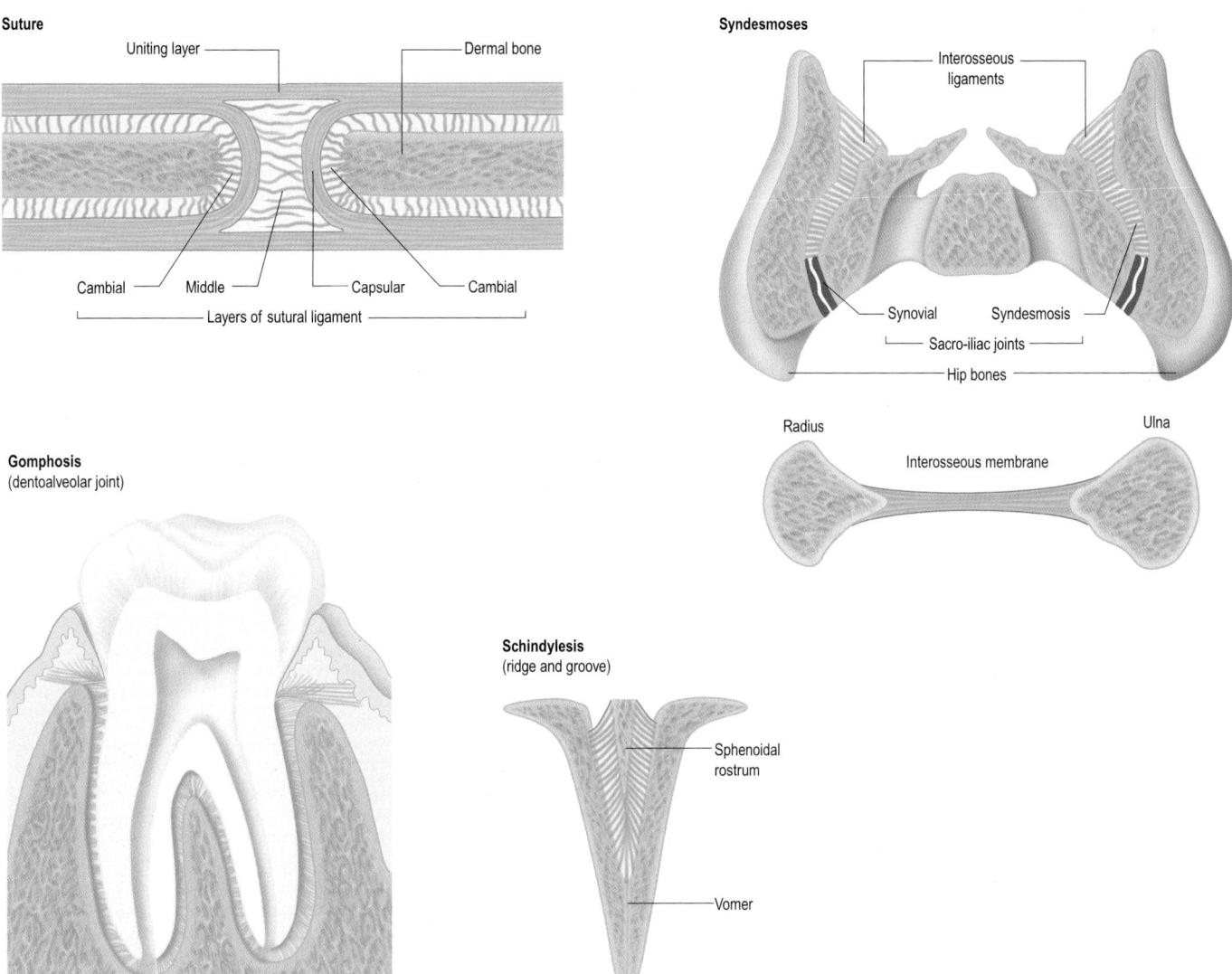

Fig. 6.33 Examples of the principal varieties of fibrous joints, each shown in section. Note that schindyleses are not regarded by some as sufficiently distinct from sutures to merit classification into a separate group. Syndesmoses are difficult to define because of the large numbers and great variety of fibrous interosseous structures. The official (internationally) recognized list has changed several times over the years: the massive sacroiliac ligament illustrated is not yet in the list.

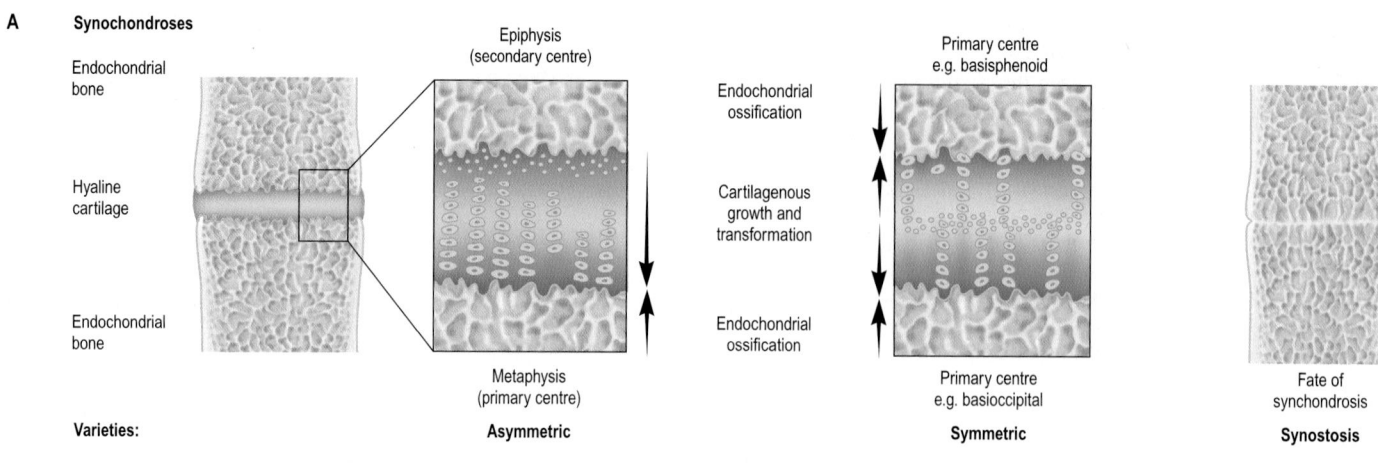

A **Synochondroses**

Endochondrial bone

Hyaline cartilage

Endochondrial bone

Epiphysis (secondary centre)

Metaphysis (primary centre)

Endochondral ossification

Cartilagenous growth and transformation

Endochondral ossification

Primary centre e.g. basisphenoid

Primary centre e.g. basioccipital

Fate of synchondrosis

Varieties: **Asymmetric**   **Symmetric**   **Synostosis**

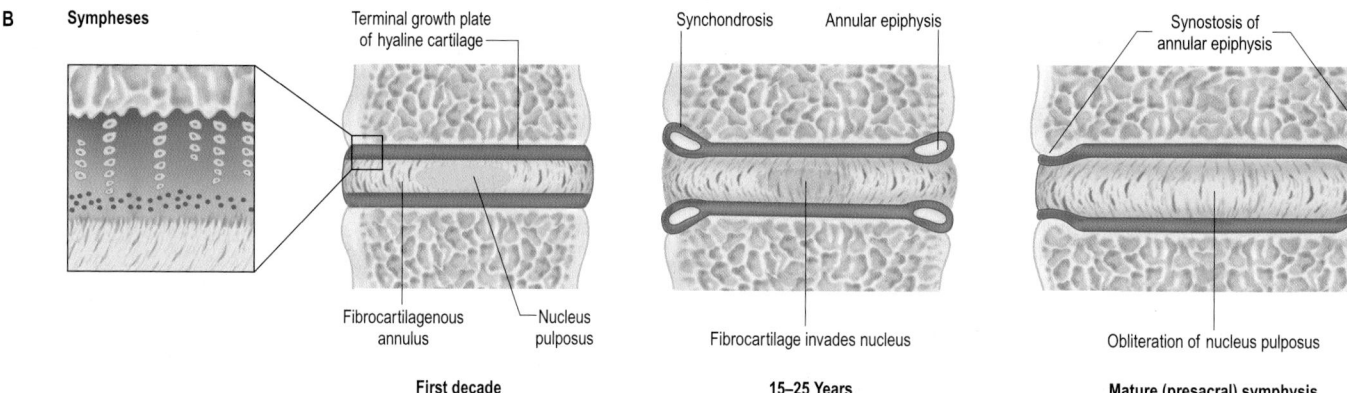

B **Sympheses**

Terminal growth plate of hyaline cartilage

Fibrocartilagenous annulus

Nucleus pulposus

First decade

Synchondrosis   Annular epiphysis

Fibrocartilage invades nucleus

15–25 Years

Synostosis of annular epiphysis

Obliteration of nucleus pulposus

Mature (presacral) symphysis

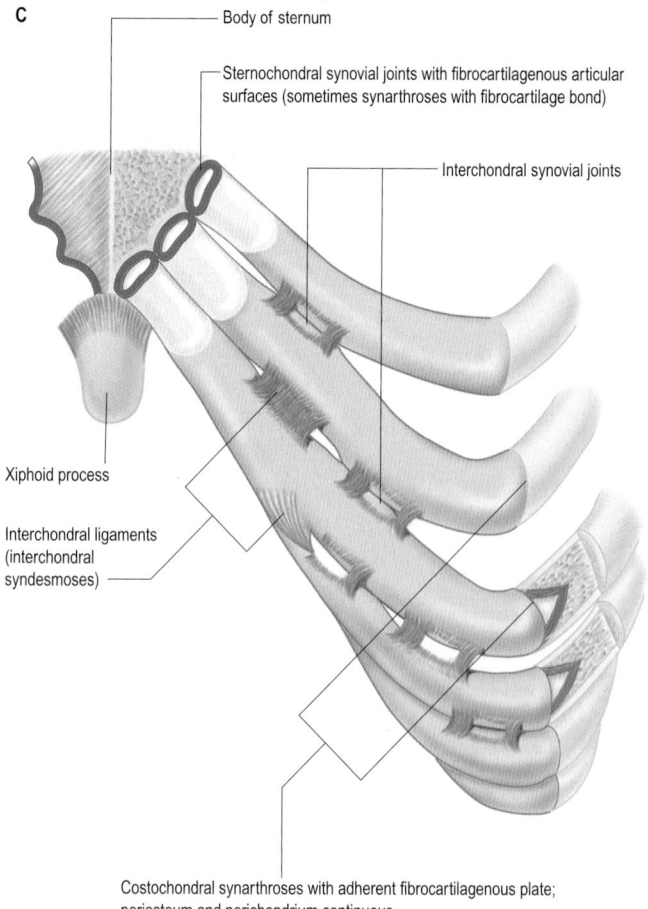

C

Body of sternum

Sternochondral synovial joints with fibrocartilagenous articular surfaces (sometimes synarthroses with fibrocartilage bond)

Interchondral synovial joints

Xiphoid process

Interchondral ligaments (interchondral syndesmoses)

Costochondral synarthroses with adherent fibrocartilagenous plate; periosteum and perichondrium continuous

General periosteum and perichondrium omitted

Fig. 6.34 Examples of varieties of cartilaginous joints. **A,** Sectional view of the principal tissues involved, more detailed architecture and main growth patterns of symmetrical and asymmetrical synchondroses. Lesser degrees of asymmetry occur in some locations. Synostosis is the normal fate of almost all synchondroses when endochondral growth has ceased. **B,** Intervertebral symphyses (presacral), shown in section, displaying age-related changes. Partial or complete synostosis is the normal fate of sacral and coccygeal symphyses. **C,** Less common interchondral and osseochondral junctions: see text for other locations.

fibrous periosteum adherent to the bones crosses the interval between them, uniting the external and internal layers which enclose the sutural ligament and adding to its strength. During active growth the orientation of collagen fibres within sutural membranes responds to several factors, particularly to the direction of growth of minute bone spicules.

When cranial growth ends, including growth at sutures, osteogenic cells usually complete the ossification of sutural ligaments, which ultimately leads to their obliteration and rigid synostosis. This is a slow process, and does not begin until the late twenties. However, it is clearly necessary that sutures should cease to be slightly flexible joints as soon as possible after birth. Sutural ligaments may create an almost immovable bond between large areas of bone, especially where they show reciprocally adapted irregularities, even when these are very fine, e.g. the intermaxillary junction. This immobility cannot be produced at narrow edges of bones in the cranial vault, and here bony margins develop spikes and recesses which interlock so well that the bones are difficult to separate even when stripped of all fibrous connective tissue. Where the edges are saw-like, e.g. the sagittal suture, the junction is a serrate suture. A denticulate suture, e.g. much of the lambdoid suture, has small tooth-like projections, often widening towards their ends to provide even more effective interlocking. When united by sutural ligament and periosteum, these sutures are almost completely immobile. Where bones overlap, as at the temporoparietal suture, a squamous suture is formed; the adjacent bone surfaces are reciprocally bevelled and, if mutually ridged or serrated, the junction is sometimes termed a limbous suture. Simple apposition of contiguous surfaces, usually rough and reciprocally irregular, is inappropriately named a plane suture, e.g. the sutures between the palatine bones; between the maxillae; and at the palatomaxillary sutures. Although surface demarcations between such bones show none of the interlocking which is evident at serrate or denticulate sutures, their irregular surfaces of contact are united by wide expanses of sutural ligament and provide considerable resistance to shearing or torsion: like other sutures they are, for all practical purposes, immovable.

Schindylesis – A schindylesis is a specialized suture where a ridged bone fits into a groove on a neighbouring element, e.g. the cleft between the alae of the vomer, which receives the rostrum of the sphenoid.

GOMPHOSIS

A gomphosis is a peg-and-socket joint and is restricted to the fixation of teeth in their alveolar sockets in the mandible and maxillae. The collagen of the periodontium connects dental cement with alveolar bone.

SYNDESMOSIS

A syndesmosis is a fibrous articulation in which bony surfaces are bound together by an interosseous ligament, a slender fibrous cord or an aponeurotic membrane, which usually allows slight, but occasionally more extensive, movement between them. The term was at one time restricted to the inferior tibiofibular joint alone. However, interosseous fibrous connections occur frequently and in a variety of forms. Though not usually so described, the dorsal part of the sacroiliac junction, through its massive interosseous sacroiliac ligaments, is a syndesmosis (**Figs 6.33, 6.34**). The sacroiliac joints proper, primarily synovial, are also often invaded by fibrous tissue late in life and may become entirely fibrous articulations, differing little from syndesmoses. The inferior tibiofibular joint, long accepted as a typical syndesmosis, could alternatively be considered little more than an interosseous ligament adjacent to the ankle joint, or to a synovial extension of the joint when this exists, as it occasionally does in man and regularly in other primates. The term syndesmosis could then be extended to many other interosseous ligaments, e.g. the carpus and tarsus, and also include the interosseous membranes of the forearm and calf, especially since these are already described as intermediate joints in the radio-ulnar and tibiofibular series. Since ligaments are almost all interosseous, it becomes difficult to restrict use of the term syndesmosis, unless only very short extrinsic ligaments close to a synovial joint are so designated. Intrinsic and intracapsular ligaments of synovial joints are, of course, excluded.

Cartilaginous joints

Cartilaginous joints are themselves classified into synchondroses (primary cartilaginous joints) and symphyses (secondary cartilaginous joints) (**Figs 6.33, 6.34**). When fully formed, each group shares common features and also has distinctive structural and functional features. The terms primary and secondary are only useful in the instances of certain symphyses which, developmentally, are preceded by synchondroses within which further differentiation occurs.

In most instances the distinction between fibrous and cartilaginous joints is clear, but at a number of sites, where a predominantly fibrous articulation contains occasional islands of cartilage or conversely a predominantly cartilaginous articulation contains aligned dense bundles of collagen, some admixture occurs.

SYNCHONDROSES

Synchondroses occur where originally separate, but adjacent, centres of ossification appear within a continuous mass of hyaline cartilage. As ossification spreads it invades the actively growing zone of cartilage which occupies the interval between the contiguous osseous surfaces. A synchondrosis therefore consists of two ossifying fronts closely bonded by a specialized hyaline growth cartilage which contains successive recognizable zones. Passing towards an ossifying surface there are zones of relative quiescence, proliferation and interstitial growth, transformation into columns (with cell hypertrophy), matrix calcification and cell death, ossification (involving chondrolysis, vascularization and

osteogenesis). Where the rate of ossification of both surfaces forming a synchondrosis is approximately equal (e.g. in the cranial base), the growth cartilage has a central quiescent zone equidistant from the surfaces, and the zones proceed symmetrically towards both surfaces. Where the growth rates are unequal, the growth cartilage structure is correspondingly asymmetrical. Extreme examples are synchondroses between the diaphysis and terminal epiphyses of long bones, where growth and progressive ossification are mainly (but not exclusively) diaphyseal. In the latter, the quiescent zone lies near the epiphyseal bone, and the ossification zone extends towards the diaphysis. The cartilaginous growth plate grows in girth by interstitial and subperichondral appositional mechanisms: activity varies at different radial distances from its centre. In this way the overall shape of the cartilage and its associated bones are changed, sometimes profoundly. Thus, the early epiphysis of the femoral head is separated from the femoral neck, which is an extension of the diaphysis, by a relatively simple horizontal plate of growth cartilage. With differential growth, the capitular tip of the neck becomes increasingly conical, and is tightly bound to a conical growth cartilage which fits into a deep conical recess in the inferolateral part of the otherwise spheroidal ossifying femoral head.

Functionally, synchondroses are primarily growth mechanisms. Although they contribute slightly to the more flexible skeleton of youth, their growth potential is combined with the ability to successfully resist forces, whether of compression, tension, shear or torsion. Thus they permit growth to continue, while free, but controlled and often powerful, movements can be executed at neighbouring synovial joints, or more restricted movements can occur at symphyses and some fibrous joints. With the exception of the clavicle and areas of subperiosteal bone accretion, all postcranial centres of ossification are endochondral. Synchondroses are present in all postcranial bones derived from two or more centres, i.e. the majority of postcranial bones. However, the carpal, and most tarsal, bones each develops from a single endochondral centre; as their ossifying surfaces advance, they invade a complete encasement of growing cartilage, parts of which persist as the specialized articular surfaces of the synovial carpal and tarsal joints. Elsewhere, the bone approaches the perichondrium (now periosteum) providing attachment for fibrous joint capsules, tendon sheaths, interosseous ligaments, fascial septa and muscles. Clearly, these relatively small bones possess no synchondroses but their essential growth mechanisms have much in common with that of epiphyses.

Most postcranial synchondroses have not been given specific topographical names, but they can be classified into general morphological groups. They may be epiphysiodiaphyseal (or more precisely epimetaphyseal, or epicorporeal); intraepiphyseal, in compound epiphyses; multiplex, in compound bones with multiple primary centres. Some of the last group are named: the triradiate acetabular cartilage of the developing hip bone; sternales between growing sternebrae; manubriosternalis (juvenile only, before transformation to a symphysis); xiphiosternalis; vertebrales (confined to individual vertebrae); sacrales centrales (juvenile only, soon to be temporary symphyses); and laterales (between centra, neural arches and costal processes).

In fibrous epiphyseal (growth) plates, e.g. the proximal growth plate of the tibia, the almost flat condylar parts are crossed by regularly aligned horizontal bundles of collagen which lie at right angles to the long axis of the bone, and suffer lateral compression during weight bearing. Where the epiphysis descends anteriorly to form the tibial tuberosity it is subjected to shearing stress caused by the oblique pull of quadriceps femoris, and the growth plate cartilage is almost completely replaced by oblique dense collagen. The fates of both postcranial and cranial synchondroses are considered below, together with some unclassified or inappropriately classified junctions involving cartilage.

Cranial synchondroses occur between neighbouring endochondral centres of ossification which develop in the chondrocranium. Some regions of the chondrocranium remain unossified. These are the lateral, alar and septal nasal cartilages and remnants which occupy and lie near the foramen lacerum. In contrast, the largely endochondral auditory ossicles articulate via specialized synovial joints, while the malleus and stapes are connected to the temporal bone by equally specialized fibrous arrangements, the fibrous stratum of the tympanic membrane and the anular ligament respectively. The endochondral centres of ossification are: inferior nasal concha (single); ethmoid (three); sphenoid (multiple pre- and postsphenoidal centres for the body, conchae, lesser wings and roots of greater wings); temporal (multiple centres for each petromastoid part and styloid process); and occipital (multiple centres for basilar, condylar and squamous parts up to the superior nuchal lines). The sites of basicranial synchondroses are numerous, some are within individual bones, others between them, and all contribute to some extent to basicranial growth. Those which persist for limited periods and coalesce early are unnamed, while those that make substantial contributions to growth are named. Omitting the prefix synchondrosis, these are: sphenoethmoidalis, spheno-occipitalis, sphenopetrosa, petro-occipitalis, intraoccipitalis anterior and intraoccipitalis posterior.

Although they are not officially named, presumably because of their relatively early fusion, it seems appropriate to include the main intrinsic synchondroses of the sphenoid. These occur in the midline between the pre- and postsphenoidal parts of the body, and bilaterally, separating the body from the conjoined greater wings and pterygoid processes. The cranial synchondroses are approximately symmetrical in structure and their zones of growth and differentiation pass from the centre towards both ossifying surfaces.

When growth between parts of a bone or between individual bones joined by a synchondrosis nears completion, classic cartilaginous growth, transformation and endochondral ossification ceases. For a period the cartilaginous plate is relatively quiescent, but it becomes irregularly thinned. Complex histological changes then follow which involve the cartilage from both osseous surfaces. The synchondrosis is ultimately entirely replaced by complete bony union between the originally separate osseous surfaces, forming a synostosis. It therefore loses its cartilaginous growth potential and mechanical properties, but acquires the maximal rigidity of bone. This enhances the effectiveness of postcranial bones in resisting a variety of powerful stresses, either in almost static postures, or during movement patterns which involve synovial and (to more limited degrees) median symphyseal or fibrous joints. Rigidity of the neurocranium, both during and after completion of growth, is functionally essential: it provides protective support and encasement of the brain and special sense organs, and of the associated vascular and ventricular systems.

ATYPICAL CARTILAGINOUS JOINTS

A number of junctions have many features of joints but do not fit within the general classification of joints. They occur where substantial masses of cartilage either remain unossified in normal development, or develop irregular patches of calcification in later decades. These junctions may be between bone (either endochondral or intramembranous) and cartilage; between two adjacent cartilages; or a cartilage may join with a fibrous suture or a synchondrosis. The junctions are similar to either fibrous joints or to synovial joints. The nasal, laryngeal and costal cartilages, and those of the auditory tube and auricle (pinna), come into this category. Fibrous junctions occur between the borders of contiguous nasal cartilages. The septal cartilage is, in part, continuous with the lateral nasal cartilage, but elsewhere fibrous bonds extend to the internasal suture, perpendicular plate of the ethmoid, the vomer, the nasal crest (and intermaxillary suture) and anterior nasal spine of the maxillae, and the septal process of the lateral nasal cartilage. At these junctions perichondria fuse or perichondrium and periosteum (and in some sites sutural ligament) blend.

A fibrous junction joins the perichondrium of the elastic auricular fibrocartilage and the periosteum of the roughened outer rim of the external acoustic meatus. A similar fibrous union suspends the perichondrium of the superior curved border of the cartilage of the auditory tube and the inferior perichondrium of the sphenopetrosal synchondrosis (this becomes periosteum after synostosis, the upper attachment spreading on to the petrous quadrate area). The larynx and hyoid bone are further examples of specialized and uncommon varieties of connection and junction. Most extensively, the laryngeal cartilages are connected to each other, and the thyroid and epiglottic cartilages to the hyoid bone, by three-dimensional complexes of fibroelastic membranes and their ligamentous thickenings. These interchondral and osseochondral structures are not officially listed as syndesmoses, but they may be regarded as such. In addition, the cricoid cartilage bears four discrete articular surfaces, one bilateral pair on the sloping superior border of its lamina, and a lateral pair at the junction of each lamina and arch. These articulate with the articular surface on the base of each arytenoid cartilage, and with the medial aspects of the tips of the inferior cornua of the thyroid cartilage respectively. The cricoarytenoid and cricothyroid articulations to which these surfaces contribute are interchondral synovial joints.

The costal cartilages are often considered as unossified cartilaginous extensions of the ribs: the first to seventh reach the sternum, the eighth to tenth reach the cartilage above, and the eleventh and twelfth are short blunt cones with free intermuscular tips. The cartilages are, however, traditionally described as separate topographical entities and, depending on its level, each engages in from one to five different types of junction. The costochondral junctions are unusual joints in which the convex tip of the cartilage is received by a complementary recess in the tip of the rib; the perichondrium and periosteum are continuous, as are the collagenous elements of bone and cartilage. The sternochondral joints (often called sternocostal joints) vary; the second to seventh are often synovial, with fibrocartilaginous articular surfaces on both chondral and sternal aspects. Quite frequently, synovial cavities are absent in some or all these joints, in which case a thin dense lamina of tightly adherent fibrocartilage is interposed between cartilage and bone, forming an unclassified variety of joint. This type of junction is usually present at the manubrial end of the first costal cartilage. It should be noted that it is commonplace for the whole first costal cartilage and attached rib and sternum, or the manubriochondral junction alone, to be incorrectly classified as a synchondrosis. The fifth to ninth costal cartilages carry a variable number of simple interchondral synovial joints, as well as irregular syndesmoses in the form of short interchondral ligaments between their borders or apices (particularly cartilages eight to ten), which anchor their tips to the border of the cartilage above.

SYMPHYSIS

Topographically, all symphyses are median and, with one exception, are confined to the axial skeleton. They include the following named joints: manubriosternalis, between manubrium and sternal body; intervertebralis between successive vertebral bodies (these are regionally grouped into cervical, thoracic, lumbar, sacral and coccygeal); symphysis menti between the bilateral halves of the fetal mandible (which continues only into the first postnatal year, when synostosis supervenes); symphysis pubis between the medial surfaces of the bodies of the pubes. Histologically, the mental junction is unlike other symphyses, however the use of its name is so widespread that retention seems inevitable.

The surface areas of the articulating endochondral bones are usually well defined, and vary from a few millimetres to over a centimetre apart, bound together by strong, tightly adherent, solid connective tissues. Each bony surface is firmly attached to a thin layer of hyaline cartilage, which in turn blends with the surface of a thick, strong, but deformable pad (or disc) of fibrocartilage. Collagenous ligaments extend from the periostea across the symphysis and blend with the hyaline and fibrocartilaginous perichondria. They do not form a complete capsule (as in synovial joints), but are similar in containing plexuses of afferent nerve terminals, which also penetrate the periphery of the fibrocartilage. The combined strength of the ligaments and of the hyaline and fibrocartilage exceeds that of the associated bones, and so they can easily withstand a range of stresses (compression, tension, shear and torsion). Tears are usually the result of sudden, massive unexpected stresses occurring with the body in an inappropriate posture. The architecture of the fibrocartilaginous tissues is such that it combines strength with limited degrees of elastic deformability, thus allowing a restricted but appreciable range of movement which characterizes symphyses. Fibrocartilaginous disc compression narrows the interosseous interval, while tension increases it; when these occur simultaneously in opposite sectors of a disc it becomes cuneiform (wedge-shaped) and the attached bones become relatively inclined (angulated).

Torsional stresses increase or decrease the spiralization of collagenous fibres within the disc and permit slight relative rotation. The range of movement possible at a symphysis is not great, since it is primarily determined by its intrinsic anatomy. It is further limited by the additional articulations and ligaments which involve the bones, but which are extrasymphyseal, e.g. the numerous syndesmoses and synovial zygapophyseal joints between adjacent vertebrae; articulations of the clavicles and costal cartilages with the sternum; the sacroiliac joints and the interosseous sacroiliac, sacrotuberous and sacrospinous ligaments. All these features profoundly affect movement patterns at their related symphyses.

Solid specialized connective tissues, typical of synarthroses, characterize the thoracolumbar and sacrococcygeal series of intervertebral symphyses. However, significant proportions of the remainder develop a single central or a bilateral pair of narrow fluid-filled clefts in (or near) their fibrocartilaginous pads. Over 30% of manubriosternal symphyses develop a central horizontal elongate cleft and over 50% of interpubic discs develop a median elongated cleft in the oblique long axis of the disc. The second to sixth (occasionally seventh) cervical intervertebral discs develop laterally placed small fluid-filled cavities in the fibrous tissue between the bevelled inferolateral edge of the vertebral body above and the superolateral lip of the vertebral body below. Some regard these cavities as being in the peripheral parts of the discs and non-synovial in character; others regard them as small synovial joints near, but external to, the discs. The synovial or non-synovial nature of all the above clefts remains controversial; they perhaps reflect a stage in the evolution of synovial joints. Distinct possibilities seem to be translations at the cervical cavities during spinal movements and translation with distraction at the interpubic cleft, particularly during the later stages of pregnancy.

The statement that synchondroses are temporary and concerned with growth, whereas symphyses are permanent and concerned with movement, is an oversimplification and only partly correct: there are notable exceptions. Both types of joint are concerned with strength and the ability to withstand and transmit considerable stresses and also with growth. In contrasting ways, both contribute either directly or indirectly to the total movement patterns of the parts involved. The strength and mechanical properties of cartilaginous joints need little further comment, except to re-emphasize that the rigidity of synchondroses increases the efficiency of positive movements at related syndesmoses, symphyses and particularly synovial joints. It must be remembered that the movements at symphyses are not a simple extrapolation of the mechanical properties of a fibrocartilaginous pad or disc. For example, movement of a vertebra relative to its neighbour is a three-dimensional summation of the properties of all its intervertebral joints (syndesmoses and synovial joints, in addition to the complex symphysis) acting in concert, each with its particular array of stresses. During their growth phases, the mechanical properties of the intravertebral synchondroses are also significant.

The cervical, thoracic, lumbar and lumbosacral intervertebral symphyses, the pubic symphysis and c.90% of manubriosternal symphyses are normally permanent, but exhibit age-related changes. In contrast, the joints between successive sacral bodies, between sacrum and coccyx and between coccygeal segments, after preliminary stages, form well-developed symphyses; however, their normal fate is partial or complete synostosis. The process is slow and lengthy. After 30 years of age c.10% of manubriosternal symphyses develop partial or complete synostosis; it is a slow and lengthy change.

The prominent role of synchondroses in skeletal growth is widely recognized, whereas growth of symphyses has received less attention.

Symphyseal growth may, for convenience, be considered from two interrelated aspects, namely intrinsic growth of the fibrocartilaginous disc, and growth of the hyaline cartilaginous plates into which endochondral ossification progresses and later 'anular' epiphyses form. At the manubriosternal symphysis, the limiting plates of proliferative hyaline cartilage are progressively invaded by the ossifying fronts of the manubrium and first sternebra, and normally no epiphyses are formed. However, at the pubic symphysis, the growth plates of hyaline cartilage which are involved with endochondral ossification on the symphyseal aspects of the bodies of the pubes after puberty commonly develop scale-like epiphyses, usually anterosuperiorly. The occurrence of intervertebral and pubic epiphyses complicates the traditional description of symphyses. At these latter sites the epiphyses appear at, or soon after, puberty, and continue slow growth for about a decade before synostosis with the main bone. During this period the epiphysis is completely encased by proliferative hyaline cartilage, its interosseous lamina is a narrow (epiphysiocorporeal) synchondrosis, and its symphyseal lamina a simple extension of the terminal plate of hyaline growth cartilage. The latter is originally derived from the early embryonic cartilaginous vertebral model.

These growth plates are the proliferative source of cartilage into which all endochondral ossification of the vertebral bodies occurs cranially and caudally, constituting c.80% of the length of the mature vertebral column. The remaining 20% is provided by growth of the fibrocartilaginous discs. Where the fibrocartilage blends with the lamina of hyaline cartilage, some bundles of collagen pass without interruption from the fibrocartilage to interlace within the matrix of the hyaline cartilage.

Both clinically and radiologically the term intervertebral symphysis is seldom used. Instead it is called an intervertebral disc, or simply a disc. Radiologically the disc space is often used to indicate all tissues between the vertebral bodies. Formally, the fibrocartilaginous intervertebral disc is regarded as part of a symphysis, and is completed by paired laminae of terminal growth cartilages and their associated ossifying or mature osseous surfaces.

Synovial joints

Synovial articulations operate differently from non-synovial fibrous and cartilaginous joints (**Figs 6.35, 6.36**). Although the bones involved are linked by a fibrous capsule which usually has intrinsic ligamentous thickenings, and often by internal or external accessory ligaments, the osseous surfaces concerned are not in continuity. They are covered by articular cartilage of varying thickness and precise topology, and contact is strictly limited between these cartilaginous surfaces, which have a

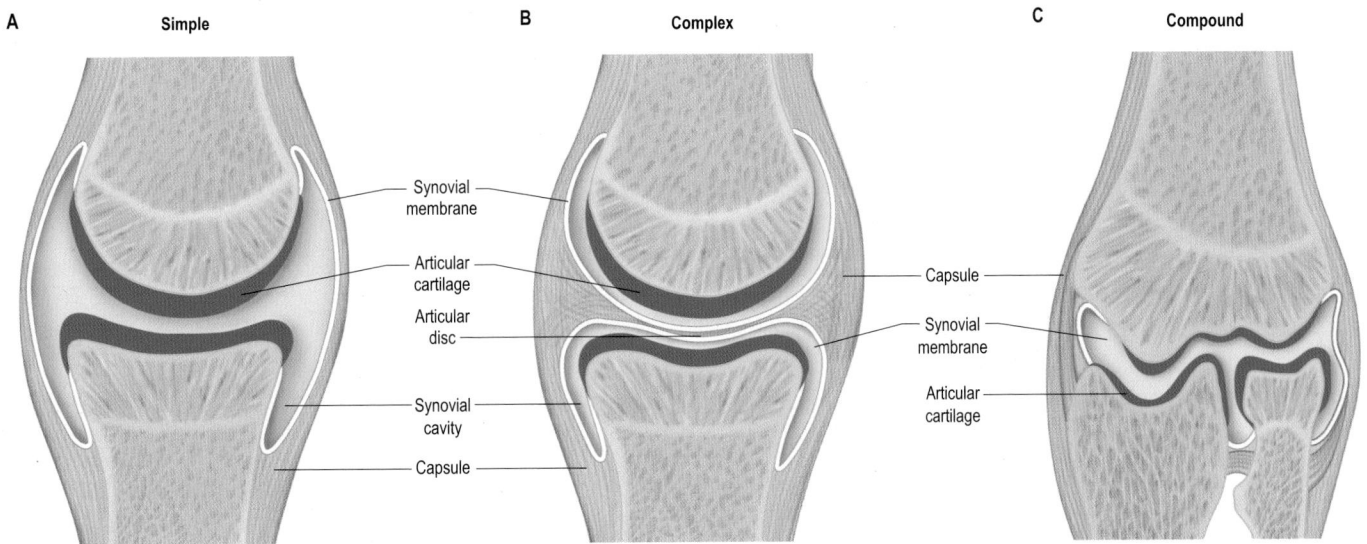

Fig. 6.35 Synovial joints, some main structural features and one elementary type of classification: **A**, simple; **B**, complex; **C**, compound joints. For clarity, the articular surfaces are artificially separated. A and B are purely diagrammatic and not related to particular joints. C, however, is a simplified representation of some features of an elbow joint but the complicated contours due to the olecranon, coronoid and radial fossae and profiles of articular fat pads present in a true section have been omitted.

very low coefficient of friction. Sliding contact is facilitated by viscous synovial fluid (synovia), which acts like a lubricant in some respects, but is also concerned with maintenance of living cells in the articular cartilages.

ARTICULAR SURFACES

Articular surfaces are mostly formed by a special variety of hyaline cartilage, reflecting their preformation as parts of cartilaginous models in embryonic life. Exceptionally, surfaces of the sternoclavicular and acromioclavicular joints and both temporomandibular surfaces are covered by dense fibrous tissue which contains isolated groups of chondrocytes and little surrounding matrix – a legacy of their formation by intramembranous ossification. Articular cartilage has a wear-resistant, low-frictional, lubricated surface, which is slightly compressible and elastic and is thus ideally constructed for easy movement over a similar surface. It is also able to absorb large forces of compression and shear generated by gravity and muscular power.

The thickness of articular cartilage is said to range from 1 to 2 mm, but this is more typical of small bones in aged individuals; in youth it may reach 5–7 mm in larger joints. Young cartilages are typically white, smooth, glistening and compressible, whereas ageing cartilages are thinner, less cellular, firmer and more brittle, with a less regular surface and a yellowish opacity.

Articular cartilages are moulded to bone, and variations in thickness often accentuate subjacent osseous surface shape. Typically, convex surfaces are thickest centrally, thinning peripherally, and concave surfaces are the reverse. The precise configuration, degree of congruence in various positions and the dispositions of the surrounding capsule and ligaments are all related to the types and ranges of movement permitted at a joint.

Articular cartilage has no nerves or blood vessels (except occasional vascular loops which reach and even penetrate the calcified zone from the osseous side). Nutrition is considered to depend on a peripheral vascular plexus in the synovial membrane (circulus vasculosus articuli) and synovial fluid and blood vessels in adjacent marrow spaces: the relative importance of these contributions is uncertain.

The zone of articular cartilage next to the joint cavity is mainly a layer of collagen fibres arranged in various planes with small, oval chondrocytes lying in the matrix deep to it. Transmission electron microscopy of heavy metal stained preparations shows an interrupted electron-dense surface coat of a particulate or filamentous material, generally 0.03–0.1 µm thick, covering the cartilage, and occasionally separated from it by an intervening layer of proteoglycan particles and associated filaments. Synovial fluid and lipidic debris, the product of chondrocytic necrosis, may contribute to a surface coat which is ephemeral in nature; the stable, permanent, articular surface is bounded by the most superficial collagen fibres. The 'lamina splendens' which appears as a bright line at the free surface of articular cartilage when oblique sections are examined by negative phase contrast microscopy, is an artefact arising at the border between regions of different refractive index and cannot be taken as evidence for an anatomically distinct surface layer.

With advancing age, undulations of articular surfaces deepen and develop minute, ragged projections perhaps due to wear and tear. Erosion occurs in pathologically 'dry' joints and where synovial viscosity is altered; but in healthy joints changes are extremely slow. Replacement

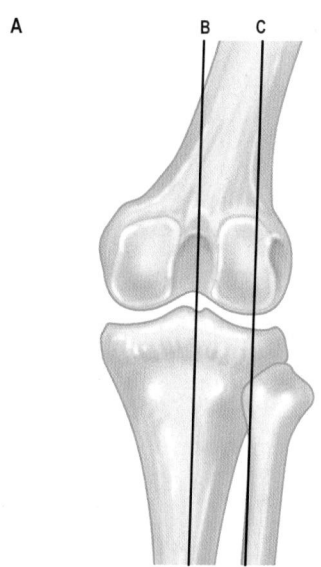

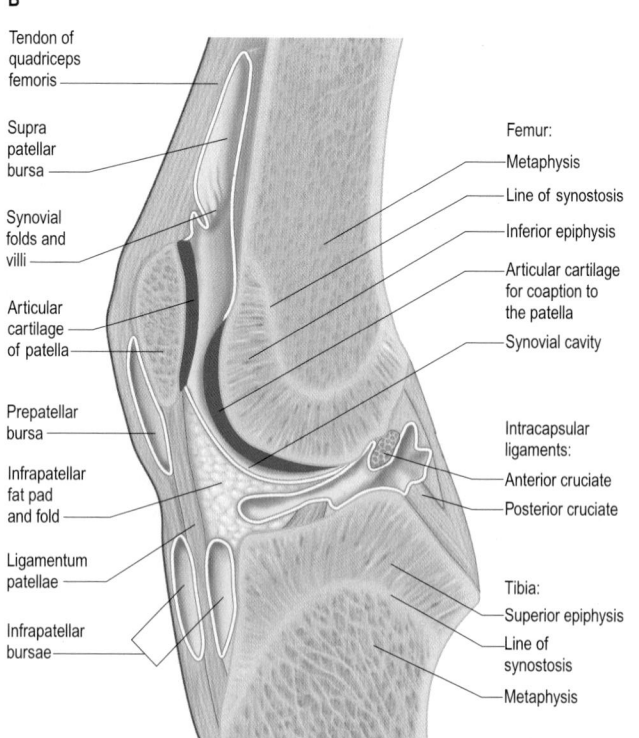

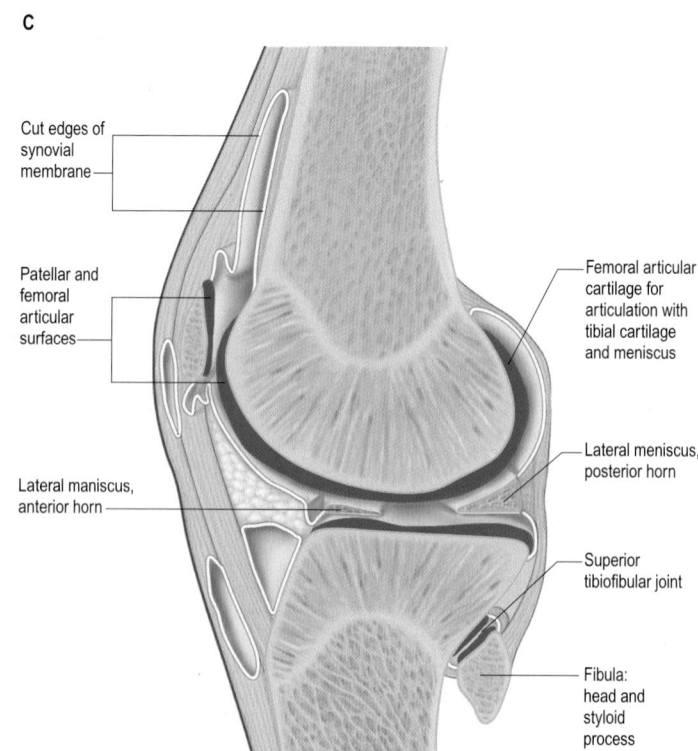

Fig. 6.36 Principal structural features of the left knee joint, which is synovial and both compound and complex. **A,** The posterior aspect showing the planes of parasagittal section **B** and **C**. The synovial cavity and bursae are, for clarity, shown as slightly distended: the articular surfaces of the patella, femur and tibia and the meniscal surfaces are thus artificially separated.

of an eroded surface by proliferation of deeper layers is uncertain: mitoses are absent from adult articular cartilage.

Ultrastructural observations have revealed a highly complex, three-dimensional reticulum of interconnected fibrils in articular cartilage, with obvious functional implications.

FIBROUS CAPSULE

A fibrous capsule completely encloses a joint except where it is interrupted by synovial protrusions; the exceptions are described with the individual joints. The capsule is composed of parallel but interlacing bundles of white collagen fibres which form a cuff whose ends are attached continuously round the articular ends of the bones concerned. In small bones this attachment is usually near the peripheries of the articular surfaces, but it varies considerably in long bones, where part or all of the attachment may be a significant distance from the articular surface. The capsule is perforated by vessels and nerves and may have apertures through which synovial membrane protrudes as bursae. The capsule is lined by synovial membrane, which also covers all non-articular surfaces including non-articular osseous surfaces, tendons and ligaments partly or wholly within the fibrous capsule, as at the shoulder and knee. Where a tendon is attached inside a joint and issues from it, a prolongation of synovial membrane usually accompanies it beyond the capsule. Some extracapsular tendons are separated from the capsule by a synovial bursa continuous with the interior of the joint. Such protrusions are potential avenues for the spread of infection into joints.

The capsule usually exhibits local thickenings of parallel fibre bundles; these capsular (intrinsic) ligaments are named by their attachments. Some capsules are reinforced or replaced by tendons of nearby muscles or expansions from them. Accessory ligaments are separate from capsules and may be extracapsular or intracapsular in position.

All ligaments, although yielding little to tension, are pliant and do not resist normal actions, being designed to check excessive or abnormal movements. Ligaments are taut at the normal limit of a particular movement. However, they are slightly elastic and protected from excessive tension by reflex contraction of appropriate muscles.

SYNOVIAL MEMBRANE (Fig. 6.37)

Synovial membrane is derived from embryonic mesenchyme. It covers all non-articular regions where movement occurs between apposed surfaces, lubricated by a fluid which is secreted and absorbed by the membrane. In joints it therefore lines fibrous capsules and covers exposed osseous surfaces, intracapsular ligaments, bursae and tendon sheaths. It is absent from intra-articular discs or menisci and stops

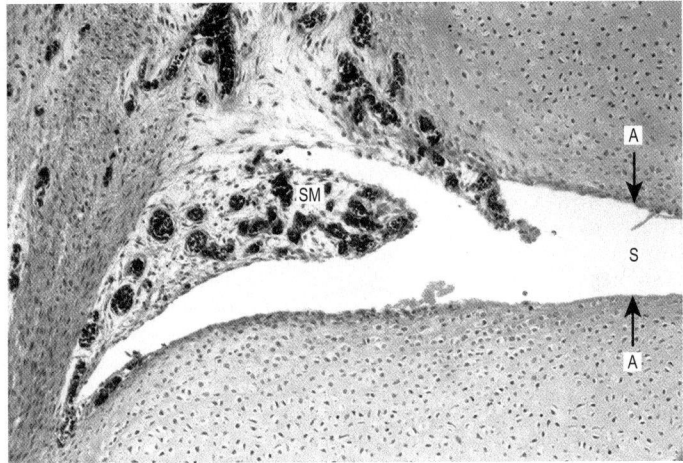

Fig. 6.37 A section of a synovial joint and its associated highly vascular (red) synovial membrane in a fetal hand. The two articular cartilage surfaces (A, arrowed) are separated on the right by a layer of synovial fluid (S) secreted by the synovial membrane (SM) which extends a short distance into the joint space from the capsule (left). (Photograph by Sarah-Jane Smith.)

at the margins of articular cartilages, the peripheral few millimetres of which are a structural transitional zone between synovial membrane and articular cartilage.

Pink, smooth and shining, the internal synovial surface displays a few small synovial villi which increase in size and number with age. Elsewhere, folds and fringes may project into a joint cavity: some are sufficiently constant to be named, e.g. the alar folds and ligamentum mucosum of the knee. Accumulations of adipose tissue (articular fat pads) occur in the synovial membrane in many joints. These pads, folds and fringes are flexible, elastic and deformable cushions occupying the potential spaces and irregularities in joints which are not wholly filled by synovial fluid; during movement they accommodate to the changing shape and volume of the irregularities. They increase synovial area and may promote the distribution of lubricant over articular surfaces (cf. intra-articular discs and menisci). Synovial villi are normally few, but they are more numerous where the membrane rests on areolar tissue near articular margins and on the surfaces of folds and fringes. They increase with age and become prominent in some pathological states.

Synovial membrane consists of a cellular intima resting on a fibrovascular subintimal layer (subsynovial tissue). The latter is often composed of loose, irregular connective tissue, but may contain organized lamellae of collagen and elastin fibres lying parallel to the membrane surface, interspersed with occasional fibroblasts, macrophages, mast cells and fat cells. The elastic component may prevent redundant fold formation during joint movement (folds might otherwise become compressed between articular surfaces). Subintimal adipose cells form compact lobules surrounded by very vascular fibroelastic interlobular septa, which provide firmness, deformability and elastic recoil. The subintima merges with the synovial membrane where it covers the adjacent capsule, intracapsular ligament or tendon.

The synovial intima consists of pleomorphic synovial cells embedded in a granular, amorphous, fibre-free intercellular matrix. There is considerable regional variation in cell morphology and numbers, which is apparently dependent upon the underlying subintimal tissue. The synovial cells of normal human joints form an interlacing, discontinuous layer, one to three cells and 20–40 μm deep, between the subintima and the joint cavity. They are not separated from the subintima by a basal lamina, and are distinguished from the subintimal cells only because they associate to form a superficial layer. In many locations, but particularly over loose subintimal tissue, areas free from synovial cells are commonly found. Over fibrous subintimal tissue the synovial cells may be flattened and closely packed, forming endothelioid sheets. Neighbouring cells are often separated by distinct gaps but their processes may interdigitate where they lie more closely.

Human synovial cells are generally elliptical, with numerous cytoplasmic processes but they can vary considerably in form. There are at least two morphologically distinct populations, type A and type B. Type A synovial cells are macrophage-like cells characterized by surface ruffles or lamellipodia, plasma membrane invaginations and associated pinocytotic vesicles, and a prominent Golgi apparatus but little rough endoplasmic reticulum. Type B synovial cells, which predominate, resemble fibroblasts, have abundant rough endoplasmic reticulum but contain fewer vacuoles and vesicles, and have a less ruffled plasma membrane.

The cells of the synovial intima synthesize some of the components of the synovial fluid, which can be considered as a specialized form of extracellular matrix. It is thought that some of the hyaluronan and glycoproteins of synovial fluid are synthesized by synovial type B cells, whereas the fluid component is a transudate from synovial capillaries. Type A synovial cells synthesize and release lytic enzymes and phagocytose joint debris: potential damage to joint tissues is limited by the secretion of enzyme inhibitors by type B synovial cells.

Synovial cells do not divide actively in normal synovial membranes. Their division rate increases dramatically in response to acute trauma and haemarthrosis. In such conditions the type B synovial cells divide in situ, while the type A cell population is increased by migration of bone marrow-derived precursors.

SYNOVIAL FLUID

Synovial fluid occupies synovial joints, bursae and tendon sheaths. In synovial joints it is clear or pale yellow, viscous, slightly alkaline at rest (the pH is reduced during activity), and contains a small mixed population of cells and metachromatic amorphous particles. Fluid volume is low: usually less than 0.5 ml can be aspirated even from a large joint such as the knee.

The composition of synovial fluid is consistent with it being mainly a dialysate of blood plasma. It contains protein (c.0.9 mg/100 ml) derived from blood, with the addition of hyaluronan, a sulphate-free GAG containing equimolar concentrations of glucuronic acid and N-acetylglucosamine. The viscoelastic and thixotropic (plastic) properties of synovial fluid are largely attributable to its hyaluronan content. Approximately 2% of synovial protein differs from plasma protein and is probably produced by synovial type B cells: c.0.5% of synovial fluid protein appears to consist of a specialized lubricating glycoprotein. The fluid contains a few cells (c.60 per ml in resting human joints) including monocytes, lymphocytes, macrophages, synovial intimal cells and polymorphonuclear leukocytes. Higher counts are found in young individuals. The amorphous metachromatic particles and fragments of cells and fibrous tissue found in synovial fluid are presumed to be produced by wear and tear.

INTRA-ARTICULAR MENISCI, DISCS AND FAT PADS

An articular disc or meniscus occurs between articular surfaces where congruity is low. It consists of fibrocartilage, where the fibrous element is usually predominant, and is not covered by synovial membrane. A disc may extend across a synovial joint, dividing it structurally and functionally into two synovial cavities. Discs are connected at their periphery to fibrous capsules, usually by vascularized connective tissue, so that they become invaded by vessels and afferent and motor (sympathetic) nerves; sometimes the union is closer and stronger, as in the knee and temporomandibular joints. Their main part contains few cells, but their surfaces may be covered by an incomplete stratum of flat cells, continuous at the periphery with adjacent synovial membrane.

Discs often have small perforations. The term meniscus should be reserved for incomplete discs, like those in the knee joint and occasionally the acromioclavicular joint. Complete discs occur in the sternoclavicular and inferior radio-ulnar joints; the disc in the temporo-mandibular joint may be complete or incomplete.

The function of intra-articular fibrocartilages is uncertain. Views advanced are deductions from structural or phylogenetic data, aided by mechanical analogies. The plethora of suggestions includes shock absorption, improvement of fit between surfaces, facilitation of combined movements, checking of translation at joints such as the knee, deployment of weight over larger surfaces, protection of articular margins, facilitation of rolling movements, and spread of lubricant. The temporomandibular disc has attracted particular attention because of its exceptional, perhaps unique, design and biomechanical properties.

A complete articular disc in effect creates two joints in series, comparable with concatenations of multiple joints, whose individual small ranges of movement nevertheless summate. This arrangement occurs in the carpus and tarsus.

The functions of labra and fat pads, two other quite common types of intra-articular structure, are also uncertain. A labrum is a fibrocartilaginous anular lip, usually triangular in cross-section like a meniscus, attached to an articular margin (e.g. the glenoid fossa and acetabulum) and so deepening the socket and increasing the area of contact. It may act as a lubricant spreader and, like menisci, may also reduce the synovial space to capillary dimensions, thus limiting drag. However, unlike menisci, labra are not compressed between articular surfaces. Small fibrous labra (connective tissue rims) have been described along the ventral or dorsal margins of the zygapophyseal joints at lumbar levels, as have meniscus-shaped fibroadipose meniscoids at the superior or inferior poles of the same joints. Fat pads are soft and change shape to fill joint recesses which vary in dimension according to joint position.

Neurovascular supply of joints

VASCULAR SUPPLY AND LYMPHATIC DRAINAGE

Joints receive blood from periarticular arterial plexuses whose numerous branches pierce the fibrous capsules to form subsynovial vascular plexuses. Some synovial vessels end near articular margins in an anastomotic fringe, the circulus articularis vasculosus. A lymphatic plexus in the synovial subintima drains along blood vessels to the regional deep lymph nodes.

INNERVATION

A movable joint is innervated by articular branches of the nerves which supply the muscles acting on the joint (Hilton's law). Although there is overlap between the territories of different nerves, each nerve innervates a specific part of the capsule. The region made taut by muscular contraction is usually innervated by nerves which supply the antagonists. For example, stretching the portion of the capsule of the hip joint supplied by the obturator nerve during abduction elicits reflex contraction of the adductors, usually sufficient to prevent damage. However, this is not the case at the shoulder, where the axillary nerve innervates the antero-inferior capsular region.

Myelinated axons in articular nerves innervate Ruffini endings, lamellated articular corpuscles and structures resembling the neuro-tendinous Golgi organs. Ruffini end organs respond to stretch and adapt slowly, whereas lamellated corpuscles respond to rapid movement and vibration and adapt rapidly; both types of receptor register the speed and direction of movement. Golgi end organs, innervated by the largest myelinated axons (10–15 µm diameter), are slow to adapt; they mediate position sense and are concerned in stereognosis, i.e. recognition of shape in held objects. Simple endings are numerous at the attachments of capsules and ligaments, and are thought to be the terminals of unmyelinated and thinly myelinated nociceptive axons.

Many unmyelinated postganglionic sympathetic axons terminate near vascular smooth muscle, and are probably vasomotor or vaso-sensory. There are no special end organs, or even simple endings, in synovial membrane, except near blood vessels. Synovial membrane is relatively insensitive to pain.

Classification and movements of synovial joints

The mechanical function of the synovial joints is to permit motion whilst carrying functional loads and remaining stable. Several criteria have been used to classify synovial joints and their movements. They include complexity and number of articulating surfaces, number and position of principal axes of movement, general geometry of surfaces and major movements, and association of more precise geometry with analysis of movements as bases for human kinesiology.

COMPLEXITY OF FORM

Most synovial joints have two surfaces and are simple articulations. In some, one surface is wholly convex and greater in area than its opposing concave surface, and occasionally, both surfaces are concavoconvex. A joint with more than two surfaces is compound, e.g. the elbow, where the humerus presents two distinct convexities and ulnar and radial concavities, and the radial convexity articulates with another ulnar concavity. In all compound joints articulating territories remain distinct. When a joint contains an intra-articular disc or meniscus it is complex.

DEGREES OF FREEDOM

Joint motion can be described by rotation and translation about three orthogonal axes, therefore there are three possible rotations (axial, abduction-adduction, flexion-extension) and three possible translations (proximo-distal, mediolateral, anteroposterior). Each is a degree of freedom. For most joints translations are negligible and do not need consideration (**Fig. 6.38**). A few joints have minor pure translatory movements, but all other joint motion is by rotation.

When movement is practically limited to rotation about one axis, e.g. the elbow, a joint is termed uniaxial: it has one degree of freedom. If independent movements can occur around two axes, e.g. as the knee (flexion–extension and axial rotation), it is biaxial, with two degrees of freedom. Since there are three axes for independent rotation, joints may have up to three degrees of freedom (**Fig. 6.38**). This apparently simple classification is complicated by the complexity of joint structure, and has consequent effects on motion. Even though a true 'ball and socket' joint can rotate about many chosen axes, i.e. it is multiaxial, for each position there is a maximum of three orthogonal planes, which means that it can have, as a maximum, three degrees of freedom.

For a uniaxial hinge joint with a single degree of freedom, a single unchanging axis of rotation would be predicted. However, because the shapes of joint surfaces are complex, there is a variable radius of

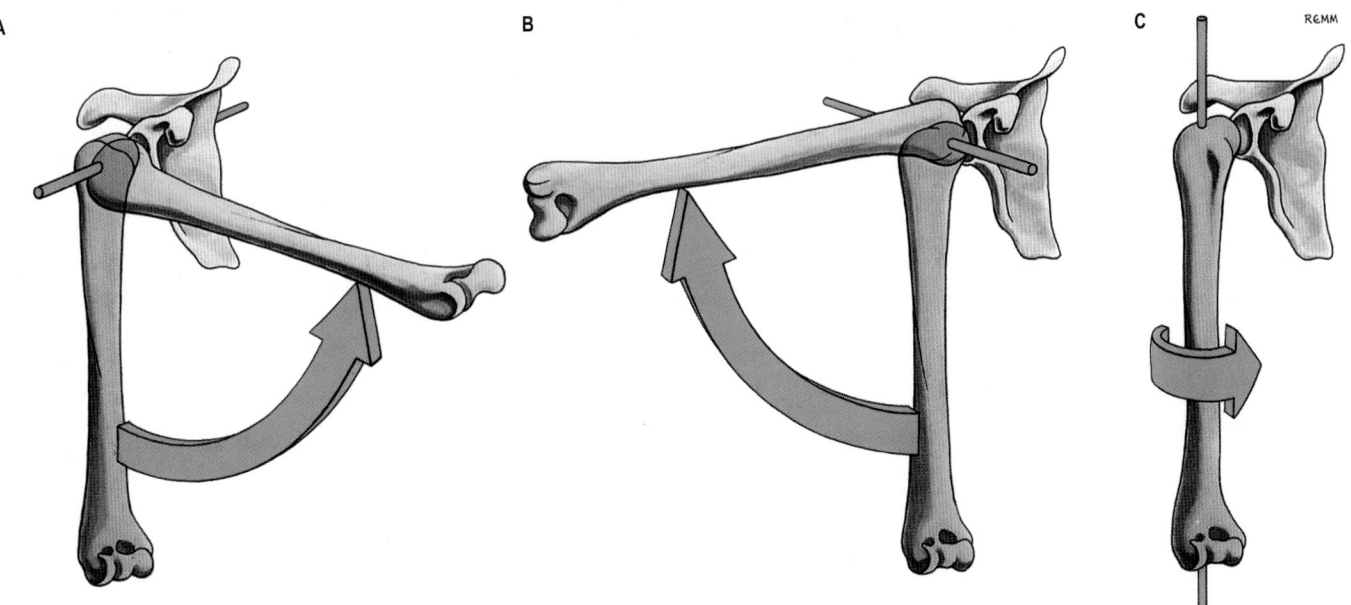

Fig. 6.38 The shoulder joint is polyaxial, and possesses three degrees of freedom. **A–C** show the three mutually perpendicular axes around which the principal movements of flexion–extension (A), abduction–adduction (B) and medial and lateral rotation (C) occur. Note that these axes are referred to the plane of the scapula and not to the coronal and sagittal planes of the erect body. Although an infinite variety of additional movements may occur at such a joint, e.g. movements involving intermediate planes or combinations, they can always be resolved mathematically into components related to the three axes illustrated.

curvature and consequently the axis of rotation will vary as joint movement progresses. When the variation is minor, e.g. the elbow, it is often appropriate to describe a mean position for the axis. In others, e.g. the knee, the situation is more complex.

Simple movements are rarely such. Often motion in one direction is linked to motion in another in an obligatory fashion. There are two varieties of rotation: conjunct (coupled), which is an integral and inevitable accompaniment of the main movement; or adjunct, which can occur independently and may or may not accompany the principal movement.

ARTICULAR MOVEMENTS AND MECHANISMS

Joint surfaces move by gliding and rotation, usually in combination, to produce gross movements at the joint (gliding, angulation, axial rotation, and circumduction). Where movement is slight, the reciprocal surfaces are of similar size; where it is wide, the habitually more mobile bone has the larger articular surface.

Translation – Translation is the simplest motion and involves sliding without appreciable angulation or rotation. Although frequently combined with other movements, it is often considered the only motion permitted in some carpal and tarsal articulations. However, cineradiography reveals that considerable rotation and angulation occur during movements of the small carpal and tarsal bones.

Angulation – Angulation implies a change in angle between the topographical axes of articulating bones, e.g. flexion and extension; abduction and adduction.

Flexion – Flexion is a widely used term, but difficult to define. It often means approximation of two ventral surfaces around a transverse axis. However, the thumb is almost at right angles to the fingers: its 'dorsal' surface faces laterally so that flexion and extension at its joints occur around anteroposterior axes. At the shoulder, flexion is referred to an oblique axis through the centre of the humeral head in the plane of the scapular body, the arm moving anteromedially forwards and hence nearer to the ventral aspect of the trunk. At the hip, which has a transverse axis, flexion brings the morphologically dorsal (but topographically ventral) surface of the thigh to the ventral aspect of the trunk.

Description of flexion at the ankle joint is complicated by the fact that the foot is set at a right angle to the leg. Elevation diminishes this angle and is usually termed flexion: since it is the approximation of two dorsal surfaces it might equally be called extension. Flexion has also been defined as the fetal posture, implying that elevation of the foot is flexion, a view supported by withdrawal reflexes in which elevation is always associated with flexion at the knee and hip. Definitions based on morphological and physiological grounds are thus contradictory: to avoid confusion, dorsiflexion and plantarflexion are used to describe ankle movements.

Abduction and adduction – Abduction and adduction occur around anteroposterior axes except at the first carpometacarpal and shoulder joints. The terms generally imply lateral or medial angulation, except in digits, where arbitrary planes are chosen (midlines of the middle digit of the hand and second digit of the foot), because these are least mobile in this respect. Abduction of the thumb occurs around a transverse axis and away from the palm. Similarly, abduction of the humerus on the scapula occurs in the scapular plane around an oblique axis at right angles to it (**Fig. 6.38**).

Axial rotation – Axial rotation is a widely, but often imprecisely, used term. Its restricted sense denotes movement around some notional 'longitudinal' axis, i.e. axial rotation, which may even be in a separate bone, e.g. the dens of the second cervical vertebra, on which the atlas rotates. An axis may be approximately the centre of the shaft of a long bone, e.g. in medial and lateral humeral rotation (**Fig. 6.38**). It may be at an angle to the topographical axis of a bone, e.g. in movement of the radius on the ulna in pronation and supination, where the axis joins the centre of the radial head to the base of the ulnar styloid process; and in medial and lateral femoral rotation, where the axis joins the centre of the femoral head to a (disputed) point in the distal femur. In these examples, rotations can be independent adjunct motion, constituting a degree of freedom, or conjunct (coupled) rotations, which always accompany some other main movement as a consequence of articular geometry. Obligatory conjunct (coupled) motion is frequently combined with a degree of voluntary adjunct motion; the latter dictates what proportion of the motion occurs above the minimum obligatory component.

Circumduction – Circumduction combines successive flexion, abduction, extension and adduction. It occurs when the distal end of a long bone circumscribes the base of a cone which has its apex at the joint in question, e.g. shoulder and hip joints.

GENERAL CLASSIFICATION OF SYNOVIAL JOINTS

Synovial joints are generally classified according to their shape. While this has some practical value, it affords no exclusive basis for separation because they are merely variations, sometimes extreme, of two basic forms.

Plane joints – Plane joints are appositions of almost flat surfaces (e.g. intermetatarsal and some intercarpal joints). Slight curvature is usual, although often disregarded, and movements are considered to be pure translations or sliding between bones. However, in precise dynamics even slight curvatures cannot be ignored.

Ginglymi (hinge) joints – Ginglymi resemble hinges and restrict movement to one plane, i.e. they are uniaxial. They have strong collateral ligaments to aid this, e.g. interphalangeal and humero-ulnar joints. The surfaces of such biological hinges differ from regular mechanical cylinders in that their profiles are not arcs but varyingly spiral, and therefore motion is not truly about a single axis.

Trochoid (pivot) joints – Trochoid joints are uniaxial. They have an osseous pivot in an osteoligamentous ring, which allows rotation only around the axis of the pivot. Pivots may rotate in rings, e.g. the head of the radius rotates within the anular ligament and ulnar radial notch; or rings may rotate around pivots, e.g. the atlas rotates around the dens of the axis.

Bicondylar joints – Bicondylar joints are largely uniaxial, with a main movement in one plane. They also display limited rotation about a second axis orthogonal to the first. Bicondylar joints are so named because they are formed of two convex condyles (knuckles) which articulate with concave or flat surfaces (sometimes inappropriately also called condyles). The condyles may lie within a common fibrous capsule, e.g. the knee, or in separate capsules which necessarily cooperate in all movements as a condylar pair, e.g. temporomandibular joints.

Ellipsoid joints – Ellipsoid joints are biaxial, and consist of an oval, convex surface apposed to an elliptical concavity, e.g. radiocarpal and metacarpophalangeal joints. Primary movements are about two orthogonal axes, e.g. flexion–extension, abduction–adduction, which may be combined as circumduction; rotation around the third axis is largely prevented by general articular shape.

Sellar (saddle) joints – Saddle joints are biaxial and have concavoconvex surfaces. Each is most convex in a particular direction, and is maximally concave at right angles to this direction. The convexity of the larger surface is apposed to the concavity of the smaller surface and vice versa. Primary movements occur in two orthogonal planes, but articular shape causes axial rotation of the moving bone. Such coupled rotation is never independent, and is functionally significant in habitual positioning and limitation of movement. The most familiar sellar joint is the carpometacarpal joint of the thumb, others include the ankle and calcaneocuboid joints.

Spheroidal joints ('ball-and-socket') – Spheroidal joints are multiaxial. They are formed by the reception of a globoid 'head' into an opposing cup, e.g. the hip and shoulder joints. Their surfaces, although resembling parts of spheres, are not strictly spherical but slightly ovoid, and consequently congruence is not perfect in most positions. Indeed, it occurs in only one position, at the end of the commonest movement.

Development of joints

The development of joints is described on page 938.

MUSCLE

Most cells are not spherical, even when they are separated from adjacent structures, and this is because they possess a cytoskeleton. Elements of the cytoskeleton are capable of lengthening or shortening, enabling the cell to undergo active changes of shape. This capacity is important in a variety of cellular functions, e.g. locomotion, phagocytosis, mitosis and extension of processes. Proteins referred to as molecular motors can effect changes of length much more rapidly than systems dependent on polymerization–depolymerization mechanisms (actin, tubulin), by using energy from the hydrolysis of adenosine 5'-triphosphate (ATP). Of these ATP-dependent systems, one of the most widespread is based on the interaction of actin and myosin.

In muscle cells the filaments of actin and myosin and their associated proteins are so abundant that they almost fill the interior of the cell. Moreover they align predominantly in one direction, so that interactions at the molecular level are translated into linear contraction of the whole cell. The ability of these specialized cells to change shape has thus become their most important property. Assemblies of contractile muscle cells, the muscles, are machines for converting chemical energy into mechanical work. The forces generated move limbs, inflate the lungs, pump blood, close and open tubes, etc. In man, muscle tissue constitutes 40–50% of the body mass.

Classification of muscle

Muscle cells (fibres) are also known as myocytes (the prefixes myo- and sarco- are frequently used in naming structures associated with muscle). They differentiate along one of three main pathways to form skeletal, cardiac or smooth muscle. Both skeletal and cardiac muscle may be called striated muscle, because their myosin and actin filaments are organized into regular, repeating elements which give the cells a finely cross-striated appearance when they are viewed microscopically. Smooth muscle, in contrast, lacks such repeating elements and thus has no striations.

Other contractile cells, including myofibroblasts and myoepithelial cells, are different in character and origin. They contain smooth muscle-like contractile proteins and are found singly or in small groups.

STRIATED MUSCLE

SKELETAL MUSCLE

Skeletal muscle is innervated by somatic motor nerves, and forms the bulk of the muscular tissue of the body. It consists of parallel bundles of long, multinucleate fibres. This type of muscle is capable of powerful contractions (c.100 watts per kilogram) by virtue of the regular organization of its contractile proteins. The price paid for this organization is a limited contractile range. Wherever a larger range of movement is required, it is achieved through the amplification provided by the lever systems of the skeleton to which the muscle is attached (hence the name skeletal muscle).

Skeletal muscle is sometimes referred to as voluntary muscle, because the movements in which it participates are often initiated under conscious control. However, this is a misleading term: skeletal muscle is involved in many movements, e.g. breathing, blinking, swallowing, and the actions of the muscles of the perineum and in the middle ear, which are usually or exclusively driven at an unconscious level.

CARDIAC MUSCLE

Cardiac muscle is found only in the heart, and in the walls of large veins where they enter the heart. It consists of a branching network of individual cells that are linked electrically and mechanically to function as a unit. Compared with skeletal muscle, cardiac muscle is much less powerful (c.3–5 watts per kilogram) but far more resistant to fatigue. It is provided with a continuous supply of energy by numerous blood vessels around the fibres, and abundant mitochondria within them. Cardiac muscle differs structurally and functionally from skeletal muscle in some important respects. It is, for example, intrinsically capable of rhythmic contraction, with a rate and strength which is nevertheless responsive to hormonal and autonomic nervous control.

Cardiac muscle is considered in detail in Chapter 7.

SMOOTH MUSCLE

Smooth muscle contains actin and myosin, but they are not organized into repeating units, and its microscopic appearance is therefore unstriated (smooth). The elongated cells are smaller than those of striated muscle, and taper at the ends. They are capable of slow but sustained contractions, and although this type of muscle is less powerful than striated muscle, the amount of shortening can be much greater. These functional attributes are well illustrated by its role in the walls of tubes and sacs, where its action regulates the size of the enclosed lumen and, in some cases, the consequent movement of luminal contents.

A smooth muscle cell may be excited in several ways, most commonly by an autonomic nerve fibre, a blood-borne neurohormone, or conduction from a neighbouring smooth muscle cell. Since none of these routes is under conscious control, smooth muscle is sometimes referred to as involuntary muscle. It is found in all systems of the body, in the walls of the viscera, including most of the gastrointestinal, respiratory, urinary and reproductive tracts, in the tunica media of blood vessels, in the dermis (as the arrector pili muscles), in the intrinsic muscles of the eye, and the dartos muscular layer of the scrotum. In some places, smooth muscle fasciculi are associated with those of skeletal muscle, e.g. the sphincters of the anus and the urinary bladder, the tarsal muscles of the upper and lower eyelids, the suspensory muscle of the duodenum, a transitional zone in the oesophagus, and fasciae and ligaments on the pelvic aspect of the pelvic diaphragm.

Skeletal muscle

SHAPE AND FIBRE ARCHITECTURE

It is possible to classify muscles based on their general shape and the predominant orientation of their fibres relative to the direction of pull (**Fig. 6.39**). Muscles with fibres that are largely parallel to the line of pull vary in form from flat, short and quadrilateral (e.g. thyrohyoid) to long and strap-like (e.g. sternohyoid, sartorius). In such muscles, individual fibres may run for the entire length of the muscle, or over shorter segments when there are transverse, tendinous intersections at intervals (e.g. rectus abdominis). In a fusiform muscle, the fibres may be close to parallel in the 'belly', but converge to a tendon at one or both ends.

Where fibres are oblique to the line of pull, muscles may be triangular (e.g. temporalis, adductor longus) or pennate (feather-like) in construction. The latter vary in complexity (see **Fig. 6.39**) from unipennate (e.g. flexor pollicis longus) and bipennate (e.g. rectus femoris, dorsal interossei) to multipennate (e.g. deltoid). In some muscles the fibres pass obliquely between deep and superficial aponeuroses, in a type of 'unipennate' form (e.g. soleus). In other sites muscle fibres start from the walls of osteofascial compartments, and converge obliquely on a central tendon in circumpennate fashion (e.g. tibialis anterior). Some muscles have a spiral or twisted arrangement (e.g. sternocostal fibres of pectoralis major and latissimus dorsi, which undergo a 180° twist between their median and lateral attachments). Others spiral around a bone (e.g. supinator, which winds obliquely around the proximal radial shaft), or contain two or more planes of fibres arranged in differing directions, a type of spiral sometimes referred to as cruciate: sternocleidomastoid, masseter and adductor magnus are all partially spiral and cruciate. Many muscles display more than one of these major types of arrangement, and show regional variations which correspond to contrasting, and in some cases independent, actions.

MUSCLE NOMENCLATURE

The names given to individual muscles are usually descriptive, based on their shape, size, number of heads or bellies, position, depth, attachments, or actions. The meanings of some of the terms used are given in **Table 6.1**.

These terms are often used in combination: thus, flexor digitorum longus (long flexor of the digits), latissimus dorsi (broadest muscle of the back). The names given to individual muscles or muscle groups are often oversimplified, and terms denoting action emphasize only one of a number of usual actions. A given muscle may play different roles in different movements, and these roles may change if the movements are assisted or opposed by gravity. The functional roles implied by names should therefore be interpreted with caution.

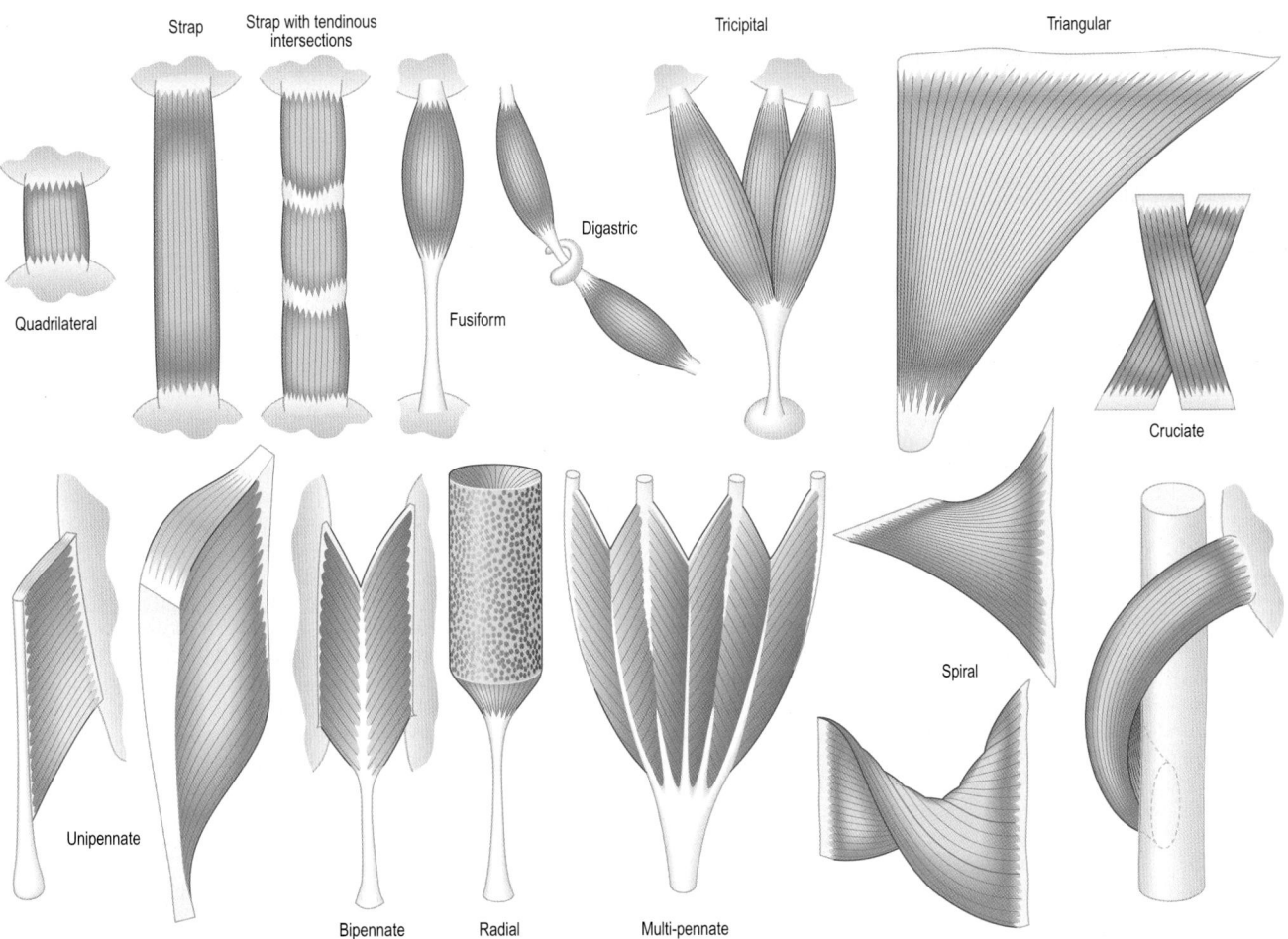

Strap

Strap with tendinous intersections

Tricipital

Triangular

Digastric

Quadrilateral

Fusiform

Cruciate

Unipennate

Spiral

Bipennate

Radial

Multi-pennate

Fig. 6.39 Morphological 'types' of muscle based on their general form and fascicular architecture.

Table 6.1 Terms used in naming muscles

Shape	Position
Deltoid (triangular)	Anterior, posterior, medial, lateral,
Quadratus (square)	superior, inferior, supra-, infra-
Rhomboid (diamond-shaped)	Interosseus (between bones)
Teres (round)	Dorsi (of the back)
Gracilis (slender)	Abdominis (of the abdomen)
Rectus (straight)	Pectoralis (of the chest)
Lumbrical (worm-like)	Brachii (of the arm)
	Femoris (of the thigh)
Size	Oris (of the mouth)
Major, minor, longus (long)	Oculi (of the eye)
Brevis (short)	
Latissimus (broadest)	**Attachment**
Longissimus (longest)	Sternocleidomastoid (from sternum
	and clavicle to mastoid process)
Number of heads or bellies	Coracobrachialis (from the coracoid
Biceps (two heads)	process to the arm)
Triceps (three heads)	
Quadriceps (four heads)	**Action**
Digastric (two bellies)	Extensor, flexor
	Abductor, adductor
Depth	Levator, depressor
Superficialis (superficial)	Supinator, pronator
Profundus (deep)	Constrictor, dilator
Externus/externi (external)	
Internus/interni (internal)	

MICROSTRUCTURE OF SKELETAL MUSCLE

The cellular units of skeletal muscle are the muscle fibres (**Fig. 6.40**). These long, cylindrical structures tend to be consistent in size within a given muscle, but in different muscles may range from 10 to 100 μm in diameter and from millimetres to many centimetres in length. Some typical skeletal muscle fibres are seen in longitudinal section in **Fig. 6.41**. Their staining characteristics are dominated by the contractile apparatus, which constitutes much of the cytoplasm or sarcoplasm. The contractile proteins are organized into cylindrical myofibrils which are too tightly packed to be visible by routine light microscopy. Of greater significance are transverse striations, which are the result of alignment across the fibre of repeating elements, the sarcomeres, within neighbouring myofibrils. These cross-striations are usually evident in sections stained conventionally, but may be demonstrated more effectively using special stains (**Fig. 6.42**).

Under polarized light, the striations are even more striking, and are seen as a pattern of alternating dark and light bands. The darker bands are birefringent, rotating the plane of polarized light strongly, and are known as anisotropic or A-bands; the lighter bands rotate the plane of polarized light to a negligible degree and are known as isotropic or I-bands. The structures responsible for this appearance are described more readily at the ultrastructural level.

The multiple nuclei are oval and located at the periphery of the fibres, under the plasma membrane or sarcolemma. They are especially numerous in the region of the neuromuscular junction (p. 64). The nuclei are moderately euchromatic and usually have one or more nucleoli. They occupy a thin transparent rim of sarcoplasm between the myofibrils and the sarcolemma, and are seen most clearly in transverse sections (**Fig. 6.43**). Other nuclei belonging to vascular endothelial cells, Schwann cells, fibroblasts, etc., may be present in the spaces between the fibres, where blood vessels and nerve fibres travel through layers of fine connective tissue, the endomysium. Nuclei of satellite cells lie between the sarcolemma and the surrounding basal lamina.

In transverse section, the profiles of the fibres are usually polygonal (**Fig. 6.43**). Some muscles, e.g. the extrinsic muscles of the larynx, tend to be less tightly packed. In such situations, as well as in conditions of generalized wasting or muscle damage, the fibres may adopt a more rounded profile, but in some normal muscles, e.g. those that close the jaw, the fibres are closely packed but have rounded profiles. The sarcoplasm often has a stippled appearance, because the transversely sectioned myofibrils are resolved as dots.

Skeletal muscle fibres are large (with a few exceptions, e.g. the laryngeal muscles) and electron micrographs, unless they are taken at very low magnification, seldom show more than part of the interior of a fibre (**Fig. 6.44A**). Myofibrils are the dominant ultrastructural feature of such micrographs. They are cylindrical structures of c.1 μm diameter, which appear as ribbons in longitudinal section. Thin, very densely stained transverse lines, which correspond to discs in the parent cylindrical structure, appear at regular intervals along these ribbons. They are called Z-lines or, more properly, Z-discs (Zwischenscheiben = between discs). They divide the myofibril into a linear series of identical contractile units, sarcomeres, each of which is c.2.2 μm long in resting muscle.

At higher power, sarcomeres are seen to consist of two types of filament, thick and thin, organized into regular arrays (**Fig. 6.44B**). The thick filaments, which are c.15 nm in diameter, are composed mainly of myosin. The thin filaments, which are 8 nm in diameter, are composed mainly of actin. The arrays of thick and thin filaments form a partially overlapping structure in which the electron density varies according to the amount of protein present. The A-band consists of the thick filaments, together with lengths of thin filaments that interdigitate with, and thus overlap, the thick filaments at either end (**Figs 6.44B, 6.45**). The central, paler region of the A-band, into which the thin filaments have not penetrated, is called the H-zone (helle = light). At their centres, the thick filaments are linked together transversely by material that constitutes the M-line (Mittelscheibe = middle (of) disc) which is visible in most muscles.

The I-band consists of the adjacent portions of two neighbouring sarcomeres in which the thin filaments are not overlapped by thick filaments. It is bisected by the Z-disc, into which the thin filaments of adjacent sarcomeres are anchored. In addition to the thick and thin filaments, there is a third type of filament composed of the elastic protein, titin. The high degree of organization of the filament arrays is equally evident in electron micrographs of transverse sections (**Figs 6.45, 6.46**). The thick myosin filaments form a hexagonal lattice; in the regions where they overlap with the thin filaments, each myosin filament is surrounded by six actin filaments at the trigonal points of the lattice. In the I-band, the thin filament pattern changes from hexagonal to square as the filaments approach the Z-disc, where they are incorporated into a square lattice structure.

The banded appearance of individual myofibrils is thus attributable to the regular alternation of the thick and thin filament arrays. However, myofibrils are at the limit of resolution of light microscopy: the fact that cross-striations are also visible at that level is the result of alignment in register of the bands in adjacent myofibrils across the breadth of the whole muscle fibre. In suitably stained, relaxed material, the A-, I- and H-bands are quite distinct, but the Z-discs, which are such a prominent feature of electron micrographs, are thin and much less conspicuous in the light microscope, and M-lines cannot be seen at all.

MUSCLE PROTEINS

Myosin, the protein of the thick filament, is the most abundant contractile protein (60% of the total myofibrillar protein). The thick filaments of skeletal (and cardiac) muscle are 1.5 μm long. Their composition from myosin heavy and light chain assemblies is described on page 17. Actin is the next most abundant contractile protein (20% of the total myofibrillar protein). In its filamentous form (F-actin), it is the principal protein of the thin filaments; the other components, the regulatory proteins tropomyosin and troponin, play a major part in the control of contraction.

The third type of long sarcomeric filament connects the thick filaments to the Z-disc, and is formed by the giant protein, titin, with a molecular mass in the millions. Single titin molecules span the half-sarcomere between the M-lines and the Z-discs, into which they are inserted, with a bound portion in the A-band and an elastic portion in the I-band. In the A-band, titin is attached to thick filaments as far as the M-line. Its physical properties endow the myosin filaments with elastic recoil after stretching.

A number of proteins which are neither contractile nor regulatory are responsible for the structural integrity of the myofibrils, particularly their regular internal arrangement. A component of the Z-disc, α-actinin, is a rod-shaped molecule which anchors the plus-ends of actin filaments from adjacent sarcomeres to the Z-disc. Nebulin inserts into the Z-disc, associated with the thin filaments, and regulates the lengths of actin filaments. An intermediate filament protein characteristic of muscle, desmin, encircles the myofibrils at the Z-disc and, with the linking molecule plectin, forms a meshwork that connects myofibrils together within the muscle fibre. Myomesin holds myosin filaments in

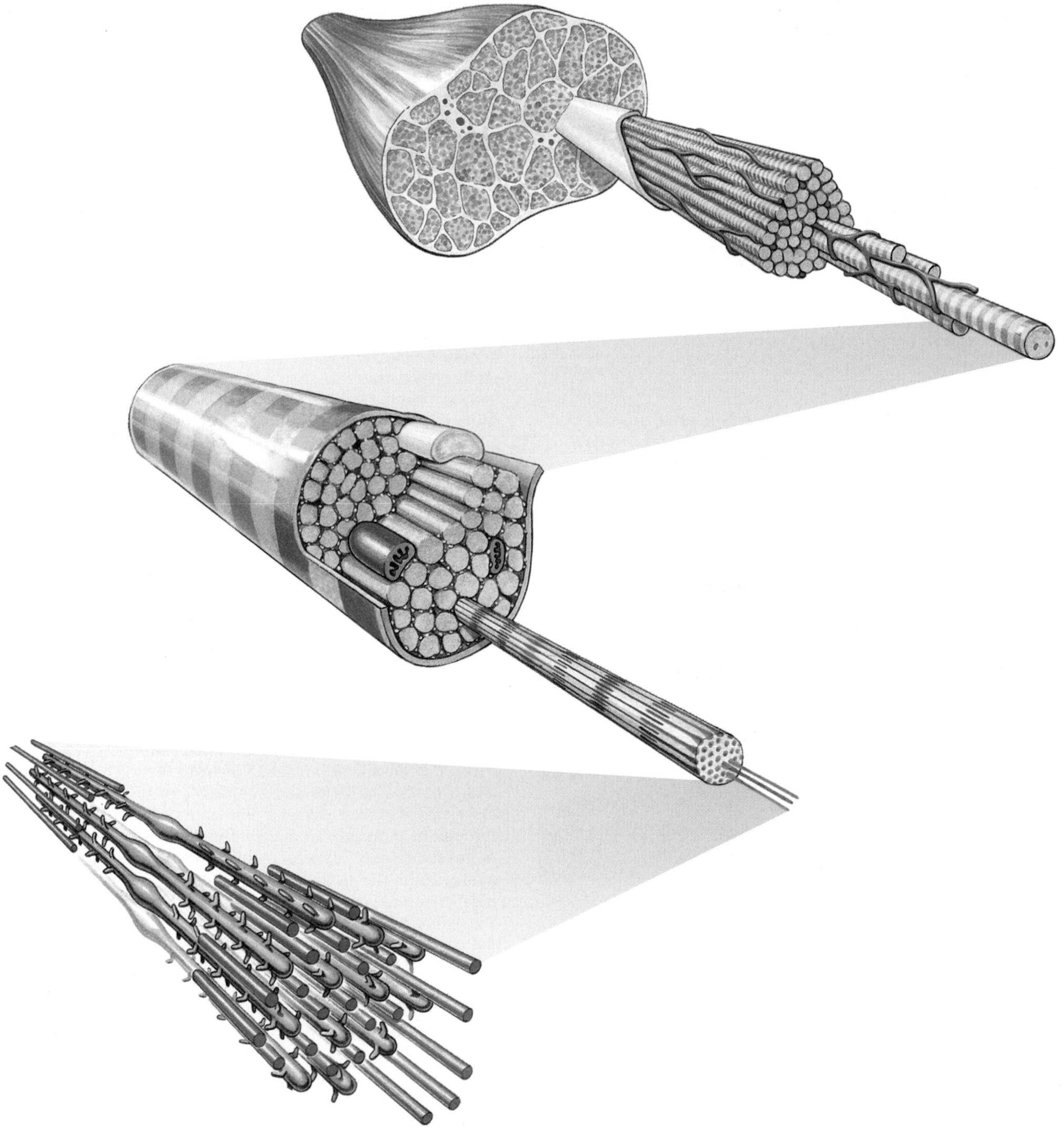

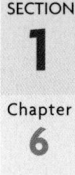

Fig. 6.40 Levels of organization within a skeletal muscle, from whole muscle to fasciculi, single fibres, myofibrils and myofilaments.

their regular lattice arrangement in the region of the M line. Dystrophin is confined to the periphery of the muscle fibre, close to the cytoplasmic face of the sarcolemma. It binds to actin intracellularly and is also associated with a large oligomeric complex of glycoproteins which spans the membrane and links specifically with merosin, the laminin isoform of the muscle basal lamina. This stabilizes the muscle fibre and transmits forces generated internally on contraction to the extracellular matrix.

Dystrophin is the product of the gene affected in Duchenne muscular dystrophy, a fatal disorder that develops when mutation of the gene leads to the absence of this protein. A milder form of the disease, Becker muscular dystrophy, is associated with a reduced size and/or abundance of dystrophin. Female carriers (heterozygous for the mutant gene) of Duchenne muscular dystrophy may also have mild symptoms of muscle weakness. At c.2500 kb, the gene is one of the largest yet discovered, which may account for the high mutation rate of Duchenne muscular dystrophy (c.35% of cases are new mutations).

OTHER SARCOPLASMIC STRUCTURES

Although myofibrils are the dominant ultrastructural feature of skeletal muscle, the fibres contain other organelles essential for cellular function, such as ribosomes, Golgi apparatus and mitochondria. Most of them are located around the nuclei, between the myofibrils and the sarcolemma and, to a lesser extent, between the myofibrils. Mitochondria, lipid droplets and glycogen provide the metabolic support needed by active muscle. The mitochondria are elongated and their cristae are closely packed. Their profiles are usually seen in longitudinal orientation between the myofibrils (**Fig. 6.44A**). The number of mitochondria in an adult muscle fibre is not fixed, but can increase or decrease quite readily in response to sustained changes in activity. Spherical lipid droplets, of c.0.25 μm diameter, are distributed uniformly throughout the sarcoplasm between myofibrils. They represent a rich source of energy which can, however, be tapped only by oxidative metabolic pathways, and they are therefore more common in fibres which have a high mitochondrial content and good capillary blood

115

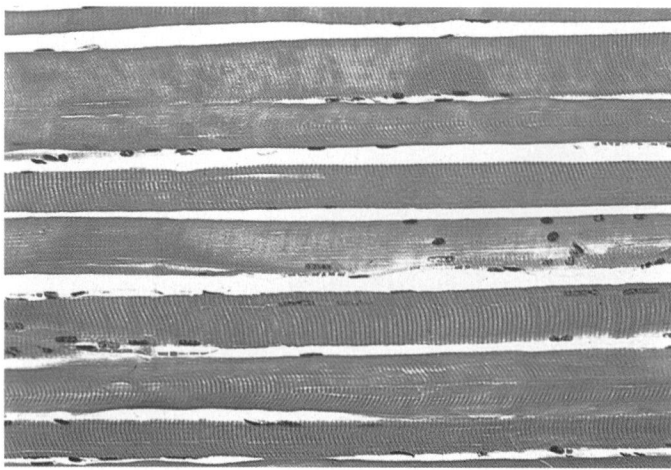

Fig. 6.41 Skeletal muscle fibres in longitudinal section. Note the numerous peripherally placed nuclei in these extremely elongated, unbranched syncytial cells and the faint transverse striations in their cytoplasm. The central fibre is sectioned in part through its periphery, close to the sarcolemma, and so several nuclei appear to be lying centrally. (By permission from Young B, Heath JW 2000 Wheater's Functional Histology. Edinburgh: Churchill Livingstone.)

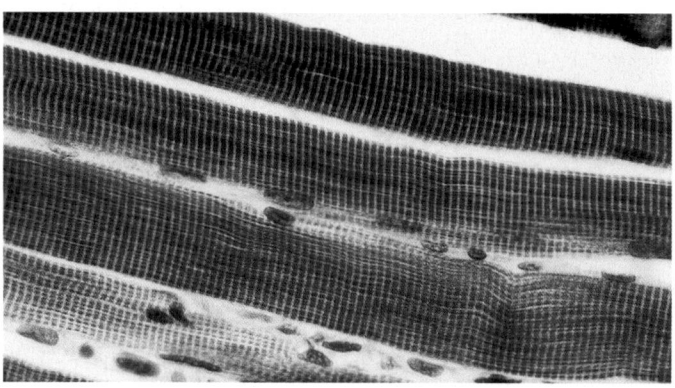

Fig. 6.42 Longitudinal section, skeletal muscle fibres. Cross-striations reflect the sarcomeric organization of actin and myosin within the myofibrils and the alignment of myofibrils in register within the cytoplasm. The nuclei between fibres are those of endomysial connective tissue and capillaries, and some may be of satellite cells. Phosphotungstic acid-stained preparation. (Photograph by Sarah-Jane Smith.)

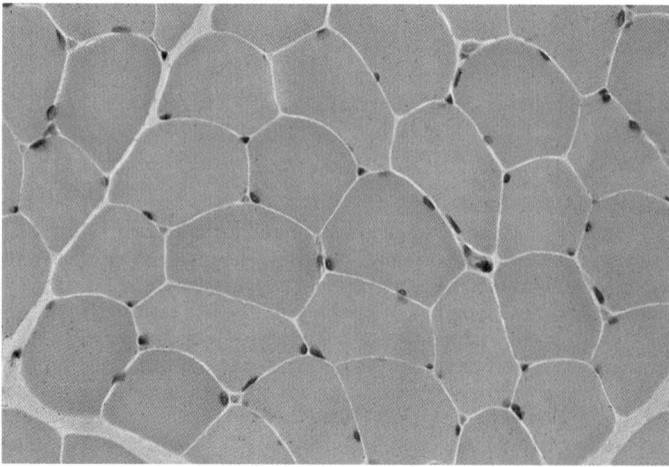

Fig. 6.43 Transverse cryostat section of adult human skeletal muscle. Note the tight packing of the fibres and the peripheral location of the dark stained nuclei. (Photograph by Stanley Salmons, from a specimen provided by Tim Helliwell, Department of Pathology, University of Liverpool.)

supply. Glycogen is distributed in small clusters of granules between myofibrils and among the thin filaments. In brief bursts of activity it provides an important source of anaerobic energy that is not dependent on nutrient blood flow to the muscle fibre.

At the ends of the muscle fibre, where force is transmitted to adjacent connective tissue structures, the sarcolemma is folded into numerous finger-like projections, which strengthen the junctional region by increasing the area of attachment. Tubular invaginations of the sarcolemma penetrate between the myofibrils in a transverse plane at the limit of each A-band (**Fig. 6.47**). The lumina of these transverse (T-) tubules is thus in continuity with the extracellular space. T-tubules play an important role in excitation–contraction coupling.

The sarcoplasmic reticulum (SR) is a specialized form of smooth endoplasmic reticulum. It consists of a plexus of anastomosing membrane cisternae which fill much of the space between myofibrils, and expand into larger sacs, the junctional sarcoplasmic reticulum or terminal cisternae, where they come into close contact with T-tubules. At this point, they form part of a structure called a triad, consisting of a central T-tubule flanked on either side by two terminal cisternae, the latter filled with dense, granular material (**Fig. 6.44B**). The membranes of the SR contain calcium–ATPase pumps. These transport calcium ions into the terminal cisternae, where the ions are bound to calsequestrin, a protein which has a high affinity for calcium, in dense storage granules. In this way, calcium can be accumulated and retained in the terminal cisternae at a much higher concentration than anywhere else in the sarcoplasm. Ca^{2+}-release channels (made of ryanodine receptor molecules) are concentrated mainly in the terminal cisternae. They form one half of the junctional 'feet' or 'pillars' which bridge the SR and T-tubules at the triads, forming a critical communication point between them. The other half of the junctional feet is the T-tubule receptor which constitutes the voltage sensor.

CONNECTIVE TISSUES OF MUSCLE

The endomysium is a delicate network of connective tissue which surrounds muscle fibres, and forms their immediate external environment. It is the site of metabolic exchange between muscle and blood, and contains capillaries and bundles of small nerve fibres. Ion fluxes associated with the electrical excitation of muscle fibres take place through its proteoglycan matrix. The endomysium is continuous with more substantial septa of connective tissue which constitute the perimysium. The latter ensheathes groups of muscle fibres to form parallel bundles or fasciculi; carries larger blood vessels and nerves; and accommodates neuromuscular spindles. Perimysial septa are themselves the inward extensions of a collagenous sheath, the epimysium, which forms part of the fascia that invests whole muscle groups.

Epimysium consists mainly of type I collagen, perimysium contains type I and type III collagen, and endomysium contains collagen types III and IV. Collagen IV is associated particularly with the basal lamina that invests each muscle fibre.

The epimysial, perimysial and endomysial sheaths coalesce where the muscles connect to adjacent structures at tendons, aponeuroses, and fasciae: this gives the attachments great strength, since the tensile forces are distributed in the form of shear stresses, which are more easily resisted. This principle is also seen at the ends of the muscle fibres, which divide into finger-like processes separated by collagen fibres. Although there are no desmosomal attachments at these myotendinous junctions, there are other specializations which assist in the transmission of force from the interior of the fibre to the extracellular matrix. Actin filaments from the adjacent sarcomeres, which would normally insert into a Z-disc at this point, penetrate instead into a dense, subsarcolemmal filamentous matrix that provides attachment to the plasma membrane. This matrix is similar in character to the cytoplasmic face of an adherens junction (p. 7). The structure as a whole is homologous to the intercalated discs of cardiac muscle. Beyond the surface of the sarcolemma, fine junctional microfibrils, c.5–10 nm thick, and of unknown composition, bridge across the lamina lucida to the prominent lamina densa of the junctional basal lamina. This in turn adheres closely to collagen and reticular fibres (type III collagen) of the adjacent tendon or other connective tissue structure.

ATTACHMENTS OF SKELETAL MUSCLES

The forces developed by skeletal muscles are transferred to bones by connective tissue structures: tendons, aponeuroses and fasciae. The microstructure of tendons is considered below.

A

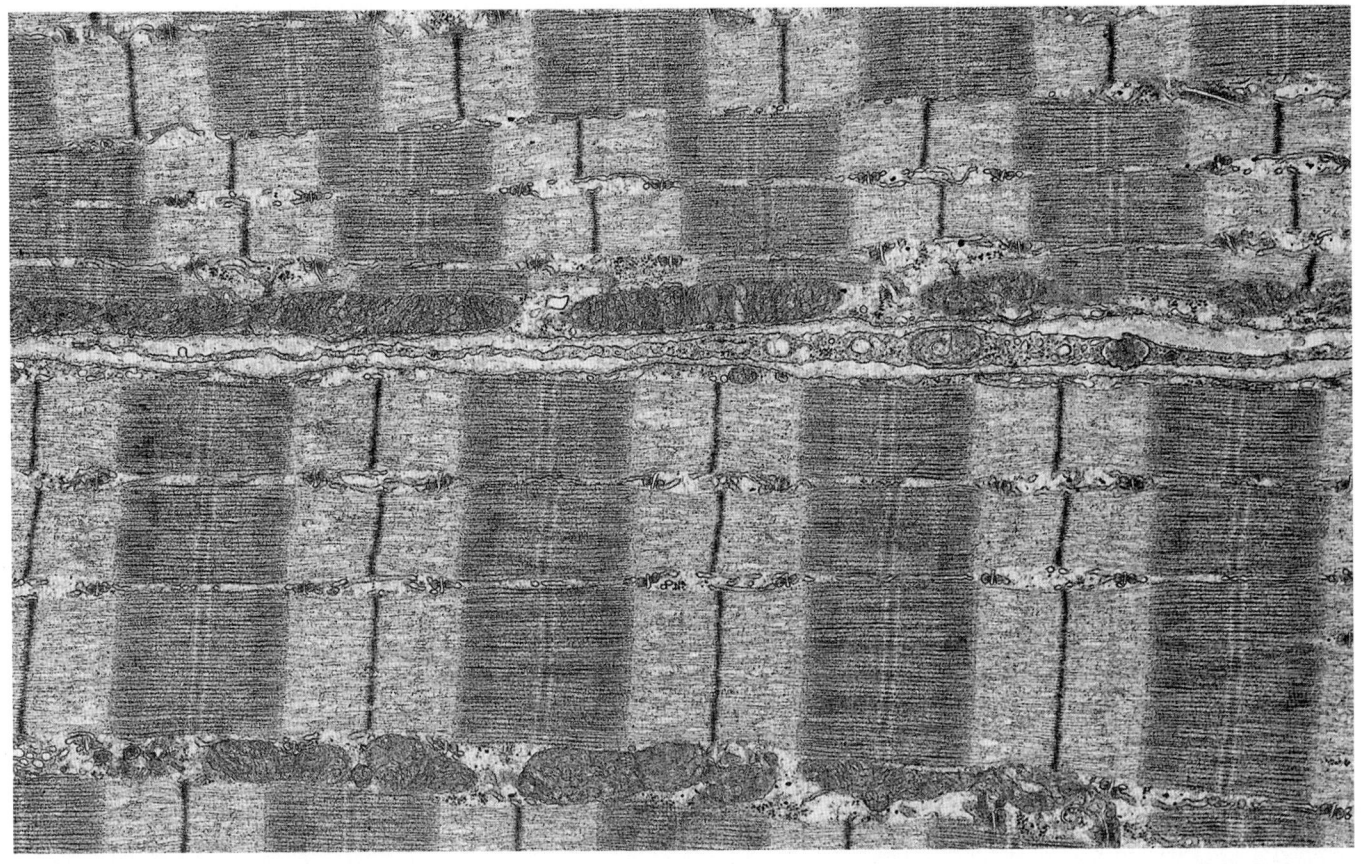

B

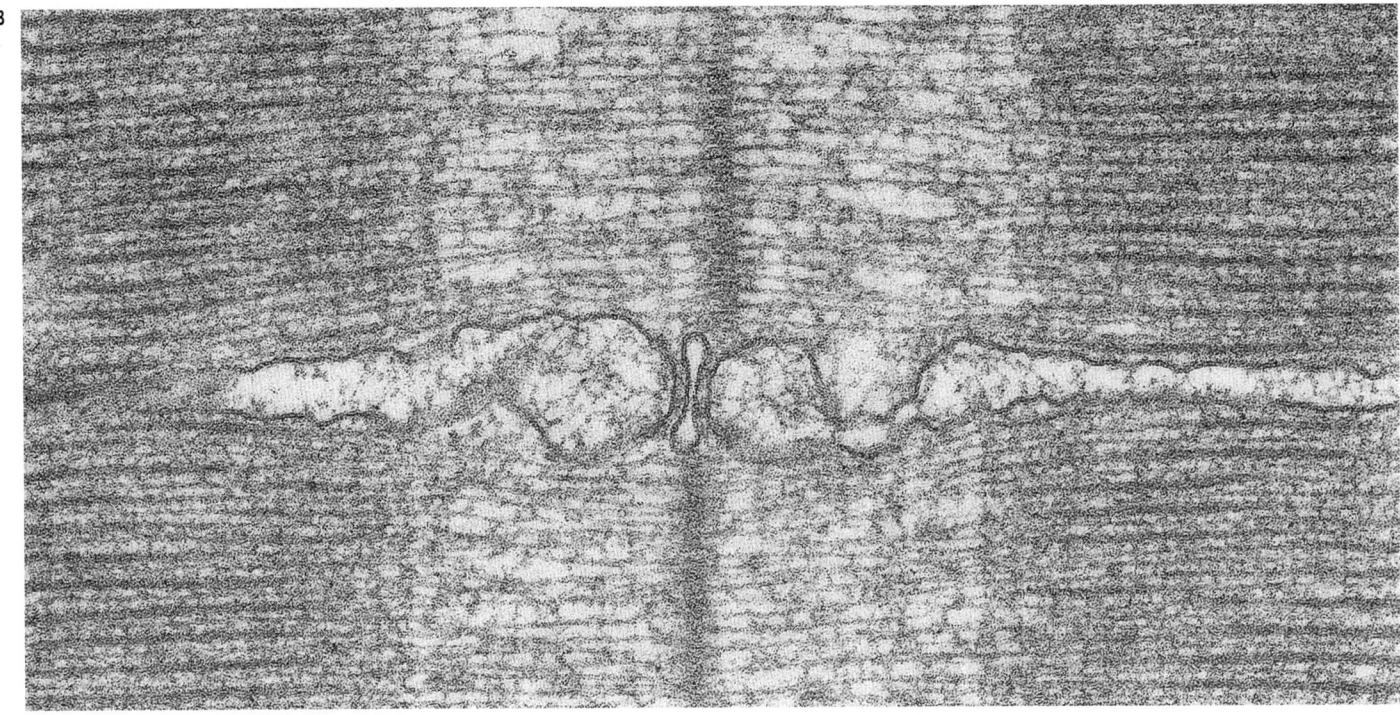

Fig. 6.44 A, Low-power electron micrograph of parts of two skeletal muscle fibres in longitudinal section. **B**, High-power electron micrograph of frog skeletal muscle in longitudinal section, showing a triad, thick and thin filaments and cross-bridges bridging the spaces between them. Note the overlap of thin filaments within the Z-disc at the top of the micrograph. (The human triad lies at the junction between the A and I bands, not at the Z-disc as shown above.) (Photographs by Brenda Russell, Department of Physiology and Biophysics, University of Illinois at Chicago.)

Tendons (Fig. 6.48)

Tendons take the form of cords or straps of round or oval cross-section, and consist of dense, regular connective tissue. They contain fascicles of type I collagen, orientated mainly parallel to the long axis, but are to some extent interwoven. The fasciculi may be conspicuous enough to give tendons a longitudinally striated appearance to the unaided eye. Tendons generally have smooth surfaces, although large tendons may be ridged longitudinally by coarse fasciculi (e.g. the osseous aspect of the angulated tendon of obturator internus). Loose connective tissue between fascicles provides a pathway for small vessels and nerves, and condenses on the surface as a sheath or epitendineum, which may contain elastic and irregularly arranged collagen fibres. The loose attachments between this sheath and the surrounding tissue present little resistance to movements of the tendon, but in situations where greater

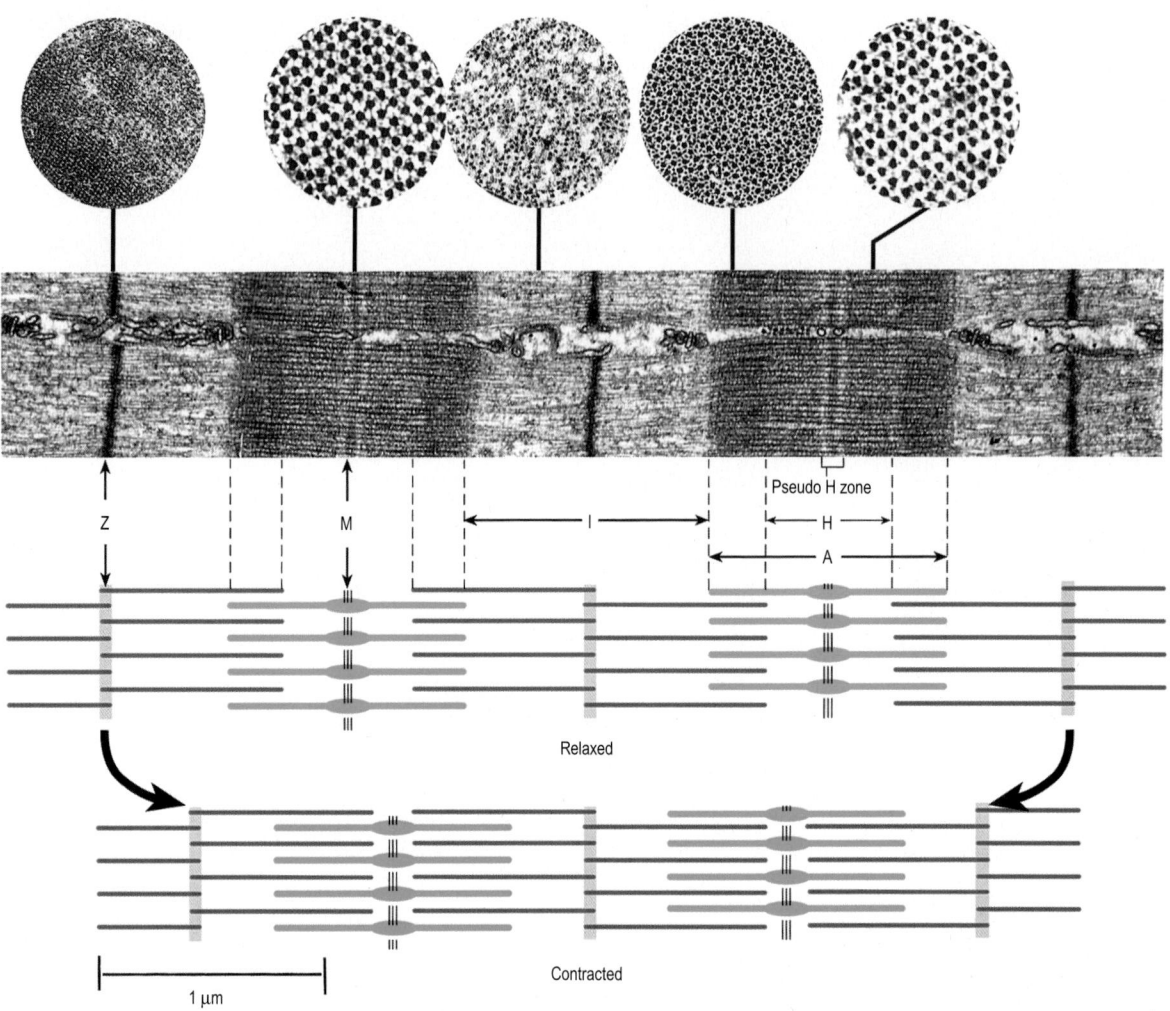

Pseudo H zone

Z M I H A

Relaxed

Contracted

1 μm

Fig. 6.45 Sarcomeric structures. The drawings below the electron micrograph (of two myofibrils sectioned longitudinally) indicate the corresponding arrangements of thick and thin filaments. Relaxed and contracted states are shown to illustrate the changes which occur during shortening. Insets at the top show the electron micrographic appearance of transverse sections through the sarcomere at the levels shown. Note that the packing geometry of the thin filaments changes from a square array at the Z-disc to a hexagonal array where they interdigitate with thick filaments in the A-band. (Photographs by Brenda Russell, Department of Physiology and Biophysics, University of Illinois at Chicago; artwork by Lesley Skeates.)

freedom of movement is required, a tendon is separated from adjacent structures by a synovial sheath.

Tendons are strongly attached to bones, both at the periosteum and through fasciculi (extrinsic collagen fibres), which continue deep into the bone cortex. Sections of fresh bone show that at sites of tendinous attachment there is often a smooth plate of white fibrocartilage, which may cushion and reinforce the attachment zone. Tendons are slightly elastic and may be stretched by up to 6% of their length without damage. Recovery of the elastic energy stored in tendons can make movement more economical. Although they resist extension, tendons are flexible. They can, therefore, be diverted around osseous surfaces or deflected under retinacula to redirect the angle of pull.

Since tendons are composed of collagen and their vascular supply is sparse, they appear white. However, the blood supply to tendons is not unimportant: small arterioles from adjacent muscle tissue pass longitudinally between the fascicles, branching and anastomosing freely, and accompanied by venae comitantes and lymphatic vessels. This longitudinal plexus is augmented by small vessels from adjacent loose connective tissue or synovial sheaths. Vessels rarely pass between bone and tendon at osseous attachments, and the junctional surfaces are usually devoid of foramina. A notable exception is the calcaneal tendon (Achilles tendon), which receives a blood supply across the osseotendinous junction. During postnatal development, tendons enlarge by interstitial growth, particularly at myotendinous junctions, where there are high concentrations of fibroblasts. Growth decreases along the tendon from the muscle to the osseous attachments. The thickness finally attained by a tendon depends on the size and strength of the associated muscle, but appears also to be influenced by additional factors, e.g. the degree of pennation of the muscle. The metabolic rate of tendons is very low but increases during infection or injury. Repair involves the initial proliferation of fibroblasts followed by interstitial deposition of new fibres.

The nerve supply to tendons is largely sensory, and there is no evidence of any capacity for vasomotor control. Specialized endings that are sensitive to force (Golgi tendon organs, see p. 62) are found near myotendinous junctions; their large myelinated afferent axons run centrally within branches of muscular nerves or in small rami of adjacent peripheral nerves.

NEUROVASCULAR SUPPLY OF SKELETAL MUSCLE

VASCULAR SUPPLY AND LYMPHATIC DRAINAGE

In most muscles the major source artery enters on the deep surface, frequently in close association with the principal vein and nerve, which together form a neurovascular hilum. The vessels course and branch within the connective tissue framework of the muscle. The smaller arteries and arterioles ramify in the perimysial septa and give off capillaries which run in the endomysium. Although the smaller vessels lie mainly parallel to the muscle fibres, they also branch and anastomose around the fibres, forming an elongated mesh.

Mathes & Nahai (1981) have classified the gross vascular anatomy of muscles into five types according to the number of vascular pedicles which enter the muscle, and their relative dominance (**Fig. 6.49**). This classification has important surgical relevance in determining which

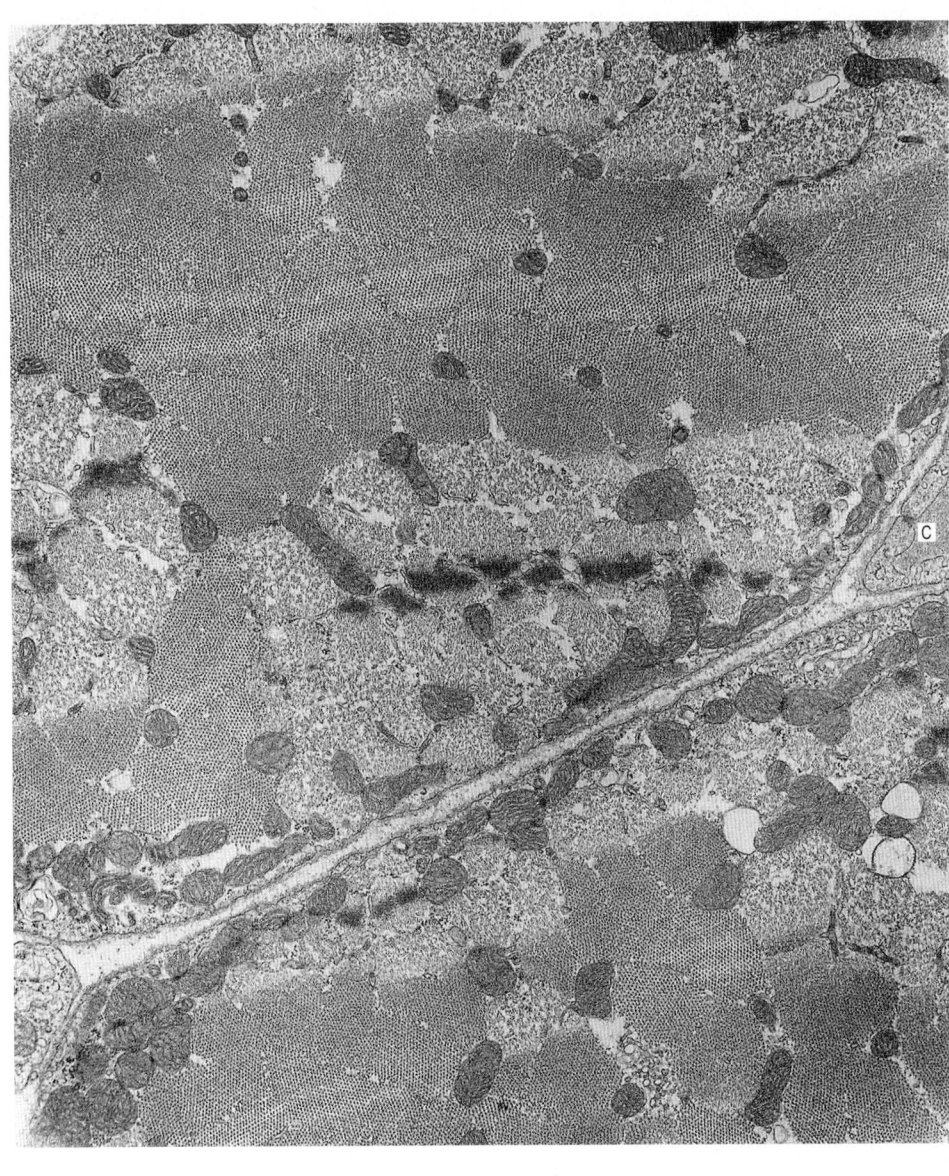

Fig. 6.46 Electron micrograph of skeletal muscle in transverse section, showing parts of two muscle fibres. Part of a capillary (C) is seen in transverse section in the endomysial space (right). The variation in the appearance of myofibrils in cross-section is explained in **Fig. 6.45**. (Photograph by Brenda Russell, Department of Physiology and Biophysics, University of Illinois at Chicago.)

muscles will survive and therefore be useful for pedicled or free tissue transfer procedures using techniques of plastic and reconstructive surgery. Type I muscles possess a single vascular pedicle supplying the muscle belly, e.g. tensor faciae latae (supplied by the ascending branch of the lateral circumflex femoral artery) and gastrocnemius (supplied by the sural artery). Type II muscles are served by a single dominant vascular pedicle and several minor pedicles, and can be supported on a minor pedicle as well as the dominant pedicle, e.g. gracilis (supplied by the medial circumflex femoral artery in the dominant pedicle). Type III muscles are supplied by two separate dominant pedicles each from different source arteries, e.g. rectus abdominus (supplied by the superior and inferior epigastric arteries) and gluteus maximus (supplied the superior and inferior gluteal arteries). Type IV muscles have multiple small pedicles which, in isolation, are not capable of supporting the whole muscle, e.g. sartorius and tibialis anterior: c.30% survive reduction onto a single vascular pedicle. Type V muscles have one dominant vascular pedicle and multiple secondary segmental pedicles, e.g. latissimus dorsi (supplied by the thoracodorsal artery as the primary pedicle, and thoracolumbar perforators from the lower six intercostal arteries and the lumbar arteries as the segmental supply), and pectoralis major (supplied by the pectoral branch of the thoracoacromial axis as the dominant pedicle, and anterior perforators from the internal thoracic vessels as the segmental supply).

In muscle cross-sections, the number of capillary profiles found adjacent to fibres usually varies from 0 to 3. Fibres that are involved in sustained activities, such as posture, are served by a denser capillary network than fibres which are recruited only infrequently. It is common for muscles to receive their arterial supply via more than one route. The accessory arteries penetrate the muscle at places other than the hilum, and ramify in the same way as the principal artery, forming vascular territories. The boundaries of adjacent territories are spanned by anastomotic vessels, sometimes at constant calibre, but more commonly through reduced-calibre arteries or arterioles which are referred to as 'choke vessels'. These arterial arcades link the territories into a continuous network.

Veins branch in a similar way, forming venous territories that correspond closely to the arterial territories. In the zones where the arterial territories are linked by choke vessels, the venous territories are linked by anastomosing veins, in this case without change of calibre. On either side of these venous bridges, the valves in the adjacent territories direct flow in opposite directions towards their respective pedicles, but the connecting veins themselves lack valves, and therefore permit flow in either direction.

Because of the potential for relative movement within muscle groups, vessels tend not to cross between muscles; rather, they radiate to them from more stable sites or cross at points of fusion. Where a muscle underlies the skin, vessels bridge between the two. These may be primarily cutaneous vessels, supplying the skin directly, but contributing small branches to the muscle as they pass through it, or they may be the terminal branches of intramuscular vessels, which leave the muscle to supplement the blood supply to the skin. The latter are less frequent where the muscle is mobile under the deep fascia. The correspondence between the vascular territories in the skin and underlying tissues has given rise to the concept of angiosomes, which are composite blocks of tissue supplied by named distributing arteries and drained by their companion veins.

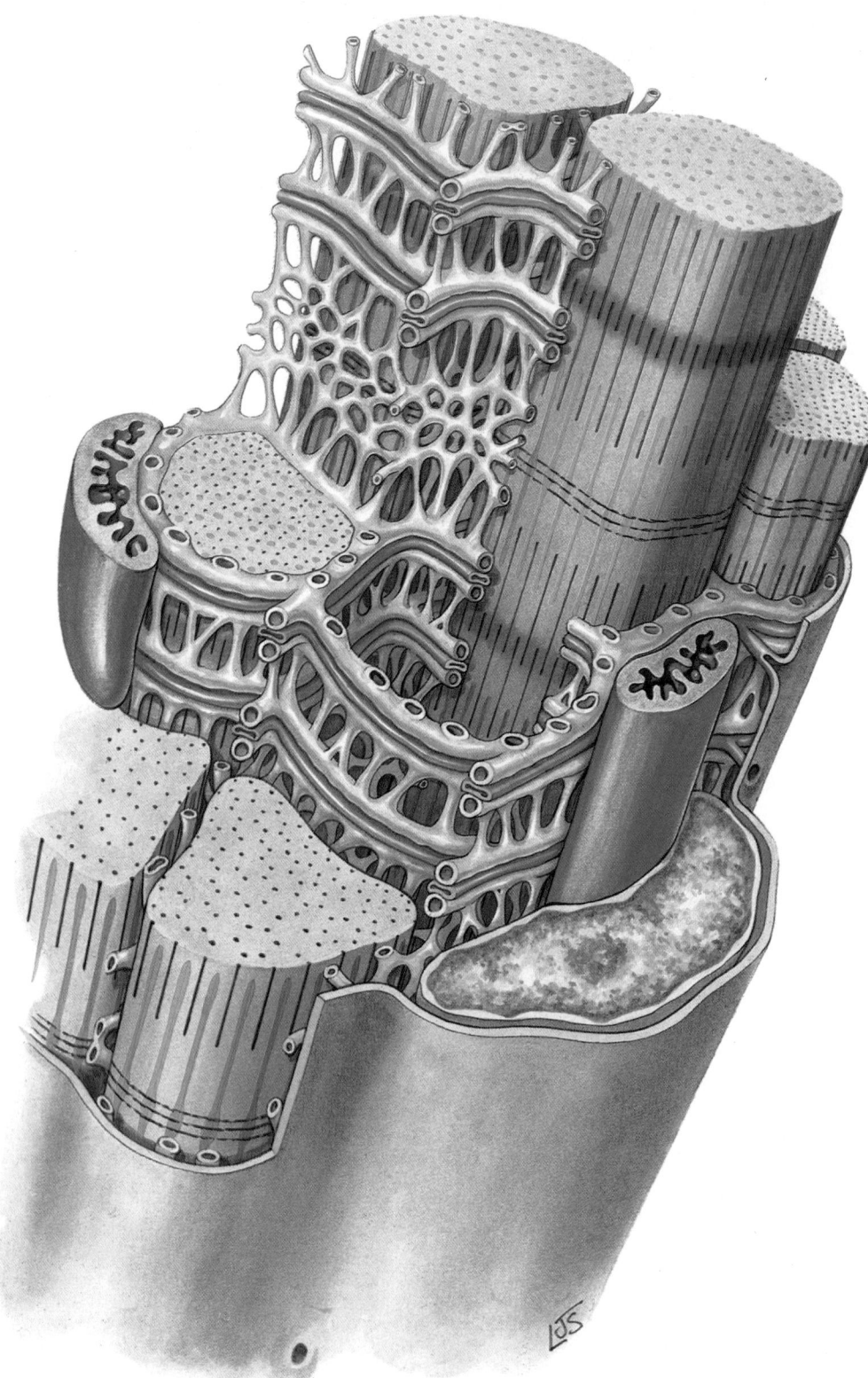

Fig. 6.47 Three-dimensional reconstruction of a mammalian skeletal muscle fibre, showing in particular the organization of the transverse tubules (orange) and sarcoplasmic reticulum (buff). Mitochondria (blue) lie between the myofibrils and a muscle nucleus (green) at the periphery. Note that transverse tubules are found at the level of the A/I junctions, where they form triads with the terminal cisternae of the sarcoplasmic reticulum. (Artist: Lesley Skeates.)

The pressure exerted on valved intramuscular veins during muscular contraction enables them to function as a 'muscle pump', promoting venous return to the heart. In some cases this role appears to be amplified by veins which pass through the muscle after originating elsewhere in superficial or deep tissues (Chapter 110). The extent to which the muscle capillary bed is perfused can be varied in accordance with functional demand. Arteriovenous anastomoses, through which blood can be returned directly to the venous system without traversing the capillaries, provide an alternative, regulated pathway.

The lymphatic drainage of muscles begins as lymphatic capillaries in epimysial and perimysial, but not endomysial, sheaths. These converge to form larger lymphatic vessels which accompany the veins, and drain to the regional lymph nodes.

INNERVATION

Every skeletal muscle is supplied by one or more nerves. In the limbs, face and neck there is usually a single nerve, although its axons may be derived from neurones in several spinal cord segments. Muscles such as those of the abdominal wall, which originate from several embryonic segments, are supplied by more than one nerve. In most cases, the nerve travels with the principal blood vessels within a neurovascular bundle, approaches the muscle near to its least mobile attachment, and enters the deep surface at a position which is more or less constant for each muscle.

Nerves supplying muscle are frequently referred to as 'motor nerves', but they contain both motor and sensory components. The motor component is mainly composed of large, myelinated α-efferent axons,

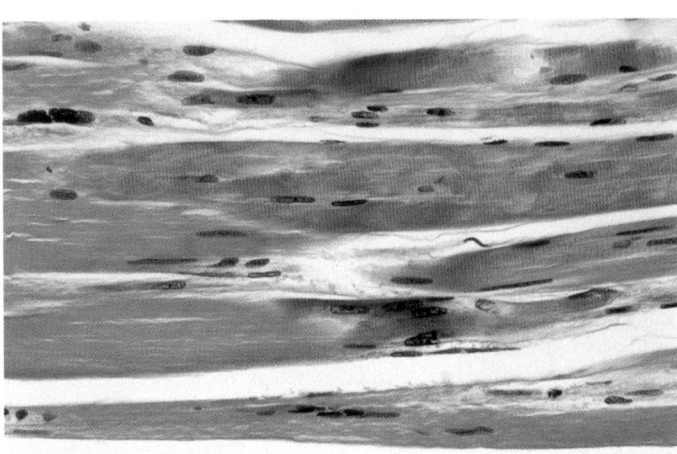

Fig. 6.48 Attachment of a tendon (orange) to skeletal muscle (pink). The regular dense connective tissue of the tendon consists of parallel bundles of type I collagen fibres which are orientated in the long axis of the tendon and the muscle to which it is attached. A few elongated fibroblast nuclei are visible. (Photograph by Sarah-Jane Smith.)

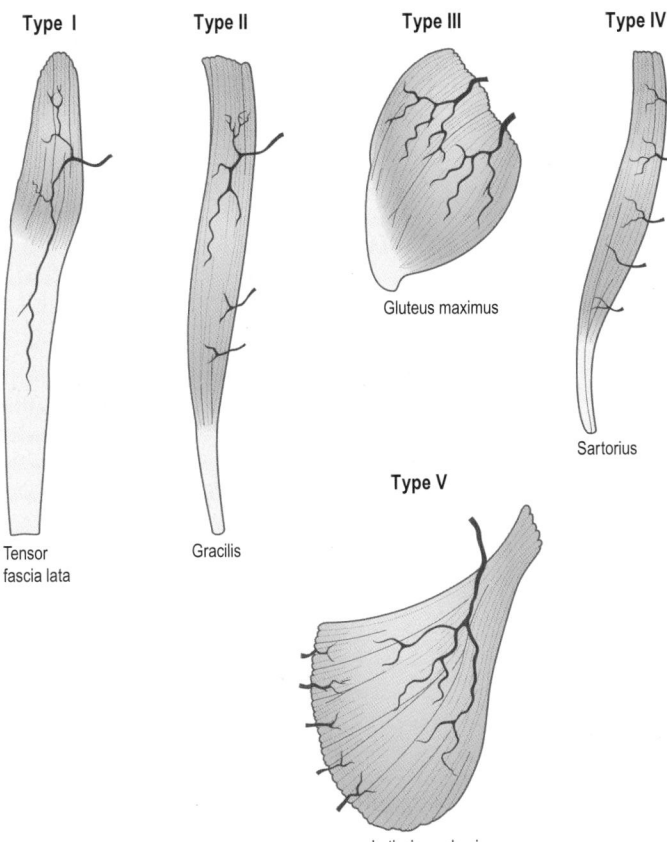

Type I — Tensor fascia lata

Type II — Gracilis

Type III — Gluteus maximus

Type IV — Sartorius

Type V — Latissimus dorsi

Fig. 6.49 Classification of muscles according to their blood supply. (By permission from Cormack GC, Lamberty BGH 1994 The Arterial Anatomy of Skin Flaps, 2nd edn. Edinburgh: Churchill Livingstone.)

which supply the muscle fibres, supplemented by small, thinly myelinated γ-efferents, or fusimotor fibres, which innervate the intrafusal muscle fibres of neuromuscular spindles, and fine, non-myelinated autonomic efferents (C fibres), which innervate vascular smooth muscle. The sensory component consists of large, myelinated IA and smaller group II afferents from the neuromuscular spindles, large myelinated IB afferents from the Golgi tendon organs, and fine myelinated and non-myelinated axons which convey pain and other sensations from free terminals in the connective tissue sheaths of the muscle. For further detail see page 56.

Within muscles, nerves follow the connective tissue sheaths, coursing in the epimysial and perimysial septa before entering the fine endomysial tissue around the muscle fibres. α-Motor axons branch repeatedly before they lose their myelinated sheaths and terminate near the middle of muscle fibres. These terminals tend to cluster in a narrow zone towards the centre of the muscle belly known as the motor point. Clinically, this is the place on the muscle from which it is easiest to elicit a contraction with stimulating electrodes. Long muscles generally have two or more terminals, or end-plate bands, because many muscle fibres do not run the full length of the anatomical muscle.

A specialized synapse, the neuromuscular junction, is formed where the terminal branch of an α-motor axon contacts the muscle fibre. The axon terminal gives off several short, tortuous branches each ending in an elliptical area, the motor end plate. Within the underlying discoidal patch of sarcolemma, the sole plate or subneural apparatus, the sarcolemma is thrown into deep synaptic folds (p. 64). This discrete type of neuromuscular junction is an example of an en plaque ending and is found on muscle fibres which are capable of propagating action potentials. A different type of ending is found on slow tonic muscle fibres, which do not have this capability, e.g. in the extrinsic ocular muscles, where these fibres form a minor component of the muscle. In this case the propagation of excitation is taken over by the nerve terminals, which branch over an extended distance to form a number of small neuromuscular junctions (en grappe endings). Some muscle fibres of this type receive the terminal branches of more than one motor neurone. The terminals of the γ-efferents that innervate the intrafusal muscle fibres of the neuromuscular spindle also take a variety of different forms.

The terminal branches of α-motor axons are normally in a 'one-to-one' relationship with their muscle fibres: a muscle fibre receives only one branch, and any one branch innervates only one muscle fibre. When a motor neurone is excited, an action potential is propagated along the axon and all of its branches to all of the muscle fibres that it supplies. The motor neurone and the muscle fibres that it innervates can therefore be regarded as a functional unit, the motor unit, which accounts for the more or less simultaneous contraction of a number of fibres within the muscle.

The size of a motor unit varies considerably. In muscles which are employed for precision tasks, e.g. extraocular muscles, interossei and intrinsic laryngeal muscles, each motor neurone innervates only c.10 muscle fibres, whereas in a large limb muscle, a motor neurone may innervate several hundred muscle fibres. Within a muscle, the fibres belonging to one motor unit are distributed over a wide territory, without regard to fascicular boundaries, and intermingle with the fibres of other motor units. The motor units become larger in cases of nerve damage, because denervated fibres induce collateral or terminal sprouting of the remaining axons. Each new branch can reinnervate a fibre, thus increasing the territory of its parent motor neurone.

MUSCLE CONTRACTION: BASIC PHYSIOLOGY

The arrival of an action potential at the motor end plate causes acetylcholine (ACh) to be released from storage vesicles into the 30–50 nm synaptic cleft that separates the nerve ending from the sarcolemma. ACh is rapidly bound by receptor molecules located in the junctional folds, triggering an almost instantaneous increase in the permeability, and hence conductance, of the postsynaptic membrane. This generates a local depolarization (the end-plate potential), which initiates an action potential in the surrounding area of sarcolemma. The activity of the neurotransmitter is rapidly terminated by the enzyme acetylcholinesterase (AChE), which is bound to the basal lamina in the sarcolemmal junctional folds. The sarcolemma is an excitable membrane, and action potentials generated at the neuromuscular junction propagate rapidly over the entire surface of the muscle fibre.

The action potentials are conducted radially into the interior of the fibre via the T-tubules, extensions of the sarcolemma: this ensures that all parts of the muscle fibre are activated rapidly and almost synchronously. Excitation–contraction coupling is the process whereby an action potential triggers the release of calcium from the terminal cisternae of the sarcoplasmic reticulum into the cytosol. This activates a calcium-sensitive switch in the thin filaments and so initiates contraction. At the end of excitation, the T-tubular membrane repolarizes, calcium release ceases, calcium ions are actively transported back to the calsequestrin stores by the calcium–ATPase pumps, and the muscle relaxes.

Electron microscopy shows that the lengths of the thick and thin filaments do not change during muscle contraction. The sarcomere shortens by the sliding of thick and thin filaments past one another, which draws the Z-discs towards the middle of each sarcomere (**Fig. 6.45**). As the overlap increases, the I- and H-bands narrow to extinction, while the width of the A-bands remains constant. Filament sliding depends on the making and breaking of bonds (cross-bridge cycling) between myosin head regions and the actin filaments. Myosin heads 'walk' along actin filaments (sliding the filaments past each other) using a series of short power strokes, each resulting in a relative movement of 5–10 nm. Actin filament binding sites for myosin are revealed only in the presence of calcium, which is released into the sarcoplasm from the sarcoplasmic reticulum, with the consequent repositioning of the troponin–tropomyosin complex on actin (the calcium-sensitive switch). Both myosin head binding and release are energy dependent (ATP binding is required for detachment of bound myosin heads as part of the normal cycle). In the absence of ATP (as occurs postmortem) the bound state is maintained, and is responsible for the muscle stiffness known as rigor mortis.

The summation of myosin power strokes leads to an average sarcomere shortening of up to 1 μm: because each muscle has thousands of sarcomeres in series along its length, the anatomical muscle shortens by a centimetre or more, depending on the muscle. For further details of actin–myosin interactions in muscle contraction, see Alberts et al (2002) and Pollard & Earnshaw (2002) (see Bibliography of selected titles for publication details).

SLOW TWITCH VS FAST TWITCH

The passage of a single action potential through a motor unit elicits a twitch contraction where peak force is reached within 25–100 ms, depending on the motor unit type involved. However, the motor neurone can deliver a second nervous impulse in less time than it takes for the muscle fibres to relax. When this happens, the muscle fibres contract again, building the tension to a higher level. Because of this mechanical summation, a sequence of impulses can evoke a larger force than a single impulse and, within certain limits, the higher the impulse frequency, the more force is produced ('rate recruitment'). The other strategy is to recruit more motor units. In practice, the two mechanisms appear to operate in parallel, but their relative importance may depend on the size and/or function of the muscle: in large muscles with many motor units, motor unit recruitment is probably the more important mechanism.

With the exception of rare tonic fibres, skeletal muscles are composed entirely of fibres of the twitch type. These fibres can all conduct action potentials but they are not the same in other respects. Some fibres obtain their energy very efficiently by aerobic oxidation of substrates, particularly of fats and fatty acids. They have large numbers of mitochondria and contain myoglobin, an oxygen-transport pigment related to haemoglobin. They are supported by a well-developed network of capillaries, which maintains a steady nutrient supply of oxygen and substrates. Such fibres are well suited to functions such as postural maintenance, in which moderate forces need to be sustained for prolonged periods. At the other extreme are fibres that have few mitochondria, little myoglobin, and a sparse capillary network. Their immediate energy requirements are met largely through anaerobic glycolysis, a route that provides prompt access to energy stores but is less sustainable than oxidative metabolism. Such fibres are capable of brief bursts of intense activity, but these must be separated by extended quiescent periods during which intracellular pH and phosphate concentrations, perturbed in fatigue, are restored to normal values and glycogen and other reserves are replenished.

These types of fibre tend to be segregated into different muscles in some animals; thus some muscles have a conspicuously red appearance, derived from the rich blood supply and high myoglobin content associated with a predominantly aerobic metabolism, whereas others have a much paler appearance, reflecting a more anaerobic character. These variations in colour led to the early classification of red and white muscles.

In man, all muscles are, in fact, mixed, with fibres that are specialized for aerobic working conditions intermingled with fibres of a more anaerobic or intermediate metabolic character. The different types of fibre are not readily distinguished in routine histological preparations but are clear when specialized enzyme histochemical techniques are used. On the basis of metabolic differences the individual fibres can be classified as predominantly oxidative, slow twitch (red) fibres, or glycolytic, fast twitch (white) fibres. Muscles composed mainly of oxidative, slow twitch fibres thus correspond to the red muscles of classical descriptions. This classification has now been largely superseded by myosin-based typing and the presence of specific disease-related enzymes (see below).

Muscles that are predominantly oxidative in their metabolism contract and relax more slowly than muscles relying on glycolytic metabolism. This difference in contractile speed is due in part to the activation mechanism (volume density of sarcotubular system and proteins of the calcium 'switch' mechanism), and in part to molecular differences between the myosin heavy chains of these types of muscle, which affect the ATPase activity of the myosin head; this in turn alters the kinetics of its interaction with actin, and hence the rate of cross-bridge cycling. Differences between myosin isoforms may be detected histochemically: ATPase histochemistry continues to play a significant role in diagnostic typing (**Table 6.2**). Two main categories have been described: type I fibres, which are slow-contracting, and type II, which are fast-contracting. Molecular analyses have revealed that type II fibres may be further subdivided according to their content of myosin heavy-chain isoforms into types IIA, IIB and IIX (Schiaffino & Reggiani, 1996). There is a correlation between categories and metabolism, and therefore with fatigue resistance, such that type I fibres are generally oxidative (slow oxidative) and resistant to fatigue, type IIA are moderately oxidative, glycolytic (fast oxidative glycolytic) and fatigue resistant, and IIB largely rely on glycolytic metabolism (fast glycolytic) and so are easily fatigued.

Fibre type transformation (Table 6.2)

The fibre type proportions in a named muscle may vary between individuals of different age or athletic ability. Fibre type grouping, where fibres with similar metabolic and contractile properties aggregate, increases after nerve damage and with age. It occurs as a result of reinnervation episodes, where denervated fibres are 'taken over' by a sprouting motor neurone and their type properties transformed under direction of the new motor neurone. If the nerves to fast white and slow red muscles are cut and cross-anastomosed in experimental animals, so that each muscle is reinnervated by the other's nerve, the fast muscle becomes slower-contracting, and the slow muscle faster-contracting (Buller et al 1960). These results were initially interpreted as the effects of neuronally delivered trophic factors on reinnervated muscle. However there is evidence that fibre type transformation may be a response to the patterns of impulse traffic in the nerves innervating the muscles. If fast muscles are stimulated continuously for several weeks at 10 Hz, which is a pattern similar to that normally experienced by slow muscles, they develop slow contractile characteristics and acquire a red appearance and a resistance to fatigue even greater than that of slow muscles.

Since the early 1970s, histochemical and biochemical studies have provided an increasingly detailed account of the phenotypic changes responsible for these stimulation-induced changes in contractile speed and fatigue resistance. The initial phase of slowing can be explained by less rapid cycling of calcium, the result of a reduction in the extent of the sarcoplasmic reticulum and changes in the amount and molecular type of proteins involved in calcium transport and binding. Chronic stimulation also triggers the synthesis of myosin heavy and light chain isoforms of the slow muscle type: the associated changes in cross-bridge kinetics result in a lower intrinsic speed of shortening. The muscle becomes more resistant to fatigue through changes in the metabolic pathways responsible for the generation of ATP. These consist of a reduced dependence on anaerobic glycolysis and a switch to oxidative pathways, particularly those involved in the breakdown of fat and fatty acids. There is an associated increase in capillary density and in the fraction of the intracellular volume occupied by mitochondria. These changes take place in an orderly sequence and bring about a complete transformation of fibre type. If stimulation is discontinued, the sequence of events is reversed and the muscle regains, over a period of weeks, all of its original characteristics. The reversibility of transformation is one of several lines of evidence that the changes take place within existing fibres, and not by a process of degeneration and regeneration.

Many of the changes in the protein profile of a muscle that are induced by stimulation are now known to be the result of regulatory events taking place at a pretranslational stage. For example, analysis

Table 6.2 Physiological, structural and biochemical characteristics of the major histochemical fibre types

Characteristics	Fibres types		
	Type I	**Type IIA**	**Type IIB**
Phyiological			
Function	Sustained forces, as in posture	—Powerful, fast movements—	
Motor neurone firing threshold	Low	Intermediate	High
Motor unit size	Small	Large	Large
Firing pattern	Tonic, low-frequency	—Phasic, high-frequency—	
Maximum shortening velocity	Slow	Fast	Fast
Rate of relaxation	Slow	Fast	Fast
Resistance to fatigue	Fatigue-resistant	Fatigue-resistant	Fatigue-susceptible
Power output	Low	Intermediate	High
Structural			
Capillary density	High		Low
Mitochondrial volume	High	Intermediate*	Low
Z-band	Broad	Narrow	Narrow
T and SR systems	Sparse		Extensive
Biochemical			
Myosin ATPase activity	Low		High
Oxidative metabolism	High	Intermediate*	Low
Anaerobic glycolysis	Low	Intermediate*	High
Calcium transport ATPase	Low		High

*Metabolic characteristics vary between species, and may show considerable overlap between fibre types. (See text for further detail and references.)

of the messenger RNA species encoding myosin heavy chain isoforms shows that expression of the fast myosin heavy chain mRNA is substantially suppressed within a few days of the onset of chronic stimulation, while the slow myosin heavy chain mRNA undergoes a corresponding increase.

Although myosin expression is responsive to the radical increase in use brought about by chronic stimulation, it tends to be stable under physiological conditions unless these involve a sustained departure from normal postural or locomotor behaviour. Other protein systems can change more easily: increases in enzymes of oxidative metabolism, for example, may be induced not only by chronic stimulation but also by exercise programmes, such as endurance training. These observations suggest that some muscle properties are continuously regulated by contractile activity, whereas myosin isoform transitions tend not to occur unless certain threshold levels of activity are crossed. Such a concept could help to explain how the influence of a parameter as variable as the pattern of activity reaching a muscle fibre can be reconciled with the existence of histochemically distinct classes of fibre.

The transformation of fibre type induced by increased contractile activity may be interpreted as evidence of a natural adaptive capacity of skeletal muscle fibres. According to this hypothesis, fibres subjected to sustained high levels of use tend to develop properties at the slow, fatigue-resistant end of the spectrum. These properties are suited to postural activity that involves maintenance of tension with little change of muscle length: the slow type of myosin is more energy efficient under these conditions, and a well-developed aerobic metabolism provides the capacity for generating ATP on a continuous basis. Fibres which are less active retain, or revert to, a native fast state. Their properties are suited to dynamic activity, for which instantaneous power is more important than endurance. The concept emerges of a machine which can optimize its properties to suit the type of work most often demanded of it. The functional matching of the neural and muscular elements of a motor unit may have its origins in connections that are established during development. There seems little doubt that it is finely tuned throughout adult life by the ability of the muscle fibres to adapt continuously to changes in their pattern of use.

The increased fibre type grouping which occurs with advancing age is probably neurogenic, and a consequence of a progressive reduction in the number of functioning motor units.

DEVELOPMENT OF SKELETAL MUSCLE

Most information about the early development of the skeletal musculature in man has been derived from other vertebrate species, principally chick, mouse, rat and sheep. However, where direct com-

parisons with the developing human embryo have been made, the patterns and mechanisms of muscle formation have been found to be the same, and the animal studies may therefore be assumed to provide an appropriate model.

A myogenic lineage, denoted by the expression of myogenic determination factors, can be demonstrated transitorily in some cells shortly after their ingression through the primitive streak. Skeletal muscle found throughout the body is derived from this paraxial mesenchyme, which is formed from ingression at the streak and subsequently segmented into somites (*see also* the origin of extraocular muscles, Chapter 43).

Skeletal muscle originates from a pool of premyoblastic cells which arise in the dermatomyotome of the maturing somite and begin to differentiate into myoblasts at 4–5 weeks of gestation. By 6 weeks, cells have migrated from the dermatomyotomal compartment to form the myotome in the centre of the somite (**Fig. 47.3**). These myotomal precursor cells are identified by the expression of myogenic determination factors; they will eventually differentiate within the somite to form the axial (or epaxial) musculature (erector spinae). A distinct cohort of precursor cells migrates away from the somite to invade the lateral regions of the embryo; there they form the muscles of the limbs, limb girdles and body wall (hypaxial musculature; see **Fig. 47.3**). Virtually all cells in the lateral half of the newly formed somite are destined to migrate in this way. Myogenic determination factors are not expressed in these cells until the muscle masses coalesce. The appearance of myotomal myoblasts, and the migration of myoblasts to the prospective limb region, occurs first in the occipital somites. Thereafter these processes follow the general craniocaudal progression of growth, differentiation and development of the embryo. The myoblastic cells from which the limb muscles develop do not arise in situ from local limb bud mesenchyme, as was once thought, but migrate from the ventrolateral border of those somites adjacent to the early limb buds.

MYOGENIC DETERMINATION FACTORS

The myogenic determination factors Myf-5, myogenin, MyoD and Myf-6 (herculin) are a family of nuclear phosphoproteins. They have in common a 70-amino-acid, basic helix-loop-helix (bHLH) domain that is essential for protein–protein interactions and DNA binding. Outside the bHLH domain there are sequence differences between the factors which probably confer some functional specificity. The myogenic bHLH factors play a crucial role in myogenesis. Forced expression of any of them diverts non-muscle cells to the myogenic lineage. They activate transcription of a wide variety of muscle-specific genes by binding directly to conserved DNA sequence motifs (–CANNTG– known as E-boxes) which occur in the regulatory regions (promoters and enhancers) of these genes. Their effect may be achieved cooperatively, and can be repressed, e.g. by some proto-oncogene products. Some of the bHLH proteins can activate their own expression. Accessory regulatory factors, whose expression is induced by the bHLH factors, provide an additional tier of control.

The myogenic factors do not all appear at the same stage of myogenesis (Buckingham et al 2003). In the somites *Myf-5* is expressed early, before myotome formation, and is followed by expression of myogenin. *MyoD* is expressed relatively late together with the contractile protein genes. *Myf-6* is expressed transitorily in the myotome and becomes the major transcript postnatally. Whether this specific timing is important for muscle development is not yet clear. The creation of mutant mice deficient in the bHLH proteins (gene 'knock-out') has shown that *myogenin* is crucial for the development of functional skeletal muscle, and that while neither *Myf-5* nor *MyoD* is essential to myogenic differentiation on their own, lack of both results in a failure to form skeletal muscle. In the limb bud the pattern of expression of the bHLH genes is generally later than in the somite: *Myf-5* is expressed first but transitorily, followed by *myogenin* and *MyoD*, and eventually *Myf-6*. These differences provide evidence at the molecular level for the existence of distinct muscle cell populations in the limb and somites. It may be that the myogenic cells which migrate to the limb differ at the outset from those that form the myotome, or their properties may diverge subsequently under the influence of local epigenetic factors.

FORMATION OF MUSCLE FIBRES

In both myotomes and limb buds, myogenesis proceeds in the following way. Myoblasts become spindle-shaped and begin to express muscle-specific proteins. The mononucleate myoblasts aggregate and fuse to form multinucleate cylindrical syncytia, or myotubes, with the nuclei aligned in a central chain (**Figs 6.50, 6.51**). These primary myotubes attach at each end to the tendons and developing skeleton. The initiation of fusion does not depend on the presence of nerve fibres, since these do not penetrate muscle primordia until after the formation of primary myotubes.

Although fusion of myoblasts is not a prerequisite for the synthesis of the contractile machinery, synthesis proceeds much more rapidly after fusion. Sarcomere formation begins at the Z-disc, which binds actin filaments to form I–Z–I complexes. The myosin filaments assemble on the I–Z–I complexes to form A-bands. Nebulin and titin are among the first myofibrillar proteins to be incorporated into the sarcomere, and may well determine the length and position of the contractile filaments. Intermediate filaments connect the Z-discs to the sarcolemma at an early stage, and these connections are retained.

Myogenic cells continue to migrate and to divide, and during weeks 7–9 there is extensive de novo myotube formation. Myoblasts aggregate near the midpoint of the primary myotubes and fuse with each other to form secondary myotubes, a process which may be related to early neural contact. Several of these smaller diameter myotubes may be aligned in parallel with each of the primary myotubes. Each develops a separate basal lamina and makes independent contact with the tendon. Initially, the primary myotube provides a scaffold for the longitudinal growth of the secondary myotubes, but eventually they separate. At the time of their formation, the secondary myotubes express an 'embryonic' isoform of the myosin heavy chains, whereas the primary myotubes express a 'slow' muscle isoform apparently identical to that found in adult slow muscle fibres. In both primary and secondary myotubes, sarcomere assembly begins at the periphery of the myotube and progresses inwards towards its centre. Myofibrils are added constantly and lengthen by adding sarcomeres to their ends. T-tubules are formed, and grow initially in a longitudinal direction. Since they contain specific proteins not found in plasma membranes, they are probably assembled via a different pathway from that which supports the growth of the sarcolemma. The sarcoplasmic reticulum wraps around the myofibrils at the level of the I-bands.

By 9 weeks, the primordia of most muscle groups are well defined, contractile proteins have been synthesized and the primitive beginnings of neuromuscular junctions can be observed, confined initially to the primary myotubes. Although some secondary fibre formation can take place in the absence of a nerve, most is initiated at sites of innervation of the primary myotubes. The pioneering axons subsequently branch and establish contact with the secondary myotubes. By 10 weeks the nerve–muscle contacts have become functional neuromuscular junctions and the muscle fibres contract in response to impulse activity in the motor nerves. Under this new influence the secondary fibres express

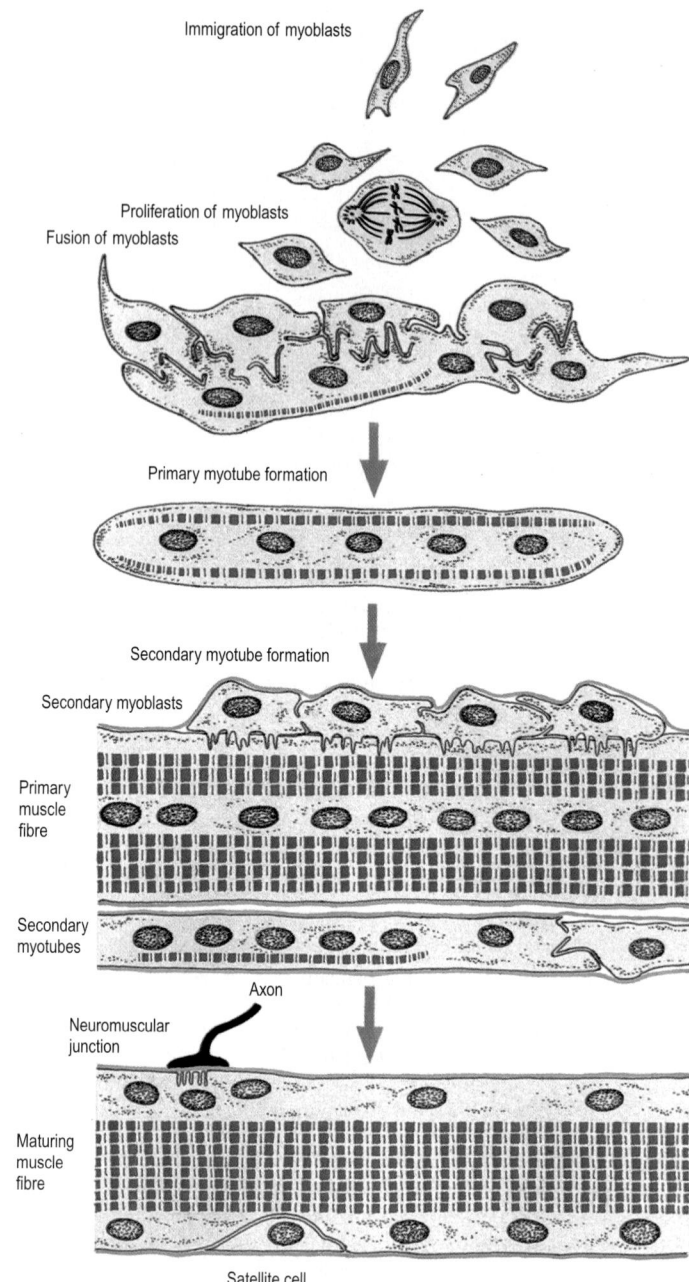

Fig. 6.50 Stages in formation of skeletal muscle. Mononucleate myoblasts fuse to form multinucleate primary myotubes, characterized initially by central nuclei. Midway along the primary myotubes other myoblasts begin to fuse, forming secondary myotubes. As the contractile apparatus is assembled, the nuclei move to the periphery, cross-striations become visible and primitive features of the neuromuscular junction emerge. Later, small adult-type myoblasts – satellite cells – can be seen lying between the basal lamina and the plasmalemma of the muscle fibre. (By permission from Terry Partridge, Department of Histology, Charing Cross Medical School, and Yvonne Edwards, MRC Human Biochemical Genetics Unit, University College, London.)

'fetal' (sometimes referred to as 'neonatal') isoforms of the myosin heavy chains. At this stage several crucial events take place which may be dependent on, or facilitated by, contractile activity. As the myofibrils encroach on the centre of the myotube, the nuclei move to the periphery, and the characteristic morphology of the adult skeletal muscle myofibre is established. The myofibrils become aligned laterally, and cross-striations are visible at the light microscopic level. T-tubules change from a longitudinal to a transverse orientation and adopt their adult positions: they may be guided in this process by the sarcoplasmic reticulum, which is more strongly bound to the myofibrils.

The myotubes and myofibres are grouped into fascicles by growing connective tissue sheaths, and the fascicles are assembled to build up

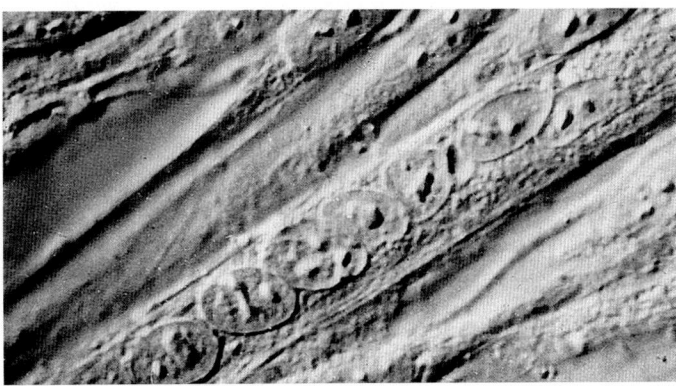

Fig. 6.51 Cultured muscle cells, showing the fusion of myoblasts to form myotubes. Note the chain of centrally placed nuclei. (Photograph reproduced by permission from Jones DA, Round JM 1990 Skeletal muscle in health and disease. Manchester: Manchester University Press.)

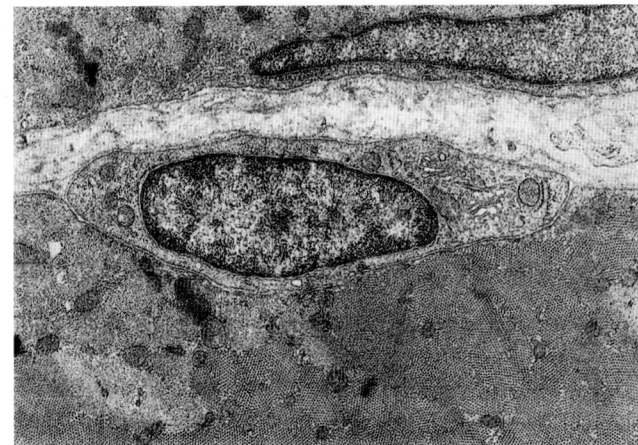

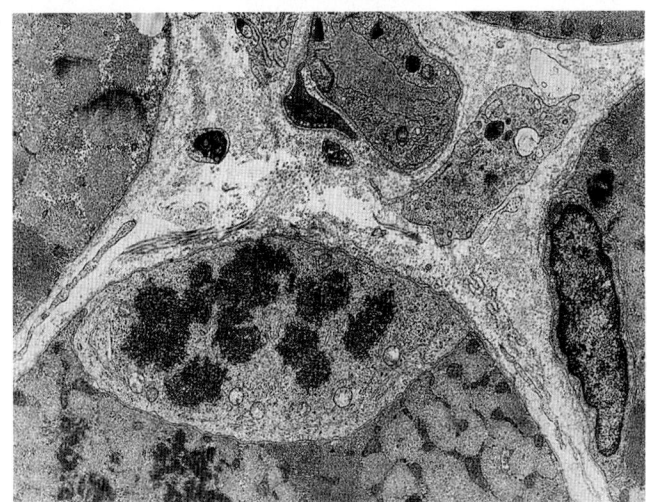

Fig. 6.52 A, A satellite cell. Note the two plasma membranes that separate the cytoplasm of the satellite cell from that of the muscle fibre, and the basal lamina of the muscle fibre, which continues over the satellite cell (see also **Fig. 6.40**). Compare this appearance with the normal muscle nucleus which is seen in the adjacent fibre. **B,** A satellite cell in mitosis. Normal skeletal muscle nuclei are incapable of division. A second, non-mitotic satellite cell is seen in the adjacent fibre on the right. (Photographs by Michael Cullen, School of Neurosciences, University of Newcastle upon Tyne.)

entire muscles. As development proceeds, the increase in intramuscular volume is accommodated by remodelling of the connective tissue matrix.

At 14–15 weeks, primary myotubes are still in the majority, but by 20 weeks the secondary myotubes predominate. During weeks 16–17, tertiary myotubes appear: they are small and adhere to the secondary myotubes, with which they share a basal lamina. They become independent by 18–23 weeks, their central nuclei move to the periphery, and they contribute a further generation of myofibres. The secondary and tertiary myofibres are always smaller and more numerous than the primary myofibres. In some large muscles, higher order generations of myotubes may be formed.

Late in fetal life, a final population of myoblasts appears which become the satellite cells of adult muscle. These normally quiescent cells lie outside the sarcolemma beneath the basal lamina (**Figs 6.50, 6.52A**). M-cadherin, a cell adhesion protein of possible regulatory significance, occurs at the site of contact between a satellite cell and its muscle fibre. In a young individual, there is one satellite cell for every 5–10 myonuclei. Myonuclei are incapable of DNA synthesis and mitosis, and satellite cells are therefore important as the sole source of additional myonuclei during postnatal growth of muscle (to maintain the normal ratio of cytoplasmic volume per nucleus) (**Fig. 6.52B**). After satellite cells divide, one of the daughter cells fuses with the growing myofibres, the other remains as a satellite cell capable of further rounds of division. Similar events may take place to support exercise-induced hypertrophy of adult skeletal muscle. Satellite cells provide a reservoir of myoblasts capable of initiating regeneration of an adult muscle after damage. Other stem cell populations may also be induced to begin a myogenic differentiation pathway, e.g. bone marrow stem cells and processed lipoaspirate cells (Mizuno et al, 2002).

The development of fibre types

Developing myotubes express an embryonic isoform of myosin which is subsequently replaced by fetal and adult myosin isoforms. The major isoform of sarcomeric actin in fetal skeletal muscle is cardiac α-actin; only later is this replaced by skeletal α-actin. The significance of these developmental sequences is not known.

The pattern of expression is fibre-specific as well as stage-specific. In primary myotubes, embryonic myosin is replaced by adult slow myosin from c.9 weeks onwards. In secondary and higher order myotubes the embryonic myosin isoform is superseded first by fetal and then by adult fast myosin, and a proportion go on to express adult slow myosin. Other fibre-specific, tissue-specific and species-specific patterns of myosin expression have been described in mammalian limb muscles and jaw muscles.

The origin of this diversity in the temporal patterns of expression of different fibres – even within the same muscle – is far from clear. It has been suggested that intrinsically different lineages of myoblast emerge at different stages of myogenesis or in response to different extracellular cues. If this is the case, their internal programmes may be retained or overridden when they fuse with other myoblasts or with fibres that have already formed. The fibres that emerge from this process go on to acquire

a phenotype that will depend on the further influence of hormones and neural activity.

In man, unlike many smaller mammals, muscles are histologically mature at birth, but fibre type differentiation is far from complete. In postural muscles the expression of type I myosin increases significantly over the first few years of life; during this period the fibre type proportions in other muscles become more divergent. The presence in adult muscles of a small proportion of fibres with an apparently transitional combination of protein isoforms reinforces the view that changes in fibre type continue to some extent in all muscles and throughout adult life.

Fibre type transitions also occur in relation to damage or neuromuscular disease; under these conditions, the developmental sequence of myosins may be recapitulated in regenerating fibres.

Growth and regulation of fibre length

Muscle fibres grow in length by addition of sarcomeres to the ends of the myofibrils. It is important that the number of sarcomeres is regulated throughout life, so that the mean sarcomere length, and hence filament overlap, is optimized for maximum force. This is achieved by addition or removal of sarcomeres in response to any prolonged change of length. For example, if a limb is immobilized in a plaster cast, the fibres of muscles which have been fixed in a shortened position lose sarcomeres, while those which have been fixed in a lengthened position add sarcomeres; the reverse process occurs after the cast has been removed.

FORM AND FUNCTION IN SKELETAL MUSCLES

DIRECTION OF ACTION (Figs 6.39, 6.53)

Although muscles differ in their internal architecture, the resultant force is directed along the line of the tendon: any forces transverse to this direction must therefore be in balance. In strap-like muscles, the transverse component is negligible. In fusiform, bipennate and multipennate muscles, symmetry in the arrangement of the fibres produces a balanced opposition between transverse components, whereas the fibres in asymmetrical, e.g. unipennate, muscles generate an unopposed lateral component of force which is balanced by intramuscular pressure.

Muscles which incorporate a twist in their geometry unwind it as they contract, so that they tend not only to approximate their attachments but also to bring them into the same plane. Muscles which spiral around a bone tend to reduce the spiral on contraction, imparting rotational force.

FORCE AND RANGE OF CONTRACTION

The force developed by an active muscle is the summation of the tractive forces exerted by millions of cross-bridges as they work asynchronously in repeated cycles of attachment and detachment. This force depends on the amount of contractile machinery that is assembled in parallel, and therefore on the cross-sectional area of the muscle. The phrase 'contractile machinery' has been chosen deliberately here. Mechanically, it matters little that the myofilaments are assembled into myofibrils, the myofibrils into fibres, and the fibres into fascicles: it is the total area occupied by myofilamentous arrays that determines force (**Fig. 6.40**). If the fibres are small, the force will be influenced only to the extent that more of the cross-sectional area will be occupied by non-contractile elements, e.g. endomysial connective tissue. If there are many small fascicles, the amount of perimysial connective tissue in the cross-section will increase.

The range of contraction generated by an active muscle depends on the relative motion that can take place between the overlapping arrays of thick and thin filaments in each sarcomere. In vertebrate muscle, the construction of the sarcomere sets a natural limit to the amount of shortening that can take place: from the minimum overlap to the maximum overlap of the thick and thin filaments represents a shortening of c.30%. Since the sarcomeres are arranged in series, the muscle fibres shorten by the same percentage. The actual movement that takes place at the ends of the fibres will depend on the number of sarcomeres in series, i.e. it will be proportional to fibre length. By way of illustration, compare the behaviour of two muscles, fixed at one end, with fibres parallel to the line of pull and the same cross-sectional area. If one muscle is twice as long as the other, then the force developed by each muscle will be the same, but the maximum movement produced at the free ends will be twice as much for the longer muscle. Muscles in which the fibres are predominantly parallel to the line of pull are often long and thin (strap-like): they develop rather low forces, but are capable of a large range of contraction. Where greater force is required the cross-sectional area must be increased, as occurs in a pennate construction (**Fig. 6.54**). Here, the fibres are set at an angle to the axis of the tendon (the angle of pennation). The range of contraction produced by such a muscle will be less than that of a strap-like muscle of the same mass, because the fibres are short and a smaller fraction of the shortening takes place in the direction of the tendon. The obliquely directed force can be resolved vectorially into two components, one acting along the axis of the tendon, and one at 90° to this. In symmetrical forms, such as that illustrated in **Fig. 6.54**, the transverse force is balanced by fibres on the opposite side of the tendon. The functionally significant component is the one acting along the axis of the tendon. As the lengths of the vectors show, less force is available in this direction than is developed by the fibres themselves. In practice, this loss is not very great: angles of pennation are usually less than 30°, and so the force in the direction of the tendon may be 90% or more of that in the fascicles (cos 30° = 0.87). Angulation of a set of fibres reduces both the force and range of contraction along the axis of the tendon. However, these negative consequences are outweighed by the design advantage conferred by pennation, i.e. the opportunity to extend the tendinous aponeurosis, and so increase the area available for the attachment of muscle fibres. A given mass of muscle can then be deployed as a large number of short fibres, increasing the total cross-sectional area, and hence the force, available. In a multipennate muscle, the effective cross-sectional area is larger still, and the fibres tend to be even shorter. The 'gearing' effect of

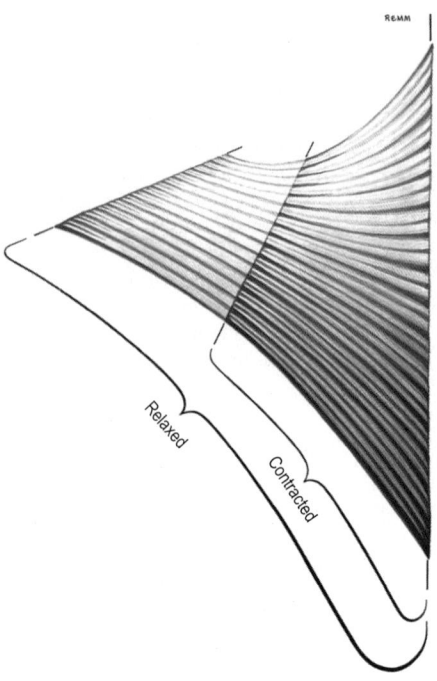

Fig. 6.53 The 'detorsion' or untwisting which results from the contraction of a spirally arranged muscle.

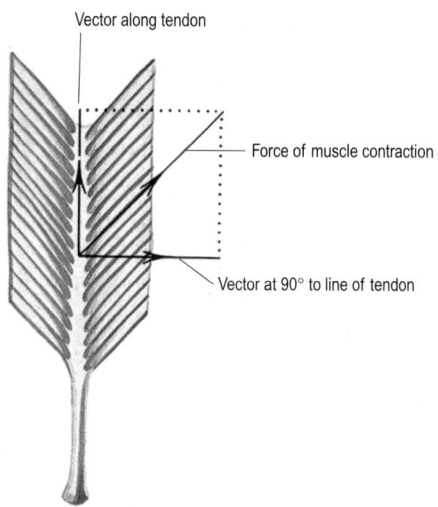

Fig. 6.54 Force vectors in an idealized pennate muscle. The increase in effective cross-sectional area made possible by this architecture outweighs the small reduction in the component of force acting in the direction of the tendon.

pennation on a muscle therefore results from an internal exchange of fibre length for total fibre area: this allows much greater forces to be developed, but at the expense of a reduced range of contraction.

Although the terms power and strength are often used interchangeably with force, they are not synonymous. Power is the rate at which a muscle can perform external work and is equal to force × velocity. Since force depends on the total cross-sectional area of fibres, and velocity (the rate of shortening) depends on their length, power is related to the total mass of a muscle. Strength is usually measured on intact subjects in tasks which require the participation of several muscles, when it is as much an expression of the skillful activation and coordination of these muscles as it is a measure of the forces which they contribute individually. Thus it is possible for strength to increase without a concomitant increase in the true force-generating capacities of the muscles involved, especially during the early stages of training.

MUSCLES AND MOVEMENT

Historically, attempts were made to elucidate the actions of muscles by gross observation. The attachments were identified by dissection, and the probable action deduced from the line of pull. With the use of localized electrical stimulation it became possible to study systematically the actions of selected muscles in the living subject. This approach was pioneered above all by Duchenne de Boulogne (1867). Such knowledge is necessarily incomplete: a study of isolated muscles, whether by dissection postmortem or stimulation *in vivo*, cannot reveal the way in which those muscles behave in voluntary movements, in which several muscles may participate in a variety of synergistic and stabilizing roles. Duchenne appreciated this, and supplemented his use of the induction coil with clinical observations on patients with partial paralysis to make more accurate deductions about the way in which muscles acted together in normal movement. Manual palpation can be used to detect contraction of muscles during the performance of a movement, but tends to be restricted to superficially placed muscles, with examination taking place under quasi-static conditions. Modern knowledge of muscle action has been acquired almost entirely by recording the electrical activity which accompanies mechanical contraction, a technique known as electromyography (EMG). This technique can be used to study voluntary activation of deep as well as superficial muscles, under static or dynamic conditions. Multiple channels of EMG can be used to examine coordination between the different muscles which participate in a movement. These data can be further supplemented by adding transducers such as goniometers and force plates to monitor joint angle and ground reaction force, and by recording the movement simultaneously on videotape or with a full three-dimensional motion analysis system.

Actions of muscles

Conventionally, the action of a muscle is defined as the movement that takes place when it contracts. However, this is an operational definition: equating 'contraction' with shortening, and 'relaxation' with lengthening, is too simple in the context of whole muscles and real movements. Whether a muscle approximates its attachments on contraction depends on the degree to which it is activated, and the forces against which it has to act. The latter are generated by gravity and inertia; any external contact or impact; actively, by opposing muscles; and passively, by the elastic and viscous resistance of all the structures which undergo extension and deformation, some within the muscle itself, others in joints, inactive muscles and soft tissues. Depending on the conditions, an active muscle may therefore maintain its original length or shorten or lengthen, and during this time its tension may increase, decrease or stay the same. Movements that involve shortening of the active muscle are termed concentric, e.g. biceps/brachialis contraction raising a weight and flexing the elbow; movements in which the active muscle undergoes lengthening are termed eccentric, e.g. lowering the weight previously mentioned. As the elbow extends so the biceps/brachialis 'pays out' length. Eccentric contractions are associated with increased risk of muscle tears, especially in the hamstrings. Muscle contraction which does not involve change in muscle length is isometric.

Natural movements are accomplished by groups of muscles. Each muscle may be classified, according to its role in the movement, as a prime mover, antagonist, fixator or synergist.

It is usually possible to identify one or more muscles which are consistently active in initiating and maintaining a movement: they are its prime movers. Muscles which wholly oppose the movement, or initiate and maintain the opposite movement, are antagonists, e.g. brachialis has the role of prime mover in elbow flexion, and triceps is the antagonist. To initiate a movement, a prime mover must overcome passive and active resistance and impart an angular acceleration to a limb segment until the required angular velocity is reached; it must then maintain a level of activity sufficient to complete the movement. Antagonists may be transiently active at the beginning of the movement, and thereafter they remain electrically quiescent until the deceleration phase, when units are activated to arrest motion. During the movement, the active prime movers are not completely unrestrained, and are balanced against the passive, inertial and gravitational forces mentioned above.

When prime movers and antagonists contract together they behave as fixators, stabilizing the corresponding joint by increased transarticular compression, and creating an immobile base on which other prime movers may act, e.g. flexors and extensors of the wrist co-contract to stabilize the wrist when an object is grasped tightly in the fingers. In some cases, sufficient joint stability can be afforded by gravity, acting either on its own, e.g. knee and hip joints when they are in or near the close-packed position in the erect posture, or in conjunction with a single prime mover, e.g. the shoulder joint when it is stabilized with supraspinatus with the arm pendent. In other cases, and whenever strong external forces are encountered, prime movers and antagonists contract together, holding the joint in any required position.

Acting across a uniaxial joint, a prime mover produces a simple movement. Acting at multiaxial joints, or across more than one joint, prime movers may produce more complex movements which contain elements that have to be eliminated by contraction of other muscles. The latter assist in accomplishing the movement, and are considered to be synergists, although they may act as fixators, or even as partial antagonists of the prime mover. For example, flexion of the fingers at the interphalangeal and metacarpophalangeal joints is brought about primarily by the long flexors, superficial and deep. However, these also cross intercarpal and radiocarpal joints, and if movement at these joints was unrestrained, finger flexion would be less efficient. Synergistic contraction of the carpal extensors eliminates this movement, and even produces some carpal extension, which increases the efficiency of the desired movement at the fingers.

In the context of different movements, a given muscle may act as a prime mover, antagonist, fixator or synergist. Even the same movement may involve a muscle in different ways if it is assisted or opposed by gravity. For example, in thrusting out the hand, triceps is the prime mover responsible for extending the forearm at the elbow, and the flexor antagonists are largely inactive. However, when the hand lowers a heavy object, the extensor action of the triceps is replaced by gravity, and the movement is controlled by active lengthening, i.e. eccentric contraction, of the flexors. It is important to remember that all movements take place against the background of gravity, and its influence must not be overlooked.

BIOMECHANICS

Two fields of study are relevant here: osseokinematics, which deals primarily with overall bone movements with little reference to joints, and arthrokinematics, which is concerned with the analysis of articular movements. For further details, see Panjabi & White (2001).

SHAPE OF ARTICULAR SURFACES

Although the usual classification of synovial joints into seven types is based on shape, this does not entail a like number of fundamentally different surface shapes. Articular surfaces are never truly flat, nor exactly parts of spheres, cylinders, cones or ellipsoids (**Fig. 6.55**). They are more nearly parts of surfaces of ovoids (**Fig. 6.55**) or compounded of more than one such surface. When these are either convex or concave, they may be termed ovoid articular surfaces. Sellar surfaces are convex in one plane and concave at approximately right angles to this plane – the curvatures are convex or concave ovoid profiles. Articular profiles vary from nearly flat to nearly spheroidal: evidence increasingly indicates that all are ovoid or sellar (**Fig. 6.56**).

Certain terms which are applied to ovoid surfaces and their properties are relevant to the movements of articular surfaces and of whole bones. Two points on an ovoid may be joined by a chord, a curved line which is the shortest distance between them, or by an arc, which is any line longer than a chord (**Fig. 6.57**). Any point moving on an ovoid surface traces a chordal or an arcuate line, or a succession of lines, as will be considered further below. (This usage of chord and arc may be unfamiliar to the reader because the terms are usually applied to circles on plane surfaces. To clarify the concept, imagine two points on a plane but deformable surface. The shortest route which joins them is a straight line or chord (geodesic); any longer route is an arc (non-geodesic). Even if the plane surface is now formed into a sphere, cylinder, ovoid, sellar surface, etc., the relation between chord and arc is preserved.)

A figure enclosed by three chords is a triangle (**Fig. 6.57**). The sum of its angles is more than 180° on an ovoid surface, less than 180° on a sellar surface, and precisely 180° when it is flat. The extent of deviation from 180° depends on the degree of curvature, an important concept in

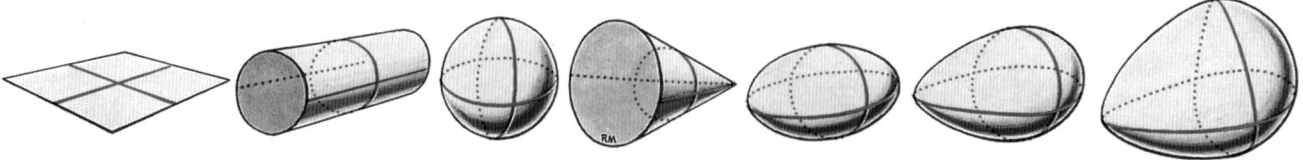

Fig. 6.55 A variety of geometric figures to which reference is commonly made in simple classifications of synovial joints. However, such comparisons are rough approximations only: no synovial joint possesses articular surfaces which are truly plane, cylindrical, spherical, conical or ellipsoid. Commonplace simple and compounded ovoids are included for comparison.

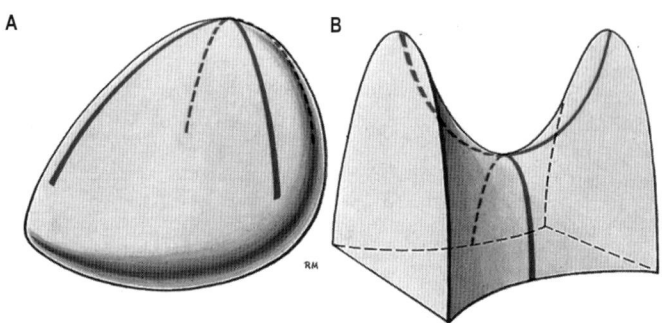

Fig. 6.56 The two fundamental geometric types of articular surface. (Note that ovoid surfaces may be 'almost flat' or 'almost spherical': the majority show intermediate grades of curvature and marked variation in change of radius from place to place. Sellar surfaces may also be compound and have a marked asymmetry, e.g. at the ankle and patellofemoral joints.) **A**, Ovoid, which may be convex or concave. The compound solid body illustrated presents different ovoid profiles in two planes at right angles, and that the curvatures of the two may be different. **B**, Sellar or saddle-shaped surfaces, which are concavoconvex. In practice, the curvature of both types of surface may show considerable variation.

MECHANICAL AXES OF BONES

Bones are irregular, and their articular surfaces bear no simple or symmetrical relation to their form. The concept of a mechanical axis enables accurate comparisons of the movements of the individual bones which articulate at a joint. In **Fig. 6.59A**, a hypothetical symmetrical long bone is shown with a terminal joint in the mid-range of movement. A rod through the bone, ending perpendicular to the articular centre, is its mechanical axis: it can represent the bone when articular movements are considered. In this special case of symmetry, the mechanical axis coincides with the shaft. In **Fig. 6.59B**, the joint is again in the mid-range of movement, but the bone is not symmetrical, and consequently the mechanical axis and shaft diverge widely. Thus articular movements result in similar displacements relative to the mechanical axis, whereas movement of the shaft is different. (See below for varieties of 'spin' and 'swing'.) Despite the usefulness of referring to a mechanical axis in some analyses, in others it is less helpful because it is difficult to define a 'central articular point' with precision. Definition of a single mechanical axis in spheroidal multiaxial joints may be an insufficient datum point for the many possible combinations of potential movements. The mechanical axis might be better defined as the axis of the most habitual conjunct rotation, which is limited by the close-packed position of the joint concerned.

MOVEMENTS OF BONES

Apart from passive accessory movements caused by external forces, all other movements are rotations. This term is often used in a restricted sense, and has acquired an associated terminology. Any bone which rotates only around its stationary mechanical axis is said to show pure spin, and any point on the bone, outside the axis, describes an arc of a circle, with the axis as its centre (**Fig. 6.59**). All other displacements of bone and axis are swings, which may be pure (**Fig. 6.59C**) or impure, when spin also occurs (**Fig. 6.59D**). (In a spheroidal joint virtually pure spin is theoretically possible around many alternative 'mechanical axes'.)

Another useful concept is the so-called ovoid of motion. During any swing, a point on the mechanical axis, distant from its related joint, describes a curved path in space: all such possible paths (**Fig. 6.60**) are on part of the surface of an ovoid (as would be expected, since they are generated from such an articular surface). The area and shape of ovoids of motion vary for individual bones and articular surfaces. During any

arthrokinematics (see below). Any three-sided figure in which at least one side is an arc is a trigone.

Sectional profiles of ovoid surfaces reveal two properties. First, the radius of curvature varies continuously. A profile is considered to be a series of short segments of circles of different radii, and a line joining their centres is the evolute of the profile (**Fig. 6.58A**). When a bone rotates by sliding on such a profile the movement is referred not to one axis, but to successive points on the evolute. Second, if a segment of a concave surface slides on a larger but similarly curved convex ovoid surface, the two will fit perfectly only in one position (**Fig. 6.58B**) (cf. close-packed position, described below). In all other positions, the surfaces are not perfectly congruent, the area of contact is much reduced, and cuneiform intervals separate them elsewhere. (Theoretically, in a 'perfect', incompressible ovoid, contact would be linear; in reality contact is over an area due to surface undulations and deformability of articular cartilage.)

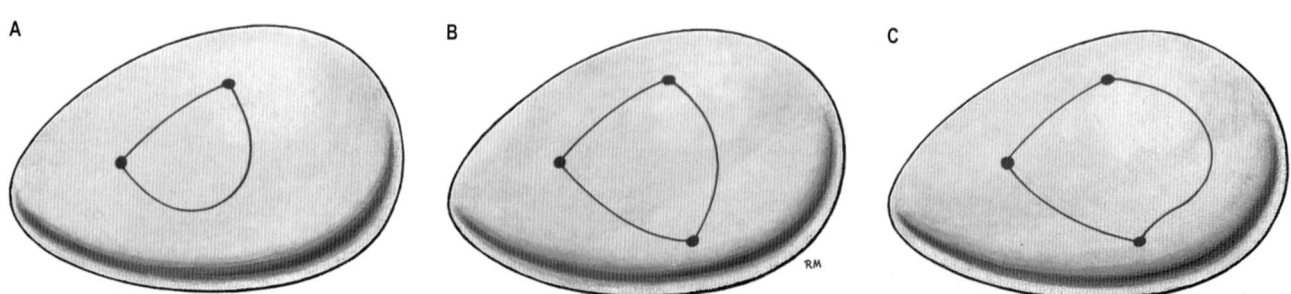

Fig. 6.57 Geometric paths across ovoid surfaces, and three-sided figures enclosed by such paths. **A**, A chord (the shortest path between two points) and one example of an arc (any longer path between the points). **B**, A triangle enclosed by three chords. **C**, A trigone, a three-sided figure in which one or more sides is an arc.

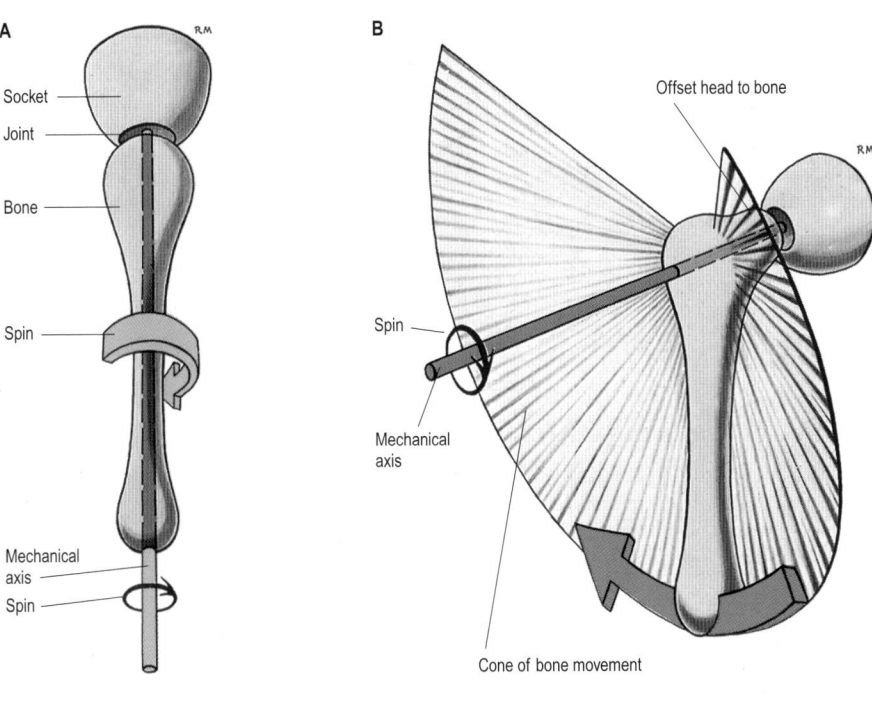

Fig. 6.58 **A**, Profile of a section through an ovoid surface showing that it may be considered as a series of segments of circles of changing radius. The (dashed) line joining the centres of the circles is the evolute of the profile. **B**, A small section of an ovoid profile (red) in various positions, in relation to a more extensive profile (black). The two fit perfectly (i.e. are fully congruent) in only one position.

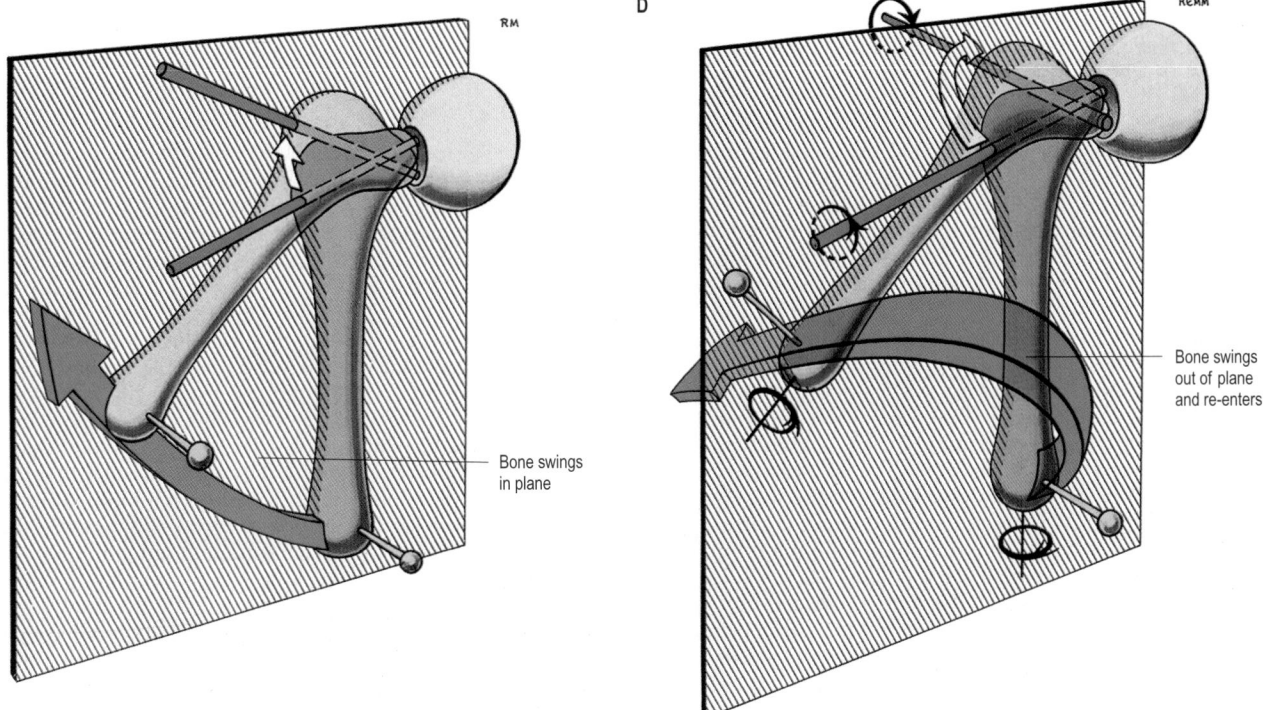

Fig. 6.59 **A**, The mechanical axis in a hypothetically simple, symmetrical long bone with a terminal joint: a 'spin' occurs around the axis. **B**, The mechanical axis in a bone with an offset head: a similar 'spin' occurs between the articular surfaces, but the shaft of the bone traces part of the surface of a cone. **C**, A cardinal swing. Note that the mechanical axis moves in one plane. (Its proximal end traces a chordal path at the joint, and its distal end traces a chordal path on the ovoid of motion.) There is no spin. **D**, An arcuate swing. Note that the bone moves out of the plane illustrated and then returns to it. The ends of the mechanical axis trace arcuate paths at the joint and on the ovoid motion. There is an associated spin or conjunct rotation around the mechanical axis (and a rotation around the long axis of the bone shaft).

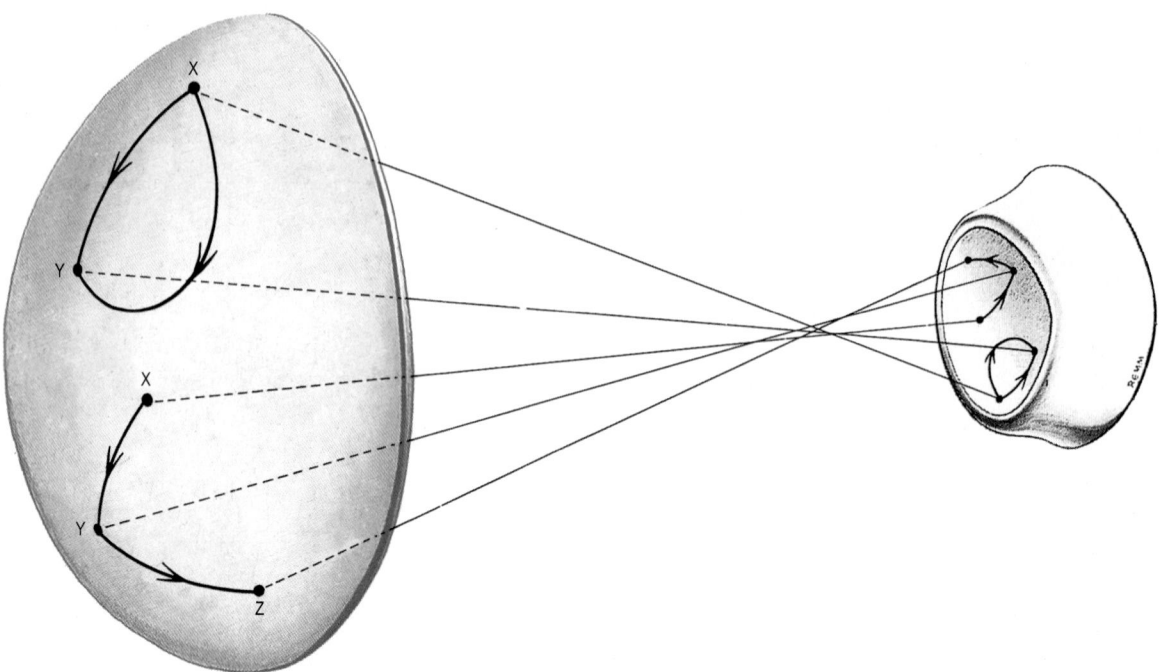

Fig. 6.60 The ovoid of motion represents an imaginary surface which would include all possible paths of a point on the mechanical axis at some distance from its related joint. Two points on the ovoid of motion are joined by a chordal and by an arcuate path, and the reciprocal movements of the end of the axis at the joint surface are shown. A succession of two movements at an angle to each other (i.e. a diadochal movement) is also illustrated.

particular swing, a point on the mechanical axis moves from X to Y on the ovoid of motion either along a chord (a cardinal swing) or by a longer route from X to Y (an arcuate swing). Synchronously the articular end of the axis traces a reciprocal chord or arc across its opposing articular surface. During a cardinal swing along a chord (an unusual movement) there is no associated spin; in an arcuate swing there must be some spin which is functionally significant (see below). Spin also occurs if a movement involves two chords in series at an angle to each other (one form of diadochal movement), e.g. X to Y and Y to Z in **Fig. 6.60**.

Spin was long undetected in some apparently simple swings of bones. That it occurs can be predicted mathematically, and it is usually verifiable by careful inspection or cineradiography. In **Fig. 6.61A**, three points, A, B and C, are on the surface of a sphere, and AB, BC, and CD are the chords between them. AB and AC are 'lines of longitude' which meet the equator at 90° at B and C. A model limb moves successively along chords A–B, B–C, C–A; it has 'spun' 90° (which is the amount by which the sum of angles of 'triangle' ABC exceeds 180°) between its initial and final positions. **Fig. 6.61B** shows intermediate 'lines of longitude'; in each case spin equals the sum of the three angles minus 180°. This relation holds mathematically for all ovoid or sellar surfaces. Spin is imparted during the B–C movement (i.e. along a second chord at an angle to the first). An arcuate path may be analysed as a series of chords which change angle. These spins, inevitable in certain swings, are conjunct (coupled) rotations and characteristic of sellar and most ovoid joints. Habitual movements at all joints always involve some demonstrable conjunct rotation.

Other rotations are adjunct, as a consequence of the interplay of gravity, external forces and muscle action. They occur only in joints with two or more degrees of freedom, and may be associated with conjunct rotation. Where there is no conjunct rotation, factors causing adjunct rotation may generate pure spin. Where conjunct rotation occurs, the effects of adjunct rotation may be in the same sense (additive), e.g. both 'clockwise', which increases rotation and is therefore termed a co-spin. Alternatively, an adjunct rotation may be in the opposite sense, which reduces or nullifies the effects of conjunct rotation and is termed an anti-spin. Thus a bone starting one or a succession of arcuate swings which, if unmodified, would involve some conjunct rotation, may also be subjected to nullifying anti-spin: the latter may be gradual, applied throughout a movement, or sudden, and near its end. While the path of the bone is a more or less complex

arcuate swing, it is modified to become quasichordal, because there is no net spin.

MOVEMENTS AT ARTICULAR SURFACES

The 'fit' of ovoid surfaces is precise only at one end of the most common excursion of the joint, which is a feature of the close-packed position. In all other positions the surfaces are not fully congruent, and the joint is 'loose-packed'. Changes in congruity at the shoulder joint are illustrated in **Fig. 6.62**.

Where articular surfaces are not fully congruent, movements can be analysed into spin, slide and roll (**Fig. 6.63**). In most natural movements these are combined. With a moving convex surface, slide and roll are simultaneous but opposite; with a moving concave surface they are in the same direction. Both combinations increase possible angulation, without a comparable increase in articular surface area, and so maximize the potential range of motion for a given joint.

JOINT POSITIONS

Ovoid or sellar surfaces are fully congruent in only one position, which is at one extreme of the most habitual articular movement, e.g. full extension at the knee, wrist and interphalangeal joints, dorsiflexion at the ankle, abduction with lateral rotation at the shoulder. As full congruence is approached, the attachments of the fibrous capsule and ligaments increasingly separate and become taut, and the conjunct rotation of all natural movements imposes a spiral twist in them. In final close-packing, surfaces are fully congruent, in maximal contact and tightly compressed or 'screwed-home'. The fibrous capsule and ligaments are maximally spiralized and tensed, and no further movement is possible. Close-packed surfaces cannot be separated by normal external force (as they may be in other positions), and bones can be regarded as temporarily locked, as if no joint existed. Close-packing is a final, limiting position, and any force which tends to further change can only be resisted by contraction of appropriate muscles. Failure to stop further movement results in injury to joint structures. Therefore movement just short of close-packing is physiologically most important. Ligaments and articular cartilage are to a small degree elastically deformable: in the final stages of close-packing the articular position is an equilibrium between the external torque applied (often gravity) and resistance to tissue deformation by the tense, twisted capsule and

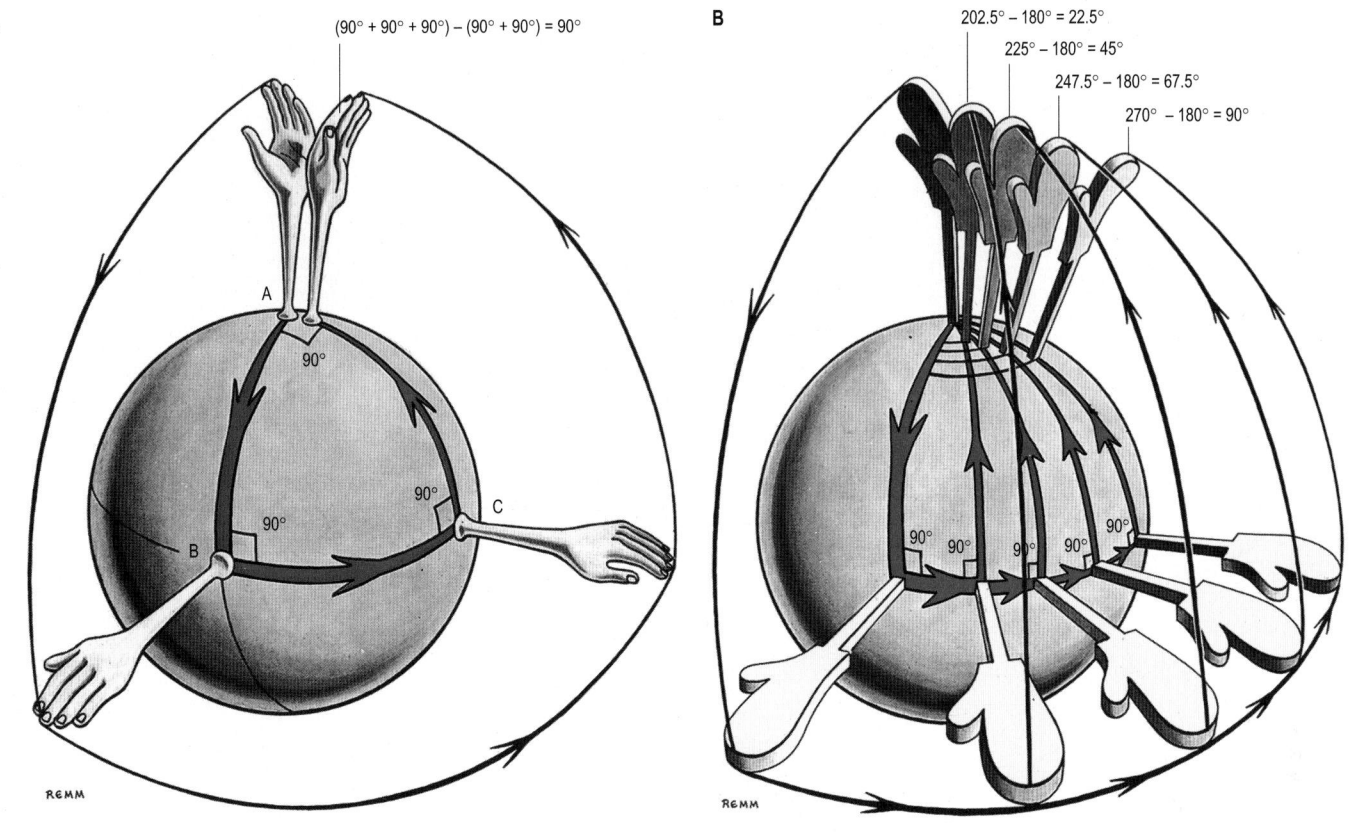

A (90° + 90° + 90°) – (90° + 90°) = 90°

B 202.5° – 180° = 22.5°
225° – 180° = 45°
247.5° – 180° = 67.5°
270° – 180° = 90°

Fig. 6.61 The 'spin' or conjunct rotation which accompanies a diadochal movement. A model hand and arm moves over the surface of a sphere, first along a line of longitude, then one of latitude to return along a line of longitude. **A**, The arm traverses three chordal paths which enclose a 'triangle' with three right angles (i.e. the sum of the angles = 270°). Note that as it passes along the line of latitude from B to C, a spin of 90° is imparted. **B**, The amount of spin imparted during a diadochal movement varies with the length and angulation of the second stage of the movement.

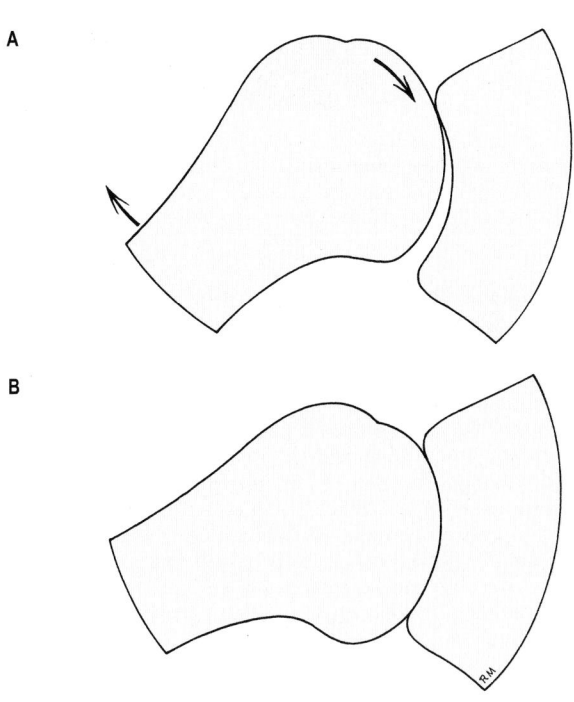

Fig. 6.62 Congruence of articular surfaces. **A**, In loose-packed positions of a joint, e.g. the shoulder, the surfaces are not congruent (this has been over-emphasized for clarity). **B**, The close-packed position of a joint with close-fitting, or full congruence, of the surfaces.

compressed cartilage surfaces. In symmetrical standing, the knee and hip joints approach close-packed positions sufficiently to maintain an erect posture with minimal energy.

In all other positions the articular surfaces are not congruent and parts of the capsule are lax; the joint is said to be loose-packed. Capsules are sufficiently lax near the mid-range of many movements to allow separation of the articulating surfaces by external forces. Congruence in which a convex surface has a smaller radius than a concave one is advantageous because it allows combined spin, roll and slide; contact area is greatly reduced and variable – which may diminish friction and erosion, although increasing joint surface contact pressures; small cuneiform intervals between the surfaces around the contact areas contain synovial fluid (their shape is perhaps a factor in maintaining efficient lubrication and nutrition of avascular articular cartilages); a combination of sliding and rolling increases the effective range of movement. Movements requiring slide or roll alone can be achieved only when articulating surfaces are more extensive.

According to MacConaill & Basmajian (1977) the close- and loose-packed positions of joints are as shown in Table 6.3.

Opinions may vary in connection with some of the positions in Table 6.3, e.g. a 'close-packed' position may possibly occur in occasional joints at both extremes of the range of movement. It is difficult to assess the situation in small tarsal and carpal joints and the first carpometacarpal joints. Intervertebral movements are the result of integrated simultaneous changes at all elements which make up the intervertebral articular complex, and perhaps should not be included in **Table 6.3**. However, most of the positions given above do correspond with postures adopted when maximal stress is encountered.

ACCESSORY MOVEMENTS

Movements actively performed at any joint do not always include all that its structure permits. Certain movements, which are either

131

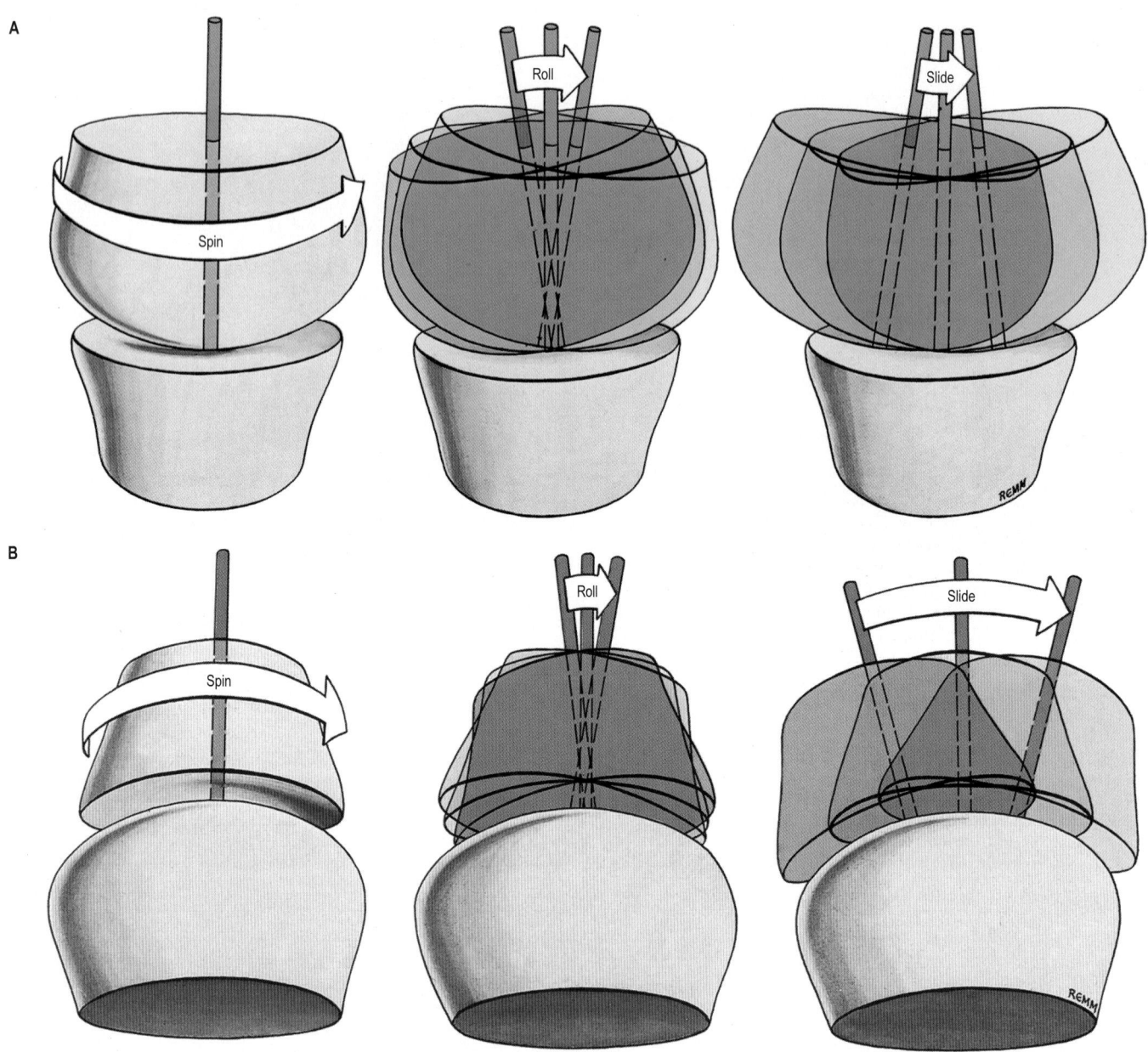

Fig. 6.63 An analysis of the types of movement which occur, usually in combination, between articular surfaces when a convex surface moves over a stationary concave surface (**A**); and a concave surface moves on a stationary convex surface (**B**).

Table 6.3 The close- and loose-packed positions of joints (Data from MacConaill MA, Basmajian JV 1977 Muscles and Movements, 2nd edn. New York: Kriger.)

Joint	Close-packed position	Loose-packed position
Shoulder	Abduction + lateral rotation	Semiabduction
Ulnohumeral	Extension	Semiflexion
Radiohumeral	Semiflexion + semipronation	Extension + supination
Wrist	Dorsiflexion	Semiflexion
2nd–5th metacarpo-phalangeal	Full flexion	Semiflexion + ulnar deviation
Interphalangeal (fingers)	Extension	Semiflexion
1st carpometacarpal	Full opposition	Neutral position of thumb
Hip	Extension + medial rotation	Semiflexion
Knee	Full extension	Semiflexion
Ankle	Dorsiflexion	Neutral position
Tarsal joints	Full supination	Semipronation
Metatarsophalangeal	Dorsiflexion	Neutral position
Interphalangeal (toes)	Dorsiflexion	Semiflexion
Intervertebral	Extension	Neutral position

voluntarily impossible or limited in range, can only be produced maximally when resistance to active movements occurs (accessory movements, first type), e.g. the fingers can only be maximally rotated at the metacarpophalangeal joints when a solid object is grasped in the hand. (However, a moderate degree of rotation of the non-grasping fingers towards the centre of the palm during flexion and its converse during extension is commonplace.) Some movements can be produced only passively (accessory movements, second type), and their widest range is obtained when the muscles of a joint are relaxed, e.g. when the supported arm is passively abducted at the shoulder, the humerus can be distracted from the glenoid cavity. These movements are commonly termed 'passive', but all movements, active or not, can be made passively when the muscles concerned are relaxed. The term 'accessory' will be used for all movements which are impossible in the absence of resistance.

LIMITATION OF MOVEMENTS/STABILITY

Movements are limited by several factors, of which tension in the joint capsule and ligaments is probably the most obvious, e.g. during attempted hyperextension of the unfixed cadaveric knee or hip.

Increasing ligamentous tension, balanced by increased compression between opposed articular surfaces, are integral factors in producing close-packing, and they limit most habitual movements. The tension of antagonistic muscles is equally important and involves passive elastic components of the muscles and other periarticular soft tissues, and reflex contraction of the muscles (when stimulation of mechanoreceptors in articular and periarticular tissues reaches a critical level). For example, flexion at the hip is much more limited in range when the knee is extended. When the knee is flexed, the hamstring muscles are relaxed and this allows flexion of the thigh to the abdominal wall. Approximation of soft parts also limits some movements, e.g. flexion at the elbow and knee. Contact (occlusion) of teeth obviously limits mandibular elevation, and contact between the bones making a joint will limit excursion, e.g. between the posterior femur and posterior tibia during knee flexion.

Joints are always subject to forces in multiple directions, such as from applied loads, gravity and muscle activity. Joint stability is essential to prevent injury and provide an efficient fulcrum for muscle action. Static stability is a function of joint configuration, i.e. joint surfaces and intra-articular structures such as menisci; the capsule and ligaments; and passive tension in the muscles and tendons crossing the joint. In some joints a negative intra-articular pressure, i.e. a vacuum, might assist achievement of stability. Dynamic stability is provided by the coordinated activity of the muscles acting on the joint which provide a net joint compression. Even when a joint would be expected to be distracted, e.g. at the dependent wrist when holding a suitcase, the joint surface is subject to compression by the stabilizing action of muscles. Posture can be actively manipulated to enhance stability. This is especially true at the shoulder, when the scapula is rotated to best position the inclination of the glenohumeral joint to maintain stability.

For each joint there is an interplay between static and dynamic stability. The price of static stability tends to be a reduced range of motion. Comparison of the hip and shoulder illustrates this well. It is not surprising that the highly mobile glenohumeral joint is commonly associated with clinical problems related to instability, or that physiotherapy rehabilitation programmes play a very important role in the treatment of glenohumeral instability.

ATTACHMENTS AND LEVERS: THE BIOMECHANICS OF MOVEMENT

Skeletal muscles have a limited range of contraction, for two reasons. First, the fibres themselves must work within inherent limits imposed by their sarcomeric construction. Second, the internal design of many muscles can reduce the excursion at the tendon still further if short, oblique fibres have been used to deliver force at the expense of range of contraction. Where it is necessary to produce a greater range of movement, this is achieved through the action of the muscles on the bony levers of the skeleton.

To produce a large range of movement, force has to be applied close to the axis of a joint. An example of this is given in **Fig. 6.64A**, based on the action of triceps on the olecranon, which produces extension at the elbow. The closeness of the muscle attachment to the joint produces a large arc of motion at the hand. However, this motion could be prevented by applying to the hand a force very much less than that developed by the muscle. In fact, the force available at any point along the forearm, wrist and hand is reduced by the same factor as the range of motion is increased. (Note, however, that the action of triceps surae on the calcaneus to produce plantar flexion of the non-weightbearing foot represents a first-class lever system.) This type of lever, in which force is applied on one side of the joint axis, and loads which resist motion appear on the other, is known as a lever of the first class. In levers of the second class, the load appears between the force and the joint axis. This is illustrated in **Fig. 6.64B**, where plantar flexion of the weight-bearing foot raises the body. The principle involved is similar to raising the handles of a loaded wheelbarrow. In contrast to the previous example, the range of motion of the load is actually less than that produced by the muscle, and the force is multiplied by the same factor. The nutcracker action of molar teeth is obtained in a similar way. In levers of the third class, the force is applied between the load and the joint axis. This is illustrated in **Fig. 6.64C**, based on the contribution to flexion at the elbow produced by the action of biceps brachii. The effect is similar to that in the first example, i.e. an increase in the range of motion, but a decrease in the available force.

Most of the levers of the body are of the first and third class: in each case they are arranged to produce a magnified version of the movement at the muscle tendon, either in the opposite sense (first class) or in the same sense (third class), and in each case this is achieved at the expense of a reduction in usable force. This effect is greater when the moving muscle attachment is closer to the joint. At first sight it seems paradoxical that the fibre architecture of so many muscles should be designed to maximize force at the expense of overall shortening, when their force has then to be scaled down by levers in order to achieve the desired range of motion. There are, however, biological advantages to such an arrangement. For example, it is far more compact, which means that the limbs can be lighter and more slender. This trend is most obvious in fast-moving animals, such as horses, in which lever lengths are increased by running on the toes, and the powerful muscle masses lie close to the body, where they do not add significantly to the inertia of the extremities.

In **Fig. 6.64A–C**, the force is shown acting approximately at 90° to the lever in each case. A force in this direction produces the greatest turning effect. However, it is more usual for only part of the force exerted by a muscle to be directed in this way. The general case is illustrated in **Fig. 6.65**; a muscle is shown crossing the joint between the two bones, one fixed and one mobile.

The force exerted by the muscle has two main consequences:

Turning effect

The tendency of the force (F) to turn the bones about a joint is measured in terms of the turning moment (M). This is simply the product: $M = F \times L$ where L is the moment arm (**Fig. 6.65A**). Note that the latter is not the distance between the muscle attachment and the joint: it is the perpendicular distance between the line of pull of the muscle and the instantaneous centre of rotation. Thus the turning moment takes account of the magnitude of the force exerted by the muscle, the positions of the muscle attachments relative to the joint, the degree of angulation of the joint, and the shape of the articulating surfaces. The turning effect of the force (F) can be regarded as that of a smaller force directed at right angles to the axis of the mobile bone (blue arrow in **Fig. 6.65B**), referred to in some analyses as the transaxial, swing, or spurt component.

This description of the turning effect of a single muscle is complete only when movement takes place in one plane. The muscle may be attached to the mobile bone at a point which lies to one side or other of this plane. In this case contraction will introduce an additional turning effect, sometimes referred to as the spin component. In **Fig. 6.65B**, this component will tend to rotate the shaft of a bone about its axis.

Reaction at a joint

Newton's Third Law demands that the force on a bone is balanced by an equal and opposite reactive force generated at a joint. The reactive force can be resolved into components which are normal and tangential to the surfaces at the principal point of contact (**Fig. 6.65C**).

The normal (i.e. perpendicular) component (Fc) results from compression of the articulating surfaces. The presence of this component contributes to the stability of a joint by helping to maintain articular contact, particularly during rapid swings, when an unresisted centrifugal force would tend to separate the joint surfaces (MacConaill & Basmajian 1977). It is referred to in some analyses as the transarticular, paraxial, or shunt component.

The tangential component (Fs) represents the reaction to a shear force. If this shear force were unopposed, it would tend to produce translation of the articulating surfaces. A degree of translational movement is a normal feature of movement at some joints, but ultimately it must be resisted or disarticulation will occur. The tangential component supplies the required balancing force. In practice, it is a composite generated by gravitational and inertial forces; the elastic and viscous resistance of structures in and around the joint, including the ligaments, articular capsule and surrounding soft tissues, which are translated, stretched or compressed by the movement; and the restraining action of other muscles.

Normally more than one muscle acts at a joint. Each contributes a turning moment, and these turning moments can be added arithmetically. The resultant moment may impart angular acceleration to the mobile bone in either a clockwise direction (flexion in **Fig. 6.65A**)

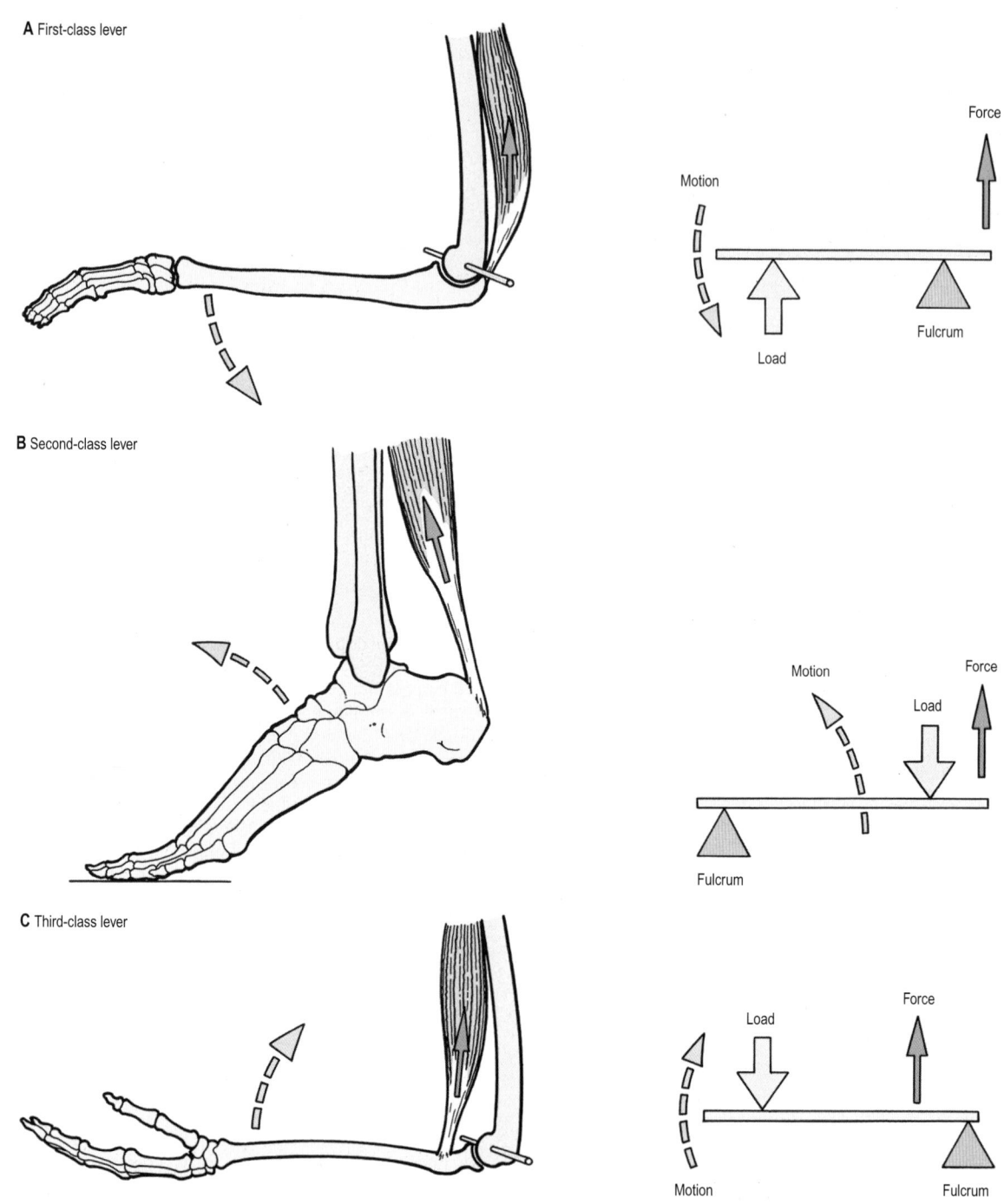

A First-class lever

Force

Motion

Load

Fulcrum

B Second-class lever

Motion

Force

Load

Fulcrum

C Third-class lever

Force

Load

Motion

Fulcrum

Fig. 6.64 The types of lever found in the body. **A**, First-class levers. **B**, Second-class levers. **C**, Third-class levers.

or an anti-clockwise direction. Similarly, summation of the spin components yields a resultant moment which may maintain the position of the shaft or rotate it about its axis in either direction. Each muscle also generates a reactive force at a joint, and these have to be added vectorially. Stability of a joint demands that when this resultant force is taken together with the gravitational and passive components already mentioned, and with the forces generated by any external contact or impact, the overall effect is neutral.

As an example, many of these elements may be seen in the actions of muscles around the shoulder joint when the arm is raised. During the initial stages of abduction, the force exerted by the acromial fibres of deltoid has a strong shear component which, if unresisted, would translate the humeral head upwards in the glenoid cavity. This is counteracted in part by gravity, but more importantly by the downward pull of subscapularis, infraspinatus and teres minor. The turning moment exerted by deltoid on the humeral shaft then adds to the moment exerted by supraspinatus to abduct the arm. The value of the

analytical approach outlined briefly here is that it enables the progression from such a verbal description to a quantitative understanding of the biomechanics of movement (Panjabi & White 2001).

Many muscles work in the manner indicated in **Fig. 6.65**, from a more stable attachment to a more mobile one. The stable attachment, which would normally be part of a heavier and more proximal structure, is commonly referred to as the origin, and the more mobile attachment, which would typically be lighter and more distal, is referred to as the insertion. Thus, in a muscle such as latissimus dorsi, the aponeurotic attachments to the vertebral column, pelvis and ribs constitute the origin, and the tendinous attachment to the highly mobile humerus constitutes the insertion. Although the relative mobility of these attachments can be reversed, e.g. during climbing, there is little difficulty about defining habitual use. For other muscles, such as rectus abdominis, it is less easy to identify the more mobile attachment. It is not, therefore, functionally meaningful to try to define an 'origin' and 'insertion' for every muscle.

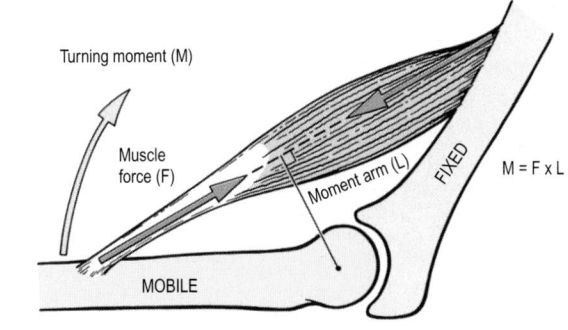

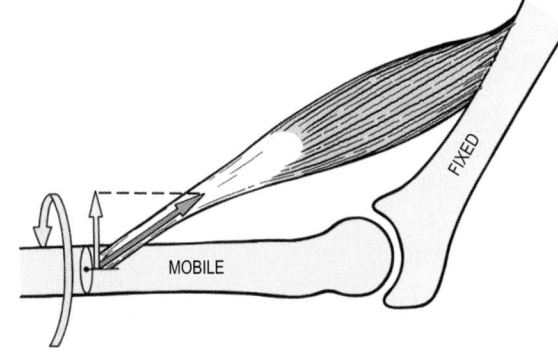

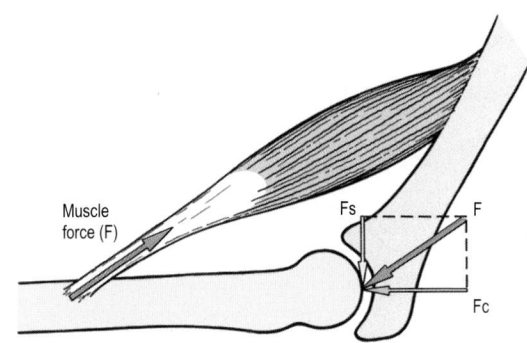

Fig. 6.65 A generalized example to illustrate the biomechanical effects of the force generated by a muscle. The muscle (which does not represent a specific anatomical muscle) arises from a fixed base or 'origin', crosses a single multiaxial joint, and is attached at its 'insertion' to a mobile bone. **A**, The turning moment about the joint. **B**, The spin component which results from off-axis attachment. **C**, The reactive force (F) at the joint can be resolved into a normal component (Fc), which represents the reaction to compression, and a tangential component (Fs), which represents the reaction to shear.

An interesting, and puzzling, feature of the mechanics of joint movement is the sheer number of muscles which are involved, even in quite simple movements. It is fairly clear that there is little actual redundancy in the system, and this is well illustrated by attempts to synthesize gait in paraplegic patients by electrical stimulation of the intact motor nerves. Early attempts produced a gait that was jerky and robotic; at least 30 channels of stimulation appear to be needed to achieve a more coordinated and fluid motion. Certainly some of these muscles act as fixators and synergists, providing a stable base for the action of other muscles and eliminating unwanted components of movement. The combination of variously directed forces may also provide more scope for achieving a balanced reaction at a joint, so that stability is less heavily dependent on passive connective tissue elements, such as ligaments and the articular capsule. Failure to provide this would lead to chronic overload of the soft tissues with their consequent stretching and failure. The limited range over which muscles can operate effectively may mean that a sequence of contractions, involving several muscles which work optimally at different joint angles, is the only way to deliver adequate force over the full arc of movement.

Any comprehensive explanation needs to take into account the dynamic, as well as the static, aspects of movement at a joint. The knowledge of integrated biomechanics can be applied in a mathematical model to stimulate the dynamic movement of a limb under the action of a muscle. Such a model predicts the different sets of attachment sites needed to maximize, say, velocity or power. It suggests that a joint acted upon by multiple muscles, each with different attachment sites, would be more versatile in terms of the available strategies.

REFERENCES

BONE, CARTILAGE AND JOINTS

Brueton RN, Revell WJ, Brookes M 1993 Haemodynamics of bone healing in model stable fracture. In: Shoutens A, Arlet J, Gardiniers JWM, Hughes SPF (eds) Bone Circulation and Vascularization in Normal and Pathological Conditions. New York: Plenum Press: 121–8.

Hall BK (ed) 1983 Cartilage. Vols 1–3. New York: Academic Press.

Maroudas A, Stockwell R, Nachemson A, Urban J 1975 Factors involved in the nutrition of the human lumbar intervertebral disc: cellularity and diffusion of glucose in vitro. J Anat 120: 113–30.

SKELETAL MUSCLE

Bishopric NH, Gahlmann R, Wade R, Kedes L 1991 Gene expression during skeletal and cardiac muscle development. In: Fozzard HA, Haber E, Jennings RB, Katz AM, Morgan HE (eds) The Heart and Cardiovascular System, 2nd edn. New York: Raven Press: 1587–98.

Brand-Saberi B, Christ B 2000 Evolution and development of distinct cell lineages derived from somites. Current Topics in Developmental Biology, Vol 48. New York: Academic Press.

Buckingham M, Bajard L, Chang T et al 2003 The formation of skeletal muscle: from somite to limb. J Anat 202: 59–68.

Buller AJ, Eccles JC, Eccles RM 1960 Interactions between motoneurones and muscles in respect of the characteristic speeds of their responses. J Physiol 150: 417–39.

Edgerton VR, Roy RR, Allen DL, Monti RJ 2002 Adaptations in skeletal muscle disuse or decreased-use atrophy. Am J Phys Med Rehabil 81(11 Suppl): S127–47.

Goldring K, Partridge T, Watt D 2002 Muscle stem cells. J Pathol 197: 457–67. *Reviews the role of the satellite cell in growth and repair of muscle fibres*

Ko C-P, Thompson WJ (guest eds) 2003 The Neuromuscular Junction. J Neurocytol 32: 421–1037.

Lieber RL, Friden J 2000 Functional and clinical significance of skeletal muscle architecture. Muscle Nerve 23: 1647–66.

Maltin CA, Delday MI, Sinclair KD, Steven J, Sneddon AA 2001 Impact of manipulations of myogenesis in utero on the performance of adult skeletal muscle. Reproduction 122: 359–74.

Mathes SJ, Nahai F 1981 Classification of the vascular anatomy of muscles: experimental and clinical correlation. Plast Reconstr Surg 67: 177–87.

Mizuno H, Zuk PA, Zhu M, Lorenz HP, Benhaim P, Hedrick MH 2002 Myogenic differentiation by human processed lipoaspirate cells. Plast Reconstr Surg 109:199–209.

Muntoni F, Brown S, Sewry C, Patel K 2002 Muscle development genes: their relevance in neuromuscular disorders. Neuromuscul Disord 12: 438–46.

Salmons S 1967 An implantable muscle stimulator. J Physiol 188: 13P–14P.

Schiaffino S, Reggiani C 1996 Molecular diversity of myofibrillar proteins: gene regulation and functional significance. Physiol Rev 76: 371–423.

BIOMECHANICS

Crompton RH, Günther M 2004 Humans and other bipeds: the evolution of bipedality. J Anat 204: 317–20. *This issue of the journal is devoted to the evolution of bipedal gait.*

MacConaill MA, Basmajian JV 1977 Muscles and Movements. A Basis for Human Kinesiology, 2nd edn. New York: Krieger.

Panjabi MM, White III AA 2001 Biomechanics in the Musculoskeletal System. Edinburgh: Churchill Livingstone.

Smooth muscle and the cardiovascular and lymphatic systems

The cardiovascular system carries blood from the heart to all parts of the body through a series of tubes, all but the smallest of which are muscular. The muscle lining these tubes is of two types: smooth muscle is characteristic of the walls of blood vessels and cardiac muscle provides the walls of the heart chambers with their powerful contractile pumping action. The general characteristics and classification of muscle tissues are given on page 112. Smooth muscle forms an important contractile element in the walls of many other organ systems of the body.

SMOOTH MUSCLE

In smooth muscle tissue the contractile proteins actin and myosin are not organized into regular sarcomeres, visible as transverse striations (p. 114), so the cytoplasm has a smooth (unstriated) appearance. Smooth muscle is also referred to as involuntary muscle, because its activity is neither initiated nor monitored consciously. It is more variable, in both form and function, than either striated or cardiac muscle, a reflection of its varied roles in different systems of the body.

Smooth muscle cells (fibres) are smaller than those of striated muscle. Their length can range from 15 µm in small blood vessels to 200 µm, and even to 500 µm or more in the uterus during pregnancy. The cells are spindle-shaped (**Fig. 7.1**), tapering towards the ends from a central diameter of 3–8 µm. The nucleus is single, located at the mid-point, and often twisted into a corkscrew shape by the contraction of the cell (**Fig. 7.2A**). Smooth muscle cells aggregate with their long axes parallel and staggered longitudinally, so that the wide central portion of one cell lies next to the tapered end of another. Such an arrangement achieves both close packing and a more efficient transfer of force from cell to cell. In transverse section, smooth muscle is seen as an array of circular or slightly polygonal profiles of very varied size, and nuclei are present only in the centres of the largest profiles (**Fig. 7.2B**). This appearance contrasts markedly with that of skeletal muscle cells, which show a consistent diameter in cross-section and peripherally placed nuclei throughout their length.

Smooth muscle is typically found in the walls of tubular structures and hollow viscera. It regulates diameter (e.g. in blood vessels, and branches of the bronchial tree); propels liquids or solids (e.g. in the ureter, hepatic duct, and intestines); or expels the contents (e.g. in the urinary bladder and uterus). The actual arrangement of the cells varies with the tissue. The account that follows will therefore be concerned with the generic properties of smooth muscle. The more specialized morphologies of smooth muscle are described in the appropriate regional chapters.

Smooth muscle has no attachment structures equivalent to the fasciae, tendons and aponeuroses associated with skeletal muscle. There is a special arrangement for transmitting force from cell to cell and, where necessary, to other soft tissue structures. Within a fascicle, the cells are separated by a gap of 40–80 nm. Each cell is covered almost entirely by a prominent basal lamina which merges with a reticular layer consisting of a network of fine elastin, reticular fibres (collagen type III) and type I collagen fibres (**Fig. 7.3**). These elements bridge the gaps between adjacent cells and provide mechanical continuity throughout the fascicle. At the boundaries of fascicles, the connective tissue fibres become interwoven with those of interfascicular septa, so that the contraction of different fascicles is communicated throughout the tissue and to neighbouring structures. The components of the reticular network, the ground substance and collagen and elastic fibres, are synthesized by the smooth muscle cells themselves, not by fibroblasts or other connective tissue cells, which are rarely found within fasciculi.

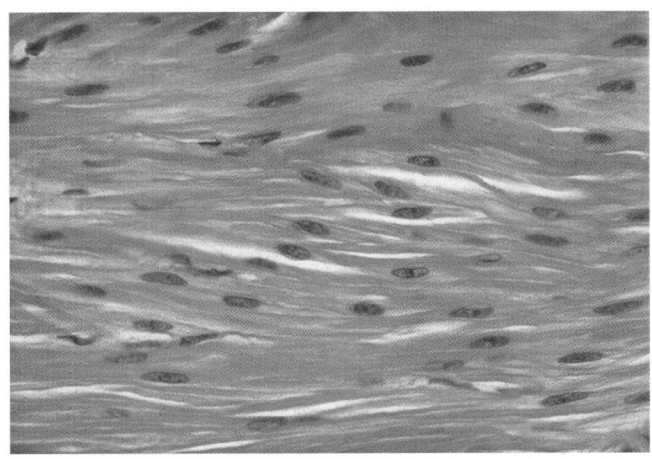

Fig. 7.1 Longitudinal section of smooth muscle fibres.

In some blood vessels, notably those of the pulmonary circulation, and in the airways, and possibly in other smooth muscle types, there is evidence for heterogeneity of cell type. Some myofibroblast-like cells have a function that is more secretory than contractile. The secretory phenotype is often increased in disease (e.g. chronic severe asthma, pulmonary hypertension) and is associated with increased proliferation and remodelling.

Discontinuities occur in the basal lamina between adjacent cells, and here the cell membranes approach to 2–4 nm of one another to form a gap junction (**Fig. 7.2B**). These junctions are believed to be structurally similar to their counterparts in cardiac muscle. They provide a low-resistance pathway through which electrical excitation can pass between cells, producing a coordinated wave of contraction. The incidence of gap junctions varies with the anatomical site of the tissue: they appear to be more abundant in the type of smooth muscle which generates rhythmic (phasic) activity.

Although some smooth muscles can generate as much force per unit cross-sectional area as skeletal muscle, the force always develops much more slowly than in striated muscle. Smooth muscle can contract by more than 80%, a much greater range of shortening than the 30% or so to which striated muscle is limited. The significance of this property is illustrated by the urinary bladder, which is capable of emptying completely from an internal volume of 300 ml or more. Smooth muscles can maintain tension for long periods with very little expenditure of energy. For example, the muscular wall of an artery can maintain vascular tone despite the complete absence of a capillary supply. Many smooth muscle structures are able to generate spontaneous contractions: examples are found in the walls of the intestines, ureter and uterine tube.

MICROSTRUCTURE OF SMOOTH MUSCLE AND THE CONTRACTILE MECHANISM

Although electron microscopy revealed the presence of filaments in smooth muscle some years ago (**Fig. 7.2A**), this observation alone provided little insight into their mode of function because of the lack of any obvious organization of the filaments. More recent work (North et al 1994), in which specific proteins were localized by high-resolution

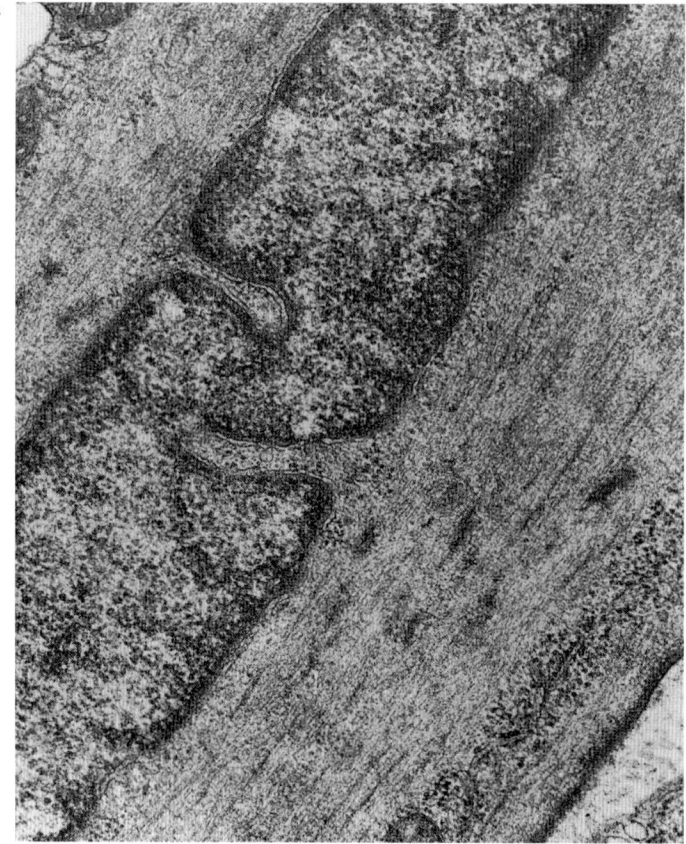

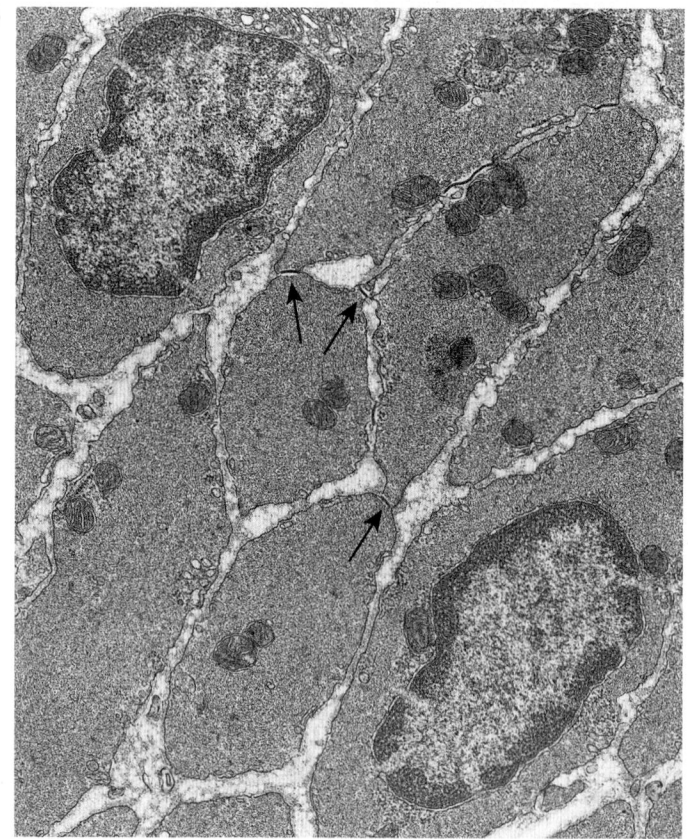

Fig. 7.2 **A**, A smooth muscle fibre in longitudinal section, showing its nucleus twisted into a corkscrew shape by contractile forces. Myofilaments and cytoplasmic dense bodies are also seen. **B**, Smooth muscle fibres in transverse section, two at the level of a single central nucleus. In several places, the plasma membranes of adjacent cells are closely approximated at gap junctions (arrows).

immunocytochemistry, has revealed further details of the internal architecture of the cell and suggested a structural basis for contractile function. The model, which is illustrated in **Fig. 7.3**, depends on the mutual interaction of two systems of filaments, one forming the cytoskeleton and the other the contractile apparatus.

Excluding the perinuclear region, the cytoplasm of a smooth muscle cell effectively consists of two structural domains. The cytoskeleton forms a structural framework that maintains the spindle-like form of the cell and provides an internal scaffold with which other elements can interact. Its major structural component is the intermediate filament desmin, with the addition of vimentin (which may also be present alone) in vascular smooth muscle. The intermediate filaments are arranged mainly in longitudinal bundles, but some filaments interconnect the bundles with each other and with the sarcolemma to form a three-dimensional network. The bundles of intermediate filaments insert into focal, electron-dense bodies, c.0.1 μm in diameter, which are distributed uniformly throughout the cytoplasm (**Fig. 2.14**) and are also attached to dense plaques underlying the plasma membrane.

The cytoplasmic dense bodies and plaques are equivalent to the Z-discs of striated muscle cells. They contain the actin-binding protein α-actinin and thus also anchor the actin filaments of the contractile apparatus. These form a lattice of obliquely arranged bundles throughout the cytoplasm, which transmit force to the plasma membrane and basal lamina. Other regulatory proteins associate specifically with actin, such as caldesmon and calponin. The ratio of actin to myosin is eight times greater in smooth compared to striated muscle, reflecting the greater length of actin filaments in smooth muscle.

Smooth muscle myosin filaments are c.1.5–2 μm long, somewhat longer than those of striated muscle. Although smooth muscle cells contain less myosin, the longer filaments are capable of generating considerable force. The myosin filaments of smooth muscle are also assembled differently, such that their head regions lie symmetrically on either side of a ribbon-like filament, rather than imposing a bipolar organization on the filament. Actin filaments, to which they bind, can thus slide along the whole length of the myosin filament during contraction. This difference underpins the ability of smooth muscle to undergo much greater changes in length than striated muscle. Actin–myosin filament sliding generates tension which transmits to focal regions of the plasma membrane, changing the cell shape in the manner of a concertina, from an elongated spindle to a more rounded and pleated shape.

Caveolae, cup-like invaginations of the plasma membrane with a resemblance to endocytotic vesicles, are a characteristic feature of smooth muscle cells. They are associated with many receptors, ion channels and kinases, and may act as loci for highly localized signalling pathways. They may also act as specialized pinocytotic structures involved in fluid and electrolyte transport into the cell. Other organelles (mitochondria, ribosomes etc.) are largely confined to the filament-free perinuclear cytoplasm, although in some smooth muscle types, including vascular smooth muscle, peripheral mitochondria are closely associated with the peripheral sarcoplasmic reticulum and cell membrane, which may be important in the regulation of intracellular calcium.

VASCULAR SUPPLY

The blood supply of smooth muscle is less extensive than that of striated muscle. Where the tissue is not too densely packed, afferent and efferent vessels gain access via connective tissue septa, and capillaries run in the connective tissue between small fascicles. However, unlike striated muscle, capillaries are not found in relation to individual cells.

INNERVATION

Smooth muscle may contract in response to nervous, hormonal or electrical depolarization transferred from neighbouring cells. Some muscles receive a dense innervation which precisely defines their contractile activity, e.g. in the iris, specific nervous control can produce either pupillary constriction or dilation. These muscles are often referred to as multi-unit smooth muscles. Other muscles are more sparsely innervated. They tend to display myogenic activity, initiated spontaneously or in response to stretch, which spreads from cell to cell via gap junctions and may be markedly influenced by hormones. In these muscles, which include those in the walls of the gastrointestinal tract, urinary bladder, ureter, uterus and uterine tube, innervation tends to exert a more global influence on the rate and force of intrinsically

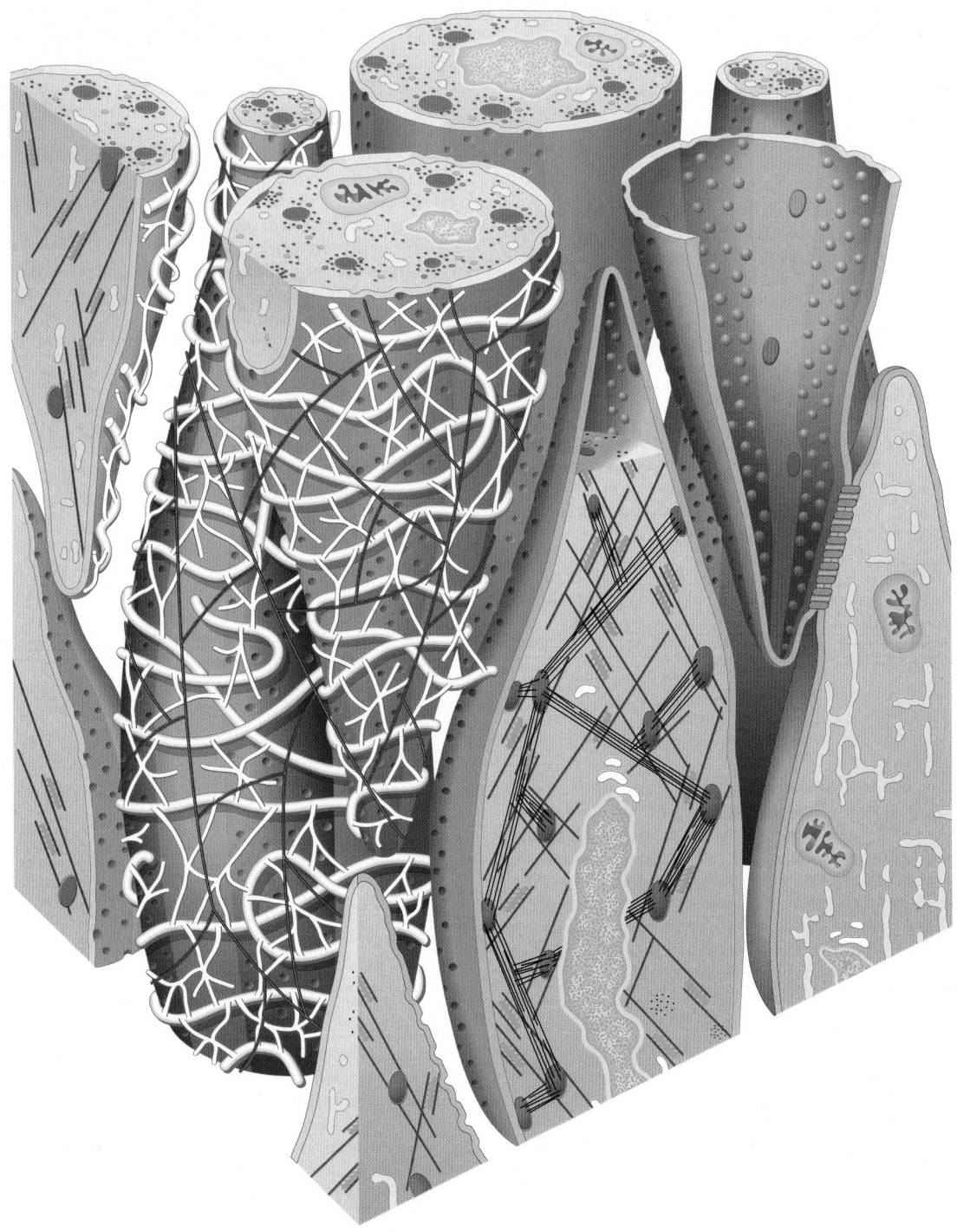

Fig. 7.3 Three-dimensional representation of smooth muscle cells. For clarity, some structural features have been separated for illustration in different cells. The spindle-shaped cells interdigitate with their long axes parallel; mechanical continuity between the cells is provided by a reticular layer (left). The cytoskeletal framework (front) consists of intermediate filaments (grey) and thin filaments of cytoplasmic actin (olive) organized into longitudinal bundles in association with dense bodies (light brown). The contractile apparatus (front) consists of oblique filaments of myosin (green) and actin, which interact with the cytoskeleton to produce contraction of the cell. The sarcolemma contains alternating domains of anchoring adherens junctions and caveolae (top right). There is a sparse sarcoplasmic reticulum (yellow, bottom right). (Artist: Lesley Skeates.)

generated contractions. These muscles have been referred to as unitary smooth muscles. The terms multi-unit and unitary smooth muscles are widely used, but in practice such distinctions are better regarded as the extremes of a continuous spectrum.

Smooth muscles are innervated by unmyelinated axons whose cell bodies are located in autonomic ganglia, either in the sympathetic chain or, in the case of parasympathetic fibres, closer to the point of innervation. They ramify extensively, spreading over a large area of the muscle and sending branches into the muscle fasciculi. The terminal portion of each axonal branch is beaded, and consists of expanded portions, varicosities, packed with vesicles and mitochondria, separated by thin, intervaricose portions. Each varicosity is regarded as a transmitter release site, and, in the functional sense, is therefore a nerve ending. In this way the axonal arborization of a single autonomic neurone bears a very large number of nerve endings (up to tens of thousands), as opposed to a maximum of a few hundred in somatic motor neurones. The neuromuscular terminals of autonomic efferents are considered in more detail on page 65.

The neuromuscular junctions in smooth muscles do not show the consistent appearance seen in skeletal muscles. The neurotransmitter diffuses across a gap that can vary from 10 to 100 nm: even separations up to 1 μm may still allow neuromuscular transmission to take place, although more slowly. The nerve ending is packed with vesicles, but the adjacent area of the muscle cell is not structurally differentiated from that of non-junctional regions.

Intramuscular afferent nerves are the peripheral processes of small sensory neurones in the dorsal root ganglia. Since they are unmyelinated, contain axonal vesicles and have a beaded appearance, they are difficult to distinguish from efferent fibres.

EXCITATION–CONTRACTION COUPLING IN SMOOTH MUSCLE

Excitation–contraction coupling in smooth muscle may be electro-mechanical or pharmacomechanical. Electromechanical coupling involves depolarization of the cell membrane by an action potential, and may be generated when a membrane receptor, usually linked with an ion channel, is occupied by a neurotransmitter, hormone or other blood-borne substance. Alternatively, it may be initiated by direct transmission of electrical excitation from an adjacent cell via a gap junction. In some types of smooth muscle, depolarization may be the consequence of other stimuli, such as cooling, stretching, and even light.

Pharmacomechanical coupling is a receptor-mediated process in which transmitters or drugs can bring about an increase in intracellular calcium, without depolarization of the membrane, either by opening calcium channels in the sarcolemma, or by triggering the formation of inositol triphosphate, which acts as a signal for intracellular calcium release from the sarcoplasmic reticulum.

The regulation of contraction of smooth muscle is largely calcium-dependent. Calcium is sequestered in the sarcoplasmic reticulum, but also enters the cell from outside through both voltage-gated and voltage-independent calcium channels. Different types of smooth muscle use these pathways to differing extents. For example, drugs that block calcium release from intracellular stores mainly affect vascular smooth muscle, whereas intestinal smooth muscle is more responsive to blockade of plasma membrane calcium channels. In the cytoplasm, calcium binds to calmodulin. The complex so formed regulates the activity of myosin light chain kinase which phosphorylates myosin regulatory light chains and initiates the myosin-actin ATPase cycle (p. 17). The process is therefore inherently slow. Unphosphorylated myosin II of smooth muscle cannot initiate actin binding, although it can maintain contraction, with little energy expenditure. Myosin phosphatase dephosphorylates myosin light chains, and thus promotes relaxation. Inhibition of the phosphatase increases phosphorylation for any level of calcium (i.e. increases calcium sensitivity). This is now believed to be a very important component of the response to many constrictor agonists.

DEVELOPMENT

It was thought that all smooth muscle cells developed *in situ* exclusively from the splanchnopleuric mesenchyme composing the walls of the anlagen of the viscera and around the endothelium of blood vessels. However, recent experimental studies which have traced the progeny of cells proliferating from the epithelial plate of the somite, have identified endothelial and tunica media smooth muscle cells arising from individual somites. The origin of the smooth muscle of the iris is still unclear. This region of the eye develops from the optic cup, and so the smooth muscle which arises there is derived either from the neurectoderm of the original optic cup or from the neural crest mesenchyme which later invades the iris.

Following a period of proliferation, clusters of myoblasts become elongated in the same orientation. Dense bodies, associated with actin and cytoskeletal filaments, appear in the cytoplasm, and the surface membrane starts to acquire its specialized features, i.e. caveolae, adherens junctions and gap junctions. Cytoskeletal filaments extend to insert into the submembranous densities. Thick filaments are seen a few days after the first appearance of thin filaments and intermediate filaments, and from this time the cells are able to contract. During development, dense bodies increase in number and further elements of the cytoskeleton are added. In addition to synthesizing the cytoskeleton and contractile apparatus, the differentiating cells express and secrete components of the extracellular matrix.

In a developing smooth muscle all the cells express characteristics of the same stage of differentiation, and there are no successive waves of differentiation. From its earliest appearance to maturity, a smooth muscle increases several hundredfold in mass, partly by a 2 to 4-fold increase in the size of individual cells, but mainly by a very large increase in cell number. Growth occurs by division of cells in every part

of the muscle, not just at its surface or ends. Mitoses occur in cells in which differentiation is already well advanced, as evidenced by the presence of myofilaments and membrane specializations. Mitotic smooth muscle cells may be found at any stage of life, but their numbers peak before birth, at a time that differs for different muscles; they are rare in the adult unless the tissue is stimulated to hypertrophy or to repair. (The ability of mature cells to undergo mitosis therefore differs between the three major types of muscle: skeletal muscle cells cannot divide at all after differentiation; cardiac muscle cells can divide, but only before birth; and smooth muscle cells appear to remain capable of division throughout life.)

During the early stages of development, smooth muscle expresses embryonic and non-muscle isoforms of myosin. The proportions of these isoforms decrease progressively. Initially, SM-1 is the dominant or exclusive smooth muscle heavy chain isoform: the SM-2 isoform becomes more established later.

THE CARDIOVASCULAR AND LYMPHATIC SYSTEMS

GENERAL ORGANIZATION

Cells of peripheral blood, suspended in plasma, circulate through the body in the blood vascular system. Interstitial fluid from peripheral tissues returns to the blood vascular system via the lymphatic system, which also provides a channel for the migration of leukocytes (p. 71) and the absorption of certain nutrients from the gut.

The cardiovascular system carries nutrients, oxygen, hormones, etc. throughout the body and the blood redistributes and disperses heat. As a consequence of the pulse pressure, the system also has mechanical effects, such as maintaining tissue turgidity and counteracting the effects of gravity. Blood circulates within a fast, high capacity system made up of the heart, which is the central pump and main motor of the system; arteries, which lead away from the heart and carry the blood to the peripheral parts of the body; and veins which return the blood to the heart. The heart can be thought of as a pair of muscular pumps, one feeding a minor loop (pulmonary circulation), which serves the lungs and oxygenates the blood, the other feeding a major loop (systemic circulation), which serves the rest of the body. With limited exceptions, each loop is a closed system of tubes, so that blood *per se* does not usually leave the circulation.

From the centre to the periphery, the vascular tree shows three main modifications. The arteries increase in number by repeated bifurcation and by sending out side branches, in both the systemic and the pulmonary circulation. For example, the aorta, which carries blood from the heart to the systemic circulation, gives rise to about 4×10^6 arterioles and four times as many capillaries. The arteries also decrease in diameter, although not to the same extent as their increase in number, so that a hypothetical cross-section of all the vessels at a given distance will increase in total area with increasing distance from the heart. At its emergence from the heart, the aorta of an adult man has an outer diameter of c.30 mm (sectional area of nearly 7 cm^2). The diameter decreases along the arterial tree until it is as little as 10 μm in arterioles (each with a sectional area of c.80 μm^2). However, given the enormous number of arterioles, the total cross-sectional area at this level is c.150 cm^2, more than 200 times that of the aorta. As a result, blood flow is faster near the heart than at the periphery.

The walls of arteries decrease in thickness towards the periphery, although this is not as substantial as the reduction in vessel diameter. Consequently, in the smallest arteries (arterioles), the thickness of the wall represents about half the outer radius of the vessel, whereas in a large vessel it represents between one-fifteenth and one-fifth, e.g. in the thoracic aorta the radius is c.17 mm and the wall thickness 1.1 mm.

Venules, which return blood from the periphery, converge on each other forming a progressively smaller number of veins of increasingly larger size. As with arteries, the hypothetical total cross-sectional area of all veins at a given level reduces nearer to the heart. Eventually, only the two largest veins, the superior and inferior vena cava, open into the heart from the systemic circulation. A similar pattern is found in the pulmonary circulation, but here the vascular loop is shorter and has fewer branch points, and consequently, the number of vessels is smaller than in the systemic circulation.

Arteries are usually more deeply situated than veins, although there are several superficial or subcutaneous arteries, such as the occipital, temporal, frontal and epigastric arteries. Arteries are located on the flexor surface near limb joints, transverse vessels usually providing a collateral circulation over the lateral parts of the joint. Arteries are usually separated from bones by muscles and fasciae: when they are in contact with bone, they leave an imprint or vascular groove, e.g. the subclavian artery on the first rib.

Large arteries, such as the thoracic aorta, subclavian, axillary, femoral and popliteal arteries, lie close to a single vein which drains the same territory as that supplied by the artery. Other arteries are usually flanked by two veins, satellite veins (venae comitantes), which lie on either side of the artery, and have numerous cross-connections: the whole is enclosed in a single connective tissue sheath. The artery and the two satellite veins are often associated with a nerve, and when they are surrounded by a common connective tissue sheath they form a neurovascular bundle.

The close association between the larger arteries and veins in the limbs allows the counterflow exchange of heat to take place. This mechanism promotes heat transfer from arterial to venous blood, and thus helps to preserve body heat. Counterflow heat exchange systems are found in other organs, e.g. in the testis, where the pampiniform plexus of veins surrounds the testicular artery (this arrangement not only conserves body heat, but also maintains the temperature of the testis below average body temperature) (p. 1306). Counterflow ion exchange mechanisms are found in the microcirculation, as in the arterial and venous sinusoids of the vasa recta in the renal medulla. Here, countercurrent exchange retains sodium ions at a high concentration in the medullary interstitium (p. 1277), and efferent venous blood transfers sodium ions to the afferent arterial supply.

Arteries and veins are named primarily according to their anatomical position. In functional terms, three main classes of vessel are described: resistance vessels (arteries, but mainly arterioles), exchange vessels (capillaries, sinusoids and small venules) and capacitance vessels (veins). Structurally, arteries can also be divided into elastic and muscular types. Although muscle cells and elastic tissue are present in all arteries, the relative amount of elastic material is greatest in the largest vessels, whereas the relative amount of smooth muscle increases progressively towards the smallest arteries.

Arteries may also be subdivided into conducting and distributing, as well as resistance vessels. The large conducting arteries which arise from the heart, together with their main branches, are characterized by the predominantly elastic properties of their walls. Distributing vessels are smaller arteries supplying the individual organs, and their wall is characterized by a well-developed muscular component. Resistance vessels are mainly arterioles. Small and muscular, they provide the main source of the peripheral resistance to blood flow, and they cause a marked drop in the pressure of blood which flows into the capillary beds within tissues.

Capillaries, sinusoids and small (postcapillary) venules are collectively termed exchange vessels. Their walls allow exchange between blood and the interstitial tissue fluid which surrounds all cells: this is the essential function of a circulatory system. Arterioles, capillaries and venules constitute the microvascular bed, the structural basis of the microcirculation.

Larger venules and veins form an extensive, but variable, large-volume, low-pressure system of vessels conveying blood back to the heart. The high capacitance of these vessels is due to the distensibility (compliance) of their walls, so that the content of blood is high even at low pressures. This part of the vascular bed contains the greatest proportion of blood, reflecting the large relative volume of veins.

Blood from the abdominal part of the digestive tube (with the exception of the lower part of the anal canal), and from the spleen, pancreas and gallbladder, drains to the liver via the portal vein. The portal vein ramifies within the substance of the liver like an artery and ends in the hepatic sinusoids (p. 1222). These drain into the hepatic veins which in turn drain into the inferior vena cava. Blood supplying the abdominal organs thus passes through two sets of capillaries before it returns to the heart. The first provides the organs with oxygenated blood, and the second carries deoxygenated blood, rich in absorption products from the intestine, through the liver parenchyma. A venous portal circulation also connects the median eminence and infundibulum of the hypothalamus with the adenohypophysis (p. 380). In essence, a venous portal system is a capillary network that lies between two veins, instead of between an artery and a vein, which is the more usual arrangement in the circulation. A capillary network may also be interposed

between two arteries, e.g. in the renal glomeruli (p. 1277), where the glomerular capillary bed lies between afferent and efferent arterioles. This maintains a relatively high pressure system, which is important for renal filtration.

A parallel circulatory system in the body is provided by the lymphatic vessels and lymph nodes (p. 75). Lymphatic vessels originate in peripheral tissues as blind-ended endothelial tubes which collect excess fluid from the interstitial spaces between cells and conduct it as lymph. Lymph is returned to the blood vascular system via lymphatic vessels which converge on the large veins in the root of the neck.

The development of blood vessels is described on page 1042.

General features of vessel walls

Blood vessels, irrespective of size, and with the exception of capillaries and venules, have walls consisting of three concentric layers (tunicae) (Fig. 7.4). The intima (tunica intima), is the innermost layer. Its main component, the endothelium, lines the entire vascular tree, including the heart, and the lymphatic vessels. The media (tunica media) is made of muscle tissue, elastic fibres and collagen. While it is by far the thickest layer in arteries, the media is absent in capillaries and is comparatively thin in veins. The adventitia (tunica adventitia) is the outer coat of the vessel, and consists of connective tissue, nerves and vessel capillaries. It links the vessels to the surrounding tissues. Vessels differ in the relative thicknesses and detailed compositions of their layers and, in the smallest vessels, the number of layers represented.

Large elastic arteries (Fig. 7.5)

The aorta and its largest branches (brachiocephalic, common carotid, subclavian and common iliac arteries) are large elastic arteries which conduct blood to the medium-sized distributing arteries.

The intima is made of an endothelium, resting on a basal lamina, and a subendothelial connective tissue layer. The endothelial cells are flat, elongated and polygonal in outline, with their long axes parallel to the direction of blood flow (see Fig. 7.7). The subendothelial layer is well developed, contains elastic fibres and type I collagen fibrils, fibroblasts and small, smooth muscle-like myointimal cells. The latter accumulate lipid with age and in an extreme form, this feature contributes to atherosclerotic changes in the intima. Thickening of the intima progresses with age and is more marked in the distal than in the proximal segment of the aorta.

A prominent internal elastic lamina, sometimes split, lies between intima and media (see Fig. 7.17). This lamina is smooth, measures c.1 μm in thickness, and, with the elastic lamellae of the media, is stretched under the effect of systolic pressure, recoiling elastically in diastole. Elastic arteries thus have the effect of sustaining blood flow despite the pulsatile cardiac output. They also smooth out the cyclical pressure wave. The media has a markedly layered structure, in which fenestrated layers of elastin (elastic lamellae) alternate with interlamellar muscle cells, collagen and fine elastic fibres. The arrangement is very regular, such that each elastic lamella and adjacent interlamellar zone is regarded as a 'lamellar unit' of the media. In the human aorta there are c.52 lamellar units, measuring c.11 μm in thickness. Number and thickness of lamellar units increases during development, from c.40 at birth.

The adventitia is well developed. In addition to collagen and elastic fibres, it contains flattened fibroblasts with extremely long thin processes, macrophages and mast cells, nerve bundles and lymphatic vessels. The vasa vasorum are usually confined to the adventitia.

Muscular arteries (Fig. 7.6, 7.17)

Muscular arteries are characterized by the predominance of smooth muscle in the media. The intima consists of an endothelium, similar to that of elastic arteries (Fig. 7.7), which rests on a basal lamina and subendothelial connective tissue. The internal elastic lamina (Figs 7.4, 7.6, see Fig. 7.18) is a distinct, thin layer, and is occasionally absent. Some 75% of the mass of the media consists of smooth muscle cells which run spirally or circumferentially around the vessel wall. The relative amount of extracellular matrix is therefore less than in large arteries, however, fine elastic fibres which run mainly parallel to the muscle cells are present. An external elastic lamina, composed of sheets of elastic fibres, forms a less compact layer than the internal lamina, and separates the media from the adventitia in the larger muscular arteries. The adventitia is mainly collagenous connective tissue, and can be as thick as the media in the smaller arteries.

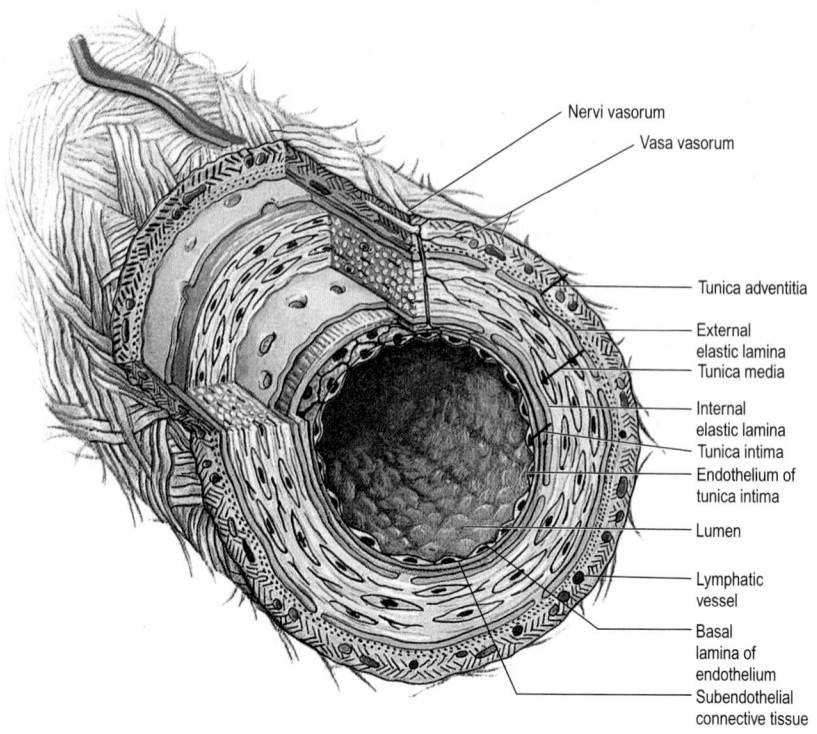

Fig. 7.4 The principal structural features of the larger blood vessels as seen in a muscular artery.

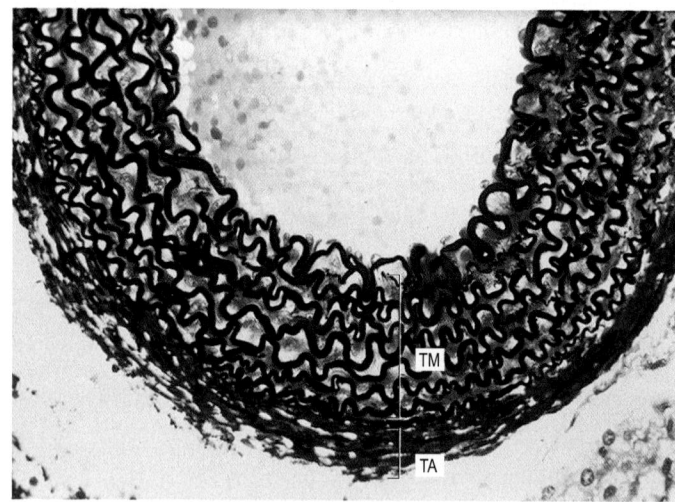

Fig. 7.5 Small elastic artery stained with Gomori trichrome showing numerous folded elastic lamellae in the tunica media (TM) and collagenous material in the tunica adventitia (TA). (By permission from Dr JB Kerr, Monash University, from Kerr JB 1999 Atlas of Functional Histology. London: Mosby.)

Arterioles (Fig. 7.8)

In arterioles the endothelial cells are smaller than in large arteries, but their nuclear region is thicker and often projects markedly into the lumen. The nuclei are elongated and orientated parallel to the vessel length, as is the long axis of the cell. The basal surface of the endothelium contacts a basal lamina, but an internal elastic lamina is either absent or is highly fenestrated and traversed by the cytoplasmic processes of muscle cells or endothelial cells.

The muscle cells are larger in cytoplasmic volume than those of large arteries and they form a layer one or two cells thick. They are arranged circumferentially and are tightly wound around the endothelium. In the smallest arterioles each cell makes several turns, producing extensive apposition between parts of the same cell. Their contractility controls

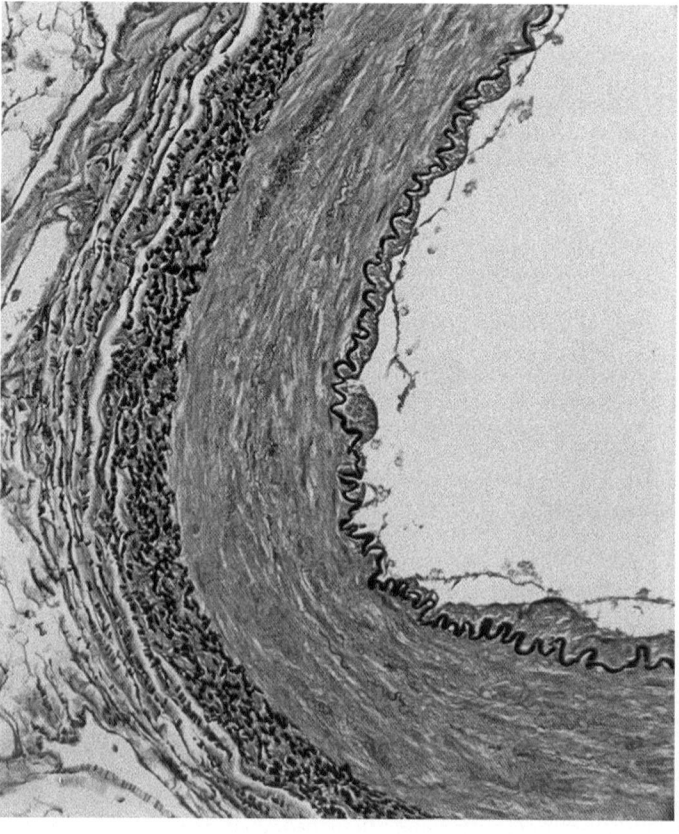

Fig. 7.6 Small muscular artery, stained to show elastin (blue-black) in the internal and external elastic laminae but little in the media, which is largely smooth muscle tissue.

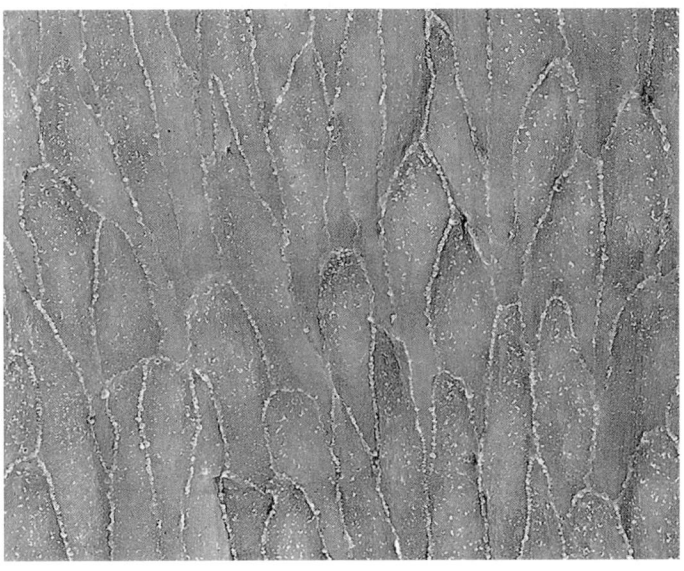

Fig. 7.7 Scanning electron micrograph of the luminal surface of the basilar artery. The tightly packed endothelial cells are elongated in the direction of blood flow. (Provided by Masoud Alian, University College, London.)

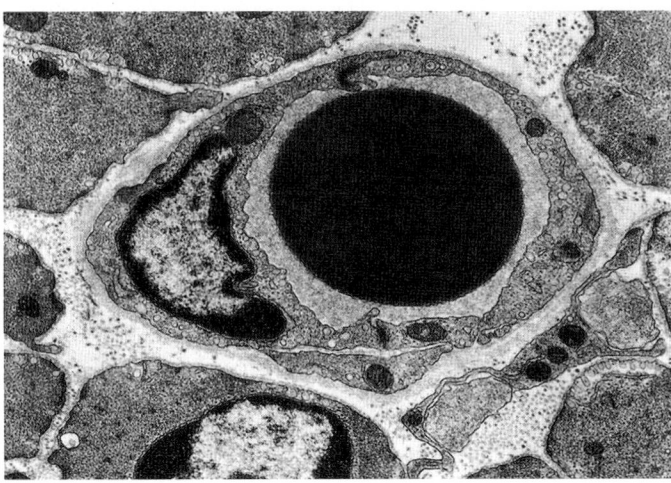

Fig. 7.9 Capillary in muscle tissue, containing a red blood cell that almost fills the lumen.

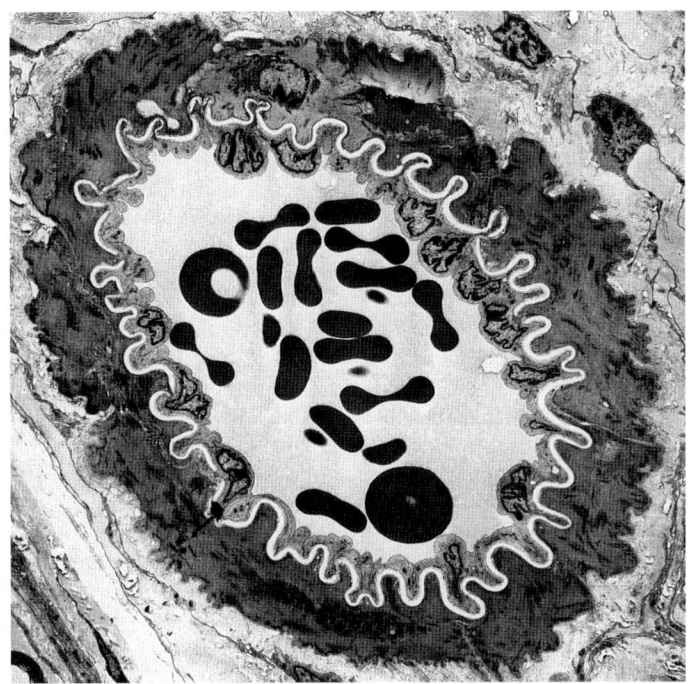

Fig. 7.8 A small arteriole in the epineurium of a peripheral nerve. The vessel lumen contains red blood cells and is lined by endothelial cells (with nuclei projecting into the lumen); note the electron-lucent internal elastic lamina (pale, wavy line), the media containing densely filamentous smooth muscle cells and the connective tissue of the adventitia merging with that of the epineurium.

Capillaries (Fig. 7.9)

The capillary wall is formed by an endothelium and its basal lamina, plus a few isolated pericytes. Capillaries are the vessels closest to the tissue they supply and their wall is a minimal barrier between blood and the surrounding tissues. Capillary structure varies in different locations. Capillaries measure 4–8 μm in diameter (much more in the case of sinusoids) and are hundreds of microns long. Their lumen is just large enough to admit the passage of single blood cells, usually with considerable deformation (p. 69). However, the true bottleneck of the circulatory system occurs at the level of the arterioles, where muscle contraction can obliterate the lumen.

Typically a single endothelial cell forms the wall of a capillary, so that the junctional complex occurs between extensions of the same cell (p. 146). The endothelial cells of some capillaries have fenestrations, or pores, through their cytoplasm. Fenestrations are approximately circular, 50–100 nm in diameter, and at their edge the luminal and abluminal membranes of the endothelial cell come into contact with each other. The fenestration itself is usually occupied by a thin electron-dense diaphragm of unknown molecular composition. Fenestrated capillaries occur in renal glomeruli, where they lack a diaphragm, in intestinal mucosae, and in endocrine and exocrine glands. Fenestrations are almost invariably present in capillaries which lie close to an epithelium, including the skin.

Capillaries without fenestrations, such as those in the brain, striated and smooth muscles, lung and connective tissues, are known as continuous capillaries. Capillary permeability varies greatly among tissues, and this can be correlated partly with the type of endothelium. Where efficient barriers to diffusion of large molecules occur, e.g. brain, thymic cortex and testis, continuous capillary endothelial cells are joined by tight junctions.

Sinusoids – Sinusoids are expanded capillaries, and are large and irregular in shape. They have true discontinuities in their walls, allowing intimate contact between blood and the parenchyma. The discontinuities are formed by gaps between endothelial cells, which are also fenestrated, such that the sinusoidal lining, and sometimes also the basal lamina, is incomplete. Sinusoids occur in large numbers in the liver (where a basal lamina is completely absent), spleen, bone marrow and suprarenal medulla.

Venules

When two or more capillaries converge, the resulting vessel is larger (10–30 μm) and is known as a venule (postcapillary venule). Venules are essentially tubes of flat, oval or polygonal endothelial cells surrounded by basal lamina and, in the larger vessels, by a delicate adventitia of a few fibroblasts and collagen fibres mainly running longitudinally. Pericytes (*see* **Fig. 7.19**) support the walls of these venules.

Postcapillary venules are sites of leukocyte migration. In venules of mucosa-associated lymphoid tissue (MALT, p. 77), particularly of the gut and bronchi, and in the lymph nodes and thymus, endothelial cells

the flow of blood into the capillary bed, and they act functionally as precapillary sphincters. Closure of the sphincter is thought to be under myogenic, rather than neurogenic, control and is responsive to local vasoactive and metabolic factors. Arteriolar adventitia is very thin.

Arterioles are usually densely innervated by sympathetic fibres, via small bundles of varicose axons packed with transmitter vesicles, mostly of the adrenergic type (p. 44). The distance between axolemma and muscle cell membrane can be as little as 50–100 nm and the gap is occupied only by a basal lamina. Autonomic neuromuscular junctions are very common in arterioles.

143

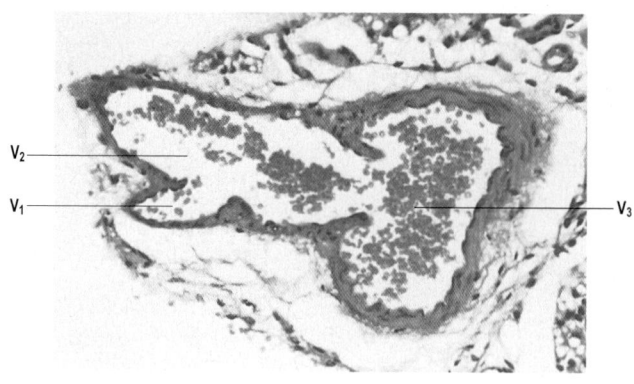

Fig. 7.10 The confluence of a small muscular venule, V₁, with a larger muscular venule, V₂, which then joins a small vein, V₃, cut in transverse section. Note the valve at the junction with the vein. (By permission from Young B, Heath JW 2000 Wheater's Functional Histology. Edinburgh: Churchill Livingstone.)

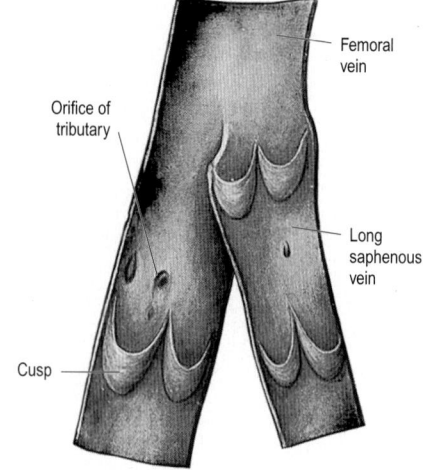

Fig. 7.11 The upper portions of the femoral and long saphenous veins laid open to show the valves. About two-thirds of the natural size.

are taller and have intercellular junctions through which lymphocytes and other blood components can readily pass. These are known as high endothelial venules (HEV) (see **Fig. 7.15**). Elsewhere, venules are believed to be a major site where migration of neutrophils, macrophages and other leukocytes into extravascular spaces occurs, and where neutrophils may temporarily attach, forming marginated pools (p. 146).

In general, the endothelium of venules has few tight junctions, and is relatively permeable. The intercellular junctions of venules are sensitive to inflammatory agents which increase their permeability to fluids and defensive cells, and facilitate leukocyte extravasation by diapedesis.

Venules do not acquire musculature until they are c.50 μm in outer diameter, when they are known as muscular venules (**Fig. 7.10**). This distinction is important, because postcapillary venules, which lack muscle in their walls, are as permeable to solutes as capillaries and are thus part of the microcirculatory bed. At the level of the postcapillary venule the cross-sectional area of the vascular tree is at its maximum, and there is a dramatic fall in pressure (from 25 mmHg in the capillary to c.5 mmHg). Muscular venules converge to produce a series of veins of progressively larger diameter. Venules and veins are capacitance vessels, i.e. they have thin distensible walls which can hold a large volume of blood and accommodate luminal pressure changes.

Veins

Veins are characterized by a relatively thin wall in comparison to arteries of similar size (**Fig. 7.6**) and by a large capacitance. Wall thickness is not correlated exactly to the size of the vein, and varies in different regions, e.g. the wall is thicker in veins of the leg than it is in veins of a similar size in the arm.

The structural plan of the wall is similar to that of other vessels, except that the amount of muscle is considerably less than in arteries, while collagen and, in some veins, elastic fibres, predominate. In most veins, e.g. those of the limbs, the muscle is arranged approximately circularly. Longitudinal muscle is present in the iliac, brachiocephalic, portal and renal veins and in the superior and inferior vena cavae. Muscular tissue is absent in the maternal placental veins, dural venous sinuses and pial and retinal veins, veins of trabecular bone and the venous spaces of erectile tissue. These veins consist of endothelium supported by variable amounts of connective tissue. Distinction between the media and adventitia layers is often difficult, and a discrete internal elastic lamina is absent.

Tethering of some veins to connective tissue fasciae and other surrounding tissues may prevent collapse of the vessel even under negative pressure. Pressure within the venous system does not normally exceed 5 mmHg, and it decreases as the veins grow larger and fewer in number, approaching zero close to the heart. Because they contain only a small amount of muscle, veins have limited influence on blood flow. However, during a sudden fall in blood pressure, e.g. following a haemorrhage, elastic recoil and reflex constriction in veins compensate for the blood loss and tend to maintain venous return to the heart. Vasoconstriction in cutaneous veins in response to cooling is important in thermoregulation.

Most veins have valves to prevent reflux of blood (**Fig. 7.11**). A valve is formed by an inward projection of the tunica intima, strengthened by collagen and elastic fibres, and covered by endothelium which differs in orientation on its two surfaces. Surfaces facing the vessel wall have transversely arranged endothelial cells, whereas on the luminal surface of the valve, over which the main stream of blood flows, cells are arranged longitudinally in the direction of flow. Most commonly two, or occasionally three, valves lie opposite one another, sometimes only one is present. They are found in small veins or where tributaries join larger veins. The valves are semilunar (cusps) and attached by their convex edges to the venous wall. Their concave margins are directed with the flow and lie against the wall as long as flow is towards the heart. When blood flow reverses, the valves close and blood fills an expanded region of the wall, a sinus, on the cardiac side of the closed valve. This may give a 'knotted' appearance to the distended veins, if these have many valves. In the limbs, especially the legs where venous return is against gravity, valves are of great importance to venous flow. Blood is moved towards the heart by the intermittent pressure produced by contractions of the surrounding muscles. Valves are absent in veins of the thorax and abdomen.

VASCULAR SHUNTS AND ANASTOMOSES (Figs 7.12, 7.13)

Arteriovenous shunts and anastomoses

Communications between the arterial and venous systems are found in many regions of the body. In some parts of the microcirculation (e.g. mesentery), the capillary circulation can be bypassed by wider thoroughfare channels formed by metarterioles. These have similarities to both capillaries and the smallest arterioles, and have a discontinuous layer of smooth muscle in their walls. Metarterioles can deliver blood directly to venules or to a capillary bed, according to local demand and conditions. When functional demand is low, blood flow is largely limited to the bypass channel, with most precapillary sphincters, i.e. the smooth muscle of distal arteriole and metarteriole walls, closed. Periodic opening and closing of different sphincters irrigates different parts of the capillary network. The number of capillaries in individual microvascular units and the size of their mesh determine the degree of vascularity of a tissue: the smallest meshes occur in the lungs and the choroid of the eye.

Arteriovenous anastomoses are direct connections between smaller arteries and veins. Connecting vessels may be straight or coiled, and often possess a thick muscular tunic. Under sympathetic control, the vessel is able to close completely, diverting blood into the capillary bed. When patent, the vessel carries blood from artery to vein, partially or completely excluding the capillary bed from the circulation. Simple arteriovenous anastomoses are widespread and occur notably in the skin of the nose, lips and ears, nasal and alimentary mucosae, erectile tissue, tongue, thyroid gland and sympathetic ganglia. In the newborn child, there are few arteriovenous anastomoses, but they develop rapidly during the early years. In old age they atrophy, sclerose and diminish in number. These factors may contribute to the less efficient temperature regulation which occurs at the two extremes of age.

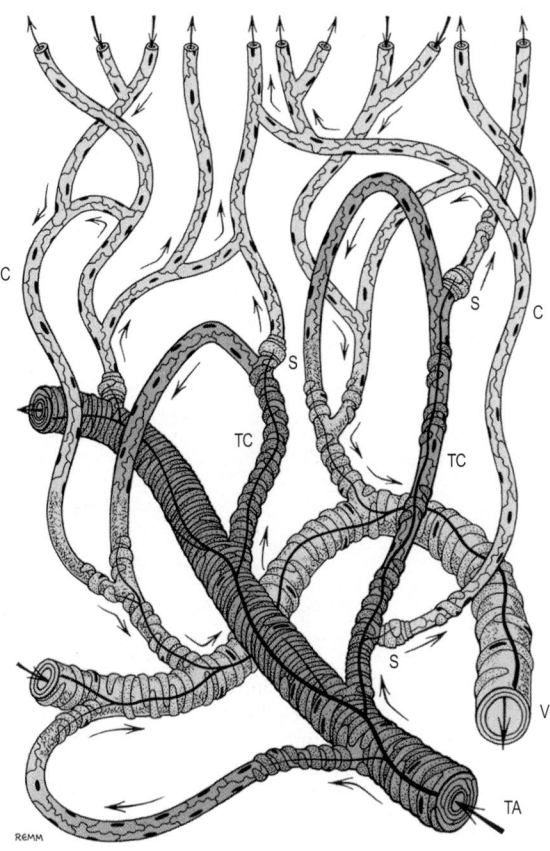

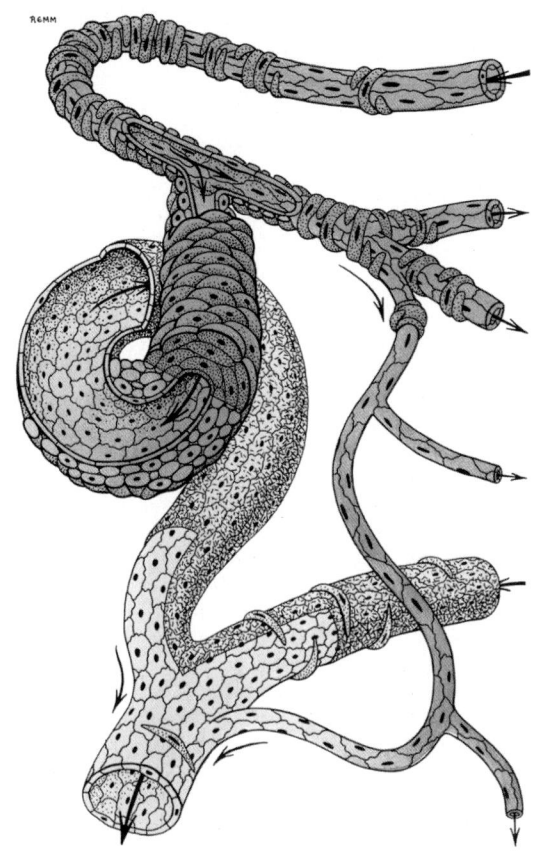

Fig. 7.12 A microcirculatory unit, showing a terminal arteriole (TA), thoroughfare channels (TC), capillaries (C) and collecting venule (V). The distribution of smooth muscle cells and precapillary sphincters (S) is also shown.

Fig. 7.13 An arteriovenous anastomosis. Note the thick wall of the anastomotic channel composed of layers of modified smooth muscle cells.

In the skin of the hands and feet, especially in digital pads and nail beds (**Fig. 8.19**), anastomoses form a large number of small units termed glomera. Each glomus organ has one or more afferent arteries, stemming from branches of cutaneous arteries which approach the surface. The afferent artery gives off a number of fine periglomeral branches and then immediately enlarges, makes a sinuous curve, and narrows again into a short funnel-shaped vein which opens at right angles into a collecting vein (**Fig. 7.14**).

Arterial anastomoses

Arteries can be joined to each other by an anastomosis, so that one can supply the territory of the other. An end-to-end anastomosis occurs when two arteries communicate directly, e.g. the vaginal and ovarian arteries, the right and the left gastroepiploic arteries, the ulnar artery and the superficial palmar branch of the radial artery. Anastomosis by convergence occurs when two arteries converge and merge, as happens when the vertebral arteries form the basilar artery at the base of the brain. A transverse anastomosis occurs when a short arterial vessel links two large arteries transversely, e.g. the anastomoses between the two anterior cerebral arteries; the posterior tibial artery and the peroneal artery; and the radial and ulnar arteries at the wrist.

The angiosome concept and vascular territories

An angiosome is a three-dimensional block of tissue (known as an anatomical territory) supplied by a source artery and its accompanying veins (Salmon 1994). It can be a composite of skin, underlying fascia, muscle and bone. These blocks of tissue form a complex three-dimensional jigsaw puzzle: some pieces have a predominantly cutaneous component while others are predominantly muscular. Each angiosome is made up of arteriosomes and venosomes and they are linked to neighbouring angiosomes by either simple anastomoses composed of similar calibre vessels or reduced calibre vessels termed choke vessels. The anastomoses between adjacent angiosomes can occur within the skin or within muscle. Some muscles are supplied by a single artery and its accompanying veins and therefore lie within one angiosome, while other muscles are

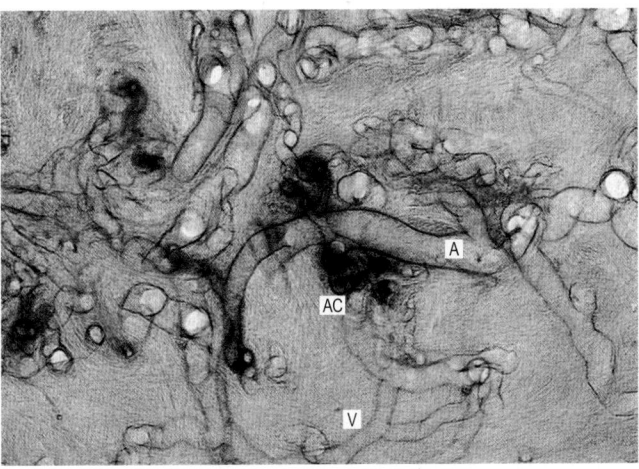

Fig. 7.14 Digital arteriovenous anastomosis prepared by intravascular perfusion of stain in a full thickness specimen of skin, followed by clearance. The heavily stained, thick-walled, tortuous anastomotic channels (AC) contrast with the central arterial stem (A) and the thin-walled venous (V) outflow channels. (Provided by RT Grant, GKT School of Medicine, London.)

supplied by more than one vessel and therefore cross more than one angiosome.

The clinical relevance of the angiosome concept is reflected in the potential connections of adjacent vascular territories. Should the source vessels for one angiosome become blocked or damaged, then that anatomical territory can be 'rescued' by receiving a blood supply from the immediately neighbouring angiosome via the connecting simple and choke vessel anastomoses. A detailed knowledge of angiosomes and vascular territories is essential for plastic and reconstructive surgeons when designing and surgically raising flaps of tissue which can reliably be moved from one part of the body to another without disrupting their blood supply.

FUNCTIONAL MICROSTRUCTURE OF VESSELS

Intima

The intimal lining of blood vessels consist of an endothelium, and a variable amount of subendothelial connective tissue, depending on the vessel.

Endothelium

The endothelium is a monolayer of flattened polygonal cells which extends continuously over the luminal surface of the entire vascular tree (see **Figs 7.7, 7.8, 7.9**). Its structure varies in different regions of the vascular bed.

The endothelium is a key component of the vessel wall, and subserves several major physiological roles. Endothelial cells are in contact with the bloodstream and thus influence blood flow. They regulate the diffusion of substances and migration of cells out of and into the circulating blood. In the brain, endothelial cells of small vessels actively transport substances, e.g. glucose, into the brain parenchyma. Endothelial cells participate in the formation of blood clots (by secreting clot-promoting factors – von Willebrand factor); in minimizing clot formation (by secreting prostacyclin, thrombomodulin); and in the process of clot dissolution or fibrinolysis (by secreting tissue plasminogen activator). They have selective phagocytic activity and are able to extract substances from the blood. For example, the endothelium of pulmonary vessels removes and inactivates several polypeptides, biogenic amines, bradykinin, prostaglandins and lipids from the circulation. Endothelial cells secrete nitric oxide (NO, relaxing factor) and endothelin (a vasoconstrictor) which affect the tone of smooth muscle in vessel walls. They are sensitive to the dilation of vessels imposed by the pulse, via stretch-sensitive ion channels in the cell membrane. Endothelial cells synthesize components of the basal lamina. They proliferate to provide new cells during the growth in size of a blood vessel, to replace damaged endothelial cells, and to provide solid cords of cells which develop into new blood vessels (angiogenesis). Angiogenesis, which may be stimulated by endothelial production of autocrine growth factors in response to locally low oxygen tension, is important in wound healing, and in the growth of tumours.

Endothelial cells are thin but extend over a relatively large surface area. They are generally elongated in the direction of blood flow, especially in arteries (see **Fig. 7.7**). They adhere firmly to each other at their edges, such that the lining of the lumen presents no discontinuity, other than in sinusoids. The thickness of endothelial cells is maximal at the level of their nucleus, where it can reach 2–3 μm, and this part of the cell often bulges slightly into the lumen (**Fig. 7.8**). Elsewhere, the endothelial cell is thinner and laminar: in capillaries, these portions of the cell often measure as little as 0.2 μm in thickness.

Transcytotic (pinocytotic) vesicles are present in all endothelial cells, but are particularly numerous in exchange vessels. They shuttle small amounts of extracellular fluid or blood plasma across the endothelial cytoplasm and thus facilitate the bulk exchange of dissolved gases, nutrients and metabolites between these compartments. In spite of the factors known to be released by endothelial cells, they do not have the morphological characterisitics of secretory cells.

An organelle which characterizes endothelial cells is the Weibel–Palade body, an elongated cytoplasmic vesicle, 0.2×2–3 μm in length, which contains regularly spaced tubular structures parallel to its long axis. Weibel–Palade bodies store the adehesion molecule, P-selectin, and a large glycoprotein known as von Willebrand factor, which is released into the subendothelial connective tissue where it mediates the binding of platelets to the extracellular matrix after vascular injury. Von Willebrand factor is also produced by megakaryocytes and is stored in platelets. Plasma von Willebrand factor binds factor VIII clotting protein, which is secreted into the bloodstream by hepatocytes.

Endothelial cells adhere to adjacent cells through the junctional complex, an area of apposition where adherent and tight junctions are found. They also communicate via gap junctions. Tight junctions are most marked in continuous capillaries. Cell contacts between endothelial cells and smooth muscle cells are common in arterioles, where the separation between endothelium and media is reduced and the inner elastic lamina is either very thin or absent.

Endothelial–leukocyte interactions – The luminal surface of endothelial cells does not normally support the adherence of leukocytes or platelets. However, many functions of human vascular endothelial cells are dynamic rather than fixed. Activated endothelial cells and the characteristic endothelium of high endothelial venules (HEV) of lymphoid tissues, are sites of leukocyte attachment and diapedesis.

HEV (**Fig. 7.15**) are located within the T cell domains, between and around lymphoid follicles in all secondary lymphoid organs and tissues (p. 74), except the spleen. They are specialized venules of 7–30 μm diameter, which possess a conspicuous cuboidal endothelial lining. The luminal aspect of HEVs shows a cobblestone appearance. The endothelial cells rest on a basal lamina and are supported by pericytes and a small amount of connective tissue (**Fig. 7.16**). They are linked by

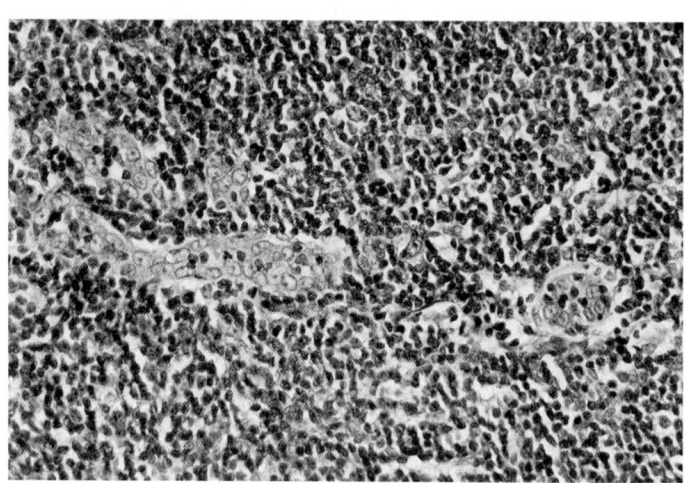

Fig. 7.15 High endothelial venules, lined by pale-stained cuboidal endothelium, in tonsillar lymphoid tissue. A vessel is sectioned longitudinally on the left (centre field) and transversely to the right. Other transversely sectioned vessels (or tributaries of the same vessel) are seen above. (Photograph by Sarah-Jane Smith.)

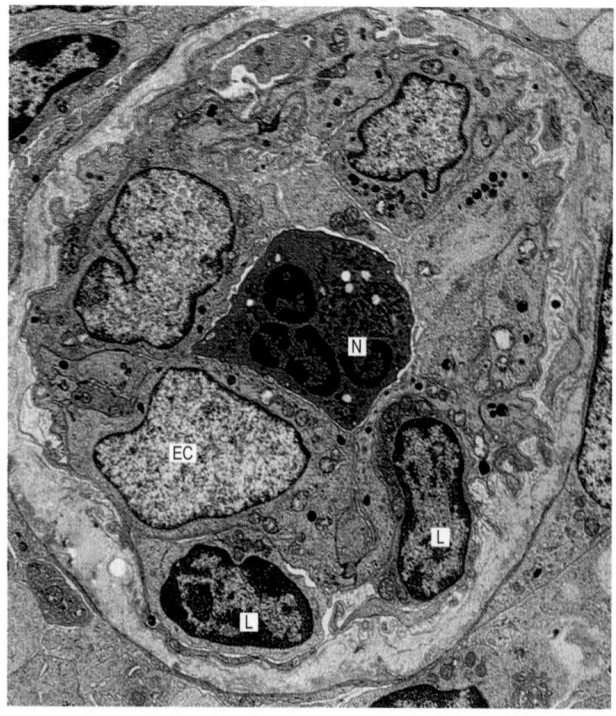

Fig. 7.16 A high endothelial venule in transverse section in the palatine tonsil. The lumen is completely filled by a neutrophil (N). Cuboidal endothelial cells (EC) line the vessel. Two lymphocytes (L) with heterochromatic nuclei are seen below, in transit within the wall of the vessel.

discontinuous adhesive junctions at their apical and basal aspects: the junctions are circumnavigated by migrating lymphocytes. Ultrastructurally, the endothelial cells have the characteristics of metabolically active secretory cells. They contain large, rounded euchromatic nuclei with one or two nucleoli, prominent Golgi complexes, many mitochondria, ribosomes and pinocytotic vesicles. Typically, they also possess Weibel–Palade bodies in which P-selectin is stored.

Many of the adhesion molecules which mediate interactions between blood leukocytes and HEVs or cytokine-activated endothelium have been identified. They can be divided into three general families: selectins, integrins and the immunoglobulin supergene family. Selectins and integrins are expressed on leukocytes and mediate adhesion of circulating cells to the endothelium, which expresses selectins and members of the immunoglobulin supergene family. Regulated expression of these molecules by both cell types provides the means by which leukocytes recognize the vessel wall (leukocyte homing antigens, vascular addressins), adhere to it and subsequently leave the circulation.

The first step in this cascade is the loose binding or tethering of leukocytes, and is initiated via L-, P- or E-selectin. This weak reversible adhesion allows leukocytes to roll along the endothelial surface of a vessel lumen at low velocity, making and breaking contact, and sampling the endothelial cell surfaces. Recognition of chemokines (chemotactic signalling molecules) presented by the endothelium leads to 'inside-out' signalling and conversion of integrins at the leukocyte surface into actively adhesive configurations which bind strongly to their endothelial ligands, resulting in stable arrest. Finally, the leukocyte migrates through the vessel wall (diapedesis), passing between endothelial cells, across the basal lamina and into the surrounding tissue by mechanisms which involve CD31 antigen (p. 73) and matrix metalloproteinases.

Cell adhesion molecules – Three members of the selectin family of adhesive proteins are currently recognized. They are L-selectin (also known as lymphocyte homing receptor), E-selectin and P-selectin. L-selectin is expressed on most leukocytes. Endothelial cells of HEVs in lymphoid organs express its oligosaccharide ligand, although other molecules such as mucins may be alternative ligands. Thus, L-selectin mediates homing of lymphocytes, especially to peripheral lymph nodes, but also promotes the accumulation of neutrophils and monocytes at sites of inflammation. E-selectin is an inducible adhesion molecule which mediates adhesion of leukocytes to inflammatory cytokine-activated endothelium, and is only transiently expressed on endothelium. P-selectin is rapidly mobilized from Weibel–Palade bodies, where it is stored, to the endothelial surface after endothelial activation. It binds to ligands expressed on neutrophils, platelets, and monocytes and, like E-selectin, tethers leukocytes to endothelium at sites of inflammation. However, since P-selectin is quickly endocytosed by the endothelial cells, its expression is short-lived.

The integrins (p. 7) are a large family of molecules which mediate cell-to-cell adhesion as well as interactions of cells with extracellular matrix. Certain β1 integrin heterodimers are expressed on lymphocytes 2–4 weeks after antigenic stimulation (very late antigens, VLA), and bind to the extracellular matrix. Additionally, VLA-4 present on resting lymphocytes (the expression increases after activation), monocytes and eosinophils, binds to the vascular cell adhesion molecule 1 (VCAM-1), the ligand on activated endothelium. In contrast to β1 integrins, which many cells express, the expression of β2 integrins is limited to white blood cells. Although the leukocyte integrins are not constitutively adhesive, they become highly adhesive after cell activation and therefore play a key role in the events required for cell migration. The endothelial ligands for one such β2 integrin are the intercellular adhesion molecules 1 and 2 (ICAM-1 and ICAM-2), which belong to the immunoglobulin superfamily.

Three members of the large immunoglobulin superfamily of proteins are involved in leukocyte-endothelial adhesion, providing integrin counter-receptors on the endothelial cell membrane. ICAM-1 and ICAM-2 are constitutively expressed but upregulated by inflammatory cytokines. VCAM-1 is absent from resting endothelium but is induced by cytokines on activated endothelium and promotes extravasation of lymphocytes at sites of inflammation.

Subendothelial connective tissue

The subendothelial connective tissue, also termed the lamina propria, is a thin but variable layer. It is largely absent in the smallest vessels, where the endothelium is supported instead by pericytes. It contains a typical fibrocollagenous extracellular matrix, a few fibroblasts and occasional smooth muscle cells. Endothelial von Willebrand factor concentrates in this layer and participates in the clotting process when the overlying endothelium is damaged.

Media

The media consists chiefly of concentric layers of circumferentially or helically arranged smooth muscle cells with variable amounts of elastin and collagen.

Smooth muscle

Smooth muscle forms most of the media of arteries (**Fig. 7.17**) and arterioles. A thinner layer of smooth muscle is also found in venules and veins, with the exception of small segments of the pulmonary veins, where striated cardiac muscle is present in the portions nearest to the heart (p. 81). Contraction of the smooth muscle in arteries and arterioles reduces the calibre of the vessel lumen, which reduces blood flow through the vessel and raises the pressure on the proximal side. This role is particularly effective in small resistance vessels where the wall is thick, relative to the diameter of the vessel. Smooth muscle can also alter the rigidity of the wall, without causing constriction (isometric contraction), and this affects the distensibility of the wall and propagation of the pulse.

The smooth muscle cells synthesize and secrete elastin, collagen and other extracellular components of the media which bear directly on the mechanical properties of the vessels. The mechanics of the musculature of the media are complex. Distensibility, strength, self-support, elasticity, rigidity, concentric constriction etc., are interrelated functions and are finely balanced in the different regions of the vascular bed.

In large arteries, where the blood pressure is high, the muscle cells are shorter (60–200 μm) and smaller in volume than in visceral muscle. In arterioles and veins, smooth muscle cells more closely resemble visceral muscle cells. The cells are packed with myofilaments and other elements of the cytoskeleton, including intermediate filaments. Vascular muscle cells have intermediate filaments of either vimentin alone or both vimentin and desmin. In visceral smooth muscle the intermediate filaments are formed exclusively of desmin. Intercellular junctions are mainly of the adhesive (adherens) type and provide mechanical coupling between the cells. In addition, there are gap (communicating) junctions which couple cells electrically (p. 7). Junctions between muscle cells and the connective tissue matrix are particularly numerous, especially in arteries.

The muscle cells of the arterial media can be regarded as multifunctional mesenchymal cells. After damage to the endothelium, muscle cells migrate into the intima and proliferate, forming bundles of longitudinally oriented cells which reform the layer. In certain pathological

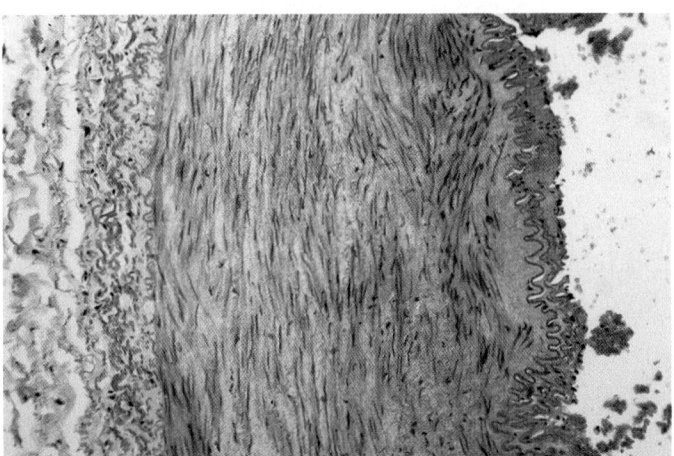

Fig. 7.17 The wall of a muscular artery showing its three layers: the innermost intima faces the lumen (right) and is separated from the media by an internal elastic lamina, seen in routine preparations (as here) as a wavy, refractile, pink line, which may be split in places. The media is composed of tightly packed smooth muscle fibres oriented spirally or circumferentially. The looser connective tissue of the adventitia is seen to the left. (Photograph by Sarah-Jane Smith.)

conditions, muscle cells undergo fatty degeneration and participate in the formation of atheromatous plaques.

Collagen and elastin

Components of the extracellular matrix are major constituents of vessel walls, and in large arteries and veins they make up more than half of the mass of the wall, mainly in the form of collagen and elastin. Other fibrous components such as fibronectin, and amorphous proteoglycans and glycosaminoglycans, are present in the interstitial space.

Elastin is found in all arteries and veins and is especially abundant in elastic arteries (**Fig. 7.5**). Individual elastic fibres (0.1–1.0 μm in diameter) anastomose with each other to form net-like structures, which extend predominantly in a circumferential direction. More extensive fusion produces lamellae of elastic material, which though usually perforated and thus incomplete, separate the layers of muscle cells. A conspicuous elastic lamella, the internal elastic lamina, is seen in arteries, between intima and media. This is a tube of elastic material which allows the vessel to recoil after distension. When the intraluminal pressure falls below physiological limits (postmortem), the inner elastic lamina is compressed and it coils up into a regular corrugated shape (**Fig. 7.18**): in these conditions the lumen is much reduced but is not obliterated, and the profile of the artery remains circular. Fenestrations in the elastic lamina, which may also be split in thickness, allow materials to diffuse between intima and media. An outer elastic lamina, similar in appearance to, but markedly less well developed and less compact than the internal elastic lamina, lies at the outer aspect of the media at its boundary with the adventitia. These laminae are less evident in elastic arteries, where elastic fibres occupy much of the media.

Collagen fibrils are found in all three vessel layers. Type III collagen (reticulin) occupies much of the interstitial space between the muscle cells of the media, and is also found in the intima. Collagen is abundant in the adventitia, where type I collagen fibres form large bundles which increase in size from the junction with the media to the outer limit of the vessel wall. In veins, collagen is the main component of the vessel wall, and accounts for more than half its mass.

In general terms, collagen and elastic fibres in the media run parallel to, or at a small angle to, the axes of the muscle cells, and they are therefore mainly circumferentially arranged. In contrast, the predominant arrangement of collagen fibres in the adventitia is longitudinal. This arrangement imposes constraints on length change in large vessels under pressure, e.g. in large arteries, the radial distension under the effect of the pulse far exceeds the longitudinal distension. The outer sheath of type I collagen in the adventitia therefore has a structurally supportive role. The more delicate type III collagen network of the media provides attachment to the muscle cells and its role is to transmit force around the circumference of the vessel. In a distended vessel, the elastic fibres store energy and, by recoiling, help to restore the resting length and calibre.

The extracellular material of the media, including collagen and elastin, is produced by the muscle cells. Its turnover is slow compared to that in other tissues. In the adventitia, collagen is synthesized and secreted by fibroblasts, as in other connective tissues. During postnatal development, while vessels increase in diameter and wall thickness, there is an increase in elastin and collagen content. Subsequent changes in vessel structure, seen during ageing, include an increase in the collagen-to-elastin ratio, with a reduction in vessel elasticity.

Adventitia

This layer is formed of general connective tissue, varying in the thickness and density of its collagen fibre bundles.

Vasa vasorum

In smaller vessels, the nourishment of the tissues of the vessel wall is provided by diffusion from the blood circulating in the vessel itself. Large vessels have their own vascular supply within the adventitia (**Fig. 7.4**), in the form of a network of small vessels, mainly of the microcirculation, which are called the vasa vasorum. The wall thickness at which simple diffusion from the lumen becomes insufficient is c.1 mm.

The vasa vasorum originate from, and drain into, adjacent vessels which are peripheral branches of the vessel they supply. They ramify within the adventitia and, in the largest of arteries, penetrate the outermost part of the media. The larger veins are also supplied by vasa vasorum, but these may penetrate the wall more deeply, perhaps because of the lower oxygen tension.

Nervi vasorum

Blood vessels are innervated by efferent autonomic fibres which regulate the state of contraction of the musculature (muscular tone), and thus

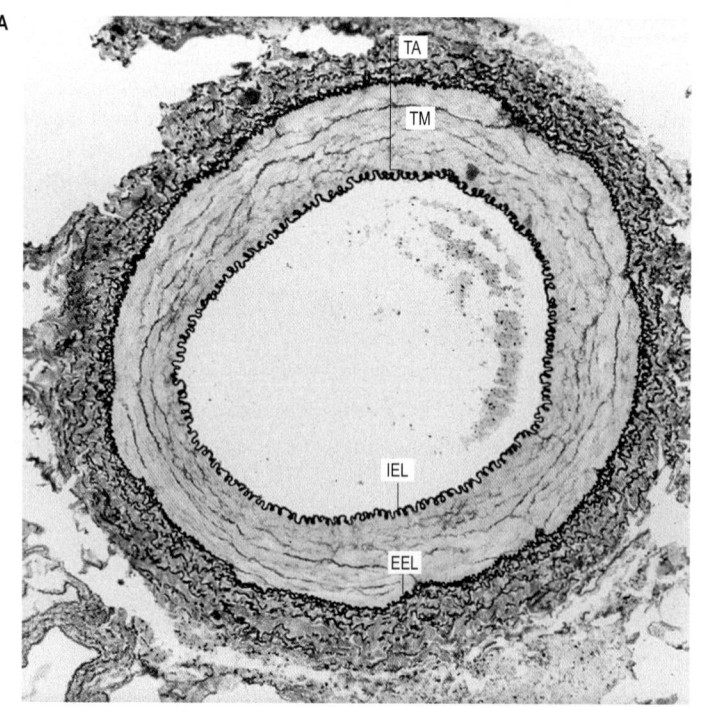

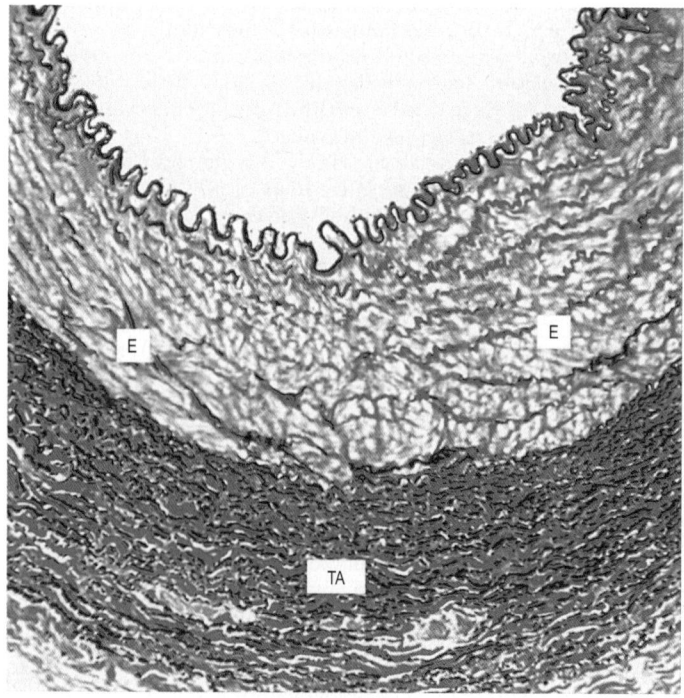

Fig. 7.18 Muscular arteries. **A** A medium-sized muscular artery stained for elastin showing the internal elastic lamina (IEL) and external elastic lamina (EEL). The tunica media (TM) contains little elastin, but the tunica adventitia (TA) contains rather more in the form of discontinuous profiles. **B** Higher magnification of a muscular artery, with discontinuous elastic lamellae (E) in the tunica media, which consists mainly of smooth muscle. The collagen-rich connective tissue of the thick tunica adventitia (TA) supports the vessel wall. (By permission from Dr JB Kerr, Monash University, from Kerr JB 1999 Atlas of Functional Histology. London: Mosby.)

the diameter of the vessels, particularly the arteries and arterioles. These perivascular nerves branch and anastomose within the adventitia of an artery, forming a meshwork around it. In some of the large muscular arteries, nerves are occasionally found within the outermost layers of the media.

Nervi vasorum are small bundles of axons, which are almost invariably unmyelinated and typically varicose. Most are postganglionic fibres which issue from sympathetic ganglion neurones. Some vessels in the brain (Chapter 17) may be innervated by intrinsic cerebral neurones although neural control of brain vessels is of minor importance compared with metabolic and autoregulation (local response to stretch stimuli). The density of innervation varies in different vessels and in different areas of the body: it is usually sparser in veins and larger lymphatic vessels. Large veins with a pronounced muscle layer, such as the hepatic portal vein, are well-innervated.

The control of vascular smooth muscle is complex. Vasoconstrictor adrenergic fibres act on adrenoceptors in the muscle cell membrane. In addition, circulating hormones and factors such as nitric oxide and endothelins, which are released from endothelial cells, exert a powerful effect on the muscle cells. The neurotransmitters reach the muscle from the adventitial surface of the media, and hormonal and endothelial factors diffuse from the intimal surface. In some tissues sympathetic cholinergic fibres inhibit smooth muscle contraction and induce vasodilation.

Most arteries are accompanied by nerves which travel in parallel with them to the peripheral organs which they supply. However, these paravascular nerves are quite independent, and do not innervate the vessels they accompany.

Pericytes

Pericytes are present at the outer surface of capillaries and the smallest venules (postcapillary venules), where an adventitia is absent and there are no muscle cells. They are elongated cells, whose long cytoplasmic processes are wrapped around the endothelium. Pericytes are scattered in a discontinuous layer around the outer circumference of capillaries. They are generally absent from fenestrated capillaries, but form a more continuous layer around postcapillary venules (Fig. 7.19). They are gradually replaced by smooth muscle cells as vessels converge and increase in diameter.

Pericytes are enclosed by their own basal lamina, which merges in places with that of the endothelium. Most pericytes display areas of close apposition with endothelial cells, and occasionally form adherens junctions where their basal laminae are absent. Pericyte cytoplasm contains actin, myosin, tropomyosin and desmin, which suggests that these cells are capable of contractile activity. They also have the potential to act as mesenchymal stem cells, and they participate in repair processes by proliferating and giving rise to new blood vessel and connective tissue cells.

Cerebral vessels
(See also Ch. 17.)

Major branches of cerebral arteries which lie in the subarachnoid space over the surface of the brain have a thin outer coating of meningeal cells, usually one layer thick, where adjacent meningeal cells are joined by desmosomes and gap junctions. These arteries have a smooth muscle media and a distinct elastic lamina. Veins on the surface of the brain have very thin walls, and the smooth muscle layers in the wall are often discontinuous. They are coated externally by a monolayer of meningeal cells.

As arteries enter the subpial space and penetrate the brain, they lose their elastic laminae, and consequently the cerebral cortex and white matter typically contain only arterioles, venules and capillaries. The exceptions are the large penetrating vessels in the basal ganglia, where many arteries retain their elastic laminae and thick smooth muscle media. Enlarged perivascular spaces form around these large arteries in ageing individuals. Arterioles and venules in the cortex and white matter can be distinguished from each other because arterioles are surrounded by a smooth muscle coat, and the veins and venules have larger lumina and thinner walls.

Cerebral capillaries are the site of the blood–brain barrier (p. 51). They are lined by endothelial cells which are joined by tight junctions. The endothelial cytoplasm contains a few pinocytotic vesicles. The cells are surrounded by a basal lamina (Fig. 4.11): at points of contact with perivascular astrocytes the intervening basal lamina is formed by

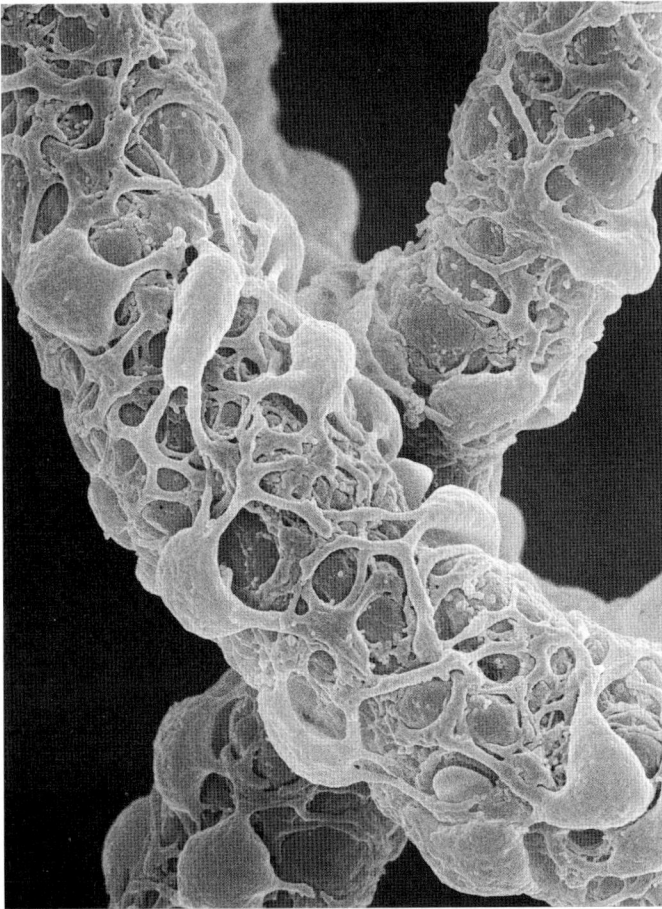

Fig. 7.19 Scanning electron micrograph of two postcapillary venules, showing pericytes supporting their walls. (From T. Fujiwara, Y. Uehara, Copyright © 1984 Am J Anat 170: 39–54. Reprinted by permission from Wiley-Liss, Inc.)

fusion of the endothelial and glial basal laminae. Pericytes, completely surrounded by basal lamina, are present around capillaries. Perivascular macrophages are attached to the outer walls of capillaries and to other vessels: they are phenotypically distinct from parenchymal microglia, which are also of monocytic origin. A thin layer of meningeal cells derived from the pia mater surrounds arterioles but disappears at the level of capillaries.

LYMPHATIC VESSELS

Lymphatic capillaries form wide-meshed plexuses in the extracellular matrices of most tissues. They begin as dilated, blind-ended tubes with larger diameters and less regular cross-sectional appearances than those of blood capillaries. A basal lamina is incomplete or absent and they lack associated pericytes. The smaller lymphatic vessels are lined by endothelial cells which have numerous transcytotic vesicles within their cytoplasm, and so they resemble blood capillaries. However, unlike capillaries, their endothelium is generally quite permeable to much larger molecules: they are readily permeable to large colloidal proteins and particulate material such as cell debris and microorganisms, and also to cells. Permeability is facilitated by gaps between the endothelial cells, which lack tight junctions, and by pinocytosis.

Lymph is formed from interstitial fluid, which is derived from blood plasma via the microcirculation. Much of this fluid is returned to the venous system. Lymphatic vessels take up the excess (about one tenth) by passive diffusion and the transient negative pressures in their lumina which are generated intrinsically by contractile activity in lymphatic vessel walls, and extrinsically, by movements of other tissues (muscles, arteries) locally. The unidirectional flow of lymph is maintained by the presence of valves in the larger vessels (see **Fig. 7.20**). Lymphatic capillaries are prevented from collapsing by anchoring filaments which tether their walls to surrounding connective tissue structures and exert radial traction.

In most tissues, lymph is clear and colourless. In contrast, the lymph from the small intestine is dense and milky, reflecting the presence of lipid droplets (chylomicrons) derived from fat absorbed by the mucosal epithelium. The terminal lymphatic vessels in the mucosa of the small intestine are known as lacteals (see **Fig. 72.5**) and the lymph as chyle. Lymphatic capillaries are not ubiquitous: they are not present in cornea, cartilage, thymus, the central or peripheral nervous system or bone marrow, and there are very few in the endomysium of skeletal muscles.

Lymphatic capillaries join into larger vessels which pass to local lymph nodes (p. 75). Typically, lymph percolates through a series of nodes before reaching a major collecting duct. There are exceptions to this arrangement: the lymph vessels of the thyroid gland and oesophagus, and of the coronary and triangular ligaments of the liver, all drain directly to the thoracic duct without passing through lymph nodes. In the larger vessels, a thin external connective tissue coat supports the endothelium. The largest lymphatic vessels (>200 μm) have three layers, like small veins, although their lumen is considerably larger than is the case in veins with a similar wall thickness. The tunica media contains smooth muscle cells, mostly arranged circumferentially. Elastic fibres are sparse in the tunica intima, but form an external elastic lamina in the tunica adventitia.

The larger lymphatic vessels differ from small veins in having many more valves (**Fig. 7.20**). The valves are semilunar, generally paired and composed of an extension of the intima. Their edges point in the direction of the current, and the vessel wall downstream is expanded into a sinus, which gives the vessels a beaded appearance when they are distended. Valves are important in preventing the backflow of lymph.

Deep lymphatic vessels usually accompany arteries or veins, and almost all reach either the thoracic duct or the right lymphatic duct, which usually join the left or right brachiocephalic veins respectively at the root of the neck.

The thoracic duct is structurally similar to a medium-sized vein, but the smooth muscle in its tunica media is more prominent (Chapter 59). Most lymphatic vessels anastomose freely, and larger ones have their own plexiform vasa vasorum and accompanying nerve fibres. If their walls are acutely infected (lymphangitis) this vascular plexus becomes congested, marking the paths of superficial vessels by red lines, which are visible through the skin, and tender to the touch.

Lymphatic vessels repair easily and new vessels readily form after damage. They begin as solid cellular sprouts from the endothelial cells of persisting vessels and later become canalized.

CARDIAC MUSCLE

In cardiac muscle, as in skeletal muscle, the contractile proteins are organized structurally into sarcomeres which are aligned in register across the fibres, producing fine cross-striations that are visible in the light microscope. They both contain the same contractile proteins (although many are cardiac isoforms), which are assembled in a similar way, and the molecular basis for contraction, but not its regulation, is the same (p. 121). Release of calcium into the sarcoplasm triggers contraction, which corresponds to cardiac systole, the pumping phase of the heart cycle. Reuptake of calcium produces relaxation, which corresponds to cardiac diastole, the filling phase of the cycle.

Despite the similarities, there are major functional, morphological and developmental differences between cardiac and skeletal muscle. Some of the ways in which cardiac muscle differs morphologically from skeletal muscle are described below, before consideration of other features that are unique to cardiac muscle.

MICROSTRUCTURE

The myocardium, the muscular component of the heart, constitutes the bulk of its tissues. It consists predominantly of cardiac muscle cells, which are usually c.120 μm long and 20–30 μm in diameter in a normal adult. Each cell has one or two large nuclei, occupying the central part of the cell, whereas skeletal muscle has multiple, peripherally placed nuclei. The cells are branched at their ends, and the branches of adjacent cells are so tightly associated that the light microscopic appearance is of a network of branching and anastomosing fibres (**Fig. 7.21**). Ultrastructurally, cells are bound together by elaborate junctional complexes (**Fig. 7.22, 7.23**), which means that, unlike skeletal muscle, the fibres of cardiac muscle are not single syncytial cells with a common cytoplasm.

Fine fibrocollagenous connective tissue is found between cardiac muscle fibres. Although this is equivalent to the endomysium of skeletal muscle, it is less regularly organized because of the complex three-dimensional geometry imposed by the branching cardiac cells. Numerous capillaries and some nerve fibres are found within this layer. Coarser connective tissue, equivalent to the perimysium of skeletal muscle, separates the larger bundles of muscle fibres, and is particularly well developed near the condensations of dense fibrous connective tissue that form the 'skeleton' of the heart (p. 996). The ventricles of the heart are composed of spiralling layers of fibres which run in different directions. Consequently, microscope sections of ventricular muscle inevitably contain the profiles of cells cut in a variety of orientations. A linear arrangement of cardiac muscle fibres is found only in the papillary muscles and trabeculae carneae.

Electron micrographs of cardiac muscle cells in longitudinal section (**Fig. 7.24**) show that the myofibrils separate before they pass around the nucleus, leaving a zone that is occupied by organelles, including sarcoplasmic reticulum, Golgi complex, mitochondria, lipid droplets, and glycogen. At the light microscopic level, these zones appear in longitudinal sections as unstained areas at the poles of each nucleus. They often contain lipofuscin granules, which accumulate there in

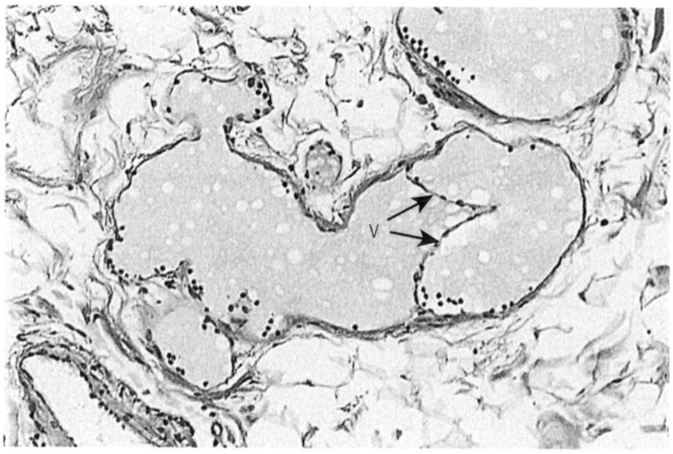

Fig. 7.20 A lymphatic vessel in longitudinal section with a valve (V) projecting into its lumen. The supporting tissue core of the valve consists of reticular (collagen type III) fibres and a little ground substance. Note the presence of lymphocytes at the periphery of the lumen. (By permission from Young B, Heath JW 2000 Wheater's Functional Histology. Edinburgh: Churchill Livingstone.)

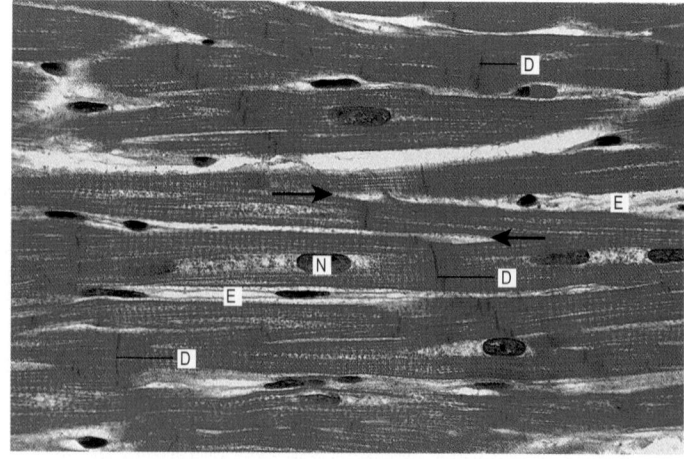

Fig. 7.21 Cardiac muscle fibres, with branched ends (arrows), sectioned longitudinally. Faint fine cross-striations indicate the intracellular organization of sarcomeres around the centrally situated nuclei (N). The darker transverse lines (some appear stepped) are intercalated discs (D). Endomysium (E) contains nuclei of endothelial cells and fibroblasts. (By permission from Dr JB Kerr, Monash University, from Kerr JB 1999 Atlas of Functional Histology. London: Mosby.)

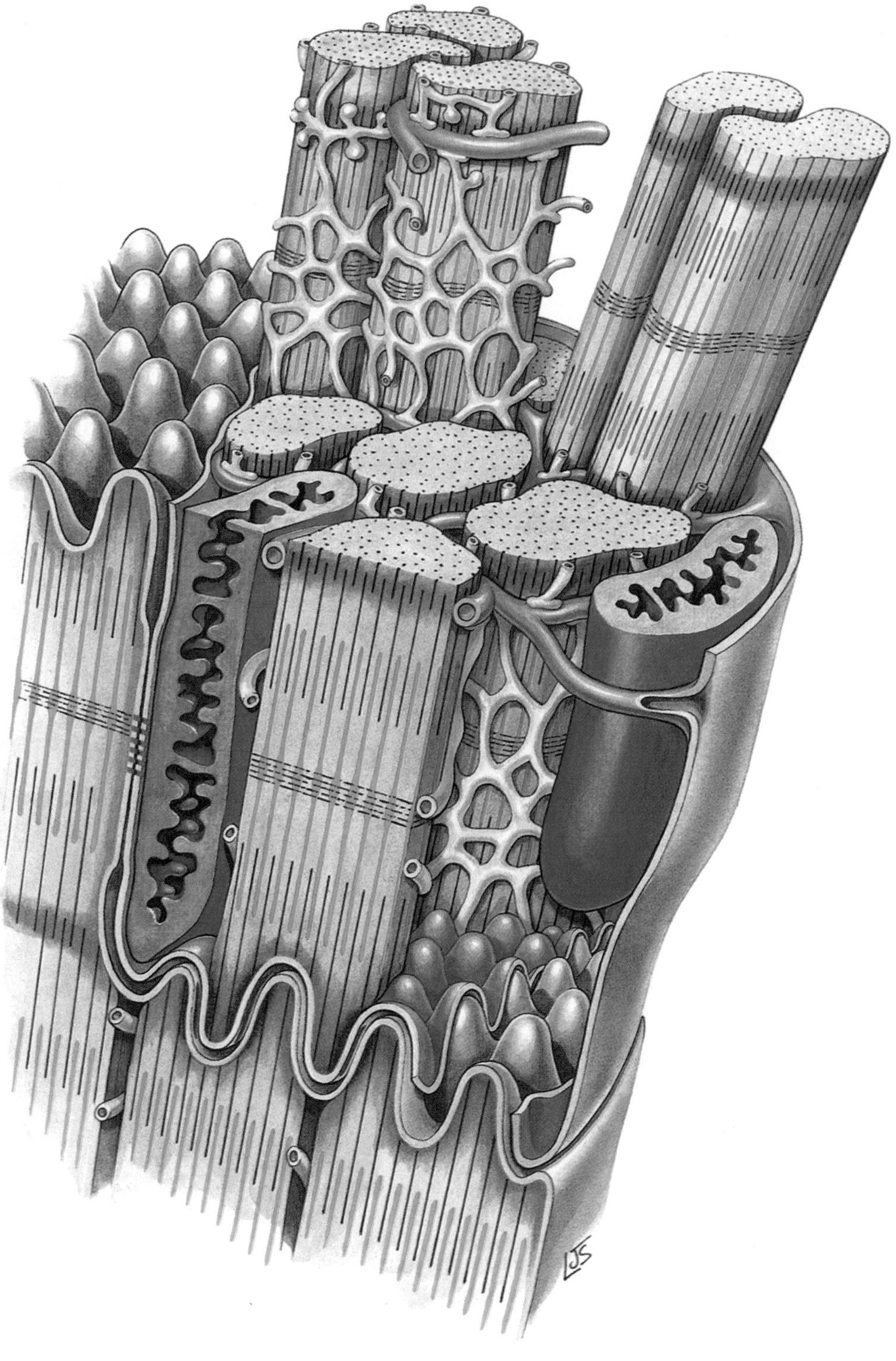

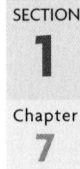

Fig. 7.22 Three-dimensional reconstruction of cardiac muscle cells, showing the organization of the transverse tubules (orange) and sarcoplasmic reticulum (buff). An intercalated disc is illustrated at the bottom and left, between adjacent cells. (Artist: Lesley Skeates.)

individuals over the age of 10; the reddish-brown pigment may be visible even in unstained longitudinal sections.

The cross-striations of cardiac muscle are less conspicuous than those of skeletal muscle. This is because the contractile apparatus of cardiac muscle lies within an abundant mitochondria-rich sarcoplasm. The myofibrils are less well delineated than they are in skeletal muscle: in transverse sections they often fuse into a continuous array of myofilaments, irregularly bounded by mitochondria and longitudinal elements of sarcoplasmic reticulum. The large mitochondria, with their closely spaced cristae, reflect the highly developed oxidative metabolism of cardiac tissue. The proportion of the cell volume occupied by mitochondria (c.35%) is even greater in cardiac muscle than it is in slow

twitch skeletal muscle fibres. The high demand for oxygen is also reflected in high levels of myoglobin and an exceptionally rich network of capillaries around the fibres.

The force of contraction is transferred through the ends of the cardiac muscle cells via the junctional strength provided by the intercalated discs. As in skeletal muscle, force is also transmitted laterally to the sarcolemma and extracellular matrix via vinculin-containing elements which bridge between the Z-discs of peripheral myofibrils and the plasma membrane.

Atrial muscle cells are smaller than ventricular cells. The cytoplasm near the Golgi complexes at the poles of the nuclei exhibits dense membrane-bound granules, which contain the precursor of atrial

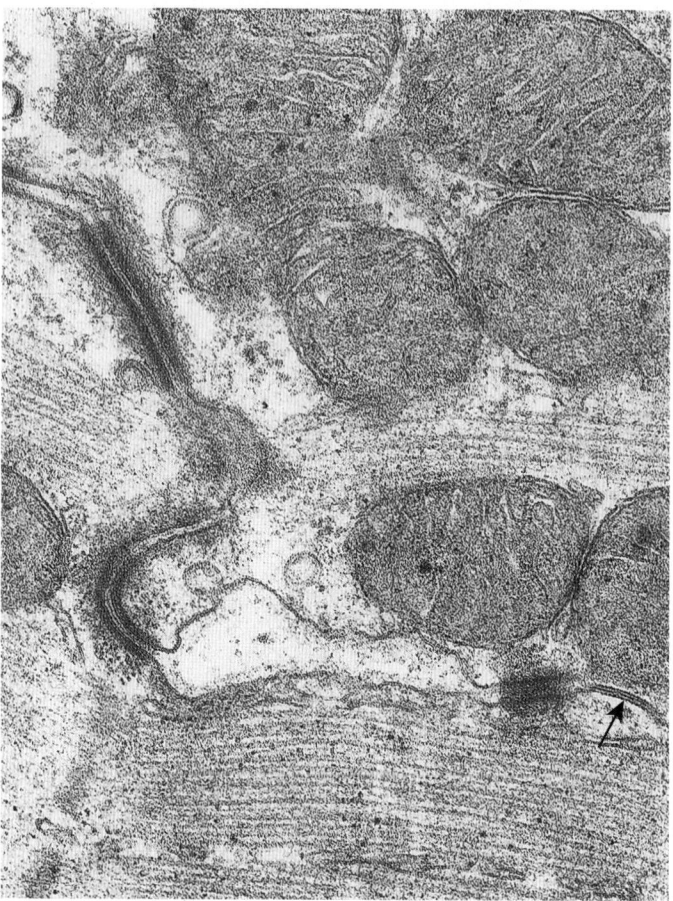

Fig. 7.23 An intercalated disc in cardiac muscle, with several zones of electron dense fascia adherens and a gap junction (arrow). (Provided by Brenda Russell, Department of Physiology and Biophysics, University of Illinois at Chicago.)

natriuretic factor. This is a hormone whose action is to promote loss of sodium chloride and water in the kidneys, reducing body fluid volume and thereby lowering blood pressure. It is released in response to stretch of the atrial wall. The actions of atrial natriuretic factor are normally balanced by the opposing effects of aldosterone and antidiuretic hormone.

The sarcolemma of ventricular cardiac muscle cells invaginates to form T-tubules with a wider lumen than those of skeletal muscle: atrial muscle cells have few or no T-tubules. Unlike skeletal muscle, the T-tubules penetrate the sarcoplasm at the level of the Z-discs (**Fig. 7.22**). The T-tubules are interconnected at intervals by longitudinal branches. They probably serve a similar function in skeletal and cardiac muscle, i.e. to carry the wave of depolarization into the core of the cells.

The sarcoplasmic reticulum is a membrane-bound tubular plexus which surrounds, and defines, sometimes incompletely, the outlines of individual myofibrils. Its main role, as in skeletal muscle, is the storage, release and reaccumulation of calcium ions. It comes into close contact with the T-tubules, leaving a 15 nm gap that is spanned by structures termed junctional processes. These processes are thought to be the cytoplasmic part of the calcium release channels (ryanodine receptors); similar processes are found in skeletal muscle at the junctional surface of the terminal cisternae. Sarcoplasmic reticulum which bears junctional processes has been termed junctional sarcoplasmic reticulum, to distinguish it from the free sarcoplasmic reticulum, which forms a longitudinal network. Junctional sarcoplasmic reticulum makes contact with both the T-tubules and the sarcolemma (of which the T-tubules are an extension). Sarcoplasmic reticulum forms small globular extensions (corbular sarcoplasmic reticulum) in the vicinity of the Z-discs, but not in immediate relation to T-tubules or the sarcolemma. Since the junctions between T-tubules and sarcoplasmic reticulum usually involve only one structure of each type, the corresponding profiles in electron micrographs are referred to as dyads, rather than triads as in skeletal muscle.

Intercalated discs

Intercalated discs are unique to cardiac muscle. In the light microscope they are seen as dark, transverse lines crossing the tracts of cardiac cells (**Fig. 7.21**). They may step irregularly within or between adjacent tracts, and may appear to jump to a new position as the plane of focus is altered. At the ultrastructural level these structures, which are complex junctions between the cardiac muscle cells, are seen to have transverse and lateral portions (**Figs 7.22, 7.23**). The transverse portions occur wherever myofibrils abut the end of the cell, and each takes the place of the last Z-disc. At this point the actin filaments of the terminal sarcomere insert into a dense subsarcolemmal matrix which anchors them, together with other cytoplasmic elements such as intermediate filaments, to the plasma membrane. Prominent desmosomes, often with a dense line in the intercellular space, occur at intervals along each transverse portion. This junctional region is homologous with, and probably similar in composition to, the structure found on the cytoplasmic face of the myotendinous junction, and is a type of fascia adherens junction. It provides firm adhesion between cells, and a route for the transmission of contractile force from one cell to the next.

The lateral portions of the intercalated disc run parallel to the myofilaments, and the long axis of the cell, for a distance which corresponds to one or two sarcomeres before it turns again to form another transverse portion. It is therefore responsible for the stepwise progression of the intercalated disc which can be seen microscopically. The lateral portions contain gap junctions, which are responsible for the electrical coupling between adjacent cells (**Fig. 7.23**). Conductance channels within these junctions enable the electrical impulse to propagate from one cell to the next, spreading excitation and contraction rapidly along the branching tracts of interconnected cells. In this way the activity of the individual cells of the heart is coordinated so that they function as if they were a syncytium.

VASCULAR SUPPLY AND LYMPHATIC DRAINAGE

The activity of the heart is equivalent to a constant power expenditure of c.1.3 watts under basal conditions, and escalates to 3 watts or more during physical exertion. Cardiac muscle cells contain glycogen, which is a reserve during peaks of activity, but the majority of their energy requirement is continuous and supplied only through a highly developed oxidative metabolism, as is evident from the high proportion of the cell volume which is occupied by mitochondria. This metabolism has to be supported by a rich blood supply. Myocardium has a very high perfusion rate of 0.5 ml/min/g of tissue (c.5 times that of liver and 15 times that of resting skeletal muscle). No cardiac muscle cell is more than c.8 μm from a capillary, and vascular channels occupy a high proportion of the total interstitial space. Heart muscle is supplied by the coronary vessels (p. 1014). Although there is some variation in the detailed distribution of the arterial branches, the left ventricle, which has the highest workload, consistently receives the highest arterial blood flow. Branches run in the myocardium along the coarser aggregations of connective tissue and ramify extensively in the endomysial layer, creating a rich plexus of anastomosing vessels. This plexus includes lymphatic as well as blood capillaries, which is not the case in skeletal muscle.

The high oxygen requirement of the myocardium makes it vulnerable to ischaemic damage arising from atheroma or embolism in the coronary arteries. Arterial anastomoses, often more than 100 μm in diameter, are found throughout the heart and are an important factor in determining whether an adequate collateral circulation can develop after a coronary occlusion.

INNERVATION

Although the impulse-generating and conducting system of the heart establishes an endogenous rhythm, the rate and force of contraction are under neural influence. Both divisions of the autonomic nervous system supply non-myelinated postganglionic fibres to the heart. The innervation is derived bilaterally, but it is functionally asymmetrical. Activation of the left stellate ganglion (sympathetic) has little effect on heart rate but increases ventricular contractility, whereas activation of the right stellate ganglion influences both rate and contractility. Activation of the right vagus nerve (parasympathetic) slows heart rate mainly through its influence on the sinoatrial (SA) node, whereas activation of the left vagus slows propagation of the impulse mainly through its effect on the atrioventricular (AV) node. Vagal activity has little direct effect on ventricular contractility.

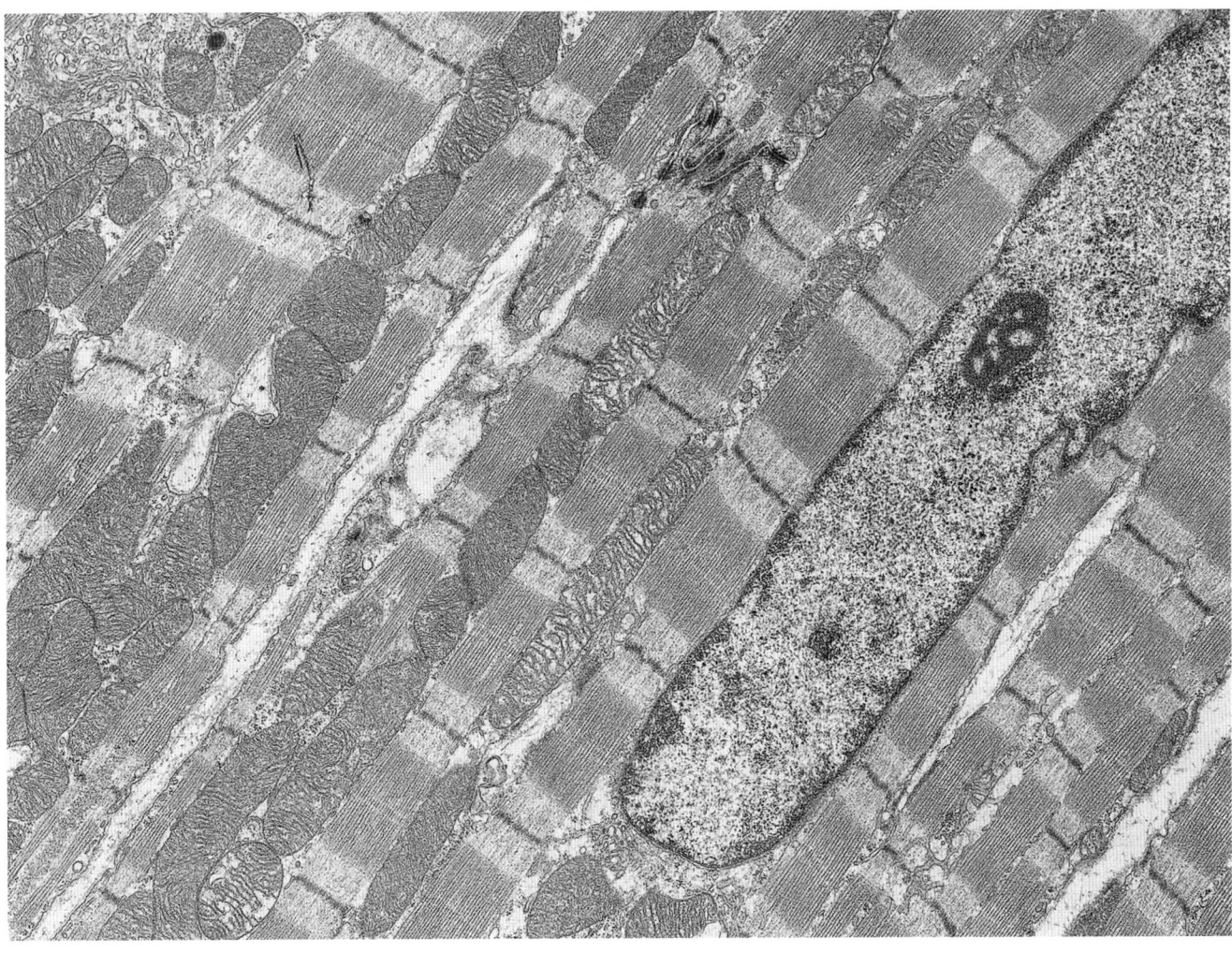

Fig. 7.24 Low power electron micrograph of cardiac muscle in longitudinal section. Note the centrally placed nucleus, abundant large mitochondria between myofibrils, and an intercalated disc. (Provided by Brenda Russell, Department of Physiology and Biophysics, University of Illinois at Chicago.)

Sympathetic nerve fibres from the cervical sympathetic ganglia reach the heart via the cardiac nerves. Parasympathetic fibres in the heart originate in ganglion cells that are innervated by efferent fibres of the vagus nerve. Adrenergic, cholinergic and peptidergic endings have been demonstrated in the myocardium. Fibres often end close to muscle cells and blood vessels, but junctional specializations are not seen, and a gap of at least 110 nm remains between cell and nerve fibre. It is probable that neurotransmitters diffuse across this gap to the adjacent cells. Some of the endings represent efferent nerve terminals, others function as pain, mechano- or chemoreceptors.

EXCITATION–CONTRACTION COUPLING IN CARDIAC MUSCLE

The molecular interaction between actin and myosin that underlies the generation of force is initiated in the same way in cardiac and skeletal muscle. However, differences in the physical arrangement and molecular composition of these contractile elements have a profound influence on contractile function in cardiac muscle.

The calcium release channels of the sarcoplasmic reticulum are sensitive to the concentration of free calcium in the gap between the T-tubule and sarcoplasmic reticulum membranes. This underlies 'calcium-induced calcium release', which is believed to be the principal, and probably the only, mechanism involved in the liberation of calcium from the sarcoplasmic reticulum during physiological activation. The passage of an action potential depolarizes the sarcolemma and thereby opens sarcolemmal L-type calcium channels, which allows some calcium to enter from the extracellular space. This produces a localized rise in the intracellular free calcium concentration near the calcium release channels, which consequently open, allowing calcium ions to flow down their concentration gradient from the

sarcoplasmic reticulum into the cytosol. The rise in cytosolic calcium concentration then activates the contractile machinery.

Systolic activation is terminated by re-uptake of calcium from the cytosol. Although both the sarcolemma and the mitochondrial membrane have some capacity for calcium transport, the main route of uptake is into the sarcoplasmic reticulum, via a high-affinity, calcium-transporting ATPase. The activity of this ATPase controls the rate of decay of the calcium transient and is therefore a determinant of the rate of relaxation of the heart. The sarcoplasmic reticulum contains a cardiac form of calsequestrin, a distant homologue of the protein found in skeletal muscle. This calcium-binding protein buffers the free calcium concentration inside the sarcoplasmic reticulum, allowing it to store considerable amounts of total calcium without increasing the gradient against which the calcium-ATPase must pump.

One of the major functional differences between cardiac and skeletal muscle is the way in which contractile force is regulated. Smoothness and gradation of contraction in a skeletal muscle depend on the recruitment and asynchronous firing of different numbers of motor units. Individual motor units can also build up a contraction through a brief series of re-excitations. In the heart, the entire mass of muscle must be activated almost simultaneously, and mechanical summation by re-excitation is not possible, because the cells are electrically refractory until mechanical relaxation has taken place.

In cardiac muscle cells, as in skeletal muscle cells, contraction is initiated when calcium binds to troponin-C, a component of the regulatory protein complex on the thin filaments. During basal activity of the heart, the amount of calcium bound to troponin-C during each systole induces less than half-maximal activation of the contractile apparatus. There is therefore the potential for producing more force by increasing the amount of calcium bound to troponin-C. This can be achieved by controlling the amount of free calcium that is released into the cytosol during systole.

A special feature of the cardiac cell is the long duration of its action potential. The long-lasting plateau of depolarization allows a prolonged inward flux of calcium to take place via the L-type calcium channels in the sarcolemma. The calcium is then actively pumped into the sarcoplasmic reticulum: the extent to which the sarcoplasmic reticulum is loaded is crucially dependent on this entry of extracellular calcium. The greater the amount of calcium that is stored in the sarcoplasmic reticulum, the more is available for release during subsequent contractions. These calcium movements provide an automatic mechanism for matching any increase in heart rate with a progressive increase in contractile force. At higher heart rates, more calcium enters per unit time and is pumped into the sarcoplasmic reticulum. Each systole is then more forceful, because the amount of calcium that can be delivered into the cytosol is greater.

The most potent physiological means of enhancing cardiac contractility is through the action of β-adrenergic agents, such as adrenaline (epinephrine) and noradrenaline (nonepinephrine). These increase calcium taken up by the sarcoplasmic reticulum in two ways. Firstly, β-adrenergic stimulation increases the amount of calcium that enters during depolarization by opening more L-type calcium channels. Secondly, β-adrenergic stimulation can enhance the activity of the calcium-pumping ATPase by phosphorylating an associated protein, phospholamban. This enables the calcium pump to lower the cytosolic free calcium more rapidly, which contributes to the accelerated relaxation produced by β-adrenergic agonists. In a coordinated manner, phosphorylation of troponin-I on the thin filament increases the rate of cross-bridge cycling to aid the acceleration of relaxation.

Because of the clinical significance of positive inotropic agents (substances which increase the strength of cardiac contraction), generally now used only in severe end-stage heart failure, there is great interest in the multiple control sites which might provide targets for pharmacological intervention. Some of these are related to another important set of ionic fluxes through the sarcolemma via the sodium-potassium pump and the bidirectional sodium–calcium exchange and sodium-hydrogen exchange transporter proteins.

DEVELOPMENT

Cardiac myocytes differentiate from the splanchnic coelomic cells of the pericardium initially subjacent to the endoderm (p. 1029). Myogenic activity begins at the beginning of stage 10, c.22 days gestation, when the embryo has c.4 somites. At this time the presumptive cardiac myocytes express myosin, actin, troponin and other contractile proteins. The cardiac myocytes do not fuse with their neighbours to form a syncytium as occurs in skeletal muscle, but remain mononucleated, branched cells connected via intercellular junctions.

Presumptive myocardial cells form a continuous sheet of cuboidal cells which line the ventral splanchnic wall of the pericardial cavity in stage 9 (unfolded) embryos. From this time, an endocardial plexus forms between the splanchnopleuric coelomic epithelium and the endoderm. The plexus cells coalesce to establish bilateral, hollow tubular structures which fuse in the midline to form a single endocardial tube. After head folding, the endocardium is separated from the myocytes of the primitive heart tube by a fine extracellular reticulum, formerly referred to as cardiac jelly, which is secreted by the myocardial cells. The extracellular matrix of the heart contains inductive signals, also secreted by the myocardial cells, which transform competent cells of the endocardial epithelium into free mesenchymal cells. Thus during cardiac development, presumptive myocardial cells engage in several processes at once: they divide and differentiate to form a functional myocardium; they secrete matrix and inductive factors that will modify the differentiation of other cells; and they participate in the bending and rotation of the primitive heart tube, and differential growth within its walls, which will ultimately produce the four-chambered adult heart.

Overt differentiation of the primitive myocardial cells begins at about the time of fusion of the endocardial tube. As the primitive heart tube is formed, the presumptive myocardial cells start to express genes that encode characteristic myocardial proteins, including myosin, actin, troponin and other components of the contractile apparatus. Myofibrils begin to appear in the developing muscle cells, and the first functional heart beats start soon afterwards.

The regulatory mechanisms underlying differentiation of cardiac muscle appear to be distinct from those of skeletal muscle. Although it is anticipated that counterparts will be found for the transcriptional factors Myf-5, myogenin, MyoD and Myf-6, which are responsible for inducing differentiation of skeletal muscle, the corresponding factors for cardiac myogenesis have yet to be identified. During fetal maturation, successive changes in gene expression give rise to the characteristics of fetal, neonatal and adult myocardium and are responsible for the divergence of the properties of atrial and ventricular muscle cells.

Committed cardiac myoblasts do not fuse to form multinucleated myotubes as occurs in skeletal muscle, but remain as single cells coupled physically and electrically through intercellular junctions. Moreover, differentiated cardiac muscle cells continue to divide during fetal development, and withdraw from the cell cycle only after birth. This is markedly different from skeletal muscle development, in which differentiation, including the activation of muscle-specific genes, coincides with withdrawal from the cell cycle.

Concurrent with development of the contractile proteins of cardiac muscle, cardiac muscle cells develop numerous specific heart granules which contain substances shown to induce natriuresis and diuresis, and a family of polypeptides generally known as atrial natriuretic peptides. Specific heart granules develop from the Golgi complex in both atria and ventricles during fetal life, but become restricted to atrial muscle in the adult. Atrial natriuretic peptide is measurable when the heart is recognizably four-chambered. Within the atria almost all cells are capable of its synthesis.

Contractile protein isoforms of cardiac muscle

As in skeletal muscle, the contractile proteins of cardiac muscle exist in a number of tissue- and stage-specific forms. The cardiac isoform of α-actin is not identical to the skeletal muscle form, and is encoded by a different gene, although the two are so similar as to be functionally interchangeable. Both skeletal and cardiac isoforms of sarcomeric actin are expressed in fetal ventricular muscle. The mRNA for skeletal α-actin increases postnatally and exceeds that of cardiac actin in the adult.

The myosin heavy chain of human cardiac muscle exists in two isoforms, α and β, both of which are present in the fetal heart. The α-form persists as the adult isoform in atrial muscle, whereas the β-form (which is associated with a slower rate of contraction) predominates in ventricular muscle. Interestingly, the β-form of myosin heavy chain in cardiac muscle is identical to the isoform in slow twitch skeletal muscle. This identity between cardiac and slow twitch skeletal protein isoforms is true of several proteins, including ventricular myosin light chains and cardiac troponin-C. Other proteins, such as troponin-I and -T, exist in cardiac specific forms in the adult, although skeletal isoforms are expressed in the fetus and neonate.

Under some experimental conditions the contractile protein isoforms expressed by mature cardiac muscle may change in the adult mammal. Two established influences in this respect are thyroid hormone, and mechanical stretch induced by pressure overload. Transitions in both the heavy chains and light chains of myosin have been shown to take place in the human heart under conditions of pathological overload, but the functional significance of these changes is not clear.

Development of the impulse-conducting tissues

The impulse-generating and conducting system of the heart is formed from muscle cells that differ in their morphology from the working cardiac cells which make up the bulk of the myocardium (p. 1037). Cells of the mature conduction system retain some similarities to the myocardium of the early heart tube, and share with that embryonic tissue a distinctive pattern of expression of many genes, including those encoding contractile proteins and acetylcholinesterase. This suggests that divergence of conducting tissues and working myocardium takes place at an early embryonic stage. A cytological marker specific for the conduction system, the sulphate-3-glucuronyl carbohydrate moiety of glycoproteins, is expressed by 32 days of development and is downregulated during the later stages of cardiac septation. Its distribution strongly suggests that the conduction tissue in man originates in a ring of specialized myocardial cells located at the interventricular foramen of the early heart (p. 1037).

Lack of regeneration of cardiac muscle

In skeletal muscle, a population of precursor cells, satellite cells, is retained in adult life, and constitutes a pool of myoblasts which is capable of dividing, fusing with existing muscle fibres, and initiating regeneration after damage. Cardiac muscle contains no equivalent of these cells, and is therefore incapable of regeneration. There is experi-mental evidence that temporary ischaemia injures cardiac cells in a reversible manner (Schwanger et al 1987), whereas longer periods of ischaemia produce irreversible damage.

REFERENCES

North AJ, Gimona M, Lando Z, Small JV 1994 Actin isoform compartments in chicken gizzard smooth muscle cells. J Cell Sci 107: 445–55.
Describes the distribution of different actin filament populations and proposes a model for the structural organization and contractile mechanism in smooth muscle cells.

Schwanger M, Fishbein MC, Block M, Wijns W, Selin C, Phelps ME, Schelbert HR 1987 Metabolic and ultrastructural abnormalities during ischemia in canine myocardium: noninvasive assessment by positron emission tomography. Mol Cell Cardiol 19: 25–89.

Taylor GI, Razaboni RM (eds) 1994 Michel Salmon: Anatomic Studies. Book 1, Arteries of the Muscles of the Extremities and the Trunk. Book 2, Arterial Anastomotic Pathways of the Extremities. St Louis: Quality Medical Publishing.
Contains the translated work of Dr Michel Salmon describing the blood supply to muscle and the anastomotic pathways in the limbs.

Skin and its appendages

In this chapter, the types and functions of skin in different parts of the body are described first, followed by the microstructure of the epidermis and dermis, and the appendages of skin including the pilosebaceous units and the sweat glands and nails. The development of skin, natural skin lines and age-related changes, and clinical aspects of skin, e.g. grafts, surgical skin flaps and wound healing, are also described. The integumental system includes the skin and its derivatives, hairs, nails, sweat and sebaceous glands; subcutaneous fat and deep fascia; the mucocutaneous junctions around the openings of the body orifices; and the breasts. Mucocutaneous junctions and breast tissues are covered in the appropriate regional sections.

TYPES AND FUNCTIONS OF SKIN

The skin covers the entire external surface of the body, including the external auditory meatus, the lateral aspect of the tympanic membrane and the vestibule of the nose. It is continuous with the mucosae of the alimentary, respiratory and urogenital tracts at their respective orifices, where the specialized skin of mucocutaneous junctions is present. It also fuses with the conjunctiva at the margins of the eyelids, and with the lining of the lachrymal canaliculi at the lachrymal puncta. Skin forms c.8% of the total body mass, and its surface area varies with height and weight; in an individual of 1.8 m and weighing 90 kg, it is c.2.2 m^2. Its thickness ranges from c.1.5–4.0 mm; these variations reflect maturation, ageing and regional specializations.

The skin forms a self-renewing interface between the body and its environment, and is a major site of intercommunication between the two. Within limits, it forms an effective barrier against microbial invasion, and has properties which can protect against mechanical, chemical, osmotic, thermal and UV radiation damage. It is an important site of immune surveillance against the entry of pathogens and the initiation of primary immune responses. Skin carries out many biochemical synthetic processes, including the formation of vitamin D under the influence of ultraviolet B (UVB) radiation and synthesis of cytokines and growth factors. Skin is the target of a variety of hormones. These activities can affect the appearance and function of individual skin components, such as the sebaceous glands, the hairs and the pigment-producing cells.

Control of body temperature is an important function of skin, and is effected mainly by regulation of heat loss from the cutaneous circulation (p. 144) through the rapid increase or reduction in the flow of blood to an extensive external surface area: the process is assisted by sweating. Skin is involved in sociosexual communication and, in the case of facial skin, can signal emotional states by means of muscular and vascular responses. It is a major sense organ, richly supplied by nerve terminals and specialized receptors for touch, temperature, pain and other stimuli. The segmental arrangement of the spinal nerves is reflected in the sensory supply of the skin: a dermatome is the area supplied by an individual spinal nerve (see **Fig. 8.28**).

Skin has good frictional properties, assisting locomotion and manipulation by its texture. It is elastic, and can be stretched and compressed within limits. The outer surface is covered by various markings, some of them are large and conspicuous and others are microscopic, or are only revealed after manipulation or incision of the skin. These markings are often referred to collectively as skin lines.

The colour of human skin is derived from, and varies with, the amount of blood (and its degree of oxygenation) in the cutaneous circulation, the thickness of the cornified layer, and the activity of specialized cells which produce the pigment melanin. Melanin has a protective role against ultraviolet radiation, and acts as a scavenger of harmful free radicals. Racial variations in colour are mainly due to differences in the amount, type and distribution of melanin, and are genetically determined.

The appearance of skin is affected by many other factors, e.g. size, shape and distribution of hairs and of skin glands (sweat, sebaceous and apocrine), changes associated with maturation, ageing, metabolism, pregnancy. The general state of health is reflected in the appearance and condition of the skin, and the earliest signs of many systemic disorders may be apparent in the skin. Examination of the skin, therefore, is of importance in the diagnosis of more than just skin disease.

CLASSIFICATION OF SKIN

Although skin in different parts of the body is fundamentally of similar structure, there are many local variations in parameters such as thickness, mechanical strength, softness, flexibility, degree of keratinization (cornification), sizes and numbers of hairs, frequency and types of glands, pigmentation, vascularity, innervation. Two major classes of skin are distinguished: they cover large areas of the body and show important differences of detailed structure and functional properties. These are thin, hairy (hirsute) skin, which covers the greater part of the body, and thick, hairless (glabrous) skin, which forms the surfaces of the palms of the hands, soles of the feet, and flexor surfaces of the digits (**Figs 8.1**, **8.2**, **8.4**).

SKIN AND SKIN APPENDAGES

EPIDERMIS

The epidermis (**Figs 8.2**, **8.3**) is a compound tissue consisting mainly of a continuously self-renewing, keratinized, stratified squamous epithelium: the principal cells are called keratinocytes. Non-keratinocytes within the mature epidermis include melanocytes (pigment-forming cells from the embryonic neural crest), Langerhans cells which are antigen-presenting cells derived from bone marrow, and lymphocytes (p. 82). Merkel cells, which may function as sensory mechanoreceptors or possibly as part of the dispersed neuroendocrine system, are associated with nerve endings. Free sensory nerve endings are sparsely present within the epidermis. In routine histological preparations, the non-keratinocytes and Merkel cells are almost indistinguishable, and appear as clear cells surrounded by a clear space produced by shrinkage during processing. Their cytoplasm lacks keratin (cytokeratin) filament bundles.

The population of keratinocytes undergoes continuous renewal throughout life: a mitotic layer of cells at the base replaces those shed at the surface. As they move away from the base of the epidermis, keratinocytes undergo progressive changes in shape and content. They transform from polygonal living cells to non-viable flattened squames full of intermediate filament proteins (keratins) embedded in a dense matrix of cytoplasmic proteins to form mature keratin. The process is known as keratinization or, more properly, cornification.

The epidermis can be divided into a number of layers from deep to superficial as follows: basal layer (stratum basale), spinous or prickle cell layer (stratum spinosum), granular layer (stratum granulosum), clear layer (stratum lucidum) and cornified layer (stratum corneum) (**Fig. 8.4**). The first three of these layers are metabolically active compartments through which cells pass and change their form as they progressively differentiate. The more superficial layers of cells undergo terminal keratinization, or cornification, which involves not only structural changes in keratinocytes, but also alterations in their relationships with each other and with non-keratinocytes, and molecular changes within the intercellular space.

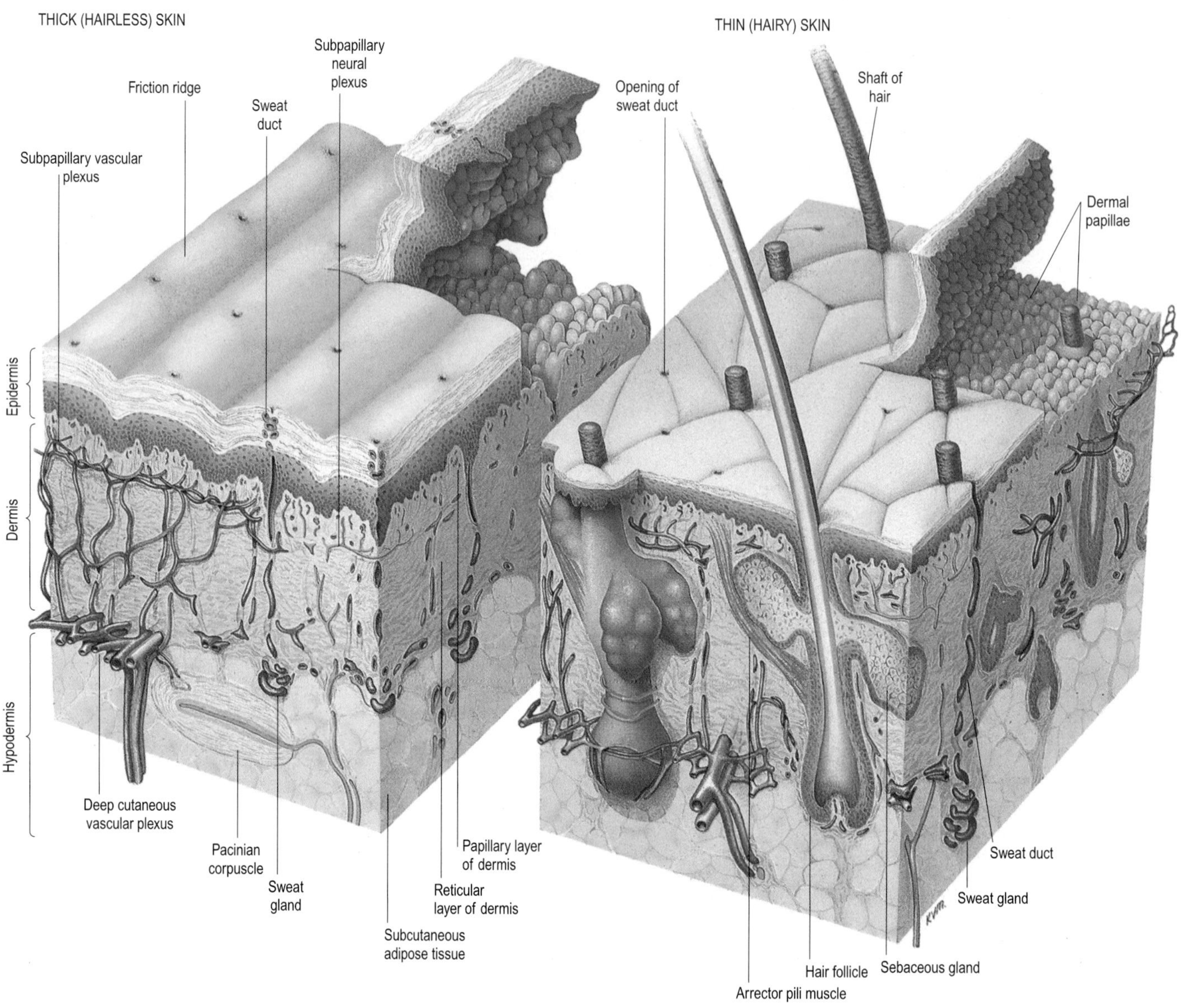

THICK (HAIRLESS) SKIN

THIN (HAIRY) SKIN

Subpapillary
neural
plexus

Friction ridge

Sweat
duct

Shaft of
hair

Opening of
sweat duct

Subpapillary vascular
plexus

Dermal
papillae

Epidermis

Dermis

Hypodermis

Deep cutaneous
vascular plexus

Pacinian
corpuscle

Sweat
gland

Papillary layer
of dermis

Reticular
layer of dermis

Subcutaneous
adipose tissue

Sweat duct

Sweat gland

Hair follicle

Sebaceous gland

Arrector pili muscle

Fig. 8.1 The organization of skin, comparing the structures found in thick, hairless (plantar and palmar) skin with thin, hairy (hirsute) skin. The epidermis has been partially peeled back to show the interdigitating dermal and epidermal papillae.

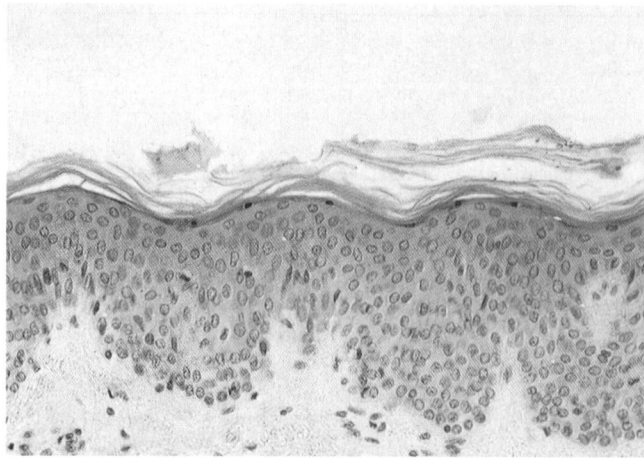

Fig. 8.2 The interfollicular epidermis of thin (scalp) skin. Note the thin cornified layer in comparison with **Figs 8.4** and **8.10**.

The epidermal appendages (pilosebaceous units, sweat glands and nails) are formed developmentally by ingrowth of the general epidermis, and the latter is thus referred to as the interfollicular epidermis.

Keratinocytes (Fig. 8.6)

Basal layer

The basal or deepest layer of cells, adjacent to the dermis, is the layer where cell proliferation in the epidermis takes place. This layer contacts a basal lamina (**Figs 8.5, 2.5, 3.13**), which is a thin layer of specialized extracellular matrix, not usually visible by light microscopy. By routine electron microscopy the basal lamina appears as a clear lamina lucida (adjacent to the basal cell plasma membrane) and a darker lamina densa. The basal plasma membrane of the basal keratinocytes, together with the extracellular basal lamina (lamina lucida and lamina densa) and anchoring fibrils within the subjacent dermal matrix (the lamina fibroreticularis), which insert into the lamina densa and loop around bundles of collagen, collectively form the basement membrane zone (BMZ) which constitutes the dermo-epidermal junction (**Fig. 8.5**). This is a highly convoluted interface, particularly in thick, hairless skin, where dermal papillae (rete ridges) project superficially into the epidermal region, interlocking with adjacent downward projections of the epidermis (rete pegs) (**Fig. 8.4**).

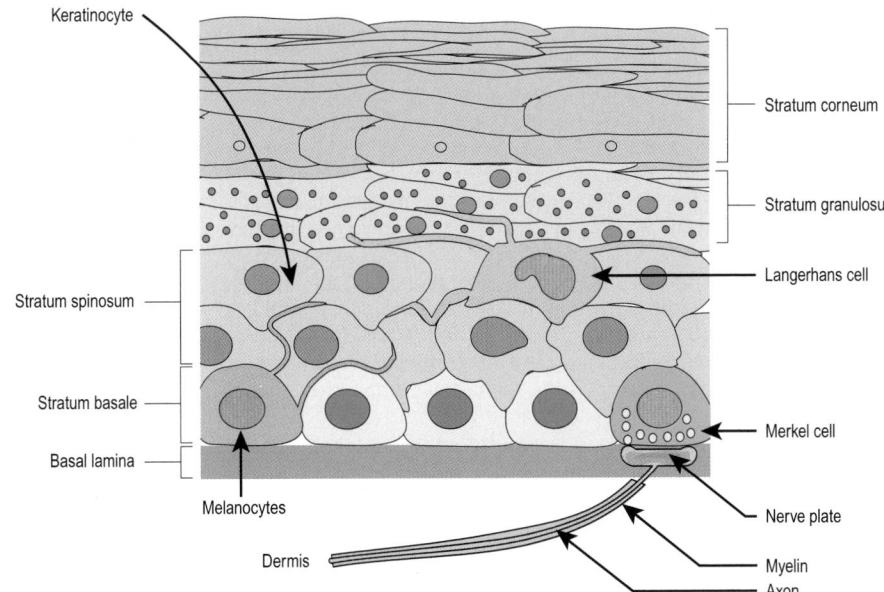

Fig. 8.3 The main features of the epidermis, including its cell layers and different cell types. Melanocytes and Merkel cells are derived from the neural crest and Langerhans cells are derived from bone marrow precursor cells. (By permission from Kierszenbaum AL 2002 Histology and Cell Biology. St Louis: Mosby.)

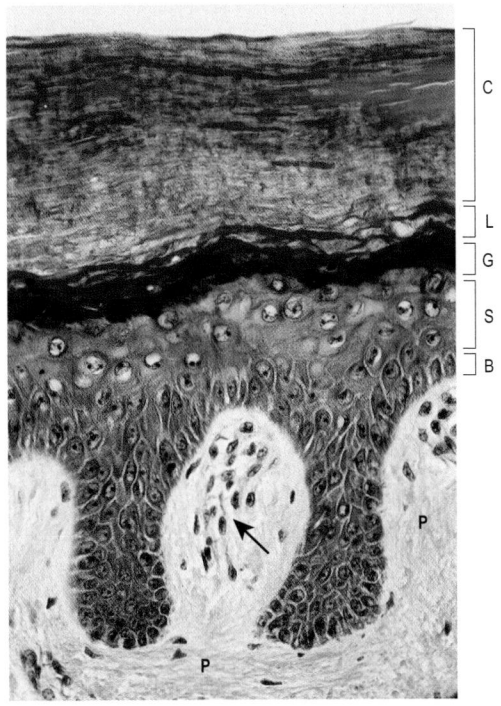

Fig. 8.4 The epidermis and papillary dermis (P) of thick skin, stained with acidic dyes to show the stratum corneum (C), the clear layer (L), the deeply stained granular layer (G, stratum granulosum), the prickle layer (S, stratum spinosum) and the stratum basale (B). The lightly stained area at the base of layer C is a histological artefact, and should not be confused with the stratum lucidum. A capillary loop (arrow) is seen entering the deep papilla (rete ridge) of the dermis (below, centre field), between two epidermal rete pegs. (Photograph by Sarah-Jane Smith.)

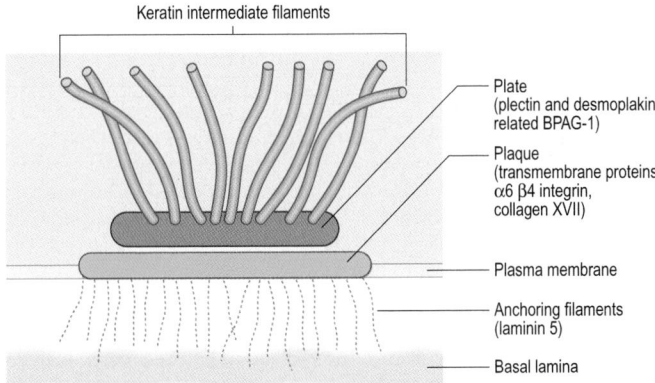

Fig. 8.5 The major features of the basement membrane zone (BMZ) of skin, including some of the important molecules involved. (By permission from Kierszenbaum AL 2002 Histology and Cell Biology. St Louis: Mosby.)

The majority of basal layer cells are columnar to cuboidal in shape, with large (relative to their cytoplasmic volume) mainly euchromatic nuclei and prominent nucleoli. The cytoplasm contains variable numbers of melanosomes and, characteristically, keratin filament bundles corresponding to the tonofilaments of classic electron microscopy. In the basal keratinocytes these keratins are mostly K5 and K14 proteins. The plasma membranes of apposed cells are connected by desmosomes, and the basal plasma membrane is linked to the basal lamina at intervals by hemidesmosomes (p. 7). Melanocytes, Langerhans cells and occasional Merkel cells are interspersed among the basal keratinocytes. Merkel cells are connected to keratinocytes by desmosomes, but melanocytes

and Langerhans cells lack these specialized contacts. Intraepithelial lymphocytes are present in small numbers.

At any one time the basal layer of the epidermis contains keratinocytes with different fates. These include multipotent stem cells. On division these may self-renew or produce a daughter cell which is committed to differentiate after undergoing further transit amplifying cell divisions. The activity of stem cells and transit (or transient) amplifying cells in the basal layer provide a continuous supply of differentiating cells which enter the prickle cell layer. The great majority of these cells are postmitotic, although some cell division may occur in the more basal regions of the prickle cell layer. Stem cells are thought to reside mainly in the troughs of rete pegs, and in the outer root sheath bulge of the hair follicle, but they cannot easily be distinguished morphologically.

The organization of the basal layer and overlying progeny cells is thought to form a series of columns. Several layers of prickle and granular cells overlie a cluster of six to eight basal cells, forming a columnar proliferative unit. Each group of basal cells consists of a central stem cell with an encircling ring of transit amplifying proliferative cells and postmitotic maturing cells. From the periphery of this unit, postmitotic cells transfer into the prickle cell layer. The normal total epidermal turnover time is between 52 and 75 days. In some pathologies of skin, turnover rates and transit times can be exceedingly rapid, e.g. in psoriasis, total epidermal turnover time may be as little as 8 days. The control of keratinocyte proliferation and differentiation is beyond the scope of this publication but is reviewed in Niemann and Watt (2002) and Byrne et al (2003).

Prickle cell layer

The prickle cell layer consists of several layers of closely packed keratinocytes that interdigitate with each other by means of numerous cell surface projections which are linked by desmosomes (**Figs 8.3, 8.4**). The latter provide tensile strength and cohesion to the layer. These suprabasal cells are committed to terminal differentiation and gradually move upwards towards the stratum corneum as more cells are produced in the basal layer. When skin is processed for routine light microscopy, the cells tend to shrink away from each other except where they are joined by desmosomes, which gives them their characteristic spiny appearance. Prickle cell cytoplasm contains prominent bundles of keratin filaments, (mostly K1 and K10 keratin proteins) arranged concentrically around a euchromatic nucleus, and attached to the dense plaques of desmosomes. The cytoplasm also contains melanosomes, either singly or aggregated within membrane-limited organelles (compound melanosomes). Langerhans cells and the occasional associated lymphocyte are the only non-keratinocytes present in the prickle cell layer.

Granular layer

Extensive changes in keratinocyte structure occur in the three to four layers of flattened cells in the granular layer. The nuclei become pyknotic and begin to disintegrate; membrane-bound organelles such as mitochondria, Golgi membranes and ribosomes degenerate; and keratin filament bundles become more compact and associated with irregular, densely staining keratohyalin granules (**Fig. 8.6**). Small round granules (100 × 300 nm) with a lamellar internal structure (lamellar granules, Odland bodies, membrane-coating granules) also appear in the cytoplasm. Keratohyalin granules contain a histidine-rich, sulphur-poor protein (profilaggrin) which, when the cell reaches the cornified layer, becomes modified to filaggrin. The lamellar granules are concentrated deep to the plasma membrane, with which they fuse, releasing their lipid contents into the intercellular space within the layer and also between it and the cornified layer. They form an important component of the permeability barrier of the epidermis.

Clear layer

The clear layer is only found in thick palmar or plantar skin. It represents a poorly understood stage in keratinocyte differentiation. It stains more strongly than the cornified layer with acidic dyes (**Fig. 8.4**), is more refractile optically, and often contains nuclear debris. Ultrastructurally, its cells resemble the incompletely keratinized cells which are occasionally seen in the innermost part of the cornified layer of thin skin.

Cornified layer

The cornified layer is the final product of epidermal differentiation, or cornification. It consists of closely packed layers of flattened polyhedral squames (**Fig. 8.7**), ranging in surface area from c.800 to 1100 μm². These cells overlap at their lateral margins and interlock with cells of apposed layers by ridges, grooves and microvilli. In thin skin this layer may be only a few cells deep, but in thick skin it may be more than 50 cells deep. The plasma membrane of the squame appears thicker than that of other keratinocytes, partly due to the cross-linking of a soluble precursor, involucrin, at the cytoplasmic face of the plasma membrane. The outer surface is also covered by a monolayer of bound lipid. The intercellular region contains extensive lamellar sheets of glycolipid derived from the lamellar granules of the granular layer. The cells lack a nucleus and membranous organelles, and consist solely of a dense array of keratin filaments embedded in a cytoplasmic matrix which is partly composed of filaggrin derived from keratohyalin granules.

Under normal conditions the production of epidermal keratinocytes in the basal layer is matched by loss of cells from the cornified layer. Desquamation of these outer cells is normally imperceptible. When excessive, it appears in hairy regions as dandruff, and more extensively in certain diseases and, to a lesser extent, after sunburn, as peeling, scaling and exfoliation. The thickness of the cornified layer can be influenced by local environmental factors, particularly abrasion, which can lead to a considerable thickening of the whole epidermis including the cornified layer. The soles of the feet become much thickened if an individual habitually walks barefoot, and cornified pads develop in areas of frequent pressure, e.g. corns from tight shoes, palmar calluses in manual workers, and digital calluses in guitar players.

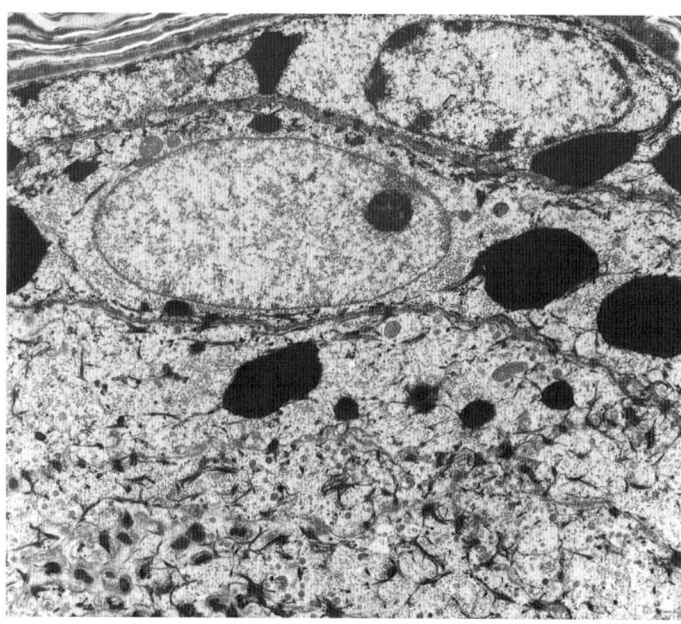

Fig. 8.6 The superficial layers of keratinocytes in thin skin. Below is a keratinocyte in the prickle cell layer, with prominent keratin filament bundles and desmosomes (nucleus not visible). Above are two squamous cells of the granular layer. Note the large, electron-dense keratohyalin granules. Most superficially (left) are the flattened cells of the cornified layer. (By kind permission from Dr Andrew Kent, King's College London.)

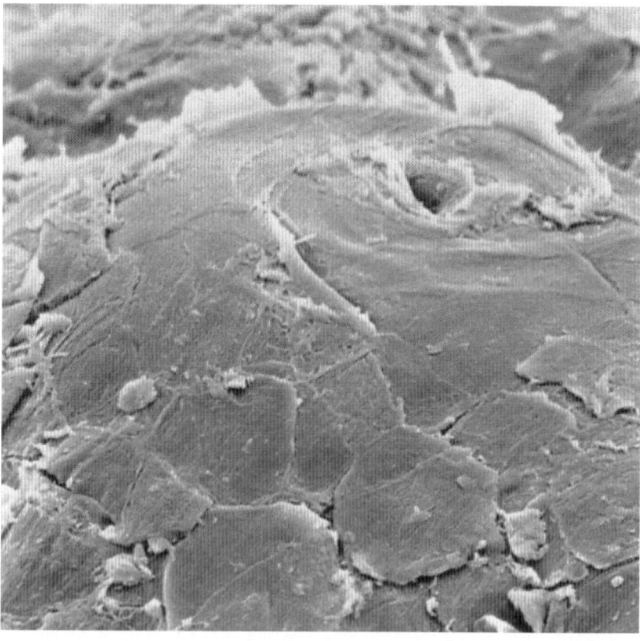

Fig. 8.7 The epidermal surface surrounding the aperture of a sweat duct. Several polygonal, scale-like keratinocytes (squames) of the superficial cornified layer are visible in this scanning electron micrograph.

Keratins

Epidermal keratinization has historically been the term applied to the final stages of keratinocyte differentiation and maturation, during which cells are converted into tough cornified squames. However, this is now regarded as ambiguous because the term keratin is assumed to refer to the protein of epithelial intermediate filaments, rather than (as previously) to the whole complement of proteins in the terminally differentiated cell of the stratum corneum.

Keratins are the intermediate filament proteins found in all epithelial cells. There are two types, type I (acidic) and type II (neutral/basic);

they form heteropolymers, are coexpressed in specific pairs and are assembled into 10 nm intermediate filaments (p. 17). Up to 49 different keratin gene sequences have been recognized and their protein products are numbered according to molecular weight. Different keratin pairs are expressed according to epithelial cell differentiation; antibodies to individual keratins are useful analytical tools. Keratins K5 and K14 are expressed by basal keratinocytes. New keratins, K1 and K10, are synthesized suprabasally. In the granular layer the filaments become associated with keratohyalin granules containing profilaggrin, a histidine-rich phosphorylated protein. As the cells pass into the cornified layer, profilaggrin is cleaved by phosphatases into filaggrin which causes aggregation of the filaments and forms the matrix in which they are embedded. Other types of keratin expression occur elsewhere, particularly in hair and nails, where highly specialized hard, or trichocyte, keratin is expressed. This becomes chemically modified and is much tougher than in the general epidermis.

Epidermal lipids

The epidermis serves as an important barrier to the loss of water and other substances through the body surface (apart from sweating and sebaceous secretion). A variety of lipids are present and synthesized in the epidermis, including triglycerides and fatty acids, phospholipids, cholesterol, cholesterol esters, glycosphingolipids and ceramides. An intermediate in the synthesis of cholesterol, 7-dehydrocholesterol, is the precursor of vitamin D, which is also synthesized in the skin. The content and composition of epidermal lipids change with differentiation. Phospholipids and glycolipids at first accumulate within keratinocytes above the basal layer, but higher up they are broken down and are practically absent from the cornified layer. Cholesterol and its esters, fatty acids and ceramides accumulate towards the surface, and are abundant in the cornified layer. The lamellar arrangement of the extracellular lipids is a major factor in their barrier function.

Melanocytes (Figs 8.8, 8.9)

Melanocytes are melanin pigment-forming cells derived from the neural crest. They are present in the epidermis and its appendages, in oral epithelium, some mucous membranes, the uveal tract (choroid coat) of the eyeball, parts of the middle and internal ear and in the pial and arachnoid meninges at the base of the brain. The cells of the retinal pigment epithelium, developed from the outer wall of the optic cup, also produce melanin, and neurones in different locations within the brainstem (e.g. the locus coeruleus and substantia nigra) synthesize a variety of melanin called neuromelanin. True melanins are high molecular weight polymers attached to a structural protein. In humans there are two classes, the brown-black eumelanin, and the red-yellow phaeomelanin, both derived from the substrate tyrosine. Most natural melanins are mixtures of eumelanin and phaeomelanin, and phaeomelanic pigments, trichochromes, occur in red hair.

Melanocytes are dendritic cells, and lack desmosomal contacts with apposed keratinocytes, though hemidesmosomal contacts with the basal lamina are present. In routine tissue preparations, melanocytes appear as clear cells in the basal layer of the epidermis; numbers per unit area of epidermis range from 2300 per mm^2 in cheek skin to 800 per mm^2 in abdominal skin. It is estimated that a single melanocyte may be in functional contact via its dendritic processes with up to 30 keratinocytes. The nucleus is large, round, and euchromatic, and the cytoplasm contains intermediate filaments, a prominent Golgi complex and vesicles and associated rough endoplasmic reticulum, mitochondria, and coated vesicles, together with a characteristic organelle, the melanosome.

The melanosome is a membrane-bound structure which undergoes a sequence of developmental stages during which melanin is synthesized and deposited within it by a tyrosine–tyrosinase reaction. Mature melanosomes move into the dendrites along the surfaces of microtubules and are transferred to keratinocytes through their phagocytic activity. Keratinocytes engulf and internalize the tip of the dendrite with the subsequent pinching off of melanosomes into the keratinocyte cytoplasm. Here, they may exist as individual granules in heavily pigmented skin, or be packaged within secondary lysosomes as melanosome complexes in lightly pigmented skin. In basal keratinocytes they can be seen to accumulate in a crescent-shaped cap over the distal part of the nucleus. As the keratinocytes progress towards the surface of the epidermis, melanosomes undergo degradation, and melanin remnants in the cornified layer form dust-like particles. Melanosomes

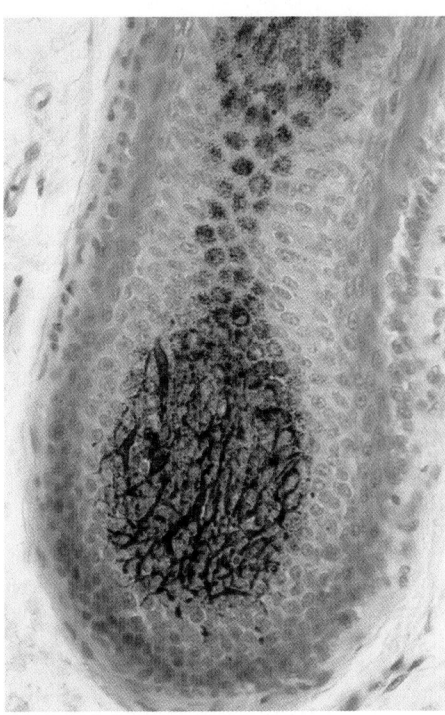

Fig. 8.8 Melanocytes in the germinal matrix of a hair bulb, sectioned tangentially. The pigmented melanocytes extend dendritic branches between proliferating keratinocytes and into the layers of differentiating cells, passing melanosomes to the keratinocytes, seen here as rounded pigmented cells (above) forming the hair cuticle. (Photograph by Sarah-Jane Smith.)

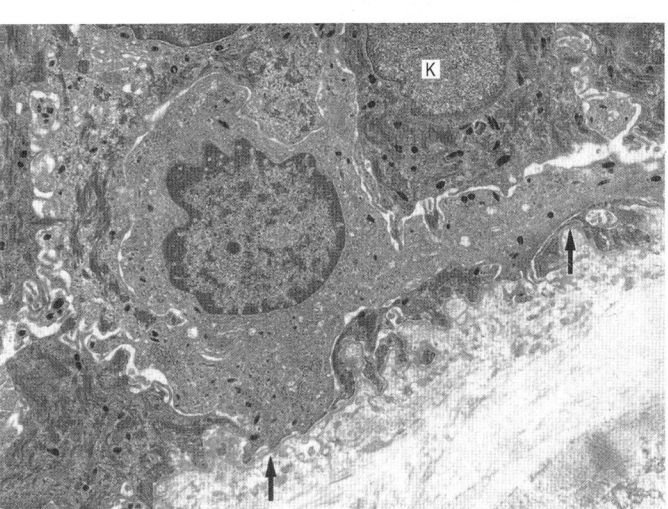

Fig. 8.9 A basal epidermal melanocyte. There are no desmosomes connecting it with apposed keratinocytes (K), the cytoplasm contains no keratin filaments, and only a few melanosomes are present as individual granules in the cytoplasm; most have been passed on to the keratinocytes. A melanocyte dendrite extends towards the right. Arrows mark the dermo-epidermal junction.

are degraded more rapidly in Caucasian skin than in dark-skinned races, where melanosomes persist in cells of the more superficial layers.

Melanin has biophysical and biochemical properties related to its functions in skin. It protects against the damaging effects of UV radiation on DNA and is also an efficient scavenger of damaging free radicals. However a high concentration of melanin may adversely affect synthesis of vitamin D in darker-skinned individuals living in northern latitudes. Melanin pigmentation is both constitutive and facultative. Constitutive pigmentation is the intrinsic level of pigmentation and is genetically determined, whereas facultative pigmentation represents reversible changes induced by environmental agents, e.g. UV and X-radiation, chemicals, and hormones. Racial variations in pigmentation are due to differences in melanocyte morphology and activity rather than to differences in frequency or distribution. In naturally heavily pigmented skins the cells tend to be larger, more dendritic, and to contain more large, late-stage melanosomes than melanocytes of paler skins. The keratinocytes in turn contain more melanosomes, individually dispersed, whereas in light skins, the majority are contained within secondary lysosomes to form melanosome complexes.

Response to UV light includes immediate tanning, pigment darkening, which can occur within a matter of minutes, probably due to photo-oxidation of pre-existing melanin. Delayed tanning occurs after c.48 hours, and involves stimulation of melanogenesis within the melanocytes, and transfer of additional melanosomes to keratinocytes. There may also be some increase in size of active melanocytes, and in their apparent numbers, mainly through activation of dormant cells. Freckles in the skin of red-haired individuals are usually thought to be induced by UV, though they do not appear until several years after birth, despite exposure. Paradoxically, melanocytes are significantly fewer in freckles than in adjacent paler epidermis, but they are larger and more active. What determines the onset of freckles, or their individual location, is not known.

Adrenocorticotrophin (ACTH) is thought to affect melanocyte activity, and is probably responsible for the hyperpigmentation associated with pituitary and adrenal disorders. In pregnancy, higher levels of circulating oestrogens and progesterone are responsible for the increased melanization of the face, abdominal and genital skin, and the nipple and areola, much of which may remain permanently.

In albinism, the tyrosinase required for melanin synthesis is either absent or inactive, and melanocytes, though present, are relatively quiescent cells in an otherwise normal epidermis. Melanocytes decrease significantly in numbers in old age, and are absent from grey-white hair.

Langerhans cells

Langerhans cells are immature dendritic antigen-presenting cells (p. 82) regularly distributed throughout the basal and prickle cell layers of the epidermis and its appendages, apart from the sweat gland. They are also present in other stratified squamous epithelia, including the buccal, tonsillar and oesophageal epithelia, as well as the cervical and vaginal mucosae and the transitional epithelium of the bladder. They are found in the conjunctiva, but not in the cornea. In routine preparations they appear as clear cells, relatively high in the stratified layer. They enter the epidermis from the bone marrow during development to establish the postnatal population (460–1000/mm^2, 2–3% of all epidermal cells, with regional variations), and this is maintained by continual replacement from the marrow.

The nucleus is euchromatic and markedly indented and the cytoplasm contains a well-developed Golgi complex, lysosomes (which often contain ingested melanosomes), and a characteristic organelle, the Birbeck granule. The latter are discoid, cup-shaped, or have a distended vesicle resembling the head of a tennis racket; in section they often appear as a cross-striated rod 0.5 μm long and 30 nm wide. When stimulated by antigen, Langerhans cells migrate out of the epidermis to lymphoid tissues. Their numbers are increased in chronic skin inflammatory disorders, particularly of an immune aetiology, such as some forms of dermatitis.

Merkel cells

Merkel cells are present as clear oval cells, singly or in groups, in the basal layer of the epidermis, especially of thick skin. They are also present in the outer root sheath of some large hair follicles. Merkel cells are derived embryologically from the neural crest and are not related developmentally to keratinocytes, as was once thought. They can be distinguished histologically from other clear cells (melanocytes and Langerhans cells) only by immunohistochemical and ultrastructural criteria.

Short, stiff processes of their plasma membrane interdigitate with adjacent basal keratinocytes, to which the Merkel cell is attached by small desmosomes. The cytoplasm contains numerous closely-packed intermediate filaments (simple epithelial keratins, mostly K8 and K18 but also K19 and K20), and characteristic 80–110 μm dense-core granules. The basal plasma membrane is closely apposed to the membrane of an axonal terminal. Merkel cells are thought to function as neuroendocrine sensory receptors (p. 61), and are slowly adapting mechanoreceptors which respond to directional deformations of the epidermis and direction of hair movement by releasing a transmitter from their dense-core cytoplasmic granules.

DERMIS

The dermis (Figs 8.1, 8.10) is an irregular, moderately dense connective tissue. It has a matrix composed of an interwoven collagenous and elastic

network in an amorphous ground substance of glycosaminoglycans, glycoproteins, and bound water, which accommodates nerves, blood vessels, lymphatics, epidermal appendages and a changing population of cells (p. 36). Mechanically, the dermis provides considerable strength to the skin by virtue of the number and arrangement of its collagen fibres (which give it tensile strength), and its elastic fibres (which give it elastic recoil). The density of its fibre meshwork, and therefore its physical properties, varies within an area, in different parts of the body, and with age and sex. The dermis is vital for the survival of the epidermis, and important morphogenetic signals are exchanged at the interface between the two both during development and postnatally. The dermis can be divided into two zones, a narrow superficial papillary layer, and a deeper reticular layer: the boundary between them is indistinct.

Adult dermal collagen is mainly of types I and III, in proportions of 80–85% and 15–20% respectively. The coarser-fibred type I is predominant in the deeper, reticular dermis, and the finer type III is found in the papillary dermis and around blood vessels. Type IV collagen is found in the basal lamina between epidermis and dermis, around Schwann cells of peripheral nerves and endothelial cells of vessels. Types V, VI and VII are minor collagenous components of the dermis. Elastic fibres form a fibrous network interwoven between the collagen bundles throughout the dermis, and are more prominent in some regions, e.g. the axilla.

Two major categories of cell are present in postnatal dermis, permanent and migrant, as is typical of all general connective tissues

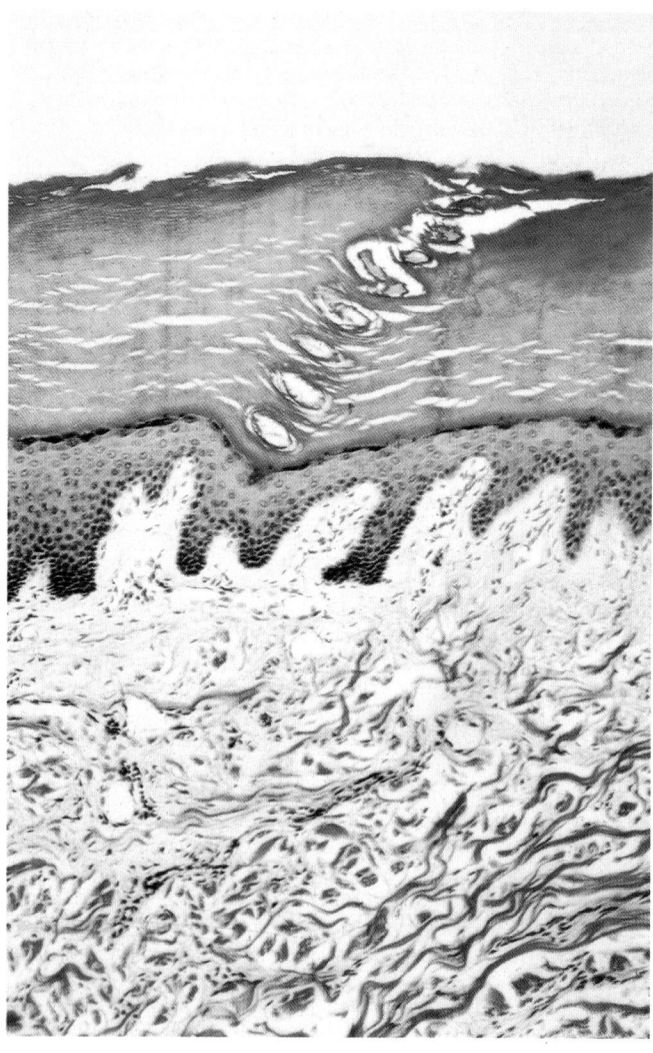

Fig. 8.10 The dermis of thick skin on the sole of the foot, sectioned vertically (trichrome-stained). Note the pale-staining papillary layer of the dermis with delicate collagen fibril bundles, compared with the thick bundles of collagen (orange) in the reticular dermis below. The epidermis is above. The thick cornified layer (orange) contains the profiles of a sweat duct spiralling towards the surface.

(p. 36). The permanent resident cells include cells of organized structures such as nerves, vessels and cells of the arrector pili muscles, and the fibroblasts, which synthesize all components of the dermal extracellular matrix. The migrant cells originate in the bone marrow and include macrophages, mast cells, eosinophils, neutrophils, T and B cells (including antibody-secreting plasma cells), and dermal interstitial dendritic cells which are capable of immune surveillance and antigen presentation (p. 81).

Layers of the dermis

Papillary layer
The papillary layer is immediately deep to the epidermis (**Figs 8.4, 8.10**), and is specialized to provide mechanical anchorage, metabolic support, and trophic maintenance to the overlying epidermis, as well as supplying sensory nerve endings and blood vessels. The cytoskeleton of basal epidermal keratinocytes is linked to the fibrous matrix of the papillary dermis through the attachment of keratin filament bundles to hemidesmosomes, then via anchoring filaments of the basal lamina, to the anchoring fibrils of type VII collagen which extend deep into the papillary dermis. This arrangement provides a mechanically stable substratum for the epidermis.

The superficial surface of the dermis is shaped into numerous papillae or rete ridges, which interdigitate with rete pegs in the base of the epidermis and form the dermo-epidermal junction at their interface. The papillae have round or blunt apices which may be divided into several cusps. In thin skin, especially in regions with little mechanical stress and minimal sensitivity, papillae are few and very small, while in the thick skin of the palm and sole of the foot they are much larger, closely aggregated, and arranged in curved parallel lines following the pattern of ridges and grooves on these surfaces (**Fig. 8.1**). Lying under each epidermal ridge are two longitudinal rows of papillae, one on either side of the epidermal rete pegs through which the sweat ducts pass on the way to the surface. Each papilla contains densely interwoven, fine bundles of types I and III collagen fibres and some elastic fibrils. Also present is a capillary loop (**Fig. 8.4**), and in some sites, especially in thick hairless skin, Meissner's corpuscle nerve endings (p. 61).

Reticular layer
The reticular layer merges with the deep aspect of the papillary layer. Its bundles of collagen fibres are thicker than those in the papillary layer and interlace with them and with each other to form a strong but deformable three-dimensional lattice, in which many fibres are parallel to each other, and which contain a variable number of elastic fibres. The predominant orientation of the collagen fibres may be related to the local mechanical forces on the dermis and thus may be involved in the development of skin lines.

Hypodermis
Also known as the superficial fascia, the hypodermis is a layer of loose connective tissue of variable thickness which merges with the deep aspect of the dermis. It is often adipose, particularly between the dermis and musculature of the body wall. It mediates the increased mobility of the skin, and the adipose component contributes to thermal insulation, acts as a shock absorber and constitutes a store of metabolic energy. Subcutaneous nerves, vessels and lymphatics travel in the hypodermis, their main trunks lying in its deepest part, where adipose tissue is scant. In the head and neck, the hypodermis also contains muscles, such as platysma, which are remnants of more extensive sheets of skin-associated musculature found in other mammals.

The quantity and distribution of subcutaneous fat differs in the sexes. It is generally more abundant and widely distributed in females. In males it diminishes from the trunk to the extremities, and this distribution is more obvious in middle age, when the total amount increases in both sexes. The amount of adipose tissue in the hypodermis, as elsewhere, reflects the quantity of lipid stored in its adipocytes rather than a change in the number of cells. There is an association with climate (rather than race), and superficial fat is more abundant in colder geographical regions. The hypodermis is most distinct on the lower anterior abdominal wall, where it contains much elastic tissue and appears many-layered as it passes through the inguinal regions into the thighs. It is similar in the limbs and the perineum, but is thin where it passes over the dorsal aspects of the hands and feet, the sides of the neck and face, around the anus, and over the penis and scrotum. It is

almost absent from the external ears but is particularly dense in the scalp, palms and soles, where it is crossed by numerous strong connective tissue bands binding the hypodermis and skin to underlying structures: these are part of the deep fascia, but are known regionally as aponeuroses of the scalp, palm and sole.

PILOSEBACEOUS UNIT
The pilosebaceous unit consists of the hair and its follicle with an associated arrector pili muscle, sebaceous gland, and sometimes an apocrine gland (**Figs 8.1, 8.11**). Not all elements of the unit occur together in all body regions.

Hairs
Hairs are filamentous cornified structures present over almost all of the body surface. They grow out of the skin at a slant (**Fig. 45.1**) as is evident in the sloping of the hairs on the dorsum of forearm, hand and fingers towards the ulnar side. Hairs are absent from several areas of the body, including the thick skin of the palms, soles, the flexor surfaces of the digits, the umbilicus, nipples, glans penis and clitoris, the labia minora and the inner aspects of the labia majora and prepuce. The presence, distribution and relative abundance of hair in certain regions such as the face (in males), pubis and axillae, are secondary sexual characteristics which play subtle roles in sociosexual communication. There are racial variations in density, form, distribution and pigmentation, as well as individual variations. Hairs assist minimally in thermoregulation: on the scalp they provide some protection against injury and the harmful effects of solar radiation. They have a sensory function.

Hairs vary from c.600 per cm^2 on the face to 60 per cm^2 on the rest of the body. In length they range from less than a millimetre to more than a metre, and in width from 0.005 to 0.6 mm. They vary in form, being straight, coiled, helical or wavy, and differ in colour depending on the type and degree of pigmentation. Curly hairs tend to have a flattened cross-section, and are weaker than straight hairs. In general, body hairs are longest and coarsest in Caucasians and least noticeable in Mongolian races. Over most of the body surface hairs are short and narrow (vellus hairs) and in some areas these hairs do not project

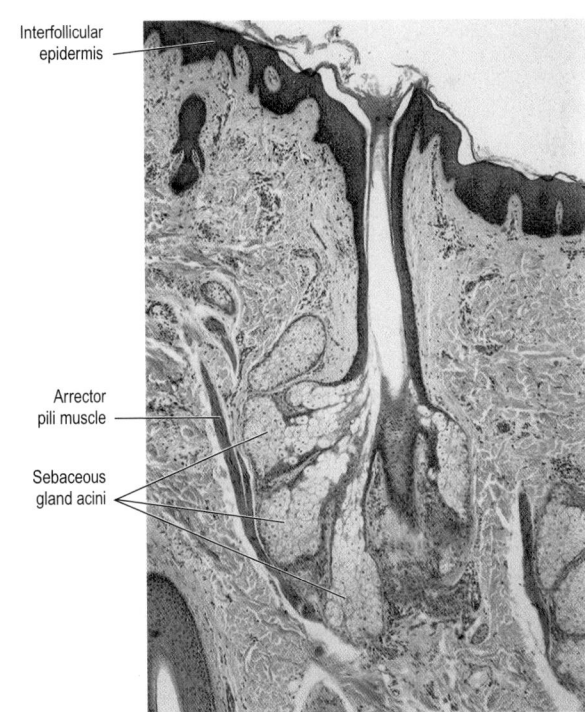

Interfollicular epidermis

Arrector pili muscle

Sebaceous gland acini

Fig. 8.11 A pilosebaceous unit in thin, hairy skin seen at low magnification. The hair follicle and hair shaft extend almost vertically through the field, the follicle joining the interfollicular epidermis (top). To the left of the follicle are the acini of a sebaceous gland, also sectioned tangentially through its capsule (centre bottom, below the portion of the hair follicle in section); the gland opens into the follicle in centre field. The associated arrector pili smooth muscle (thin red fibre bundle) is seen to the left of the sebaceous gland, following its contours. (Photograph by Sarah-Jane Smith.)

beyond their follicles, e.g. in eyelid skin. In other regions they are longer, thicker and often heavily pigmented (terminal hairs); these include the hairs of the scalp, the eyelashes and eyebrows and the postpubertal skin of the axillae and pubis, and the moustache, beard and chest hairs of males. The presence in females of coarse terminal hairs in a male-like pattern is termed hirsutism and is usually a sign of an endocrine disorder and excess androgen production (Azziz 2003).

Hair follicle

The hair follicle (Figs 8.1, 8.11, 8.12) is a downgrowth of the epidermis containing a hair, which may extend deeply (3 mm) into the hypodermis, or may be more superficial (1 mm) within the dermis. Typically, the long axis of the follicle is oblique to the skin surface; with curly hairs it is also curved. There are cycles of hair growth and loss, during which the follicle presents different appearances. In the anagen phase the hair is actively growing and the follicle is at its maximum development. In the involuting or catagen phase hair growth ceases and the follicle shrinks. During the resting or telogen phase the inferior segment of the follicle is absent. This is succeeded by the next anagen phase. Further details of the hair growth cycle are given below, after the description of the anagen follicle and hair.

Anagen follicle

The anagen follicle has several regions. The deepest is the inferior segment which includes the hair bulb region extending up to the level of attachment of the arrector pili muscle at the follicular bulge. Between this point and the site of entry of the sebaceous duct is the isthmus, above which is the infundibulum, or dermal pilary canal, which is continuous with the intraepidermal pilary canal. Below the sebaceous duct, the hair shaft and follicular wall are intimately connected, and it is only towards the upper end of the isthmus that the hair becomes free in the pilary canal. Below the infundibulum the follicle is surrounded by a thick perifollicular dermal coat containing type III collagen, elastin, sensory nerve fibres and blood vessels, and into which the arrector pili muscle fibres blend. A thick, specialized basal lamina, the glassy membrane, marks the interface between dermis and the epithelium of large hair follicles.

Hair bulb

The hair bulb forms the lowermost portion of the follicular epithelium and encloses the dermal papilla of connective tissue cells (Fig. 8.13). The dermal papilla is an important cluster of inductive mesenchymal cells which is required for hair follicle growth in each cycle throughout adult life: it is a continuation of the layer of adventitious mesenchyme that follows the contours of the hair follicle. The hair bulb generates the hair and its inner root sheath. A hypothetical line drawn across the widest part of the hair bulb divides it into a lower germinal matrix and an upper bulb. The germinal matrix is formed of closely packed, mitotically active pluripotential keratinocytes, among which are interspersed melanocytes, and some Langerhans cells. The upper bulb consists of cells arising from the matrix. These migrate apically and differentiate along several lines. Those arising centrally form the hair medulla. Radially, successive concentric rings of cells give rise to the cortex and cuticle of the hair and outside this, to the three layers of the inner root sheath. The latter are, from within out, the cuticle of the inner root sheath, Huxley's layer and Henle's layer. Henle's layer is surrounded by the outer root sheath, which forms the cellular wall of the follicle (Fig. 8.12, 8.14). Differentiation of cells in the various layers of the hair and its inner root sheath begins at the level of the upper bulb and is asynchronous, beginning earliest in Henle's layer and Huxley's layer.

Structure of hair and its sheaths

A fully developed hair shaft consists of three concentric zones which are, from outwards in, the cuticle, cortex and medulla. Each has different types of keratin filament proteins and different patterns of cornification. In finer hairs the medulla is usually absent. The cuticle forms the hair surface and consists of several layers of overlapping cornified squames directed apically and slightly outwards (Fig. 8.15). Immature cuticle cells have dense amorphous granules aligned predominantly along the outer plasma membrane with a few filaments. The cortex forms the greater part of the hair shaft and consists of numerous closely packed, elongated squames which may contain nuclear remnants and melanosomes (Fig. 8.14). Immature cortical cells contain bundles of closely packed filaments but no dense granules, and when fully cornified, they have a characteristic thumb-print appearance with filaments

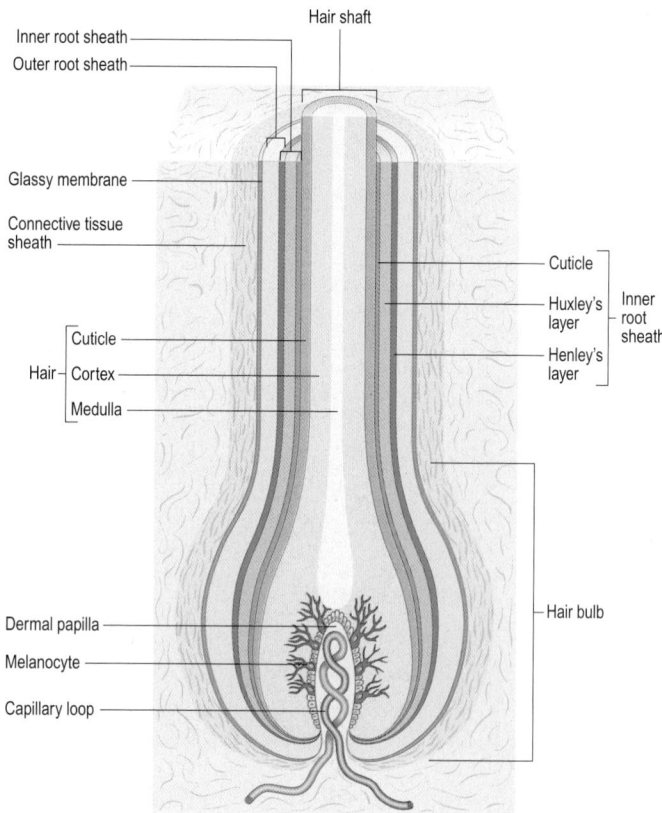

Fig. 8.12 The major structural features of the base of a hair follicle, showing the organization of the major layers of the hair and surrounding sheath, arising from the hair bulb. A dermal papilla invaginates the bulb, and along the basal layer of the epidermis, at its interface with the dermis, melanocytes insert their dendrites among the keratinocytes forming the hair.

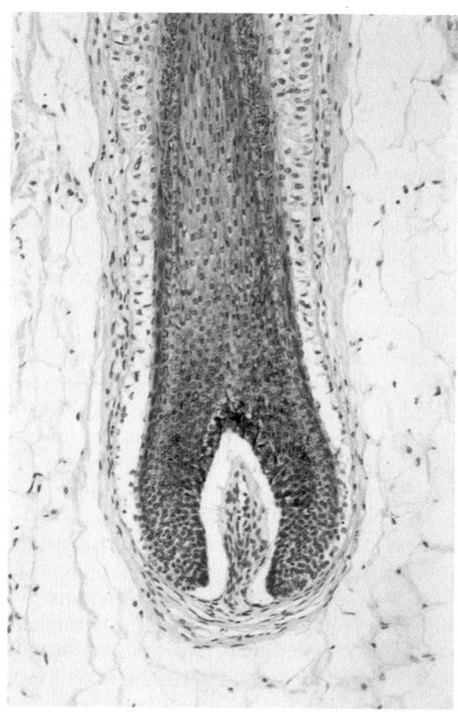

Fig. 8.13 The hair bulb at the base of the follicle. The dermal papilla invaginates the bulb from its fibrous outer sheath, carrying a loop of capillaries. Melanocytes in the germinal matrix (equivalent to the basal layer of interfollicular epidermis) extend dendrites into the adjacent layers of keratinocytes, to which they pass melanosomes. The layers of the root sheath are also visible (see **Fig. 8.12**). (Photograph by Sarah-Jane Smith.)

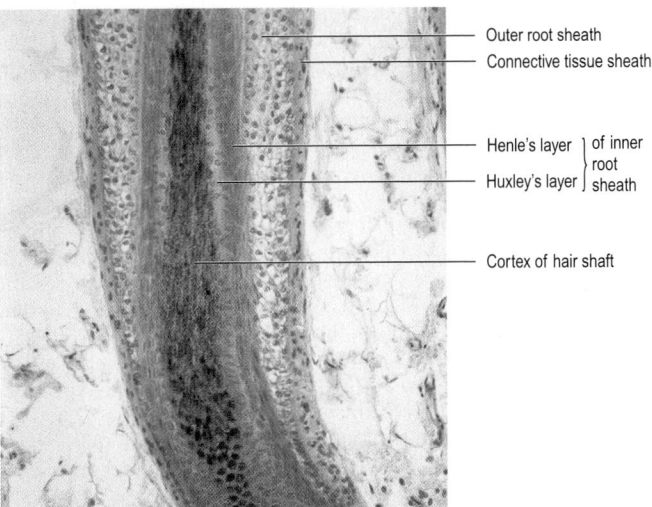

Outer root sheath
Connective tissue sheath

Henle's layer] of inner
] root
Huxley's layer] sheath

Cortex of hair shaft

Fig. 8.14 Melanosomes (dark pigment) in cortical cells of the hair shaft. The layers of the root sheath are also visible (see **Fig. 8.12**). The bulb is out of the field of view, below. (Photograph by Sarah-Jane Smith.)

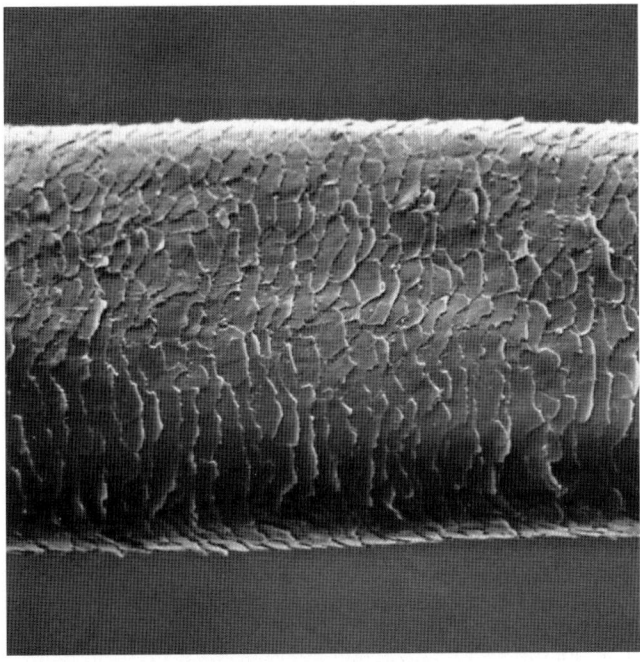

Fig. 8.15 A scalp hair showing details of surface structure. Note that the cuticular cells overlap each other; their free ends point towards the apex of the hair. (By kind permission from Michael Crowder.)

arranged in whorls. The medulla, when present, is composed of loosely aggregated and often discontinuous columns of partially disintegrated cells containing vacuoles, scattered filaments, granular material and melanosomes. Air cavities lie between the cells or even within them.

Henle's layer and Huxley's layer of the inner root sheath contain irregular dense keratohyalin granules and associated filaments in the precornified state. At the level of the upper bulb Henle's layer begins to cornify, as does Huxley's layer at the middle of the inferior follicle. When fully differentiated, cells of both layers have a thickened cornified envelope enclosing keratin filaments embedded in a matrix. The cells of the inner root sheath cuticle undergo terminal differentiation at a level closer to the hair bulb than that of Huxley's layer, but lack a clear-cut filament pattern such as is seen in the cortical cells of the hair shaft. As they cornify, the cuticle cells of the inner root sheath and hair become interlocked. At about the level of entry of the sebaceous duct, above the

isthmus, the inner root sheath undergoes fragmentation, and the hair then lies free in the pilary canal.

The outer root sheath, beginning at the level of the upper bulb, is a single or double layer of undifferentiated cells containing glycogen. Higher up the follicle it becomes multilayered. At the isthmus all remaining cell layers of the follicle sheath become flattened, compressed and attenuated. On emerging from the isthmus, the outer root sheath assumes the stratified, differentiating characteristics of interfollicular epidermis, with which it becomes continuous. At the level of entry of the sebaceous duct, it forms the wall of the pilary canal.

Hair cycle and growth of hair

Recurrent cyclic activity of hair follicles involves growth, rest, and shedding of hair in phases. In humans, these occur in irregular cycles of variable duration: there are regional and other variations in the length of the individual phases. In the growing or anagen phase, follicle and hair are as described above. Melanocytes are active only in mid-anagen, and are capable of producing both phaeo- and eumelanosomes, which they pass to precortical and medullary keratinocytes. Changes in hair colour of an individual, usually in adolescence, are due to alterations in the dominant type of melanosome produced.

Anagen is followed by the involuting or catagen phase during which mitotic activity of the germinal matrix ceases, the base of the hair condenses into a club which moves upwards to the level of the arrector pili muscle, and the whole inferior segment of the follicle degenerates. The dermal papilla also ascends and remains close to the base of the shortened follicle and its enclosed club hair, a situation which persists during the resting or telogen phase. During telogen, melanocytes become amelanotic and can be identified only ultrastructurally. At the beginning of the next anagen, the epithelial cells at the base of the follicle divide to form a secondary hair rudiment which envelops the dermal papilla to form a new hair bulb. This grows downwards, reforming the inferior segment of the follicle, from which a new hair grows up alongside the club hair, which is eventually shed.

Postnatally, hairs exhibit regional asynchrony of cycle duration and phase leading to an irregular pattern of growth and replacement. In some regions, such as the scalp, the cycle is measured in years; in others, such as general body hair, the cycle is much shorter and hairs are therefore limited in length. At puberty, hair growth and generation of much thicker hairs occurs on the pubes and axillae in both sexes, and on the face and trunk in males. The actions of hormones on hair growth are complex, and involve not only sex hormones, but also those of the thyroid, suprarenal cortex and pituitary glands. Androgens stimulate facial and general body hair formation. After about the first 30 years, they tend to cause the thick terminal hairs of the scalp to change to small vellus hairs, which produces recession from the forehead and sometimes almost complete male pattern baldness. In females, oestrogens tend to maintain vellus hairs: postmenopausal reduction of oestrogens may permit stronger facial and bodily hair growth. In mid-pregnancy, hair growth may be particularly active but later, often post-partum, an unusually large number of hairs enter the telogen phase and are shed before the growth cycle recommences. In older men, growth of hairs on the eyebrows and within the nostrils and external ear canals increases, whereas elsewhere on the body growth slows and the hairs become much finer.

Measurements of the rate of growth of individual hairs vary considerably, probably because of the influence of the factors mentioned above. A rate of 0.2–0.44 mm per 24 hours in males is usually given: the higher rate occurs on the scalp. Contrary to popular myth, shaving does not appear to affect the growth rate and hair ceases growth after death.

Sebaceous glands

Sebaceous glands are small saccular structures (**Figs 8.1, 8.11, 8.16**) lying in the dermis; together with the hair follicle and arrector pili muscle, they constitute the pilosebaceous unit. They are present over the whole body except the thick hairless skin of the palm, soles and flexor surfaces of digits. Typically, they consist of a cluster of secretory acini which open by a short common duct into the dermal pilary canal of the hair follicle. They release their lipid secretory product, sebum, into the canal by a holocrine mechanism (p. 34). In some areas of thin skin which lack hair follicles, their ducts open instead directly on to the skin surface, e.g. on the lips and corners of the mouth, the buccal mucosa, nipples, female breast areolae, penis, inner surface of the prepuce, clitoris and labia minora. At the margins of the eyelids, the

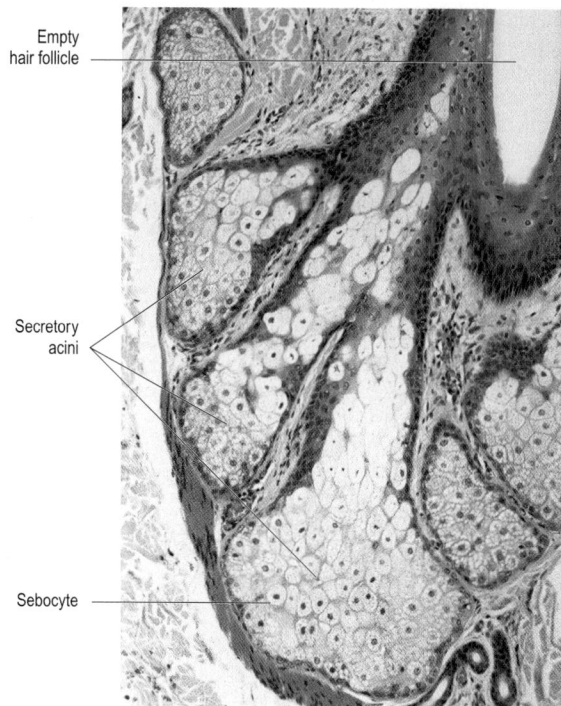

Empty hair follicle

Secretory acini

Sebocyte

Fig. 8.16 A sebaceous gland, showing a group of secretory acini opening into a hair follicle (top right). The distended sebocytes are filled with their oily secretion (sebum), which is discharged into the hair follicle by the holocrine disintegration of secretory cells. (Photograph by Sarah-Jane Smith.)

large complex palpebral tarsal glands (meibomian glands) are of this type. They are also present in the external auditory meatus.

In general, numbers of sebaceous glands in any given area reflect the distribution of hair follicles, ranging from an average of c.100/cm² over most of the body to as many as 400–900/cm² on the face and scalp. They are also numerous in the midline of the back. Individual sebaceous glands are particularly large on the face, around the external auditory meatus, chest and shoulders, and on the anogenital surfaces. Those on the face are often related to very small vellus hairs whose follicles have particularly wide apertures.

Microscopically, the glandular acini are enclosed in a basal lamina supported by a thin dermal capsule and a rich capillary network. Each acinus is lined by a single layer of small, flat, polygonal epithelial cells (sebocytes) which ultrastructurally resemble undifferentiated basal keratinocytes of interfollicular epidermis. They possess euchromatic nuclei and large nucleoli, scattered keratin filaments, free ribosomes, smooth endoplasmic reticulum and rounded mitochondria, and are attached to each other by desmosomes. Functionally, they are mitotically active stem cells whose progeny move gradually towards the centre of the acinus, increasing in volume and accumulating increasingly large lipid vacuoles. The nuclei become pyknotic as the cells mature. The huge distended cells ultimately disintegrate, filling the central cavity and its duct with a mass of fatty cellular debris (**Fig. 8.16**). The process takes 2–3 weeks. The secretory products pass through a wide duct lined with keratinized stratified squamous epithelium into the infundibulum of the hair follicle and then to the surface of the hair and the general epidermis.

The normal functions of sebum are the provision of a protective coating on hairs, possibly helping to waterproof the epidermis, discouragement of ectoparasites and contribution to a characteristic body odour. When first formed, sebum is a complex mixture of over 50% di- and triglycerides, with smaller proportions of wax esters, squalene, cholesterol esters, cholesterol and free fatty acids. At birth, sebaceous glands are quite large, regressing later until stimulated again at puberty. At that time, sebaceous gland growth and secretory activity increase greatly in both males and females, under the influence of androgens (testicular and suprarenal), which act directly on the gland. Excessive amounts of sebum may become impacted within the duct, and this, associated with hyperkeratinization, may lead to blockage and formation of a comedone. This may become infected and inflamed, and is the primary lesion of acne. Oestrogens have an effect opposite to that of androgens, and sebum secretion is considerably lower in women, becoming greatly decreased after the age of 50 years.

Apocrine glands

Apocrine glands are particularly large glands of the dermis or hypodermis, classed as a type of sweat gland. Since they develop as outgrowths of the hair follicle and discharge secretion into the hair canal, they are considered here. In the adult, they are present in the axillae, perianal region, areolae, periumbilical skin, prepuce, scrotum, mons pubis and labia minora. Ceruminous glands of the external auditory meatus and the ciliary glands of the palpebral margins (glands of Moll) are also usually included in this category, but their secretions are quite different and they should be considered as distinct, specialized subtypes.

An apocrine gland consists of a basal secretory coil and a straight duct which opens into either the pilary canal above the duct of the sebaceous gland, or directly onto the skin surface if there is no associated hair. The secretory region may be as much as 2 mm wide and its coils often anastomose to form a labyrinthine network. Each coil is lined by cuboidal secretory cells whose apical cytoplasm projects into the lumen and basally is in contact with a layer of myoepithelial cells within a thick basal lamina. The secretory cells contain vacuoles, vesicles and dense granules of varying size and internal structure: the numbers and character vary with the cycle of synthesis and discharge. The mechanism of secretion is still not clear, but may involve merocrine secretion of granules, apocrine secretion or complete holocrine disintegration of the cells.

Apocrine activity is minimal before puberty, after which it is androgen dependent and responsive to emotional stimuli. It is controlled by adrenergic nerves, and is sensitive to adrenaline (epinephrine) and noradenaline (nonepinephrine). The secretion is initially sterile and odourless, but it undergoes bacterial decomposition to generate potent odorous, musky compounds, including short-chain fatty acids, and steroids such as 5α-androstenone. In many animals these are potent pheromonal signals but their role in humans is less certain.

Arrector pili muscles

The arrector pili muscles are small bundles of closely packed smooth muscle cells which form diagonal links between the dermal sheaths of hair follicles and the papillary layer of the dermis (**Figs 8.1, 8.11**). They show the typical features of smooth muscle cells and are separated by narrow spaces containing collagen fibres and unmyelinated noradrenergic sympathetic axons.

The muscles are attached to the bulge region of the follicles by elastin fibrils, and are directed obliquely and towards the side to which the hair slopes superficially. The sebaceous gland occupies the angle between the muscle and the hair follicle, and muscle contraction helps to expel the gland contents. Contraction tends to pull the hair into a more vertical position and to elevate the epidermis surrounding it into a small hillock, dimpling the skin surface where the muscle is inserted superficially. Arrector pili muscles are absent from facial, axillary, and pubic hairs, from eyelashes and eyebrows, and from the hairs around the nostrils and the external auditory meatuses.

SWEAT GLANDS (Fig. 8.17)

The vast majority of sweat glands are often classified as eccrine, although their mode of secretion includes typical merocrine mechanisms (p. 34). They are long unbranched tubular structures, each with a highly coiled, secretory portion up to 0.4 mm in diameter, situated deep in the dermis or hypodermis. From there, a narrower, straight or slightly helical ductal portion emerges (**Fig. 8.1**). The walls of the duct fuse with the base of epidermal rete pegs and the lumen passes between the keratinocytes, often in a tight spiral particularly in thick hairless skin (**Fig. 8.18**), and opens via a rounded aperture (pore) onto the skin surface (**Fig. 8.7**). In thick hairless skin, sweat glands discharge along the centres of friction ridges, incidentally providing fingerprint patterns for forensic analysis. Sweat glands have an important thermoregulatory function, they contribute significantly to excretion and their secretion enhances grip and sensitivity of the palms and soles.

Sweat glands are absent from the tympanic membrane, margins of the lips, nail bed, nipple, inner preputial surface, labia minora, penis and clitoris, where apocrine glands are located. Elsewhere they are

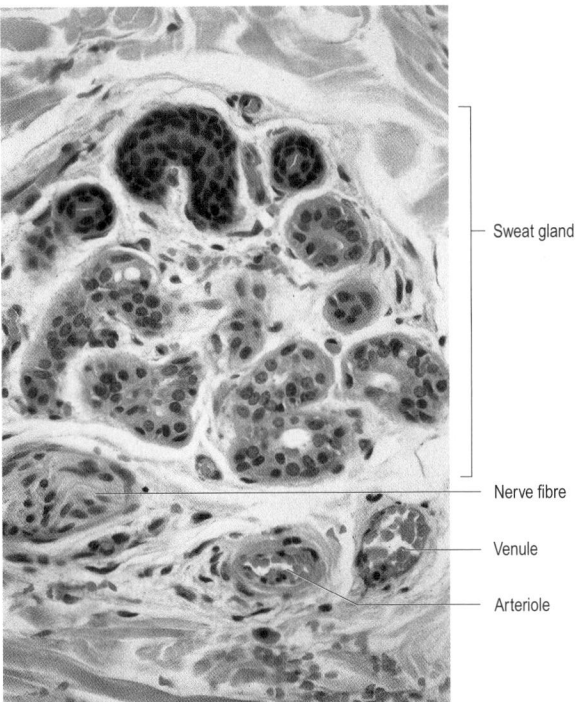

Fig. 8.17 The coiled secretory portion of a sweat gland in the reticular dermis. The deeper-stained profiles (above) are the origins of the duct. An autonomic nerve fibre and accompanying arteriole and venule are seen below. (Photograph by Sarah-Jane Smith.)

Sweat gland

Nerve fibre

Venule

Arteriole

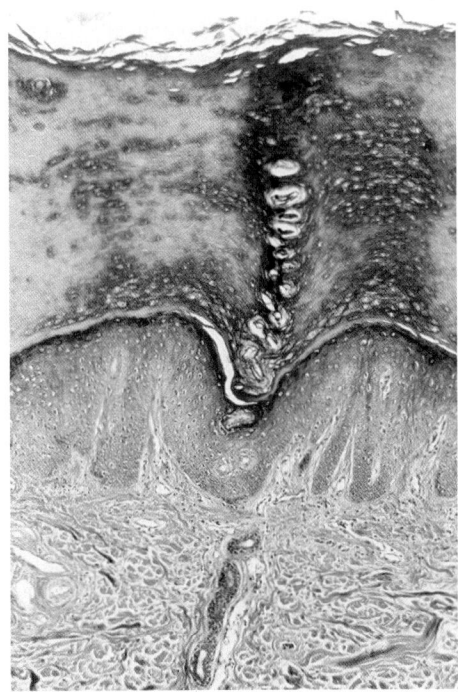

Fig. 8.18 A sweat duct in thick skin (trichrome-stained), spiralling through the dermis and epidermis, visible most clearly in the cornified superficial layer.

mately pyramidal in shape, and their bases rest on the basal lamina or contact myoepithelial cells. Their apical plasma membranes line lateral intercellular canaliculi which connect with the main lumen. The baso-lateral plasma membranes are highly folded, interdigitating with apposed clear cells, and they have the basal membrane infoldings typical of cells involved in fluid and ion transport. Their cytoplasm contains glycogen granules, mitochondria, rough endoplasmic reticulum and a small Golgi complex, but few other organelles. The nucleus is round and moderately euchromatic. Dark cells are pyramidal, and lie closer to the lumen such that their broad ends form its lining. Their cytoplasm contains a well-developed Golgi complex, numerous vacuoles and vesicles and dense glycoprotein granules which they secrete by a typical merocrine mechanism. Myoepithelial cells resemble those associated with secretory acini of the salivary glands and breast, and contain abundant myofilaments.

The intradermal sweat duct is formed of an outer basal layer and an inner layer of luminal cells connected by numerous desmosomes. The intraepidermal sweat duct (acrosyringium) is coiled, and consists of two layers of cells which, developmentally, are different from the surrounding keratinocytes and can be distinguished from them by the presence of keratin K19. The outer cells near the surface contain keratohyalin granules and lamellar granules, and undergo typical cornification. The inner cells, from a midepidermal level, contain numerous vesicles, undergo an incomplete form of cornification, and are largely shed into the lumen at the level of the cornified epidermal layer.

Sweat is a clear, odourless fluid, hypotonic to tissue fluid, and contains mainly sodium and chloride ions, but also potassium, bicarbonate, calcium, urea, lactate, amino acids, immunoglobulins and other proteins. Excessive sweating can lead to salt depletion. Heavy metals and various organic compounds are eliminated in sweat, the greater part of which is thought to be produced by the clear cells. When initially secreted, the fluid is similar in composition to interstitial fluid. It is modified as it passes along the duct by the action mainly of the basal cells, which resorb sodium and chloride and some water. The hormone aldosterone enhances this activity. The sweat glands are capable of producing up to 10 litres of sweat per day, in response to thermal, emotional and taste stimuli, mediated by unmyelinated sympathetic cholinergic fibres; the glands also respond to adrenaline. Thermo-regulation involves a heat centre in the hypothalamus which reacts to changes in blood temperature and afferent stimuli from the skin, by controlling cutaneous blood supply and the rate and volume of sweat secretion for evaporation at the surface.

NAIL APPARATUS (Fig. 8.19)

Nails are homologous with the cornified layer of the general epidermis. They consist of compacted, anucleate, keratin-filled squames in two or three horizontal layers. Ultrastructurally, the squames contain closely packed filaments which lie transversely to the direction of proximodistal growth, and are embedded in a dense protein matrix. Unlike the general epidermis, squames are not shed from the nail plate surface. A variety of mineral elements are present in nail, including calcium. Calcium is not responsible for the hardness of nail: this is determined by the arrangement and cohesion of the layers of squames, and their internal fibres. The water content of nail is low, but nail is 10 times more perme-able to water than the general epidermis. The softness and elasticity of the nail plate is related to its degree of hydration.

The nail apparatus consists of the nail plate, proximal and lateral nail folds, nail matrix, nail bed and hyponychium.

Nail plate

The nail plate is embedded within the proximal and lateral nail folds. It is approximately rectangular in shape and is mostly convex in both longitudinal and transverse axes: there is considerable inter- and intra-individual variation (**Fig. 8.19**). The thickness of the plate increases proximodistally from c.0.7 mm to 1.6 mm: the terminal thickness varies between individuals. The surface of the nail plate may show fine longitudinal ridges, and its undersurface is grooved by corresponding ridges in the nail bed. Disturbances of growth pattern or disease may lead to transverse ridging or grooves, and minute trapped air bubbles may produce white flecks. These defects move distally with growth of the plate.

The nail plate arises from compacted cornified epithelial cells derived from the dorsal, intermediate and ventral nail matrices. It is densely adherent to the matrices on its undersurface, but becomes a free

numerous, their frequency ranging from 80 to over 600/cm^2, depending on position and genetic variation. The total number lies between 1.6 and 4.5 million, and is greatest on the plantar skin of the feet. There are many sweat glands on the face and flexor aspects of the hands, and fewest on the surfaces of the limbs. Racial groups indigenous to warmer climates tend to have more sweat glands than those indigenous to cooler regions.

Microscopically the secretory coil consists of a pseudostratified epithelium enclosing a lumen. Three types of cell have been described: clear cells from which most of the secretion derives, dark cells which share the same lumen, and myoepithelial cells. Clear cells are approxi-

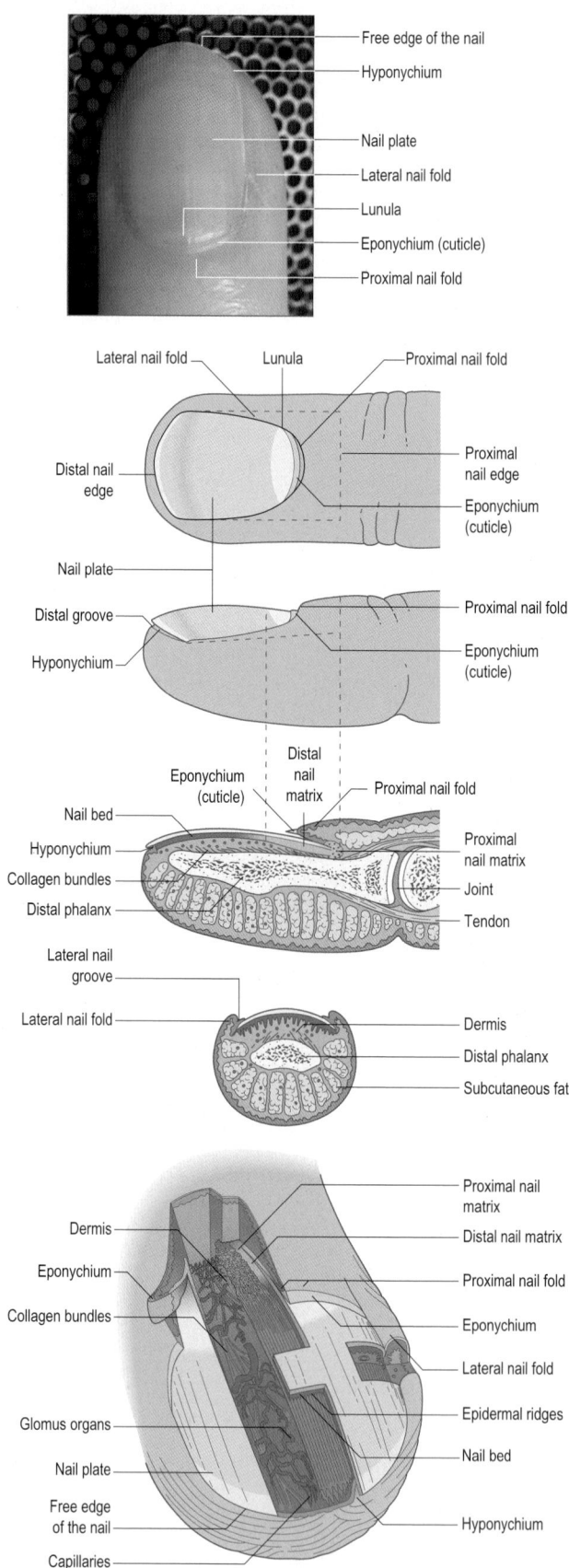

Fig. 8.19 The organization and terminology of the structures associated with a fingernail. (By permission from Paus R, Peker S 2003 Biology of hair and nails. In: Bolognia JL, Jorizzo JL, Rapini RP (eds) Dermatology. London: Mosby.)

structure distal to the onychodermal band. The dorsal aspect of the nail plate originates from the more proximal regions of the germinal matrix, i.e. dorsal and intermediate matrices, whereas the deeper, volar aspect of the plate originates from the ventral matrix.

Nail folds

The sides of the nail plate are bordered by lateral nail folds which are continuous with the proximal fold (**Fig. 8.19**). The lateral nail folds enclose the lateral free edges of the nail plate and are bounded by the attachment of the skin to the lateral aspect of the distal phalanx margin and the lateral nail. The proximal nail fold provides the visible proximal border to the nail apparatus. It consists of two epidermal layers, superficial and deep, separated by a core of dermis. The epidermis of the superficial layer lacks hair follicles and epidermal ridges: its cornified distal margin extends over the nail plate for a little distance as the cuticle or eponychium. The deep layer merges with the nail matrix.

The eponychium is bounded by the fascial attachment of the skin to the base of the distal phalanx, distal to the insertion of the extensor tendon, and its distal free edge. It adheres to the dorsal aspect of the nail plate and overlies the root of the nail.

Nail matrix

The nail matrix is the source of the nail plate, and can be divided into three parts. Proximally, the dorsal matrix is defined as the volar surface (undersurface) of the proximal nail fold. The intermediate matrix (germinal matrix) starts where the dorsal matrix folds back on itself and extends as far as the distal portion of the lunule. The ventral matrix (sterile matrix) is the remainder of the nail bed: it starts at the distal border of the lunule and ends at the hyponychium.

The matrix epithelium consists of typical basal and prickle cell layer keratinocytes, among which are scattered melanocytes and Langerhans cells. Cornified cells of the dorsal and ventral aspects of the matrix are steadily extruded distally to form the nail plate: the proximal 50% of the nail matrix contributes 80% of the nail plate. This process continues into the nail bed at the distal edge of the lunule, which is formed where the distal portion of the ventral matrix underlies the nail plate.

The lunule is pale, opaque and convex and is more prominent in the thumb than the other digits. It is not known why the lunule is so pale compared with the more distal translucent pink nail bed. The lack of colour may reflect the thickness of the epidermis in the lunule and/or a paucity of capillaries in the dermis of the lunule.

Nail bed

The nail bed epidermis extends from the distal margin of the lunule to the hyponychium. The distal margin of the nail bed, at which point the nail plate becomes free of the nail bed, is called the onychodermal band. The surface of the nail bed is ridged and grooved longitudinally, corresponding to a similar pattern on the undersurface of the nail plate. This results in a tight interlocking of the two which prevents the invasion of microbes and the impaction of debris underneath the nail. The epidermis of the nail bed is thin and lacks a stratum granulosum. It consists of two to three layers of nucleated cells which lack keratohyalin granules, and a thin cornified layer which moves distally with the growing nail plate. It contains an occasional sweat gland distally.

The dermis of the nail bed is anchored to the periosteum of the distal phalanx without any intervening subcutaneous layer. It forms a distinct compartment, which means that infections of the nail bed, or other local causes of a rise of pressure (e.g. haematoma) may cause severe pain which is only relieved by excision of part or all of the nail plate. The dermis is richly vascularized. The blood vessels are arranged longitudinally and display numerous glomus bodies, which are encapsulated arteriovenous anastomoses involved in the physiological control of peripheral blood flow in relation to temperature (Chs 7, 53). The dermis is well-innervated, and contains numerous sensory nerve endings, including Merkel endings and Meissner's corpuscles.

Nail bed cells differentiate towards the nail plate, contributing to it ventrally.

Hyponychium

The hyponychium is the area under the free nail between the onychodermal band proximally and the distal groove. It is an epidermal ridge which demarcates the junction between the finger pulp and the subungual structures.

Growth of nail

Nail growth is determined by the turnover rate of the matrix cells, which varies with digit, age, environmental temperature and season, time of day, nutritional status, trauma and various diseases. Generally, its speed is related to the length of the digit, being fastest (c.0.1 mm per day) in the middle finger of the hand, and slowest in the little finger. Fingernails grow three to four times faster than toenails, quicker in summer than in winter, and faster in the young than in the old. A fingernail grows out in c.6 months, whereas a toenail is replaced, on average, in c.18 months.

Genetic keratin disorders (Irvine & McLean 1999) may lead to nail dystrophies such as pachyonychia, where the nails become grossly thickened.

VASCULAR SUPPLY, LYMPHATIC DRAINAGE AND INNERVATION

Vascular supply and lymphatic drainage

The metabolic demands of the skin are not great, and yet, under normal conditions, its blood flow exceeds nutritional requirements by 10 times, and may amount to 5% of the cardiac output. This is because the cutaneous circulation has an important thermoregulatory function, and is arranged so that its capacity can be increased or decreased rapidly by as much as 20 times, in response to the required loss or conservation of heat.

The blood supply to the skin originates from three main sources, the direct cutaneous system, the musculocutaneous system and the fasciocutaneous system. The direct cutaneous system of vessels is derived from the main arterial trunks and accompanying veins. Vessels course in the subcutaneous fat parallel to the skin surface, and are confined to certain areas of the body, e.g. the supraorbital artery, the superficial circumflex iliac artery and the dorsalis pedis artery. The musculocutaneous perforators arise from the intramuscular vasculature, pass through the surface of the muscle, and pierce the deep fascia to reach the skin by spreading out in the subcutaneous tissues. The fasciocutaneous system consists of perforating branches from deeply located vessels (deep to the deep fascia) which pass along intermuscular septa and then fan out at the level of the deep fascia to reach the skin. Examples include the fasciocutaneous perforating vessels from the radial and ulnar arteries.

The direct cutaneous vessels, the musculocutaneous perforators and the fasciocutaneous perforators each contribute to six anastomosing horizontal reticular plexi of arterioles (**Fig. 8.20**) which have vascular connections between them and which ultimately provide the blood supply to the skin. Three plexi are located in the skin itself and supply all elements including the sweat glands and pilosebaceous units. The subpapillary plexus is located at the junction of the papillary and reticular layers of the dermis. It gives off small branches which form capillary loops in the dermal papillae (usually one loop per papilla) which are perpendicular to the skin surface (**Figs 8.1, 8.4, 8.21**). The reticular dermal plexus is located in the middle portion of the dermis and is primarily venous. The deep dermal plexus is located in the deepest part of the reticular dermis and on the undersurface of the dermis. The close association between arteriolar and venous plexi permits exchange of heat between blood in vessels at different temperatures flowing in opposite directions (counter-current heat exchange).

The remaining three plexi are the subcutaneous plexus, and two plexi associated with the deep fascia. The deep fascia has a plexus on its deep surface and a more extensive plexus on its superficial surface. This arrangement is much more pronounced in the limbs than it is in the trunk.

The general structure and arrangement of the microvasculature is described in detail on pages 140 and 146, and so only features particular to skin will be considered here. In the deeper layers of the dermis, arteriovenous anastomoses are common, particularly in the extremities (hands, feet, ears, lips, nose), where, as glomera, they are surrounded by thick muscular coats. Under autonomic vasomotor control, these vascular shunts, when relaxed, divert blood away from the superficial plexus and so reduce heat loss, while at the same time ensuring some deep cutaneous circulation and preventing anoxia of structures such as nerves. Extensive capillary anastomoses are present. Generally, cutaneous blood flow is regulated according to thermoregulatory need, and also, in some areas of the body, according to emotional state. In very cold conditions, the peripheral circulation is greatly reduced by vasoconstriction, but intermittent spontaneous vasodilatation results in periodic increases in temperature which prevent cooling to the level at which frostbite might occur. This is thought to be due to a direct effect of oxygen lack on the arteriolar constrictor muscle, rather than to a neural influence.

The lymphatics of the skin, as elsewhere, are small terminal vessels which collect interstitial fluid and macromolecules for return to the circulation via larger vessels. They also convey lymphocytes, Langerhans cells and macrophages to regional lymph nodes. They begin as blind endothelial-lined tubes or loops just below the papillary dermis. These drain into a superficial plexus below the subpapillary venous plexus,

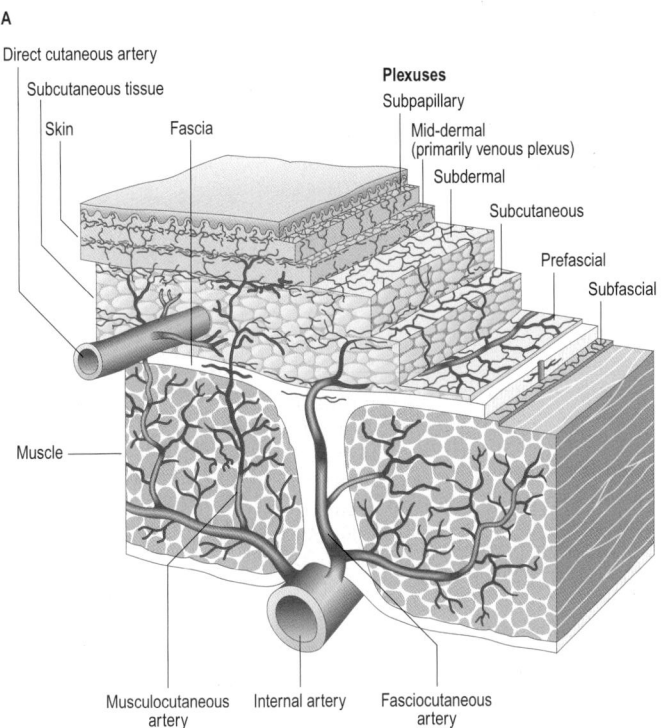
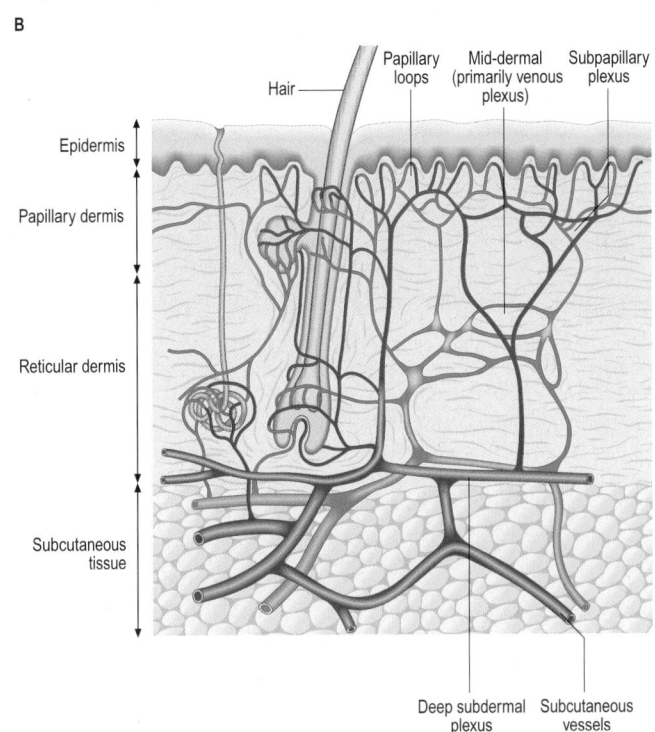

Fig. 8.20 Vascular supply to the skin. **A**, Note the various horizontal plexuses fed by direct cutaneous, fasciocutaneous and musculocutaneous arteries. **B**, Close-up of vascular supply. (**A**, by permission from McCarthy JG (ed) Chapter 9 in Plastic Surgery, Vol 1. Philadelphia: Saunders. **B**, by permission from Cormack GC, Lamberty BGH 1994 The Arterial Anatomy of Skin Flaps, 2nd edition. Edinburgh: Churchill Livingstone.)

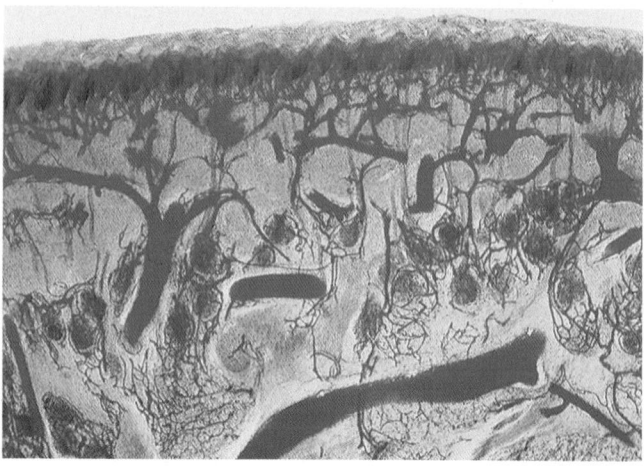

Fig. 8.21 A thick vertical section through palmar skin, the arteries, arterioles and capillaries of which have been injected with red gelatin to demonstrate the pattern of dermal vascularization. At the base of the dermis a broad flat arterial plexus supplies a more superficial papillary plexus, which in turn gives off capillary loops which enter the dermal papillae.

which drains via collecting vessels into a deeper plexus at the junction of the reticular dermis and subcutis, and this, in turn, drains into the larger subcutaneous channels.

Innervation

Skin is a major sensory surface, with regional variations in sensitivity to different stimuli. It has a rich nerve supply, which is also concerned with autonomic functions, particularly related to thermoregulation. Cutaneous sense provides information about the external environment through receptors responsive to stimuli which may be mechanical (rapid or sustained touch, pressure, vibration, stretching, bending of hairs, etc.), thermal (hot and cold), or noxious (perceived as itching, discomfort or pain). Pacinian corpuscles (p. 61) subserve deep pressure and vibrational sensation, and are located deep in the dermis or in the hypodermis, particularly of the digits. Meissner's corpuscles (p. 61) are located in dermal papillae, close to the dermo-epidermal junction, and are sensitive to touch sensation. These receptors are particularly suited to detecting shape and texture during active exploratory touch.

The primary input is transmitted by neurones whose cell bodies lie in the spinal and cranial ganglia, and whose myelinated or unmyelinated axons are terminally distributed, mainly within the dermis. Efferent autonomic fibres are unmyelinated and noradrenergic or cholinergic. They innervate the arterioles, arrector pili muscles, and the myoepithelial cells of sweat and apocrine glands. In the scrotum, labia minora, perineal skin and nipples they also supply smooth muscle fasciculi of the dermis and adjacent connective tissue. Except in the nipples and genital area, activity of the autonomic efferent nerves is mainly concerned with regulation of heat loss by vasodilation and vasoconstriction, sweat production, and pilo-erection (although this is a minor function in humans).

On reaching the dermis, nerve fasciculi branch extensively to form a deep reticular plexus which serves much of the dermis, including most sweat glands, hair follicles and the larger arterioles. Many small fasciculi pass from this plexus to ramify in another superficial papillary plexus at the junction between the reticular and papillary layers of the dermis. Branches from this pass superficially into the papillary layer, ramifying horizontally and vertically, and terminate either in relation to encapsulated receptors, or as terminals reaching the level of the basal lamina. In some instances, they enter the epidermis as free endings, responsive to light pressure and touch sensation or to nociceptive stimuli. As these latter fasciculi terminate, they lose their epineurial and perineurial sheaths, leaving Schwann cell axonal complexes or naked axons enveloped by basal lamina, in direct contact with the matrix. These naked distal axonal terminals may be vulnerable to pathogens entering via a skin abrasion.

The detailed structure and classification of sensory endings are described in detail on page 59.

DEVELOPMENT OF SKIN AND SKIN APPENDAGES

Skin is developed from the surface ectoderm and its underlying mesenchyme. Surface ectoderm gives rise to the cornifying general surface epidermis and its appendages, the pilosebaceous units, sweat glands and nail units, depending on interactions with the mesenchyme. Interactions between ectoderm and mesenchyme also give rise to the internal epithelium of the buccal cavity and the teeth and the nasal epithelia. The differentiated descendants of ectodermal cells are keratinocytes. Immigrant cells of different developmental origin constitute an important component of the epithelial sheet formed by the keratinocytes. The non-keratinocytes are melanocytes and Merkel cells derived from the neural crest, Langerhans cells of bone-marrow origin, and lymphocytes.

The dermis, composed of irregular connective tissue and some of the connective tissue sheaths of peripheral nerves, is derived from somatopleuric mesenchyme (in the limbs and trunk), and possibly somitic mesenchyme (covering the epaxial musculature), and from neural crest (in the head). Angiogenic mesenchyme gives rise to the blood vessels of the dermis. Nerves and associated Schwann cells, of neural crest origin, enter and traverse the dermis to reach their peripheral terminations during development.

EPIDERMIS AND APPENDAGES

General (interfollicular) epidermis

In the first 4–5 weeks, embryonic skin consists of a single layer of ectodermal cells overlying a mesenchyme containing cells of stellate dendritic appearance interconnected by slender processes and sparsely distributed in a loosely arranged microfibrillar matrix (**Fig. 8.22**). The interface between ectoderm and mesenchyme, known as the basement membrane zone (BMZ), is an important site of mutual interactions upon which the maintenance of the two tissues depends, both in prenatal and postnatal life (p. 172). Ectodermal cells, which characteristically contain glycogen deposits, contact each other at gap and tight junctions. The layer so formed soon develops into a bilaminar epithelium, and desmosomes also appear. The basal germinative layer gives rise to the definitive postnatal epidermis, and the superficial layer to the periderm, a transient layer confined to fetal life. The periderm maintains itself, expresses different keratin polypeptides, and grows by the mitotic activity of its own cells, independent of those of the germinative layer. Originally flattened, the periderm cells increase in depth: the central area containing the nucleus becomes elevated and projects as a globular elevation towards the amniotic cavity. The plasma membrane develops numerous surface microvilli with an extraneous coat of glycosaminoglycans, and cytoplasmic vesicles become prominent deep to it. These developments reach a peak over the period 12–18 weeks, at which time the periderm is a major source of the amniotic fluid to which it may contribute glucose; it also has an absorptive function. From c.20 weeks onwards, the globular protrusions become undermined and pinched off to float free in the amniotic fluid. The now flattened periderm cells undergo a type of terminal differentiation to form what is regarded as a temporary protective layer for the underlying developing epidermis proper, against an amniotic fluid of changing composition as a result of the accumulation of products of fetal renal excretion. Up to parturition, periderm squames continue to be cast off into the amniotic fluid, and they contribute to the vernix caseosa, a layer of cellular debris which covers the fetal skin at birth.

Proliferation in the germinative layer leads to a stratified appearance with successive layers of intermediate cells between it and the periderm. From an early stage, cells of all layers are packed with glycogen granules, presumably a source of energy during this early replicative stage of differentiation. Differentiation of these layers is not synchronous throughout all regions of the developing skin, being more advanced cranially than caudally, and progressing on the body from the midaxillary line ventrally. Reduction in glycogen content of the cells is associated with a shift towards biosynthetic activity connected with terminal (cornifying) differentiation, manifested by the presence of different enzymes and expression of keratins. Simple epithelial keratins present from before implantation (K8 and K18) are replaced by typical keratinocyte basal cell keratins (K5 and K14), followed in the first suprabasal cell layer by those of higher molecular weight associated with differentiation (K1 and K10) at c.10–12 weeks. This is soon followed by expression of

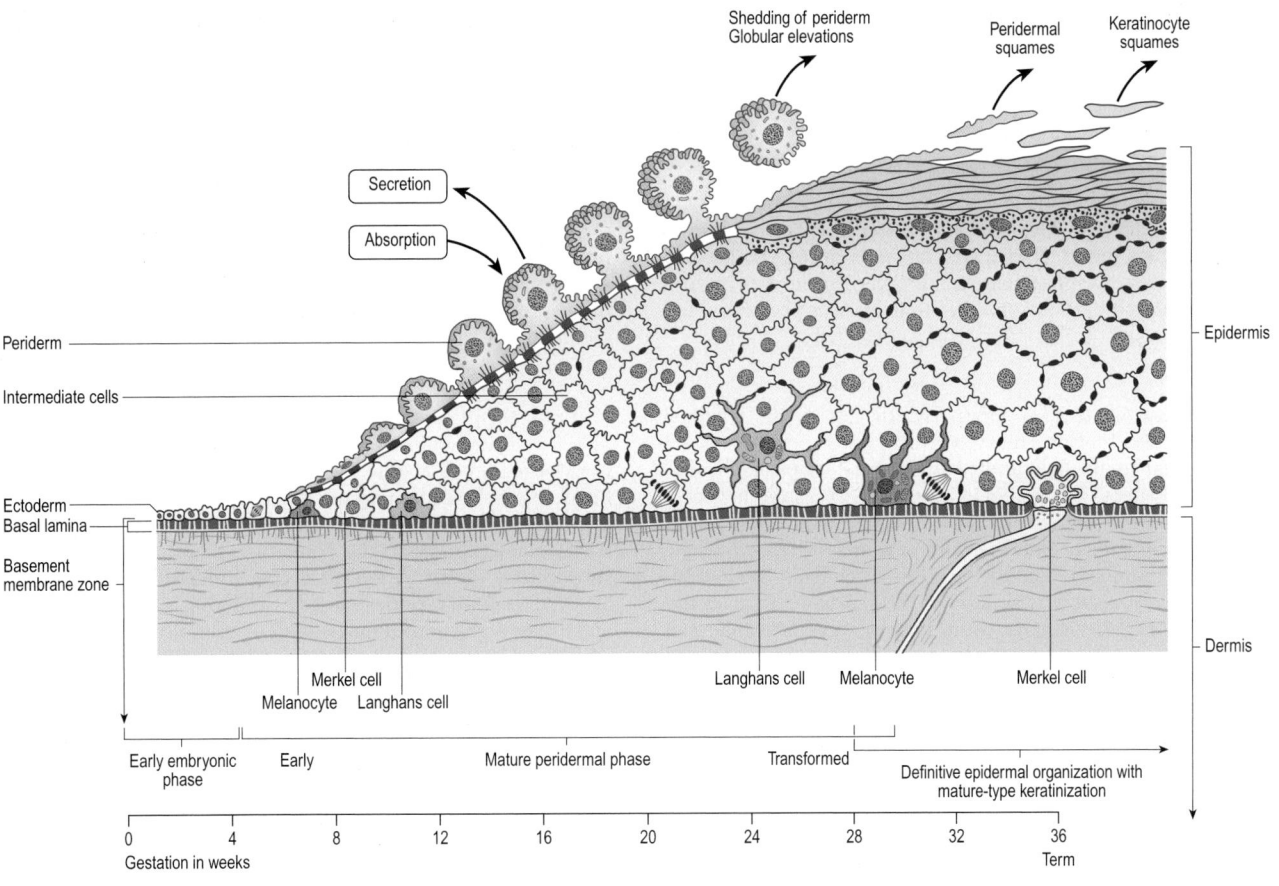

Fig. 8.22 Development of the skin. (After an idea of V. Uazzaro.)

profillagrin and fillagrin, and the appearance of keratohyalin granules among filamentous bundles of the uppermost intermediate layer cells at c. 20 weeks. The first fully differentiated keratinocytes appear shortly afterwards. By 24–26 weeks a definite stratum corneum exists in some areas, and by 30 weeks or so, apart from some lingering glycogen in intermediate cells, the interfollicular epidermis is essentially similar to its postnatal counterpart (see Holbrook and Odland 1980, for further details).

Non-keratinocytes are present in developing epidermis from c.8 weeks. Langerhans cells can be seen in the epidermis by 5–6 weeks and are fully differentiated by 12–14 weeks. Their numbers increase at least partially by mitotic division *in situ*, but at 6 months are only 10–20% of those in the adult. It is not known if the Langerhans cell functions in immune surveillance in fetal skin. Melanocytes, of neural crest origin, are present in the bilaminar epidermis of cephalic regions as early as 8 weeks. By 12–14 weeks they can reach a density of 2300 per mm^2 reducing to 800 per mm^2 just before birth. Keratinocytes regulate the final ratio between themselves and melanocytes via growth factors, cell surface molecules and other signals. Fetal melanocytes produce melanized melanosomes and transfer them to keratinocytes: these are intrinsic activities clearly independent of ultraviolet (UV) irradiation, and suggest functions of melanin other than photoprotection.

Merkel cells originate from migratory neural crest cells (Szeder et al 2003) and begin to appear in the epidermis of the palm and sole of the foot between 8 and 12 weeks, and later in association with some hairs and with dermal axonal–Schwann cell complexes.

Pilosebaceous unit
Pilosebaceous units develop at c.9 weeks, first in the regions of the eyebrows, lips, and chin, and at progressively later stages elsewhere, proceeding caudally. The first rudiment is a crowding of cells in the basal layer of the epidermis, the hair placode, adjacent to a local concentration of mesenchymal cells which will become the dermal papilla. Further proliferation and elongation of the cells leads to a hair germ, which protrudes downwards into the mesenchyme in association with the primitive dermal papilla during weeks 13–15. With continued downward growth in a slanted direction, the hair germ becomes a hair

peg, and when its bulbous lower end envelops the dermal papilla it is known as a bulbous peg. Melanocytes are individually present at the hair peg stage, and abundantly so and quite active in the bulbous peg. At this stage (approximately week 15) two or three swellings appear on the posterior wall. The uppermost is the rudiment of the apocrine gland (present only in some follicles), the middle forms the sebaceous gland and the lower one is the bulb, to which the arrector pili muscle (arising from underlying mesenchyme) later becomes attached, and where it is believed the main reservoir of hair follicle stem cells resides. The cells of the lowermost region of the bulb, the matrix, divide actively and produce a pointed hair cone. This grows upwards to canalize a developing hair tract, along which the fully formed hair, derived by further differentiation of cells advancing from the matrix, reaches the surface at approximately week 18 of gestation.

Sebaceous glands develop independently of hair follicles in the nostrils, eyelids (as tarsal glands) and in the anal region. Apocrine sweat glands are formed at the same time as eccrine (merocrine) sweat glands and are at first distributed widely over the body. Their number diminishes from 5 months' gestation, producing the distribution seen in the adult.

Hairs produced prenatally are called lanugo hairs; they are short and downy, lack a medulla, and in certain parts of the body are arranged in a vortex-like manner into tracts. Late in pregnancy, lanugo hairs are replaced by vellus hairs, and these in turn by intermediate hairs, which are the predominant type until puberty. New follicles do not develop in postnatal skin.

Eccrine sweat glands
Eccrine (merocrine) sweat glands are one type of sudoriferous gland. Sweat gland rudiments appear in the second and third months as cell buds associated with the primary epidermal ridges of the finger and toe pads of terminal digits. They elongate into the dermis and by 16 weeks the lower end begins to form the secretory coil, within which, by 22 weeks, secretory and myoepithelial cells are evident. The solid cord of cells connecting the coil to the epidermis becomes the intradermal duct, and the lumina of both are formed by dissolution of desmosomal contacts between the cells. The intraepidermal duct is foreshadowed by a coiled column of concentrically arranged inner and outer cells,

within which, by fusion of lysosomal vacuoles, a lumen is formed which opens on the surface at 22 weeks. As with hair follicles, no new eccrine sweat glands develop postnatally. Emotional sweating, detected by skin conductance changes, occurs in preterm infants from 29 weeks' gestational age.

Epidermal ridges

The epidermal ridges are foreshadowed as regularly spaced small downgrowths of epidermal cells which appear in finger and toe pads during the second and third months. They are known as primary epidermal ridges, separated by corresponding dermal ridges. In the fifth month secondary ridges develop, the pattern becomes evident on the surface, and is finalized through further remodelling postnatally.

Nails

Fields of proliferative ectoderm appear on the tips of the terminal segments of the digits. They progressively reach a dorsal position, where at c.9 weeks a flattened nail field limited by proximal, distal, and lateral nail grooves is apparent. The nail field ultimately forms the nail bed, and the primordium of the nail is formed of a wedge of cells which grows diagonally, proximally and deeply into the mesenchyme from the proximal groove towards the underlying terminal phalanx. The deeper cells of this wedge form the primordium of the matrix which gives rise to the nail plate. The latter emerges from under a, now proximal, nail fold at c.14 weeks and grows distally over an already keratinized nail bed. The nail matrix is usually considered to have dorsal and ventral (intermediate) components, but there are conflicting opinions as to the extent to which each contributes to the nail, both in ontogeny and postnatally: it is generally agreed that the ventral matrix contributes the major part. It has been claimed that the nail bed additionally contributes up to 20% of the postnatal nail plate, but embryological studies to date are not clear on this matter. Most texts state that keratohyalin is not involved in the cornification of nail. However, up to at least 16 weeks, the dorsal matrix granulosa cells which contribute cornified cells to the nail plate and eponychium (cuticle) contain typical keratohyalin granules, and the cells of the ventral matrix next to the nail plate contain single and compound granules similar to those present in granulosa cells of oral epithelia. Similar granules have been reported in matrix cells of postnatal human toenail.

At 20 weeks, the nail plate entirely covers the nail field (nail bed), now limited distally by a distal ridge, which, when the plate projects beyond the tip, becomes the hyponychium beneath it. At birth, the microstructure of the main nail unit components is similar to that postnatally; the nail is long and overhanging, and easily falls off during cleansing.

Abnormalities of the epidermis

Anomalous development of the epidermis and its derivatives is relatively common. Excessive or diminished growth, or even complete absence, may affect sebaceous or sudoriferous glands and hair, either locally or generally. Similarly, the epidermis may be excessively pigmented (melanism). Excessive production of stratum corneum leads to ichthyosis. A naevus or mole is a benign proliferation of melanocytes which is found in the basal layer of the epidermis. Ectodermal dysplasia is a rare condition characterized by fine blond and scanty hair, reduced or absent eyelashes and eyebrows. The skin has deficient sweat and sebaceous glands. Teeth are usually peg- or cone-shaped, and absence of major salivary glands may occur. For information on keratin diseases, see Irvine & McLean 1999.

DERMIS

The embryonic dermis is far richer in cells than the adult dermis, and many of these mesenchymal cells are involved in an essential signalling dialogue which regulates ectodermal differentiation. The mesenchymal cells underlying the surface ectoderm and early bi- and trilaminar epidermis contact each other by slender processes to form an intercommunicating network. They secrete a matrix which is rich in ions, water, and macromolecules, proteoglycan/glycosaminoglycans, fibronectin, collagenous proteins of various types and elastin. Further development of these intrinsic components involves the differentiation of individual cell types, fibroblasts, endothelial cells, mast cells, etc. and the assembly of matrix components into organized fibrillar collagen fibres and elastic fibres. During embryogenesis, the matrix is heterogeneous with regard to its biochemical and macromolecular components. The main

glycosaminoglycans of embryonic and fetal skin are glycuronic acid and dermatan sulfate. Collagens type I, III, V, and VI are distributed more or less uniformly regardless of fetal age, and there are some local concentrations of III and V, the levels of which are higher than in postnatal skin. Collagens type IV and VII are found predominantly in the basement membrane zone.

The progressive morphological differentiation of the dermis involves its separation from the subcutis at about the third month; changes in composition and size of collagen fibrils and their organization into bundles amongst which cells become relatively fewer; downgrowth of epidermal appendages; the organization of nervous and vascular plexuses, and the relatively late appearance of elastic networks. The papillary and reticular regions are said to be evident as early as 14 weeks, but the overall organization of the dermis continues postnatally.

Vascular supply and lymphatic drainage

The dermal vasculature is generally thought to be developed *in situ* by transformation of angiogenic mesenchymal cells. Closed endothelial-lined channels containing nucleated red cells are present by 6 weeks underneath the ectoderm, and by the eighth week are arranged in a single plane parallel to the epidermis: they will ultimately form the subpapillary plexus. A second deeper horizontal plexus is evident by 50–70 days. Both plexuses extend by budding as development proceeds, and they give rise to the final patterns of arterioles, venules and capillaries which are established shortly after birth. Pericytes also develop from mesenchymal cells. Lymphatic vessels are formed by mesenchymal cells which become organized to enclose pools of proteinaceous fluid leaking from the developing capillaries.

Innervation

Sensory cutaneous nerves (axons and Schwann cells) are derived by outgrowth from the neural crest (via dorsal root ganglia). Motor fibres to vessels and glands arise from cells of sympathetic ganglia. As individual parts of the embryo grow, the nerves grow and lengthen with them. Small axons are present superficially at a stage when the epidermis is bilaminar, and by 8 weeks' gestation there is already a functioning cutaneous plexus. By the fourth gestational month, the dermal plexuses are very richly developed, and Meissner and Pacinian corpuscles have appeared. The outer lamellar cells of Pacinian corpuscles in the dermis are homologous with the perineurium (p. 56), but the source of the laminar cells of the Meissner corpuscle is unclear.

EPITHELIAL–MESENCHYMAL INTERACTIONS IN DEVELOPING SKIN

Epidermal–mesenchymal (dermal) interactions at the basement membrane zone (BMZ) occur during development and throughout life. At the ectodermal stage, the BMZ consists of the basal plasma membrane of the ectodermal cell, paralleled on its cytoplasmic side by various cytoskeletal filaments, and beneath it, by a layer (0.1–0.2 μm) of microfibrillar-amorphous material deposited by the cell. At the bilaminar stage, a definite continuous lamina densa is present, separated from the basal plasma membrane by a lamina lucida traversed by loosely fibrillar material: similar filaments extend from the lamina densa into the mesenchymal matrix (**Fig. 8.23**).

Hemidesmosomes begin to appear at 8 weeks as stratification starts, and anchoring fibrils at 9–10 weeks. By the end of the third month the basic morphology of the interfollicular BMZ is essentially similar to that of the postnatal BMZ.

Laminin and collagen type IV are present in the developing basal lamina at 6 weeks, and bullous pemphigoid antigen (in hemidesmosomes) and anchoring fibril proteins are expressed later. These immunocytochemical and morphological observations are of importance for prenatal diagnosis of genetically determined diseases, e.g. epidermolysis bullosa. The basal lamina provides a physical supporting substrate and attachment for the developing epidermis, and is thought to be selectively permeable to macromolecules and soluble factors regulating epidermal–dermal morphogenetic interactions.

NEONATAL GROWTH

The surface area of the skin increases with growth. It has been estimated that the surface area of a premature neonate weighing 1505 g is c.1266 cm², whereas a neonate of 2980 g has a surface area of 2129 cm². The skin of the neonate is thinner than that of older infants and children. It cornifies over a period of 2–3 weeks which provides

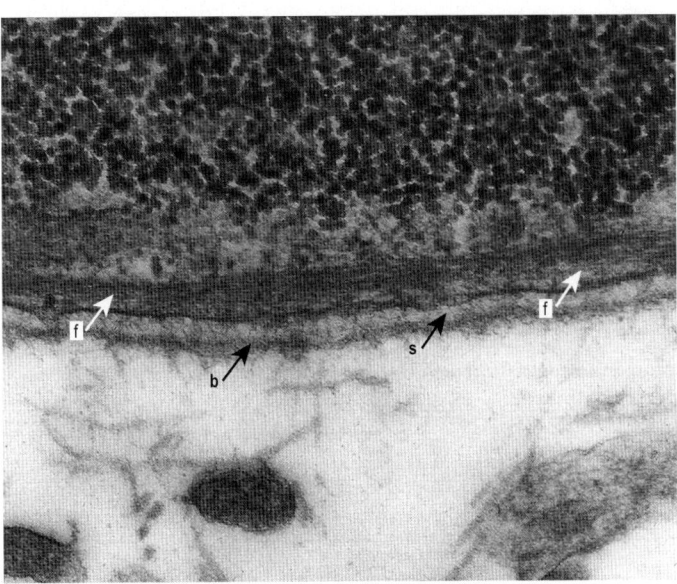

Fig. 8.23 Interface between basal germinative cells of the bilaminar epidermis and mesenchyme of arm skin of a 6-week embryo. Note basal lamina (b), reticulofilamentous material in lucid interval (s) between the plasma membrane and basal lamina, and skein of filaments (f) lying parallel to the plasma membrane which lacks hemidesmosomes at this stage. The cytoplasm of the cell is packed with densely staining glycogen granules. (From Breathnach AS 1981 Ultrastructural morphology of Langerhans cells of normal epidermis. In: Marks R, Christophers E (eds) The Epidermis in Disease. Lancaster: MTP Press.)

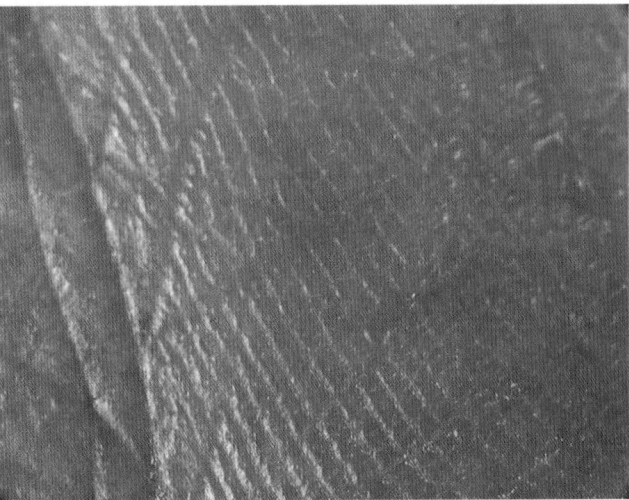

Fig. 8.24 The surface of hairless skin from the palm of the hand, showing epidermal friction (papillary) ridges and larger flexure lines (left).

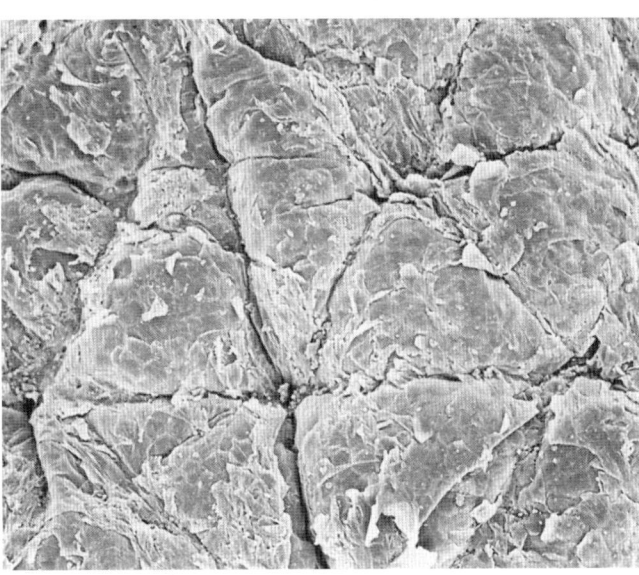

Fig. 8.25 Scanning electron micrograph of the surface of thin skin of the back, showing an interlacing network of fine creases and predominantly triangular areas between them.

protection; however, in the premature infant the thin epidermal layer allows absorption of a variety of substances, e.g. chlorhexidine and boric acid and also permits a significantly higher transepidermal water loss than occurs in full term neonates. At birth the skin is richly vascularized by a dense subepidermal plexus. The mature pattern of capillary loops and of the subpapillary venous plexus is not present at birth but develops as a result of capillary budding with migration of endothelia at some sites and the absorption of vessels from other sites. Some regions mature faster than others. With the exceptions of the palms, soles and nail beds, the skin of the neonate has almost no papillary loops. It has a disordered capillary network which becomes more orderly from the second week when papillary loops appear; defined loops are not present until the fourth or fifth week, and all areas possess loops by 14–17 weeks postnatally.

Neonates exhibit a regional sequence of eccrine gland maturation. The earliest sweating occurs on the forehead, followed by the chest, upper arm and, later, more caudal areas. Acceleration of maturation of the sweating response occurs in premature babies after delivery.

NATURAL SKIN CREASES AND WRINKLES

SKIN LINES

The surface of the skin and its deeper structures show various linear markings, seen as grooves, raised areas and preferred directions of stretching. Some of these are clearly evident in intact skin, others only appear after some sort of intervention.

Surface pattern lines, tension lines and skin creases (Figs 8.24, 8.25)

Externally visible skin lines are related to various patterns of epidermal creasing, ridge formation, scarring and pigmentation. A simple lattice pattern of creases occurs on all major areas of the body other than the thick skin of volar and plantar surfaces. The lattice pattern typically consists of polygons formed by relatively deep primary creases visible to the naked eye, which are irregularly divided by finer secondary creases into triangular areas. These, in turn, are further subdivided by tertiary creases limited to the cornified layer of the epidermis, and, finally, at the microscopic level, by quaternary lines which are simply the outlines of individual squames (**Fig. 8.7**). Apart from the quaternary lines, all the others increase the surface area of the skin, permit considerable stretching and recoil and distribute stresses more evenly. Details of the pattern vary according to the region of the body; e.g. on the cheek the primary creases radiate from the hair follicles, on the scalp they form hexagons, while on the calf and thigh they form parallelograms. There is a relationship between type of pattern and local skin extensibility.

Wrinkle lines

Wrinkle lines are caused by contraction of underlying muscles and are usually perpendicular to their axis of shortening. On the face they are known as lines of expression, and with progressive loss of skin elasticity due to ageing, they become permanent. Occupational lines are creases produced by repeated muscular contractions associated with particular trades or skills. Contour lines are lines of division at junctions of body planes, e.g. the cheek with the nose, and lines of dependency are produced by the effect of gravity on loose skin or fatty tissue, e.g. the creases associated with the pendulous fold beneath the chin in older age.

Flexure (joint) lines

Flexure (joint) lines are major markings found in the vicinity of synovial joints, where the skin is attached strongly to the underlying deep fascia (**Fig. 8.24**). They are conspicuous on the flexor surfaces of the palms, soles, and digits, and in combination with associated skin

173

folds, they facilitate movement. The skin lines do not necessarily co-incide with the associated underlying joint line. For example, the flexure lines demarcating the extended fingers from the palm lie approximately half an inch distal to the metacarpophalangeal joints, the positions of which are more closely related to the distal palmar crease (heart-line of palmistry). The patterns of flexure lines on the palms and soles may vary and are to some extent genetically determined. In Down's syndrome, the distal and middle palmar creases tend to be united into a prominent single transverse crease, a sign which is of diagnostic importance.

Papillary ridges

Papillary ridges are confined to the palms and soles and the flexor surfaces of the digits, where they form narrow parallel or curved arrays separated by narrow furrows (**Figs 8.26, 8.27**). The apertures of sweat ducts open at regular intervals along the summit of each ridge. The epidermal ridges correspond to an underlying interlocking pattern of dermal papillae, an arrangement which helps to anchor the two components firmly together. The pattern of dermal papillae determines the early development of the epidermal ridges. This arrangement is stable throughout life, unique to the individual, and therefore significant as a means of identification. The ridge pattern can be affected by certain abnormalities of early development, including genetic disorders such as Down's syndrome, and skeletal malformations such as polydactyly. Absence of epidermal ridges is extremely rare. Functionally, epidermal ridges increase the gripping ability of hands and feet, preventing slipping. The great density of tactile nerve endings beneath them means that they are also important sensory structures.

The analysis of ridge patterns by studying prints of them (finger-prints) is known as dermatoglyphics and is of considerable forensic importance. Measurable parameters include the frequency of ridges in particular patterns and the disposition of tri-radii, which are junctional areas where three sets of parallel ridges meet. Fingerprint ridge patterns can be separated into three major types (**Fig. 8.26**), arches (5%), loops (70%), and whorls (25%). Arches have no tri-radii, one loop, and two or more whorls. Whorl finger patterns are more common on the right hand, and males generally have more whorls and fewer arches than females, in whom the ridges are relatively narrower. The frequency of individual patterns varies with particular fingers. Similar patterns are seen on the toes.

The precise positions, numbers and ridge-counts associated with the tri-radii have an inherited basis: in general the genetics are multi-factorial and highly complex. However, the total ridge-count of all 10 digits of the hand appears to have a simpler inheritance.

If the mechanical demands placed on the skin are greater than the skin creases and the dermis can accommodate, the lateral cohesion of dermal collagen fibres is disrupted, and there is associated haemorrhage and cellular reaction, and eventually, formation of poorly vascularized scar tissue. These changes can be termed intrinsic, to distinguish them from scars formed by external wounding. Sites of dermal rupture are visible externally as lines or striae. They are initially pink in colour, later widen and become a vivid purple or red (striae rubrae), and eventually fade, becoming paler than the surrounding intact skin (striae albae). They develop on the anterior abdominal wall of some women in pregnancy when they are termed striae gravidarum (stretch marks).

Variation in pigmentation can also produce externally visible lines on the surface of the skin. Voigt lines mark differences in pigmentation between the darker extensor and paler flexor surfaces of the arms, and occur along the anterior axial lines, extending from the sternum to the wrist. They are more common in darker-skinned races.

Lines detectable after manipulation or incision

In certain regions of the body, surgical wounds heal with a better and less conspicuous scar if they are lying in a particular direction. This finding is related to a number of factors including skin tension and naturally formed wrinkle lines. Skin is normally under tension and the direction in which this is greatest varies regionally. Tension is dependent on the protrusion of underlying structures, the direction of underlying muscles, and on joint movements. Many anatomists and surgeons have therefore attempted to produce a body map to indicate the best direction in which to make an elective incision to obtain the most aesthetic scar. These maps frequently differ, especially in the region of the face (p. 498).

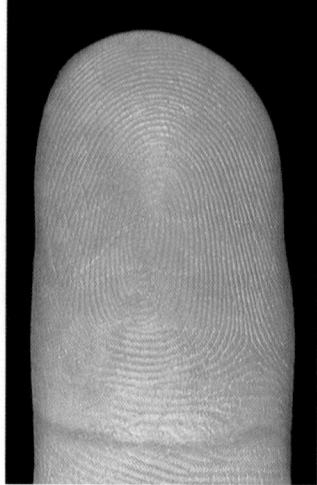

Fig. 8.26 The palmar aspect of a terminal phalanx to show fingerprint ridges. Note interphalangeal flexure lines.

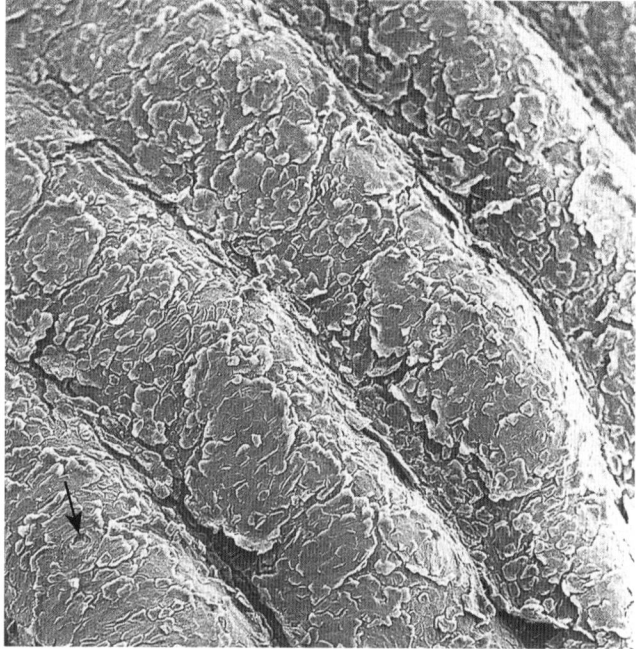

Fig. 8.27 Scanning electron micrograph of the surface of thick hairless skin from the volar surface of a human digit, showing friction ridges along which lines of sweat ducts open as pores (one pore is arrowed). (By kind permission from Lawrie Bannister and Caroline Wigley.)

Out of the multitude of described cleavage lines, the most commonly referred to are relaxed skin tension lines (RSTLs), Langer's lines, and Kraissl's lines (Borges 1984). Of these, the RSTLs and Kraissl's lines are probably more appropriate lines for surgical incision.

Relaxed skin tension lines – Relaxed skin tension lines (RSTLs) are those which correspond to the directional pull (which forms furrows) when the skin is relaxed: they do not always correspond to wrinkle lines. The tension across the RSTL is constant even during sleep but can be altered (increased, decreased or abolished) by underlying muscle contraction. The direction of the RSTLs can be determined by pinching the skin in different directions. Pinching at right angles to the RSTLs will result in fewer and higher furrows than pinching parallel to these lines.

Lines of Langer and Kraissl (See also Ch. 29) – Langer (1861) punctured the skin of cadavers with a circular awl and noted the subsequent elliptical-shaped openings. By connecting the long axis of these holes, he produced the cleavage lines named after him. These lines represent skin tension in rigor mortis but frequently do not relate to the lines of choice in making elective incisions. Indeed Langer's lines often run at right angles to the RSTLs in the face.

Kraissl's lines are essentially exaggerated wrinkle lines obtained by studying the loose skin of elderly faces whilst contracting the muscles of facial expression. These lines for the most part correspond to RSTLs, but slight variation exists on the face, especially on the lateral side of the nose, the lateral aspect of the orbit, and the chin.

Blaschko lines – Blaschko lines refer to the way in which patterns of naevi and related dermatological pathologies are distributed or develop along certain preferred cutaneous pathways. They do not appear to correspond to vascular or neural elements of the skin, and may be related to earlier developmental boundaries of a 'mosaic' nature.

AGE-RELATED SKIN CHANGES

Two main factors, chronological and environmental, are involved in skin ageing. Chronological changes are physiological or intrinsic in origin. A major environmental factor is chronic exposure to the sun, referred to as photoageing: emphasis is laid upon differences between the two because photoageing is to some extent preventable.

Intrinsic ageing

From about the third decade onwards there are gradual changes in the appearance and mechanical properties of the skin which reflect natural ageing processes. These become very marked in old age. Normal ageing is accompanied by epidermal and dermal atrophy, which result in some changes in the appearance, microstructure and function of the skin. Alterations include wrinkling, dryness, loss of elasticity, thinning and a tendency towards purpura on minor injury. Epidermal atrophy is expressed by general thinning and loss of the basal rete pegs with flattening of the dermo-epidermal junction, and this results in a reduction in contact area between the two which may affect epidermal nutrition. Flattening of the junction decreases resistance to shear, leading to poor adhesion of epidermis and its separation following minor injury. The thickness of the cornified layer is not reduced in old age, and its permeability characteristics seem little affected. Epidermal proliferative activity and rate of cell replacement decline with age, being reduced by up to 50% in elderly skin. Synthesis of vitamin D is also reduced. After middle age there is a 10–20% decline in the number of melanocytes, and Langerhans cells become sparser, which is associated with a reduction in immune responsiveness. Depigmentation and loss of hair, and some local increases (eyebrows, nose and ears in males, and face and upper lip in females) are commonly observed. Alterations in non-keratinocytes may be aggravated by chronic exposure to UV irradiation.

Dermal changes are mainly responsible for the appearance of aged skin, its stiffness, flaccidity and wrinkling, and loss of extensibility and elasticity. Its general thickness diminishes as a result of decline in collagen synthesis by a reduced population of fibroblasts, though the relative proportion of type III collagen increases. Senile elastosis is a degenerative condition of collagen which may be partly due to excessive exposure to sun. Vascularization of the skin is reduced, the capillary loops of the dermal papillae are particularly affected, and the tendency towards small spontaneous purpuric haemorrhages indicates a general fragility of the cutaneous microvasculature. A decrease in sensitivity of sensory perception associated with some loss of specialized receptors occurs.

Photoageing

Photoageing is a major concern because of an association with epidermal cancer. The effects of chronic sun exposure on melanocytes (stimulatory) and Langerhans cells (destructive) are thought to be connected with the increasing incidence of malignant melanoma in some groups of individuals, where reduction in tumour monitoring activity by Langerhans cells may be a factor.

DERMATOMES (Fig. 8.28)

The cutaneous area supplied by one spinal nerve, through both rami, is a dermatome. Typically, dermatomes extend round the body from the posterior to the anterior median line. The upper half of each zone is supplemented by the nerve above, the lower half by the nerve below.

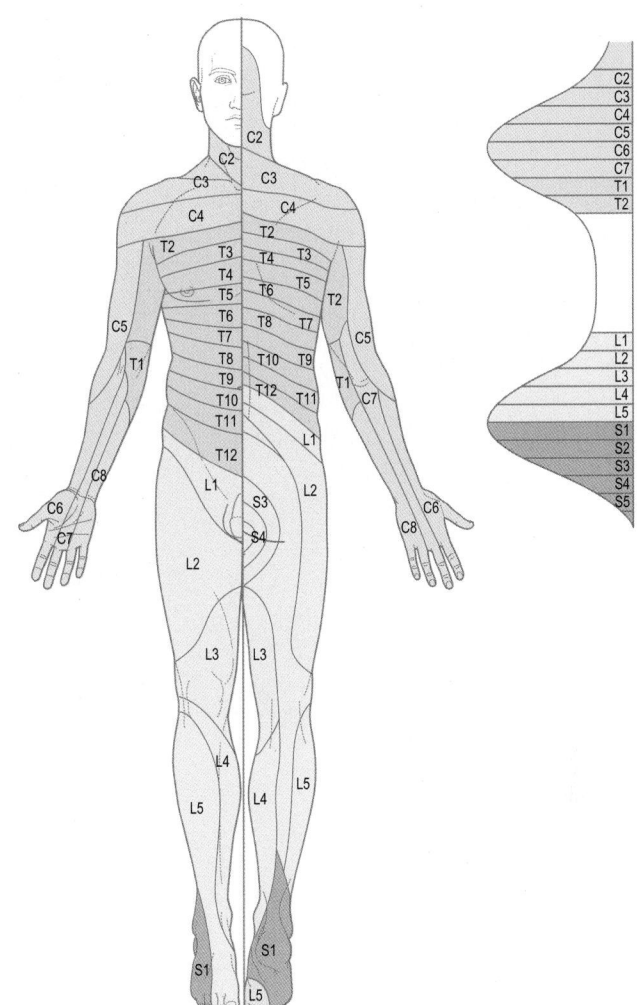

Fig. 8.28 Dermatomes. The small diagram shows the regular arrangement of dermatomes in the upper and lower limbs of the embryo. (By permission from Moffat DB 1993 Lecture Notes on Anatomy, 2nd edn. Oxford: Blackwell Scientific.)

The area supplied by dorsal rami is limited laterally by the dorsolateral line, which descends laterally from the occiput to the medial end of the acromion, continues to the posterior aspect of the greater trochanter and curves medially to the coccyx. Cutaneous strips supplied by dorsal rami do not correspond exactly to those served by ventral rami, and differ both in breadth and position. Dermatomes of adjacent spinal nerves overlap markedly, particularly in the segments least affected by development of the limbs, i.e. the second thoracic to the first lumbar. In some regions, e.g. the upper anterior thoracic wall, cutaneous nerves supplying adjoining areas are not from consecutive spinal nerves and the overlap is minimal. When the second thoracic spinal ramus is severed, anaesthesia is sharply demarcated but some overlap for awareness of painful and thermal stimuli may exist. Likewise, after section of a peripheral nerve (e.g. the ulnar nerve at the wrist) the area of tactile loss is always greater than that for pain and temperature sensation. Hence the area of total anaesthesia and analgesia following section of peripheral nerves is always less than might be anticipated from their anatomical distribution.

DERMAL REPAIR

Dermal repair is divisible into three overlapping phases, which are inflammation, proliferation and remodelling (**Fig. 8.29**).

INFLAMMATION

Acute inflammation begins with the activation of platelets and mast cells as an immediate response to injury. During inflammation, haemostasis is achieved, removal of damaged tissue occurs and factors which start the

175

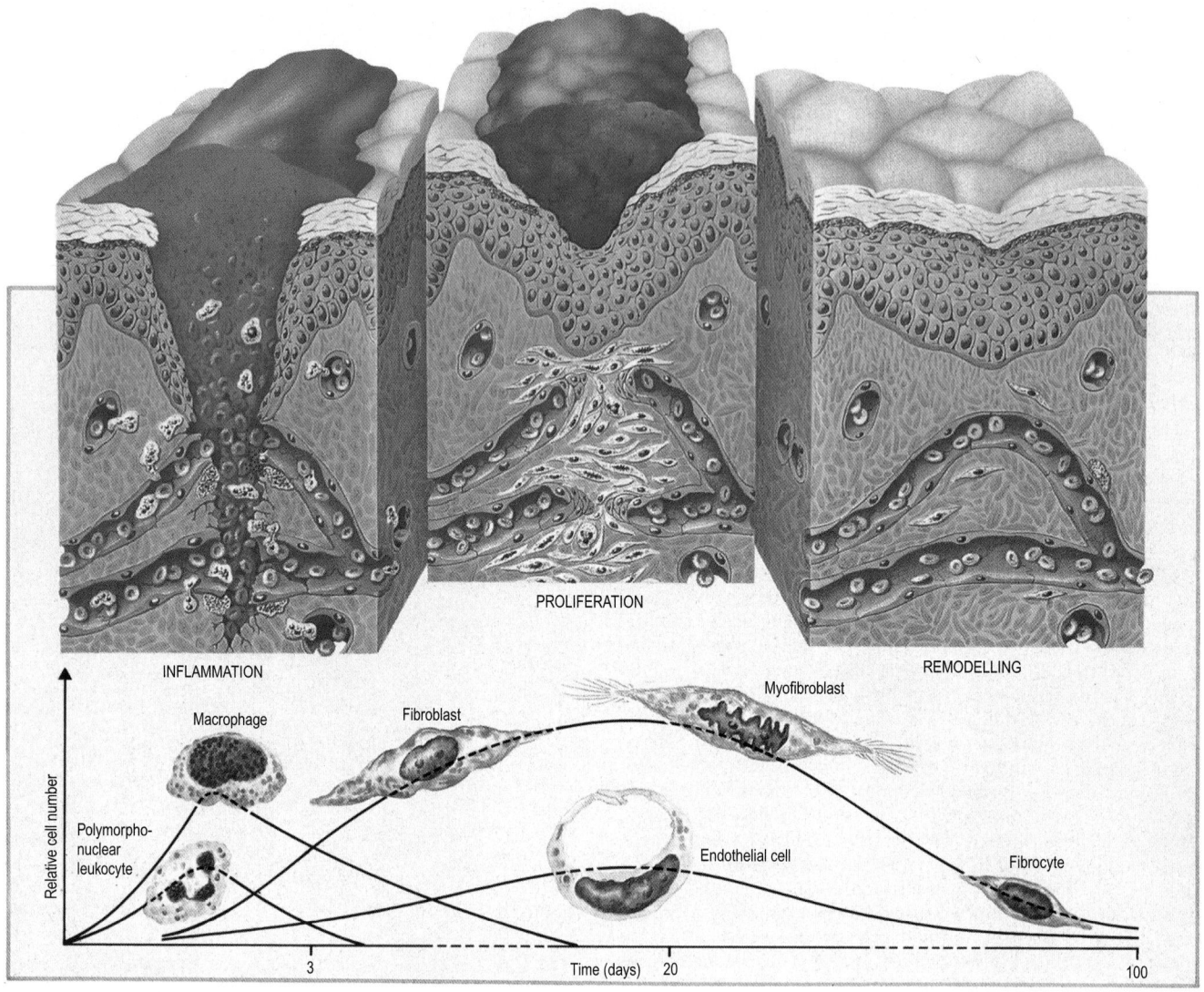

Fig. 8.29 The normal response of skin to incision, showing the changes in relative numbers of different cell types during inflammation, proliferation and remodelling.

formation of granulation tissue are released or deposited in the wound. Neutrophils infiltrate the wound and phagocytose pathogenic bacteria. When this has been achieved, neutrophil infiltration stops and the early inflammatory phase of repair is at an end. In contrast, monocytes, which develop into macrophages on entering the wound bed, remain throughout the entire inflammatory phase. Macrophages are not only phagocytic but also release a host of biologically active materials, including growth factors essential for the initiation and propagation of granulation tissue during the next, proliferative, phase of repair.

PROLIFERATION

During this stage, cells and intercellular substances increase greatly to form granulation tissue. This is a highly vascular tissue consisting largely of macrophages, pluripotent pericytes, fibroblasts and endothelial cells lining capillaries, all embedded in a matrix of fibronectin, proteoglycans rich in hyaluronic acid, and collagen, which at first is mainly type III, changing later to type I. The profuse assemblies of capillaries, which are the main type of blood vessel, give this tissue its 'granular' appearance when incised, hence its name.

Granulation tissue forms a nutritive substrate over which the regenerating epidermis can migrate and is gradually replaced by scar tissue. Macrophages, fibroblasts and blood capillaries migrate into the wound bed as a mutually dependent unit termed a wound module. In the lead are activated macrophages, followed in sequence by newly differentiated fibroblasts, dividing fibroblasts and capillaries. The macro-

phages release chemotactic agents which attract pericytes, fibroblasts and endothelial cells into the wound. As the fibroblasts mature they produce a matrix through which other cells can readily migrate and from which delicate new capillaries can obtain mechanical support. As each capillary loop becomes functional it brings nutrients and oxygen to nearby cells, enabling the fibroblasts to secrete materials for the matrix, through which macrophages and other cells can migrate further. These proliferative and migratory processes are repeated sequentially until the wound bed is filled with granulation tissue.

During the proliferative phase of repair, fibroblasts of the granulation tissue develop into myofibroblasts which are responsible for wound contraction, the centripetal movement of the wound margin, and the consequent reduction of the size of the wound. Myofibroblasts are similar to smooth muscle cells, contain peripherally located micro-filaments and become linked together by intercellular contacts.

Angiogenesis – Angiogenesis is a vital part of the proliferative phrase of dermal repair. Without it invasion of the wound bed by macrophages and fibroblasts would cease through lack of oxygen and nutrients. *In vitro* studies have shown that capillary endothelial cells release collagenase in response to angiogenic factors. These degrade the collagen of the basal lamina which subsequently fragments, permitting migration of endothelial cells into the perivascular spaces, where they form buds which are augmented by the proliferation of cells within and near the parent vessel. During dermal repair these buds grow rapidly towards the free surface, where they branch at their tips and unite to form functional capillary loops. New buds then develop on these loops so that a superficial capillary plexus rapidly forms in the granulation tissue.

REMODELLING

Just as the proliferative overlaps the inflammatory phase, so remodelling overlaps proliferation. During remodelling the highly cellular, highly vascular, granulation tissue is gradually replaced by scar tissue which contains few cells or blood vessels. During the protracted process of remodelling, which may occupy months or even years, most of the fibronectin is removed from the matrix and there is a slow accumulation of large bundles of type I collagen fibres. The latter, as they form cross-links, increase the tensile strength of the scar tissue. When collagen first appears in the granulation tissue of the wound bed it forms randomly arranged fibrils, and these gradually develop into large irregular masses which lack fibrillar substructure. The absence of the characteristic pattern found in uninjured dermis may be associated with the decreased extensibility and tensile strength which are typical of scar tissue. During subsequent remodelling, the orientation of fibres becomes less random and the strength of the scar tissue increases. This change may be caused by the action of mechanical forces exerted on the scar during normal usage which produce orientation of the collagen fibrils in the scar tissue and improve its mechanical function, so that it more closely resembles uninjured dermis.

EPIDERMAL REGENERATION

One of the most important characteristics of the epidermis is its capacity to seal any breeches rapidly. Changes in the epidermis leading to re-epithelialization begin within a few hours of the formation of a cutaneous wound. They include the synthesis of new keratins, K6 and K16, in suprabasal cells; changes in cell adhesion molecules; and reorganization of the actin cytoskeleton at the wound edge. Intact keratinocytes at the free edge of the cut epidermis begin to migrate across the defect. Cells superficial to the basal layer at the edges of the wound elongate laterally and crawl over each other until they make contact with the wound bed. They then cease to move and begin to divide, producing a new supply of cells, some of which add to the thickness of the regenerating epidermis. Meanwhile other cells migrate over the first cells, reach the wound bed, where they divide and repeat the process in 'leap-frog' fashion until prevented from doing so by contact inhibition. Thus no single keratinocyte moves more than about four or five cell diameters (c.40 μm) from its original position during epidermal regeneration. Within 48 hours of injury the basal keratinocytes of the new epidermis begin to divide, generating more cells capable of migration. In shallow, partial thickness wounds of thin skin, each cut hair follicle also acts as a source of reparative epidermal stem cells to accelerate the wound healing process. Once the wound has closed, the suprabasal keratinocytes downregulate production of K6 and K16 and revert to synthesizing K1 and K10.

SKIN GRAFTS AND FLAPS

GRAFTS

A graft is a piece of tissue which has been detached from its blood supply and therefore needs to regain a blood supply from the bed in which it is placed in order to survive. This process involves an outgrowth of capillary buds from the bed which unite with the free cut edges of the capillaries on the undersurface of the graft, and an ingrowth of vessels from the bed into the graft substance. The graft can be composed of skin, fat, fascia or bone, either separately or together as a composite piece of tissue. Skin grafts are commonly used in plastic and reconstructive surgery and are either full thickness grafts or split thickness grafts. Full thickness grafts consist of the epidermis and the full thickness of the dermis. Split thickness grafts consist of the epidermis and a variable quantity of the dermis. They have different properties and so are used in different clinical situations: an essential difference is that the donor site following the harvest of a full thickness graft has no epidermal elements from which new skin can regenerate. These grafts therefore tend to be taken from sites of the body where the donor defect can be primarily closed. The donor site from split thickness grafting contains adnexal remnants such as pilosebaceous follicles and sweat glands, which have the propensity to divide and regenerate new epidermis and so resurface the donor defect. Split thickness grafts therefore tend to be harvested when large areas of skin are required for reconstruction as is the case for burn victims.

FLAPS

A flap is a piece of tissue which is surgically raised and transferred from one location in the body to another whilst maintaining its blood supply, which enters the base (pedicle) of the flap when it is transplanted. A graft, in contrast to a flap, has no such blood supply. Flaps are used surgically to reconstruct areas of the body where tissue is missing as a result of, for example, trauma or following resection of malignancies. They are named according to the type of tissue transferred, e.g. a fasciocutaneous flap contains skin and fascia, a musculocutaneous flap contains both muscle and the overlying skin, whereas a skin flap, fascial flap and muscle flap contain only the separate elements as their names imply. The blood supply to a skin flap can be randomly orientated, which limits the flap length to breadth proportions to no more than 2:1 (except on the face, where much longer flaps can be raised). Much longer skin flaps can be raised elsewhere if the blood supply to the flap is a direct cutaneous artery and vein: these are called axial pattern flaps.

A free flap (free tissue transfer) is a specific type of flap in which the tissue, whether skin, fascia, muscle, bone or a combination, is completely removed from its original location in the body along with a single identifiable artery and vein and transferred to a remote site. The blood vessels in the flap are anastomosed to vessels located in the new site using microsurgical techniques. This often allows for greater flexibility in performing reconstructive surgery.

REFERENCES

Borges AF 1984 Relaxed skin tension lines (RSTL) versus other skin lines. Plast Reconstr Surg 73: 144–50.
A mini-review of skin lines which also highlights the shortfalls in using some of these lines when planning elective skin incisions.

Byrne C, Hardman M and Nield K 2002 Covering the limb – formation of the integument. In: Lane EB, Tickle C (eds) Symposium issue: how to make a hand. J Anat 1: 113–24.
Current views on the differentiation of skin and its appendages during embryogenesis.

Holbrook KA, Odland GF 1980 Regional development of the human epidermis in the first trimester embryo and the second trimester fetus (ages related to the timing of amniocentesis and fetal biopsy). J Dermatol 4(3):161–8.

Irvine AD, McLean WHI 1999 Human keratin diseases: increasing spectrum of disease and subtlety of phenotype–genotype correlation. Br J Dermatol 140: 815–28.
Reviews the molecular basis of skin and other epithelial tissue disorders which are the result of abnormalities in keratin genes.

Montagna W, Kligman AM, Carlisle KS 1992 Atlas of Normal Human Skin. New York: Springer-Verlag.

Niemann C, Watt FM 2002 Designer skin: lineage commitment in postnatal epidermis. Trends Cell Biol 12 (4): 185–92.
Summarizes current understanding of epidermal stem cell biology and commitment to alternative differentiation pathways.

Szeder V, Grim M, Halata Z, Sieber-Blum M 2003 Neural crest origin of mammalian Merkel cells. Dev Biol 253: 258–63.

Endocrine system: principles of hormone production and secretion

The activities of cells in the various tissue and organ systems of the body are tightly regulated by the coordinated activity of the autonomic and endocrine systems. Endocrine signals (hormones) reach cells in interstitial fluid, often via blood plasma, and together with autonomic nervous signals they ensure that the body responds to normal physiological stimuli and adjusts to changes in the external environment. In addition to the cells of specialized ductless endocrine glands (e.g. pituitary, pineal, thyroid and parathyroid), hormone-producing cells also form components of other organ systems. These include the cells of the pancreatic islets, specific thymic and renal cells, circumventricular organs, interstitial testicular (Leydig) cells, interstitial follicular and luteal ovarian cells and, in pregnancy, placental cells. Some cardiac myocytes, particularly in the walls of the atria, also have endocrine functions. The dispersed neuroendocrine system, particularly of the gut and lung, is an important part of the endocrine system. It consists of scattered cells in most parts of the body which have endocrine, paracrine or neurocrine signalling functions (p. 9).

Hormones function in cell–cell signalling (p. 9). Hormonal messenger molecules are released from an endocrine cell into its surrounding interstitial fluid and ultimately interact with target cells via their specific hormone receptors. According to classic definitions, hormones are secreted into interstitial fluid by cells within ductless glands and act on distant target cells, which they reach through the bloodstream. It is now recognized that some endocrine signalling molecules also act more locally and may reach their target cells by diffusion through interstitial fluid alone. This type of action is described as paracrine if the target cell type differs from the secretory cell, or autocrine if a signalling molecule acts on cells of the same type, including the secretory cell itself. Hormone receptors may be located at the target cell surface as integral plasma membrane molecules, or they may be intracellular, either cytoplasmic or nuclear.

HORMONES, SECRETORY REGULATION, FEEDBACK LOOPS AND ENDOCRINE AXES

A wide variety of molecular species function as hormones. Many are peptides, proteins or glycoproteins. They are synthesized in the rough endoplasmic reticulum and Golgi complex and stored, before release, within cytoplasmic secretory granules. Examples are insulin, growth hormone, the hypothalamic releasing hormones (which act on the adenohypophysis) and oxytocin and vasopressin (which are released by neurosecretion from nerve terminals in the neurohypophysis). Many cells of the dispersed neuroendocrine system secrete peptide hormones, e.g. gastrin is released in the stomach.

Some hormones are steroids, synthesized in the smooth endoplasmic reticulum and mitochondria. They include androgens, oestrogens and corticosteroids of the suprarenal cortex. Steroid hormones are nonpolar molecules derived from cholesterol, and are released by diffusion and carried in the bloodstream complexed to a binding protein. Steroid-secreting cells are often quite eosinophilic (**Fig. 9.1**), and typically contain lipid droplets, which are related metabolically to the pathways of steroid synthesis.

Yet other hormones are monoamines (amino-acid derivatives).They include the tyrosine-based catecholamines (adrenaline [epinephrine], noradrenaline [norepinephrine]), which are released by chromaffin cells of the suprarenal medulla (**Fig. 9.2**), and thyroid hormones, which are iodinated tyrosine derivatives complexed to the protein thyroglobulin for extracellular storage in thyroid follicles. The indoleamine, serotonin (5-hydroxytryptamine) and histamine are monoamines secreted by cells of the dispersed neuroendocrine system, e.g. serotonin-secreting cells in the lungs and histamine-secreting cells in the stomach. Like the catecholamines, these molecules are known primarily for their function

as neurotransmitters or neuromodulators in the nervous system. Details of hormone storage and release by different endocrine cells are included in the regional descriptions of their microstructure.

Hormone secretion is controlled in a number of ways, e.g. by neural control, regulatory feedback loops or according to various cyclical, rhythmical or pulsatile patterns of release. Endocrine glands have a rich vascular supply (**Fig. 9.3**). Their blood flow is controlled by autonomic vasomotor nerves, which can modify glandular activity. Capillaries or larger sinusoids, lined by an endothelium that is typically fenestrated

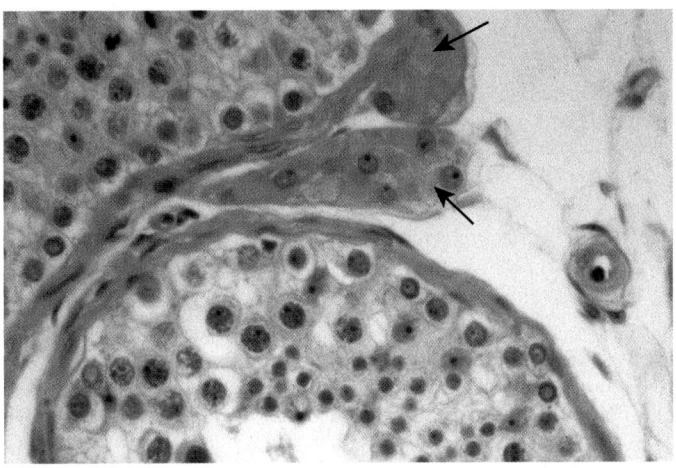

Fig. 9.1 Testosterone-secreting Leydig cells in the testis. These are the eosinophilic cells (arrows) with round nuclei, clustered in the interstitium between seminiferous tubules. A small blood vessel is seen to the right. (Photograph by Sarah-Jane Smith.)

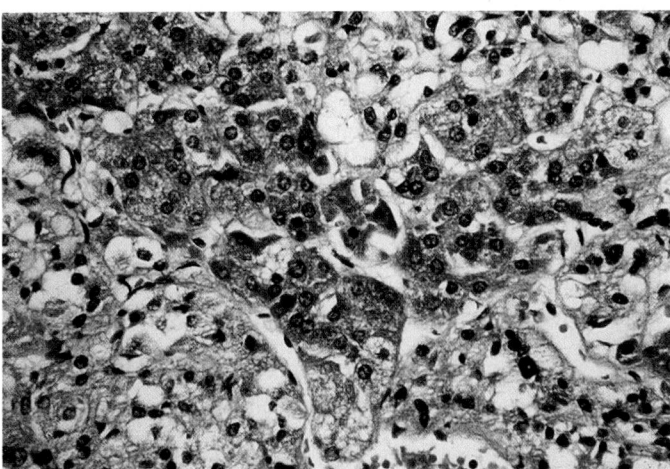

Fig. 9.2 Chromaffin cells in the suprarenal medulla, seen as clusters of large cells with rounded nuclei and greyish, vacuolated cytoplasm. Basal laminae and connective tissues of the medulla are stained green in this trichrome preparation. (Photograph by Sarah-Jane Smith.)

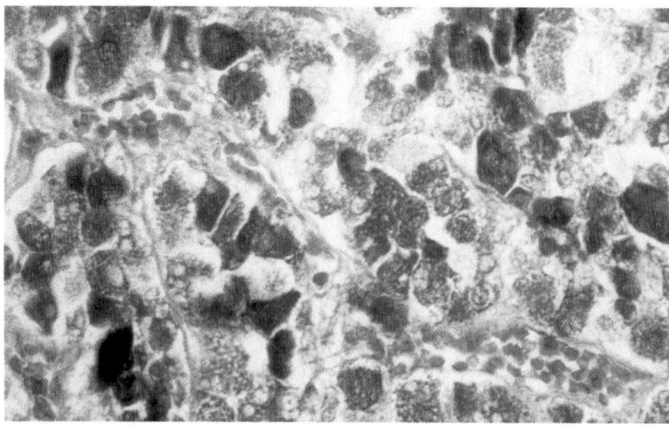

Fig. 9.3 Expanded sinusoids typical of endocrine glands, seen here containing erythrocytes (orange) in the adenohypophysis. Secretory endocrine cells are stained dark red (acidophils) or purple (basophils), or are poorly staining (chromophobes) in this trichrome-stained preparation. (Photograph by Sarah-Jane Smith.)

and thus highly permeable, surround clusters, cords or, in the thyroid gland, follicles, of secretory endocrine cells. Glandular cells can also be controlled directly or indirectly by autonomic secretomotor fibres, which may either form synapses at their bases (e.g. the suprarenal (adrenal) medulla), or release neuromediators in the vicinity of the cells and so reach them by diffusion. Neural control may act indirectly through an intermediary cell type, e.g. histamine released neurogenically from one cell type potentiates the functions of another (G cell, see below) in the gastric lining. Paracrine influences from neuroendocrine cells are important in the bronchial glands.

The consequences of hormonal stimulation alter some aspects of the metabolism of the target cell. Nuclear receptors change gene transcription and translation. Cell surface or cytoplasmic receptors activate cell functions more directly, often via cyclic AMP as the second messenger. The affected functions may include the synthesis and secretion of other hormones, or of proteins under endocrine control, e.g. casein in breast epithelium. Hormones may act in concert to produce their effect, each contributing synergistically to a process that neither alone can induce, e.g. spermatogenesis, which depends on both testosterone and follicle stimulating hormone. In many endocrine glands, regulatory hormones from the adenohypophysis stimulate synthesis and secretion in their target cells; these glands therefore respond to, in addition to generating, hormonal signals.

The hypothalamus and adenohypophysis are central to most regulatory feedback loops within the endocrine system. Loops can be either positive or negative, e.g. the hypothalamus stimulates release of follicle stimulating hormone by the adenohypophysis, which in turn stimulates ovarian follicular maturation and secretion of oestradiol, which acts on breast and endometrial target tissues. Oestradiol, in this case, also acts back on the adenohypophysis and hypothalamus to reinforce their function positively in a feedback loop. In contrast, hypothalamic and adenohypophyseal stimulation of testicular production of testosterone, which acts on targets such as skeletal muscle, are negatively regulated in a feedback loop generated by circulating testosterone.

Negative feedback regulation is a widely utilized mechanism. For instance, secretion of thyroid stimulating hormone (TSH, thyrotropin) by the adenohypophysis stimulates thyroid hormone synthesis and secretion, under the overall control of hypophyseal thyrotropin-releasing hormone and, indirectly, of neural input to hypothalamic centres. Thyroid hormone released into the circulation feeds back negatively on both adenohypophyseal and hypothalamic activity in a delicate balance of thyroid-controlled metabolic activity throughout the body.

The pituitary gland, in particular the adenohypophysis, is often termed the master gland, because of its central role in endocrine physiological processes. It provides the means by which the central nervous system regulates and integrates, by non-neural mechanisms, the widespread functions of the body. In particular, the thyroid, gonads and suprarenal cortex are pituitary-dependent endocrine glands: they are directly regulated by the hypothalamus and adenohypophysis in an integrated neuroendocrine network.

RELATIONSHIPS BETWEEN THE ENDOCRINE AND NERVOUS SYSTEMS

Although both the endocrine and nervous systems operate by intercellular communication, they differ in the mode, speed and degree or localization of the effects produced. The autonomic nervous system uses impulse conduction and neurotransmitter release to transmit information; the responses induced are rapid and localized. The dispersed neuroendocrine system uses only secretion. It is slower and the induced responses are less localized, because the secretions, e.g. neuromediators, can act either on contiguous cells, on groups of nearby cells reached by diffusion, or on distant cells via the bloodstream. Many of its effector molecules operate in both the nervous system and the neuroendocrine system. The endocrine system proper, which consists of clusters of cells and discrete, ductless, hormone-producing glands, is even slower and less localized, although its effects are specific and often prolonged. These regulatory systems overlap in function, and can be considered as a single neuroendocrine regulator of the metabolic activities and internal environment of the organism, acting to provide conditions in which it can function successfully.

Neural and neuroendocrine axes appear to cooperate to modulate some forms of immunological reaction: the extensive system of vessels, circulating hormones and nerve fibres that link the brain with all viscera has been termed the 'hard-wired neuroimmune network' (Downing & Miyan 2000).

DISPERSED NEUROENDOCRINE SYSTEM

Certain cells are able to take up and decarboxylate amine precursor compounds. They are characterized by dense-core granules in their cytoplasm, similar to the neurotransmitter vesicles seen in some types of neuronal terminal (p. 44). This group includes cells described as chromaffin cells (phaeochromocytes), which are derived from neuroectoderm and innervated by preganglionic sympathetic nerve fibres. Chromaffin cells synthesize and secrete catecholamines (dopamine, noradrenaline or adrenaline). Their name refers to the finding that their cytoplasmic store of catecholamines is sufficiently concentrated to give an intense yellow-brown colouration, the positive chromaffin reaction, when they are treated with aqueous solutions of chromium salts, particularly potassium dichromate. Classic chromaffin cells include: clusters of cells in the suprarenal medulla (**Fig. 9.2**); the para-aortic bodies, which secrete noradrenaline; paraganglia; certain cells in the carotid bodies; small groups of cells irregularly dispersed among the paravertebral sympathetic ganglia, splanchnic nerves and prevertebral autonomic plexuses. Distribution of the classic chromaffin tissues in newborn infants is shown in **Fig. 9.4**.

The alimentary tract, particularly the stomach, small intestine, bile and pancreatic ducts, contains numerous cells of a similar type in its wall (**Figs 9.5, 9.6**). (These cells were previously called enterochromaffin cells). The neonatal respiratory tract contains a prominent system of dispersed and aggregated (as neuroepithelial bodies) neuroendocrine cells, which decline in number during childhood. The glandular epithelium of the prostate gland includes numerous serotonin-rich neuroendocrine cells: like the cells in the lung, their numbers decline after middle age. Merkel cells in the basal epidermis of the skin can also be classed as neuroendocrine, since they store neuropeptides which they release to associated nerve endings in response to pressure.

Amine-storing cells are also present in the connective tissues of the gut, pancreas and liver, and in paraneurones. They share many features with chromaffin cells in sympathetic ganglia. It is therefore appropriate to consider all these cells as part of a dispersed neuroendocrine system. Other descriptions and terms that were applied to cells of this system in the older literature include: clear cells (reflecting their poor staining properties in routine preparations); argentaffin cells (which reduce silver salts); argyrophil cells (which absorb silver); small intensely fluorescent cells; peptide-producing cells (particularly of the hypothalamus, hypophysis, pineal, parathyroid glands and placenta); Kulchitsky cells in the lungs. Many cells of the dispersed neuroendocrine system are derived embryologically from the neural crest. Some, in particular cells from the

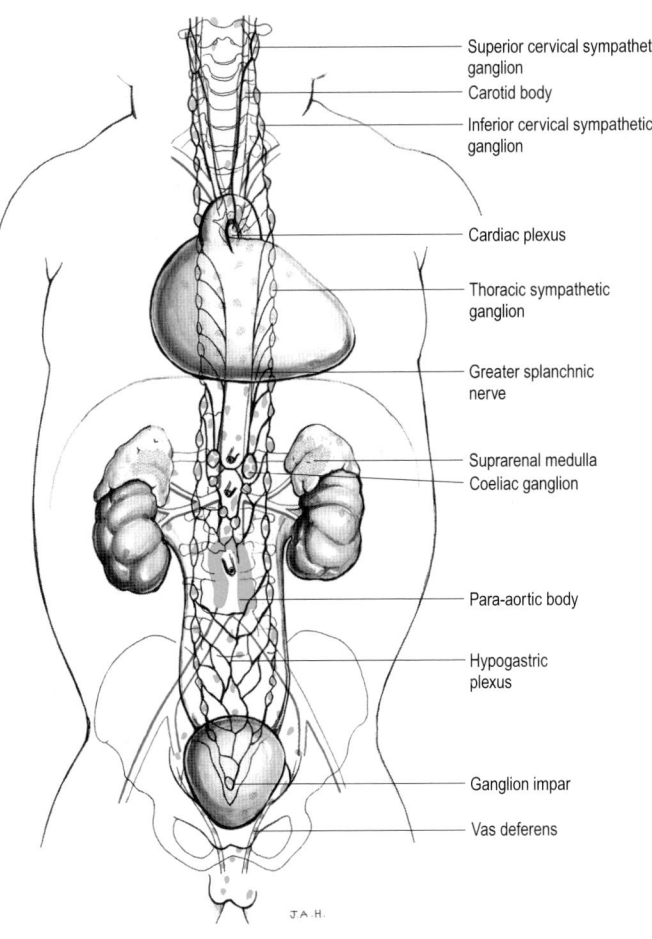

Fig. 9.4 The principal aggregations of 'classic' chromaffin tissue in the human neonate. The aggregates in stippled blue lie deep to overlying structures.

Labels on figure:
- Superior cervical sympathetic ganglion
- Carotid body
- Inferior cervical sympathetic ganglion
- Cardiac plexus
- Thoracic sympathetic ganglion
- Greater splanchnic nerve
- Suprarenal medulla
- Coeliac ganglion
- Para-aortic body
- Hypogastric plexus
- Ganglion impar
- Vas deferens

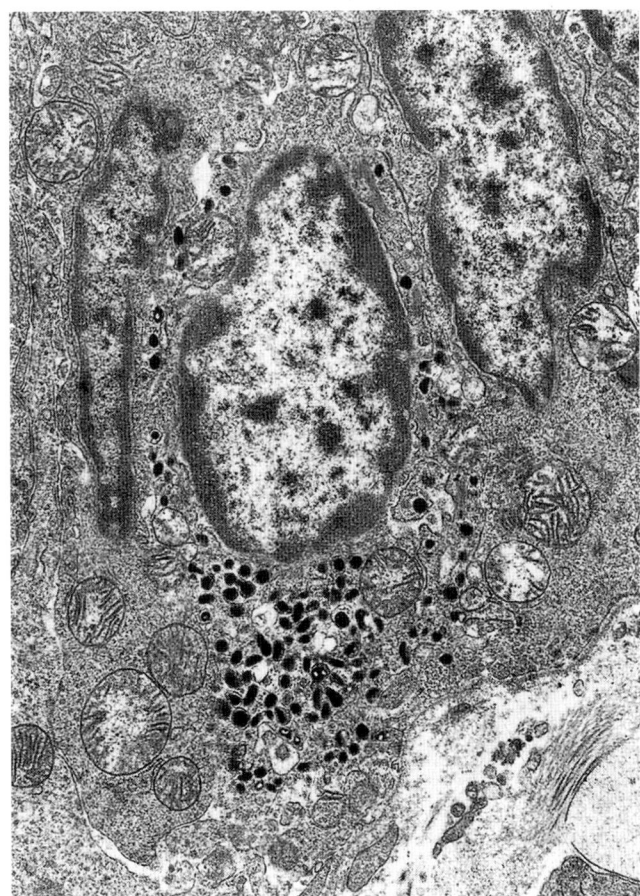

Fig. 9.5 A neuroendocrine cell of the epithelium lining the colon (rat). Secretory vesicles can be seen towards the basal aspect of the cell. Absorptive columnar cells lie on either side of the neuroendocrine cell. (By kind permission from Michael Crowder.)

alimentary system, are now known to be endodermal in origin, and Merkel cells in the skin are believed to be ectodermal. More than 40 different cell types have been included in the dispersed neuroendocrine system, including peptide-secreting myoendocrine cells of the heart, which are modified cardiac muscle cells.

Cells of the dispersed neuroendocrine system are also called paraneurones, forming a third division of the nervous system that supports, modifies or amplifies the actions of neurones in the autonomic and somatic divisions. Their effects are slower in onset and longer in duration than those of autonomic neurones, which have a similar functional relation to the faster somatic neurones. Secretions of the dispersed neuroendocrine system cells may act on immediately adjacent cells, on groups of cells locally, or on more distant cells via the blood. They may be considered to be intermediate between the short-range transmitters produced by neurones, and remote-acting endocrine secretions, so that the dispersed neuroendocrine system complements and coordinates the nervous and endocrine systems.

Neuroendocrine cells are scattered, generally within a mucosal epithelium. Their bases often rest on the basal lamina. In response to an external stimulus, they secrete their product basally into interstitial fluid. A typical neuroendocrine cell is shown in **Fig. 9.5**. The secretory granules vary in shape, size and ultrastructure in the different cell types, many of which take the name of their secretion (**Fig. 9.6B**). PP cells, common in the pancreatic islets, but rare in the exocrine pancreas, store pancreatic polypeptide in granules of 150–170 nm. G cells in the stomach synthesize gastrin, which stimulates acid secretion by parietal cells and is stored in large granules with floccular contents. D cells (an exception to the nomenclature) in the stomach and small intestine contain granules about 140–190 nm in diameter and store somatostatin, which inhibits gastrin release. S cells are scattered in duodenojejunal mucosa and produce secretin, which stimulates pancreatic bicarbonate and fluid secretion, reduces stomach acid secretion, and stimulates the release of

pepsinogen by chief cells. M cells release motilin under neural control, cyclically every 90 minutes during fasting, and this stimulates gastrointestinal motility. ECL (enterochromaffin-like) cells store histamine in granules with intensely argyrophilic cores. I (CCK) cells are most frequent in the duodenum and jejunum but rare in the ileum, and are sources of cholecystokinin, which stimulates contraction of the gallbladder in the presence of fat in the intestine. K cells in the duodenum and jejunum contain large (350 nm) granules and produce gastric inhibitory peptide, formerly called urogastrone. Gastric inhibitory peptide inhibits gastric secretion and stimulates the release of insulin when serum glucose concentrations are high. N cells have granules that are c.300 nm in diameter and contain neurotensin.

The numbers of the various neuroendocrine cells in the gastrointestinal mucosa generally decrease progressively in an anal direction (**Fig. 9.9B**). Their functions, some specific examples of which are given above, generally modulate neural control of gut motility and regulate gut secretions. In the lung, neuropeptides may be involved in lung development, but in adult life, when numbers of such cells are low, their principal action is on bronchiolar smooth muscle.

PARAGANGLIA

Paraganglia are extrasuprarenal aggregations of chromaffin tissue (**Fig. 9.4**), distributed near to or within the autonomic nervous system. Cells like those in paraganglia also occur in the sympathetic ganglia of various viscera and in a variety of retroperitoneal and mediastinal sites. All are derived from the neural crest, and their cells synthesize and store catecholamines. Their functions differ with location. Intraneural cells act as interneurones, the remainder as sources of neuroendocrine secretion. Paraganglionic catecholamine release occurs mainly in response to chemical rather than to neural stimuli, e.g. in the suprarenal medulla.

Extrasuprarenal chromaffin tissue is prominent in the fetus, where it is the main source of catecholamines while the suprarenal medulla is immature. Although many paraganglia degenerate soon after birth, others persist into adulthood, often as microscopic paraganglia.

Paraganglia are well-vascularized and their secretory cells are usually close to one or more fenestrated capillaries. Most, like the suprarenal medullary chromaffin cells, have a sympathetic innervation and act as endocrine organs. Some, like the carotid body, are associated with the parasympathetic system and their secretions probably have activities on local nerve endings. Paraganglia produce regulatory peptides, particularly enkephalins, and store them as cytoplasmic granules until stimulated to release them. Their secretions may exert a local paracrine action on nearby cells, in addition to having remote endocrine effects.

OTHER HORMONE-SECRETING TISSUES

There are cells within other tissues that secrete hormone-like products into interstitial fluid, and which do not fit readily into the categories described above. These include the renin-secreting cells of the kidney juxtaglomerular apparatus, which release renin in an endocrine manner to regulate, via the renin–angiotensin system, the volume of extracellular fluid. Erythropoietin-secreting cells, also in the kidney, function to regulate the oxygen-carrying capacity of the blood through their distant action on bone marrow erythropoiesis. Placental hormones (p. 1347) influence the uterine lining, the functioning of the ovarian corpus luteum, development of the breast and the onset of labour. Gonadal hormones, chiefly sex steroids, are secreted by specialized cells of the ovary and testis. These are all described within the appropriate regional sections.

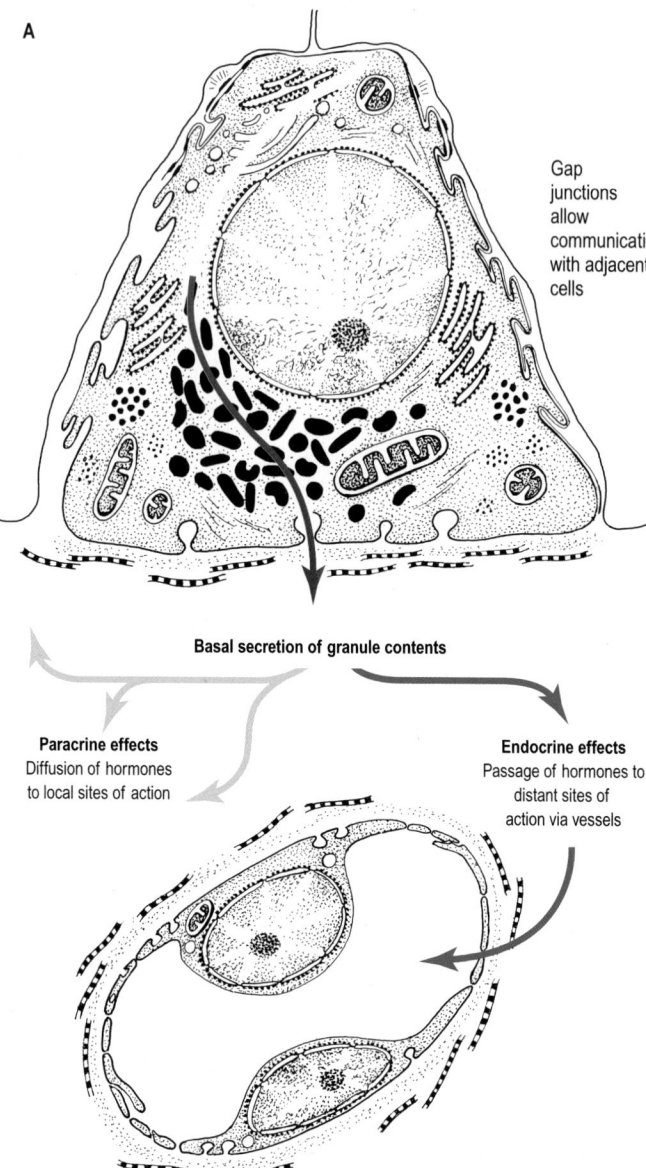

A

Gap junctions allow communication with adjacent cells

Basal secretion of granule contents

Paracrine effects
Diffusion of hormones to local sites of action

Endocrine effects
Passage of hormones to distant sites of action via vessels

Fig. 9.6 A, Ultrastructure and possible modes of action of a neuroendocrine cell. (After Bloom SR, Polack JM 1978 Gut hormone overview. In Bloom SR (ed) Gut hormones. Edinburgh: Churchill Livingstone.)

B

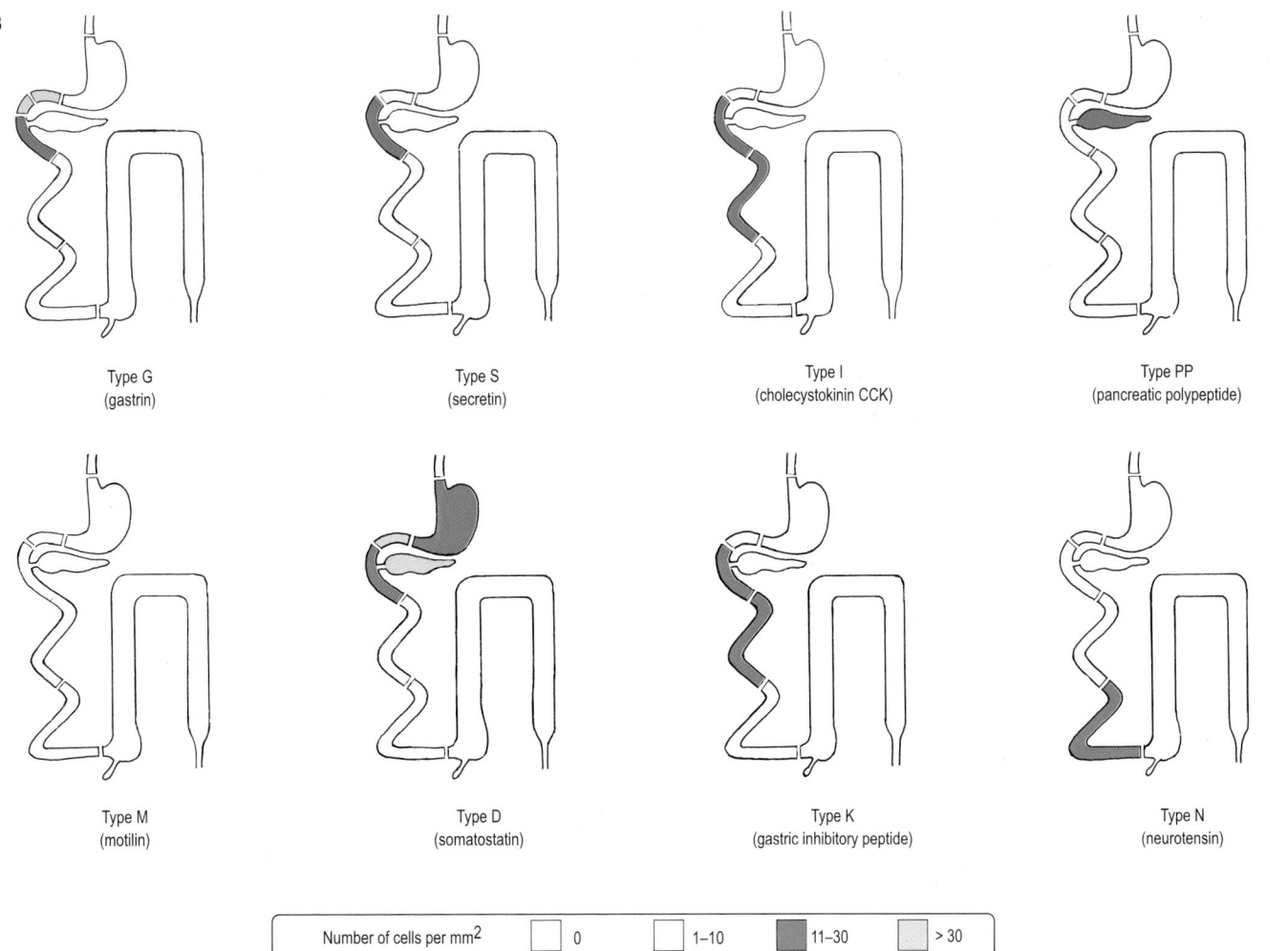

Type G
(gastrin)

Type S
(secretin)

Type I
(cholecystokinin CCK)

Type PP
(pancreatic polypeptide)

Type M
(motilin)

Type D
(somatostatin)

Type K
(gastric inhibitory peptide)

Type N
(neurotensin)

| Number of cells per mm^2 | 0 | 1–10 | 11–30 | > 30 |

Fig. 9.6 (*Cont'd*) **B**, Approximate quantitative distribution in the gastrointestinal tract of a selection of human neuroendocrine cells (highly diagrammatic). (After Bloom SR, Polak JM 1978 Gut hormone overview. In: Bloom SR (ed) Gut hormones. Edinburgh: Churchill Livingstone.)

REFERENCES

Downing JE, Miyan JA 2000 Neural immunoregulation: emerging roles for nerves in immune homeostasis and disease. Immunol Today 21: 281–9.
Reviews evidence for neural mechanisms that contribute to specific categories of host defence. Complements the established view of neuroendocrine–immune modulation.

Embryogenesis

Understanding the spatial and temporal developmental processes that take place within an embryo as it develops from a single cell into a recognizable human is the challenge of embryology. The control of these processes resides within the genome: fundamental questions remain concerning the genes and interactions involved in development.

FERTILIZATION

The central feature of reproduction is the fusion of the two gamete pronuclei at fertilization. In humans the male gametes are spermatozoa, which are produced from puberty onwards. Female gametes are released as secondary oocytes in the second meiotic metaphase, usually singly, in a cyclical fashion. The signal for the completion of the second meiotic division is fertilization, which stimulates the cell division cycle to resume, completing meiosis and extruding the second polar body (the second set of redundant meiotic chromosomes).

Fertilization normally occurs in the ampullary region of the uterine tube, probably within 24 hours of ovulation. Very few spermatozoa reach the ampulla to achieve fertilization. They must undergo capacitation, a process which is still incompletely understood, and which may involve modifications of membrane sterols or surface proteins. They traverse the cumulus oophorus and corona radiata, then bind to specific glycoprotein receptors on the zona pellucida, ZP3 and ZP2. Interaction of ZP3 with the sperm head induces the acrosome reaction, in which fusion of membranes on the sperm head releases enzymes, such as acrosin, which help to digest the zona around the sperm head, allowing the sperm to reach the perivitelline space. In the perivitelline space, the spermatozoon fuses with the oocyte microvilli, possibly via two disintegrin peptides in the sperm head and integrin in the oolemma (Figs 10.1, 10.2A).

Fusion of the sperm with the oolemma causes a weak membrane depolarization and leads to a calcium wave, which is triggered by the sperm at the site of fusion and crosses the egg within 5–20 seconds. The calcium wave amplifies the local signal at the site of sperm–oocyte interaction and distributes it throughout the oocyte cytoplasm. The increase in calcium concentration is the signal that causes the oocyte to resume cell division, initiating the completion of meiosis II and setting off the developmental programme that leads to embryogenesis. The pulses of intracellular calcium that occur every few minutes for the first few hours of development also trigger the fusion of cortical granules with the oolemma. The cortical secretory granules release an enzyme that hydrolyses the ZP3 receptor on the zona pellucida and so prevents other sperm from binding and undergoing the acrosome reaction, thus establishing the block to polyspermy. The same cortical granule secretion may also modify the vitelline layer and oolemma, making them less susceptible to sperm–oocyte fusion and providing a further level of polyspermy block.

The sperm head undergoes its protamine → histone transition as the second polar body is extruded. The two pronuclei grow, move together and condense in preparation for syngamy and cleavage after 24 hours (Fig. 10.2B). Nucleolar rRNA, and perhaps some mRNA, is synthesized in pronuclei. A succeeding series of cleavage divisions produces eight even-sized blastomeres at 2.5 days, when embryonic mRNA is transcribed.

Several examples of cells, ootids, which contain male and female pronuclei have been described. Pronuclear fusion as such does not occur; the two pronuclear envelopes disappear and the two chromosome groups move together to assume positions on the first cleavage spindle. Thus there is no true zygote stage containing a membrane-bound nucleus.

The presence of the pronuclei from both parental origins is crucial for spatial organization and the controlled growth of cells, tissues and organs. Embryos in which the paternal pronucleus has been removed and replaced with a second maternal pronucleus develop to a relatively advanced stage (25 somites), in the mouse, but with limited development of the trophoblast and extraembryonic tissues. In contrast, embryos in which the maternal pronucleus has been replaced by a second paternal pronucleus develop very poorly, forming embryos of only six to eight somites, but with extensive trophoblast. Thus it seems that the maternal genome is relatively more important for the development of the embryo, whereas the paternal genome is essential for the development of the extraembryonic tissues that would lead to placental formation.

This functional inequivalence of homologous parental chromosomes is called parental imprinting. The process of parental imprinting causes the expression of particular genes to be dependent on their parental origin, with some genes being expressed only from the maternally inherited chromosome and others from the paternally inherited chromosome. The genes involved are called imprinted genes. The requirement for both parental genomes is limited to a subset of the chromosomes. Uniparental disomy can arise through meiotic and mitotic non-disjunction events, and results in individuals who are completely disomic or who exhibit mosaicism of disomic and non-disomic cells. If imprinted genes reside on the affected chromosomes, then the uniparental disomic cells will either express a double dose of the gene or have both copies repressed. For example, the gene encoding the embryonal mitogen insulin-like growth factor II is expressed from the paternally inherited chromosome, and repressed when maternally inherited.

IN-VITRO FERTILIZATION

Fertilization of human gametes in vitro (IVF) is a successful way of overcoming most forms of infertility. Controlled stimulation of the ovaries (e.g. pituitary downregulation using gonadotrophin-releasing hormone superactive analogues, followed by stimulation with purified follicle stimulating hormone or urinary menopausal gonadotrophins) enables many preovulatory oocytes (often 10 or more) to be recruited and matured, and then aspirated either by laparoscopy or transvaginally using ultrasound guidance, 34–38 hours after injection of human chorionic gonadotrophin (which is given to mimic the luteinizing hormone surge). These oocytes are then incubated overnight with motile spermatozoa in a specially formulated culture medium, to achieve successful fertilization in vitro. In cases of severe male-factor infertility, in which there are insufficient normal spermatozoa to achieve fertilization in vitro, individual spermatozoa can be directly injected into the oocyte in a process known as intracytoplasmic injection of sperm, which is as successful as routine in-vitro fertilization. In cases in which there are no spermatozoa in the ejaculate, suitable material can sometimes be directly aspirated from the epididymis or surgically retrieved from the testes and the extracted sperm then used for intracytoplasmic injection of sperm. It is also now possible, in some cases, to test embryos for the presence of a particular genetic or chromosomal abnormality in a process known as preimplantation genetic diagnosis. A sample (biopsy) is removed from the oocyte polar body, the cleavage stage embryo (blastomere) or the blastocyst (small piece of trophectoderm), and subjected to a specific genetic test. Unaffected embryos can then be identified for transfer to the patient. Embryos that are surplus to immediate therapeutic requirements can also be cryopreserved in liquid nitrogen for later use. Propanediol or dimethylsulphoxide is used as a cryoprotectant for early stage embryos, and glycerol for blastocysts. Conception rates per cycle using ovarian stimulation, in-vitro fertilization and successive

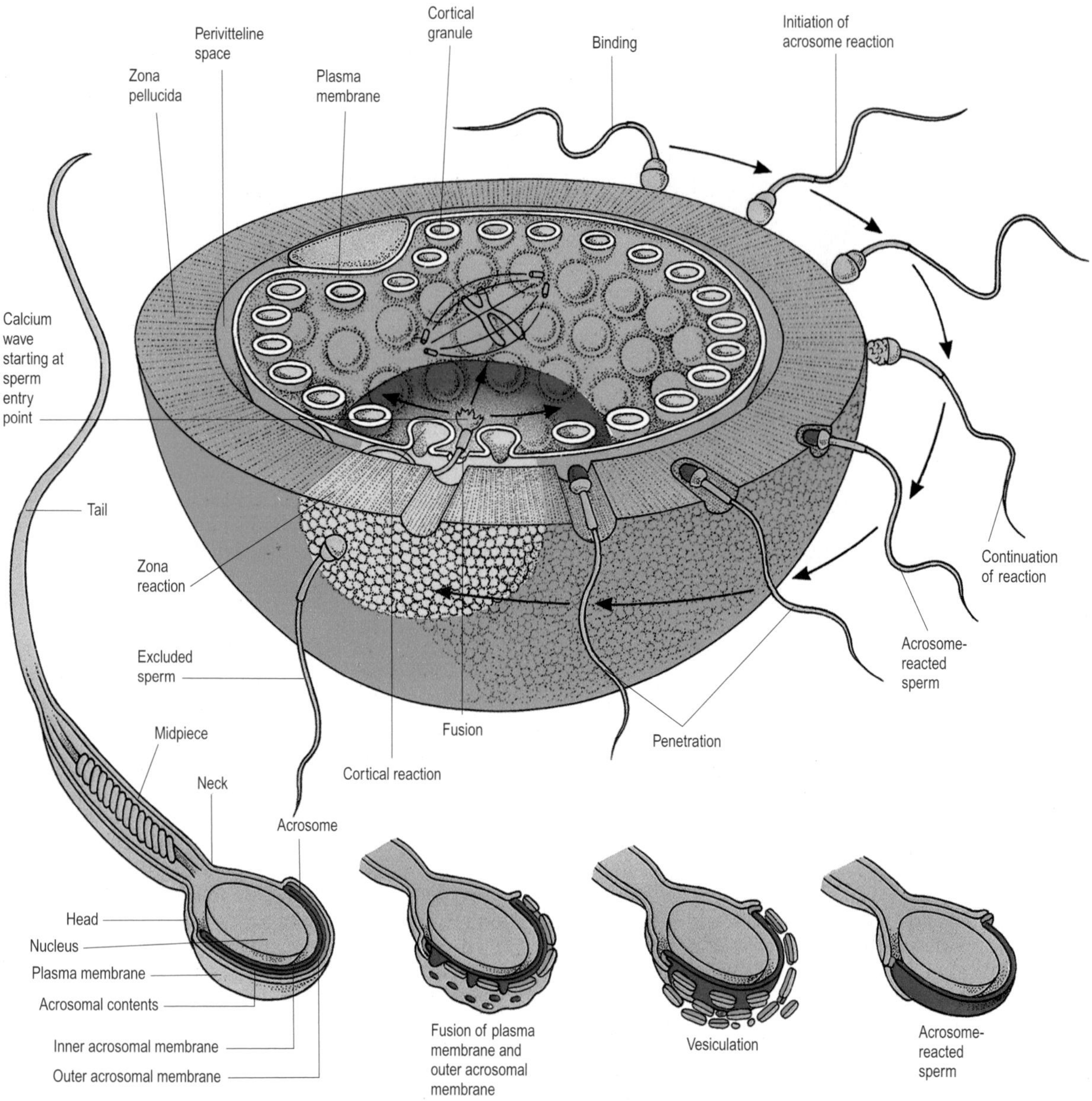

Cortical
granule

Perivitelline
space

Plasma
membrane

Binding

Initiation of
acrosome reaction

Zona
pellucida

Calcium
wave
starting at
sperm
entry
point

Tail

Zona
reaction

Continuation
of reaction

Excluded
sperm

Acrosome-
reacted
sperm

Midpiece

Fusion

Penetration

Neck

Cortical reaction

Acrosome

Head

Nucleus

Plasma membrane

Acrosomal contents

Inner acrosomal membrane

Outer acrosomal membrane

Fusion of plasma
membrane and
outer acrosomal
membrane

Vesiculation

Acrosome-
reacted
sperm

Fig. 10.1 Fertilization pathway: a succession of steps. After a sperm binds to the zona pellucida, the acrosome reaction takes place (see detail at bottom). The outer acrosomal membrane (blue), an enzyme-rich organelle in the anterior of the sperm head, fuses at many points with the plasma membrane surrounding the sperm head. Then those fused membranes form vesicles, which are eventually sloughed off from the head, exposing the acrosomal enzymes (red). The enzymes digest a path through the zona pellucida, enabling the sperm to advance. Eventually, the sperm meets and fuses with the plasma membrane of the egg, fertilizing the egg. Completion of the pathway triggers the cortical and zona reactions. First, enzyme-rich cortical granules in the cytoplasm of the egg release their contents (yellow) into the zona pellucida, starting at the point of fusion and progressing right and left. Next, in the zona reaction, the enzymes modify the zona pellucida, transforming it into an impenetrable barrier to sperm as a guard against polyspermy (multiple fertilization). (From Wassarman P 1988 Scientific American 259: 78–84, with permission from illustrator Neil O Hardy.)

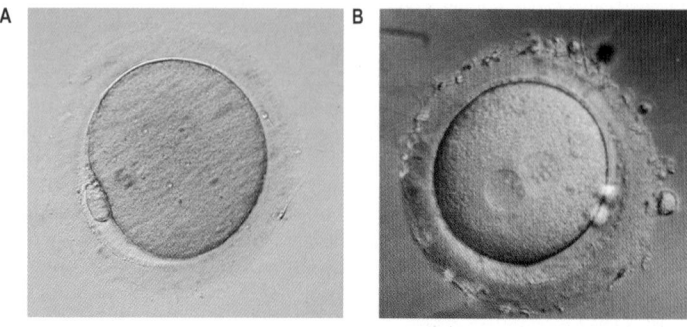

A B

Fig. 10.2 A, An unfertilized human secondary oocyte surrounded by the zona pellucida; the first polar body can be seen. Spermatozoa can be seen outside the zona pellucida. **B**, Fertilized human ootid before fusion of the pronuclei. Two polar bodies can be seen beneath the zona pellucida.

transfers of fresh and cryopreserved embryos, far outstrip those obtained during non-assisted conception.

PREIMPLANTATION DEVELOPMENT

CLEAVAGE

The first divisions of the zygote are termed cleavage. They distribute the cytoplasm approximately equally among daughter blastomeres, so although the cell number of the preimplantation embryo increases, its total mass actually decreases slightly (**Fig. 10.3**). The cell cycle is quite long, the first two cell cycles being around 24 hours each, thereafter reducing to 12–18 hours. Cell division is asynchronous and daughter cells may retain a cytoplasmic link through much of the immediately subsequent cell cycle via a midbody, as a result of the delayed completion of cytokinesis. No centrioles are present until the 16- to 32-cell stage, but amorphous pericentriolar material is present and serves to organize the mitotic spindles, which are characteristically more barrel- than spindle-shaped at these stages.

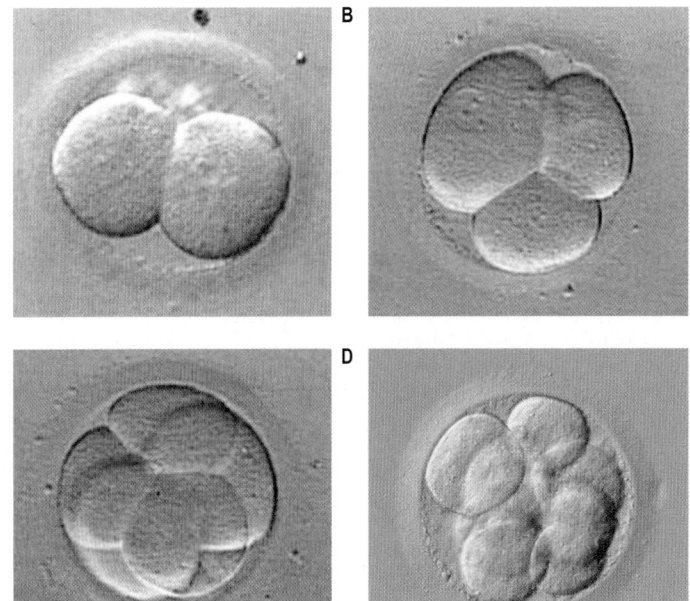

Fig. 10.3 Successive stages of cleavage of a human ootid. **A**, Two-cell stage; **B**, three-cell stage; **C**, five-cell stage; **D**, eight-cell stage.

All cleavage divisions after fertilization are dependent upon continuing protein synthesis. In contrast, passage through the earliest cycles, up to eight cells, is independent of mRNA synthesis. Thereafter, experimental inhibition of transcription blocks further division and development, indicating that activation of the embryonic genome is required. There is also direct evidence for the synthesis of embryonically encoded proteins at this stage. At the same time as the genes of the embryo first become both active and essential, the previously functional maternally derived mRNA is destroyed. However, protein made on these maternal templates does persist at least to the blastocyst stage. Spontaneous developmental arrest of embryo culture *in vitro* seems to occur during the cell cycle of gene activation, but it is not caused by total failure of that activation process. The early cleavage stages, up to around the eight-cell stage, require pyruvate or lactate as metabolic substrates, but thereafter more glucose is metabolized and may be required.

The earliest stage at which different types of cells can be identified within the cleaving embryo tends to be around the 8- to 16-cell stage. Up to the early eight-cell stage, cells are essentially spherical, touch each other loosely, and have no specialized intercellular junctions or significant extracellular matrix; the cytoplasm in each cell is organized in a radially symmetric manner around a centrally located nucleus. During the eight-cell stage, a process of compaction occurs. Cells flatten on each other to maximize intercellular contact, initiate the formation of gap and focal tight junctions, and radically reorganize their cytoplasmic conformation from a radially symmetric to a highly asymmetric phenotype. This latter process includes the migration of nuclei towards the centre of the embryo, the redistribution of surface microvilli and an underlying mesh of microfilaments and microtubules to the exposed surface, and the localization of endosomes beneath the apical cytoskeletal mesh. As a result of the process of compaction, the embryo forms a primitive protoepithelial cyst, which consists of eight polarized cells, in which the apices face outward and basolateral surfaces face internally. The focal tight junctions, which align to become increasingly linear, are localized to the boundary between the apical and basolateral surfaces. Gap junctions form between apposed basolateral surfaces and become functional.

The process of compaction involves the cell surface and calcium-dependent cell–cell adhesion glycoprotein, E-cadherin (also called L-CAM or uvomorulin). Neutralization of its function disturbs all three elements of compaction. The entire process can function in the absence of both mRNA and protein synthesis. Post-translational controls are sufficient and seem to involve regulation through protein phosphoryl-

ation. Significantly, although E-cadherin is not synthesized and present on the surface of cleaving blastomeres, it first becomes phosphorylated early during the eight-cell stage at the initiation of compaction.

The process of compaction is important for the generation of cell diversity in the early embryo. As each polarized cell divides, it retains significant elements of its polar organization, so that its daughter cells inherit cytocortical domains, the nature of which reflects their origin and organization in the parent eight-cell. Thus, if the axis of division is aligned approximately at right angles to the axis of cell polarity, the more superficially placed daughter cell inherits all the apical cytocortex and some of the basolateral cytocortex and is polar, whereas the more centrally placed cell inherits only basolateral cytocortex and is apolar. In contrast, if the axis of division is aligned approximately along the axis of the cell polarity, two polar daughter cells are formed. In this way, two-cell populations are formed in the 16-cell embryo that differ in phenotype (polar, apolar) and position (superficial, deep). The number of cells in each population in any one embryo will be determined by the ratio of divisions along, and at right angles to, the axis of eight-cell polarity. The theoretical and observed limits of the polar to apolar ratio are 16:0 and 8:8. The outer polar cells contribute largely to the trophectoderm, whereas the inner apolar cells contribute almost exclusively to the inner cell mass in most embryos.

In cleavage the generation of cell diversity, to either trophectoderm or inner cell mass, occurs in the 16-cell morula and precedes the formation of the blastocyst. During the 16-cell cycle, the outer polar cells continue to differentiate an epithelial phenotype, and display further aspects of polarity and intercellular adhesion typical of epithelial cells, while the inner apolar cells remain symmetrically organized. During the next cell division (16- to 32-cell stage), a proportion of polar cells again divide differentiatively as in the previous cycle, each yielding one polar and one apolar progeny, which enter the trophectoderm and inner cell mass lineages, respectively. Although differentiative division at this stage is less common than at the 8- to 16-cell transition, it has the important function of regulating an appropriate number of cells in the two tissues of the blastocyst. Thus, if differentiative divisions were relatively infrequent at the 8- to 16-cell transition, they will be more frequent at the 16- to 32-cell transition, and *vice versa*.

After division to the 32-cell stage, the outer polar cells complete their differentiation into a functional epithelium, and display structurally complete zonular tight junctions and begin to form desmosomes. The nascent trophectoderm engages in vectorial fluid transport in an apical to basal direction to generate a cavity that expands in size during the 32- to 64-cell cycles and converts the ball of cells, the morula, to a sphere, the blastocyst (**Fig. 10.4**). By the blastocyst stage, the diversification of the trophectoderm and inner cell mass lineages is complete, and trophectoderm differentiative divisions no longer occur. In the late blastocyst, the trophectoderm is referred to as the trophoblast. It can be

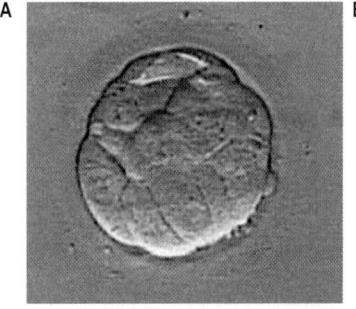

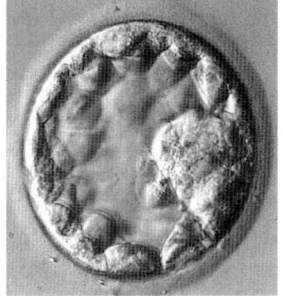

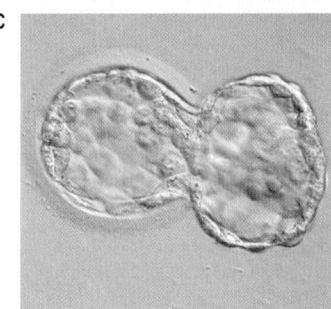

Fig. 10.4 Photographs of human embryos. Formation of a morula and blastocyst within the zona pellucida and blastocyst hatching from the zona pellucida. **A**, A ball of cells, the morula, with the cells undergoing compaction; **B**, the blastocyst cavity is developing and the inner cell mass can be seen on one side of the cavity; **C**, the blastocyst is beginning to hatch from the zona pellucida.

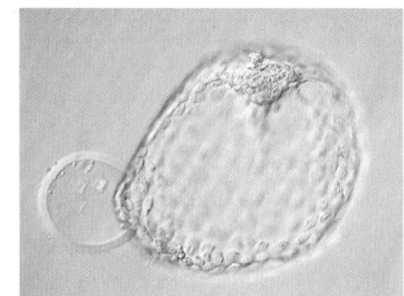

Fig. 10.5 Human blastocyst nearly completely hatched from the zona pellucida. The blastocyst can now expand to its full size.

divided into polar trophoblast, which lies in direct contact with the inner cell mass, and mural trophoblast, which surrounds the blastocyst cavity (**Fig. 10.5**).

STAGING OF EMBRYOS

For the purposes of embryological study, prenatal life is divided into an embryonic period and a fetal period. The embryonic period covers the first 8 weeks of development (weeks following ovulation and fertilization resulting in pregnancy). The ages of early human embryos have previously been estimated by comparing their development with that of monkey embryos of known postovulatory ages. Because embryos develop at different rates and attain different final weights and sizes, a classification of human embryos into 23 stages occurring during the first 8 weeks after ovulation was developed most successfully by Streeter (1942). The task was continued by O'Rahilly and Muller (1987). An embryo was initially staged by comparing its development with that of other embryos. On the basis of correlating particular maternal menstrual histories and the known developmental ages of monkey embryos, growth tables were constructed so that the size of an embryo (specifically, the greatest length) could be used to predict its presumed age in postovulatory days. Streeter believed such estimations could be ± 1 day for any given stage. Within this staging system, embryonic life commences with fertilization at stage 1; stage 2 encompasses embryos from two cells, through compaction and early segregation, to the appearance of the blastocoele. The developmental processes occurring during the first 10 stages of embryonic life are shown in **Fig. 10.12**.

Much of our knowledge of the early developmental processes is derived from experimental studies on amniote embryos, particularly the chick, mouse and rat. **Fig. 10.6** shows the comparative timescales of development of these species and human development up to stage 12. The size and age, in postovulatory days, of human development from stage 10 to stage 23 is given in **Fig. 10.7**.

Information on developmental age after that time is shown in **Fig. 11.3**, which juxtaposes the developmental staging used throughout this text alongside the obstetric estimation of gestation used clinically.

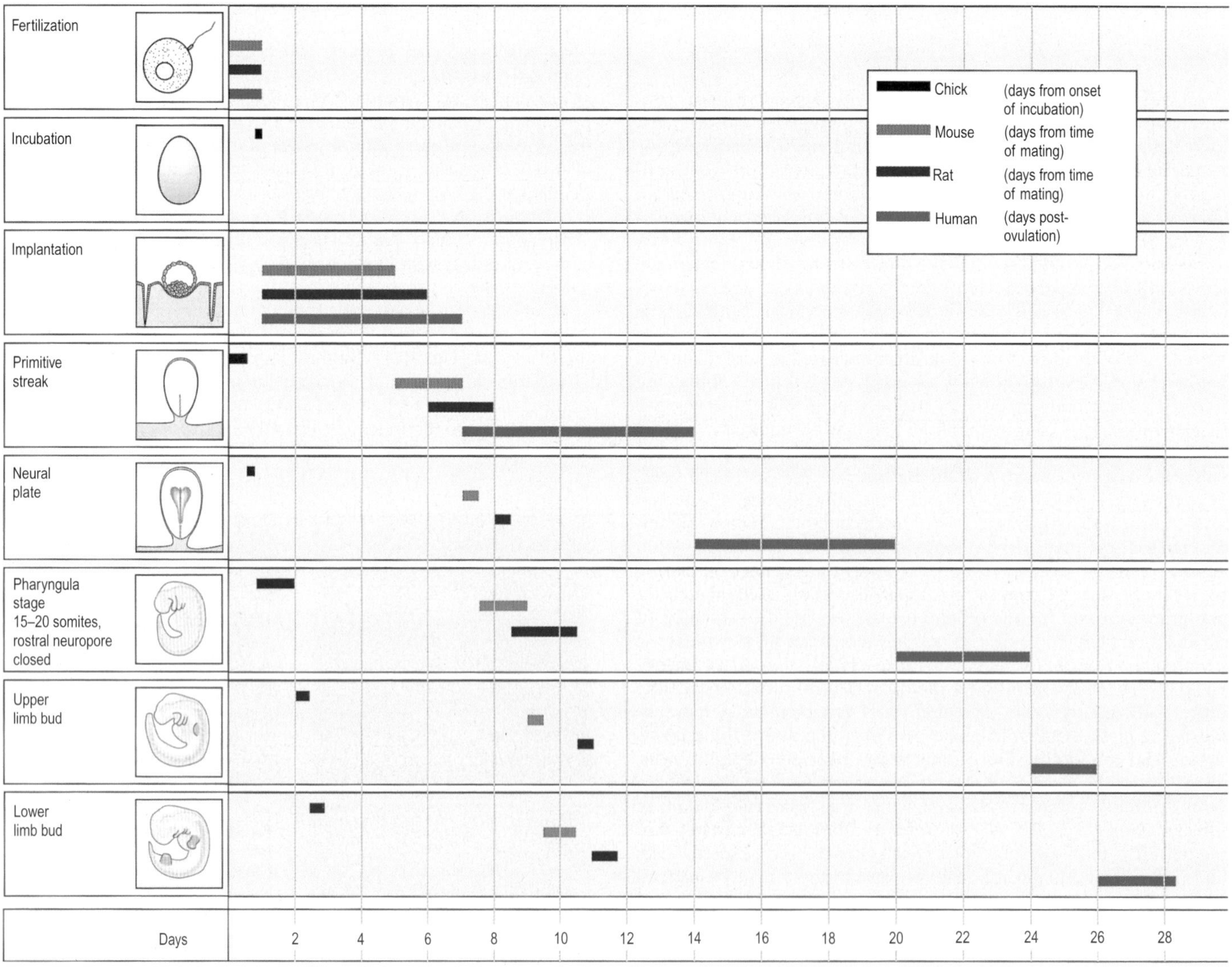

Fig. 10.6 Within developmental biology, evidence concerning the nature of developmental processes has come mainly from studies in vertebrate embryos, most commonly amniote embryos of the chick, mouse and rat. This chart illustrates the comparative timescale of development of these animals and the human.

A critique of staging terminology and the hazards of the concurrent use of gestational age and embryonic age is given in Chapter 11 (p. 216). Sizes and ages of fetuses towards the end of gestation are illustrated in **Fig. 11.4**.

THE BLASTOCYST

The blastocyst 'hatches' from its zona pellucida at 6–7 days, possibly assisted by an enzyme similar to trypsin (**Figs 10.4C, 10.5**). Trophoblast oozes out of a small slit; many embryos form a figure-of-eight shape, bisected by the zona pellucida, especially if it has been hardened during oocyte maturation and cleavage. Such half-hatching could result in the formation of identical twins. Hatched blastocysts expand and differentiation of the inner cell mass proceeds (**Fig. 10.5**).

The free, unattached blastocyst is assigned to stage 3 of development at approximately 4 days postovulation, whereas implantation (before villus development) occurs within a period of 7–12 days postovulation and over the next two stages of development. Even at this early stage, cells of the inner cell mass are already arranged into an upper layer (i.e. closest to the polar trophoblast), the epiblast, which will give rise to the embryonic cells, and a lower layer, the hypoblast, which has an extra-embryonic fate. Thus the dorsoventral axis of the developing embryo and a bilaminar arrangement of the inner cell mass is established at or before implantation. (The earliest primordial germ cells may also be defined at this stage.).

IMPLANTATION

On the sixth postovulatory day the blastocyst adheres to the uterine mucosa and the events leading to the specialized, intimate contact of trophoblast and endometrium commence. Implantation, which is the term used for this complicated process, includes the following stages: dissolution of the zona pellucida; orientation and adhesion of the blastocyst onto the endometrium; trophoblastic penetration into the endometrium; migration of the blastocyst into the endometrium; spread and proliferation of the trophoblast, which envelops and specifically disrupts and invades the maternal tissues.

The embryo is drawn into a tight association with the uterine epithelium; uterine fluid is withdrawn by progesterone-sensitive pinopods, and short-range forces enable embryos to adhere to epithelia. Trophoblast cells express L-selectin, whereas the maternal epithelium upregulates selectin oligosaccharide-based ligands.

The trophoblast from stages 4 and 5 onwards has two distinct cellular arrangements: the cytotrophoblast, cuboidal cells that form the mural and polar trophoblast and, externally, syncytial trophoblast (syncytiotrophoblast), a multinucleated mass of cytoplasm that forms initially in areas near the inner cell mass after apposition of the blastocyst to the uterine mucosa. Flanges of syncytial trophoblast penetrate the cell junctions of the uterine luminal epithelium (**Fig. 10.8**), without apparent damage to the maternal cell membranes or disruption of the intercellular junctions; instead, shared junctions are formed with many of the uterine epithelial cells. As the blastocyst burrows more deeply into the endometrium, syncytial trophoblast forms over the mural cytotrophoblast, but never achieves the thickness of the syncytial trophoblast over the embryonic pole (**Figs 10.9, 10.10**). Further details of placental development are given on page 1341.

The site of implantation is normally in the endometrium of the posterior wall of the uterus, nearer to the fundus than to the cervix, and may be in the median plane or to one or other side. Implantation may occur elsewhere in the uterus, or in an extrauterine or ectopic site. Implantation near the internal os results in the condition of placenta praevia, with its attendant risk of severe antepartum haemorrhage.

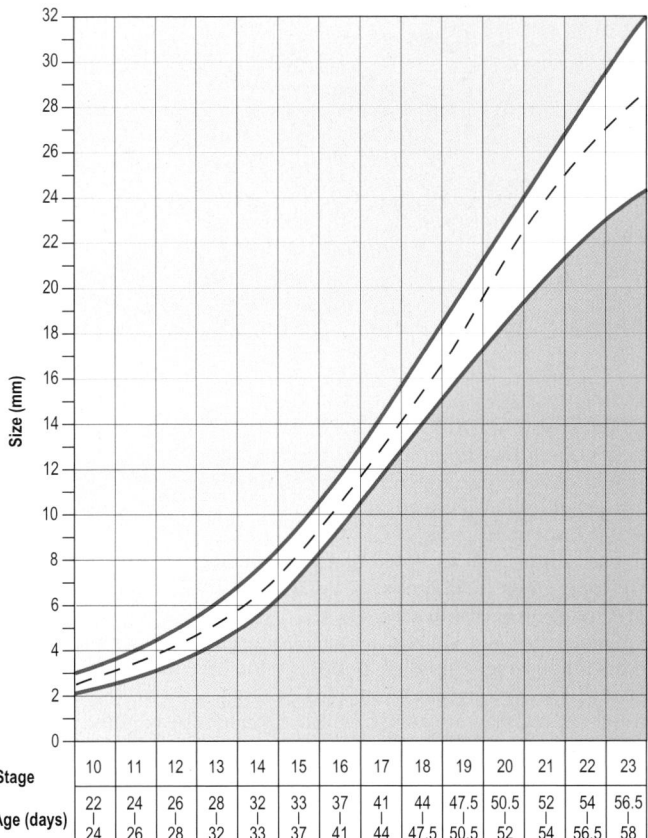

Fig. 10.7 Chart of human developmental stages 10–23.

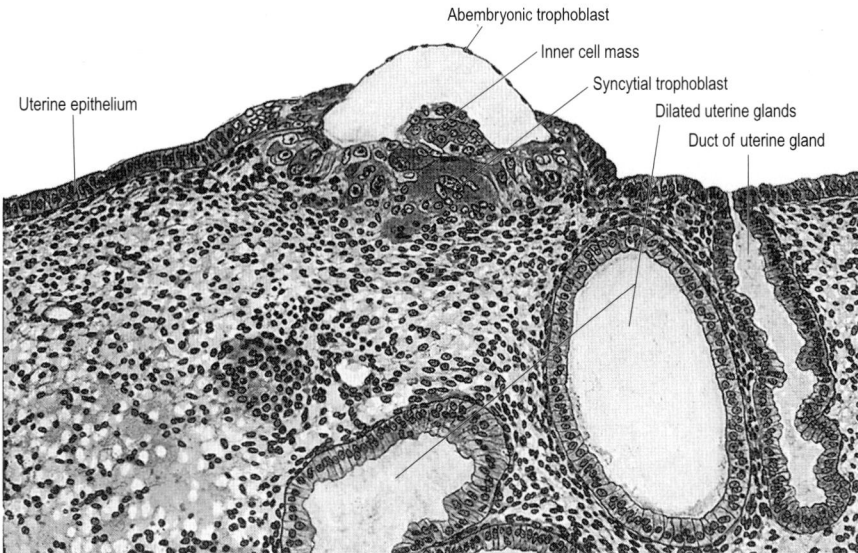

Fig. 10.8 A human blastocyst (Carnegie 8020) at stage 5a of development (7–7.5 days after ovulation) in the process of embedding in the uterine mucosa. In the actual specimen, the abembryonic trophoblast had collapsed on the inner cell mass but, for clarity, it has been shown projecting into the uterine cavity. (By permission from Rock J, Hertig AT 1942 Some aspects of early human development. Am J Obstet Gynecol 44: 973–983, and from Rock J, Hertig AT 1944 Information regarding time of human ovulation derived from study of 3 unfertilized and 11 unfertilized ova. Am J Obstet Gynecol 47: 343–356.)

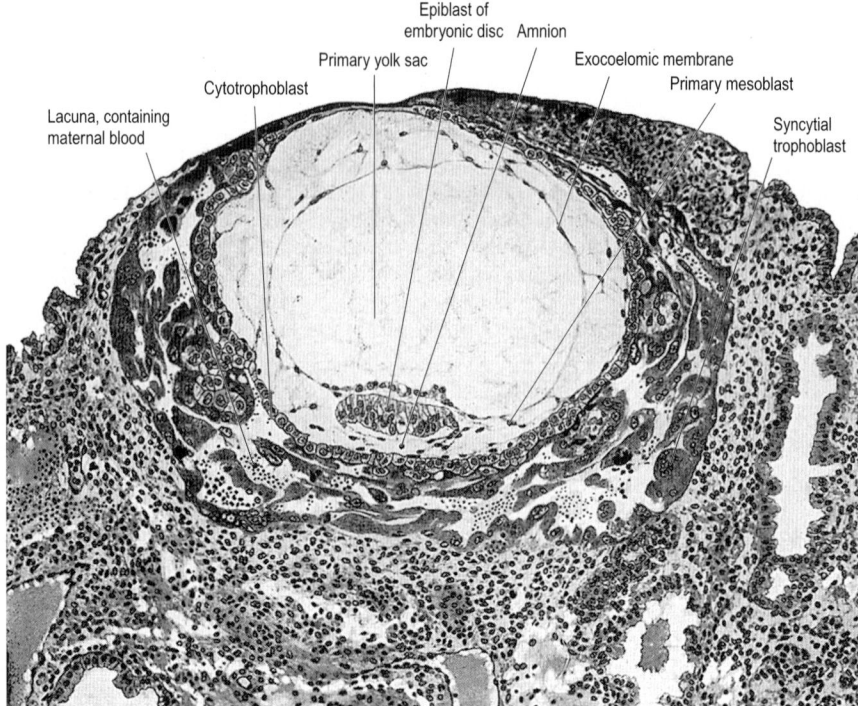

Epiblast of embryonic disc
Amnion
Primary yolk sac
Exocoelomic membrane
Cytotrophoblast
Primary mesoblast
Lacuna, containing maternal blood
Syncytial trophoblast

Fig. 10.9 A human conceptus (Carnegie 7700) at stage 5c of development (12–12.5 days postovulation), embedded in the stratum compactum of the endometrium. Compare with **Fig. 10.8**. Note lacunae in the syncytiotrophoblast, many containing maternal blood; also that the primary yolk sac, surrounded by the exocoelomic membrane, does not fill the blastocyst cavity. The epiblast cells are now columnar and, with the underlying hypoblast, constitute the early bilaminar embryonic disc. (By permission from Hertig AT, Rock J 1941 Two human ova of the pre-villous stage. Contrib Embryol Carnegie Inst Washington 29: 127–156. Drawn from a photomicrograph by AT Hertig.)

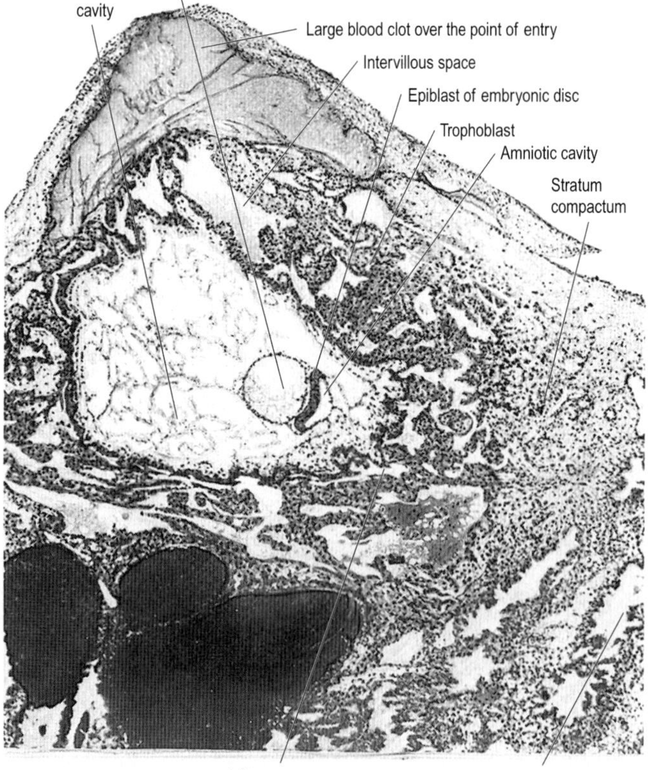

Strands of coagulum in chorionic cavity
Secondary yolk sac
Large blood clot over the point of entry
Intervillous space
Epiblast of embryonic disc
Trophoblast
Amniotic cavity
Stratum compactum
Villous stems
Uterine gland

Fig. 10.10 A human conceptus (Carnegie 7801) at stage 6 of development, embedded in the stratum compactum. (By permission from Rock J, Hertig AT 1942 Some aspects of early human development. Am J Obstet Gynecol 44: 973–983.)

ECTOPIC IMPLANTATION

The conceptus may be arrested at any point during its migration through the uterine tube and implant in its wall. Previous pelvic inflammation damages the tubal epithelium and may predispose to such delay in tubal transport. The presence of an intrauterine contraceptive device or the use of progesterone-based oral contraceptives may also predispose to ectopic pregnancy, probably because of alteration in the normal tubal transport mechanisms.

Nidation of the embryo as an ectopic pregancy most frequently occurs in the wider ampullary portion of the uterine tube, but may also occur in the narrow intramural part or even in the ovary itself. Most ectopic pregnancies are anembryonic, although the continuing growth of the trophoblast will produce a positive pregnancy test, and may cause rupture of the uterine tube and significant intraperitoneal haemorrhage. Ectopic pregnancies with a live embryo are the most dangerous, because they grow rapidly and may be detected only when they have eroded the uterine tube wall and surrounding blood vessels, as early as 8 weeks of pregnancy. Similarly, cornual ectopics (in the intramural part of the tube) may present with catastrophic haemorrhage, as there is a substantial blood supply in the surrounding muscularis.

Ovarian or abdominal pregnancies are exceptionally rare. Although some are presumed to have been caused by fertilization occurring in the vicinity of the ovary (primary), most are probably caused secondarily and result from an extrusion of the conceptus through the abdominal ostium of the tube.

Apart from their important clinical implications, these conditions emphasize the fact that the conceptus can implant successfully into tissues other than a normal progestational endometrium. Further, prolonged development can occur in such sites and is usually terminated by a mechanical or vascular accident and not by a fundamental nutritive or endocrine insufficiency or by an immune maternal response. Abdominal implantation may occur on any organ, e.g. bowel, liver, omentum. If such a pregnancy continues, this makes removal of the placenta at delivery or abortion hazardous as a result of haemorrhage, and consequently the placenta is usually left *in situ* to degenerate spontaneously.

TWINNING

Spontaneous twinning occurs once in about every 80 births. Monozygotic twins arise from a single ovum fertilized by a single sperm. At some stage up to the establishment of the axis of the embryonic area and the development of the primitive streak, the embryonic cells separate into two parts, each of which gives rise to a complete embryo. The process of hatching of the blastocyst from the zona pellucida may result in constriction of the emerging cells and separation into two discrete entities. There is a gradual decrease in the average thickness of the zona pellucida with increasing maternal age, which may be causally related to the increase in frequency of monozygotic twinning with increased maternal age. The resultant twins have the same genotype, but the description 'identical twins' is best avoided, as most monozygotic twins have differences in phenotypes. Late separation of twins from a single conceptus may result in conjoined twins; these may be equal, as in some varieties of so called 'Siamese twins', or unequal as in acardia. After twinning, monozygotic embryos enter a period of intense catch-up growth. Despite starting out at half the size, each twin embryo or fetus is of a size comparable to a singleton fetus in the second trimester of pregnancy, but declines in relative size in the last 10 weeks of pregnancy. The sex of monozygotic twins will be the same. Monoamniotic, monochorionic, monozygotic twins are most likely to be female, as are acardiac twins. The male:female ratio for all monozygotic twins is 0.487, and for monoamniotic, monochorionic it is 0.231.

The most frequent form of twinning is dizygotic. Dizygotic twins result from multiple ovulations, which can be induced by gonado-trophins or drugs commonly used in patients with infertility. Dizygotic twins may be different sexes; however, like-sex pairs are more common. The male:female ratio is 0.518. Multiple births greater than twinning, such as triplets or quadruplets, can arise from multiple ovulations, a single ovum, or both. It is most likely to be seen in women treated with drugs to stimulate ovulation.

The range of separation of twin embryos is reflected in the separation of the extraembryonic membranes. The types of placentation that can occur are shown in **Fig. 10.11**. Monoamniotic, monochorionic placentae are associated with the greatest perinatal mortality (50%), caused both by entanglement of the umbilical cords impeding the blood supply and by various vascular shunts between the placentae, which may divert blood from one fetus to the other. Artery–artery anastomoses are the most common, followed by artery–vein anastomoses. If the shunting of blood across the placentae from one twin to the other is balanced by more than one vascular connection, development may proceed unimpaired. However, if this is not the case, one twin may receive blood from the other, leading to cardiac enlargement, increased urination and hydramnios in the recipient, and anaemia, oligohydramnios and atrophy in the donor.

Dizygotic twins have either completely separate chorionic sacs or sacs that have fused. Such placentae are separated by four membranes, two amnia and two choria; in addition such placentae have a ridge of firmer tissue at the base of the dividing membranes, caused by the abutting of two expanding placental tissues against each other.

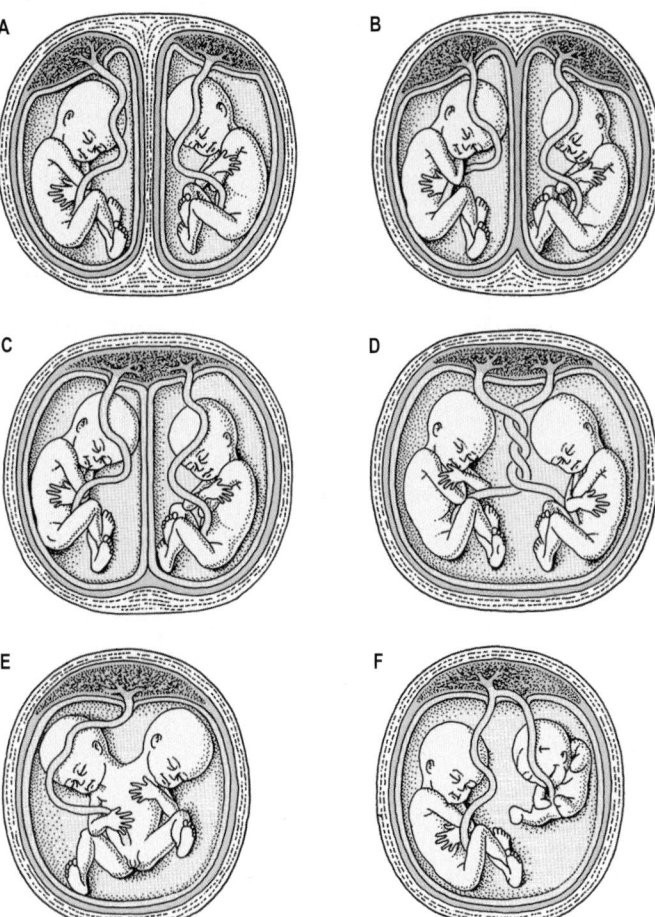

Fig. 10.11 Relationships of the extraembryonic membranes in different types of twinning. **A**, Diamnionic, dichorionic separated; i.e. separation of the first two blastomeres results in separate implantation sites. **B**, Diamnionic, dichorionic fused; here the chorionic membranes are fused, but the fetuses occupy separate choria. **C**, Diamnionic, monochorionic; reduplication of the inner cell mass can result in a single placenta and chorionic sacs, but separate amniotic cavities. **D**, Monoamnionic, monochorionic; duplication of the embryonic axis results in two embryos sharing a single placenta, chorion and amnion. **E**, Incomplete separation of the embryonic axis results in conjoined twins ('Siamese twins'). **F**, Unequal division of the embryonic axis or unequal division of the blood supply may result in an acardiac monster.

FORMATION OF EXTRAEMBRYONIC TISSUES

The earliest developmental processes in mammalian embryos involve the production of the extraembryonic structures, which will support and nourish the embryo during development. Production of these layers begins before implantation is complete. At present it is unclear where the extraembryonic cell lines arise. The trophoblast was considered to be a source, but evidence now points to the inner cell mass as the site of origin. **Fig. 10.12** shows the sequence of development of various tissues in the early embryo.

EPIBLAST AND AMNIOTIC CAVITY
Epiblast cells, which are closest to the implanting face of the trophoblast, have a definite polarity, being arranged in a radial manner with extensive junctions near the centre of the mass of cells, supported by supranuclear organelles. A few epiblast cells are contiguous with cytotrophoblast cells; however, apart from this contact a basal lamina surrounds what is now, initially, a spherical cluster of epiblast cells and isolates them from all other cells. Those epiblast cells adjacent to the hypoblast become taller and more columnar than those adjacent to the trophoblast; this causes the epiblast sphere to become flattened and the centre of the sphere to be shifted towards the polar trophoblast. Amniotic fluid accumulates at the eccentric centre of the now lenticular epiblast mass, which is bordered by apical junctional complexes and microvilli. As further fluid accumulates, an amniotic cavity forms, roofed by low cuboidal cells that possess irregular microvilli. The cells share short apical junctional complexes and associated desmosomes and rest on an underlying basal lamina. The demarcation between true

amnion cells and those of the remaining definitive epiblast is clear. The columnar epiblast cells are arranged as a pseudostratified layer with microvilli, frequently a single cilium, clefted nuclei and large nucleoli; the cells have a distinct, continuous basal lamina. Cell division in the epiblast tends to occur near the apical surface, causing this region to become more crowded than the basal region. At the margins of the embryonic disc, the amnion cells are contiguous with the epiblast; there is a gradation in cell size from columnar to low cuboidal within a two- to three-cell span (**Figs 10.9, 10.10**). Further development of the amnion and amniotic fluid is described on page 1340.

HYPOBLAST AND YOLK SAC
Hypoblast is the term used to delineate the lower layer of cells of the early bilaminar disc, most commonly in avian embryos. This layer is also termed anterior, or distal, visceral endoderm in the mouse embryo. Just before implantation, the hypoblast consists of a layer of squamous cells only slightly larger in extent than the epiblast. The cells exhibit polarity, with apical microvilli facing the cavity of the blastocyst and apical junctional complexes, but they lack a basal lamina. During early implantation, the hypoblast extends beyond the edges of the epiblast and can now be subdivided into those cells in contact with the epiblast basal lamina, the visceral hypoblast, and those cells in contact with the mural trophoblast, the parietal hypoblast. The parietal hypoblast cells are squamous, and may share adhesion junctions with the mural trophoblast and, rarely, gap junctions. The visceral hypoblast cells are

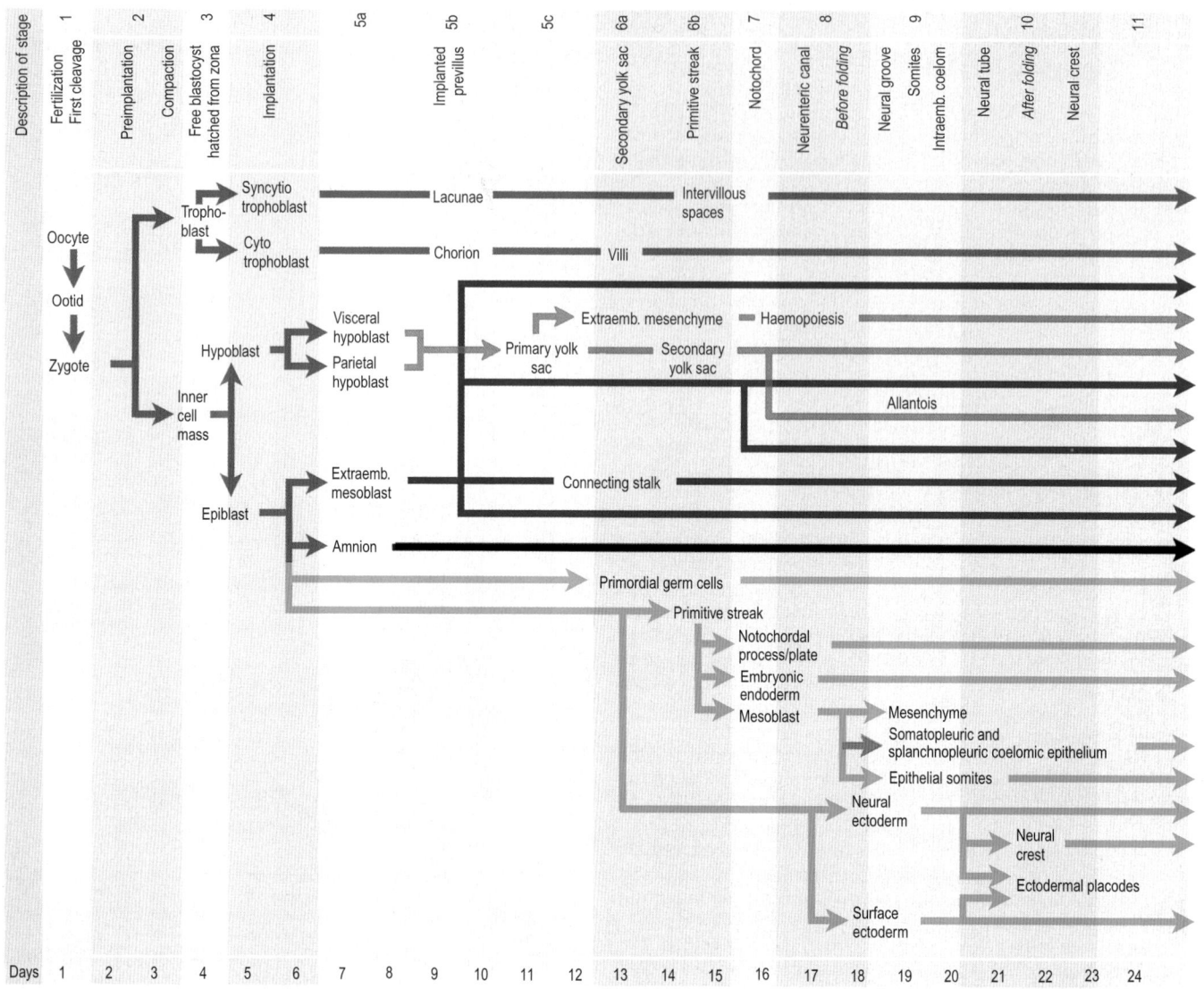

Fig. 10.12 Developmental processes occurring during the first 10 stages of development. In the early stages, a series of binary choices determine the cell lineages. Generally, the earliest stages are concerned with formation of the extraembryonic tissues, whereas the later stages see the formation of embryonic tissues.

cuboidal; they have a uniform apical surface towards the blastocyst cavity, but irregular basal and lateral regions, with flanges and projections underlying one another and extending into intercellular spaces. There is no basal lamina subjacent to the visceral hypoblast, and the distance between the hypoblast cells and the epiblast basal lamina is variable.

A series of modifications of the original blastocystic cavity develops beneath the hypoblast later than those developing above the epiblast. Whilst the amniotic cavity is enlarging within the sphere of epiblast cells, the parietal hypoblast cells are proliferating and spreading along the mural trophoblast until they extend most of the way around the circumference of the blastocyst, converging towards the abembryonic pole; at the same time, a space appears between the parietal hypoblast and the mural trophoblast limiting the circumference of the hypoblastic cavity. A variety of terms have been applied to the parietal hypoblast layer: extraembryonic hypoblast and later extraembryonic endoderm or the exocoelomic (Heuser's) membrane. The cavity that the layer initially surrounds is termed the primary yolk sac, or alternatively the primary umbilical vesicle. The resultant smaller cavity lined by hypoblast is termed the secondary yolk sac. It has been suggested to form in a variety of ways, including: cavitation of visceral hypoblast, a method similar to formation of the amnion; rearrangement of proliferating visceral hypoblast; folding of the parietal layer of the primary yolk sac into the secondary yolk sac. Further development of the yolk sac is described on page 1340.

The visceral hypoblast cells are now believed to be important in many aspects of early specification of cell lines. The cells induce the formation of the primitive streak, thus establishing the first axis of the embryonic disc. They are also believed to be necessary for successful induction of the head region and for the successful specification of the primordial germ cells. With the later formation of the embryonic cell layers from the epiblast, the visceral hypoblast appears to be sequestered into the secondary yolk sac wall by the expansion of the newly formed embryonic endoderm beneath the epiblast. Hypoblastic cells remain beneath the primitive streak; their removal causes multiple embryonic axes to form.

After the formation of the secondary yolk sac, a diverticulum of the visceral hypoblast – the allantois – forms towards one end of the embryonic region and extends into the local extraembryonic mesoblast. It passes from the roof of the secondary yolk sac to the same plane as the amnion. Further development of the allantois is described on page 1341.

EXTRAEMBRYONIC MESOBLAST

By definition, extraembryonic tissues encompass all tissues that do not contribute directly to the future body of the definitive embryo and, later, the fetus. At stage 5, blastocysts are implanted but not yet villous; they range from 7 to 12 days in age (**Fig. 10.9**). A feature of this stage is the first formation of extraembryonic mesoblast, which will come to cover the amnion, secondary yolk sac and the internal wall of the mural trophoblast, and will form the connecting stalk of the embryo with its contained allanto-enteric diverticulum. The origin of this first mesoblastic extraembryonic layer is by no means clear, and it may arise from several sources, including the caudal region of the epiblast, the parietal hypoblast and subhypoblastic cells. The trophoblastic origin of extraembryonic mesoblast is questioned, because there is always a complete basal lamina underlying the trophoblast. The migration of cells out of an epithelium is usually associated with previous disruption of the basal lamina. Certainly, the origin of extraembryonic cells will change over time as new germinal populations are established.

The fate of the first mesoblastic extraembryonic layer is at least twofold. It gives rise to the layer known as extraembryonic mesoblast, arranged as a mesothelium with underlying extraembryonic mesenchymal cells; this also appears to form an extracellular structure corresponding to the magma reticulare, between the mural trophoblast and the primary yolk sac in the stage 5 embryo. Later extraembryonic mesoblast populations mushroom beneath the cytotrophoblastic cells at the embryonic pole, forming the cores of the developing villus stems, and villi, and the angioblastic cells that will give rise to the capillaries within them and the earliest blood cells (p. 1341).

Initially, the extraembryonic mesoblast connects the amnion to the chorion over a wide area. Continued development and expansion of the extraembryonic coelom means that this attachment becomes increasingly circumvented to a connecting stalk, which is a permanent connection between the future caudal end of the embryonic disc and the chorion. The connecting stalk forms a pathway along which vascular anastomoses around the allantois establish communication with those of the chorion.

CONCEPTUS WITH A BILAMINAR EMBRYONIC DISC

At stage 6 the conceptus is composed of the walls of three cavities: the large chorionic cavity is surrounded by a meshwork of trophoblast and developing villi and lined with extraembryonic mesoblast. The chorion, trophoblast and extraembryonic mesoblast enclose the extraembryonic coelom and contain the much smaller amniotic cavity and yolk sac (Fig. 10.10). These latter cavities abut at the embryonic bilaminar disc where the epithelial epiblast and visceral hypoblast are approximated. A fourth cavity, the allantois, will form as a hypoblastic diverticulum in stage 7. The 'bilaminar disc' commonly referred to in embryology texts does not yet possess the definitive embryonic ectoderm and endoderm layers that will give rise to embryonic structures. Only the epiblast will give rise to the embryo; all other layers produced so far are extraembryonic. The amnion and chorion (and surrounding mesoblast) are part of the extraembryonic somatopleure, whereas the yolk sac, allantois and surrounding extraembryonic mesoblast constitute extraembryonic splanchnopleure. At the junctional zone surrounding the margins of the embryonic area, where the walls of the amnion and yolk sac converge, the somatopleuric and splanchnopleuric layers of extraembryonic mesoblast are continuous.

The terms epiblast and hypoblast are used to make the distinction between the earliest bilaminar disc layers and the later embryonic layers. Epiblast and hypoblast contain mixed populations of cells with little restriction, which establish the placental structures and extraembryonic tissues before the production of embryonic cell lines at gastrulation. The older terminology depicting three germ layers that give rise to the skin, gut lining and intervening tissues is thus incorrect for the bilaminar embryonic disc. The application and the retention of this aged terminology for the early stages of embryology causes confusion and inhibits the development of more pertinent descriptive language to describe these early events.

FORMATION OF INTRAEMBRYONIC TISSUES

At early stage 6, the epiblast is producing extraembryonic mesenchyme from its caudal margin. With the appearance of the primitive streak, a process is begun whereby cells of the epiblast either pass deep to the epiblast layer to form the populations of cells within the embryo, or remain on the dorsal aspect of the embryo to become the embryonic ectoderm. The primitive streak marks the beginning of gastrulation, a period when gross alterations in morphology and complex rearrangements of cell populations occur. During this time, the epiblast will give rise to a complex multilaminar structure with a defined craniocaudal axis. By the end of gastrulation, cell populations from different, often widely separated, regions of the embryonic disc will become closely related and the embryonic shape will have been produced.

PRIMITIVE STREAK AND NODE

Seen from the dorsal (epiblastic) aspect, at stage 6, the embryonic disc appears elongated. The primitive streak is first seen in the caudal region of the embryonic disc at this stage, orientated along its long axis, conferring the future craniocaudal axis of the embryo (Figs 10.13, 10.14). Although the future cranial and caudal regions of the embryo are well within the boundaries of the embryonic disc, it has become the practice to term the region of the disc closest to the streak 'caudal', and the region of the disc furthest from the streak 'cranial' or 'rostral'. With the development of the streak, the terms medial and lateral can be used. The relative dimensions of the primitive streak and the fates of the cells that pass through it change with the developmental stage. Thus the streak extends half way along the disc in the stage 6 embryo, reaches its greatest relative length in stage 7 and its maximum length in stage 8. It is still present in stage 11 embryos, but relatively fewer cells pass through it at this stage compared with the early stages.

Formation of the primitive streak is induced by the underlying visceral hypoblast; this remains beneath the streak even at late-streak stages. The primitive streak may be considered to be generally homologous with the blastopore of lower vertebrates (e.g. amphibia), with the nodal region corresponding to the dorsal lip. Experiments clearly show

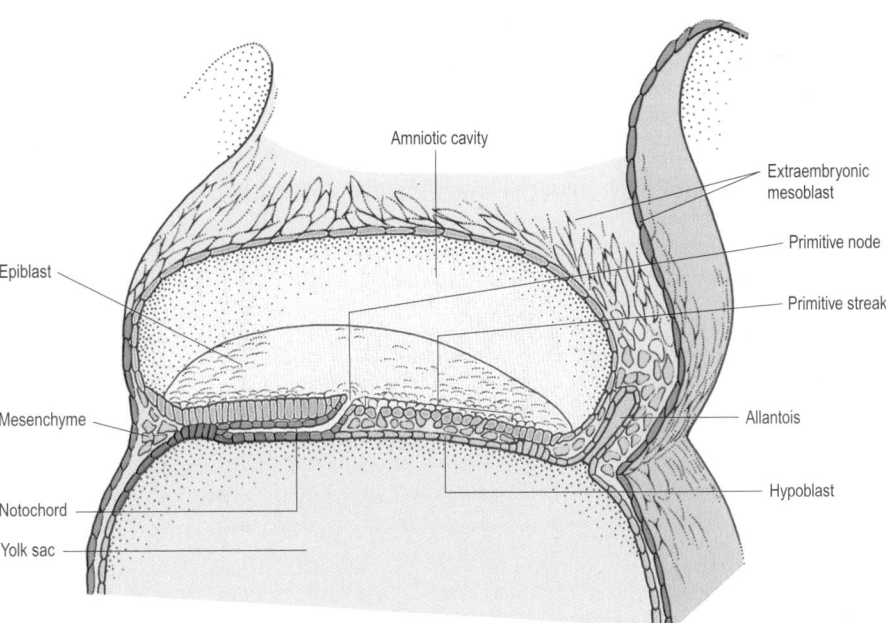

Fig. 10.13 Section through an early conceptus. Ingression of mesoblast is occurring at the primitive streak and the notochord is ingressing via the primitive (Hensen's) node.

Amniotic cavity

Extraembryonic mesoblast

Primitive node

Primitive streak

Epiblast

Mesenchyme

Notochord

Yolk sac

Allantois

Hypoblast

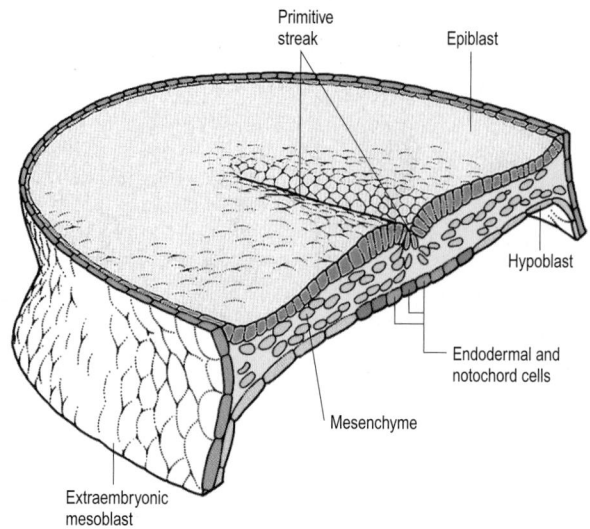

Fig. 10.14 Transverse section through the embryonic plate at the level of the primitive streak to show the early movement of mesoblast between the epiblast and underlying hypoblast.

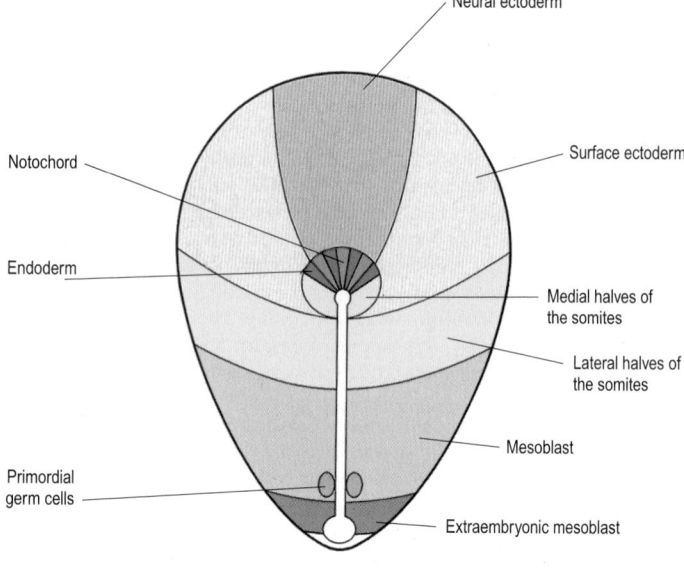

Fig. 10.15 The predictive fates of the epiblast cell population at the time the primitive streak is present.

the lip of the blastopore to be a dynamic wave front on which cells are carried into the interior to form the roof of the archenteron, a situation analogous to ingression through the node of the prechordal plate and endoderm. The primitive streak similarly may be considered analogous to the coapted, or fused, lateral lips of the blastopore. Finally, the cloacal membrane and its immediate environs are considered analogous to the ventral lip of the blastopore.

At the primitive streak, epiblast cells undergo a period of intense proliferation, the rate of division being much faster than that of blastomeres during cleavage. Streak formation is associated with the local production of several cell layers, extensive disruption of the basal lamina, increase in adhesive plaques and gap junctions, synthesis of vimentin, and loss of cytokeratins by the emerging cells.

As the epiblast cells proliferate, two ridges are formed on each side of the primitive streak, which appears to sink between them. The lower midline portion of the streak is termed the primitive groove. The process by which cells become part of the streak and then migrate away from it beneath the epiblast is termed ingression.

The primitive node, or Hensen's node, is the most rostral region of the primitive streak. It appears as a curved ridge of cells similar in shape to the top of an old-fashioned keyhole. Cells ingressing from the ridge pass into the primitive pit (the most rostral part of the primitive groove), and then migrate rostrally beneath the epiblast. The primitive node has been recorded in all stage 7 human embryos. The primitive node produces axial cell populations, the prechordal plate, notochord, embryonic endoderm and the medial halves of the somites. Removal of the node results in complete absence of the notochord and a loss of neurulation.

POSITION AND TIME OF INGRESSION THROUGH THE PRIMITIVE STREAK

Studies of cell fate have shown that epiblast cells which will pass through the streak are randomly located within the epiblast layer before their ingression, and that epiblast fate is determined at or before the time of ingression through the streak, indicating that passage through the primitive streak is the most important factor for future differentiation. The position and time of ingression through either streak or node directly affect the developmental fate of cells. The embryonic disc grows at a very high rate during the primitive streak stage. In the mouse, the embryonic axis increases 3.5-fold in length between the prestreak and neural plate stages. At each stage of development, the streak is slightly different, as is the embryo, therefore descriptions of streak-stage embryos, and of cells ingressing through the streak, must specify the stage of streak development and the position of ingression. The primitive streak stage is subdivided into early, mid- or late streak stages. Passage through the streak is specified according to position, e.g. via the node, or rostral,

middle or caudal regions of the streak. Cells that ingress through the primitive node give rise to the axial cell lines, the prechordal mesenchyme and notochord, and to the endoderm and the medial halves of the somites. The rostral portion of the primitive streak produces cells for the lateral halves of the somites, whereas the middle streak produces the lateral plate mesoblast. The adjacent caudal portion of the streak gives rise to the primordial germ cells, which can be distinguished histologically and histochemically at mid-streak stages, and the most caudal portion of the streak contributes cells to the extraembryonic mesoblast until the early somite stage. A composite of the information on the position of ingression through the streak and node is shown in **Fig. 10.15**. The epiblast cells that do not pass through the streak but remain within the epiblast population give rise to the neural and surface ectoderm of the embryo.

PRECHORDAL PLATE

The earliest cells migrating through the primitive node and streak give rise to both the embryonic endoderm and the notochord. The prechordal plate is defined as a localized thickening of the endoderm rostral to the notochordal process. As such, it represents the first population of endoderm cells to ingress through the primitive node. There is some confusion over the limits and fate of the prechordal plate (sometimes called the prochordal plate). The term has been used to describe a variety of structures: it has been applied to an area of endoderm, the buccopharyngeal membrane, and an accumulation of mesenchymal cells immediately rostral to the notochord. The first and most rostral ingression through the primitive node gives rise to a local prechordal region up to eight cells thick, and the cells become both epithelial and mesenchymal. The epithelial cells form the endodermal layer of the buccopharyngeal membrane, the preoral gut and probably all the foregut epithelium. The mesenchymal cells form the most cranial axial mesenchyme population, the prechordal mesenchyme.

NOTOCHORD

The notochord, also called chordamesoderm, the head process or chorda, arises from epiblast cells of the medial part of the primitive node. It passes through several stages during development. The cells of the early notochordal process express myogenic markers transitorily as they migrate beneath the epiblast, but later they become epithelial, forming junctions and a basal lamina. The notochordal cells are intimately mixed with endodermal cells, as both cells lines ingress at the same time (**Figs 10.13, 10.14, 10.16**). In the stage 8 embryo, the ingressing notochordal cells remain in the midline along the cephalocaudal axis. They form a rostral part, which is composed of a cell mass continuous with the prechordal mesenchyme, a mid portion in which cells are arranged in a tube with a central notochordal canal, and a caudal

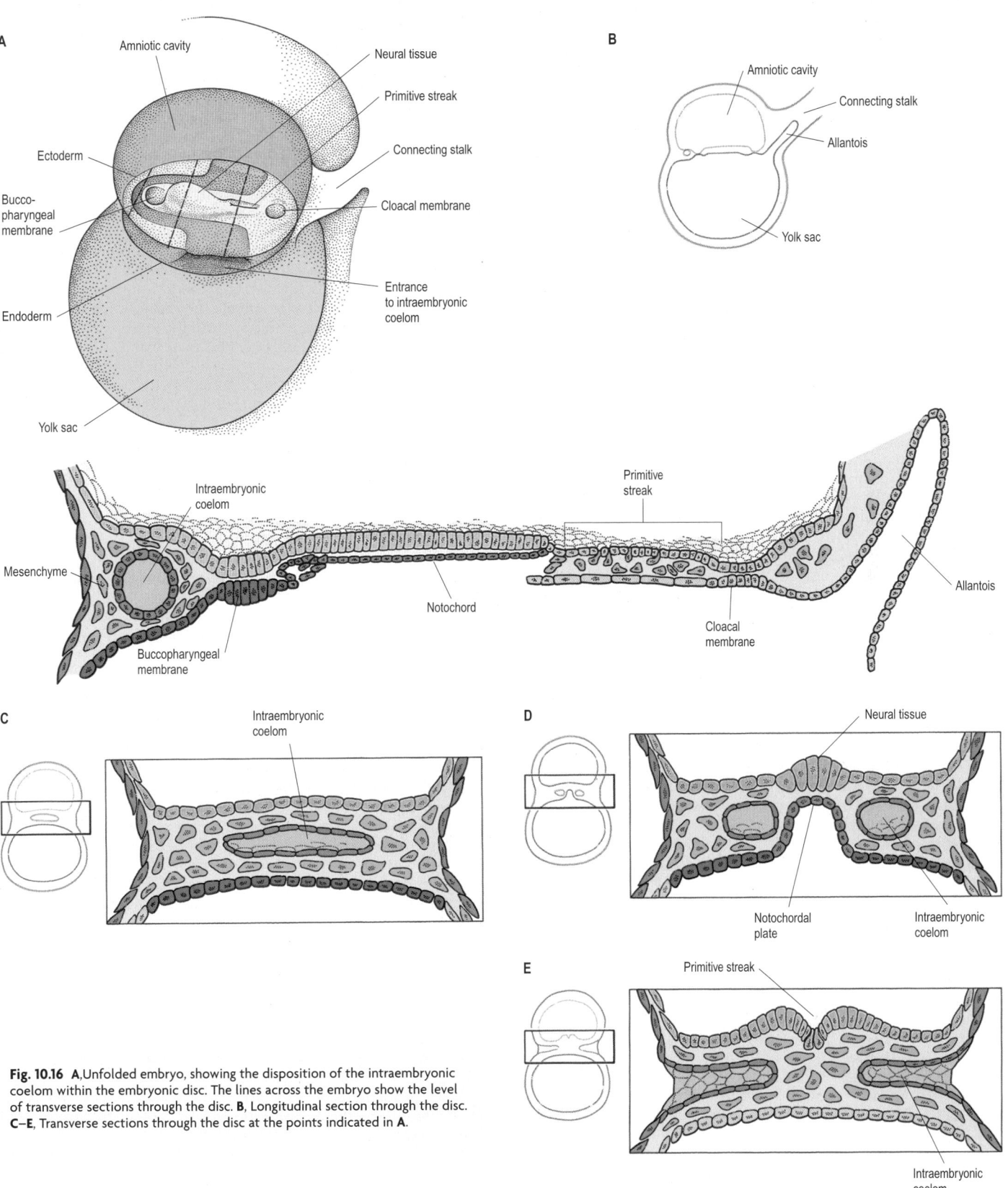

Fig. 10.16 A,Unfolded embryo, showing the disposition of the intraembryonic coelom within the embryonic disc. The lines across the embryo show the level of transverse sections through the disc. **B**, Longitudinal section through the disc. **C–E**, Transverse sections through the disc at the points indicated in **A**.

epithelial layer of cells, the notochordal plate, which is contiguous with the embryonic endoderm and forms a roof to the secondary yolk sac. There is a transitory opening between the primitive node and the secondary yolk sac called the neurenteric canal (so named because its upper opening is in the future caudal floor of the neural groove, and its lower opening is into the archenteron, the primitive gut); it may still be found at stage 9, and the site of the neurenteric canal can be recognized in stage 10 embryos. The ingression of notochordal cells at the primitive node is matched by specification of the overlying neural ectodermal

cells, and the notochordal plate is thus matched in length by the future neural floor plate. Both the notochord and the region of the floor plate of the neural tube may arise from a common progenitor cell. The early notochord is important for the maintenance and subsequent development of the neural floor plate and the induction of motor neurones. Removal of the notochord results in elimination of the neural floor plate and motor neurones, and expression of sensory cells types (p. 243). The caudal portions of the notochord which form later in development, when secondary neurulation processes commence, arise from the cell populations within the tail bud termed the caudoneural hinge (p. 241). This tissue is thicker and more advanced in differentiation than the tissues derived from the early streak.

EMBRYONIC ENDODERM

Before ingression, definitive embryonic endoderm cells are found in the epiblast located at the primitive node and rostral primitive streak. By the mid-streak stage, in the mouse, the endodermal cells are beneath the epiblast mainly in the midline, interspersed with presumptive noto-chordal cells, forming the roof of the secondary yolk sac. The ingressing endoderm displaces the visceral hypoblast into the secondary yolk sac wall by a dramatic territorial expansion that is brought about by a change in the morphology of the cells (Figs 10.13, 10.14, 10.16). The putative endoderm cells are cuboidal epithelial cells within the node, but they become squamous in the endoderm layer; this could result in a four-fold increase in the surface area covered by the cells. A complete replacement of the visceral hypoblast has not yet been confirmed, and there may be a mixed population of cells in the endodermal layer in the early stages. Ingression of cells through the streak and node in the human is apparent at stage 6, and by stage 7 a population of endoderm and notochord cells is present beneath the epiblast (Figs 10.13, 10.14, 10.16). During stages 6–11, the midline roof of the secondary yolk sac becomes populated mainly by the notochordal plate, which remains in direct lateral continuity with the endodermal cells. It is not until stage 11, after the definitive notochord is formed, that the endoderm cells can join across the midline. For the developmental fate of the embryonic endoderm, see Fig. 10.28.

INTRAEMBRYONIC MESOBLAST (MESENCHYME)

Epiblast cells ingress through the cranial and middle parts of the streak individually, maintaining their apical epithelial contacts while elongating ventrally. The cells become flask-shaped, with thin attenuated apical necks and broad basal regions. The basal and lateral surfaces form lamellipodia and filopodia and the apical contact is released. The cells are now free mesoblast cells, their fibroblastic, stellate morphology reflecting the release from the epithelial layer. Once through the streak, the cells migrate away from it, using the basal lamina of the overlying epiblast and extracellular matrix as a substratum. The cells contact one another by filopodia and lamellipodia, with which they also contact the basal lamina. Gap junctions have been observed between filopodia and cell bodies. With the appearance of the mesoblast, spaces form between the epiblast and visceral hypoblast that are filled with extracellular matrix rich in glycosaminoglycans. The migrating mesoblast has a leading edge of cells that open up the migration routes, and the following cells seem to be pulled along behind in a coordinated mass movement. Mesoblast formed by cells migrating through the primitive node and rostral primitive streak will form the paraxial mesenchyme, whereas cells migrating through the middle to caudal streak will form the lateral plate mesenchyme (Figs 10.13, 10.14, 10.16).

EMBRYONIC ECTODERM

When the ingression of cells through the primitive streak is completed, the epithelial cells remaining in the epiblast layer are termed embryonic ectoderm cells. This layer still contains a mixed population, because both surface ectoderm cells and neural ectoderm cells are present. It is believed that these cells were originally in the cranial half of the disc at the early streak stage, at which time the neural-fated cells were closest to the streak, and the surface ectoderm cells were most cranial (Fig. 10.15). The process of neurulation relocates most of the neuroepithelial cells (see below).

PRIMORDIAL GERM CELLS

Although early studies on human embryos have reported primordial germ cells, and described their development from the early endoderm of the yolk sac and allantois, it is now clear from animal experimentation that the primordial germ cells arise from epiblast ingressing at the caudal end of the primitive streak (Fig. 10.15). Whether these cells originate from rostral regions that migrate to the streak, or from local caudal regions, is not known. Extremely early segregation of the germ cells, when the epiblast layer consists of only 10–13 cells, has been demonstrated. It has been suggested that the primordial germ cells remain sequestered in the extraembryonic mesenchyme at the caudal end of the embryo until the embryonic endoderm has been produced and gastrulation completed, and that they start to migrate along the

allantoic and hindgut endoderm as the folding of the embryo begins. The formation of the tail fold brings the proximal portion of the allantois within the body, so reducing the final distance over which the cells migrate to the genital ridges. Further development of the germ cells is described on page 1381.

TRILAMINAR DISC

The stage 8 embryo is termed a trilaminar disc; however, as the middle, mesoblast, layer is several cells thick with intervening extracellular matrix, the concept of three epithelial layers forming a trilaminar disc is not correct. The embryo at this stage, c.18–19 days after ovulation, is pear-shaped, and broader cranially than caudally (Fig. 10.14). The upper epiblast cells are tall, and form a pseudostratified columnar epithelial layer with a basal lamina, except at the primitive streak, where the cells are ingressing to form the other layers. The more cranially placed epiblast will give rise to the surface ectoderm. The extent of the future neural plate can be assessed: it is correlated with the length and width of the notochordal plate directly beneath. The lower embryonic endoderm, a simple squamous layer with a developing basal lamina, is not always complete at this stage, particularly in the midline caudal to the pre-chordal plate, which is still occupied by the notochordal process or plate.

The middle, mesoblast, layer is composed of free cells migrating cranially, laterally and caudally from the primitive streak. They produce extracellular matrix, which separates the epiblast and endoderm of the embryonic area and permits their passage. The streams of mesoblast extend between the epiblast and endoderm over all of the disc area except cranially at the prechordal plate, a portion of which will become the buccopharyngeal membrane, and caudally at the cloacal membrane, which is a patch of thickened endoderm, similar to the prechordal plate, caudal to the primitive streak.

Mesoblast that passes in a cranial direction flanks the notochordal plate and passes around the prechordal plate region, converging medially to fuse in the midline beyond its cephalic border. This transmedian mass is the cardiogenic mesoblast in which the heart and periardium will develop. The cardiogenic mesoblast fuses with the junctional zone of extraembryonic mesoblast around the extreme cephalic margin of the embryonic area. This region will eventually form the septum trans-versum and primitive ventral mesentery of the foregut. Mesoblast pass-ing laterally from the streak soon approaches and becomes confluent with the extraembryonic mesoblast around the margins of the disc, i.e. at the junctional zone where the splanchnic and somatic strata of extra-embryonic mesoblast merge. Mesoblast that streams caudally from the primitive streak skirts the margins of the cloacal membrane and then converges towards the caudal midline extremity of the embryonic disc to become continuous with the extraembryonic mesoblast of the connecting stalk. It is unclear if the lower layer of the cloacal membrane consists of visceral hypoblast, like the more cranial primitive streak (the hypoblast is necessary for maintaining the streak), or if it is replaced by migrating embryonic endoderm, or if there is a region for ingression of endoderm at the caudal end of the streak, similar to the node cranially.

Still further caudally, the embryonic disc develops a midline diver-ticulum adjacent to the cloacal membrane. This diverticulum, the allantois, projects into the extraembryonic connecting stalk (Figs 10.16, 10.21). There is little information about which cells form the allantois, i.e. whether it is composed of visceral hypoblast, parietal hypoblast or embryonic endoderm. The allantois later develops a rich anastomotic blood supply around it, in the manner of the yolk sac.

NEURULATION

The generation of cells at the primitive node produces midline endo-derm, notochord and the floor plate of the future neural tube. As the notochord grows and elongates, there is a matched growth of neural floor plate cells until both cell lines extend to the buccopharyngeal membrane. The epiblast lateral to the midline contains both future surface and neural ectoderm. The latter becomes arranged between the primitive node and buccopharyngeal membrane: cells destined to be in the neural plate lie medially, and those destined for the neural crest lie laterally (Fig. 10.17). A smaller subpopulation of neuronal cells, the ectodermal placodes, are arranged either close to the neural crest or within the rostral limit of the neural plate itself.

Buccopharyngeal
membrane

Neural
plate

Cloacal membrane

Fig. 10.17 Extent and shape of the neural plate in an unfolded embryo. The buccopharyngeal and cloacal membranes are indicated.

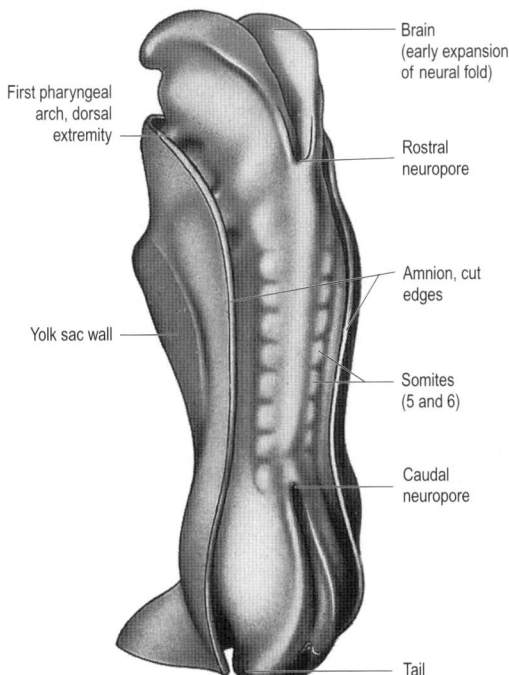

First pharyngeal
arch, dorsal
extremity

Yolk sac wall

Brain
(early expansion
of neural fold)

Rostral
neuropore

Amnion, cut
edges

Somites
(5 and 6)

Caudal
neuropore

Tail

Fig. 10.19 A human embryo at stage 10, 2.1 mm long, with nine somites: left lateral and dorsal aspects. Nearly all the yolk sac and the caudal amnion have been excised to show the tail region. (From a model by Eternod.)

Proliferation of the neural ectoderm matches the underlying migration of mesoblast from the primitive streak, so that the neural plate covers the paraxial mesenchyme each side of the notochord (**Fig. 10.21E**). As the paraxial mesenchyme undergoes somitogenesis (p. 789), the formation of the epithelial somites elevates the edges of the neural plate and starts neurulation (**Figs 10.18, 10.21F**). The plate itself undergoes concurrent morphological changes. The most medial cells become wedge-shaped, forming the neural groove. Further elevation of the edges of the neural groove permits fusion of the neuronal populations in the dorsal midline to form the neural tube. The surface ectoderm forms the putative dorsal epidermis (**Fig. 10.19, 10.21G**). The neural crest cells remain as a linearly arranged mesenchymal population between these two epithelia. The ectodermal placodes remain within the surface ectoderm at this stage.

The process described above is primary neurulation. It commences in the future cervical region of the embryo and proceeds rostrally and caudally. Primary neurulation continues caudally to about the level of somite 27, from which the process of neural tube formation occurs by secondary neurulation. Neurulation is described further in Chapter 14 (p. 241).

A

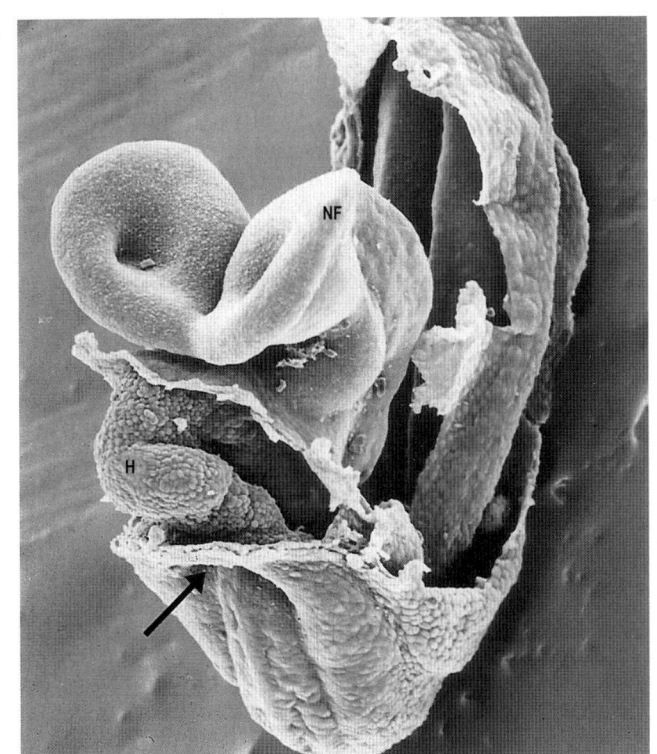

B

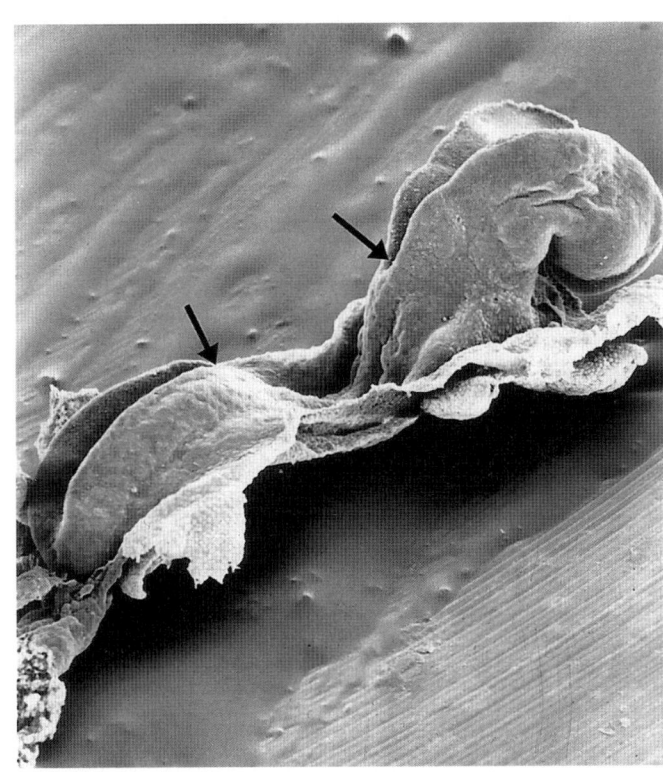

Fig. 10.18 Scanning electron micrographs of rat embryos at the time of neurulation. **A**, Ventral view, showing the neural fold (NF), and the heart (H) with the somatopleuric pericardial membrane and surface ectoderm removed; the arrow indicates the entrance to the foregut via the cranial intestinal portal. **B**, Dorsolateral view; the arrows indicate the extent of rostral (to the right) and caudal (to the left) neural tube formation. (Photographs by P Collins; printed by S Cox, Electron Microscopy Unit, Southampton General Hospital.)

Cells of the neural plate give rise to all of the central nervous system and the motor neurones, whereas the neural crest gives rise to most of the peripheral nervous system, i.e. autonomic, enteric and sensory neurones and Schwann cells.

NEURAL CREST

Neural crest is the name given to the band of cells at the outermost edges of the neural plate, adjacent to the presumptive epidermis (**Fig. 10.17**). Neural crest cells from the head region assume a mesenchymal morphology and begin migration before closure of the neural tube. In the trunk, the cells remove themselves from the epithelium as the neural tube closes. They lie on the dorsal part of the newly formed neural tube for some time before migration. Neural crest cells can migrate over considerable distances. They contribute a major population of mesenchyme to the head, and also to a wide range of different cell lines in the trunk. They are referred to either as neural crest cells or as ectomesenchyme, to acknowledge their derivation from the ectoderm. They do not usually give rise to epithelial tissues, but give rise to much of the peripheral nervous system and the sensory nerves.

ECTODERMAL PLACODES

The ectodermal placodes are initially small local aggregates of ectoderm remaining within the surface ectoderm, which pass deep to the surface ectoderm sometime after neurulation. These cells give rise to non-nervous and nervous structures. The former produce the paired optic placodes, which give rise to the lens in each eye (p. 721). Similar specializations of the ectoderm on the frontonasal, maxillary and mandibular processes give rise to the outer coating of the teeth (p. 612). The neuronal placodes may invaginate *in toto* to form a vesicle, they may remain as a neuronal layer, or they may contribute to neuronal structures with cells of other origins. The paired otic placodes overlying the rhombencephalon at the lateral portion of the second pharyngeal arch invaginate to form the otic vesicles, which give rise to the membranous labyrinth of the ear (p. 679). The midline adenohypophyseal placode, which is initially on the rostral margin of the neural plate, invaginates as Rathke's pouch immediately rostral to the buccopharyngeal membrane (p. 246). The olfactory placodes, which are also found, bilaterally, on the rostral edges of the neural plate, remain as the special olfactory sensory epithelia at the top of the nasal cavity (p. 610). Placodal cells in the lateral regions of the pharyngeal arches remove themselves individually from the ectoderm at stage 10–11 and become associated with the neural crest cells within the cranial sensory ganglia supplying these arches. In summary, the ectodermal placodes give rise to elements of the special senses and the cranial sensory nerves (p. 245).

FOLDING OF THE EMBRYO

In a diagrammatic representation of the trilaminar disc viewed from the ectodermal aspect, all of the future external surface of the body is delimited (see **Fig. 10.17**). The ends of the gut tube are specified on the ectodermal surface at the buccopharyngeal and cloacal membranes, which are regions where the ectoderm and underlying endoderm are apposed without intervening mesoblast. In the midline between these membranes, the neural tube will form from fusion of the lateral edges of the neural plate, and the surface ectoderm will fuse in the midline to constitute the future skin of the back.

The representation of a person on the trilaminar disc (**Fig. 10.20**) shows, to some extent, the way in which the positions of the main body structures are already specified in the unfolded embryo. The portion of the disc between the buccopharyngeal membrane and the edge of the disc will become the anterior thoracic wall and the anterior abdominal wall cranial to the umbilicus. Further caudally, midway along the neural axis, the lateral portions of the disc will become the lateral and anterior abdominal walls of the trunk. The portion of the disc beyond the cloacal membrane will form the anterior abdominal wall caudal to the umbilicus. The circumference of the disc, where the embryonic tissue meets the extraembryonic membranes, will become restricted to the connection between the anterior abdominal wall and the umbilical cord, i.e. the umbilicus.

Head folding begins at stage 9, when the fusing cranial neural plate rises above the surface ectoderm and the portion of the disc rostral to the buccopharyngeal membrane (which contains the cardiogenic mesenchyme), moves to lie ventral to the developing brain (**Fig. 10.21**).

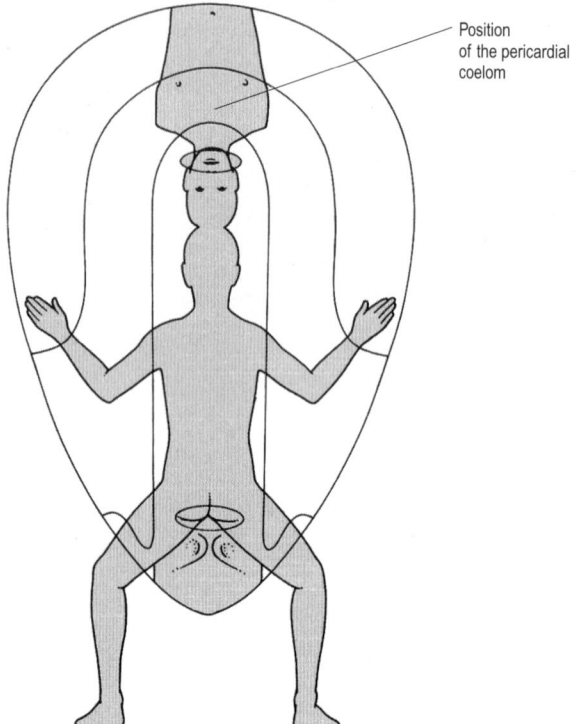

Position of the pericardial coelom

Fig. 10.20 Representation of a person on the flat embryonic disc. The position of the central nervous system has been matched to the dimensions of the neural plate, and the position of the heart in the thorax to the position of the pericardial coelom. The limbs, although represented in this diagram, are not present on the disc at this stage. The usefulness of this diagram lies in its illustration of the extent of the anterior body wall both rostral to the buccopharyngeal membrane and caudal to the cloacal membrane. The future dorsal regions of the body are found medially on the disc, while the ventral regions of the body are situated laterally and peripherally on the disc. After head and tail folding and lateral folding, the peripheral edge of the disc becomes constricted as the edge of the umbilicus.

The prosencephalon and buccopharyngeal membrane are now the most rostral structures of the embryo. The previously flat region of endoderm, the prechordal plate, is now modified into a deep tube, the primitive foregut. Tail folding can be seen in stage 10 embryos, when the entire embryo comes to rise above the level of the yolk sac. Similar movement of the part of the disc caudal to the cloacal membrane results in its repositioning ventral to the neural plate. Generally, as the embryo rises above the edges of the disc, the lateral regions of the disc are drawn ventrally and medially, contributing to the lateral folding of the embryo. For a full understanding of this process, it is necessary to study the diagrams in **Figs 10.21** and **10.22**.

FORMATION OF THE INTRAEMBRYONIC COELOM

At and just before stage 9 (before formation of the head fold), vesicles appear between the mesenchymal cells cranial to the buccopharyngeal membrane and within the cranial lateral plate mesenchyme. At the periphery of the vesicles, the mesenchymal cells develop junctional complexes and apical polarity, and form an epithelium. The vesicles become confluent to form a horse-shoe shaped tube, the intraembryonic coelom, which extends caudally to the level of the first somite and laterally into the lateral plate mesenchyme towards the extraembryonic mesenchyme. The intra- and extraembryonic coeloms do not communicate at this stage. The lateral plate mesenchyme thus develops somatopleuric coelomic epithelium subjacent to the ectoderm, and a splanchnopleuric coelomic epithelium next to the embryonic endoderm (**Fig. 10.16**).

During development of the head fold, the morphological movements that organize the foregut and buccopharyngeal membrane have a similarly profound effect on the shape of the intraembryonic coelom.

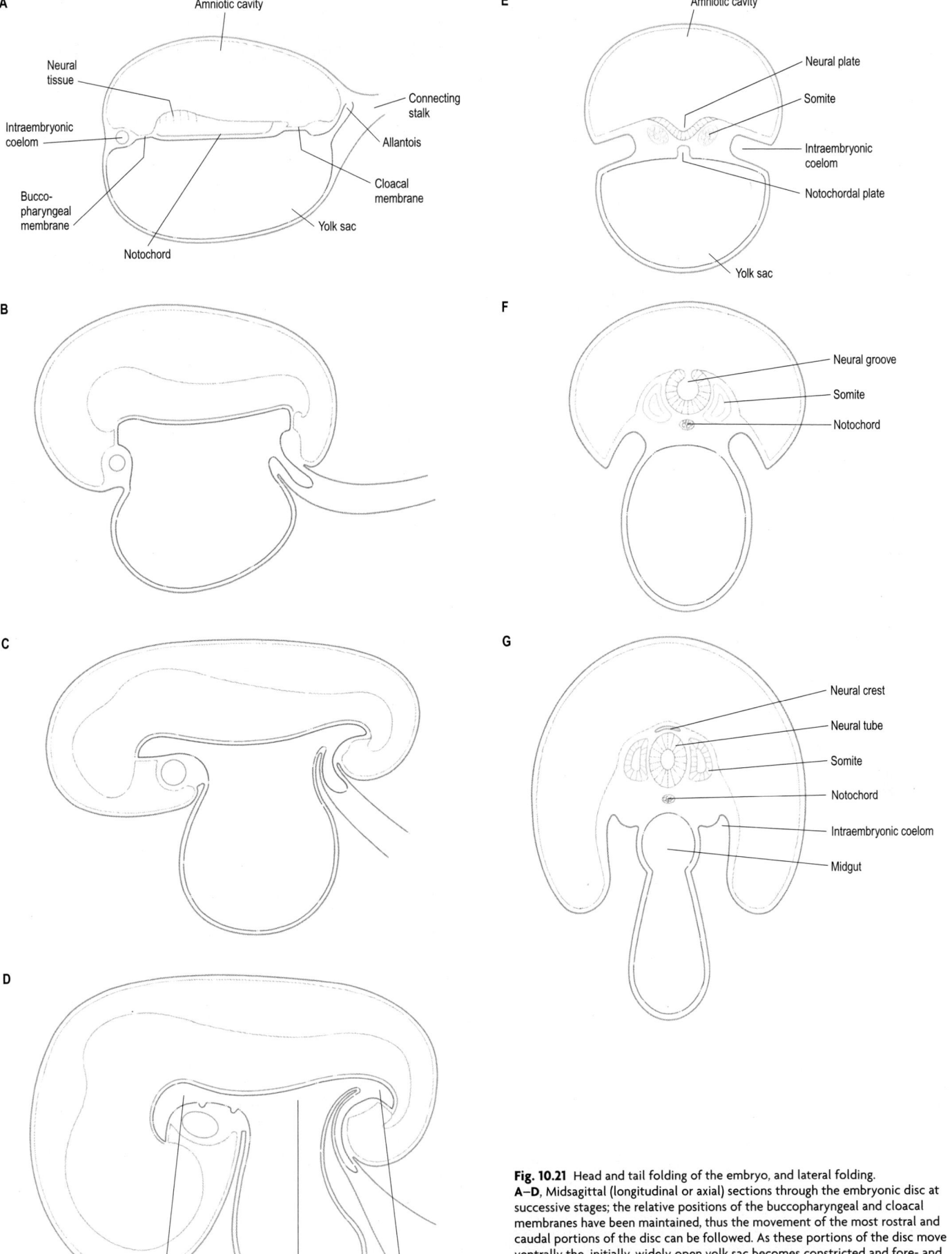

Fig. 10.21 Head and tail folding of the embryo, and lateral folding.
A–D, Midsagittal (longitudinal or axial) sections through the embryonic disc at successive stages; the relative positions of the buccopharyngeal and cloacal membranes have been maintained, thus the movement of the most rostral and caudal portions of the disc can be followed. As these portions of the disc move ventrally the, initially, widely open yolk sac becomes constricted and fore- and hindgut divisions can be seen; the midgut is that region which remains in wide connection to the yolk sac. **E–G**, Transverse sections through the midpoint of the embryonic disc at successive stages to illustrate lateral folding. This occurs as neurulation proceeds.

199

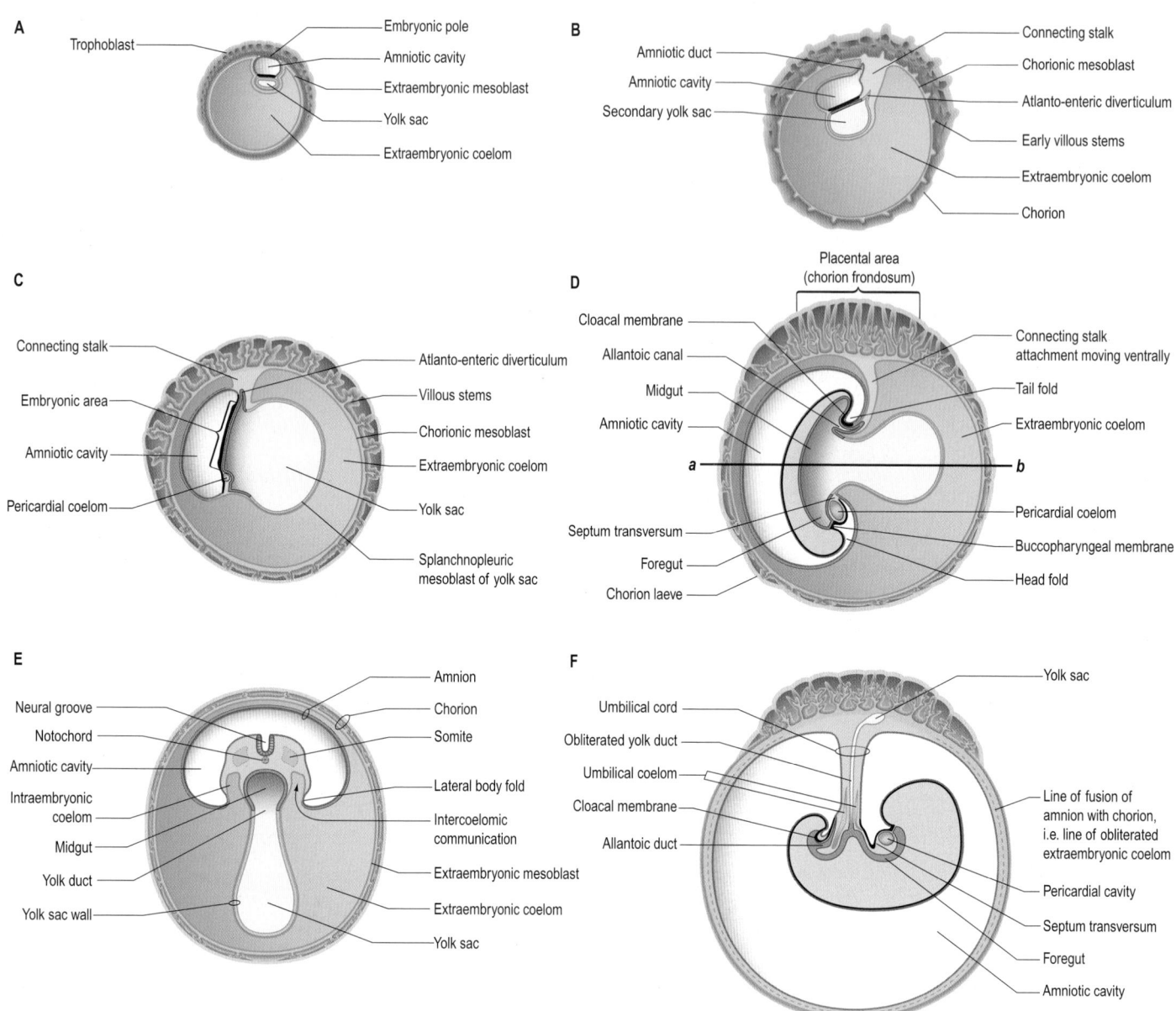

Fig. 10.22 A, An early stage in development of the human blastocyst. **B,** Blastocyst sectioned through the longitudinal axis of the embryo, showing the early formation of the allantois and the connecting stalk. **C,** Longitudinal section of embryo at a later stage of development; the amniotic cavity can be see at the most rostral part of the embryonic area. **D,** Longitudinal section of embryo at a later stage, showing formation of the head and tail folds, the expansion of the amnion and the delimitation of the umbilicus. **E,** Transverse section along the line a–b in **D**; observe that the intraembryonic coelom communicates freely with the extraembryonic coelom. **F,** Longitudinal section of embryo at a later stage, showing full expansion of the amniotic cavity and the umbilical cord.

The midline portion of the originally flat, horse-shoe shaped coelom moves ventrally, leaving the caudal arms of the horse-shoe in their original position. In this way the midline part of the coelom, which was originally just rostral to the buccopharyngeal membrane, comes to lie anterior (ventral) to the foregut (caudal to the buccopharyngeal membrane), and the two lateral extensions of the coelom pass close to the lateral walls of the foregut on each side. The caudal portions of the coelom (the two arms of the horse-shoe), which in the unfolded disc communicated laterally with the extraembryonic coelom, turn 90° to lie lateral to the gut, and communicate with the extraembryonic coelom ventrally.

Compartments of the coelom that will later in development give rise to the body cavities can already be seen. The midline ventral portion, caudal to the buccopharyngeal membrane, becomes the pericardial cavity. The canals lateral to the foregut (pericardioperitoneal canals) become the pleural cavities and the uppermost part of the peritoneal cavity. The remaining portion of the coelom becomes the peritoneal cavity. By stage 11, the intraembryonic coelom within the lateral plate mesenchyme extends caudally to the level of the caudal wall of the yolk

sac. The intra- and extraembryonic coeloms communicate widely each side of the midgut along the length of the embryo from the level of the 4th somite (**Figs 10.22, 10.23**).

In the early embryo, the intraembryonic coelom provides a route for the circulation of coelomic fluid and, with the beating of the heart tube, functions as a primitive circulation that takes nutritive fluid deep into the embryo, until it is superseded by the blood vascular system. The coelomic channel, and the primitive circulation that passes through it, is of paramount importance up to stage 13. Whereas the superficial tissues of the embryo can receive nutrients via the amniotic sac and yolk sac fluids, the deeper tissues are, until the formation of the coelom, under conditions similar to tissue culture. From stage 10, however, exocoelomic fluid, propelled by the first contractions of the developing heart, is brought into contact with the deeply placed mesenchyme. This early 'circulation' ensures that an adequate supply of nutrients reaches the rapidly increasing amount of embryonic tissue, and meets most of the requirements of the deeper mesenchymal derivatives. From stage 12 the endothelial system expands and fills rapidly with plasma, which passes across the locally thinned coelomic epithelium into the large

A

B

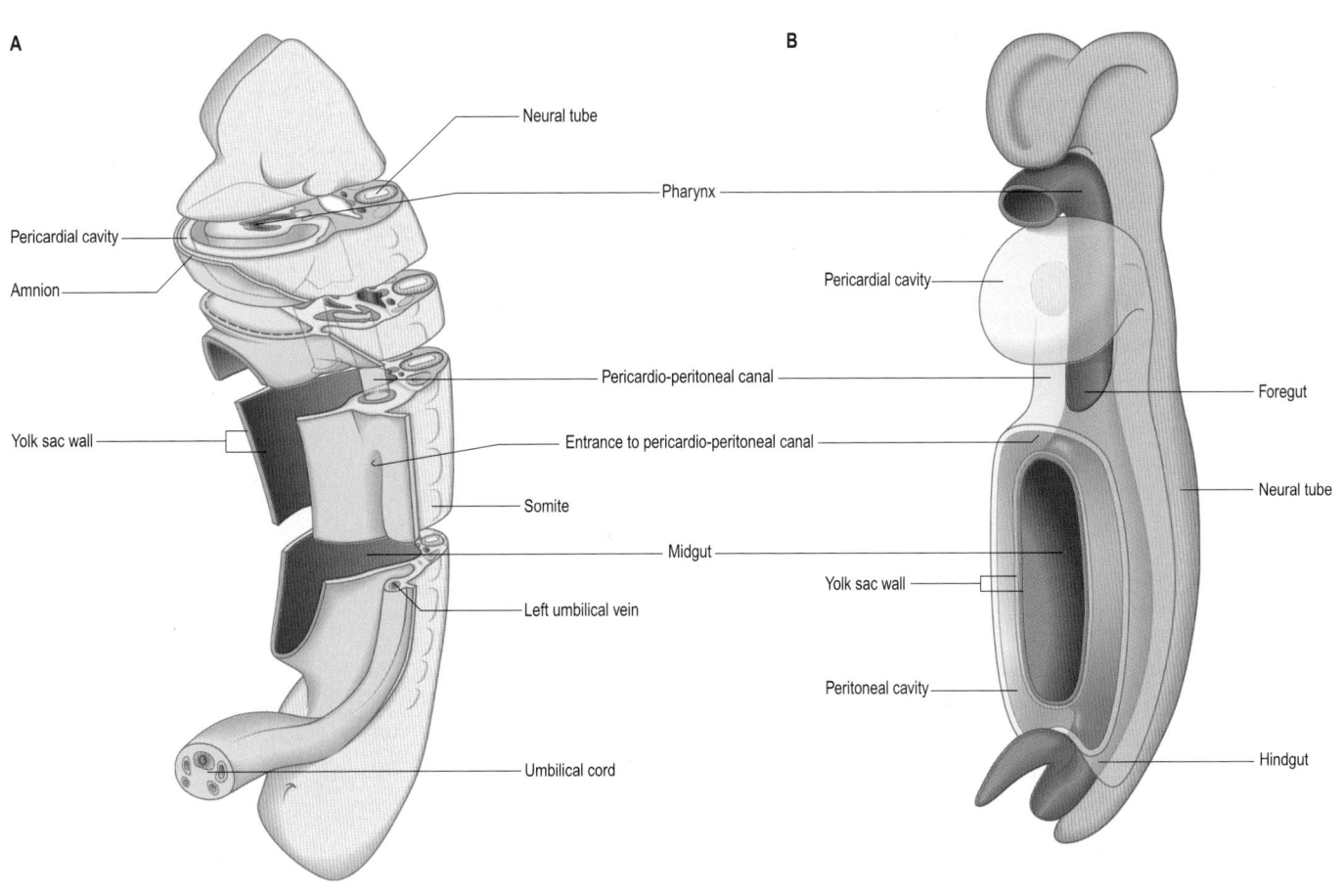

- Neural tube
- Pharynx
- Pericardial cavity
- Amnion
- Pericardio-peritoneal canal
- Foregut
- Yolk sac wall
- Entrance to pericardio-peritoneal canal
- Neural tube
- Somite
- Midgut
- Yolk sac wall
- Left umbilical vein
- Peritoneal cavity
- Umbilical cord
- Hindgut

Fig. 10.23 **A**, Embryo at stage 11, showing the position of the intraembryonic coelom (contained by the walls coloured blue). **B**, The three major epithelial populations within a stage 11 embryo, viewed from a ventrolateral position. The neural tube lies dorsal to the gut; ventrally, the intraembryonic coelom crosses the midline at the level of the foregut and hindgut, but is lateral to the midgut and a portion of the foregut. (**A**, after Streeter.)

hepatocardiac channels that project into the pericardioperitoneal canals at the level of the seventh somite.

In spite of the importance of the coelom in defining the body cavities, and of the coelomic epithelium in the production of the major mesenchymal populations of the trunk (**Fig. 10.24**), only a few workers have considered the overall contribution of the coelom and its epithelium to the embryo (Streeter 1942, Langemeijer 1976). The coelom can be described as a single, tubular organ which is comparable to the neural tube, in that it possesses a specialized wall that encloses a cavity. Certainly, the proliferating coelomic epithelium has many similarities to the neural ectoderm. It is pseudostratified columnar epithelium with an inner germinal layer from which cellular progeny migrate. After the germinal phase, both epithelia ultimately form the lining of a cavity, i.e. ependyma for the neural epithelium and mesothelium for the coelomic epithelium. The coelomic epithelium, like the neural epithelium, produces cells destined for different fates from different sites and at different developmental times. Coelomic cells are like the neural epithelium, in that they have apical epithelial specializations and tapering basal processes that are in direct contact with the underlying mesenchyme, without an intervening basal lamina. The possibility of the tapering processes forming directional signals for migrating progeny, similar to radial glia of the neural tube, has not been examined.

EMBRYONIC CELL POPULATIONS AT GASTRULATION

After gastrulation, the cells of the embryo contribute to two fundamental types of tissue, namely epithelial and mesenchymal. Differentiation of specialized circulating blood cells and other cell types occurs in sequence. Embryonic and fetal cell types are replaced later in development or after birth.

EPITHELIA

Epithelial populations in the embryo have many of the morphological characteristics of differentiated epithelia, i.e. they are composed of sheets of closely packed cells, with narrow intercellular clefts containing minimal extracellular material, and a developed basal lamina containing specific proteins synthesized by the epithelium itself (p. 29). The cells usually show juxtaluminal intercell surface specializations such as desmosomes, tight junctions, gap junctions, etc., and specializations of the apical surface, which may exhibit microvilli or cilia. Characteristically, epithelia clothe internal and external surfaces as simple or compound cellular sheets that separate phases of differing composition (e.g. the external environment and the subepithelial tissue fluids, intravascular and extravascular fluids, etc.). Traffic of materials in the intercellular clefts between cells is limited. Traffic occurs across the cells: their limiting membranes, which function as energy-dependent selective barriers, enhance the passage of some materials and impede the passage of others.

Embryonic epithelia differ from those in the fetus and adult. Two distinct types of embryonic epithelia can be identified. Early germinal epithelia give rise to epithelial or mesenchymal populations of the embryo and confer their early patterning; such epithelia are termed organizers, e.g. the primitive streak. Later germinal epithelia give rise to system-specific progenitor populations, e.g. the ventricular zone of the neural tube. All epithelia other than special germinal epithelia divide to produce embryonic growth throughout development and may retain stem cells, which will divide throughout life.

MESENCHYME

The terms mesoblast and mesenchyme are used in this text in a specific manner and not interchangeably. Previously, cells forming a population between the epiblast and hypoblast were termed mesoderm and, more recently, mesenchyme. The terms primary and secondary mesenchyme have been used to distinguish between those cells which arise from

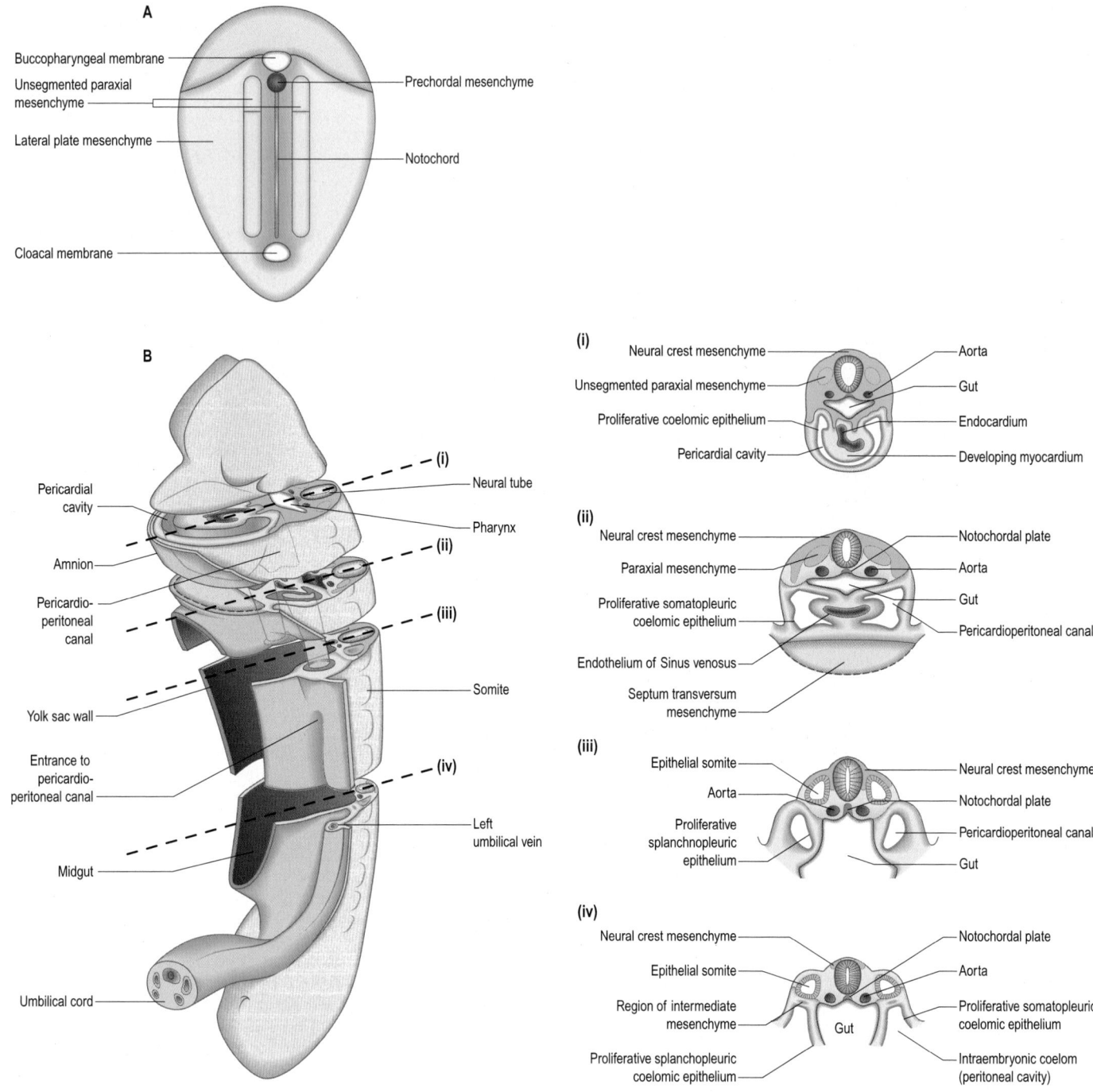

Fig. 10.24 A, Mesoblast populations within the early embryonic disc. **B**, Stage 11 embryo, showing the position of the intraembryonic coelom (contained by the walls coloured blue) and the positions of the sections **C–F**, which are shown to the right. **C–F**, Transverse sections, arranged cranial to caudal, from a stage 11 embryo. The populations of mesenchyme and the sites of mesenchymal proliferation are indicated. (After Streeter.)

ingression through the primitive streak and those which arise from neural crest ingression. Primary mesenchymal cells revert to epithelia at their destinations. However, whereas some primary mesenchymal cells may become epithelial within a short time frame, e.g. somites and lateral plate, other cells may transform later, e.g. the epithelium lining blood vessels. To cope with these conflicts in terminology, the mixed population of epiblast cells that ingress through the primitive streak and come to lie between the epiblast and embryonic endoderm is termed mesoblast until they have migrated to their final position, at which time the populations of mesenchyme can be identified and their fates inferred.

Mesoblastic and mesenchymal cells have no polarity. They form junctional complexes, which are not exclusively juxtaluminal, and they produce extracellular matrix molecules and fibres from the entire cell surface. Mesenchymal populations are formed from a range of germinal

epithelia and by proliferation of mesenchymal cells directly. They occupy all the regions between the various epithelial layers described above. The term mesoderm is reserved for the coelomic epithelia that later form mesothelia.

Mesenchymal cells support epithelia throughout the developing body, both locally where they contribute to the basement membrane and form the lamina propria and smooth muscle of tubes, and generally where they differentiate into connective tissue. Specific mesenchymal populations control the patterning of local regions of epithelium (e.g. the zone of polarizing activity on the postaxial limb border posterior to the apical ectodermal ridge; p. 937).

EXTRACELLULAR MATRIX

The space beneath epithelia and between mesenchyme cells is filled with extracellular matrix. Extracellular matrix molecules and their receptors are synthesized by both epithelial and mesenchymal cells. Epithelial cells produce a two-dimensional basal lamina, which contains a variety of matrix molecules including laminin, fibronectin, type IV collagen and various proteoglycans. The particular molecules can vary during development according to spatial and temporal patterns and this results in changes in the behaviour of the underlying mesenchymal cells (e.g. in patterning of the basal regions of the skull; p. 493). Mesenchymal cells produce extracellular matrix molecules in three dimensions. Those adjacent to an epithelial layer will connect with its basal lamina, forming a basement membrane that secures the epithelial layer to the underlying tissue. Cells deep within a mesenchymal population may synthesize matrix molecules (fibrillar or granular) to separate cells locally, open migration routes or leave information within the matrix to act on cell populations passing at a later time.

Molecules of the extracellular matrix are complex: they include more than 19 individual types of collagen (some of which are capable of being individually spliced to give more than 100 variants), proteoglycans and glycoproteins (which come in a wide variety of forms, with and without binding proteins) and elastic fibres (p. 38). Of particular interest is hyaluronic acid, a glycosaminoglycan. Because of its vast capacity to bind water molecules, it creates and structures the space between the mesenchymal cells, producing much of the overall shape of an embryo. Experimental removal of hyaluronic acid prevents the formation of cell migration routes, removes the support for overlying epithelia, and disrupts the normal branching of glandular systems.

Fibronectin deposited extracellularly along a migration pathway will affect cells that touch it later, causing realignment of their intracellular actin filaments and thus of their orientation; it induces cell migration. The receptors for extracellular matrix molecules such as fibronectin and laminin were termed integrins because they integrate (via α and β subunits that span the cell membrane) extracellular proteins and intracellular cytoskeletal elements, allowing them to act together. The binding preference of integrins depends upon their combination of subunits and environmental conditions (p. 38).

Epithelial and mesenchymal cell populations can structure the space around them by secretion of particular matrix molecules or growth factors, which in turn can organize the cells that contact them. The extracellular matrix is structured rather than random. Cell–matrix interactions and matrix–cell interactions control the position of migration routes and cellular 'decisions' to migrate or to begin to differentiate. Matrix molecules propagate developmental instructions from cell to cell and form a far-reaching four-dimensional (spatial and temporal) mechanism of communication.

TRANSITION BETWEEN EPITHELIAL AND MESENCHYME STATES

Transformations of cell morphology from epithelium to mesenchyme, and the reverse, occur in specific places and times during development: they can be seen as ways of dispersing germinal centres with increasing restriction. The first epithelial-to-mesenchyme transition occurs at the primitive streak, a germinal epithelium which confers embryonic specification on the resultant mesoblast population. The mesoblast so formed migrates and the cells undergo mesenchyme-to-epithelial transitions when they reach their final destinations. Series of small epithelial germinal centres, the somites, are formed, as are larger, more extensive, germinal epithelial sheets which line the walls of the intraembryonic coelom. The coelomic walls, especially those derived from somatopleure and splanchnopleure, form germinal epithelia that give rise to the major mesenchymal populations forming the viscera. The early epithelial somites undergo further local epithelial-to-mesenchyme transitions, to form the sclerotomes, and subsequently form several germinal epithelia in the epithelial plate of each somite. Later mesenchyme-to-epithelium transitions are not associated with the formation of germinal epithelia; the most common involve the transition of mesenchyme into the endothelium of the vascular system (pp. 1029 and 797). The nephrons of the mesonephric (p. 1375) and metanephric (p. 1375) systems also form from mesenchyme-to-epithelial transition.

EMBRYONIC INDUCTION AND CELL DIVISION

Cell populations within the embryo interact to provide the developmental integration and fine control necessary to achieve tissue-specific morphogenesis. In the early embryo, such interactions may occur only if particular regions of the embryo are present, e.g. signalling centres or organizers. As the embryo matures, so interactions tend to occur between adjacent cell populations, e.g. epithelium and mesenchyme, and later between adjacent differentiating tissues, e.g. between nerves and muscle, or muscle and skeletal elements. The interactions between adjacent epithelia and underlying connective tissue continue throughout embryonic and fetal life and extend into postnatal life. In the adult, these interactions also permit the metaplastic changes that tissue can undergo in response to local environmental conditions.

Tissue interactions result in changes or reorganization of one or both tissues, which would not occur in the absence of the tissue interactions. The process of tissue interaction is also called induction, i.e. one tissue is said to induce another. The ability of a tissue to respond to inductive signals is called competence, and denotes the ability of a cell population to develop in response to the environments present in the embryo at that particular stage. After a cell population has been induced to develop along a certain pathway, it will lose competence and become restricted. Once restricted, cells are set on a particular pathway of development; after a number of binary choices (further restrictions) they are said to be determined. Determined cells are programmed to follow a process of development that will lead to differentiation. The determined state is a heritable characteristic of cells, and is the final step in restriction. Once a cell has become determined, it will progress to a differentiated phenotype if the environmental factors are suitable.

The process of determination and differentiation within embryonic cell populations is reflected by the ability of these populations to produce specific proteins. Primary proteins (colloquially termed housekeeping proteins) are considered essential for cellular metabolism, whereas proteins synthesized as cells become determined; those specific to the state of determination are termed secondary proteins – for example, liver and kidney cells, but not muscle cells, produce arginase. Fully differentiated cells produce tertiary proteins, which no other cell line can synthesize, e.g. haemoglobin in erythrocytes.

As populations of cells become progressively determined, they can be described within a hierarchy of cellular development as transiently amplifying cells, progenitor cells, stem cells and terminally differentiated cells.

Transiently amplifying cells – are cells undergoing proliferative cell mitosis and producing equally determined cells. At some stage these cells will, as a result of an inductive stimulus, enter a quantal cycle that culminates in a quantal mitosis. This will result in an increase in the restriction of their progeny, which continue to undergo proliferative mitoses at a progressive level of determination. The quantal mitosis corresponds to the time of binary choice when the commitment of the progeny is different from that of the parent.

Progenitor cells – are already determined along a particular pathway. They may individually follow that differentiation pathway, or may proliferate and produce large numbers of similarly determined progenitor cells that subsequently differentiate. Examples of progenitor cells are neuroblasts or myoblasts.

Stem cells – are cells that individually, or as a population, can both produce determined progeny and reproduce themselves. It is generally believed that, whereas proliferative cells division may be symmetric, producing derived cells with identical determination, stem cells undergo asymmetric divisions, in which one daughter cell remains as a stem cell, while the other proceeds along a differentiation pathway.

Terminally differentiated cells – by virtue of their extreme specialization, can no longer divide, e.g. erythrocytes and neurones. Apoptosis is a particular variety of terminal differentiation in which the final outcome is the death of the individual cells or cell populations. It occurs in the developing limb, where cells die along the pre- and postaxial limits of the apical ectodermal ridge, and so limit its extent, and between the digits, and so permit their separation (p. 937).

Tissue interactions

There are two types of cell and tissue interaction, namely, permissive and instructive.

In a permissive interaction, a signal from an apposing tissue is necessary for the successful self-differentiation of the responding tissue. This means that a particular cell population (or the matrix molecules secreted by the cells that it contains) will maintain mitotic activity in an adjacent cell population. As a variety of different cell populations may permit a specific cell population to undergo mitosis and cell differentiation, no specific instruction or signal, which may limit the developmental options of the responding tissue, is involved. Thus this signal does not influence the developmental pathway selected and there is no restriction. The responding tissue has the intrinsic capacity to develop, and only needs appropriate environmental conditions in order to express this capacity. Permissive interactions often occur later in development, when a tissue, the fate of which has already been determined, is maintained and stabilized by another.

An instructive (directive) interaction (induction) changes the cell type of the responding tissue, which means that the cell population becomes restricted. Wessells (1977) proposed four general principles in most instructive interactions:

1 In the presence of tissue A, responding tissue B develops in a certain way
2 In the absence of tissue A, responding tissue B does not develop in that way
3 In the absence of tissue A, but in the presence of tissue C, tissue B does not develop in that way
4 In the presence of tissue A, a tissue D, which would normally develop differently, is changed to develop like B

Principles 1–4 are exemplified in induction of the lens vesicle by the optic cup (Ch. 43, p. 721). An example of principle 4 is the experimental association of chicken flank ectoderm with mouse mammary mesenchyme, which results in the morphogenesis of mammary-gland-like structures: chickens do not normally develop mammary glands.

Tissue interactions continue into adult life and are probably responsible for maintaining the functional heterogeneity of adult tissues and organs. For example, there is complex tissue heterogeneity, with sharply compartmentalized boundaries in the oral cavity. The junctions between the attached gingiva, the alveolar mucosa of the floor of the mouth and the lips, the vermilion border and the skin are all sharp and distinct boundaries of specific epithelial and mesenchymal differentiation, and are almost certainly maintained by continuing epithelial–mesenchymal interactions in adult life. Perturbation of these interactions throughout the body may underlie a wide variety of adult diseases, including susceptibility to cancer and proliferative disorders.

Signalling between embryonic cells and tissues
Cellular interactions may be signalled by four principle mechanisms: direct cell–cell contact; cell adhesion molecules and their receptors; extracellular matrix molecules and their receptors; growth factors and their receptors. Many of these mechanisms interact, and it is likely that combinations of them are involved in development. **Fig. 10.25** illustrates diagrammatically some ways by which mesenchymal cells could signal to epithelial cells. An additional set of identical mechanisms could operate for epithelial-to-mesenchymal signalling. Clearly, these mechanisms would increase in complexity, e.g. by reciprocal interactions, or by the divergent effects of a single molecule on epithelial and mesenchymal cells.

Direct cell–cell contact permits the construction of gap junctions, which are important for communication and transfer of information between cells. The transient production of gap junctions is seen as epithelial somites are formed, between neuroepithelial cells within rhombomeres, and in the tunica media of the outflow tract of the heart. Endogenous electrical fields are also believed to have a role in cell–cell communication. Such fields have been demonstrated in a range of amphibian embryos, and in vertebrate embryos during primitive streak ingression. Neuroepithelial cells are electrically coupled, regardless of their position relative to interrhombomeric boundaries.

Cell adhesion molecules (or cadherins) are a feature of epithelial populations. An early response of groups of cells to embryonic induction is the production of these molecules. The spatial and temporal distribution of a variety of cell adhesion molecules have been localized in the early embryo. Other molecules found in the extracellular matrix, e.g. fibronectin and laminin, *inter alia* can modulate cell adhesion by their degree of glycosylation. Self-assembly or cross-linking by matrix molecules may affect cell adhesiveness by increasing the availability of binding sites or by obscuring them.

Extracellular matrix molecules include localized molecules of the basal lamina, e.g. laminin, fibronectin, and much larger complex associations of collagen, glycosaminoglycans, proteoglycans and glycoproteins between the mesenchyme cells. Mutations of the genes that code for extracellular matrix molecules give rise to a number of congenital disorders: e.g. mutations in type I collagen produce osteogenesis imperfecta; mutations in type II collagen produce disorders of cartilage; mutations in fibrillin are associated with Marfan's syndrome.

Growth factors are distinguished from extracellular matrix molecules. They can be delivered to, and act upon, cells in a variety of ways: endocrine, autocrine, paracrine, intracrine, juxtacrine and matricrine (**Fig. 10.26**). Interestingly, many growth factors are secreted in a latent form, e.g. associated with a propeptide (latency-associated peptide) in the case of transforming growth factor β, or attached to a binding protein, in the case of insulin-like growth factors.

Morphogenesis and pattern formation
Morphogenesis may be described as the assumption of form by the whole, or part, of a developing embryo. As a term, it is used to denote the movement of cell populations and the changing shape of an embryo, particularly during early development. The most obvious examples of morphogenesis are the large migrations that occur during gastrulation; local examples include branching morphogenesis.

The development of branches from a tubular duct occur over a period of time. In this case, an interaction between the proliferating epithelium of the duct and its surrounding mesenchyme and extracellular matrix results in a series of clefts that produce a characteristic branching pattern (**Fig. 10.27**). During tubular and acinar development, hyaluronidase secreted by the underlying mesenchymal cells breaks down the basal lamina produced by the epithelial cells: this increases epithelial mitoses locally and results in an expanding acinus. Cleft formation is initiated by the mesenchyme, which produces collagen III fibrils within putative clefts. (If the collagen is removed, no clefts develop, whereas if excess collagen is not removed, supernumerary clefts appear.) The collagen acts to protect the basal lamina from the effects of the hyaluronidase, which means that the overlying epithelia have a locally reduced rate of mitosis. The region of rapid mitoses at the tip of the acinus is therefore split into two, and two branches develop from this point. This mechanism of branching morphogenesis is seen throughout the systems, from lungs to kidney, and includes most glandular organs.

Pattern formation concerns the processes whereby the individual members of a mass of cells, initially apparently homogeneous, follow a number of different avenues of differentiation which are precisely related to each other in an orderly manner in space and time. The patterns embraced by the term apply not only to regions of regular geometric order, e.g. the crystalline lens, but also to asymmetric structures such as the limb. For such a process to occur, individual cells must be informed of their position within the embryo, and utilize that information for appropriate differentiation. Patterning of regions is seen in: the progress zone and zone of polarizing activity within the limbs; the fates of the medial and lateral and later the cranial and caudal halves of the somites; the neural crest mesenchyme within the pharyngeal arches. For details of patterning in vertebrate development, see Tickle (2003).

Hox genes in development
Two related themes have emerged from experimental studies of development. First, that the control of embryonic morphology has been highly conserved in evolution between vertebrates and invertebrates, and second, that this control involves families of genes coding for proteins that act as transcriptional regulators.

The fruit fly, *Drosophila*, possesses eight homeotic genes that specify the structures developing on each body segment. These genes have been identified in vertebrates, raising the possibility that they have similar functions in development. They are termed homeobox genes, abbreviated to Hox in the mouse and HOX in humans, and are found on four clusters known as A, B, C and D. Individual genes are numbered from 1 to 13: 1 is a cephalic gene and 13 is a more caudally placed gene.

Homeobox genes are believed to be responsible, at least in part, for the evolutionary origin of the embryonic body plan (Robert 2001). Experimental study of transgenic animals in which the homeobox genes have been knocked out provide some evidence of their function: as developmental processes permit significant recovery from insult, some of the outcomes cannot be directly interpreted as demonstrating the effect of such gene loss.

Experimental approaches to embryology
One of the most exciting techniques to provide information on cell movements and fates during development is the use of chimeric embryos. Small portions of an embryo are excised and replaced with

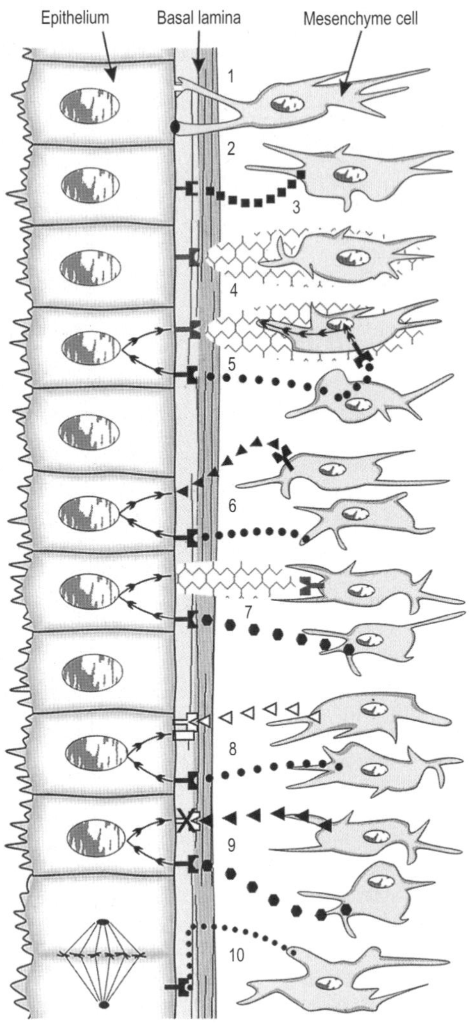

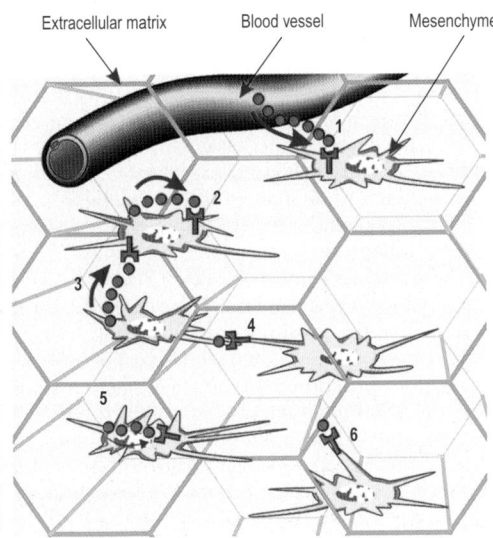

Fig. 10.25 The many ways by which mesenchyme cells could signal to epithelial cells. Precisely the same mechanisms can operate in reverse, i.e. epithelium to mesenchyme.

1   Direct cell–cell contact by gap junctions.

2   Cell–cell contact by cell adhesion molecules.

3   A soluble factor (growth factor) reacting with a receptor for that factor on the epithelial cells.

4   Extracellular matrix molecule secreted by the mesenchyme cells interacting with a receptor on the epithelial cell.

5   A soluble factor (growth factor) secreted by a mesenchymal cell having a biphasic action interacting (i) with a receptor on an epithelial cell, causing it to express a specific extracellular matrix molecule receptor; (ii) with a receptor on a mesenchyme cell, causing it to secrete a specific extracellular matrix molecule which then interacts with the induced epithelial receptor.

6   A soluble factor (growth factor) secreted by a mesenchyme cell interacting with a receptor on an epithelial cell, causing it to express a receptor, or secrete a factor, which interacts with another factor synthesized, or receptor expressed, by another mesenchyme cell.

7   A soluble factor secreted by a mesenchyme cell interacting with a receptor on an epithelial cell, causing it to synthesize an extracellular matrix molecule (or a receptor for such a molecule) which then interacts with a specific receptor for that molecule on another mesenchyme cell.

8   A soluble factor secreted from a mesenchyme cell interacting with a receptor on an epithelial cell, causing it to synthesize a molecule which stabilizes or enhances the interaction between a mesenchymal-derived factor and its epithelial receptor.

9   A soluble factor secreted by a mesenchyme cell interacting with a receptor on an epithelial cell, causing the inhibition of synthesis/assembly of a factor or receptor.

10 A soluble factor secreted by a mesenchyme cell binding to the extracellular matrix of the basal lamina, where it remains active and subsequently interacts with a receptor on an epithelial cell which appears at a later developmental time.

1   **Endocrine**   Delivery of growth factor by the bloodstream from a distant biosynthetic site to the target mesenchyme cell.

2   **Autocrine**   Synthesis of growth factor by the cell, its secretion, binding and activation of a surface receptor elsewhere on its own surface.

3   **Paracrine**   Synthesis of growth factor by the cell, its secretion and diffusion to an adjacent cell (or group of cells) where it binds to and activates a cell surface receptor.

4   **Juxtacrine**   Synthesis of growth factor by the cell. The growth factor remains on the cell surface and binds to and activates a receptor on an immediately adjacent cell.

5   **Intracrine**   Synthesis of growth factor within the cytoplasm of the cell. The growth factor moves to the nucleus and binds and activates its own nuclear receptors.

6   **Matricrine**   Synthesis and export of growth factor from the cell. The growth factor binds to the extracellular matrix where it remains active and subsequently binds to and activates a receptor for that growth factor on the same or a different cell.

Fig. 10.26 Cells can also communicate by the reception, production and secretion of growth factors. A typical embryonic mesenchyme cell could receive and produce growth factors in this way.

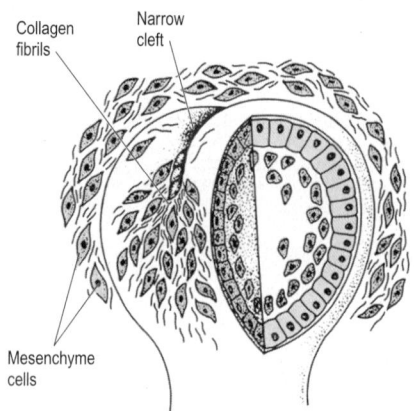

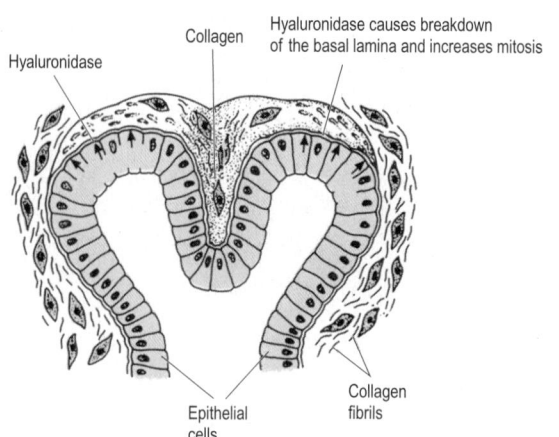

Fig. 10.27 Branching of a tubular duct may occur as a result of an interaction between the proliferating epithelium of the duct and its surrounding mesenchyme and extracellular matrix. Mesenchymal cells initiate cleft formation by producing collagen III fibrils locally within the development clefts and hyaluronidase over other parts of the epithelium. Collagen III prevents local degradation of the epithelial basal lamina by hyaluronidase and slows the rate of mitosis of the overlying epithelial cells. In regions where no collagen III is produced, hyaluronidase breaks down the epithelial basal lamina and locally increases epithelial mitoses, forming an expanded acinus. (From Gilbert SF 1991 Developmental Biology. Sunderland, MA: Sinauer Associates.)

similar portions of an embryo from a different species at the same stage. The resulting development is then studied. This technique has been particularly effective using chick and quail embryos, because the nucleolus is especially prominent in all quail cells, whereas it is not prominent in chick cells. This means that quail cells may be easily identified within a chick embryo after chimeric transplantation (Le Douarin 1969). Chimeric transplantation also confirms the reciprocity of tissue interaction between the embryonic species: this had previously been illustrated, for a limited period, in co-cultures of embryonic avian and mammalian tissues. Most recently, somite development and vertebral formation have been studied in mouse–chick chimeras (Fontaine-Pérus 2000).

SPECIFICATION OF THE BODY AXES AND THE BODY-PLAN STAGE

Embryos may be thought of as being constructed with three orthogonal spatial axes (cephalocaudal, dorsoventral and laterolateral), plus a temporal axis. In mammalian embryos, axes cannot be specified at very early stages. Embryonic axes can be defined only after the early extra-embryonic structures have been formed and the inner cell mass can be seen. The position of the future epiblast can be predicted in human embryos when the hollow blastocyst has formed. The inner cell mass becomes (seemingly) randomly located on the inside of the trophectoderm and forms a population of epiblast cells subjacent to the trophoblast. This region implants first. It is not known whether the trophectoderm in contact with the inner cell mass initiates implantation, so that the future dorsal surface of the embryo is closest to the disrupted maternal vessels at the implantation site, or whether the inner cell mass can travel around the inside of the trophoblast to gain a position subjacent to the implantation site once implantation has started.

Axes may be conferred on the whole embryonic disc, which is initially flat and mainly two-dimensional. However, their subsequent orientation in the folded three-dimensional embryo will be completely different. The dorsal structures of the folded embryo form from a circumscribed central ellipse of the early flat embryonic disc (**Fig. 10.17**). Lateral and ventral structures form from the remainder of the disc, and the peripheral edge of the disc eventually becomes constricted at the umbilicus (**Figs 10.20, 10.22**). Although the appearance of part of the epiblast is taken to specify the dorsal surface of the embryo, the inner layer – i.e. the hypoblast – is not by default a ventral embryonic structure.

The primary, cephalocaudal, axis is conferred by the appearance of the primitive streak in the bilaminar disc. The primitive streak patterns cells during ingression, and so also specifies the dorsoventral axis after embryonic folding. The position of ingression through the streak confers axial, medial or lateral characteristics on the forming mesenchyme cells. The axial and medial populations remain as dorsal structures in the

folded embryo, and the surface ectoderm above them will exhibit dorsal characteristics. The lateral plate mesenchyme will assume lateral and ventral positions after embryonic folding, and the surface ectoderm above this population will gain ventral characteristics.

The third and last spatial axis is the bilateral, or laterolateral axis, which appears as a consequence of the development of the former two axes. Initially, the right and left halves of the embryonic body are bilaterally symmetric. Lateral projections, the upper and lower limbs, develop in two places on each side of the body wall (somatopleure).

With the last axis established, the temporal modification of the original embryonic axes can be seen. The segmental arrangement of the cephalocaudal axis is very obvious in the early embryo and is retained in many structures in adult life. Similarly, dorsal embryonic structures remain dorsal and undergo relatively little change. However, structures that were originally midline and ventral, especially those derived from splanchnopleuric mesenchyme, e.g. the cardiovascular system and the gut, are subject to extensive shifts, and change from a bilaterally symmetric arrangement to an entire body that is now chiral, i.e. has distinct left and right sides.

The development of all the body systems, organogenesis, begins after the dramatic events of gastrulation, when the embryo has attained the body plan, or pharyngula, stage. In human embryos this corresponds to the end of stage 10 (**Fig. 10.23**). The head and tail folds are well formed, with enclosure of the foregut and hindgut (proenteron and metenteron), although the midgut (mesenteron) is only partly constricted from the yolk sac. The forebrain projection dominates the cranial end of the embryo, and the buccopharyngeal membrane and cardiac prominence are caudal and ventral to it. The cardiac prominence contains the transmedian pericardial cavity, which communicates dorsocaudally with right and left pericardioperitoneal canals. These pass dorsally to the transverse septum mesenchyme and open caudally into the extraembryonic coelom on each side of the midgut The intra-embryonic mesenchyme has begun to differentiate and the paraxial mesenchyme is being segmented into somites. Neural groove closure is progressing caudally, so that a neural tube is forming between the newly segmenting somites. Rostrally, the early brain regions, which have not yet fused, can be discerned. The neuroepithelium is separated from the dorsal aspect of the gut by the notochord. The earliest blood vessels have appeared, and a primitive tubular heart occupies the pericardium. The chorionic circulation is soon to be established, after which the embryo rapidly becomes completely dependent upon the maternal bloodstream for its requirements. The embryo is connected to the developing placenta by a mesenchymal connecting stalk in which the umbilical vessels develop. This stalk also contains a hindgut diverticulum, the allantois. The lateral body walls are still widely separated. The embryo has contact with three different vesicles: the amnion, which is in contact with the surface ectoderm, the yolk sac, which is in contact with the endoderm, and the chorionic cavity, containing the extra-embryonic coelom, which is in contact with the intraembryonic coelomic lining. The development of all body systems and regions that are described elsewhere in this book begins at this stage.

The early body plan of the embryo is segmented. The boundaries between the segments are maintained by the differential expression of genes and proteins that restrict cell migration in these regions. Organogenetic processes either retain the segmental plan (e.g. spinal nerves), or replace it locally (e.g. the modifications of somatic intersegmental vessels by the development of longitudinal anastomoses). Abnormalities may result from improper specification of segments along the cephalocaudal axis, in addition to failure to produce the appropriately modified segmental plan.

The degree to which vertebrate embryos are developmentally constrained at this period of development is controversial. Comparative studies on the timing at which specific embryonic structures appear, heterochrony, have shown that other embryonic species do not follow the same developmental sequence as humans (Richardson & Keuck 2002). Although some developmental mechanisms are highly conserved, e.g. the homeobox gene codes, others may have been dissociated and modified in different vertebrate species during evolution.

EMBRYONIC CELL POPULATIONS AT THE START OF ORGANOGENESIS

The developmental processes operating in the embryo between stages 5 and 9 enabled the construction of the bi- and trilaminar embryonic disc, the intraembryonic coelom and new proliferative epithelia. From the end of stage 10, a range of local epithelial and mesenchymal populations now interact to produce viscera and appendages. The inductive influences on these tissues and their repertoire of responses are very different from those seen at the onset of gastrulation. The range of tissues present at the body-plan stage, i.e. at the start of organogenesis, is given below. For a summary of the fates of the embryonic cell populations, see **Fig. 10.28**.

EPITHELIAL POPULATIONS IN THE EMBRYO AT THE BODY-PLAN STAGE

Surface ectoderm

During embryogenesis, the surface ectoderm shows regional differences in thickness. Ectoderm over the dorsal region of the head and trunk is thin, as is the pericardial covering; this has been interpreted as resulting from the expansion of this epithelium over structures that are enlarging rapidly as development proceeds. The ectoderm on the head and lateral borders of the embryo shows a zone of epithelial thickening, which has been termed the ectodermal ring; it seems likely that the thickened regions within the ectodermal ring are zones of ectoderm that will be involved in a number of epithelial–mesenchymal interactions. The ectodermal ring can be discerned from stage 10 and is completed by stage 12.

The most rostral region is the site of the adenohypophyseal placode, which later invaginates. From there, the ectodermal ring passes bilaterally and encompasses the olfactory and optic placodes, then the pharyngeal arches. The placodal cells of the lens and epibranchial placodes will move deep to the epithelium. The pharyngeal arches undergo developmental processes similar to those of the limbs, as the frontonasal, maxillary and mandibular primordia arise (p. 609). Local thickenings will later give rise to the teeth (p. 612). The ectodermal ring then passes over the occipital and cervicothoracic parts of the embryo, superficial to the four occipital somites and later to the occipito–cervical junction. Further caudally it is associated with the upper limb field, where it will give rise to the apical ectodermal ridge (p. 937). O'Rahilly and Muller (1985) have called the portion of the ring between the upper and lower limbs the intermembral part. It overlies the underlying intraembryonic coelom, and later (between stages 12 and 13), the mesonephric duct and ridge. In stages 14 and 15, this portion of the ectodermal ring gives rise to the mammary line (p. 973). Caudal to the lower limb field, in the unfolded embryo, the ring passes distal to the cloacal membrane. This region becomes superior to the cloacal membrane in the folded embryo and corresponds to the ectoderm associated with the external genitalia, particularly the genital tubercle and urogenital swellings (p. 1393). After the ectoderm has completed these early interactions it forms the periderm, which remains throughout fetal life and differentiates into epidermis (p. 170).

Neural ectoderm

The neuroepithelium at the time of primary neurulation is pseudostratified. It has a midline hinge region which, with concomitant wedging of the cells in the lateral wall of the neural groove, promotes neural tube formation (p. 241). The processes of the neuroepithelium abut onto internal and external limiting membranes. This epithelium proliferates to form all the cell lines of the central nervous system and, via the production of neural crest, all the cell lines of the peripheral nervous system. The ectodermal placodes may be considered to be neuroepithelial cells that remain within the surface ectoderm until central nervous system development has progressed sufficiently for their inclusion into sensory epithelia and cranial nerve ganglia (pp. 245, 246, 610, 679).

Notochord

During stage 10, the notochordal plate undergoes a process which is similar to, but a mirror image of, neurulation, and forms an epithelial tube from caudal to rostral, ending with the pharynx. The notochordal plate forms a deep groove, the vertical edges of the groove move medially and touch, and then the endodermal epithelium from each side fuses ventral to the notochord. The cells swell and develop an internal pressure (turgor) that confers rigidity on the notochord. The notochord is surrounded by a basal lamina, which is initially referred to as a perinotochordal sheath, but this term is subsequently applied to mesenchymal populations surrounding the notochord. After stage 11, the tubular notochord is in contact with the neural tube dorsally and the endoderm ventrally. It is not a proliferative epithelium, but it has inductive effects on the overlying neural tube, the adjacent somites and later provides a focus for sclerotomal migration.

Endoderm

The craniocaudal progression of development means that the endoderm of the early stomodeum develops ahead of other portions of the endodermal epithelium. The development of the pharyngeal arches and pouches (pp. 449, 617) is closely associated with the development of the neural epithelium and proliferation of the neural crest. The respiratory diverticulum arises slightly later when the postpharyngeal gut may also be distinguished (p. 1251). The endoderm gives rise to the epithelial lining of the respiratory and gastrointestinal tracts, the biliary system (p. 1378), and the bladder (p. 1392) and urethra (p. 1392).

Coelomic epithelium

The coelomic epithelium lines the intraembryonic coelom, which is subdivided into a midline pericardial cavity, two bilateral pericardioperitoneal canals, and the initially bilateral peritoneal cavities, which are continuous with the extraembryonic coelom. The coelomic epithelium is a germinal epithelium that produces the myocardium (p. 1029) and connective tissue populations for the viscera (p. 1251). It also gives rise to the supporting cells for the germ cells (pp. 1386, 1386), the epithelial lining of the urogenital tracts (p. 1382) and the mesothelial lining of the pericardial, pleural (p. 1092) and peritoneal cavities (p. 1261).

The relative dispositions of the neural epithelium, endodermal and coelomic epithelia are shown in **Fig. 10.23**.

MESENCHYMAL POPULATIONS IN THE EMBRYO AT THE BODY-PLAN STAGE

In the stage 10 embryo, the major mesenchymal populations are in place. Mesoblast is still being generated at the primitive streak and moving into the presomitic mesenchymal population adjacent to the notochord. Some mesoblast is also contributing to the lateral regions of the embryo. The different mesenchymal populations within the embryo from the body-plan stage onwards are given below. The relative dispositions of the early mesenchymal populations are shown in **Fig. 10.24**.

Axial mesenchyme

The first epiblast cells to ingress through the primitive streak form the endoderm and notochord. These cells initially occupy a midline position. The earliest endodermal cells form the prechordal plate (p. 194), but later the notochordal cells remain medially and the endodermal cells flatten and spread laterally. A population of cells that remain mesenchymal just rostral to the notochordal plate is termed prechordal mesenchyme (**Fig. 26.5**). These axial mesenchyme cells are tightly

Endoderm epithelium	Coelomic wall epithelium	Mesenchyme
Primitive gut	**Walls of intraembryonic coelom**	**Paraxial mesenchyme (somites and somitomeres)**
Foregut – recesses, diverticula and glands of the pharynx.	**Primitive pericardium** – myocardium, parietal pericardium.	*Sclerotome* – vertebrae and portions of the neurocranium, axial skeleton.
General mucous glandular and duct-lining cells and the main follicular cells of the thyroid.	**Pericardioperitoneal canals** – visceral, parietal and mediastinal pleura, pleuroperitoneal membranes contributing to diaphragm.	*Myotome* – all voluntary muscles of the head, trunk and limbs. *Dermatome* – dermis of skin over dorsal regions.
Epithelium of pharyngeal pouches (tonsil, middle ear cavity, thymus, parathyroids 3 and 4, C-cells of thyroid), adenoids, epithelial lining of the auditory tube, tympanic cavity, tympanic antrum, internal lamina of the tympanic membrane.	*Splanchnopleuric epithelium* – visceral peritoneum of stomach, peritoneum of lesser and greater omenta, falciform ligament, lienorenal and gastrosplenic ligaments.	**Intermediate mesenchyme** – connective tissue of gonads, mesonephric and metanephric nephrons, smooth muscle and connective tissues of the reproductive tracts. **Septum transversum** – epicardium, fibrous pericardium, portion of diaphragm, oesophageal mesentery, sinusoids of liver, tissue within lesser omentum and falciform ligament.
Respiratory tract – epithelial lining, secretory and duct-lining cells of the trachea, bronchi, bronchioles and alveolar sacs.	*Somatopleuric epithelium* – parietal peritoneum. **Primitive peritoneal cavity** Splanchnopleuric epithelium – visceral peritoneal covering of mid- and hindgut, the mesentery, transverse and sigmoid mesocolon.	**Lateral plate mesenchyme** *Splanchnopleuric layer* – smooth muscle and connective tissues of respiratory tract and associated glands.
Epithelial lining, secretory and duct-lining cells of the oesophagus, stomach and duodenum.		Smooth muscle and connective tissues of intestinal tract, associated glands and abdominal mesenteries.
Hepatocytes of liver, biliary tract, exocrine and endocrine cells of the pancreas.	Pronephros, epithelial lining of mesonephric ducts, was deferens, epididymis, seminal vesicles, ejaculatory duct, ureters, vesical trigone.	Smooth muscle and connective tissue of blood vessels (also see below). *Somatopleuric layer* – appendicular skeleton, connective tissue of limbs and trunk, including cartilage, ligaments and tendons.
Midgut – epithelial lining, glandular and duct-lining cells of the duodenum, jejunum, appendix, caecum, part of transverse colon.	Müllerian ducts, epithelial lining of uterine tubes, body and cervix of uterus, vagina, broad ligament of uterus.	Dermis of ventral body wall and limbs. Mesenchyme of external genitalia.
Hindgut – epithelial lining, glandular and duct-lining cells of part of the transverse, descending and sigmoid colon, rectum, upper part of anal canal.	Germinal epithelium of gonad (note the germ cells are not included on this chart because of their early sequestration into the extraembryonic tissues). Germinal epithelium forming cortex of suprarenal gland.	**Angiogenic mesenchyme** Endocardium of heart, endothelium of blood and lymphatic vessels, vessels of choroid plexus, sinusoids of liver and spleen, circulating blood cells, microglia, tissue macrophages.
Allantois – urinary bladder, vagina, urethra, secretory cells of the prostate and urethral glands.	*Somatopleuric epithelium* – parietal peritoneum, tunica vaginalis of testis.	

Surface ectoderm epithelium	Neural plate epithelium	Neural crest
Ectodermal placodes Adenohypophysis.	**CNS – Brain and spinal cord** Neurohypophysis.	**Neural derivatives** Sensory neurones of the cranial ganglia V, VII, VIII, IX, X.
Cranial sensory ganglia of nerves V, VII, VIII, IX, X.	Prosencephalon (telencephalon and diencephalon) – cerebral hemispheres, basal nuclei.	Sensory neurones of the spinal dorsal root ganglia and their peripheral sensory receptors.
Olfactory receptor cells and olfactory epithelium.	Mesencephalon – cerebral peduncles, tectum, tegmentum.	Satellite cells in all sensory ganglia. Sympathetic ganglia and plexuses: neurones and satellite cells.
Epithelial walls of the membranous labyrinth, the cochlear organ of Corti.	Rhombencephalon (metencephalon and myelencephalon) – cerebellum, pons, medulla oblongata.	Parasympathetic ganglia and plexuses: neurones and satellite cells.
Lens of the eye.		Enteric plexuses: neurones and glial cells.
Enamel organs of the teeth.	Spinal cord.	Schwann cells of all the peripheral nerves.
Cranial structures Secretory and duct-lining cells of the lacrimal nasal, labial, palatine, oral and salivary glands.	All cranial and spinal motor nerves.	Medulla of the suprarenal gland. Chromaffin cells. Carotid body type I cells (and type II, satellite type cells). Calcitonin-producing cells (C- cells).
Epithelia of the cornea and conjunctiva.	All CNS neurones, including preganglionic efferent neurones, with somata within the CNS.	Melanocytes.
Epithelial lining of the external acoustic meatus and external epithelium of the tympanic membrane.	Astrocytes and oligodendrocytes.	**Mesenchymal derivatives in the head** Frontal, parietal, squamous temporal, nasal, vomer, palatine bones, maxillae and mandible, etc.
Epithelial lining of the lacrimal canaliculi and nasolacrimal duct.	Ependyma lining the cerebral ventricles, aqueduct and central canal of brain and spinal cord, tanycytes, cells covering the choroid plexuses, circumventricular cells.	Meninges. Choroid and sclera of eye.
Epithelial lining of the paranasal sinuses, lips, cheeks, gums and palate.		Connective tissue of lacrimal, nasal, labial, palatine, oral and salivary glands.
Epidermal structures Most of the cutaneous epidermal cells, the secretory, duct-lining and myoepithelial cells of the sweat, sebaceous and mammary glands.	Retina and optic nerve (II), epithelium of the iris, ciliary body and processes.	Dentine of teeth. Connective tissues of head, including cartilage, ligaments and tendons.
Hair and nails.		Connective tissues of thyroid gland and of the pharyngeal pouches, i.e. parathyroid glands, thymus.
Proctodeal epithelium and epithelium of the terminal male urethra.		Tunica media of the outflow tract of the heart and the great vessels.

Fig. 10.28 Structures that will be derived from specific epithelial and mesenchymal populations in the early embryo. Abbreviation: CNS, central nervous system.

packed, unlike the more lateral paraxial cells, but are not contained in an extracellular sheath, unlike the notochord. They are displaced laterally at the time of head flexion and become associated with the local paraxial mesenchyme. Orthotopic grafting has demonstrated that these cells leave the edges of the prechordal mesenchyme and migrate laterally into the periocular mesenchyme, and that they give rise to all the extrinsic ocular muscles (p. 723).

Paraxial mesenchyme

Epiblast cells that migrate through the primitive node and rostral primitive streak during gastrulation form mesoblast cells which migrate to a position lateral to the notochord and beneath the developing neural plate. Cells that ingress through the primitive node form the medial part of this paraxial mesenchyme, and cells that ingress through the rostral streak form the lateral part (**Fig. 10.15**). The paraxial mesenchyme extends cranially from the primitive streak to the prechordal plate immediately rostral to the notochord. Before somite formation it is also termed presomitic or unsegmented mesenchyme in mammals (segmental plate in birds). Somitogenesis commences caudal to the otic vesicles on each side of the rhombencephalon, thus somites are postotic. Paraxial mesenchyme rostral to the otic vesicle was believed not to segment. However, the mesenchyme in this region shows concentric rings of cells bodies and processes that form paired, bilateral cylinders, termed somitomeres. These structures have been identified in a wide range of vertebrate embryos; they form the skeletal muscle in the head.

Caudal to the otic vesicle, the paraxial mesenchyme segments into somites as the neural folds elevate and neurulation commences (p. 789). During somitogenesis the mesenchyme cells show changes in shape, and in cell–cell adhesion, and become organized into epithelial somites. This begins at the eighth somitomere, which is just caudal to the midpoint of the notochordal plate. The first somite so formed is the first occipital. Somites can be seen on each side of the fusing neural tube in the human embryo from stage 9. As development proceeds in a craniocaudal direction, presomitic mesenchyme is a transient structure. It forms somites from its cranial end, whilst mesenchyme, patterned into somitomeres, is added to its caudal end by the regressing primitive streak. Somites give rise to the base of the skull (p. 123); the vertebral column and ribs (p. 123); and the skeletal muscle of the body, including that in the limbs (p. 938).

Septum transversum

Early mesenchyme that invaginates through the middle part of the primitive streak comes to lie rostral to the buccopharyngeal membrane, where the cells form the epithelial wall of the pericardial coelom. As this epithelium proliferates, the visceral pericardial wall gives rise to the myocardium (p. 1029). The parietal pericardial wall forms mesenchyme, initially termed precardiac, or cardiac, mesenchyme, which is able to induce proliferation of hepatic endodermal epithelium. With further proliferation, the mesenchyme forms a ventral mass caudal to the heart which separates the foregut endoderm from the pericardial coelom, and is called the septum transversum (**Fig. 10.24**). By stage 11 the septum transversum extends dorsally on each side of the developing gut, to become continuous with the mesenchymal populations proliferating from the walls of the pericardioperitoneal canals. Cells of the septum transversum give rise to the sinusoids of the liver (p. 1255), the central portions of the diaphragm (p. 1093) and the epicardium (p. 1029).

Lateral plate

Lateral plate is the term for the early unsegmented mesoblast population lateral to the paraxial mesenchyme. Mesoblastic cells, which arise from the middle of the primitive streak (primary mesenchyme), migrate cranially, laterally and caudally to their destinations, where they revert to epithelium and form a continuous layer that adheres to the ectoderm dorsally and the endoderm ventrally. The epithelium faces a new intra-embryonic cavity, the intraembryonic coelom, which becomes confluent with the extraembryonic coelom and provides a route for the circulation of coelomic fluid through the embryo. Cells in the epithelial coelomic wall thus formed proliferate and rapidly produce a thick layer of mesenchymal cells. The mesenchymal population subjacent to the ectoderm is termed somatopleuric mesenchyme, and is produced by the somatopleuric coelomic epithelium. The mesenchymal population surrounding the endoderm is termed splanchnopleuric mesenchyme, and is produced by the splanchnopleuric coelomic epithelium (**Fig. 10.24**).

It is important to note that these terms are relevant only caudal to the third pharyngeal arch. Rostral to this there is a sparse mesenchymal population between the pharynx and the surface ectoderm (before migration of the head neural crest), and there are no landmarks with which to demarcate lateral from paraxial mesenchyme. This unsplit lateral plate is believed to contribute to the cricoid and arytenoid cartilages, the tracheal rings and the associated connective tissue.

Somatopleuric mesenchyme – produces a mixed population of connective tissues and has a significant organizing effect opposite the limbs. The pattern of limb development is controlled by information contained in the somatopleuric mesenchyme. Regions of the limb are specified by interaction between the surface ectoderm (apical ectodermal ridge) and underlying somatopleuric mesenchyme; together these tissues form the progress zone of the limb (p. 937). The somatopleuric mesenchyme in the limb bud further specifies the postaxial border of the developing limb (p. 937). The somatopleuric mesenchyme thus gives rise to the connective tissue elements of the appendicular skeleton, including the pectoral and pelvic girdles and the bones and cartilage of the limbs and their associated ligaments and tendons. (Muscles of the limbs are derived from paraxially derived somitic precursor muscle cells.) Somatopleuric mesenchyme gives rise to the dermis of the skin of the ventral and lateral body walls and of the limbs.

Splanchnopleuric mesenchyme – surrounding the developing gut and respiratory tubes contributes connective tissue cells to the lamina propria and submucosa, and smooth muscle cells to the muscularis mucosae and muscularis externa. It has a patterning role in endodermal development. Splanchnopleuric mesenchyme specifies the region and villus type in the gut (p. 1251), and the branching pattern in the respiratory tract (p. 1088).

Intermediate mesenchyme

Intermediate mesenchyme is a loose collection of cells found between the somites and the lateral plate (**Fig. 10.24**). Its development is closely related to the progress of differentiation of the somites and the proliferating coelomic epithelium from which it is derived. Intermediate mesenchyme is not present before somitogenesis or the formation of the eighth somite. In embryos with eight to ten somites, it is present lateral to the sixth somite, but does not extend cranially. The mesenchyme cells are arranged as layers, one continuous with the dorsal side of the paraxial mesenchyme and the somatopleure, the other with the ventral side of the paraxial mesenchyme and the splanchnopleure.

As development proceeds, the intermediate mesenchyme forms a loosely packed dorsolateral cord of cells, which lengthens at the caudal end and ultimately joins the cloaca. It gives rise to the nephric system, gonads and reproductive ducts (pp. 1373, 1381).

Angioblastic mesenchyme

Mesoblastic cells give rise to the blood vascular and lymphatic systems of the embryo. They form the endothelial lining, smooth muscle coat and connective tissue adventitia (although the last of these may alternatively arise from splanchnopleuric mesenchyme). The vascular systems have to function precociously to fulfil the needs of the embryo, and also develop in preparation for independent life after birth. The early endothelial channels form complex anastomotic links, which may supply structures valuable to embryonic life, or develop along redundant phylogenetic lines until they are converted to vessels appropriate for later stages of development.

The specific origin of endothelium is proving very difficult to establish, in spite of the newer techniques of chimera production and immunocytochemical labelling. The extreme rapidity with which embryos are vascularized, and the associated constant modelling and remodelling of vessels that this involves, confound systematic study. Certainly, during vascular reorganization, the direction of blood flow in many vessels may reverse several times, so that it is difficult to determine which vessels are veins and which are arteries: vessels may be both. It is only after the tunica media has developed that histological criteria can be used to identify the status of vessels.

Numerous theories have supported the extraembryonic development of blood vessels. Blood islands appear in the yolk sac wall between the yolk sac endoderm and the extraembryonic mesoblast, and they fuse to provide the early yolk sac circulation. As vasculogenesis is seen in the body of an embryo only after the formation of extraembryonic blood islands, it was believed that all intraembryonic vessels were derived from extraembryonic yolk sac endothelial populations that grew into the embryo. This led to the conclusion that there were no angiogenic precursor cells within the embryo. However, recent evidence suggests a local origin for endothelia from the somites. Chimera experiments have demonstrated that angioblastic cells are highly invasive, and are able to migrate in every direction throughout embryonic mesenchymal tissues. They do not enter the neural epithelium, but form a plexus of endothelial capillaries around the brain.

The ultimate position of endothelial vessels is believed to be patterned, like other tissues, by the mesenchymal populations of neural crest in the head, somatopleuric mesenchyme in the limbs and splanchnopleuric mesenchyme around the viscera.

Neural crest

Neural crest cells arise from cells that lie initially at the outermost edges of the neural plate, between the presumptive epidermis and the neural tube. They are committed to a neural crest lineage before the neural plate begins to fold. The neural crest is unique because it appears after the formation of mesoblast from the primitive streak, as an additional and separate pool of mesenchyme cells in the embryo. It has only a transitory existence as a recognizable entity. It develops at the time of closure of the neural tube; however, soon afterwards, crest cells disperse, in some cases migrating over considerable distances, to a variety of different developmental fates. Unlike mesoblast, which is produced from the primitive streak, none of the cells that arise from the neural crest become arranged as epithelia. As both the development and fate of head and trunk neural crest cells are very different, they will be considered separately.

Trunk neural crest – is formed as the neural tube closes, initially in the cervical region, then proceeding caudally. Consequently, various stages of crest development can be found in the more caudal regions of an embryo. As the neural tube begins to fuse dorsally in the midline, the neural crest cells lose their epithelial characteristics and junctional connections. They form a band of loosely arranged mesenchyme cells immediately dorsal to the neural tube and beneath the ectoderm. Initially, most of the crest cells lie with their long axes perpendicular to the long axis of the neural tube. Later, the cell population expands laterally and around the neural tube as a sheet. Trunk neural crest cells migrate via three routes from their position dorsal to the neural tube (**Fig. 14.11**). They migrate dorsolaterally to form the dorsal root ganglia throughout the trunk (p. 252), ventrally to form sympathetic ganglia (p. 254), enteric nerves (p. 254) and the suprarenal medulla, and in a rostrocaudal direction along the aorta to form the preaortic ganglia (p. 314). In a second migration route, crest cells pass dorsolaterally between the ectoderm and the epithelial plate of the somite into the somatopleure, where they eventually form the skin melanocytes (p. 170).

Head neural crest – unlike that in the trunk, migrates before the neural tube closes. Two populations of crest cells develop. Some retain a neuronal lineage and contribute to the somatic sensory and parasympathetic ganglia in the head and neck (pp. 252, 254). Others produce extensive mesenchymal populations; indeed, the crest cell population arising from the head is larger than that found at any trunk level. Each brain region has its own crest population that migrates dorsolaterally around the sides of the neural tube to reach the ventral side of the head. Crest cells surround the prosencephalic and optic vesicles and occupy each of the pharyngeal arches (p. 447). They provide mesenchyme cells which will produce the connective tissue in parts of the neurocranium, and the viscerocranium (pp. 447, 447). All cartilage, bone, ligament, tendon, dermal components and glandular stroma in the head are derived from the head neural crest. Head neural crest also contributes to the tunica media of the aortic arch arteries.

START OF ORGANOGENESIS

Embryonic development has so far been considered holistically. However, this approach is less helpful as the embryo grows; indeed, it becomes so complicated that it impedes the clarity of appreciation of the events that occur. Although it is both conventional and convenient to consider the further development of systems on an individual basis, it should be remembered that thinking about the development of an entire organism in this way, however attractive on morphological and functional grounds, is largely a product of the sequential nature of human perception. Not only do the several systems into which we divide the organism develop simultaneously, they also interact and modify each other. This necessary interdependence is supported by the evidence of experimental embryology and reinforced by the phenomena of growth anomalies, which cut across the artificial boundaries of systems in most instances. For these reasons, it is recommended that the development of an individual system should be studied in relation to others, especially those most closely associated with it, whether spatiotemporally or causally.

REFERENCES

Fontaine-Pérus J 2000 Mouse–chick chimera: an experimental system for study of somite development. Curr Top Dev Biol 48: 269–300.
Earliest description of the experimental production of mouse–chick chimeras.

Langemeijer RATM 1976 Le coelome et son revêtement comme organoblasteme. Bull Ass Anat 60: 547–58.
Langemeijer conceptualizes a coelomic organ, an epithelium surrounding a cavity, which serves as the blastema for the development of the thoracic organs.

Le Douarin NM 1969 Particularités du noyau interphasique chez la Caille japonaise (Coturnix coturnix japonica). Utilisation de ces particularités comme 'marquage biologique' dans les recherches sur les interactions tissulaires et les migrations cellulaires au cours de l'ontogenèse. Bull Biol Fr Belg 103: 435–52.
Sets out the technique for the production of a quail–chick chimera.

O'Rahilly R, Muller F 1985 The origin of the ectodermal ring in staged human embryos of the first 5 weeks. Acta Anat 122: 145–57.
Describes and illustrates a zone of surface ectoderm that is involved in interactions with the underlying mesenchyme, apart from epidermal development.

O'Rahilly R, Muller F 1987 Developmental Stages in Human Embryos. Washington: Carnegie Institution.
Provides the most comprehensive and detailed morphological account of human development during the first 8 weeks of life. It sets out the basis for the staging system used for human embryos.

Richardson MK, Keuck G 2002 Haeckel's ABC of evolution and development. Biol Rev Camb Philos Soc 77: 495–528.
Discusses the limitations of the evolutionary recapitulation concept of development that was promoted in the early 20th century, and which still informs current thinking about embryological mechanisms.

Robert JS 2001 Interpreting the homeobox: metaphors of gene action and activation in development and evolution. Evol Dev 3: 287–95.
An analysis of the assumptions made about the homeobox and its role in development.

Streeter GL 1942 Developmental horizons in human embryos. Descriptions of age group XI, 13 to 20 somites, and age group XII, 21 to 29 somites. Contrib Embryol Carnegie Inst Washington 30: 211–45.
Streeter's works provide the baseline for all studies on human embryology at this time.

Tickle C 2003 Patterning in Vertebrate Development. Oxford: Oxford University Press.
Presents an overview of patterning and considers the patterning of the body plan, somites, the nervous system and the limb.

Wessells NK 1977 Tissue Interaction and Development. Menlo Park CA: Benjamin.

Prenatal and neonatal growth

PRENATAL STAGES

The absolute size of an embryo or fetus does not afford a reliable indication of either its true age or the stage of structural organization, even though graphs based on large numbers of observations have been constructed to provide averages. All such data suffer from the difficulty of equating dimensions and degree of differentiation with the actual time of conception, which can rarely, if ever, be established with complete exactness. The life of the individual really commences with fertilization, but this date cannot normally be established exactly in humans. It has long been customary to compute the age, whether in a normal birth or an abortion, from the first day of the last menstrual period of the mother but, as ovulation usually occurs near the fourteenth day of a menstrual cycle, this 'menstrual age' is an overestimate of about 2 weeks. Where a single coitus can be held to be responsible for conception, a 'coital age' can be established and the 'fertilization age' cannot be much less than this, because of the limited viability of both gametes. It is usually held that the difference may be several days, which is a highly significant interval in the earlier stages of embryonic development. Even if the time of ovulation and coitus were known in instances of spontaneous abortion, not only would some uncertainty still persist with regard to the time of fertilization, but there would also remain an indefinable period between the cessation of development and the actual recovery of the conceptus.

To overcome these difficulties, early embryos have been graded or classified, on the basis of both internal and external features, into developmental stages or 'horizons'. The studies of the Carnegie collection of embryos by Streeter (1942, 1945, 1948) and the continuation of this work by O'Rahilly and Muller (1987) to this day have provided, and continue to provide, a sound foundation for embryonic study and a means of comparing stages of human development with those of the animals used for experimental study: the chick, mouse and rat. Recent use of ultrasound for the examination of embryos and fetuses *in utero* has confirmed much of the staging data.

The development of a human from fertilization to birth is divided into two periods, embryonic and fetal. The embryonic period has been defined by Streeter as 8 weeks postfertilization, or 56 days. This timescale is divided into 23 Carnegie stages, a term introduced by O'Rahilly & Muller (1987) to replace developmental 'horizons'. The designation of stage is based on external and internal morphological criteria and not on length or age.

EMBRYONIC STAGES

Embryonic stages 1–10 are shown in detail in (**Fig. 10.12**). **Fig. 11.1** shows the external appearance of embryos from stage 6 to stage 23, with details of their size and age in days. Although the use of the stages is the most appropriate for comparative descriptions of development, only by constant study and usage do the stages come to be related to the morphological features of embryos. Therefore, in the earliest stages of development, external features are also used to describe the stage. This means that, in the earliest stages, somites are the main means of identification, and somite number conveys a means of distinguishing embryos. Once the number of somites is too great to count with accuracy, the number of pharyngeal arches present is often used. With the appearance of the limb buds, external staging becomes more obvious. The upper limb bud is clearly visible at stage 13, and by stage 16 the acquisition of a distal paddle on the upper limb bud is characteristic. At stage 18 the lower limb bud now has a distal paddle, whereas the upper limb bud has digit rays that are beginning to separate. By stage 23, the embryo has a head that is almost erect and rounded, and eyelids are beginning to form. The limbs look far more in proportion and fingers and toes are separate. At this stage the external genitalia are well developed, although they may not be sufficiently developed for the accurate determination of the sex.

The external characteristics of the embryo may be correlated with internal development. The stages of development reflect all aspects of morphogenetic change that occur within the embryo. **Fig. 11.2** shows the correlation between the external appearance of the embryo and the state of development of individual systems.

Historically, the onset of bone marrow formation in the humerus was adopted by Streeter as the conclusion of the embryonic and the beginning of the fetal period of prenatal life. The fetal period occupies the remainder of intrauterine life. In this phase of development growth is accentuated, although differentiative processes continue up to and beyond birth. Overall, the fetus increases in length from c.30 mm to 500 mm, and increases in weight from c.2–3 g to more than 3000 g.

FETAL STAGING

Whereas development of a human from fertilization to full term averages 266 days, or 9.5 lunar months (28 day units), staging of fetal development and growth is based on an estimate of the duration of a pregnancy. The commencement of gestation is traditionally determined clinically by counting the date from the last menstrual period. Estimated in this manner, it averages 280 days, or 10 lunar months (40 weeks). **Fig. 11.3** shows the embryonic timescale used in all descriptions of embryonic development and the obstetric timescale used to gauge the stage of pregnancy. Studies that discuss fetal development and the gestational age of neonates, particularly those born before 40 weeks' gestation, use the clinically estimated stages and age unless they specifically correct for this. If a fetal ageing system is used, it must be remembered that the age of the fetus may be 2 weeks more than a comparable fetus that has been aged from postovulatory days.

O'Rahilly and Muller (1999, 2000) recommend that the words 'gestation', 'gestational age' and 'gestational weeks' are ambiguous and should be avoided. They further recommend that the 'ageing' of fetuses by measuring crown–rump length is also unsatisfactory for a multitude of reasons, e.g. the two points used for this measurement either do not exist or may not be evident in young embryos, and their relative positions may change during development.

O'Rahilly and Muller (2000) recommend the use of greatest length, exclusive of lower limbs, as this measurement is similar to that routinely taken in ultrasound examination. O'Rahilly and Muller also recommend that the term 'crown–rump length' should be replaced by greatest length in ultrasound examination. They predict that, in future years, the confusion concerning prenatal age will disappear as ambiguous terminology is abandoned.

Although accurate morphological stages are not available for the fetal period, the developmental progression is broadly clear. During the fourth and fifth months, the fetus has a head and upper limbs that are still disproportionately large. The trunk and lower limbs begin to catch up by increased rates of growth during the remainder of uterine life, but the same disproportion is present after birth and, to a diminishing degree, throughout childhood and on into the years of puberty. A covering of primary hair, lanugo, appears and towards the end of this period sebaceous glands become active. The sebum that is secreted blends with desquamated epidermal cells to form a cheesy covering to the skin, the vernix caseosa, usually considered to protect the skin from maceration by the amniotic fluid. About this time the mother becomes conscious of fetal movement, which was formerly termed 'quickening'.

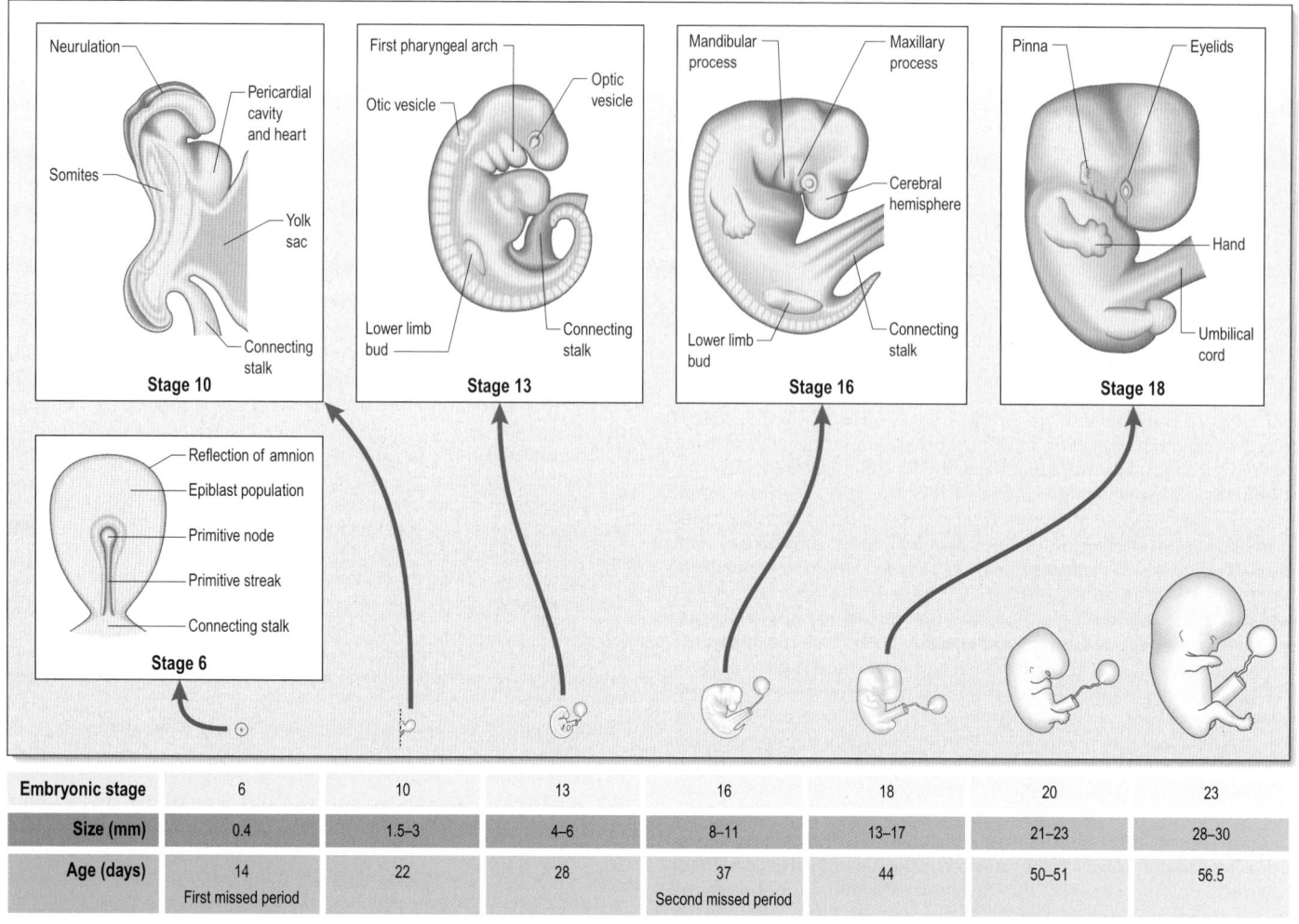

Fig. 11.1 The external appearance and size of embryos between stages 6 and 23. Early in development, external features are used to describe the stage, e.g. somites, pharyngeal arches or limb buds. (By permission from Rodeck CH, Whittle MJ 1999 Fetal Medicine. London: Churchill Livingstone.)

In the sixth month, the lanugo darkens, the vernix caseosa is more abundant and the skin becomes markedly wrinkled. The eyelids and eyebrows are now well developed. During the seventh month, the hair of the scalp is lengthening and the eyebrow hairs and the eyelashes are well developed. The eyelids themselves separate and the pupillary membrane disappears. The body becomes more plump and rounded in contour and the skin loses its wrinkled appearance as a result of the increased deposition of subcutaneous fat. Its length has increased to c.350 mm and it weighs c.1.5 kg. Towards the end of this month the fetus is viable, and if born prematurely is able to survive without the technological assistance found in Neonatal Intensive Case Units. The future postnatal development of such individuals can proceed normally.

Throughout the remaining lunar months of normal gestation, the covering of vernix caseosa is prominent. There is a progressive loss of lanugo, except for the hairs on the eyelids, eyebrows and scalp. The bodily shape is becoming more infantile but, despite some acceleration in its growth, the leg has not quite equalled the arm in length proportionally, even at the time of birth. The thorax broadens relative to the head, and the infra-umbilical abdominal wall shows a relative increase in area, so that the umbilicus gradually becomes more centrally situated. Average lengths and weights for the eighth, ninth and tenth months are 40, 45 and 50 cm and 2, 2.5 and 3–3.5 kg, respectively. The rate of growth of fetuses slows from c.36 to 40 weeks in response to the limiting influence of the maternal uterus. Birth weight thus reflects the maternal environment more than the genotype of the child. This slowing of the growth rate enables a genetically larger child developing within a small mother to be delivered successfully. After birth, the growth rate of the neonate picks up and, in weight, reaches a peak some 2 months postnatally.

Just before birth, the lanugo almost disappears, the umbilicus is central and the testes, which begin to descend with the processus vaginalis of peritoneum during the seventh month and are approaching the scrotum in the ninth month, are usually scrotal in position. The ovaries are not yet in their final position at birth: although they have attained their final relationship to the uterine folds, they are still above the level of the pelvic brim.

OBSTETRIC STAGES

In obstetric practice the duration of the period of gestation is regarded as nine calendar months, which is approximately 270 days. The period of pregnancy is divided into thirds, termed trimesters. The first and second trimesters each cover a period of 12 weeks, and the third trimester covers the period from 24 weeks to delivery. Although the expected date of delivery is computed at 40 weeks of pregnancy, the term of the pregnancy, i.e. its completion resulting in delivery, is considered normal between 37 and 42 weeks. Neonates delivered before 37 weeks are called preterm (or premature); those delivered after 42 weeks are postterm. The period immediately before, and up to 7 days after, birth is termed the perinatal period. It begins from the end of week 24, so that infants born from this stage of pregnancy are classed as stillborn and contribute to the statistics of perinatal mortality, if they die. In contrast, those fetuses which are delivered and die before this time are considered to be miscarriages of pregnancy. The technological advances in neonatal care can now assist the delivery and support of infants younger than 24 weeks. The neonatal period extends from birth to 28 days postnatally, and is divided into an early neonatal period from birth to 7 days, and a late neonatal period from 7 to 28 days.

THE NEONATE

Immediately after parturition the fetus, once it has been exposed to the environment external to the maternal uterus, becomes a neonate. In Western societies, technological advances have enabled successful

Fig. 11.2 Timetable of development of the body systems.

	Week 1	Week 2	Week 3	Week 4	Week 5	Week 6	Week 7	Week 8	Week 9	Week 10	Week 11	Week 12
Embryonic stages			7 8 9	10 11 12	13 14	15	16 17	18 19 20 21 22	23			
Length (mm)			2	5		10	15	20	30			55
External appearance			Head and tail folding	Pharyngeal arches		Upper lip / Palate	Digits on hand / External ear	Eyelids fuse				
Nervous			Neurulation / First neural crest cells	Otic vesicle / Optic cup		Anterior lobe pituitary	Posterior lobe pituitary / Membranous labyrinth					
Respiratory			Trachea	Lung buds / Primary bronchi			Further division of bronchi					
Gastrointestinal			Fore-mid-hind-gut	Thyroid / Liver / Urorectal septum	Pharyngeal pouches dorsal and ventral / Pancreas / Rotation of stomach		Midgut loop rotating					Midgut loop returns to abdomen
Urinary			Mesonephros / Mesonephric duct	Ureteric bud		Metanephric nephrons / Major calyces	Minor calyces	Kidneys ascend				
Reproductive			Germ cells in allantois wall	Indifferent gonad	Mullerian ducts / Testis differentiating / External genitalia indifferent			Uterus and uterine tubes / Vagina		Testis at inguinal canal / Prostate / External genitalia differentiating		
Cardiovascular			Primitive vascular system / Heart tube	Septum primum / Heart beats	Septation of ventricles / Spleen		Septum secondum					
Musculoskeletal			Somite period 20 days .... 30 days / Forelimb bud		Forelimb digit rays / Hindlimb bud	Cartilaginous part of skull		Membranous part of skull				

Fig. 11.2 Timetable of development of the body systems. The development of individual systems can be seen progressing from left to right. Embryonic stages, weeks of development and embryo length are shown. Embryonic stages are associated with external and internal morphological features rather than embryonic length. To identify the systems and organs at risk at any time of development, follow a vertical progression from top to bottom.

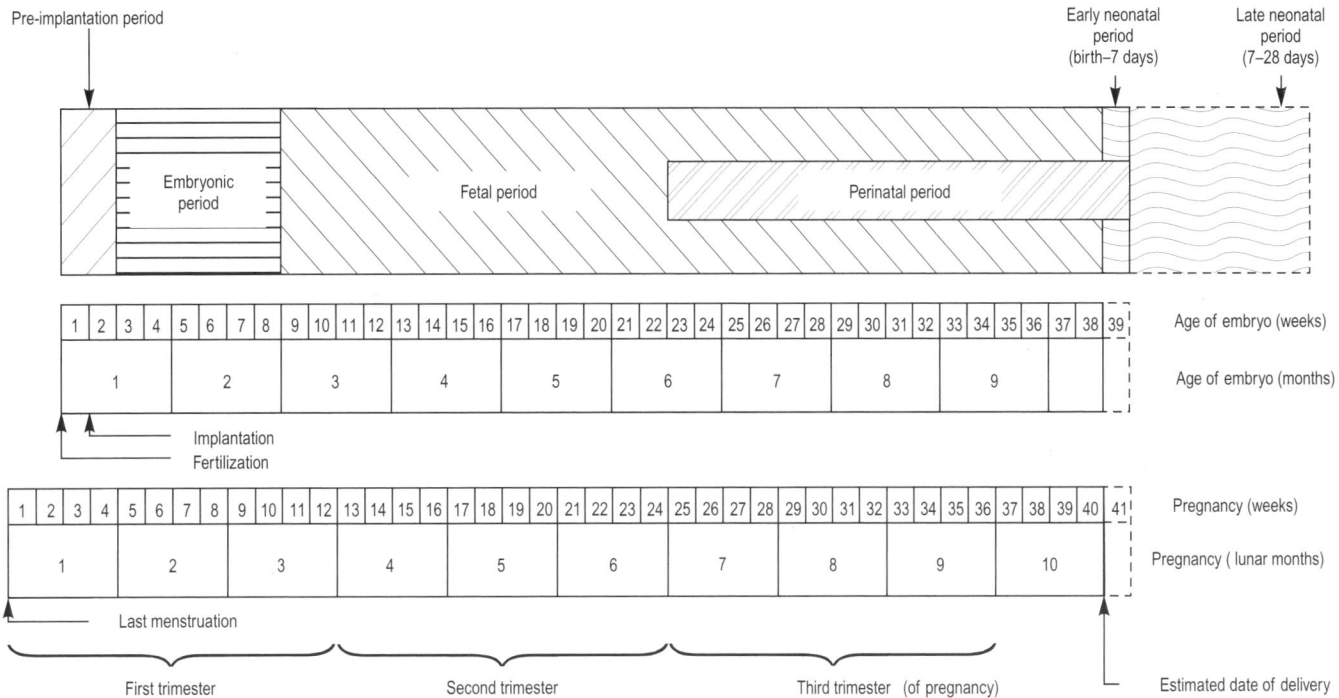

Fig. 11.3 The two timescales used to depict human development. Embryonic development, in the upper scale, is counted from fertilization (or from ovulation, i.e. in postovulatory days; see O'Rahilly & Muller 1987). Throughout this book, times given for development are based on this scale. The clinical estimation of pregnancy is counted from the last menstrual period and is shown on the lower scale; throughout this book, fetal ages relating to neonatal anatomy and growth will have been derived from the lower scale. Note that there is a 2 week discrepancy between these scales. The perinatal period is very long, because it includes all preterm deliveries.

213

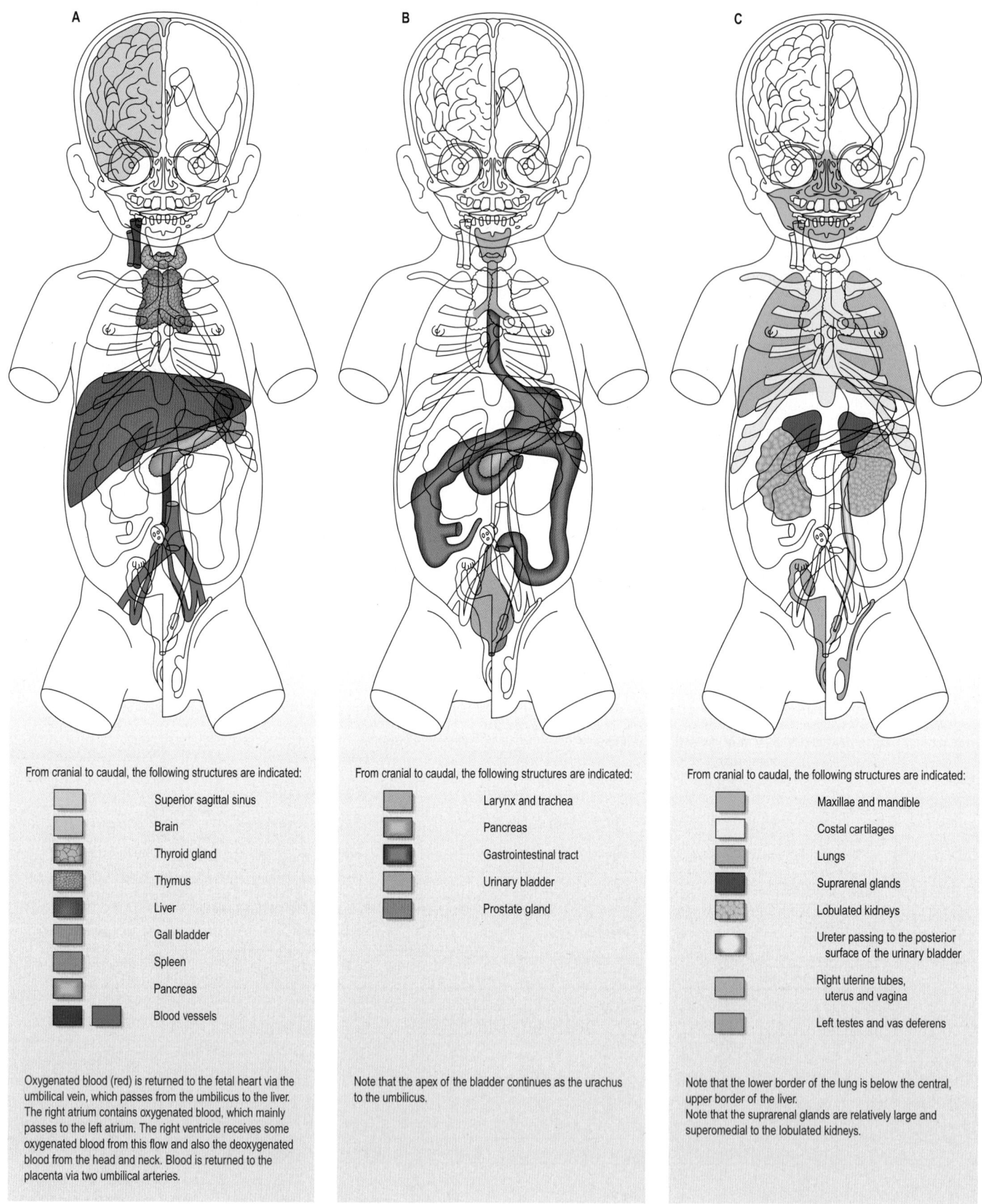

A

From cranial to caudal, the following structures are indicated:

Superior sagittal sinus

Brain

Thyroid gland

Thymus

Liver

Gall bladder

Spleen

Pancreas

Blood vessels

Oxygenated blood (red) is returned to the fetal heart via the umbilical vein, which passes from the umbilicus to the liver. The right atrium contains oxygenated blood, which mainly passes to the left atrium. The right ventricle receives some oxygenated blood from this flow and also the deoxygenated blood from the head and neck. Blood is returned to the placenta via two umbilical arteries.

B

From cranial to caudal, the following structures are indicated:

Larynx and trachea

Pancreas

Gastrointestinal tract

Urinary bladder

Prostate gland

Note that the apex of the bladder continues as the urachus to the umbilicus.

C

From cranial to caudal, the following structures are indicated:

Maxillae and mandible

Costal cartilages

Lungs

Suprarenal glands

Lobulated kidneys

Ureter passing to the posterior surface of the urinary bladder

Right uterine tubes, uterus and vagina

Left testes and vas deferens

Note that the lower border of the lung is below the central, upper border of the liver.
Note that the suprarenal glands are relatively large and superomedial to the lobulated kidneys.

Fig. 11.4 Topographical representation of the anatomy of a full-term neonate. The surface markings of all organs are shown, with some coloured and others only in outline. The female genital tract is shown on the right of the body in **C**, with the male tract on the left.

management of preterm infants, many at ages that were considered non-viable a decade or two previously. Now, the study of neonatology very much overlaps the later stages of fetal development. Preterm infants, although obviously past organogenetic processes, are still engaged in maturational processes with local interactions and pattern formation driving development at local and body-system levels. The sudden release of such fetuses into a gaseous environment, of variable temperature, with full gravity and a range of microorganisms promotes the rapid maturation of some systems and the compensatory growth, in terms of effect of gravity or enteral feeding or exposure to microorganisms, of others. To understand this multitude of mechanisms operating within a newly delivered fetus, as much information as possible concerning normal embryological and fetal development is required.

Details of the relative positions of the viscera and the skeleton in a full term neonate are shown in **Figs 11.4**, **11.5**, **11.6**. The newborn infant is not a miniature adult, and extremely preterm infants are not the same as full-term infants. Thus, just as there are immense differences in the relations of some structures between the full-term neonate, child and adult, so there are also major differences between the 20 week gestation fetus and the 40 week fetus, just before birth. The study of fetal anatomy at 20, 25, 30 and 35 weeks is vital for the investigative and life-saving procedures carried out on preterm infants today.

Neonatal measurements and period of time in utero

The 10th to 90th centile ranges for length of full-term neonates are c.48 cm to c.53 cm (**Fig. 11.7A**). Length of the newborn is measured from crown to heel. *In utero*, length has been estimated either from crown–rump length, i.e. the greatest distance between the vertex of the skull and the ischial tuberosities, with the fetus in the natural curved position, or from the greatest length exclusive of the lower limbs. Greatest length is independent of fixed points and thus much simpler to measure. It is generally taken to be the sitting height in postnatal life. This measurement is recommended by O'Rahilly and Muller (2000) as the standard in ultrasound examination. The 10th to 90th centile ranges for weight of the full-term infant at parturition ranges are c.2700 g to c.3800 g (**Fig. 11.7B**), the average being 3400 g; 75–80% of this weight is body water and a further 15–28% is composed of adipose tissue. After birth, there is a general decrease in the total body water, but a relative increase in intracellular fluid. Normally, the newborn loses c.10% of the birth weight by 3–4 days postnatally, because of loss of excess extracellular fluid and meconium. By 1 year, total body water makes up 60% of the body weight. Two populations of neonates are at particular risk, namely those who are preterm, and those who are small-for-dates, some of whom have suffered 'intrauterine growth restriction'.

Low birth weight has been defined as less than 2500 g, very low birth weight as less than 1500 g, and extremely low birth weight as less than 1000 g. Infants may weigh less than 2500 g but not be premature by gestational age. Measurement of the range of weights fetuses may attain before birth has led to the production of weight charts, which allow babies to be described according to how appropriate their birth weight is for their gestational age, e.g. small for gestational age, appropriate for gestational age and large for gestational age (**Fig. 11.8**). Small for gestational age infants, also termed 'small-for-dates', are often the outcome of intrauterine growth retardation. The causes of growth restriction are many and various and beyond the scope of this text.

For both premature and growth-retarded infants, an assessment of gestational age, which correlates closely with the stage of maturity, is desirable. Gestational age at birth is predicted by its proximity to the estimated date of delivery and the results of ultrasonographic examinations during pregnancy. It is currently assessed in the neonate by evaluation of a number of external physical and neuromuscular signs. Scoring of these signs results in a cumulative score of maturity that is usually within ± 2 weeks of the true age of the infant. The scoring scheme has been devised and improved over many years. For an account of methods of assessing gestational age in neonates, consult Gandy (1992).

GROWTH

Growth is a term widely used in everyday conversation and applied to both living and inanimate objects. It commonly implies an increase in mass or size. However, this definition is too simplistic in the context of examining the growth of the cells, tissues or organs that make up a

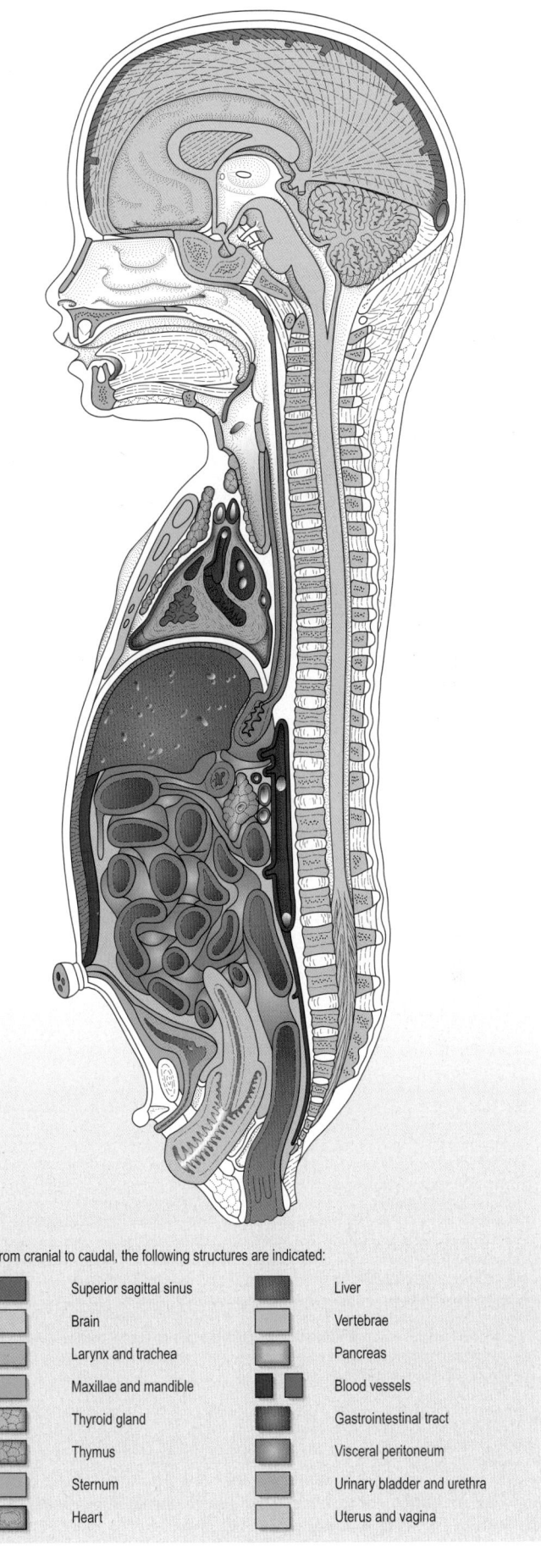

From cranial to caudal, the following structures are indicated:

	Superior sagittal sinus		Liver
	Brain		Vertebrae
	Larynx and trachea		Pancreas
	Maxillae and mandible		Blood vessels
	Thyroid gland		Gastrointestinal tract
	Thymus		Visceral peritoneum
	Sternum		Urinary bladder and urethra
	Heart		Uterus and vagina

Fig. 11.5 Topographical representation of the anatomy of a full-term female neonate. The cut surfaces of the organs are the same colours as in Fig. 11.4.

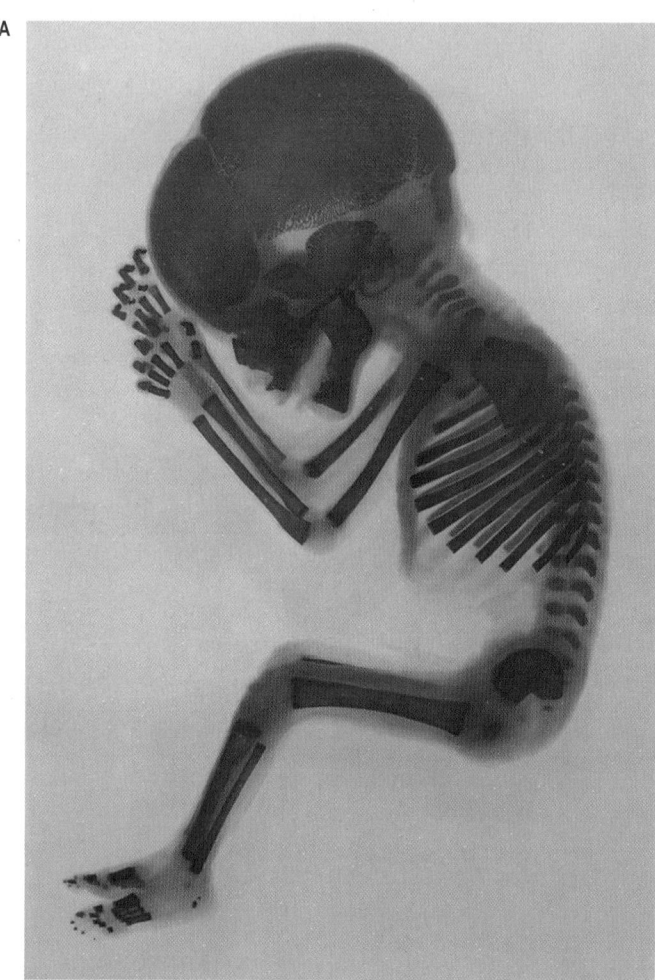

Fig. 11.6 A, Alizarin stained and cleared human fetus of c.14 weeks *in utero*. Note the degree of progression of ossification from primary centres, which is endochondral in the appendicular and axial skeletons, except for the clavicles, and the intramembranous centres for the majority of the cranial bones which are visible. The carpus and tarsus are wholly cartilaginous, except for the primary centre of the calcaneus, as are the epiphyses of all the long bones.The central and neural arches of the vertebrae are septate. The sternum is still unossified. The membranous anterolateral and posterolateral fontanelles are particularly obvious. **B**, The extent of the ossified skeleton in the full term neonate. Note the derivation of the parts of the skeleton: the skull is derived from paraxial mesenchyme and neural crest mesenchyme; the axial skeleton, vertebrae and ribs are derived from paraxial mesenchyme; skeletal elements in the limbs are derived from the somatopleuric mesenchyme, which forms the limb buds. (**A**, specimen prepared by Roslyn Holthouse; photograph by Kevin Fitzpatrick on behalf of GKT School of Medicine, London.)

Neural crest mesenchyme

Paraxial mesenchyme

Somatopleuric mesenchyme

whole animal. In order to appreciate the complex nature of the process, and the exquisite control mechanisms involved, it is necessary to distinguish between different types of growth

TYPES OF GROWTH

At the cellular level, distinctions can be made between cellular hyperplasia, i.e. protein and DNA synthesis that leads to an increase in cell number by mitotic division, and cellular hypertrophy, in which synthesis of protein and cellular material without mitotic division leads to an increase in cell size. At this level, growth may also be described with reference to the amount of extracellular matrix produced by the cells, which is termed accretionary growth, or by the position in which cells and extracellular matrix are added (either within a tissue or to its surface), which is termed appositional growth.

Cellular hyperplasia

Within the normal life cycle, hyperplasia or multiplicative growth is seen during the developmental stages of embryogenesis, organogenesis

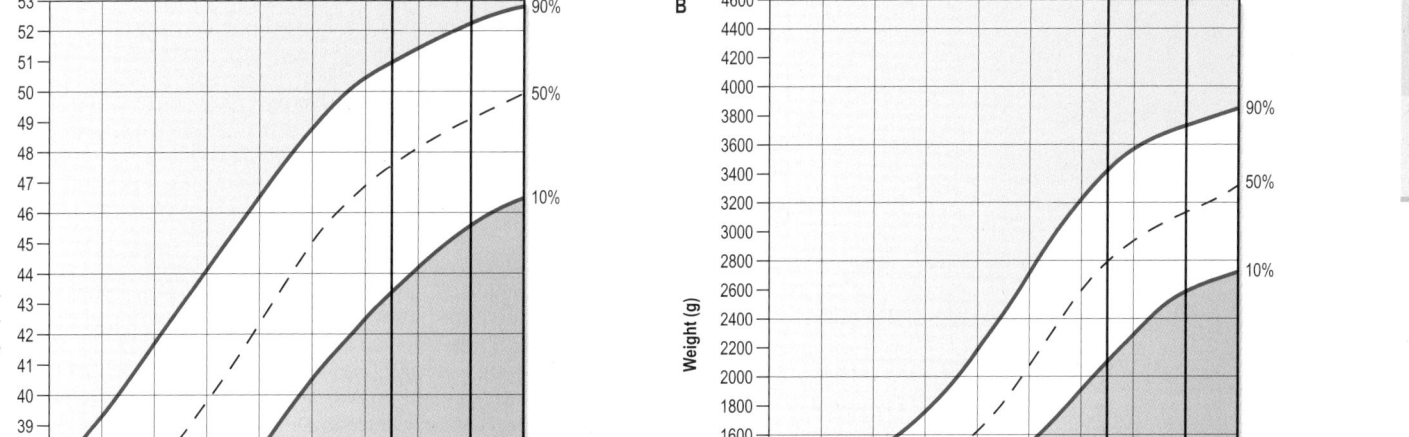

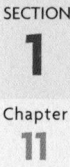

Fig. 11.7 Standardized graphs of (**A**) fetal length and (**B**) weight from 24 weeks of pregnancy, showing the 10th, 50th and 90th centiles.

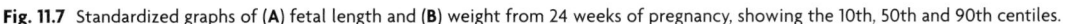

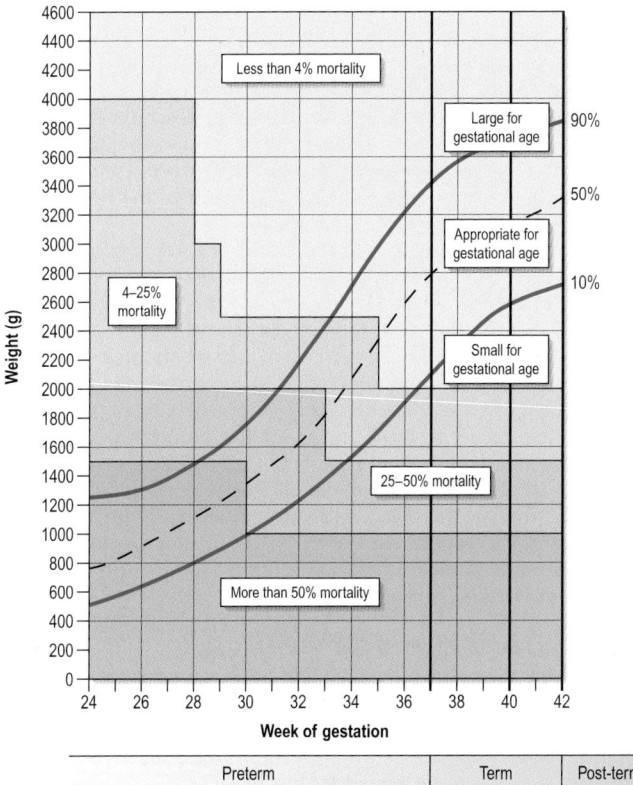

Fig. 11.8 Intrauterine growth status and its appropriateness for gestational age. Gestational age is more closely related to maturity than birth weight. The mortality for the weight ranges is indicated.

and growth *in utero*, and also in infancy and childhood. Generally, hyperplastic growth decreases as the individual approaches sexual maturity. However, each cell lineage normally remains in multiplicative growth for differing periods of time. Some cells, e.g. neurones, complete their mitotic proliferative phase *in utero*; other cells, e.g. type I alveolar epithelial cells, continue to divide during childhood; and yet others, e.g. stem cells for blood production, divide continuously for the lifetime of the individual (**Fig. 11.9**).

Cell division is controlled at two main levels, extrinsic and intrinsic, which may be correlated with the distance that effector substances have to travel to exert their effect. Extrinsic control of cell division depends on factors derived from other tissues (a hormonal effect), whereas intrinsic control depends on factors produced locally by the cells themselves (a paracrine effect).

Cellular hypertrophy

Hypertrophic or auxetic growth involves an increase in the size of the specific cells that characterize a tissue, without their division. It is usually seen in cells that can no longer undergo mitosis and is therefore mainly a feature of postnatal life. Obvious examples are the vast postnatal increase in both surface area and cytoplasmic volume in many neurones and glial cells, growing striated muscle fibres, oocytes, myelinating Schwann cells, and the smooth muscle cells of the pregnant uterus. The majority of tissues show limited hypertrophic growth. Sometimes, continued multiplicative growth is accompanied by a reduction in cell volume, e.g. granule cells of the cerebellar cortex, and small lymphocytes in lymphoid tissue.

It is widely held that the general nucleo:cytoplasmic ratio to which most of the cells of the body roughly approximate reflects the fixed quantity of DNA in their diploid nuclei, as this imposes a rate limitation on the replacement of cytoplasmic proteins, each of which has a characteristic turnover rate. Thus, with continuing auxetic growth, the cytoplasmic volume of a cell eventually reaches a point beyond which its structural genes cannot effectively replace the protein that is undergoing continual degradation. In some cases, growth ceases at this point, or nuclear replication with cell division occurs. The cases of hypertrophic growth cited above, however, often proceed far beyond the usual ratio of cytoplasmic volume to nuclear material and, in these cells, various

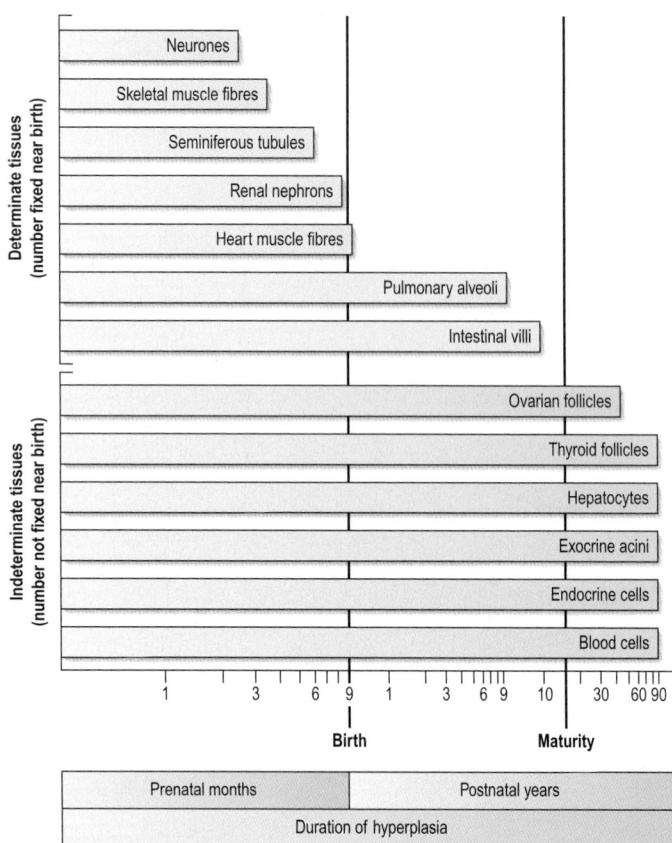

Fig. 11.9 The duration of multiplicative growth for various human tissues.

methods of providing auxiliary nuclear support have emerged. The striated muscle fibre and other 'giant' cells such as megakaryocytes are multinucleate syncytia. The enlarging oocyte and neurone, possessing but a single haploid and a single diploid nucleus, respectively, have their surfaces clothed by numerous satellite cells (follicular or glial cells, respectively). These satellite cells probably provide auxiliary metabolic and nuclear support for the enlarged central cell, i.e. the two are functionally interlocked as a cytophysiological unit.

Hypertrophic growth can be induced; for example, muscle fibres enlarge when exercised, and adipose cells enlarge with fat deposition in obesity.

Accretionary growth
Accretionary growth denotes an increase in the amount of extracellular matrix between tissue cells, rather than an increase in either cell number or cell size. Bone and cartilage are the most commonly cited examples. Other less obvious examples are the other fibrous connective tissues, tendons, joint capsules, aponeuroses, fasciae and the cornea.

Appositional growth
Appositional growth is a specific type of growth in which new generations of cells and extracellular matrix are added to the surface of the tissue by the repeated division of the cells of a cambial layer that surrounds the tissue, e.g. periosteum and perichondrium.

Interstitial growth
Interstitial growth is seen where multiplicative, and sometimes accretionary, growth continues throughout the thickness of a tissue mass, which consequently grows as a whole, and expands from within.

Meristematic growth
Meristematic growth describes growth from a tip that contains populations of dividing cells. As division occurs, the tip moves distally, leaving behind populations of cells from its earlier divisions. An example of meristematic growth is seen in the limb buds, in which the progress zone initially produces cells of the shoulder, and then is moved distally to produce populations of the arm, and so on.

Compensatory growth
Tissue and organ growth are normally under some sort of control. A balance is achieved between loss through 'wear and tear' and the maintenance of functional tissue integrity. Large-scale loss can be compensated for either through regeneration of the tissue itself, as in the liver, or by compensatory growth elsewhere, as occurs after the loss of one kidney. However, compensatory growth appears to be strictly regulated: once the regenerating liver has regained its approximate original size, growth ceases.

Integration of types of growth
In the later prenatal months and in the postnatal period, all the types of growth described above occur in various patterns, and with differential growth rates and directions in different regions. For example, in the developing limb the production of the mesenchymal populations occurs by meristematic growth, whereas the overlying ectoderm grows interstitially. Generally speaking, differential patterns of growth (with either random or preferentially polarized directions of mitotic division), together with alterations in cell size, shape and surface consistency, are central features of embryonic development. Collectively, they are responsible for the moulding of tissues into specific shapes, whether they are solid masses, hollow balls, tubes or sheets. Equally important in some regions is a process of tissue regression, which involves tissue degeneration, and cell death and removal.

PATTERNS OF GROWTH
In describing growth patterns of an entire body, two types of growth can be considered. These are isometric growth and allometric growth.

Isometric growth
True isometric growth would imply a progressive proportional increase in all organs and systems with time. Clearly, isometry does not occur in developing embryos, in which differential rates of growth obtain. This process is termed allometric growth.

Allometric growth
Allometric growth describes the differences in the relative rates of growth between one part of the body and another. It is most clearly seen in the changes in body proportion between fetuses, neonates, children and adults. Between 6 and 7 weeks after fertilization, the head is nearly one-half of the total embryonic length. Subsequently, the head grows proportionally more slowly, and at birth it is one-quarter of the entire length. During childhood, this pattern of growth continues with lengthening of the torso and limbs until, in adults, the head is one-eighth the length (**Fig. 11.10**).

Allometric growth can be considered to be responsible for the variation of the vertebrate body plan, especially in skull development in mammals. It has been suggested that a basic pattern for the base of the skull is specified by the basal layer of the neural tube (p. 493). The initial stimulus to chondrogenesis is provided by the neuroepithelial cells. The migration of the underlying mesenchymal cells is arrested, and the pattern of arrest forms the template for the base of the skull. In mammals there is some modification of the skull before birth, but generally the mammalian skull is globular, which assists passage along the birth canal. After birth, specific skull shapes develop by allometric growth, and produce the flat, neotenous human skull, the more prognathous skulls of lower primates, or the relatively extreme elongation of skulls in horses or anteaters. In humans, much of the postnatal growth of the skull is viscerocranial (**Fig. 34.9**).

GROWTH HORMONES AND GROWTH FACTORS
Growth during the embryonic, fetal and postnatal period is controlled by a variety of processes which are not yet understood. Postnatal growth is profoundly affected by the circulating concentrations of growth hormone (somatotropin), growth hormone releasing hormone and somatostatin. These hormones have not been shown to control fetal growth.

Growth hormones
Growth hormone can be detected in fetal serum by 100 days. The concentration increases in concentration up to 30 weeks but decreases in the last trimester, although the amount at birth is still increased compared with that of the mother. The concentration of growth hormone remains fairly constant from birth until the end of the first postnatal year.

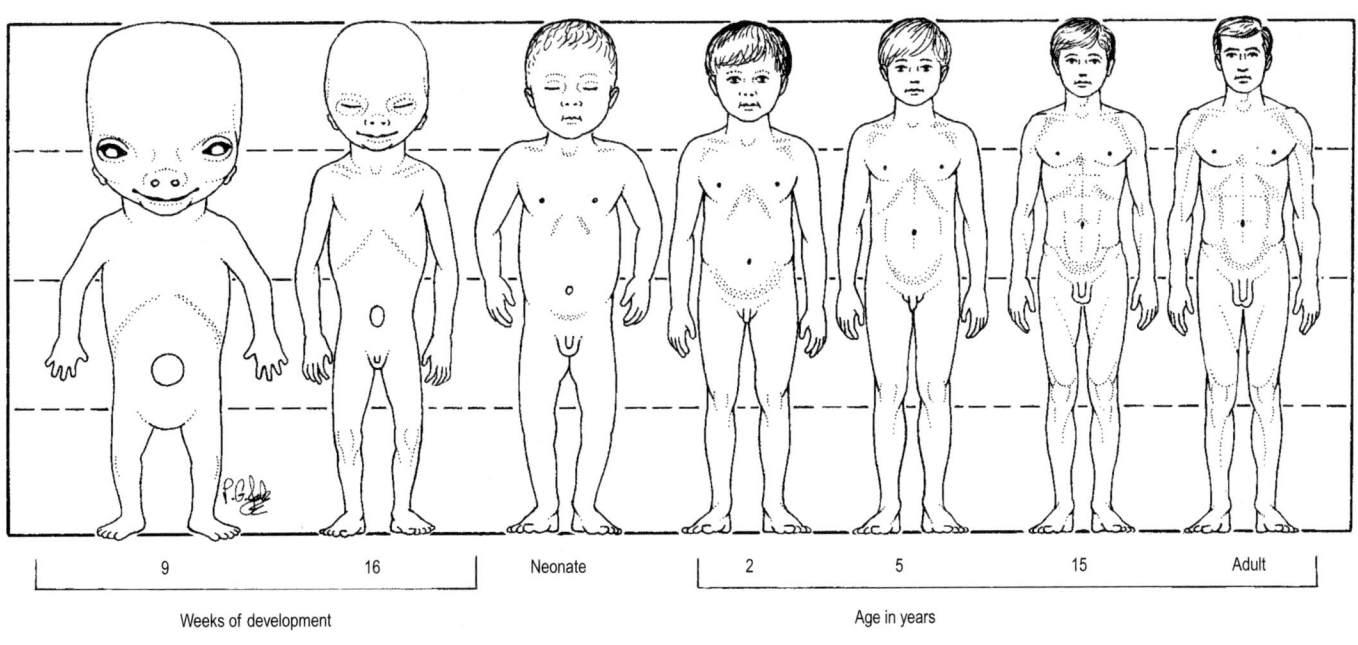

Fig. 11.10 Allometric growth in humans. The head is very large in proportion to the rest of the body during the embryonic period. After this time the head grows more slowly than the torso and limbs and by adulthood the head is only one-eighth of the body length.

9   16   Neonate   2   5   15   Adult

Weeks of development   Age in years

The role of growth hormone in the fetus is unclear. Because anencephalic babies and those with genetically determined growth hormone deficiencies attain lengths within normal limits, it has been assumed that fetal growth is independent of pituitary growth hormone. However, this may not be the case.

It is clear from epidemiological studies that growth hormone is necessary after the first 2–3 months, if not before. All tissues respond to growth hormone, and produce a proportional body growth that slows after puberty when secretion of the hormone decreases. The effects of growth hormone are seen particularly on the epiphyseal growth plates of the long bones. Continued secretion of growth hormone will result in gigantism, and lack of the hormone produces proportional dwarfism. In cases of acromegaly, in which growth hormone is abnormally secreted (after the epiphyseal growth plates have fused), the presenting symptoms develop over many years: there is enlargement of the heart and liver, thickening of the bones (especially the maxilla and mandible) and thickening of the skin. In this case, all the cells and tissues that are normally responsive to growth hormone continue proliferating after puberty.

Somatomedins: insulin-like growth factors

At the cellular level, growth hormone acts by stimulating the synthesis of somatomedin by the liver. Somatomedins are a family of insulin-like growth factors including insulin-like growth factor I (IGF-I or somatomedin C) and insulin-like growth factor II (IGF-II or somatomedin A).

In the human embryo, IGF-I concentrations are low. Administration of growth hormone does not affect growth at this time. IGF-II concentrations are increased in the fetus and are not influenced by growth hormone. Thus it is believed that the regulation of growth in the fetus is regulated mainly by IGF-II, which, in turn, may be controlled by placental lactogen. Because of its widespread expression in the embryo and fetus, IGF-II is believed to be the major paracrine growth factor *in vivo*, and a major determinant of fetal growth.

There is a positive correlation between birth weight and plasma concentrations of IGFs at delivery: decreased concentrations of IGFs are observed in children who are small-for-dates. The concentrations of growth hormone, IGF-I and IGF-II increase during the growth spurt of adolescence.

Other growth factors

Platelet-derived growth factor stimulates division of fibroblasts, smooth muscle and glioblasts. Epidermal growth factor promotes division in, *inter alia*, epidermis, mammary gland epithelium and skeletal muscle.

A wide range of growth factors are secreted in breast milk. Epidermal growth factor is the major growth factor in human milk (cow's milk does not contain this factor). Human milk contains low concentrations of insulin: IGF-I concentrations are 10% of those in normal human serum. The concentrations of these growth factors change during lactation. They are maximal in day 1 colostrum and decline during the first week, to reach a plateau at which concentrations of epidermal growth factor and insulin are 10% of their concentrations in colostrum. The total growth factor delivery to the baby remains nearly constant throughout lactation. As endogenous production of epidermal growth factor is undetectable in the neonatal period, human milk may provide the only source for the baby. However, neonates maintained entirely on artificial formulae develop at apparently normal rates, and so it seems unlikely that growth factors in milk are essential requirements for normal growth.

GROWTH IN UTERO

Poor nutrition at critical stages of fetal life may permanently alter the normal developmental pattern of a range of organs and tissues, e.g. the endocrine pancreas, liver and blood vessels, and this results in their pathological responses to certain conditions in later adult life (Barker et al 1993). An increase in placental size occurs in pregnancy as an adaptive response to both high altitude and mild undernutrition, particularly during midpregnancy. However, although a larger placenta may be better able to deliver the full nutritional requirements of the fetus, the perfusion of a larger placenta is not without problems. It may produce changes in fetal blood flow and placental enzymes, and in the normal structure of the fetal vessel wall or of its responses to circulating trophins, e.g. catecholamines or angiotensin II, which will continue into adult life. Undernutrition in later pregnancy does not produce the same sequelae and placental enlargement does not occur. However, fetal growth slows and fetal wasting may occur as oxygen, glucose and aminoacids are redistributed to the placenta to maintain its function.

Maternal starvation during pregnancy decreases fetal IGF-I concentrations, which may, along with a general hypoglycaemia, impair the development of the fetal β cells of the pancreas. Generally, fetal undernutrition may induce insulin resistance in the tissues. The coexistence of insulin resistance and impaired β-cell development in the fetus appears to be important in the pathogenesis of non-insulin-dependent diabetes. The risk of developing this 'type 2' diabetes is greatest in those individuals with low weight at birth and at 1 year, and who become obese as adults, thus challenging an already impaired glucose–insulin metabolism. Fetal IGF-I concentrations are also lower in infants who are short at birth as a result of a long period of maternal undernutrition. These individuals have exaggerated responses to growth

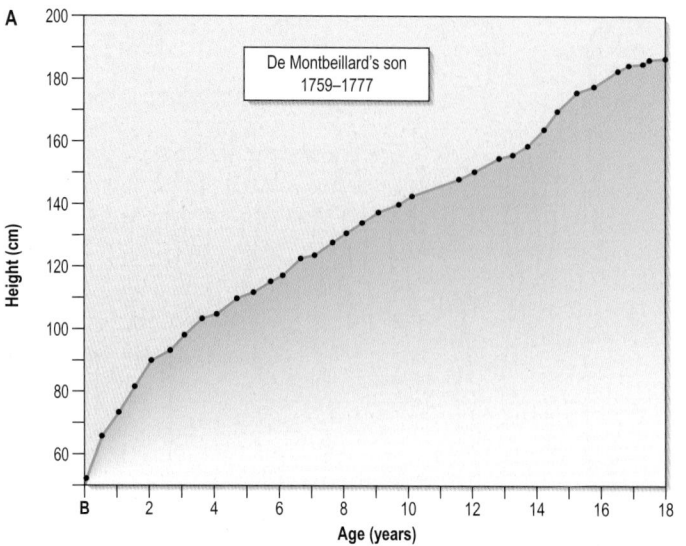
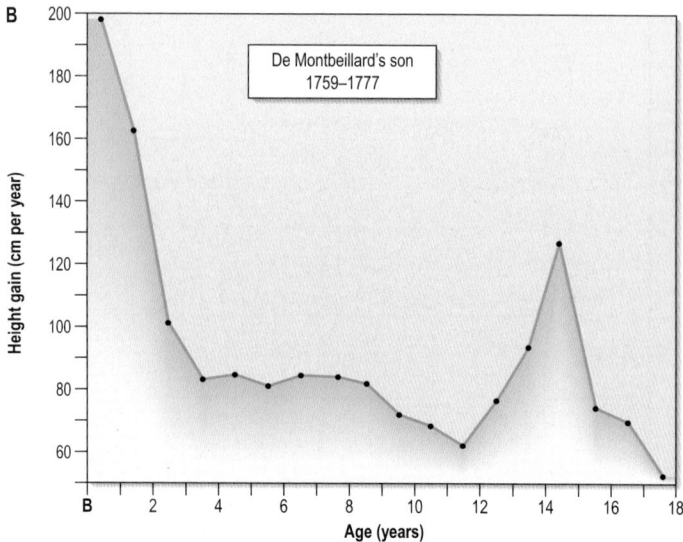

Fig. 11.11 A longitudinal study of growth. **A**, The height of de Montbeillard's son (1759–1777) from birth to 18 years. **B**, A growth velocity curve, plotting increments in height from year to year. (After D'Arcy Thompson, On Growth and Form, 1942, Cambridge University Press.)

hormone-releasing factor, which, together with low IGF-I concentrations, suggests a degree of growth hormone resistance.

Different birth phenotypes have been correlated with different pathological sequelae. Infants who are thin at birth, with a low ponderal index (weight/length^3), tend to develop a combination of insulin resistance, hypertension, non-insulin-dependent diabetes and lipid disorders, whereas those who are short in relation to head size tend to develop hypertension and high plasma fibrinogen concentrations (Barker et al 1993). These associations occurred in babies born small for dates, rather than in those born prematurely. However, some babies of average weight also developed later cardiovascular pathology. They were either small at birth in relation to the size of their placenta, and thin at birth or, although of average weight, were short in relation to head size and had below-average weight gain during the first year.

In summary, it appears that alterations in the availability of nutrients to the fetus at particular stages of pregnancy cause adaptive responses by the fetus that ensure fetal coping, but which lead on to pathology in adult life when different conditions operate. The implications of these findings is that the nutritional status of pregnant women is of fundamental importance for the health of the next generation.

GROWTH IN CHILDHOOD

The rates of prenatal and postnatal growth can be indicated by increments in body length or weight which, when plotted, form a growth curve (**Fig. 11.7**). Growth curves can be plotted for individuals if accurate measurements are taken, preferably by the same person, for the entire period of growth, i.e. a longitudinal study. An alternative method is to collect a series of averages for each year of age obtained from different individuals, i.e. a cross-sectional study. Cross-sectional studies are valuable for the construction of standards for height and weight attained by healthy children at specific ages, and can establish percentile limits of normal growth, but they cannot reveal individual differences in either the rate of growth or the timing of particular phases of growth.

The data from longitudinal and cross-sectional studies can also be used to plot the increments in height or weight from one age to the next. This produces a velocity curve, which reflects a child's state at any particular time much better than the growth curve, in which each point is dependent on the preceding one. The oldest published longitudinal study, still of great value today, was made by Count Philibert de Montbeillard on his son (**Fig. 11.11**). It shows that the velocity of growth in height decreases from birth onwards, with a marked acceleration of growth from 13 to 15 years – the adolescent growth spurt.

Cross-sectional data have enabled comparison of prenatal and postnatal growth. Childhood growth charts are used to predict normal childhood development. The velocity curve for the prenatal and postnatal period (**Fig. 11.12**) shows that the peak velocity for length is reached at c.4 months (note that these prenatal charts use the obstetric measurements of gestational time, in which fetal age is estimated from the last

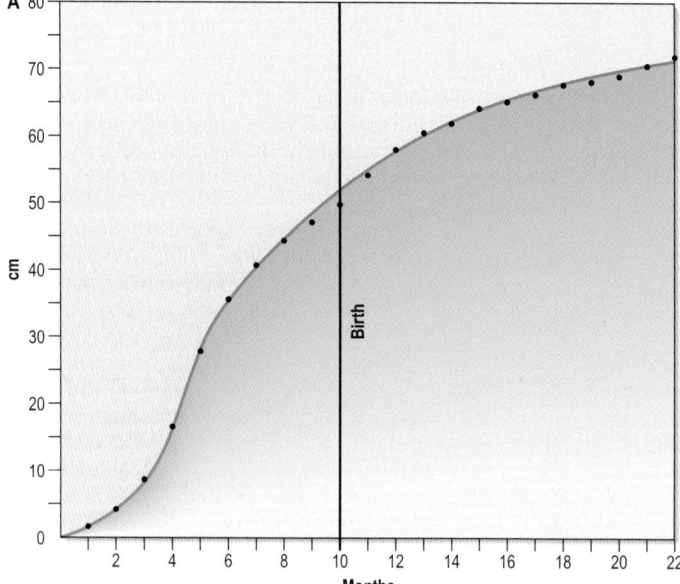

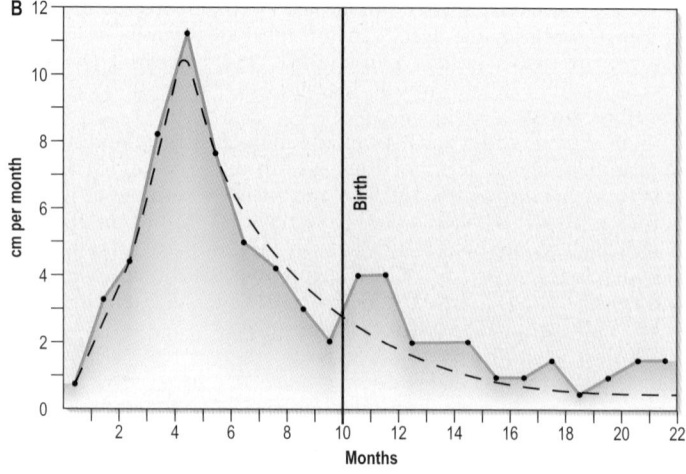

Fig. 11.12 Cross-sectional data showing growth in length in the prenatal and early postnatal period (**A**) and the corresponding velocity curve for this period (**B**). (After D'Arcy Thompson, On Growth and Form, 1942, Cambridge University Press.)

menstrual period, 2 weeks before fertilization). Growth in weight usually reaches its peak velocity after birth.

Growth has always been regarded as a regular process. Tanner (in Harrison et al 1964) stated that growth does not proceed in fits and starts, and noted that, the more carefully the measurements are taken, the more regular is the succession of points on a growth curve. However, a longitudinal study of growth measured weekly, semi-weekly and daily (Lampl 2002), recorded that growth in length and head circumference occurred by saltatory increments, with a mean amplitude of 1.01 cm for length.

Charts of height and weight correlated to age are compiled from extensive cross-sectional growth studies. Such charts show the mean height or weight attained at each age, termed the 50th centile, and also the centile lines for the 75th, 90th and 97th centiles, in addition to the 25th, 9th and 2nd centiles. The data shown in **Fig. 11.13** are derived from United Kingdom cross-sectional references. Any comparison of an

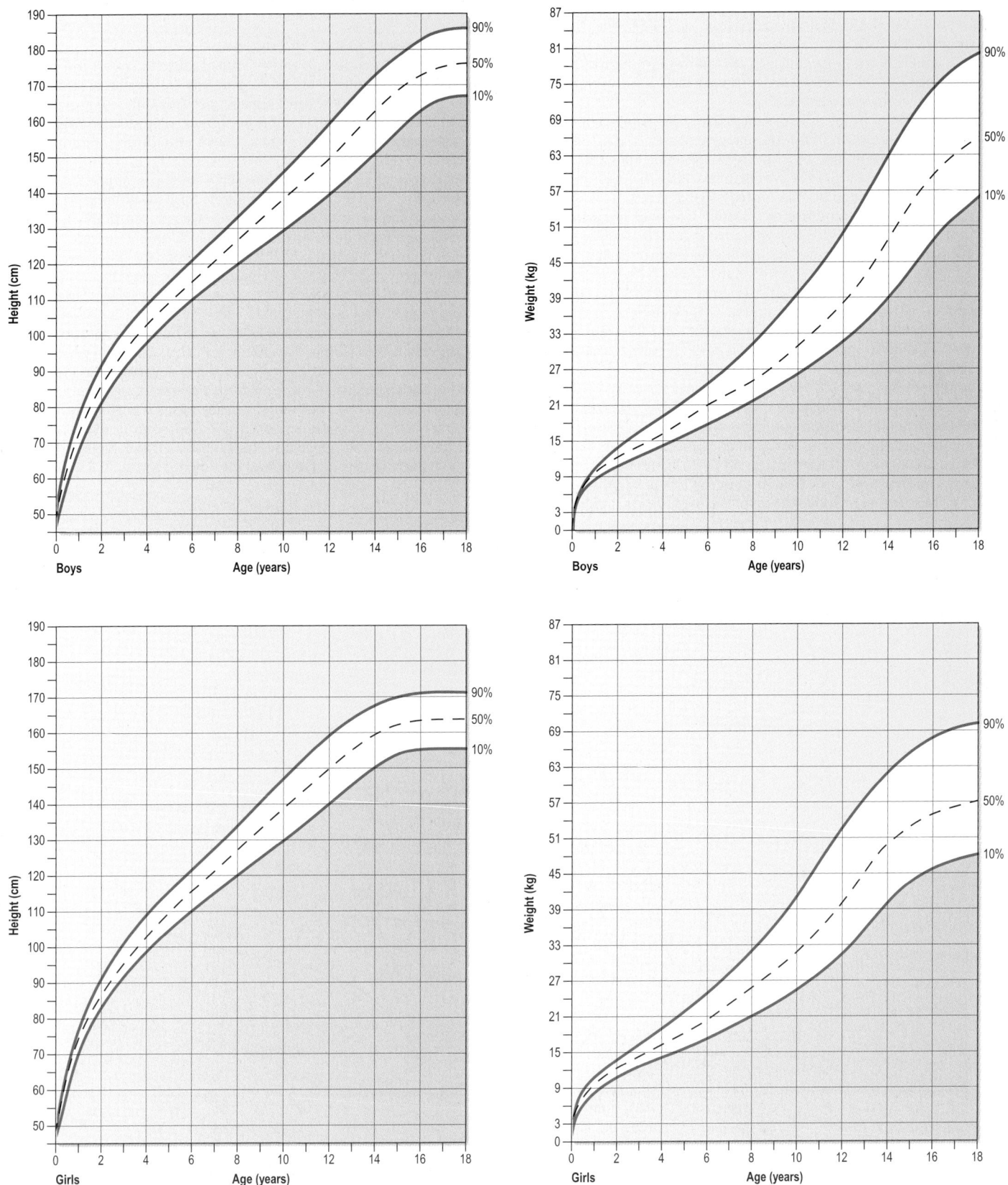

Fig. 11.13 Standard growth charts of boys and girls showing the 90th, 50th and 10th centiles. (© Child Growth Foundation.)

individual growth curve with these data should also take into account ethnicity and the nutritional and family history of an individual.

Adolescent growth spurt

Growth charts reveal that body length increases from a neonatal range of 48–53 cm to about 75 cm during the first year after birth, and increases by 12–13 cm in the second year. Thereafter, 5–6 cm is added each year. In individual longitudinal growth curves, an increase in the velocity of growth occurs between 10.5 and 11 years in girls, and 12.5 and 13 years in boys. This rapid increase in growth is termed the adolescent growth spurt (**Figs 11.13, 11.14**). In both sexes it lasts for 2–2.5 years. Girls gain c.16 cm in height during the spurt, with a peak velocity at 12 years of age. Boys gain c.20 cm in height (mostly by growth of the trunk), with a peak velocity at 14 years of age, during which time they may be growing at the rate of 10 cm a year.

Humans seem to be the only species to have a long quiescent interval between the rapid growth that takes place immediately after birth and the adolescent growth spurt. It has been suggested that this period allows the brain to mature, and learning to take place, before individuals pass through puberty and become sexually active.

Growth in height continues at a slower rate after the adolescent growth spurt. Noticeable growth is said to stop at c.18 years in females and 20 years in males (longitudinal studies have indicated that an average figure for this is 16.25 years for girls and 17.75 years for boys, with a normal variation of ± 2 years (Harrison et al 1964). After this time, any increments that occur as a result of appositional growth at the cranial and caudal ends of the vertebral bodies and intervening intervertebral discs are so small as to be difficult to measure. There is a loss of height after middle age.

The phenomenal growth rates of adolescence are most obvious in the increase in height. Weight gain is more variable. At birth, weight reflects the maternal environment, the number of conceptuses, the sex of the baby and the parity of the mother. Generally, full-term female babies are lighter than full-term males, twins are lighter than singletons, and later children tend to be heavier than the first-born. Although the birth weight seems to be independent of the maternal diet, unless there

has been severe malnutrition, mothers in a low socioeconomic group have smaller babies than those with a higher rating, and small mothers tend to have small babies.

The birth weight is normally tripled by the end of the first year, and quadrupled by the end of the second year. Thereafter, weight increases by 2.25–2.75 kg annually until the adolescent growth spurt, when boys may add 20 kg to their weight and girls 16 kg. The peak velocity for weight gain lags behind the peak velocity for height by about 3 months. Body weight does not reach adult values until some time after adult height is attained.

Growth rates of tissues and organs

Although the dimensions of organs such as the liver, spleen and kidneys, and skeletal and muscular tissues generally follow the growth curves given for the entire body, other tissues have very different growth rates. Thus the brain and skull, lymphoid tissues, reproductive organs and subcutaneous fat all show differing growth rates during childhood and adolescence (**Fig. 11.15**).

Subcutaneous fat deposits are measured by calipers applied to a fold of fat pinched up from the underlying muscles. Such measurements are taken over triceps and beneath the angle of the scapula. Fat begins to be laid down in the fetus from c.34 weeks, after which time it increases to birth, and from birth to 9 months. After 9 months, when the velocity is zero, the subcutaneous fat decreases (i.e. it has a negative growth velocity), until 6–8 years, when it begins to increase again. This early decrease in fat is less marked in girls than in boys so that, after 1 year, girls have more fat than boys. From 7 years the increase in fat occurs in both sexes. At adolescence, the limb fat in boys (triceps measurement) decreases, and is not regained until the late 20s, whereas girls show a slight slowing of the increase in limb fat, but no loss. At this time the trunk fat (subscapular measurement) stops increasing in boys, but shows a steady increase in girls. Postpubertal girls, but not boys, show fat deposits in a secondary sexual distribution, i.e. in the breasts, over the upper arms, lower abdomen and thighs. Adult men are more likely to deposit fat around the anterior abdominal wall.

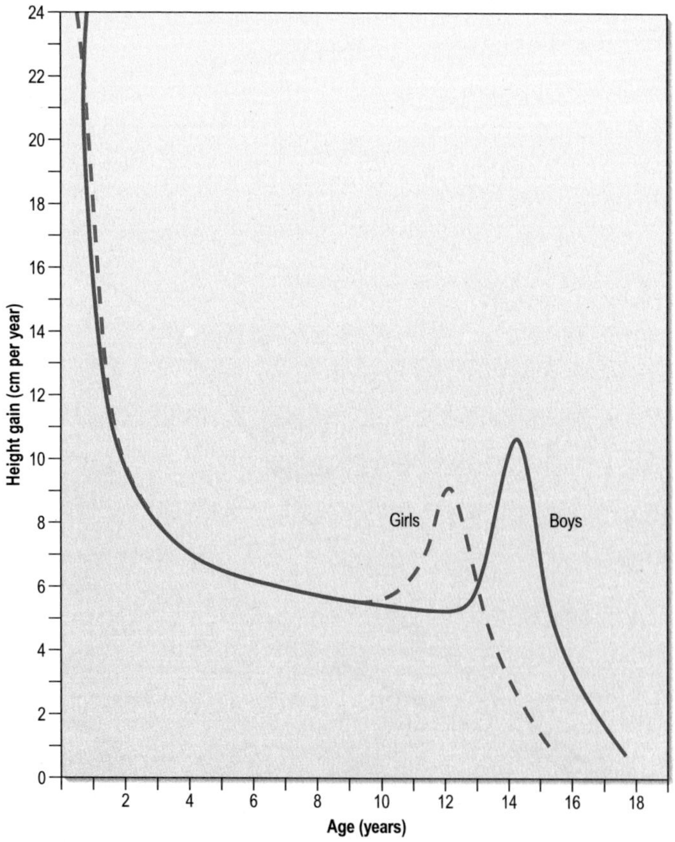

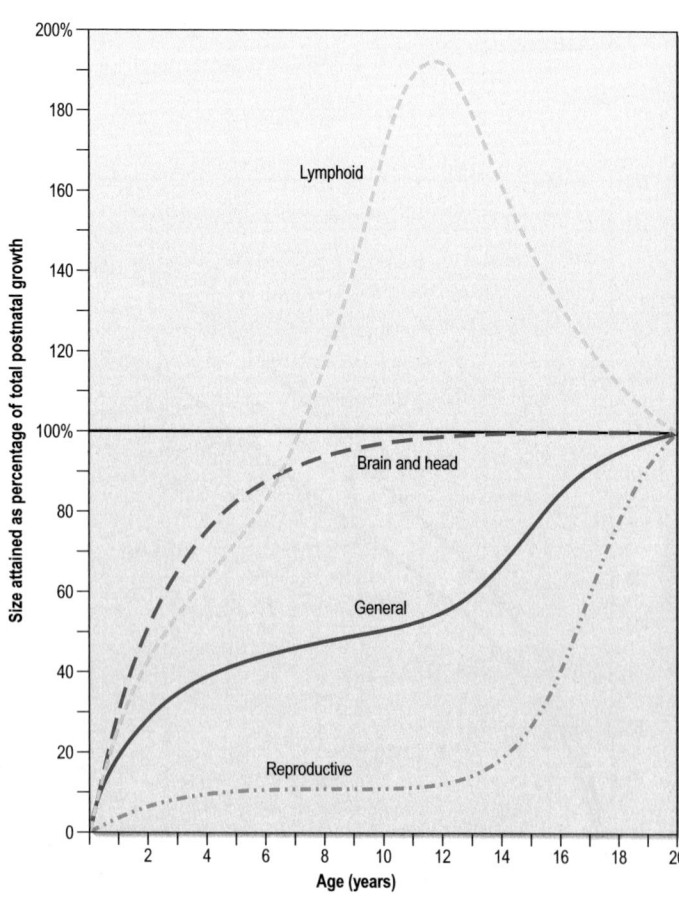

Fig. 11.14 Typical individual velocity curves for height: English boys and girls. (After Tanner JM, Whitehouse RH, Takaishi IM 1966 Standards from birth to maturity for height, weight, height velocity and weight velocity. Arch Dis Child 41: 454–471, with permission from BMJ Publishing.)

Fig. 11.15 Growth curves of different tissues, regions of the body and systems. Note that the growth of lymphoid tissue, thymus, lymph nodes and intestinal lymph masses decreases after puberty. (Adapted with permission from Tanner JM 1962 Growth at Adolescence, 2nd edn. Oxford: Blackwell Publishing.)

REFERENCES

Barker DJP, Osmond C, Simmonds SJ, Wield GA 1993 The relation of head size and thinness at birth to death from cardiovascular disease in adult life. BMJ 306: 422–6.
Provides evidence for a link between birth weight and size and predictions of later cardiovascular pathology.

Gandy GM 1992 Examination of the neonate including gestational assessment. In: Robertson NRC (ed) Textbook of Neonatology. Edinburgh: Churchill Livingstone: 199–215.
Presents the maturation dates of physical characteristics used in the assessment of gestational age.

Harrison GA, Weiner JS, Tanner JM, Barnicot NA 1964 Human Biology, ch 19. Clarendon Press: Oxford.
Presents data on the human growth curve.

Lampl M 2002 Saltation and stasis. In: Cameron N (ed) Human Growth and Development. New York: Academic Press, Ch. 12.
Presents the evidence for saltatory growth in humans.

O'Rahilly R, Muller F 1987 Developmental Stages in Human Embryos. Washington: Carnegie Institution.
Provides the most comprehensive and detailed morphological account of human development during the first 8 weeks of life. It sets out the basis for the staging system used for human embryos.

O'Rahilly, Muller F 1999 Mini review: prenatal ages and stages – measures and errors. Teratology 61: 382–4.

O'Rahilly, Muller F 2000 Mini review: summary of the initial development of the human nervous system. Teratology 60: 39–41.
Continues Streeter's work on the Carnegie collections of embryos and reviews early nervous system development.

Streeter GL 1942 Developmental horizons in human embryos. Descriptions of age group XI, 13 to 20 somites, and age group XII, 21 to 29 somites. Contrib Embryol Carnegie Inst Washington 30: 211–45.

Streeter GL 1945 Developmental horizons in human embryos. Description of age group XIII, embryos of about 4 or 5 millimeters long, and age group XIV, period of indentation of the lens vesicle. Contrib Embryol Carnegie Inst Washington 31: 27–63.

Streeter GL 1948 Developmental horizons in human embryos. Description of age groups XV, XVI, XVII, and XVIII, being the third issue of a survey of the Carnegie collection. Contrib Embryol Carnegie Inst Washington 32: 133–203.

NEUROANATOMY

Editors:

Susan Standring *(Lead Editor)*

Alan R Crossman *(Editor)*

MJ Turlough FitzGerald *(Editor, chapter 20)*

Patricia Collins *(Embryology, Growth and Development)*

With specialist contributions on clinical and functional anatomy by

Leila Abbas *(chapter 14)*, **Wolfgang Hamann** *(18)*, **Stephen McMahon** *(18)*

Critical reviewers:

Tipu Aziz *(chapters 13, 23)*, **Paul Griffiths** *(17)*, **Alan Jackson** *(15, 16)*, **Andrez Lozano** *(21)*, **David Neary** *(12, 13, 22)*

Overview of the organization of the nervous system

The human nervous system is the most complex product of biological evolution. The constantly changing patterns of activity of its billions of interactive units represent the fundamental physical basis of every aspect of human behaviour and experience. Many thousands of scientists and clinicians around the world, whether driven by intellectual curiosity or the quest for better methods of disease prevention and treatment, have studied the nervous system over many years. However, our understanding of complex neural organization and function is still quite rudimentary, as is our ability to deal with its many pathologies. Multidisciplinary research into the nervous system is one of the most active areas of contemporary biology and medicine and rapid advances across a range of fronts bring with them the realistic prospect of better methods for the prevention and treatment of many neurological disorders in the future.

The functional capabilities of the nervous system are a product of its vast population of intercommunicating nerve cells or neurones, estimated to number in the order of 10^{10} (p. 43). Neurones encode information, conduct it, sometimes over considerable distances and then transmit it to other neurones or to non-neural tissues (muscles or

glandular cells). Most neurones consist of a central mass of cytoplasm within a limiting cell membrane (the cell body or soma) from which extend a number of branched processes termed neurites (**Fig. 12.1**). One of these, the axon, is usually much longer than the others and normally conducts information away from the cell body. The other processes are termed dendrites and these typically conduct information towards the soma. The nerve cell membrane is polarized, the inside of the cell being around − 70 mV negative with respect to the outside. Information is coded in the form of patterns of transient depolarizations and repolarizations of this membrane potential, known as nerve impulses or action potentials. These are conducted along the axon, which may have collateral branches that permit information to be distributed simultaneously to several targets (**Fig. 12.2**). Axons possess specialized endings, or axon terminals, which come into close apposition with the membrane of the target cell at synapses (p. 44), where information passes from one cell to another. Axon terminals may form synaptic contacts with dendrites (axodendritic), cell bodies (axosomatic), other axons (axoaxonic) or non-neural tissue such as

Axon

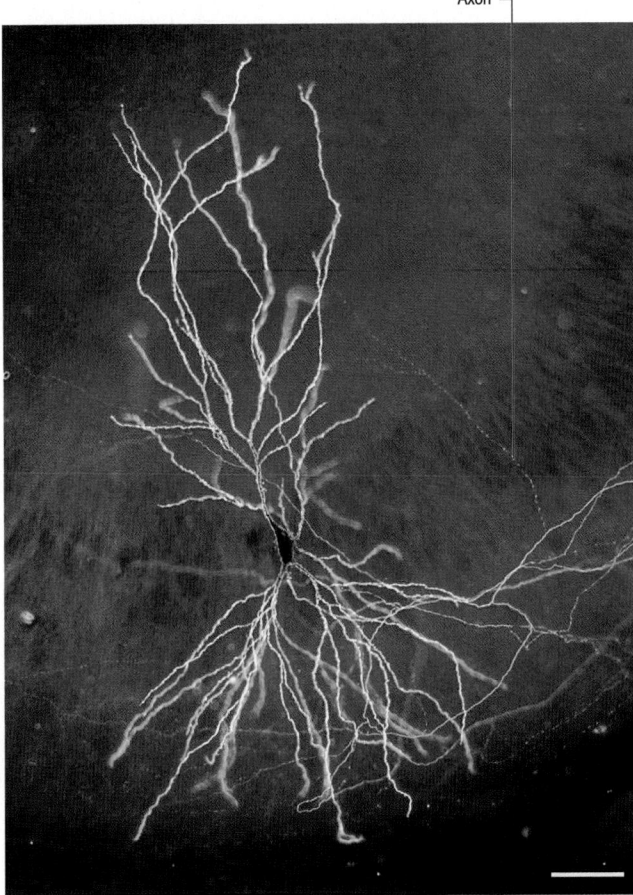

Fig. 12.1 A dark-field illuminated micrograph of a CA3 pyramidal cell in a hippocampal slice culture, intracellularly injected with the dye biocytin. Scale bar 50 μm. (By kind permission from Mathias Abegg and R Anne McKinney, Brain Research Institute, University of Zurich.)

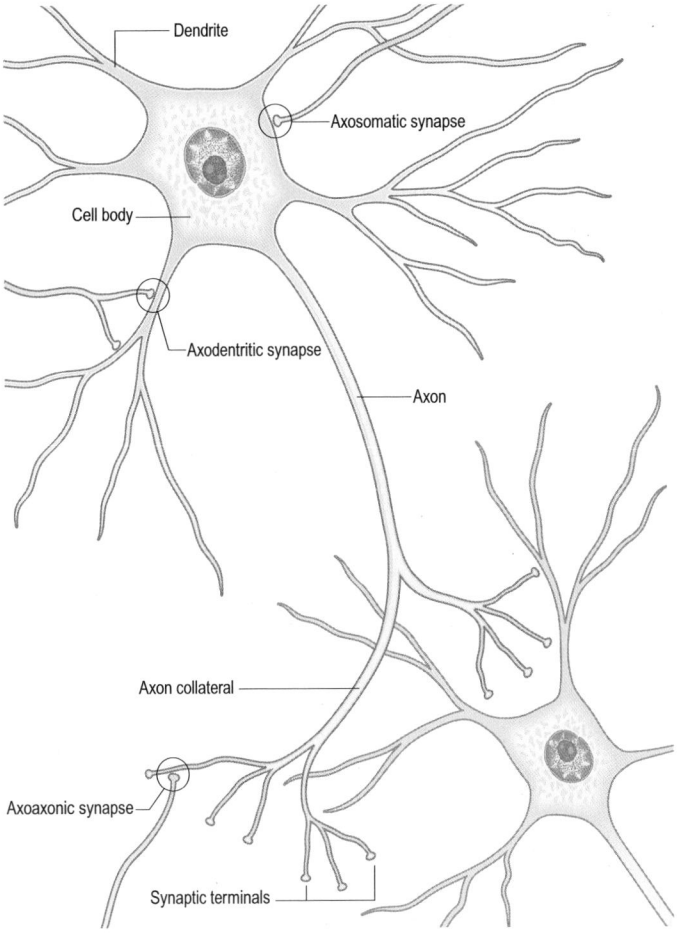

Fig. 12.2 The structure of a typical neurone.

muscle cells (neuromuscular junction). Transmission of information to other cells is brought about when action potentials cause the release of specific neurotransmitter substances, stored in synaptic vesicles within the presynaptic nerve terminal. Specialized receptors are located on the postsynaptic target cell membrane. The neurotransmitter binds to these and, depending upon the nature of the chemical and the receptor, either elicits an excitatory (depolarizing) or inhibitory (hyperpolarizing) response, or may modulate intracellular second messenger systems.

The huge complexity of the nervous system reflects the fact that individual neurones may make synaptic contact with hundreds, or even thousands, of other neurones via profuse axonal and dendritic branching (arborization). This is exemplified by the extensive dendritic field of the cerebellar Purkinje cell, which is traversed by thousands of axons, each of which makes synaptic contact as it passes. At the level of the individual neurone, competing incoming excitatory and inhibitory synaptic potentials are summated in time (temporal summation) and between synapses (spatial summation). If the postsynaptic neurone is depolarized above a certain threshold it fires action potentials which are conducted along the axon to the next target cells.

The nervous system contains far more supporting cells (neuroglia) than neurones. Glia are responsible for creating and maintaining an appropriate environment in which the neurones can operate efficiently (p. 50); they are not electrically excitable in the same way as neurones.

The nervous system consists of three basic functional types of neurone, namely afferent (sensory), efferent (motor) and interneurones. At the simplest level of interpretation, they allow the nervous system to detect changes in the internal and external environment and to respond appropriately. The sensory elements are able to detect a wide range of stimuli and subserve the general senses (touch, pressure, temperature, etc.) and the special senses (vision, hearing, smell, taste, and vestibular sensation). Motor neurones send axons from the central nervous system to effector organs, chiefly muscles and glands. Neurones that are confined to the central nervous system and which possess neither sensory nor motor terminals are called interneurones. They greatly outnumber sensory and motor neurones and confer on the nervous system its prodigious capacity to analyse, integrate and store information.

The nervous system is customarily divided into two major parts, the central nervous system (CNS) and the peripheral nervous system (PNS). The CNS consists of the brain and spinal cord. The PNS is composed of cranial nerves and spinal nerves together with their ramifications and certain groupings of cell bodies which constitute the peripheral ganglia. Another convention divides the nervous system into somatic and autonomic components. Anatomically, both of these have elements in the CNS and PNS. The autonomic nervous system, which consists of sympathetic and parasympathetic divisions, is made up of neurones concerned primarily with control of the internal environment, through innervation of secretory glands, cardiac and smooth muscle. It is considered in detail in Chapter 13. The wall of the gastrointestinal tract contains neurones capable of sustaining local reflex activity independent of the CNS, which are known as the enteric nervous system.

CENTRAL NERVOUS SYSTEM

The brain and spinal cord (**Fig. 12.3**) contain the great majority of neuronal cell bodies in the nervous system. In many parts of the CNS the cell bodies of neurones are grouped together and are, more or less, segregated from axons. The generic term for such collections of cell bodies is grey matter. Smaller aggregations of neuronal cell bodies, which usually share a common functional role, are termed nuclei. It follows that neuronal dendrites and synaptic interactions are mostly confined to grey matter. Axons tend to be grouped together to form white matter, so called because axons are often ensheathed in myelin (p. 56) which confers a paler colouration. Axons which pass between similar sources or destinations within the CNS tend to run together in defined pathways or tracts. These often cross the midline (decussate), which means that one half of the body is, in many respects, controlled by, and sends information to, the opposite side of the brain.

Some groups of neurones in the spinal cord and brain stem which subserve similar functions are organized into longitudinal columns. The neurones in these columns may be concentrated into discrete discontinuous nuclei in some areas, e.g. the cranial nerve nuclei of the brain stem, or they may form more or less continuous longitudinal bands, as in much of the spinal cord (**Fig. 12.4**). Efferent neurones

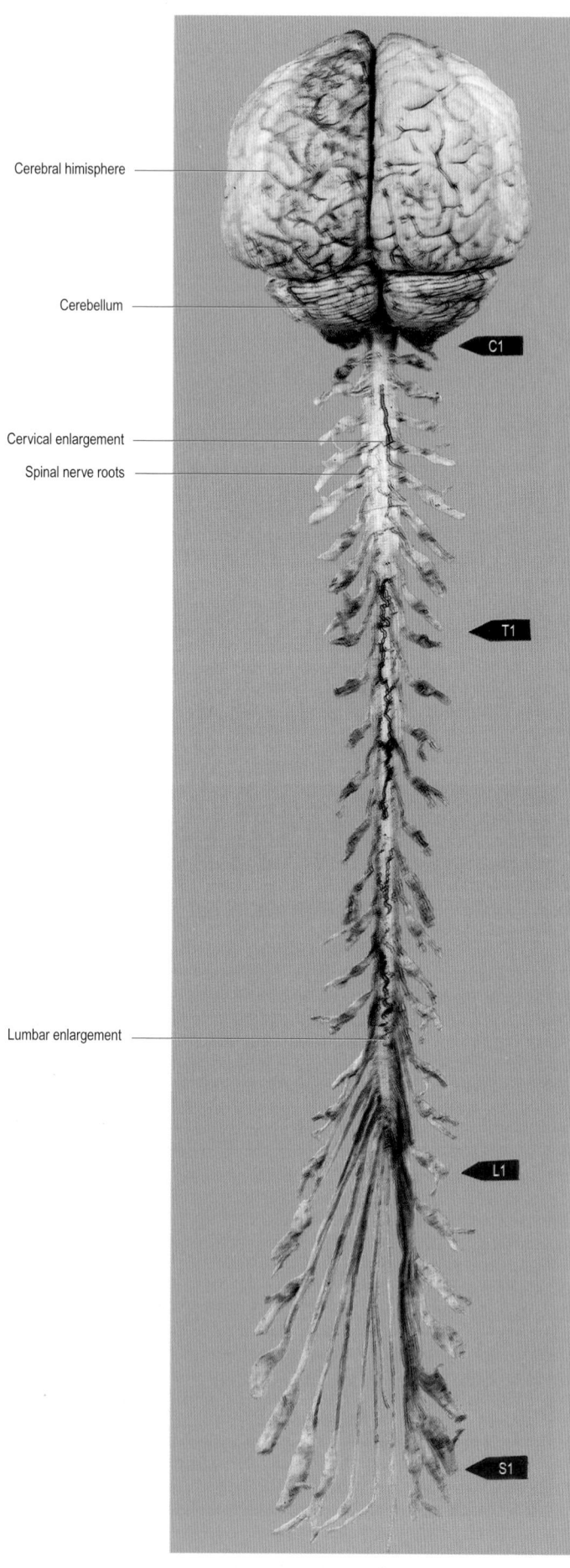

Cerebral himisphere

Cerebellum

C1

Cervical enlargement

Spinal nerve roots

T1

Lumbar enlargement

L1

S1

Fig. 12.3 The brain and spinal cord with attached spinal nerve roots and dorsal root ganglia, photographed from the dorsal aspect. (Photograph by Kevin Fitzpatrick on behalf of GKT School of Medicine, London.)

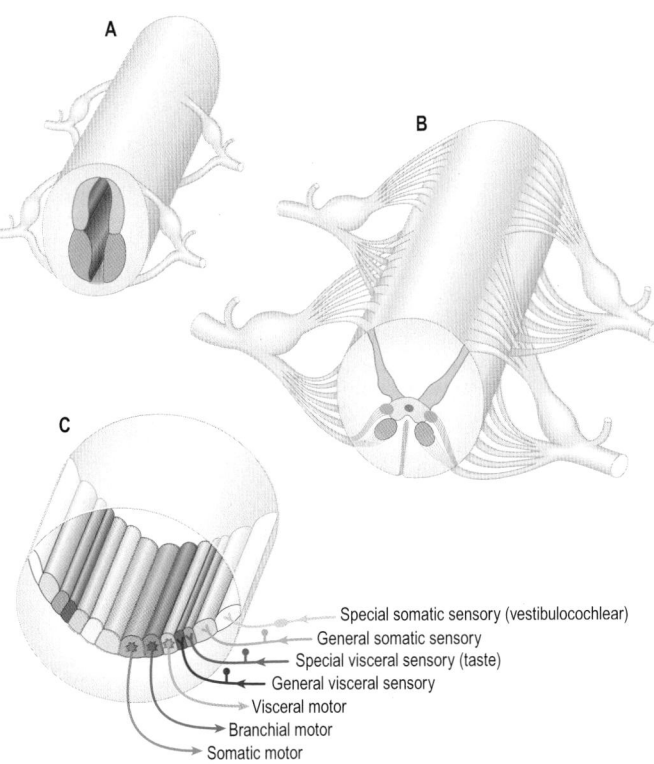

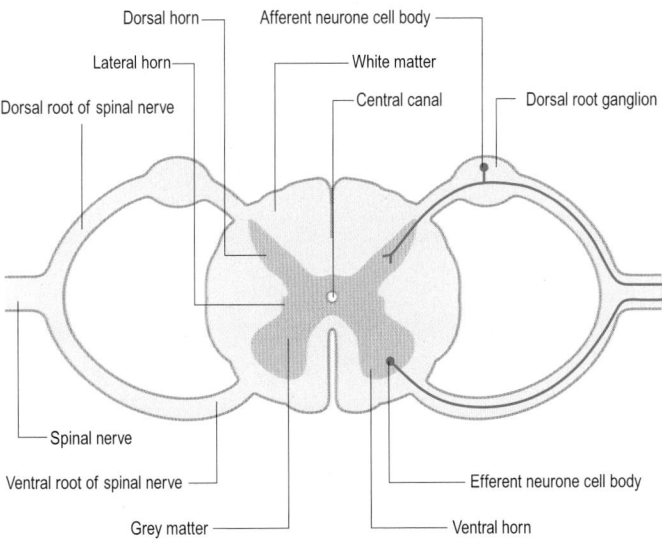

Fig. 12.5 Transverse section through the spinal cord illustrating the disposition of grey and white matter and the attachment of dorsal and ventral spinal nerve roots.

Fig. 12.4 The arrangement of sensory and motor cell columns in the spinal cord and brain stem. **A** shows the organization of the primitive spinal cord with a dorsal sensory column (blue), a ventral column (red), and segmentally arranged dorsal and ventral nerve roots. **B** depicts the arrangement of adult spinal cord serving the thorax, with sensory and somatic motor columns colour coded in the same way, and an additional intermediate (lateral) visceral motor column (orange). **C** indicates the arrangement of multiple longitudinal columns in the brain stem, where the motor column is now subdivided into three, and the sensory column into four. For further information about the embryological aspects of the early nervous system consult Chapter 14. Consult also **Fig. 19.1**.

constitute three such columns. The somatic motor column contains motor neurones the axons of which serve muscles derived from head somites. The two other columns are related to specialized features of head morphology. Of these, the branchial motor column innervates muscles derived from the wall of the embryonic pharynx (branchial muscles) whilst the visceral motor column supplies preganglionic parasympathetic fibres to glands and visceral smooth muscle. There are four longitudinal cell columns related to sensory functions. The general somatic sensory column essentially deals with information from the head. Special somatic sensory neurones are related to the special senses and receive vestibular and auditory input. General visceral sensory neurones deal with information from widespread and varied visceral sensory endings whilst special visceral sensory neurones are related to the special sense of taste.

The brain and spinal cord receive information from, and send it to, the rest of the body through cranial and spinal nerves, respectively. These contain afferent fibres carrying information from sensory receptors and efferent fibres running to effector organs. Through inherent connections of varying complexity between afferent and efferent components of spinal and cranial nerves, the spinal cord and brain stem have the innate capacity to control many aspects of body function and respond to external and internal stimuli by reflex action. Such functions are under the modulatory influence of rich descending connections from the brain. In addition, afferent input to the spinal cord and brain stem is channelled into various ascending pathways, some of which eventually impinge upon the cerebral cortex, conferring conscious awareness.

To sustain the energy required by constant neuronal activity, the CNS has a high metabolic rate, and a rich blood supply (Chs 17, 46). The blood–brain barrier controls the neuronal environment and imposes severe restrictions on the types of substances which can pass from the bloodstream into nervous tissue (p. 51).

SPINAL CORD

The spinal cord is located within the vertebral column, lying in the upper two-thirds of the vertebral canal (Ch. 46). It is continuous rostrally with the medulla oblongata. For the most part, the spinal cord controls the functions of, and receives afferent input from, the trunk and limbs. Afferent and efferent connections travel in 31 pairs of segmentally arranged spinal nerves. These attach to the cord as dorsal and ventral rootlets which unite to form the spinal nerves proper (**Fig. 12.5**). The dorsal and ventral roots are functionally distinct. Dorsal roots carry primary afferent nerve fibres from cell bodies located in dorsal root ganglia (p. 58). Ventral roots carry efferent fibres from cell bodies located in the spinal grey matter.

Internally, the spinal cord is differentiated into a central core of grey matter surrounded by white matter. The grey matter is configured in a characteristic H, or butterfly, shape that has projections known as dorsal and ventral horns (**Fig. 12.6**). In general, neurones situated in the dorsal horn are primarily concerned with sensory functions and those in the ventral horn are mostly associated with motor activities. At certain levels of the spinal cord a small lateral horn is additionally present, marking the location of the cell bodies of preganglionic sympathetic neurones. The central canal, which is a vestigial component of the ventricular system, lies at the centre of the spinal grey matter and runs the length of the cord. The white matter of the spinal cord consists of ascending and descending axons which link spinal cord segments to one another and the spinal cord to the brain.

BRAIN

The brain (encephalon) lies within the cranium (Ch. 28). It receives information from, and controls the activities of, the trunk and limbs mainly through rich connections with the spinal cord. It possesses 12 pairs of cranial nerves through which it communicates mostly with structures of the head and neck. The brain is divided into major regions on the basis of ontogenetic growth in individuals (Ch. 12) and phylogenetic principles (**Figs 12.7, 12.8, 12.9, 17.8**). Ascending in sequence from the spinal cord, the principal divisions are the rhombencephalon or hindbrain, the mesencephalon or midbrain, and the prosencephalon or forebrain.

The rhombencephalon is subdivided into the myelencephalon or medulla oblongata, metencephalon or pons, and the cerebellum. The medulla oblongata, pons and midbrain are collectively referred to as the brain stem which lies upon the basal portions of the occipital and sphenoid bones (clivus). The medulla oblongata is the most caudal part of the brain stem and is continuous with the spinal cord below the level of the foramen magnum. The pons lies rostral to the medulla and is distinguished by a mass of transverse nerve fibres which connect it to the cerebellum. The midbrain is a short segment of brain stem, rostral

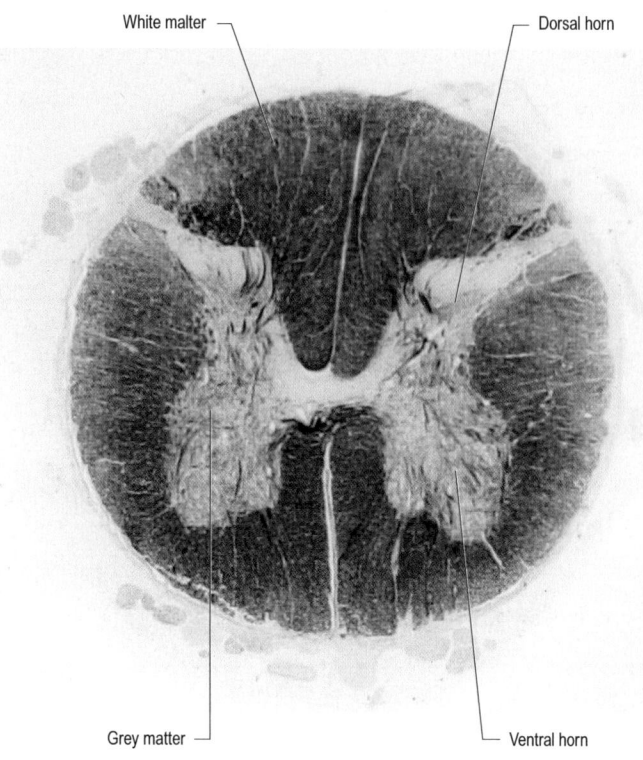

Fig. 12.6 Transverse section through the human spinal cord at the lumbar level, stained to demonstrate myelinated nerve fibres in the white matter (blue-black). Grey matter remains relatively unstained. (Figure enhanced by B Crossman.)

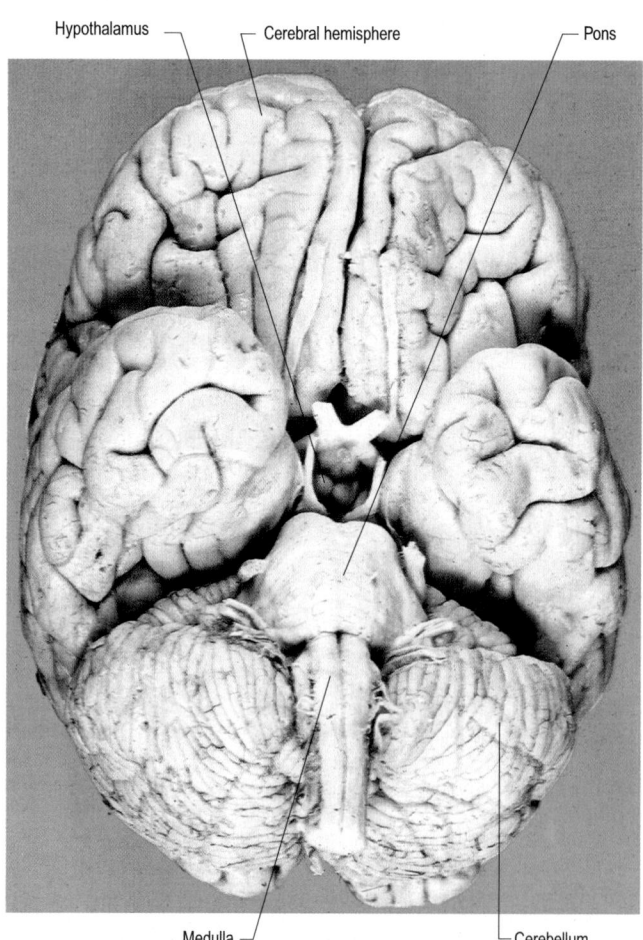

Fig. 12.8 The base of the brain. The midbrain, lying between the pons and hypothalamus, cannot be seen in this photograph. (Photograph by Kevin Fitzpatrick on behalf of GKT School of Medicine, London.)

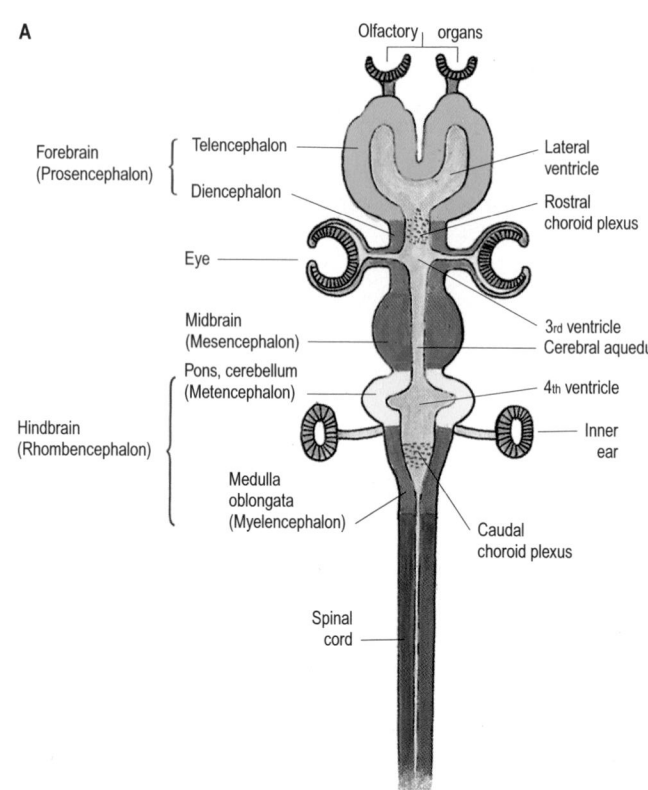

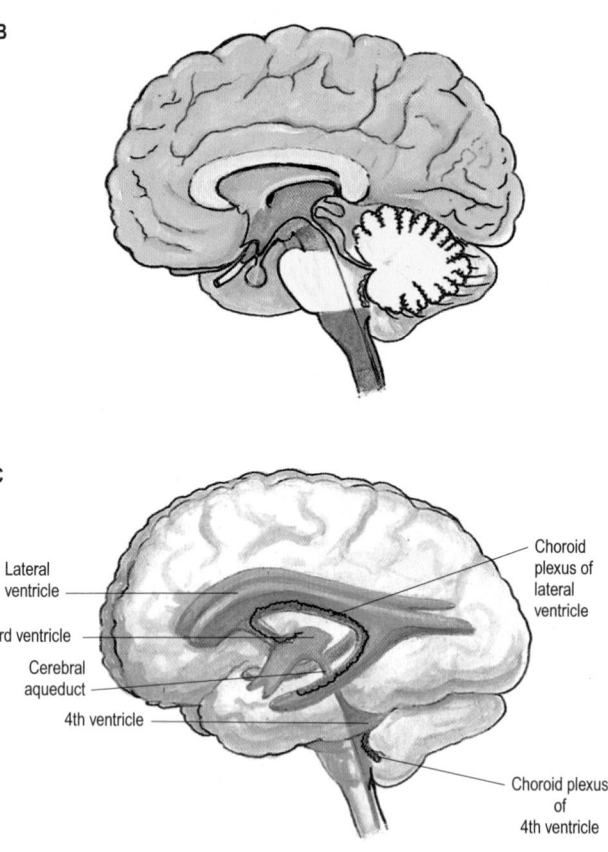

Fig. 12.7 The nomenclature and arrangement of the different areas of the brain. A depicts the major features of the basic brain plan, including the relationships of its parts to the major special sensory organs of the head. B shows how the same regions are arranged in the adult brain, seen in sagittal section. C illustrates the organization of the ventricular system in the brain.

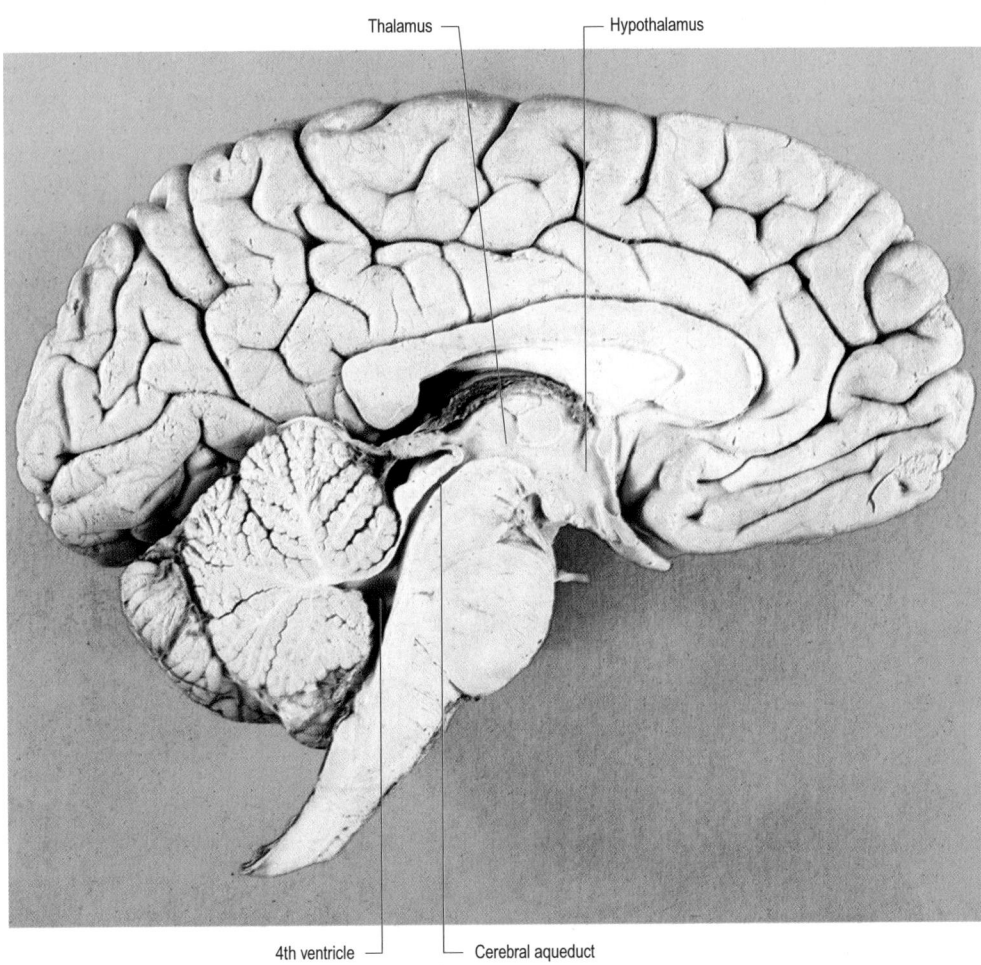

Thalamus — Hypothalamus

4th ventricle — Cerebral aqueduct

Fig. 12.9 A sagittal section of the brain. (Photograph by Kevin Fitzpatrick on behalf of GKT School of Medicine, London.)

to the pons. The cerebellum consists of paired hemispheres united by a median vermis and lies within the posterior cranial fossa, dorsal to the pons, medulla and caudal midbrain, with all of which it has rich fibre connections.

The prosencephalon may be subdivided into the diencephalon and the telencephalon. The diencephalon equates mostly to the thalamus and hypothalamus, but also includes the smaller epithalamus and subthalamus. The telencephalon is mainly composed of the two cerebral hemispheres or cerebrum. The diencephalon is almost completely embedded in the cerebrum and is therefore largely hidden. The human cerebrum constitutes the major fraction of the volume of the brain. It occupies the anterior and middle cranial fossae and is directly related to the cranial vault. It consists of two cerebral hemispheres. The surface of each hemisphere is convoluted into a complex pattern of ridges (gyri) and furrows (sulci). Internally, each hemisphere has an external layer of grey matter, the cerebral cortex, beneath which lies a dense mass of white matter (**Fig. 12.10**). One of the most important components of the cerebral white matter, the internal capsule, contains nerve fibres which pass to and from the cerebral cortex. Several large nuclei of grey matter, usually referred to as the basal ganglia, are partly embedded in the subcortical white matter. Connections between corresponding areas of the two sides of the brain cross the midline within commissures. By far the largest commissure is the corpus callosum, which links the two cerebral hemispheres.

During prenatal development, the walls of the neural tube thicken greatly, but never completely obliterate the central lumen. Although the latter remains in the spinal cord as the narrow central canal, it becomes greatly expanded in the brain to form a series of interconnected cavities called the ventricular system (Ch. 16). In two regions, the fore- and hindbrains, parts of the neural tube roof do not generate nerve cells but become thin, folded sheets of highly vascular secretory tissue, the choroid plexuses. These secrete cerebrospinal fluid which fills the ventricles. The cavity of the rhombencephalon becomes expanded to form the fourth ventricle, which lies dorsal to the pons and upper half of the medulla. Caudally, the fourth ventricle is continuous with a canal in the caudal medulla and, through this, with the spinal central canal. At its rostral

extent, the fourth ventricle is continuous with a narrow channel, the cerebral aqueduct, which passes through the midbrain. The rostral end of the cerebral aqueduct opens out into the median third ventricle, a narrow slit-like cavity bounded laterally by the diencephalon. At the rostral end of the third ventricle, a small aperture on each side leads into the large lateral ventricle which is located within each cerebral hemisphere.

OVERVIEW OF ASCENDING SENSORY PATHWAYS

Sensory modalities are conventionally described as either special senses or general senses. The special senses are olfaction, vision, taste, hearing and vestibular function. Afferent information is encoded by highly specialized sense organs and transmitted to the brain in certain cranial nerves (I, II, VII, VIII and IX). The special senses are described in Chapter 24.

The general senses include touch, pressure, vibration, pain, thermal sensation and proprioception (perception of posture and movement). Stimuli from the external and internal environments activate a diverse range of receptors in the skin, viscera, muscles, tendons and joints (p. 59). Afferent impulses from the trunk and limbs are conveyed to the spinal cord in spinal nerves whilst those from the head are carried to the brain in cranial nerves. The detailed anatomy of the complex pathways by which the various general senses impinge upon conscious levels is better understood with reference to certain overall organizational principles. Whilst undoubtedly oversimplified and subject to many exceptions, this schema is helpful in emphasizing the essential similarities which exist between the ascending sensory systems.

In essence, ascending sensory projections related to the general senses consist of a sequence of three neurones extending from the peripheral receptor to the contralateral cerebral cortex (**Fig.12.11**). These are often referred to as primary, secondary and tertiary sensory (afferent) neurones or first-, second- and third-order neurones, respectively. Primary afferents have peripherally located sensory endings and their cell bodies lie in dorsal root ganglia or the ganglia associated with certain of the cranial nerves. Their axons enter the CNS through ipsilateral spinal or trigeminal nerves. Within the CNS they terminate

231

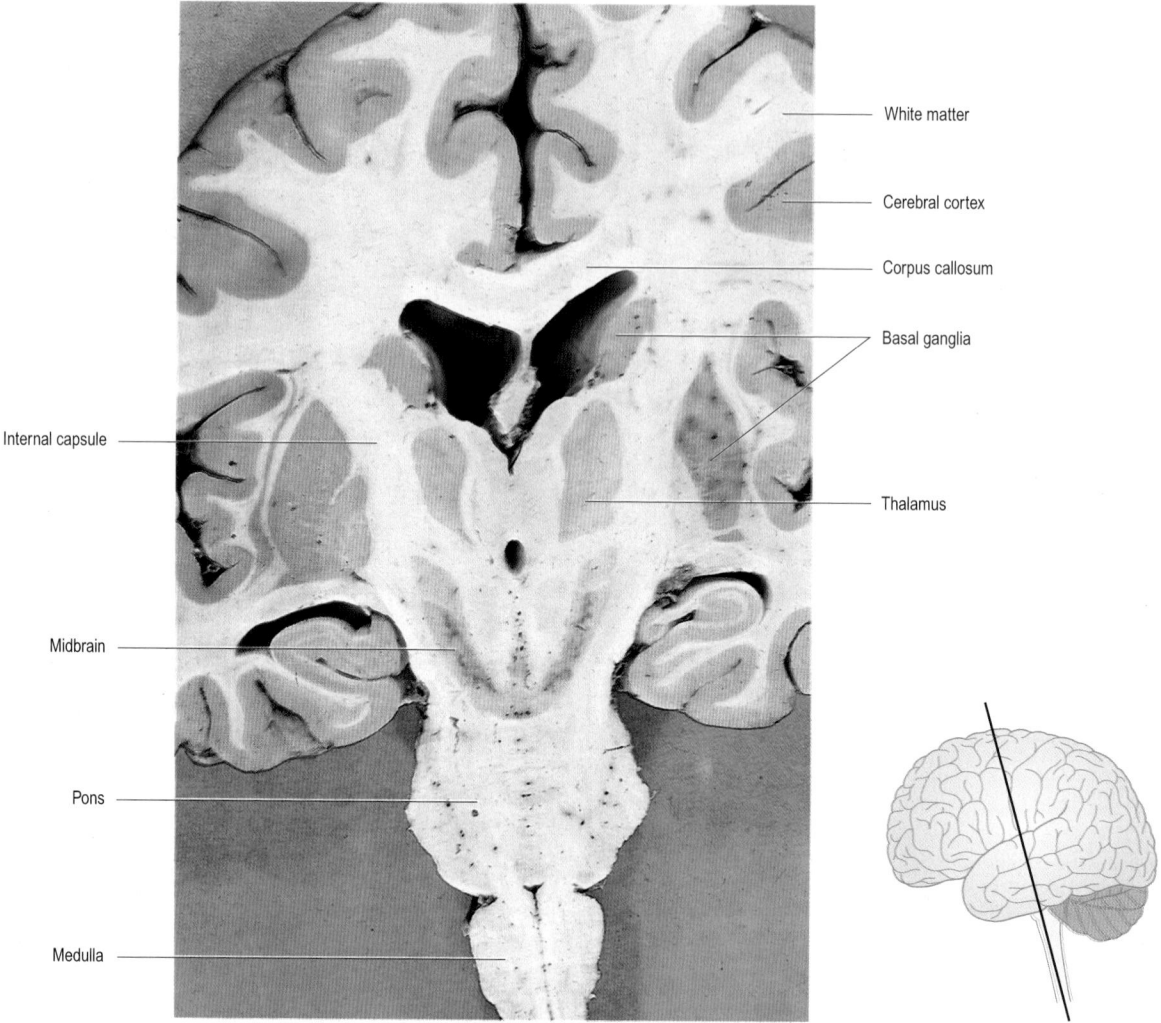

White matter

Cerebral cortex

Corpus callosum

Basal ganglia

Thalamus

Internal capsule

Midbrain

Pons

Medulla

Fig. 12.10 Section through the cerebral hemisphere and brain stem showing the disposition of grey and white matter, the basal ganglia and the internal capsule. (Photograph by Kevin Fitzpatrick on behalf of GKT School of Medicine, London.)

ipsilateral to their side of entry, upon the cell bodies of second-order neurones. The precise location of this termination depends upon the modality.

Primary afferent fibres carrying pain, temperature and coarse touch/ pressure information from the trunk and limbs terminate in the dorsal horn of the spinal grey matter, near their point of entry into the spinal cord. Homologous fibres from the head terminate in the trigeminal sensory nucleus of the brain stem. The cell bodies of second-order neurones are located in the dorsal horn and trigeminal sensory nucleus. Their axons decussate and ascend to the thalamus. The ascending second-order axons from the spinal cord form the spinothalamic tract. Those from the trigeminal sensory nucleus constitute the trigemino-thalamic tract.

Primary afferent fibres carrying proprioceptive information and fine (discriminative) touch from the trunk and limbs ascend ipsilaterally in the spinal cord without synapse. The ascending fibres constitute the dorsal columns (fasciculus gracilis and fasciculus cuneatus). They end in the dorsal column nuclei (nucleus gracilis and nucleus cuneatus) of the medulla. The dorsal column nuclei contain the cell bodies of second-order neurones. Their axons decussate in the medulla and then ascend as the medial lemniscus. Similarly, an homologous projection exists for afferents derived from the head.

Within the thalamus, ascending second-order sensory neurones terminate in the ventral posterior nucleus, making synaptic contact with the cell bodies of third-order neurones. The axons of third-order neurones pass through the internal capsule to reach the cerebral cortex, where they terminate in the postcentral gyrus of the parietal lobe, also known as the primary somatosensory cortex.

OVERVIEW OF DESCENDING MOTOR PATHWAYS

The concept of upper and lower motor neurones is fundamental to the clinical description of the effects of lesions of the motor system. The term 'lower motor neurones' refers to the alpha motor neurones which innervate the extrafusal muscle fibres of skeletal muscle. The term 'upper motor neurones' in theory refers collectively to all the descending pathways which impinge upon the activity of lower motor neurones. In common parlance, however, the term is often equated with the corticospinal (pyramidal) tract (**Fig. 12.12**). This pathway originates from widespread regions of the cerebral cortex, including the primary motor cortex of the frontal lobe where the opposite half of the body is represented in a detailed somatotopic fashion. Corticofugal fibres descend through the internal capsule and pass into the brain stem, where some of them (designated corticobulbar fibres) terminate. Corticobulbar fibres control the activity of brain stem neurones, including motor neurones within the cranial nerve nuclei. Corticospinal fibres descend through the brain stem. The majority of them cross to the contralateral side in the pyramidal decussation of the medulla and continue as the lateral corticospinal tract of the spinal cord. This terminates in association with interneurones and motor neurones of the spinal grey matter. The principal function of the corticospinal and corticobulbar tracts is the control of fine, fractionated movements, particularly of those parts of the body where delicate muscular control is required. These tracts are particularly important in speech (corticobulbar tract) and movement of the hand (corticospinal tract).

The terms upper and lower motor neurone lesion are used clinically to distinguish, for example, between the effects of a stroke in the internal capsule (a typical upper motor neurone lesion) and those of motor

232

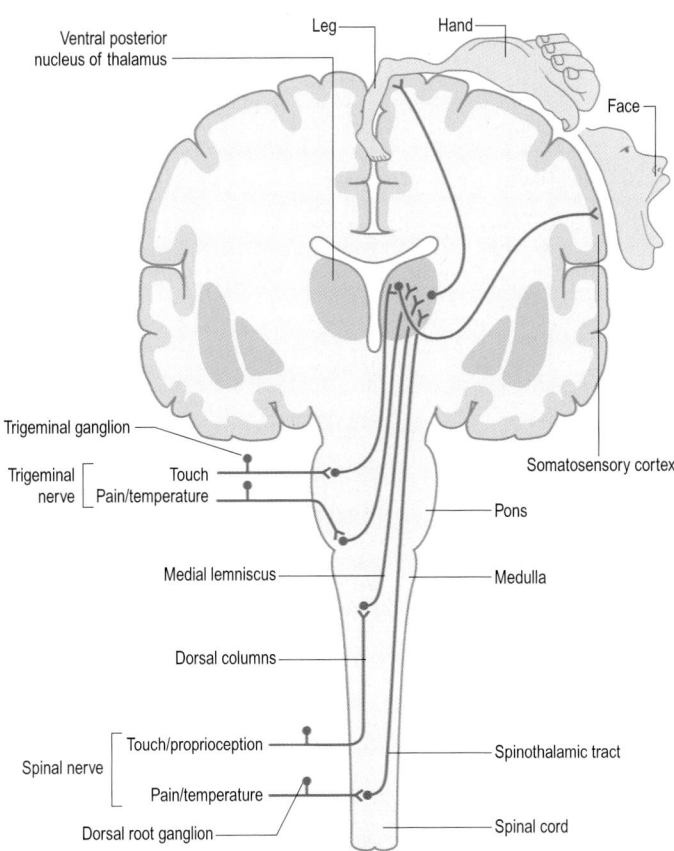

Fig. 12.11 The organization of general sensory pathways showing first-order (green), second-order (blue) and third-order (red) neurones.

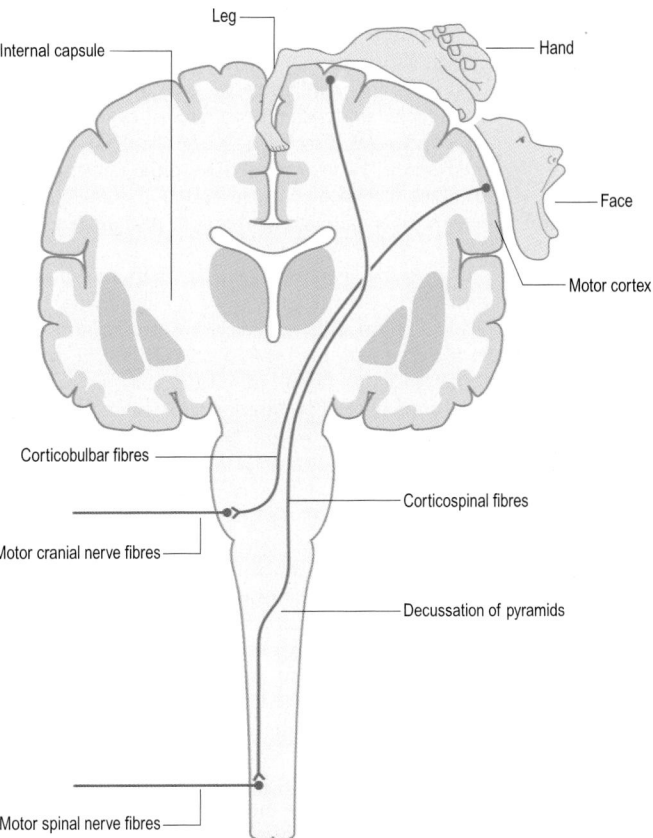

Fig. 12.12 The corticospinal and corticobulbar tracts.

neurone disease (a typical lower motor neurone lesion). These produce very different signs and symptoms (summarized below), which are indicative of the anatomical site of the lesion.

Lower motor neurone lesions cause paralysis or paresis of specific muscles due to: loss of innervation; loss or reduction of tendon reflex activity of muscles; reduced muscle tone; spontaneous muscular contractions (fasciculation); and atrophy of muscles over time. Upper motor neurone lesions cause paralysis or paresis of movements due to: loss of higher control; increased tendon reflex activity of muscles; increased muscle tone; no atrophy of muscles; and positive plantar reflex. The combination of paralysis, increased tendon reflex activity and hypertonia is referred to as spasticity.

The pathophysiology of upper motor neurone lesions is complex. This is because many descending pathways other than the corticospinal tract exist and they also influence lower motor neurone activity. These pathways include rich corticofugal projections to the brain stem (e.g. corticoreticular and corticopontine) which traverse the internal capsule and numerous pathways which originate within the brain stem itself (e.g. reticulospinal, vestibulospinal). Clearly, these pathways may be compromised to varying extents which are determined by the site of a lesion. Their involvement is believed to be important in the pathophysiological mechanisms which underlie the generation of spasticity. Pure corticospinal tract lesions, which are exceedingly rare in man because corticospinal tract fibres lie in close relationship to other pathways throughout most of their course, are believed to cause deficits in delicate, fractionated movements and to induce the positive plantar reflex.

Two other major systems which contribute to the control of movement are the basal ganglia and the cerebellum. The basal ganglia are a group of large subcortical nuclei, the major components of which are the caudate nucleus, putamen and globus pallidus (**Fig. 12.10**; Ch. 23). These structures have important connections with the cerebral cortex, certain diencephalic nuclei of the thalamus and subthalamus and with the brain stem. They appear to be involved in the selection of appro-

priate movements and the suppression of inappropriate ones. Disorders of the basal ganglia cause either too little movement (akinesia) or abnormal involuntary movements (dyskinesia) as well as tremor and abnormalities of muscle tone. The basal ganglia are sometimes described as being part of the so-called 'extrapyramidal (motor) system'. This term is used to distinguish between the effects of basal ganglia disease and those of damage to the 'pyramidal' (corticospinal) system. However, the progressive elucidation of the anatomy of the basal ganglia and of the pathophysiology of motor disorders has revealed the close functional interrelationship between the two 'systems', and has rendered the terms which distinguish them largely obsolete (Brodal 1981). The cerebellum (Ch. 20) has rich connections with the brain stem, particularly the reticular and vestibular nuclei, and with the thalamus. It is concerned with the coordination of movement. Cerebellar disorders cause ataxia, intention tremor and hypotonia.

PERIPHERAL NERVOUS SYSTEM

The PNS is composed mainly of spinal nerves, cranial nerves, their ganglia and their ramifications which carry afferent and efferent neurones between the CNS and the rest of the body. It also includes the peripheral part of the autonomic nervous system (Ch. 13), notably the sympathetic trunks and ganglia, and the enteric nervous system which is composed of plexuses of nerve fibres and cell bodies in the wall of the alimentary tract.

SPINAL NERVES

Spinal nerves are the means by which the CNS receives information from, and controls the activities of, the trunk and limbs. Spinal nerves are considered in detail elsewhere on a regional basis (Sections 4, 5, 7 and 8).

In brief, there are 31 pairs of spinal nerves (8 cervical, 12 thoracic, 5 lumbar, 5 sacral, 1 coccygeal) which contain a mixture of sensory and motor fibres. They originate from the spinal cord as continuous lines of dorsal and ventral nerve rootlets. Adjacent groups of rootlets fuse to form dorsal and ventral roots which then merge to form the spinal nerves proper. The dorsal roots of spinal nerves contain afferent nerve fibres from cell bodies located in dorsal root ganglia. These cells give off both centrally and peripherally directed processes and do not have synapses on their cell bodies. The ventral roots of spinal nerves contain efferent fibres from cell bodies located in the spinal grey matter. They include motor neurones innervating skeletal muscle and preganglionic autonomic neurones.

Spinal nerves exit from the vertebral canal via their corresponding intervertebral foramina. They then divide to form a large ventral ramus and a much smaller dorsal ramus. In general terms, the ventral ramus innervates the limbs together with the muscles and skin of the anterior part of the trunk. The posterior ramus innervates the post-vertebral muscles and the skin of the back. The anterior rami serving the upper and lower limbs are redistributed within brachial and lumbosacral plexuses, respectively.

CRANIAL NERVES

Cranial nerves are the means by which the brain receives information from, and controls the activities of, the head and neck and to a lesser extent the thoracic and abdominal viscera. The component fibres, their route of exit from the cranial cavity, their subsequent peripheral course and the distribution and functions of the cranial nerves, are considered in detail elsewhere on a regional basis (Sections 3, 6, 7). Their origins, destinations and connections within the CNS are considered in this section.

Briefly, there are 12 pairs of cranial nerves. They are individually named and numbered (using Roman numerals) in a rostrocaudal sequence (**Table 12.1**). Unlike spinal nerves, only some are mixed in function, and so carry both sensory and motor fibres. Others are purely sensory or purely motor. The first cranial nerve (I; olfactory) has an ancient lineage and is derived from the forerunner of the cerebral hemisphere. It retains this unique position through the connections of the olfactory bulb, and is the only sensory cranial nerve that projects directly to the cerebral cortex rather than via the thalamus, as do all other sensory modalities. The areas of cerebral cortex involved have a primitive cellular organization and are an integral part of the limbic system, which is concerned with the emotional aspects of behaviour (p. 404). The second cranial nerve (II; optic) consists of the axons of second order visual neurones and terminates in the thalamus. The other ten pairs of cranial nerves attach to the brain stem. Most of the component fibres originate from, or terminate in, named cranial nerve nuclei (Ch. 19).

The sensory fibres in individual spinal and cranial nerves have characteristic, but often overlapping, peripheral distributions. As far as the innervation of the body surface is concerned, the area which is

Table 12.1 Summary of cranial nerves.

Number	Name	Function
I	Olfactory	Olfaction
II	Optic	Vision
III	Oculomotor	Eye movement Parasympathetic innervation of eye
IV	Trochlear	Eye movement
V	Trigeminal	General sensation from head Motor to muscles of mastication
VI	Abducens	Eye movement
VII	Facial	Taste Facial movement Parasympathetic innervation of salivary and lacrimal glands
VIII	Vestibulocochlear	Vestibular sense Hearing
IX	Glossopharyngeal	Taste General sensory and motor innervation of pharynx Visceral innervation from carotid body and sinus Parasympathetic innervation of salivary gland
X	Vagus	General sensory and motor innervation of pharynx, larynx and oesophagus Visceral innervation from thorax and abdomen, including aortic body and arch Parasympathetic innervation of thoracic and abdominal viscera
XI	Accessory	Movement of head and shoulders
XII	Hypoglossal	Movement of tongue

supplied by a particular spinal or cranial nerve is referred to as a dermatome. Detailed dermatome maps are described on a regional basis (p. 175). The motor axons of individual spinal and cranial nerves tend to innervate anatomically and functionally related groups of skeletal muscles, which are referred to as myotomes.

REFERENCES

Brodal A 1981 Neurological Anatomy in Relation to Clinical Medicine. 3rd edition. Oxford: Oxford University Press.
Unconventional but highly-readable text of neuroanatomy with an emphasis on clinical relevance. Particularly good account of motor pathways.
Crossman AR, Neary D 2000 Neuroanatomy. An Illustrated Colour Text. 2nd edition. Edinburgh: Churchill Livingstone.

England MA, Wakely J 1991 A Colour Atlas of the Brain and Spinal Cord. London: Wolfe Publishing Ltd.
Haines DE 2000 Neuroanatomy. An Atlas of Structures, Sections and Systems. 5th edition. Philadelphia: Lippincott Williams & Wilkins.

Autonomic nervous system

The autonomic nervous system represents the visceral component of the nervous system. It consists of neurones located within both the central nervous system (CNS) and the peripheral nervous system (PNS) and which are concerned with the control of the internal environment, through innervation of secretory glands, and both cardiac and smooth muscle. The term 'autonomic' is a convenient rather than appropriate title, since the functional autonomy of this part of the nervous system is illusory. Rather, its functions are normally closely integrated with changes in somatic activities, although the anatomical bases for such interactions are not always clear.

Visceral afferent pathways resemble somatic afferent pathways. The cell bodies of origin are unipolar neurones located in cranial and dorsal root ganglia. Their peripheral processes are distributed through autonomic ganglia or plexuses, or possibly through somatic nerves, without interruption. Their central processes (axons) accompany somatic afferent fibres through cranial nerves or dorsal spinal roots into the CNS where they establish connections which mediate autonomic reflexes and visceral sensation.

Visceral efferent pathways differ from their somatic equivalents in that the former are interrupted by peripheral synapses, there being a sequence of at least two neurones between the CNS and the target structure (**Fig. 13.1**). These are referred to as preganglionic and postganglionic neurones. The somata of preganglionic neurones are located in the visceral efferent nuclei of the brain stem and in the lateral grey columns of the spinal cord. Their axons, which are usually finely myelinated, exit from the CNS in certain cranial and spinal nerves and then pass to peripheral ganglia, where they synapse with the postganglionic neurones. The axons of postganglionic neurones are usually non-myelinated. Postganglionic neurones are more numerous than preganglionic ones; one preganglionic neurone may synapse with 15 to 20 postganglionic neurones, which permits the wide diffusion of many autonomic effects.

The autonomic nervous system can be divided into three major parts: sympathetic; parasympathetic; and enteric. These differ in organization and structure but are closely integrated functionally. Most, but not all, structures innervated by the autonomic nervous system receive both sympathetic and parasympathetic fibres, whereas the enteric nervous system is a network of neurones intrinsic to the wall of the gastrointestinal tract.

Two long-held assumptions about the sympathetic and parasympathetic nervous systems are that they are functionally antagonistic (because activation of their respective efferents has opposing actions upon target structures), and that sympathetic reactions are mass responses whereas parasympathetic reactions are usually localized. A more realistic notion is that these sets of neurones represent an integrated system for the coordinated neural regulation of visceral and homeostatic functions. Moreover, even though widespread activation of the sympathetic nervous system may occur, e.g. in association with fear or rage, it is now recognized that the sympathetic nervous system is also capable of discrete activation, and many different patterns of activation of sympathetic nerves throughout the body occur in response to a wide variety of stimuli. Thus, sympathetic activity may result in the general constriction of cutaneous arteries (increasing blood supply to the heart, muscles and brain), cardiac acceleration, an increase in blood pressure, contraction of sphincters and depression of peristalsis, all of which mobilize body energy stores for dealing with increased activity. Parasympathetic activity results in cardiac slowing and an increase in intestinal glandular and peristaltic activities, which may be considered to conserve body energy stores.

Autonomic activity is not initiated or controlled solely by the reflex connections of general visceral afferent pathways, nor do impulses in these pathways necessarily activate general visceral efferents. For example, in many situations demanding general sympathetic activity the initiator is somatic and typically arises either from the special senses or the skin. Rises in blood pressure and pupillodilatation may result from the stimulation of somatic receptors in the skin and other tissues. Peripheral autonomic activity is integrated at higher levels in the brain stem and cerebrum, including various nuclei of the brain stem reticular formation, thalamus and hypothalamus, the limbic lobe and prefrontal neocortex, together with the ascending and descending pathways which interconnect these regions.

The traditional concept of autonomic neurotransmission is that preganglionic neurones of both sympathetic and parasympathetic systems are cholinergic and that postganglionic parasympathetic neurones are also cholinergic while those of the sympathetic nervous system are noradrenergic. The discovery of neurones which do not use either acetylcholine or noradrenaline (norepinephrine) as their primary transmitter, and the recognition of a multiplicity of substances in autonomic nerves which fulfil the criteria for a neurotransmitter or neuromodulator, have greatly complicated neuropharmacological concepts of the autonomic nervous system. Thus, adenosine 5'-triphosphate (ATP), numerous peptides and nitric oxide have all been implicated in the mechanisms of cell signalling in the autonomic nervous system. The principal cotransmitters in sympathetic nerves are ATP and neuropeptide Y, vasoactive intestinal polypeptide (VIP) in parasympathetic nerves and ATP, VIP and substance P in enteric nerves.

SYMPATHETIC NERVOUS SYSTEM

The sympathetic trunks are two ganglionated nerve cords which extend from the cranial base to the coccyx (pp. 991, 1126). The ganglia are joined to spinal nerves by short connecting nerves called white and grey rami communicantes. Preganglionic axons join the trunk through the white rami communicantes while postganglionic axons leave the trunk in the grey rami. In the neck each sympathetic trunk lies posterior to the carotid sheath and anterior to the transverse processes of the cervical vertebrae. In the thorax the trunks are anterior to the heads of the ribs; in the abdomen they lie anterolateral to the bodies of the lumbar vertebrae; and in the pelvis they are anterior to the sacrum and medial to the anterior sacral foramina. Anterior to the coccyx the two trunks meet in a single, median, terminal ganglion. Cervical sympathetic ganglia are usually reduced to three by fusion. The internal carotid nerve, a continuation of the sympathetic trunk, issues from the cranial pole of the superior ganglion and accompanies the internal carotid artery through its canal into the cranial cavity. There are from 10 to 12 (usually 11) thoracic ganglia, 4 lumbar ganglia and 4 or 5 ganglia in the sacral region.

The cell bodies of preganglionic sympathetic neurones are located in the lateral horn of the spinal grey matter of all thoracic segments and the upper two or three lumbar segments (**Fig. 13.2**). Their axons are myelinated, with diameters of 1.5–4 µm. These leave the cord in corresponding ventral nerve roots and pass into the spinal nerves, but soon leave in white rami communicantes to join the sympathetic trunk (**Fig. 13.3**). Neurones like those in the lateral grey column exist at other levels of the cord above and below the thoracolumbar outflow and small numbers of their fibres leave in other ventral roots. Preganglionic sympathetic neurones release acetylcholine as their principal neurotransmitter.

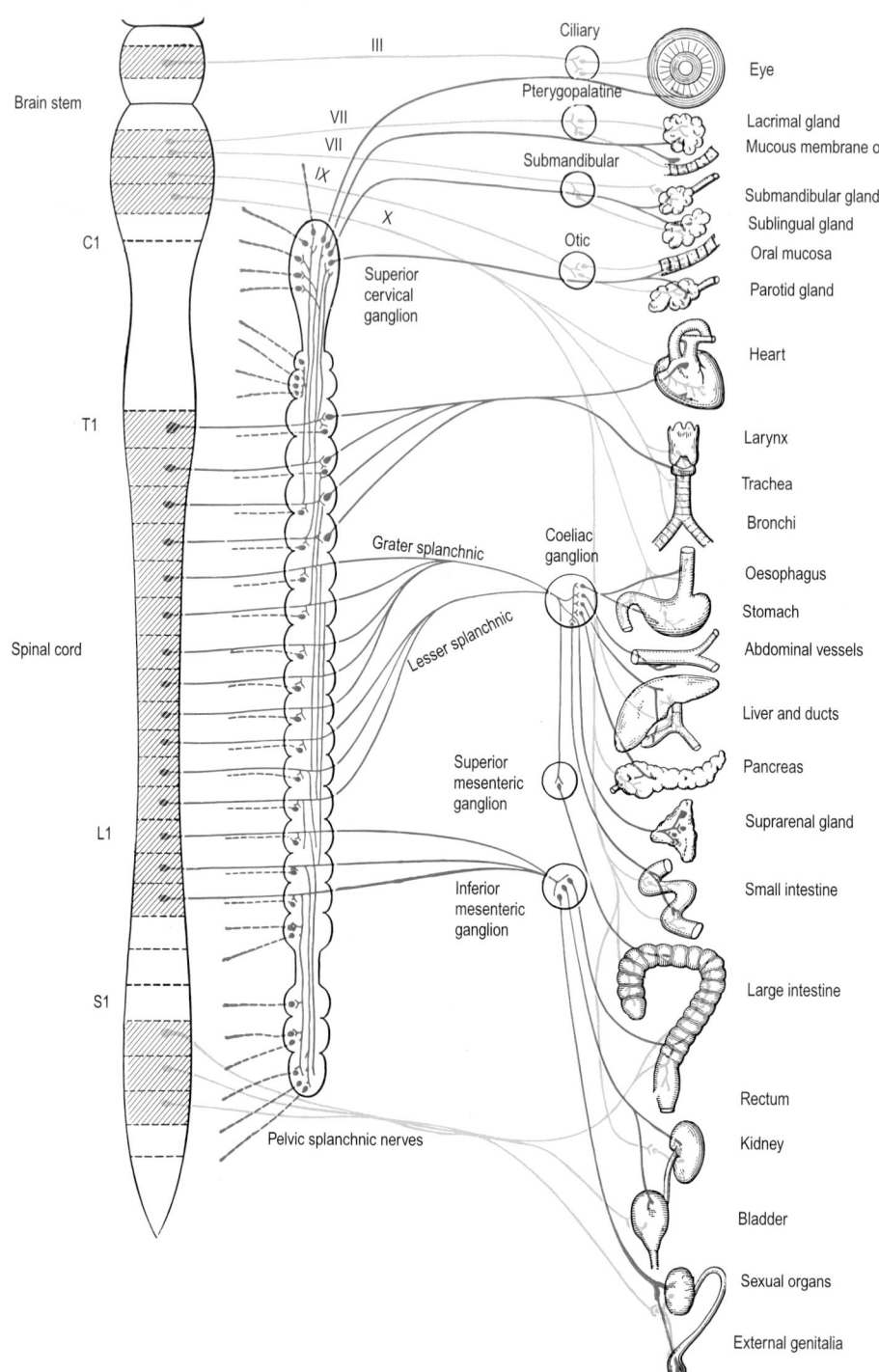

Fig. 13.1 The efferent pathways of the autonomic nervous system. The parasympathetic pathways are represented by blue and the sympathetic by red lines. The interrupted red lines indicate postganglionic rami to the cranial and spinal nerves. (After Meyer and Gottlieb.)

On reaching the sympathetic trunk, preganglionic fibres may behave in one of several ways (**Fig. 13.3**). They may synapse with neurones in the nearest ganglion, or traverse the nearest ganglion and ascend or descend in the sympathetic chain to end in another ganglion. A preganglionic fibre may terminate in a single ganglion or, through collateral branches, synapse with neurones in several ganglia. Preganglionic fibres may traverse the nearest ganglion, ascend or descend and, without synapsing, emerge in one of the medially-directed branches of the sympathetic trunk to synapse in the ganglia of autonomic plexuses (mainly situated in the midline, e.g. around the coeliac and mesenteric arteries). More than one preganglionic fibre may synapse with a single postganglionic neurone. Uniquely, the suprarenal gland is innervated directly by preganglionic sympathetic neurones which traverse the sympathetic trunk and coeliac ganglion without synapse.

The somata of sympathetic postganglionic neurones are located mostly in ganglia of the sympathetic trunk or ganglia in more peripheral plexuses. The axons of postganglionic neurones are, therefore, generally longer than those of preganglionic neurones, an exception being some

of those that innervate pelvic viscera. The axons of ganglionic cells are non-myelinated. They are distributed to target organs in various ways. Those from a ganglion of the sympathetic trunk may return to the spinal nerve of preganglionic origin through a grey ramus communicans, which usually joins the nerve just proximal to the white ramus, and are then distributed through ventral and dorsal spinal rami to blood vessels, sweat glands, hairs, etc., in their zone of supply. Segmental areas vary in extent and overlap considerably. The extent of innervation of different effector systems, e.g. vasomotor, sudomotor, etc., by a particular nerve may not be the same. Alternatively, postganglionic fibres may pass in a medial branch of a ganglion direct to particular viscera, or innervate adjacent blood vessels, or pass along them externally to their peripheral distribution. They may ascend or descend before leaving the sympathetic trunk as above. Many fibres are distributed along arteries and ducts as plexuses to distant effectors.

The principal neurotransmitter released by postganglionic sympathetic neurones is noradrenaline. The sympathetic system has a much wider distribution than the parasympathetic. It innervates all sweat

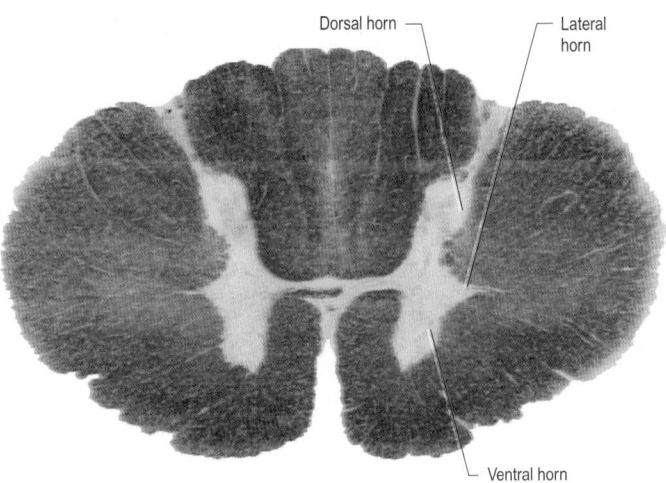

Fig. 13.2 Transverse section through the thoracic spinal cord showing the lateral horn where preganglionic sympathetic neurones are located. (Figure enhanced by B Crossman.)

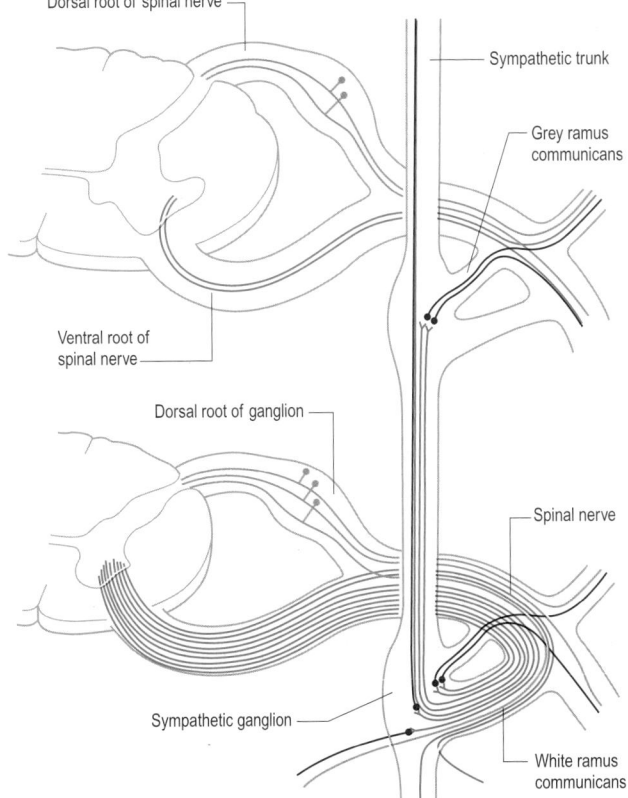

Fig. 13.3 The relationship between spinal nerves and the sympathetic trunk. The somatic components of spinal nerve roots are illustrated in the upper part of the diagram and the visceral components are shown in the lower part. Somatic and preganglionic sympathetic fibres are coloured red; somatic and visceral afferent fibres blue; and postganglionic sympathetic fibres black.

glands, the arrector pili muscles, the muscular walls of many blood vessels, the heart, lungs and respiratory tree, the abdominopelvic viscera, the oesophagus, the muscles of the iris, and the non-striated muscle of the urogenital tract, eyelids and elsewhere.

Postganglionic sympathetic fibres which return to the spinal nerves are vasoconstrictor to blood vessels, secretomotor to sweat glands and motor to the arrector pili muscles within their dermatomes. Those which accompany the motor nerves to voluntary muscles are probably

only dilatatory. Most, if not all, peripheral nerves contain postganglionic sympathetic fibres. Those reaching the viscera are concerned with general vasoconstriction, bronchial and bronchiolar dilatation, modification of glandular secretion, pupillary dilatation, inhibition of alimentary muscle contraction, etc. A single preganglionic fibre probably synapses with the postganglionic neurones in only one effector system, which means that effects such as sudomotor and vasomotor actions can be separate.

PARASYMPATHETIC NERVOUS SYSTEM

Preganglionic parasympathetic neurone cell bodies are located in certain cranial nerve nuclei of the brain stem (**Fig. 16.6**) and in the grey matter of the second to fourth sacral segments of the spinal cord. Efferent fibres, which are myelinated, emerge from the CNS only in certain cranial nerves (oculomotor, facial, glossopharyngeal, vagus) and the second to fourth sacral spinal nerves. The preganglionic parasympathetic neurones are cholinergic.

The cell bodies of postganglionic parasympathetic neurones are mostly sited distant from the CNS, either in discrete ganglia located near the structures innervated, or dispersed in the walls of viscera. In the cranial part of the parasympathetic system there are four small peripheral ganglia, namely ciliary, pterygopalatine, submandibular and otic, which are all described on a regional basis. These are solely efferent parasympathetic ganglia, unlike the trigeminal, facial, glossopharyngeal and vagal ganglia, all of which are concerned exclusively with afferent impulses and contain the cell bodies of sensory neurones. However, the cranial parasympathetic ganglia are traversed by afferent fibres, postganglionic sympathetic fibres, and, in the case of the otic ganglion, even by branchial efferent fibres, but none of these are interrupted in the ganglia. Postganglionic parasympathetic fibres are usually nonmyelinated and shorter than those in the sympathetic system, because the ganglia in which the former synapse are in or near the viscera they supply. In contrast to the sympathetic system, postganglionic parasympathetic neurones are cholinergic.

Oculomotor preganglionic parasympathetic fibres originate in the Edinger–Westphal nucleus of the midbrain (p. 342) and travel in the nerve along its branch to the inferior oblique, reaching the ciliary ganglion where they synapse. Postganglionic fibres, which are thinly myelinated, travel in the short ciliary nerves which pierce the sclera to run forwards in the perichoroidal space to the ciliary muscle and the sphincter pupillae (p. 709). Their activation mediates accommodation of the eye to near objects and pupillary constriction.

The facial nerve contains preganglionic parasympathetic axons of neurones with their somata in the superior salivatory nucleus (p. 342). The fibres emerge from the brain stem in the nervus intermedius, leave the main facial nerve trunk above the stylomastoid foramen and travel in the chorda tympani, which subsequently joins the lingual nerve (p. 523). In this way, preganglionic fibres are conveyed to the submandibular ganglion, where they synapse on ganglionic neurones. Postganglionic fibres innervate the submandibular and sublingual salivary glands and are said to travel in the lingual nerve. Some preganglionic fibres may synapse around cells in the hilum of the submandibular gland. Stimulation of the chorda tympani dilates the arterioles in both glands in addition to having a direct secretomotor effect. The facial nerve also contains efferent parasympathetic lacrimal secretomotor axons, which travel in its greater petrosal branch and thence via the nerve of the pterygoid canal, to relay in the pterygopalatine ganglion. Postganglionic axons are thought to travel by the zygomatic nerve to the lacrimal gland (p. 685) and by ganglionic branches to the nasal and palatal glands.

The glossopharyngeal nerve contains preganglionic parasympathetic secretomotor fibres for the parotid gland. These originate in the inferior salivatory nucleus (p. 342) and travel in the glossopharyngeal nerve and its tympanic branch. They traverse the tympanic plexus and lesser petrosal nerve to reach the otic ganglion where they synapse. Postganglionic fibres pass by communicating branches to the auriculotemporal nerve, which conveys them to the parotid gland. Stimulation of the lesser petrosal nerve produces vasodilator and secretomotor effects.

The vagal nucleus (dorsal motor nucleus of the vagus) in the medulla is a major source of preganglionic parasympathetic fibres. Efferent fibres travel in the vagus nerve and its pulmonary, cardiac, oesophageal, gastric, intestinal and other branches. They synapse in minute ganglia in the visceral walls. Cardiac branches, which act to slow the cardiac cycle, join the cardiac plexuses and fibres relay in ganglia distributed over both atria. Pulmonary branches contain fibres which relay in ganglia of the pulmonary plexuses. They are motor to the circular non-striated muscle fibres of the bronchi and bronchioles and are bronchoconstrictor in function. With the exception of the pyloric sphincter, gastric branches are secretomotor and motor to the non-striated muscle of the stomach, which they inhibit. Intestinal branches have a corresponding action in the small intestine, caecum, vermiform appendix, ascending colon, right colic flexure and most of the transverse colon. They are secretomotor to the glands and motor to the intestinal muscular coats, but inhibitory to the ileocaecal sphincter. Their synaptic relays with postganglionic neurones are situated in the myenteric (Auerbach's) and submucosal (Meissner's) plexuses.

Pelvic splanchnic nerves to the pelvic viscera travel in anterior rami of the second, third and fourth sacral spinal nerves. These nerves unite with branches of the sympathetic pelvic plexuses. Minute ganglia occur at the points of union and in the visceral walls, and sacral preganglionic parasympathetic fibres relay synaptically in these ganglia. The pelvic splanchnic nerves are motor to the muscle of the rectum and bladder wall but inhibitory to the vesical sphincter. They supply vasodilator fibres to the erectile tissue of the penis and clitoris and are probably also vasodilator to the testes, ovaries, uterine tubes and uterus. Filaments from the pelvic splanchnic nerves ascend in the hypogastric plexus and are visceromotor to the sigmoid and descending colon, the left colic flexure and terminal transverse colon.

ENTERIC NERVOUS SYSTEM

The traditional view of the autonomic nervous system was that intrinsic neurones in peripheral organs such as the heart, airways and bladder were postganglionic parasympathetic neurones, which acted as simple cholinergic relay stations. However, many peripheral ganglia contain circuits that are capable of sustaining and modulating visceral activities by local reflex mechanisms. Large populations of intrinsic neurones exist which are derived from the neural crest, and are independent of sympathetic and parasympathetic nerves. The enteric nervous system consists of ganglionated plexuses localized in the wall of the gastro-intestinal tract. It contains reflex pathways through which the contractions of the muscular coats of the alimentary tract, the secretion of gastric acid, intestinal transport of water and electrolytes, mucosal blood flow and other functions are controlled. While complex interactions occur between the enteric and sympathetic and parasympathetic nervous systems, the enteric nervous system is capable of sustaining local reflex activity independent of the CNS. Thus, since intrinsic neurones survive following section of the extrinsic sympathetic and parasympathetic nerves, organs which are transplanted are not truly denervated. It is worth noting that separation from their autonomic input often has no obvious impact on the non-striated muscle or glands innervated by autonomic fibres – contraction may be unaffected and no structural changes ensue. This has been variously attributed to the continued activity of local plexuses or the intrinsic activity of visceral muscle. In some important instances, however, denervation does result in cessation of activity, e.g. in sweat glands, pilomotor muscle, orbital non-striated muscle and the suprarenal medulla.

VISCERAL AFFERENT PATHWAYS

General visceral afferent fibres from the viscera and blood vessels accompany their efferent counterparts, and are the peripheral processes of unipolar cell bodies located in some cranial nerve and dorsal root ganglia. They are contained in the vagus, glossopharyngeal, and possibly other cranial nerves; the second to fourth sacral spinal nerves, distributed with the pelvic splanchnic nerves; and in thoracic and upper lumbar spinal nerves, distributed through rami communicantes and alongside the efferent sympathetic innervation of viscera and blood vessels.

The cell bodies of vagal general visceral afferent fibres are in the superior and inferior vagal ganglia. Their peripheral processes are distributed to terminals in the pharyngeal and oesophageal walls where, acting synergistically with glossopharyngeal visceral afferents in the pharynx, they are concerned with swallowing reflexes. Vagal afferents are also believed to innervate the thyroid and parathyroid glands. In the heart, vagal afferents innervate the walls of the great vessels, the aortic

bodies and pressor receptors, where they are stimulated by raised intravascular pressure. In the lungs they are distributed via the pulmonary plexuses. They supply bronchial mucosa, where they are probably involved in cough reflexes; bronchial muscle, where they encircle myocytes and end in tendrils, which are sometimes regarded as 'muscle spindles' and which are believed to be stimulated by change in the length of myocytes; interalveolar connective tissue, where their knob-like endings, together with terminals on myocytes, may evoke Hering–Breuer reflexes; the adventitia of pulmonary arteries, where they may be pressor receptors; and the intima of pulmonary veins, where they may be chemoreceptors. Vagal visceral afferent fibres also end in the gastric and intestinal walls, digestive glands, and the kidneys. Fibres ending in the gut and its ducts respond to stretch or contraction. Gastric impulses may evoke sensations of hunger and nausea.

The cell bodies of glossopharyngeal general visceral afferents are in the glossopharyngeal ganglia. Their peripheral processes innervate the posterior lingual region, the tonsils and pharynx, but they do not innervate taste buds. They also innervate the carotid sinus and the carotid body, which contain receptors sensitive to tension and changes in chemical composition of the blood. Impulses from these receptors are essential to circulatory and respiratory reflexes.

Visceral afferents which enter the spinal cord through spinal nerve roots terminate in the spinal grey matter. The central processes of vagal and glossopharyngeal afferent fibres end in the vagal nucleus or the nucleus solitarius of the medulla. Visceral afferents establish connections within the CNS that mediate autonomic reflexes. In addition, afferent impulses probably mediate visceral sensations such as hunger, nausea, sexual excitement, vesical distension, etc. Visceral pain fibres may follow these routes. Although viscera are insensitive to cutting, crushing or burning, excessive tension in smooth muscle and some pathological conditions produce visceral pain. In visceral disease, vague pain may be felt near the viscus itself (visceral pain) or in a cutaneous area or other tissue whose somatic afferents enter spinal segments receiving afferents from the viscus, a phenomenon known as referred pain. If inflammation spreads from a diseased viscus to the adjacent parietal serosa (e.g. the peritoneum), somatic afferents will be stimulated, causing local somatic pain, which is commonly spasmodic. Referred pain is often associated with local cutaneous tenderness.

Afferent fibres in pelvic splanchnic nerves innervate pelvic viscera and the distal part of the colon. Vesical receptors are widespread: those in muscle strata are associated with thickly myelinated fibres and are believed to be stretch receptors, possibly activated by contraction. Pain fibres from the bladder and proximal urethra traverse both pelvic splanchnic nerves and the inferior hypogastric plexus, hypogastric nerves, superior hypogastric plexus and lumbar splanchnic nerves to reach their cell bodies in ganglia on the lower thoracic and upper lumbar dorsal spinal roots. The significance of this dual sensory pathway is uncertain. Lesions of the cauda equina abolish pain from vesical overdistension but hypogastric section is ineffective. Pain fibres from the uterus traverse the hypogastric plexus and lumbar splanchnic nerves to reach somata in the lowest thoracic and upper lumbar spinal ganglia; hypogastric division may relieve dysmenorrhoea. However, afferents from the uterine cervix traverse the pelvic splanchnic nerves to somata in the upper sacral spinal ganglia. Stretch of the cervix uteri causes pain but cauterization and biopsy excisions do not.

In general, afferent fibres which accompany pre- and postganglionic sympathetic fibres have a segmental arrangement. They end in spinal cord segments from which preganglionic fibres innervate the region or viscus concerned. General visceral afferents entering thoracic and upper lumbar spinal segments are largely concerned with pain. Nociceptive impulses from the pharynx, oesophagus, stomach, intestines, kidneys, ureter, gallbladder and bile ducts seem to be carried in sympathetic pathways. Cardiac nociceptive impulses enter the spinal cord via the first to fifth thoracic spinal nerves, mainly in the middle and inferior cardiac nerves, but a few pass directly to the spinal nerves. It is said that there are no general visceral afferents in the superior cardiac nerves. Peripherally, the fibres pass through the cardiac plexuses and along the coronary arteries. Myocardial anoxia may evoke symptoms of angina pectoris in which pain is typically presternal, and is also referred to much of the left chest, and radiates to the left shoulder, the medial aspect of the left arm, along the left side of the neck to the jaw and occiput, and down to the epigastrium. Cardiac afferents carried in vagal cardiac branches are concerned with the reflex depression of cardiac activity. Ureteric pain fibres, also running with sympathetic fibres, are presumably involved in the agonizing renal colic that follows obstruction by calculi. Afferent fibres from the testis and ovary run through the corresponding plexuses to somata in the tenth and eleventh thoracic dorsal root ganglia.

Certain primary afferent nerve fibres, which have their cell bodies in cranial and dorsal root ganglia, also have an efferent function (so-called sensory–motor nerves). The importance of sensory–motor nerve regulation in many organs, such as the gut, lungs, heart and blood vessels, is now recognized. While most such nerves are, presumably, purely sensory, certain of them have been termed sensory–motor

because they release transmitter from their peripheral endings during the axon reflex and have a motor rather than a sensory role. The primary substances so released are substance P, calcitonin gene-related peptide (CGRP) and ATP. These substances act on target cells to produce several biological actions which include vasodilatation, increased venular permeability, changes in smooth muscle contractility, degranulation of mast cells and a variety of effects on leukocytes and fibroblasts, a process collectively known as 'neurogenic inflammation'. The local release of such substances may play a trophic role in the maintenance of tissue integrity and repair in response to injury.

REFERENCES

Björklund A, Hökfelt T, Owman C (eds) 1988 The Peripheral Nervous Systems. Handbook of Chemical Neuroanatomy. Vol. 6. Amsterdam: Elsevier.
Description of sensory–motor nerves.

Burnstock G 1990 Co-transmission. The fifth Heymans lecture. Arch Int Pharmacodyn Ther 304: 7–33.
A review of neurotransmission in the autonomic nervous system.

Burnstock G (ed) 1992–95 The Autonomic Nervous System. Vols 1–14. Switzerland: Harwood Academic Publishers.
Contains extensive material on the neurotransmitters of the autonomic nervous system.

Maggi CA 1991 The pharmacology of the efferent function of sensory nerves. J Auton Pharmacol 11: 173–208.

Vinken PJ, Bruyn GW (eds) 1999 The Autonomic Nervous System. Part 1. Normal Functions. Appenzeller O (volume ed). Amsterdam and London: Elsevier Science Publishers.

Vinken PJ, Bruyn GW (eds) 2000 The Autonomic Nervous System. Part 2. Dysfunctions. Appenzeller O (volume ed). Amsterdam and London: Elsevier Science Publishers.

Development of the nervous system

The entire nervous system and the special sense organs originate from three sources, each derived from specific cell populations of the early epiblast termed neural ectoderm. The first source to be clearly delineated is the neural plate, which gives rise to the central nervous system, the somatic motor nerves and the preganglionic autonomic nerves. The second source is from cells at the perimeter of the neural plate, which remove themselves by epithelial/mesenchymal transition from the plate just prior to its fusion as a neural tube. These are the neural crest cells and they form nearly all the peripheral nervous system, including the somatic sensory nerves, the somatic and autonomic ganglia, post-ganglionic autonomic nerves and adrenal and chromaffin cells. They also give rise to significant mesenchymal populations in the head. The third source is from ectodermal placodes, a group of cells which originate at the edge of the neural plate but which remain in the surface ectoderm after neural tube formation, undergoing epithelial/mesenchymal transformation after the neural crest cells have started their migration. Ectodermal placodes contribute to the cranial sensory ganglia, to the hypophysis, the inner ear and, by a non-neuronal contribution, to the lens of the eye.

With the initiation of gastrulation, the first populations of epiblast cells to invaginate through the primitive streak form the prechordal plate, embryonic endoderm and notochord. These cells invaginate through the rostral end of the primitive streak (Hensen's node in the chick). The node gives rise concomitantly to the midline floor plate of the neural plate, which extends with the subjacent notochord to the bucco-pharyngeal membrane. The neural plate is a thickened epithelium, roughly oval but wider rostrally and narrowed caudally (**Fig. 10.17**). It extends over the paraxial mesenchyme invaginating from the more caudal regions of the primitive streak.

NEURULATION

Primary neurulation begins at stage 9 (**Fig. 14.1**). The process, although continuous spatially and temporally, has been envisaged as four stages. It begins with local elongation of the ectoderm cells in a midline zone of the disc and their reorganization into a pseudostratified epithelium, the neural plate. This is followed by reshaping of the neural plate and bending of the plate into a neural groove. The latter is closed to form into a neural tube bidirectionally from the midportion to its cranial and caudal ends. A continuous surface ectoderm forms dorsal to the tube.

The regions of rostral and caudal fusion are termed rostral and caudal neuropores respectively. However, there may be more than one region of fusion. Primary neurulation occurs contemporaneously with somitogenesis: its success depends on the cellular changes and movements of the paraxial mesenchyme. The neural ectodermal cells become elongated and then wedge-shaped. It has been suggested that the forces needed to shape the neural tube are intrinsic to the cells of the neurecto-derm. When the neural tube is closing, its walls consist of a single layer of columnar neural epithelial cells, whose extremities abut on internal and external limiting membranes. The columnar cells increase in length and develop numerous longitudinally disposed microtubules. The borders of their luminal ends are firmly attached to adjacent cells by junctional complexes, and the cytoplasmic aspect of the complexes are associated with a dense paraluminal web of microfilaments. The nuclei assume basal positions which, together with the disposition of organelles, impart a slight wedge conformation on some of the cells, and create a hinge point.

The position of hinge points within the neural plate confers different characteristics on the formed neural tube. With a median hinge point,

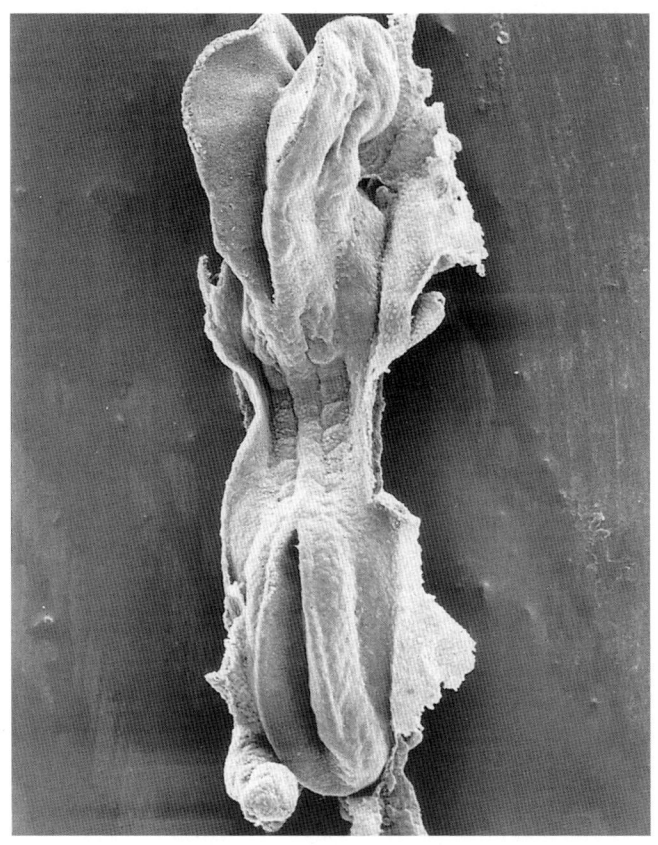

Fig. 14.1 Scanning electron micrograph of a neurulating rat embryo comparable to a stage-10 human embryo (22–24 days). Somite formation occurs as neurulation proceeds caudally. (Photograph by P Collins; printed by S Cox, Electron Microscopy Unit, Southampton General Hospital.)

the neural folds remain relatively straight and the tube in this position has a slit-shaped lumen: this can be seen from the initial region of fusion rostralward. If dorsolateral hinge points are added, the resulting neural tube is rhombic, as can be seen from the initial region of fusion, caudally. If all the neuroepithelial cells exhibit some apical narrowing, then the resulting tube has a circular lumen. The rostral slit-shaped profile of the neural tube may depend more on support from adjacent tissues than the caudal end of the tube, where neurulation is generated by the neuroepithelium. The transition from primary to secondary neurulation continues the production of a neural tube with a circular lumen.

Secondary neurulation is a process which has only recently received more extensive study. Primary neurulation ceases when the neural tube has closed completely: the rostral neuropore closes during stage 11 (24 days) and the caudal neuropore during stage 12. There is some discrepancy in the literature about the level of the caudal neuropore at the start and end of closure. It is expressed as a somite level, ranging from somite 25 to somite 31. The level is significant because the junction of primary and secondary neurulation is seen as a site of future anomalies of neural development. Somite 27 participates in the formation of thoracic vertebra 12 and lumbar vertebra 1, and somite 31 corresponds to sacral vertebra 2. When the caudal neuropore reaches a certain level, the cell populations for these caudal somites have already been produced from the unsegmented paraxial mesenchyme, which compounds the difficulty of specifying the level.

At the time of caudal neuropore closure the midline cells located caudally are generically termed the tail bud. A specific population called the caudoneural hinge shares the same molecular markers as the primitive node. These cells aggregate at the midline and undergo mesenchymal/epithelial transformation which produces a cellular cylinder contiguous with the caudal end of the neural tube. Further elongation of the caudal neural tube involves cavitation of the neural cylinder. Neural crest cells delaminate from the dorsal surface of the cylinder in a rostrocaudal direction. Concurrently, the paraxial mesenchyme undergoes somitogenesis.

The main difference between primary and secondary neurulation is that the latter leads to the formation of a neural tube in the absence of a neural plate. Close to the level of the caudal neuropore these processes overlap both temporally and spatially.

EARLY VESICLES AND FLEXURES OF THE NEURAL TUBE

Prior to the closure of the neural tube, the neural folds become considerably expanded in the head region, as a first indication of a brain. After the rostral neuropore closes these regional expansions form three primary cerebral vesicles (**Fig. 14.2**). The term 'vesicle' may be rather a misnomer, since it suggests an exaggerated view of these localized accelerations of growth in the wall of the brain. The bulging is not initially marked, and the vesicles are more like gently fusiform tubes. The three regions are named prosencephalon (forebrain), mesencephalon (midbrain), and rhombencephalon (hindbrain), the last being continuous caudally with the spinal cord. As a result of unequal growth of their different regions, the prosencephalon and rhombencephalon enlarge more than the mesencephalon and can be subdivided. The prosencephalon gives rise to a midline diencephalon and bilateral telencephalon; the rhombencephalon gives rise to the metencephalon and myelencephalon. A summary of the derivative of the cerebral vesicles is given on page 256.

The elongation of the brain occurs at the same time as the appearance of three flexures which are also developing prior to the closure of the neural tube; two are concave ventrally and one concave dorsally. During stages 13 and 14 the brain bends at the mesencephalon (mesencephalic flexure) so that the prosencephalon bends in a ventral direction around the cephalic end of the notochord and foregut until its floor lies almost parallel with that of the rhombencephalon (**Fig. 14.2**). A bend also appears at the junction of the rhombencephalon and spinal cord (cervical flexure). This increases from the fifth to the end of the seventh week, by which time the rhombencephalon forms nearly a right angle to the spinal cord. However, after the seventh week, extension of the head takes place and the cervical flexure diminishes and eventually disappears. The third bend, the pontine flexure, is directed ventrally between the metencephalon and myelencephalon. It does not substantially affect the outline of the head. In this region, the roof plate thins until it is composed only of a single layer of cells and pia mater, the tela choroidea. The flexure of the neural tube at this point produces a rhombic shape in the roof which later forms the medullary velum.

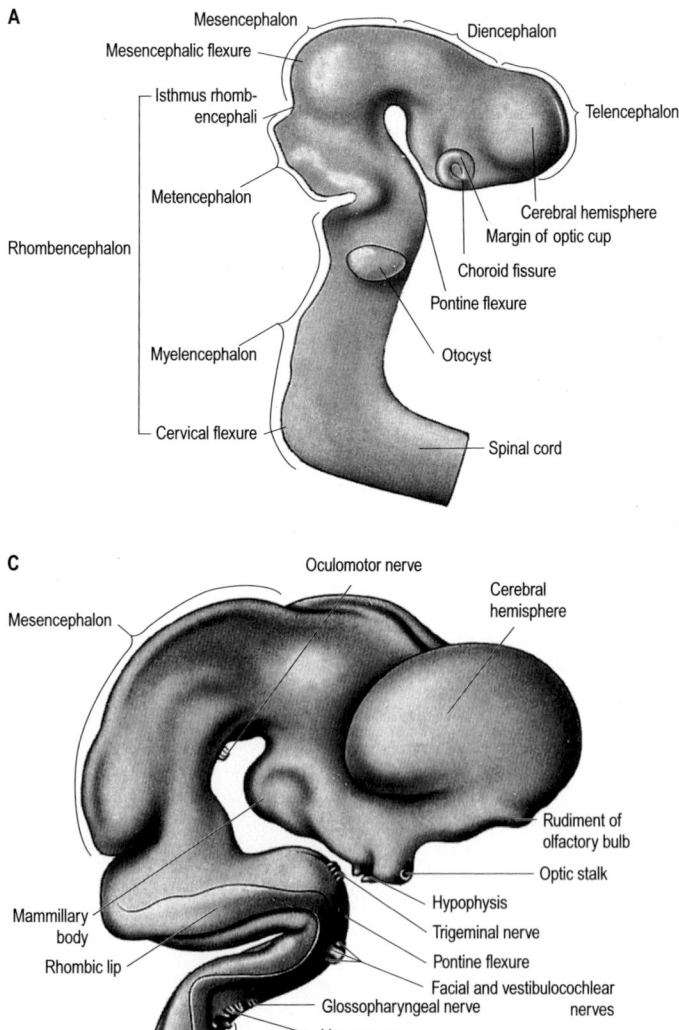

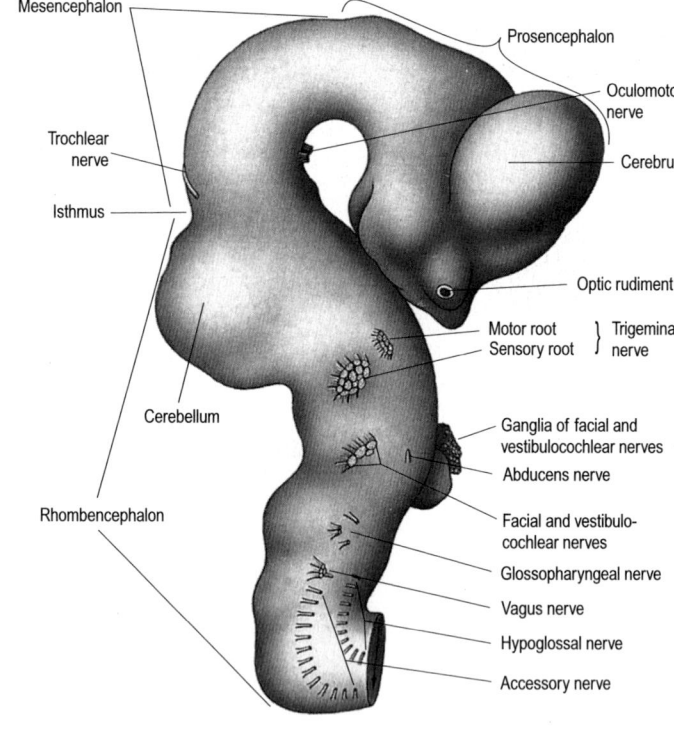

Fig. 14.2 A, The right side of the brain of a human embryo, 9 mm long. **B,** The brain of a human embryo c.10.2 mm long: right lateral surface. **C,** The right side of the brain of a human embryo, 13.6 mm long. The roof of the hindbrain has been removed.

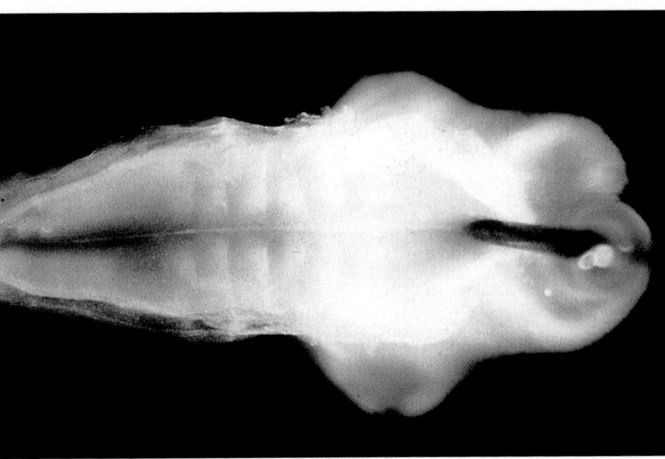

Fig. 14.3 Rhombomeric segmentation. Rostral is toward the right. (By kind permission from Professor Lumsden.)

In addition to these gross divisions, a number of ridges and depressions are present transiently on the inner surface of the brain. Prominent among these are the serial bulges that appear very early in the rhombencephalon, before the main flexures of the neural tube develop (**Fig. 14.3**). These bulges are termed rhombomeres.

EARLY CELLULAR ARRANGEMENT OF THE NEURAL TUBE

Histologically the early neural tube is composed of a pseudostratified neuroepithelium. It extends from the inner aspect of the tube to the outer limiting basal lamina and surrounding neural crest, which will form the pia mater. The epithelium contains stem cells which will give rise to populations of neuroblasts and glioblasts. A population of radial glia differentiates very early and provides a scaffold for later cells to follow. As development proceeds, three zones or layers develop (**Figs 14.4, 14.5, 14.6**). These are: an internal ventricular zone (variously termed the germinal, primitive ependymal or matrix layer), in which mitosis occurs, and which contains the nucleated parts of the columnar cells and rounded cells undergoing mitosis; a middle, mantle zone (also termed the intermediate zone) which contains the migrant cells from the divisions occurring in the ventricular zone; and an outer, marginal zone, which initially consists of the external cytoplasmic processes of

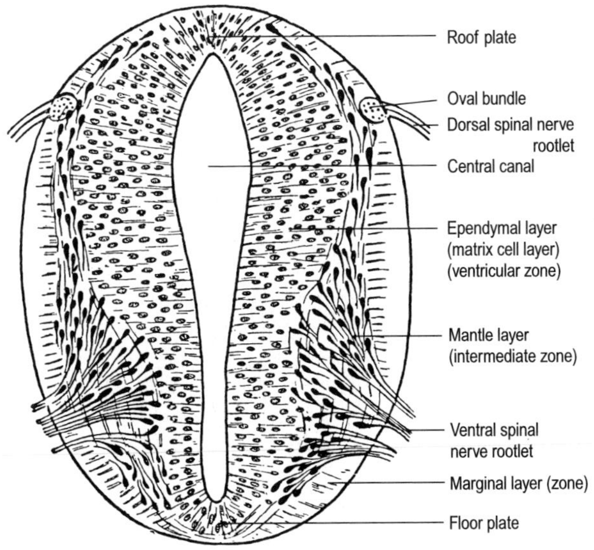

Fig. 14.4 Transverse section through the developing spinal cord of a 4-week-old human embryo. Historically early terminology is retained; more recent terms are in parentheses.

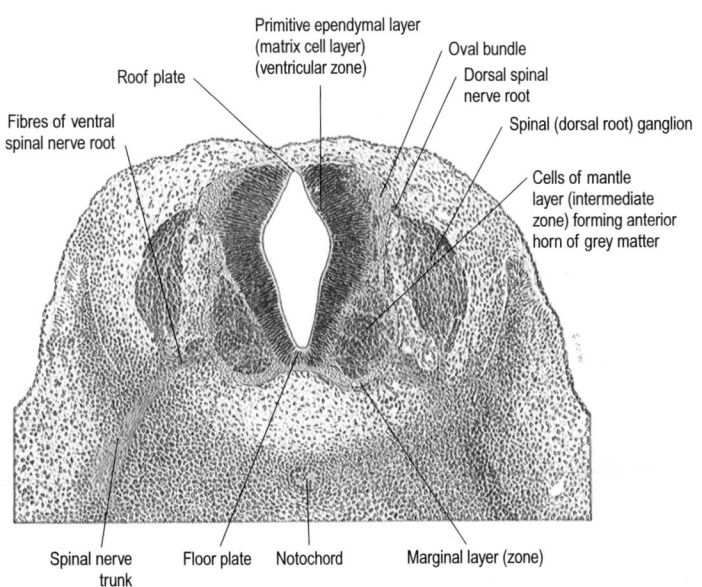

Fig. 14.6 Transverse section of the developing spinal cord in the cervical region of a human embryo early in the sixth week; CR length 8 mm.

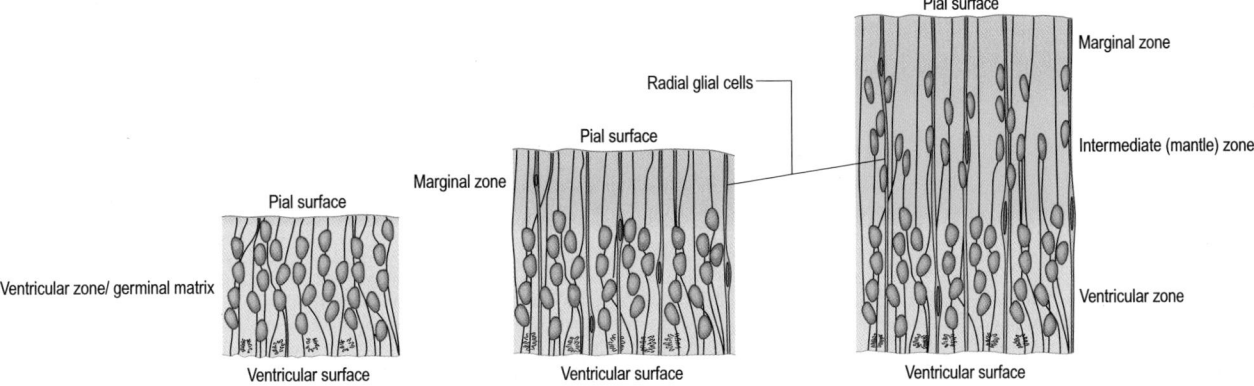

Fig. 14.5 Early development of the neural tube. Three layers can be delineated in the spinal cord and brain stem.

the radial glia and the neuroepithelial stem cells. The latter is soon invaded by tracts of axonal processes which grow from neuroblasts developing in the mantle zone, together with varieties of non-neuronal cells (glial cells and later vascular endothelium and perivascular mesenchyme). For further development of these layers see page 248.

At first the neural tube caudal to the brain is oval in transverse section and its lumen is narrow and slit-like (Fig. 14.4). The original floor plate and the dorsal site of fusion of the tube initially contain non-neural cells. With cellular proliferation, the lateral walls thicken and the lumen, now the central canal, widens in its dorsal part and is somewhat diamond-shaped on cross-section (Fig. 14.6). The widening of the canal is associated with the development of a longitudinal sulcus limitans on each side. This divides the ventricular and mantle (intermediate) zones in each lateral wall into a ventrolateral lamina or basal plate and a dorsolateral lamina or alar plate. This separation indicates a fundamental functional difference.

Throughout the neural tube there is a generic pattern in the position of the neurones which is specified by the juxtaposition of the notochord to the neural tube. Lateral or dorsal grafting of a notochord results in the induction of a floor plate overlying the grafted notochord and the induction of ectopic dorsal motor neurones. Similarly, lateral or dorsal grafts of a floor plate also result in the induction of a new floor plate overlying the graft and the induction of ectopic dorsal motor neurones. Removal of the notochord results in the elimination of the floor plate and the motor neurones and the differentiation of dorsal cell types in the ventral region of the cord (Fig. 14.7).

The basal plate is normally concerned predominantly with motor function, and contains the cell bodies of motor neurones of the future anterior and lateral grey columns. The alar plate receives sensory inflow from external dorsal root ganglia. Motor and sensory axons combine to form the mixed nerves.

FAILURE OF NEURULATION

Failure of neurulation produces the conditions of craniorachischisis totalis (where the entire neural tube is unfused in the dorsal midline) cranioschisis or anencephaly (where the neural tube is fused dorsally to form the spinal cord but is not fused dorsally in the brain), and spina bifida (where local regions of the spinal neural tube is unfused, or there is failure of formation of the vertebral neural arches). (Fig. 14.8; see also p. 797). Anencephalic fetuses display severe disturbances in the shape, position and ossification of the basichondrocranium and in the course of the intracranial notochord.

NEURAL CREST

The neuronal populations of the early epiblast become arranged in the medial region of the embryonic disc as the neural plate. Laterally, neural folds or crests indicate the transitional region between neural and surface ectoderm. Along most of the neuraxis the cells at the tips of the neural folds undergo an epithelial/mesenchyme transformation. They acquire migratory properties and leave the epithelium just prior to its fusion with the contralateral fold in the dorsal midline. The migratory cells so formed are collectively termed the neural crest (Brown, Keynes & Lumsden 2001). Cells within the rostral prosencephalic neural fold and smaller populations of cells in bilateral sites along the early brain do not form migratory neural crest cells, but remain within the surface epithelium as ectodermal placodes.

Neural crest populations arise from the neural folds as primary neurulation proceeds and simultaneously progress rostrally and caudally. Crest cells migrate from the neural folds of the brain prior to tube closure. Caudally, from somite 27, secondary neurulation processes produce the most caudal neural crest. Two distinct populations of neural crest cells are formed: a neuronal population produced throughout the brain and spinal cord which gives rise to sensory and autonomic neurones and glia, and a non-neuronal mesenchymal population which arises only from the brain (Figs 14.9, 14.10). Melanocytes develop from a subpopulation of neural crest cells derived from both the head and trunk. They form one of the three pigment cell types (the others being retinal pigment epithelium and pigment cells of the pineal organ, which both originate from the diencephalon).

In the trunk the migration patterns of neural crest cells is channelled by the somites (p. 790). As the crest cells move laterally and ventrally they can pass between the somites and within the rostral sclerotomal half of each somite, but they cannot penetrate the caudal moiety of the sclerotomal mesenchyme. Thus the segmental distribution of the spinal and sympathetic ganglia is imposed on the neural crest cells by a pre-pattern that exists within the somitic paraxial mesenchyme (Fig. 14.11).

Rostral to the otic vesicle, neural crest cells arise from specific regions of the brain. Within the rhombencephalon a number of transverse subdivisions perpendicular to the long axis of the brain can be seen early in development. These are termed rhombomeres (neuromeres) to note their segmental arrangement (Muller & O'Rahilly 1997). At stage 9, six primary rhombomeres can be seen. Up to 16 secondary segments can be identified at stage 14. Eight main rhombomeres are recognized extending from the midbrain–hindbrain boundary, rostrally to the spinal cord caudally (Fig. 14.3). Rhombomeres 8 and 7 give rise to crest cells which migrate into the fourth and sixth pharyngeal arches; rhombomere 6 crest invades pharyngeal arch three. Rhombomere 4 crest migrates into arch 2, whereas rhombomeres 5 and 3 give rise to a very small number of neural crest cells which migrate rostrally and caudally to enter the adjacent even-numbered neighbours. Rhombomeres 1 and 2 produce crest which invades the first pharyngeal arch. In each case mesenchymal populations and the sensory and autonomic ganglia are formed from the crest cells.

Further rostrally, neural crest from the mesencephalon migrates into the first arch maxillary and mandibular processes. Crest cells are produced from the diencephalon up to the level of the epiphysis. Neural crest cells

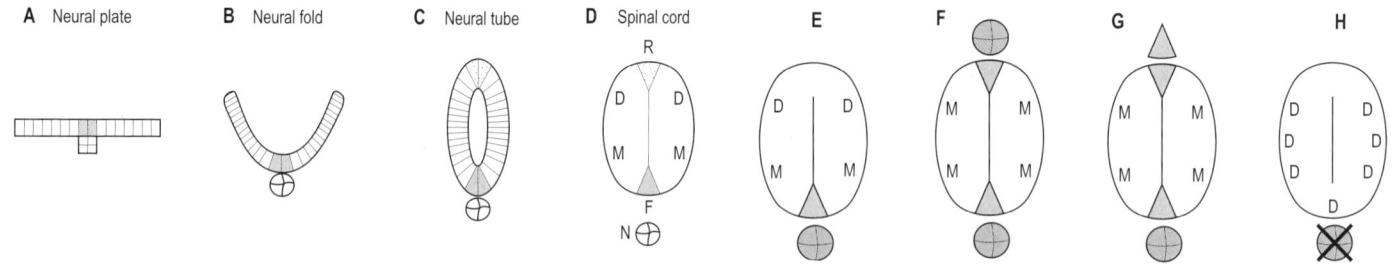

Fig. 14.7 A–B, Successive stages in the development of the neural tube and spinal cord. **A,** The neural plate consists of epithelial cells. Cells in the midline of the neural plate are contacted directly by the notochord. More lateral regions of the neural plate overlie the paraxial mesenchyme (not shown). **B,** During neurulation, the neural plate bends at its midline and this elevates the lateral edges of the plate as the neural folds. Contact between the midline of the neural plate and the notochord is maintained at this stage. **C,** The neural tube is formed when the dorsal tips of the neural folds fuse. Cells in the region of fusion form the roof plate which is a specialized group of dorsal midline cells. **D,** Cells at the ventral midline of the neural tube retain proximity to the notochord and differentiate into the floor plate. After neural tube closure neuroepithelial cells continue to proliferate and eventually differentiate into defined classes of neurones at different dorsoventral positions within the spinal cord. For example, sensory relay, commissural and other classes of dorsal neurones (D) differentiate near to the roof plate (R), and motor (M) neurones differentiate ventrally near to the floor plate (F), which by this time is no longer in contact with the notochord (N). **E–H,** A summary of the results obtained from experiments in chick embryos in which a notochord or floor plate is grafted to the dorsal midline of the neural tube or where the notochord is removed before neural tube closure. **E,** The normal condition, showing the ventral location of motor neurones (M) and the dorsal location of sensory relay neurones (D). **F,** Dorsal grafts of a notochord result in the induction of a floor plate in the dorsal midline and ectopic dorsal motor neurones. **G,** Dorsal grafts of a floor plate induce a new floor plate in the dorsal midline and ectopic dorsal motor neurones. **H,** Removal of the notochord results in the elimination of the floor plate and the motor neurones and the expression of dorsal cells types (D) in the ventral region of the spinal cord. (After Jessell and Dodd 1992, WB Saunders.)

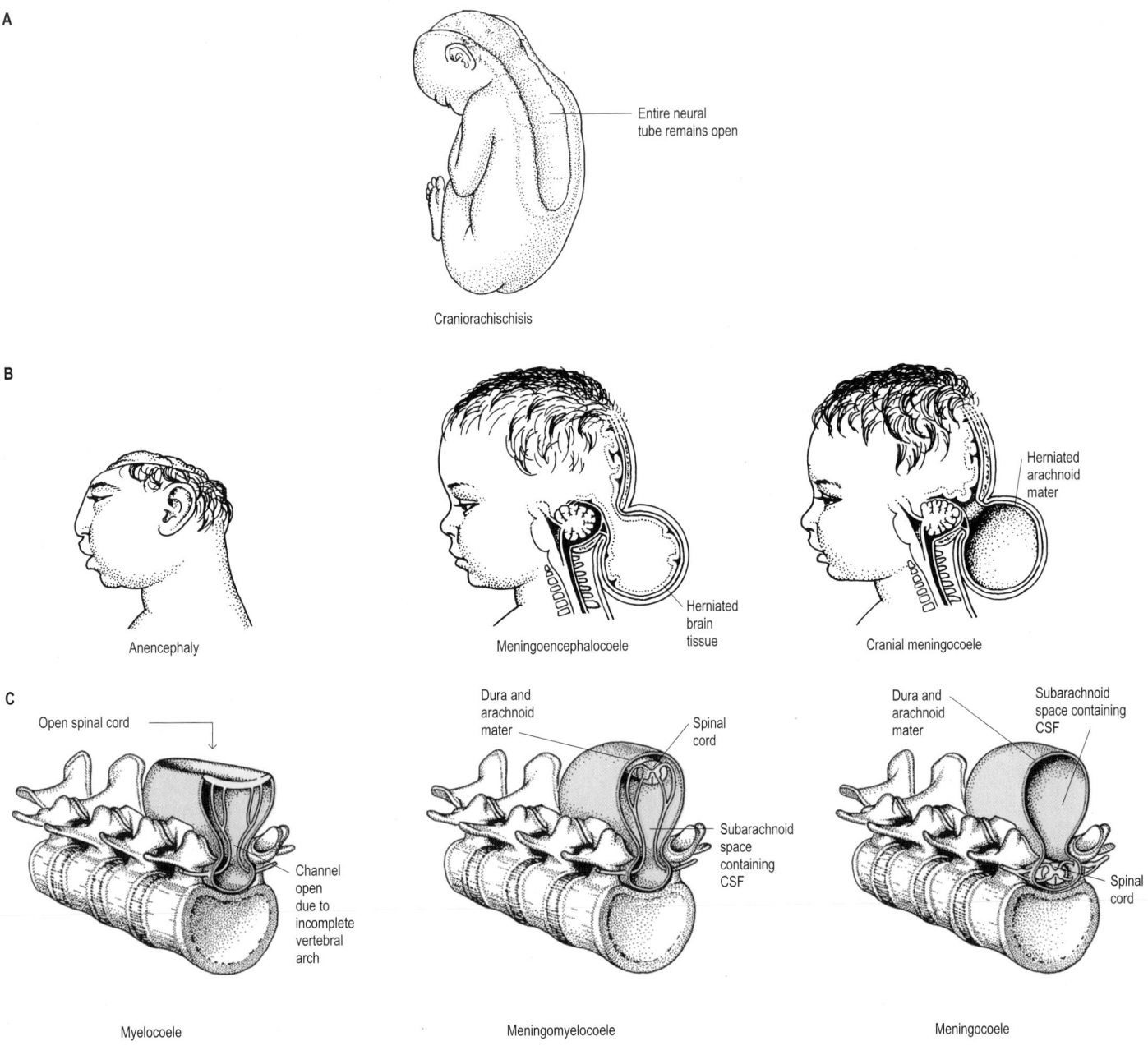

A

Entire neural
tube remains open

Craniorachischisis

B

Anencephaly

Herniated
brain
tissue

Meningoencephalocoele

Herniated
arachnoid
mater

Cranial meningocoele

C

Open spinal cord

Channel
open
due to
incomplete
vertebral
arch

Myelocoele

Dura and
arachnoid
mater

Spinal
cord

Subarachnoid
space
containing
CSF

Meningomyelocoele

Dura and
arachnoid
mater

Subarachnoid
space containing
CSF

Spinal
cord

Meningocoele

Fig. 14.8 Defects caused by failure of neural tube formation. **A**, Total failure of neurulation. **B**, Failure of rostral neurulation. **C**, Failure of caudal neurulation.

which are produced from this rostral portion of the brain contribute mesenchymal populations to the frontonasal process. The most rostral prosencephalic neural fold does not give rise to neural crest and produces cells which either remain epithelial as placodes, or form the epithelial lining of the nasal cavity.

ECTODERMAL PLACODES

Prior to neural tube closure, the elevating neural folds contain two distinctive neuronal populations. The larger population of neural crest cells migrates from the neural epithelium prior to neural tube fusion. A smaller population of neuroepithelial cells becomes incorporated into the surface ectoderm after neural tube closure. These areas of neuro-epithelium within the surface ectoderm have been termed ectodermal placodes. Although the majority of the ectodermal placodes form nervous tissue, non-neurogenic placodes also occur (Begbie & Graham 2001). After an appropriate inductive stimulus, local clusters of placodal cells remove themselves from the surrounding surface ectoderm either by epithelial/mesenchymal transition or by invagination of the whole placodal region to form a vesicle beneath the remaining surface ectoderm.

Neurogenic placodes undergo both processes. Paired non-neurogenic placodes invaginate to form the lens vesicles under the inductive influence of the optic vesicles (p. 721).

The neural folds meet in the rostral midline adjacent to the bucco-pharyngeal membrane. This rostral neural fold does not generate neural crest but gives rise to the hypophyseal placode, i.e. the future Rathke's pouch, which remains within the surface ectoderm directly rostral to the buccopharyngeal membrane. The rostral neural fold also gives rise to the olfactory placodes (p. 610) (which remain as paired) laterally placed placodes, and to the epithelium of the nasal cavity (**Fig. 14.10**).

Further caudally, similar neurogenic placodes can be identified and divided into three categories: ventrolateral or epibranchial; dorsolateral; and intermediate (**Fig. 14.12**). The epibranchial placodes appear in the surface ectoderm immediately dorsal to the area of pharyngeal (branchial) cleft formation. The first epibranchial placode is located at the level of the first pharyngeal groove and contributes cells to the distal (geniculate) ganglion of the facial nerve; the second and third epibranchial placodes contribute cells to the distal ganglia of the glosso-pharyngeal (petrosal) and vagus (nodose) nerves respectively. Generally these placodes thicken and cells begin to detach from the epithelium soon after the pharyngeal pouches have contacted the overlying ectoderm.

245

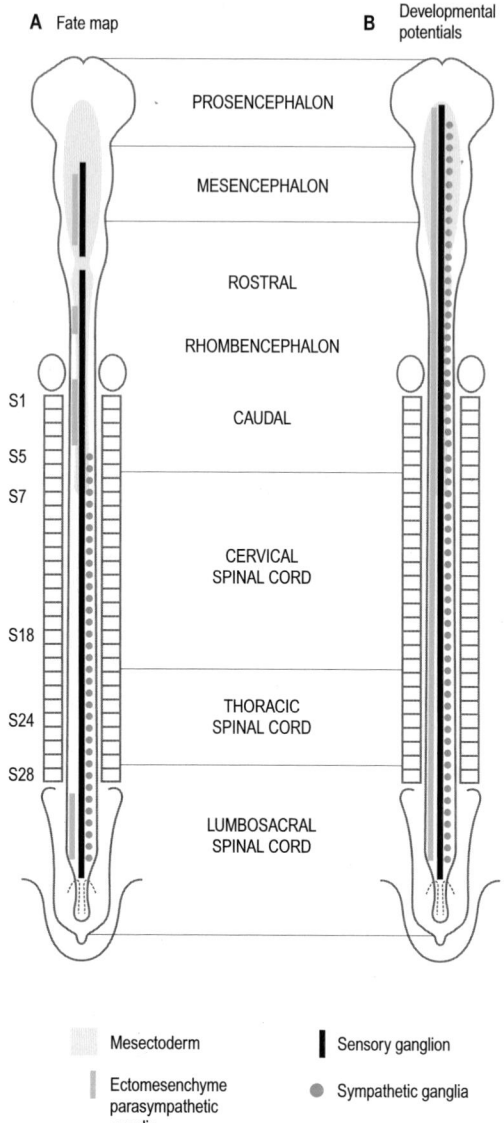

A Fate map   **B** Developmental potentials

PROSENCEPHALON

MESENCEPHALON

ROSTRAL

RHOMBENCEPHALON

CAUDAL

S1

S5

S7

CERVICAL SPINAL CORD

S18

THORACIC SPINAL CORD

S24

S28

LUMBOSACRAL SPINAL CORD

Mesectoderm   ▌ Sensory ganglion

▐ Ectomesenchyme parasympathetic ganglia   ● Sympathetic ganglia

Fig. 14.9 **A**, Fate map along the neural crest of the presumptive territories which yield the ectomesenchyme, the sensory, parasympathetic and sympathetic ganglia and neural crest derived mesenchyme in normal development. **B**, Developmental potentials for the same cell types. If neural crest cells from any level of the neural axis are implanted into the appropriate sites of a host embryo, they can give rise to almost all the cell types forming the various kinds of PNS ganglia. This is not true for the neural crest derived mesenchyme whose precursors are confined to the cephalic area of the crest down to the level of somite 5. S, somite.

Concurrently the neural crest cells reach and move beyond these lateral extensions of the pharynx. Cells budding off placodes show signs of early differentiation into neurones including the formation of neurites. Epibranchial placodes may have their origins in the neurones which innervate the taste buds in fishes.

Dorsolateral placodes may be related evolutionarily to the sensory receptors of the lateral line system of lower vertebrates. They are represented by the otic placodes, located lateral to the myelencephalon, and invaginate to form otic vesicles from which the membranous labyrinth of the ear develops. Neurones of the vestibulocochlear nerve ganglia arise by budding off the ventromedial aspect of the otic cup after which they can be distinguished in the acoustic and vestibular ganglia.

Intermediate between the epibranchial and dorsolateral placodes are the profundal and trigeminal placodes which fuse in man to form a single entity. Prospective neuroblasts migrate from foci dispersed throughout the surface ectoderm lateral and ventrolateral to the caudal

mesencephalon and metencephalon to contribute to the distal portions of the trigeminal ganglia.

PITUITARY GLAND (HYPOPHYSIS CEREBRI)

The hypophysis cerebri consists of the adenohypophysis and the neurohypophysis. Prior to neurulation the cell populations which give rise to these two portions of the pituitary gland are found next to each other within the rostral portion of the floor of the neural plate and the contiguous midline neural fold. As neurulation proceeds the future neurohypophysis remains within the floor of the prosencephalon. The cells of the future adenohypophysis are displaced into the surface ectoderm, where they form the hypophyseal placode in close apposition and adherent to the overlying prosencephalon.

The most rostral portion of the neural plate, which will form the hypothalamus, is in contact rostrally with the future adenohypophysis in the rostral neural ridge, and caudally with the neurohypophysis, in the floor of the neural plate (**Fig. 14.10**). After neurulation the cells of the anterior neural ridge remain in the surface ectoderm and form the hypophyseal placode which is in close apposition and adherent to the overlying prosencephalon.

Neural crest mesenchyme later moves between the prosencephalon and surface ectoderm except at the region of the placode. Before rupture of the buccopharyngeal membrane, proliferation of the periplacodal mesenchyme means that the placode forms the roof and walls of a saccular depression. This hypophyseal recess (pouch of Rathke; **Figs 14.13, 14.14**) is the rudiment of the adenohypophysis. It lies immediately ventral to the dorsal border of the buccopharyngeal membrane, extending in front of the rostral tip of the notochord, and retaining contact with the ventral surface of the prosencephalon. It is constricted by continued proliferation of the surrounding mesenchyme to form a closed vesicle, but remains for a time connected to the ectoderm of the stomodeum by a solid cord of cells, which can be traced down the posterior edge of the nasal septum. Masses of epithelial cells form mainly on each side and in the ventral wall of the vesicle, and the development of the adenohypophysis progresses by the ingrowth of a mesenchymal stroma. Differentiation of epithelial cells into stem cells and three differentiating types is said to be apparent during the early months of fetal development. It has been suggested that different types of cells arise in succession, and that they may be derived in differing proportions from different parts of the hypophyseal recess. A craniopharyngeal canal, which sometimes runs from the anterior part of the hypophyseal fossa of the sphenoid to the exterior of the skull, is often said to mark the original position of the hypophyseal recess. Traces of the stomodeal end of the recess are usually present at the junction of the septum of the nose with the palate. Others have claimed that the craniopharyngeal canal itself is a secondary formation caused by the growth of blood vessels, and is quite unconnected with the stalk of the anterior lobe.

A small endodermal diverticulum, named Seessel's pouch, projects towards the brain from the cranial end of the foregut, immediately caudal to the buccopharyngeal membrane. In some marsupials this pouch forms a part of the hypophysis, but in man it apparently disappears entirely.

Just caudal to, but in contact with, the adenohypophyseal recess, a hollow diverticulum elongates towards the stomodeum from the floor of the neural plate just caudal to the hypothalamus (**Fig. 14.14B**); this region of neural outgrowth is the neurohypophysis. It forms an infundibular sac, the walls of which increase in thickness until the contained cavity is obliterated except at its upper end, where it persists as the infundibular recess of the third ventricle. The neurohypophysis becomes invested by the adenohypophysis, which extends dorsally on each side of it. The adenohypophysis gives off two processes from its ventral wall which grow along the infundibulum and fuse to surround it, coming into relation with the tuber cinereum and forming the tuberal portion of the hypophysis. The original cavity of Rathke's pouch remains first as a cleft, and later as scattered vesicles, and can be identified readily in sagittal sections through the mature gland. The dorsal wall of Rathke's pouch, which remains thin, fuses with the adjoining part of the neurohypophysis as the pars intermedia.

At birth the hypophysis is about one-sixth the weight of the adult gland; it increases in weight to become about one-half the weight of the adult gland at 7 years, and attains adult weight at puberty. Throughout postnatal life the gland appears larger in females, in both size and weight.

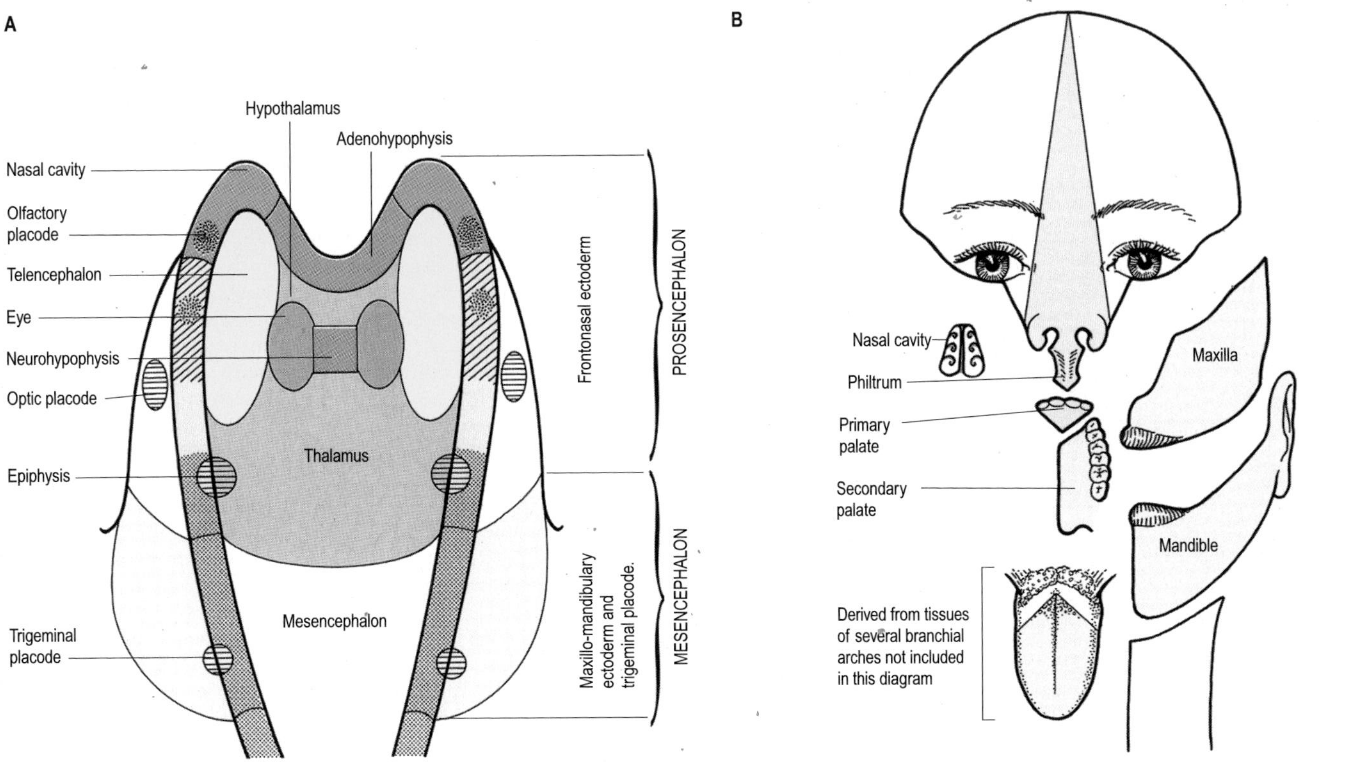

A

Hypothalamus

Adenohypophysis

Nasal cavity

Olfactory placode

Telencephalon

Eye

Neurohypophysis

Optic placode

Epiphysis

Thalamus

Trigeminal placode

Mesencephalon

Frontonasal ectoderm

PROSENCEPHALON

Maxillo-mandibulary ectoderm and trigeminal placode.

MESENCEPHALON

B

Nasal cavity

Philtrum

Primary palate

Secondary palate

Maxilla

Mandible

Derived from tissues of several branchial arches not included in this diagram

Fig. 14.10 Fate map of the rostral region of the neural primordium as established by the quail–chick chimera system. **A**, The various territories yielding rostral head are indicated on the neural plate and neural fold of a 1–3 somite embryo. **B**, The results obtained in the avian embryo have been extrapolated to the human head. Thus, the neural fold area coloured green yields the epithelium of the rostral roof of the mouth, the nasal cavities and part of the frontal area.

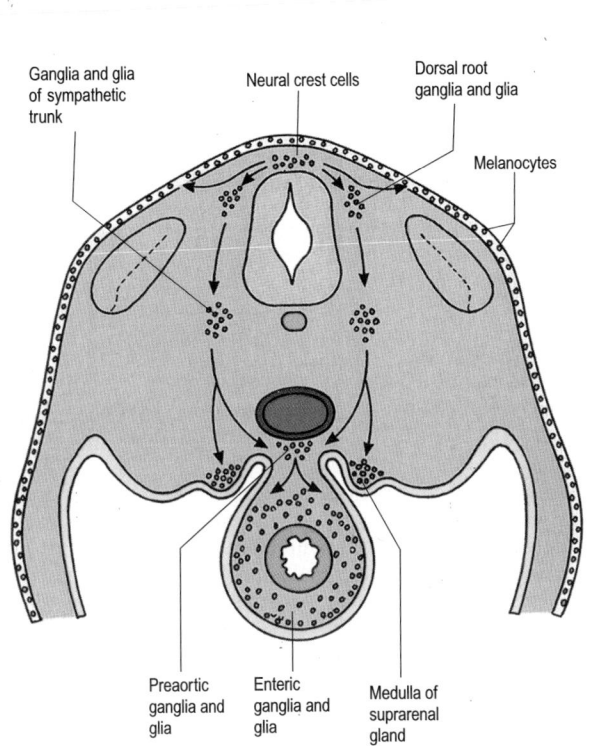

Ganglia and glia of sympathetic trunk

Neural crest cells

Dorsal root ganglia and glia

Melanocytes

Preaortic ganglia and glia

Enteric ganglia and glia

Medulla of suprarenal gland

Fig. 14.11 The migration routes taken by neural crest cells in the trunk.

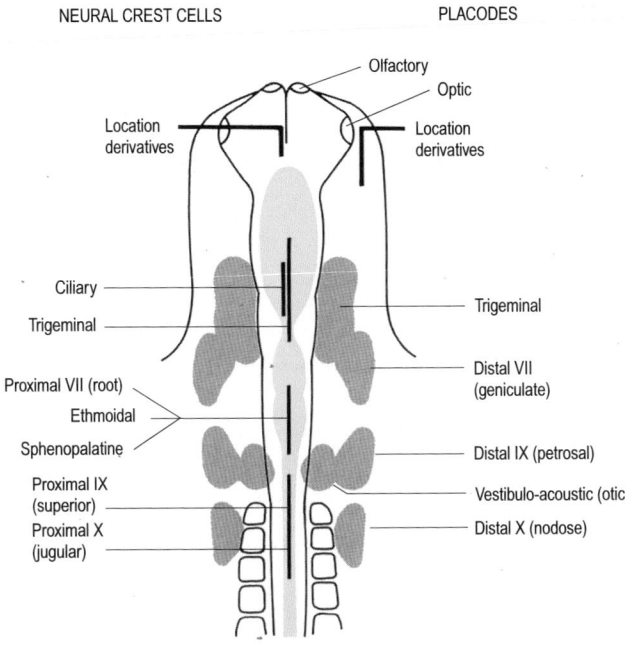

NEURAL CREST CELLS

PLACODES

Olfactory

Optic

Location derivatives

Location derivatives

Ciliary

Trigeminal

Proximal VII (root)

Ethmoidal

Sphenopalatine

Proximal IX (superior)

Proximal X (jugular)

Trigeminal

Distal VII (geniculate)

Distal IX (petrosal)

Vestibulo-acoustic (otic)

Distal X (nodose)

Fig. 14.12 The positions of neural crest and placodal cells in a 9.5-stage chick embryo. Neural crest cells are shown in the midline in green. Placodes are more laterally placed in grey. The otic placode is dorsolateral to the rhombencephalon, the trigeminal placode is placed intermediately and the epibranchial placodes (for facial, glossopharyngeal and vagus cranial nerves) are placed ventrolaterally and dorsal to the future pharyngeal grooves. (From Am J Anat 166: 445–468, D'Amico-Martel A, Noden DM, 1983, Wiley. Reprinted by permission of Wiley-Liss, Inc.)

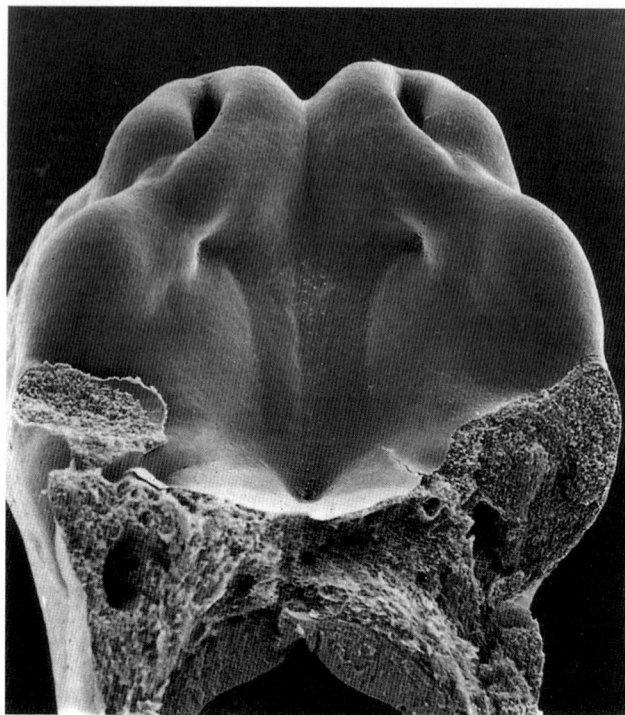

Fig. 14.13 Scanning electron micrograph of the roof of the pharynx showing the invagination of placodal ectoderm to form the adenohypophysis (Rathke's pouch). (Photograph by P Collins; printed by S Cox, Electron Microscopy Unit, Southampton General Hospital.)

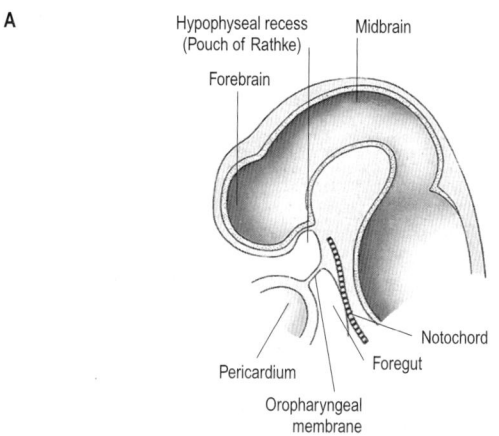

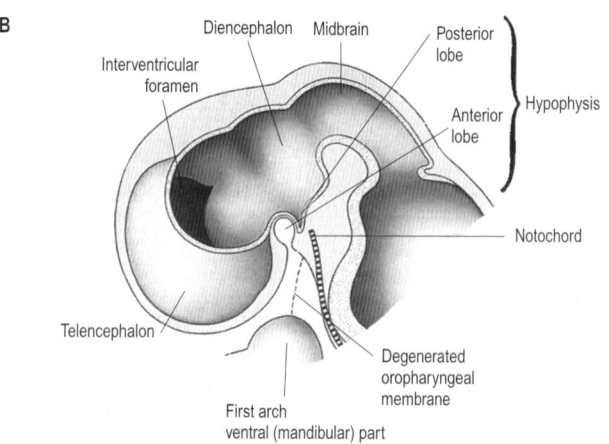

Fig. 14.14 Sagittal sections of heads of early embryos showing first stages in the development of the hypophysis.

NEUROGLIA

Glial cells which support neurones in the CNS and PNS are derived from three lineages: the neuroectoderm of the neural tube; the neural crest; and angioblastic mesenchyme. In the CNS, cells of the proliferating ventricular zone give rise to astrocyte and oligodendrocyte cell lines. After the proliferative phase the cells remaining at the ventricular surface differentiate into ependymal cells, which are specialized in many regions of the ventricular system as circumventricular organs. In the PNS, neural crest cells produce Schwann cells and astrocyte-like support cells in the enteric nervous system. Angioblastic mesenchyme gives rise to a variety of blood cell types including circulating monocytes which infiltrate the brain as microglial cells later in development.

The ventricular zone lining the early central canal of the spinal cord and the cavities of the brain gives rise to neurones and glial cells (**Figs 14.4, 14.5**). One specialized form of glial cell is the radial glial cell, whose radial processes extend both outwards to form the outer limiting membrane deep to the pia mater, and inwards, to form the inner limiting membrane around the central cavity. The geometry of these cells may provide contact guidance paths for cell migrations, both neuroblastic and glioblastic. A secondary radial glial scaffold is formed in the late developing cerebellum and dentate gyrus and serves to translocate neuroblasts, formed in secondary germinal centres, to their definitive adult locations. Radial glia eventually lose their connections with both inner and outer limiting membranes, except those persisting in the retina as Müller cells, in the cerebellum as Bergmann glia and in the hypothalamus as tanycytes. They can differentiate into neurones as well as astrocytes. They may partially clothe the somata of neighbouring developing neurones (between presumptive synaptic contacts), or similarly enwrap the intersynaptic surfaces of their neurites. Glial processes may expand around intraneural capillaries as perivascular end-feet. Other glioblasts retain an attachment (or form new expansions) to the pia mater, the innermost stratum of the meninges, as pial end-feet. Glioblasts also line the central canal and cavities of the brain as generalized or specialized ependymal cells, but lose their peripheral attachments. In some situations, as in the anterior median fissure of the spinal cord, ependymal cells retain their attachments to both the inner and outer limiting membranes. Thus, glia function as perineuronal satellites, and provide cellular channels interconnecting extracerebral and intraventricular cerebrospinal fluid, the cerebral vascular bed, the intercellular crevices of the neuropil and the cytoplasm of all neural cell varieties.

Microglia appear in the CNS after it has been penetrated by blood vessels and invade it in large numbers from certain restricted regions, whence they spread in what have picturesquely been called 'fountains of microglia', to extend deeply amongst the nervous elements.

MECHANISMS OF NEURAL DEVELOPMENT

For more than a century the mechanisms that operate during the development of the nervous system have been studied experimentally. Whilst much has been established, answers to many fundamental questions still remain obscure. In recent years, significant advances in our understanding of the development of vertebrates have come from work on amphibian, chicken, mouse and fish embryos and from the production of embryonic chimera (Le Douarin, Teillet & Catala 1998). A combination of genetic, embryological, biochemical and molecular techniques has been used to elucidate the mechanisms operating with early neural populations.

The CNS has a fundamental structure of layers and cells which are all derived from a pluripotential neuroepithelium. Developing neuroblasts produce axons which traverse great distances to reach their target organs. Within the CNS, they form myriad connections with other neuroblasts in response to locally secreted neurotrophins. The brain and spinal cord reveal an intrinsic metamerism, induced rostrally by genes and caudally by inductive influences from adjacent structures.

HISTOGENESIS OF THE NEURAL TUBE

The wall of the early neural tube consists of an internal ventricular zone (sometimes termed the germinal matrix) abutting the central lumen. It contains the nucleated parts of the pseudostratified columnar neuroepithelial cells and rounded cells undergoing mitosis. The early ventricular zone also contains a population of radial glial cells whose processes pass from the ventricular surface to the pial surface, thus forming the internal and external glia limitans (glial limiting membrane). As development proceeds the early pseudostratified epithelium proliferates and an outer layer, the marginal zone, devoid of nuclei but containing the external cytoplasmic processes of cells, is delineated. Subsequently a middle, mantle layer (intermediate zone) forms as the progeny from the ventricular zone migrate ventriculofugally (see **Fig. 14.5**).

Most CNS cells are produced in the proliferative zone adjacent to the future ventricular system, and in some regions this area is the only actively mitotic zone. According to the monophyletic theory of neurogenesis it is assumed to produce all cell types. The early neural epithelium, including the deeply placed ventricular mitotic zone, consists of a homogeneous population of pluripotent cells whose varying appearances reflect different phases in a proliferative cycle. The ventricular zone is considered to be populated by a single basic type of progenitor cell and to exhibit three phases. The cells show an 'elevator movement' as they pass through a complete mitotic cycle, progressively approaching and then receding from the internal limiting membrane (**Fig. 14.15**). DNA replication occurs while the cells are extended and their nuclei approach the pial surface; they then enter a premitotic resting period while the cells shorten and their nuclei pass back towards the ventricular surface. The cells now become rounded close to the internal limiting membrane and undergo mitosis. They then elongate and their nuclei move towards the outer edge during the postmitotic resting period, after which DNA synthesis commences once more and the cycle is repeated. The cells so formed may then either start another proliferative cycle or migrate outwards (i.e. radially) and differentiate into neurones as they approach and enter the adjacent stratum. This differentiation may be initiated as they pass outwards during the postmitotic resting period. The proliferative cycle continues with the production of clones of neuroblasts and glioblasts. This sequence of events has been called inter-kinetic nuclear migration: it eventually declines. At the last division two postmitotic daughter cells are produced and they differentiate at the ventricular surface into ependyma.

The progeny of some of these divisions move away from the ventricular zone to form an intermediate zone of neurones. The early spinal cord and much of the brain stem shows only these three main layers, i.e. ventricular, intermediate and marginal zones. However, in the telencephalon the region of cellular proliferation extends deeper than the ventricular zone where the escalator movement of interkinetic migration is seen, and a subventricular zone appears between the ventricular and intermediate layers (**Fig. 14.5**). Here cells continue to multiply to provide further generations of neurones and glia which subsequently migrate into the intermediate and marginal zones. In some regions of the nervous system (e.g. the cerebellar cortex) some mitotic subventricular stem cells migrate across the entire neural wall to form a subpial population, and establish a new zone of cell division

and differentiation. Many cells formed in this site remain subpial in position, but others migrate back towards the ventricle through the developing nervous tissue, and finish their migrations in various definitive sites where they differentiate into neurones or macroglial cells. In the cerebral hemispheres, a zone termed the cortical plate is formed outside the intermediate zone by radially migrating cells from the ventricular zone. The most recently formed cells migrate to the outermost layers of the cortical plate, so that earlier formed and migrating cells become subjacent to those migrating later. In the forebrain there is an additional transient stratum deep to the early cortical plate, the subplate zone.

LINEAGE AND GROWTH IN THE NERVOUS SYSTEM

Neurones come from two major embryonic sources: CNS neurones originate from the pluripotential neural plate and tube, whereas ganglionic neurones originate from the neural crest and ectodermal placodes. The neural plate also provides ependymal and macroglial cells. Peripheral Schwann cells and chromaffin cells arise from the neural crest. The origins and lineages of cells in the nervous system have been determined experimentally by the use of autoradiography, microinjection or retroviral labelling of progenitor cells, and in cell culture.

During development, neurones are formed before glial cells. The timing of events differs in various parts of the CNS and between species. Most neurones are formed prenatally in mammals but some postnatal neurogenesis does occur, e.g. the small granular cells of the cerebellum, olfactory bulb and hippocampus, and neurones of the cerebral cortex. Gliogenesis continues after birth in periventricular and other sites. Autoradiographic studies have shown that different classes of neurones develop at specific times. Large neurones such as principal projection neurones tend to differentiate before small ones such as local circuit neurones. However, their subsequent migration appears to be independent of the times of their initial formation. Neurones can migrate extensively through populations of maturing, relatively static cells, to reach their destination, e.g. cerebellar granule cells pass through a layer of Purkinje cells en route from the external pial layer to their final central position. Later, the final form of their projections, cell volume and indeed their continuing survival, depend on the establishment of patterns of functional connection.

Initially immature neurones, termed neuroblasts, are rotund or fusiform. Their cytoplasm contains a prominent Golgi apparatus, many lysosomes, glycogen and numerous unattached ribosomes. As maturation proceeds, cells send out fine cytoplasmic processes which contain neurofilaments, microtubules and other structures, often including centrioles at their bases where microtubules form. Internally, endoplasmic reticulum cisternae appear and attached ribosomes and mitochondria proliferate, whereas the glycogen content progressively diminishes. One process becomes the axon and other processes establish a dendritic tree. Axonal growth, studied in tissue culture, may be as much as 1 mm per day.

Growth cones

Ramón y Cajal (1890) was the first to recognize that the expanded end of an axon, the growth cone, is the principal sensory organ of the neurone. The growing tips of neuroblasts have been studied extensively in tissue culture. Classically, the growth cone is described as an expanded region that is constantly active, changing shape, extending and withdrawing small filopodia and lamellipodia that apparently 'explore' the local environment for a suitable surface along which extension may occur. These processes are stabilized in one direction, determining the direction of future growth, and following consolidation of the growth cone, the exploratory behaviour recommences. This continuous cycle resembles the behaviour at the leading edge of migratory cells such as fibroblasts and neutrophils. The molecular basis of this behaviour is the transmission of signals external to the growth cone via cell surface receptors to the scaffolding of microtubules and neurofilaments within the axon. Growing neuroblasts have a cortex rich in actin associated with the plasma membrane, and a core of centrally located microtubules and sometimes neurofilaments. The assembly of these components, along with the synthesis of new membrane, occurs in segments distal to the cell body and behind the growth cone, though some assembly of microtubules may take place near the cell body.

The driving force of growth cone extension is uncertain. One possible mechanism is that tension applied to objects by the leading edge of the growth cone is mediated by actin, and that local accumulations of F-actin redirect the extension of microtubules. Under some culture

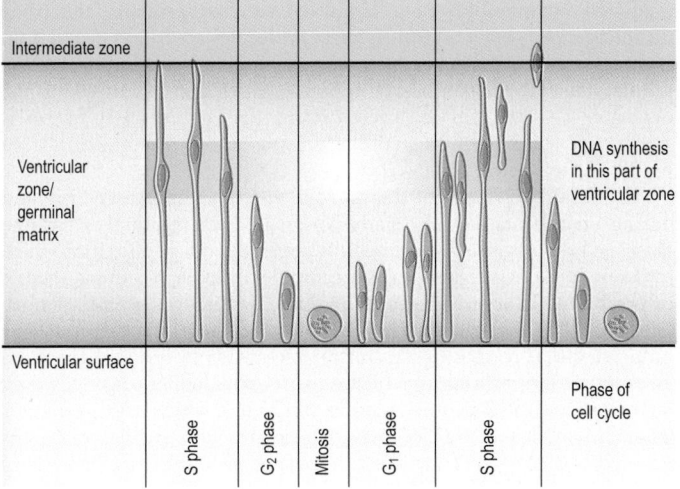

Intermediate zone

Ventricular zone/ germinal matrix

DNA synthesis in this part of ventricular zone

Ventricular surface

| S phase | G₂ phase | Mitosis | G₁ phase | S phase | Phase of cell cycle |

Fig. 14.15 The cell cycle in the ventricular zone of the developing neural tube. The nuclei of the proliferating stem cells show interkinetic migration. (From *Journal of Comparative Neurology*, 120: 37–42, S Fujita, 1963. Reprinted by permission from Wiley-Liss, Inc.)

conditions, growth cones can develop mechanical tension, pulling against other axons or the substratum to which they are attached. Possibly, tension in the growth cone acts as a messenger to mediate the assembly of cytoskeletal components. Adhesion to the substratum appears to be important for consolidation of the growth cone and elaboration of the cytoskeleton in that direction.

During development, the growing axons of neuroblasts navigate with precision over considerable distances, often pursuing complex courses to reach their targets. Eventually they make functional contact with their appropriate end organs (neuromuscular endings, secretomotor terminals, sensory corpuscles or synapses with other neurones). During the outgrowth of axonal processes the earliest nerve fibres are known to traverse appreciable distances over an apparently virgin landscape, often occupied by loose mesenchyme. A central problem for neurobiologists, therefore, has been understanding the mechanisms of axon guidance (Gordon-Weeks 2000). Axon guidance is thought to involve short-range, local guidance cues and long-range diffusible cues, any of which can be either attractive and permissive for growth, or repellent and hence inhibitory. Short-range cues require factors which are displayed on cell surfaces or in the extracellular matrix, e.g. axon extension requires a permissive, physical substrate, the molecules of which are actively recognized by the growth cone. They also require negative cues which inhibit the progress of the growth cone. Long-range cues come from gradients of specific factors diffusing from distant targets, which cause neurones to turn their axons towards the source of the attractive signal. The evidence for this has come from *in vitro* co-culture studies. The floor plate of the developing spinal cord exerts a chemotropic effect on commissural axons that later cross it, whereas there is chemo-repulsion of developing motor axons from the floor plate. These forces are thought to act *in vivo* in concert in a dynamic process to ensure the correct passage of axons to their final destinations and to mediate their correct bundling together en route.

Dendritic tree

Once growth cones have arrived in their general target area, they then have to form terminals and synapses. In recent years, much emphasis has been placed on the idea that patterns of connectivity depend on the death of inappropriate cells. Programmed cell death or apoptosis occurs during the period of synaptogenesis if neurones fail to acquire sufficient amounts of specific neurotrophic factors. Coincident firing of neighbouring neurones that have found the appropriate target region might be involved in eliciting release of factor(s), thus reinforcing correct connections. Such mechanisms may explain the numerical correspondence between neurones in a motor pool and the muscle fibres innervated. On a subtler level, pruning of collaterals may give rise to mature neuronal architecture. The projections of pyramidal neurones from the motor and visual cortex, for example, start out with similar architecture: the mature repertoire of targets is produced by the pruning of collaterals leading to loss of projections to some targets.

The final growth of dendritic trees is also influenced by patterns of afferent connections and their activity. If deprived of afferents experimentally, dendrites fail to develop fully and, after a critical period, may become permanently affected even if functional inputs are restored, e.g. in the visual systems of young animals which have been visually deprived. This is analogous to the results of untreated amblyopia in infants. Metabolic factors also affect the final branching patterns of dendrites, e.g. thyroid deficiency in perinatal rats results in a small size and restricted branching of cortical neurones. This may be analogous to the mental retardation of cretinism.

Once established, dendritic trees appear remarkably stable and partial deafferentation affects only dendritic spines or similar small details. As development proceeds plasticity is lost, and soon after birth a neurone is a stable structure with a reduced rate of growth.

Neurotrophins

If neurones lose all afferent connections or are totally deprived of sensory input, there is atrophy of much of the dendritic tree and even the whole soma. Different regions of the nervous system vary quantitatively in their response to such anterograde transneuronal degeneration. Similar effects occur in retrograde transneuronal degeneration. Thus neurones are dependent on peripheral structures for their survival. Loss of muscles or sensory nerve endings, e.g. in the developing limb, will result in reduction in numbers of motor and sensory neurones. The specific factor which these target organs produce is termed nerve growth factor (NGF). NGF is taken into nerve endings and transported back to the neuronal somata. It is necessary for the survival of many types of neurone during early development and for growth of their axons and dendrites, and promotes the synthesis of neurotransmitters and enzymes. Antibodies to NGF cause the death of neuronal subsets at times when they have reached their targets, and added NGF rescues neurones that would otherwise die. Since the discovery of NGF, several other trophic factors have been identified, including brain derived neurotrophic factor (BDNF), neurotrophin-3 (NT-3) and NT-4/5.

Neurotrophins exert their survival effects selectively on particular subsets of neurones. NGF is specific to sensory ganglion cells from the neural crest, sympathetic postganglionic neurones and basal forebrain cholinergic neurones. BDNF promotes the survival of retinal ganglion cells, motor neurones, sensory proprioceptive and placode-derived neurones, such as those of the nodose ganglion, that are unresponsive to NGF. NT-3 has effects on motor neurones, and both placode and neural crest-derived sensory neurones. Other growth factors found to influence the growth and survival of neural cells include the fibroblast growth factors (FGFs) and ciliary neurotrophic factor (CNTF), all of which are unrelated in sequence to the NGF family. Members of the FGF family support the survival of embryonic neurones from many regions of the CNS. CNTF may control the proliferation and differentiation of sympathetic ganglion cells and astrocytes.

Each of the neurotrophins binds specifically to certain receptors on the cell surface. The receptor termed $p75^{NTR}$ binds all the neurotrophins with similar affinity. By contrast, members of the family of receptor tyrosine kinases (Trks) bind with higher affinity and display binding preferences for particular neurotrophins. However, the presence of a Trk receptor seems to be required for $p75^{NTR}$ function.

Nervous tissue influences the metabolism of its target tissues. If during development a nerve fails to connect with its muscle, both degenerate. If the innervation of slow (red) or fast (white) skeletal muscle is exchanged, the muscles change structure and properties to reflect the new innervation, indicating that the nerve determines muscle type and not vice versa.

INDUCTION AND PATTERNING OF THE BRAIN AND SPINAL CORD

The generation of neural tissue involves an inductive signal from the underlying chordamesoderm (notochord, see p. 194), termed the 'organizer'. The observation by Spemann in 1925 that, in intact amphibian embryos, the presence of an organizer caused ectodermal cells to form nervous tissue, whereas in its absence they formed epidermis, led to the discovery of neural induction. However, experiments performed much later in the century revealed that when ectodermal cells were dissociated they also gave rise to neural tissue. The paradox was resolved by the finding that intact ectodermal tissue is prevented from becoming neural by an inhibitory signal(s) that is diluted out when cells are dissociated. Many lines of evidence now indicate that this inhibitory signal is mediated by members of a family of secreted proteins, the bone morphogenetic proteins (BMP). These molecules are found throughout ectodermal tissue during early development, and their inhibitory effect is antagonized by several neural inducers which are present within the organizer, i.e. noggin, chordin and follistatin. Each of these factors is capable of blocking BMP signalling, in some cases by preventing it from binding to its receptor(s).

The regional pattern of the nervous system is induced before and during neural tube closure. Early concepts about regional patterning envisaged that regionalization within mesenchymal populations which transmit inductive signals to the ectoderm impose a similar mosaic of positional values on the overlying neural plate. For example, translantation of caudal mesenchyme beneath the neural plate in *Amphibia* induced spinal cord, whereas rostral mesenchyme induced brain, as assessed by the morphology of the neuroepithelial vesicles. However, later work indicated a more complex scenario in which organizer grafts from early embryos induced mainly head structures, while later grafts induced mainly trunk structures. Subsequent molecular data have tended to support a model in which neural-inducing factors released by the organizer such as noggin, chordin and follistatin, neuralize the ectoderm and promote a mainly rostral neural identity. Later secreted signals then act to caudalize this rostral neural tissue, setting up an entire array of axial values along the neural tube. Candidates for these later, caudalizing, signals have been shown to be retinoic acid, fibroblast growth factors and the WNT secreted proteins, which are present in the paraxial mesenchyme and later in its derivatives, the somites. This combination of signals does not seem to be sufficient to produce the most rostral, forebrain structures. Other secreted proteins resident in the rostralmost part of the earliest ingressing axial populations of endoderm and mesenchyme are also capable of inducing markers of forebrain identity from ectodermal cells (Withington, Beddington & Cooke 2001).

As the neural tube grows and is modified in shape, a number of mechanisms refine the crude rostrocaudal pattern which has been imposed during neurulation. Molecules which diffuse from tissues adjacent to the neural tube such as the somites have patterning influences. The neural tube possesses a number of intrinsic signalling centres, such as the midbrain–hindbrain boundary, which produce diffusible molecules capable of influencing tissue development at a distance. In this way extrinsic and intrinsic factors serve to subdivide the neural tube into a number of fairly large domains, on which local influences can then act. Domains are distinguished by their expression of particular transcription factors, which in many cases have been causally related to the development of particular regions. Examples of such genes are the *Hox* family which are expressed in the spinal cord and hindbrain, and the *Dlx*, *Emx* and *Otx* families of genes which are expressed in various regions of the forebrain. All of these are developmental control genes which lie high up in the hierarchy, and are capable of initiating cascades of expression of other genes to create a more fine-grained pattern of cellular differentiation. In contrast to the aforementioned secreted molecules, these genes encode proteins which are retained in the cell nucleus, and so can act on DNA to induce or repress further gene expression.

Segmentation in the neural tube

One mechanism which is involved in the process of regional differentiation of cell populations within the neural tube is segmentation, which is conspicuous in man and other vertebrates in the serial arrangement of the vertebrae and axial muscles and in the periodicity of the spinal nerves. In the last century, the possibility that the neural tube might be divided into segments or neuromeres was entertained, but some contended that bulges observed in the lateral walls of the neural tube were artifacts, or caused by mechanical deformation of the tube by adjacent structures. Recent years have seen a resurgence of interest in this subject, and to a detailed evaluation of the significance of neuromeres. A series of eight prominent bulges which appear bilaterally in the rhombencephalic wall early in development have been termed rhombomeres (**Fig. 14.3**). (While the term neuromere applies generally to putative 'segments' of the neural tube, the term rhombomere applies specifically to the rhombencephalon.) Many aspects of the patterning of neuronal populations and the elaboration of their axon tracts conform to a segmental plan, and rhombomeres have now been shown to constitute crucial units of pattern formation. Domains of expression of developmental control genes abut rhombomere boundaries, and perhaps most importantly, single cell labelling experiments have revealed that cells within rhombomeres form segregated non-mixing populations (**Fig. 14.16**). The neural crest also shows intrinsic segmentation in the hindbrain, and is segregated into streams at its point of origin in the dorsal neural tube. This may represent a mechanism whereby morphogenetic specification of the premigratory neural crest cells is conveyed to the pharyngeal arches. Although these segmental units lose their morphological prominence with subsequent development, they represent the fundamental ground plan of this part of the neuraxis, creating a series of semi-autonomous units within which local variations in patterning can then develop. The consequences of early segmentation for events later in development, such as the formation of definitive neuronal nuclei within the brain stem, and of peripheral axonal projections remain to be explored.

Other brain regions are not segmented in quite the same way as the hindbrain. However, morphological boundaries, domains of cell lineage restriction and of cell mixing, and regions of gene expression that abut sharp boundaries, are found in the diencephalon and telencephalon. It is thus likely that compartmentation of cell groups with some, if not all, the features of rhombomeres plays an important role in the formation of various brain regions.

The significance of intrinsic segmentation in the hindbrain is underlined by the absence of overt segmentation of the adjacent paraxial mesenchyme. There is no firm evidence for intrinsic segmentation in the spinal cord. Instead, segmentation of the neural crest, motor axons, and thus eventually the spinal nerves, is dependent on the segmentation

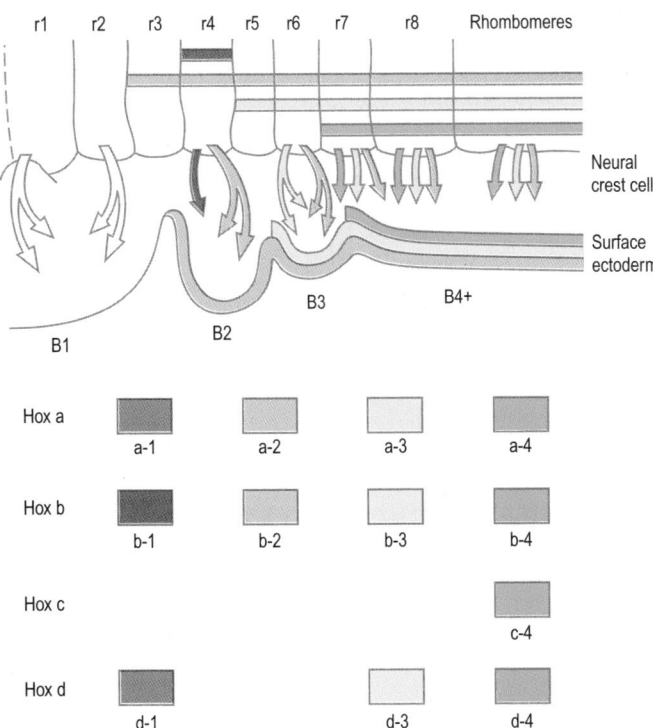

Fig. 14.16 *Hox* gene expression domains in the branchiorhombomeric area in the mouse embryo at E9.5. The arrows indicate neural crest cells migrating from the rhombencephalon and midbrain. At the former level they are shaded to indicate the *Hox* genes they express. The same combination of *Hox* genes is expressed in the rhombomeres and in the superficial ectoderm of the pharyngeal arches at the corresponding rostrocaudal levels. The four *Hox* clusters are represented below. (Modified by permission from the Annual Review of Cell and Developmental Biology, Volume 8, 1992 by Annual Reviews www.annualreviews.org.)

of the neighbouring somites. Both neural crest cell migration and motor axon outgrowth occur through only the rostral and not the caudal sclerotome of each somite, so that dorsal root ganglia form only at intervals. The caudal sclerotome possesses inhibitory properties that deter neural crest cells and motor axons from entering. This illustrates the general principle that the nervous system is closely interlocked, in terms of morphogenesis, with the 'periphery', i.e. surrounding non-nervous structures, and each is dependent upon the other for its effective structural and functional maturation.

Genes such as the *Hox* and *Pax* gene families, which encode transcription factor proteins, show intriguing expression patterns within the nervous system. Genes of the *Hox-b* cluster, for example, are expressed throughout the caudal neural tube, and up to discrete limits in the hindbrain that coincide with rhombomere boundaries. The ordering of these genes within a cluster on the chromosome (5'–3') is the same as the caudal to rostral limits of expression of consecutive genes. This characteristic pattern is surprisingly similar in fish, frogs, birds and mammals. *Hox* genes play a role in patterning not only of the neural tube but also of much of the head region, consistent with their expression in neural crest cells, and within the pharyngeal arches. Disruption of *Hox a-3* gene in mice mimics DiGeorge's syndrome, a congenital human disorder characterized by the absence (or near absence) of the thymus, parathyroid and thyroid glands, by the hypotrophy of the walls of the arteries derived from the aortic arches, and by subsequent conotruncal cardiac malformations. Some *Pax* genes are expressed in different dorsoventral domains within the neural tube. *Pax-3* is expressed in the alar lamina, including the neural crest, while *Pax-6* is expressed in the intermediate plate. The *Pax-3* gene has the same chromosomal localization as the mouse mutation Splotch and the affected locus in the human Waardenburg's syndrome, both of which are characterized by neural crest disturbances with pigmentation disorders and occasional neural tube defects. Both *Hox* and *Pax* genes have restricted expression patterns with respect to the rostrocaudal and the dorsoventral axes of the neural tube, consistent with roles in positional specification. (For reviews of the expression patterns of these genes see Krumlauf et al 1993.)

Whilst craniocaudal positional values are probably conferred on the neuroepithelium at the neural plate or early neural tube stage, dorsoventral positional values may become fixed later. The development of the dorsoventral axis is heavily influenced by the presence of the underlying notochord. The notochord induces the ventral midline of the neural tube, the floor plate. This specialized region consists of a strip of non-neural cells with distinctive adhesive and functional properties. Notochord and floor plate together participate in inducing the differentiation of the motor columns. Motor neurone differentiation occurs early, giving some grounds for the idea of a ventral to dorsal wave of differentiation. The notochord/floor plate complex may also be responsible for allotting the values of more dorsal cell types within the tube (Fig. 14.7). For example, the dorsal domain of expression of *Pax-3* extends more ventrally in embryos experimentally deprived of notochord and floor plate, while grafting an extra notochord adjacent to the dorsal neural tube leads to a repression of *Pax-3* expression.

PERIPHERAL NERVOUS SYSTEM

SOMATIC NERVES

Spinal nerves

Each spinal nerve is connected to the spinal cord by a ventral root and a dorsal root (Fig. 14.17). The fibres of the ventral roots grow out from cell bodies in the anterior and lateral parts of the intermediate zone. These pass through the overlying marginal zone and external limiting membrane. Some enter the myotomes of the somites, and some penetrate the somites, reaching the adjacent somatopleure, and in both sites they ultimately form the α-, β- and γ-efferents. At appropriate levels these are accompanied by the outgrowing axons of preganglionic sympathetic neuroblasts (segments T1–L2), or preganglionic parasympathetic neuroblasts (S2–S4).

The fibres of the dorsal roots extend from cell somata in dorsal root ganglia (DRG) into the spinal cord and also extend into the periphery. Neural crest cells are produced continuously along the length of the spinal cord, but gangliogenic cells migrate only into the rostral part of each somitic sclerotome where they condense and proliferate to form a bilateral series of oval-shaped primordial spinal ganglia (dorsal root ganglia) (Fig. 14.11). Negative factors in the caudal sclerotome deter neural crest from entering (p. 790). The rostral sclerotome has a mitogenic effect on the crest cells that settle within it. From the ventral region of each ganglion a small part separates to form sympathochromaffin cells (p. 255), while the remainder becomes a definitive spinal ganglion (dorsal root ganglion). The spinal ganglia are arranged symmetrically at the sides of the neural tube and, except in the caudal region, are equal in number to the somites. The cells of the ganglia, like the cells of the intermediate zone of the early neural tube, are glial and neuronal precursors. The glial precursors develop into satellite cells (which become closely applied to the ganglionic nerve cell somata), Schwann cells, and possibly other cells. The neuroblasts, at first round or oval, soon become fusiform, and their extremities gradually elongate into central and peripheral processes. The central processes grow into the neural tube as the fibres of dorsal nerve roots, while the peripheral processes grow ventrolaterally to mingle with the fibres of the ventral root, thus forming a mixed spinal nerve. As development proceeds the original bipolar form of the cells in the spinal ganglia changes and the two processes become approximated until they ultimately arise from a single stem to form a unipolar cell. The bipolar form is retained in the ganglion of the vestibulocochlear nerve.

Cranial nerves

Cranial nerves may contain motor, sensory or both types of fibres. With the exception of the olfactory and optic nerves, the cranial nerves develop in a manner similar in some respects to components of the spinal nerves. The somata of motor neuroblasts originate within the neuroepithelium, while those of sensory neuroblasts are derived from the neural crest with the addition in the head of contributions from ectodermal placodes (Figs 14.18; 26.5).

The motor fibres of the cranial nerves which project to striated muscle are the axons of cells originating in the basal plate of the midbrain and hindbrain. The functional and morphological distinction between the neurones within these various nerves is based on the types of muscle innervated. In the trunk, the motor roots of the spinal nerves all emerge from the spinal cord close to the ventral midline to supply the muscles derived from the somites.

In the head the motor outflow is traditionally segregated into two pathways (Figs 14.2B, 14.18). General somatic efferent neurones exit ventrally in a similar manner to those of the spinal cord. Thus the oculomotor, trochlear, abducens and hypoglossal nerves parallel the organization of the somatic motor neurones in the spinal cord. The second motor component, special branchial efferent, consists of the motor parts of the trigeminal, facial, glossopharyngeal and vagus nerves which supply the pharyngeal (branchial) arches and the accessory nerve. These nerves all have nerve exit points more dorsally placed than the somatic motor system.

The cranial nerves also contain general visceral efferent neurones (parasympathetic preganglionic) which travel in the oculomotor, facial, glossopharyngeal and vagus nerves and leave the hindbrain via the same exit points as the special branchial efferent fibres. All three categories of motor neurones probably originate from the same region of the basal plate, adjacent to the floor plate. The definitive arrangement of nuclei reflects the differential migration of neuronal somata. It is not known whether all these cell types share a common precursor within the rhombencephalon, however, in the spinal cord somatic motor and preganglionic autonomic neurones are linearly related.

These motor neurone types have been designated according to the types of muscles or structures they innervate. General somatic efferent nerves supply striated muscle derived from the cranial (occipital) somites and prechordal mesenchyme. Myogenic cells from the ventrolateral edge of the epithelial plate of occipital somites give rise to the intrinsic

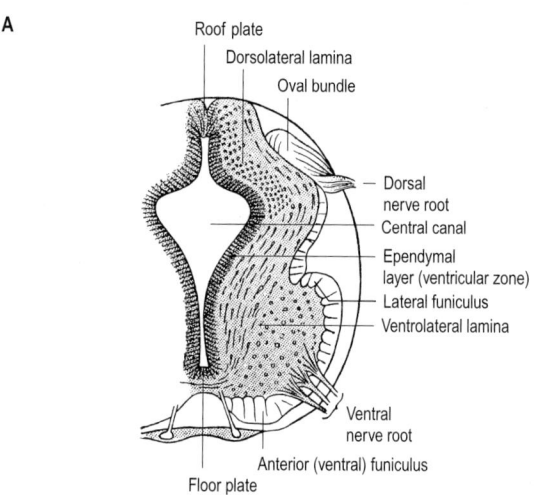

A

Roof plate
Dorsolateral lamina
Oval bundle
Dorsal nerve root
Central canal
Ependymal layer (ventricular zone)
Lateral funiculus
Ventrolateral lamina
Ventral nerve root
Anterior (ventral) funiculus
Floor plate

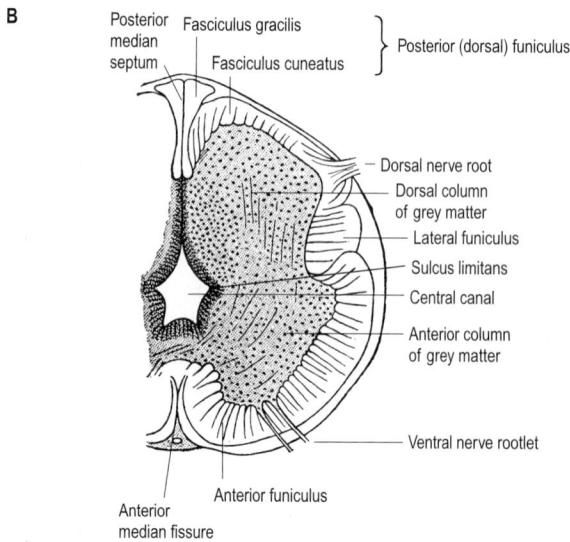

B

Posterior median septum
Fasciculus gracilis
Fasciculus cuneatus
Posterior (dorsal) funiculus
Dorsal nerve root
Dorsal column of grey matter
Lateral funiculus
Sulcus limitans
Central canal
Anterior column of grey matter
Ventral nerve rootlet
Anterior funiculus
Anterior median fissure

Fig. 14.17 Transverse sections through the developing spinal cord of human embryos: **A**, c.6 weeks old; **B**, c.3 months old.

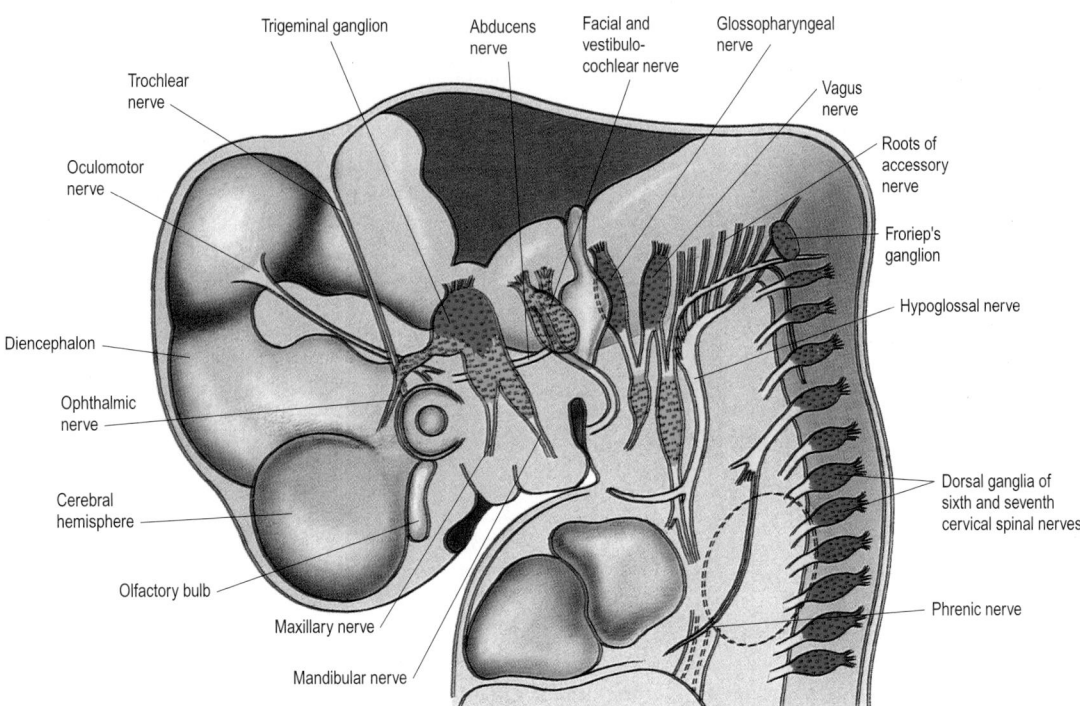

Fig. 14.18 The brain and cranial nerves of a human embryo, 10.2 mm long. Note also the ganglia (stippled) associated with the trigeminal, facial vestibulocochlear, glossopharyngeal, vagus and spinal accessory nerves. Froriep's ganglion, an occipital dorsal root ganglion, is inconstant and soon disappears.

muscles of the tongue, while the prechordal mesenchyme gives rise to the extrinsic ocular muscles. Special branchial efferent nerves supply the striated muscles developing within the pharyngeal (branchial) arches (**Fig. 26.5**) which are derived from parachordal mesenchyme between the occipital somites and the prechordal mesenchyme. All the voluntary muscles of the head originate from axial (prechordal) or paraxial mesenchyme which renders the distinction between somatic efferent supply and branchial efferent supply somewhat artificial. However, the obviously special nature of the arch musculature, its patterning by the neural crest cells, its particularly rich innervation for both voluntary and reflex activity, and the different origins from the basal plate of the branchial efferent nerves compared to the somatic efferent nerves, make the retention of a distinction between the two of some value.

General visceral efferent neurones (parasympathetic preganglionic) innervate glands of the head, the sphincter pupillae and ciliary muscles, and the thoracic and abdominal viscera.

The cranial sensory ganglia are derived in part from the neural crest, and in part from cells of the ectodermal placodes (**Figs 14.12, 14.18**). Generally, neurones distal to the brain are derived from placodes while proximal ones are derived from the neural crest (**Figs 14.18**). Supporting cells of all sensory ganglia arise from the neural crest. The most rostral sensory ganglion, the trigeminal, contains both neural crest and placode-derived neurones that mediate general somatic afferent functions. In the case of more caudal cranial nerves (the facial, glossopharyngeal and vagus), the same applies, but the two cell populations form separate ganglia in the case of each nerve. The proximal series of ganglia is neural crest derived (forming the proximal ganglion of the facial nerve, the superior ganglion of the glossopharyngeal nerve and the jugular ganglion of the vagus) while the distal series is derived from placodal cells (forming the geniculate ganglion of the facial nerve, the petrosal ganglion of the glossopharyngeal nerve and the nodose ganglion of the vagus). These ganglia contain neurones which mediate special, general visceral and somatic afferent functions. The vestibulocochlear nerve has a vestibular ganglion which contains both crest and placodal cells and an acoustic ganglion from placodal neurones only: it conveys special somatic afferents.

The neurones and supporting cells of the cranial autonomic ganglia in the head and the trunk originate from neural crest cells. Caudal to the ganglion of the vagus the occipital region of the neural crest is concerned with the 'ganglia' of the accessory and hypoglossal nerves.

Rudimentary ganglion cells may occur along the hypoglossal nerve in the human embryo; they subsequently regress. Ganglion cells are found on the developing spinal root of the accessory nerve and these are believed to persist in the adult. The central processes of the cells of these various ganglia, where they persist, form some sensory roots of the cranial nerves and enter the alar lamina of the hindbrain. Their peripheral processes join the efferent components of the nerve to be distributed to the various tissues innervated. Some incoming fibres from the facial, glossopharyngeal and vagus nerves collect to form an oval bundle, the tractus solitarius, on the lateral aspect of the myelencephalon. This bundle is the homologue of the oval bundle of the spinal cord, but in the hindbrain it becomes more deeply placed by the overgrowth, folding and subsequent fusion of tissue derived from the rhombic lip on the external aspect of the bundle.

AUTONOMIC NERVOUS SYSTEM

Autonomic nerves, apart from the preganglionic motor axons arising from the CNS, are formed by the neural crest. The autonomic nervous system includes the sympathetic and parasympathetic neurones in the peripheral ganglia and their accompanying glia, the enteric nervous system and glia, and the suprarenal medulla.

In the trunk at neurulation, neural crest cells migrate from the neural epithelium to lie transitorily on the fused neural tube. Thereafter crest cells migrate laterally and then ventrally to their respective destinations (**Fig. 14.11**). Within the head the neural crest cells migrate prior to neural fusion, producing a vast mesenchymal population as well as autonomic neurones.

The four major regions of neural crest cell distribution to the autonomic nervous system are cranial, vagal, trunk and lumbosacral. The cranial neural crest gives rise to the cranial parasympathetic ganglia, whereas the vagal neural crest gives rise to the thoracic parasympathetic ganglia. The trunk neural crest gives rise to the sympathetic ganglia, mainly the paravertebral ganglia, and suprarenomedullary cells. This category is often referred to as the sympathoadrenal lineage.

Neurones of the enteric nervous system are described as arising from the vagal crest, i.e. neural crest derived from somite levels 1–7, and sacral crest, caudal to the 28th somite. At all of these levels the crest cells also differentiate into glial-like support cells alongside the neurones (**Fig. 14.19**).

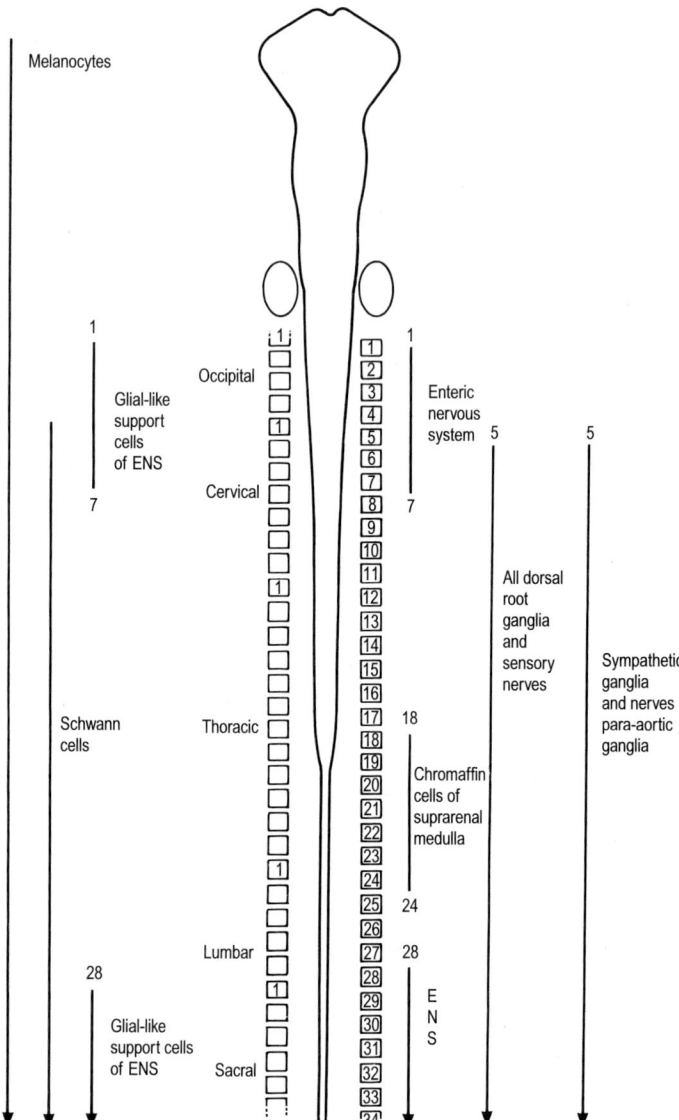

Fig. 14.19 The derivatives of neural crest cells in the trunk. The somites are indicated on the right and vertebral levels are indicated on the left. The fate of crest cells arising at particular somite levels is shown.

Parasympathetic ganglia

Neural crest cells migrate from the region of the mesencephalon and rhombencephalon prior to neural tube closure. From rostral to caudal, three populations of neural crest have been noted: cranial neural crest, cardiac neural crest and vagal neural crest. The migration of the sacral neural crest and the formation of the caudal parasympathetic ganglia have attracted little research interest.

Neural crest cells from the caudal third of the mesencephalon and the rostral metencephalon migrate along or close to the ophthalmic branch of the trigeminal nerve and give rise to the ciliary ganglion. Cells migrating from the nucleus of the oculomotor nerve may also contribute to the ganglion; a few scattered cells are always demonstrable in postnatal life along the course of this nerve. Preotic myelencephalic neural crest cells give rise to the pterygopalatine ganglion, which may also receive contributions from the ganglia of the trigeminal and facial nerves. The otic and submandibular ganglia are also derived from myelencephalic neural crest and may receive contributions from the glossopharyngeal and facial cranial nerves respectively (**Fig. 26.5**).

Neural crest from the region located between the otic placode and the caudal limit of somite 3 has been termed cardiac neural crest. Cells derived from these levels migrate through pharyngeal arches 3, 4, and 6 where they provide, inter alia, support for the embryonic aortic arch arteries, cells of the aorticopulmonary septum and truncus arteriosus. Some of these neural crest cells also differentiate into the neural anlage

of the parasympathetic ganglia of the heart. Sensory innervation of the heart is from the inferior ganglion of the vagus, which is derived from the nodose placodes. Neural crest cells migrating from the level of somites 1–7 are collectively termed vagal neural crest; they migrate to the gut along with sacral neural crest.

Sympathetic ganglia

Neural crest cells migrate ventrally within the body segments to penetrate the underlying somites and continue to the region of the future paravertebral and prevertebral plexuses, notably forming the sympathetic chain of ganglia, as well as the major ganglia around the ventral visceral branches of the abdominal aorta (**Figs 14.11, 14.19**).

There is cell specific recognition of postganglionic neurones and the growth cones of sympathetic preganglionic neurones. They meet during their growth, and this may be important in guidance to their appropriate target. The position of postganglionic neurones, and the exit point from the spinal cord of preganglionic neurones, may influence the types of synaptic connections made, and the affinity for particular postganglionic neurones. When a postganglionic neuroblast is in place it extends axons (and dendrites) and synaptogenesis occurs. The earliest axonal outgrowths from the superior cervical ganglion occur at about stage 14: although the axon is the first cell process to appear, the position of the neurones does not apparently influence the appearance of the cell processes.

The local environment is the major factor which controls the appropriate differentiation of the presumptive autonomic ganglion neurones. The identity of the factors responsible for subsequent adrenergic, cholinergic or peptidergic phenotype has yet to be elucidated, though it has been proposed that fibronectin and basal lamina components initiate adrenergic phenotypic expression at the expense of melanocyte numbers. Cholinergic characteristics are acquired relatively early and the appropriate phenotypic expression may be promoted by cholinergic differentiation factor and ciliary neurotrophic factor.

Neuropeptides are expressed by autonomic neurones *in vitro* and may be stimulated by various target tissue factors in sympathetic and parasympathetic neurones. Some neuropeptides are expressed more intensely during early stages of ganglion formation.

Enteric nervous system

The enteric nervous system is different from the other components of the autonomic nervous system because it can mediate reflex activity independently of control by the brain and spinal cord. The number of enteric neurones which develop is believed to be of the same magnitude as the number of neurones in the spinal cord. The number of preganglionic fibres which supply the intestine, and therefore modulate the enteric neurones, is much fewer.

The enteric nervous system is derived from the neural crest. The axial levels of crest origin are shown in **Fig. 14.19**. Premigratory neural crest cells are not prepatterned for specific axial levels, rather they attain their axial value as they leave the neuraxis. Once within the gut wall there is a regionally specific pattern of enteric ganglia formation which may be controlled by the local splanchnopleuric mesenchyme. Cranial neural crest from somite levels 1–7 contributes to the enteric nervous system, forming both neuroblasts and glial support cells.

The most caudal derivatives of neural crest cells, from the lumbosacral region, somites 28 onwards, form components of the pelvic plexus after migrating through the somites towards the level of the colon, rectum and cloaca. Initially the cells come to lie within the developing mesentery, then transiently between the layers of the differentiating muscularis externa, before finally forming a more substantial intramural plexus characteristic of the adult enteric nervous system.

Of the neural crest cells that colonize the bowel, some in the foregut may acquire the ability to migrate outwards and colonize the developing pancreas.

Hirschsprung's disease appears to result from a failure of neural crest cells to colonize the gut wall appropriately. The condition is characterized by a dilated segment of colon proximally and lack of peristalsis in the segment distal to the dilatation. Infants with Hirschsprung's disease show delay in the passage of meconium, constipation, vomiting and abdominal distension. In humans, Hirschsprung's disease is often seen associated with other defects of neural crest development, e.g. Waardenburg type II syndrome, which includes deafness and facial clefts with megacolon.

CHROMAFFIN CELLS

Chromaffin cells are derived from the neural crest and found at numerous sites throughout the body. They are the classic chromaffin cells of the suprarenal medulla, bronchial neuroepithelial cells, dispersed epithelial endocrine cells of the gut (formerly known as argentaffin cells), carotid body cells, and the paraganglia.

The sympathetic ganglia, suprarenal medulla and chromaffin cells are all derived from the cells of the sympathoadrenal lineage. In the suprarenal medulla these cells differentiate into a number of types consisting of small and intermediate-sized neuroblasts or sympathoblasts and larger, initially rounded phaeochromocytoblasts.

Large cells with pale nuclei, thought to be the progenitors of chromaffin cells, can be detected from 9 weeks in human fetuses, and clusters of small neuroblasts are evident from 14 weeks.

Intermediate-sized neuroblasts differentiate into the typical multipolar postganglionic sympathetic neurones (which secrete noradrenaline at their terminals) of classic autonomic neuroanatomy. The smaller neuroblasts have been equated with the small intensely fluorescent (SIF) cells, types I and II, which store and secrete dopamine type I and are thought to function as true interneurones, synapsing with the principal postganglionic neurones. Type II probably operate as local neuroendocrine cells, secreting dopamine into the ganglionic microcirculation. Both types of SIF cells can modulate preganglionic/postganglionic synaptic transmission in the ganglionic neurones. The large cells differentiate into masses of columnar or polyhedral phaeochromocytes (classic chromaffin cells) which secrete either adrenaline (epinephrine) or noradrenaline (norepinephrine). These cell masses are termed paraganglia and may be situated near, on the surface of, or embedded in, the capsules of the ganglia of the sympathetic chain, or in some of the large autonomic plexuses. The largest members of the latter are the para-aortic bodies which lie along the sides of the abdominal aorta in relation to the inferior mesenteric artery. During childhood the para-aortic bodies and the paraganglia of the sympathetic chain partly degenerate and can no longer be isolated by gross dissection, but even in the adult, chromaffin tissue can still be recognized microscopically in these various sites. Both phaeochromocytes and SIF cells belong to the amine precursor uptake and decarboxylation (APUD) series of cells and are paraneuronal in nature.

CENTRAL NERVOUS SYSTEM

SPINAL CORD

In the future spinal cord the median roof plate (dorsal lamina) and floor plate (ventral lamina) of the neural tube do not participate in the cellular proliferation which occurs in the lateral walls and so remain thin. Their cells contribute largely to the formation of the ependyma.

The neuroblasts of the lateral walls of the tube are large and at first round or oval (apolar). Soon they develop processes at opposite poles and become bipolar neuroblasts. However, one process is withdrawn and the neuroblast becomes unipolar, although this is not invariably so in the case of the spinal cord. Further differentiation leads to the development of dendritic processes and the cells become typical multipolar neurones. In the developing cord they occur in small clusters representing clones of neurones. The development of a longitudinal sulcus limitans on each side of the central canal of the cord divides the ventricular and intermediate zones in each lateral wall into a basal (ventrolateral) plate or lamina and an alar (dorsolateral) plate or lamina (**Fig. 14.17**). This separation indicates a fundamental functional difference. Neural precursors in the basal plate include the motor cells of the anterior (ventral) and lateral grey columns, while those of the alar plate exclusively form 'interneurones' (which possess both short and long axons), some of which receive the terminals of primary sensory neurones. Caudally the central canal of the cord ends as a fusiform dilatation, the terminal ventricle.

Anterior (ventral) grey column

The cells of the ventricular zone are closely packed at this stage and arranged in radial columns (**Fig. 14.6**). Their disposition may be determined in part by contact guidance along the earliest radial array of glial fibres which cross the full thickness of the early neuroepithelium. The cells of the intermediate zone are more loosely packed. They increase in number initially in the region of the basal plate. This enlargement outlines the anterior (ventral) column of the grey matter and causes a

ventral projection on each side of the median plane: the floor plate remains at the bottom of the shallow groove so produced. As growth proceeds these enlargements, which are further increased by the development of the anterior funiculi (tracts of axons passing to and from the brain), encroach on the groove until it becomes converted into the slit-like anterior median fissure of the adult spinal cord (**Fig. 14.17**). The axons of some of the neuroblasts in the anterior grey column cross the marginal zone and emerge as bundles of ventral spinal nerve rootlets on the anterolateral aspect of the spinal cord. These constitute, eventually, both the α-efferents which establish motor end plates on extrafusal striated muscle fibres and the γ-efferents which innervate the contractile polar regions of the intrafusal muscle fibres of the muscle spindles.

Lateral grey column

In the thoracic and upper lumbar regions some intermediate zone neuroblasts in the dorsal part of the basal plate outline a lateral column. Their axons join the emerging ventral nerve roots and pass as preganglionic fibres to the ganglia of the sympathetic trunk or related ganglia, the majority eventually myelinating to form white rami communicantes. The axons within the rami synapse on the autonomic ganglionic neurones, and axons of some of the latter pass as postganglionic fibres to innervate smooth muscle cells, adipose tissue or glandular cells. Other preganglionic sympathetic efferent axons pass to the cells of the suprarenal medulla. An autonomic lateral column is also laid down in the midsacral region. It gives origin to the preganglionic parasympathetic fibres which run in the pelvic splanchnic nerves.

The anterior region of each basal plate initially forms a continuous column of cells throughout the length of the developing cord. This soon develops into two columns (on each side): one is medially placed and concerned with innervation of axial musculature, and the other is laterally placed and innervates the limbs. At limb levels the lateral column enlarges enormously, but regresses at other levels.

Axons arising from ventral horn neurones, i.e. α-, β- and γ-efferent fibres, are accompanied at thoracic, upper lumbar and midsacral levels by preganglionic autonomic efferents from neuroblasts of the developing lateral horn. Numerous interneurones develop in these sites (including Renshaw cells): it is uncertain how many of these differentiate directly from ventrolateral lamina (basal plate) neuroblasts and how many migrate to their final positions from the dorsolateral lamina (alar plate).

In the human embryo, the definitive grouping of the ventral column cells, which characterizes the mature cord, occurs early, and by the fourteenth week (80 mm) all the major groups can be recognized. As the anterior and lateral grey columns assume their final form the germinal cells in the ventral part of the ventricular zone gradually stop dividing. The layer becomes reduced in thickness until ultimately it forms the single-layered ependyma which lines the ventral part of the central canal of the spinal cord.

Posterior (dorsal) grey column

The posterior (dorsal) column develops later; consequently the ventricular zone is for a time much thicker in the dorsolateral lamina (alar plate) than it is in the ventrolateral lamina (basal plate) (**Fig. 14.6**).

While the columns of grey matter are being defined, the dorsal region of the central canal becomes narrow and slit-like, and its walls come into apposition and fuse with each other (**Fig. 14.17**). In this way the central canal becomes relatively reduced in size and somewhat triangular in outline.

About the end of the fourth week advancing axonal sprouts invade the marginal zone. The first to develop are those destined to become short intersegmental fibres from the neuroblasts in the intermediate zone, and fibres of dorsal roots of spinal nerves which pass into the spinal cord from neuroblasts of the early spinal ganglia. The earlier dorsal root fibres that invade the dorsal marginal zone arise from small dorsal root ganglionic neuroblasts. By the sixth week they form a well-defined oval bundle near the peripheral part of the dorsolateral lamina (**Figs 14.6, 14.17**). This bundle increases in size and, spreading towards the median plane, forms the primitive posterior funiculus of fine calibre. Later, fibres derived from new populations of large dorsal root ganglionic neuroblasts join the dorsal root: they are destined to become fibres of much larger calibre. As the posterior funiculi increase in thickness, their medial surfaces come into contact separated only by the posterior medial septum, which is ependymal in origin and neuroglial in nature. It is thought that the displaced primitive posterior funiculus may form the basis of the dorsolateral tract or fasciculus (of Lissauer).

Maturation of the spinal cord

Long intersegmental fibres begin to appear at about the third month and corticospinal fibres are seen at about the fifth month. All nerve fibres at first lack myelin sheaths. Myelination starts in different groups at different times, e.g. the ventral and dorsal nerve roots about the fifth month, the corticospinal fibres after the ninth month. In peripheral nerves the myelin is formed by Schwann cells (derived from neural crest cells) and in the CNS by oligodendrocytes (which develop from the ventricular zone of the neural tube). Myelination persists until overall growth of the CNS and PNS has ceased. In many sites, slow growth continues for long periods, even into the postpubertal years.

The cervical and lumbar enlargements appear at the time of the development of their respective limb buds.

In early embryonic life, the spinal cord occupies the entire length of the vertebral canal and the spinal nerves pass at right angles to the cord. After the embryo has attained a length of 30 mm the vertebral column begins to grow more rapidly than the spinal cord and the caudal end of the cord gradually becomes more cranial in the vertebral canal. Most of this relative rostral migration occurs during the first half of intrauterine life. By the twenty-fifth week the terminal ventricle of the spinal cord has altered in level from the second coccygeal vertebra to the third lumbar, a distance of nine segments. As the change in level begins rostrally, the caudal end of the terminal ventricle, which is adherent to the overlying ectoderm, remains *in situ*, and the walls of the intermediate part of the ventricle and its covering pia mater become drawn out to form a delicate filament, the filum terminale. The separated portion of the terminal ventricle persists for a time, but it usually disappears before birth. It does, however, occasionally give rise to congenital cysts in the neighbourhood of the coccyx. In the definitive state, the upper cervical spinal nerves retain their position roughly at right angles to the cord. Proceeding caudally, the nerve roots lengthen and become progressively more oblique.

During gestation the relationship between the conus medullaris and the vertebral column changes, such that the conus medullaris gradually ascends to lie at higher vertebral levels. By 19 weeks of gestation the conus is adjacent to the fourth lumbar vertebra, and by full term (40 weeks) it is at the level of the second lumbar vertebra. By 2 months postnatally the conus medullaris has usually reached its permanent position at the level of the body of the first lumbar vertebra.

In performing a lumbar puncture it is important to enter the spinal canal below the level of the tip of the conus medullaris. While this is usually at or above the level of the second lumbar vertebra, in some individuals the cord may, rarely, extend as low as the third lumbar vertebral. It is advisable, therefore, for the needle to enter the canal below this level.

BRAIN

A summary of the derivatives of the cerebral vesicles from caudal to rostral is given in Table 14.1.

Rhombencephalon

By the time the midbrain flexure appears, the length of the hindbrain is greater than that of the combined extent of the other two brain vesicles. Rostrally it exhibits a constriction, the isthmus rhombencephali (**Fig. 14.2B**), best viewed from the dorsal aspect. Ventrally the hindbrain is separated from the dorsal wall of the primitive pharynx only by the notochord, the two dorsal aortae and a small amount of mesenchyme; on each side it is closely related to the dorsal ends of the pharyngeal arches (**Fig. 26.4**).

The pontine flexure appears to 'stretch' the thin, epithelial roof plate which becomes widened. The greatest increase in width corresponds to the region of maximum convexity, so that the outline of the roof plate becomes rhomboidal. By the same change the lateral walls become separated, particularly dorsally, and the cavity of the hindbrain, subsequently the fourth ventricle, becomes flattened and somewhat triangular in cross-section. The pontine flexure becomes increasingly acute until, at the end of the second month, the laminae of its cranial (metencephalic) and caudal (myelencephalic) slopes are opposed to each other (see **Fig. 14.21**) and, at the same time, the lateral angles of the cavity extend to form the lateral recesses of the fourth ventricle.

Table 14.1 Derivatives of the cerebral vesicles from caudal to rostral

Rhombencephalon (or hindbrain)

1.	Myelencephalon	Medulla oblongata
		Caudal part of the 4th ventricle
		Inferior cerebellar peduncles
2.	Metencephalon	Pons
		Cerebellum
		Middle part of the 4th ventricle
		Middle cerebellar peduncles
3	Isthmus rhombencephali	Superior medullary velum
		Superior cerebellar peduncles
		Rostral part of the 4th ventricle

Mesencephalon (or midbrain)

	Cerebral peduncles
	Tegmentum
	Tectum
	Aqueduct

Prosencephalon (or forebrain)

1.	Diencephalon	Thalamus
		Metathalamus
		Subthalamus
		Epithalamus
		Caudal part of the hypothalamus
		Caudal part of the 3rd ventricle
2.	Telencephalon	Rostral part of the hypothalamus
		Rostral part of the 3rd ventricle
		Cerebral hemispheres
		Lateral ventricles
		Cortex (archaeocortex, palaeocortex, neocortex)
		Corpus striatum

About the end of the fourth week, when the pontine flexure is first discernible, a series of seven transverse rhombic grooves appears in the ventrolateral laminae (basal plate) of the hindbrain. Between the grooves, the intervening masses of neural tissue are termed rhombomeres. These are closely associated with the pattern of the underlying motor nuclei of certain cranial nerves. The general pattern of distribution of motor nuclei seems to be as follows: rhombomere 1 contains the trochlear nucleus, rhombomeres 2 and 3 the trigeminal nucleus, rhombomeres 4 and 5 the facial nucleus, rhombomere 5 the abducens nucleus, rhombomeres 6 and 7 the glossopharyngeal nucleus, and rhombomeres 7 and 8 the vagal, accessory and hypoglossal nuclei. Rhombomeric segmentation represents the ground plan of development in this region of the brain stem and is pivotal for the development of regional identity (**Fig. 26.5**). With further morphogenesis, however, the obvious constrictions of the rhombomere boundaries disappear, and the medulla once again assumes a smooth contour. The differentiation of the lateral walls of the hindbrain into basal (ventrolateral) and alar (dorsolateral) plates has a similar significance to the corresponding differentiation in the lateral wall of the spinal cord, and ventricular, intermediate and marginal zones are formed in the same way.

Cells of the basal plate (ventrolateral lamina)

Cells of the basal plate form three elongated, but interrupted, columns positioned ventrally and dorsally with an intermediate column between (**Fig. 14.20**).

The most ventral column is continuous with the anterior grey column of the spinal cord and will supply muscles considered 'myotomic' in origin. It is represented in the caudal part of the hindbrain by the hypoglossal nucleus, and it reappears at a higher level as the nuclei of the abducens, trochlear and oculomotor nerves, which are somatic efferent nuclei. The intermediate column is represented in the upper part of the spinal cord and caudal brainstem (medulla oblongata and pons) and is for the supply of branchial (pharyngeal) and postbranchial musculature. It is interrupted and forms the elongated nucleus ambiguus in the caudal brainstem, which gives fibres to the ninth, tenth and eleventh cranial nerves. The latter continues into the cervical spinal cord as the origin of the spinal accessory nerve. At higher levels parts of this column give origin to the motor nuclei of the facial and trigeminal nerves. These three nuclei are termed branchial (special visceral) efferent nuclei. The most dorsal column of the basal plate (represented in the spinal cord by the lateral grey column) innervates viscera. It is interrupted also, its large caudal part forming some of the dorsal nucleus of the vagus and its cranial part the salivatory nucleus. These are termed general visceral (general splanchnic) efferent nuclei and their neurones give rise to preganglionic, parasympathetic nerve fibres.

It should be noted here that the neurones of the basal plate and their three columnar derivatives are only motor in the sense that some of their number form either motor neurones or preganglionic parasympathetic neurones. The remainder, which greatly outnumber the former, differentiate into functionally related interneurones and, in some loci, neuroendocrine cells.

Cell columns of the alar plate (dorsolateral lamina)

Cell columns of the alar plate are interrupted and give rise to general visceral (general splanchnic) afferent, special visceral (special splanchnic) afferent, general somatic afferent, and special somatic afferent nuclei (their relative positions, in simplified transverse section, are shown in **Fig. 14.20**). The general visceral afferent column is represented by a part of the dorsal nucleus of the vagus, the special visceral afferent column by the nucleus of the tractus solitarius, the general somatic afferent column by the afferent nuclei of the trigeminal nerve and the special somatic afferent column by the nuclei of the vestibulocochlear nerve. (The relatively simple functional independence of these afferent columns implied by the foregoing classification is, in the main, an aid to elementary learning. The emergent neurobiological mechanisms are in fact much more complex and less well understood.) Although they tend to retain their primitive positions, some of these nuclei are later displaced by differential growth patterns and by the appearance and growth of neighbouring fibre tracts, and possibly by active migration.

It has been suggested that a neurone tends to remain as near as possible to its predominant source of stimulation and that when the possibility of separation arises, as a result of the development of neighbouring structures, it will migrate in the direction from which the greatest density of stimuli come – a phenomenon termed neurobiotaxis. The curious courses of the fibres arising from the facial nucleus and the nucleus ambiguus have been held to illustrate this phenomenon. In the 10 mm embryo, the facial nucleus lies in the floor of the fourth ventricle, occupying the position of the special visceral efferent column, and it is placed at a higher level than the abducens nucleus. As growth proceeds, the facial nucleus migrates at first caudally and dorsally, relative to the abducens nucleus, and then ventrally to reach its adult position. As it migrates, the axons to which its somata give rise elongate and their subsequent course is assumed to map out the pathway along which the facial nucleus has travelled. Similarly the nucleus ambiguus arises initially immediately deep to the ventricular floor, but in the adult it is more deeply placed and its efferent fibres pass first dorsally and medially before curving laterally to emerge at the surface of the medulla oblongata.

MYELENCEPHALON

The caudal slope of the embryonic hindbrain constitutes the myelencephalon, which develops into the medulla oblongata (**Fig. 14.2**). The nuclei of the ninth, tenth, eleventh and twelfth cranial nerves develop in the positions already indicated and afferent fibres from the ganglia of the ninth and tenth nerves form an oval marginal bundle in the region overlying the alar (dorsolateral) lamina. Throughout the rhombencephalon, the dorsal edge of this lamina is attached to the thin expanded roof plate and is termed the rhombic lip. (The inferior rhombic lip is confined to the myelencephalon; the superior rhombic lip to the metencephalon.) As the walls of the rhombencephalon spread outwards, the rhombic lip protrudes as a lateral edge which becomes folded over the adjoining area. The rhombic lip may later become adherent to this area, and its cells migrate actively into the marginal zone of the basal plate. In this way the oval bundle which forms the tractus solitarius becomes buried. Alar plate cells which migrate from the rhombic lip are believed to give rise to the olivary and arcuate nuclei and the scattered grey matter of the nuclei pontis. While this migration is in progress, the floor plate is invaded by fibres which cross the median plane (accompanied by neurones that cluster in and near this plane), and it becomes thickened to form the median raphe. Some of the migrating cells from the rhombic lip in this region do not reach the basal plate and form an oblique ridge: the corpus pontobulbare (nucleus of the circumolivary bundle) across the dorsolateral aspect of the inferior cerebellar peduncle.

The lower (caudal half) part of the myelencephalon takes no part in the formation of the fourth ventricle and, in its development, it closely resembles the spinal cord. The gracile and cuneate nuclei, and some reticular nuclei, are derived from the alar plate, and their efferent arcuate fibres and interspersed neurones play a large part in the formation of the median raphe.

At about the fourth month the descending corticospinal fibres invade the ventral part of the medulla oblongata to initiate formation of the pyramids. Contemporaneously, dorsally, the inferior cerebellar peduncle is formed by ascending fibres from the spinal cord, and by olivocerebellar and parolivocerebellar fibres, external arcuate fibres, and two-way reticulocerebellar and vestibulocerebellar interconnections. (The reticular nuclei of the lower medulla probably have a dual origin from both basal and alar plates.) In the neonate the brain stem is more oblique and has a distinct bend as it passes through the foramen magnum to become the spinal cord.

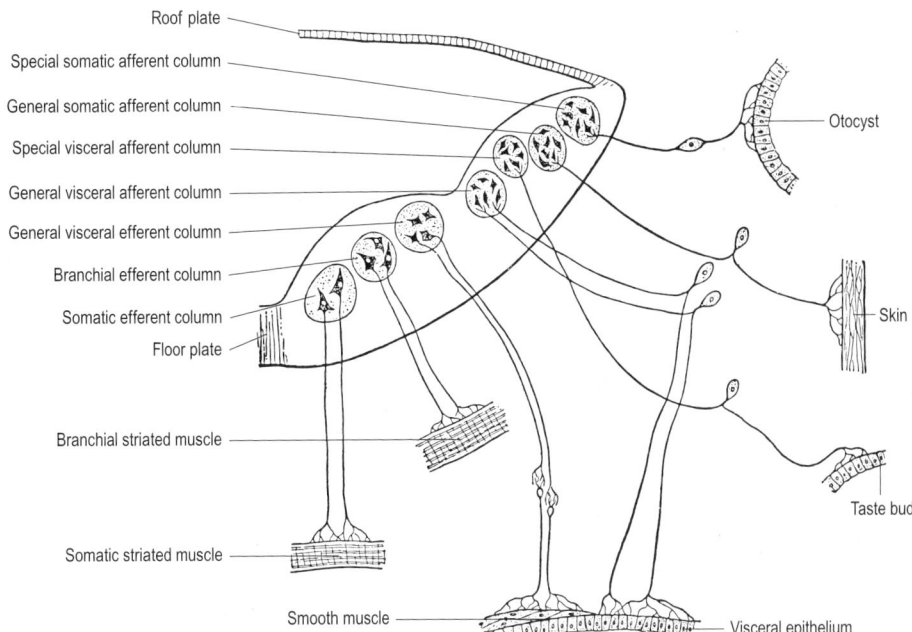

Fig. 14.20 Transverse section through the developing hindbrain of a human embryo 10.5 mm long, to show the relative positions of the columns of grey matter from which the nuclei associated with the different varieties of nerve components are derived. Postganglionic neurones are associated with the general visceral efferent column, bipolar neurones are associated with the otocyst and unipolar afferent neurones are associated with the other alar lamina columns.

Roof plate
Special somatic afferent column
General somatic afferent column
Special visceral afferent column
General visceral afferent column
General visceral efferent column
Branchial efferent column
Somatic efferent column
Floor plate
Branchial striated muscle
Somatic striated muscle
Smooth muscle
Otocyst
Skin
Taste bud
Visceral epithelium

METENCEPHALON

The rostral slope of the embryonic hindbrain is the metencephalon, from which both the cerebellum and pons develop. Before formation of the pontine flexure, the dorsolateral laminae of the metencephalon are parallel with one another. After its formation the roof plate of the hindbrain becomes rhomboidal and the dorsal laminae of the metencephalon lie obliquely. They are close at the cranial end of the fourth ventricle, but widely separated at the level of its lateral angles (**Fig. 14.21**). Accentuation of the flexure approximates the cranial angle of the ventricle to the caudal, and the alar plates of the metencephalon now lie almost horizontally.

The basal plate of the metencephalon becomes the pons. Ventricular, intermediate and marginal zones are formed in the usual way, and the nuclei of the trigeminal, abducens and facial nerves develop in the intermediate layer. It is possible that the grey matter of the formatio reticularis is derived from the basal plate and that of the nuclei pontis from the alar plate by the active migration of cells from the rhombic lip. However, about the fourth month the pons is invaded by cortico-pontine, corticobulbar and corticospinal fibres, becomes proportionately thicker, and takes on its adult appearance: it is relatively smaller in the full-term neonate.

The region of the isthmus rhombencephali undergoes a series of changes which are notoriously difficult to interpret, but which result in the incorporation of the greater part of the region into the caudal end of the midbrain. Only the roof plate, in which the superior medullary velum is formed, and the dorsal part of the alar plate, which becomes invaded by converging fibres of the superior cerebellar peduncles, remain as recognizable derivatives in the adult. Early in development,

the decussation of the trochlear nerves is caudal to the isthmus, but as growth changes occur it is displaced rostrally until it reaches its adult position.

Fourth ventricle and choroid plexus

Caudal to the developing cerebellum the roof of the fourth ventricle remains epithelial, and covers an approximately triangular zone from the lateral angles of the rhomboid fossa to the median obex (**Fig. 14.21**). Nervous tissue fails to develop over this region and vascular pia mater is closely applied to the subjacent ependyma. At each lateral angle and in the midline caudally the membranes break through forming the lateral (Luschka) and median (Magendie) apertures of the roof of the fourth ventricle. These become the principal routes by which cerebrospinal fluid, produced in the ventricles, escapes into the sub-arachnoid space. The vascular pia mater (tela choroidea), in an inverted V formation cranial to the apertures, invaginates the ependyma to form vascular fringes which become the vertical and horizontal parts of the choroid plexuses of the fourth ventricle.

Cerebellum

The cerebellum develops from the rhombic lip, the dorsal part of the alar plate of the metencephalon, which constitutes the rostral margin of the diamond-shaped fourth ventricle. Two rounded swellings develop which at first project partly into the ventricle (**Fig. 14.21**), forming the rudimentary cerebellar hemispheres. The most rostral part of the roof of the metencephalon originally separates the two swellings, but it becomes invaded by cells derived from the alar plate, which form the rudiments of the vermis. At a later stage, extroversion of the cerebellum occurs, its intraventricular projection is reduced and the dorsal extra-ventricular prominence increases. The cerebellum now consists of a bilobar (dumb-bell shaped) swelling stretched across the rostral part of the fourth ventricle (**Fig. 14.21**). It is continuous rostrally with the superior medullary velum, formed from the isthmus rhombencephali, and caudally with the epithelial roof of the myelencephalon. With growth, a number of transverse grooves appear on the dorsal aspects of the cerebellar rudiment: these are the precursors of the numerous fissures which characterize the surface of the mature cerebellum (**Fig. 14.22**).

The first fissure to appear on the cerebellar surface (**Fig. 14.22**) is the lateral part of the posterolateral fissure which forms the border of a caudal region corresponding to the flocculi of the adult. The right and left parts of this fissure subsequently meet in the midline, where they form the boundary between the most caudal vermian lobule, the nodule, and the rest of the vermis. The flocculonodular lobe can now be recognized as the most caudal cerebellar subdivision at this stage and it serves as the attachment of the epithelial roof of the fourth ventricle.

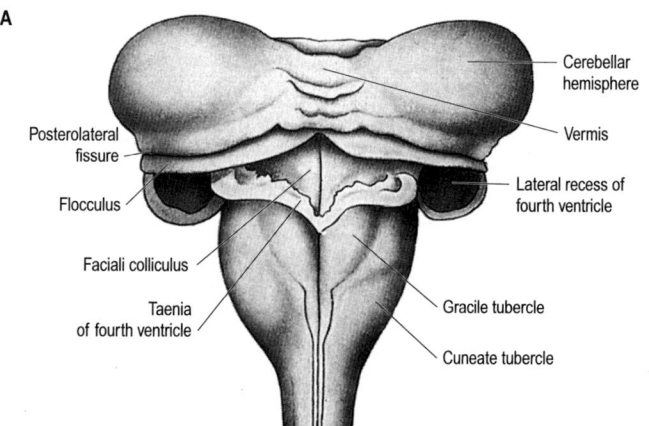

A

Cerebellar hemisphere

Posterolateral fissure

Vermis

Flocculus

Lateral recess of fourth ventricle

Faciali colliculus

Taenia of fourth ventricle

Gracile tubercle

Cuneate tubercle

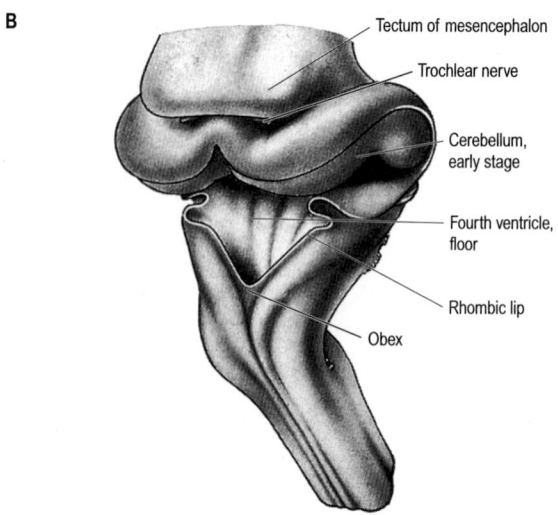

B

Tectum of mesencephalon

Trochlear nerve

Cerebellum, early stage

Fourth ventricle, floor

Rhombic lip

Obex

Fig. 14.21 A, The cerebellum of a fetus in the fifth month. **B**, The dorsal aspect of the hindbrain of a human fetus c.3 months old, viewed from and partly from the right side.

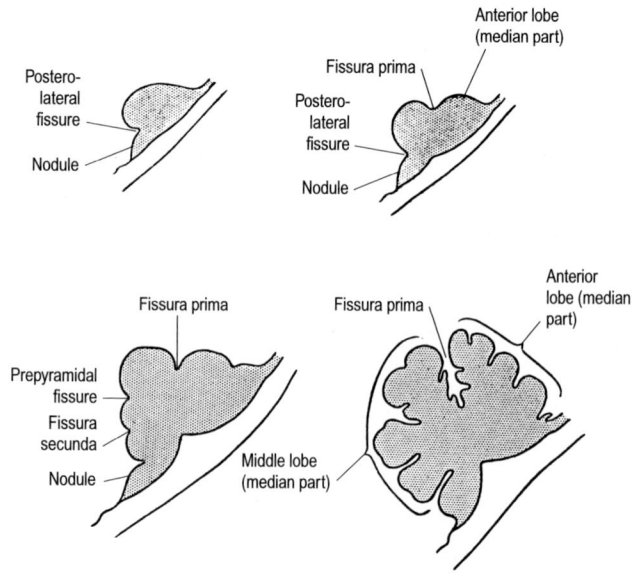

Anterior lobe (median part)

Fissura prima

Postero-lateral fissure

Nodule

Postero-lateral fissure

Nodule

Fissura prima

Prepyramidal fissure

Fissura secunda

Nodule

Fissura prima

Anterior lobe (median part)

Middle lobe (median part)

Fig. 14.22 Median sagittal sections through the developing cerebellum, showing four different stages.

Because of the expansion of the other divisions of the cerebellum, the flocculonodular lobe comes to occupy an anteroinferior position in adults. At the end of the third month a transverse sulcus appears on the rostral slope of the cerebellar rudiment and deepens to form the fissura prima. This cuts into the vermis and both hemispheres, and forms the border between the anterior and posterior lobes. Contemporaneously, two short transverse grooves appear in the caudal vermis. The first is the fissura secunda (postpyramidal fissure), which forms the rostral border of the uvula; the second, the prepyramidal fissure, demarcates the pyramid (Fig. 14.22). The cerebellum now grows dorsally, rostrally, caudally and laterally, and the hemispheres expand much more than the inferior vermis, which therefore becomes buried at the bottom of a deep hollow, the vallecula. Numerous other transverse grooves develop, the most extensive being the horizontal fissure.

Cellular development of the cerebellum

The cerebellum consists of a cortex beneath which are buried a series of deep nuclei. The organization of the cerebellar cortex is similar to that of the cerebral cortex, except that the latter has six layers, while the former has only three. However, whereas in the cerebral cortex neuroblasts originate from the ventricular zone and migrate ventriculofugally towards the pial surface (in an 'inside-out' fashion), early in cerebellar development a layer of cells derived exclusively from the metencephalic rhombic lip initially migrates ventriculofugally to form a layer beneath the glia limitans over the surface of the developing cerebellum. These cells form the external germinative layer and later in development their progeny will migrate ventriculopetally (in an 'outside-in' manner), into the cerebellum. Thus, the cerebellum has an intraventricular portion (cells proliferating from the ventricular zone) and an extraventricular portion (cells proliferating from the external germinative layer) during development. The extraventricular portion becomes larger at the expense of the intraventricular part, the so-called extroversion of the cerebellum. Before the end of the third month the main mass of the cerebellum is extraventricular.

The developed cerebellar cortex contains three layers, namely the molecular layer, the Purkinje layer, and the granular layer. The early bilateral expansion of the ventricular surface reflects the production, by the metencephalic alar plate ventricular epithelium, of neuroblasts which will give rise to the radial glia, cerebellar nuclei, and efferent neurones of the cerebellar cortex (the Purkinje cells) (Fig. 14.23). The radial glia play a role in guiding the Purkinje cells to the meningeal surface of the cerebellar anlage. During this early stage of cerebellar development, which is dominated by the production and migration of efferent cerebellar neurones, the surface of the cerebellar anlage remains smooth. The extroversion of the cerebellum begins later when cells of the external granular layer, also termed the superficial matrix, begin proliferation and migration. These cells produce the granule cells, which migrate inward along the radial glia, through the layers of Purkinje cells, settling deep to them in the granular layer. This stage coincides with the emergences of the transverse folial pattern. Proliferation and migration of granule cells leads to a great rostrocaudal expansion of the meningeal surface of the cerebellum, forming the transverse fissures and transforming the multicellular layer of Purkinje cells into a monolayer. Purkinje cells and nuclear cells are formed prior to the granule cells, and granule cells serve as the recipient of the main afferent (mossy fibre) system of the cerebellum. Thus the development of the efferent neurones of the cerebellar cortex and nuclei precedes the development of its afferent organization.

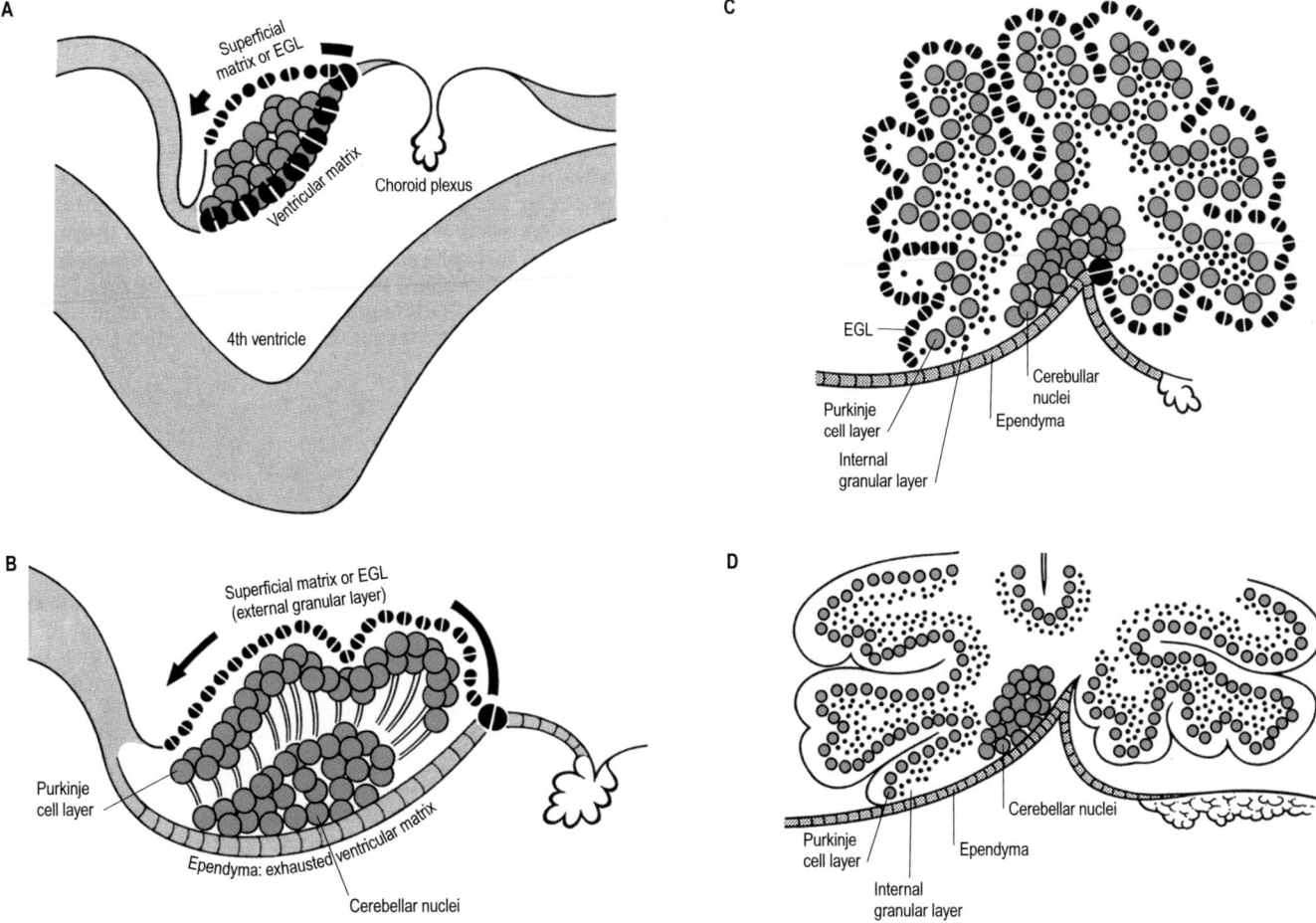

Fig. 14.23 Four stages in the histogenesis of the cerebellar cortex and the cerebellar nuclei. **A,** Purkinje cells and cells of the cerebellar nuclei are produced by the ventricular epithelium and are in the process of migration to their future positions. The cells of the superficial matrix (the external granular layer) take their origin from the ventricular epithelium at the caudal pole of the cerebellar anlage and migrate rostrally over its surface. **B,** After migration the Purkinje cells constitute a multicellular layer beneath the external granular layer. Cell production in the ventricular epithelium has stopped. The remaining cells transform into ependymal cells. **C,** Granule cells are produced by the external granular layer and migrate inwards through the Purkinje cell layer to their position in the granular layer. Purkinje cells spread into a monolayer. **D,** Adult position of cortical and nuclear neurones.

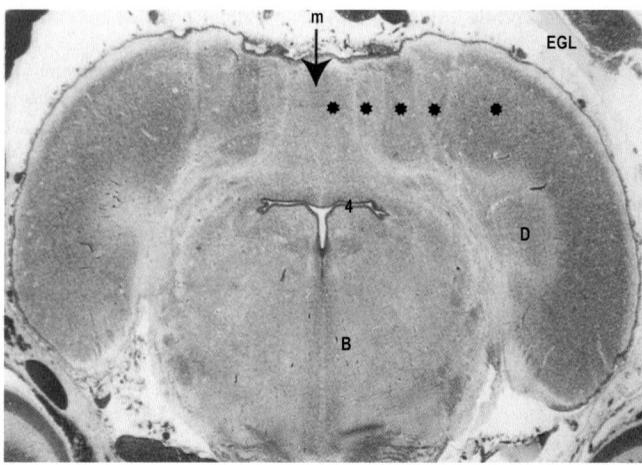

Fig. 14.24 Coronal section through the cerebellum and the brain stem of 65 mm human fetus. The Purkinje cells are located in five multicellular clusters (stars) on both sides of the midline. The anlage of the dentate nucleus occupies the centre of the most lateral Purkinje cell cluster. Abbreviations: B, brain stem; D, dentate nucleus; EGL, external granular layer; m, midline; 4, fourth ventricle. (By kind permission from the Schenk Collection, Dr Johan M Kros, Division of Neuropathology, Department of Pathology, Erasmus Medical Centre, Rotterdam, The Netherlands.)

The early bilateral cerebellar anlage is changed into a unitary structure by fusion of the bilateral intraventricular bulges and the disappearance of the ependyma at this site, the merging of the left and right primitive cerebellar cortex over the midline, and the development of the cerebellar commissure by ingrowth of afferent fibres and outgrowth of efferent axons of the medial cerebellar nucleus.

When the external germinative layer is initially formed, the multicellular Purkinje cell layer beneath is not uniform, but subdivided into clusters which form rostrocaudally extending columns (**Fig. 14.24**). The medial Purkinje cell clusters develop into the future vermis. These Purkinje cells will grow axons which connect to neurones in the vestibular nuclei and the fastigial nucleus. The lateral clusters belong to the future hemispheres and will grow axons terminating in the interposed and dentate nuclei. The sharp border in the efferent projections from the vermis and hemispheres is thus established at an early age. These clusters will give rise to Purkinje cell zones in the adult cerebellum which project to a single vestibular or cerebellar nucleus.

Mesencephalon

The mesencephalon or midbrain is derived from the intermediate primary cerebral vesicle. It persists for a time as a thin-walled tube enclosing a cavity of some size, separated from that of the prosencephalon by a slight constriction and from the rhombencephalon by the isthmus rhombencephali (**Figs 14.2, 14.25**). Later, its cavity becomes relatively reduced in diameter, and in the adult brain it forms the cerebral aqueduct. The basal (ventrolateral) plate of the midbrain increases in thickness to form the cerebral peduncles, which are at first of small size, but enlarge rapidly after the fourth month, when their numerous fibre tracts begin to appear in the marginal zone. The neuroblasts of the basal plate give rise to the nuclei of the oculomotor nerve and some grey masses of the tegmentum, while the nucleus of the trochlear nerve remains in the region of the isthmus rhombencephali. The cells which give rise to the trigeminal mesencephalic nucleus arise either side of the dorsal midline, from the isthmus rhobencephali rostrally across the roof of the mesencephalon. Recent studies have shown that the progenitors of these cells do not express neural crest cell markers.

The cells of the dorsal part of the alar (dorsolateral) plates proliferate and invade the roof plate, which therefore thickens and is later divided into corpora bigemina by a median groove. Caudally this groove becomes a median ridge, which persists in the adult as the frenulum veli. The corpora bigemina are later subdivided into the superior and inferior colliculi by a transverse furrow. The red nucleus, substantia nigra and reticular nuclei of the midbrain tegmentum may first be defined at the end of the third month. Their origins are probably mixed from neuroblasts of both basal and alar plates.

The detailed histogenesis of the tectum and its main derivatives, the colliculi, will not be followed here, but in general the principles outlined

for the cerebellar cortex, the palaeopallium and neopallium also apply to this region. A high degree of geometric order exists in the developing retinotectal projection (the equivalent of the retinogeniculate projection), and in the tectospinal projection.

Prosencephalon

At an early stage, a transverse section through the forebrain shows the same parts as are displayed in similar sections of the spinal cord and medulla oblongata, i.e. thick lateral walls connected by thin floor and roof plates. Moreover, each lateral wall is divided into a dorsal area and a ventral area separated internally by the hypothalamic sulcus (**Fig. 14.25**). This sulcus ends anteriorly at the medial end of the optic stalk. In the fully developed brain it persists as a slight groove extending from the interventricular foramen to the cerebral aqueduct. It is analogous to, if not the homologue of, the sulcus limitans. The thin roof plate remains epithelial, but invaginated by vascular mesenchyme, the tela choroidea of the choroid plexuses of the third ventricle. Later, the lateral margins of the tela undergo a similar invagination into the medial walls of the cerebral hemispheres. The floor plate thickens as the nuclear masses of the hypothalamus and subthalamus develop.

At a very early period, before the closure of the rostral neuropore, two lateral diverticula, the optic vesicles, appear, one on each side, about the level of the prosencephalon. For a time they communicate with the cavity of the prosencephalon by relatively wide openings. The distal parts of the optic vesicles expand, while the proximal parts become the tubular optic stalks. (Their further development is described in Chapter 43.) The optic vesicles (which are described with the development of the eye in Chapter 43) are derived from the lateral walls of the prosencephalon before the telencephalon can be identified. They are usually regarded as derivatives of the diencephalon, and the optic chiasma is often regarded as the boundary between diencephalon and telencephalon.

As the most rostral portion of the prosencephalon enlarges it curves ventrally, and two further diverticula rapidly expand from it, one on each side. These diverticula are rostrolateral to the optic stalks and subsequently form the cerebral hemispheres. Their cavities are the rudiments of the lateral ventricles and they communicate with the median part of the forebrain cavity by relatively wide openings which ultimately become the interventricular foramina. The anterior limit of the median part of the forebrain consists of a thin sheet, the lamina terminalis (**Fig. 14.25A–C**), which stretches from the interventricular foramina to the recess at the base of the optic stalks. The anterior part of the forebrain, including the rudiments of the cerebral hemispheres, is the telencephalon (endbrain) and the posterior part of the diencephalon (between brain). Both contribute to the formation of the third ventricle, although the latter predominates. The fate of the lamina terminalis is described below.

DIENCEPHALON

The diencephalon is broadly divided by the hypothalamic sulcus into dorsal (pars dorsalis diencephali) and ventral (pars ventralis diencephali) parts; these, however, are composite and each contributes to diverse neural structures. The dorsal part develops into the (dorsal) thalamus and metathalamus along the immediate suprasulcal area of its lateral wall, whilst the highest dorsocaudal lateral wall and roof form the epithalamus. The thalamus (**Fig. 14.25A–C**) is first visible as a thickening which involves the anterior part of the dorsal area. Caudal to the thalamus the lateral and medial geniculate bodies, or metathalamus, are recognizable at first as surface depressions on the internal aspect and as elevations on the external aspect of the lateral wall. With the enlargement of the thalami as smooth ovoid masses, the wide interval between them gradually narrows into a vertically compressed cavity which forms the greater part of the third ventricle. After a time these medial surfaces may come into contact and become adherent over a variable area, the connection (single or multiple) constituting the interthalamic adhesion or massa intermedia. The caudal growth of the thalamus excludes the geniculate bodies from the lateral wall of the third ventricle.

At first the lateral aspect of the developing thalamus is separated from the medial aspect of the cerebral hemisphere by a cleft, but with growth the cleft becomes obliterated (**Fig. 14.26**) as the thalamus fuses with the part of the hemisphere in which the corpus striatum is developing. Later, with the development of the projection fibres (corticofugal and corticopetal) of the neocortex, the thalamus becomes related to the internal capsule, which intervenes between it and the

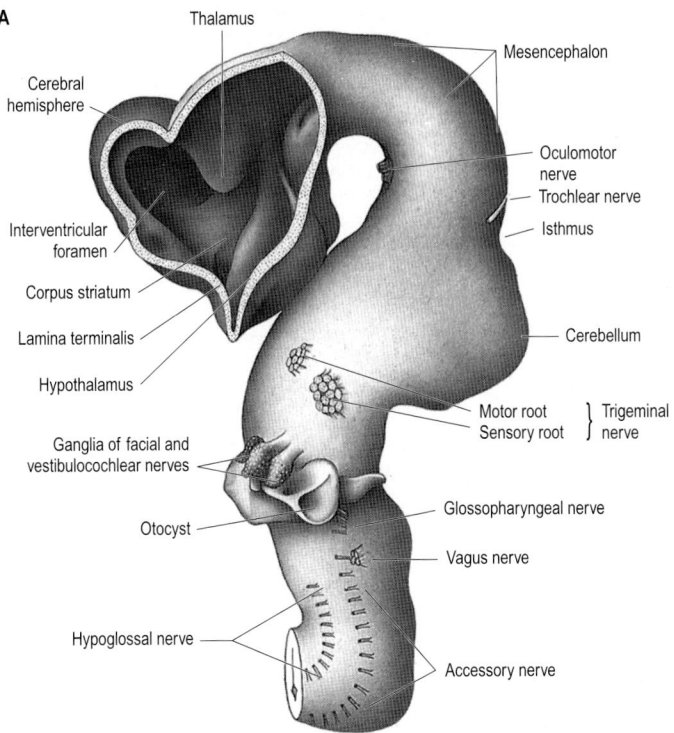

A

Thalamus
Mesencephalon
Cerebral hemisphere
Oculomotor nerve
Trochlear nerve
Isthmus
Interventricular foramen
Corpus striatum
Lamina terminalis
Cerebellum
Hypothalamus
Motor root \} Trigeminal
Sensory root \} nerve
Ganglia of facial and vestibulocochlear nerves
Glossopharyngeal nerve
Otocyst
Vagus nerve
Hypoglossal nerve
Accessory nerve

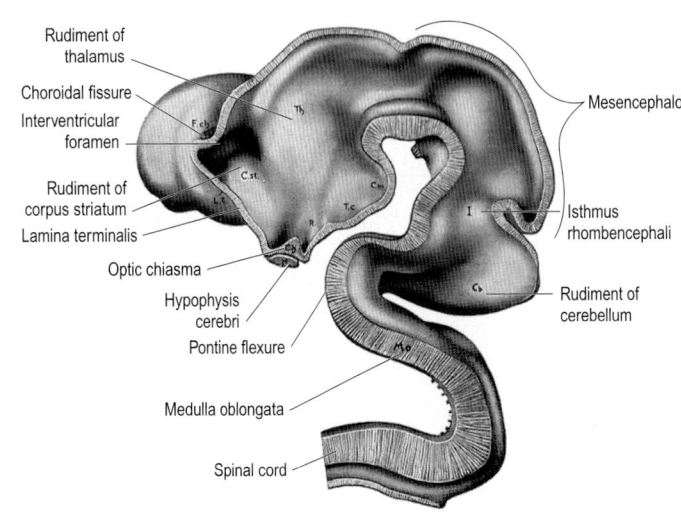

B

Rudiment of thalamus
Choroidal fissure
Interventricular foramen
Mesencephalon
Rudiment of corpus striatum
Isthmus rhombencephali
Lamina terminalis
Optic chiasma
Rudiment of cerebellum
Hypophysis cerebri
Pontine flexure
Medulla oblongata
Spinal cord

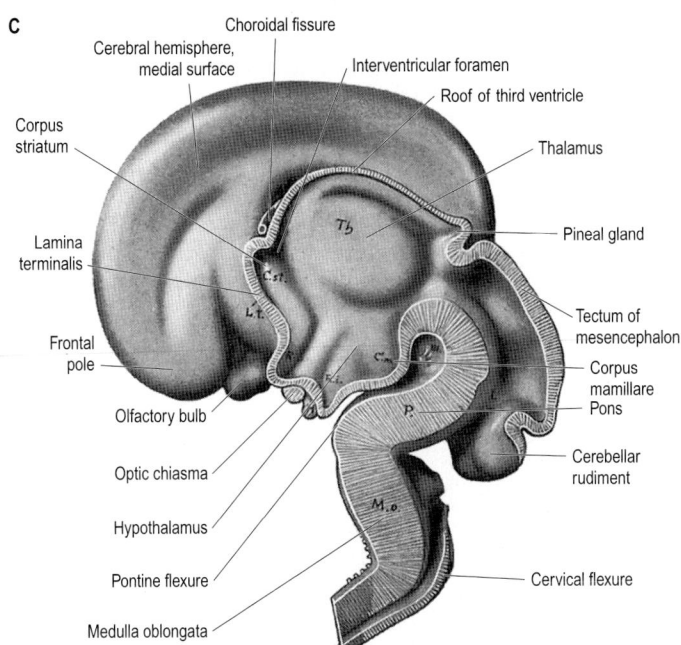

C

Choroidal fissure
Cerebral hemisphere, medial surface
Interventricular foramen
Roof of third ventricle
Corpus striatum
Thalamus
Pineal gland
Lamina terminalis
Frontal pole
Tectum of mesencephalon
Olfactory bulb
Corpus mamillare
Pons
Optic chiasma
Cerebellar rudiment
Hypothalamus
Pontine flexure
Cervical flexure
Medulla oblongata

Fig. 14.25 **A**, The brain of a human embryo, c.10.2 mm long. **B**, The brain of a human embryo, 13.6 mm long: medial surface of right half. The roof of the hindbrain has been removed. **C**, Medial surface of the right half of the brain of a human fetus, c.3 months old.

lateral part of the corpus striatum (lentiform nucleus). Ventral to the hypothalamic sulcus, the lateral wall of the diencephalon, in addition to median derivatives of its floor plate, forms a large part of the hypothalamus and subthalamus.

The epithalamus, which includes the pineal gland, the posterior and habenular commissures and the trigonum habenulae, develops in association with the caudal part of the roof plate and the adjoining regions of the lateral walls of the diencephalon. At an early period (12–20 mm CR length), the epithalamus in the lateral wall projects into the third ventricle as a smooth ellipsoid mass, larger than the adjacent mass of the (dorsal) thalamus and separated from it by a well-defined epithalamic sulcus. In subsequent months, growth of the thalamus rapidly overtakes that of the epithalamus and the intervening sulcus is obliterated. Thus, structures of epithalamic origin are ultimately topographically relatively diminutive.

The pineal gland arises as a hollow outgrowth from the roof plate, immediately adjoining the mesencephalon. Its distal part becomes solid by cellular proliferation, but its proximal stalk remains hollow,

containing the pineal recess of the third ventricle. In many reptiles the pineal outgrowth is two-fold. The anterior outgrowth (parapineal organ) develops into the pineal or parietal eye while the posterior outgrowth is glandular in character. It is the posterior outgrowth which is homologous with the pineal gland in man. The anterior outgrowth also develops in the human embryo but soon disappears entirely.

The nucleus habenulae, which is the most important constituent of the trigonum habenulae, develops in the lateral wall of the diencephalon and is at first in close relationship with the geniculate bodies, from which it becomes separated by the dorsal growth of the thalamus. The habenular commissure develops in the cranial wall of the pineal recess. The posterior commissure is formed by fibres which invade the caudal wall of the pineal recess from both sides.

The ventral part of the diencephalon forms the subsulcal lateral walls of the third ventricle and takes part in the formation of the hypothalamus, including the mammillary bodies, the tuber cinereum and infundibulum of the hypophysis. The mammillary bodies arise as a single thickening, which becomes divided by a median furrow during the

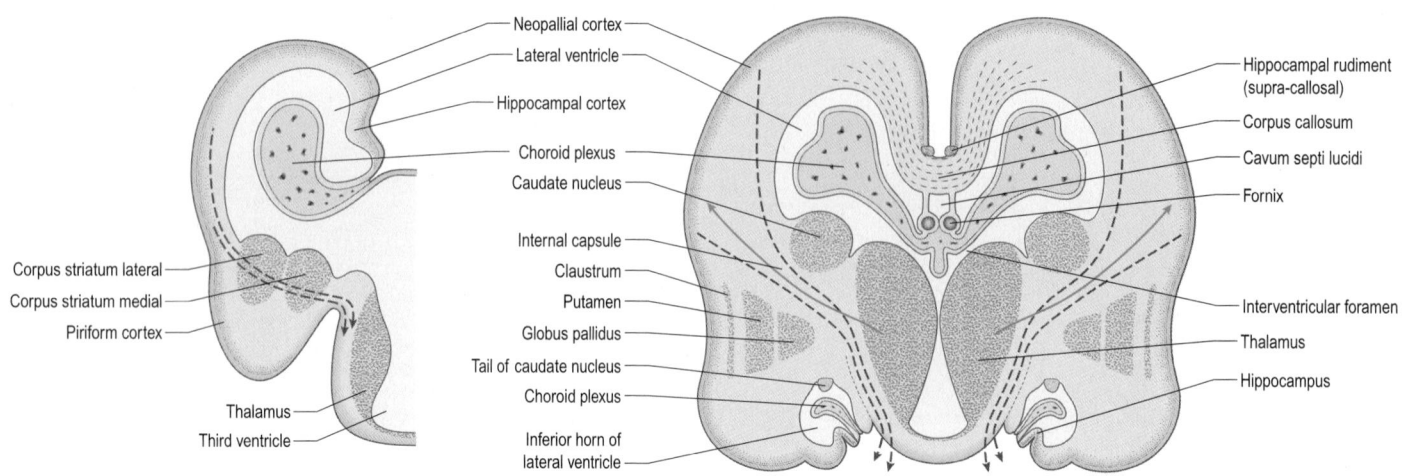

Fig. 14.26 The development of the basal nuclei and internal capsule. (Redrawn by permission from Hamilton WJ, Boyd JD, Mossman HW 1972 Human Embryology: Prenatal Development of Form and Function. Baltimore: Williams and Wilkins.)

third month. Anterior to them the tuber cinereum develops as a cellular proliferation which extends forwards as far as the infundibulum. In front of the tuber cinereum a wide-mouthed diverticulum forms in the floor of the diencephalon. It grows towards the stomodeal roof and comes into contact with the posterior aspect of a dorsally directed ingrowth from the stomodeum (Rathke's pouch). These two diverticula together form the hypophysis cerebri (**Fig. 14.14**). An extension of the third ventricle persists in the base of the neural outgrowth as the infundibular recess. The remaining caudolateral walls and floor of the ventral diencephalon are an extension of the midbrain tegmentum, the subthalamus. This forms the rostral limits of the red nucleus, substantia nigra, numerous reticular nuclei and a wealth of interweaving, ascending, descending and oblique nerve fibre bundles, which have many origins and destinations.

Third ventricle and choroid plexus

The roof plate of the diencephalon, rostral to the pineal gland (and continuing over the median telencephalon) remains thin and epithelial in character and is subsequently invaginated by the choroid plexuses of the third ventricle (**Fig. 14.27**). Before the development of the corpus callosum and the fornix it lies at the bottom of the longitudinal fissure, between and reaching the two cerebral hemispheres. It extends as far rostrally as the interventricular foramina and lamina terminalis. Here, and elsewhere, choroid plexuses develop by the close apposition of vascular pia mater and ependyma without intervening nervous tissue. With development, the vascular layer is infolded into the ventricular cavity and develops a series of small villous projections, each covered by a cuboidal epithelium derived from the ependyma. The cuboidal cells carry numerous microvilli on their ventricular surfaces while basally their plasma membrane becomes complexly folded into the cell. The early choroid plexuses secrete a protein-rich cerebrospinal fluid into the ventricular system which may provide a nutritive medium for the developing epithelial neural tissues. As the latter becomes increasingly vascularized the histochemical reactions of the cuboidal cells and the character of the fluid change to the adult type. In addition to choroid plexus formation, the remaining lining of the third ventricle does not simply form generalized ependymal cells. Many regions become highly specialized, developing concentrations of tanycytes or other modified cells, e.g. those of the subfornical organ, the organum vasculosum (intercolumnar tubercle) of the lamina terminalis, the subcommissural organ and those lining the pineal, suprapineal, and infundibular recesses, which are collectively termed the circumventricular organs.

TELENCEPHALON

The telencephalon (endbrain) consists of two lateral diverticula connected by a median region (the telencephalon impar). The anterior part of the third ventricle develops from the impar, and is closed below and in front by the lamina terminalis. The lateral diverticula are outpouchings of the lateral walls of the telencephalon, which may correspond to the alar lamina, although this is uncertain. Their cavities are the future lateral ventricles, and their walls are formed by the presumptive nervous

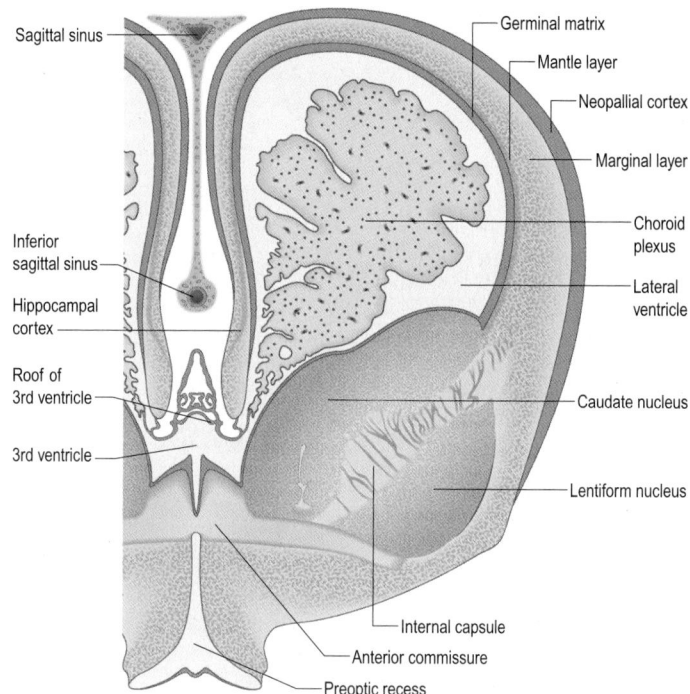

Fig. 14.27 Coronal section of the left cerebral hemisphere in a 73 mm fetus. (Redrawn by permission from Hamilton WJ, Boyd JD, Mossman HW 1972 Human Embryology: Prenatal Development of Form and Function. Baltimore: Williams and Wilkins.)

tissue of the cerebral hemispheres. The roof plate of the median part of the telencephalon remains thin and is continuous behind with the roof plate of the diencephalon (**Fig. 14.25**). The anterior parts of the hypothalamus, which include the optic chiasma, optic recess and related nuclei, develop in the floor plate and lateral walls of the prosencephalon, ventral to the primitive interventricular foramina. The chiasma is formed by the meeting, and partial decussation, of the optic nerves in the ventral part of the lamina terminalis. The optic tracts subsequently grow backwards from the chiasma to end in the diencephalon and midbrain.

Cerebral hemispheres

The cerebral hemispheres arise as diverticula of the lateral walls of the telencephalon, with which they remain in continuity around the margins of the initially relatively large interventricular foramina, except caudally, where they are continuous with the anterior part of the lateral wall of the diencephalon (**Figs 14.2, 14.25**). As growth proceeds the hemisphere enlarges forwards, upwards and backwards and acquires an oval outline, medial and superolateral walls, and a floor. As a result the medial surfaces approach, but are separated by, a vascularized mesenchyme and pia mater which fills the median longitudinal fissure (**Fig. 14.27**). At this stage the floor of the fissure is the epithelial roof plate of the telencephalon, which is directly continuous caudally with the epithelial roof plate of the diencephalons.

At the early oval stage of hemispheric development, regions are named according to their future principal derivatives. The rostromedial and ventral floor becomes linked with the forming olfactory apparatus and is termed the primitive olfactory lobe. The floor (ventral wall, or base) of the larger remainder of the hemisphere forms the anlage of the primitive corpus striatum and amygdaloid complex including its associated rim of lateral and medial walls; this is the striate part of the hemisphere. The rest of the hemisphere i.e. the medial, lateral, dorsal and caudal regions, is the suprastriate part of the hemisphere. Although the largest in terms of surface area, initially it possesses comparatively thin walls. The rostral end of the oval hemisphere becomes the definitive frontal pole. As the hemisphere expands, its original posterior pole moves relatively in a caudoventral and lateral direction, following a curve like a ram's horn: it curves towards the orbit in association with the growth of the caudate nucleus (and other structures) to form the definitive temporal pole. A new posterior part persists as the definitive occipital pole of the mature brain (**Fig. 14.28**). The great expansion of the cerebral hemispheres is characteristic of mammals and especially of man. In their subsequent growth they overlap, successively, the diencephalon and the mesencephalon, and then meet the rostral surface of the cerebellum. The temporal lobes embrace the flanks of the brain stem.

Olfactory bulb

A longitudinal groove appears in the anteromedial part of the floor of each developing lateral ventricle about the fifth week of embryonic development. This groove deepens and forms a hollow diverticulum which is continuous with the hemisphere by a short stalk. The diverticulum becomes connected on its ventral or inferior surface to the olfactory placode (pp. 245, 609). Placodal cells give rise to afferent axons which terminate in the walls of the diverticulum. As the head increases in size the diverticulum grows forwards and, subsequently losing its cavity, becomes converted into the solid olfactory bulb. The forward growth of the bulb is accompanied by elongation of its stalk,

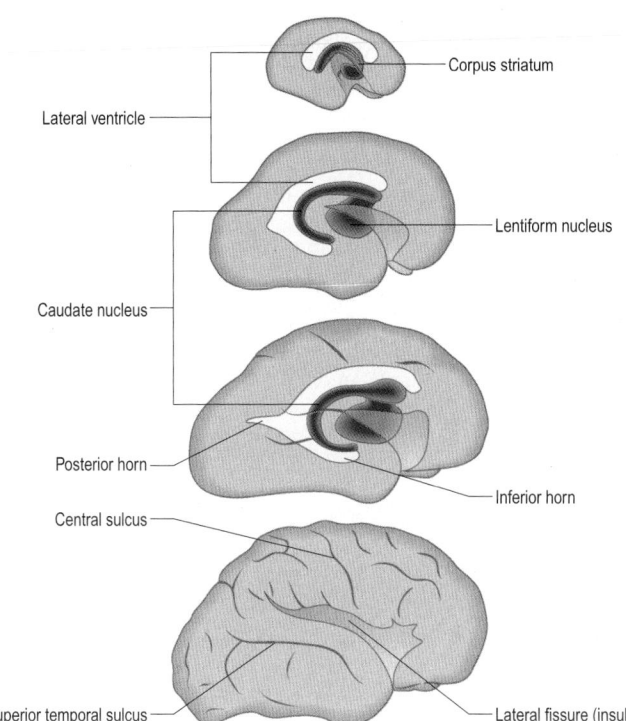

Fig. 14.28 Formation of the basal nuclei and lateral ventricles as the telencephalon develops. (Redrawn by permission from Hamilton WJ, Boyd JD, Mossman HW 1972 Human Embryology: Prenatal Development of Form and Function. Baltimore: Williams and Wilkins.)

which forms the olfactory tract. The part of the floor of the hemisphere to which the tract is attached constitutes the piriform area.

Lateral ventricles and choroid plexus

The early diverticulum or anlage of the cerebral hemisphere initially contains a simple spheroidal lateral ventricle which is continuous with the third ventricle via the interventricular foramen. The rim of the foramen is the site of the original evagination. The expanding ventricle develops the ram's horn shape of the surrounding hemisphere, becoming first roughly ellipsoid and then a curved cylinder, which is convex dorsally (**Fig. 14.28**). The ends of the cylinder expand towards, but do not reach, the frontal and (temporary) occipital poles: differentiating and thickening neural tissues separate the ventricular cavities and pial surfaces at all points, except along the line of the choroidal fissure. Pronounced changes in ventricular form accompany the emergence of a temporal pole. The original caudal end of the curved cylinder expands within its substance and the temporal extensions in each hemisphere pass ventrolaterally to encircle both sides of the upper brain stem. Another extension may develop from the root of the temporal extension in the substance of the definitive occipital pole and pass caudomedially; it is quite variable in size, often asymmetrical on the two sides, and one or both may be absent. Although the lateral ventricle is a continuous system of cavities, specific parts are now given regional names. The central part (body) extends from the interventricular foramen to the level of the posterior edge (splenium) of the corpus callosum. Three cornua (horns) diverge from the body: anterior towards the frontal pole, posterior towards the occipital pole, and inferior towards the temporal pole.

At these early stages of hemispheric development the term pole is preferred, in most instances, to lobe. Lobes are defined by specific surface topographical features which will appear over several months, and differential growth patterns persist for a considerable period.

The pia mater which covers the epithelial roof of the third ventricle at this stage is itself covered with loosely arranged mesenchyme and developing blood vessels. These vessels subsequently invaginate the roof of the third ventricle on each side of the median plane to form its choroid plexuses. The lower part of the medial wall of the cerebral hemisphere, which immediately adjoins the epithelial roof of the interventricular foramen and the anterior extremity of the diencephalon, also remains epithelial. It consists of ependyma and pia mater; elsewhere the walls of the hemispheres are thickening to form the pallium. The thin part of the medial wall of the hemisphere is invaginated by vascular tissue which is continuous in front with the choroid plexus of the third ventricle and constitutes the choroid plexus of the lateral ventricle. This invagination occurs along a line which arches upwards and backwards, parallel with and initially limited to, the anterior and upper boundaries of the interventricular foramen. This curved indentation of the ventricular wall, where no nervous tissue develops between ependyma and pia mater, is termed the choroidal fissure (**Figs 14.25C, 14.26**). The subsequent assumption of the definitive form of the choroidal fissure depends on related growth patterns in neighbouring structures. Of particular importance are the relatively slow growth of the interventricular foramen, the secondary 'fusion' between the lateral diencephalon and medial hemisphere walls, the encompassing of the upper brain stem by the forward growth of the temporal lobe and its pole towards the apex of the orbit, and the massive expansion of two great cerebral commissures (the fornix and corpus callosum). The choroidal fissure is now clearly a caudal extension of the much reduced interventricular foramen, which arches above the thalamus and is here only a few millimetres from the median plane. Near the caudal end of the thalamus it diverges ventrolaterally, its curve reaching and continuing in the medial wall of the temporal lobe over much of its length (i.e. to the tip of the inferior horn of the lateral ventricle). The upper part of the arch will be overhung by the corpus callosum and, throughout its convexity, it is bordered by the fornix and its derivatives.

Basal nuclei

At first growth proceeds more actively in the floor and the adjoining part of the lateral wall of the developing hemisphere, and elevations formed by the rudimentary corpus striatum encroach on the cavity of the lateral ventricle (**Figs 14.25, 14.26**). The head of the caudate nucleus appears as three successive parts, medial, lateral and intermediate, which produce elevations in the floor of the lateral ventricle. Caudally these merge to form the tail of the caudate nucleus and the amygdaloid complex, which both remain close to the temporal pole of the hemisphere. When the occipital pole grows backwards, and the general enlargement of the hemisphere carries the temporal pole downwards and forwards, the tail of the caudate is continued from the floor of the central part (body) of the ventricle into the roof of its temporal extension, the future inferior horn. The amygdaloid complex encapsulates its tip. Anteriorly the head of the caudate nucleus extends forwards to the floor of the interventricular foramen, where it is separated from the developing anterior end of the thalamus by a groove; later, the head expands in the floor of the anterior horn of the lateral ventricle. The lentiform nucleus develops from two laminae of cells, medial and lateral, which are continuous with both the medial and lateral parts of the caudate nucleus. The internal capsule appears first in the medial lamina and extends laterally through the outer lamina to the cortex. It divides the laminae into two, the internal parts join the caudate nucleus and the external parts form the lentiform nucleus. In the latter, the remaining medial lamina cells give rise mainly to the globus pallidus and the lateral lamina cells to the putamen. The putamen subsequently expands concurrently with the intermediate part of the caudate nucleus.

Fusion of diencephalic and telencephalic walls

As the hemisphere enlarges, the caudal part of its medial surface overlaps and hides the lateral surface of the diencephalon (thalamic part), from which it is separated by a narrow cleft occupied by vascular connective tissue. At this stage (about the end of the second month) a transverse section made caudal to the interventricular foramen would pass from the third ventricular cavity successively through the developing thalamus, the narrow cleft just mentioned, the thin medial wall of the hemisphere, and the cavity of the lateral ventricle, with the corpus striatum in its floor and lateral wall (**Fig. 14.26**).

As the thalamus increases in extent it acquires a superior surface in addition to medial and lateral surfaces. The lateral part of its superior surface fuses with the thin medial wall of the hemisphere so that this part of the thalamus is finally covered with the ependyma of the lateral ventricle immediately ventral to the choroidal fissure. As a result the corpus striatum is approximated to the thalamus and is separated from it only by a deep groove which becomes obliterated by increased growth along the line of contact. The lateral aspect of the thalamus is now in continuity with the medial aspect of the corpus striatum so that a secondary union between the diencephalon and the telencephalon is affected over a wide area, providing a route for the subsequent passage of projection fibres to and from the cortex (**Fig. 14.26**).

Development of the cortex

The migration and differentiation of neural progenitors to form nuclei is either minimal or limited throughout the brain stem, as it is in the spinal cord. Their progeny remain immediately extra-ependymal or partially displaced towards the pial exterior, and are arrested deeply embedded in the myelinated fibre 'white matter' of the region. In marked contrast, proliferation and migration of neuroblasts in the cerebral hemisphere produces a superficial layer of grey matter. This occurs in both the striate and suprastriate regions, but not in the central areas of the original medial wall, where secondary fusion of the diencephalon occurs. The superficial layer of grey matter consists of neuronal somata, dendrites, the terminations of incoming (afferent) axons, the stems of (or the whole of) efferent axons, and glial cells and endothelial cells. Successive generations of neuroblasts migrate through the layers of earlier generations to attain subpial positions, so that the surface of the cerebral hemispheres expands at a rate greater than the hemispheres as a whole. Subsequent differentiation results in a highly organized subpial surface coat of grey matter termed the cortex or pallium.

The terminology used to describe regions of the cortex is based on evolutionary concepts. The oldest portions of cortex receive information concerned with olfaction; they are termed the archicortex (archipallium) and paleocortex (paleopallium), and both are subdivisions of an overall allocortex. The archicortex is the forerunner of the hippocampal lobe, and the paleocortex gives rise to the piriform area. The remaining cortical surface expands greatly in mammals forming the neocortex (young cortex) which displaces the earlier cortices so that they come to lie partially internally in each hemisphere.

Formation of the insula

At the end of the third month, while the corpus striatum is developing there is a relative restriction of growth between the frontal and temporal lobes. The region lateral to the striatum becomes depressed to form a lateral cerebral fossa with a portion of cortex, the insula, at its base (**Fig. 14.28**). As the temporal lobe continues to protrude towards the orbit, and with more rapid growth of the temporal and frontal cortices, the surface of the hemisphere expands at a rate greater than the hemisphere as a whole and the cortical areas become folded, forming gyri and sulci. The insula is gradually overgrown by these adjacent cortical regions, and they overlap it forming the opercula, the free margins of which form the anterior part of the lateral fissure. This process is not completed until after birth. The lentiform nucleus remains deep to and coextensive with the insula.

Olfactory nerve, limbic lobe and hippocampus

The growth changes in the temporal lobe which help to submerge the insula produce important changes in the olfactory and neighbouring limbic areas. As it approaches the hemispheric floor, the olfactory tract diverges into lateral, medial and (variable) intermediate striae. The medial stria is clothed with a thin archaeocortical medial olfactory gyrus. This curves up into further archaeocortical areas anterior to the lamina terminalis (paraterminal gyrus, prehippocampal rudiment, parolfactory gyrus, septal nuclei) and these continue into the indusium griseum. The lateral stria, clothed by the lateral olfactory gyrus, and, when present, the intermediate stria, terminate in the rostral parts of the piriform area. This includes the olfactory trigone and tubercle, anterior perforated substance and uncus (hook) and entorhinal area of the anterior part of the future parahippocampal gyrus. Its lateral limit is indicated by the rhinal sulcus. The forward growth of the temporal pole and the general expansion of the neocortex cause the lateral olfactory gyrus to bend laterally, the summit of the convexity lying at the antero-inferior corner of the developing insula (**Fig. 14.29A–G**). During the fourth and fifth months, much of the piriform area becomes submerged by the adjoining neocortex and in the adult only a part of it remains visible on the inferior aspect of the cerebrum.

The limbic (bordering) lobe is the first part of the cortex to differentiate and at first it forms a continuous, almost circular strip on the medial and inferior aspects of the hemisphere. Below and in front, where the stalk of the olfactory tract is attached, it constitutes a part of the piriform area. The portion outside the curve of the choroid fissure (**Fig. 14.30**) constitutes the hippocampal formation. In this region the neural progenitors of the developing cortex proliferate and migrate, and the wall of the hemisphere thickens and produces an elevation which projects into the medial side of the ventricle: this elevation is the hippocampus. It appears first on the medial wall of the hemisphere in the area above and in front of the lamina terminalis (paraterminal area) and gradually extends backwards, curving into the region of the temporal pole where it adjoins the piriform area. The marginal zone in the neighbourhood of the hippocampus is invaded by neuroblasts to form the dentate gyrus. Both extend from the paraterminal area backwards above the choroid fissure and follow its curve downwards and forwards towards the temporal pole, where they continue into the piriform area. A shallow groove (the hippocampal sulcus) crosses the medial surface of the hemisphere throughout the hippocampal formation.

The efferent fibres from the cells of the hippocampus collect along its medial edge and run forwards immediately above the choroid fissure. Anteriorly they turn ventrally and enter the lateral part of the lamina terminalis to gain the hypothalamus, where they end in and around the mammillary body and neighbouring nuclei. These efferent hippocampal fibres form the fimbria hippocampi and the fornix.

Projection fibres, internal capsule

The growth of the neocortex and its enormous expansion during the latter part of the third month are associated with the initial appearance of corticofugal and corticopetal projection fibres and the pathway they follow, the internal capsule. These fibres follow the route provided by the apposition of the lateral aspect of the thalamus with the medial aspect of the corpus striatum, and, as they do so, they divide the latter, almost completely, into a lateral part, the lentiform nucleus, and a medial part, the caudate nucleus; these two nuclei remain confluent only in their anteroinferior regions (**Figs 14.26, 14.28**). The corticospinal tracts begin to develop in the ninth week of fetal life and have reached their caudal limits by the twenty-ninth week. The fibres destined for the cervical and upper thoracic regions and involved in the innervation of the upper limbs are in advance of those concerned with the lower limbs, which, in turn, are in advance of those concerned with the face.

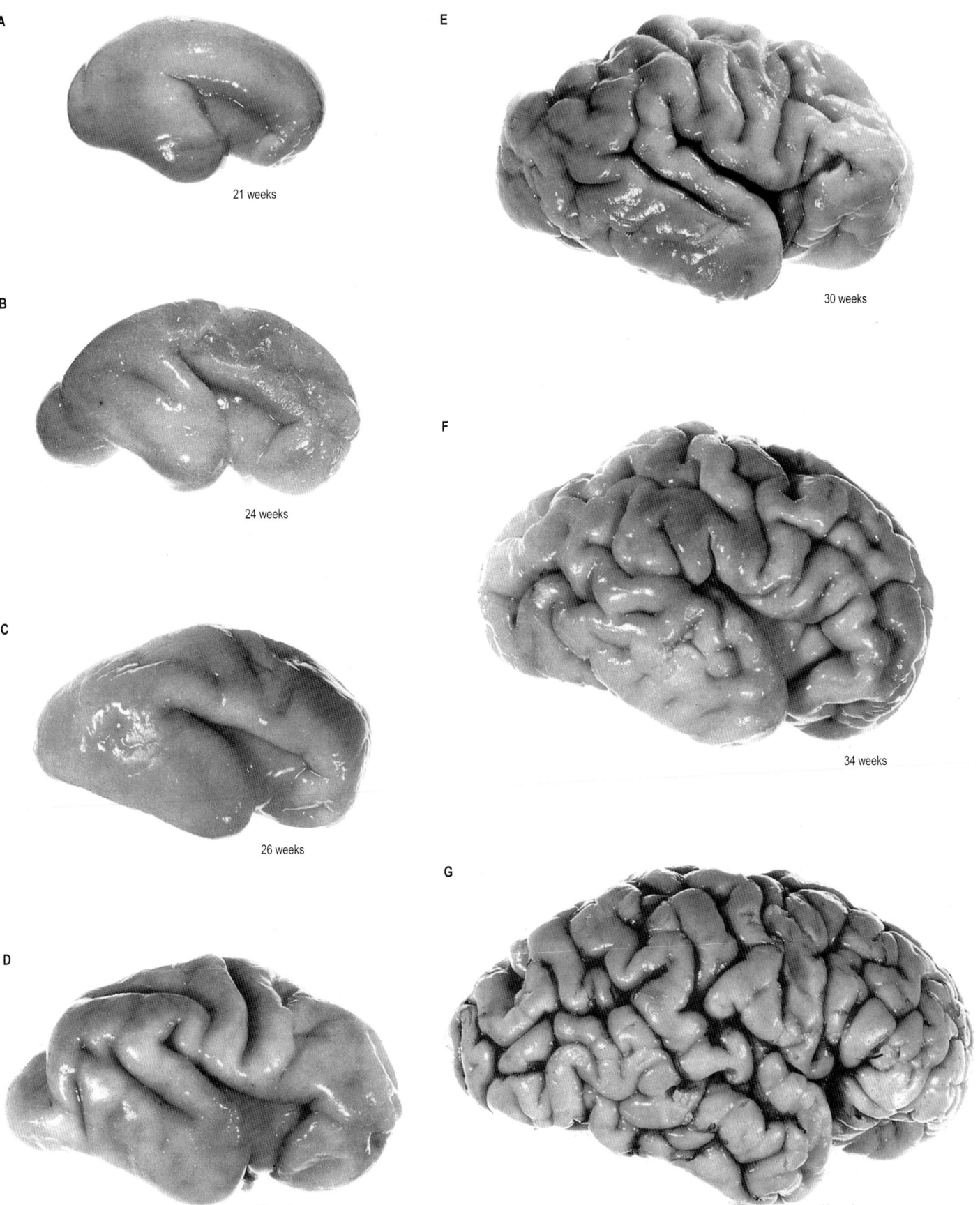

A 21 weeks

B 24 weeks

C 26 weeks

D 28 weeks

E 30 weeks

F 34 weeks

G 40 weeks

Fig. 14.29 The superolateral surfaces of human fetal cerebral hemispheres at the ages indicated, showing the changes in size, profile and the emerging pattern of cerebral sulci with increasing maturation. Note the changing prominence and relative positions of the frontal, occipital and particularly the temporal pole of the hemisphere. At the earliest stage (A) the lateral cerebral fossa is already obvious; its floor covers the developing corpus striatum in the depths of the hemisphere and progressively matures into the cortex of the insula. The fossa is bounded by overgrowing cortical regions, the frontal, temporal and parietal opercula, which gradually converge to bury the insula; their approximation forms the lateral cerebral sulcus. By the sixth month the central, pre- and postcentral, superior temporal, intraparietal and parieto-occipital sulci are all clearly visible. In the subsequent stages shown all the remaining principal and subsidiary sulci rapidly appear and by 40 weeks all the features which characterize the adult hemisphere in terms of surface topography are present in miniature. (Photographs provided by Dr Sabina Strick, The Maudsley Hospital, London.)

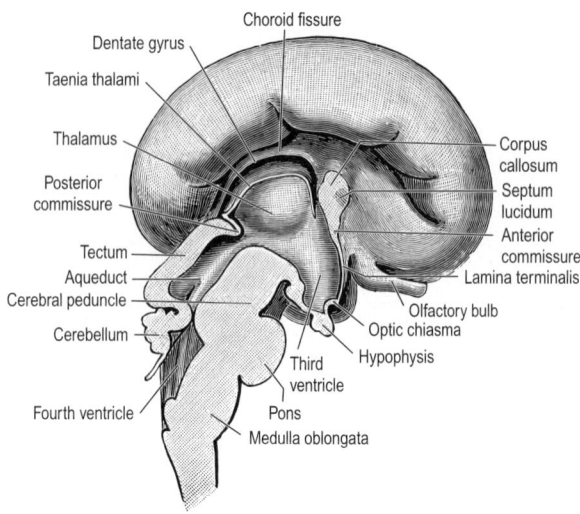

Fig. 14.30 The brain of a human fetus, 16 weeks old: medial aspect of left half.

The appearance of reflexes in these three parts of the body shows a comparable sequence.

The majority of subcortical nuclear masses receive terminals from descending fibres of cortical origin. These are joined by thalamocortical, hypothalamocortical and other afferent ascending bundles. The internal capsular fibres pass lateral to the head and body of the caudate nucleus, the anterior cornu and central part of the lateral ventricle, the rostroventral extensions and body of the fornix, the dorsal thalamus and dorsal choroidal fissure, and medial to the lentiform nucleus (**Fig. 14.26**).

Formation of gyri and sulci

Apart from the shallow hippocampal sulcus and the lateral cerebral fossa, the surfaces of the hemisphere remain smooth and uninterrupted until early in the fourth month (**Fig. 14.29**). The parieto-occipital sulcus appears about that time on the medial aspect of the hemisphere. Its appearance seems associated with an increase in the number of splenial fibres in the corpus callosum. Over the same period the posterior part of the calcarine sulcus appears as a shallow groove extending forwards from a region near the occipital pole. It is a true infolding of the cortex in the long axis of the striate area and produces an elevation, the calcar avis, on the medial wall of the posterior horn of the ventricle.

During the fifth month the cingulate sulcus appears on the medial aspect of the hemisphere, and sulci appear on the inferior and superolateral aspects in the sixth month. The central, precentral and postcentral sulci appear, each in two parts, upper and lower, which usually coalesce shortly afterwards, although they may remain discontinuous. The superior and inferior frontal, the intraparietal, occipital, superior and inferior temporal, occipitotemporal, collateral and rhinal sulci all make their appearance during the same period. By the end of the eighth month all the important sulci can be recognized (**Fig. 14.29**).

Development of commissures

The development of the commissures causes a very profound alteration of the medial wall of the hemisphere. At the time of their appearance the two hemispheres are connected to each other by the median part of the telencephalon. The roof plate of this area remains epithelial, whilst its floor becomes invaded by the decussating fibres of the optic nerves and developing hypothalamic nuclei. These two routes are thus not available for the passage of commissural fibres passing from hemisphere to hemisphere across the median plane, and these fibres therefore pass through the anterior wall of the interventricular foramen, i.e. the lamina terminalis. The first commissures to develop are those associated with the palaeocortex and archicortex. Fibres of the olfactory tracts cross in the ventral or lower part of the lamina terminalis and, together with fibres from the piriform and prepiriform areas and the amygdaloid bodies, form the anterior part of the anterior commissure (**Figs 14.30, 14.31**). In addition the two hippocampi become interconnected by transverse fibres which cross from fornix to fornix in the upper part of the lamina terminalis as the commissure of the fornix.

Various other decussating fibre bundles (known as the supraoptic commissures, although they are not true commissures) develop in the lamina terminalis immediately dorsal to the optic chiasma, between it and the anterior commissure.

The commissures of the neocortex develop later and follow the pathways already established by the commissures of the limbic system. Fibres from the tentorial surface of the hemisphere join the anterior commissure and constitute its larger posterior part. All the other commissural fibres of the neocortex associate themselves closely with the commissure of the fornix and lie on its dorsal surface. These fibres increase enormously in number and the bundle rapidly outgrows its neighbours to form the corpus callosum (**Figs 14.30, 14.31**).

The corpus callosum originates as a thick mass connecting the two cerebral hemispheres around and above the anterior commissure. (This site has been called the precommissural area, but this use has been rejected here because of increasing use of the adjective precommissural to denote the position of parts of the limbic lobe, i.e. prehippocampal rudiment, septal areas and nuclei and strands of the fornix, in relation to the anterior commissure of the mature brain.) The upper end of this neocortical commissural area extends backwards to form the trunk of the corpus callosum. The rostrum of the corpus callosum develops later

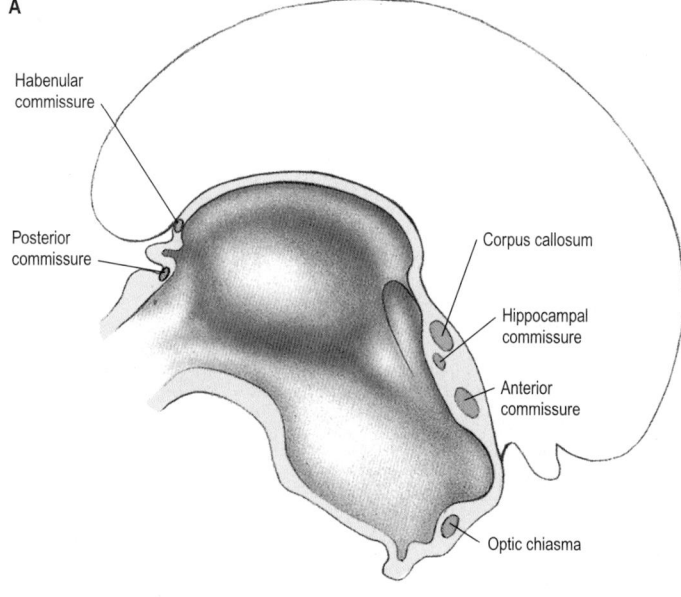

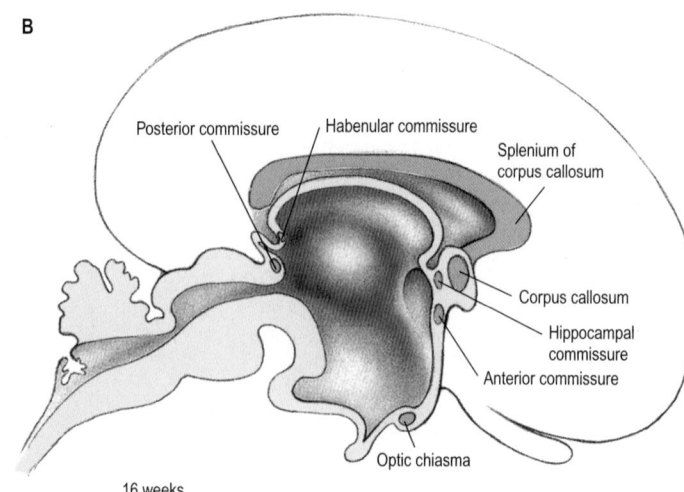

Fig. 14.31 Formation of the commissures. The telencephalon gives rise to commissural tracts that integrate the activities of the left and right cerebral hemispheres. These include the anterior and hippocampal commissures and the corpus callosum. The small posterior and habenular commissures arise from the epithalamus. **A**, 10 weeks; **B**, 16 weeks. (By permission from Larsen.)

and separates some of the rostral end of the limbic area from the remainder of the cerebral hemisphere. Further backward growth of the trunk of the corpus callosum then results in the entrapped part of the limbic area becoming stretched out to form the bilateral septum pellucidum. As the corpus callosum grows backwards it extends above the choroidal fissure, carrying the commissure of the fornix on its under surface. In this way a new floor is formed for the longitudinal fissure, and additional structures come to lie above the epithelial roof of the third ventricle. In its backward growth the corpus callosum invades the area hitherto occupied by the upper part of the archaeocortical hippocampal formation, and the corresponding parts of the dentate gyrus and hippocampus are reduced to vestiges, the indusium griseum and the longitudinal striae (**Figs 14.30, 14.31**). However, the posteroinferior (temporal) archaeocortical regions of both dentate gyrus and hippocampus persist and enlarge.

Cellular development of the cerebrum

The wall of the earliest cerebral hemisphere consists of a pseudostratified epithelium, whose cells exhibit interkinetic nuclear migration as they proliferate to form clones of germinal cells. The columnar cells elongate and their non-nucleated peripheral processes now constitute a marginal zone, whilst their nucleated, paraluminal and mitosing regions constitute the ventricular zone. Some of their progeny leave the ventricular zone and migrate to occupy an intermediate zone. The proliferative phase continues for a considerable period of fetal life. Ultimately, groups of progenitor cells form, at first, generations of definitive neurones and, later, glial cells which migrate to, and mature in, their final positions. These phases of proliferation, migration, differentiation and maturation overlap each other in space and time, and are not precisely sequential.

The earliest migration of neuronal precursors from the ventricular and intermediate zones occurs radially until they approach, but do not reach, the pial surface. Their somata become arranged as a transient cortical plate. Subsequently, proliferation wanes in the ventricular zone but persists for considerable periods in the immediately subjacent subventricular zone. From the pial surface inwards, the following zones may be defined marginal, cortical plate, subplate, intermediate, subventricular and ventricular (**Fig. 14.5**). The marginal zone gives rise to the outermost layer of the cerebral cortex, and the neuroblasts of the cortical plate and subplate form the neurones of the remaining cortical laminae (the complexity varies in different locations and with further additions of neurones from the deeper zones). The intermediate zone gradually transforms into the white matter of the hemisphere. Meanwhile other deep progenitor cells produce generations of glioblasts which also migrate into the more superficial layers. As proliferation wanes and finally ceases in the ventricular and subventricular zones their remaining cells differentiate into general or specialized ependymal cells, tanycytes or subependymal glial cells.

The phases of proliferation vary spatiotemporally with location and cell type. The first groups of cells to migrate are destined for the deep cortical laminae and later groups pass through them to more superficial regions. The subplate zone, a transient feature that is most prominent during mid-gestation, contains neurones surrounded by a dense neuropil: it is the site of the most intense synaptogenesis in the cortex. The cumulative effect of this radial and tangential growth is evident in a marked increase in cortical thickness and surface area.

In the pallial walls of the mammalian cerebral hemisphere the phylogenetically oldest regions, which are the first to differentiate during ontogeny, are those that border the interventricular foramen and its extension the choroidal fissure, the lamina terminalis and the piriform lobe. An increasingly complex level of organization, from three to six tangential laminae, is encountered in passing from the dentate gyrus and cornu ammonis through the subiculum to the general neocortex. (Many investigators find the simple progression from three to six major laminae a gross oversimplification, and numerous subdivisions have been proposed.)

Mechanisms of cortical development

Rakic (1971) initially demonstrated the migration of neuroblasts along radial glial processes, and this has subsequently been seen to occur in three phases. First, the neuroblasts become apposed to the radial glial cells and establish an axis of polarity away from the ventricular surface. Next, they are propelled along the glial surface until they 'recognize' their final destination, whereupon they cease locomotion and detach from the glial processes. They then continue to differentiate according

to their final position, and later-born neuroblasts migrate past them towards the pial surface (**Figs 14.5, 14.32, 14.33**). Cortical neurones or cerebellar granule cells appear equally capable of migrating on hippocampal or cerebellar Bergmann glia, indicating conservation of migration mechanisms in different brain regions.

Various lines of evidence support the proposal that the laminar fate of neurones is determined prior to migration. In the mutant reeler mouse, laminar formation is inverted so that layers form in outside-in rather than inside-out array, yet axonal connections and neuronal properties appear normal, suggesting that the cells differentiate according to their time of origin rather than their location. Likewise, the prevention of neuronal migration by irradiation leads to the production of cells which remain apposed to the ventricular surface but which develop an appropriate phenotype and efferent projections. Transplantation of labelled cells has suggested that commitment to a particular cortical lamina occurs shortly after S-phase. Neurones of pre-existing laminae that have begun axonogenesis may provide a feedback on the forming cortical layers, providing a sort of developmental clock for histogenesis.

In a plane perpendicular to its laminae, i.e. tangentially/circumferentially, the cortex is divided up into a number of areas, displaying a hierarchy of organization. These include primary areas, such as the motor cortex, unimodal association areas concerned with the integration of information from one of the primary areas, and multimodal association areas that integrate information from more than one modality. There are also the areas concerned with functions that are even less understood, such as the frontal lobes, concerned with goal-orientation responsibility and long-term planning. The primary areas are further divided into somatotopic maps. At the finest level, the cortex is known to consist of a series of 'columns', 50–500 μm wide, within which cells on a vertical traverse display common features of modality and electrophysiological responses to stimuli, e.g. the ocular dominance columns of the visual cortex. Despite the precise stacking of neurones in these columns, only 80–85% of cells are thought to migrate radially along the glial cells: a subpopulation is thought to move tangentially in the intermediate zone (O'Rourke et al 1995). Moreover, some neurones may also migrate tangentially on the radial glial cells, as a result of glial cell branching in the cortical plate. The ventricular zone is not the only source of cortical neurones, since striatal and GABAergic neurones are known to migrate from the lateral ganglionic eminence into the developing cortex.

Two models have been proposed to explain the development of the complexity of cortical organization. The 'protocortex' model assumes that the proliferative ventricular epithelium is a 'tabula rasa' which generates homogeneous layers of neurones that are patterned solely by the ingrowth of processes from the thalamus. The 'protomap' hypothesis proposes that the intrinsic differences between the different areas are specified prior to cell migration (Rakic 1988, 2003). The radial glial cells translate this map from the ventricular zone to the cortical plate where the pattern is refined by innervating axons. In this 'radial unit' model, the tangential co-ordinates of the different areas are determined by the position of their ventricular ancestors, whereas their radial position is determined by their time of birth and rate of migration.

But what would constitute such a 'protomap'? The investigation of gene expression patterns shows that the early cortex is not homogeneous, and that it expresses some markers that are transient and some which persist into the adult. For example, the mouse gene *Id2* marks the transition between the motor and somatosensory cortices in the embryo, whereas limbic associated membrane protein (LAMP) delineates the limbic cortex throughout life. LAMP expression is regulated by transforming growth factor-α, which is expressed by the lateral ganglionic eminence at the lateral edge of the cortex; the medial edge or cortical hem expresses signalling molecules of the Wnt and BMP families. Any, if not all, of these may be the components of short range signalling centres along the edges of the cortex. Coupled with the gradients of transcription factors such as Emx2 and Lhx2, there is therefore evidence to support the 'protomap' hypothesis (Donoghue and Rakic 1999).

However, studies of cell migration are consistent with the idea that cortical areas might not be rigidly determined. Manipulations of the developing cortex by deafferentation or manipulation of inputs give some indication of the state of commitment of cortical areas. In two independent sets of experiments, somatosensory or auditory cortex was induced to process visual information by misrouting retinal axons to somatosensory thalamus or auditory thalamus (von Melchner, Pallas &

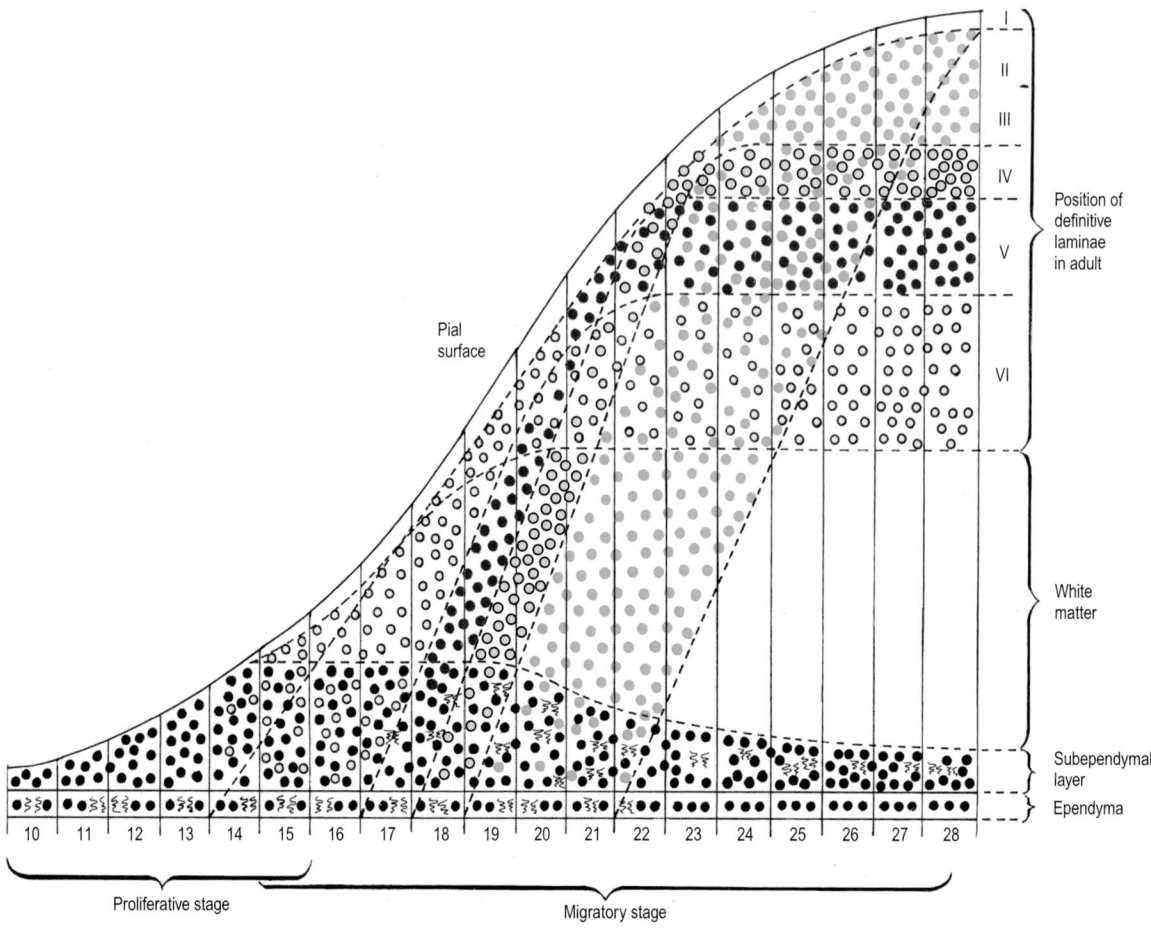

Fig. 14.32 The dynamics of neuroblast migrations during transformation of the early cranial neural tube to form the cerebral neocortex of the rat through days 10 to 28. Note the successive waves of migration. Symbolic metaphase chromosomes: mitotic cells; full black discs: ventricular and subventricular zone neuroblasts; full yellow discs: infragranular neuroblasts destined for lamina VI; full magenta discs: infragranular neuroblasts destined for lamina V; open black circles: granular neuroblasts destined for lamina IV; full blue discs: supragranular neuroblasts destined for laminae III and II. (Redrawn and colour coded from data provided by Professor M Berry (1974) of the Anatomy Department, Guy's Hospital Medical School, London.)

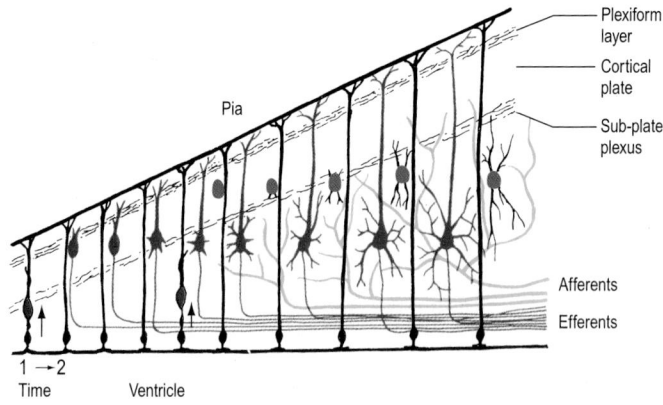

Fig. 14.33 The initial stages of formation of apical and basal dendrites of pyramidal neurones, also of stellate neurone dendrites in the cortical plate. Note radial glial cells (black) extending from internal to external limiting membrane; these provide contact guidance paths for neuroblasts. 1, Migration of a presumptive pyramidal neurone (magenta). 2, Migration of a presumptive stellate neurone (purple). Time increments from left to right. (After Berry M 1982 Cellular differentiation. Neurosci Res Program Bull 20: 451–461.)

Sur 2000). When the lateral geniculate nucleus and the visual cortex were ablated and space was created in the medial geniculate by ablating the inferior colliculus, cells in the somatosensory or auditory cortex were visually driven, and receptive field and response properties resembled that seen in the visual cortex. These results suggest that the modality of a sensory thalamic nucleus or cortical area can be specified by inputs during development.

The development of cortical projections has been investigated both in terms of laminar and area-specific connectivity. Recently, attention has focused on the idea that connections might be influenced by the existence of a transient population of subplate neurones, which later dies. The cortex develops within a preplate, consisting of corticopetal nerve fibres and the earliest generated neurones. This zone is then split into two zones, the subplate underneath the cortical plate, and the marginal zone at the pial surface, by the arrival of cortical neurones. Subplate neurones extend axons via the internal capsule to the thalamus and superior colliculus at times before other cortical neurones have been born.

How are region-specific projections generated? Layer 5 neurones in various cortical areas extend axons to different repertoires of targets. For instance, layer 5 neurones of the visual cortex project to the tectum, pons and mesencephalic nuclei, while those in the motor cortex project to mesencephalic and pontine targets, the inferior olive and dorsal column nuclei and the spinal cord. An interesting feature of these cortical projections is that they arise by collateral formation rather than by projection of the primary axon, or by growth cone bifurcation. In the case of the corticopontine projection, collaterals are elicited by a diffusible, chemotrophic agent. Retrograde labelling of neurones at various times in development has shown that rather than being generated *de novo*, these patterns seem to arise by pruning of collaterals from a more widespread projection. Visual cortical neurones possess a projection to the spinal cord early in development, which is later eliminated. This late emergence of the specificity of projections could be driven by intrinsic programming of the neurones to be pruned, or a response to position-dependent factors. There is evidence that the latter is the case. When pieces of visual cortex were transplanted into motor areas, and the resulting layer 5 projections labelled at later times in development, projections to the spinal cord persisted, rather than being eliminated as in normal development. Thus position plays an important role in the modelling of cortical projections, implying that the same classes of neurones exist in different tangential regions of the cortex. Regressive events such as axon and synapse elimination and neuronal death thus play an important part in modelling the cortex. For example in rodents c.30% of cortical neurones die, and the number of cells in layer 4 is governed by thalamic input.

Human cortical malformations are thought to arise as neuronal migration disorders (NMDs). A broad class of NMDs is lissencephaly, in which the cortex has a normal thickness, but a decreased number of neurones and a smoothened surface with a decreased number of gyri. The mutated protein in some forms of the disorder, LIS-1, is expressed in the ventricular neuroepithelium and is responsible for regulating the levels of the lipid messenger platelet activating factor (PAF). How this translates into a cell migration defect remains as yet obscure. Conversely, polymicrogyria manifests as a highly convoluted cerebrum, with a nearly normal surface area but a thinner cortex. It is thought that the normal number of proliferative units and thus ontogenetic columns are established, but each column contains fewer neurones, implying either a reduced rate of proliferation and/or cell migration, or an enhanced level of cell death.

Neonatal brain and reflexes
The brain of the full-term neonate ranges from 300–400 g with an average of 350 g; the brains of neonatal males are slightly heavier than those of females. Because the head is large at birth, measuring one quarter the total body length, the brain is also proportionally larger, and constitutes 10% of the body weight compared with 2% in the adult. At birth the volume of the brain is 25% of its volume in adult life. The greater part of the increase occurs during the first year, at the end of which the volume of the brain has increased to 75% of its adult volume. The growth can be accounted for partly by increase in the size of nerve cell somata, the profusion and dimensions of their dendritic trees, axons and their collaterals and by growth of the neuroglial cells and cerebral blood vessels, but it mainly reflects the acquisition of myelin sheaths by the axons. The sensory pathways, visual, auditory and somatic, myelinate first, the motor fibres later. During the second and subsequent years, growth proceeds much more slowly. The brain reaches 90% of its adult size by the fifth year, and 95% by 10 years. The brain attains adult size by the seventeenth or eighteenth year. This is largely due to continued myelination of various groups of nerve fibres.

The sulci of the cerebral hemispheres appear from the fourth month of gestation (**Fig. 14.29**) and at full term the general arrangement of sulci and gyri are present, but the insula is not completely covered. The central sulcus is situated further rostrally and the lateral sulcus is more oblique than in the adult. Most of the developmental stages of sulci and gyri have been identified in the brains of premature infants. Of the cranial nerves, the olfactory and the optic at the chiasma are much larger than in the adult, whereas the roots of the other nerves are relatively smaller.

The brain occupies 97.5% of the cranial cavity from birth to 6 years of age after which the space between the brain and skull increases in volume until the adult brain occupies only 92.5% of the cranial cavity. Although the cerebral ventricles are larger in the neonate than in the adult, the newborn has a total of 10–15 ml of cerebrospinal fluid when delivered vaginally and 30 ml when delivered by caesarean section.

Myelination
Myelination occurs over a protracted period beginning during the second trimester in the peripheral nervous system (PNS). Motor roots myelinate before sensory roots in the PNS whereas the sensory nerves myelinate before the motor systems. The cranial nerves of the midbrain, pons and medulla oblongata begin myelination at about 6 months' gestation. Myelination is not complete at birth; its most rapid phase occurs during the first 6 months of postnatal life, after which it continues at a slower rate up to puberty and beyond. The sequence of myelination of the motor pathways may explain, at least partially, the order of development of muscle tone and posture in the premature infant and neonate. Myelination of the various subcorticospinal pathways, i.e. vestibulospinal, reticulospinal, olivospinal and tectospinal (often grouped as bulbospinal tracts) occurs from 24–30 weeks' gestation for

the medial groups, and extends to 28–34 weeks' gestation for the lateral groups. Myelination of the corticospinal tracts occurs some 10–14 days after birth in the internal capsule and cerebral peduncles, and then proceeds simultaneously in both tracts. Longer axons appear to myelinate first. Thus, in the preterm infant, axial extension precedes flexion, whereas finger flexion precedes extension. By term the neonate at rest has a strong flexor tone accompanied by adduction of all limbs. Neonates also display a distinct preference for a head position facing to the right, which appears to be independent of handling practices and may reflect the normal asymmetry of cerebral function at this age.

Reflexes present at birth
A number of reflexes are present at birth and their demonstration is used to indicate normal development of the nervous system and responding muscles. Five tests of neurological development are most useful in determining gestational age. The pupillary reflex is consistently absent before 29 weeks' gestation and present after 31 weeks; the glabellar tap, a blink in response to a tap on the glabella, is absent before 32 weeks and present after 34 weeks; the neck righting reflex appears between 34 and 37 weeks; the traction response, where flexion of the neck or arms occurs when the baby is pulled up by the wrists from the supine position appears after 33 weeks; head turning in response to light appears between 32 and 36 weeks. The spinal reflex arc is fully developed by the eighth week of gestation and lower limb flexor tone is detectable from about 29 weeks. The Babinski response, which involves extension of the great toe with spreading of the remaining toes in response to stimulation of the lateral aspect of the sole of the foot, is elicited frequently in neonates; it reflects poor cortical control of motor function by the immature brain. Generally reflexes develop as muscles gain tone. They appear in a sequential manner from caudal to cephalic, i.e. in the lower limb before the upper, and centripetally, i.e. distal reflexes appear before proximal ones (Allen & Capute 1990).

The usual reflexes which can be elicited in the neonate include Moro, asymmetric tonic neck response, rooting–sucking, grasp, placing (contacting the dorsum of the foot with the edge of a table produces a 'stepping over the edge' response), stepping, and trunk incurvation (elicited by stroking down the paravertebral area with the infant in the prone position). Examination of the motor system and evaluation of these reflexes allows assessment of the nervous system in relation to gestational age. The neonate also exhibits complex reflexes such as nasal reflexes and sucking and swallowing.

Nasal reflexes produce apnoea via the diving reflex, sneezing, sniffing, and both somatic and autonomic reflexes. Stimulation of the face or nasal cavity with water or local irritants produces apnoea in neonates. Breathing stops in expiration, with laryngeal closure, and infants exhibit bradycardia and a lowering of cardiac output. Blood flow to the skin, splanchnic areas, muscles and kidneys decreases, whereas flow to the heart and brain is protected. Different fluids produce different effects when introduced into the pharynx of preterm infants. A comparison of the effects of water and saline in the pharynx showed that apnoea, airway obstruction, and swallowing occur far more frequently with water than with saline, suggesting the presence of an upper airway chemoreflex. Reflex responses to the temperature of the face and nasopharynx are necessary to start pulmonary ventilation. Midwives have for many years blown on the faces of neonates to induce the first breath.

Sucking and swallowing are a particularly complex set of reflexes, partly conscious and partly unconscious. As a combined reflex sucking and swallowing require the coordination of several of the 12 cranial nerves. The neonate can, within the first couple of feeds, suck at the rate of once per second, swallow after five or six sucks, and breathe during every second or third suck. Air moves in and out of the lungs via the nasopharynx, and milk crosses the pharynx en route to the oesophagus without apparent interruption of breathing and swallowing, or significant misdirection of air into the stomach or fluids in the trachea.

Swallowing movements are first noted at about 11 weeks' gestation; in utero fetuses swallow 450 ml of amniotic fluid per day. Sucking and swallowing in premature infants (1700 g) is not associated with primary peristaltic waves in the intestine; however, in older babies and full-term neonates, at least 90% of swallows will initiate primary peristaltic waves.

Sucking develops, generally, slightly later than swallowing, although mouthing movements have been detected in premature babies as early as 18–24 weeks' gestation, and infants delivered at 29–30 weeks' gestation make sucking movements a few days after birth. Coordinated activities are not noted before 33–34 weeks. The concept of non-nutritive and nutritive sucking has been introduced to account for the different rates of sucking seen in the neonate. Non-nutritive sucking, when rhythmic negative intraoral pressures are initiated which do not result in the delivery of milk, can be spontaneous or stimulated by an object in the mouth. This type of sucking tends to be twice as fast as nutritive sucking: the sucking frequency for non-nutritive sucking is 1.7 sucks/second in 37–38 week premature babies, two sucks/second in term neonates, and 2.7 sucks/second at 7–9 months postnatally. Corresponding times for nutritive sucking are about one suck/second in term neonates, increasing to 1.5 sucks/second by 7 months postnatally.

The taste of the fluid as well as nutrient content affects the efficiency of nutritive sucking in the early neonatal period. There is more sucking with milk than with 5% dextrose; however, sucking activities increase with solutions that are determined to be sweet by adult appraisal.

In full-term neonates, the placing of a spoon or food onto the anterior part of the tongue elicits an extrusion reflex: the lips are pursed and the tongue pushes vigorously against the object. By 4–6 months the reflex changes and food deposited on the anterior part of the tongue is moved to the back of the tongue, into the pharynx, and swallowed. Rhythmic biting movements occur by 7–9 months postnatally, even in the absence of teeth.

Difficulties in sucking and swallowing in infancy may be an early indication of disturbed nervous system function. There is an interesting correlation between feeding styles of neonates and later eating habits. Children who were obese at 1 and 2 years of age, as measured by triceps skin-fold thickness, had a feeding pattern in the first month of life that was characterized by sucking more rapidly, producing higher pressures during prolonged bursts of sucking, and having shorter periods between bursts of sucking. Fewer feeds and higher sucking pressure seem to be associated with greater adiposity.

MENINGES

The meningeal layers originate from paraxial mesenchyme in the trunk and caudal regions of the head and from neural crest in regions rostral to the mesencephalon (the prechordal plate has also been suggested to make a contribution). Those skull bones which are formed from neural crest, e.g. the base of the skull rostral to the sella turcica, and the frontal, parietal and squamous temporal bones, overlie meninges which are also formed from crest cells.

The meninges may be divided in development into the pachymeninx (dura mater) and leptomeninges (arachnoid mater, subarachnoid space with arachnoid cells and fibres, and pia mater). All meningeal layers are derived from loose mesenchyme which surrounds the developing neural tube, termed meninx primitiva, or primary meninx. (For a detailed account of the development of the meninges in the human consult O'Rahilly & Muller 1986.)

The first indication of pia mater, containing a plexus of blood vessels which forms on the neural surface, is seen at stage 11 (24 days), around the caudal-most part of the medulla; this extends to the mesencephalic level by stage 12. Mesenchymal cells projecting from the rostral end of the notochord, and those in the region of the prechordal plate, extend rostrally into the mesencephalic flexure and form the earliest cells of the tentorium cerebelli; at the beginning of its development the medial part of the tentorium is predominantly leptomeningeal. By stage 17 (41 days) dura mater can be seen in the basal areas where the future chondrocranium is also developing. The precursors of the venous sinuses lie within the pachymeninx at stage 19 (48 days), and by stage 20, cell populations in the region of the future falx cerebri are proliferating, although the dorsal regions of the brain are not yet covered with putative meninges.

By stage 23 (57 days) the dura is almost complete over the rhombencephalon and mesencephalon, but is only present laterally around the prosencephalon. Subarachnoid spaces and most of the cisternae are present from this time, after the arachnoid mater becomes separated from the primitive dura mater by the accumulation of cerebrospinal fluid (which now has a net movement out of the ventricular system). The medial part of the tentorium is becoming thinner. A dural component of the tentorium is seen from stage 19. The earlier medial portion disappears leaving an incomplete partition which separates a subarachnoid area containing the telencephalon and diencephalon from one containing the cerebellum and rhombencephalon.

There is a very close relationship, during development, between the mesenchyme from which the cranial dura mater is formed and that which is either chondrified and ossified, or ossified directly, to form the skull. These layers are only clearly differentiated as the venous sinuses develop. The relationship between the developing skull and the underlying dura mater continues during postnatal life while the bones of the calvaria are still growing.

The growth of the cranial vault is initiated from ossification centres within the desmocranial mesenchyme. A wave of osteodifferentiation moves radially outward from these centres stopping when adjacent bones meet at regions where sutures are induced to form. Once sutures are formed, a second phase of development occurs in which growth of the cranial bones occurs at the sutural margins. This growth forms most of the skull. A number of hypotheses have been generated to explain the process of sutural morphogenesis. It has been suggested that the dura mater contains fibre tracts which extend from fixed positions in the cranial base to sites of dural reflection underlying each of the cranial sutures and that the tensional forces so generated would dictate the position of the sutures and locally inhibit precocious ossification. Other hypotheses support the concept of local factors in the calvaria which regulate suture morphogenesis. Following removal of the entire calvaria the skull regenerates and sutures and bones develop in anatomically correct positions, suggesting that the dura can dictate suture position at least in regeneration of the neonatal calvaria. In transplants of sutures in which the fetal dura mater was left intact, a continuous fibrous suture remained between developing vault bones, whereas in transplants in which the fetal dura mater was removed bony fusion occurred (Opperman et al 1993).

The presence of fetal dura is not required for initial suture morphogenesis, which appears to be controlled by mesenchymal cell proliferation and fibrous extracellular matrix synthesis induced by the overlapping of the advancing osteoinductive fronts of the calvarial bones. It is thought that following overlap of the bone fronts, a signal is transferred to the underlying dura which induces changes in localized regions beneath the sutures. Once a suture has formed, it serves as a primary site for cranial bone growth, but constant interaction with the dura is required to avoid ossiferous obliteration.

CRANIAL ARTERIES

The internal carotid artery is formed progressively from the third arch artery (**Fig. 34.11**), the dorsal aorta cranial to this, and a further forward continuation which differentiates, at the time of regression of the first and second aortic arches, from the capillary plexus extending to the walls of the forebrain and midbrain. At its anterior extremity this primitive internal carotid artery divides into cranial and caudal divisions. The former terminates as the primitive olfactory artery, and supplies the developing regions implied. The latter sweeps caudally to reach the ventral aspect of the midbrain, its terminal branches are the primitive mesencephalic arteries. Simultaneously bilateral longitudinal channels differentiate along the ventral surface of the hindbrain from a plexus fed by intersegmental and transitory presegmental branches of the dorsal aorta and its forward continuation. The most important of the presegmental branches is closely related to the fifth nerve, the primitive trigeminal artery. Otic and hypoglossal presegmental arteries occur and may persist. The longitudinal channels later connect cranially with the caudal divisions of the internal carotid arteries (each of which gives rise to an anterior choroidal artery supplying branches to the diencephalon, including the telae choroideae and midbrain) and caudally with the vertebral arteries through the first cervical intersegmental arteries. Fusion of the longitudinal channels results in the formation of the basilar artery, whilst the caudal division of the internal carotid artery becomes the posterior communicating artery and the stem of the posterior cerebral artery. The remainder of the posterior cerebral artery develops comparatively late, probably from the stem of the posterior choroidal artery which is annexed by the caudally expanding cerebral hemisphere, its distal portion becoming a choroidal branch of the posterior cerebral artery. The posterior choroidal artery supplies the tela choroidea at the future temporal end of the choroidal fissure; its rami advance through the tela to become confluent with branches of the anterior choroidal artery. The cranial division of the internal carotid artery gives rise to anterior choroidal, middle cerebral and anterior cerebral arteries. The stem of the primitive olfactory artery remains as a small medial striate branch of the anterior cerebral artery. The cerebellar arteries, of which the superior is the first to differentiate, emerge from the capillary plexus on the wall of the rhombencephalon.

The source of the blood supply to the territory of the trigeminal nerve varies at different stages in development. When the first and second aortic arch arteries begin to regress, the supply to the corresponding arches is derived from a transient ventral pharyngeal artery, which grows from the aortic sac. It terminates by dividing into mandibular and maxillary branches.

Meningeal arteries

At stage 20–23 (7–8 weeks), further expansion of the cerebral hemispheres produces the completion of the circle of Willis, with the development of the anterior communicating arteries by 8 weeks' gestation. An annular network of meningeal arteries originates, mainly from each middle cerebral artery, and passes over each developing cerebral hemisphere. Caudally, similar meningeal branches arise from the vertebral and basilar arteries and embrace the cerebellum and brain stem. The further development of the telencephalon somewhat obscures this early pattern over the cerebrum.

The meningeal arteries so formed have been classified into three groups: paramedian, short circumferential and long circumferential arteries. They can be described both supratentorially and infratentorially: all give off fine side branches and end as penetrating arteries. Of the supratentorial vessels, the paramedian arteries have a short course prior to penetrating the cerebral neuropil (e.g. branches of the anterior cerebral artery); the short circumferential arteries have a slightly longer course before becoming penetrating arteries (e.g. the striate artery); and the long circumferential arteries reach the dorsal surface of the hemispheres. Infratentorial meningeal arteries are very variable. The paramedian arteries, after arising from the basilar or vertebral arteries, penetrate the brain stem directly. The short circumferential arteries end at the lateral surface of the brain before penetration and the long circumferential arteries later form the range of cerebellar arteries. These vessels, arranged as a series of loops over the brain, arise from the circle of Willis and brain stem vessels on the base of the brain.

At 16 weeks' gestation, the anterior, middle and posterior cerebral arteries contributing to the formation of the circle of Willis are well-established. The meningeal arteries arising from them display a simple pattern with little tortuosity and very few branches. With the increasing age of the fetus and acquisition of the gyral pattern on the surface of the brain, their tortuosity, diameter and number of branches all increase. The branching pattern is completed by 28 weeks' gestation and the number of branches does not increase further. Numerous anastomoses (varying in size from 200–760 μm) occur between the meningeal arteries in the depths of the developing sulci, nearly always in the cortical boundary zones of the three main cerebral arteries supplying each hemisphere. The number, diameter and location of these anastomoses changes as fetal growth progresses, reflecting the regression and simplification of the complex embryonic cerebral vascular system. The boundary zones between the cerebral arteries may be the sites of inadequate perfusion in the premature infant.

Vascularization of the brain

The brain becomes vascularized by angiogenesis (angiotrophic vasculogenesis; p. 1051) rather than by direct invasion by angioblasts. Blood vessels form by sprouting from vessels in the pial plexus which surrounds the neural tube from an early stage. These sprouts form branches which elongate at the junction between the ventricular and marginal zones; the branches project laterally within the inter-rhombomeric boundaries and longitudinally adjacent to the median floorplate. Subsequently, additional sprouts penetrate the inter-rhombomeric regions on the walls and floor of the hindbrain. Branches from the latter elongate towards and join the branches in the inter-rhombomeric junctions, forming primary vascular channels between rhombomeres and longitudinally on each side of the median floorplate. Later additional sprouts invade the hindbrain within the rhombomeres, anastomosing in all directions.

The meningeal perforating branches pass into the brain parenchyma as cortical, medullary and striate branches (Fig. 14.34). The cortical vessels supply the cortex via short branches which may form precapillary anastomoses, whereas the medullary branches supply the white matter. The latter converge towards the ventricle but rarely reach it; they often follow a tortuous course as they pass around bundles of nerves. The striate branches which penetrate into the brain through the anterior perforated substance, supply the basal nuclei and internal capsule via a sinuous course: they are larger than the medullary branches and the longest of them reach close to the ventricle. The periventricular region and basal nuclei are also supplied by branches from the tela choroidea,

which develops from the early pial plexus but becomes medially and deeply placed as the telencephalon enlarges.

The cortical and medullary branches irrigate a series of cortico-subcortical cone-shaped areas, centred around a sulcus containing an artery. They supply a peripheral portion of the cerebrum and are grouped as ventriculopetal arteries. Striate branches, on the other hand, arborize close to the ventricle and supply a more central portion of the cerebrum: together with branches from the tela choroidea, they give rise to ventriculofugal arteries. The latter supply the ventricular zone (germinal matrix of the brain) and send branches towards the cortex. The ventriculopetal and ventriculofugal arteries run towards each other but they do not make any connections or anastomoses (Fig. 14.34), however, the ventriculopetal arteries form networks of small arterioles. The ventriculopetal vessels supply relatively more mature regions of the brain compared to the ventriculofugal, which are subject to constant remodelling and do not develop tunicae mediae until ventricular zone proliferation is completed. The boundary zone between these two systems (an outer centripetal and inner centrifugal) has practical implications related to the location of ischaemic lesions (periventricular leukomalacia, PVL) in the white matter of premature infant brains. Although it was thought that the distribution of ischaemic lesions in PVL coincided with the demarcation zone between the centrifugal and centripetal vascular arterial systems, this is now not thought to provide the complete answer. Three major interacting factors contribute to the pathology seen in PVL, the incomplete state of development of the vasculature in the ventricular zone, the maturation-dependent impairment of the cerebral blood flow regulation in premature infants, and the vulnerability of oligodendroblasts in the periventricular region, which are particularly affected by swings in cerebral ischaemia and reperfusion (Volpe 2001).

The same pattern of centripetal and centrifugal arteries develops around the fourth ventricle. The ventriculofugal circulation is more extensive in the cerebellum than in the telencephalon. The arteries arise from the various cerebellar arteries and course, with the cerebellar peduncles, directly to the centre of the cerebellum, by-passing the cortex. The ventriculopetal arteries are derived from the meningeal vessels over the cerebellar surface, and most terminate in the white matter.

At 24 weeks of gestation, there is a relatively well-developed blood supply to the basal nuclei and internal capsule, through a prominent Heubner's artery (arteria recurrens anterior), a branch of the anterior cerebral artery. The cortex and the white matter regions are rather poorly vascularized at this stage. The distribution of arteries and veins on the lateral aspect of the cerebral hemispheres is affected by the formation of the lateral fissure and development of cerebral sulci and gyri. Between 12 and 20 weeks' gestation the middle cerebral artery and its branches are relatively straight, branching in an open-fan pattern. At the end of 20 weeks, the arteries become more curved as the opercula begin to appear and submerge the insular cortex. The area supplied by the middle cerebral artery becomes dominant when compared to the territories supplied by the anterior and posterior cerebral arteries. Early arterial anastomoses appear around 16 weeks of gestation and increase in size with advancing age. The sites of anastomoses between the middle and anterior cerebral arteries move from the convexity of the brain towards the superior sagittal sinus. Anastomotic connections between the middle and posterior cerebral arteries shift towards the basal aspect of the brain.

By 32–34 weeks, marked involution of the ventricular zone (germinal matrix) has occurred and the cortex acquires its complex gyral pattern and an increased vascular supply. Ventricular zone capillaries are gradually remodelled to blend with the capillaries of the caudate nucleus. Heubner's artery eventually supplies only a small area at the medial aspect of the head of the caudate nucleus. In the cortex there is progressive elaboration of cortical blood vessels (Fig. 14.34) and, towards the end of the third trimester, the balance of cerebral circulation shifts from one which is central and basal nuclei-oriented, to one which predominantly serves the cortex and white matter. These changes in the pattern of cerebral circulation are of major significance in the pathogenesis and distribution of hypoxic/ischaemic lesions in the developing human brain. In a premature brain, the majority of ischaemic lesions occur in the boundary zone between the centripetal and centrifugal arteries, i.e. in the periventricular white matter. In the full-term infant the cortical boundary zones and watershed areas between different arterial blood supplies are similar to those in adults.

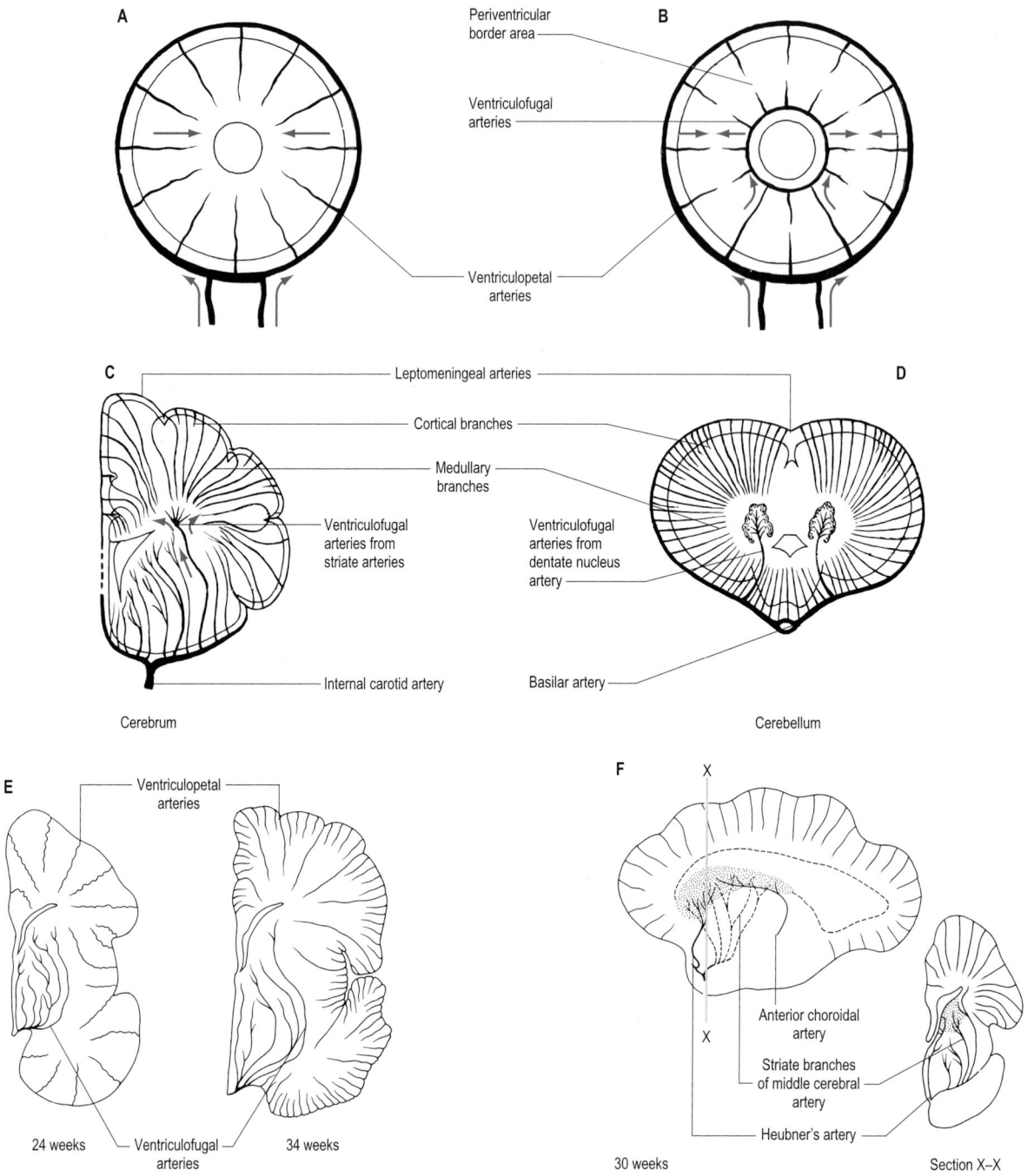

Fig. 14.34 Development of cerebral blood vessels. **A**, The brain is surrounded by a system of leptomeningeal arteries from afferent trunks at the base of the brain. Intracerebral arteries arise from this system and converge (ventriculopetally) towards the ventricle (the inner circle in this diagram). **B**, A few deep penetrating vessels supply the brain close to the ventricle and send ventriculofugal arteries towards the ventriculopetal vessels without making anastomoses. **C**, The arrangement of ventriculopetal and ventriculofugal vessels around a cerebral hemisphere. **D**, The similar arrangement of vessels around the cerebellum. **E**, Changes in the arterial pattern of the human cerebrum between 24 and 34 weeks' gestation. **F**, Arterial supply to the basal nuclei at 30 weeks' gestation. (**A–D**, by permission from Van den Bergh R, Van der Eecken H 1968 Anatomy and embryology of cerebral circulation. Prog Brain Res 30: 1–25; **E** and **F**, by permission from the BMJ Publishing Group from Hambleton G, Wigglesworth J S 1976 Origin of intraventricular haemorrhage in the preterm infant. Arch Dis Child 51: 651–659.)

Vessels of the ventricular zone (germinal matrix)

The germinal matrix (ventricular zone) is the end zone or border zone between the cerebral arteries and the collection zone of the deep cerebral veins. The germinal matrix is probably particularly prone to ischaemic injury in the immature infant because of its unusual vascular architecture. The subependymal veins (septal, choroidal, thalamostriate and posterior terminal) flow towards the interventricular foramen, with a sudden change of flow at the level of the foramen, where the veins recurve at an acute angle to form the paired internal cerebral veins. The capillary channels in the germinal matrix open at right angles directly into the veins, and it has been postulated that these small vessels may be points of vascular rupture and the site of subependymal haemorrhage.

The capillary bed in the ventricular zone is supplied mainly by Heubner's artery and terminal branches of the lateral striate arteries from the middle cerebral artery. The highly cellular structure of the ventricular zone is a temporary feature, and the vascular supply to this area displays some primitive features. It has the capacity to remodel when the ventricular zone cells migrate and the remaining cells differentiate as ependyma towards the end of gestation.

Vessel density is relatively low in the ventricular zone suggesting that this area may normally have a relatively low blood flow. Immature vessels, without a complex basal lamina or glial sheet, have been described up to 26 weeks' gestation in the zone: the endothelium of these vessels is apparently thinner than in the cortical vessels. In infants of less than 30 weeks' gestation, the vessels in the ventricular zone contain no smooth muscle, collagen or elastic fibres. Collagen and smooth muscle are seen in other regions after 30 weeks, but are not detected in the remains of the germinal matrix. The lack of these components could make the vessels in this zone vulnerable to changes in the intraluminal pressure, and the lack of smooth muscle would preclude them from participating in autoregulatory processes. Cerebral vessels in premature infants lack elastic fibres and have a disproportionately small number of reticulin fibres. Comparison of the cortical and germinal plate blood vessels shows that in infants of between 25 and 32 weeks' gestation the germinal matrix vessels consist commonly of 1–2 endothelial cells with an occasional pericyte, and the capillary lumina are larger than those of the vessels in the cortex. In more mature infants the basal lamina is thicker and more irregular when compared to cortical vessels.

Glial fibrillary acidic protein (GFAP) positive cells have been detected around blood vessels in the germinal matrix from 23 weeks' gestation. Glial cells may contribute to changes in the nature of endothelial intercellular junctions in brain capillaries.

Cerebral veins

From 16 weeks onwards, cerebral veins can be identified. The superior, middle, inferior, anterior and posterior cerebral veins appear more tortuous than meningeal arteries. Veins draining the cortex, white matter and deeper structures are recognized in the midtrimester. Subcortical veins drain the deep white matter, deep cortical and subcortical superficial tissue: they terminate together with cortical veins which drain the cortex in the meningeal veins. The deep white matter and central nuclei are drained by longer veins, which meet and join subependymal veins from the ventricular zone. Anastomoses between various groups of cortical veins can be recognized by 16 weeks' gestation. The inferior anastomotic vein (of Labbe), an anastomosis between the middle cerebral and inferior cerebral veins, becomes recognizable at 20 weeks, but the superior anastomotic vein (of Trolard), connecting the superior and middle cerebral veins, does not appear before the end of 30 weeks.

Rapid cortical development is correlated with the regression of the middle cerebral vein and its tributaries, and development of ascending and descending cortical veins and intraparenchymal (medullary) arteries and veins.

Cerebral venous drainage in a full-term baby is essentially composed of two principal venous arrays, the superficial veins and the deep Galenic venous system. Anastomoses between these two systems persist into adult life.

VEINS OF THE HEAD

The earliest vessels form a transitory primordial hindbrain channel which drains into the precardinal vein. This is soon replaced by the primary head vein which runs caudally from the medial side of the trigeminal ganglion, lateral to the facial and vestibulocochlear nerves and otocyst, then medial to the vagus nerve, to become continuous with the precardinal vein. A lateral anastomosis subsequently brings it lateral to the vagus nerve. The cranial part of the precardinal vein forms the internal jugular vein.

The primary capillary plexus of the head becomes separated into three fairly distinct strata by the differentiation of the skull and meninges. The superficial vessels, draining the skin and underlying soft parts, eventually discharge in large part into the external jugular system. They retain some connections with the deeper veins through so-called emissary veins. Deep to this is the venous plexus of the dura mater, from which the dural venous sinuses differentiate. This plexus converges on each side into anterior, middle and posterior dural stems (**Fig. 14.35**). The anterior stem drains the prosencephalon and mesencephalon and enters the primary head vein rostral to the trigeminal ganglion. The middle stem drains the metencephalon and empties into the primary head vein caudal to the trigeminal ganglion, while the posterior stem drains the myelencephalon into the start of the precardinal vein. The deepest capillary stratum is the pial plexus from which the veins of the brain differentiate. It drains at the dorsolateral aspect of the neural tube into the adjacent dural venous plexus. The primary head vein also receives, at its cranial end, the primitive maxillary vein which drains the maxillary prominence and region of the optic vesicle.

The vessels of the dural plexus undergo profound changes, largely accommodating the growth of the cartilaginous otic capsule of the membranous labyrinth and expansion of the cerebral hemispheres. With growth of the otic capsule the primary head vein is gradually reduced and a new channel joining anterior, middle and posterior dural

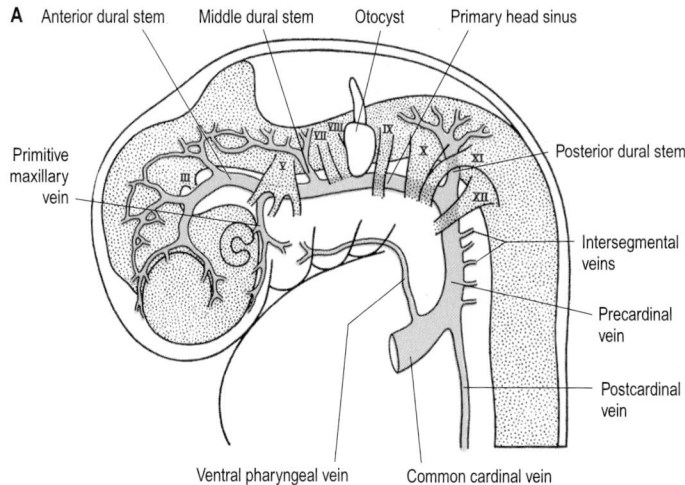

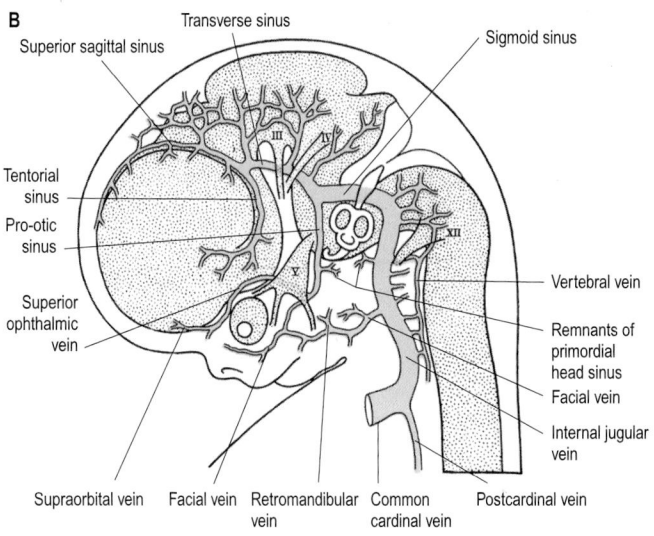

Fig. 14.35 Successive stages in the development of the veins of the head and neck. **A**, At c.8 mm CR length; **B**, at c.24 mm CR length.

stems appears dorsal to the cranial nerve ganglia and the capsule. Where this new vessel joins the middle and posterior stems, together with the posterior dural stem itself (**Fig. 14.35B**), the adult sigmoid sinus is formed.

A curtain of capillary veins, the sagittal plexus, forms between the growing cerebral hemispheres and along the dorsal margins of the anterior and middle plexuses, in the position of the future falx cerebri. Rostrodorsally this plexus forms the superior sagittal sinus. It is continuous behind with the anastomosis between the anterior and middle dural stems, which forms most of the transverse sinus. Ventrally the sagittal plexus differentiates into the inferior sagittal and straight sinuses and the great cerebral vein, and drains, more commonly, into the left transverse sinus.

The vessels along the ventrolateral edge of the developing cerebral hemisphere form the transitory tentorial sinus, which drains the convex surface of the cerebral hemisphere and basal ganglia, and the ventral aspect of the diencephalon, to the transverse sinus. With expansions of the cerebral hemispheres, and in particular the emergence of the temporal lobe, the tentorial sinus becomes elongated, attenuated and eventually disappears, and its territory is drained by enlarging anastomoses of pial vessels. The latter become the basal veins, which are radicles of the great cerebral vein.

The anterior dural stem disappears and the caudal part of the primary head vein dwindles: it is represented in the adult by the inferior petrosal sinus. The cranial part of the primary head vein, medial to the trigeminal ganglion, persists and still receives the stem of the primitive maxillary vein. The latter has now lost most of its tributaries to the anterior facial vein, and its stem becomes the main trunk of the primitive

273

supraorbital vein, which will form the superior ophthalmic vein of the adult. The main venous drainage of the orbit and its contents is now carried via the augmented middle dural stem, the pro-otic sinus, into the transverse sinus and, at a later stage, into the cavernous sinus. The cavernous sinus is formed from a secondary plexus, derived from the primary head vein and lying between the otic and basioccipital cartilages. The plexus forms the inferior petrosal sinus which drains through the primordial hindbrain channel into the internal jugular vein. The superior petrosal sinus arises later from a ventral metencephalic tributary of the pro-otic sinus and it communicates secondarily with the cavernous sinus. The pro-otic sinus meanwhile has developed a new and more caudally situated stem draining into the sigmoid sinus: this new stem is the petrosquamosal sinus. With progressive ossification of the skull, the pro-otic sinus becomes diploic in position. The development of the venous drainage and portal system of the hypophysis cerebri is closely associated with that of the venous sinuses.

REFERENCES

Allen MC, Capute AJ 1990 Tone and reflex development before term. J Pediatrics 85: 393–9.
Provides details of the development of reflexes in extremely premature infants.

Begbie J, Graham A 2001 The ectodermal placodes: a dysfunctional family. Phil Trans R Soc Lond B Biol Sci 356: 1655–60.
Challenges the view of ectodermal placodes as a coherent group and discusses their early development, induction and evolution.

Brown M, Keynes R, Lumsden A 2001 The Developing Brain. Oxford: Oxford University Press.
Covers the main mechanisms of neural development from neurulation to synaptic reorganization.

Donoghue MJ, Rakic P 1999 Molecular gradients and compartments in the embryonic primate cerebral cortex. Cereb Cortex 9: 586–600.
Presents evidence for the existence of an intrinsic protomap which predicts the functional map of the mature cerebral cortex.

Gordon-Weeks PR 2000 Neuronal Growth Cones. Cambridge: Cambridge University Press.

Krumlauf R, Marshall H, Studer M, Nonchev S, Sham MH, Lumsden A 1993. Hox homeobox genes and regionalisation of the nervous system. J Neurobiol 24:1328–40.
Discusses the influence of the Hox family of homeobox-containing genes on the patterning of rhombomeres and neural crest.

Le Douarin N, Teillet M, Catala M 1998 Neurulation in amniote vertebrates: a novel view deduced from the use of quail–chick chimeras. Int J Dev Biol 42: 909–916.
Explores the mechanisms which contribute to secondary neurulation using chimeric techniques.

Muller F, O'Rahilly R 1997 The timing and sequence of appearance of neuromeres and their derivatives in staged human embryos. Acta Anat (Basel) 158: 83–99.

Opperman LA, Sweeney TM, Redmon J, Persing JA, Ogle RC 1993 Tissue interactions with underlying dura mater inhibit osseous obliteration of developing cranial sutures. Dev Dynam 198: 312–22.
Examines the role of the dura mater in the development of the skull bones and sutures.

O'Rahilly R, Muller F 1986 The meninges in human development. J Neuropath Exp Neurol 45: 588–608.

O'Rourke NA, Sullivan DP, Kaznowski CE, Jacobs AA, McConnell SK 1995 Tangential migration of neurons in the developing cerebral cortex. Development 121: 2165–76.

Rakic P 1988 Specification of cerebral cortical areas. Science 241: 170–6.
Discusses the radial unit hypothesis as a framework for exploring cerebral evolution and the causes of some cortical disorders in humans.

Rakic P 2003 Developmental and evolutionary adaptations of cortical radial glia. Cereb Cortex. 13 :541–9.
Discusses cortical development and evolution and the pathogenesis of some genetic and acquired cortical anomalies.

Volpe JJ 2001 Neurobiology of periventricular leukomalacia in the premature infant. Pediatr Res 50: 553–62.

von Melchner L, Pallas SL, Sur M 2000 Visual behaviour mediated by retinal projections directed to the auditory pathway. Nature 404: 820–1.
Describes the consequences of successful routing of visual projections into non-visual structures in the brain.

Withington S, Beddington R, Cooke J 2001 Foregut endoderm is required at head process stage for anteriormost neural patterning in chick. Development 128: 309–20.
Presents evidence for an early system of neuroepithelial patterning by the most rostral endoderm, the region of the prechordal plate.

Cranial meninges

The brain and spinal cord are entirely enveloped by three concentric membranes, the meninges, which provide support and protection. The outermost meningeal layer is the dura mater (pachymeninx). Beneath this lies the arachnoid mater. The innermost layer is the pia mater. The dura is an opaque, tough, fibrous coat. It incompletely divides the cranial cavity into compartments and accommodates the dural venous sinuses. It is separated from the arachnoid by a narrow subdural space. The arachnoid mater and pia mater are sometimes referred to collectively as the leptomeninges and they share many similarities. The arachnoid is much thinner than the dura and is mostly translucent. It surrounds the brain loosely, spanning over depressions and concavities. Beneath the arachnoid lies the subarachnoid space which contains cerebrospinal fluid, secreted by the choroid plexuses of the cerebroventricular system. The pia mater is a transparent, microscopically thin, membrane which follows the contours of the brain and is closely adherent to its surface. The subarachnoid space thus varies greatly in depth, the larger expanses being termed subarachnoid cisterns. Cerebrospinal fluid circulates within the subarachnoid space and is reabsorbed into the venous system through arachnoid villi and granulations associated with the dural venous sinuses. Cranial and spinal meninges are continuous through the foramen magnum. Only the cranial meninges are described in this section. An account of the spinal meninges is given elsewhere (p. 778).

DURA MATER

The dura mater is a thick, dense, fibrous membrane, composed of densely packed fascicles of collagen fibres arranged in laminae. The fascicles run in different directions in adjacent laminae, producing a lattice-like appearance. This is particularly obvious in the tentorium cerebelli and around the defects or perforations that sometimes occur in the anterior portion of the falx cerebri. There is little histological difference between the endosteal and meningeal layers of the dura. The dura is largely acellular, but it contains fibroblasts, which are distributed throughout, and osteoblasts, which are confined to the endosteal layer. Focal calcification may occur in the falx cerebri.

The cranial dura differs from the spinal dura mainly in its relationship to the surrounding bones. The cranial dura lines the cranial cavity. It is composed of two layers; an inner, or meningeal, layer and an outer, or endosteal, layer. They are united except where they separate to enclose the venous sinuses that drain blood from the brain (p. 277). The dura mater adheres to the internal surfaces of the cranial bones and fibrous bands pass from it into the bones. Adhesion of the dura to the bones is firmest at the sutures, the cranial base and around the foramen magnum. In children it is difficult to remove the dura from the suture lines, but in adults the dura becomes separated from the suture lines as they fuse. With increasing age the dura becomes thicker, less pliable, and more firmly adherent to the inner surface of the skull, particularly that of the calvaria. The endosteal layer of the dura is continuous through the cranial sutures and foramina with the pericranium and through the superior orbital fissure with the orbital periosteum. The meningeal layer provides tubular sheaths for the cranial nerves as they pass out through the cranial foramina, and these sheaths fuse with the epineurium as the nerves emerge from the skull. The dural sheath of the optic nerve is continuous with the ocular sclera (p. 701). At sites where major vessels, such as the internal carotid and vertebral arteries, pierce the dura to enter the cranial cavity, the dura is firmly fused with the adventitia of the vessels.

The inner aspect of the dura mater is closely applied to the arachnoid mater over the surface of the brain. They are easily separated, however, and are physically joined only at sites where either veins pass from the brain into venous sinuses, e.g. the superior sagittal sinus, or where they connect the brain to the dura, e.g. at the anterior pole of the temporal lobe.

The anatomical organization of the dura, and its relationships to the major venous sinuses, sutures and blood vessels, have significant pathological implications. In the case of head trauma, separation of the dura from the underlying periosteum requires significant force, and consequently occurs only when high-pressure arterial bleeding occurs into the virtual space. This can result from damage to any arterial vessel, commonly following skull fracture. The classic site for such injury is along the course of the middle meningeal artery where a direct blow causing a bone fracture can rupture the artery and cause rapid collection of an extradural haematoma. The haematoma is under considerable pressure due to the arterial blood pressure feeding it and the resistance of the strong adhesion between dura and periosteum. As a result of these factors, an extradural haematoma acts as a rapidly expanding intracranial mass lesion and forms a classic medical emergency requiring immediate diagnosis and surgery.

DURAL PARTITIONS

The meningeal layer of the dura is reflected inwards to form four septa that partially divide the cranial cavity into compartments in which subdivisions of the brain are lodged.

Falx cerebri

Falx cerebri is a strong, crescent-shaped sheet of dura mater lying in the sagittal plane and occupying the great longitudinal fissure between the two cerebral hemispheres (**Figs 15.1, 15.2**). The crescent is narrow in front, where the falx is fixed to the crista galli, and broad behind, where it blends into the midline with the tentorium cerebelli. The anterior part of the falx is thin and may have a number of irregular perforations (**Fig.15.2**). Its convex upper margin is attached to the internal cranial surface on each side of the midline, as far back as the internal occipital protuberance. The superior sagittal sinus (p. 277) runs within the dura along this margin, in a cranial groove, and the falx is attached to the lips of this groove. At its lower edge, the falx is free and concave and contains the inferior sagittal sinus. The straight sinus runs along the line of attachment of the falx to the tentorium cerebelli (**Fig. 15.1**).

Tentorium cerebelli

Tentorium cerebelli (**Figs 15.1, 15.2, 15.3**) is a sheet of dura mater which has a peaked configuration reminiscent of a single-poled tent, from which its name is derived. It covers the cerebellum and passes under the occipital lobes of the cerebral hemispheres. Its concave anterior edge is free; between it and the dorsum sellae of the sphenoid bone is a large curved hiatus (the tentorial incisure or notch), which is occupied by the midbrain and the anterior part of the superior aspect of the cerebellar vermis. The tentorium divides the cranial cavity into supratentorial and infratentorial compartments, which contain the forebrain and hindbrain respectively. The convex outer limit of the tentorium is attached posteriorly to the lips of the transverse sulci of the occipital bone and the posterior-inferior angles of the parietal bones, where it encloses the transverse sinuses. Laterally, the tentorium is attached to the superior borders of the petrous temporal bones, where it contains the superior petrosal sinuses (**Fig. 15.3**). Near the apex of the petrous temporal bone, the lower layer of the tentorium is evaginated anterolaterally under the superior petrosal sinus to form a recess between the endosteal and meningeal layers in the middle cranial fossa. This recess is the trigeminal cave and contains the roots and

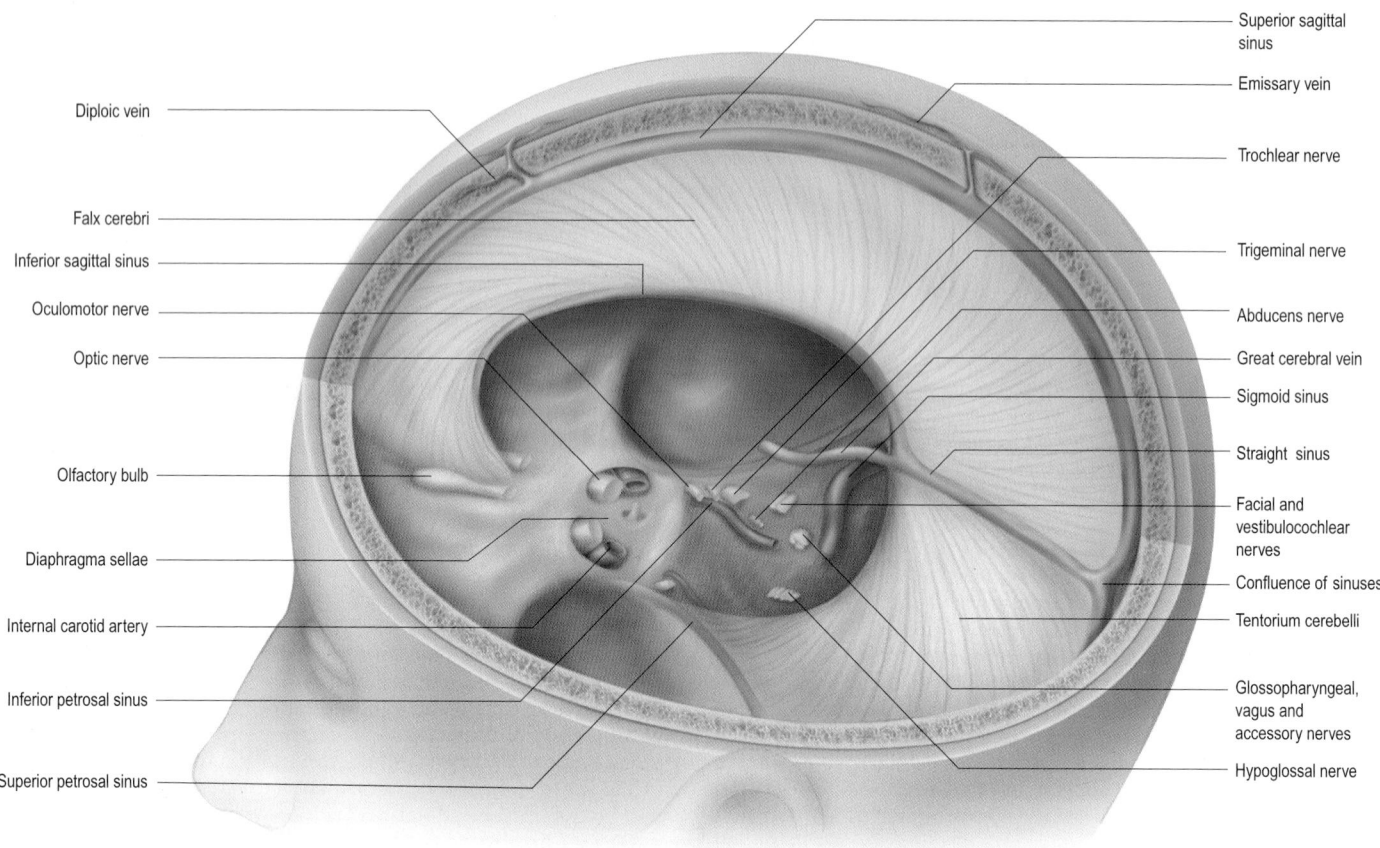

Fig. 15.1 The cerebral dura mater, its reflections and major venous sinuses.

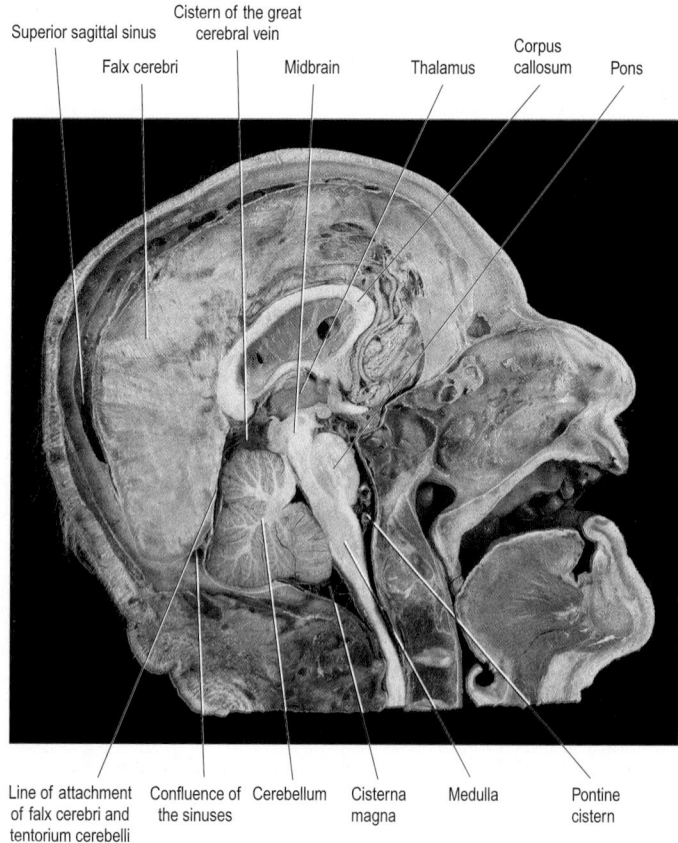

Fig. 15.2 Parasagittal section of the head showing the disposition of the falx cerebri, together with some of the dural venous sinuses and subarachnoid cisterns. (Figure enhanced by B Crossman.)

ganglion of the trigeminal nerve. The evaginated meningeal layer fuses in front with the anterior part of the trigeminal ganglion. At the apex of the petrous temporal bone, the free border and attached periphery of the tentorium cross each other (**Fig. 15.3**). The anterior ends of the free border are fixed to the anterior clinoid processes and the attached periphery to the posterior clinoid processes. The oculomotor nerve lies in the groove between them on each side.

Falx cerebelli
Falx cerebelli is a small midline fold of dura mater lying below the tentorium cerebelli. It projects forward into the posterior cerebellar notch between the cerebellar hemispheres. Its base is directed upwards and attached to the posterior part of the inferior surface of the tentorium cerebelli in the midline. Its posterior margin is attached to the internal occipital crest and contains the occipital sinus. The apex of the falx cerebelli frequently divides into two small folds, which disappear at the sides of the foramen magnum. Frequently the falx is double.

Diaphragma sellae
Diaphragma sellae (**Fig. 15.1**) is a small, circular, horizontal sheet of dura mater which forms a roof to the sella turcica and, in many cases, almost completely covers the pituitary gland (hypophysis). The central opening in the diaphragma allows the infundibulum and pituitary stalk to pass into the pituitary fossa. There is wide individual variation in the size of the central opening. The diaphragma sellae was an important landmark structure in pituitary surgery in the past – extension of a pituitary tumour above it was an indication for a subfrontal approach through a craniotomy. However, a transsphenoidal approach is currently the first preferred option, irrespective of whether there is suprasellar extension.

The arrangement of the dura mater in the central part of the middle cranial fossa is complex (**Fig. 15.3**). The tentorium cerebelli forms a large part of the floor of the middle cranial fossa, and fills much of the gap between the ridges of the petrous temporal bones. On both sides, the rim of the tentorial incisure is attached to the apex of the petrous temporal bone and continues forward as a ridge of dura mater to attach

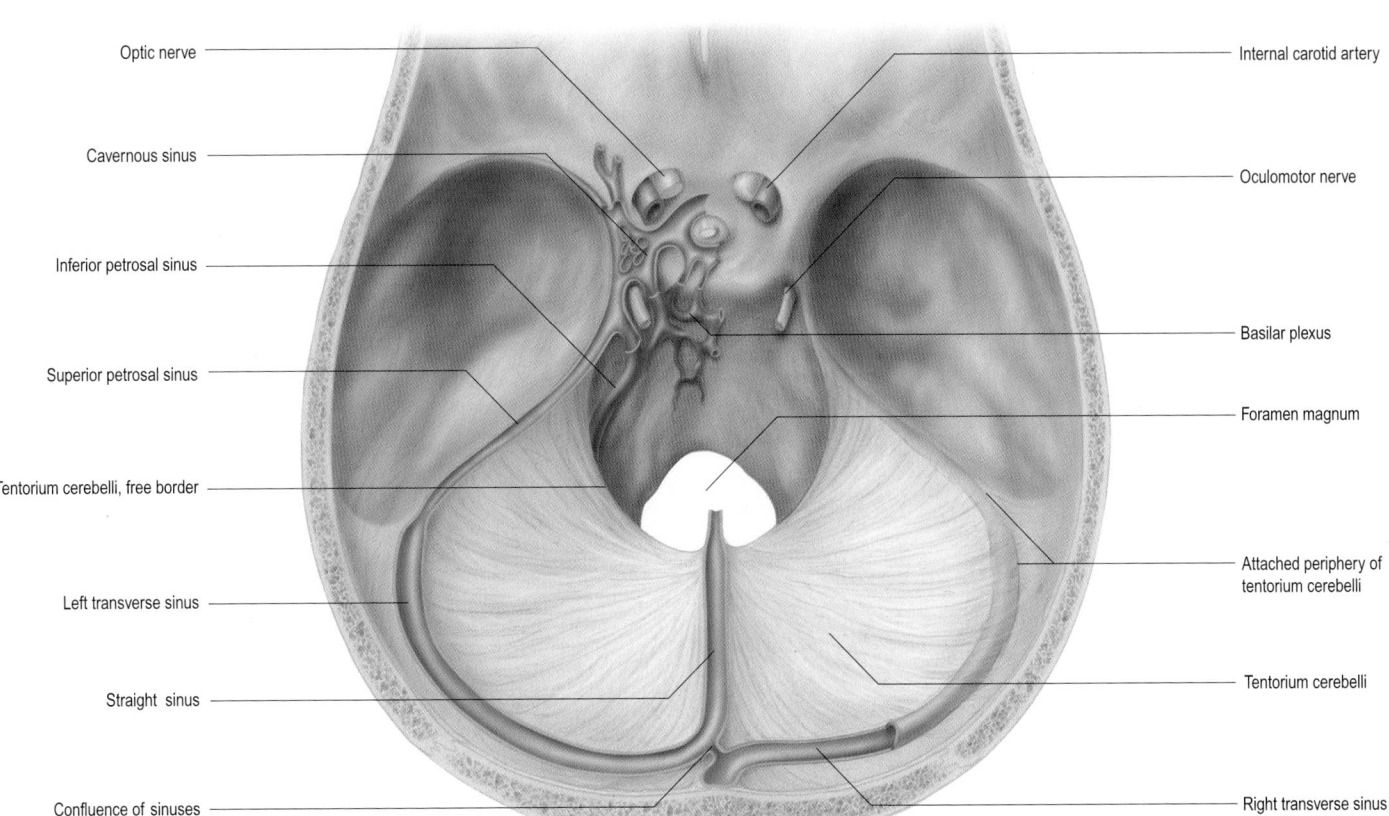

Optic nerve

Cavernous sinus

Inferior petrosal sinus

Superior petrosal sinus

Tentorium cerebelli, free border

Left transverse sinus

Straight sinus

Confluence of sinuses

Internal carotid artery

Oculomotor nerve

Basilar plexus

Foramen magnum

Attached periphery of tentorium cerebelli

Tentorium cerebelli

Right transverse sinus

Fig. 15.3 The dura mater of the floor of the cranial cavity and the superior aspect of the tentorium cerebelli. Representation of the cavernous sinus and its venous relationships are greatly simplified and are shown on the left only. Note that the trochlear and abducens nerves have not been shown (see **Fig. 15.5**).

to the anterior clinoid process. This ridge marks the junction of the roof and the lateral part of the cavernous sinus (**Figs.15.1, 15.3, 15.4, 15.5**). The periphery of the tentorium cerebelli is attached to the superior border of the petrous temporal bone, crosses under the free border of the tentorial incisure, and continues forward to the posterior clinoid processes as a rounded, indefinite ridge of the dura mater. Thus, an angular depression exists between the anterior parts of the peripheral attachment of the tentorium and the free border of the tentorial incisure (**Figs. 15.1, 15.3**). This depression in the dura mater is part of the roof of the cavernous sinus and is pierced in front by the oculomotor and behind by the trochlear nerves, which proceed antero-inferiorly into the lateral wall of the cavernous sinus (**Fig. 15.6**). In the anteromedial part of the middle cranial fossa, the dura mater ascends as the lateral wall of the cavernous sinus. It reaches the ridge produced by the anterior continuation of the free border of the tentorium and runs medially as the roof of the cavernous sinus, where it is pierced by the internal carotid artery (**Figs. 15.1, 15.3**). Medially, the roof of the sinus is continuous with the upper layer of the diaphragma sellae. At, or just below, the opening in the diaphragma for the infundibulum and pituitary stalk, the dura, arachnoid and pia mater blend with each other and and with the capsule of the pituitary gland. It is not possible to distinguish the layers of the meninges within the sella turcica, and the subarachnoid space is obliterated.

Through its projections as the falx cerebri and tentorium cerebelli, the dura may act to stabilize the brain within the cranial cavity. However, this arrangement causes problems when there is focal brain swelling or a focal space-occupying lesion within the brain or cranial cavity. Herniation of the brain may consequently occur under the falx cerebri or, more significantly, through the tentorial incisure, which will compress the oculomotor nerve, midbrain and arteries on the inferior medial surface of the temporal lobe. This process of transtentorial coning is particularly dangerous because of the risk of secondary vascular compression and often represents the terminal event in patients with supratentorial space-occupying lesions. Similarly, space-occupying lesions in the small infratentorial compartment may cause upward herniation

through the tentorial hiatus or downward herniation through the foramen magnum.

DURAL VENOUS SINUSES

Dural venous sinuses (**Fig. 17.14**) are a complex of venous channels which lie between the two layers of dura mater, draining blood from the brain and cranial bones. They are lined by endothelium, have no valves, and their walls are devoid of muscular tissue. Developmentally, the venous sinuses emerge as venous plexuses and most sinuses preserve a plexiform arrangement to a variable degree, rather than being simple vessels with a single lumen. Browder and Kaplan (1976) examined human venous sinuses in hundreds of corrosion casts, and observed vascular plexuses adjoining the superior and inferior sagittal and straight sinuses and, with a lesser incidence, the transverse sinuses. There was much individual variation, and departures from 'average' patterns were frequent in earlier years, e.g. in infancy the falx cerebelli may contain large plexiform channels and venous lacunae, augmenting the occipital sinus. These variations cannot be detailed in a general text. They must be established for the individual by angiography when clinical necessity arises. However, it is important to emphasize the wide variation that may occur in the structure of cranial venous sinuses, together with their plexiform nature and wide connections with cerebral and cerebellar veins. Another kind of connection has been shown experimentally. Parts of sinuses (and even diploic veins) can be filled by forcible internal carotid injection, suggesting the existence of arteriovenous shunts (Browder & Kaplan 1976). A connection between the middle meningeal arteries and the superior sagittal sinus has been demonstrated in this way, although the sites of communication are unknown.

Superior sagittal sinus

The superior sagittal sinus runs in the attached, convex margin of the falx cerebri, and grooves the internal surface of the frontal bone, the adjacent margins of the two parietal bones and the squamous part of the occipital bone (**Figs 15.1, 17.14, 15.7**). It begins near the crista

277

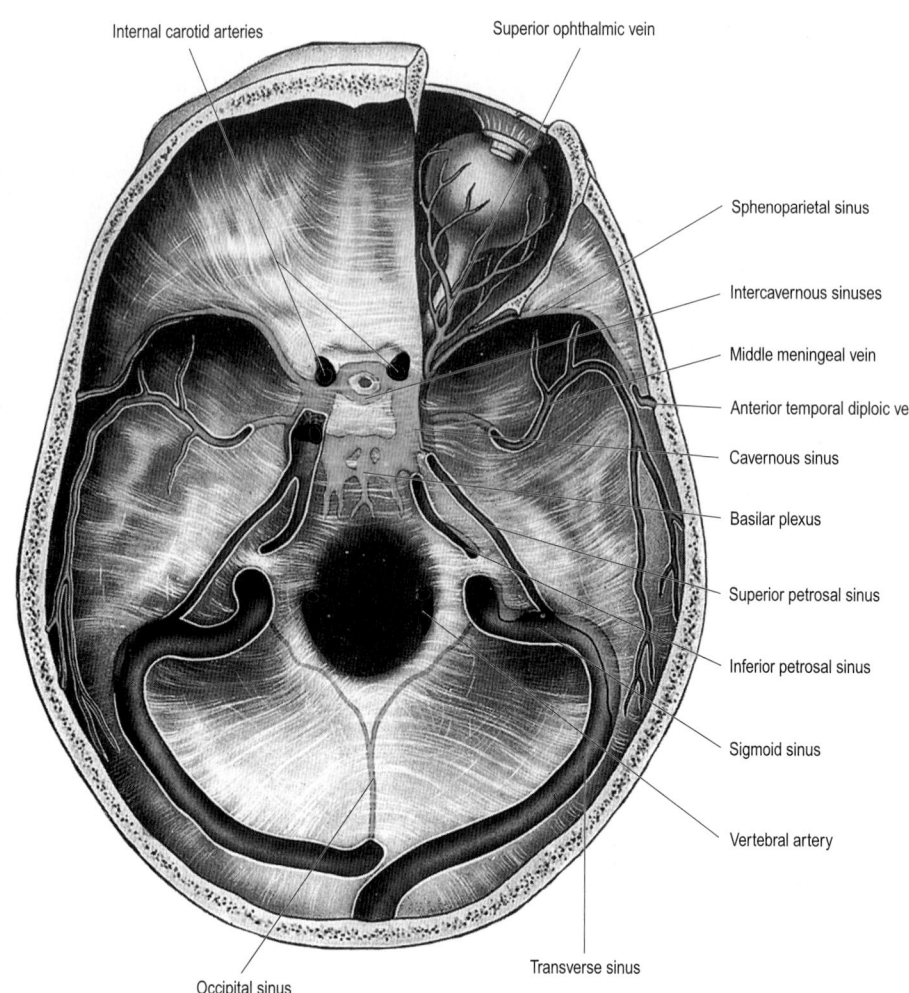

Internal carotid arteries

Superior ophthalmic vein

Sphenoparietal sinus

Intercavernous sinuses

Middle meningeal vein

Anterior temporal diploic vein

Cavernous sinus

Basilar plexus

Superior petrosal sinus

Inferior petrosal sinus

Sigmoid sinus

Vertebral artery

Transverse sinus

Occipital sinus

Fig. 15.4 The sinuses at the base of the skull. The sinuses coloured dark blue have been opened up.

galli, a few millimetres posterior to the foramen caecum, and receives primary tributaries from cortical veins of the frontal lobes, the ascending frontal veins. Narrow anteriorly, the sinus runs backwards, gradually widening to c.1 cm. Near the internal occipital protuberance it deviates, usually to the right, and continues as a transverse sinus. Triangular in cross-section, the interior of the superior sagittal sinus possesses the openings of superior cerebral veins and projecting arachnoid granulations. It is traversed by many fibrous bands. It also communicates by small orifices with irregular venous lacunae, situated in the dura mater near the sinus. There are usually two or three of these on each side – a small frontal, a large parietal and an occipital which is intermediate in size. In the elderly, the lacunae tend to become confluent, so that there is one elongated lacuna on each side. Fine fibrous bands cross them, and numerous arachnoid granulations project into them. The superior sagittal sinus receives the superior cerebral veins and, near the posterior end of the sagittal suture, veins from the pericranium, which pass through the parietal foramina. The lacunae also drain the diploic veins and meningeal veins (p. 281).

Lateral lacunae are often so complex as to be almost plexiform and are rarely simple venous spaces. Plexiform arrays of small veins adjoin the sagittal, transverse and straight sinuses and ridges of such 'spongy' venous tissue often project into the lumina of the superior sagittal and transverse sinuses. The superior sagittal sinus is also invaded, in its intermediate third, by variable bands and projections from its dural walls, which even extend as horizontal shelves that divide its lumen into superior and inferior channels. Such variable features make it impossible to give a simple description of this or other venous sinuses, and individual variations can only be shown by radiological investigations.

The dilated posterior end of the superior sagittal sinus is referred to as the confluence of the sinuses (**Fig. 15.3**). This is situated to one side (usually the right) of the internal occipital protuberance, where the superior sagittal sinus turns to become a transverse sinus. It also connects with the occipital and contralateral transverse sinus. The size and degree of communication of the channels meeting at the confluence are highly variable. In more than half of subjects all venous channels that converge towards the occiput interconnect, including the straight and occipital sinuses. In many instances, however, communication is absent or tenuous. Any sinus involved may be duplicated, narrowed, or widened near the confluence.

Inferior sagittal sinus

The inferior sagittal sinus is located in the posterior half or two-thirds of the free margin of the falx cerebri (**Fig. 15.1**). It increases in size posteriorly, and ends in the straight sinus. It receives veins from the falx and sometimes from the medial surfaces of the cerebral hemispheres.

Straight sinus

The straight sinus lies in the junction of the falx cerebri with the tentorium cerebelli (**Figs 15.1, 15.3**). It runs posteroinferiorly as a continuation of the inferior sagittal sinus into the transverse sinus. It is not (or only tenuously) continuous with the superior sagittal sinus. Its tributaries include the great cerebral vein (**Figs 15.1, 17.14**) and some superior cerebellar veins. Internally, the straight sinus is triangular in cross-section.

Transverse sinus

The transverse sinuses begin at the internal occipital protuberance (**Figs 15.3, 15.4**). One, usually the right, is directly continuous with the superior sagittal sinus, the other with the straight sinus. On both sides the sinuses run in the attached margin of the tentorium cerebelli, first on the squama of the occipital bone, then on the mastoid angle of the parietal bone. Each follows a gentle anterolateral curve, increasing in size as it does so, to the posterolateral part of the petrous temporal bone. Here it turns down as a sigmoid sinus, which ultimately becomes continuous with the internal jugular vein. Transverse sinuses are triangular in section and usually unequal in size; the one draining the superior sagittal sinus is the larger. They receive the inferior cerebral, inferior cerebellar, diploic and inferior anastomotic veins, and are

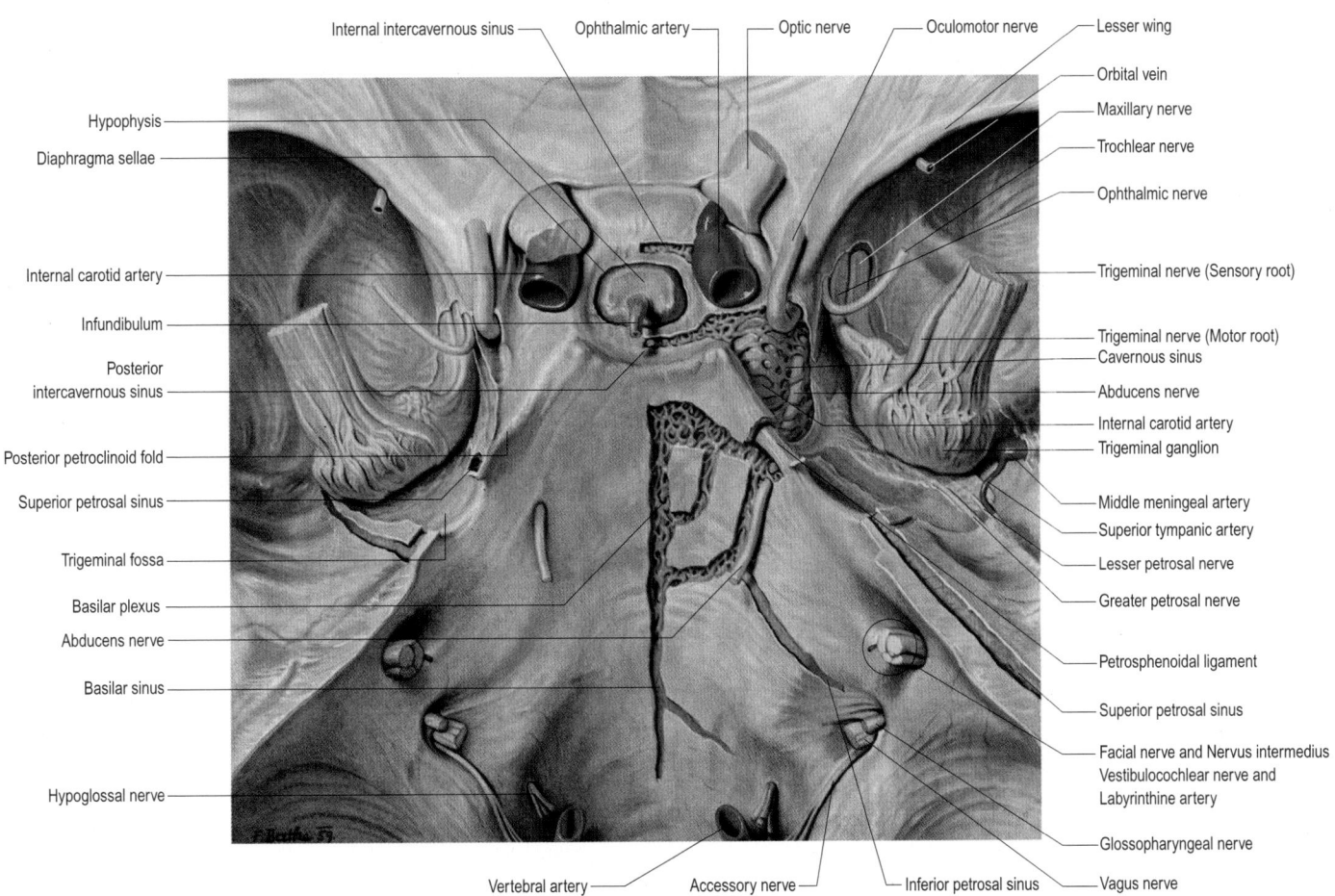

Internal intercavernous sinus — Ophthalmic artery — Optic nerve — Oculomotor nerve — Lesser wing

Hypophysis

Diaphragma sellae

Internal carotid artery

Infundibulum

Posterior
intercavernous sinus

Posterior petroclinoid fold

Superior petrosal sinus

Trigeminal fossa

Basilar plexus

Abducens nerve

Basilar sinus

Hypoglossal nerve

Orbital vein

Maxillary nerve

Trochlear nerve

Ophthalmic nerve

Trigeminal nerve (Sensory root)

Trigeminal nerve (Motor root)
Cavernous sinus

Abducens nerve

Internal carotid artery
Trigeminal ganglion

Middle meningeal artery
Superior tympanic artery

Lesser petrosal nerve

Greater petrosal nerve

Petrosphenoidal ligament

Superior petrosal sinus

Facial nerve and Nervus intermedius
Vestibulocochlear nerve and
Labyrinthine artery

Glossopharyngeal nerve

Vertebral artery — Accessory nerve — Inferior petrosal sinus — Vagus nerve

Fig. 15.5 The middle cranial fossa, viewed from above to show the cavernous and related sinuses. These have been exposed by partial removal of the dura matter. The trigeminal, trochlear and oculomotor nerves have been reflected forwards on both sides.

joined by the superior petrosal sinuses where they continue as sigmoid sinuses.

Petrosquamous sinus

The petrosquamous sinus runs back in a groove, which posteriorly sometimes becomes a canal, along the junction of the squamous and petrous parts of the temporal bone, and opens behind into the transverse sinus. Anteriorly it connects with the retromandibular vein through a postglenoid or squamous foramen. The sinus may be absent or it may drain entirely into the retromandibular vein.

Sigmoid sinus

The sigmoid sinuses are continuations of the transverse sinuses, beginning where these leave the tentorium cerebelli (**Figs 15.4, 15.8**). Each sigmoid sinus curves inferomedially in a groove on the mastoid process of the temporal bone, crosses the jugular process of the occipital bone and turns forward to the superior jugular bulb, lying posterior in the jugular foramen. Anteriorly, a thin plate of bone separates its upper part from the mastoid antrum and air cells. It connects with pericranial veins via mastoid and condylar emissary veins.

Occipital sinus

The occipital sinus is the smallest of the sinuses. It lies in the attached margin of the falx cerebelli (**Fig. 15.4**) and is occasionally paired. It commences near the foramen magnum in several small channels, one joining the end of the sigmoid sinus, and connects with the internal vertebral plexuses. It ends in the confluence of the sinuses.

Cavernous sinus

The cavernous sinus is a large venous plexus that lies on both sides of the body of the sphenoid bone (**Figs 15.4, 15.5, 15.6**). The sinus extends from the superior orbital fissure to the apex of the petrous temporal bone, with an average length of 2 cm and width of 1 cm. The sphenoidal

air sinus and pituitary gland are medial to the cavernous sinus. The trigeminal cave is near the inferoposterior part of its lateral wall, and extends posteriorly beyond it to enclose the trigeminal ganglion. The uncus of the temporal lobe is also lateral to the sinus.

The internal carotid artery, and associated sympathetic plexus, passes forward through the sinus together with the abducens nerve, which lies lateral to the artery. The oculomotor and trochlear nerves and the ophthalmic and maxillary divisions of the trigeminal nerve all lie in the lateral wall of the sinus (**Fig. 15.6**). They are of such diameters that they project into the lumen and are usually covered medially by little more than endothelium. Propulsion of blood in the cavernous sinus is partly due to pulsation of the internal carotid artery, but it is also influenced by gravity, and hence by the position of the head.

Tributaries of the cavernous sinus are the superior ophthalmic vein, a branch from the inferior ophthalmic vein (or sometimes the whole vessel), the superficial middle cerebral vein, inferior cerebral veins and sphenoparietal sinus. The central retinal vein and frontal tributary of the middle meningeal vein sometimes drain into it. The sinus drains to the transverse sinus via the superior petrosal sinus, to the internal jugular vein via the inferior petrosal sinus and a plexus of veins on the internal carotid artery, to the pterygoid plexus by veins traversing the emissary sphenoidal foramen, foramen ovale and foramen lacerum, and to the facial vein via the superior ophthalmic vein.

Caroticocavernous sinus fistula and cavernous sinus thrombosis

The unique location of the internal carotid artery within a venous structure occasionally gives rise to direct communication between the two structures such that a caroticocavernous sinus fistula (CCF) is established, either as a result of severe head trauma or degenerative or aneurysmal vessel disease. A CCF causes proptosis, which may be pulsatile, together with vascular dilatation in the tissues of the orbit and globe and combinations of third, fourth and sixth cranial nerve palsies. These changes can cause permanent blindness. CCFs are most commonly

279

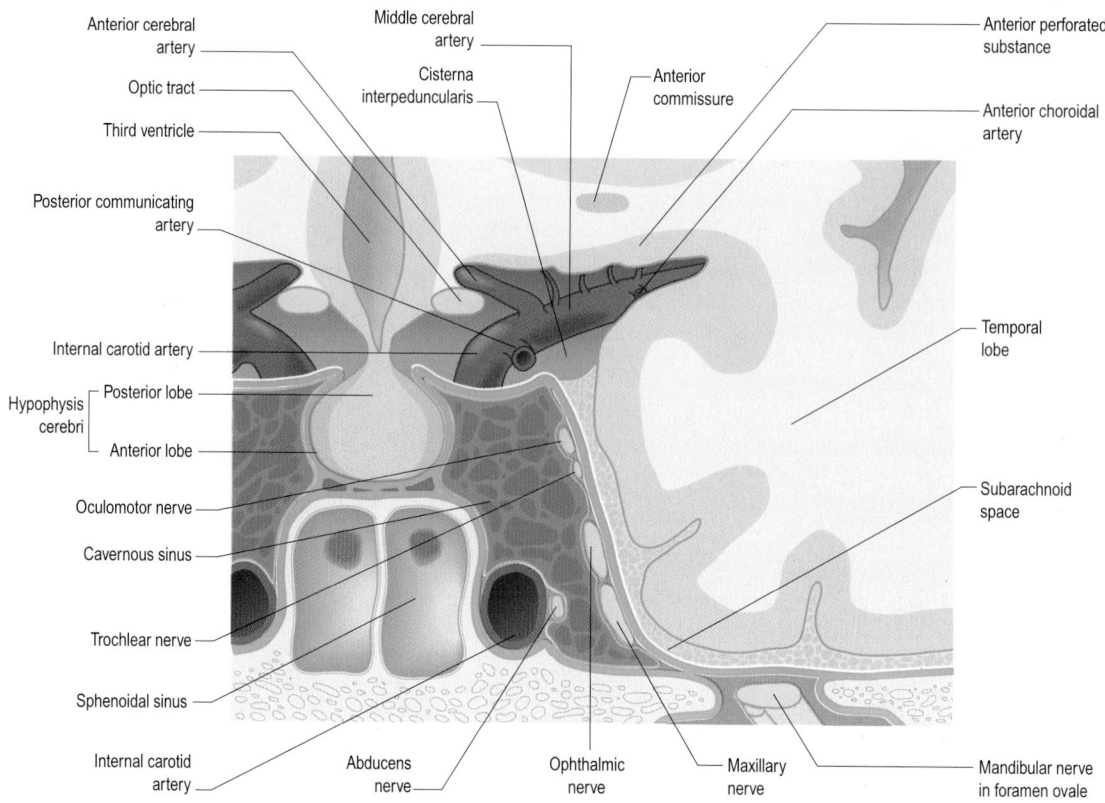

Anterior cerebral artery

Middle cerebral artery

Cisterna interpeduncularis

Anterior commissure

Anterior perforated substance

Optic tract

Third ventricle

Posterior communicating artery

Anterior choroidal artery

Internal carotid artery

Hypophysis cerebri
  Posterior lobe
  Anterior lobe

Oculomotor nerve

Cavernous sinus

Trochlear nerve

Sphenoidal sinus

Internal carotid artery

Abducens nerve

Ophthalmic nerve

Maxillary nerve

Mandibular nerve in foramen ovale

Temporal lobe

Subarachnoid space

Fig. 15.6 Coronal, slightly oblique section through the middle cranial fossa, showing the cavernous and cerebral portions of the internal carotid artery and the cavernous sinus. Pia mater: mauve; arachnoid mater: white; layers of dura mater (the mesothelium of the dura mater is not indicated): green; endothelium of cavernous sinus: blue.

treated by passing a catheter up the carotid into the fistula, and then occluding it with dilatable balloons or flexible metal coils. Any spreading infection involving the upper nasal cavities, paranasal sinuses, cheek (especially near the medial canthus), upper lip, anterior nares or even an upper incisor or canine tooth, may very rarely lead to septic thrombosis of the cavernous sinuses as infected thrombi pass from the facial vein or pterygoid venous complex into the sinus (via either ophthalmic veins or emissary veins that enter the cranial cavity through the foramen ovale). This is a critical medical emergency with a high risk of disseminated cerebritis and cerebral venous thrombosis.

Intercavernous sinuses

The two cavernous sinuses are connected by anterior and posterior intercavernous sinuses (**Fig. 15.4**) and the basilar plexus (**Fig. 15.5**). The intercavernous sinuses lie in the anterior and posterior attached borders of the diaphragma sellae and they thus form a complete circular venous sinus (**Fig. 15.5**). All connections are valveless and the direction of flow in them is reversible. Small irregular sinuses inferior to the pituitary gland drain into the intercavernous sinuses. Such inferior intercavernous sinuses are plexiform in nature and important in a surgical transnasal approach to the pituitary.

Superior petrosal sinus

This small narrow sinus drains the cavernous sinus into the transverse sinus on either side (**Figs 15.3, 15.4, 15.5**). It leaves the posterosuperior part of the cavernous sinus, runs posterolaterally in the attached margin of the tentorium cerebelli, and crosses above the trigeminal nerve to lie in a groove on the superior border of the petrous part of the temporal bone. It ends by joining a transverse sinus where this curves down to become the sigmoid. It receives cerebellar, inferior cerebral and tympanic veins, and connects with the inferior petrosal sinus and the basilar plexus.

Inferior petrosal sinus

The inferior petrosal sinus drains the cavernous sinus into the internal jugular vein (**Figs 17.14, 15.4**). It begins at the posteroinferior aspect of the cavernous sinus and runs back in a groove between the petrous

temporal and basilar occipital bones. It traverses the anterior part of the jugular foramen and ends in the superior jugular bulb. It receives labyrinthine veins via the cochlear canaliculus and the vestibular aqueduct and tributaries from the medulla oblongata, pons and inferior cerebellar surface. The sinus is often a plexus and sometimes drains by a vein in the hypoglossal canal to the suboccipital vertebral plexus.

There is a complex relationship between structures in the jugular foramen. The inferior petrosal sinus is anteromedial with a meningeal branch of the ascending pharyngeal artery, and it descends obliquely backwards. The sigmoid sinus is situated at the lateral and posterior part of the foramen with a meningeal branch of the occipital artery. Between the sinuses are, in succession posterolaterally, the glossopharyngeal, vagus and accessory nerves.

Sphenoparietal sinus

The sphenoparietal sinus is located below the periosteum of the lesser wing of the sphenoid bone, near its posterior edge (**Fig. 15.4**). It curves medially to open into the anterior part of the cavernous sinus. It receives small veins from the adjacent dura mater and sometimes the frontal ramus of the middle meningeal vein. It may also receive connecting rami, in its middle course, from the superficial middle cerebral vein, and veins from the temporal lobe and the anterior temporal diploic vein. When these connections are well developed, the sphenoparietal sinus is a large channel.

Basilar sinus and plexus

The basilar sinus and plexus consist of interconnecting channels between layers of dura mater on the clivus (**Fig. 15.5**). The basilar venous plexus interconnects the inferior petrosal sinuses and joins with the internal vertebral venous plexus. It also usually connects with the cavernous and superior petrosal sinuses at its anterior end. When veins around the foramen magnum (so-called marginal sinuses) are large they communicate anteriorly with the plexus, and this produces an almost complete circular venous channel around the foramen magnum, connecting the basilar plexus intracranially to the inferior petrosal, sigmoid and occipital sinuses, and extracranially to variable vertebral plexuses in the suboccipital region.

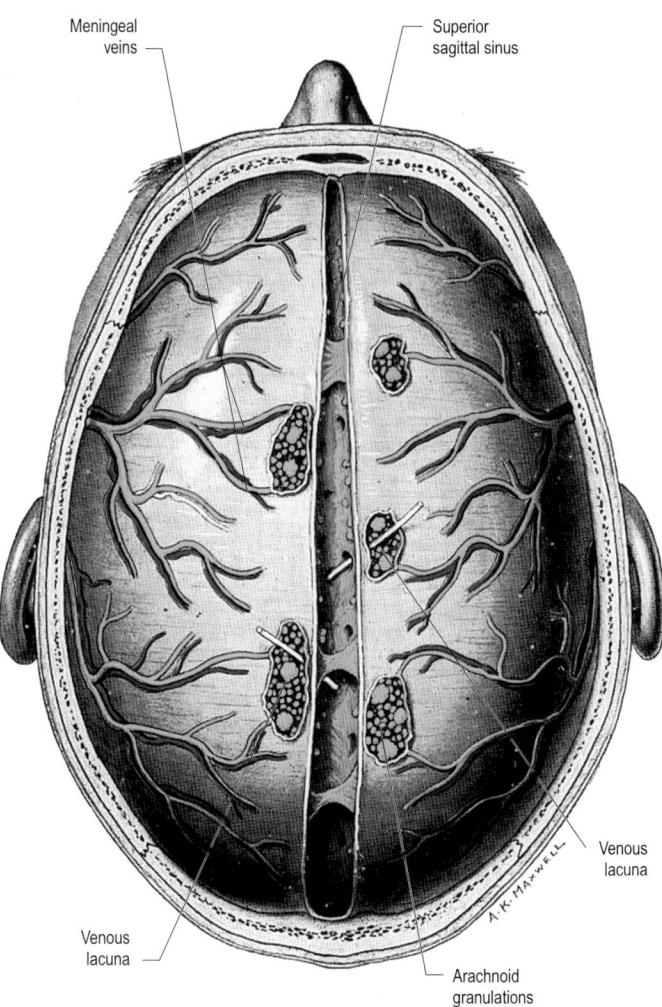

Fig. 15.7 The superior sagittal sinus laid open after removal of the cranial vault. Some of the fibrous bands which cross the sinus are shown (from two of the venous lacunae). Markers are passed into the sinus.

Labels on figure: Meningeal veins; Superior sagittal sinus; Venous lacuna; Venous lacuna; Arachnoid granulations

Middle meningeal vein (sinus)

Tributaries of the middle meningeal vein communicate with the superior sagittal sinus through its venous lacunae. Below, they converge and unite as frontal and parietal trunks, which accompany branches of the middle meningeal arteries in grooves on the internal parietal surfaces. The veins lie closer to the bone than the arteries, and may occupy separate grooves. This situation makes them particularly liable to tear in cranial fractures. Their termination is variable. The parietal trunk may traverse the foramen spinosum to the pterygoid venous plexus. The frontal trunk may also reach this plexus via the foramen ovale or it may end in the sphenoparietal or cavernous sinus (**Fig. 15.4**). The middle meningeal vein receives meningeal tributaries and small inferior cerebral veins, and connects with the diploic and superficial middle cerebral veins. It frequently bears arachnoid granulations.

The diploic veins constitute a hypothetical fourth venous tier. However, since they drain into dural veins they are here grouped with them, following Browder and Kaplan (1976). It is to be noted that intracranial veins communicate at many points with extracranial vessels via emissary and other veins.

Emissary veins

Emissary veins traverse cranial apertures and make connections between intracranial venous sinuses and extracranial veins. Some emissary veins are relatively constant, others sometimes absent. These connections are of clinical significance in the spread of infection from extracranial foci to venous sinuses. The success of a ligature of the internal jugular vein, to limit the spread of some oral and pharyngeal pathologies, depends on the adequacy of the collateral drainage. The following emissary veins are recognized. A mastoid emissary vein in the mastoid foramen, which

unites the sigmoid sinus with the posterior auricular or occipital veins. A parietal emissary vein which traverses the parietal foramen to connect the superior sagittal sinus with the veins of the scalp. The venous plexus of the hypoglossal canal, which is occasionally a single vein, and which runs between the sigmoid sinus and the internal jugular vein. A (posterior) condylar emissary vein which runs between the sigmoid sinus and veins in the suboccipital triangle via the (posterior) condylar canal. A plexus of emissary veins (venous plexus of foramen ovale) which links the cavernous sinus to the pterygoid plexus via the foramen ovale. Two or three small veins which traverse the foramen lacerum and run between the cavernous sinus and the pharyngeal veins and pterygoid plexus. A vein in the emissary sphenoidal foramen (of Vesalius) which connects the cavernous sinus with the pharyngeal veins and pterygoid plexus. The internal carotid venous plexus, which passes through the carotid canal, and connects the cavernous sinus to the internal jugular vein. The petrosquamous sinus which connects the transverse sinus with the external jugular vein. A vein may traverse the foramen caecum (which is patent in c.1% of adult skulls) and connect nasal veins with the superior sagittal sinus. An occipital emissary vein usually connects the confluence of sinuses with the occipital vein through the occipital protuberance, and also receives the occipital diploic vein. The occipital sinus connects with variably developed veins around the foramen magnum (so-called marginal sinuses) and thus with the vertebral venous plexuses. This is an alternative venous drainage when the jugular vein is blocked or tied. The ophthalmic veins are potentially emissary, since they connect intracranial to extracranial veins. However, parietal emissary veins, included here, are usually minute and do not appear to connect with veins of the scalp in corrosion casts.

ARTERIAL SUPPLY AND VENOUS DRAINAGE OF THE CRANIAL DURA MATER

The arterial supply of the dura mater is derived from numerous vessels. In the anterior cranial fossa, the dura is supplied by the anterior meningeal branches of the anterior and posterior ethmoidal and internal carotid arteries and a branch of the middle meningeal artery. In the middle cranial fossa, it is supplied by the middle and accessory meningeal branches of the maxillary artery, a branch of the ascending pharyngeal artery (entering via the foramen lacerum), branches of the internal carotid and a recurrent branch of the lacrimal artery. Dura mater in the posterior fossa is supplied by the meningeal branches of the occipital artery (one enters the skull by the jugular foramen and another by the mastoid foramen), the posterior meningeal branches of the vertebral artery and occasional small branches of the ascending pharyngeal artery, which enter by the jugular foramen and hypoglossal canal. The cranial meningeal arteries are chiefly distributed to bone. In contrast to the arterial supply of the spinal dura mater, only very fine arterial branches are distributed to the cranial dura mater *per se*. The smaller branches of the meningeal vessels are, therefore, mainly in the endosteal layer of dura.

The middle meningeal is the largest of the meningeal arteries. It passes between the roots of the auriculotemporal nerve and may lie lateral to the tensor veli palatini before entering the cranial cavity through the foramen spinosum. It then runs in an anterolateral groove on the squamous part of the temporal bone, dividing into frontal and parietal branches. The larger frontal (anterior) branch crosses the greater wing of the sphenoid, reaches a groove or canal in the sphenoidal angle of the parietal bone and divides into branches between the dura mater and cranium, some ascending to the vertex, others to the occipital region. One ascending branch grooves the parietal bone c.15 mm behind the coronal suture, corresponding approximately to the precentral sulcus (**Fig. 15.8**). The parietal (posterior) branch curves back on the squamous temporal bone, reaching the lower border of the parietal bone anterior to its mastoid angle and dividing to supply the posterior parts of the dura mater and cranium. These branches anastomose with their fellows and with the anterior and posterior meningeal arteries.

In the cranial cavity the artery has several branches. Numerous ganglionic branches supply the trigeminal ganglion and roots. A petrosal branch enters the hiatus for the greater petrosal nerve and supplies the facial nerve, geniculate ganglion and tympanic cavity, anastomosing with the stylomastoid artery. A superior tympanic artery runs in the canal for tensor tympani, supplying both muscle and the mucosa lining the canal.

Temporal branches traverse minute foramina in the greater wing of the sphenoid and anastomose with deep temporal arteries. An

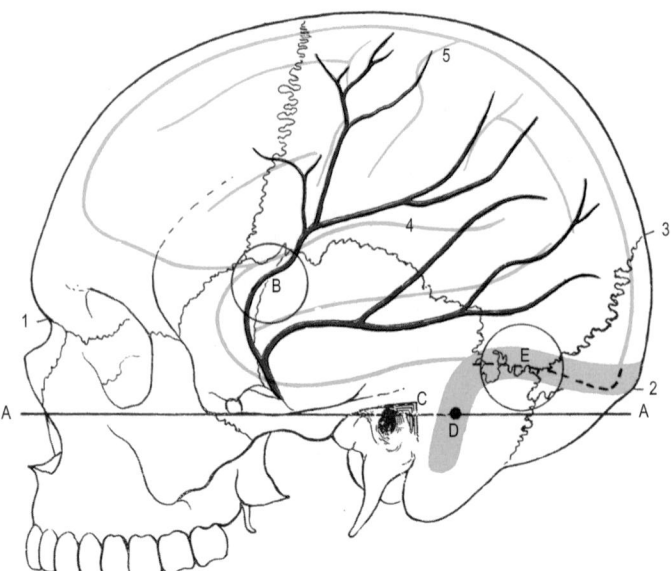

Fig. 15.8 The relations of the brain, the middle meningeal artery and the transverse and sigmoid sinuses to the surface of the skull. Nasion: 1; inion: 2; lambda: 3; lateral cerebral sulcus: 4; central sulcus: 5. Frankfurt plane, which traverses the lower margin of the orbital opening and the upper margin of the external acoustic meatus: AA; area (including the pterion) for trephining over the frontal branch of the middle meningeal artery and the cerebral Sylvian point: B; suprameatal triangle: C; sigmoid sinus: D; area for trephining over the transverse sinus, exposing the dura mater of both cerebrum and cerebellum: E. The outline of the cerebral hemisphere and its major sulci are indicated in blue; the course of the middle meningeal artery is in red. A mental image of this arrangement allows safe planning of craniotomies to avoid injuring major vessels and in trauma to predict which vessels might be injured when there is an intracranial clot.

anastomotic branch enters the orbit laterally in the superior orbital fissure, and anastomoses with a recurrent branch of the lacrimal artery – enlargement of this anastomosis explains an occasional origin of the lacrimal from the middle meningeal artery.

Apart from these branches, and a supply to the dura mater, the middle meningeal artery is predominantly periosteal, and supplies bone and red bone marrow.

The accessory meningeal artery may arise from the maxillary or the middle meningeal artery. It enters the cranial cavity through the foramen ovale, and supplies the trigeminal ganglion, dura mater and bone. However, its main distribution is extracranial, principally to medial pterygoid, lateral pterygoid (upper head), tensor veli palatini, the greater wing and pterygoid processes of the sphenoid bone, mandibular nerve and otic ganglion. It is sometimes replaced by separate small arteries.

Meningeal veins begin from plexiform vessels in the dura mater and drain into efferent vessels in the outer dural layer. The latter connect with lacunae of the superior sagittal sinus and with other cranial sinuses, including those accompanying the middle meningeal arteries, and with diploic veins.

INNERVATION OF THE CRANIAL DURA MATER

The innervation of the cranial dura mater is derived mainly from the three divisions of the trigeminal nerve, the first three cervical spinal nerves, and the cervical sympathetic trunk. Less well-established meningeal branches have been described arising from the vagus and hypoglossal nerves and possibly from the facial and glossopharyngeal nerves.

In the anterior cranial fossa, the dura is innervated by meningeal branches of the anterior and posterior ethmoidal nerves and anterior filaments of the meningeal rami of the maxillary (nervus meningeus medius) and mandibular (nervus spinosus) trigeminal divisions. Nervi meningeus medius and spinosus are, however, largely distributed to the dura of the middle cranial fossa, which also receives filaments from the trigeminal ganglion. The nervus spinosus re-enters the cranium through

the foramen spinosum with the middle meningeal artery, and divides into anterior and posterior branches, which accompany the main divisions of the artery and supply the dura mater in the middle cranial fossa and, to a lesser extent, the anterior fossa and calvarium. The anterior branch communicates with the meningeal branch of the maxillary nerve, while the posterior branch also supplies the mucous lining of the mastoid air cells. The nervus spinosus also contains sympathetic postganglionic fibres from the middle meningeal plexus. A recurrent tentorial nerve (a branch of the ophthalmic division of the trigeminal) supplies the tentorium cerebelli. The dura in the posterior cranial fossa is innervated by ascending meningeal branches of the upper cervical nerves, which enter through the anterior part of the foramen magnum (second and third cervical nerves) and through the hypoglossal canal and jugular foramen (first and second cervical nerves). Meningeal branches of both the vagus and hypoglossal nerves have been described. Those from the vagus apparently start from the superior vagal ganglion and are distributed to the dura mater in the posterior cranial fossa. Those from the hypoglossal leave the nerve in its canal to supply the diploë of the occipital bone, the dural walls of the occipital and inferior petrosal sinuses, and much of the floor and anterior wall of the posterior cranial fossa. These meningeal rami may not contain vagal or hypoglossal fibres but ascending, mixed sensory and sympathetic fibres from the upper cervical nerves and superior cervical sympathetic ganglion. All meningeal nerves contain a postganglionic sympathetic component, either from the superior cervical sympathetic ganglion or by communication with its perivascular intracranial extensions.

The brain itself, the arachnoid mater, and the pia mater, do not contain sensory nerve endings. These are restricted to the dura mater and cerebral blood vessels. Stimulation of such nerve endings causes pain and is the basis of certain forms of headache. The role of the autonomic nerve supply of the cranial dura mater is uncertain.

ARACHNOID MATER

The arachnoid mater and the pia mater together are referred to as the leptomeninges. They share many similarities, including their cellular structure. The arachnoid and pia are composed of the same basic cell type embedded in bundles of collagen. The cells share a common embryological origin from mesenchyme surrounding the developing nervous system. They are flattened or cuboidal and have oval nuclei, usually with a single small but prominent nucleolus. Joined together by desmosomes, gap junctions and, in the outer layer of the arachnoid, by tight junctions, these cells are not surrounded by basement membrane, except where they are in contact with collagen in the inner layers of the arachnoid and on the deep aspects of the pia mater.

The outer layer of the arachnoid, the dura–arachnoid interface, is formed from five or six layers of cells joined by numerous desmosomes and tight junctions. This layer forms a barrier that normally prevents permeation of CSF through the arachnoid into the subdural space. The central portion of the arachnoid is closely apposed to the outer layer, and is formed from tightly packed polygonal cells, which are joined by desmosomes and gap junctions. The cells are more loosely packed in the inner layer of the arachnoid, where they intermingle with bundles of collagen continuous with the trabeculae that cross the subarachnoid space.

The arachnoid and pia are separated by the subarachnoid space and joined by trabeculae (**Fig. 15.9**). The anatomical relationships of the arachnoid and pia differ to some extent in the cerebral and spinal regions.

The cerebral part of the arachnoid mater invests the brain loosely but does not enter the sulci or fissures, except for the great longitudinal fissure between the cerebral hemispheres. The arachnoid also coats the superior surface of the pituitary fossa. In young individuals the arachnoid on the upper surface of the brain is transparent but in older people it may become white and opaque, particularly near the midline. The arachnoid is thicker on the basal aspect of the brain and is also slightly opaque where it extends between the temporal lobes and the front of the pons, producing a large space between arachnoid and pia mater, which is one of the subarachnoid cisterns. The arachnoid is easily separated from the dura over the surface of the brain. However, at the sites where the internal carotid and the vertebral arteries enter the subarachnoid space, the arachnoid mater is adherent to the adventitia

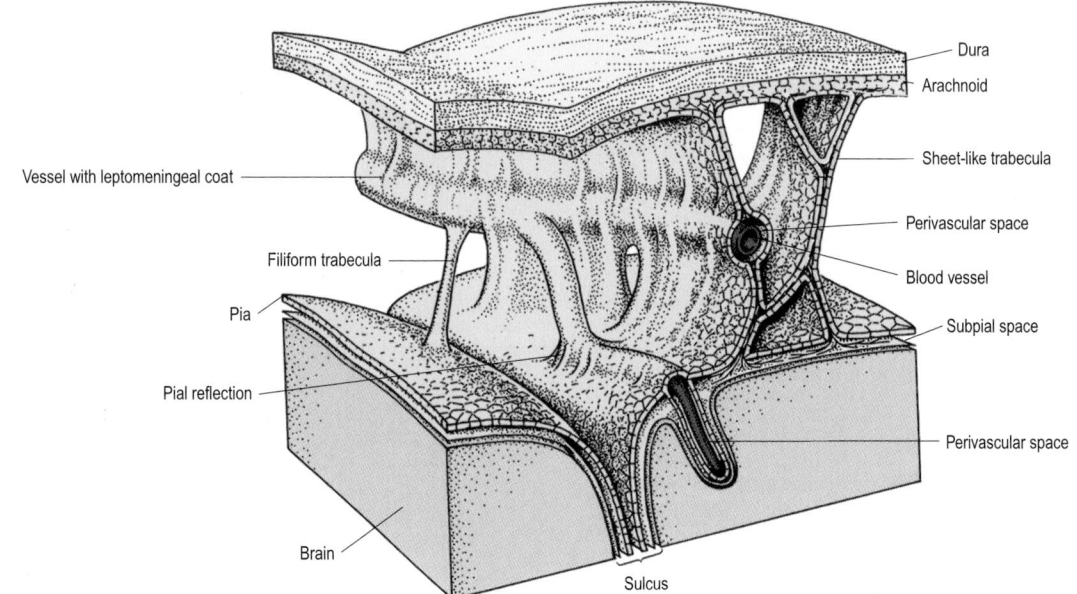

Fig. 15.9 Relationships of pia and arachnoid mater to the dura, brain and vessels. (Modified from Alcolado et al. 1988 according to Zhang ET, Inman CBE, Weller RO 1990 Interrelationships of the pia mater and the perivascular (Virchow–Robin) spaces in the human cerebrum. J Anat 170: 111-123, by permission from Blackwell Science.)

of the vessels. It is then reflected onto the surface of blood vessels in the subarachnoid space and is eventually continuous with the pia mater.

Separation of the arachnoid and dura mater is easily achieved and requires little physical force. Damage to small bridging veins in the space can give rise to subdural haematoma following even relatively mild head trauma. The characteristics of a subdural haematoma differ from the extradural haematoma described above. Clinically the accumulation is often of relatively low pressure and seldom presents as a medical emergency. In many cases there is some predisposing factor, such as cerebral atrophy or increased size of the underlying subarachnoid space, and even sizeable accumulations may be tolerated on a chronic basis with mild or no symptoms. The distinction between subdural and extradural haematoma on a computed tomography (CT) scan relies on the anatomical features of the space. Extradural collections tend to be lentiform in shape due to the pressure required to separate the dura and periosteum. They will pass deep to any major dural sinuses and cannot extend along the falx cerebri or tentorium cerebelli. Subdural haematomas tend to be biconcave in shape and more extensive, often following the line of the dura along the falx or tentorium and always lying superficial to the deep venous sinuses.

SUBARACHNOID SPACE

The subarachnoid space lies between the arachnoid and the pia mater. It contains cerebrospinal fluid (CSF) and the larger arteries and veins which traverse the surface of the brain. Arachnoid and pia mater are in close apposition over the convexities of the brain, such as the cortical gyri, whereas concavities are followed by the pia but spanned by the arachnoid. This arrangement produces a subarachnoid space of greatly variable depth that is location-dependent. The more expansive spaces are identified as subarachnoid cisterns (**Fig. 15.10**). Cisterns are continuous with each other through the general subarachnoid space of which they are dilatations.

The largest cistern, the cisterna magna or cerebellomedullary cistern, is formed where the arachnoid bridges the interval between the medulla oblongata and the inferior surface of the cerebellum. The cistern is continuous above with the lumen of the fourth ventricle through its median aperture, the foramen of Magendie, and below with the subarachnoid space of the spinal cord. The pontine cistern is an extensive space ventral to the pons, continuous below with the spinal subarachnoid space, behind with the cisterna magna and, rostral to the pons, with the interpeduncular cistern. The basilar artery runs through the pontine cistern into the interpeduncular cistern. As the arachnoid mater spans between the two temporal lobes it is separated from the cerebral peduncles and structures within the interpeduncular fossa by the interpeduncular cistern, which contains the circulus arteriosus (circle of Willis). Anteriorly, the interpeduncular cistern extends to the optic chiasma. The cistern of the lateral fossa is formed by the arachnoid

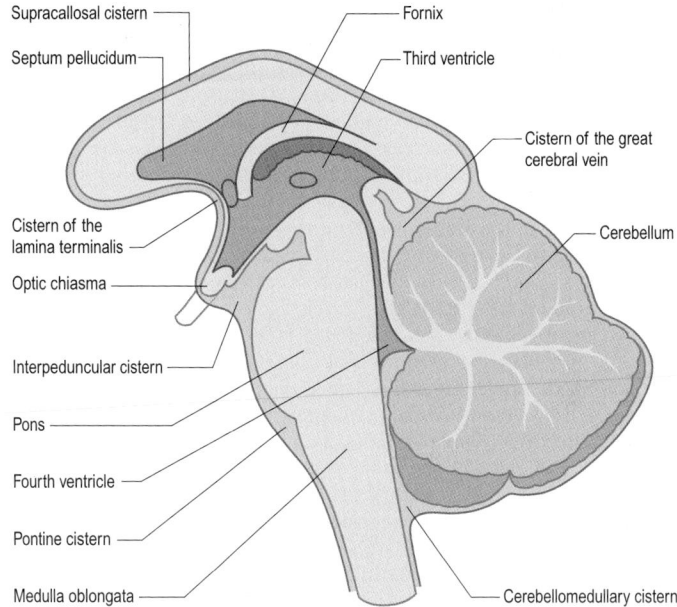

Fig. 15.10 Sagittal section of the brain illustrating the positions of the principal subarachnoid cisterns. Ventricular system and subarachnoid space: blue.

as it bridges the lateral sulcus between the frontal, parietal and temporal opercula, and contains the middle cerebral artery. The cistern of the great cerebral vein (cisterna ambiens or superior cistern) lies posterior to the brain stem and third ventricle, and occupies the interval between the splenium of the corpus callosum and the superior cerebellar surface. The great cerebral vein traverses this cistern and the pineal gland protrudes into it.

Several smaller cisterns have been described, including the prechiasmatic and postchiasmatic cistern related to the optic chiasma, the cistern of the lamina terminalis and the supracallosal cistern, all of which are extensions of the interpeduncular cistern and contain the anterior cerebral arteries. The subarachnoid space also extends along the optic nerves to the back of the globe where the dura fuses with the sclera of the eye. There is a connection between the subarachnoid space and the inner ear through the cochlear duct.

The cerebral subarachnoid space is connected with the fourth ventricle of the brain by three openings, through which CSF flows. The

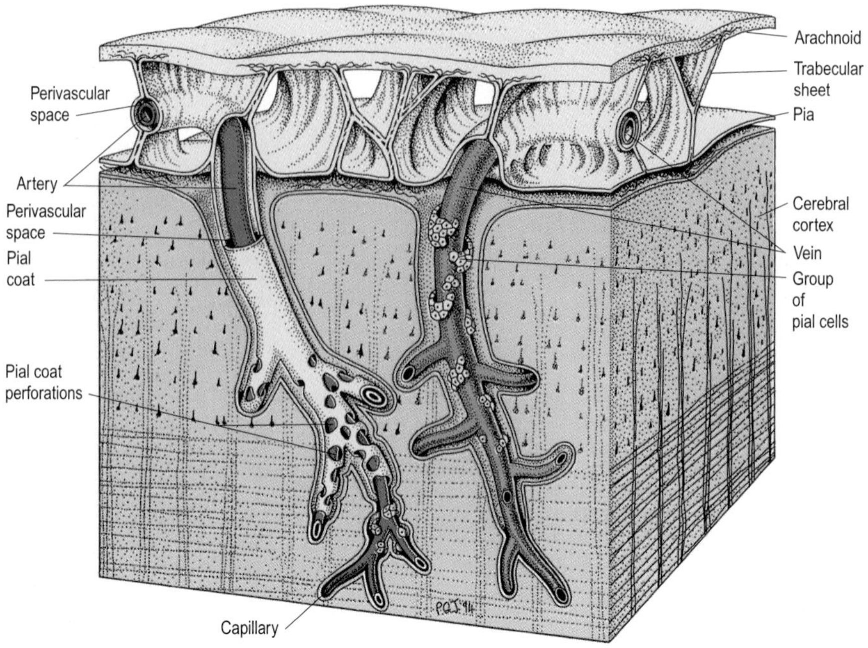

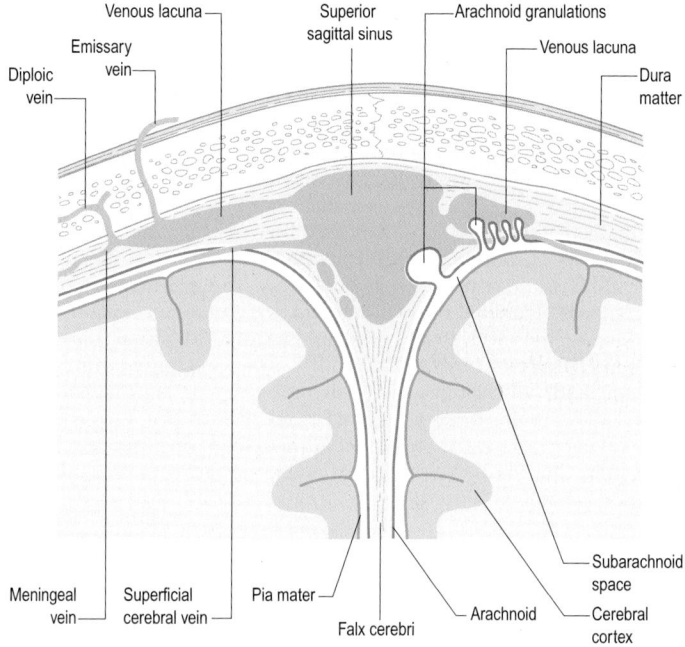

Fig. 15.11 The inter-relationships between leptomeninges and blood vessels entering and leaving the cerebral cortex. The subarachnoid space is divided by trabeculae and, as the artery enters the cortex, a layer of pia mater accompanies the vessel into the brain. With decreasing size of the vessel, the pial coating becomes perforated and finally disappears at capillary level. The perivascular space between the artery and the pia mater inside the brain is continuous with the perivascular space around the meningeal vessel. Veins do not have a similar coating of pia mater. (Reproduced and modified from Zhang ET, Inman CBE, Weller RO 1990 Interrelationships of the pia mater and the perivascular (Virchow–Robin) spaces in the human cerebrum. J Anat 170: 111-123, by permission from Blackwell Science.)

median aperture, or foramen of Magendie, lies in the median plane in the inferior part of the roof of the fourth ventricle and provides communication with the cisterna magna. The paired lateral apertures, or foramina of Luschka, are located at the ends of the lateral recesses of the fourth ventricle, and open into the subarachnoid space at the cerebellopontine angle, behind the upper roots of the glossopharyngeal nerves (**Fig. 16.9**).

Trabeculae, in the form of sheets or fine filiform structures, traverse the subarachnoid space from the deep layers of the arachnoid mater to the pia mater and are also attached to large blood vessels within the subarachnoid space (**Figs 15.9, 15.11**). Each trabecula has a core of collagen and is coated by leptomeningeal cells. Subarachnoid trabeculae are long and filamentous and cross the subarachnoid cisterns. The topography of trabeculae which cross the subarachnoid space may, in effect, form compartments, particularly in the perivascular regions, enabling directional flow of CSF through the subarachnoid space.

Arteries and veins in the subarachnoid space are coated by a thin layer of leptomeninges, often only one cell thick. The pia mater, the blood vessels and the arachnoid mater are connected by collagenous trabeculae and sheets, which are also coated by leptomeningeal cells (**Fig. 15.9**). Cranial and spinal nerves that traverse the subarachnoid space to pass out of cranial or intervertebral foramina are coated by a thin layer of leptomeninges, which fuses with the arachnoid at the exit foramina.

ARACHNOID VILLI AND GRANULATIONS

Arachnoid villi and the larger arachnoid granulations represent extensions of the arachnoid mater and subarachnoid space through the wall of dural venous sinuses. As such they present an exchange surface to the sinus endothelium (**Fig. 15.12**), which constitutes the major pathway for the passage of CSF from the subarachnoid space into the blood. They are, therefore, an essential step in the normal circulation and reabsorption of CSF.

These structures are most prominent along the margins of the great longitudinal fissure, where they project into the superior sagittal sinus (**Fig. 15.7**). Arachnoid villi are also found in association with other cerebral venous sinuses, such as the transverse sinus. Microscopic villi are present in the superior sagittal sinus of the fetus and newborn infant. These hypertrophy to form granulations which are visible by the age of 18 months in the parieto-occipital region of the superior sagittal sinus, and by the age of 3 years in the laterally-located sinuses of the posterior fossa. The arachnoid granulations become more lobulated and complex with increasing age. They may become calcified, when they are known as Pacchionian bodies.

At the base of each arachnoid granulation, a thin neck of arachnoid mater projects through an aperture in the dural lining of the venous

Fig. 15.12 Coronal section through the vertex of the skull showing the relationships between the superior sagittal sinus, meninges and arachnoid granulations.

sinus and expands to form a core of collagenous trabeculae and interwoven channels (**Fig. 15.13**). The core is surmounted by an apical cap of arachnoid cells, some 150 μm thick. Channels extend through the cap to reach the subendothelial regions of the granulation. The cap region of each granulation is attached to the endothelium of the sinus over an area some 300 μm in diameter, whereas the rest of the granulation core is separated from the endothelium by a fibrous dural cupola.

PIA MATER

The pia mater is a delicate membrane which closely invests the surface of the brain, from which it is separated by a microscopic subpial space

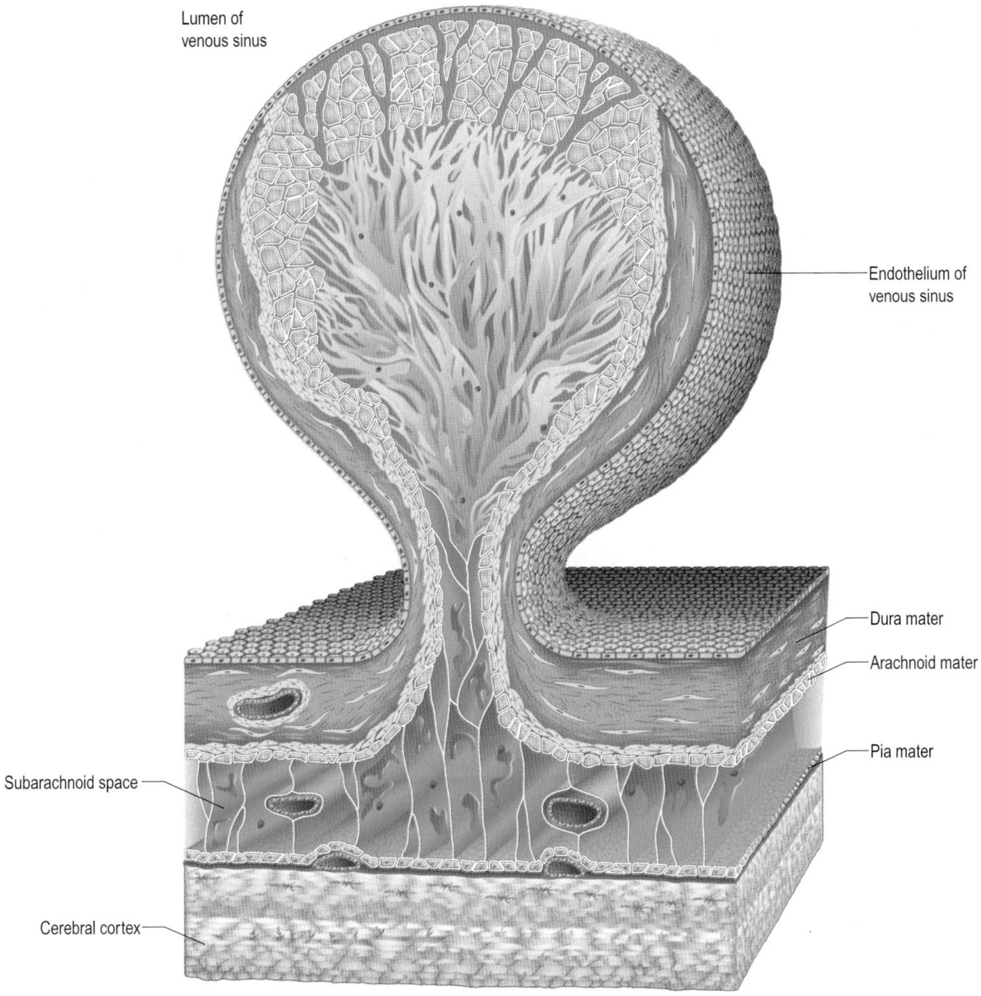

Lumen of
venous sinus

Endothelium of
venous sinus

Dura mater

Arachnoid mater

Pia mater

Subarachnoid space

Cerebral cortex

Fig. 15.13 An arachnoid granulation. The subarachnoid space between the arachnoid and pia mater is highly trabeculated and is continuous with the channel in the centre of the granulation. Narrow channels traverse the cap region of the granulation to come into contact with the endothelium of the venous sinus. The fluid finally drains through the endothelium. (Modified by permission from Springer-Verlag, Principles of Pediatric Neurosurgery, Vol 4: Morphology of CSF drainage pathways in man. Raimondi (ed), Kida and Weller 1994.)

(Fig. 15.9). It follows the contours of the brain into concavities and into the depths of fissures and sulci. During development, it becomes apposed to the ependyma in the roof of the telencephalon and fourth ventricle to form the stroma of the choroid plexus (p. 54).

The pia mater shares a common embryological origin and structural similarity with the arachnoid mater. Their common features are described under arachnoid mater (p. 282).

Pia mater is formed from a layer of leptomeningeal cells, which is often only 1 to 2 cells thick. The cells are joined by desmosomes and gap junctions but few, if any, tight junctions and are continuous with the coating of the subarachnoid trabeculae. They are separated from the basal lamina of the glia limitans by collagen bundles, fibroblast-like cells, and arteries and veins lying in the subpial space (Fig. 15.11).

Despite its delicate and thin nature, the pia mater appears to form a regulatory interface between the subarachnoid space and the brain. Not only does it separate the subarachnoid space from the subpial and perivascular spaces, but cells of the pia mater exhibit pinocytotic activity and ingest particles up to 1 μm in diameter. They contain enzymes such as catechol-O-methyltransferase and glutamine synthetase which will degrade neurotransmitters. Further evidence of effectiveness of the pia as a barrier is seen in subarachnoid haemorrhages and in subpial haemorrhages in infants – in neither of these instances do red blood cells penetrate the pia mater.

It was long thought that the subarachnoid space connected directly with the perivascular spaces (Virchow–Robin spaces) surrounding blood vessels in the brain. However, it is now recognized that the pia mater is reflected from the surface of the brain onto the surface of blood vessels in the subarachnoid space. Thus, the subarachnoid space is separated by a layer of pia from the subpial and perivascular spaces of the brain (Figs 15.9, 15.11).

REFERENCES

Browder J, Kaplan HA 1976 Cerebral Dural Sinuses and their Tributaries. Springfield, Illinois: Thomas.
Describes variations in the form of the superior sagittal and other venous sinuses.
Kida S, Weller RO 1994 Morphology of CSF drainage pathways in man. In: Raimondi A (ed) Principles of Pediatric Neurosurgery, vol 4. Berlin: Springer.
Describes the morphology and relationships of the subarachnoid space including the structure of arachnoid granulations.

Klintworth GK 1967 The ontogeny and growth of the human tentorium cerebelli. Anat Rec 158: 433–42.
Zhang ET, Inman CBE, Weller RO 1990 Interrelationships of the pia mater and the perivascular (Virchow–Robin) spaces in the human cerebrum. J Anat 170: 111–23.

Ventricular system and cerebrospinal fluid

The cerebral ventricular system consists of a series of interconnecting spaces and channels within the brain which are derived from the central lumen of the embryonic neural tube and the cerebral vesicles to which it gives rise (Ch. 14). Within each cerebral hemisphere lies a large C-shaped lateral ventricle (**Figs 16.1, 16.2**). Near its rostral end the lateral ventricle communicates through the interventricular foramen (foramen of Monro) with the third ventricle, which is a midline, slit-like cavity lying between the right and left halves of the thalamus and hypothalamus. Caudally, the third ventricle is continuous with the cerebral aqueduct, a narrow tube that passes the length of the midbrain, and which is continuous in turn with the fourth ventricle, a wide tent-shaped cavity lying between the brain stem and cerebellum. Caudally, the fourth ventricle is continuous with the vestigial central canal of the spinal cord.

The ventricular system contains cerebrospinal fluid (CSF), which is mostly secreted by the choroid plexuses located within the lateral, third and fourth ventricles. CSF flows from the lateral to the third ventricle, through the cerebral aqueduct and into the fourth ventricle. It leaves the fourth ventricle through three apertures to reach the subarachnoid space surrounding the brain.

TOPOGRAPHY AND RELATIONS OF THE VENTRICULAR SYSTEM

LATERAL VENTRICLE

Viewed from its lateral aspect, the lateral ventricle has a roughly C-shaped profile, with an occipital tail. (**Fig. 16.1**). The shape is a consequence of the developmental expansion of the frontal, parietal and occipital regions of the hemisphere (p. 262), which displaces the temporal lobe inferiorly and anteriorly. Both the caudate nucleus and the fornix, which lie in the wall of the ventricle, have adopted a similar morphology, so that the tail of the caudate nucleus encircles the thalamus in a C-shape, and the fornix traces the outline of the ventricle forwards to the interventricular foramen.

The lateral ventricle is customarily divided into a body and anterior, posterior and inferior horns (**Figs 16.1, 16.3**). The anterior (frontal) horn lies within the frontal lobe. It is bounded anteriorly by the posterior aspect of the genu and rostrum of the corpus callosum, and its roof is formed by the anterior part of the body of the corpus callosum. The anterior horns of the two ventricles are separated by the septum pellucidum. The coronal profile of the anterior horn is roughly that of a flattened triangle in which the rounded head of the caudate nucleus forms the lateral wall and floor (**Fig. 16.4**). The anterior horn extends back as far as the interventricular foramen. The body lies within the frontal and parietal lobes and extends from the interventricular foramen to the splenium of the corpus callosum. The bodies of the lateral ventricles are separated by the septum pellucidum, which contains the columns of the fornices in its lower edge. The coronal profile of the body of the ventricle is a flattened triangle with an inward bulging lateral wall, formed by the thalamus inferiorly and the tail of the caudate nucleus superiorly. The boundary between the thalamus and caudate nucleus is marked by a groove (**Fig. 16.3**), which is occupied by a fascicle of nerve fibres, the stria terminalis, and by the thalamostriate vein. The inferior limit of the body of the ventricle and its medial wall are formed by the body of the fornix. The fornix is separated from the thalamus by the choroidal fissure. The choroid plexus occludes the choroidal fissure and covers part of the thalamus and fornix. The body of the lateral ventricle widens posteriorly to become continuous with the posterior and inferior horns at the collateral trigone or atrium. The posterior (occipital) horn curves posteromedially into the occipital lobe. It is usually diamond-shaped or square in outline, and the two sides are often asymmetrical. Fibres of the tapetum of the corpus callosum separate the ventricle from the optic radiation, and form the roof and lateral wall of the posterior horn. Fibres of the splenium of the corpus callosum (forceps major) pass medially as they sweep back into the occipital lobe, and produce a rounded elevation in the upper medial wall of the posterior horn. Lower down, a second elevation, the calcar avis, corresponds to the deeply infolded cortex of the anterior part of the calcarine sulcus. The inferior (temporal) horn is the largest

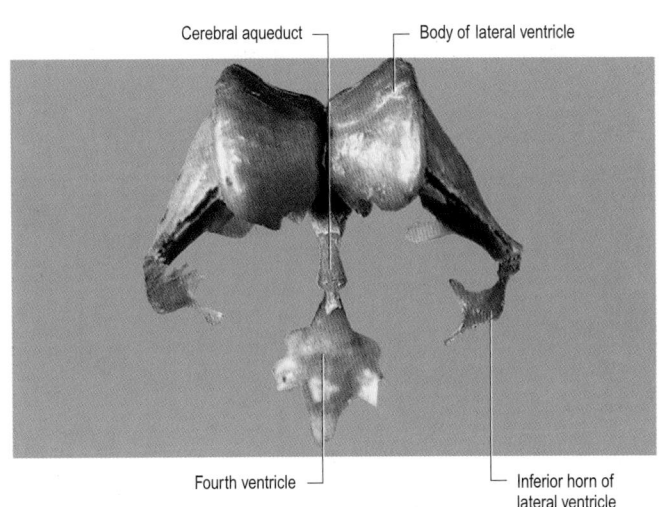

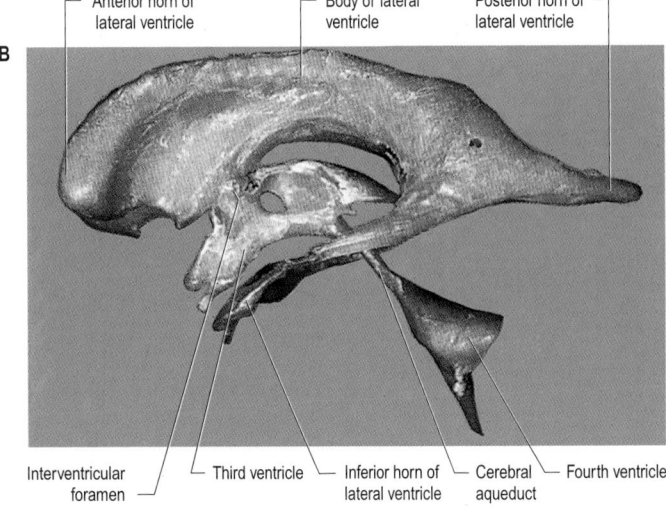

Cerebral aqueduct — Body of lateral ventricle

A

Fourth ventricle — Inferior horn of lateral ventricle

Anterior horn of lateral ventricle — Body of lateral ventricle — Posterior horn of lateral ventricle

B

Interventricular foramen — Third ventricle — Inferior horn of lateral ventricle — Cerebral aqueduct — Fourth ventricle

Fig. 16.1 Resin casts of the ventricular system of the human brain. **A**, anterior view. **B**, left lateral view. (Prepared by DH Tompsett of the Royal College of Surgeons of England.)

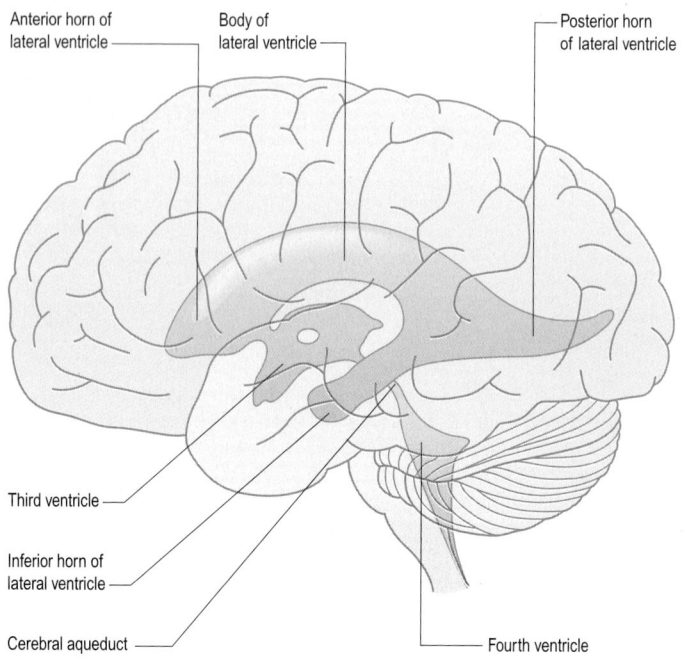

Fig. 16.2 Projection of the ventricles onto the left surface of the brain.

compartment of the lateral ventricle and extends forwards into the temporal lobe. It curves round the posterior aspect of the thalamus (pulvinar) and at first passes downwards and posterolaterally and then curves anteriorly to end within 2.5 cm of the temporal pole, near the uncus. Its position relative to the surface of the hemisphere usually corresponds to the superior temporal sulcus. The roof of the inferior horn is formed mainly by the tapetum of the corpus callosum, but also by the tail of the caudate nucleus and the stria terminalis, which extend forwards in the roof to terminate in the amygdala at the anterior end of the ventricle. The floor of the ventricle consists of the hippocampus medially and the collateral eminence, formed by the infolding of the collateral sulcus, laterally. The inferior part of the choroid fissure lies between the fimbria (a distinct bundle of efferent fibres that leaves the hippocampus) and the stria terminalis in the roof of the temporal horn (**Fig. 16.5**). The temporal extension of the choroid plexus fills this fissure and covers the outer surface of the hippocampus.

THIRD VENTRICLE

The third ventricle is a midline, slit-like cavity, which is derived from the primitive forebrain vesicle (**Figs 16.1, 16.2, 16.6–16.8**). The upper part of the lateral wall of the ventricle is formed by the medial surface of the anterior two-thirds of the thalamus, and the lower part is formed by the hypothalamus anteriorly and the subthalamus posteriorly. An indistinct hypothalamic sulcus extends horizontally on the ventricular wall between the interventricular foramen and the cerebral aqueduct, and marks the boundary between the thalamus and hypothalamus. Dorsally, the lateral wall is limited by a ridge covering the stria medullaris thalami. The lateral walls of the third ventricle are joined by an interthalamic adhesion, or massa intermedia, a band of grey matter which extends from one thalamus to the other.

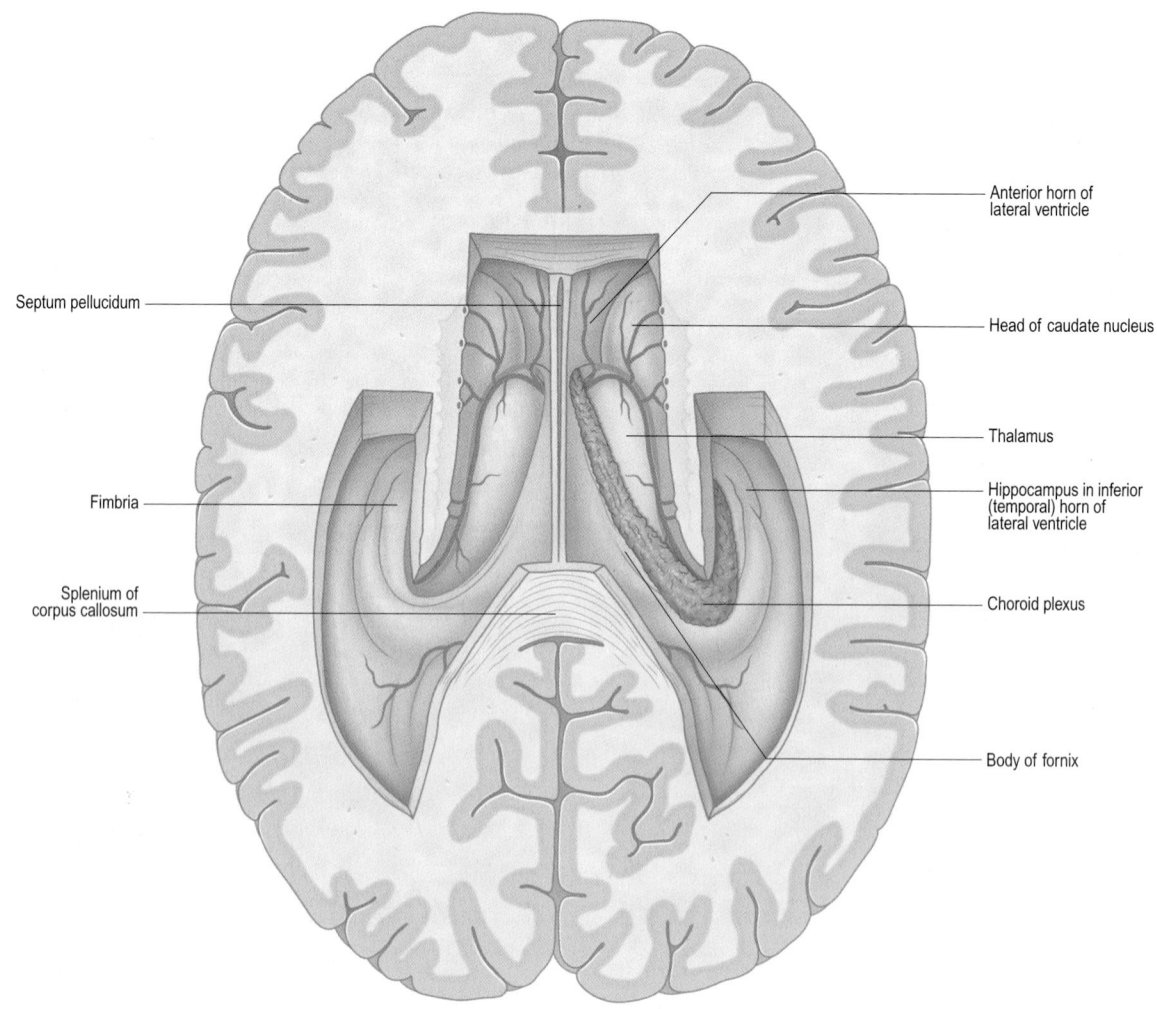

Fig. 16.3 Horizontal section of the cerebrum dissected to remove the roofs of the lateral ventricles.

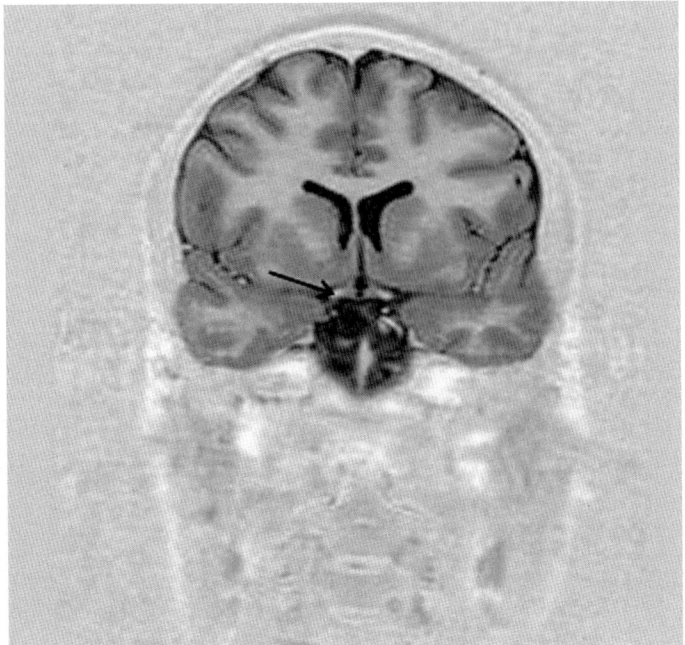

Fig. 16.4 Transverse MRI scan, at the level of the anterior horn of the lateral ventricle. (By kind permission from Professor Alan Jackson, Professor of Neuroradiology, University of Manchester.)

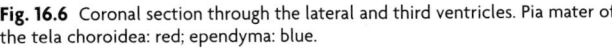

Body of lateral ventricle — Body of fornix — Corpus callosum

Choroid plexus

Caudate nucleus

Anterior part of thalamus

Right internal cerebral vein

Medial part of thalamus

Lateral part of thalamus

Third ventricle

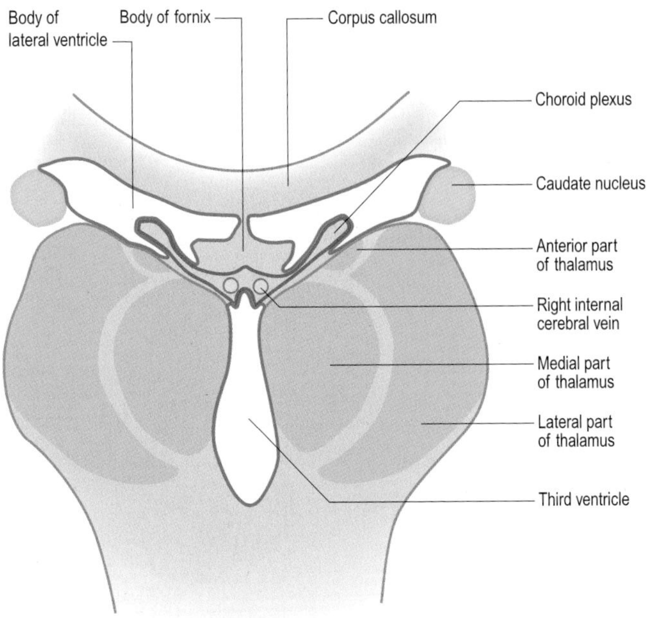

Fig. 16.6 Coronal section through the lateral and third ventricles. Pia mater of the tela choroidea: red; ependyma: blue.

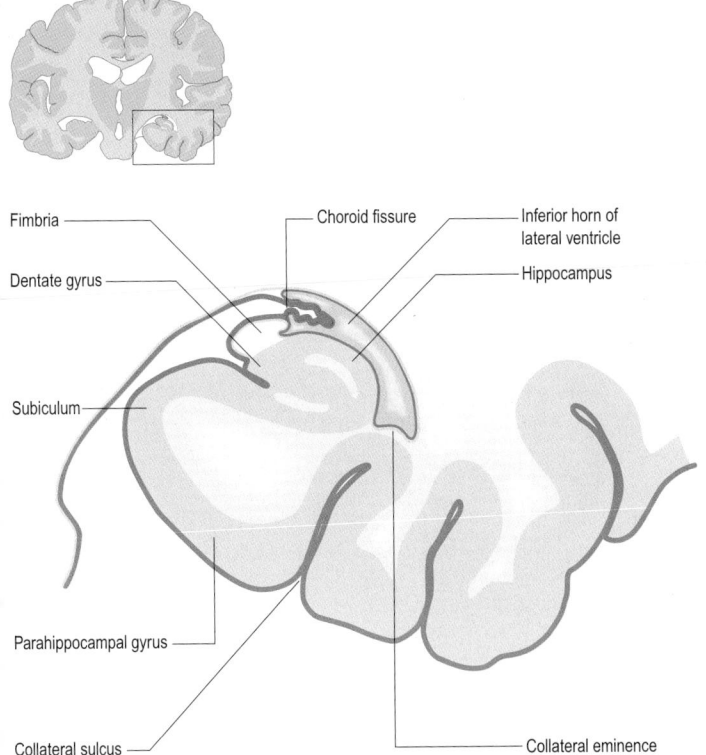

Fimbria

Dentate gyrus

Subiculum

Choroid fissure

Inferior horn of lateral ventricle

Hippocampus

Parahippocampal gyrus

Collateral sulcus

Collateral eminence

Fig. 16.5 Coronal section through the inferior horn of the lateral ventricle. Pia mater: red; ependyma: blue.

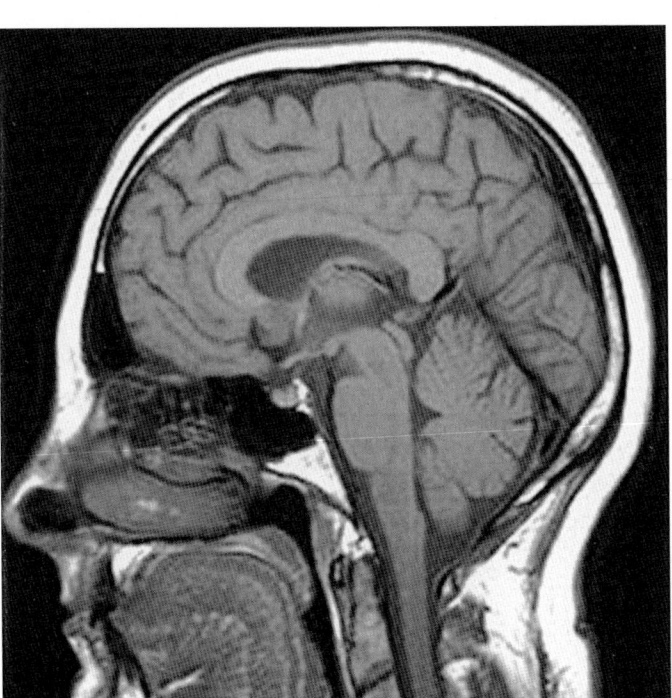

Fig. 16.7 MRI scan of head in sagittal plane. (By kind permission from Professor Alan Jackson, Professor of Neuroradiology, University of Manchester.)

Anteriorly, the third ventricle extends to the lamina terminalis (Fig.16.8). This thin structure stretches from the optic chiasma to the rostrum of the corpus callosum and represents the rostral boundary of the embryonic neural tube. The lamina terminalis forms the roof of the small virtual cavity lying immediately below the ventricle called the cistern of the lamina terminalis. This is important because it contains the anterior communicating artery and aneurysm formation at this site may cause intraventricular haemorrhage through the thin membrane of the lamina terminalis. Above this, the anterior wall is formed by the diverging columns of the fornices and the transversely orientated anterior commissure, which crosses the midline. The anterior and posterior commissures are important neuroradiological landmarks.

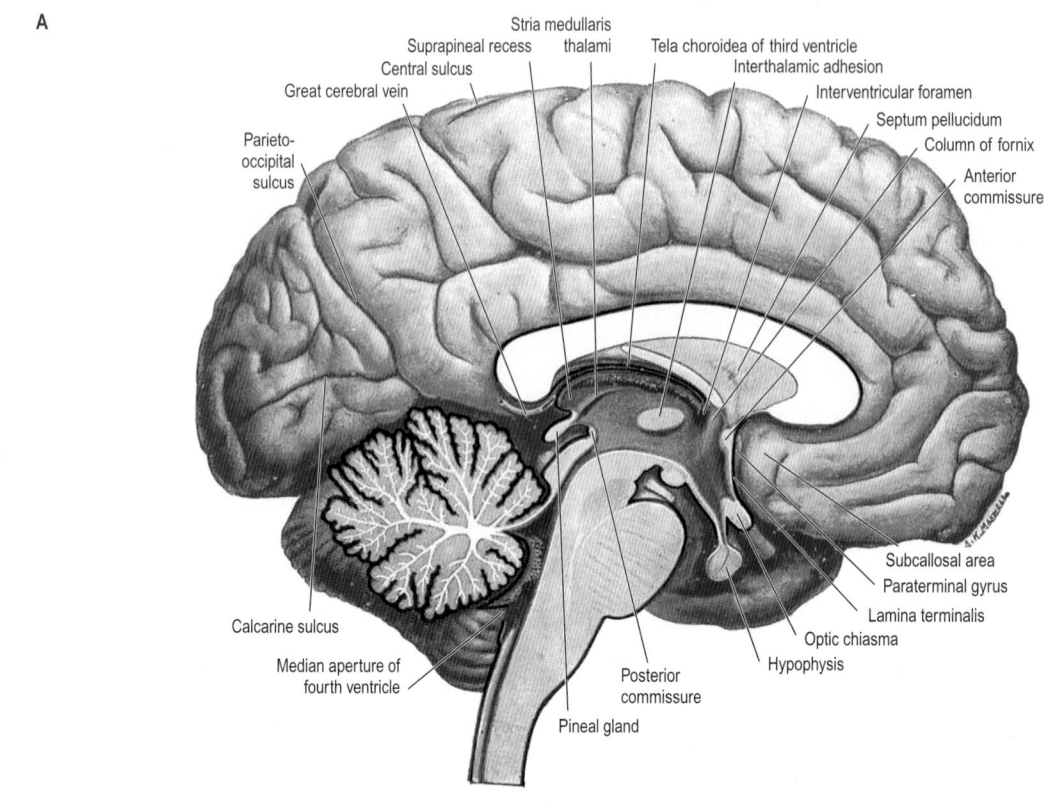

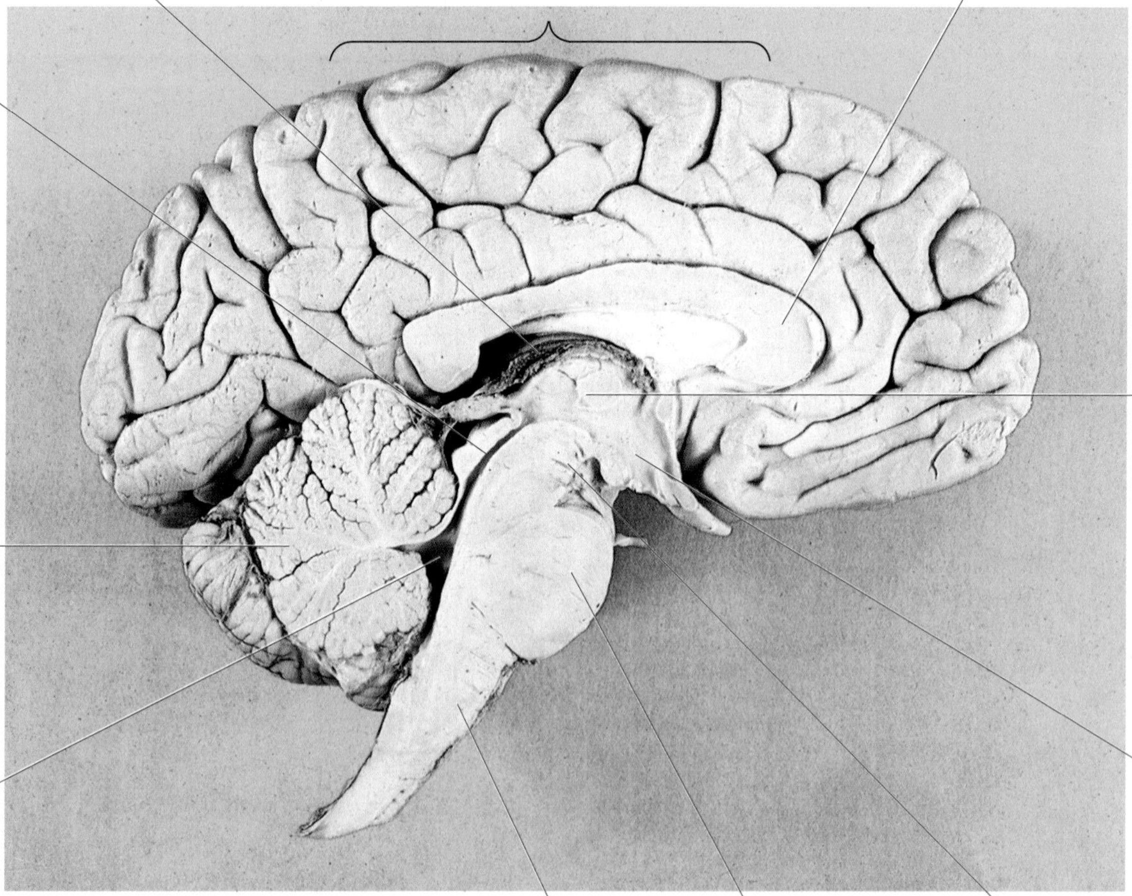

A

Stria medullaris
thalami

Suprapineal recess

Central sulcus

Great cerebral vein

Tela choroidea of third ventricle

Interthalamic adhesion

Interventricular foramen

Septum pellucidum

Column of fornix

Anterior
commissure

Parieto-
occipital
sulcus

Calcarine sulcus

Median aperture of
fourth ventricle

Pineal gland

Posterior
commissure

Hypophysis

Optic chiasma

Lamina terminalis

Paraterminal gyrus

Subcallosal area

Choroid plexus
of third ventricle

Cerebral hemisphere

Corpus
callosum

B

Cerebral
aqueduct

Cerebellum

Fourth
ventricle

Thalamus

Hypothalamus

Medulla

Pons

Midbrain

Fig. 16.8 **A**, Sagittal hemisection of the brain to show the third and fourth ventricles. Pia mater: red; ependyma: blue. **B**, Sagittal hemisection through the brain. (Hemisection by EL Rees; photograph by Kevin Fitzpatrick on behalf of GKT School of Medicine, London.)

Prior to the introduction of modern imaging techniques the anterior and posterior commissures could be identified by ventriculography. This led to the use of these two landmarks as the markers of the baseline used for stereotaxic surgical procedures. This convention is now universal and the positions of the anterior and posterior commissures are used as the basic reference points for most surgical atlases of brain anatomy. The narrow interventricular foramen is located immediately posterior to the column of the fornix and separates the fornix from the anterior nucleus of the thalamus.

There is a small, angular, optic recess at the base of the lamina terminalis, just dorsal to and extending into the optic chiasma. Behind it, the anterior part of the floor of the third ventricle is formed mainly by hypothalamic structures. Immediately behind the optic chiasma lies the thin infundibular recess, which extends into the pituitary stalk. Behind this recess, the tuber cinereum and the mammillary bodies form the floor of the ventricle.

The roof of the third ventricle is a thin ependymal layer that extends from its lateral walls to the choroid plexus, which spans the choroidal fissure (**Fig. 16.6**). Above this is the body of the fornix. The posterior boundary of the ventricle is marked by a suprapineal recess above the pineal gland, a pineal (epiphyseal) recess, which extends into the pineal stalk, and by the posterior commissure. Below the commissure the ventricle is continuous with the cerebral aqueduct of the midbrain.

CEREBRAL AQUEDUCT

The cerebral aqueduct is a small tube, roughly circular in transverse section and c.2 mm in diameter. It extends throughout the dorsal quarter of the midbrain in the midline and is surrounded by the central, periaqueductal, grey matter (**Fig. 16.8**). Rostrally, it commences immediately behind and below the posterior commissure, where it is continuous with the caudal aspect of the third ventricle. Caudally, it is continuous with the lumen of the fourth ventricle at the junction of the midbrain and pons. The superior and inferior colliculi are dorsal to the aqueduct and the midbrain tegmentum is ventral.

FOURTH VENTRICLE

The fourth ventricle lies between the brain stem and the cerebellum (**Figs 16.2, 16.7–16.10**). Rostrally it is continuous with the cerebral aqueduct, and caudally with the central canal of the spinal cord. In sagittal section, the fourth ventricle has a characteristic triangular profile, and the apex of its tented roof protrudes into the inferior aspect of the cerebellum. The ventricle is at its widest at the level of the pontomedullary junction, where a lateral recess on both sides extends to the lateral border of the brain stem. At this point the lateral aperture of the fourth ventricle (foramen of Luschka) provides access to the sub-arachnoid space at the cerebellopontine angle, and CSF flows through it into the lateral extension of the pontine cistern. Occasionally, a lateral recess may not open.

The floor of the fourth ventricle is a shallow diamond-shaped, or rhomboidal, depression (rhomboid fossa) on the dorsal surfaces of the pons and the rostral half of the medulla. It consists largely of grey matter and contains important cranial nerve nuclei. The precise location of some nuclei is discernable from surface features. The superior part of the ventricular floor is triangular in shape and is limited laterally by the superior cerebellar peduncles as they converge towards the cerebral aqueduct. Its posterior limit is called the obex. The inferior part of the ventricular floor is also triangular in shape. It is bounded caudally by the gracile and cuneate tubercles, which contain the dorsal column nuclei, and, more rostrally, by the diverging inferior cerebellar peduncles. A longitudinal median sulcus divides the floor of the fourth ventricle. Each half is itself divided, by an often indistinct sulcus limitans, into a medial region known as the medial eminence and a lateral region known as the vestibular area. The vestibular nuclei lie beneath the vestibular area. In the superior part of the ventricular floor, the medial eminence is represented by the facial colliculus, a small elevation produced by an underlying loop of efferent fibres from the facial nucleus, which covers the abducens nucleus. Between the facial colliculus and the vestibular area the sulcus limitans widens into a small depression, the superior fovea. In its upper part, the sulcus limitans constitutes the lateral limit of the floor of the fourth ventricle. Here a small region of bluish-grey pigmentation denotes the presence of the subjacent locus coeruleus. Inferior to the facial colliculus, at the level of the lateral recess of the ventricle, a variable group of nerve fibre fascicles, known as the striae medullaris, runs transversely across the ventricular

floor and passes into the median sulcus. In the inferior area of the floor of the fourth ventricle, the medial eminence is represented by the hypoglossal triangle (trigone), which lies over the hypoglossal nucleus. Laterally, the sulcus limitans widens to produce an indistinct inferior fovea. Caudal to the inferior fovea, between the hypoglossal triangle and the vestibular area, is the vagal triangle (trigone), which covers the dorsal vagal nucleus. The triangle is crossed below by a narrow translucent ridge, the funiculus separans, which is separated from the gracile tubercle by the small area postrema. The funiculus and area postrema are both covered by thickened ependyma, containing tanycytes; the area postrema also contains neurones. The blood–brain barrier is modified in both sites.

The roof of the fourth ventricle is formed by the superior and inferior medullary veli. Superiorly, a thin sheet of tissue, the superior medullary velum, stretches across the ventricle between the converging superior cerebellar peduncles (**Fig. 16.9**). The superior medullary velum is continuous with the cerebellar white matter and is covered dorsally by the lingula of the superior vermis. The inferior medullary velum is more complex and is mostly composed of a thin sheet, devoid of neural tissue, formed by ventricular ependyma and the pia mater of the tela choroidea, which covers it dorsally. A large median aperture (foramen of Magendie) is present in the roof of the ventricle as a perforation in the posterior medullary velum, just inferior to the nodule of the cerebellum. CSF flows from the ventricle through the foramen into the cerebellomedullary cistern.

CIRCUMVENTRICULAR ORGANS

The walls of the ventricular system are lined with ependymal cells (p. 53) beneath which lies a subependymal layer of glia. At certain sites, collectively referred to as circumventricular organs (**Fig. 16.11**), specialized ependymal cells called tanycytes are also present. Ependyma and tanycytes may be involved in secretion into the CSF; transport of neurochemicals from subjacent neurones, glia or vessels to the CSF; transport of neurochemicals from CSF to the same subjacent structures; chemoreception. In addition, in the adult, the ependymal and subependymal glial cell layers are the source of undifferentiated stem cells (Mercier et al 2002), currently under intensive study for their potential neurorestorative properties.

The circumventricular organs are midline sites in the ventricular walls (McKinley et al 2003) where the blood–brain barrier (p. 51) is absent. They include the vascular organ (organum vasculosum), subfornical organ, neurohypophysis, median eminence, subcommissural organ, pineal gland and area postrema.

The vascular organ – lies in the lamina terminalis between the optic chiasma and the anterior commissure. Its external zone contains a rich fenestrated vascular plexus, which covers glia and a network of nerve fibres. The ependymal cells of the vascular organ, like those of other circumventricular organs, are flattened and have few cilia. The major inputs appear to come from the subfornical organ, locus coeruleus and a number of hypothalamic nuclei, and the vascular organ projects to the median preoptic and supraoptic nuclei. The vascular organ is involved in the regulation of fluid balance and may also have neuroendocrine functions.

The subfornical organ – lies at the level of the interventricular foramen. It contains many neurones, glial cells and a dense fenestrated capillary plexus, and is covered by flattened ependyma. It is believed to have widespread hypothalamic interconnections and to function in the regulation of fluid balance and drinking.

The neurohypophysis (posterior pituitary) – is the site of termination of neurosecretory projections from the supraoptic and paraventricular nuclei of the hypothalamus. These neurones release vasopressin and oxytocin, respectively, into the capillary bed of the neurohypophysis where the hormones gain access to the general circulation.

The median eminence – contains the terminations of axons of hypothalamic neurosecretory cells. Peptides released from these axons control the hormonal secretions of the anterior pituitary via the pituitary portal system of vessels.

The subcommissural organ – lies ventral to and below the posterior commissure (i.e. near the inferior wall of the pineal recess). The ependymal

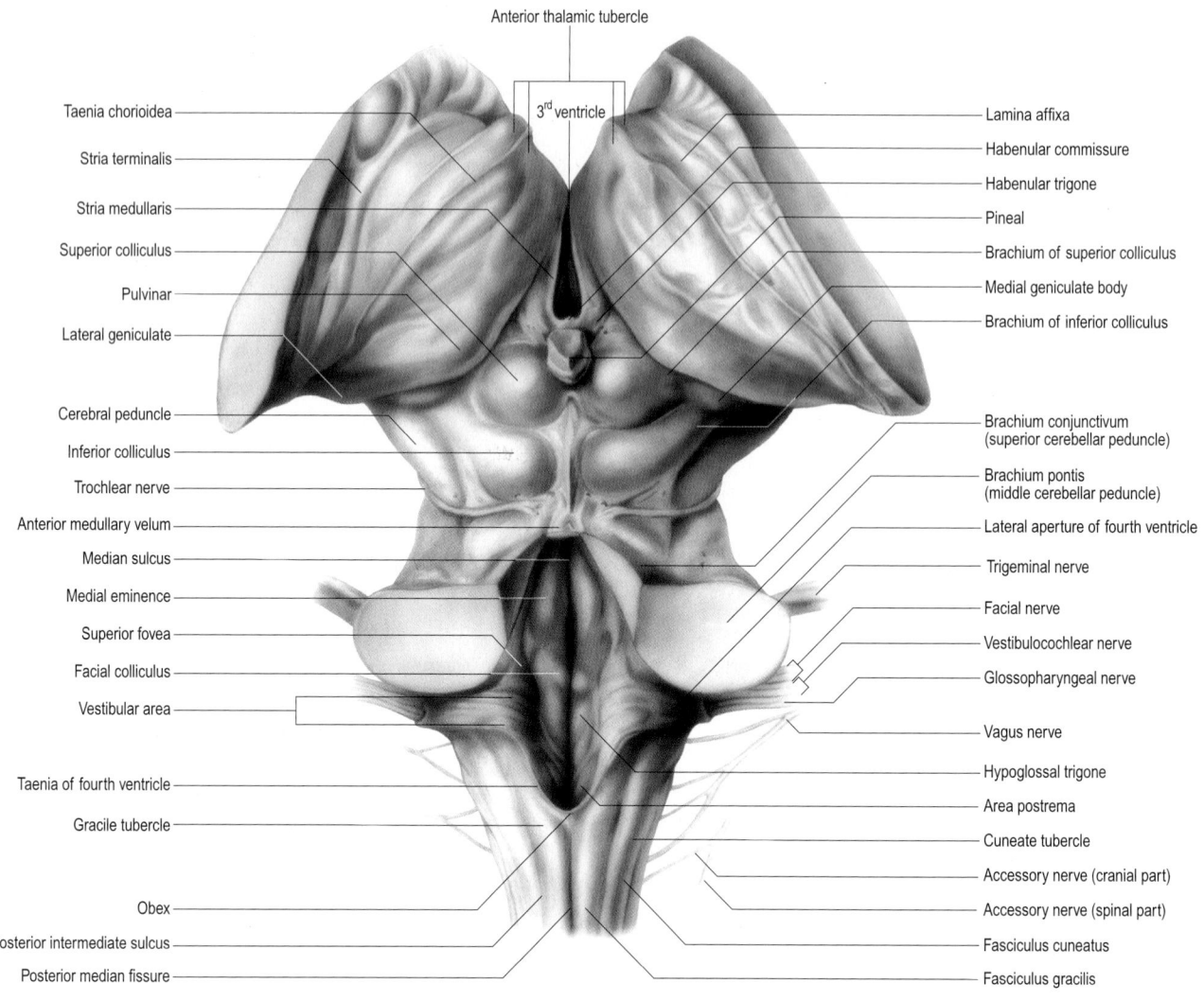

Anterior thalamic tubercle

Taenia chorioidea

Stria terminalis

Stria medullaris

Superior colliculus

Pulvinar

Lateral geniculate

Cerebral peduncle

Inferior colliculus

Trochlear nerve

Anterior medullary velum

Median sulcus

Medial eminence

Superior fovea

Facial colliculus

Vestibular area

Taenia of fourth ventricle

Gracile tubercle

Obex

Posterior intermediate sulcus

Posterior median fissure

3rd ventricle

Lamina affixa

Habenular commissure

Habenular trigone

Pineal

Brachium of superior colliculus

Medial geniculate body

Brachium of inferior colliculus

Brachium conjunctivum
(superior cerebellar peduncle)

Brachium pontis
(middle cerebellar peduncle)

Lateral aperture of fourth ventricle

Trigeminal nerve

Facial nerve

Vestibulocochlear nerve

Glossopharyngeal nerve

Vagus nerve

Hypoglossal trigone

Area postrema

Cuneate tubercle

Accessory nerve (cranial part)

Accessory nerve (spinal part)

Fasciculus cuneatus

Fasciculus gracilis

Fig. 16.9 The dorsal aspect of the brain stem. The floor of the fourth ventricle has been exposed by cutting the cerebellar peduncles and removing the cerebellum. (By permission from Neuroanatomy by FA Mettler (1948) 2nd edn; St Louis: The CV Mosby Company.)

cells on the dorsal aspect of the cerebral aqueduct are tall, columnar and ciliated, with granular basophilic cytoplasm. They may be involved in the secretion of materials into the CSF from adjoining axonal terminals or capillaries.

The pineal gland – is part of the epithalamus, located beneath the splenium of the corpus callosum. It secretes melatonin and is involved in the regulation of the circadian rhythm.

The area postrema – a bilaterally-paired structure located at the caudal limit of the floor of the fourth ventricle, is an important chemoreceptive area that triggers vomiting in response to the presence of emetic substances in the blood.

CHOROID PLEXUS AND CEREBROSPINAL FLUID

CHOROID PLEXUS

In the roofs of the third and fourth ventricles, and in the medial wall of the lateral ventricle along the line of the choroid fissure, the vascular pia mater lies in close apposition to the ependymal lining of the ventricles, without any intervening brain tissue. It forms the tela choroidea, which gives rise to the highly vascularized choroid plexuses from which CSF is secreted into the ventricles.

Choroid plexuses are located in the lateral ventricles, the third ventricle and the fourth ventricle (**Figs 16.3, 16.5, 16.6**).

In the lateral ventricle, the choroid plexus extends anteriorly as far as the interventricular foramen, through which it is continuous across the third ventricle with the plexus of the opposite lateral ventricle. From the interventricular foramen, the plexus passes posteriorly, in contact with the thalamus, curving round its posterior aspect to enter the inferior horn of the ventricle and reach the hippocampus. Throughout the body of the ventricle, the choroid fissure lies between the fornix superiorly and the thalamus inferiorly (**Fig. 16.6**).

From above, the tela choroidea is triangular with a rounded apex between the interventricular foramina, often indented by the anterior columns of the fornices (**Fig. 16.3**). Its lateral edges are irregular, and contain choroid vascular fringes. At the posterior basal angles of the tela, these fringes continue and curve on into the inferior horn of the ventricle, while centrally the pial layers depart from each other as described above. When the tela is removed, a transverse slit (the transverse fissure) is left between the splenium and the junction of the ventricular roof with the tectum. It marks the posterior limit of the extracerebral space enclosed by the posterior extensions of the corpus callosum above the third ventricle. The latter contains the roots of the choroid plexus of the third ventricle and of the lateral ventricles, enclosed between the two layers of pia mater (**Fig. 16.6**). The choroid plexus of the third ventricle is attached to the tela choroidea which is, in effect, the thin roof of the third ventricle as it develops during fetal life. In coronal sections of the cerebral hemispheres, the choroid plexus of the third ventricle can be seen in continuity with the choroid plexus of the lateral ventricles (**Fig. 16.6**).

The choroid plexus of the fourth ventricle is similar in structure to that of the lateral and third ventricles. Thus, the roof of the inferior part of the fourth ventricle develops as a thin sheet in which the pia mater is in direct contact with the ependymal lining of the ventricle. This thin sheet forms the tela choroidea of the fourth ventricle, lying between the

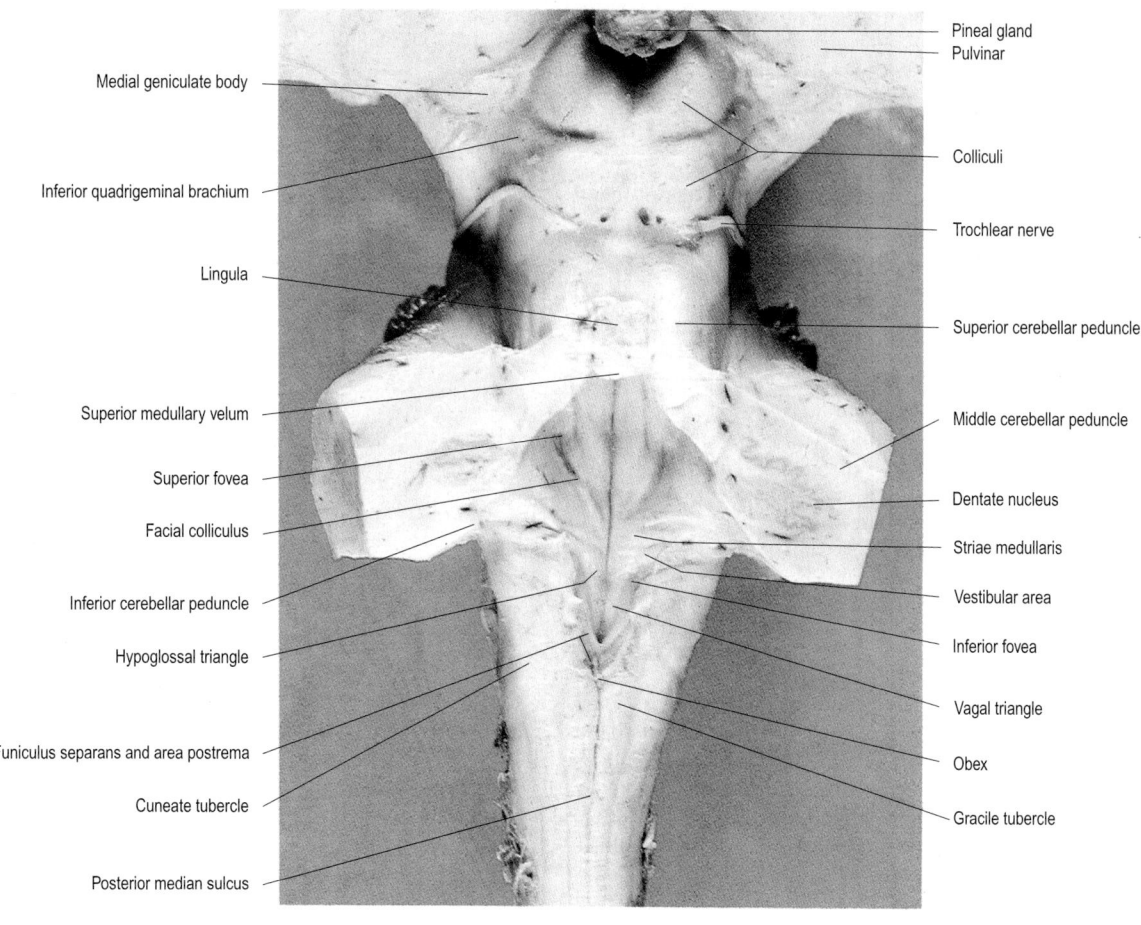

Pineal gland
Pulvinar
Colliculi
Trochlear nerve
Superior cerebellar peduncle
Middle cerebellar peduncle
Dentate nucleus
Striae medullaris
Vestibular area
Inferior fovea
Vagal triangle
Obex
Gracile tubercle

Medial geniculate body
Inferior quadrigeminal brachium
Lingula
Superior medullary velum
Superior fovea
Facial colliculus
Inferior cerebellar peduncle
Hypoglossal triangle
Funiculus separans and area postrema
Cuneate tubercle
Posterior median sulcus

Fig. 16.10 The dorsal aspect of the brain stem including the floor of the fourth ventricle.

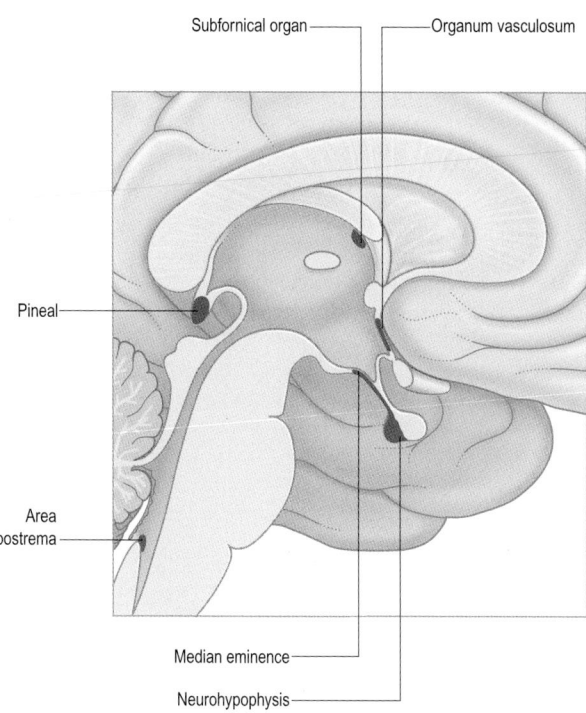

Subfornical organ
Organum vasculosum
Pineal
Area postrema
Median eminence
Neurohypophysis

Fig. 16.11 Median sagittal section of the brain indicating the locations of the circumventricular organs.

of Magendie) and are often prolonged on to the ventral aspect of the cerebellar vermis. The horizontal limbs of the plexus project into the lateral recesses of the ventricle. Small tufts of plexus pass through the lateral apertures (foramina of Luschka) and emerge, still covered by ependyma, in the subarachnoid space of the cerebellopontine angle.

The blood supply of the choroid plexus in the tela choroidea of the lateral and third ventricles is usually via a single vessel from the anterior choroidal branch of the internal carotid artery and several choroidal branches of the posterior cerebral artery. The two sets of vessels anastomose to some extent. Capillaries drain into a rich venous plexus served by a single choroidal vein. The blood supply of the fourth ventricular choroid plexus is from the inferior cerebellar arteries.

CEREBROSPINAL FLUID

Composition and secretion
CSF is a clear, colourless, liquid. In normal individuals CSF contains a very small amount of protein and differs from blood in its electrolyte content. It is not simply an ultrafiltrate of blood but is actively secreted by the choroid plexus epithelium. Choroid plexus epithelial cells have the characteristics of transport and secretory cells. Their apical surfaces, from which CSF is secreted, possess microvilli, and their basal surfaces exhibit interdigitations and folding. There are tight junctions at the apical ends of the epithelial cells, which are permeable to small molecular weight substances. Fenestrated capillaries in the stroma of the choroid plexus lie just beneath the epithelial cells. A blood–CSF barrier is sited at the choroid plexus epithelium.

Circulation and drainage
Most of the CSF is secreted by the choroid plexuses in the lateral, third and fourth ventricles. However, there is also a small contribution from the ependymal lining of the ventricles and from the extracellular fluid from the brain parenchyma.

The total CSF volume is c.150 ml, of which 125 ml is intracranial. The ventricles contain c.25 ml (almost all of which is in the later ventricles), and the remaining 100 ml is located in the cranial arachnoid space. CSF is secreted at a rate of 0.35–0.40 ml per m

cerebellum and the inferior part of the roof of the ventricle. The choroid plexus of the fourth ventricle is T-shaped, having vertical and horizontal limbs, but this form varies widely. The vertical (longitudinal) limb is double, flanks the midline and is adherent to the roof of the ventricle. The limbs fuse at the superior margin of the median aperture (foramen

which means that normally c.50% of the total volume of CSF is replaced every five to six hours. An effective means of removal from the cranial cavity is thus essential. CSF flows from the lateral ventricles to the third ventricle and then through the cerebral aqueduct to the fourth ventricle. Mixing of CSF from different choroidal sources occurs and is probably assisted by cilia on the ependymal cells lining the ventricles and by arterial pulsations. CSF leaves the fourth ventricle through the medial and lateral apertures to enter the subarachnoid space of the cisterna magna and subarachnoid cisterns over the front of the pons, respectively. The movement of CSF in the extra-axial space is complex and is characterized by a fast-flow component and a much slower bulk-flow component. During systole, the major arteries lying in the basal cisterns and other extra-axial intracranial spaces dilate significantly and exert pressure effects on the CSF, which cause rapid CSF flow around the brain out of the cranial cavity and into the upper cervical spine. The pressure wave which causes this outflow of CSF is dispersed through the spinal CSF space, which acts as a capacitance vessel. As the blood within the major arteries passes into the brain in late systole and diastole, CSF re-enters the skull from the spine. This CSF flow occurs at rapid rates and is repeated during every heart cycle. In addition, there is a slow bulk flow of CSF, with a time course measured in hours, which results in circulation of CSF over the cerebral surface in a superolateral direction. CSF is absorbed into the venous system through arachnoid villi associated with the major dural venous sinuses, predominantly the superior sagittal sinus.

Hydrocephalus

Obstruction of the circulation of CSF leads to accumulation of fluid (hydrocephalus), which causes compression of the brain (**Fig. 16.12**). Within the brain, critical points at which obstruction may occur correspond to the narrow foramina and passages of the ventricular system. Thus, obstruction of the interventricular foramen causes enlargement of the lateral ventricles. Obstruction of the cerebral aqueduct leads to enlargement of both the lateral ventricles and the third ventricle. Obstruction or congenital absence of the apertures of the fourth ventricle leads to enlargement of the entire ventricular system. Obstruction or restriction of CSF circulation can also occur within the subarachnoid space as a result of meningeal adhesions caused by meningitis. When this occurs at the level of the tentorial notch, passage of CSF from the posterior fossa to its sites of reabsorption is restricted.

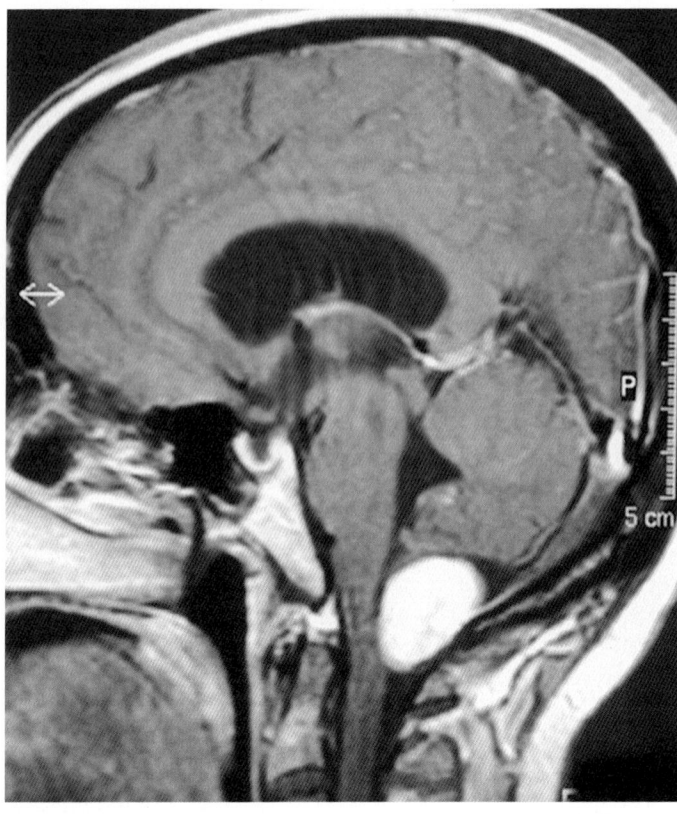

Fig. 16.12 MR scan showing an enhancing mass which is a meningioma growing from the meninges at the edge of the foramen magnum. The tumour is benign but is causing compression of the brain stem and secondary hydrocephalus. (By kind permission from Professor Alan Jackson, Professor of Neuroradiology, University of Manchester.)

REFERENCES

McKinley MJ, McAllen RM, Davern P, Giles ME, Penschow J, Sunn N, Uschakov A, Oldfield BJ 2003 The sensory circumventricular organs of the mammalian brain. Adv Anat Embryol Cell Biol 172: III–XII, 1–122.

Mercier F, Kitasako JT, Hatton GI. 2002 Anatomy of the brain neurogenic zones revisited: fractones and the fibroblast/macrophage network. J Comp Neurol 451(2): 170–88.
Describes the structure and ultrastructure of the basal laminae and subependymal layer.

Paulson OB 2002 Blood–brain barrier, brain metabolism and cerebral blood flow. Eur Neuropsychopharmacol 12(6): 495–501.

Strazielle N, Ghersi-Egea JF 2000 Choroid plexus in the central nervous system: biology and physiopathology. J Neuropathol Exp Neurol 59(7): 561–74.
Describes choroid plexus functions in brain development, transfer of neuro-humoral information, brain/immune system interactions, brain aging, and cerebral pharmacotoxicology.

Wolburg H, Lippoldt A. 2002 Tight junctions of the blood–brain barrier: development, composition and regulation. Vascul Pharmacol 38(6): 323–37.
Reviews the molecular properties of the tight junctions between endothelial cells which constitute the blood–brain barrier.

Vascular supply of the brain

Chapter

17

The brain is a highly vascular organ, its profuse blood supply characterized by a densely branching arterial network (**Fig. 17.1**). It has a high metabolic activity due in part to the energy requirements of constant neural activity. It demands about 15% of the cardiac output and utilizes 25% of the total oxygen consumption of the body. The brain is supplied by two internal carotid arteries and two vertebral arteries which form a complex anastomosis (circulus arteriosus, circle of Willis) on the base of the brain. Vessels diverge from this anastomosis to supply the various cerebral regions. In general, the internal carotid arteries and the vessels arising from them supply the forebrain, with the exception of the occipital lobe of the cerebral hemisphere, whereas the vertebral arteries and their branches supply the occipital lobe, the brain stem and the cerebellum. Venous blood from the brain drains into sinuses within the dura mater. Acute interruption of the blood supply to the brain for more than a few minutes causes permanent neurological damage. Such ischaemic strokes along with intracranial haemorrhage are major contemporary sources of morbidity and mortality.

ARTERIAL SUPPLY OF THE BRAIN

The arterial supply of the brain is derived from the internal carotid and vertebral arteries, which lie, together with their proximal branches, within the subarachnoid space at the base of the brain.

INTERNAL CAROTID ARTERY (Figs 17.2, 17.3)

The internal carotid arteries and their major branches (sometimes referred to as the internal carotid system) essentially supply blood to the forebrain, with the exception of the occipital lobe.

The internal carotid artery (Figs 17.2, 17.3) arises from the bifurcation of the common carotid artery, ascends in the neck and enters the carotid canal of the temporal bone. Its subsequent course is said to have petrous, cavernous and cranial parts.

Petrous part

The petrous part of the internal carotid artery ascends in the carotid canal, and curves anteromedially and then superomedially above the cartilage filling the foramen lacerum, to enter the cranial cavity. It lies at first anterior to the cochlea and tympanic cavity, and is separated from the latter and the pharyngotympanic tube by a thin, bony lamella which is cribriform in the young and partly absorbed in old age. Further anteriorly it is separated from the trigeminal ganglion by the thin roof of the carotid canal, although this is often deficient. The artery is surrounded by a venous plexus and the carotid autonomic plexus, which is derived from the internal carotid branch of the superior cervical ganglion. The petrous part of the artery gives rise to two branches. The caroticotympanic artery is a small, occasionally double, vessel which enters the tympanic cavity by a foramen in the carotid canal and anastomoses with the anterior

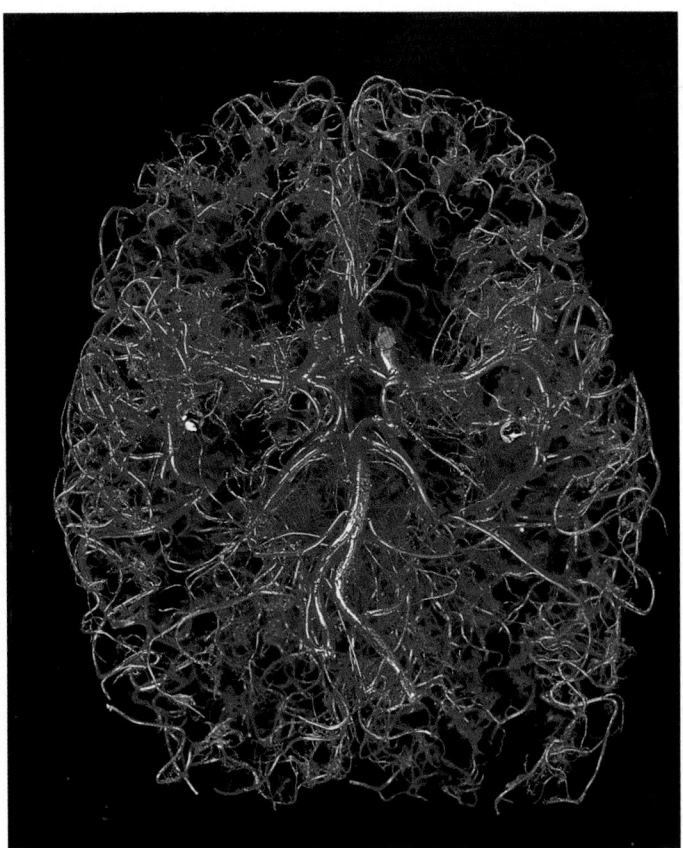

Fig. 17.1 Resin cast of the arterial supply of the brain. (Photograph by Sarah-Jane Smith.)

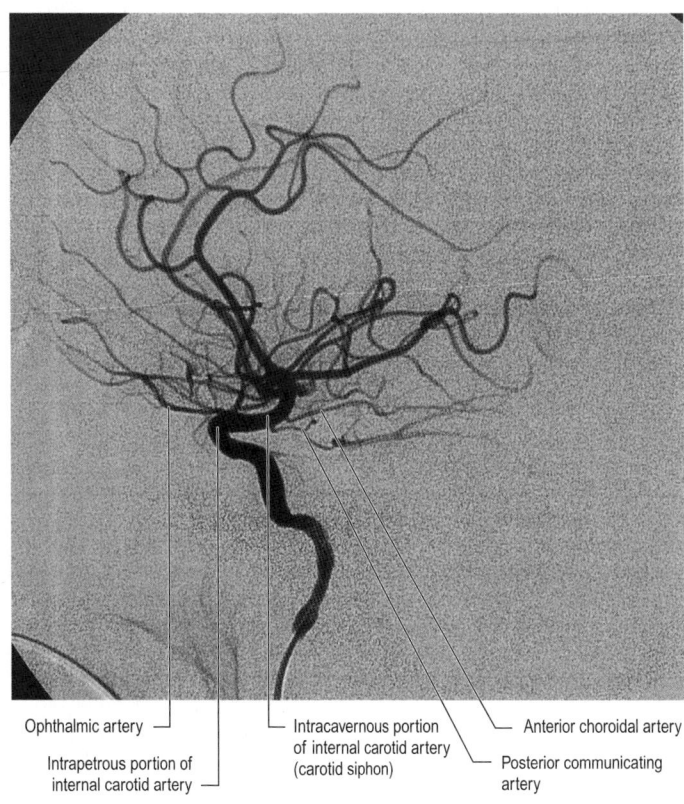

Ophthalmic artery

Intrapetrous portion of internal carotid artery

Intracavernous portion of internal carotid artery (carotid siphon)

Anterior choroidal artery

Posterior communicating artery

Fig. 17.2 Internal carotid arteriogram. This image is a lateral projection obtained by intra-arterial digital subtraction angiography. (By kind permission from Professor PD Griffiths, Academic Unit of Radiology, The University of Sheffield.)

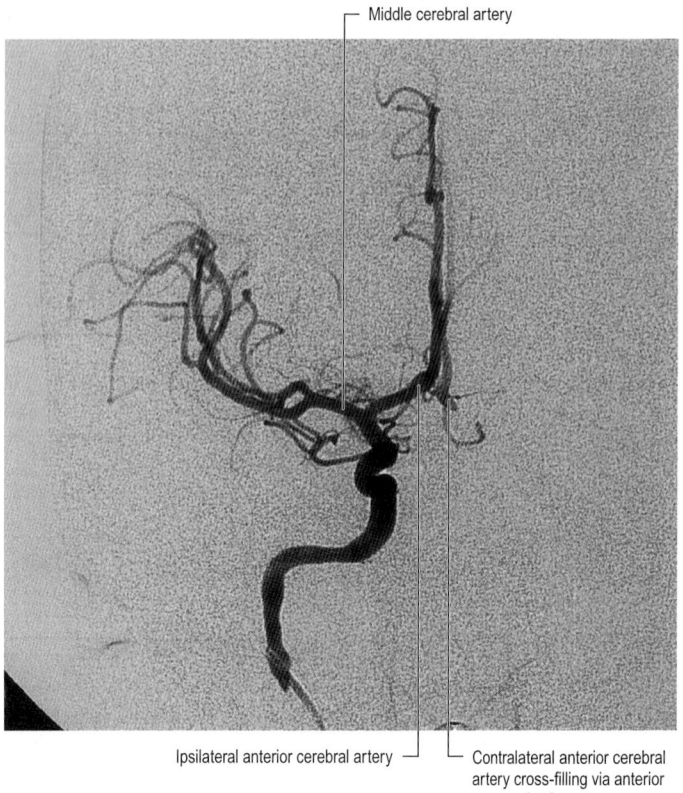

Middle cerebral artery

Ipsilateral anterior cerebral artery

Contralateral anterior cerebral artery cross-filling via anterior communicating artery

Fig. 17.3 Internal carotid arteriogram. This image is a Towne's projection obtained by intra-arterial digital subtraction angiography. (By kind permission from Professor PD Griffiths, Academic Unit of Radiology, The University of Sheffield.)

tympanic branch of the maxillary artery and the stylomastoid artery. The pterygoid artery is inconsistent. When present, it enters the pterygoid canal with the nerve of the same name, and anastomoses with a (recurrent) branch of the greater palatine artery.

Cavernous part

The cavernous part of the internal carotid artery ascends to the posterior clinoid process. It turns anteriorly to the side of the sphenoid within the cavernous sinus and then curves up medial to the anterior clinoid process, to emerge through the dural roof of the sinus. Occasionally, the two clinoid processes form a bony ring round the artery, which is also surrounded by a sympathetic plexus. The oculomotor, trochlear, ophthalmic and abducens nerves are lateral to it (p. 279).

This part of the artery gives off a number of small vessels. Cavernous branches supply the trigeminal ganglion, the walls of the cavernous and inferior petrosal sinuses and the nerves contained therein. A minute meningeal branch passes over the lesser sphenoid wing to supply the dura mater and bone in the anterior cranial fossa and also anastomoses with a meningeal branch of the posterior ethmoidal artery. Numerous small hypophyseal branches supply the neurohypophysis, and are of particular importance because they form the pituitary portal system (p. 382).

Cerebral part

After piercing the dura mater, the internal carotid artery turns back below the optic nerve to run between the optic and oculomotor nerves. It reaches the anterior perforated substance at the medial end of the lateral cerebral fissure and terminates by dividing into large anterior and middle cerebral arteries.

Several preterminal vessels leave the cerebral portion of the internal carotid. The ophthalmic artery arises from the internal carotid as it leaves the cavernous sinus, often at the point of piercing the dura, and enters the orbit through the optic canal. The posterior communicating artery (**Figs 17.4, 17.5, 17.6**) runs back from the internal carotid above the oculomotor nerve, and anastomoses with the posterior

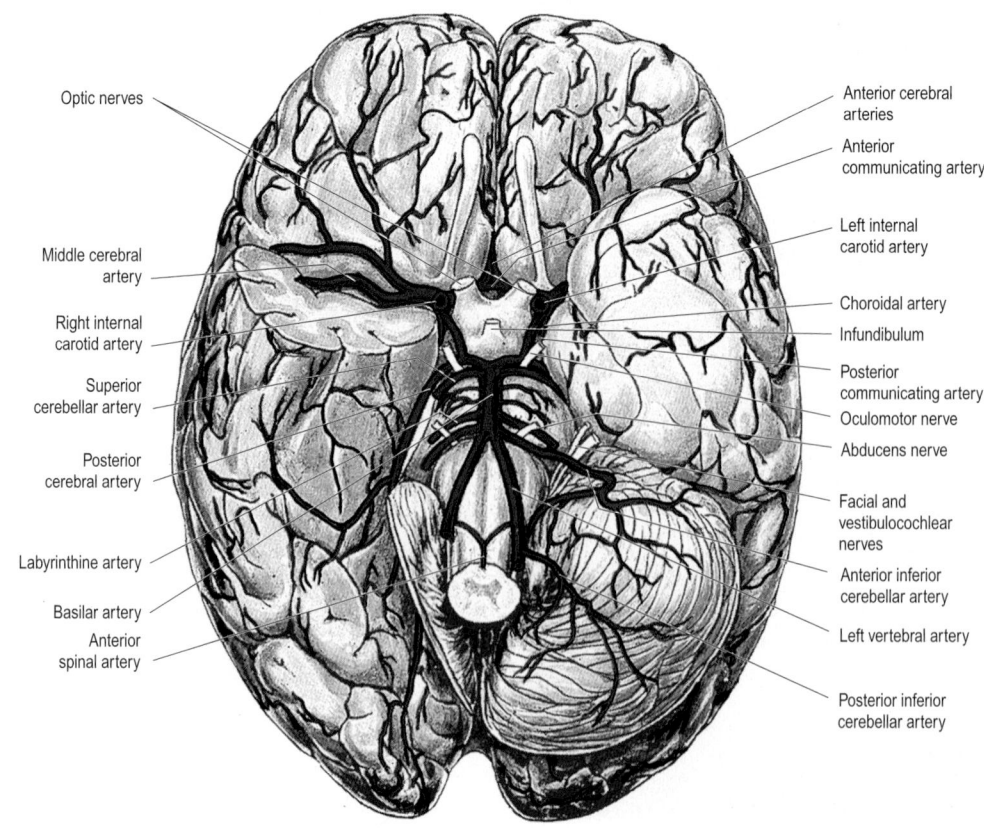

Optic nerves

Middle cerebral artery

Right internal carotid artery

Superior cerebellar artery

Posterior cerebral artery

Labyrinthine artery

Basilar artery

Anterior spinal artery

Anterior cerebral arteries

Anterior communicating artery

Left internal carotid artery

Choroidal artery

Infundibulum

Posterior communicating artery

Oculomotor nerve

Abducens nerve

Facial and vestibulocochlear nerves

Anterior inferior cerebellar artery

Left vertebral artery

Posterior inferior cerebellar artery

Fig. 17.4 The arteries on the base of the brain. The anterior part of the right temporal lobe has been removed to display the initial course of the middle cerebral artery within the lateral fissure.

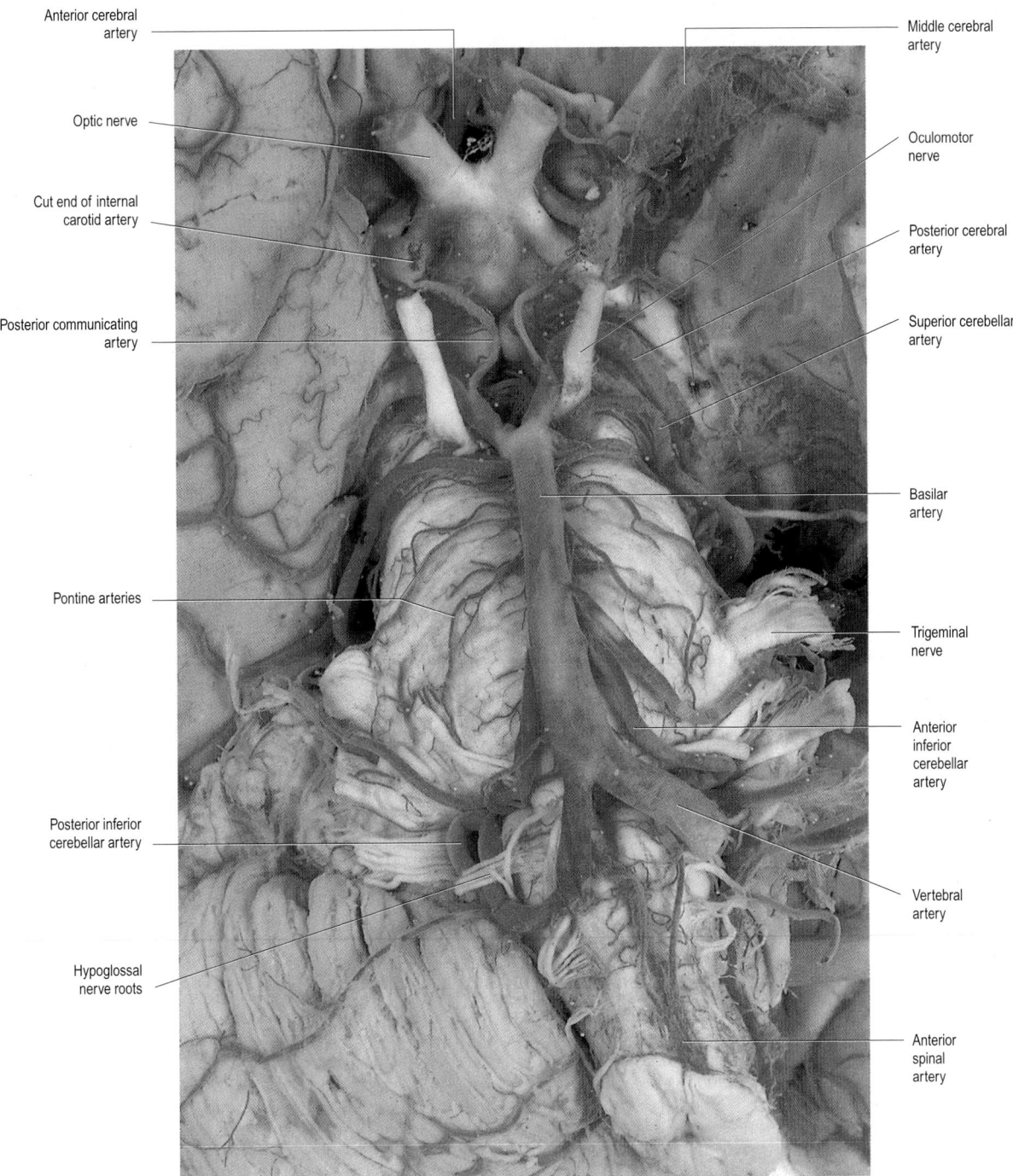

Anterior cerebral artery

Optic nerve

Cut end of internal carotid artery

Posterior communicating artery

Pontine arteries

Posterior inferior cerebellar artery

Hypoglossal nerve roots

Middle cerebral artery

Oculomotor nerve

Posterior cerebral artery

Superior cerebellar artery

Basilar artery

Trigeminal nerve

Anterior inferior cerebellar artery

Vertebral artery

Anterior spinal artery

Fig. 17.5 Arteries on the base of the brain injected with resin. (By permission from Crossman AR, Neary D 2000 Neuroanatomy, 2nd edn. Edinburgh: Churchill Livingstone.)

cerebral artery (which is a terminal branch of the basilar artery), thereby contributing to the circulus arteriosus around the interpeduncular fossa. The posterior communicating artery is usually very small. Sometimes, however, it is so large that the posterior cerebral artery is supplied via the posterior communicating artery rather than from the basilar artery ('fetal posterior communicating artery'). It is often larger on one side. Small branches from its posterior half pierce the posterior perforated substance together with branches from the posterior cerebral artery. Collectively they supply the medial thalamic surface and walls of the third ventricle. The anterior choroidal artery leaves the internal carotid near its posterior communicating branch and passes back above the medial part of the uncus. It crosses the optic tract to reach and supply the crus cerebri of the midbrain, then turns laterally, recrosses the optic tract, and gains the lateral side of the lateral geniculate body, which it supplies with several branches. It finally enters the inferior horn of the lateral ventricle via the choroidal fissure and ends in the choroid plexus. This small, but important, vessel also contributes to the

blood supply of the globus pallidus, caudate nucleus, amygdala, hypothalamus, tuber cinereum, red nucleus, substantia nigra, posterior limb of the internal capsule, optic radiation, optic tract, hippocampus and the fimbria of the fornix.

ANTERIOR CEREBRAL ARTERY

The anterior cerebral artery is the smaller of the two terminal branches of the internal carotid (**Figs 17.5, 17.6**).

The surgical nomenclature divides the vessel into three parts: A_1 – from the termination of the internal carotid artery to the junction with the anterior communicating artery; A_2 – from the junction with the anterior communicating artery to the origin of the callosomarginal artery; and A_3 – distal to the origin of the callosomarginal artery. This segment is also known as the pericallosal artery.

The anterior cerebral artery starts at the medial end of the stem of the lateral cerebral fissure and passes anteromedially above the optic nerve to the great longitudinal fissure where it connects with its fellow

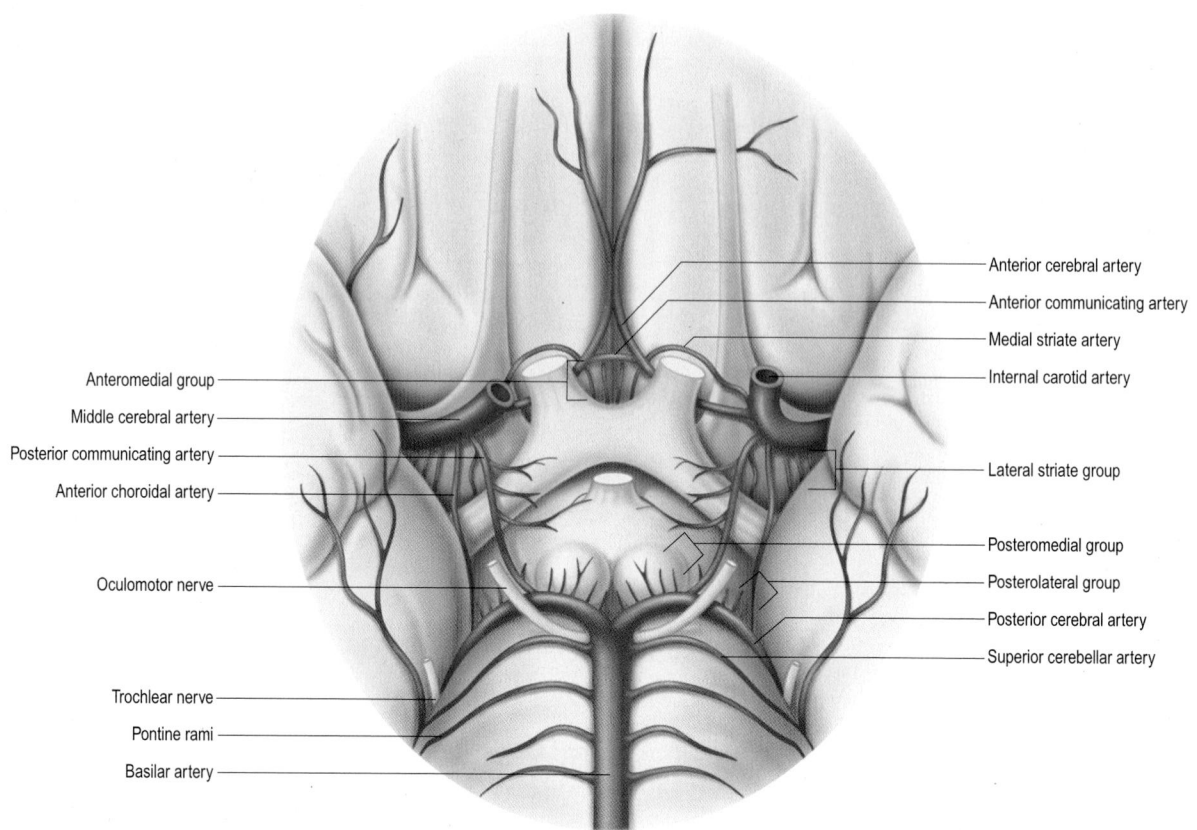

Anterior cerebral artery
Anterior communicating artery
Medial striate artery
Internal carotid artery

Anteromedial group
Middle cerebral artery
Posterior communicating artery
Anterior choroidal artery

Lateral striate group

Oculomotor nerve

Posteromedial group
Posterolateral group
Posterior cerebral artery
Superior cerebellar artery

Trochlear nerve
Pontine rami
Basilar artery

Fig. 17.6 The circulus arteriosus on the base of the brain showing the distribution of central (perforating or ganglionic) branches. The anteromedial, posteromedial, posterolateral and anterolateral (lateral striate) vessels are shown. The medial striate and anterior choroidal arteries are also shown.

by a short transverse anterior communicating artery. The anterior communicating artery is c.4 mm in length and may be double. It gives off numerous anteromedial central branches which supply the optic chiasma, lamina terminalis, hypothalamus, para-olfactory areas, anterior columns of the fornix and the cingulate gyrus.

The two anterior cerebral arteries travel together in the great longitudinal fissure. They pass around the curve of the genu of the corpus callosum (**Fig. 17.7**) and then along its upper surface to its posterior end, where they anastomose with posterior cerebral arteries. They give off cortical and central branches.

The cortical branches of the anterior cerebral artery are named by distribution. Two or three orbital branches ramify on the orbital surface of the frontal lobe and supply the olfactory cortex, gyrus rectus and medial orbital gyrus. Frontal branches supply the corpus callosum, cingulate gyrus, medial frontal gyrus and paracentral lobule. Parietal branches supply the precuneus, while the frontal and parietal branches both send twigs over the superomedial border of the hemisphere to supply a strip of territory on the superolateral surface (**Fig. 17.8**). Cortical branches of the anterior cerebral artery therefore supply the areas of the motor and somatosensory cortices which represent the lower limb (p. 389).

Central branches of the anterior cerebral artery arise from its proximal portion and enter the anterior perforated substance (**Fig.17.6**) and lamina terminalis. Collectively, they supply the rostrum of the corpus callosum, the septum pellucidum, the anterior part of the putamen, the head of the caudate nucleus and adjacent parts of the internal capsule. Immediately proximal or distal to its junction with the anterior communicating artery, the anterior cerebral artery gives rise to the medial striate artery which supplies the anterior part of the head of the caudate nucleus and adjacent regions of the putamen and internal capsule.

MIDDLE CEREBRAL ARTERY

The middle cerebral artery is the larger terminal branch of the internal carotid.

The surgical nomenclature identifies four subdivisions: M_1 – from the termination of the internal carotid artery to the bi/trifurcation, this segment is also known as the sphenoidal; M_2 – the segment running in the lateral (Sylvian) fissure, also known as the insular; M_3 – coming out of the lateral fissure, also known as the operator; and M_4 – cortical portions.

The middle cerebral artery runs first in the lateral cerebral fissure, then posterosuperiorly on the insula, and divides into branches distributed to this and the adjacent lateral cerebral surface (**Figs 17.5, 17.6, 17.8**). Like the anterior cerebral, it has cortical and central branches.

Cortical branches send orbital vessels to the inferior frontal gyrus and the lateral orbital surface of the frontal lobe. Frontal branches supply the precentral, middle and inferior frontal gyri. Two parietal branches are distributed to the postcentral gyrus, the lower part of the superior parietal lobule and the whole inferior parietal lobule. Two or three temporal branches supply the lateral surface of the temporal lobe. Cortical branches of the middle cerebral therefore supply the motor and somatosensory cortices representing the whole of the body other than the lower limb, the auditory area (p. 400) and the insula.

Small central branches of the middle cerebral artery, the lateral striate or lenticulostriate arteries, arise at its commencement and enter the anterior perforated substance together with the medial striate artery. Lateral striate arteries ascend in the external capsule over the lower lateral aspect of the lentiform complex, then turn medially, traverse the lentiform complex and the internal capsule and extend as far as the caudate nucleus.

VERTEBRAL ARTERY

The vertebral arteries and their major branches (sometimes referred to as the 'vertebrobasilar system') essentially supply blood to the upper spinal cord, the brain stem, cerebellum and occipital lobe of the cerebrum (**Figs 17.9, 17.10**). In addition, other branches have a wider distribution.

The vertebral arteries are derived from the subclavian arteries. They ascend through the neck in the foramina transversaria of the upper six cervical vertebrae and enter the cranial cavity through the foramen magnum, close to the anterolateral aspect of the medulla (**Fig. 17.5**). They converge medially as they ascend the medulla and unite to form

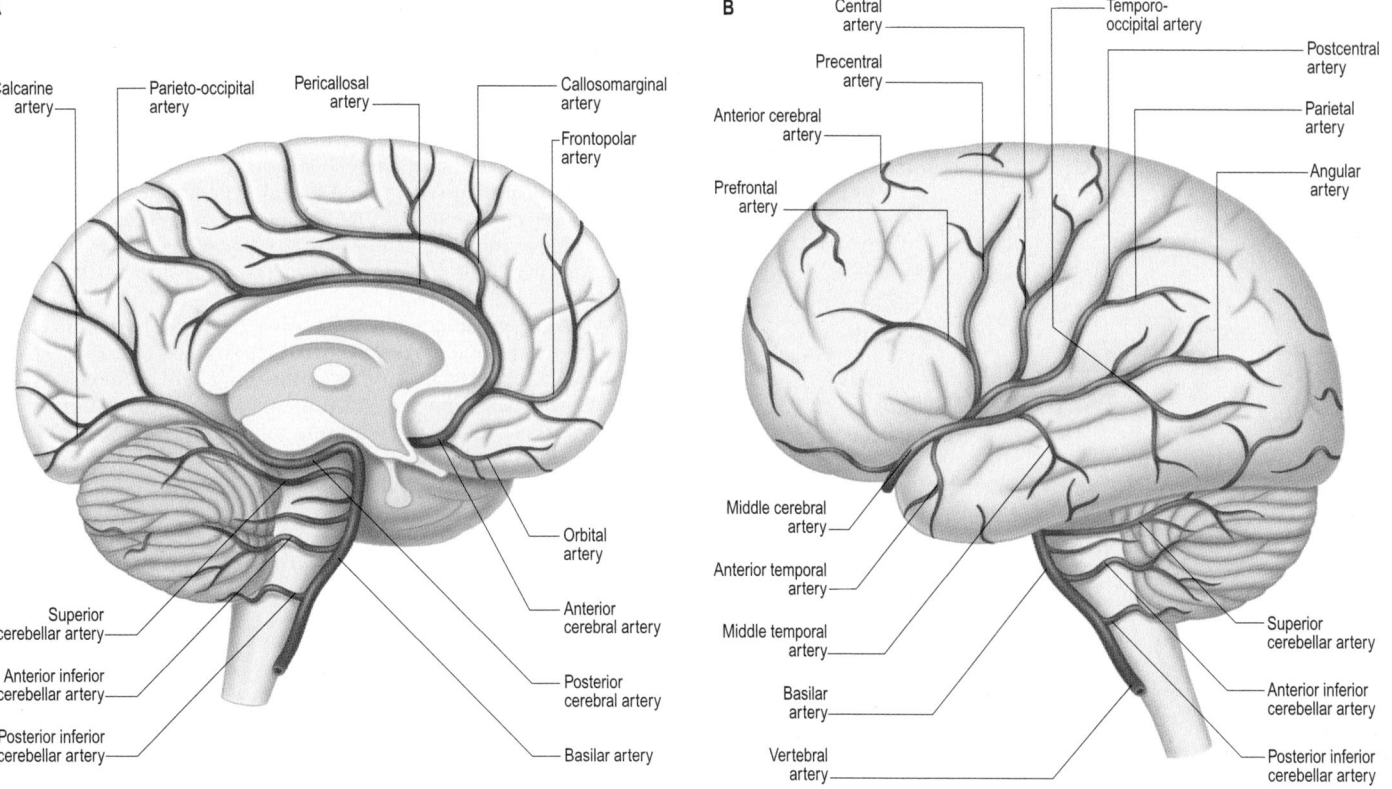

Fig. 17.7 Major arteries of the brain. **A,** medial aspect; **B,** lateral aspect.

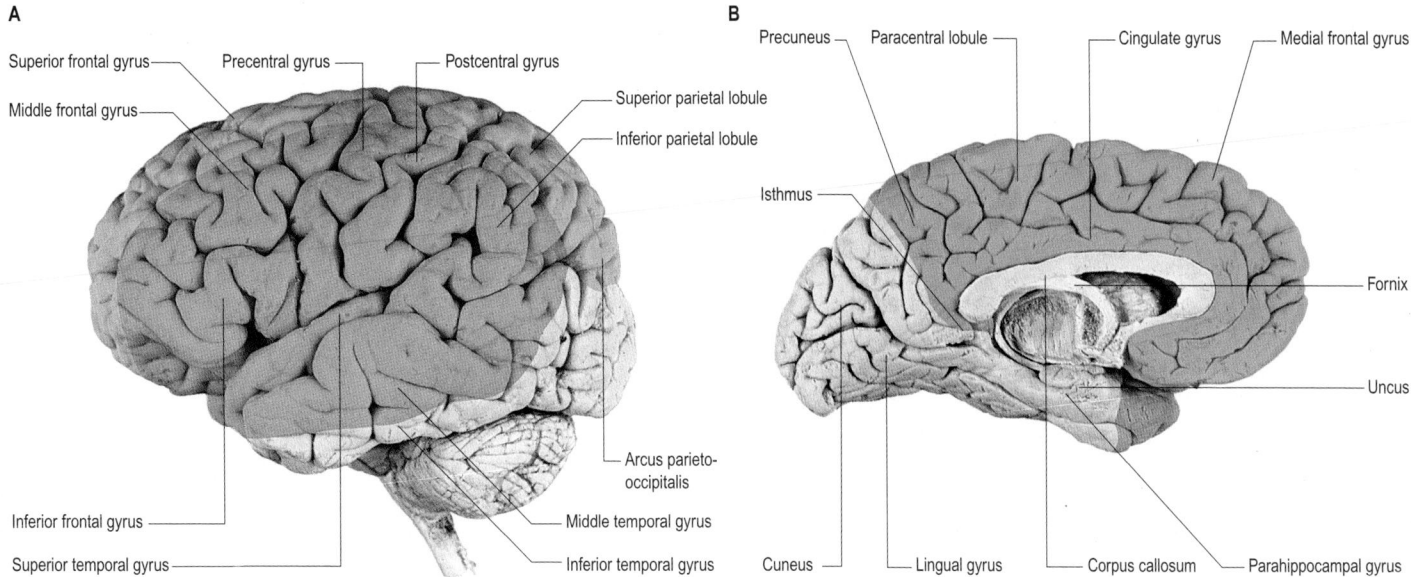

Fig. 17.8 **A,** The lateral surface of the left cerebral hemisphere, showing the areas supplied by the cerebral arteries. **B,** The medial surface of the left cerebral hemisphere, showing the areas supplied by the cerebral arteries. In these figures the area supplied by the anterior cerebral artery is coloured blue, that by the middle cerebral artery pink and that by the posterior cerebral artery is yellow.

the midline basilar artery at approximately the level of the junction between medulla and pons.

One or two meningeal branches arise from the vertebral artery near the foramen magnum. These ramify between the bone and dura mater in the posterior cranial fossa, and supply bone, diploë and the falx cerebelli.

A small anterior spinal artery arises near the end of the vertebral artery, and descends anterior to the medulla oblongata to unite with its fellow from the opposite side at mid-medullary level. The single trunk then descends on the ventral midline of the spinal cord, and is reinforced

sequentially by small spinal rami from the vertebral, ascending cervical, posterior intercostal and first lumbar arteries, which all enter the vertebral canal via intervertebral foramina (Ch. 46). Branches from the anterior spinal arteries and the beginning of their common trunk are distributed to the medulla oblongata.

The largest branch of the vertebral artery is the posterior inferior cerebellar artery. It arises near the lower end of the olive, which it curves back around, and then ascends behind the roots of the glossopharyngeal and vagus nerves to reach the inferior border of the pons. Here it curves and descends along the inferolateral border of the fourth ventricle before

299

Basilar artery — Posterior cerebral artery

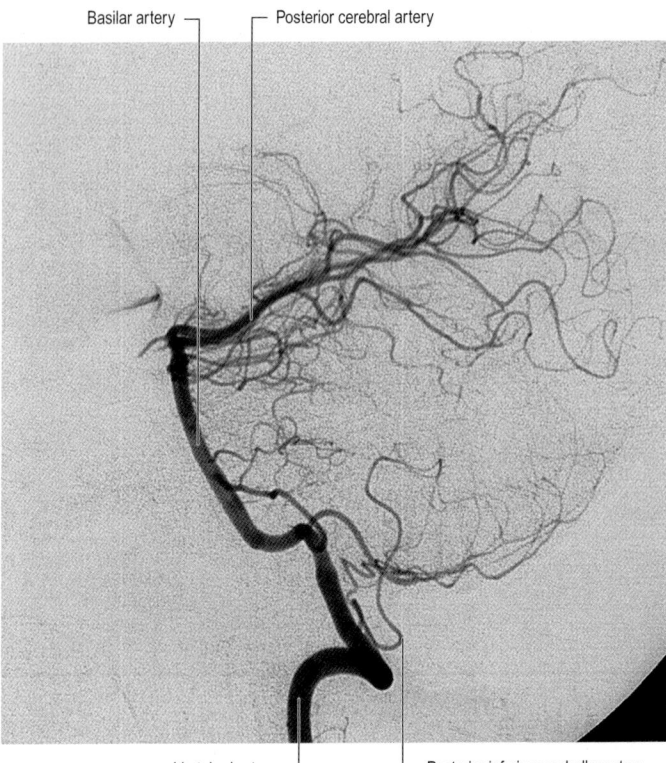

Vertebral artery — Posterior inferior cerebellar artery

Fig. 17.9 Vertebral arteriogram. This image is a lateral projection obtained by intra-arterial digital subtraction angiography. (By kind permission from Professor PD Griffiths, Academic Unit of Radiology, The University of Sheffield.)

Right posterior cerebral artery — Superior cerebellar artery

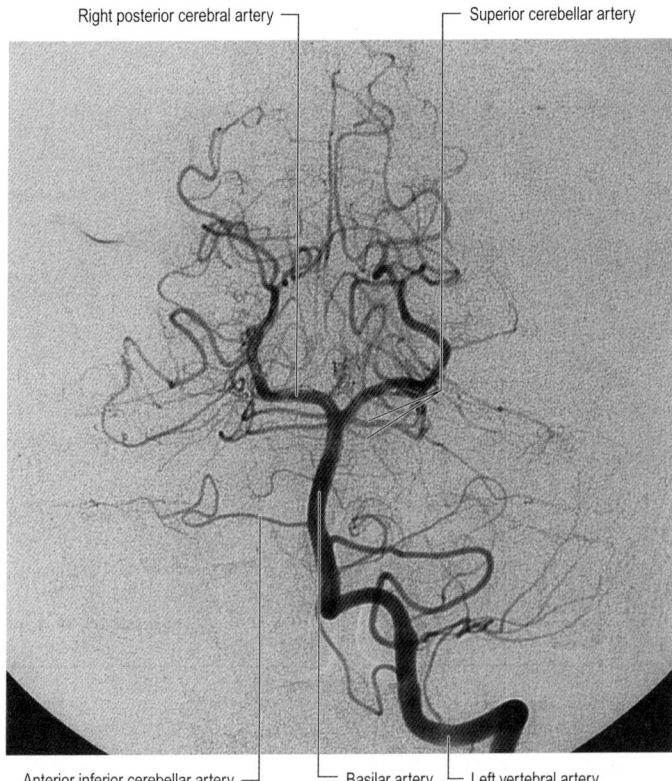

Anterior inferior cerebellar artery — Basilar artery — Left vertebral artery

Fig. 17.10 Vertebral arteriogram. This image is a Towne's projection obtained by intra-arterial digital subtraction angiography. (By kind permission from Professor PD Griffiths, Academic Unit of Radiology, The University of Sheffield.)

it turns laterally into the cerebellar vallecula between the hemispheres, and divides into medial and lateral branches. The medial branch runs back between the cerebellar hemisphere and inferior vermis, and supplies both. The lateral branch supplies the inferior cerebellar surface as far as its lateral border and anastomoses with the anterior inferior and superior cerebellar arteries (from the basilar artery). The trunk of the posterior inferior cerebellar artery supplies the medulla oblongata dorsal to the olivary nucleus and lateral to the hypoglossal nucleus and its emerging nerve roots. It also supplies the choroid plexus of the fourth ventricle and sends a branch lateral to the cerebellar tonsil to supply the dentate nucleus. The posterior inferior cerebellar artery is sometimes absent.

A posterior spinal artery usually arises from the posterior inferior cerebellar artery but it may come directly from the vertebral artery near the medulla oblongata. It passes posteriorly and descends as two branches which lie anterior and posterior to the dorsal roots of the spinal nerves. These are reinforced by spinal twigs from the vertebral, ascending cervical, posterior intercostal and first lumbar arteries, all of which reach the vertebral canal by the intervertebral foramina, thereby sustaining the posterior spinal arteries to the lower spinal levels (Ch. 46).

Minute medullary arteries arise from the vertebral artery and its branches and are distributed widely to the medulla oblongata.

BASILAR ARTERY

This large median vessel is formed by the union of the vertebral arteries at the mid-medullary level and extends to the upper border of the pons (**Figs 17.5, 17.6**). It lies in the pontine cistern, and follows a shallow median groove on the ventral pontine surface. The basilar artery terminates by dividing into two posterior cerebral arteries at a variable level but most frequently in the interpeduncular cistern, behind the dorsum sellae.

Numerous small pontine branches arise from the front and sides of the basilar artery along its course and supply the pons. The long and slender labyrinthine (internal auditory) artery has a variable origin. It usually arises from the anterior inferior cerebellar artery, but variations in its origin include the lower part of the basilar artery, the superior cerebellar artery or, occasionally, the posterior inferior cerebellar artery. The labyrinthine artery accompanies the facial and vestibulocochlear nerves into the internal acoustic meatus and is distributed to the internal ear.

The anterior inferior cerebellar artery (**Fig. 17.6**) is given off from the lower part of the basilar artery and runs posterolaterally, usually ventral to the abducens, facial and vestibulocochlear nerves. It commonly exhibits a loop into the internal acoustic meatus below the nerves, and when this occurs, the labyrinthine artery may arise from the loop. The anterior inferior cerebellar artery supplies the inferior cerebellar surface anterolaterally and anastomoses with the posterior inferior cerebellar branch of the vertebral artery. A few branches supply the inferolateral parts of the pons and occasionally also supply the upper medulla oblongata.

The superior cerebellar artery (**Fig. 17.6**) arises near the distal portion of the basilar artery, immediately before the formation of the posterior cerebral arteries. It passes laterally below the oculomotor nerve, which separates it from the posterior cerebral artery, and curves round the cerebral peduncle below the trochlear nerve to gain the superior cerebellar surface. Here it divides into branches which ramify in the pia mater and supply this aspect of the cerebellum, and also anastomose with branches of the inferior cerebellar arteries. The superior cerebellar artery supplies the pons, pineal body, superior medullary velum and tela choroidea of the third ventricle.

POSTERIOR CEREBRAL ARTERY

The posterior cerebral artery (**Figs 17.5, 17.6**) is a terminal branch of the basilar artery.

The surgical nomenclature identifies three segments: P_1 – from the basilar bifurcation to the junction with the posterior communicating artery; P_2 – from the junction with the posterior communicating artery to the portion in the perimesencephalic cistern; and P_3 – the portion running in the calcarine fissure.

The posterior cerebral artery is larger than the superior cerebellar artery, from which it is separated near its origin by the oculomotor nerve, and, lateral to the midbrain, by the trochlear nerve. It passes laterally, parallel with the superior cerebellar artery, and receives the posterior communicating artery. It then winds round the cerebral peduncle and reaches the tentorial cerebral surface, where it supplies the temporal and occipital lobes. Like the anterior and middle cerebral arteries, the posterior cerebral artery has cortical and central branches.

The cortical branches of the posterior cerebral artery are named by distribution. Temporal branches, usually two, are distributed to the uncus, parahippocampal, medial and lateral occipitotemporal gyri. Occipital branches supply the cuneus, lingual gyrus and posterolateral surface of the occipital lobe. Parieto-occipital branches supply the cuneus and precuneus. The posterior cerebral artery supplies the visual areas of the cerebral cortex (p. 403) and other structures in the visual pathway.

The central branches supply subcortical structures. Several small posteromedial central branches arise from the beginning of the posterior cerebral artery (**Fig. 17.6**), and, together with similar branches from the posterior communicating artery, pierce the posterior perforated substance and supply the anterior thalamus, subthalamus, lateral wall of the third ventricle and the globus pallidus. One or more posterior choroidal branches pass over the lateral geniculate body and supply it before entering the posterior part of the inferior horn of the lateral ventricle via the lower part of the choroidal fissure. Branches also curl round the posterior end of the thalamus and pass through the transverse fissure, or go to the choroid plexus of the third ventricle, or traverse the upper choroidal fissure. Collectively these supply the choroid plexuses of the third and lateral ventricles and the fornix. Small posterolateral central branches arise from the posterior cerebral artery beyond the cerebral peduncle, and supply the peduncle and the posterior thalamus, superior and inferior colliculi, pineal gland and medial geniculate body.

CIRCULUS ARTERIOSUS

The circulus arteriosus (circle of Willis) is a large arterial anastomosis which unites the internal carotid and vertebrobasilar systems (**Figs 17.5, 17.6**). It lies in the subarachnoid space within the deep interpeduncular cistern, and surrounds the optic chiasma, the infundibulum and other structures of the interpeduncular fossa. Anteriorly, the anterior cerebral arteries, which are derived from the internal carotid arteries, are joined by the small anterior communicating artery. Posteriorly, the two posterior cerebral arteries, which are formed by the division of the basilar artery, are joined to the ipsilateral internal carotid artery by a posterior communicating artery. In the majority of instances, the posterior communicating arteries are very small, however, and a limited flow is possible between the anterior and posterior circulations. This is important because the primary purpose of the vascular circle is to provide anastomotic channels if one vessel is occluded. The normal-sized posterior communicating artery cannot usually fulfil this role.

There is considerable individual variation in the pattern and calibre of vessels which make up the circulus arteriosus. Although a complete circular channel almost always exists, one vessel is usually sufficiently narrowed to reduce its role as a collateral route. Cerebral and communicating arteries individually may all be absent, variably hypoplastic, double or even triple. The circle is rarely functionally complete.

The haemodynamics of the circle is influenced by variations in the calibre of communicating arteries and in the segments of the anterior and posterior cerebral arteries which lie between their origins and their junctions with the corresponding communicating arteries. The greatest variation in calibre between individuals occurs in the posterior communicating artery. Commonly, the diameter of the precommunicating part of the posterior cerebral artery is larger than that of the posterior communicating artery; in which case the blood supply to the occipital lobes is mainly from the vertebrobasilar system. Sometimes, however, the diameter of the precommunicating part of the posterior cerebral artery is smaller than that of the posterior communicating artery, in which case the blood supply to the occipital lobes is mainly from the internal carotids via the posterior communicating arteries. Agenesis or hypoplasia of the initial segment of the anterior cerebral artery are more frequent than anomalies in the anterior communicating artery and contribute to defective circulation in about a third of individuals.

Cerebral aneurysms

Aneurysms are balloon-like swellings which occur on arteries as a result of defects in the vessel wall. They are most commonly found on the vessels of the circulus arteriosus, particularly at or near the junctions of vessels. Aneurysms on the internal carotid artery near its termination may compress the lateral aspect of the optic chiasma, and compromise axons

derived from the temporal side of the ipsilateral retina, which causes a defect in the nasal visual field. Aneurysms in the vicinity of the third (oculomotor) cranial nerve, on the posterior communicating artery, superior cerebellar artery or basilian tip, can cause third nerve palsy by compression. (**Figs 17.11, 17.12**). A complete third nerve palsy consists of paralysis of the extraocular muscles except the lateral rectus and superior oblique. The unopposed actions of these muscles causes the eye to be deviated laterally and inferiorly. The eyelid droops (ptosis) because of the involvement of levator palpebrae. The pupil is dilated and the pupillary light reflex is lost because of involvement of parasympathetic fibres.

In some clinical situations, the third nerve palsy may be incomplete. Diabetic patients have a high incidence of partial third nerve palsies inasmuch as the nerve supply to the extraocular muscles is lost but the pupil is spared. In this case, the central part of the third nerve is infarcted by the microvascular disease but the peripherally sited parasympathetic fibres are not involved.

CENTRAL OR PERFORATING ARTERIES

Numerous small central (perforating or ganglionic) arteries arise from the circulus arteriosus, or from vessels near it (**Fig. 17.6**). Many of these enter the brain through the anterior and posterior perforated substances (**Fig. 21.9**). Central branches supply nearby structures on or near the base of the brain together with the interior of the cerebral hemisphere including the internal capsule, basal ganglia and thalamus They form four principal groups. The anteromedial group arises from the anterior cerebral and anterior communicating arteries and passes through the medial part of the anterior perforated substance. These arteries supply the optic chiasma, lamina terminalis, anterior, preoptic and supraoptic areas of the hypothalamus, septum pellucidum, paraolfactory areas, anterior columns of the fornix, cingulate gyrus, rostrum of the corpus callosum and the anterior part of the putamen and the head of the caudate nucleus. The posteromedial group comes from the entire length of the posterior communicating artery and from the proximal portion of the posterior cerebral artery. Anteriorly, these arteries supply the hypothalamus and pituitary, and the anterior and medial parts of the thalamus via thalamoperforating arteries. Caudally, branches of the

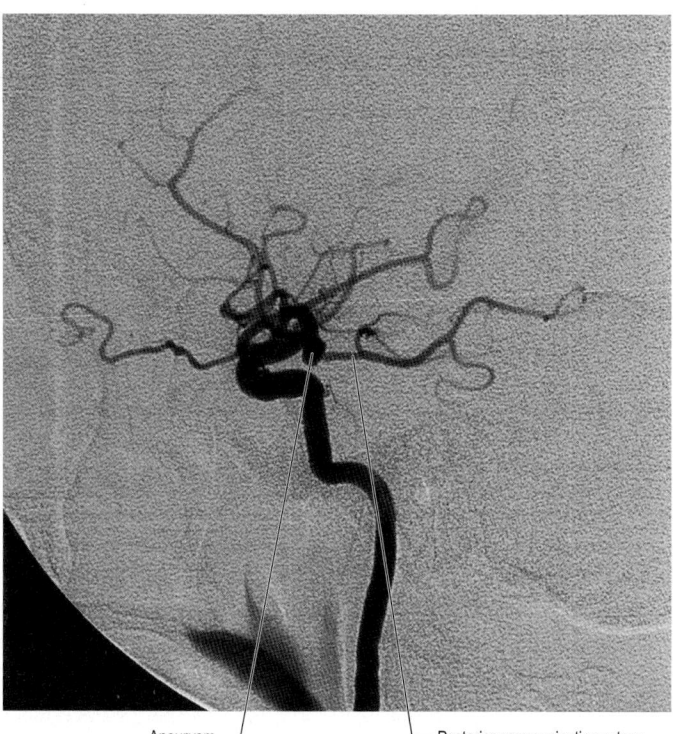

Aneurysm ⎯⎯   ⎯⎯ Posterior communicating artery

Fig. 17.11 Intra-arterial digital subtraction angiogram of the right internal carotid artery in a patient with a complete right IIIrd nerve palsy. Lateral projection. Note the difference in the size of the posterior communicating artery in comparison to that in **Fig. 17.2**. (By kind permission from Professor PD Griffiths, Academic Unit of Radiology, The University of Sheffield.)

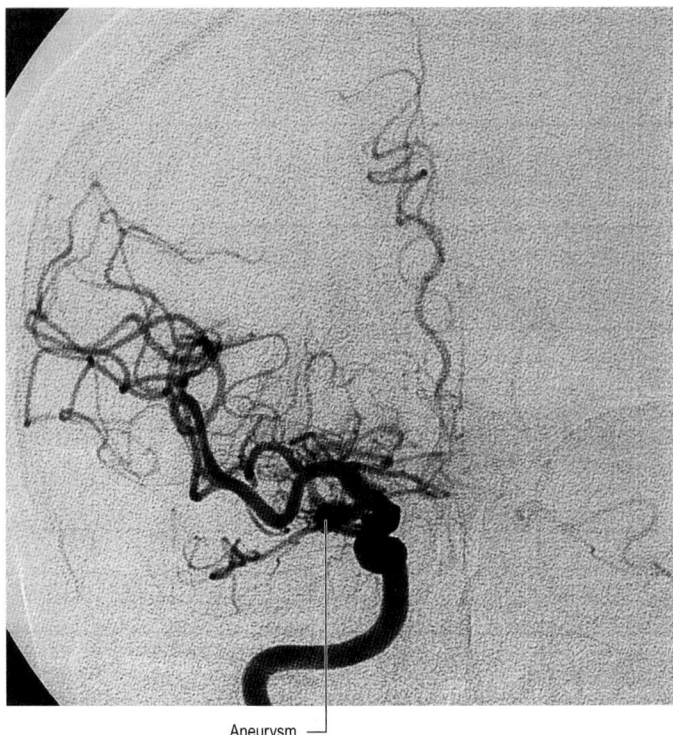

Fig. 17.12 Intra-arterial digital subtraction angiogram of the right internal carotid artery in a patient with a complete right IIIrd nerve palsy. Towne's projection. (By kind permission from Professor PD Griffiths, Academic Unit of Radiology, The University of Sheffield.)

Aneurysm

posteromedial group supply the mammillary bodies, subthalamus, the lateral wall of the third ventricle including the medial thalamus, and the globus pallidus. The anterolateral group is mostly comprised of branches from the proximal part of the middle cerebral artery, and they are also known as striate, lateral striate or lenticulostriate arteries. They enter the brain through the anterior perforated substance and supply the posterior striatum, lateral globus pallidus and the anterior limb, genu and posterior limb of the internal capsule. The medial striate artery, which is derived from the middle or anterior cerebral arteries, supplies the rostral part of the caudate nucleus and putamen and the anterior limb and genu of the internal capsule. The posterolateral group is derived from the posterior cerebral artery distal to its junction with the posterior communicating artery, and supplies the cerebral peduncle, colliculi, pineal gland and, via thalamogeniculate branches, the posterior thalamus and medial geniculate body.

The territories supplied by the central branches are described in detail in the sections dealing with the anterior, middle and posterior cerebral arteries (pp. 297, 298, 300).

REGIONAL ARTERIAL SUPPLY OF THE BRAIN

Brain stem
The medulla oblongata is supplied by the branches of the vertebral, anterior and posterior spinal, posterior inferior cerebellar and basilar arteries, which enter along the anterior median fissure and the posterior median sulcus. Vessels which supply the central substance enter along the rootlets of the glossopharyngeal, vagus, accessory and hypoglossal nerves. There is an additional supply via a pial plexus from the same main arteries (see also p. 298).

The pons is supplied by the basilar artery and the anterior inferior and superior cerebellar arteries. Direct branches from the basilar artery enter the pons along the ventral medial groove (basilar sulcus). Other vessels enter along the trigeminal, abducens, facial and vestibulocochlear nerves and from the pial plexus.

The midbrain is supplied by the posterior cerebral, superior cerebellar and basilar arteries. The crura cerebri are supplied by vessels entering on their medial and lateral sides. The medial vessels enter the medial side of the crus and also supply the superomedial part of the tegmentum,

including the oculomotor nucleus, and lateral vessels supply the lateral part of the crus and the tegmentum. The colliculi are supplied by three vessels on each side from the posterior cerebral and superior cerebellar arteries. An additional supply to the crura, and the colliculi and their penduncles comes from the posterolateral group of central branches of the posterior cerebral artery.

Cerebellum
The cerebellum is supplied by the posterior inferior, anterior inferior and superior cerebellar arteries. Their courses and territories are described in detail elsewhere (pp. 298, 300). The cerebellar arteries form superficial anastomoses on the cortical surface. Anastomoses between deeper, subcortical, branches have been postulated.

The choroid plexus of the fourth ventricle is supplied by the posterior inferior cerebellar arteries.

Optic chiasma, tract and radiation
The blood supplies of the optic chiasma, tract and radiation are of considerable clinical importance. The chiasma is supplied in part by the anterior cerebral arteries but its median zone depends upon rami from the internal carotid arteries reaching it via the stalk of the hypophysis. The anterior choroidal and posterior communicating arteries supply the optic tract, and the optic radiation receives blood through deep branches of the middle and posterior cerebral arteries.

Diencephalon
The thalamus is supplied chiefly by branches of the posterior communicating, posterior cerebral and basilar arteries. A contribution from the anterior choroidal artery is often noted, but this has been disputed. The medial branch of the posterior choroidal artery supplies the posterior commissure, habenular region, pineal gland and medial parts of the thalamus, including the pulvinar. Small central branches, which arise from the circulus arteriosus and its associated vessels, supply the hypothalamus. The pituitary gland is supplied by hypophyseal arteries derived from the internal carotid artery (p. 296), and the anterior cerebral and anterior communicating arteries supply the lamina terminalis.

The choroid plexuses of the third and lateral ventricles are supplied by branches of the internal carotid and posterior cerebral arteries.

Basal ganglia
The majority of the arterial supply to the basal ganglia comes from the striate arteries, which are branches from the roots of the anterior and middle cerebral arteries (**Fig. 17.13**). They enter the brain through the anterior perforated substance and also supply the internal capsule. The caudate nucleus receives blood additionally from the anterior and

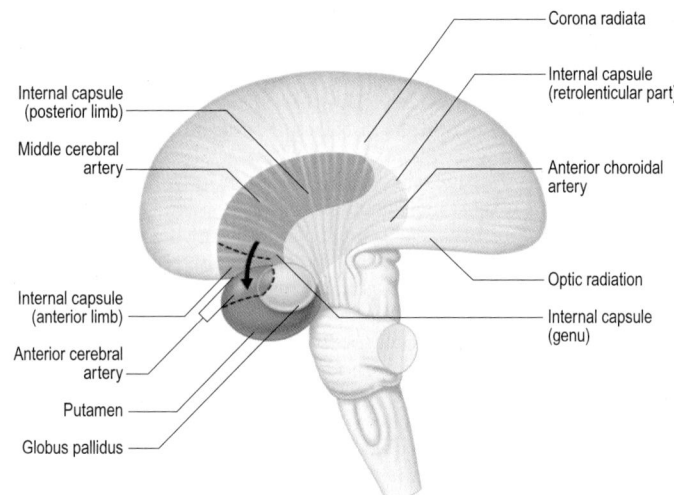

Internal capsule (posterior limb)

Middle cerebral artery

Internal capsule (anterior limb)

Anterior cerebral artery

Putamen

Globus pallidus

Corona radiata

Internal capsule (retrolenticular part)

Anterior choroidal artery

Optic radiation

Internal capsule (genu)

Fig. 17.13 Arterial supply to the internal capsule and parts of the basal ganglia of the left cerebral hemisphere. The outer layers of the hemisphere have been removed to reveal these structures. The putamen and globus pallidus are displaced downwards to display the internal capsule. Territory supplied by branches of the anterior and middle cerebral arteries is shown in red. Territory supplied by the anterior choroidal artery is shown in green.

posterior choroidal arteries. The posteroinferior part of the lentiform complex is supplied by the thalamostriate branches of the posterior cerebral artery. The anterior choroidal artery, a preterminal branch of the internal carotid artery (p. 296), contributes to the blood supply of both segments of the globus pallidus and the caudate nucleus. Famously, the ligation of this vessel during a neurosurgical procedure on a patient suffering from Parkinson's disease led to alleviation of the Parkinsonian symptoms, presumably as a consequence of infarction of the globus pallidus. This chance observation led to the initiation of pallidal surgery (pallidotomy) for this condition (see also p. 428).

Internal capsule

The internal capsule is supplied by central, or perforating, arteries which arise from the circulus arteriosus and its associated vessels (**Fig. 17.13**). These include the lateral and medial striate arteries, which come from the middle and anterior cerebral arteries and also supply the basal ganglia. The lateral striate arteries supply the anterior limb, genu and much of the posterior limb of the internal capsule and are commonly involved in ischaemic and haemorrhagic stroke. One of the larger striate branches of the middle cerebral artery is known as 'Charcot's artery of cerebral haemorrhage'.

The medial striate artery, a branch of the proximal part of the middle or anterior cerebral, supplies the anterior limb and genu of the internal capsule and the basal ganglia. The anterior choroidal artery also contributes to the supply of the ventral part of the posterior limb and the retrolenticular (retrolentiform) part of the internal capsule.

Stroke – Embolic or haemorrhagic events commonly involve the perforating arteries because of their small diameter and fragile nature. The internal capsule, therefore, is frequently the site of a stroke. The often devastating consequences of a stroke reflect the fact that the internal capsule is effectively the only route between the cerebral cortex and other regions of the neuraxis. All major cortical efferent motor pathways pass through the internal capsule, as do third-order thalamo-cortical sensory fibres (p. 414). The neurological deficits which occur following stroke damage to these fibres will include contralateral spastic hemiparesis and contralateral hemisensory loss as well as psychological deficits. The precise nature and distribution of the deficits will be determined by the regions involved. Thus, for example, infarction of the retrolenticular part of the internal capsule damages the optic radiation and produces homonomous hemianopia.

Cerebral cortex

The entire blood supply of the cerebral cortex comes from cortical branches of the anterior, middle and posterior cerebral arteries. In general, long branches traverse the cortex and penetrate the subjacent white matter for 3 or 4 cm without communicating. Short branches are confined to the cerebral cortex, and form a compact network in the middle zone of the grey matter, whereas the outer and inner zones are sparingly supplied. Although adjacent vessels anastomose on the surface of the brain, they become end arteries as soon as they enter it. In general, superficial anastomoses only occur between microscopic branches of the cerebral arteries, and there is little evidence that they can provide an effective alternative circulation after the occlusion of larger vessels.

The lateral surface of the hemisphere is mainly supplied by the middle cerebral artery (**Fig. 17.14**). This includes the territories of the motor and somatosensory cortices which represent the whole of the body, apart from the lower limb, and also the auditory cortex and language areas. The anterior cerebral artery supplies a strip next to the superomedial border of the hemisphere, as far back as the parieto-occipital sulcus. The occipital lobe and most of the inferior temporal gyrus (excluding the temporal pole) are supplied by the posterior cerebral artery.

Medial and inferior surfaces of the hemisphere are supplied by the anterior, middle and posterior cerebral arteries. The area supplied by the anterior cerebral artery is the largest, and extends almost to the parieto-occipital sulcus and includes the medial part of the orbital surface. The rest of the orbital surface and the temporal pole are supplied by the middle cerebral artery, and the remaining medial and inferior surfaces are supplied by the posterior cerebral artery.

Near the occipital pole, the junctional zone between the territories of the middle and posterior cerebral arteries corresponds to the visual (striate) cortex which receives information from the macula. When the posterior cerebral artery is occluded, a phenomenon known as 'macular sparing' may occur in which vision with the central part of the retina is

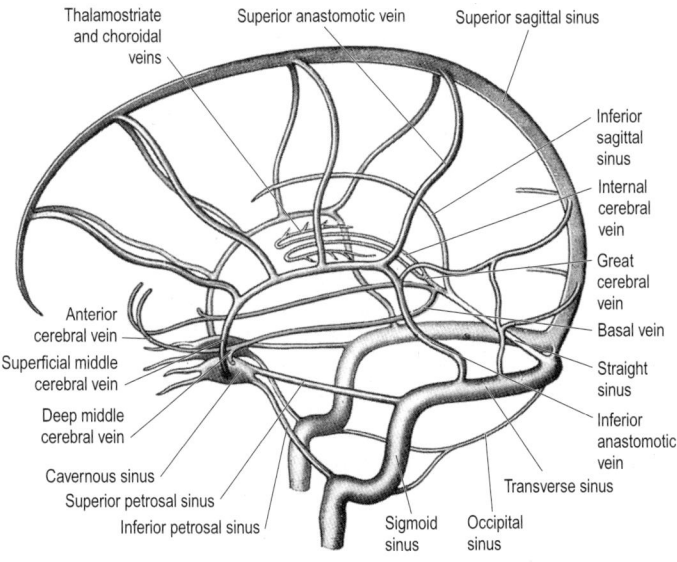

Fig. 17.14 The cerebral venous system (viewed from the left side) showing the principal superficial and deep veins of the brain and their relationship to the dural venous sinuses. The more deeply placed veins are shown in blue and those inside the brain are shown in interrupted blue.

preserved. Collateral circulation of blood from branches of the middle cerebral artery into those of the posterior cerebral artery may account for this phenomenon. Indeed, in some individuals, the middle cerebral artery may itself supply the macular area.

Cerebral blood flow

The brain is devoid of either glucose stores or a means of storing oxygen and is, therefore, dependent minute-by-minute upon an adequate blood supply. It has a high metabolic rate in comparison to other organs, which reflects the metabolic demands of constant neural activity. The blood supply of grey matter is more copious than that of white matter.

Cerebral blood flow in the human brain is approximately $50 \text{ ml g}^{-2} \text{ min}^{-1}$. Global cerebral blood flow is autoregulated, i.e. it remains constant in normal individuals despite variations in mean arterial blood pressure over a range of approximately 8.7–18.7 kPa, (65–140 mmHg). If the blood pressure falls below this range, cerebral blood flow decreases. Alternatively, if the pressure rises above this range, cerebral blood flow may increase. Arterial and arteriolar intraluminal pressure directly control contraction of intramural muscle, so that an increase in arterial pressure, for example, causes arterial constriction, and blood flow remains constant.

Although autoregulation normally ensures that global cerebral blood flow remains constant, regional blood flow varies in response to the level of neural activity and, thus, to local metabolic demand. This has been demonstrated for many brain areas including the motor and sensory cortical regions, areas involved in convulsive activity and even cortical areas involved in complex thought processes. The principal local factors affecting regional blood flow are the local hydrogen ion (H^+) or carbon dioxide concentration which cause arterial dilatation.

Not all substances circulating in arterial blood have access to the brain parenchyma. Particulate matter, such as bacteria, is excluded. In general, lipophilic molecules and small molecules, such as oxygen and carbon dioxide, can cross the blood–brain barrier but hydrophilic ones (excluding glucose) cannot. The cellular basis for the blood–brain barrier is discussed in Chapter 4 (p. 51).

VENOUS DRAINAGE OF THE BRAIN

The venous drainage of the brain occurs through a complex system of deep and superficial veins. These veins possess no valves and have thin walls devoid of muscular tissue. They pierce the arachnoid mater and the inner layer of the dura mater to open into the dural venous sinuses (p. 277).

VEINS OF THE BRAIN STEM

The veins of the brain stem form a superficial venous plexus deep to the arteries.

Veins of the medulla oblongata drain into the veins of the spinal cord or the adjacent dural venous sinuses, or into variable radicular veins which accompany the last four cranial nerves to either the inferior petrosal or occipital sinuses, or to the superior bulb of the jugular vein. Anterior and posterior median medullary veins may run along the anterior median fissure and posterior median sulcus, to become continuous with the spinal veins in corresponding positions. Pontine veins, which may include a median vein and a lateral vein on each side, drain into the basal vein, cerebellar veins, the petrosal sinuses, transverse sinus or the venous plexus of the foramen ovale. Veins of the midbrain join the great cerebral vein or basal vein.

VEINS OF THE CEREBELLUM

The veins of the cerebellum drain mainly into sinuses adjacent to them or, from the superior surface, into the great cerebral vein. The cerebellar veins course on the cerebellar surface, and comprise superior and inferior groups. Superior cerebellar veins either run anteromedially across the superior vermis to the straight sinus or great cerebral vein, or they run laterally to the transverse and superior petrosal sinuses. Inferior cerebellar veins include a small median vessel running backwards on the inferior vermis to enter the straight or sigmoid sinus. Laterally coursing vessels join the inferior petrosal and occipital sinuses.

VEINS OF THE CEREBRAL HEMISPHERE

External and internal cerebral veins (**Figs 17.14–17.18**) drain the surfaces and the interior of the cerebral hemisphere.

External cerebral veins may be divided into three groups, namely superior, middle and inferior.

Eight to twelve superior cerebral veins drain the superolateral and medial surfaces of each hemisphere. They mainly follow the sulci,

although some do pass across gyri. They ascend to the superomedial border of the hemisphere, where they receive small veins from the medial surface, and then open into the superior sagittal sinus. Superior cerebral veins in the anterior part of the hemisphere join the sinus almost at right angles. The larger posterior veins are directed obliquely

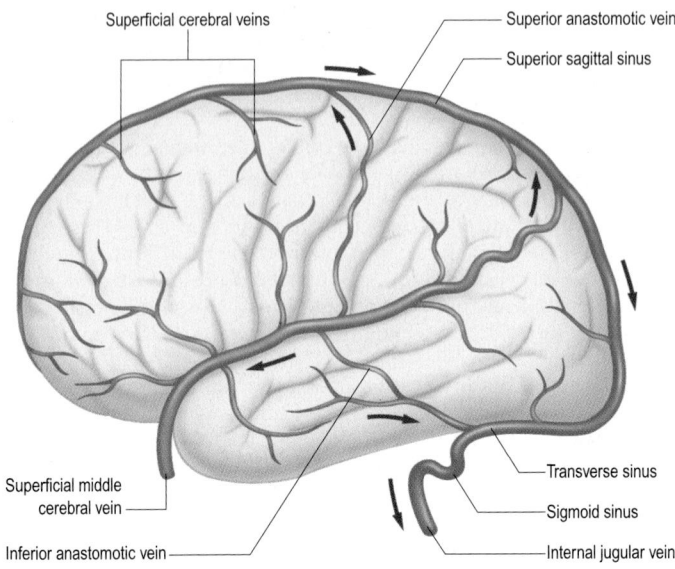

Fig. 17.15 The external (superficial) cerebral veins of the left hemisphere and their relationship to the dural venous sinuses.

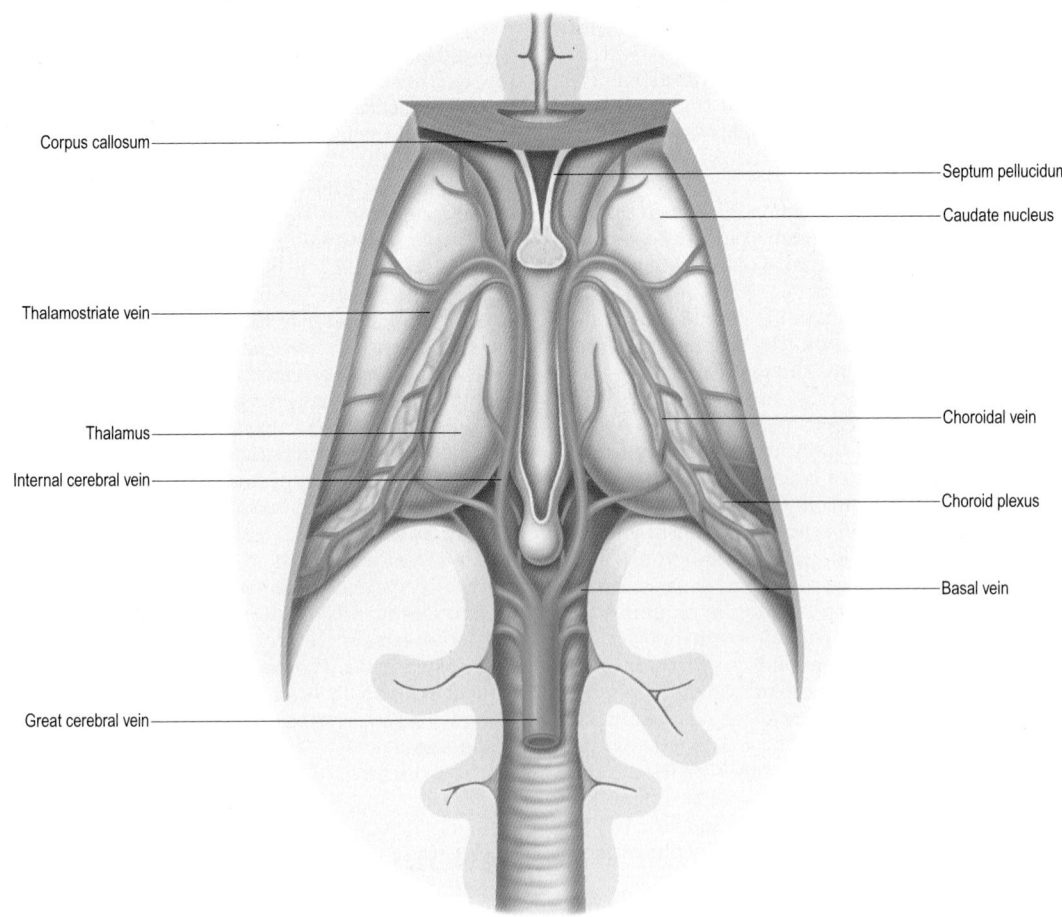

Fig. 17.16 The internal (deep) cerebral veins, viewed from above after removal of the central portion of the corpus callosum.

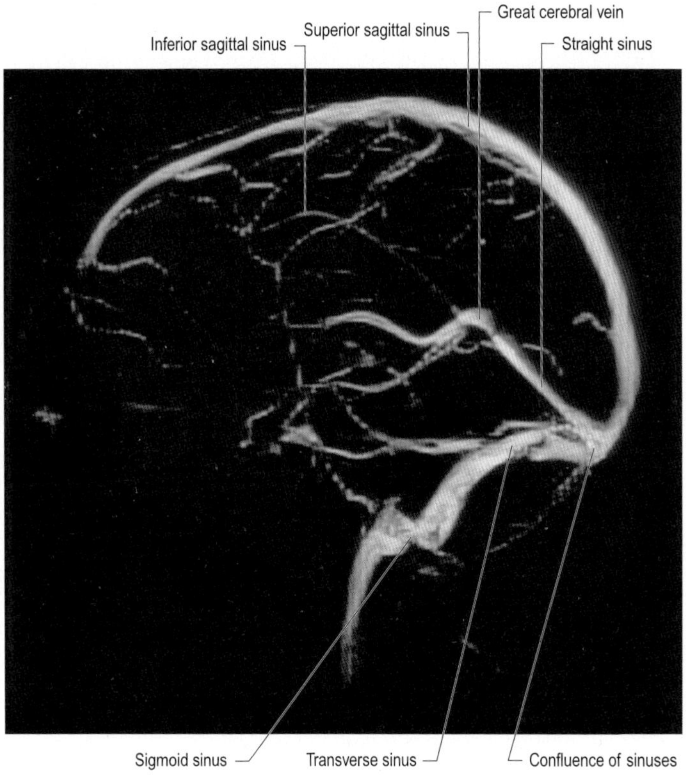

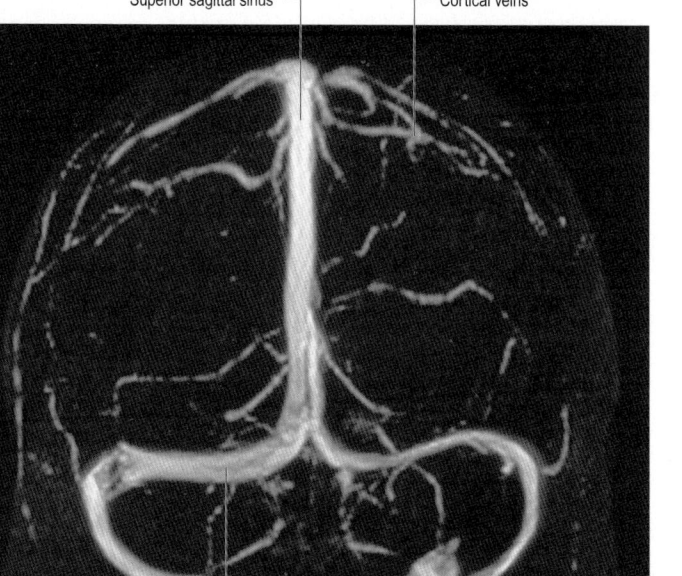

Inferior sagittal sinus — Superior sagittal sinus — Great cerebral vein — Straight sinus

Sigmoid sinus — Transverse sinus — Confluence of sinuses

Fig. 17.17 Lateral projection from a magnetic resonance venogram using time-of-flight methods. (By kind permission from Professor PD Griffiths, Academic Unit of Radiology, The University of Sheffield.)

Superior sagittal sinus — Cortical veins

Transverse sinus — Sigmoid sinus

Fig. 17.18 Frontal projection from a magnetic resonance venogram using time-of-flight methods. (By kind permission from Professor PD Griffiths, Academic Unit of Radiology, The University of Sheffield.)

forwards, against the direction of flow in the sinus, an arrangement which may resist their collapse when intracranial pressure is raised.

The superficial middle cerebral vein drains most of the lateral surface of the hemisphere, and follows the lateral fissure to end in the cavernous sinus. A superior anastomotic vein runs posterosuperiorly between the superficial middle cerebral vein and the superior sagittal sinus, thus connecting the superior sagittal and cavernous sinuses. An inferior anastomotic vein courses over the temporal lobe and connects the superficial middle cerebral vein to the transverse sinus. The deep middle cerebral vein drains the insular region and joins the anterior cerebral and striate veins to form a basal vein. Regions drained by the anterior cerebral and striate veins correspond approximately to those supplied by the anterior cerebral artery and the central branches which enter the anterior perforated substance. The basal veins pass back alongside the interpeduncular fossa and midbrain, receive tributaries from this vicinity and join the great cerebral vein.

Inferior cerebral veins on the orbital surface of the frontal lobe join the superior cerebral veins and thus drain to the superior sagittal sinus. Those on the temporal lobe anastomose with basal veins and middle cerebral veins, and drain to the cavernous, superior petrosal and transverse sinuses.

The basal vein begins at the anterior perforated substance by the union of a small anterior cerebral vein, which accompanies the anterior cerebral artery, a deep middle cerebral vein, which receives tributaries

from the insula and neighbouring gyri and runs in the lateral cerebral fissure, and striate veins, which emerge from the anterior perforated substance. The basal vein passes back round the cerebral peduncle to the great cerebral vein (**Fig. 17.14**), and receives tributaries from the interpeduncular fossa, inferior horn of the lateral ventricle, parahippocampal gyrus and midbrain.

The internal cerebral vein drains the deep parts of the hemisphere and the choroid plexuses of the third and lateral ventricles. It is formed near the interventricular foramen, behind the column of the fornix, primarily by union of the thalamostriate and choroidal (choroid) veins, although numerous smaller veins from surrounding structures also converge here. The thalamostriate vein runs anteriorly, between the caudate nucleus and thalamus, and receives many tributaries from both. The choroidal vein runs a convoluted course along the whole choroid plexus, and receives veins from the hippocampus, fornix, corpus callosum and adjacent structures. After their formation, the two internal cerebral veins travel back parallel to one another, beneath the splenium of the corpus callosum, where they unite to form the great cerebral vein. The great cerebral vein is a short median vessel, which curves sharply up around the splenium of the corpus callosum and opens into the anterior end of the straight sinus after receiving the right and left basal veins.

REFERENCES

Duvernoy HM, Delon S, Vannson JL 1981 Cortical blood vessels of the human brain. Brain Res Bull 7: 519–79.

Duvernoy H, Delon S, Vannson JL 1983 The vascularization of the human cerebellar cortex. Brain Res Bull 11(4): 419–80.

Kaplan HA, Ford DH 1966 The Brain Vascular System. Amsterdam: Elsevier.

Plets C, De Reuck J, Vander Eecken H, Van den Bergh R 1970 The vascularization of the human thalamus. Acta Neurol Belg 70(6): 687–770.

Puchades-Orts A, Nombela-Gomez M, Ortuño-Pacheco G 1976 Variation in form of the circle of Willis. Some anatomical and embryological considerations. Anat Rec 185: 119–23.

Sengupta RP, McAllister VL (eds) 1986 Subarachnoid Haemorrhage. Berlin: Springer-Verlag: 9–31.
Includes details on variations of the circle of Willis.

Spinal cord

The spinal cord provides innervation for the trunk and limbs through the paired spinal nerves and their peripheral ramifications. Through them it receives primary afferent fibres from peripheral receptors located in widespread somatic and visceral structures. It also sends motor axons to skeletal muscle and provides autonomic innervation of cardiac and smooth muscle and secretory glands. Many functions are regulated by intraspinal, reflex connections. Profuse ascending and descending pathways link the spinal cord with the brain. They allow higher centres to monitor and perceive external and internal stimuli and modulate and control spinal efferent activity.

EXTERNAL FEATURES AND RELATIONS

The topographical anatomy of the spinal cord, its external features and relations are described in more detail in Chapter 46. The spinal cord lies within the vertebral canal, and is continuous rostrally with the medulla oblongata just below the level of the foramen magnum (**Fig. 12.3**). Caudally, it terminates as the conus medullaris, which is continuous with the filum terminale, and is anchored to the dorsum of the coccyx. It is ensheathed by spinal meninges, which are continuous with the cranial meninges through the foramen magnum. The spinal cord is approximately circular in cross-section and its diameter varies according to the level. It bears two enlargements, cervical and lumbar, from which the innervation of the upper and lower limbs, respectively, arises.

The spinal cord is essentially a segmental structure. It gives rise to 31 pairs of segmentally arranged spinal nerves, which are attached to the cord by a linear series of dorsal and ventral rootlets. Dorsal rootlets contain afferent nerve fibres and ventral rootlets contain efferent fibres (**Fig. 12.5**). Groups of adjacent rootlets coalesce to form dorsal or ventral nerve roots. These cross the subarachnoid space and unite to form functionally mixed spinal nerves as they pass through the intervertebral foramina. The dorsal roots bear dorsal root ganglia, which contain the cell bodies of primary afferent neurones.

INTERNAL ORGANIZATION

In transverse section, the spinal cord is incompletely divided into symmetrical halves by a dorsal (posterior) median septum and a ventral (anterior) median sulcus (**Fig. 46.5**). It consists of an outer layer of white matter and an inner core of grey matter. The dimensions and relative volumes of white matter and centrally aggregated neurone cell bodies vary according to the level (**Fig. 18.1**). The amount of grey matter at any level is a function of the amounts of muscle, skin and other tissues innervated by neurones at that level. It is, therefore, largest by proportion in the cervical and lumbar enlargements, since neurones in these segments of the cord innervate the limbs, and is attenuated at thoracic levels. The absolute amount of white matter is greatest at cervical levels, and decreases progressively at lower levels, because descending tracts shed fibres as they descend and ascending tracts accumulate fibres as they ascend.

In the centre of the spinal grey matter, the central canal extends the whole length of the spinal cord. Rostrally, the central canal extends into the caudal half of the medulla oblongata where it opens into the fourth ventricle. Caudally, in the conus medullaris, it expands as a fusiform 'terminal ventricle' 8–10 mm in length, which contains cerebrospinal fluid (CSF), and is lined by columnar, ciliated epithelium (ependyma). The terminal ventricle is obliterated at c.40 years.

SPINAL GREY MATTER

In three dimensions, the spinal grey matter is shaped like a fluted column (**Fig. 46.6**). In transverse section (**Fig. 18.1**) the column is often described as being 'butterfly shaped' or resembling the letter 'H'. It consists of four cellular masses, referred to as the dorsal and ventral horns (or columns), which project dorsolaterally and ventrolaterally towards the surface. The grey matter which immediately surrounds the central canal and unites the two sides is termed the dorsal and ventral grey commissure. The dorsal horns are the site of termination of primary afferent fibres, which enter via the dorsal roots of spinal nerves. The tip of the dorsal horn is separated from the surface of the cord by a thin dorsolateral tract (tract of Lissauer) (**Figs 18.2, 18.3**) in which primary afferents ascend and descend for a short distance before terminating in the subjacent grey matter. The dorsal horn may be described in terms of a head, neck and base, the individual constituents of which are described in more detail below. The ventral horns contain efferent neurones whose axons leave the spinal cord in ventral nerve roots. A small intermediate lateral horn is present at thoracic and upper lumbar levels – it contains the cell bodies of preganglionic sympathetic neurones.

Spinal grey matter (**Fig. 18.4**) is a complex mixture of neuronal cell bodies (somata), their processes (neurites) and synaptic connections, neuroglia and blood vessels. Neurones in the grey matter are multipolar, and vary in size and other features, particularly the length and the arrangement of their axons and dendrites. Many are Golgi type I and II neurones. Axons of Golgi type I neurones pass out of the grey matter into ventral spinal roots or spinal tracts. Axons and dendrites of Golgi type II neurones are largely confined to the nearby grey matter. Neurones may be intrasegmental, i.e. deployed within a single segment, or intersegmental, i.e. spread through several segments, in distribution.

Neuronal cell groups of the spinal cord

Viewed from the perspective of its longitudinal columnar organization, the grey matter of the spinal cord consists of a series of discontinuous cell groupings associated with their corresponding segmentally arranged spinal nerves. At any particular spinal level (as seen in transverse section) the spinal grey matter is considered to consist of ten layers, Rexed's laminae, which are defined on the basis of neuronal size, shape, cytological features and density. The laminae are numbered sequentially in a dorsoventral sequence (**Fig. 18.5**).

Laminae I–IV correspond to the head of the dorsal horn, and are the main receiving areas for cutaneous primary afferent terminals and collateral branches. Many complex polysynaptic reflex paths (ipsilateral, contralateral, intrasegmental and intersegmental) start from this region and many long ascending tract fibres which pass to higher levels arise from it. Lamina I (lamina marginalis) is a very thin layer with an ill-defined boundary at the dorsolateral tip of the dorsal horn. It has a reticular appearance, reflecting its content of intermingling bundles of coarse and fine nerve fibres. It contains small, intermediate and large neuronal somata, many of which are fusiform in shape. Lamina II occupies most of the head of the dorsal horn and consists of densely packed small neurones responsible for its dark appearance in Nissl-stained sections. With myelin stains, Lamina II is characteristically distinguished from adjacent laminae by the almost total lack of myelinated fibres. Lamina II corresponds to the substantia gelatinosa. Lamina III consists of somata which are mostly larger, more variable and less closely packed than those in lamina II. It also contains many myelinated fibres. Some workers consider that the substantia gelatinosa contains part or all of lamina III as well as lamina II. The ill-defined nucleus proprius of the dorsal horn corresponds to some of the cell

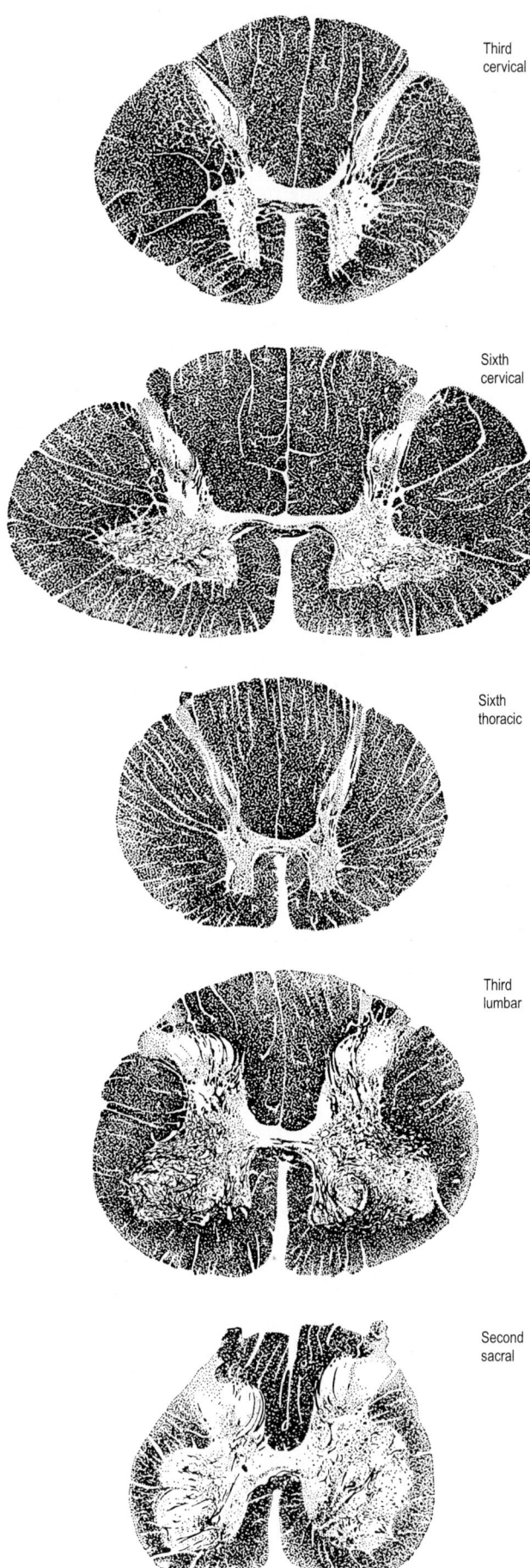

Fig. 18.1 Transverse sections through the spinal cord at representative levels. Note changes in overall profile and the relative changes in grey and white regions, their shape, size and proportions. Magnification ×5.

Third cervical

Sixth cervical

Sixth thoracic

Third lumbar

Second sacral

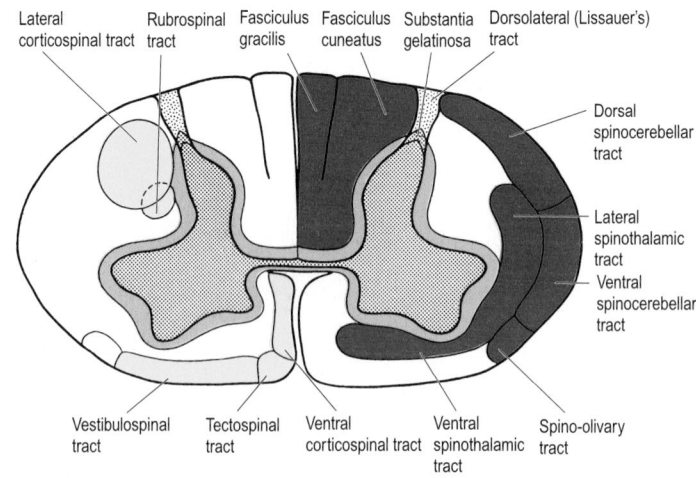

Fig. 18.2 Simplified diagram of the main tracts of the spinal cord. The ascending tracts are shown in red on the right side of the figure; the descending tracts are shown in yellow on the left side; the 'intersegmental' tracts are in orange on both sides. Many tracts are omitted (*see* **Fig. 18.3A, B**).

constituents of laminae III and IV. Lamina IV is a thick, loosely packed, heterogeneous zone permeated by fibres. Its neuronal somata vary considerably in size and shape, from small and round, through intermediate and triangular, to very large and stellate.

Laminae V and VI receive most of the terminals of proprioceptive primary afferents and profuse corticospinal projections from the motor and sensory cortex and subcortical levels, which suggests their intimate involvement in the regulation of movement. Lamina V is a thick layer which includes the neck of the dorsal horn. It is divisible into a lateral third and medial two-thirds. Both have a mixed cell population but the former contains many prominent well-staining somata interlaced by numerous bundles of transverse, dorsoventral and longitudinal fibres. Lamina VI is most prominent in the limb enlargements. It has a densely staining medial third of small, densely packed neurones and a lateral two-thirds containing larger, more loosely packed, triangular or stellate somata. Lamina VI corresponds approximately to the base of the dorsal horn.

Laminae VII–IX show a variety of complex forms in the limb enlargements (**Fig. 18.5**). Lamina VII includes much of the intermediate (lateral) horn. It contains prominent neurones of Clarke's column (nucleus dorsalis, nucleus thoracis, thoracic nucleus) and intermediomedial and intermediolateral cell groupings (**Fig. 18.6**). The lateral part of lamina VII has extensive ascending and descending connections with the midbrain and cerebellum (via the spinocerebellar, spinotectal, spinoreticular, tectospinal, reticulospinal and rubrospinal tracts) and is thus involved in the regulation of posture and movement. Its medial part has numerous propriospinal reflex connections with the adjacent grey matter and segments concerned both with movement and autonomic functions. Lamina VIII spans the base of the thoracic ventral horn but is restricted to its medial aspect in limb enlargements. Its neurones display a heterogeneous mixture of sizes and shapes from small to moderately large. Lamina VIII is a mass of propriospinal interneurones. It receives terminals from the adjacent laminae, many commissural terminals from the contralateral lamina VIII, and descending connections from the interstitiospinal, reticulospinal and vestibulospinal tracts and the medial longitudinal fasciculus. The axons from these interneurones influence motor neurones bilaterally, perhaps directly but more probably by excitation of small neurones supplying γ efferent fibres to muscle spindles. Lamina IX is a complex array of cells (**Fig. 18.7**) consisting of α and γ motor neurones and many interneurones. The large α motor neurones supply motor end-plates of extrafusal muscle fibres in striated muscle. Recording techniques have demonstrated tonic and phasic α motor neurones. The former have a lower rate of firing and lower conduction velocity and tend to innervate type S muscle units. The latter have higher conduction velocity and tend to supply fast twitch (type FR, FF) muscle units. The smaller γ motor neurones give rise to

A

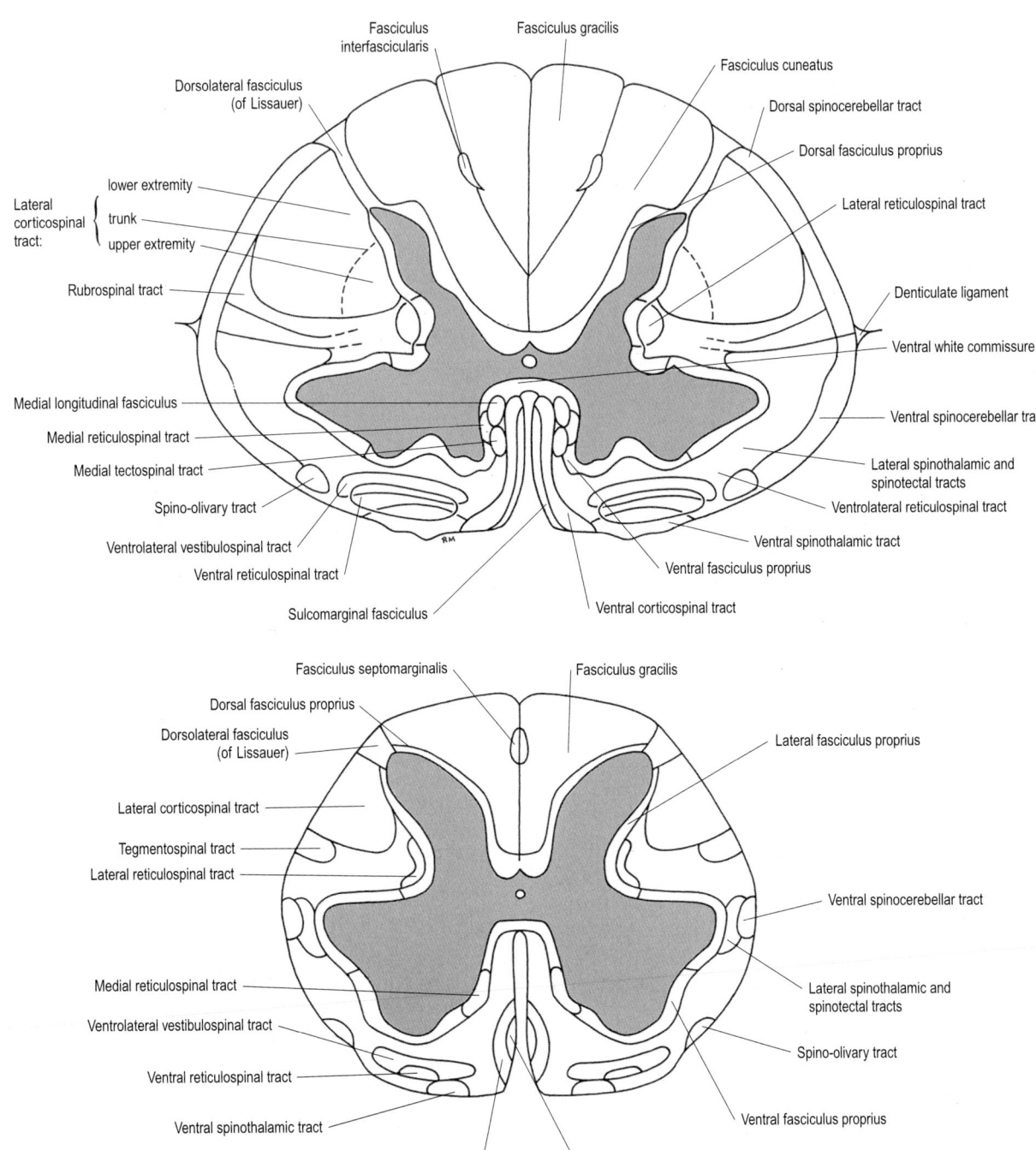

Fasciculus interfascicularis

Fasciculus gracilis

Fasciculus cuneatus

Dorsal spinocerebellar tract

Dorsal fasciculus proprius

Dorsolateral fasciculus (of Lissauer)

Lateral reticulospinal tract

Lateral corticospinal tract:
- lower extremity
- trunk
- upper extremity

Rubrospinal tract

Denticulate ligament

Ventral white commissure

Medial longitudinal fasciculus

Medial reticulospinal tract

Ventral spinocerebellar tract

Medial tectospinal tract

Lateral spinothalamic and spinotectal tracts

Spino-olivary tract

Ventrolateral reticulospinal tract

Ventrolateral vestibulospinal tract

Ventral spinothalamic tract

Ventral reticulospinal tract

Ventral fasciculus proprius

Sulcomarginal fasciculus

Ventral corticospinal tract

B

Fasciculus septomarginalis

Fasciculus gracilis

Dorsal fasciculus proprius

Dorsolateral fasciculus (of Lissauer)

Lateral fasciculus proprius

Lateral corticospinal tract

Tegmentospinal tract

Lateral reticulospinal tract

Ventral spinocerebellar tract

Medial reticulospinal tract

Lateral spinothalamic and spinotectal tracts

Ventrolateral vestibulospinal tract

Spino-olivary tract

Ventral reticulospinal tract

Ventral fasciculus proprius

Ventral spinothalamic tract

Ventral corticospinal tract

Sulcomarginal fasciculus

Fig. 18.3 The approximate relative positions of nerve fibre tracts of the human spinal cord at mid-cervical (A) and lumbar (B) levels. (Adapted from Crosby et al 1962. www.nature.com.)

small-diameter efferent axons (fusimotor fibres), which innervate the intrafusal muscle fibres in muscle spindles. There are several functionally distinct types of γ motor neurone. The 'static' and 'dynamic' responses of muscle spindles have separate controls mediated by static and dynamic fusimotor fibres, which are distributed variously to nuclear chain and nuclear bag fibres.

Lamina X surrounds the central canal and consists of the dorsal and ventral grey commissures.

Dorsal horn

The dorsal horn is a major receptive zone (zone of termination) of primary afferent fibres, which enter the spinal cord through the dorsal roots of spinal nerves. Dorsal root fibres contain numerous molecules, which are either known, or suspected, to fulfil a neurotransmitter or neuromodulator role. These include glutamate, substance P, calcitonin gene-related peptide (CGRP), bombesin, vasoactive intestinal polypeptide (VIP), cholecystokinin (CCK), somatostatin, dynorphin and

angiotensin II. Dorsal root afferents carry exteroceptive, proprioceptive and interoceptive information. Laminae I–IV are the main cutaneous receptive areas; lamina V receives fine afferents from the skin, muscle and viscera; and lamina VI receives proprioceptive and some cutaneous afferents. Most, if not all, primary afferent fibres divide into ascending and descending branches on entering the cord. These then travel for variable distances in the tract of Lissauer, near the surface of the cord, and send collaterals into the subjacent grey matter. The formation, topography and division of dorsal spinal roots have all been confirmed in man.

At the dorsolateral tip of the dorsal horn, deep to the tract of Lissauer, lies a thin lamina of neurones, the lamina marginalis. Beneath this lies the substantia gelatinosa (laminae II and III), which is present at all levels, and consists mostly of small Golgi type II neurones, together with some larger neurones. It receives afferents via the dorsal roots and is the site of origin of the spinothalamic tract complex. The large cells of the nucleus proprius lie ventral to the substantia gelatinosa (**Fig. 18.6**).

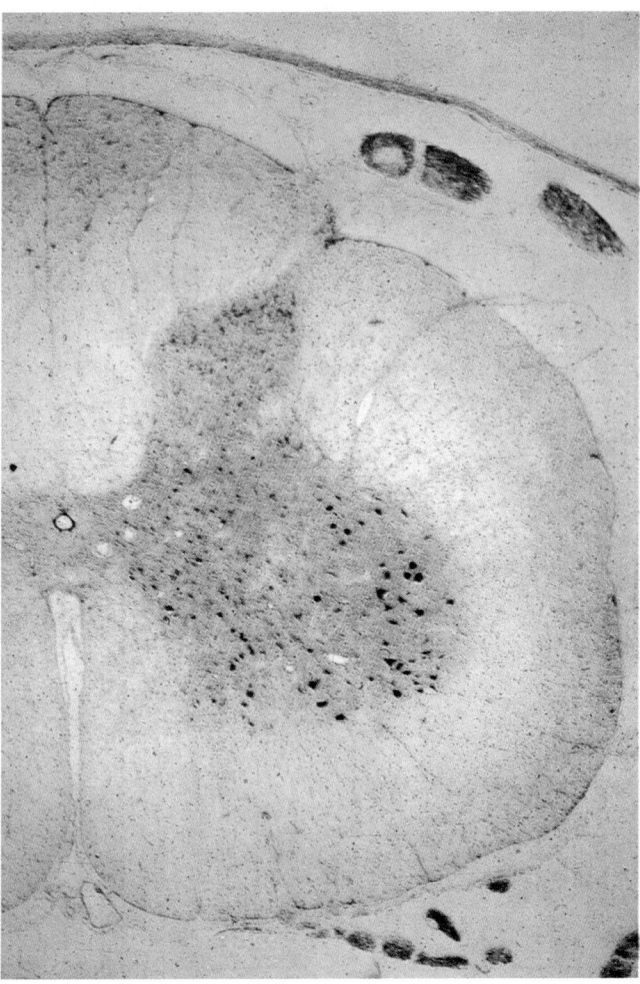

Fig. 18.4 Transverse section of left half of human spinal cord at a midlumbar level. Note dorsal and ventral grey columns and commissural grey mass. The larger motor neurones in the ventral grey column are visibly grouped. Stained with cresyl fast violet.

These propriospinal neurones link segments for the mediation of intraspinal coordination.

Clarke's column lies at the base of the dorsal horn. At most levels, it is near the dorsal white funiculus and may project into it. In the human spinal cord, it can usually be identified from the eighth cervical to the third or fourth lumbar segments. Neurones of Clarke's column vary in size, but most are large, especially in the lower thoracic and lumbar segments. Some send axons into the dorsal spinocerebellar tracts and others are interneurones.

Lateral horn

The lateral horn is a small lateral projection of grey matter located between the dorsal and ventral horns. It is present from the eighth cervical or first thoracic segment to the second or third lumbar segment. It contains the cell bodies of preganglionic sympathetic neurones. These develop in the embryonic cord dorsolateral to the central canal and migrate laterally, forming intermediomedial and intermediolateral cell columns. Their axons travel via ventral spinal roots and white rami communicantes to the sympathetic trunk. A similar cell group is found in the second to fourth sacral segments, but unlike the thoracolumbar lateral cell column, it does not form a visible lateral projection. It is the source of the sacral outflow of parasympathetic preganglionic nerve fibres.

Ventral horn

Neurones in the ventral horn vary in size. The largest cell bodies, which may exceed 25 μm in diameter, are those of α motor neurones whose axons emerge in ventral roots to innervate extrafusal fibres in striated skeletal muscles. Large numbers of smaller neurones, 15–25 μm in diameter, are also present. Some of these are γ motor neurones, which innervate intrafusal fibres of muscle spindles, and the rest are interneurones. The motor neurones utilize acetylcholine as their neurotransmitter.

Considered longitudinally, ventral horn neurones are arranged in elongated groups, and form a number of separate columns, which extend through several segments. These are seen most easily in transverse sections (**Fig. 18.4**). The ventral horn is essentially divided into medial, central and lateral cell columns, which all exhibit subdivision at certain levels, usually into dorsal and ventral parts. As can be seen in **Fig. 18.6**, the medial group extends throughout the cord, but may be absent in the fifth lumbar and first sacral segments. In the thoracic and the upper four lumbar segments, it is subdivided into ventromedial and dorsomedial groups. In segments cranial and caudal to this region, the medial group has only a ventromedial moiety, except in the first cervical segment, where only the dorsomedial group exists.

The central group of cells is the least extensive, and is found only in some cervical and lumbosacral segments. The third to seventh cervical segments contain the centrally situated phrenic nucleus – abundant experimental and clinical evidence shows that its neurones innervate the diaphragm. Neurones whose axons are thought to enter the spinal accessory nerve form an irregular accessory group in the upper five or six cervical segments at the ventral border of the ventral horn (**Fig. 18.6**).

The lateral group of cells in the ventral horn is subdivided into ventral, dorsal and retrodorsal groups, largely confined to the spinal segments which innervate the limbs. Their extents are indicated in **Fig. 18.6**. The nucleus of Onuf, which is thought to innervate the perineal striated muscles, is a ventrolateral group of cells in the first and second sacral segments.

The motor neurones of the ventral horn are somatotopically organized. The basic arrangement is that medial cell groups innervate the axial musculature, and lateral cell groups innervate the limbs. The basic building block of the somatic motor neuronal populations is represented by a longitudinally disposed group of neurones, which innervate a given muscle, and in which the α and γ motor neurones are intermixed. The various groups innervating different muscles are aggregated into two major longitudinal columns, medial and lateral. In transverse section these form the medial and lateral cell groups in the ventral horn (**Fig. 18.8**).

The medial longitudinal motor column extends throughout the length of the spinal cord. Its neurones innervate epaxial and hypaxial muscle groups. Basically, epaxial muscles include the erector spinae group (which extend the head and vertebral column), while hypaxial muscles include prevertebral muscles of the neck, intercostal and anterior abdominal wall muscles (which flex the neck and the trunk). The epaxial muscles are innervated by branches of the dorsal primary rami of the spinal nerves, and the hypaxial muscles by branches of the ventral primary rami. In the medial column, motor neurones supplying epaxial muscles are sited ventral to those supplying hypaxial muscles.

The lateral longitudinal motor column is found only in the enlargements of the spinal cord. The motor neurones in this column in the cervical and lumbar enlargements innervate muscles of the upper and lower limbs, respectively. In the cervical enlargement, motor neurones which supply muscles intrinsic to the upper limb are situated dorsally in the ventral grey column, and those innervating the most distal (hand) muscles are sited further dorsally. Motor neurones of the girdle muscles lie in the ventrolateral part of the ventral horn (**Fig. 18.8**). There is a further somatotopic organization in that the proximal muscles of the limb are supplied from motor cell groups located more rostrally in the enlargement than those supplying the distal muscles. For example, motor neurones innervating intrinsic muscles of the hand are sited in segments C8 and T1, while motor neurones of shoulder muscles are in segments C5 and 6. A similar overall arrangement of motor neurones innervating lower limb muscles applies in the lumbosacral cord (**Fig. 18.9**).

The main afferent connections to motor neurones are direct monosynaptic connections from proprioceptive dorsal root afferents in the same or nearby segments; connections from axonal collaterals of dorsal horn and other interneurones; and direct monosynaptic connections from the vestibulospinal and corticospinal tracts.

Spinal reflexes

The intrinsic connections of the spinal cord and brain stem subserve a number of reflexes by which the functions of peripheral structures are modulated in response to afferent information in a relatively automatic

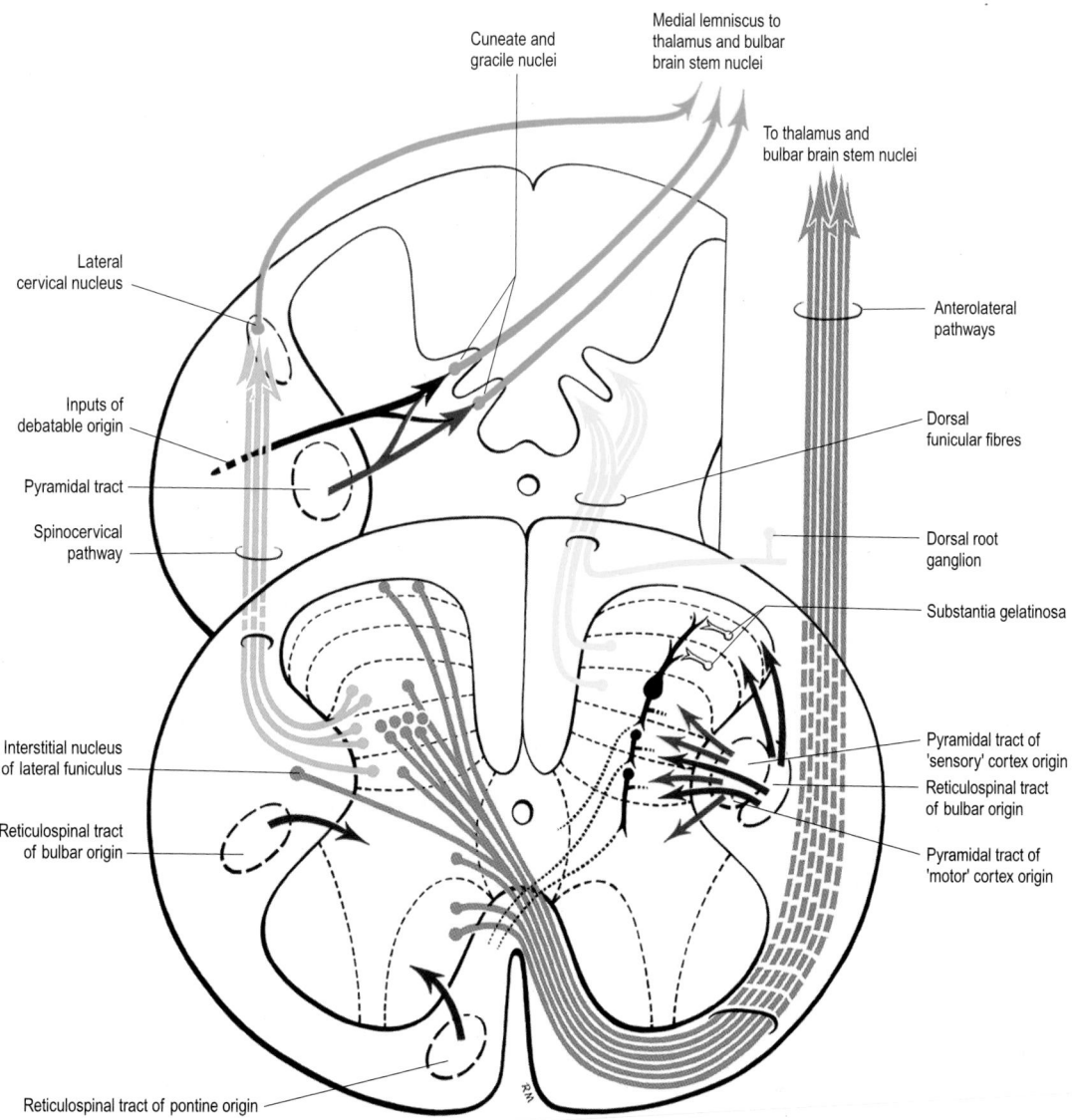

Fig. 18.5 The principal somaesthetic pathways. Descending corticospinal and reticulospinal tracts involved in sensory modulation are also indicated. (Modified from data provided by KE Webster, GKT School of Medicine, London.)

or autonomous fashion. The fundamental components of such reflex 'arcs' are thus an afferent and an efferent neurone. However, in all but the simplest of reflexes, interneurones intervene between the afferent and efferent components and confer the capacity to increase the versatility and complexity of reflex responses. Reflexes, by their very nature, are relatively fixed and stereotyped in form. Nevertheless they are strongly influenced and modulated by descending connections. In the case of spinal reflexes these descending controls come from both the brain stem and the cerebral cortex. Pathology of descending supraspinal pathways commonly causes abnormalities of spinal reflex activity, which are routinely tested for in neurological examination. During development, descending control mechanisms suppress what may be regarded as 'primitive' reflex responses. However, these may be released or uncovered in certain pathological conditions, e.g. the plantar (Babinski) and grasp reflexes.

Stretch reflex – The stretch reflex is the mechanism by which stretch applied to a muscle elicits its reflex contraction. It is essential for the maintenance of both muscle tone and an upright stance (via the innervation of the postural muscles of the neck, back and lower limbs). Anatomically it is the simplest of reflexes – it consists of an afferent and an efferent neurone. The afferent component arises from stretch receptors associated with intrafusal muscle fibres located within muscle spindles, the primary or anulospiral endings of which give rise to primary afferent fibres, which enter the spinal cord where they make

excitatory synaptic contact directly onto α motor neurones innervating the same muscle (**Fig. 18.10**). The α motor neurones of antagonistic muscles are simultaneously inhibited via collateral connections to inhibitory interneurones.

Gamma reflex – As well as α motor neurones innervating extrafusal muscle fibres, muscles also receive γ motor neurones, which innervate intrafusal muscle fibres. Activation of γ motor neurones increases the sensitivity of the intrafusal fibres to stretch (**Fig. 18.11**). Therefore, changes in γ activity have a profound effect upon the stretch reflex and upon muscle tone. Like α motor neurones, γ motor neurones are under the influence of descending pathways from the brain stem and cerebral cortex. Changes in the activity of the stretch reflex and of muscle tone are commonly found in disorders of the CNS as well as the PNS.

Flexor reflex – Painful stimulation of the limbs leads to reflex flexion withdrawal mediated by a polysynaptic reflex (**Fig. 18.12**) in which interneurones are interposed between afferent and efferent elements. Thus, activation of nociceptive primary afferents indirectly causes activation of limb flexor motor neurones. Collateralization of fibres to nearby spinal segments mediates flexion of a limb at several joints, depending on the intensity of the stimulus. Decussating connections to the contralateral side of the cord activate α motor neurones innervating corresponding extensor muscles, which produces the so-called crossed extensor reflex. In principle, virtually any cutaneous stimulus has the

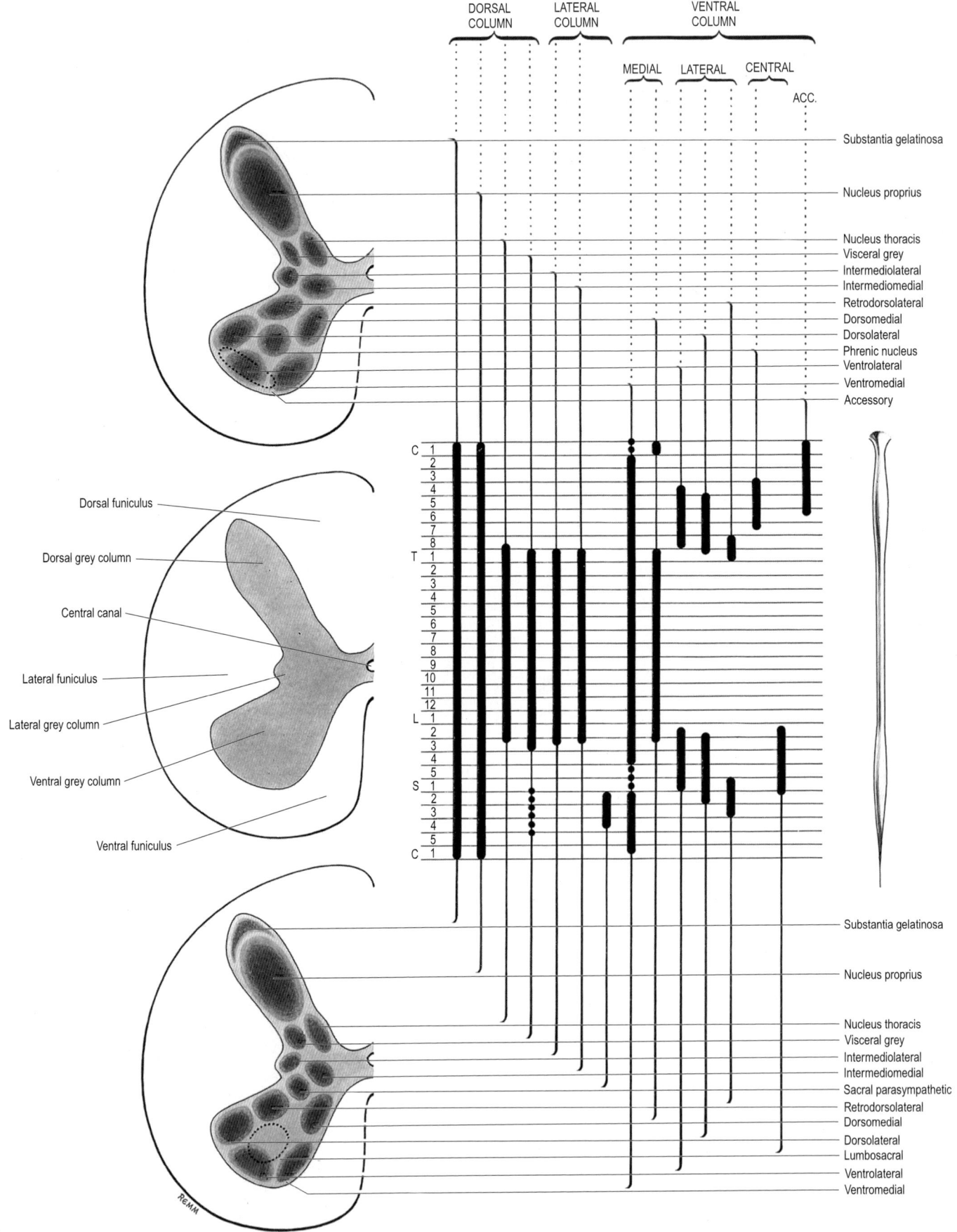

Fig. 18.6 The groups or nuclei of nerve cells in the grey columns of the human spinal cord as generally accepted. Relative positions of these columnar groups, as well as their extension through varying series of spinal segments, are indicated. ACC = accessory group. (Modified with the permission of Simon & Schuster from Correlative Anatomy of the Nervous System by E. Crosby, T. Humphrey, E. Lauer. Copyright © 1962 Macmillan Publishing Company.)

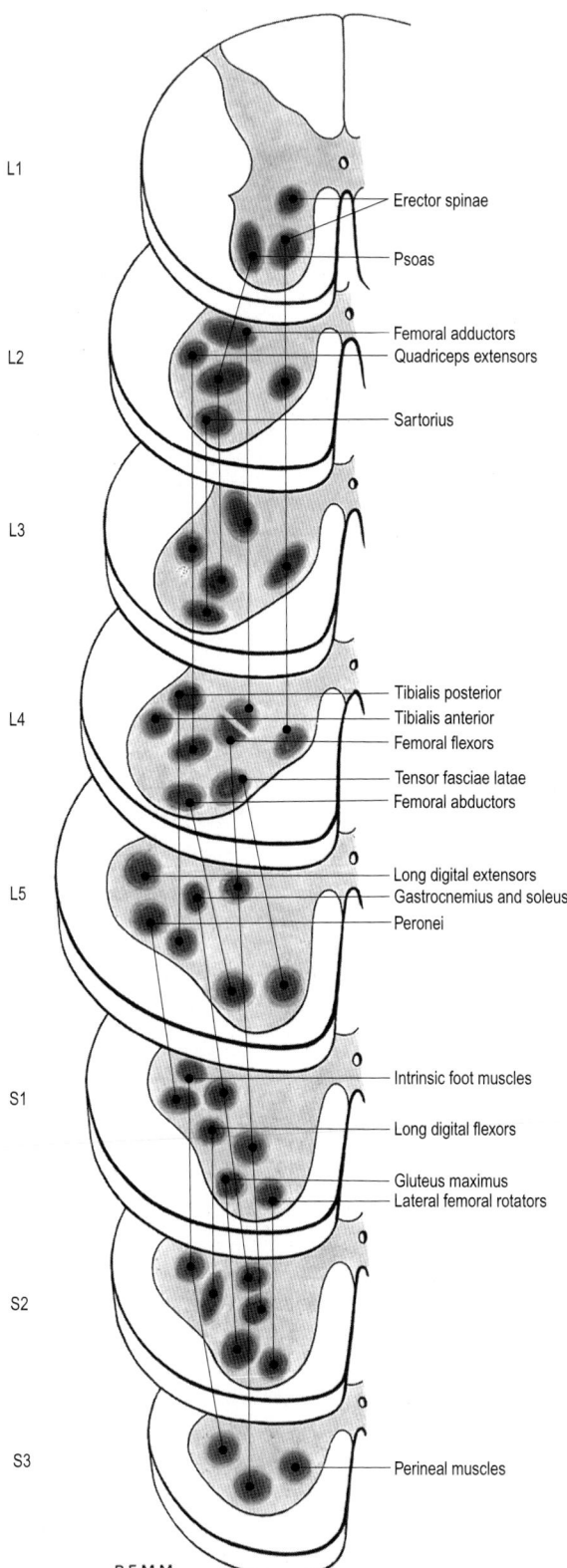

L1
— Erector spinae
— Psoas

L2
— Femoral adductors
— Quadriceps extensors
— Sartorius

L3

L4
— Tibialis posterior
— Tibialis anterior
— Femoral flexors
— Tensor fasciae latae
— Femoral abductors

L5
— Long digital extensors
— Gastrocnemius and soleus
— Peronei

S1
— Intrinsic foot muscles
— Long digital flexors
— Gluteus maximus
— Lateral femoral rotators

S2

S3
— Perineal muscles

R.E.M.M.

Fig. 18.7 The approximate location in the transverse plane and in longitudinal extent, of the nerve cell groups innervating muscles, chiefly in the leg, in the lumbosacral segments of the human spinal cord. Based on clinicopathological studies of poliomyelitis. (By permission from Sharrard WJW 1955 the distribution of the permanent paralysis in the lower limb in poliomyelitis. J Bone Jt Surg 37B: 540–558.)

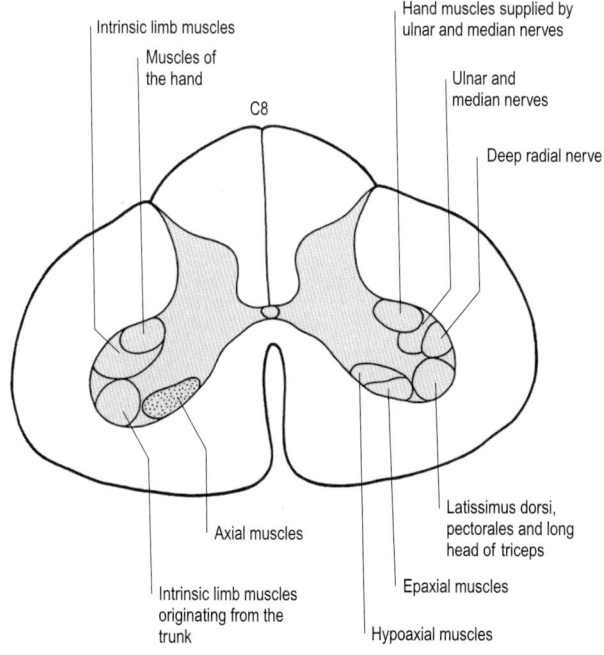

Intrinsic limb muscles

Muscles of the hand

Hand muscles supplied by ulnar and median nerves

Ulnar and median nerves

C8

Deep radial nerve

Latissimus dorsi, pectorales and long head of triceps

Axial muscles

Epaxial muscles

Intrinsic limb muscles originating from the trunk

Hypoaxial muscles

Fig. 18.8 Schematic overview of the location of motor cell groups at C8 segmental level of the spinal cord. The left side of the figure shows the subdivision of the lateral and medial longitudinal motor columns, while the right side depicts these in more detail. (Redrawn and modified from Holstege G 1991 Descending motor pathways and the spinal motor system: limbic and non-limbic components. Prog Brain Res 87: 307–421.)

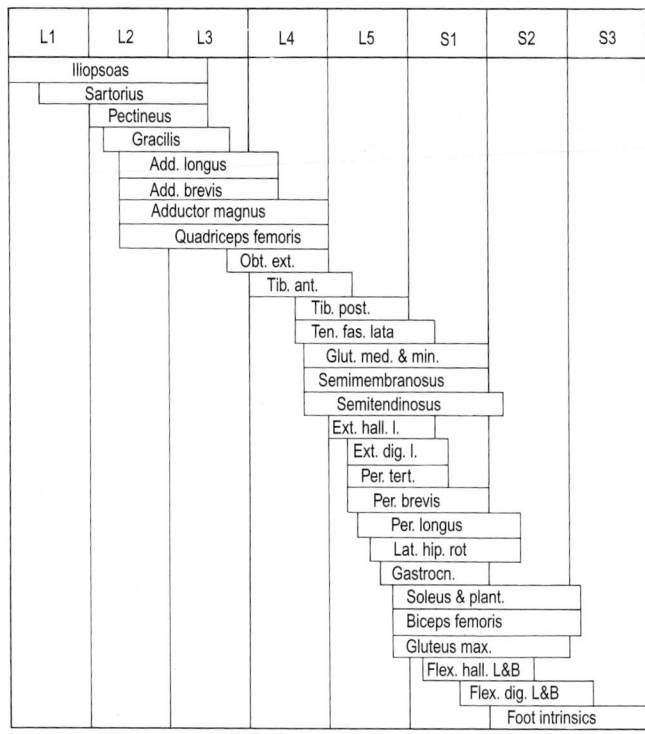

L1	L2	L3	L4	L5	S1	S2	S3
Iliopsoas							
Sartorius							
Pectineus							
Gracilis							
Add. longus							
Add. brevis							
Adductor magnus							
Quadriceps femoris							
Obt. ext.							
Tib. ant.							
Tib. post.							
Ten. fas. lata							
Glut. med. & min.							
Semimembranosus							
Semitendinosus							
Ext. hall. l.							
Ext. dig. l.							
Per. tert.							
Per. brevis							
Per. longus							
Lat. hip. rot							
Gastrocn.							
Soleus & plant.							
Biceps femoris							
Gluteus max.							
Flex. hall. L&B							
Flex. dig. L&B							
Foot intrinsics							

Fig. 18.9 The segmental arrangement of the innervation of the lower limb muscles. (From Sharrard 1964.)

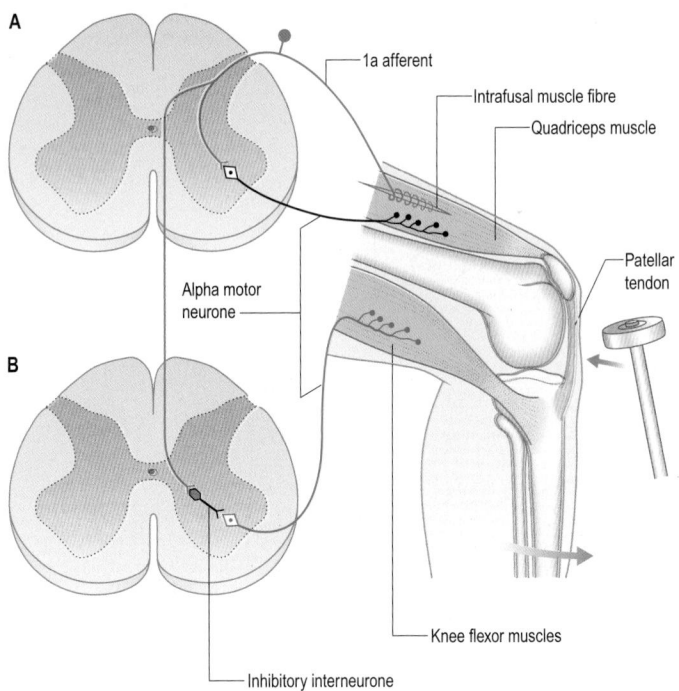

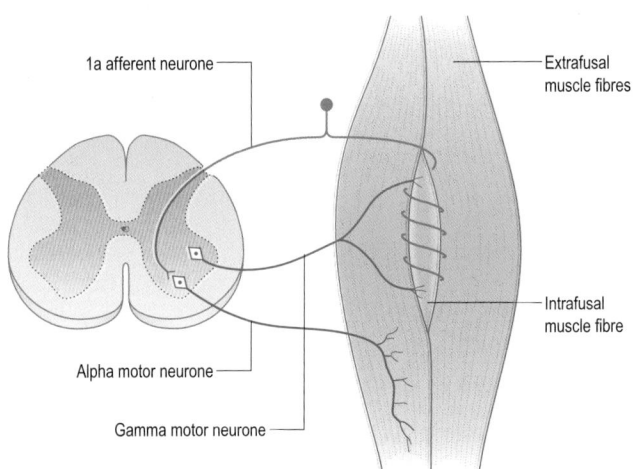

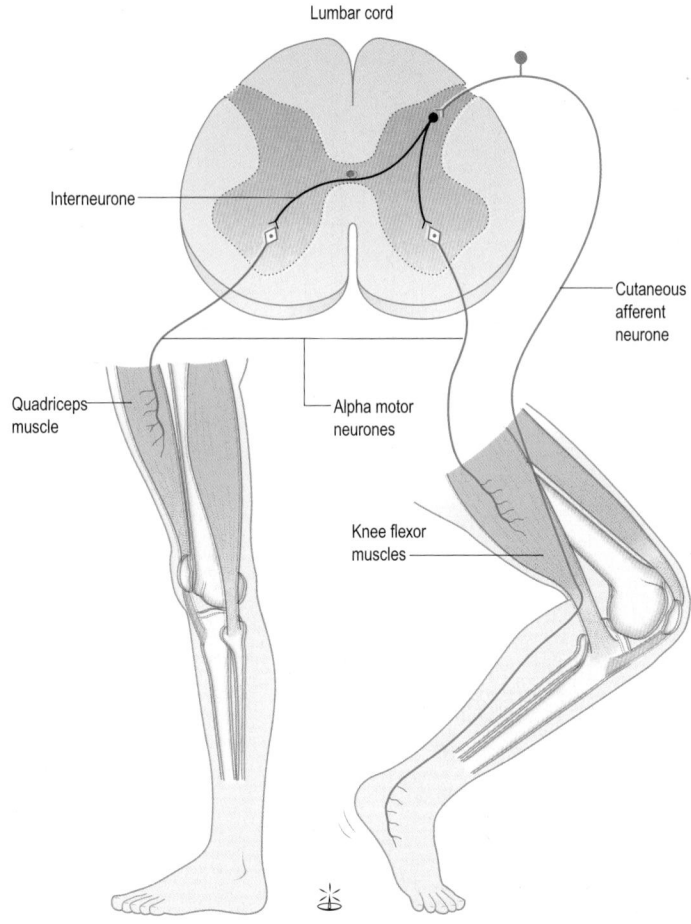

Fig. 18.10 The stretch reflex. (By permission from Crossman AR, Neary D 2000 Neuroanatomy, 2nd edn. Edinburgh: Churchill Livingstone.)

Fig. 18.11 The gamma reflex. (By permission from Crossman AR, Neary D 2000 Neuroanatomy, 2nd edn. Edinburgh: Churchill Livingstone.)

Fig. 18.12 The flexor reflex and crossed extensor reflex. (By permission from Crossman AR, Neary D 2000 Neuroanatomy, 2nd edn. Edinburgh: Churchill Livingstone.)

potential to induce a flexor reflex, but, other than in the case of noxious stimuli, this response is normally inhibited by descending pathways. When descending influences are lost, even harmless cutaneous stimulation can elicit flexion of the limbs. The Babinski (extensor plantar) reflex, which is generally regarded as pathognomonic of damage to the corticospinal tract, is part of a flexion withdrawal of the lower limb in response to stimulation of the sole of the foot.

SPINAL WHITE MATTER

The spinal white matter surrounds the central core of grey matter. It contains nerve fibres, neuroglia and blood vessels. Most of the nerve fibres run longitudinally. They are arranged in three large masses, the dorsal, lateral and ventral funiculi, on either side of the cord (**Fig. 46.5**). Fibres of related function and those with common origins or destinations are grouped to form ascending and descending tracts within the funiculi. Narrow dorsal and ventral white commissures run between the two halves of the cord. In the following account, the tracts are considered under three main headings: ascending; descending; and propriospinal. Ascending tracts contain primary afferent fibres, which enter by dorsal

roots, and fibres derived from intrinsic spinal neurones, which carry afferent impulses to supraspinal levels. Descending tracts contain long fibres, which descend from various supraspinal sources to synapse with spinal neurones. Propriospinal tracts, both ascending and descending, contain the axons of neurones which are localized entirely to the spinal cord, and link nearby and distant spinal segments. They mediate intra-segmental and intersegmental coordination.

Fibres in the white matter vary in calibre. Many are small and lightly, or non-, myelinated. Most regions contain a wide spectrum of fibre diameters, from 1 μm or less to 10 μm. Some tracts typically contain only small fibres, e.g. the dorsolateral tract, fasciculus gracilis and central part of the lateral funiculus. The fasciculus cuneatus, anterior funiculus and peripheral zone of the lateral funiculus all contain many large-diameter fibres.

Whilst the ascending and descending tracts are to a large extent discrete and regularly located, significant overlap between adjacent tracts occurs. The following account of spinal tracts is concerned with the human cord, and reference to findings in animals is only made where adequate clinicopathological data are unavailable in man. The general disposition of the major tracts is shown in **Fig. 18.2** and in greater detail at two transverse levels in **Fig. 18.3**. Some features are further summarized in **Figs 18.5, 18.13**.

Ascending tracts

Dorsal columns

The dorsal funiculus on each side of the cord consists of two large ascending tracts, the fasciculus gracilis and fasciculus cuneatus (**Fig. 18.14**), separated by a posterointermediate septum. They are also known as the dorsal columns. The dorsal columns contain a high proportion of myelinated fibres carrying proprioception (position sense and kinaesthesia) and exteroceptive (touch-pressure) information, including vibratory sensation, to higher levels. These fibres come from

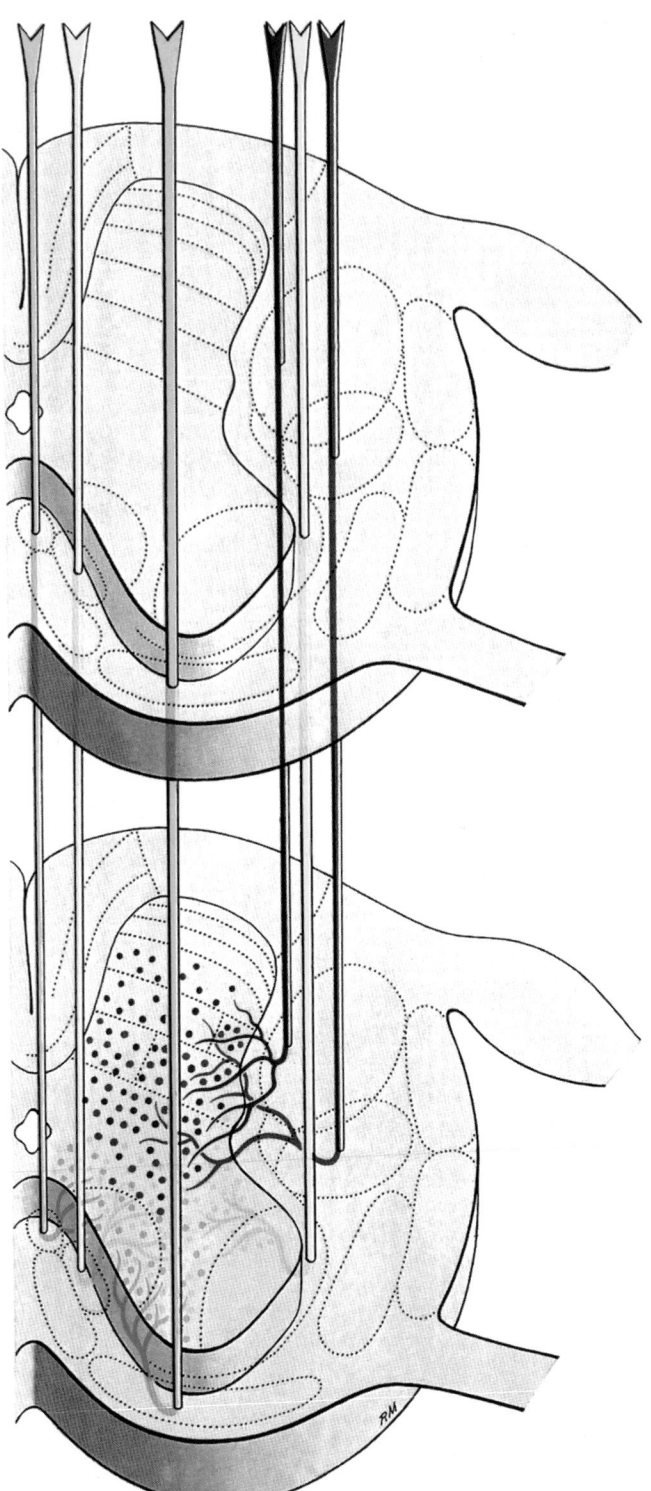

Fig. 18.13 A simplified scheme of some of the major descending tract systems of the spinal cord including their overlapping zones of termination in the grey matter. Within the grey matter the dotted lines show the laminar pattern, while within the white matter they are an approximate guide to the topography of the tracts. Corticospinal tract: mauve; rubrospinal tract: magenta; reticulospinal tracts: yellow; vestibulospinal tracts: blue.

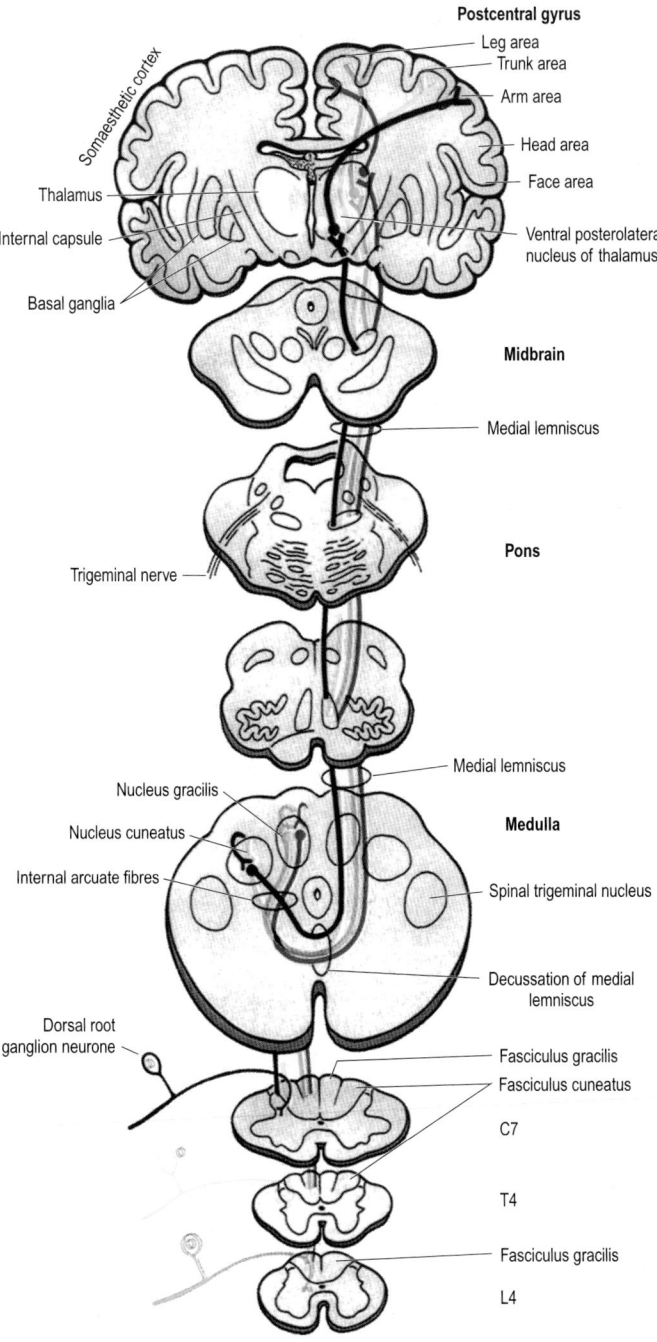

Fig. 18.14 The dorsal column system. Primary afferent fibres from different levels and their associated second- and third-order neurones are depicted in different colours (sacral: red; lumbar: blue; thoracic: yellow; cervical: black). (From Carpenter MB 1991 Core Text of Neuroanatomy, 4th edn. Baltimore: Williams and Wilkins, by permission of author and publisher.)

several sources, namely: long primary afferent fibres which enter the cord in the dorsal roots of spinal nerves and ascend to the dorsal column nuclei in the medulla oblongata; shorter primary afferent fibres projecting to neurones of Clarke's column and other spinal neurones; and axons from secondary neurones of the spinal cord ascending to the dorsal column nuclei. The dorsal columns also contain axons of propriospinal neurones.

The fasciculus gracilis begins at the caudal end of the spinal cord. It contains long ascending branches of primary afferents, which enter the cord through ipsilateral dorsal spinal roots and ascending axons of secondary neurones in laminae IV to VI of the ipsilateral dorsal horn. As the fibres ascend, they are joined by axons of successive dorsal roots. Fibres entering in coccygeal and lower sacral regions are shifted medially by successive additions of fibres entering at higher levels.

The fasciculus gracilis lies medial to the fasciculus cuneatus in the upper spinal cord (**Fig. 18.3**). At upper cervical levels the fasciculus gracilis contains a larger proportion of afferents from cutaneous receptors than from deep proprioceptors because many of the latter leave the fasciculus at lower segments to synapse in Clarke's column. Indeed, proprioception from the lower limb mostly reaches the thalamus by relaying in Clarke's column and then again in the nucleus Z. Axons of the fasciculus gracilis, from both primary and secondary neurones, terminate in the nucleus gracilis of the dorsal medulla.

The fasciculus cuneatus (**Fig. 18.14**) begins at midthoracic level and lies lateral to the fasciculus gracilis. It is composed mostly of primary afferent fibres of the upper thoracic and cervical dorsal roots. At upper cervical levels it contains a large population of afferents from both deep and cutaneous receptors of the upper limb. In addition, some of its axons arise from secondary neurones in laminae IV–VI of the ipsilateral dorsal horn. Many axons (both primary and secondary) that ascend in the fasciculus cuneatus terminate in the nucleus cuneatus of the dorsal medulla. Some also end in the lateral (external or accessory) cuneate nucleus, whose neurones project to the cerebellum via the cuneocerebellar pathway.

Many ascending fibres of the fasciculus gracilis and fasciculus cuneatus terminate by synapsing on neurones of the dorsal column nuclei (nucleus gracilis and nucleus cuneatus, respectively) in the medulla oblongata. (The connections of the dorsal column nuclei are described further with the medulla oblongata, p. 333). Axons arising from neurones in the dorsal column nuclei arch ventromedially round the central grey matter of the medulla as internal arcuate fibres (**Fig. 19.6**) and decussate in the sensory or lemniscal decussation. As the medial lemniscus, they ascend to the ventral posterolateral nucleus of the thalamus, from where neurones project to the somatosensory cortex in the postcentral gyrus of the parietal lobe (areas 3, 1 and 2). Some neurones of the dorsal column nuclei form posterior external arcuate fibres, which enter the cerebellum.

The high degree of somatotopic organization that is present in the dorsal columns is preserved as the pathways ascend through the dorsal column nuclei and thalamus to reach the primary somatosensory cortex. In the dorsal column nuclei, the lower limb is represented in the nucleus gracilis, the upper limb in the nucleus cuneatus, and the trunk lies between. Fibres are also segregated by modality in the dorsal columns. Fibres from hair receptors are most superficial, while those from tactile and vibratory receptors lie in deeper layers.

Spinocerebellar tracts

There are two principal spinocerebellar tracts, dorsal or posterior and ventral or anterior. They occupy the periphery of the lateral aspect of the spinal white matter (**Fig. 18.15**) and carry proprioceptive and cutaneous information to the cerebellum for the coordination of movement. Both tracts contain large-diameter myelinated fibres, but there are more in the posterior tract. Finer-calibre fibres are associated with the anterior tract.

The dorsal spinocerebellar tract lies lateral to the lateral corticospinal tract (**Fig. 18.2**). It begins about the level of the second or third lumbar segment and enlarges as it ascends. Axons of the tract originate ipsilaterally from the larger neurones of Clarke's column, in lamina VII throughout spinal segments T1–L2. Clarke's column receives input from collaterals of long ascending primary afferents of the doral columns and terminals of shorter ascending primary afferents of the dorsal columns. Many of these afferent fibres ascend from segments caudal to L2. In the medulla, the dorsal spinocerebellar tract passes through the inferior cerebellar peduncle to terminate ipsilaterally in the rostral and caudal parts of the cerebellar vermis.

The ventral spinocerebellar tract (**Fig. 18.15**) lies immediately ventral to the dorsal spinocerebellar tract (**Fig. 18.2**). The cells of origin are in laminae V–VII of the lumbosacral cord and the tract carries information from the lower limb. Axons forming the tract mostly decussate – a few remain ipsilateral. The tract begins in the upper lumbar region and ascends through the medulla oblongata to reach the upper pontine level, from where it descends in the dorsal part of the superior cerebellar peduncle to terminate, mainly contralaterally, in the anterior cerebellar vermis.

The spinocerebellar tracts are laminated, such that fibres from lower segments are superficial. Both tracts convey proprioceptive and exteroceptive information, but they are functionally different. Neurones of Clarke's column are excited monosynaptically by Ia and Ib primary afferent fibres (from muscle spindles and tendon organs, respectively) and also by group II muscle afferents, and cutaneous touch and pressure afferents. The proprioceptive impulses often arise from a single muscle or from synergistic muscles acting at a common joint. Thus, the dorsal spinocerebellar tract transmits modality-specific and space-specific information that is used in the fine coordination of individual limb muscles. On the other hand, the cells of the ventral tract are activated monosynaptically by Ib afferents and transmit information from large receptive fields that include different segments of a limb. The ventral tract

lacks subdivisions for different modalities and transmits information for the coordinated movement and posture of the entire lower limb.

Since Clarke's column diminishes rostrally (**Fig. 18.6**) and does not extend above the lowest cervical segment, it follows that the dorsal spinocerebellar tract carries information from the trunk and lower limb. Proprioceptive and exteroceptive information from the upper limb travels in primary afferent fibres of the fasciculus cuneatus. These fibres end somatotopically in the accessory (external or lateral) cuneate nucleus and the adjoining part of the cuneate nucleus situated in the medulla oblongata. Cells of these nuclei give rise to the posterior external arcuate fibres that form the cuneocerebellar tract (**Fig. 18.15**), which enters the cerebellum via the ipsilateral inferior cerebellar peduncle. The accessory cuneate nucleus and the lateral part of the cuneate nucleus are considered to be homologous to the cells of Clarke's column. The cuneocerebellar tract is therefore functionally allied to the dorsal spinocerebellar tract, and is its upper limb equivalent.

Axons of all the spinocerebellar tracts and the cuneocerebellar tract form part of the 'mossy-fibre system'. They end in the cerebellar cortex in a highly organized, somatotopical and functional pattern (p. 357).

Spinothalamic tracts

The spinothalamic tracts consist of second-order neurones which convey pain, temperature, coarse (non-discriminative) touch and pressure information to the somatosensory region of the thalamus. Axons arise from neurones in diverse laminae in all segments of the cord. Tract fibres decussate in the ventral white commissure. Pain and temperature fibres do so promptly, within about one segment of their origin, whilst fibres carrying other modalities may ascend for several segments before crossing. Spinothalamic fibres mostly ascend in the white matter ventrolateral to the ventral horn, partly intermingled with ascending spinoreticular fibres and descending reticulospinal fibres. Some authorities describe two spinothalamic tracts (lateral and ventral) with more-or-less distinct anatomical locations and functions. However, it should be noted that physiological studies in animals support the notion that these tracts are best considered as a structural and functional continuum.

The lateral spinothalamic tract (**Fig. 18.16**) is sited in the lateral funiculus, lying medial to the ventral spinocerebellar tract (**Fig. 18.2**). Clinical evidence indicates that it subserves pain and temperature sensations. The ventral spinothalamic tract (**Fig. 18.17**) lies in the anterior funiculus medial to the point of exit of the ventral nerve roots and dorsal to the vestibulospinal tract (**Fig. 18.2**), which it overlaps. On the basis of clinical evidence, it subserves coarse tactile and pressure modalities.

A dorsolateral spinothalamic tract has been described in animals, arising mainly from lamina I neurones whose axons cross to ascend in the contralateral dorsolateral funiculus. These neurones respond maximally to noxious, mechanical and thermal cutaneous stimuli. That such a projection exists in man is suggested by examples of clinical pain relief following dorsolateral cordotomy.

On reaching the lower brain stem, spinothalamic tract axons separate. Axons in the ventral tract join the medial lemniscus. Axons in the lateral tract continue as the spinal lemniscus.

There is clear somatotopic organization of the fibres in the spinothalamic tracts throughout their extent. Fibres crossing at any cord level join the deep aspect of those that have already crossed, which means that both tracts are segmentally laminated (**Fig. 18.18**). Somatotopy is maintained throughout the medulla oblongata and pons. In the midbrain, fibres in the spinal lemniscus conveying pain and temperature sensation from the lower limb extend dorsally, while those from the trunk and upper limb are more ventrally placed. Both lemnisci ascend to end in the thalamus (**Figs 18.16, 18.17**). The major spinothalamic projections in man are to the ventral posterolateral nucleus, and also to the centrolateral intralaminar nucleus of the thalamus.

Neurones of the spinothalamic tract

The specific localization of spinothalamic tract cell bodies in man is poorly documented. In animal studies, about a third are localized to the upper three cervical segments. About 20% are located in lower cervical segments, 20% in the thoracic region (mostly in segments T1–3), 20% in the lumbar region and 10% in the sacrococcygeal cord. Cells are located in laminae I and IV–VIII, and the greatest concentration is in laminae VI and VII. Cell bodies giving rise to spinothalamic tract axons are predominantly contralateral. A relatively small number (10%) are

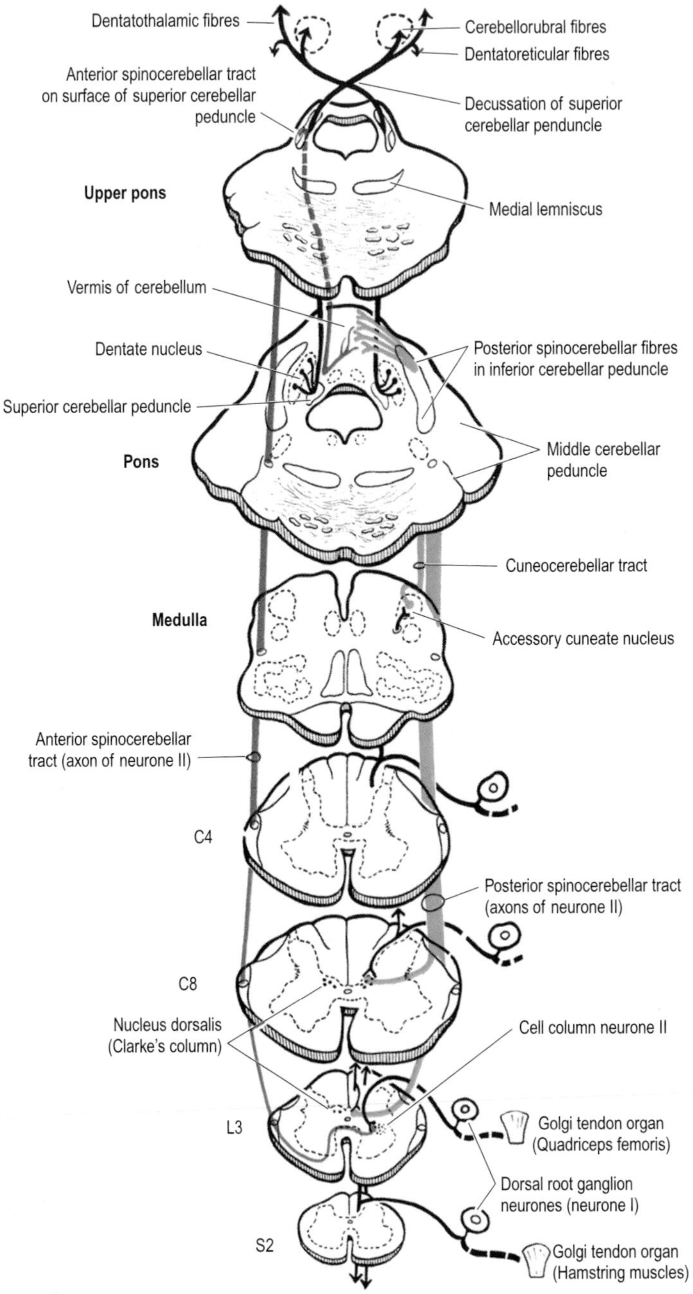

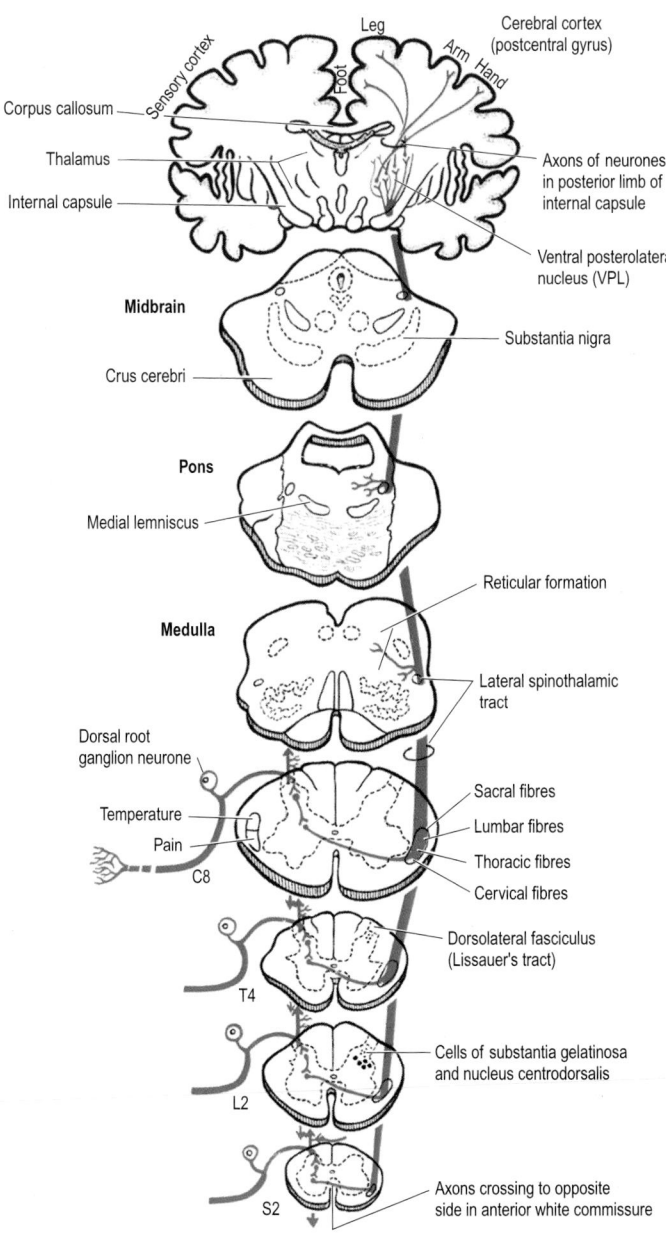

Fig. 18.15 The spinocerebellar tracts. The cells of the dorsal spinocerebellar tract and cuneocerebellar tract are shown in blue; the cells of the ventral spinocerebellar tract are shown in red. (From Carpenter MB 1991 Core Text of Neuroanatomy, 4th edn. Baltimore: Williams and Wilkins, by permission of author and publisher.)

Fig. 18.16 The lateral spinothalamic tract. (From Carpenter MB 1991 Core Text of Neuroanatomy, 4th edn. Baltimore: Williams and Wilkins, by permission of author and publisher.)

ipsilateral, of which the majority are in the upper three cervical segments.

Neurones of the spinothalamic tract have very different receptive fields. Specificity of separate channels, as it exists in the dorsal column nuclei, is absent in the laminae of the cord. Convergence of different functional types of afferent fibres onto an individual tract cell is a common feature in the cord. On the basis of laminar site, functional properties, and specific thalamic termination of their axons, spino-thalamic tract neurones may be divided into three separate groups. These are the apical cells of the dorsal grey column (lamina I), deep dorsal column cells (laminae IV–VI), and cells in the ventral grey column (laminae VII, VIII). There are species differences, the data given below pertain to the monkey.

Lamina I cells which project to the thalamus show the following characteristics. In essence they respond maximally to noxious or thermal cutaneous stimulation, and consist mainly of high-threshold, but also some wide-dynamic-range, units. Their receptive fields are usually small, representing a part of a digit or a small area of skin involving several

digits. Lamina I spinothalamic tract neurones receive input from Aδ and C fibres, and some respond to convergent input from deep somatic and visceral receptors. Spinothalamic tract cells in the thoracic cord display marked viscerosomatic convergence. Lamina I spinothalamic tract neurones project preferentially to the ventroposterolateral nucleus of the thalamus, with limited projections to the centrolateral and mediodorsal thalamic nuclei. The population of deep dorsal column (laminae IV–VI) spinothalamic neurones of the lumbar cord contains wide-dynamic-range (60%), high-threshold (30%), and low-threshold (10%) type units. They can code accurately both innocuous and noxious cutaneous stimuli. Some cells also respond to input from deep somatic and visceral receptors. In the lumbar cord their receptive fields are small or medium sized, they are larger than the area of the foot, but smaller than the entire leg. In the thoracic cord the fields of these laminar cells are larger, and often include the entire upper limb plus part of the chest. Many of the deep dorsal column spinothalamic tract neurones in the thoracic segments receive convergent input from sympathetic afferent fibres. Laminae IV–VI spinothalamic tract units project either to the ventroposterolateral (VPL) nucleus or to the centrolateral nucleus of the thalamus, and sometimes to both. Units projecting to the ventro-posterolateral nucleus receive input from all classes (Aβ, Aδ and C) of cutaneous fibres.

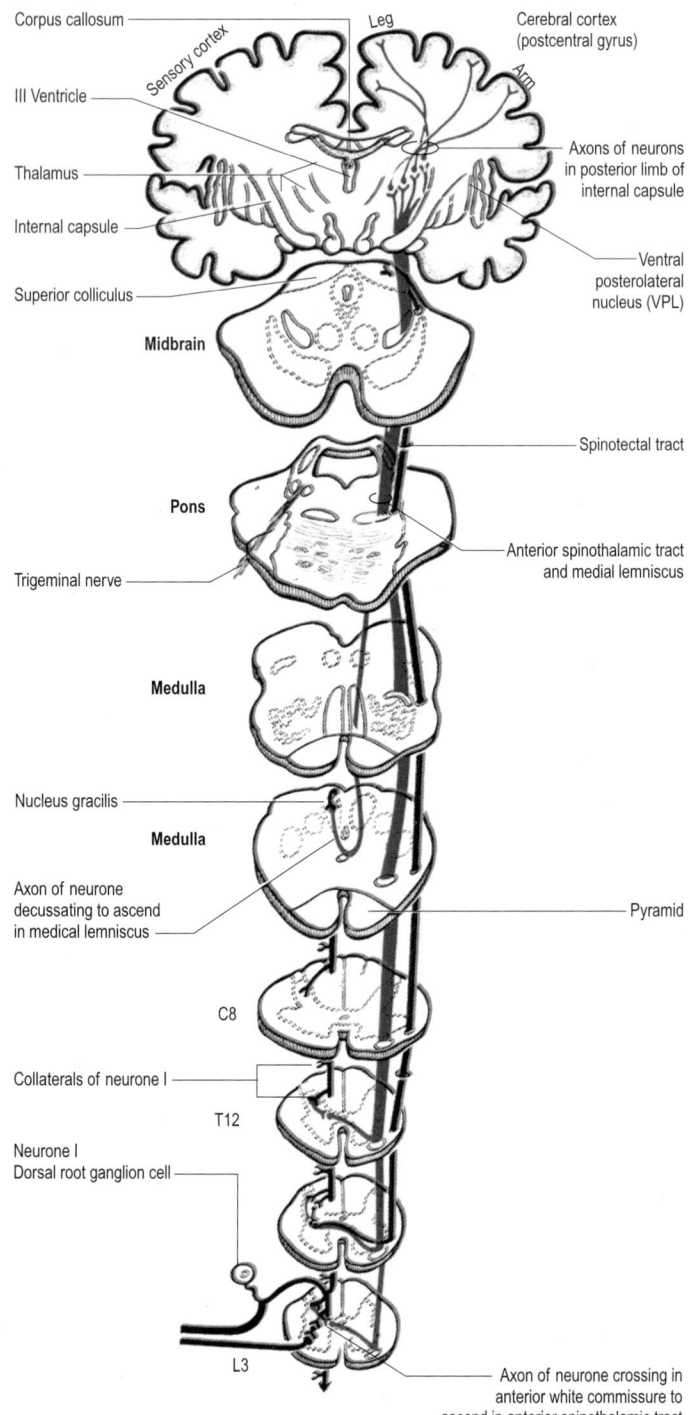

Fig. 18.17 The ventral (anterior) spinothalamic tract. (From Carpenter MB 1991 Core Text of Neuroanatomy, 4th edn. Baltimore: Williams and Wilkins, by permission of author and publisher.)

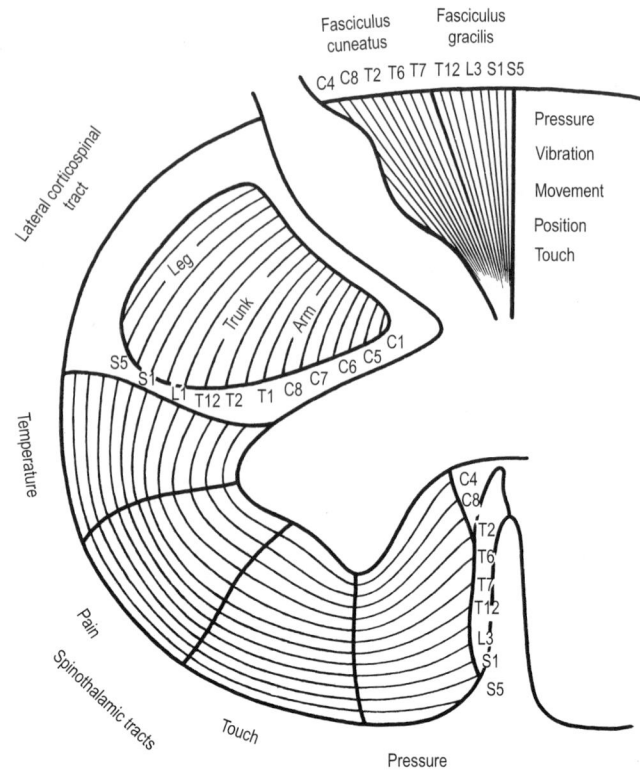

Fig. 18.18 General plan of the segmental organization of fibres in the dorsal funiculus, the lateral corticospinal tract and the spinothalamic tracts. The probable cross-sectional areas of these tracts are schematically enlarged. This general plan applies to all segmentally organized tracts whether ascending, descending, ipsilateral or contralateral. (After Foerster O 1936 Motorische Felder und Bahnen. In: Bumke O, Foerster O (eds) Handbuch der Neurologie, Vol. 6. Berlin: Springer-Verlag, by permission.)

different intensities of painful stimulation. It has been suggested that the spinothalamic projection to the ventroposterolateral nucleus is concerned with the discriminative aspects of pain perception, whereas the projection to other thalamic regions, particularly the intralaminar nuclei, may be involved in arousal and/or aversive behaviour.

The activity of spinothalamic tract neurones may be selectively modulated by pathways descending from the brain to the spinal cord. Many studies show that the response of spinothalamic tract cells to noxious stimuli is inhibited by stimulation of certain regions of the brain. This is obviously of considerable clinical interest in the treatment of chronic, intractable, pain. In the brain stem, these regions include the nucleus raphe magnus, the periaqueductal grey matter, and parts of the mesencephalic and medullary reticular formation including the parabrachial region. These neuronal groups and their connections constitute the endogenous analgesic system. Forebrain sites, which inhibit spinothalamic tract cells on stimulation, include the periventricular grey matter, the ventral posterolateral nucleus of the thalamus, and the primary sensory (SI) and posterior parietal cortices. Inhibition of spinothalamic tract neurones is also produced by electrical stimulation of peripheral nerves, the most effective being volleys from Aδ fibres. In contrast, some spinothalamic tract cells are excited by stimulation of the medullary reticular formation, and the primary motor cortex (this latter effect is probably mediated by the corticospinal tract).

Spinoreticular pathway
Spinoreticular fibres are intermingled with those of the spinothalamic tracts, and ascend in the ventrolateral quadrant of the spinal cord (**Fig. 18.19**). Evidence from animal studies suggests that cells of origin occur at all levels of the spinal cord, particularly in the upper cervical segments. Most neurones are in lamina VII, some are in lamina VIII, and others are in the dorsal horn, especially lamina V. Most axons in the lumbar and cervical enlargements cross the midline, but there is a large uncrossed component in cervical regions. Most axons are myelinated. The pattern of anterograde degeneration, in both human postmortem studies and in experimental animals following anterolateral cordotomy, indicates spinoreticular projections to many nuclei of the medial pontomedullary

Ventral grey column (laminae VII and VIII) spinothalamic tract cells respond mainly to deep somatic (muscle and joint) stimuli, but also to innocuous and/or noxious cutaneous stimuli. In the thoracic regions of the spinal cord they also receive convergent input from visceral sources. The majority of laminae VII and VIII spinothalamic tract neurones have large, complex receptive fields (often bilateral), which encompass widespread areas of the body. Cells of this group, which project exclusively to the medial thalamus, receive input from Aβ, Aδ and C classes of afferent fibres, and many respond to convergent input from receptors of deep structures. This population of neurones contains wide-dynamic-range (25%), high-threshold (63%), and low-threshold or deep (12%) units. Most of the spinothalamic tract cells in the ventral grey column project to the intralaminar nuclei of the thalamus. Wide-dynamic-range type neurones are particularly effective for discriminating between

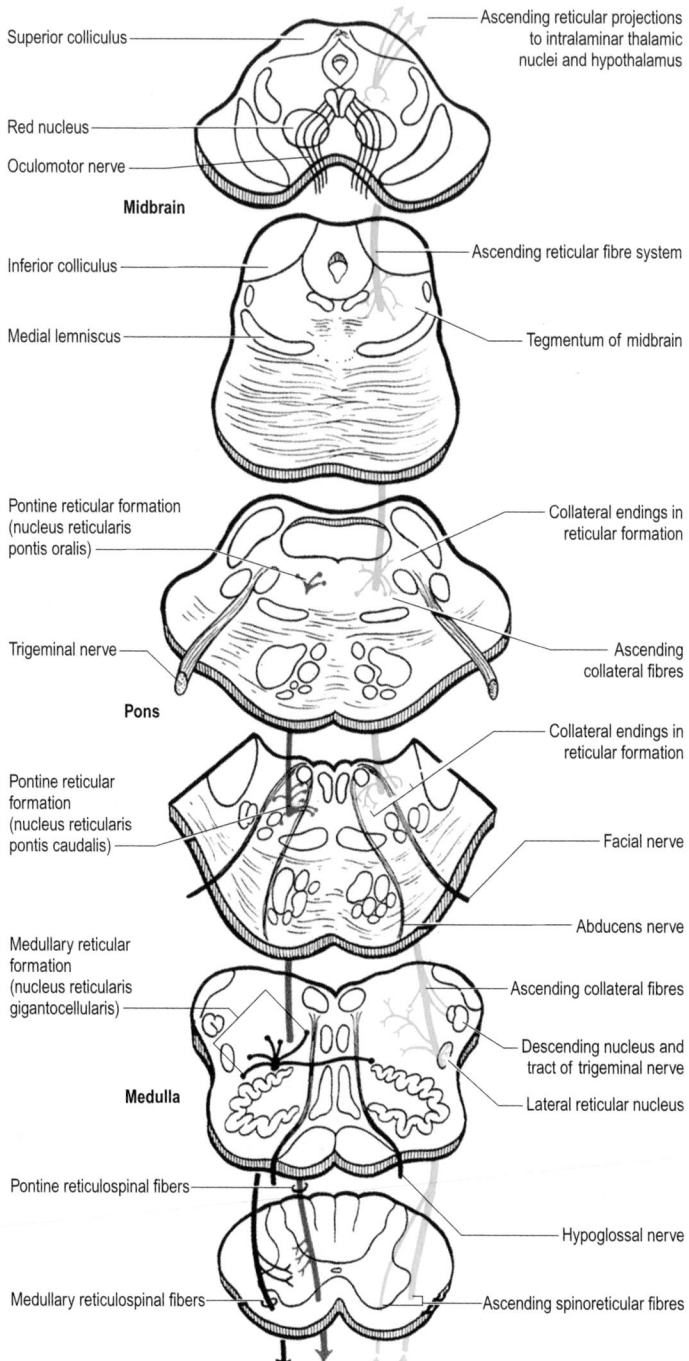

Superior colliculus

Ascending reticular projections to intralaminar thalamic nuclei and hypothalamus

Red nucleus

Oculomotor nerve

Midbrain

Inferior colliculus

Ascending reticular fibre system

Medial lemniscus

Tegmentum of midbrain

Pontine reticular formation (nucleus reticularis pontis oralis)

Collateral endings in reticular formation

Trigeminal nerve

Ascending collateral fibres

Pons

Collateral endings in reticular formation

Pontine reticular formation (nucleus reticularis pontis caudalis)

Facial nerve

Medullary reticular formation (nucleus reticularis gigantocellularis)

Abducens nerve

Ascending collateral fibres

Medulla

Descending nucleus and tract of trigeminal nerve

Lateral reticular nucleus

Pontine reticulospinal fibers

Hypoglossal nerve

Medullary reticulospinal fibers

Ascending spinoreticular fibres

Fig. 18.19 Reticular tracts. Ascending: blue; descending: red; medullary: black. (From Carpenter MB 1991 Core Text of Neuroanatomy, 4th edn. Baltimore: Williams and Wilkins, by permission of author and publisher.)

reticular formation. There is also a projection to the lateral reticular nucleus (a precerebellar relay nucleus). No somatotopic arrangement has been reported. Spinoreticular neurones respond to inputs from the skin or deep tissues. Innocuous cutaneous stimuli may inhibit or excite a particular cell, whereas noxious stimuli are often excitatory. A spino–reticulo–thalamo–cortical pathway has been proposed as an important route serving pain perception. Like other ascending pathways, the tract cells are influenced by descending control. For example, electrical stimulation of the periaqueductal grey matter inhibits the responses of certain spinoreticular cells to input from cardiopulmonary afferents. Stimulation of the reticular formation also alters the activity of spino-reticular neurones.

Spinocervicothalamic pathway

The lateral cervical nucleus is small in man. It lies in the lateral funiculus, ventrolateral to the dorsal horn in the upper two cervical segments. In some human cord specimens the nucleus was not distinctly defined, and was possibly incorporated into the dorsal horn. It receives axons from the spinocervical tract, which ascends in the dorsolateral funiculus. The tract cells are found in laminae III–V at all levels of the spinal cord, ipsilateral to the nucleus. Most neurones of the nucleus project to the contralateral thalamus via the medial lemniscus, and some project to the contralateral midbrain. Specific thalamic targets include the ventral posterolateral nucleus and part of the posterior complex. Spinocervical tract neurones respond to hair movement, pressure, pinch and thermal stimuli and to high-threshold muscle input; many also respond to noxious stimuli. Like tract cells of other ascending pathways, they are under tonic descending inhibitory control.

Spinomesencephalic pathway

The spinomesencephalic pathway consists of a number of tracts ascending from the spinal cord to various regions of the midbrain. It includes the spinotectal tract projecting to the superior colliculus, neurones synapsing in the periaqueductal grey matter, and other spinal cord projections which terminate in the parabrachial nucleus, the pretectal nuclei and the nucleus of Darkschewitsch. Cells of origin are located throughout the length of the spinal cord, particularly in the cervical segments and the lumbosacral enlargement, mostly in lamina I, but they are also present in laminae IV–VIII, where they are concentrated in lamina V. Most are contralateral, but a prominent ipsilateral group is also found at upper cervical levels. Fibres of the spinomesencephalic tract are mostly myelinated and ascend in the white matter of the ventrolateral quadrant of the spinal cord, in association with the spinothalamic and spinoreticular tracts.

Spinomesencephalic tract neurones are of low-threshold, wide-dynamic-range, or high-threshold classes. Their receptive fields may be small, or very complex and encompass large surface areas of the body. Many spinomesencephalic tract cells are nociceptive and are likely to be involved in the motivational-affective component of pain. Electrical stimulation of their site of termination in the periaqueductal grey matter results in severe pain in man. Furthermore, the cells of the deeper layers of the superior colliculus, where spinotectal fibres synapse, are activated by noxious stimuli.

Spino-olivary tract

The spino-olivary tract is described in animals as arising from neurones in the deeper laminae of grey matter. Axons forming the tract cross and then ascend superficially at the junction of the anterior and lateral white funiculi, to end in the 'spinal' regions of the dorsal and medial accessory olivary nuclei. The tract carries information from muscle and tendon proprioceptors, and also from cutaneous receptors. A function-ally similar route, the dorsal spino-olivary tract, ascends in the dorsal white funiculi, and relays in the dorsal column nuclei to the contra-lateral inferior olive. Information on these tracts in primates is scant, but postmortem evidence following cordotomies in man has revealed degenerating axonal terminals in the inferior olive.

Pain mechanisms

The ascending connections through which sensory information reaches higher centres should not be regarded as simple relays. Because it is known that they are subject to modulation by complex intraspinal influences and by descending pathways from the brain stem and cerebral cortex. This is particularly important in relation to the spino-thalamic and spinoreticular pathways and the perception of pain.

Presynaptic inhibition influences many, possibly all, primary afferent terminals. A much-investigated site of presynaptic effects is the sub-stantia gelatinosa. It has been proposed that impulses from cutaneous (and other) afferents are here subjected to tonic control by presynaptic modulation of primary afferent terminals, mediated by small neurones of the substantia gelatinosa.

The 'gate control theory' (Melzack & Wall 1965) defined a possible mechanism for modulating the inflow of information along nociceptive and other afferent pathways (**Fig. 18.20**). The proposition was that large-diameter afferents (e.g. from hairs and touch corpuscles) are excitatory to the large neurones of lamina IV, from which spinothalamic fibres arise, and to interneurones in the substantia gelatinosa. In contrast, fine non-myelinated afferents are excitatory to tract cells but inhibitory to the interneurones. The axons of substantia gelatinosa interneurones are presumed to inhibit presynaptically the terminals of all afferents that synapse with tract cells. In such a system, low activity in the fine afferents

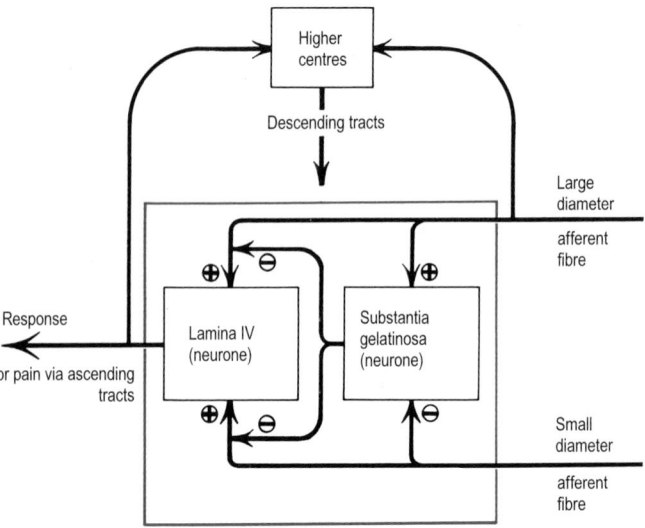

Fig. 18.20 The basic arrangement of the sensory 'gate' mechanism in the dorsal laminae of the grey matter of the spinal cord. (Redrawn with permission from Melzack R, Wall PD Pain mechanisms: a new theory. Science 150: 971–979. Copyright 1965 American Association for the Advancement of Science.)

inhibits the interneurones, and so prevents them inhibiting tract cells, hence the 'gate' to T cells in lamina IV is open to transmit intermittent small volleys of impulses from the large fibres. A prolonged high-frequency volley of impulses in the large-diameter afferents would be transmitted to lamina IV tract cells initially, but this would soon cease as activity in the interneurones closed the gate. Conversely, a persistent high activity in the fine afferents would open the gate resulting in massive bombardment of neurones of lamina IV (which include some neurones of high threshold that are only activated by such bombardment). It was assumed that onward transmission in the lateral spinothalamic tract would evoke pain at supraspinal centres. Pain, therefore, would result from an imbalance between the varieties of afferent impulses when there was a disproportionately large traffic along the fine afferents.

The overall sensitivity of the gate may be varied by descending supraspinal control systems. These originate within three principal, interconnected, regions in the midbrain, hindbrain and spinal cord, each of which receives a variety of afferents and contains an array of neuromediators.

The midbrain regions are the periaqueductal grey matter, dorsal raphe nucleus, and part of the cuneiform nucleus. Neurones in these sites contain serotonin (5-HT), γ-aminobutyric acid (GABA), substance P, CCK, neurotensin, enkephalin and dynorphin. The periaqueductal grey matter receives afferents from the frontal somatosensory and cingulate neocortex, the amygdala, numerous local reticular nuclei and the hypothalamus. Afferents from the latter are separate bundles, which carry histamine, luteinizing hormone-releasing hormone (LHRH), vasopressin, oxytocin, adrenocorticotrophic hormone (ACTH), melanocyte-stimulating hormone (γ-MSH), endorphin, and angiotensin II. Some fibres descend from the periaqueductal grey matter to rhombencephalic centres, others pass directly to the spinal cord.

In the rhombencephalon, the raphe magnus nucleus and the medial reticular column constitute an important multineuromediator centre. Neurones in these sites contain serotonin, substance P, CCK, thyrotrophin-releasing hormone (TRH), enkephalin and dynorphin. Some neurones contain two or even three neuromediators. Descending bulbospinal fibres pass to the nucleus of the spinal tract of the trigeminal nerve and its continuation, the substantia gelatinosa. The latter extends throughout the length of the cord and contains populations of neurones expressing many different neuromediators, e.g. GABA, substance P, neurotensin, enkephalin and dynorphin. There is abundant physiological and pharmacological evidence that all of these regions are intimately concerned with the control of nociceptive (and probably other modality) inputs.

Descending pathways

Descending pathways to the spinal cord originate primarily in the cerebral cortex and in numerous sites within the brain stem (**Figs 18.19,**

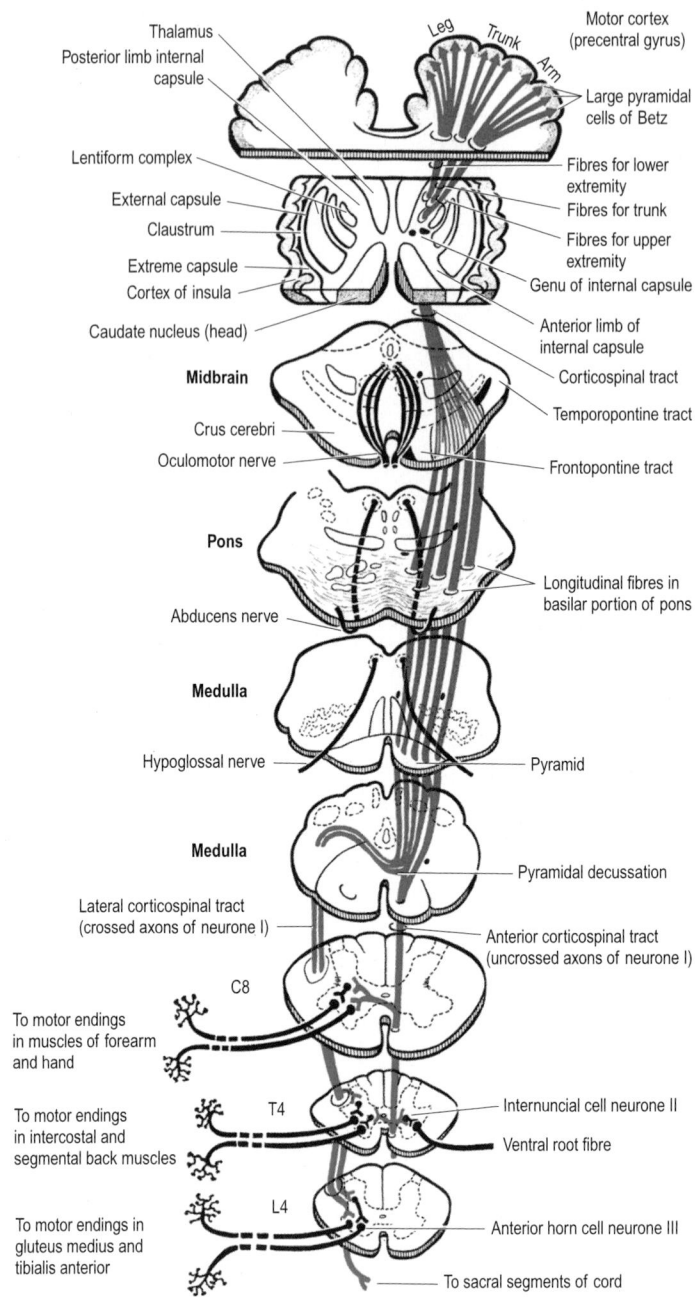

Fig. 18.21 The corticospinal tracts. (From Carpenter MB 1991 Core Text of Neuroanatomy, 4th edn. Baltimore: Williams and Wilkins, by permission of author and publisher.)

18.21, 18.22). They are concerned with the control of movement, muscle tone and posture; the modulation of spinal reflex mechanisms; and the transmission of afferent information to higher levels. They also mediate control over spinal autonomic neurones.

Corticospinal tract

Corticospinal fibres arise from neurones of the cerebral cortex. They project, in a somatotopically organized fashion, to neurones that are mostly located in the contralateral side of the spinal cord (**Fig. 18.21**). The majority of corticospinal fibres arise from cells situated in the upper two-thirds of the precentral motor cortex (area 4), and from the premotor cortex (area 6). A small contribution of fibres stems from cells of the postcentral gyrus (somatosensory cortex, areas 3, 1, and 2) and the adjacent parietal cortex (area 5). In the monkey, 30% of corticospinal fibres arise from area 4, 30% from area 6, and 40% from the parietal regions. Cells of origin of corticospinal fibres vary in size in the different cortical areas and are clustered into groups or strips. The largest cells (giant pyramidal neurones, or Betz cells) are in the precentral cortex.

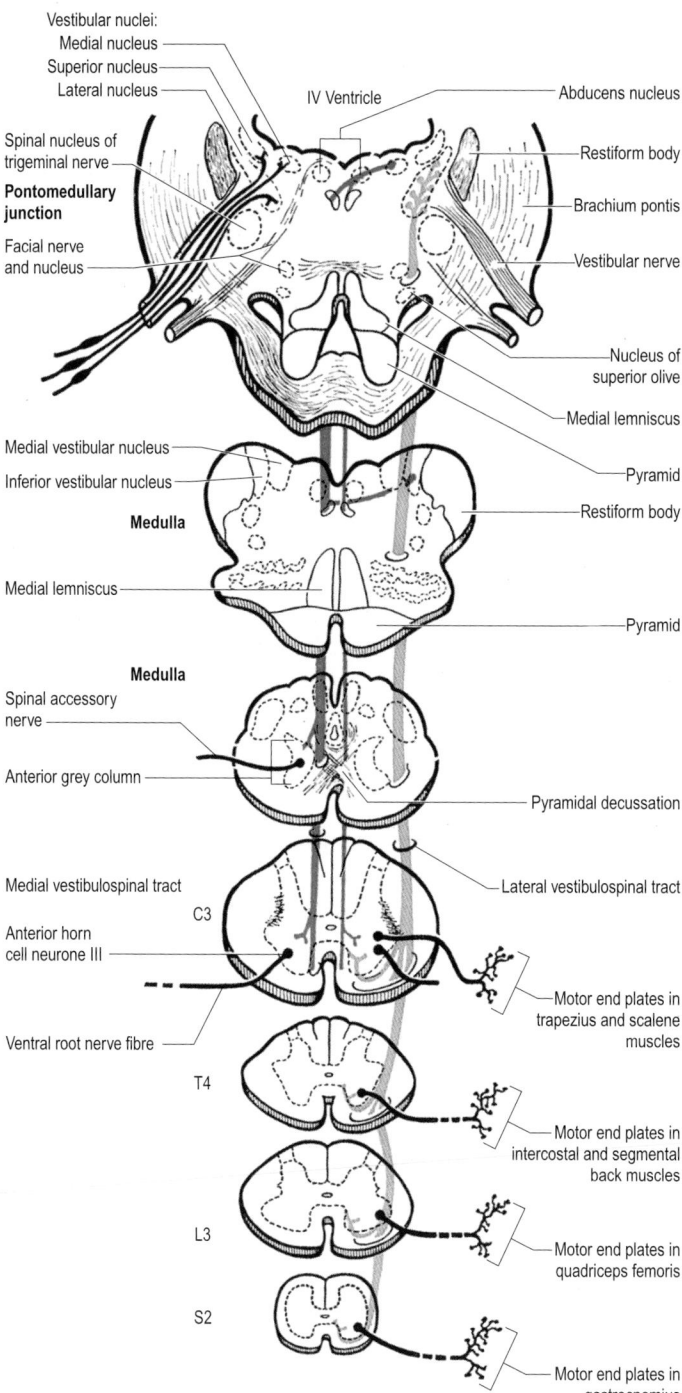

Fig. 18.22 The vestibulospinal tracts. (From Carpenter MB 1991 Core Text of Neuroanatomy, 4th edn. Baltimore: Williams and Wilkins, by permission of author and publisher.)

Corticospinal fibres descend at first through the subcortical white matter and enter the posterior limb of the internal capsule. They then pass through the ventral part of the midbrain in the cerebral peduncle or crus cerebri. As they continue caudally through the pons they are separated from its ventral surface by transversely running ponto-cerebellar fibres. In the medulla oblongata, they form a discrete bundle, the pyramid (**Fig. 19.3**), which forms a prominent longitudinal column on the ventral surface of the medulla. The corticospinal tracts are therefore also referred to as the pyramidal tracts. However, this term is often used to embrace not only corticospinal fibres, but also corticobulbar fibres, which diverge above this level and end in association with cranial motor nuclei. Each pyramid contains about a million axons of varying diameter. The majority (70%) are myelinated: most (90%) have a diameter of 1–4 μm; 9% have diameters of 5–10 μm; and less than 2% have diameters of 11–22 μm. The largest diameter axons arise from the giant Betz cells.

Just rostral to the level of the spinomedullary junction, c.75–90% of the corticospinal fibres in the pyramid cross the median plane in the pyramidal decussation (decussation of the pyramids) and continue caudally as the lateral corticospinal tract. The rest of the fibres continue uncrossed as the ventral corticospinal tract. The lateral tract also contains some uncrossed corticospinal fibres. The lateral corticospinal tract (**Fig. 18.21**) descends in the lateral funiculus throughout most of the length of the spinal cord. It occupies an oval area, ventrolateral to the dorsal horn and medial to the dorsal spinocerebellar tract (**Fig. 18.3**). In the lumbar and sacral regions, where the dorsal spinocerebellar tract is absent, the lateral corticospinal tract reaches the dorsolateral surface of the cord. As it descends, the lateral corticospinal tract progressively diminishes in size until about the fourth sacral spinal segment. Its axons terminate on ipsilateral spinal neurones.

The smaller ventral corticospinal tract (**Fig. 18.21**) descends in the ventral funiculus. It lies close to the ventral median fissure, and is separated from it by the sulcomarginal fasciculus (**Fig. 18.3**). The ventral corticospinal tract diminishes as it descends and usually disappears completely at midthoracic cord levels. It may either be absent or, very rarely, contain almost all the corticospinal fibres. Near their termination, most fibres of the tract cross the median plane in the ventral white commissure to synapse with contralateral neurones. The vast majority of corticospinal fibres, irrespective of the tract in which they descend, therefore terminate in the spinal cord on the side contralateral to their cortical origin.

Knowledge of the detailed termination of corticospinal fibres is based largely upon animal studies, but is supplemented by data from postmortem studies on human brains using anterograde degeneration methods. Most corticospinal fibres are believed to terminate contralaterally on interneurones in the lateral parts of laminae IV–VI and both lateral and medial parts of lamina VII. Some are also distributed to lamina VIII bilaterally. Terminals are also associated with contralateral motor neuronal cell groups in lamina IX, in the dorsolateral group and the lateral parts of both central and ventrolateral groups (**Fig. 18.13**).

Corticospinal fibres from the frontal cortex, including motor and premotor areas 4 and 6, terminate mostly on interneurones in laminae V–VIII, with the densest concentration laterally in lamina VI. They influence α and γ motor neurones of lamina IX via these interneurones. Because the widespread dendrites of multipolar neurones in lamina IX penetrate lamina VII, direct monosynaptic axodendritic contacts also occur on large α motor neurones. Direct termination on motor neurones is most abundant in the spinal enlargements.

Experimental evidence shows that precentral corticospinal axons influence the activities of both α and γ motor neurones, facilitating flexor muscles and inhibiting extensors, which are the opposite effects to those mediated by lateral vestibulospinal fibres. Evidence from animal studies shows that direct projections from the precentral cortical areas to spinal motor neurones are concerned with highly fractionated, precision movements of the limbs. Accordingly, in primates, precentral corticospinal fibres are mainly distributed to motor neurones supplying the distal limb muscles. Corticospinal projections may use glutamate or aspartate, often co-localized, as excitatory neurotransmitters.

Corticospinal fibres from parietal sources end mainly in the contralateral dorsal horn, in the lateral parts of laminae IV–VI and lamina VII. Phylogenetically these fibres represent the oldest part of the corticospinal system. Axons from the sensory cortex terminate chiefly in laminae IV and V. They are concerned with the supraspinal modulation of the transmission of afferent impulses to higher centres, including the motor cortex.

Experimental studies in primates indicate that isolated transection of corticospinal fibres at the level of the pyramid (pyramidotomy) results in flaccid paralysis or paresis of the contralateral limbs and loss of independent hand and finger movements. Destruction of corticospinal fibres at the level of the internal capsule, commonly caused by a cerebral vascular accident or 'stroke', results in a contralateral hemiplegia. The paralysis is initially flaccid, but later becomes spastic, and is most marked in the distal muscles of the extremities, especially those concerned with individual movements of the fingers and hand. Associated signs on the paralysed side are: hyperactive deep tendon reflexes; hypertonicity; the loss of superficial abdominal and cremasteric reflexes; and the appearance of dorsiflexion of the toes (Babinski's sign) in response to stroking the sole of the foot. The latter is usually interpreted as pathognomonic of corticospinal damage, but it is not always present in patients with confirmed corticospinal lesions. Moreover,

Babinski's sign is normally present in human infants up to about 2 years of age – its subsequent disappearance may reflect the completion of myelination of the corticospinal fibres and/or the establishment of direct cortical connections to lower motor neurones.

Some of the sequelae of stroke damage in the internal capsule, in particular hyperreflexia and hypertonia, are due to the involvement of other pathways in addition to the corticospinal tract. These include descending cortical fibres to brain stem nuclei, such as the vestibular and reticular nuclei, that themselves give rise to descending projections which influence motor neurone activity.

Rubrospinal tract

The rubrospinal tract arises from neurones in the caudal magnocellular part of the red nucleus (an ovoid mass of cells situated centrally in the midbrain tegmentum (p. 344). This part of the nucleus contains some 150–200 large neurones, interspersed with smaller neurones.

The origin, localization, termination and functions of rubrospinal connections are poorly defined in man, and the tract appears to be rudimentary. Rubrospinal fibres cross in the ventral tegmental decussation and descend in the lateral funiculus of the cord, where they lie ventral to, and intermingled with, fibres of the lateral corticospinal tract (**Fig. 18.3**). In animals the tract descends as far as lumbosacral levels, whereas in man it appears to project only to the upper three cervical cord segments. Rubrospinal fibres are distributed to the lateral parts of laminae V–VI and the dorsal part of lamina VII of the spinal grey matter. The terminal zones of the tract correspond to those of corticospinal fibres from the motor cortex. Animal studies demonstrate that the effects of rubrospinal fibres on α and γ motor neurones are similar to those of corticospinal fibres.

Tectospinal tract

The tectospinal tract arises from neurones in the intermediate and deep layers of the superior colliculus of the midbrain. It crosses ventral to the periaqueductal grey matter in the dorsal tegmental decussation and descends in the medial part of the ventral funiculus of the spinal cord (**Fig. 18.2**). Fibres of the tract project only to the upper cervical cord segments, ending in laminae VI–VIII. They make polysynaptic connections with motor neurones serving muscles in the neck, facilitating those that innervate contralateral muscles and inhibiting those that innervate ipsilateral ones. In animals, turning of the head to the contralateral side results from unilateral, electrical stimulation of the superior colliculus, and is mainly effected through the tectospinal tract.

Vestibulospinal tracts

The large vestibular nuclear complex lies in the lateral part of the floor of the fourth ventricle around the pontomedullary junction of the brain stem. It gives rise to the lateral and ventral vestibulospinal tracts, which are functionally and topographically distinct (**Fig. 18.22**).

The lateral vestibulospinal tract arises from small and large neurones of the lateral vestibular nucleus (Deiters' nucleus). It descends ipsilaterally, initially in the periphery of the ventrolateral spinal white matter but subsequently shifting into the medial part of the ventral funiculus at lower spinal levels. Fibres of this tract are somatotopically organized. Thus, fibres projecting to the cervical, thoracic and lumbosacral segments of the cord arise from neurones in the rostroventral, central and dorsocaudal parts, respectively, of the lateral vestibular nucleus. Lateral vestibulospinal fibres end ipsilaterally, mostly in the medial part of the ventral horn in lamina VIII and the medial part of lamina VII. Axons of the lateral vestibulospinal tract excite, through mono- and polysynaptic connections, motor neurones of extensor muscles of the neck, back and limbs; γ motor neurones are also probably facilitated. Lateral vestibulospinal tract axons also inhibit, disynaptically, motor neurones of flexor limb muscles, via 1a inhibitory interneurones.

The medial vestibulospinal tract arises mainly from neurones in the medial vestibular nucleus, but some are also located in the inferior and lateral vestibular nuclei. The medial vestibulospinal tract (**Fig. 18.22**) descends in the medial longitudinal fasciculus into the ventral funiculus of the spinal cord where it lies close to the midline in the so-called sulcomarginal fasciculus (**Fig. 18.3**). Unlike the lateral tract it contains both crossed and uncrossed fibres, and does not extend beyond the midthoracic cord level. Fibres of the medial tract project mainly to the cervical cord segments, ending in lamina VIII and the adjacent dorsal part of lamina VII. Data from stimulation of the vestibular nuclei in animals indicate that axons of the medial tract monosynaptically inhibit the motor neurones that innervate axial muscles of the neck and upper part of the back.

Reticulospinal tracts

The reticulospinal tracts pass from the brain stem reticular formation to the spinal cord. Detailed knowledge of their origins and connections has been obtained mainly from studies in animals.

The medial reticulospinal tract (**Fig. 18.19**) originates from the medial tegmental fields of the pons and medulla. The main sources are the oral and caudal pontine reticular nuclei and the gigantocellular reticular nucleus in the medulla. Pontine fibres descend, mainly ipsilaterally, in the ventral funiculus of the cord. Medullary fibres descend, both ipsilaterally and contralaterally, in the ventral funiculus and the ventral part of the lateral funiculus. These fibres have many collaterals, and two-thirds of the reticulospinal neurones that reach the cervical cord also descend to lumbosacral levels. The terminals of reticulospinal fibres are distributed to lamina VIII, and the central and medial parts of lamina VII. The medullary reticulospinal terminals are more widely distributed, ending additionally in the lateral parts of laminae VI and VII and also directly on motor neurones. From animal studies, it appears that terminations of reticulospinal fibres, that originate in the medulla are, in general, more dorsally placed than those that originate in the pons, although there is considerable overlap.

Both α and γ motor neurones are influenced by reticulospinal fibres, through polysynaptic and monosynaptic connections. Physiological evidence shows that reticulospinal fibres from pontine sources excite motor neurones of axial and limb muscles, while medullary fibres excite, or inhibit motor neurones of cervical muscles and excite motor neurones of axial muscles. Functionally, the medial reticulospinal tract is concerned with posture, the steering of head and trunk movements in response to external stimuli, and crude, stereotyped movements of the limbs.

The lateral reticulospinal tract lies in the lateral funiculus of the spinal cord, closely associated with the rubrospinal and lateral corticospinal tracts (**Fig. 18.3**). Its fibres arise from neurones of the ventrolateral tegmental field of the pons. The fibres cross in the rostral medulla oblongata and project, with a high degree of collateralization, throughout the length of the spinal cord. Axons of this tract terminate in laminae I, V and VI, and also bilaterally in the lateral cervical nucleus. Evidence suggests that this pathway is involved in the control of pain perception and in motor functions.

Interstitiospinal tract

The interstitiospinal tract arises from neurones in the interstitial nucleus (of Cajal) and the immediate surrounding area, and descends via the medial longitudinal fasciculus into the ventral funiculus of the spinal cord. Its fibres project, mainly ipsilaterally, as far as lumbosacral levels, and are mostly distributed to the dorsal part of lamina VIII and the dorsally adjoining part of lamina VII. They establish some monosynaptic connections with motor neurones supplying neck muscles, but their main connections are disynaptic with motor neurones supplying limb muscles.

Solitariospinal tract

The solitariospinal tract is a small group of mostly crossed fibres which arises from neurones in the ventrolateral part of the nucleus solitarius of the medulla. Descending in the ventral funiculus and ventral part of the lateral funiculus of the cord, these axons terminate on phrenic motor neurones supplying the diaphragm and thoracic motor neurones which innervate intercostal muscles. A pathway with somewhat similar course and terminations to that of the solitariospinal tract originates from the nucleus retroambiguus. Both pathways subserve respiratory activities by driving inspiratory muscles, and some descending axons from the nucleus retroambiguus facilitate expiratory motor neurones. There is clinical evidence that bilateral ventrolateral cordotomy at high cervical levels abolishes rhythmic ventilatory movements.

Hypothalamospinal fibres

Hypothalamospinal fibres exist in animals. They arise from the paraventricular nucleus and other areas of the hypothalamus and descend ipsilaterally, mainly in the dorsolateral region of the cord, to be distributed to sympathetic and parasympathetic preganglionic neurones in the intermediolateral column. Fibres from the paraventricular nucleus show oxytocin and vasopressin immunoreactivity. They are also distributed to laminae I and X. Descending fibres from the dopaminergic cell group (A11) situated in the caudal hypothalamus innervate sympathetic preganglionic neurones and neurones in the dorsal horn. That similar pathways exist in man may be inferred from ipsilateral sympathetic deficits (e.g. Horner's syndrome), which follow lesions of the hypothalamus, the lateral tegmental brain stem, or the lateral funiculus of the cord.

Monoaminergic spinal pathways

Monoaminergic cell groups utilize dopamine, adrenaline (epinephrine), noradrenaline (norepinephrine) and 5-HT (5-hydroxytryptamine, serotonin) as neurotransmitters. They occur widely throughout the brain stem and in the hypothalamus. They project rostrally to many forebrain areas and caudally to the spinal cord and appear to be concerned with the modulation of sensory transmission, and the control of autonomic and somatic motor neuronal activities.

The projections to the spinal cord arise from several sources. Coeruleospinal projections originate from noradrenergic cell groups A4 and A6 in the locus coeruleus complex in the pons and descend via the ventrolateral white matter to innervate all cord segments bilaterally. They end in the dorsal grey matter (laminae IV–VI) and the intermediate and ventral horns. They also project extensively to preganglionic parasympathetic neurones in the sacral cord. Descending noradrenergic fibres, which arise from the lateral tegmental cell groups A5 and A7 of the pons, travel in the dorsolateral white matter. They are distributed to laminae I–III, and particularly to the intermediate grey horn. Descending fibres from adrenergic cell groups C1 and C3 of the medulla oblongata have been traced into the anterior funiculus of the cord and are extensively distributed to the intermediolateral column. Dopaminergic fibres projecting to the spinal cord travel in the hypothalamospinal pathway.

The raphe nuclei pallidus (B1), obscurus (B2) and magnus (B3) in the brain stem give rise to two serotoninergic descending bundles. The lateral raphe spinal bundle, from B3 neurones, is concerned with the control of nociception. It descends close to the lateral corticospinal tract and ends in the dorsal horn (laminae I, II and V). The ventral bundle, composed mainly of axons from B1 neurones, travels in the medial part of the ventral white column and ends in the ventral horn (laminae VIII and IX). It facilitates extensor and flexor motor neurones. Some descending serotoninergic fibres project to sympathetic preganglionic neurones and are concerned with the central control of cardiovascular function.

Summary of major descending brain stem tracts

In an analysis of the descending tracts in mammals, Kuypers (1981) subdivided the descending brain stem pathways into groups, A and B, on the basis of their terminal distribution and functional attributes.

Group A (ventromedial brain stem pathways) consists of both vestibulospinal tracts, together with the medial reticulospinal, tectospinal and interstitiospinal tracts, all of which pass through the medial and ventral parts of the lower brain stem tegmentum to descend in the ventral and ventrolateral funiculi of the spinal cord. Fibres of these tracts end, often with a bilateral distribution, in the ventromedial part of the intermediate zone (laminae V–VII) of the spinal grey matter. The fibres of most of these tracts are highly collateralized. Some make monosynaptic connections with motor neurones innervating muscles of the limbs. The neurones from which group A axons arise receive cortical projections mainly from areas rostral to the precentral gyrus. Functionally, this system is concerned with the maintenance of posture, the integration of movements of the body and limbs, and synergistic whole-limb movements, but it also subserves the orientation movements of the body and head.

Group B (lateral brain stem pathways) consists of the rubrospinal tract and the lateral reticulospinal tract. These tracts descend through the ventrolateral part of the lower brain stem tegmentum and continue in the dorsolateral funiculus of the spinal cord. They terminate, mainly ipsilaterally, in the dorsal and lateral parts of the intermediate zone of spinal grey matter (laminae V–VII). Rubrospinal fibres in non-human primates also establish monosynaptic connections with motor neurones innervating distal limb muscles. Rubrospinal neurones receive cortical afferent fibres mainly from the precentral gyrus. Group B pathways provide the capacity for independent, flexion-biased movements of the limbs and shoulder and especially of the elbow and hand. They supplement the motor control mediated by group A pathways. The termination of the two groups of brain stem pathways is largely overlapped by that of the corticospinal pathway arising from motor areas of the frontal lobe. Functionally, this part of the corticospinal system enhances the brain stem controls. In addition, it provides the capacity for fractionation of movements, as exemplified by individual finger movements, which are probably executed through direct corticospinal connections with motor neurones.

Propriospinal pathways

Propriospinal pathways, or tracts, are also sometimes referred to as the fasciculi proprii. Propriospinal neurones are confined to the spinal cord, i.e. their ascending and descending fibres begin and end within the spinal grey matter. They connect neurones within the same segment and/or other neurones in more distant segments of the spinal cord and so subserve intrasegmental and intersegmental integration and coordination. The majority of spinal neurones are propriospinal neurones, most of which lie in laminae V–VIII. Propriospinal fibres are mainly concentrated around the margins of the grey matter (**Fig. 18.2**), but are also dispersed diffusely in the white funiculi.

The propriospinal system plays important roles in spinal functions. Descending pathways end on specific subgroups of propriospinal neurones and these, in turn, relay to motor neurones and other spinal neurones. The system mediates all those automatic functions which continue after transection of the spinal cord, e.g. sudomotor and vasomotor activities, bowel and bladder functions.

Some propriospinal axons are very short, and span only one segment, while others run the entire length of the cord. The shortest axons lie immediately adjacent to the grey matter, and the longer ones are situated more peripherally. Propriospinal neurones can be categorized according to the length of their axons as long, intermediate, or short neurones. Long propriospinal neurones distribute their axons throughout the length of the cord, mainly via the ventral and lateral funiculi; their cell bodies are in lamina VIII and the dorsally adjoining part of lamina VII. Axons from the long propriospinal neurones of the cervical cord descend bilaterally, whereas those from the corresponding lumbosacral neurones ascend mainly contralaterally. Most of the fibres are fine (less than 3 µm in diameter). Some are the first spinal tract axons to become myelinated. Intermediate propriospinal neurones occupy the central and medial parts of lamina VII and project mainly ipsilaterally. Short propriospinal neurones are found in the lateral parts of laminae V–VIII and their axons run ipsilaterally in the lateral funiculus.

Propriospinal fibres in the different parts of the white funiculi are distributed preferentially to specific regions of the spinal grey matter. In the spinal enlargements, the propriospinal fibres in the dorsolateral funiculus project to the dorsal and lateral parts of the intermediate zone, and also to spinal motor neurones which supply distal limb muscles, especially those of the hand and the foot. The propriospinal fibres in the ventral part of the ventrolateral funiculus are distributed to the central and medial parts of lamina VII and to motor neurones of proximal limb and girdle muscles. Other propriospinal fibres run in the medial part of the ventral funiculus and travel mainly to the ventromedial part of the intermediate zone, which characteristically contains long propriospinal neurones, and to motor neurones innervating axial and girdle muscles.

The tract of Lissauer

The tract of Lissauer, or the dorsolateral tract, lies between the apex of the dorsal horn and the surface of the spinal cord, where it surrounds the incoming dorsal root fibres. It is present throughout the spinal cord, and is most developed in the upper cervical regions.

The tract consists of fine myelinated and non-myelinated axons. Many are the branches of axons in the lateral bundles of the dorsal roots. These axons bifurcate into ascending and descending branches as they enter the cord. The branches travel in the tract of Lissauer for one or two segments and give off collaterals, which end on and around neurones in the dorsal horn. The tract also contains propriospinal fibres, some of which are short axons of small substantia gelatinosa neurones, which re-enter the dorsal horn.

SPINAL CORD LESIONS

Mechanical compression and secondary ischaemic damage to underlying nervous tissue cause surgically relevant spinal cord disease (myelopathy). The site and the level of damage to the cord determine the particular clinical syndrome, e.g. whether the lesion involves the upper or lower cervical, thoracic or lumbosacral spinal cord. At each of these levels, symptoms and signs are determined by direct destruction of segmental tissue, i.e. transversely distributed damage, and disconnection of suprasegmental ascending and descending tracts above and below the level of a lesion, i.e. longitudinally distributed damage (**Fig. 18.23**). For example, a lower cervical spinal cord lesion damages the segmental sensory and motor contributions to the nerve roots and brachial plexus causing sensory loss, weakness and wasting of the muscles and loss of tendon reflexes in the upper limbs. Disruption of the ascending sensory pathways in the lateral and dorsal columns of the cervical spinal cord leads to loss of sensation to pain and temperature (lateral spinothalamic tracts) and touch and proprioception (dorsal fasciculi) below the 'sensory level' corresponding to the segment of the spinal cord.

Damage to the descending corticospinal tracts in the lateral columns of the spinal cord produces a spastic paraparesis, i.e. increased tone of the muscles, weakness of movements of flexion, exaggerated tendon reflexes and abnormal superficial reflexes, e.g. extensor plantar responses and absent abdominal reflexes. Descending pathways to the bladder are interrupted, and this produces a 'neurogenic bladder'.

The same principles apply to lesions at other levels of the spinal cord and they are illustrated in diagrammatic form in **Fig. 18.23**.

The precise clinical syndrome is determined by anatomical site alone and not by pathology. However, it is of practical use to classify lesions on the basis of their anatomical relationship to the spinal cord and meninges, i.e. whether they are extradural, intradural or intramedullary (*see* table). This anatomic classification provides a guide to the diagnostic probabilities as well as an aid to neuroradiological interpretation prior to neurosurgical intervention. For example, neurofibromas are common in the cervical spinal canal, meningiomas in the thoracic spinal canal, and ependymomas in the lumbosacral spinal canal. Degenerative disease of the vertebral column is common in the cervical and lumbosacral vertebrae, but rare in the thoracic vertebrae. Discrete anterior and

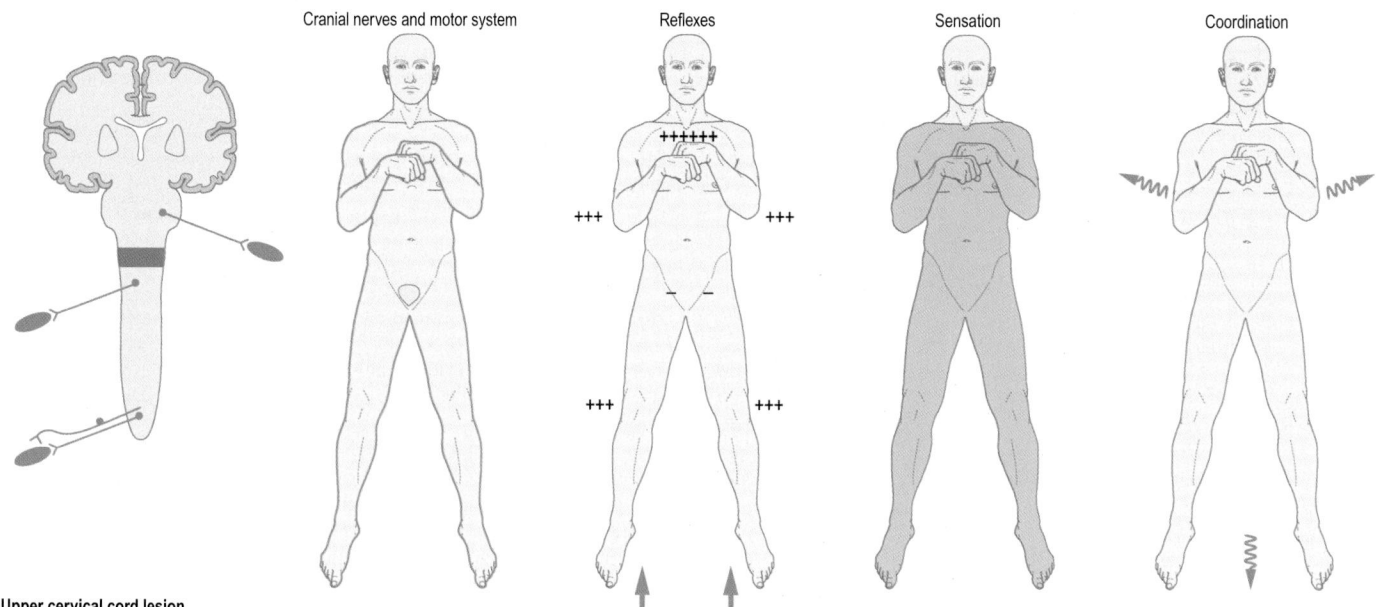

Upper cervical cord lesion
A high cervical cord lesion causes spastic tetraplegia with hyperreflexia, extensor plantar responses (upper motor neurone lesion), incontinence, sensory loss below the level of the lesion and 'sensory' ataxia.

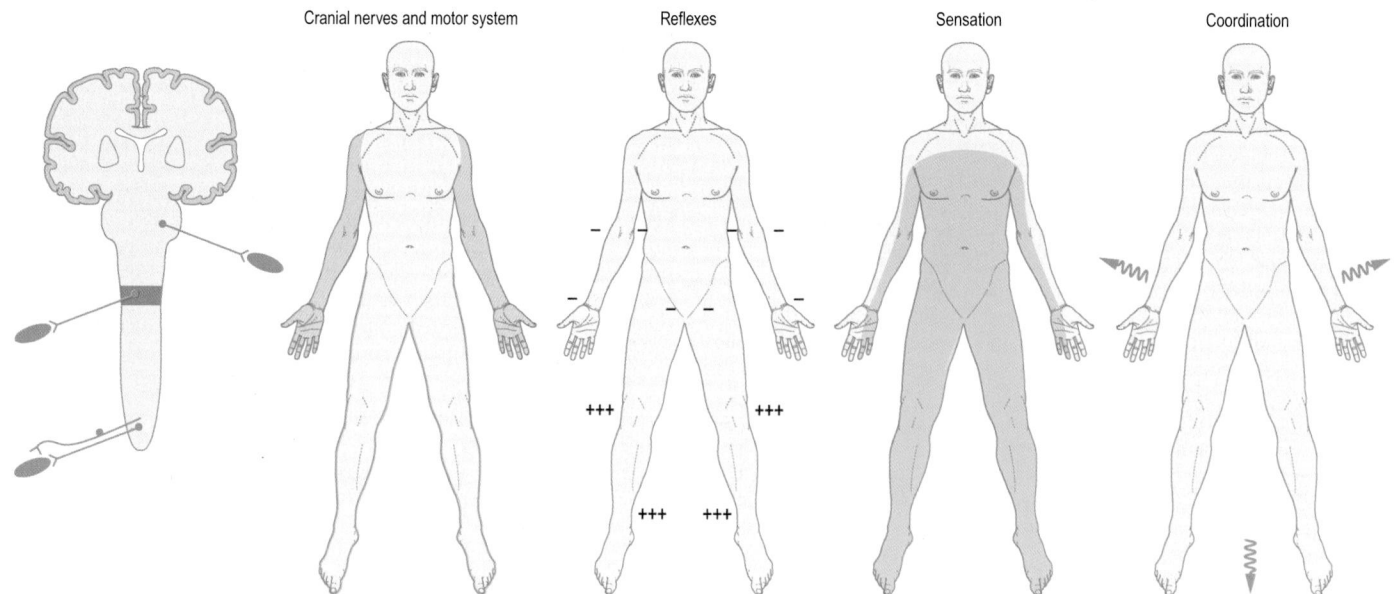

Lower cervical cord lesion
A lower cervical cord lesion causes weakness, wasting and fasciculation of muscles and areflexia of the upper limbs (lower motor neurone lesion). In addition, there is spastic paraparesis, hyperreflexia and extensor plantar responses (upper motor neurone lesion) in the lower limbs, incontinence, sensory loss below the level of the lesion and 'sensory' ataxia.

Fig. 18.23 Lesions of the spinal cord. (By permission from Crossman AR, Neary D 2000 Neuroanatomy, 2nd edn. Edinburgh: Churchill Livingstone.)

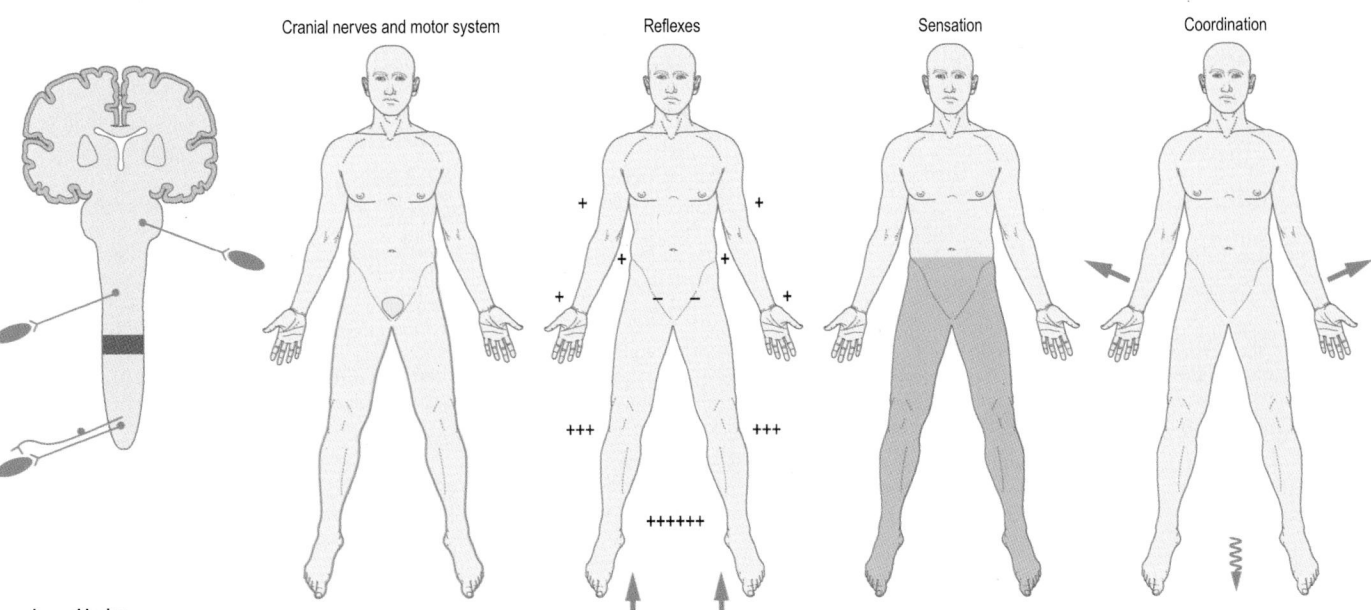

Thoracic cord lesion
A thoracic cord lesion causes a spastic paraparesis, hyperreflexia and extensor plantar responses (upper motor neurone lesion), incontinence, sensory loss below the level of the lesion and 'sensory' ataxia.

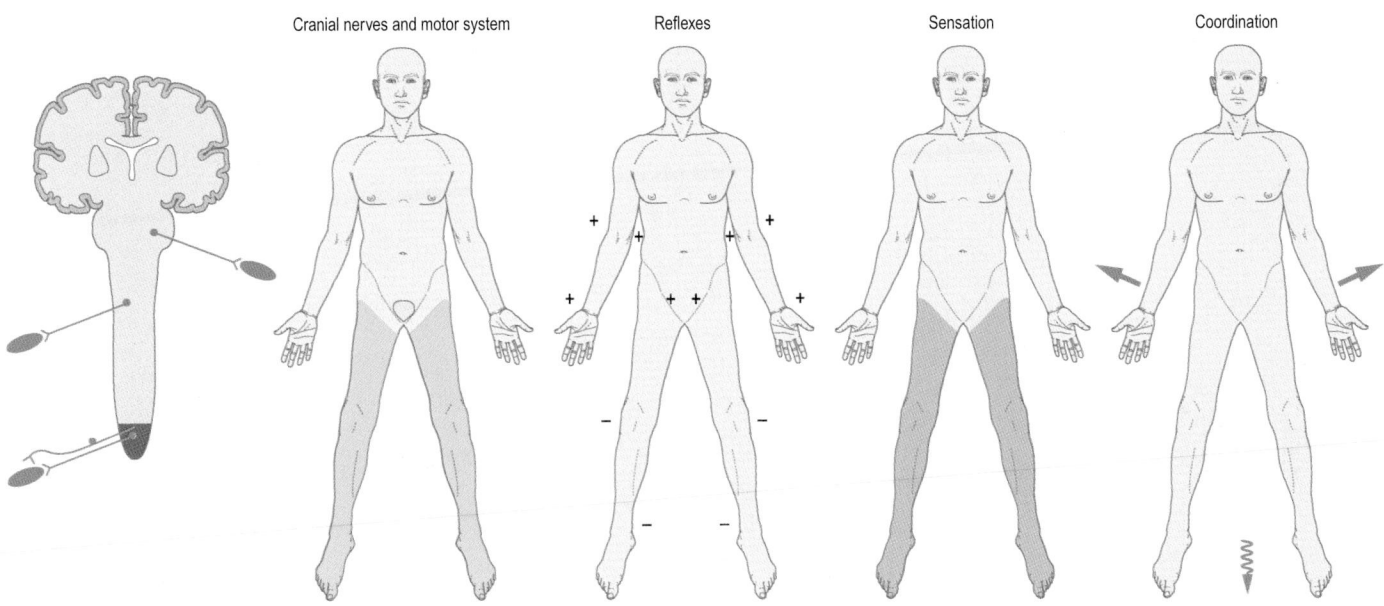

Lumbar cord lesion
A lumbar cord lesion causes weakness, wasting and fasciculation of muscles, areflexia of the lower limbs (lower motor neurone lesion), incontinence, sensory loss below the level of the lesion and 'sensory' ataxia.

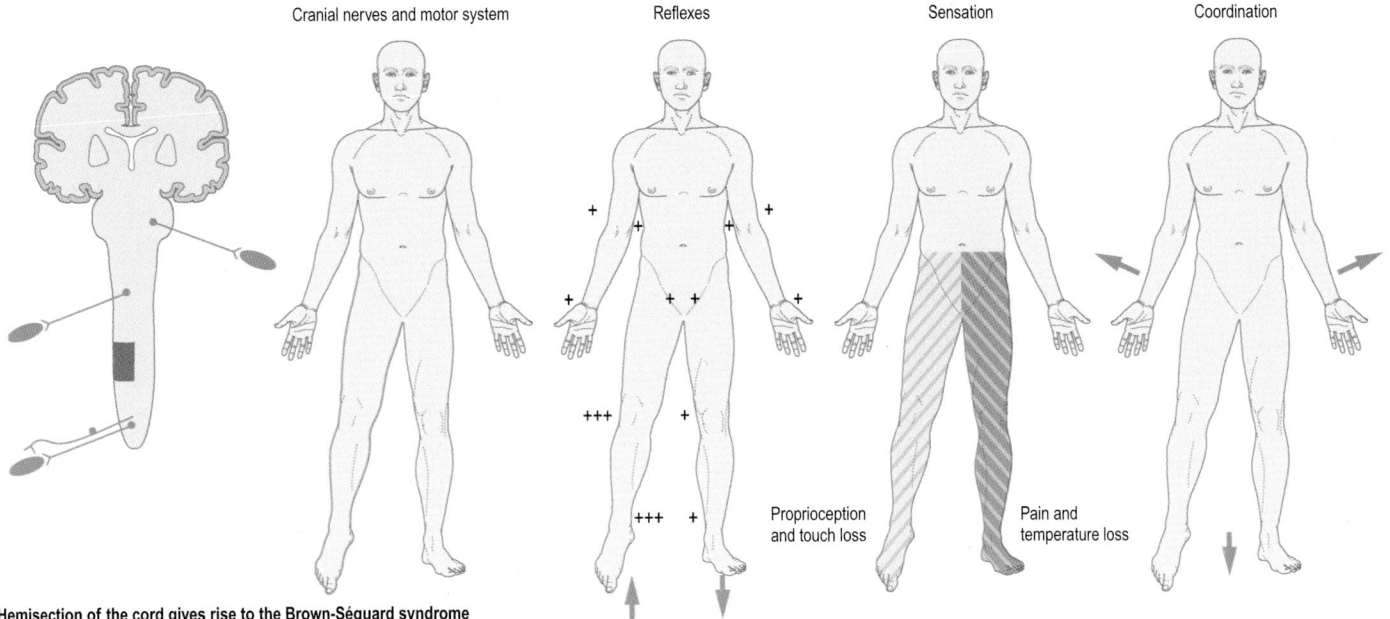

Hemisection of the cord gives rise to the Brown-Séquard syndrome
This is characterised by ipsilateral loss of proprioception and upper motor neurone signs (hemiplegia/monoplegia) plus contralateral loss of pain and temperature sensation.

Fig. 18.23 *(Cont'd)* Lesions of the spinal cord.

325

Extradural lesions	A. Disorder of the vertebral column	Degenerative osteoarthritis (osteophytes and prolapsed intervertebral disc)
		Infection (tuberculosis)
		Tumour (chordoma, sarcoma, metastatic tumour)
	B. Abscess	(Carcinoma, myeloma, lymphoma)
	C. Haematoma	(Complication of bleeding diathesis or anticoagulation)
Intradural lesions		Meningioma, neurofibroma, lipoma, angioma
Intramedullary lesions		Syringomyelia (Arnold–Chiari malformation), angioma, glioma, ependymoma, epidermoid tumour

central intramedullary lesions, e.g. due to syringomyelia and angiomas respectively, preferentially destroy the spinothalamic pathways in the anterolateral columns and central areas of the spinal cord. This leads to a characteristic 'dissociated' sensory loss, i.e. loss of pain and temperature sensation, but with preservation of touch sensation and proprioception at and below the level of the lesion.

REFERENCES

Boyd IA, Gladden MH 1985 The Muscle Spindle. London: Macmillan.

Kuypers HGJM 1981 Anatomy of descending pathways. In: Brookhart JM, Mountcastle VB et al (eds) Handbook of Physiology, vol 2 Motor Control, pt 1. Bethesda, MD: Am Physiol Soc: 597–666.

Melzack R, Wall PD 1965 Pain mechanisms: a new theory. Science 150: 971–9.

Rexed B 1952 The cytoarchitectonic organization of the spinal cord in the cat. J Comp Neurol 96: 415–95.

Schoenen J, Faull RLM 1990 Spinal cord: cytoarchitectural, dendroarchitectural and myeloarchitectural organization. In: Paxinos G (ed) The Human Nervous System. San Diego, CA: Academic Press: 19–53.

Brain stem

The brain stem consists of the medulla oblongata, pons and midbrain. It is sited in the posterior cranial fossa, and its ventral surface lies on the clivus. It contains numerous intrinsic neurone cell bodies and their processes, some of which are the brain stem homologues of spinal neuronal groups. These include the sites of termination and cells of origin of axons that enter or leave the brain stem through the cranial nerves. They provide the sensory, motor and autonomic innervation of structures that are mostly in the head and neck. Autonomic fibres, which arise from the brain stem, are distributed more widely. Additional groups of neurones receive input related to the special senses of hearing, vestibular function and taste (Ch. 24). The reticular formation is an extensive and often ill-defined network of neurones that extends throughout the length of the brain stem, and is continuous caudally with its spinal counterpart. Some of its nuclei are concerned with cardiac, respiratory and alimentary control, others are involved in aspects of many neural activities, while yet more provide or receive massive afferent and efferent cerebellar projections.

The brain stem is the site of termination of numerous ascending and descending fibres and is traversed by many others. The spinothalamic (spinal lemniscal), medial lemniscal and the trigeminal systems ascend through the brain stem to reach the thalamus (**Figs 18.14, 19.17**). Prominent corticospinal projections descend through the brain stem while corticobulbar projections end within it (**Fig. 18.21**).

Clinically, damage to the brain stem is often devastating and life threatening. This is because it is a structurally and functionally compact region, where even small lesions can destroy vital cardiac and respiratory centres, disconnect forebrain motor areas from brain stem and spinal motor neurones, and sever incoming sensory fibres from higher centres of consciousness, perception and cognition. Irreversible cardiac and respiratory arrest follow complete destruction of the neural respiratory and cardiac centres in the medulla. Clinically this is called brain stem death, a condition that requires accurate diagnosis since it may occur in patients on life-support machines whose respiratory and cardiac functions can be artificially maintained indefinitely.

The following account starts with a brief systematic overview of the cranial nerves that attach to the brain stem, their central origins and connections within the cranial nerve nuclei. The major subdivisions of the brain stem are then described. Many structures, including nuclei and tracts, extend longitudinally across their boundaries. The structure and function of the most notable of these are dealt with in detail once only, at the most appropriate point. As is customary, transverse sections of the brain stem are included in order to illustrate the relationships between structures and the regional variation that occurs at different levels.

OVERVIEW OF CRANIAL NERVES AND CRANIAL NERVE NUCLEI

The cranial nerves are the conduits by which the brain receives information directly from, and controls the functions of, structures which are mainly, but not exclusively, within the head and neck. All but two of the twelve pairs of cranial nerves attach to the brain stem; this chapter is therefore an appropriate place to describe their structure and function.

The cranial nerves are individually named and numbered (using Roman numerals) in a rostro–caudal sequence (*see* summary in Ch.12, p. 234). The first cranial nerve (olfactory) terminates directly in cortical and subcortical areas of the frontal and temporal lobes. It is closely associated functionally with the limbic system and is described in that context (p. 405). The fibres of the second cranial nerve (optic) pass into the optic chiasma and emerge as the optic tract, which terminates in the lateral geniculate nucleus of the thalamus. Cranial nerves III (oculomotor) and IV (trochlear) attach to the midbrain. Cranial nerve V (trigeminal) attaches to the pons, medial to the middle cerebellar peduncle. Cranial nerves VI (abducens), VII (facial) and VIII (vestibulocochlear) attach to the brain stem at, or close to, the junction of the pons with the medulla. Cranial nerves IX (glossopharyngeal), X (vagus), the cranial part of XI (accessory) and XII (hypoglossal) all attach to the medulla.

Cranial nerves III–XII, which attach to the brain stem, are associated with a number of cell groupings of varying size, referred to collectively as the cranial nerve nuclei (**Fig. 19.1**). The nuclei are either the origin of efferent cranial nerve fibres or the site of termination of cranial nerve afferents. They are conveniently considered to be organized into six discontinuous, longitudinal cell columns, which correspond to columns that may be identified in the embryo (**Fig. 12.4**). Three columns are 'sensory' and three are 'motor' in function.

The trigeminal sensory nucleus, which extends throughout the length of the brain stem and into the cervical spinal cord, represents a general somatic afferent cell column. Its principal afferents are carried in the trigeminal nerve. General visceral afferents carried by the facial, glossopharyngeal and vagus nerves end in the nucleus solitarius of the medulla. The special visceral afferent column corresponds to the vestibular and cochlear nuclei, which are located beneath the vestibular area of the floor of the fourth ventricle.

The general somatic efferent cell column consists of four nuclei that lie near the midline and give rise to motor fibres which run in nerves of the same name. From rostral to caudal, these are the oculomotor, trochlear and abducens nuclei which innervate the extraocular muscles, and the hypoglossal nucleus, which innervates all but one of the muscles of the tongue. The general visceral efferent, or parasympathetic, cell column is made up of the Edinger–Westphal nucleus of the midbrain, salivary nuclei of the pons, and vagal nucleus of the medulla. Cells in the special visceral efferent column innervate muscles derived from the branchial arches, and lie in the trigeminal motor nucleus, the facial nucleus and the nucleus ambiguus.

MEDULLA OBLONGATA

EXTERNAL FEATURES AND RELATIONS

The medulla oblongata extends from the lower pontine margin to a transverse plane, above the first pair of cervical spinal nerves, which intersects the upper border of the atlas dorsally and the centre of the dens ventrally (**Fig. 19.2**). It is c.3 cm in length and 2 cm in diameter at its widest. The ventral surface of the medulla is separated from the basilar part of the occipital bone and apex of the dens by the meninges and occipito-axial ligaments. Caudally, the dorsal surface of the medulla occupies the midline notch between the cerebellar hemispheres.

The ventral and dorsal surfaces of the medulla (**Figs 16.10, 19.3**) possess a longitudinal median fissure and sulcus, respectively, which are continuous with their spinal counterparts. Caudally, the ventral median fissure is interrupted by the obliquely crossing fascicles of the pyramidal decussation. Rostrally, it ends at the pontine border in a diminutive depression, the foramen caecum. Immediately lateral to the ventral median fissure there is a prominent elongated ridge named the pyramid, which contains descending pyramidal, or corticospinal, axons (**Fig. 19.3**). The lateral margin of the pyramid is indicated by a shallow

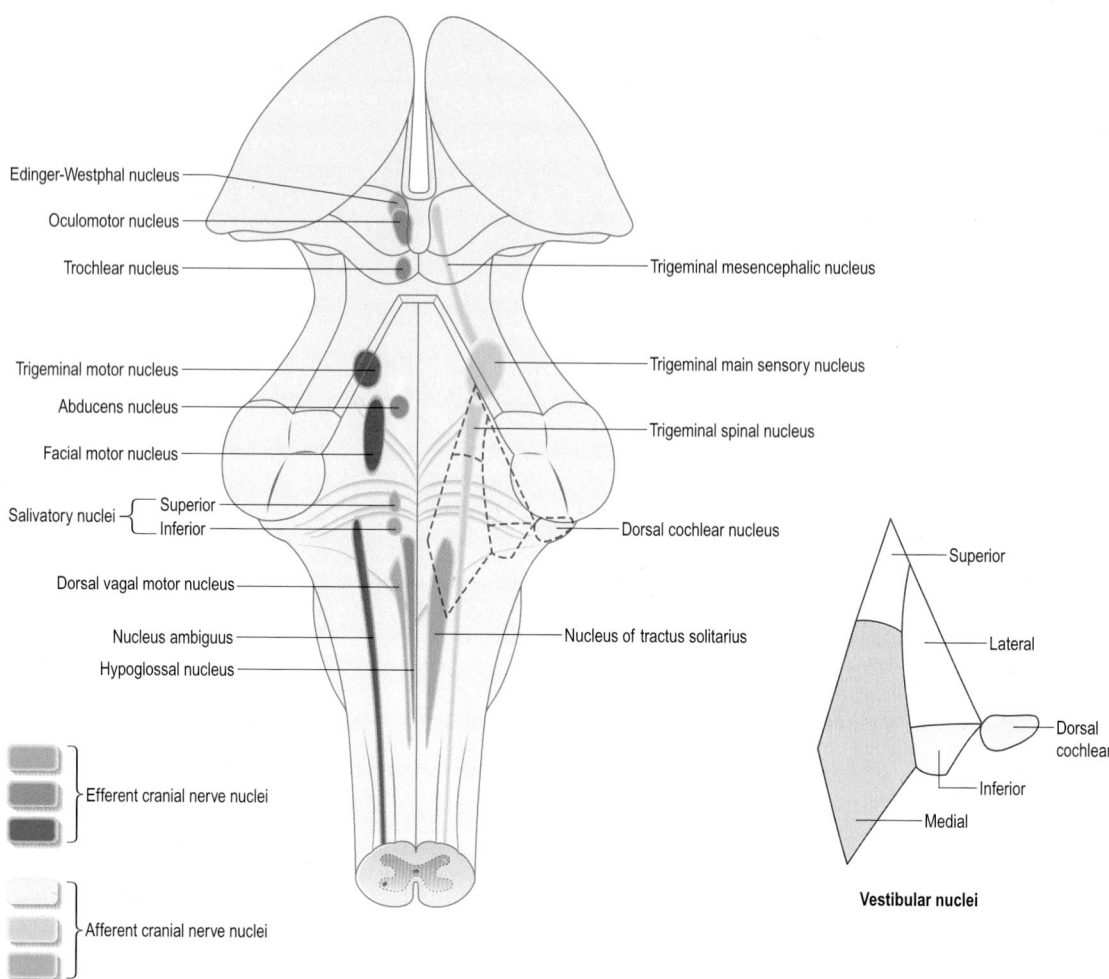

Fig. 19.1 The cranial nerve nuclei.

ventrolateral sulcus. From this emerges, in line with the ventral spinal nerve roots, a linear series of rootlets which constitute the hypoglossal nerve. The abducens nerve emerges at the slightly narrowed rostral end of the pyramid, where it adjoins the pons. Caudally the pyramid tapers into the spinal ventral funiculus. Lateral to the pyramid and the ventrolateral sulcus there is an oval prominence, the olive (**Figs 19.3, 19.4**), which contains the inferior olivary nucleus. Lateral to the olive is the posterolateral sulcus. The glossopharyngeal, vagus and accessory nerves join the brain stem along the line of this sulcus, in line with the dorsal spinal nerve roots.

The spinal central canal extends into the caudal half of the medulla, migrating progressively more dorsally until it opens out into the lumen of the fourth ventricle. This divides the medulla into a closed part, which contains the central canal, and an open part, which contains the caudal half of the fourth ventricle (**Figs 19.2, 16.10**).

In the closed part of the medulla, a shallow postero-intermediate sulcus on either side of the dorsal median sulcus, continuous with its cervical spinal counterpart, indicates the location of the ascending dorsal columns (fasciculus gracilis and fasciculus cuneatus). The ascending fasciculi are at first parallel to each other, but at the caudal end of the fourth ventricle they diverge, and each develops an elongated swelling, the gracile and cuneate tubercles, produced by the subjacent nuclei gracilis and cuneatus respectively (**Figs 19.5, 19.6**). Most fibres in the fasciculi synapse with neurones in their respective nuclei, and these project to the contralateral thalamus, which, in turn, projects to the primary somaesthetic cortex (**Fig. 18.14**). The inferior cerebellar peduncle forms a rounded ridge between the caudal part of the fourth ventricle and the glossopharyngeal and vagal rootlets. The two peduncles diverge and incline to enter the cerebellar hemispheres, where they are crossed by the striae medullares which run to the median ventricular sulcus (**Fig. 16.10**). Here also the peduncles form

the anterior and rostral boundaries of the lateral recess of the fourth ventricle. This becomes continuous with the subarachnoid space through the lateral apertures of the fourth ventricle, the foramina of Luschka. A tuft of choroid plexus, continuous with that of the fourth ventricle, protrudes from the foramina on either side. The fibre composition of the inferior cerebellar peduncle is described on page 354.

INTERNAL STRUCTURE

Transverse section of the medulla at the level of the pyramidal decussation

A transverse section across the lower medulla oblongata (**Fig. 19.5**) intersects the dorsal, lateral and ventral funiculi, which are continuous with their counterparts in the spinal cord. The ventral funiculi are separated from the central grey matter by corticospinal fibres, which cross in the pyramidal decussation to reach the contralateral lateral funiculi (**Fig. 19.9**). The decussation displaces the ventral intersegmental tract, the central grey matter and the central canal dorsally. Continuity between the ventral grey column and central grey matter, which is maintained throughout the spinal cord, is lost. The column subdivides into the supraspinal nucleus (continuous above with that of the hypoglossal nerve), which is the efferent source of the first cervical nerve, and the spinal nucleus of the accessory nerve, which provides some spinal accessory fibres and merges rostrally with the nucleus ambiguus.

The dorsal grey column is also modified at this level as the nucleus gracilis appears as a grey lamina in the ventral part of the fasciculus gracilis. The nucleus begins caudal to the nucleus cuneatus, which invades the fasciculus cuneatus from its ventral aspect in similar fashion.

The spinal nucleus and spinal tract of the trigeminal nerve are visible ventrolateral to the dorsal columns. They are continuous with the substantia gelatinosa and tract of Lissauer of the spinal cord.

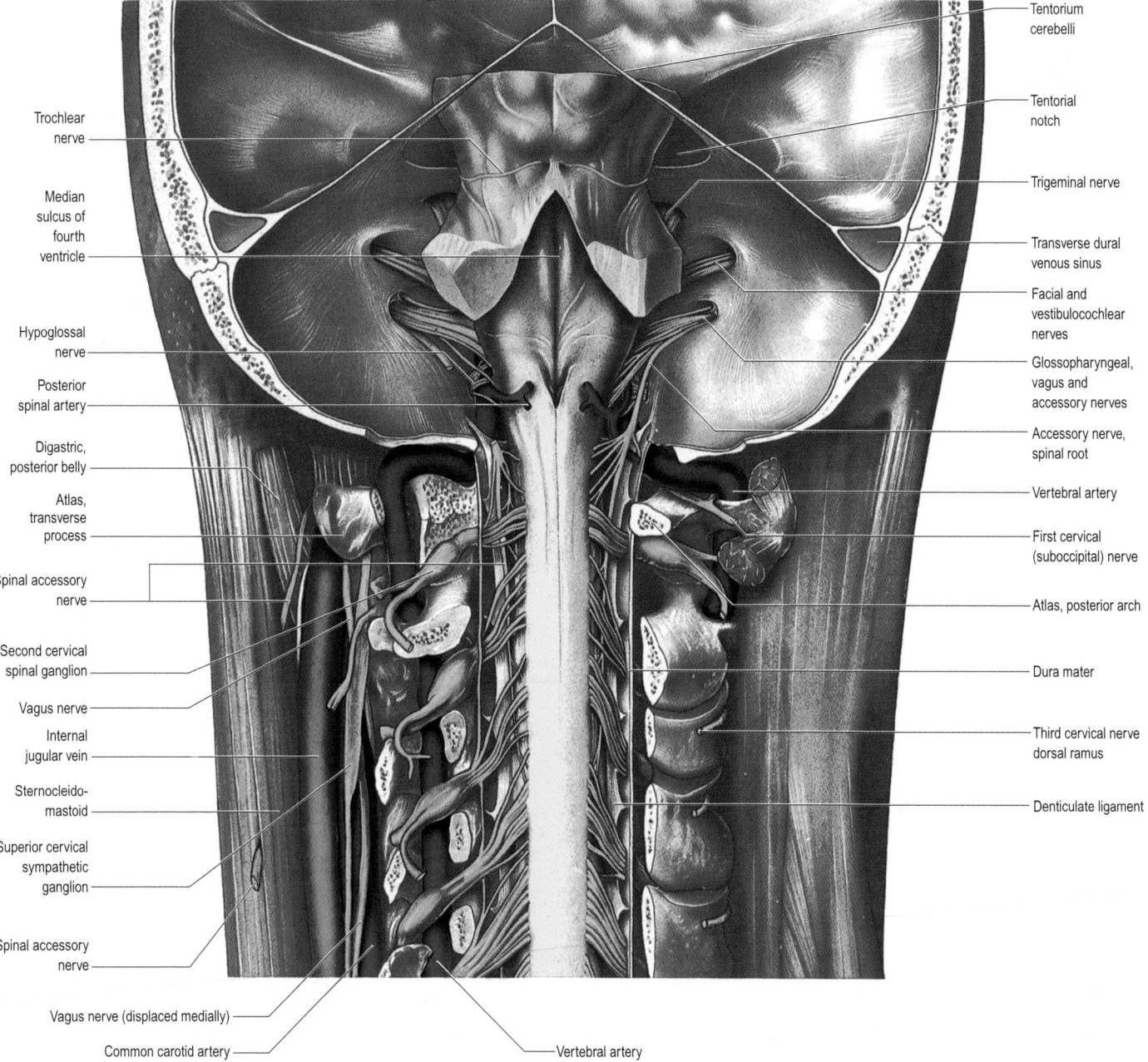

Trochlear nerve

Median sulcus of fourth ventricle

Hypoglossal nerve

Posterior spinal artery

Digastric, posterior belly

Atlas, transverse process

Spinal accessory nerve

Second cervical spinal ganglion

Vagus nerve

Internal jugular vein

Sternocleido-mastoid

Superior cervical sympathetic ganglion

Spinal accessory nerve

Vagus nerve (displaced medially)

Common carotid artery

Tentorium cerebelli

Tentorial notch

Trigeminal nerve

Transverse dural venous sinus

Facial and vestibulocochlear nerves

Glossopharyngeal, vagus and accessory nerves

Accessory nerve, spinal root

Vertebral artery

First cervical (suboccipital) nerve

Atlas, posterior arch

Dura mater

Third cervical nerve dorsal ramus

Denticulate ligament

Vertebral artery

Fig. 19.2 Dissection exposing the brain stem and upper five cervical spinal segments after removal of large portions of the occipital and parietal bones, and the cerebellum and the roof of the fourth ventricle. On the left, the foramina transversaria of the atlas and the third, fourth and fifth cervical vertebrae have been opened to expose the vertebral artery. On the right, the posterior arch of the atlas and the laminae of the succeeding cervical vertebrae have been removed.

Transverse section of the medulla at the level of the decussation of the medial lemniscus

The medullary white matter is rearranged above the level of the pyramidal decussation (**Fig. 19.6**). The pyramids contain ipsilateral corticospinal and corticonuclear fibres, the latter distributed to nuclei of cranial nerves and other medullary nuclei. At this level, they form two large ventral bundles flanking the ventral median fissure. The accessory olivary nuclei and lemniscal decussation are dorsal.

The nucleus gracilis is broader at this level and the fibres of its fasciculus are located on its dorsal, medial and lateral surfaces. The nucleus cuneatus is well developed. Both nuclei retain continuity with the central grey matter at this level, but this is subsequently lost. First-order gracile and cuneate fascicular fibres, which have ascended ipsilaterally and uninterrupted from their origin in the spinal cord, synapse upon neurones in their respective nuclei. Second-order axons emerge from the nuclei as internal arcuate fibres, at first curving ventrolaterally around the central grey matter and then ventromedially

between the trigeminal spinal tract and the central grey matter. They decussate to form an ascending contralateral tract, the medial lemniscus. The lemniscal decussation is located dorsal to the pyramids and ventral to the central grey matter. The latter is, therefore, more dorsally displaced than in the previous section.

The medial lemniscus ascends from the lemniscal decussation on each side as a flattened tract near the median raphe. As the tracts ascend, they increase in size because fibres join from upper levels of the decussation. Corticospinal fibres are ventral, and the medial longitudinal fasciculus and tectospinal tract are dorsal. Fibres are rearranged in the decussation, so that those from the nucleus gracilis come to lie ventral to those from the nucleus cuneatus. Above this, the medial lemniscus is also rearranged, ventral (gracile) fibres becoming lateral, and dorsal (cuneate) fibres medial. At this level, medial lemniscal fibres show a laminar somatotopy on a segmental basis, in that fibres from C1 to S4 spinal segments are segregated sequentially from medial to lateral, respectively.

329

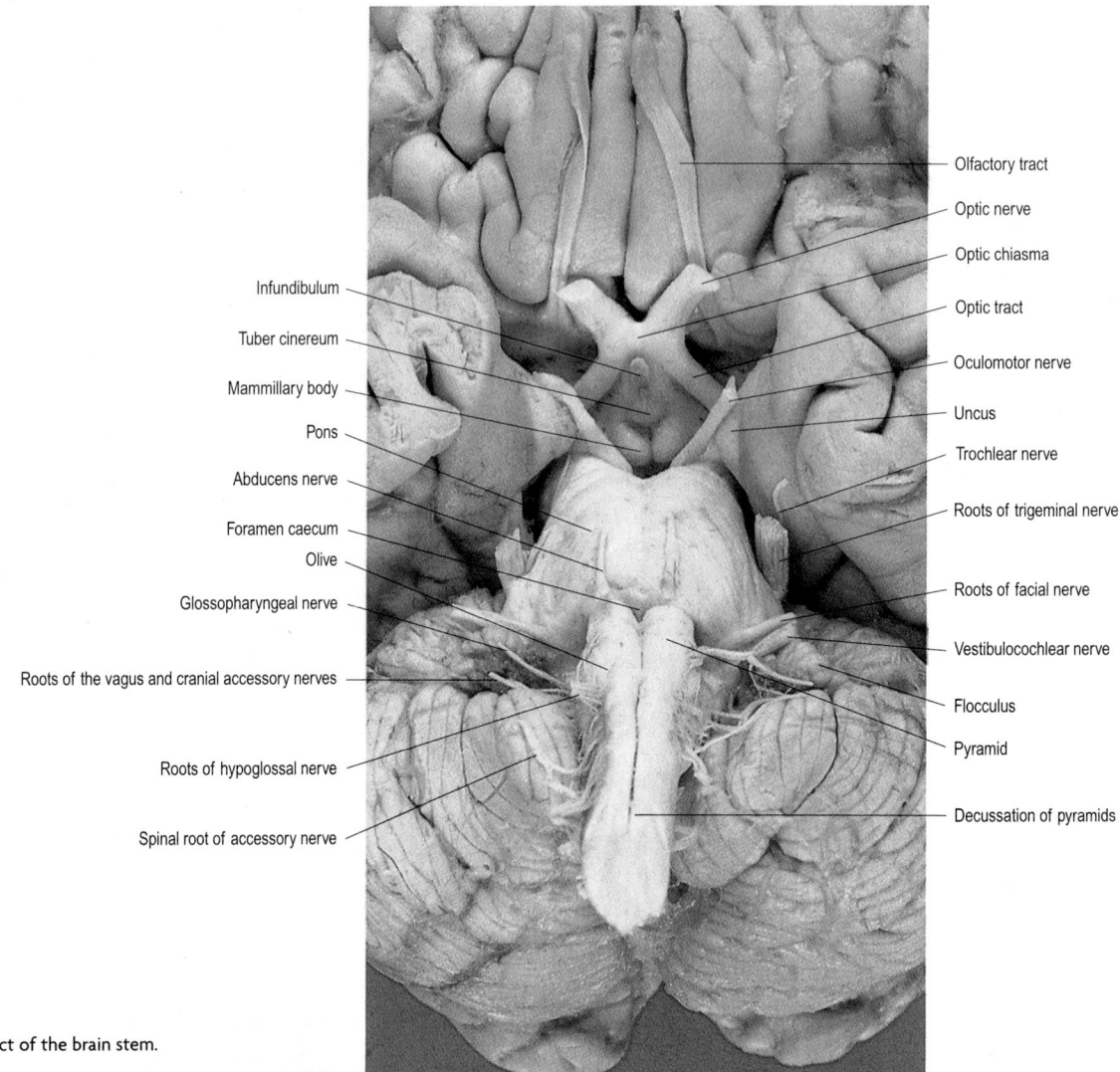

Infundibulum

Tuber cinereum

Mammillary body

Pons

Abducens nerve

Foramen caecum

Olive

Glossopharyngeal nerve

Roots of the vagus and cranial accessory nerves

Roots of hypoglossal nerve

Spinal root of accessory nerve

Olfactory tract

Optic nerve

Optic chiasma

Optic tract

Oculomotor nerve

Uncus

Trochlear nerve

Roots of trigeminal nerve

Roots of facial nerve

Vestibulocochlear nerve

Flocculus

Pyramid

Decussation of pyramids

Fig. 19.3 Ventral aspect of the brain stem.

Pineal body

Superior colliculus

Inferior colliculus

Inferior quadrigeminal brachium

Medial geniculate body

Superior medullary velum

Lateral lemniscus

Superior cerebellar peduncle

Middle cerebellar peduncle

Dorsolateral sulcus

Roots of spinal accessory nerve

Olive

Pyramid

Roots of vagus and glossopharyngeal nerves

Corona radiata

Pulvinar

Superior quadrigeminal brachium

Lateral geniculate body

Lentiform complex

Trochlear nerve

Optic tract

Base of cerebral peduncle

Oculomotor nerve

Pons

Trigeminal nerve (sensory and motor roots)

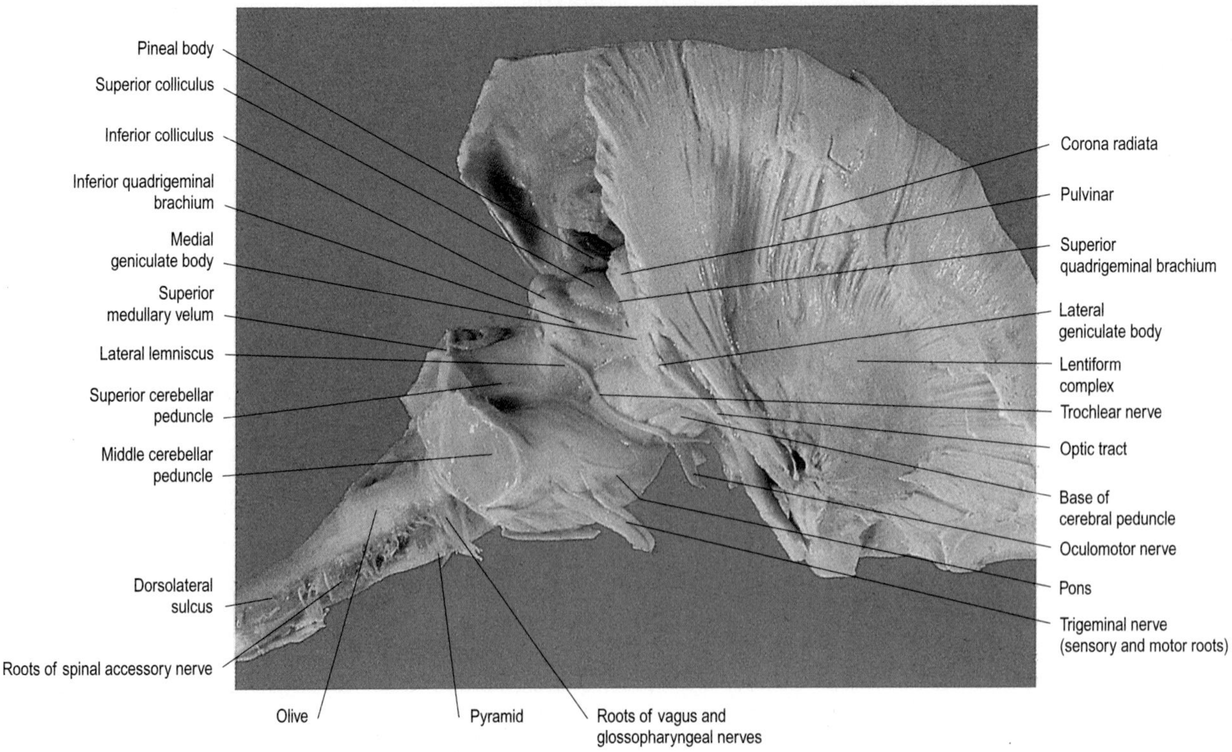

Fig. 19.4 Lateral aspect of the brain stem.

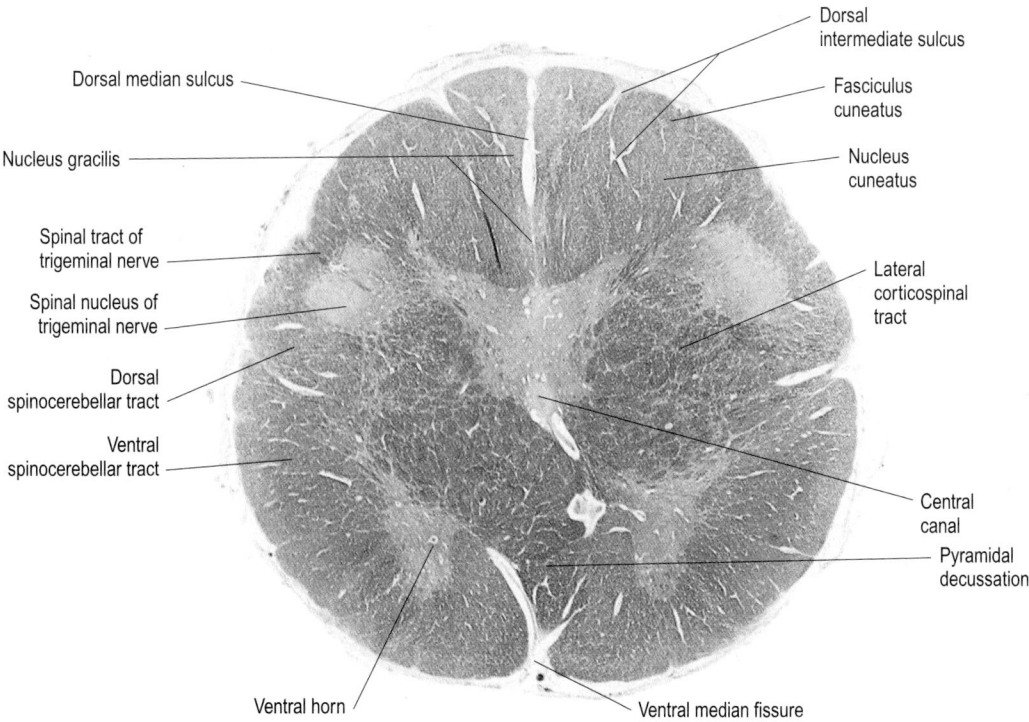

Dorsal median sulcus

Nucleus gracilis

Spinal tract of
trigeminal nerve

Spinal nucleus of
trigeminal nerve

Dorsal
spinocerebellar tract

Ventral
spinocerebellar tract

Ventral horn

Dorsal
intermediate sulcus

Fasciculus
cuneatus

Nucleus
cuneatus

Lateral
corticospinal
tract

Central
canal

Pyramidal
decussation

Ventral median fissure

Fig. 19.5 Transverse section through the medulla oblongata at the level of the pyramidal decussation.

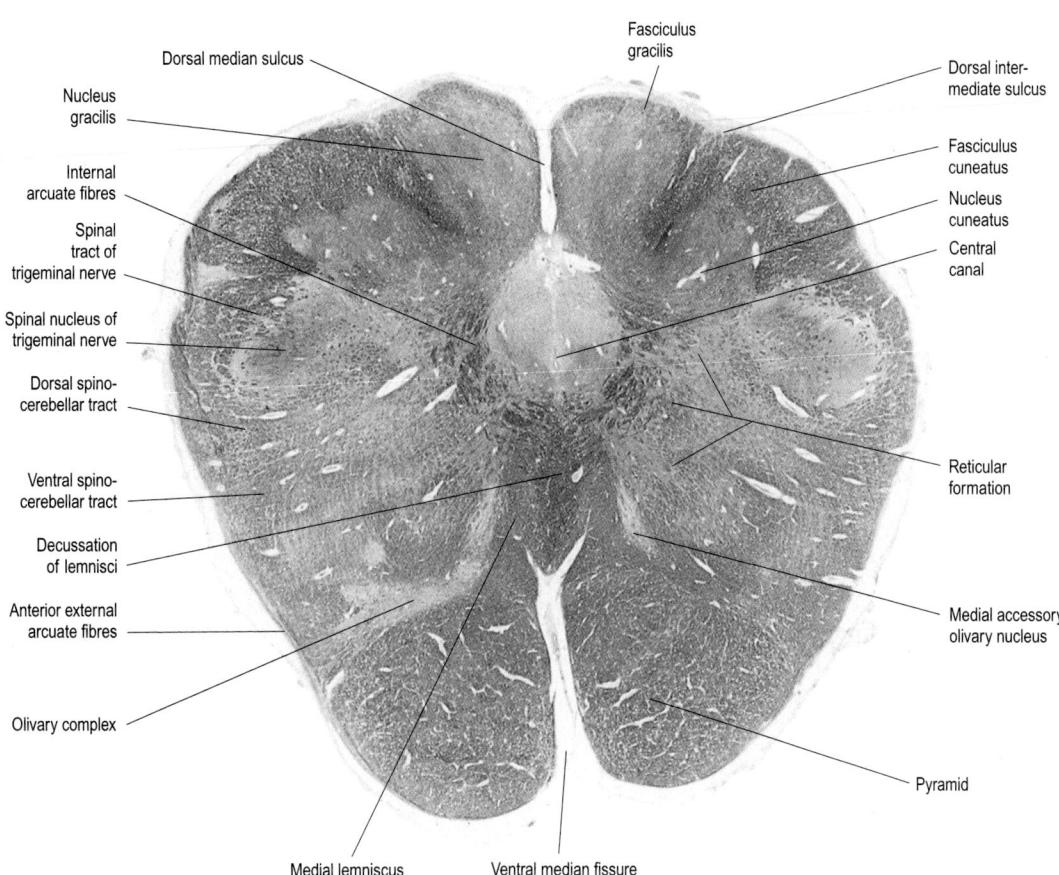

Fasciculus
gracilis

Dorsal median sulcus

Nucleus
gracilis

Internal
arcuate fibres

Spinal
tract of
trigeminal nerve

Spinal nucleus of
trigeminal nerve

Dorsal spino-
cerebellar tract

Ventral spino-
cerebellar tract

Decussation
of lemnisci

Anterior external
arcuate fibres

Olivary complex

Dorsal inter-
mediate sulcus

Fasciculus
cuneatus

Nucleus
cuneatus

Central
canal

Reticular
formation

Medial accessory
olivary nucleus

Pyramid

Medial lemniscus

Ventral median fissure

Fig. 19.6 Transverse section through the medulla oblongata at the level of the decussation of the medial lemniscus.

331

The nucleus of the spinal tract of the trigeminal nerve (**Fig. 19.17**) is separated from the central grey matter by internal arcuate fibres, and from the lateral medullary surface by the trigeminal spinal tract, which ends in it, and by some dorsal spinocerebellar tract fibres. The latter progressively incline dorsally, and enter the inferior cerebellar peduncle at a higher level.

Two other nuclei occur at this level. One is dorsolateral to the pyramid, the other medial to it and near the median plane. These are parts of the precerebellar medial accessory olivary nucleus, described with the inferior olivary nuclear complex (p. 336). Precerebellar nuclei of the vestibular, pontine and reticular system are described on page 362.

Transverse section of the medulla at the caudal end of the fourth ventricle

A transverse section level with the lower end of the fourth ventricle (**Fig. 19.7**) shows some new features together with most of those already described. The total area of grey matter is increased by the presence of the large olivary nuclear complex and nuclei of the vestibulocochlear, glossopharyngeal, vagus and accessory nerves.

A smooth, oval elevation, the olive, lies between the ventrolateral and dorsolateral sulci of the medulla. It is formed by the underlying inferior olivary complex of nuclei, and lies lateral to the pyramid, separated from it by the ventrolateral sulcus and emerging hypoglossal nerve fibres. The roots of the facial nerve emerge between its rostral end and the lower pontine border, in the cerebellopontine angle. The arcuate nuclei are curved, interrupted bands, ventral to the pyramids, and are said to be displaced pontine nuclei. Anterior external arcuate fibres and those of the striae medullares are derived from them. They project mainly to the contralateral cerebellum through the inferior cerebellar peduncle (**Fig. 19.8**).

The inferior olivary nucleus is a hollow, irregularly crenated grey mass. It has a longitudinal medial hilum, and is surrounded by myelinated fibres which form the olivary amiculum. Dorsolateral to the pyramid, it underlies the olive but ascends within the pons. It is described more fully on page 336.

The central grey matter at this level constitutes the ventricular floor. It contains (sequentially from medial to lateral): the hypoglossal nucleus; dorsal vagal nucleus; nucleus solitarius; and the caudal ends of the inferior and medial vestibular nuclei.

The tractus solitarius and its associated circumferential nucleus solitarius extend throughout the length of the medulla. The tract is composed of general visceral afferents from the vagus and glossopharyngeal nerves. The nucleus and its central connections with the reticular formation subserve the reflex control of cardiovascular, respiratory and cardiac functions. The rostral fibres of the tract consist of gustatory fibres from the facial, glossopharyngeal and vagal nerves that project to the rostral pole of the nucleus solitarius, which is sometimes referred to as the gustatory nucleus.

The medial longitudinal fasciculus, a small compact tract near the midline and ventral to the hypoglossal nucleus, is continuous with the ventral vestibulospinal tract. At this medullary level it is displaced dorsally by the pyramidal and lemniscal decussations. It ascends in the pons and midbrain, maintaining its relationship to the central grey matter and midline, and is therefore near the somatic efferent nuclear column. Fibres from a variety of sources course for short distances in the tract.

The spinocerebellar, spinotectal, vestibulospinal, rubrospinal and lateral spinothalamic (spinal lemniscal) tracts all lie in the ventrolateral area of the medulla at this level. The tracts are limited dorsally by the spinal trigeminal nucleus, and ventrally by the pyramid.

Numerous islets of grey matter are scattered centrally in the ventrolateral medulla, an area intersected by nerve fibres that run in all directions. This is the reticular formation, which exists throughout the medulla and extends into the pontine tegmentum and midbrain (p. 347).

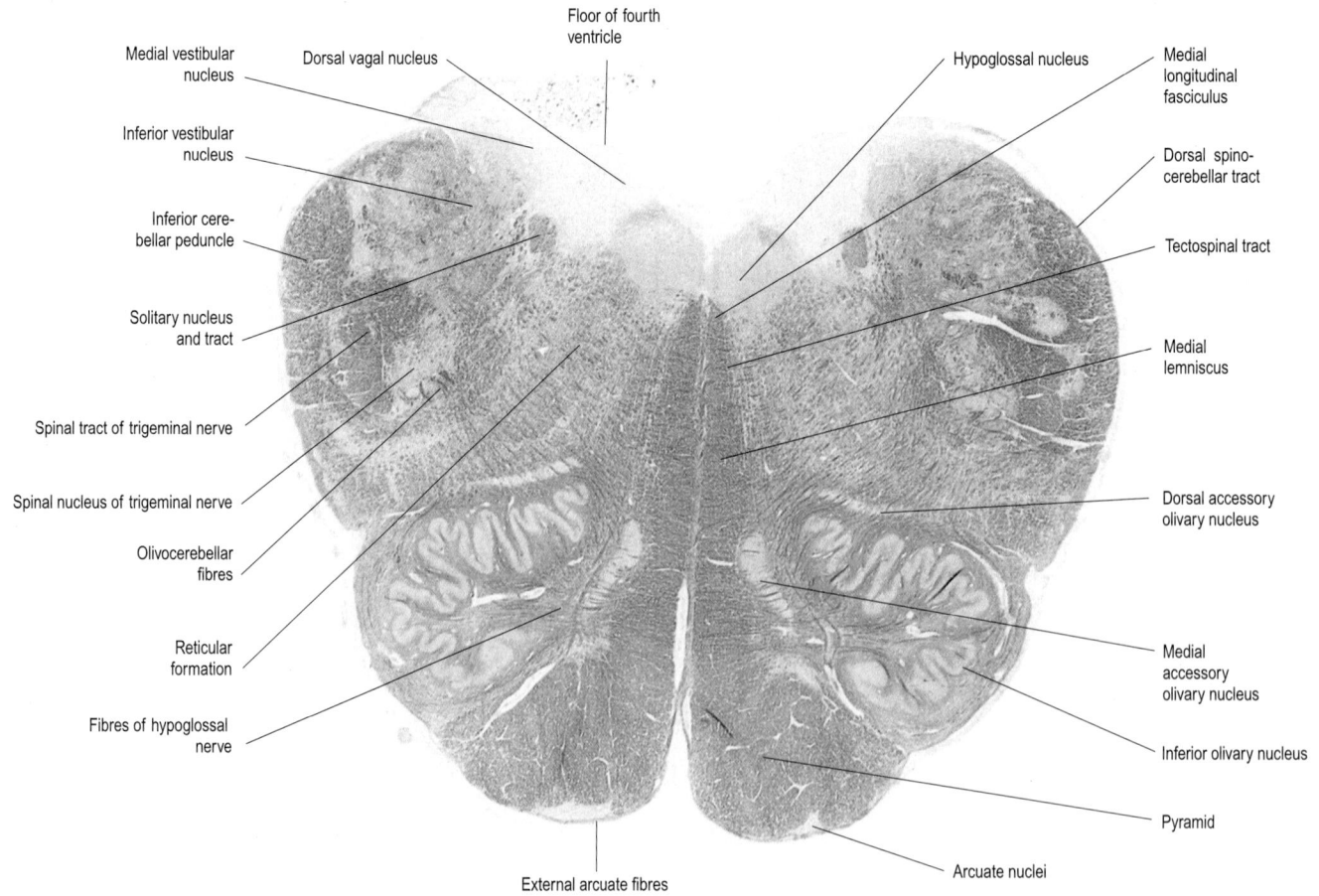

Medial vestibular nucleus
Dorsal vagal nucleus
Floor of fourth ventricle
Hypoglossal nucleus
Medial longitudinal fasciculus
Inferior vestibular nucleus
Dorsal spino-cerebellar tract
Inferior cere-bellar peduncle
Tectospinal tract
Solitary nucleus and tract
Medial lemniscus
Spinal tract of trigeminal nerve
Spinal nucleus of trigeminal nerve
Dorsal accessory olivary nucleus
Olivocerebellar fibres
Reticular formation
Medial accessory olivary nucleus
Fibres of hypoglossal nerve
Inferior olivary nucleus
Pyramid
Arcuate nuclei
External arcuate fibres

Fig. 19.7 Transverse section through the medulla oblongata at the caudal end of the fourth ventricle.

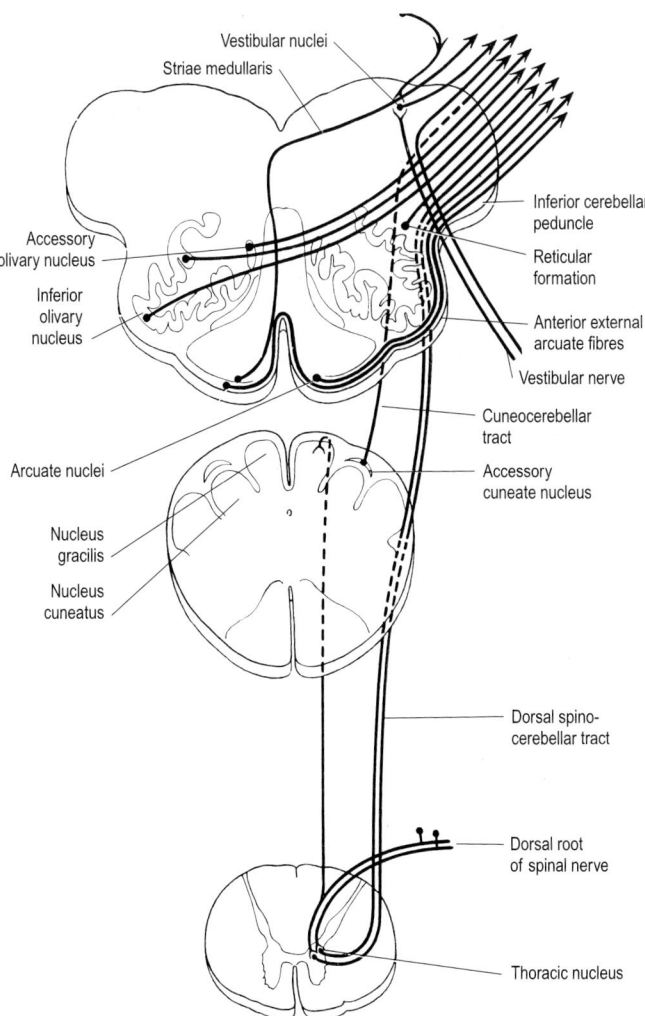

Fig. 19.8 Some of the afferent components of the inferior cerebellar peduncles. The efferent components have been omitted.

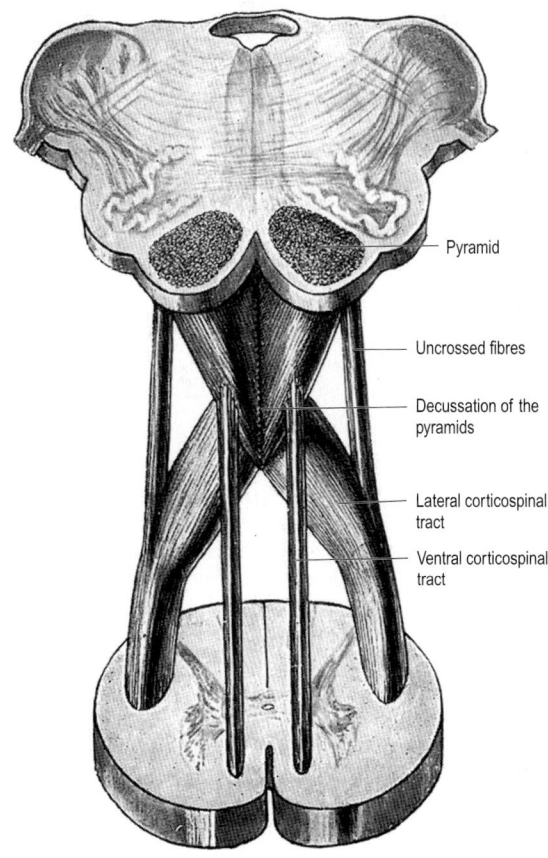

Fig. 19.9 Schematic dissection to show the decussation of the pyramids.

Pyramidal tract

Each pyramid contains descending corticospinal fibres, derived from the ipsilateral cerebral cortex, which have traversed the internal capsule, midbrain and pons (**Fig. 19.9**). Approximately 70–90% of the axons leave the pyramids in successive bundles, crossing in and deep to the ventral median fissure as the pyramidal decussation. In the rostral medulla fibres cross by inclining ventromedially, whereas more caudally they pass dorsally, decussating ventral to the central grey matter. The decussation is orderly, such that fibres destined to end in the cervical segments cross first. They continue to pass dorsally as they descend, and reach the contralateral spinal lateral funiculus as the crossed lateral corticospinal tract. Most uncrossed corticospinal fibres descend ventromedially in the ipsilateral ventral funiculus, as the ventral corticospinal tract. A minority run dorsolaterally to join the lateral corticospinal tracts as a small uncrossed component. The corticospinal tracts display somatotopy at almost all levels. In the pyramids the arrangement is like that at higher levels, in that the most lateral fibres subserve the most medial arm and neck movements. Similar somatotopy is ascribed to the lateral corticospinal tracts within the spinal cord.

Dorsal column nuclei

The nuclei gracilis and cuneatus are part of the pathway that is considered to be the major route for discriminative aspects of tactile and locomotor sensation. The upper regions of both nuclei are reticular and contain small and large multipolar neurones with long dendrites. The lower regions contain clusters of large round neurones with short and profusely branching dendrites. Upper and lower zones differ in their connections but both receive terminals from the dorsal spinal roots at all levels. Dorsal funicular fibres from neurones in the spinal grey matter terminate only in the superior, reticular zone. Variable ordering and overlap of terminals, on the basis of spinal root levels, occur in both zones. The lower extremity is represented medially, the trunk ventrally, and the digits dorsally. There is modal specificity, i.e. lower levels respond to low-threshold cutaneous stimuli, and upper reticular levels to inputs from fibres serving receptors in the skin, joints and muscles. The cuneate nucleus is divided into several parts. Its middle zone contains a large pars rotunda, in which rostrocaudally elongated medium-sized neurones are clustered between bundles of densely myelinated fibres. The reticular poles of its rostral and caudal zones contain scattered, but evenly distributed, neurones of various sizes. The pars triangularis is smaller and laterally placed.There is a somatotopic pattern of termination of cutaneous inputs from the upper limb upon the cell clusters of the pars rotunda. Terminations are diffuse in the reticular poles.

The gracile and cuneate nuclei serve as relays between the spinal cord and higher levels. Primary spinal afferents synapse with multipolar neurones in the nuclei to form the major nuclear efferent projection. The nuclei also contain interneurones, many of which are inhibitory. Descending afferents from the somatosensory cortex reach the nuclei through the corticobulbar tracts, and appear to be restricted to the upper, reticular zones. Since these afferents both inhibit and enhance activity, the nuclear region is clearly one of sensory modulation. The reticular zones also receive connections from the reticular formation. Feedback from the gracile and cuneate nuclei to the spinal cord probably occurs.

Neurones of dorsal column nuclei receive terminals of long, uncrossed, primary afferent fibres of the fasciculi gracilis and cuneatus, which carry information concerning deformation of skin, movement of hairs, joint movement and vibration. Unit recording of the neurones in dorsal column nuclei shows that their tactile receptive fields (i.e. the skin area in which a response can be elicited) vary in size, although they are mostly small, and are smallest for the digits. Some fields have excitatory centres and inhibitory surrounds, which means that stimulation just outside its excitatory field inhibits the neurone. Neurones in the nuclei are spatially organized into a somatotopic map of the

333

periphery (in accord with the similar localization in the dorsal columns). In general, specificity is high. Many cells receive input from one or a few specific receptor types, e.g. hair, type I and II slowly adapting receptors and Pacinian corpuscles, and some cells respond to Ia muscle spindle input. However, some neurones receive convergent input from tactile pressure and hair follicle receptors.

A variety of control mechanisms can modulate the transmission of impulses through the dorsal column–medial lemniscus pathway. Concomitant activity in adjacent dorsal-column fibres may result in presynaptic inhibition by depolarization of the presynaptic terminals of one of them. Stimulation of the sensory–motor cortex also modulates the transmission of impulses by both pre- and postsynaptic inhibitory mechanisms, and sometimes by facilitation. These descending influences are mediated by the corticospinal tract. Modulation of transmission by inhibition also results from stimulation of the reticular formation, raphe nuclei and other sites.

The accessory cuneate nucleus, dorsolateral to the cuneate, is part of the spinocerebellar system of precerebellar nuclei (**Fig. 19.8**) and contains large neurones like those in the spinal thoracic nucleus. These form the posterior external arcuate fibres, which enter the cerebellum by the ipsilateral inferior peduncle. The nucleus receives the lateral fibres of the fasciculus cuneatus, carrying proprioceptive impulses from the upper limb (which enter the cervical spinal cord rostral to the thoracic nucleus). Its efferent fibres form the cuneocerebellar tract. A group of neurones, nucleus Z, identified in animals between the upper pole of the nucleus gracilis and the inferior vestibular nucleus, is said to be present in the human medulla. Its input is probably from the dorsal spinocerebellar tract, which carries proprioceptive information from the ipsilateral lower limb, and it projects through internal arcuate fibres to the contralateral medial lemniscus.

Trigeminal sensory nucleus

The trigeminal sensory nucleus receives the primary afferents of the trigeminal nerve. It is a large nucleus, and extends caudally into the cervical spinal cord and rostrally into the midbrain. The principal and largest division of the nucleus is located in the pontine tegmentum.

On entering the pons, the fibres of the sensory root of the trigeminal nerve run dorsomedially towards the principal sensory nucleus, which

is situated at this level (**Fig. 19.10**). Before reaching the nucleus c.50% of the fibres divide into ascending and descending branches – the others ascend or descend without division. The descending fibres, of which 90% are less than 4 µm in diameter, form the spinal tract of the trigeminal nerve, which reaches the upper cervical spinal cord. The tract embraces the spinal trigeminal nucleus (**Figs 19.5, 19.6, 19.7, 19.11, 19.12**). There is a precise somatotopic organization in the tract. Fibres from the ophthalmic root lie ventrolaterally, those from the mandibular root lie dorsomedially, and the maxillary fibres lie between them. The tract is completed on its dorsal rim by fibres from the sensory roots of the facial, glossopharyngeal and vagus nerves. All of these fibres synapse in the nucleus caudalis.

The detailed anatomy of the trigeminospinal tract excited early clinical interest because it was recognized that dissociated sensory loss could occur in the trigeminal area. For example, in Wallenberg's syndrome, occlusion of the posterior inferior cerebellar branch of the vertebral artery leads to loss of pain and temperature sensation in the ipsilateral half of the face with retention of common sensation. Neurosurgery in the 1890s originated largely in attempts to alleviate paroxysmal trigeminal neuralgia. The introduction of medullary tractotomy confirmed that dissociated thermoanalgesia of the face was associated with destruction of the tract.

There are conflicting opinions on the pattern of termination of the fibres in the spinal nucleus. It has long been held that fibres are organized rostrocaudally within the tract. According to this view, ophthalmic fibres are ventral and descend to the lower limit of the first cervical spinal segment, maxillary fibres are central and do not extend below the medulla oblongata, whilst mandibular fibres are dorsal and do not extend much below the mid-medullary level. The results of section of the spinal tract in cases of severe trigeminal neuralgia support this distribution. It was found that a section 4 mm below the obex rendered the ophthalmic and maxillary areas analgesic but tactile sensibility, apart from the abolition of 'tickle', was much less affected. To include the mandibular area it was necessary to section at the level of the obex. More recently, it has been proposed that fibres are arranged dorsoventrally within the spinal tract. There appear to be sound anatomico-physiological and clinical reasons for believing that all divisions terminate throughout the whole nucleus, although the ophthalmic division may not project fibres as far caudally as the maxillary and mandibular

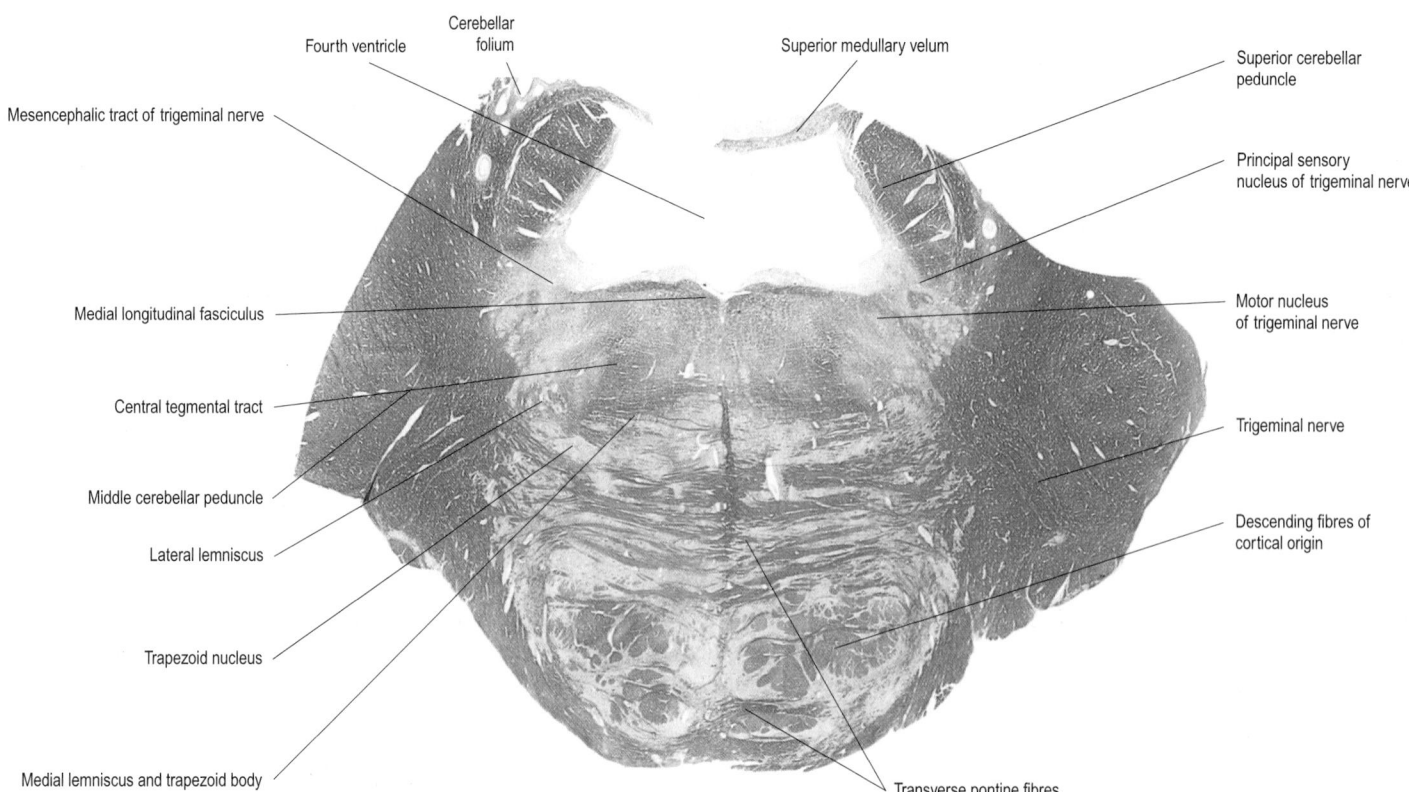

Fig. 19.10 Transverse section of the pons at the level of the trigeminal nerve.

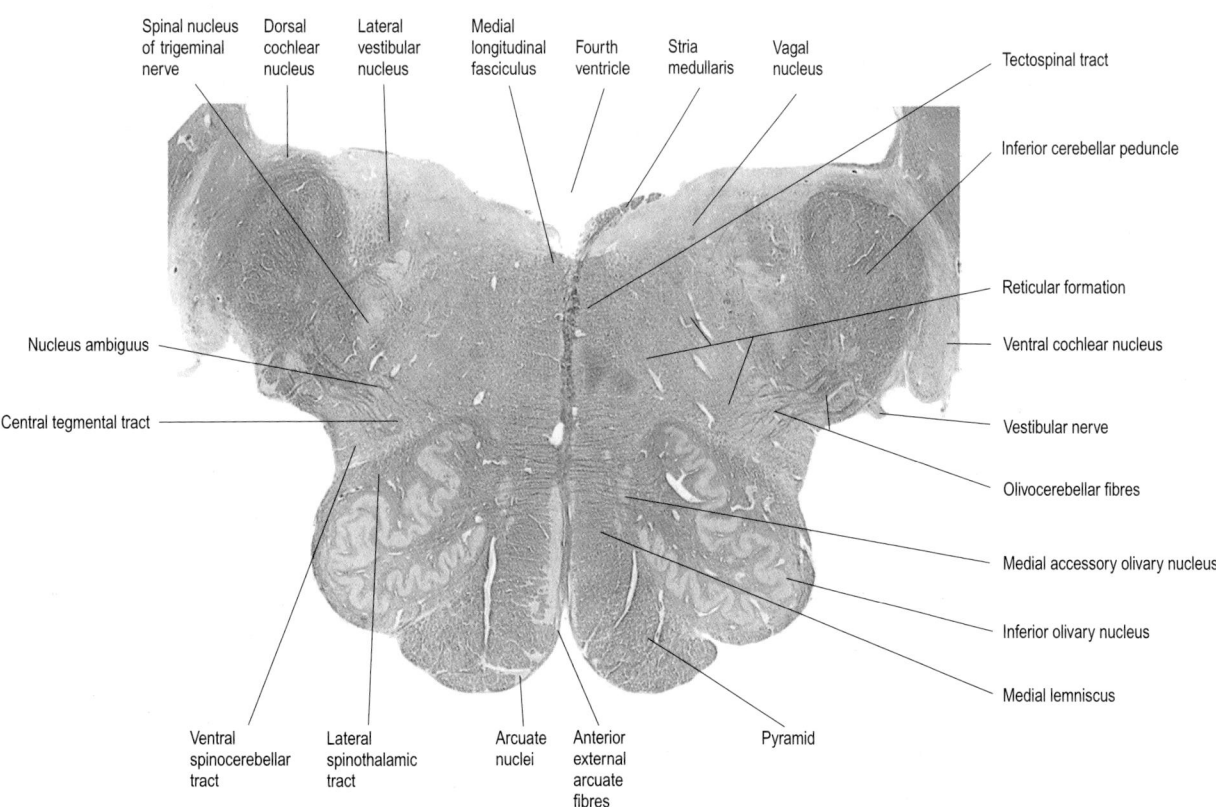

Fig. 19.11 Transverse section through the superior half of the medulla oblongata at the level of the inferior olivary nucleus.

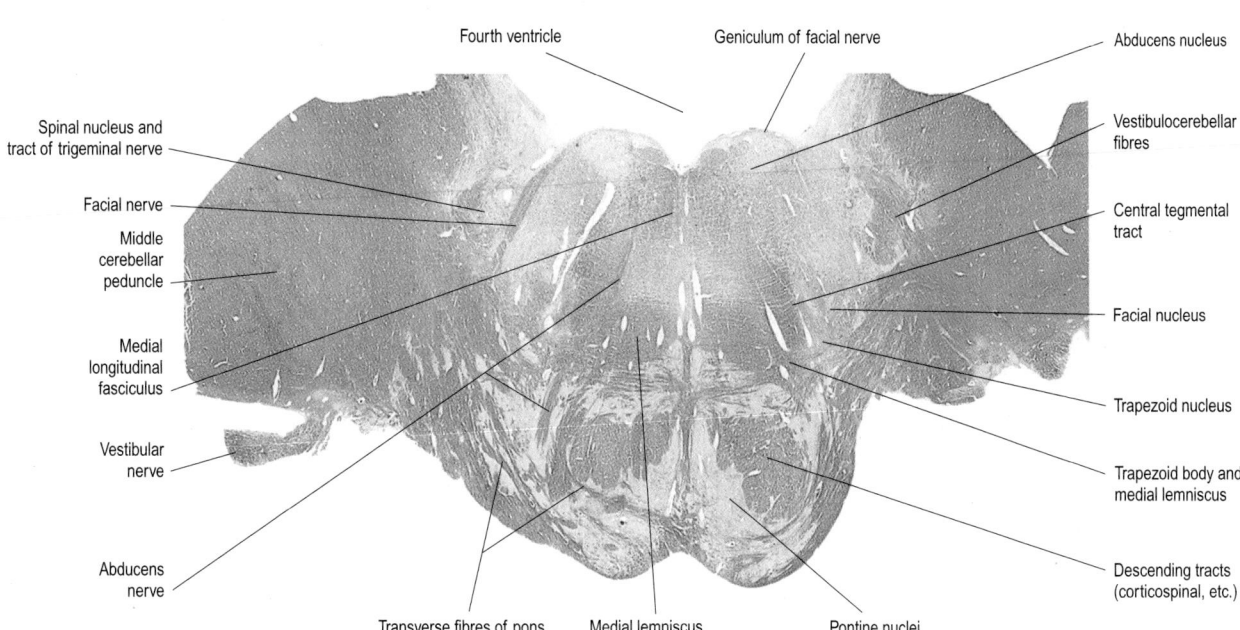

Fig. 19.12 Transverse section through the pons at the level of the facial colliculus.

divisions. Fibres from the posterior face (adjacent to C2) terminate in the lower (caudal) part, whilst those from the upper lip, mouth and nasal tip terminate at a higher level. This can give rise to a segmental (cross-divisional) sensory loss in syringobulbia. Tractotomy of the spinal tract, if carried out at a lower level, can spare the perioral region, a finding that would accord with the 'onion-skin' pattern of loss of pain sensation. However, in clinical practice, the progression of anaesthesia on the face is most commonly 'divisional' rather than onion-skin in distribution.

Fibres of the glossopharyngeal, vagus and facial nerves subserving common sensation (general visceral afferent) form a column dorsally within the spinal tract of the trigeminal nerve and synapse with cells in the lowest part of the spinal trigeminal nucleus. Consequently, operative section of the dorsal part of the spinal tract results in analgesia that extends to the mucosa of the tonsillar sinus, the posterior third of the tongue and adjoining parts of the pharyngeal wall (glossopharyngeal nerve), and the cutaneous area supplied by the auricular branch of the vagus.

335

Other afferents that reach the spinal nucleus are from the dorsal roots of the upper cervical nerves and from the sensorimotor cortex.

The spinal nucleus is considered to consist of three parts: the subnucleus oralis (which is most rostral and adjoins the principal sensory nucleus); the subnucleus interpolaris; and the subnucleus caudalis (which is the most caudal part and is continuous below with the dorsal grey column of the spinal cord). The structure of the subnucleus caudalis is different from that of the other trigeminal sensory nuclei. It has a structure analogous to that of the dorsal horn of the spinal cord, with a similar arrangement of cell laminae, and is involved in trigeminal pain perception. Cutaneous nociceptive afferents and small-diameter muscle afferents terminate in layers I, II, V and VI of the subnucleus caudalis. Low-threshold mechanosensitive afferents of Aβ neurones terminate in layers III and IV of the subnucleus caudalis and rostral (interpolaris, oralis and main sensory) nuclei.

Many of the neurones in the subnucleus caudalis that respond to cutaneous or tooth-pulp stimulation are also excited by noxious electrical, mechanical or chemical stimuli derived from the jaw or tongue muscles. This indicates that convergence of superficial and deep afferent inputs via wide-dynamic-range or nociceptive-specific neurones occurs in the nucleus. Similar convergence of superficial and deep inputs occurs in the rostral nuclei and may account for the poor localization of trigeminal pain, and for the spread of pain, which often makes diagnosis difficult.

There are distinct subtypes of cells in lamina II. Afferents from 'higher-centres' arborize within it, as do axons from nociceptive and low-threshold afferents. Descending influences from these higher centres include fibres from the periaqueductal grey matter and from the nucleus raphe magnus and associated reticular formation.

The nucleus raphe magnus projects directly to the subnucleus caudalis, probably via enkephalin, noradrenaline and 5-HT-containing terminals. These fibres directly or indirectly (through local interneurones) influence pain perception. Stimulation of periaqueductal grey matter or nucleus raphe magnus inhibits the jaw opening reflex to nociception, and may induce primary afferent depolarization in tooth-pulp afferents and other nociceptive facial afferents. Neurones in the subnucleus caudalis can be suppressed by stimuli applied outside their receptive field, particularly by noxious stimuli. The subnucleus caudalis is an important site for relay of nociceptive input and functions as part of the pain 'gate-control'. However, rostral nuclei also have a nociceptive role. Tooth-pulp afferents via wide-dynamic-range and nociceptive-specific neurones may terminate in rostral nuclei, which all project to the subnucleus caudalis.

Most fibres arising in the trigeminal sensory nuclei cross the midline and ascend in the trigeminal lemniscus. They end in the contralateral thalamic nucleus ventralis posterior medialis, from which third-order neurones project to the cortical postcentral gyrus (areas 1, 2 and 3). However, some trigeminal nucleus efferents ascend to the nucleus ventralis posterior medialis of the ipsilateral thalamus.

Fibres from the subnucleus caudalis, especially from laminae I, V and VI, also project to the rostral trigeminal nuclei, cerebellum, periaqueductal grey of the midbrain, parabrachial area of the pons, the brain stem reticular formation and the spinal cord. Fibres from lamina I project to the subnucleus medius of the medial thalamus.

Vagal nucleus

The vagal nucleus (also known as the dorsal motor nucleus of the vagus) lies dorsolateral to the hypoglossal nucleus, from which it is separated by the nucleus intercalatus. It extends caudally to the first cervical spinal segment and rostrally to the open part of the medulla under the vagal triangle (Fig. 19.2).

The vagal nucleus is a general visceral efferent nucleus and is the largest parasympathetic nucleus in the brain stem. Most (80%) of its neurones give rise to the preganglionic parasympathetic fibres of the vagus nerve. The remainder are interneurones or project centrally. Its fibres control the non-striated muscle of the viscera of the thorax (heart, bronchi, lungs and oesophagus) and abdomen (stomach, liver, pancreas, spleen, small intestine and proximal part of the colon). Neurones within the nucleus are heterogeneous and can be classified into nine subnuclei, which are regionally grouped into rostral, intermediate and caudal divisions. Topographic maps of visceral representation in animals suggest that the heart and lungs are represented in the caudal and lateral part of the nucleus, the stomach and pancreas in intermediate regions, and the remaining abdominal organs in the rostral and medial part of the nucleus.

There may be a sparse sensory afferent supply, which arises in the nodose ganglion and projects directly to the nucleus and possibly beyond into the nucleus tractus solitarius.

Hypoglossal nucleus

The prominent hypoglossal nucleus lies near the midline in the dorsal medullary grey matter. It is c.2 cm long. Its rostral part lies beneath the hypoglossal triangle in the floor of the fourth ventricle, and its caudal part extends into the closed part of the medulla (Figs 19.2, 19.6, 16.10).

The hypoglossal nucleus consists of large motor neurones interspersed with myelinated fibres. It is organized into dorsal and ventral nuclear tiers, each divisible into medial and lateral subnuclei. There is a musculotopic organization of motor neurones within the nuclei that corresponds to the structural and functional divisions of tongue musculature. Thus, motor neurones innervating tongue retrusor muscles are located in dorsal/dorsolateral nuclei, whereas motor neurones innervating the main tongue protrusor muscle are located in ventral/ventromedial regions of the nucleus. Although relatively little is known about the organization of motor neurones innervating the intrinsic muscles of the tongue, experimental evidence suggests that motor neurones of the medial division of the hypoglossal nucleus innervate tongue muscles that are oriented in planes transverse to the long axis of the tongue (transverse and vertical intrinsics and genioglossus), whereas motor neurones of the lateral division innervate tongue muscles that are oriented parallel to this axis (styloglossus, hyoglossus, superior and inferior longitudinal).

Several smaller groups of cells lie near the hypoglossal nucleus. They are perhaps misnamed as the 'perihypoglossal complex' or 'perihypoglossal grey', for none is known for certainty to be connected with the hypoglossal nerve or nucleus. They include the nucleus intercalatus, sublingual nucleus, nucleus prepositus hypoglossi and nucleus paramedianus dorsalis (reticularis). Gustatory and visceral connections are attributed to the nucleus intercalatus.

Hypoglossal fibres emerge ventrally from their nucleus, traverse the reticular formation lateral to the medial lemniscus, pass medial to (sometimes through) the inferior olivary nucleus, and curve laterally to emerge superficially as a linear series of 10–15 rootlets in the ventrolateral sulcus between the pyramid and olive (Fig. 19.3).

The hypoglossal nucleus receives corticonuclear fibres from the precentral gyrus and adjacent areas of (mainly) the contralateral hemisphere. They either synapse on motor neurones of the nucleus directly or on interneurones. Evidence indicates that the most medial hypoglossal subnuclei receive projections from both hemispheres. The nucleus may connect with the cerebellum via adjacent perihypoglossal nuclei, and perhaps also with the medullary reticular formation, the trigeminal sensory nuclei and the solitary nucleus.

Inferior olivary nucleus

The olivary nuclear complex consists of the large inferior olivary nucleus and the much smaller medial accessory and dorsal accessory olivary nuclei. They are the so-called precerebellar nuclei, a group that also includes the pontine, arcuate, vestibular, reticulocerebellar and spinocerebellar nuclei, all of which receive afferents from specific sources and project to the cerebellum. The inferior olivary nucleus contains small neurones, most of which form the olivocerebellar tract, which emerges either from the hilum or through the adjacent wall, to run medially and intersect the medial lemniscus (Fig. 19.8). Its fibres cross the midline, and sweep either dorsal to, or through, the opposite olivary nucleus. They intersect the lateral spinothalamic and rubrospinal tracts and the spinal trigeminal nucleus, and enter the contralateral inferior cerebellar peduncle, where they constitute its major component. Fibres from the contralateral inferior olivary complex terminate on Purkinje cells in the cerebellum as climbing fibres – there is a one-to-one relationship between Purkinje cells and neurones in the complex. Afferent connections to the inferior olivary nucleus are both ascending and descending. Ascending fibres, mainly crossed, arrive from all spinal levels in the spino-olivary tracts and via the dorsal columns. Descending ipsilateral fibres come from the cerebral cortex, thalamus, red nucleus and central grey of the midbrain. In part the two latter projections make up central tegmental tract (fasciculus) that forms the olivary amiculum.

The medial accessory olivary nucleus is a curved grey lamina, concave laterally, between the medial lemniscus and pyramid and the ventromedial aspect of the inferior olivary nucleus. The dorsal accessory olivary nucleus is a similar lamina dorsomedial to the inferior olivary nucleus. Both nuclei are connected to the cerebellum. The accessory nuclei are phylogenetically older than the inferior, and connected with the paleocerebellum. In all connections, cerebral, spinal and cerebellar, the olivary nuclei sometimes display very specific somatotopy, particularly in their cerebellar connections, which are described in detail on page 362.

Nucleus solitarius

The nucleus solitarius (solitary nucleus, nucleus of the solitary tract) lies ventrolateral to the vagal nucleus and is almost coextensive with it. A neuronal group ventrolateral to the nucleus solitarius has been termed the nucleus parasolitarius. The nucleus solitarius is intimately related to, and receives fibres from, the tractus solitarius, which carries afferent fibres from the facial, glossopharyngeal and vagus nerves. These fibres enter the tract in descending order and convey gustatory information from the lingual and palatal mucosa. They may also convey visceral impulses from the pharynx (glossopharyngeal and vagus) and from the oesophagus and abdominal alimentary canal (vagus). There is some overlap in this vertical representation.

Termination of special visceral gustatory afferents within the nucleus shows a viscerotopic pattern, predominantly in the rostral region. Experimental evidence suggests that fibres from the anterior two-thirds of the tongue and the roof of the oral cavity (which travel via the chorda tympani and greater petrosal branches of the facial nerve) terminate in the extreme rostral part of the solitary complex. Those from the circumvallate and foliate papillae of the posterior third of the tongue, tonsils, palate and pharynx (which travel via the lingual branch of the glossopharyngeal nerve) are distributed throughout the rostrocaudal extent of the nucleus, predominantly rostral to the obex. Gustatory afferents from the larynx and epiglottis (which travel via the superior laryngeal branch of the vagus) have a more caudal and lateral distribution. The nucleus solitarius may also receive fibres from the spinal cord, cerebral cortex and cerebellum.

Medial and commissural subnuclei in the caudal part of the nucleus appear to be the primary site of termination for gastrointestinal afferents. Ventral and interstitial subnuclei probably receive tracheal, laryngeal and pulmonary afferents and play an important role in both respiratory control and possibly rhythm generation. The carotid sinus and aortic body nerves terminate in the dorsal and dorsolateral region of the nucleus solitarius, which may be involved in cardiovascular regulation.

The nucleus solitarius is thought to project to the sensory thalamus with a relay to the cerebral cortex. It may also project to the upper levels of the spinal cord through a solitariospinal tract. Secondary gustatory axons cross the midline. Many subsequently ascend the brain stem in the dorsomedial part of the medial lemniscus and synapse on the most medial neurones of the thalamic nucleus ventralis posterior medialis (in a region sometimes termed the accessory arcuate nucleus). Axons from the nucleus ventralis posterior medialis radiate through the internal capsule to the anteroinferior area of the sensorimotor cortex and the insula. It is thought that other ascending paths end in a number of the hypothalamic nuclei, and so mediate the route by which gustatory information may reach the limbic system and allow appropriate autonomic reactions to be made.

Swallowing and gag reflexes

During the normal processes of eating and drinking, passage of material to the rear of the mouth stimulates branches of the glossopharyngeal nerve in the oropharynx (**Fig. 19.13**). This information is relayed via the nucleus solitarius to the nucleus ambiguus, which contains the motor neurones innervating the muscles of the palate, pharynx, and larynx. The nasopharynx is closed off from the oropharynx by elevation of the soft palate. The larynx is raised, its entrance narrowed and the glottis is closed. Peristaltic activity down the oesophagus to the stomach is mediated through the pharyngeal plexus (p. 630).

If stimulation of the oropharynx occurs other than during swallowing, the gag reflex may be initiated. There is a reflex contraction of the muscles of the pharynx, soft palate, and fauces that, if extreme, may result in retching and vomiting.

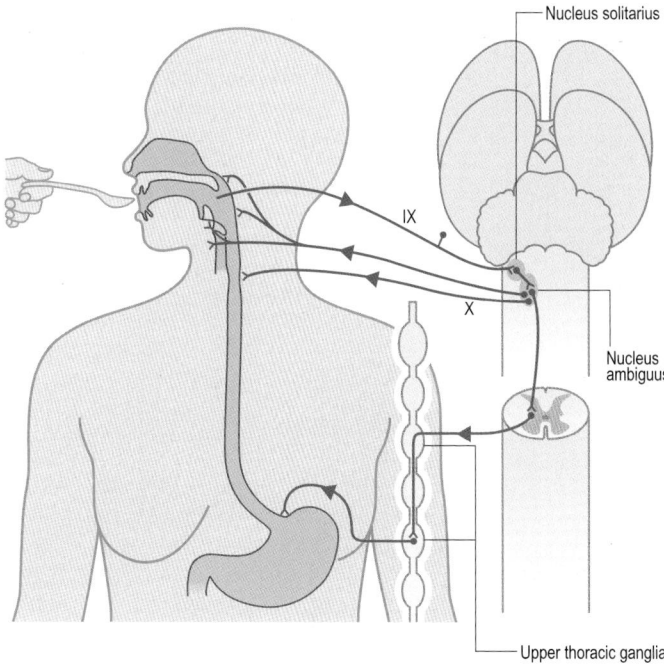

Fig. 19.13 Swallowing and gag reflexes. (Redrawn from Oxford Textbook of Functional Anatomy, Vol 3 Head and Neck, MacKinnon P, Morris J (eds), 1990. By permission of Oxford University Press.)

Nucleus ambiguus

The nucleus ambiguus is a group of large motor neurones, situated deep in the medullary reticular formation. It extends rostrally as far as the upper end of the vagal nucleus while caudally it is continuous with the nucleus of the spinal accessory nerve. Fibres emerging from it pass dorsomedially, then curve laterally. Rostral fibres join the glossopharyngeal nerve. Caudal fibres join the vagus and cranial accessory nerves and are distributed to the pharyngeal constrictors, intrinsic laryngeal muscles and striated muscles of the palate and upper oesophagus.

The nucleus ambiguus contains several cellular subgroups, and some topographical representation of the muscles innervated has been established. Individual laryngeal muscles are innervated by relatively discrete groups of cells in more caudal zones. Neurones that innervate the pharynx lie in the intermediate area, and neurones that innervate the oesophagus and soft palate are rostral.

The nucleus ambiguus is connected to corticonuclear tracts bilaterally and to many brain stem centres. At its upper end, a small retrofacial nucleus intervenes between it and the facial nucleus. Although the nucleus ambiguus lies in line with the special visceral efferent nuclei, it is a reputed source of general visceral efferent vagal fibres.

Cough and sneeze reflexes

Irritation of the larynx or trachea is conveyed via laryngeal branches of the vagus nerve to the trigeminal sensory nucleus of the brain stem. Impulses are relayed to medullary respiratory centres and to the nucleus ambiguus. More-or-less energetic exhalation (coughing) occurs, caused by contraction of intercostal and abdominal wall muscles after a build-up of pressure against a closed glottis.

A similar mechanism underlies sneezing (**Fig. 19.14**) except that the stimulus arises from the nasal mucosa and afferent impulses are conveyed by the ophthalmic or maxillary divisions of the trigeminal nerve to the trigeminal sensory nucleus. After sharp inhalation, explosive exhalation occurs with closure of the oropharyngeal isthmus by the action of palatoglossus, which diverts air through the nasal cavity and so expels the irritant.

PONS

EXTERNAL FEATURES AND RELATIONS

The pons lies rostral to the medulla and caudal to the midbrain. Ventrally, the site of transition with the medulla is demarcated superficially by a transverse sulcus. Laterally, in a region known as the

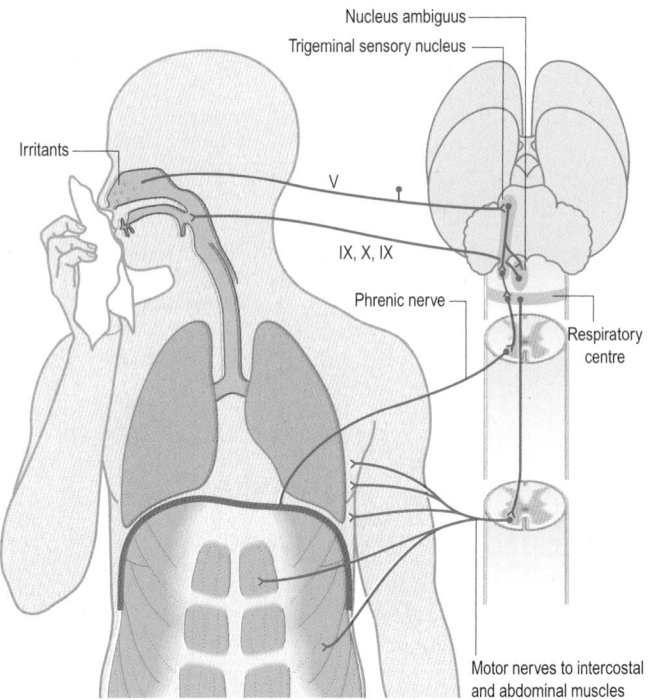

Fig. 19.14 Sneeze and cough reflexes. (Redrawn from Oxford Textbook of Functional Anatomy, Vol 3 Head and Neck, MacKinnon P, Morris J (eds), 1990. By permission of Oxford University Press.)

cerebellopontine angle (**Figs 19.2, 19.3**), the facial, vestibulocochlear and glossopharyngeal roots and the nervus intermedius all lie on the choroid plexus of the fourth ventricle (which protrudes from the foramen of Luschka into the subarachnoid space). The ventral surface of the pons (**Fig. 19.3**) is separated from the clivus (basisphenoid and dorsum sellae) by the cisterna pontis. It is markedly convex transversely, less so vertically, and grooves the petrous part of the temporal bone laterally up to the internal acoustic meatus. The surface has a shallow vertical median sulcus, in which the basilar artery runs, bounded bilaterally by prominences that are formed partly by underlying corticospinal fibres as they descend through the pons. Bundles of transverse fibres, bridging the midline and originating from nuclei in the basal pons (nuclei pontis), converge on each side into the large middle cerebellar peduncle and project to the cerebellum. The trigeminal nerve emerges near the midpontine level. It has a small superomedial motor root and a large inferolateral sensory root.

The dorsal surface of the pons is hidden by the cerebellum which covers the rostral half of the rhomboid fossa, into which the aqueduct of the midbrain empties. The roof of the fossa is formed by a thin sheet of tissue, the superior medullary velum, and is overlain by the lingula of the vermis of the cerebellum. The velum is attached on each side to the superior cerebellar peduncles and is enclosed by pia mater above and ependyma below (**Fig. 16.10**). The abducens nerves decussate in the velum.

INTERNAL STRUCTURE

Transverse sections of the pons

Transverse sections (**Figs 19.10, 19.12**) reveal that the pons consists of a dorsal tegmentum, which is a continuation of the medulla (excluding the pyramids), and a ventral (basilar) part. The latter contains bundles of longitudinal descending fibres, some of which continue into the pyramids, while others end in the many pontine or medullary nuclei. It also contains numerous transverse fibres and scattered pontine nuclei.

Ventral pons

The ventral pons is similar in structure at all levels. The longitudinal fibres of the corticopontine, corticonuclear and corticospinal tracts descend from the crus cerebri of the midbrain and enter the pons compactly. They rapidly disperse into fascicles, which are separated by the pontine nuclei and transverse pontine fibres. Corticospinal fibres run through the pons to the medullary pyramids, where they again con-

verge into compact tracts. They are accompanied by corticonuclear fibres, some of which diverge to contralateral (and some ipsilateral) nuclei of cranial nerves and other nuclei in the pontine tegmentum, while others reach reach the pyramids. Clinical evidence supports the view that the facial and other nuclei receive ipsilateral corticonuclear fibres.

Corticopontine fibres, from the frontal, temporal, parietal and occipital cortices end in the pontine nuclei (**Fig. 19.12**). Axons from the latter constitute the transverse pontine (pontocerebellar) fibres, which, after decussation, continue as the contralateral middle cerebellar peduncle. Frontopontine axons end in the pontine nuclei above the level of the emerging trigeminal roots, and are relayed to the contralateral cerebellum in the upper transverse pontine fibres. All pontocerebellar fibres end as mossy fibres in the cerebellar cortex, and a degree of somatotopy is maintained in these connections.

The precerebellar pontine nuclei include all the neurones that are scattered in the ventral pons. In man, there are some 20 million pontine neurones. They are probably all glutamatergic, and most project to the cerebellar cortex, with some input to the deep cerebellar nuclei. Corticopontine fibres arise mainly from neurones in layer V of the premotor, somatosensory, posterior parietal, extrastriate visual and cingulate neocortices. Projections from prefrontal, temporal and striate cortices are sparse. The terminal fields, although divergent, form topographically segmented patterns resembling overlapping columns, slabs or lamellae within the pons. Subcortical projections to the pontine nuclei include those from the superior colliculus to the dorsolateral pons, and the medial mammillary nucleus to the rostromedial pons and pretectal nuclei. The lateral geniculate nucleus, dorsal column nuclei, trigeminal nuclei, hypothalamus and intracerebellar nuclei also project to restricted neurones of the pons. Functionally related subcortical and cerebrocortical afferents converge, e.g. those from the somatosensory cortex, dorsal column nuclei medial mammillary nucleus. There is also non-specific input from the reticular formation, raphe nuclei, locus coeruleus and paraqueductal grey matter.

Pontine tegmentum

The pontine tegmentum varies in cytoarchitecture at different levels. A transverse section through the lower pontine tegmentum transects the facial colliculi (**Figs 19.12, 19.15**). Each colliculus contains the motor nucleus of the abducens nerve and the geniculum of the facial nerve. More deeply placed are the facial nuclei, the nearby vestibular and cochlear nuclei and other isolated neuronal groups. The medial vestibular nucleus continues a little from the medulla into the pontine tegmentum, and is separated from the inferior cerebellar peduncle by the lateral vestibular nucleus.

The vestibular nuclei are laterally placed in the rhomboid fossa of the fourth ventricle, subjacent to the vestibular area, which spans the rostral medulla and caudal pons (**Fig. 19.1**). They consist of medial,

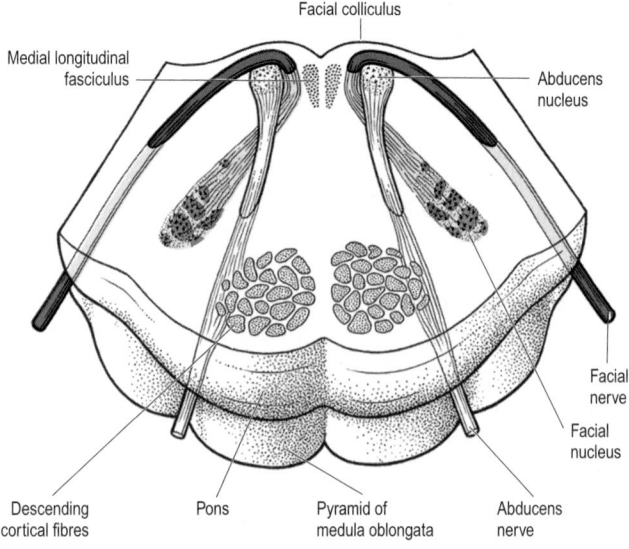

Fig. 19.15 The central course of the fibres of the facial nerve in a transverse section of the pons, viewed from the rostral aspect.

lateral (Deiters' nucleus), superior and inferior vestibular groups. They all receive fibres from the vestibulocochlear nerve and send axons to the cerebellum, medial longitudinal fasciculus, spinal cord and lateral lemniscus. Evidence suggests that the vestibular apparatus is spatially represented in the nuclei. The medial vestibular nucleus broadens, then narrows as it ascends from the upper olivary level into the lower pons, where it separates the vagal nucleus from the floor of the fourth ventricle. It is crossed by the striae medullares nearer the floor. Below, it is continuous with the nucleus intercalatus. The inferior vestibular nucleus (which is the smallest) lies between the medial vestibular nucleus and inferior cerebellar peduncle, from the level of the upper end of the nucleus gracilis to the pontomedullary junction. It is crossed by descending fibres of the vestibulocochlear nerve and the vestibulospinal tract. The lateral vestibular nucleus lies just above the inferior nucleus, and ascends almost to the level of the abducens nucleus. It is composed of large multipolar neurones, which are the main source of the vestibulospinal tract. The superior vestibular nucleus is small and lies above the medial and lateral nuclei.

Vestibular fibres of the vestibulocochlear nerve enter the medulla between the inferior cerebellar peduncle and the trigeminal spinal tract, and approach the vestibular area, where they bifurcate into descending and ascending branches. The former descend medial to the inferior cerebellar peduncle and end in medial, lateral and inferior vestibular nuclei, and the latter enter the superior and medial nuclei. A few vestibular fibres enter the cerebellum directly through the inferior peduncle (superficially in the juxtarestiform body), and end in the fastigial nucleus, flocculonodular lobe and uvula. Vestibular nuclei project extensively to the cerebellum and also receive axons from the cerebellar cortex and the fastigial nuclei. Their uncrossed spinal projections run in the vestibulospinal tracts. Vestibular axons also reach the spinal cord in the medial longitudinal fasciculus (Figs 18.22, 19.21). Some reach cerebral levels, possibly for bilateral cortical representation. The vestibular nuclear complex projects to the pontine reticular nuclei and to motor nuclei of the ocular muscles in the medial longitudinal fasciculus.

Fibres of the cochlear division of the vestibulocochlear nerve partially encircle the inferior cerebellar peduncle laterally and end in the dorsal and ventral cochlear nuclei. The dorsal cochlear nucleus forms a bulge, the auditory tubercle, on the posterior surface of the peduncle, and is continuous medially with the vestibular area in the rhomboid fossa. The ventral cochlear nucleus is ventrolateral to the dorsal cochlear nucleus, and lies between the cochlear and vestibular fibres of the vestibulocochlear nerve.

The striae medullares of the fourth ventricle (Figs 16.10, 19.11) are an aberrant cerebropontocerebellar connection, in which the arcuate nuclei and external arcuate fibres are involved. Axons from arcuate nuclei spread round the medulla, above and below the inferior olive, where they are superficially visible as the circumolivary fasciculus. All these fibres, which collectively are known as the external arcuate fibres, enter the inferior cerebellar peduncle (Fig. 19.8). Some fibres from arcuate nuclei pass dorsally through the medulla near its midline, decussate near the floor of the fourth ventricle, then turn laterally under the ependyma and enter the cerebellum through the inferior peduncle.

In addition to the tracts already noted at lower levels, the lower pontine tegmentum contains the trapezoid body, lateral lemniscus and emerging fibres of the abducens and facial nerves. The medial lemniscus is ventral, its transverse outline now a flat oval. It extends laterally from the median raphe (Figs 19.10, 19.12) and is laterally related to the lateral spinothalamic tract and trigeminal lemniscus. The fibres of the latter originate from neurones of the contralateral spinal nucleus, serving pain and thermal sensibility in facial skin and mucosae of the conjunctiva, tongue, mouth, nose, etc. Here the lemnisci together form a transverse band which is composed, in lateral order from the midline, of the medial and trigeminal lemnisci, the lateral spinothalamic tract and the lateral lemniscus.

The trapezoid body contains cochlear fibres, mainly from the ventral cochlear and trapezoid nuclei. They ascend transversely in the ventral tegmentum, pass either through or ventral to the vertical medial lemniscal fibres, and decussate with the contralateral fibres in the median raphe. Below the emerging facial axons, the trapezoid fibres turn up into the lateral lemniscus. As the lateral lemniscus ascends it lies near the dorsolateral surface of the brain stem. Above, its fibres enter the inferior colliculus and medial geniculate body. The ascending auditory pathway is described in detail on page 436.

The medial longitudinal fasciculus is paramedian, ventral to the fourth venticle, near the abducens nucleus from which it is separated by facial nerve fibres. It is the main intersegmental tract in the brain stem, particularly for interactions between nuclei of cranial nerves innervating the extraocular muscles and the vestibular system (Fig. 19.21). In the lower pons it receives fibres from vestibular, and perhaps dorsal trapezoid, nuclei. Its greater part is formed by vestibulocochlear contributions.

A transverse section at an upper pontine tegmental level contains trigeminal elements (Fig. 19.10), but otherwise shows little notable alteration from a section through a lower pontine tegmental level. Its dorsolateral parts are invaded by the superior cerebellar peduncles. The small lateral lemniscal nucleus is medial to its tract in the upper pons, and receives some lemniscal terminals. Some of its efferent fibres enter the medial longitudinal fasciculus, others return to the lemniscus. The lateral lemniscal nucleus is a relay station in the auditory pathway associated with the trapezoid nucleus.

The medial lemniscus (Figs 19.10, 18.14) retains its paramedian position in the ventral pontine tegmentum, where it lies a little lateral to the median raphe, and is joined medially by fibres from the principal trigeminal sensory nucleus. The trigeminal lemniscus, lateral spinothalamic tract, and the lateral lemniscus and its nucleus all lie dorsolaterally.

Cochlear nuclei

Cochlear nerve fibres, which are derived from neuronal somata in the spiral ganglion, bifurcate on entering the brain stem and terminate in both dorsal and ventral cochlear nuclei.

The ventral cochlear nucleus has a complex cytoarchitecture. It contains many neuronal types with distinct dendritic field characteristics. Marked topographical order has been demonstrated in cochlear nerve terminals within the nucleus. Different parts of the spiral ganglion and differing stimulation frequencies are related to neurones that are serially arrayed anteroinferiorly in the ventral nucleus. All cochlear nerve fibres enter the nucleus. There are c.25,000 axons in the human cochlear nerve, and they project onto a much larger number of neurones in the cochlear nucleus. The number of cochlear fibres in the lateral lemniscus greatly exceeds that in the cochlear nerve. A minor fraction of the cochlear neurones receive terminals from the nerve, though each fibre may connect with several neurones. Terminals are limited to the anteroinferior region of the ventral nucleus, where the neurones are probably mostly local interneurones.

The dorsal cochlear nucleus is almost continuous with the ventral nucleus, from which it is only separated by a thin stratum of nerve fibres. Giant cells predominate, and their dendritic fields are aligned with the incoming auditory fibres.

Though the cellular origins are not precisely known, axons of most neuronal types in the cochlear nuclei leave to end at pontine levels in the superior olivary, trapezoid and lateral lemniscal nuclei (Fig. 19.10). They leave the cochlear nuclei by three routes. The largest group of axons lies ventrally and decussates as the trapezoid body, level with the pontomedullary junction (Figs 19.10, 19.12). Most of these axons ascend slightly, decussate and relay in the contralateral nuclei. A few do not cross, and synapse in the ipsilateral superior olivary nuclei. From both nuclei, the next order axons ascend in the corresponding lateral lemniscus. Occasional decussating fibres traverse the contralateral superior olive and enter the lateral lemniscus to relay in lemniscal nuclei.

Some axons from ventral cochlear neurones pass dorsally, superficial to descending trigeminal spinal fibres, cerebellar fibres in the inferior peduncle, and axons of the dorsal cochlear nucleus. This bundle of ventral cochlear fibres is smaller than that of the trapezoid decussation. It swerves ventromedially across the midline, ventral to the medial longitudinal fasciculus, as the intermediate acoustic striae. Its further path is uncertain, but it probably ascends in the contralateral lateral lemniscus.

The most dorsally placed axons issue from the dorsal cochlear nucleus. They curve dorsomedially round the inferior cerebellar peduncle towards the midline as the dorsal acoustic striae, ventral to the striae medullares. They incline ventromedially and cross the midline to ascend in the contralateral lateral lemniscus, probably relaying in its nuclei.

The superior olivary complex is sited in the tegmentum of the caudal pons, lateral in the reticular formation at the level of the pontomedullary junction. The superior complex includes several named nuclei and nameless smaller groups. In humans, the lateral superior olivary nucleus is made up of some six small cellular clusters. The medial (accessory) superior olivary nucleus is large and compact. The trapezoid nucleus is medial. A retro-olivary group, the reputed origin of some efferent cochlear fibres, is dorsal. Some internuclear connections have been described. The medial superior olivary nucleus receives impulses from both spiral organs, and may be involved in auditory sound source localization. The superior olivary complexes and the trapezoid nuclei are relay stations in the ascending auditory projection. These intricate connections have not been well established in man.

The medial nucleus of the trapezoid body is small in man. It has a ventral component, which consists of large neurones scattered among the trapezoid fascicles, and a more compact dorsal nucleus, medial to the superior olivary complex. The nucleus lies at the level of the exiting abducens nerve roots, anterior to the central tegmental tract. It is not known whether the human trapezoid nuclei function in the auditory relay. Some trapezoid axons may enter the medial longitudinal fasciculus, and ascend to end in trigeminal, facial, oculomotor, trochlear and abducens nuclei, where they mediate reflexes involving tensor tympani, stapedius and oculogyric muscles, respectively.

The nucleus of the lateral lemniscus consists of small groups of neurones that lie among the fibres of the lateral lemniscus. Dorsal, ventral and intermediate groups probably receive afferent axons from both cochlear nuclei. Their efferents enter the midbrain along the lateral lemniscus and terminate in the inferior colliculi (**Fig. 19.4**). Total neuronal counts of 18,000 to 24,000 have been recorded in human lemniscal nuclei.

Efferent cochlear axons travel in the cochlear nerves to the spiral organ. Though few in number, they may be involved in hearing, perhaps by modulating sensory transduction through reflexes via cochlear nuclei. The neurones of origin are located at the hilus and along the lateral border of the lateral superior olivary nucleus and lateral edge of the ventral trapezoid nucleus. Fibres from both sides proceed to both cochleae.

Vestibular nuclei

The vestibular nuclear complex contains medial, lateral, inferior and superior nuclei. The medial vestibular nucleus is the largest subdivision, and extends up from the medulla oblongata into the pons. It lies under the vestibular area of the floor of the fourth ventricle, and is crossed dorsally by the striae medullares. The inferior vestibular nucleus is lateral to the medial nucleus, and extends to a lower medullary level. It lies between the medial nucleus and the inferior cerebellar peduncle. Descending branches of afferent vestibular fibres end among its cells. The lateral nucleus is ventrolateral to the upper part of the medial nucleus and is characterized by its large neurones. Its rostral end is continuous with the caudal end of the superior nucleus, which extends higher into the pons than other subdivisions, and occupies the upper part of the vestibular area.

All vestibular nuclei receive fibres from the vestibulocochlear nerve and also from the spinal cord and the reticular formation. Vestibulo-cerebellar fibres from the nuclei travel via the inferior cerebellar peduncle mainly to the flocculus and nodule. Some afferent fibres bypass the nuclei and reach the flocculus and nodule directly via the inferior cerebellar peduncle. Cerebellovestibular fibres pass to the nuclei in the inferior cerebellar peduncle. They arise mainly in the flocculus and nodule (posterior lobe), but some fibres are derived from the anterior lobe and fastigial nucleus.

In summary, the vestibular nuclear complex is a relay station on an afferent cerebellar path, and a distributing station for vestibulocerebellar fibres. Fibres from vestibular nuclei also enter the medial longitudinal fasciculus (**Fig. 19.21**), and ascend or descend to motor nuclei of the oculogyric and nuchal muscles. It is suggested that excitatory and inhibitory projections exist, mediating complex and subtle integration between vestibular signals and eye movements. From the vestibular nuclei, and from the lateral nucleus in particular, fibres descend in the ventral funiculus of the spinal cord as the vestibulospinal tracts. Information from the vestibular nuclei also reaches the cerebral cortex by way of the thalamus (probably via posterior parts of the ventroposterior complex and the medial pulvinar). The primary vestibular cortical area is located in the parietal lobe at the junction between the intraparietal and the postcentral sulci, which is adjacent to that portion of the postcentral gyrus where the head is represented. This makes sense functionally because this region of the somatosensory cortex is concerned with conscious appreciation of body position. There may be an additional representation of the vestibular system in the superior temporal gyrus near the auditory cortex. Through its connections, the vestibular system influences movements of the eyes and head, and of the muscles of the trunk and limbs, in order to maintain equilibrium.

Abducens nucleus

The abducens nucleus occupies a paramedian position in the central grey matter, in line with the trochlear, oculomotor and hypoglossal nuclei, with which it forms a somatic motor column (**Fig. 19.1**). It lies ventromedial to the medial longitudinal fasciculus, which is the means by which vestibular, cochlear and other cranial nerve nuclei, especially the oculomotor, connect with the abducens. The abducens nucleus contains large motor neurones and small multipolar interneurones, which are intermixed, although the latter are most heavily concentrated in its lateral and ventral aspects. Axons from the motor neurones cross the midline at the level of the nucleus and ascend in the medial longitudinal fasciculus to all three medial rectus subnuclei of the oculomotor nucleus. The total number of neurones in the nucleus is c.6500.

Efferent abducens axons pass ventrally, descend through the reticular formation, trapezoid body and medial lemniscus, and traverse the ventral pons to emerge at its inferior border (**Fig. 19.15**).

The abducens nucleus receives afferent connections from cortico-nuclear fibres (which are principally contralateral, some of the fibres being aberrant corticospinal fibres that descend from the midbrain to this level in the medial lemniscus); the medial longitudinal fasciculus (by which it is connected to oculomotor, trochlear and vestibular nuclei); the tectobulbar tract (from the deep layers of the superior colliculus); the paramedian pontine reticular formation (which lies rostral and caudal to the nucleus); the nucleus prepositus hypoglossi; and the contralateral medullary reticular formation.

Facial nucleus

The facial (motor) nucleus lies in the caudal pontine reticular formation, posterior to the dorsal trapezoid nucleus and ventromedial to the trigeminal spinal tract and nucleus. Groups of facial neurones form columns, which innervate individual muscles or which correspond to branches of the facial nerve. Neurones innervating muscles in the scalp and upper face are dorsal, and those supplying the lower facial musculature are ventral.

Efferent fibres of the large motor neurones of the facial nucleus form the motor root of the facial nerve. The motor nucleus represents the branchial efferent column, but it lies much more deeply in the pons than might be expected, and its axons have a most unusual course (**Fig. 19.15**). At first they incline dorsomedially towards the fourth ventricle, below the abducens nucleus, and ascend medial to it, near the medial longitudinal fasciculus. They then curve round the upper pole of the abducens nucleus and descend ventrolaterally through the reticular formation. Finally, they pass between their own nucleus medially and the spinal trigeminal nucleus. They emerge between the olive and the inferior cerebellar peduncle at the cerebellopontine angle (**Fig. 19.3**).

The facial nucleus receives corticobulbar fibres for volitional control. Neurones that innervate muscles in the scalp and upper face are believed to receive bilateral corticobulbar fibres, while those supplying lower facial musculature only receive a contralateral innervation. Clinically, upper and lower motor neurone lesions of the facial nerve can be differentiated because the former results in paralysis that is confined to the contralateral lower face, and the latter in a complete ipsilateral paralysis (Bell's palsy).

The facial nucleus also receives ipsilateral rubroreticular tract fibres and afferents from its own sensory root (via the nucleus solitarius) and from the spinal trigeminal nucleus. These infracortical afferents complete local reflex loops.

Some efferent fibres of the facial nerve originate from neurones in the superior salivatory nucleus, which is said to be in the reticular formation dorsolateral to the caudal end of the motor nucleus. These preganglionic parasympathetic neurones belong to the general visceral efferent column. They send fibres into the sensory root of the facial nerve. These travel via the chorda tympani to the submandibular ganglion and via the greater petrosal nerve and the nerve of the pterygoid canal to the pterygopalatine ganglion.

Corneal reflex – Touching the cornea or shining a bright light into the eye elicits reflex closure of the eye. The former action stimulates nasociliary branches of the ophthalmic nerve, and the latter stimulates the retina and optic pathway. In both cases, afferent impulses enter the central nervous system and spread via interneurones to activate neurones in the facial motor nucleus in the pons (**Fig. 19.16**). The efferent impulses pass along the facial nerve to activate the palpebral component of orbicularis oculi, which contracts, producing a 'blink'. The sweep of the eyelids will carry lacrimal secretions across the eye, and this helps to remove any irritating particles (p. 681).

Trigeminal sensory nucleus

On entering the pons, the fibres of the sensory root of the trigeminal nerve run dorsomedially towards the principal sensory nucleus (**Fig. 19.10**). About 50% of the fibres divide into ascending and descending branches, the others ascend or descend without division. The descending fibres form the spinal tract of the trigeminal, which terminates in the subjacent spinal nucleus of the trigeminal nerve. The spinal nucleus is described in detail on page 334.

Some ascending trigeminal fibres, many of them heavily myelinated, synapse around the small neurones in the principal sensory nucleus (**Fig. 19.17**), which lies lateral to the motor nucleus and medial to the middle cerebellar peduncle, and is continuous inferiorly with the spinal nucleus. The principal nucleus is considered to be mainly concerned with tactile stimuli.

Other ascending fibres enter the mesencephalic nucleus, a column of unipolar cells whose peripheral branches may convey proprioceptive impulses from the masticatory muscles, and possibly also from the teeth and the facial and oculogyric muscles. Its neurones are unique in being the only primary sensory neurones with somata in the CNS. It is the relay for the 'jaw-jerk', which is the only supraspinal monosynaptic reflex. Nerve fibres that ascend to the mesencephalic nucleus may give collaterals to the motor nucleus of the trigeminal nerve and to the cerebellum.

Jaw-jerk reflex – Rapid stretching of the muscles that close the jaw (masseter, temporalis, medial pterygoid) activates muscle spindle afferents, which travel via the mandibular division of the trigeminal nerve to the brain stem (**Fig. 19.18**). The cell bodies of these primary afferent neurones are located in the mesencephalic nucleus of the trigeminal. Collaterals project monosynaptically to the motor nucleus of the trigeminal nerve in the pons. From here motor axons of the mandibular nerve innervate the muscles that close the jaw.

Most fibres that arise in the trigeminal sensory nuclei cross the midline and ascend in the trigeminal lemniscus. They end in the contralateral thalamic nucleus ventralis posterior medialis, from which third-order neurones project to the cortical postcentral gyrus (areas 1, 2 and 3). Some trigeminal nucleus efferents ascend to the nucleus ventralis posterior medialis of the ipsilateral thalamus.

Trigeminal motor nucleus

The trigeminal motor nucleus is ovoid in outline and lies in the upper pontine tegmentum, under the lateral part of the floor of the fourth ventricle (**Fig. 19.1**). It lies medial to the principal sensory nucleus, and

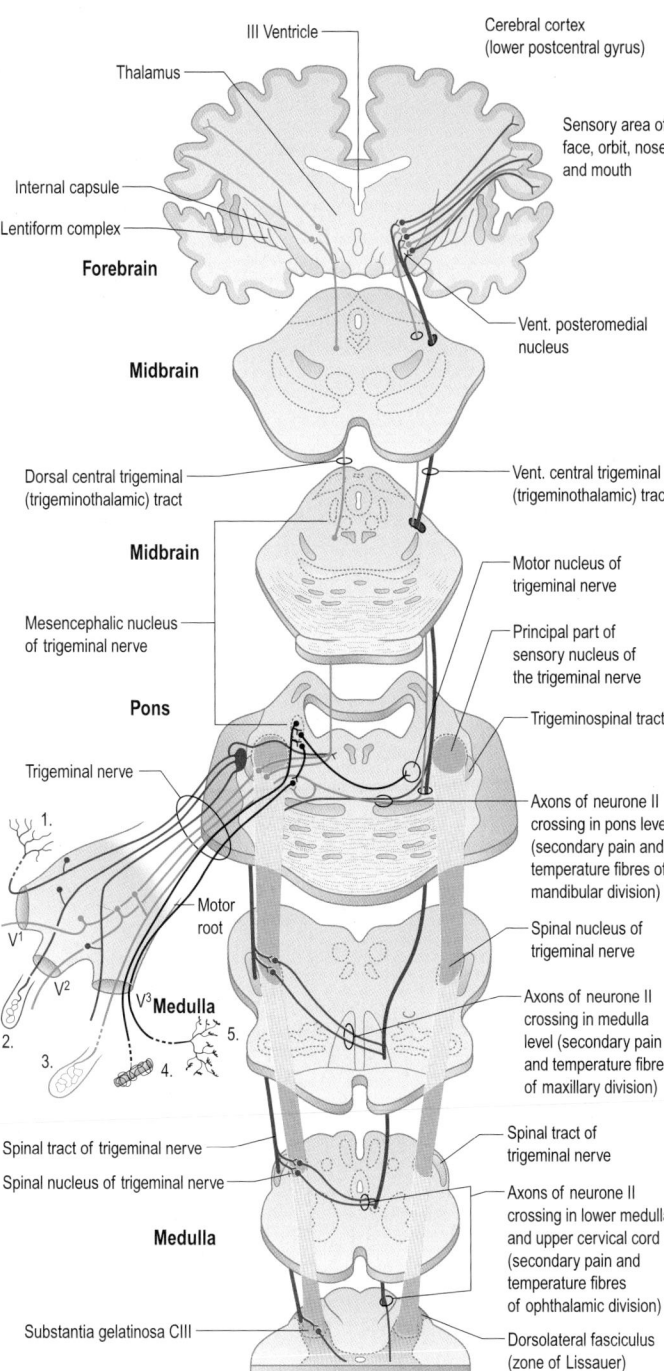

Fig. 19.17 The trigeminal nerve and its central connections.

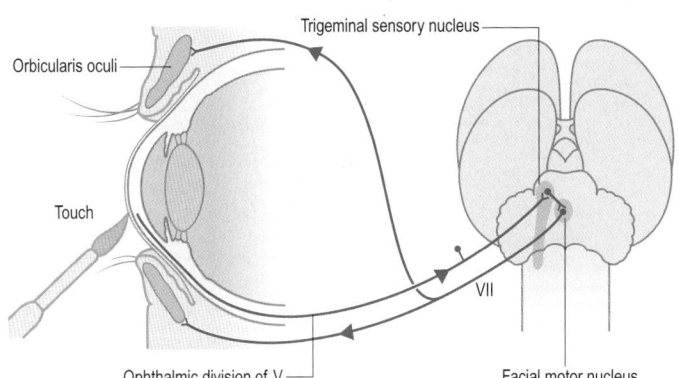

Fig. 19.16 Corneal reflex. (Redrawn from Oxford Textbook of Functional Anatomy, Vol 3 Head and Neck, MacKinnon P, Morris J (eds), 1990. By permission of Oxford University Press.)

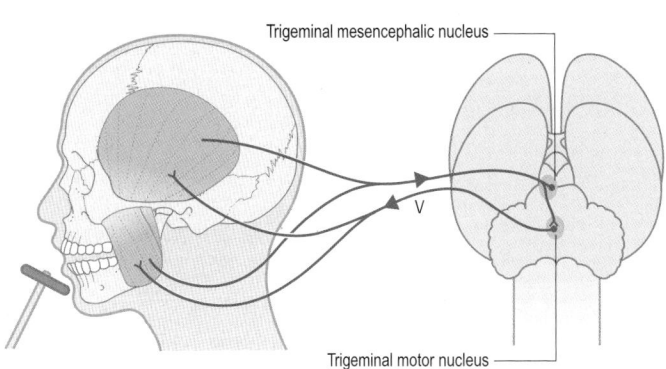

Fig. 19.18 Jaw jerk reflex. (Redrawn from Oxford Textbook of Functional Anatomy, Vol 3 Head and Neck, MacKinnon P, Morris J (eds), 1990. By permission of Oxford University Press.)

is separated from it by fibres of the trigeminal nerve. It occupies the position of the branchial (special visceral) efferent column.

The motor nucleus contains characteristic large multipolar neurones interspersed with smaller multipolar cells. The neurones are organized into a number of relatively discrete subnuclei, the axons from which innervate individual muscles. It receives fibres from both corticobulbar tracts. These fibres leave the tracts at the nuclear level or higher in the pons (aberrant corticospinal fibres), and descend in the medial lemniscus. They may end on motor neurones or interneurones. The motor nucleus receives afferents from the sensory nuclei of the trigeminal nerve, possibly including some from the mesencephalic nucleus, which form monosynaptic reflex arcs for proprioceptive control of the masticatory muscles. It also receives afferents from the reticular formation, red nucleus and tectum, the medial longitudinal fasciculus and possibly from the locus coeruleus. Collectively these represent pathways by which salivary secretion and mastication may be coordinated.

Tensor tympani and stapedius reflex – Loud sound elicits reflex contraction of tensor tympani and stapedius, which attenuates movement of the tympanic membrane and middle ear ossicles. Afferent impulses travel in the cochlear nerve to the cochlear nuclei in the brain stem. Efferent fibres to tensor tympani arise in the trigeminal motor nucleus and travel in the mandibular division of the trigeminal nerve. Efferent fibres to stapedius originate in the facial nucleus and travel in the facial nerve.

Salivary nucleus

The salivary (salivatory) nucleus is near the upper pole of the vagal nucleus, just above the pontomedullary junction and near the inferior pole of the facial nucleus. It is customarily divided into superior and inferior salivary nuclei, which send preganglionic parasympathetic fibres into the facial and glossopharyngeal nerves for the control of the salivary and lacrimal glands.

MIDBRAIN

EXTERNAL FEATURES AND RELATIONS

The midbrain traverses the hiatus in the tentorium cerebelli, and connects the pons and cerebellum with the forebrain. It is the shortest brain stem segment, not more than 2 cm in length, and most of it lies in the posterior cranial fossa. Lateral to it are the parahippocampal gyri, which hide its sides when the inferior surface of the brain is examined. Its long axis inclines ventrally as it ascends. For descriptive purposes, it may be divided into a dorsal tectum and right and left cerebral peduncles, each of which is further divided into a ventral crus cerebri and a dorsal tegmentum by a pigmented lamina, the substantia nigra. The two crura are separate, whereas the tegmental parts are united and traversed by the cerebral aqueduct that connects the third and fourth ventricles. The tectum lies dorsal to an oblique coronal plane which includes the aqueduct, and consists of the pretectal area and the corpora quadrigemina (the paired superior and inferior colliculi).

The crura cerebri are superficially corrugated and emerge from the cerebral hemispheres. They converge as they descend and meet as they enter the pons, where they form the caudolateral boundaries of the interpeduncular fossa (**Figs 19.19, 19.20**). At the level of the tentorial incisure, the basilar artery divides in the interpeduncular fossa into the right and left posterior cerebral arteries. The superior cerebellar arteries branch from the basilar artery immediately distal to this bifurcation. The posterior cerebral and superior cerebellar arteries both run laterally around the ventral (basilar) crural surfaces. The former passes above the tentorium cerebelli, the latter below. The oculomotor and trochlear nerves lie between the two arteries. The roots of the oculomotor nerve emerge from a medial sulcus on each crus (**Figs 19.3, 19.19, 19.20**). The posterior communicating artery joins the posterior cerebral artery on the medial surface of the peduncle in the interpeduncular fossa. The median caudal part of the interpeduncular fossa is a greyish area, the posterior perforated substance, which is pierced by central branches of the posterior cerebral arteries. The optic tract winds dorsolaterally around the crus near the crural entry into the hemispheres. Its lateral

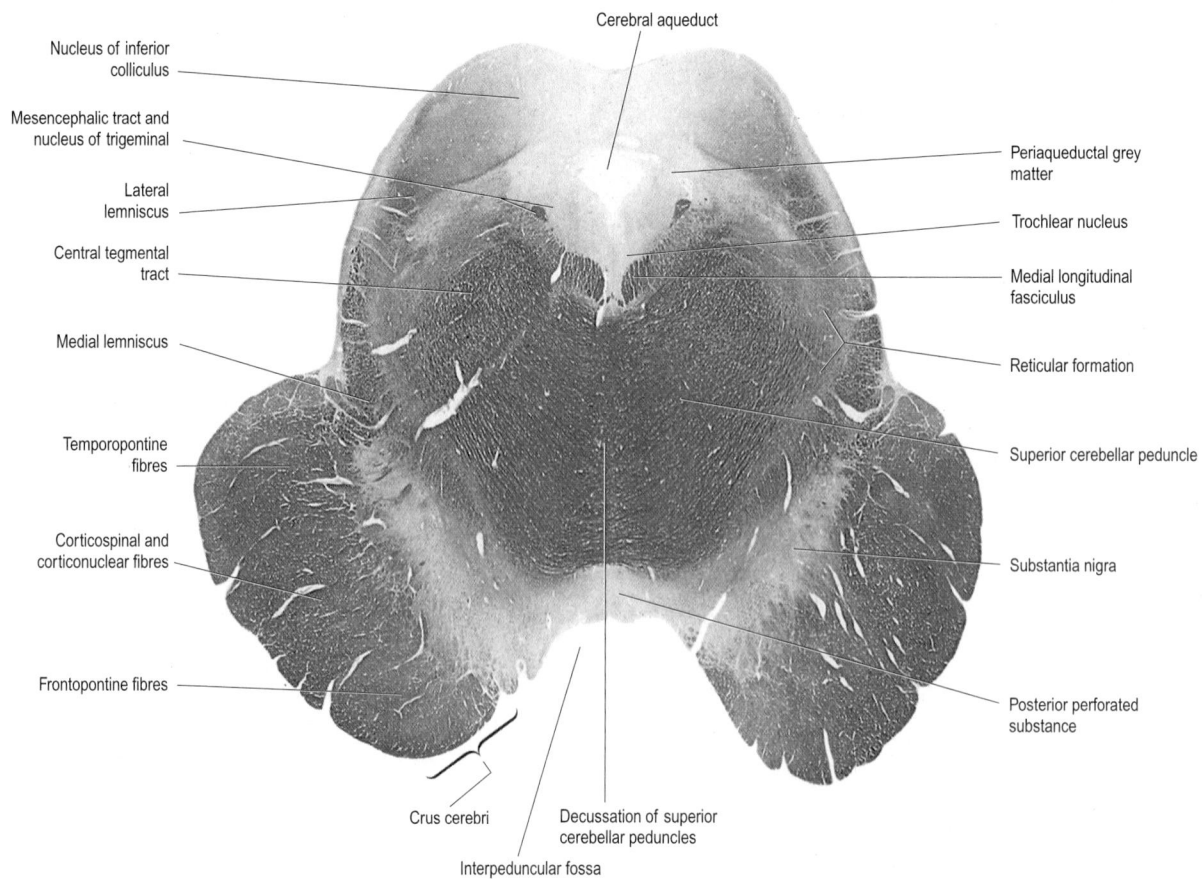

Fig. 19.19 Transverse section of the midbrain at the level of the inferior colliculi.

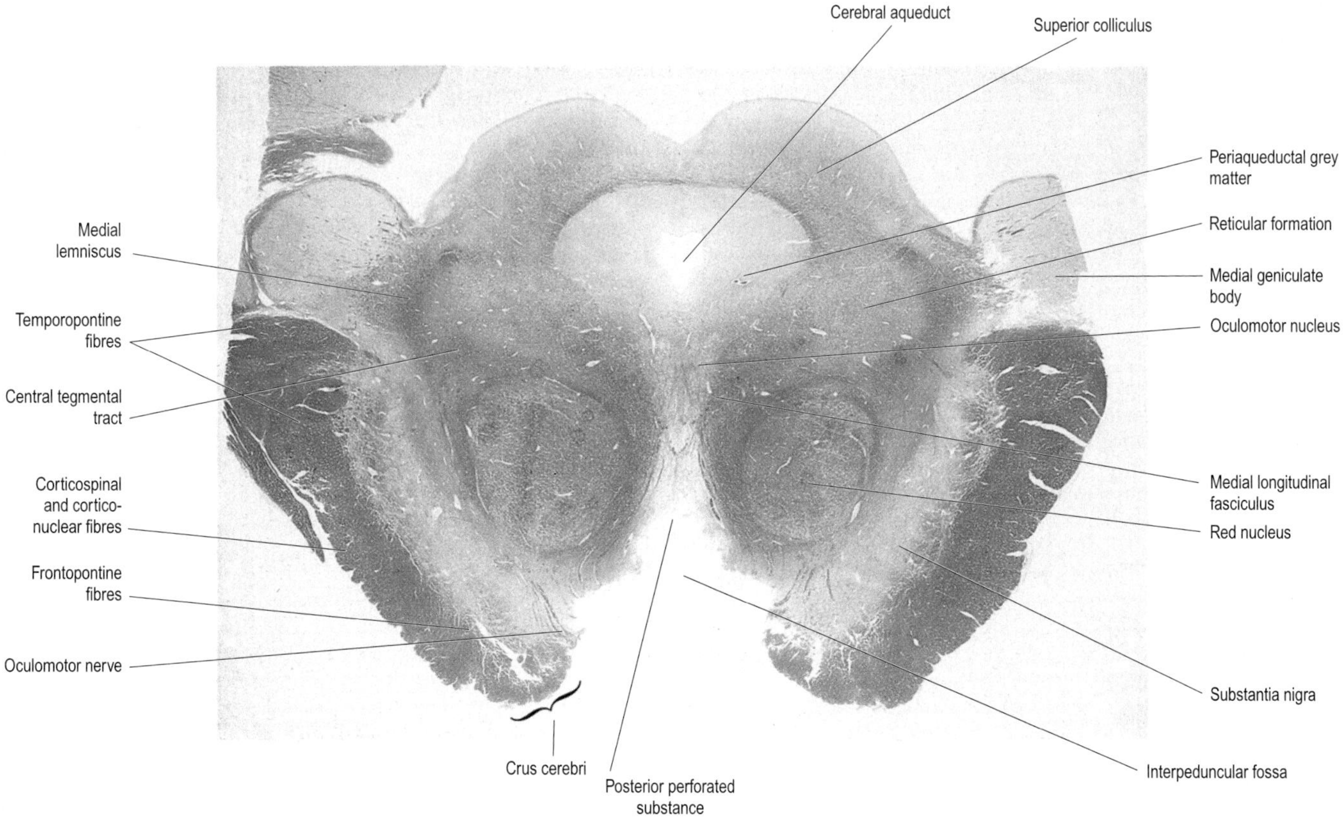

Fig. 19.20 Transverse section of the midbrain at the level of the superior colliculi.

Labels on figure: Cerebral aqueduct · Superior colliculus · Periaqueductal grey matter · Reticular formation · Medial geniculate body · Oculomotor nucleus · Medial longitudinal fasciculus · Red nucleus · Substantia nigra · Interpeduncular fossa · Medial lemniscus · Temporopontine fibres · Central tegmental tract · Corticospinal and cortico-nuclear fibres · Frontopontine fibres · Oculomotor nerve · Crus cerebri · Posterior perforated substance

surface adjoins the parahippocampal gyrus and is crossed by the trochlear nerve (**Figs 16.10, 19.4**). It bears a longitudinal lateral sulcus in which fibres of the lateral lemniscus reach and form a surface elevation. The latter inclines rostrodorsally, and part joins the inferior colliculus, while the rest continues into the inferior quadrigeminal brachium.

The colliculi or corpora quadrigemina are two paired eminences (**Figs 16.10, 19.4**). They lie rostral to the superior medullary velum, inferior to the pineal gland and caudal to the posterior commissure, the whole sloping ventrally as it ascends. Below the splenium of the corpus callosum they are partly overlapped on each side by the pulvinar of the dorsal thalamus. The superior and inferior colliculi are separated by a cruciform sulcus. The upper limit of the sulcus expands into a depression for the pineal gland, and a median frenulum veli is prolonged from its caudal end down over the superior medullary velum. The trochlear nerves emerge lateral to the frenulum. They pass ventrally over the lateral aspects of the cerebral peduncles and traverse the interpeduncular cistern to the petrosal end of the cavernous sinus. The superior colliculi, larger and darker than the inferior, are stations for visual responses. The inferior colliculi, smaller but more prominent, are associated with auditory paths. The difference in colour is attributed to the presence of superficial layers of neurones in the superior colliculi.

A brachium ascends ventrolaterally from the lateral aspect of each colliculus (**Figs 16.10, 19.4**). The brachium of the superior colliculus (superior quadrigeminal brachium) passes below the pulvinar, partly overlapping the medial geniculate body, and continues partly into the lateral geniculate body and partly into the optic tract. It conveys fibres from the retina and optic radiation to the superior colliculus. The brachium of the inferior colliculus (inferior quadrigeminal brachium) ascends ventrally. It conveys fibres from the lateral lemniscus and inferior colliculus to the medial geniculate body.

INTERNAL STRUCTURE

Transverse sections of the midbrain

In transverse section, the cerebral peduncles are seen to be composed of dorsal and ventral regions separated by the substantia nigra (**Figs 19.19, 19.20**). On each side, the dorsal region is the tegmentum and the ventral part is the crus cerebri. The tegmenti are continuous across the midline but the crura are separated.

Crus cerebri

Each crus cerebri is semilunar in section. It contains corticospinal, corticonuclear and corticopontine fibres. Corticonuclear and cortico-spinal fibres occupy the middle two-thirds of the crura, and descend via the pons and medulla. Corticonuclear fibres end in the nuclei of the cranial nerves and other brain stem nuclei, while corticospinal fibres continue into the medullary pyramid (**Fig. 18.21**). Corticopontine fibres arise in the cerebral cortex and form two groups, both of which end in the pontine nuclei. The frontopontine fibres from the frontal lobe, principally areas 6 and 4, traverse the internal capsule and then occupy the medial sixth of the ipsilateral crus cerebri. The temporopontine fibres, which are largely from the posterior region of the temporal lobe, traverse the internal capsule but occupy the lateral sixth of the ipsilateral crus. Parietopontine and occipitopontine fibres are also described in the crus, lying medial to the temporopontine fibres. There are few fibres from the primary sensory cortex in corticopontine projections.

Mesencephalic tegmentum

The mesencephalic tegmentum is directly continuous with the pontine tegmentum and contains the same tracts. At inferior collicular levels, grey matter is restricted to scattered collections of neurones in the reticular formation and the tectum near the cerebral aqueduct. The trochlear nucleus is in the ventral grey matter near the midline, in a position corresponding to the abducens and hypoglossal nuclei at other levels. It extends through the lower half of the midbrain, just caudal to the oculomotor nucleus and immediately dorsal to the medial longitudinal fasciculus.

The trigeminal mesencephalic nucleus occupies a lateral position in the central grey matter. It ascends from the upper pole of the main trigeminal sensory nucleus in the pons to the level of the superior colliculus in the midbrain, and is accompanied by a tract of both peripheral and central branches from its axons. Its large ovoid neurones are unipolar, like those in peripheral sensory ganglia. They are arranged in many small groups, which extend as curved laminae on the lateral margins of the periaqueductal grey matter. Neurones are most numerous in its lower level.

Apart from these nuclei, the mesencephalic tegmentum contains many other scattered neurones, most of which are included in the reticular formation.

The white matter contains all the tracts mentioned in the pontine tegmentum. The decussation of the superior cerebellar peduncles is particularly prominent. Fibres enter the tegmentum and pass ventromedially round the central grey matter to the median raphe, where most cross in the decussation of the superior cerebellar penduncles, and then separate into ascending and descending fascicles. Some ascending fibres either end in, or give collaterals to, the red nucleus, which they encapsulate and penetrate. Many other fibres ascend to the nucleus ventralis lateralis of the thalamus. Some uncrossed fibres are believed to end in the periaqueductal grey matter and reticular formation, interstitial nucleus and posterior commissural nucleus (the nucleus of Darkschewitsch). The latter nucleus may send efferent fibres to the medial longitudinal fasciculus and posterior commissure. Descending fascicles end in the pontine and medullary reticular formation, the olivary complex and, possibly, cranial motor nuclei.

The medial longitudinal fasciculus adjoins the somatic efferent column, dorsal to the decussating superior cerebellar peduncles (**Fig. 19.21**). The medial, trigeminal, lateral and spinal lemnisci form a curved band dorsolateral to the substantia nigra. Fibres in the medial, spinal and trigeminal lemnisci continue a rostral course to synapse with neurones in the lateral and medial ventral posterior nuclei of the thalamus, respectively (**Figs 18.15, 19.17**). Some fibres of the lateral lemniscus end in the nucleus of the inferior colliculus, encapsulating it and synapsing with its neurones. The remaining fibres (direct lemniscal) join inferior colliculus-derived fibres and enter the inferior quadrigeminal brachium, which starts at this level, and which carries them to the medial geniculate body. Some fibres to the inferior colliculus are collaterals of direct lemniscal fibres.

Superiorly, level with the superior colliculus, the tegmentum contains the red nucleus, which extends into the subthalamic region. The ventromedial central grey matter around the aqueduct contains the oculomotor nucleus, which is elongated, related ventrolaterally to the medial longitudinal fasciculus, and caudally reaches the trochlear nucleus. The oculomotor nucleus is divisible into neuronal groups which are partially correlated with the motor distribution of the oculomotor nerve. A group of preganglionic parasympathetic neurones, the accessory oculomotor (Edinger–Westphal) nucleus, which controls the activity of smooth muscle within the eyeball (p. 435), lies dorsal to the oculomotor nucleus.

Substantia nigra

The substantia nigra is a lamina of many multipolar neurones that extends through the whole midbrain, from the medial to the lateral crural sulcus, and from the pons to the subthalamic region. It is connected massively with the basal ganglia, but has other projections.

The substantia nigra is semilunar in transverse section, concave dorsally and thicker medially, where it is traversed by oculomotor axons as they stream ventrally to their point of exit in the interpeduncular fossa. Extensions from its convex ventral surface pass between fibres of the crus cerebri. The substantia nigra is subdivided into a dorsal pars compacta and a ventral pars reticulata (reticularis), and the cells of these two parts have different connections. The pars compacta consists of many darkly pigmented neurones, which contain neuromelanin granules. Their arrangement is irregular and they partially penetrate the subjacent pars reticulata. The pigmentation is easily visible in transverse or coronal sections, and is related to the aminergic status of the neurones (**Figs 19.19, 19.20**). Pigmentation increases with age, is most abundant in primates, maximal in man, and present even in albinos. The pigmented pars compacta neurones synthesize dopamine as their neurotransmitter and project to the corpus striatum of the basal ganglia and other sides.

The pars compacta of the substantia nigra corresponds to the dopaminergic cell group A9 (**Fig. 23.10**). Two other dopaminergic cell groups are found in the ventral tegmentum: cell group A10 in the rostromedial region, which constitutes the ventral tegmental area (of Tsai); and cell group A8 in the dorsolateral reticular area, which forms the nucleus parabrachialis pigmentosus. The whole ventral tegmental system of dopaminergic neurones appears to act as an integrative centre for adaptive behaviour. It projects via a number of pathways, mainly through ipsilateral fibres in the medial forebrain bundle. These pathways are: a mesodiencephalic system, which terminates in thalamic and hypothalamic nuclei; a mesostriatal projection; a mesolimbic (mesorhombic) pathway to the nucleus accumbens, olfactory tubercle, lateral septum, interstitial nucleus of the stria terminalis, amygdala and entorhinal cortex; and mesocortical fibres to most cortical areas, particularly the prefrontal, orbitofrontal and cingulate cortex.

The pars compacta projects heavily to the caudate nucleus and putamen in a topographically organized fashion (nigrostriatal fibres). Lesser projections end in the globus pallidus and subthalamic nucleus. In Parkinson's disease, the levels of dopamine in the substantia nigra and striatum decrease dramatically as a result of the degeneration of pars compacta neurones (p. 428).

The ventral pars reticulata of the substantia nigra contains clusters of neurones, most of which are GABAergic, that intermingle with fibres of the crus cerebri. The pars reticulata extends rostrally as far as the subthalamic region, and is considered to be homologous with the medial segment of the globus pallidus, which it resembles structurally. The neurones in both contain high levels of iron.

There are reciprocal connections between the substantia nigra and the basal ganglia. Efferent fibres from the basal ganglia end largely, but by no means exclusively, in the pars reticulata. Topographically organized striatonigral fibres originate from the caudate nucleus and putamen and project to the pars reticulata. The head of the caudate nucleus projects to the rostral third of the substantia nigra, while the putamen projects to all parts. The fibres end in axodendritic synapses. A small number of GABAergic pallidonigral fibres from the lateral segment of the globus pallidus end mostly in the pars reticulata. The subthalamic nucleus sends an important glutamatergic projection to the pars reticulata and to the globus pallidus. Subthalamonigral and subthalamopallidal projections are important in the pathophysiology of movement disorders such as Parkinson's disease and dyskinesias (p. 428).

GABAergic neurones in the pars reticulata project through a nigrothalamic tract to the ventral anterior and dorsomedial thalamic nuclei, and a nigrotegmental tract to the pedunculopontine nucleus and reticular formation, whence impulses are relayed to spinal ventral column neurones. A pars lateralis of the substantia nigra is recognizable, but small, in man. It projects to the ipsilateral superior colliculus, which may control saccadic eye movements.

Corticonigral fibres arise from precentral and probably postcentral gyri. A few terminate on neurones in the pars reticulata, while many more are fibres of passage to the red nucleus and reticular formation.

Red nucleus

The red nucleus is an ovoid mass c.5 mm in diameter, with a pink tinge, dorsomedial to the substantia nigra (**Fig. 19.20**). The tint appears only in fresh material and is caused by a ferric iron pigment in its multipolar neurones. The latter are of varying size. Their proportions and arrangements vary between species, e.g. in primates the magnocellular element is decreased, and there is a reciprocal increase in the size of the parvocellular component. Small multipolar neurones occur in all parts of the nucleus. In man, the larger neurones are restricted to the caudal part of the nucleus and have been estimated to be as few as 200 in number. The magnocellular element is considered phylogenetically old, which accords with the parvocellular predominance in primates. Rostrally, the red nucleus is poorly demarcated, and it blends into the reticular formation and caudal pole of the interstitial nucleus. It is traversed and surrounded by fascicles of nerve fibres, including many from the oculomotor nucleus.

Principal afferent connections of the red nucleus travel via corticorubral and cerebellorubral fibres. Uncrossed corticorubral fibres originate from primary somatomotor and somatosensory areas. In animals, the red nucleus receives fibres from the contralateral nucleus interpositus (which corresponds to the human globose and emboliform nuclei), and dentate nucleus, via the superior cerebellar peduncle. It has bilateral, probably reciprocal, connections with the superior colliculi. In man, the rubrospinal tract is small and originates from the caudal magnocellular part of the red nucleus. Few fibres reach the cervical cord. The fibres decussate and then run obliquely laterally in the ventral tegmental decussation, ventral to the tectospinal decussation, and dorsal to the medial lemniscus. On reaching the grey matter ventral to the inferior cerebellar peduncle, the tract turns caudally to enter the lateral part of the lateral lemniscus. It continues descending ventral to the tract and nucleus of the trigeminal nerve throughout the medulla, and enters the upper part of the cervical cord intermingled with fibres of the lateral corticospinal tract (p. 322). Some efferent axons form a rubrobulbar tract to motor nuclei of the trigeminal, facial, oculomotor, trochlear and abducens nerves.

The largest group of efferents from the red nucleus in man is found in the massive uncrossed central tegmental tract (fasciculus), which lies in the ventral part of the midbrain. Initially it lies lateral to the medial longitudinal fasciculus and dorsolateral to both the red nucleus and the decussation of the superior cerebellar peduncles (Figs 19.10, 19.11, 19.12, 19.19). Most fibres arise from the parvocellular part of the red nucleus and join the tract as it traverses the nucleus on its way to the ipsilateral inferior olivary nucleus in the medulla. Some tract fibres terminate in the brain stem reticular nuclei. Ascending and descending axons from the brain stem reticular formation run in the central tegmental tract. Their collaterals and terminals innervate other 'reticular' or adjacent 'specific' nuclei. These axons include dorsal and ventral ascending noradrenergic bundles, a ventral ascending serotoninergic bundle, and some fibres of dorsal and ventral ascending cholinergic bundles.

Lesions of the corticospinal system in man result in permanent paresis. In monkeys, although initially complete, the paralysis disappears and good recovery ensues. The explanation for this interprimate variability in recovery of corticospinal lesions could lie in the differential capacity of the rubrospinal system to compensate for loss of corticospinal drive. Monkeys never fully recover from combined lesions of both the corticospinal and rubrospinal tracts, which suggests that the two systems are functionally interrelated in the control of movement. Both systems encode force, velocity and direction parameters, but the rubrospinal system primarily directs activity both during the terminal phase of a movement and preceding a movement. There is thus overlap of activity in the two systems for all parameters during movements of limbs and even of individual digits. The corticospinal system is most active during the learning of new movements, whereas the rubrospinal system is most active during the execution of learnt automated movements.

The rubro-olivary projection, which travels in the central tegmental tract, connects the red nucleus directly to the contralateral cerebellar cortex and indirectly to the ipsilateral motor cortex, which is where both the corticospinal and central tegmental tracts originate. The cerebellum is thought to play a role in motor learning, and so the rubro-olivary system could switch the control of movements from the corticospinal to the rubrospinal system for programmed automation. The relative absence of a rubrospinal system in man could explain the poor recovery of motor function after stroke.

Oculomotor nucleus

The nuclear complex from which the efferent fibres of the oculomotor nerve arise consists of several groups of large motor neurones and smaller preganglionic parasympathetic neurones. On each side, the large-celled motor neurone groups innervate, in dorsoventral order, the ipsilateral inferior rectus, inferior oblique and medial rectus. There is also a medially placed column, almost in the long axis of the midbrain, which innervates the contralateral superior rectus. The axons from this nucleus decussate in its caudal part. The medial rectus subnucleus consists of three anatomically distinct subpopulations. The ventral portion, which contains the largest number of motor neurones, occupies the rostral two-thirds. A subpopulation of smaller diameter motor neurones lies dorsally throughout the rostral two-thirds of the nucleus and innervates the small orbital fibres of the medial rectus. They are thought to be involved in vergence movements. Another subpopulation lies dorsolaterally in the caudal two-thirds of the nucleus.

A median nucleus of large neurones, the caudal central nucleus, lies at the caudal pole of the oculomotor nucleus adjacent to the superior rectus and medial rectus subnuclei. In experimental primates, c.30% of the motor neurones in this subnucleus innervate levator palpebrae superioris bilaterally, which is a unique condition among all paired skeletal muscles.

The Edinger–Westphal nucleus lies dorsal to the main oculomotor nucleus. It is composed of small, multipolar, preganglionic parasympathetic neurones, which give rise to axons that travel in the oculomotor nerve and relay in the ciliary ganglion.

Separate fascicles from these subnuclei course forward in the midbrain and emerge on the surface of the brain stem in the interpeduncular fossa. The fascicles are most probably arranged from medial to lateral subserving the pupil, inferior rectus, medial rectus, levator palpebrae superioris and superior rectus, and inferior oblique. The human oculomotor nerve contains c.15,000 axons.

Afferent inputs to the oculomotor nuclear complex include fibres from the rostral interstitial nucleus of the medial longitudinal fasciculus and the interstitial nucleus of Cajal (INC), both of which are involved in the control of vertical and torsional gaze; the nuclei of the posterior commissure, both directly and via the INC, and, via these nuclei, from the frontal eye fields, the superior colliculus, the dentate nucleus and other cortical areas; the medial longitudinal fasciculus (including fibres from the trochlear, abducens and vestibular nuclei); the medial and lateral vestibular nuclei to the medial rectus subnucleus; the superior colliculus; and the nucleus prepositus hypoglossi, primarily to the medial rectus subnucleus.

Afferent inputs to the Edinger–Westphal nucleus come from the pretectal nuclei (primarily the pretectal olivary nucleus) bilaterally, and mediate the pupillary light reflex. Afferents also come from the visual cortex, mediating accommodation. Efferent fibres relay through the ciliary ganglion in the orbit.

The oculomotor nucleus also contains neurones connected with other nuclei concerned with ocular motor function. In particular, reciprocal connections exist between the oculomotor and abducens nuclei, both ipsilateral and contralateral. These internuclear connections are predictable on the basis of the results of experimental stimulation of, or damage to, the medial longitudinal fasciculus, and from clinicopathological data derived from cases of internuclear ophthalmoplegia.

Trochlear nucleus

The trochlear nucleus lies in the grey matter in the floor of the cerebral aqueduct, level with the upper part of the inferior colliculus (Figs 19.1, 19.19). It is in line with the ventromedial part of the oculomotor nucleus, in the position of the somatic efferent column. The medial longitudinal fasciculus is ventral and lateral to it. The oculomotor and trochlear nuclei often overlap slightly but can be distinguished by the smaller size of the trochlear neurones.

The afferent inputs to the trochlear nucleus are similar to those described for the oculomotor nucleus.

Trochlear efferent fibres pass laterodorsally round the central grey matter, then descend medial to the trigeminal mesencephalic nucleus to reach the upper end of the superior medullary velum, where they decussate and emerge lateral to the frenulum. A few fibres remain ipsilateral.

Medial longitudinal fasciculus

The medial longitudinal fasciculus (Fig. 19.21) is a heavily myelinated composite tract, lying near the midline, ventral to the periaqueductal grey matter. It ascends to the interstitial nucleus (of Cajal), which lies in the lateral wall of the third ventricle, just above the cerebral aqueduct. The fasciculus retains its position relative to the central grey matter through the midbrain, pons and upper medulla, but is displaced ventrally by successive decussations of the medial lemnisci and lateral corticospinal tracts. At spinal levels it is synonymous with the medial vestibulospinal tract.

The medial longitudinal fasciculus interconnects the oculomotor, trochlear, abducens, Edinger–Westphal, vestibular, reticular and spinal accessory nuclei, coordinating conjugate eye movements and associated movements of the head and neck. Lesions cause internuclear ophthalmoplegia. All four vestibular nuclei contribute ascending fibres. Those from the superior nucleus remain uncrossed, while the others are partly crossed. Some fibres reach the interstitial and posterior commissural nuclei, and some decussate to the contralateral nuclei. Descending axons, from the medial vestibular nuclei and perhaps the lateral and inferior nuclei, partially decussate and descend in the fasciculus as the medial vestibulospinal tract (Fig. 18.22). Fibres join from the dorsal trapezoid, lateral lemniscal and posterior commissural nuclei, which means that both the cochlear and vestibular components of the vestibulocochlear nerve may influence movements of the eyes and head via the medial longitudinal fasciculus. Some vestibular fibres may ascend in the medial longitudinal fasciculus as far as the thalamus.

Tectum

Inferior colliculus

The inferior colliculus (Fig. 19.19) has a central, ovoid, main nucleus, which is continuous with the periaqueductal grey matter. It is surrounded

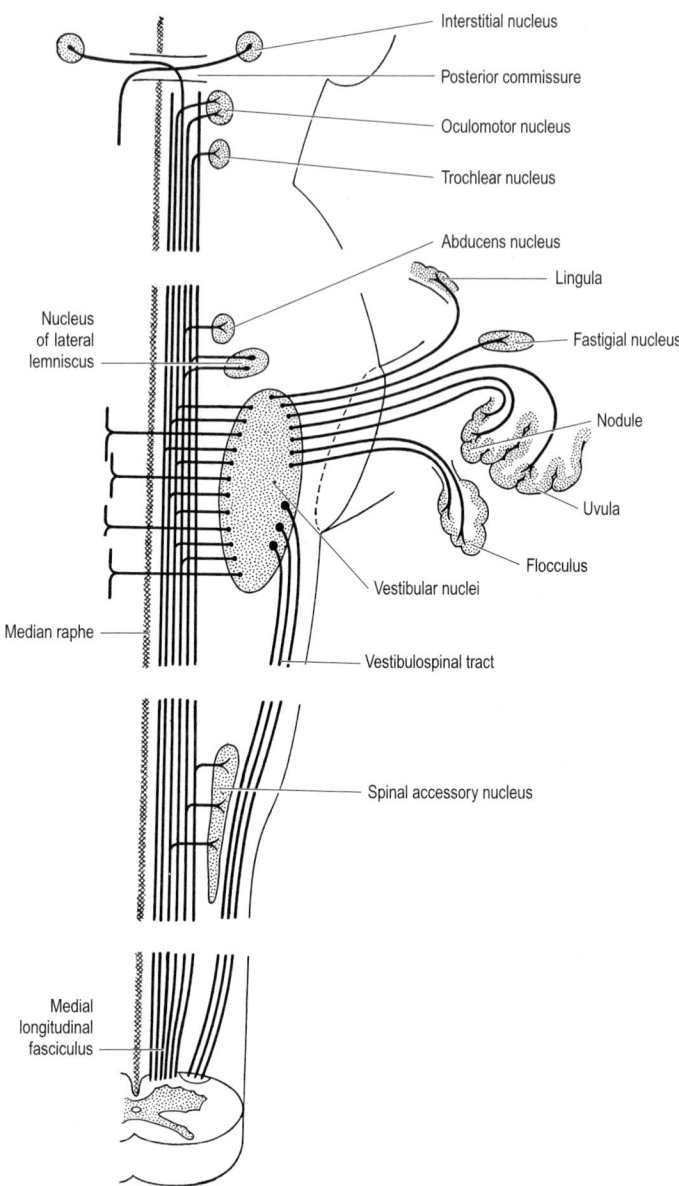

Interstitial nucleus

Posterior commissure

Oculomotor nucleus

Trochlear nucleus

Abducens nucleus

Lingula

Nucleus of lateral lemniscus

Fastigial nucleus

Nodule

Uvula

Flocculus

Vestibular nuclei

Median raphe

Vestibulospinal tract

Spinal accessory nucleus

Medial longitudinal fasciculus

Fig. 19.21 Some of the fibre components of the medial longitudinal fasciculus.

by a lamina of nerve fibres, many from the lateral lemniscus, which terminate in it. The central nucleus has dorsomedial and ventrolateral zones, which are covered by a dorsal cortex. In humans, the cortex has four cytoarchitectonic layers: layer I contains small neurones with flattened radial dendritic fields; layer II, medium-sized neurones with ovoid dendritic fields aligned parallel with the collicular surface; layer III, medium-sized neurones with spherical dendritic fields; and layer IV, large neurones with variably shaped dendritic fields. The central nucleus is laminated. Bands of cells with disc-shaped or stellate dendritic fields orthogonally span the fibre layers in which the terminals of lateral lemniscal fibres ramify. The neurones are sharply tuned to frequency, and the laminae may represent the structural basis of tonal discrimination. Experimental studies have found cells driven by low frequencies in the dorsal laminae, and others driven by high frequencies in the ventral laminae. Neurones are broadly frequency-tuned in the dorsal cortex and lateral nucleus.

Most efferent fibres travel via the inferior brachium to the ipsilateral medial geniculate body. Lemniscal fibres relay only in the central nucleus, and some pass without relay to the medial geniculate body. In man, the ventral division of the medial geniculate body receives a topographic projection from the central nucleus and the dorsal division receives a similar projection from the dorsal cortex. Some colliculogeniculate fibres do not relay in the geniculate body, but continue, with those that do, via the auditory radiation to the auditory cortex area. A

descending projection from the auditory cortex reaches the inferior colliculus via the medial geniculate body. Some fibres may traverse this projection without relay. This descending path may produce effects at levels from the medial geniculate body downwards, and it probably links with efferent cochlear fibres, through the superior olivary and cochlear nuclei.

Inferior collicular projections to the brain stem and spinal cord appear to traverse the superior colliculi before they descend. In this way they connect with the origins of the tectospinal and tectotegmental tracts. These projections are relatively small and probably mediate reflex turning of the head and eyes in response to sounds.

In experimental animals, lesions of either the inferior colliculus or its brachium produce defects in tonal discrimination, sound localization and auditory reflexes. The effects of such lesions are poorly documented in man.

The inferior colliculus is part of the ascending auditory pathway which is described further on page 436.

Superior colliculus

The superior colliculi are laminated structures. At successive depths from the external surface, each superior colliculus may be divided into a stratum zonale, cinereum, opticum and lemnisci. The stratum lemnisci may be subdivided into the stratum griseum medium, album medium, griseum profundum and album profundum. These seven layers have also been termed zonal, superficial grey, optic, intermediate grey, deep grey, deep white and periventricular strata. The two schemes do not completely accord, but, as a generalization, layers may be considered to be composed alternately of neuronal somata or their processes. The zonal layer consists chiefly of myelinated and non-myelinated fibres from the occipital cortex (areas 17, 18 and 19), which arrive as the external corticotectal tract. It also contains a few small neurones, which are horizontally arrayed. The superficial grey layer (stratum cinereum) forms a crescentic lamina over the deeper layers and contains many small multipolar interneurones, on which cortical fibres synapse. The optic layer consists partly of fibres from the optic tract. As they terminate, they permeate the entire anterior–posterior extent of the superficial layers with numerous collateral branches. This arrangement provides a retinotopic map of the contralateral visual field, in which the fovea is represented anterolaterally. Retinal axons terminate in clusters from specific retinotectal neurones and as collaterals of retinogeniculate fibres. The layer also contains some large multipolar neurones. Efferent fibres to the retina are said to start in this layer.

The intermediate grey and white layers collectively constitute the main reception zone. The main afferent input is the medial corticotectal path from layer V neurones of the ipsilateral occipital cortex (area 18), and from other neocortical areas that are concerned with ocular following movements. Afferent fibres are also received from the contralateral spinal cord (via spinotectal and spinothalamic routes), the inferior colliculus, and the locus coeruleus and raphe nuclei (from noradrenergic and serotoninergic neurones). The deep grey and deep white layers adjacent to the periaqueductal grey matter are collectively called the parabigeminal nucleus. They contain neurones whose dendrites extend into the optic layer, and whose axons of which form many of the collicular efferents.

The superior colliculus receives afferents from many sources including the retina, spinal cord, inferior colliculus and occipital and temporal cortices. The first three of these pathways convey visual, tactile and probably thermal, pain and auditory impulses. Collicular efferents pass to the retina, lateral geniculate nucleus, pretectum, parabigeminal nucleus, the inferior, medial and lateral pulvinar, and to numerous sites in the brain stem and spinal cord. Fibres passing from the pulvinar are relayed to primary and secondary visual cortices and form an extrageniculate retinocortical pathway for visual orientation and attention.

The tectospinal and tectobulbar tracts start from neurones in the superior colliculi. They sweep ventrally round the central grey matter to decussate ventral to the oculomotor nuclei and medial longitudinal fasciculi as part of the dorsal tegmental decussations. The tectospinal tract descends ventral to the medial longitudinal fasciculus as far as the medial lemniscal decussation in the medulla, where it diverges ventrolaterally to reach the spinal ventral white column near the ventral lip of the ventral median fissure. Tectospinal fibres descend to cervical segments. The tectobulbar tract, mainly crossed, descends near the tectospinal tract, and ends in the pontine nuclei and motor nuclei of the cranial nerves, particularly those innervating the oculogyric muscles. It subserves reflex ocular movements. Other tectotegmental fibres reach various tegmental reticular nuclei in the ipsilateral mesencephalic and contralateral pontomedullary reticular formation (gigantocellular reticular, caudal pontine reticular, oral pontine reticular nuclei), and the substantia nigra and red nucleus. Tectopontine fibres, which probably descend with the tectospinal tract, terminate in dorsolateral pontine nuclei, with a relay to the cerebellum. A tecto-olivary projection, from deeper collicular laminae to the upper third of the medial accessory olivary nucleus, exists in primates it is crossed and links with the posterior vermis.

In animals, central collicular stimulation produces contralateral head movement as well as movements involving the eyes, trunk and limbs, which implicates the superior colliculus in complex integrations between vision and widespread bodily activity.

Pretectal nucleus

The pretectal nucleus is a poorly defined mass of neurones at the junction of the mesencephalon and diencephalon. It extends from a position dorsolateral to the posterior commissure caudally towards the superior colliculus, with which it is partly continuous. It receives fibres from the visual cortex via the superior quadrigeminal brachium, the lateral root of the optic tract from the retina, and the superior colliculus. Its efferent fibres reach both parasympathetic Edinger–Westphal nuclei. Those which decussate pass ventral to the aqueduct or through the posterior commissure. In this way, sphincter pupillae contract in both eyes in response to impulses from either eye. This bilateral light reflex may not be the sole activity of the pretectal nucleus. Some of its efferents project to the pulvinar and deep laminae of the superior colliculus, and provide another extrageniculate path to the cerebral cortex.

BRAIN STEM RETICULAR FORMATION

The brain stem contains extensive fields of intermingled neurones and nerve fibres, which are collectively termed the reticular formation. The reticular regions are often regarded as phylogenetically ancient, representing a primitive nerve network upon which more anatomically organized, functionally selective, connections have developed during evolution. However, the most primitive nervous systems show both diffuse and highly organized regions, which cooperate in response to different demands.

The general characteristics of reticular regions may be summarized as follows. They tend to be ill-defined collections of neurones and fibres with diffuse connections. Their conduction paths are difficult to define, complex and often polysynaptic, and they have ascending and descending components that are partly crossed and uncrossed. Their components subserve somatic and visceral functions. They include distinct chemoarchitectonic nuclear groups, including clusters of serotoninergic neurones (group B cells), which synthesize the indolamine 5-hydroxytryptamine (serotonin); cholinergic neurones (group Ch cells), which contain acetyltransferase, the enzyme which catalyses the synthesis of acetylcholine; and three catecholaminergic groups composed of noradrenergic (group A), adrenergic (group C), and dopaminergic (group A) neurones, which synthesize noradrenaline (norepinephrine), adrenaline (epinephrine) and dopamine respectively as neurotransmitters.

Studies with the Golgi technique show that few brain stem reticular neurones are classic Golgi type II neurones (i.e. with short axons that branch locally). In contrast, they have long dendrites that spread across the long axis of the brain stem in transverse sheets. These radiating dendrites may spread into 50% of the cross-sectional area of their half of the brain stem, and they are intersected by, and may synapse with, a complex of ascending and descending fibres. Many axons of the reticular neurones ascend or descend, or bifurcate to do both. They travel far, perhaps through the whole brain stem and often beyond. As an example, a bifurcating axon from a cell in the magnocellular medullary nucleus may project rostrally into the upper medulla, pons, midbrain tegmentum, subthalamus, hypothalamus, dorsal thalamus, septum, limbic system and neocortex, while its descending branch innervates the reticular core of the lower medulla and may reach the cervical spinal intermediate grey matter (laminae V and VI). Many reticular neurones have unidirectional, shorter axons, which synapse with the radiating dendrites of innumerable other neurones *en route*, and give off collaterals, which synapse with cells in 'specific' brain stem nuclei or cortical formations, such as the cerebellum. Multitudes of afferent fibres converging on individual neurones and their myriad synapses and destinations provide the structural basis for the polymodal responses elicited by experiment, and also for such terms as 'diffuse', 'non-specific' polysynaptic systems.

A contrasting dendritic form is also found, in which dendrites are short, sinuous or curved, branch profusely and pursue re-entrant courses at the perimeter of a nuclear group, defining a boundary between it and its environs. Neurones with an intermediate dendritic complexity occur in and near such nuclei and vary in density in much of the remaining reticular formation. In different zones, the proportion of different sizes of neuronal somata varies. Some regions contain only small to intermediate multipolar cells ('parvocellular' regions). However, there are a few areas where these mingle with large multipolar neurones in 'gigantocellular' or 'magnocellular' nuclei.

In general terms the reticular formation is a continuous core that traverses the whole brain stem, and is continuous below with the reticular intermediate spinal grey laminae. It is divisible, on the basis of cytoarchitectonic, chemoarchitectonic and functional criteria, into three bilateral longitudinal columns: median; medial, containing mostly large reticular neurones; and lateral, containing mostly small to intermediate neurones (**Fig. 19.22**).

MEDIAN COLUMN OF RETICULAR NUCLEI

The median column of reticular nuclei extends throughout the medulla, pons and midbrain and contains neurones that are largely aggregated in bilateral, vertical sheets, blended in the midline and occupying the paramedian zones. Collectively they are called the nuclei of the raphe, or raphe nuclei (**Fig. 19.22**). Many neurones in raphe nuclei are serotoninergic and are grouped into nine clusters, B1–9. The raphe pallidus nucleus and associated raphe obscurus nucleus lie in the upper two-thirds of the medulla and cross the pontomedullary junction. The raphe magnus nucleus, corresponding to many B3 neurones, partly overlaps them, and ascends into the pons. Above it is the pontine raphe nucleus, which is formed by the cell group B5. Also located in the pons is the central superior raphe nucleus, which contains parts of cell groups B6 and B8. The dorsal (rostral) raphe nucleus, approximating to cell group B7, ascends – it expands, then narrows, through much of the midbrain.

The serotoninergic raphe system ramifies extensively throughout the entire CNS. Although many of these fibres may be diffusely distributed, recent work has revealed substantial preferential innervation by discrete parts of the system. For example, whereas the central superior raphe nucleus projects divergently to all areas of the cortex, different neurones in the dorsal raphe nucleus not only project specifically to circumscribed regions of the frontal, parietal and occipital cortex, but also to functionally related regions of the cerebellar cortex. Similarly, the caudate nucleus and putamen receive a preferential input from the dorsal raphe nucleus, whereas the hippocampus, septum and hypothalamus are innervated mainly by cells in the central superior mesencephalic raphe nucleus.

All raphe nuclei provide mainly serotoninergic descending projections, which terminate in the brain stem and spinal cord. Brain stem connections are multiple and complex. For example, the dorsal raphe nucleus, in addition to sending a large number of fibres to the locus coeruleus, projects to the dorsal tegmental nucleus and most of the rhombencephalic reticular formation, together with the central superior, pontine raphe and raphe magnus nuclei.

Raphe spinal serotoninergic axons originate mainly from neurones in the raphe magnus, pallidus and obscurus nuclei. They project as ventral, dorsal and intermediate spinal tracts in the ventral and lateral funiculi, and terminate respectively in the ventral horns and laminae I, II and V of the dorsal horns of all segments, and in the thoracolumbar intermediolateral sympathetic and sacral parasympathetic preganglionic cell columns. The dorsal raphe spinal projections function as a pain-control pathway that descends from the mesencephalic pain-control centre, which is located in the periaqueductal grey matter, dorsal raphe and cuneiform nuclei. The intermediate raphe spinal projection is inhibitory, and, in part, modulates central sympathetic control of cardiovascular function. The ventral raphe spinal system excites ventral horn cells and could function to enhance motor responses to nociceptive stimuli and to promote the flight and fight response.

Principally, the mesencephalic serotoninergic raphe system is reciprocally interconnected rostrally with the limbic system, septum, prefrontal cortex and hypothalamus. Efferents ascend and form a large

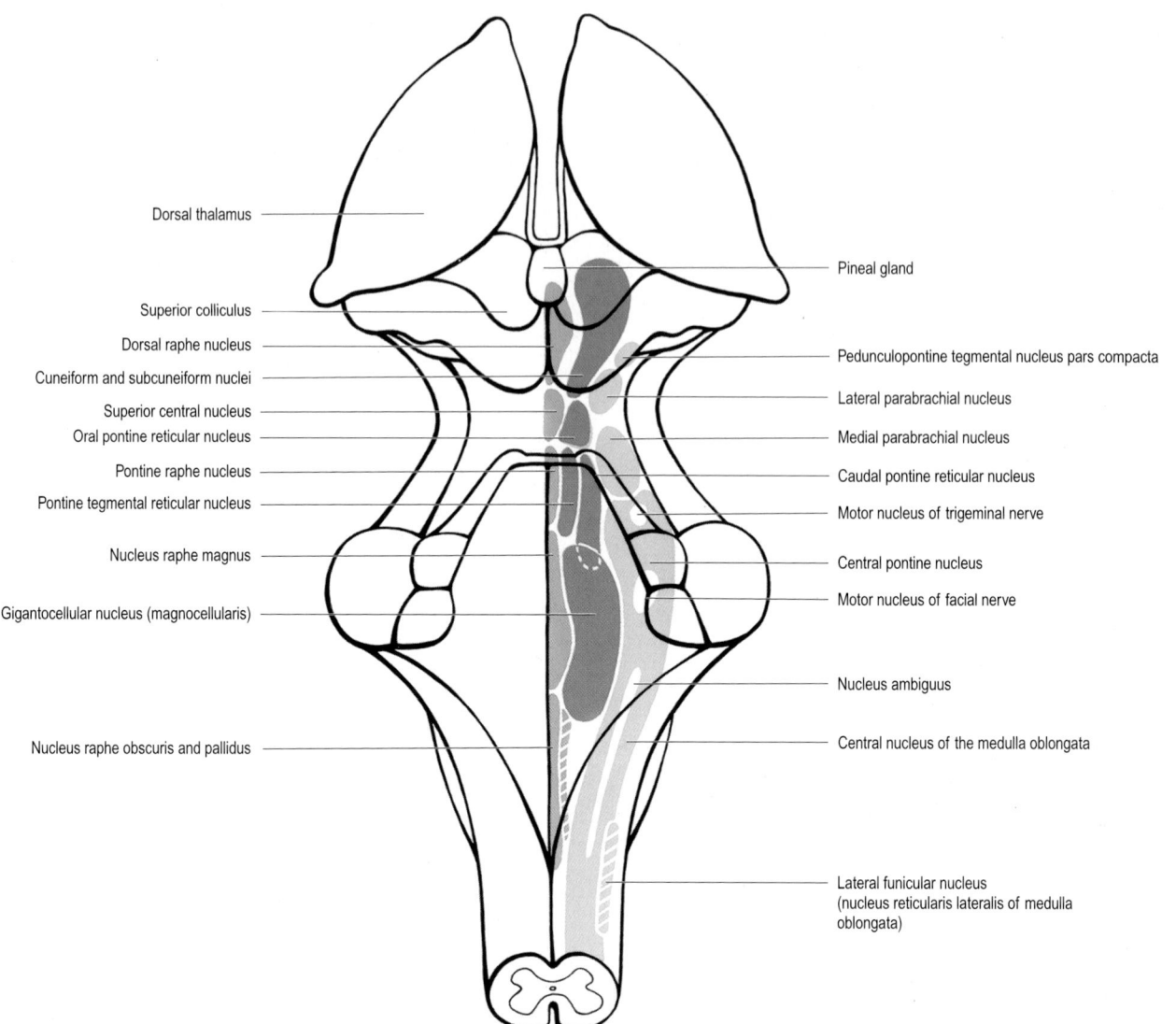

Dorsal thalamus

Superior colliculus

Dorsal raphe nucleus

Cuneiform and subcuneiform nuclei

Superior central nucleus

Oral pontine reticular nucleus

Pontine raphe nucleus

Pontine tegmental reticular nucleus

Nucleus raphe magnus

Gigantocellular nucleus (magnocellularis)

Nucleus raphe obscuris and pallidus

Pineal gland

Pedunculopontine tegmental nucleus pars compacta

Lateral parabrachial nucleus

Medial parabrachial nucleus

Caudal pontine reticular nucleus

Motor nucleus of trigeminal nerve

Central pontine nucleus

Motor nucleus of facial nerve

Nucleus ambiguus

Central nucleus of the medulla oblongata

Lateral funicular nucleus
(nucleus reticularis lateralis of medulla
oblongata)

Fig. 19.22 An outline of the human brain stem (black) extending from the caudal end of the medulla to the dorsal thalami. Note the margins of the rhomboid fossa, the lateral angles of which indicate the pontomedullary junction. Note also the profiles of the transected surfaces of the cerebellar penducles, the colliculi and pineal gland. The principal nuclear derivatives of the brain stem reticular formation are indicated in approximate outline. Those from the median and paramedian nuclear column are in magenta; medial column derivatives are purple, lateral column derivatives blue. In reality, considerable overlap of the nuclear profiles would be present when the third dimension is considered. A number of 'non-reticular' nuclei are also included.

ventral and a diminutive dorsal pathway. Both originate from neurones in the dorsal and central superior raphe nuclei. The raphe magnus nucleus also contributes to the dorsal ascending serotoninergic pathway, which is at first incorporated into the dorsal longitudinal fasciculus (of Schütz). A few fibres terminate in the central mesencephalic grey matter and posterior hypothalamus, but most continue into the medial forebrain bundle and merge with the axons of the ventral pathway, which are distributed to the same targets. The fibres of the ventral ascending serotoninergic pathway exit the ventral aspect of the mesencephalic raphe nuclei, and then course rostrally through the ventral tegmentum from where fibres pass to the ventral tegmental area, substantia nigra and interpeduncular nucleus. A large number of fibres then enter the habenulointerpeduncular tract and run rostrally to innervate the habenular nucleus, intralaminar, midline, anterior, ventral and lateral dorsal thalamic nuclei, and the lateral geniculate body. The ventral ascending serotoninergic pathway enters the median forebrain bundle in the lateral hypothalamic area and splits to pass medially and laterally. The fibres in the medial tract terminate in the mammillary body, dorsomedial, ventromedial, infundibular, anterior and lateral hypothalamic, medial and lateral preoptic and suprachiasmatic nuclei. Those in the lateral tract take the ansa peduncularis–ventral amygdalofugal path to the amygdala, striatum and caudal neocortex. The medial forebrain bundle carries the remaining ventral ascending serotoninergic axons

into the medullary stria, stria terminalis, fornix, diagonal band, external capsule, cingulate fasciculus and medial olfactory stria, to terminate in all the structures that these systems interconnect.

Major afferents into the mesencephalic raphe nuclei include those from the interpeduncular nucleus linking the limbic and serotoninergic systems; the lateral habenular nucleus linking the septum, preoptic hypothalamus and prefrontal cortex via the habenulointerpeduncular tract and the medial forebrain bundle; and the pontine central grey matter.

The ascending raphe system probably functions to moderate forebrain activities, particularly limbic, septal and hypothalamic activities. Recent demonstrations of specific connectivity suggest that it exerts precise, as well as tonal, control.

MEDIAL COLUMN OF RETICULAR NUCLEI

The medial column of reticular nuclei is composed predominantly of neurones of medium size, although very large neurones are found in some regions, and most have processes orientated in the transverse plane (**Fig. 19.22**). In the lower medulla the column is indistinct, and is perhaps represented by a thin lamina lateral to the raphe nuclei. However, in the upper medulla it expands into the medullary gigantocellular (magnocellular) nucleus, which lies ventrolateral to the hypoglossal nucleus, ventral to the vagal nuclei and dorsal to the inferior olivary complex. Ascending further, the column continues as the pontine gigantocellular (magnocellular) nucleus, which lies medially in the tegmentum. Its neurones suddenly diminish in size to form, in rostral order, the almost coextensive caudal and oral pontine tegmental reticular nuclei. It then expands into the cuneiform nucleus and subcuneiform nucleus, before fading away in the midbrain tegmentum.

Axons of medial reticular column neurones form a multisynaptic ascending and descending system within the column, and ultimately enter the spinal cord and diencephalon. Descending fibres form the pontospinal (lateral reticulospinal), and bulbospinal (medial reticulo-spinal) tracts. Pontospinal axons arise from neurones in the caudal and oral parts of the pontine reticular nucleus, descend uncrossed in the ventral spinal funiculus, and terminate in spinal cord laminae VII, VIII and IX. Bulbospinal axons descend bilaterally to end in laminae VII, VIII, IX, and X, and ipsilaterally to end in laminae IV, V and VI. The system modulates spinal motor function and segmental nociceptive input.

Afferent components to the medial reticular nuclear column include the spinoreticular projection and collaterals of centrally projecting spinal trigeminal, vestibular and cochlear fibres. Spinoreticular fibres arise from neurones in the intermediate grey matter of the spinal cord. They decussate in the ventral white commissure, ascend in the ventro-lateral funiculus, usually via several neurones, and terminate not only at all levels of the medial column of reticular nuclei but also in the intralaminar nuclei of the thalamus. Three areas of the medial reticular zone receive particularly high densities of terminations. These are the combined caudal and rostral ends of the gigantocellular and central nuclei respectively; and the caudal pontine reticular nucleus; and the pontine tegmentum. Retinotectal and tectoreticular fibres relay visual information and the medial forebrain bundle transmits olfactory impulses.

Efferents from the medial column of reticular nuclei project through a multisynaptic pathway within the column to the thalamus. Areas of maximal termination of spinoreticular fibres also project directly to the intralaminar thalamic nuclei. The multisynaptic pathway is integrated into the lateral column of reticular nuclei with cholinergic neurones in the lateral pontine tegmentum. The intralaminar thalamic nuclei project directly to the striatum and neocortex.

LATERAL COLUMN OF RETICULAR NUCLEI

The lateral column of reticular nuclei contains six nuclear groups. These are the parvocellular reticular area; superficial ventrolateral reticular area; lateral pontine tegmental noradrenergic cell groups A1, A2, A4–A7 (A3 is absent in primates); adrenergic cell groups C1–C2; and cholinergic cell groups Ch5–Ch6. The column descends through the lower two-thirds of the lateral pontine tegmentum and upper medulla, where it lies between the gigantocellular nucleus medially, and the sensory trigeminal nuclei laterally. It continues caudally, and expands to form most of the reticular formation lateral to the raphe nuclei. It abuts the superficial ventrolateral reticular area, nucleus solitarius, nucleus ambiguus and vagal nucleus, and there contains the adrenergic cell group C2, and the noradrenergic group A2.

The lateral paragigantocellular nucleus lies at the rostral pole of the diffuse superficial ventrolateral reticular area (at the level of the facial nucleus). The zone extends caudally as the nucleus retroambiguus and descends into the spinal cord. It contains noradrenergic cell groups A1, A2, A4 and A5, and the adrenergic cell group C1. The ventrolateral reticular area is involved in cardiovascular, respiratory, vasoreceptor and chemoreceptor reflexes, and in the modulation of nociception. The A2 or noradrenergic dorsal medullary cell group lies in the nucleus of the tractus solitarius, vagal nucleus and adjoining parvocellular reticular area. Adrenergic group C1 lies rostral to the A2 cell group. Noradrenergic cell group A4 extends into the lateral pontine tegmentum, along the sub-ependymal surface of the superior cerebellar peduncle. Noradrenergic group A5 forms part of the paragigantocellular nucleus in the caudolateral pontine tegmentum. Noradrenergic cell group A5 and adrenergic cell group C1 probably function as centres of vasomotor control. The entire region is subdivided into functional areas on the basis of stimulation experiments in animals, in which vasoconstrictor, cardioaccelerator, depressor, inspiratory, expiratory and sudomotor effects have been elicited.

The lateral pontine tegmental reticular grey matter is related to the superior cerebellar peduncle and forms the medial and lateral para-brachial nuclei and the ventral Kölliker-Fuse nucleus, a pneumotaxic centre. The locus coeruleus (noradrenergic cell group A6), area sub-

coeruleus, noradrenergic cell group A7, and cholinergic group Ch5 in the pedunculopontine tegmental nucleus, are all located in the lateral pontine and mesencephalic tegmental reticular zones. The mesen-cephalic group Ch5 is continuous caudally with cell group Ch6 in the pontine central grey matter.

Cell group A6 contains all the noradrenergic cells in the central region of the locus coeruleus. Group A6 has ventral (nucleus sub-coeruleus, A6 Sc), rostral and caudolateral extensions, the latter merges with the A4 group. The locus coeruleus probably functions as an attention centre, focusing neural functions to prevailing needs. The noradrenergic A7 group occupies the rostroventral part of the pontine tegmentum and is continuous with groups A5 and A1 through the lateral rhombencephalic tegmentum. The A7, A5, A1 complex is also connected by noradrenergic cell clusters with group A2, caudally, and group A6, rostrally. The A5 and A7 groups lie mainly within the medial parabrachial and Kölliker-Fuse nuclei. Reticular neurones in the lateral pontine tegmental reticular area, like those of the ventrolateral zone, function to regulate respiratory, cardiovascular and gastrointestinal activity. Two micturition centres are located in the dorsomedial and ventrolateral parts of the lateral pontine tegmentum.

The connections of the lateral column reticular nuclei are complex. The short ascending and descending axons of the parvocellular reticular area constitute bulbar reflex pathways, which connect all branchio-motor nuclei and the hypoglossal nucleus with central afferent cranial nerve complexes through a propriobulbar system. The area also receives descending afferents from the contralateral motor cortex via the cortico-tegmental tract, and from the contralateral red nucleus via the rubro-spinal tract. The longitudinal catacholamine bundle passes through the parvocellular reticular formation.

The superficial ventrolateral reticular area receives some input from the spinal cord, insular cortex and amygdala, but the principal projection is from the nucleus solitarius and subserves cardiovascular, baroreceptor, chemoreceptor and respiratory reflexes. Reticulospinal afferents from the region terminate bilaterally on sympathetic preganglionic neurones in the thoracic spinal cord. Afferents from the pneumotaxic centre project to an inspiratory centre in the ventrolateral part of the nucleus solitarius, and a mixed expiratory–inspiratory centre in the superficial ventrolateral reticular area. Inspiratory neurones in both centres mono-synaptically project to the phrenic and intercostal motor neurones. Axons of expiratory neurones terminate on lower motor neurones which innervate intercostal and abdominal musculature.

The superficial ventrolateral area is also the seat of the visceral alerting response. Fibres from the hypothalamus, periaqueductal grey matter and midbrain tegmentum mediate increased respiratory activity, raised blood pressure, tachycardia, vasodilation in skeletal muscle and renal and gastrointestinal vasoconstriction. Ascending efferents from the superficial ventrolateral area synapse on neurones of the supraoptic and paraventricular hypothalamic nuclei. Excitation of these neurones causes release of vasopressin from the neurohypophysis. Medullary nor-adrenergic cell groups A1 and A2 also innervate (directly and indirectly) the median eminence, and control the release of growth hormone, luteinizing hormone and adrenocorticotrophic hormone (ACTH).

The lateral pontine tegmentum, particularly the parabrachial region, is reciprocally connected to the insular cortex. It shares reciprocal projections with the amygdala through the ventral amygdalofugal path-way, medial forebrain bundle and central tegmental tract, and with the hypothalamic, median preoptic and paraventricular nuclei, which prefer-entially project to the lateral parabrachial nucleus and the micturition centres. It also shares reciprocal bulbar projections, many from the pneumotaxic centre, with the nucleus solitarius and superficial ventro-lateral reticular area.

Reticulospinal fibres descend from the lateral pontine tegmentum. A mainly ipsilateral subcoeruleospinal pathway is distributed to all spinal segments of the cord through the lateral spinal funiculus. Crossed pontospinal fibres descend from the ventrolateral pontine tegmentum, decussate in the rostral pons and occupy the contralateral dorsolateral spinal funiculus. They terminate in laminae I, II, V and VI of all spinal segments of the cord. Fibres from the pneumotaxic centre innervate the phrenic nucleus and T1–T3 sympathetic preganglionic neurones bilaterally through this projection system.

Bilateral projections from the micturition centres travel in the lateral spinal funiculus. They terminate on preganglionic parasympathetic neurones in the sacral cord (which innervate the detrusor muscle in the urinary bladder), and on neurones in the nucleus of Onuf (which innervate the musculature of the pelvic floor and the anal and urethral sphincters).

Descending fibres of the A6 noradrenergic neurones of the locus coeruleus project into the longitudinal dorsal fasciculus (as the caudal limb of the dorsal periventricular pathway), and into the caudal limb of the dorsal noradrenergic bundle (as part of the longitudinal catecholamine bundle). In this way they innervate, mainly ipsilaterally, all other rhombencephalic reticular areas, principal and spinal trigeminal nuclei, pontine nuclei, cochlear nuclei, nuclei of the lateral lemniscus, and, bilaterally, all spinal preganglionic autonomic neurones and the ventral region of the dorsal horn in all segments of the spinal cord. Other axons that contribute to the longitudinal catecholamine bundle originate from cell groups C1, A1, A2, A5 and A7. The main projection is a descending one from cell groups C1 and A5, which are sudomotor neural control centres and innervate preganglionic sympathetic neurones.

Most ascending fibres from the locus coeruleus pass in the dorsal noradrenergic (or tegmental) bundle; others run in either the rostral limb of the dorsal periventricular pathway or in the superior cerebellar peduncle. The latter fibres terminate on the deep cerebellar nuclei. The dorsal noradrenergic bundle is large and runs through the ventrolateral periaqueductal grey matter to join the medial forebrain bundle in the hypothalamus, from where fibres continue forward to innervate all rostral areas of the brain. The pathway contains efferent and afferent axons that reciprocally connect the locus coeruleus with adjacent structures along its course, e.g. central mesencephalic grey matter, dorsal raphe nucleus, superior and inferior colliculi, interpeduncular nucleus, epithalamus, dorsal thalamus, habenular nuclei, amygdala, septum, olfactory bulb and anterior olfactory nucleus, entire hippocampal formation and neocortex. Fibres from the locus coeruleus which travel in the rostral limb of the dorsal periventricular pathway, ascend in the ventromedial periaqueductal grey matter adjacent to the longitudinal dorsal fasciculus and terminate in the parvocellular part of the paraventricular nucleus in the hypothalamus.

The functions of the locus coeruleus and related tegmental noradrenergic cell groups are poorly understood, largely because the afferent neurones that drive them have yet to be identified. The diversity of their rostral and caudal projections suggests a holistic role in central processing. In animals, firing rates of locus coeruleus neurones peak during wakefulness and decrease during sleep – they cease almost completely during rapid eye movement (REM) sleep. During wakefulness, firing rates are augmented when novel stimuli are presented. The locus coeruleus may, therefore, function to control the level of attentiveness. Other functions that have been ascribed to the locus coeruleus include control of the wake–sleep cycle, regulation of blood flow, and maintenance of synaptic plasticity.

The A1, A2, A5 and A7 noradrenergic cell groups project rostrally, mainly through the central tegmental tract. Their axons constitute a major longitudinal catecholamine pathway that continues through the medial forebrain bundle and ends in the amygdala, lateral septal nucleus, bed nucleus of the stria terminalis, nucleus of the diagonal band and the hypothalamus. The ascending dorsal periventricular pathway contains a few non-coerulean noradrenergic fibres, which terminate in the periventricular region of the thalamus.

Propriobulbar projections receive a contribution from the diffusely organized dorsal medullary and lateral tegmental noradrenergic cell groups. These interconnect cranial nerve nuclei and other reticular cell groups, particularly those of the vagus, facial and trigeminal nerves, and the rhombencephalic raphe and parabrachial nuclei.

Three precerebellar nuclei, the lateral and paramedian reticular nuclei and the nucleus of the pontine tegmentum, are involved in the relay of spinal information into the vermis and paravermal regions of the ipsilateral cerebellar hemisphere. They receive inputs from the contralateral primary motor and sensory neocortices, and the ipsilateral cerebellar and vestibular nuclei and spinal cord (the latter through the ascending spinoreticular pathway). This system augments the dorsal and ventral spinocerebellar, cuneocerebellar, accessory cuneocerebellar and trigeminocerebellar tracts.

BRAIN STEM LESIONS (Figs 19.23, 19.24)

Unilateral brain stem lesions may arise as a result of extrinsic compression of the brain stem by space occupying tumours (e.g. meningioma, acoustic neuroma or metastatic carcinoma) or may be caused by intrinsic disease (e.g. glioma, demyelination or stroke). The clinical syndrome is determined by the neuroanatomical site of the lesion. At the segmental level, an ipsilateral cranial nerve palsy occurs. Below the level of the lesion, there is a contralateral loss of power and sensation in the limbs (corresponding to dysfunction of the decussating corticospinal and ascending sensory pathways), and ipsilateral incoordination of the limbs (as a result of the interruption of efferent and afferent cerebellar connections).

The ipsilateral cranial nerve dysfunction reflects the segmental level of the lesion in the midbrain, pons and medulla. Midbrain lesions cause ophthalmoplegia, pupillary dilatation and ptosis (oculomotor nerve palsy) and impaired upward gaze (e.g. due to a pinealoma). Pontine lesions (e.g. an acoustic neuroma in the cerebellopontine angle) lead to ophthalmoplegia (abducens nerve lesion), loss of facial sensation and weakness of masticatory muscles (trigeminal nerve lesion), weakness of facial muscles (facial nerve lesion), deafness and

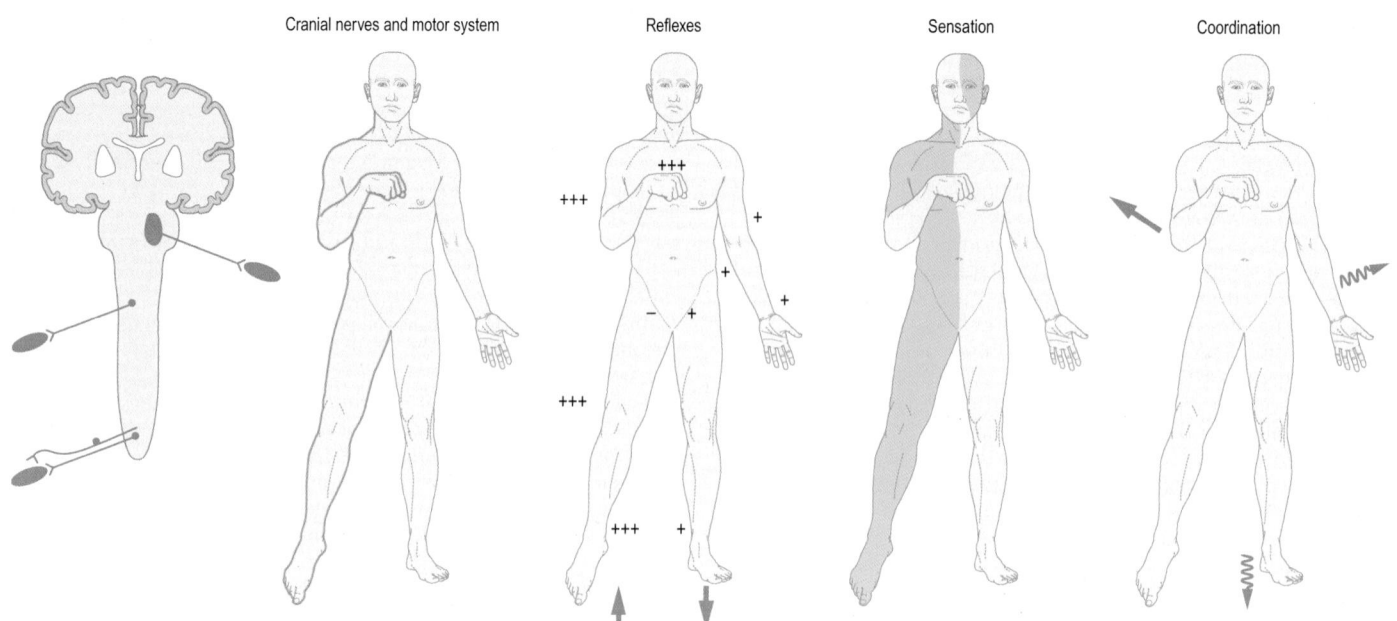

Cranial nerves and motor system   Reflexes   Sensation   Coordination

Fig. 19.23 Brain stem lesions. (By permission from Crossman AR, Neary D 2000 Neuroanatomy, 2nd edn. Edinburgh: Churchill Livingstone.)

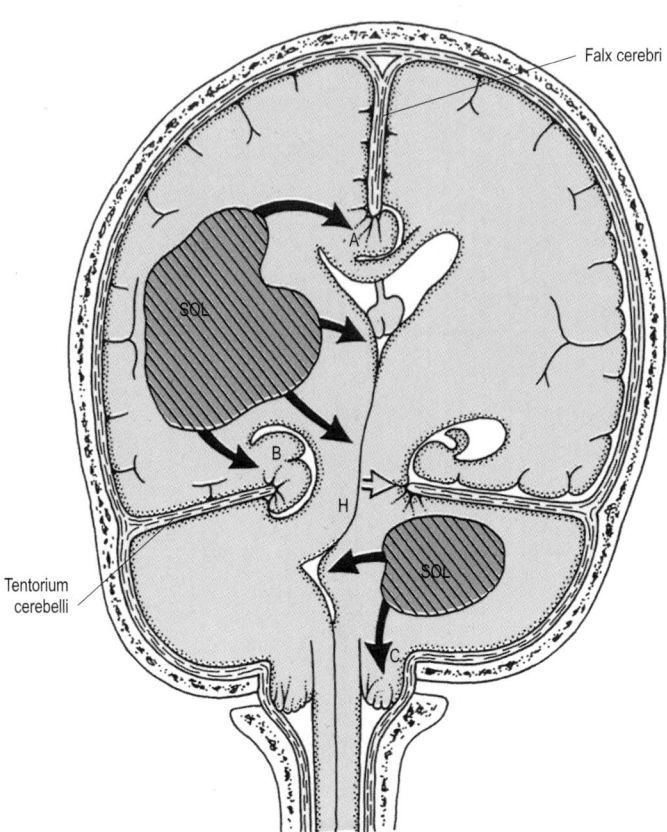

Falx cerebri

Tentorium
cerebelli

Fig. 19.24 Consequences of a space-occupying lesion (SOL). **A**, Herniation of the cingulate gyrus under the falx. **B**, Tentorial herniation of the parahippocampal gyrus. **C**, Herniation of cerebellar tonsils through the foramen magnum. Haemorrhage into the midbrain: H; compression of cerebral peduncle against the free edge of the tentorium cerebelli: open arrow.

vertigo (vestibulocochlear nerve lesion). Medullary lesions cause a 'bulbar palsy', i.e. dysarthria, dysphagia and dysphonia, with wasting of the hemi-tongue and palate (glossopharyngeal, vagal and hypoglossal nerve lesions) and weakness and wasting of sternocleidomastoid and trapezius (accessory nerve lesion).

In addition to this focal brain stem syndrome, blockage of the outflow of CSF from the fourth ventricle via the foramina of Magendie and Luschka (e.g. by extrinsic tumours) produces hydrocephalus, which is characterized by headache, papilloedema and progressive stupor and coma.

Bilateral destructive lesions of the brain stem are fatal if untreated, because of damage to 'centres' in the medulla that control respiration, heart rate and blood pressure. Impairment of the reticular activating system in the core of the brain stem leads to progressive impairment of consciousness, followed by stupor and coma. In this state of 'brain stem death', life can only be supported artificially. This is the fate of all untreated expanding space-occupying lesions in the cranium (e.g. haematoma, abscess, tumour, whether extrinsic or intrinsic to the brain, and cerebral oedema). A space-occupying lesion within the unyielding skull raises the intracranial pressure directly and also indirectly by obstruction of CSF flow, which causes headache and papilloedema. The brain is distorted and displaced downward (rostro-caudally) within the skull and meningeal framework. The brain stem is vulnerable to compression at two critical sites, which are determined by the neuro-anatomical relationship of the meningeal tentorium and foramen magnum to the cerebral hemisphere (supratentorial) and brain stem (infratentorial). The downward displacement of the cerebral hemisphere leads to herniation of the ipsilateral medial temporal lobe (uncus) through the tentorial notch. There may be direct ipsilateral compression of the midbrain and emergent oculomotor and trochlear cranial nerves or contralateral compression of the upper brain stem by the abutting sharp edge of the tentorium. The ipsilateral posterior cerebral artery is vulnerable to compression at this site. Unilateral herniation is heralded by a progressive oculomotor nerve palsy (ophthalmoplegia, pupillary dilatation and ptosis), contralateral limb weakness, falling level of consciousness, and, if treatment is long delayed, a contralateral homonymous hemianopia. Compression of the contralateral brain stem by the tentorium leads to ipsilateral 'false localizing' signs.

Further progressive rostro-caudal displacement of the brain ultimately leads to herniation of the medulla through the foramen magnum and into the spinal canal. This is accompanied by bilateral cranial nerve dysfunction, quadriplegia, deepening coma and finally apnoea, i.e. brain stem death. These neuroanatomical and functional processes underlie the diagnosis and management of the traumatically brain injured patient, and the complications of intracranial haematomas (extradural, subdural and intracerebral) and cerebral oedema.

REFERENCES

Brodal P, Bjaalie JG 1992 Organization of the pontine nuclei. Neurosci Res 13: 83–118.

Ciriello J 1983 Brainstem projections of aortic baroreceptor afferent fibres in the rat. Neurosci Lett 36: 37–42.

Dahlström A, Fuxe K 1964 Evidence for the existence of monamine-containing neurones in the central nervous system. Acta Physiol Scand Suppl 232: 1–55.

Dahlström A, Fuxe K 1965 Evidence for the existence of monoamine neurones in the central nervous system. II. Experimentally induced changes in the intraneuronal amine levels of bulbospinal neurone systems. Acta Physiol Scand Suppl 247: 1–36.

Hamilton RB, Norgren R 1984 Central projections of gustatory nerves in the rat. J Comp Neurol 222: 560–77.

Johnston JB 1909 The morphology of the forebrain vesicle in vertebrates. J Comp Neurol 19: 458–539.

Millar J, Basbaum AI 1975 Topography of the projection of the body surface of the cat to cuneate and gracile nuclei. Exp Neurol 49(1 pt 1): 281–90.

Nathan PW, Smith MC 1982 The rubrospinal and central tegmental tracts in man. Brain 105: 223–69.

Nieuwenhuys R, Voogd J, Huijzen C van 1988 The human central nervous system. A synopsis and atlas, 3rd edition. Berlin: Springer Verlag.

Olszewski J 1950 On the anatomical and functional organization of the spinal trigeminal nucleus. J Comp Neurol 92: 401–9.

Cerebellum

The cerebellum, the largest part of the hindbrain, is dorsal to the pons and medulla, and its median region is separated from them by the fourth ventricle. It is joined to the brain stem by three pairs of cerebellar peduncles, which contain afferent and efferent fibres. The cerebellum occupies the posterior cranial fossa, where it is covered by the tentorium cerebelli. It is roughly spherical, but somewhat constricted in its median region, and flattened – its greatest diameter is transverse. In adults the weight ratio of cerebellum to cerebrum is c.1:10, in infants c.1:20.

The cerebellum is a central part of the major circuitry that links sensory to motor areas of the brain, and is required for the coordination of fine movement. In health, it provides corrections during movement, which are the basis for precision and accuracy, and it is critically involved in motor learning and reflex modification. It receives sensory information through spinal, trigeminal and vestibulocerebellar pathways and, via the pontine nuclei, from the cerebral cortex and the tectum. Cerebellar output is mainly to those structures of the brain that control movement.

The basic internal organization of the cerebellum is of a superficial, highly convoluted cortex (a laminated sheet of neurones and supporting cells) overlying a dense core of white matter. The latter contains deep cerebellar nuclei, which give rise to the efferent cerebellar projections. Although the human cerebellum makes up approximately one-tenth of the entire brain by weight, the surface area of the cerebellar cortex, if unfolded, would be about half that of the cerebral cortex. The great majority of cerebellar neurones are small granule cells, which are so densely packed that the cerebellar cortex contains many more neurones than the cerebral cortex. Unlike the cerebral cortex, where a large number of diverse cell types are arranged differently in different regions, the cerebellar cortex contains a relatively small number of different cell types, which are interconnected in a highly stereotyped way. Consequently, one region of the cerebellar cortex looks very much like another.

Disease processes affecting the cerebellum or its connections lead to incoordination. Movements of the eyes, speech apparatus, individual limbs and balance are usually affected, which results in nystagmus, dysarthria, incoordination, and ataxia. Although all of these movements become defective in widespread disease of the cerebellum or its connections, topographical arrangements within the cerebellum lead to a variety of clinically recognizable disease patterns. Thus, in cerebellar hemisphere disease, the ipsilateral limbs show rhythmical tremor during movement, but not at rest. The tremor increases as the target is approached, so reaching and accurate movements of the arm are especially difficult. Diseases that affect the ascending spinocerebellar pathways or the midline vermis have a disproportionate effect on axial structures, leading to severe loss of balance. Lesions of outflow tracts in the superior cerebellar peduncles result in a wide amplitude, severely disabling, proximal tremor, which interferes with all movements and may even disturb posture, leading to rhythmic oscillations of the head or trunk so that the patient is unable to stand or sit without support. However, although cerebellar lesions may initially cause profound motor impairment, a considerable degree of recovery is possible. There are clinical reports that the initial symptoms of large cerebellar lesions (caused by trauma or surgical excision) have improved progressively over time.

Although the basic structure of the cerebellum and its importance for normal movement have long been recognized, many of the details of how it functions remain obscure. The main goal of this chapter is to describe the known structure and connections of the cerebellum.

EXTERNAL FEATURES AND RELATIONS
(Figs 20.1, 20.2, 20.3)

The cerebellum consists of two large, laterally located hemispheres which are united by a midline vermis. The superior surface of the cerebellum, which would constitute the anterior part of the unrolled cerebellar cortex, is relatively flat. The paramedian sulci are shallow and the borders between vermis and hemispheres are indicated by kinks in the transverse fissures. The superior surface adjoins the tentorium cerebelli and projects beyond its free edge. The transverse sinus borders the cerebellum at the point where the superior and inferior surfaces meet. The inferior surface is characterized by a massive enlargement of the cerebellar hemispheres, which extends medially to overlie some of the vermis. Deep paramedian sulci demarcate the vermis from the hemispheres. Posteriorly the hemispheres are separated by a deep vallecula, which contains the dural falx cerebelli. The inferior cerebellar surface lies against the occipital squama. The shape of the surface facing the brain stem is irregular. It forms the roof of the fourth ventricle and the lateral recesses on each side of it, while the cerebellar peduncles define the diamond shape of the ventricle when viewed from behind. Anterolaterally the cerebellum lies against the posterior surface of the petrous part of the temporal bone.

The cerebellar surface is divided by numerous curved transverse fissures which separate its folia and give it a laminated appearance. Deeper fissures divide it into lobules. One conspicuous fissure, the horizontal fissure, extends around the dorsolateral border of each hemisphere from the middle cerebellar peduncle to the vallecula, separating the superior and inferior surfaces. Although the horizontal fissure is prominent, it appears relatively late in embryological development and does not mark the boundary between major functional subdivisions of the cortex. The deepest fissure in the vermis is the primary fissure, which curves ventrolaterally around the superior surface of the cerebellum to meet the horizontal fissures. It appears early in embryological development and marks the boundary between the anterior and posterior lobes.

Because the cerebellar cortex has a roughly spherical shape, the true relations between its parts can sometimes be obscured. Thus, the most anterior lobule of the cerebellar vermis, the lingula, lies very close to the most posterior lobule, the nodule. Deep fissures divide the superior vermis into lobules. The lobules of the superior vermis that belong to the anterior lobe are the lingula, central lobule and culmen. The lingula is a single lamina of four or five shallow folia. Its white core is continuous with the anterior medullary velum. It is separated from the central lobule by the precentral fissure. The central lobule and culmen are continuous bilaterally with an adjoining wing (ala) in each hemisphere. The central lobule is separated from the culmen by the preculminary fissure. The culmen (with attached anterior quadrangular lobules) lies between the preculminary and primary fissures.

Between the primary and the horizontal fissure are the simple lobule (with attached posterior quadrangular lobules) and the folium (with attached superior semilunar lobules). These two lobule sets are separated by the posterior superior fissure.

From the back forward, the inferior vermis is divided into the tuber, pyramis, uvula and nodule, in that order (**Fig. 20.3C**). The tuber is continuous laterally with the inferior semilunar lobules and separated from the pyramis by the lunogracile fissure. The pyramis and attached biventral lobules (containing an intrabiventral fissure) are separated

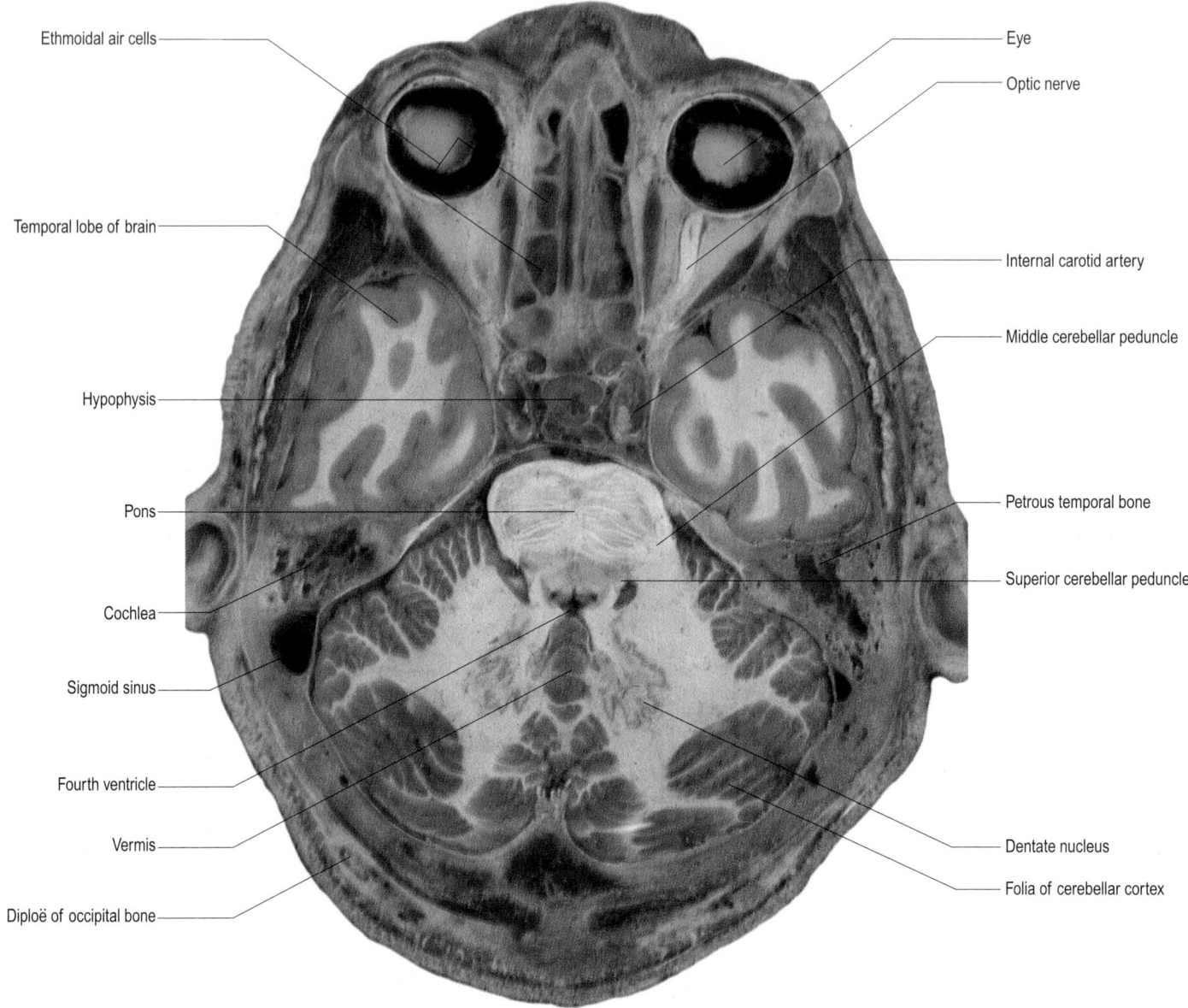

Ethmoidal air cells

Temporal lobe of brain

Hypophysis

Pons

Cochlea

Sigmoid sinus

Fourth ventricle

Vermis

Diploë of occipital bone

Eye

Optic nerve

Internal carotid artery

Middle cerebellar peduncle

Petrous temporal bone

Superior cerebellar peduncle

Dentate nucleus

Folia of cerebellar cortex

Fig. 20.1 Horizontal section through the cerebellum and brain stem. (By kind permission from Dr GJA Maart.)

from the uvula and attached cerebellar tonsils by the secondary fissure. Behind the uvula, and separated from it by the median part of the posterolateral fissure, is the nodule. The tonsils are roughly spherical and overhang the foramen magnum on each side of the medulla oblongata.

The nodule and attached flocculi constitute a separate flocculonodular lobe, which is separated from the uvula and tonsils by the deep posterolateral fissure. This lobe is richly interconnected with the vestibular nucleus, which is located at the lateral margin of the fourth ventricle.

FUNCTIONAL DIVISIONS OF THE CEREBELLUM (Fig. 20.4)
The cerebellum is divided functionally into a body, with inputs mainly from the spinal cord and pontine nuclei, and a flocculonodular lobe, which has strong afferent and efferent connections with the vestibular nuclei. The body is subdivided into a series of regions dominated by their spinal or pontine inputs. The anterior lobe, simple lobule, pyramis and biventral lobules are the main recipients of spinal and trigeminal cerebellar afferents. Pontocerebellar input dominates in the folium, tuber and uvula, and in the entire hemisphere, including those regions that receive afferents from the spinal cord.

The mediolateral subdivision of the cerebellum into vermis and hemispheres represents a functional subdivision that is closely related to its output. In mammals, a great increase in the size of the cerebellar

hemispheres parallels the development of the cerebral cortex, and reflects the importance of the corticopontocerebellar input and of the efferent projections of the cerebellar hemispheres (through the dentate and interposed cerebellar nuclei and the thalamus) to the cerebral cortex.

CEREBELLAR PEDUNCLES (Figs 20.5, 20.6)
Three peduncles connect the cerebellum with the rest of the brain The middle cerebellar peduncle is the most lateral and by far the largest of the three. It passes obliquely from the basal pons to the cerebellum and is composed almost entirely of fibres arising from the contralateral basal pontine nuclei, with a small addition from nuclei in the pontine tegmentum. The inferior cerebellar peduncle is located medial to the middle peduncle. It consists of an outer, compact fibre tract, the restiform (Latin: rope-like) body and a medial, juxtarestiform body. The restiform body is a purely afferent system. It receives the posterior spinocerebellar tract from the spinal cord and the trigeminocerebellar, cuneocerebellar, reticulocerebellar and olivocerebellar tracts from the medulla oblongata. The juxtarestiform body is mainly an efferent system. Apart from primary afferent fibres of the vestibular nerve and secondary afferent fibres from the vestibular nuclei, it is made up almost entirely of efferent Purkinje cell axons from the vestibulocerebellum, on their way to the vestibular nuclei, and the uncrossed fibres from the fastigial nucleus. The crossed fibres from the fastigial nucleus, after passing dorsal to the superior

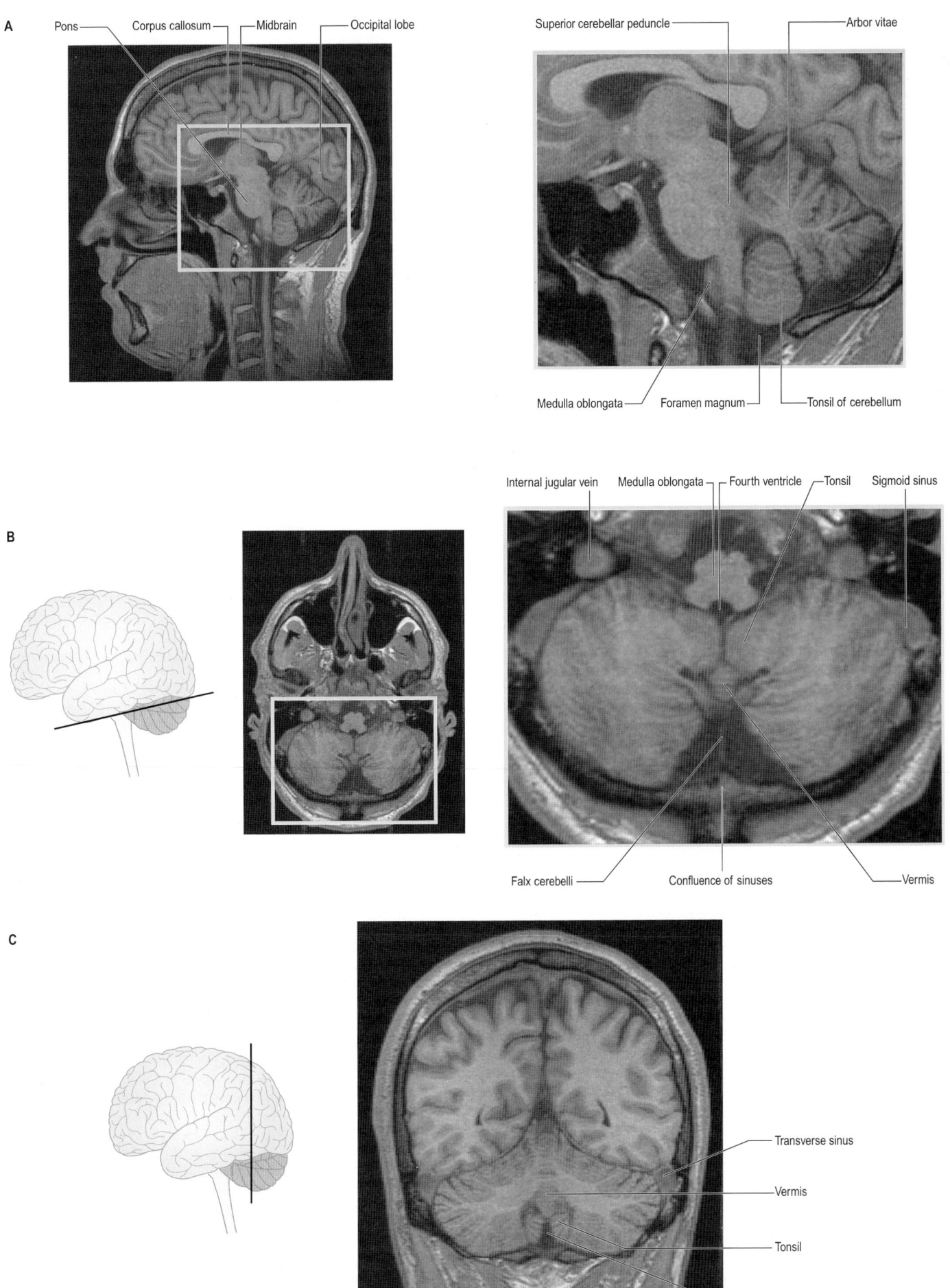

Fig. 20.2 Magnetic resonance images of the cerebellum of a 16-year-old female. **A**, sagittal slice. **B**, coronal slice. **C**, axial slice. (By kind permission from Drs JP Finn and T Parrish, Northwestern University School of Medicine, Chicago.)

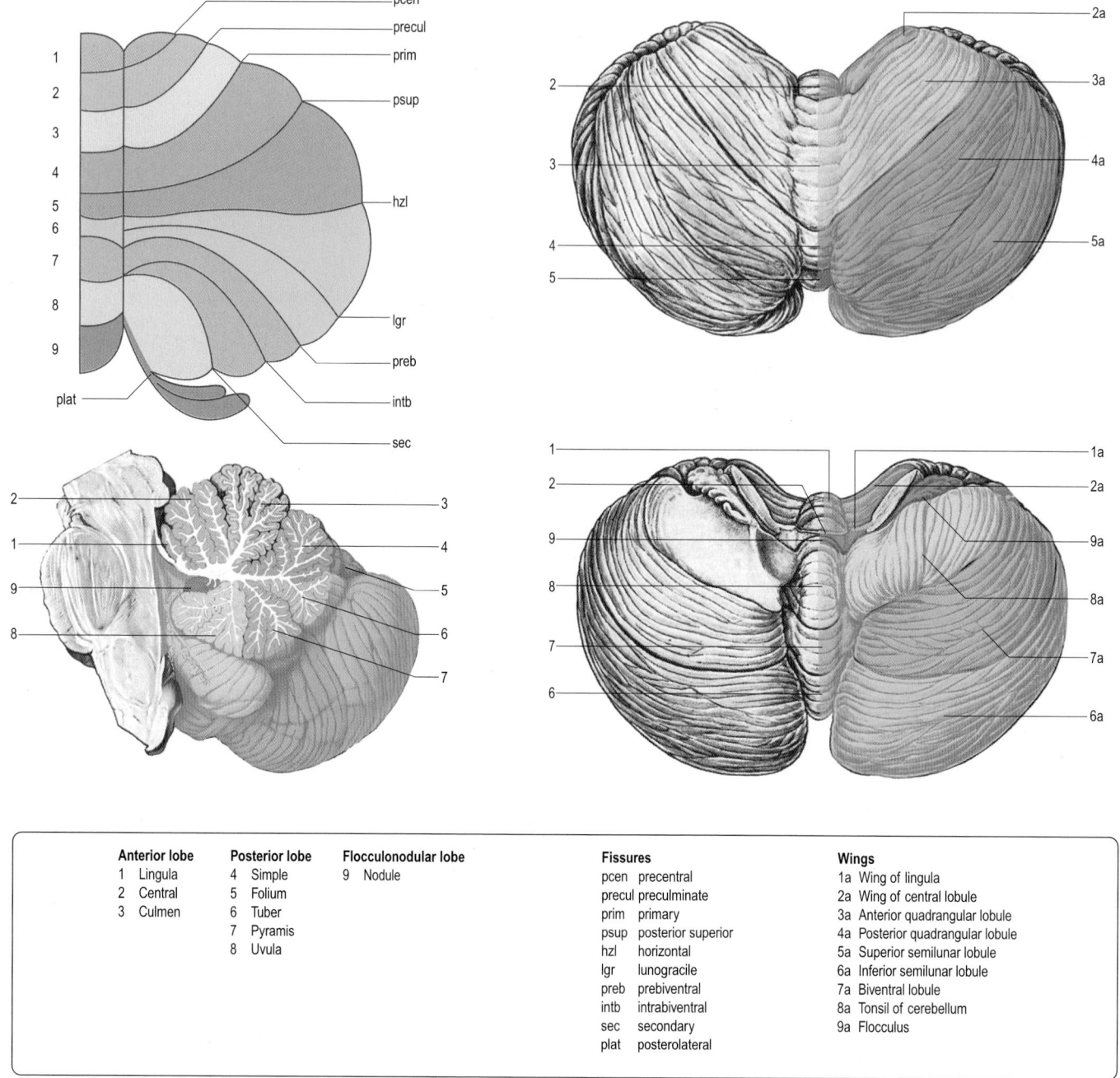

Fig. 20.3 Terminology of cerebellar lobes and fissures, using a schematic 'unrolled' diagram as a frame of reference. **A**, Unrolled cerebellar cortex. The lobules are labelled by numbers and the fissures between the wings are listed. **B**, Cerebellum viewed from above. **C**, Median sagittal section of cerebellum. The nodules and wings are numbered and listed. **D**, Cerebellum viewed from below.

cerebellar peduncle, enter the brain stem as the uncinate fasciculus at the border of the juxtarestiform and restiform body.

The superior cerebellar peduncle contains all of the efferent fibres from the dentate, emboliform and globose nuclei and a small fascicle from the fastigial nucleus. It decussates with its opposite number in the caudal mesencephalon, on its way to synapse in the contralateral red nucleus and thalamus. The anterior spinocerebellar tract reaches the upper part of the pontine tegmentum before looping down within this peduncle to join the spinocerebellar fibres entering through the restiform body.

INTERNAL STRUCTURE

The white core of the cerebellum branches in diverging medullary laminae, which occupy the central part of the lobules and are covered by the cerebellar cortex. In a sagittal section through the cerebellum the

highly branched pattern of medullary laminae is known as the arbor vitae. The white core consists of the efferents (Purkinje cell axons) and afferents of the cerebellar cortex. Fibres crossing the midline in the white core of the cerebellum and the anterior medullary velum constitute the cerebellar commissure. This consists of an efferent portion, containing decussating fibres from the fastigial nucleus, and an afferent portion, containing fibres of the restiform body and the middle cerebellar peduncle. (In neuroanatomy the word commissure may have two meanings. In one sense a commissure, such as the corpus callosum, connects homotopic points on the two sides of the brain. However, in the cerebellum commissural afferent and efferent fibres are simply crossing the midline. The cerebellum has no callosum-like commissure connecting homotopic points on the two sides.)

Laterally, the medullary laminae merge into a large, central white mass, which contains the four cerebellar nuclei. These are the dentate, anterior (emboliform) and posterior (globose) interposed and fastigial nuclei (**Fig. 20.4**). The dentate is the most lateral and largest and is an

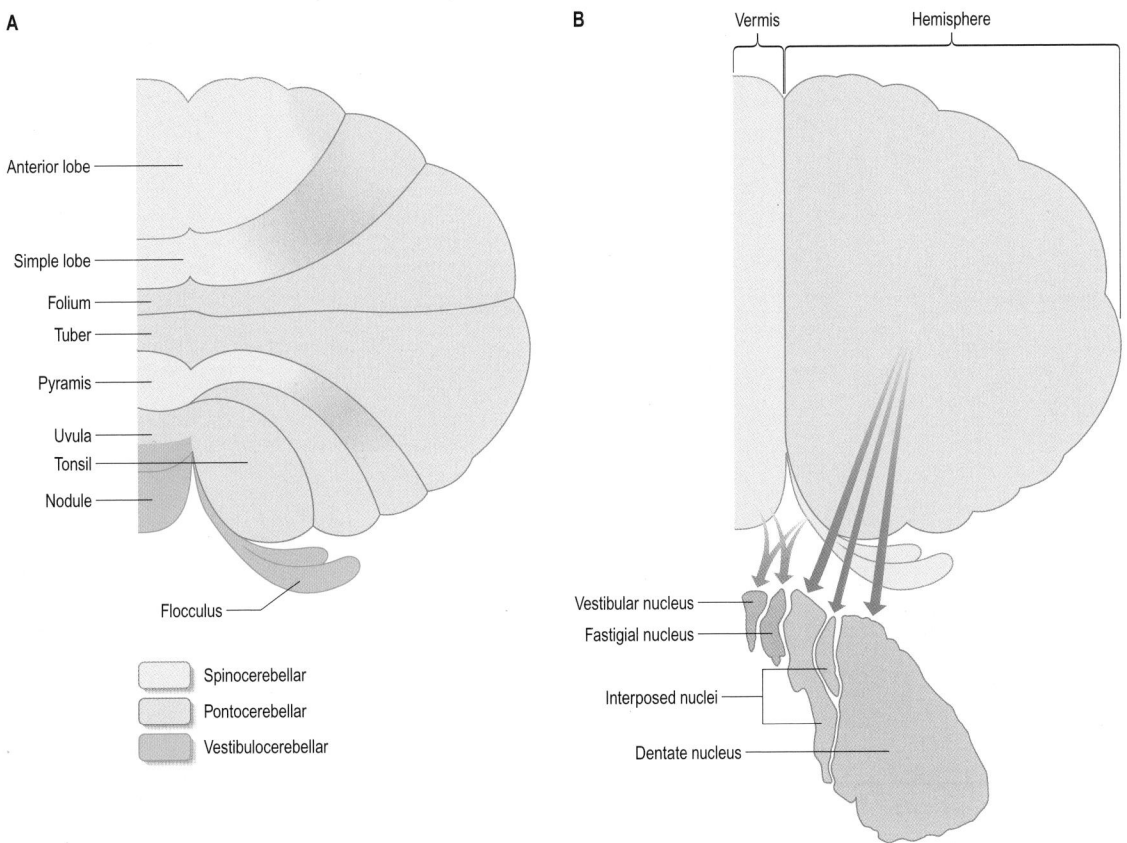

A

Anterior lobe

Simple lobe

Folium

Tuber

Pyramis

Uvula

Tonsil

Nodule

Flocculus

Spinocerebellar

Pontocerebellar

Vestibulocerebellar

B

Vermis   Hemisphere

Vestibular nucleus

Fastigial nucleus

Interposed nuclei

Dentate nucleus

Fig. 20.4 Diagrams of the flattened cerebellar surface. **A,** Transverse lobular organization of the afferent spino-, ponto- and vestibulocerebellar connections of the cortex. **B,** Longitudinal zonal organization of the vermis and hemispheres with the cerebellar and vestibular nuclei.

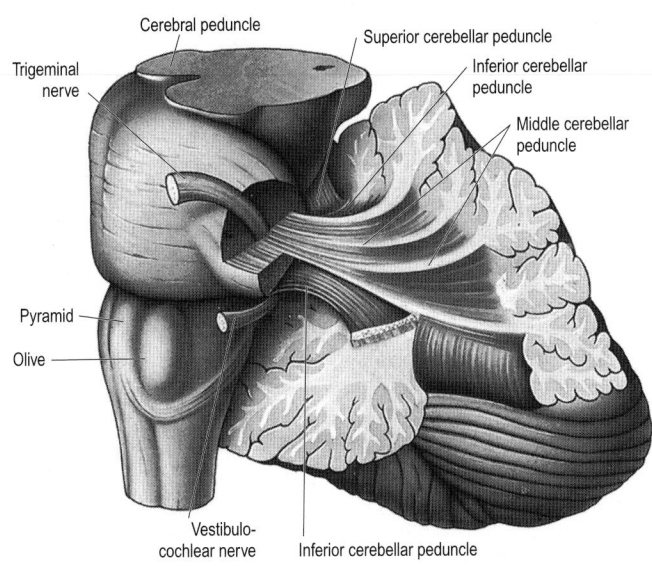

Cerebral peduncle

Trigeminal nerve

Superior cerebellar peduncle

Inferior cerebellar peduncle

Middle cerebellar peduncle

Pyramid

Olive

Vestibulo-cochlear nerve   Inferior cerebellar peduncle

Fig. 20.5 Dissection of the left cerebellar hemisphere and its peduncles. By kind permission from Dr EB Jamieson, University of Edinburgh.)

irregularly folded sheet of neurones, which encloses a mass of fibres mainly derived from dentate neurones. It resembles a leather purse, the opening of which is directed medially. Fibres stream out through this so-called 'hilum' to form the bulk of the superior cerebellar peduncle. The anterior and posterior interposed and fastigial nuclei lie medial to the dentate nucleus. The anterior interposed nucleus is continuous laterally with the dentate. The posterior interposed nucleus is medial to the anterior nucleus, and is continuous with the fastigial nucleus, which

is located next to the midline, bordering on the fastigium (roof) of the fourth ventricle. Efferent fibres from the interposed nuclei join the superior cerebellar peduncle. A large proportion of the efferent fibres from the fastigial nucleus cross within the cerebellar white matter of the cerebellar commissure. After their decussation they constitute the uncinate fasciculus (hook bundle), which passes dorsal to the superior cerebellar peduncle to enter the vestibular nuclei of the opposite side (**Fig. 20.6**). Uncrossed fastigiobulbar fibres enter the vestibular nuclei by passing along the lateral angle of the fourth ventricle. Some fibres of the fastigial nucleus ascend in the superior cerebellar peduncle.

CEREBELLAR CORTEX

The elements of the cerebellar cortex possess a precise geometric order, which is arrayed relative to the tangential, longitudinal and transverse planes in individual folia. The cortex contains the terminations of afferent 'climbing' and 'mossy' fibres, five varieties of neurone (granular, stellate, basket, Golgi and Purkinje), neuroglia and blood vessels.

There are three main layers: molecular; Purkinje cell; and granular (**Fig. 20.7**). The main circuit of the cerebellum involves granule cells, Purkinje cells and neurones in the cerebellar nuclei. Granule cells receive the terminals of the mossy fibre afferents (i.e. all afferent systems except the olivocerebellar fibres). The axons of the granule cells ascend to the molecular layer, where they bifurcate into parallel fibres (so called because they are oriented parallel to the transverse fissures and perpendicular to the dendritic trees of the Purkinje cells on which they terminate). Purkinje neurones are large and are the sole output cells of the cerebellar cortex. Their axons terminate in the cerebellar nuclei and in the vestibular nuclei. In addition to the dense array of parallel fibres, the dendritic trees of Purkinje cells receive terminals from climbing fibres, the neurones of origin of which are in the inferior olivary nucleus. The cerebellar cortex thus receives two distinct types of input: olivocerebellar climbing fibres, which synapse directly on Purkinje neurones; and mossy fibres, which connect to the Purkinje cells via granular neurones, the axons of which are the parallel fibres.

357

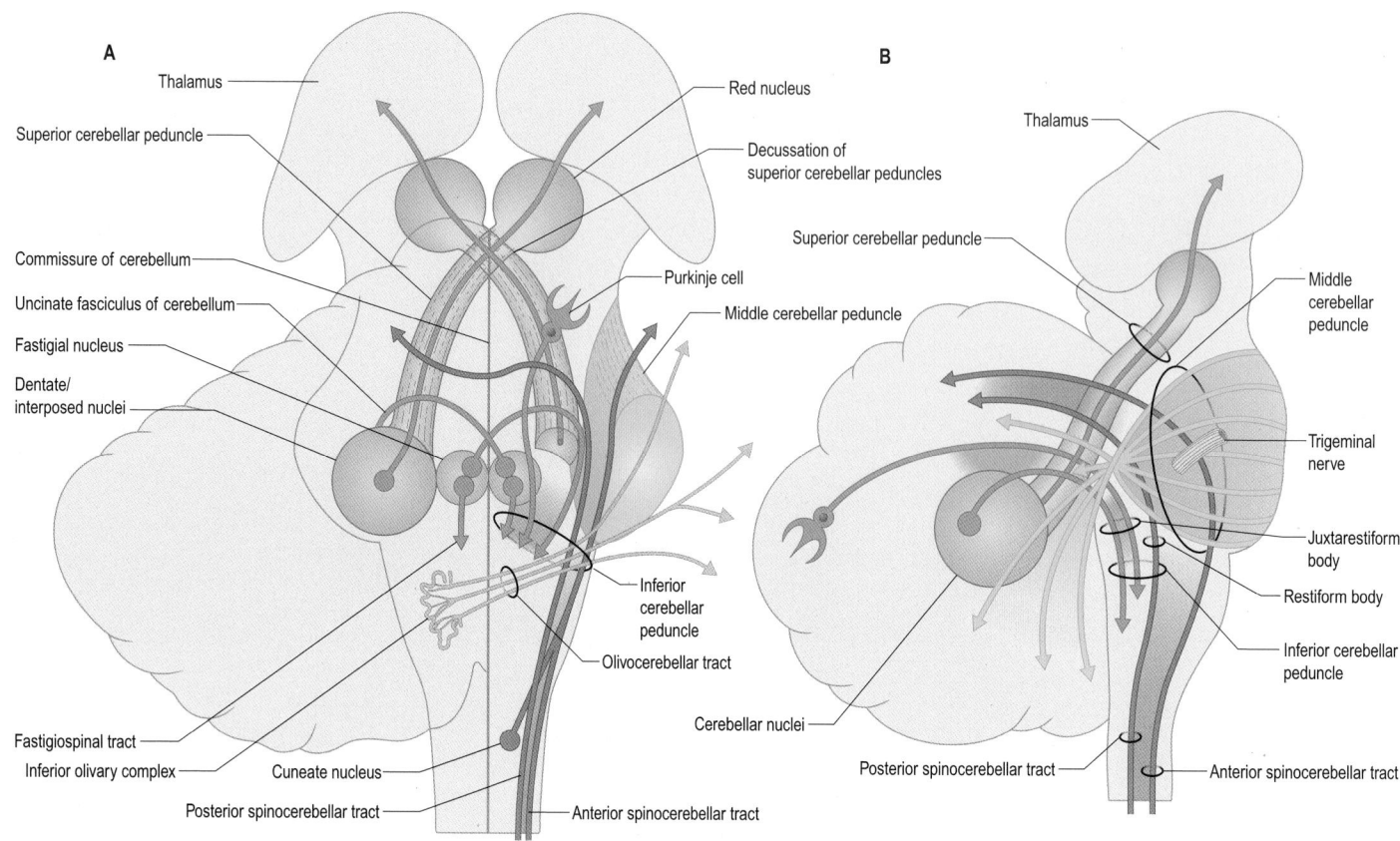

Fig. 20.6 Diagram illustrating the composition of the cerebellar peduncles. **A**, dorsal view. **B**, lateral view.

Both parallel and climbing fibres excite the Purkinje cells, but they differ greatly in their firing characteristics and their effect on them. Purkinje cell axons inhibit their target neurones in the cerebellar nuclei. The cerebellar nuclei project to all the major motor control centres in the brain stem and cerebrum. The stellate, basket and Golgi cells are inhibitory interneurones, which connect the cortical elements in complex geometrical patterns.

The molecular layer is c.300–400 μm thick. It contains a sparse population of neurones, dendritic arborizations, non-myelinated axons and radial fibres of the neuroglial cells. Purkinje cell dendritic trees extend towards the surface and spread out in a plane perpendicular to the long axis of the cerebellar folia. Purkinje cell dendrites are flattened. The lateral extent of the Purkinje cell dendrites is c.30 times greater in the transverse plane than it is in a plane parallel to the cerebellar folia. Parallel fibres are the axons of granule cells, the stems of which ascend into the molecular layer where they bifurcate at T-shaped branches. The two branches extend in opposite directions as parallel fibres along the axis of a folium. Parallel fibres terminate on the dendrites of the Purkinje cells and Golgi cells, which they pass on their way, and on the basket and stellate cells of the molecular layer. Dendritic trees of Golgi neurones reach towards the surface. Unlike the flattened dendritic tree of the Purkinje cell, Golgi cell dendrites span the territory of many Purkinje neurones longitudinally as well as transversely. These dendrites receive synapses from parallel fibres. Some Golgi cell dendrites enter the granular layer, where they contact mossy fibre terminals. The cell bodies of Golgi neurones lie below, in the superficial part of the granular layer. The molecular layer also contains the somata, dendrites and axons of stellate neurones (which are located superficially within the molecular layer) and of basket cells (whose somata lie deeper within the molecular layer). Climbing fibres, which are the terminals of olivo-cerebellar fibres, ascend through the granular layer to contact Purkinje dendrites in the molecular layer. Radiating branches from large epithelial (Bergmann) glial cells give off processes that surround all neuronal elements, except at the synapses. At the surface of the cerebellum their conical expansions join to form an external limiting membrane.

The Purkinje cell layer contains the large, pear-shaped somata of the Purkinje cells and the smaller somata of epithelial (Bergmann) glial cells. Clumps of granule cells and occasional Golgi cells penetrate between the Purkinje cell somata.

The granular layer (**Fig. 20.7**) is c.100 μm thick in the fissures and 400–500 μm on foliar summits. There are c.2.7 million granular neurones per cubic millimetre. It has been estimated that the human cerebellum contains a total of c.4.6×10^{10} granule cells, and that there are c.3000 granule cells for each Purkinje cell.

In summary, the granular layer consists of the somata of granule cells and the start of their axons; dendrites of granule cells; branching terminal axons of afferent mossy fibres; climbing fibres passing through the granular layer *en route* to the molecular layer; and the somata, basal dendrites and complex axonal ramifications of Golgi neurones. Cerebellar glomeruli are synaptic rosettes consisting of a mossy fibre terminal that forms excitatory synapses upon the dendrites of both granule cells and Golgi cells (**Fig. 20.8**).

Of the five cell types to be described, the first four are inhibitory, liberating γ-aminobutyric acid (GABA), and the fifth is excitatory, liberating L-glutamate. **Fig. 20.9** summarizes their main connections.

Purkinje cells have a specific geometry, which is conserved in all vertebrate classes (**Fig. 20.7**). They are arranged in a single layer between the molecular and granular layers. Individual Purkinje cells are separated by c.50 μm transversely and 50–100 μm longitudinally. Their somata measure c.50–70 μm vertically and 30–35 μm transversely. The sub-cellular structure of the Purkinje cell is similar to that of other neurones. One distinguishing feature is subsurface cisterns, often associated with mitochondria, which are present below the plasmalemma of somata and dendrites and may penetrate into the spines. They are intracellular calcium stores, which are important links in the second messenger systems of the cell.

One, sometimes two, large primary dendrites arise from the outer pole of a Purkinje cell. From these an abundant arborization, with several orders of subdivision, extends towards the surface. Branches of each neurone are confined to a narrow sheet in a plane transverse to the long axis of the folium. Proximal first- and second-order dendrites

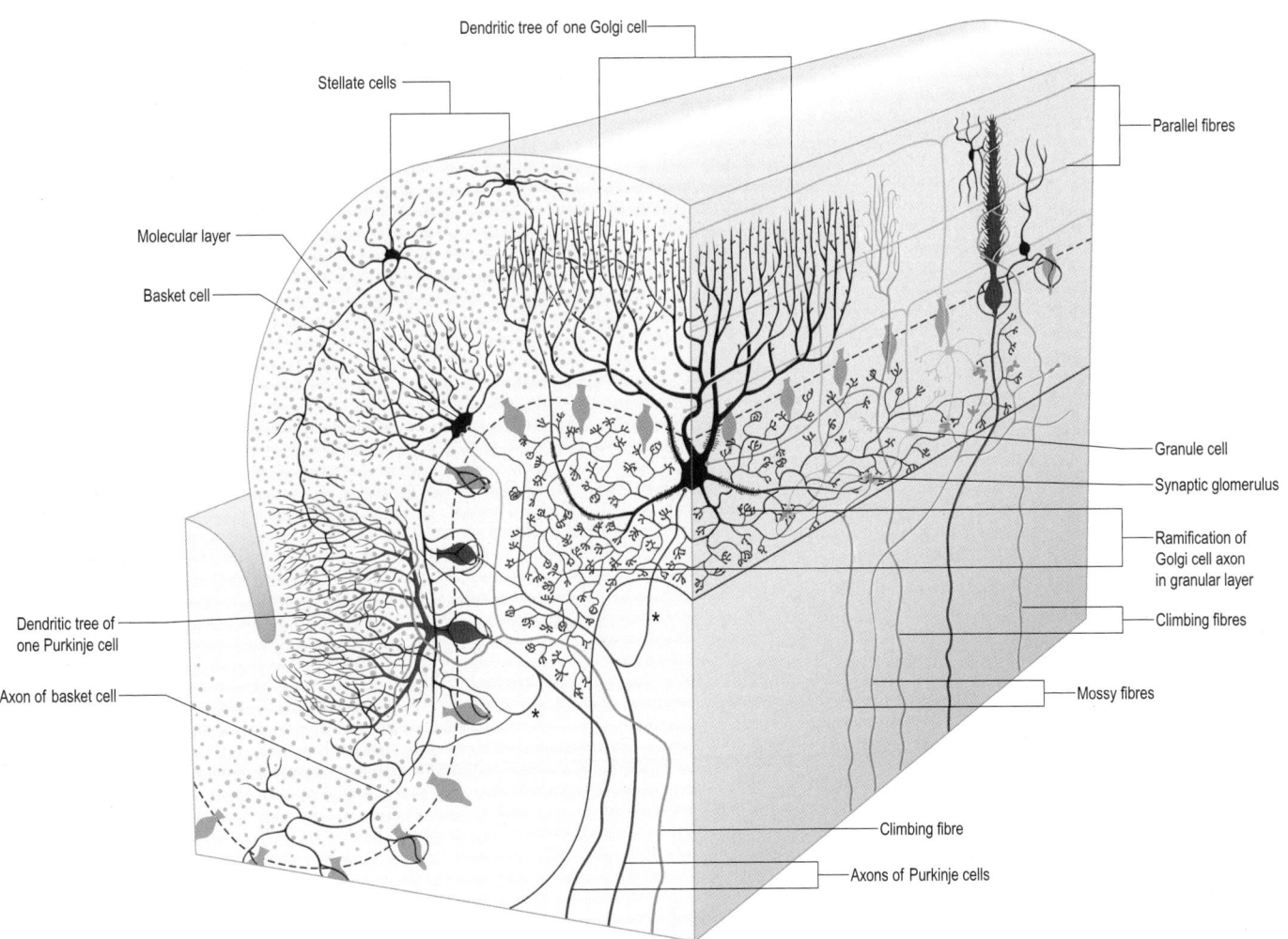

Fig. 20.7 The general organization of the cerebellar cortex. A single folium has been sectioned vertically, both in its longitudinal axis (right part of diagram) and transversely. The two asterisks on the left face indicate recurrent collateral branches of Purkinje cell axons.

have smooth surfaces with short, stubby spines, and are contacted by climbing fibres. Distal branches show a dense array of dendritic spines, which receive synapses from the terminals of parallel fibres. Inhibitory synapses are received from basket and stellate cells and from the recurrent collaterals of Purkinje cell axons, which contact the shafts of the proximal dendrites. The total number of dendritic spines per Purkinje neurone is c.180,000.

The axon of a Purkinje cell leaves the inner pole of the soma and crosses the granular layer to enter the subjacent white matter. The initial axon segment receives axo-axonic synaptic contacts from distal branches of basket cell axons. Beyond the initial segment, the axon enlarges, becomes myelinated, and gives off collateral branches. The main axon ultimately forms a plexus in one of the cerebellar or vestibular nuclei. The recurrent collateral branches end on other Purkinje cells and on basket and Golgi neurones.

Basket and stellate cells are the neurones of the molecular layer. Their sparsely branched dendritic trees and the ramifications of their axons lie in a plane approximately perpendicular to the long axis of the folium, i.e. in the same plane as the Purkinje cell dendritic tree. Stellate cells are located in the superficial molecular layer and their axons synapse with the shafts of Purkinje cell dendrites. Both stellate and basket cells receive excitatory synapses from parallel fibres passing through their dendritic tree. Basket cells lie in the lower third of the molecular layer. Their somata receive synapses from Purkinje cell recurrent collaterals, climbing and mossy fibres as well as from the parallel fibres. Basket cell axons increase in size away from their somata and run deep in the molecular layer just above the Purkinje cells. Continuing for c.1 mm, each covers the territories of 10 to 12 Purkinje neurones. Collaterals of the basket cell axons ascend along Purkinje cell dendrites, and descend

towards Purkinje cell somata and initial axonal segments forming peri-cellular networks, or 'baskets', around them. Branches from each basket cell axon also extend in the direction of the long axis of the folium to a further 3 to 6 rows of Purkinje neurones, flanking the axon. It follows that as many as 72 Purkinje cell neurones may receive synapses from a single basket neurone.

Most Golgi cell somata occupy the superficial zone of the granular layer, adjoining the Purkinje cell somata. Their dendrites radiate into the molecular layer. Unlike Purkinje cells, the dendritic trees of Golgi cells are not flattened, appearing much the same in transverse and longitudinal foliar section. In both planes they overlap the territories of several neighbouring Purkinje and Golgi cells. Some Golgi dendrites, however, divide in the granular layer and join cerebellar glomeruli, where they receive excitatory synaptic contacts from mossy fibres. The axon of the Golgi cell arises from the base of the cell body or proximal dendrite and immediately divides into a profuse arborization which extends through the entire thickness of the granular layer. The territory occupied by the axonal ramifications is of a volume that corresponds approximately to its dendritic tree in the molecular layer, and which overlaps with the axonal arborizations of adjacent Golgi cells. The main synaptic input to Golgi cell dendrites is from parallel fibres in the molecular layer. Purkinje cell recurrent collaterals and mossy and climbing fibres also terminate on their proximal dendrites and, more sparsely, on their somata.

Each granule cell has a spherical nucleus, 5–8 μm in diameter, with a mere shell of cytoplasm containing a few small mitochondria, ribosomes and a diminutive Golgi complex. Granule cells give rise to 3 to 5 short dendrites, which end in claw-like terminals within the synaptic glomeruli. The fine axons of granule cells enter the molecular layer and branch at a T-junction to form parallel fibres passing in opposite

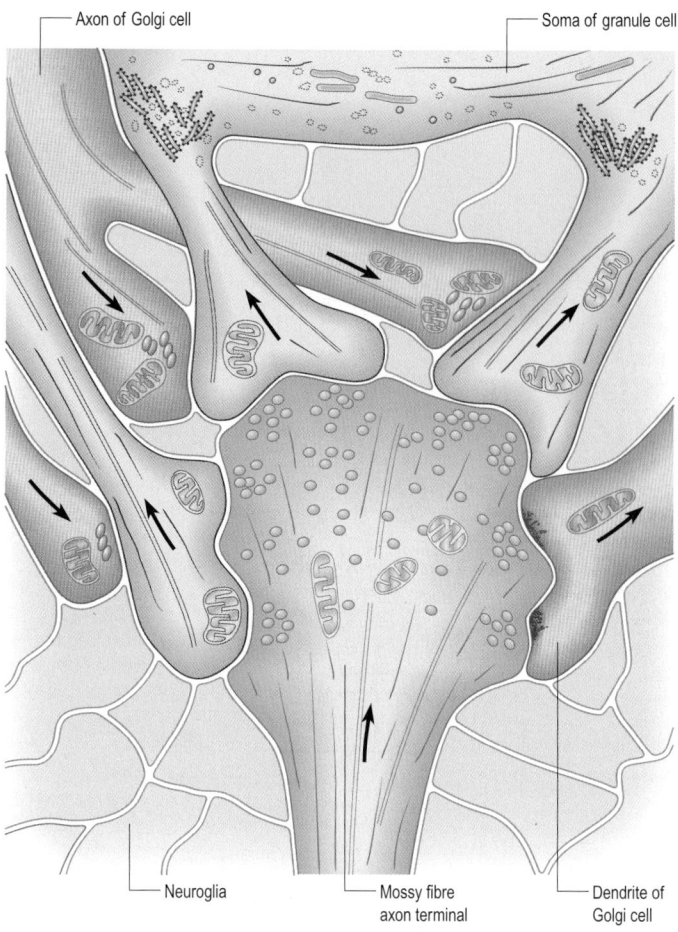

Axon of Golgi cell

Soma of granule cell

Neuroglia

Mossy fibre axon terminal

Dendrite of Golgi cell

Fig. 20.8 A cerebellar synaptic glomerulus. Arrows indicate directions of impulse conduction. (From The Cerebellum as a Neuronal Machine, Eccles et al, 1967, © Springer-Verlag.)

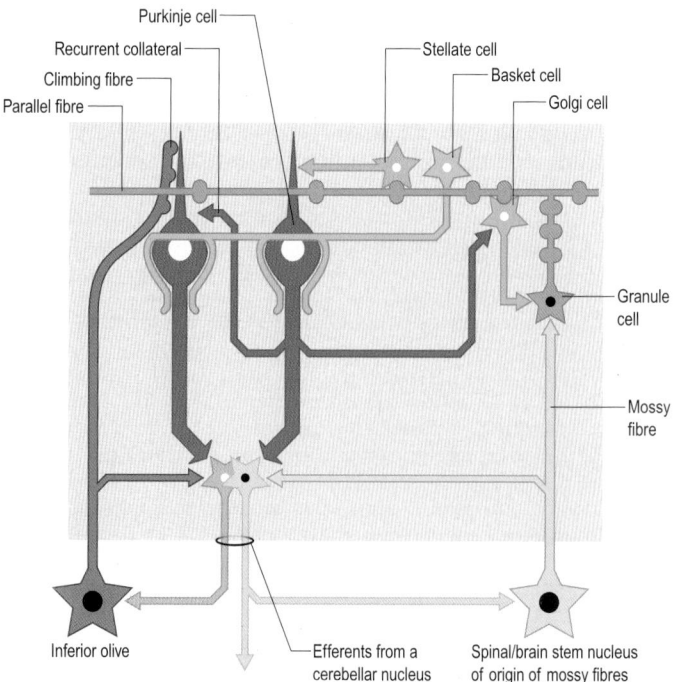

Purkinje cell

Recurrent collateral

Climbing fibre

Parallel fibre

Stellate cell

Basket cell

Golgi cell

Granule cell

Mossy fibre

Inferior olive

Efferents from a cerebellar nucleus

Spinal/brain stem nucleus of origin of mossy fibres

Fig. 20.9 Diagrammatic representation of the main circuits of the cerebellar cortex. The cortex is indicated by the grey background.

directions over a distance of several millimetres. Terminals located along the parallel fibres give them a beaded appearance and are sites of synapses upon the dendrites of Purkinje, stellate, basket and Golgi cells in the molecular layer. Most numerous are the synapses with Purkinje dendritic spines. It had been estimated that c.250,000 parallel fibres cross a single Purkinje dendritic tree, although every parallel fibre may not synapse with the dendritic tree that it crosses.

Two very different excitatory inputs serve the cerebellar cortex, namely climbing fibres and mossy fibres.

Climbing fibres arise only from the inferior olivary nucleus. Olivo-cerebellar fibres cross the white matter and enter the granular layer where they branch to form climbing fibres. Each climbing fibre innervates a single Purkinje cell. There are about ten times as many Purkinje cells as there are cells in the inferior olive and so each olivocerebellar fibre branches into c.10 climbing fibres. Individual climbing fibres pass alongside the soma of a Purkinje cell, and then branch to make numerous synapses on the short, stubby spines that protrude from the proximal segments of Purkinje cell dendrites.

Mossy fibres take their origin from the spinal cord, the trigeminal, dorsal column, and reticular nuclei of the medulla, and the pontine tegmentum and basal pons. Like climbing fibres they are excitatory, but they contrast sharply in their anatomical distribution and physiological properties. As each mossy fibre traverses the white matter its branches diverge to enter several adjacent folia. Within each folium these branches expand into grape-like synaptic terminals (mossy fibre rosettes), which occupy the centre of cerebellar glomeruli.

Noradrenergic and serotoninergic fibres form a rich plexus in all layers of the cerebellar cortex. The aminergic fibres are fine, varicose and form extensive cortical plexuses: their release of noradrenaline (norepinephrine) and serotonin is assumed to be non-synaptic, and their effects paracrine, involving volumes of tissue. The serotoninergic afferents of the cerebellum take their origin from neurones in the medullary reticular formation, other than the raphe nuclei. The noradrenergic, coeruleocerebellar projection, when active, inhibits Purkinje cell firing not by direct action but via β-adrenergic-receptor-mediated inhibition of adenylate cyclase in the Purkinje cells. The presence of dopamine in elements of the cerebellar cortex is still disputed. Cerebellar afferents have been traced from dopaminergic cells in the ventral tegmental area, and dopamine D2 and D3 receptors are present in the molecular layer. A similar plexus of thin, ChAT-containing fibres is centred on the Purkinje cell layer. The origin of this cholinergic plexus is not known.

The connections of the cerebellum are organized in two perpendicular planes, corresponding to the planar organization of the cerebellar cortex. Efferent connections of the cortex are disposed in parasagittal sheets or bundles, which connect longitudinal strips of Purkinje cells with specific cerebellar or vestibular nuclei. The climbing fibre afferents to a Purkinje cell zone from the inferior olive display a similar zonal disposition. Cerebellar output is organized in modules, where a module consists of one or more Purkinje cell zones, their cerebellar or vestibular target nucleus, and their olivocerebellar climbing fibre input. Modular function is determined by the brainstem projections of the cerebellar or vestibular target nucleus. A general feature of the modular organization of the cerebellum is that GABAergic neurones in the cerebellar nuclei project to the subnuclei of the contralateral inferior olive, which give rise to their respective climbing fibre afferents. These recurrent connections are known as nucleo-olivary pathways.

Mossy fibre afferent systems from precerebellar nuclei in the spinal cord and the brain stem terminate in the granular layer of certain lobules in transversely oriented terminal fields. The transverse lobular arrangement of the mossy fibre afferents is enforced by the transverse orientation of the parallel fibres, which are axons of the granule cells and constitute the second link in the mossy fibre–parallel fibre input of the Purkinje cells. Parallel fibres cross and terminate on Purkinje cells belonging to several successive modules as they course through the molecular layer.

Purkinje cells can be activated in two different ways. Granule cell activity generates simple spikes, which resemble the response of other neurones in the brain, whereas activation by a climbing fibre produces a prolonged depolarization upon which several spike-like waves are superimposed. The rate of firing of single and complex spikes also differs markedly. While the Purkinje cell may fire simple spikes at a rate of hundreds per second, complex spikes occur at very low frequencies, seldom more than three or four per second.

Purkinje cell activity is regulated by local Golgi, basket and stellate cells. Like Purkinje cells, Golgi cells have a rich dendritic tree which extends through the molecular layer. Unlike Purkinje cells, the Golgi cell dendrites are not restricted to a plane transverse to the folia and their axons do not leave the cerebellar cortex. Golgi cells regulate firing by presynaptic inhibition of the mossy fibre afferents, and so act as a governor, or rate limiter, of Purkinje cell activity. Stellate and basket cells synapse directly on Purkinje cells and are powerful inhibitors of their activity.

Structural and functional cerebellar localization

Since the cerebellar cortex is largely uniform in microstructure and microcircuitry, it seems likely that its basic mode of operation is also uniform. The most obvious input for this operation is provided by the mossy fibre afferents, which carry information from all levels of the spinal cord, and specialized sensory and motor information relayed from the cerebral cortex and subcortical motor centres. The most obvious output from the cerebellum is directed at motor systems. Purkinje cells are organized in modules, i.e. discrete, parallel zones that converge upon different cerebellar output nuclei coupled to different motor systems in the brain stem, spinal cord and cerebral cortex. Cerebellar function is therefore determined by temporal and spatial factors, e.g. inhibitory interneurones of the cerebellar cortex, which regulate the access of a particular combination of mossy fibre–parallel fibre inputs to an appropriate output. Plastic changes in the response properties of Purkinje cells, in the form of long-term depression of the parallel fibre–Purkinje cell synapses, may also contribute. Short-term and long-term changes in the response properties of Purkinje cells are under the influence of the climbing fibres.

A double, mirrored, localization exists in the anterior and posterior cerebellum (**Fig. 20.10**). The anterior lobe, simple lobule, pyramis and the adjoining lobules of the hemisphere of the posterior lobe all receive branches from the same mossy and climbing fibres and project to the same cerebellar nuclei. The efferent pathways of these regions monitor the activity in the corticospinal tract and in the subcortical motor systems descending from the vestibular nuclei and reticular formation. The inputs to the cerebellum and the outputs from it are organized according to the same somatotopical patterns, but the orientation of these patterns is reversed. The representation of the head is found principally in the simple lobule, and caudally in a corresponding region of the posterior lobe. The double representation of the body follows in rough somatotopic order. Vestibular connections of the cerebellum display a similar double representation in the most rostral lobules of the anterior lobe and far caudally in the vestibulocerebellum (**Fig. 20.11**).

The folium, tuber, uvula, tonsil and posterior biventral lobule all receive an almost pure pontine mossy fibre input. Climbing fibres from the inferior olive and mossy fibres from the basilar and tegmental pontine nuclei relay visual and acoustic information from the respective cerebral association areas and midbrain tectum to the folium and tuber thought to represent a vermal visual/acoustic area (**Fig. 20.10**). The efferent connections of this area travel via the fastigial nucleus to gaze centres in the pons and midbrain.

AFFERENT CONNECTIONS OF THE CEREBELLUM

Afferent connections of the cerebellum include the mossy fibres and the climbing fibres. Mossy fibre systems terminate bilaterally in transversely oriented 'lobular' areas. The terminations of different mossy fibre systems overlap considerably (**Fig. 20.4**). Climbing fibres from different subnuclei of the inferior olive terminate contralaterally, on discrete longitudinal strips of Purkinje cells. This longitudinal pattern closely corresponds with the zonal arrangement in the corticonuclear projection (**Fig. 20.12**).

Spinocerebellar and trigeminocerebellar fibres

The spinal cord is connected to the cerebellum through the spinocerebellar and cuneocerebellar tracts and through indirect mossy fibre pathways relayed by the lateral reticular nucleus in the medulla oblongata. These pathways are all excitatory in nature and give collaterals to the interposed and fastigial nuclei before ending on cortical granule cells.

The posterior spinocerebellar tract takes its origin from the posterior thoracic nucleus at the base of the dorsal horn in all thoracic segments of the spinal cord (**Fig. 20.13**). It enters the inferior cerebellar peduncle, gives collaterals to the cerebellar nuclei, and terminates, mainly ipsilaterally, in the vermis and adjoining regions of the anterior lobe and in the pyramis and adjoining lobules of the posterior lobe. The posterior thoracic nucleus receives primary afferents of all kinds from the muscles and joints of the lower limbs, which reaches the nucleus via the gracile fasciculus. It also receives collaterals from cutaneous sensory neurones. Accordingly, the tract transmits proprioceptive and exteroceptive information about the ipsilateral lower limb. Very fast conduction is required to keep the cerebellum informed about ongoing movements. The axons in the posterior spinocerebellar tract are the largest in the CNS, measuring 20 μm in external diameter. The upper limb equivalent of the posterior spinocerebellar tract is the cuneocerebellar tract.

The anterior spinocerebellar tract is a composite pathway. It informs the cerebellum about the state of activity of spinal reflex arcs related to the lower limb and lower trunk. Its fibres originate in the intermediate grey matter of the lumbar and sacral segments of the spinal cord (**Fig. 20.13**). They cross near their origin, and ascend close to the surface as far as the lower midbrain before looping down in the superior cerebellar peduncle. Most fibres cross again in the cerebellar commissure, thus their distributions to the cerebellar nuclei and cortex appear to be the same as those of the posterior tract.

The rostral spinocerebellar tract originates from cell groups of the intermediate zone and horn of the cervical enlargement. Although considered to be the upper limb and upper trunk counterpart of the anterior spinocerebellar tract, most of its fibres remain ipsilateral throughout their course. It enters the inferior cerebellar peduncle and terminates in the same cerebellar nuclei and folia as the cuneocerebellar tract.

The cuneocerebellar tract contains exteroceptive and proprioceptive components which originate from the cuneate and external cuneate nuclei respectively. The primary afferents travel in the cuneate fasciculus. The tract itself is predominantly uncrossed and ends in the posterior half of the anterior lobe. Exteroceptive and proprioceptive mossy fibre components of the tract terminate differentially in the apical and basal part of the folia. The exteroceptive component overlaps the pontocerebellar mossy fibre projection in the apices of the folia of the anterior lobe.

Comparable sets of ipsilateral proprioceptive and interoceptive cerebellar projections exist for the extensive territory of the trigeminal brain stem nuclei. These nuclei also project to the ipsilateral inferior olive, relaying there to the contralateral cerebellar cortex and deep nuclei. The cortical representation of the head is directly behind the primary fissure.

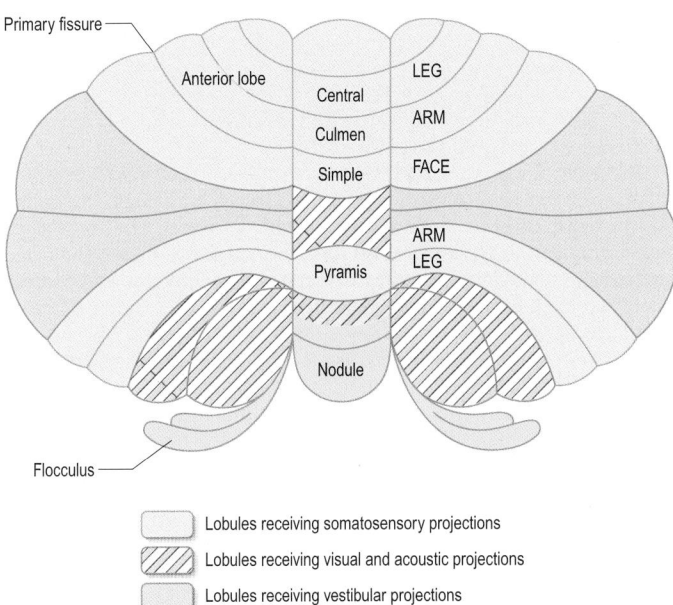

Fig. 20.10 Diagram of localizations in the cerebellar cortex. Somatosensory: pink; visual and acoustic: blue; vestibular: yellow.

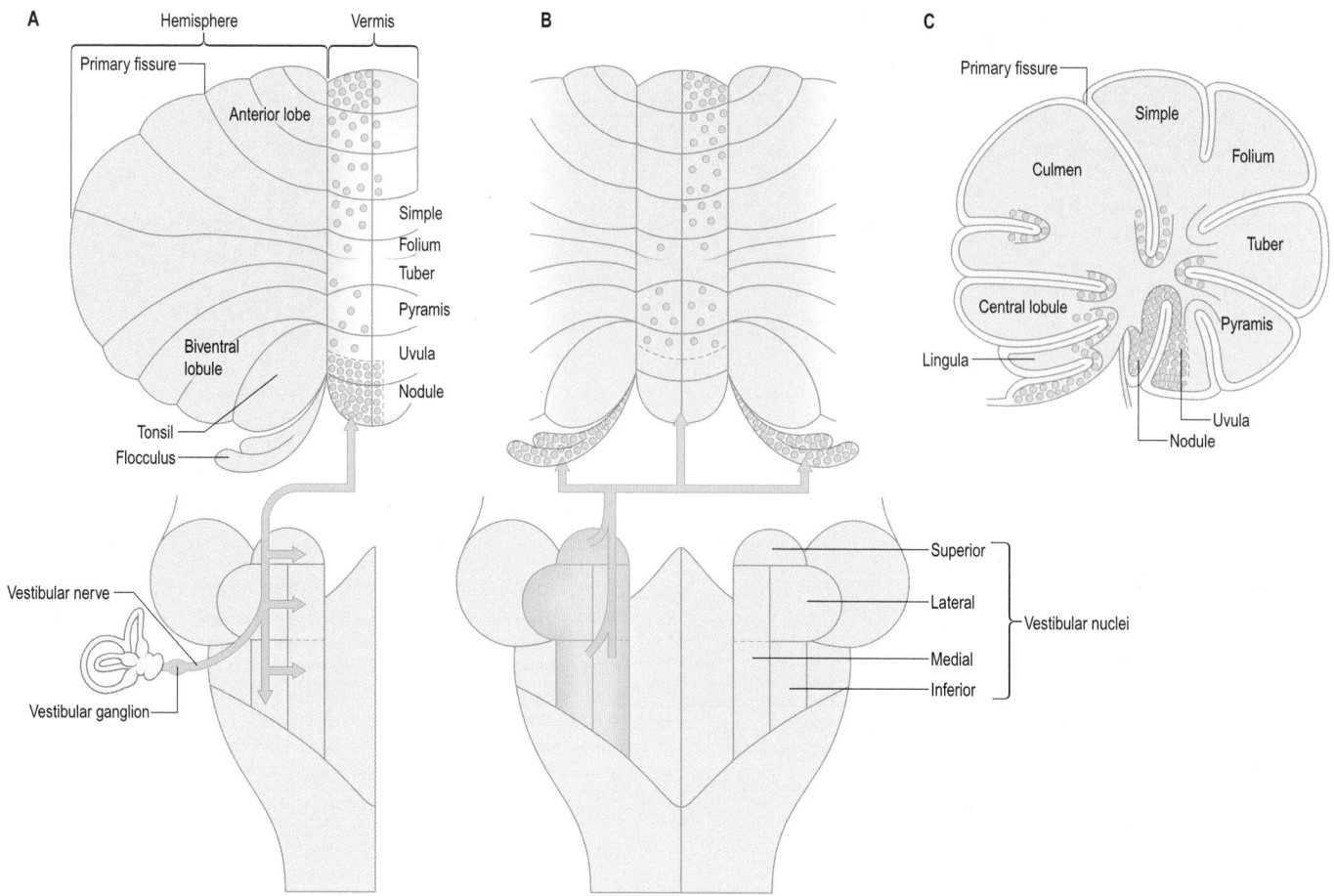

Fig. 20.11 Vestibulocerebellar mossy fibre projections. **A**, Primary vestibulocerebellar projections from the bipolar neurones of the vestibular ganglion. **B**, Secondary vestibulocerebellar projections from the vestibular nuclei. **C**, Sagittal section showing distribution of both sets of afferents.

Olivocerebellar fibres

Localization in the olivocerebellar system: zones and microzones

Climbing fibres originate exclusively from the contralateral inferior olivary complex. Projections from the different subnuclei of the inferior olive terminate as climbing fibres on longitudinal strips of Purkinje cells in the cerebellar cortex. Collaterals end on the cerebellar or vestibular target nuclei of these Purkinje cells. A longitudinal zonal arrangement is therefore characteristic of the organization of the olivocerebellar projection (**Fig. 20.12**). Moreover, the olivocerebellar projection zones correspond precisely to the corticonuclear projection zones already described. Climbing fibres from the inferior olive are able to modify the cerebellar output in such a way that cells within each subnucleus of the inferior olivary complex monitor the output of a single cerebellar module.

The inferior olivary complex and its climbing fibres can be activated by tactile, proprioceptive, visual and vestibular stimulation, and from the sensory, motor and visual cortices and their brain stem relays. A somatotopic arrangement of body parts, matching the olivary projections on to the cerebellar cortex, has been detected in animal experiments.

Olivocerebellar climbing fibre connections

The inferior olivary complex can be subdivided into a convoluted principal olivary nucleus, and posterior and medial accessory olivary nuclei. Olivary fibres form the olivocerebellar projection to the contralateral cerebellar cortex, and give off collaterals to the lateral vestibular nucleus and to the cerebellar nuclei. Climbing fibres terminate on longitudinal strips of Purkinje cells. The zonal patterns of the olivo–cerebellar and Purkinje–nuclear projections correspond precisely. The accessory olivary nuclei project to the vermis and the adjacent hemispheres. The caudal halves of the posterior and medial accessory nuclei innervate the vermis. The caudal part of the posterior accessory nucleus

projects to Deiters' nucleus and to the B zone of the anterior vermis. The caudal half of the medial accessory olive gives rise to a projection to the fastigial nucleus and provides climbing fibres to the A zone. The rostral halves of the accessory olives project to the pars intermedia. Climbing fibres from the rostral dorsal accessory olive give collateral projections to the emboliform nucleus and terminate in zones C1 and C3. Zone C2 receives terminals from the rostral medial accessory olive, which provides a collateral projection to the globose nucleus. The principal nucleus projects to the contralateral hemisphere (D zone), and gives collaterals to the dentate nucleus.

The inferior olivary complex receives afferent connections from the spinal cord and from sensory relay nuclei in the brain stem, including the posterior column and sensory trigeminal nuclei. It also receives descending connections from the superior colliculus, parvicellular red nucleus and related nuclei in the midbrain and a GABAergic projection, mainly crossed, from the cerebellar nuclei and certain vestibular nuclei. This latter nucleo-olivary pathway is topically organized. The dentate nucleus projects to the principal nucleus, the emboliform nucleus to the rostral posterior accessory nucleus, and the globose nucleus to the rostral medial accessory nucleus. The fastigial nucleus is connected with the caudal medial accessory olive, but the connections are less numerous. The caudal posterior accessory olive receives a nucleo-olivary projection from the lateral vestibular nucleus.

The posterior accessory olive and the caudal half of the medial accessory olive receive an input from the spinal cord and sensory relay nuclei. The middle region of the medial accessory olive receives a projection from the superior colliculus and projects to folium and vermis. The parvocellular red nucleus and related nuclei project to the olive through the ipsilateral descending central tegmental tracts, which terminate in the rostral half of the medial accessory olive and the principal olive. The parvocellular red nucleus receives converging projections from the cerebellar nuclei and from the motor and premotor cortex. Direct pathways from the cerebral cortex to the

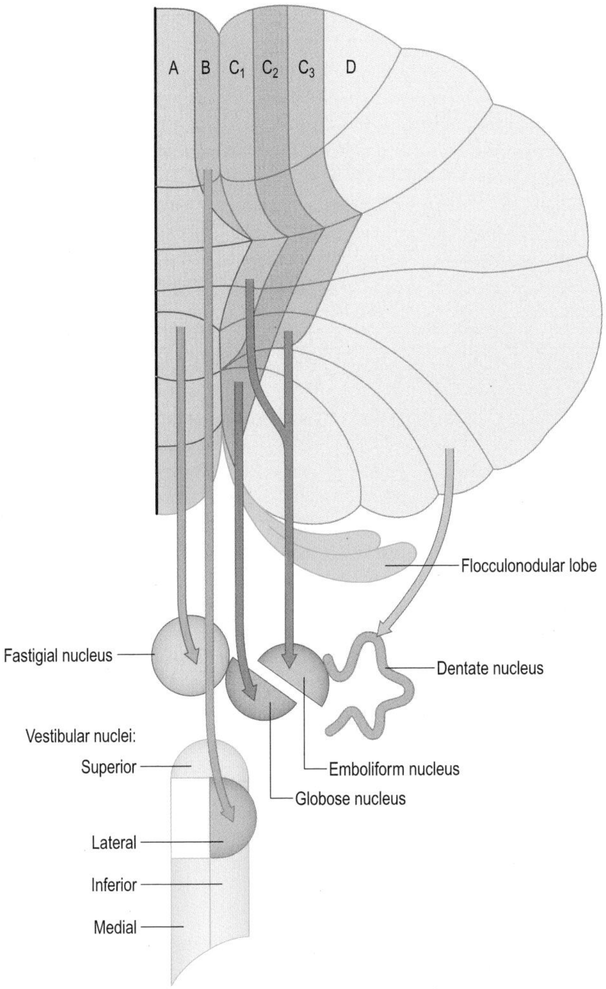

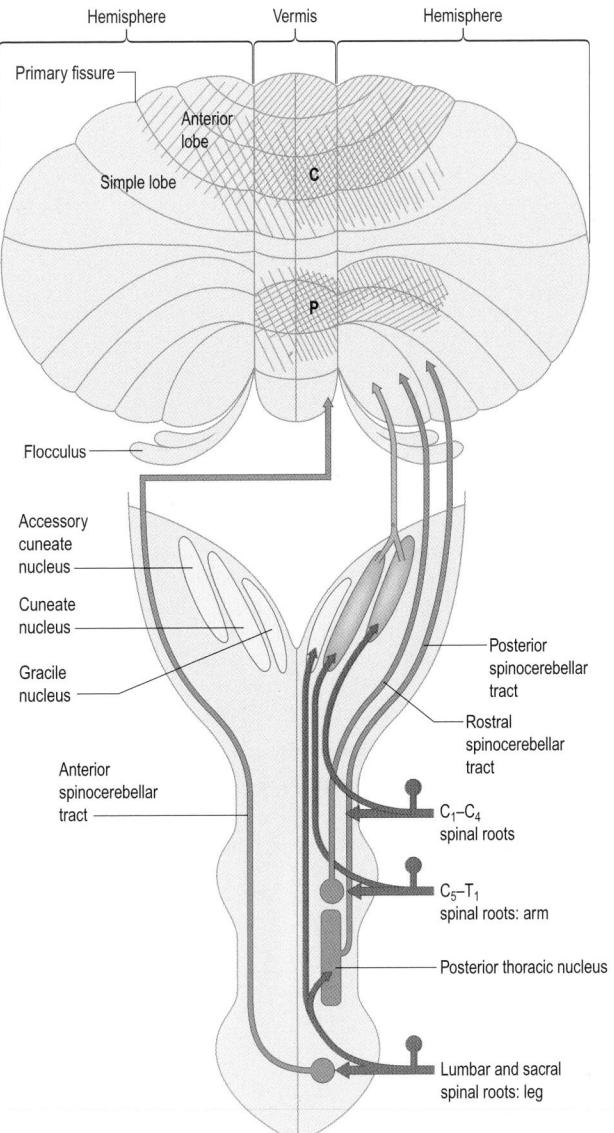

Fig. 20.12 Cerebellar corticonuclear and corticovestibular projections. The widespread projection from flocculonodular lobe to vestibular nucleus is not arrowed but is indicated in green. (Based on data from Voogd J 1964 The cerebellum of the cat. Proefschr. Van Gorcum: Assen, and from Voogd J, Bigaré F 1980 Topographic distribution of olivary and corticonuclear fibers in the cerebellum: a review. In: Courville J, de Mountigny I, y Latha RE (eds) The Inferior Olivary Nucleus. New York: Raven Press, pp 207–234.)

Fig. 20.13 Spinocerebellar (red) and cuneocerebellar (blue) mossy fibre projections overlap extensively in the culmen (C), pyramis (P) and related intermediate areas of the cortex.

inferior olive are sparse. The indirect pathways via the parvicellular red nucleus are much stronger.

Climbing fibres, which terminate in the vestibulocerebellum (flocculus and nodule), are derived from neurones of the medial accessory olive, which receive a strong descending afferent connection from optokinetic centres in the midbrain. Optokinetic information is used by the flocculus in long-term adaptation of compensatory eye movements. Neighbouring neurones are under vestibular control and project to the nodule and the adjoining uvula.

Vestibulocerebellar fibres

Primary vestibulocerebellar mossy fibres are fibres of the vestibular branch of the vestibulocochlear nerve. They enter the cerebellum with the ascending branch of the vestibular nerve, and pass through the superior vestibular nucleus and the juxtarestiform body. They terminate, mainly ipsilaterally, in the granular layer of the nodule, caudal part of the uvula, ventral part of the anterior lobe and bottom of the deep fissures of the vermis (**Fig. 20.11A**). Secondary vestibulocerebellar mossy fibres arise from the superior vestibular nucleus and the caudal portions of the medial and inferior vestibular nuclei. They terminate bilaterally not only in the same regions that receive primary vestibulocerebellar fibres but also in the flocculus, which lacks a primary vestibulocerebellar projection (**Fig. 20.11B**). Some of the mossy fibres from the medial and inferior vestibular nuclei are cholinergic.

Reticulocerebellar fibres

The lateral reticular nucleus of the medulla oblongata, and the paramedian reticular and tegmental reticular nuclei of the pons, give rise to mossy fibres. The latter nuclei also supply major collateral projections to the cerebellar nuclei. Spinoreticular fibres terminate in a somatotopical pattern within the entire lateral reticular nucleus, where they overlap with collaterals from the rubrospinal and lateral vestibulospinal tracts and a projection from the cerebral cortex.

The lateral reticular nucleus projects bilaterally to the vermis and hemispheres of the cerebellum. The projection from the dorsal part of the nucleus, which receives collaterals from the rubrospinal tract in addition to spinal afferents, is centred on the ipsilateral hemisphere. The ventral part of the nucleus, which receives a strong projection from the spinal cord and a collateral projection from the lateral vestibulospinal tract, projects bilaterally, mainly to the vermis. The lateral reticular nucleus provides a strong projection to the superior fastigial nucleus, the emboliform nucleus and the medial pole of the globose nucleus.

The paramedian reticular nucleus consists of cell groups at the lateral border of the medial longitudinal fasciculus. It receives fibres from the vestibular nuclei and the interstitiospinal and tectospinal tracts (which descend in the medial longitudinal fasciculus), and from the spinal cord and the cerebral cortex. It projects to the entire cerebellum.

The tegmental reticular nucleus of the pons is located next to the midline in the caudal half of the tegmentum. It receives afferent connections from the cerebral cortex, tectum, nucleus of the optic tract and cerebellar nuclei via the crossed descending branch of the superior cerebellar peduncle. Efferents from the tegmental reticular nucleus reach

363

the cerebellum through the middle cerebellar peduncle. Some terminate superficially in the cortex of the anterior lobe, but many more end in the simple lobule, folium, tuber, vermis and adjoining flocculus. Additional efferents terminate in the caudal fastigial nucleus, dentate nucleus and lateral parts of the globose nucleus.

Pontocerebellar fibres

The cerebral cortex is the largest single source of fibres that project to the pontine nuclei. Fibres from the pontine nuclei access the cerebellum via the middle cerebellar peduncle, which is the largest afferent system of the human cerebellum. Many corticopontine fibres are collaterals of axons that project to other targets in the brain or spinal cord, e.g. it is likely that all corticospinal fibres give off collaterals to the pontine nuclei. Although corticopontine axons arise from lamina V pyramidal cells, the projection from different areas of the cerebral cortex is highly uneven. The areas of cerebral cortex that project to the pontine nuclei are those that are particularly involved in the control of movement. For example, in the case of visual areas, the input arises from extrastriate visual areas in the parietal lobe, whose cells are responsive to movement, and function as important links in the visual guidance of movement. Dorsal pontine nuclei receive collateral branches from corticotectal fibres that project to the superior and inferior colliculi from the parietal, temporal and frontal areas of the cerebral cortex, and from tectopontine relays. The onward pontocerebellar projections are to the simple lobule and to the folium and tuber of the vermis.

Fibres of the pontine reticular nuclei are distributed bilaterally, with ipsilateral predominance, to all lobules of the cerebellum other than the lingula and nodule.

More than 90% of fibres in the middle cerebellar peduncle belong to the corticopontocerebellar pathway. Corticopontine fibres travel in the cerebral peduncle. Fibres from the frontal lobe occupy the medial part of the peduncle, and fibres from the parietal, occipital and temporal lobes occupy the lateral part. They synapse on some 20 million neurones in corresponding regions of the basilar pons. The onward pontocerebellar mossy fibre projection is predominantly to the lateral regions of the posterior and anterior lobes, but collaterals are given off to the dentate nucleus (**Fig. 20.4A**).

EFFERENT CONNECTIONS OF THE CEREBELLUM

The output of the cerebellum consists of the inhibitory projections of the Purkinje cells to the cerebellar and vestibular nuclei, and the efferent connections of the cerebellar nuclei to motor centres in the brain stem and, through the thalamus, the motor cortex. Their effects on movement are always indirect, as there are no direct projections from the cerebellar nuclei to motor neurones. Disynaptic connections of the Purkinje cells in the anterior vermis and vestibulocerebellum with motor neurones controlling oculogyric and proximal limb muscles are mediated by the vestibular nuclei. The vermis also influences these motor neurones bilaterally through multisynaptic pathways that involve the fastigial and vestibular nuclei and the reticular formation (**Fig. 20.14**). The

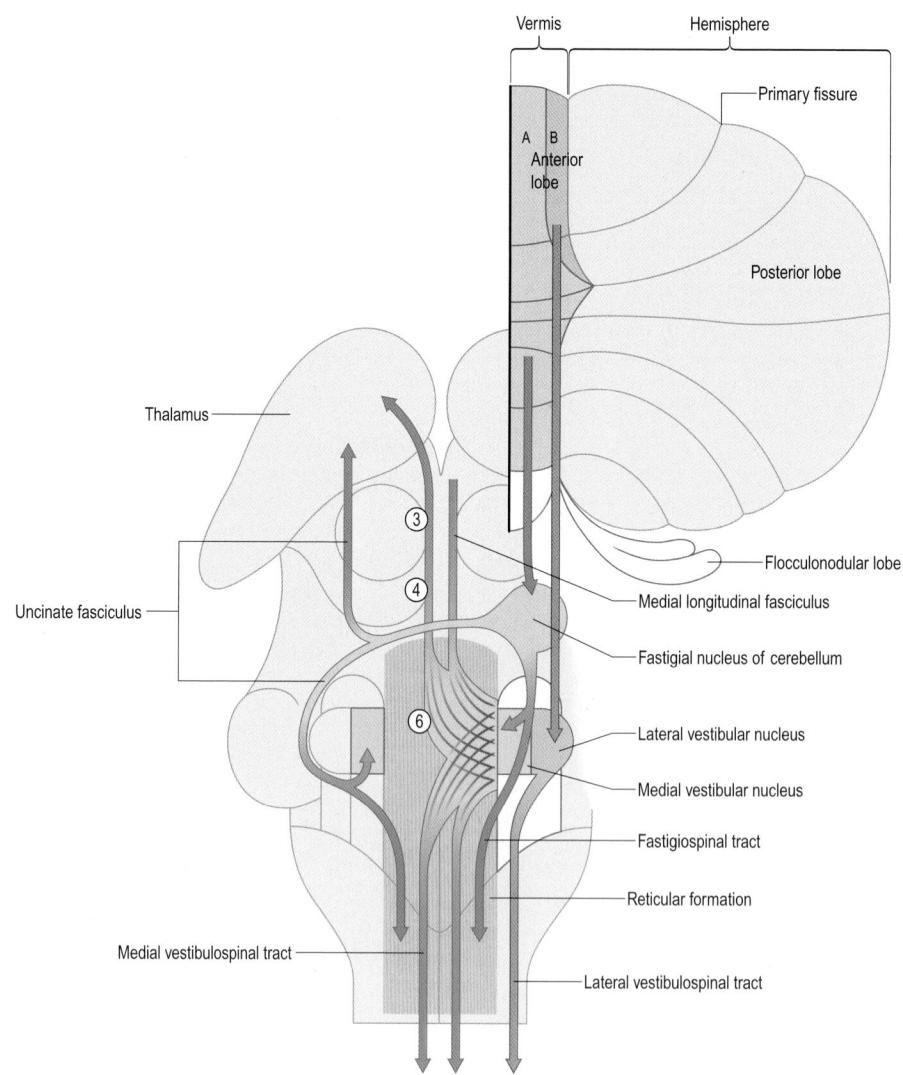

Fig. 20.14 Efferent connections of the vermis. Connections of the A zones of the vermis and flocculonodular lobe with the fastigial nucleus are indicated, also those of the B zone with the lateral vestibular nucleus. Some vestibular efferents ascend bilaterally to the ocular motor nuclei and thalamus, others descend to the spinal cord. Motor nuclei of the 3rd, 4th and 6th cranial nerves: 3; 4; 6.

vermis cannot be considered as a single module. Each half of the vermis is composed of several modules (each made up of a longitudinal Purkinje cell zone and a target nucleus) and their supporting climbing fibre afferent projections.

Each cerebellar hemisphere influences movements of the ipsilateral extremities by way of projections to the dentate and interposed (emboliform and globose) nuclei, which in turn project to the contralateral red nucleus, thalamus and motor cortex (**Fig. 20.15**).

Corticonuclear and corticovestibular fibres

Purkinje cells of each hemivermis project to the ipsilateral fastigial and vestibular nuclei. Purkinje cells of the hemisphere project to the interposed and dentate nuclei. Although the cerebellar cortex is organized in strips of Purkinje cell zones, which project to different cerebellar and vestibular nuclei, the borders between these strips are not apparent in the structure of the cortex when it is examined histologically using conventional staining methods. The vermis of the anterior lobe and simple lobule consist of two parallel strips, A and B, of Purkinje cells (**Figs 20.12, 20.14**). The medial strip (A zone) projects to the rostral pole of the fastigial nucleus, and the lateral strip (B zone) projects to the lateral vestibular nucleus. The B zone does not continue beyond the simple lobule. The cortex of the entire caudal vermis, which projects to the fastigial nucleus, is included in the A zone. The folium and tuber, which represent a region of the cerebellum that receives a visual input and which are involved in the accurate calibration of saccades, project to the caudal pole of the fastigial nucleus. The pyramis, uvula and nodule can be subdivided into several Purkinje cell zones. However, the significance of their connections with the cerebellar and vestibular nuclei is not well understood. Corticovestibular projections to the superior, medial and inferior vestibular nuclei, but not to the lateral nucleus, take their origin from the nodule and the adjacent region of the uvula.

The intermediate region consists of two strips of Purkinje cells (C1 and C3 zones), which project to the anterior interposed nucleus. They flank a single zone (C2) that projects to the posterior interposed nucleus (**Figs 20.12, 20.15**). The rest of the hemisphere projects to the dentate nucleus. There are indications for a subdivision of the hemisphere into two zones that project to the caudolateral zone and rostromedial parts of the dentate nucleus. The neurones of the caudolateral dentate are generally smaller than those of the rostromedial dentate and the convolutions are broader. The efferent connections of the flocculus are mainly with the superior, medial and inferior vestibular nuclei and resemble those from the nodule and uvula.

Cerebellovestibular and cerebelloreticular fibres

Efferent connections of the fastigial nucleus

The fastigial nucleus is connected bilaterally with the vestibular nuclei and the medullary and pontine reticular formation (**Figs 20.12, 20.15**). Smaller crossed connections either ascend to the midbrain and diencephalon or descend into the spinal cord. Small GABAergic neurones give rise to nucleo-olivary fibres, which terminate in the medial accessory olive. The uncinate fasciculus is the major efferent pathway of the fastigial nucleus. Its fibres cross in the rostral part of the cerebellar commissure, and pass dorsal to the superior cerebellar peduncle, to

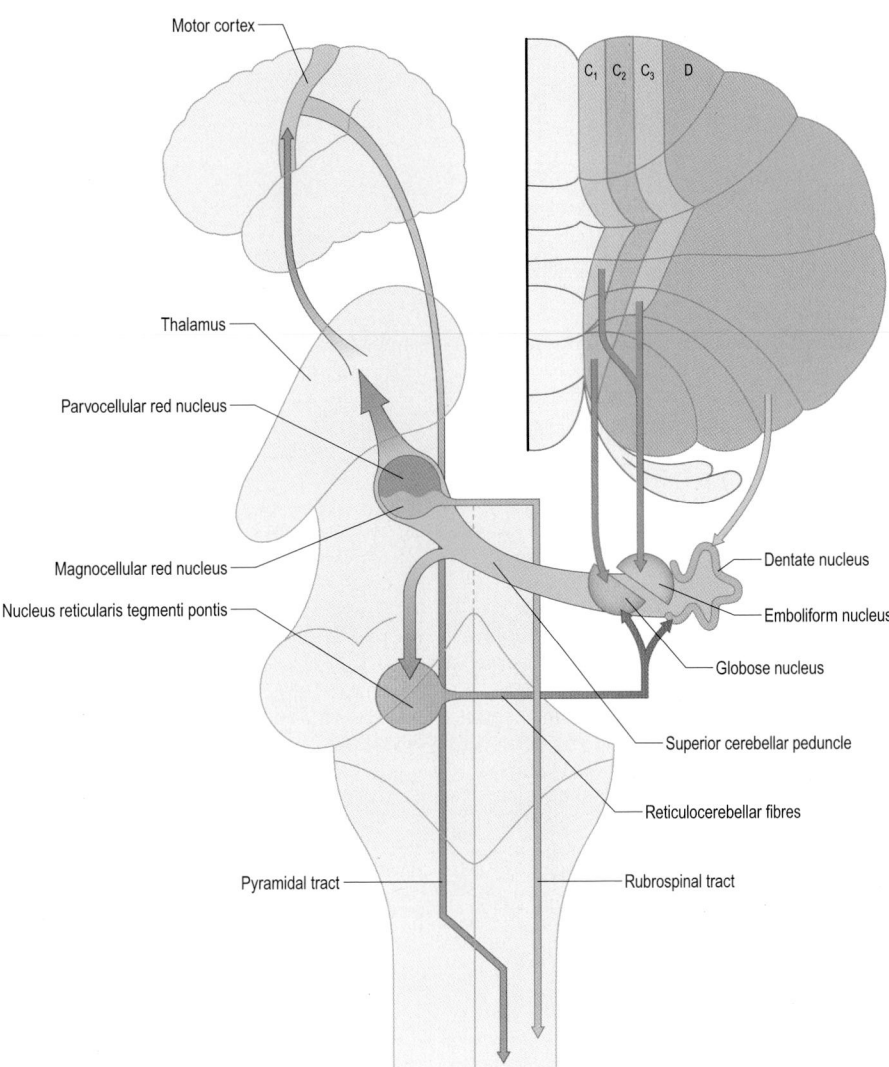

Fig. 20.15 Efferent connections of the cerebellar hemisphere. Purkinje cell zones and their target nuclei are indicated with the same colours. Efferent fibres from the motor cortex and from the very small magnocellular red nucleus recross and descend to the upper part of the spinal cord.

enter the vestibular nuclei from their lateral side. Uncrossed fibres enter the vestibular nuclei through the juxtarestiform body (**Fig. 20.6**). The distribution of the fastigial projection is bilateral, but with a contralateral preponderance (**Fig. 20.14**). Crossed and uncrossed projections end in the medial and inferior vestibular nuclei. They also cross these nuclei to terminate in the medial reticular formation. Some crossed fibres can be traced caudally into the spinal cord. A small fascicle of crossed fibres from the fastigial nucleus ascends along the superior cerebellar peduncle and is distributed bilaterally to the dorsal tegmentum, central grey matter and deep layers of the superior colliculus and the nuclei of the posterior commissure. Fibres terminate bilaterally in the ventrolateral nucleus and the intralaminar nuclei of the thalamus.

Cerebellovestibular connections

The relationship between the cerebellum and the vestibular nuclei is complex (**Fig. 20.14**). In addition to the vestibulocerebellum (nodule, adjacent folia of the uvula and flocculus), the main vermis and the fastigial nucleus also project to the vestibular nuclei. The vestibulocerebellum projects to the superior, medial and inferior vestibular nuclei. Neurones of these nuclei, which receive an input from the vestibular nerve and project to the nuclei controlling eye movements (vestibulo-ocular relay cells), are among the main targets of the Purkinje cells of the nodule and flocculus. Through these connections with vestibulo-ocular relay neurones, the flocculus is involved in the long-term adaptation of compensatory eye movements, the generation of smooth eye movements used to pursue an object, and the suppression of the vestibulo-ocular reflex during smooth pursuit. The function of the nodule in the control of eye movement is less well understood.

The vestibular nuclei are the main source of mossy fibre afferents to the nodule. Their projection to the flocculus is relatively minor. Most mossy fibres which terminate in the flocculus arise from the reticular formation and relay optokinetic and visual information.

The lateral vestibular nucleus, which lacks an input from the labyrinth and receives Purkinje cell axons from the B zone of the anterior vermis, can be regarded as a displaced cerebellar nucleus. It gives rise to the lateral vestibulospinal tract, which descends to all levels of the spinal cord. It is avoided by the efferent pathways from the fastigial nucleus, which terminate more ventrally on large neurones in the magnocellular part of the medial vestibular nucleus and in the medial reticular formation. The medial and inferior vestibular nuclei receive a major input from the vestibular nerve. They give rise to bilaterally ascending and descending tracts, which course in the medial longitudinal fasciculus. The ascending tract is composed predominantly of the axons of vestibulo-ocular relay cells. The descending fibres form the medial vestibulospinal tract, which is particularly involved in head righting reflexes when the trunk is tilted.

Fastigial fibres, which terminate in the reticular formation, stimulate the bilaterally descending medullary reticulospinal tracts. The A zone of the vermis exerts a bilateral influence on ventromedially located spinal interneurones and motor neurones that innervate axial, truncal and proximal limb muscles. Some fibres of the uncinate tract descend as far as the cervical cord, where they terminate on the same motor neurones. The B zone exerts an influence on ipsilateral interneurones and motor neurones of the same system through its projection to the lateral vestibular nucleus and the lateral vestibulospinal tract.

The projections of the fastigial nucleus to the thalamus are relatively minor. They are bilateral, as a result of the recrossing of the crossed ascending fibres of the uncinate fasciculus. Their targets include parts of the ventrolateral nucleus and the intralaminar, centrolateral and parafascicular nuclei. Fibres that terminate in the ventrolateral nucleus lie medial to the terminations of fibres from the dentate and interposed nuclei. This region of the ventrolateral nucleus projects to the upper region of the motor cortex and sends collaterals to the medullary reticular formation, which influences ventromedial interneurones and motor neurones in lumbar and sacral segments of the spinal cord via the medullary reticulospinal tracts.

The caudal region of the fastigial nucleus receives Purkinje cell axons from the folium and tuber, an area of the vermis that receives visual inputs. It projects to the contralateral horizontal gaze centre, or paramedian pontine reticular formation (PPRF), and the vertical gaze centre, or rostral interstitial nucleus of the medial longitudinal fascicle (riMLF), and, bilaterally, to deep layers of the superior colliculus. These projections probably mediate the adaptation of saccades by the vermal visual area.

The cerebellum influences visceromotor systems via the projections of the fastigial nucleus to the parasolitary nucleus (a region bordering the viscerosensory nuclei of the solitary tract), the dorsal visceromotor nucleus of the vagus, the central grey matter, the serotoninergic raphe nuclei of the pons and medulla, and the noradrenergic nucleus of the locus coeruleus.

Other pathways from the cerebellar nuclei terminate on precerebellar relay nuclei that give rise to mossy or climbing fibres. Recurrent circuits involving the fastigial nucleus include the nucleus reticularis tegmenti pontis and a projection from the fastigial nucleus to the medial accessory olive. Nucleo-olivary projections arise from all the cerebellar nuclei, are crossed, and contain GABA as a neurotransmitter. The connections of the fastigial nucleus with the reticular nuclei are excitatory.

Cerebellar nuclei also project to the contralateral interstitial nucleus (of Darkschewitsch), which lies at the boundary between the midbrain and diencephalon. This nucleus projects to the medial accessory olive via the central tegmental tract. The fastigial nucleus controls the climbing fibre output of the medial accessory olive, both via its nucleo-olivary projection and by its connection to the nucleus of Darkschewitsch.

Cerebellorubral and cerebellothalamic fibres

The axons of neurones in the dentate and interposed nuclei leave the cerebellum in the superior cerebellar peduncle. The superior peduncles, including their nucleo-olivary component, decussate in the caudal midbrain (**Fig. 20.15**). Each peduncle then gives off a small descending branch carrying fibres that terminate in the medial reticular formation of the pons and medulla and the pontine tegmental reticular nucleus (**Fig. 20.15**). The nucleo-olivary fibres join this descending branch and terminate in the inferior olive in a strictly orderly manner. The ascending branch is distributed to the midbrain and diencephalon, mainly to the red nucleus and thalamus. The anterior interposed nucleus projects to the magnocellular part of the red nucleus. In humans this projection is very small and it gives rise to a relatively trivial rubrospinal tract, which crosses in the caudal midbrain and terminates on lateral medullary interneurones and a small number of motor neurones in the upper cervical spinal cord.

The anterior interposed nucleus projects to lateral parts of the ventrolateral nucleus of the thalamus, which are connected with elements of the motor cortex projecting to axial and proximal limb muscles, and to the reticular formation of the pons and medulla. It also projects to the pontine tegmental reticular nucleus and to basal pontine nuclei, both of which give rise to mossy fibres. Its nucleo-olivary efferents terminate in the rostral half of the dorsal accessory olive.

The projections of the posterior interposed nucleus are very similar to those of the fastigial nucleus. The two nuclei share projections to the cord, the superior colliculus, the central grey matter and the raphe nuclei. Nucleo-olivary projections from the globose nucleus and the recurrent globose nucleus–interstitial nucleus–inferior olivary nucleus pathway converge upon the rostral half of the medial accessory olive. The thalamic projections overlap those from the fastigial and anterior interposed nuclei.

The dentate nucleus projects to the contralateral parvicellular red nucleus and the thalamus. The central tegmental tract takes its origin from the parvocellular red nucleus and terminates on the principal nucleus of the olive. The thalamic projection to the ventrolateral nucleus overlaps those of the other cerebellar nuclei. The inferior and lateral parts of the dentate nucleus project into the most medial region of the ventrolateral nucleus, which in turn projects to the premotor area of the frontal lobe.

The thalamus receives a massive input from other major motor systems, in addition to the input it receives from the cerebellum. In particular, the output of the basal ganglia is relayed to the thalamus by a projection from the globus pallidus. Available evidence suggests that these two great subcortical motor systems terminate on different regions in the ventral thalamus and project to different targets in the motor and premotor cortex.

CEREBELLAR FUNCTIONS

ANTICIPATORY FUNCTION

The vermis of the cerebellum is involved in taking anticipatory action in order to maintain upright posture when objects are picked up. For example, when a book is taken down from a shelf, the first muscle groups to be activated are not the flexors of shoulder, elbow or fingers, but the plantar flexors of the ankle. Contraction of the ankle flexors causes the forefeet to push the lower limbs and trunk backwards at the moment the hand grasps the book. Once the lift gets under way, the erector spinae muscles correct for the combined weights of the book and the reaching arm, in order to prevent forward sway of the head and trunk. Labyrinthine receptors simultaneously inform the cerebellum of any forward movement of the head, and appropriate antigravity thrust is exerted via one or both lateral vestibulospinal tracts. Damage to the vermis may cause total loss of the anticipatory function of the trunk musculature, with the result that any reaching movement may cause the patient to fall in the direction of reach (p. 367). Damage to the anterior lobe may also compromise the anticipatory function, in this case by deterioration or severance of its linkage with the pontine and medullary reticular nuclei, with resultant gait ataxia.

POSTURAL FIXATION

The posterolateral region of the cerebellum is required to prevent oscillation of distal limb parts caused by the viscoelastic properties of the muscles in response to sudden movements. If a volunteer is instructed to exert rapid wrist extension and to maintain the extended posture for two seconds, electromyographic records taken from the prime movers and antagonists reveal that the antagonists begin to contract prior to completion of the movement, and that they continue to contract and relax several times in alternating fashion with the prime movers, although with much less force, during the measured fixation period. This 'freeze' control of the wrist can be disrupted by disease of the contralateral posterior lobe, resulting in an action tremor.

MOTOR LEARNING

Experiments with monkeys have shown that when a novel motor skill is being learned, the olivocerebellar climbing fibre system becomes active when errors are made. The inferior olivary complex appears to be involved in correction, based on receipt of a copy of the intended movement from collateral branches of the corticospinal tract. Cerebellar output via the superior cerebellar peduncle is also copied on to the parvicellular red nucleus and projected from there to the inferior olive, where it can be compared with the original. Short bursts of climbing fibre activity depress the Purkinje cells responsible for producing the errors. Most human cerebellar disorders involve the anterior and/or

posterior lobes or their outflows, causing the monitoring system to be lost, and learned movements to become clumsy.

Many motor skills require precise timing, which involves an extreme degree of cooperation between prime movers and their antagonists. For example, reading a printed page requires that the scanning eyes snap back to the beginning of a line, time after time. Even small errors may result in dyslexia, where slight incoordination of eye movements may cause the letters of a word to appear jumbled. Clinical testing of timing can be performed easily by checking the ability to perform rhythmic movements such as repetitive pronation/supination (**Fig. 20.16**).

HIGHER FUNCTIONS

The cerebellum is currently believed to participate in higher brain functions. This is not unexpected in view of the two-way linkages (via the thalamus) that exist between the cerebellum and the association and paralimbic areas of the cerebral cortex. Its role appears to be one of assistance rather than of generation. For example, during speech, the right posterolateral region of the cerebellum is active bilaterally, which reflects its role in coordinating the muscles involved. However, there is a right-sided predominance, which is consistent with a possible linkage (via the thalamus) with the motor speech area of the left frontal cortex. Moreover, because right lateral cerebellar activity is even greater during functional naming, e.g. 'dig', 'fly', than during object identification, e.g. 'shovel', 'airplane', cognitive as well as motor functions are compromised by cerebellar disorders.

CEREBELLAR DYSFUNCTION

MIDLINE LESIONS: TRUNCAL ATAXIA

Isolated lesions of the vermis are produced in children by medulloblastomas in the roof of the fourth ventricle. In the recumbent position there may be no abnormality of motor coordination in the limbs, but there is a progressive inability to stand upright without support, a state known as truncal ataxia. These tumours, which are highly sensitive to radiotherapy, attack the pathway from the vermis to the nuclei of the vestibular nerves. The ataxia reflects malfunction of the linkage between the vermis and the lateral vestibular nucleus, which means that the antigravity support normally driven by the lateral vestibulospinal tract is lost or impaired. Nystagmus can be elicited during visual tracking of the examiner's finger from side to side, and reflects disruption of the

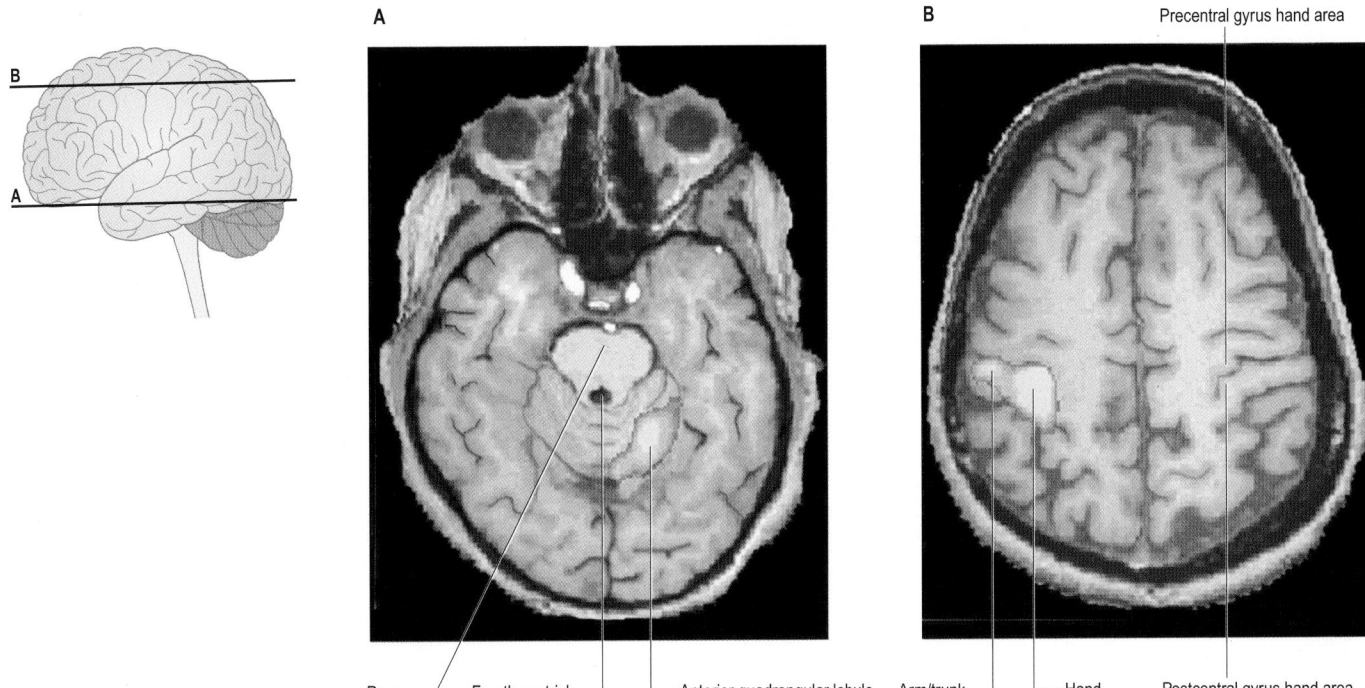

A B Precentral gyrus hand area

Pons — Fourth ventricle — Anterior quadrangular lobule Arm/trunk — Hand Postcentral gyrus hand area

Fig. 20.16 fMRI (functional magnetic resonance imaging) of a volunteer executing repetitive finger movements of the right hand. The arm/trunk areal activity is attributable to a stabilization function. (By kind permission from Drs JP Finn and T Parrish, Northwestern University School of Medicine, Chicago.)

labyrinthine connections. Scanning movements of the eye are inaccurate because the vermis no longer controls the gaze centres effectively.

ANTERIOR LOBE LESIONS: GAIT ATAXIA

Disease of the anterior lobe is most often observed in chronic alcoholics and results from prolonged thiamine deficiency. Postmortem studies reveal pronounced shrinkage of the cortex of the anterior lobe. There can be losses of up to 10% of granule cells, 20% of Purkinje cells, and a 30% reduction in the thickness of the molecular layer. The principal anatomical effect is atrophy of the connections between the anterior lobe and interposed nuclei and the reticulospinal pathways involved in normal locomotion. Incoordination of the lower limbs leads to a staggering gait, and inability to perform heel to toe walking.

Tendon reflexes may be depressed in the lower limbs because of the loss of tonic stimulation of fusimotor neurones via the pontine reticulospinal tract. This causes a reduction of monosynaptic reflex activity during walking, which may eventually produce stretching of soft tissues, a phenomenon that can result in hyperextension of the knee joint during standing.

NEOCEREBELLAR LESIONS: INCOORDINATION OF VOLUNTARY MOVEMENTS

Disease of the neocerebellar cortex, dentate nucleus, or white matter of the superior cerebellar peduncle, leads to incoordination of voluntary movements, particularly in the upper limb. When fine purposive movements are attempted, an 'action tremor' or 'intention tremor' develops: the hand and forearm quiver as the target is approached because of faulty agonist/antagonist muscle synergies around the elbow and wrist. The hand may travel past the target ('overshoot'). The normal smooth trajectory of reaching movements may be replaced by stepped flexions, abductions, etc. ('decomposition of movement'). Rapid alternating movements performed under command, such as pronation/supination, become irregular as a consequence of the loss of the timing function of the cerebellum. The 'finger-to-nose' and 'heel-to-knee' tests are performed with equal clumsiness whether the eyes are open or closed. This is in contrast to performance of these tasks in posterior column disease, where performance is adequate when the eyes are open. Speech is impaired both with regard to phonation and to articulation. Phonation (production of vowel sounds) is uneven and often tremulous, reflecting the loss of smoothness of contraction of the expiratory muscles. Articulation is slurred ('cerebellar dysarthria') because of faulty coordination of the groups of muscles that move the lips, tongue and soft palate, and which act on the temporomandibular joint. Signs of neocerebellar disorder sometimes originate in the midbrain or pons rather than in the cerebellum itself. Such lesions are usually vascular and interrupt one or other cerebellothalamic pathway (or both, if the decussation of the superior cerebellar peduncles is affected).

'Cerebellar cognitive affective syndrome' is the term used to indicate cerebral functional deficits that follow sudden severe damage to the cerebellum, e.g. after thrombosis of one of the three pairs of cerebellar arteries, or surgical removal of a cerebellar tumour. Such patients show cognitive defects in the form of diminished reasoning power, inattention, grammatical errors of speech, poor spatial sense, and patchy memory loss. If the vermis is included in the lesion, affective (emotional) symptoms appear, in the form of flatness of affect (dulling of emotional responses) or of aberrant emotional behaviour. There may be a reduced blood flow (on PET) in one or more of the associated areas linked to the cerebellum by corticopontocerebellar fibres.

REFERENCES

Bastian AJ, Mugnaini E, Thach WT 1999 Cerebellum. In: Zigmond MJ, Bloom FE, Landis SC, Roberts JL, Squire LR (eds) Fundamental Neuroscience. San Diego: Academic Press: 973–92.

Jueptner M, Kruckenberg M 2001 Anatomic basis of functional magnetic resonance imaging. Motor system. Neuroimage Clin N Am 11: 203–19.

Rae C, Haresty JA, Dzendrowskyj TE et al 2002 Cerebellar morphology in developmental dyslexia. Neuropsychologia 40: 1285–92.

Schmahmann JD, Sherman JC 1998 The cerebellar cognitive affective syndrome. Brain 121: 561–79.

Ivry RB, Spencer RM, Zelaznik HN, Diedrichsen J 2002 The cerebellum and event timing. Ann NY Acad Sci 978: 302–17.

Gebhart AL, Petersen SE, Thach WT 2002 Role of the posterolateral cerebellum in language. Ann NY Acad Sci 978: 318–33.

One of several studies using fMRI which have indicated that the right posterolateral cerebellum is involved during word retrieval and syntax generation.

Topka H, Mescheriakov S, Boose A et al 1999 A cerebellar-like terminal and postural tremor induced in normal man by transcranial magnetic stimulation. Brain 122: 1551–62.

Diencephalon

The diencephalon is part of the prosencephalon (forebrain), which develops from the foremost primary cerebral vesicle and differentiates into a caudal diencephalon and rostral telencephalon. The cerebral hemispheres develop from the sides of the telencephalon, each containing a lateral ventricle. The sites of evagination become the interventricular foramina, through which the two lateral ventricles and midline third ventricle communicate. The diencephalon corresponds largely to the structures that develop lateral to the third ventricle.

The lateral walls of the diencephalon form the epithalamus most superiorly, the thalamus centrally and the subthalamus and hypothalamus most inferiorly. The epithalamus in the mature brain contains the anterior and posterior paraventricular nuclei, the medial and lateral habenular nuclei, the stria medullaris thalami and the pineal gland. The thalamus undergoes proliferation to form numerous nuclear masses, which have extensive reciprocal connections with the cerebral cortex. The subthalamic region consists of the subthalamic nucleus, zona incerta and the fields of Forel. The subthalamic nucleus is closely related to the basal ganglia and is considered with them (Ch. 23). The hypothalamic rudiment gives rise to most of the subdivisions of the adult hypothalamus.

THALAMUS

The thalamus is an ovoid nuclear mass, c.4 cm long, which borders the dorsal part of third ventricle (**Figs 21.1–21.3, Fig. 12.10**). The narrow anterior pole lies close to the midline, and forms the posterior boundary of the interventricular foramen. Posteriorly, an expansion, the pulvinar, extends beyond the third ventricle to overhang the superior colliculus (**Fig. 21.4**). The brachium of the superior colliculus (superior quadrigeminal brachium) separates the pulvinar above from the medial geniculate body below. A small oval elevation, the lateral geniculate body, lies lateral to the medial geniculate.

The superior (dorsal) surface of the thalamus (**Fig. 21.2**) is covered by a thin layer of white matter, the stratum zonale. It extends laterally from the line of reflection of the ependyma (taenia thalami), and forms the roof of the third ventricle. This curved surface is separated from the overlying body of the fornix by the choroid fissure with the tela choroidea within it. More laterally it forms part of the floor of the lateral ventricle. The lateral border of the superior surface of the thalamus is marked by the stria terminalis and overlying thalamostriate vein, which separate the thalamus from the body of the caudate nucleus. Laterally, a slender sheet of white matter, the external medullary lamina, separates the main body of the thalamus from the reticular nucleus. Lateral to this, the thick posterior limb of the internal capsule lies between the thalamus and the lentiform complex.

The medial surface of the thalamus is the superior (dorsal) part of the lateral wall of the third ventricle (**Fig. 16.8**). It is usually connected to the contralateral thalamus by an interthalamic adhesion behind the interventricular foramina. The boundary with the hypothalamus is marked by an indistinct hypothalamic sulcus, which curves from the upper end of the cerebral aqueduct to the interventricular foramen. The thalamus is continuous with the midbrain tegmentum, the subthalamus and the hypothalamus.

Internally, the thalamus is divided into anterior, medial and lateral nuclear groups by a vertical Y-shaped sheet of white matter, the internal medullary lamina, (**Figs 21.5, 21.6**). In addition, intralaminar nuclei lie embedded within, and surrounded by, the internal medullary lamina. Midline nuclei either abut the ependyma of the lateral walls of the third ventricle medially, or lie adjacent to, and to some extent within, the

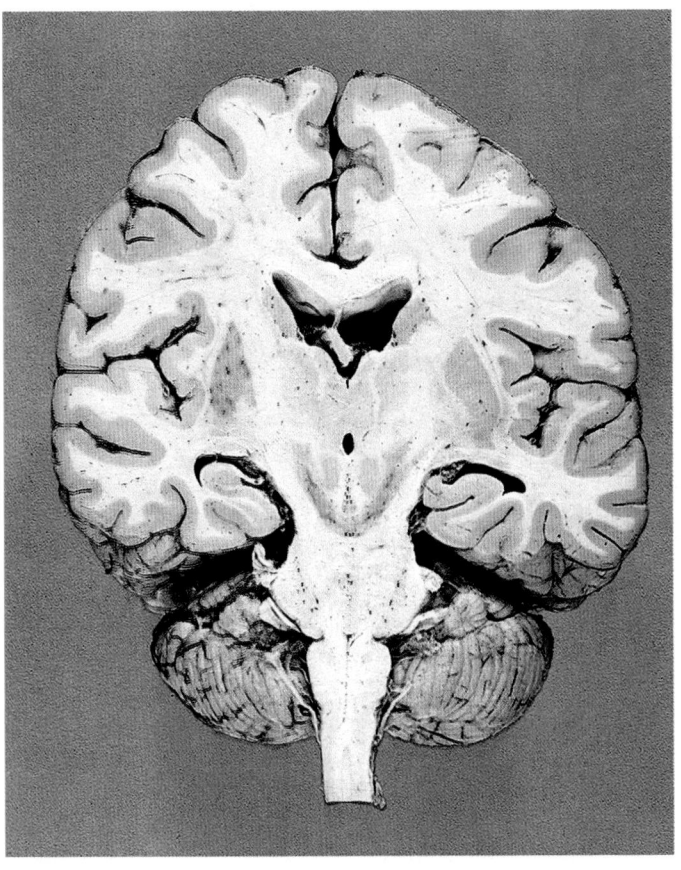

Fig. 21.1 The dorsal half of a brain sectioned in an oblique coronal plane that passes through the cerebral hemispheres, diencephalon, midbrain, pons and medulla oblongata, to show the general disposition of main structures, some of which are labelled in **Fig. 21.3**. Compare also with **Fig. 12.10**. (Photograph by Kevin Fitzpatrick on behalf of GKT School of Medicine, London.)

interthalamic adhesion. Reticular nuclei lie lateral to the main nuclear mass, separated from it by the external medullary lamina.

In general, thalamic nuclei both project to and receive fibres from the cerebral cortex (**Fig. 21.6**). The whole cerebral cortex, not only neocortex but also the phylogenetically older paleocortex of the piriform lobe and archicortex of the hippocampal formation, is reciprocally connected with the thalamus. The thalamus is the major route by which subcortical neuronal activity influences the cerebral cortex, and the greatest input to most thalamic nuclei comes from the cerebral cortex.

The projection to the thalamus from the cortex is precisely reciprocal; each cortical area projects in a topographically organized manner to all sites in the thalamus from which it receives an input. Corticothalamic fibres which reciprocate 'specific' thalamocortical pathways arise from modified pyramidal cells of layer VI, whereas those reciprocating 'non-specific' inputs arise from typical pyramidal cells of layer V, and may in part be axon collaterals of other cortico–subcortical pathways.

It is customary to consider thalamic nuclei as either 'specific' nuclei, which mediate finely-organized and precisely-transmitted sensory information to discrete cortical sensory areas, or as 'non-specific' nuclei, which are part of a general arousal system. The specific nuclei are

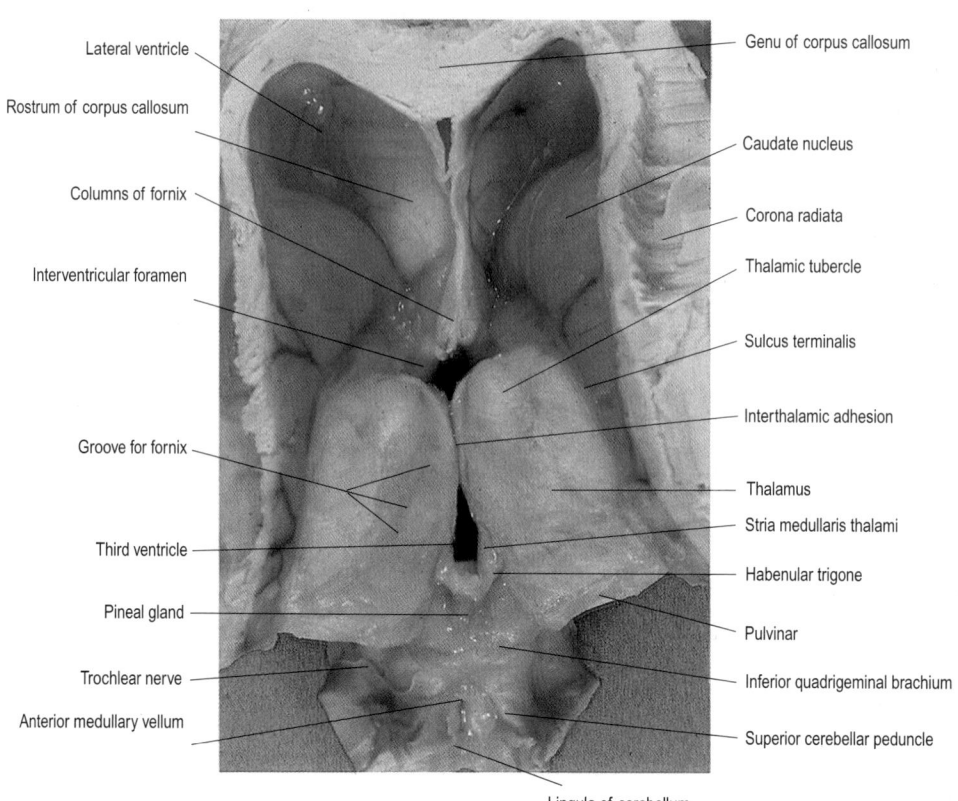

Fig. 21.2 Dorsal aspect of the caudate nuclei, thalami, pineal gland and tectum, revealed by removal of most of the corpus callosum, the body of the fornix and of the tela choroidea.

Labels (clockwise from top left): Lateral ventricle, Rostrum of corpus callosum, Columns of fornix, Interventricular foramen, Groove for fornix, Third ventricle, Pineal gland, Trochlear nerve, Anterior medullary vellum, Lingula of cerebellum, Superior cerebellar peduncle, Inferior quadrigeminal brachium, Pulvinar, Habenular trigone, Stria medullaris thalami, Thalamus, Interthalamic adhesion, Sulcus terminalis, Thalamic tubercle, Corona radiata, Caudate nucleus, Genu of corpus callosum

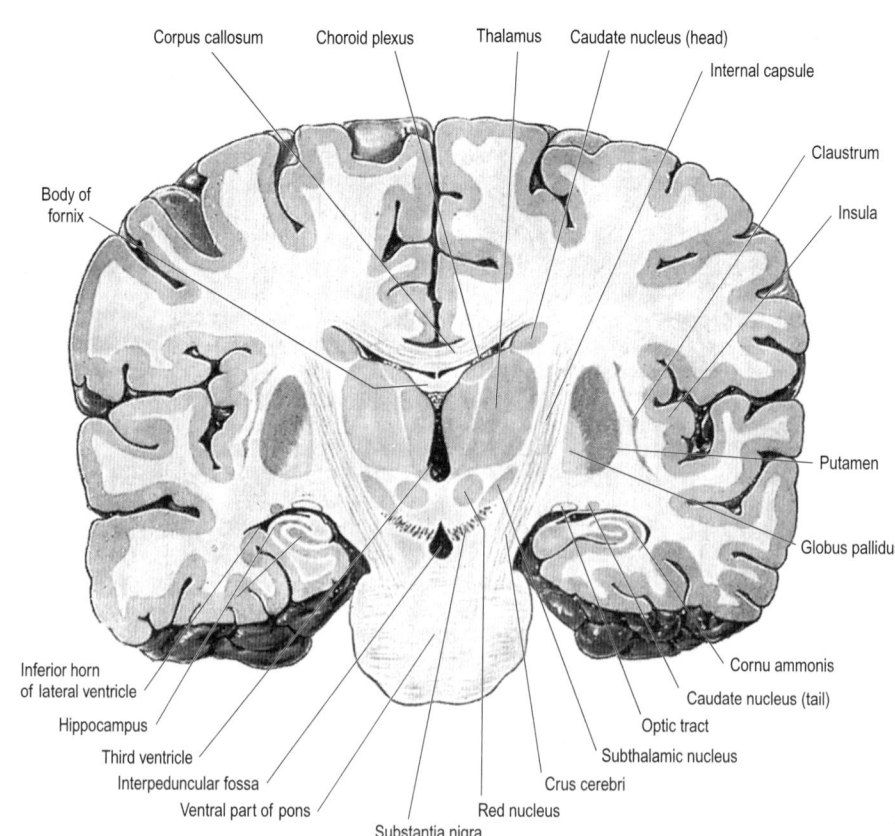

Fig. 21.3 Coronal section of the brain showing the principal parts of the diencephalon and basal ganglia. Compare also with **Fig. 12.10**.

Labels: Corpus callosum, Choroid plexus, Thalamus, Caudate nucleus (head), Internal capsule, Claustrum, Insula, Putamen, Globus pallidus, Cornu ammonis, Caudate nucleus (tail), Optic tract, Subthalamic nucleus, Crus cerebri, Red nucleus, Substantia nigra, Ventral part of pons, Interpeduncular fossa, Third ventricle, Hippocampus, Inferior horn of lateral ventricle, Body of fornix

further subdivided into relay nuclei and association nuclei. However, many nuclei classified as specific may also send non-specific projections to widespread cortical areas. Similarly, the division of thalamic nuclei into relay and association groups rests upon the assumption that relay nuclei receive a major subcortical pathway, whereas association nuclei receive their principal non-cortical input from other thalamic nuclei. There is little evidence of significant intrathalamic connectivity, but increasing indications of non-cortical afferent pathways linked to so-called association nuclei.

ANTERIOR GROUP OF THALAMIC NUCLEI

The anterior group of nuclei are enclosed between the arms of the Y-shaped internal medullary lamina, and underlie the anterior thalamic tubercle (**Fig. 21.2**). Three subdivisions are recognized. The largest is the

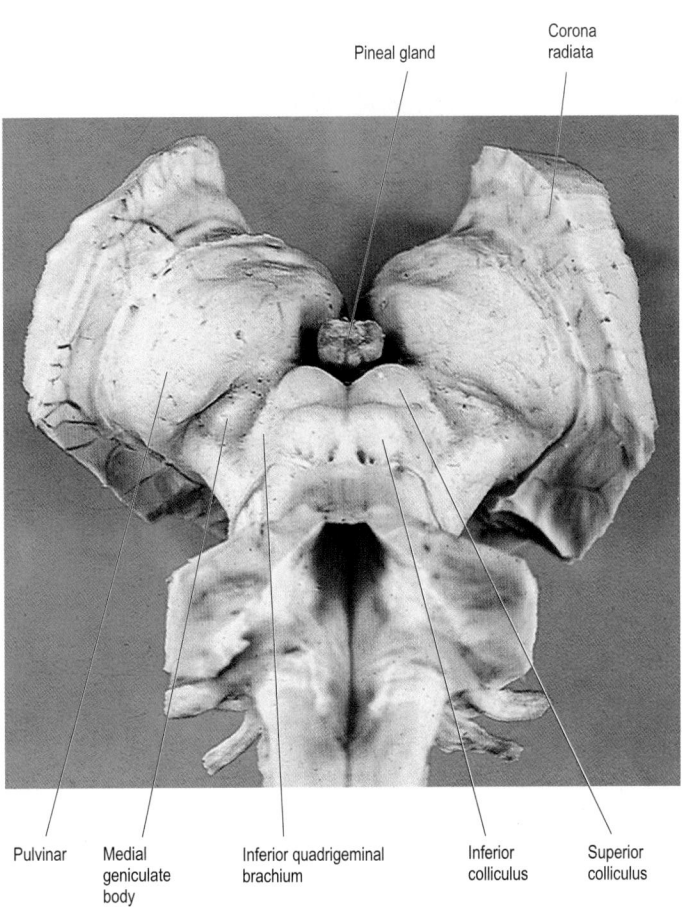

Fig. 21.4 An oblique view of the dorsal aspect of the brain stem and thalamus. (Photograph by Kevin Fitzpatrick on behalf of GKT School of Medicine, London.)

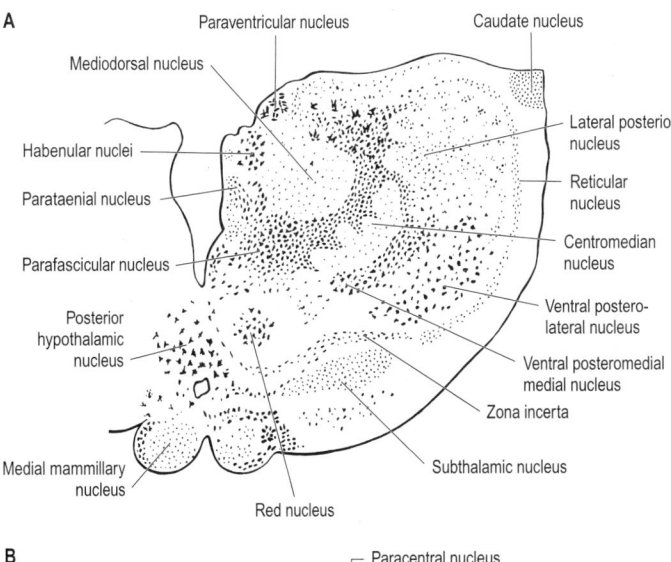

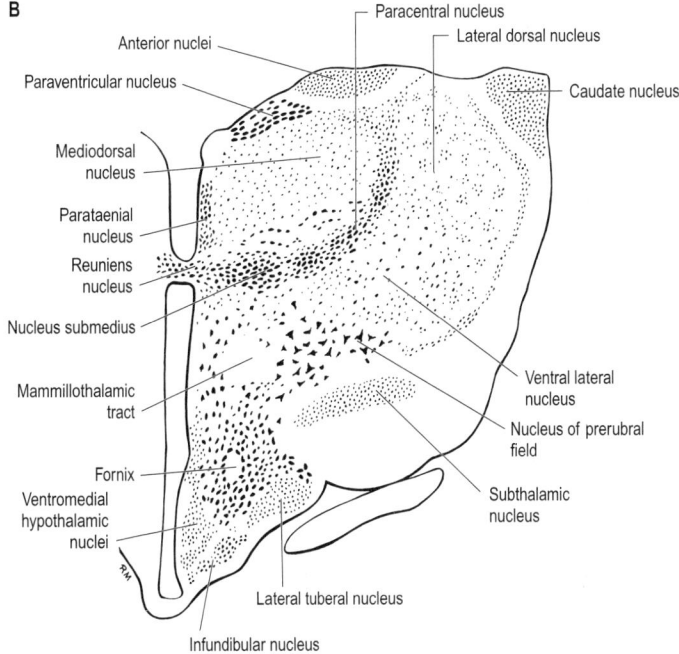

Fig. 21.5 Coronal sections through the diencephalon showing the main nuclear aggregations of nerve cell bodies. **A,** at the level of the mammillary bodies. **B,** at the level of the tuber cinereum. Note the variations in cell size, shape and packing density, which characterize the nuclear masses of the thalamus, subthalamus and hypothalamus at these levels.

anteroventral nucleus, the others are the anteromedial and anterodorsal nuclei.

The anterior nuclei are the principal recipients of the mammillothalamic tract, which arises from the mammillary nuclei of the hypothalamus. The mammillary nuclei receive fibres from the hippocampal formation via the fornix. The medial mammillary nucleus projects to the ipsilateral anteroventral and anteromedial thalamic nuclei, and the lateral mammillary nucleus projects bilaterally to the anterodorsal nuclei. The nuclei of the anterior group also receive a prominent cholinergic input from the basal forebrain and the brain stem.

The cortical targets of efferent fibres from the anterior nuclei of the thalamus lie largely on the medial surface of the hemisphere. They include the anterior limbic area (in front of and inferior to the corpus callosum), the cingulate gyrus, and the parahippocampal gyrus (including the medial entorhinal cortex and the pre- and para-subiculum). These thalamocortical pathways are reciprocal. There also appear to be minor connections between the anterior nuclei and the dorsolateral prefrontal and posterior areas of neocortex. The anterior thalamic nuclei are believed to be involved in the regulation of alertness and attention and in the acquisition of memory.

MEDIAL GROUP OF THALAMIC NUCLEI

The single component of this thalamic region is the mediodorsal or dorsomedial nucleus, which is particularly large in man. Laterally it is limited by the internal medullary lamina and intralaminar nuclei. Medially, it abuts the midline parataenial and reuniens (medioventral) nuclei. It may be divided into anteromedial magnocellular, and posterolateral parvocellular, parts.

The small magnocellular division receives olfactory input from the piriform and adjacent cortex, the ventral pallidum, and the amygdala. The mediobasal amygdaloid nucleus projects to the dorsal part of the anteromedial magnocellular nucleus, and the lateral nuclei project to the more central and anteroventral regions. The anteromedial magnocellular nucleus projects to the anterior and medial prefrontal cortex, notably to the lateral posterior and central posterior olfactory areas on

the orbital surface of the frontal lobe. In addition, fibres pass to the ventromedial cingulate cortex and a few to the inferior parietal cortex and anterior insula. These cortical connections are reciprocal.

The larger, posterolateral, parvocellular division connects reciprocally with the dorsolateral and dorsomedial prefrontal cortex, the anterior cingulate gyrus and the supplementary motor area. In addition, efferent fibres pass to the posterior parietal cortex.

The mediodorsal nucleus appears to be involved in a wide variety of higher functions. Damage may lead to a decrease in anxiety, tension, aggression or obsessive thinking. There may also be transient amnesia, with confusion developing particularly over the passage of time. Much of the neuropsychology of medial nuclear damage reflects defects in functions similar to those performed by the prefrontal cortex, with which it is closely linked. The effects of ablation of the mediodorsal nuclei parallel, in part, the results of prefrontal lobotomy.

LATERAL GROUP OF THALAMIC NUCLEI

The lateral nuclear complex, lying lateral to the internal medullary lamina, is the largest major division of the thalamus. It is divided into dorsal and ventral tiers of nuclei. The lateral dorsal nucleus, lateral

SUPEROLATERAL SURFACE OF HEMISPHERE   MEDIAL SURFACE OF HEMISPHERE

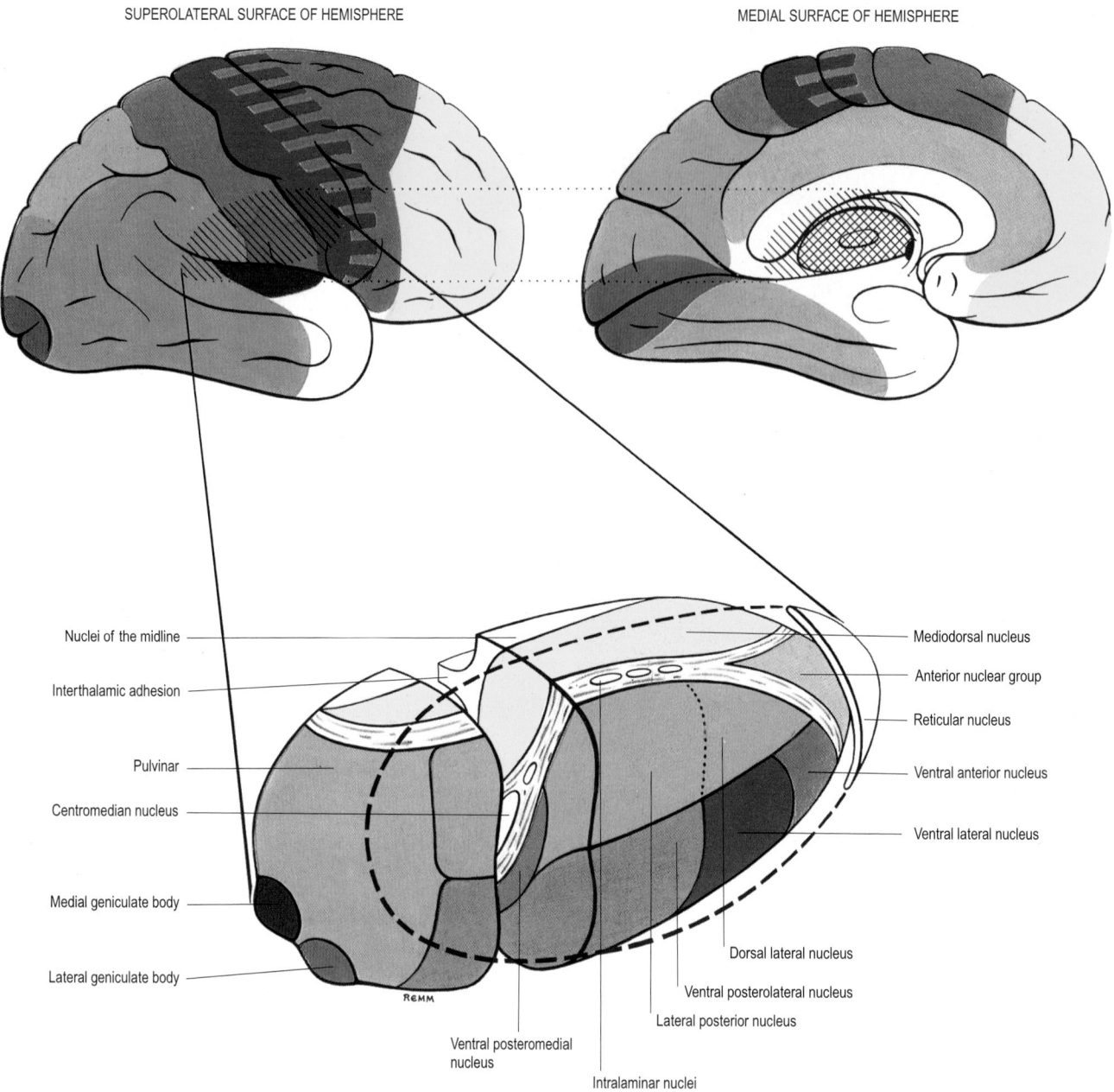

Nuclei of the midline

Interthalamic adhesion

Pulvinar

Centromedian nucleus

Medial geniculate body

Lateral geniculate body

Ventral posteromedial nucleus

Intralaminar nuclei

Mediodorsal nucleus

Anterior nuclear group

Reticular nucleus

Ventral anterior nucleus

Ventral lateral nucleus

Dorsal lateral nucleus

Ventral posterolateral nucleus

Lateral posterior nucleus

Fig. 21.6 The main nuclear masses of the thalamus (viewed from the lateral aspect in the lower illustration) have been labelled and colour coded and the same colours have been used to indicate the areas of cerebral neocortex interconnected with these nuclei. The lack of colour in the centromedian, intralaminar and reticular nuclei and in restricted areas of the frontal and temporal lobes are not related to the colour code.

posterior nucleus and the pulvinar all lie dorsally. The lateral and medial geniculate nuclei lie inferior to the pulvinar near the posterior pole of the thalamus. The ventral tier nuclei are the ventral anterior, ventral lateral and ventral posterior nuclei.

Ventral anterior nucleus

The ventral anterior (VA) complex lies at the anterior pole of the ventral nuclear group. It is limited anteriorly by the reticular nucleus, posteriorly by the ventral lateral nucleus, and lies between the external and internal medullary laminae. It consists of a principal part (VApc) and a magnocellular part (VAmc). The subcortical connections to this region are largely ipsilateral from the internal segment of the globus pallidus and the pars reticulata of the substantia nigra. The terminal fields from these origins do not overlap. Fibres from the globus pallidus end in VApc. The substantia nigra projects to VAmc. Corticothalamic fibres from premotor cortex (area 6) terminate in VApc and fibres from the frontal eye field (area 8) terminate in VAmc. VA thalamus does not appear to receive fibres directly from the motor cortex. The efferent projections from VA are incompletely known. Some pass to intralaminar thalamic nuclei

and others project to widespread regions of the frontal lobe and to the anterior parietal cortex. Their functions are unclear. The VA thalamus appears to play a central role in the transmission of the cortical 'recruiting response', a phenomenon in which stimulation of the thalamus can initiate long-lasting, high voltage repetitive negative electrical waves over much of the cerebral cortex.

Ventral lateral nucleus

The ventral lateral (VL) thalamus consists of two major divisions with distinctly different connections and functions. The anterior division or pars oralis (VLo) receives topographically organized fibres from the internal segment of the ipsilateral globus pallidus. The posterior division or pars caudalis (VLc) receives topographically organized fibres from the contralateral deep cerebellar nuclei. Additional subcortical projections have been reported from the spinothalamic tract and the vestibular nuclei. Numerous cortical afferents to both VLo and VLc originate from precentral motor cortical areas, including both area 4 and area 6.

VLo nucleus sends efferent fibres to the supplementary motor cortex on the medial surface of the hemisphere and to the lateral premotor cortex. The VLc nucleus projects efferent fibres to the primary motor cortex where they end in a topographically arranged fashion. The head region of area 4 receives fibres from the medial part of VLc, and the leg region receives fibres from lateral VLc.

Responses can be recorded in VL thalamus during both passive and active movement of the contralateral body. The topography of its connections, and recordings made within the nucleus, suggest that VLc contains a body representation comparable to that in the ventral posterior nucleus. Stereotaxic surgery of the ventral lateral nucleus is sometimes used in the treatment of essential tremor. In the past, thalamotomy was used extensively for the treatment of Parkinson's disease. However the internal segment of the globus pallidus and the subthalamic nucleus are now the preferred neurosurgical targets for Parkinson's disease (p. 428).

Ventral posterior nucleus

The ventral posterior (VP) nucleus is the principal thalamic relay for the somatosensory pathways. It is thought to consist of two major divisions, the ventral posterolateral (VPl) and ventral posteromedial (VPm) nuclei. The VPl nucleus receives the medial lemniscal and spinothalamic pathways, and the VPm nucleus receives the trigeminothalamic pathway. Connections from the vestibular nuclei and lemniscal fibres terminate along the ventral surface of the VP nucleus.

There is a well-ordered topographic representation of the body in the ventral posterior nucleus. The VPl is organized so that sacral segments are represented laterally and cervical segments medially. The latter abut the face area of representation (trigeminal territory) in VPm. Taste fibres synapse most anteriorly and ventromedially within the ventral posterolateral nucleus.

At a more detailed level, single body regions are represented as curved lamellae of neurones, parallel to the lateral border of the ventral posterior nucleus, such that there is a continuous overlapping progression of adjacent receptive fields from dorsolateral to ventromedial. Considerably less change in location of receptive field on the body is seen when passing anteroposteriorly through the nucleus. While not precisely dermatomal in nature, these curvilinear lamellae of cells probably derive from afferents related to a few adjacent spinal segments. There is considerable distortion of the body map within the nucleus, reflecting the differences in the density of peripheral innervation which occur in different body regions, e.g. many more neurones respond to stimulation of the hand than of the trunk. Within a single lamella, neurones in the anterodorsal part of the nucleus respond to deep stimuli, including movement of joints, tendon stretch, and manipulation of muscles. Most ventrally, neurones once again respond to deep stimuli, particularly tapping. Intervening cells within a single lamella respond only to cutaneous stimuli. This organization has been confirmed by recordings made in the human ventral posterior nucleus.

Single lemniscal axons have an extended anteroposterior terminal zone within the nucleus. Rods of cells running the length of the anteroposterior, dorsoventrally oriented, lamellae respond with closely similar receptive field properties and locations, derived from a small bundle of lemniscal afferents. It appears, therefore, that each lamella contains the complete representation of a single body part, e.g. a finger. Lamellae consist of multiple narrow rods of neurones, oriented anteroposteriorly, each of which receives input from the same small region of the body that is represented within the lamella, and from the same type of receptors. These thalamic 'rods' form the basis for both the place- and modality-specific input to columns of cells in the somatic sensory cortex. Spinothalamic tract afferents to the ventral posterolateral nucleus terminate throughout the nucleus. The neurones from which these axons originate appear to be mainly of the 'wide dynamic range' class, with responses to both low threshold mechanoreceptors and high threshold nociceptors. A smaller proportion are solely high-threshold nociceptors. Some neurones respond to temperature changes. There is evidence that spinothalamic tract neurones carrying nociceptive and thermal information terminate in a distinct nuclear area, identified as the posterior part of the ventral medial nucleus (VMpo).

The VP nucleus projects to the primary somatic sensory cortex (SI) of the postcentral gyrus and to the second somatic sensory area (SII) in the parietal operculum. VMpo projects to the insular cortex. Within the primary sensory cortex, the central cutaneous core of the VP nucleus projects solely to area 3b; dorsal and ventral to this, a narrow band of cells projects to both 3b and area 1. The most dorsal and ventral deep

stimulus receptive cells project to areas 3a and 2. The whole nucleus projects to the second somatic sensory area.

Medial geniculate nucleus

The medial geniculate nucleus, which is a part of the auditory pathway (p. 436), is located within the medial geniculate body, a rounded elevation situated posteriorly on the ventrolateral surface of the thalamus, and separated from the pulvinar by the superior quadrigeminal brachium. It receives fibres travelling in the inferior quadrigeminal brachium. Three major subnuclei, medial, ventral and dorsal, are recognized within it. The inferior brachium separates the medial (magnocellular) nucleus, which consists of sparse, deeply staining neurones, from the lateral nucleus, which is made up of medium-sized, densely packed and darkly staining cells. The dorsal nucleus overlies the ventral nucleus and expands posteriorly, therefore it is sometimes known as the posterior nucleus of the medial geniculate. It contains small- to medium-sized, pale-staining cells, which are less densely packed than those of the lateral nucleus. The ventral nucleus receives fibres from the central nucleus of the ipsilateral inferior colliculus via the inferior quadrigeminal brachium and also from the contralateral inferior colliculus. The nucleus contains a complete tonotopic representation. Low-pitched sounds are represented laterally, and progressively higher-pitched sounds are encountered as the nucleus is traversed from lateral to medial. The dorsal nucleus receives afferents from the pericentral nucleus of the inferior colliculus and from other brain stem nuclei of the auditory pathway. A tonotopic representation has not been described in this subdivision and cells within the dorsal nucleus respond to a broad range of frequencies. The magnocellular medial nucleus receives fibres from the inferior colliculus and from the deep layers of the superior colliculus. Neurones within the magnocellular subdivision may respond to modalities other than sound. However, many cells respond to auditory stimuli, usually to a wider range of frequencies than neurones in the ventral nucleus. Many units show evidence of binaural interaction, with the leading effect arising from stimuli in the contralateral cochlea. The ventral nucleus projects primarily to the primary auditory cortex. The dorsal nucleus projects to auditory areas surrounding the primary auditory cortex. The magnocellular division projects diffusely to auditory areas of the cortex and to adjacent insular and opercular fields.

Lateral geniculate nucleus

The lateral geniculate body, which is part of the visual pathway (p. 432), is a small ovoid ventral projection from the posterior thalamus (**Fig. 21.7**). The superior quadrigeminal brachium enters the posteromedial part of the lateral geniculate body dorsally, lying between the medial geniculate body and the pulvinar.

The lateral geniculate nucleus is an inverted, somewhat flattened, U-shaped nucleus and is laminated. Its internal organization is usually described on the basis of six laminae, although seven or eight may be present. The laminae are numbered 1 to 6, from the innermost ventral to the outermost dorsal (**Fig. 21.8**). Laminae 1 and 2 consist of large cells, the magnocellular layers, whereas layers 4 to 6 have smaller neurones, the parvocellular laminae. The apparent gaps between laminae are called the interlaminar zones. Most ventrally an additional superficial, or S, lamina is recognized.

The lateral geniculate nucleus receives a major afferent input from the retina (p. 710). The contralateral nasal retina projects to laminae 1, 4 and 6, whereas the ipsilateral temporal retina projects to laminae 2, 3 and 5. The parvocellular laminae receive axons predominantly of X-type retinal ganglion cells, i.e. more slowly conducting cells with sustained responses to visual stimuli. The faster conducting, rapidly adapting Y-type retinal ganglion cells project mainly to the magnocellular laminae 1 and 2, and give off axonal branches to the superior colliculus. A third type of retinal ganglion cell, the W cells, which have large receptive fields and slow responses, project to both the superior colliculus and the lateral geniculate nucleus, where they terminate particularly in the interlaminar zones and in the S lamina.

The lateral geniculate nucleus is organized in a visuotopic manner and it contains a precise map of the contralateral visual field. The vertical meridian is represented posteriorly, the peripheral anteriorly, the upper field laterally, and the lower field medially (p. 432). Similar precise point-to-point representation is also found in the projection of the lateral geniculate nucleus to the visual cortex. Radially arranged inverted pyramids of neurones in all laminae respond to a single, small

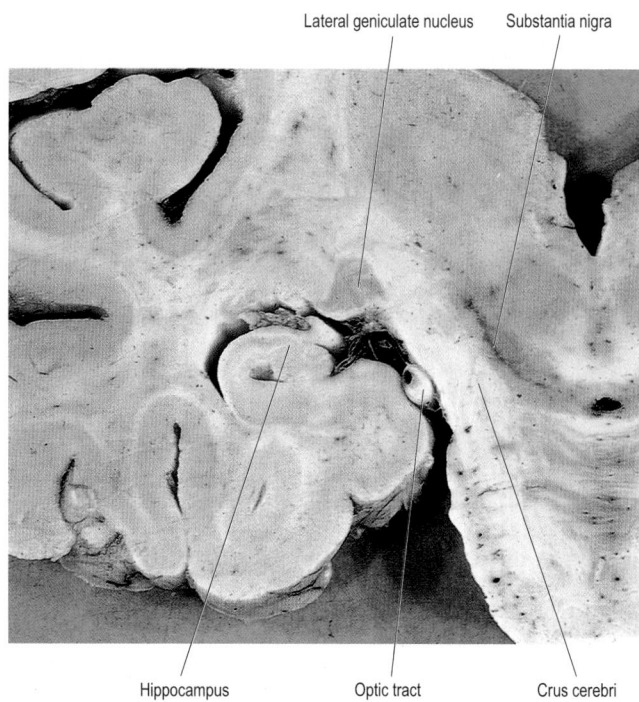

Lateral geniculate nucleus   Substantia nigra

Hippocampus   Optic tract   Crus cerebri

Fig. 21.7 Coronal section through the brain showing the lateral geniculate nucleus. (Photograph by Kevin Fitzpatrick on behalf of GKT School of Medicine, London.)

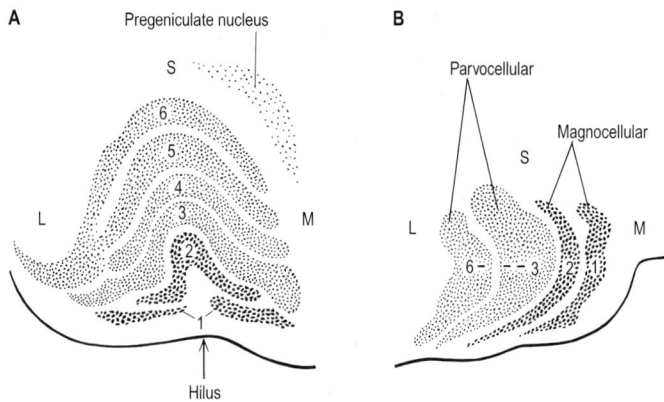

A   Pregeniculate nucleus

S

6

5

4

3

2

1

Hilus

L   M

B   Parvocellular

Magnocellular

S

6   3   2 1

L   M

Fig. 21.8 Coronal sections through the lateral geniculate nucleus near its central region (**A**); its posterior pole (**B**). (Photograph by Kevin Fitzpatrick on behalf of GKT School of Medicine, London.)

area of the contralateral visual field and project to a circumscribed area of cortex. The termination of geniculocortical axons in the visual cortex is considered in detail elsewhere (p. 403).

Aside from retinal afferents, the lateral geniculate nucleus receives a major corticothalamic projection, the axons of which ramify densely in the interlaminar zones.

The major part of this projection arises from the primary visual cortex, Brodmann's area 17, but smaller projections from extrastriate visual areas pass to the magnocellular and S laminae. Other afferents include: fibres from the superficial layer of the superior colliculus (which terminate in the interlaminar zone between laminae 1 and 2, 2 and 3, and around lamina S); noradrenergic fibres from the locus coeruleus; serotoninergic afferents from the midbrain raphe nuclei; and cholinergic fibres from the pontine and mesencephalic reticular formation.

The efferent fibres of the lateral geniculate nucleus pass principally to the primary visual cortex (area 17) in the banks of the calcarine sulcus. It is possible that additional small projections pass to extrastriate visual areas in the occipital lobe, possibly arising primarily in the interlaminar zones.

Lateral dorsal nucleus

The lateral dorsal nucleus is the most anterior of the dorsal tier of lateral nuclei. Its anterior pole lies within a splitting of the internal medullary lamina. Posteriorly, it merges with the lateral posterior nucleus. Subcortical afferents to the lateral dorsal nucleus are from the pretectum and superior colliculus. It is connected with the cingulate, retrosplenial and posterior parahippocampal cortices, the presubiculum of the hippocampal formation, and the parietal cortex.

Lateral posterior nucleus

The lateral posterior nucleus, which lies dorsal to the ventral posterior nucleus, receives its subcortical afferents from the superior colliculus. It is reciprocally connected with the superior parietal lobe. Additional connections have been reported with the inferior parietal, cingulate and medial parahippocampal cortex.

Pulvinar

The pulvinar corresponds to the posterior expansion of the thalamus, which overhangs the superior colliculus. It has three major subdivisions, which are the medial, lateral and inferior pulvinar nuclei. The medial pulvinar nucleus is dorsomedial and consists of compact, evenly spaced, neurones. The inferior pulvinar nucleus lies laterally and inferiorly, and is traversed by bundles of axons in the mediolateral plane, an arrangement which confers a fragmented appearance of horizontal cords or sheets of cells separated by fibre bundles. The inferior pulvinar nucleus lies most inferiorly and laterally and is a more homogeneous collection of cells.

The subcortical afferents to the pulvinar are uncertain. Medial and lateral pulvinar nuclei may receive fibres from the superior colliculus. It has been suggested that the inferior pulvinar nucleus receives fibres both from the superior colliculus and directly from the retina and that it contains a complete retinotopic representation.

The cortical targets of efferent fibres from the pulvinar are widespread. In essence, the medial pulvinar nucleus projects to association areas of the parietotemporal cortex, whereas lateral and inferior pulvinar nuclei project to visual areas in the occipital and posterior temporal lobes. Thus, the inferior pulvinar nucleus connects with the striate and extrastriate cortex in the occipital lobe, and with visual association areas in the posterior part of the temporal lobe. The lateral pulvinar nucleus connects with extrastriate areas of the occipital cortex, with posterior parts of the temporal association cortex, and with the parietal cortex. The medial pulvinar nucleus connects with the inferior parietal cortex, with the posterior cingulate gyrus and with the widespread areas of the temporal lobe, including the posterior parahippocampal gyrus, perirhinal and entorhinal cortex. It also has extensive connections with prefrontal and orbitofrontal cortices. Similarly, the lateral pulvinar nucleus may also connect with the rostromedial prefrontal cortex.

Little is known of the functions of the pulvinar. The inferior pulvinar nucleus contains a complete retinotopic representation, and lateral and medial pulvinar nuclei also contain visually responsive cells. However, the latter nucleus, at least, is not purely visual – other modality responses can be recorded, and some cells may be polysensory. Given the complexity of functions of the association areas to which they project, particularly in the temporal lobe (e.g. perception, cognition and memory), it is likely that the role of the pulvinar in modulating these functions is equally complex.

Anteriorly, the major subdivisions of the pulvinar blend into a poorly differentiated region, within which several nuclear components have been recognized, including the anterior or oral pulvinar, the suprageniculate/limitans and the posterior nuclei. The connectivity of this complex is also not well understood. It is recognized that different components receive subcortical afferents from the spinothalamic tract and the superior and inferior colliculi. Cortical connections centre primarily on the insula and adjacent parts of the parietal operculum posteriorly. Stimulation of this region has been reported to elicit pain, and large lesions may alleviate painful conditions. Similarly, excision of its cortical target in the parietal operculum, or small infarcts in this cortical region, may result in hypoalgesia.

INTRALAMINAR NUCLEI

The term intralaminar nuclei refers to collections of neurones within the internal medullary lamina of the thalamus. Two groups of nuclei are recognized. The anterior (rostral) group are subdivided into central medial, paracentral and central lateral nuclei. The posterior (caudal) intralaminar group consists of the centromedian and parafascicular nuclei. The designations central medial and centromedian are open to confusion, however they are an accepted part of the terminology of thalamic nuclei in common usage. The centromedian nucleus is much larger, is considerably expanded in man in comparison with other species, and is importantly related to the globus pallidus, deep cerebellar nuclei and motor cortex. Anteriorly, the internal medullary lamina separates the mediodorsal nucleus from the ventral lateral complex. It is occupied by the paracentral nucleus laterally, and the central medial nucleus ventromedially, as the two laminae converge towards the midline. A little more posteriorly, the central lateral nucleus appears dorsally in the lamina as the latter splits to enclose the lateral dorsal nucleus. More posteriorly, at the level of the ventral posterior nucleus, the lamina splits to enclose the ovoid centromedian nucleus. The smaller parafascicular nucleus lies more medially.

The anterior intralaminar nuclei, i.e. central medial, paracentral and central lateral, have reciprocal connections with widespread cortical areas. There is some evidence of areal preference. Thus, the central lateral nucleus projects mainly to parietal and temporal association areas, the paracentral nucleus to occipitotemporal and prefrontal cortex, and the central medial nucleus to orbitofrontal and prefrontal cortex and to the cortex on the medial surface. In contrast, the posterior nuclei, i.e. centromedian and parafascicular, have more restricted connections, principally with the motor, premotor and supplementary motor areas. Both anterior and posterior intralaminar nuclei also project to the striatum. Many cells throughout the anterior nuclei have branched axons, which pass to both the cortex and the striatum. Dual projections are less frequent in the posterior nuclei. The thalamostriate projection is topographically organized. The posterior intralaminar nuclei receive a major input from the internal segment of the globus pallidus. Additional afferents come from the pars reticulata of the substantia nigra, the deep cerebellar nuclei, the pedunculopontine nucleus of the midbrain, and possibly the spinothalamic tract. The anterior nuclei have widespread subcortical afferents. The central lateral nucleus receives afferents from the spinothalamic tract, and all component nuclei receive fibres from the brain stem reticular formation, the superior colliculus and several pretectal nuclei. Afferents to all intralaminar nuclei from the brain stem reticular formation include a prominent cholinergic pathway.

The precise functional role of the intralaminar nuclei is unclear. They appear to mediate cortical activation from the brain stem reticular formation, and to play a part in sensorimotor integration. Damage to the intralaminar nuclei may contribute to thalamic neglect, i.e. the unilateral neglect of stimuli originating from the contralateral body or extrapersonal space. This may arise particularly from unilateral damage to the centromedian–parafascicular complex. The latter has been targeted in humans for the neurosurgical control of pain and epilepsy. Bilateral injury to the posterior intralaminar nuclei leads to a kinetic mutism with apathy and loss of motivation. A second syndrome associated with damage involving the intralaminar nuclei is that of unilateral motor neglect, in which there is contralateral paucity of spontaneous movement and motor activity.

MIDLINE NUCLEI

There is considerable divergence between different authors as to which elements of the medial diencephalon constitute the nuclei of the midline thalamic group. In the present account, the midline group of nuclei includes those medial thalamic structures ventral to the central medial nucleus, i.e. the rhomboid and reuniens nuclei together with the parataenial nuclei more dorsolaterally.

The midline nuclei receive subcortical afferent fibres from the hypothalamus, the periaqueductal grey matter of the midbrain, the spinothalamic tract and the medullary and pontine reticular formation. They are the major thalamic target of ascending noradrenergic and serotoninergic axons from the locus coeruleus and raphe nuclei respectively, and they also receive a cholinergic input from the midbrain. Efferents from the midline nuclei pass to the hippocampal formation, the amygdala and the nucleus accumbens. Additional thalamocortical axons reach the cingulate, and possibly orbitofrontal, cortex. The dual cortical and basal nuclear relationship of these nuclei has often led to their being considered a part of the intralaminar system. The cortical projections are reciprocal. The relationships of the midline nuclei clearly identify them as part of the limbic system. There is some evidence that they may play a role in memory and arousal, and, pathologically, may be important in the regulation of seizure activity.

RETICULAR NUCLEUS

The reticular nucleus is a curved lamella of large, deeply staining fusiform cells that wraps around the lateral margin of the thalamus, separated from it by the external medullary lamina. Anteriorly, it curves around the rostral pole of the thalamus to lie between it and the prethalamic nuclei, notably the bed nucleus of the stria terminalis. The nucleus is so named because it is criss-crossed by bundles of fibres which, as they pass between thalamus and cortex, produce a reticular appearance.

The nucleus is thought to receive collateral branches of cortico-thalamic, thalamocortical and probably thalamostriatal and pallido-thalamic fibres as they traverse it. It receives an additional, probably cholinergic, afferent pathway from the nucleus cuneiformis of the midbrain. Broadly speaking, the afferents from the cortex and thalamus are topographically arranged. The reticular nucleus contains visual, somatic and auditory regions, each with a crude topographic representation of the sensorium concerned. Cells within these regions respond to visual, somatic or auditory stimuli with a latency suggesting that these properties arise from activation by thalamocortical axon collaterals. Only in areas where representations abut do cells show modality convergence.

The efferent fibres from the reticular nucleus pass into the body of the thalamus and are GABAergic. The projections into the main thalamic nuclei broadly, but not entirely, reciprocate the thalamoreticular connections. There may also be projections to the contralateral dorsal thalamus. The reticular nucleus is believed to function in gating information relayed through the thalamus.

HYPOTHALAMUS

The hypothalamus consists of only 4 cm^3 of neural tissue, or 0.3% of the total brain. Nevertheless, it contains the integrative systems that, via the autonomic and endocrine effector systems, control fluid and electrolyte balance, food ingestion and energy balance, reproduction, thermoregulation, and immune and many emotional responses.

The hypothalamus extends from the lamina terminalis to a vertical plane posterior to the mammillary bodies, and from the hypothalamic sulcus to the base of the brain beneath the third ventricle. It lies beneath the thalamus and anterior to the tegmental part of the subthalamus and the mesencephalic tegmentum (**Fig. 16.8**). Laterally, it is bordered by the anterior part of the subthalamus, internal capsule and optic tract. Structures in the floor of the third ventricle reach the pial surface in the interpeduncular fossa (**Fig. 21.9**). From anterior to posterior they are the optic chiasma, the tuber cinereum, tuberal eminences and the infundibular stalk, the mammillary bodies and the posterior perforated substance. The latter lies in the interval between the diverging crura cerebri, pierced by small central branches of posterior cerebral arteries. Within it is the small interpeduncular nucleus, which receives terminals of the fasciculus retroflexus of both sides, and has other connections with the mesencephalic reticular formation and mammillary bodies.

The mammillary bodies are smooth, hemispherical, pea-sized eminences, lying side by side, anterior to the posterior perforated substance, each with nuclei enclosed in white fascicles derived largely from the fornix. The tuber cinereum, between the mammillary bodies and the optic chiasma, is a convex mass of grey matter. From it, the median, conical, hollow infundibulum becomes continuous ventrally with the posterior lobe of the pituitary. Around the base of the infundibulum is the median eminence, which is demarcated by a shallow tubero-infundibular sulcus.

Hypothalamic lesions have long been linked with widespread and bizarre endocrine syndromes and with metabolic, visceral, motor and emotional disturbances. The hypothalamus has major interactions with the neuroendocrine system and the autonomic nervous system, integrating responses to both internal and external afferent stimuli with the complex analysis of the world provided by the cerebral cortex.

The hypothalamus controls the endocrine system in a variety of ways: through magnocellular neurosecretory projections to the posterior pituitary; through parvocellular neurosecretory projections to the median eminence (these control the endocrine output of the anterior pituitary and thereby the peripheral endocrine organs); and via the autonomic nervous system. The posterior pituitary neurohormones, vasopressin and oxytocin, are primarily involved in the control of osmotic homeostasis and various aspects of reproductive function, respectively. Through its effects on the anterior pituitary, the hypothalamus influences the thyroid gland (thyroid stimulating hormone, TSH), suprarenal cortex

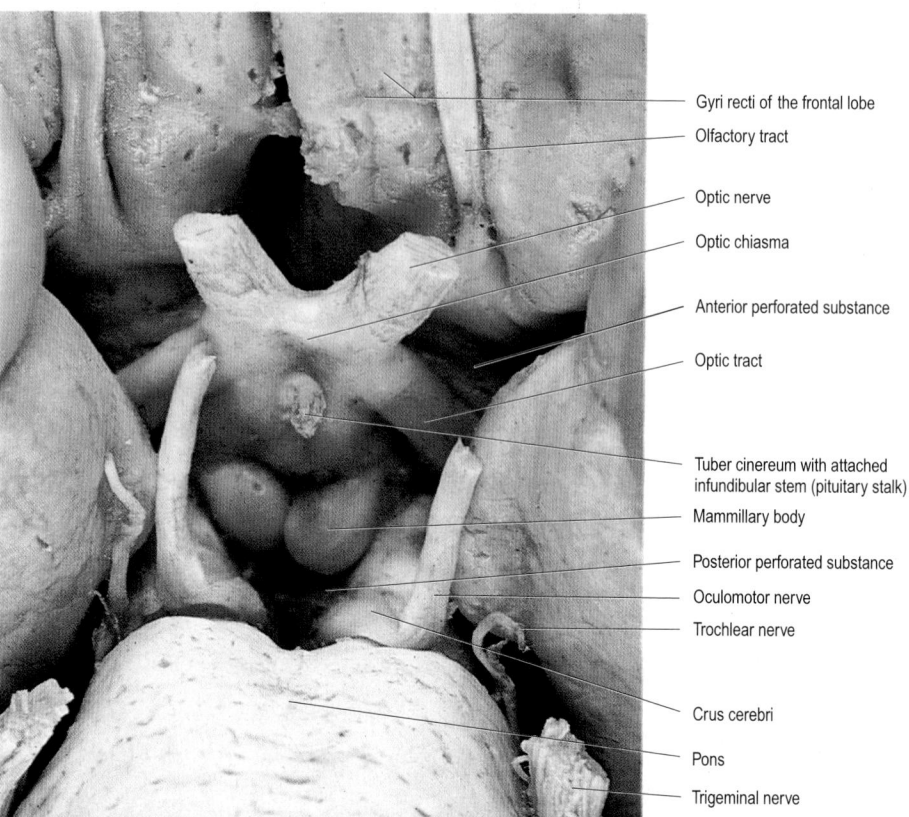

Fig. 21.9 The interpeduncular fossa and surrounding structures. (Photograph by Kevin Fitzpatrick on behalf of GKT School of Medicine, London.)

Labels:
- Gyri recti of the frontal lobe
- Olfactory tract
- Optic nerve
- Optic chiasma
- Anterior perforated substance
- Optic tract
- Tuber cinereum with attached infundibular stem (pituitary stalk)
- Mammillary body
- Posterior perforated substance
- Oculomotor nerve
- Trochlear nerve
- Crus cerebri
- Pons
- Trigeminal nerve

(adrenocorticotrophic hormone, ACTH), gonads (luteinizing hormone, LH; follicle stimulating hormone, FSH, prolactin), mammary gland (prolactin), and the processes of growth and metabolic homeostasis (growth hormone, GH).

The hypothalamus influences both parasympathetic and sympathetic divisions of the autonomic nervous system. In general, parasympathetic effects predominate when the anterior hypothalamus is stimulated – sympathetic effects depend more on the posterior hypothalamus.

Stimulation of the anterior hypothalamus and paraventricular nucleus can cause decreased blood pressure and decreased heart rate. Stimulation in the anterior hypothalamus induces sweating and vaso-dilatation (and thus heat loss) via projections that pass through the medial forebrain bundle to autonomic centres in the brain stem and cord. Damage to the anterior hypothalamus, e.g. during surgery for suprasellar extensions of pituitary tumours, can result in an uncontrollable rise in body temperature. Projections to the ventromedial hypothalamus conjointly regulate food intake. Stimulation in the posterior part of the hypothalamus induces sympathetic arousal with vasoconstriction, piloerection, shivering and increased metabolic heat production. Circuitry mediating shivering is located in the dorsomedial posterior hypothalamus. This does not imply the existence of discrete parasympathetic and sympathetic 'centres'. Stimuli in many different parts of the hypothalamus can cause profound changes in heart rate, cardiac output, vasomotor tone, peripheral resistance, differential blood flow in organs and limbs, the frequency and depth of respiration, motility and secretion in the alimentary tract, erection and ejaculation.

HYPOTHALAMIC NUCLEI

The hypothalamus contains a number of neuronal groups that have been classified on phylogenetic, developmental, cytoarchitectonic, synaptic and histochemical grounds into named nuclei, many of which are not very clearly delimited, especially in the adult. While it contains a few large myelinated tracts, many of the connections are diffuse and unmyelinated, and the precise paths of many afferent, efferent, and intrinsic connections are uncertain.

The hypothalamus can be divided anteroposteriorly into chiasmatic (supraoptic), tuberal (infundibulo-tuberal) and posterior (mammillary) regions, and mediolaterally into periventricular, intermediate (medial), and lateral zones. Between the intermediate and lateral zones is a paramedian plane, which contains the prominent myelinated fibres of

the column of the fornix, the mammillothalamic tract and the fasciculus retroflexus. For this reason, some authors group the periventricular and intermediate zones as a single medial zone. These divisions are artificial and functional systems cross them. The main nuclear groups and myelinated tracts are illustrated in Figs 21.10, 21.11.

The periventricular zone of the hypothalamus borders the third ventricle. In the anterior wall of the ventricle is the vascular organ of the lamina terminalis (OVLT, organum vasculosum), which is continuous dorsally with the median preoptic nucleus and subfornical organ. On each side in the chiasmatic region are: part of the preoptic nucleus; the small, sexually dimorphic suprachiasmatic nucleus; periventricular neurones, which are medial to, and blend with, the paraventricular nucleus. In the tuberal region, the periventricular cell group expands around the base of the third ventricle to form the arcuate nucleus, which overlies the median eminence. In the posterior region, the narrow periventricular zone is continuous laterally with the posterior hypothalamic area and behind that with midbrain periaqueductal grey matter. The periventricular zone also contains a prominent periventricular fibre system.

Suprachiasmatic nucleus

Although it contains only a few thousand neurones, the suprachiasmatic nucleus is a remarkable structure. It appears to be the neural substrate for day–night cycles in motor activity, body temperature, plasma concentration of many hormones, renal secretion, sleeping and waking, and many other variables. Lesions of the suprachiasmatic region lead to a disordered sleep–wake cycle.

The suprachiasmatic nucleus has two principal subdivisions. Retinal fibres terminate in a ventrolateral subdivision, characterized by neurones immunoreactive for vasoactive intestinal polypeptide (VIP). This appears to be a general input zone, which also receives afferents from the midbrain raphe and parts of the lateral geniculate nucleus of the thalamus. The dorsomedial subdivision has relatively sparse afferent innervation, and characteristically contains parvocellular neurones immunoreactive for arginine vasopressin (AVP). Neurones within the suprachiasmatic nuclei that receive direct retinal input do not respond to pattern, movement or colour. Instead, they operate as luminance detectors, responding to the onset and offset of light, and their firing rates vary in proportion to light intensity, thereby synchronizing to the light–dark cycle.

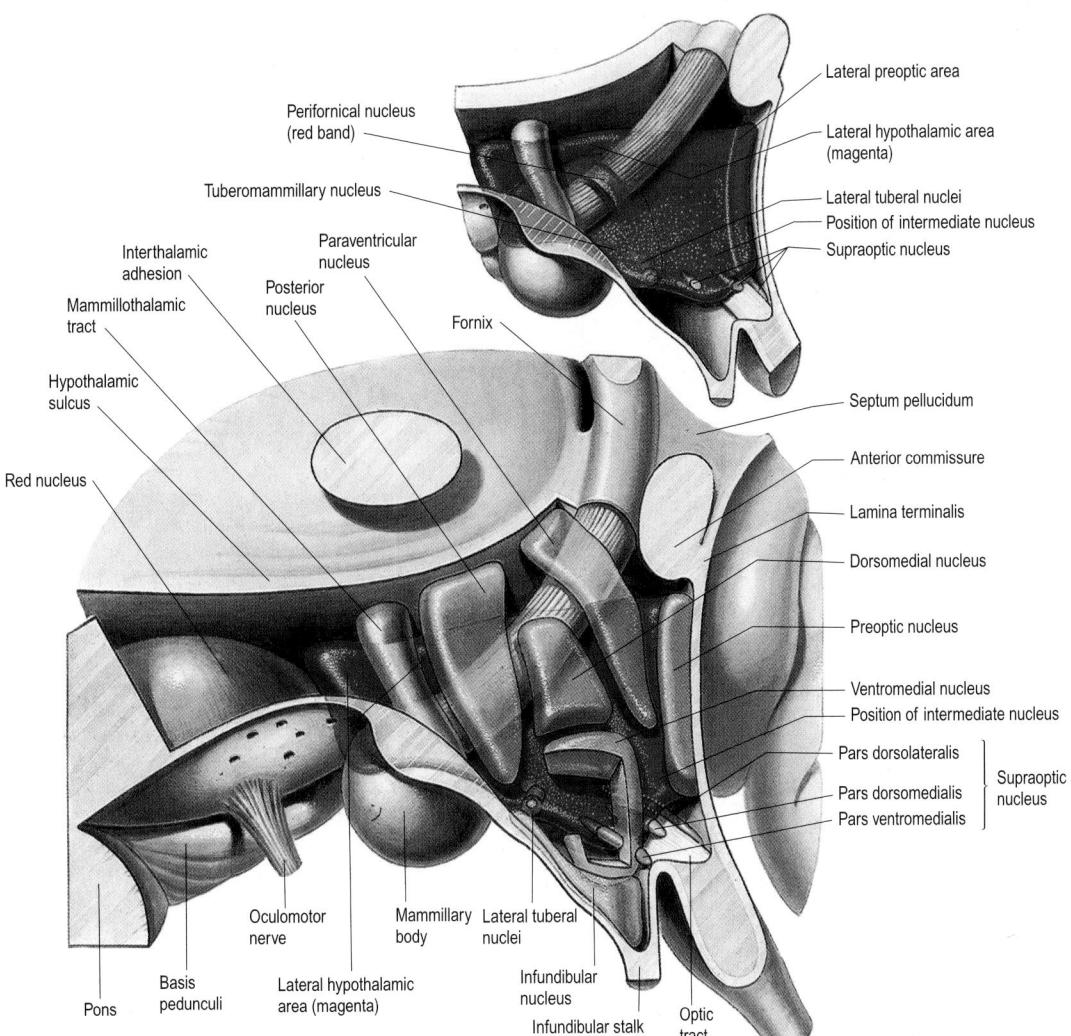

Perifornical nucleus
(red band)

Tuberomammillary nucleus

Interthalamic
adhesion

Mammillothalamic
tract

Posterior
nucleus

Paraventricular
nucleus

Hypothalamic
sulcus

Red nucleus

Fornix

Lateral preoptic area

Lateral hypothalamic area
(magenta)

Lateral tuberal nuclei

Position of intermediate nucleus

Supraoptic nucleus

Septum pellucidum

Anterior commissure

Lamina terminalis

Dorsomedial nucleus

Preoptic nucleus

Ventromedial nucleus

Position of intermediate nucleus

Pars dorsolateralis

Pars dorsomedialis   Supraoptic
                       nucleus

Pars ventromedialis

Pons   Basis   Oculomotor   Mammillary   Lateral tuberal   Infundibular   Optic
         pedunculi nerve   body   nuclei   nucleus   tract

Lateral hypothalamic   Infundibular stalk
area (magenta)

Fig. 21.10 The hypothalamic region of the left cerebral hemisphere viewed from the medial aspect and dissected to display the major hypothalamic nuclei. In the upper diagram the medially placed nuclear groups have been removed; in the lower diagram both lateral and medial groups are included. Lateral to the fornix and the mammillothalamic tract is the lateral hypothalamic region (magenta), in which the tuberomammillary nucleus is situated posteriorly, and the lateral preoptic nucleus rostrally. Surrounding the fornix is the perifornical nucleus (red band), which joins the lateral hypothalamic area with the posterior hypothalamic nucleus. The medially placed nuclei (yellow) fill in much of the region between the mammillothalamic tract and the lamina terminalis, but also project caudally to the tract. The lateral tuberal nuclei (blue) are situated ventrally, largely in the lateral hypothalamic area. The supraoptic nucleus (green) may form three rather separate parts. The intermediate nuclei form three groups between the supraoptic and paraventricular nuclei. (Modified from Nauta WJH, Haymaker W 1969 Hypothalamic nuclei and fiber connections. In: Haymaker W, Anderson E, Nauta WJH (eds) The Hypothalamus, by permission of Charles C Thomas Publisher, Ltd, Springfield, Illinois.)

The nucleus receives glutamatergic afferents from retinal ganglion cells that entrain the rhythm to the light–dark cycle, but these are not essential for the production of the rhythm, which persists in the blind. The suprachiasmatic nucleus contains many different neurotransmitters including vasopressin, VIP, neuropeptide Y (NPY) and neurotensin. Axons from the suprachiasmatic nuclei pass to many other hypothalamic nuclei including the paraventricular, ventromedial, dorsomedial and arcuate nuclei.

The suprachiasmatic nucleus also influences the activity of preganglionic sympathetic neurones at C8–T1 level. These project to superior cervical ganglion neurones, which, in turn, project to the pineal gland. In the pineal, which contains modified photoreceptors, circadian variation in the postganglionic sympathetic input causes parallel variation in pineal N-acetyltransferase activity and thus pineal melatonin production. The role of the pineal gland in man is uncertain – pineal tumours can influence reproductive development, and administration of melatonin has been advocated to alleviate jet-lag.

Parvocellular neurosecretory neurones lie within the periventricular zone, in particular the medial parvocellular part of the paraventricular nucleus, and the arcuate nucleus. The arcuate nucleus is median in the postinfundibular part of the tuber cinereum. It extends forward into the median eminence and almost encircles the infundibular base, but does not meet anteriorly, where the infundibulum adjoins the median part of the optic chiasma. Its numerous neurones are all small and round in

coronal section, and oval or fusiform in sagittal section. No glial layer intervenes between the nucleus and the ependymal tanycytes lining the infundibular recess of the third ventricle. Circadian variation in the secretion of all anterior pituitary hormones suggests that projections from the suprachiasmatic nucleus must reach parvocellular neurosecretory neurones. Afferents from the limbic system probably mediate the widespread effects of stress, and serotonin and noradrenaline from the brain stem influence the output of most anterior pituitary hormones. The axons of parvocellular neurones converge on the infundibulum, forming a tubero-infundibular tract, which ends on the capillary loops that form the hypophysiel portal vessels.

Neurones producing growth hormone-releasing hormone (GHRH) are largely restricted to the arcuate nucleus. Some extend dorsally into the periventricular nucleus and laterally into the retrochiasmatic area. Their fibres run through the periventricular region to the neurovascular zone of the median eminence. The neurones receive afferent information from glucose receptors in the ventromedial nucleus. Inputs from the hippocampal–amygdala–septal complex could explain the release of GH during stress. In man, midline defects such as septo-optic dysplasia are associated with defective growth hormone secretion. Dopamine has a stimulatory effect.

Neurones producing somatostatin (growth hormone release-inhibiting hormone) are located in the periventricular nucleus. GHRH and somatostatin are secreted in intermittent (3–5 hour) reciprocal

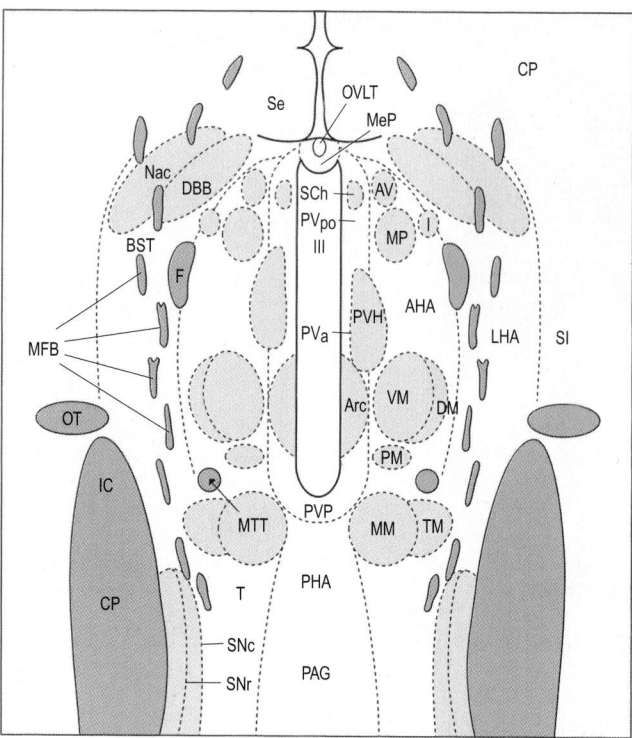

Fig. 21.11 Schematic horizontal section to show the major cell groups and tracts in and around the hypothalamus. Abbreviations: AH, anterior hypothalamic area; Arc, arcuate nucleus; AV, anteroventral preoptic nucleus; BST , bed nucleus of stria terminalis; CP, caudate nucleus and putamen; DBB, nucleus of diagonal band; DM, dorsomedial nucleus; LHA, lateral hypothalamic area; MB, mammillary body (mainly medial mammillary nucleus); MeP, median preoptic nucleus; MP, medial preoptic nucleus; NAc, nucleus accumbens; OVLT, vascular organ of the lamina terminalis; PAG, periaqueductal grey matter; PHA, posterior hypothalamic area; PV, periventricular nucleus (PVpo, preoptic part; PVa, anterior part; PVp, posterior part); PVH, paraventricular (hypothalamic) nucleus; Se, septal cortex; SCh, suprachiasmatic nucleus; T, midbrain tegmentum; TM, tuberomammillary nucleus; VM, ventromedial nucleus; VTA, ventral tegmental area. Fibre tracts (shaded): CP, cerebral peduncle; F, fornix; MFB, medial forebrain bundle; MTT, mammillothalamic tract; OT, optic tract. (Modified with permission from Elsevier. Progress in Brain Research, vol 87, Swanson LW, Biochemical switching in hypothalamic circuits mediating responses to stress, pp 181–200, 1991.)

pulses, but the origin of the pulses is unclear. A large pulse of GH is secreted at the onset of slow wave sleep. Somatostatin also inhibits release of pituitary thyroid-stimulating hormone (TSH).

Neurones producing GHRH and projecting to the median eminence are also located in the periventricular and arcuate nuclei. Other GHRH neurones are found in the periventricular preoptic area, but these appear to project to the vascular organ of the lamina terminalis. Luteinizing hormone (LH) and follicle-stimulating hormone (FSH) are secreted in circhoral (hourly) pulses, which are stimulated by GHRH, and are influenced by central monoamine and GABA, by oestrogen and progesterone acting indirectly through other neurones, by corticotrophin-releasing factor, and by endogenous opioids.

Corticotrophin-releasing hormone (CRH) neurones are located primarily in parvocellular paraventricular neurones. They are profoundly stimulated by neurogenic (limbic input) and hypoglycaemic (ventromedial nucleus) stress, and are also controlled by negative feedback by cortisol.

Thyrotrophin-releasing hormone (TRH) neurones are rather more widely distributed in the periventricular, ventromedial and dorsomedial nuclei. TRH release is influenced by core temperature, sensed in the anterior hypothalamus, and by negative feedback of thyroid hormones. It stimulates release of pituitary TSH and also acts to excite cold-sensitive, and to inhibit warm-sensitive neurones in the preoptic area.

Other tubero-infundibular arcuate neurones contain neuropeptide Y (NPY) and neurotensin. Arcuate neurones containing pro-opiomelanocortin peptides project to the periventricular nucleus rather than the median eminence.

In addition to these peptide-containing cells, dopamine neurones in the arcuate nucleus (A12 group) have terminals in the median eminence and infundibulum. Dopamine acts as the principal prolactin-release inhibiting hormone, and also inhibits secretion of TSH (likewise, TSH acts as a prolactin-releasing hormone). Noradrenergic terminals are found in the median eminence, where they may act largely in a paracrine manner.

The intermediate zone of the hypothalamus contains the best differentiated nuclei. These are: the paraventricular and supraoptic nuclei; 'intermediate' nuclear groups, which show sexual dimorphism; ventromedial and dorsomedial nuclei; the mammillary body; and tuberomammillary nuclei. Magnocellular neurosecretory neurones are found in the supraoptic nucleus, paraventricular nucleus, and as isolated clusters of cells between them.

Supraoptic and paraventricular nuclei

The supraoptic nucleus, curved over the lateral part of the optic chiasma, contains a uniform population of large neurones. Behind the chiasma, a thin plate of cells in the floor of the brain forms the retrochiasmatic part.

Supraoptic neurones synthesise vasopressin, and they all appear to project to the neurohypophysis. The magnocellular vasopressin neurones detect as little as 1% increase in the osmotic pressure of the blood and stimulate release of vasopressin from the posterior pituitary. A fall in blood volume or blood pressure of greater than 5–10% stimulates the release of vasopressin and the urge to drink via volume receptors in the walls of the great veins and atria and baroreceptors in the carotid sinus. These project via the vagus and glossopharyngeal nerves to the nucleus tractus solitarius and thence to the magnocellular nuclei. A biochemical defect in vasopressin production, or interruption of the supraopticohypophysiel pathway (e.g. due to a head injury), can cause cranial diabetes insipidus.

The paraventricular nucleus extends from the hypothalamic sulcus downward across the medial aspect of the column of the fornix, its ventrolateral angle reaching towards the supraoptic nucleus. Its neurones are more diverse. Magnocellular neurones, which project to the neurohypophysis, tend to lie laterally; parvocellular neurones, which project to the median eminence and infundibulum, lie more medially; and intermediate-sized neurones, which may project caudally, lie posteriorly. The axons of the paraventricular magnocellular neurones pass towards the supraoptic nucleus (paraventriculo-hypophysiel tract), where they join axons of supraoptic neurones to form a supraopticohypophysiel tract. This runs down the infundibulum, superficially, and into the neural lobe, where the axons are distended and branch repeatedly around the capillaries. Vasopressin and oxytocin are produced by separate neurones. Vasopressin neurones tend to cluster in the ventrolateral part of the paraventricular nucleus and the oxytocin cells lie around them.

The hypothalamus is essential for the control of pituitary oxytocin, gonadotrophin and prolactin secretion. The release of oxytocin from neurosecretory nerve terminals in the neurohypophysis induces contraction of both the uterus, at term, and the myoepithelial cells that surround the mammary gland alveoli. Two neuroendocrine reflexes are involved. Stretching of the cervix of the uterus during childbirth stimulates a multisynaptic afferent pathway that passes via the pelvic plexus, anterolateral column and brain stem to the magnocellular oxytocin neurones (the Ferguson reflex). This is a positive feedback mechanism, which is terminated by the birth of the child. The milk ejection reflex involves stimulation of the intercostal nerves, which innervate the nipples, by suckling, and a similar central pathway. It can be both conditioned to a baby's cry and inhibited by stress.

At the tuberal level, the ventromedial nucleus is well defined by a surrounding neurone-poor zone, but the dorsomedial nucleus above it is much less distinct. The ventromedial nucleus contains neurones receptive to plasma levels of glucose and other nutrients and receives visceral somatic afferents via the nucleus tractus solitarius. The lateral hypothalamus receives olfactory afferents, which act as important food signals. Both areas receive extensive inputs from limbic structures. Stimulation and lesion experiments, together with human case studies, suggest that the ventromedial nuclei act together as a 'satiety centre'. Bilateral ventromedial nucleus damage promotes overeating (hyperphagia), and restricting food intake may provoke rage-like outbursts. The resultant obesity is usually coupled with hyposexuality (Fröhlich syndrome). Interestingly, in infants, ventromedial damage can lead to emaciation despite apparent normal feeding. Experimental lesions in the lateral hypothalamus promote hypophagia or aphagia, while stimulation can prolong feeding, supporting the concept of a lateral hypothalamic 'feeding centre'.

The ventromedial nucleus, lateral hypothalamic area and paraventricular nucleus also influence intermediate metabolism through the autonomic and endocrine systems. These appear to complement the effects on feeding behaviour. Thus, ventromedial stimulation facilitates glucagon release and increases glycogenolysis, gluconeogenesis and lipolysis, whereas lateral hypothalamic stimulation causes insulin release and opposite metabolic effects. Lesions of the ventromedial nucleus also cause increased vagal and decreased sympathetic tone.

The medial mammillary nuclei, which form the bulk of the mammillary bodies, are very prominent. The composition of a lateral mammillary nucleus is controversial, though a group of larger cells can be distinguished along the lateral border of the medial mammillary nucleus. Lateral to this lies the tuberomammillary nucleus, which gives rise to widespread axons that diffusely innervate the entire cerebral cortex, hypothalamus and brain stem.

The lateral zone of the hypothalamus forms a continuum that runs from the preoptic nucleus through the lateral hypothalamic area to the posterior hypothalamus. In the tuberal region, the lateral tuberal nuclei are large and well defined and surrounded by fine fibres.

CONNECTIONS OF THE HYPOTHALAMUS

The hypothalamus has afferent and efferent connections with the rest of the body via two (possibly three) quite distinct routes: neural connections; the bloodstream; and (probably) the CSF.

Some hypothalamic neurones have specific receptors that sense the temperature, osmolarity, glucose, free fatty acid, and hormone content of the blood. Neurosecretory neurones secrete neurohormones into the blood. These control the anterior pituitary and act on organs such as the kidney, breast, uterus and blood vessels. Some of these neural connections, especially those to the mammillary bodies, form discrete myelinated fascicles, but most are diffuse, unmyelinated and their origin and termination are uncertain. Most pathways are multisynaptic, which means that the majority of synapses on any hypothalamic neurone are derived from hypothalamic interneurones.

Broadly, neural inputs to the hypothalamus are derived from the ascending visceral and somatic sensory systems, the visual and olfactory systems, and numerous tracts from the brain stem, thalamus, 'limbic' structures and neocortex. Efferent neural projections are reciprocal to most of these sources and, in particular, they impinge on and control the central origins of autonomic nerve fibres. The hypothalamus therefore exerts control via the autonomic and endocrine systems and through its connections to the telencephalon.

Afferent connections

The hypothalamus receives visceral, gustatory and somatic sensory information from the spinal cord and brain stem. It receives largely polysynaptic projections from the nucleus tractus solitarius, probably directly and indirectly via the parabrachial nucleus and medullary noradrenergic cell groups (ventral noradrenergic bundle); collaterals of lemniscal somatic afferents (to the lateral hypothalamus); and projections from the dorsal longitudinal reticular formation. Many enter via the medial forebrain bundle (**Fig. 21.11**) and periventricular fibre system. Others converge in the midbrain tegmentum, forming the mammillary peduncle to the mammillary body.

The major forebrain inputs to the hypothalamus are derived from structures in the limbic system, including the hippocampal formation, amygdala and septum, and from the piriform lobe and adjacent neocortex. These connections, which are reciprocal, form prominent fibre systems, i.e. the fornix, stria terminalis, and ventral amygdalofugal tracts.

The hippocampal formation, in particular the subiculum and CA1, is reciprocally connected to the hypothalamus by the fornix, a complex tract that also contains commissural connections. As the fornix curves ventrally towards the anterior commissure it is joined by fascicles from the cingulate gyrus, indusium griseum and the septal areas. It divides around the anterior commissure into pre- and postcommissural parts. The precommissural fornix is distributed to the septum and preoptic hypothalamus, and the septum in turn sends numerous fibres to the hypothalamus. The postcommissural fornix passes ventrally and posteriorly through the hypothalamus to the medial mammillary nucleus. In its course it gives off many fibres to the medial and lateral hypothalamic nuclei.

The amygdala innervates most hypothalamic nuclei anterior to the mammillary bodies. Its corticomedial nucleus innervates preoptic and anterior hypothalamic areas and the ventromedial nucleus. The central nuclei project to the lateral hypothalamus. The fibres reach the hypothalamus by two routes. The short ventral amygdalofugal path passes medially over the optic tract, beneath the lentiform complex, to reach the hypothalamus. The long curved stria terminalis runs parallel to the fornix, separated from it by the lateral ventricle, passes through the bed nucleus of the stria terminalis, and is then distributed to the anterior hypothalamus via the medial forebrain bundle.

Olfactory afferents reach the hypothalamus largely via the nucleus accumbens and septal nuclei, and most terminate in the lateral hypothalamus. Visual afferents leave the optic chiasma and pass dorsally into the suprachiasmatic nucleus. No auditory connections have been identified, though it is clear that such stimuli influence hypothalamic activity. However, many hypothalamic neurones respond best to complex sensory stimuli, suggesting that sensory information reaching the neocortex has converged and been processed by the amygdala, hippocampus and neocortex. Neocortical corticohypothalamic afferents to the hypothalamus are poorly defined, but probably arise from frontal and insular cortices. Some may relay in the mediodorsal thalamic nucleus and project into the hypothalamus via the periventricular route. Other direct corticohypothalamic fibres may end in lateral, dorsomedial, mammillary and posterior hypothalamic nuclei, but all these connections are questioned.

Like the rest of the forebrain, the hypothalamus also receives diffuse aminergic inputs from the locus coeruleus – noradrenaline (norepinephrine), and raphe nuclei – serotonin (5-hydroxytryptamine; 5-HT). In addition, it receives a cholinergic input from the ventral tegmental ascending cholinergic pathway; a noradrenergic input to dorsomedial, periventricular, paraventricular, supraoptic and lateral hypothalamic nuclei from the ventral tegmental noradrenergic bundle; and dopamine fibres from the mesolimbic dopaminergic system. Group A11 innervates the medial hypothalamic nuclei, and groups A13 and A14 supply the dorsal and rostral hypothalamic nuclei. Many of these fibres also run in the medial forebrain bundle.

The medial forebrain bundle is a loose grouping of fibre pathways that mostly run longitudinally through the lateral hypothalamus (**Fig. 21.11**). It connects forebrain autonomic and limbic structures with the hypothalamus and brain stem, receiving and giving small fascicles throughout its course. It contains descending hypothalamic afferents from the septal area and orbitofrontal cortex, ascending afferents from the brain stem, and efferents from the hypothalamus.

Efferent connections

Hypothalamic efferents include reciprocal paths to the limbic system, descending polysynaptic paths to autonomic and somatic motor neurones, and neural and neurovascular links with the pituitary.

Septal areas and the amygdaloid complex have reciprocal hypothalamic connections along the paths described above. The medial preoptic and anterior hypothalamic areas give short projections to nearby hypothalamic groups. The ventromedial nucleus has more extensive projections that pass via the medial forebrain bundle to the bed nucleus of the stria terminalis, basal nucleus of Meynert, central nucleus of the amygdala, and midbrain reticular formation. The posterior hypothalamus projects largely to midbrain central grey matter. Some tuberal and posterior lateral hypothalamic neurones project directly to the entire neocortex and appear to be essential for maintaining cortical arousal, but the topography of these projections is unclear.

Hypothalamic neurones projecting to autonomic neurones are found in the paraventricular nucleus (oxytocin and vasopressin neurones), perifornical and dorsomedial nuclei (atrial natriuretic peptide neurones), lateral hypothalamic area (α-melanocyte-stimulating hormone; α-MSH neurones), and zona incerta (dopamine neurones). These fibres run through the medial forebrain bundle into the tegmentum, ventrolateral medulla and dorsal lateral funiculus of the spinal cord. In the brain stem, fibres innervate the parabrachial nucleus, nucleus ambiguus, nucleus of the solitary tract and dorsal motor nucleus of the vagus. In the spinal cord, they end on sympathetic and parasympathetic preganglionic neurones in the intermediolateral column. Both oxytocin- and vasopressin-containing fibres can be traced to the most caudal spinal autonomic neurones.

The medial mammillary nucleus gives rise to a large ascending fibre bundle, which diverges into mammillothalamic and mammillotegmental tracts (**Fig. 21.11**). The mammillothalamic tract ascends through the lateral hypothalamus to reach the anterior thalamic nuclei, whence massive projections radiate to the cingulate gyrus. The mammillo-tegmental tract curves inferiorly into the midbrain ventral to the medial longitudinal fasciculus, and is distributed to tegmental reticular nuclei.

PITUITARY GLAND (Figs 16.8, 21.12)

The pituitary gland, or hypophysis cerebri, is a reddish-grey, ovoid body, c.12 mm in transverse and 8 mm in anteroposterior diameter, and weighing c.500 mg. It is continuous with the infundibulum, a hollow, conical, inferior process from the tuber cinereum of the hypothalamus. It lies within the pituitary fossa of the sphenoid bone, where it is covered superiorly by a circular diaphragma sellae of dura mater. The latter is pierced centrally by an aperture for the infundibulum, and separates the anterior superior aspect of the pituitary from the optic chiasma. The pituitary is flanked by the cavernous sinuses and their contents. Inferiorly, it is separated from the floor of the pituitary fossa by a venous sinus that communicates with the circular sinus. The meninges blend with the pituitary capsule and are not separate layers.

The pituitary has two major parts, neurohypophysis and adeno-hypophysis, which differ in their origin, structure and function. The neurohypophysis is a diencephalic downgrowth connected with the hypothalamus. The adenohypophysis is an ectodermal derivative of the stomatodeum. Both include parts of the infundibulum (whereas the older terms 'anterior lobe' and 'posterior lobe' do not). The infundibulum has a central infundibular stem, which contains neural hypophyseal connections and is continuous with the median eminence of the tuber cinereum. Thus, the term neurohypophysis includes the median eminence, infundibular stem and neural lobe or pars posterior. Surrounding the infundibular stem is the pars tuberalis, a component of the adenohypophysis. The main mass of the adenohypophysis may be divided into the pars anterior (pars distalis) and the pars intermedia, which are separated in fetal and early postnatal life by the hypophyseal cleft, a vestige of Rathke's pouch, from which it develops. Usually obliterated in childhood, remnants may persist in the form of cystic cavities often present near the adenoneurohypophyseal frontier and sometimes invading the neural lobe. The human pars intermedia is rudimentary. It may be partially displaced into the neural lobe, and so it has been included in the anterior and posterior parts by different observers. Apart from this equivocation, of little significance in view of the exiguous status of the human pars intermedia, the pars anterior and pars posterior may be equated with the anterior and posterior lobes. When the associated infundibular parts continuous with these lobes are included, the names adenohypophysis and neurohypophysis become appropriate, and will be used here as follows. Neurohypophysis includes the pars posterior (pars nervosa, posterior or neural lobe), infundibular stem and median eminence. Adenohypophysis includes the pars anterior (pars distalis or glandularis), pars intermedia and pars tuberalis.

Neurohypophysis

In early fetal life the neurohypophysis contains a cavity continuous with the third ventricle. Axons arising from groups of hypothalamic neurones (e.g. the magnocellular neurones of the supraoptic and paraventricular nuclei) terminate in the neurohypophysis. The long magnocellular axons pass to the main mass of the neurohypophysis. They form the neurosecretory hypothalamohypophyseal tract and terminate near the sinusoids of the posterior lobe. Some smaller parvocellular neurones in the periventricular zone have shorter axons, and end in the median eminence and infundibular stem among the superior capillary beds of the venous portal circulation. These small neurones produce releasing and inhibitory hormones, which control the secretory activities of the adenohypophysis via its portal blood supply.

The neurohormones stored in the main part of the neurohypophysis are vasopressin (antidiuretic hormone; ADH), which controls reabsorption of water by renal tubules (p. 1277), and oxytocin, which promotes the contraction of uterine smooth muscle (p. 1334) in childbirth and the ejection of milk from the breast during lactation. Storage granules containing active hormone polypeptides bound to a transport glycoprotein, neurophysin, pass down axons from their site of synthesis in the neuronal somata. The granules are seen as swellings along the axons and at their terminals, which can reach the size of erythrocytes (**Fig. 21.13**).

The thin, non-myelinated axons of the neurohypophysis (**Figs 21.14, 21.15**) are ensheathed by typical astrocytes in the infundibulum. Near the posterior lobe, astrocytes are replaced by pituicytes, which constitute most of the non-excitable tissue in the neurohypophysis. Pituicytes are dendritic neuroglial cells of variable appearance, often with long processes running parallel to adjacent axons. Typically, their cytoplasmic processes end on the walls of capillaries and sinusoids between nerve terminals. Axons also end in perivascular spaces. Although they are close to the walls of sinusoids, they remain separated from them by two basal laminae, one around the nerve endings and the other underlying the fenestrated endothelial cells. Fine collagen fibrils occupy the spaces between basal laminae.

Adenohypophysis

The adenohypophysis is highly vascular. It consists of epithelial cells of varying size and shape arranged in cords or irregular follicles, between which lie thin-walled vascular sinusoids supported by a delicate reticular connective tissue (**Figs 21.13, 21.14, 21.15**). Most of the hormones synthesized by the adenohypophysis are trophic. They include the peptides, growth hormone (GH), involved in the control of body growth, and prolactin (PRL), which stimulates both growth of breast tissue and milk secretion. Glycoprotein trophic hormones are the large pro-opiomelanocortin precursor of adrenocorticotrophin (ACTH), which controls the secretion of certain suprarenal cortical hormones; thyroid-stimulating hormone (TSH); follicle-stimulating hormone (FSH), which

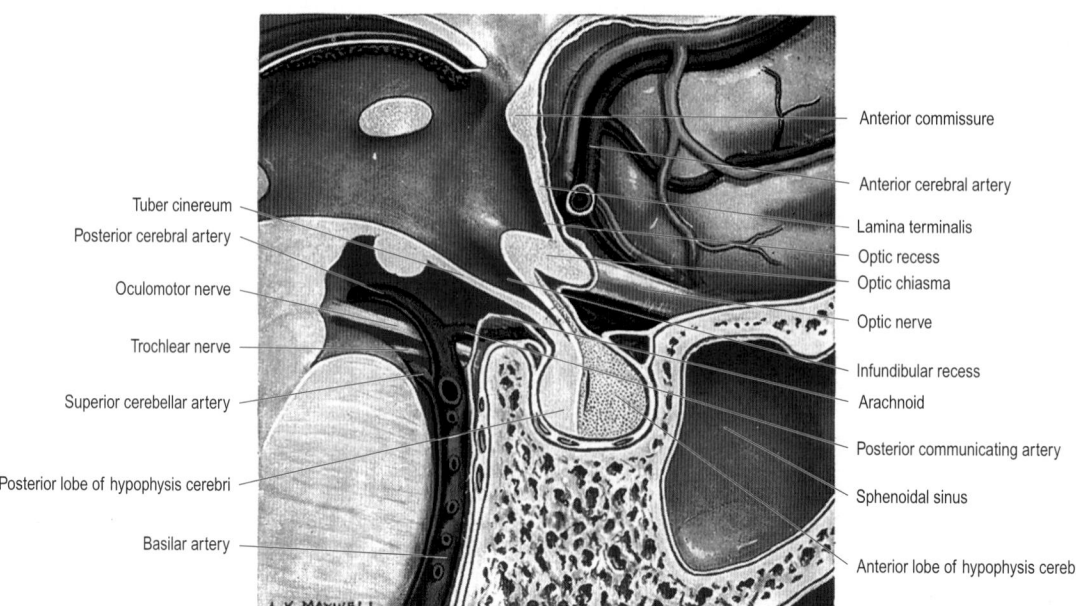

Fig. 21.12 Median section through the hypophysis cerebri.

Tuber cinereum
Posterior cerebral artery
Oculomotor nerve
Trochlear nerve
Superior cerebellar artery
Posterior lobe of hypophysis cerebri
Basilar artery

Anterior commissure
Anterior cerebral artery
Lamina terminalis
Optic recess
Optic chiasma
Optic nerve
Infundibular recess
Arachnoid
Posterior communicating artery
Sphenoidal sinus
Anterior lobe of hypophysis cerebri

A.K. MAXWELL

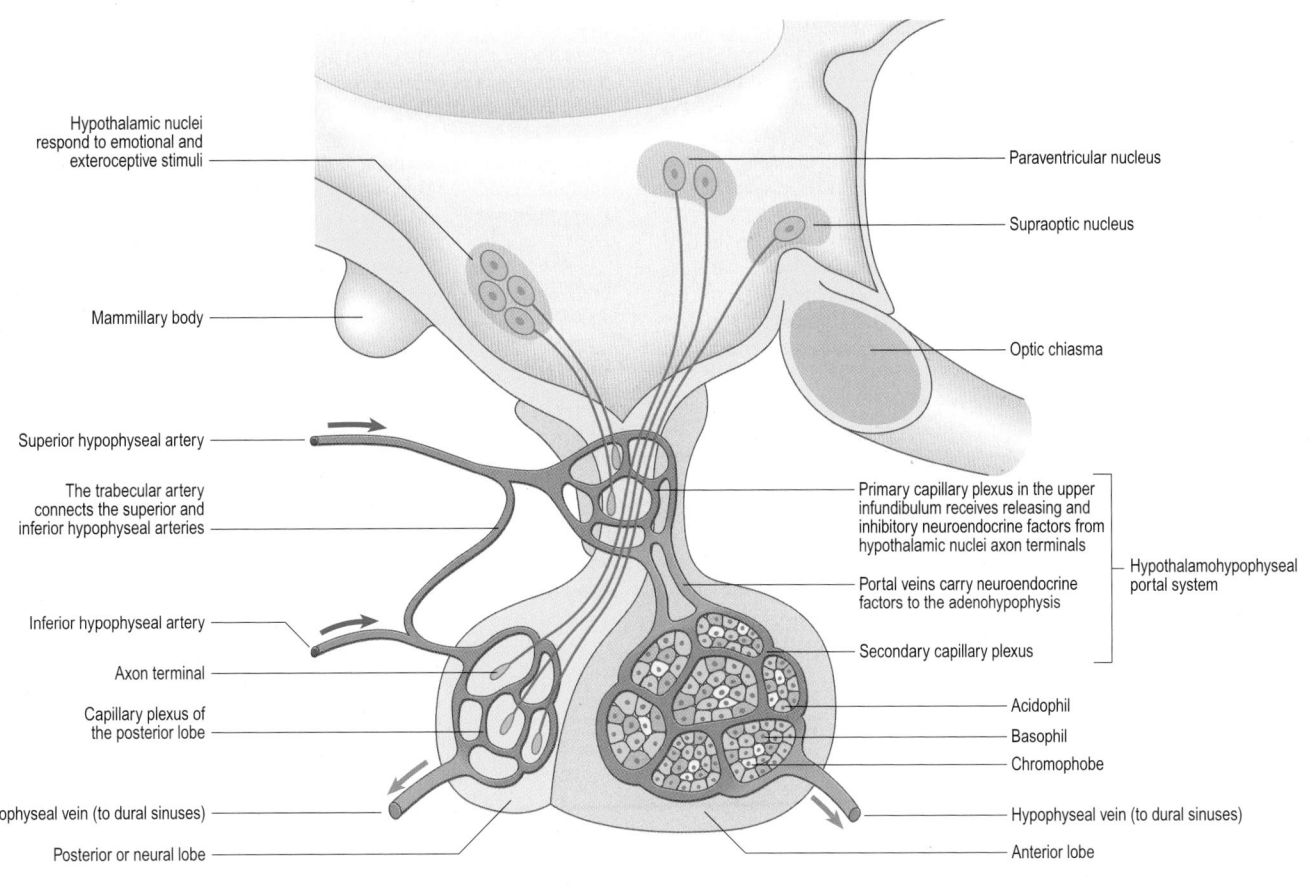

Hypothalamic nuclei respond to emotional and exteroceptive stimuli

Paraventricular nucleus

Supraoptic nucleus

Mammillary body

Optic chiasma

Superior hypophyseal artery

The trabecular artery connects the superior and inferior hypophyseal arteries

Primary capillary plexus in the upper infundibulum receives releasing and inhibitory neuroendocrine factors from hypothalamic nuclei axon terminals

Portal veins carry neuroendocrine factors to the adenohypophysis

Hypothalamohypophyseal portal system

Inferior hypophyseal artery

Axon terminal

Secondary capillary plexus

Acidophil

Capillary plexus of the posterior lobe

Basophil

Chromophobe

Hypophyseal vein (to dural sinuses)

Hypophyseal vein (to dural sinuses)

Posterior or neural lobe

Anterior lobe

Fig. 21.13 The main systems controlling the endocrine secretory activities of the pituitary gland.

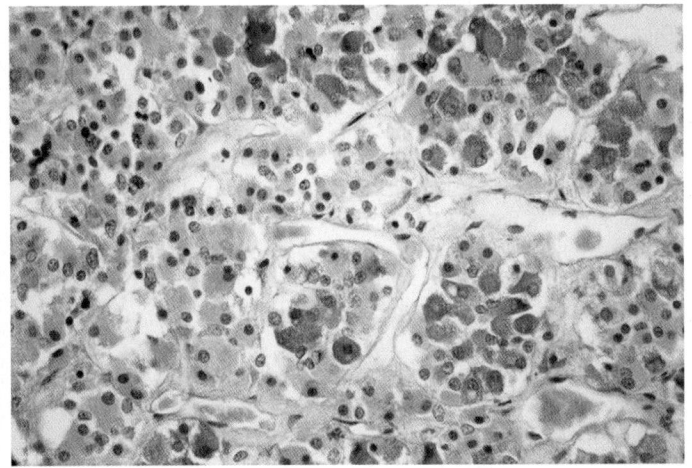

Fig. 21.14 The pituitary gland (trichrome-stained) showing the endocrine cells of the adenohypophysis. Chromophils can be distinguished as acidophils (yellow) and basophils (pink). Chromophobes are pale-staining cells. A network of sinusoids is seen between clusters of secretory cells. (Photograph by Sarah-Jane Smith.)

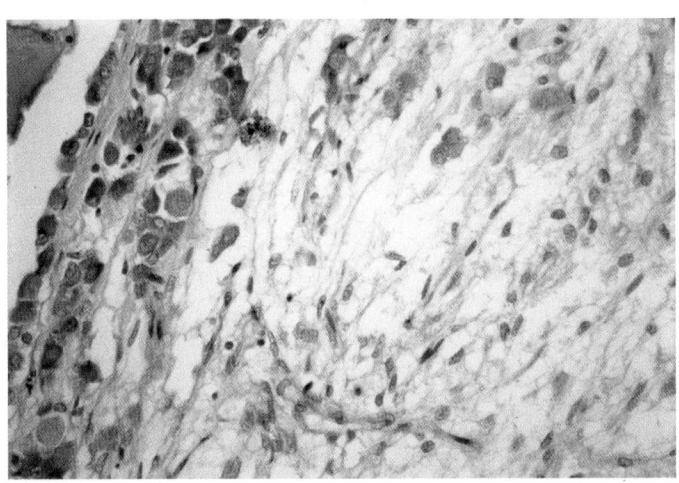

Fig. 21.15 The pituitary neurohypophysis (right), with nerve fibres and pituicytes. To the left is the pars intermedia with scattered, deeper staining secretory cells and a cyst containing colloid (top left), representing the remnants of Rathke's pouch. (Photograph by Sarah-Jane Smith.)

stimulates growth and secretion of oestrogens in ovarian follicles and spermatogenesis (acting on testicular Sertoli cells); and luteinizing hormone (LH), which induces progesterone secretion by the corpus luteum and testosterone synthesis by Leydig cells in the testis. Proopiomelanocortin is cleaved into a number of different molecules including ACTH. β-Lipotropin is released from the pituitary, but its lipolytic function in humans is uncertain. β-Endorphin is another cleavage product released from the pituitary (p. 43).

The epithelial endocrine cells, which secrete the different adenohypophyseal hormones, are distinguished in part by their differing affinities for acidic and basic dyes. Cells staining strongly are described as chromophils, those with low affinity for dyes are chromophobes. Chromophils that stain strongly with acidic dyes are classed as acidophils, whereas basophils stain strongly with basic dyes; the latter are more prevalent in the central part of the gland. Classification according to the hormones synthesized divides cells into somatotrophs (GH-secreting acidophils, the most numerous chromophil type); lactotrophs (prolactin-secreting acidophils, which are dominant in pregnancy and hypertrophy during lactation); gonadotrophs (FSH- and LH-secreting basophils); thyrotrophs (TH-secreting basophils); and corticotrophs (ACTH-secreting basophils). Chromophobes are thought to be quiescent or degranulated chromophils, or immature precursor cells – they constitute up to half of the cells of the adenohypophysis.

Neurones that secrete the peptides and amines that control the anterior lobe are widely distributed within the hypothalamus. They are situated mainly in the medial zone, in the arcuate nucleus, medial parvocellular part of the paraventricular nucleus, and periventricular nucleus.

The pars intermedia contains follicles of chromophobe cells that surround cyst-like structures lined by epithelium and filled, to varying degrees, with glycosylated colloidal material. Secretory products of this region may include cleavage products of pro-opiomelanocortin but their functional significance is uncertain. The pars tuberalis contains a large number of blood vessels, between which are cords or clusters of gonadotrophs and undifferentiated cells.

A small collection of adenohypophyseal tissue lies in the mucoperiosteum of the human nasopharyngeal roof. By 28 weeks *in utero* it is well vascularized and capable of secretion, receiving blood from the systemic vessels of the nasopharyngeal roof. At this stage it is covered posteriorly by fibrous tissue. This is replaced in the second half of fetal life by venous sinuses, and a transsphenoidal portal venous system develops, bringing the nasopharyngeal tissue under the same hypothalamic control as the cranial adenohypophyseal tissue. The peripheral vascularity of the pharyngeal hypophysis persists until about the fifth year. The organ is then reinvested by fibrous tissue and presumed to be again controlled by factors present in systemic blood. Though it does not change in size after birth in males, in females it becomes smaller, returning to natal volume during the fifth decade, when once again it may be controlled via a transsphenoidal extension of the hypothalamohypophyseal portal venous system. The human pharyngeal hypophysis may be a reserve of potential adenohypophyseal tissue, which may be stimulated, particularly in females, to synthesize and secrete adenohypophyseal hormones in middle age, when intracranial adenohypophyseal tissue is beginning to fail.

Vessels of the pituitary

The arteries of the pituitary arise from the internal carotid arteries via a single inferior and several superior hypophyseal arteries on each side (Fig. 21.16). The former come from the cavernous part of the internal carotid artery, the latter from its supraclinoid part and from the anterior and posterior cerebral arteries. The inferior hypophyseal arteries divide into medial and lateral branches, which anastomose across the midline and form an arterial ring around the infundibulum. Fine branches from this circular anastomosis enter the neurohypophysis to supply its

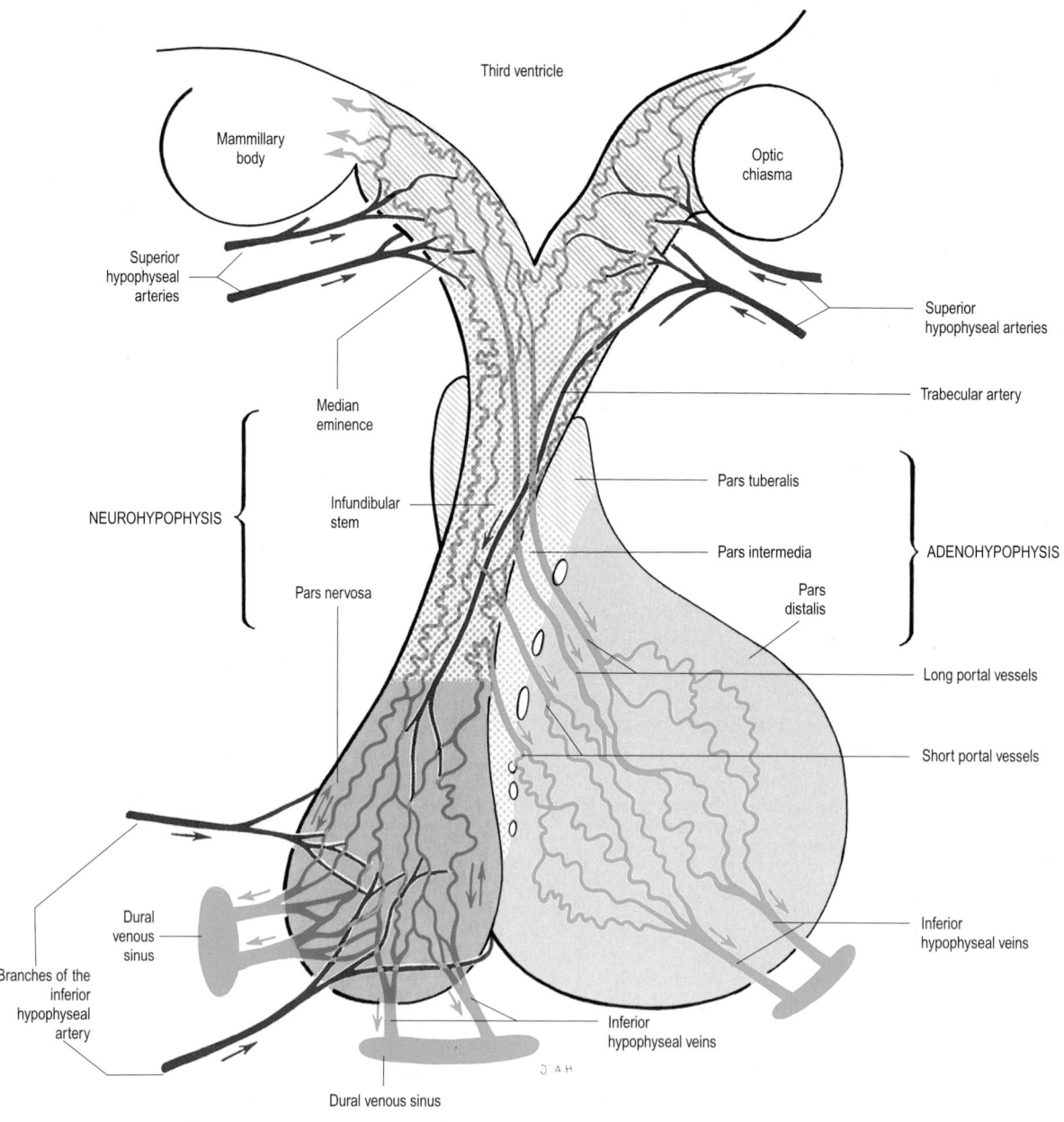

Fig. 21.16 A summary of the vasculature of the hypothalamic median eminence, infundibulum and the other regimes of the hypophysis cerebri.

capillary bed. The superior hypophyseal arteries supply the median eminence, upper infundibulum and, via arteries of the trabeculae, the lower infundibulum. A confluent capillary net, extending through the neurohypophysis, is supplied by both sets of hypophyseal vessels. Reversal of flow can occur in cerebral capillary beds lying between the two supplies.

The arteries of the median eminence and infundibulum end in characteristic sprays of capillaries, which are most complex in the upper infundibulum. In the median eminence these form an external or 'mantle' plexus and an internal or 'deep' plexus. The external plexus, fed by the superior hypophyseal arteries, is continuous with the infundibular plexus and is drained by long portal vessels, which descend to the pars anterior. The internal plexus lies within and is supplied by the external plexus. It is continuous posteriorly with the infundibular capillary bed and, like the external plexus, is drained by long portal vessels. Short portal vessels run from the lower infundibulum to the pars anterior. Both types of portal vessel open into vascular sinusoids, which lie between the secretory cords in the adenohypophysis and provide most of its blood. There is no direct arterial supply. The portal system carries hormone-releasing factors, probably elaborated in parvocellular groups of hypothalamic neurones, and these control the secretory cycles of cells in the pars anterior. The pars intermedia appears to be avascular.

There are three possible routes for venous drainage of the neurohypophysis. These are: to the adenohypophysis, via long and short portal vessels; into the dural venous sinuses, via the large inferior hypophyseal veins; and to the hypothalamus, via capillaries passing to the median eminence. The venous drainage carries hypophyseal hormones from the gland to their targets and also facilitates feedback control of secretion. However, venous drainage of the adenohypophysis appears restricted. Few vessels connect it directly to the systemic veins so the routes by which blood leaves remain obscure.

SUBTHALAMUS

The subthalamus is a complex region of nuclear groups and fibre tracts (Fig. 21.17). The main nuclear groups are the subthalamic nucleus, the reticular nucleus, the zona incerta, the fields of Forel and the pregeniculate nucleus. The rostral poles of the red nucleus and substantia nigra also extend into this area.

The main subthalamic tracts are: the upper parts of the medial, spinal and trigeminal lemnisci and the solitariothalamic tract, all approaching their terminations in the thalamic nuclei; the dentatothalamic tract from the contralateral superior cerebellar peduncle accompanied by ipsilateral rubrothalamic fibres; the fasciculus retroflexus; the fasciculus lenticularis; the fasciculus subthalamicus; the ansa lenticularis; fascicles from the prerubral field (H field of Forel); the continuation of the fasciculus lenticularis (in the H$_2$ field of Forel); the fasciculus thalamicus (the H$_1$ field of Forel).

SUBTHALAMIC NUCLEUS

The subthalamic nucleus is intimately connected with the basal ganglia and is considered with them (p. 428).

ZONA INCERTA AND FIELDS OF FOREL

The zona incerta is an aggregation of small cells that lies between the ventral part of the external medullary lamina of the thalamus and the cerebral peduncle. It is linked to the reticular nucleus dorsolaterally. More medially is a scattered group of cells in a matrix of fibres known as the H field of Forel. Field H$_1$ of Forel consists of the thalamic fasciculus, which lies dorsal to the zona incerta. Field H$_2$ of Forel contains the fasciculus lenticularis, and lies ventrally, between the zona incerta and the subthalamic nucleus (Fig. 21.17).

The zona incerta receives fibres from the sensorimotor cortex, the pregeniculate nucleus, the deep cerebellar nuclei, the trigeminal nuclear complex and the spinal cord. It projects to the spinal cord and the pretectal region. Its functions are unknown.

The neurones of the H field of Forel receive afferents from the internal segment of the globus pallidus, the spinal cord and the reticular formation of the brain stem. They may project to the spinal cord. Like the zona incerta, their functions are unknown.

In addition to terminal parts of the lemniscal, dentatothalamic and rubrothalamic tracts, the subthalamus contains massive fibre tracts derived from the globus pallidus. The fasciculus lenticularis is the dorsal component of pallidofugal fibres that traverse the internal capsule. It

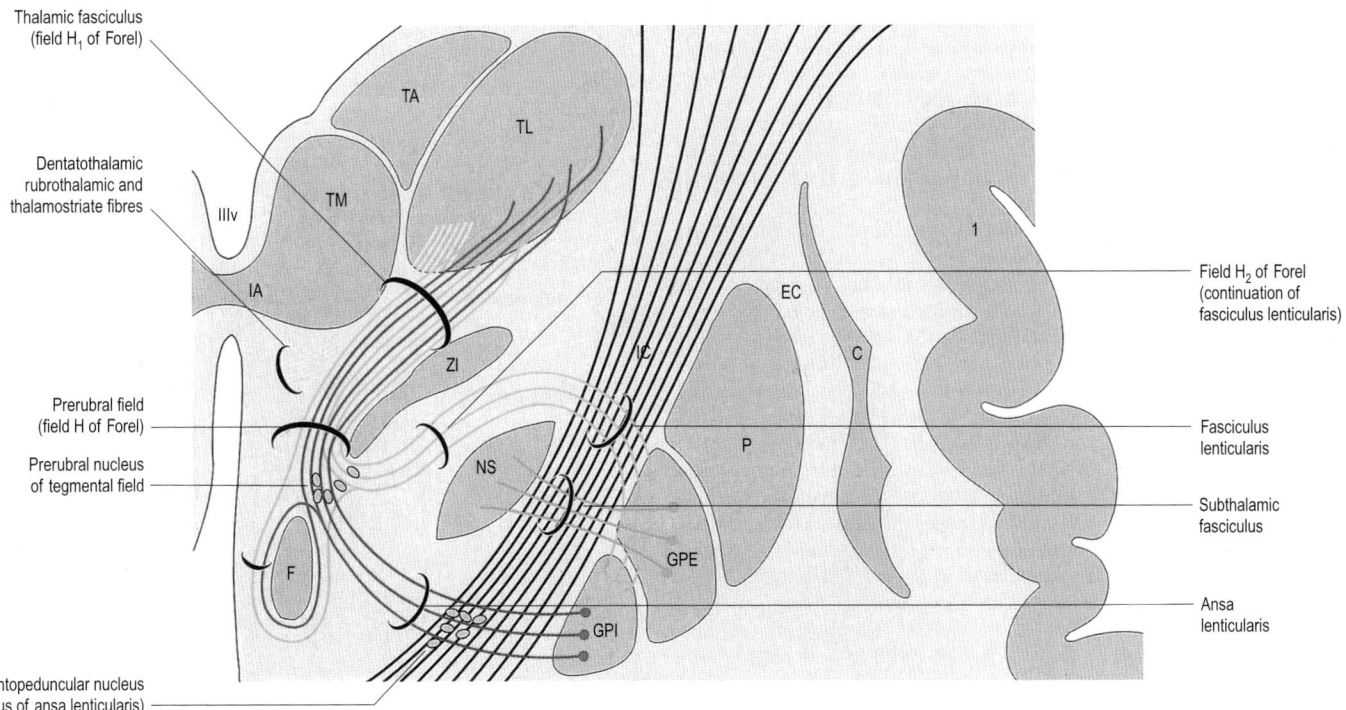

Fig. 21.17 The nuclear masses and fibre tract systems associated with, or closely related topographically to, parts of the thalamus, subthalamus and globus pallidus. Abbreviations: C, claustrum; EC, external capsule; F, column of fornix; GPI and GPE, internal and external parts of globus pallidus; I, cortex of insula; IA, interthalamic adhesion; IC, internal capsule; IIIv, third ventricle; M, medial nuclear group of thalamus; NS, subthalamic nucleus; P, putamen; TA, anterior nuclear group of thalamus; TL, lateral nuclear group of thalamus; ZI, zona incerta.

turns medially near the medial aspect of the capsule, partly intermingled with the dorsal zone of the subthalamic nucleus and the ventral part of the zona incerta, where the fasciculus traverses the H_2 field of Forel. Reaching the medial border of the zona incerta, the fasciculus intermingles with fibres of the ansa lenticularis, scattered elements of the prerubral nucleus, and dentatothalamic and rubrothalamic fibres. This merging of diverse pathways and associated cell groups is variously called the prerubral, tegmental or H field of Forel.

The ansa lenticularis has a complex origin from both parts of the globus pallidus and possibly other adjacent structures. It curves medially round the ventral border of the internal capsule, and continues dorsomedially to mingle with other fibres in the prerubral field. Some fibres in the fasciculus lenticularis and ansa lenticularis synapse in the subthalamic nucleus, prerubral field and zona incerta. The remainder continue laterally, with other fascicles, into the thalamic nuclei, particularly the ventral anterior, ventral lateral and centromedian nuclei.

The thalamic fasciculus extends from the prerubral field – its territory is sometimes termed the H_1 field of Forel. It lies dorsal to, and also partly traverses, the zona incerta, and is related dorsally to the ventral thalamic nuclei. It contains continuations of the fasciculus lenticularis and ansa lenticularis, and dentatothalamic, rubrothalamic and thalamostriate fibres.

The subthalamic fasciculus connects the subthalamic nucleus with the globus pallidus. It contains an abundant two-way array of fibres which traverse the internal capsule, interweaving with it at right angles.

EPITHALAMUS

The epithalamus consists of the anterior and posterior paraventricular nuclei, the medial and lateral habenular nuclei, the stria medullaris thalami, posterior commissure and the pineal body.

HABENULAR NUCLEI AND STRIA MEDULLARIS

The habenular nuclei lie posteriorly at the dorsomedial corner of the thalamus, immediately deep to the ependyma of the third ventricle, with the stria medullaris thalami above and laterally. The medial habenular nucleus is a densely packed, deeply staining, mass of cholinergic neurones, whereas the lateral nucleus is more dispersed and paler staining. The habenulo-interpenduncular tract, or fasciculus retroflexus, emerges from the ventral margin of the nuclei and courses ventrally, skirts the inferior zone of the thalamic mediodorsal nucleus, and traverses the superomedial region of the red nucleus to reach the interpeduncular nucleus. The habenular nuclear complex is limited laterally by a fibrous lamina, which enters the habenulo-interpeduncular tract. Posteriorly, the nuclei of the two sides and the internal medullary laminae are linked across the midline by the habenular commissure. The tela choroidea of the third ventricle usually arises from the ependyma at the superolateral corner of the medial habenular nucleus.

Afferent fibres to the habenular nuclei travel in the stria medullaris from the prepiriform cortex bilaterally, the basal nucleus of Meynert, and the hypothalamus. Afferents from the internal segment of the globus pallidus ascend through the thalamus, and may be collaterals of pallidothalamic axons. Additional inputs come from the pars compacta of the substantia nigra, the midbrain raphe nuclei and the lateral dorsal tegmental nucleus. The afferent pathways mostly end in the lateral habenular nucleus. The only identified afferent fibres to the medial habenular nucleus come from the septofimbrial nucleus.

The medial habenular nucleus sends efferent fibres to the interpeduncular nucleus of the midbrain. The lateral habenular nucleus sends fibres to the raphe nuclei and the adjacent reticular formation of the midbrain, the pars compacta of the substantia nigra and the ventral tegmental area, and to the hypothalamus and basal forebrain.

The main habenular outflow reaches the interpeduncular nucleus, mediodorsal thalamic nucleus, mesencephalic tectum and reticular formation, the largest component constituting the habenulo-interpeduncular tract to the interpeduncular nucleus. The latter provides relays to the midbrain reticular formation, from which tectotegmentospinal tracts and dorsal longitudinal fasciculi connect with autonomic preganglionic neurones controlling salivation, gastric and intestinal secretory activity and motility, and motor nuclei for mastication and deglutition.

The stria medullaris crosses the superomedial thalamic aspect, skirts medial to the habenular trigone and sends many fibres into the ipsilateral

habenula. Other fibres cross in the anterior pineal lamina, and decussate, as the habenular commissure, to reach the contralateral habenula. Some fibres are really commissural and interconnect the amygdaloid complexes and hippocampal cortices. They are accompanied by crossed tectohabenular fibres. Serotonin-containing fibres from the ventral ascending tegmental serotoninergic bundle, which join the habenulo-interpeduncular tract to reach the nuclei, may control neurones of the habenulopineal tract, and thus influence innervation of pinealocytes. Similarly, habenular nuclear afferents from the dorsal ascending tegmental noradrenergic bundle may influence pinealocytes.

Little is known of the physiological functions of the habenular nuclei. It has been suggested that they may be involved in the control of sleep mechanisms. Though the human habenula is relatively small, it is a focus of integration of diverse olfactory, visceral and somatic afferent paths. Lesions that include this area of the medial diencephalon indicate that it plays a role in the regulation of visceral and neuroendocrine functions. Ablation of the habenula causes extensive changes in metabolism, and endocrine and thermal regulation.

POSTERIOR COMMISSURE

The posterior commissure, which is of unknown constitution in man, is a small fasciculus which decussates in the posterior pineal lamina. Various small nuclei are associated with it. Among these are the interstitial nuclei of the posterior commissure, the nucleus of Darkschewitscz in the periaqueductal grey matter, and the interstitial nucleus of Cajal near the upper end of the oculomotor complex, closely linked with the medial longitudinal fasciculus. Fibres from all these nuclei and the fasciculus cross in the posterior commissure. It also contains fibres from thalamic and pretectal nuclei and the superior colliculi, together with fibres that connect the tectal and habenular nuclei. The destinations and functions of many of these fibres are obscure.

PINEAL GLAND

The pineal gland or epiphysis cerebri (**Figs 16.8, 21.18**) is a small, reddish-grey organ, occupying a depression between the superior colliculi. It is inferior to the splenium of the corpus callosum, from which it is separated by the tela choroidea of the third ventricle and the contained cerebral veins. It is enveloped by the lower layer of the tela, which is reflected from the gland to the tectum. The pineal is c.8 mm in length. Its base, directed anteriorly, is attached by a peduncle, which divides into inferior and superior laminae, separated by the pineal recess of the third ventricle, and containing the posterior and habenular

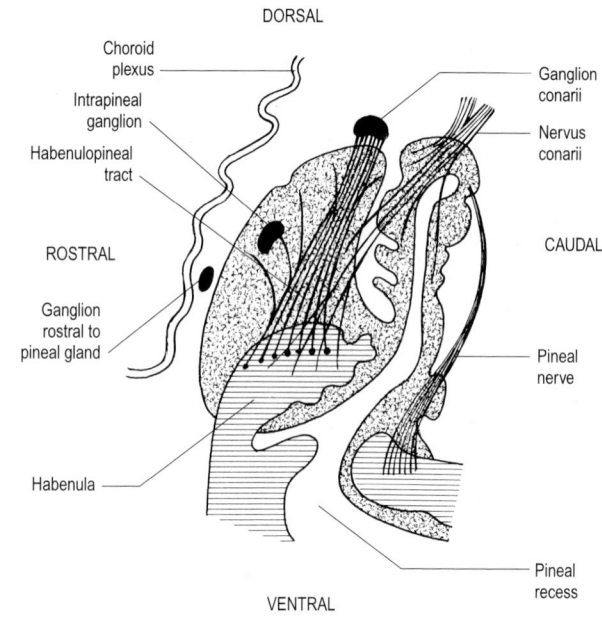

Fig. 21.18 The principal neural pathways which have been described in connection with the human fetal pineal gland.

commissures respectively. Aberrant commissural fibres may invade the gland but do not terminate near parenchymal cells.

Septa extend into the pineal gland from the surrounding pia mater. They divide the gland into lobules and carry blood vessels and fine unmyelinated sympathetic axons. The gland has a rich blood supply. The pineal arteries are branches of the medial posterior choroidal arteries, which are branches of the posterior cerebral artery. Within the gland, branches of the arteries supply fenestrated capillaries whose endothelial cells rest on a tenuous and sometimes incomplete basal lamina. The capillaries drain into numerous pineal veins, which open into the internal cerebral veins and/or into the great cerebral vein.

Postganglionic adrenergic sympathetic axons (derived from the superior cervical ganglion) enter the dorsolateral aspect of the gland from the region of the tentorium cerebelli as the nervus conarii, which may be single or paired. The nerve lies deep to the endothelium of the wall of the straight sinus. It is associated with blood vessels and parenchymal cells within the pineal.

The pineal gland contains cords and clusters of pinealocytes, associated with astrocyte-like neuroglia. Neuroglia are the main cellular component of the pineal stalk. Pinealocytes are highly modified neurones. They contain multiple synaptic ribbons (p. 44), randomly distributed between adjacent cells, and are coupled by gap junctions. Two or more processes extend from each cell body and end in bulbous expansions near capillaries or, less frequently, on ependymal cells of the pineal recess. These terminal expansions contain rough endoplasmic reticulum, mitochondria and dense-cored vesicles which store melatonin. Melatonin, and its precursor serotonin, are synthesized from tryptophan by the pinealocytes, and secreted into the surrounding network of fenestrated capillaries.

The pineal is an endocrine gland of major regulatory importance. It modifies the activity of the adenohypophysis, neurohypophysis, endocrine pancreas, parathyroids, adrenal cortex, adrenal medulla and gonads. Its effects are largely inhibitory. Indoleamine and polypeptide hormones secreted by pinealocytes are believed to reduce the synthesis and release of hormones by the pars anterior, either by direct action on its secretory cells or indirectly by inhibiting production of hypothalamic releasing factors. Pineal secretions may reach their target cells via the cerebrospinal fluid or the bloodstream. Some pineal indoleamines, including melatonin and enzymes for their biosynthesis (e.g. serotonin *N*-acetyltransferase) show circadian rhythms in concentration. The level rises during darkness, and falls during the day, when secretion may be inhibited by sympathetic activity. It is thought that the intrinsic rhythmicity of an endogenous circadian oscillator in the suprachiasmatic nucleus of the hypothalamus governs cyclical pineal behaviour (p. 376).

From the second decade, calcareous deposits accumulate in pineal extracellular matrix, where they are deposited concentrically as corpora arenacea or 'brain sand' (**Fig. 21.19**). Calcification is often detectable in skull radiographs, when it can provide a useful indicator of a space-occupying lesion if the gland is significantly displaced from the midline.

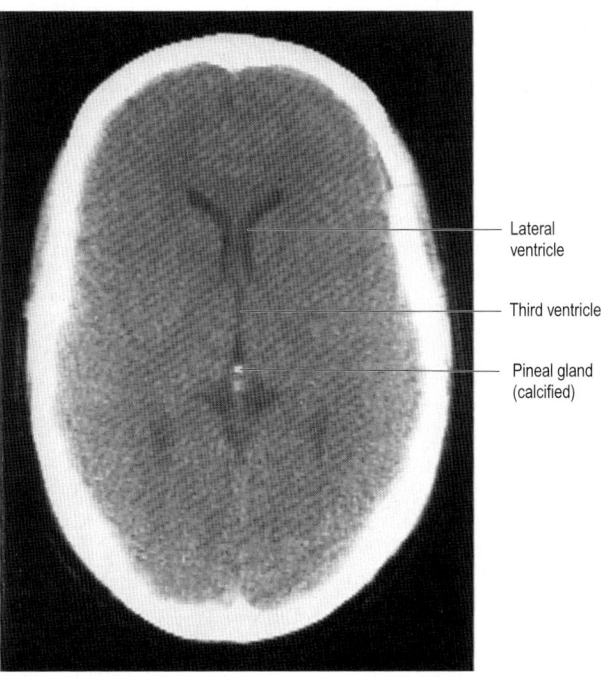

Lateral ventricle

Third ventricle

Pineal gland (calcified)

Fig. 21.19 Computed tomogram of the head in the horizontal plane at the level of the pineal gland. (Provided by Shaun Gallagher, GKT School of Medicine, London; photograph by Sarah-Jane Smith.)

REFERENCES

Jones EG 1985 The Thalamus. New York: Plenum Press: 403–11.
  Describes the nomenclature and connections of thalamic nuclei
Macchi G, Jones EG 1997 Toward an agreement on terminology of nuclear and subnuclear divisions of the motor thalamus. J Neurosurg 86(4): 670–85.
  Compares the different nomenclatures for motor thalamic nuclei in humans and monkeys and proposes a common terminology.
Nieuwenhuys R 1985 Chemoarchitecture of the Brain. Berlin: Springer-Verlag.
  Describes the connections and neurochemistry of the hypothalamus.

Cerebral hemisphere

The cerebral hemispheres are the largest part of the brain. They each have an external highly convoluted cortex, beneath which lies an extensive internal mass of white matter that contains the basal ganglia. Each hemisphere also contains a lateral ventricle, continuous with the third ventricle through the interventricular foramen. The two hemispheres are linked by the commissural fibres of the corpus callosum.

The cerebral hemisphere contains primary motor and sensory areas. These represent the highest level at which motor activities are controlled and the highest level to which general and special sensory systems project, providing the neural substrate for conscious experience of sensory stimuli. Association areas are modality-specific and also multi-modal, and they enable complex analysis of the internal and external environment and the relationship of the individual to the external world. Parts of the hemisphere, termed the limbic system, have an ancient lineage. They are concerned with memory and the emotional aspects of behaviour, providing an affective patina to conscious experience and interfacing with subcortical areas, such as the hypothalamus, through which widespread physiological activities are integrated. Other areas, primarily within the frontal region, are concerned with the highest aspects of cognitive function, and contribute to personality, foresight and planning.

The cerebral cortex is often divided into a phylogenetically old allocortex, consisting of the archicortex and paleocortex, and a newer neocortex.

The cerebral hemispheres are separated by a deep median cleft, the great longitudinal fissure, which contains a crescentic fold of the dura mater, the falx cerebri. Each cerebral hemisphere presents superolateral, medial and inferior surfaces or aspects.

The superolateral surface follows the concavity of the cranial vault. The medial surface is flat and vertical, separated from its fellow by the great longitudinal fissure and falx cerebri. The inferior (basal) surface is irregular and divided into orbital and tentorial regions. The orbital part of the frontal lobe is concave and lies above the orbital and nasal roofs. The tentorial region is the inferior surface of the temporal and occipital lobes. Anteriorly it is adapted to its half of the middle cranial fossa, and

posteriorly it lies above the tentorium cerebelli, which is interposed between it and the superior surface of the cerebellum. The anterior and posterior hemispheric extremities are the frontal and occipital poles respectively, and the temporal pole is the anterior extremity of the temporal lobe.

GYRI, SULCI AND LOBES

The surface of the cerebral hemisphere shows a complex pattern of convolutions, or gyri, which are separated by furrows of varying depth known as fissures, or sulci. Some of these are consistently located, others less so. They partly provide the basis for division of the hemisphere into lobes. The frontal, parietal, temporal and occipital lobes approximately correspond in surface extent to the cranial bones from which they take their names. The insula is a cortical region hidden within the depths of the lateral fissure by overhanging parts (opercula) of the frontal, parietal and temporal lobes. A complex of gyri on the medial aspect of the hemisphere makes up the limbic lobe.

The area of the cerebral cortex is c.2200 cm². Its convoluted nature increases the cortical volume to three times what it would be if the surface were smooth.

On the superolateral cerebral surface two prominent furrows, the lateral (Sylvian) fissure and the central sulcus, are the main features that determine its surface divisions (**Figs 22.1, 22.3**).

The lateral fissure is a deep cleft on the lateral and inferior surfaces. It separates the frontal and parietal lobes above from the temporal lobe below. It has a short stem, which divides into three rami. The stem commences inferiorly at the anterior perforated substance, extending laterally between the orbital surface of the frontal lobe and the anterior pole of the temporal lobe and accommodating the sphenoparietal venous sinus. Reaching the lateral surface of the hemisphere it divides into anterior horizontal, anterior ascending and posterior rami. The anterior ramus runs forwards for 2.5 cm or less into the inferior frontal gyrus, while the ascending ramus ascends for an equal distance into the

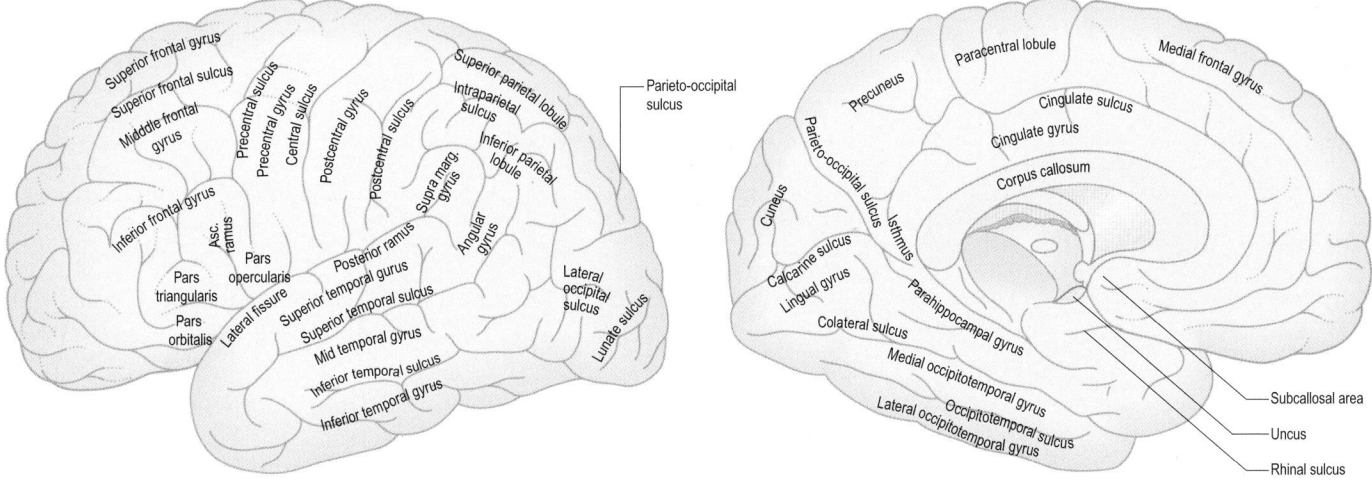

Fig. 22.1 Lateral aspect of the left cerebral hemisphere indicating the major gyri and sulci.

Fig. 22.2 Sagittal section of the brain, with the brain stem removed, showing the medial aspect of the left cerebral hemisphere.

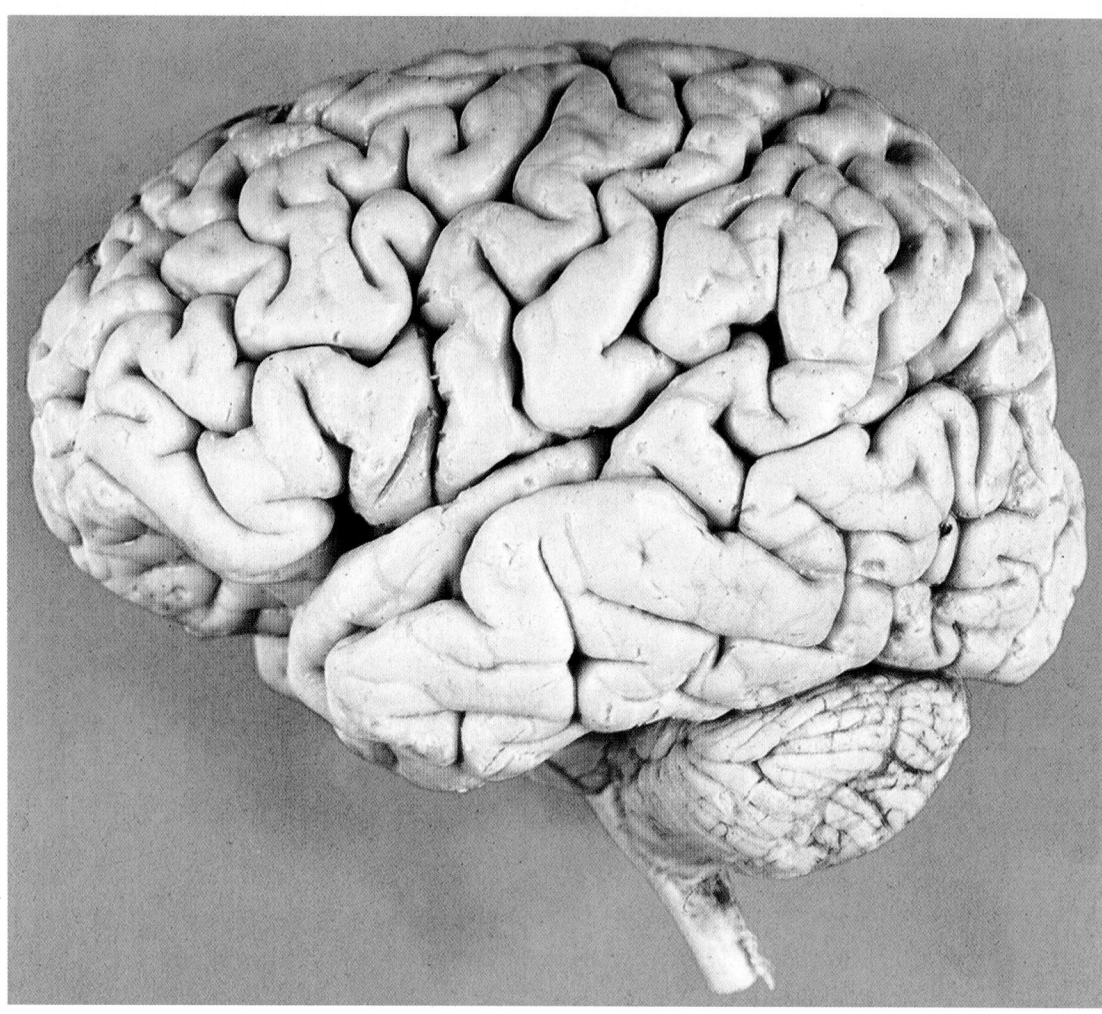

Fig. 22.3 Left lateral aspect of the brain. (Dissection by EL Rees; photograph by Kevin Fitzpatrick on behalf of GKT School of Medicine, London.)

same gyrus. The posterior ramus is the largest. It runs posteriorly and slightly upwards, across the lateral surface of the hemisphere for c.7 cm, and turns up to end in the parietal lobe. Its floor is the insula, and it accommodates the middle cerebral vessels.

The central sulcus (**Figs 22.1, 22.3**) is the boundary between the frontal and parietal lobes. It starts in or near the superomedial border of the hemisphere, a little behind the midpoint between the frontal and occipital poles. It runs sinuously downwards and forwards for c.8–10 cm to end a little above the posterior ramus of the lateral sulcus, from which it is always separated by an arched gyrus. Its general direction makes an angle of c.70° with the median plane. It demarcates the primary motor and somatosensory areas of the cortex, located in the precentral and postcentral gyri, respectively.

The superior frontal gyrus, above the superior frontal sulcus, is continuous over the superomedial margin with the medial frontal gyrus. It may be incompletely divided. The middle frontal gyrus is between the superior and inferior frontal sulci. The inferior frontal gyrus is below the inferior frontal sulcus and is invaded by the anterior and ascending rami of the lateral fissure. In the left hemisphere, the areas around these rami make up the motor speech area (Broca's area; areas 44 and 45).

The medial cerebral surface (**Figs 22.2, 22.4**) lies within the great longitudinal fissure. The commissural fibres of the corpus callosum lie in the depths of the fissure. The curved anterior part of the corpus callosum is the genu, continuous below with the rostrum and narrowing rapidly as it passes back to the upper end of the lamina terminalis. The genu continues above into the trunk or body, the main part of the commissure, which arches up and back to a thick, rounded posterior extremity, the splenium. The bilateral vertical laminae of the septum pellucidum are attached to the concave surfaces of the trunk, genu and rostrum, occupying the interval between them and the fornix. In front of the lamina terminalis, and almost coextensive with it, is the paraterminal gyrus, a narrow triangle of grey matter separated from the rest of the cortex by a shallow posterior parolfactory sulcus. A short vertical sulcus, the anterior parolfactory sulcus, may occur a little anterior to the paraterminal gyrus. The cortex between these two sulci is the subcallosal area (parolfactory gyrus).

The anterior region of the medial surface is divided into outer and inner zones by the curved cingulate sulcus, starting below the rostrum and passing first forwards, then up and finally backwards, conforming to the callosal curvature. Its posterior end turns up to the superomedial margin c.4 cm behind its midpoint, and is posterior to the upper end of the central sulcus. The outer zone, except for its posterior extremity, is part of the frontal lobe, subdivided into anterior and posterior areas by a short sulcus, which ascends from the cingulate sulcus above the midpoint of the corpus callosum. The larger anterior area is the medial frontal gyrus, the posterior is the paracentral lobule. The superior end of the central sulcus usually invades the paracentral lobule posteriorly and the precentral gyrus is continuous with the lobule. This area is concerned with movements of the contralateral lower limb and perineal region – clinical evidence suggests that it exercises voluntary control over defaecation and micturition.

The zone under the cingulate sulcus is the cingulate gyrus. Starting below the rostrum, this gyrus follows the callosal curve, separated by the callosal sulcus. It continues round the splenium to the inferior surface, and then into the parahippocampal gyrus through the narrow isthmus.

The posterior region of the medial surface is traversed by the parieto-occipital and the calcarine sulci. These two deep sulci converge anteriorly to meet a little posterior to the splenium. The parieto-occipital sulcus marks the boundary between parietal and occipital lobes. It starts on the superomedial margin of the hemisphere c.5 cm anterior to the occipital pole, sloping down and slightly forwards to the calcarine sulcus. The calcarine sulcus starts near the occipital pole. Though usually restricted to the medial surface, its posterior end may reach the lateral surface. Directed anteriorly, it joins the parieto-occipital sulcus at an acute angle behind the splenium. Continuing forwards, it crosses the inferomedial margin of the hemisphere, and forms the inferolateral boundary of the isthmus, which connects the cingulate with the

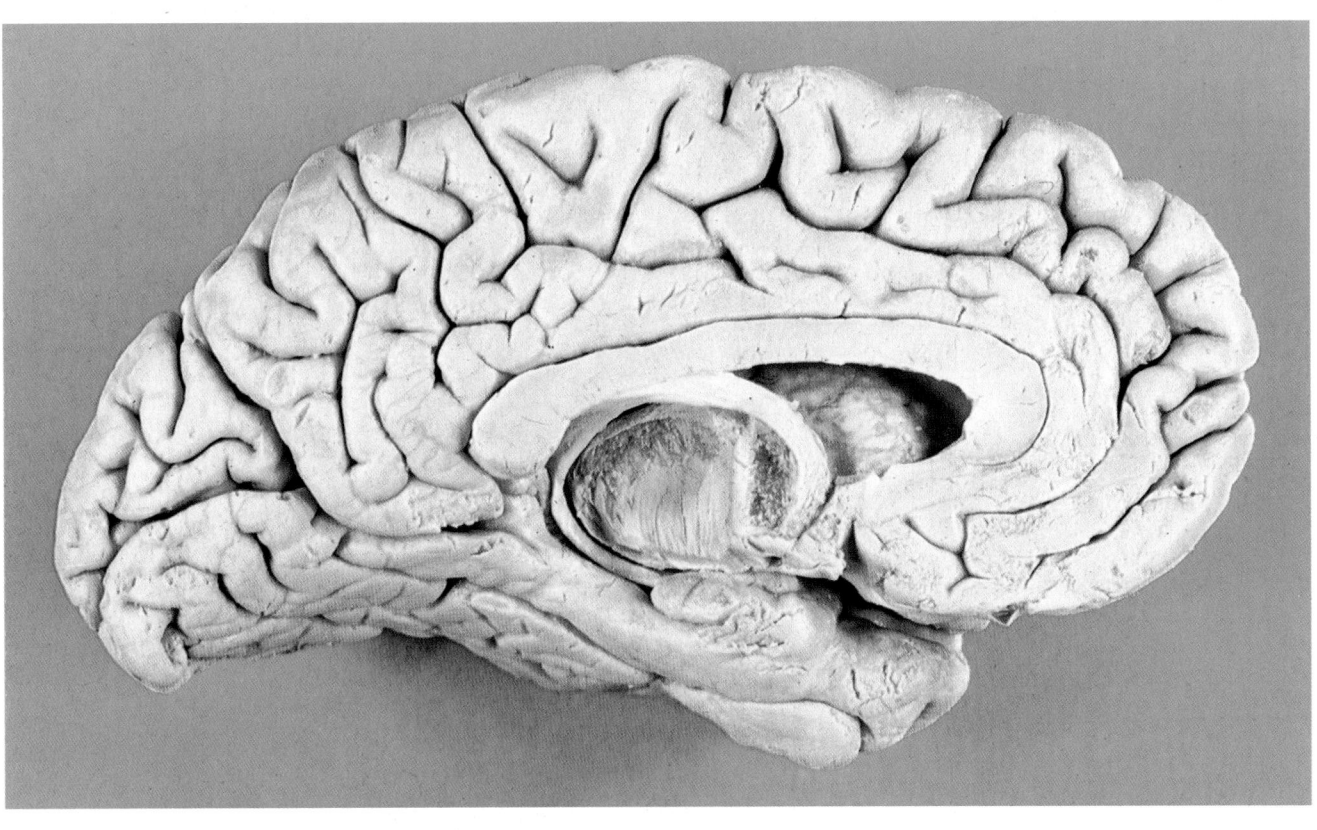

Fig. 22.4 The medial surface of the left cerebral hemisphere after sagittal section of the brain, followed by removal of the brain stem and septum pellucidum. (Photograph by Kevin Fitzpatrick on behalf of GKT School of Medicine, London.)

parahippocampal gyrus. The visual cortex lies above and below the posterior part of the calcarine sulcus, behind the junction with the parieto-occipital. The calcarine is deep and produces an elevation, the calcar avis, in the wall of the posterior horn of the lateral ventricle.

The area posterior to the upturned end of the cingulate sulcus, and anterior to the parieto-occipital sulcus, is the precuneus. It forms the medial surface of the parietal lobe with the part of the paracentral lobule behind the central sulcus. The medial surface of the occipital lobe is formed by the cuneus, a wedge of cortex bounded in front by the parieto-occipital sulcus, below by the calcarine sulcus, and above by the superomedial margin.

The inferior cerebral surface is divided by the stem of the lateral fissure into a small anterior and larger posterior part (**Figs 12.8, 22.5, 22.6**). The anterior is the orbital region of the inferior surface. It is transversely concave and lies above the cribriform plate of the ethmoid, the orbital plate of the frontal, and the lesser wing of the sphenoid. A rostrocaudal olfactory sulcus traverses it near its medial margin, overlapped by the olfactory bulb and tract. The medial strip thus demarked is the gyrus rectus. The rest of this surface bears irregular orbital sulci, generally H-shaped, which divide it into the anterior, medial, posterior and lateral orbital gyri.

The larger, posterior region of the inferior cerebral surface is partly superior to the tentorium but also to the middle cranial fossa, and traversed by the anteroposterior collateral and occipitotemporal sulci (**Figs 22.2, 22.4**). The collateral sulcus starts near the occipital pole, and extends anteriorly and parallel to the calcarine sulcus, separated from it by the lingual gyrus. Anteriorly it may continue into the rhinal sulcus, but they are usually separate. The rhinal sulcus (fissure) runs forwards in the line of the collateral, separating the temporal pole from the hook-shaped uncus posteromedial to it. This sulcus is the lateral limit of the piriform lobe (**Fig. 22.7**).

The occipitotemporal sulcus is parallel to the collateral sulcus and lateral to it. It usually does not reach the occipital pole and is frequently divided.

The lingual gyrus, between the calcarine and collateral sulci, passes into the parahippocampal gyrus, which begins at the isthmus where it is continuous with the cingulate gyrus and passes forwards medial to the collateral and rhinal sulci. Anteriorly the parahippocampal gyrus

continues into the uncus, its medial edge lying lateral to the midbrain. The uncus is the anterior end of the parahippocampal gyrus and is the posterolateral boundary of the anterior perforated substance. It is part of the piriform lobe of the olfactory system, which is phylogenetically one of the oldest parts of the cortex.

The medial occipitotemporal gyrus extends from the occipital to the temporal poles. It is limited medially by the collateral and rhinal sulci and laterally by the occipitotemporal sulcus. The lateral occipitotemporal gyrus is continuous, round the inferolateral margin of the hemisphere, with the inferior temporal gyrus.

CEREBRAL CORTEX

The microscopic structure of the cerebral cortex is an intricate blend of nerve cells and fibres, neuroglia and blood vessels. The principal cell types are described here, while their laminar organization within the cortex is described on page 391.

MICROSTRUCTURE

The neocortex essentially consists of three neuronal cell types. The most abundant are pyramidal cells. Non-pyramidal cells, also called stellate or granule cells, are divided into spiny and non-spiny neurones. All types have been subdivided on the basis of size and shape (**Fig. 22.8**).

Pyramidal cells (**Fig. 22.9**) have a flask-shaped or triangular cell body ranging from 10 to 80 μm in diameter. The soma gives rise to a single thick apical dendrite and multiple basal dendrites. The apical dendrite ascends towards the cortical surface, tapering and branching, to end in a spray of terminal twigs in the most superficial lamina, the molecular layer. From the basal surface of the cell body, dendrites spread more horizontally, for distances up to 1 mm for the largest pyramidal cells. Like the apical dendrite, the basal dendrites branch profusely along their length. All pyramidal cell dendrites are studded with a myriad of dendritic spines. These become more numerous as distance from the parent cell soma increases. A single slender axon arises from the axon hillock, which is usually situated centrally on the basal surface of the pyramidal neurone. Ultimately, in the vast majority of, if not in all, cases, the axon leaves the cortical grey matter to enter the white matter.

389

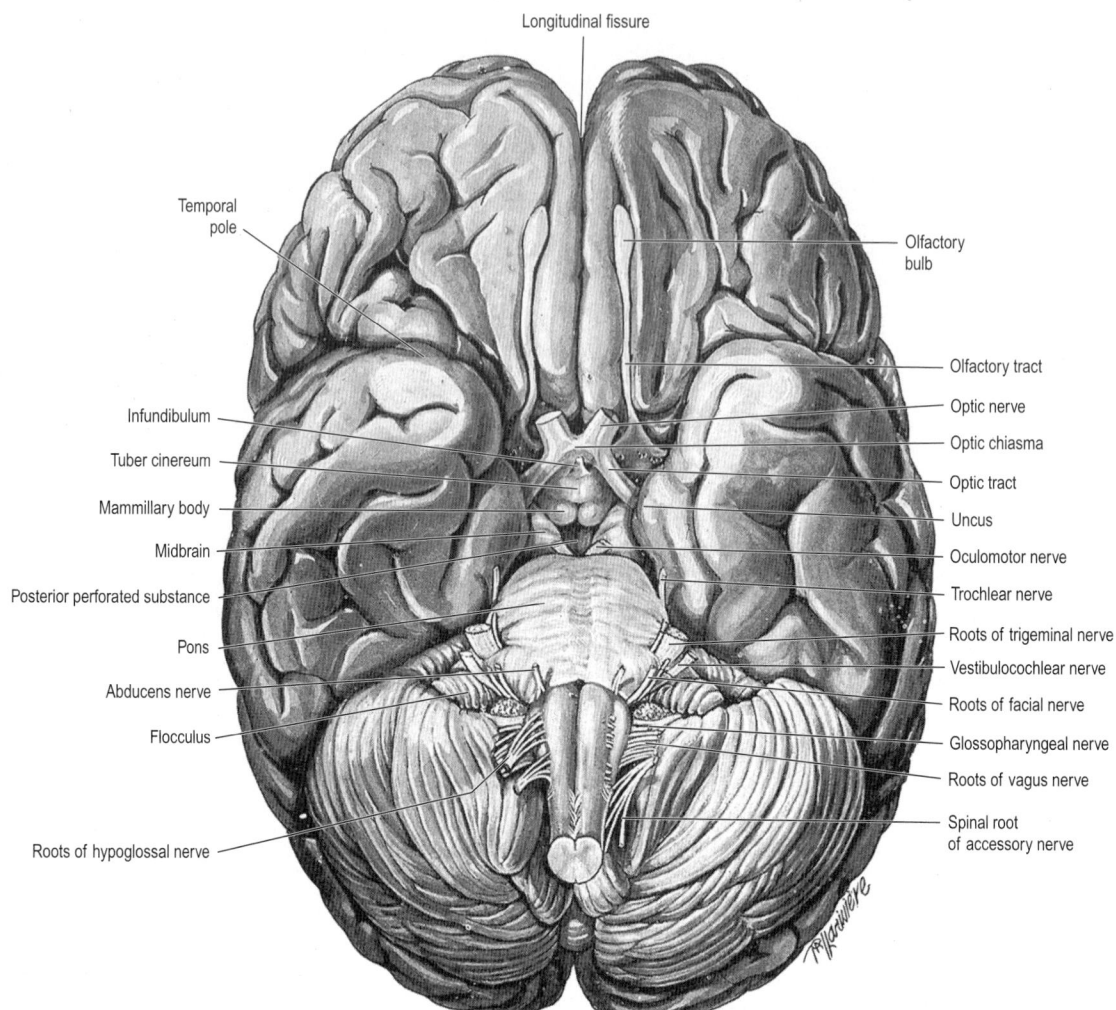

Longitudinal fissure

Temporal pole

Infundibulum

Tuber cinereum

Mammillary body

Midbrain

Posterior perforated substance

Pons

Abducens nerve

Flocculus

Roots of hypoglossal nerve

Olfactory bulb

Olfactory tract

Optic nerve

Optic chiasma

Optic tract

Uncus

Oculomotor nerve

Trochlear nerve

Roots of trigeminal nerve

Vestibulocochlear nerve

Roots of facial nerve

Glossopharyngeal nerve

Roots of vagus nerve

Spinal root of accessory nerve

Fig. 22.5 Basal aspect of the brain.

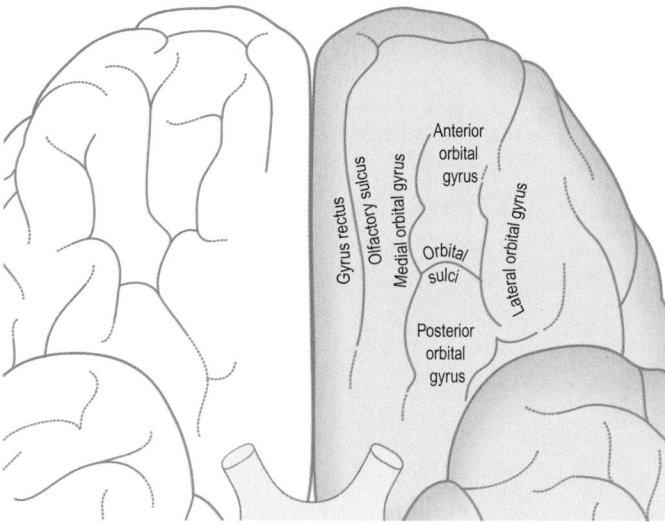

Gyrus rectus

Olfactory sulcus

Medial orbital gyrus

Orbital sulci

Anterior orbital gyrus

Lateral orbital gyrus

Posterior orbital gyrus

Fig. 22.6 The orbital suface of the left frontal lobe.

Pyramidal cells are thus, perhaps universally, projection neurones. They appear to use excitatory amino acids, either glutamate or aspartate, exclusively as their neurotransmitters.

Spiny stellate cells are the second most numerous cell type in the neocortex and for the most part occupy lamina IV. They have relatively small multipolar cell bodies, commonly 6 to 10 μm in diameter. Several primary dendrites, profusely covered in spines, radiate for variable distances from the cell body. Their axons ramify within the grey matter predominantly in the vertical plane. Spiny stellate cells are likely to use glutamate as their neurotransmitter.

The smallest group comprises the heterogeneous non-spiny or sparsely spinous stellate cells. All are interneurones, and their axons are confined to grey matter. In morphological terms, this is not a single class of cell, but a multitude of different forms, including basket, chandelier, double bouquet, neurogliaform, bipolar/fusiform and horizontal cells. Various types may have horizontally, vertically or radially ramifying axons.

Neurones with mainly horizontally dispersed axons include basket and horizontal cells. Basket cells have a short, vertical axon, which rapidly divides into horizontal collaterals, and these end in large terminal sprays synapsing with the somata and proximal dendrites of pyramidal cells. The cell bodies of horizontal cells lie mainly at the superficial border of lamina II, occasionally deep in lamina I (the molecular or plexiform layer). They are small and fusiform, and their dendrites spread short distances in two opposite directions in lamina I. Their axons often stem from a dendrite, then divide into two branches, which travel away from each other for great distances in the same layer.

Neurones with an axonal arborization predominantly perpendicular to the pial surface include chandelier, double bouquet and bipolar/fusiform cells. Chandelier cells have a variable morphology, although most are ovoid or fusiform and their dendrites arise from the upper and lower poles of the cell body. The axonal arborization, which emerges from the cell body or a proximal dendrite, is characteristic and identifies these neurones. A few cells in the more superficial laminae (II and IIIa) have descending axons, deeper cells (laminae IIIc and IV) have ascending axons, and intermediate neurones (IIIb) often have both. The axons ramify close to the parent cell body and terminate in numerous vertically oriented strings, which run alongside the axon hillocks of pyramidal cells with which they synapse. Double bouquet (or bitufted) cells are found in laminae II and III and their axons traverse laminae II and V. Generally, these neurones have two or three main dendrites, which

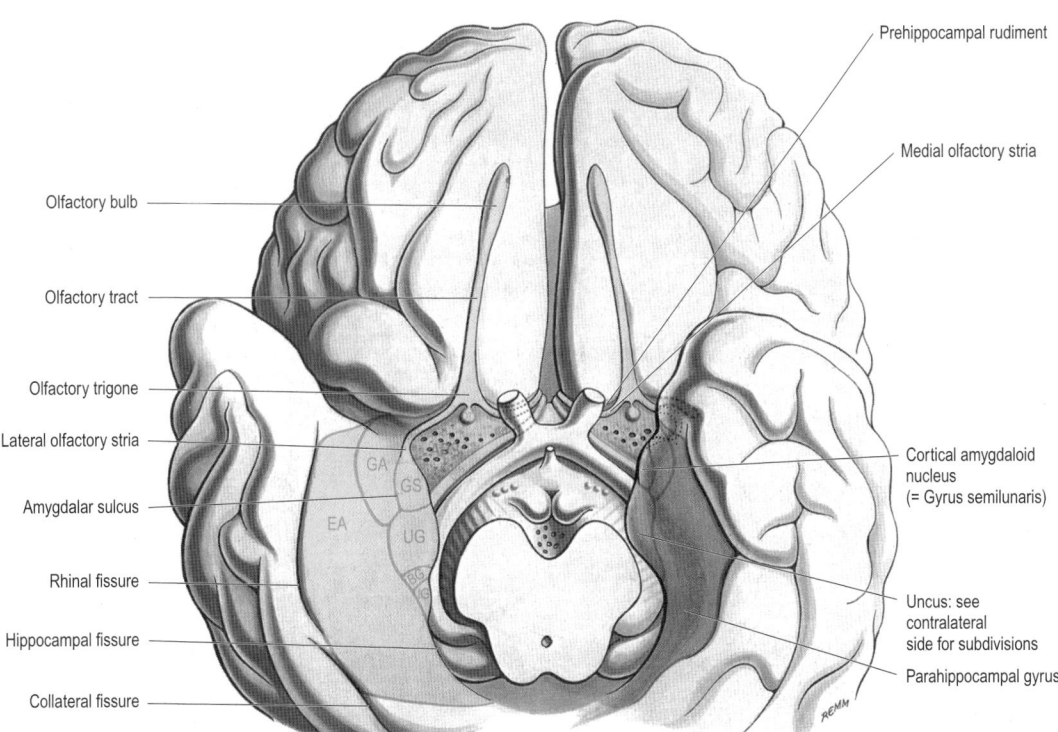

Olfactory bulb

Olfactory tract

Olfactory trigone

Lateral olfactory stria

Amygdalar sulcus

Rhinal fissure

Hippocampal fissure

Collateral fissure

Prehippocampal rudiment

Medial olfactory stria

Cortical amygdaloid
nucleus
(= Gyrus semilunaris)

Uncus: see
contralateral
side for subdivisions

Parahippocampal gyrus

Fig. 22.7 Inferior aspect of the brain with the brain stem removed. The right temporal pole has been displaced laterally to expose underlying structures. Structures related to the olfactory and limbic systems are coloured blue. OT, olfactory tubercle; APS, anterior perforated substance; DBB, diagonal band of Broca. The uncus is divided into three areas: IG, the intralimbic gyrus; BG, the band of Giacomini; UG, the uncinate gyrus. The lateral olfactory stria continues into the gyrus semilunaris (GS); this is bordered laterally by the gyrus ambiens (GA); whilst further laterally is the entorhinal area (EA), which is the rostral extension of the parahippocampal gyrus. (After Kuhlenbeck. From Haymaker W, Anderson E, Nauta WJH (eds) The Hypothalamus, by permission of Charles C Thomas Publisher, Ltd, Springfield, Illinois.)

give rise to a superficial and deep dendritic tuft. A single axon arises usually from the oval or spindle-shaped cell soma and rapidly divides into an ascending and descending branch. These branches collateralize extensively, but the axonal arbor is confined to a perpendicularly extended, but horizontally confined, cylinder, c.50 to 80 μm across. Bipolar cells are ovoid with a single ascending and a single descending dendrite, which arise from the upper and lower poles, respectively. These primary dendrites branch sparsely. Their branches run vertically to produce a narrow dendritic tree, rarely more than 100 μm across, which may extend through most of the cortical thickness. Commonly, the axon originates from one of the primary dendrites, and rapidly branches to give a vertically elongated, horizontally confined, axonal arbor, which closely parallels the dendritic tree in extent.

The principal recognizable neuronal type is the neurogliaform or spiderweb cell. These small spherical cells, 10 to 12 μm in diameter, are found mainly in laminae II to IV, depending on cortical area. Seven to ten thin dendrites typically radiate out from the cell soma, some branching once or twice to form a spherical dendritic field of c.100 to 150 μm diameter. The slender axon arises from the cell body or a proximal dendrite. Almost immediately, it branches profusely within the vicinity of the dendritic field (and usually somewhat beyond), to give a spherical axonal arbor up to 350 μm in diameter.

The majority of non-spiny or sparsely spinous non-pyramidal cells probably use GABA as their principal neurotransmitter. This is almost certainly the case for basket, chandelier, double bouquet, neurogliaform and bipolar cells. Some are also characterized by the coexistence of one or more neuropeptides, including neuropeptide Y, vasoactive intestinal polypeptide (VIP), cholecystokinin, somatostatin and substance P. Acetylcholine is present in a subpopulation of bipolar cells, which may additionally be GABAergic and contain VIP.

LAMINAR ORGANIZATION

The most apparent microscopical feature of the neocortex stained for cell bodies or for fibres is its horizontal lamination. Its value for understanding cortical functional organization is debatable, but the use of cytoarchitectonic description to identify regions of cortex is common.

Typical neocortex is described as having six layers or laminae lying parallel to the surface (**Figs 22.10, 22.11, 22.12**).

I   The molecular or plexiform layer is cell sparse, containing only scattered horizontal cells and their processes enmeshed in a compacted mass of tangential, principally horizontal axons and dendrites. These are afferent fibres, which arise from outside the cortical area, together with intrinsic fibres from cortical interneurones, and the apical dendritic arbors of virtually all pyramidal neurones of the cerebral cortex. In histological sections stained to show myelin, layer I appears as a narrow horizontal band of fibres.

II   The external granular lamina contains a varying density of small neuronal cell bodies. These include both small pyramidal and non-pyramidal cells; the latter may predominate. Myelin fibre stains show mainly vertically arranged processes traversing the layer.

III   The external pyramidal lamina contains pyramidal cells of varying sizes, together with scattered non-pyramidal neurones. The size of the pyramidal cells is smallest in the most superficial part of the layer and greatest in the deepest part. This lamina is frequently further subdivided into IIIa, IIIb and IIIc, with IIIa most superficial and IIIc deepest. As in layer II, myelin stains reveal a mostly vertical organization of fibres.

IV   The internal granular lamina is usually the narrowest of the cellular laminae. It contains densely packed, small, round cell bodies of non-pyramidal cells, notably spiny-stellate cells and some small pyramidal cells. Within the lamina, in myelin stained sections, a prominent band of horizontal fibres (outer band of Baillarger) is seen.

V   The internal pyramidal (ganglionic) lamina typically contains the largest pyramidal cells in any cortical area, though actual sizes vary considerably from area to area. Scattered non-pyramidal cells are also present. In myelin stains, the lamina is traversed by ascending and descending vertical fibres, and also contains a prominent central band of horizontal fibres (inner band of Baillarger).

VI   The multiform (or fusiform/pleiomorphic) layer consists of neurones with a variety of shapes, including recognizable pyramidal, spindle, ovoid and many other shaped somata. Typically, most cells are small to medium in size. This lamina blends gradually with the underlying white matter, and a clear demarcation of its deeper boundary is not always possible.

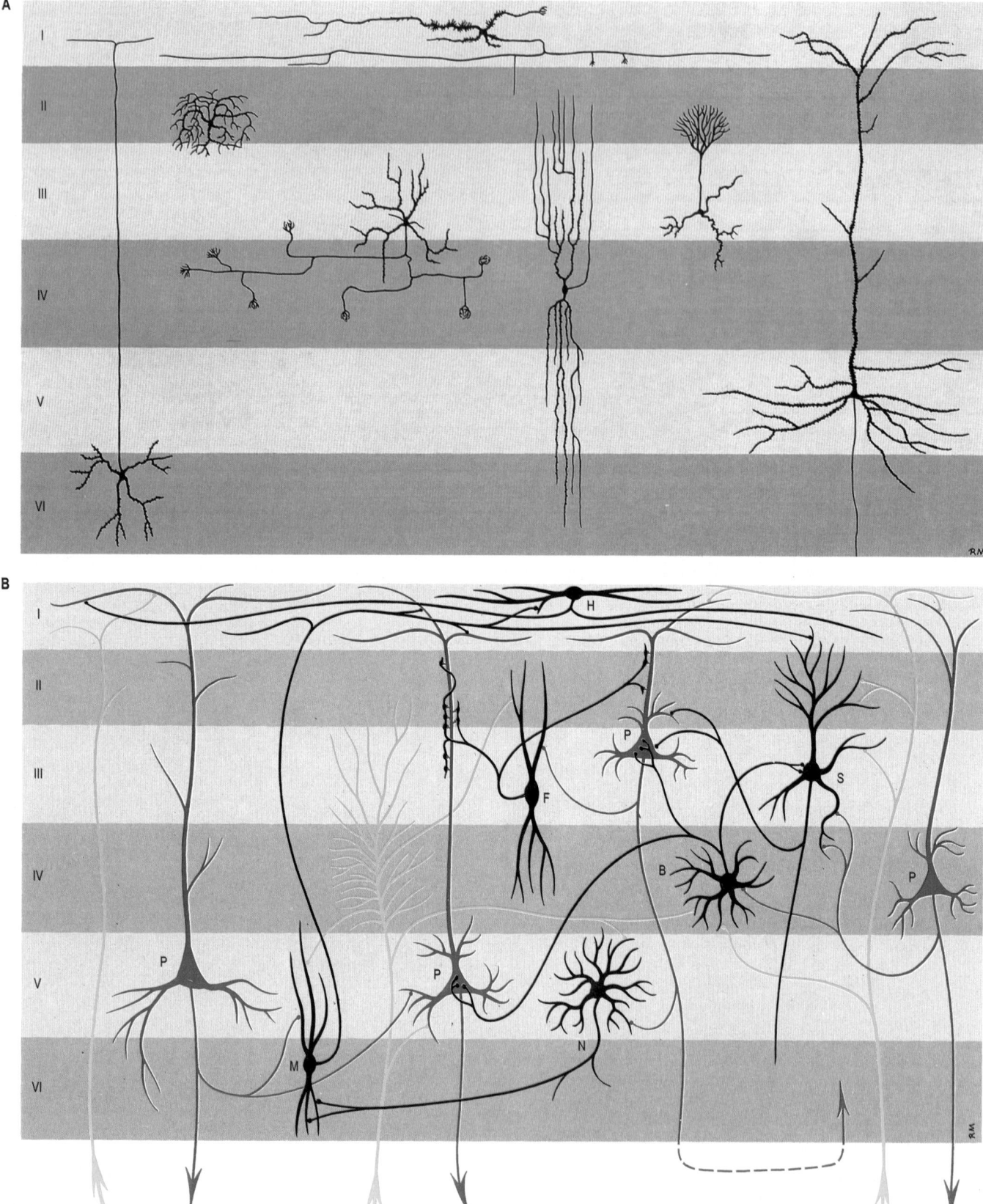

Fig. 22.8 A, Characteristic neocortical neurones. From left to right are shown Martinotti, neurogliaform, basket, horizontal, fusiform, stellate and pyramidal types of neurone. **B**, The most frequent types of neocortical neurone, showing typical connections with each other and with afferent fibres (blue). Neurones limited to the cortex in their distribution are indicated in black. Efferent neurones are in magenta. The right and left afferent fibres are association or corticocortical connections, the central afferent is a specific sensory fibre. Neurones are shown in their characteristic lamina, but many have somata in more than one layer. Abbreviations: B, basket; F, fusiform; H, horizontal; M, Martinotti; N, neurogliaform; P, pyramidal; S, stellate.

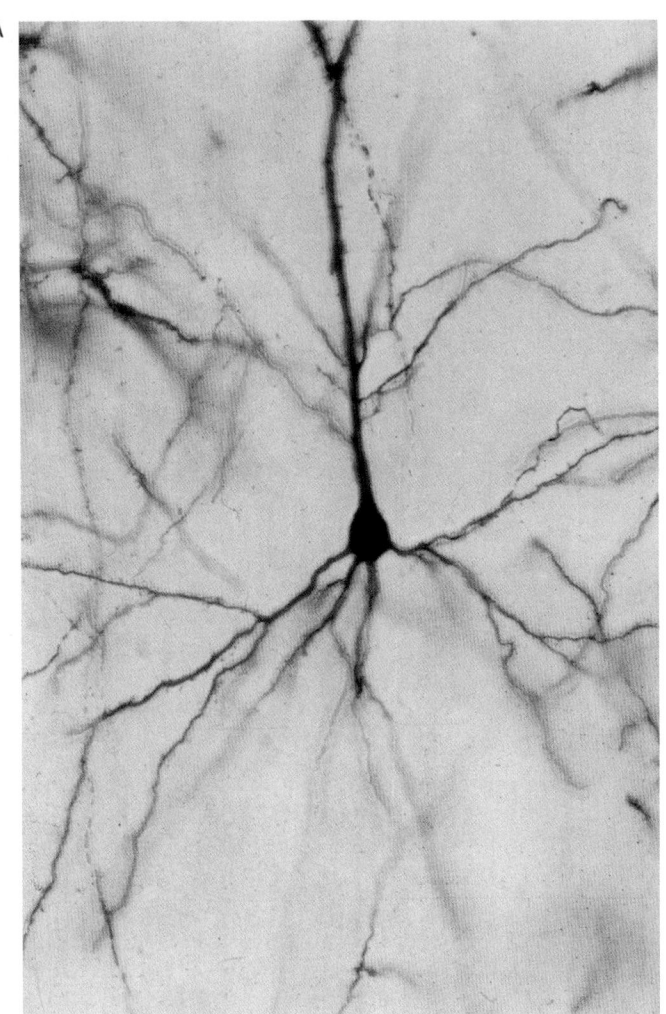

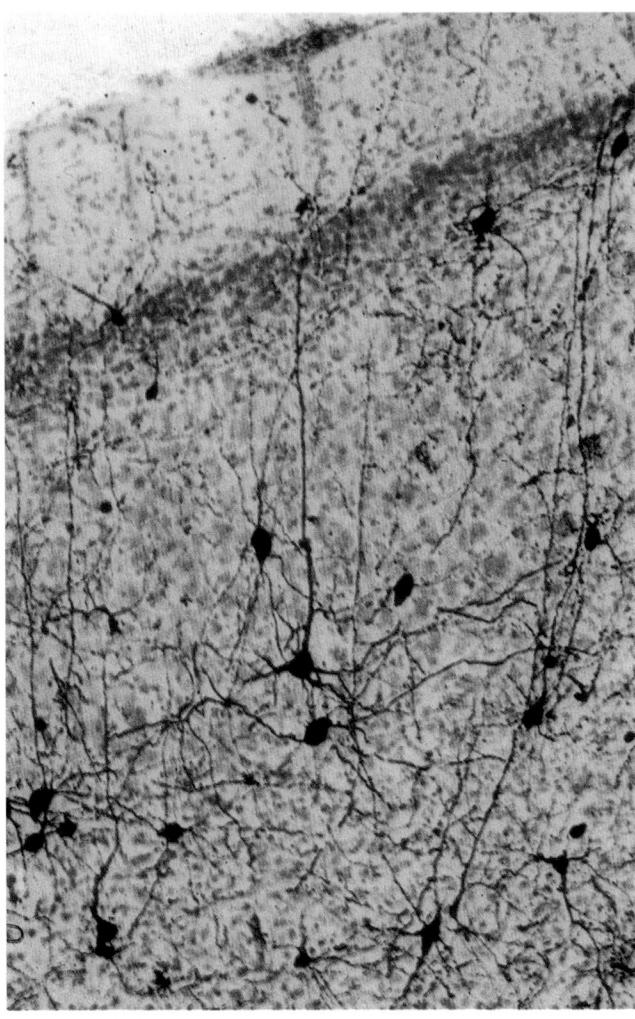

Fig. 22.9 Neurones in the cerebral cortex. **A**, A single pyramidal cell stands out amongst many unstained elements. **B**, Isolated Golgi-stained neurones are prominent among the Nissl-stained cortical elements. (Preparations provided by AR Lieberman, Department of Anatomy, University College, London.)

Five regional variations are described in neocortical structure (**Fig. 22.11**). While all are said to develop from the same six-layered pattern, two types, granular and agranular, are regarded as virtually lacking certain laminae, and are referred to as heterotypical. Homotypical variants, in which all six laminae are found, are called frontal, parietal and polar, names that link them with specific cortical regions in a somewhat misleading manner (e.g. the frontal type also occurs in parietal and temporal lobes).

The agranular type is considered to have diminished, or absent, granular laminae (II and IV), but always contains scattered stellate somata. Large pyramidal neurones are found in the greatest densities in agranular cortex, which is typified by the numerous efferent projections of pyramidal cell axons. Although it is often equated with motor cortical areas such as the precentral gyrus (area 4), agranular cortex also occurs elsewhere, e.g. areas 6, 8 and 44 and parts of the limbic system.

In the granular type of cortex the granular layers are maximally developed, and contain densely packed stellate cells, amongst which small pyramidal neurones are dispersed. Laminae III and IV are poorly developed or unidentifiable. This type of cortex is particularly associated with afferent projections. However it does have efferent fibres, derived from the scattered pyramidal cells, although they are less numerous than elsewhere. Granular cortex occurs in the postcentral gyrus (somatosensory area), striate area (visual area) and superior temporal gyrus (acoustic area), and in small parts of the parahippocampal gyrus. Despite its very high density of stellate cells, especially in the striate area, it is almost the thinnest of the five main types. In the striate cortex the external band of Baillarger (lamina IV) is well defined as the stria (white line) of Gennari.

The other three types of cortex are intermediate forms. In the frontal type, large numbers of small- and medium-sized pyramidal neurones appear in laminae III and V, and granular layers (II and IV) are less

prominent. The relative prominence of these major forms of neurone vary reciprocally wherever this form of cortex exists.

The parietal type of cortex contains pyramidal cells, which are mostly smaller in size than in the frontal type. The granular laminae are, on the contrary, wider and contain more of the stellate cells. This kind of cortex occupies large areas in the parietal and temporal lobes. The polar type is classically identified with small areas near the frontal and occipital poles. It is the thinnest form of cortex. All six laminae are represented but the pyramidal layer (III) is reduced in thickness and not so extensively invaded by stellate cells as it is in the granular type of cortex. In both polar and granular types, the multiform layer (VI) is more highly organized than in other types.

For almost 100 years it has been customary to refer to discrete cortical territories not only by their anatomical location in relation to gyri and sulci, but also in relation to their cytoarchitectonic characteristics as originally descried by Brodmann (**Fig. 22.12**). Some of the areas so defined, e.g. the primary sensory and motor cortices, have clear relevance in terms of anatomical connections and functional significance, others less so.

OVERVIEW OF CORTICAL CONNECTIVITY

All neocortical areas have axonal connections with other cortical areas on the same side (ipsilateral corticocortical or association connections), the opposite side (contralateral corticocortical or commissural connections), and with subcortical structures.

The primary somatic sensory, visual and auditory areas give rise to ipsilateral corticocortical connections to the association areas of the parietal, occipital and temporal lobes, respectively, which then progressively project towards the medial temporal limbic areas, notably the parahippocampal gyrus, entorhinal cortex, and hippocampus. Thus,

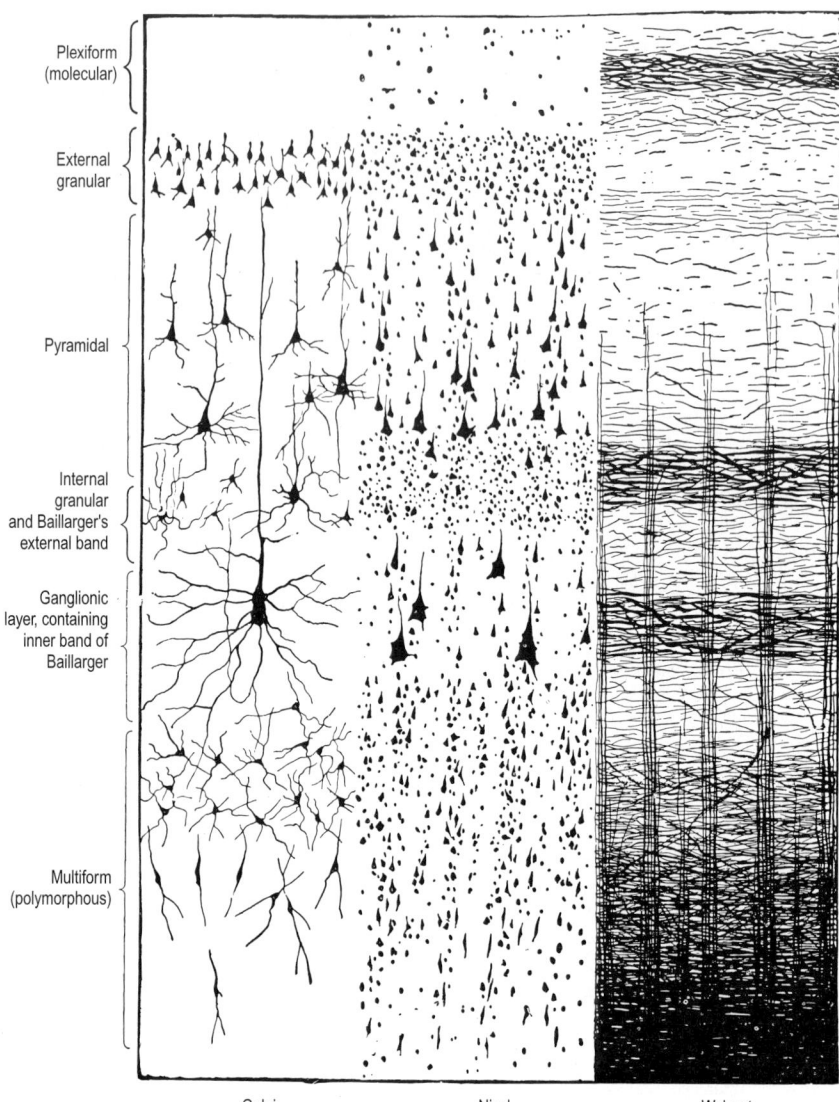

Plexiform
(molecular)

External
granular

Pyramidal

Internal
granular
and Baillarger's
external band

Ganglionic
layer, containing
inner band of
Baillarger

Multiform
(polymorphous)

Golgi   Nissl   Weigert

Fig. 22.10 The layers of the cerebral cortex. The three vertical columns represent the disposition of cellular elements as revealed by the staining techniques of Golgi (impregnating whole neurones), Nissl (staining cell bodies) and Weigert (staining nerve fibres).

the first somatic sensory area (SI) projects to the superior parietal cortex (Brodmann's area 5), which in turn projects to the inferior parietal cortex (area 7). From here connections pass to cortex in the walls of the superior temporal sulcus, and so on to the posterior parahippocampal gyrus, and on into limbic cortex. Similarly, for the visual system, the primary visual cortex (area 17) projects to the parastriate cortex (area 18), which in turn projects to the peristriate region (area 19). Information then flows to inferotemporal cortex (area 20), to cortex in the walls of the superior temporal sulcus, then to medial temporal cortex in the posterior parahippocampal gyrus, and so to limbic areas. The auditory system shows a similar progression from primary auditory cortex to temporal association cortex and so to the medial temporal lobe.

In addition to this stepwise outward progression from sensory areas through posterior association cortex, connections also occur at each stage with parts of the frontal cortex. Thus, taking the somatic sensory system as an example, primary somatic sensory cortex (SI) in the postcentral gyrus is reciprocally connected with the primary motor cortex (area 4) in the precentral gyrus. The next step in the outward progression, the superior parietal lobule (area 5), is interconnected with the premotor cortex (area 6), and this in turn is connected with area 7 in the inferior parietal lobule. This has reciprocal connections with prefrontal association cortex on the lateral surface of the hemisphere (areas 9 and 46), and temporal association areas, which connect with more anterior prefrontal association areas, and, ultimately in the sequence, with orbitofrontal cortex. Similar stepwise links exist between areas on the visual and auditory association pathways in the occipitotemporal lobe and areas of the frontal association cortex. The connections between sensory and association areas are reciprocal.

All neocortical areas are connected with subcortical regions although their density varies between areas. First among these are connections with the thalamus (p. 370). All areas of the neocortex receive afferents from more than one thalamic nucleus, and all such connections are reciprocal. The vast majority of, if not all, cortical areas project to the striatum, tectum, pons and brain stem reticular formation. Additionally, all cortical areas are reciprocally connected with the claustrum; the frontal cortex connects with the anterior part and the occipital lobe with the posterior part.

All cortical areas receive a topographically organized cholinergic projection from the basal forebrain, which is profoundly affected by the neurodegenerative processes of Alzheimer's disease. Similarly, noradrenergic fibres pass to all cortical areas from the locus coeruleus, as do serotoninergic fibres from the midbrain raphe nuclei, histaminergic fibres from the posterior hypothalamus, and dopaminergic fibres from the ventral midbrain.

Different cortical areas have widely different afferent and efferent connections. Some have connections that are unique, e.g. the corticospinal motor projection (the corticospinal tract) from pyramidal cells in a restricted area around the central sulcus.

Widely separated, but functionally interconnected, areas of cortex share common patterns of connections with subcortical nuclei, and within the neocortex. For example, contiguous zones of the striatum, thalamus, claustrum, cholinergic basal forebrain, superior colliculus and pontine nuclei connect with anatomically widely separated areas in the prefrontal and parietal cortex, which are themselves interconnected. In contrast, other cortical regions, which are functionally distinct, e.g. areas in the temporal and parietal cortex, do not share such contiguity in their subcortical connections.

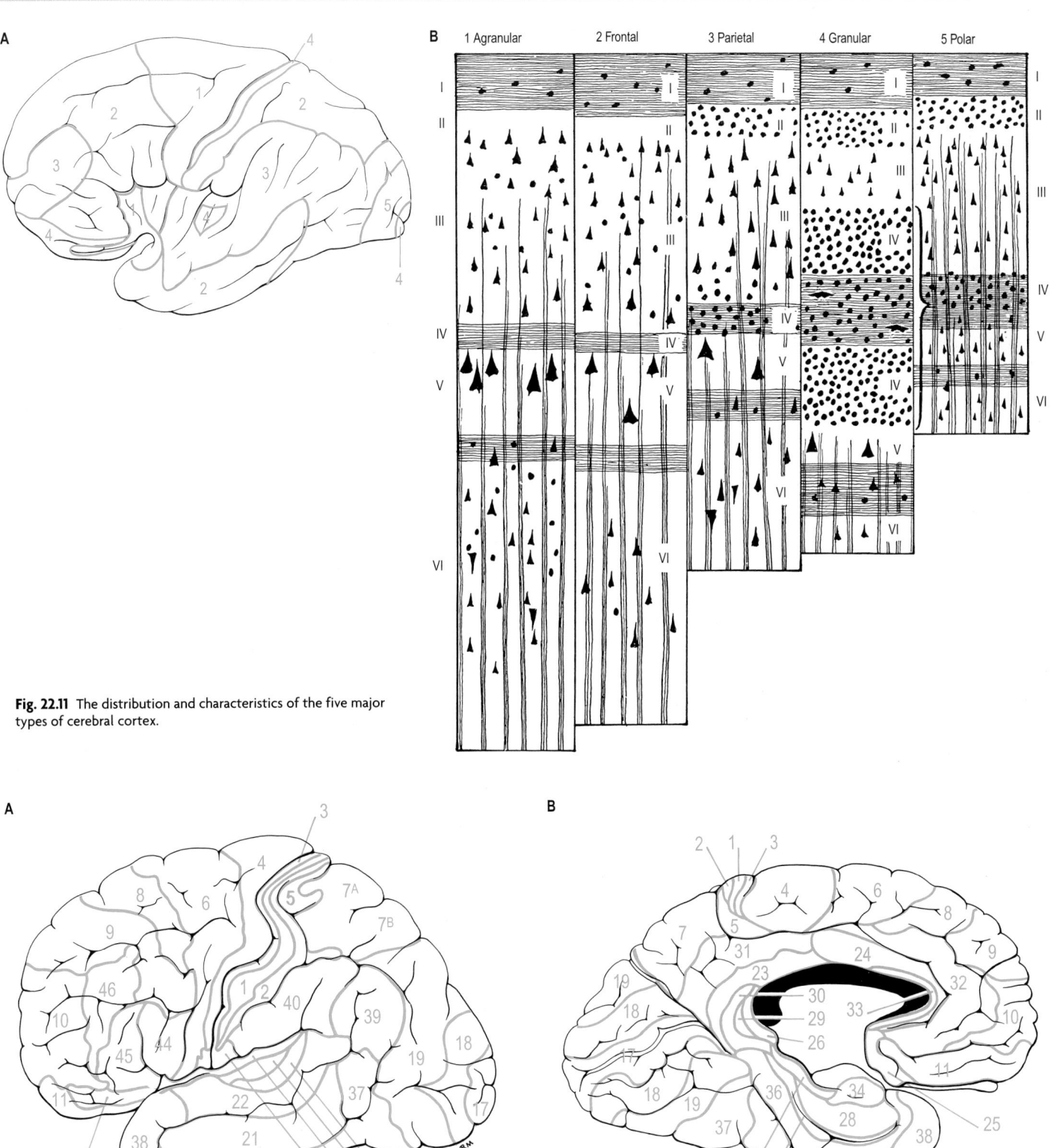

Fig. 22.11 The distribution and characteristics of the five major types of cerebral cortex.

Fig. 22.12 The lateral (**A**) and medial (**B**) surfaces of the left cerebral hemisphere depicting Brodmann's areas.

Cortical lamination and cortical connections

The cortical laminae represent, to some extent, horizontal aggregations of neurones with common connections. This is most clearly seen in the lamination of cortical efferent (pyramidal) cells. The internal pyramidal lamina, layer V, gives rise to corticosubcortical fibres, notably corticostriate, corticobulbar, corticopontine, and corticospinal axons. In addition, a significant proportion of feedback corticocortical axons arise from cells in this layer, as do some corticothalamic fibres. Layer VI, the multiform lamina, is the major source of corticothalamic fibres. Supragranular pyramidal cells, predominantly layer III, but also lamina II, give rise primarily to both ipsilateral (association) and contralateral (commissural) corticocortical pathways. Short corticocortical fibres arise more superficially, and long corticocortical (both association and commissural) axons come from cells in the deeper parts of layer III. Major afferents to a cortical area tend to terminate in layers I, IV and VI. Quantitatively lesser projections end either in the intervening laminae II/III and V, or sparsely throughout the depth of the cortex. Numerically, the major single input to a cortical area tends to have its main termination field in layer IV. This pattern of termination is seen in the major thalamic input to visual and somatic sensory cortex. In general, non-thalamic subcortical afferents to the neocortex, which are shared by widespread areas, tend to terminate throughout all cortical layers, but the laminar pattern of their endings still varies considerably from area to area.

Columns and modules

Experimental physiological and connectional studies have demonstrated an internal organization of the cortex, which is at right angles to the pial surface, with vertical columns or modules running through the depth of the cortex. The term column refers to the observation that all cells encountered by a microelectrode penetrating and passing perpendicularly through the cortex respond to a single peripheral stimulus, a phenomenon first identified in the somatosensory cortex. In the visual cortex narrow (50 μm) vertical strips of neurones respond to a bar stimulus of the same orientation (orientation columns), and wider strips (500 μm) respond preferentially to stimuli detected by one eye (ocular dominance columns). Adjacent orientation columns aggregate within an ocular dominance column to form a hypercolumn, responding to all orientations of stimulus for both eyes for one point in the visual field. Similar functional columnar organization has been described in widespread areas of neocortex, including motor cortex and so-called association areas.

FRONTAL LOBE

The frontal lobe is the rostral region of the hemisphere, anterior to the central sulcus and above the lateral fissure. On the superolateral surface, extending onto the medial surface, is the precentral gyrus running parallel to the central sulcus and limited anteriorly by the precentral sulcus. The area of the frontal lobe anterior to the precentral sulcus is divided into the superior, middle and inferior frontal gyri (**Figs 22.1, 22.3**). In front of these gyri lies the frontal pole. The ventral surface of the frontal lobe overlies the bony orbit and is the orbitofrontal cortex. The medial surface extends from the frontal pole anteriorly to the paracentral lobule behind. It consists of the medial frontal cortex and the anterior cingulate cortex.

Primary motor cortex

The primary motor cortex (MI) corresponds to the precentral gyrus (area 4). It is the area of cortex with the lowest threshold for eliciting contralateral muscle contraction by electrical stimulation. The primary motor cortex contains a detailed topographically organized map (motor homunculus) of the opposite body half, with the head represented most laterally, and the legs and feet represented on the medial surface of the hemisphere in the paracentral lobule (**Fig. 22.13**). A striking feature is the disproportionate representation of body parts in relation to their physical size. Thus, large areas represent the muscles of the hand and face, which are capable of finely controlled or fractionated movements.

The cortex of area 4 is agranular, and layers II and IV are difficult to identify. The most characteristic feature is the presence in lamina V of some extremely large pyramidal cell bodies, the Betz cells, which may approach 80 μm in diameter. These neurones project their axons into the corticospinal and corticobulbar tracts.

The major thalamic connections of area 4 are with the ventral posterolateral nucleus (VPL), which in turn receives afferents from the deep cerebellar nuclei. The VPL nucleus also contains a topographic representation of the contralateral body, which is preserved in its point-to-point projection to area 4, where it terminates largely in lamina IV. Other thalamic connections of area 4 are with the centromedian and parafascicular nuclei. These appear to provide the only route through which output from the basal ganglia, routed via the thalamus, reaches the motor cortex, since the projection of the internal segment of the globus pallidus to the ventrolateral nucleus of the thalamus is confined to the anterior division, and there is no overlap with cerebellothalamic territory. The anterior part of the ventrolateral nucleus projects to the

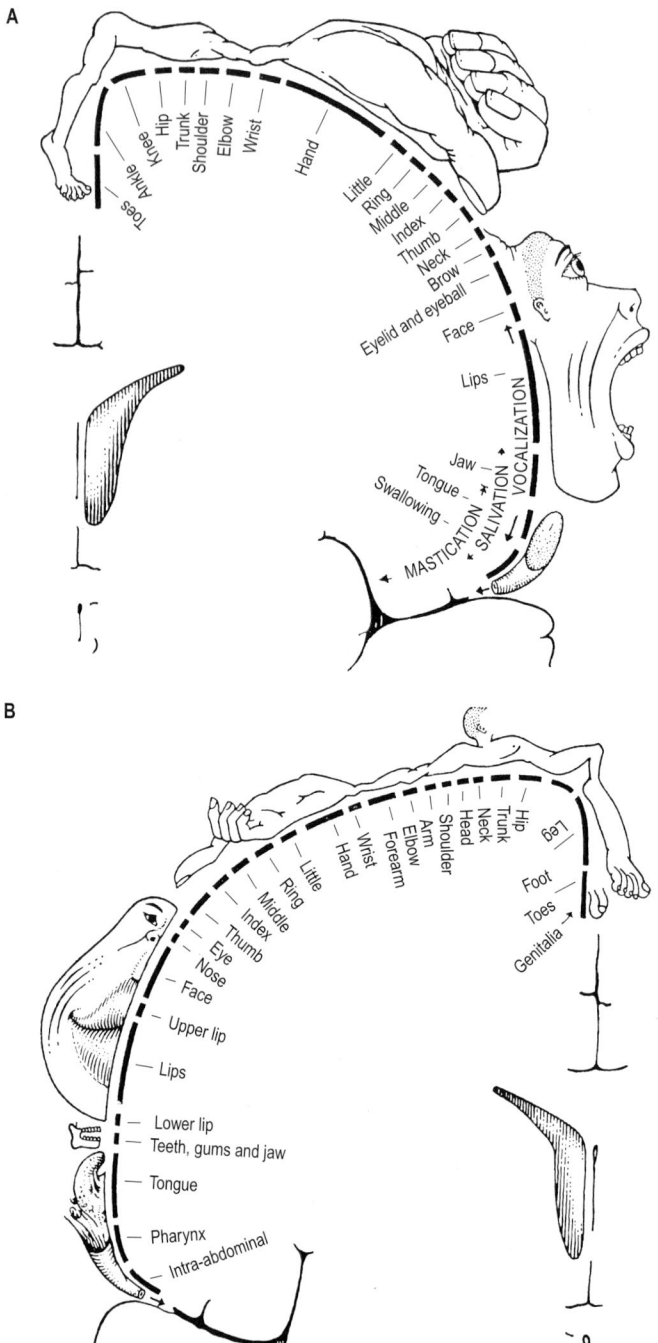

Fig. 22.13 A, The motor homunculus showing proportional somatotopical representation in the main motor area. **B**, The sensory homunculus showing proportional somatotopical representation in the somaesthetic cortex. (After Penfield W, Rasmussen T 1950 The Cerebral Cortex of Man. New York: Macmillan.)

premotor and supplementary motor areas of cortex with no projection to area 4.

The ipsilateral somatosensory cortex (SI) projects in a topographically organized way to area 4, and the connection is reciprocal. The projection to the motor cortex arises in areas 1 and 2, with little or no contribution from area 3b. Fibres from SI terminate in layers II and III of area 4, where they contact mainly pyramidal neurones. Evidence suggests that neurones activated monosynaptically by fibres from SI, as well as those activated polysynaptically, make contact with layer V pyramidal cells, which give rise to corticospinal fibres, including Betz cells. Movement-related neurones in the motor cortex which can be activated from SI tend to have a late onset of activity, mainly during the execution of movement. It has been suggested that this pathway plays a role primarily in making motor adjustments during a movement.

Additional ipsilateral corticocortical fibres to area 4 from behind the central sulcus come from the second somatic sensory area (SII).

Neurones in area 4 are responsive to peripheral stimulation, and have receptive fields similar to those in the primary sensory cortex. Cells located posteriorly in the motor cortex have cutaneous receptive fields, whereas more anteriorly situated neurones respond to stimulation of deep tissues.

The motor cortex receives major frontal lobe association fibres from the premotor cortex and the supplementary motor area and also fibres from the insula. It is probable that these pathways modulate motor cortical activity in relation to the preparation, guidance and temporal organization of movements. Area 4 sends fibres to, and receives fibres from, its contralateral counterpart, and also projects to the contralateral supplementary motor cortex.

Apart from its contribution to the corticospinal tract, the motor cortex has diverse subcortical projections. The connections to the striatum and pontine nuclei are heavy. It also projects to the subthalamic nucleus. The motor cortex sends projections to all nuclei in the brain stem, which are themselves the origin of descending pathways to the spinal cord, namely the reticular formation, the red nucleus, the superior colliculus, the vestibular nuclei and the inferior olivary nucleus.

Corticospinal tract

The corticospinal or pyramidal tract provides direct control by the cerebral cortex over motor centres of the spinal cord. An homologous pathway to the brain stem, the corticobulbar or corticonuclear projection, fulfils a similar function in relation to motor nuclei of the brain stem. The corticospinal tract does not originate solely from the motor cortex, but is conveniently considered in conjuction with it.

The percentage of corticospinal fibres that arise from the primary motor cortex may actually be quite small, probably in the region of 20 to 30%. They arise from pyramidal cells in layer V and give rise to the largest diameter corticospinal axons. There is also a widespread origin from other parts of the frontal lobe, including the premotor cortex and the supplementary motor area. Many axons from the frontal cortex, notably the motor cortex, terminate in the ventral horn of the spinal cord. In cord segments mediating dexterous hand and finger movements they terminate in the lateral part of the ventral horn, in close relationship to motor neuronal groups. A small percentage establish direct monosynaptic connections with α motor neurones.

Between 40 and 60% of pyramidal tract axons arise from parietal areas, including area 3a, area 5 of the superior parietal lobe, and SII in the parietal operculum. The majority of parietal fibres to the spinal cord terminate in the deeper layers of the dorsal horn.

Corticomotor neuronal cells are active in relation to agonist muscle force of contraction; their relation to amplitude of movement is less clear. Their activity precedes the onset of electromyographic activity by 50 to 100 milliseconds, suggesting a role for cortical activation in generating rather than monitoring movement.

Premotor cortex

Immediately in front of the primary motor cortex lies Brodmann's area 6 (**Fig. 22.14**). Area 6 extends onto the medial surface, where it becomes contiguous with area 24 in the cingulate gyrus, anterior and inferior to the paracentral lobule. A number of functional motor areas are contained within this cortical region. Lateral area 6, the area over most of the lateral surface of the hemisphere, corresponds to the premotor cortex.

The premotor cortex is divided into a dorsal and a ventral area (PMd and PMv respectively) on functional grounds, and on the basis of ipsilateral corticocortical association connections.

The major thalamic connections of the premotor cortex are with the anterior division of the ventrolateral nucleus and with the centromedian, parafascicular and centrolateral components of the intralaminar nuclei. Subcortical projections to the striatum and pontine nuclei are prominent, and this area also projects to the superior colliculus and the reticular formation. Both dorsal and ventral areas contribute to the corticospinal tract. Commissural connections are with the contralateral premotor, motor and superior parietal (area 5) cortex. Ipsilateral corticocortical (association) connections with area 5 in the superior parietal cortex, and inferior parietal area 7b are common to both dorsal and ventral subdivisions of the premotor cortex, and both send a major projection to the primary motor cortex. The dorsal premotor area also receives fibres from the posterior superior temporal cortex and projects to the supplementary motor cortex. The frontal eye field (area 8) projects to the dorsal subdivision. Perhaps the greatest functionally significant difference in connectivity between the two premotor area subdivisions is that the dorsal premotor area receives from the dorsolateral prefrontal cortex, whereas the ventral subdivision receives from the ventrolateral prefrontal cortex. All of these association connections are likely to be, or are known to be, reciprocal.

Neuronal activity in the premotor cortex in relation to both preparation for movement and movement itself has been extensively studied experimentally. Direction selectivity for movement is a common feature of many neurones. In behavioural tasks, neurones in the dorsal premotor cortex show anticipatory activity and task-related discharge as well as direction selectivity, but little or no stimulus-related changes. The dorsal premotor cortex is probably important in establishing a motor set or intention, contributing to motor preparation in relation to internally guided movement. In contrast, ventral premotor cortex is more related to the execution of externally (especially visually) guided movements in relation to a specific external stimulus.

Frontal eye field

The frontal eye field lies predominantly within Brodmann's area 8, anterior to the superior premotor cortex. It receives its major thalamic projection from the parvocellular mediodorsal nucleus, with additional afferents from the medial pulvinar, the ventral anterior nucleus and the suprageniculate–limitans complex. It connects with the paracentral

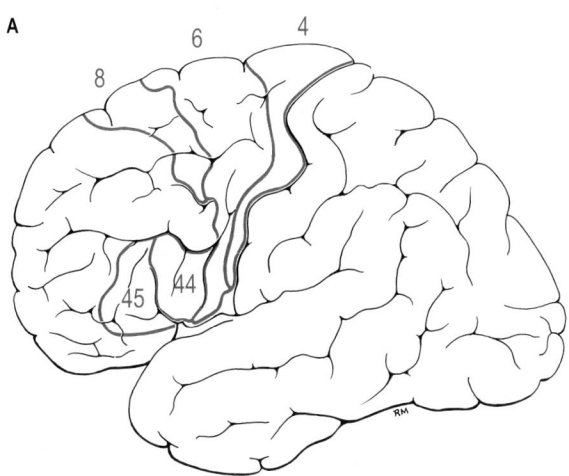

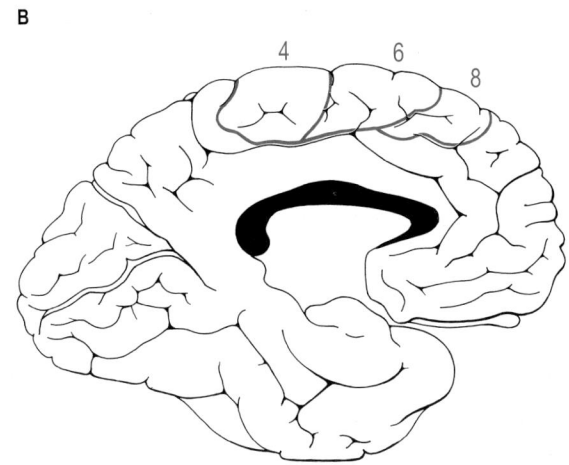

Fig. 22.14 Lateral (**A**) and medial (**B**) surfaces of the left cerebral hemisphere, showing approximate correspondence of Brodmann's areas to the primary motor cortex (area 4), the premotor area (areas 6, 8) and motor speech area (areas 44, 45).

nucleus of the intralaminar group. The thalamocortical pathways to the frontal eye field form part of a pathway from the superior colliculus, the substantia nigra and the dentate nucleus of the cerebellum. The frontal eye field has extensive ipsilateral corticocortical connections, receiving fibres from several visual areas in the occipital, parietal and temporal lobes, including the medial temporal area (V5) and area 7a. There is also a projection from the superior temporal gyrus, which is auditory rather than visual in function. From within the frontal lobe, the frontal eye field receives fibres from the ventrolateral and dorsolateral prefrontal cortices. It projects to the dorsal and ventral premotor cortices and to the medial motor area, probably to the supplementary eye field adjacent to the supplementary motor area proper. It projects prominently to the superior colliculus, to the pontine gaze centre within the pontine reticular formation, and to other oculomotor related nuclei in the brain stem. As its name implies, it is important in the control of eye movements. Lesions of the frontal eye field cause ipsilateral conjugate deviation of the eyes, whereas stimulation induces contralateral deviation.

Supplementary motor cortex

The supplementary motor area (SMA; MII) lies medial to area 6, and extends from the most superolateral part to the medial surface of the hemisphere. Area 24 in the cingulate gyrus adjacent to area 6 contains several motor areas, which are termed cingulate motor areas. An additional functional subdivision, the preSMA, lies anterior to the supplementary motor area on the medial surface of the cortex. For the purposes of the present discussion, these additional medial motor areas will be included with the supplementary motor cortex.

The supplementary motor area receives its major thalamic input from the anterior part of the ventral lateral nucleus, which in turn is the major recipient of fibres from the internal segment of the globus pallidus. Additional thalamic afferents are from the ventral anterior nucleus, the intralaminar nuclei, notably the centrolateral and centromedial nuclei, and also from the mediodorsal nucleus. The connections with the thalamus are reciprocal. The supplementary motor cortex receives connections from widespread regions of the ipsilateral frontal lobe, including from the primary motor cortex, the dorsal premotor area, the dorsolateral and ventrolateral prefrontal, medial prefrontal and orbitofrontal cortex and the frontal eye field. These connections are reciprocal, but the major ipsilateral efferent pathway is to the motor cortex. Parietal lobe connections of the supplementary motor cortex are with the superior parietal area 5 and possibly inferior parietal area 7b. Contralateral connections are with the supplementary motor area, and motor and premotor cortices of the contralateral hemisphere. Subcortical connections, other than with the thalamus, pass to the striatum, subthalamic nucleus and pontine nuclei, the brain stem reticular formation and the inferior olivary nucleus. The supplementary motor area makes a substantial contribution to the corticospinal tract, contributing as much as 40% of the fibres from the frontal lobe.

The supplementary motor area contains a representation of the body in which the leg is posterior and the face anterior, with the upper limb between them. Its role in the control of movement is primarily in complex tasks, which require temporal organization of sequential movements and retrieval of motor memory. The consequences of damage to the supplementary motor area bear some striking similarities to the effects of basal ganglia dysfunction – akinesia is common, and there may be problems with the performance of sequential, complex movements. Stimulation of the supplementary motor area in conscious patients has been reported to elicit the sensation of an urge to move, or of anticipation that a movement is about to occur. A region anterior to the supplementary motor area for face representation is important in vocalization and speech production.

Prefrontal cortex

The prefrontal cortex on the lateral surface of the hemisphere comprises predominantly Brodmann's areas 9, 46 and 45 (**Figs 22.12, 22.14, 22.15**). In non-human primates, two subdivisions of the lateral prefrontal cortex are recognized, a dorsal area equivalent to area 9, and perhaps including the superior part of area 46, and a ventral area, consisting of the inferior part of area 46 and area 45. Areas 44 and 45 are particularly notable in man since, in the dominant hemisphere, they constitute the motor speech area (Broca's area). Both the dorsolateral and ventrolateral prefrontal areas receive their major thalamic afferents from the mediodorsal nucleus, and there are additional contributions from the medial pulvinar, the ventral anterior nucleus and from the

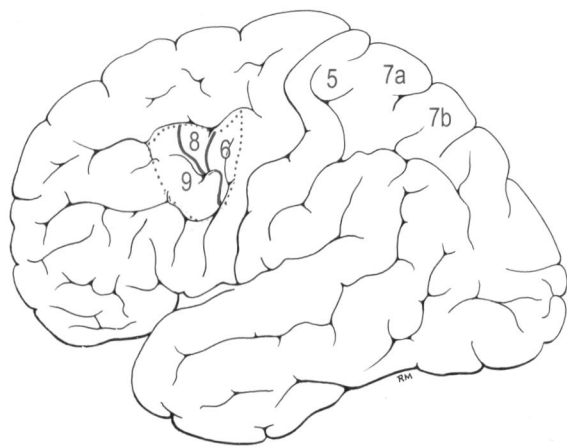

Fig. 22.15 Lateral surface of the left cerebral hemisphere showing the frontal eye field, corresponding to parts of Brodmann's areas 6, 8 and 9. The perimeter of this area is delineated by an interrupted line to indicate uncertainty as to its precise extent.

paracentral nucleus of the anterior intralaminar group. The dorsolateral area receives long association fibres from the posterior and middle superior temporal gyrus, including auditory association areas; from parietal area 7a; and from much of the middle temporal cortex. From within the frontal lobe it also receives projections from the frontal pole (area 10), and from the medial prefrontal cortex (area 32) on the medial surface of the hemisphere. It projects to the supplementary motor area, the dorsal premotor cortex and the frontal eye field. All these thalamic and corticocortical connections are reciprocal. Commissural connections are with the homologous area, and with the contralateral inferior parietal cortex. The ventrolateral prefrontal area receives long association fibres from both area 7a and area 7b of the parietal lobe, from auditory association areas of the temporal operculum, from the insula and from the anterior part of the lower bank of the superior temporal sulcus. From within the frontal lobe it receives fibres from the anterior orbitofrontal cortex and projects to the frontal eye field and the ventral premotor cortex. It connects with the contralateral homologous area via the corpus callosum. These connections are probably all reciprocal.

The cortex of the frontal pole (area 10) receives thalamic input from the mediodorsal nucleus, the medial pulvinar and the paracentral nucleus. It is reciprocally connected with the cortex of the temporal pole, the anterior orbitofrontal cortex, and the dorsolateral prefrontal cortex. The orbitofrontal cortex connects with the mediodorsal, anteromedial, ventral anterior, medial pulvinar, paracentral and midline nuclei of the thalamus. Cortical association pathways come from the inferotemporal cortex, the anterior superior temporal gyrus and the temporal pole. Within the frontal lobe it has connections with the medial prefrontal cortex, the ventrolateral prefrontal cortex and medial motor areas. Commissural and other connections follow the general pattern for all neocortical areas.

The medial prefrontal cortex is connected with the mediodorsal, ventral anterior, anterior medial pulvinar, paracentral, midline and supragenicul ate–limitans nuclei of the thalamus. It receives fibres from the anterior cortex of the superior temporal gyrus. Within the frontal lobe, it has connections with the orbitofrontal cortex, and the medial motor areas of the dorsolateral prefrontal cortex.

Information on the detailed functions of the subregions of the prefrontal cortex is sparse. The dorsolateral prefrontal cortex is important for spatial processing of afferent information and for the organization of self-ordered working memory tasks, including verbal working memory. The ventrolateral prefrontal cortex is concerned with mnemonic processing of objects.

Evidence from surgical lesions (prefrontal lobotomy) or pathological damage suggests a role for the prefrontal cortex in the appreciation or understanding of time, the normal expression of emotions (affect) and the ability to predict the consequences of actions. Both hemispheres interact in these functions, so deficits following unilateral damage may be relatively slight. Medial prefrontal cortex as a whole is important in auditory and visual associations and widespread changes in prefrontal activation are associated with calculating, thinking and decision making.

PARIETAL LOBE

The parietal lobe lies posterior to the central sulcus. On the medial aspect of the hemisphere its boundary with the occipital lobe is clearly demarcated by the deep parieto-occipital sulcus. On the lateral aspect of the hemisphere its boundaries with the occipital and temporal lobes are less distinct and somewhat arbitrary. The inferior boundary is the posterior ramus of the lateral fissure and its imaginary posterior prolongation.

The lateral aspect of the parietal lobe is divided into three areas by postcentral and intraparietal sulci (**Fig. 22.1**). The postcentral sulcus, often divided into upper and lower parts, is posterior and parallel to the central sulcus. Inferiorly, it ends above the posterior ramus of the lateral fissure. The postcentral gyrus or primary somatosensory cortex lies between the central and postcentral sulci. Posterior to the postcentral sulcus there is a large area, subdivided by the intraparietal sulcus. It usually starts in the postcentral sulcus near its midpoint and extends posteroinferiorly across the parietal lobe, dividing it into superior and inferior parietal lobules. Posteriorly, its occipital ramus extends into the occipital lobe, joining the transverse occipital sulcus at right angles.

The superior parietal lobule, between the superomedial margin of the hemisphere and the intraparietal sulcus, is continuous anteriorly with the postcentral gyrus round the upper end of the postcentral sulcus; posteriorly it often joins the arcus parieto-occipitalis, surrounding the lateral part of the parieto-occipital sulcus.

The inferior parietal lobule, below the intraparietal sulcus and behind the lower part of the postcentral sulcus, is divided into three. The anterior part is the supramarginal gyrus, which arches over the upturned end of the lateral fissure. It is continuous anteriorly with the lower part of the postcentral gyrus and posteroinferiorly with the superior temporal gyrus. The middle part of the inferior parietal lobule, called the angular gyrus, arches over the end of the superior temporal sulcus and is continuous posteroinferiorly with the middle temporal gyrus. The posterior part of the inferior parital lobule arches over the upturned end of the inferior temporal sulcus on to the occipital lobe, forming an arcus temporo-occipitalis.

Somatosensory cortex

The postcentral gyrus corresponds to the primary somtosensory cortex (SI; Brodmann's areas 3a, 3b, 1 and 2). Area 3a lies most anteriorly, apposing area 4, the primary motor cortex of the frontal lobe; area 3b is buried in the posterior wall of the central sulcus; area 1 lies along the posterior lip of the central sulcus; and area 2 occupies the crown of the postcentral gyrus.

The primary somatosensory cortex contains within it a topographical map of the contralateral half of the body. The face, tongue and lips are represented inferiorly, the trunk and upper limb are represented on the superolateral aspect, and the lower limb on the medial aspect of the hemisphere, giving rise to the familiar 'homunculus' map (**Fig. 22.13**).

The somatosensory properties of SI depend on its thalamic input from the ventral posterior nucleus of the thalamus, which in turn receives the medial lemniscal, spinothalamic and trigeminothalamic pathways. The nucleus is divided into a ventral posterolateral part, which receives information from the trunk and limbs, and a ventral posteromedial part, in which the head is represented. Within the ventral posterior nucleus, neurones in the central core respond to cutaneous stimuli and those in the most dorsal anterior and posterior parts, which arch as a 'shell' over this central core, respond to deep stimuli. This is reflected in the differential projections to SI: the cutaneous central core projects to 3b; the deep tissue-responsive neurones send fibres to areas 3a and 2; and an intervening zone projects to area 1. Within the ventral posterior nucleus, anteroposterior rods of cells respond with similar modality and somatotopic properties. They appear to project to restricted focal patches in SI of c.0.5 mm, which form narrow strips mediolaterally along SI. The laminar termination of thalamocortical axons from the ventral posterior nucleus is different in the separate cytoarchitectonic subdivisions of SI. In 3a and 3b these axons terminate mainly in layer IV and the adjacent deep part of layer III, whereas in areas 1 and 2 they end in the deeper half of layer III, avoiding lamina IV. Additional thalamocortical fibres to SI arise from the intralaminar system, notably the centrolateral nucleus.

There is a complex internal connectivity within SI. An apparently stepwise hierarchical progression of information processing occurs from area 3b through area 1 to area 2. Outside the postcentral gyrus, SI has ipsilateral corticocortical association connections with a second somatosensory area (SII); area 5 in the superior parietal lobe; area 4, the motor cortex, in the precentral gyrus; and the supplementary motor cortex in the medial part of area 6 of the frontal lobe.

SI has reciprocal commissural connections with its contralateral homologue, with the exception that the cortices containing the representation of the distal extremities are relatively devoid of such connections. Callosal fibres in SI arise mainly from the deep part of layer III and terminate in layers I to IV. Callosally projecting pyramidal cells receive monosynaptic thalamic and commissural connections.

SI has reciprocal subcortical connections with the thalamus and claustrum, and receives afferents from the basal nucleus of Meynert, the locus coeruleus and the midbrain raphe. It has other prominent subcortical projections. Corticostriatal fibres, arising in layer V, pass mainly to the putamen of the same side. Corticopontine and corticotectal fibres from SI arise in layer V. SI projects to the main pontine nuclei, and to the pontine tegmental reticular nucleus. In addition, axons arising in SI pass to the dorsal column nuclei and the spinal cord. Corticospinal pyramidal cells are found in layer V of SI. The topographical representation in the cortex is preserved in terms of the spinal segments to which different parts of the postcentral gyrus project. Thus, the arm representation projects to the cervical enlargement, the leg representation to the lumbosacral enlargement, and so on. Within the grey matter of the spinal cord, fibres from SI terminate in the dorsal horn, Rexed's laminae 3 to 5. Fibres from 3b and 1 end more dorsally, and those from area 2 more ventrally.

The second somatosensory area (SII) lies along the upper bank of the lateral fissure, posterior to the central sulcus. SII contains a somatotopic representation of the body, with the head and face most anteriorly, adjacent to SI, and the sacral regions most posteriorly. SII is reciprocally connected with the ventral posterior nucleus of the thalamus in a topographically organized fashion. Some thalamic neurones probably project to both SI and SII via axon collaterals. Other thalamic connections of SII are with the posterior group of nuclei and with the intralaminar central lateral nucleus. SII also projects to laminae IV to VII of the dorsal horn of the cervical and thoracic spinal cord, the dorsal column nuclei, the principal trigeminal nucleus, and the periaqueductal grey matter of the midbrain.

Within the cortex, SII is reciprocally connected with SI in a topographically organized manner, and projects to the primary motor cortex. SII also projects in a topographically organized way to the lateral part of area 7 (area 7b) in the superior parietal lobe, and makes connections with the posterior cingulate gyrus. Across the corpus callosum, both right and left SII areas are interconnected, although distal limb representations are probably excluded. There are additional callosal projections to SI and area 7b.

Experimental studies show that neurones in SII respond particularly to transient cutaneous stimuli, e.g. brush strokes or tapping, which are characteristic of the responses of Pacinian corpuscles in the periphery. They show little response to maintained stimuli.

Superior and inferior parietal lobules

Posterior to the postcentral gyrus, the superior part of the parietal lobe is composed of areas 5, 7a and 7b (**Figs 22.12, 22.16**). Area 5 receives a dense feedforward projection from all cytoarchitectonic areas of SI in a topographically organized manner. The thalamic afferents to this area come from the lateral posterior nucleus and from the central lateral nucleus of the intralaminar group. Ipsilateral corticocortical fibres from area 5 go to area 7, the premotor and supplementary motor cortices, the posterior cingulate gyrus, and the insular granular cortex. Commissural connections between area 5 on both sides tend to avoid the areas of representation of the distal limbs. The response properties of cells in area 5 are more complex than in SI, with larger receptive fields and evidence of submodality convergence. Area 5 contributes to the corticospinal tract.

In non-human primates, the inferior parietal lobe is area 7. In man, this area is more superior, and areas 39 and 40 intervene inferiorly. The counterparts for the latter areas in monkeys are unclear and little experimental evidence is available on their connections and functions. Their role in human cerebral processing is discussed below. In the monkey, area 7b receives somatosensory inputs from area 5 and SII.

Connections pass to the posterior cingulate gyrus (area 23), insula and temporal cortex. Area 7b is reciprocally connected with area 46 in the prefrontal cortex and the lateral part of the premotor cortex. Commissural connections of area 7b are with the contralateral homologous area, and with SII, the insular granular cortex and area 5. Thalamic connections are with the medial pulvinar nucleus and the intralaminar paracentral nucleus.

In monkeys, area 7a is not related to the cortical pathways for somatosensory processing, but instead forms part of a dorsal cortical pathway for spatial vision. The major ipsilateral corticocortical connections to area 7a are derived from visual areas in the occipital and temporal lobes. In the ipsilateral hemisphere, area 7a has connections with the posterior cingulate cortex (area 24) and with areas 8 and 46 of the frontal lobe. Commissural connections are with its contralateral homologue. Area 7a is connected with the medial pulvinar and intralaminar paracentral nuclei of the thalamus. In experimental studies, neurones within area 7a are visually responsive. They relate largely to peripheral vision, respond to stimulus movement, and are modulated by eye movement.

Injury of the superior parietal cortex in man can lead to the inability to recognize the shape of objects by touch (astereognosis); difficulty with assimilation of spatial perception of the body (amorphosynthesis); and sensory neglect of the contralateral body (asomatognosia), which causes a variety of syndromes, including dressing apraxias. More complex perceptional disturbances follow damage of the inferior parietal cortex, including areas 39 and 40. These include difficulties in language, since Wernicke's speech area includes parts of the inferior parietal lobe of the dominant hemisphere (Fig. 22.16), and dyscalculia, if the nondominant hemisphere is involved. Contralateral sensory neglect extends to include the visual appreciation of the world, e.g. the omission of one side of a drawing when the patient is asked to copy a sketch of a clock face. Difficulties with complex orientation in space, such as map reading, are also seen.

TEMPORAL LOBE

The temporal lobe is inferior to the lateral fissure. It is limited behind by an arbitrary line from the preoccipital incisure to the parieto-occipital sulcus, which meets the superomedial margin of the hemisphere c.5 cm from the occipital pole. Its lateral surface is divided into three parallel gyri by two sulci.

The superior temporal sulcus begins near the temporal pole and slopes slightly up and backwards parallel to the posterior ramus of the lateral sulcus. Its end curves up into the parietal lobe. The inferior temporal sulcus is subjacent and parallel to the superior and is often broken into two or three short sulci. Its posterior end also ascends into the parietal lobe, posterior and parallel to the upturned end of the superior sulcus.

Thus the lateral surface is divided into three parallel gyri: superior (area 22); middle (area 21); and inferior (area 20) temporal gyri. The temporal pole (area 38) lies in front of the termination of these gyri. Along its superior margin the superior temporal gyrus is continuous with gyri in the floor of the posterior ramus of the lateral sulcus. These vary in number, and extend obliquely anterolaterally from the circular sulcus around the insula as transverse temporal gyri of Heschl (Fig. 22.17). The anterior transverse temporal gyrus and adjoining part of the superior temporal gyrus are auditory in function, and are considered to be Brodmann's area 42. The anterior gyrus is approximately area 41.

Cortex of the medial temporal lobe includes major subdivisions of the limbic system, such as the hippocampus and entorhinal cortex. Areas of neocortex adjacent to these limbic regions are grouped together as medial temporal association cortex. The temporal and frontal lobes are expanded enormously in man. This poses the problem of relating physiological and anatomical studies of non-human primates to human brain topography. In general, the commonly studied old world monkeys lack a middle temporal gyrus.

Auditory cortex

The temporal operculum houses the primary auditory cortex, AI (Fig. 22.18). This is coextensive with the granular area 41 in the transverse temporal gyri. Surrounding areas constitute auditory association cortex. The primary auditory cortex is reciprocally connected with all subdivisions of the medial geniculate nucleus, and may receive additional thalamocortical projections from the medial pulvinar. The geniculocortical fibres terminate densely in layer IV. AI contains a tonotopic representation of the cochlea in which high frequencies are represented posteriorly, and low frequencies anteriorly. Single-cell responses are to single tones of a narrow frequency band. Cells in single vertical electrode penetrations share an optimum frequency response.

The auditory cortex interconnects with prefrontal cortex, though the projections from AI are small. In general, posterior parts of the operculum project to areas 8 and 9. Central parts project to areas 8, 9 and 46. More anterior regions project to areas 9 and 46, to area 12 on the orbital surface of the hemisphere, and to the anterior cingulate gyrus on the medial surface. Contralateral corticocortical connections are with the same and adjacent regions in the other hemisphere. Onward connections of the auditory association pathway converge with those of the other sensory association pathways in cortical regions within the superior temporal sulcus.

Injury of the auditory cortex in man produces a variety of manifestations, including cortical deafness, verbal auditory agnosia and nonverbal auditory agnosia. The markedly bilateral nature of the auditory

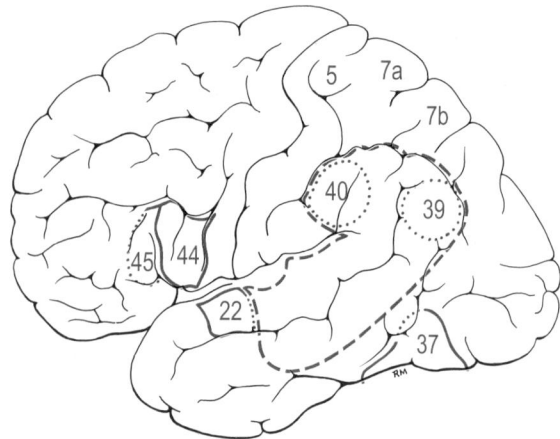

Fig. 22.16 Lateral surface of the left hemisphere showing the motor speech area (44, 45), and areas 5, 7a and 7b. Wernicke's area is variously depicted by different authorities and is tentatively indicated by the large parietotemporal area enclosed in an interrupted outline, which includes areas 39 and 40. Areas 22 and 37 are considered by some to be respectively auditory and visuo-auditory areas associated with speech and language.

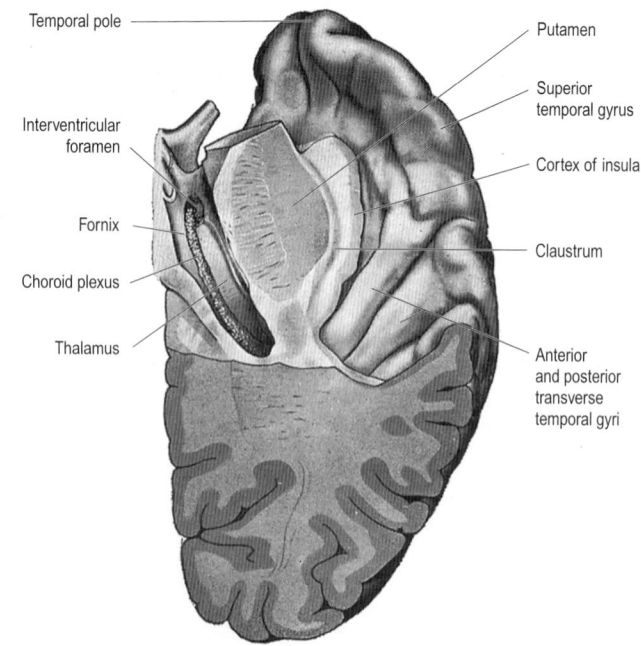

Fig. 22.17 Horizontal section showing the left temporal lobe, viewed from below.

pathway means that noticeable deficits occur only when there is bilateral damage. Damage of the temporoparietal junction has effects on auditory selective attention.

Evidence suggests that in man area 21, the middle temporal cortex, is polysensory, and that it connects with auditory, somatosensory and visual cortical association pathways. The auditory association areas of the superior temporal gyrus project in a complex ordered fashion to the middle temporal gyrus, as does the parietal cortex. The middle temporal gyrus connects with the frontal lobe – the most posterior parts project to posterior prefrontal cortex, areas 8 and 9, while intermediate regions connect more anteriorly with areas 19 and 46. Further forwards, the middle temporal region has connections with anterior prefrontal areas 10 and 46, and with anterior orbitofrontal areas 11 and 14. The most anterior middle temporal cortex is connected with the posterior orbitofrontal cortex, area 12, and with the medial surface of the frontal pole. Further forwards, this middle temporal region projects to the temporal pole and the entorhinal cortex. Thalamic connections are with the pulvinar nuclei and the intralaminar group. Other subcortical connections follow the general pattern for all cortical areas. Some projections (e.g. to the pons), particularly from anteriorly in the temporal lobe, are minimal. Physiological responses of cells in this middle temporal region show convergence of different sensory modalities, and many neurones respond to faces. In line with this complexity, lesions of the temporal lobe in man can lead to considerable disturbance of intellectual function, particularly when the dominant hemisphere is involved. These disturbances can include visuospatial difficulties, prosopagnosia, hemiagnosia and severe sensory dysphasia.

The inferior temporal cortex, area 20, is a higher visual association area. The posterior inferior temporal cortex receives major ipsilateral corticocortical fibres from occipitotemporal visual areas, notably V4. It contains a coarse retinotopic representation of the contralateral visual field, and sends a major feedforward pathway to the anterior part of the inferior temporal cortex. The anterior inferior temporal cortex projects onto the temporal pole and to paralimbic areas on the medial surface of the temporal lobe. Additional ipsilateral association connections of the inferior temporal cortex are with the anterior middle temporal cortex, in the walls of the superior temporal gyrus, and with visual areas of the parietotemporal cortex. Frontal lobe connections are with area 46 in the dorsolateral prefrontal cortex (posterior inferior temporal), and with the orbitofrontal cortex (anterior inferior temporal). The posterior area also connects with the frontal eye fields. Reciprocal thalamic connections are with the pulvinar nuclei; the posterior part is related mainly to the inferior and lateral nuclei, and the anterior part to the medial and adjacent lateral pulvinar. Intralaminar connections are with the paracentral and central medial nuclei. Other subcortical connections conform to the general pattern of all cortical regions. Callosal connections are between corresponding areas and the adjacent visual association areas of each hemisphere.

The cortex of the temporal pole receives feedforward projections from widespread areas of temporal association cortex which are immediately posterior to it. The dorsal part receives predominantly auditory input from the anterior part of the superior temporal gyrus. The inferior part receives visual input from the anterior area of the inferior temporal cortex. Other ipsilateral connections are with the anterior insular, the posterior and medial orbitofrontal, and the medial prefrontal cortices. The temporal pole projects onwards into limbic and paralimbic areas. Thalamic connections are mainly with the medial pulvinar nucleus, and with intralaminar and midline nuclei. Other subcortical connections are as for the cortex in general, although some projections, such as that to the pontine nuclei, are very small. Physiological responses of cells in this and more medial temporal cortex correspond particularly to behavioural performance and to the recognition of high-level aspects of social stimuli.

Nuclei of the amygdala (p. 409) project to, and receive fibres from, neocortical areas, predominantly of the temporal lobe, and possibly inferior parietal cortex. The density of these pathways increases towards the temporal pole.

INSULA (Figs 22.17, 22.18, 22.19, 22.20)

The insula lies deep in the floor of the lateral fissure, almost surrounded by a circular sulcus, and overlapped by adjacent cortical areas, the opercula. The frontal operculum is between the anterior and ascending rami of the lateral fissure, forming a triangular division of the inferior frontal gyrus. The frontoparietal operculum, between ascending and

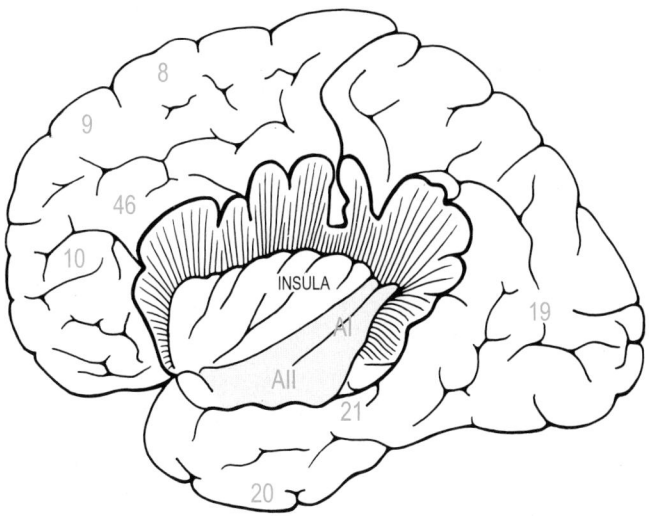

Fig. 22.18 Lateral aspect of the left cerebral hemisphere. The opercula have been cut away to expose the insula and the adjoining anterior and posterior transverse temporal gyri and their continuity with the superior temporal gyrus.

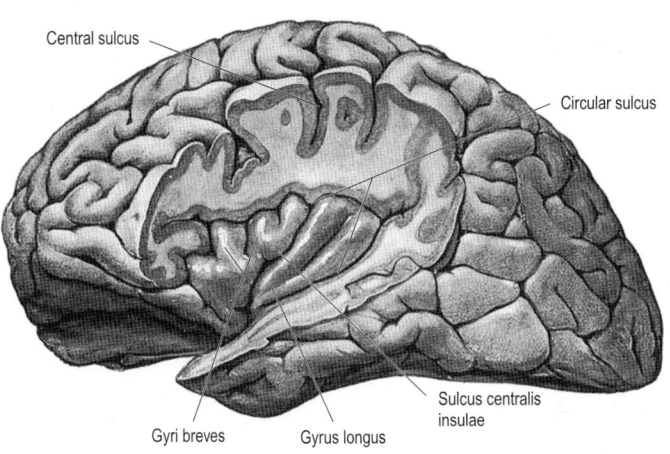

Fig. 22.19 The insula, exposed by removal of the opercula.

posterior rami of the lateral fissure, consists of the posterior part of the inferior frontal gyrus, the lower ends of the precentral and postcentral gyri, and the lower end of the anterior part of the inferior parietal lobule. The temporal operculum, below the posterior ramus of the lateral fissure, is formed by superior temporal and transverse temporal gyri. Anteriorly, the inferior region of the insula adjoins the orbital part of the inferior frontal gyrus.

When the opercula are removed, the insula appears as a pyramidal area, its apex beneath and near the anterior perforated substance, where the circular sulcus is deficient (**Figs 22.19, 22.20**). The medial part of the apex is termed the limen insulae (gyrus ambiens). A central insular sulcus, which slants posterosuperiorly from the apex, divides the insular surface into a large anterior and a small posterior part. The anterior part is divided by shallow sulci into three or four short gyri, whereas the posterior part is one long gyrus, often divided at its upper end. The cortex of the insula is continuous with that of its opercula in the circular sulcus. The insula is approximately coextensive with the subjacent claustrum and putamen.

Cytoarchitectonically, three zones are recognized within the insula. Anteriorly, and extending caudally into the central insula, the cortex is agranular. It is surrounded by a belt of dysgranular cortex, in which laminae II and III can be recognized, and this in turn is surrounded by an outer zone of homotypical granular cortex, which extends to the caudal limit of the insula.

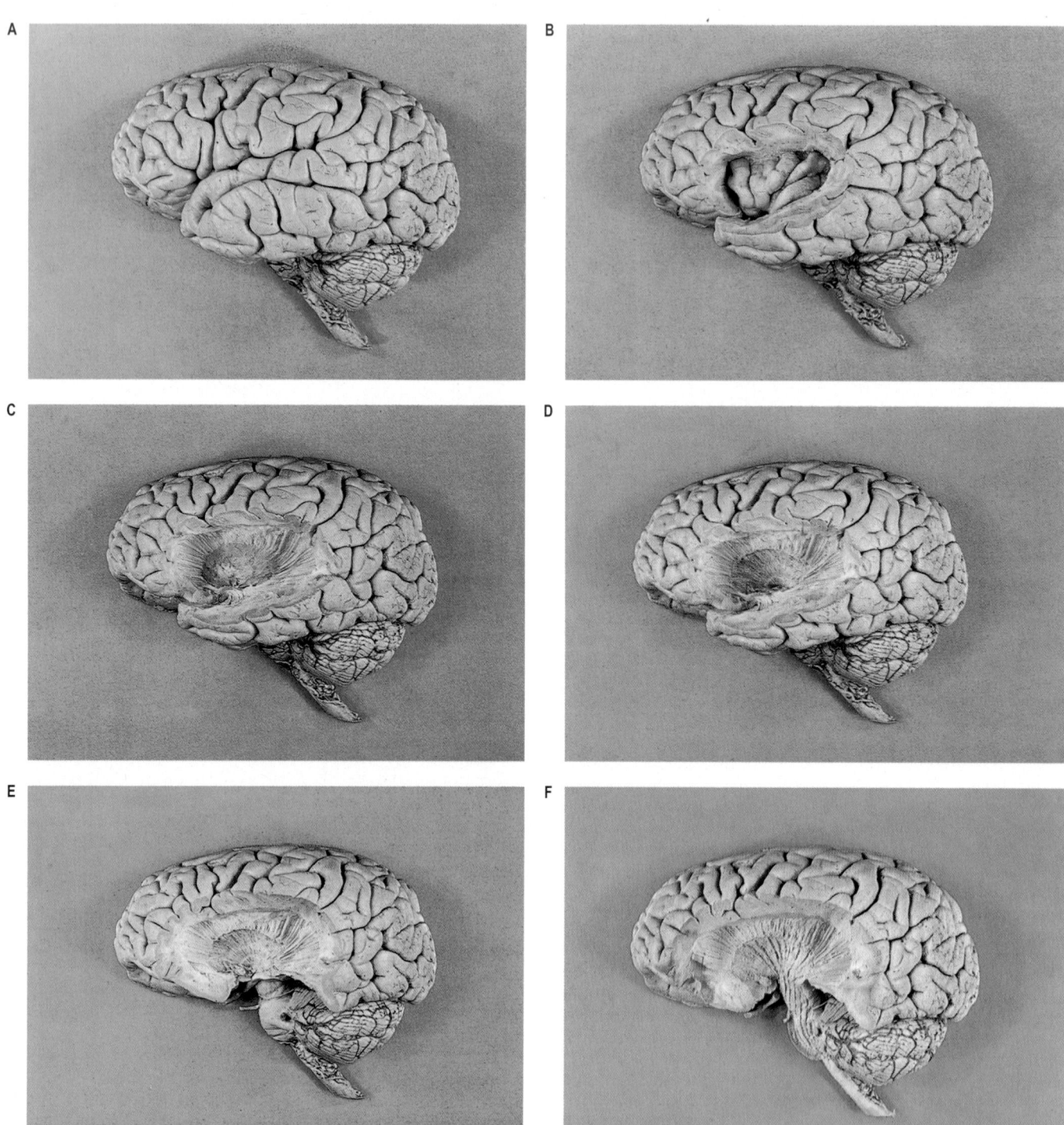

Fig. 22.20 A series of dissections of the left cerebral hemisphere at progressively deeper levels to demonstrate the insula and subjacent structures. **A**, the intact brain; **B**, the cortical gyri of the insula exposed by removal of the frontal, temporal and parietal opercula; **C**, the removal of the insular cortex, extreme capsule, claustrum and external capsule to expose the lateral aspect of the putamen; **D**, removal of the lentiform complex to display fibres of the internal capsule; **E**, removal of part of the temporal lobe to show the internal capsule fibres converging on the crus cerebri of the midbrain; **F**, removal of the optic tract, and superficial dissection of the pons and upper medulla, emphasizing the continuity of the corona radiata, internal capsule, crus cerebri, longitudinal pontine fibres and the medullary pyramid. (Dissection by EL Rees; photograph by Kevin Fitzpatrick on behalf of GKT School of Medicine, London.)

Thalamic afferents to the insula come from subdivisions of the ventral posterior nucleus and of the medial geniculate body, from the oral and medial parts of the pulvinar, the suprageniculate nucleus limitans complex, the mediodorsal nucleus and the nuclei of the intralaminar and midline groups. It appears that the anterior (agranular) cortex is connected predominantly with the mediodorsal and ventroposterior nuclei, while the posterior (granular) cortex is connected predominantly with the pulvinar and the ventral posterior nuclei. The other nuclear groups appear to connect with all areas.

Ipsilateral cortical connections of the insula are diverse. Somatosensory connections are with SI, SII and surrounding areas, area 5 of the superior parietal lobe and area 7b of the inferior parietal lobe. The insular cortex also has connections with the orbitofrontal cortex. Several auditory regions in the temporal lobe interconnect with the posterior granular insula and the dysgranular cortex more anteriorly. Connections with visual areas are virtually absent. The anterior agranular cortex of the insula appears to have connections primarily with olfactory, limbic and paralimbic structures, including, most prominently, the amygdala. Little is known about the functions of the human insula. However, the somatosensory functions of the posterior part are clearly present in man, and anterior insular cortex appears to have a role in olfaction and taste. The insula appears to be a key station in the discriminative-touch pathway, which passes via SII, at least for the somatosensory pathway. The posterior region of the insula has also been implicated in language functions, which resonates with the possibility that higher order auditory association pathways may pass via areas in the insula.

Claustrum

The claustrum (**Figs 22.33, 22.38**) is a thin sheet of grey matter lying deep to the insula. It is approximately coextensive with the insula, from which it is separated by the extreme capsule. Medially, the claustrum is separated from the putamen by the external capsule. It is thickest anteriorly and inferiorly, where it becomes continuous with the anterior perforated substance, amygdala and prepiriform cortex. In animals, it has reciprocal, topographically organized, connections with many regions of the neocortex. Little is known about the connections and functional significance of the claustrum in the human brain.

OCCIPITAL LOBE

The occipital lobe lies behind an arbitrary line joining the preoccipital incisure and the parieto-occipital sulcus. The transverse occipital sulcus descends from the superomedial margin of the hemisphere, behind the parieto-occipital sulcus, and is joined about its midpoint by the intra-parietal sulcus. The lateral occipital sulcus divides the lobe into superior and inferior occipital gyri (**Figs 22.1, 22.2**). The lunate sulcus, when present, lies just in front of the occipital pole. It is placed vertically and is occasionally joined to the calcarine sulcus. Its lips separate striate from peristriate areas; the parastriate area is buried in the sulcus between the other two striate areas. The lunate sulcus is posterior to the gyrus descendens, which is behind the superior and inferior occipital gyri. Curved superior and inferior polar sulci often appear near the ends of the lunate sulcus. The superior polar sulcus arches up on to the medial occipital surface near the upper limit of the lunate sulcus. The inferior polar sulcus arches down and forwards on to the inferior cerebral surface from the lower limit of the lunate sulcus. These polar sulci enclose semilunar extensions of the striate area, and indicate the extent of the visual cortex associated with the macula.

The occipital lobe comprises almost entirely Brodmann's areas 17, 18 and 19. Area 17, the striate cortex, is the primary visual cortex (VI). A host of other distinct visual areas reside in the occipital and temporal cortex. Functional subdivisions V2, V3 (dorsal and ventral) and V3A lie within Brodmann's area 18. Other functional areas at the junction of the occipital cortex with the parietal or temporal lobes lie wholly or partly in area 19.

The primary visual cortex is mostly located on the medial aspect of the occipital lobe, and is coextensive with the subcortical nerve fibre stria of Gennari in layer IV, hence its alternative name, the striate cortex. It occupies the upper and lower lips and depths of the posterior part of the calcarine sulcus and extends into the cuneus and lingual gyrus (**Fig. 22.21**). Posteriorly it is limited by the lunate sulcus, and by polar sulci above and below this sulcus. It extends to the occipital pole.

The primary visual cortex receives afferent fibres from the lateral geniculate nucleus (**Figs 21.7, 21.8**) via the optic radiation. The latter curves posteriorly and spreads through the white matter of the occipital lobe. Its fibres terminate in strict point-to-point fashion in the striate area. The cortex of each hemisphere receives impulses from two half-retinae, which represent the contralateral half of the binocular visual field. Superior and inferior retinal quadrants are connected with corresponding areas of the striate cortex. Thus, the superior retinal quadrants (representing the inferior half of the visual field) are connected with the visual cortex above the calcarine sulcus, and the inferior retinal quadrants (representing the upper half of the visual field) are connected with the visual cortex below the calcarine sulcus. The peripheral parts of the retinae activate the most anterior parts in the visual cortex. The macula impinges upon a disproportionately large posterior part.

The striate cortex is granular. Layer IV, bearing the stria of Gennari, is commonly divided into three sublayers. Passing from superficial to deep, these are IVA, IVB (which contains the stria), and IVC. The densely cellular IVC is further subdivided into a superficial IVCα and a deep IVCβ. Layer IVB contains only sparse, mainly non-pyramidal, neurones. The input to area 17 from the lateral geniculate nucleus terminates predominantly in layers IVA and IVC. Other thalamic afferents, from the inferior pulvinar nucleus and the intralaminar group, pass to layers I and VI. Geniculocortical fibres terminate in alternating bands. Axons from geniculate laminae, which receive information from the ipsilateral eye (laminae 2, 3 and 5), are segregated from those of laminae receiving input from the contralateral eye (laminae 1, 4 and 6). Neurones within layer IVC are monocular, i.e. they respond to stimulation of either the ipsilateral or contralateral eye, but not both. This horizontal segregation forms the anatomical basis of the ocular dominance column in that neurones encountered in a vertical strip from pia to white matter, although binocular outside layer IV, exhibit a preference for stimulation of one or other eye. The other major functional basis for visual cortical columnar organization is the orientation column. This describes the observation that an electrode passing through the depth of the cortex at right angles to the plane from pia to white matter, encounters neurones that all respond preferentially to either a stationary or a moving straight line of a given orientation within the visual field. Cells with simple, complex and hypercomplex receptive fields occur in area 17. Simple cells respond optimally to lines in a narrowly defined position. Complex cells respond to a line anywhere within a receptive field, but with a specific orientation. Hypercomplex cells are similar to complex cells except that the length of the line or bar stimulus is also critical for an optimal response. There is a relationship between the complexity of response and the position of cells in relation to the cortical laminae. Simple cells are mainly in layer IV and complex and hypercomplex cells predominate in either layers II and III or layers V and VI.

Ipsilateral corticocortical fibres pass from area 17 to a variety of functional areas in areas 18 and 19 and in the parietal and temporal

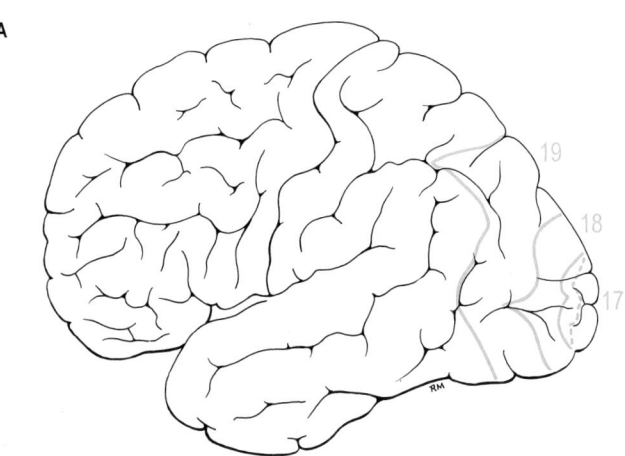

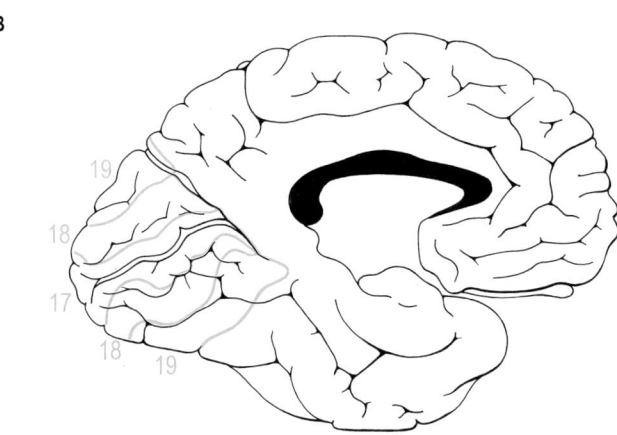

Fig. 22.21 Lateral (**A**) and medial (**B**) surfaces of the left cerebral hemispheres showing the visual areas in the occipital lobe. The striate (17), parastriate (18) and peristriate (19) areas correspond approximately to the Brodmann areas as indicated and also to visual areas VI, V2 and V3.

cortices. Fibres from area 17 pass to area 18 (which contains visual areas V2, V3 and V3a); area 19 (which contains V4); the posterior intra-parietal and the parieto-occipital areas; and to parts of the posterior temporal lobe, the middle temporal area and the medial superior temporal area. Subcortical efferents of the striate cortex pass to the superior colliculus, pretectum and parts of the brain stem reticular formation. Projections to the striatum (notably the tail of the caudate nucleus), and to the pontine nuclei, are sparse, but do exist. Geniculo- and claustrocortical projections are reciprocated by prominent descending projections, which arise in layer VI.

The second visual area (V2) occupies much of area 18 but is not coextensive with it. It contains a complete retinotopic representation of the visual hemifield, which is a mirror image of that in area 17, with the vertical meridian represented most posteriorly along the border between areas 17 and 18. The major ipsilateral corticocortical feedforward projection to V2 comes from V1. Feedforward projections from V2 pass to several other visual areas (and are reciprocated by feedback connections) including the third visual area (V3) and its various subdivisions (V3/V3d; VP/V3v; V3a); the fourth visual area (V4); areas in the temporal and parietal association cortices; and the frontal eye fields. Thalamic afferents to V2 come from the lateral geniculate nucleus, the inferior and lateral pulvinar nuclei and parts of the intralaminar group of nuclei. Additional subcortical afferents are as for cortical areas in general. Subcortical efferents arise predominantly in layers V and VI. They pass to the thalamus, claustrum, superior colliculus, pretectum, brain stem reticular formation, striatum and pons. As for area 17, the callosal connections of V2 are restricted predominantly to the cortex, which contains the representation of the vertical meridian.

The third visual area (V3) is a narrow strip adjoining the anterior margin of V2, probably still within area 18 of Brodmann. V3 has been subdivided into dorsal (V3/V3d) and ventral (VP/V3v) regions on the basis of its afferents from area V1, myeloarchitecture, callosal and association connections, and receptive field properties. The dorsal subdivision receives from V1, whereas the ventral does not. Functionally, the dorsal part shows less wavelength selectivity, greater direction selectivity and smaller receptive fields than does the ventral subdivision. Both areas receive a feedforward projection from V2, and are interconnected by association fibres. A further visual area, area V3a, lies anterior to the dorsal subdivision of V3. It receives afferent association connections from V1, V2, V3/V3d and VP/V3v, and has a complex and irregular topographic organization. All subdivisions project to diverse visual areas in the parietal, occipital and temporal cortices, including V4, and to the frontal eye fields.

The fourth visual area, V4, lies within area 19 anterior to the V3 complex. It receives a major ipsilateral feedforward projection from V2. Colour selectivity as well as orientation selectivity may be transmitted to V4 and bilateral damage causes achromatopsia. V4 is more complex than a simple colour discrimination area because it is also involved in the discrimination of orientation, form and movement. It sends a feed-forward projection to the inferior temporal cortex and receives a feed-back projection. It also connects with other visual areas that lie more dorsally in the temporal lobe, and in the parietal lobe. Thalamocortical connections are with the lateral and inferior pulvinar and the intra-laminar nuclei. Other subcortical connections conform to the general pattern for all cortical areas. Callosal connections are with the contra-lateral V4 and other occipital visual areas.

A fifth visual area, V5 or the middle temporal area, is found in non-human primates towards the posterior end of the superior temporal sulcus. It receives ipsilateral association connections from areas VI, V2, V3 and V4, in a topographically organized way. Other lesser projections are received from widespread visual areas in the temporal and parieto-occipital lobes and from the frontal eye fields. V5 is primarily a move-ment detection or discrimination area, and contains a high proportion of movement-sensitive, direction-selective, cells. Feedforward projections go to surrounding temporal and parietal areas, and to the frontal eye field. Thalamic connections are with the lateral and inferior pulvinar and intralaminar group of nuclei. Other connections follow the general pattern of all neocortical areas.

Current concepts of visual processing in inferior temporal and temporoparietal cortices suggest that two parallel pathways (dorsal and ventral) emanate from the occipital lobe. The dorsal pathway, concerned primarily with visuospatial discrimination, projects from V1 and V2 to the superior temporal and surrounding parietotemporal areas and ultimately to area 7a of the parietal cortex. Damage to these pathways disrupts motion perception and causes optic ataxia and may also disrupt learning of visuospatial tasks. The fourth visual area, V4, is a key relay station for the ventral pathway, which is related to perception and object recognition. Its connections pass sequentially along the inferior temporal gyrus in a feedforward manner, from V4 to posterior, inter-mediate and then anterior, inferior temporal cortices. Ultimately they feed into the temporal polar and medial temporal areas and so interface with the limbic system.

LIMBIC LOBE (Fig. 22.22)

The limbic lobe includes large parts of the cortex on the medial wall of the hemisphere, principally the subcallosal, cingulate and para-hippocampal gyri. It also includes the hippocampal formation, which consists of the hippocampus proper (Ammon's horn or 'cornu ammonis'), the dentate gyrus, the subicular complex (subiculum, pre-subiculum, parasubiculum) and the entorhinal cortex (area 28). There is a close relationship between these phylogenetically old cortical structures and the termination of the olfactory tract in the frontal and medial temporal lobes.

On the basis of emotional disturbances displayed by patients who presented with damage to the hippocampus and cingulate gyrus, Papez (1937) described a closed circuit (the Papez circuit), which linked the hippocampus with the cingulate cortex, via the mammillary bodies and anterior thalamus. He proposed that emotional expression is organized in the hippocampus, experienced in the cingulate gyrus and expressed via the mammillary bodies. The hypothalamus was considered to be the site where hippocampal processes gain access to the autonomic outflow that controls the peripheral expression of emotional states. The Papez circuit is now widely accepted to be involved with cognitive processes, including mnemonic functions and spatial short-term memory.

Later the term 'limbic system' became popular to describe the limbic lobe, together with closely associated subcortical nuclei including the amygdala, septum, hypothalamus, habenula, anterior thalamic nuclei and parts of the basal ganglia.

The cingulate gyrus may be divided rostrocaudally into several cytoarchitectonically discrete areas. These are the prelimbic (area 32) and infralimbic (area 25) cortices, the anterior cingulate cortex (areas 23 and 24) and part of the posterior cingulate or retrosplenial cortex (area 29).

The cingulate gyrus, which is related to the medial surfaces of the frontal lobe, contains specific motor areas, and has extensive connections with neocortical areas of the frontal lobe. The cingulate gyrus on the medial surface of the parietal lobe has equally extensive connections with somatosensory and visual-association areas of the parietal, occipital and temporal lobes. These afferents to the cingulate gyrus are predominantly from neocortical areas on the lateral surface of the hemisphere. Within the cingulate cortex, most projections pass caudally, ultimately into the posterior parahippocampal gyrus. Through this system, afferents from widespread areas of association cortex converge upon the medial temporal lobe and hippocampal formation. There are other parallel stepwise routes to these targets through cortical areas on the lateral surface.

The cingulate gyrus is the area that shows the most consistent pain-evoked changes in synaptic activity related to regional cerebral blood flow (rCBF) as measured by either positron emission tomography (PET) or functional magnetic resonance imaging (fMRI) (Derbyshire et al 1997). It must be remembered that pain evokes a multidimensional response in the brain including cognitive, emotional, autonomic and motor components, and so it is not always possible to assign specific functions to parts of the brain that generate PET or fMRI signals in response to pain (Peyron et al 2000). However, in many experimental paradigms a combination of signals from the cingulate gyrus, somato-sensory area SII and the insula appears to be involved in the conscious appreciation of nociception and neuropathic pain.

The complex parahippocampal gyrus includes areas 27, 28 (entorhinal cortex), 35, 36, 48, 49 and temporal cortical fields. The rich interconnections within the cingulate and parahippocampal cortices, and with the hippocampal formation, are schematically represented in **Fig. 22.23**. Only a few will be described in detail here. In monkeys, the infralimbic cortex (area 25) has been shown to project to areas 24a and 24b. Area 25 also has reciprocal connections with the entorhinal cortex. Projections between the paralimbic area 32 and the limbic cortex (anterior, retrosplenial and entorhinal cortex) are somewhat less prominent. Areas 24 and 29 are connected with the paralimbic posterior

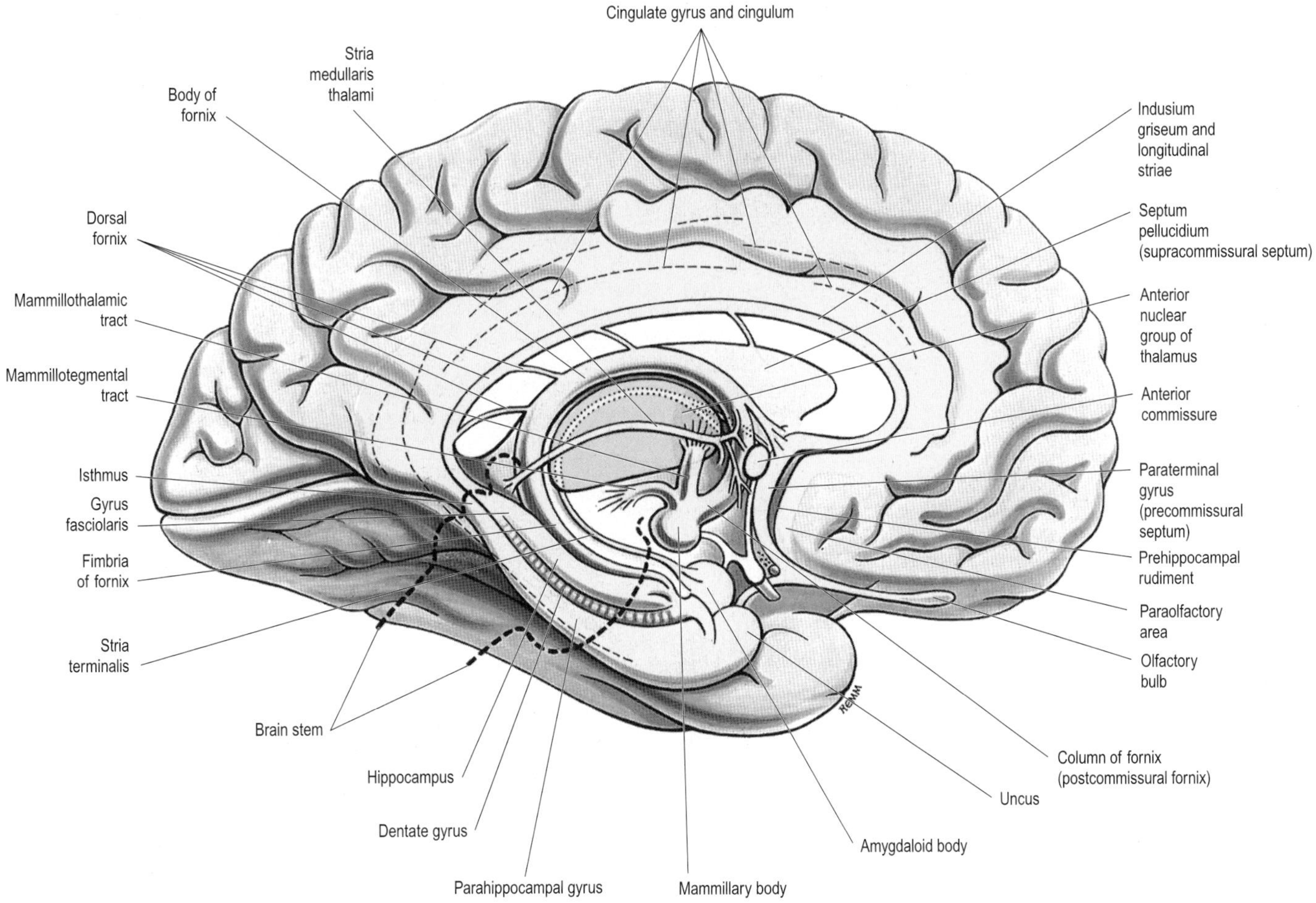

Cingulate gyrus and cingulum

Stria
medullaris
thalami

Body of
fornix

Indusium
griseum and
longitudinal
striae

Dorsal
fornix

Septum
pellucidium
(supracommissural septum)

Mammillothalamic
tract

Anterior
nuclear
group of
thalamus

Mammillotegmental
tract

Anterior
commissure

Isthmus

Paraterminal
gyrus
(precommissural
septum)

Gyrus
fasciolaris

Fimbria
of fornix

Prehippocampal
rudiment

Paraolfactory
area

Stria
terminalis

Olfactory
bulb

Brain stem

Hippocampus

Column of fornix
(postcommissural fornix)

Uncus

Dentate gyrus

Amygdaloid body

Parahippocampal gyrus   Mammillary body

Fig. 22.22 The medial aspect of the left cerebral hemisphere demonstrating some limbic structures (yellow). The anterior nuclear group of the thalamus is coloured orange and the rest of the thalamus is magenta. The approximate position of the brain stem is outlined in a heavy interrupted line.

cingulate area 23. The strong connections between subicular and entorhinal areas will be discussed in the context of the hippocampal formation itself. Reference to **Fig. 22.23** emphasizes the way that the pro-isocortical cingulate and related areas (32, 24c, 23, 29d, 35b, 36) interface between the limbic-archicortex and peri-archicortex and widespread areas of the neocortex. This pattern of cortical connection, i.e. outwards from the hippocampus, via the entorhinal cortex to the perirhinal cortex, caudal parahippocampal gyrus and posterior cingulate gyrus, has assumed enormous functional importance so far as the hippocampus is concerned, as will be discussed below. The parahippocampal gyrus projects to virtually all association areas of the cortex in primates and also provides the major funnel through which polymodal sensory inputs converge on the hippocampus.

Olfactory pathways
The olfactory pathways include the olfactory nerves, olfactory bulb and olfactory tract, together with its central connections in the frontal and temporal lobes. These are primarily described in Ch. 24. The close association of these structures with limbic regions is shown in **Fig. 22.7**.

Hippocampal formation
The hippocampal formation includes the dentate gyrus, hippocampus, subicular complex and entorhinal cortex.

The hippocampus lies above the subiculum and medial parahippocampal gyrus, forming a curved elevation, c.5 cm long, along the floor of the inferior horn of the lateral ventricle (**Fig. 22.24**). Its anterior end is expanded, and here its margin may present two or three shallow grooves that give a paw-like appearance, the pes hippocampi. The ventricular aspect is convex. It is covered by ependyma, beneath which fibres of the alveus converge medially on a longitudinal bundle of fibres, the fimbria of the fornix (**Fig. 22.25**). Passing medially from the

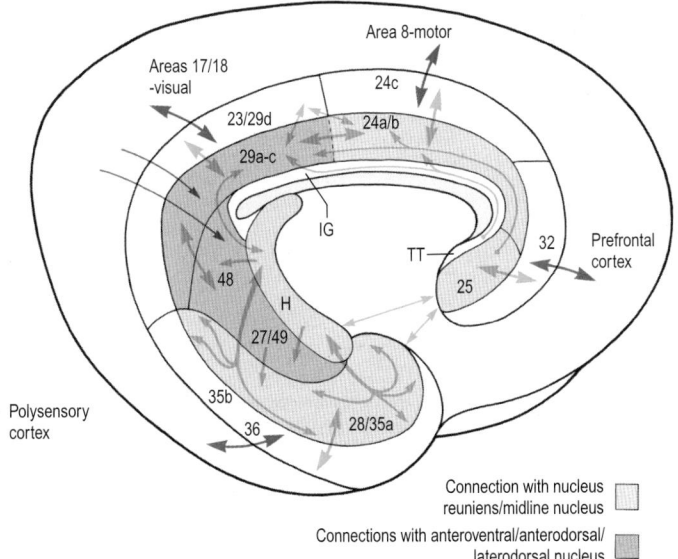

Fig. 22.23 The left limbic cortex illustrating the major interconnections between areas as well as connections with major thalamic areas and extralimbic cortex. (Redrawn from Lopes da Silva FH, Witter MP, Beoijinga PH et al 1990 Anatomic organization and physiology of the limbic cortex. Physiol Rev 70: 453–511, by permission from the American Physiological Society.)

collateral sulcus, the neocortex of the parahippocampal gyrus merges with the transitional juxtallocortex of the subiculum. The latter curves superomedially to the inferior surface of the dentate gyrus, then laterally to the laminae of the hippocampus. This continues the curvature, first

405

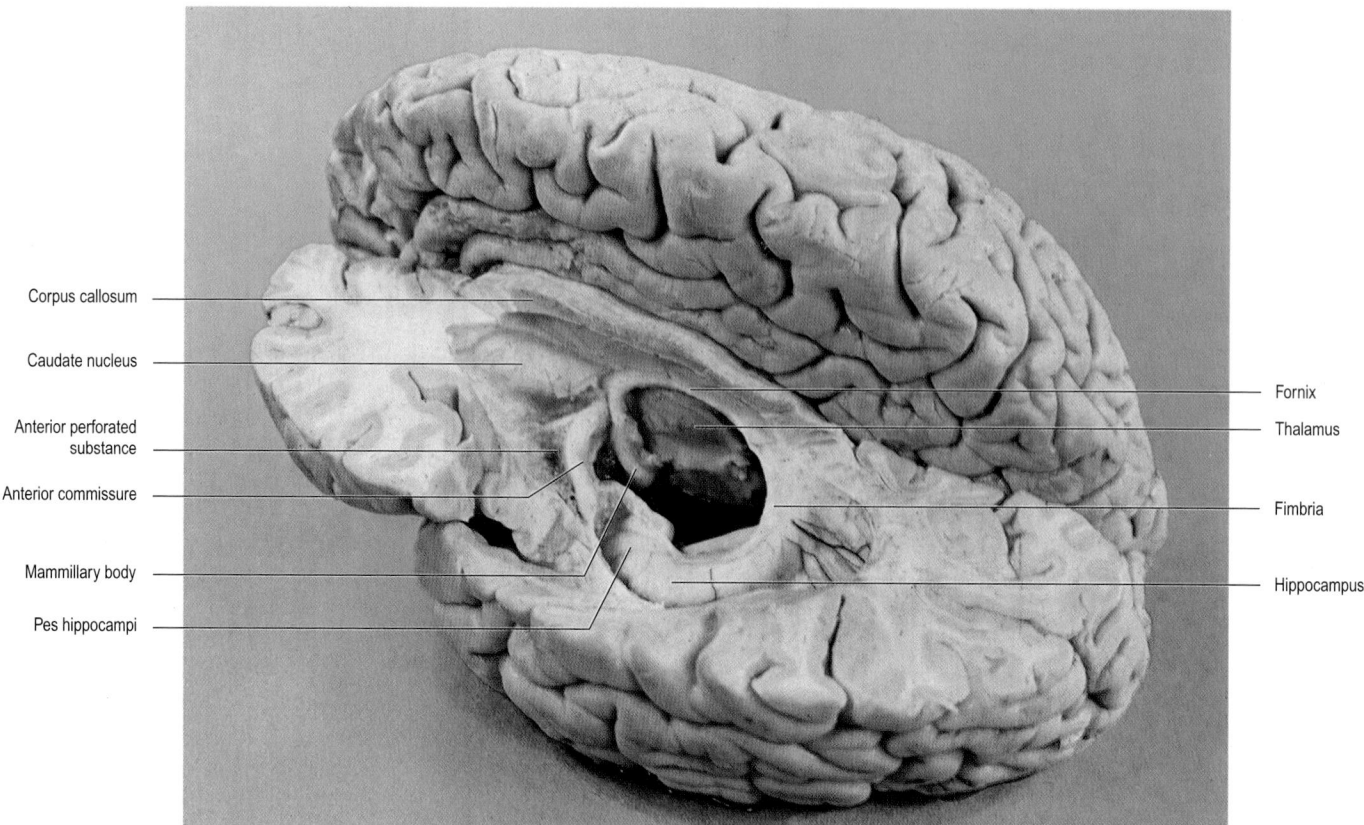

Corpus callosum

Caudate nucleus

Anterior perforated substance

Anterior commissure

Mammillary body

Pes hippocampi

Fornix

Thalamus

Fimbria

Hippocampus

Fig. 22.24 Dissection of the left cerebral hemisphere demonstrating structures of the limbic system. The body of the corpus callosum has been divided sagitally. The frontal, temporal and occipital lobes have been sectioned horizontally and their superior parts removed. The left lentiform complex and thalamus have been removed and the floor of the inferior horn of the lateral ventricle opened. (Dissection by AM Seal; photograph by Kevin Fitzpatrick on behalf of GKT School of Medicine, London.)

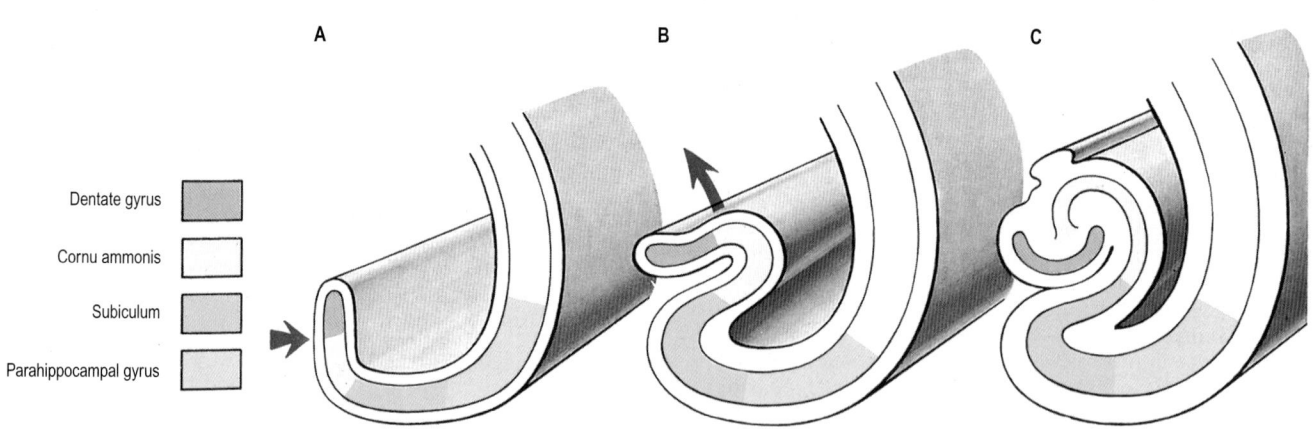

A   B   C

Dentate gyrus

Cornu ammonis

Subiculum

Parahippocampal gyrus

Fig. 22.25 Coronal sections of the temporal lobe and inferior horn of the lateral ventricle illustrating the hippocampus and related structures. **A**, **B** and **C** are a series of diagrams to assist understanding of the relative positions of the dentate gyrus, cornu ammonis, subiculum and parahippocampal gyrus in the floor of the inferior horn.

superiorly, then medially above the dentate gyrus, and ends pointing towards the centre of the superior surface of the dentate gyrus. The dentate gyrus is a crenated strip of cortex related inferiorly to the subiculum, laterally to the hippocampus and, more medially, to the fimbria of the fornix (**Figs 22.25, 22.26**). The form of the fimbria is quite variable, but medially it is separated from the crenated medial margin of the dentate gyrus by the fimbriodentate sulcus (**Fig. 22.27**). The hippocampal sulcus, of variable depth, lies between the dentate gyrus and the subicular extension of the parahippocampal gyrus. Posteriorly, the dentate gyrus is continuous with the gyrus fasciolaris and thus with the indusium griseum. Anteriorly, it is continued into the notch of the uncus, turning medially across its inferior surface, as the tail of the dentate gyrus (band of Giacomini), and vanishes on the

medial aspect of the uncus (**Fig. 22.26**). The tail separates the inferior surface of the uncus into an anterior uncinate gyrus and posterior intralimbic gyrus.

The trilaminar cortex of the dentate gyrus is the least complex of the hippocampal fields, and its major cell type is the granule cell, found in the dense granule-cell layer. Granule cells (c.9 × 10^6 in the human dentate gyrus) have unipolar dendrites that extend into the overlying molecular layer, which receives most of the afferent projections to the dentate gyrus (primarily from the entorhinal cortex). The granule cell and molecular layers are sometimes referred to as the fascia dentata. The polymorphic layer, or hilus of the dentate gyrus, contains cells that give rise primarily to ipsilateral association fibres. They remain within the dentate gyrus and do not extend into other hippocampal fields.

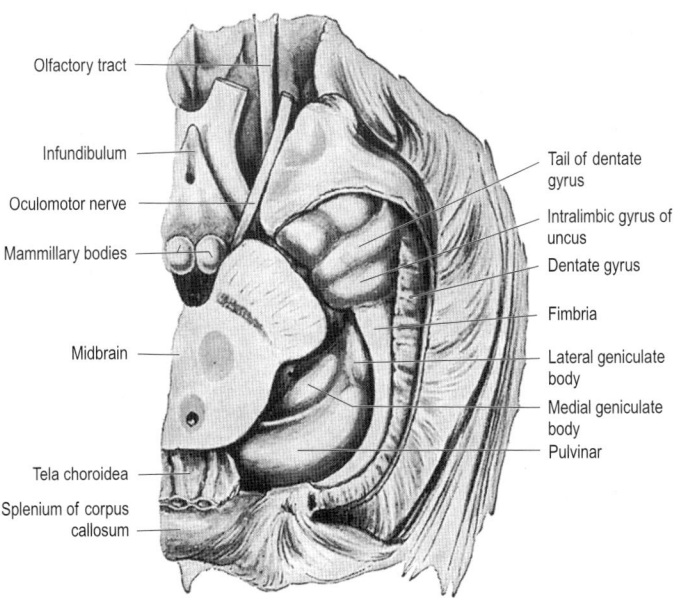

Fig. 22.26 Basal aspect of the brain dissected to display the dentate gyrus, uncus and fimbria on the left.

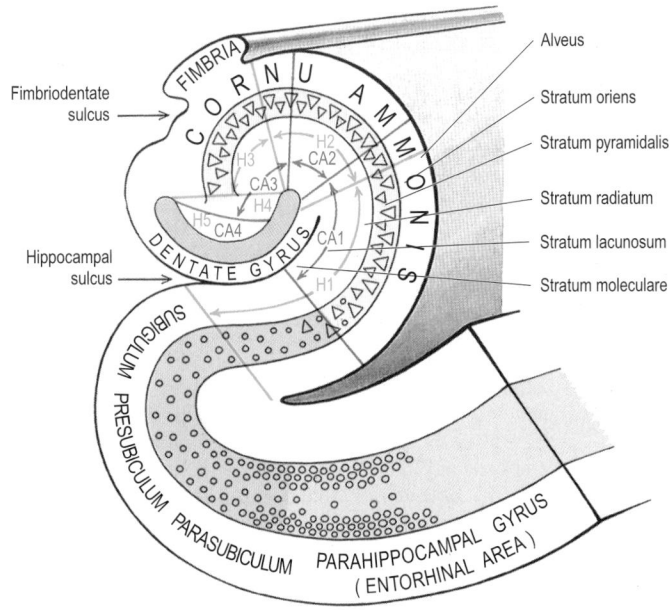

Fig. 22.28 The hippocampal formation showing the disposition of the various cell fields. Dentate gyrus: pink; hippocampus proper (cornu ammonis): yellow; areas of the subicular complex: green; entorhinal cortex: blue. CA1–3, hippocampal cell fields.

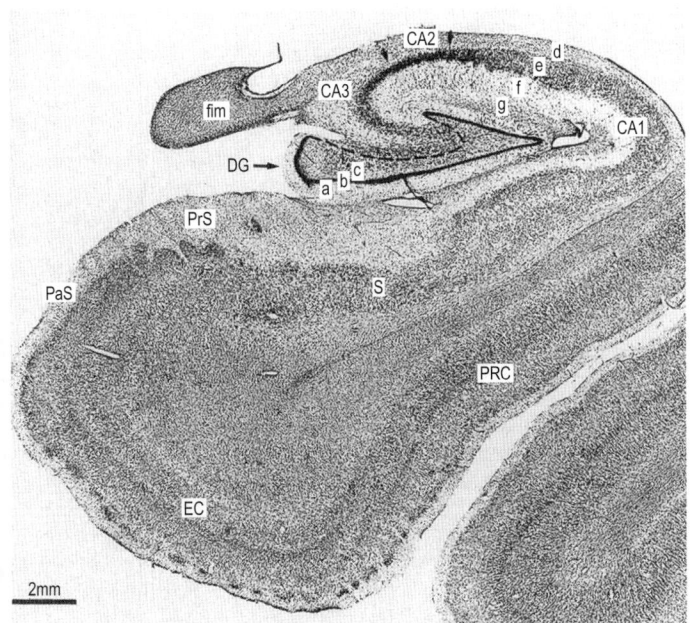

Fig. 22.27 Coronal, thionin-stained section of the human hippocampal formation. Abbreviations: a, molecular layer of the dentate gyrus; b, granule cell layer of the dentate gyrus; c, plexiform layer of the dentate gyrus; CA1–3, fields of the hippocampus; d, stratum oriens layer of the hippocampus; DG, dentate gyrus; e, pyramidal cell layer of the hippocampus; EC, entorhinal cortex; f, stratum radiatum of the hippocampus; fim, fimbria; g, stratum lacunosum-molecular of the hippocampus; PaS, parasubiculum; PRC, perirhinal cortex; PrS, presubiculum; S, subiculum. (Photomicrograph by kind permission from David Amaral.)

The hippocampus is trilaminar archicortex. It consists of a single pyramidal cell layer, with plexiform layers above and below it. It may best be divided into three distinct fields, CA1, CA2 and CA3 (**Figs 22.27, 22.28**). Field CA3 borders the hilus of the dentate gyrus at one end, and field CA2 at the other. Field CA3 pyramidal cells are the largest in the hippocampus and the whole pyramidal cell layer in this field is c.10 cells thick. The most important feature of pyramidal cells in CA3 is that they receive the mossy fibre input from dentate granule cells on their proximal dendrites. The border between CA3 and CA2 is not well

marked because the pyramidal cells of the former appear to extend under the border of the latter for some distance. The CA2 field has the most compact layer of pyramidal cells. It completely lacks a mossy fibre input from dentate granule cells and receives a major input from the supramammillary region of the hypothalamus. Field CA1 is usually described as the most complex of the hippocampal subdivisions and its appearance varies along its transverse and rostrocaudal axes. The CA1/CA2 border is not sharp, and at its other end CA1 overlaps the subiculum for some distance. The thickness of the pyramidal cell layer varies from c.10 to more than 30 cells. Approximately 10% of neurones in this field are interneurones.

It is common to describe several strata within the layers of the hippocampus (**Figs 22.27, 22.28**). Starting from the ventricular aspect, these are: the alveus (contains subicular and hippocampal pyramidal cell axons converging on the fimbria of the fornix); stratum oriens (mainly the basal dendrites of pyramidal cells and some interneurones); stratum pyramidalis; stratum lucidum (contains mossy fibres which make contact with the proximal dendrites of pyramidal cells in field CA3); and the stratum radiatum and stratum lacunosum-moleculare. The stratum lucidum is not as prominent in man as it is in other primates, and is not present in fields CA1 and CA2.

In the stratum radiatum and stratum oriens, CA3 and CA2 cells receive associational connections from other rostrocaudal levels of the hippocampus, as well as afferents from subcortical structures, e.g. the septal nuclei and supramammillary region. The projections from pyramidal cells of fields CA3 and CA2 to CA1, often called Schaffer collaterals, also terminate in the stratum radiatum and stratum oriens. The projections from the entorhinal cortex to the dentate gyrus (the perforant pathway) travel in the stratum lacunosum-moleculare, where they make synaptic contact *en passant* with the distal apical dendrites of hippocampal pyramidal cells.

The subicular complex is generally subdivided into subiculum, presubiculum and parasubiculum (**Figs 22.27, 22.28**). The major subcortical projections of the hippocampal formation (to the septal nuclei, mammillary nuclei, nucleus accumbens and anterior thalamus), and to the entorhinal cortex, all arise from pyramidal neurones of the subicular complex. The subiculum consists of a superficial molecular layer containing apical dendrites of subicular pyramidal cells, a pyramidal cell layer that is c.30 cells thick, and a deep polymorphic layer. The presubiculum is medial to the subiculum and is distinguished by a densely packed superficial layer of pyramidal cells. There is a plexiform layer superficial to this dense cell layer. Cells deep to it are best regarded as either a medial extension of the subiculum or a lateral extension of the deep layers of the entorhinal cortex. The parasubiculum also has a superficial plexiform layer and a primary cell layer. It forms the boundary between the subicular complex as a whole and the entorhinal cortex. The cell layers deep to the parasubiculum are indistinguishable from the deep layers of the entorhinal cortex.

The entorhinal cortex (Brodmann's area 28; Figs 22.7, 22.27, 22.28) extends rostrally to the anterior limit of the amygdala. Caudally it overlaps a portion of the hippocampal fields. The more primitive levels of the entorhinal cortex (below the amygdala) receive projections from the olfactory bulb. More caudal regions do not generally receive primary olfactory inputs.

The entorhinal cortex is divisible into six layers and is quite distinct from other neocortical regions. Layer I is acellular and plexiform. Layer II is a narrow cellular layer, which consists of islands of large pyramidal and stellate cells. These cell islands are a distinguishing feature of the entorhinal cortex. They form small bumps on the surface of the brain that can be seen by the naked eye (verrucae hippocampae), and provide an indication of the boundaries of the entorhinal cortex. Layer III consists of medium-sized pyramidal cells. There is no internal granular layer (another classic feature of entorhinal cortex); in its place is an acellular region of dense fibres called the lamina dissecans, which is sometimes called layer IV. Layers III and V are apposed in regions where the lamina dissecans is absent. Layer V consists of large pyramidal cells five or six deep. Layer VI is only readily distinguishable from layer V close to the border with the perirhinal cortex. Its cells continue around the angular bundle (subcortical white matter deep to the subicular complex made up largely of perforant path axons) to lie beneath the pre- and parasubiculum.

Glutamate and/or aspartate appears to be the major excitatory transmitter in three pathways in the hippocampal formation, namely the perforant pathway (which arises in the entorhinal cortex and terminates primarily in the dentate gyrus); the mossy fibres, which run from the dentate granule cells to the pyramidal cells of the CA3 field; and in the Schaffer collaterals of CA3 pyramidal cells, which terminate on CA1 pyramidal cells.

GABAergic neurones are found in the deep portions of the granule cell layer in the dentate gyrus (basket cells). The highest concentration of GABA receptors is found in the molecular layer of the dentate gyrus. In the hippocampus proper, GABAergic cells are found mostly in the stratum oriens, but also in the pyramidal cell layer and stratum radiatum.

There are many peptide-containing neurones in the hippocampal formation. Granule cells in the dentate gyrus appear to contain the opioid peptide dynorphin, which is also present in mossy fibres running to the CA3 field. Enkephalin, or a related peptide, may be present in fibres arising in the entorhinal cortex. There is a dense plexus of somatostatin-immunoreactive fibres in the molecular layer of the dentate gyrus and also in the stratum lacunosum-moleculare of the hippocampus. The polymorphic layer of the dentate gyrus, stratum oriens of the hippocampus and the deep layers of the entorhinal cortex, all contain somatostatin-immunoreactive neurones. Vasoactive intestinal polypeptide (VIP)-immunoreactive neurones are plentiful in many hippocampal fields, especially in the superficial layers of the entorhinal cortex. Cells containing cholecystokinin (CCK)-immunoreactivity are found in the hilar region of the dentate gyrus, in all layers of the hippocampus, especially in the pyramidal cell layer, and also throughout the subicular complex and entorhinal cortex. There are also substantial plexuses of CCK-immunoreactive fibres in the stratum lacunosum-moleculare, subicular complex and entorhinal cortex. Hippocampal CCK-immunoreactive cells may give rise to extrinsic projections, e.g. to the lateral septum and medial mammillary nucleus, because CCK-immunoreactive fibres are found in the fimbria/fornix.

The dentate gyrus is the point of entry into the hippocampal circuitry. It receives fibres via the perforant path projections from layers II and III of the entorhinal cortex. The axons terminate in the outer two-thirds of the molecular layer of the dentate gyrus, on the dendritic spines of granule cells. These cells project heavily via their mossy fibres onto the proximal dendrites of CA3 pyramidal cells. The latter give rise, via the so-called Schaffer collaterals, to a projection that terminates mainly in the stratum radiatum of the CA1 hippocampal field. The CA1 field projects heavily to the subicular complex, which projects to the entorhinal cortex.

The subiculum, rather than the hippocampus, projects to the mammillary complex, whereas the hippocampus gives rise principally to

efferents destined for the septal complex. Summaries of hippocampal circuitry and connections are shown schematically in Fig. 22.29.

The medial septal complex and the supramammillary area of the posterior hypothalamus are the two major sources of subcortical afferents to the hippocampal formation. There are also projections from the amygdaloid complex and claustrum (to the subicular complex and entorhinal cortex), as well as monoaminergic projections from the ventral tegmental area, the mesencephalic raphe nuclei and the locus coeruleus. The noradrenergic and serotoninergic projections reach all hippocampal fields, but are especially dense in the dentate gyrus.

The projections from the septal complex arise in the medial septal and vertical limb nuclei of the diagonal band. They travel via the dorsal fornix, fimbria, supracallosal striae and a ventral route through the amygdaloid complex. While these projections reach all hippocampal fields, the most prominent terminations are in the dentate gyrus, field CA3, presubiculum, parasubiculum and entorhinal cortex. Many of these medial septal/diagonal band neurones are GABAergic or cholinergic, and they form part of the topographically organized basal forebrain cholinergic system (cell groups Ch1 and Ch2).

Neurones in the supramammillary area also provide a significant innervation of the hippocampal formation. They arrive partly through the fornix and partly through a ventral route, and terminate most heavily in the dentate gyrus, and fields CA2 and CA3 of the cornu ammonis.

All divisions of the anterior thalamic nuclear complex and associated lateral dorsal nucleus project to the hippocampal formation, and are directed predominantly to the subicular complex. Some midline thalamic nuclei, particularly the parataenial, central medial and reuniens

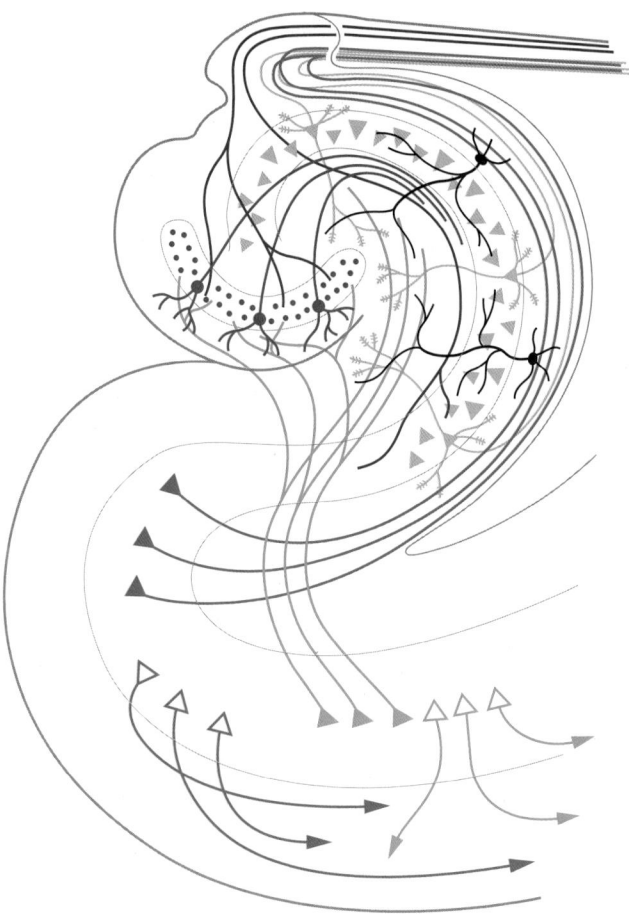

Fig. 22.29 Neuronal organization and connections of the dentate gyrus, hippocampus (cornu ammonis), subiculum and parahippocampal gyrus. Cell somata, dendrites and axons of the pyramidal neurones of the cornu ammonis: yellow; the axons form the efferent hippocampal fibres of the alveus and fimbria; afferent fibres to the cornu ammonis from the fimbria: purple; afferents from the entorhinal cortex via the perforant path: blue; basket neurones: black; neurones of the dentate gyrus and their axons, which form the mossy fibres of the hippocampus: magenta; subicular efferents to the fornix via the alveus: green.

nuclei, also project to the hippocampal formation, especially to the entorhinal cortex.

In humans the fornix contains c.1.2 million fibres. Cells in the CA3 field project bilaterally to the lateral nucleus of the septal complex, via the precommissural fornix. They give rise to the Schaffer collaterals to CA1 cells and to the commissural projections to the contralateral hippocampus. Neurones in the subicular complex and entorhinal cortex give rise to projections to the nucleus accumbens and to parts of the caudate nucleus and putamen. The subicular complex gives rise to the major, postcommissural fibre system of the fornix. The presubiculum, in particular, projects to the anterior thalamic nuclear complex (anteromedial, anteroventral and laterodorsal nuclei). Both the subiculum and presubiculum provide the major extrinsic input to the mammillary complex. Both the lateral and the medial mammillary nuclei receive afferents from the subicular complex.

Several fields in the temporal lobe neocortex, especially TF and TH of the parahippocampal gyrus, the dorsal bank of the superior temporal gyrus, the perirhinal cortex (Brodmann's area 35) and the temporal polar cortex, together with the agranular insular cortex and posterior orbitofrontal cortex, all project to the entorhinal cortex. Projections to the entorhinal cortex also arise from the dorsolateral prefrontal cortex (Brodmann's areas 9, 10, 46), the medial frontal cortex (Brodmann's areas 25, 32), the cingulate cortex (Brodmann's areas 23, 24), and retrosplenial cortex. The subicular complex receives direct cortical inputs, e.g. from the temporal polar cortex, perirhinal cortex, parahippocampal gyrus, superior temporal gyrus and dorsolateral prefrontal cortex. The entorhinal cortex projects to the perirhinal cortex as well as to temporal polar cortex, caudal parahippocampal and cingulate gyri. In monkeys, the subicular complex also projects to a number of cortical areas, including perirhinal cortex, parahippocampal gyrus, caudal cingulate gyrus, medial frontal and medial orbitofrontal cortex.

Septum

The septum is a midline and paramedian structure (Figs 22.22, 23.6). Its upper portion corresponds largely to the bilateral laminae of fibres, sparse grey matter and neuroglia, known as the septum pellucidum, which separates the lateral ventricles. Below this, the septal region is made up of four main nuclear groups: dorsal; ventral; medial; and caudal. The dorsal group is essentially the dorsal septal nucleus; the ventral group consists of the lateral septal nucleus; the medial group contains the medial septal nucleus and the nucleus of the diagonal band of Broca; and the caudal group contains the fimbrial and triangular septal nuclei.

The major afferents to the region terminate primarily in the lateral septal nucleus. They include fibres carried in the fornix that arise from hippocampal fields CA3 and CA1, and the subiculum. There are also afferents arising from the preoptic area, anterior, paraventricular and ventromedial hypothalamic nuclei, and the lateral hypothalamic area. The lateral septum receives a rich monoaminergic innervation, including noradrenergic afferents from the locus coeruleus and medullary cell groups (A1, A2); serotoninergic afferents from the midbrain raphe nuclei; and dopaminergic afferents from the ventral tegmental area (A10).

Projections from the lateral septum run to the medial and lateral preoptic areas, anterior hypothalamus, supramammillary and midbrain ventral tegmental area, via the medial forebrain bundle. There is also a projection to the medial habenular nucleus and some midline thalamic nuclei via the stria medullaris thalami, which runs on the dorsomedial wall of the third ventricle. The projections from the habenula via the fasciculus retroflexus to the interpeduncular nucleus and adjacent ventral tegmental area in the midbrain provide a route through which forebrain limbic structures can influence midbrain nuclear groups.

A large proportion of the medial septal/diagonal band neurones are cholinergic or GABAergic. They project to the hippocampal formation and cingulate cortex.

Amygdala

The amygdaloid nuclear complex is made up of lateral, central and basal nuclei, which lie in the dorsomedial temporal pole, anterior to the hippocampus, and close to the tail of the caudate nucleus (Fig. 22.22). Collectively the nuclei form the ventral, superior and medial walls of the tip of the inferior horn of the lateral ventricle. The amygdala is partly continuous above with the inferomedial margin of the claustrum. Fibres of the external capsule and substriatal grey matter, including the cholinergic magnocellular nucleus basalis (of Meynert), incompletely

separate it from the putamen and globus pallidus. Laterally, it is close to the optic tract. It is partly deep to the gyrus semilunaris, gyrus ambiens and uncinate gyrus (Fig. 22.7).

The lateral nucleus has dorsomedial and ventrolateral subnuclei. The central nucleus has medial and lateral subdivisions. The basal nucleus is commonly divided into a dorsal magnocellular basal nucleus, an intermediate parvicellular basal nucleus, and a ventral band of darkly staining cells usually referred to as the paralaminar basal nucleus, because it borders the white matter ventral to the amygdaloid complex. The accessory basal nucleus lies medial to the basal nuclear divisions. It is usually divided into dorsal, magnocellular, and ventral, parvicellular, parts. The lateral and basal nuclei are often referred to collectively as the basolateral area (nuclear group) of the amygdaloid complex.

It has been suggested that the basolateral complex of nuclei (lateral, basal, accessory basal) shares several characteristics with the cortex, and that it may be considered as a quasi-cortical structure. Although it lacks a laminar structure, it has direct, often reciprocal, connections with adjacent temporal and other areas of cortex, and it projects to the motor or premotor cortex. It receives a direct cholinergic and non-cholinergic input from the magnocellular corticopetal system in the basal forebrain, and has reciprocal connections with the mediodorsal thalamus. The distribution of small peptidergic neurones in the basolateral nuclear complex, e.g. those containing neuropeptide-Y (NY), somatostatin (SOM) and CCK, are also similar in form and density to those found in the adjacent temporal lobe cortex. Projection neurones from this part of the amygdala appear to utilize, at least in part, the excitatory amino acids glutamate or aspartate as a transmitter. Moreover, they project to the ventral striatum rather than to hypothalamic and brain stem sites. Thus, it may be appropriate to consider this part of the amygdaloid complex as a polymodal cortex-like area, which is separated from the cerebral cortex by fibres of the external capsule.

The central nucleus is present through the caudal half of the amygdaloid complex, lying dorsomedial to the basal nucleus. It is divided into medial and lateral parts. The medial part, which contains larger cells than the lateral part, resembles the adjacent putamen. The medial and central nuclei appear to have an extension across the basal forebrain, as well as within the stria terminalis, which merges with the bed nucleus of the stria terminalis. This extensive nuclear complex, sometimes referred to as the 'extended amygdala', is illustrated in Fig. 22.30. It can be considered as a macrostructure formed by the centromedial amygdaloid complex (medial nucleus, medial and lateral parts of the central nucleus), the medial bed nucleus of the stria terminalis, and the cell columns that traverse the sublenticular substantia innominata, which lies between them. It has been suggested that portions of the medial nucleus accumbens may be included in the extended amygdala.

A consistent feature of the intrinsic connections among amygdaloid nuclei is that they arise primarily in lateral and basal nuclei, and terminate in the central and medial nuclei, which suggests a largely unidirectional flow of information. In brief, the lateral nucleus projects to all divisions of the basal nucleus, accessory basal nucleus, paralaminar and anterior cortical nuclei, and less heavily to the central nucleus. The lateral nucleus receives few afferents from other nuclei. The magnocellular, parvicellular and intermediate parts of the basal nucleus project to the accessory basal, central (especially the medial part) and medial nuclei, as well as to the periamygdaloid cortex and the amygdalohippocampal area. The accessory basal nucleus projects densely to the central nucleus, especially its medial division, as well as to the medial and cortical nuclei. Its major intra-amygdaloid afferents arise from the lateral nucleus. The medial nucleus projects to the accessory basal, anterior cortical and central nuclei as well as to the periamygdaloid cortex and amygdalohippocampal area, while afferents arise especially from the lateral nucleus. The intrinsic connections of the cortical nucleus are not very well understood. The posterior part of the cortical nucleus projects to the medial nucleus, but it has been difficult to differentiate this projection from that arising in the amygdalohippocampal area. The central nucleus projects to the anterior cortical nucleus and the various cortical transition zones. It forms an important focus for afferents from many of the amygdaloid nuclei, especially the basal and accessory basal nuclei, and it has major extrinsic connections.

The organization of the extensive subcortical and cortical interconnections and connections of the amygdala are consistent with a role in emotional behaviour. It receives highly processed unimodal and multimodal sensory information from the thalamus, sensory and

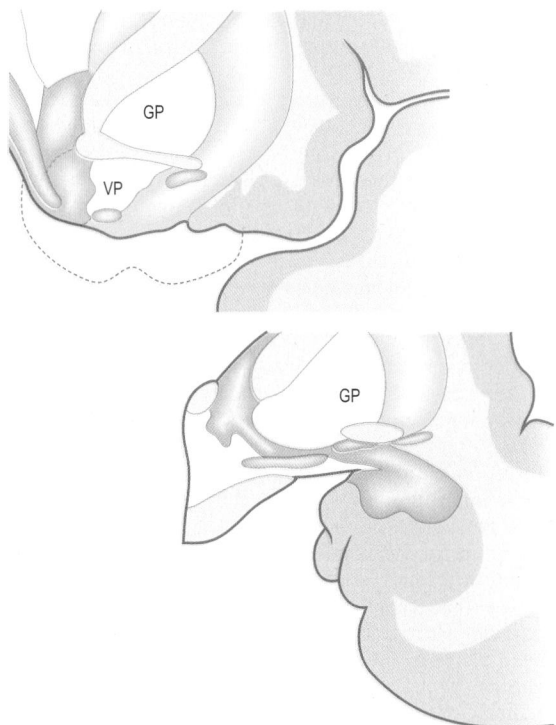

Fig. 22.30 Coronal section through the basal forebrain and temporal pole, illustrating the relationship between the striatum (yellow); globus pallidus (GP, dorsal globus pallidus; VP, ventral pallidum); extended amygdala (blue); and the magnocellular corticopetal basal forebrain system (magenta). Note that the medial part of the nucleus accumbens–olfactory tubercle area (green) may possibly be a mixed zone of the ventral striatopallidal system and the extended amygdala.

association cortices, and olfactory information from the bulb and piriform cortex, and visceral and gustatory information relayed via brain stem structures and the thalamus. Its projections reach widespread areas of the brain, including the endocrine and autonomic domains of the hypothalamus and brain stem.

Afferent connections

The heaviest brain stem projection to the amygdala arises in the peripeduncular nucleus. The parabrachial nuclei also project to the central nucleus. The amygdala receives a rich monoaminergic innervation. The noradrenergic projection arises primarily from the locus coeruleus, serotonergic fibres arise from the dorsal and, to some extent the median, raphe nuclei, and the dopaminergic innervation arises primarily in the midbrain ventral tegmental area (A10). The basal and parvicellular accessory basal nuclei, the amygdalohippocampal area and nucleus of the lateral olfactory tract receive a very dense cholinergic innervation arising from the magnocellular nucleus basalis of Meynert.

The amygdala has rich interconnections with allocortical, juxtallocortical and, especially, neocortical areas. In addition to direct projections from the olfactory bulb to the nucleus of the lateral olfactory tract, anterior cortical nucleus and the periamygdaloid cortex (piriform cortex), there are also associational connections between all parts of the primary olfactory cortex and these same superficial amygdaloid structures. The amygdaloid complex has particularly extensive and rich connections with many areas of the neocortex in unimodal and polymodal regions of the frontal, cingulate, insular and temporal neocortices.

The anterior temporal lobe provides the largest proportion of the cortical input to the amygdala, predominantly to the lateral nucleus. Rostral parts of the superior temporal gyrus, which may represent unimodal auditory association cortex, project to the lateral nucleus. There are also projections from polymodal sensory association cortices of the temporal lobe, including perirhinal cortex (areas 35 and 36), the caudal half of the parahippocampal gyrus, the dorsal bank of the superior temporal sulcus, and both the medial and lateral areas of the cortex of the temporal pole.

The CA1 field of the hippocampus and adjacent subiculum, and possibly the entorhinal cortex, project to the amygdala, mainly to the parvicellular basal nucleus.

The rostral insula projects heavily to the lateral, parvicellular basal and medial nuclei. The caudal insula, which is reciprocally connected with the second somatosensory cortex, also projects to the lateral nucleus, thus providing a route by which somatosensory information reaches the amygdala. The caudal orbital cortex projects to the basal, magnocellular accessory basal and lateral nuclei. The medial prefrontal cortex projects to the magnocellular divisions of the accessory and basal nuclei.

Efferent connections

The central nucleus provides the major relay for projections from the amygdala to the brain stem and receives many of the return projections. It projects to the periaqueductal grey matter, ventral tegmental area, substantia nigra pars compacta, peripeduncular nucleus and tegmental reticular formation (midbrain); the parabrachial nuclei (pons); the nucleus of the solitary tract and the dorsal motor nucleus of the vagus (medulla).

The central nucleus is the major relay for amygdaloid projections to the hypothalamus. Amygdaloid fibres reach the bed nucleus of the stria terminalis primarily via the stria terminalis, but also via the ventral amygdalofugal pathway. In general, central and basal nuclei project to the lateral part of the bed nucleus, while medial and posterior cortical nuclei project to the medial bed nucleus. Anterior cortical and medial nuclei project largely to the medial preoptic area and anterior medial hypothalamus, including the paraventricular and supraoptic nuclei. There is a particularly prominent projection to the ventromedial and premammillary nuclei. The amygdala projects to the rostrocaudal extent of the lateral hypothalamus. The majority of the fibres originate in the central nucleus and run principally in the ventral amygdalofugal pathway and medial forebrain bundle.

There is a rich projection to the mediodorsal nucleus of the thalamus, which gives access to the prefrontal cortex, and also complements direct projections from the amygdala to the same cortical domain. The projection to the mediodorsal nucleus arises from most amygdaloid nuclei, but particularly from the lateral, basal and accessory basal nuclei and the periamygdaloid cortex. The major termination of amygdaloid afferents is in the medial, magnocellular part of the mediodorsal nucleus, especially rostrally. This part of the mediodorsal nucleus projects to the identical medial and orbital prefrontal cortical areas that receive amygdaloid afferents directly. However, this projection to the mediodorsal nucleus is not reciprocated. The central and medial nuclei do not project to the mediodorsal nucleus, but to the midline nuclei, especially the nucleus centralis and nucleus reuniens.

The parvicellular division of the basal nucleus, magnocellular accessory basal nucleus (but not the magnocellular basal nucleus), and the central nucleus all project to basal forebrain cholinergic cell groups, notably the nucleus basalis of Meynert and the horizontal limb nucleus of the diagonal band.

The striatum, and particularly the nucleus accumbens, receives prominent projections from the amygdaloid complex. The basal and accessory basal nuclei are the most important contributors to this projection. The ventral striatum sends many fibres to the ventral pallidum, which in its turn projects to the mediodorsal nucleus of the thalamus. Thus, the ventral striatopallidal system provides a second route through which the amygdala can influence mediodorsal thalamic–prefrontal cortical processes.

The lateral, magnocellular accessory basal and parvicellular basal nuclei contribute the largest proportion of efferents to the hippocampal formation. The main projection is from the lateral nucleus to the rostral entorhinal cortex, but many fibres also terminate in the hippocampus proper and the subiculum. There appears to be marked polarity in amygdalohippocampal connections – the amygdala has a greater influence on hippocampal processes than vice versa.

The amygdaloid nuclear complex projects to widely dispersed neocortical fields. Amygdalocortical projections principally originate in the basal nucleus, and to a smaller extent in the lateral and cortical nuclei.

The amygdala projects to virtually all levels of the visual cortex in both temporal and occipital lobes. The largest component of these projections arises from the magnocellular basal nucleus. The amygdala also reciprocates projections to the auditory cortex in the rostral half of the superior temporal gyrus. Projections to the polymodal sensory areas of the temporal lobe generally reciprocate the amygdalopetal projections. Efferents from the lateral and accessory basal nuclei are directed to the temporal pole, particularly the medial perirhinal area.

The insular cortex is heavily innervated by the amygdaloid medial and anterior cortical nuclei. The orbital cortex and medial frontal cortical areas 24, 25 and 32, including parts of the anterior cingulate gyrus, also receive a heavy projection. Areas 8, 9, 45 and 46 of the dorsolateral prefrontal cortex, as well as the premotor cortex (area 6), receive a patchy innervation. The basal nucleus is an important source of these projections, which are augmented by contributions from the accessory basal (magnocellular and parvicellular divisions) and lateral nuclei.

Lesions of the amygdala

The amygdala is important in evaluating the significance of environmental events, most particularly the association between environmental stimuli and reinforcement. Such stimulus–reward associations are markedly impaired following lesions of the amygdala, e.g. the Klüver–Bucy syndrome.

WHITE MATTER OF CEREBRAL HEMISPHERE

The nerve fibres which make up the white matter of the cerebral hemispheres are categorized on the basis of their course and connections. They are either association fibres, which link different cortical areas in the same hemisphere; commissural fibres, which link corresponding cortical areas in the two hemispheres; or projection fibres, which connect the cerebral cortex with the corpus striatum, diencephalon, brain stem and the spinal cord.

ASSOCIATION FIBRES (Figs 22.31, 22.32)

Association fibres may be either short association (arcuate or 'U') fibres, which link adjacent gyri, or long association fibres, which connect more widely separated gyri.

Short association fibres may be entirely intracortical. Many pass subcortically between adjacent gyri, some merely pass from one wall of a sulcus to the other.

Long association fibres are grouped into bundles, e.g. uncinate fasciculus, cingulum, superior longitudinal fasciculus, inferior longitudinal fasciculus and fronto-occipital fasciculus.

The uncinate fasciculus connects the motor speech (Broca's) area and orbital gyri of the frontal lobe with the cortex in the temporal pole. The fibres follow a sharply curved course across the stem of the lateral sulcus, near the anteroinferior part of the insula. The cingulum is a long, curved fasciculus, which lies deep to the cingulate gyrus. It starts in the medial cortex below the rostrum of the corpus callosum, follows the curve of the cingulate gyrus, enters the parahippocampal gyrus and spreads into the adjoining temporal lobe. The superior longitudinal fasciculus is the largest of the long association fasciculi. It starts in the anterior frontal region and arches back, above the insular area, contributing fibres to the occipital cortex (areas 18 and 19). It curves down and forwards, behind the insular area, to spread out in the temporal lobe. The inferior longitudinal fasciculus starts near the occipital pole. Its fibres, probably derived mostly from areas 18 and 19, sweep forwards, separated from the posterior horn of the lateral ventricle by the optic radiation and tapetal commissural fibres, and are distributed throughout the temporal lobe. The fronto-occipital fasciculus starts at the frontal pole. It passes back deep to the superior longitudinal fasciculus, separated from it by the projection fibres in the corona radiata. It lies lateral to the caudate nucleus near the central part of the lateral ventricle. Posteriorly, it fans out into the occipital and temporal lobes, lateral to the posterior and inferior horns of the lateral ventricle.

COMMISSURAL FIBRES

Commissural fibres cross the midline, many linking corresponding areas in the two cerebral hemispheres. By far the largest commissure is the corpus callosum. Others include the anterior, posterior and habenular commisures, and the commissure of the fornix.

Corpus callosum (Figs 22.3, 22.4, 22.33, 22.34)

The corpus callosum is the largest fibre pathway of the brain. It links the cerebral cortex of the two cerebral hemispheres, and it roofs much of the lateral ventricles. It forms an arch c.10 cm in length, with an anterior

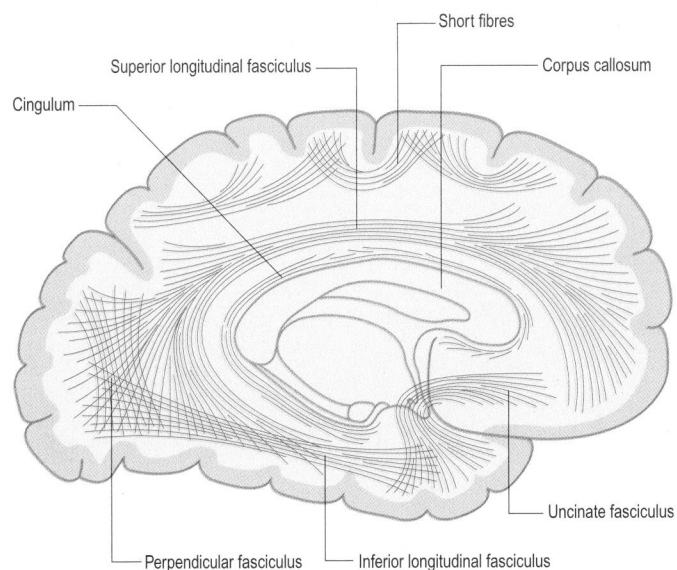

Fig. 22.31 The principal association fibres of the cerebral hemisphere.

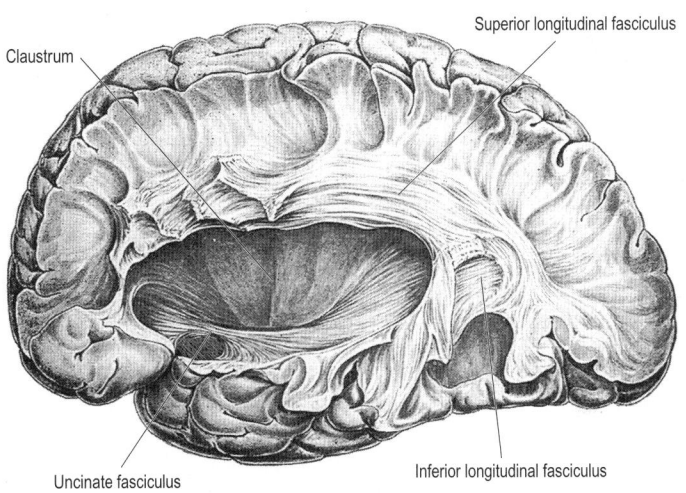

Fig. 22.32 Some of the long association fasciculi of the left cerebral hemisphere.

end c.4 cm from the frontal poles and a posterior end c.6 cm from the occipital poles. Its anterior portion is known as the genu. This recurves posteroinferiorly in front of the septum pellucidum, then diminishes rapidly in thickness and is prolonged to the upper end of the lamina terminalis as the rostrum. The trunk of the corpus callosum arches back and is convex above. It ends posteriorly in the expanded splenium, which is its thickest part.

The median region of the trunk of the corpus callosum forms the floor of the great longitudinal fissure. Here, it lies close to the anterior cerebral vessels and the lower border of the falx cerebri, which may contact it behind. On each side, the trunk is overlapped by the cingulate gyrus, separated from it by the callosal sulcus. The inferior surface of the corpus callosum is concave in its long axis. The septum pellucidum is attached to it anteriorly. Posteriorly, it is fused with the fornix and its commissure.

The superior surface of the callosal trunk (**Fig. 22.34**) is covered by a thin layer of grey matter, the indusium griseum. This extends anteriorly around the genu then, on the inferior aspect of the rostrum, continues into the paraterminal gyrus. It contains narrow longitudinal bundles of fibres on each side, the medial and lateral longitudinal striae. Posteriorly, the indusium griseum is continuous with the dentate gyrus and hippocampus through the gyrus fasciolaris (**Fig. 22.35**).

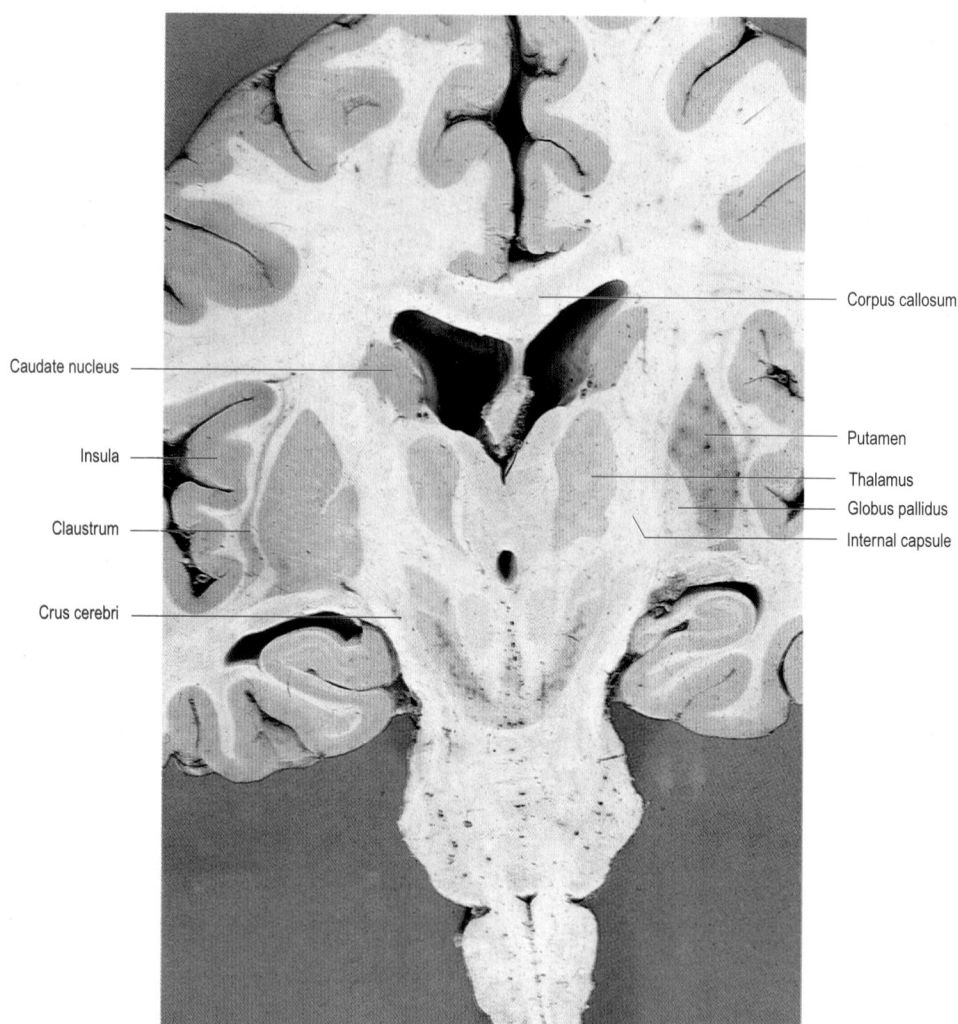

Corpus callosum

Caudate nucleus

Insula

Claustrum

Crus cerebri

Putamen

Thalamus

Globus pallidus

Internal capsule

Fig. 22.33 Oblique coronal section of the brain. (Dissection by EL Rees; photograph by Kevin Fitzpatrick on behalf of GKT School of Medicine, London.)

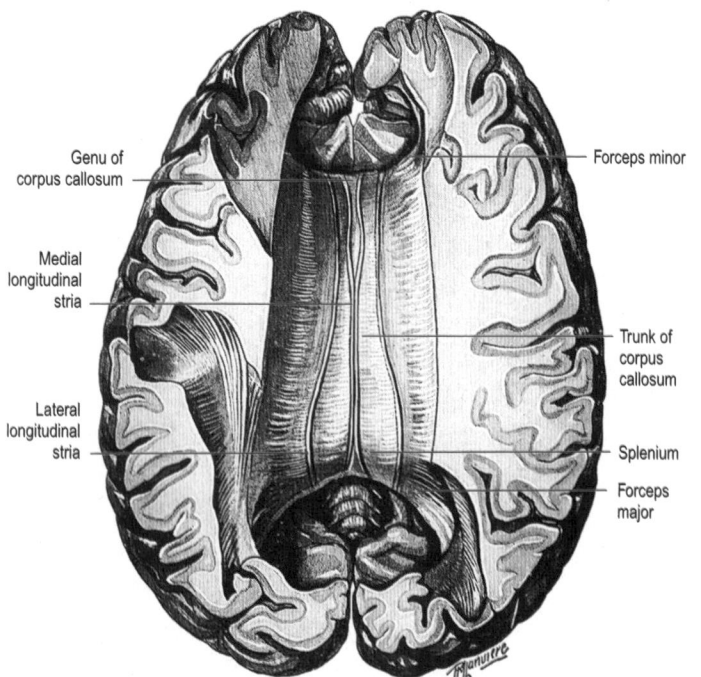

Genu of corpus callosum

Medial longitudinal stria

Lateral longitudinal stria

Forceps minor

Trunk of corpus callosum

Splenium

Forceps major

Fig. 22.34 The superior aspect of the corpus callosum revealed by partial removal of the cerebral hemispheres.

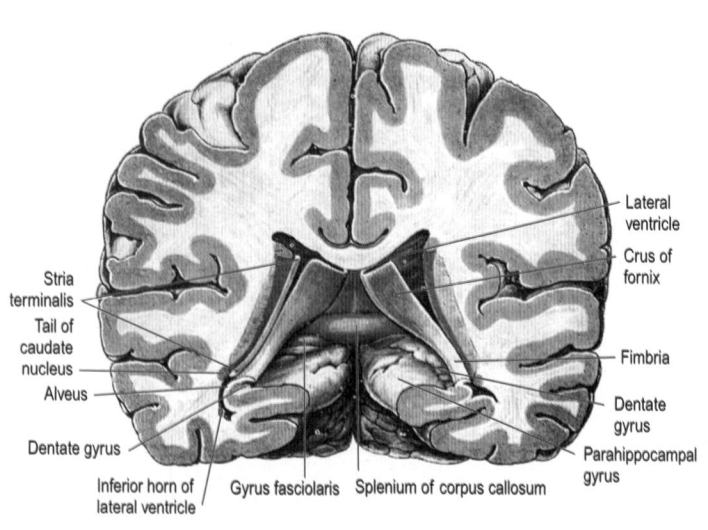

Stria terminalis

Tail of caudate nucleus

Alveus

Dentate gyrus

Inferior horn of lateral ventricle

Gyrus fasciolaris

Splenium of corpus callosum

Lateral ventricle

Crus of fornix

Fimbria

Dentate gyrus

Parahippocampal gyrus

Fig. 22.35 Anterior aspect of a coronal section of the cerebrum. The posterior parts of the thalami have been removed to reveal the splenium of the corpus callosum.

The splenium of the corpus callosum overhangs the posterior ends of the thalami, the pineal gland and tectum, but is separated from them by several structures. On each side the crus of the fornix and gyrus fasciolaris curve up to the splenium. The crus continues forwards on the inferior surface of the callosal trunk, but the gyrus fasciolaris skirts above the splenium, then rapidly diminishes into the indusium griseum. The tela choroidea of the third ventricle advances below the splenium through the transverse fissure, and the internal cerebral veins emerge between its two layers to form the great cerebral vein. Posteriorly the splenium is near the tentorium cerebelli, great cerebral vein and the start of the straight sinus.

Nerve fibres of the corpus callosum radiate into the white matter core of each hemisphere, thereafter dispersing to the cerebral cortex. Commissural fibres forming the rostrum extend laterally, below the anterior horn of the lateral ventricle, connecting the orbital surfaces of the frontal lobes. Fibres in the genu curve forwards, as the forceps minor, to connect the lateral and medial surfaces of the frontal lobes. Fibres of the trunk pass laterally, intersecting with the projection fibres of the corona radiata to connect wide neocortical areas of the hemispheres (**Figs 22.36, 22.37**). Fibres of the trunk and splenium, which form the roof and lateral wall of the posterior horn and the lateral wall of the inferior horn of the lateral ventricle, constitute the tapetum. The remaining fibres of the splenium curve back into the occipital lobes as the forceps major.

Interhemispheric connections through the corpus callosum do not all represent a simple linking of loci in one hemisphere with the same loci in the other. In areas containing a clear representation of a contralateral sensorium (e.g. body surface, visual field), only those areas that are functionally related to midline representation are linked to the contralateral hemisphere. This is most clearly seen for the visual areas, where the cortex containing the representation of each midline retinal zone is linked to its counterpart on the contralateral side. A similar arrangement is seen in somatic areas, where the trunk representation is callosally linked, but the peripheral limb areas (hand and foot) are not.

Connections that link the same, or similar, areas on each side are termed homotopic connections. The corpus callosum also interconnects heterogeneous cortical areas on the two sides (heterotopic connections). These may serve to connect functionally similar, but anatomically different, loci in the two hemispheres, and/or to connect functional areas

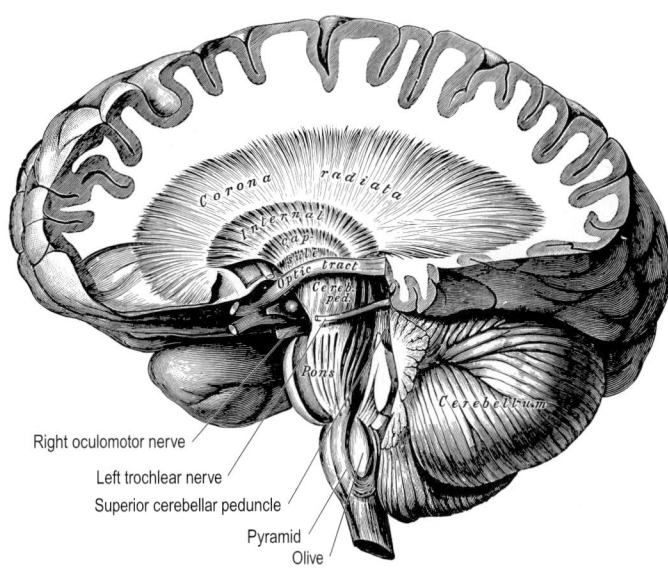

Right oculomotor nerve
Left trochlear nerve
Superior cerebellar peduncle
Pyramid
Olive

Fig. 22.37 Lateral aspect of the left side of the brain showing the convergence of cortical projection fibres through the corona radiata into the cerebral peduncles and pons.

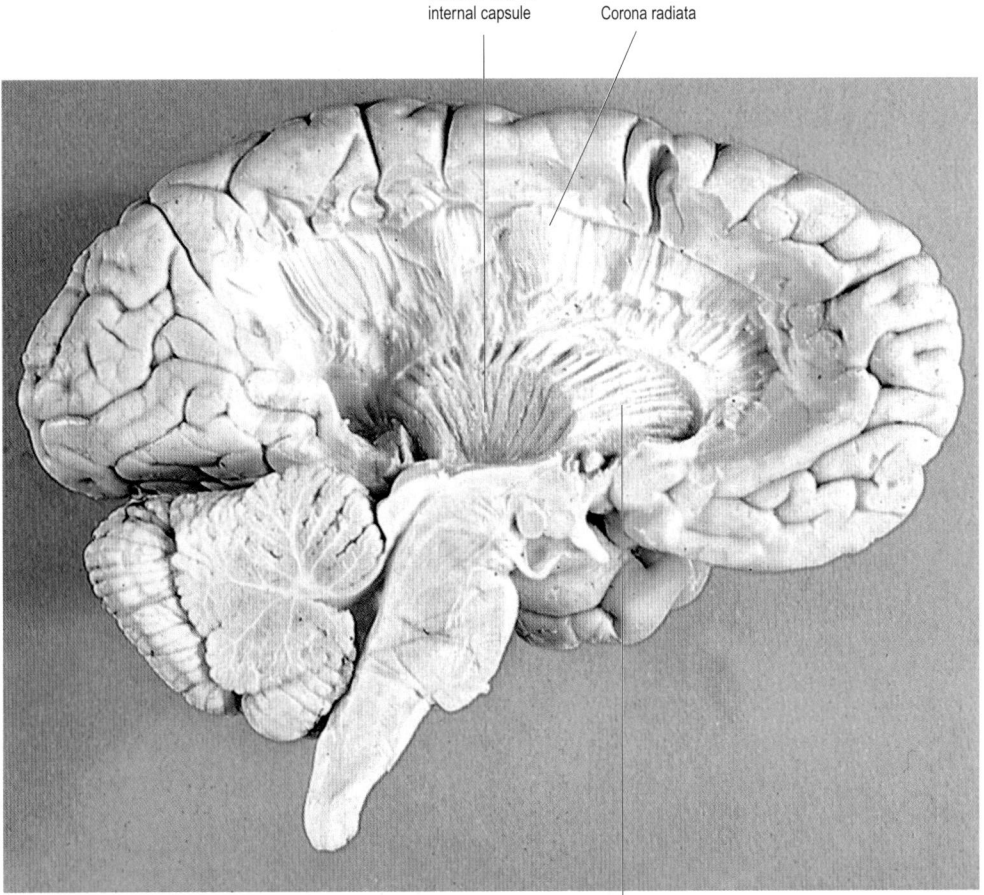

Posterior limb of internal capsule

Corona radiata

Anterior limb of internal capsule

Fig. 22.36 The left cerebral hemisphere dissected from its medial aspect to display the fibre bundles of the corona radiata and internal capsule. (Dissection by AM Seal; photograph by Kevin Fitzpatrick on behalf of GKT School of Medicine, London.)

in one hemisphere with regions that are specialized for a unilaterally confined function in the other.

Congenital absence of the corpus callosum is rare. When it occurs the clinical history usually lacks diagnostic features. This is perhaps not surprising since apparently little disturbance of function occurs when large parts, and in some cases all, of the corpus callosum have been surgically divided for the control of intractable epilepsy. The studies of Sperry (1974, 1984) on the effects of the division of the human corpus callosum revealed its function in the transfer of information (including memorized data) across the midline of the cerebrum and confirmed a long-suspected asymmetry of function, leading to a concept of 'dominance', usually by the left hemisphere (p. 414).

Anterior commissure

The anterior commissure is a compact bundle of myelinated nerve fibres, which crosses anterior to the columns of the fornix and is embedded in the lamina terminalis, where it is part of the anterior wall of the third ventricle (**Fig. 22.22**). In sagittal section it is oval, its long (vertical) diameter is c.1.5 mm. Laterally it splits into two bundles. The smaller anterior bundle curves forwards on each side to the anterior perforated substance and olfactory tract. The posterior bundle curves posterolaterally on each side in a deep groove on the anteroinferior aspect of the lentiform complex, and subsequently fans out into the anterior part of the temporal lobe, including the parahippocampal gyrus. Areas thought to be connected via commissural fibres include: the olfactory bulb and anterior olfactory nucleus; the anterior perforated substance, olfactory tubercle and diagonal band of Broca; the prepiriform cortex; the entorhinal area and adjacent parts of the parahippocampal gyrus; part of the amygdaloid complex (especially the nucleus of the lateral olfactory stria); the bed nucleus of the stria terminalis and the nucleus accumbens; the anterior regions of the middle and inferior temporal gyri.

PROJECTION FIBRES

Projection fibres connect the cerebral cortex with lower levels in the brain and spinal cord. They include large numbers of both corticofugal and corticopetal projections. Corticofugal projection fibres converge from all directions to form the dense subcortical white matter mass of the corona radiata. Large numbers of fibres pass to the corpus striatum and the thalamus, intersecting commissural fibres of the corpus callosum en route (**Fig. 22.37**). The corona radiata is continuous with the internal capsule, which contains the majority of the cortical projection fibres.

Internal capsule

In horizontal cerebral sections the internal capsule appears as a broad white band, with a lateral concavity, which accommodates the lentiform complex (**Figs 22.33, 22.36, 22.38, 22.39, 22.40**). It has an anterior limb, genu, posterior limb, and retrolenticular (retrolentiform) and sublenticular (sublentiform) parts. Both anterior and posterior limbs are medial to the lentiform complex. The head of the caudate nucleus is medial to the anterior limb, and the thalamus is medial to the posterior limb. Cortical efferent fibres of the internal capsule continue to converge as they descend. Fibres derived from the frontal lobe tend to pass posteromedially, while temporal and occipital fibres pass anterolaterally. Many, but not all, corticofugal fibres pass into the crus cerebri of the ventral midbrain. Here, corticospinal and corticobulbar fibres are located in the middle half of the crus. Frontopontine fibres are located medially, whereas corticopontine fibres from temporal, parietal and occipital cortices are found laterally.

The anterior limb of the internal capsule contains frontopontine fibres, which arise from the cortex in the frontal lobe. They synapse with cells in the pontine nuclei. Axons of these cells enter the opposite cerebellar hemisphere through the middle cerebellar peduncle. Anterior thalamic radiations interconnect the medial and anterior thalamic nuclei and various hypothalamic nuclei and limbic structures with the frontal cortex.

The genu of the internal capsule is usually regarded as containing corticonuclear (corticobulbar) fibres, which are mainly derived from area 4 and terminate mostly in the contralateral motor nuclei of cranial nerves. Anterior fibres of the superior thalamic radiation, between the thalamus and cortex, also extend into the genu.

The posterior limb of the internal capsule includes the corticospinal tract. The fibres concerned with the upper limb are anterior. More posterior regions contain fibres representing the trunk and lower limbs.

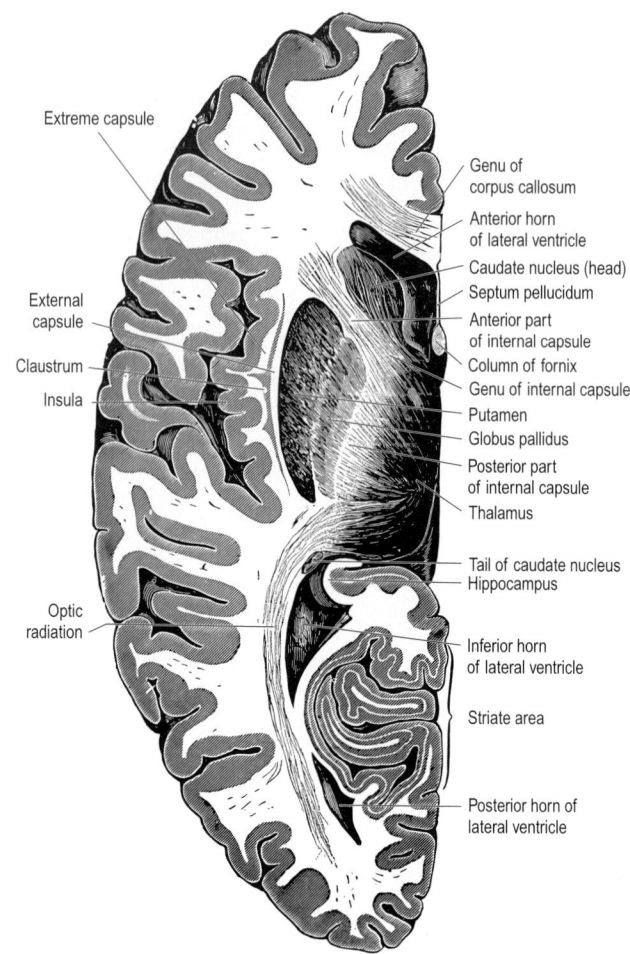

Fig. 22.38 Superior aspect of a horizontal section through the left cerebral hemisphere.

Labels on figure:
Extreme capsule
External capsule
Claustrum
Insula
Optic radiation
Genu of corpus callosum
Anterior horn of lateral ventricle
Caudate nucleus (head)
Septum pellucidum
Anterior part of internal capsule
Column of fornix
Genu of internal capsule
Putamen
Globus pallidus
Posterior part of internal capsule
Thalamus
Tail of caudate nucleus
Hippocampus
Inferior horn of lateral ventricle
Striate area
Posterior horn of lateral ventricle

Other descending axons include frontopontine fibres, particularly from areas 4 and 6, and corticorubral fibres, which connect the frontal lobe to the red nucleus. Most of the posterior limb also contains fibres of the superior thalamic radiation (the somaesthetic radiation) ascending to the postcentral gyrus.

The retrolenticular part of the internal capsule contains parietopontine, occipitopontine, and occipitotectal fibres. It also includes the posterior thalamic radiation and the optic radiation, and interconnections between the occipital and parietal lobes and caudal parts of the thalamus, especially the pulvinar.

The optic radiation arises in the lateral geniculate body. It sweeps backwards, intimately related to the superolateral aspect of the inferior horn and the lateral aspect of the posterior horn of the lateral ventricle, from which it is separated by the tapetum.

The sublenticular part of the internal capsule contains temporopontine and some parietopontine fibres, the acoustic (auditory) radiation from the medial geniculate body to the superior temporal and transverse temporal gyri (areas 41 and 42), and a few fibres that connect the thalamus with the temporal lobe and insula. Fibres of the acoustic radiation sweep anterolaterally below and behind the lentiform complex to reach the cortex.

CEREBRAL ASYMMETRY

The two human cerebral hemispheres are not simply mirror images of each other.

In 1861 Broca described a case of expressive aphasia resulting from an infarct in the left posterior inferior frontal lobe, which became known as Broca's area. The later discovery of Wernicke's area in the left posterior temporal and inferior parietal lobe provided unequivocal evidence of another lateralized function, and demonstrated an asymmetry for language comprehension as well as for speech production. The

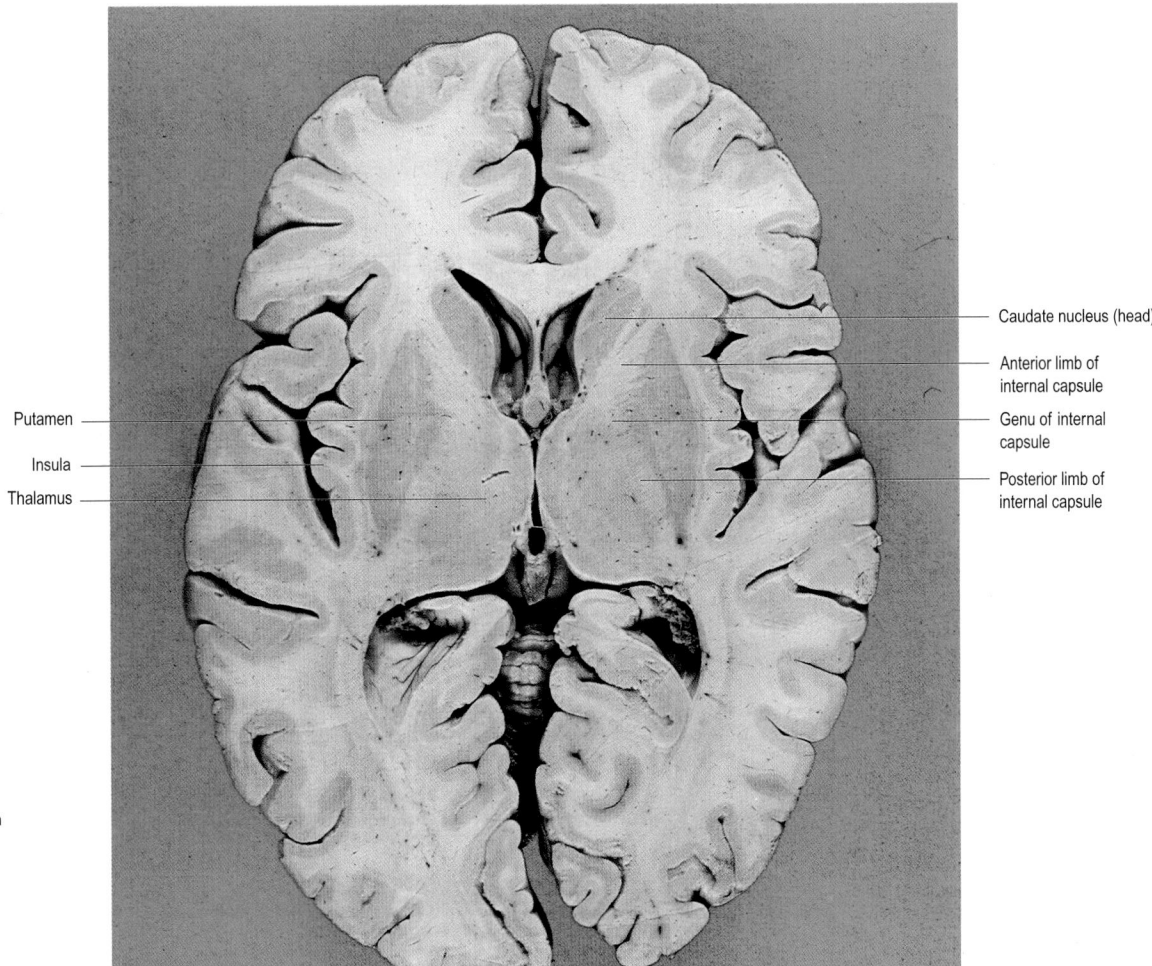

Caudate nucleus (head)

Anterior limb of
internal capsule

Genu of internal
capsule

Posterior limb of
internal capsule

Putamen

Insula

Thalamus

Fig. 22.39 Horizontal section of the brain through the frontal and occipital poles of the cerebral hemispheres. (Dissection by EL Rees; photograph by Kevin Fitzpatrick on behalf of GKT School of Medicine, London.)

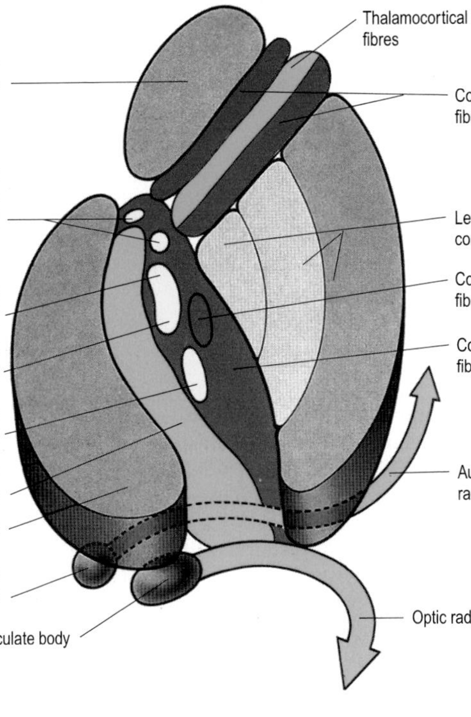

Thalamocortical
fibres

Head of caudate
nucleus

Corticofugal
fibres

Corticonuclear and
corticospinal fibres
(Head and neck)

Lentiform
complex

Corticospinal fibres
(Upper limb)

Corticorubral
fibres

Corticospinal fibres
(Trunk)

Corticofugal
fibres

Corticospinal fibres
(Lower limb)

Thalamocortical
fibres

Auditory
radiation

Thalamus

Medial geniculate
body

Lateral geniculate body

Optic radiation

Fig. 22.40 Horizontal section through the internal capsule illustrating its main fibre components. Descending motor fibres: yellow; corticofugal fibres to the thalamus and pons: red; ascending fibres: blue. (From Truex RC (ed) Strong and Elwyn's Human Neuroanatomy, 4th edn. London: Baillière Tindall and Cox, and from Kretschmann H-J 1998 Localization of the corticospinal fibres in the internal capsule in man. J Anat (Lond) 160: 219–225.)

association of language impairment with left hemisphere lesions leads to the more general concept of a dominant left and a minor right hemisphere.

Much information on the lateralization of cerebral function has come from studying patients in whom the corpus callosum had been divided (commissurotomy) as a treatment for intractable epilepsy, and rare subjects who lack part, or all, of their corpus callosum. Commissurotomy produces the 'split-brain' syndrome (**Fig. 22.41**), which has provided evidence supporting the notion that abilities or functions are predominantly associated with one or other hemisphere. Knowledge of such lateralization of function has been advanced more recently by functional brain imaging techniques such as positron emission tomography (PET).

The left hemisphere usually prevails for verbal and linguistic functions, for mathematical skills and for analytical thinking. The right hemisphere is mostly non-verbal. It is more involved in spatial and holistic or 'Gestalt' thinking, in many aspects of musical appreciation, and in some emotions. Memory also shows lateralization. Thus, verbal memory is primarily a left hemisphere function, whilst non-verbal memory is represented in the right hemisphere. These asymmetries are relative, not absolute, and vary in degree according to the function and individual concerned. Moreover, they apply primarily to right-handed men. Those men with left-hand preference, or mixed handedness, make up a heterogeneous group, which (as an approximation) shows reduced or anomalous lateralization, rather than a simple reversal of the situation in right handers. For example, speech representation can occur in either or both hemispheres. Women show less functional asymmetry, on average, than men.

Certain cerebral anatomical asymmetries are apparent at both the macroscopic and histological levels. One of the most notable is in the

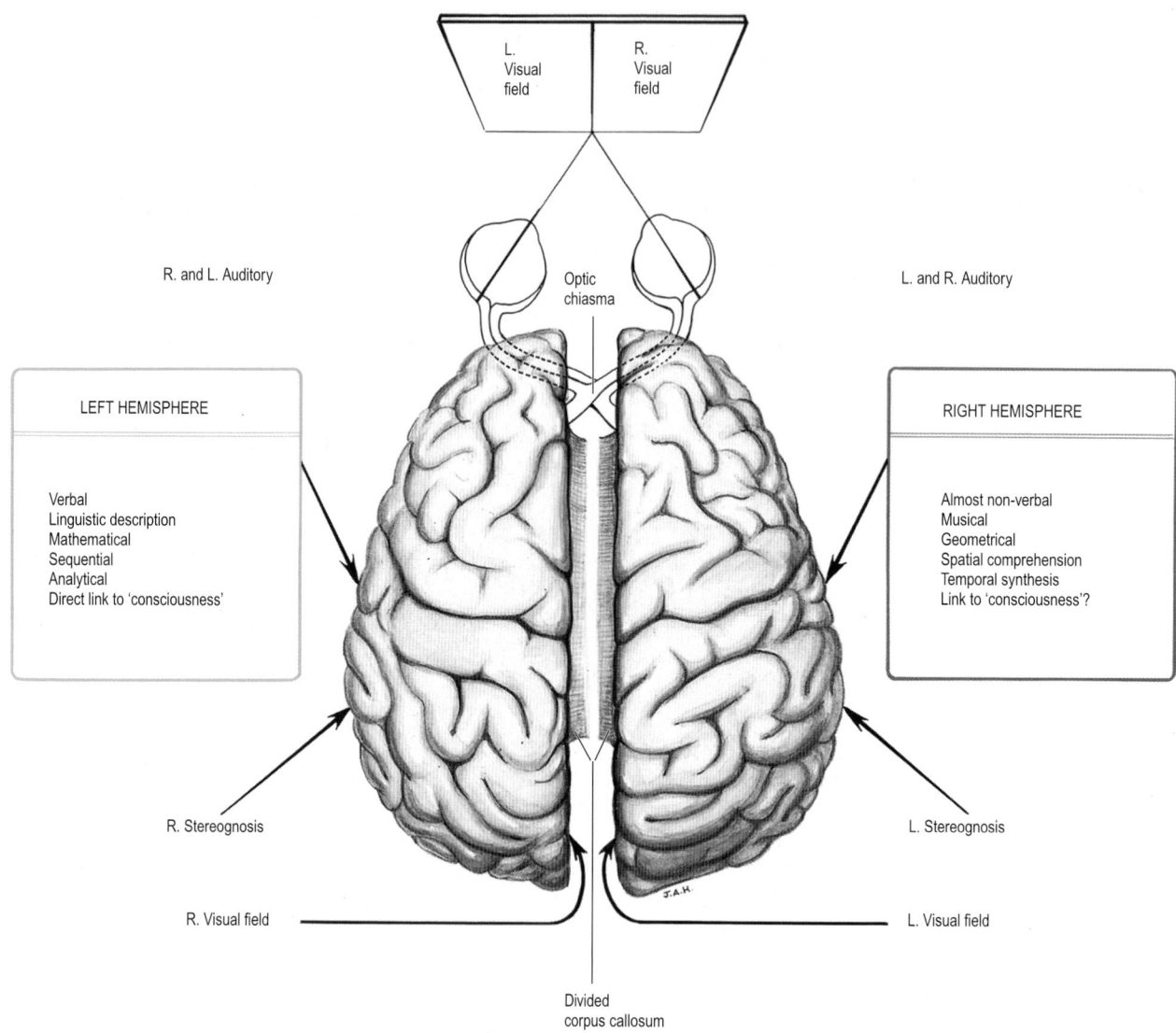

Fig. 22.41 A summary of Sperry's split-brain schema, showing the functions that are lateralized to one or other hemisphere. Split-brain patients have been studied by presenting stimuli selectively to one or other hemisphere and comparing the subject's responses to them. For instance, a stimulus presented briefly to one visual field, or placed in one hand, is only accessible to the opposite hemisphere (since the projections are contralateral and all commissural connections have been severed). Objects in the right visual field or right hand are recognized and named easily by the 'verbal' left hemisphere. In contrast, patients cannot name, and appear to lack knowledge of, objects placed in the left visual field or left hand, as these are available only to the 'non-verbal' right hemisphere. However, the object has undoubtedly been identified correctly since the person can later point to it from a selection of objects. These functional specializations are relative and apply to people with left hemisphere language representation. Subsequent studies since this original formulation have added more detail and complexity. Overall, split-brain work has been central in establishing the extent and nature of functional asymmetries. Its importance was highlighted by the award of a Nobel prize to Sperry in 1981. For more extensive discussion see Sperry (1974, 1984). (From Neuropsychologia, vol 17, Sperry RW, Consciousness, personal identity and the divided brain, pp 153–166, 1984, modified with permission from Elsevier, and from Sperry RW, The Neurosciences, Lateral specialisation in the surgically separated hemispheres, pp5-19, 1974, MIT Press.)

planum temporale, which is usually larger on the left than the right side (**Fig. 22.42**). Probably as a result of this, the lateral fissure is longer and more horizontal in the left hemisphere, an observation which, together with the orientation of the overlying vasculature, provides a surface marker of temporal lobe asymmetry. The limits of asymmetry in the superior temporal lobe remain uncertain, but appear to include Heschl's gyrus and some other structures adjacent to (and sometimes considered to be an extension of) the planum temporale.

There is evidence that planum temporale asymmetry originates almost entirely from right–left differences in the size of a cyto-architectonic subfield called Tpt (**Fig. 22.42**). Subtle asymmetries in the superior temporal lobe have been demonstrated in terms of overall size and shape, sulcal pattern, cytoarchitecture and at the neuronal level. It seems reasonable to assume that these differences underlie some of the functional asymmetry for language representation.

Asymmetries in areal size, cytoarchitecture or neurocytology occur elsewhere in the cerebral cortex as well as subcortically. A few recent examples will be given here. Many brains have a wider right frontal pole and a wider left occipital pole. Brodmann's area 45 in the inferior frontal

lobe, corresponding to Broca's area, contains a population of large pyramidal neurones that are found only on the left side. The cortical surface surrounding the central sulcus is larger in the left hemisphere, especially in the areas containing the primary somatosensory and motor maps of the arm, suggesting that one cerebral manifestation of hand preference is a larger amount of neural circuitry in the relevant parts of the cortex. Histological asymmetries are also found in areas that are not usually considered to be closely related either to language or handedness. The left entorhinal cortex has significantly more neurones than the right.

The most interesting clinical implications of cerebral asymmetry occur where disturbed lateralization appears to be inherent in the nature and even aetiology of a disorder. This relationship is most striking in schizophrenia. A number of studies suggest that the disease is associated with a failure to develop normal structural and functional cerebral asymmetry, and that its pathology is characterized by a greater affliction of the left than the right hemisphere. Other putative neurodevelopmental disorders, including dyslexia and autism, may also be associated with asymmetrical cerebral abnormalities.

A

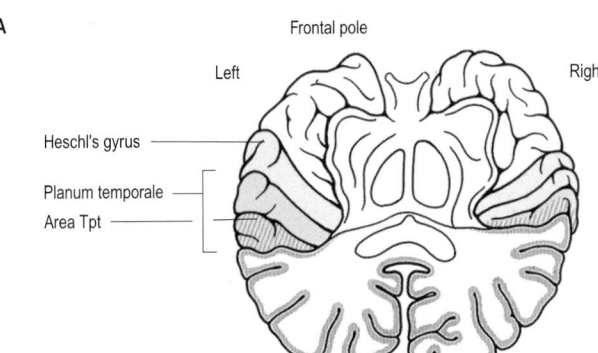

B

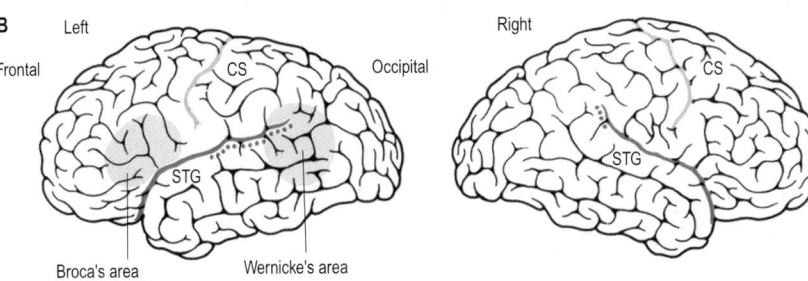

Fig. 22.42 Examples of anatomical asymmetries in the cerebral cortex. **A**, Horizontal section showing the exposed upper surface of the temporal lobes. The planum temporale (shown stippled in red) forms the upper posterior part of the temporal lobe, bordered anteriorly by Heschl's gyrus (stippled in blue), laterally by the Sylvian fissure, and posteriorly by the end of the Sylvian fissure. The brain shown here demonstrates a marked asymmetry in size of the planum temporale, which is larger on the left in a majority of brains. This brain also shows asymmetry of Heschl's gyrus. The asymmetrical length of the lateral border of the planum temporale underlies the asymmetries in the Sylvian fissure itself (see also **B**). Asymmetry of the planum temporale arises mostly from differences in the size of the cytoarchitectonic field Tpt (shown shaded in green). Tpt forms much of the posterior part of the planum temporale, though it also extends on to the lateral surface of the posterior superior temporal gyrus. **B**, Lateral views of the left and right hemispheres emphasizing differences between the two Sylvian fissures, in red. Compared to the left hemisphere, the right Sylvian fissure is shorter and turns upwards. This reflects planum temporale asymmetries (represented by the adjacent red stippling). CS, central sulcus; STG, superior temporal gyrus. The approximate locations of Broca's and Wernicke's areas in the left hemisphere are indicated. However, much of Wernicke's area is buried within the sulcal folds and is not visible on a lateral view. (Adapted from Geschwind N, Levitsky W 1968 Human brain. Science 161: 186–187, by permission from AAAS.)

REFERENCES

Alheid GF, Heimer L 1988 New perspectives in basal forebrain organization of special relevance for neuropsychiatric disorders: the striatopallidal, amygdaloid and corticopetal components of the substantia innominata. Neuroscience 27: 1–39.
Provides evidence that the region of the 'substantia innominata' in the basal forebrain is composed of parts of three forebrain structures: the ventral striatopallidal system; the extended amygdala; and the magnocellular corticopetal system.

Derbyshire SW, Jones AK, Gyulai F, Clark S, Townsend D, Firestone LL (1997) Pain processing during three levels of noxious stimulation produces differential patterns of central activity. Pain. 73: 431–45.

Papez JW 1937 A proposed mechanism of emotion. Arch Neurol Psychiat 38: 725–43.
The now classic description of the mechanism of emotion in man.

Passingham RE 1993 The Frontal Lobes and Voluntary Action. Oxford: Oxford University Press.

Penfield W, Rasmussen T 1950. The Cerebral Cortex of Man. New York: Macmillan.
The now classic description of the organization of sensory and motor homunculi in the human cerebral cortex.

Peyron R, Laurent B, Garcia-Larrea L (2000) Functional imaging of brain responses to pain. A review and meta-analysis. Neurophysiologie Clinique. 30: 263–88.

Sperry RW 1974 Lateral specialization in the surgically separated hemisphere. In: Schmidt FO, Worden FG (eds) The Neurosciences. Third study program. Cambridge, MASS,: MIT Press: 5–19.

Sperry RW 1984 Consciousness, personal identity and the divided brain. Neuropsychologia 17: 153–66.

Basal ganglia

The term basal ganglia is used to denote a number of subcortical nuclear masses that lie in the inferior part of the cerebral hemisphere, lateral to the thalamus (**Figs 23.1, 23.2**). They have traditionally been regarded as including the corpus striatum, the claustrum, and the amygdaloid complex. More recently, however, the working definition has been narrowed to signify the corpus striatum and its associated structures in the diencephalon and midbrain. This is because they form a functional complex that is involved in the control of movement and motivational aspects of behaviour. The claustrum is of unknown function (p. 403). The amygdala is more closely related to the limbic system and is described elsewhere (p. 409).

The corpus striatum consists of the caudate nucleus, putamen and globus pallidus (**Fig. 23.3**). Because of their close proximity, the putamen and globus pallidus have historically been considered as an entity, termed the lentiform complex or nucleus. With increasing knowledge of their structure and function, however, it has become clear that the putamen is more correctly considered to be in unity with the caudate nucleus, with which it shares common chemocytoarchitecture and connections. The putamen and caudate nucleus are together referred to as the neostriatum or simply the striatum.

The striatum is considered as the principal 'input' structure of the basal ganglia since it receives the majority of afferents from other parts of the neuraxis. Its principal efferent connections are to the globus pallidus and pars reticulata of the substantia nigra. The globus pallidus and, more particularly, its medial segment, together with the pars reticulata of the substantia nigra (p. 344) is regarded as the main

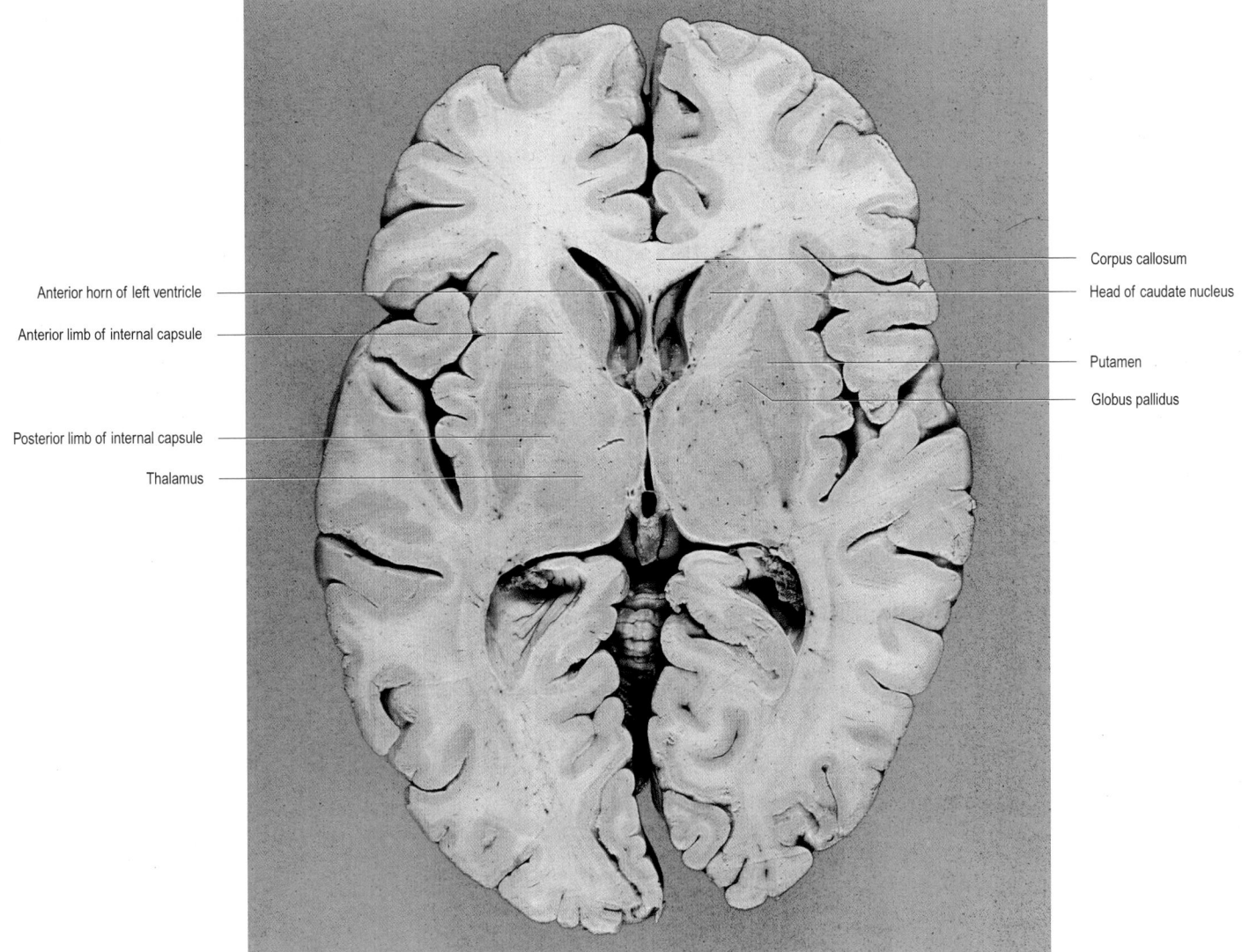

Anterior horn of left ventricle

Anterior limb of internal capsule

Posterior limb of internal capsule

Thalamus

Corpus callosum

Head of caudate nucleus

Putamen

Globus pallidus

Fig. 23.1 Horizontal section of the brain. (Dissection by EL Rees; photograph by Kevin Fitzpatrick on behalf of GKT School of Medicine, London.)

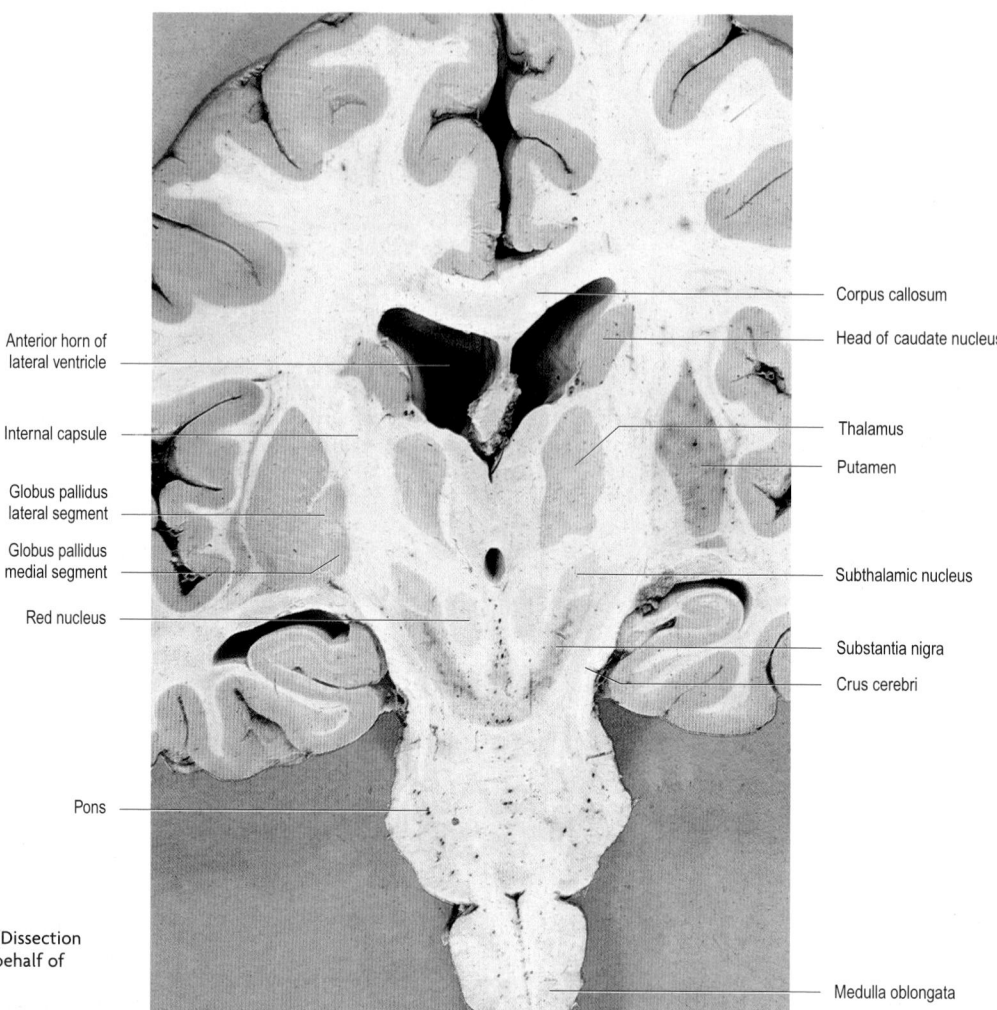

Corpus callosum

Head of caudate nucleus

Anterior horn of
lateral ventricle

Thalamus

Internal capsule

Putamen

Globus pallidus
lateral segment

Globus pallidus
medial segment

Subthalamic nucleus

Red nucleus

Substantia nigra

Crus cerebri

Pons

Medulla oblongata

Fig. 23.2 Oblique coronal section of the brain. (Dissection by EL Rees; photograph by Kevin Fitzpatrick on behalf of GKT School of Medicine, London.)

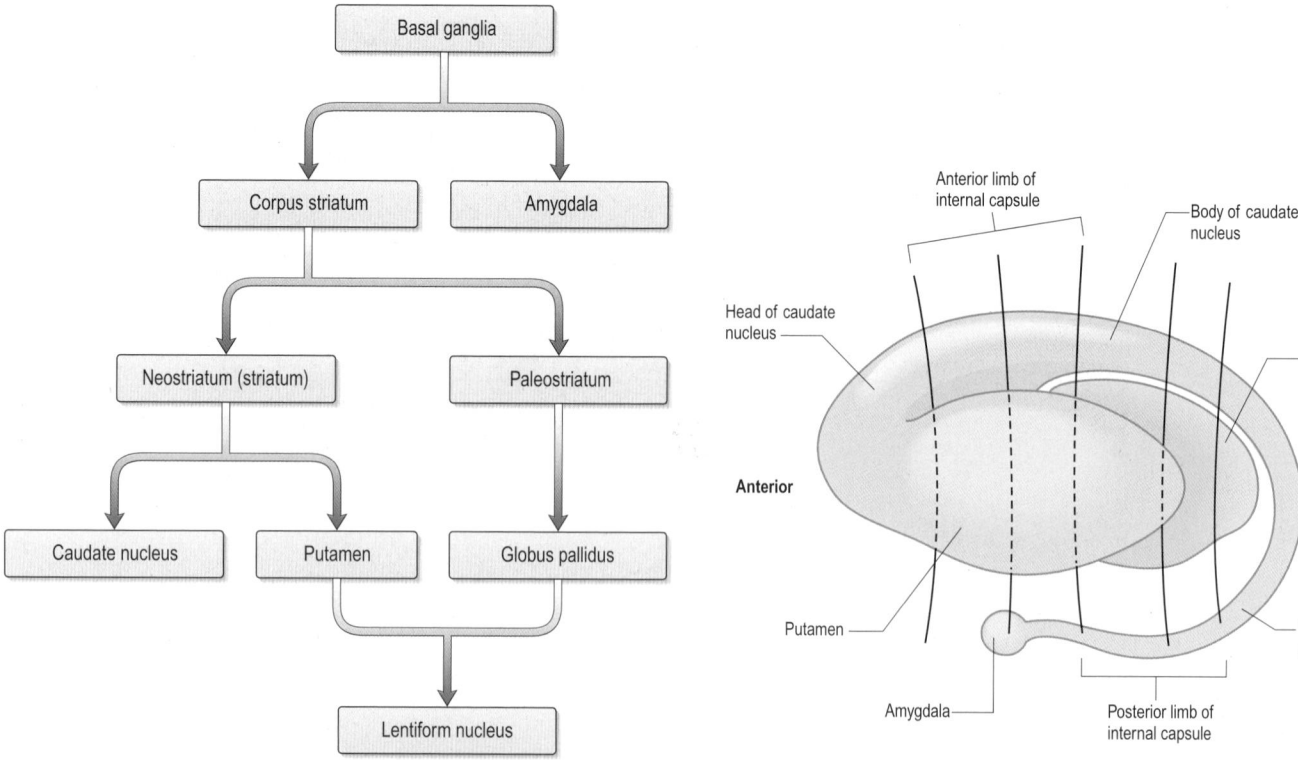

Fig. 23.3 Relationships of structures forming the basal ganglia.

Fig. 23.4 The striatum within the left cerebral hemisphere. (By permission from Crossman AR, Neary D 2000 Neuroanatomy, 2nd edn. Edinburgh: Churchill Livingstone.)

'output' structure because it is the source of massive efferent fibre projections, mostly directed to the thalamus.

Disorders of the basal ganglia are principally characterized by abnormalities of movement, muscle tone and posture. There is a wide spectrum of clinical presentations ranging from poverty of movement and hypertonia at one extreme (typified by Parkinson's disease) to abnormal involuntary movements (dyskinesias) at the other. The underlying pathophysiological mechanism that mediates these disorders has been much studied in recent years and is better understood than that for any other type of complex neurological dysfunction. This has led to the introduction of new rational therapeutic strategies for both medical and neurosurgical treatment of movement disorders.

The caudate nucleus is a curved, tadpole-shaped mass. It has a large anterior head, which tapers to a body, and a down-curving tail (**Fig. 23.4**). The head is covered with ependyma and lies in the floor and lateral wall of the anterior horn of the lateral ventricle, in front of the interventricular foramen. The tapering body is in the floor of the body of the ventricle, and the narrow tail follows the curve of the inferior horn, and so lies in the ventricular roof, in the temporal lobe. Medially, the greater part of the caudate nucleus abuts the thalamus, along a junction that is marked by a groove, the sulcus terminalis. The sulcus contains the stria terminalis, lying deep to the ependyma (**Figs 16.3, 23.5**). The stria terminalis forms one margin of the choroid fissure of the lateral ventricle, the hippocampal fimbria and fornix form the other margin. The sulcus terminalis is especially prominent anterosuperiorly (because of the large size of the head and body of the caudate nucleus relative to the tail), and here the stria terminalis is accompanied by the thalamostriate vein.

The corpus callosum lies above the head and body of the caudate nucleus. The two are separated laterally by the fronto-occipital bundle, and medially by the subcallosal fasciculus, a bundle of axons that caps the nucleus (**Figs 23.5, 23.6**). The caudate nucleus is largely separated from the lentiform complex by the anterior limb of the internal capsule (**Figs 23.1, 23.6, 23.7**). However, the inferior part of the head of the caudate becomes continuous with the most inferior part of the putamen immediately above the anterior perforated substance. This junctional region is sometimes known as the fundus striati (**Fig. 23.6**). Variable bridges of cells connect the putamen to the caudate nucleus for most of its length. They are most prominent anteriorly, in the region of the fundus striati and the head and body of the caudate nucleus, where they break up the anterior limb of the internal capsule (**Figs 23.6, 23.7**). In the temporal lobe, the anterior part of the tail of the caudate nucleus becomes continuous with the posteroinferior part of the putamen. The vast bulk of the caudate nucleus and putamen are often referred to as the dorsal striatum. A smaller inferomedial part of the rostral striatum is referred to as the ventral striatum, and includes the nucleus accumbens.

The lentiform complex lies deep to the insular cortex, with which it is roughly coextensive, although the two are separated by a thin layer of white matter and the claustrum (**Figs 23.2, 23.8**). The claustrum splits

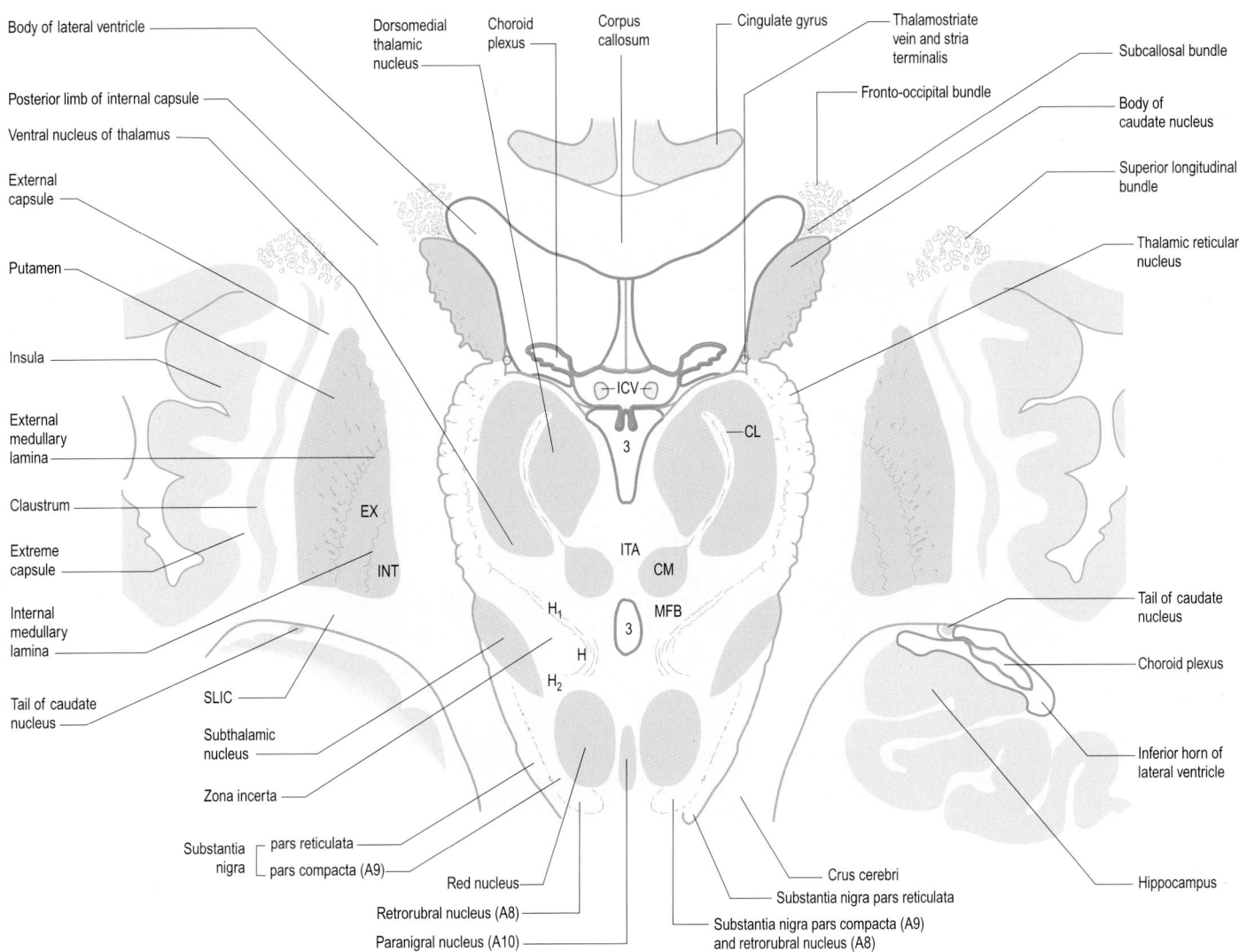

Fig. 23.5 An oblique section through the diencephalon and basal ganglia. Abbreviations: A8, 9, 10, dopaminergic cell groups; AL, ansa lenticularis; CL, centrolateral nucleus of thalamus; CM, centromedian nucleus of thalamus; EX, external pallidal segment; FS, fasciculus subthalamicus; H, H₁, H₂, subthalamic fields of Forel; ICV, internal cerebral veins in the transverse fissure; INT, internal pallidal segment; ITA, interthalamic adhesion; MFB, median forebrain bundle; SLIC, sublentiform internal capsule; 3, 3rd ventricle.

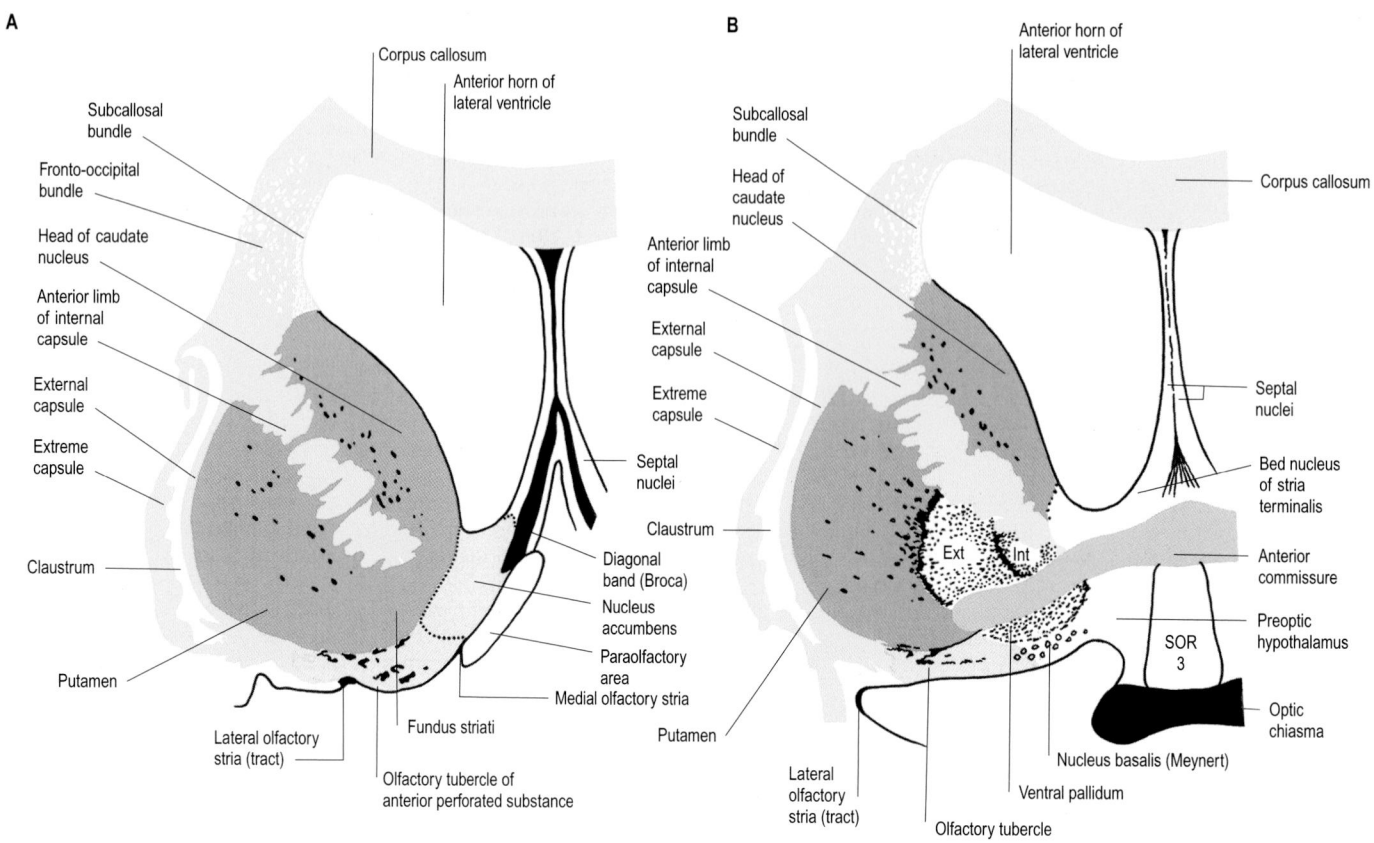

A

Subcallosal bundle

Fronto-occipital bundle

Head of caudate nucleus

Anterior limb of internal capsule

External capsule

Extreme capsule

Claustrum

Putamen

Corpus callosum

Anterior horn of lateral ventricle

Septal nuclei

Diagonal band (Broca)

Nucleus accumbens

Paraolfactory area

Medial olfactory stria

Lateral olfactory stria (tract)

Fundus striati

Olfactory tubercle of anterior perforated substance

B

Subcallosal bundle

Head of caudate nucleus

Anterior limb of internal capsule

External capsule

Extreme capsule

Claustrum

Putamen

Lateral olfactory stria (tract)

Anterior horn of lateral ventricle

Corpus callosum

Septal nuclei

Bed nucleus of stria terminalis

Anterior commissure

Preoptic hypothalamus

Optic chiasma

Ext   Int

SOR 3

Nucleus basalis (Meynert)

Ventral pallidum

Olfactory tubercle

Fig. 23.6 Coronal sections through the corpus striatum and anterior perforated substance. **A** is anterior to **B**. The pallidum is shown in **B**. EX, external segment; INT, internal segment; SOR3, supraoptic recess of the third ventricle.

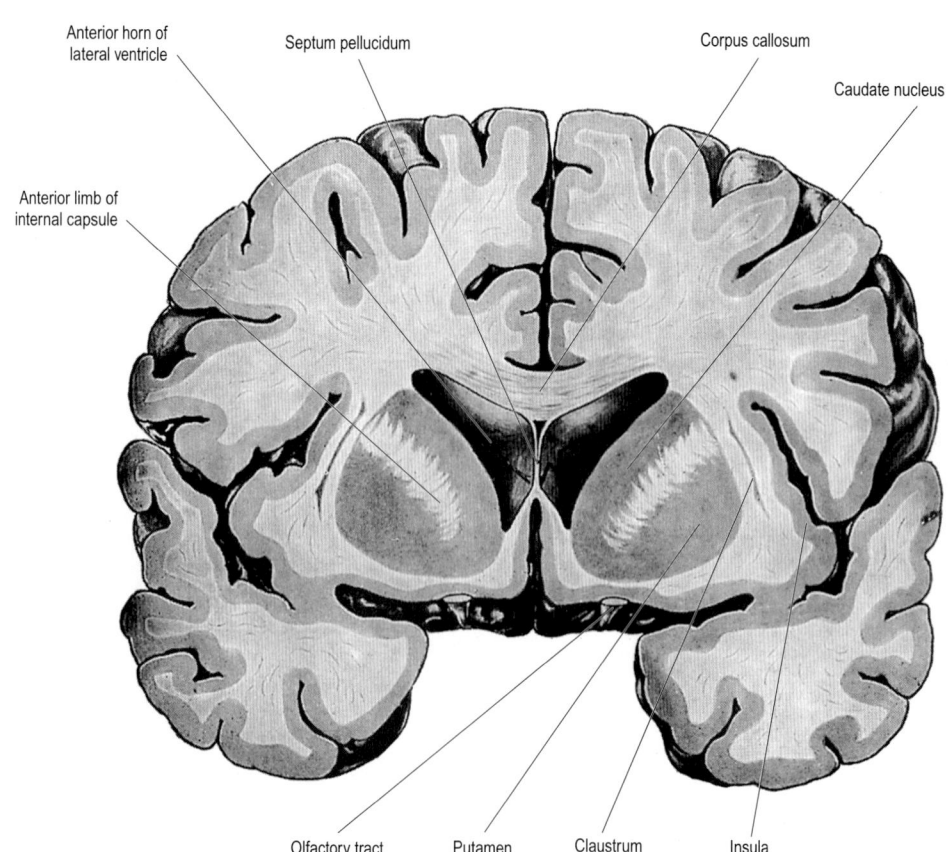

Anterior horn of lateral ventricle

Septum pellucidum

Corpus callosum

Caudate nucleus

Anterior limb of internal capsule

Olfactory tract

Putamen

Claustrum

Insula

Fig. 23.7 Posterior aspect of a coronal section through the anterior horn of the lateral ventricles.

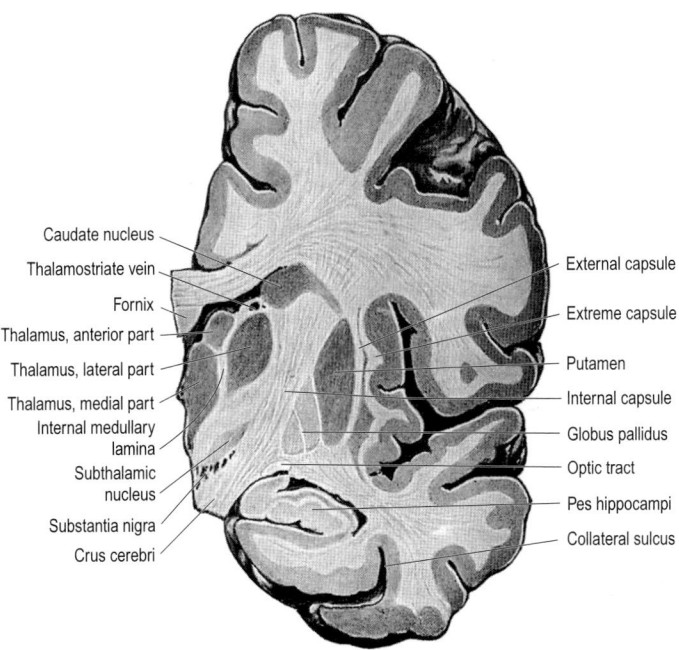

Caudate nucleus
Thalamostriate vein
Fornix
Thalamus, anterior part
Thalamus, lateral part
Thalamus, medial part
Internal medullary lamina
Subthalamic nucleus
Substantia nigra
Crus cerebri

External capsule
Extreme capsule
Putamen
Internal capsule
Globus pallidus
Optic tract
Pes hippocampi
Collateral sulcus

Fig. 23.8 Anterior aspect of a coronal section through the left cerebral hemisphere.

the insular subcortical white matter to create the extreme and external capsules. The latter separates the claustrum from the putamen (**Figs 22.39, 23.1, 23.2, 23.8**). The lentiform complex is separated from the caudate nucleus by the internal capsule.

The lentiform complex consists of the laterally placed putamen and the more medial globus pallidus (pallidum), which are separated by a thin layer of fibres, the lateral or external medullary lamina. The globus pallidus is itself divided into two segments, a lateral (or external) segment and a medial (or internal) segment, separated by an internal (or medial) medullary lamina. The two segments have distinct afferent and efferent connections.

Inferiorly, a little behind the fundus striati, the lentiform complex is grooved by the anterior commissure, which connects inferior parts of the temporal lobes and the anterior olfactory cortex of the two sides (**Fig. 23.6**). The area above the commissure is referred to as the dorsal pallidum, and that below it as the ventral pallidum.

STRIATUM

The striatum consists of the caudate nucleus, putamen and ventral striatum, which are all highly cellular and well vascularized. The caudate and putamen are traversed by numerous small bundles of thinly myelinated, or non-myelinated, small-diameter axons, which are mostly striatal afferents and efferents. They radiate through the striatal tissue as though converging on, or radiating from, the globus pallidus. The bundles are occasionally referred to by the archaic term 'Wilson's pencils' and they account for the striated appearance of the corpus striatum.

Neurones of both dorsal and ventral striatum are mainly medium-sized multipolar cells. They have round, triangular or fusiform somata, mixed with a smaller number of large multipolar cells. The ratio of medium to large cells is at least 20:1. The large neurones have extensive spherical or ovoid dendritic trees up to 600 µm across. The medium-sized neurones also have spherical dendritic trees, c.200 µm across, which receive the synaptic terminals of many striatal afferents. The dendrites of both medium and large striatal cells may be either spiny or non-spiny. The most common neurone (usually 75% of the total) is a medium-sized cell with spiny dendrites. These cells utilize γ-aminobutyric acid (GABA) as their transmitter and also express the genes coding for either enkephalin or substance P/dynorphin. Enkephalinergic neurones appear to express D2 dopamine receptors. Substance P/dynorphin neurones have D1 receptors. These neurones are the major, and perhaps exclusive, source of striatal efferents to the pallidum and substantia nigra pars

reticulata. The remaining medium-sized striatal neurones are aspiny, and are intrinsic cells that contain acetylcholinesterase (AChE), choline acetyltransferase (CAT) and somatostatin. Large neurones with spiny dendrites contain AChE and CAT. Most, perhaps all, are intrinsic neurones, as are aspiny large neurones.

Intrinsic synapses are probably largely asymmetric (Type II), while those derived from external sources are symmetric (Type I). The aminergic afferents from the substantia nigra, raphe and locus coeruleus all end as profusely branching axons with varicosities, which contain dense-core vesicles (the presumed store of amine transmitters). Many of these varicosities have no conventional synaptic membrane specializations, and may release transmitter in a way analogous to that found in peripheral postsynaptic sympathetic axons.

Neuroactive chemicals, whether intrinsic or derived from afferents, are not distributed uniformly in the striatum. For example, serotonin and glutamic acid decarboxylase (GAD) concentrations are highest caudally, while substance P, acetylcholine (ACh) and dopamine are highest rostrally. However, there is a finer grain neurochemical organization that informs the view of the striatum as a mosaic of islands or striosomes (sometimes referred to as patches), each 0.5–1.5 mm across, packed into a background matrix. Striosomes contain substance P and enkephalin. During development, the first dopamine terminals from the substantia nigra are found in striosomes. Although this exclusivity does not persist after birth, striosomes in the caudate nucleus still contain a higher concentration of dopamine than the matrix. The latter contains ACh and somatostatin and is the target of thalamostriate axons. Receptors for at least some neurotransmitters are also differentially distributed. For example, opiate receptors are found almost exclusively within striosomes, and muscarinic receptors predominantly so. Moreover, the distribution of neuroactive substances within the striosomes is not uniform. In humans, the striosome/matrix patchwork is less evident in the putamen, where it appears to consist predominantly of matrix, than it is in the caudate nucleus.

All afferents to the striatum terminate in a mosaic manner. The size of a cluster of terminals is usually 100–200 µm across. Some afferent terminal clusters are not arranged in register with the clear striosome/matrix distributions seen in nigrostriatal and thalamostriatal axons. In general, afferents from neocortex end in striatal matrix and those from allocortex end in striosomes. However, the distinction is not absolute. Thus although afferents from the neocortex arise in layers V and VI, those from the superficial part of layer V end predominantly in striatal matrix, whereas those from deeper neocortex project to striosomes. Striatal cell bodies, which are the sources of efferents, also form clusters, but again are not uniformly related to striosomes. For example, the cell bodies of some striatopallidal and striatonigral axons lie clustered within striosomes, and others lie outside them, but still in clusters. The neurones and neuropil of the ventral striatum are essentially similar to those of the dorsal striatum, but the striosomal/matrix organization is less well-defined, and seems to consist predominantly of striosomes.

The major connections of the striatum are summarized in **Fig. 23.9**. Although the connections of the dorsal and ventral divisions overlap, the generalization can be made that the dorsal striatum is predominantly connected with motor and associative areas of the cerebral cortex, whilst the ventral striatum is connected with the limbic system and orbitofrontal and temporal cortices. For both dorsal and ventral striatum, the pallidum and substantia nigra pars reticulata are key efferent structures. The fundamental arrangement is the same for both divisions. The cerebral cortex projects to the striatum, which in turn projects to the pallidum and substantia nigra pars reticulata. From these, efferents leave to influence the cerebral cortex (either the supplementary motor area or prefrontal and cingulate cortices via the thalamus) and the superior colliculus.

The entire neocortex sends glutamatergic axons to the ipsilateral striatum. For a long time, these axons were thought to be collaterals of other cortical efferents, but it is now known that they arise exclusively from small pyramidal cells in layers V and VI. It has also been suggested that some of the cells of origin lie in the supragranular 'cortical association' layers II and III. The projection is organized topographically. The greater part of the input from the cerebral cortex to the dorsal striatum is derived from the frontal and parietal lobes, and that from the occipitotemporal cortex is relatively small. Thus, the orbitofrontal association cortex projects to the inferior part of the head of the caudate nucleus, which lies next to the ventral striatum. The dorsolateral frontal association cortex and frontal eye fields project to the rest of the head

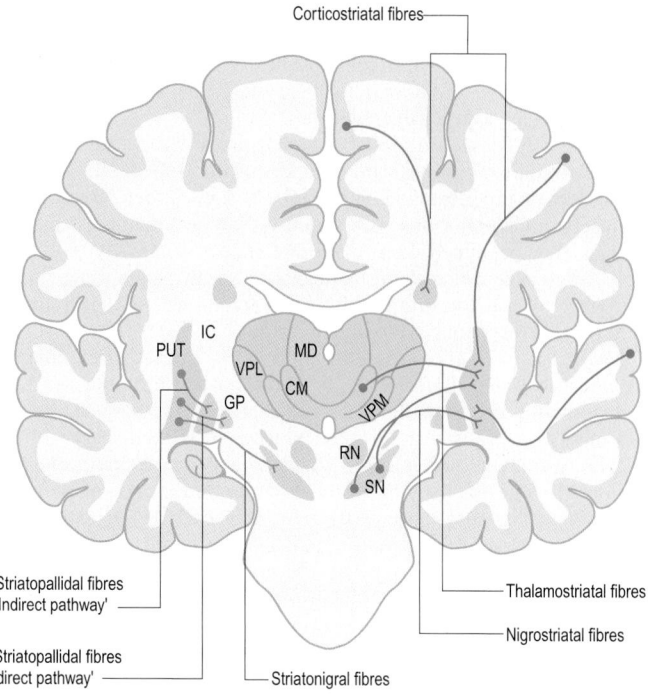

Fig. 23.9 Connections of the striatum. The major afferent projections to the striatum are shown on the left and major efferent projections from the striatum on the right.

of the caudate nucleus, and much of the parietal lobe projects to the body of the nucleus. The somatosensory and motor cortices project predominantly to the putamen. Their afferents establish a somatotopic pattern, in which the lower body is represented laterally and the upper body is represented medially. The motor cortex is unique in sending axons through the corpus callosum to the opposite putamen, where they end with the same spatial ordering. The occipital and temporal cortices project to the tail of the caudate nucleus and to the inferior putamen.

The striatum also receives afferents, which are more crudely spatially organized, from the polysensory intralaminar thalamus. The cerebello-receptive nucleus centralis lateralis projects to the anterior striatum (especially the caudate nucleus), and the cerebello- and pallido-receptive centromedian nucleus projects to the putamen.

The aminergic inputs to the caudate and putamen are derived from the substantia nigra pars compacta (dopaminergic group A9; **Figs 23.10, 23.11**); the retrorubral nucleus (dopaminergic group A8; **Fig. 23.5**); the dorsal raphe nucleus (serotoninergic group B7; **Fig. 23.10**); and the locus coeruleus (noradrenergic group A6). The nigrostriatal input is sometimes referred to as the 'mesostriatal' dopamine pathway. It reaches the striatum by traversing the H fields of the subthalamus. These aminergic inputs appear to modulate the responses of the striatum to cortical and thalamic afferent influences.

Efferents from the striatum pass to both segments of the globus pallidus and to the substantia nigra pars reticulata, where they end in a topically ordered fashion. Fibres ending in either the lateral or medial pallidal segment originate from different striatal cells (**Figs 23.9, 23.12**). Those to the lateral pallidum come from neurones which co-localize GABA and enkephalin and give rise to the so-called 'indirect pathway'. This name refers to the fact that these striatal neurones influence the activity of basal ganglia output neurones in the medial pallidum via the intermediary of the subthalamic nucleus. Other striatal neurones, which co-localize GABA and substance P/dynorphin, project directly to the medial pallidum and are, therefore, described as the 'direct pathway'.

A second outflow is established from the striatum to the pars reticulata of the substantia nigra. This also has both direct and indirect components, via the lateral pallidum and subthalamic nucleus (**Fig. 23.13**). The axons of the direct striatonigral projection constitute the laterally placed 'comb' system, which is spatially quite distinct from the ascending dopaminergic nigrostriatal pathway. Striatonigral fibres end in a spatially ordered way in the pars reticulata.

The ventral striatum is the primary target of cortical afferents from limbic cortices, including allocortex, and from limbic associated regions (**Fig. 23.13**). Thus, the hippocampus (through the fornix) and orbito-frontal cortex (through the internal capsule) project to the nucleus accumbens, and the olfactory, entorhinal, anterior cingulate and temporal visual cortices project to both the nucleus accumbens and olfactory tubercle in varying degrees. The tubercle also receives afferents from the amygdala. The contiguities of the cortical areas, which project to the ventral striatum and neighbouring dorsal striatum, emphasize the imprecise nature of the boundaries between the two divisions. All the cortical regions overlap and abut one another, and they project to neighbouring parts of the dorsal striatum as well as to the ventral striatum. The fundus striati and ventromedial caudate nucleus abut the olfactory tubercle and nucleus accumbens (**Fig. 23.6**), and receive connections from the orbitofrontal cortex and, to a lesser extent, from

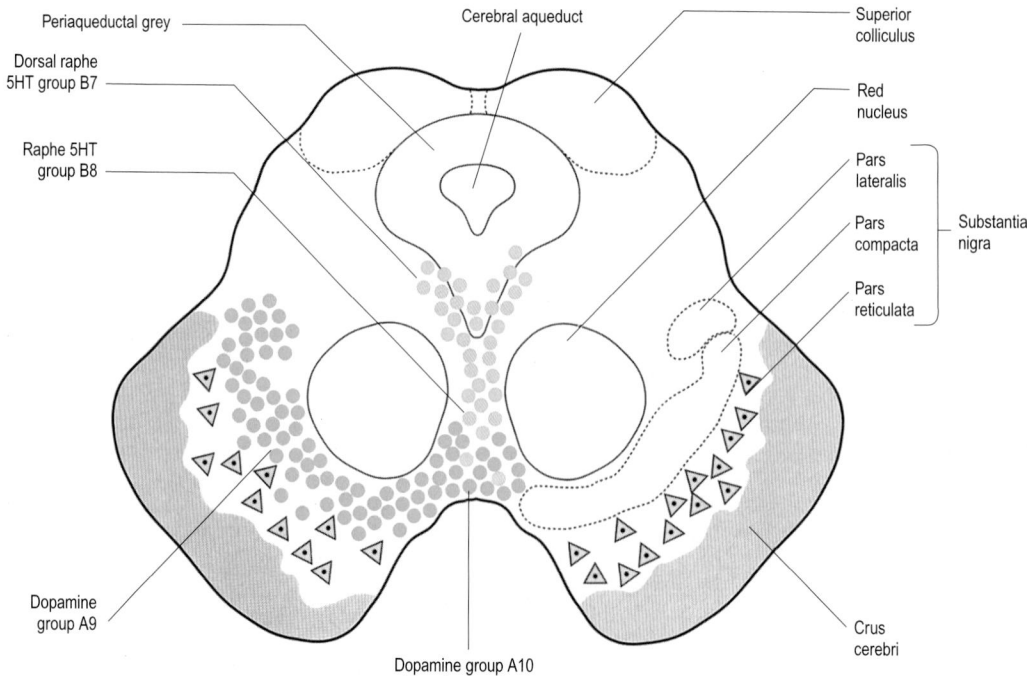

Fig. 23.10 Transverse section through the midbrain to show the arrangement of dopaminergic cell groups A9 and A10 in the substantia nigra (left) and serotoninergic cell groups B7 and B8 in the raphe.

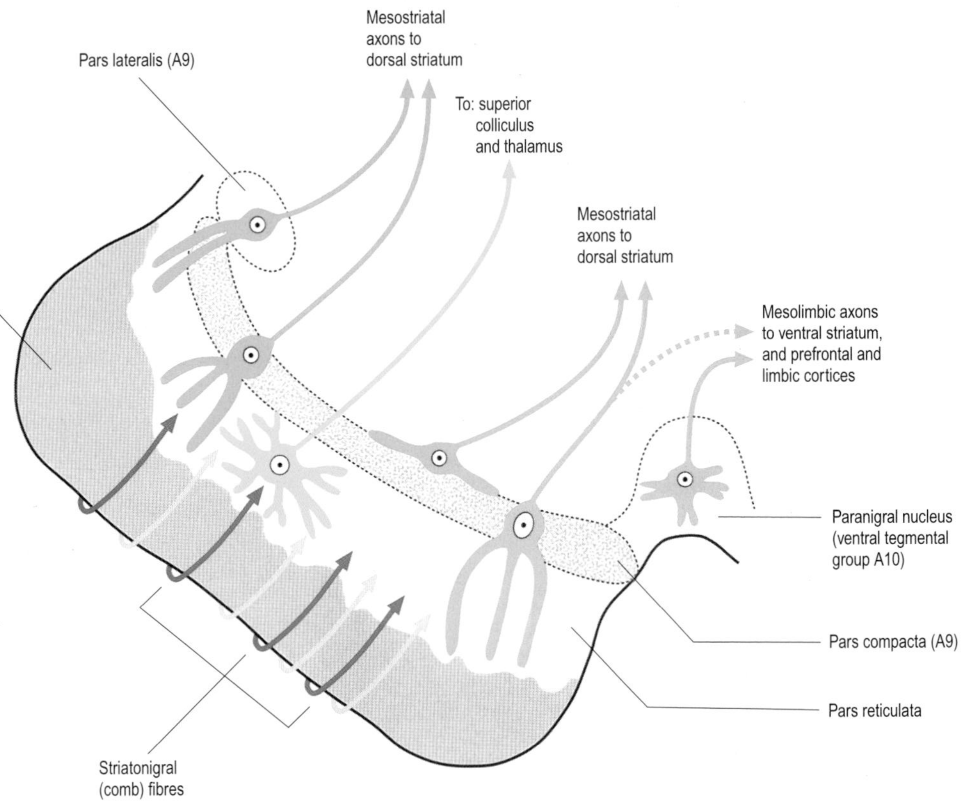

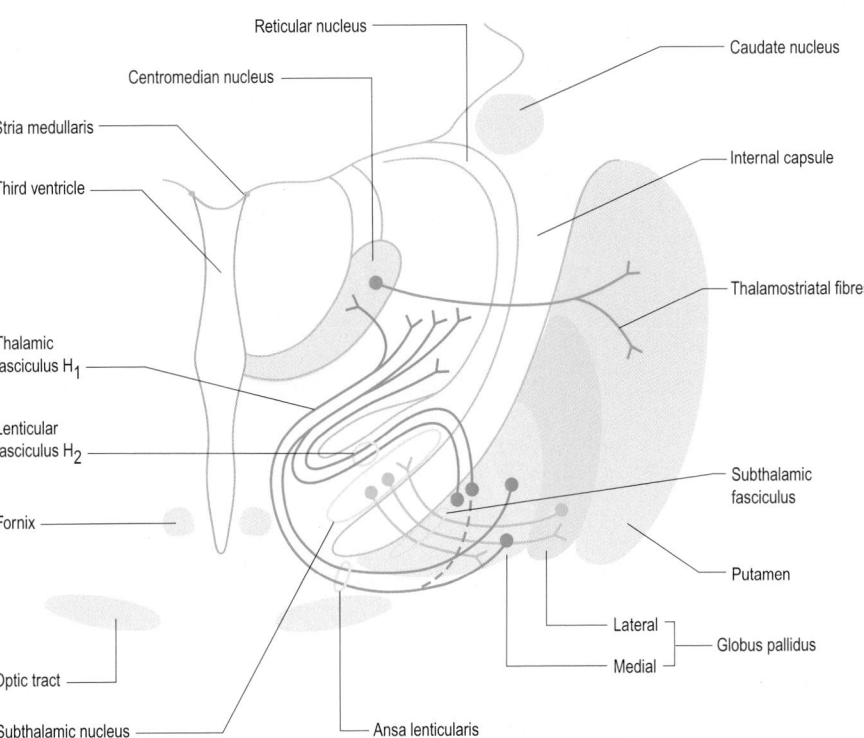

Pars lateralis (A9)

Mesostriatal
axons to
dorsal striatum

To: superior
colliculus
and thalamus

Crus cerebri

Mesostriatal
axons to
dorsal striatum

Mesolimbic axons
to ventral striatum,
and prefrontal and
limbic cortices

Fig. 23.11 A scheme of the organization of
the substantia nigra in transverse section.
Compare with **Fig. 23.10**. Medially, there is no
sharp distinction between dopaminergic cells
projecting to the dorsal striatum (pars
compacta, A9) and those projecting to the
ventral striatum and limbic system (paranigral
nucleus, A10). Dendrites of dopaminergic
neurones intrude into the pars reticulata. Note
the distinctive projection systems from the
pars reticulata. (From The Human Nervous
System, Vol 1, Webster (Paxinos ed), 889–944,
1990. Modified with permission from Elsevier.)

Paranigral nucleus
(ventral tegmental
group A10)

Pars compacta (A9)

Pars reticulata

Striatonigral
(comb) fibres

Reticular nucleus

Caudate nucleus

Centromedian nucleus

Internal capsule

Stria medullaris

Third ventricle

Thalamostriatal fibres

Thalamic
fasciculus H$_1$

Lenticular
fasciculus H$_2$

Subthalamic
fasciculus

Fornix

Putamen

Lateral

Globus pallidus

Medial

Optic tract

Subthalamic nucleus

Ansa lenticularis

Fig. 23.12 Major interconnections of the basal ganglia.

the lateral prefrontal and anterior cingulate cortices (which also project
to the contiguous head of the caudate nucleus).

This continuity of the ventral and dorsal striata, as revealed by the
arrangements of corticostriate projections, is reinforced by consideration
of the aminergic inputs to the ventral striatum. They are derived from
the dorsal raphe (serotoninergic group B7); the locus coeruleus (noradrenergic group A6); and from the paranigral nucleus (dopamine
group A10), as well as the most medial part of the substantia nigra pars
compacta (A9) (**Figs 23.10, 23.11**). The dopamine projections constitute

the so-called mesolimbic dopamine pathway, which also projects to the
septal nuclei, hippocampus and amygdala and prefrontal and cingulate
cortices through the medial forebrain bundle. The lateromedial
continuity of cell groups A9 and 10 (**Fig. 23.10**) is thus reflected in the
relative positions of their ascending fibres in the subthalamus and
hypothalamus (the H fields and median forebrain bundle, respectively),
as well as in the lateromedial topography of the dorsal and ventral striata
(**Fig. 23.6**), which in turn have contiguous and overlapping sources of
cortical afferents.

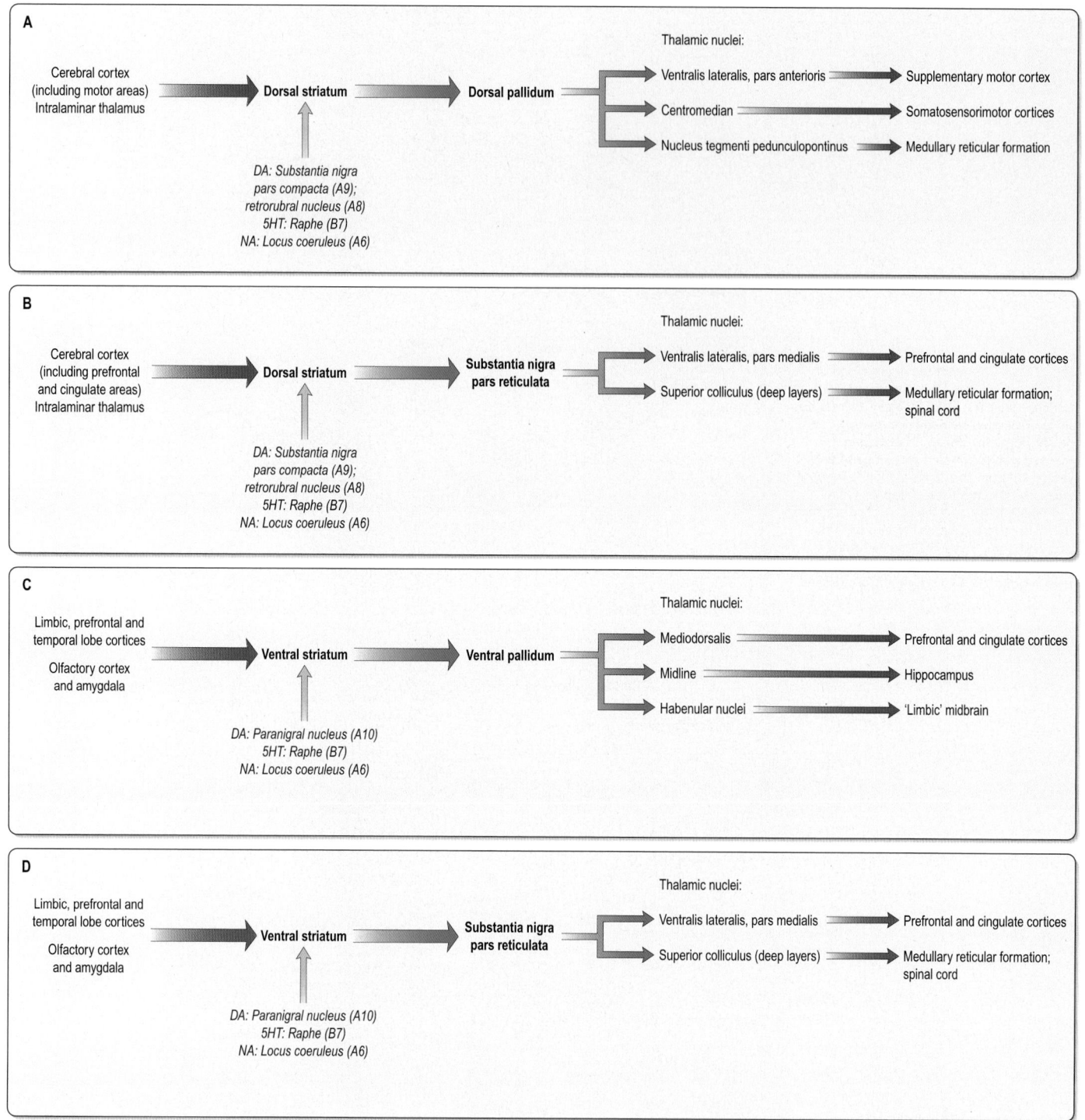

Fig. 23.13 Schemes of the principal output connections of the basal ganglia derived from dorsal (**A**, **B**) and ventral (**C**, **D**) divisions of the striatum. In each case pathways established through the pallidum are distinguished from those passing through the substantia nigra pars reticulata. Abbreviations: DA, dopamine; NA, noradrenaline (norepinephrine); 5HT, 5-hydroxytryptamine.

As for the dorsal striatum, efferents from the ventral striatum project to the pallidum (in this case the ventral pallidum) and the substantia nigra pars reticulata (**Figs 23.13, 23.14**). In the latter case, the connection is both direct and indirect via the subthalamic nucleus. The projections from the pars reticulata are as described for the dorsal system, but axons from the ventral pallidum reach the thalamic mediodorsal nucleus (which projects to cingulate and prefrontal association cortex) and midline nuclei (which project to the hippocampus). Ventral pallidal axons also reach the habenular complex of the limbic system.

The brain areas beyond the basal nuclei, substantia nigra and subthalamic nucleus, to which both ventral and dorsal systems appear to project, are, therefore, the prefrontal association and cingulate cortices and the deep superior colliculus.

NUCLEUS ACCUMBENS

The ventral striatum consists of the nucleus accumbens and the olfactory tubercle. In front of the anterior commissure, much of the grey matter of the anterior perforated substance, and especially the olfactory tubercle, is indistinguishable from, and continuous with, the fundus striati, in terms of cellular composition, histochemistry and interconnections. The caudate nucleus is continuous medially with the nucleus accumbens (**Fig. 23.6**), which abuts the nuclei of the septum, close by the paraolfactory area, diagonal band of Broca and the fornix.

The nucleus accumbens receives a dopaminergic innervation from the midbrain ventral tegmental area (cell group A10). It is believed to represent the neural substrate for the rewarding effects of several classes of drugs of abuse and is, therefore, a major determinant of their addic-

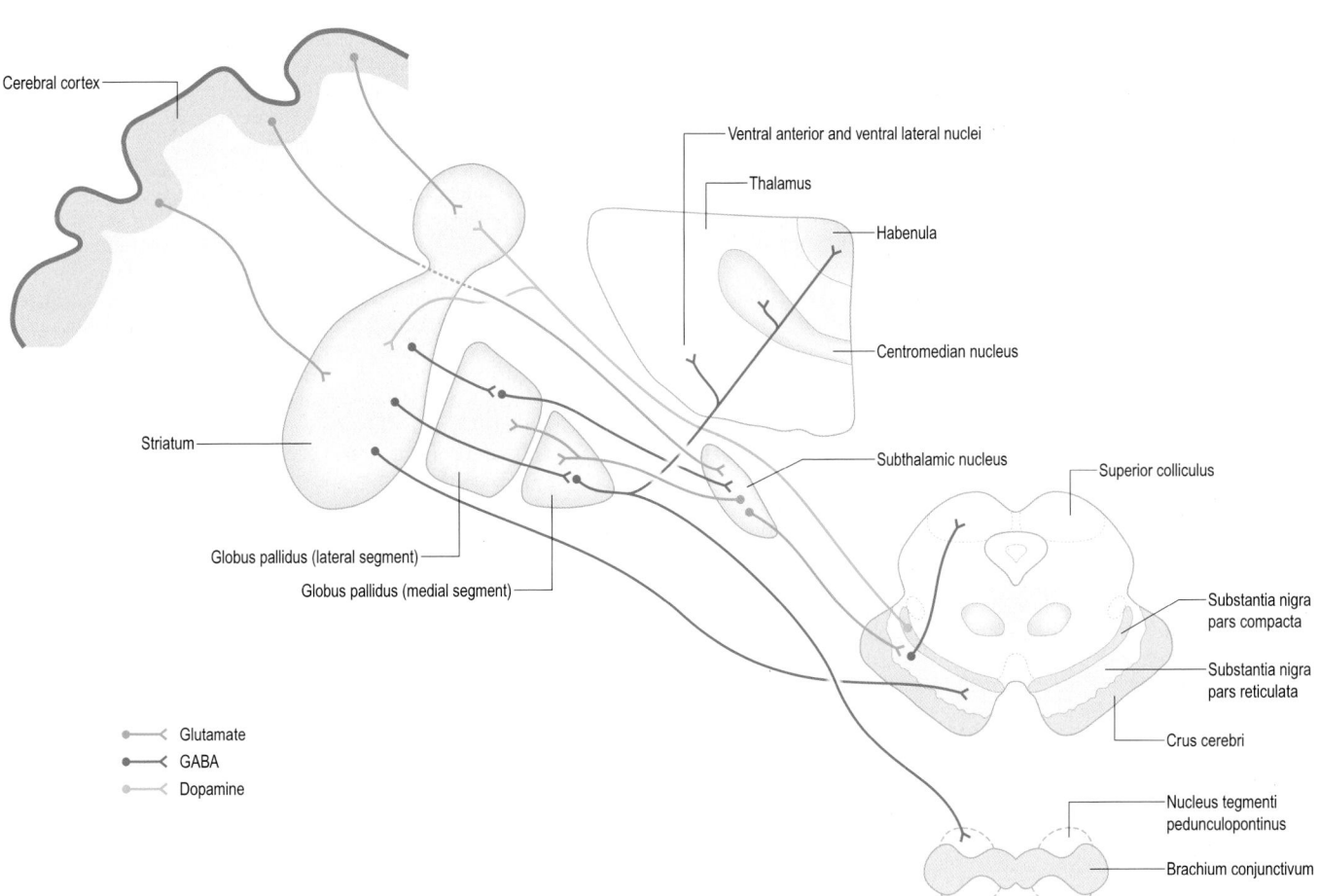

Fig. 23.14 Transverse section through the basal ganglia showing the principal connections of the globus pallidus with the thalamus and subthalamic nucleus.

tive potential. The experimental observation that the locomotor activating effects of psychomotor stimulant drugs such as amphetamine and cocaine (which act presynaptically on dopaminergic neurones to enhance dopamine release or block its reuptake, respectively) are dependent on dopamine transmission in the nucleus accumbens, led to the hypothesis that the reinforcing or rewarding properties of these drugs are mediated by the mesolimbic dopamine system.

GLOBUS PALLIDUS

The globus pallidus lies medial to the putamen and lateral to the internal capsule. It consists of two segments, lateral (external) and medial (internal), which are separated by an internal medullary lamina, and which have substantially different connections. Both segments receive large numbers of fibres from the striatum and subthalamic nucleus. The lateral segment projects reciprocally to the subthalamic nucleus as part of the 'indirect pathway'. The medial segment is considered to be a homologue of the pars reticulata of the substantia nigra, with which it shares similar cellular and connectional properties. Together, these segments constitute the main output of the basal ganglia to other levels of the neuraxis, principally to the thalamus and superior colliculus.

The cell density of the globus pallidus is less than one-twentieth of that of the striatum. The morphology of the majority of cells is identical in the two segments. They are large multipolar GABAergic neurones that closely resemble those of the substantia nigra pars reticulata. The dendritic fields are discoid, with planes at right angles to incoming striatopallidal axons, each of which, therefore, potentially contacts many pallidal dendrites *en passant*. This arrangement, coupled with the diameters of the dendritic fields (>500 μm), suggests that a precise topographical organization is unlikely within the pallidum.

Striatopallidal fibres are of two main types. They project either to the lateral or the medial pallidal segment. Those projecting to the lateral segment constitute the beginning of the so-called 'indirect pathway'. They

utilize GABA as their primary transmitter and also contain enkephalin. Efferent axons from neurones in the lateral segment pass through the internal capsule in the subthalamic fasciculus, and travel to the subthalamic nucleus (**Fig. 21.17**).

Striatopallidal axons destined for the medial pallidum constitute the so-called 'direct pathway'. Like the indirect projection, these also utilize GABA as their primary transmitter but they also contain substance P and dynorphin, rather than enkephalin. Efferent axons from the medial pallidal segment project through the ansa lenticularis and fasciculus lenticularis (**Figs 21.17, 23.12**). The former runs round the anterior border of the internal capsule and the latter penetrates the capsule directly. Having traversed the internal capsule, both pathways unite in the subthalamic region, where they follow a horizontal hairpin trajectory, and turn upwards to enter the thalamus as the thalamic fasciculus. The trajectory circumnavigates the zona incerta and creates the so-called 'H' fields of Forel (**Figs 21.17, 23.5, 23.12**). Within the thalamus, pallidothalamic fibres end in the ventral anterior and ventral lateral nuclei and in the intralaminar centromedian nucleus. These in turn project excitatory (presumed glutamatergic) fibres primarily to the frontal cortex, including the primary and supplementary motor areas. The medial pallidum also projects fibres caudally to the pedunculopontine nucleus (**Fig. 23.14**). This lies at the junction of the midbrain and the pons, close to the superior cerebellar peduncle, and corresponds approximately to the physiologically identified 'mesencephalic locomotor region'.

SUBSTANTIA NIGRA

The substantia nigra is a nuclear complex deep to the crus cerebri in each cerebral peduncle of the midbrain. It consists of a pars compacta and a pars reticulata (**Figs 23.10, 23.11**). The pars compacta, together with the smaller pars lateralis, corresponds to the dopaminergic cell group A9. With the retrorubral nucleus (A8), it makes up most of the dopaminergic neurone population of the midbrain and is the source of the mesostriatal dopamine system that projects to the striatum. The pars compacta of each side is continuous with its opposite counterpart through the ventral tegmental dopamine group A10, which is sometimes known as the paranigral nucleus. This is the source of the mesolimbic dopamine system, which supplies the ventral striatum and neighbouring parts of the dorsal striatum, as well as the prefrontal and anterior cingulate cortices. The dopaminergic neurones of the pars compacta (A9) and paranigral nucleus (ventral tegmental group A10) also contain cholecystokinin (CCK) or somatostatin.

The pars reticulata contains large multipolar cells, which are very similar to those of the pallidum. Together they constitute the output neurones of the basal ganglia system. Their disc-like dendritic trees, like those of the pallidum, are orientated at right angles to afferents from the striatum, probably making *en-passant* contacts. Like the striatopallidal axons, of which they may be collaterals, striatonigral axons utilize GABA and substance P (SP) or enkephalin. They distribute differentially in the pars reticulata, such that the enkephalinergic axons terminate in the medial part, whereas substance P axons terminate throughout.

The efferent neurones of the pars reticulata are GABAergic. They project to the deep (polysensory) layers of the superior colliculus and to the brain stem reticular formation, including the pedunculopontine nucleus. The pathway from the striatum to the superior colliculus, via the substantia nigra pars reticulata, is thought to function in the control of gaze in a manner analogous to the pathway that initiates general body movement via the pallidum, thalamus and supplementary motor cortex. The uncontrolled or fixed-gaze disturbances of advanced Parkinson's disease, progressive supranuclear palsy (PSP) and Huntington's disease tend to support this.

SUBTHALAMIC NUCLEUS

The subthalamic nucleus is a biconvex, lens-shaped nucleus in the subthalamus of the diencephalon. It lies medial to the internal capsule, immediately rostral to the level at which the latter becomes continuous with the crus cerebri of the midbrain (**Figs 23.2, 23.5, 23.8**). Within its substance, small interneurones intermingle with large multipolar cells with dendrites, which extend for about one-tenth the diameter of the nucleus. It is encapsulated dorsally by axons, many of which are derived from the subthalamic fasciculus, and which carry a major GABAergic projection from the lateral segment of the globus pallidus as part of the indirect pathway. It also receives afferents from the cerebral cortex. The subthalamic nucleus is unique in the intrinsic circuitry of the basal ganglia in that its cells are glutamatergic. They project excitatory axons to both the globus pallidus and substantia nigra pars reticulata. Within the pallidum, subthalamic efferent fibres end predominantly in the medial segment but many also end in the lateral segment.

The subthalamic nucleus plays a central role in the normal function of the basal ganglia and in the pathophysiology of basal ganglia-related disorders. Destruction of the nucleus, which occurs rarely as a result of stroke, results in the appearance of violent, uncontrolled involuntary movements, known as ballism (ballismus). The subthalamic nucleus is also crucially involved in the pathophysiology of Parkinson's disease and is a target for functional neurosurgical therapy of the condition.

PATHOPHYSIOLOGY OF BASAL GANGLIA DISORDERS

The normal functions of the basal ganglia are difficult to summarize succinctly. As far as their role in movement control is concerned, however, a reasonable definition is that they function to promote and support patterns of behaviour and movement that are appropriate in the prevailing circumstances and to inhibit unwanted or inappropriate behaviour and movements. This is exemplified by disorders of the basal ganglia, which are characterized, depending on the underlying pathology, by an inability to initiate and execute wanted movements (as in Parkinson's disease) or an inability to prevent unwanted movements (as in Huntington's disease).

Parkinson's disease is the most common pathological condition affecting the basal ganglia. This is characterized by akinesia, muscular rigidity and tremor. It is due to degeneration of the dopaminergic neurones of the substantia nigra pars compacta. As a consequence, dopamine levels in the striatum are depleted. This has been amply

confirmed by post-mortem studies. Furthermore, in parkinsonian patients, positron emission tomography (PET) reveals a deficit of dopamine storage and reuptake, due to loss of nigrostriatal terminals, but intact dopamine receptors, which are located upon the medium spiny neurones, the target of the nigrostriatal pathway.

Dopamine appears to have a dual action on medium spiny striatal neurones. It inhibits those of the indirect pathway and excites those of the direct pathway. Consequently, when dopamine is lost from the striatum, the indirect pathway becomes overactive and the direct pathway becomes underactive (**Fig. 23.15**). Overactivity of the striatal projection to the lateral pallidum results in inhibition of pallidosubthalamic neurones and, consequently, overactivity of the subthalamic nucleus. Subthalamic efferents mediate excessive excitatory drive to the medial globus pallidus and substantia nigra pars reticulata. This is exacerbated by underactivity of the GABAergic, inhibitory direct pathway. Overactivity of basal ganglia output then inhibits the motor thalamus and its excitatory thalamocortical connections. While this description is little more than a first approximation of the underlying pathophysiology, this model of the basis of parkinsonian symptoms has led to the introduction of new neurosurgical approaches to the treatment of Parkinson's disease, based upon lesioning and deep brain stimulation of the medial globus pallidus and subthalamic nucleus (see below).

The current medical treatment for Parkinson's disease relies upon levodopa (L-DOPA; L-dihydroxyphenylalanine), the immediate metabolic precursor of dopamine, or dopamine agonists. Whilst these usually provide good symptomatic relief for many years, they eventually lead to the development of side-effects, including dyskinesias. The involuntary movements that occur as a consequence of long-term treatment of Parkinson's disease resemble those seen in Huntington's disease, tardive dyskinesia and ballism. Experimental evidence suggests that these may

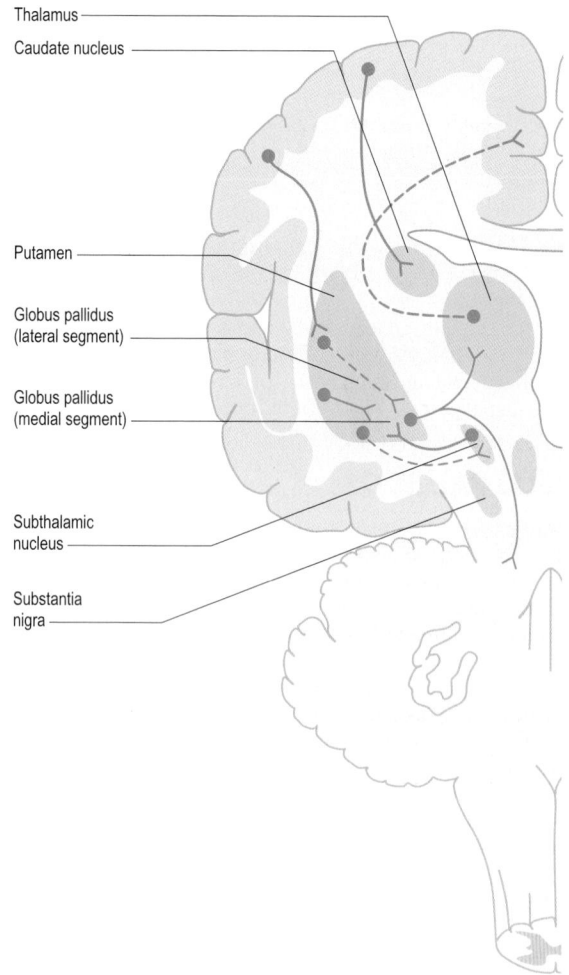

Fig. 23.15 Pathophysiology of Parkinson's disease. Dotted lines indicate dysfunctional pathways. (By permission from Crossman AR, Neary D 2000 Neuroanatomy, 2nd edn. Edinburgh: Churchill Livingstone.)

share a common neural mechanism (**Fig. 23.16**). Thus, the indirect pathway becomes underactive, e.g. due to the effects of dopaminergic drugs in Parkinson's disease or the degeneration of the striatopallidal projection to the lateral pallidum in Huntington's disease. This leads to physiological inhibition of the subthalamic nucleus by overactive pallidosubthalamic neurones. The involvement of the subthalamic nucleus explains why the dyskinetic movements of levodopa-induced dyskinesia and Huntington's disease resemble those of ballism produced by lesion of the subthalamic nucleus. Underactivity of the subthalamic nucleus removes the excitatory drive from medial pallidal neurones, which are known to be underactive in dyskinesias. Once again this is an oversimplification. Whilst it is true that underactivity of the medial globus pallidus is associated with dyskinesias, it is also known that lesions of the globus pallidus alleviate them. This suggests that the dynamic aspects of pallidal and nigral efferent activity are important factors in the generation of dyskinesia.

Another manifestation of basal ganglia dysfunction is dystonia, which is characterized by increased muscle tone and abnormal postures. This may occur as a consequence of levodopa treatment in Parkinson's disease or inherited disease (e.g. idiopathic torsion, or Oppenheim's dystonia). The pathophysiological basis of dystonia is unclear. Like dyskinesias it is probably caused by underactivity of basal ganglia output, and so deep-brain stimulation of the globus pallidus may be beneficial.

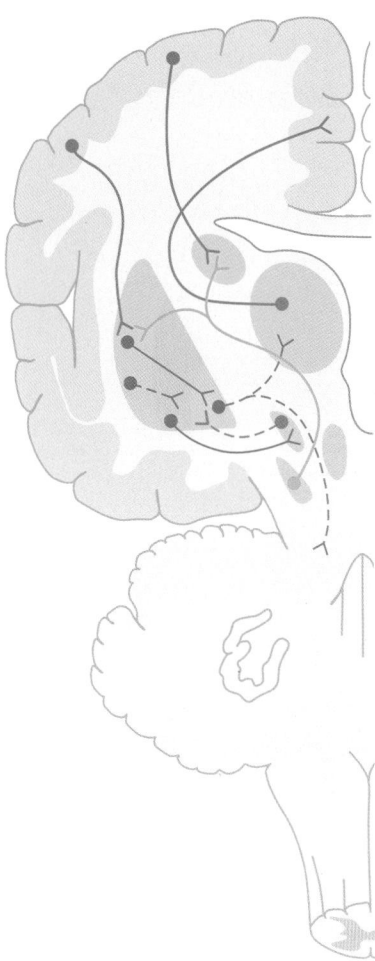

Fig. 23.16 Pathophysiology of dyskinesias. Dotted lines indicate dysfunctional pathways. (By permission from Crossman AR, Neary D 2000 Neuroanatomy, 2nd edn. Edinburgh: Churchill Livingstone.)

There is evidence that dysfunction of the basal ganglia is involved in other complex, less well-understood, behavioural disorders. In animal experiments, lesions of the basal ganglia, especially of the caudate nucleus, induce uncontrollable hyperactivity (e.g. obstinate progression, incessant pacing and other constantly repeated behaviour). This and other evidence has led to the notion that the corpus striatum enables the individual to make motor choices and to avoid 'stimulus-bound' behaviour. PET scanning studies in man have shown that sufferers from obsessive-compulsive disorder (OCD), which is characterized by repeated ritualistic motor behaviour and intrusive thoughts, exhibit abnormal activity in the prefrontal cortex and caudate nuclei. There are similar suggestive observations in the hyperactive child syndrome. In this respect it may be significant that the basal ganglia, besides receiving connections from the frontal lobe and limbic cortices, also have an ascending influence on the prefrontal and cingulate cortices through the substantia nigra pars reticulata and dorsomedial and ventromedial thalamus (**Fig. 23.13B,C,D**).

Before the advent of levodopa, neurosurgery for Parkinson's disease was commonplace. The globus pallidus and thalamus were favoured targets for chemical or thermal lesions. Pallidotomy and thalamotomy often improved rigidity and tremor, but they produced little consistent beneficial effect upon akinesia. With the arrival of levodopa therapy, which had a profound effect upon akinesia, the surgical treatment of Parkinson's disease underwent progressive decline. However, it soon became clear that long-term use of levodopa was associated with a number of side-effects such as dyskinesias, 'wearing-off', and the 'on–off' phenomenon. More recent advances in understanding the pathophysiology of movement disorders, and in particular Parkinson's disease, have stimulated a renaissance in the use of neurosurgery to treat movement disorders.

In primates that had been made parkinsonian experimentally with the neurotoxin MPTP, lesioning the subthalamic nucleus alleviated tremor, rigidity and bradykinesia. This finding raised the possibility that the subthalamic nucleus could be used as a clinical target. Indeed, lesions of the subthalamic nucleus in humans exert a powerful effect in alleviating tremor, rigidity and bradykinesia. However, the likelihood of side-effects is not trivial (the subthalamic nucleus is a small structure wrapped by fibres of passage and close to the hypothalamus and internal capsule), and relatively few centres perform this procedure.

In 1992, Laitinen et al reintroduced pallidotomy for the treatment of end-stage Parkinson's disease, but confined the lesions to the posteroventral part of the internal pallidal segment. These lesions were found to be extremely reliable in abolishing contralateral rigidity and drug-induced dyskinesias, with slightly less efficacy on tremor and bradykinesia.

Implantation of deep-brain electrodes through which high-frequency pulses generated by a pacemaker could inhibit cells in the vicinity has been a concept since the early 1970s, but did not become a widespread reality until the late 1980s, as a result of technological advances. The introduction of this technique, which avoids making permanent lesions, made bilateral surgery safer. There have been numerous reports of the effectiveness of both bilateral pallidal and subthalamic nucleus stimulation (**Figs 23.17, 23.18**). Subthalamic nucleus stimulation is favoured by most groups because, unlike pallidal stimulation, it allows patients to reduce their anti-parkinsonian medication.

Serendipity also has a role in such surgery. Clinically, parkinsonian patients can develop painful dystonic posturing of their limbs which responds dramatically to bilateral pallidal stimulation. This has led to preliminary studies of bilateral pallidal stimulation for dystonia with very promising results. Since it is held that in dystonia the pallidal neurones fire at rates below normal, this presents quite a puzzle as it is open to question how stimulation works. It also would appear that the neural mechanism that underlies this therapeutic effect on dystonia may differ from that in Parkinson's disease and tremor, because in dystonia the improvement may take weeks to emerge, whereas it is immediate in the case of Parkinson's disease.

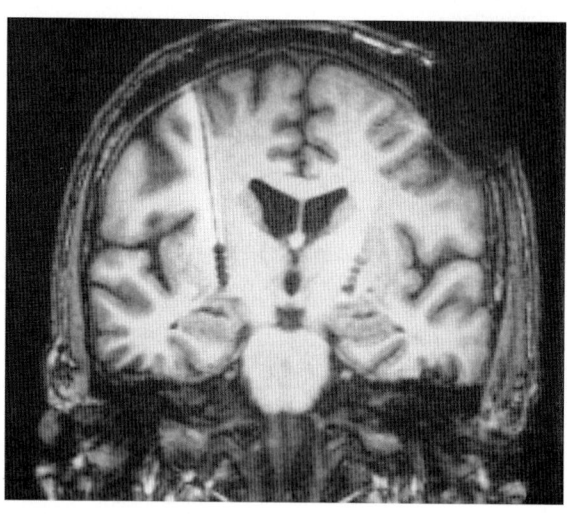

Fig. 23.17 MRI image showing placement of deep brain stimulating electrodes bilaterally in the globus pallidus of a patient with Parkinson's disease. (By kind permission from Professor TZ Aziz, Radcliffe Infirmary, Oxford and Charing Cross Hospital, London.)

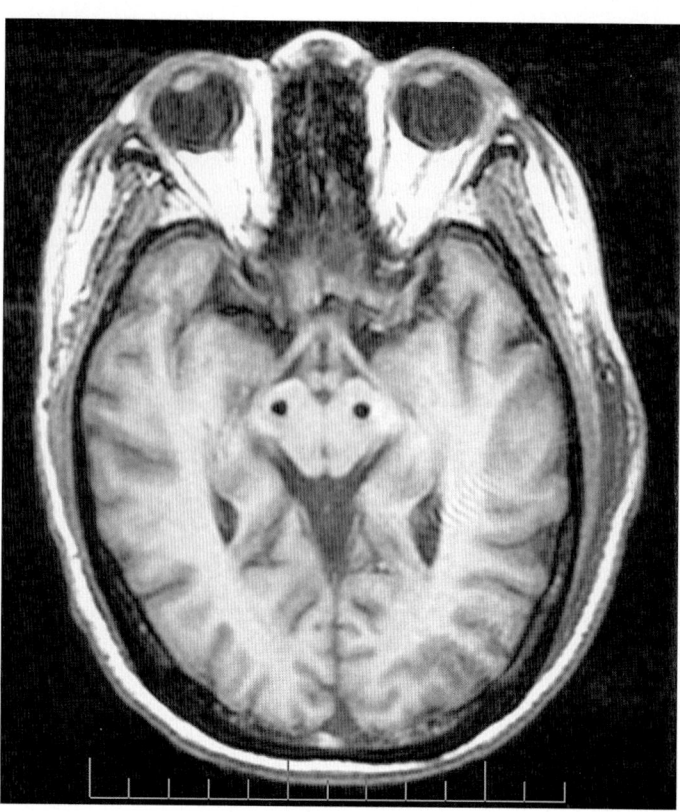

Fig. 23.18 MRI image showing placement of deep brain stimulating electrodes bilaterally in the subthalamic nucleus of a patient with Parkinson's disease. (By kind permission from Professor AM Lozano, Toronto Western Hospital.)

REFERENCES

Alexander GE, DeLong MR, Strick PL 1986 Parallel organization of functionally segregated circuits linking basal ganglia and cortex. Ann Rev Neurosci 9: 357–82.
A landmark publication setting out a conceptual framework for the way in which the basal ganglia and cerebral cortex process different types of information through largely distinct parallel circuits based upon known anatomical connectivity.

Crossmann AR 1990 A hypothesis on the pathophysiological mechanisms that underlie levodopa- or dopamine agonist-induced dyskinesia in Parkinson's disease: implications for future strategies in treatment. Mov Disord 5: 100–108.

Krack P, Batir A, Van Blercom N et al 2003 Five-year follow-up of bilateral stimulation of the subthalamic nucleus in advanced Parkinson's disease. N Engl J Med 349: 1925–1934.
Reviews the long-term outcome of deep brain stimulation of the subthalamic nucleus in Parkinson's disease.

Laitinen LV, Bergenheim AT, Hariz MI 1992 Ventroposterolateral pallidotomy can abolish all Parkinsonian symptoms. Stereotact Funct Neurosurg 58: 14–21.
A key paper which ignited widespread interest in functional neurosurgery for Parkinson's disease.

Penney JB Jr, Young AB 1986 Striatal inhomogeneities and basal ganglia function. Mov Disord 1: 3–15.
A landmark publication, introducing some of the basic concepts behind current models of the pathophysiology of Parkinson's disease and Huntington's disease.

Special senses

The special senses of olfaction, vision, taste, hearing and balance are conveyed to the brain in cranial nerves. In each case, highly specialized peripheral receptors respond to stimuli in the external environment or our relationship to it. The olfactory system has an ancient lineage, reflected by the fact that afferent olfactory pathways proceed directly to the cerebral cortex and bypass the thalamus. Its terminal fields are, likewise, primitive cortical areas in a phylogenetic sense and are considered to be parts of the limbic system. All other special senses have a thalamic representation which projects to specialized regions of the neocortex.

OLFACTION

Olfactory pathways subserving the sense of smell are described in this section. Details of the relationship between the olfactory pathways and the limbic system are shown in **Fig. 22.7**.

The olfactory nerves arise from olfactory receptor neurones in the olfactory mucosa. The axons collect into c.20 bundles and enter the anterior cranial fossa by passing through the foramina in the cribriform plate. They attach to the inferior surface of the olfactory bulb, which is situated at the anterior end of the olfactory sulcus on the orbital surface

of the frontal lobe, and terminate in the bulb. Apparently unique in the nervous system, olfactory receptor neurones are continually replaced throughout life by differentiation of stem cells in the olfactory mucosa. The olfactory bulb is continuous posteriorly with the olfactory tract, through which the output of the bulb passes directly to the olfactory cortex.

There is a clear laminar structure in the olfactory bulb (**Fig. 24.1**). From the surface inwards the laminae are the olfactory nerve layer, glomerular layer, external plexiform layer, mitral cell layer, internal plexiform layer and granule cell layer.

The olfactory nerve layer consists of unmyelinated axons of the olfactory neurones. The continuous turnover of receptor cells means that axons in this layer are at different stages of growth, maturity or degeneration. The glomerular layer consists of a thin sheet of glomeruli where the incoming olfactory axons divide and synapse on terminal dendrites of secondary olfactory neurones, i.e. mitral, tufted and periglomerular cells. The external plexiform layer contains the principal and secondary dendrites of mitral and tufted cells. The mitral cell layer is a thin sheet composed of the cell bodies of mitral cells, each of which sends a single principal dendrite to a glomerulus, secondary dendrites to the external plexiform layer, and a single axon to the olfactory tract.

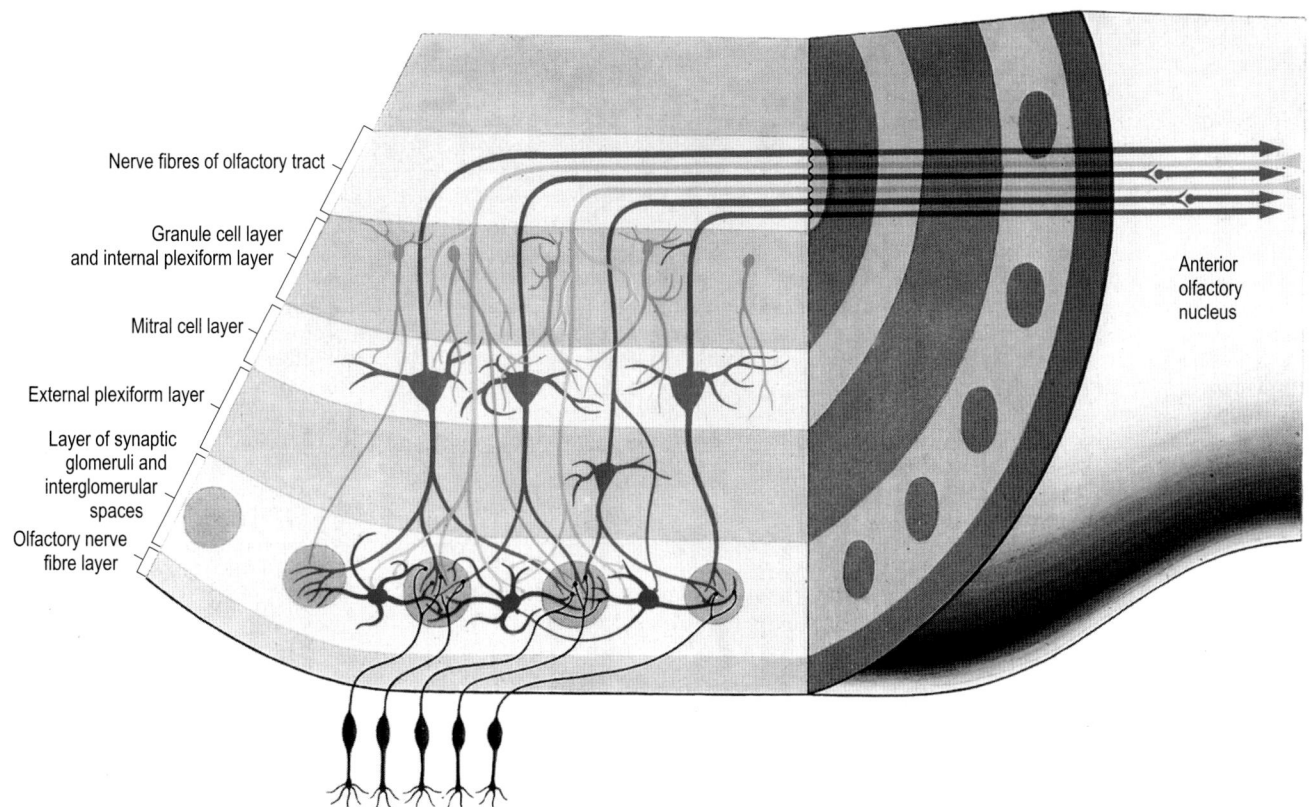

Nerve fibres of olfactory tract

Granule cell layer
and internal plexiform layer

Mitral cell layer

External plexiform layer

Layer of synaptic
glomeruli and
interglomerular
spaces

Olfactory nerve
fibre layer

Anterior
olfactory
nucleus

Fig. 24.1 Organization of the olfactory bulb. The radial organization of the bulb into 'layers', with their principal neurone types, and an indication of their main connections is shown. Red: mitral and tufted neurones and their processes; light blue: internal granule neurones; dark blue: dopaminergic periglomerular neurones; black: olfactory receptor neurones and their processes. The olfactory tract consists of (1) centripetal axons of mitral and tufted cells, some of which synapse with neurones in the anterior olfactory nucleus and (2) centrifugal axons (yellow) which terminate in the different zones indicated.

It also contains a few granule cell bodies. The internal plexiform layer contains axons, recurrent and deep collaterals of mitral and tufted cells, and granule cell bodies. The granule cell layer contains the majority of the granule cells and their superficial and deep processes, together with numerous centripetal and centrifugal nerve fibres which pass through the layer.

The principal neurones in the olfactory bulb are the mitral and tufted cells: their axons form its output via the olfactory tract. These cells are morphologically similar and most use an excitatory amino acid, probably glutamate or aspartate, as their neurotransmitter. The mitral cell spans the layers of the bulb, and receives the sensory input superficially at its glomerular tuft. The axons of mitral and tufted cells appear to be parallel output pathways from the olfactory bulb. It is not known whether they receive inputs from different olfactory sensory neurones.

The main types of intrinsic neurone in the olfactory bulb are periglomerular cells and granule cells. The majority of periglomerular cells are dopaminergic (cell group A15); some are GABAergic. Their axons are distributed laterally and terminate within extraglomerular regions. Granule cells are similar in size to periglomerular cells. Their most characteristic feature is the absence of an axon, and they therefore resemble amacrine cells in the retina. Granule cells have two principal spine-bearing dendrites which pass radially in the bulb, to ramify and terminate in the external plexiform layer. They appear to be GABAergic. The granule cell is likely to be a powerful inhibitory influence on the output neurones of the olfactory bulb.

Centrifugal inputs to the olfactory bulb arise from a variety of central sites. Neurones of the anterior olfactory nucleus and collaterals of pyramidal neurones in the olfactory cortex project to the granule cells of the olfactory bulb. Cholinergic neurones in the horizontal limb nucleus of the diagonal band of Broca, part of the basal forebrain cholinergic system, project to the granule cell layer and also to the glomerular layer. Other afferents to the granule cell layer and the glomeruli arise from the pontine locus coeruleus and the mesencephalic raphe nucleus.

The olfactory tract leaves the posterior pole of the olfactory bulb to run along the olfactory sulcus on the orbital surface of the frontal lobe (Fig. 22.7). The granule cell layer of the bulb is extended into the olfactory tract as scattered medium-sized multipolar neurones which constitute the anterior olfactory nucleus. They continue into the olfactory striae and trigone to the grey matter of the prepiriform cortex, the anterior perforated substance and precommissural septal areas. Many centripetal axons from mitral and tufted cells relay in, or give collaterals to, the anterior olfactory nucleus; the axons from the nucleus continue with the remaining direct fibres from the bulb into the olfactory striae.

As the olfactory tract approaches the anterior perforated substance it flattens and splays out as the olfactory trigone. Fibres of the tract continue from the caudal angles of the trigone as diverging medial and lateral olfactory striae, which border the anterior perforated substance. An intermediate stria sometimes passes from the centre of the trigone to end in a small olfactory tubercle. The lateral olfactory stria follows the anterolateral margin of the anterior perforated substance to the limen insulae, where it bends posteromedially to merge with an elevated region, the gyrus semilunaris, at the rostral margin of the uncus in the temporal lobe (Fig. 22.7). The lateral olfactory gyrus forms a tenuous grey layer covering the lateral olfactory stria: it merges laterally with the gyrus ambiens, part of the limen insulae. The lateral olfactory gyrus and gyrus ambiens form the prepiriform region of the cortex, passing caudally into the entorhinal area of the parahippocampal gyrus. The prepiriform and periamygdaloid regions and the entorhinal area (area 28) together make up the piriform cortex. The medial olfactory stria, covered thinly by the grey matter of the medial olfactory gyrus, passes medially along the rostral boundary of the anterior perforated substance towards the medial continuation of the diagonal band of Broca. Together, they curve up on the medial aspect of the hemisphere, anterior to the attachment of the lamina terminalis. The diagonal band enters the paraterminal gyrus. The medial stria becomes indistinct as it approaches the boundary zone, which includes the paraterminal gyrus, parolfactory gyrus and, between them, the prehippocampal rudiment (Fig. 22.7).

The olfactory cortex receives a direct input from the olfactory bulb, which arrives via the olfactory tract without relay in the thalamus. The largest cortical olfactory area is the piriform cortex. The anterior olfactory nucleus, olfactory tubercle, regions of the entorhinal and insular cortex and amygdala also receive direct projections from the olfactory bulb.

The entorhinal cortex (Brodmann's area 28) is the most posterior part of the piriform cortex, and is divided into medial and lateral areas (areas 28a and 28b). The lateral parts receive fibres mainly from the olfactory bulb, and also from the piriform and periamygdaloid cortices.

Projections from the piriform olfactory cortex are widespread, and include the neocortex (especially the orbitofrontal cortex), thalamus (especially the medial dorsal thalamic nucleus), hypothalamus, amygdala and hippocampal formation.

VISION

The anatomy of the eye is described in Chapters 41 and 42. The visual pathway is illustrated in Fig. 24.2. The first-order neurone of the visual system is a bipolar cell which is contained entirely within the retina. The second-order neurone is a ganglion cell whose axon enters the optic nerve.

The optic nerves pass posteromedially into the cranial cavity and meet in the midline, forming the optic chiasma, a flat mass of decussating fibres which lies at the junction of the anterior wall and floor of the third ventricle. The tuber cinereum and infundibulum lie posterior to the chiasma, and the third ventricle is dorsal to them. The termination of the internal carotid artery and anterior perforated substance are lateral relations. The optic recess of the third ventricle passes over its superior surface to reach the lamina terminalis.

Optic nerve fibres arising from the nasal half of each retina, including half of the macula, cross in the chiasma to enter the contralateral optic tract. Fibres from the temporal hemiretinae continue into the ipsilateral optic tract. Decussating fibres loop a little backwards into their ipsilateral optic nerve before crossing and then pass forwards into the contralateral optic tract after crossing. Macular fibres, and those from an adjacent central area, occupy almost two-thirds of the central chiasma, dorsal to all peripheral decussating fibres. The most ventral axons are nasal fibres concerned with monocular fringes of the binocular field. They lie beneath fibres from the extramacular parts of both nasal hemiretinae, which occupy an intermediate position in the chiasma.

The optic chiasma is supplied with blood from a pial plexus which receives branches from the superior hypophyseal, internal carotid, posterior communicating, anterior cerebral and anterior communicating arteries. The venous drainage of the chiasma is into the basal and anterior cerebral venous system.

Behind the optic chiasma, the optic tracts diverge dorsolaterally, each passing between the anterior perforated substance and tuber cinereum. The tract curves around the cerebral peduncle, to which it adheres. Optic tract fibres terminate primarily in the lateral geniculate nucleus of the thalamus, but also in the superior colliculus, pretectal area, suprachiasmatic nucleus of the hypothalamus and inferior pulvinar.

Axons from third-order visual neurones in the lateral geniculate nucleus run in the retrolenticular part of the internal capsule and form the optic radiation, which curves dorsomedially to the occipital cortex. Fibres representing the lower half of the visual field sweep superiorly to reach the visual cortex above the calcarine sulcus. Those representing the upper half of the visual field curve inferiorly into the temporal lobe (Meyer's loop) before reaching the visual cortex below the calcarine sulcus.

Some neurones in the occipital cortex send descending axons to the superior colliculus, which therefore receives cortical and retinal afferents. From here fibres travel by tectobulbar tracts to motor nuclei of the third, fourth, sixth and eleventh cranial nerves and the ventral horn of the spinal cord.

Visual field defects

Plotting visual field loss frequently reveals the approximate location of the causative lesion in the visual pathway and sometimes its nature. Since retinal lesions can be visualized using an ophthalmoscope, these aids might appear to be redundant, but visual field measurement is still helpful in assessing the extent of the damage and may be the key factor in confirming a diagnosis. Glaucoma serves as an example. Field defects in glaucoma, occurring as a consequence of damage to the nerve fibre bundles at the optic nerve head, may be detectable ophthalmoscopically, but confirmation of the diagnosis frequently depends on field assessment. An initial constriction of the visual field is of little

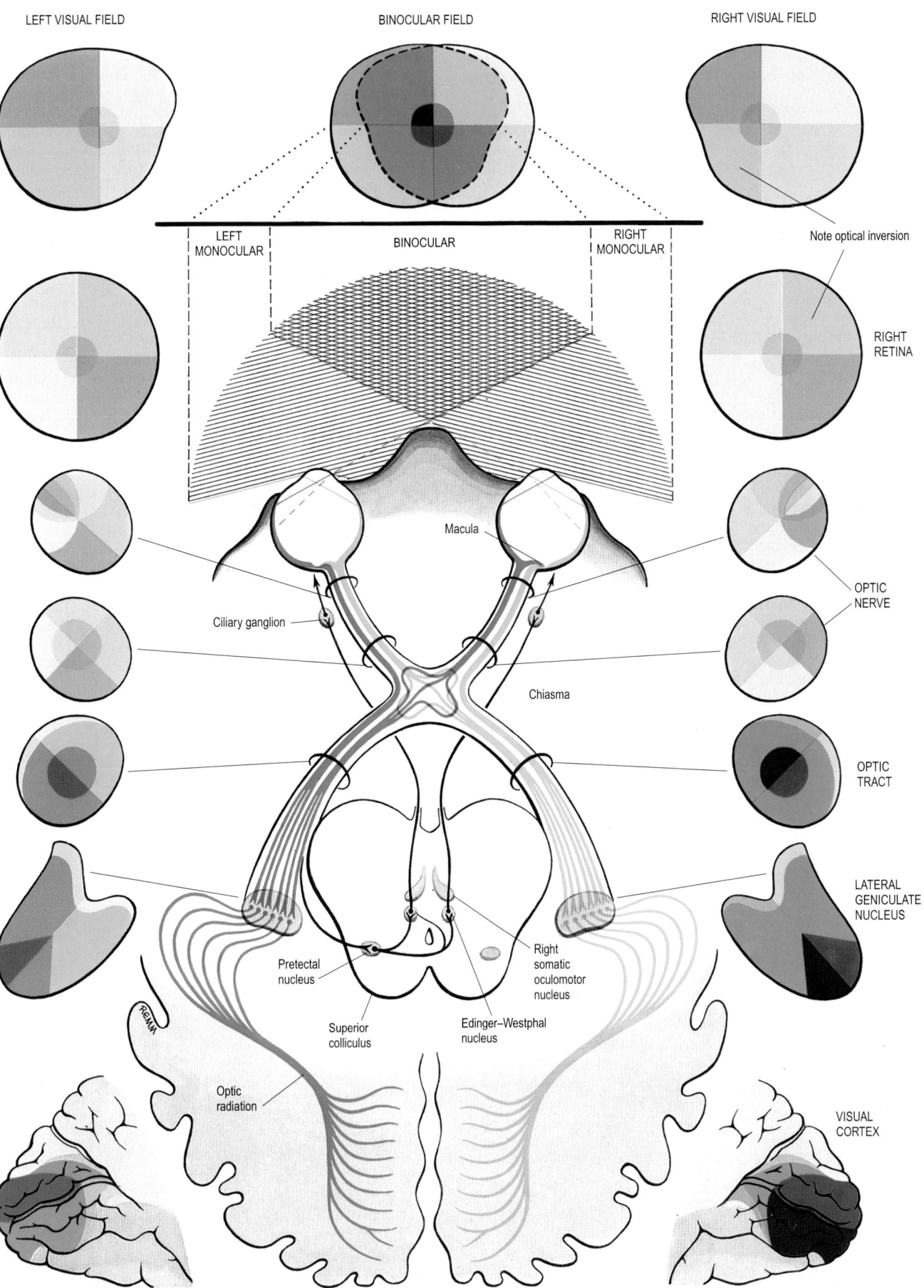

LEFT VISUAL FIELD

BINOCULAR FIELD

RIGHT VISUAL FIELD

LEFT
MONOCULAR

BINOCULAR

RIGHT
MONOCULAR

Note optical inversion

RIGHT
RETINA

Macula

OPTIC
NERVE

Ciliary ganglion

Chiasma

OPTIC
TRACT

LATERAL
GENICULATE
NUCLEUS

Pretectal
nucleus

Right
somatic
oculomotor
nucleus

Superior
colliculus

Edinger–Westphal
nucleus

Optic
radiation

VISUAL
CORTEX

Fig. 24.2 The visual pathway, showing the spatial arrangement of neurones and their fibres in relation to the quadrants of the retinae and visual fields. The proportions at various levels are not exactly to scale and in particular the macula is exaggerated in size in the visual fields and retinae. In each quadrant of the visual field, and the parts of the visual pathway subserving it, two shades of the respective colour are used, the paler for the peripheral fields and a darker shade for the macular part of the quadrant. From the optic tract onwards these two shades are both made more saturated to denote intermixture of neurones from both retinae, the palest shade being reserved for parts of the visual pathway concerned with monocular vision. The pathway subserving the pupillary light reflex is also indicated.

clinical significance but later defects, characteristic of the disease, consist of a scotoma between 10 and 20 degrees of the fixation area, extending upwards, or less commonly downwards, from the blind spot. This later elongates circumferentially along the arcuate nerve fibres and subsequently extends further. The field defect forms a linear limit or step along the horizontal meridian nasally, the loss continuing to blindness.

So far as the location of lesions central to the retina are concerned, deficits in the vision of one eye are usually attributable to optic nerve lesions. Lesions of the optic chiasma, involving crossing nerve fibres, produce a bilateral field loss as exemplified by a pituitary adenoma. The tumour expands upwards from the pituitary fossa, compressing the inferior midline of the chiasma, and eventually produces bitemporal hemianopia, starting with an early loss in the upper temporal quadrants. Field defects in the rare instances of optic tract lesions are distinctive. The tract contains contralateral nasal and ipsilateral temporal retinal projections and damage will cause a homonymous contralateral loss of field with substantial incongruity (dissimilar defects in the two fields). Incongruity probably results from a delay in achieving coincidence between retinal topographical projections of the two inputs of the visual pathway, as contiguous projections adjust their location, gradually achieving coincidence. It also likely reflects the reorganization of fibres which occurs normally in the optic tracts, as some fibres leave the tract in the superior brachium and others progress to the lateral geniculate nucleus. The two defective fields may display incongruency as a result of lesions above the level of the chiasma. It is most marked in optic tract defects, less obvious in optic radiation defects, and is usually absent in cortically induced field defects, thus providing an additional clue in assessing location of the cause.

Lesions of the optic radiations are usually unilateral, and commonly vascular in origin. Field defects therefore develop abruptly, in contrast to the slow progression of defects associated with tumours. Resulting hemifield loss follows the general rule that visual field defects central to the chiasma are on the opposite side to the lesion. Little or no incongruity is seen in visual cortical lesions but they commonly display the phenomenon of macula sparing, the central 5–10° field being retained in an otherwise hemianopic defect.

Neural control of gaze

Neural control systems are required to coordinate the movements of the eyes so that the image of the object of interest is simultaneously held on both foveae, despite movement of the object or the observer. A number of separate neural systems are involved: first, to shift gaze to the object of interest using rapid movements, called saccades; and second, to stabilize the image on the fovea either during movement of the object of interest (the smooth pursuit system), and/or during movement of the head or body (the vestibulo-ocular and optokinetic systems). Although the detailed anatomical substrates for these systems differ, they share common circuitry which lies mainly in the pons and midbrain, for horizontal and vertical gaze movements respectively (**Fig. 24.3**).

The common element for all types of horizontal gaze movements is the abducens nucleus. This contains motor neurones which innervate the ipsilateral lateral rectus. It also contains interneurones which project via the medial longitudinal fasciculus (MLF) to the contralateral oculomotor nucleus controlling medial rectus. A lesion of the abducens nucleus leads to a total loss of ipsilateral horizontal conjugate gaze. A lesion of the MLF produces slowed or absent adduction of the ipsilateral eye, usually associated with jerky movements (nystagmus) of the abducting eye, a syndrome called internuclear ophthalmoplegia.

The gaze motor command involves specialized areas of the reticular formation of the brain stem which receive a variety of supranuclear inputs. The main region for horizontal gaze is the paramedian pontine reticular formation (PPRF), which is located on each side of the midline in the central paramedian part of the tegmentum, and extends from the pontomedullary junction to the pontopeduncular junction. Each PPRF contains excitatory neurones which discharge at high frequencies just prior to and during ipsilateral saccades. Pause neurones, which are located in a midline caudal pontine nucleus called the nucleus raphe interpositus, discharge tonically except just before and during saccades. They appear to exert an inhibitory influence on the burst neurones and so prevent extraneous saccades occurring during fixation.

The vestibular nuclei and the perihypoglossal complex (especially the nucleus prepositus hypoglossi) project directly to the abducens

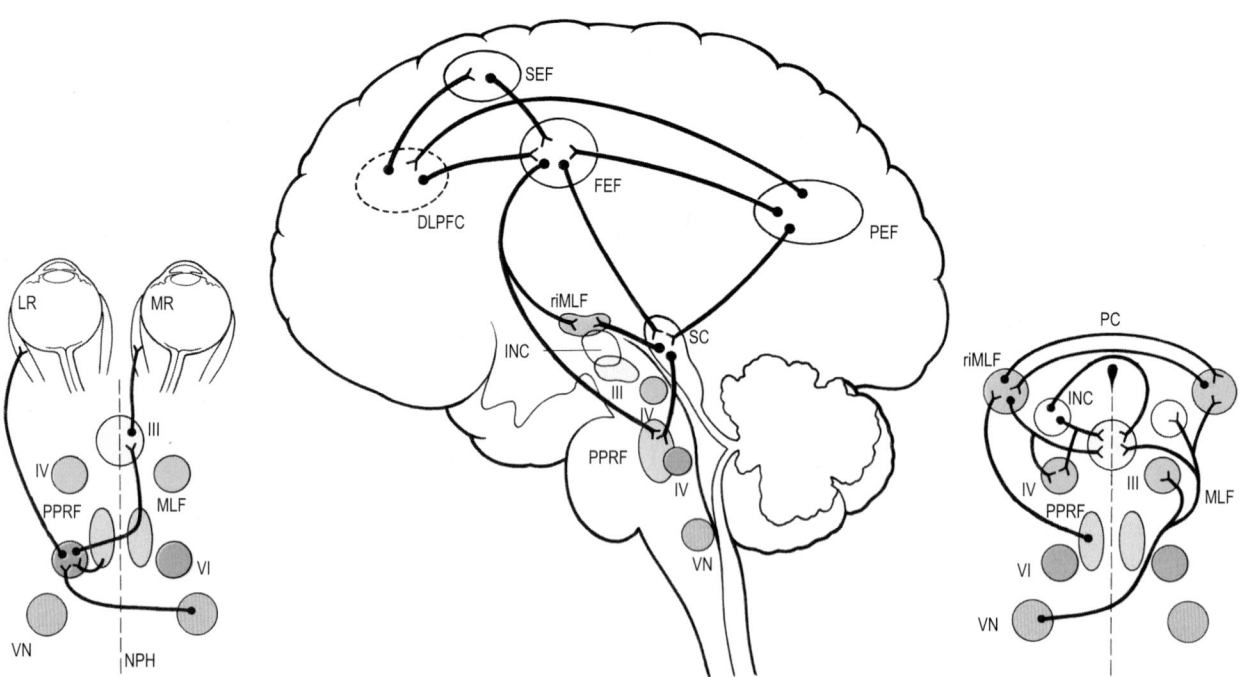

Fig. 24.3 Summary of eye movement control. The central drawing shows the supranuclear connections from the frontal eye field (FEF) and the posterior eye field (PEF) to the superior colliculus (SC), rostral interstitial nucleus of the medial longitudinal fasciculus (riMLF), and the paramedian pontine reticular formation (PPRF). The FEF and SC are involved in the production of saccades, while the PEF is thought to be important in the production of pursuit. The drawing on the left shows the brain stem pathways for horizontal gaze. Axons from the PPRF travel to the ipsilateral abducens nucleus innervating lateral rectus (LR). Abducens internuclear axons cross the midline and travel in the medial longitudinal fasciculus (MLF) to the portion of the oculomotor nucleus (III) innervating medial rectus (MR) of the contralateral eye. The drawing on the right shows the brain stem pathways for vertical gaze. Important structures include the riMLF, PPRF, the interstitial nucleus of Cajal (INC), and the posterior commissure (PC). Other abbreviations: DLPFC, dorsolateral prefrontal cortex; IV, trochlear nucleus; SEF, supplementary eye field; VN, vestibular nucleus.

nuclei. These projections probably carry both smooth pursuit signals, via the cerebellum, and vestibular signals. In addition, these nuclei, via reciprocal innervation with the PPRF, contain integrator neurones which control the step change in innervation required to maintain the eccentric position of the eye against the viscoelastic forces in the orbit. These forces tend to move the eyeball back to the position of looking straight ahead, i.e. the primary position, after a saccade.

The final common pathway of vertical gaze movements is formed by the oculomotor and trochlear nuclei. The rostral interstitial nucleus of the medial longitudinal fasciculus (riMLF) contains neurones that discharge in relation to up-and-down vertical saccadic movements. The riMLF projects through the posterior commissure to its equivalent on the other side of the mesencephalon, as well as directly to the oculomotor nucleus. Therefore, lesions within the posterior commissure give rise to disturbance in vertical gaze, especially up-gaze. Lesions placed more ventrally in the region of the riMLF give rise to vertical gaze disorders which may be mixed up-and-down, or mainly down-gaze. Slightly caudal to the riMLF, and directly connected to it, lies the interstitial nucleus of Cajal. It contains neurones which appear to be involved in vertical gaze in holding the vertical pursuit.

The cerebral hemispheres are extremely important for the programming and coordination of both saccadic and pursuit conjugate eye movements. There appear to be four main cortical areas in the cerebral hemispheres involved in the generation of saccades (**Fig. 24.3**). These are: the frontal eye field (FEF), which lies laterally at the caudal end of the second frontal gyrus in the premotor cortex (Brodmann area 8); the supplementary eye field (SEF), which lies at the anterior region of the supplementary motor area in the first frontal gyrus (Brodmann area 6); the dorsolateral prefrontal cortex (DLPFC), which lies anterior to the FEF in the second frontal gyrus (Brodmann area 46); and a posterior eye field (PEF), which lies in the parietal lobe, possibly in the superior part of the angular gyrus (Brodmann area 39), and the adjacent lateral intraparietal sulcus. These areas all appear to be interconnected with each other and to send projections to the superior colliculus and the brain stem areas controlling saccades.

It appears that there are two parallel pathways involved in the cortical generation of saccades. An anterior system originates in the FEF and projects both directly, and via the superior colliculus, to the brain stem saccadic generators. This pathway also passes indirectly via the basal ganglia to the superior colliculus. Projections from the frontal cortex influence cells in the pars reticulata of the substantia nigra, via a relay in the caudate nucleus. An inhibitory pathway from the pars reticulata projects directly to the superior colliculus. This appears to be a gating circuit related to volitional saccades, especially of the memory-guided type. A posterior pathway originates in the PEF and passes to the brain stem saccadic generators via the superior colliculus.

To maintain foveation of a moving target, the smooth pursuit system has developed relatively independently of the saccadic oculomotor system, although there are inevitable interconnections between the two. The first task is to identify and code the velocity and direction of a moving target. This is carried out in the extrastriate visual area known as the middle temporal visual area (MT; also called visual area V5), which contains neurones sensitive to visual target motion. In man, this lies immediately posterior to the ascending limb of the inferior temporal sulcus at the occipitotemporal border. Area MT send this motion signal to the medial superior temporal visual area (MST), which is thought to lie superior and a little anterior to area MT within the inferior parietal lobe. Damage to this area results in an impairment of smooth pursuit of targets moving towards the damaged hemisphere.

Both area MST and FEF send direct projections to a group of nuclei which lie in the basal part of the pons. In the monkey, the dorsolateral and lateral groups of pontine nuclei receive direct cortical inputs related to smooth pursuit. Lesions of similarly located nuclei in man result in abnormal pursuit. These nuclei transfer the pursuit signal bilaterally to the posterior vermis, contralateral flocculus and fastigial nuclei of the cerebellum. The pursuit signal ultimately passes from the cerebellum to the brain stem, specifically to the medial vestibular nucleus and nucleus propositus hypoglossi, thence to the PPRF and possibly directly to the ocular motor nuclei. This circuitry therefore involves a double decussation, firstly at the level of the midpons (pontocerebellar neurones) and secondly in the lower pons (vestibuloabducens neurones).

The vestibulo-ocular reflex maintains coordination of vision during movement of the head. It results in a compensatory conjugate eye movement which is equal but opposite to the movement of the head.

This is essentially a three-neurone arc. It consists of primary vestibular neurones which project to the vestibular nuclei, secondary neurones which project from these nuclei directly to the abducens nucleus, and tertiary neurones which are abducens motor neurones.

The optokinetic response is another visually mediated reflex which stabilizes retinal imagery during rotational movement. As the visual scene changes, the eyes follow, holding the retinal image steady until they shift rapidly in the opposite direction to another area of the visual scene. The full field of vision, rather than small objects within it, is the stimulus, and the alternating slow and fast phases of movement generated, describes optokinetic nystagmus. The optokinetic reflex functions in collaboration with the rotational vestibulo-ocular reflex. Because of the mechanical arrangements of the semicircular canals, in the sustained rotations of the body described above the vestibulo-ocular reflex fades. In darkness the reflex, which is initially compensatory, loses velocity, and after c.45 seconds the eyes become stationary.

Pupillary light reflex

The pupillary light reflex is a dynamic system for controlling the amount of light reaching the retina (**Fig. 24.4**). Illumination of the retina causes reflex constriction of the pupil (miosis). There is a direct component of the light reflex which mediates the constriction of the pupil of the ipsilateral eye, and a consensual component which elicits simultaneous constriction of the contralateral pupil.

A light stimulus acting upon the retinal photoreceptors gives rise to activity in retinal ganglion cells, the axons of which form the optic nerve. Activity is conducted through the optic chiasma and along the optic tract, and the majority of fibres end in the lateral geniculate nucleus of the thalamus. However, a small number of fibres leave the optic tract before it reaches the thalamus and synapse in the pretectal nucleus. The information is relayed from the pretectal nucleus by short neurones which synapse bilaterally with preganglionic parasympathetic neurones in the Edinger–Westphal nucleus of the oculomotor nerve complex in the rostral midbrain. Efferent impulses pass along parasympathetic fibres of the oculomotor nerve to the orbit where they synapse in the ciliary ganglion. Postganglionic fibres (short ciliary nerves) pass to the eyeball to supply sphincter pupillae, which reduces the size of the pupil when it contracts.

There is also a connection to the spinal sympathetic centre controlling the dilator pupillae. The preganglionic fibres arise from neurones in the lateral column of the first and second thoracic segments, and pass via the sympathetic trunk to the superior cervical ganglion where they synapse on postganglionic neurones. Postganglionic fibres arising from these neurones are distributed to the cavernous plexus, whence they travel mainly through the long ciliary nerves to the anterior part of the eye where they supply the dilator pupillae.

Since pupillary size results from the balanced action of these two innervations, the pupil dilates when the parasympathetic stimulus ceases. The pupil dilates also in response to painful stimulation of almost any part of the body. Presumably fibres of sensory pathways connect with the sympathetic preganglionic neurones described above.

Accommodation reflex

When focussing on a nearby object, the eyes converge, the lens becomes more convex, and the pupils constrict (**Fig. 24.4**).

Information from the retina passing to the visual cortex does not constitute the afferent limb of a simple reflex in the usual sense of the term, but permits the visual areas to assess the clarity of objects in the visual field. Cortical efferent information passes to the pretectal area and thence to the Edinger–Westphal nucleus, which contains preganglionic parasympathetic neurones whose axons travel in the oculomotor nerve. Efferent impulses pass in the oculomotor nerve to the orbit where they synapse in the ciliary ganglion. Postganglionic fibres (short ciliary nerves) pass to the eyeball and stimulate contraction of the ciliary muscle, which slackens the ligament of the lens and increases the curvature of the lens for near vision. Contraction of sphincter pupillae and relaxation of dilator pupillae constrict the pupil. Simultaneously, contraction of the medial, superior, and inferior recti (all innervated by the oculomotor nerve) converges the eyes on the near target. The pupillary changes may be secondary to the convergence.

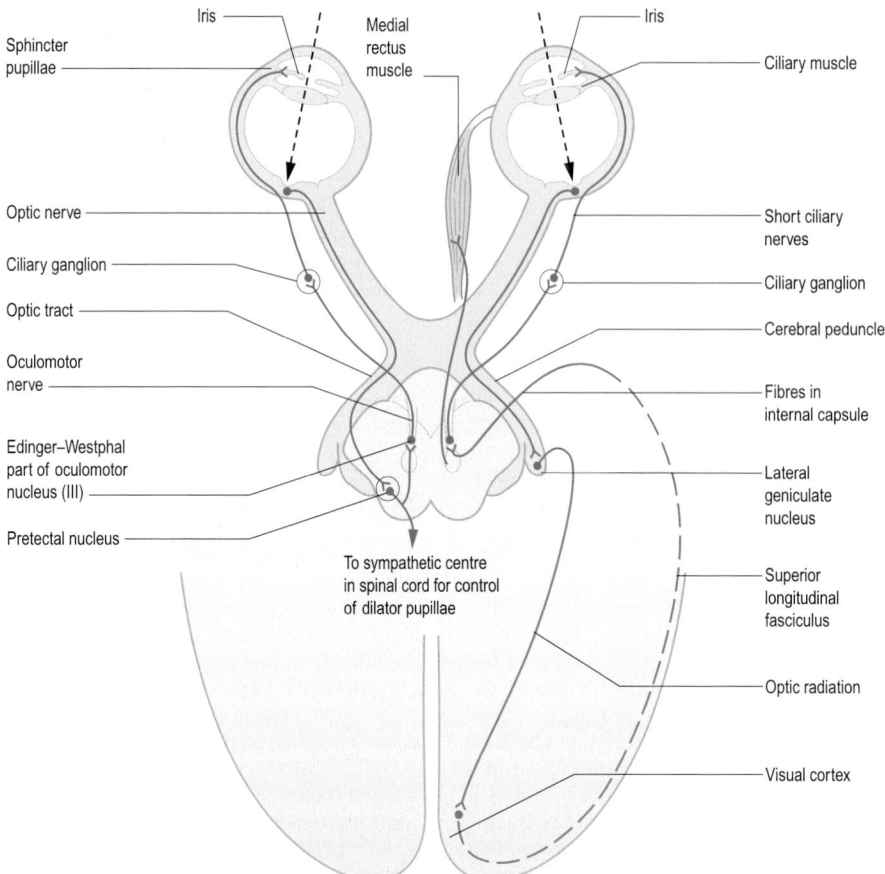

Fig. 24.4 The pupillary light reflex and accommodation reflex. (From Oxford Textbook of Functional Anatomy, Vol 3 Head and Neck, MacKinnon P, Morris J (eds), 1990. By permission of Oxford University Press.)

In certain central nervous diseases (e.g. tabes dorsalis) the pupillary light reflex may be lost, but pupilloconstriction as part of the accommodation reflex is retained (the Argyll Robertson pupil). The site of a lesion producing such an effect is unclear, but may involve the periaqueductal grey matter.

TASTE

Afferent nerve fibres carrying taste information are the peripheral processes of neuronal cell bodies in the geniculate ganglion of the facial nerve and in the inferior ganglia of the glossopharyngeal and vagus nerves. Taste from the anterior two-thirds of the tongue, excluding the vallate papillae, and from the inferior surface of the palate, is carried in the sensory root of the facial nerve (nervus intermedius). Taste buds in the vallate papillae, posterior third of the tongue, palatoglossal arches, oropharynx and, to some extent, the palate, are innervated by the glossopharyngeal nerve. Those in the extreme pharyngeal part of the tongue and the epiglottis are innervated by fibres of the vagus nerve.

On entering the brain stem, these afferent fibres constitute the tractus solitarius, and they terminate in the rostral third of the nucleus solitarius of the medulla. Second-order neurones arising from the nucleus solitarius cross the midline and many ascend through the brain stem in the dorsomedial part of the medial lemniscus. They terminate in the medial part of the ventral posteromedial (VPm) nucleus of the thalamus. From the ventral posteromedial nucleus, third-order neurones project through the internal capsule to the anteroinferior part of the sensory cortex and to the limen insulae. Other ascending projections to the hypothalamus have been described which may represent the pathway by which gustatory information reaches the limbic system.

HEARING

The primary afferents of the auditory pathway arise from cell bodies in the spiral ganglion of the cochlea. The axons constitute the auditory component of the vestibulocochlear nerve, which enters the brain stem at the cerebellopontine angle. Afferent fibres bifurcate, and terminate in the dorsal and ventral cochlear nuclei. Onward connections make up the ascending auditory pathway (**Fig. 24.5**). The dorsal cochlear nucleus projects via the dorsal acoustic stria to the contralateral inferior colliculus. The ventral cochlear nucleus projects via the trapezoid body or the intermediate acoustic stria to relay centres in either the superior olivary complex, the nuclei of the lateral lemniscus, or the inferior colliculus. The superior olivary complex is dominated by the medial superior olivary nucleus which receives direct input from the ventral cochlear nucleus on both sides, and is involved in localization of sound by measuring the time difference between afferent impulses arriving from the two ears.

The inferior colliculus consists of a central nucleus and two cortical areas. The dorsal cortex lies dorsomedially, and the external cortex lies ventromedially. Secondary and tertiary fibres ascend in the lateral lemniscus. They converge in the central nucleus, which projects to the ventral division of the medial geniculate body of the thalamus. The external cortex receives both auditory and somatosensory input. It projects to the medial division of the medial geniculate body, and, together with the central nucleus, also projects to olivocochlear cells in the superior olivary complex and to cells in the cochlear nuclei. The dorsal cortex receives an input from the auditory cortex and projects to the dorsal division of the medial geniculate body. Connections also run from the nucleus of the lateral lemniscus to the deep part of the superior colliculus, to coordinate auditory and visual responses.

The ascending auditory pathway crosses the midline at several points both below and at the level of the inferior colliculus. However, the input to the central nucleus of the inferior colliculus and higher centres has a clear contralateral dominance. The medial geniculate body is connected reciprocally to the primary auditory cortex, which is located in the superior temporal gyrus, buried in the lateral fissure.

BALANCE

The vestibular sensory pathways are concerned with perception of the position of the head in space and movement of the head. They also

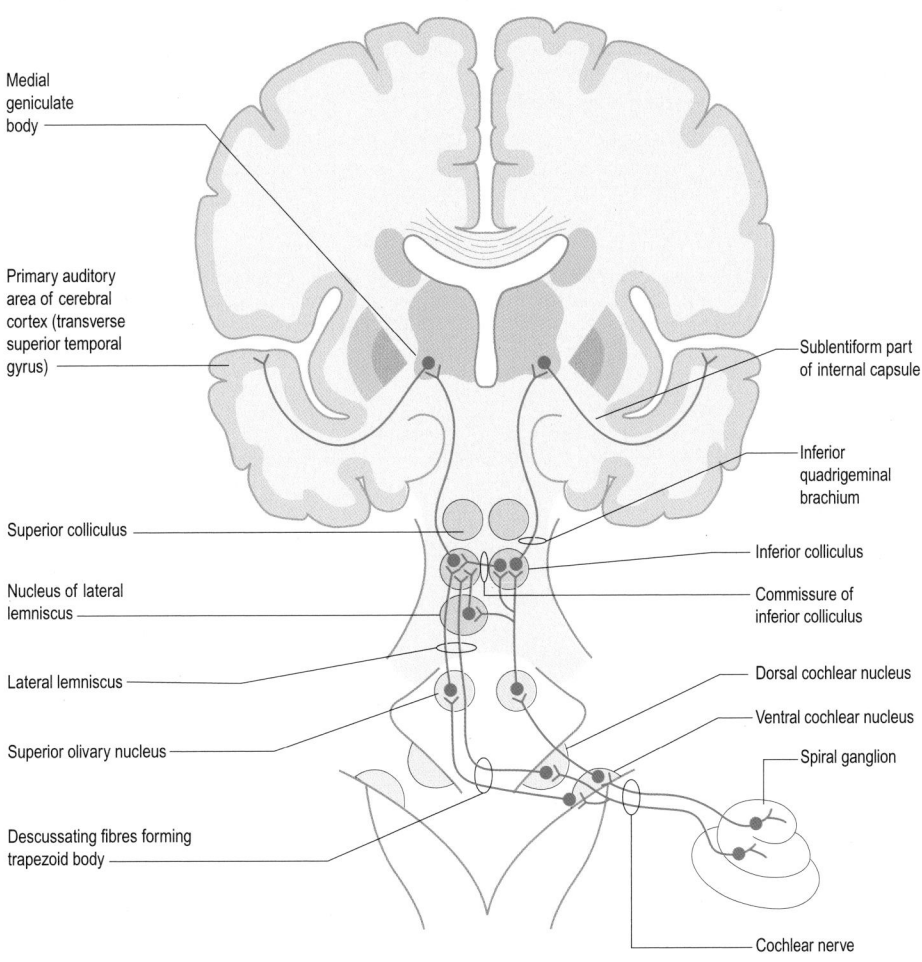

Medial
geniculate
body

Primary auditory
area of cerebral
cortex (transverse
superior temporal
gyrus)

Superior colliculus

Nucleus of lateral
lemniscus

Lateral lemniscus

Superior olivary nucleus

Descussating fibres forming
trapezoid body

Sublentiform part
of internal capsule

Inferior
quadrigeminal
brachium

Inferior colliculus

Commissure of
inferior colliculus

Dorsal cochlear nucleus

Ventral cochlear nucleus

Spiral ganglion

Cochlear nerve

Fig. 24.5 Ascending auditory pathway.

establish important connections for reflex movements governing the equilibrium of the body and the fixity of gaze.

Functionally, the vestibular apparatus is customarily divided into two components. These are the kinetic labyrinth, which provides information about acceleration and deceleration of the head, and the static labyrinth which detects the orientation of the head in relation to the pull of gravity. In terms of structure, the kinetic labyrinth consists of the semicircular canals and their ampullary cristae, while the static labyrinth consists of the maculae of the utricle and saccule. However, the saccular macula also responds to head movements, and both maculae can be stimulated by low frequency sound, and may, therefore, have minor auditory functions.

Angular acceleration and deceleration of the head cause a counterflow of endolymph in the semicircular canals, which deflects the cupola of each crista and bends the stereocilial/kinocilial bundles. This causes a change in the membrane potential of the receptor cell, which is signalled to the brain as a change in the firing frequency of the vestibular nerve afferents (either an increase or a decrease of the basal resting discharge, depending on the direction of stimulation). When a steady velocity of head movement is reached, the endolymph rapidly adopts the same velocity as the surrounding structures because of friction with the canal walls, so that the cupula and receptor cells return to their resting state. Since the three semicircular canals are orientated at right angles to each other, all possible directions of acceleration can be detected. In addition, the labyrinths on both sides of the head provide complementary information which is integrated centrally.

In the maculae, the weight of the otoconial crystals creates a gravitational pull on the otoconial membrane and thus on the stereocilial bundles of the sensory cells which are inserted into its base. Because of this, they are able to detect the static orientation of the head with respect to gravity. They also detect shifts in position according to the extent to which the stereocilia are deflected from the perpendicular. As the two maculae are set at right angles to each other, and the cells of both

maculae are orientated functionally in opposite directions across their striolar boundaries, this system is very sensitive to orientation. Moreover, because the otoconia have a collective inertia/momentum, linear acceleration and deceleration along the anteroposterior axis can be detected by the lag or overshoot of the otoconial membrane with respect to the epithelial surface, and so the saccular macula is able to signal these changes of velocity. Similarly, the macular receptors can be stimulated by low frequency sound which sets up vibratory movements in the otoconial membrane, although this appears to require relatively high sound levels. Efferent synapses on the afferent endings of the type I sensory cells and on the bases of type II cells receive inputs from the brain stem which appear to be inhibitory. They serve to reduce the activity of the afferent fibres either indirectly, in the case of the type I cells, or directly, for the type II cells.

The information gathered by these various receptors is carried to the CNS in the vestibular nerve, which enters the brain stem at the cerebellopontine angle, and terminates in the vestibular nuclear complex. Neurones in this complex project to motor nuclei in the brain stem and upper spinal cord, and to the cerebellum and thalamus. Thalamic efferent projections pass to a cortical vestibular area which is probably located near the intraparietal sulcus in area 2 of the primary somatosensory cortex.

Another major function of the vestibular system is the control of visual reflexes, which allow the fixation of gaze on an object in spite of movements of the head, and require the coordinated movements of the eye, neck and upper trunk. Constant adjustments of the visual axes are achieved chiefly through the medial longitudinal fasciculus, which connects the vestibular nuclear complex with neurones in the oculomotor, trochlear and abducens nuclei and with upper spinal motor neurones (**Fig. 19.21**), and also by the vestibulospinal tracts.

Abnormal activity of the vestibular input or central connections has various effects on these reflexes, e.g. the production of nystagmus. This can be elicited by a clinical test of vestibular function by syringing the external auditory meatus with water above or below body temperature, a procedure which appears to stimulate the cristae of the lateral semi-circular canal directly. Spontaneous high activity in the afferent fibres of the vestibular nerve is seen in Ménière's disease, in which those affected experience a range of disturbances including the sensation of dizziness and nausea, the latter reflecting the vestibular input to the vagal reflex pathway.

REFERENCES

Cagan RH (ed) 1989 Neural Mechanisms in Taste. Boca Raton, FL: CRC Press

Hubel DH 1988 Eye, brain and vision. Scientific American Library Series No. 22

Kandel ER, Schwartz JH, Jessel TM (eds) 2000 Principles of Neural Science, 4th edn. New York; McGraw-Hill

Oertel D, Fay RR, Popper AN (eds) 2002 Integrative Functions in the Mammalian Auditory Pathway. Springer Handbook of Auditory Research, vol. 15. New York: Springer

Zeki S 1993 A Vision of the Brain. Oxford: Blackwell Scientific

HEAD AND NECK

Editors:

Susan Standring (Lead Editor)

Barry KB Berkovitz (Editor)

Carole M Hackney (Editor, chapter 39)

The late Gordon L Ruskell (Editor, chapters 41, 42)

Patricia Collins (Embryology, Growth and Development)

Caroline Wigley (Microstructure)

With specialist contributions on clinical and functional anatomy by

Martin E Atkinson (chapter 36), **Simon A Hickey** (32, 35, 36, 38, 39), **John D Langdon** (25, 27, 29–31, 33–35), **Daniel E Lieberman** (27), **V Mahadev** (29), **BJ Moxham** (27, 33), **Jeff Osborn** (30), and **Allan Thexton** (30, 35)

Critical reviewers:

Paul Cartwright (chapter 25), **Michael Dilkes** (31), **Peter Morgan** (29 & 33), **BJ Moxham** (30)

Surface anatomy of the head and neck

To avoid repetition, additional information related to clinical and surgical anatomy is provided in the appropriate chapters in this section.

HEAD

SKELETAL SURFACE LANDMARKS (Figs 25.1, 25.2)

The skeletal surface landmarks of the head can be examined from the back, from the side and from the front. The palpable bony landmarks of the calvarium are visible in bald people but more commonly they have to be palpated through the hair. The anterior fontanelle, at the junction of the coronal and sagittal sutures, may be palpated until c.18 months after birth.

Most of the superficial aspect of the skull is covered by skin, subcutaneous tissue and thin muscles, and so it is relatively easy to feel the bony prominences and surfaces. The pericraniocervical line demarcates the head from the neck. It runs from the midpoint of the chin anteriorly to the external occipital protuberance posteriorly. Starting anteriorly from the midline, where the mental tubercles may be felt, the lower border of the body of the mandible may be traced to the mandibular angle (the angle is often everted in the male, incurved in the female). An oblique line joins the mental tubercle to the lower end of the anterior border of the ramus of the mandible. The teeth can be easily felt (when present) by palpating the superior border of the body of the mandible through the cheek. The mental foramen, which transmits the mental nerve and vessels, lies below the level of the premolar teeth, c.2 fingers' breadth from the median plane and c.1 finger's breadth above the lower border of the mandible. It is worth noting that the supraorbital, infraorbital and mental foramina all lie in approximately the same vertical plane.

The posterior border of the ramus of the mandible may be palpated up to the neck of the condylar process, which lies just under the lobule of the ear. The ramus is easily palpable, although mostly covered by masseter. With the mouth loosely open, the mandibular notch between condylar and coronoid processes can be felt through masseter. As the mouth is opened and closed, articulation at the temporomandibular joint may be appreciated as the condylar process slides up and down the articular eminence of the temporal bone; anteriorly the coronoid process can be felt to move from its resting position under the zygomatic arch as the mouth is opened. A finger probing inwards just behind

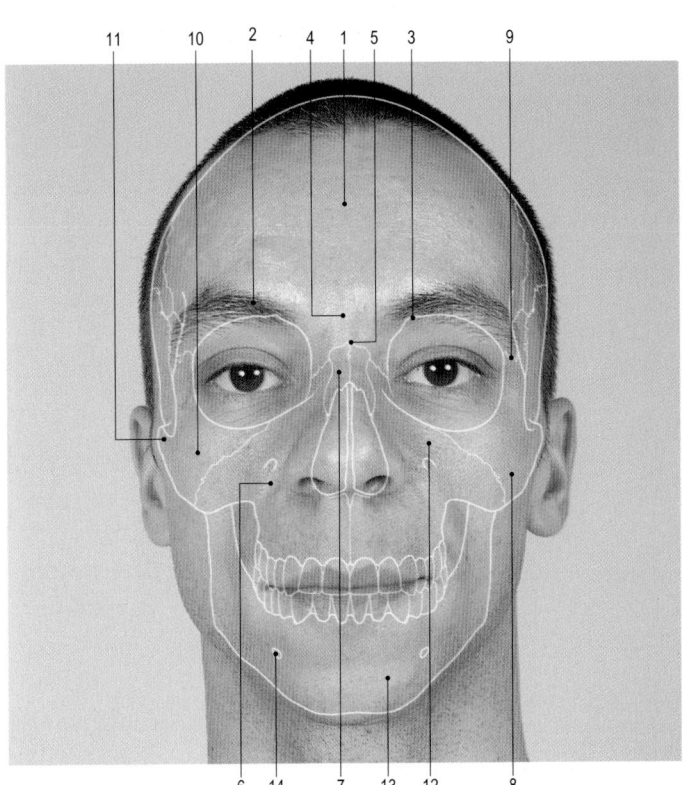

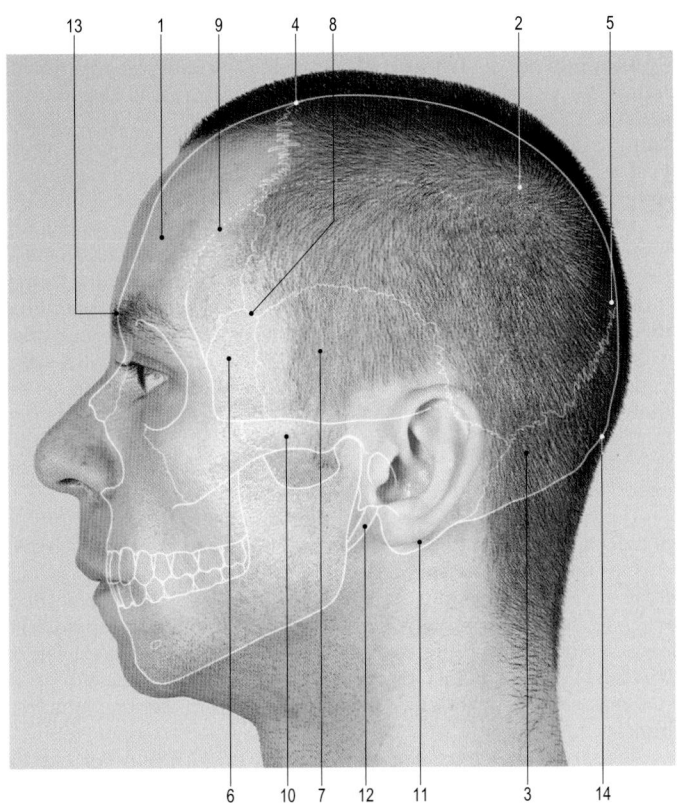

1. Frontal bone. **2.** Superciliary arch. **3.** Supraorbital notch. **4.** Glabella. **5.** Nasion.
6. Maxilla. **7.** Nasal bone. **8.** Zygomatic bone. **9.** Frontozygomatic suture.
10. Prominence of cheek. **11.** Zygomatic arch. **12.** Infraorbital foramen. **13.** Mandible.
14. Mental foramen.

Fig. 25.1 Anterior aspect of the head: bones. (Photograph by Sarah-Jane Smith. Artwork modified from Lumley JSP 2002 Surface Anatomy, 3rd edn. Edinburgh: Churchill Livingstone.)

1. Frontal. **2.** Parietal. **3.** Occipital. **4.** Bregma (anterior fontanelle).
5. Lambda (posterior fontanelle). **6.** Greater wing of sphenoid. **7.** Squamous temporal.
8. Pterion. **9.** Temporal lines. **10.** Zygomatic arch. **11.** Mastoid process.
12. Styloid process. **13.** Glabella. **14.** External occipital protruberance.

Fig. 25.2 Lateral aspect of the head: bones. (Photograph by Sarah-Jane Smith. Artwork modified from Lumley JSP 2002 Surface Anatomy, 3rd edn. Edinburgh: Churchill Livingstone.)

the condylar process enters the small retromandibular fossa where, anteriorly, the mandibular neck, and superiorly, the inferior wall of the external acoustic meatus, may be felt. The meatus is bounded anteriorly by the tragus, a small curved flap that partly projects over the orifice of the meatus. Palpating behind the meatus, first the anterolateral aspect and tip of the mastoid process, and, on deeper palpation, a somewhat indistinct resistance offered by the styloid process and its attached structures, will be encountered. If the examining finger is then taken posteriorly over the convexity of the mastoid process, the lateral part of the superior nuchal line is felt. This curves upwards to meet the contralateral superior nuchal line at a bony midline prominence, the external occipital protuberance, which is an important surface marking for the confluence of the underlying dural venous sinuses.

The lateral aspect of the face consists of the temporal region above, the cheek in the middle, and the lower jaw below. The temporal region lies in front of the external ear and above the zygomatic arch. It is demarcated superiorly by the temporal lines, which indicate the upper limit of temporalis. The temporal lines (superior and inferior) curve downwards anteriorly and posteriorly and help to delineate the temporal fossa. Below, the temporal fossa is bounded laterally by the zygomatic arch, which consists of the zygomatic process of the temporal bone behind and the temporal process of the zygomatic bone in front. The body of the zygomatic bone, which accounts for the variably prominent 'cheekbone', forms the anterior part of the arch. If the sharp posterior margin of the frontal process of the zygomatic bone is followed upwards, it fuses with the zygomatic process of the frontal bone. Continuing posteriorly, in the line of a gentle arch, the temporal lines may be palpated. The lower temporal line terminates by curving downwards and forwards to end just above the root of the mastoid process as the supramastoid crest on the squamous part of the temporal bone. The pterion is a small circular area within the temporal fossa which contains the junction of the frontal, sphenoid, parietal and temporal sutures. It usually lies 4 cm above the zygomatic arch and 3.5 cm behind the frontozygomatic suture, and marks the anterior branch of the middle meningeal artery and the Sylvian point of the brain. Its position can be estimated roughly by a shallow palpable hollow, c.3.5 cm above the centre of the zygomatic bone.

The prominence of the cheek is formed by the underlying zygomatic bone. The suprameatal triangle lies above and behind the external acoustic meatus and overlies the lateral wall of the mastoid (tympanic) antrum. It is bounded above by the supramastoid crest, in front by the posterosuperior margin of the meatus, and behind by a vertical tangent to the posterior border of the meatus.

The forehead extends from the hair margin of the scalp to the eyebrows. The superciliary arch is usually palpable above the orbit and is better marked in the male than the female. Above it the rounded frontal tuberosity may be felt c.3 cm above the midpoint of each supraorbital margin. Between the superciliary arches there is a small horizontal ridge called the glabella, again easily palpable. Below the glabella the nasal bones meet the frontal bone in a small depression, the nasion, at the root of the nose. With a little finger inserted into the nostril, the bony margins of the anterior nasal aperture can be felt: they are formed by the inferior border of the nasal bone, the sharp margins of the nasal notch, and the coapted nasal spines of the maxillae.

The orbital opening is somewhat quadrangular. The supraorbital margin is formed entirely by the frontal bone and is easily palpable. At the junction of its sharp lateral two-thirds and rounded medial third (c.2 fingers' breadth from the median plane) the supraorbital notch, if present, may be felt. This notch transmits the supraorbital nerve and vessels, and pressure exerted here with the fingernail can be painful. A frontal notch may also be found towards the bridge of the nose and is associated with the supratrochlear neurovascular bundle.

The lateral margin of the orbit consists of the frontal process of the zygomatic bone and the zygomatic process of the frontal bone. The frontozygomatic suture between them may be felt as a palpable depression. Approximately 1 cm below this suture a tubercle (Whitnall's tubercle) may be palpated within the orbital opening: it gives attachment to the lateral palpebral and cheek ligaments. The inferior border of the orbit is formed by the zygomatic bone laterally and the maxilla medially. It blends into the less obvious medial margin formed above by the frontal bone and below by the lacrimal crest of the frontal process of the maxilla. A shallow fossa behind the lower part of the medial wall houses the nasolacrimal sac. The infraorbital foramen, which transmits the infraorbital nerve and vessels, lies c.0.5 cm below the

infraorbital margin, a finger's breadth from the side of the nose and above the canine fossa.

The anterior surface of the maxilla is extensive and may be palpated between the infraorbital margin and the alveolar processes that bear the upper teeth (when present). The canine eminence overlies the roots of the canine tooth and separates the incisive fossa anteriorly from the deeper canine fossa posteriorly. The palatine process of the maxilla (which forms the greater part of the roof of the mouth) is easily palpable within the mouth.

UNDERLYING SOFT TISSUES AND VISCERA

The muscular, fatty and cutaneous features which so clearly differentiate individuals are readily apparent on inspection. The external features of the eyelids and eyebrows are described on page 681. The tympanic membrane may be examined under direct vision using an auroscope. The retinal vascular supply may be examined directly by ophthalmoscopy (p. 716).

Two important masticatory muscles are palpable when the jaw is clenched, but are difficult to define when relaxed (**Fig. 25.3**). Temporalis, which lies in the temporal fossa and is covered by the temporal fascia, is palpable if the flat of the hand is placed on the side of the head and the jaw is clenched and unclenched. Masseter is similarly easily palpable with the jaw clenched, when its anterior border stands out. The palatine tonsil can be represented by an oval area over the lower part of masseter, just above and in front of the angle of the mandible.

The parotid gland is soft and indistinct and lies largely below the external acoustic meatus, wedged between the ramus of the mandible, the mastoid process and sternocleidomastoid (**Fig. 25.4**). The anterior border of the gland is represented by a line descending from the mandibular condyle to a point just above the middle of the masseter and then to a point c.2 cm below and behind the angle of the mandible. Its concave upper border corresponds to a curve traced from the mandibular

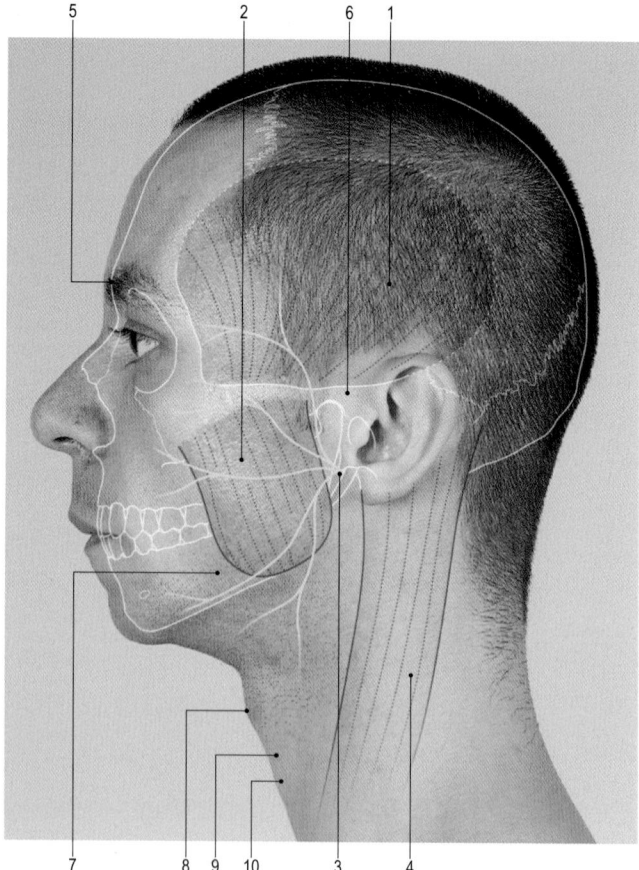

1. Temporalis. **2.** Masseter. **3.** Divisions of the facial nerve. **4.** Sternocleidomastoid.
5. Glabella. **6.** Pulse of superficial temporal artery. **7.** Pulse of facial artery.
8. Laryngeal prominence. **9.** Anterior (median) cricothyroid ligament. **10.** Cricoid cartilage.

Fig. 25.3 Lateral aspect of the head and neck: soft tissues. (Photograph by Sarah-Jane Smith. Artwork modified from Lumley JSP 2002 Surface Anatomy, 3rd edn. Edinburgh: Churchill Livingstone.)

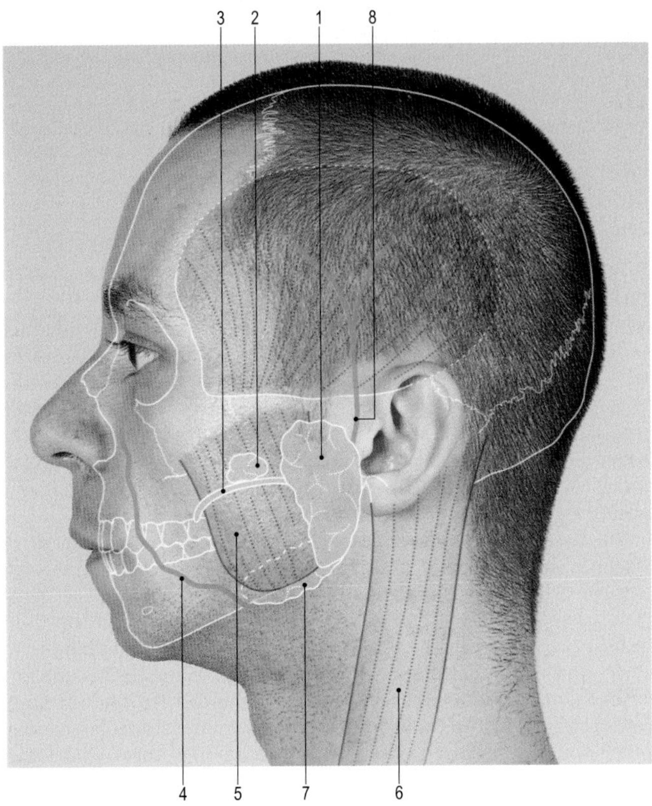

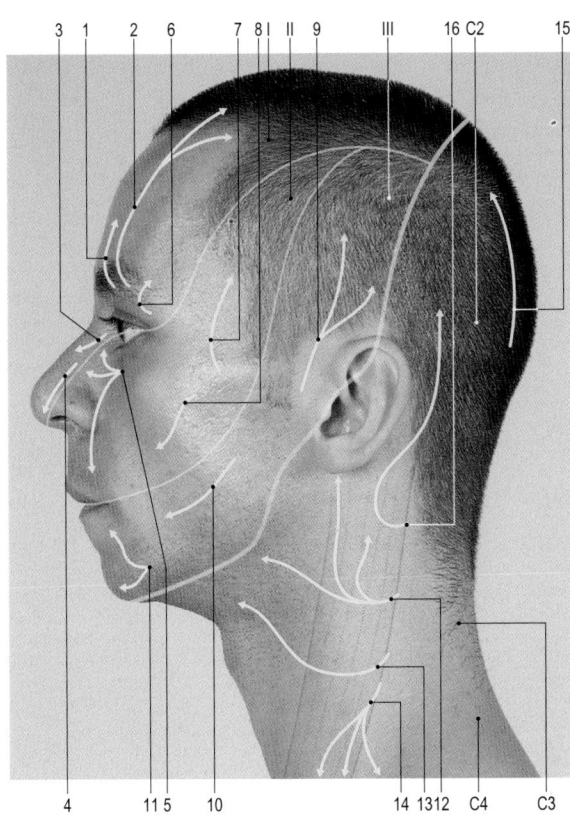

1. Parotid gland. **2.** Accessory part of parotid gland. **3.** Parotid duct. **4.** Facial artery.
5. Masseter. **6.** Sternocleidomastoid. **7.** Submandibular gland. **8.** Superficial temporal artery.

Fig. 25.4 Parotid gland. (Photograph by Sarah-Jane Smith. Artwork modified from Lumley JSP 2002 Surface Anatomy, 3rd edn. Edinburgh: Churchill Livingstone.)

1. Supratrochlear. **2.** Supraorbital. **3.** Infratrochlear. **4.** External nasal.
5. Infraorbital. **6.** Lacrimal. **7.** Zygomaticotemporal. **8.** Zygomaticofacial.
9. Auriculotemporal. **10.** Buccal. **11.** Mental. **12.** Greater auricular.
13. Transverse cervical. **14.** Supraclavicular. **15.** Greater occipital.
16. Lesser occipital. I, II, III Ophthalmic, maxillary and mandibular divisions of the trigeminal nerve.

Fig. 25.5 Cutaneous innervation of the head and neck. (Photograph by Sarah-Jane Smith. Artwork modified from Lumley JSP 2002 Surface Anatomy, 3rd edn. Edinburgh: Churchill Livingstone.)

condyle across the lobule of the ear to the mastoid process. The posterior border corresponds to a line drawn between the posterior ends of the anterior and upper borders. The parotid duct arises from the gland just above half-way along its anterior margin. It runs over masseter to its anterior border where it bends sharply to pierce the underlying buccinator. The orifice of the duct is visible as a small papilla within the cheek opposite the second upper molar tooth. The duct can be represented by the middle third of a line drawn from the lower border of the tragus of the auricle to a point midway between the ala of the nose and labial margin of the upper lip. It can be felt on the face (or more easily in the vestibule of the mouth) and rolled on the anterior border of masseter by pressing the finger backwards on it (preferably with the teeth clenched, to tense masseter).

With the mouth open it is possible to examine all the teeth and the palatine tonsils (when present), and to inspect and palpate the orifice of the parotid duct. The tongue may be examined for its general appearance and any abnormalities of movement, which may reflect neuronal damage.

Course of vessels

Two main arteries, the facial and superficial temporal arteries, can be palpated on the face (**Fig. 25.4**). The pulsation of the facial artery can be felt as it crosses the lower margin of the body of the mandible immediately in front of masseter and again just over a centimetre from the angle of the mouth, between a finger placed within the mouth and a thumb placed on the skin surface. If the lateral part of the lip is gripped in a similar manner the pulsation of the labial artery can be felt beneath the mucous surface c.0.5 cm from the free margin of the lip. The facial artery subsequently runs a tortuous course towards the medial corner of the eye.

The superficial temporal artery arises within the parotid gland and passes upwards across the zygomatic process of the temporal bone, immediately in front of the tragus of the auricle. Compression at this point allows palpation of a superficial temporal pulse. This is of special value during anaesthesia when access to the patient is frequently restricted to the head. The artery branches into frontal and parietal divisions c.2.5 cm above the zygomatic arch.

Course of nerves (Fig. 25.5)

The facial nerve exits the skull at the stylomastoid foramen and therefore is deep to the posterior margin of the external acoustic meatus. The surface marking of the cranial exit of the facial nerve is a point immediately in front of the intertragic notch (situated between the tragus and the antitragus of the auricle). From here the nerve crosses the styloid process to enter the substance of the parotid salivary gland, where it divides into five main branches which radiate out across the face (p. 514). The distribution of the trigeminal dermatomes is described on page 512.

NECK

SKELETAL SURFACE LANDMARKS (Fig. 25.6)

The superior limit of the neck is the pericraniocervical line. Inferiorly the neck blends with the thorax and upper limb at the level of the clavicle and scapula. Several skeletal features are easily palpable. At the back of the neck the cervical vertebrae may be felt in the midline. The transverse process of the first cervical vertebra (atlas) may be palpated in the uppermost part of the neck, in the hollow between the mastoid process of the temporal bone and the external ear. Just below, the transverse process of the second cervical vertebra (axis) can be felt on deep palpation. Inferiorly the spine of the seventh cervical vertebra (vertebra prominens) is especially prominent, particularly when the neck is flexed. The remaining cervical spines are indistinct because they are covered by the ligamentum nuchae, which separates the postvertebral musculature on both sides. However, the spines of the second, fifth and sixth cervical vertebrae may be felt on deeper palpation. The hyoid bone may be felt a few centimetres below and behind the chin, especially if the neck is extended. It may be palpated between finger and thumb and moved from side to side. The hyoid bone lies approximately at the level of the third cervical vertebra. The most obvious palpable feature in the front of the neck below the hyoid bone is the thyroid

443

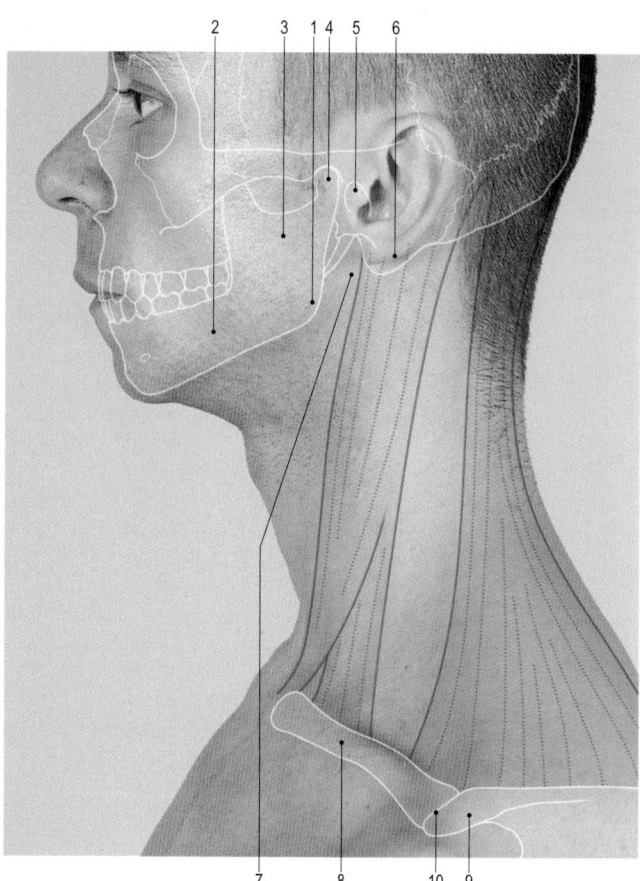

1. Angle of mandible. 2. Body of mandible. 3. Ramus of mandible.
4. Temporomandibular joint. 5. External acoustic meatus. 6. Mastoid process.
7. Tip of transverse process of atlas. 8. Clavicle. 9. Acromion. 10. Acromioclavicular joint.

Fig. 25.6 Lateral aspect of the head and neck. (Photograph by Sarah-Jane Smith. Artwork modified from Lumley JSP 2002 Surface Anatomy, 3rd edn. Edinburgh: Churchill Livingstone.)

cartilage, and the prominent midline subcutaneous laryngeal prominence or Adam's apple, which indicates the line of fusion of the two thyroid laminae. In the male, the prominence is usually clearly visible, whereas in the female it is not usually apparent, even when the neck is viewed from the side. The curved upper border of the thyroid cartilage and the thyroid notch are easily palpable. The middle part of the thyroid cartilage lies at the level of the fifth cervical vertebra. The anterior arch of the cricoid cartilage can be felt below the inferior border of the thyroid cartilage. The cricoid cartilage lies at the level of the sixth cervical vertebra. The groove between the thyroid and cricoid cartilages, filled by the anterior (median) cricothyroid ligament, is a useful site for emergency access to the airway if there is obstruction at or above the vocal cords (cricothyroid puncture). In the child the laryngeal structures lie at a higher level.

The trachea can be palpated inferior to the cricoid cartilage. It normally lies in the midline but may be deviated by disease. The upper tracheal cartilages may be impalpable if they are covered by the thyroid isthmus, which joins the two lobes of the gland across the midline of the neck.

The clavicle is a sigmoid-shaped bone which is easily visible in thin people and palpable in all except the morbidly obese. Its medial two-thirds are rounded and convex forwards and the lateral third is flat and concave forwards. The suprasternal (jugular) notch lies between the medial expanded ends of the clavicles: its inferior border is the superior edge of the manubrium sterni. For much of its length the clavicle may be almost encircled by two fingers, but medially its massive ligamentous attachments make definition more difficult. The posterior end of the first rib may sometimes be felt rather indistinctly as it lies in the supraclavicular fossa in the root of the neck, between sternocleidomastoid and trapezius and above the clavicle.

It should be remembered that the head and neck are extremely mobile but, with the head held in the anatomical position, the following vertebral levels should be noted:

C1	Dens, level of nasopharynx
C2	Level of oropharynx and dependent soft palate with the mouth open
C3	Level of body of hyoid and its greater cornu
C3–4 junction	Level of upper border of thyroid cartilage and bifurcation of common carotid artery
C4–5	Level of thyroid cartilage
C6	Level of cricoid cartilage

UNDERLYING SOFT TISSUES AND VISCERA

From the front and side (**Fig. 25.7**) the neck is obviously divided into two major portions by sternocleidomastoid. These are the anterior and posterior cervical triangles, both of which may be subdivided. The anterior cervical triangle may be divided into a submental triangle, a muscular triangle, a carotid triangle and a digastric triangle. The posterior cervical triangle may be split into the occipital triangle and the supraclavicular triangle. The structures that form the boundaries of some of the lesser triangles are not readily palpable or visible.

The base of the anterior triangle is formed by the base of the mandible and a line from its angle to the mastoid process, and the sides are formed by the midline anteriorly and the anterior edge of sternocleidomastoid laterally. The triangle is best inspected from the front, but best examined bimanually with the examiner standing behind the subject and using the fingers of both hands to examine the structures within the triangle. Inspection reveals the rounded tendinous oblique head of sternocleidomastoid, which arises from the superolateral angle of the manubrium, and the more vertical muscular portion, which arises from the upper surface of the medial third of the clavicle. Between these two heads there is usually a hollow in which the internal jugular vein lies just before it joins the subclavian vein posterior to the clavicle.

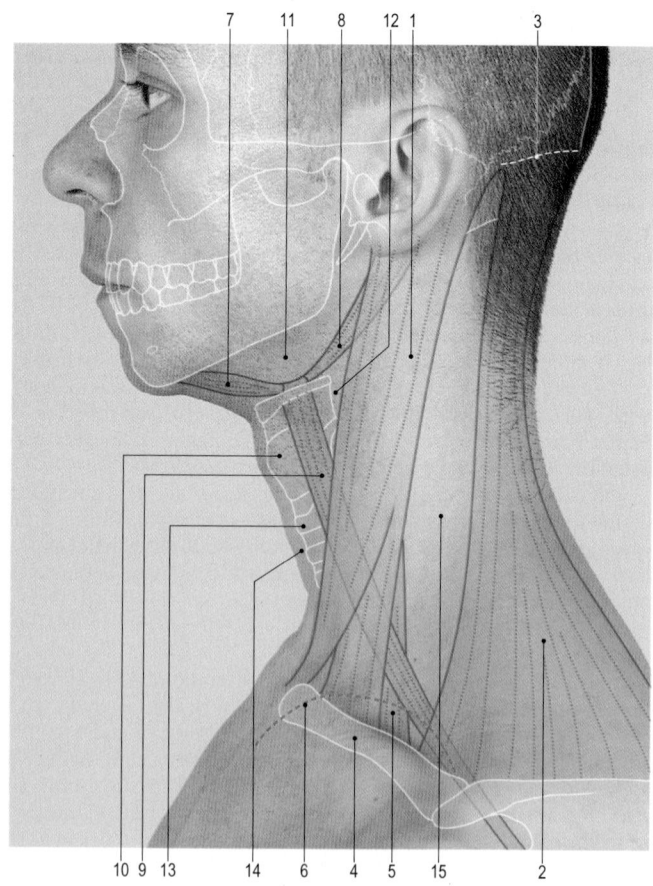

1. Sternocleidomastoid. 2. Trapezius. 3. Superior nuchal line. 4. Clavicle.
5. Scalenus anterior. 6. Apex of lung. 7. Anterior belly of digastric.
8. Posterior belly of digastric. 9. Omohyoid. 10. Thyroid cartilage. 11. Digastric triangle.
12. Carotid triangle. 13. Cricoid cartilage. 14. Muscular triangle. 15. Posterior triangle.

Fig. 25.7 Anterior and posterior triangles of the neck. (Photograph by Sarah-Jane Smith. Artwork modified from Lumley JSP 2002 Surface Anatomy, 3rd edn. Edinburgh: Churchill Livingstone.)

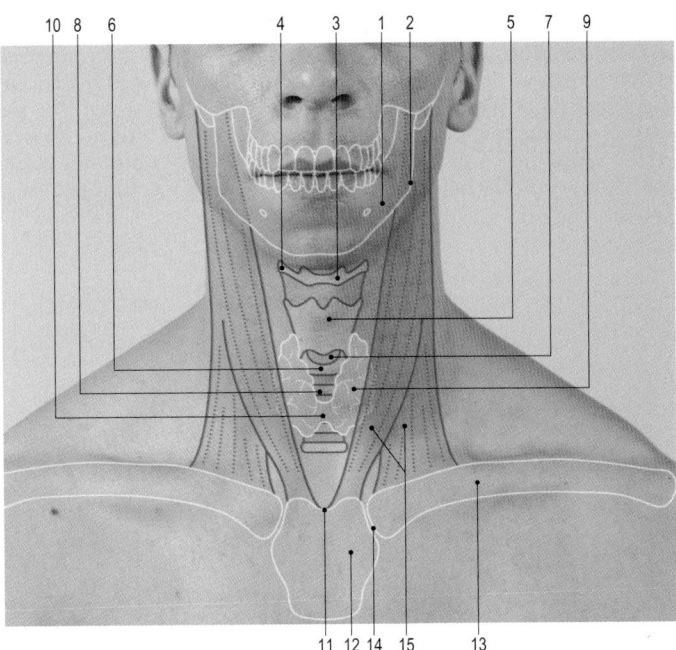

1. Body of mandible.   **2.** Angle of mandible.   **3.** Body of hyoid bone.
4. Greater horn of hyoid bone.   **5.** Thyroid cartilage.   **6.** Cricoid cartilage.
7. Anterior (median) cricothyroid ligament.   **8.** First tracheal ring.
9. Lobe of the thyroid gland.   **10.** Isthmus of thyroid gland.   **11.** Sternal notch.
12. Manubrium.   **13.** Clavicle.   **14.** Sternoclavicular joint.
15. Sternocleidomastoid – sternal and clavicular heads.

Fig. 25.8 Anterior aspect of the neck: bones and muscles; larynx and thyroid gland. (Photograph by Sarah-Jane Smith. Artwork modified from Lumley JSP 2002 Surface Anatomy, 3rd edn. Edinburgh: Churchill Livingstone.)

The trachea and its cartilaginous 'rings' can be palpated inferior to the cricoid cartilage. If the examining finger is moved laterally, the lobes of the thyroid gland may be felt, particularly if the subject is asked to swallow. The thyroid gland consists of two lobes lying either side of the thyroid cartilage and joined in the midline of the neck by an isthmus (**Fig. 25.8**). The upper border of each lobe lies alongside the lower half of the lamina of the cartilage. The lower border reaches towards the sternal end of the clavicle. The isthmus, c.2 cm wide, lies in front of the trachea just below the cricoid cartilage and usually overlies the second and third tracheal 'rings'.

Taken superiorly, an examining finger will enter either the submental or submandibular triangle, in which enlarged lymph nodes or salivary glands may be felt. The submandibular gland extends c.2 cm beneath the lower border of the mandible and reaches the approximate level of the hyoid bone. Its posterior border is level with the angle of the mandible; its anterior border extends forwards c.4 cm.

It should be noted that above the hyoid bone the musculature runs in a predominantly horizontal or oblique direction, and below the hyoid it runs in a vertical direction. Lymph nodes above the hyoid bone tend to be disposed in a horizontal plane and lie mainly just below the pericraniocervical line, whereas the deep cervical nodes run vertically and are related to the internal jugular vein. Apart from a few retrovisceral nodes and some deep to sternocleidomastoid, members of all of the groups of lymph nodes in the head and neck are clinically palpable when enlarged.

The boundaries of the posterior triangle are the posterior border of sternocleidomastoid, the middle third of the superior surface of the clavicle, which forms the base, and the anterior margin of trapezius. The apex is the point where sternocleidomastoid and trapezius approximate to each other at the superior nuchal line. The lower portion of the posterior triangle forms the supraclavicular fossa, a very important clinical area, which lies just above and behind the clavicle at the confluence of the thoracic inlet and the aditus to the axilla and arm. It is better inspected from in front, but palpated from behind, when a right-handed examiner stands behind and to the right of the subject. When inspecting the supraclavicular fossa, the pulsation of the great veins may be seen if the central venous pressure is raised. The external jugular vein, a prominent feature, may be distended due to kinking, raised venous pressure or

obstruction. The supraclavicular fossa is a common site in which to feel pathologically enlarged lymph nodes. In particular, cancers of the upper gastrointestinal tract and of the lung frequently spread to the supraclavicular group of nodes. The posterior end of the first rib may be felt as a fullness in the posterior aspect of the fossa. The subclavian artery can be felt pulsating as it crosses the first rib, and the trunks of the brachial plexus may be felt above and behind it. A point c.2.5 cm above the middle of the medial third of the clavicle marks the level of the neck of the first rib and thus the surface marking for the apex of the dome of the cervical pleura and lung.

Course of vessels

In the neck, the common carotid artery and its continuation, the internal carotid artery, may be represented by a more or less straight line from the sternoclavicular joint to a point just behind the condyle of the mandible. At the level of the upper border of the thyroid cartilage (approximately at a level between the third and fourth cervical vertebrae) the common carotid artery divides into the external and internal carotid arteries. The transverse process of the sixth cervical vertebra is prominent (Chassaignac's tubercle), and the common carotid artery may be compressed here. Above this level the artery is superficial and its pulsation can be readily felt beneath the anterior border of sternocleidomastoid. The pulse is produced as much by the roots of the main branches as it is by the internal and external carotid arteries themselves, and this is therefore one of the prime sites in the body to feel for a pulse.

The subclavian artery enters the root of the neck behind the sternoclavicular joint. It arches upwards to reach a point c.2 cm above the clavicle deep to the posterior border of sternocleidomastoid, and then passes across the upper surface of the first rib behind the middle region of the clavicle. A pulse may be felt at this point when the artery is compressed against the first rib.

The anterior jugular vein runs downwards beneath the chin approximately a finger's breadth from the midline. It turns laterally c.2.5 cm from the sternal end of the clavicle and passes beneath sternocleidomastoid to drain into the external jugular vein. The veins of each side join to form a jugular arch just above the manubrium sterni.

The external jugular vein lies superficial to sternocleidomastoid and can be represented by a line which starts just below and behind the angle of the mandible and runs down to the clavicle near the posterior border of sternocleidomastoid (**Fig. 29.8**). It drains into the subclavian vein after penetrating the investing layer of deep cervical fascia. The vein may be kinked at this point. If the proximal part of the vein is damaged it may be held open by the surrounding fascia: air can then be sucked in, resulting in an air embolus. The external jugular vein can be distended if venous pressure is raised, e.g. by performing Valsalva's manoeuvre (forced expiration against a closed mouth and blocked nostrils) or by supraclavicular digital pressure.

The internal jugular vein runs in the carotid sheath, lying just lateral to the arteries. It therefore has similar surface markings to those described for the common and internal arteries and is represented in surface projection by a broad band from the lobule of the ear to the medial end of the clavicle, where it joins the subclavian vein. The inferior bulb of the internal jugular vein lies in the lesser supraclavicular fossa (the depression between the sternal and clavicular heads of sternocleidomastoid): this site is one of several at which the internal jugular vein may be accessed for central vein cannulation (see p. 948). Pulsation of the great veins may be seen in this region if the central venous pressure is raised.

The subclavian vein runs just below the subclavian artery.

Course of nerves

The course of the spinal accessory nerve can be indicated by a line that crosses the floor of the posterior triangle passing from the tragus of the auricle to the junction of the lower and middle thirds of the anterior border of trapezius. This line will also cross the (palpable) transverse process of the atlas c.1 cm below the mastoid process and the junction of the upper and middle thirds of the posterior border of sternocleidomastoid. The sensory nerves of the cervical plexus, which supply the skin of the neck, emerge from behind the posterior border of sternocleidomastoid just below the spinal accessory nerve (**Fig. 25.5**). The roots and trunks of the brachial plexus can be represented by a line passing between the middle of the posterior border of sternocleidomastoid and the middle of the clavicle. With the head held to the opposite side, the upper trunk of the plexus is palpable. The trunks lie above and behind the subclavian artery. The divisions of the brachial plexus are situated behind the clavicle near the lateral border of the first rib.

The cervical sympathetic chain has three ganglia and lies at the side of the neck behind the common and internal carotid arteries. The superior cervical ganglion lies slightly anterior to the (palpable) transverse process of the second cervical vertebra, while the middle cervical ganglion lies just in front of the transverse process of the sixth cervical vertebra (which is difficult to palpate). The inferior cervical ganglion may be fused with the first thoracic cervical ganglion, forming the stellate ganglion. Stellate ganglion block is often employed to perform a sympathetic nerve block to the head and neck, or to the arm: the surface marking is approximately at the level of the transverse process of the seventh cervical vertebra (situated two finger's breadths above the sterno-clavicular joint when the neck is fully extended) (Ellis & Feldman, 1997).

Overview of the development of the head and neck

Head development is distinct from that of the trunk, utilizing region-specific genes, signalling mechanisms and morphogenetic processes. Evolution of the vertebrate head was made possible by the origin of a novel cell population, the neural crest (Gans & Northcutt 1983). Cranial neural crest cells emigrate from the neural folds before cranial neurulation is complete, and also differ from those of the trunk in having the potential to form connective and skeletal tissues; they make major contributions to the skull. Sensory placodes form the nasal pits, the lens, and the otocyst. These are areas in which the otherwise squamous epithelium develops a pseudostratified structure before undergoing morphogenesis to form a pit and then (for the lens and otic pits) a closed cyst. Epibranchial placodes are similar pseudostratified epithelial thickenings within the proximal ectoderm of each pharyngeal arch; they contribute cells by epithelial-mesenchymal transformation to underlying neural crest cell condensations to form the cranial sensory ganglia (there is no functional difference between the ganglion cells of each origin).

Three separate populations of neural crest cells migrate from the cranial neural folds (**Fig. 26.5**). The first of these populations originates from the diencephalic region of the forebrain, the midbrain, and the first two rhombomeres of the hindbrain. They migrate to surround the telencephalon and nasal region (frontonasal mesenchyme), and the maxillary and mandibular regions of the first arch (Jiang et al., 2002). The other two populations contribute anterior neck structures. They migrate from rhombomeres 3-8, into the second and subsequent pharyngeal arches (**Fig. 26.5**). The segmental organization of the embryonic head caudal to rhombomere 2 is related to the expression of evolutionarily conserved *HOX* genes in the rhombomeres and their derived neural crest.

THE SKULL

The skull is composed of the neurocranium, which surrounds the brain, eyes and inner plus middle ears, and the viscerocranium, which is derived from the frontonasal and first arch mesenchyme and forms the facial skeleton. The whole of the viscerocranium is neural crest-derived; the neurocranium (skull vault and the skull base) is derived from mesenchyme of both neural crest and mesodermal origin. Bone anlagen first form as mesenchymal condensations, which may either ossify directly (intramembranous ossification) or via a cartilaginous precursor (endochondral ossification). There is no correspondence between the tissue origin and the type of ossification process. The neural crest- and mesoderm-derived components of the skull vault both form by intramembranous ossification, corresponding to the dermal bones that protect the brain of ancestral fishes. Similarly, tissues of both origins contribute to the endochondral skull base. (For details of skull development, see Chapter 28.)

THE EMBRYONIC PHARYNX

The embryonic pharynx forms the template for the future face (except for the nasal region, which is derived from frontonasal mesenchyme), palate, and anterior neck structures. Its development from neural crest, surface ectoderm and foregut endoderm involves spatiotemporal integration of cell movement, tissue growth and tissue interactions.

PHARYNGEAL APPARATUS (Figs 26.1, 26.2, 26.3, 26.4)

After head fold formation, the stomodeum, or primitive mouth, lies between the maxillary and mandibular parts of the first pharyngeal arch; these are bounded rostrally by the projecting forebrain and caudally by the cardiac prominence (**Fig. 26.1**). The neck, which will subsequently intervene between the developing jaws and thorax, is absent: it is formed later by modification of the second and subsequent pairs of branchial (pharyngeal) arches anteriorly and the neural tube and somite-derived structures posteriorly (**Figs 26.2, 26.3, 26.4**), and by descent of the heart. There are five pairs of pharyngeal arches in mammals, numbered 1,2,3,4, and 6 by analogy with their evolutionary origin, the fifth arch having been lost. In the earliest jawless vertebrates (Agnatha), the branchial arches were a uniform series of bars behind the gill clefts. However, long before the evolution of the terrestrial vertebrates remarkable adaptations occurred. Structures commonly regarded as the first pair of arches became the upper and lower jaws of the jaw-bearing vertebrates (Gnathostomata).

The term 'mandibular arch' is widely used to describe the first arch but is not entirely appropriate because numerous maxillofacial and palatopharyngeal structures are derived from its proximal end. (The evolutionary origin of the jaws is currently controversial, but some authorities suggest that the trabeculae cranii, probably represented by the interorbitonasal cartilage of the human embryo, are derived from a pair of ancestral premandibular skeletal structures.) The second branchial arch is the hyoid arch, whose skeletal derivatives form the varied hyoid elements present in all jawed vertebrates. The most dorsal of these elements, the hyomandibula, is already present in cartilaginous fishes as a strut between the skull and the jaw joint: it reduces the cleft between the mandibular and hyoid arches to a small opening, the spiracle. Further evolution of this region occurred in land animals in connection with the auditory apparatus.

At first the arches produce rounded ridge-like prominences of both the overlying ectoderm and of the endodermal lining of the lateral walls and floor of the pharynx. Ectoderm and endoderm are in virtual contact in the depressions between these prominences, i.e. the ectodermal clefts and endodermal pouches. The thin membranes so formed break down permanently in gill-breathing vertebrates, and transiently in reptile embryos, but persist in mammals, in which open channels or 'true clefts' are not formed. The region of the embryo which contains the rostral foregut surrounded by mesenchyme and ectoderm of the branchial arches constitutes the embryonic pharynx, and the stage of development at which the arches are prominent has been termed the pharyngula stage (p. 206). The first arch, which forms most of the face, is composed largely of ectoderm, both on the outer and inner surfaces and within the arch (neural crest mesenchyme). Technically speaking therefore, the first arch is not a pharyngeal structure, unlike the subsequent arches which are composed of ectoderm externally, pharyngeal endoderm internally and neural crest mesenchyme within the arches. The arch musculature is mesodermal in origin.

Since the term "branchial" means "of the gills", the term "pharyngeal arch" will be used in the following account of human embryology.

In general, each pharyngeal arch consists of a mesenchymal core covered by epithelium (**Figs 26.2, 26.3**). The latter may be entirely ectodermal (as in the first arch), or ectodermal externally and endodermal internally (as in the remaining arches). The mesenchymal core is derived from neural crest, paraxial mesoderm and angiogenic mesenchyme, which give rise to region-specific structures. Consequently each

A

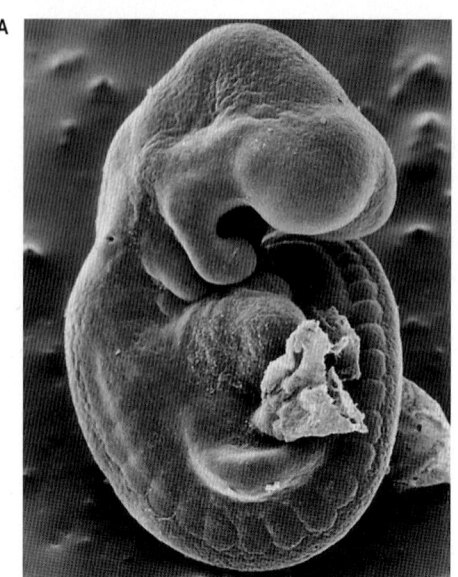

B

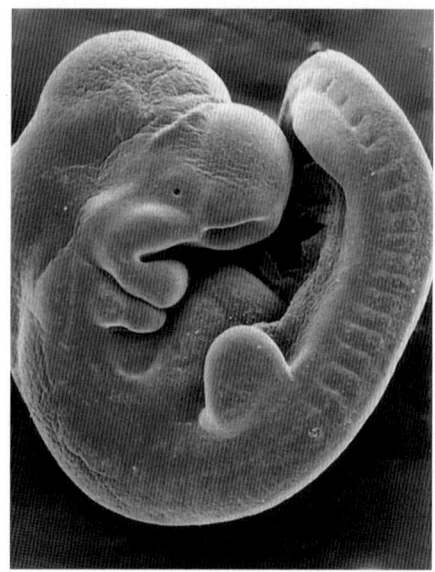

C

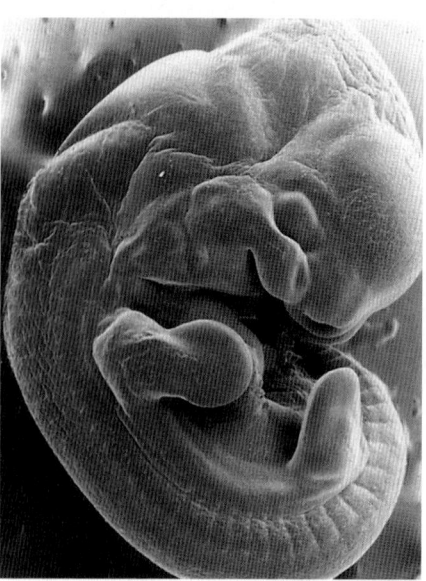

Fig. 26.1 Series of scanning electron micrographs of rat embryos at days 11, 12 and 13: lateral view. **A**, Day 11, the pharyngula stage; the otic vesicle is still open but the lens vesicle has yet to invaginate; the first, second and third pharyngeal arches are present; an upper limb bud is present dorsal to the heart. **B**, Day 12, the lens vesicle has invaginated but is still open; the maxillary process has developed and is beneath the eye; the upper limb is becoming paddle-shaped and the lower limb is present. **C**, Day 13, the eyelids are beginning to develop; the maxillary process is merging with the lateral nasal process; both limb buds are well developed. The relative size and number of somites can be seen at each age. (Photographs by P Collins; printed by S Cox, Electron Microscopy Unit, Southampton General Hospital.)

arch contains a skeletal element derived from neural crest mesenchyme; associated striated muscle from paraxial mesoderm; an arch artery from angiogenic mesenchyme and motor and sensory nerves from arch-specific cranial nerves.

The epithelium covering each arch is patterned by the underlying mesenchyme and endoderm. Patterning is arch-specific and produces keratinized stratified squamous epithelium (hair, sweat, sebaceous and ceruminous glands); pseudostratified columnar epithelium (teeth, salivary, mucous and lacrimal glands); glandular epithelia (thyroid, parathyroids, thymus); and lymphoid tissues of the oro- and nasopharynx.

The skeletal element is formed by condensation of neural crest mesenchyme, which subsequently chondrifies either wholly or in part of its length. If chondrification is complete then the element extends dorsally until it comes into contact with the mesenchymatous cranial base lateral to the hindbrain. The arch cartilage, entirely or in part, may remain as cartilage, undergo endochondral ossification, be replaced completely by intramembranous ossification, or become ligamentous. Neural crest also gives rise to the ligaments, tendons and connective tissues in the arches and the dermis underlying the surface ectoderm, which becomes the epidermis.

The striated muscle of each arch, sometimes termed branchial musculature to denote its origin, is derived from the rostral continuation of the paraxial mesenchyme (in the trunk this becomes segmented to form somites). The paraxial mesoderm of the head is unsegmented, although a segmental pattern of seven cranial somitomeres has been described (Meier 1979). Clear segmentation equivalent to the somites of the trunk is seen only in the paraxial mesoderm of the occipital region, which gives rise to the occipital part of the skull and the extrinsic musculature of the tongue. The organization of cranial muscles formed from the more rostral unsegmented paraxial mesoderm is illustrated in **Fig. 26.5**. Myoblasts migrate from the paraxial mesoderm to sites of future muscle differentiation and form premuscle condensations prior to the development of any skeletal elements. The pattern of primary myotube alignment for any one muscle is specified by the surrounding neural crest mesenchyme and is not related to the source of the myoblasts. The rate and pattern of muscle maturation are closely associated with the development of the skeletal elements but remain unattached until an appropriate stage. Figure 26.5 shows the relation-

ship between the notional somitomeres and the muscle masses migrating to each arch. An arch artery develops in each arch either by vasculogenesis, where angioblastic mesenchyme migrates into a region and initiates vessel development *in situ*, or by angiogenesis, where vessels develop by sprouting from the endothelium of pre-existing vessels. The paired arch arteries arise from the aortic sac at the rostral end of the truncus arteriosus and pass laterally each side of the pharynx to join the dorsal aortae.

The nerves associated with each arch arise from the adjacent hindbrain (**Figs 14.2, 14.18**). The motor nerves grow out from the basal plate of the midbrain and hindbrain to innervate the striated muscle of the arches: they are termed special branchial efferent nerves because they innervate branchial musculature. Sensory nerves form from midbrain- and hindbrain-derived neural crest, extending from cranial sensory ganglia, but also have a placodal component (see above); they convey general and special somatic afferent axons. Each arch is innervated by a mixed nerve, but each nerve also has a purely sensory branch that innervates the arch rostral to its "own" arch; this sensory nerve is called the pretrematic branch, because it lies rostral to the cleft or trema between the two arches, while the mixed branch may be referred to as the post-trematic branch (**Fig. 26.2**). Hence the mandibular division of the trigeminal nerve is the post-trematic nerve of the first arch; the chorda tympani and greater petrosal nerves – branches of the facial nerve – are usually regarded as the pretrematic nerves of the arch. The facial nerve supplies the second arch; the glossopharyngeal is the nerve of the third arch; the superior laryngeal branch of the vagus supplies the fourth arch; and the recurrent laryngeal branch of the vagus is the nerve of the sixth arch. The tympanic branch of the glossopharyngeal and the auricular branch of the vagus have also been described as pretrematic nerves, but this attribution is not widely accepted.

The difference in the courses of the right and left recurrent laryngeal nerves can be explained by the development of the aortic arch arteries. The arch nerve for arches 1–4 enters rostral to its aortic arch artery, whereas it enters the sixth arch caudal to the aortic arch artery. The sixth arch artery retains this position on the left side, where it lies caudal to and then loops round the ligamentum arteriosum in the adult. However, on the right, the dorsal part of the sixth aortic arch arteries disappear, and so the nerve loops round the caudal aspect of the fourth aortic arch artery, i.e. the subclavian artery.

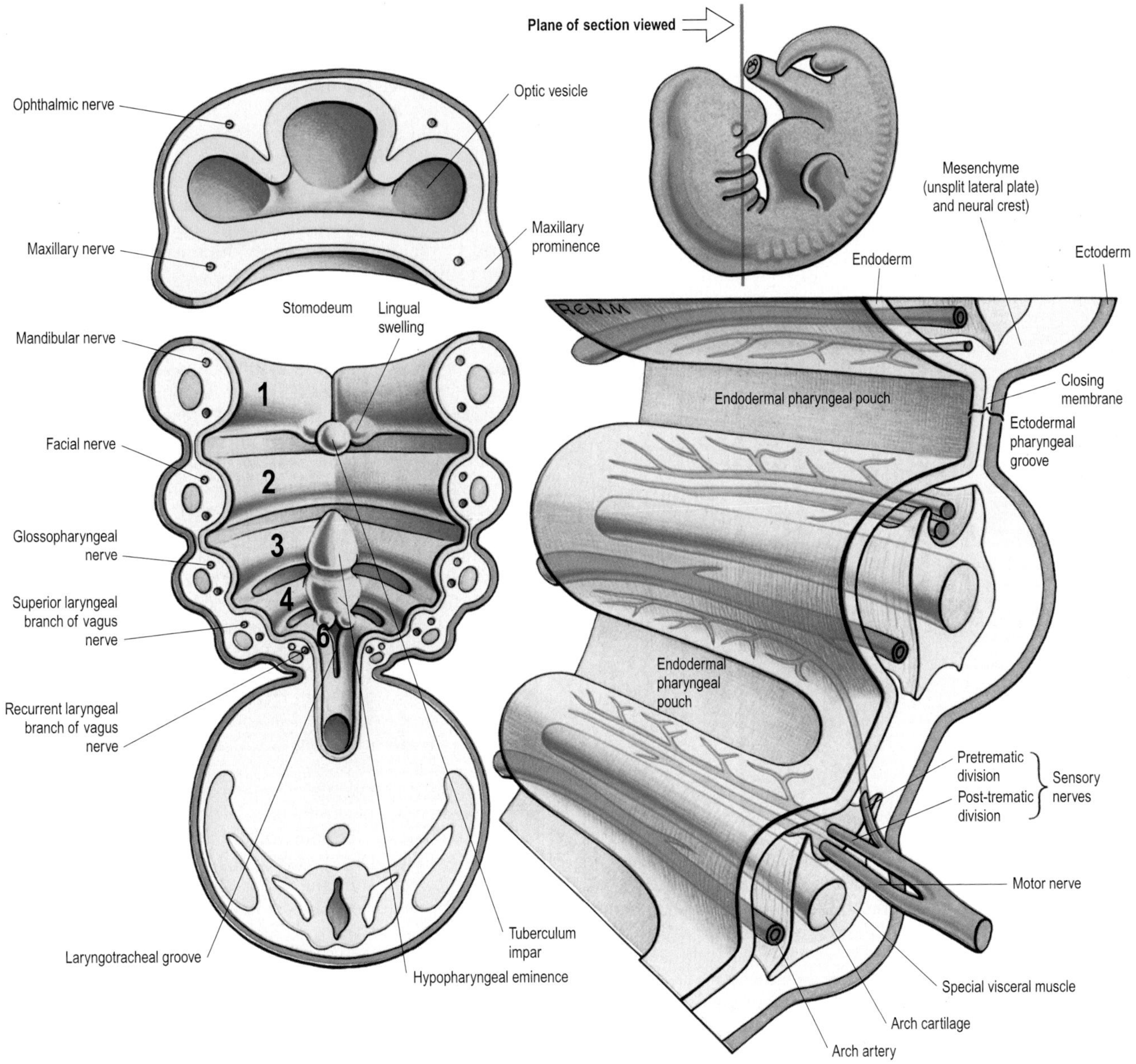

Plane of section viewed

Ophthalmic nerve

Optic vesicle

Maxillary nerve

Maxillary
prominence

Mesenchyme
(unsplit lateral plate)
and neural crest)

Endoderm

Ectoderm

Stomodeum   Lingual
swelling

Mandibular nerve

Closing
membrane

Endodermal pharyngeal pouch

Ectodermal
pharyngeal
groove

Facial nerve

Glossopharyngeal
nerve

Endodermal
pharyngeal
pouch

Superior laryngeal
branch of vagus
nerve

Recurrent laryngeal
branch of vagus
nerve

Pretrematic
division
Post-trematic
division

Sensory
nerves

Motor nerve

Laryngotracheal groove

Tuberculum
impar

Special visceral muscle

Hypopharyngeal eminence

Arch cartilage

Arch artery

Fig. 26.2 Developing pharyngeal region showing (left) the pharyngeal floor and sectioned lateral walls, viewed from the dorsal aspect, and (right) details of generalized pharyngeal constituents, including arches, endodermal pouches and ectodermal grooves. (Modified with permission from Williams PL, Wendell-Smith CP, Treadgold S 1969 Basic Human Embryology, 2nd edn. Philadelphia: Lippincott.)

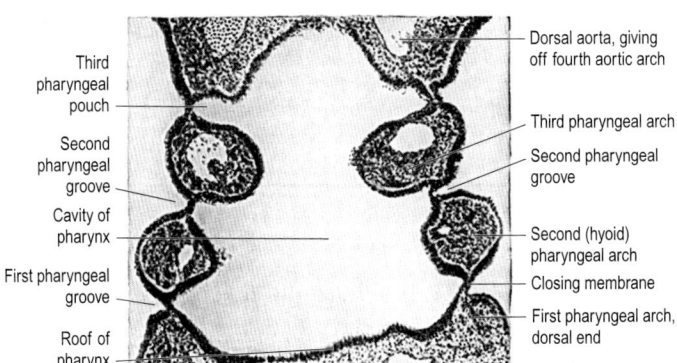

Third
pharyngeal
pouch

Second
pharyngeal
groove

Cavity of
pharynx

First pharyngeal
groove

Roof of
pharynx

Dorsal aorta, giving
off fourth aortic arch

Third pharyngeal arch

Second pharyngeal
groove

Second (hyoid)
pharyngeal arch

Closing membrane

First pharyngeal arch,
dorsal end

Roof of
pharynx

Fig. 26.3 Oblique section through the pharynx of a human embryo of CR length 2 mm. (Modified with permission from Norris EH 1938 The morphogenesis and histogenesis of the thymus gland in man. Contrib Embryol Carnegie Inst Washington 27: 191–207.)

DEVELOPMENT OF THE PHARYNGEAL ARCHES

On each side, the human circumoral first pharyngeal arch (**Figs 26.1, 26.2**) consists of a ventral part or mandibular process (prominence) and a dorsal part or maxillary process (prominence). Each mandibular process, first seen at stage 10 (22 postovulatory days), grows ventromedially in the floor of the pharynx to meet its fellow in the midline, and is situated between the primitive mouth and the cardiac (pericardial) prominence. The maxillary processes are not seen until stage 13: their enlargement coincides with the proliferation of neural crest mesenchyme between the ectoderm and prosencephalon which forms the frontonasal process. The enlargement of the first arch is rostral to the site of the buccopharyngeal membrane and so the inner and outer aspects of this arch are covered with ectoderm. The second or hyoid arches, seen from stage 11, are caudal to the maxillomandibular; they also grow ventrally to meet and fuse in the midline. The third arches are seen at stage 12 (26 days) and the fourth arches by stage 13 (28 days). The fourth arches are not especially prominent, since they are largely sunk in a depression produced by the caudal overlapping of the hyoid arch. The sixth arch cannot be recognized externally and can only be identified by the arrangement of the mesenchyme and by a slight projection on the pharyngeal aspect.

449

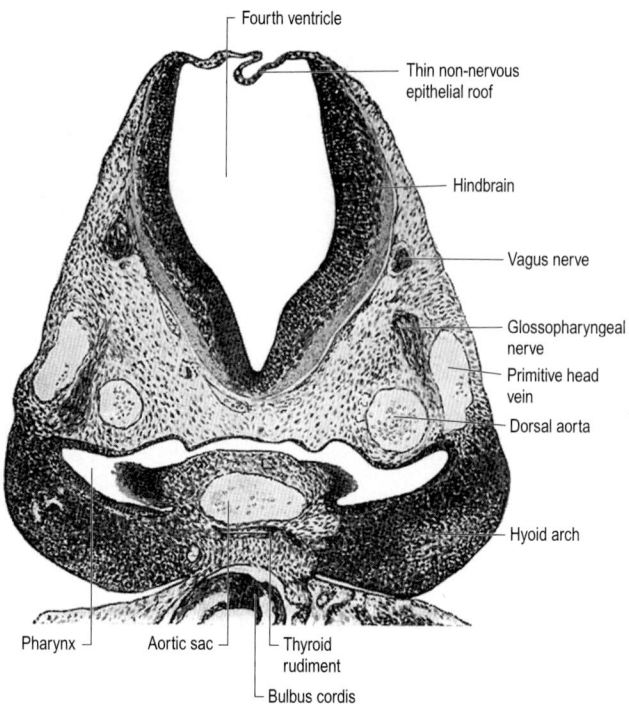

Fourth ventricle

Thin non-nervous
epithelial roof

Hindbrain

Vagus nerve

Glossopharyngeal
nerve

Primitive head
vein

Dorsal aorta

Hyoid arch

Pharynx

Aortic sac

Thyroid
rudiment

Bulbus cordis

Fig. 26.4 Oblique section through the head of a mole embryo, 4.5 mm long. The section passes through the hindbrain, the pharynx, the second (hyoid) and a part of the third pharyngeal arches.

First pharyngeal arch

The first pharyngeal arch is sufficiently different from the subsequent arches, in both structure and development, to merit separate examination. Unlike the other arches it possesses dorsal and ventral processes, and appears C-shaped in lateral view (see **Fig. 26.1**). The dorsal (maxillary) processes interact with overlying ectodermal epithelium and adjacent frontonasal mesenchyme, and generally form more extensive skeletal structures than the other arches. Indeed, these skeletal elements fuse with the neurocranium (**Fig. 26.6**). The first arch is completely clothed with ectoderm, unlike the caudal arches which are dependent on the proximity of pharyngeal endoderm for their development. The ectoderm originates from a territory lateral to the rostral rhombencephalic neural folds (future rhombomeres 1 and 2). It includes the first epibranchial placode, which, together with the rhombomere 1- and 2-derived neural crest cells, forms the trigeminal ganglion. The neural crest of this level streams into the mandibular and maxillary prominences.

The first arch contains a dorsal and ventral cartilage on each side. The former represents the palatopterygoquadrate bar, which forms part of the upper jaw in earlier vertebrates, but is much reduced in mammals. The ventral cartilage (of Meckel, **Fig. 26.7**) extends from the developing middle ear into the mandibular prominence, where it meets its fellow at its ventral end. The dorsal end of Meckel's cartilage, which becomes separated, was once thought to form the rudiments of both malleus and incus. However, there is strong palaeontological and comparative anatomical evidence that at least part of the incus should be regarded as a homologue of the quadrate bone of reptiles. It is therefore probably more correct to consider the incus to be a derivative of the palatopterygoquadrate cartilage, which may also contribute to the greater wing of the sphenoid bone and to the roots of its pterygoid plates. Other than contributing the rudiment of the malleus, the intermediate part of Meckel's cartilage disappears, while its sheath persists as the anterior malleolar and sphenomandibular ligaments. The ventral part, which is much the largest, is enveloped by the developing mandible as it undergoes intramembranous ossification. The portion which extends from the mental foramen almost to the site of the future symphysis, probably becomes ossified from, and incorporated into, invading mandibular tissue, and the remainder of the cartilage is ultimately absorbed.

The cells which give rise to the muscle of the first arch arise from the paraxial mesenchyme localized to the putative somitomeres 2 and 3. The muscle mass of the mandibular part of the first arch forms tensor tympani, tensor veli palatini, mylohyoid, anterior belly of digastric, and the masticatory muscles (**Fig. 26.8**). Tensor tympani retains its connection with the skeletal element of the arch through its attachments to the malleus, and tensor veli palatini remains attached to the base of the medial pterygoid process – which may be derived from the dorsal cartilage of the first arch. However, the masticatory muscles transfer to the mandible, which is mainly a dermal bone. All of these muscles are supplied by the mandibular nerve, the mixed 'post-trematic' nerve of the first arch.

Second pharyngeal arch

The ectoderm covering the outer aspect of the second pharyngeal arch originates from a strip of ectoderm lateral to the metencephalic neural fold, as does the otic placode. The cartilaginous element of the second arch (Reichert's cartilage) extends from the otic capsule to the midline on each side (**Fig. 26.6**). Its dorsal end separates and becomes enclosed in the developing tympanic cavity as the stapes. The cartilage also gives rise to the styloid process, stylohyoid ligament, and the lesser cornu and cranial rim of the body of the hyoid bone (**Fig. 26.7**). The remainder of the hyoid bone derives from the third arch.

The fully formed hyoid bone has a relatively higher and more anterior position in the neonate; it has a small ossification centre in the body of the bone, which is mainly cartilaginous at birth. Its two constituent parts, derived from the second and third pharyngeal arch cartilages, can be identified from the horizontal groove present along the body. The length of the hyoid bone from greater cornu to greater cornu is 3 cm. The stylohyoid ligament attached to the lesser cornu of the hyoid bone passes to a more horizontally inclined styloid process. In infancy the hyoid bone descends with the larynx to a lower position in the neck. The muscles of the second arch derive from somitomeres 4 and 5. For the most part the muscle mass migrates widely, but retains its original nerve supply from the facial nerve: migration is facilitated by the early obliteration of some of the first groove (cleft) and pouch. Stapedius, stylohyoid and posterior belly of digastric remain attached to the hyoid skeleton, but the facial musculature, platysma, auricular muscles and epicranius all lose connection with it (**Fig. 26.8**).

Third, fourth and sixth pharyngeal arches

The ectoderm adjacent to the myelencephalic neural fold, down to the level of somite 3, develops to cover the third and fourth pharyngeal arches, and consequently has a much smaller distribution than that of the more rostral arches. The ectoderm in this region also gives rise to placodal cells which contribute to the petrosal (distal IXth) and nodose ganglia. Chondrification does not occur in the dorsal parts of the skeletal elements of the third to sixth arches. The ventral cartilage of the third arch becomes the greater cornu of the hyoid bone and the caudal part of the body of the hyoid.

The final adaptations of the cartilages of the skeletal elements in the fourth and sixth arches are a source of disagreement, but the following represents a fairly general view. The thyroid cartilage develops from the fourth arch, which may also give rise to the arytenoid, corniculate and cuneiform cartilages. The cricoid cartilage may be derived from the sixth arch cartilage, or it may be a modified tracheal cartilage. The epiglottis is developed in the substance of the hypobranchial eminence and is probably not derived from 'true' branchial cartilage (**Fig. 23.8**).

The paraxial mesenchyme from somitomeres 6 and 7 migrates to the third arch, while somitomere 7 alone appears to invade the fourth arch. The muscle masses are adapted to form the musculature of the pharynx, larynx and soft palate. Stylopharyngeus is a third arch muscle, cricothyroid develops in the fourth arch (**Fig. 23.8**), and the rest of the laryngeal muscles are derived from the sixth arch. The precise origin of the remaining palatal muscles and the pharyngeal constrictors is uncertain. Sternocleidomastoid and trapezius are thought to be derived partly from paraxial mesenchyme and partly from adjacent myotomes.

PHARYNGEAL GROOVES

The external contours of the arches are modified as the skeletal and muscular elements develop. The modification of the external pharyngeal grooves or clefts produces the smooth contour of the neck. The concurrent development of the internal pharyngeal pouches also contributes to this process.

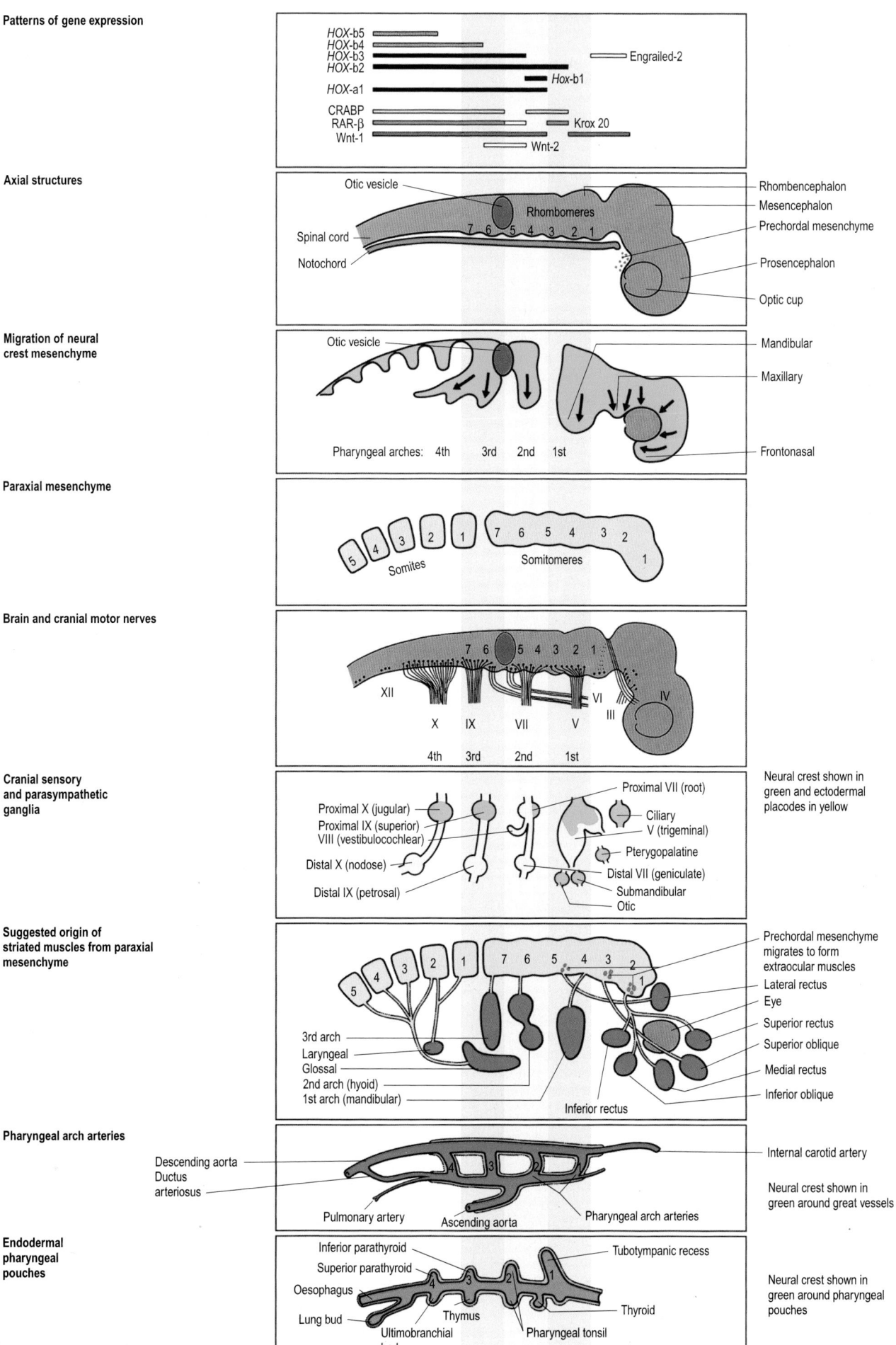

Patterns of gene expression

HOX-b5
HOX-b4
HOX-b3
HOX-b2
HOX-a1
CRABP
RAR-β
Wnt-1

Engrailed-2
Hox-b1
Krox 20
Wnt-2

Axial structures

Otic vesicle
Rhombomeres
Spinal cord
Notochord
7 6 5 4 3 2 1

Rhombencephalon
Mesencephalon
Prechordal mesenchyme
Prosencephalon
Optic cup

Migration of neural crest mesenchyme

Otic vesicle

Mandibular
Maxillary

Pharyngeal arches: 4th 3rd 2nd 1st

Frontonasal

Paraxial mesenchyme

5 4 3 2 1   7 6 5 4 3 2 1
Somites   Somitomeres

Brain and cranial motor nerves

7 6 5 4 3 2 1
XII
X IX VII V
VI
III
IV
4th 3rd 2nd 1st

Cranial sensory and parasympathetic ganglia

Proximal X (jugular)
Proximal IX (superior)
VIII (vestibulocochlear)
Distal X (nodose)
Distal IX (petrosal)

Proximal VII (root)
Ciliary
V (trigeminal)
Pterygopalatine
Distal VII (geniculate)
Submandibular
Otic

Neural crest shown in green and ectodermal placodes in yellow

Suggested origin of striated muscles from paraxial mesenchyme

5 4 3 2 1   7 6 5 4 3 2 1

3rd arch
Laryngeal
Glossal
2nd arch (hyoid)
1st arch (mandibular)
Inferior rectus

Prechordal mesenchyme migrates to form extraocular muscles
Lateral rectus
Eye
Superior rectus
Superior oblique
Medial rectus
Inferior oblique

Pharyngeal arch arteries

Descending aorta
Ductus arteriosus
4 3 1
Pulmonary artery   Ascending aorta
Pharyngeal arch arteries

Internal carotid artery

Neural crest shown in green around great vessels

Endodermal pharyngeal pouches

Inferior parathyroid
Superior parathyroid
Oesophagus
4 3 2 1
Lung bud
Ultimobranchial body
Thymus
Pharyngeal tonsil
Tubotympanic recess
Thyroid

Neural crest shown in green around pharyngeal pouches

Fig. 26.5 The organization of the head and pharynx in an embryo at about stage 14. The individual tissue components have been separated but are aligned in register through the numbered zones. (After Noden.)

451

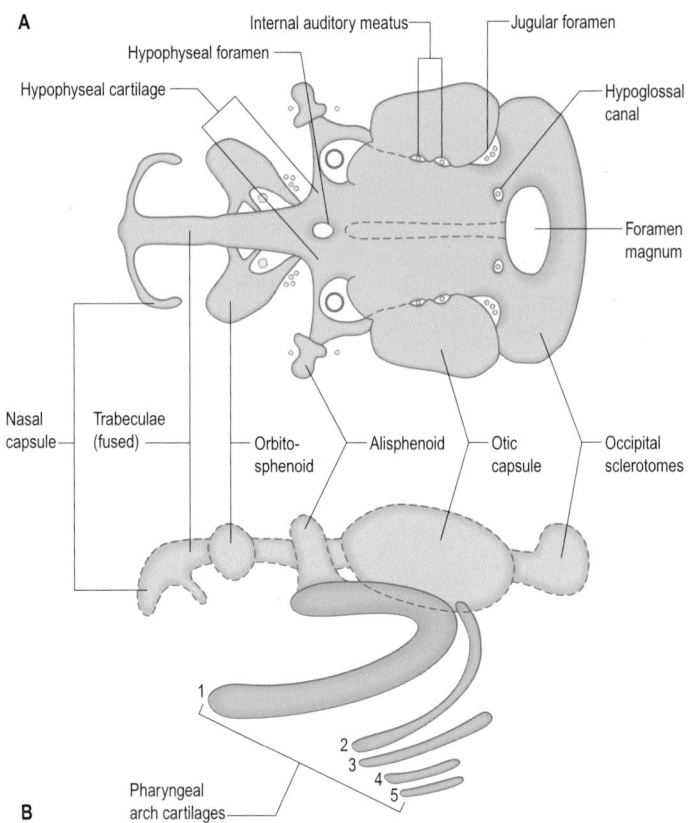

Fig. 26.6 **A**, Cartilaginous components of the base of the neurocranium from above. **B**, Cartilaginous components of the skull from the lateral aspect. The basal components of the neurocranium are in register with those in A. The pharyngeal arch cartilages of the viscerocranium are also shown.

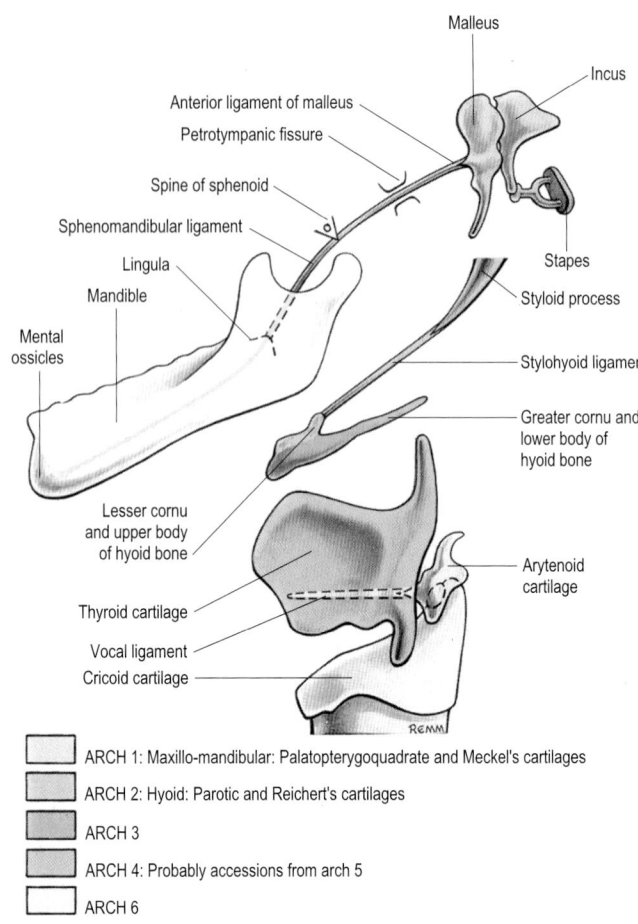

ARCH 1: Maxillo-mandibular: Palatopterygoquadrate and Meckel's cartilages

ARCH 2: Hyoid: Parotic and Reichert's cartilages

ARCH 3

ARCH 4: Probably accessions from arch 5

ARCH 6

Fig. 26.7 The skeletal derivatives (osseous and cartilaginous) of the pharyngeal arches (viscerocranium). (Modified with permission from Williams PL, Wendell-Smith CP, Treadgold S 1969 Basic Human Embryology, 2nd edn. Philadelphia: Lippincott.)

The first pharyngeal groove is obliterated ventrally; its dorsal end deepens to form the epithelium of the external acoustic meatus and the external surface of the tympanic membrane. Thickened patches of ectoderm, the epibranchial placodes, appear at the dorsal ends of the first, second and fourth pharyngeal grooves. They are closely related to the developing ganglia of the facial, glossopharyngeal and vagus nerves, to which they contribute. Together with dorsolateral and suprabranchial placodal cells, the epibranchial placodes also contribute to the trigeminal and vestibulocochlear ganglia (**Fig. 14.12**).

At the end of the fifth week the third and fourth arches are sunk in a retrohyoid depression, the cervical sinus. Cranially the sinus is bounded by the hyoid arch, dorsally by a ridge produced by ventral extensions from the occipital myotomes and by mesenchyme developing into sternocleidomastoid and trapezius. Caudally, the smaller epipericardial ridge separates the sinus from the pericardium: it curves cranially near the midline and then with its opposite fellow reaches the lingual swelling of the mandibular prominence and the hypobranchial eminence. The cervical sinus may be obliterated by caudal growth of the hyoid arches to fuse with the cardiac elevation, so excluding the succeeding arches from any part in the formation of the skin of the neck. Alternatively, the sinus may be reduced by gradual approximation of its walls from within outwards. There is a view that the surface course of the second groove persists as the curved submandibular cervical flexure line. Whatever the mechanism, the neck becomes covered with a smooth layer of epidermis. Platysma (a second arch muscle), bounded both superficially and deep by superficial fascia, passes along the neck to the anterior thoracic wall.

PHARYNGEAL POUCHES

The first four pharyngeal pouches appear in sequence craniocaudally during stages 10–13. The rostral pharynx – primitive rostral foregut – is wide and the endoderm of the pouches approaches the ectoderm of the overlying pharyngeal grooves to form thin closing membranes (**Figs 26.2, 26.3**). It is compressed dorsoventrally which means that there is limited, or virtually no, true lateral wall. The close proximity of the ectoderm and endoderm between the first cleft and pouch is maintained as the tympanic membrane: there is minimal mesenchyme between the layers. The first pouch, and possibly the dorsal part of the second pouch, expand as the tubotympanic recess which gives rise to the middle ear system.

The relationship between subsequent clefts and pouches diverges as mesenchyme intervenes between ectoderm and endoderm. The blind recesses of the second, third and fourth pouches are prolonged dorsally and ventrally as angular, wing-like diverticula. The endoderm of the pouches thickens and evaginates into localized regions of neural crest and undivided lateral plate mesenchyme. The second pouch is much reduced in dimensions compared to the first, and its ventral part is the focus of lymphoid development as the palatine tonsil (p. 614). A generalized ring of lymphoid tissue develops in the primitive foregut at this region (Matsunaga & Rahman 2001). The third pouch gives rise to the thymus ventrally and the parathyroid III dorsally, whereas the fourth pouch produces the parathyroid IV and an ultimobranchial body. The dorsal and ventral portions of the fourth pouch together with the lower ultimobranchial body are collectively termed the caudal pharyngeal complex (**Fig. 34.1**).

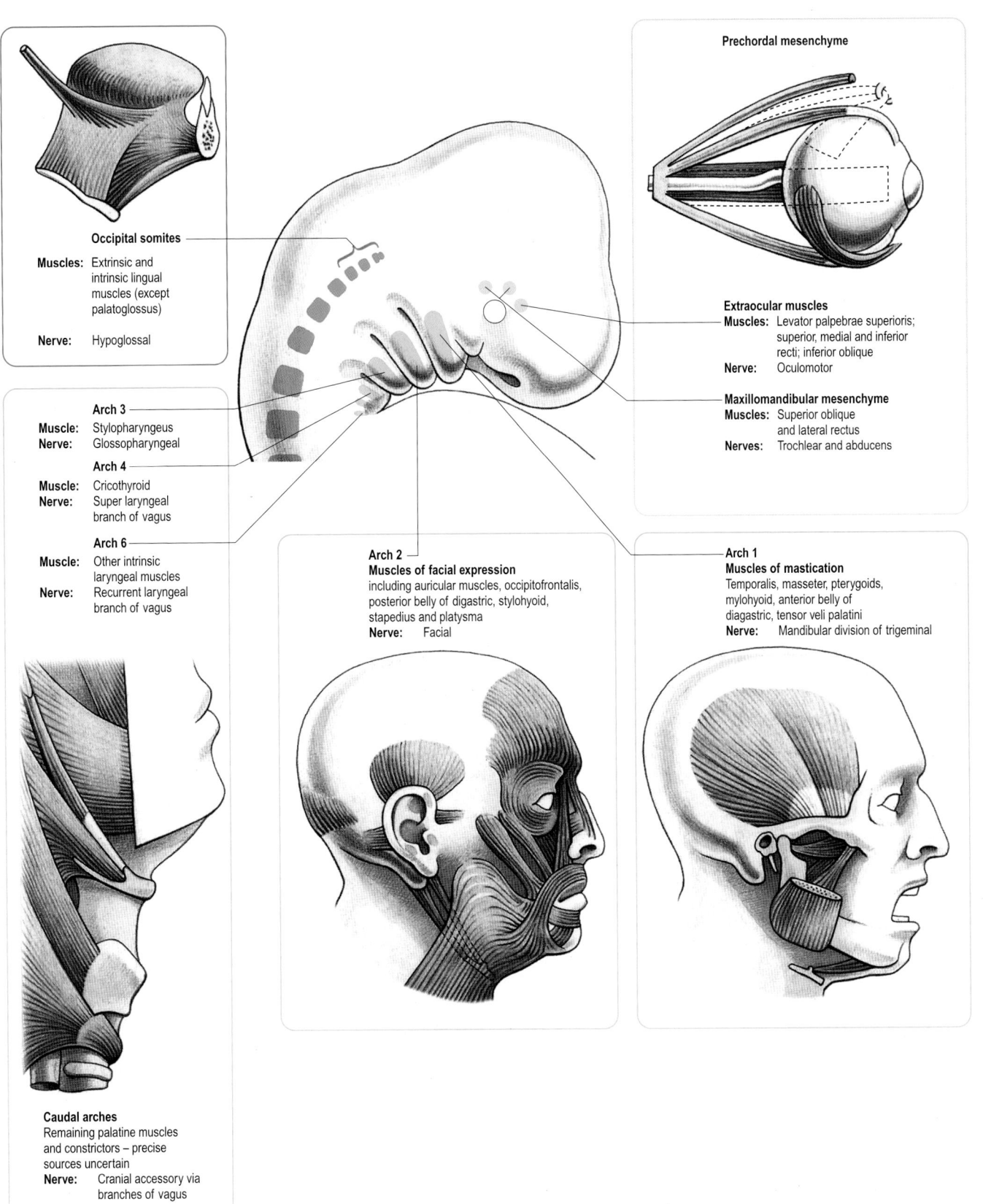

Occipital somites

Muscles: Extrinsic and intrinsic lingual muscles (except palatoglossus)

Nerve: Hypoglossal

Prechordal mesenchyme

Extraocular muscles
Muscles: Levator palpebrae superioris; superior, medial and inferior recti; inferior oblique
Nerve: Oculomotor

Maxillomandibular mesenchyme
Muscles: Superior oblique and lateral rectus
Nerves: Trochlear and abducens

Arch 3
Muscle: Stylopharyngeus
Nerve: Glossopharyngeal

Arch 4
Muscle: Cricothyroid
Nerve: Super laryngeal branch of vagus

Arch 6
Muscle: Other intrinsic laryngeal muscles
Nerve: Recurrent laryngeal branch of vagus

Arch 2
Muscles of facial expression
including auricular muscles, occipitofrontalis, posterior belly of digastric, stylohyoid, stapedius and platysma
Nerve: Facial

Arch 1
Muscles of mastication
Temporalis, masseter, pterygoids, mylohyoid, anterior belly of diagastric, tensor veli palatini
Nerve: Mandibular division of trigeminal

Caudal arches
Remaining palatine muscles and constrictors – precise sources uncertain
Nerve: Cranial accessory via branches of vagus

Fig. 26.8 The muscular derivatives of the prechordal mesenchyme, unsegmented paraxial mesenchyme and rostral somites. (Modified with permission from Williams PL, Wendell-Smith CP, Treadgold S 1969 Basic Human Embryology, 2nd edn. Philadelphia: Lippincott.)

REFERENCES

Gans C, Northcutt RG 1983 Neural crest and the origin of vertebrates: a new head. Science 220: 268–74.
Matsunaga T, Rahman A 2001 In search of the origin of the thymus: the thymus and GALT may be evolutionarily related. Scand J Immunol 53: 1–6.

Meier S 1979 Development of chick mesoblast. Formation of the embryonic axis and the establishment of the metameric pattern. Dev Biol 73: 24–45.

Skull and mandible

The skull is the bony skeleton of the head and is the most complex osseous structure in the body. It is protective, shielding the brain, the organs of special sense and the cranial parts of the respiratory and digestive systems, and also provides attachments for many of the muscles of the head and neck, thus allowing for movement. Of particular importance is movement of the lower jaw (mandible) which occurs at the temporomandibular joint. The marrow within the skull bones is a site of haemopoiesis, at least in the young skull.

The skull is composed of 28 separate bones, of which most are paired, but some in the median plane are single. Many of the bones are flat bones, consisting of two thin plates of compact bone enclosing a narrow layer of cancellous bone containing bone marrow. In terms of shape, however, the bones are far from flat and can show pronounced curvatures. The term diploë is used to describe the cancellous bone within the flat bones of the skull. The inner table is thinner and more brittle; the outer table is generally very resilient. Many bones are so thin that the tables are fused, for example the vomer and pterygoid plates. The skull bones vary in thickness in different regions, but tend to be thinner where they are covered by muscles, for example in the temporal and posterior cranial fossae. The skull is thicker in some races, but no relationship exists between this and cranial capacity which, on average is c.1400 ml. In all races, the bone is thinner in women and children when compared with adult males.

The majority of bones in the skull are held firmly together by fibrous joints termed sutures. In the developing skull sutures allow for growth. There are three main arrangements: the margins of adjacent bones of a suture may be smooth and meet end-to-end, giving a simple (butt-end) suture (e.g. median palatine suture); the margins of adjacent bones may be bevelled, so that the border of one bone overlaps the other (e.g. zygomaticomaxillary suture); or the margins of adjacent bones may present numerous projections that interlock, giving a serrated appearance (e.g. sagittal suture). The complexity of serrated sutures increases from the inner to the outer surface. Fusion across sutures (synostosis) commences at c.30 years, although its variability precludes using this information to age skulls. The process of fusion commences on the internal surface of the cranium and the sagittal suture is one of the first affected. At c.40 years of age the sphenofrontal, lambdoid and occipitomastoid sutures close. In the facial region, the posterior part of the median palatine suture starts to close at c.30 years, followed by the sutures around the nose. The squamosal, zygomaticofrontal and anterior part of the intermaxillary suture rarely exhibit synostosis. Premature fusion of sutures during the early growth phase of the skull will result in various cranial abnormalities.

The bones forming the base of the skull develop endochondrally and play an important part in growth. In this region, therefore, primary cartilaginous joints are encountered during growth: one of the most important is the spheno-occipital synchondrosis that disappears at c.14–16 years of age. The skull articulates with the first cervical vertebra at the synovial atlanto-occipital joints. These joints allow for flexion and extension of the skull. Rotation of the skull does not directly involve any joints of the skull but occurs at the atlanto-axial joint between the first and second cervical vertebrae.

Many important nerves and vessels pass in and out of the skull via openings termed foramina. The skull is a prime site for fractures resulting from trauma, and these structures can be damaged as a result of head injury. Detailed clinical examination should reveal signs and symptoms that, together with radiological examination, should provide information regarding the extent and seriousness of a traumatic incident. In addition to main foramina, irregular emissary foramina allow veins situated externally on the face and scalp to communicate with those lying intra-

cranially: spread of infection along these routes can have serious clinical consequences.

For ease of navigation, the skull can be subdivided into cranium and mandible, based upon the fact that, whereas most of the bones of the skull articulate by relatively fixed joints, the mandible is easily detached. The cranium may then itself be subdivided into a number of regions. These are: the cranial vault, which is the upper, dome-like part of the skull and includes the skullcap or calvaria; the cranial base, which consists of the inferior surface of the skull extracranially and the floor of the cranial cavity intracranially; the facial skeleton, which includes the orbital cavities and the nasal fossae; the tooth-bearing bones or jaws; the acoustic cavities which contain the middle and inner ears; and the cranial cavity which houses the brain. Alternatively, the skull can be divided into neurocranium and viscerocranium. The neurocranium is defined as that part of the skull which houses and protects the brain and the organs of special sense, while the viscerocranium is associated with the cranial parts of the respiratory and digestive tracts.

In the account of the skull that follows, a generalized account of a number of standard views of the skull as a whole will be given first, followed by a more detailed account of each individual disarticulated bone.

EXTERNAL APPEARANCE OF ARTICULATED SKULL (Figs 27.1, 27.2)

FRONTAL (ANTERIOR) VIEW

The upper part of the facial region is formed by the frontal bone. Supero-medial to each orbit is a rounded superciliary arch (better marked in males) between which is a median elevation, the glabella. The glabella may show the remains of the inter-frontal (metopic) suture, which is present in c.9% of adult skulls, where it ascends to the coronal suture, indicating that the frontal bone is the result of fusion of two halves that ossify independently. Above each superciliary arch is a slightly elevated frontal tuber or tuberosity. Below, where the nasal bones meet the frontal bone, is a depression marking the root of the nose. Just below the glabella, the frontal bone meets the two nasal bones at the frontonasal sutures. The point at which the frontonasal and internasal sutures meet is the nasion.

Each orbital opening is approximately quadrangular. The upper, supraorbital, margin is formed entirely by the frontal bone, interrupted at the junction of its sharp lateral two-thirds and rounded medial third by the supraorbital notch or foramen, which transmits the supraorbital vessels and nerve. The lateral margin of the orbit is formed largely by the frontal process of the zygomatic bone, completed above by the zygomatic process of the frontal bone: the suture between them is a palpable depression. The lower, infraorbital, margin is formed by the zygomatic bone laterally and maxilla medially. Both lateral and infraorbital margins are sharp and palpable. The medial margin of the orbit is formed above by the frontal bone and below by the lacrimal crest of the frontal process of the maxilla. The osteology of the orbit is considered in detail on page 688.

The central part of the face is occupied mainly by the maxillary bones, and the anterior nasal aperture lies between them. Each maxilla therefore contributes to the upper jaw, the bridge of the nose, the floor of the orbital cavity, the nasal aperture and the bone of the cheek. The medial surface of the maxilla forms the nasal notch which is the lower and partly lateral border of the anterior nasal aperture. The prominent anterior nasal spine surmounts the intermaxillary suture at the lower margin of the anterior nasal aperture and is palpable in the nasal

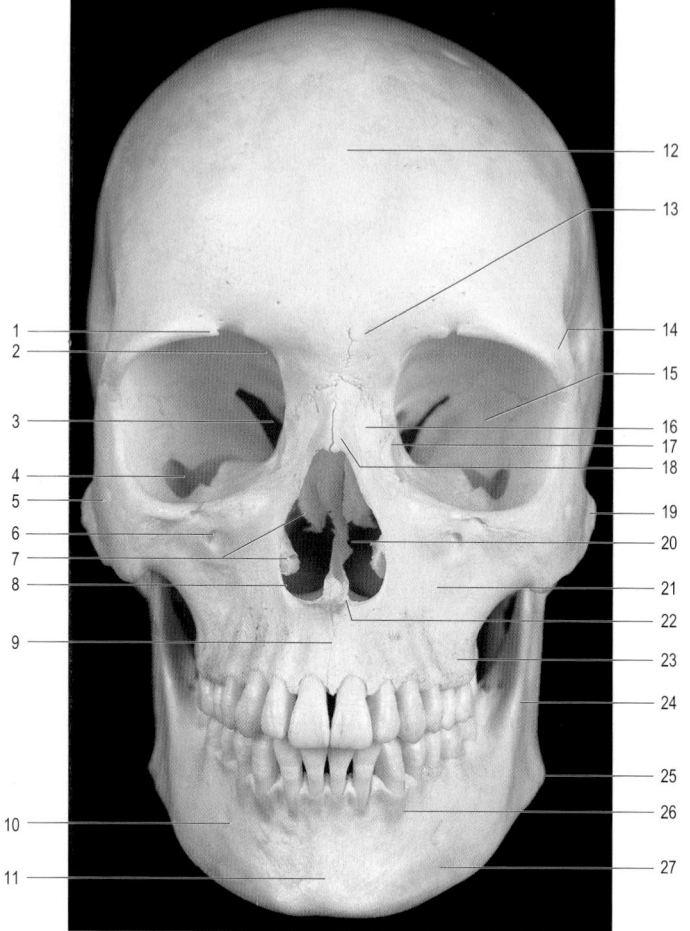

1. Supraorbital notch.
2. Frontal notch.
3. Superior orbital fissure.
4. Inferior orbital fissure.
5. Zygomaticofacial foramen.
6. Infraorbital foramen.
7. Nasal conchae.
8. Anterior nasal aperture.
9. Intermaxillary suture.
10. Mental foramen.
11. Mental protuberance.
12. Frontal bone.
13. Glabella.
14. Zygomatic process of frontal bone.

15. Greater wing of sphenoid bone.
16. Frontal process of maxilla.
17. Lacrimal bone.
18. Nasal bone.
19. Zygomatic bone.
20. Nasal septum.
21. Body of maxilla.
22. Anterior nasal spine.
23. Alveolus of maxilla (upper jaw).
24. Ramus of mandible.
25. Angle of mandible.
26. Alveolus of mandible (lower jaw).
27. Body of mandible.

Fig. 27.1 Front view of skull. (By permission from Berkovitz and Moxham, 1994.)

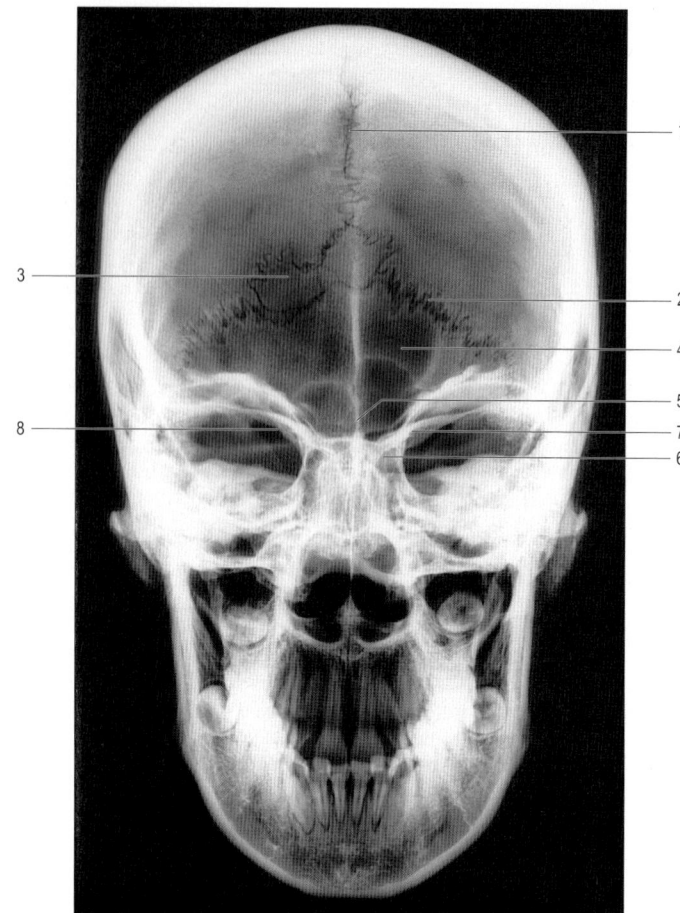

1. Sagittal suture.
2. Lambdoid suture.
3. Sutural bone.
4. Frontal sinus.
5. Crista galli.
6. Ethmoidal air cells.
7. Lesser wing of sphenoid bone.
8. Superior orbital fissure.

Fig. 27.2 Anteroposterior radiograph of skull. (By permission from Berkovitz and Moxham, 1989.)

septum. The infraorbital foramen which transmits the infraorbital vessels and nerve lies c.1 cm below the infraorbital margin. The maxillary alveolar process contains sockets for the upper teeth. The short, thick zygomatic process of the maxilla has an oblique upper surface that articulates with the zygomatic bone at the zygomaticomaxillary suture. The frontal process of the maxilla ascends posterolateral to the nasal bone to reach the frontal bone.

The anterior nasal aperture is piriform, wider below, and bounded by the nasal bones and maxillae: these bones articulate with each other, with their contralateral fellows, and with the frontal bone above. The upper boundary of the aperture is formed by the nasal bones; the remainder is formed by the maxillary bones. In life, various cartilages (septal, lateral nasal, major and minor alar) help to delineate two nasal cavities: however, the macerated skull contains a single anterior nasal aperture because these cartilages are lost during preparation.

The lower part of the face is formed by the body of the mandible. In the midline the mental protuberance produces the characteristic prominence of the chin. The mental foramen, which transmits the mental nerve and accompanying vessels, lies in the same vertical plane as the supraorbital and infraorbital foramina.

POSTERIOR VIEW (Fig. 27.3)

When the skull is viewed from behind, the occipital bone is the most prominent bone, and consequently this is sometimes termed the occipital view. The superolateral parts are formed by the parietal bones, while the temporal bones contribute the mastoid processes to the inferolateral parts of the back of the skull. The parietal bones are separated from the occipital bone by the lambdoid suture; the latter also meets the occipitomastoid and the parietomastoid sutures above and behind the mastoid process. Sutural bones are islands of bone commonly found within the lambdoid suture: they arise from separate centres of ossification and have no clinical significance.

The external occipital protuberance is a midline ridge or a distinct process on the occipital bone. Superior nuchal lines extend laterally from the protuberance to a point above the mastoid processes. Inferior nuchal lines run parallel to, and below, the superior nuchal lines, while supreme nuchal lines may sometimes be seen above the superior nuchal lines. The external occipital protuberance, nuchal lines and roughened external surface of the occipital bone between the nuchal lines all afford attachment to muscles.

SUPERIOR VIEW (Fig. 27.4)

Seen from above, the contour of the cranial vault varies greatly but is usually ellipsoid, or more strictly, a modified ovoid. Its greatest width lies nearer to its occipital pole. It is formed by four bones separated by three prominent sutures. The squamous part of the frontal bone is anterior, and the squamous part of the occipital bone is posterior. The two parietal bones lie between the frontal and occipital bones. The maximal parietal convexity on each site is palpable at the parietal tuber or tuberosity. The superior and inferior temporal lines run close to the tuberosity but are best seen in a lateral view.

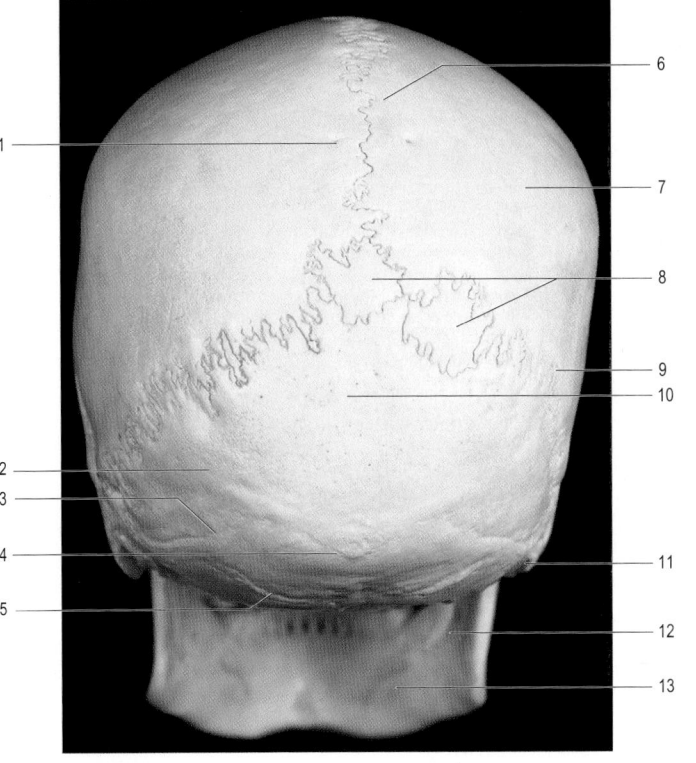

1. Parietal foramen.
2. Supreme nuchal line.
3. Superior nuchal line.
4. External occipital protuberance.
5. Inferior nuchal line.
6. Sagittal suture.
7. Parietal bone.

8. Sutural bones in region of lambda.
9. Lambdoid suture.
10. Occipital bone (squamous part).
11. Mastoid process of temporal bone.
12. Styloid process.
13. Mandible.

Fig. 27.3 Posterior view of skull. (By permission from Berkovitz and Moxham, 1994.)

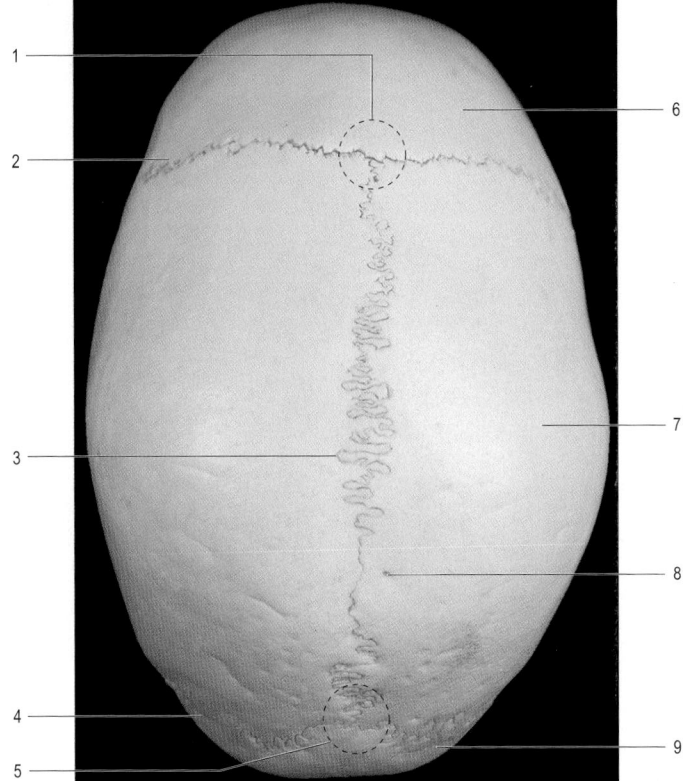

1. Bregma.
2. Coronal suture.
3. Sagittal suture.
4. Lambdoid suture.
5. Lambda.

6. Frontal bone (squamous part).
7. Parietal bone.
8. Parietal foramen.
9. Occipital bone (squamous part).

Fig. 27.4 Superior view of skull. (By permission from Berkovitz and Moxham, 1994.)

The coronal suture marks the junction of the posterior margin of the frontal bone with the anterior margins of the two parietal bones, and it descends around and forwards across the cranial vault. The sagittal suture runs in the midline between the two parietal bones. The lambdoid suture delineates the junction between the posterior borders of the right and left parietal bones and the superior border of the occipital bone, and it descends laterally across the cranial vault. The coronal and sagittal sutures meet at the bregma: in the fetal skull, together with the temporary interfrontal suture, they form the boundaries of a diamond-shaped membrane-filled anterior fontanelle that persists until c.18 months after birth. The lambda, at the junction of the sagittal and lambdoid sutures, is the site of the posterior fontanelle, which closes c.2 months after birth.

A parietal foramen may pierce either or both parietal bones near the sagittal suture c.3.5 cm anterior to the lambda. It transmits a small emissary vein from the superior sagittal sinus.

LATERAL VIEW (Figs 27.5, 27.6)

The skull, viewed from the side, can be subdivided into three zones: face (anterior); temporal and infratemporal fossae and zygomatic arch (intermediate); occipital region (posterior).

The temporal fossa is related to the temple of the head (where greying of the hair first denotes the passage of time). It is bounded inferiorly by the zygomatic arch, superiorly and posteriorly by the temporal lines on the calvaria, and anteriorly by the frontal process of the zygomatic bone. It continues beneath the zygomatic arch into the infratemporal fossa. The temporal lines often present anteriorly as distinct ridges, but become much less prominent as they arch across the parietal bone. Indeed, the superior line usually disappears posteriorly. The inferior temporal line becomes distinct once more as it curves down the squamous part of the temporal bone, forming a supramastoid crest at the base of the mastoid process. The superior temporal line gives attachment to the

temporal fascia. The inferior temporal line provides attachment for temporalis.

The floor of the temporal fossa is formed by the frontal and parietal bones, the greater wing of the sphenoid, and the squamous part of the temporal bones. All four bones meet on each side at an H-shaped junction of sutures termed the pterion. This is an important landmark on the side of the skull because it overlies both the anterior branch of the middle meningeal artery and the lateral (Sylvian) cerebral fissure intracranially (it is also known as the Sylvian point). The pterion corresponds to the site of the anterolateral (sphenoidal) fontanelle on the neonatal skull, which disappears about three months after birth.

The suture between the temporal and parietal bones is called the squamosal suture. The sphenosquamosal suture lies between the greater wing of the sphenoid and the squamous part of the temporal bone.

The lateral surface of the ramus of the mandible will be described briefly here. The ramus is a plate of bone projecting upwards from the back of the body of the mandible. It bears two prominent processes superiorly, the coronoid and condylar processes separated by the mandibular notch. The coronoid process is the site for the insertion of temporalis. The condylar process articulates with the mandibular fossa of the temporal bone at the temporomandibular joint and is the site of attachment of lateral pterygoid. The inferior and posterior borders of the ramus meet at the angle of the mandible.

The zygomatic arch stands clear of the rest of the skull, and the temporal and infratemporal fossae communicate via the gap thus created. The bones of the cheek are the zygomatic bone together with the zygomatic processes of the frontal, maxillary and temporal bones; the term zygomatic arch is generally restricted to the temporal process of the zygomatic bone and the zygomatic process of the temporal bone which meet at the zygomaticotemporal suture. The suture between the zygomatic process of the frontal bone and the frontal process of the zygomatic bone is the frontozygomatic suture, that between the

457

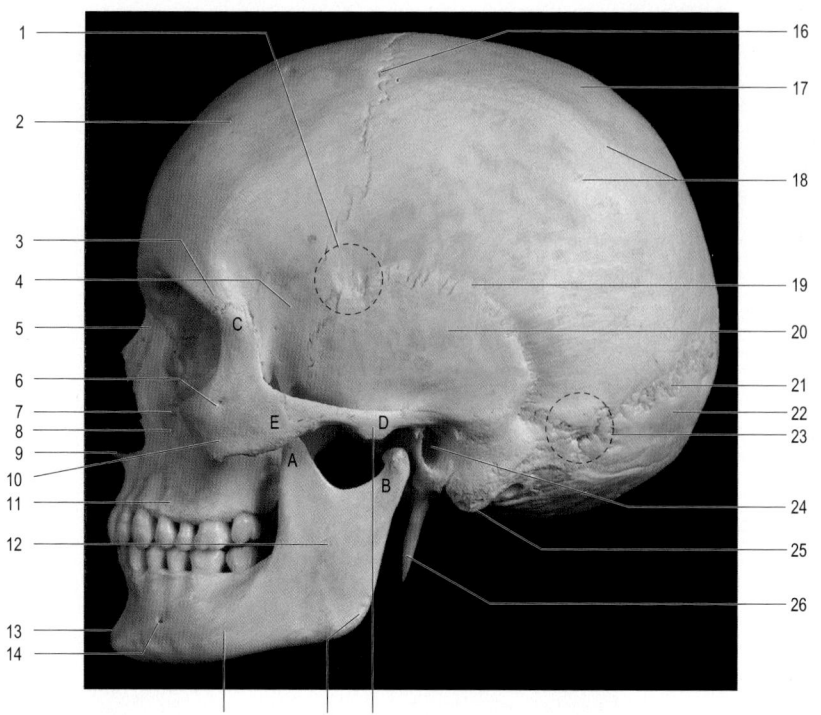

1. Pterion.
2. Frontal bone.
3. Zygomatic process of frontal bone.
4. Greater wing of sphenoid bone.
5. Nasal bone.
6. Zygomaticofacial foramen.
7. Infraorbital foramen.
8. Zygomatic process of maxilla.
9. Anterior nasal spine.
10. Zygomatic bone.
11. Maxilla.
12. Ramus of mandible.
13. Mental protuberance.
14. Mental foramen.
15. Body of mandible.
16. Coronal suture.
17. Parietal bone.
18. Superior and inferior temporal lines.
19. Squamosal suture.
20. Squamous part of temporal bone.
21. Lambdoid suture.
22. Occipital bone.
23. Asterion.
24. External acoustic meatus and tympanic plate.
25. Mastoid process of temporal bone.
26. Styloid process of temporal bone.
27. Zygomatic arch (zygomatic process of temporal bone).
28. Angle of mandible.
   A. Coronoid process of mandible.
   B. Condylar process of mandible in mandibular fossa.
   C. Frontal process of zygomatic bone.
   D. Articular eminence.
   E. Temporal process of zygomatic bone.

Fig. 27.5 Lateral view of skull. (By permission from Berkovitz and Moxham, 1994.)

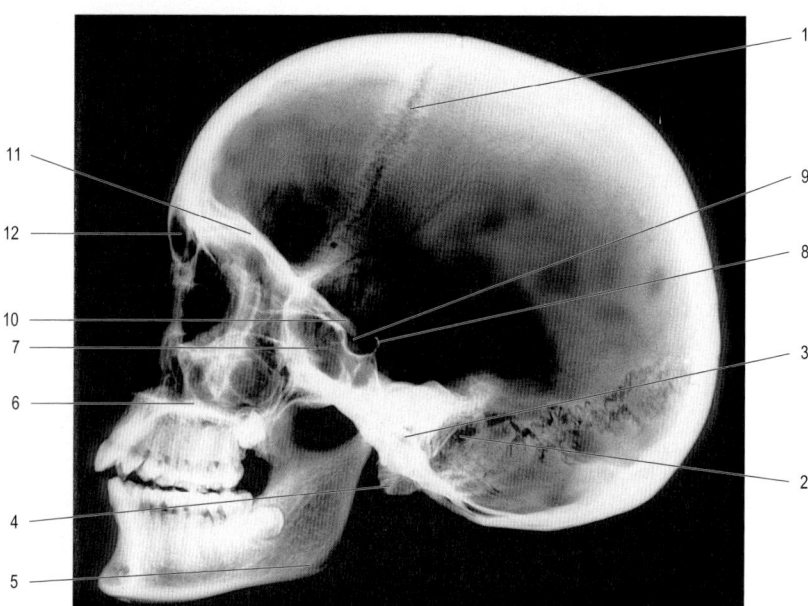

1. Coronal suture.
2. Mastoid air cells.
3. External acoustic meatus.
4. Mastoid process.
5. Angle of mandible.
6. Hard palate.
7. Sphenoidal sinus.
8. Posterior clinoid process.
9. Pituitary fossa.
10. Anterior clinoid process.
11. Floor of anterior cranial fossa.
12. Frontal sinus.

Fig. 27.6 Lateral radiograph of skull. (By permission from Berkovitz and Moxham, 1989.)

maxillary margin of the zygomatic bone and the zygomatic process of the maxillary bone is the zygomaticomaxillary suture, and between the sphenoid and zygomatic is the sphenozygomatic suture. As the zygomatic process of the temporal bone passes posteriorly, it becomes associated with the mandibular fossa and the supramastoid crest. Two small foramina, the zygomaticofacial and zygomaticotemporal, lie on the outer and inner surfaces respectively, of the zygomatic bone: they transmit similarly named nerves and vessels onto the face.

The temporal bone is a prominent structure on the lateral aspect of the skull. Its squamous part lies in the floor of the temporal fossa and its zygomatic process contributes to the bones of the cheek. Additional components visible in the lateral view of the skull are the mandibular fossa and its articular eminence (tubercle), the tympanic plate, the external acoustic meatus, and the mastoid and styloid processes.

The mandibular (glenoid) fossa is the part of the temporomandibular joint into which the condylar process of the mandible articulates. It is bounded in front by the articular eminence and behind by the tympanic plate. The articular eminence is important functionally as it provides a

surface down which the mandibular condyle glides during mandibular movements.

The tympanic plate of the temporal bone contributes most of the margin of the external acoustic meatus, and the squamous part forms the posterosuperior region. The external margin is roughened to provide an attachment for the cartilaginous part of the meatus. Above and behind the meatus lies a small depression, the suprameatal triangle, which is related to the lateral wall of the mastoid antrum.

The mastoid process is a small inferior projection of the temporal bone, which lies posteroinferior to the external acoustic meatus. It is in contact behind with the posteroinferior angle of the parietal bone at the parietomastoid suture and with the squamous part of the occipital bone at the occipitomastoid suture. These two sutures meet the lateral end of the lambdoid suture at the asterion. The asterion coincides with the site of the posterolateral fontanelle in the neonatal skull: this fontanelle closes during the second year. A mastoid foramen may be found near or in the occipitomastoid suture and transmits an emissary vein from the sigmoid sinus. Sutural bones may appear in the parietomastoid suture.

The styloid process lies anterior and medial to the mastoid process and gives attachment to several muscles and ligaments. Its base is partly ensheathed by the tympanic plate and it descends anteromedially, its tip usually reaching a point medial to the posterior margin of the mandibular ramus. However, the styloid process is very variably developed, and ranges in length from a few millimetres to a few centimetres. Often approximately straight, it is on occasion curved, when an anteromedial concavity is common, whereas a posterior concavity is rare.

The infratemporal fossa is an irregular postmaxillary space located deep to the ramus of the mandible, which communicates with the temporal fossa deep to the zygomatic arch. It is best visualized, therefore, when the mandible is removed but, for completeness, is considered here. Its roof is the infratemporal surface of the greater wing of the sphenoid. The lateral pterygoid plate lies medial to the fossa, and the ramus of the mandible and styloid process lie laterally and posteriorly respectively. The infratemporal fossa has no anatomical floor. Its anterior and medial walls are separated above by the pterygomaxillary fissure lying between the lateral pterygoid plate and the posterior wall of the maxilla. The infratemporal fossa communicates with the pterygopalatine fossa through this fissure.

INFERIOR (BASAL) SURFACE (Fig. 27.7)

The inferior surface of the skull, the base of the cranium, is complex and extends from the upper incisor teeth in front to the superior nuchal lines of the occipital bone behind. The region contains many of the foramina through which structures enter and exit the cranial cavity. The inferior surface can be conveniently subdivided into anterior, middle, posterior and lateral parts. The anterior part contains the hard palate and the dentition of the upper jaw, and lies at a lower level than the rest of the cranial base. The middle and posterior parts can be arbitrarily divided by a transverse plane passing through the anterior margin of the foramen magnum. The middle part is occupied mainly by the base of the sphenoid bone, the petrous processes of the temporal bones and the basilar part of the occipital bone. The lateral part contains the zygomatic arches and the mastoid and styloid processes. Whereas the middle and posterior parts are directly related to the cranial cavity (the middle and posterior cranial fossae), the anterior part (the palate) is some distance from the anterior cranial fossa, being separated from it by the nasal cavities.

Anterior part of cranial base

The bony palate within the superior alveolar arch is formed by the palatine processes of the maxillae and the horizontal plates of the palatine bones, which meet at a cruciform system of sutures. The median palatine suture runs anteroposteriorly and divides the palate into right and left halves. This suture is continuous with the intermaxillary suture between the maxillary central incisor teeth. The transverse palatine (palatomaxillary) sutures run transversely across the palate between the maxillary and the palatine bones. The palate is arched sagittally and transversely: its depth and breadth are variable but are always greatest in the molar region, the average width between the maxillary first molars being c.50 mm. The incisive fossa lies behind the central incisor teeth, and the lateral incisive foramina, through which incisive canals pass to the nasal cavity lie in its lateral walls. Median incisive foramina, present in some skulls, open on the anterior and posterior walls of the fossa. The incisive fossa transmits the nasopalatine nerve and the termination of the greater palatine vessels. When median incisive foramina occur, the left nasopalatine nerve traverses the anterior foramen, and the right nerve traverses the posterior foramen. The greater palatine foramen lies near the lateral palatal border of the transverse palatine suture, and a vascular groove which is deep posteriorly, leads forwards from it. The lesser palatine foramina, usually two, lie behind the greater palatine foramen, and pierce the pyramidal process of the palatine bone which is wedged between the lower ends of the medial and lateral pterygoid plates. The palate is pierced by many other small foramina and is marked by pits for palatine glands. Variably prominent palatine crests extend medially from behind the greater palatine foramina. The posterior border projects back as a median posterior nasal spine. The alveolar arch has 16 sockets or alveoli for teeth, varying in size and depth, some single, some divided by septa in adaptation to tooth roots.

The nasal fossae, separated in the midline by the nasal septum, lie above the hard palate. The two posterior nasal apertures (choanae) are located where the nasal fossae end. The posterior part of the septum is formed by the vomer. The upper border of the vomer is applied to the

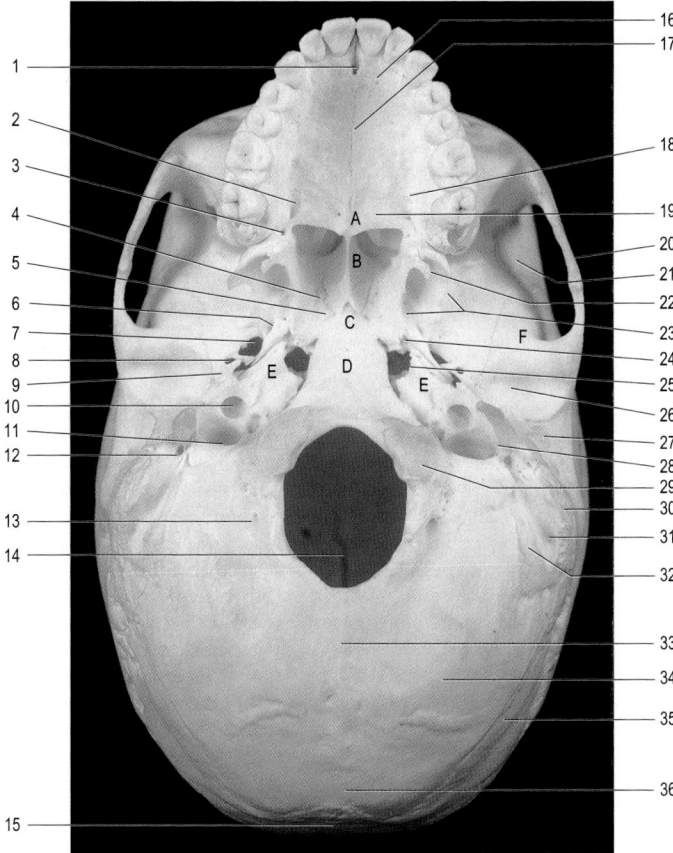

1. Incisive fossa.
2. Greater palatine foramen.
3. Lesser palatine foramen.
4. Palatovaginal canal.
5. Vomerovaginal canal.
6. Sphenoidal foramen.
7. Foramen ovale.
8. Foramen spinosum.
9. Spine of sphenoid.
10. Carotid canal.
11. Jugular foramen.
12. Stylomastoid foramen.
13. Condylar canal.
14. Foramen magnum.
15. External occipital protuberance.
16. Palatine process of maxilla.
17. Median palatine suture.
18. Transverse palatine suture.
19. Horizontal plate of palatine bone.
20. Zygomatic arch.
21. Greater wing of sphenoid.
22. Pterygoid hamulus.
23. Medial and lateral pterygoid plates of sphenoid bone.
24. Opening of pterygoid canal.
25. Foramen lacerum.
26. Mandibular fossa.
27. External acoustic meatus.
28. Styloid process of temporal bone.
29. Occipital condyle.
30. Mastoid process of temporal bone.
31. Mastoid notch.
32. Groove for occipital artery.
33. External occipital crest.
34. Inferior nuchal line.
35. Superior nuchal line.
36. Squamous part of occipital bone.
   A. Posterior nasal spine.
   B. Vomer contributing to nasal septum.
   C. Body of sphenoid.
   D. Basilar part of occipital bone.
   E. Petrous processes of temporal bones.
   F. Articular eminence.

Fig. 27.7 Inferior view of skull. (By permission from Berkovitz and Moxham, 1994.)

inferior aspect of the body of the sphenoid, where it expands into an ala on each side. The lateral border of each ala reaches a thin vaginal process which projects medially from the medial pterygoid plate. The two may either touch or the vaginal process may overlap the ala of the vomer inferiorly. The inferior surface of the vaginal process bears an anteroposterior groove, which is converted into a canal anteriorly by the superior aspect of the sphenoidal process of the palatine bone. This palatovaginal canal opens anteriorly into the pterygopalatine fossa and transmits a pharyngeal branch of the pterygopalatine ganglion and a pharyngeal branch from the third part of the maxillary artery. An inconstant vomerovaginal canal may lie between the ala of the vomer and the vaginal process of the sphenoid bone, medial to the palatovaginal canal, and lead into the anterior end of the palatovaginal canal. It transmits the pharyngeal branch of the third part of the maxillary artery.

Middle part of cranial base

The middle part of the cranial base is made up by the occipital, sphenoid and temporal bones. The body of the sphenoid bone lies anteriorly, and the basilar part of the occipital bone lies posteriorly, just in front of the foramen magnum. Where these meet in the growing skull, the junction between the two bones is a primary cartilaginous joint, the spheno-occipital synchondrosis. This joint is important for growth of the skull in an anteroposterior direction, and ossifies at c.14–16 years of age. The basilar part of the occipital bone bears a small midline pharyngeal tubercle, which gives attachment to the pharyngeal raphe and the highest attachment of the superior pharyngeal constrictor.

The middle part of the cranial base is completed by the petrous processes of the two temporal bones, which pass from the lateral sides of the base of the skull towards the site of union of the sphenoid and occipital bones. Each petrous process meets the basilar part of the occipital bone at a petro-occipital suture, which is deficient posteriorly at the jugular foramen. The petrosphenoidal suture and the groove for the pharyngotympanic tube lie between the petrous process and the infratemporal surface of the greater wing of the sphenoid. The apex of the petrous process does not meet the spheno-occipital suture and the deficit so produced is called the foramen lacerum.

Each pterygoid process of the sphenoid bone bears medial and lateral pterygoid plates separated by a pterygoid fossa. Anteriorly the plates are fused, except below, where they are separated by the pyramidal process of the palatine bone. Sutures are usually discernible at this site. Laterally the pterygoid plates are separated from the posterior maxillary surface by the pterygomaxillary fissure, which leads into the pterygopalatine fossa. The posterior border of the medial pterygoid plate is sharp, and bears a small projection near the midpoint, above which it is curved and attached to the pharyngeal end of the pharyngotympanic tube. Above, the medial pterygoid plate divides to enclose the scaphoid fossa, while below it projects as a slender pterygoid hamulus, which curves laterally and is grooved anteriorly by the tendon of tensor veli palatini. The pterygoid hamulus gives origin to the pterygomandibular raphe. The lateral pterygoid plate projects posterolaterally and its lateral surface forms the medial wall of the infratemporal fossa. Superiorly and laterally the pterygoid process is continuous with the infratemporal surface of the greater wing of the sphenoid bone that forms part of the roof of the infratemporal fossa. This surface forms the posterolateral border of the inferior orbital fissure and bears an infratemporal crest associated with the origin of the upper part of lateral pterygoid. The infraorbital and zygomatic branches of the maxillary nerve and accompanying vessels pass through the inferior orbital fissure. Laterally the greater wing of the sphenoid bone articulates with the squamous part of the temporal bone. Features associated with the pterygoid plate region may be assessed radiographically (**Fig. 27.8**).

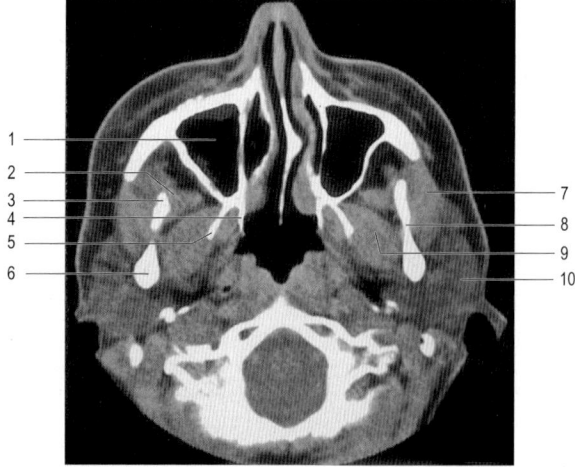

1. Maxillary sinus.
2. Temporalis.
3. Coronoid process.
4. Medial pterygoid plate.
5. Lateral pterygoid plate.
6. Neck of mandible.
7. Masseter.
8. Ramus of mandible.
9. Lateral pterygoid muscle.
10. Parotid gland.

Fig. 27.8 Horizontal CT at level of upper part of ramus of mandible showing relationships of the pterygoid plates. (By permission from Berkovitz and Moxham, 1994.)

A thin-walled depression in the temporal bone, the mandibular fossa, may be inspected when the mandible is removed, in front of which the zygomatic arch extends laterally. A distinct ridge, the articular eminence, is anterior to the fossa, and three fissures can be distinguished behind it. The squamotympanic fissure extends from the spine of the sphenoid, between the mandibular fossa and the tympanic plate of the temporal bone, and curves up the anterior margin of the external acoustic meatus. A thin wedge of bone forming the inferior margin of the tegmen tympani lies within the fissure and divides the squamotympanic fissure into petrotympanic and petrosquamous fissures. The petrotympanic fissure transmits the chorda tympani branch of the facial nerve from the skull into the infratemporal fossa.

The foramen lacerum is bounded in front by the body and adjoining roots of the pterygoid process and greater wing of the sphenoid bone, posterolaterally by the apex of the petrous part of the temporal bone, and medially by the basilar part of the occipital bone. Although it is nearly 1 cm long, no large structure completely traverses it. A large, almost circular, foramen, the carotid canal, lies behind and posterolateral to the foramen lacerum in the petrous part of the temporal bone. The internal carotid artery enters the skull through this foramen, ascends in the carotid canal, and turns anteromedially to reach the posterior wall of the foramen lacerum. It ascends through the upper end of the foramen lacerum with its venous and sympathetic nerve plexuses. Meningeal branches of the ascending pharyngeal artery, and emissary veins from the cavernous sinus also traverse the foramen lacerum. In life, the lower part of the foramen lacerum is partially occluded by cartilaginous remnants of the developmental chondrocranium. The pterygoid canal can be seen on the base of the skull at the anterior margin of the foramen lacerum, above and between the pterygoid plates of the sphenoid bone. It leads into the pterygopalatine fossa and contains the nerve of the pterygoid canal and accompanying blood vessels.

The foramen ovale and the foramen spinosum lie lateral to the foramen lacerum on the infratemporal surface of the greater wing of the sphenoid bone. The foramen ovale, near the posterior margin of the lateral pterygoid plate, transmits the mandibular nerve as well as the lesser petrosal nerve, the accessory meningeal branch of the maxillary artery, and an emissary vein which connects the cavernous venous sinus to the pterygoid venous plexus in the infratemporal fossa. Posterolaterally, the smaller and rounder foramen spinosum transmits the middle meningeal artery and a meningeal branch of the mandibular nerve. The irregular spine of the sphenoid projects posterolateral to the foramen spinosum. The medial surface of the spine is flat and forms, with the adjoining posterior border of the greater wing of the sphenoid, the anterolateral wall of a groove that is completed posteromedially by the petrous part of the temporal bone. This groove contains the cartilaginous pharyngotympanic (auditory) tube and leads posterolaterally into the bony portion of the tube lying within the petrous part of the temporal bone. Occasionally the foramen ovale and foramen spinosum are confluent. The posterior edge of the foramen spinosum may be defective. A small foramen, the sphenoidal emissary foramen (of Vesalius), is sometimes found between the foramen ovale and scaphoid fossa. When present, it contains an emissary vein linking the pterygoid venous plexus in the infratemporal fossa with the cavernous sinus in the middle cranial fossa.

The zygomaticotemporal foramen passes up and backwards from the posterior surface of the zygomatic bone in the anterior wall of the infratemporal fossa. It transmits the zygomaticotemporal nerve and a small accompanying artery.

Posterior part of cranial base

The posterior part of the cranial base is formed by the occipital and temporal bones. Prominent features are the foramen magnum and associated occipital condyles; jugular foramen; mastoid and styloid processes of the temporal bone; stylomastoid foramen; mastoid notch and squamous part of the occipital bone up to the external occipital protuberance and the superior nuchal lines; hypoglossal canals (anterior condylar canals) and condylar canals (posterior condylar canals).

The foramen magnum lies in an anteromedian position. It is oval, wider behind, with its greatest diameter being anteroposterior. It contains the lower end of the medulla oblongata, the vertebral arteries and the spinal accessory nerve. Anteriorly, the margin of the foramen magnum is slightly overlapped by the occipital condyles which project down to articulate with the superior articular facets on the lateral masses of the atlas. Each occipital condyle is oval in outline and oriented obliquely so that its anterior end lies nearer the midline. It is markedly convex anteroposteriorly, less so transversely, and its medial aspect is roughened by ligamentous attachments. The hypoglossal canal, directed laterally and slightly forwards, traverses each condyle and transmits the hypoglossal nerve, a meningeal branch of the ascending pharyngeal artery and an emissary vein from the basilar plexus. A depression, the condylar fossa, lies immediately posterior to the condyle and sometimes contains a (posterior) condylar canal for an emissary vein from the sigmoid sinus. A jugular process joins the petrous part of the temporal bone lateral to each condyle, and its anterior border forms the posterior boundary of the jugular foramen.

Laterally, the occipital bone joins the petrous part of the temporal bone anteriorly at the petro-occipital suture, and the mastoid process of the temporal bone more posteriorly at the petromastoid suture. The jugular foramen, a large irregular hiatus, lies at the posterior end of the petro-occipital suture between the jugular process of the occipital bone and the jugular fossa of the petrous part of the temporal bone. A number of important structures pass through this foramen: inferior petrosal sinus (anterior); glossopharyngeal, vagus and accessory nerves (midway); internal jugular vein (posterior). A mastoid canaliculus runs through the lateral wall of the jugular fossa and transmits the auricular branch of the vagus nerve. The canaliculus for the tympanic nerve – a branch of the glossopharyngeal nerve to the cavity of the middle ear – lies on the ridge between the jugular fossa and the opening of the carotid canal. A small notch, related to the inferior glossopharyngeal ganglion, may be found medially, on the upper boundary of the jugular foramen (it is more easily identified internally). The orifice of the cochlear canaliculus may be found at the apex of the notch.

The stylomastoid foramen lies between the mastoid and styloid processes of the temporal bone on the lateral aspect. It transmits the facial nerve and the stylomastoid artery. A groove, the mastoid notch, lies medial to the mastoid process and gives origin to the posterior belly of digastric. A groove related to the occipital artery often lies medial to the mastoid notch. A mastoid foramen may be present near or in the occipitomastoid suture and, when present, it transmits an emissary vein from the sigmoid sinus. The external acoustic meatus lies in front of the mastoid process. It is surrounded inferiorly by the tympanic plate which partly ensheathes the base of the styloid process.

The squamous part of the occipital bone exhibits the external occipital protuberance, supreme, superior and inferior nuchal lines, and the external occipital crest, all of which lie in the midline, posterior to the foramen magnum. The region is roughened for the attachment of muscles whose primary function is extension of the skull.

INTERNAL APPEARANCE OF ARTICULATED SKULL

The cranial cavity contains the brain, the intracranial portions of cranial and spinal nerves, blood vessels, meninges and cerebrospinal fluid. It is formed by the frontal, parietal, sphenoid, temporal and occipital bones, and a part of the ethmoid bone. All the bones are lined by fibrous endocranium, the external layer of the dura mater, a tough connective tissue which traverses various foramina to join the external periosteum, the pericranium. Both membranes fuse with sutural ligaments or cartilages in the narrow interosseous intervals.

INTERNAL SURFACE OF CRANIAL VAULT (Fig. 27.9)
The gradual obliteration of the sutures that occurs with age commences on the intracranial surface.

The internal surface includes most of the frontal and parietal bones and the squamous part of the occipital bone. The bones are united at the coronal, sagittal and lambdoid sutures (unless fusion has obliterated them). Parietal foramina may occur near the sagittal sulcus, c.3.5 cm anterior to the lambdoid suture, for the passage of emissary veins associated with the superior sagittal sinus. The cranial vault, deeply concave, presents numerous vascular furrows. The frontal branch of the middle meningeal vein, and sometimes the artery, groove the bone deeply just behind the coronal suture. Branches of both these vessels and their parietal branches ascend backwards, and groove the internal surface of the parietal bone. Smaller grooves may mark the frontal and occipital bones. Impressions for cerebral gyri are less distinct on the vault than on the cranial base.

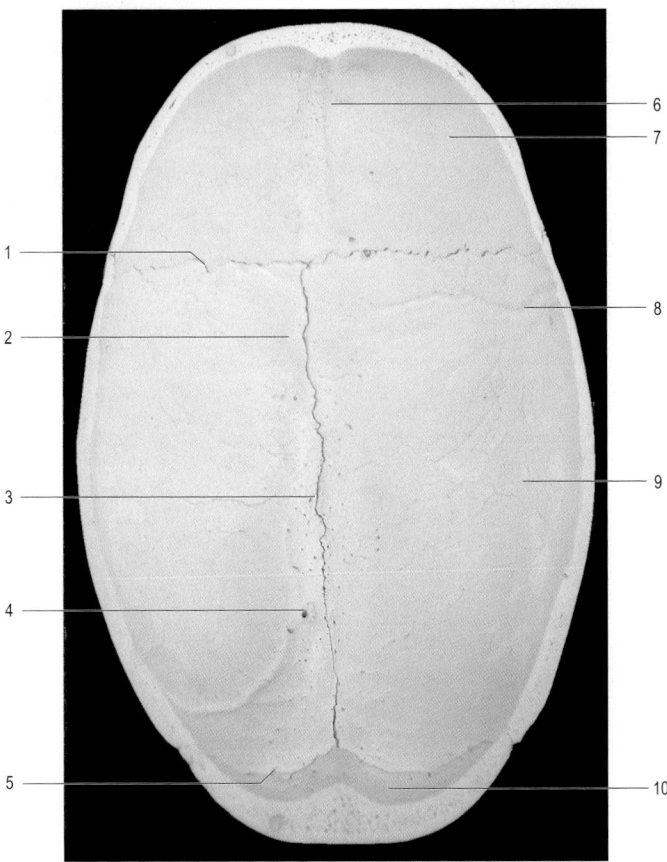

1. Coronal suture.	**6.** Frontal crest.
2. Groove for superior sagittal sinus.	**7.** Frontal bone.
3. Sagittal suture.	**8.** Groove for middle meningeal vessels.
4. Parietal foramen.	**9.** Parietal bone.
5. Lambdoid suture.	**10.** Occipital bone.

Fig. 27.9 Internal surface of cranial vault. (By permission from Berkovitz and Moxham, 1994.)

An anteromedian frontal crest projects backwards and gives attachment to the falx cerebri, a dural partition that passes between the two cerebral hemispheres of the brain. The crest exhibits a groove related to the origin of the sagittal sulcus that accommodates the superior sagittal sinus. This groove widens as it passes back below the sagittal suture. Irregular depressions, granular foveolae, which become larger and more numerous with age, lie on either side of the sulcus and are adapted to arachnoid granulations.

CRANIAL FOSSAE (ANTERIOR, MIDDLE, POSTERIOR) (Fig. 27.10)
The base of the cranial cavity is divided into three distinct fossae, the anterior, middle and posterior cranial fossae (**Fig. 27.10**). The floor of the anterior cranial fossa is at the highest level and the floor of the posterior fossa is at the lowest.

Anterior cranial fossa
The anterior cranial fossa is formed at the front and sides by the frontal bone, while its floor contains the orbital plate of the frontal bone, the cribriform plate and crista galli of the ethmoid bone, and the lesser wings and anterior part of the body of the sphenoid. Unlike the other cranial fossae, it does not directly communicate with the inferior surface of the cranium but instead is related to the roofs of the orbits and the nasal fossae.

A perforated plate of bone, the cribriform plate of the ethmoid bone, spreads across the midline between the orbital plates of the frontal bone, and is depressed below them, forming part of the roof of the nasal cavity. Olfactory nerves pass from the nasal mucosa to the olfactory bulb of the brain through numerous small foramina in the cribriform plate. Anteriorly a spur of bone, the crista galli, projects upwards between the cerebral hemispheres. A depression between the crista galli and the crest of the frontal bone is crossed by the fronto-ethmoidal suture

461

The posterior border of each lesser wing fits the stem of the lateral cerebral sulcus and may be grooved by the sphenoparietal sinus. Above is the inferior surface of the frontal lobe of the cerebral hemisphere and medially is the anterior perforated substance. Inferiorly the lesser wing bounds the superior orbital fissure, and completes the orbital roof. Each anterior clinoid process gives attachment to the free margin of the tentorium cerebelli and is grooved medially by the internal carotid artery as it leaves the cavernous sinus. It may be connected to the middle clinoid process by a thin osseous bar, completing a caroticoclinoid foramen around the artery.

Middle cranial fossa

The middle cranial fossa is deeper and more extensive than the anterior cranial fossa, particularly laterally. It is bounded in front by the lesser wings and part of the body of the sphenoid, behind by the superior borders of the petrous part of the temporal bone and the dorsum sellae of the sphenoid, and laterally by the squamous parts of the temporal bone, parietal bone and greater wings of the sphenoid. This region corresponds with the middle part of the cranial base.

Centrally the floor is narrower and formed by the body of the sphenoid bone. The hollowed out area is the site of the hypophysial (pituitary) gland and is therefore termed the hypophysial (pituitary) fossa. The area has the shape of a Turkish saddle, and so is also known as the sella turcica. The anterior edge of the hypophysial fossa is completed laterally by a middle clinoid process, the floor forms the roof of the sphenoidal air sinuses, and the posterior boundary presents a vertical pillar of bone, the dorsum sellae. The superolateral angles of the dorsum are expanded as the posterior clinoid processes. A fold of dura, the diaphragma sella, is attached to the anterior and posterior clinoid processes and roofs over the hypophysial fossa. The smooth upper part of the anterior wall of the fossa is the jugum sphenoidale which is bounded behind by the anterior border of the grooved sulcus chiasmatis leading laterally to the optic canals. The optic nerve and ophthalmic artery pass through the optic canal, and the optic chiasma usually lies posterosuperior to the sulcus chiasmatis. Below the sulcus chiasmatis is the tuberculum sellae. The cavernous sinus lies lateral to the hypophysial fossa, and the lateral wall of the body of the sphenoid contains a shallow carotid groove related to the internal carotid artery as it ascends from the carotid canal and runs through the cavernous sinus. Posterolaterally the groove may be deepened by a small projecting lingula.

Laterally the middle cranial fossa is deep and supports the temporal lobes of the cerebral hemispheres. Anteriorly are the orbits, laterally the temporal fossae, and inferiorly the infratemporal fossae. The middle cranial fossa communicates with the orbits by the superior orbital fissures, each bounded above by a lesser wing, below by a greater wing, and medially by the body of the sphenoid bone. Each fissure is wider medially, and has a long axis sloping inferomedially and forwards. Many nerves and vessels pass through it, namely, the oculomotor, trochlear and abducens nerves, and the lacrimal, frontal and nasociliary branches of the ophthalmic division of the trigeminal nerve, together with filaments from the internal carotid plexus (sympathetic), the ophthalmic veins, the orbital branch of the middle meningeal artery, and the recurrent branch of the lacrimal artery.

Three foramina can be identified in the greater wing of the sphenoid bone. The foramen rotundum is situated just below and behind the medial end of the superior orbital fissure, and leads forwards into the pterygopalatine fossa, to which it conducts the maxillary nerve. Behind the foramen rotundum is the foramen ovale which transmits the mandibular nerve. The foramen spinosum is posterolateral to the foramen ovale and transmits the middle meningeal artery. The latter, with companion veins, ascends lateral to the squamous part of the temporal bone, and turns anterolaterally across the sphenosquamosal suture to the greater wing of the sphenoid bone where it divides into frontal and parietal branches. The frontal branch ascends across the pterion to the anterior part of the parietal bone; at or near the pterion it is often in a bony canal. The parietal branch runs back and up on to the squamous part of the temporal bone, crossing the squamosal suture to gain the parietal bone. These arteries and veins groove the floor and lateral wall of the middle cranial fossa. The foramen ovale and foramen spinosum connect with the underlying infratemporal fossa.

The foramen lacerum is situated at the posterior end of the carotid groove, posteromedial to the foramen ovale. Its boundaries and contents have already been considered when describing the intermediate part of the cranial base. A small foramen may occur at the root of the greater

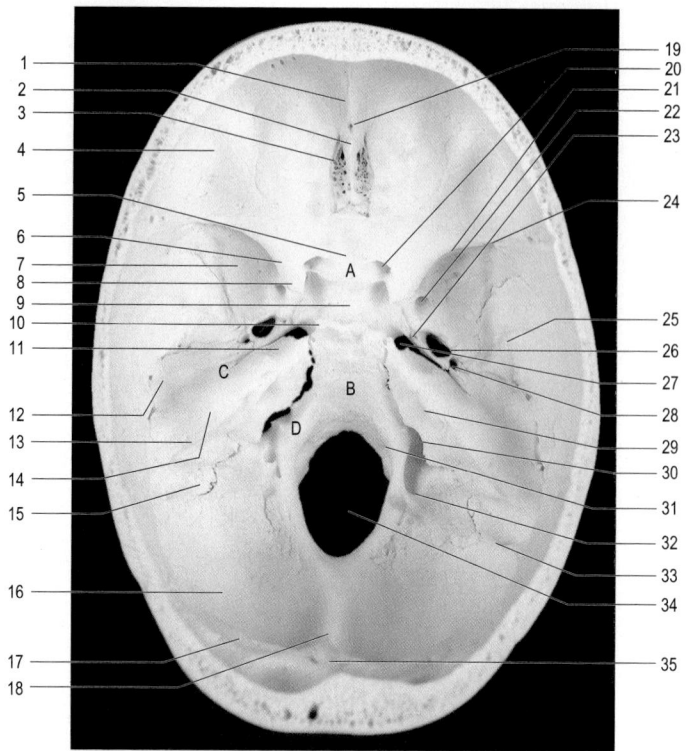

1. Frontal crest.
2. Crista galli.
3. Cribriform plate of ethmoid.
4. Orbital part of frontal bone.
5. Jugum of sphenoid bone.
6. Lesser wing of sphenoid.
7. Greater wing of sphenoid.
8. Anterior clinoid process.
9. Pituitary fossa in body of sphenoid.
10. Posterior clinoid process on dorsum sellae.
11. Trigeminal impression.
12. Squamous part of temporal bone.
13. Groove associated with superior petrosal sinus.
14. Petrous part of temporal bone.
15. Groove associated with sigmoid sinus.
16. Squamous part of occipital bone.
17. Groove associated with transverse sinus.
18. Internal occipital crest.
19. Foramen caecum.
20. Optical canal.
21. Superior orbital fissure.
22. Foramen rotundum.
23. Sphenoidal foramen.
24. Openings of canal for middle meningeal vessels.
25. Groove associated with middle meningeal vessels.
26. Foramen ovale.
27. Foramen lacerum.
28. Foramen spinosum.
29. Internal acoustic meatus.
30. Jugular foramen.
31. Hypoglossal canal.
32. Condylar canal.
33. Mastoid foramen.
34. Foramen magnum.
35. Internal occipital.
   A. Prechiasmatic groove.
   B. Basilar part of occipital bone.
   C. Hiatus and groove for greater petrosal nerve.
   D. Petro-occipital fissure.

Fig. 27.10 Floor of cranial cavity showing the cranial fossae. (By permission from Berkovitz and Moxham, 1994.)

and bears the foramen caecum, which is usually a small blind-ended depression, but which occasionally accommodates a vein draining from the nasal mucosa to the superior sagittal sinus. The anterior ethmoidal nerve enters the cranial cavity where the cribriform plate meets the orbital part of the frontal bone and then passes into the roof of the nose via a small foramen by the side of the crista galli: the nerve grooves the crista galli. The anterior ethmoidal vessels accompany the nerve. The posterior ethmoidal canal, which transmits the posterior ethmoidal nerve and vessels, opens at the posterolateral corner of the cribriform plate and is overhung by the sphenoid bone.

The convex cranial surface of the frontal bone separates the brain from the orbit and bears impressions of cerebral gyri and small grooves for meningeal vessels. Posteriorly, it joins the anterior border of the lesser wing of the sphenoid bone which forms the posterior boundary of the anterior cranial fossa. The medial end of the lesser wing constitutes the anterior clinoid process. The lesser wing joins the body of the sphenoid body by two roots which are separated by the optic canal. The anterior root, broad and flat, is continuous with the jugum sphenoidale, while the smaller and thicker posterior root joins the body of the sphenoid bone near the posterior bank of the sulcus chiasmatis. The frontosphenoid and sphenoethmoidal sutures divide the sphenoid from the adjacent bones.

wing of the sphenoid medial to the foramen lacerum, when present; this emissary sphenoidal foramen transmits a vein from the cavernous sinus.

A shallow trigeminal impression, adapted to the trigeminal ganglion, is situated posterior to the foramen lacerum on the anterior surface of the petrous part of the temporal bone near its apex. Posterolateral to this impression is a shallow pit, limited posteriorly by a rounded arcuate eminence which is produced by the anterior semicircular canal. Lateral to the trigeminal impression a narrow groove passes posterolaterally into the hiatus for the greater petrosal nerve, and even further laterally is the hiatus for the lesser petrosal nerve. The anterior surface of the petrous part of the temporal bone is formed by the tegmen tympani, a thin osseous lamina in the roof of the tympanic cavity, which extends anteromedially above the auditory tube, anterolateral to the arcuate eminence. The posterior part of the tegmen tympani roofs the mastoid antrum, lateral to the eminence. The superior border of the petrous part of the temporal bone separates the middle and the posterior cranial fossae, and is grooved by the superior petrosal sinus. In young skulls, a petrosquamous suture may be visible at the lateral limit of the tegmen tympani but it is obliterated in adults. The tegmen tympani then turns down as the lateral wall of the osseous auditory tube and its lower border may appear in the squamotympanic fissure. Lateral to the anterior part of the tegmen tympani, the squamous part of the temporal bone is thin over a small area that coincides with the deepest part of the mandibular fossa.

A smooth trigeminal notch leads into the trigeminal impression and lies on the upper border of the petrous temporal, anteromedial to the groove for the superior petrosal sinus. At this point, the trigeminal nerve separates the sinus from bone. The petrosphenoidal ligament is attached to a tiny bony spicule, directed anteromedially at the anterior end of the trigeminal notch. The abducent nerve bends sharply across the upper petrous border, passing between the ligament and the dorsum sellae anterior to the petrosphenoidal ligament.

Posterior cranial fossa

The posterior cranial fossa is the largest and deepest of the cranial fossae. It is bounded in front by the dorsum sellae, posterior aspects of the sphenoidal body and basilar part of occipital bone; behind by the squamous part of the occipital bone; laterally by the petrous and mastoid parts of the temporal bone and by the lateral parts of the occipital bone, and above and behind by the mastoid angles of the parietal bones. The posterior cranial fossa contains the cerebellum, pons and medulla oblongata. The region corresponds extracranially with the posterior part of the cranial base.

The most prominent feature in the floor of the posterior cranial fossa is the foramen magnum in the occipital bone. A sloping surface, the clivus, formed successively by the basilar part of the occipital bone, the posterior part of the body and then the dorsum sellae of the sphenoid bone, lies anterior to the foramen magnum. The clivus is gently concave from side to side. On each side it is separated from the petrous part of the temporal bone by a petro-occipital fissure, filled by a thin plate of cartilage and limited behind by the jugular foramen. Its margins are grooved by the inferior petrosal sinus. The spheno-occipital synchondrosis is evident on the clivus of a growing child.

A large jugular foramen, sited at the posterior end of the petro-occipital fissure, lies above and lateral to the foramen magnum. Its upper border is sharp and irregular, and contains a notch for the glossopharyngeal nerve. The cochlear canaliculus, which contains the perilymphatic 'duct' is sited in the deepest part of the notch. The lower border of the jugular foramen is smooth. Posteriorly it is grooved by the sigmoid sinus which continues into the foramen as the internal jugular vein. The accessory, vagus and glossopharyngeal nerves pass through the anterior part of the jugular foramen from behind forwards, and may groove the jugular tubercle as they enter the foramen. The hypoglossal (anterior condylar) canal lies medial to and below the lower border of the jugular foramen at the junction of the basilar and lateral parts of the occipital bone. This canal transmits the hypoglossal nerve (and its recurrent branch), the meningeal branch of the ascending pharyngeal artery and an emissary vein linking the basilar plexus intracranially with the internal jugular vein extracranially. If a posterior condylar canal is present behind the occipital condyle, its internal orifice is posterolateral to that of the hypoglossal canal and contains a sigmoid emissary vein (associated with the occipital veins) and a meningeal branch of the occipital artery. The occipital condyles lie within the anterior aspect of the

foramen magnum: their medial aspects are roughened for the attachments of the alar ligaments associated with the atlanto-axial joints.

The posterior surface of the petrous part of the temporal bone forms much of the anterolateral wall of the posterior cranial fossa. It contains the internal acoustic meatus, which lies anterosuperior to the jugular foramen, and transmits the facial and vestibulocochlear nerves, the nervus intermedius, and labyrinthine vessels.

The mastoid part of the temporal bone lies behind the petrous part of the temporal bone in the lateral wall of the posterior cranial fossa. Anteriorly it is grooved by a wide sigmoid sulcus (groove) running forwards and downwards, then downwards and medially, and finally forwards to the jugular foramen. It contains the sigmoid sinus. Superiorly, where the groove touches the mastoid angle of the parietal bone, it is continuous with a groove transmitting the transverse sinus; it next crosses the parietomastoid suture, and then descends behind the mastoid antrum. A mastoid foramen for an emissary vein from the sigmoid sinus and a meningeal branch of the occipital artery, sometimes large enough to groove the squamous part of the occipital bone, may be sited here. The lowest part of the sigmoid sulcus crosses the occipitomastoid suture and grooves the jugular process of the occipital bone. The right sigmoid sulcus is usually larger than the left.

A thin plate with an irregularly curved margin projects back behind the internal acoustic meatus and bounds a slit containing the opening of the vestibular aqueduct (which contains the saccus and ductus endolymphaticus and a small artery and vein). A small subarcuate fossa lies between the internal acoustic meatus and the aqueductal opening. It contains dura mater. Near the superior border of the petrous part of the temporal bone it is pierced by a small vein. In infants the fossa is a relatively large blind tunnel under the anterior semicircular canal.

The squamous part of the occipital bone displays a median internal occipital crest, which runs posteriorly from the foramen magnum to an internal occipital protuberance and gives attachment to the falx cerebelli. The internal occipital crest may be grooved by the occipital sinus. The internal occipital protuberance is close to the confluence of the sinuses and is grooved bilaterally by the transverse sinuses. The latter curve laterally with an upward convexity to the mastoid angles of the parietal bones. The groove for the transverse sinus is usually deeper on the right, where it is generally a continuation of the superior sagittal sinus, while on the left it is frequently a continuation of the straight sinus. On both sides the transverse sulcus is continuous with the sigmoid sulcus. Below the transverse sulcus the internal occipital crest separates two shallow fossae, adapted to the cerebellar hemispheres. The margins of the grooves for the transverse sinus and superior petrosal sinus, together with the posterior clinoid process, all provide anchorage for the attached margin of the tentorium cerebelli.

DISARTICULATED INDIVIDUAL BONES

OCCIPITAL BONE (Fig. 27.11)

The occipital bone forms much of the back and base of the cranium. It is trapezoid, internally concave and encloses the foramen magnum. It has four parts, namely, basilar (basioccipital), which is the quadrilateral part in front of the foramen magnum; squamous, which is the expanded plate posterosuperior to the foramen; and lateral (condylar or exoccipital), on each side of the foramen magnum. The foramen magnum is situated in an anteromedian position, and is oval, being wider behind and with its greatest diameter being anteroposterior.

Squamous part

The squamous part is convex externally and concave internally. On the external surface the external occipital protuberance lies midway between its summit and the foramen magnum. On each side, two curved lines extend laterally from this protuberance. The upper, faintly marked and often almost imperceptible, is the highest nuchal line, to the medial part of which the epicranial aponeurosis is attached, and the lower is the superior nuchal line. The lateral part of the highest nuchal line gives attachment to the occipital part of occipitofrontalis. The median external occipital crest, often faint, descends from the external occipital protuberance to the foramen magnum. On each side an inferior nuchal line spreads laterally from the midpoint of the crest.

The internal surface of the squamous part is divided into four deep fossae by an irregular internal occipital protuberance and by ridged sagittal and horizontal extensions from it. The two superior fossae are

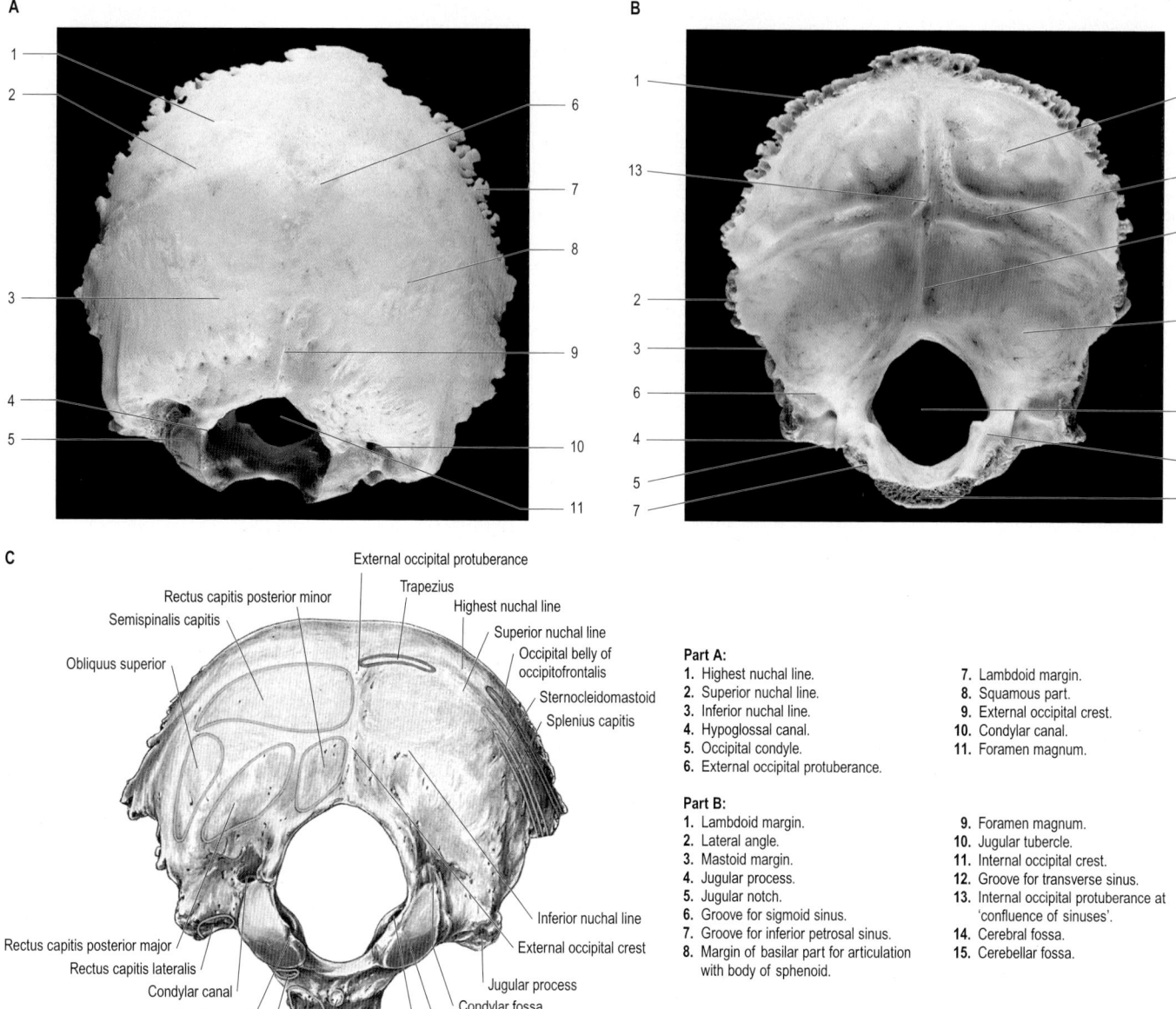

A

1
2
6
7
8
3
9
4
5
10
11

B

1
13
2
3
6
4
5
7
14
12
11
15
9
10
8

C

Semispinalis capitis
Rectus capitis posterior minor
Obliquus superior
External occipital protuberance
Trapezius
Highest nuchal line
Superior nuchal line
Occipital belly of occipitofrontalis
Sternocleidomastoid
Splenius capitis
Rectus capitis posterior major
Rectus capitis lateralis
Condylar canal
Alar ligament
Rectus capitis anterior
Longus capitis
Pharyngeal tubercle
Condyle
Hypoglossal canal
Condylar fossa
Jugular process
External occipital crest
Inferior nuchal line

Part A:
1. Highest nuchal line.
2. Superior nuchal line.
3. Inferior nuchal line.
4. Hypoglossal canal.
5. Occipital condyle.
6. External occipital protuberance.

7. Lambdoid margin.
8. Squamous part.
9. External occipital crest.
10. Condylar canal.
11. Foramen magnum.

Part B:
1. Lambdoid margin.
2. Lateral angle.
3. Mastoid margin.
4. Jugular process.
5. Jugular notch.
6. Groove for sigmoid sinus.
7. Groove for inferior petrosal sinus.
8. Margin of basilar part for articulation with body of sphenoid.

9. Foramen magnum.
10. Jugular tubercle.
11. Internal occipital crest.
12. Groove for transverse sinus.
13. Internal occipital protuberance at 'confluence of sinuses'.
14. Cerebral fossa.
15. Cerebellar fossa.

Fig. 27.11 Occipital bone. **A,** External surface; **B,** internal surface; **C,** muscle attachments. (By permission from Berkovitz and Moxham, 1994.)

triangular and adapted to the occipital poles of the cerebral hemispheres; the inferior fossae are quadrilateral and shaped to accommodate the cerebellar hemispheres. A wide groove with raised banks, the superior sagittal sulcus, ascends from the protuberance to the superior angle of the squamous part. The posterior part of the falx cerebri is attached to the margins of the sulcus. A prominent internal occipital crest descends from the protuberance and bifurcates near the foramen magnum, providing an attachment for the falx cerebelli. The occipital sinus, sometimes double, lies in this attachment. A small vermian fossa may exist, at the lower end of the internal occipital crest; when present, it is occupied by part of the inferior cerebellar vermis. On each side a wide sulcus for the transverse sinus extends laterally from the internal occipital protuberance. The tentorium cerebelli is attached to the margins of these sulci. The right sulcus is usually larger, passing into the sulcus for the superior sagittal sinus, the left being a continuation of the straight sinus. The position of this confluence of sinuses is indicated by a depression on one side of the protuberance.

The position of the fetal posterior fontanelle coincides with the junction between the superior angle of the squamous part of the occipital bone and the occipital angles of the parietal bones. The lateral angles of the squamous part are marked internally by the ends of the transverse sulci and project between the parietal and temporal bones. The lambdoid borders extend from superior to lateral angles and are serrated for articulation with the occipital borders of the parietal bones

at the lambdoid suture. The mastoid borders extend from the lateral angles to the jugular processes, articulating with the mastoid parts of the temporal bones. A variety of sutural bones (ossicles) may occur at or near the lambda, e.g. the 'interparietal' (Inca bone or ossicle of Goethe).

Basilar part

The basilar part extends anterosuperiorly from the foramen magnum, fusing with the sphenoid bone in adults. In young skulls a rough and uneven surface is joined to the body of the sphenoid by a growth cartilage (spheno-occipital synchondrosis). By the twenty-fifth year, this plate has fully ossified and the occipital and sphenoid bones are fused.

The inferior surface of the basilar part bears a small pharyngeal tubercle for attachment of the fibrous pharyngeal raphe c.1 cm in front of the foramen magnum. Longus capitis is attached anterolateral to the tubercle, and rectus capitis anterior is attached to a small depression immediately anterior to the occipital condyle. This depression may occasionally be replaced by a small precondylar tubercle. The anterior atlanto-occipital membrane is attached to the anterior margin of the foramen magnum.

The superior surface of the basilar part is a broad groove and forms part of the clivus that ascends anteriorly from the foramen magnum, and on which rest the medulla oblongata and lower pons. Sulci of the inferior petrosal sinuses are on its lateral margins, which articulate below with the petrous part of the temporal bones.

Lateral (condylar) parts

The lateral (condylar) parts of the occipital bone flank the foramen magnum. On their inferior surfaces are occipital condyles for articulation with the superior articular facets of the atlas vertebra. The condyles are oval or reniform, their long axes converging anteromedially. The articular surfaces, wholly convex, face inferolaterally. They are occasionally constricted and a condyle may be in two parts (as may be the reciprocal surfaces of the atlas vertebra). A tubercle gives attachment to an alar ligament medial to each articular facet. The hypoglossal (anterior condylar) canal, which is situated anteriorly above each condyle, starts internally a little above the anterolateral part of the foramen magnum and continues anterolaterally. It may be partly or wholly divided by a spicule of bone and transmits the hypoglossal nerve and a meningeal branch of the ascending pharyngeal artery. A condylar fossa, behind each condyle, fits the posterior margin of the superior facet of the atlas vertebra in full extension of the skull. Its floor is sometimes perforated by a posterior condylar canal for a sigmoid emissary vein.. A quadrilateral plate, the jugular process, projects laterally from the posterior half of each condyle, and contributes the posterior part of the jugular foramen. The inferior surface of the jugular process is roughened by the attachment of rectus capitis lateralis. The jugular process is indented in front by a jugular notch, which is sometimes partly divided by a small intrajugular process that projects anterolaterally. A paramastoid process sometimes projects down and may even articulate with the transverse process of the atlas vertebra. Laterally, the jugular process has a rough quadrilateral or triangular area that is joined to the jugular surface of the temporal bone by cartilage: it begins to ossify at c.25 years.

An oval jugular tubercle overlies the hypoglossal canal on the superior surface of the occipital condyle. Its posterior part often bears a shallow furrow for the glossopharyngeal, vagus and accessory nerves. A deep groove containing the end of the sigmoid sinus curves anteromedially around a hook-shaped process to end at the jugular notch. The posterior condylar canal opens into the posterior cranial fossa near the medial end of the groove.

Ossification

Above the highest nuchal lines the squamous part of the occipital bone is developed in a fibrous membrane and is ossified from two centres (one on each side) from about the second fetal month. This part of the occipital bone may remain separate as the interparietal bone. The remainder of the occipital bone is preformed in cartilage. Below the highest nuchal lines, the squamous part ossifies from two centres, appearing in about the seventh week and soon uniting. The two components of the squamous part unite in the third postnatal month, but the line of union is recognizable at birth. The remainder of the cartilage of the occipital is ossified from five centres, two each for the lateral parts during the eighth week and one for the basilar part commencing around the sixth week.

At birth the occipital bone consists of four separate parts (**Fig. 27.12**), a basilar part, two lateral parts and a squamous part, all joined by cartilage and forming a ring around the foramen magnum. The squamous and lateral parts fuse together from the second year. The lateral parts fuse with the basilar part during years 3 and 4, but fusion may be delayed until the 7th year.

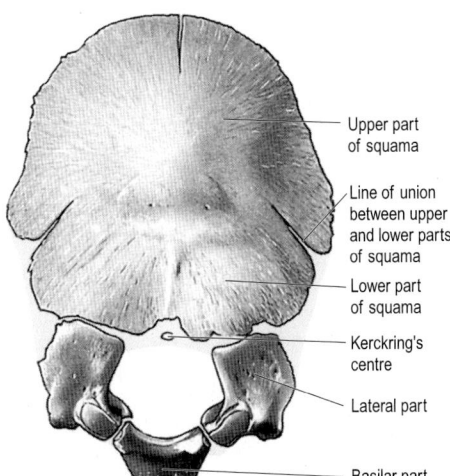

Fig. 27.12 The occipital bone of a newborn child: external surface. Parts of the chondrocranium which are still unossified are shown in blue.

Upper part of squama

Line of union between upper and lower parts of squama

Lower part of squama

Kerckring's centre

Lateral part

Basilar part

s.w.w

SPHENOID BONE (Fig. 27.13)

The sphenoid bone lies in the base of the skull between the frontal, temporal and occipital bones. It has a central body, paired greater and lesser wings that spread laterally from the body, and two pterygoid processes that descend from the junction of the body and greater wings. The body contains the sphenoidal air sinuses while immediately above it is a depression which contains the hypophysis cerebri (pituitary gland).

Body

The body is cuboidal and contains two sphenoidal air sinuses, separated by a septum. The cerebral or superior surface articulates in front with the cribriform plate of the ethmoid bone. Anteriorly is the smooth jugum sphenoidale, related to gyri recti and olfactory tracts. The jugum is bounded behind by the anterior border of the sulcus chiasmatis that leads laterally to the optic canals. Posteriorly is the tuberculum sellae, behind which is the deeply concave sella turcica. In life the sella turcica contains the hypophysis cerebri in the hypophysial fossa. The anterior edge of the sella turcica is completed laterally by two middle clinoid processes. Posteriorly the sella turcica is bounded by a square dorsum sellae, the superior angles of which bear variable posterior clinoid processes. The clinoid process is related to the attachment of the diaphragma sella and the tentorium cerebelli. On each side, below the dorsum sellae, a small petrosal process articulates with the apex of the petrous part of the temporal bone. The body of the sphenoid slopes directly into the basilar part of the occipital bone posterior to the dorsum sellae, and together these bones form the clivus. In the growing child this is the site of the spheno-occipital synchondrosis.

The lateral surfaces of the body are united with the greater wings and the medial pterygoid plates. A broad carotid sulcus accommodates the internal carotid artery and a series of cranial nerves associated with the cavernous sinus above the root of each wing. The sulcus is deepest posteriorly, overhung medially by the petrosal part of the temporal and has a sharp lateral margin, the lingula. The lingula continues back over the posterior opening of the pterygoid canal.

A median triangular, bilaminar sphenoidal crest on the anterior surface of the body of the sphenoid makes a small contribution to the nasal septum. The anterior border of the crest joins the perpendicular plate of the ethmoid bone, and a sphenoidal sinus opens on each side of it. The sphenoidal sinuses, which are two large, irregular cavities within the body, are usually separated by an asymmetrical septum. Each sinus varies in form and size and is partially divided by bony laminae. A lateral recess may extend into the greater wing and lingula and may even invade the basilar part of the occipital bone almost to the foramen magnum. The morphology of the sphenoidal sinus is of clinical importance in relation to the trans-sphenoidal surgical approach to the hypophysis cerebri. Sphenoidal sinuses may be classified according to size into three main types: sellar, the commonest type, where the sinus extends for a variable distance beyond the tuberculum sellae; presellar, where the sinus occasionally extends posteriorly towards, but not beyond, the tuberculum sellae; conchal, the rarest type, where a small sinus is separated from the sella turcica by c.10 mm of trabecular bone. In the articulated state the sphenoidal sinuses are closed anteroinferiorly by the sphenoidal conchae, which are largely destroyed when disarticulating a skull. Each half of the anterior surface of the body of the sphenoid possesses a superolateral depressed area joined to the ethmoid labyrinth, which completes the posterior ethmoidal sinuses; a lateral margin which articulates with the orbital plate of the ethmoid above and the orbital process of the palatine bone below; and an inferomedial, smooth, triangular area, which forms the posterior nasal roof and near whose superior angle is the orifice of a sphenoidal sinus.

The inferior surface of the body of the sphenoid bears a median triangular sphenoidal rostrum, embraced above by the diverging lower margins of the sphenoidal crest. The narrow anterior end of the rostrum fits into a fissure between the anterior parts of the alae of the vomer, and posterior ends of the sphenoidal conchae flank the rostrum, articulating with its alae. A thin vaginal process projects medially from the base of the medial pterygoid plate on each side of the posterior part of the rostrum, behind the apex of the sphenoidal concha.

Greater wings

The greater wings of the sphenoid bone curve broadly superolaterally from the body. Posteriorly each is triangular, fitting the angle between the petrous and squamous parts of the temporal bone at a sphenosquamosal suture. The cerebral surface contributes to the anterior part of the

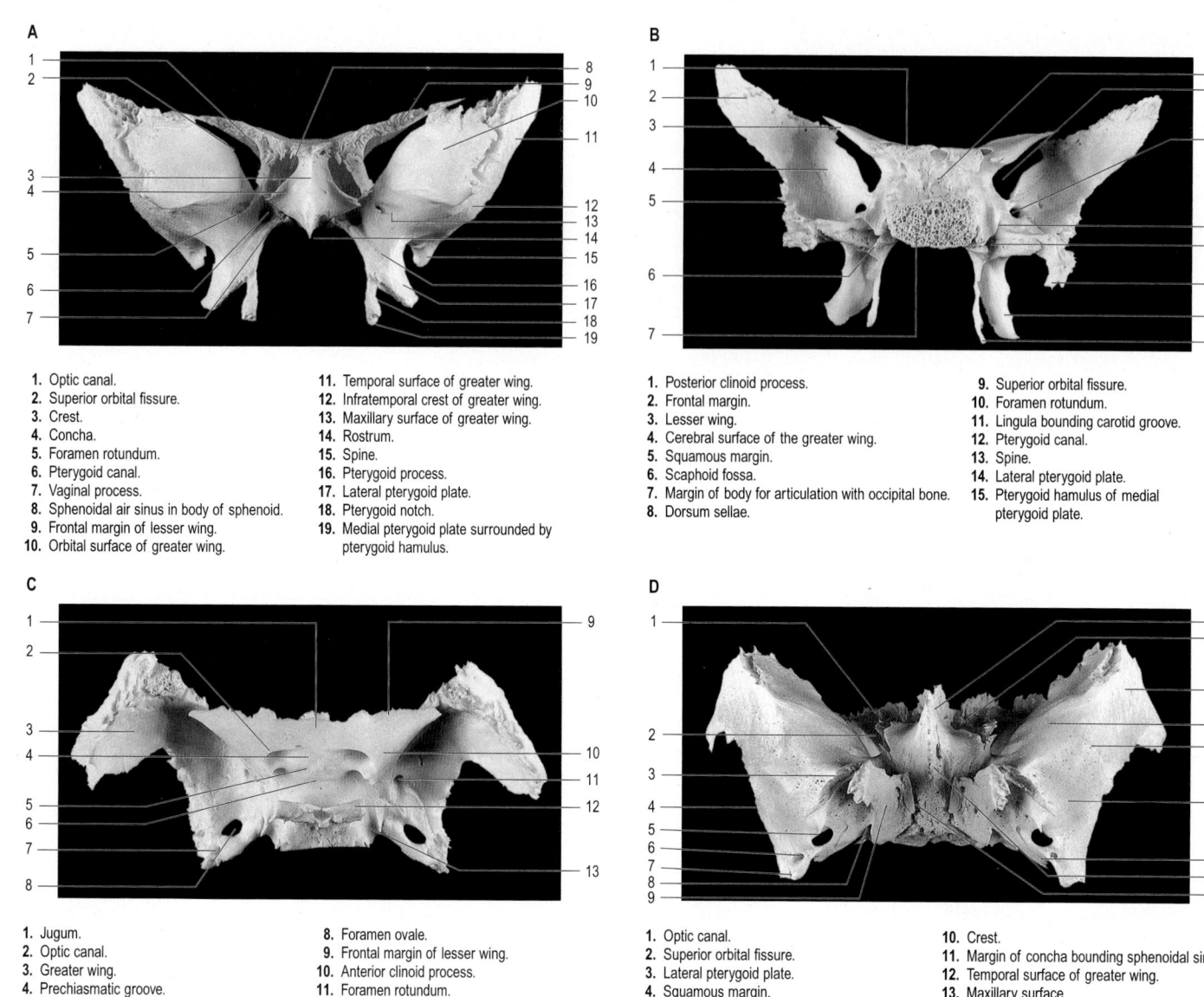

A

1. Optic canal.
2. Superior orbital fissure.
3. Crest.
4. Concha.
5. Foramen rotundum.
6. Pterygoid canal.
7. Vaginal process.
8. Sphenoidal air sinus in body of sphenoid.
9. Frontal margin of lesser wing.
10. Orbital surface of greater wing.
11. Temporal surface of greater wing.
12. Infratemporal crest of greater wing.
13. Maxillary surface of greater wing.
14. Rostrum.
15. Spine.
16. Pterygoid process.
17. Lateral pterygoid plate.
18. Pterygoid notch.
19. Medial pterygoid plate surrounded by pterygoid hamulus.

B

1. Posterior clinoid process.
2. Frontal margin.
3. Lesser wing.
4. Cerebral surface of the greater wing.
5. Squamous margin.
6. Scaphoid fossa.
7. Margin of body for articulation with occipital bone.
8. Dorsum sellae.
9. Superior orbital fissure.
10. Foramen rotundum.
11. Lingula bounding carotid groove.
12. Pterygoid canal.
13. Spine.
14. Lateral pterygoid plate.
15. Pterygoid hamulus of medial pterygoid plate.

C

1. Jugum.
2. Optic canal.
3. Greater wing.
4. Prechiasmatic groove.
5. Tuberculum sellae.
6. Pituitary fossa.
7. Foramen spinosum.
8. Foramen ovale.
9. Frontal margin of lesser wing.
10. Anterior clinoid process.
11. Foramen rotundum.
12. Posterior clinoid process on dorsum sellae.
13. Carotid groove.

D

1. Optic canal.
2. Superior orbital fissure.
3. Lateral pterygoid plate.
4. Squamous margin.
5. Foramen ovale.
6. Foramen spinosum.
7. Spine.
8. Pterygoid canal.
9. Medial pterygoid plate.
10. Crest.
11. Margin of concha bounding sphenoidal sinus.
12. Temporal surface of greater wing.
13. Maxillary surface.
14. Infratemporal crest.
15. Infratemporal surface.
16. Groove for pharyngotympanic tube.
17. Rostrum.
18. Vaginal process.

Fig. 27.13 Sphenoid bone. **A**, Anterior view; **B**, posterior view; **C**, superior view; **D**, inferior view. (By permission from Berkovitz and Moxham, 1994.)

middle cranial fossa. Deeply concave, its undulating surface is adapted to the anterior gyri of the temporal lobe of the cerebral hemisphere. The foramen rotundum for the maxillary nerve lies anteromedially. Posterolateral to the foramen rotundum is the foramen ovale, which transmits the mandibular nerve, accessory meningeal artery and sometimes the lesser petrosal nerve, although the latter nerve may have its own canaliculus innominatus medial to the foramen spinosum. A small emissary sphenoidal foramen which transmits a small vein from the cavernous sinus is present medial to the foramen ovale (on one or both sides) in c.40% of skulls. Behind the foramen ovale is the foramen spinosum, which transmits the middle meningeal artery and meningeal branch of the mandibular nerve.

The lateral surface is vertically convex and divided by a transverse infratemporal crest into temporal (upper) and infratemporal (lower) surfaces. Temporalis is attached to the temporal surface. The infratemporal surface is directed downwards and, with the infratemporal crest, is the site of attachment of the upper fibres of lateral pterygoid. It contains the foramen ovale and foramen spinosum. The small downward projecting spine of the sphenoid lies posterior to the foramen spinosum. The sphenomandibular ligament, a remnant of the first branchial arch cartilage, is attached to the tip of the spine of the sphenoid. The medial side of the spine has a faint anteroinferior groove for the chorda tympani

nerve and appears in the lateral wall of the sulcus for the auditory tube. A ridge which forms a posterior boundary of the pterygomaxillary fissure descends to the front of the lateral pterygoid plate medial to the anterior end of the infratemporal crest.

The quadrilateral orbital surface of the greater wing faces anteromedially, and forms the posterior part of the lateral wall of the orbit. It has a serrated upper edge which articulates with the orbital plate of the frontal bone, and a serrated lateral margin which articulates with the zygomatic bone. Its smooth inferior border is the posterolateral edge of the inferior orbital fissure, and its sharp medial margin forms the inferolateral edge of the superior orbital fissure, on which a small tubercle gives partial attachment to the common annular ocular tendon. Below the medial end of the superior orbital fissure a grooved area forms the posterior wall of the pterygopalatine fossa, which is pierced by the foramen rotundum.

The irregular margin of the greater wing, from the body of the sphenoid to the spine, is an anterior limit of the foramen lacerum, in its medial half. It also displays the posterior aperture of the pterygoid canal. Its lateral half articulates with the petrous part of the temporal bone at a sphenopetrosal synchondrosis. Inferior to this the sulcus tubae contains the cartilaginous auditory tube. Anterior to the spine of the sphenoid the concave squamosal margin is serrated – bevelled internally below, externally above – for articulation with the squamous part of the temporal bone. The tip of the greater wing, bevelled internally, articulates with the sphenoidal angle of the parietal bone at the pterion. Medial to this, a triangular rough area articulates with the frontal bone: its medial angle is continuous with the inferior boundary of the superior orbital fissure, and its anterior angle joins the zygomatic bone by a serrated articulation.

Lesser wings

The lesser wings are triangular, pointed plates that protrude laterally from the anterosuperior regions of the body. The superior surface of each wing is smooth and related to the frontal lobe of the cerebral hemisphere. The inferior surface is a posterior part of the orbital roof and upper boundary of the superior orbital fissure, and overhangs the middle cranial fossa. The posterior border projects into the lateral fissure of the cerebral hemisphere. The medial end of the lesser wing forms the anterior clinoid process. The anterior and middle clinoid processes are sometimes united to form a caroticoclinoid foramen. The lesser wing is connected to the body by a thin flat anterior root and a thick triangular posterior root, between which lies the optic canal. Growth of the posterior root is closely associated with variations in the canal. The cranial opening of the canal may be duplicated, or more commonly, the division is incomplete.

Superior orbital fissure

The superior orbital fissure connects the cranial cavity with the orbit. It is bounded medially by the body of the sphenoid, above by the lesser wing of the sphenoid, below by the medial margin of the orbital surface of the greater wing, and laterally, between greater and lesser wings, by the frontal bone.

Pterygoid processes

The pterygoid processes descend perpendicularly from the junctions of the greater wings and body. Each consists of a medial and lateral plate, whose upper parts are fused anteriorly. The plates are separated below by the angular pterygoid fissure, whose margins articulate with the pyramidal process of the palatine bone. They diverge behind, and medial pterygoid and tensor veli palatini lie in the cuneiform pterygoid fossa between them. Above is a small, oval, shallow scaphoid fossa, formed by division of the upper posterior border of the medial plate. Part of tensor veli palatini is attached to the fossa. The anterior surface of the root of the pterygoid process is broad and triangular. It forms the posterior wall of the pterygopalatine fossa which is pierced by the anterior opening of the pterygoid canal.

Lateral pterygoid plate

The lateral pterygoid plate is broad, thin and everted. Its lateral surface forms part of the medial wall of the infratemporal fossa and gives origin to the lower part of lateral pterygoid. Its medial surface is the lateral wall of the pterygoid fossa, and most of the deep head of medial pterygoid is attached to it. The upper part of its anterior border is a posterior boundary of the pterygomaxillary fissure and the lower part articulates with the palatine bone. Its posterior border is free.

Medial pterygoid plate

The medial pterygoid plate is narrower and longer than the lateral. Its lower end curves to the lateral, unciform pterygoid hamulus. The tendon of tensor veli palatini winds around the hamulus, and the pterygomandibular raphe is attached to it. The lateral surface is the medial wall of the pterygoid fossa. The medial surface is a lateral boundary of the posterior nasal aperture. The medial plate is prolonged above on the inferior aspect of the body of the sphenoid as a thin vaginal process, which articulates anteriorly with the sphenoidal process of the palatine bone and medially with the ala of the vomer. Inferiorly it bears a furrow, which is converted into the palatovaginal canal anteriorly by the sphenoidal process of the palatine bone. This canal transmits pharyngeal branches of the maxillary artery and pterygopalatine ganglion. The pharyngobasilar fascia is attached to the whole of the posterior margin of the medial plate, and the superior pharyngeal constrictor is attached to its lower end. At its upper end, just below the posterior opening of the pterygoid canal, is a small pterygoid tubercle. The processus tubarius, which supports the cartilaginous pharyngeal end of the pharyngotympanic tube, projects back near the midpoint of the margin of the medial pterygoid plate. The plate articulates with the posterior border

of the perpendicular plate of the palatine bone in the lower part of its anterior margin.

Sphenoidal conchae

The sphenoidal conchae are two thin, curved platelets, attached anteroinferiorly to the body of the sphenoid bone. The superior concave surface of each forms the anterior wall and part of the floor of a sphenoidal sinus. They are largely destroyed in disarticulating a skull. *In situ*, each has vertical quadrilateral anterior and horizontal triangular posterior parts. The anterior part consists of a superolateral depressed area, which completes the posterior ethmoidal sinuses and joins below with the orbital process of a palatine bone; and a smooth and triangular inferomedial area, which forms part of the nasal roof and is perforated above by the round opening connecting the sphenoidal sinus and sphenoethmoidal recess.

Anterior parts of the two bones meet in the midline, and protrude as the sphenoidal crest. The horizontal part appears in the nasal roof and completes the sphenopalatine foramen. Its medial edge articulates with the rostrum of the sphenoid and the ala of the vomer. Its apex, directed posteriorly, is superomedial to the vaginal process of the medial pterygoid plate and joins the posterior part of the ala. A small conchal part sometimes appears in the medial wall of the orbit, lying between the orbital plate of the ethmoid in front, the orbital process of the palatine bone below and the frontal bone above.

Ossification

Until the seventh or eighth month *in utero* the sphenoid body has a presphenoidal part, anterior to the tuberculum sellae, with which the lesser wings are continuous, and a postsphenoidal part, comprising the sella turcica and dorsum sellae, and integral with the greater wings and pterygoid processes. Much of the bone is preformed in cartilage. There are six ossification centres for the presphenoidal, and eight for postsphenoidal, parts.

Presphenoidal part – About the ninth week of fetal life, a centre appears in each wing, lateral to the optic canal, and a little later two bilateral centres appear in the presphenoidal body. Each sphenoidal concha has a centre, appearing superoposteriorly in the nasal capsule in the fifth month *in utero*. As this enlarges it partly surrounds a posterosuperior expansion of the nasal cavity, which becomes the sphenoidal sinus. The posterior conchal wall is absorbed and the sinus invades the presphenoid component. In the fourth year the concha fuses with the ethmoidal labyrinth and before puberty it fuses with the sphenoid and palatine bones. Its anterior deficiency persists as an opening for the sphenoidal sinus.

Postsphenoidal part – The first centres appear in the greater wings about the eighth week of fetal life, one in the basal cartilage of each wing below the foramen rotundum. These centres only contribute to the root of the greater wing (near the foramen rotundum and pterygoid canal). The remainder of the greater wing is ossified in mesenchyme, spreading also into the lateral pterygoid plate. About the fourth month of fetal life two centres appear, flanking the sella turcica, and soon fuse. The medial pterygoid plates are also ossified in 'membrane', a centre in each probably appearing about the ninth or tenth week. The hamulus is chondrified during the third fetal month and at once begins to ossify. Medial and lateral pterygoid plates join about the sixth fetal month. During the fourth month, a centre appears for each lingula, soon joining the body. The optic canal in the neonate is relatively large and has a keyhole or 'figure of eight' shape rather than the circular profile seen in the adult.

Postnatal details – Presphenoidal and postsphenoidal parts fuse about the eighth month *in utero*, but an unciform cartilage persists after birth in lower parts of the junction. At birth the bone is tripartite (**Fig. 27.13**) and consists of a central part (body and lesser wings) and two lateral parts (each comprising a greater wing and pterygoid process). During the first year the greater wings and body unite around the pterygoid canals and the lesser wings extend medially above the anterior part of the body, meeting to form the smooth, elevated jugum sphenoidale. By the twenty-fifth year, sphenoid and occipital bones are completely fused. An occasional vascular foramen, often erroneously termed the craniopharyngeal canal, is occasionally seen in the anterior part of the hypophysial fossa. Although the sphenoidal sinus can be identified in the fourth month of fetal life as an evagination of the posterior part of the nasal capsule, by birth it represents an outgrowth of the sphenoethmoidal recess. Pneumatization of the body of the sphenoid bone commences in the second or third year and spreads first into the presphenoid, and later invades the postsphenoid, part. It reaches full size in adolescence, but often enlarges further by absorption of its walls as age advances.

Certain sphenoidal parts are connected by ligaments that occasionally ossify, e.g. the pterygospinous, between the sphenoid spine and upper part of lateral pterygoid plate; the interclinoid, joining the anterior to the posterior clinoid process; and the caroticoclinoid, connecting the anterior to the middle clinoid process.

Premature synostosis of the junction between pre- and postsphenoidal parts, or of the spheno-occipital suture, produces a characteristic appearance, obvious in profile, of an abnormal depression of the nasal bridge (hypertelorism).

TEMPORAL BONE (Fig. 27.14)

Each temporal bone consists of four components: the squamous, petromastoid and tympanic parts and the styloid process. The squamous part has a shallow mandibular fossa associated with the temporomandibular joint. The petromastoid part is relatively large. Its petrous portion houses the auditory apparatus and is formed of compact bone. In contrast, the mastoid process is trabecular and variably pneumatized. The tympanic part has the form of a thin and incomplete ring whose ends are fused with the squamous part. The styloid process gives attachment to the styloid group of muscles. Two canals are associated with the temporal bone. The external acoustic meatus, visible on the lateral surface, conveys sound waves to the tympanic membrane. The internal acoustic meatus, evident on the medial surface, conveys the facial and vestibulocochlear nerves.

Squamous part

The squamous part lies anterosuperiorly and is thin and partly translucent. Its external temporal surface is smooth, slightly convex, and forms part of the temporal fossa for attachment of temporalis. Above the external acoustic meatus, it is grooved vertically by the middle temporal artery. The supramastoid crest curves backwards and upwards across its posterior part and gives attachment to the temporal fascia. The junction between the squamous and mastoid parts is c.1.5 cm below this crest and traces of the squamomastoid suture may persist. The suprameatal triangle, a depression marking the position of the mastoid antrum (medial to it at a depth of c.1.25 cm), lies between the anterior end of the supramastoid crest and the posterosuperior quadrant of the external acoustic meatus. The triangle usually contains a small suprameatal spine anteriorly.

The internal cerebral surface of the squamous part is concave and contains depressions corresponding to convolutions of the temporal lobe of the cerebral hemisphere. This surface is grooved by the middle meningeal vessels. Its lower border is fused to the anterior region of the petrous part, but traces of a petrosquamosal suture often appear in adult bones. The superior border is thin, bevelled internally and overlaps the inferior border of the parietal bone at the squamosal suture. Posteriorly it forms an angle with the mastoid element. The anteroinferior border, thin above and thick below, meets the greater wing of the sphenoid bone: above it is bevelled internally, below it is bevelled externally.

The squamous part has a zygomatic process and a mandibular fossa.

Zygomatic process

The zygomatic process juts forwards from the lower region of the squamous part. Its triangular posterior part has a broad base directed laterally, presenting superior and inferior surfaces. The zygomatic process then twists anteromedially, so that its surfaces become medial and lateral.

The superior surface of the posterior part is concave. The inferior surface is bounded by anterior and posterior roots, converging into the anterior part of the process. At the junction of the roots the tubercle of the zygomatic root gives attachment to the lateral temporomandibular ligament. The posterior root is prolonged forwards above the external acoustic meatus, its upper border continues into the supramastoid crest. Very rarely the squamous part is perforated above the posterior root by a squamosal foramen, transmitting the petrosquamous sinus. The anterior root juts almost horizontally from the squamous part. Its inferior surface, with an anteroposterior convexity, forms a short semicylindrical articular tubercle and comes in contact with the articular disc of the temporomandibular joint. The tubercle forms the anterior limit of the mandibular fossa.

The anterior part of the zygomatic process is thin and flat and the temporal fascia is attached to its superior border. The inferior border is short and arched and gives origin to some fibres of masseter. The lateral surface is convex. The medial surface is concave and provides further attachment for part of masseter. The anterior end is deeply serrated and slopes obliquely posteroinferiorly to articulate with the temporal process of the zygomatic bone, forming the zygomatic arch. Anterior to the articular tubercle, a small triangular area forms part of the roof of the infratemporal fossa. It is continuous behind with the anterior root and in front with the infratemporal crest of the greater wing of the sphenoid.

Mandibular fossa

The mandibular fossa is limited in front by the articular eminence of the zygomatic process. It presents an anterior articular area, formed by the squamous part, and a posterior non-articular area, formed by the tympanic element. The articular surface is smooth, oval and concave and contacts the articular disc of the temporomandibular joint. Unlike most other synovial joints, it is lined by fibrous tissue rather than hyaline cartilage, reflecting its intramembranous development. The non-articular area sometimes contains part of the parotid gland. A small, conical postglenoid tubercle separates the articular surface laterally from the tympanic plate.

Posteriorly, the mandibular fossa is separated from the tympanic part by the squamotympanic fissure. Rarely, a postglenoid foramen exists anterior to the external acoustic meatus in the line of fusion of the squamous and tympanic parts. It then replaces the squamosal foramen noted above and transmits the petrosquamous sinus. Medially, a projection from the petrous part of the temporal bone (tegmen tympani) comes to lie within the squamotympanic fissure, further dividing it into petrotympanic and petrosquamous fissures. The petrotympanic fissure leads into the tympanic cavity and contains an anterior malleolar ligament and the anterior tympanic branch of the maxillary artery. At the medial end of the fissure is the anterior opening of the anterior canaliculus for the chorda tympani nerve.

Petromastoid part

The petromastoid part of the temporal bone, although morphologically one element, is more conveniently described as two parts, the mastoid and petrous parts.

Mastoid part

This is the posterior region of the temporal bone. It has an outer surface roughened by attachments of the occipital belly of occipitofrontalis and auricularis posterior. A mastoid foramen, of variable size and position, and traversed by a vein from the sigmoid sinus and a small dural branch of the occipital artery, frequently lies near its posterior border. The foramen may be in the occipital or occipitotemporal suture; parasutural (40–50% of crania); or may be absent.

The mastoid part projects down as the conical mastoid process, and is larger in adult males. Sternocleidomastoid, splenius capitis and longissimus capitis are attached to its lateral surface. There is a deep mastoid notch on the medial aspect to which the posterior belly of digastric is attached. The occipital artery runs in a shallow occipital groove medial to this notch.

The internal surface of the mastoid process bears a deep, curved sigmoid sulcus for the sigmoid venous sinus. The sulcus is separated from the underlying innermost mastoid air cells by a thin lamina of bone. The air cells and mastoid antrum are described in Chapter 38.

The superior border of the mastoid part is thick and serrated for articulation with the mastoid angle of the parietal bone. The posterior border is also serrated and articulates with the inferior border of the occipital bone between its lateral angle and jugular process. The mastoid element is fused with the descending process of the squamous part: below, it appears in the posterior wall of the tympanic cavity.

Petrous part

This mass of bone is wedged between the sphenoid and occipital bones in the cranial base, and is inclined superiorly and anteromedially. It has a base, apex, three surfaces (anterior, posterior and inferior) and three borders (superior, posterior and anterior), and contains the acoustic labyrinth.

The base would correspond to the part that lies on the base of the skull and is separated from the squamous part by a suture. However, this suture disappears soon after birth. The subsequent development of

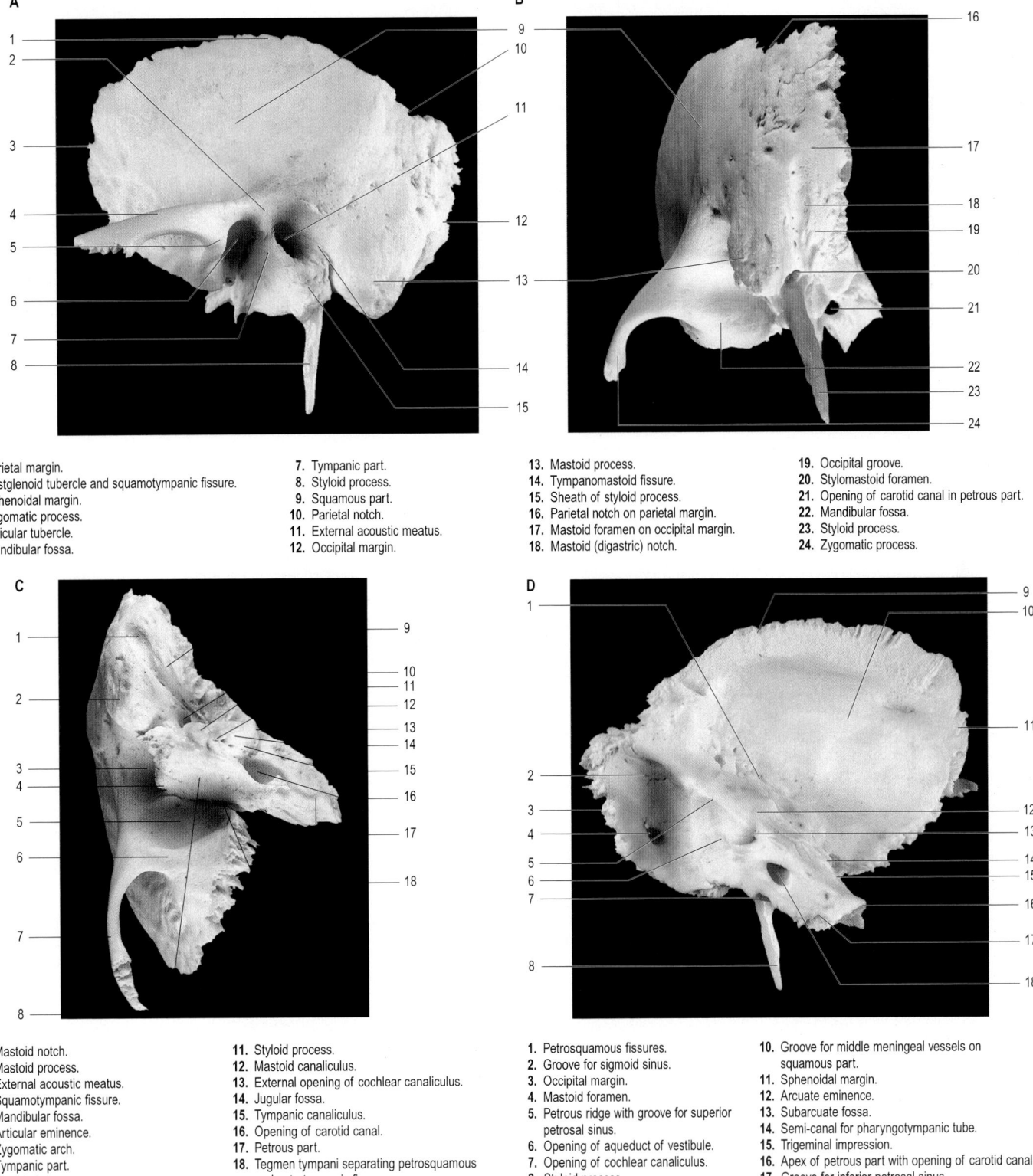

A

1. Parietal margin.
2. Postglenoid tubercle and squamotympanic fissure.
3. Sphenoidal margin.
4. Zygomatic process.
5. Articular tubercle.
6. Mandibular fossa.
7. Tympanic part.
8. Styloid process.
9. Squamous part.
10. Parietal notch.
11. External acoustic meatus.
12. Occipital margin.

B

13. Mastoid process.
14. Tympanomastoid fissure.
15. Sheath of styloid process.
16. Parietal notch on parietal margin.
17. Mastoid foramen on occipital margin.
18. Mastoid (digastric) notch.
19. Occipital groove.
20. Stylomastoid foramen.
21. Opening of carotid canal in petrous part.
22. Mandibular fossa.
23. Styloid process.
24. Zygomatic process.

C

1. Mastoid notch.
2. Mastoid process.
3. External acoustic meatus.
4. Squamotympanic fissure.
5. Mandibular fossa.
6. Articular eminence.
7. Zygomatic arch.
8. Tympanic part.
9. Occipital groove.
10. Stylomastoid foramen.
11. Styloid process.
12. Mastoid canaliculus.
13. External opening of cochlear canaliculus.
14. Jugular fossa.
15. Tympanic canaliculus.
16. Opening of carotid canal.
17. Petrous part.
18. Tegmen tympani separating petrosquamous and petrotympanic fissures.

D

1. Petrosquamous fissures.
2. Groove for sigmoid sinus.
3. Occipital margin.
4. Mastoid foramen.
5. Petrous ridge with groove for superior petrosal sinus.
6. Opening of aqueduct of vestibule.
7. Opening of cochlear canaliculus.
8. Styloid process.
9. Parietal margin.
10. Groove for middle meningeal vessels on squamous part.
11. Sphenoidal margin.
12. Arcuate eminence.
13. Subarcuate fossa.
14. Semi-canal for pharyngotympanic tube.
15. Trigeminal impression.
16. Apex of petrous part with opening of carotid canal.
17. Groove for inferior petrosal sinus.
18. Internal acoustic meatus.

Fig. 27.14 Temporal bone. **A**, External view; **B**, posterior/oblique view; **C**, inferior view; **D**, internal view. (By permission from Berkovitz and Moxham, 1994.)

the mastoid processes means that the precise boundaries of the base are no longer identifiable.

The apex, blunt and irregular, is angled between the posterior border of the greater wing of the sphenoid and the basilar part of the occipital bone. It contains the anterior opening of the carotid canal and limits the foramen lacerum posterolaterally.

The anterior surface contributes to the floor of the middle cranial fossa and is continuous with the cerebral surface of the squamous part

(although the petrosquamosal suture often persists late in life). The whole surface is adapted to the inferior temporal gyri. Behind the apex is a trigeminal impression for the trigeminal ganglion. Bone antero-lateral to this roofs the anterior part of the carotid canal, but is often deficient. A ridge separates the trigeminal impression from another hollow behind, which partly roofs the internal acoustic meatus and cochlea. This in turn is limited behind by the arcuate eminence raised by the anterior semicircular canal. Laterally, it roofs the vestibule and,

469

partly, the facial canal. Between the squamous part laterally and the arcuate eminence and the hollows just described medially, the anterior surface is formed by the tegmen tympani. This thin plate of bone forms the roof of the mastoid antrum, extending forwards above the tympanic cavity and the canal for tensor tympani. Its lateral margin meets the squamous part at the petrosquamosal suture, turning down in front as the lateral wall of the canal for the tensor tympani and the osseous part of the pharyngotympanic tube: its lower edge is in the squamotympanic fissure. Anteriorly the tegmen bears a narrow groove related to the greater petrosal nerve which passes posterolaterally to enter the bone by a hiatus anterior to the arcuate eminence. The groove passes forwards to the foramen lacerum. A smaller and similar hiatus and groove may be found more laterally and are related to the lesser petrosal nerve. This nerve runs to the foramen ovale. The posterior slope of the arcuate eminence overlies the posterior and lateral semicircular canals. Lateral to the eminence the posterior part of the tegmen tympani roofs the mastoid antrum.

The posterior surface contributes to the anterior part of the posterior cranial fossa and is continuous with the internal surface of the mastoid part. The opening of the internal acoustic meatus lies near its centre. A small slit leading to the vestibular aqueduct lies behind the opening of the meatus, almost hidden by a thin plate of bone. This contains the saccus and ductus endolymphaticus together with a small artery and vein. The terminal half of the saccus endolymphaticus protrudes through the slit between the periosteum and dura mater. The subarcuate fossa lies above these openings.

The irregular inferior surface is part of the exterior of the cranial base. Near the apex of the petrous part, there is a quadrilateral area which is partly associated with the attachment of levator veli palatini and the cartilaginous pharyngotympanic tube, and partly connected to the basilar part of the occipital bone by dense fibrocartilage. Behind this region is the large, circular opening of the carotid canal, and behind the opening of the canal is the jugular fossa, which is of variable depth and size and contains the superior jugular bulb. The inferior ganglion of the glossopharyngeal nerve lies in a triangular depression anteromedial to the jugular fossa (below the internal acoustic meatus). At its apex is a small opening into the cochlear canaliculus, occupied by the perilymphatic duct (a tube of dura mater) and a vein draining from the cochlea to the internal jugular vein. A canaliculus for the tympanic nerve from the glossopharyngeal nerve lies on the ridge between the carotid canal and the jugular fossa. The mastoid canaliculus for the auricular branch of the vagus nerve is laterally positioned in the jugular fossa. Behind the jugular fossa, the rough quadrilateral jugular surface is covered by cartilage which joins it to the jugular process of the occipital bone.

The superior border, the longest, is grooved by the superior petrosal sinus. The attached margin of the tentorium cerebelli is fixed to the edges of the groove except at its medial end, where it is crossed by the roots of the trigeminal nerve. The posterior border, intermediate in length, bears a sulcus medially which forms, together with the occipital bone, a gutter for the inferior petrosal sinus. Behind this the jugular fossa contributes (together with the occipital bone) to the jugular foramen and is notched by the glossopharyngeal nerve. Bone on either or both sides of the jugular notch may meet the occipital bone and divide the jugular foramen into two or three parts. The anterior border is joined laterally to the squamous part of the temporal bone at the petrosquamosal suture; medially it articulates with the greater wing of the sphenoid bone.

At the junction of the petrous and squamous parts two canals exist, one above the other, which are separated by a thin osseous plate. Both lead to the tympanic cavity; the upper canal contains tensor tympani, the lower canal is the pharyngotympanic tube.

Tympanic part

The tympanic part of the temporal bone is a curved plate below the squamous part and anterior to the mastoid process. Internally it fuses with the petrous part and appears between this and the squamous part, where it is inferolateral to the auditory orifice. Behind, it fuses with the squamous part and mastoid process and is the anterior limit of the tympanomastoid fissure. Its concave posterior surface forms the anterior wall, floor and part of the posterior wall of the external acoustic meatus. A narrow tympanic sulcus on the medial surface serves for the attachment of the tympanic membrane. The quadrilateral concave anterior surface is the posterior wall of the mandibular fossa and may contact the parotid gland. Its rough lateral border forms most of the margin of the external acoustic meatus and is continuous with its cartilaginous part. Laterally

the upper border is fused with the back of the postglenoid tubercle; medially it is the posterior edge of the petrotympanic fissure. The inferior border is sharp, splitting laterally to form, at its root, the sheath of the styloid process (vaginal process). Centrally the tympanic part is thin, and is often perforated. The stylomastoid foramen lies between the styloid and mastoid processes: it represents the external end of the facial canal and transmits the facial nerve and stylomastoid artery.

Styloid process

The styloid process is slender, pointed and projects anteroinferiorly from the inferior aspect of the temporal bone. Its length is variable, ranging from a few millimetres to an average of c.2.5 cm. Often approximately straight, it can show a curvature, an anteromedial concavity being most common. Its proximal part (tympanohyal) is ensheathed by the tympanic plate, especially anterolaterally, while muscles and ligaments are attached to its distal part (stylohyal). *In vivo*, its relationships are important. The styloid process is covered laterally by the parotid gland; the facial nerve crosses its base; the external carotid artery crosses its tip, embedded in the parotid; and medially the process is separated from the beginning of the internal jugular vein by the attachment of stylopharyngeus.

External acoustic meatus

The temporal bone contains the bony part of the external acoustic meatus. This is c.16 mm long and slopes down anteromedially while its floor is convex upwards. In sagittal section it is oval or elliptical, with a long axis directed down and slightly back. The anterior wall, floor and lower posterior wall are formed by the tympanic plate; the roof and upper posterior wall are formed by the squamous part, and the medial end is closed by the tympanic membrane. The outer wall of the meatus is bounded above by the posterior zygomatic root, below which there may be a suprameatal spine. The cartilaginous part of the external acoustic meatus is attached to the lateral surface of the bony part.

Ossification

The four temporal components ossify independently (**Fig. 27.15**). The squamous part is ossified in a sheet of condensed mesenchyme from a single centre near the zygomatic roots, which appear in the seventh or eighth week *in utero*. The petromastoid part has several centres appearing in the cartilaginous otic capsule during the fifth month. As many as 14 have been described, variable in order of appearance. Several are small and inconstant, soon fusing with others. The otic capsule is almost fully ossified by the end of the sixth month. The tympanic part is also ossified in mesenchyme from a centre identifiable about the third month; at birth it is an incomplete tympanic ring, deficient above, its concavity grooved by a tympanic sulcus for the tympanic membrane. Inclined obliquely downwards and forwards across the medial aspect of the anterior part of the ring is the malleolar sulcus for the anterior malleolar process, chorda tympani and anterior tympanic artery. The styloid process develops from two centres at the cranial end of cartilage in the second visceral or hyoid arch: a proximal centre for the tympanohyal, appearing before birth and another, for the distal stylohyal, after birth. The tympanic ring unites with the squamous part shortly before birth, and the petromastoid fuses with it and the tympanohyal during the first year. The stylohyal does not unite with the rest of the process until after puberty and may never do so.

Once ossified, the tympanic cavity, mastoid antrum and the posterior end of the pharyngotympanic tube become surrounded by bone. The petrous part forms the roof, floor and medial wall of the cavity, while the squamous and tympanic parts, together with the tympanic membrane, form its lateral wall. At birth the middle and inner ears are adult size, and the tympanic cavity, mastoid antrum, tympanic membrane and auditory ossicles are all almost adult size. The anterior process does not join the malleus until 6 months later. The internal acoustic meatus is c.6 mm in horizontal diameter, 4 mm in vertical diameter and 7 mm in length at birth: the adult diameters are 7.7 mm and 11 mm respectively.

After birth and apart from general growth, the tympanic ring extends posterolaterally to become cylindrical, growing into a fibrocartilaginous tympanic plate, which forms the adjacent part of the external acoustic meatus at this stage. This growth is not equal but is rapid in the anterior and posterior regions, which meet and blend. Thus, for a time, there is in the floor an opening (foramen of Huschke), usually closed at about the fifth year, but sometimes permanent (in 5–46% of adult crania from

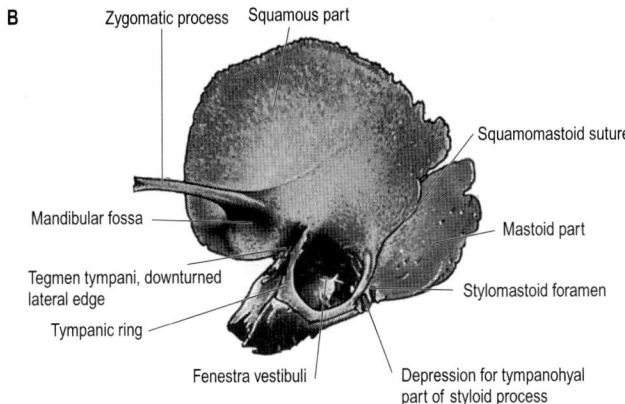

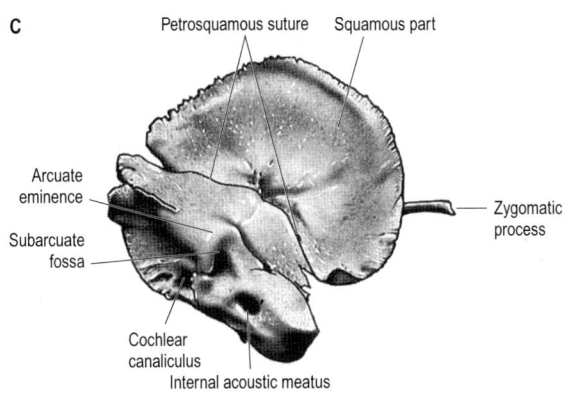

Fig. 27.15 The left temporal bone at birth. **A,** The three principal parts are, from left to right, petromastoid part (lateral aspect), tympanic ring (medial aspect) and squama (medial aspect). **B,** Lateral aspect with the rudimentary styloid process removed (yellow: tympanic part; brown: squamous part; uncoloured: petromastoid part). **C,** Medial aspect.

ancient and modern populations). The external acoustic meatus is relatively as long in children as it is in adults, but the canal is fibro-cartilaginous, whereas its medial two-thirds are osseous in adults. Surgical access to the tympanic cavity is via the mastoid antrum, and in children it is necessary to remove only a thin scale of bone in the supra-meatal triangle to reach the antrum. The tympanic plate ensheathes the styloid process by posterior extension, and extends medially over the petrous bone to the carotid canal.

Initially, the mandibular fossa is shallow, facing more laterally, but it then deepens and ultimately faces downwards. Posteroinferiorly the squamous part grows down behind the tympanic ring to form the lateral wall of the mastoid antrum. The mastoid part is at first flat, so that the stylomastoid foramen and rudimentary styloid process are immediately behind the tympanic ring. The mastoid part becomes invaded by air cells, especially at puberty. The lateral mastoid region grows downwards and forwards to form the mastoid process, so that the styloid process and stylomastoid foramen become inferior. Descent of the foramen lengthens the facial canal. The mastoid process is not perceptible until

late in the second year. The subarcuate fossa gradually fills and is almost obliterated.

In the neonate the petrous and squamous parts of the temporal bone are usually partially separated by the petrosquamous fissure which opens directly into the mastoid antrum of the middle ear. The fissure closes in 4% of infants during the first year, but it remains unclosed in 20–40% up to the age of 19 years. It is a route for the spread of infection from the middle ear to the meninges.

In the neonate the internal acoustic meatus is about half the length of that of the adult. Its opening from the middle ear cavity is as large as it is in the adult, but the pharyngeal opening in the nasal part of the pharynx is relatively smaller. The course of the pharyngotympanic tube is horizontal in the newborn, whereas in the adult it passes from the middle ear downward, forward and medially.

PARIETAL BONE (Fig. 27.16)

The two parietal bones form most of the cranial roof and sides of the skull. Each is irregularly quadrilateral and has two surfaces, four borders and four angles.

The external surface is convex and smooth, with a central parietal tuber (tuberosity). Curved superior and inferior temporal lines cross it and form posterosuperior arches. The temporal fascia is attached to the superior line or arch and the inferior line or arch indicates the upper limit of attachment of temporalis. The epicranial aponeurosis (galea aponeurotica) lies above these lines, and part of the temporal fossa lies below. Posteriorly, close to the sagittal (superior) border, an inconstant parietal foramen transmits a vein from the superior sagittal sinus and sometimes a branch of the occipital artery.

The internal surface is concave and marked by cerebral gyri and grooves for the middle meningeal vessels. The vessels ascend, inclining backwards, from the sphenoidal (anteroinferior) angle and posterior half (or more) of its inferior border. A groove for the superior sagittal sinus lies along the sagittal border, and is completed by the groove on the opposite parietal bone. The falx cerebri is attached to the edges of the groove. Granular foveolae for arachnoid granulations flank the sagittal sulcus, being most pronounced in old age.

The dentated sagittal border, longest and thickest, articulates with the opposite parietal bone at the sagittal suture. In the squamosal (inferior) border the anterior part is short, thin and truncated, bevelled externally and overlapped by the greater wing of the sphenoid. The middle part of the inferior border is arched, bevelled externally and overlapped by the squamous part of the temporal bone. The posterior part of the inferior border is short, thick and serrated for articulation with the mastoid part.

The frontal border is deeply serrated, bevelled externally above, internally below, and articulates with the frontal bone to form one half of the coronal suture. The occipital border, deeply dentated, articulates with the occipital, forming one half of the lambdoid suture.

The frontal (anterosuperior) angle, c.90°, is at the bregma, the meeting of the sagittal and coronal sutures. In the neonatal skull, this is the site of the anterior fontanelle. The sphenoidal (anteroinferior) angle is between the frontal bone and greater wing of the sphenoid. Its internal surface is marked by a deep groove or sometimes even a canal related to the frontal branches of the middle meningeal vessels. The frontal bone sometimes meets the squamous part of the temporal bone which means that the parietal bone then fails to reach the greater wing of the sphenoid bone. These four bones meet at the pterion. The rounded occipital (posterosuperior) angle is at the lambda, the meeting of the sagittal and lambdoid sutures. In the neonatal skull this marks the site of the posterior fontanelle. The blunt mastoid (posteroinferior) angle articulates with the occipital bone and the mastoid portion of the temporal bones. This is the site of the asterion. Internally it bears a broad, shallow groove for the junction of the transverse and sigmoid sinuses.

Ossification

Each parietal bone is ossified from two centres which appear in dense mesenchyme near the tuberosity, one above the other, at about the seventh week *in utero*. These two centres unite early and the ossification radiates towards the margins. This means that the angles are the last to be ossified and so fontanelles occur at these sites. At birth the temporal lines are low down, and they only reach their final position after the eruption of the molar teeth. Occasionally the parietal bone is divided by an anteroposterior suture.

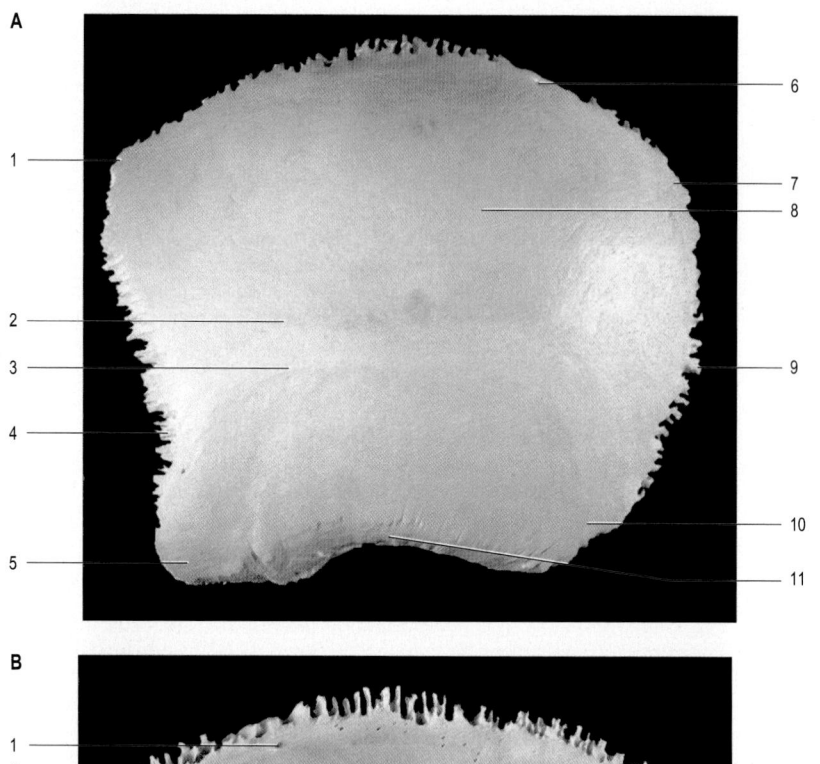

A

1. Frontal (anterosuperior) angle.
2. Superior temporal line.
3. Inferior temporal line.
4. Frontal margin (for coronal suture).
5. Sphenoidal (anteroinferior) angle.
6. Parietal foramen on sagittal margin (for sagittal suture).
7. Occipital (posterosuperior) angle.
8. Parietal tuberosity.
9. Occipital margin (for lambdoid suture).
10. Mastoid (posteroinferior) angle.
11. Squamous margin (for squamosal suture).

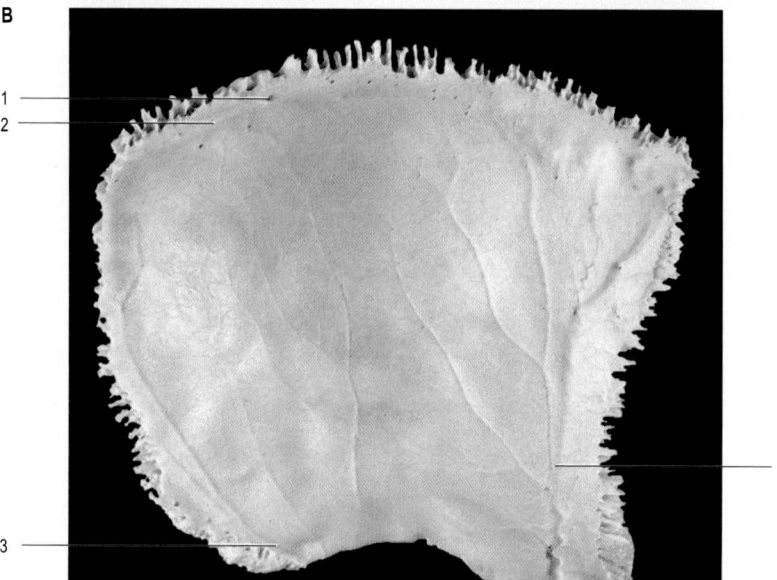

B

1. Parietal foramen.
2. Groove for superior sagittal sinus.
3. Groove for sigmoid sinus.
4. Groove for middle meningeal vessels.

Fig. 27.16 Left parietal bone. **A,** External view; **B,** internal view. (By permission from Berkovitz and Moxham, 1994.)

FRONTAL BONE (Fig. 27.17)

The frontal bone is like half a shallow, irregular cap forming the forehead or frons. It has three parts, and contains two cavities, which are the frontal sinuses.

Squamous part of the frontal bone

This forms the major portion of the bone. The external surface has a rounded frontal tuber (tuberosity) c.3 cm above the midpoint of each supraorbital margin. These tubera vary, but are especially prominent in young skulls and more so in adult females than males. Below them and separated by a shallow groove, are two curved superciliary arches, medially prominent and joined by a smooth median elevated glabella. The arches are more prominent in males, depending partly on the size of the frontal sinuses; but prominence is occasionally associated with small sinuses. The curved supraorbital margins of the orbital openings lie inferior to the superciliary arches. The lateral two-thirds of each margin are sharp, the medial third rounded, and a supraorbital notch (or foramen), which transmits the supraorbital vessels and nerve, lies at the junction between them. A small frontal notch or foramen occurs medial to it in 50% of skulls. A supraorbital notch or foramen occurs equally in some populations, whereas the appearance of a frontal foramen is more variable (15–87% in various ethnic groups). Both features show sexual dimorphism. The supraorbital margin ends laterally in a strong, prominent zygomatic process that meets the zygomatic bone.

From here a line curves posterosuperiorly, and divides into superior and inferior temporal lines, which are continued on the squamous part of the temporal bone. The area of the frontal bone below and behind the temporal lines is known as the temporal surface and forms the anterior part of the temporal fossa; it gives an attachment to temporalis. The parietal (posterior) margin is thick, deeply serrated, bevelled internally above and externally below. Inferiorly it becomes a rough, triangular surface for the greater wing of the sphenoid.

The internal surface is concave. Its upper, median part has a vertical sulcus for the sagittal sinus, the edges of which unite below as the frontal crest. The sulcus contains the anterior part of the superior sagittal sinus, and part of the falx cerebri is attached to its margins and frontal crest. The crest ends in a small notch, which is completed by the ethmoid bone to form a foramen caecum. The internal surface shows impressions of cerebral gyri and small furrows for meningeal vessels. Several granular foveolae for arachnoid granulations usually exist near the sagittal sulcus.

Nasal part of the frontal bone

The region between the supraorbital margins is the nasal part. A serrated nasal notch articulates with the nasal bones inferiorly and with the frontal processes of the maxillae and the lacrimal bones laterally. From the centre of the notch posteriorly the bone projects anteroinferiorly behind the nasal bones and the frontal processes of the maxillae, and supports the nasal bridge. The region ends in a sharp nasal spine, on

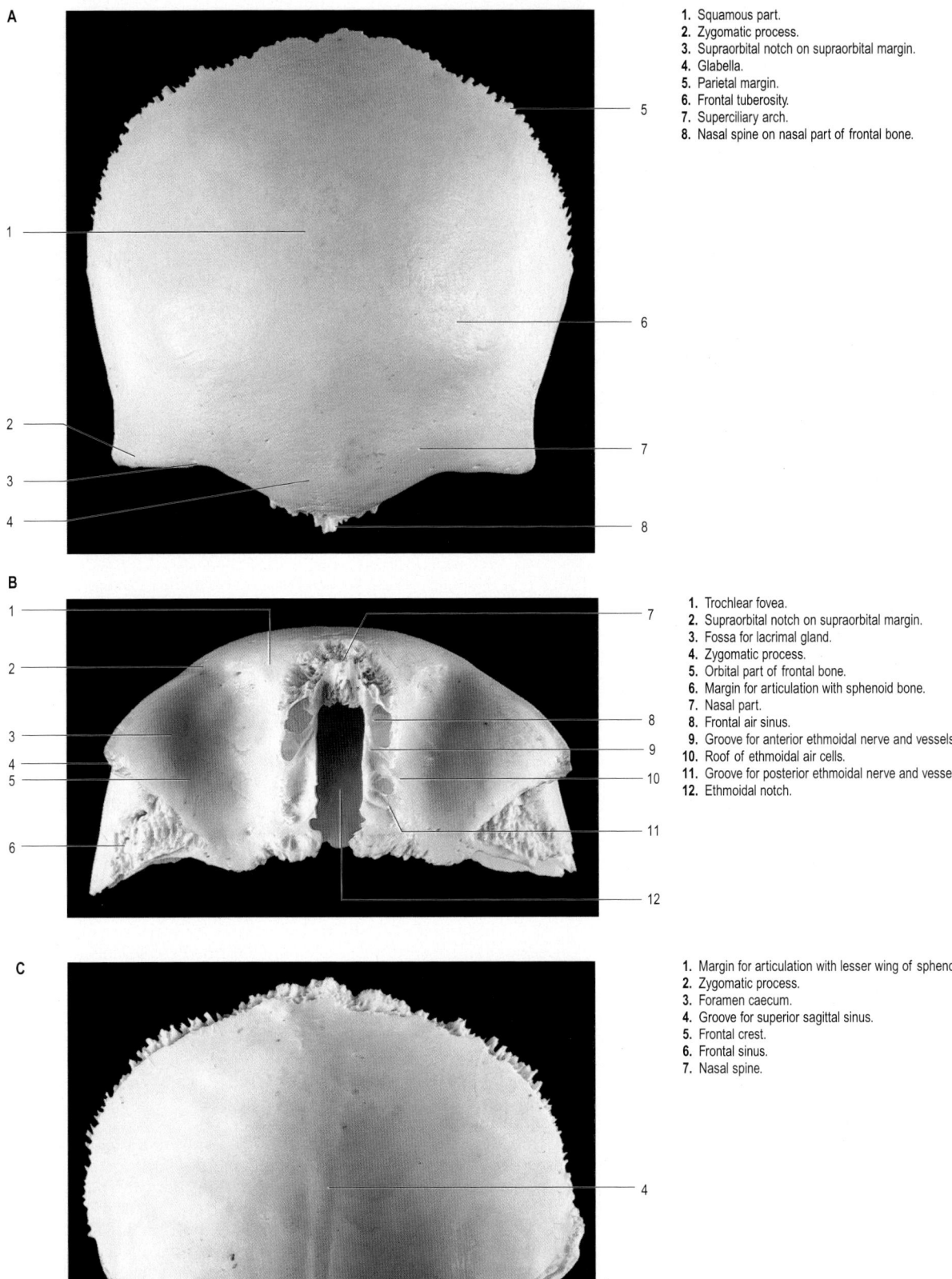

A

1. Squamous part.
2. Zygomatic process.
3. Supraorbital notch on supraorbital margin.
4. Glabella.
5. Parietal margin.
6. Frontal tuberosity.
7. Superciliary arch.
8. Nasal spine on nasal part of frontal bone.

B

1. Trochlear fovea.
2. Supraorbital notch on supraorbital margin.
3. Fossa for lacrimal gland.
4. Zygomatic process.
5. Orbital part of frontal bone.
6. Margin for articulation with sphenoid bone.
7. Nasal part.
8. Frontal air sinus.
9. Groove for anterior ethmoidal nerve and vessels.
10. Roof of ethmoidal air cells.
11. Groove for posterior ethmoidal nerve and vessels.
12. Ethmoidal notch.

C

1. Margin for articulation with lesser wing of sphenoid.
2. Zygomatic process.
3. Foramen caecum.
4. Groove for superior sagittal sinus.
5. Frontal crest.
6. Frontal sinus.
7. Nasal spine.

Fig. 27.17 Frontal bone. **A,** External view; **B,** inferior view; **C,** internal view. (By permission from Berkovitz and Moxham, 1994.)

473

each side of which a small grooved surface partly roofs the ipsilateral nasal cavity. The nasal spine makes a very small contribution to the nasal septum. In front it articulates with the crest of the nasal bones and behind with the perpendicular plate of the ethmoid bone.

Orbital parts of the frontal bone

The orbital parts of the frontal bone are two thin, curved, triangular laminae which form the largest part of the orbital roofs and are separated by a wide ethmoidal notch. Most of the frontal bone is thick, and displays trabecular tissue lying between two compact laminae. In contrast, the orbital plates consist entirely of compact bone and are thin and often translucent posteriorly, indeed they may be partly absorbed in old age.

The orbital surface of each plate is smooth and concave, and bears a shallow anterolateral fossa for the lacrimal gland. Below and behind the medial end of the supraorbital margin, midway between the supra-orbital notch and frontolacrimal suture, is the trochlear fovea (or spine) for attachment of a fibrocartilaginous trochlea for superior oblique. The convex cerebral surface is marked by frontal gyri and faint grooves for meningeal vessels.

The quadrilateral ethmoidal notch is occupied by the cribriform plate of the ethmoid bone. Inferior to its lateral margins, the bone articulates with the labyrinths of the ethmoid bone and impressions of the eth-moidal air cells can be seen on this surface. Two transverse grooves across each margin are converted into anterior and posterior ethmoidal canals by articulation with the ethmoid bone. These canals open on the medial orbital wall, transmitting anterior and posterior ethmoidal nerves and vessels.

Openings of the frontal sinuses are anterior to the ethmoidal notch and lateral to the nasal spine. These two irregular cavities ascend postero-laterally for a variable distance between the frontal laminae, separated by a thin septum and usually deflected from the median plane. The sinuses are consequently rarely symmetrical, are variable in size, and larger in males. Each communicates with the middle meatus in the ipsilateral nasal cavity by a frontonasal canal. The degree of development is linked to the prominence of the superciliary arches, which is thought to be a response to masticatory stresses. The posterior borders of the orbital plates are thin and serrated to articulate with the lesser wings of the sphenoid; their lateral parts usually appear in the middle cranial fossa between greater and lesser wings.

Ossification

The frontal bone is ossified in fibrous mesenchyme from two primary centres that appear in the eighth week *in utero*, one near each frontal tuber. Ossification extends superiorly to form half of the main part of the bone; posteriorly to form the orbital part, and inferiorly to form nasal parts (**Fig. 27.18**). Two secondary centres occur for the nasal spine, and appear about the tenth year. At birth the bone consists of two halves, and the median suture usually disappears by about 8 years. However, it may persist as the metopic suture. Such metopism has been assessed at 0–7.4% of individuals in various ethnic groups.

The sinuses are rudimentary at birth and can barely be distinguished. Growth is slow in the early years but it can be detected radiographically by 6 years. The sinuses show a primary expansion with eruption of the first deciduous molars at c.1½ years, and again when the permanent molars begin to appear in the sixth year. They reach full size after puberty, although with advancing age osseous absorption may lead to further enlargement.

ETHMOID BONE (Fig. 27.19)

The ethmoid bone is cuboidal and fragile, and lies anteriorly in the cranial base. It contributes to the medial orbital walls, nasal septum, and the roof and lateral walls of the nasal cavity. It has a horizontal, perforated cribri-form plate, a median perpendicular plate, and two lateral labyrinths which contain the ethmoidal air cells.

Cribriform plate

The cribriform plate fills the ethmoidal notch of the frontal bone and forms a large part of the nasal roof. It derives its name from the fact that it is penetrated by numerous foramina containing branches of the olfactory nerves and their associated meninges. A thick, smooth, tri-angular, median crista galli projects up from the horizontally aligned plate of bone. The falx cerebri is attached to its thin and curved posterior border. Its shorter, thick, anterior border joins the frontal

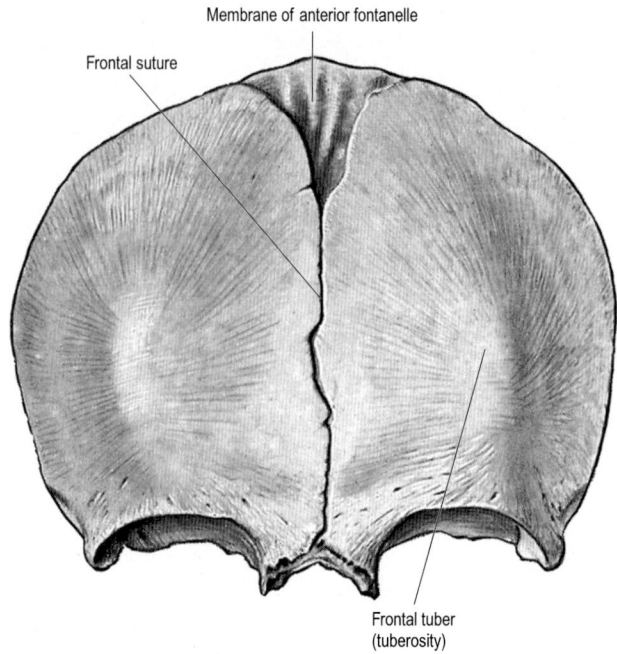

Fig. 27.18 The frontal bone at birth: anterior aspect. Note that at this stage the bone consists of right and left halves connected by the frontal suture.

bone by two small alae, to complete the foramen caecum. Its sides are generally smooth, but may show slight bulges related to underlying ethmoidal air cells. On both sides of the crista galli, the cribriform plate is narrow and depressed: it is related to the gyrus rectus and the olfactory bulb which lie above it. On each side of the crista anteriorly there is a small slit occupied by dura mater, and just anterolateral to the slit, a foramen which transmits the anterior ethmoidal nerve and vessels to the nasal cavity: a groove runs forwards to the foramen caecum from the anterior ethmoidal canal.

Perpendicular plate

The perpendicular plate is thin, flat, quadrilateral and median, and it descends from the cribriform plate to form the upper part of the nasal septum, usually deviating slightly from the midline. Its anterior border meets the nasal spine of the frontal bone and the crests of the nasal bones. Its posterior border joins the crest of the body of the sphenoid bone above and vomer below. The thick inferior border is attached to the nasal septal cartilage. Its surfaces are smooth, except above, where numerous grooves and canals lead to medial foramina in the cribriform plate for filaments of the olfactory nerves.

Ethmoidal labyrinths

The ethmoidal labyrinths consist of thin-walled ethmoidal air cells between two vertical plates and are arranged in anterior, middle and posterior groups. On average there are c.11 anterior ethmoidal air cells, 3 middle, and 6 posterior. The lateral surface (orbital plate) of the labyrinth is part of the medial orbital wall. In the disarticulated bone, many air cells are open, but in life these are closed when articulated with adjoining bones, except where they open into the nasal cavity. The superior surface shows open air cells that will be covered by the edges of the ethmoidal notch of the frontal bone. It is crossed by two grooves that will be converted into anterior and posterior ethmoidal canals by the frontal bone. On the posterior surface open air cells are present that will be covered by the sphenoidal conchae and the orbital process of the palatine bone. The thin, smooth, oblong orbital plate covers the middle and posterior ethmoidal air cells. It articulates superiorly with the orbital plate of the frontal bone, inferiorly with the maxilla and orbital process of the palatine bone, anteriorly with the lacrimal bone and posteriorly with the sphenoid bone. The walls of the air cells lying anterior to the orbital plate are completed by the lacrimal bone and frontal process of the maxilla.

A thin, curved uncinate process, variable in size, projects postero-inferiorly from the labyrinth. The upper edge of this process is a medial

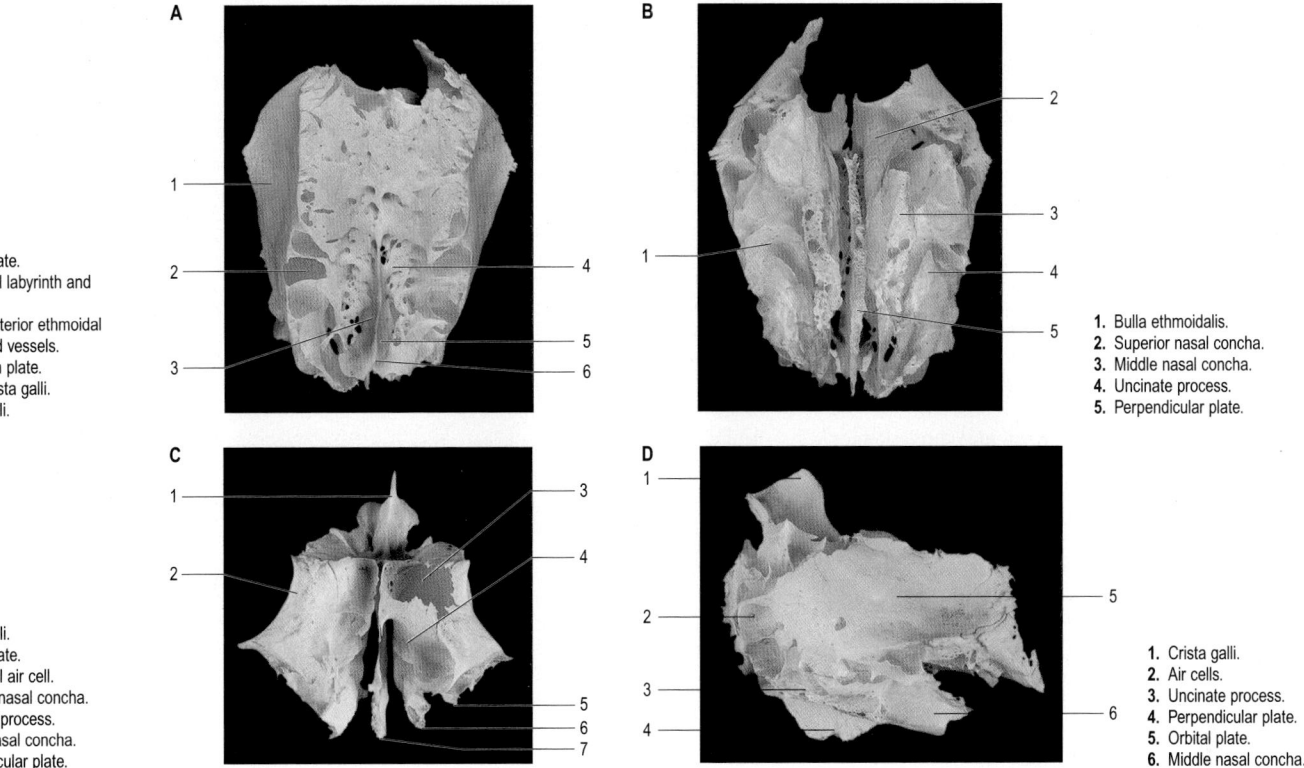

A

1. Orbital plate.
2. Ethmoidal labyrinth and air cells.
3. Slit for anterior ethmoidal nerve and vessels.
4. Cribriform plate.
5. Ala of crista galli.
6. Crista galli.

B

1. Bulla ethmoidalis.
2. Superior nasal concha.
3. Middle nasal concha.
4. Uncinate process.
5. Perpendicular plate.

C

1. Crista galli.
2. Orbital plate.
3. Ethmoidal air cell.
4. Superior nasal concha.
5. Uncinate process.
6. Middle nasal concha.
7. Perpendicular plate.

D

1. Crista galli.
2. Air cells.
3. Uncinate process.
4. Perpendicular plate.
5. Orbital plate.
6. Middle nasal concha.

Fig. 27.19 Ethmoid bone. **A,** Superior view; **B,** inferior view; **C,** posterior view; **D,** lateral view. (By permission from Berkovitz and Moxham, 1994.)

boundary of the hiatus semilunaris in the middle meatus. The uncinate process appears in the medial wall of the maxillary sinus as it crosses the ostium of the maxillary sinus to join the ethmoidal process of the inferior nasal concha.

The medial surface of the labyrinth forms part of the lateral nasal wall as a thin lamella descending from the inferior surface of the cribriform plate to end as the convoluted middle nasal concha. Above this the surface contains many vertical grooves for olfactory nerves. Posteriorly it is divided by the narrow, oblique superior meatus, bounded above by the thin, curved superior nasal concha. Posterior ethmoidal air cells open into this meatus. Anteroinferior to the superior meatus, the convex surface of the middle nasal concha extends along the entire medial surface of the labyrinth, its lower edge being thick. Its lateral surface is concave and forms part of the middle meatus. Middle ethmoidal air cells produce a swelling (bulla ethmoidalis) on the lateral wall of the middle meatus. These air cells open into the meatus, on the bulla or above it. A curved infundibulum extends up and forwards from the middle meatus and communicates with the anterior ethmoidal sinuses. In more than 50% of crania it continues up as the frontonasal duct to include the drainage point for the frontal sinus.

Ossification

The ethmoid bone ossifies in the cartilaginous nasal capsule from three centres, one in the perpendicular plate, and one in each labyrinth. The latter two appear in the orbital plates between the fourth and fifth months

in utero, and extend into the ethmoid conchae. At birth, the labyrinths, although ill-developed, are partially ossified, and the remainder are cartilaginous. During the first year the perpendicular plate begins to ossify from the median centre, and fuses with the labyrinths early in the second year. The cribriform plate is ossified partly from the perpendicular plate, and partly from the labyrinths. The crista galli ossifies during the second year. The parts of the ethmoid bone unite to form a single bone at c.3 years of age. Ethmoidal air cells begin to develop c.3 months *in utero.* Although present at birth, they are difficult to visualize radiographically until the end of the first year. They grow slowly and have almost reached adult size by the age of 12 years.

INFERIOR NASAL CONCHA (Fig. 27.20)

The inferior nasal conchae are curved horizontal laminae in the lateral nasal walls. Each has two surfaces (medial and lateral), two borders (superior and inferior) and two ends (anterior and posterior). The medial surface is convex, much perforated, and longitudinally grooved by vessels. The lateral surface is concave and part of the inferior meatus. The superior border, thin and irregular, may be divided into three regions, namely, an anterior region articulating with the conchal crest of the maxilla, a posterior region articulating with the conchal crest of the palatine bone, and a middle region with three processes, which are variable in size and form. The lacrimal process is small and pointed and lies towards the front, and articulates apically with a descending process from the lacrimal bone. It also articulates at its margins

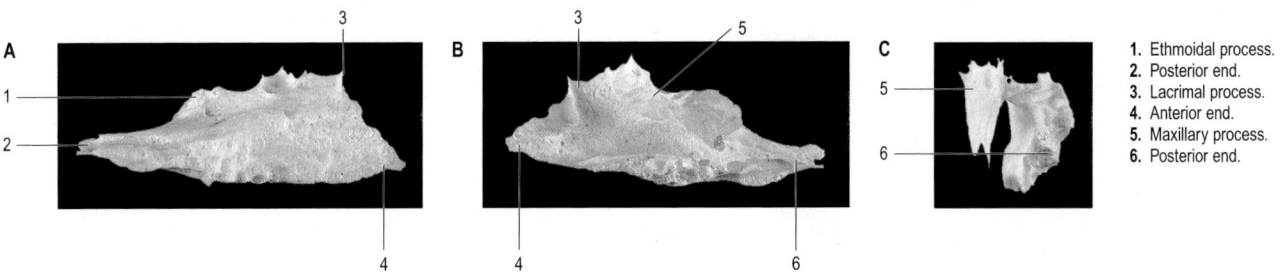

A

1
2

B

3

C

5
6

1. Ethmoidal process.
2. Posterior end.
3. Lacrimal process.
4. Anterior end.
5. Maxillary process.
6. Posterior end.

Fig. 27.20 Inferior nasal concha. **A,** Medial view; **B,** lateral view; **C,** posterior view. (By permission from Berkovitz and Moxham, 1994.)

with the edges of the nasolacrimal groove on the medial surface of the maxilla, and so helps complete the nasolacrimal canal. Most posteriorly, a thin ethmoidal process ascends to meet the uncinate process of the ethmoid bone. An intermediate thin maxillary process curves inferolaterally to articulate with the medial surface of the maxilla at the opening of the maxillary sinus. The inferior border is thick and spongiose, especially in its midpart. Both anterior and posterior ends of the inferior nasal concha are more or less tapered, the posterior more than the anterior.

Ossification

Ossification is from one centre which appears at about the fifth month *in utero* in the incurved lower border of the cartilaginous lateral wall of the nasal capsule. It loses continuity with the capsule during ossification.

LACRIMAL BONE (Fig. 27.21)

The lacrimal bones, the smallest and most fragile of the cranial bones, lie anteriorly in the medial walls of the orbits. Each has two surfaces (medial and lateral) and four borders (anterior, posterior, superior and inferior). The lateral (orbital) surface is divided by a vertical posterior lacrimal crest. There is a vertical groove anterior to the crest, and the anterior edge of this groove meets the posterior border of the frontal process of the maxilla to complete the fossa for the lacrimal sac. The medial wall of the groove is prolonged by a descending process that contributes to the formation of the nasolacrimal canal by joining the lips of the nasolacrimal groove of the maxilla and the lacrimal process of the inferior nasal concha. A smooth part of the medial orbital wall lies behind the posterior lacrimal crest: the lacrimal part of orbicularis oculi is attached to this surface and crest. The surface ends below in the lacrimal hamulus which, together with the maxilla, completes the upper opening of the nasolacrimal canal. The hamulus may appear as a separate lesser lacrimal bone. The anteroinferior region of the medial (nasal) surface is part of the middle meatus. Its posterosuperior part meets the ethmoid to complete some anterior ethmoidal air cells. The anterior lacrimal border articulates with the frontal process of the maxilla, the posterior border with the orbital plate of the ethmoid bone, the superior border with the frontal bone, and the inferior border with the orbital surface of the maxilla.

Ossification

Ossification is from a centre that appears at about the twelfth week *in utero* in mesenchyme around the nasal capsule. In later life the lacrimal bone is subject to patchy erosion.

NASAL BONE (Fig. 27.22)

The nasal bones are small, oblong, variable in size and form, and placed side by side between the frontal processes of the maxillae. They jointly form the nasal bridge. Each nasal bone has two surfaces (external and internal) and four borders (superior, inferior, lateral and mesial). The external surface has a descending concavo-convex profile and is transversely convex. It is covered by procerus and nasalis and perforated centrally by a small foramen traversed by a vein. The internal surface, transversely concave, is traversed by a longitudinal groove for the anterior ethmoidal nerve. The superior border, thick and serrated, articulates with the nasal part of the frontal bone. The inferior border, thin and notched, is continuous with the lateral nasal cartilage. The lateral border joins the frontal process of the maxilla. The medial border, thicker above, meets its fellow and projects behind as a vertical crest, so forming a small part of the nasal septum. It articulates from above with

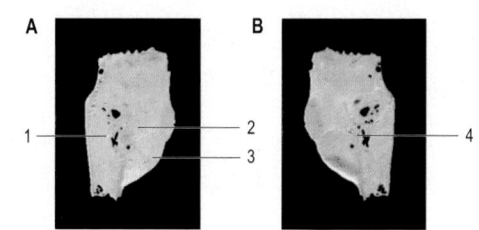

1. Lacrimal groove.
2. Posterior lacrimal crest.
3. Orbital surface.
4. Nasal surface.

Fig. 27.21 Lacrimal bone. **A,** External view; **B,** internal view. (By permission from Berkovitz and Moxham, 1994.)

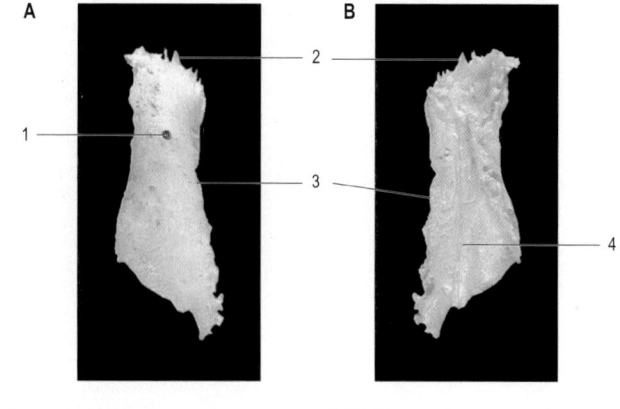

1. Vascular foramen.
2. Frontal margin.
3. Maxillary margin.
4. Groove for anterior ethmoidal nerve.

Fig. 27.22 Left nasal bone. **A,** External view; **B,** internal view. (By permission from Berkovitz and Moxham, 1994.)

the nasal spine of the frontal bone, the perpendicular plate of the ethmoid bone, and the nasal septal cartilage.

Ossification

Ossification is from a centre that appears early in the third month *in utero* in mesenchyme overlying the cartilaginous anterior part of the nasal capsule.

VOMER (Fig. 27.23)

The vomer is thin, flat, and almost trapezoid. It forms the posteroinferior part of the nasal septum and presents two surfaces and four borders. Both surfaces are marked by grooves for nerves and vessels, and a prominent groove for the nasopalatine nerve and vessels lies obliquely in an anteroinferior plane. The superior border is thickest, and possesses a deep furrow between projecting alae which fits the rostrum of the body of the sphenoid bone. The alae articulate with the sphenoidal conchae, the vaginal processes of the medial pterygoid plates of the sphenoid bone, and the sphenoidal processes of the palatine bones. Where each ala lies between the body of the sphenoid and the vaginal process, its inferior surface helps to form the vomerovaginal canal. The inferior border articulates with the median nasal crests of the maxilla and palatine bones. The anterior border is the longest, and articulates in its upper half with the perpendicular plate of the ethmoid bone. Its lower half is cleft to receive the inferior margin of the nasal septal cartilage. The posterior border is concave, separating the posterior nasal apertures. It is thick and bifid above, thin below. The anterior extremity of the vomer articulates with the posterior margin of the maxillary incisor crest and descends between the incisive canals.

Ossification

The nasal septum is at first a plate of cartilage, part of which is ossified above to form the perpendicular plate of the ethmoid. Its anteroinferior region persists as septal cartilage. The vomer is ossified in a layer of connective tissue which covers cartilage on each aspect in its postero-inferior part. About the eighth week *in utero*, two centres appear flanking the midline, and in the twelfth week these unite below the cartilage, to form a deep groove for the nasal septal cartilage. Union of the bony lamellae progresses anterosuperiorly while intervening cartilage is absorbed. By puberty they are almost united, but the bilaminar origin remains in the everted alae and anterior marginal groove.

ZYGOMATIC BONE (Fig. 27.24)

Each zygomatic bone forms the prominence of a cheek, contributes to the floor and lateral wall of the orbit and the walls of the temporal and infratemporal fossae, and completes the zygomatic arch. It is roughly quadrangular and is described as having three surfaces, five borders and two processes.

The lateral (facial) surface is convex and is pierced near its orbital border by the zygomaticofacial foramen, which is often double and occasionally absent, for the zygomaticofacial nerve and vessels. This surface gives attachment to zygomaticus major posteriorly and

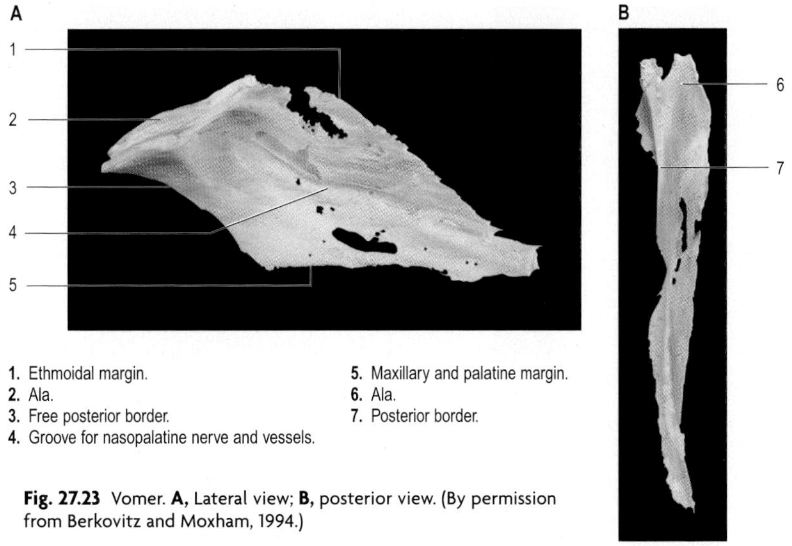

1. Ethmoidal margin.
2. Ala.
3. Free posterior border.
4. Groove for nasopalatine nerve and vessels.

5. Maxillary and palatine margin.
6. Ala.
7. Posterior border.

Fig. 27.23 Vomer. **A,** Lateral view; **B,** posterior view. (By permission from Berkovitz and Moxham, 1994.)

zygomaticus minor anteriorly. The posteromedial (temporal) surface has a rough anterior area for articulation with the zygomatic process of the maxilla, and a smooth, concave posterior area that extends up posteriorly on its frontal process as the anterior aspect of the temporal fossa. It also extends back on the medial aspect of the temporal process as an incomplete lateral wall for the infratemporal fossa. The zygomaticotemporal foramen pierces this surface near the base of the frontal process. The smooth and concave orbital surface forms the anterolateral part of the orbital floor and adjoining lateral wall, and extends up on the medial aspect of its frontal process. It usually bears zygomatico-orbital foramina which represent the openings of canals leading to zygomaticofacial and zygomaticotemporal foramina.

The smoothly concave anterosuperior (orbital) border forms the inferolateral circumference of the orbital opening, and separates the orbital and lateral surfaces of the bone. The anteroinferior (maxillary) border articulates with the maxilla. Its medial end tapers to a point above the infraorbital foramen. A part of levator labii superioris is attached at this surface. The posterosuperior (temporal) border is sinuous, convex above and concave below, and is continuous with the posterior border of the frontal process and upper border of the zygomatic arch. The temporal fascia is attached to this border. There is often a small, easily palpable, marginal tubercle below the frontozygomatic suture. The posteroinferior border is roughened for the attachment of masseter. The serrated posteromedial border articulates with the greater wing of the sphenoid bone above, and the orbital surface of the maxilla below. Between these serrated regions a short, concave, non-articular part usually forms the lateral edge of the inferior orbital fissure. Occasionally absent, the fissure is then completed by junction of the maxilla and sphenoid bones (or with a small sutural bone between them).

The frontal process, thick and serrated, articulates above with the zygomatic process of the frontal bone and behind with the greater wing of the sphenoid bone. A tubercle of varying size and form, Whitnall's tubercle, is usually present on its orbital aspect, within the orbital opening and c.1 cm below the frontozygomatic suture. This tubercle provides attachment for the lateral palpebral ligament, the suspensory ligament of the eye, and part of the aponeurosis of levator palpebrae superioris. The temporal process, directed backwards, has an oblique, serrated end that articulates with the zygomatic process of the temporal bone to complete the zygomatic arch.

Ossification

Ossification is from one centre, which appears in fibrous tissue about the eighth week *in utero*. The bone is sometimes divided by a horizontal suture into a larger upper and smaller lower part.

MAXILLA (Fig. 27.25)

The maxillae are the largest of the facial bones, other than the mandible, and jointly form the whole of the upper jaw. Each bone forms the greater part of the floor and lateral wall of the nasal cavity, and of the floor of the orbit. It contributes to the infratemporal and pterygopalatine fossae and bounds the inferior orbital and pterygomaxillary fissures. The maxilla has a body and four processes, namely the zygomatic, frontal, alveolar and palatine processes.

Body

The body of the maxilla is roughly pyramidal, and has anterior, infra-temporal (posterior), orbital and nasal surfaces that enclose the maxillary sinus.

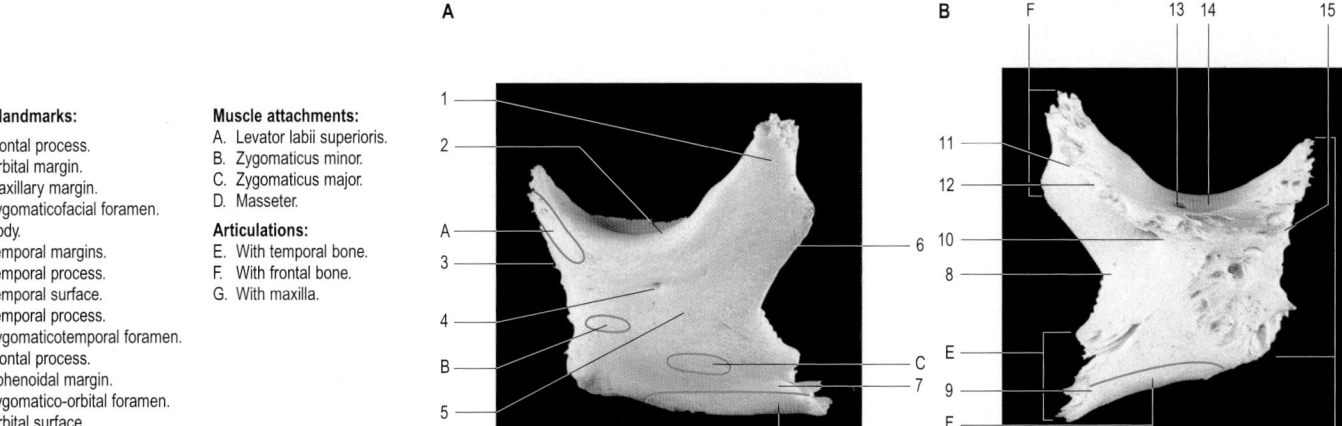

Bone landmarks:

1. Frontal process.
2. Orbital margin.
3. Maxillary margin.
4. Zygomaticofacial foramen.
5. Body.
6. Temporal margins.
7. Temporal process.
8. Temporal surface.
9. Temporal process.
10. Zygomaticotemporal foramen.
11. Frontal process.
12. Sphenoidal margin.
13. Zygomatico-orbital foramen.
14. Orbital surface.
15. Maxillary margin.

Muscle attachments:

A. Levator labii superioris.
B. Zygomaticus minor.
C. Zygomaticus major.
D. Masseter.

Articulations:

E. With temporal bone.
F. With frontal bone.
G. With maxilla.

Fig. 27.24 Left zygomatic bone. **A,** External view; **B,** internal view. (By permission from Berkovitz and Moxham, 1994.)

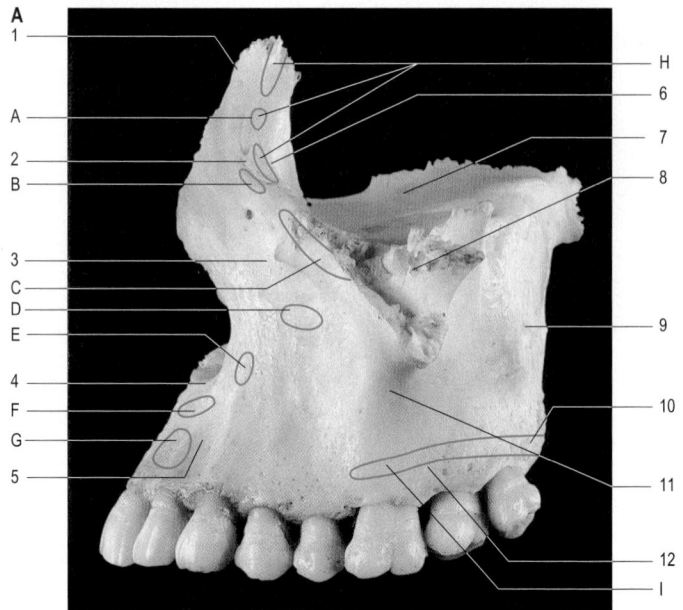

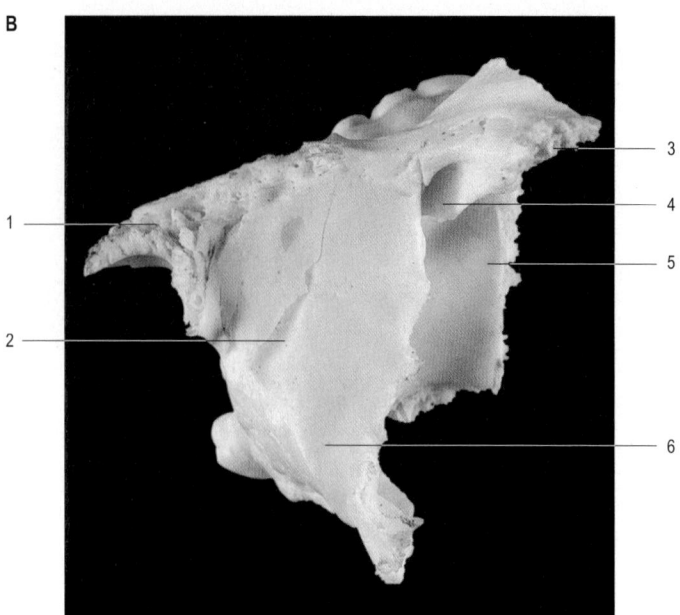

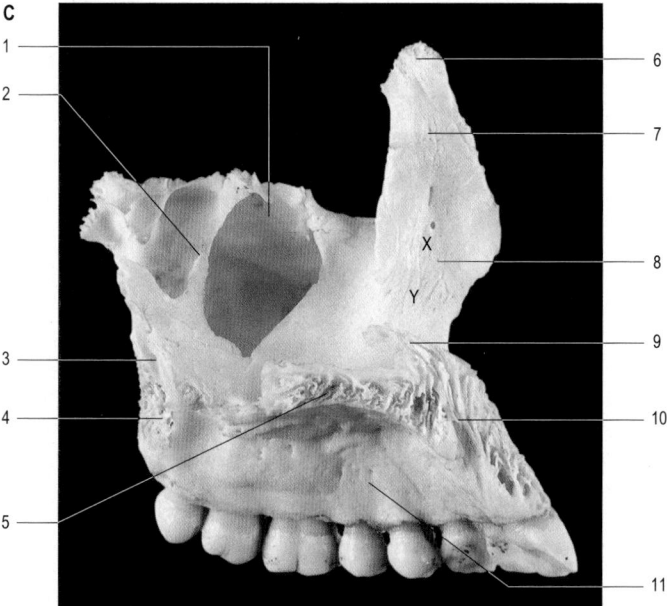

Bone landmarks:

1. Frontal process.
2. Anterior lacrimal crest.
3. Infraorbital foramen.
4. Site of anterior nasal spine.
5. Canine eminence.
6. Lacrimal groove.
7. Orbital surface.
8. Zygomatic process.
9. Infratemporal surface.

10. Tuberosity.
11. Jugal crest.
12. Alveolar process and teeth.

Muscle and ligament attachments:

A. Medial palpebral ligament.
B. Levator labii superioris alaeque nasi.
C. Levator labii superioris.
D. Levator anguli oris.
E. Nasalis, transverse part.
F. Nasalis, alar part.
G. Depressor septi.
H. Orbicularis oculi.
I. Buccinator.

1. Zygomatic process.
2. Infraorbital groove running into infraorbital canal.
3. Frontal process.

4. Lacrimal groove.
5. Palatine process.
6. Orbital surface.

1. Maxillary sinus.
2. Bony partition in sinus.
3. Greater palatine groove.
4. Tuberosity.
5. Palatine process.
6. Frontal process.

7. Ethmoidal crest.
8. Conchal crest.
9. Nasal crest.
10. Incisive canal emerging at incisive fossa.
11. Alveolar process and teeth.

X. Middle meatus.
Y. Inferior meatus.

Fig. 27.25 Left maxilla. **A,** Lateral view; **B,** superior view; **C,** medial view. (By permission from Berkovitz and Moxham, 1994.)

Anterior surface

This surface faces anterolaterally and displays inferior elevations overlying the roots of teeth. There is a shallow incisive fossa above the incisors to which depressor septi is attached. A slip of orbicularis oris is attached to the alveolar border below this fossa, and nasalis is attached superolateral to it. Lateral to the incisive fossa is a larger, deeper canine fossa and levator anguli oris is attached to the bone of this fossa. The incisive

and canine fossae are separated by the canine eminence, which overlies the socket of the canine tooth. The infraorbital foramen lies above the fossa and transmits the infraorbital vessels and nerve. Above the foramen a sharp border separates the anterior and orbital surfaces of the bone and contributes to the infraorbital margin. Levator labii superioris is attached here above the infraorbital foramen and levator anguli oris below it. Medially the anterior surface ends at a deeply concave nasal notch, and terminates in a pointed process which, with its fellow of the opposite side, forms the anterior nasal spine. Nasalis and depressor septi are attached to the anterior surface near the notch.

Infratemporal surface

This surface is concave and faces posterolaterally, forming the anterior wall of the infratemporal fossa. It is separated from the anterior surface by the zygomatic process and a ridge (jugal crest) that ascends to it from the first molar socket. Near its centre are the openings of two or three alveolar canals, which transmit posterior superior alveolar vessels and nerves. Posteroinferior is the maxillary tuberosity which is roughened superomedially where it meets the pyramidal process of the palatine bone. A few fibres of medial pterygoid are attached here. Above the tuberosity the smooth anterior boundary of the pterygopalatine fossa is grooved by the maxillary nerve as it passes laterally and slightly upwards into the infraorbital groove on the orbital surface.

Orbital surface

This surface is smooth and triangular, and forms most of the floor of the orbit. Anteriorly its medial border bears a lacrimal notch, behind which it articulates with the lacrimal bone, the orbital plate of the ethmoid and, posteriorly, with the orbital process of the palatine bone. Its posterior border is smoothly rounded, and forms most of the anterior edge of the inferior orbital fissure. The infraorbital groove lies centrally. The anterior border is part of the orbital margin, and is continuous medially with the lacrimal crest of the frontal process of the maxilla. The infraorbital groove transmits similarly named vessels and a nerve, and begins midway on the posterior border, where it is continuous with a groove on the posterior surface. It passes forwards into the infraorbital canal which opens on the anterior surface below the infraorbital margin. Near its midpoint, the infraorbital canal has a small lateral branch, the canalis sinuosus, for the anterior superior alveolar nerve and vessels. The canalis sinuosus descends in the orbital floor lateral to the infraorbital canal and curves medially in the anterior wall of the maxillary sinus. It then passes below the infraorbital foramen to the margin of the anterior nasal aperture in front of the anterior end of the inferior concha. Here it follows the lower margin of the aperture to open near the nasal septum in front of the incisive canal. The site of the attachment of inferior oblique may be indicated by a small depression in the bone at the anteromedial corner of the orbital surface, lateral to the lacrimal groove.

Nasal surface

This surface displays posterosuperiorly the large, irregular maxillary hiatus leading into the maxillary sinus. Parts of air sinuses which are completed by articulation with the ethmoid and lacrimal bones lie at the upper border of the hiatus. The smooth concave surface below the hiatus is part of the inferior meatus. Posteriorly, the surface is roughened where it meets the perpendicular plate of the palatine bone. This surface is traversed by a groove which descends forwards from the midposterior border, and is converted into a greater palatine canal by the perpendicular plate. Anterior to the hiatus, a deep groove, the nasolacrimal groove, which is continuous above with the lacrimal groove, makes up about two-thirds of the circumference of the nasolacrimal canal. The rest is contributed by the descending part of the lacrimal bone and the lacrimal process of the inferior nasal concha. This canal leads the nasolacrimal duct to the inferior meatus. More anterior is an oblique conchal crest which articulates with the inferior nasal concha. The concavity below it is part of the inferior meatus, while the surface above it is part of the atrium of the middle meatus.

Zygomatic process

Anterior, infratemporal and orbital surfaces converge at a pyramidal projection, the zygomatic process. Anteriorly, the process merges into the facial surface of the body of the maxilla. Posteriorly, it is concave and continuous with the infratemporal surface. Superiorly, it is roughly serrated for articulation with the zygomatic bone. Inferiorly, a bony arched ridge, the zygomaticoalveolar ridge or jugal crest, separates the facial (anterior) and infratemporal surfaces.

Frontal process

The frontal process projects posterosuperiorly between the nasal and lacrimal bones. Its lateral surface is divided by a vertical anterior lacrimal crest which gives attachment to the medial palpebral ligament and is continuous below with the infraorbital margin. A small palpable tubercle at the junction of the crest and orbital surface is a guide to the lacrimal sac. The smooth area anterior to the lacrimal crest merges below with the anterior surface of the body of the maxilla. Parts of orbicularis oculi and levator labii superioris alaeque nasi are attached here. Behind the crest, a vertical groove combines with one on the lacrimal bone to complete the lacrimal fossa. The medial surface is part of the lateral nasal wall. A rough subapical area articulates with the ethmoid, and closes anterior ethmoidal air cells. Below this an oblique ethmoidal crest articulates posteriorly with the middle nasal concha, and anteriorly underlies the agger nasi, which is a ridge anterior to the concha on the lateral nasal wall. The ethmoidal crest forms the upper limit of the atrium of the middle meatus. The frontal process articulates above with the nasal part of the frontal bone. Its anterior border articulates with the nasal bone and its posterior border articulates with the lacrimal bone.

Alveolar process

The alveolar process is thick and arched, wide behind, and socketed for the roots of the upper teeth. The eight sockets on each side vary according to the tooth type. The socket for the canine is deepest, the sockets for molars are widest and subdivided into three by septa, those for incisors and second premolar are single, and that for the first premolar usually double. Buccinator is attached to the external alveolar aspect as far forwards as the first molar. In articulated maxillae the processes form the alveolar arch. Occasionally a variably prominent longitudinal maxillary torus is present on the palatal aspect of the process near the molar sockets.

Palatine process

The palatine process, thick and horizontal, projects medially from the lowest part of the medial aspect of the maxilla. It forms a large part of the nasal floor and hard palate and is much thicker in front. Its inferior surface is concave and uneven, and it forms with its contralateral fellow the anterior three-fourths of the osseous (hard) palate. The palatine process displays numerous vascular foramina and depressions for palatine glands and, posterolaterally, two grooves that transmit the greater palatine vessels and nerves. The infundibular incisive fossa is placed between the two maxillae, behind the incisor teeth. The median intermaxillary palatal suture runs posterior to the fossa, and although a little uneven, is usually relatively flat on its oral aspect. Its bony margins are sometimes raised into a prominent longitudinal palatine torus. Two lateral incisive canals, each ascending into its half of the nasal cavity, open in the incisive fossa: they transmit the terminations of the greater palatine artery and nasopalatine nerve. Two additional median openings, anterior and posterior incisive foramina, are occasionally present: they transmit the nasopalatine nerves, the left passing through the anterior and the right through the posterior foramen. On the inferior palatine surface a fine groove, sometimes termed the incisive suture, and prominent in young skulls, may be observed in adults. It extends anterolaterally from the incisive fossa to the interval between the lateral incisor and canine teeth. The superior surface of the palatine process is smooth, concave transversely, and forms most of the nasal floor. The incisive canal lies anteriorly, near its median margin. The lateral border is continuous with the body of the maxilla. The medial border, thicker in front, is raised into a nasal crest that, with its contralateral fellow, forms a groove for the vomer. The front of this ridge rises higher as an incisor crest, prolonged forwards into a sharp process which, with its fellow, forms an anterior nasal spine. The posterior border is serrated for articulation with the horizontal plate of the palatine bone.

Maxillary sinus

The maxillary sinus is the largest of the paranasal sinuses and is situated in the body of the maxilla. Pyramidal in shape, the base (medial wall) forms part of the lateral wall of the nose, while the apex extends into the zygomatic process of the maxilla. The floor is formed by the alveolar process and part of the palatine process of the maxilla, and the roof contributes the major part of the floor of the orbit. The facial and infratemporal surfaces of the maxilla form its anterior and posterior walls respectively. The sinus may be partially divided by bony septa.

The medial wall of the maxilla sinus bears the opening (ostium) of the sinus. The infraorbital nerve and vessels lie within the infraorbital canal in the roof. The floor of the sinus lies below the level of the floor of the nose, and is related to the roots of the cheek teeth, although this relationship is variable according to the size of the sinus. Usually, at least the upper second premolar and first molar are related to the floor of the sinus, however the sinus may extend anteriorly to the first premolar tooth – and sometimes even to the canine – and posteriorly to the third molar tooth. The anterior superior alveolar nerve and vessels that arise within the infraorbital canal pass downwards in a fine canal (canalis sinuosus) in the anterior wall of the maxillary sinus, to be distributed to the anterior upper teeth. The posterior superior alveolar nerve and vessels pass through canals in the posterior surface of the sinus.

In an isolated maxillary, the ostium of the maxillary sinus appears large. However, in life, the size of the ostium is considerably reduced by portions of the perpendicular plate of the palatine bone, the uncinate process of the ethmoid bone, the inferior nasal concha and the lacrimal bone, and by the overlying nasal mucosa. The ostium lies high up at the back of the medial wall of the maxillary sinus, where it is unfavourably situated for drainage. It usually opens into the posterior part of the ethmoidal infundibulum, and thence into the hiatus semilunaris of the middle meatus of the lateral wall of the nose. An accessory ostium is sometimes present behind the major ostium.

Ossification

The maxilla ossifies from a single centre in a sheet of mesenchyme that appears above the canine fossa at about the sixth week *in utero* and spreads into the rest of the maxilla and its processes. The pattern of spread of ossification may initially leave an unmineralized zone in a region roughly corresponding to a site where a premaxillary suture may occur. However, this deficiency is soon ossified and there is no evidence of a separate centre of ossification for the incisor-bearing portion of the maxilla (i.e. premaxilla).

The maxillary sinus appears as a shallow groove on the nasal aspect at about the fourth month *in utero*. Though small at birth, the sinus is identifiable radiologically. After birth the maxillary sinus enlarges with the growing maxilla, though it is only fully developed following the eruption of the permanent dentition. The infraorbital vessels and nerve are for a time in an open groove in the orbital floor, and the anterior part is subsequently converted into a canal by a lamina that grows in from the lateral side.

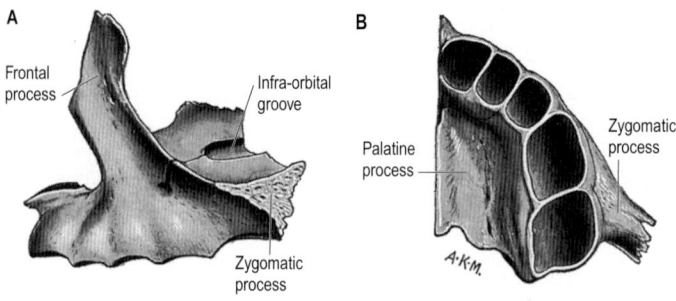

Fig. 27.26 Maxilla at birth.

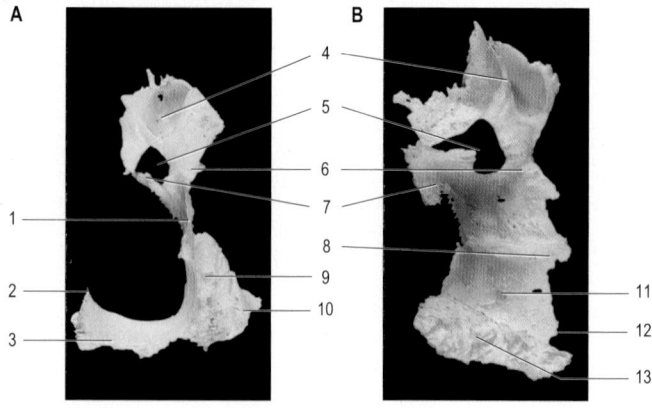

1. Perpendicular plate.
2. Nasal crest.
3. Horizontal plate.
4. Orbital process with air cell.
5. Sphenopalatine notch.

6. Ethmoidal crest.
7. Sphenoidal process.
8. Conchal crest.
9. Greater palatine groove.

10. Pyramidal process.
11. Perpendicular plate.
12. Maxillary process.
13. Horizontal plate.

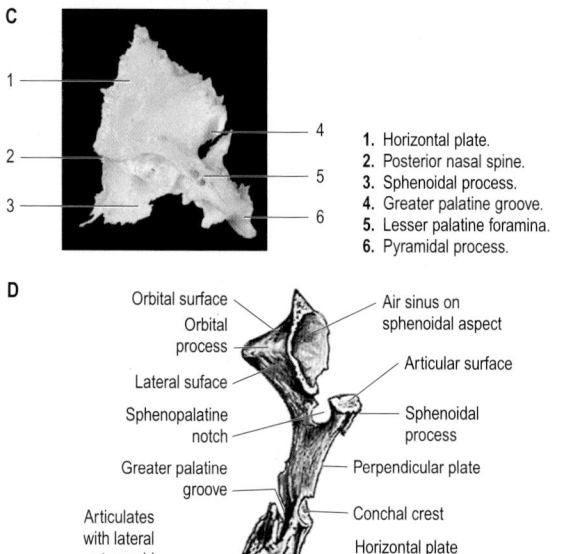

1. Horizontal plate.
2. Posterior nasal spine.
3. Sphenoidal process.
4. Greater palatine groove.
5. Lesser palatine foramina.
6. Pyramidal process.

Fig. 27.27 Left palatine bone. A, Anterior view; B, medial view; C, Inferior view; D, Posterior view and muscle attachment. (By permission from Berkovitz and Moxham, 1994.)

Age changes in the maxilla

At birth the transverse and sagittal maxillary dimensions are greater than the vertical. The frontal process is prominent, but the body is little more than an alveolar process, since the alveoli reach almost to the orbital floor (**Fig. 27.26**). In adults the vertical dimension is greatest, reflecting the development of the alveolar process and enlargement of the sinus. When teeth are lost, the bone reverts towards its infantile shape. Thus, its height diminishes, the alveolar process is absorbed, and the lower parts of the bone contract and become reduced in thickness at the expense of the labial wall.

PALATINE BONE (Fig. 27.27)

The palatine bones are posteriorly placed in the nasal cavity between the maxillae and the pterygoid processes of the sphenoid bones. They contribute to the floor and lateral wall of the nose, to the floors of the palate and orbit, to the pterygopalatine and pterygoid fossae, and to the inferior orbital fissures. Each has two plates (horizontal and perpendicular plates) arranged as an L-shape, and three processes (pyramidal, orbital and sphenoidal).

Horizontal plate

The horizontal plate is quadrilateral, with two surfaces (nasal and palatine) and four borders (anterior, posterior, lateral and medial). The nasal surface, transversely concave, forms the posterior nasal floor. The palatine surface forms, with its fellow, the posterior quarter of the bony palate. There is often a curved palatine crest near its posterior margin. The posterior border is thin and concave: the expanded tendon of tensor veli palatini is attached to it and its adjacent surface behind the palatine crest. Medially, with its fellow from the opposite side, the posterior border forms a median posterior nasal spine to which the uvular muscle is attached. The serrated anterior border articulates with the palatine process of the maxilla. The lateral border is continuous with the perpendicular plate of the palatine bone and is marked by a greater palatine groove. The medial border, thick and serrated, articulates with its fellow in the midline, and forms the posterior part of the nasal crest which articulates with the posterior part of the lower edge of the vomer.

Perpendicular plate

The perpendicular plate is thin and oblong, and has two surfaces (nasal and maxillary) and four borders (anterior, posterior, superior and inferior). The nasal surface bears two crests (conchal and ethmoidal) and shows areas which contribute to the inferior middle and superior meatuses. Inferiorly, the nasal surface is concave where it contributes to part of the inferior meatus. Above this is a horizontal conchal crest that articulates with the inferior concha. Above the conchal crest the surface presents a shallow depression which forms part of the middle meatus. This depression is limited above by an ethmoidal crest for the middle nasal concha, above which a narrow, horizontal groove forms part of the superior meatus.

The maxillary surface is largely rough and irregular and articulates with the nasal surface of the maxilla. Posterosuperiorly it forms a smooth medial wall to the pterygopalatine fossa. Its anterior area, also smooth, overlaps the maxillary hiatus from behind to form a posterior part of the medial wall of the maxillary sinus. A deep, obliquely descending greater palatine groove – converted into a canal by the maxilla – lies posteriorly on this maxillary surface and transmits the greater palatine vessels and nerve.

The anterior border is thin and irregular. Level with the conchal crest, a pointed lamina projects below and behind the maxillary process of the inferior concha: it articulates with it and so appears in the medial wall of the maxillary sinus. The posterior border has a serrated suture with the medial pterygoid plate. It is continuous above with the sphenoidal process of the palatine bone and expands below into its pyramidal process. Orbital and sphenoidal processes project from the superior border, and are separated by the sphenopalatine notch (converted into a foramen by articulation with the body of the sphenoid). This foramen connects the pterygopalatine fossa to the posterior part of the superior meatus, and transmits sphenopalatine vessels and the posterior superior nasal nerves. The inferior border is continuous with the lateral border of the horizontal plate and bears the lower end of the greater palatine groove in front of the pyramidal process.

Pyramidal process

The pyramidal process slopes down posterolaterally from the junction of the horizontal and perpendicular palatine plates into the angle between the pterygoid plates of the sphenoid bone. On its posterior surface a smooth, grooved triangular area, limited on each side by rough articular furrows which articulate with the pterygoid plates, completes the lower part of the pterygoid fossa. Anteriorly the lateral surface articulates with the maxillary tuberosity. This area gives attachment to fibres of the superficial head of medial pterygoid. Posteriorly a smooth triangular area appears low in the infratemporal fossa between the tuberosity and lateral pterygoid plate. The inferior surface, near its union with the horizontal plate, bears the lesser palatine foramina for the corresponding nerves and arteries.

Orbital process
The orbital process is directed superolaterally from in front of the perpendicular plate, and has a constricted 'neck'. It encloses an air sinus and presents three articular and two non-articular surfaces. Of the articular surfaces, the oblong anterior, or maxillary, surface faces down and anterolaterally to articulate with the maxilla; the posterior, or sphenoidal, surface, directed up and posteromedially, bears the opening of an air sinus. It usually communicates with the sphenoidal sinus, and is completed by a sphenoidal concha. The medial, or ethmoidal, surface, faces anteromedially and articulates with the labyrinth of the ethmoid bone. The sinus of the orbital process sometimes opens on the surface, and communicates with the posterior ethmoidal air cells. More rarely it opens on both the ethmoidal and sphenoidal surfaces, and communicates with both posterior ethmoidal air cells and the sphenoidal sinus.

Of the non-articular surfaces, the triangular superior or orbital surface is directed superolaterally to the posterior part of the orbital floor. The lateral surface is oblong, faces the pterygopalatine fossa and is separated from the orbital surface by a rounded border that forms a medial part of the lower margin of the inferior orbital fissure. This surface may present a groove, directed superolaterally, for the maxillary nerve and is continuous with the groove on the upper posterior surface of the maxilla. The border between the lateral and posterior surfaces descends anterior to the sphenopalatine notch.

Sphenoidal process
The sphenoidal process is a thin plate that is smaller and lower than the orbital process, and is directed superomedially. Its superior surface articulates with the sphenoidal concha and, above it, the root of the medial pterygoid plate. It carries a groove that contributes to the formation of the palatovaginal canal. The concave inferomedial surface forms part of the roof and lateral wall of the nose. Posteriorly the lateral surface articulates with the medial pterygoid plate, while its smooth anterior region forms part of the medial wall of the pterygopalatine fossa. The posterior border articulates with the vaginal process of the medial pterygoid plate. The anterior border is the posterior edge of the sphenopalatine notch. The medial border articulates with the ala of the vomer. The sphenopalatine notch, between the two processes, becomes a foramen by articulation with the body of the sphenoid bone.

Ossification
Ossification is in mesenchyme from one centre in the perpendicular plate that appears during the eighth week *in utero*. From this, ossification spreads into all parts. At birth the height of the perpendicular plate equals the width of the horizontal plate, but in adults it is almost twice as great, a change in proportions that accords with those that occur in the maxilla.

MANDIBLE (Fig. 27.28)
The mandible is the largest, strongest and lowest bone in the face. It has a horizontally curved body that is convex forwards, and two broad rami, that ascend posteriorly. The body of the mandible supports the mandibular teeth within the alveolar process. The rami bear the coronoid and condylar processes, and the latter articulate with the temporal bones at the temporomandibular joints.

Body
The body, is somewhat U-shaped, and has external and internal surfaces separated by upper and lower borders. Anteriorly, the upper external surface shows an inconstant faint median ridge, which indicates fusion of the halves of the fetal bone at the symphysis menti. Inferiorly this ridge divides to enclose a triangular mental protuberance; its base is centrally depressed but raised on each side as a mental tubercle. The mental protuberance and mental tubercles constitute the chin. The mental foramen, from which the mental nerve and vessels emerge, lies below either the interval between the premolar teeth, or the second premolar tooth. The posterior border of the foramen is smooth, and accommodates the nerve which emerges posterolaterally. A faint external oblique line ascends backwards from each mental tubercle, and sweeps below the foramen: it becomes more marked as it continues into the anterior border of the ramus.

The lower border of the body, the base, extends posterolaterally from the mandibular symphysis into the lower border of the ramus behind the third molar tooth. Near the midline, on each side, is a rough digastric fossa that gives attachment to the anterior belly of digastric. Behind the fossa the base is thick and rounded, and has a slight anteroposterior convexity. This changes to a gentle concavity as the ramus is approached, which gives the base a sinuous profile.

The upper border, the alveolar part, contains 16 alveoli for the roots of the lower teeth. It consists of buccal and lingual plates of bone joined by interdental and inter-radicular septa. Near the second and third molar teeth the external oblique line is superimposed upon the buccal plate. Like the maxilla, the form and depth of the tooth sockets is related to the morphology of the roots of the mandibular teeth. Usually, the sockets of the incisors, canines and premolar teeth contain a single root, while those for the three molar teeth each contain two roots. The external surface of the alveolus adjacent to the molar teeth gives attachment to buccinator. A number of muscles of facial expression are attached to the lateral surface of the mandible.

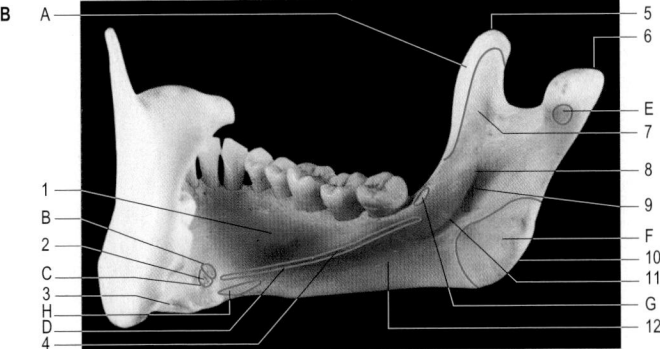

Bone landmarks:

1. Alveolar process and teeth.	7. Mandibular notch.
2. Incisive fossa.	8a. Head.
3. Mental protuberance.	8b. Neck.
4. Mental foramen.	9. Ramus.
5. Body.	10. External oblique line.
6. Coronoid process.	11. Angle.

Muscle attachments:

A. Temporalis.
B. Mentalis.
C. Depressor labii inferioris.
D. Depressor anguli oris.
E. Masseter.
F. Buccinator.
G. Platysma (part).

Bone landmarks:

1. Sublingual fossa.	7. Temporal crest.
2. Mental spines (genial tubercles).	8. Lingula.
3. Digastric fossa.	9. Mandibular foramen.
4. Mylohyoid (internal oblique) line.	10. Angle.
5. Coronoid process.	11. Mylohyoid groove.
6. Head of condyle.	12. Submandibular fossa.

Muscle attachments:

A. Temporalis.
B. Genioglossus.
C. Geniohyoid.
D. Mylohyoid.
E. Lateral pterygoid.
F. Medial pterygoid.
G. Superior constrictor.
H. Digastric, anterior belly.

Fig. 27.28 Mandible. **A,** Lateral view; **B,** medial view. (By permission from Berkovitz and Moxham, 1994.)

The internal surface of the mandible is divided by an oblique mylohyoid line to which mylohyoid is attached (as are, above its posterior end, the superior pharyngeal constrictor, some retromolar fascicles of buccinator, and the pterygomandibular raphe behind the third molar). This line, which extends from a point a centimetre from the upper border behind the third molar to the mental symphysis, is sharp and distinct near the molars, but faint in front. A slightly concave submandibular fossa related to the submandibular gland lies below the mylohyoid line. The area above the line widens anteriorly into a triangular sublingual fossa related to the sublingual gland. The bone is covered by oral mucosa above the sublingual fossa as far back as the third molar. Above the anterior ends of the mylohyoid lines, the posterior symphyseal aspect bears a small elevation, often divided into upper and lower parts, the mental spines (genial tubercles). The upper part gives attachment to genioglossus, the lower part to geniohyoid. Posteriorly the mylohyoid groove extends downwards and forwards from the ramus below the posterior part the mylohyoid line and contains the mylohyoid nerve and vessels. Superior to the mental spines, most mandibles display a lingual (genial) foramen that opens into a canal which traverses the bone to c.50% of the buccomandibular dimension of the mandible: it contains a branch of the lingual artery. As yet its development is uncertain, although it is a useful radiological landmark (see also accessory mandibular foramina). A rounded torus mandibularis sometimes occurs above the mylohyoid line, medial to the molar roots.

Ramus

The mandibular ramus is quadrilateral, and has two surfaces (lateral and medial), four borders (superior, inferior, anterior and posterior) and two processes (coronoid and condylar). The lateral surface is relatively featureless and bears the (external) oblique ridge in its lower part. The medial surface presents, a little above centre, an irregular mandibular foramen, that leads into the mandibular canal. This canal curves downwards and forwards into the body to the mental foramen. Anteromedially the mental foramen is overlapped by a thin, triangular lingula. The mylohyoid groove descends forwards from behind the lingula. The inferior border, continuous with the mandibular base, meets the posterior border at the angle. This is typically everted in males, but in females is frequently inverted. The thin superior border bounds the mandibular incisure, surmounted in front by the somewhat triangular, flat, coronoid process and behind by the condylar process. The posterior border, thick and rounded, extends from the condyle to the angle, being gently convex backwards above, and concave below. The anterior border is thin above where it is continuous with that of the coronoid process, and thicker below where it is continuous with the external oblique line. The temporal crest is a ridge that runs down from the tip of the coronoid process on its medial side to the bone just behind the third molar tooth. The triangular depression between the temporal crest and the anterior border of the ramus is called the retromolar fossa.

Coronoid process

The coronoid process projects upwards and slightly forwards as a triangular plate of bone. Its posterior border bounds the mandibular incisure, and its anterior border continues into that of the ramus. The temporal crest is a ridge that runs down from the tip of the coronoid process on its medial side.

Condylar process

The mandibular condyle varies considerably both in size and shape. When viewed from above, the condyle is roughly ovoid in outline, the anteroposterior dimension of the condyle (c.1 cm) being approximately half the mediolateral dimension. The medial aspect of the condyle is wider than the lateral. However, the long axis of the condyle is not at right angles to the ramus, but diverges posteriorly from a strictly coronal plane. Thus, the lateral pole of the condyle lies slightly anterior to the medial, and if the long axes of the two condyles are extended, they meet at an obtuse angle (c.145°) at the anterior border of the foramen magnum. The articular head of the condyle joins the ramus through a thin bony projection, the neck of the condyle. A small depression situated on the anterior surface of the neck, below the articular surface, termed the pterygoid fovea, receives part of the attachment of lateral pterygoid.

The condyle is composed of a core of cancellous bone covered by a thin layer of compact bone. During the period of growth a layer of hyaline cartilage forms a secondary condylar cartilage and lies immediately beneath the fibrous articulating surface of the condyle.

The ramus and its processes provide attachment for the four primary muscles of mastication. Masseter is attached to the lateral surface, medial pterygoid is attached to the medial surface, temporalis is inserted into the coronoid process and lateral pterygoid is attached to the condyle. The sphenomandibular ligament is attached to the lingula.

Accessory foramina of the mandible

These are usually unnamed and infrequently described, yet they are numerous. Accessory foramina of the mandible are common. They may transmit auxiliary nerves to the teeth (from facial, mylohyoid, buccal, transverse cervical cutaneous and other nerves), and their occurrence is significant in dental anaesthetic blocking techniques.

Ossification

The mandible forms in dense fibromembranous tissue lateral to the inferior alveolar nerve and its incisive branch, and also in the lower parts of Meckel's cartilage. Each half is ossified from a centre that appears near the mental foramen about the sixth week *in utero*. From this site, ossification spreads medially and posterocranially to form the body and ramus, first below, and then around, the inferior alveolar nerve and its incisive branch. It then spreads upwards, initially forming a trough, and later crypts, for developing teeth. By the tenth week, Meckel's cartilage below the incisor rudiments is surrounded and invaded by bone. Secondary cartilages appear later (**Fig. 27.29**): a conical mass, the condylar cartilage, extends from the mandibular head downwards and forwards in the ramus, and contributes to its growth in height. Although it is largely replaced by bone by midfetal life, its proximal end persists as proliferating cartilage under the fibrous articular lining until about the third decade. Another secondary cartilage, which soon ossifies, appears along the anterior coronoid border, and disappears before birth. One or two cartilaginous nodules also occur at the symphysis menti. At about the seventh month *in utero* these may ossify as variable mental ossicles in symphyseal fibrous tissue, and unite to adjacent bone before the end of the first postnatal year.

Age changes in the mandible (Fig. 27.30)

At birth the two halves of the mandible are united by a fibrous symphysis menti. Anterior ends of both rudiments are covered by cartilage,

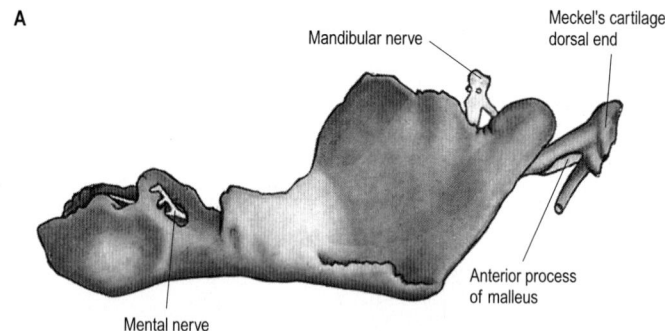

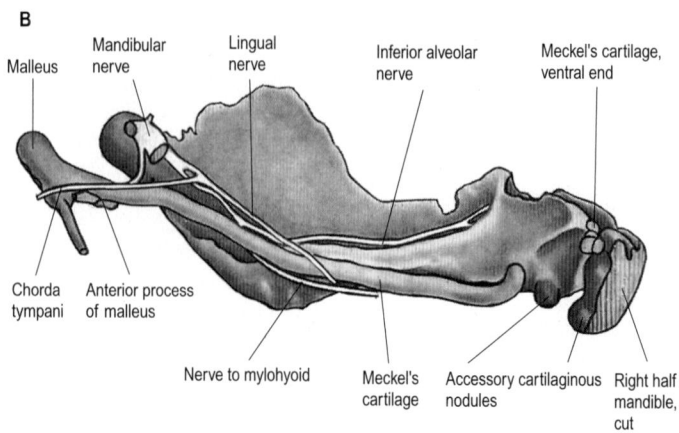

Fig. 27.29 The left half of the mandible of a human embryo, 95 mm long. **A**, Lateral aspect; **B**, medial aspect. Blue: cartilage; yellow: bone. (By kind permission from A Low.)

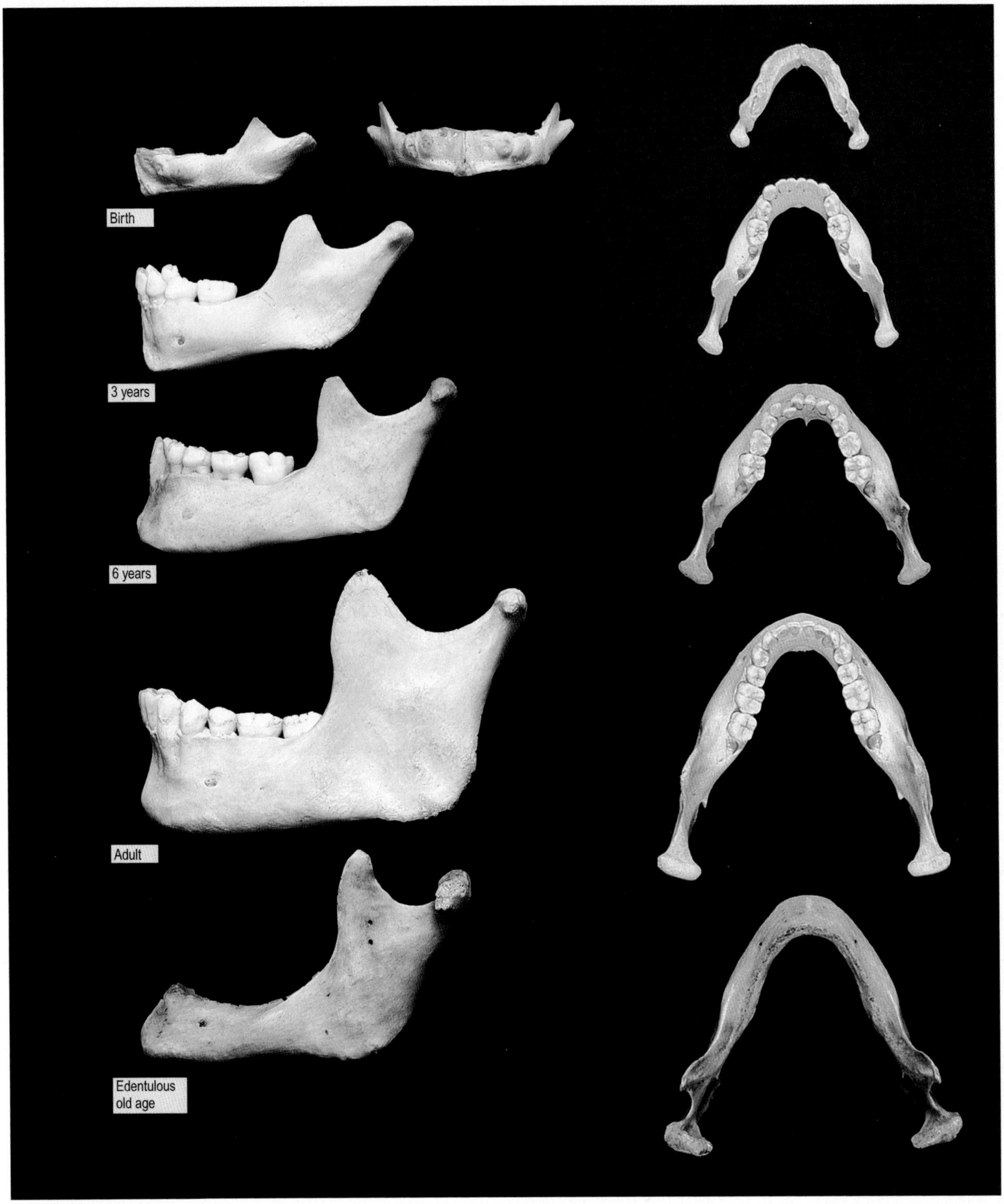

Fig. 27.30 The mandible at different ages. (Photographs by Andrew Dyer.)

separated only by a symphysis. Until fusion occurs new cells are added to each cartilage from symphyseal fibrous tissue, and ossification on its mandibular side proceeds towards the midline. When the latter process overtakes the former, and ossification extends into median fibrous tissue, the symphysis fuses. At this stage the body is a mere shell which encloses the imperfectly separated sockets of deciduous teeth. The mandibular canal is near the lower border, and the mental foramen opens below the first deciduous molar and is directed forwards. The coronoid process projects above the condyle.

In the first to third postnatal years the two halves join at their symphysis from below upwards, although separation near the alveolar margin may persist into the second year. The body elongates, especially behind the mental foramen, providing space for three additional teeth. During the first and second years, as a chin develops, the mental foramen alters direction from facing forwards to facing backwards, as in adult mandibles, to accommodate a changing direction of the emerging mental nerve.

In general terms, increase in height of the body of the mandible occurs primarily by formation of alveolar bone associated with the developing and erupting teeth, although some bone is deposited on the lower border. Increase in length of the mandible is accomplished by deposition of bone on the posterior surface of the ramus with compensatory resorption on its anterior surface (accompanied by deposition of bone on the posterior surface of the coronoid process and resorption on the anterior surface of the condylar process). Increase in width of the mandible is produced by deposition of bone on the outer surface of the mandible and resorption on the inner surface. An increase in the comparative size of the ramus compared with the body of the mandible occurs during postnatal growth and tooth eruption.

There is some controversy concerning the role of the condylar cartilages in mandibular growth. One view states that continued proliferation of this cartilage is primarily responsible for the increase in both the mandibular length and the height of the ramus. Alternatively, there is experimental evidence which supports the view that proliferation of the condylar cartilage is a response to growth and not its cause. In adults, alveolar and subalveolar regions are about equal in depth, the mental foramen appears midway between the upper and lower borders, and the mandibular canal nearly parallels the mylohyoid line. If the teeth are lost, alveolar bone is resorbed and the mandibular canal and mental foramen come to lie nearer the superior border. Indeed, both may disappear, so that the nerves lie just beneath the oral mucosa.

JOINTS

The general characteristics of cranial sutures and the detailed anatomy of the temporomandibular joint are described in Chapters 6 and 30, respectively. Sutural bones are described on page 486.

NEONATAL, PAEDIATRIC AND SENESCENT ANATOMY

THE SKULL AT BIRTH

At birth the skull is large in proportion to other skeletal parts, but the facial region is relatively small, and constitutes only about one-eighth of the neonatal cranium, compared with half in adult life. Smallness of the face at birth is due to the rudimentary stage of the mandible and maxillae, non-eruption of the teeth, and the small size of the maxillary sinuses and the nasal cavity. The latter is almost entirely between the orbits, the lower border of the piriform nasal aperture being only slightly below the orbital floors. The large size of the calvaria, especially the cranial vault, is related to precocious cerebral growth. The cranial base is relatively short and narrow and, although the middle and internal auditory parts are almost adult in size, the petrous temporal bones are generally far from adult dimensions. Bones of the cranial vault are unilaminar and without diploë. Frontal and parietal tuberosities are prominent and in norma verticalis the greatest width is between the parietal tuberosities. The glabella, superciliary arches and mastoid processes are not developed.

Ossification is incomplete, and many bones are still in several elements united by fibrous tissue or cartilage. The 'os incisivum' is continuous with the maxilla; pre- and postsphenoids have just united, but the halves of frontal bone and mandible, and the squamous, lateral and basilar parts of the occipital bone are all separate. A second styloid centre (stylohyal) has not appeared and parts of the temporal bones are separate except for the commencing fusion of the tympanic with the petrous and squamous parts. The fibrous membrane, forming the cranial vault before ossification, is unossified at the angles of the parietal bones, leaving six fonticuli (fontanelles), two median (anterior and posterior) and two lateral pairs (sphenoidal and mastoid). The anterior fontanelle (**Fig. 27.31**), the largest, at the junction of the sagittal, coronal and frontal sutures, and hence rhomboid in shape, is c.4 cm in anteroposterior and 2.5 cm in transverse dimensions. The posterior fontanelle, at the junction of the sagittal and lambdoid sutures, is hence triangular. The sphenoidal (anterolateral) and mastoid (posterolateral) fontanelles (**Fig. 27.31**) are small, irregular and at the sphenoidal and mastoid angles of the parietal bones.

At birth the orbits are large and the germs of the developing teeth are near their orbital floors. Temporal bones differ greatly from their adult form. The internal ear, tympanic cavity, auditory ossicles and mastoid antrum are almost adult in size, the tympanic plate is an incomplete ring, and the mastoid process is absent. Hence the external acoustic meatus is short, straight, unossified and wholly fibrocartilaginous. The external aspect of the tympanic membrane faces down rather than laterally, in accord with the basal cranial contour. The stylomastoid foramen is exposed on the lateral surface of the skull; the styloid process has not fused with the temporal bone; the mandibular fossa is flat and more

lateral, and its articular tubercle undeveloped. Paranasal sinuses are rudimentary or absent; only the maxillary sinuses are usually identifiable.

During birth the skull is moulded by slow compression. That part of the scalp which is more central in the birth canal is often temporarily oedematous as a result of interference with venous return, and is called the caput succedaneum. Fontanelles and the width of the sutures allow bones of the cranial vault some overlap. The skull is compressed in one plane with compensatory elongation orthogonal to this. These effects disappear within the first week.

POSTNATAL GROWTH

Coordinated postnatal growth of the calvarial and facial skeleton proceeds at different rates and periods, that of the cranial cavity being related to cerebral growth, the facial skeleton to the development of the teeth, muscles of mastication and tongue. Growth of the cranial base is not at the same rate as that of the vault. Therefore the three regions must be considered separately. The anterior part of the cranial base is a zone of interaction between facial and cerebral growth.

Growth of the vault

Growth of the vault is rapid during the first year and then slower to the seventh, by which time it has reached almost adult dimensions. For most of this period expansion is largely concentric; form is determined early in the first year, remaining thereafter largely unaltered. That shape of the vault is not directly related to cerebral growth but to genetic factors is supported by the great range of cranial indices and shapes in racial groups. During the first and early second years, growth of the vault is mainly by ossification at apposed margins of bones – which possess an osteogenic layer – accompanied by some accretion and absorption of bone at surfaces to adapt to continually altering curvatures. Growth in breadth occurs at the sagittal, sphenofrontal, sphenotemporal and occipitomastoid sutures and petro-occipital cartilaginous joints. Growth in height occurs at the frontozygomatic and squamosal sutures, pterion and asterion. During this period fontanelles are closed by ossification of the bones around them, but separate centres may convert them into sutural bones. The sphenoidal and posterior fontanelles 'fill in' within 2 or 3 months of birth; mastoid fontanelles usually near the end of the first year; and the anterior fontanelle at about the middle of the second, by which time calvarial bones have interlocked at sutures, a process which commences early in the first year. Further expansion is chiefly by accretion and absorption on external and internal surfaces respectively. Meanwhile the bones thicken, although not uniformly. At birth the vault is unilaminar. Tables and intervening diploë appear about the fourth year, with maximal differentiation at about 35 years, when diploic veins are prominent in radiograms. Thickening of the vault and development of external muscular markings reflect the development of the masticatory and neck muscles. The mastoid process is a visible bulge in the second year, and is invaded by air cells in the sixth year.

Growth of the base

This is responsible for much of the cranial lengthening, mostly at cartilaginous joints between the sphenoid and ethmoid, and especially between the sphenoid and occipital bones. Largely independent of cerebral growth, it continues at the occipitosphenoid synchondrosis until the eighteenth to twenty-fifth year, a period prolonged by continued expansion of the jaws to accommodate erupting teeth, and by growth in the muscles of mastication and those of the nasopharynx. However, there is some evidence that growth may cease at about 15 years. A pubertal growth spurt has been ascribed to both sexes, about 2 years earlier in females; considerable postpubertal growth, up to 17.5 years in males, has been described. Multivariate analysis of Cartesian coordinates of cranial landmarks in Polynesian crania suggests that there is considerable independence in the growth and positioning of the segments noted above.

Growth of the face

Growth of the face occupies a longer period than does that of the calvaria. Much information has been derived from serial radiography. The ethmoid and the orbital and upper nasal cavities have almost completed growth by the seventh year. Orbital and upper nasal growth is achieved by sutural accretion, with deposition of bone on the facial aspects of the margins. The maxilla is carried downwards and forwards by expansion

A

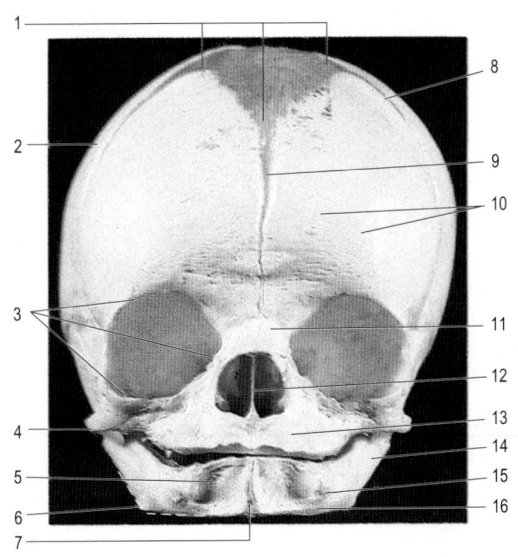

B

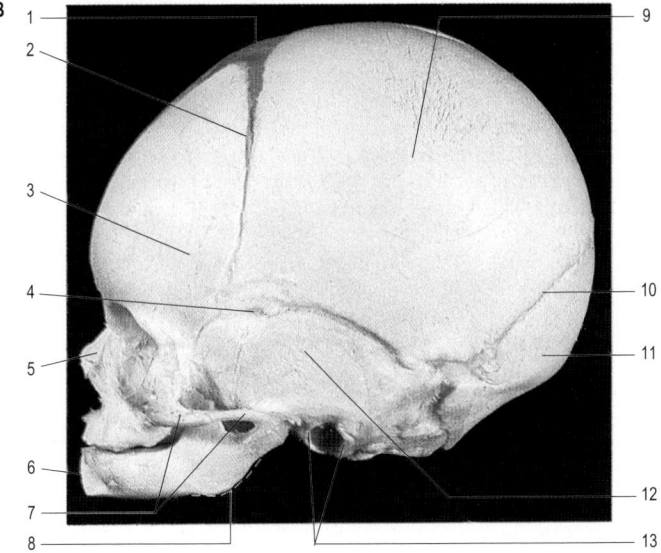

1. Anterior fontanelle.
2. Parietal bone.
3. Orbital margins.
4. Zygomatic bone.
5. Mandible: large alveolar process.
6. Obtuse mandibular angle.
7. Symphysis menti.
8. Coronal suture.
9. Frontal (metopic) suture.
10. Frontal bone and tuber.
11. Nasal bone.
12. Nasal septum.
13. Maxilla.
14. Mandibular ramus.
15. Mental foramen.
16. Mandible: small base.

1. Anterior fontanelle.
2. Coronal suture.
3. Left frontal bone.
4. Future pterion: closing sphenoidal fontanelle.
5. Nasal bone.
6. Symphysis menti.
7. Zygomatic arch.
8. Gonial contour.
9. Parietal tuber.
10. Lambdoid suture.
11. Occipital squama.
12. Temporal squama.
13. Tympanic ring.

C

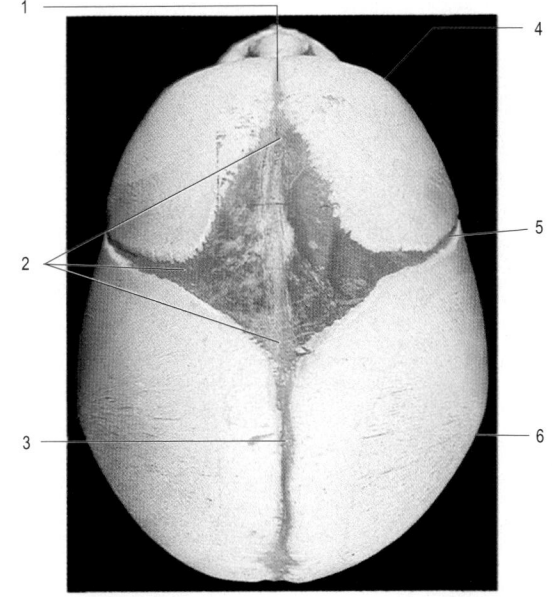

D

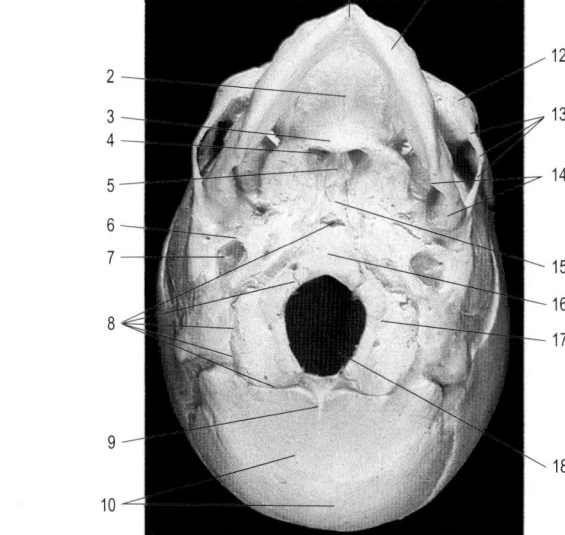

1. Frontal (metopic) suture.
2. Anterior fontanelle.
3. Sagittal suture.
4. Frontal bone and tuber.
5. Coronal suture.
6. Parietal bone and tuber.

1. Frontal (metopic) symphysis.
2. Hard palate: intermaxillary suture.
3. Palatine bone.
4. Posterior choana.
5. Vomer (nasal septum).
6. Tympanic ring.
7. Handle of malleus.
8. Synchondroses.
9. External occipital crest.
10. Occipital squama.
11. Base of mandible.
12. Zygomatic bone.
13. Zygomatic arch.
14. Gonial contour: head of mandible.
15. Basisphenoid.
16. Basiocciput.
17. Exocciput.
18. Foramen magnum.

E

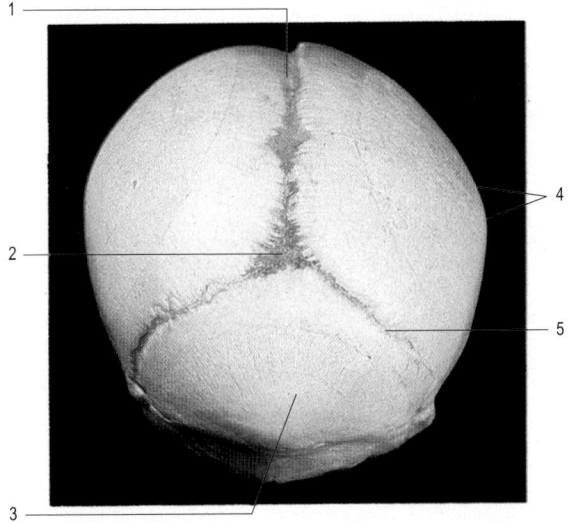

1. Sagittal suture.
2. Lambda, posterior fontanelle.
3. Squamous part of occipital bone.
4. Parietal bone and tuber.
5. Lambdoid suture.

Fig. 27.31 Skull of a newborn infant. **A,** Anterior aspect; **B,** lateral aspect; **C,** superior aspect; **D,** basal aspect; **E,** posterior occipital aspect. (Photographs by Kevin Fitzpatrick on behalf of GKT School of Medicine, London.)

485

of the orbits and nasal septum and by sutural growth, especially at the fontanelles and zygomaticomaxillary and pterygomaxillary sutures. In the first year, growth in width occurs at the symphysis menti and mid-palatal, internasal and frontal sutures; but such growth diminishes or even ceases when the symphysis menti and frontal suture close during the first few years, even though the midpalatal suture persists until mature years. Facial growth in this period continues to puberty and later, linked with the eruption of the permanent teeth. After sutural growth, near the end of the second year, expansion of the facial skeleton is by surface accretion on the face, alveolar processes and palate, and there is resorption in the walls of the maxillary sinuses, the upper surface of the hard palate and the labial aspect of the alveolar process. Co-ordinated growth and divergence of the pterygoid processes is due to deposition and resorption of bone on appropriate surfaces. Mandibular growth is described on page 482.

Obliteration of the calvarial sutures progresses with age, commencing between 30 and 40 years internally, and 10 years later on the exterior. Closure times vary greatly. Obliteration usually begins at the bregma, extending into the sagittal, coronal and lambdoid sutures, in that order. In old age the skull becomes thinner and lighter, but occasionally the reverse may occur. The most striking senile feature is diminution in size of the mandible and maxillae following the loss of teeth and absorption of alveolar bone. This reduces the vertical depth of the face and increases the mandibular angles.

Sutural bones

Additional ossificatory centres may occur in or near sutures, giving rise to isolated sutural bones (**Fig. 27.32**). Usually irregular in size and shape, and most frequent in the lambdoid suture, they sometimes occur at fontanelles, especially the posterior. They may represent a pre-interparietal element, a true interparietal, or some composite. An isolated bone at the lambda is sometimes dubbed the Inca bone or Goethe's ossicle. One or more pterion ossicles or epipteric bones may appear between the sphenoidal angle of the parietal and the greater wing of the sphenoid, varying much in size, but more or less symmetrical. Sutural bones usually have little morphological significance. However, they appear in great numbers in hydrocephalic skulls (**Figs 27.32, 16.12**), and they have therefore been linked with rapid cranial expansion: this is unproven. For a detailed analysis of these and other epigenetic variations in adult crania, consult Berry and Berry (1967) and (Berry 1975).

Craniosynostosis

Sutural growth makes an important contribution to growth of the skull, especially during the first few years of life. The reasons for premature fusion of sutures (synostosis) are varied, but many occur as a result of small brain size or failure of the development of dural bands between the sutures. Premature fusion may occur in one or more of the cranial sutures. When the sutures around the skull base are involved in premature fusion, severe limitation of facial bone growth will occur. Metabolic disorders such as rickets and familial hypophosphatasia can also result in synostosis. Raised intracranial pressure with or without hydrocephalus, visual deterioration and mental retardation may result. Scaphocephaly (sagittal craniosynostosis) is the commonest and leads to lengthening of the vault in an anteroposterior direction. Sagittal craniosynostosis occurs in conjunction with other sutures, e.g. Crouzon's syndrome. Coronal synostosis, either unilateral (plagiocephaly) or bilateral (brachycephaly/oxycephaly) is the next most frequently seen. Premature fusion of the coronal suture results in reduced anteroposterior development with marked supraorbital recession. When it is unilateral the face develops asymmetrically and is rotated away from the side with premature fusion. Metopic craniosynostosis (trigonocephaly) and pansynostosis (turricephaly, where both the coronal and sphenofrontal sutures are involved) are much less common.

Treatment of these premature sutural fusions is critical to prevent abnormalities of skull growth. It is usually carried out between 3–6 months of age. Early release of the synostosis is also indicated to relieve increased intracranial pressure. Treatment consists of release of the sutures involved and the prevention of refusion. This is usually achieved by covering the bone edges with silastic sheeting after the radical removal of bone from either side of the suture line. Simultaneous expansion and reshaping of the skull is often required, particularly if diagnosis has been delayed. It is usually necessary to advance the

A

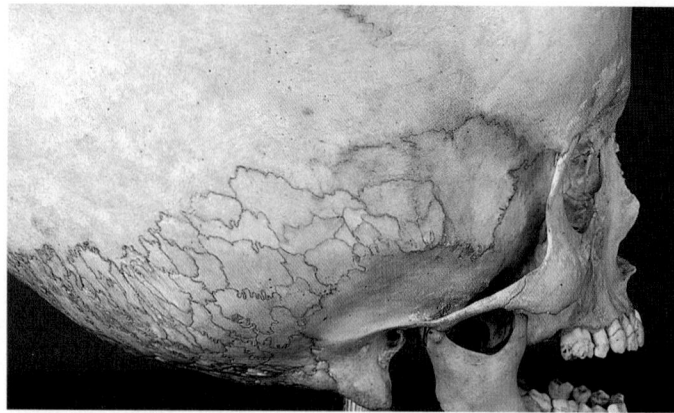

B

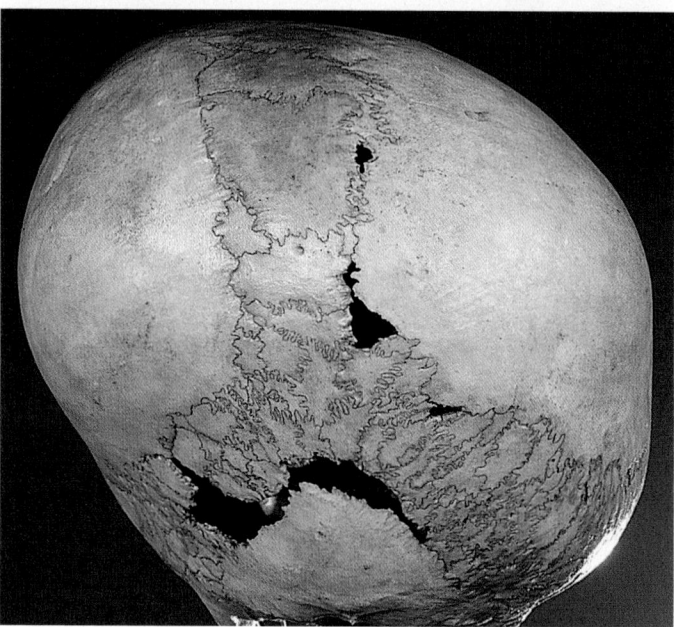

Fig. 27.32 Lateral (**A**) and posterior (**B**) views of the hydrocephalic skull of a 25-year old male showing numerous sutural bones. Courtesy of the Museum of the Royal College of Surgeon of England. (Photographer Mr J Carr).

supraorbital ridge and to straighten it if there is asymmetrical growth (as seen in plagiocephaly).

The craniofacial dysostosis syndromes such as Crouzon's, Apert's, Saethre–Chotzen, Pfeiffer's and Carpenter's, show a varying degree of calvarial synostoses, which are usually accompanied by a significant lack of growth in the mid-face. Early release of the calvarial synostoses does not result in normal facial growth, and a midfacial osteotomy at the Le Fort III level is usually required later in life. When significant orbital hypertelorism develops, a transcranial bipartitioning procedure is needed in order to bring the two orbits together.

Skull deformities can also be derived deliberately by affecting sutural growth using binding and other pressure, as has been practised in certain tribal regions of the world (**Fig. 27.33**).

CONGENITAL ANOMALIES AFFECTING THE SKULL

A large number of malformations and anomalies affect the bones and associated soft tissue structures of the skull. They result from a localized error of morphogenesis during embryological development. Many of these are recognized patterns of malformation which are presumed to have the same aetiology. They do not arise as the result of just one isolated error in morphogenesis, and are described as syndromes.

Hemifacial microsomia (Goldenhar syndrome)

The term hemifacial microsomia is used to describe patients with unilateral microtia, macrostomia and varying degrees of failure of

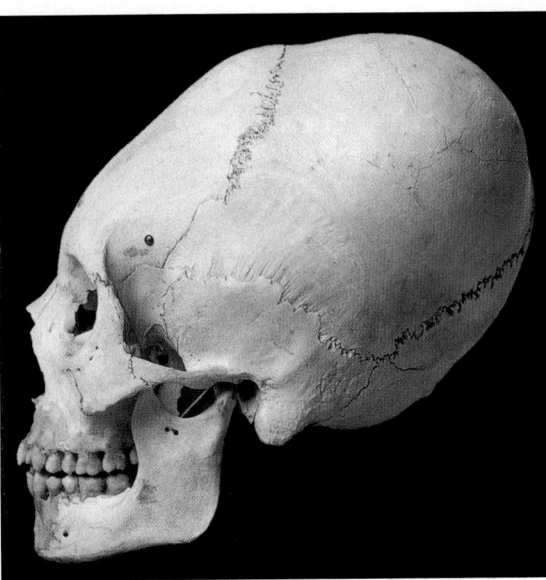

Fig. 27.33 Skull binding. Egyptian Copts. (Provided by John Langdon.)

formation of the mandibular ramus and condyle. Vertebral anomalies and epibulbar dermoids are common. Most cases are sporadic, but familial instances have been described.

The facies are strikingly asymmetric as a result of hypoplasia or displacement of the ear. The maxilla, temporal and zygomatic bones show varying degrees of hypoplasia on the affected side. The mandible similarly shows varying degrees of hypoplasia ranging from mild asymmetry to major failure of development of the ramus and condyle. The mastoid process also shows degrees of hypoplasia. Often there is frontal bossing. Ten per cent of cases are bilateral, but invariably one side is more severely affected.

There is concomitant hypoplasia of the main masticatory muscles on the affected side, and occasionally the muscles of facial expression are involved. In 10% of cases there is a lower motor neurone weakness of the facial nerve. Mental retardation is unusual. The ear deformities vary from complete aplasia to minor distortions of the pinna, which is displaced anteriorly and inferiorly. Absence of the external auditory meatus is common, as are middle ear deficiencies, which result in conduction deafness. Supernumerary eartags are present and occur anywhere along a line from the tragus to the angle of the mouth.

Epibulbar dermoids occur and are usually located at the limbus or lower outer quadrant. A coloboma of the upper lid is present in most cases. Unilateral microphthalmia or anophthalmia can occur and is associated with mental retardation. Vertebral anomalies are common and include occipitalization of the atlas, cuneiform vertebrae, and fusion of several adjacent vertebrae. A variety of cardiac anomalies have been described ranging from ventricular septal defects to Fallot's tetralogy. Pulmonary hypoplasia and renal anomalies have been recorded.

Mandibulofacial dysostosis (Treacher Collins syndrome)

Mandibulofacial dysostosis mainly involves structures derived from the first branchial arch, groove and pouch. It is inherited as an autosomal dominant trait with variable penetration. The facial appearance is characteristic. There are downward sloping palpebral fissures, depressed cheek prominences, deformed ears, mandibular hypoplasia and a large fishlike mouth. The hairline often shows a tongue-shaped extension toward the cheek.

Clinically the skull vault appears normal, but on imaging it is seen that the supraorbital ridges are poorly developed and despite normal sutural development there may be increased digital markings (copper beating) on the inner table. The zygomatic bones may be totally absent, or more frequently are grossly deficient in a symmetrical manner with failure of fusion of the zygomatic arches. The mastoid processes are not pneumatized and may be sclerotic. The paranasal sinuses are frequently abnormally small or even absent. The infraorbital rims are also poorly developed.

There may be various eye anomalies. Colobomas affecting the lateral third of the lower eyelid are present in 75% of cases. Microphthalmia may also be present. The ears are usually severely deformed, have a crumpled appearance and are often wrongly positioned. In a third of patients the external auditory meatus is absent and there may be ossicular defects resulting in conduction deafness. Additional ear tags and blind fistulae may be present anywhere between the tragus and the angle of the mouth. The nasofrontal angle is usually obliterated and the bridge of the nose elevated. The alar cartilages are hypoplastic and choanal atresia may be present. The mandible is almost always hypoplastic, the angle is obtuse and the ramus deficient. The coronoid and condylar processes may also be hypoplastic. A cleft palate is present in 30% of cases and there is a high arched palate. Mental retardation is common.

Distraction osteogenesis

The pioneering Russian orthopaedic surgeon Ilizaroff demonstrated that long bones could be lengthened by performing osteotomies in the axial plane and then slowly separating the two parts of the bone. If the distraction is performed slowly, bone morphogenetic proteins are released and new bone is formed between the sectioned bone ends. When the desired length has been achieved, the long bone is immobilized in its desired position. After a period of a few weeks the initial woven bone is replaced by normal mature bone and the resulting lengthened bone is stable and functional.

These techniques are now applied to the bones of the skull. Mandibular distraction is commonly used, particularly when there is asymmetry of the mandible as seen in hemifacial microsomia. By performing the osteotomies at the angles of the mandible, and using carefully adjusted distraction devices, the mandible can be lengthened in the vertical and anteroposterior planes. Distraction is usually performed at one millimetre per day, and the jaw can be lengthened indefinitely until the distraction is stopped and the callus matures and unites. Using complicated frames bolted onto the skull vault, distraction techniques have now been applied to the middle third of the facial skeleton. The technique is particularly useful for the management of the craniofacial syndromes such as Crouzon's, in which the facial bones which articulate with the sphenoid fail to develop normally. If the facial bones can be released at an early age and the mobilized bones distracted, the facial profile can develop normally.

SEXUAL AND GEOGRAPHIC VARIATION IN THE SKULL

MEASUREMENT OF SHAPE AND SIZE (Fig. 27.34)

Metrical studies are used to compare shapes and sizes of skulls. Frequently, these analyses are accomplished using internationally standard techniques of craniometry in which linear (chord) or surface (arc) distances were measured between a variety of defined cranial and mandibular landmarks (**Fig. 27.34**). For example, the calvarial part of the skull is measured (usually to the nearest millimetre) as follows:

A.	Maximal cranial length	Summit of glabella to furthest occipital point
B.	Maximal cranial breadth	Greatest breadth, at right angles to median plane
C.	Cranial height	From basion (median point on anterior rim of foramen magnum) to bregma

From these three dimensions, three indices are calculated: B/A, C/A and C/B and expressed as percentages. The most frequently used, the breadth/length ratio, is called the cranial index (cephalic index in the living), and has often been used to classify skull types because of its high degree of variability both within and between populations. By convention, skulls with a cranial or cephalic index (CI) below 75.0 were classified as dolichocranic or dolichocephalic; skulls with a CI between 75.0 and 79.9 were classified as mesocranic or mesocephalic; and skulls with a CI greater than 80.0 were classified as brachycranic or brachycephalic. Variations in the CI have little utility in distinguishing skulls from different geographic regions, and mostly reflect interactions between the width of the cranial base and the volume of the brain (Lieberman et al 2000).

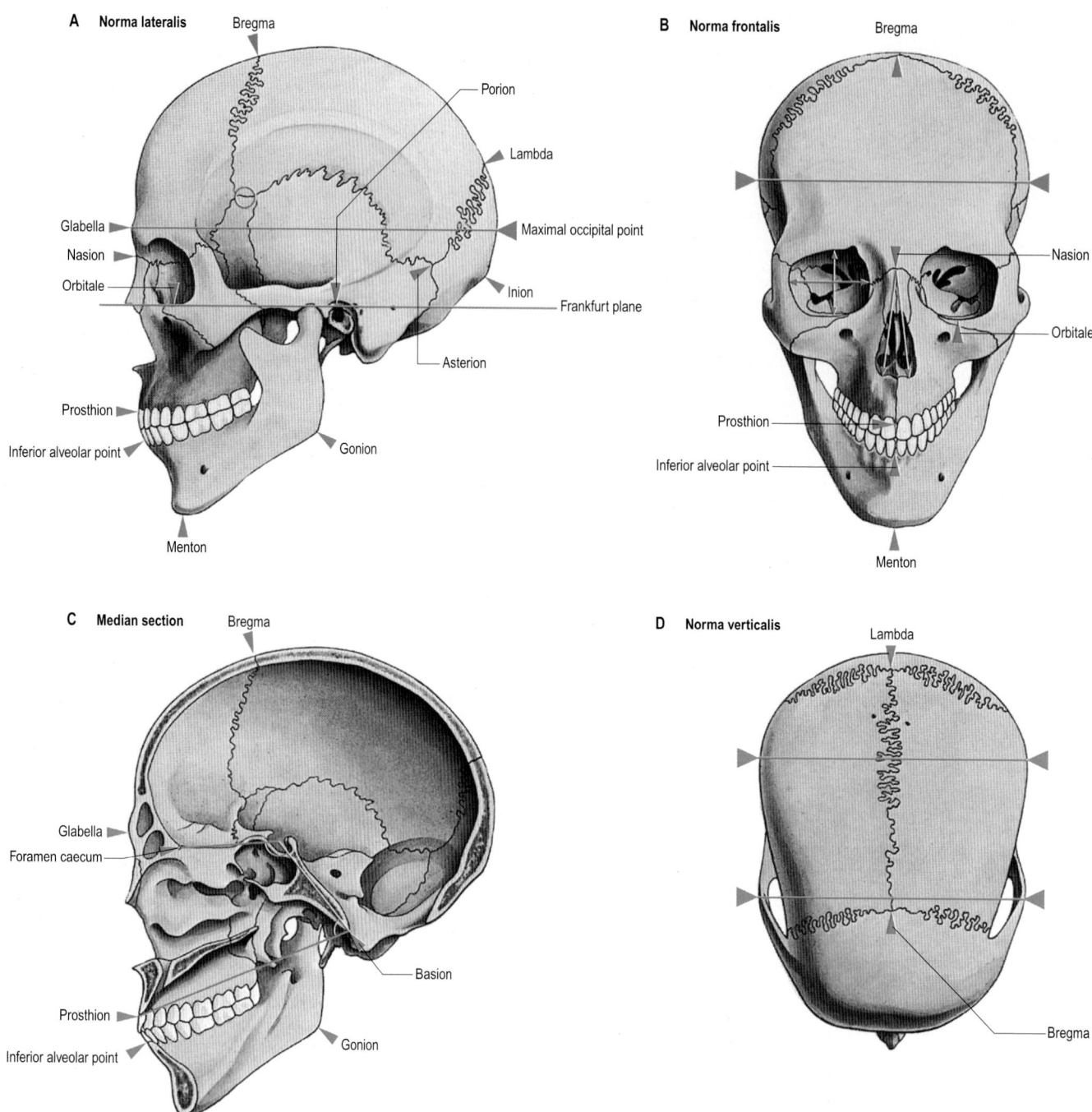

Fig. 27.34 The cranial points used, by international agreement, in making linear and certain angular measurements in anthropometry. In all four views (A–D) the skull is in the standard orientation, that is, with the Frankfurt plane as a horizontal.

Other indices in common use are:

(a) Total facial index = (nasion–gnathion height/bizygomatic breadth) × 100
The nasion is the point where the internasal suture meets the frontal bone. The gnathion is the midpoint of the lower mandibular border

(b) Upper facial index = (nasion–prosthion length/bizygomatic breadth) × 100
The prosthion is the midpoint of the maxillary alveolar rim, between the central incisors. The bizygomatic breadth is the greatest distance measured by trial between zygomatic arches on external aspects

(c) Nasal index   = (nasal breadth/nasal height) × 100
Breadth is the horizontal maximum across the nasal aperture, and height is from nasion to the mean between the two lowest points on the lower border of the aperture

(d) Orbital index   = (maximal orbital height/maximal orbital breadth) × 100

(e) Palatal index   = (maximal palatal breadth/maximal palatal length) × 100

(f) Gnathic index   = (basion–prosthion/basion–nasion) × 100

Similar measurements are frequently taken on mandibles between landmarks including the superoinferior height and anteroposterior thickness of the symphysis; the anteroposterior length of the mandibular body; the anteroposterior length and superoinferior height of the ramus; bigonial width, the bicondylar width; and so on. In addition, a variety of radiographic measurements using landmarks visible in radiographs make it possible to extend classic craniometry to measure certain angles directly, e.g. the gnathic angle (between the basion–nasion and basion–prosthion lines). The cranial base angle is of special interest and represents the orientation of the anterior cranial base relative to the posterior cranial base. The cranial base angle can be measured in many ways. The most common measurement, the angle between the chord from the sella to the foramen caecum relative to the chord between the sella and basion, has an average value in humans of about 135°, which it attains by flexion c.2 years after birth (Lieberman & McCarthy 1999). The cranial base angle is an important determinant of craniofacial form because it influences the position of the face relative to the neurocranium, the protrusion of the mandible relative to the maxilla and the shape of the pharynx.

Another important variable, cranial capacity which is correlated to brain volume can be assessed directly by filling the cavity with lead shot, millet seed or other particulate materials suitable for volumetric measurement when poured out again. Cranial capacity can also be measured using CT scans. In addition, several formulae have also been calculated to estimate cranial capacity from linear measurements of the length, breadth and height of the cranium (in millimetres). Examples are:

Males : 0.000337 (L−11) (B−11) (H−11) + 406.01 cc
Females : 0.000400 (L−11) (B−11) (H−11) + 206.60 cc

In these formulae, L and B are length and breadth, and H is the auricular height, measured to the vertex from the external acoustic meatus. Such methods involve some inaccuracy.

Variations in skull shape and form have most commonly been analysed using multivariate statistical methods using many measurements taken on large sets of individuals. Radiographic and three-dimensional imaging technology, especially computer tomography (CT) and magnetic resonance imaging (MRI), in combination with new methods of analysing shape from three-dimensional landmarks have revolutionized the ability to study the shapes of skulls by including information about the relative position between multiple landmarks in multivariate space. Several analytical techniques are most commonly used, including Euclidean distance matrix analysis (EDMA), which examines variations in size and shape (hence form, which is shape corrected by size) by comparing matrices of all the interlandmark distances between individuals or sets of individuals (Lele & Richtsmeier 1993). Another set of techniques, termed geometric morphometrics, analyses the relative spatial arrangements of landmarks between individuals or sets of individuals, allowing the full three-dimensionality of form differences to be modelled, compared and visualized.

SEXUAL VARIATION

Until puberty there is little sexual difference in skulls. Adult males tend to be larger than females in a number of features due to a combination of faster rates of growth during puberty and longer period of growth. However, ranges of variation between sexes overlap considerably. In general, the adult male cranium has c.11% larger cranial capacity than females, mostly reflecting larger male body mass. In terms of shape differences, the male cranium tends to have thicker bones in the neurocranial vault; and more marked muscle origins and insertions, e.g. the temporal and nuchal lines; the frontal sinuses are larger, as are the glabella and the superciliary arches; the external occipital protuberance and the mastoid processes are more prominent; the superior margin of the orbits tends to be squarer; and the mandibular and maxillary arches are larger, in part due to larger tooth size. In addition, the male mandible tends to have larger coronoid processes; larger, more flared, gonial regions; longer rami; and a more pronounced mental eminence. Because variation is greater within than between sexes, diagnosis of sex is difficult or impossible for many crania, and is most accurately assessed using multivariate statistical techniques such as discriminant function analysis.

GEOGRAPHIC VARIATION

Several major studies have assessed variation in cranial shape among and between populations (Howells 1973; Lahr 1996). As with the genotype, variation in human cranial shape is far greater within than between populations (Relethford 1994). Nonetheless some tendencies are evident when comparing average cranial shapes from populations of different geographic origin. Summarizing these studies, there is more variation in Africa than elsewhere, with marked differences between Bushmen, Bantu, and other groups. On average, African crania are broader, with taller upper faces, more inferiorly positioned nasal regions, and more prognathic mandibular and maxillary arches than crania from other parts of the globe. European skulls tend to be narrow, with concomitantly narrow faces, retracted zygomatic arches, tall nasal regions, and prominent midfaces. Europeans and American Indians share many cranial similarities. Asian skulls are typically wide (brachycephalic), with wide faces, a high degree of facial flatness, and flat supranasal regions. Australian aborigines are often characterized by narrow skulls (dolichocephaly), and large, low projecting faces with prominent subnasal regions.

Attempts to differentiate crania by region of geographic origin using multivariate methods such as discriminant function analysis can have accuracies of over 90%.

FRACTURES OF THE FACIAL SKELETON

Fractures affecting the jaw bones are common. They result from road traffic accidents, sports injuries, accidents at work and increasingly as a result of interpersonal violence. Many of these injuries are sustained by those intoxicated with alcohol or are as a result of an assailant who is drunk.

Given that the majority of people are right-handed, most jaw fractures resulting from assault affect either the left cheek bone (zygomaticomaxillary complex) or the left angle of the mandible. Because of the shape and structure of the jaw bones, skull fractures tend to adopt well-recognized patterns, which are determined by the concentration of stresses and lines of weakness in the bones affected.

Although in severe injuries the fractures are often complex, it is convenient to describe them as arising in the upper, middle and lower thirds of the face. Often a subject will have sustained fractures involving more than one of these areas.

UPPER THIRD OF FACE (NASOETHMOIDAL COMPLEX)

Fractures in the upper third of the face are almost invariably comminuted and involve many bones. The skeletal foundation of the nasoethmoidal complex consists of a strong triangular-shaped frame. However, all these structures are fragile and any force sufficient to fracture the frame results in severe comminution and displacement. A severe impact delivered to the midface, particularly over the bridge of the nose, may result in these structures being driven backwards between the orbits. This may result in traumatic hypertelorism, producing an increase in distance between the pupils. Associated displacement of the medial canthal ligaments results in traumatic telecanthus. Comminution of the cribriform plates of the ethmoid results in dural tears and cerebrospinal rhinorrhoea. Often these fractures are combined with more extensive fractures of the frontal bone. Such fractures involve the orbital roofs and, if displaced significantly, will in turn displace the globe of the eye. Fractures that involve both the inner and outer walls of the frontal sinus carry a risk of both early and delayed intracranial infection, and often it is necessary to obliterate the frontal sinuses in order to prevent this complication.

MIDDLE THIRD OF THE FACE

The middle third of the face is defined as that area bounded above by a transverse line connecting the two zygomaticofrontal sutures, passing through the frontomaxillary and frontonasal sutures, and limited below by the occlusal plane of the maxillary teeth. Posteriorly the region is limited by the sphenoethmoidal junction, but it includes the free margins of the pterygoid plates inferiorly. Fractures of the middle third of the facial skeleton may involve the two maxillae, the two palatine bones, the two zygomatic bones, the zygomatic processes of the temporal bones, the two nasal bones, the vomer, the ethmoid bone together with its nasal conchae and the body and greater and lesser wings of the sphenoid bone. They are divided into those involving the central block and those involving the lateral middle thirds.

Central middle third of the face

The majority of the skeleton of the central middle third is composed of wafer thin sheets of cortical bone with stronger reinforcements, i.e. the palate and alveolar process; the lateral rim of the piriform aperture extending upwards (via the canine fossa) to the medial orbital rim, and finally to the glabella; the zygomatic buttress and its connections to the inferior and lateral orbital margins and the zygomatic arch; the orbital rims and the pterygoid plates. The strength lies in the facial surface of the skeleton which, although thin in most areas, is cross-braced. The design is ideally suited to transmit occlusal forces vertically to the skull base.

The fracture lines of the central middle third are customarily described with respect to the Le Fort lines. Although comminuted fractures are common in this region, the various fracture lines do follow the Le Fort lines.

Le Fort I fractures (Guerin's fracture) – Le Fort I fractures consist of a horizontal fracture line above the level of the floor of the nose involving the lower third of the nasal septum. The mobile segment consists of the palate, the alveolar process and the lower thirds of the pterygoid plates.

Le Fort II fractures (pyramidal fracture) – Le Fort II fractures are pyramidal fractures involving the maxillary bones. From the nasal bridge, the fracture enters the medial wall of the orbit to involve the lacrimal bone and then crosses the inferior orbital rim, usually at the junction of the medial and lateral two-thirds, and often involves the infraorbital foramen. The fracture line then runs beneath the zygomaticomaxillary suture, traversing the lateral wall of the maxillary sinus to extend posteriorly horizontally across the pterygoid plates. The zygomatic bones and arches remain attached to the skull base.

Le Fort III fractures – Le Fort III fractures run parallel with the base of the skull, separating the entire mid-facial skeleton from the cranial base. The fracture extends through the nasal base and continues posteriorly across the ethmoid bone. The fracture then crosses the lesser wing of the sphenoid and, on occasion, involves the optic foramen. Usually, however, it slopes down medially passing below the optic foramen to reach the pterygomaxillary fissure and pterygopalatine fossa. From the base of the inferior orbital fissure the fracture runs laterally and upwards, separating the greater wing of the sphenoid from the zygomatic bone, to reach the frontozygomatic suture. It also extends downwards and backwards across the pterygopalatine fossa to involve the root of the pterygoid plates. The zygomatic arch is usually fractured at the zygomaticotemporal suture.

Frequently these fractures do not occur as bilateral symmetrical fractures but occur in various combinations, e.g. both together, on the same side, and involving both sides. Typically these fractures arise from force applied anteriorly over a wide area. Such injuries are seen in road traffic accidents where, e.g. a driver or passenger is thrown forwards on to the steering wheel or dashboard. The direction of the applied force determines the displacement of these fractures. With the possible exception of the relatively weak lateral pterygoids, muscle pull plays a relatively small part. As the fractures are generally displaced backwards, because of the angulation of the strong skull base, there is also a downward component, which results clinically in a lengthening of the face and a dished-in appearance. There may be airway obstruction if this downwards and backwards displacement is severe.

Lateral middle third of the face

Fractures of the lateral middle third involve the zygomaticomaxillary complex. The zygomatic bone forms the prominence of the cheek and so is subject to direct trauma to the side of the face. As the most common cause of a zygomatic fracture is a blow from a fist, depressed fractures of the zygomaticomaxillary complex are a common injury. There is separation at both the zygomaticofrontal and zygomaticotemporal sutures. The major damage is at the lateral wall of the maxilla, which is usually comminuted. Displacement of the zygomatic bone into the lateral wall of the maxilla leads to damage to the infraorbital nerve. Isolated fractures of the zygomatic arch are relatively unusual.

Orbital fractures – The orbit is invariably involved in depressed fractures of the zygomatic bone and in Le Fort II and III fractures. The orbit is also involved in fractures of the frontal bone and in extensive nasal complex injuries. A fracture of the orbital floor without associated rim involvement is known as a 'blow-out' fracture. Fortunately the optic foramen which is situated within the lesser wing of the sphenoid bone is surrounded by dense bone and is only rarely involved in fractures. Direct injury to the optic nerve is therefore unusual.

LOWER THIRD OF FACE (MANDIBLE)

The bone of the lower third of the face is the mandible, which is essentially a tubular bone bent into a blunt V-shape. This basic configuration is modified by sites of muscle attachments, notably masseter and medial pterygoid around the angle, and temporalis around the coronoid process. The presence of teeth, particularly those with long roots such as the canines, or unerupted teeth, produces lines of weakness in the mandible. When the teeth are lost, or fail to develop, the subsequent progressive resorption of the alveolar bone means that the mandible reverts to its underlying tubular structure. Like all tubular bones, the strength of the mandible resides in a dense cortical plate, thickened anteriorly and at the lower border of the mandible. It follows that the mandible is strongest anteriorly in the midline and is progressively weaker posteriorly towards the condylar processes. Again, like all tubular bones, the mandible has great resistance to compressive forces, but fractures at sites of tensile strain. The mandible is liable to particular patterns of distribution of tensile strain when forces are applied to it. Anterior forces applied to the mental symphysis, or over the body of the mandible, lead to strain at the condylar necks and also along the lingual cortical plates on the contralateral side in the molar region. In order of frequency, fractures occur most commonly at the neck of the condyle, the angle, the parasymphyseal region and the body of the mandible. Most often the mandible fractures occur at two of these sites: isolated fractures are relatively unusual.

Condylar process – The condyle is protected from direct injury by the zygomatic arches. Fractures occur usually by the transmission of force following a blow to the front of the mandible or to the contralateral body. Except in children most condylar fractures are not intracapsular, and occur in the neck. They typically run obliquely downwards and backwards from the mandibular notch. The condyle is usually displaced anteromedially (because of the attachment of lateral pterygoid to the temporomandibular joint disc, capsule and anterior border of the neck of the condyle).

Angle of the mandible – The majority of fractures at the angle of the mandible run vertically downwards and backwards from the alveolar bone to the angle. When a third molar tooth is present the fracture line will pass through its socket. The presence of the tooth results in a line of weakness. A fracture at the angle prevents the powerful elevator muscles (masseter, medial pterygoid and temporalis) from having any direct effect on the tooth-bearing part of the jaw. Thus, the posterior fragment is typically displaced upwards, forwards and inwards as a result of the unopposed pull of these powerful muscles.

Ramus and coronoid process – Fractures at the ramus exhibit very little displacement due to the splinting activity of medial pterygoid medially and masseter laterally. These two bulky muscles are widely attached to the ramus and their attachments extend across the fracture lines. Similarly the coronoid process is rarely significantly displaced because it is splinted by the tendinous insertion of temporalis.

Body of the mandible – Most fractures of the body of the mandible occur as the result of direct trauma and tend to be concentrated in the first molar or canine region. The further forward the site of the fracture, the more the upward displacement of the elevators is counter-acted by the downward pull of geniohyoid and the anterior belly of digastric. When teeth are present displacement is limited by the dental occlusion, since further displacement is resisted by the lower and upper teeth. Displacement may be considerable in the edentulous patient.

CRANIAL BASE

The cranial base – composed of the frontal, ethmoid, sphenoid and occipital bones – is a relatively solid platform inclined at an angle of 45° to the maxillary occlusal plane. Fractures of the cranial base are not readily visible on normal radiographs. They result in bleeding in the floor of the middle cranial fossa. This often presents as bruising over the mastoid process and is known as Battle's sign. Such fractures also result in escape of cerebrospinal fluid which may be seen leaking from a ruptured tympanic membrane. Alternatively, if this membrane remains intact it will be seen as blue and bulging, possibly with a transmitted pulsation.

SKELETAL ACCESS SURGERY

The craniofacial skeleton has an excellent blood supply, and so can be dismantled as a series of osteoplastic flaps. The surgical disarticulation of the craniofacial skeleton has been used to gain access to otherwise inaccessible sites in order to allow the surgeon to attend to pathology in the skull base, cervical spine and anterior and posterior cranial fossae. The aim is to provide increased and more direct exposure of both the pathology and the adjacent vital structures without the need to resect uninvolved structures. The craniofacial skeleton can be divided into a series of modular osteotomies, which permit both independent and conjoined mobilization.

The zygomatic and nasal bones and the maxilla may be exposed and mobilized, pedicled on the overlying soft tissues either unilaterally or bilaterally. These approaches improve access to the nasal cavity, maxillary, ethmoid and sphenoid sinuses, the soft palate and nasopharynx, and the infratemporal fossa and pharyngeal space. The exposures may be extended to gain access to the anterior and middle cranial fossae, cavernous sinus, clivus, craniocervical junction and upper cervical vertebrae.

A variety of different access osteotomies have been described and found to be useful in specific clinical situations. Most of the osteotomies described follow the conventional patterns of facial fractures described above. The entire hemimaxilla and zygoma can be mobilized, and pedicled on the soft tissues of the face by making bone cuts that follow the lines of a Le Fort II fracture on one side. The osteotomy is completed by dividing the upper alveolus and palate just to the side of the nasal septum and perpendicular plate of the vomer. The maxilla may be mobilized at the Le Fort I level and downfractured, pedicled on the palatoglossal muscles and soft tissue attachments. This gives good access to the nasopharynx, clivus and upper cervical spine, particularly if the palate is divided in the midline.

Lateral zygomatic osteotomies may be performed to gain access to the orbital apex and infratemporal fossa. The surgical approach is from behind using a hemi- or bicoronal flap. The zygomatic complex is mobilized inferiorly pedicled on masseter. When combined with a mandibular ramus osteotomy, access is gained to the retromaxillary area and pterygoid space as well as to the infratemporal fossa. In combination with a frontotemporal craniotomy, the zygomatic osteotomy has been used for access to the middle cranial fossa, cavernous sinus, apex of the petrous temporal bone and the interpeduncular cistern.

Dividing the lower lip in the midline, and dividing the mandible either in the midline or just in front of the mental foramen, allows the hemimandible to be swung laterally. The technique is used to give improved access to the floor of the mouth, the base of the tongue, tonsillar fossa, soft palate, oropharynx, posterior pharyngeal wall, supraglottic larynx and pterygomandibular region. By extending the dissection laterally access is gained to the pterygoid space, infratemporal fossa and parapharyngeal space. By dissecting more medially access is gained to the nasopharynx, lower part of the clivus and all seven of the cervical vertebrae. A modification of the mandibular swing procedure increases access up to the skull base, by combining the classic mandibular swing with a horizontal osteotomy of the mandibular ramus above the level of the lingula.

REFERENCES

Berkovitz BKB, Moxham BJ 1989 Colour atlas of the skull. London: Mosby-Wolfe

Berkovitz BKB, Moxham BJ 1994 Color atlas of the skull. London: Mosby-Wolfe

Berry AC 1975 Factors affecting the incidence of non-metrical skeletal variants. J Anat 120: 519–35.

Berry AC, Berry RJ 1967 Epigenetic variation in the human cranium. J Anat 101: 361–80.

Howells WW 1973 Cranial Variation in Man. Cambridge MA: Papers of the Peabody Museum of Archaeology and Ethnography, vol 67.

Lahr MM 1996 The Evolution of Modern Human Diversity: A Study of Cranial Variation. Cambridge: Cambridge University Press.

Lele S, Richtsmeier JT 1991 Euclidean distance matrix analysis: a coordinate-free approach for comparing biological shapes using landmark data. Am J Phys Anthropol 86: 415–27.

Lieberman DE, McCarthy RC 1999 The ontogeny of cranial base angulation in humans and chimpanzees and its implications for reconstructing pharyngeal dimensions. J Hum Evol 36:487–517.

Lieberman DE, Pearson OM, Mowbray KM 2000 Basicranial influence on overall cranial shape. J Hum Evol 38(2): 291–315.

Moos KF, Baker AW 1998 Craniofacial surgery. Assessment and techniques. In: Langdon JD, Patel MF (eds) Operative Maxillofacial Surgery. London: Chapman & Hall, 407–436.
A detailed description of the various craniosynostoses.

Relethford JH. 1994 Craniometric variation among modern human populations. Am J Phys Anthropol 95(1): 53–62.

Sperber GH 2001 Craniofacial Development, 4th edn. Edinburgh: Churchill Livingstone.

Vidarsdottir US, O'Higgins P, Stringer C 2002 A geometric morphometric study of regional differences in the ontogeny of the modern human facial skeleton. J Anat 201: 211–29.

Williams JL 1994 Rowe and Williams' Maxillofacial Injuries. Edinburgh: Churchill Livingstone.

Development of the skull

BASAL REGIONS OF THE SKULL

PATTERNING OF THE BASAL REGION OF THE SKULL

The skull base forms entirely by endochondral ossification. The pattern of the initial chondrogenic anlagen is closely related to that of the brain and olfactory epithelium and may involve an epithelial-mesenchymal interaction between these structures, which transiently express type II collagen, and the adjacentskeletogenic mesenchyme (Thorogood, 1988). This intimate relationship between brain and skull during development means that evolutionary changes in the brain and skull are co-ordinated. After neural expression of type II collagen has ceased, chondrogenesis is initiated in the mesenchyme. The skeletogenic mesenchyme of the skull base is of neural crest origin rostral to the tip of the notochord and of mesodermal origin more caudally, i.e. in the notochordal region.

CARTILAGINOUS NEUROCRANIUM

Differentiation of the endochondral component of the skull is initiated in several centres: in the prechordal region, rostral to the notochord; in the parachordal region, from the caudal end of the rhombencephalon to the tip of the notochord (caudal to the hypophysis); and in sense capsules, around the olfactory pits and otocyst. In mammals, a complete optic cartilaginous capsule does not differentiate, but a partial capsule is represented by the orbital wing of the sphenoid. The initial sites of chondrogenesis fuse to form a continuous cartilaginous framework prior to endochondral ossification Cranial chondrification begins in the second month. Cartilaginous foci appear in the occipital plate, one on each side of the notochord (parachordal cartilages), and fuse at the end of the seventh week to surround the notochord. The otic capsules, presphenoid, bases of the greater and lesser wings of the sphenoid, and the nasal capsules, become chondrified in sequence (**Figs 26.6, 28.1**).

Prechordal region

The rostral neural crest mesenchyme on a level with, and in front of, the hypophysis develops two pairs of centres of chondrogenic differentiation. The front pair form the trabeculae cranii which fuse to form the trabecular cartilage. The other pair form the polar hypophyseal cartilages on each side of the craniopharyngeal duct (remnant of Rathke's pouch) which leads to the hypophysis. They unite at first behind, then in front, to enclose the craniopharyngeal canal which contains the hypophyseal diverticulum. The canal is usually obliterated by the third month. The hypophyseal cartilage derives from both paraxial mesenchyme and neural crest. The neural crest forms the more rostral portion of the sella turcica, whereas the paraxial mesenchyme contributes to the caudal part, and forms each side of the rostral end of the notochord (Couly et al 1993).

Two chondrogenic centres for the sphenoid appear lateral to the trabecular cartilage. The orbitosphenoid forms part of the back of the orbit and lesser wing of the sphenoid. Medial processes extend around the optic nerve and fuse with the trabecular cartilage to form the optic canal. The alisphenoid is separated from the orbitosphenoid by the oculomotor, trochlear and abducens cranial nerves and by the first and second divisions of the trigeminal nerve. Posteriorly the alisphenoid is separated from the otic capsule by the mandibular division of the trigeminal nerve and the internal carotid artery. The mandibular nerve becomes surrounded by cartilage to form the foramen ovale. A large portion of the alisphenoid forms the greater wing of the sphenoid by membranous ossification.

Parachordal region

Immediately caudal to the hypophysis, the unsegmented paraxial mesenchyme gives rise to a sclerotomal component. This condenses to form an unpaired, plate-like parachordal cartilage which lies at first between the notochord and brain stem. The region of fusion of the hypophyseal and parachordal cartilages corresponds to the spheno-occipital synchondrosis, which is a site of growth until up to 20 years of age. More caudally, the segmented portion of paraxial mesenchyme gives rise to four occipital somites. Although the most rostral is rudimentary and does not form a clear sclerotome, the next three occipital somites produce sclerotomes which fuse rostrally with the parachordal cartilage and caudally with each other to form the clivus. The hypoglossal canal forms between the lower occipital somites. In the region of the foramen magnum the occipital sclerotomes extend dorsally to enclose the neural tube like the neural arch of a vertebra.

Sense capsules

Each otic vesicle is surrounded by skeletogenic mesenchyme which becomes chondrified to form the otic capsule (Chapter 40). Each capsule lies lateral to the parachordal cartilage and fuses with its lateral margin, except caudally, where fusion is incomplete at the site of the jugular foramen. The capsule is pierced medially by the internal auditory meatus.

A cartilaginous nasal capsule develops within the frontonasal mesenchyme around each olfactory pit (Chapter 34). These capsules unite with each other and with the trabecular cartilage. The whole nasal capsule is well-developed by the end of the third month, and consists of a common median septal part – sometimes initially termed the interorbitonasal septum – and two lateral regions. The free caudal borders of the lateral regions incurve to form the interior nasal conchae: these ossify during the fifth month and become separate elements. Posteriorly, each lateral part of the nasal capsule becomes ossified as the ethmoidal labyrinth. This bears ridges on its medial surface which will become the middle and superior conchae. Part of the rest of the capsule remains cartilaginous as the septal and alar cartilages of the nose, and part is replaced by the mesenchymatous vomer and nasal bones.

OSSIFICATION OF THE BASE OF THE SKULL

Ossification starts before the chondrocranium has fully developed, and bone replaces cartilage until little of the chondrocranium remains. However, at birth unossified chondrocranium persists in the alae, lateral nasal cartilage and septum of the nose; the spheno-ethmoidal junction; the spheno-occipital and sphenopetrous junctions; the apex of the petrous bone (foramen lacerum), and also between ossifying elements of the sphenoid bone and between elements of the occipital bone. Most of these regions function as growth cartilages and are termed synchondroses. Small areas of unossified cartilage remain in the adult skull.

VAULT OR UPPER REGIONS OF THE SKULL

The vault of the neurocranium is formed entirely by intramembranous ossification and its elements are frequently described as dermal bones. They are the frontal and parietal bones, the squamous part of the temporal bones and the upper part (interparietal) of the occipital bone. The frontal and squamous temporal bones are of neural crest origin

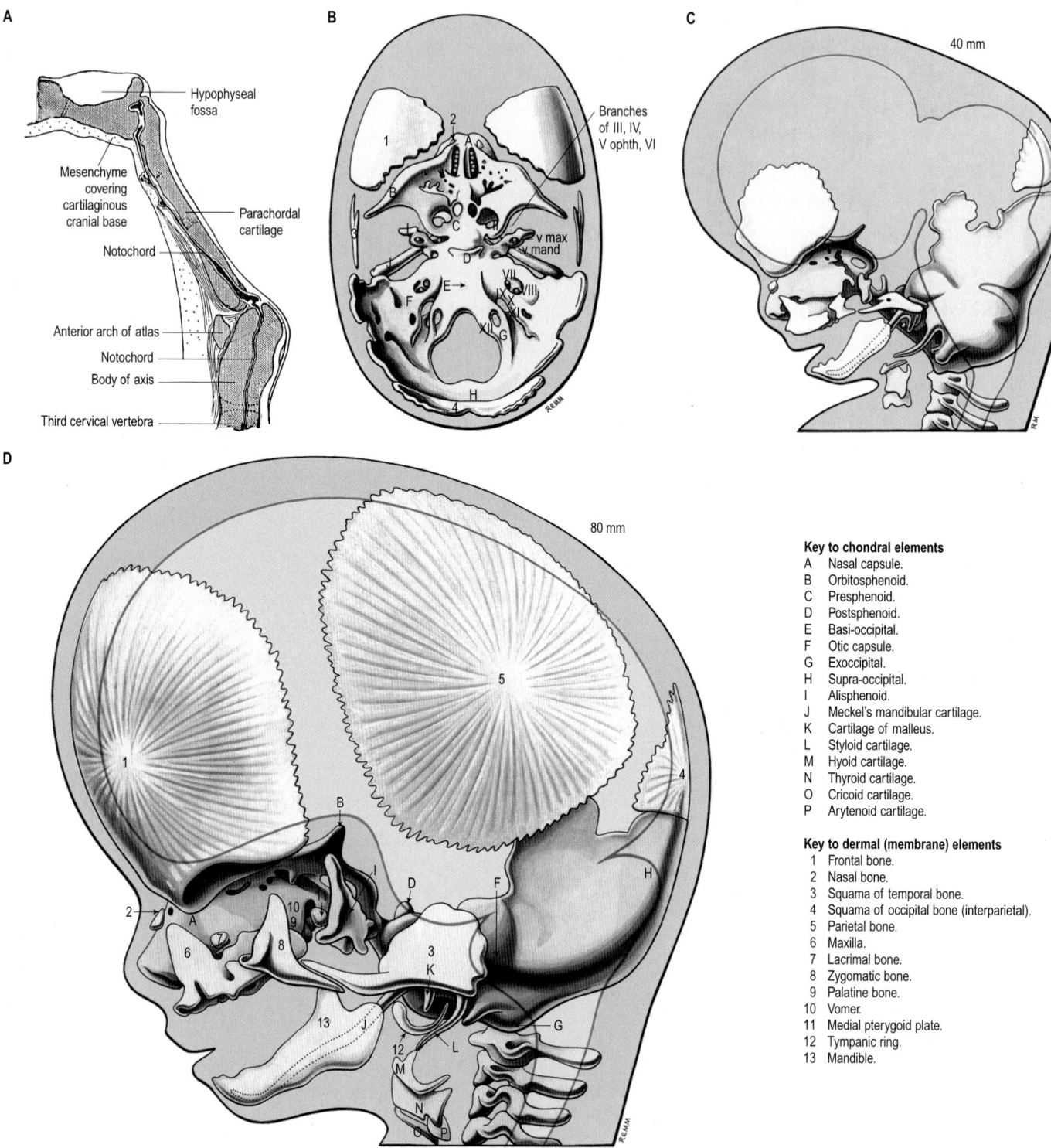

Key to chondral elements

A   Nasal capsule.
B   Orbitosphenoid.
C   Presphenoid.
D   Postsphenoid.
E   Basi-occipital.
F   Otic capsule.
G   Exoccipital.
H   Supra-occipital.
I   Alisphenoid.
J   Meckel's mandibular cartilage.
K   Cartilage of malleus.
L   Styloid cartilage.
M   Hyoid cartilage.
N   Thyroid cartilage.
O   Cricoid cartilage.
P   Arytenoid cartilage.

Key to dermal (membrane) elements

1   Frontal bone.
2   Nasal bone.
3   Squama of temporal bone.
4   Squama of occipital bone (interparietal).
5   Parietal bone.
6   Maxilla.
7   Lacrimal bone.
8   Zygomatic bone.
9   Palatine bone.
10   Vomer.
11   Medial pterygoid plate.
12   Tympanic ring.
13   Mandible.

Fig. 28.1 Representative stages in the development of the cranium. In all the diagrams the chondrocranium and cartilaginous stages of vertebrae are shown in blue, except where ossification is occurring and here the colour is green. The desmocranium, consisting of elements ossifying directly in mesenchyme, is shown in yellow. Cranial nerves are indicated by the appropriate Roman numeral. **A**, Sagittal section through the cranial end of the developing axial skeleton in an early human embryo of c.10 mm, showing the extent of the notochord. **B**, Superior aspect of cranium of human embryo at 40 mm. **C**, Lateral aspect of B. **D**, Lateral aspect of cranium of human embryo at 80 mm.

and the parietals are of mesodermal origin; the interparietal is mixed (Jiang et al., 2002). The coronal suture thus forms at the neural crest-mesoderm interface, as does the sagittal suture, due to a small tongue of neural crest tissue lying between the two developing bones. These tissue interfaces may be significant for initiating the signaling system that governs growth of the skull vault. The bones of the vault of the skull first appear at about day 30. They consist of curved plates of mesenchyme at the sides of the skull which gradually extend towards each other, and towards the cartilaginous base of the skull (**Fig. 28.1**).

The dermal bones are formed by the initiation of a wave of osteo-differentiation which extends radially from ossification centres within the desmocranial (skeletogenic) mesenchyme. When the paired bones meet in the midline, metopic and sagittal suture formation is induced. In contrast, the coronal suture, between the frontal and parietal bones, is present from the onset of ossification. Once sutures have been established and the fibrous desmocranium has been replaced by mineralized bone, growth continues within the sutural growth centres until growth of the brain is complete.

There is a close association between the developing meninges, particularly the dura mater, and the calvarial bones. Transplants of sutures in which the fetal dura mater is left intact result in a continuous fibrous suture between developing vault bones, whereas in transplants in which the fetal dura mater is removed, bony fusion occurs. This interaction of underlying dura mater with the developing calvarial bones has been demonstrated experimentally in the rabbit, showing that the dura not only promotes the position and maintenance of sutures, but also that dura can re-pattern both the appearance and position of the bones and sutures of the cranial vault after removal of the calvaria in the neonate (Opperman et al 1993). At the site of a developing suture the osteogenic fronts of two adjacent bones meet and overlap. Initially there is a highly cellular suture blastema between the bones which later becomes more dense and acellular. In the mature suture there is a narrow overlap of compact bone which contains a dense, narrow band of cells continuous with the periosteum.

POSTNATAL GROWTH OF THE SKULL

The brain, skull, eyes and ears all develop earlier than other parts of the body. After birth, the skull thickens with age and continues ossification towards the sutures. The face is relatively underdeveloped at birth and undergoes profound changes throughout childhood and at the adolescent spurt, in response to the eruption of the deciduous and permanent teeth, the formation of the sinuses, and the elongation of the maxilla and mandible (**Fig. 34.9**).

REFERENCES

Couly GF, Coltey PM, Le Douarin NM 1993 The triple origin of the skull in higher vertebrates: a study in quail–chick chimeras. Development 117: 409–29.

Jiang,X, Iseki S, Maxson RE, Sucov HM, Morriss-Kay GM 2002. Tissue origins and interactions in the mammalian skull vault. Developmental Biology 241, 106–116.

Opperman LA, Sweeney TM, Redmon J, Persing JA, Ogle RC 1993 Tissue interactions with underlying dura mater inhibit osseous obliteration of developing cranial sutures. Dev Dyn 198: 312–22.

Thorogood P 1988 The developmental specification of the vertebrate skull. Development 103 (suppl): 141–53.

Face and scalp

SKIN

The scalp and buccolabial tissues are described here. The structure of the eyelids is described on page 681.

SCALP

The scalp extends from the top of the forehead in front to the superior nuchal line behind. Laterally it projects down to the zygomatic arch and external acoustic meatus. It consists of five layers: skin, subcutaneous tissue, occipitofrontalis (epicranius) and its aponeurosis, subaponeurotic areolar tissue and pericranium (**Fig. 29.1**).

The skin of the scalp contains the hair and associated glands. There are many sebaceous glands, and the scalp is the commonest site for sebaceous cysts. The dense subcutaneous connective tissue has the richest cutaneous blood supply in the body. The third layer contains occipitofrontalis whose anterior and posterior muscular components are connected by a tough, fibrous, epicranial aponeurosis, and consequently this layer is called the aponeurotic layer (galea aponeurotica). Beneath the aponeurotic layer is a layer of loose connective tissue over which the upper three layers of the scalp can easily slide. The deepest layer is the periosteum of the skull. It is very easy to raise a scalp flap within the plane between the galea and the pericranium without compromising the blood or nerve supply of the scalp, because all of these structures lie in the superficial fascia. Scalp flaps are used in craniofacial surgery – e.g. for the correction of congenital deformity, for the release of craniosynostoses and for the treatment of craniofacial fractures – and also for repairing scalp defects following the excision of skin tumours. An anteriorly based scalp flap gives excellent access to the frontal bone and upper facial skeleton including the orbits and the infratemporal fossa and temporomandibular joint. Similar flaps are seen in traumatic scalp avulsions, which occur when the hair is trapped in moving machinery, and are also used electively in surgery.

The arterial blood supply to the scalp is particularly rich, and there are free anastomoses between branches of the occipital and superficial temporal vessels. Scalp lacerations continue to bleed profusely because the elastic fibres of the underlying galea aponeurotica prevent initial vessel retraction: these wounds may be associated with significant blood loss which can result in clinical shock. When suturing scalp lacerations it is essential to control all the bleeding points before repairing the scalp itself. Usually it is necessary to tie off any larger arterioles and use bipolar diathermy to control smaller arterioles and veins. Failure to control the bleeding as a separate step can result in significant haematomas, often subgaleal, leading to breakdown of the original wound and sometimes necessitating surgical drainage. Repair of scalp lacerations usually requires full thickness tension sutures because the galea aponeurotica will otherwise gape as the occipital and frontal muscle bellies contract. However, a wound that does not involve epicranius or its aponeurosis does not gape.

Eyebrows

The eyebrows are two arched eminences of skin which surmount the orbits. Numerous short, thick hairs are set obliquely in them. Fibres of orbicularis oculi, corrugator and the frontal part of occipitofrontalis are inserted into the dermis of the eyebrows.

BUCCOLABIAL TISSUE

Cheeks

The cheeks are continuous in front with the lips. The external junction is indicated by the nasolabial groove (sulcus) (see **Fig. 29.6**), and further laterally by the nasolabial fold, which descends from the side of the nose to the angle of the mouth. The cheek is covered on the outer surface by skin and on the inner surface by mucosa. Each cheek contains the buccinator muscle, and a variable, but usually considerable, amount of adipose tissue often encapsulated to form a biconcave mass, the buccal fat pad (of Bichat), which is particularly evident in infants. Indeed, this fat was originally named the suctorial pad, although its association with suckling is far from obvious. The walls of the cheek also contain fibrous connective tissue, vessels, nerves and numerous small buccal mucous (salivary) glands.

Lips

The lips are two fleshy folds surrounding the oral orifice (see **Fig. 29.6**). The centre of each lip contains a thick fibrous strand, consisting of

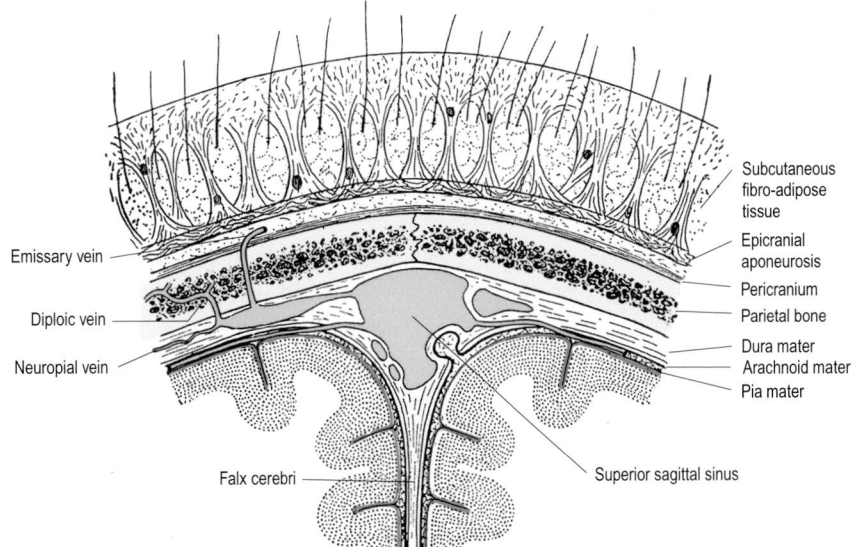

Fig. 29.1 Coronal section through the scalp, skull and brain. Note: loculated fat between fibrous septa blending with dermis and epicranial aponeurosis (galea aponeurotica); loose subaponeurotic areolar tissue; emissary, diploic, dural and neuropial veins. The superior sagittal sinus and lateral lacunae are more complex than depicted here.

Subcutaneous fibro-adipose tissue

Epicranial aponeurosis

Pericranium

Parietal bone

Dura mater

Arachnoid mater

Pia mater

Emissary vein

Diploic vein

Neuropial vein

Falx cerebri

Superior sagittal sinus

parallel bundles of skeletal muscle fibres (orbicularis oris, together with incisivus superior and inferior, and the direct labial tractors (p. 508), and their attachments to skin, mucosa or other muscle fibres. The free external surface of each lip is covered by a thin keratinized epidermis, and is continuous with the mucosa at the vermilion (red) zone of the lip. The dermis is well vascularized and accommodates numerous hair follicles (many of them large in the male), sebaceous glands and sweat glands. Subcutaneous adipose tissue is scanty. The internal mucous surfaces are lined with a thick non-keratinizing stratified squamous epithelium, and the submucosa is well vascularized and accommodates numerous labial mucous glands, which may be several millimetres in diameter, the largest being palpable with the tip of the tongue.

Because of the thickness of its semi-opaque epithelium, the mucosa of the everted lip appears moist, glistening and pink. Between the skin and mucosa, the vermilion zone is covered with a specialized keratinized stratified squamous epithelium which is thin near the skin, increases in thickness slightly as the mucosa is approached, and then thickens abruptly when true mucosa is reached. The epithelium is covered with transparent, dead squames and its deep surface is highly convoluted, interdigitating with abundant long dermal papillae. The latter carry a rich capillary plexus which imparts a dusky red colour. These surfaces are hairless, their dermis carries no sebaceous, sweat or mucous glands, and they are moistened with saliva by the tip of the tongue. The dense innervation of the lips is consistent with their acute sensitivity to light touch sensation. This is due mainly to the increased density of Meissner's corpuscles (p. 61) in the dermal papillae.

The size and curvature of the exposed red lip surfaces is subject to considerable individual, gender, and ethnic variation. The line of contact between the lips, the oral fissure, lies just above the cutting edges of the maxillary incisor teeth. On each side a labial commissure forms the angle (corner) of the mouth, usually near the first premolar tooth. The labial epithelia and internal tissues radiate over the boundaries of the commissure to become continuous with those of the cheek. With age, buccolabial (labiomarginal) grooves appear at the corners of the mouth. On each side the upper lip is separated from the cheek laterally by the nasolabial groove and is continuous above the nasal ala with the circumalar groove (sulcus). The lower lip is separated from the chin by the mentolabial groove (sulcus).

Externally, the central region in the upper lip presents a shallow vertical groove, the philtrum, which ends below in a slight tubercle limited by lateral ridges. The lower lip shows a small depression in the midline that corresponds to the tubercle. The junction between the external, hair-bearing skin and the red, hairless surface of the upper lip almost invariably takes the form of a double-curved Cupid's bow. From the centre it rises rapidly on each side to an apex that corresponds to the lower end of each ridge of the philtrum. It then slopes gently downwards and usually ends horizontally but sometimes curves slightly upwards

(infrequently downwards). The line of contact between the red lip surfaces is often almost horizontal but quite frequently takes the form of a much less wavy Cupid's bow. In the lower lip the junction between the skin and the red lip varies greatly between individuals in its vertical depth at the centre, whereas the lateral extremities descend medially for a few millimetres in all individuals.

In the upper lip, a narrow band of smooth tissue related to the subnasal maxillae marks the point at which labial mucosa becomes continuous with gingival mucosa. The corresponding reflexion in the lower lip coincides approximately with the mentolabial sulcus, and here the lip is continuous with mental tissues. The upper and lower lips differ in cross-sectional profile in that neither is a simple fold of uniform thickness. The upper lip has a bulbous asymmetrical profile, the skin and red-lip having a slight external convexity, and the adjoining red-lip and mucosa a pronounced internal convexity, creating a mucosal ridge or shelf that can be wrapped around the incisal edges of the parted teeth. The lower lip is on a more posterior plane than the upper lip. In the position of neutral lip contact, the external surface of the lower lip is concave, and there is minimal or no elevation of the internal mucosal surface. The profile of the lips can be modified by muscular activity (p. 508).

RELAXED SKIN TENSION LINES AND SKIN FLAPS ON THE FACE

The direction in which facial skin tension is greatest varies regionally. Skin tension lines which follow the furrows formed when the skin is relaxed are known as 'relaxed skin tension lines' (p. 173) (Borges & Alexander 1962). In the living face, these lines frequently (but not always) coincide with wrinkle lines (**Fig. 29.2**) and can therefore act as a guide in planning elective incisions.

When lesions on the face such as scars, pigmented lesions and skin cancers are excised, the dimensions of these lesions often permit excision as an ellipse, so that the resulting defect can be closed as a straight line. If the resulting scar is to be aesthetically acceptable it is important to make the long axis of the ellipse parallel to the natural relaxed skin tension lines, so that the scar will look like a natural skin crease. If the excision line runs contrary to the skin tension lines, the scar may be more conspicuous and will tend to stretch transversely as a result of natural expressive facial movements.

When larger lesions are excised it may be necessary to advance or rotate other adjacent soft tissue to fill the defect. The ability to raise these skin flaps is entirely dependent on the regional blood supply and both random pattern and axial pattern skin flaps (p. 169) are used surgically. Because of the richness of the subdermal plexus in the face, random pattern flaps can be raised with a greater length:breadth ratio than in any other area of the body.

The following are examples of axial pattern flaps that can be used to reconstruct defects on the face and scalp. Supratrochlear/supraorbital

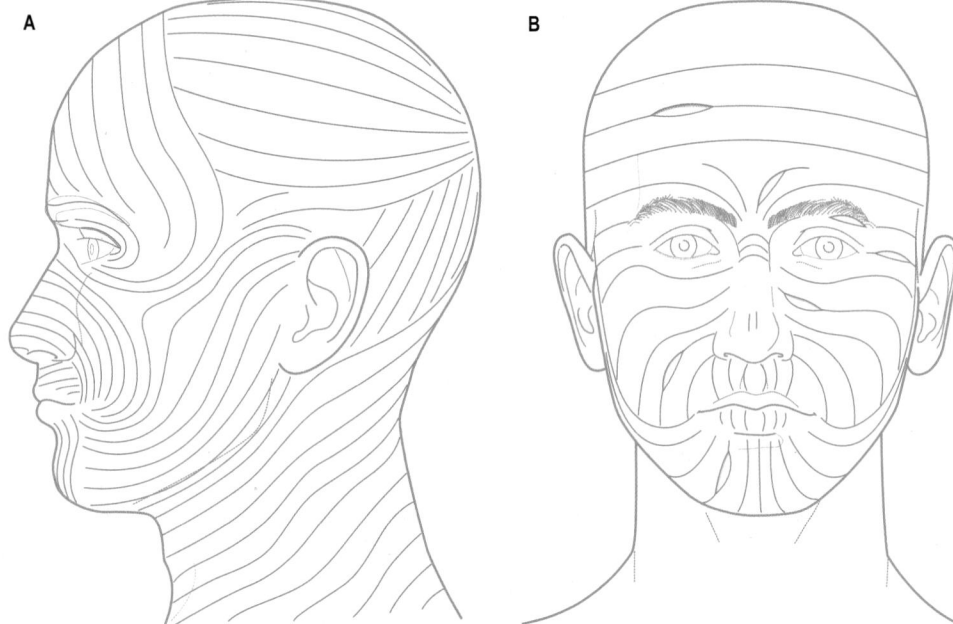

Fig. 29.2 A, Distribution of relaxed skin tension lines (Kraissl's lines) lateral view. **B**, Anterior view.

arteries support forehead flaps that are useful for nasal reconstruction. There is usually enough skin laxity to allow the majority of the donor site to be closed directly. The frontal branch of the superficial temporal artery anastomoses in the midline with its opposite number, and consequently the entire forehead skin can be raised on a narrow pedicle based on just one of the superficial temporal arteries. These flaps can be used to repair many facial defects and also intraoral defects, but the donor site defect cannot be closed directly and must be covered by a skin graft. The parietal branch of the superficial temporal artery and the occipital artery can support hair-bearing flaps from the scalp which are useful for reconstructing defects involving the scalp. The nasolabial flap utilizes the lax skin just lateral to the nasolabial groove. It is not supplied by a named axial artery but rather its blood supply is provided by many small branches from the underlying facial artery, which run perpendicular to the skin surface, allowing these flaps to be raised with their base either superior or inferior.

SOFT TISSUE

FASCIAL LAYERS

Fascia of scalp

The superficial fascia of the scalp is firm, dense and fibroadipose, and adheres closely to both skin and the underlying epicranius including its epicranial aponeurosis, the galea aponeurotica. Posteriorly it is continuous with the superficial fascia of the back of the neck, and laterally it is prolonged into the temporal region, where it is looser in texture.

FASCIAL LAYERS AND TISSUE PLANES IN THE FACE

On the basis of gross dissection and complementary histological studies, four distinct tissue planes are recognized on the face superficial to the plane of the facial nerve and its branches. From superficial to deep, these layers are the skin; a subcutaneous layer of fibro–adipose tissue; the superficial musculo-aponeurotic system (SMAS); and the parotid–masseteric fascia.

Subcutaneous fibroadipose tissue

This homogeneous layer is present throughout the face, although the degree of adiposity varies in different parts of the face. Anteriorly, it crosses the nasolabial fold onto the lip, and superiorly it crosses the zygomatic arch. In both locations the layer is more fascial than fatty. The fat content of the subcutaneous tissue in the cheek accounts for the cheek mass: part of the subcutaneous adipose tissue is the malar fat pad, a more or less discrete aggregation of fatty tissue inferolateral to the orbital margin.

Superficial musculo-aponeurotic system (SMAS)

This is described as a single tissue plane in the face. In some areas it is composed of muscle fibres, and elsewhere it is composed of fibrous or fibroaponeurotic tissue: it is not directly attached to bone. When traced below the level of the lower border of the mandible it becomes continuous with platysma in the neck. Microdissection has revealed that the SMAS becomes indistinct on the lateral aspect of the face c.1 cm below the level of the zygomatic arch. Anteromedially, the SMAS layer becomes continuous with some of the mimetic muscles including zygomaticus major, frontalis and the peri-orbital fibres of orbicularis oculi.

In most areas of the face, a distinct sub-SMAS plane can be defined deep to SMAS. It is continuous with the plane between platysma and the underlying investing layer of deep cervical fascia in the neck. However, where it overlies the parotid gland, the SMAS is firmly blended with the superficial layer of the parotid fascia, which means that a clear sub-SMAS plane is difficult, if not impossible, to define in the region of the parotid.

Parotid–masseteric fascia

This is a filmy areolar layer that overlies the filamentous branches of the facial nerve and the parotid duct as these structures lie on the surface of masseter. Further anteriorly the parotid–masseteric fascia overlies the buccal fat pad which lies superficial to buccinator. Having crossed the surface of the buccal fat pad, the fascia blends with the epimysium on the surface of buccinator. Below the lower border of the mandible, it is continuous with the investing layer of deep cervical fascia.

Parotid fascia (capsule)

The parotid gland is surrounded by a fibrous capsule called the parotid fascia or capsule. Traditionally this has been described as an upward continuation of the investing layer of deep cervical fascia in the neck which splits to enclose the gland within a superficial and a deep layer. The superficial layer is attached above to the zygomatic process of the temporal bone, the cartilaginous part of the external acoustic meatus, and the mastoid process. The deep layer is attached to the mandible, and to the tympanic plate, styloid and mastoid processes of the temporal bone. The prevailing view is that the deep layer of the parotid gland is derived from the deep cervical fascia. However, the superficial layer of the parotid capsule appears to be continuous with the fascia associated with platysma, and is now regarded as a component of the SMAS (Mitz & Peyronie 1976, Wassef 1987, Gosain et al 1993). It varies in thickness from a thick fibrous layer anteriorly to a thin translucent membrane posteriorly. It may be traced forwards as a separate layer which passes over the masseteric fascia (itself derived from the deep cervical fascia), separated from it by a cellular layer which contains branches of the facial nerve and the parotid duct. Histologically, the parotid fascia is atypical in that it contains muscle fibres which parallel those of platysma, especially in the lower part of the parotid capsule. Although thin fibrous septa may be seen in the subcutaneous layer at the histological level, macroscopically there is little evidence of a distinct layer of superficial fascia.

The deep fascia covering the muscles forming the parotid bed (digastric and styloid group of muscles) contains the stylomandibular and mandibulostylohyoid ligaments. The stylomandibular ligament passes from the styloid process to the angle of the mandible. The more extensive mandibulostylohyoid ligament (angular tract) passes between the angle of the mandible and the stylohyoid ligament for varying distances, generally reaching the hyoid bone (**Fig. 29.3**). It is thick posteriorly but thins anteriorly in the region of the angle of the mandible (Ziarah & Atkinson 1981, Shimada & Gasser 1988). There is some dispute as to whether the mandibulostylohyoid ligament is part of the deep cervical fascia (Ziarah and Atkinson 1981), or lies deep to it (Shimada & Gasser 1988). The stylomandibular and mandibulostylohyoid ligaments separate the parotid gland region from the superficial part of the submandibular gland, and so are landmarks of surgical interest.

Temporo-parietal and temporal fasciae

Above the level of the zygomatic arch, on the lateral side of the head, the temporo-parietal fascia (superficial temporal fascia) constitutes a fascial layer which lies in the same plane as, but is not continuous with, the SMAS. It is quite separate from, and superficial to, the temporal fascia (deep temporal fascia). More superiorly, it blends with the galea aponeurotica. The plane between the temporo-parietal fascia and the underlying deep temporal fascia contains loose areolar tissue and a small amount of fat. This tissue plane, the temporo-parietal fat pad, is continuous superiorly with the subgaleal plane of loose areolar tissue in the scalp. Running superiorly in the temporo-parietal fascia or just deep to it are the superficial temporal vessels, the auriculotemporal nerve and its branches, and the temporal branch of the facial nerve. The temporal fascia (deep temporal fascia) is a dense aponeurotic layer which lies deep to the temporo-parietal fat pad and covers temporalis: the deep surface of the fascia affords attachment to the superficial fibres of temporalis. Above, it is a single layer attached along the length of the superior temporal line where it blends with the periosteum. Below, at approximately the level of the superior orbital rim, it splits into superficial and deep laminae which run downwards to attach to the lateral and medial margins of the upper surface of the zygomatic arch respectively. The fat enclosed between these two layers is termed the superficial temporal fat pad, and contains the zygomatico-orbital branch of the superficial temporal artery and a cutaneous nerve, the zygomatico-temporal branch of the maxillary nerve. The temporal fascia is overlapped by auriculares anterior and superior, the epicranial aponeurosis and part of orbicularis oculi; the superficial temporal vessels and the auriculotemporal nerve ascend over it.

Buccopharyngeal fascia

Buccinator is covered by a thin layer of fascia, the buccopharyngeal fascia, which also covers the superior constrictor of the pharynx.

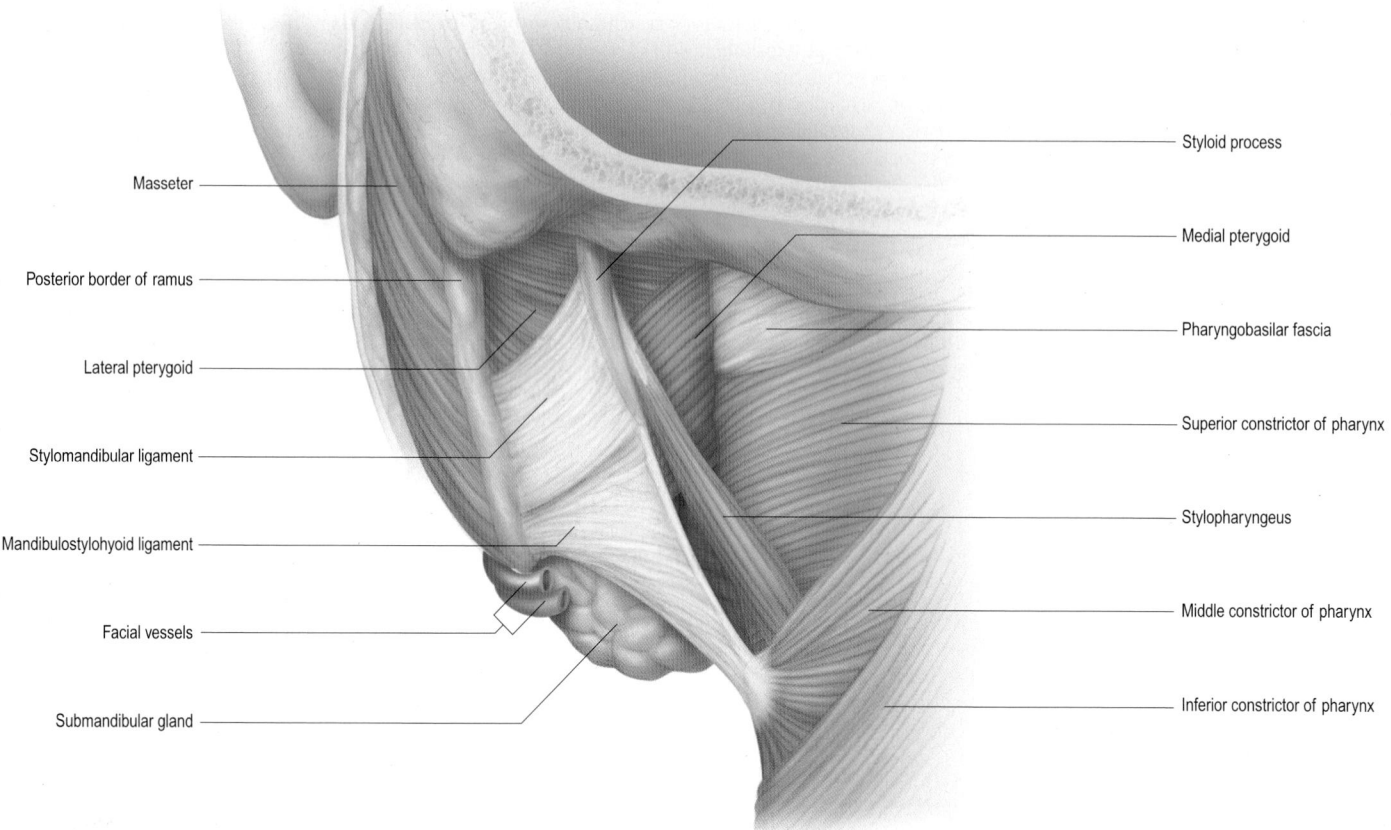

Masseter

Posterior border of ramus

Lateral pterygoid

Stylomandibular ligament

Mandibulostylohyoid ligament

Facial vessels

Submandibular gland

Styloid process

Medial pterygoid

Pharyngobasilar fascia

Superior constrictor of pharynx

Stylopharyngeus

Middle constrictor of pharynx

Inferior constrictor of pharynx

Fig. 29.3 The mandibulostylohyoid ligament.

Retaining ligaments of the face

These ligaments are fascial bands at specific sites which serve to anchor the skin to the underlying bone. The general cutaneous laxity that attends the ageing process renders facial skin subject to gravitational pull. However, at sites where retaining ligaments are present, the effect of gravitational pull is resisted. When performing facelift procedures, these ligaments must be surgically divided in order to facilitate redraping of facial skin. Examples of retaining ligaments in the face are the zygomatic ligament (also known as McGregor's patch) and the mandibular ligament.

FASCIAL SPACES

Two tissue spaces on the face may be involved in spread of odontogenic infection. They are the buccal tissue space, lying between the skin and surface of buccinator, and the infraorbital tissue space, lying between the bony attachments of levator labii superioris and levator anguli oris.

CRANIOFACIAL MUSCLES (Fig. 29.4)

Muscles of the head can be divided into craniofacial and masticatory groups. Craniofacial muscles are often referred to, not very accurately, as 'muscles of facial expression', and are related mainly to the orbital margins and eyelids, the external nose and nostrils, the lips, cheeks and mouth, the pinna, scalp and cervical skin. Masticatory muscles are concerned primarily with movements of the temporomandibular joint. This division of head musculature reflects differences in embryonic origin and innervation. In functional terms, activities such as mastication, deglutition, vocalization, communication, emotional expression, respiration, ocular, aural and nasal action reflect the close cooperation and interdependence between muscles in the two groups.

The organization of the muscles of facial expression differs from that of muscles in most other regions of the body because there is no deep membranous fascia beneath the skin. Instead, many small slips of muscle attached to the facial skeleton insert directly into the skin. Although the muscles can cause movement of the facial skin that reflects emotions, because they are grouped mainly around the orifices of the face, it is often argued that their primary function is to act as sphincters and dilators of the facial orifices and that the function of facial expression has developed secondarily. Embryologically, they are derived from the mesenchyme of the second branchial arch and so are innervated by the facial nerve. Topographically and functionally the muscles of facial expression may be subdivided into epicranial, circumorbital and palpebral, nasal, and buccolabial groups (**Fig. 29.5**).

EPICRANIAL MUSCLE GROUP

Epicranius

Epicranius consists of occipitofrontalis and temporoparietalis.

Occipitofrontalis (Fig. 29.5)

Occipitofrontalis covers the dome of the skull from the highest nuchal lines to the eyebrows. It is a broad, musculofibrous layer consisting of four thin, muscular quadrilateral parts, two occipital and two frontal, connected by the epicranial aponeurosis. Each occipital part (occipitalis) arises by tendinous fibres from the lateral two-thirds of the highest nuchal line of the occipital bone and the adjacent region of the mastoid part of the temporal bone, and extends forwards to join the aponeurosis. The gap between the two occipital parts is occupied by an extension of the epicranial aponeurosis. Each frontal part (frontalis) is adherent to the superficial fascia, particularly of the eyebrows. Although frontalis has no bony attachments of its own, its fibres blend with those of adjacent muscles – procerus, corrugator supercilii and orbicularis oculi – and ascend to join the epicranial aponeurosis in front of the coronal suture.

Vascular supply – Occipitofrontalis is supplied by branches of the superficial temporal, ophthalmic, posterior auricular and occipital arteries.

Innervation – The occipital part of occipitofrontalis is supplied by the posterior auricular branch of the facial nerve and the frontal part is supplied by the temporal branches of the facial nerve.

A

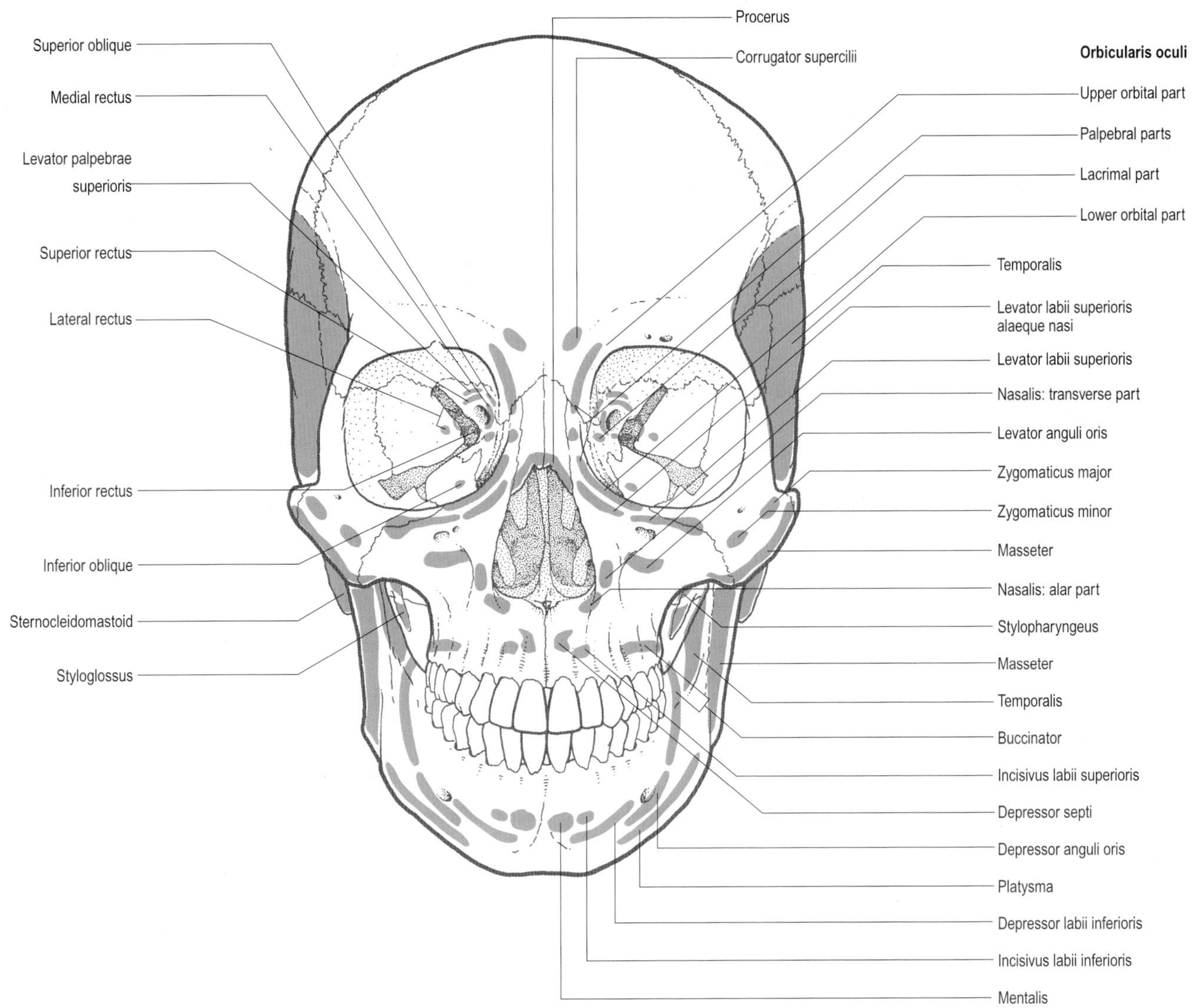

Superior oblique

Medial rectus

Levator palpebrae
superioris

Superior rectus

Lateral rectus

Inferior rectus

Inferior oblique

Sternocleidomastoid

Styloglossus

Procerus

Corrugator supercilii

Orbicularis oculi

Upper orbital part

Palpebral parts

Lacrimal part

Lower orbital part

Temporalis

Levator labii superioris
alaeque nasi

Levator labii superioris

Nasalis: transverse part

Levator anguli oris

Zygomaticus major

Zygomaticus minor

Masseter

Nasalis: alar part

Stylopharyngeus

Masseter

Temporalis

Buccinator

Incisivus labii superioris

Depressor septi

Depressor anguli oris

Platysma

Depressor labii inferioris

Incisivus labii inferioris

Mentalis

Fig. 29.4 A, Anterior view of the skull, showing muscle attachments.

Actions – Acting from above, the frontal parts raise the eyebrows and the skin over the root of the nose (e.g. as in expressions of surprise or horror). Acting from below, the frontal parts draw the scalp forwards, throwing the forehead into transverse wrinkles. The occipital parts draw the scalp backwards. Acting alternately, the occipital and frontal parts can move the entire scalp backwards and forwards.

Variations – A thin muscular slip, transversus nuchae, is present in c.25% of people. It arises from the external occipital protuberance or from the superior nuchal line, either superficial or deep to trapezius. It is frequently inserted with auricularis posterior, but may blend with the posterior edge of sternocleidomastoid.

The epicranial aponeurosis (Fig. 29.5) – The epicranial aponeurosis covers the upper part of the cranium and, with the epicranial muscle, forms a continuous fibromuscular sheet extending from the occiput to the eyebrows. Posteriorly, between the occipital parts of occipitofrontalis, it is attached to the external protuberance and highest nuchal line of the occipital bone. Anteriorly it splits to enclose the frontal parts and sends a short narrow prolongation between them. Laterally, the anterior and superior auricular muscles are attached to it, and the aponeurosis is thinner, and continues over the temporal fascia to the zygomatic arch. It is united to the skin lying over the cranial vault by fibrous superficial fascia, but it is connected more loosely to the underlying pericranium by areolar tissue, and this arrangement allows it to move freely, carrying with it the skin of the scalp.

Temporoparietalis
Temporoparietalis is a variably developed sheet of muscle which lies between the frontal parts of occipitofrontalis and the anterior and superior auricular muscles.

CIRCUMORBITAL AND PALPEBRAL MUSCLE GROUP
The circumorbital and palpebral group of muscles are orbicularis oculi, corrugator supercilii and levator palpebrae superioris. The first two are described here and levator palpebrae superioris is described in the context of the eye (p. 691).

Orbicularis oculi (Fig. 29.5)
Orbicularis oculi is a broad, flat, elliptical muscle which surrounds the circumference of the orbit and spreads into the adjacent regions of the eyelids, anterior temporal region, infraorbital cheek and superciliary region. It has orbital, palpebral and lacrimal parts.

The orbital part arises from the nasal component of the frontal bone, the frontal process of the maxilla and from the medial palpebral ligament. The fibres form complete ellipses, without interruption on the lateral side, where there is no bony attachment. The upper orbital fibres blend with the frontal part of occipitofrontalis and the corrugator supercilii. Many of them are inserted into the skin and subcutaneous tissue of the eyebrow, constituting depressor supercilii. Inferiorly and medially, the ellipses overlap or blend to some extent with adjacent muscles (levator labii superioris alaeque nasi, levator labii superioris and zygomaticus minor). At the extreme periphery, sectors of complete,

501

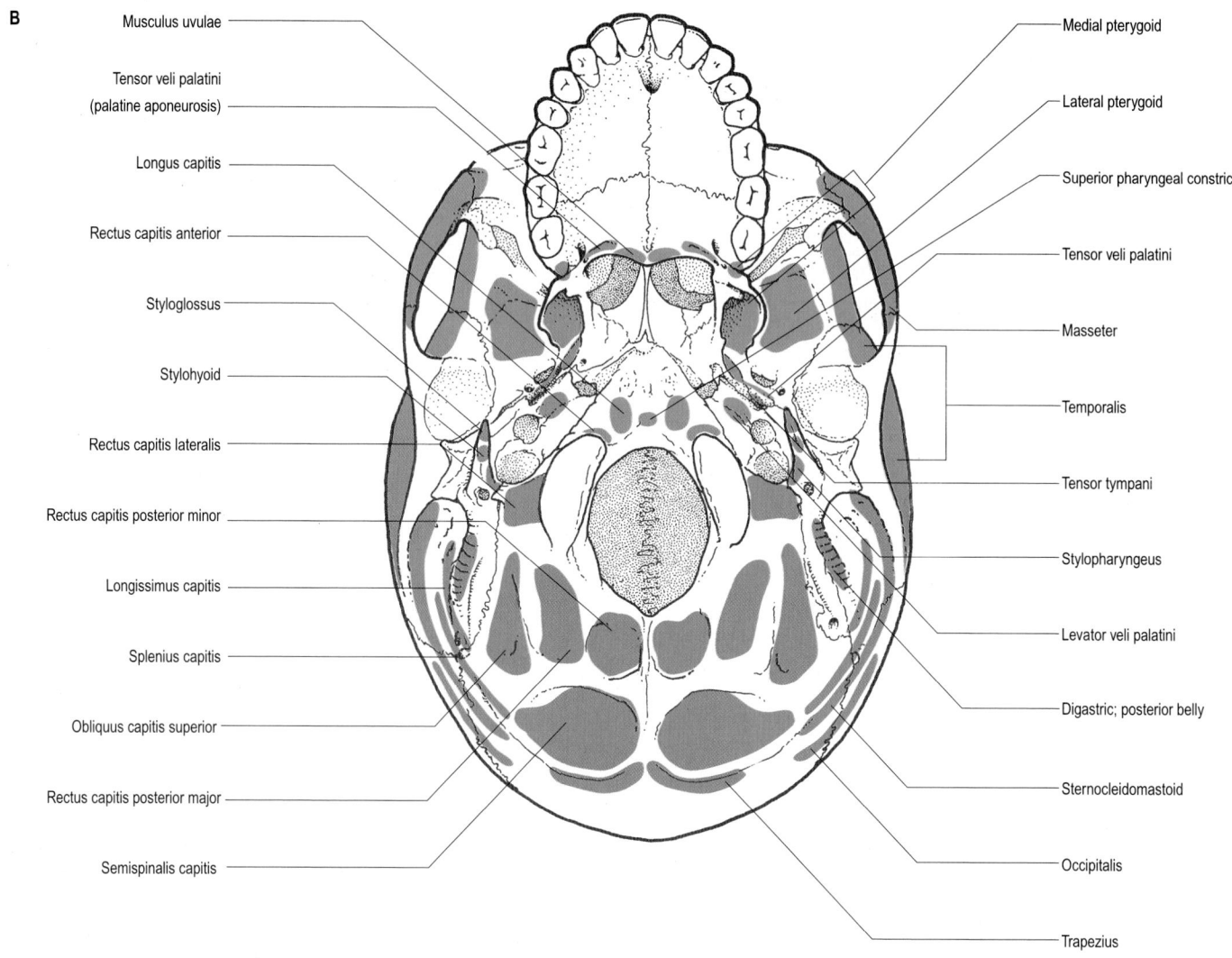

B

Musculus uvulae

Tensor veli palatini (palatine aponeurosis)

Longus capitis

Rectus capitis anterior

Styloglossus

Stylohyoid

Rectus capitis lateralis

Rectus capitis posterior minor

Longissimus capitis

Splenius capitis

Obliquus capitis superior

Rectus capitis posterior major

Semispinalis capitis

Medial pterygoid

Lateral pterygoid

Superior pharyngeal constrictor

Tensor veli palatini

Masseter

Temporalis

Tensor tympani

Stylopharyngeus

Levator veli palatini

Digastric; posterior belly

Sternocleidomastoid

Occipitalis

Trapezius

Fig. 29.4 B, Basal view of the skull, showing muscle attachments.

and sometimes incomplete, ellipses have a loose areolar connection with the temporal extension of the epicranial aponeurosis.

The palpebral part arises from the medial palpebral ligament, mainly from its superficial surface, and from the bone immediately above and below the ligament. The fibres sweep across the eyelids anterior to the orbital septum, interlacing at the lateral commissure to form the lateral palpebral raphe. A small group of fine fibres, close to the margin of each eyelid behind the eyelashes, constitutes the ciliary bundle.

The lacrimal part arises from the upper part of the lacrimal crest, and the adjacent lateral surface, of the lacrimal bone. It passes laterally behind the nasolacrimal sac (where some fibres are inserted into the associated fascia), and divides into upper and lower slips. Some fibres are inserted into the tarsi of the eyelids close to the lacrimal canaliculi, but most continue across in front of the tarsi and interlace in the lateral palpebral raphe.

Vascular supply – Orbicularis oculi is supplied by branches of the facial, superficial temporal, maxillary and ophthalmic arteries.

Innervation – Orbicularis oculi is supplied by temporal and zygomatic branches of the facial nerve.

Actions – Orbicularis oculi is the sphincter muscle of the eyelids and plays an important role in facial expression and various ocular reflexes. The orbital portion is usually activated under voluntary control. Contraction of the upper orbital fibres produces vertical furrowing above the bridge of the nose, narrowing of the palpebral fissure, and bunching and protrusion of the eyebrows, which reduces the amount of light entering the eyes. Eye closure is largely affected by lowering of the upper

eyelid, but there is also considerable elevation of the lower eyelid. The palpebral portion can be contracted voluntarily, to close the lids gently as in sleep, or reflexly, to close the lids protectively in blinking. The palpebral part has upper depressor and lower elevator fascicles. The lacrimal part of the muscle draws the eyelids and the lacrimal papillae medially, exerting traction on the lacrimal fascia and may aid drainage of tears by dilating the lacrimal sac. It may also influence pressure gradients within the lacrimal gland and ducts. This activity may assist in the sinuous flow of tears across the cornea, direct the lacrimal punctum into the lacus lacrimalis, and express secretions of the ciliary and tarsal glands. When the entire orbicularis oculi muscle contracts, the skin is thrown into folds which radiate from the lateral angle of the eyelids. Such folds, when permanent, cause wrinkles in middle age (the so-called 'crow's feet').

Corrugator supercilii (Fig. 29.5)

Corrugator supercilii is a small pyramidal muscle located at the medial end of each eyebrow. It lies deep to the frontal part of occipitofrontalis and orbicularis oculi, with which it is partially blended. Its fibres arise from bone at the medial end of the superciliary arch and pass laterally and slightly upwards to exert traction on the skin above the middle of the supraorbital margin.

Vascular supply – Corrugator supercilii is supplied by branches from adjacent arteries, mainly from the superficial temporal and ophthalmic arteries.

Innervation – Corrugator supercilii is innervated by temporal branches of the facial nerve.

C

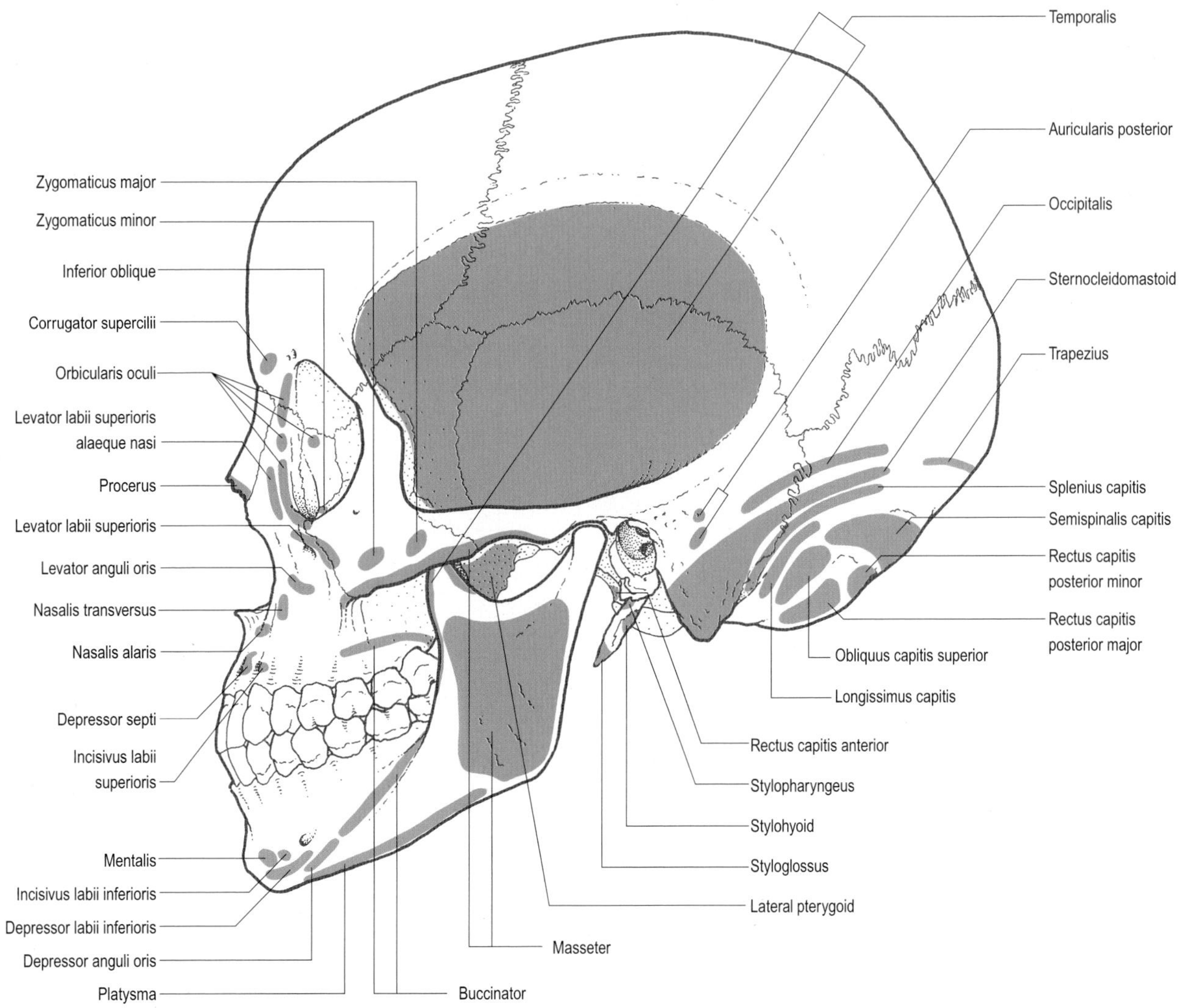
Temporalis
Auricularis posterior
Occipitalis
Sternocleidomastoid
Trapezius
Splenius capitis
Semispinalis capitis
Rectus capitis posterior minor
Rectus capitis posterior major
Obliquus capitis superior
Longissimus capitis
Rectus capitis anterior
Stylopharyngeus
Stylohyoid
Styloglossus
Lateral pterygoid
Masseter
Buccinator
Zygomaticus major
Zygomaticus minor
Inferior oblique
Corrugator supercilii
Orbicularis oculi
Levator labii superioris alaeque nasi
Procerus
Levator labii superioris
Levator anguli oris
Nasalis transversus
Nasalis alaris
Depressor septi
Incisivus labii superioris
Mentalis
Incisivus labii inferioris
Depressor labii inferioris
Depressor anguli oris
Platysma

Fig. 29.4 **C**, Lateral view of the skull, showing muscle attachments.

Actions – Corrugator supercilii cooperates with orbicularis oculi, drawing the eyebrows medially and downwards to shield the eyes in bright sunlight. It is also involved in frowning. The combined action of the two muscles produces mainly vertical wrinkles on the supranasal strip of the forehead.

BUCCOLABIAL MUSCLE GROUP

The nasal muscle group comprises procerus, nasalis and depressor septi.

Procerus (Fig. 29.5)

Procerus is a small pyramidal slip close to, and often partially blended with, the medial side of the frontal part of occipitofrontalis. It arises from a fascial aponeurosis covering the lower part of the nasal bone and the upper part of the lateral nasal cartilage. It is inserted into the skin over the lower part of the forehead between the eyebrows. Normally its lower aponeurosis blends with that of the transverse part of nasalis. A few muscle fascicles of procerus occasionally continue to the nasal ala, some even reaching the upper lip.

Vascular supply – Procerus is supplied mainly by branches from the facial artery.

Innervation – Procerus is supplied by temporal and lower zygomatic branches from the facial nerve (although a supply from the buccal branch has been described).

Actions – Procerus draws down the medial angle of the eyebrow and produces transverse wrinkles over the bridge of the nose. It is active in frowning and 'concentration', and helps to reduce the glare of bright sunlight.

Nasalis (Fig. 29.5)

Nasalis consists of transverse and alar parts that may be continuous at their origins. The transverse part (compressor naris) arises from the maxilla just lateral to the nasal notch. Its fibres pass upwards and medially and expand into a thin aponeurosis. At the bridge of the nose, the aponeuroses of the paired muscles merge with each other and with the aponeurosis of procerus. The alar part (dilatator naris) arises from the maxilla below and medial to the transverse part, with which it partly merges, and is attached to the cartilaginous ala nasi.

Vascular supply – Nasalis is supplied by branches from the facial artery and the infraorbital branch of the maxillary artery.

Innervation – Nasalis is supplied by the buccal branch of the facial nerve, although there may also be a contribution from the zygomatic branch.

Actions – The transverse part of nasalis compresses the nasal aperture at the junction of the vestibule of the nose with the nasal cavity. The alar part draws the ala downwards and laterally and so assists in widening the anterior nasal aperture. These actions accompany deep inspiration, and are thus associated with exertion, and also with some emotional states.

Depressor septi

Depressor septi is often regarded as part of dilatator naris. It arises from the maxilla above the central incisor tooth and ascends to attach to the

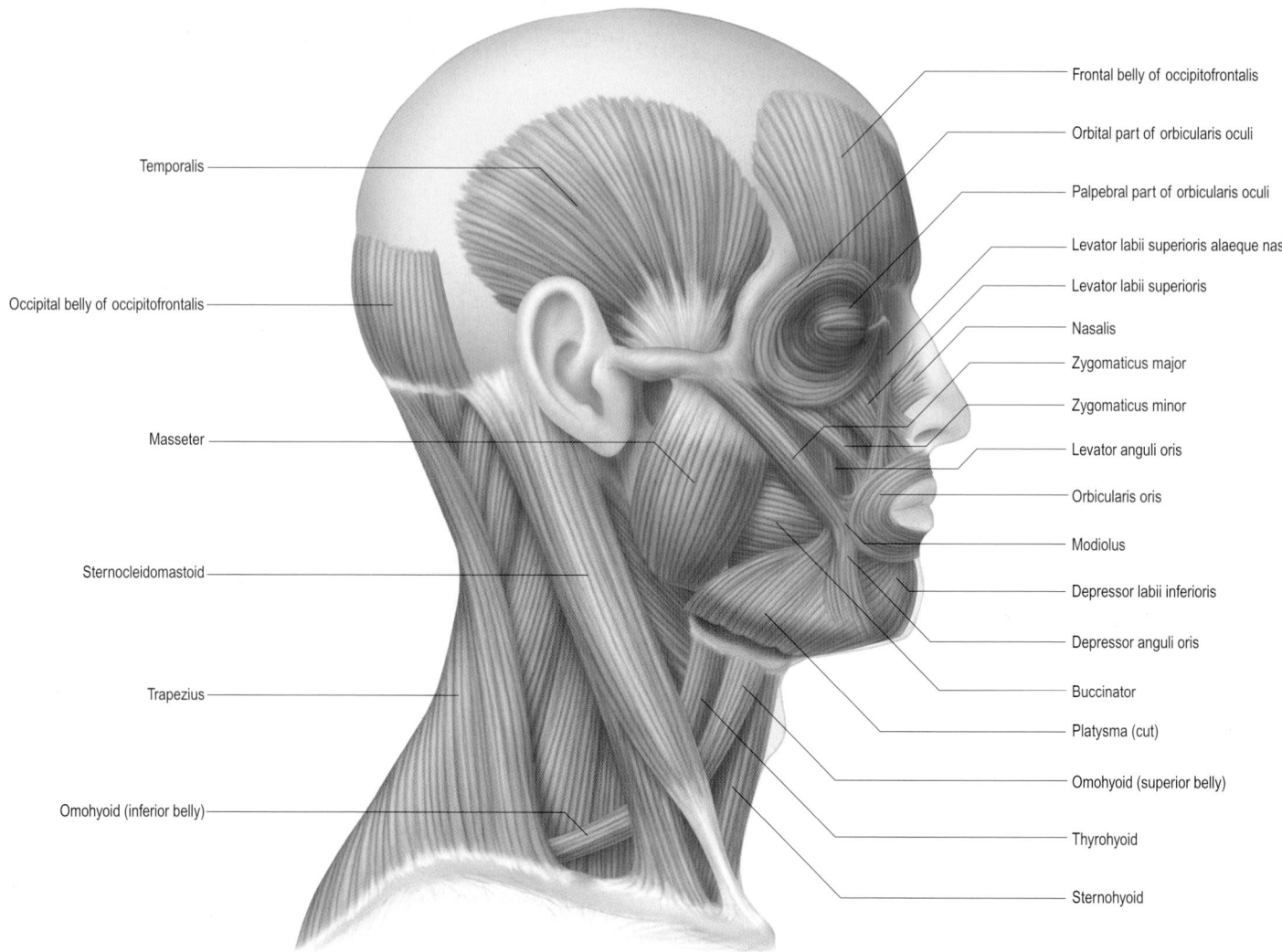

Temporalis

Occipital belly of occipitofrontalis

Masseter

Sternocleidomastoid

Trapezius

Omohyoid (inferior belly)

Frontal belly of occipitofrontalis

Orbital part of orbicularis oculi

Palpebral part of orbicularis oculi

Levator labii superioris alaeque nasi

Levator labii superioris

Nasalis

Zygomaticus major

Zygomaticus minor

Levator anguli oris

Orbicularis oris

Modiolus

Depressor labii inferioris

Depressor anguli oris

Buccinator

Platysma (cut)

Omohyoid (superior belly)

Thyrohyoid

Sternohyoid

Fig. 29.5 The superficial muscles of the head and neck.

mobile part of the nasal septum. It is immediately deep to the mucous membrane of the upper lip.

Vascular supply – Depressor septi is supplied by the superior labial branch of the facial artery.

Innervation – Depressor septi is innervated by the buccal branch, and sometimes by the zygomatic branch, of the facial nerve.

Actions – Depressor septi pulls the nasal septum downwards and, with the alar part of nasalis, widens the nasal aperture.

BUCCOLABIAL GROUP OF MUSCLES
The shape of the mouth and the posture of the lips are controlled by a complex three-dimensional assembly of muscular slips. These include elevators, retractors and evertors of the upper lip (levator labii superioris alaeque nasi, levator labii superioris, zygomaticus major and minor, levator anguli oris and risorius); depressors, retractors and evertors of the lower lip (depressor labii inferioris, depressor anguli oris, and mentalis); a compound sphincter (orbicularis oris, incisivus superior and inferior); buccinator.

Levator labii superioris alaequae nasi (Fig. 29.5)
Levator labii superioris alaequae nasi arises from the upper part of the frontal process of the maxilla and, passing obliquely downwards and laterally, divides into medial and lateral slips. The medial slip is inserted into the greater alar cartilage of the nose and the skin over it. The lateral slip is prolonged into the lateral part of the upper lip, where

it blends with levator labii superioris and orbicularis oris. Superficial fibres of the lateral slip curve laterally across the front of levator labii superioris and attach along the floor of the dermis at the upper part of the nasolabial furrow and ridge.

Vascular supply – Levator labii superioris alaequae nasi is supplied by the facial artery and the infraorbital branch of the maxillary artery.

Innervation – Levator labii superioris alaequae nasi is innervated by zygomatic and buccal branches of the facial nerve.

Actions – The lateral slip raises and everts the upper lip and raises, deepens and increases the curvature of the top of the nasolabial furrow. The medial slip dilates the nostril, displaces the circumalar furrow laterally, and modifies its curvature.

Levator labii superioris (Fig. 29.5)
Levator labii superioris starts from the infraorbital margin, where it arises from the maxilla and zygomatic bone above the infraorbital foramen. Its fibres converge into the muscular substance of the upper lip between the lateral slip of levator labii superioris alaequae nasi and zygomaticus minor.

Vascular supply – Levator labii superioris is supplied by the facial artery and the infraorbital branch of the maxillary artery.

Innervation – Levator labii superioris is innervated by the zygomatic and buccal branches of the facial nerve.

Actions – Levator labii superioris elevates and everts the upper lip. Acting with other muscles, it modifies the nasolabial furrow. In some faces, this furrow is a highly characteristic feature and it is often deepened in expressions of sadness or seriousness.

Zygomaticus major (Fig. 29.5)

Zygomaticus major arises from the zygomatic bone, just in front of the zygomaticotemporal suture, and passes to the angle of the mouth where it blends with the fibres of levator anguli oris, orbicularis oris and more deeply placed muscular bands.

Vascular supply – Zygomaticus major is supplied by the superior labial branch of the facial artery.

Innervation – Zygomaticus major is innervated by the zygomatic and buccal branches of the facial nerve.

Actions – Zygomaticus major draws the angle of the mouth upwards and laterally as in laughing.

Zygomaticus minor (Fig. 29.5)

Zygomaticus minor arises from the lateral surface of the zygomatic bone immediately behind the zygomaticomaxillary suture, and passes downwards and medially into the muscular substance of the upper lip. Superiorly it is separated from levator labii superioris by a narrow triangular interval, and inferiorly it blends with this muscle.

Vascular supply – Zygomaticus minor is supplied by the superior labial branch of the facial artery.

Innervation – Zygomaticus minor is innervated by the zygomatic and buccal branches of the facial nerve.

Actions – Zygomaticus minor elevates the upper lip, exposing the maxillary teeth. It also assists in deepening and elevating the nasolabial furrow. Acting together, the main elevators of the lip – levator labii superioris alaequae nasi, levator labii superioris and zygomaticus minor – curl the upper lip in smiling, and in expressing smugness, contempt or disdain.

Levator anguli oris (Fig. 29.5)

Levator anguli oris arises from the canine fossa of the maxilla, just below the infraorbital foramen and inserts into and below the angle of the mouth. Its fibres mingle there with other muscle fibres (zygomaticus major, depressor anguli oris, orbicularis oris). Some superficial fibres curve anteriorly and attach to the dermal floor of the lower part of the nasolabial furrow. The infraorbital nerve and accompanying vessels enter the face via the infraorbital foramen between the origins of levator anguli oris and levator labii superioris.

Vascular supply – Levator anguli oris is supplied by the superior labial branch of the facial artery and the infraorbital branch of the maxillary artery.

Innervation – Levator anguli oris is innervated by the zygomatic and buccal branches of the facial nerve.

Actions – Levator anguli oris raises the angle of the mouth in smiling, and contributes to the depth and contour of the nasolabial furrow.

Malaris

Malaris is a thin sheet of muscle that is sometimes found covering and blending with zygomaticus major and minor and the levator labii superioris muscles. It is subject to considerable variation. When present it is continuous with the inferior limit of orbicularis oculi, from which it is possibly derived. Its fibres incline medially and downwards. Some of its superficial fascicles have a dermal attachment to the nasolabial ridge and sulcus, and others pass directly to the angle of the mouth and to the outer third of the upper lip to intersect with bundles of orbicularis oris.

Mentalis

Mentalis is a conical fasciculus lying at the side of the frenulum of the lower lip. The fibres arise from the incisive fossa of the mandible and descend to attach to the skin of the chin.

Vascular supply – Mentalis is supplied by the inferior labial branch of the facial artery and the mental branch of the maxillary artery.

Innervation – Mentalis is innervated by the mandibular branch of the facial nerve.

Actions – Mentalis raises the lower lip, wrinkling the skin of the chin. Since it raises the base of the lower lip, it helps in protruding and everting the lower lip in drinking and also in expressing doubt or disdain.

Depressor labii inferioris (Fig. 29.5)

Depressor labii inferioris is a quadrilateral muscle that arises from the oblique line of the mandible, between the symphysis menti and the mental foramen. It passes upwards and medially into the skin and mucosa of the lower lip, blending with the paired muscle from the opposite side and with orbicularis oris. Below and laterally it is continuous with platysma.

Vascular supply – Depressor labii inferioris is supplied by the inferior labial branch of the facial artery and the mental branch of the maxillary artery.

Innervation – Depressor labii inferioris is innervated by the mandibular branch of the facial nerve.

Actions – Depressor labii inferioris draws the lower lip downwards and a little laterally in masticatory activity, and may assist in eversion of the lower lip. It contributes to the expressions of irony, sorrow, melancholy and doubt.

Depressor anguli oris (Fig. 29.5)

Depressor anguli oris has a long, linear origin from the mental tubercle of the mandible and its continuation, the oblique line, below and lateral to depressor labii inferioris. It converges into a narrow fasciculus that blends at the angle of the mouth with orbicularis oris and risorius. Some fibres continue into the levator anguli oris muscle. Depressor anguli oris is continuous below with platysma and cervical fasciae. Some of its fibres may pass below the mental tubercle and cross the midline to interlace with their contralateral fellows; these constitute the transversus menti (the 'mental sling').

Vascular supply – Depressor anguli oris is supplied by the inferior labial branch of the facial artery and the mental branch of the maxillary artery.

Innervation – Depressor anguli oris is innervated by the buccal and mandibular branches of the facial nerve.

Actions – Depressor anguli oris draws the angle of the mouth downwards and laterally in opening the mouth and in expressing sadness. During opening of the mouth the mentolabial sulcus becomes more horizontal and its central part deeper.

Buccinator (Fig. 29.5)

The muscle of the cheek, buccinator, is a thin quadrilateral muscle which occupies the interval between the maxilla and the mandible. Its upper and lower boundaries are attached respectively to the outer surfaces of the alveolar processes of the maxilla and mandible opposite the molar teeth. Its posterior border is attached to the anterior margin of the pterygomandibular raphe. In addition, a few fibres spring from a fine tendinous band that bridges the interval between the maxilla and the pterygoid hamulus, between the tuberosity of the maxilla and the upper end of the pterygomandibular raphe. On its way to the soft palate the tendon of tensor veli palatini pierces the pharyngeal wall in the small gap that lies behind this tendinous band. The posterior part of buccinator is deeply placed, internal to the mandibular ramus and in the plane of the medial pterygoid plate. Its anterior component curves out behind the third molar tooth to lie in the submucosa of the cheek and lips. The fibres of buccinator converge towards the modiolus near the angle of the mouth. Here the central (pterygomandibular) fibres intersect, those from below crossing to the upper part of orbicularis oris, and those from above crossing to the lower part. The highest (maxillary) and lowest (mandibular) fibres of buccinator continue forward to enter their corresponding lips without decussation. As buccinator courses through the cheek and modiolus substantial numbers of its fibres are diverted internally to attach to submucosa.

Relations – Posteriorly, buccinator lies in the same plane as the superior pharyngeal constrictor, which arises from the posterior margin of the pterygomandibular raphe, and is covered there by the buccopharyngeal fascia. Superficially, the buccal pad of fat separates the posterior part of buccinator from the ramus of the mandible, masseter and part of temporalis. Anteriorly, the superficial surface of buccinator is related to zygomaticus major, risorius, levator and depressor anguli oris, and the parotid duct. It is crossed by the facial artery, facial vein and branches of the facial and buccal nerves. The deep surface of buccinator is related to the buccal glands and mucous membrane of the mouth. The parotid duct pierces buccinator opposite the third upper molar tooth, and lies on the deep surface of the muscle before opening into the mouth opposite the maxillary second molar tooth.

Vascular supply – Buccinator is supplied by branches from the facial artery and the buccal branch of the maxillary artery.

Innervation – Buccinator is supplied by the buccal branch of the facial nerve.

Actions – Buccinator compresses the cheek against the teeth and gums during mastication, and assists the tongue in directing food between the teeth. As the mouth closes, the teeth glide over the buccolabial mucosa, which must be retracted progressively from their occlusal surfaces by buccinator and other submucosally attached muscles. When the cheeks have been distended with air, the buccinators expel it between the lips, an activity important when playing wind instruments, accounting for the name of the muscle (Latin *buccinator* = trumpeter).

Pterygomandibular raphe – The pterygomandibular raphe is a thin band of tendinous fibres that stretches from the hamulus of the medial pterygoid plate down to the posterior end of the mylohyoid line of the mandible. It is easily palpated medially, where it is covered by the mucous membrane of the mouth, and laterally it is separated from the ramus of the mandible by a quantity of adipose tissue. It gives attachment posteriorly to the superior constrictor of the pharynx, and anteriorly to the central part of buccinator.

Orbicularis oris (Figs 29.5, 29.6)

Orbicularis oris is so named because it was once assumed that the oral fissure was surrounded by a series of complete ellipses of striated muscle which acted together in the manner of a sphincter. However, it is now recognized that the muscle actually consists of four substantially independent quadrants (upper, lower, left and right), each of which contains a larger pars peripheralis and a smaller pars marginalis. Marginal and peripheral parts are apposed along lines that correspond externally to the lines of junction between the vermilion zone of the lip and the skin. Thus, orbicularis oris is composed of eight segments, each of which is named systematically according to its location. Each segment resembles a fan that has its stem at the modiolus and is open in peripheral segments and almost closed in marginal segments.

Pars peripheralis – Pars peripheralis has, in each quadrant, a lateral stem attached to the labial side of the modiolus over its full thickness, from apex to base, including the corresponding upper or lower cornu. Most of these stem fibres are thought to originate within the modiolus (although it is possible that some are direct continuations from the other modiolar muscles). The consensus view is that stem fibres are reinforced directly by fibres from buccinator (upper fibres and decussating lower central fibres), levator anguli oris and the superficial part of zygomaticus major in the upper lip, and from buccinator (lower fibres and decussating upper central fibres), and depressor anguli oris in the lower lip.

The fibres of orbicularis oris enter their respective superior and inferior labial areas and diverge to form triangular muscular sheets. These are thickest at the junctions between skin and the vermilion zone and become progressively thinner as they reach the limits of the labial region (as defined above). The greater part of each sheet enters the free lip, where its fibres aggregate into cylindrical bundles orientated parallel to the vermilion zone. Fibres of the direct labial tractors pass to their submucosal attachments between these cylindrical bundles and between pars peripheralis and pars marginalis. In the upper lip, the highest fibres run near the nasolabial sulcus, a few fibres attach to the sulcus, and a few to the nasal ala and septum. In the lower lip, the lowest fibres reach and attach to the mentolabial sulcus. A small proportion of the main body of fibres is thought to end in the labial connective tissue, dermis or submucosa as it traverses its quadrant of free lip. Most fibres continue towards the median plane and cross some 5 mm into the opposite half-lip. At this point the fibres from the two sides interlace on their way to their dermal insertions, creating the ridges of the philtrum of the upper lip and the less marked corresponding depression in the lower lip.

Pars marginalis – Pars marginalis of orbicularis oris is developed to a unique extent in human lips and is closely associated with speech and the production of some kinds of musical tone. In each quadrant the pars marginalis consists of a single (occasionally double) band of narrow diameter muscle fibres lodged within the tissues of each vermilion zone. At their medial end, the marginal fibres meet and interlace with their contralateral fellows and then attach to the dermis of the vermilion zone a few millimetres beyond the median plane in a manner similar to pars peripheralis. At their lateral ends, the fibres converge and attach to the deepest part of the modiolar base along a horizontal strip level with the buccal angle.

The relations between pars marginalis and pars peripheralis are complex. In a full thickness section of an upper lip at right angles to the vermilion zone, the cylindrical bundles of peripheralis fibres form an S-shape, with an external convexity above, and an internal convexity below: the classic analogy is to the shank and initial curved part of a hook. Beyond peripheralis, the hook-shape is completed by the blunted triangular profile of marginalis, which occupies the core of the vermilion zone with its base adjacent to peripheralis and its apex reaching upwards and anteriorly towards the junction between vermilion zone and skin. In a similar section through the lower lip, peripheralis bundles form a continuous curve that is concave towards the external surface. This is surmounted by the flattened triangular profile of marginalis, which curves anteriorly, its apex again nearing the vermilion/cutaneous junction. Thus, throughout the vermilion zones of both lips, marginalis lies substantially anterior to the adjacent bundles of peripheralis. However, as the muscles are traced laterally beyond the vermilion zone and across the buccal angle, this relationship alters and marginalis becomes inverted as it wraps progressively around the adjacent edge of peripheralis to reach its deep (submucosal) surface, and maintains this position up to its attachment at the modiolar base.

Vascular supply – Orbicularis oris is supplied mainly by the superior and inferior labial branches of the facial artery, the mental and infra-orbital branches of the maxillary artery and the transverse facial branch of the superficial temporal artery.

Nerve supply – Orbicularis oris is supplied by the buccal and mandibular branches of the facial nerve.

Actions – The actions of orbicularis oris are considered in detail on page 508.

Incisivus labii superioris

Incisivus labii superioris has a bony origin from the floor of the incisive fossa of the maxilla above the eminence of the lateral incisor tooth. Initially it lies deep to orbicularis oris pars peripheralis superior. Arching laterally, its fibre bundles become intercalated between, and parallel to, the orbicular bundles. Approaching the modiolus, it segregates into superficial and deep parts: the former blends partially with levator anguli oris and attaches to the body and apex of the modiolus and the latter is attached to the superior cornu and base of the modiolus.

Incisivus labii inferioris

Incisivus labii inferioris, an accessory muscle of the orbicularis oris muscle complex, has many features in common with incisivus labii superioris. Its osseous attachment is to the floor of the incisive fossa of the mandible, lateral to mentalis and below the eminence of the lateral incisor tooth. Curving laterally and upwards, it blends to some extent with orbicularis oris pars peripheralis inferior before reaching the modiolus, where superficial bundles attach to the apex and body, and deep bundles attach to the base and inferior cornu.

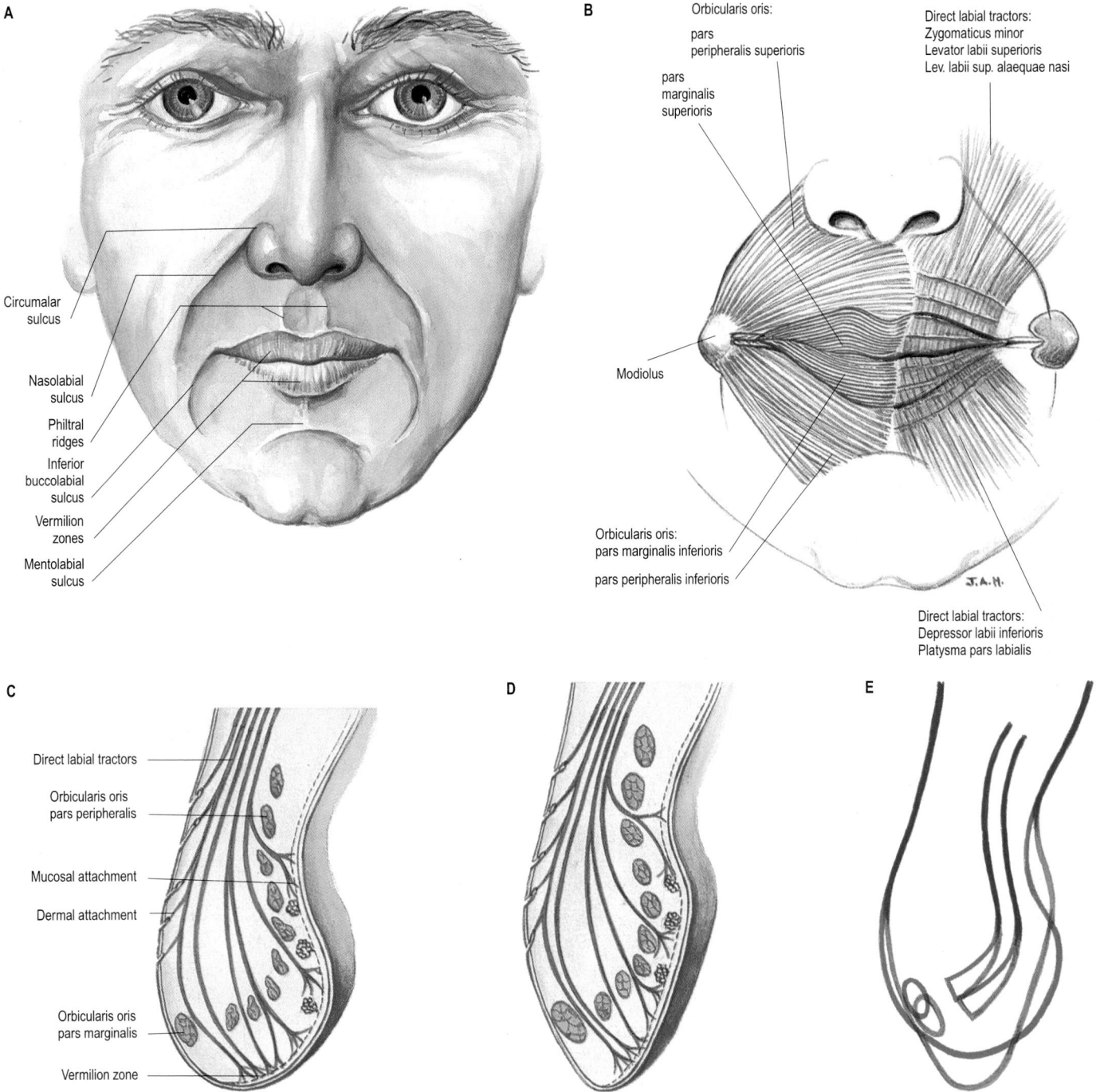

A

Circumalar
sulcus

Nasolabial
sulcus

Philtral
ridges

Inferior
buccolabial
sulcus

Vermilion
zones

Mentolabial
sulcus

B

Orbicularis oris:

pars
peripheralis superioris

pars
marginalis
superioris

Direct labial tractors:
Zygomaticus minor
Levator labii superioris
Lev. labii sup. alaequae nasi

Modiolus

Orbicularis oris:
pars marginalis inferioris

pars peripheralis inferioris

J.A.H.

Direct labial tractors:
Depressor labii inferioris
Platysma pars labialis

C

Direct labial tractors

Orbicularis oris
pars peripheralis

Mucosal attachment

Dermal attachment

Orbicularis oris
pars marginalis

Vermilion zone

D

E

Fig. 29.6 A, The principal sulci, creases and ridges of the face referred to at various points in the text. Note particularly those defining the 'labial hexagon' (see text). **B**, The disposition of the modiolus and orbicularis oris pars peripheralis and pars marginalis (on the left); the successively transected laminae of the direct labial tractors of both upper and lower lips (on the right). **C**, Parasagittal section of the upper lip in repose. On the left is thin skin with oblique hair follicles; on the right is thick mucosa with mucous glands and mucosal shelf; between them is the vermilion zone. **D**, as C but slightly contracted, forming a narrowed profile (labial cord). **E**, Superimposed outlines of C (magenta) and D (blue).

Platysma (Fig. 29.5)

Platysma is described as a muscle of the neck (p. 535) but it is considered here as a contributor to the orbicularis oris muscle complex. The pars mandibularis attaches to the lower border of the body of the mandible. Posterior to this attachment, a substantial flattened bundle separates and passes superomedially to the lateral border of depressor anguli oris, where a few fibres join this muscle. The remainder continue deep to depressor anguli oris and reappear at its medial border. Here they continue within the tissue of the lateral half of the lower lip, as a direct labial tractor, platysma pars labialis. Pars labialis occupies the interval between depressor anguli oris and depressor labii inferioris and is in the same plane as these muscles. The adjacent margins of all three muscles blend and they have similar labial attachments. Platysma pars

modiolaris constitutes all the remaining bundles posterior to pars labialis, other than a few fine fascicles that end directly in buccal dermis or submucosa. Pars modiolaris is posterolateral to depressor anguli oris and passes superomedially, deep to risorius, to apical and subapical modiolar attachments.

Risorius

Risorius is a highly variable muscle that ranges from one or more slender fascicles to a wide, thin superficial fan. Its peripheral attachments may include some or all of the following: the zygomatic arch, parotid fascia, fascia over the masseter anterior to the parotid, fascia enclosing pars modiolaris of platysma, and fascia over the mastoid process. Its fibres converge to apical and subapical attachments at the modiolus.

507

Vascular supply – Risorius is supplied mainly by the superior labial branch of the facial artery.

Nerve supply – Risorius is supplied by buccal branches of the facial nerve.

Actions – Risorius pulls the corner of the mouth laterally in numerous facial activities, including grinning and laughing.

MOVEMENTS OF THE FACE AND LIPS

Direct labial tractors (Fig. 29.6)

Direct labial tractors, as their name suggests, pass directly into the tissues of the lips and not via the modioli. In broad terms, the force exerted by tractors is directed vertically at an approximate right angle to the oral fissure. Their action will therefore elevate and/or evert the whole, or part, of the upper lip and depress and/or evert the whole, or part, of the lower lip. The tractors are, from medial to lateral: the labial part of levator labii superioris alaequae nasi, levator labii superioris and zygomaticus minor in the upper lip, and depressor labii inferioris and platysma pars labialis in the lower lip.

In both upper and lower lips the tractors blend into a continuous sheet that divides into a series of superimposed coronal sheets which are anterior to the muscle bundles of pars peripheralis orbicularis oris as they enter the free lip. The sheets may be divided into three groups at increasing depths from the skin surface, each with a distinct zone of attachment. The superficial group comprises a succession of fine fibre bundles which curve anteriorly a short distance before attaching in a series of horizontal rows to the dermis between the hair follicles, sebaceous glands and sweat glands. The intermediate group attaches to the dermis of the vermilion zone, which they reach by two routes: the more superficial bundles continue past the skin/vermilion junction, then curve posteriorly over pars marginalis orbicularis oris to punctate attachments on the ventral half of the dermis of the vermilion zone; the deeper bundles first pass posteriorly between pars peripheralis and pars marginalis, then curve anteriorly to punctate attachments on the dorsal half of the dermis of the vermilion zone. The deep group is closely applied to the anterior surface of pars peripheralis orbicularis oris, and sends fine tractor fibres between its parallel bundles to attach posteriorly into the submucosa and periglandular connective tissue.

Movements of the lips

The various groups of direct labial tractors may act together or individually, and their effects may involve a complete labial quadrant, or be restricted to a short segment. For example, partial contraction of the superior labial tractors can result in localized elevation of a segment of the upper lip, in a postural expression reminiscent of the 'canine snarl'. Normally, however, the activity of the tractors is modified by the superimposed activity of orbicularis oris and the modiolar muscles. The resultant actions range from delicate adjustments of the tension and profile of the lip margins to large increases of the oral fissure with eversion of the lips.

Lip protrusion is passive in its initial stages. It may be suppressed by powerful contraction of the whole of orbicularis oris or enhanced by selective activation of parts of the direct labial tractors. However, lip movements must accommodate separation of the teeth brought about by mandibular depression at the temporomandibular joints. Beyond a certain range of mouth opening, labial movements are almost completely dominated by mandibular movements. Thus over the last 2.5–3 cm interincisal distance of wide jaw separation, strong contraction of orbicularis oris cannot effect lip contact, and instead it causes full-thickness inflection of upper and lower lips, including the vermilion zone, towards the oral cavity, wrapping them around the incisal edges, canine cusps and premolar occlusal surfaces. The involvement of the lips in speech is described elsewhere, but some aspects relevant to the actions of orbicularis oris pars marginalis will be described here. Contraction of marginalis is considered to alter the cross-sectional profile of the free margin of the vermilion zone such that both the gentle bulbous profile of the upper lip and the smooth posterosuperior convexity of the lower lip change to a narrow, symmetrical triangular profile. The transformed rims, whose length and tension can be delicately controlled, have been named labial cords. They are known to be involved in the production of some consonantal (labial) sounds. A labial cord may also function as a 'vibrating reed' in whistling or playing a wind instrument such as the trumpet.

The modiolus and its role in facial movements

Modiolus

On each side of the face a number of muscles converge towards a focus just lateral to the buccal angle, where they interlace to form a dense, compact, mobile, fibromuscular mass called the modiolus (**Fig. 29.6B**). This can be palpated most effectively by using the opposed thumb and index finger to compress the mucosa and skin simultaneously. At least nine muscles, depending on the classification employed, are attached to each modiolus. Moreover, the muscles lie in different planes, their modiolar stems are often spiralized, and most divide into two bundles, some into three or four, each of them interlacing and attaching in a distinctive way. Not surprisingly, therefore, the three-dimensional organization of the modiolus has proved difficult to analyse.

The shape and dimensions of the modiolus are given approximately because they are subject to individual, age, sexual and ethnic variation. Furthermore the modiolus has no precise histological boundaries, and is an irregular zone where dense, compact interlacing tissue grades into the stems of individually recognizable muscles. The modiolus has the rough form of a blunt cone. The base of the cone (basis moduli) is adjacent and adherent to the mucosa. It is roughly elliptical in outline and extends vertically c.20 mm above and 20 mm below a horizontal line through the buccal angle. It also extends laterally a similar distance from the angle. The blunt apex of the cone (apex moduli) is c.4 mm across, and is centred c.12 mm lateral to the buccal angle. From mucosa to dermis the thickness of the mass is c.10 mm, divided approximately equally into basal, central and apical parts. The central body has an oblique fibrous cleft or channel that transmits the facial artery, an arrangement that may limit the extent to which it is compressed by contraction of the buccolabial musculature. The cone shape is modified by two round-edged flanges (or cornua) that extend into the lateral free lip tissues above and below the corner of the mouth. The tip of the superior cornu extends 5–5 mm medial to the buccal angle, the tip of the inferior cornu only 3–5 mm. With these additions, the modiolar base becomes kidney-shaped, with the buccal angle projecting towards the hilum.

The apex of the modiolus is deep and adherent to the panniculus carnosus, which extends posteromedially as a thin sloping sheet down to the buccal angle. There, its free border forms a crescentic, narrow, flexible, subcutaneous fibroelastic cord that accommodates the varying postures of the modioli, lips, mouth and jaws.

Modiolar movements

Controlled three-dimensional mobility of the modioli enables them to integrate the activities of the cheeks, lips and oral fissure, the oral vestibule and the jaws. Such activities include biting, chewing, drinking, sucking, swallowing, changes in vestibular contents and pressure, the innumerable subtle variations involved in speech, the modulation (and occasional generation) of musical tones, production of harsher sounds in shouting and screaming, crying, and all the permutations of facial expression, ranging from mere hints to gross distortion, symmetrical or asymmetrical. Major modiolar movements appear to involve many, if not all, of its associated muscles, and there is little value in considering the actions of the individual muscles in isolation. While the most obvious determinant of modiolar position and mobility is the balance between the forces exerted by muscles that are directly attached to it, another influential factor is the degree of separation or 'gape' between the upper and lower teeth. Starting from the occlusal position, and with the lips maintained in contact, the teeth can be separated by c.1.25 cm near the midline, and the mentolabial sulcus descends by a similar distance. With further separation the lips part, and as gape increases to its maximum, interlabial and interdental distances approach 4 cm, at which point the mentolabial sulcus has descended a further 2 cm. In this posture the modiolus has descended c.1 cm to lie over the interdental space, into which its basal and surrounding buccal mucosa projects a few millimetres, and its cornua diverge into their respective lips at an obtuse angle to each other, the dispositions of the modiolar muscles being correspondingly modified. The general hexagonal shape of the labial area changes as the mouth and jaws open progressively. In maximal opening, the distance between the superior and inferior boundaries has increased by 3–3.5 cm at the centre; the transverse distance between its lateral angles has decreased by c.1 cm and the angles are obtuse; the nasolabial sulci are longer, straighter and more vertical; and the inferior buccolabial sulci are less deep and curved. These soft tissue changes radiate from the bilateral modioli.

With the lips in contact and the teeth in tight occlusion, the modiolus can move a few millimetres in all directions. However, mobility is maximal when there is 2–3 mm clearance between the teeth: the apex of the modiolus may then move vertically upwards c.10 mm, downwards 5 mm, posterolaterally 10 mm, and anteromedially 10 mm, these movements occurring in the curved planes of the cheek and lips. Specific movements of the modiolus may occur to any point, and along any path, within the boundaries of the envelope of movement thus defined. When the mouth is opened wide, the modiolus becomes immobile. From the neutral position the modiolus may be displaced superficially along its apicobasal axis for up to 5–10 mm by liquids or solids in the vestibule, or by an increase in air pressure that 'balloons' the cheeks and lips.

Many activities take place in three phases. Initially, a particular modiolar muscle group becomes dominant over its antagonists and the modiolus is rapidly relocated. Next, the modiolus is transiently fixed in this new site by simultaneous contraction of modiolar muscles, principally zygomaticus major, levator anguli oris, depressor anguli oris, platysma pars modiolaris, and this provides a fixed base from which the main physiological effectors, buccinator and orbicularis oris, carry out their specific actions. These actions are usually integrated with partial separation or closure of the jaws, and with varying degrees of activity in the direct labial tractors. All these factors combine to determine the positions of the lips and oral fissure from moment to moment. Modiolar movements may be bilaterally symmetrical, unilateral or asymmetrical.

MUSCLES OF MASTICATION

Two muscles of mastication are to be seen on the face; masseter, which covers the ramus of the mandible and on which the parotid gland lies, and temporalis, which lies over the temporal fossa. These muscles are described in detail with the other main muscles of mastication on pages 519 and 520.

VASCULAR SUPPLY AND LYMPHATIC DRAINAGE

ARTERIAL SUPPLY TO THE FACE

The main arterial supply to the face is derived from the facial and superficial temporal arteries. Blood is also supplied by branches of the maxillary and ophthalmic arteries. The back of the scalp is supplied by the posterior auricular and occipital arteries. There are numerous anastomoses between the branches.

FACIAL ARTERY (Fig. 29.7)

The facial artery arises in the neck from the external carotid artery. It passes onto the face at the anteroinferior border of masseter (where its pulse can be felt as it crosses the mandible). It is superficial and at first lies beneath platysma. It is covered by skin, the fat of the cheek and, near the angle of the mouth, by zygomaticus major and risorius. It pursues a tortuous course – that presumably allows it to stretch when the face is distorted during jaw opening – by the side of the nose towards the medial corner of the eye. Buccinator and levator anguli oris lie deep to the facial artery, and it may pass over or through levator labii superioris. At its termination it is embedded in levator labii superioris alaequae nasi. Occasionally, the facial artery barely extends beyond the angle of the mouth, in which case its normal territory beyond this region is taken over by an enlarged transverse facial branch from the superficial temporal artery, and by branches from the contralateral facial artery. The facial vein is posterior, running a more direct course across the face. At the anterior border of masseter, the two vessels are in contact, but in the neck the vein is superficial. The facial artery supplies branches to the adjacent muscles and skin of the face. Its named branches on the face are the premasseteric artery, the superior and inferior labial arteries and the lateral nasal artery. The part of the artery distal to its terminal branch is called the angular artery.

Premasseteric artery – This small inconstant artery passes upwards along the anterior border of masseter and supplies the adjacent tissue.

Inferior labial artery – The inferior labial artery arises near the angle of the mouth, passes upwards and forwards under depressor anguli oris, penetrates orbicularis oris and runs sinuously near the margin of the lower lip, between the muscle and the mucous membrane. It supplies the inferior labial glands, mucous membrane and muscles, and anastomoses with its fellow of the opposite side and with the mental branch of the inferior alveolar artery.

Superior labial artery – Larger and more tortuous than the inferior labial artery, the superior labial artery has a similar course along the superior labial margin, between the mucous membrane and orbicularis oris. It anastomoses with its fellow of the opposite side, and supplies the upper

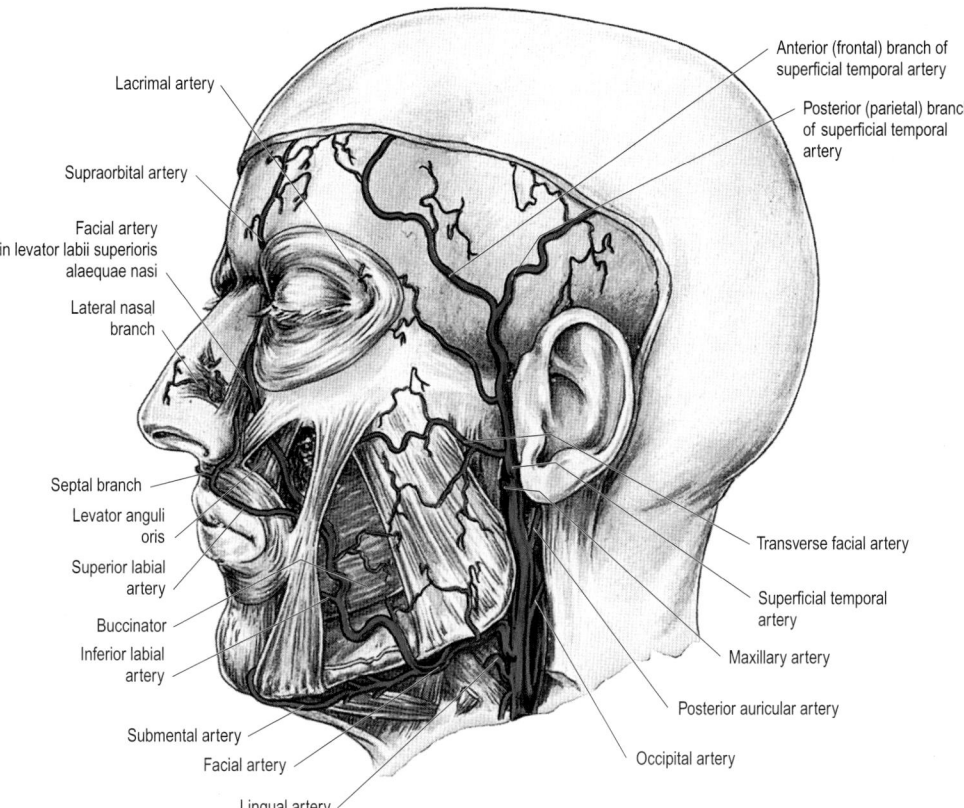

Fig. 29.7 The arteries of the left side of the face and their main branches.

Lacrimal artery

Supraorbital artery

Facial artery in levator labii superioris alaequae nasi

Lateral nasal branch

Septal branch

Levator anguli oris

Superior labial artery

Buccinator

Inferior labial artery

Submental artery

Facial artery

Lingual artery

Anterior (frontal) branch of superficial temporal artery

Posterior (parietal) branch of superficial temporal artery

Transverse facial artery

Superficial temporal artery

Maxillary artery

Posterior auricular artery

Occipital artery

lip. It gives off a septal branch, which ramifies anteroinferiorly in the nasal septum, and an alar branch.

Lateral nasal artery – This is given off by the side of the nose and supplies the dorsum and alae of nose, and anastomoses with its fellow of the opposite side. It may be replaced by a branch from the superior labial artery.

SUPERFICIAL TEMPORAL ARTERY (Fig. 29.7)
This is the smaller terminal branch of the external carotid artery. It arises in the parotid gland behind the neck of the mandible, where it is crossed by temporal and zygomatic branches of the facial nerve. Initially deep, it becomes superficial as it passes over the posterior root of the zygomatic process of the temporal bone, where its pulse can be felt. It then runs up the scalp for c.4cm and divides into frontal (anterior) and parietal (posterior) branches. It is accompanied by corresponding veins, and the auriculotemporal nerve lies just posterior to it. The superficial temporal artery supplies skin and muscles at the side of the face and in the scalp, the parotid gland and the temporo-mandibular joint. Its named branches are the transverse facial, auricular, zygomatico-orbital, middle temporal, frontal and parietal arteries. There are variations in the relative sizes of the frontal, parietal and transverse facial branches, in that the frontal and parietal branches may be absent, and the transverse facial may replace a shortened transverse facial artery.

Transverse facial artery – The transverse facial artery arises before the superficial temporal artery emerges from the parotid gland. It traverses the gland, crosses masseter between the parotid duct and the zygomatic arch (accompanied by one or two facial nerve branches) and divides into numerous branches that supply the parotid gland and duct, masseter and adjacent skin. The branches anastomose with the facial, masseteric, buccal, lacrimal and infraorbital arteries, and may have a direct origin from the external carotid artery.

Auricular artery – The branches of the auricular artery are distributed to the lobule and lateral surface of the auricle and the external acoustic meatus.

Zygomatico-orbital artery – The zygomatico-orbital artery may arise independently from the superficial temporal artery or from its middle temporal or parietal branches. It runs close to the upper border of the zygomatic arch, between the two layers of temporal fascia, to the lateral orbital angle. It supplies orbicularis oculi and anastomoses with the lacrimal and palpebral branches of the ophthalmic artery. A well-developed zygomatico-orbital artery is associated with a delayed division into frontal and parietal branches.

Middle temporal artery – The middle temporal artery arises just above the zygomatic arch and perforates the temporal fascia to supply temporalis. It anastomoses with the deep temporal branches of the maxillary artery.

Frontal (anterior) branch – The artery passes upwards towards the frontal tuberosity and supplies adjacent muscles, skin and pericranium in this region. It anastomoses with its fellow of the opposite side and with the supraorbital and supratrochlear branches of the ophthalmic artery.

Parietal (posterior) branch – The parietal branch is larger than the frontal branch of the superficial temporal artery, and curves upwards and back-wards. It remains superficial to the temporal fascia, and anastomoses with its fellow of the opposite side and with the posterior auricular and occipital arteries.

Facial branches of the maxillary artery
The maxillary artery is the larger of the two terminal branches of the external carotid artery, and has three branches that supply the face, namely the mental, buccal and infraorbital arteries.

Mental artery – The mental artery arises from the first part of the maxillary artery as a terminal branch of the inferior alveolar artery. It emerges onto the face from the mandibular canal at the mental foramen,

and supplies muscles and skin in the chin region. The mental artery anastomoses with the inferior labial and submental arteries.

Buccal artery – The buccal artery is a branch of the second part of the maxillary artery. It emerges onto the face from the infratemporal fossa and crosses buccinator to supply the cheek. The buccal artery anastomoses with the infraorbital artery and with branches of the facial artery.

Infraorbital artery – The infraorbital artery arises from the third part of the maxillary artery. It runs through the infraorbital foramen and onto the face, supplying the lower eyelid, the lateral aspect of the nose and the upper lip. The infraorbital artery has extensive anastomoses with the transverse facial and buccal arteries and branches of the ophthalmic and facial arteries.

Facial branches of the ophthalmic artery
The ophthalmic artery is a branch of the internal carotid artery. Its supra-trochlear, supraorbital, lacrimal, medial palpebral, dorsal nasal and external nasal branches supply the face.

Supratrochlear artery – The supratrochlear artery emerges from the orbit onto the face at the frontal notch. It supplies the medial parts of the upper eyelid, forehead and scalp. The supratrochlear artery anastomoses with the supraorbital artery and with its contralateral fellow.

Supraorbital artery – The supraorbital artery leaves the orbit through the supraorbital notch (or foramen). It divides into superficial and deep branches, supplying skin and muscle of the upper eyelid, forehead and scalp. It anastomoses with the supratrochlear artery, frontal branch of the superficial temporal and its contralateral fellow. At the supraorbital margin it often sends a branch to the diploë of the frontal bone and may also supply the mucoperiosteum in the frontal sinus.

Lacrimal artery – The lacrimal artery appears on the face at the upper lateral corner of the orbit and supplies the lateral part of the eyelids. Within the orbit, it gives off a zygomatic artery which subdivides into zygomaticofacial and zygomaticotemporal arteries. The zygomaticofacial artery passes through the lateral wall of the orbit to emerge onto the face at the zygomaticofacial foramen, and supplies the region overlying the prominence of the cheek. The zygomaticotemporal artery also passes through the lateral wall of the orbit, via the zygomaticotemporal foramen, to supply the skin over the non-beard part of the temple. The lacrimal artery anastomoses with the deep temporal branch of the maxillary artery and the transverse facial branch of the superficial temporal artery.

Medial palpebral arteries – Superior and inferior medial palpebral arteries arise from the ophthalmic artery below the trochlea. They descend behind the nasolacrimal sac to enter the eyelids where each divides into two branches that course laterally along the edges of the tarsal plates to form the superior and inferior arches, and supply the eyelids. They anastomose with branches of the supraorbital, zygomatico-orbital and lacrimal arteries. The inferior arch also anastomoses with the facial artery.

External (dorsal) nasal artery – The external nasal artery is a terminal branch of the anterior ethmoidal artery from the ophthalmic artery. It supplies skin on the external nose, and emerges at the junction of the nasal bone and the lateral nasal cartilage.

Occipital artery
The occipital artery runs in a groove on the temporal bone, medial to the mastoid process. It arises in the neck from the external carotid artery, and enters the back of the scalp by piercing the investing layer of deep cervical fascia connecting the cranial attachments of trapezius and sternocleidomastoid, accompanied by the greater occipital nerve. Tortuous branches run between the skin and the occipital belly of occipitofrontalis, anastomosing with the opposite occipital, posterior auricular and superficial temporal arteries as well as the transverse cervical branch of the subclavian artery. They supply the occipital belly of occipitofrontalis and skin and pericranium associated with the scalp as far forward as the vertex. There may be a meningeal lateral branch, traversing the parietal foramen.

Posterior auricular artery

The posterior auricular artery arises in the neck from the external carotid artery, ascends between the auricle and mastoid process and gives off an auricular branch supplying the cranial surface of the auricle and an occipital branch to supply the occipital belly of occipitofrontalis and the scalp behind and above the auricle. The posterior auricular artery anastomoses with the occipital artery.

VEINS OF THE FACE (Fig. 29.8)

The veins of the face are subject to considerable variations, and therefore the following description concerns those which are relatively constant.

Supratrochlear vein

The supratrochlear vein starts on the forehead from a venous network connected to the frontal tributaries of the superficial temporal vein. Veins from this network form a single trunk, descending near the midline parallel with its fellow to the bridge of the nose. Each vein is joined by a nasal arch across the nose. The veins then diverge, each joining a supraorbital vein to form the facial vein near the medial canthus of the eye.

Supraorbital vein

The supraorbital vein begins near the zygomatic process of the frontal bone, connecting with branches of the superficial and middle temporal veins. It passes medially above the orbital opening, pierces the orbicularis oculi and unites with the supratrochlear vein near the medial canthus of the eye to form the facial vein. A branch passes through the supraorbital notch to connect with the superior ophthalmic vein. In the notch it receives veins from the frontal sinus and frontal diploë.

Facial vein

The facial vein is the main vein of the face. After receiving the supratrochlear and supraorbital veins, it travels obliquely downwards by the side of the nose, passes under zygomaticus major, risorius and platysma, descends to the anterior border and then passes over the surface of masseter. It crosses the body of the mandible, and runs in the neck to drain into the internal jugular vein. The uppermost segment of the facial vein – above its junction with the superior labial vein – is also termed the angular vein. The facial vein initially lies behind the more tortuous facial artery, but crosses it at the lower border of the mandible.

The fact that the vein lacks valves and that it is connected with the cavernous sinus is of considerable clinical significance in terms of the spread of infection.

Tributaries – Near its origin, the facial vein connects with the superior ophthalmic vein, both directly and via the supraorbital vein, and so is linked to the cavernous sinus. The facial vein receives tributaries from the side of the nose and, below this, an important deep facial vein from the pterygoid venous plexus. It also receives the inferior palpebral, superior and inferior labial, buccinator, parotid and masseteric veins, and other tributaries which join it below the mandible.

Cavernous sinus thrombosis (See also Section 2 and intracranial venous sinuses) – Any spreading infection involving the cheek, upper lip, anterior nares or even an upper incisor or canine tooth can result in cavernous sinus thrombosis (p. 279).

Superficial temporal vein

The superficial temporal vein begins in a widespread network joined across the scalp to the contralateral vein and to the ipsilateral supratrochlear, supraorbital, posterior auricular and occipital veins that all drain the same network. Anterior and posterior tributaries unite above the zygomatic arch to form the superficial temporal vein. Accompanying its artery (behind in c.70% of cases), the vein crosses the posterior root of the zygoma and enters the parotid gland. Here, the superficial temporal vein joins the maxillary vein, to form the retromandibular vein.

Tributaries

The tributaries are the parotid veins, rami draining the temporomandibular joint, anterior auricular veins and the transverse facial vein. The middle temporal vein receives the orbital vein (formed by the lateral palpebral veins), and passes back between layers of temporal fascia, which it pierces to join the superficial temporal vein just above the level of the zygomatic arch.

Buccal, mental and infraorbital veins

The buccal, mental and infraorbital veins drain the cheek and chin regions and pass into the pterygoid venous plexus

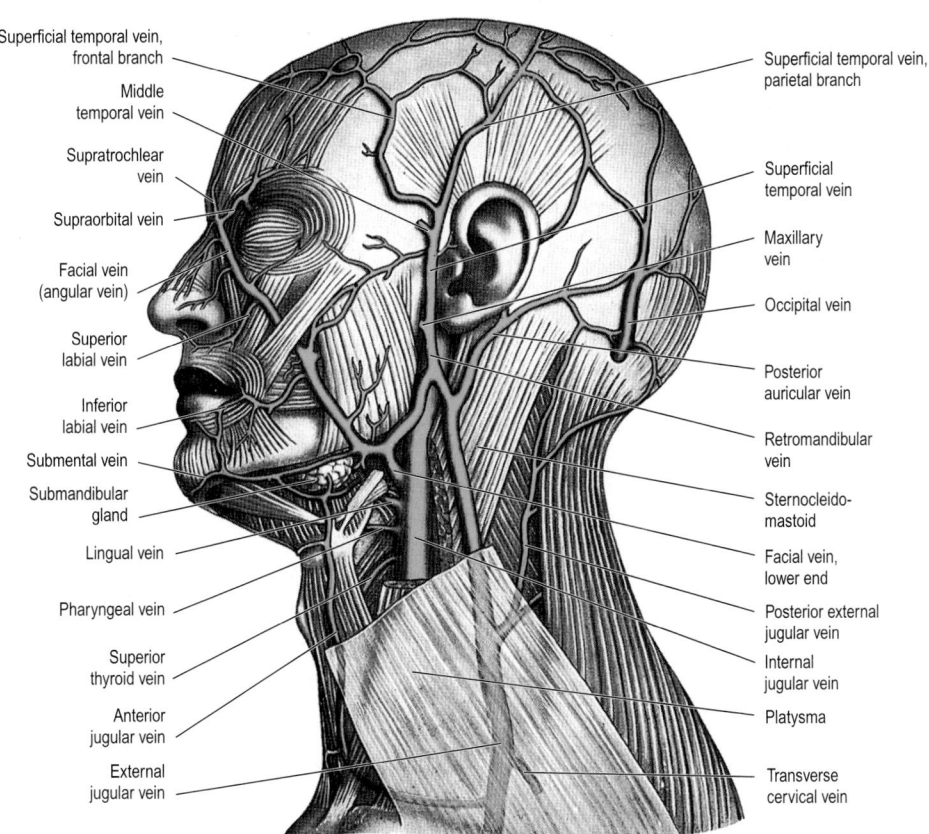

Fig. 29.8 The veins of the left side of the head and neck. Parts of the left sternocleidomastoid and platysma have been excised to expose the trunk of the internal jugular vein. The external jugular vein is visible through the lower part of platysma.

Superficial temporal vein, frontal branch
Middle temporal vein
Supratrochlear vein
Supraorbital vein
Facial vein (angular vein)
Superior labial vein
Inferior labial vein
Submental vein
Submandibular gland
Lingual vein
Pharyngeal vein
Superior thyroid vein
Anterior jugular vein
External jugular vein

Superficial temporal vein, parietal branch
Superficial temporal vein
Maxillary vein
Occipital vein
Posterior auricular vein
Retromandibular vein
Sternocleidomastoid
Facial vein, lower end
Posterior external jugular vein
Internal jugular vein
Platysma
Transverse cervical vein

Posterior auricular and occipital veins

The posterior auricular vein arises in a parieto-occipital network that also drains into tributaries of the occipital and superficial temporal veins. It descends behind the auricle to join the posterior division of the retromandibular vein in, or just below, the parotid gland, to form the external jugular vein. It receives a stylomastoid vein and tributaries from the cranial surface of the auricle, drains the region of the scalp behind the ear and drains into the external jugular vein. The occipital vein begins in a posterior network in the scalp, pierces the cranial attachment of trapezius, turns into the suboccipital triangle and joins the deep cervical and vertebral veins. It may be joined by a vein draining the diploë in the occipital bone and then passes to either the internal jugular, posterior auricular, deep cervical or vertebral veins. Emissary veins connect the occipital vein to the intracranial venous sinuses via the mastoid and parietal foramina and through the posterior condylar canal and occipital protuberances.

LYMPHATIC DRAINAGE OF THE FACE AND SCALP (Fig. 31.1)

Lymph vessels from the frontal region above the root of the nose drain to the submandibular nodes. Vessels from the rest of the forehead, temporal region, upper half of the lateral auricular aspect and anterior wall of the external acoustic meatus drain to the superficial parotid nodes, just anterior to the tragus, on or deep to the parotid fascia. These nodes also drain lateral vessels from the eyelids and skin of the zygomatic region. Their efferent vessels pass to the upper deep cervical nodes. A strip of scalp above the auricle, the upper half of the cranial aspect and margin of the auricle, and the posterior wall of the external acoustic meatus all drain to the upper deep cervical and retroauricular nodes. The retroauricular nodes, superficial to the mastoid attachment of sternocleidomastoid and deep to auricularis posterior, drain to the upper deep cervical nodes. The auricular lobule, floor of the external acoustic meatus and skin over the mandibular angle and lower parotid region are drained to the superficial cervical or upper deep cervical nodes. Superficial cervical nodes spread along the external jugular vein superficial to sternocleidomastoid. Some efferents pass round the anterior border of sternocleidomastoid to the upper deep cervical nodes; others follow the external jugular vein to the lower deep cervical nodes in the subclavian triangle.

The occipital region of the scalp is drained partly to the occipital nodes, and partly by a vessel that runs along the posterior border of sternocleidomastoid to the lower deep cervical nodes. Occipital nodes are commonly superficial to the upper attachment of trapezius, but occasionally lie in the superior angle of the posterior triangle.

There are usually three submandibular nodes, internal to the deep cervical fascia in the submandibular triangle. There is one at the anterior pole of the submandibular gland, and two flanking the facial artery as it reaches the mandible. Other nodes are often embedded in the gland or deep to it. Submandibular nodes drain a wide area, including vessels from the submental, buccal and lingual groups of nodes and their efferents pass to the upper and lower deep cervical nodes. The external nose, cheek, upper lip and lateral parts of the lower lip drain directly to the submandibular nodes; the afferent vessels may have a few buccal nodes along their course and near the facial vein. The mucous membrane of the lips and cheek drains to the submandibular nodes and the lateral part of the cheek drains to the parotid nodes.

The central part of the lower lip, buccal floor and tip of the tongue drain to the submental nodes on mylohyoid between the anterior bellies of the digastric muscles. They receive afferents from both sides, some decussate across the chin, and their efferents pass to the submandibular and jugulo-omohyoid nodes.

INNERVATION OF THE FACE AND SCALP

The numerous muscles of facial expression are supplied by the facial nerve, while the two muscles of mastication that relate to the face are innervated by the mandibular division of the trigeminal nerve. The sensory innervation is primarily from the three divisions of the mandibular nerve, with smaller contributions from the cervical spinal nerves. The detailed innervation of the auricle is considered on page 651.

TRIGEMINAL NERVE

Three large areas of the face can be mapped out to indicate the peripheral nerve fields associated with the three divisions of the trigeminal nerve. The fields are not horizontal but curve upwards (**Fig. 29.9A**), apparently because the facial skin moves upwards with growth of the brain and skull. Embryologically, each division of the trigeminal nerve is associated with a developing facial process which gives rise to a specific area of the face in the adult. Thus the ophthalmic nerve is associated with the frontonasal process, the maxillary nerve with the maxillary process and the mandibular nerve with the mandibular process.

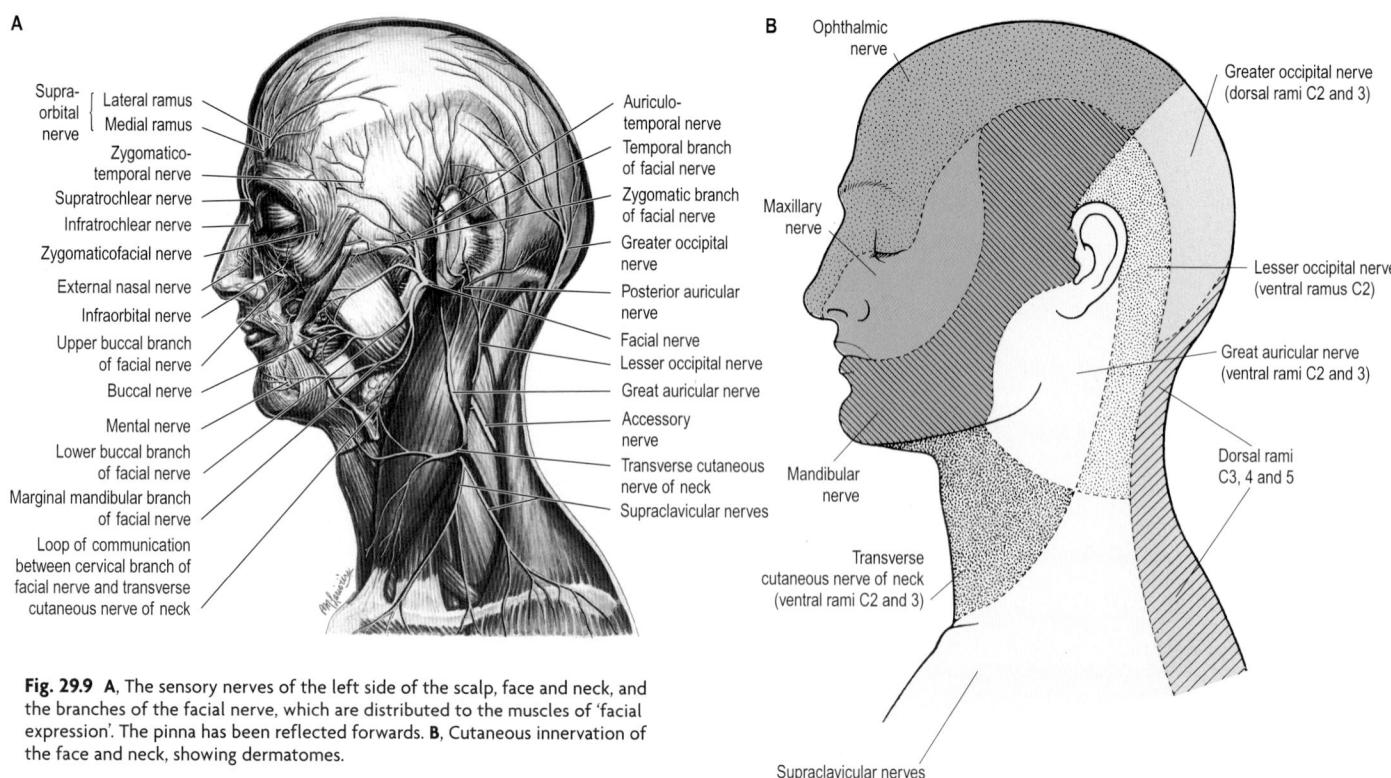

Fig. 29.9 A, The sensory nerves of the left side of the scalp, face and neck, and the branches of the facial nerve, which are distributed to the muscles of 'facial expression'. The pinna has been reflected forwards. **B**, Cutaneous innervation of the face and neck, showing dermatomes.

Ophthalmic nerve (Fig. 29.9B)

The cutaneous branches of the ophthalmic nerve supply the conjunctiva, skin over the forehead, upper eyelid and much of the external surface of the nose.

Supratrochlear nerve

The supratrochlear nerve is the smaller terminal branch of the frontal nerve. It runs anteromedially in the roof of the orbit, passes above the trochlea, and supplies a descending filament to the infratrochlear branch of the nasociliary nerve. The nerve emerges between the trochlea and the supraorbital foramen at the frontal notch, curves up on the forehead close to the bone with the supratrochlear artery and supplies the conjunctiva and the skin of the upper eyelid. It then ascends beneath the corrugator and the frontal belly of occipitofrontalis before dividing into branches which pierce these muscles to supply the skin of the lower forehead near the midline.

Supraorbital nerve

The supraorbital nerve is the larger terminal branch of the frontal nerve. It traverses the supraorbital notch or foramen and supplies palpebral filaments to the upper eyelid and conjunctiva. It ascends on the forehead with the supraorbital artery, and divides into medial and lateral branches, which supply the skin of the scalp nearly as far back as the lambdoid suture. These branches are at first deep to the frontal belly of the occipitofrontalis. The medial branch perforates the muscle to reach the skin, while the lateral pierces the epicranial aponeurosis.

Lacrimal nerve

The lacrimal nerve is the smallest of the main ophthalmic branches and pierces the orbital septum to end in the lateral region of the upper eyelid, which it supplies. It joins filaments of the facial nerve. Occasionally it is absent, in which case it is replaced by the zygomaticotemporal nerve: the relationship is reciprocal, and when the zygomaticotemporal nerve is absent it is replaced by a branch of the lacrimal nerve.

Infratrochlear nerve

The infratrochlear nerve branches from the nasociliary nerve. It leaves the orbit below the trochlea and supplies the skin of the eyelids, the conjunctiva, lacrimal sac, lacrimal caruncle and the side of the nose above the medial canthus.

External nasal nerve (Fig. 29.9A,B)

The external nasal nerve is the terminal branch of the anterior ethmoidal nerve. It descends through the lateral wall of the nose, and supplies the skin of the nose below the nasal bones, excluding the alar portion around the external nares.

Maxillary nerve

The maxillary nerve passes through the orbit to supply the skin of the lower eyelid, the prominence of the cheek, the alar part of the nose, part of the temple, and the upper lip. It has three cutaneous branches, namely the zygomaticotemporal, zygomaticofacial and infraorbital nerves.

Zygomaticotemporal nerve

The zygomaticotemporal nerve is a terminal branch of the zygomatic nerve. It traverses a canal in the zygomatic bone to emerge into the anterior part of the temporal fossa, ascends between the bone and temporalis and finally pierces the temporal fascia c.2 cm above the zygomatic arch to supply the skin of the temple. It communicates with the facial and auriculotemporal nerves. As it pierces the deep layer of the temporal fascia it sends a slender twig between the two layers of the fascia towards the lateral angle of the eye. This lacrimal ramus conveys parasympathetic postganglionic fibres from the pterygopalatine ganglion to the lacrimal gland.

Zygomaticofacial nerve

The zygomaticofacial nerve is a terminal branch of the zygomatic nerve. It traverses the inferolateral angle of the orbit, and emerges on the face through a foramen in the zygomatic bone. It next perforates orbicularis oculi to supply the skin on the prominence of the cheek. It forms a plexus with zygomatic branches of the facial nerve and palpebral branches of the maxillary nerve. Occasionally the nerve is absent.

Infraorbital nerve

The infraorbital nerve emerges onto the face at the infraorbital foramen, where it lies between levator labii superioris and levator anguli oris. It divides into three further groups of branches. The palpebral branches ascend deep to orbicularis oculi, and pierce the muscle to supply the skin in the lower eyelid and join with the facial and zygomaticofacial nerves near the lateral canthus. Nasal branches supply the skin of the side of the nose and of the movable part of the nasal septum, and join the external nasal branch of the anterior ethmoidal nerve. Superior labial branches, large and numerous, descend behind levator labii superioris, to supply the skin of the anterior part of the cheek and upper lip. They are joined by branches from the facial nerve to form the infraorbital plexus.

Mandibular nerve

The mandibular nerve supplies skin over the mandible, the lower lip, the fleshy part of the cheek, part of the auricle of the ear and part of the temple via the buccal, mental and auriculotemporal nerves.

Buccal nerve

The buccal nerve emerges onto the face from behind the ramus of the mandible and passes laterally in front of the masseter to unite with the buccal branches of the facial nerve. It supplies the skin over the anterior part of buccinator.

Mental nerve

The mental nerve is the terminal branch of the inferior alveolar nerve. It enters the face through the mental foramen, where it is directed backwards. It supplies the skin of the lower lip.

Auriculotemporal nerve

The auriculotemporal nerve emerges onto the face behind the temporomandibular joint within the superior surface of the parotid gland. It ascends posterior to the superficial temporal vessels, over the posterior root of the zygoma, and divides into superficial temporal branches. The cutaneous branches of the auriculotemporal nerve supply the tragus and part of the adjoining auricle of the ear and the posterior part of the temple. It communicates with the facial nerve, usually by two rami that pass anterolaterally behind the neck of the mandible. The communications with the temporofacial division of the facial nerve anchor the facial nerve close to the lateral surface of the condylar process of the mandible, limiting its mobility during surgery. Communications with the temporal and zygomatic branches loop around the transverse facial and superficial temporal vessels.

FACIAL NERVE

The facial nerve emerges from the base of the skull at the stylomastoid foramen. At this point the facial nerve lies c.9 mm from the posterior belly of the digastric muscle and 11 mm from the bony external acoustic meatus. It gains access to the face by passing through the substance of the parotid gland. Although mainly motor, there are some cutaneous fibres from the facial nerve which accompany the auricular branch of the vagus and which probably innervate the skin on both auricular aspects, in the conchal depression and over its eminence.

Close to the stylomastoid foramen the facial nerve gives off the posterior auricular nerve, which supplies the occipital belly of occipitofrontalis, and some of the auricular muscles, and the nerves to the posterior belly of digastric and stylohyoid. The nerve then enters the parotid gland high up on the posteromedial surface and passes forwards and downwards behind the mandibular ramus. Within the substance of the gland the facial nerve branches into the temporofacial and cervicofacial trunks, just behind (within c.5 mm) the retromandibular vein. In c.90% of cases, the two trunks lie superficial to the vein, in intimate contact with it. Occasionally the trunks pass beneath the retromandibular vein (temporofacial trunk c.9%; cervicofacial trunk c.2%). The trunks branch further to form a parotid plexus (pes anserinus), which exhibits variations in branching pattern. Five main terminal branches arise from the plexus and diverge within the gland. They leave the parotid gland by its anteromedial surface, medial to its anterior margin and supply the muscles of facial expression.

The temporal branches are generally multiple and pass across the zygomatic arch to the temple to supply intrinsic muscles on the lateral surface of the auricle, and the anterior and superior auricular muscles. They join with the zygomaticotemporal branch of the maxillary nerve and the auriculotemporal branch of the mandibular nerve. The more anterior branches supply the frontal belly of occipitofrontalis, orbicularis oculi and corrugator and join the supraorbital and lacrimal branches of the ophthalmic nerve.

Zygomatic branches are generally multiple and cross the zygomatic bone to the lateral canthus of the eye, to supply the orbicularis oculi and join filaments of the lacrimal nerve and zygomaticofacial branch of the maxillary nerve. The branches may also help supply muscles associated with the buccal branch of the facial nerve.

The buccal branch has a variable origin and passes horizontally to a distribution below the orbit and around the mouth. It is usually single, but two branches occur in 15% of cases. The buccal branch has a close relationship to the parotid duct, and usually lies below it. Superficial branches run deep to subcutaneous fat and the superficial musculo-aponeurotic system (SMAS) (p. 499). Some branches pass deep to procerus and join the infratrochlear and external nasal nerves. Upper deep branches pass under zygomaticus major and levator labii superioris, supply them and form an infraorbital plexus with the superior labial branches of the infraorbital nerve. They also supply levator anguli oris, zygomaticus minor, levator labii superioris alaeque nasi and the small nasal muscles. These branches are sometimes described as lower zygomatic branches. Lower deep branches supply the buccinator and orbicularis oris, and join filaments of the buccal branch of the mandibular nerve.

The marginal mandibular branches, of which there are usually two, run forwards towards the angle of the mandible under platysma, at first superficial to the upper part of the digastric triangle, then turning up and forwards across the body of the mandible to pass under depressor anguli oris. The branches supply risorius and the muscles of the lower lip and chin, and join the mental nerve. The marginal mandibular branch has an important surgical relationship with the lower border of the mandible, and may pass below the lower border with a reported incidence varying between 20% and 50%, the furthest distance being 1.2 cm.

The cervical branch issues from the lower part of the parotid gland and runs anteroinferiorly under platysma to the front of the neck, to supply platysma and communicate with the transverse cutaneous cervical nerve. In 20% of cases, there are two branches.

The peripheral branches of the facial nerve described above are joined by anastomotic arcades between adjacent branches to form the parotid plexus of nerves which shows considerable variation. In surgical terms these anastomoses are important, and presumably explain why accidental or essential division of a small branch often fails to result in the expected facial nerve weakness. Six distinctive anastomotic patterns were originally classified by Davis et al (1956) and these are illustrated in **Fig. 29.10**. These observations have been confirmed by others, although some variation in the frequency has been reported.

Surgery of the facial nerve

When operating on the face, a detailed understanding of the anatomy of the facial nerve is essential if iatrogenic trauma is to be avoided. Three surgical manoeuvres are used to identify the facial nerve trunk as it exits the stylomastoid foramen. The blood-free plane immediately in front of the cartilaginous external acoustic meatus can be opened up by blunt dissection, and this leads the surgeon to the skull bases just superficial to the styloid process and the stylomastoid foramen. This plane can then be gently opened up in an inferior direction by further blunt dissection until the trunk of the facial nerve is encountered. Second, the trunk of the facial nerve can be identified by exposing the anterior border of sternocleidomastoid just below its insertion into the mastoid process, and retracting the muscle posteriorly to expose the posterior belly of digastric, which is then traced upwards and backwards to the mastoid process. This point lies immediately below the stylomastoid foramen and the facial nerve trunk. A third option is to identify a terminal branch of the facial nerve peripherally – commonly the marginal mandibular branch – and to trace it back centripetally until the facial nerve trunk is identified.

Complications of facial nerve dissection

The facial nerve is routinely dissected as part of a superficial parotid-ectomy operation – typically in the treatment of parotid tumours – in

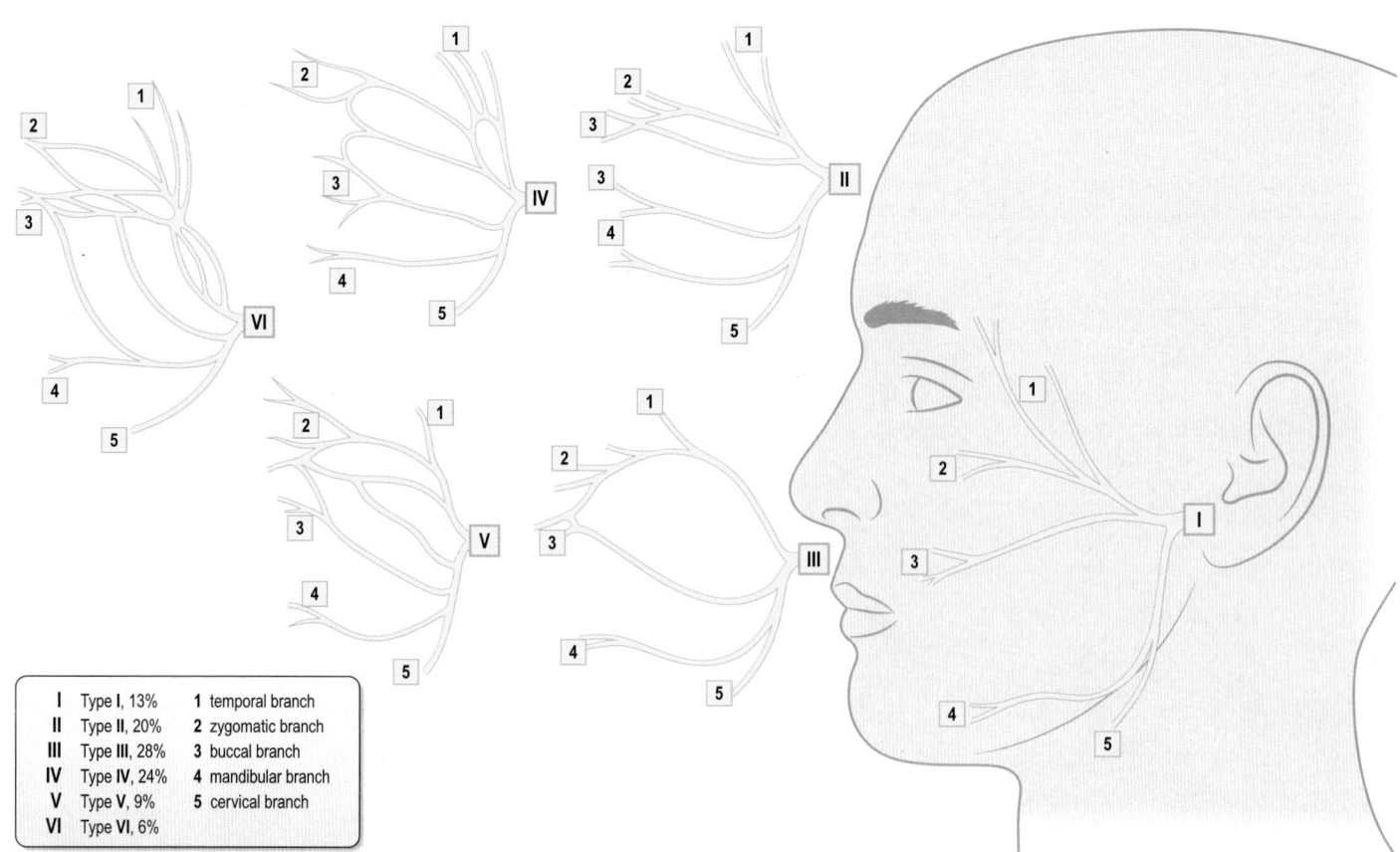

I	Type I, 13%	1	temporal branch
II	Type II, 20%	2	zygomatic branch
III	Type III, 28%	3	buccal branch
IV	Type IV, 24%	4	mandibular branch
V	Type V, 9%	5	cervical branch
VI	Type VI, 6%		

Fig. 29.10 Pattern of branching of the facial nerve. (Modified with permission from Berkovitz BKB, Moxham BJ 2002 Head and Neck Anatomy. London: Martin Dunitz, and from Davis RA, Anson BJ, Budinger JM, Kurth IE 1956 Surgical anatomy of the facial nerve and parotid gland based upon a study of 350 cervicofacial halves. Surg Gynecol Obstet 102: 385–412, with permission from the American College of Surgeons.)

which that part of the gland lying superficial to the plane of the facial nerve is removed. Although all branches of the facial nerve are preserved, there is often some postoperative facial weakness caused by bruising and ischaemia of the nerve which results in a temporary and reversible demyelination of the nerve fibres. Although this can affect all the branches of the facial nerve, the weakness is often confined to the territory innervated by the marginal mandibular branch and is manifested by a weakness of the lower lip on the affected side. This is because anastomotic arcades between the marginal mandibular branch and other branches of the facial nerve are relatively rare, whereas they are plentiful between the various branches of the temporofacial division and the buccal branch of the cervicofacial division of the facial nerve.

Facial nerve lesions

Facial nerve paralysis may be due to an upper motor neurone lesion (when frontalis is partially spared due to the bilateral innervation of the muscle of the upper part of the face), or a lower motor neurone lesion (when all branches may be involved). Bell's palsy and acoustic neuromas can produce a complete lower motor neurone facial paralysis as a result of compression of the facial nerve trunk as it passes through the middle ear. More commonly, cheek lacerations or malignant parotid tumours result in weakness in part of the face depending upon which branch of the nerve is involved. Unfortunately the presence of facial paralysis is not a reliable diagnostic sign of a malignant tumour. It is not uncommon for a facial nerve infiltrated by a malignant tumour to continue to function normally. However when paralysis does accompany a parotid mass it is certainly malignant.

CERVICAL SPINAL NERVES (Fig. 29.9A,B)

Cervical spinal nerves have cutaneous branches which supply areas of skin in the face and scalp. The named branches are the great auricular, lesser occipital and greater occipital nerves.

Great auricular nerve

The great auricular nerve forms part of the cervical plexus (p. 555) and is derived from the anterior primary rami of the second and third cervical spinal nerves. It passes up from the neck, lying on sternocleidomastoid, towards the angle of the jaw, and supplies much of the lower part of the auricle of the ear, and skin overlying the parotid gland.

Lesser occipital nerve

The lesser occipital nerve is a branch of the cervical plexus (p. 555). It ascends along the posterior border of sternocleidomastoid to supply the scalp above and behind the ear and a small area on the cranial surface of the auricle.

Greater occipital nerve

The greater occipital nerve represents the posterior primary ramus of the second cervical spinal nerve. It pierces trapezius close to its attachment to the superior nuchal line and ascends to supply the skin of the back of the scalp up to the vertex of the skull. Greater occipital neuralgia is a syndrome of pain and paraesthesiae felt in the distribution of the greater occipital nerve and is usually due to an entrapment neuropathy of the nerve as it pierces the attachment of the neck extensors to the occiput.

PAROTID SALIVARY GLAND

The paired parotid glands are the largest of the salivary glands. Each has an average weight of c.25 g and is an irregular, lobulated, yellowish mass, lying largely below the external acoustic meatus between the mandible and sternocleidomastoid. The gland also projects forwards on the surface of masseter (**Fig. 33.37**). In c.20% of cases, a small, usually detached, part called the accessory parotid gland (pars accessoria or socia parotidis) lies between the zygomatic arch above and the parotid duct below.

The overall shape of the parotid gland is variable. Viewed laterally, in c.50% of cases it is roughly triangular in outline. However in c.30% of cases the gland is more or less of even width throughout, and the upper and lower poles are rounded.

In its usual inverted pyramidal form, the parotid gland presents a small superior surface, and superficial, anteromedial and posteromedial surfaces. It tapers inferiorly to a blunt apex.

The concave superior surface is related to the cartilaginous part of the external acoustic meatus and posterior aspect of the temporomandibular joint. Here the auriculotemporal nerve curves round the neck of the mandible, embedded in the capsule of the gland. The apex overlaps the posterior belly of digastric and the carotid triangle to a variable extent.

The superficial surface is covered by skin and superficial fascia, which contains the facial branches of the great auricular nerve, superficial parotid lymph nodes and the posterior border of platysma. It extends upwards to the zygomatic arch, backwards to overlap sternocleidomastoid, downwards to its apex posteroinferior to the mandibular angle, and forwards to lie on masseter below the parotid duct.

The anteromedial surface (**Fig. 29.11**) is grooved by the posterior border of the mandibular ramus. It covers the posteroinferior part of masseter, the lateral aspect of the temporomandibular joint and the adjoining part of the mandibular ramus. It passes forwards, medial to the ramus of the mandible, to reach medial pterygoid. The gland may therefore be subdivided into a larger superficial part and a smaller part deep to the ramus, the two being joined by an isthmus. Branches of the facial nerve emerge on the face from the anterior margin of this surface.

The posteromedial surface is moulded to the mastoid process, sternocleidomastoid, posterior belly of the digastric, and the styloid process and its associated muscles. The external carotid artery grooves this surface before entering the gland, and the internal carotid artery and internal jugular vein are separated from the gland by the styloid process and its associated muscles (**Fig. 29.12**). The anteromedial and posteromedial surfaces meet at a medial margin that may project so deeply that it contacts the lateral wall of the pharynx.

Deep lobe tumours

Although it comprises only a small component of the parotid gland, the deep 'lobe' of the gland extends behind the mandibular ramus, where its deep surface lies immediately lateral to the superior constrictor of the pharynx. When a parotid tumour, either benign or malignant, occurs in the deep 'lobe', the mass presents as a swelling in the lateral wall of the pharynx and not as a facial swelling, which means that it is important to examine the oropharynx when following-up a patient who has undergone parotid surgery for the removal of a tumour.

STRUCTURES WITHIN THE PAROTID GLAND

The external carotid artery, retromandibular vein and facial nerve, either in part or in whole, traverse the gland and branch within it. The external

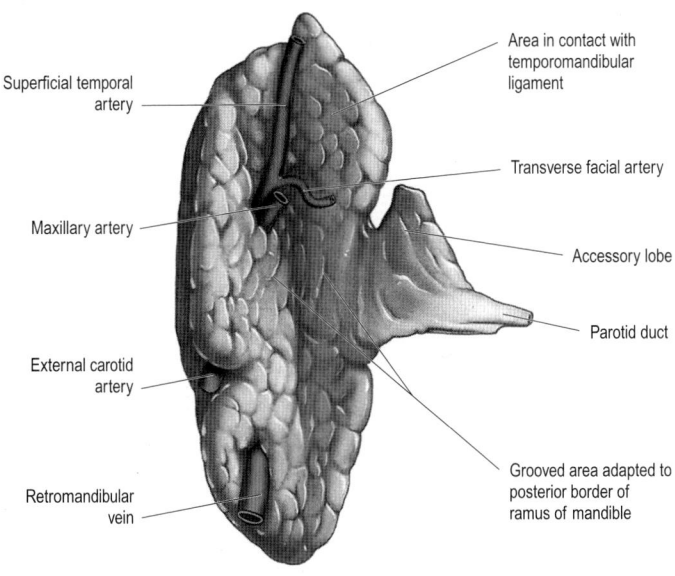

Superficial temporal artery

Maxillary artery

External carotid artery

Retromandibular vein

Area in contact with temporomandibular ligament

Transverse facial artery

Accessory lobe

Parotid duct

Grooved area adapted to posterior border of ramus of mandible

Fig. 29.11 The left parotid gland: anteromedial aspect.

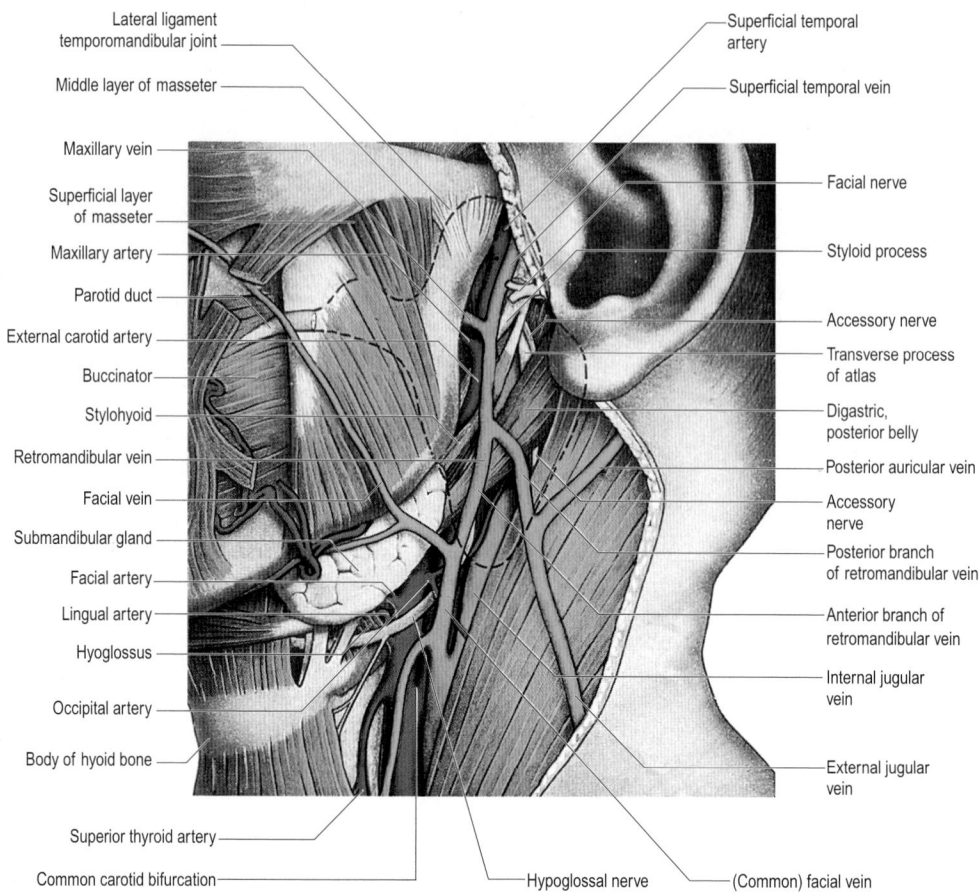

Lateral ligament
temporomandibular joint

Middle layer of masseter

Maxillary vein

Superficial layer
of masseter

Maxillary artery

Parotid duct

External carotid artery

Buccinator

Stylohyoid

Retromandibular vein

Facial vein

Submandibular gland

Facial artery

Lingual artery

Hyoglossus

Occipital artery

Body of hyoid bone

Superior thyroid artery

Common carotid bifurcation

Superficial temporal
artery

Superficial temporal vein

Facial nerve

Styloid process

Accessory nerve

Transverse process
of atlas

Digastric,
posterior belly

Posterior auricular vein

Accessory
nerve

Posterior branch
of retromandibular vein

Anterior branch of
retromandibular vein

Internal jugular
vein

External jugular
vein

Hypoglossal nerve

(Common) facial vein

Fig. 29.12 The principal immediate deep relations of the parotid gland. The outline of the parotid gland is indicated by the interrupted black line.

carotid artery enters the posteromedial surface, and divides into the maxillary artery, which emerges from the anteromedial surface, and the superficial temporal artery which gives off its transverse facial branch in the gland and ascends to leave its upper limit (**Figs 29.11, 29.12**). The posterior auricular artery may also branch from the external carotid artery within the gland, leaving by its posteromedial surface.

The retromandibular vein (**Fig. 29.12**), formed by the union of the maxillary and superficial temporal veins (which enter near the points of exit of the corresponding arteries), is superficial to the external carotid artery. It descends in the parotid gland and emerges behind the apex of the gland, where it usually divides into two branches. An anterior branch passes forwards to join the facial vein while a posterior branch joins the posterior auricular vein to form the external jugular vein. Occasionally it is not connected to the external jugular vein, which is then small, and the anterior jugular vein is often enlarged. The retromandibular vein is invariably of a reasonable size and is an important landmark for the facial nerve.

Parotid capsule

The parotid gland is enclosed within an unyielding parotid capsule, the deep part of which is derived from the investing layer of deep cervical fascia (p. 499). Any inflammation or tension within the parotid gland can cause an exquisite pain just in front of the temporomandibular joint. This is caused by stretching of the capsule and stimulation of the great auricular nerve. The pain is usually exacerbated at mealtimes when the gustatory stimulus to the gland results in further turgor within the capsule, and is seen routinely in patients suffering from mumps or with parotid duct obstruction.

Parotid duct (Figs 29.11, 29.12, 33.37)

The parotid duct begins by the confluence of two main tributaries within the anterior part of the gland. It appears at the anterior border of the upper part of the gland and passes horizontally across masseter, approximately at the level midway between the angle of the mouth and

the zygomatic arch. If the duct arises lower down, it may run obliquely upwards. It crosses masseter and turns medially at its anterior border at almost a right angle to traverse the buccal fat pad and buccinator opposite the crown of the upper third molar tooth. The duct then runs obliquely forwards for a short distance between buccinator and the oral mucosa before it opens upon a small papilla opposite the second upper molar crown. While crossing masseter it can receive the accessory parotid duct and lies between the upper and lower buccal branches of the facial nerve. The accessory part of the gland and the transverse facial artery lie above the parotid duct. The buccal branch of the mandibular nerve, emerging from beneath temporalis and masseter, is just below the duct at the anterior border of masseter. The parotid duct may be crossed by anastomosing branches between the zygomatic and buccal branches of the facial nerve. The duct is c.5 cm long and its lumen is c.3 mm wide (although narrower at its oral orifice).

The ramifications of the ductal systems, and their patterns and calibres, can be demonstrated radiographically by injecting a radio-opaque substance into the parotid duct via a cannula. The parotid duct as seen in a lateral sialogram (**Fig. 29.13**) and is formed near the centre of the posterior border of the mandibular ramus by the union of two or three ducts which ascend and descend respectively at right angles to the main duct. As it crosses the face, the main duct also receives from above five or six ductules from the accessory parotid gland. As it curves round the anterior border of the masseter muscle it is often compressed and its shadow is attenuated.

VASCULAR SUPPLY AND LYMPHATIC DRAINAGE

The arterial supply to the parotid gland is from the external carotid artery and its branches within and near the gland. The veins drain to the external jugular vein via local tributaries.

Lymph nodes are found both in the skin overlying the parotid gland (preauricular nodes) and in the substance of the parotid gland itself. There are usually 10 lymph nodes present in the gland. The majority are found in the superficial part of the gland lying above the plane related

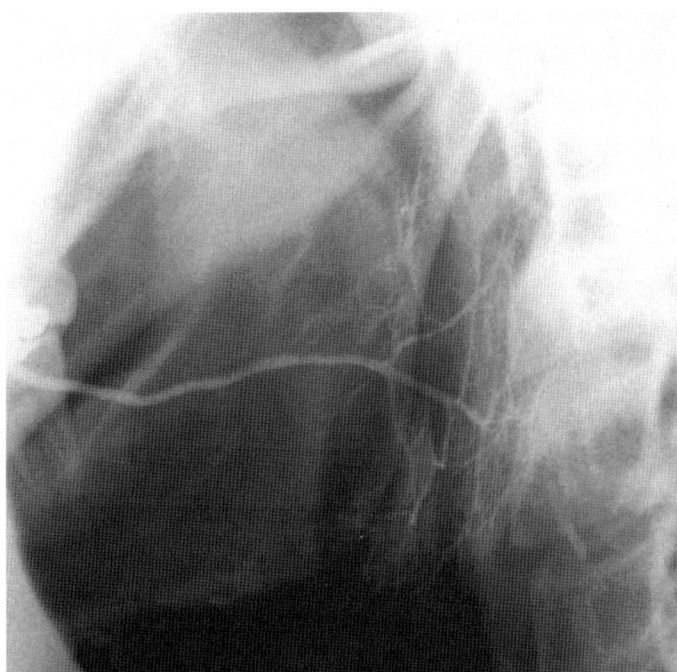

Fig. 29.13 Oblique lateral radiograph showing normal parotid duct outlined after injection of radiopaque contrast medium (sialogram) Note that here the main duct is formed by the union of three smaller ducts at the posterior border of the ramus. (By kind permission from Dr N Drage.)

to the facial nerve. The deeper part of the parotid gland beneath the branches of the facial nerve contains one or two lymph nodes. Lymph from the parotid gland drains to the upper deep cervical lymph nodes.

INNERVATION

Preganglionic nerves travel in the lesser petrosal branch of the glossopharyngeal nerve and synapse in the otic ganglion. Postganglionic fibres reach the gland via the auriculotemporal nerve.

Gustatory sweating (Frey's syndrome)

Gustatory sweating (auriculotemporal syndrome) commonly occurs following parotid surgery or other surgery or trauma that results in opening of the parotid capsule. It is thought to arise as a result of damage to the autonomic nerve fibres supplying the parotid gland and the overlying sweat glands. During the healing process parasympathetic secretomotor fibres to the parotid gland regenerate into the nerve sheaths of the sympathetic secretomotor nerves to the sweat glands. Frey's syndrome is characterized by sweating, warmth and redness of the face as a result of salivary stimulation by the smell or taste of food. The management of Frey's syndrome is difficult. Denervation by tympanic neurectomy or auriculotemporal nerve avulsion have been advocated but are often not curative. The symptoms can be managed by the subcutaneous infiltration of purified botulinum toxin into the affected area.

REFERENCES

Borges AF, Alexander JE 1962 Relaxed skin tension lines, Z-plasties on scars, and fusiform excision of lesions. Br J Plast Surg 15: 242–54.

Davis RA, Anson BJ, Budinger JM, Kurth LE 1956 Surgical anatomy of the facial nerve and parotid gland based upon a study of 350 cervicofacial halves. Surg Gynecol Obstet 102: 385–412.

Fromer J 1977 The human accessory parotid gland: its incidence, nature and significance. Oral Surg Oral Med Oral Pathol 43: 671–6.

Gosain AK, Yousif NJ, Madiedo G, Larson DL, Matloub HS, Sanger JR 1993 Surgical anatomy of the SMAS: a reinvestigation. Plast Reconstruct Surg 92: 1254–63.

Langdon JD 1998 Parotid surgery. In: Langdon JD, Patel MF (eds) Operative Maxillofacial Surgery. London: Chapman and Hall: 381–90.
A detailed account of the procedures for the safe dissection of the intraparotid part of the facial nerve.

Markus AF, Delaire J, Smith WP. Facial balance in cleft lip and palate II. Cleft lip and palate and secondary deformities. Br J Oral Maxillofac Surg 1992 30: 296–304.
Discusses the anatomical basis for the repair of cleft lip and palate deformities.

Mitz V, Peyronie M 1976 The superficial musculo-aponeurotic system (SMAS) in the parotid and cheek area. Plast Reconstruct Surg 58: 80–88.

Myint K, Azian AL, Khairul FA 1992 The clinical significance of the branching pattern of the facial nerve in Malaysian subjects. Med J Malaysia 47: 114–21.

Norman JE de, McGurk M (eds) 1995 Color Atlas and Text of the Salivary Glands. London: Mosby-Wolfe.

Park IY, Lee ME 1977 A morphological study of the parotid gland and the peripheral part of the facial nerve in Koreans. Yonsei Med J 18: 45–51.

Shimada K, Gasser RF 1988 Morphology of the mandibulo-stylohyoid ligament in human adults. Anat Rec 222: 207–210.

Wassef M 1987 Superficial fascial and muscular layers in the face and neck: a histological study. Aesth Plast Surg 11: 171–6.

Yousif NJ, Mendelson BC 1995 Anatomy of the midface. Clin Plast Surg 22, 227–40.

Ziarah HA, Atkinson ME 1981 The surgical anatomy of the mandibular distribution of the facial nerve. Br J Oral Surg 19: 159–70.

Infratemporal region and temporomandibular joint

INFRATEMPORAL FOSSA

The infratemporal fossa is the space located deep to the ramus of the mandible. It communicates with the temporal fossa deep to the zygomatic arch and the pterygopalatine fossa through the pterygomaxillary fissure (p. 578). The major structures which occupy the infratemporal fossa are the lateral and medial pterygoid muscles, the mandibular division of the trigeminal nerve, the chorda tympani branch of the facial nerve, the otic parasympathetic ganglion, the maxillary artery and the pterygoid venous plexus.

The temporomandibular joint is a synovial joint between the condyle of the mandible below and the mandibular fossa of the temporal bone above. The joint is unusual in that its articular surfaces are lined by fibrous tissue (rather than hyaline cartilage) and its joint cavity is divided into two by an articular disc.

The roof of the infratemporal fossa is the infratemporal surface of the greater wing of the sphenoid, its medial wall is formed by the lateral pterygoid plate of the sphenoid bone, separated from the maxilla by the pterygomaxillary fissure (**Fig. 30.1**) and the lateral wall is formed by the ramus of the mandible. The posterior wall shows the presence of the styloid process of the temporal bone. The infratemporal fossa has no anatomical floor.

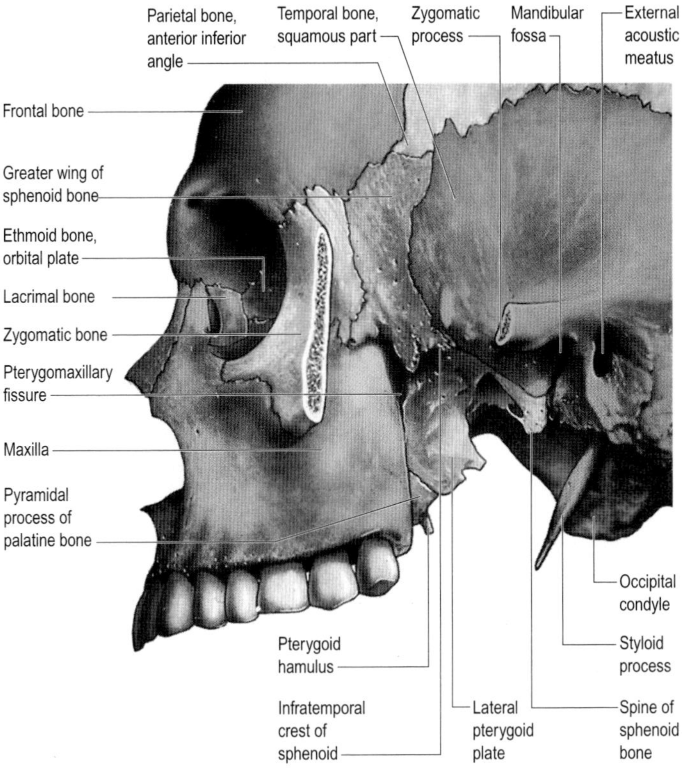

Lateral pterygoid provides a key to understanding the relationships of structures within the infratemporal fossa. This muscle lies in the roof of the fossa and runs anteroposteriorly in a more or less horizontal plane from the region of the pterygoid plates to the mandibular condyle (**Figs 30.1**, **30.2**). Branches of the mandibular nerve and the main origin of medial pterygoid are deep relations and the maxillary artery is superficial. The buccal branch of the mandibular nerve passes between the two heads of lateral pterygoid. Medial pterygoid and the lingual and inferior alveolar nerves emerge below its inferior border and the deep temporal nerves and vessels emerge from its upper border. A venous network, the pterygoid venous plexus, lies around and within lateral pterygoid.

MUSCLES

The infratemporal fossa contains two of the four principal muscles of mastication, medial and lateral pterygoid. The tendon of a third muscle, temporalis, is also found in this region. The remaining muscle, masseter, lies on the face on the lateral surface of the ramus but is considered here with the muscles of mastication. The masticatory muscles are most immediately concerned with movements of the mandible at the temporomandibular joints.

Masseter

Masseter (**Fig. 29.12**) consists of three layers which blend anteriorly. The superficial layer is the largest. It arises by a thick aponeurosis from the maxillary process of the zygomatic bone and from the anterior two-thirds of the inferior border of the zygomatic arch. Its fibres pass downwards and backwards, to insert into the angle and lower posterior half of the lateral surface of the mandibular ramus. Intramuscular tendinous septa in this layer are responsible for the ridges on the surface of the

Parietal bone, anterior inferior angle

Temporal bone, squamous part

Zygomatic process

Mandibular fossa

External acoustic meatus

Frontal bone

Greater wing of sphenoid bone

Ethmoid bone, orbital plate

Lacrimal bone

Zygomatic bone

Pterygomaxillary fissure

Maxilla

Pyramidal process of palatine bone

Occipital condyle

Styloid process

Pterygoid hamulus

Infratemporal crest of sphenoid

Lateral pterygoid plate

Spine of sphenoid bone

Fig. 30.1 The left infratemporal fossa: seen from the side after detachment of the mandible and removal of the zygomatic arch. Blue: frontal bone; yellow: sphenoid and lacrimal bones; brown: temporal and nasal bones; green: maxilla. The parts shown of the parietal, zygomatic, ethmoid and palatine bones are uncoloured.

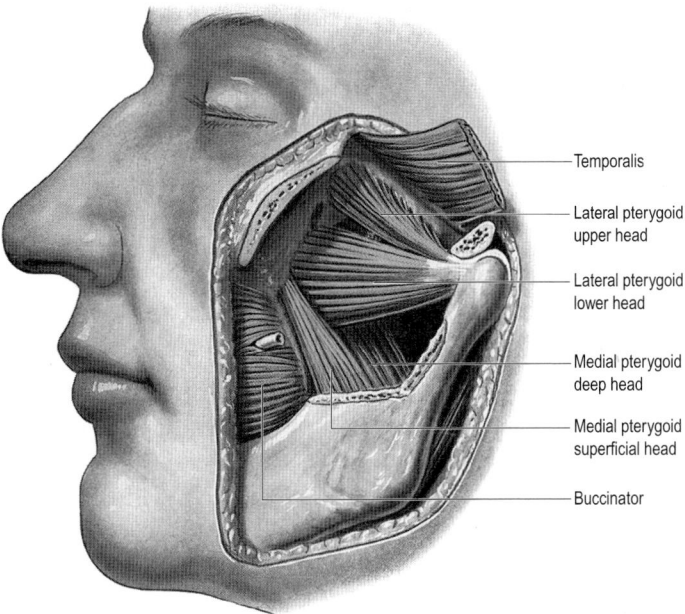

Temporalis

Lateral pterygoid upper head

Lateral pterygoid lower head

Medial pterygoid deep head

Medial pterygoid superficial head

Buccinator

Fig. 30.2 Left pterygoid muscles: the zygomatic arch and part of the ramus of the mandible have been removed, and temporalis has been reflected back.

ramus. The middle layer of masseter arises from the medial aspect of the anterior two-thirds of the zygomatic arch and from the lower border of the posterior third of this arch. It inserts into the central part of the ramus of the mandible. The deep layer arises from the deep surface of the zygomatic arch and inserts into the upper part of the mandibular ramus and into its coronoid process. There is still debate as to whether fibres of masseter are attached to the anterolateral part of the articular disc of the temporomandibular joint.

Relations – Skin, platysma, risorius, zygomaticus major, the parotid gland and duct, branches of the facial nerve and the transverse facial branches of the superficial temporal vessels are all superficial relations. Temporalis and the ramus of the mandible lie deep to masseter. The anterior margin of masseter is separated from buccinator and the buccal branch of the mandibular nerve by a buccal pad of fat and crossed by the facial vein. The posterior margin of the muscle is overlapped by the parotid gland. The masseteric nerve and artery reach the deep surface of masseter by passing over the mandibular incisure (mandibular notch).

Vascular supply – Masseter is supplied by the masseteric branch of the maxillary artery, the facial artery and the transverse facial branch of the superficial temporal artery.

Innervation – Masseter is supplied by the masseteric branch of the anterior trunk of the mandibular nerve.

Actions – Masseter elevates the mandible to occlude the teeth in mastication and has a small effect in side-to-side movements, protraction and retraction. Its electrical activity in the resting position of the mandible is minimal.

Submasseteric space infections – Sometimes infection around a mandibular third molar tooth tracks backwards, lateral to the mandibular ramus and pus localizes deep to the attachment of masseter in the submasseteric tissue space. Such an abscess, lying deep to this thick muscle produces little visible swelling, but is accompanied by profound muscle spasm and limitation of jaw opening.

Temporalis

Temporalis (**Fig. 30.3**) arises from the whole of the temporal fossa up to the inferior temporal line – except the part formed by the zygomatic

bone – and from the deep surface of the temporal fascia. Its fibres converge and descend into a tendon which passes through the gap between the zygomatic arch and the side of the skull. The muscle is attached to the medial surface, apex, anterior and posterior borders of the coronoid process and to the anterior border of the mandibular ramus almost up to the third molar tooth. The anterior fibres of temporalis are orientated vertically, the most posterior fibres almost horizontally, and the intervening fibres with intermediate degrees of obliquity, in the manner of a fan. Fibres of temporalis may occasionally gain attachment to the articular disc.

Relations – Skin, auriculares anterior and superior, temporal fascia, superficial temporal vessels, the auriculotemporal nerve, temporal branches of the facial nerve, the zygomaticotemporal nerve, the epicranial aponeurosis, the zygomatic arch and the masseter muscle are all superficial relations. Posterior relations of temporalis are the temporal fossa above and the major components of the infratemporal fossa below. Behind the tendon of the muscle, the masseteric nerve and vessels traverse the mandibular notch. The anterior border is separated from the zygomatic bone by a mass of fat.

Vascular supply – Temporalis is supplied by the deep temporal branches from the second part of the maxillary artery. The anterior deep temporal artery supplies c.20% of the muscle anteriorly, the posterior deep temporal supplies c.40% of the muscle in the posterior region and the middle temporal artery supplies c.40% of the muscle in its mid-region.

Innervation – Temporalis is supplied by the deep temporal branches of the anterior trunk of the mandibular nerve.

Actions – Temporalis elevates the mandible and so closes the mouth and approximates the teeth. This movement requires both the upward pull of the anterior fibres and the backward pull of the posterior fibres, because the head of the mandibular condyle rests on the articular eminence when the mouth is open. The muscle also contributes to side-to-side grinding movements. The posterior fibres retract the mandible after it has been protruded.

Lateral pterygoid

Lateral pterygoid (**Figs 30.2, 30.4, 30.5**) is a short, thick muscle consisting of two parts. The upper head arises from the infratemporal surface and infratemporal crest of the greater wing of the sphenoid bone. The lower head arises from the lateral surface of the lateral pterygoid plate. From the two origins, the fibres converge, and pass backwards and laterally, to be inserted into a depression on the front of the neck of the mandible (the pterygoid fovea). A part of the upper head may be attached to the capsule of the temporomandibular joint and to the anterior and medial borders of its articular disc. Unlike the other muscles of mastication, lateral pterygoid is not pennate, nor does it have a significant number of Golgi tendon organs associated with its attachments.

Relations – The mandibular ramus and masseter, the maxillary artery – which crosses either deep or superficial to the muscle – and the superficial head of medial pterygoid and the tendon of temporalis, are all superficial relations. Deep to the muscle are the deep head of medial pterygoid, the sphenomandibular ligament, the middle meningeal artery, and the mandibular nerve. The upper border is related to the temporal and masseteric branches of the mandibular nerve and the lower border is related to the lingual and inferior alveolar nerves. The buccal nerve and the maxillary artery pass between the two heads of the muscles (**Fig. 30.4**).

Vascular supply – Lateral pterygoid is supplied by pterygoid branches from the maxillary artery which are given off as the artery crosses the muscle and from the ascending palatine branch of the facial artery.

Innervation – The nerves to lateral pterygoid (one for each head) arise from the anterior trunk of the mandibular nerve, deep to the muscle. The upper head and the lateral part of the lower head receive their innervation from a branch given off from the buccal nerve. However, the medial part of the lower head has a branch arising directly from the anterior trunk of the mandibular nerve.

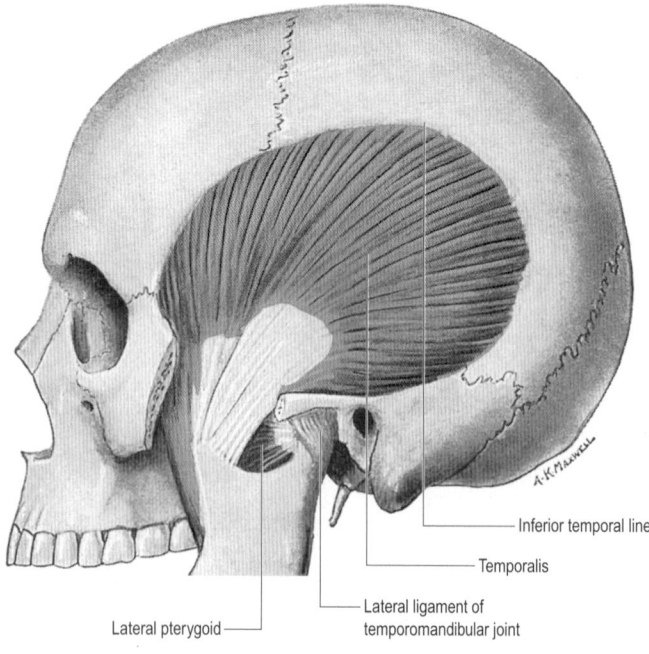

Inferior temporal line

Temporalis

Lateral ligament of temporomandibular joint

Lateral pterygoid

Fig. 30.3 Left temporalis: the zygomatic arch and masseter have been removed. Note the changing orientations of the muscle fibres, from vertical anteriorly to horizontal posteriorly.

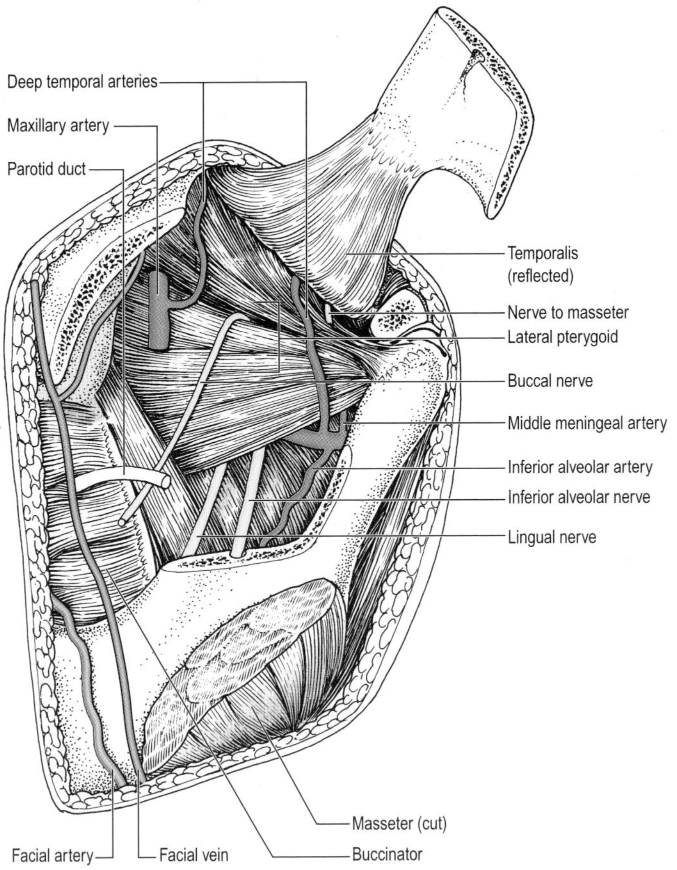

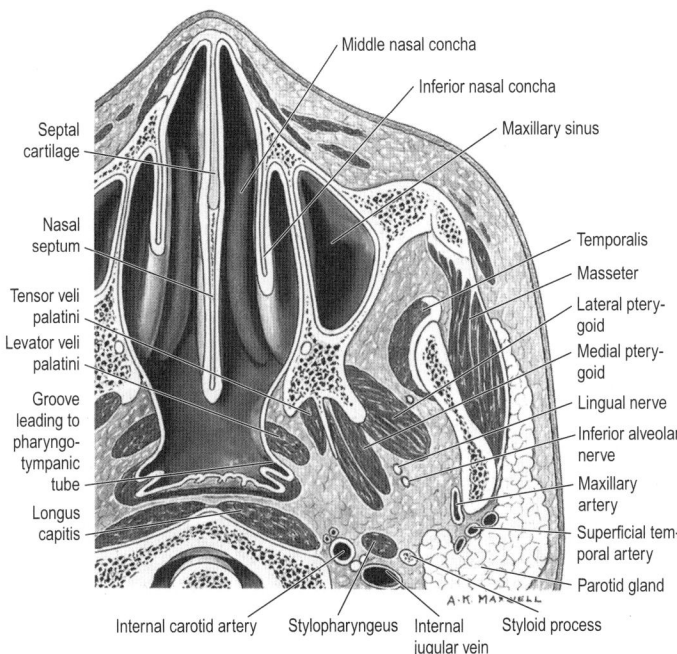

Deep temporal arteries

Maxillary artery

Parotid duct

Temporalis
(reflected)

Nerve to masseter

Lateral pterygoid

Buccal nerve

Middle meningeal artery

Inferior alveolar artery

Inferior alveolar nerve

Lingual nerve

Masseter (cut)

Buccinator

Facial artery — Facial vein

Fig. 30.4 A dissection of the left pterygoid region, showing some of the branches of the mandibular nerve and maxillary artery. Temporalis and the coronoid process of the mandible have been reflected upwards. Masseter has been removed (with the exception of a small inferior portion). The zygomatic arch has been removed.

Middle nasal concha

Inferior nasal concha

Maxillary sinus

Septal cartilage

Nasal septum

Tensor veli palatini

Levator veli palatini

Groove leading to pharyngo-tympanic tube

Longus capitis

Temporalis

Masseter

Lateral ptery-goid

Medial ptery-goid

Lingual nerve

Inferior alveolar nerve

Maxillary artery

Superficial tem-poral artery

Parotid gland

Internal carotid artery   Stylopharyngeus   Internal jugular vein   Styloid process

Fig. 30.5 A transverse section through the anterior part of the head at a level just inferior to the apex of the odontoid process: inferior aspect.

Actions – When left and right muscles contract together the condyle is pulled forward and slightly downward. This protrusive movement alone has little or no function except to assist opening the jaw. Digastric and geniohyoid are the main jaw opening muscles: unlike lateral pterygoid, when acting alone they rotate the jaw open, provided other muscles attached to the hyoid prevent if from being pulled forward. If only one lateral pterygoid contracts, the jaw rotates about a vertical axis passing roughly through the opposite condyle and is pulled medially toward the opposite side. This contraction together with that of the adjacent medial pterygoid (both attached to the lateral pterygoid plate) provides most of the strong medially directed component of the force used when grinding food between teeth of the same side. It is arguably the most important function of the inferior head of lateral pterygoid. It is often stated that the upper head is used to pull the articular disc forward when the jaw is opened. But electromyography studies have proved that the upper head is inactive during jaw opening and most active when the jaws are clenched. An explanation for this surprising activity is as follows (Osborn 1995a). Most of the power of a clenching force is due to contractions of masseter and temporalis. The associated backward pull of temporalis is greater than the associated forward pull of (superficial) masseter, and so their combined jaw closing action potentially pulls the condyle backward. This is prevented by the simultaneous contraction of the upper head of lateral pterygoid.

Medial pterygoid

Medial pterygoid (**Figs 30.2, 30.4, 30.5**) is a thick, quadrilateral muscle with two heads of origin. The major component is the deep head which arises from the medial surface of the lateral pterygoid plate of the sphenoid bone and is therefore deep to the lower head of lateral pterygoid. The small, superficial head arises from the maxillary tuberosity and the pyramidal process of the palatine bone, and therefore lies on the lower head of lateral pterygoid. The fibres of medial pterygoid descend posterolaterally and are attached by a strong tendinous lamina to the posteroinferior part of the medial surface of the ramus and angle of the mandible, as high as the mandibular foramen and almost as far forwards as the mylohyoid groove. This area of attachment is often ridged.

Relations – The lateral surface of medial pterygoid is related to the mandibular ramus, from which it is separated above its insertion by lateral pterygoid, the sphenomandibular ligament, the maxillary artery, the inferior alveolar vessels and nerve, the lingual nerve and a process of the parotid gland. The medial surface is related to tensor veli palatini and is separated from the superior pharyngeal constrictor by styloglossus and stylopharyngeus and by some areolar tissue.

Vascular supply – Medial pterygoid derives its main arterial supply from the pterygoid branches of the maxillary artery.

Innervation – Medial pterygoid is innervated by the medial pterygoid branch of the mandibular nerve.

Actions – The medial pterygoid muscles assist in elevating the mandible. Acting with the lateral pterygoids they protrude it. When the medial and lateral pterygoids of one side act together, the corresponding side of the mandible is rotated forwards and to the opposite side, with the opposite mandibular head as a vertical axis. Alternating activity in the left and right sets of muscles produces side-to-side movements, which are used to triturate food.

Pterygospinous ligament – The pterygospinous ligament, which is occasionally replaced by muscle fibres, stretches between the spine of the sphenoid bone and the posterior border of the lateral pterygoid plate near its upper end. It is sometimes ossified, and then completes a foramen which transmits the branches of the mandibular nerve to temporalis, masseter and lateral pterygoid.

VASCULAR SUPPLY AND LYMPHATIC DRAINAGE

Maxillary artery (Fig. 30.6)

The maxillary artery, the larger terminal branch of the external carotid artery, arises behind the neck of the mandible, and is at first embedded in the parotid gland. It then crosses the infratemporal fossa to enter the pterygopalatine fossa through the pterygomaxillary fissure. The artery is widely distributed to the mandible, maxilla, teeth, muscles of

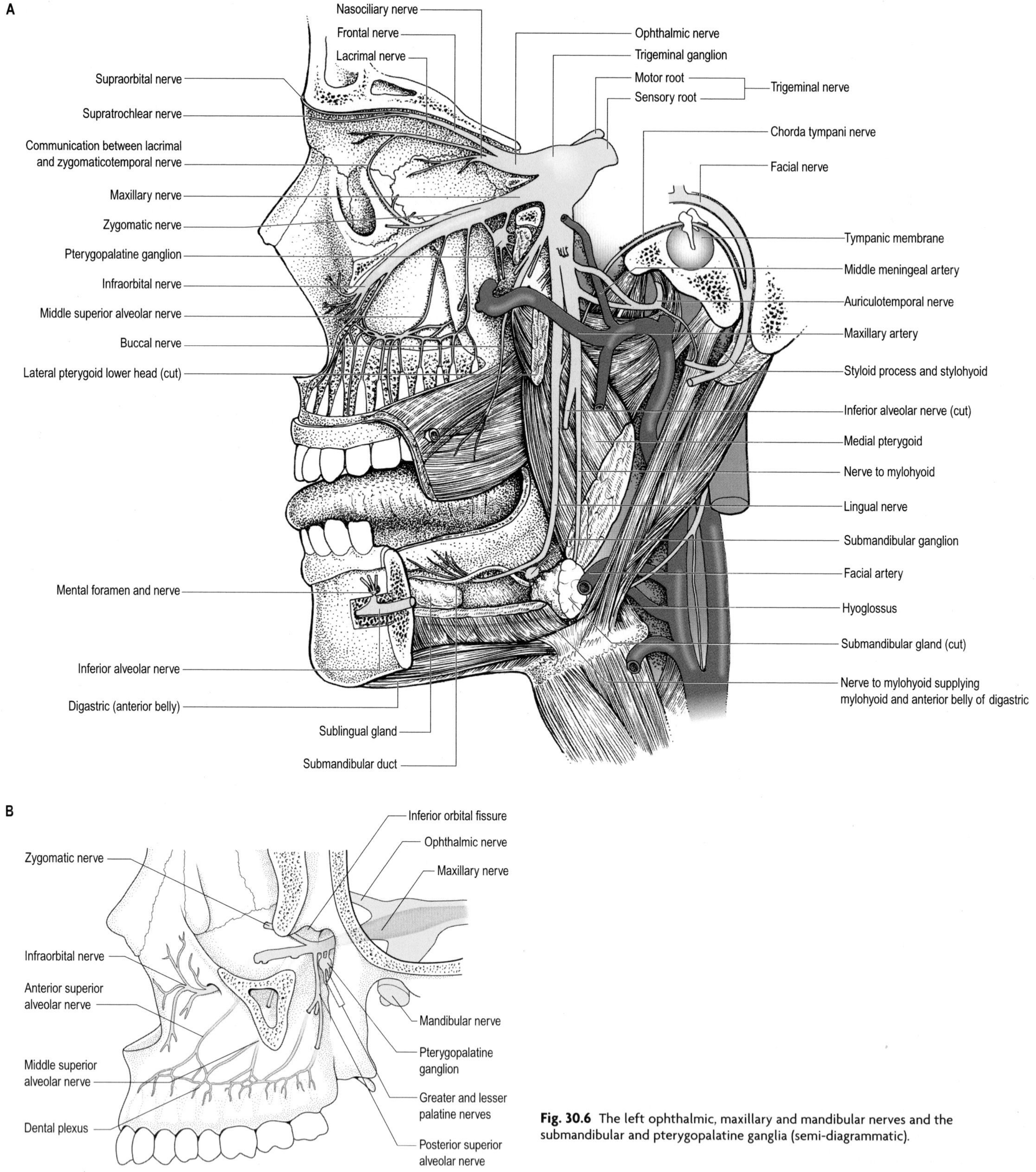

A

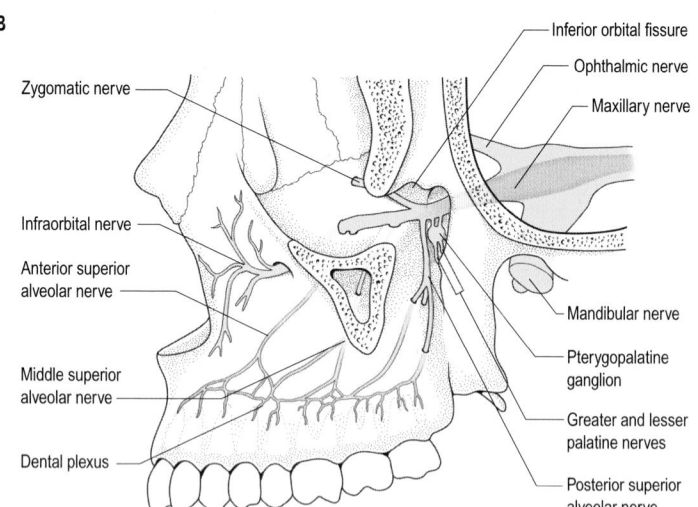

Nasociliary nerve

Frontal nerve

Lacrimal nerve

Supraorbital nerve

Supratrochlear nerve

Communication between lacrimal and zygomaticotemporal nerve

Maxillary nerve

Zygomatic nerve

Pterygopalatine ganglion

Infraorbital nerve

Middle superior alveolar nerve

Buccal nerve

Lateral pterygoid lower head (cut)

Mental foramen and nerve

Inferior alveolar nerve

Digastric (anterior belly)

Sublingual gland

Submandibular duct

Ophthalmic nerve

Trigeminal ganglion

Motor root

Sensory root

Trigeminal nerve

Chorda tympani nerve

Facial nerve

Tympanic membrane

Middle meningeal artery

Auriculotemporal nerve

Maxillary artery

Styloid process and stylohyoid

Inferior alveolar nerve (cut)

Medial pterygoid

Nerve to mylohyoid

Lingual nerve

Submandibular ganglion

Facial artery

Hyoglossus

Submandibular gland (cut)

Nerve to mylohyoid supplying mylohyoid and anterior belly of digastric

B

Zygomatic nerve

Infraorbital nerve

Anterior superior alveolar nerve

Middle superior alveolar nerve

Dental plexus

Inferior orbital fissure

Ophthalmic nerve

Maxillary nerve

Mandibular nerve

Pterygopalatine ganglion

Greater and lesser palatine nerves

Posterior superior alveolar nerve

Fig. 30.6 The left ophthalmic, maxillary and mandibular nerves and the submandibular and pterygopalatine ganglia (semi-diagrammatic).

mastication, palate, nose and cranial dura mater. It will be described in three parts, mandibular, pterygoid and pterygopalatine.

The mandibular part runs horizontally by the medial surface of the ramus. It passes between the neck of the mandible and the spheno-mandibular ligament, parallel with and slightly below the auriculotemporal nerve. It next crosses the inferior alveolar nerve and skirts the lower border of lateral pterygoid. The pterygoid part ascends obliquely forwards medial to temporalis and in c.60% cases is superficial to the lower head of lateral pterygoid. When it runs deep to lateral pterygoid it lies between the muscle and branches of the mandibular nerve, and

may project as a lateral loop between the two parts of lateral pterygoid. Asymmetry in this pattern of distribution may occur between the right and left infratemporal fossae and ethnic differences have been reported. Where the maxillary artery runs superficial to the lower head of lateral pterygoid, the commonest pattern is that the artery passes lateral to the inferior alveolar, lingual and buccal nerves. Less frequently, only the buccal nerve crosses the artery laterally, and rarely the artery passes deep to all the branches of the mandibular nerve. The pterygopalatine part passes between the two heads of lateral pterygoid to reach the pterygomaxillary fissure before it passes into the pterygopalatine fossa.

Branches

The mandibular part of the maxillary artery has five branches, namely, deep auricular, anterior tympanic, middle meningeal, accessory meningeal and inferior alveolar: they all enter bone. The pterygoid part of the maxillary artery also has five branches. They do not enter bone, but supply muscle, and include deep temporal, pterygoid, masseteric and buccal arteries. The distribution of the branches from the pterygopalatine segment is described on page 579.

Deep auricular artery – The deep auricular artery pierces the osseous or cartilaginous wall of the external acoustic meatus and supplies the skin of the external acoustic meatus and part of the tympanic membrane. A small branch contributes to the arterial supply of the temporomandibular joint.

Anterior tympanic artery – The anterior tympanic artery passes through the petrotympanic fissure to supply part of the lining of the middle ear and accompanies the chorda tympani nerve.

Middle meningeal artery – The middle meningeal artery is the main source of blood to the bones of the vault of the skull. It may arise either directly from the first part of the maxillary artery or from a common trunk with the inferior alveolar artery. When the maxillary artery lies superficial to lateral pterygoid, the middle meningeal artery is usually the first branch of the maxillary artery. However, when the maxillary artery takes a deep course in relation to the muscle this is not usually the case. The middle meningeal artery ascends between the spheno-mandibular ligament and lateral pterygoid, passes between the two roots of the auriculotemporal nerve and leaves the infratemporal fossa through the foramen spinosum to enter the cranial cavity medial to the midpoint of the zygomatic bone. Its further course is described on page 281.

Accessory meningeal artery – The accessory meningeal artery runs through the foramen ovale into the middle cranial fossa and may arise directly from the maxillary artery or as a branch of the middle meningeal artery itself. In its course in the infratemporal fossa, the accessory meningeal artery is closely related to tensor and levator veli palatini and usually runs deep to the mandibular nerve. Although it runs intracranially, its main distribution is extracranial, principally to medial pterygoid, lateral pterygoid (upper head), tensor veli palatini, the greater wing and pterygoid processes of the sphenoid, branches of the mandibular nerve and the otic ganglion. The accessory meningeal artery is sometimes replaced by separate small arteries.

Deep temporal arteries – The anterior, middle and posterior branches of the deep temporal arteries pass between temporalis and the peri-cranium, producing shallow grooves in the bone. They anastomose with the middle temporal branch of the superficial temporal artery. The anterior deep temporal artery connects with the lacrimal artery by small branches which perforate the zygomatic bone and greater wing of the sphenoid.

Masseteric artery – The masseteric artery, which is small, accompanies the masseteric nerve as it passes behind the tendon of temporalis through the mandibular incisure (notch) to enter the deep surface of masseter. Its branches can also supply the temporomandibular joint. The masseteric artery anastomoses with the masseteric branches of the facial artery and with the transverse facial branch of the superficial temporal artery.

Pterygoid arteries – The pterygoid arteries are irregular in number and origin, and are distributed to lateral and medial pterygoid.

Buccal artery – The buccal artery runs obliquely forwards between medial pterygoid and the attachment of temporalis and supplies the skin and mucosa over buccinator, accompanying the lower part of the buccal branch of the mandibular nerve. It anastomoses with branches of the facial and infraorbital arteries. A small lingual branch may be given off to accompany the lingual nerve and supply structures in the floor of the mouth.

Maxillary veins and the pterygoid venous plexus

Maxillary vein

The maxillary vein is a short trunk which accompanies the first part of the maxillary artery. It is formed from the confluence of veins from the pterygoid plexus and passes back between the sphenomandibular ligament and the neck of the mandible, to enter the parotid gland. It unites within the substance of the gland with the superficial temporal vein to form the retromandibular vein (**Fig. 29.12**).

Pterygoid venous plexus

The pterygoid plexus of veins is found partly between temporalis and lateral pterygoid and partly between the two pterygoid muscles. Sphenopalatine, deep temporal, pterygoid, masseteric, buccal, alveolar (dental), greater palatine and middle meningeal veins and a branch or branches from the inferior ophthalmic vein are all tributaries. The plexus connects with the facial vein via the deep facial vein and with the cavernous sinus through veins that pass through the sphenoidal emissary foramen, foramen ovale and foramen lacerum. Its deep temporal tributaries often connect with tributaries of the anterior diploic veins and thus with the middle meningeal veins.

INNERVATION

The infratemporal fossa contains the major subdivisions of the man-dibular branch of the trigeminal nerve, together with the chorda tympani, which enters the fossa and joins the lingual nerve, and the otic ganglion, which is functionally related to the parotid gland. The main sensory branches of the mandibular nerve extend beyond the infra-temporal fossa and their distribution to the face is described on page 512.

Mandibular nerve (Figs 29.9, 30.6, 30.7)

The mandibular nerve is the largest trigeminal division and is a mixed nerve. Its sensory branches supply the teeth and gums of the mandible, the skin in the temporal region, part of the auricle – including the external meatus and tympanic membrane – and the lower lip, the lower part of the face (**Fig. 29.9**), and the mucosa of the anterior two-thirds (presulcal part) of the tongue and the floor of the oral cavity. The motor branches innervate the muscles of mastication. The large sensory root emerges from the lateral part of the trigeminal ganglion and exits the cranial cavity through the foramen ovale. The small motor root passes under the ganglion and through the foramen ovale to unite with the sensory root just outside the skull. As it descends from the foramen ovale, the nerve is c.4 cm from the surface and a little anterior to the neck of the mandible. The mandibular nerve immediately passes between tensor veli palatini, which is medial, and lateral pterygoid, which is lateral, and gives off a meningeal branch and the nerve to medial pterygoid from its medial side. The nerve then divides into a small anterior and large posterior trunk. The anterior division gives off branches to the four main muscles of mastication and a buccal branch which is sensory to the cheek. The posterior division gives off three main sensory branches, the auriculotemporal, lingual and inferior alveolar nerves, and motor fibres to supply mylohyoid and the anterior belly of digastric (**Figs 30.6, 30.7**).

Meningeal branch (nervus spinosus) – The meningeal branch re-enters the cranium through the foramen spinosum with the middle meningeal artery. It divides into anterior and posterior branches which accompany the main divisions of the middle meningeal artery and supply the dura mater in the middle cranial fossa and, to a lesser extent, in the anterior fossa and calvarium.

Nerve to medial pterygoid – The nerve to medial pterygoid is a slender ramus which enters the deep aspect of the muscle. It supplies one or two filaments that pass through the otic ganglion without interruption to supply tensor tympani and tensor veli palatini (*see* **Fig. 30.7**).

Anterior trunk of mandibular nerve

The anterior trunk of the mandibular nerve gives rise to the buccal nerve, which is sensory, and the masseteric, deep temporal and lateral pterygoid nerves, which are all motor.

Buccal nerve – The buccal nerve (**Fig. 30.4**) passes between the two heads of lateral pterygoid. It descends deep to the tendon of temporalis,

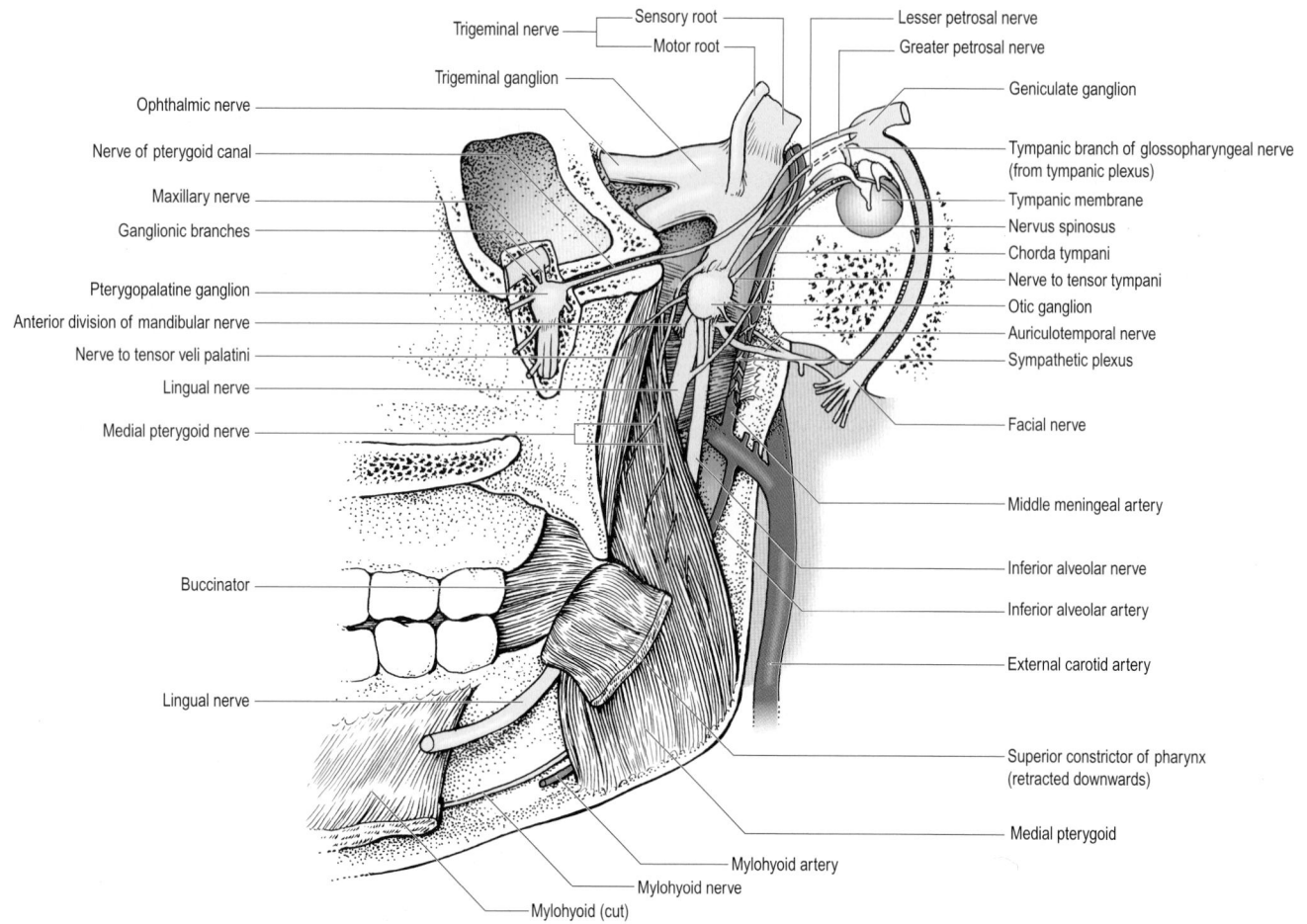

Fig. 30.7 The right otic and pterygopalatine ganglia and their branches displayed from the medial side (semi-diagrammatic).

passes laterally in front of masseter, and anastomoses with the buccal branches of the facial nerve. It carries the motor fibres to lateral pterygoid, and these are given off as the buccal nerve passes through the muscle. It may also give off the anterior deep temporal nerve. The buccal nerve supplies sensation to the skin over the anterior part of buccinator and the buccal mucous membrane, together with the posterior part of the buccal gingivae adjacent to the second and third molar teeth.

Nerve to masseter – The nerve to masseter (**Fig. 30.4**) passes laterally above lateral pterygoid, on to the skull base, anterior to the temporo-mandibular joint and posterior to the tendon of temporalis. It crosses the posterior part of the mandibular notch with the masseteric artery and ramifies on and enters the deep surface of masseter. It also provides articular branches which supply the temporomandibular joint.

Deep temporal nerves – The deep temporal nerves usually consist of two branches, anterior and posterior, although there may be a middle branch. They pass above lateral pterygoid to enter the deep surface of temporalis. The anterior nerve frequently arises as a branch of the buccal nerve. The small posterior nerve sometimes arises in common with the nerve to masseter.

Nerve to lateral pterygoid – The nerve to lateral pterygoid enters the deep surface of the muscle. It may arise separately from the anterior division of the mandibular nerve or from the buccal nerve.

Posterior trunk of mandibular nerve

The posterior trunk of the mandibular nerve is larger than the anterior and is mainly sensory, although it receives fibres from the motor root for the nerve to mylohyoid. It divides into auriculotemporal, lingual and inferior alveolar (dental) nerves.

Auriculotemporal nerve – The auriculotemporal nerve usually has two roots which encircle the middle meningeal artery (**Figs 30.6, 30.7**). It

runs back under lateral pterygoid on the surface of tensor veli palatini, passes between the sphenomandibular ligament and the neck of the mandible, and then runs laterally behind the temporomandibular joint related to the upper part of the parotid gland. Emerging from behind the joint, it ascends over the posterior root of the zygoma, posterior to the superficial temporal vessels, and divides into superficial temporal branches. It communicates with the facial nerve and otic ganglion. The rami to the facial nerve, usually two, pass anterolaterally behind the neck of the mandible to join the facial nerve at the posterior border of masseter. Filaments from the otic ganglion join the roots of the auriculotemporal nerve close to their origin (**Figs 30.7, 30.8**). The sensory distribution of the auriculotemporal nerve on the face is described on page 513.

Lingual nerve – The lingual nerve (**Figs 30.4, 30.6, 30.7**) is sensory to the mucosa of the anterior two-thirds of the tongue, the floor of the mouth and the mandibular lingual gingivae. It arises from the posterior trunk of the mandibular nerve and at first runs beneath lateral pterygoid and superficial to tensor veli palatini, where it is joined by the chorda tympani branch of the facial nerve, and often by a branch of the inferior alveolar nerve. Emerging from under cover of lateral pterygoid, the lingual nerve then runs downwards and forwards on the surface of medial pterygoid, and is thus carried progressively closer to the medial surface of the mandibular ramus. It becomes intimately related to the bone a few millimetres below and behind the junction of the vertical ramus and horizontal body of the mandible. Here it lies anterior to, and slightly deeper than, the inferior alveolar (dental) nerve. It next passes below the mandibular attachment of the superior pharyngeal constrictor and pterygomandibular raphe, closely applied to the periosteum of the medial surface of the mandible, until it lies opposite the posterior root of the third molar tooth, where it is covered only by the gingival mucoperiosteum. At this point it usually lies 2–3 mm below the alveolar crest and 0.6 mm from the bone, however in c.5% of cases it lies above the alveolar crest. It next passes medial to the mandibular

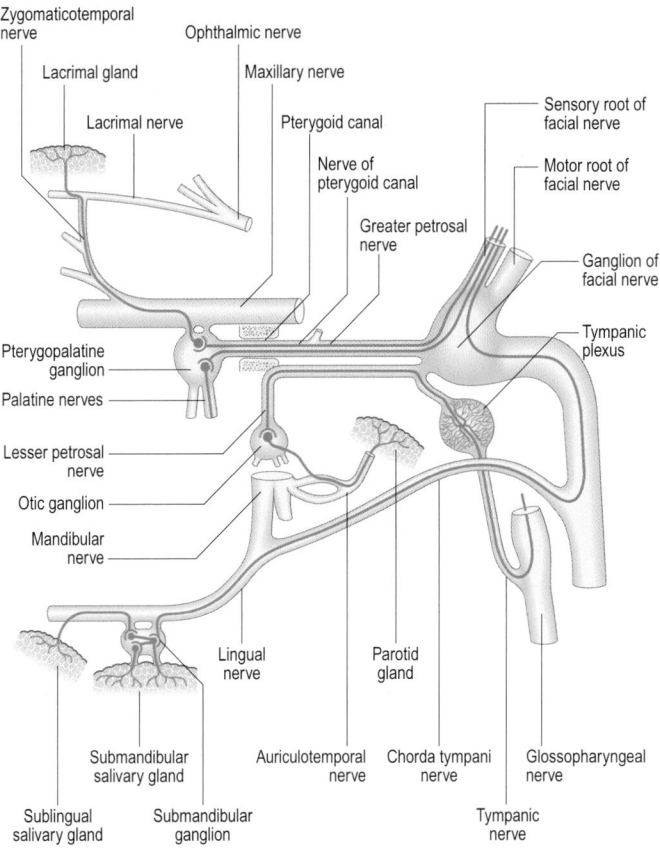

Fig. 30.8 The parasympathetic connections of the pterygopalatine, otic and submandibular ganglia. The parasympathetic fibres, both pre- and postganglionic, are shown as blue lines. The parasympathetic fibres in the palatine nerves are secretomotor to the nasal, palatine and pharyngeal glands.

origin of mylohyoid, and this carries it progressively away from the mandible, and separates it from the alveolar bone covering the mesial root of the third molar tooth. The rest of the nerve is described with the mouth and oral cavity (p. 588).

Inferior alveolar (dental) nerve – The inferior alveolar nerve descends behind lateral pterygoid. At the lower border of the muscle the nerve passes between the sphenomandibular ligament and the mandibular ramus and enters the mandibular canal via the mandibular foramen. Below lateral pterygoid it is accompanied by the inferior alveolar artery, a branch of the first part of the maxillary artery, which also enters the canal with associated veins. The subsequent course of the inferior alveolar nerve is described on page 601.

Otic ganglion

This is a small, oval, flat reddish-grey ganglion (*see* **Figs 30.7**, **30.8**) situated just below the foramen ovale. It is a peripheral parasympathetic ganglion related topographically to the mandibular nerve, but connected functionally with the glossopharyngeal nerve. Near its junction with the trigeminal motor root, the mandibular nerve lies lateral to the ganglion; tensor veli palatini lies medially, separating the ganglion from the cartilaginous part of the pharyngotympanic tube, and the middle meningeal artery is posterior to the ganglion. The otic ganglion usually surrounds the origin of the nerve to medial pterygoid.

Like all parasympathetic ganglia, there are three roots, motor, sympathetic and sensory. Only the parasympathetic fibres relay in the ganglion. The motor, parasympathetic, root of the otic ganglion is the lesser petrosal nerve, conveying preganglionic fibres from the glossopharyngeal nerve which originate from neurones in the inferior salivatory nucleus. The lesser petrosal nerve runs intracranially in the middle cranial fossa on the anterior surface of the petrous bone before passing through the foramen ovale to join the otic ganglion. The nerve synapses in the otic ganglion, and postganglionic fibres pass by a communicating branch to the auriculotemporal nerve and so to the parotid gland. The

sympathetic root is from a plexus on the middle meningeal artery. It contains postganglionic fibres from the superior cervical sympathetic ganglion which traverse the otic ganglion without relay and emerge with parasympathetic fibres in the connection with the auriculotemporal nerve to supply blood vessels in the parotid gland. The sensory fibres from the gland are derived from the auriculotemporal nerve. Clinical observations suggest that in humans the gland also receives secretomotor fibres through the chorda tympani.

Branches – A branch connects the otic ganglion to the chorda tympani nerve, while another ramus ascends to join the nerve of the pterygoid canal. These branches may form an additional pathway by which gustatory fibres from the anterior two-thirds of the tongue may reach the facial ganglion without traversing the middle ear, and they do not synapse in the otic ganglion. Motor branches to tensor veli palatini and tensor tympani, derived from the nerve to medial pterygoid, also pass through the ganglion without synapsing.

Chorda tympani nerve

The chorda tympani nerve enters the infratemporal fossa region by passing through the medial end of the petrotympanic fissure behind the capsule of the temporomandibular joint. The nerve descends medial to the spine of the sphenoid bone – which it sometimes grooves – lying posterolateral to tensor veli palatini. It is crossed medially by the middle meningeal artery, the roots of the auriculotemporal nerve and by the inferior alveolar nerve (**Fig. 30.6**). The chorda tympani joins the posterior aspect of the lingual nerve at an acute angle. It carries taste fibres for the anterior two-thirds of the tongue and efferent preganglionic parasympathetic (secretomotor) fibres destined for the submandibular ganglion in the floor of the mouth.

LE FORT AND ZYGOMATIC FRACTURES (p. 489)

Le Fort I, II or III fractures inevitably involve the infratemporal fossa. The bones of the midface transmit the forces of impact directly to the cranium. The most important strut related to the infratemporal and pterygopalatine fossae is the pterygomaxillary strut. Fractures involving this strut may extend elsewhere to involve the cranial base and orbit. The associated soft tissue damage which accompanies these fractures may damage nerves, blood vessels and muscles. Injuries to the second or third divisions of the trigeminal nerve or the chorda tympani nerve result in altered sensation to the oral cavity, face and jaws, including impaired taste. Fractures extending into the orbit may result in decreased visual acuity and ophthalmoplegia. Neural damage to motor nerves or direct damage to muscles may result in problems with chewing, swallowing, speech, middle ear function and eye movements. Injuries that involve the pterygopalatine or otic ganglia interfere with lacrimation, nasal secretions and salivation. Damage to adjacent blood vessels may result in haemorrhage, thrombosis emboli and the formation of false aneurisms or arteriovenous fistulae.

Classic zygomatic complex fractures involve the lateral wall of the orbit and cross laterally into the infratemporal fossa at the frontozygomatic suture. From this point the fracture line extends inferiorly to join the most lateral aspect of the inferior orbital fissure, continues inferiorly along the posterior surface of the zygomatic buttress – where it communicates with the lateral bulge of the maxillary antrum – and runs around the zygomatic buttress, high in the buccal sulcus in the upper molar region, and then extends upwards towards the infraorbital foramen. It finally runs laterally along the floor of the orbit to reach the lateral extension of the inferior orbital fissure.

These fractures involve the maxillary sinus and the infratemporal fossa and orbit, which means that any blood which collects in the antrum, if it becomes infected, will allow infection to spread into the infratemporal fossa. Infection in this area can have grave consequences and can rapidly spread through the foramina in the skull base into the middle cranial fossa. For this reason patients presenting with zygomatic complex fractures are placed on prophylactic antibiotic therapy to prevent infection.

SPREAD OF INFECTION FROM THE INFRATEMPORAL FOSSA (p. 607)

The majority of infected teeth in the upper jaw and those in the front part of the lower jaw will generally drain harmlessly into the oral cavity – either via the vestibule buccally, or via the palate or mouth lingually – and they are of little clinical significance. In contrast, a pericoronitis affecting a partially impacted mandibular third molar tooth, or less commonly either a dental abscess of this tooth, or an infection following tooth extraction, spreads into the infratemporal fossa. Infection may also result from an infected needle used during an inferior alveolar nerve block, or as a result of spread from an adjacent infected tissue space. The main symptom caused by infection of the pterygomandibular space is trismus – painful reflex muscle spasm – which usually affects medial pterygoid.

Infection may potentially spread some distance from the infratemporal fossa because the latter lies between the tissue spaces of the face above and the tissue spaces of the neck below. Thus infection may spread to involve the buccal tissue space, or directly around the back of the maxillary tuberosity and into the orbit via the inferior orbital fissure, which may result in a cavernous sinus thrombosis. Once in the orbit, infection may spread directly through the superior orbital fissure into the cranial cavity. Infection may also spread from the infratemporal fossa via the pterygomaxillary fissure to involve the pterygopalatine fossa and its contents, and may spread further via a number of small canals which lead from the fossa into the nose, pharynx and palate.

TEMPOROMANDIBULAR JOINT

Each joint involves the articular fossa (also known as the mandibular fossa or glenoid fossa) above and the mandibular condyle below. These have been described on page 482, and are considered here in more detail.

The articular eminence, a transversely elliptical region sinuously curved in the sagittal plane and tilted forward at c.25° to the occlusal plane, forms most of the articular surface of the articular fossa. Its steepness is variable, and it becomes flatter in the edentulous. Its anterior limit is the summit of the articular eminence, a transverse ridge that extends laterally out to the zygomatic arch as far as the articular tubercle. Articular tissue extends anteriorly beyond the articular summit and on to the preglenoid plane. Posteriorly it extends behind the depth of the fossa as far as the squamotympanic fissure. A postglenoid tubercle (at the root of the zygomatic arch, just anterior to the fissure) is usually poorly developed in human skulls.

The articular surface of the mandibular condyle is slightly curved and tilted forward at c.25° to the occlusal plane. Like the articular eminence, its slope is variable. In the coronal plane its shape varies (Osborn & Baranger 1992) from that of a gable (particularly marked in those whose diet is hard), to roughly horizontal in the edentulous.

It is probably impossible to measure the pressure developed on the articular surfaces of the human jaw joint when biting. There is, however, irrefutable theoretical evidence based on Newtonian mechanics that the jaw joint is a weight-bearing joint. With a vertical bite force of 500 N on the left first molar the right condyle must support a load of well over 300 N (Osborn 1995a). The non-working condyle is more loaded than the condyle on the working side, which may help explain why patients with a fractured condyle choose to bite on the side of the fracture.

FIBROUS CAPSULE

The lower part of the joint is surrounded by tight fibres which attach the condyle of the mandible to the disc. The upper part of the joint is surrounded by loose fibres which attach the disc to the temporal bone (Fig. 30.9). Thus the articular disc is attached separately to the temporal bone and to the mandibular condyle forming what could be considered two joint capsules. Longer fibres joining the condyle directly to the temporal bone may be regarded as reinforcing. The capsule is attached above to the anterior edge of the preglenoid plane, posteriorly to the lips of the squamotympanic fissure, between these to the edges of the articular fossa, and below to the periphery of the neck of the mandible.

LIGAMENTS

Sphenomandibular ligament

The sphenomandibular ligament (Fig. 30.9) is medial to, and normally separate from, the capsule. It is a flat, thin band that descends from the spine of the sphenoid and widens as it reaches the lingula of the mandibular foramen. Some fibres traverse the medial end of the petrotympanic fissure and attach to the anterior malleolar process. This part is a vestige of the dorsal end of Meckel's cartilage.

With the jaw closed, there is c.5 mm slack within the ligament, but it becomes taut when the jaw is about half open. Lateral pterygoid and the auriculotemporal nerve are lateral relations, the chorda tympani

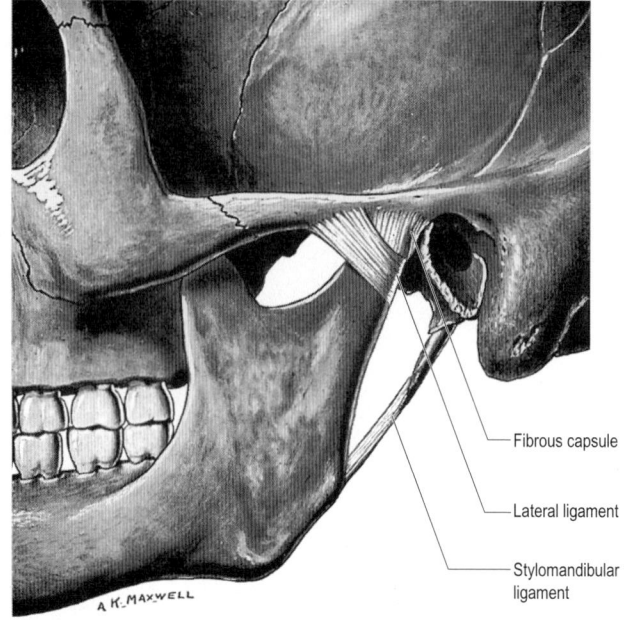

A

Fibrous capsule

Lateral ligament

Stylomandibular ligament

A.K.MAXWELL

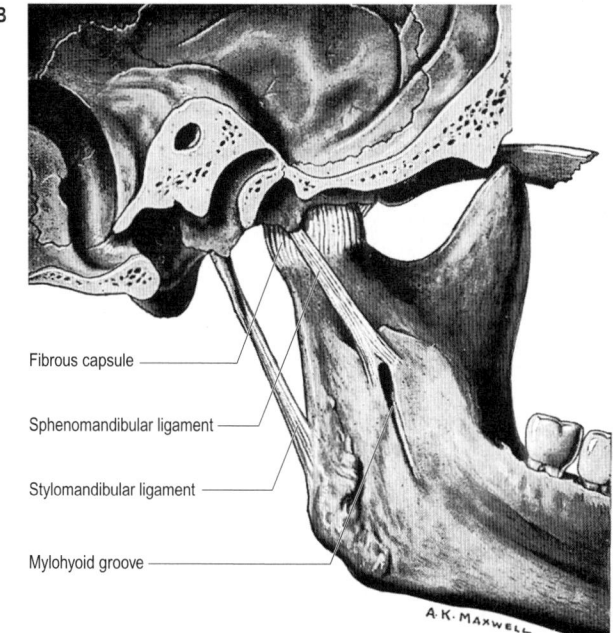

B

Fibrous capsule

Sphenomandibular ligament

Stylomandibular ligament

Mylohyoid groove

A.K.MAXWELL

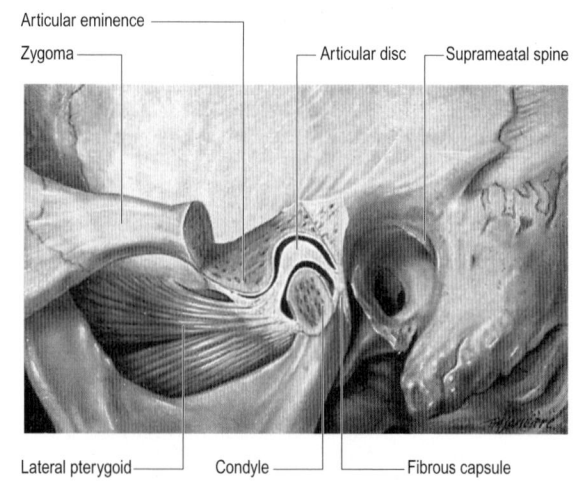

Articular eminence

Zygoma

Articular disc

Suprameatal spine

C

Lateral pterygoid

Condyle

Fibrous capsule

Fig. 30.9 The left temporomandibular joint. **A**, lateral aspect; **B**, medial aspect; **C**, sagittal section.

nerve lies medial near its upper end and medial pterygoid is an infero-medial relation. The sphenomandibular ligament is separated from the neck of the mandible below lateral pterygoid by the maxillary artery and from the ramus of the mandible by the inferior alveolar vessels and nerve and a parotid lobule. At this point the vessels and nerve to mylohyoid pierce the ligament. It is separated from the pharynx by fat and a pharyngeal vein.

Stylomandibular ligament

The stylomandibular ligament (**Fig. 30.9**) is a thickened band of deep cervical fascia that stretches from the apex and adjacent anterior aspect of the styloid process to the angle and posterior border of the mandible. Its position and orientation indicate that it cannot mechanically constrain any normal movements of the mandible and does not seem to warrant the status of a ligament of the joint.

Temporomandibular (lateral) ligament

This broad ligament (**Fig. 30.9**) is attached above to the articular tubercle on the root of the zygomatic process of the temporal bone. It extends downwards and backwards at an angle of c.45° to the horizontal, to attach to the lateral surface and posterior border of the neck of the condyle, deep to the parotid gland. It appears to be poorly developed in the edentulous. A short, almost horizontal, band of collagen connects the articular tubercle in front to the lateral pole of the condyle behind. It may function to prevent posterior displacement of the resting condyle.

SYNOVIAL MEMBRANE

The synovial membrane lines the inside of the capsule of the joint but does not extend to cover the disc or the articular surfaces.

ARTICULAR DISC

The transversely oval articular disc is composed predominantly of dense fibrous connective tissue (**Fig. 30.10**). It has a thick margin which forms a peripheral annulus and a central depression in its lower surface that accommodates the articular surface of the mandibular condyle. The depression probably develops as a mechanical response to pressure from the condyle as it rotates inside the annulus. The disc is stabilized on the condyle in three ways. Its edges are fused with the part of the capsular ligament that tightly surrounds the lower joint compartment

and is attached around the neck of the condyle. Well-defined bands in the capsular ligament attach the disc to the medial and lateral poles of the condyle. The thick annulus prevents the disc sliding off the condyle, provided that the condyle and disc are firmly lodged against the articular fossa (as is normally the case).

In sagittal section, the disc appears to possess a thin intermediate zone and thickened anterior and posterior bands, and its upper surface appears concavo-convex where it fits against the convex articular eminence and the concavity of the articular fossa. Posteriorly the disc is attached to a region of loose vascular and nervous tissue which splits into two laminae, the bilaminar region: unlike the rest of the disc, its normal function is to provide attachment rather than intra-articular support. The upper lamina, composed of fibroelastic tissue, is attached to the squamotympanic fissure, and the lower lamina, composed of fibrous non-elastic tissue, is attached to the back of the condyle. The bilaminar region contains a venous plexus, but the central part of the disc is avascular.

The collagen is crimped, and this probably serves to absorb energy when a sudden tensile force is applied, and so briefly protects the disc from potential rupture. Cells in the disc also secrete chondroitin sulphate – a glycosaminoglycan found in cartilage – which is most heavily concentrated in the centre of the disc and which probably gives the disc some of the resilience and compressive strength of cartilage. The amount increases in response to load and to age, and by the fifth decade the disc shows signs of ageing including fraying, thinning and perforation.

Functions of the articular disc

The functions of the articular disc remain controversial. It is generally believed that the disc helps to stabilize the temporomandibular joint. The articulating surfaces of the mandibular condyle and the articular fossa fit together poorly (**Fig. 30.10**) and are therefore separated by an irregular space. Muscle forces control the position of the mandible, and therefore of the condyle, in relation to the articular eminence, and these in turn set the shape and thickness of the irregular space. The position of the disc is controlled by neuromuscular forces: the upper head of lateral pterygoid anteriorly, and the elastic tissue in the bilaminar region posteriorly, together pull the disc backward or forward to keep the joint space filled and thereby stabilize the condyle. The articular disc may reduce wear, because the frictional wear on the condyle and the articular eminence is halved by separating slide and rotation into different joint compartments. It may also aid lubrication of the joint because it stores fluid that is squeezed out to create a weeping lubricant from the loaded part of the disc.

A final view is based on the fact that the addition of a slippery disc doubles the number of virtually friction free sliding surfaces suggesting that its function is to destabilize the condyle (certainly not stabilize it) in the same way that stepping on a banana skin destabilizes the foot. All other joints are most heavily loaded when their articular surfaces are closely fitted together, creating a large area of contact, and braced to prevent further movement. However the condyle of the mandible is most heavily loaded when it is required to move, sliding backward during the buccal phase of the power stroke of a masticatory cycle on the opposite side of the jaw. If the articular tissues were composed of hyaline cartilage, the small area of contact between poorly fitting surfaces would promote free sliding (**Fig. 30.11A**) but simultaneously create a potentially damaging pressure (force per unit area). Making them of compressible fibrous tissue would reduce the pressure by increasing the surface area of contact and thereby spread the load, but the compressed tissues would interfere with free sliding movements (**Fig. 30.11B**). The problem is overcome by fitting a disc between them (**Fig. 30.11C**), which therefore destabilizes the condyle. In this context it is perhaps telling that the pathological absence of a disc, and not its presence, stabilizes the condyle during grinding movements and thereby renders the articular tissues vulnerable to damage. If these tissues respond by increasing their cartilaginous properties, the increased resistance to compression reduces the area of contact and results in damagingly large articular pressures. If they respond by becoming more fibrous the sliding condyle destructively gouges through the compressed fibrous tissue on the articular eminence.

Temporomandibular joint syndrome

Symptoms arising from the temporomandibular joints and their associated masticatory muscles are very common (temporomandibular joint syndrome/internal derangement). Diffuse facial pain due to

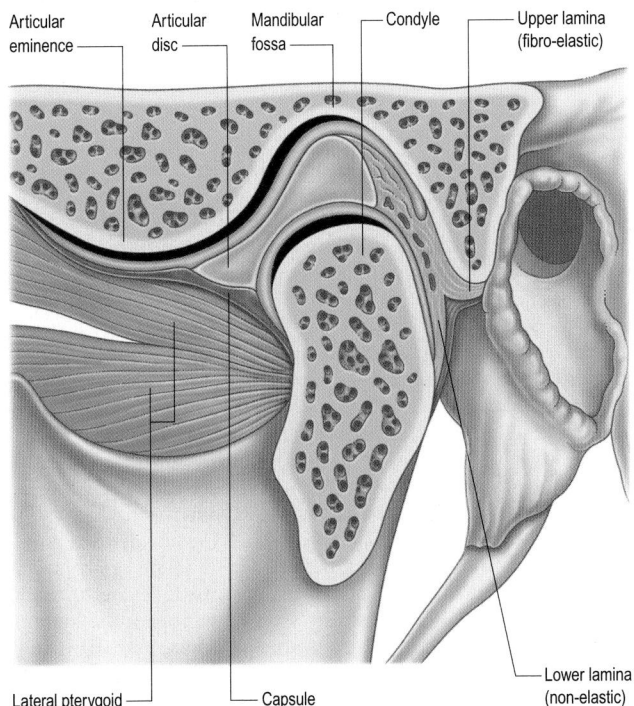

Articular eminence — Articular disc — Mandibular fossa — Condyle — Upper lamina (fibro-elastic)

Lateral pterygoid — Capsule — Lower lamina (non-elastic)

Fig. 30.10 A sagittal section of the temporomandibular joint. The upper and lower joint spaces are normally compressed. They have been widened to illustrate the anteroposterior extent of each. The bilaminar posterior region contains a venous plexus.

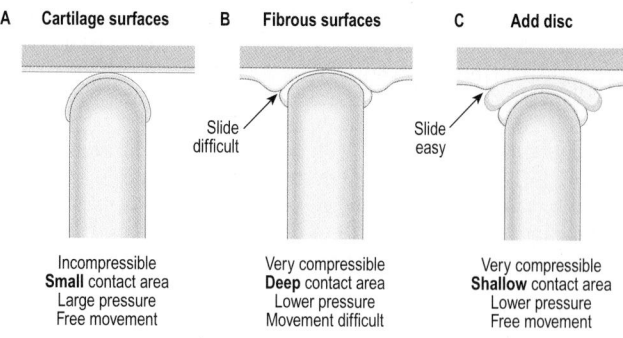

Fig. 30.11 The advantages and disadvantages of covering articular surfaces with cartilage (**A**) and fibrous tissue (**B**). The addition of a fibrous disc (**C**) decreases the intra-articular pressure while simultaneously facilitating loaded sliding movements, unique requirements of the temporomandibular joint. (By kind permission from Dr JW Osborn.)

masseteric muscle spasm, headache due to temporalis muscle spasm and jaw ache due to lateral pterygoid spasm are typical presenting symptoms. These may be associated with clicking, which is often audible whilst the patient is chewing, and sometimes locking, when the patient is unable to open fully. Changes in the normal structure of the articular disc occur and the disc does not smoothly follow the movements of the condyle. Clicking and locking occur when the attachment of the articular disc posteriorly to the squamotympanic fissure becomes stretched or detached, allowing the disc to become temporarily or permanently trapped anteriorly. These symptoms affect predominantly adolescents and young adults and affect females more frequently than males. The symptoms occur particularly when the subject is under stress. Although predisposing factors have been implicated, such as the nature of the dental occlusion, the morphology of the head of the condyle, and variations in the attachments of lateral pterygoid, the precise aetiology of temporomandibular joint syndrome awaits clarification.

VASCULAR SUPPLY AND INNERVATION

The articular tissues and the dense part of the articular disc have no nerve supply. Branches of the auriculotemporal and masseteric nerves and postganglionic sympathetic nerves supply the tissues associated with the capsular ligament and the looser posterior bilaminar extension of the disc. The temporomandibular joint capsule, lateral ligament and retroarticular tissue contain mechanoreceptors and nociceptors. The input from mechanoreceptors provides a source of proprioceptive sensation that helps control mandibular posture and movement.

The joint derives its arterial supply from the superficial temporal artery laterally and the maxillary artery medially. Penetrating vessels that supply lateral pterygoid may also supply the condyle of the mandible. Veins drain the anterior aspect of the joint and associated tissues into the plexus surrounding lateral pterygoid, and posteriorly they drain into the vascular region that separates the two laminae of the bilaminar region of the disc. Pressure produced by forward and backward movement of the condyle shunts blood between these regions. Lymphatics drain deeply to the upper cervical lymph nodes surrounding the internal jugular vein.

JAW MOVEMENTS

Muscle synergism

During opening of the mouth, the incisors of adults may be separated by 50–60 mm, and this involves c.35° rotation of the mandible. The mandible may be protruded or laterally displaced c.10 mm, although this is very variable. The adult range of movements is reached at c.10 years in females and 15 years in males.

When a jaw muscle contracts in the absence of a restraint, the mandible is pulled in the direction of the shortening muscle. The muscles have therefore been classified as protruders (lateral and medial pterygoids); retractors (posterior fibres of temporalis assisted by digastric and geniohyoid); elevators (anterior and middle fibres of temporalis, superficial and deep fibres of masseter and medial pterygoid); depressors (lateral pterygoids aided by digastric, geniohyoid and mylohyoid); lateral movers (medial and lateral pterygoids of each side). While these

descriptions are correct, they fail to explain why the jaw muscles are so powerful, and ignore the synergism of these muscles in the generation of bite force. For example, the lateral pterygoids are each capable of exerting about 160 N force, a total of 320 N, and yet less than 5% of this is used to protrude or open the jaw.

The jaw muscles normally exert large forces only during the power stroke of mastication. In general, a jaw muscle is most active when a line joining its attachments is more parallel to the bite force. Each jaw muscle has a component of force in parasagittal, coronal and horizontal planes. For example, masseter pulls the mandible upward, forward and outward. Moreover, active jaw muscles often have a component of force in one plane that is unwanted, e.g. the outward pull of the left masseter opposes a medially directed power stroke on the left molars. This wasteful lateral component must be counteracted by another muscle, even one that is poorly placed to help produce the required output force. If the activity of all the jaw muscles is analysed when they create a given bite force, it is possible to subdivide them into 'power' muscles that largely create the force, and 'balancing' muscles that largely counteract unwanted components and help to increase the output force by more than their contribution to that force. For example, the superior head of lateral pterygoid acts as a balancing muscle during clenching, even though it is very poorly placed to increase the bite force, because it allows temporalis to be much more active by balancing its unwanted backward force component. It becomes a power muscle during protrusion because its activity increases the output force by an amount equal to its contribution to a protrusive force (see Osborne 1995a).

Movements of the condyle in the temporomandibular joint

The major function of the mandible is to exert, via the teeth, the force necessary to break down food into smaller particles and so facilitate digestion. Pure vertical movements of the lower teeth create a crushing force that is ineffective in breaking up tough fibrous food. Man uses a lateral movement of the lower jaw to create a shear component of force that enhances the effectiveness of the power stroke of mastication. Bodily lateral movement of the whole jaw, the Bennet shift, is insignificant. Extensive lateral movement is only possible when the jaw is rotated horizontally about one condyle while the other condyle slides backward and forward.

The temporomandibular joint is structurally adapted to accommodate both sliding and rotation in a parasagittal plane. Sliding occurs because the capsular ligament which surrounds the upper joint compartment is loose, whereas the capsular ligament which encloses the lower joint compartment is tight, and only allows the condyle to rotate over the depression inside the annulus of the articular disc.

Symmetrical opening

Symmetrical jaw opening is associated with preparation for incising. At the start, each mandibular condyle rotates in the lower joint compartment inside the annulus of its disc. After a few degrees of opening, the condyle continues rotating inside its disc, and, in addition, both slide forward down the articular eminence of the upper joint compartment. Without this forward slide, it rapidly becomes impossible to continue opening the jaw.

There are conflicting views about the reason why forward slide occurs, probably because direct experimental testing is not possible. No other animal has an articular eminence constraint and ligaments comparable to man, which means that most supporting evidence for any theory is based on analyses of human joint dysfunction. It has been argued that a sensory input from the rotary movement, possibly from either the joint capsule or the jaw muscles, initiates a response that reflexly activates muscles that cause the slide. The fact that the condyle in a cadaver still slides forward when the jaw is rotated open suggests that it is not a neuromuscular response but is the mechanical result of physical constraints. When the jaw is rotated open the temporomandibular ligament rapidly becomes taut (Osborn 1995b). The taut ligament acts as a constraint that allows the mandible only two rotary movements: it can swing about the upper attachment of the ligament and rotate about the lower attachment. The lower end of the taut ligament acts as a moving fulcrum that converts the downward and backward pull of the opening rotary force (created at the front by digastric and geniohyoid) into one that drives the condyle upward and forward into the concavity of the overlying articular disc. This now pushes the disc forward. Swing about the upper attachment creates space above for the disc to slide further forward which is possible because the upper part of the capsular ligament is loose. The two movements, rotation and swing, are inextricably linked by the taut ligament and, via the condyle, combine to keep the disc in firm contact with the articular eminence while the jaw is opened. The disc is stabilized by its tight attachment to the condyle and by the thickened margins of its anulus that prevent it sliding through the thinner compressed region between the centre of the condyle and the articular eminence.

As forward slide of the condyle continues, the controlling influence exerted by the temporomandibular ligament diminishes. The lingula of the mandible moves away from the spine of the sphenoid, tautening the originally slack sphenomandibular ligament, which now acts in the same way as the temporomandibular ligament, to maintain the condyle against the articular eminence. Symmetrical opening thus appears to consist of at least three separate phases: an early phase controlled by the temporomandibular ligament and articular eminence; a short middle phase in which either both, or neither, temporomandibular and spheno-mandibular ligaments act to constrain movements; and a late phase controlled by the sphenomandibular ligament and articular eminence.

Eccentric jaw opening
Eccentric jaw opening is associated with preparing for the power stroke of mastication. The mandibular condyle on the non-working side slides back and forth during lateral movements associated with the power stroke on the working side. Although the jaw muscles now have the major control over mandibular movements, the temporomandibular and sphenomandibular ligaments keep the condyle firmly against its articular eminence during opening.

Eccentric and symmetrical jaw closing
The resultant of the jaw closing muscles of the mandible has a com-ponent that forces the joint surfaces together. This compresses the joint tissues and potentially shortens the ligaments so that they no longer constrain jaw movements. Under these conditions, jaw movements and the positions of the condyles are controlled by neuromuscular processes (within the limits of constraints imposed by the articular eminence, the occluding surfaces of the teeth and the presence of food between them). Note that the non-working condyle moves the furthest, and is the most heavily loaded, during the power stroke of mastication. The loads on each joint, balancing and working, drive each condyle more forcefully into its articular eminence.

Temporomandibular joint dislocation
The mandible is dislocated only forwards. With the mouth open, the mandibular condyles are on the articular eminences and sudden violence, even muscular spasm – a convulsive yawn – may displace one or both condyles onto the preglenoid plane. To reduce the dislocation the condyle must be lowered and pushed back behind the summit of the articular eminence into the articular fossa. This is achieved by first rotating the jaw closed: the chin is elevated and the lower molar region depressed by pushing down with the thumbs in the buccal sulci. Once the condyle has been lowered below the articular summit the jaw can easily be pushed back.

ANATOMY OF MASTICATION
Intake of food is carried out primarily by a series of intraoral, pharyn-geal and oesophageal transport mechanisms. Mastication is an inter-ruption in the intraoral transport process which occurs when the ingested material is not of a consistency suitable for further onward transport. It is the process, characteristic of adult mammals, in which ingested food is cut or crushed into small pieces, mixed with saliva and formed into a bolus in preparation for swallowing.

The intraoral transport of ingested food relies primarily upon tongue movements, whereas food breakage can be considered primarily a func-tion of the teeth, jaws and jaw closing muscles. Nevertheless, efficient food breakage is heavily dependent upon the ability of the tongue to select and place appropriate sized food items between the occluding teeth. Initially puncturing forces are applied by the tips of the cusps of premolar/molar teeth during a simple vertical closure of the jaw (essentially the same breakage mechanism is used by the incisors when hard food is fractured prior to ingestion during the initial stages of intraoral transport). In subsequent cycles shearing forces are generated

as the inclined planes of cusps of the premolar/molar teeth of one side move past each other: this occurs as the jaw closes, initially with a slight lateral movement and finally, after tooth–food–tooth contact, with the medial movement necessary for the shear production. Once the food has been mechanically processed to the point where it is suitable for swallowing, the jaw movements revert to cycles with a simple vertical path. During these cycles, tongue movements transport the processed food into the swallow.

Jaw closing movements are produced by contraction of masseter, temporalis and medial pterygoid. In each cycle closing movement is initially carried out largely against gravity until tooth–food–tooth contact is made, after which closure can only occur if the food is deformed or fractured. Electromyographic activity in the jaw elevator muscles increases only moderately – from the negligible level seen just prior to jaw closure – as the jaw accelerates in closure against gravity, but the activity then increases significantly as tooth–food–tooth contact is made. The recruitment of the additional muscle activity is thought to be due to sensory feedback, probably from subsets of periodontal and muscle afferents. However, a large part of the sensory feedback from periodontal afferents is associated with tooth overload protection, and inhibits the activity of the jaw-closing muscles. Jaw opening is produced by relaxation of the jaw-closing muscles associated with activation of the lateral pterygoid muscles to bring the condyles forward, and activation of submandibular muscles (including the digastric muscles).

Profiles of cycles of jaw movement (plotted as gape versus time) for hard food and for soft food are different because the former is dominated by the proportion of the cycle devoted to the breakage of food, whereas the latter is devoted to the proportion of the cycle dedicated to tongue movement (much of which occurs in opening). When a piece of hard food is being mechanically processed, the form of the jaw cycle changes as the consistency of the food item changes. When jaw movements in eating are plotted as X–Y coordinates in the coronal plane, the mandible usually moves laterally (towards the side containing the food bolus) during closure until a time which broadly corresponds to when food contact is made. After this the teeth move medially while still closing (although the extent of this movement varies, depending upon whether puncture crushing or shearing is being performed). When the food is soft, the jaw movement tends to be a simple vertical one with little or no lateral excursion. It should be noted that the profiles of naturally occurring movements in the coronal plane are not limited anatomically except by tooth contact; the anatomically limited envelope of motion is normally substantially larger.

The envelope of motion
The envelope of motion is the volume of space within which all move-ments of a point on the mandible have to occur because the limits are set by anatomical features i.e. by the shape or size of the upper and lower jaws, by tooth contacts, by the attachment and insertions of muscle and ligaments.

In consciously controlled movement of the jaw from the rest position to the fully opened position, the trajectory of the mandibular incisal edge is two-phased. The first phase is a hinge-like movement during which the condyles are retruded within the mandibular fossae. When the teeth are opened by c.25 mm, the second phase of opening occurs by anterior movement or protrusion of the condyles down the articular eminences with further rotation.

If conscious effort is used, a closure path can then be followed in which the jaw is closed to an extreme protruded tooth contact position after which it has to be retruded to the starting position. The free, habitual, unconscious movement during both jaw opening and closing has a significantly more limited trajectory. Similar considerations apply to lateral movements: mandibular rotation around a retruding condyle and the protraction of the opposite condyle are anatomically limiting factors that are again rarely encountered in normal function.

The majority of normal movements of the jaw are not consciously controlled in the sense that they are totally deliberate throughout their course. They are largely automatic, indeed, some rhythmic movements can even be performed in the absence of functioning cerebral hemi-spheres. The current view is that the rhythmic movements of the jaw are produced by a central pattern generator (CPG) in the brainstem, which is activated by sensory input from nerves of the orofacial region (e.g. by material in the mouth) and/or by intact descending influences from cerebrocortical sources. The nature of the rhythmic output from the CPG may also be subject to subsequent modification by oral sensory input and by descending influences. This helps to explain the change in cycle type as different foods are processed. In all such cyclical movements anatomical constraints can act only during tooth contact in closing and during the transition from hinge axis opening to condylar sliding. The main limitations set on rhythmic movements, so that they conform to particular profiles, are those set by neural controls.

REFERENCES

Barker BCW, Davies PL 1972 The applied anatomy of the pterygomandibular space. Br J Surg 10: 43–55.
Describes the relationships of the structures within the pterygomandibular space, with particular reference to anaesthesia associated with an inferior alveolar nerve block.

Bertilsson O, Strom D 1995 A literature survey of a hundred years of anatomic and functional lateral pterygoid muscle research. J Orofac Pain 9: 17–23.

Pogrel MA, Renaut A, Schmidt B, Ammar A 1995 The relationship of the lingual nerve to the mandibular third molar region. J Oral Maxillofac Surg 53: 1178–81.
Describes the relationships between the lingual nerve and the third molar tooth and the clinical relevance of this knowledge to the extraction of such teeth.

Lang J 1995 Clinical Anatomy of the Masticatory Apparatus and Peripharyngeal Spaces. New York: Thième Medical Publishers.
Provides detailed anatomical information (including quantitation) of the infratemporal fossa, relating such information to the clinic.

Langdon JD, Patel MF (eds) 1998 Operative Maxillofacial Surgery. London: Chapman and Hall.

Langdon JD, Berkovitz BKB, Moxham BJ 2002 The Surgical Anatomy of the Infra-temporal Fossa. London: Dunitz.
The two previous references are textbooks which contain detailed information about surgical approaches associated with the infratemporal fossa, including access to the brain.

Orchardson R, Cadden W 1998 Mastication. In: Linden RWA (ed) The Scientific Basis of Eating. Taste and Smell, Salivation, Mastication and Swallowing and their Dysfunctions. Frontiers of Oral Biology Series Vol 9. Basel: Karge: 76–121.

Turker KS 2002 Reflex control of human jaw muscles. Crit Rev Oral Biol Med 13: 85–104.
These two last papers contain detailed descriptions of the process of mastication.

Osborn JW 1985 The disc of the human temporomandibular joint: design, function and failure. J Oral Rehab 12: 279–93.
Analyses of the design, function and physical properties of the articular disc and the capsular ligament including explanations for the origin of disc displacement and clicking joints.

Osborn JW 1995a Biomechanical implications of lateral pterygoid contributions to biting and jaw opening in humans. Arch Oral Biol 40: 1099–108.

Osborn JW 1995b Internal derangement and the accessory ligaments around the temporomandibular joint. J Oral Rehab 22: 731–40.
Analyses of the anatomy of the ligaments associated with the jaw joint and how they control the movements of the condyle during border movements of the jaw associated with jaw opening and the aetiology of jaw dislocation and disc displacement.

Osborn JW, Baranger FA 1992 Observed shapes of human condyles. J Biomechan 25: 967.
Describes the shapes of human jaw joints in three dimensions, and analyses how the shapes are related to the different loads that need to be supported at the joint surfaces during biting. Includes predictions about changes in joint loads and jaw muscle activity in response to theoretical changes in joint and muscle receptors.

Neck

The neck extends from the base of the cranium and the inferior border of the mandible to the thoracic inlet. For gross descriptive purposes it can be divided into musculoskeletal, visceral and two laterally positioned neurovascular compartments, that are each delineated by fascia. The investing layer of deep cervical fascia encloses trapezius and sternocleidomastoid. Anteriorly and on each side, platysma lies between the fascia and the skin, and the infrahyoid muscles lie posterior to the fascia. The musculoskeletal compartment is posterior and contains the vertebral column and the prevertebral and postvertebral muscles, enclosed by the prevertebral fascia. The visceral compartment occupies the midline of the neck and, depending on the level, may contain the pharynx or the oesophagus; the larynx or the trachea; the thyroid and parathyroid glands. The compartment is enclosed by pretracheal fascia. The neurovascular compartments lie on each side of the neck beneath sternocleidomastoid and contain the common carotid or internal carotid artery, the internal jugular vein, and the vagus nerve, all enclosed within the carotid sheath.

SKIN

The skin in the neck is normally under tension, and the direction in which this is greatest varies regionally. In the living face, these lines often coincide with wrinkle lines. Lines of greatest tension have been termed 'relaxed skin tension lines': surgical incisions made along these lines are said to heal with minimal postoperative scarring.

Cutaneous vascular supply and lymphatic drainage

The blood vessels supplying the skin of the neck are derived chiefly from the facial, occipital, posterior auricular and subclavian arteries. They form a rich network within platysma and in the subdermal plexus, and account for the viability of the various skin flaps raised during block dissection of the neck, irrespective of whether they include platysma.

The vessels supplying the anterior skin of the neck are derived mainly from the superior thyroid artery and the transverse cervical branch of the subclavian artery. The posterior skin is supplied by branches from the occipital artery and the deep cervical and transverse cervical branches of the subclavian artery. Superiorly, the skin is supplied from the occipital artery and its upper sternocleidomastoid branch, and the submandibular and submental branches of the facial artery. Inferiorly, the skin of the neck is supplied from the transverse cervical and/or suprascapular branches of the subclavian artery.

The pattern of venous drainage of the skin of the neck mirrors the arterial supply, and drains into the jugular and facial veins.

Many lymphatic vessels draining the superficial cervical tissues skirt the borders of sternocleidomastoid to reach the superior or inferior deep cervical nodes. Some pass over sternocleidomastoid and the posterior triangle to the superficial cervical and occipital nodes (**Fig. 31.1**). Lymph from the superior region of the anterior triangle drains to the submandibular and submental nodes. Vessels from the anterior

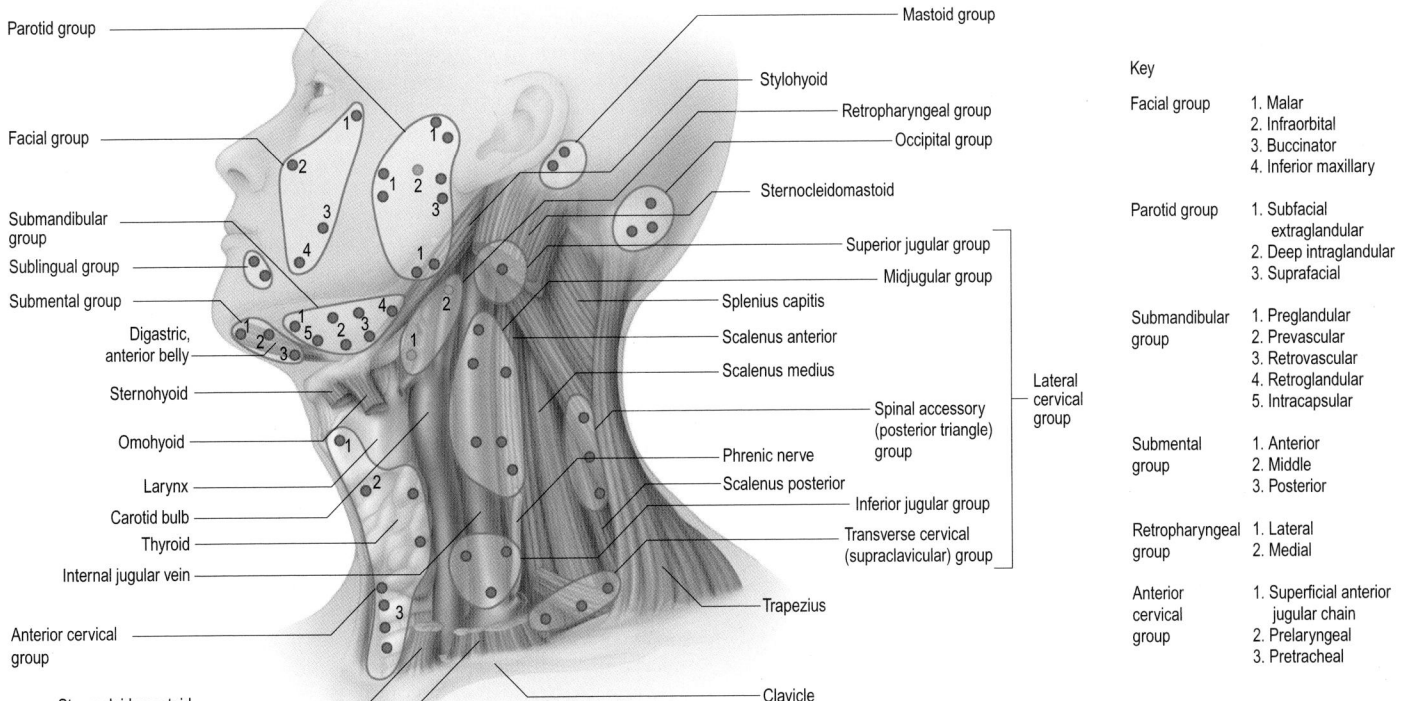

Fig. 31.1 Lymph nodes of the head and neck. Adapted from Montgomery WW 2002 Surgery of the Larynx, Trachea, Esophagus and Neck. Philadelphia: Saunders. Inset courtesy of Professor John D Langdon, GKT Schools of Medicine, Dentistry and Biomedical Sciences.

cervical skin inferior to the hyoid bone pass to the anterior cervical lymph nodes near the anterior jugular veins, and their efferents go to the deep cervical nodes of both sides, including the infrahyoid, prelaryngeal and pretracheal groups. An anterior cervical node often occupies the suprasternal space.

Cutaneous innervation (Figs 29.9, 31.2, 46.14, 45.58)

The skin of the neck is innervated by branches of cervical spinal nerves, via both dorsal and ventral rami. The dorsal rami supply skin over the back of the neck and scalp, and the ventral rami supply skin covering the lateral and anterior portions of the neck, and extend onto the face over the angle of the mandible. The dorsal rami of the first, sixth, seventh and eighth cervical nerves have no cutaneous distribution in the neck. The greater occipital nerve mainly supplies the scalp and comes from the medial branch of the dorsal ramus of the second cervical nerve. The medial branches of the dorsal rami of the third, fourth and fifth cervical nerves pierce trapezius to supply skin over the back of the neck sequentially. The ventral rami of the second, third and fourth cervical nerves supply named cutaneous branches (the lesser occipital, great auricular, transverse cutaneous and supraclavicular nerves), via the cervical plexus located deep to sternocleidomastoid. The cervical plexus is described in detail on page 555.

LESSER OCCIPITAL NERVE

The lesser occipital nerve is derived mainly from the second cervical nerve (although fibres from the third cervical nerve may sometimes contribute). It curves around the accessory nerve and ascends along the

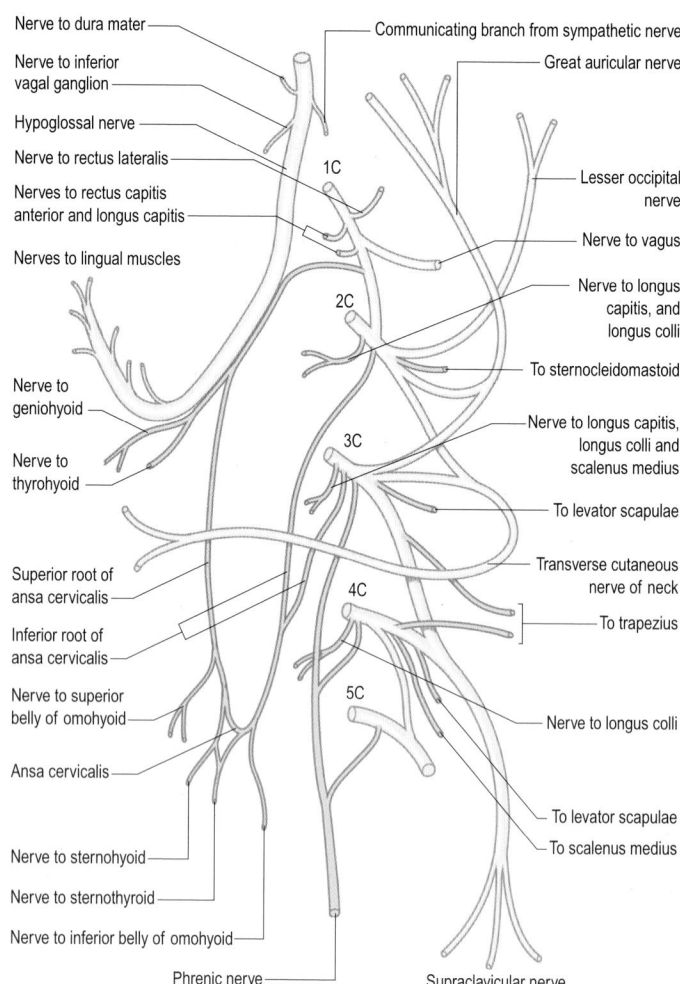

Labels on figure:
- Nerve to dura mater
- Nerve to inferior vagal ganglion
- Hypoglossal nerve
- Nerve to rectus lateralis
- Nerves to rectus capitis anterior and longus capitis
- Nerves to lingual muscles
- Nerve to geniohyoid
- Nerve to thyrohyoid
- Superior root of ansa cervicalis
- Inferior root of ansa cervicalis
- Nerve to superior belly of omohyoid
- Ansa cervicalis
- Nerve to sternohyoid
- Nerve to sternothyroid
- Nerve to inferior belly of omohyoid
- Phrenic nerve
- 1C
- 2C
- 3C
- 4C
- 5C
- Communicating branch from sympathetic nerve
- Great auricular nerve
- Lesser occipital nerve
- Nerve to vagus
- Nerve to longus capitis, and longus colli
- To sternocleidomastoid
- Nerve to longus capitis, longus colli and scalenus medius
- To levator scapulae
- Transverse cutaneous nerve of neck
- To trapezius
- Nerve to longus colli
- To levator scapulae
- To scalenus medius
- Supraclavicular nerve

Fig. 31.2 A plan of the cervical plexus.

posterior margin of sternocleidomastoid. Near the cranium it perforates the deep fascia and passes up onto the scalp behind the auricle. It supplies the skin and connects with the great auricular and greater occipital nerves and the auricular branch of the facial nerve. Its auricular branch supplies the skin on the upper third of the medial aspect of the auricle and connects with the posterior branch of the great auricular nerve. The auricular branch is occasionally derived from the greater occipital nerve.

It has been suggested that compression or stretching of the lesser occipital nerve contributes to cervicogenic headache.

GREAT AURICULAR NERVE

This is the largest ascending branch of the cervical plexus. It arises from the second and third cervical rami, encircles the posterior border of sternocleidomastoid, perforates the deep fascia and ascends on the muscle beneath platysma with the external jugular vein. It passes to the parotid gland, dividing into anterior and posterior branches. The anterior branch is distributed to the facial skin over the parotid gland, connecting in the gland with the facial nerve. The posterior branch supplies the skin over the mastoid process and on the back of the auricle (except its upper part); a filament pierces the auricle to reach the lateral surface where it is distributed to the lobule and concha. The posterior branch communicates with the lesser occipital, the auricular branch of the vagus and the posterior auricular branch of the facial nerve.

TRANSVERSE CUTANEOUS (CERVICAL) NERVE OF THE NECK

The transverse cutaneous nerve arises from the second and third cervical rami, curves round the posterior border of sternocleidomastoid near its midpoint and runs obliquely forwards, deep to the external jugular vein, to the anterior border of the muscle. It perforates the deep cervical fascia, and divides under platysma into ascending and descending branches that are distributed to the anterolateral areas of the neck. The ascending branches ascend to the submandibular region, forming a plexus with the cervical branch of the facial nerve beneath platysma. Some branches pierce platysma and are distributed to the skin of the upper anterior areas of the neck. The descending branches pierce platysma and are distributed anterolaterally to the skin of the neck, as low as the sternum.

SUPRACLAVICULAR NERVES

The supraclavicular nerves arise from a common trunk formed from rami from the third and fourth cervical nerves and emerge at the posterior border of sternocleidomastoid. Descending under platysma and the deep cervical fascia, the trunk divides into medial, intermediate and lateral (posterior) branches, which diverge to pierce the deep fascia a little above the clavicle. The medial supraclavicular nerves run infero-medially across the external jugular vein and the clavicular and sternal heads of sternocleidomastoid to supply the skin as far as the midline and as low as the second rib. They supply the sternoclavicular joint. The intermediate supraclavicular nerves cross the clavicle to supply the skin over pectoralis major and deltoid down to the level of the second rib, next to the area of supply of the second thoracic nerve. Overlap between these nerves is minimal. The lateral supraclavicular nerves descend superficially across trapezius and the acromion, supplying the skin of the upper and posterior parts of the shoulder.

TRIANGLES OF THE NECK (Figs 31.3, 31.4)

Anterolaterally the neck appears as a somewhat quadrilateral area, limited superiorly by the base of the mandible and a line continued from the angle of the mandible to the mastoid process, inferiorly by the upper border of the clavicle, anteriorly by the anterior median line, and posteriorly by the anterior margin of trapezius. This quadrilateral area can be further divided into anterior and posterior triangles by sterno-cleidomastoid, which passes obliquely from the sternum and clavicle to the mastoid process and occipital bone. It is true that these triangles and their subdivisions are somewhat arbitrary, because many major structures – arteries, veins, lymphatics, nerves, and some viscera – transgress their boundaries without interruption, nevertheless they have

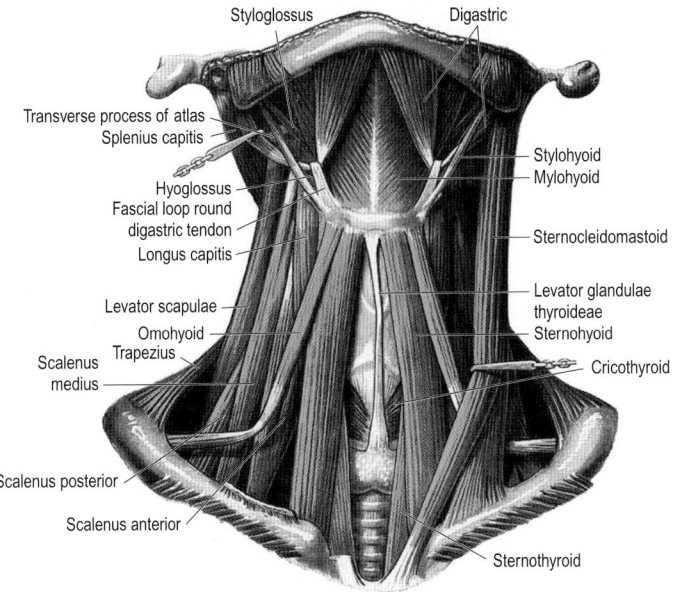

Fig. 31.3 Muscles of the front of the neck. Sternocleidomastoid has been removed on the right side. In this subject, the origin of scalenus medius is extended up to the transverse process of the atlas.

a topographical value in description. Moreover, some of their subdivisions are easily identified by inspection and palpation and provide invaluable assistance in surface anatomical and clinical examination.

Anterior triangle of the neck

The anterior triangle of the neck is bounded anteriorly by the median line of the neck and posteriorly by the anterior margin of sternocleidomastoid. Its base is the inferior border of the mandible and its projection to the mastoid process, and its apex is at the manubrium sterni. It can be subdivided into suprahyoid and infrahyoid areas above and below the hyoid bone, and into digastric, submental, muscular and carotid triangles by the passage of digastric and omohyoid across the anterior triangle.

DIGASTRIC TRIANGLE

The digastric triangle is bordered above by the base of the mandible and its projection to the mastoid process, posteroinferiorly by the posterior belly of digastric and by stylohyoid, and anteroinferiorly by the anterior belly of digastric (**Fig. 31.5**). It is covered by the skin, superficial fascia, platysma and deep fascia, which contain branches of the facial and transverse cutaneous cervical nerves. Its floor is formed by mylohyoid and hyoglossus. The anterior region of the digastric triangle contains the submandibular gland, which has the facial vein superficial to it and the facial artery deep to it. The submental and mylohyoid arteries and nerves lie on mylohyoid. The submandibular lymph nodes are variably related to the submandibular gland. The posterior region of the digastric triangle contains the lower part of the parotid gland. The external carotid artery, passing deep to stylohyoid, curves above the muscle, and overlaps its superficial surface as it ascends deep to the parotid gland before entering it. The internal carotid artery, internal jugular vein and vagus nerve lie deeper and are separated from the external carotid artery by styloglossus, stylopharyngeus and the glossopharyngeal nerve.

SUBMENTAL TRIANGLE

The single submental triangle is demarcated by the anterior bellies of both digastric muscles. Its apex is at the chin, its base is the body of the hyoid bone and its floor is formed by both mylohyoid muscles. It contains lymph nodes and small veins that unite to form the anterior jugular vein. The structures within the digastric and submental triangles are described in more detail with the floor of the mouth (p. 583).

MUSCULAR TRIANGLE

The muscular triangle is bounded anteriorly by the median line of the neck from the hyoid bone to the sternum, inferoposteriorly by the anterior margin of sternocleidomastoid and posterosuperiorly by the superior belly of omohyoid. The triangle contains omohyoid, sternohyoid, sternothyroid and thyrohyoid.

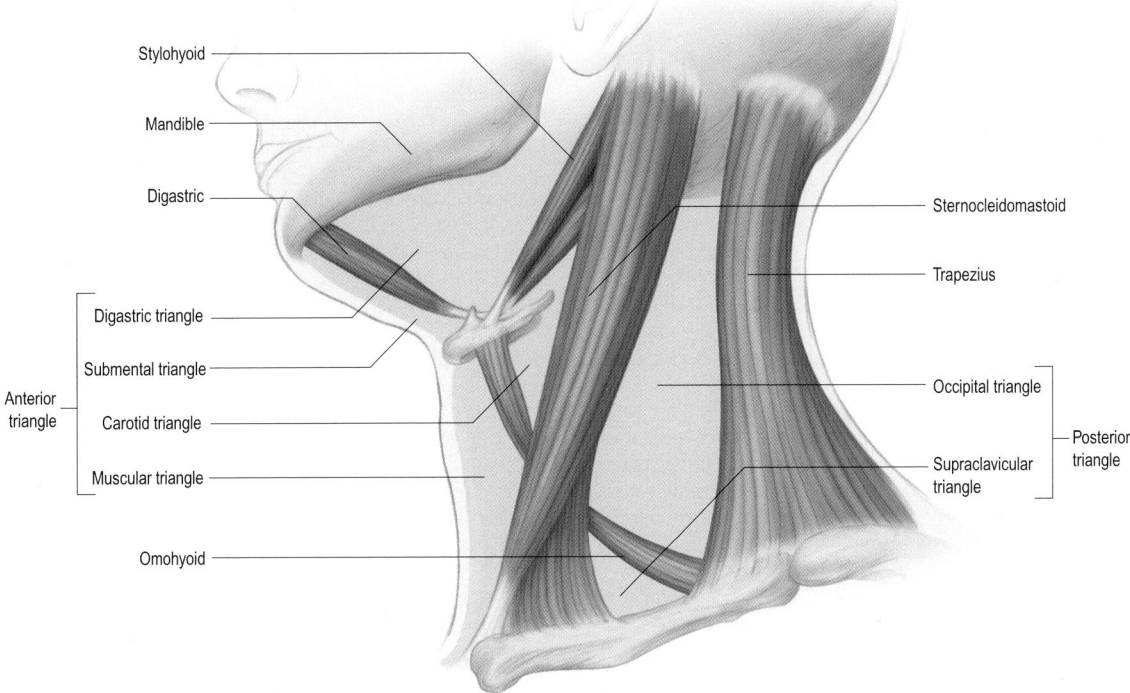

Fig. 31.4 The triangles of the left side of the neck. This is a highly schematic two dimensional representation of what in reality are non-planar trigones distributed over a waisted column.

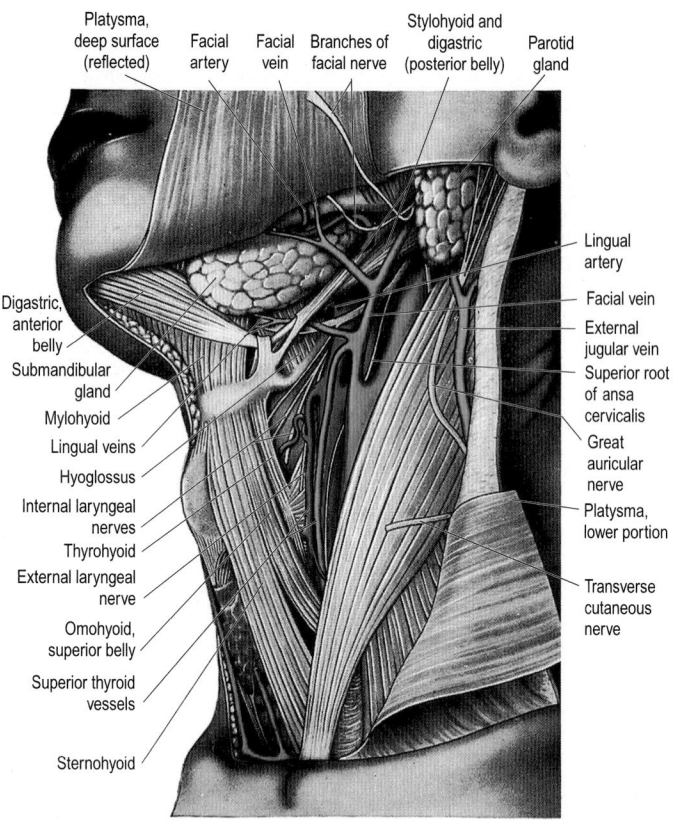

Platysma, deep surface (reflected) — Facial artery — Facial vein — Branches of facial nerve — Stylohyoid and digastric (posterior belly) — Parotid gland

Lingual artery
Facial vein
External jugular vein
Superior root of ansa cervicalis
Great auricular nerve
Platysma, lower portion
Transverse cutaneous nerve

Digastric, anterior belly
Submandibular gland
Mylohyoid
Lingual veins
Hyoglossus
Internal laryngeal nerves
Thyrohyoid
External laryngeal nerve
Omohyoid, superior belly
Superior thyroid vessels
Sternohyoid

Fig. 31.5 Dissection of the left anterior triangle. Platysma has been divided transversely: its upper part has been turned upwards on to the face, and its lower part turned backwards, exposing the lower part of sternocleidomastoid.

CAROTID TRIANGLE

The carotid triangle is limited posteriorly by sternocleidomastoid, anteroinferiorly by the superior belly of omohyoid and superiorly by stylohyoid and the posterior belly of digastric (**Fig. 31.5**). In the living (except the obese) the triangle is usually a small visible triangular depression, sometimes best seen with the head and cervical vertebral column slightly extended and the head contralaterally rotated. The carotid triangle is covered by the skin, superficial fascia, platysma and deep fascia containing branches of the facial and cutaneous cervical nerves. The hyoid bone forms its anterior angle and adjacent floor and can be located on simple inspection, verified by palpation. Parts of thyrohyoid, hyoglossus and inferior and middle pharyngeal constrictor muscles form its floor. The carotid triangle contains the upper part of the common carotid artery and its division into external and internal carotid arteries. Overlapped by the anterior margin of sternocleidomastoid, the external carotid artery is first anteromedial, then anterior to the internal carotid artery. Branches of the external carotid artery are encountered in the carotid triangle. Thus the superior thyroid artery runs anteroinferiorly, the lingual artery anteriorly with a characteristic upward loop, the facial artery anterosuperiorly, the occipital artery posterosuperiorly and the ascending pharyngeal artery medial to the internal carotid artery. Arterial pulsation greets the examining finger. The superior thyroid, lingual, facial, ascending pharyngeal and sometimes the occipital, veins, correspond to the branches of the external carotid artery, and all drain into the internal jugular vein. The hypoglossal nerve crosses the external and internal carotid arteries. It curves round the origin of the lower sternocleidomastoid branch of the occipital artery, and at this point the superior root of the ansa cervicalis leaves it to descend anteriorly in the carotid sheath. The internal laryngeal nerve and, below it, the external laryngeal nerve, lie medial to the external carotid artery below the hyoid bone. Many structures in this region, such as all or part of the internal jugular vein, associated deep cervical lymph nodes, and the vagus nerve, may be variably obscured by sternocleidomastoid, and, pedantically, are thus 'outside the triangle'.

Posterior triangle of the neck

The posterior triangle is delimited anteriorly by sternocleidomastoid, posteriorly by the anterior edge of trapezius, and inferiorly by the middle third of the clavicle. Its apex is between the attachments of sternocleidomastoid and trapezius to the occiput and is often blunted, so that the 'triangle' becomes quadrilateral. The roof of the posterior triangle is formed by the investing layer of the deep cervical fascia. The floor of the triangle is formed by the prevertebral fascia overlying splenius capitis, levator scapulae and the scalene muscles. It is crossed, c.2.5 cm above the clavicle, by the inferior belly of omohyoid, which subdivides it into occipital and supraclavicular triangles. Collectively these contain the cervical and brachial plexuses, the subclavian artery and the spinal accessory nerve. The muscles forming the floor of the posterior triangle constitute the anterior and lateral groups of the prevertebral musculature (**Fig. 31.6**).

OCCIPITAL TRIANGLE

The occipital triangle constitutes the upper and larger part of the posterior triangle, with which it shares the same borders, except that inferiorly it is limited by the inferior belly of omohyoid. Its floor is constituted, from above down, by splenius capitis, levator scapulae, and scaleni medius and posterior, and semispinalis capitis occasionally appears at the apex (**Fig. 31.4**). It is covered by the skin, superficial and deep fasciae and below by platysma. The spinal accessory nerve pierces sternocleidomastoid and crosses levator scapulae obliquely downwards and backwards to reach the deep surface of trapezius. Cutaneous and muscular branches of the cervical plexus emerge at the posterior border of sternocleidomastoid. Inferiorly, supraclavicular nerves, transverse cervical vessels and the uppermost part of the brachial plexus cross the triangle. Lymph nodes lie along the posterior border of sternocleidomastoid from the mastoid process to the root of the neck.

SUPRACLAVICULAR TRIANGLE

The supraclavicular triangle is the lower and smaller division of the posterior triangle, with which it shares the same boundaries, except that superiorly it is limited by omohyoid (**Fig. 31.4**). It corresponds in the living neck with the lower part of a deep, prominent hollow, namely, the greater supraclavicular fossa. Its floor contains the first rib, scalenus medius and the first slip of serratus anterior. Its size varies with the extent of the clavicular attachments of sternocleidomastoid and trapezius and also the level of the inferior belly of omohyoid. The triangle is covered by the skin, superficial and deep fasciae and platysma and crossed by the supraclavicular nerves. Just above the clavicle, the third part of the subclavian artery curves inferolaterally from the lateral margin of scalenus anterior across the first rib to the axilla. The subclavian vein is behind the clavicle and is not usually in the triangle; but it may rise as high as the artery and even accompany it behind scalenus anterior. The brachial plexus is partly superior, and partly posterior to the artery and is always closely related to it. The trunks of the brachial plexus may easily be palpated here if the neck is contralaterally flexed and the examining finger is drawn across the trunks at right angles to their length. With the musculature relaxed, pulsation of the subclavian artery may be felt and the arterial flow can be controlled by retroclavicular compression against the first rib. The suprascapular vessels pass transversely behind the clavicle, below the transverse cervical artery and vein. The external jugular vein descends behind the posterior border of sternocleidomastoid to end in the subclavian vein. It receives the transverse cervical and suprascapular veins, which form a plexus in front of the third part of the subclavian artery; occasionally it is joined by a small vein crossing the clavicle anteriorly from the cephalic vein. The nerve to subclavius crosses the triangle. The triangle contains some lymph nodes.

ROOT OF THE NECK (Figs 31.7, 31.8, 31.9, 31.24, 31.25, 63.5)

A number of important structures and tissue spaces pass between the neck and thorax or upper limb in the root of the neck. They include the subclavian vessels; common carotid artery; trunks of the brachial plexus; sympathetic trunk; phrenic, vagus and recurrent laryngeal nerves (on both sides); the terminal portion of the thoracic duct (on the left side only); the terminal portion of the right lymphatic duct (on the right

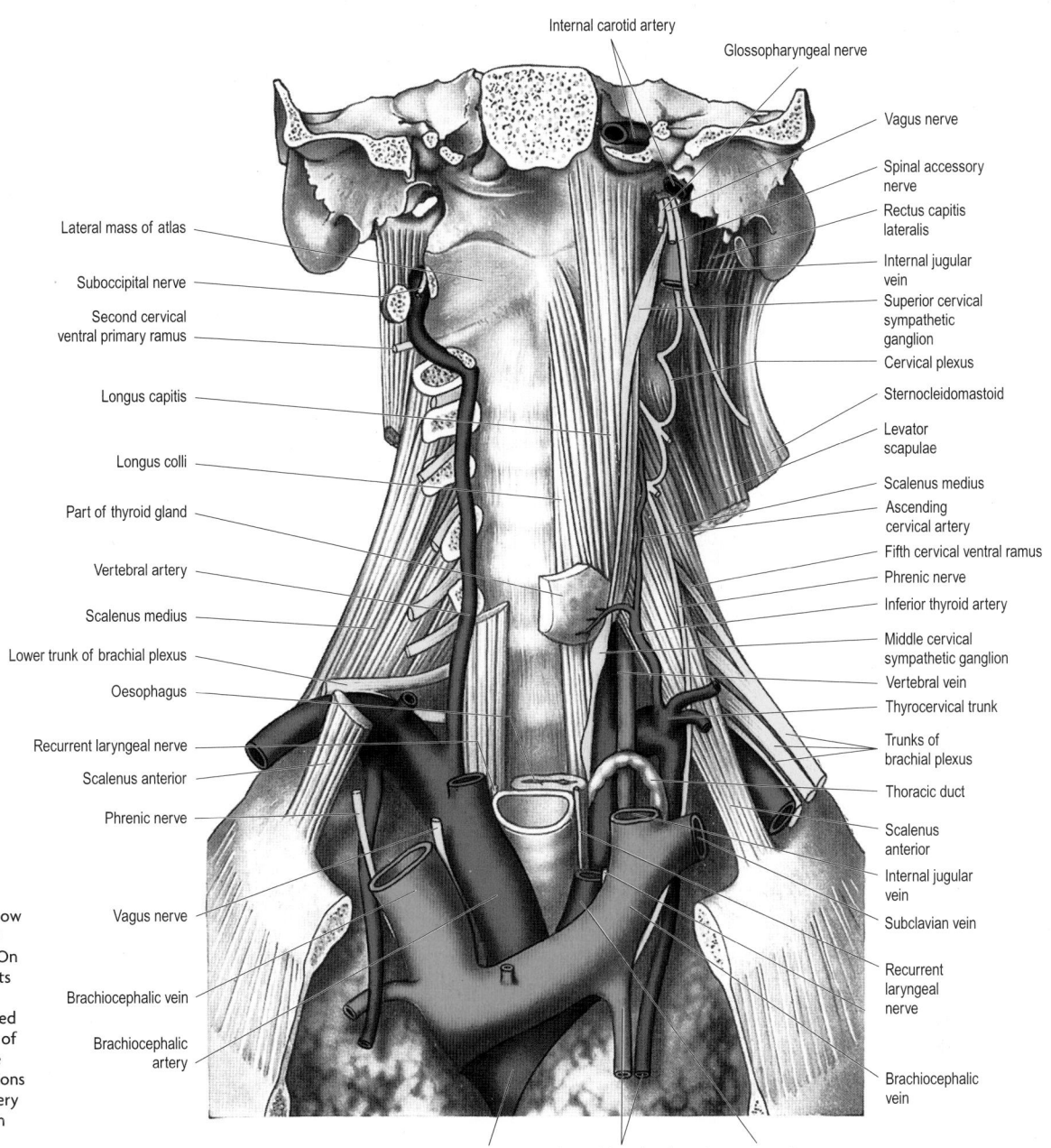

Internal carotid artery

Glossopharyngeal nerve

Vagus nerve

Spinal accessory
nerve

Rectus capitis
lateralis

Internal jugular
vein

Superior cervical
sympathetic
ganglion

Cervical plexus

Sternocleidomastoid

Levator
scapulae

Scalenus medius

Ascending
cervical artery

Fifth cervical ventral ramus

Phrenic nerve

Inferior thyroid artery

Middle cervical
sympathetic ganglion

Vertebral vein

Thyrocervical trunk

Trunks of
brachial plexus

Thoracic duct

Scalenus
anterior

Internal jugular
vein

Subclavian vein

Recurrent
laryngeal
nerve

Brachiocephalic
vein

Lateral mass of atlas

Suboccipital nerve

Second cervical
ventral primary ramus

Longus capitis

Longus colli

Part of thyroid gland

Vertebral artery

Scalenus medius

Lower trunk of brachial plexus

Oesophagus

Recurrent laryngeal nerve

Scalenus anterior

Phrenic nerve

Vagus nerve

Brachiocephalic vein

Brachiocephalic
artery

Arch of aorta   Internal thoracic vein   Common carotid artery
and artery

Fig. 31.6 A dissection to show
the prevertebral region and
the superior mediastinum. On
the right the costal elements
of the upper six cervical
vertebrae have been removed
to expose the cervical part of
the vertebral artery. On the
left most of the deep relations
of the common carotid artery
and the internal jugular vein
are exposed.

side only); and the oesophagus and trachea (in the midline). The
brachiocephalic veins are formed by the union of the internal jugular
and subclavian veins at the junction of the neck and thorax.

On each side, the apical (cervical) pleura and the apex of the lung
bulge up into the root of the neck. The height to which the apical pleura
rises – with reference to the first pair of ribs and costal cartilages – varies
in different individuals according to the obliquity of the thoracic inlet.
Posteriorly the apical pleura typically reaches the level of the neck of the
first rib, and forms a domed roof over each side of the thoracic cavity,
strengthened by the suprapleural membrane. Scalenus anterior covers
the anterolateral part of the dome of the pleura, and separates it from
the subclavian vein. The subclavian artery crosses the dome below its
summit and immediately above the vein. The internal thoracic artery
descends from the first part of the subclavian artery, passes behind the
brachiocephalic vein and, on the right side, is crossed by the phrenic
nerve. The costocervical trunk arches backwards from the subclavian
artery and crosses the summit of the dome of the lung: its superior intercostal branch descends behind the dome, between the first intercostal
nerve laterally and the first thoracic sympathetic ganglion medially. The
vagus descends anterior to the first part of the subclavian artery, and on
the right side its recurrent laryngeal branch turns around the lower
border of the artery.

CERVICAL RIB

A small extra rib (cervical rib) may develop in the root of the neck in
association with the seventh cervical vertebra. Its presence may result in
symptoms associated with compression of adjacent structures, particularly the brachial plexus and subclavian artery. Anatomical variations in
the relationship between scalenus anterior and the brachial plexus can
also give rise to compression syndromes of the brachial plexus.

MUSCLES

Superficial and lateral cervical muscles

PLATYSMA

Platysma is a broad sheet of muscle of varying prominence which arises
from the fascia covering the upper parts of pectoralis major and deltoid.
Its fibres cross the clavicle and ascend medially in the side of the neck.
Anterior fibres interlace across the midline with the fibres of the contralateral muscle, below and behind the symphysis menti. Other fibres
attach to the lower border of the mandible or to the lower lip or cross
the mandible to attach to skin and subcutaneous tissue of the lower
face.

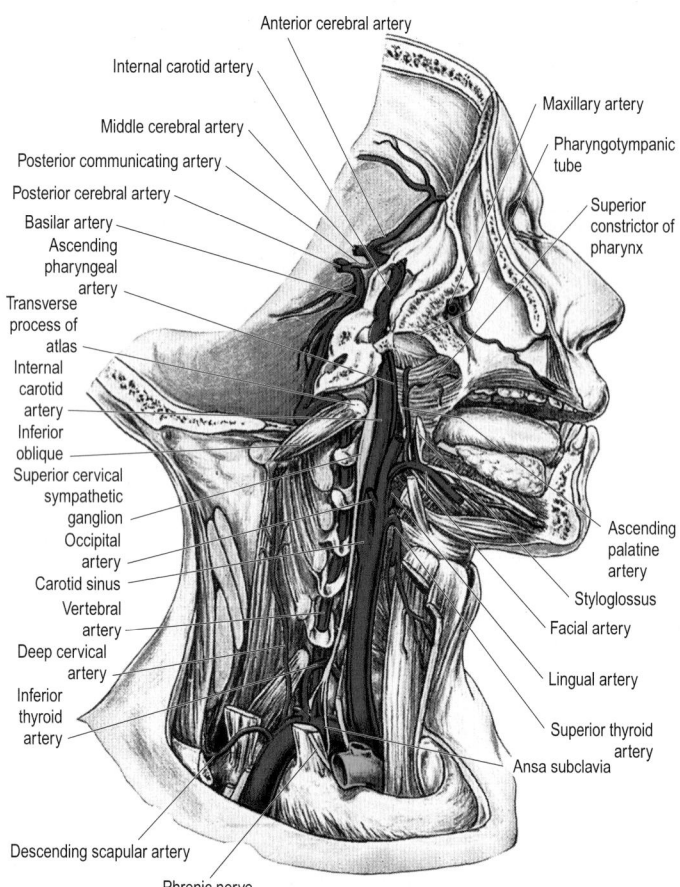

Anterior cerebral artery

Internal carotid artery

Middle cerebral artery

Posterior communicating artery

Posterior cerebral artery

Basilar artery

Ascending pharyngeal artery

Transverse process of atlas

Internal carotid artery

Inferior oblique

Superior cervical sympathetic ganglion

Occipital artery

Carotid sinus

Vertebral artery

Deep cervical artery

Inferior thyroid artery

Descending scapular artery

Phrenic nerve

Maxillary artery

Pharyngotympanic tube

Superior constrictor of pharynx

Ascending palatine artery

Styloglossus

Facial artery

Lingual artery

Superior thyroid artery

Ansa subclavia

Fig. 31.7 Dissection to show the course of the right vertebral and internal carotid arteries and some of their branches.

Vascular supply – Platysma receives its blood supply from the submental branch of the facial artery and the suprascapular artery from the thyrocervical trunk of the subclavian artery.

Innervation – Platysma is innervated by the cervical branch of the facial nerve which descends on the deep surface of the muscle close to the angle of the mandible.

Actions – Contraction diminishes the concavity between the jaw and the side of the neck and produces tense oblique ridges in the skin of the neck. Platysma may assist in depressing the mandible, and via its labial and modiolar attachments it can draw down the lower lip and corners of the mouth in expressions of horror or surprise.

STERNOCLEIDOMASTOID

Sternocleidomastoid (**Fig. 31.10**) descends obliquely across the side of the neck and forms a prominent surface landmark, especially when contracted. It is thick and narrow centrally, and broader and thinner at each end. The muscle is attached inferiorly by two heads. The medial or sternal head is rounded and tendinous, arises from the upper part of the anterior surface of the manubrium and sterni and ascends posterolaterally. The lateral or clavicular head, which is variable in width and contains muscular and fibrous elements, ascends almost vertically from the superior surface of the medial third of the clavicle. The two heads are separated near their attachments by a triangular interval which corresponds to a surface depression, the lesser supraclavicular fossa. As they ascend, the clavicular head spirals behind the sternal head and blends with its deep surface below the middle of the neck, forming a thick, rounded belly. Sternocleidomastoid inserts superiorly by a strong tendon into the lateral surface of the mastoid process from its apex to its superior border, and by a thin aponeurosis into the lateral half of the superior nuchal line. The clavicular fibres are directed mainly to the mastoid process; the sternal fibres are more oblique and superficial, and

extend to the occiput. The direction of pull of the two heads is therefore different, and the muscle may be classed as 'cruciate' and slightly 'spiralized'.

Relations – The superficial surface of sternocleidomastoid is covered by skin and platysma, between which lie the external jugular vein, the great auricular and transverse cervical nerves and the superficial lamina of the deep cervical fascia. Near its insertion the muscle is overlapped by a small part of the parotid gland. The deep surface of the muscle near its origin is related to the sternoclavicular joint and sternohyoid, sternothyroid and omohyoid. The anterior jugular vein crosses deep to it, but superficial to the infrahyoid muscles, immediately above the clavicle. The carotid sheath and the subclavian artery are deep to these muscles. Between omohyoid and the posterior belly of digastric, the anterior part of sternocleidomastoid lies superficial to the common, internal and external carotid arteries, the internal jugular, facial and lingual veins, the deep cervical lymph nodes, the vagus nerve and the rami of the ansa cervicalis. The sternocleidomastoid branch of the superior thyroid artery crosses deep to the muscle at the upper border of omohyoid. The posterior part of sternocleidomastoid is related on its internal surface to splenius capitis, levator scapulae and the scalene muscles, the cervical plexus, the upper part of the brachial plexus, the phrenic nerve and the transverse cervical and suprascapular arteries. The occipital artery crosses deep to the muscle at, or under cover of, the lower border of the posterior belly of digastric. At this point the accessory nerve passes deep to sternocleidomastoid, then pierces and supplies the muscle, before it reappears just above the middle of the posterior border. At its insertion the muscle lies superficial to the mastoid process, splenius capitis, longissimus capitis and the posterior belly of digastric.

Vascular supply – Sternocleidomastoid receives its blood supply from branches of the occipital and posterior auricular arteries (upper part of muscle), the superior thyroid artery (middle part of muscle), and the suprascapular artery (lower part of muscle). A superiorly based flap can be raised on sternocleidomastoid to include a paddle of skin supplied by perforator vessels. This flap has been used to reconstruct the lips, floor of mouth and inner aspect of the cheeks, however its use has been superseded by microvascular free transfer flaps or by conventional myocutaneous flaps such as the pectoralis major flap.

Innervation – Sternocleidomastoid is supplied by the spinal part of the accessory nerve. Branches from the ventral rami of the second, third, and sometimes fourth, cervical spinal nerves also enter the muscle. Although these cervical rami were believed to be solely proprioceptive, clinical evidence suggests that some of their fibres are motor.

Actions – Acting alone, each sternocleidomastoid will tilt the head towards the ipsilateral shoulder, simultaneously rotating the head so as to turn the face towards the opposite side. This movement occurs in an upward, sideways glance. A more common visual movement is a level rotation from side to side, and this probably represents the most frequent use of the sternocleidomastoids. Acting together from below, the muscles draw the head forwards and so help longi colli to flex the cervical part of the vertebral column, which is a common movement in feeding. The two sternocleidomastoids are also used to raise the head when the body is supine, and when the head is fixed, they help to elevate the thorax in forced inspiration.

Branchial cysts and fistulae – Branchial cysts usually present in the upper neck in early adulthood as fluctuant swellings at the junction of the upper and middle thirds of the anterior border of sternocleidomastoid. The cyst typically passes backwards and upwards through the carotid bifurcation and ends at the pharyngeal constrictor muscles, a course which brings it into intimate association with the hypoglossal, glossopharyngeal and spinal accessory nerves. Great care must be taken to avoid damage to these nerves during surgical removal of a branchial cyst.

Branchial fistulae represent a persistent connection between the second branchial pouch and the cervical sinus. The fistula typically presents as a small pit adjacent to the anterior border of the lower third of sternocleidomastoid, which may weep saliva and become intermittently infected. Excision involves following the tract of the fistula up the neck – often through the carotid bifurcation – and into the distal tonsillar fossa where it opens into the pharynx.

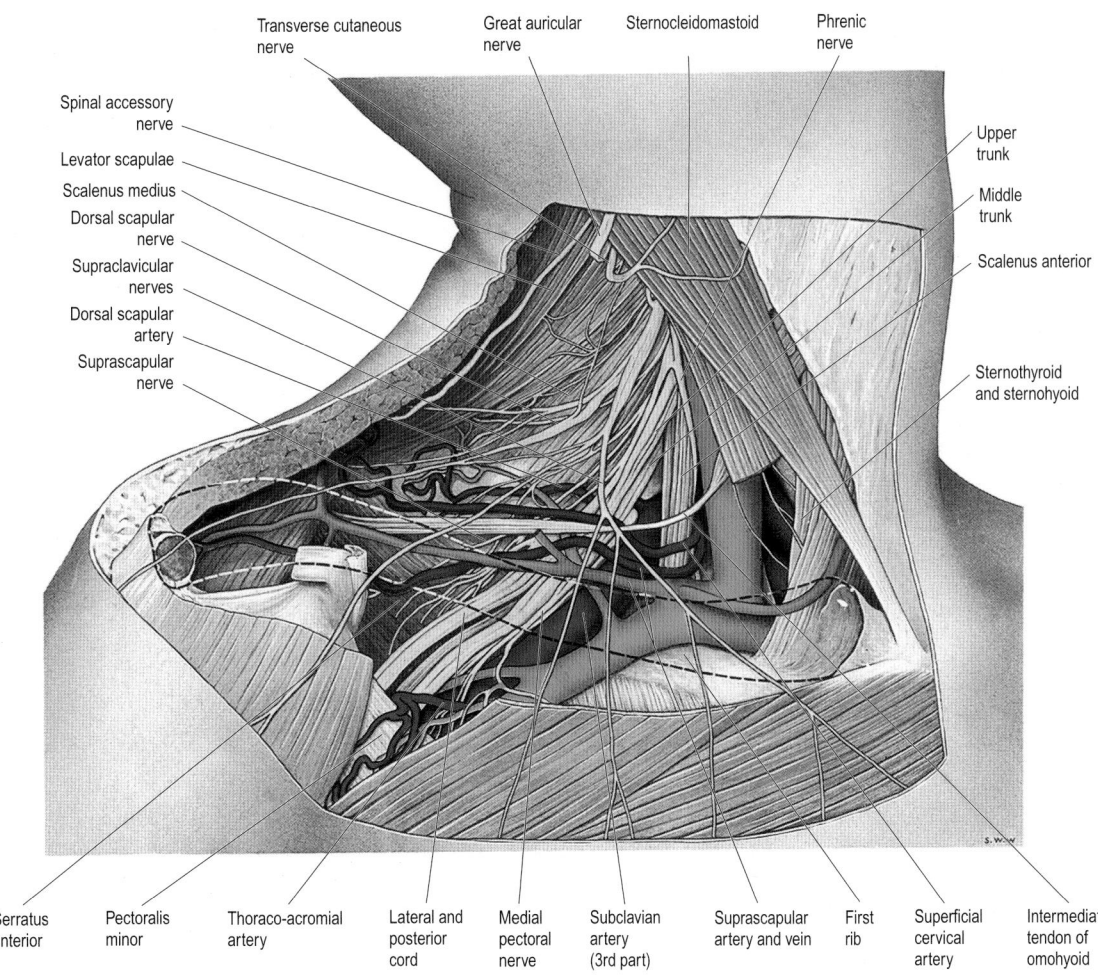

Transverse cutaneous nerve

Great auricular nerve

Sternocleidomastoid

Phrenic nerve

Spinal accessory nerve

Levator scapulae

Scalenus medius

Dorsal scapular nerve

Supraclavicular nerves

Dorsal scapular artery

Suprascapular nerve

Upper trunk

Middle trunk

Scalenus anterior

Sternothyroid and sternohyoid

Fig. 31.8 The lower part of the posterior triangle to show the relations of the third part of the right subclavian artery. The clavicle has been removed, but its outline is indicated by a dashed line. In this dissection, the middle trunk of the brachial plexus gives an unusual contribution to the medial cord.

Serratus anterior

Pectoralis minor

Thoraco-acromial artery

Lateral and posterior cord

Medial pectoral nerve

Subclavian artery (3rd part)

Suprascapular artery and vein

First rib

Superficial cervical artery

Intermediate tendon of omohyoid

Branchial cysts, sinuses and fistulae are thought to arise from inclusions of salivary gland tissue in lymph nodes: they may also occur around the parotid gland.

Muscles of the anterior triangle of the neck

Apart from the superficial neck muscles already described, the anterior triangle contains two of the suprahyoid muscles, namely digastric and stylohyoid, and the four infrahyoid strap muscles. The other suprahyoid muscles, namely mylohyoid and geniohyoid, are described with the floor of the mouth (p. 583).

DIGASTRIC

Digastric has two bellies and lies below the mandible, extending from the mastoid process to the chin (**Figs 31.3, 31.5**). The posterior belly, which is longer than the anterior, is attached in the mastoid notch of the temporal bone, and passes downwards and forwards. The anterior belly is attached to the digastric fossa on the base of the mandible near the midline, and slopes downwards and backwards. The two bellies meet in an intermediate tendon which runs in a fibrous sling attached to the body and greater cornu of the hyoid bone and is sometimes lined by a synovial sheath. The tendon perforates stylohyoid.

Variations – Digastric may lack the intermediate tendon and is then attached midway along the body of the mandible. The posterior belly may be augmented by a slip from the styloid process or arise wholly from it. The anterior belly may cross the midline and it is not uncommon for it to fuse with mylohyoid.

Relations – Superficial to digastric are platysma, sternocleidomastoid, splenius capitis, longissimus capitis and stylohyoid, the mastoid process,

the retromandibular vein and the parotid and submandibular salivary glands. Mylohyoid is medial to the anterior belly, and hyoglossus, superior oblique and rectus capitis lateralis, the transverse process of the atlas vertebra, the accessory nerve, internal jugular vein, occipital artery, hypoglossal nerve, internal and external carotid, facial and lingual arteries are all medial to the posterior belly.

Vascular supply – The posterior belly is supplied by the posterior auricular and occipital arteries. The anterior belly of digastric receives its blood supply chiefly from the submental branch of the facial artery.

Innervation – The anterior belly of digastric is supplied by the mylohyoid branch of the inferior alveolar nerve, and the posterior belly is supplied by the facial nerve. The different innervation of the two parts reflects their separate derivations from the mesenchyme of the first and second branchial arches.

Actions – Digastric depresses the mandible and can elevate the hyoid bone. The posterior bellies are especially active during swallowing and chewing.

STYLOHYOID

Stylohyoid arises by a small tendon from the posterior surface of the styloid process, near its base. Passing downwards and forwards, it inserts into the body of the hyoid bone at its junction with the greater cornu (and just above the attachment of the superior belly of omohyoid) (**Fig. 31.3**). It is perforated near its insertion by the intermediate tendon of digastric. The muscle may be absent or double. It may lie medial to the external carotid artery and may end in the suprahyoid or infrahyoid muscles.

Vascular supply – Stylohyoid receives its blood supply from branches of the facial, posterior auricular and occipital arteries.

537

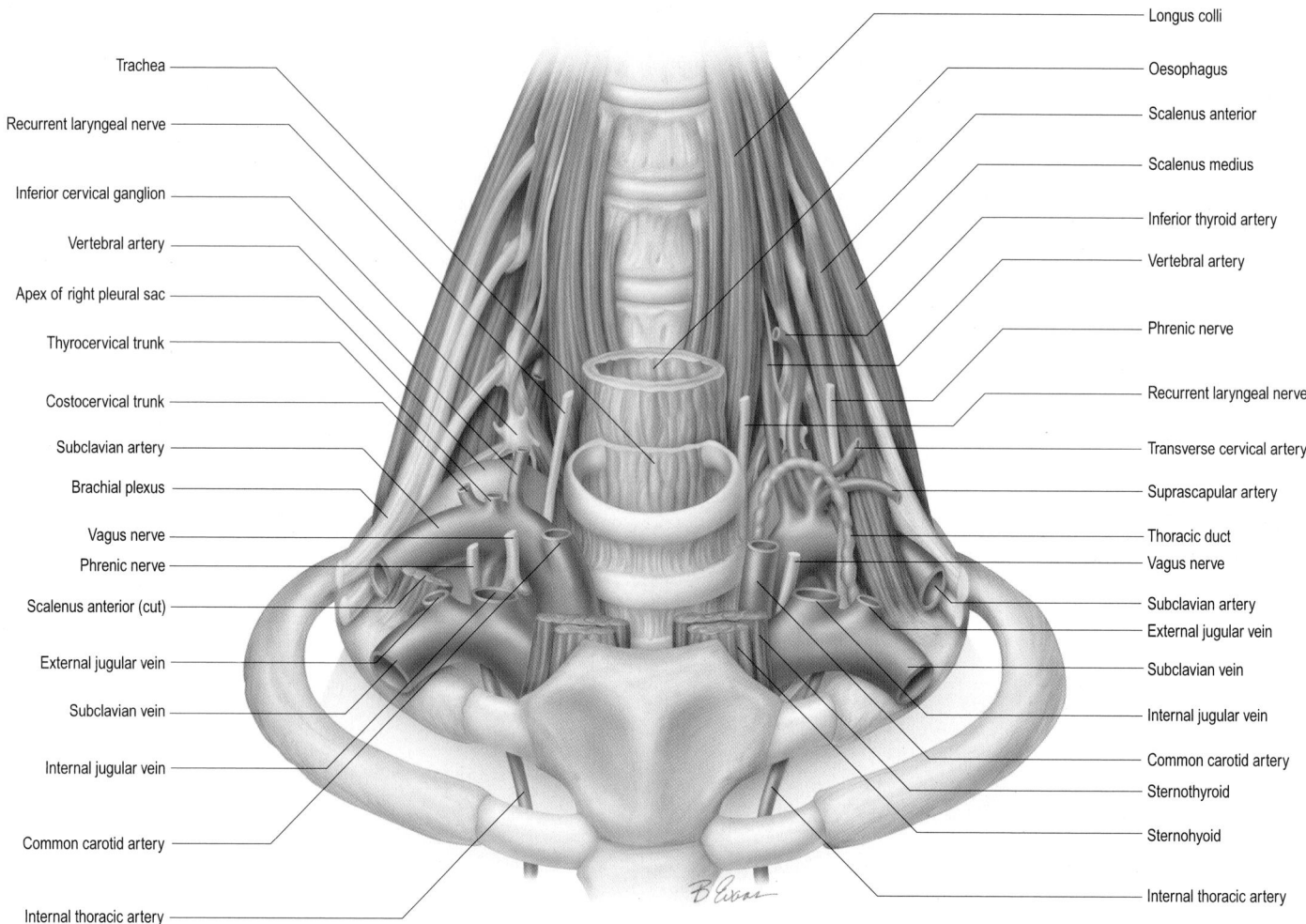

Trachea

Recurrent laryngeal nerve

Inferior cervical ganglion

Vertebral artery

Apex of right pleural sac

Thyrocervical trunk

Costocervical trunk

Subclavian artery

Brachial plexus

Vagus nerve
Phrenic nerve

Scalenus anterior (cut)

External jugular vein

Subclavian vein

Internal jugular vein

Common carotid artery

Internal thoracic artery

Longus colli

Oesophagus

Scalenus anterior

Scalenus medius

Inferior thyroid artery

Vertebral artery

Phrenic nerve

Recurrent laryngeal nerve

Transverse cervical artery

Suprascapular artery

Thoracic duct
Vagus nerve

Subclavian artery
External jugular vein

Subclavian vein

Internal jugular vein

Common carotid artery
Sternothyroid

Sternohyoid

Internal thoracic artery

Fig. 31.9 Root of the neck. (From Brash JC 1958 Cunningham's Manual of Practical Anatomy, Vol 3. Head and Neck: Brain. London: Oxford University Press. By permission of Oxford University Press.)

Innervation – Stylohyoid is innervated by the stylohyoid branch of the facial nerve, which frequently arises with the digastric branch, and enters the middle part of the muscle.

Actions – Stylohyoid elevates the hyoid bone and draws it backwards, elongating the floor of the mouth.

STYLOHYOID LIGAMENT

The stylohyoid ligament is a fibrous cord extending from the tip of the styloid process to the lesser cornu of the hyoid bone. It gives attachment to the highest fibres of the middle pharyngeal constrictor and is intimately related to the lateral wall of the oropharynx. Below, it is overlapped by hyoglossus. The ligament is derived from the cartilage of the second branchial arch, and may be partially calcified.

Infrahyoid muscles

The infrahyoid muscles are organized so that sternohyoid and omohyoid lie superficially and sternothyroid and thyrohyoid lie more deeply. The muscles are involved in movements of the hyoid bone and thyroid cartilage during vocalization, swallowing and mastication and are mainly innervated from the ansa cervicalis.

STERNOHYOID

Sternohyoid (**Fig. 31.3**) is a thin, narrow strap muscle that arises from the posterior surface of the medial end of the clavicle, the posterior sternoclavicular ligament and the upper posterior aspect of the manubrium sterni. It ascends medially and is attached to the inferior border of the body of the hyoid bone. Inferiorly, there is a considerable

gap between the muscle and its contralateral fellow, but the two usually come together in the middle of their course, and are contiguous above this. Sternohyoid may be absent or double, augmented by a clavicular slip (cleidohyoid), or interrupted by a tendinous intersection.

Vascular supply – Sternohyoid is supplied by branches from the superior thyroid artery.

Innervation – Sternohyoid is innervated by branches from the ansa cervicalis (C1, 2, 3).

Action – Sternohyoid depresses the hyoid bone after it has been elevated.

OMOHYOID

Omohyoid consists of two bellies united at an angle by an intermediate tendon (**Fig. 31.3**). The inferior belly is a flat, narrow band, which inclines forwards and slightly upwards across the lower part of the neck. It arises from the upper border of the scapula, near the scapular notch, and occasionally from the superior transverse scapular ligament. It then passes behind sternocleidomastoid and ends there in the intermediate tendon. The superior belly begins at the intermediate tendon, passes almost vertically upwards near the lateral border of sternohyoid and is attached to the lower border of the body of the hyoid bone lateral to the insertion of sternohyoid. The length and form of the intermediate tendon varies, although it usually lies adjacent to the internal jugular vein at the level of the arch of the cricoid cartilage. The angulated course of the muscle is maintained by a band of deep cervical fascia, attached below to the clavicle and the first rib, which ensheathes the tendon. A variable amount of skeletal muscle may be present in the fascial band; either belly may be absent or double; the inferior belly may be attached

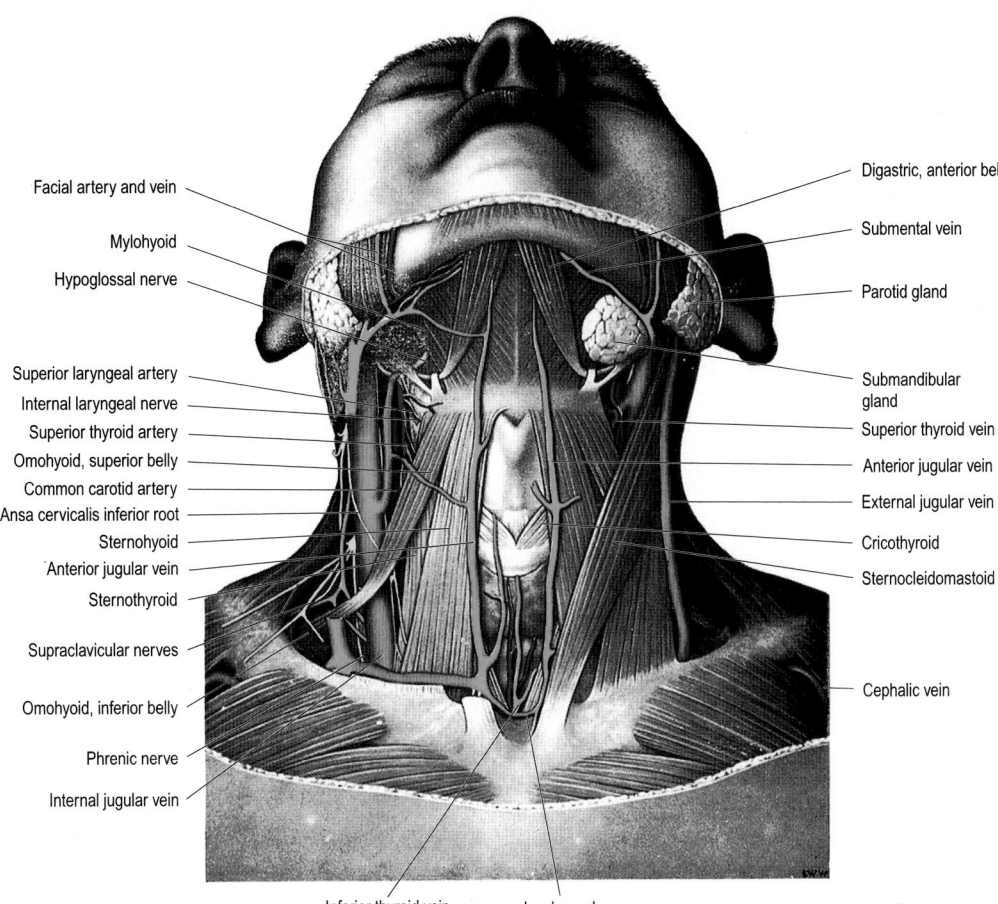

Facial artery and vein

Mylohyoid

Hypoglossal nerve

Superior laryngeal artery
Internal laryngeal nerve
Superior thyroid artery
Omohyoid, superior belly
Common carotid artery
Ansa cervicalis inferior root
Sternohyoid
Anterior jugular vein
Sternothyroid

Supraclavicular nerves

Omohyoid, inferior belly

Phrenic nerve

Internal jugular vein

Digastric, anterior belly

Submental vein

Parotid gland

Submandibular gland
Superior thyroid vein
Anterior jugular vein
External jugular vein
Cricothyroid
Sternocleidomastoid

Cephalic vein

Inferior thyroid vein   Jugular arch

Fig. 31.10 Anterior view of the veins of the neck. The head has been extended.

directly to the clavicle and the superior is sometimes fused with sternohyoid.

Vascular supply – Omohyoid is supplied by branches from the superior thyroid and lingual arteries.

Innervation – The superior belly of omohyoid is innervated by branches from the superior ramus of the ansa cervicalis (C1). The inferior belly is innervated from the ansa cervicalis itself (C1, 2 and 3).

Actions – Omohyoid depresses the hyoid bone after it has been elevated. It has been speculated that the muscle tenses the lower part of the deep cervical fascia in prolonged inspiratory efforts, reducing the tendency for soft parts to be sucked inward.

STERNOTHYROID

Sternothyroid (**Fig. 31.3**) is shorter and wider than sternohyoid, and lies deep and partly medial to it. It arises from the posterior surface of the manubrium sterni inferior to the origin of sternohyoid and from the posterior edge of the cartilage of the first rib. It is attached above to the oblique line on the lamina of the thyroid cartilage, where it delineates the upward extent of the thyroid gland. In the lower part of the neck the muscle is in contact with its contralateral fellow, but the two diverge as they ascend.

Vascular supply – Sternothyroid is supplied by branches from the superior thyroid and lingual arteries.

Innervation – Sternothyroid is innervated by branches from the ansa cervicalis (C1, 2 and 3).

Action – Sternothyroid draws the larynx downwards after it has been elevated by swallowing or vocal movements. In the singing of low notes, this downward traction would be exerted with the hyoid bone relatively fixed.

THYROHYOID

Thyrohyoid is a small, quadrilateral muscle that may be regarded as an upward continuation of sternothyroid (**Fig. 31.5**). It arises from the oblique line on the lamina of the thyroid cartilage, and passes upwards to attach to the lower border of the greater cornu and adjacent part of the body of the hyoid bone.

Vascular supply – Thyrohyoid is supplied by branches from the superior thyroid and lingual arteries.

Innervation – Unlike the other infrahyoid muscles, thyrohyoid is not innervated by the ansa cervicalis. In common with geniohyoid, it is supplied by fibres from the first cervical spinal nerve which branch off from the hypoglossal nerve beyond the descendens hypoglossi.

Actions – Thyrohyoid depresses the hyoid bone. With the hyoid bone stabilized, it pulls the larynx upwards, e.g. when high notes are sung.

Anterior vertebral muscles (Fig. 31.11)

The anterior vertebral group of muscles consists of longi colli and capitis, and recti capitis anterior and lateralis, all of which are flexors of the head and neck to varying degrees. Together with the lateral vertebral muscles they form the prevertebral muscle group.

RECTUS CAPITIS ANTERIOR

Rectus capitis anterior is a short, flat muscle situated behind the upper part of longus capitis. It arises from the anterior surface of the lateral mass of the atlas and the root of its transverse process, and ascends almost vertically to the inferior surface of the basilar part of the occipital bone immediately anterior to the occipital condyle.

Vascular supply – Rectus capitis anterior is supplied by branches from the vertebral and ascending pharyngeal arteries.

539

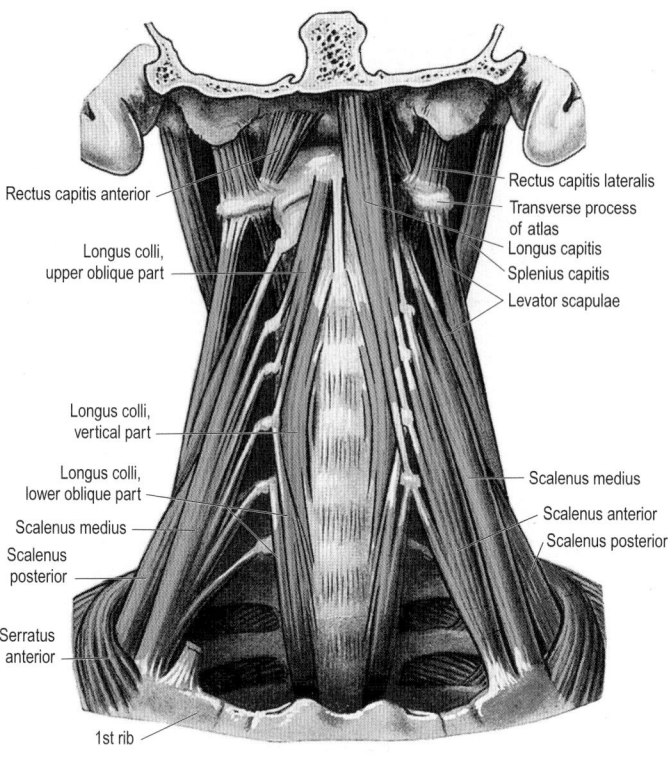

Rectus capitis anterior

Longus colli, upper oblique part

Longus colli, vertical part

Longus colli, lower oblique part

Scalenus medius

Scalenus posterior

Serratus anterior

1st rib

Rectus capitis lateralis

Transverse process of atlas

Longus capitis

Splenius capitis

Levator scapulae

Scalenus medius

Scalenus anterior

Scalenus posterior

Fig. 31.11 The anterior and lateral vertebral muscles. Scalenus anterior and longus capitis have been removed on the right side.

Innervation – Rectus capitis anterior is innervated by branches from the loop between the ventral rami of the first and second cervical spinal nerves.

Actions – Rectus capitis anterior flexes the head at the atlanto-occipital joints.

RECTUS CAPITIS LATERALIS

Rectus capitis lateralis is a short, flat muscle that arises from the upper surface of the transverse process of the atlas and inserts into the inferior surface of the jugular process of the occipital bone. In view of its attachments and its relation to the ventral ramus of the first spinal nerve, rectus capitis lateralis is regarded as homologous with the posterior intertransverse muscles.

Vascular supply – Rectus capitis lateralis is supplied by branches from the vertebral, occipital and ascending pharyngeal arteries.

Innervation – Rectus capitis lateralis is innervated by branches from the loop between the ventral rami of the first and second cervical spinal nerves.

Actions – Rectus capitis lateralis flexes the head laterally to the same side.

LONGUS CAPITIS

Longus capitis (**Fig. 31.6**) has a narrow origin from tendinous slips from the anterior tubercles of the transverse processes of the third, fourth, fifth and sixth cervical vertebrae and becomes broad and thick above, where it is inserted into the inferior surface of the basilar part of the occipital bone.

Vascular supply – Longus capitis is supplied by the ascending pharyngeal, ascending cervical branch of the inferior thyroid and the vertebral arteries.

Innervation – Longus capitis is innervated by branches from the ventral rami of the first, second and third cervical spinal nerves.

Actions – Longus capitis flexes the head.

LONGUS COLLI

Longus colli (**Fig. 31.6**) is applied to the anterior surface of the vertebral column, between the atlas and the third thoracic vertebra. It can be divided into three parts which all arise by tendinous slips. The inferior oblique part is the smallest, running upwards and laterally from the fronts of the bodies of the first two or three thoracic vertebrae to the anterior tubercles of the transverse processes of the fifth and sixth cervical vertebrae. The superior oblique part passes upwards and medially from the anterior tubercles of the transverse processes of the third, fourth and fifth cervical vertebrae to be attached by a narrow tendon to the anterolateral surface of the tubercle on the anterior arch of the atlas. The vertical intermediate part ascends from the fronts of the bodies of the upper three thoracic and lower three cervical vertebrae to the fronts of the bodies of the second, third and fourth cervical vertebrae.

Vascular supply – Longus colli is supplied by branches from the vertebral, inferior thyroid and ascending pharyngeal arteries.

Innervation – Longus colli is innervated by branches from the ventral rami of the second, third, fourth, fifth and sixth cervical spinal nerves.

Actions – Longus colli flexes the neck forwards. In addition, the oblique parts may flex it laterally, and the inferior oblique part rotates it to the opposite side. Its main antagonist is longissimus cervicis.

Lateral vertebral muscles (Figs 31.6, 31.11)

The scaleni, anterior, medius and posterior, extend obliquely between the upper two ribs and the cervical transverse processes.

SCALENUS ANTERIOR

Scalenus anterior lies at the side of the neck deep (posteromedial) to sternocleidomastoid. Above, it is attached by musculotendinous fascicles to the anterior tubercles of the transverse processes of the third, fourth, fifth and sixth cervical vertebrae. These converge, blend and descend almost vertically, to be attached by a narrow, flat tendon to the scalene tubercle on the inner border of the first rib, and to a ridge on the upper surface of the rib anterior to the groove for the subclavian artery.

Relations – Scalenus anterior forms an important landmark in the root of the neck, because the phrenic nerve passes above it, the subclavian artery below it, and the brachial plexus lies at its lateral border. The clavicle, subclavius, sternocleidomastoid and omohyoid, lateral part of the carotid sheath, transverse cervical, suprascapular and ascending cervical arteries, subclavian vein, prevertebral fascia and phrenic nerve are all anterior to scalenus anterior. Posteriorly are the suprapleural membrane, pleura, roots of the brachial plexus and the subclavian artery: the latter two separate scalenus anterior from scalenus medius. The proximity of the muscle to the brachial plexus, subclavian artery and vein can give rise to compression syndromes. Below its attachment to the sixth cervical vertebra, the medial border of the muscle is separated from longus colli by an angular interval in which the vertebral artery and vein pass to and from the foramen transversarium of the sixth cervical vertebra. The inferior thyroid artery crosses this interval from the lateral to the medial side near its apex. The sympathetic trunk and its cervicothoracic ganglion are closely related to the posteromedial side of this part of the vertebral artery. On the left side the thoracic duct crosses the triangular interval at the level of the seventh cervical vertebra and usually comes into contact with the medial edge of scalenus anterior. The musculotendinous attachments of scalenus anterior to anterior tubercles are separated from those of longus capitis by the ascending cervical branch of the inferior thyroid artery.

Innervation – Scalenus anterior is innervated by branches from the ventral rami of the fourth, fifth and sixth cervical spinal nerves.

Actions – Acting from below, scalenus anterior bends the cervical portion of the vertebral column forwards and laterally and rotates it towards the opposite side. Acting from above, the muscle helps to elevate the first rib.

SCALENUS MEDIUS

Scalenus medius, the largest and longest of the scaleni, is attached above to the transverse process of the axis and the front of the posterior tubercles of the transverse processes of the lower five cervical vertebrae. It frequently extends upwards to the transverse process of the atlas. Below it is attached to the upper surface of the first rib between the tubercle of the rib and the groove for the subclavian artery.

Relations – The anterolateral surface of the muscle is related to sternocleidomastoid. It is crossed anteriorly by the clavicle and omohyoid, and it is separated from scalenus anterior by the subclavian artery and ventral rami of the cervical spinal nerves. Levator scapulae and scalenus posterior lie posterolateral to it. The upper two roots of the nerve to serratus anterior and the dorsal scapular nerve (to the rhomboids) pierce the muscle and appear on its lateral surface.

Innervation – Scalenus medius is supplied by branches from the ventral rami of the third to eighth cervical spinal nerves.

Actions – Acting from below, scalenus medius bends the cervical part of the vertebral column to the same side. Acting from above, it helps to raise the first rib. The scalene muscles, particularly scalenus medius, are active during inspiration, even during quiet breathing in the erect attitude.

SCALENUS POSTERIOR

Scalenus posterior is the smallest and most deeply situated of the scalene muscles. It passes from the posterior tubercles of the transverse processes of the fourth, fifth, and sixth cervical vertebrae to the outer surface of the second rib, behind the tubercle for serratus anterior, where it is attached by a thin tendon.

Scalenus posterior is occasionally blended with scalenus medius. The scalene muscles vary a little in the number of vertebrae to which they are attached, in their degree of separation, and their segmental innervation.

Vascular supply – All the scalene muscles are chiefly supplied by the ascending cervical branch of the inferior thyroid artery. Scalenus posterior receives an additional supply from the superficial cervical artery.

Innervation – Scalenus posterior is innervated by branches from the ventral rami of the lower three cervical spinal nerves.

Actions – When the second rib is fixed, scalenus posterior bends the lower end of the cervical part of the vertebral column to the same side. When its upper attachment is fixed, it helps to elevate the second rib.

SCALENUS MINIMUS

Scalenus minimus (pleuralis) is associated with the suprapleural membrane and cervical pleura, and is described in that context (pp. 1065, 742).

SPLENIUS CAPITIS AND CERVICIS

Splenius capitis and splenius cervicis are described in detail in Chapter 45.

HYOID BONE

The U-shaped hyoid bone (**Fig. 31.12**) is suspended from the tips of the styloid processes by the stylohyoid ligaments. It has a body, two greater and two lesser horns, or cornua.

Body – The body is irregular, elongated and quadrilateral. Its anterior surface is convex, faces anterosuperiorly, and is crossed by a transverse ridge with a slight downward convexity. A vertical median ridge often bisects the upper part of the body; its presence on the lower part is rare. The posterior surface is smooth, concave, faces posteroinferiorly, and is separated from the epiglottis by the thyrohyoid membrane and loose areolar tissue. There is a bursa between the hyoid bone and the membrane.

Geniohyoid is attached to most of the anterior surface of the body, above and below the transverse ridge, although the medial part of hyoglossus invades the lateral geniohyoid area. The lower anterior surface gives attachment to mylohyoid; the line of attachment lies above the sternohyoid medially and omohyoid laterally. The lowest fibres of the genioglossus, the hyoepiglottic ligament and (most posteriorly) the

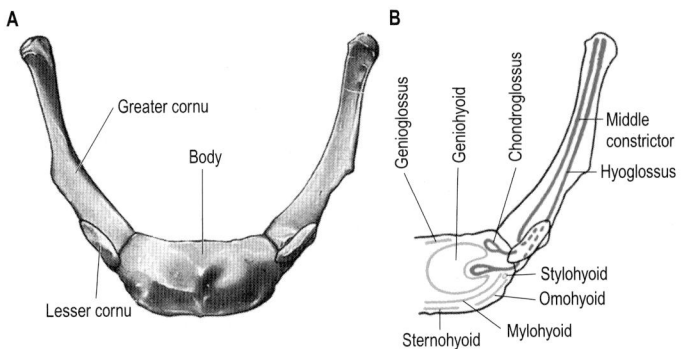

Fig. 31.12 A, B, The hyoid bone: anterosuperior aspect. B shows positions of muscular attachments.

thyrohyoid membrane are attached to the rounded superior border. Sternohyoid is attached to the inferior border medially and omohyoid laterally. Occasionally the medial fibres of thyrohyoid and of levator glandulae thyroideae, when present, are attached along the inferior border.

Greater cornua – In early life, the greater cornua are connected to the body by cartilage, but after middle age they are usually united by bone. They project backwards (curving posterolaterally) from the lateral ends of the body. They are horizontally flattened, taper posteriorly, and each ends in a tubercle. When the throat is gripped between finger and thumb above the thyroid cartilage, the greater cornua can be identified and the bone can be moved from side to side.

The middle pharyngeal constrictor and, more laterally (i.e. superficially), hyoglossus, are attached along the whole length of the upper surface of each greater cornu. Stylohyoid is attached near the junction of the cornu with the body. The fibrous loop for the digastric tendon is attached lateral and a little posterior to hyoglossus. The thyrohyoid membrane is attached to the medial border and thyrohyoid is attached to the lateral border. The oblique inferior surface is separated from the thyrohyoid membrane by fibroareolar tissue.

Lesser cornua – The lesser cornua are two small conical projections at the junctions of the body and greater cornua. At its base, each is connected to the body by fibrous tissue and occasionally to the greater cornu by a synovial joint which occasionally becomes ankylosed.

The middle pharyngeal constrictors are attached to the posterior and lateral aspects of the lesser cornua The stylohyoid ligaments are attached to their apices and are often partly calcified, and the chondroglossi are attached to the medial aspects of their bases.

Ossification – The hyoid bone develops from cartilages of the second and third pharyngeal arches, the lesser cornua from the second, the greater cornua from the third and the body from the fused ventral ends of both. Chondrification begins in the fifth fetal week in these elements, and is completed in the third and fourth months. Ossification proceeds from six centres, i.e. a pair for the body and one for each cornu. Ossification begins in the greater cornua towards the end of intrauterine life, in the body shortly before or after birth, and in the lesser cornua around puberty. The greater cornual apices remain cartilaginous until the third decade and epiphyses may occur here. They fuse with the body. Synovial joints between the greater and lesser cornua may be obliterated by ossification in later decades.

CERVICAL FASCIA
Superficial fascia

The superficial cervical fascia is usually a thin lamina covering platysma and is hardly demonstrable as a separate layer. It may, however, contain considerable amounts of adipose tissue, especially in females. Like all superficial fascia it is not a separate stratum, but merely a zone of loose connective tissue between dermis and deep fascia, and is joined to both.

Deep cervical fascia

Deep fascia in the neck is organized into an investing layer, prevertebral fascia, and pretracheal fascia (**Fig. 31.13**). The carotid sheath is a non-membranous layer of fascia that is conventionally described as part of the deep cervical fascia.

INVESTING LAYER OF DEEP FASCIA

The investing layer of deep cervical fascia is continuous behind with the ligamentum nuchae and the periosteum covering the spine of the seventh cervical vertebra. It forms a thin covering for trapezius and continues forwards from the anterior border of this muscle as a loose areolar layer roofing over the posterior triangle of the neck to the posterior border of sternocleidomastoid, where it becomes denser. It divides around sternocleidomastoid, enclosing it, and reunites at the anterior margin as a single sheet, which covers the anterior triangle of the neck and reaches forwards to the midline. Here it meets the corresponding sheet from the opposite side and adheres to the symphysis menti and the body of the hyoid bone. Superiorly, the deep fascia fuses with periosteum along the superior nuchal line of the occipital bone, over the mastoid process and along the entire base of the mandible. Between the angle of the mandible and the anterior edge of sternocleidomastoid it is particularly strong. Between the mandible and the mastoid process it is related to the parotid gland, extending beneath it to become attached to the zygomatic arch. From this region the strong stylomandibular ligament ascends to the styloid process. Inferiorly, the investing layer of deep fascia is attached to the acromion, clavicle and manubrium sterni, fusing with their periostea. A short distance above the manubrium it splits into superficial and deep layers. The superficial layer is attached to the anterior border of the manubrium, the deep layer to its posterior border and to the interclavicular ligament. Between these two layers is a slit-like interval, the suprasternal space. This contains a small amount of areolar tissue, the lower parts of the anterior jugular veins and the jugular venous arch, the sternal heads of the sternocleidomastoid muscles and sometimes a lymph node. Over the lower part of the posterior triangle, between trapezius and sternocleidomastoid, the deep fascia again divides into superficial and deep layers. The superficial layer is attached below to the superior border of the clavicle. The deep layer surrounds the inferior belly of omohyoid and, deep to sternocleidomastoid, the intermediate tendon of omohyoid. The deep layer blends inferiorly with the fascia around subclavius and the periosteum on the posterior surface of both the clavicle and anterior end of the first rib.

PRETRACHEAL FASCIA

The pretracheal layer of the deep cervical fascia is very thin. It provides a fascial sheath for the thyroid gland and lies deep to the strap muscles. Superiorly, it attaches to the arch of the cricoid cartilage, and inferiorly

it continues into the superior mediastinum along the great vessels to merge with the fibrous pericardium. The pretracheal fascia merges laterally with the investing layer of deep cervical fascia and with the carotid sheath.

PREVERTEBRAL FASCIA

The prevertebral fascia covers the anterior vertebral muscles and extends laterally on scalenus anterior, scalenus medius and levator scapulae, forming a fascial floor for the posterior triangle of the neck. As the subclavian artery and the brachial plexus emerge from behind scalenus anterior they carry the prevertebral fascia downwards and laterally behind the clavicle as the axillary sheath. The prevertebral fascia is particularly prominent in front of the vertebral column, where there may be two distinct layers of fascia. Traced laterally, it becomes thin and areolar and is lost as a definite fibrous layer under cover of trapezius. Superiorly the prevertebral fascia is attached to the base of the skull. Inferiorly it descends in front of longus colli into the superior mediastinum, where it blends with the anterior longitudinal ligament. Anteriorly the prevertebral fascia is separated from the pharynx and its covering buccopharyngeal fascia by a loose areolar zone, the retropharyngeal space. Laterally this loose tissue connects the prevertebral fascia to the carotid sheath and the fascia on the deep surface of sternocleidomastoid. All the ventral rami of the cervical nerves are initially behind the prevertebral fascia. The nerves to the rhomboids and serratus anterior and the phrenic nerve retain this position throughout their course in the neck, but the accessory nerve lies superficial to the prevertebral fascia.

CAROTID SHEATH

The carotid sheath is a condensation of deep cervical fascia around the common and internal carotid arteries, the internal jugular vein, the vagus nerve and the constituents of the ansa cervicalis. It is thicker around the arteries than the vein, an arrangement that allows the vein to expand. Peripherally the carotid sheath is connected to adjacent fascial layers by loose areolar tissue.

TISSUE SPACES AND THE SPREAD OF INFECTION

The fascial layers of the neck define a number of potential tissue 'spaces' above and below the hyoid bone. In health, the tissues within these spaces are closely applied to each other or are filled with relatively loose connective tissue. However, infection, which often arises superiorly in the region of the infratemporal fossa as a result of dental or tonsillar infections, can alter these relationships. The organisms responsible are often beta-haemolytic streptococci or a variety of anaerobes. Streptococci produce proteolytic enzymes which digest the loose connective tissue and so open up the tissue spaces. Since there are no tissue barriers running horizontally or vertically in the neck, infections which are not treated promptly can spread from the infratemporal fossa down to the mediastinum below, and can even cross the midline through the sublingual and submental spaces.

The tissue spaces above the hyoid bone are the submandibular and submental spaces beneath the inferior border of the mandible; the pharyngeal spaces; and the prevertebral space near the base of the skull. These spaces are described on pages 607 and 626. Tissue spaces around the larynx are described on page 640.

Tissue spaces below the hyoid bone are the pretracheal and retrovisceral tissue spaces in the visceral compartment of the neck; the prevertebral space in front of the vertebral column; and a space associated with the carotid sheath.

Pretracheal space – The pretracheal tissue space lies behind the pretracheal fascia and the infrahyoid strap muscles, and in front of the anterior wall of the oesophagus, and therefore immediately surrounds the trachea. It is bounded superiorly by the attachments of the infrahyoid muscles to the thyroid cartilage of the larynx. Inferiorly, it extends down into the anterior portion of the superior mediastinum. Infection usually spreads into the pretracheal space either by perforating the anterior wall of the oesophagus or from the retrovisceral space.

Retrovisceral space – The retrovisceral space is continuous superiorly with the retropharyngeal space. It is situated between the posterior wall of the oesophagus and the prevertebral fascia. Inferiorly, the retrovisceral space extends into the superior mediastinum. Should the prevertebral fascia merge with the connective tissue on the posterior surface of the

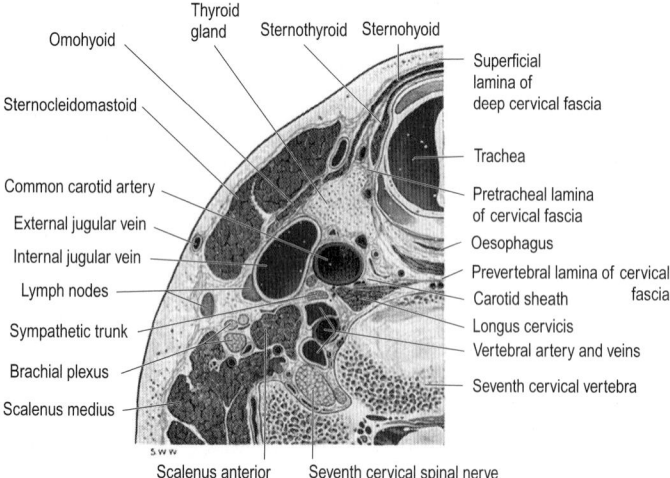

Fig. 31.13 Transverse section through the lower part of the neck at the level of the seventh cervical vertebra, showing the arrangement of the deep cervical fascia, much of which has been coloured blue. (Specimen provided by REM Bowden.)

Labels on figure:
Omohyoid — Thyroid gland — Sternothyroid — Sternohyoid
Sternocleidomastoid
Common carotid artery
External jugular vein
Internal jugular vein
Lymph nodes
Sympathetic trunk
Brachial plexus
Scalenus medius
Scalenus anterior — Seventh cervical spinal nerve

Superficial lamina of deep cervical fascia
Trachea
Pretracheal lamina of cervical fascia
Oesophagus
Prevertebral lamina of cervical fascia
Carotid sheath
Longus cervicis
Vertebral artery and veins
Seventh cervical vertebra

oesophagus – usually at the level of the fourth thoracic vertebra – the retrovisceral space then has a distinct inferior boundary.

Prevertebral space – The prevertebral tissue space has been variously described as the potential space lying between the prevertebral fascia and the vertebral column, and as the space between the two layers of the prevertebral fascia. Infection usually spreads into the space via its fascial walls from the retrovisceral area because it is closed superiorly and laterally. Inferiorly, it extends into the posterior mediastinum.

Carotid space – The carotid sheath is a layer of loose connective tissue demarcated by adjacent portions of the investing layer of deep cervical fascia, the pretracheal fascia, and the prevertebral fascia. Nevertheless, it delineates a potential space into which infections from the visceral spaces may track. Infections around the carotid sheath may be restricted because superiorly (near the hyoid bone) and inferiorly (near the root of the neck) the connective tissues adhere to the vessels.

Cellulitis in the neck – The main cause of cellulitis of the neck is infection arising from the region of the mandibular molar teeth. Several fascial spaces are accessible from this area, and several factors contribute to the spread of infection. Thus, the apices of the second and, more especially, the third, mandibular molar teeth are often close to the lingual surface of the mandible. The apices of the roots of the third mandibular molars are usually – and the second molars are often – below the attachment of mylohyoid on the inner aspect of the mandible and so drain directly into the submandibular tissue space. The posterior free border of mylohyoid is close to the sockets of the third mandibular molars, and at this point, the floor of the mouth consists only of mucous membrane covering part of the submandibular salivary gland. Any virulent periapical infection of the mandibular third molar teeth may therefore penetrate the lingual plate of the mandible and is then at the entrance to several fascial spaces, namely, the submandibular and sublingual spaces anteriorly, and the parapharyngeal and pterygoid spaces posteriorly. Infection in this area may also spread from an acute pericoronitis, particularly when the deeper tissues are opened to infection by extraction of the tooth during the acute phase.

In general, cellulitis around the jaw is only likely to develop when the tissues are infected by virulent and invasive organisms at a point where there is access to the fascial spaces. As the predisposing causes do not often coincide, cellulitis is uncommon. Cellulitis in the region of the maxilla is even more uncommon, but fascial space infections may develop in various sites as the result of infected local anaesthetic needles. It is evident that there are no barriers running vertically with respect to the tissue spaces in the neck. Thus, infection entering in this site can rapidly spread more or less unhindered down the neck and may enter the mediastinum.

VASCULAR SUPPLY AND LYMPHATIC DRAINAGE

Arteries of the neck

The common carotid, internal carotid, and external carotid arteries provide the major source of blood to the head and neck. Additional arteries arise from branches of the subclavian artery, particularly the vertebral artery.

The common, internal and external carotid arteries and accompanying veins and nerves, all lie in a cleft that is bound posteriorly by the transverse processes of cervical vertebrae and attached muscles, medially by the trachea, oesophagus, thyroid gland, larynx and pharyngeal constrictors, and anterolaterally by sternocleidomastoid and, at different levels, omohyoid, sternohyoid, sternothyroid, digastric and stylohyoid muscles. The common and internal carotid arteries lie within the carotid sheath, accompanied by the internal jugular vein and the vagus nerve.

COMMON CAROTID ARTERY (Figs 31.14, 31.15, 31.16)

The common carotid arteries differ on the right and left sides with respect to their origins. On the right, the common carotid arises from the brachiocephalic artery as it passes behind the sternoclavicular joint. On the left, the common carotid artery comes directly from the arch of

the aorta in the superior mediastinum. The right common carotid has, therefore, only a cervical part whereas the left common carotid has cervical and thoracic parts. Following a similar course on both sides, the common carotid artery ascends, diverging laterally from behind the sternoclavicular joint to the level of the upper border of the thyroid cartilage of the larynx (C3–4 junction), where it divides into external and internal carotid arteries. This bifurcation can sometimes be at a higher level. The artery may be compressed against the prominent transverse process of the sixth cervical vertebra (Chassaignac's tubercle), and above this level it is superficial and its pulsation can be easily felt.

Relations – In the lower part of the neck the common carotid arteries are separated by a narrow gap which contains the trachea. Above this, the arteries are separated by the thyroid gland, larynx and pharynx. Each artery is contained within the carotid sheath of deep cervical fascia, which also encloses the internal jugular vein and vagus nerve. The vein lies lateral to the artery, and the nerve lies between them and posterior to both.

The artery is crossed anterolaterally, at the level of the cricoid cartilage, by the intermediate tendon – sometimes the superior belly – of omohyoid. Below omohyoid it is sited deeply, covered by skin, superficial fascia, platysma, deep cervical fascia, and sternocleidomastoid, sternohyoid and sternothyroid. Above omohyoid it is more superficial, covered merely by skin, superficial fascia, platysma, deep cervical fascia and the medial margin of sternocleidomastoid, and it is crossed obliquely from its medial to lateral side by the sternocleidomastoid branch of the superior thyroid artery. The superior root of the ansa cervicalis, joined by its inferior root from the second and third cervical spinal nerves, lies anterior to, or embedded within, the carotid sheath as it crosses it obliquely. The superior thyroid vein usually crosses near the upper border of the thyroid cartilage, and the middle thyroid vein crosses a little below the level of the cricoid cartilage. The anterior jugular vein crosses the common carotid artery above the clavicle, separated from it by sternohyoid and sternothyroid. Posterior to the carotid sheath are the transverse processes of the fourth to sixth cervical vertebrae, to which are attached longus colli, longus capitis and tendinous slips of scalenus anterior. The sympathetic trunk and ascending cervical branch of the inferior thyroid artery lie between the common carotid artery and the muscles. Below the level of the sixth cervical vertebra the artery is in an angle between scalenus anterior and longus colli, anterior to the vertebral vessels, inferior thyroid and subclavian arteries, sympathetic trunk and, on the left, the thoracic duct. The oesophagus, trachea, inferior thyroid artery and recurrent laryngeal nerve and, at a higher level, the larynx and pharynx are medial to the sheath and its contents. The thyroid gland overlaps it anteromedially. The internal jugular vein lies lateral, and, in the lower neck also anterior, to the artery, while the vagus nerve lies posterolaterally in the angle between artery and vein.

On the right side, low in the neck, the recurrent laryngeal nerve crosses obliquely behind the artery. The right internal jugular vein diverges from it below but the left vein approaches and often overlaps its artery.

In c.12% of cases the right common carotid artery arises above the level of the sternoclavicular joint, or it may be a separate branch from the aorta. The left common carotid artery varies in origin more than the right and may arise with the brachiocephalic artery. Division of the common carotid may occur higher, near the level of the hyoid bone, or, more rarely, at a lower level alongside the larynx. Very rarely it ascends without division, so that either the external or internal carotid is absent, or it may be replaced by separate external and internal carotid arteries which arise directly from the aorta, on one side, or bilaterally.

Although the common carotid artery usually has no branches, it may occasionally give rise to the vertebral, superior thyroid, superior laryngeal, ascending pharyngeal, inferior thyroid or occipital arteries.

EXTERNAL CAROTID ARTERY

The external carotid artery (**Figs 31.7, 31.14, 31.15, 31.16**) begins lateral to the upper border of the thyroid cartilage, level with the intervertebral disc between the third and fourth cervical vertebrae. A little curved and with a gentle spiral, it first ascends slightly forwards and then inclines backwards and a little laterally, to pass midway between the tip of the mastoid process and the angle of the mandible. Here, in the substance of the parotid gland behind the neck of the mandible, it divides into its

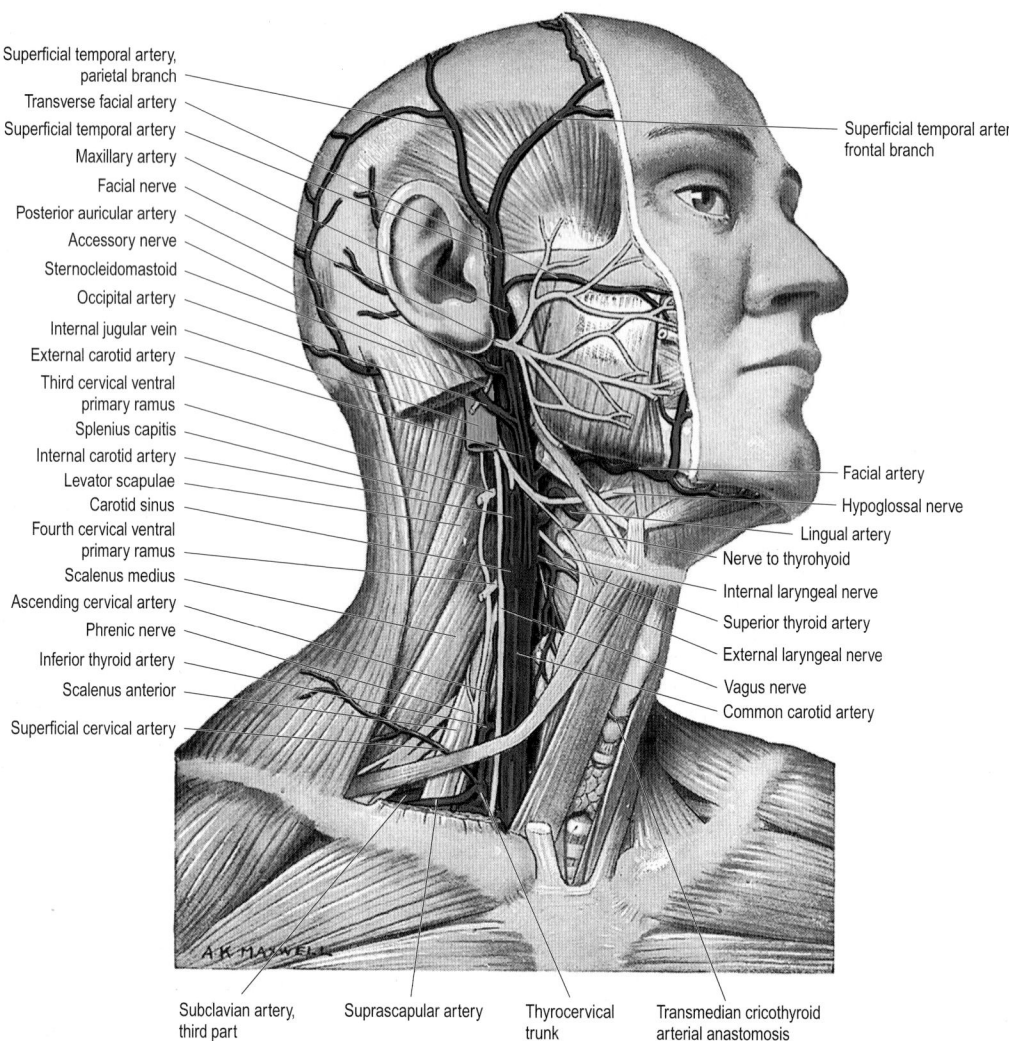

Superficial temporal artery, parietal branch

Transverse facial artery

Superficial temporal artery

Maxillary artery

Facial nerve

Posterior auricular artery

Accessory nerve

Sternocleidomastoid

Occipital artery

Internal jugular vein

External carotid artery

Third cervical ventral primary ramus

Splenius capitis

Internal carotid artery

Levator scapulae

Carotid sinus

Fourth cervical ventral primary ramus

Scalenus medius

Ascending cervical artery

Phrenic nerve

Inferior thyroid artery

Scalenus anterior

Superficial cervical artery

Superficial temporal artery, frontal branch

Facial artery

Hypoglossal nerve

Lingual artery

Nerve to thyrohyoid

Internal laryngeal nerve

Superior thyroid artery

External laryngeal nerve

Vagus nerve

Common carotid artery

Subclavian artery, third part

Suprascapular artery

Thyrocervical trunk

Transmedian cricothyroid arterial anastomosis

Fig. 31.14 Dissection of the right side of the neck, showing the carotid and subclavian arteries and their branches. The parotid and submandibular glands have been removed together with the lower part of the internal jugular vein, most of the sternocleidomastoid and the upper parts of stylohyoid and the posterior belly of digastric.

terminal branches, the superficial temporal and maxillary arteries. As it ascends, it gives off several large branches, and diminishes rapidly in calibre. In children the external carotid is smaller than the internal carotid, but in adults the two are of almost equal size. At its origin, it is in the carotid triangle and lies anteromedial to the internal carotid artery. It later becomes anterior, then lateral, to the internal carotid as it ascends. At mandibular levels the styloid process and its attached structures intervene between the vessels: the internal carotid is deep, and the external carotid superficial, to the styloid process. A fingertip placed in the carotid triangle perceives a powerful arterial pulsation, which represents the termination of the common carotid, the origins of external and internal carotids and the stems of the initial branches of the external carotid.

Relations – The skin and superficial fascia, the loop between the cervical branch of the facial nerve and the transverse cutaneous nerve of the neck, the deep cervical fascia and the anterior margin of sternocleidomastoid all lie superficial to the external carotid artery in the carotid triangle. The artery is crossed by the hypoglossal nerve and its vena comitans and by the lingual, facial and, sometimes, the superior thyroid veins. Leaving the carotid triangle, the external carotid artery is crossed by the posterior belly of digastric and by stylohyoid, and ascends between these muscles and the posteromedial surface of the parotid gland, which it next enters. Within the parotid, the artery lies medial to the facial nerve and the junction of the superficial temporal and maxillary veins. The pharyngeal wall, superior laryngeal nerve and ascending pharyngeal artery are the initial medial relations of the artery. At a higher level, it is separated from the internal carotid artery by the styloid process, styloglossus and stylopharyngeus, glossopharyngeal nerve, pharyngeal branch of vagus nerve and part of the parotid gland. The artery is equally likely to lie medial to the parotid gland, or within it.

The external carotid artery has eight named branches distributed to the head and neck. The superior thyroid, lingual and facial arteries arise

from its anterior surface, the occipital and posterior auricular arteries arise from its posterior surface and the ascending pharyngeal artery arises from its medial surface. The maxillary and superficial temporal arteries are its terminal branches within the parotid gland.

SUPERIOR THYROID ARTERY (Figs 31.7, 31.14)

The superior thyroid artery is the first branch of the external carotid artery, and arises from the anterior surface of the external carotid just below the level of the greater cornu of the hyoid bone. It descends along the lateral border of thyrohyoid to reach the apex of the lobe of the thyroid gland. Lying medially are the inferior constrictor muscle and the external laryngeal nerve: the nerve is often posteromedial, and therefore at risk when the artery is being ligatured. Occasionally it may issue directly from the common carotid.

Branches

The superior thyroid artery supplies the thyroid gland and some adjacent skin. Glandular branches are: anterior, which runs along the medial side of the upper pole of the lateral lobe to supply mainly the anterior surface; a branch which crosses above the isthmus to anastomose with its fellow of the opposite side; and posterior, which descends on the posterior border to supply the medial and lateral surfaces and anastomoses with the inferior thyroid artery. Sometimes a lateral branch supplies the lateral surface. The artery also has the following named branches: infrahyoid, superior laryngeal, sternocleidomastoid and cricothyroid.

Infrahyoid artery

The infrahyoid artery is a small branch which runs along the lower border of the hyoid bone deep to thyrohyoid and anastomoses with its fellow of the opposite side to supply the infrahyoid strap muscles.

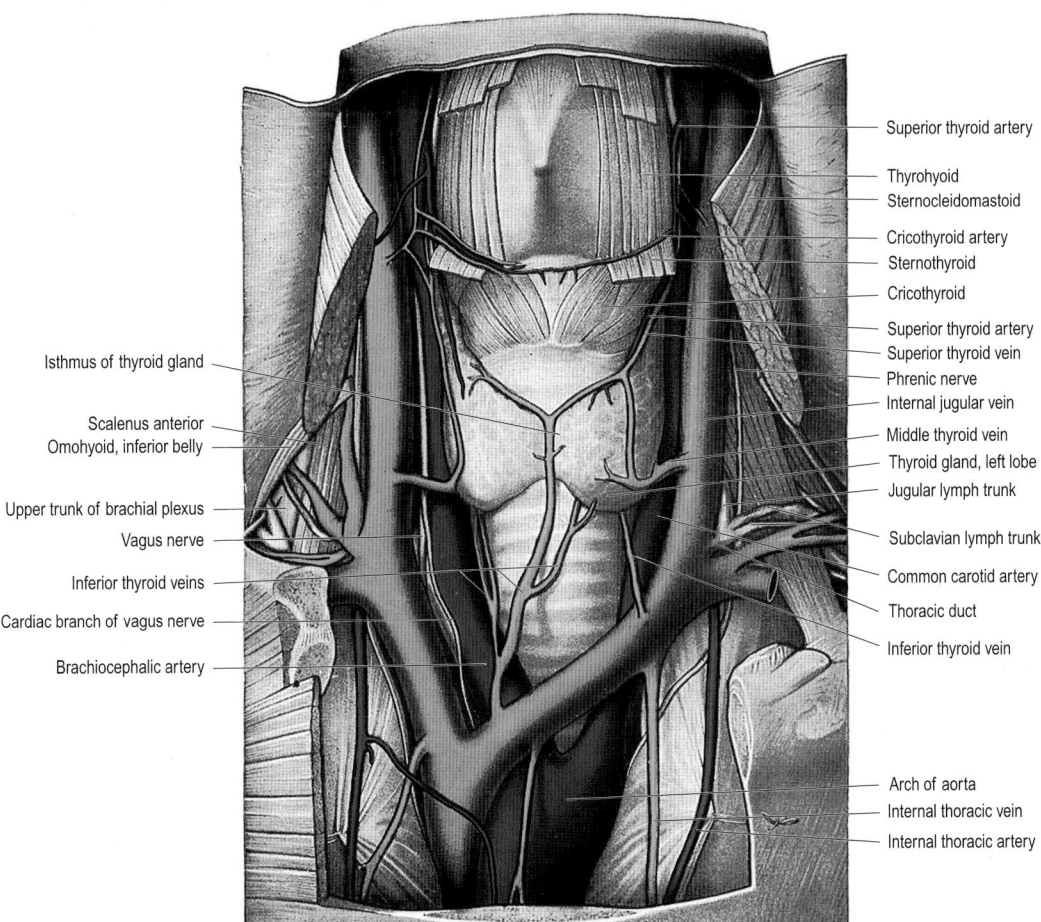

Superior thyroid artery

Thyrohyoid
Sternocleidomastoid

Cricothyroid artery
Sternothyroid

Cricothyroid

Superior thyroid artery
Superior thyroid vein
Phrenic nerve
Internal jugular vein

Middle thyroid vein

Thyroid gland, left lobe

Jugular lymph trunk

Subclavian lymph trunks

Common carotid artery

Thoracic duct

Inferior thyroid vein

Isthmus of thyroid gland

Scalenus anterior
Omohyoid, inferior belly

Upper trunk of brachial plexus

Vagus nerve

Inferior thyroid veins

Cardiac branch of vagus nerve

Brachiocephalic artery

Arch of aorta
Internal thoracic vein
Internal thoracic artery

Fig. 31.15 Dissection of the lower part of the front of the neck and the superior mediastinum. The manubrium sterni and the sternal ends of the clavicles and the first costal cartilages have been removed and the pleural sac and lung have been retracted on each side. In this specimen, each superior thyroid artery arose from the common carotid artery.

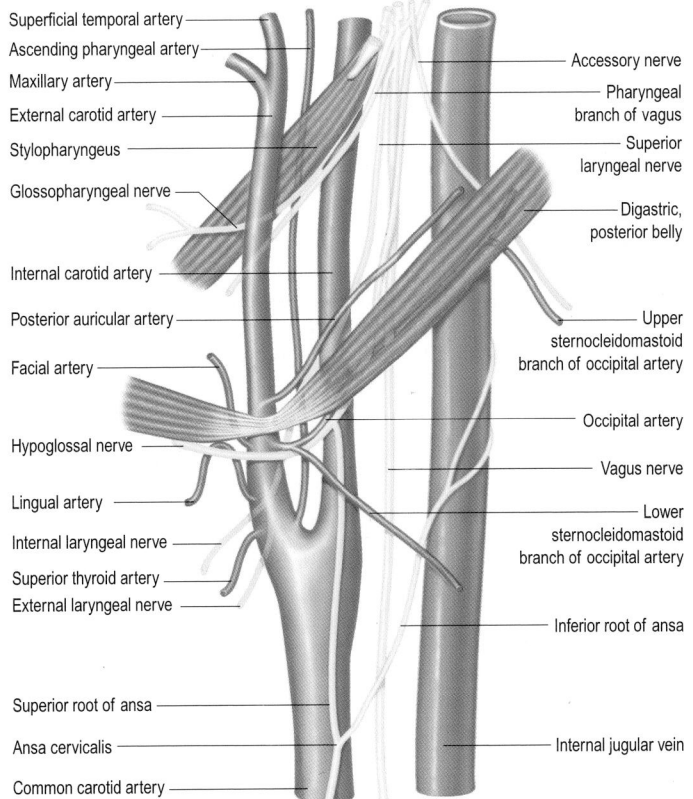

Superficial temporal artery
Ascending pharyngeal artery
Maxillary artery
External carotid artery
Stylopharyngeus
Glossopharyngeal nerve

Internal carotid artery

Posterior auricular artery

Facial artery

Hypoglossal nerve

Lingual artery

Internal laryngeal nerve
Superior thyroid artery
External laryngeal nerve

Superior root of ansa

Ansa cervicalis

Common carotid artery

Accessory nerve

Pharyngeal branch of vagus

Superior laryngeal nerve

Digastric, posterior belly

Upper sternocleidomastoid branch of occipital artery

Occipital artery

Vagus nerve

Lower sternocleidomastoid branch of occipital artery

Inferior root of ansa

Internal jugular vein

Fig. 31.16 The structures crossing the internal jugular vein and carotid arteries and those intervening between the external and internal carotid arteries.

Superior laryngeal artery (Fig. 31.10)

The superior laryngeal artery accompanies the internal laryngeal nerve. Deep to thyrohyoid it pierces the lower part of the thyrohyoid membrane to supply the tissues of the upper part of the larynx. It anastomoses with its fellow of the opposite side and with the inferior laryngeal branch of the inferior thyroid artery.

Sternocleidomastoid artery

The sternocleidomastoid artery descends laterally across the carotid sheath and supplies the middle region of sternocleidomastoid. Like the parent artery itself, it may arise directly from the external carotid artery.

Cricothyroid artery

The cricothyroid artery crosses high on the anterior cricothyroid ligament, anastomoses with its fellow of the opposite side and supplies cricothyroid.

ASCENDING PHARYNGEAL ARTERY

The ascending pharyngeal artery is the smallest branch of the external carotid. It is a long, slender vessel which arises from the medial (deep) surface of the external carotid artery near the origin of that artery. It ascends between the internal carotid artery and the pharynx to the base of the cranium. The ascending pharyngeal artery is crossed by styloglossus and stylopharyngeus, and longus capitis lies posterior to it. It gives off numerous small branches to supply longus capitis and longus colli, the sympathetic trunk, the hypoglossal, glossopharyngeal and vagus nerves and some of the cervical lymph nodes. It anastomoses with the ascending palatine branch of the facial artery and the ascending cervical branch of the vertebral artery. Its named branches are the pharyngeal, inferior tympanic and meningeal arteries.

Pharyngeal artery

The pharyngeal artery gives off three or four branches to supply the constrictor muscles of the pharynx and stylopharyngeus. A variable ramus supplies the palate, and may replace the ascending palatine branch of the facial artery. The artery descends forwards between the superior

545

border of the superior constrictor and levator veli palatini to the soft palate, and also supplies a branch to the palatine tonsil and the pharyngotympanic tube.

Inferior tympanic artery

The inferior tympanic artery is a small branch which traverses the temporal canaliculus with the tympanic branch of the glossopharyngeal nerve and supplies the medial wall of the tympanic cavity.

Meningeal branches

The meningeal branches are small vessels which supply the nerves that traverse the foramen lacerum, jugular foramen and hypoglossal canal, and the associated dura mater and adjoining bone. One branch, the posterior meningeal artery, reaches the cerebellar fossa via the jugular foramen, and is usually regarded as the terminal branch of the ascending pharyngeal artery.

LINGUAL ARTERY (Figs 31.14, 31.16)

The lingual artery provides the chief blood supply to the tongue and the floor of the mouth. It arises anteromedially from the external carotid artery opposite the tip of the greater cornu of the hyoid bone, between the superior thyroid and facial arteries. It often arises with the facial or, less often, with the superior thyroid artery. It may be replaced by a ramus of the maxillary artery. Ascending medially at first, it loops down and forwards, passes medial to the posterior border of hyoglossus and then runs horizontally forwards deep to it. The lingual artery next ascends again almost vertically, and courses sinuously forwards on the inferior surface of the tongue as far as its tip. The further course of the lingual artery is described on page 587.

Relations – Its relationship to hyoglossus naturally divides the lingual artery into descriptive 'thirds'. In its first part the lingual artery is in the carotid triangle. Skin, fascia and platysma are superficial to it, while the middle pharyngeal constrictor muscle is medial. The artery ascends a little medially, then descends to the level of the hyoid bone, and the loop so formed is crossed externally by the hypoglossal nerve. The second part passes along the upper border of the hyoid bone, deep to hyoglossus, the tendons of digastric and stylohyoid, the lower part of the submandibular gland and the posterior part of mylohyoid. Hyoglossus separates it from the hypoglossal nerve and its vena comitans. Here its medial aspect adjoins the middle constrictor muscle and it crosses the stylohyoid ligament accompanied by lingual veins. The third part is the arteria profunda linguae which turns upward near the anterior border of hyoglossus and then passes forwards close to the inferior lingual surface near the frenulum, accompanied by the lingual nerve. Genioglossus is a medial relation, and the inferior longitudinal muscle of the tongue lies lateral to it below the lingual mucous membrane. Near the tip of the tongue the lingual artery anastomoses with its fellow of the opposite side. Its named branches are the suprahyoid, dorsal lingual and sublingual arteries.

SUPRAHYOID ARTERY

The suprahyoid artery is a small branch which runs along the upper border of the hyoid bone to anastomose with the contralateral artery. It supplies adjacent structures.

DORSAL LINGUAL ARTERIES

The dorsal lingual arteries are described on page 587.

SUBLINGUAL ARTERY

The sublingual artery is described on page 587.

FACIAL ARTERY

The facial artery (**Figs 31.7, 31.14, 29.7, 29.12**) arises anteriorly from the external carotid in the carotid triangle, above the lingual artery and immediately above the greater cornu of the hyoid bone. In the neck, at its origin, it is covered only by the skin, platysma, fasciae and often by the hypoglossal nerve. It runs up and forwards, deep to digastric and stylohyoid. At first on the middle pharyngeal constrictor, it may reach the lateral surface of styloglossus, separated there from the palatine tonsil only by this muscle and the lingual fibres of the superior constrictor. Medial to the mandibular ramus it arches upwards and grooves the posterior aspect of the submandibular gland. It then turns down and

descends to the lower border of the mandible in a lateral groove on the submandibular gland, between the gland and medial pterygoid. Reaching the surface of the mandible, the facial artery curves round its inferior border, anterior to masseter, to enter the face: its further course is described on page 509. The artery is very sinuous throughout its extent. In the neck this may be so that the artery is able to adapt to the movements of the pharynx during deglutition, and similarly on the face, so that the artery can adapt to movements of the mandible, lips and cheeks. Facial artery pulsation is most palpable where the artery crosses the mandibular base, and again near the corner of the mouth. Its branches in the neck are the ascending palatine, tonsillar, submental and glandular arteries.

Ascending palatine artery (Fig. 31.7)

The ascending palatine artery arises close to the origin of the facial artery. It passes up between styloglossus and stylopharyngeus to reach the side of the pharynx, along which it ascends between the superior constrictor of the pharynx and medial pterygoid towards the cranial base. It bifurcates near levator veli palatini. One branch follows this muscle, winding over the upper border of the superior constrictor of the pharynx to supply the soft palate and to anastomose with its fellow of the opposite side and the greater palatine branch of the maxillary artery. The other branch pierces the superior constrictor muscle to supply the tonsil and pharyngotympanic tube and to anastomose with the tonsillar and ascending pharyngeal arteries.

Tonsillar artery

The tonsillar artery provides the main blood supply to the palatine tonsil, and may sometimes arise from the ascending palatine artery. It ascends between medial pterygoid and styloglossus, and penetrates the superior constrictor of the pharynx at the upper border of styloglossus to ramify in the tonsil and the musculature of the posterior part of the tongue.

Submental artery (Figs 31.14, 29.7)

The submental artery is the largest cervical branch of the facial artery. It arises as the facial artery separates from the submandibular gland and turns forwards on mylohyoid below the mandible. It supplies the overlying skin and muscles, and anastomoses with a sublingual branch of the lingual and mylohyoid branch of the inferior alveolar artery. At the chin it ascends over the mandible, and divides into superficial and deep branches, which anastomose with the inferior labial and mental arteries to supply the chin and lower lip.

Glandular branches

Three or four large vessels supply the submandibular salivary gland and associated lymph nodes, adjacent muscles and skin.

OCCIPITAL ARTERY (Figs 31.14, 31.16, 31.17)

The occipital artery arises posteriorly from the external carotid artery, c.2 cm from its origin. At its origin, the artery is crossed superficially by the hypoglossal nerve, which winds round it from behind. The artery next passes backwards, up and deep to the posterior belly of digastric, and crosses the internal carotid artery, internal jugular vein, hypoglossal, vagus and accessory nerves. Between the transverse process of the atlas and the mastoid process, the occipital artery reaches the lateral border of rectus capitis lateralis. It then runs in the occipital groove of the temporal bone, medial to the mastoid process and attachments of sternocleidomastoid, splenius capitis, longissimus capitis and digastric, and lies successively on rectus capitis lateralis, obliquus superior and semispinalis capitis. Finally, accompanied by the greater occipital nerve, it turns upwards to pierce the investing layer of the deep cervical fascia connecting the cranial attachments of trapezius and sternocleidomastoid, and ascends tortuously in the dense superficial fascia of the scalp where it divides into many branches.

The occipital artery has two main branches (upper and lower) to the upper part of sternocleidomastoid in the neck. The lower branch arises near the origin of the occipital artery, and may sometimes arise directly from the external carotid artery. It descends backwards over the hypoglossal nerve and internal jugular vein, enters sternocleidomastoid and anastomoses with the sternocleidomastoid branch of the superior thyroid artery. The upper branch arises as the occipital artery crosses the accessory nerve, and runs down and backwards superficial to the internal jugular vein. It enters the deep surface of sternocleidomastoid with the accessory nerve.

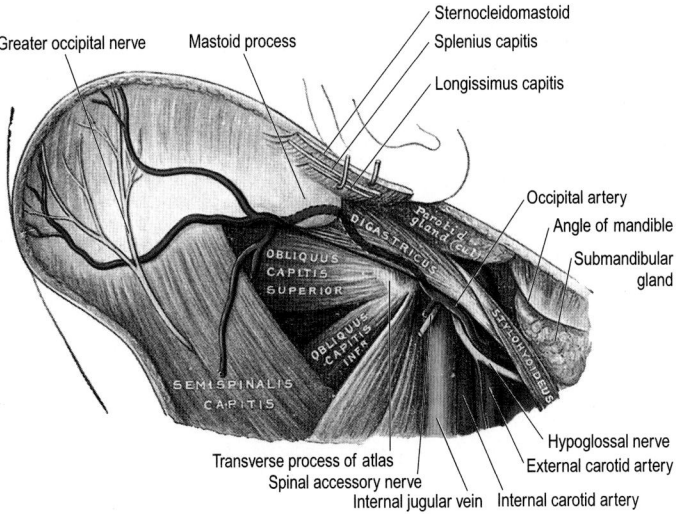

Greater occipital nerve
Mastoid process
Sternocleidomastoid
Splenius capitis
Longissimus capitis
Occipital artery
Angle of mandible
Submandibular gland
DIGASTRICUS
OBLIQUUS CAPITIS SUPERIOR
OBLIQUUS CAPITIS INFER
SEMISPINALIS CAPITIS
Transverse process of atlas
Spinal accessory nerve
Internal jugular vein
Hypoglossal nerve
External carotid artery
Internal carotid artery

Fig. 31.17 Dissection to show the course of the right occipital artery. The upper and lower sternocleidomastoid branches of the artery have been transected and are not labelled.

POSTERIOR AURICULAR ARTERY (Figs 31.14, 31.16)

The posterior auricular artery is a small vessel which branches posteriorly from the external carotid just above digastric and stylohyoid. It ascends between the parotid gland and the styloid process to the groove between the auricular cartilage and mastoid process, and divides into auricular and occipital branches which are described with the face on page 510, 511. In the neck, it provides branches to supply digastric, stylohyoid, sternocleidomastoid and the parotid gland. It also gives origin to the stylomastoid artery – described as an indirect branch of the posterior auricular artery in about a third of subjects – which enters the stylomastoid foramen to supply the facial nerve, tympanic cavity, mastoid antrum air cells and semicircular canals. In the young, its posterior tympanic ramus forms a circular anastomosis with the anterior tympanic branch of the maxillary artery.

INTERNAL CAROTID ARTERY

The internal carotid artery supplies most of the ipsilateral cerebral hemisphere, eye and accessory organs, forehead and, in part, the nose (Figs 31.14, 31.16). From its origin at the carotid bifurcation (where it usually has a carotid sinus), it ascends in front of the transverse processes of the upper three cervical vertebrae to the inferior aperture of the carotid canal in the petrous part of the temporal bone. Here it enters the cranial cavity and turns anteriorly through the cavernous sinus in the carotid groove on the side of the body of the sphenoid bone. It terminates below the anterior perforated substance by division into the anterior and middle cerebral arteries. It may be divided conveniently into cervical, petrous, cavernous and cerebral parts.

Relations – The internal carotid artery is initially superficial in the carotid triangle, then passes deeper, medial to the posterior belly of digastric. Except near the skull, the internal jugular vein and vagus nerve are lateral to it within the carotid sheath. The external carotid artery is first anteromedial, but then curves back to lie superficial. Posteriorly the internal carotid adjoins longus capitis, and the superior cervical sympathetic ganglion lies between them. The superior laryngeal nerve crosses obliquely behind it. The pharyngeal wall lies medial to the artery, which is separated by fat and pharyngeal veins from the ascending pharyngeal artery and superior laryngeal nerve. Anterolaterally the internal carotid artery is covered by sternocleidomastoid. Below the posterior belly of digastric, the hypoglossal nerve and superior root of the ansa cervicalis and the lingual and facial veins are superficial to the artery. At the level of the digastric, the internal carotid is crossed by stylohyoid and the occipital and posterior auricular arteries. Above the digastric it is separated from the external carotid artery by the styloid process, styloglossus and stylopharyngeus, the glossopharyngeal nerve and the pharyngeal branch of the vagus, and the deeper part of the parotid

gland (**Fig. 31.16**). At the base of the skull the glossopharyngeal, vagus, accessory and hypoglossal nerves lies between the internal carotid artery and the internal jugular vein, which here has become posterior. The length of the artery varies with the length of the neck and the point of the carotid bifurcation. It may arise from the aortic arch and then lies medial to the external carotid as far as the larynx, where it crosses behind it. The cervical portion is normally straight but may be very tortuous, in which case it lies closer to the pharynx than usual and very near the tonsil. Its absence has also been recorded.

The cervical portion of the internal carotid artery has no branches.

CAROTID SINUS AND CAROTID BODY

The common carotid artery shows two specialized organs near its bifurcation, the carotid sinus and the carotid body. They relay information concerning the pressure and chemical composition of the arterial blood respectively, and are innervated principally by carotid branch(es) of the glossopharyngeal nerve, with small contributions from the cervical sympathetic trunk and the vagus nerve.

The carotid sinus usually appears as a dilation of the lower end of the internal carotid, and functions as a baroreceptor.

The carotid body is a reddish-brown, oval structure, 5–7 mm in height and 2.5–4 mm in width. It lies either posterior to the carotid bifurcation or between its branches, and is attached to, or sometimes partly embedded in, their adventitia. Occasionally it takes the form of a group of separate nodules. Aberrant miniature carotid bodies, microstructurally similar but with diameters of 600 μm or less, may appear in the adventitia and adipose tissue near the carotid sinus.

The carotid body is surrounded by a fibrous capsule from which septa divide the enclosed tissue into lobules. Each lobule contains glomus (Type I) cells which are separated from an extensive network of fenestrated sinusoids by sustentacular (type II) cells (**Fig. 31.18**). Glomus cells store a number of peptides, particularly enkephalins, bombesin and neurotensin, and amines including dopamine, serotonin, adrenaline (epinephrine) and noradrenaline (norepinephrine), and are therefore regarded as paraneurones. Unmyelinated axons lie in a collagenous matrix between the sustentacular cells and the sinusoidal endothelium, and many synapse on the glomus cells. They are visceral afferents which travel in the carotid sinus nerve to join the glossopharyngeal nerve. Preganglionic sympathetic axons and fibres from the carotid sinus synapse on parasympathetic and sympathetic ganglion cells, which lie either in isolation or in small groups near the surface of each carotid body. Postganglionic axons travel to local blood vessels: the parasympathetic efferent fibres are probably vasodilatory and the sympathetic ones are vasoconstrictor.

The carotid body receives a rich blood supply from branches of the adjacent external carotid artery, which is consistent with its role as an arterial chemoreceptor. When stimulated by hypoxia, hypercapnia or increased hydrogen ion concentration (low pH) in the blood flowing through it, it elicits reflex increases in the rate and volume of ventilation via connections with brain stem respiratory centres. The bodies are most prominent in children and normally involute in older age, when they are infiltrated by lymphocytes and fibrous tissue. Individuals with chronic hypoxia, or who live at high altitude or suffer from lung disease, may have enlarged carotid bodies as a result of hyperplasia.

Other small bodies, resembling carotid bodies, and also considered to be chemoreceptors, occur near the arteries of the fourth and sixth pharyngeal arches and hence are found near the aortic arch, ligamentum arteriosum and right subclavian artery, and are supplied by the vagus nerve.

SUBCLAVIAN ARTERY (Fig. 31.19)

The right subclavian artery arises from the brachiocephalic trunk, the left from the aortic arch. For description, each is divided into a first part, from its origin to the medial border of scalenus anterior, a second part behind this muscle and a third part from the lateral margin of scalenus anterior to the outer border of the first rib, where the artery becomes the axillary artery. Each subclavian artery arches over the cervical pleura and pulmonary apex. Their first parts differ, whereas the second and third parts are almost identical.

First part of right subclavian artery

The right subclavian artery branches from the brachiocephalic trunk behind the upper border of the right sternoclavicular joint, and passes

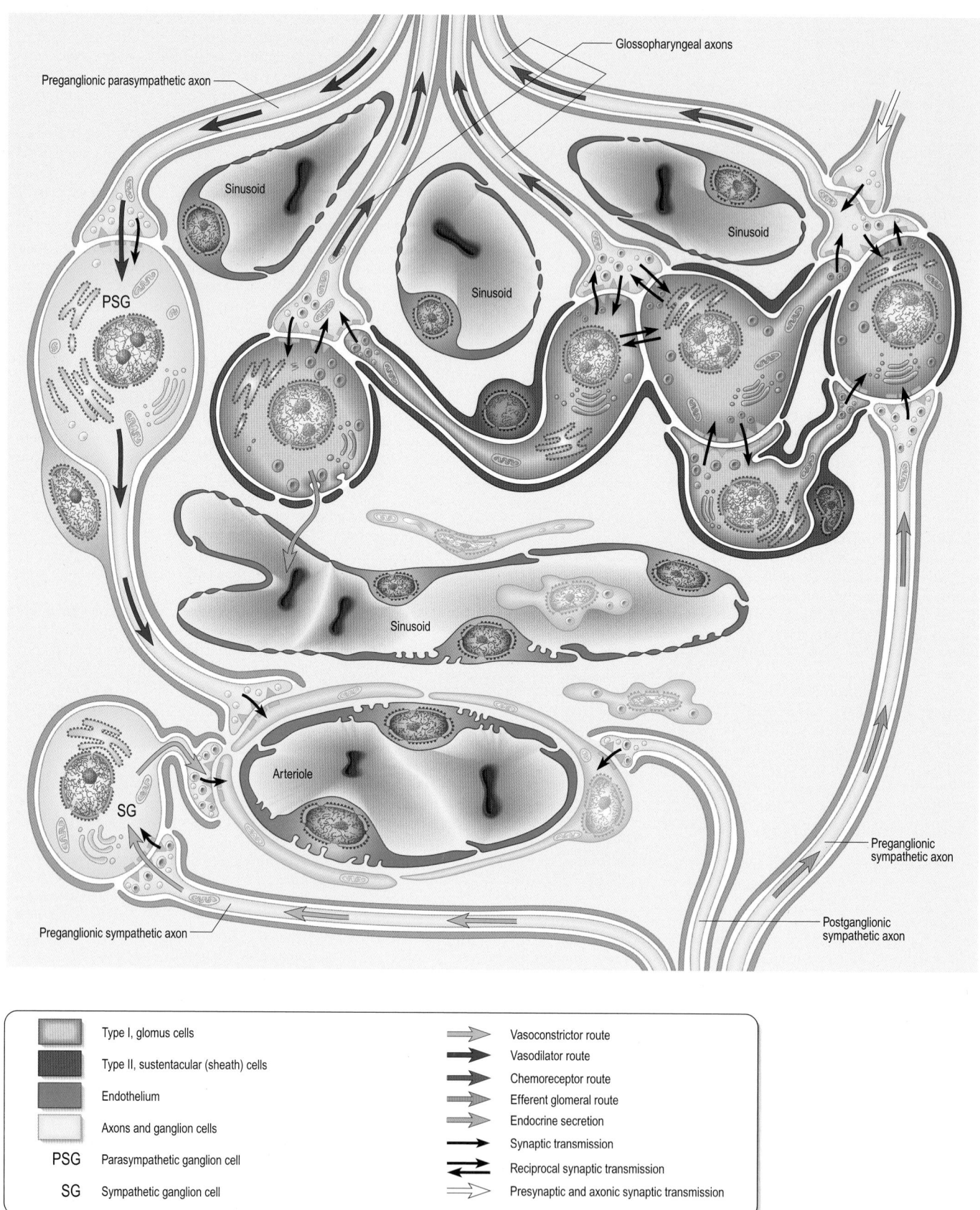

Fig. 31.18 The cellular, neural and vascular architecture of the carotid body. Functional pathways are indicated.

Legend:

- Type I, glomus cells
- Type II, sustentacular (sheath) cells
- Endothelium
- Axons and ganglion cells
- PSG Parasympathetic ganglion cell
- SG Sympathetic ganglion cell

- Vasoconstrictor route
- Vasodilator route
- Chemoreceptor route
- Efferent glomeral route
- Endocrine secretion
- Synaptic transmission
- Reciprocal synaptic transmission
- Presynaptic and axonic synaptic transmission

superolaterally to the medial margin of scalenus anterior (**Figs 31.7, 60.27**). It ascends c.2 cm above the clavicle but this varies.

Relations – The artery is deep to the skin, superficial fascia, platysma, supraclavicular nerves, deep fascia, clavicular attachment of sterno-cleidomastoid, sternohyoid and sternothyroid. It is at first behind the origin of the right common carotid artery; more laterally it is crossed by the vagus nerve, the cardiac branches of the vagus and the sympathetic chain and by internal jugular and vertebral veins; the subclavian sympathetic loop encircles it. The anterior jugular vein diverges laterally

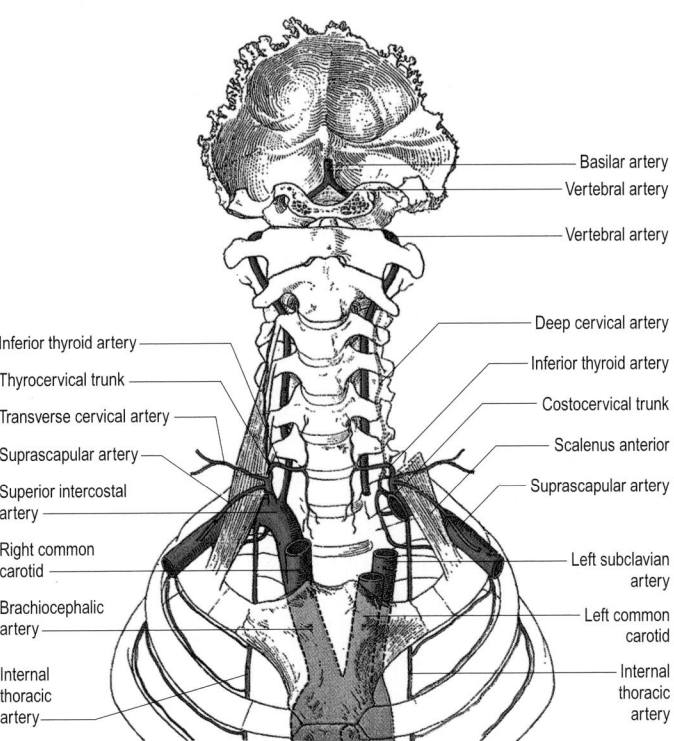

Fig. 31.19 The subclavian arteries and their branches. (From Brash JC 1979 Cunningham's Manual of Practical Anatomy, Vol 3. Head, Neck and Brain, 14th edn. London: Oxford University Press. By permission of Oxford University Press.)

Labels (left, top to bottom): Inferior thyroid artery; Thyrocervical trunk; Transverse cervical artery; Suprascapular artery; Superior intercostal artery; Right common carotid; Brachiocephalic artery; Internal thoracic artery

Labels (right, top to bottom): Basilar artery; Vertebral artery; Vertebral artery; Deep cervical artery; Inferior thyroid artery; Costocervical trunk; Scalenus anterior; Suprascapular artery; Left subclavian artery; Left common carotid; Internal thoracic artery

in front of it, separated by sternohyoid and sternothyroid. Below and behind the artery are the pleura and pulmonary apex: they are separated from the artery by the suprapleural membrane, the ansa subclavia, a small accessory vertebral vein and the right recurrent laryngeal nerve which winds round the lower and posterior part of the vessel.

First part of left subclavian artery

The first part of the left subclavian artery springs from the aortic arch, behind the left common carotid, level with the disc between the third and fourth thoracic vertebrae. It ascends into the neck, then arches laterally to the medial border of scalenus anterior.

Relations – In the neck, near the medial border of scalenus anterior, the artery is crossed anteriorly by the left phrenic nerve and the termination of the thoracic duct. Otherwise anterior relations are the same as those of the first part of the right subclavian artery. Posteriorly and inferiorly, the relations of both vessels are identical but the left recurrent laryngeal nerve, medial to the left subclavian artery in the thorax, is not directly related to its cervical part.

Second part of subclavian artery

The second part of the subclavian artery lies behind scalenus anterior; it is short and the highest part of the vessel (**Figs 31.8, 31.14**).

Relations – The skin, superficial fascia, platysma, deep cervical fascia, sternocleidomastoid and scalenus anterior are anterior. The right phrenic nerve is often described as being separated from the second part of the subclavian artery by scalenus anterior, whereas it crosses the first part of the left subclavian artery. However, both nerves may sometimes lie anterior to the muscle. The suprapleural membrane, pleura and lung and the lower trunk of the brachial plexus are posteroinferior; the upper and middle trunks of the plexus are superior; the subclavian vein is anteroinferior, separated by scalenus anterior (**Fig. 31.8**).

Third part of subclavian artery

The third part of the subclavian artery descends laterally from the lateral margin of scalenus anterior to the outer border of the first rib, where it becomes the axillary artery. It is the most superficial part of the artery

and lies partly in the supraclavicular triangle, where its pulsations may be felt and it may be compressed. The third part of the subclavian artery is the most accessible segment of the artery. Since the line of the posterior border of sternocleidomastoid approximates to the (deeper) lateral border of scalenus anterior, the artery can be felt in the anteroinferior angle of the posterior triangle. It can only be effectively compressed against the first rib: with the shoulder depressed, pressure is exerted down, back and medially in the angle between sternocleidomastoid and the clavicle. The palpable trunks of the brachial plexus may be injected with local anaesthetic allowing major surgical procedures to the arm.

Relations – The skin, superficial fascia, platysma, supraclavicular nerves and deep cervical fascia are anterior (**Figs 31.8, 60.4**). The external jugular vein crosses its medial end and here receives the suprascapular, transverse cervical and anterior jugular veins, which collectively often form a venous plexus. The nerve to subclavius descends between the veins and the artery; the latter is terminally behind the clavicle and sub-clavius, where it is crossed by the suprascapular vessels. The subclavian vein is anteroinferior and the lower trunk of the brachial plexus is posteroinferior, between the subclavian artery and the scalenus medius (and on the first rib). The upper and middle trunks of the brachial plexus (which are palpable here) and the inferior belly of omohyoid are superolateral. The first rib is inferior.

The right subclavian artery may arise above or below sternoclavicular level; it may be a separate aortic branch and be the first or last branch of the arch. When it is the first branch, it is in the position of a brachiocephalic trunk. When it is the last branch, it arises from the left end of the arch, and ascends obliquely to the right behind the trachea, oesophagus and right common carotid to the first rib. When this occurs, the right recurrent laryngeal nerve hooks round the common carotid artery. Sometimes, when the right subclavian artery is the last aortic branch, it passes between the trachea and oesophagus. It may perforate scalenus anterior, and very rarely may pass anterior to it. Sometimes the subclavian vein accompanies the artery behind scalenus anterior. The artery may ascend as high as 4 cm above the clavicle or it may reach only its upper border. The left subclavian artery is occasionally combined at its origin with the left common carotid artery

VERTEBRAL ARTERY (Figs 31.20, 31.24, 31.25)

The vertebral artery arises from the superoposterior aspect of the first part of the subclavian artery. It passes through the foramina in the transverse processes of all of the cervical vertebrae except the seventh, curves medially behind the lateral mass of the atlas and enters the cranium via the foramen magnum. At the lower pontine border it joins its fellow to form the basilar artery. Occasionally it may enter the cervical vertebral column via the fourth, fifth or seventh cervical vertebra (**Figs 31.7, 63.5**)

Relations – The first part passes back and upwards between longus colli and scalenus anterior, behind the common carotid artery and the vertebral vein. It is crossed by the inferior thyroid artery, and by the thoracic duct on the left side and the right lymphatic duct on the right side. The seventh cervical transverse process, the inferior cervical ganglion and ventral rami of the seventh and eighth cervical spinal nerves lie posterior to the artery. The second part ascends through the transverse foramina of the remaining cervical vertebrae, accompanied by a large branch from the inferior cervical ganglion and a plexus of veins which form the vertebral vein low in the neck. It lies anterior to the ventral rami of the cervical spinal nerves (C.2–C.6), and ascends almost vertically to pass through the transverse process of the axis, where it turns laterally to gain access to the transverse foramen of the atlas. The third part issues medial to rectus capitis lateralis, and curves backwards and medially behind the lateral mass of the atlas, with the first cervical ventral spinal ramus lying on its medial side. In this position it lies in a groove on the upper surface of the posterior arch of the atlas, and it enters the vertebral canal below the inferior border of the posterior atlanto-occipital membrane. This part of the artery, covered by semispinalis capitis, lies in the suboccipital triangle. The first cervical dorsal spinal ramus separates the artery from the posterior arch. The fourth part pierces the dura and arachnoid mater, and ascends anterior to the hypoglossal roots. It inclines anterior to the medulla oblongata and unites with its contralateral fellow to form the midline basilar artery at the lower border of the pons.

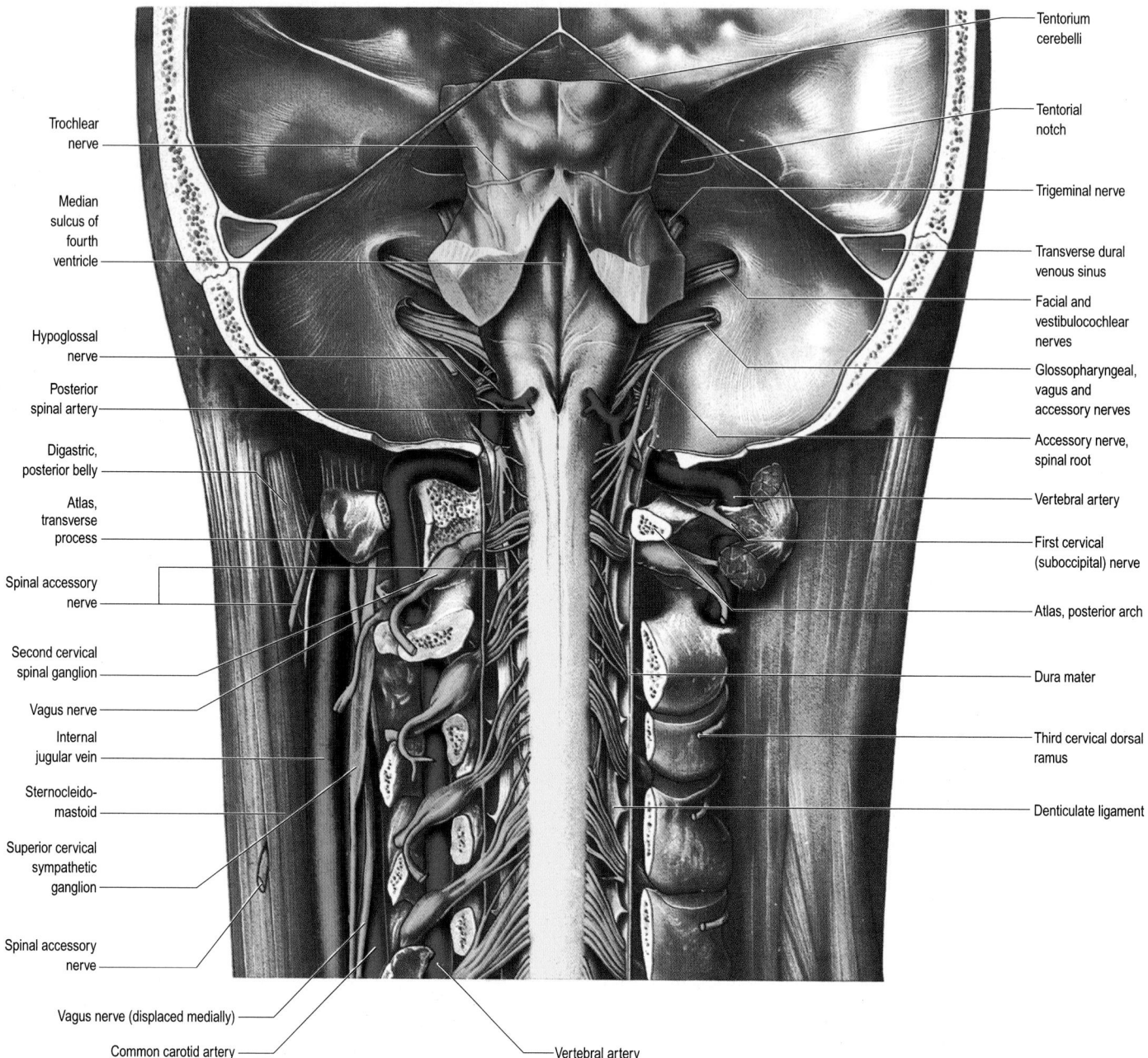

Trochlear nerve

Median sulcus of fourth ventricle

Hypoglossal nerve

Posterior spinal artery

Digastric, posterior belly

Atlas, transverse process

Spinal accessory nerve

Second cervical spinal ganglion

Vagus nerve

Internal jugular vein

Sternocleido-mastoid

Superior cervical sympathetic ganglion

Spinal accessory nerve

Vagus nerve (displaced medially)

Common carotid artery

Vertebral artery

Tentorium cerebelli

Tentorial notch

Trigeminal nerve

Transverse dural venous sinus

Facial and vestibulocochlear nerves

Glossopharyngeal, vagus and accessory nerves

Accessory nerve, spinal root

Vertebral artery

First cervical (suboccipital) nerve

Atlas, posterior arch

Dura mater

Third cervical dorsal ramus

Denticulate ligament

Fig. 31.20 A dissection of the brain stem and the upper part of the spinal cord after removal of large portions of the occipital and parietal bones, the cerebellum and the roof of the fourth ventricle. On the left side, the foramina transversaria of the atlas and the third, fourth and fifth cervical vertebrae have been opened to expose the vertebral artery. On the right side the posterior arch of the atlas and the laminae of the succeeding cervical vertebrae have been divided and have been removed together with the vertebral spines and the contralateral laminae. The tentorium cerebelli and the transverse sinuses have been divided and their posterior portions removed.

CERVICAL BRANCHES OF THE VERTEBRAL ARTERY

Spinal branches

The spinal branches enter the vertebral canal via the intervertebral foramina, and supply the spinal cord and its membranes. They fork into ascending and descending rami, which unite with those above and below, to form two lateral anastomotic chains on the posterior surfaces of the vertebral bodies near the attachment of their pedicles. Branches from these chains supply the periosteum and vertebral bodies, and others communicate with similar branches across the midline; from these connections small rami join similar ones above and below, to form a median anastomotic chain on the posterior surfaces of the vertebral bodies.

Muscular branches

Muscular branches arise from the vertebral artery as it curves round the lateral mass of the atlas. They supply the deep muscles of the suboccipital region and anastomose with the occipital, ascending and deep cervical arteries.

INTERNAL THORACIC ARTERY (Fig. 63.5)

The internal thoracic artery arises inferiorly from the first part of the subclavian artery, c.2 cm above the sternal end of the clavicle, opposite the root of the thyrocervical trunk.

THYROCERVICAL TRUNK (Fig. 31.6)

The thyrocervical trunk is a short wide artery which arises from the front of the first part of the subclavian artery near the medial border of scalenus anterior, and divides almost at once into the inferior thyroid, suprascapular and superficial cervical arteries.

Inferior thyroid artery (Figs 31.6, 31.25)

The inferior thyroid artery loops upwards anterior to the medial border of the scalenus anterior, turns medially just below the sixth cervical transverse process, then descends on longus colli to the lower border of the thyroid gland. It passes anterior to the vertebral vessels and posterior to the carotid sheath and its contents (and usually the sympathetic trunk, whose middle cervical ganglion frequently adjoins the vessel). On the left, near its origin, the artery is crossed anteriorly by the thoracic duct as the latter curves inferolaterally to its termination. Relations between the terminal branches of the artery and recurrent laryngeal nerve are very variable and of considerable surgical importance. The artery usually passes behind the nerve as it nears the gland. However, very close to the gland, the right nerve is equally likely to be anterior, posterior or amongst, the branches of the artery, and the left nerve is usually posterior. The artery is not accompanied by the inferior thyroid vein.

Muscular branches

These supply the infrahyoid muscles, longus colli, scalenus anterior and the inferior pharyngeal constrictor.

Ascending cervical artery

The ascending cervical artery is a small branch which arises as the inferior thyroid turns medially behind the carotid sheath and ascends on the anterior tubercles of the cervical transverse processes between scalenus anterior and longus capitis. It supplies the adjacent muscles and gives off one or two spinal branches which enter the vertebral canal through the intervertebral foramina to supply the spinal cord and membranes and vertebral bodies, and thereby supplement the spinal branches of the vertebral artery. The ascending cervical artery anastomoses with the vertebral, ascending pharyngeal, occipital and deep cervical arteries.

Inferior laryngeal artery

The inferior laryngeal artery ascends on the trachea with the recurrent laryngeal nerve, enters the larynx at the lower border of the inferior constrictor and supplies the laryngeal muscles and mucosa. It anastomoses with its contralateral fellow, and with the superior laryngeal branch of the superior thyroid artery.

Pharyngeal branches

These supply the lower part of the pharynx. Tracheal branches supply the trachea and anastomose with the bronchial arteries; oesophageal branches supply the oesophagus and anastomose with the oesophageal branches of the thoracic aorta; inferior and ascending glandular branches supply the posterior and inferior regions of the thyroid gland, and anastomose with the contralateral inferior and ipsilateral superior thyroid arteries. The ascending branch also supplies the parathyroid glands.

Suprascapular artery (Fig. 31.8)

The suprascapular artery descends laterally across scalenus anterior and the phrenic nerve, posterior to the internal jugular vein and sternocleidomastoid. It then crosses anterior to the subclavian artery and brachial plexus, posterior to, and parallel with, the clavicle, subclavius and the inferior belly of omohyoid, to reach the superior scapular border.

Superficial cervical artery (Fig. 31.8)

The superficial cervical artery is given off at a higher level than the suprascapular artery. It crosses anterior to the phrenic nerve, scalenus anterior and the brachial plexus and is covered by the internal jugular vein, sternocleidomastoid and platysma. It crosses the floor of the posterior triangle to reach the anterior margin of levator scapulae, and ascends deep to the anterior part of the trapezius, which it supplies, together with the adjoining muscles and the cervical lymph nodes. It anastomoses with the superficial ramus of the descending branch of the occipital artery. About a third of the superficial cervical and dorsal scapular arteries arise in common from the thyrocervical trunk, with a superficial (superficial cervical artery) and a deep (dorsal scapular artery) branch. The latter passes laterally anterior to the brachial plexus and then posterior to levator scapulae.

COSTOCERVICAL TRUNK (Fig. 63.5)

On the right, this short vessel arises posteriorly from the second part of the subclavian artery, and, on the left, from its first part (**Fig. 31.8**). It arches back above the cervical pleura to the neck of the

first rib, where it divides into superior intercostal and deep cervical branches.

Deep cervical artery

The deep cervical artery usually arises from the costocervical trunk. It is analogous in its first segment to a posterior branch of a posterior intercostal artery, and occasionally is a separate branch of the subclavian artery. It passes back above the eighth cervical spinal nerve between the transverse process of the seventh cervical vertebra and the neck of the first rib (sometimes between the transverse processes of the sixth and seventh cervical vertebrae). It then ascends between semispinales capitis and cervicis to the level of the second cervical vertebra. It supplies adjacent muscles and anastomoses with the deep branch of the descending branch of the occipital artery and branches of the vertebral artery. A spinal branch enters the vertebral canal between the seventh cervical and first thoracic vertebrae.

Dorsal scapular artery

The dorsal scapular artery arises from the third, or less often the second, part of the subclavian artery. It gives off a small branch (which sometimes arises directly from the subclavian artery), to scalenus anterior. It passes laterally through the brachial plexus in front of scalenus medius and then deep to levator scapulae to the superior scapular angle.

About a third of the superficial cervical and dorsal scapular arteries arise in common from the thyrocervical trunk as a transverse cervical artery, with a superficial (superficial cervical artery) and a deep (dorsal scapular artery) branch; the latter passes laterally anterior to the brachial plexus and then posterior to levator scapulae.

VEINS OF THE NECK

Veins in the neck show considerable variation. They are superficial or deep to the deep fascia but are not entirely separate systems. Superficial veins are tributaries, some with specific names, given below, of the anterior, external and posterior jugular veins. They drain a much smaller volume of tissue than the deep veins. The latter drain all but the subcutaneous structures, mostly into the internal jugular vein and also into the subclavian vein.

EXTERNAL JUGULAR VEIN

The external jugular vein mainly drains the scalp and face, although it also drains some deeper parts. The vein is formed by the union of the posterior division of the retromandibular vein with the posterior auricular vein and begins near the mandibular angle just below or in the parotid gland. It descends from the angle to the midclavicle, running obliquely, superficial to sternocleidomastoid, to the root of the neck. Here it crosses the deep fascia and ends in the subclavian vein, lateral or anterior to scalenus anterior. There are valves at its entrance into the subclavian, but they do not prevent regurgitation. Its wall is adherent to the rim of the fascial opening. It is covered by platysma, superficial fascia and skin, and is separated from sternocleidomastoid by deep cervical fascia. The vein crosses the transverse cutaneous nerve and lies parallel with the great auricular nerve, posterior to its upper half. In size the external jugular vein is inversely proportional to the other veins in the neck, and may be double. Between the entrance into the subclavian vein and a point c.4 cm above the clavicle, the vein is often dilated, producing a so-called sinus.

Tributaries – In addition to formative tributaries, the external jugular receives the posterior external jugular and, near its end, transverse cervical, suprascapular and anterior jugular veins. In the parotid gland it is often joined by a branch from the internal jugular. The occipital vein occasionally joins it.

POSTERIOR EXTERNAL JUGULAR VEIN

The posterior external jugular vein begins in the occipital scalp, and drains the skin and the superficial muscles which lie posterosuperior in the neck. It usually joins the middle part of the external jugular vein.

ANTERIOR JUGULAR VEIN

The anterior jugular vein arises near the hyoid bone from the confluence of the superficial submandibular veins. It descends between the midline and the anterior border of sternocleidomastoid. Turning laterally, low in the neck, deep to sternocleidomastoid but superficial to the infrahyoid strap muscles, it joins either the end of the external jugular vein or may enter the subclavian vein directly. In size it is usually inverse to the external jugular vein. It communicates with the internal jugular vein, and receives the laryngeal veins and sometimes a small thyroid vein. There are usually two anterior jugular veins, united just above the manubrium by a large transverse jugular arch, receiving the inferior thyroid tributaries. They have no valves and may be replaced by a midline trunk.

INTERNAL JUGULAR VEIN (Figs 29.8, 31.8, 31.10, 31.15, 31.16, 31.21)
The internal jugular vein collects blood from the skull, brain, superficial parts of face and much of the neck. It begins at the cranial base in the posterior compartment of the jugular foramen, where it is continuous with the sigmoid sinus. At its origin it is dilated as the superior bulb, which lies below the posterior part of the tympanic floor. The internal jugular vein descends in the carotid sheath, and unites with the subclavian vein, posterior to the sternal end of the clavicle, to form the brachiocephalic vein. Near its termination the vein dilates into the inferior bulb, above which is a pair of valves.

Relations – From above, rectus capitis lateralis, the transverse process of the atlas, levator scapulae, scalenus medius, scalenus anterior, the cervical plexus, the phrenic nerve, thyrocervical trunk, vertebral vein and the first part of the subclavian artery all lie posterior to the vein. On the left, the internal jugular crosses anterior to the thoracic duct (**Fig. 31.6**). The internal and common carotid arteries and the vagus nerve are medial to the vein: the nerve lies between vein and arteries but posterior to them. Superficially the internal jugular vein is overlapped above, then covered below, by sternocleidomastoid and is crossed by the posterior belly of digastric and the superior belly of omohyoid. Superior to digastric the parotid gland, styloid process, accessory nerve, and posterior auricular and occipital arteries cross the vein. Between digastric and omohyoid, the sternocleidomastoid arteries and inferior root of the ansa cervicalis cross it, although the nerve often passes between the vein and the common carotid artery. Below omohyoid, the

vein is covered by the infrahyoid muscles and sternocleidomastoid and is crossed by the anterior jugular vein. Deep cervical lymph nodes lie along the internal jugular, mainly on its superficial aspect. At the root of the neck the right internal jugular vein is separated from the common carotid artery, but the left usually overlaps its artery. At the base of the skull the internal carotid artery is anterior to the vein, separated from it by the ninth to twelfth cranial nerves.

Tributaries – The inferior petrosal sinus, facial, lingual, pharyngeal, superior and middle thyroid veins, and occasionally the occipital vein, are all tributaries of the internal jugular vein. The internal jugular vein may communicate with the external jugular vein. The thoracic duct opens near the union of the left subclavian and internal jugular veins, and the right lymphatic duct opens at the same site on the right.

INFERIOR PETROSAL SINUS
The inferior petrosal sinus leaves the skull through the anterior part of the jugular foramen, crosses lateral or medial to the ninth to eleventh cranial nerves and joins the superior jugular bulb.

FACIAL VEIN (Figs 29.8, 31.10)
The initial part of the facial vein as it lies on the face is described on page 511. From the face it passes over the surface of masseter, crosses the body of the mandible and enters the neck where it runs obliquely back under platysma. Here it lies superficial to the submandibular gland, digastric and stylohyoid. Just anteroinferior to the mandibular angle it is joined by the anterior division of the retromandibular vein, and then descends superficial to the loop of the lingual artery, the hypoglossal nerve and external and internal carotid arteries, to enter the internal jugular near the greater cornu of the hyoid bone, i.e. in the upper angle of the carotid triangle. Near its end a large branch often descends along the anterior border of sternocleidomastoid to the anterior jugular vein. Its uppermost segment, above its junction with the superior labial vein, is often termed the angular vein.

Tributaries – Submental, tonsillar, external palatine (paratonsillar), submandibular, vena comitans of the hypoglossal nerve (sometimes), pharyngeal and superior thyroid veins are all tributaries of the portion of the facial vein that lies below the mandible.

LINGUAL VEIN (Fig. 29.8)
The lingual veins follow two routes. The dorsal lingual veins drain the dorsum and sides of the tongue, join the lingual veins accompanying the lingual artery between hyoglossus and genioglossus, and enter the internal jugular near the greater cornu of the hyoid bone. The deep lingual vein begins near the tip of the tongue and runs back, lying near the mucous membrane on the inferior surface of the tongue. Near the anterior border of hyoglossus it joins a sublingual vein, from the sublingual salivary gland, to form the vena comitans nervi hypoglossi which runs back between mylohyoid and hyoglossus with the hypoglossal nerve to join the facial, internal jugular or lingual vein.

PHARYNGEAL VEINS (see Chapter 35)
The pharyngeal veins begin in a pharyngeal plexus external to the pharynx. They receive meningeal veins and a vein from the pterygoid canal, and usually end in the internal jugular vein, but may sometimes end in the facial, lingual or superior thyroid vein.

SUPERIOR THYROID VEIN (Figs 29.8, 31.15)
The superior thyroid vein is formed by deep and superficial tributaries corresponding to the arterial branches in the upper part of the thyroid gland (**Fig. 31.15**). It accompanies the superior thyroid artery, receives the superior laryngeal and cricothyroid veins, and ends in the internal jugular or facial vein.

MIDDLE THYROID VEIN
The middle thyroid vein drains the lower part of the gland and also receives veins from the larynx and trachea (**Fig. 31.15**). It crosses anterior to the common carotid artery to join the internal jugular vein behind the superior belly of omohyoid.

TYMPANIC BODY
The tympanic body (glomus jugulare) is ovoid, c.0.5 mm long and 0.25 mm broad, and lies in the adventitia of the upper part of the

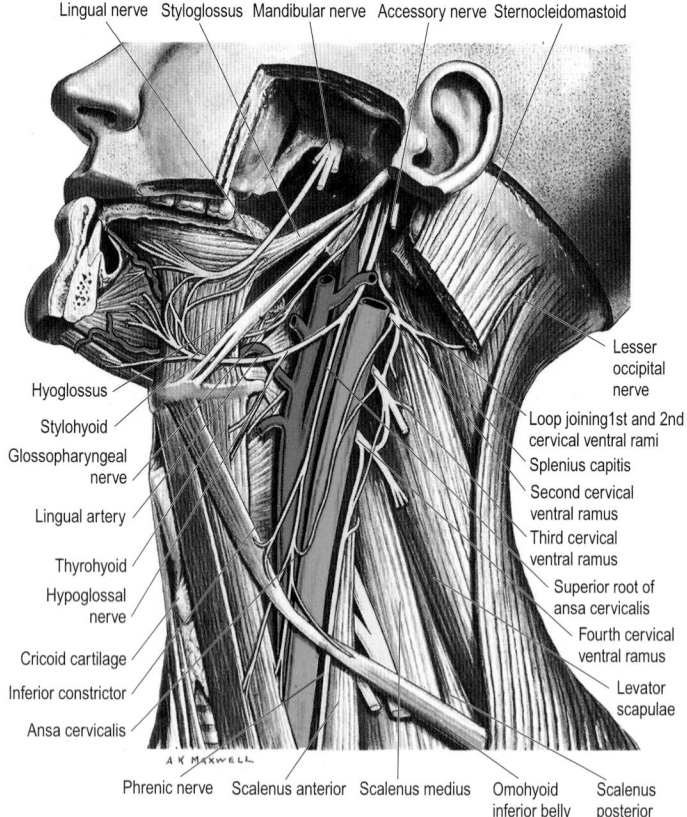

Lingual nerve Styloglossus Mandibular nerve Accessory nerve Sternocleidomastoid

Hyoglossus
Stylohyoid
Glossopharyngeal nerve
Lingual artery
Thyrohyoid
Hypoglossal nerve
Cricoid cartilage
Inferior constrictor
Ansa cervicalis

A K MAXWELL

Lesser occipital nerve
Loop joining 1st and 2nd cervical ventral rami
Splenius capitis
Second cervical ventral ramus
Third cervical ventral ramus
Superior root of ansa cervicalis
Fourth cervical ventral ramus
Levator scapulae

Phrenic nerve Scalenus anterior Scalenus medius Omohyoid inferior belly Scalenus posterior

Fig. 31.21 A dissection to show the general distribution of the left hypoglossal and lingual nerves and the position and constitution of some parts of the cervical plexus of the left side.

superior bulb of the internal jugular vein. It is similar in structure to the carotid body (p. 547) and is presumed to have a similar function. The predominant cell type has morphological similarities to adrenal chromaffin cells, and is derived from the neural crest. Cells obtained from glomus jugulare paragangliomas show spontaneous neurite outgrowth in culture, and have vasoactive intestinal peptide (VIP)-like activity. The tympanic body may be present as two or more parts near the tympanic branch of the glossopharyngeal nerve or the auricular branch of the vagus as they lie within their canals in the petrous part of the temporal bone. Tumours of tympanic bodies may involve the adjacent cranial nerves and the middle ear.

SUBCLAVIAN VEIN (Fig. 31.8)

The subclavian vein is a continuation of the axillary vein and extends from the outer border of the first rib to the medial border of scalenus anterior, where it joins the internal jugular vein to form the brachiocephalic vein. The clavicle and subclavius lie anterior to it, the subclavian artery is posterosuperior, separated by scalenus anterior and the phrenic nerve, and the first rib and pleura are inferior. The vein usually has a pair of valves, c.2 cm from its end. Its tributaries are the external jugular, dorsal scapular and sometimes the anterior jugular vein. At its junction with the internal jugular, the left subclavian vein receives the thoracic duct, and the right subclavian vein receives the right lymphatic duct.

VERTEBRAL VEIN

Numerous small tributaries from internal vertebral plexuses leave the vertebral canal above the posterior arch of the atlas and join small veins from local deep muscles in the suboccipital triangle. Their union produces a vessel which enters the foramen in the transverse process of the atlas and forms a plexus around the vertebral artery. It descends through successive transverse foramina and ends as the vertebral vein. The vein emerges from the sixth cervical transverse foramen, whence it descends, at first anterior, then anterolateral, to the vertebral artery, to open superoposteriorly into the brachiocephalic vein: the opening has a paired valve. As it descends it passes behind the internal jugular vein and in front of the first part of the subclavian artery. A small accessory vertebral vein usually descends from the vertebral plexus, traverses the seventh cervical transverse foramen and turns forwards between the subclavian artery and the cervical pleura to join the brachiocephalic vein.

Tributaries – The vertebral vein connects with the sigmoid sinus by a vessel in the posterior condylar canal, when this exists. It also receives branches from the occipital vein, prevertebral muscles, internal and external vertebral plexuses. It is joined by anterior vertebral and deep cervical veins (see below) and, sometimes near its end, by the first intercostal vein.

ANTERIOR VERTEBRAL VEIN

The anterior vertebral vein starts in a plexus around the upper cervical transverse processes, descends near the ascending cervical artery between attachments of scalenus anterior and longus capitis, and opens into the end of the vertebral vein.

DEEP CERVICAL VEIN

The deep cervical vein accompanies its artery between semispinales capitis and cervicis. It is formed in the suboccipital region by the union of communicating branches of the occipital vein; veins from suboccipital muscles; and veins from plexuses around the cervical spines. It passes forwards between the seventh cervical transverse process and the neck of the first rib to end in the lower part of the vertebral vein.

Cervical groups of lymph nodes (Fig. 31.1)

Lymph nodes in the head and neck are distributed in terminal and outlying groups. The terminal group is related to the carotid sheath and the nodes it contains are the deep cervical lymph nodes. All lymph vessels of the head and neck drain into this group, either directly from tissues or indirectly through nodes in the outlying groups. Efferents of the deep cervical nodes form the jugular trunk. The right jugular trunk collects lymph from the right arm and right half of the thorax and the right head and neck and may end in the jugulosubclavian junction or the right lymphatic duct. The left jugular trunk usually enters the thoracic duct, but it may join the internal jugular or subclavian vein.

LYMPHATIC DRAINAGE OF THE NECK (Fig. 31.1)

Many vessels draining the superficial cervical tissues skirt the borders of sternocleidomastoid to reach the superior or inferior deep cervical nodes. Others pass to the superficial cervical and occipital nodes. Lymph from the superior region of the anterior triangle drains to the submandibular and submental nodes. Vessels from the anterior cervical skin inferior to the hyoid bone pass to the anterior cervical lymph nodes near the anterior jugular veins. Their efferents go to the deep cervical nodes of both sides, including the infrahyoid, prelaryngeal and pretracheal groups. An anterior cervical node often occupies the suprasternal space. Lymph from tissues of the head and neck internal to the deep fascia drains to the deep cervical nodes directly or through outlying groups that include the retropharyngeal, paratracheal, lingual, infrahyoid, prelaryngeal and pretracheal groups. The lymphatic drainage associated with the nasal region, larynx and oral cavity is described in the appropriate regions. The deep cervical lymphatic nodes lie alongside the carotid sheath, and form superior and inferior groups.

Superior deep cervical nodes – The superior deep cervical nodes adjoin the upper part of the internal jugular vein. Most are deep to sternocleidomastoid, but a few extend beyond it. One subgroup, consisting of one large and several small nodes, is in a triangular region bounded by the posterior belly of digastric and the facial and internal jugular veins, and is known as the jugulodigastric group. It is concerned specially with drainage of the tongue. Efferents from the upper deep cervical nodes drain either to the lower group or direct to the jugular trunk.

Inferior deep cervical nodes – The inferior deep cervical nodes are partly deep to the sternocleidomastoid, and are particularly related to the lower part of the internal jugular vein. Some are closely related to the brachial plexus and subclavian vessels. The jugulo-omohyoid node lies on, or just above, the intermediate tendon of omohyoid, and is concerned especially with lymphatic drainage from the tongue. Efferents from this lower group join the jugular lymph trunk.

Retropharyngeal nodes – Retropharyngeal nodes lie between the pharyngeal and prevertebral fasciae and form a median and two lateral groups, the latter anterior to the lateral masses of the atlas along the lateral borders of longus capitis. The nodes receive afferents from the nasopharynx, pharyngotympanic tube and atlanto-occipital and atlanto-axial joints and drain to the upper deep cervical nodes.

Paratracheal nodes – The paratracheal nodes flank both trachea and oesophagus along the recurrent laryngeal nerves. Efferents pass to the corresponding deep cervical nodes.

Infrahyoid, prelaryngeal and pretracheal nodes – The infrahyoid, prelaryngeal and pretracheal nodes lie beneath the deep cervical fascia. They drain afferents from the anterior cervical nodes, and their efferents join the deep cervical nodes. Infrahyoid nodes are anterior to the thyrohyoid membrane, prelaryngeal nodes lie on the cricovocal membrane, and pretracheal nodes lie anterior to the trachea near the inferior thyroid veins.

Lingual nodes – Lingual nodes are small and inconstant, and are situated on the external surface of hyoglossus and also between the genioglossi. They drain to the upper deep cervical nodes.

SPREAD OF MALIGNANT DISEASE IN THE NECK

Cancers arising in the head and neck from regions such as the thyroid gland, larynx, oral cavity and oropharynx, nasopharynx and paranasal sinuses have predictable patterns of spread through the chains of lymph nodes in the neck. When operating on malignant disease in this region it is vitally important to understand these patterns of spread so that for any individual cancer the appropriate operation is undertaken. Clinical experience has shown that the lymph nodes in the neck fall into five distinct groups (**Fig. 31.1**). Level I nodes lie in the submandibular triangle bounded by the anterior and posterior bellies of digastric and the lower border of the mandible above. Level II (upper jugular) nodes lie around the upper portion of the internal jugular vein and the upper part of the spinal accessory nerve. They extend from the skull base to the bifurcation of the common carotid artery or the hyoid bone. Level III (middle jugular) nodes lie around the middle third of the internal jugular vein from the inferior border of level II to the superior belly of omohyoid or cricothyroid membrane. Level IV (lower jugular) nodes lie around the lower third of the internal jugular vein from the inferior border of level III to the clavicle. The anterior and posterior borders for levels II, III and IV are the lateral border of sternohyoid and the posterior border of sternocleidomastoid respectively. Level V (posterior triangle) nodes lie around the lower part of the spinal accessory nerve and the transverse cervical vessels.

Knowing which levels of nodes are likely to be involved in the metastatic spread of a particular cancer arising in the head and neck means that appropriate nodal clearance can be undertaken. The classic radical neck dissection first described by Crile in 1906 involves a thorough clearance of levels I to V including the sacrifice of sterno-cleidomastoid, the internal jugular vein and the spinal accessory nerve. Modified radical neck dissections (so-called functional neck dissections) still remove level I to V nodes, but spare either or all of sternocleido-mastoid, the internal jugular vein and the spinal accessory. Selective neck dissections remove selected groups of nodes, e.g. the supraomohyoid neck dissection removes level I to III nodes, the lateral neck dissection removes level II to IV nodes, and the posterolateral neck dissection removes level II to V nodes.

CERVICAL LYMPHOVENOUS PORTALS

Lymph is returned to the systemic venous circulation via right and left lymphovenous portals sited at, or near, the junctions of the internal jugular and subclavian veins. The arrangement of these terminations is variable. Usually, three small lymph trunks converge towards their venous junctions on either side of the body, and they are joined, on the left side only, by the larger thoracic duct.

On the right side, the three trunks are the right jugular, right sub-clavian and right bronchomediastinal. The right jugular trunk extends from the terminal lower deep cervical nodes along the ventrolateral aspect of the internal jugular vein, and conveys all the lymph from the right half of the head and neck. The right subclavian trunk drains from the terminal apical axillary group. It extends along the axillary and subclavian veins, and conveys lymph from the right upper limb and superficial tissues of the right half of the thoracoabdominal wall, down to the umbilicus anteriorly and iliac crest posteriorly (and includes much of the breast). The right bronchomediastinal trunk, ascends over the trachea towards the lymphovenous portal and conveys lymph from the thoracic walls, the right cupola of the diaphragm and subjacent liver, the right lung, bronchi and trachea, the greater part of the 'right heart' – of clinical parlance, not the geometric right half – and a proportionately small drainage from the thoracic oesophagus.

The three right lymphatic trunks usually open independently (**Fig. 31.22**). Their orifices are clustered either on the ventral aspect of the jugulo/subclavian junction, or in the nearby wall of either of the great veins. Sometimes one or more of the trunks may bifurcate (or even trifurcate) preterminally and then terminate via multiple orifices. Rarely, the three trunks fuse to form a short, single, right lymphatic duct (c.1 cm long) that inclines across the medial border of scalenus anterior at the root of the neck to reach the ventral aspect of the venous junction, where its orifice is guarded by a bicuspid semilunar valve. An incomplete right lymphatic duct may be present if the subclavian and jugular trunks, or any combination of their terminals, are fused. When this occurs, the bronchomediastinal trunk almost invariably opens separately.

On the left, the four trunks that converge on the left lymphovenous portal are the left jugular and left subclavian trunks, which have a disposition corresponding to that of their counterparts on the right; the left bronchomediastinal trunk, which has a drainage similar to the right trunk, but which drains more of the heart – the 'left' and 'right' hearts of clinical parlance – and more of the oesophagus; and the thoracic duct, which drains all of the rest of the body.

INNERVATION

The skin, joints, viscera and muscles of the neck are innervated by branches of the glossopharyngeal, vagus and spinal accessory nerves, the cervical spinal nerves and the cervical sympathetic trunk.

The first and second cervical dorsal root ganglia lie on the vertebral arches of the atlas and axis respectively. The first cervical ganglion may

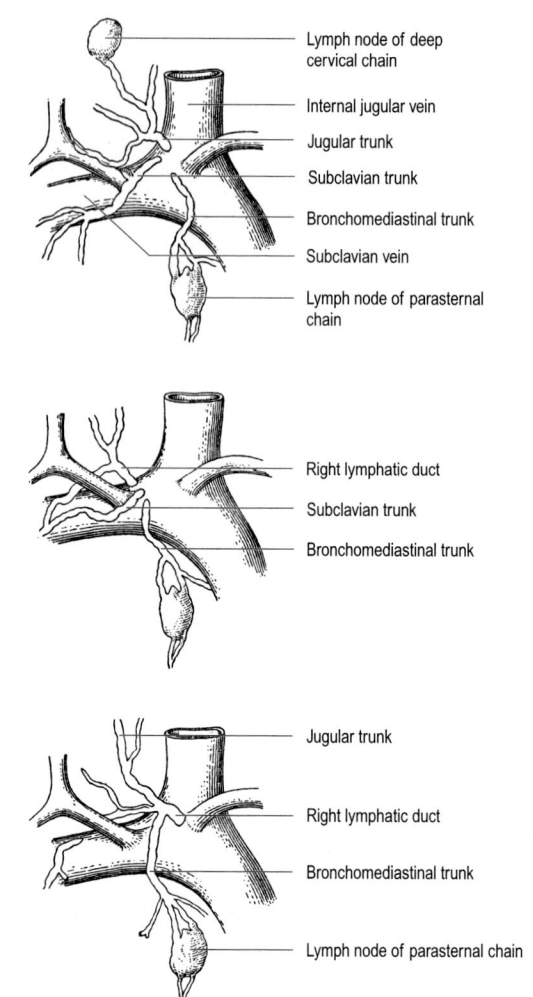

Fig. 31.22 Variation in the terminal lymphatic trunks nodes of the right side. (By permission from Poirier P, Charpy A 1901 Traite d'Anatomie Humaine. Paris: Masson et Cie.)

be absent. Smaller aberrant ganglia sometimes occur on the upper cervical dorsal roots between the ganglia and cord. The upper four cervical roots are small, the lower four are large. In general, cervical dorsal roots have a thickness ratio to the ventral roots of three to one, which is greater than is seen in other regions. The first dorsal root is an exception, being smaller than the ventral, and in c.8% cases it is absent. The first and second cervical roots are short, and run almost horizon-tally to their exit from the vertebral canal. From the third to the eighth cervical they slope obliquely down. Obliquity and length increase successively, however the distance between spinal attachment and vertebral exit never exceeds the height of one vertebra.

Cervical ventral rami

Cervical ventral rami, except the first, appear between the anterior and posterior intertransverse muscles. The upper four form the cervical plexus, and the lower four, together with most of the first thoracic ventral ramus, form the brachial plexus. Each receives at least one grey ramus communicans, the upper four from the superior cervical sympathetic ganglion, the fifth and sixth from the middle ganglion and the seventh and eighth from the cervicothoracic ganglion.

The first cervical ventral ramus, the suboccipital nerve, emerges above the posterior arch of the atlas, passes forwards lateral to its lateral mass and medial to the vertebral artery. It supplies rectus capitis lateralis, emerges medial to it, descends anterior to the transverse process of the atlas and posterior to the internal jugular vein and joins the ascending branch of the second cervical ventral ramus.

The second cervical ventral ramus issues between the vertebral arches of the atlas and axis. It ascends between their transverse processes, passes anterior to the first posterior intertransverse muscle and emerges lateral to the vertebral artery generally between longus capitis and levator scapulae. The ramus divides into an ascending branch which joins the first cervical nerve and a descending branch which joins the ascending branch of the third cervical ventral ramus.

The third cervical ventral ramus appears between longus capitis and scalenus medius. The remaining ventral rami emerge between scalenus anterior and the scalenus medius.

CERVICAL PLEXUS (Figs 31.2, 31.6, 31.21, 29.9)

The cervical plexus is formed by the ventral rami of the upper four cervical nerves, and supplies some neck muscles and the diaphragm, and areas of skin on the head, neck and chest. It is situated in the neck opposite a line drawn down the side of the neck from the root of the auricle to the level of the upper border of the thyroid cartilage. It is deep to the internal jugular vein, the deep fascia and sternocleidomastoid, and anterior to scalenus medius and levator scapulae. Each ramus, except the first, divides into ascending and descending parts, which unite in communicating loops. From the first loop (C2 and 3) superficial branches supply the head and neck; cutaneous nerves of the shoulder and chest arise from the second loop (C3 and 4). Muscular and communicating branches arise from the same nerves. The branches are superficial or deep. The superficial branches perforate the cervical fascia to supply the skin while the deep branches in general supply muscles. The superficial branches either ascend (the lesser occipital, great auricular and the transverse cutaneous nerves) or descend (supraclavicular nerves). These nerves are described in detail on page 532. The deep branches form medial and lateral series.

DEEP BRANCHES – MEDIAL SERIES

Communicating branches – Communicating branches pass from the loop between the first and second cervical rami to the vagus and hypoglossal nerves and to the sympathetic trunk. The hypoglossal branch later leaves the hypoglossal nerve as a series of branches, viz. the meningeal, superior root of ansa cervicalis, nerves to thyrohyoid and to geniohyoid. A branch also connects the fourth and fifth cervical rami. The first four cervical ventral rami each receive a grey ramus communicans from the superior cervical sympathetic ganglion.

The superior root of the ansa cervicalis (descendens hypoglossi) (Fig. 31.2) leaves the hypoglossal nerve where it curves round the occipital artery and then descends anterior to or in the carotid sheath. It contains only fibres from the first cervical spinal nerve. After giving a branch to the superior belly of omohyoid, it is joined by the inferior root of the ansa from the second and third cervical spinal nerves. The two roots form the ansa cervicalis (ansa hypoglossi), from which branches supply sternohyoid, sternothyroid and the inferior belly of omohyoid. Another branch is said to descend anterior to the vessels into the thorax to join the cardiac and phrenic nerves.

Muscular branches – Muscular branches supply rectus capitis lateralis (C1), rectus capitis anterior (C1, 2), longus capitis (C1–3) and longus colli (C2–4). The inferior root of the ansa cervicalis and the phrenic nerve are additional muscular branches.

Inferior root of the ansa cervicalis (nervus descendens cervicalis) (Fig. 31.2) – The inferior root of the ansa cervicalis is formed by the union of a branch from the second with another from the third cervical ramus. It descends on the lateral side of the internal jugular vein, crosses it a little below the middle of the neck, and continues forwards to join the superior root anterior to the common carotid artery, forming the ansa cervicalis (ansa hypoglossi), from which all infrahyoid muscles except thyrohyoid are supplied. The inferior root comes from the second and third cervical ventral rami in c.75% cases, from the second to fourth in c.15%, from the third alone in c.5%. Occasionally it may be derived from either the second alone or from the first to third.

Phrenic nerve – The phrenic nerve arises chiefly from the fourth cervical ventral ramus, but also has contributions from the third and fifth. It is formed at the upper part of the lateral border of scalenus anterior and descends almost vertically across its anterior surface behind the prevertebral fascia. It descends posterior to sternocleidomastoid, the inferior

belly of omohyoid (near its intermediate tendon), the internal jugular vein, transverse cervical and suprascapular arteries and, on the left, the thoracic duct. At the root of the neck, it runs anterior to the second part of the subclavian artery, from which it is separated by the scalenus anterior (some accounts state that on the left side the nerve passes anterior to the first part of the subclavian artery), and posterior to the subclavian vein. The phrenic nerve enters the thorax by crossing medially in front of the internal thoracic artery.

In the neck, each nerve receives variable filaments from the cervical sympathetic ganglia or their branches and may also connect with internal thoracic sympathetic plexuses.

Accessory phrenic nerve – The accessory phrenic nerve is composed of fibres from the fifth cervical ventral ramus which run in a branch of the nerve to subclavius. This lies lateral to the phrenic nerve and descends posterior (occasionally anterior) to the subclavian vein. The accessory phrenic nerve usually joins the phrenic nerve near the first rib, but may not do so until near the pulmonary hilum or beyond. The accessory phrenic nerve may be derived from the fourth or sixth cervical ventral rami or from the ansa cervicalis.

DEEP BRANCHES – LATERAL SERIES

Communicating branches – Lateral deep branches of the cervical plexus (C2, 3, 4) may connect with the spinal accessory nerve within sternocleidomastoid, the posterior triangle or beneath trapezius.

Muscular branches (Fig. 31.15) – Muscular branches are distributed to sternocleidomastoid (C2, 3, 4), trapezius (C2 and possibly C3), levator scapulae (C3, 4) and scalenus medius (C3, 4). Branches to trapezius cross the posterior triangle obliquely below the spinal accessory nerve.

BRACHIAL PLEXUS (Fig. 31.8)

The brachial plexus is formed by the union of the ventral rami of the lower four cervical nerves and the greater part of the ventral ramus of the first thoracic ventral ramus. It may also receive contributions from the fourth cervical and second thoracic spinal nerves. As its name suggests, its branches supply the muscles, joints and skin of the upper limb. The relations and distribution of the brachial plexus are described in detail in Section 5. However, it is also mentioned here because, at its origin, the brachial plexus lies in the posterior triangle of the neck, in the angle between the clavicle and the lower posterior border of sternocleidomastoid. It emerges between the scaleni anterior and medius, superior to the third part of the subclavian artery, and is covered by platysma, deep fascia and skin, through which it is palpable. It is crossed by the supraclavicular nerves, the nerve to subclavius, the inferior belly of omohyoid, the external jugular vein and the superficial ramus of the transverse cervical artery. The plexus passes posterior to the medial two-thirds of the clavicle, subclavius and the suprascapular vessels, and lies on the first digitation of serratus anterior and on subscapularis.

Cervical dorsal rami (Figs 46.14, 29.9)

Each cervical spinal dorsal ramus except the first divides into medial and lateral branches, and all innervate muscles. In general, only medial branches of the second to fourth, and usually the fifth, supply skin. Except for the first (sometimes called the suboccipital nerve) and second, each dorsal ramus passes back medial to a posterior intertransverse muscle, curving round the articular process into the interval between semispinalis capitis and semispinalis cervicis. The cervical dorsal rami are described in detail on pages 783–784.

Cranial nerves

GLOSSOPHARYNGEAL NERVE (Fig. 31.23)

The glossopharyngeal nerve (**Figs 31.16, 31.20**) supplies motor fibres to stylopharyngeus, parasympathetic secretomotor fibres to the parotid gland (derived from the inferior salivatory nucleus), sensory fibres to the tympanic cavity, pharyngotympanic tube, fauces, tonsils, nasopharynx, uvula and posterior (postsulcal) third of the tongue, and gustatory fibres for the postsulcal part of the tongue.

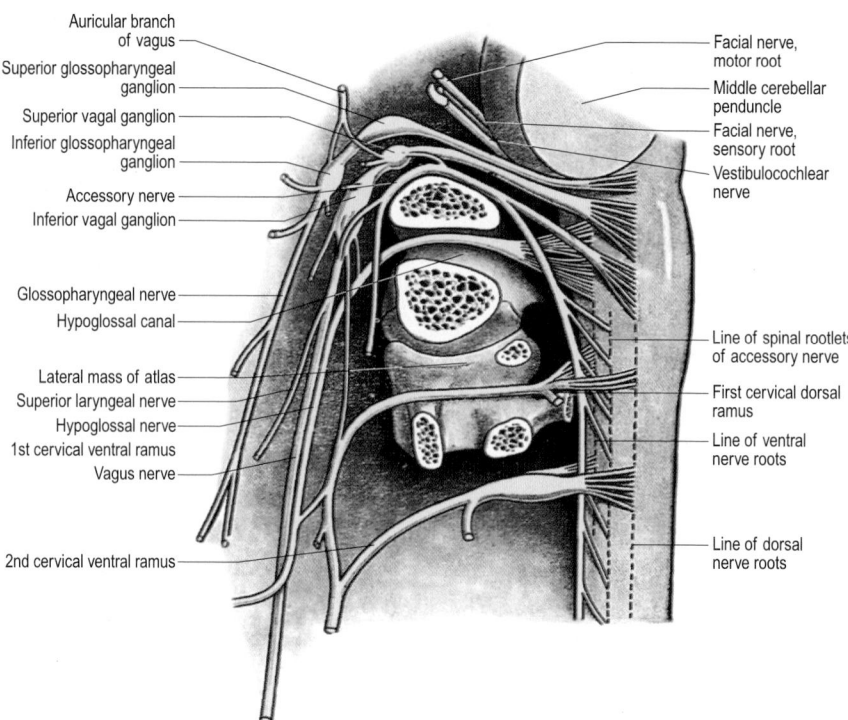

Auricular branch of vagus
Superior glossopharyngeal ganglion
Superior vagal ganglion
Inferior glossopharyngeal ganglion
Accessory nerve
Inferior vagal ganglion
Glossopharyngeal nerve
Hypoglossal canal
Lateral mass of atlas
Superior laryngeal nerve
Hypoglossal nerve
1st cervical ventral ramus
Vagus nerve
2nd cervical ventral ramus

Facial nerve, motor root
Middle cerebellar peduncle
Facial nerve, sensory root
Vestibulocochlear nerve
Line of spinal rootlets of accessory nerve
First cervical dorsal ramus
Line of ventral nerve roots
Line of dorsal nerve roots

Fig. 31.23 The communications between the last four cranial nerves of the left side viewed from the dorsolateral aspect. The hypoglossal canal has been split in its long axis and the transverse process of the atlas has been divided close to the lateral mass. The descending branch of the hypoglossal nerve is not shown.

The nerve leaves the skull through the anteromedial part of the jugular foramen, anterior to the vagus and accessory nerves, and in a separate dural sheath. In the foramen it is lodged in a deep groove leading from the cochlear aqueductal depression, and is separated by the inferior petrosal sinus from the vagus and accessory nerves. The groove is bridged by fibrous tissue, which is calcified in c.25% of skulls. After leaving the foramen, the nerve passes forwards between the internal jugular vein and internal carotid artery and then descends anterior to the latter, deep to the styloid process and its attached muscles, to reach the posterior border of stylopharyngeus. It curves forwards on stylopharyngeus and either pierces the lower fibres of the superior pharyngeal constrictor or passes between it and the middle constrictor to be distributed to the tonsil, the mucosae of the pharynx and postsulcal part of the tongue, the vallate papillae, and oral mucous glands.

Two ganglia, superior and inferior, are situated on the glossopharyngeal nerve as it traverses the jugular foramen (**Fig. 31.23**). The superior ganglion is in the upper part of the groove occupied by the nerve in the jugular foramen. It is small, has no branches and is usually regarded as a detached part of the inferior ganglion. The inferior ganglion is larger and lies in a notch in the lower border of the petrous part of the temporal bone. Its cells are typical unipolar neurones, whose peripheral branches convey gustatory and tactile signals from the mucosa of the tongue (posterior third including the sulcus terminalis and vallate papillae) and general sensation from the oropharynx, where it is responsible for initiating the gag reflex.

COMMUNICATING BRANCHES

The glossopharyngeal nerve communicates with the sympathetic trunk, vagus and facial nerves. The inferior ganglion is connected with the superior cervical sympathetic ganglion. Two filaments from the inferior ganglion pass to the vagus, one to its auricular branch and the other to its superior ganglion. A branch to the facial nerve arises from the glossopharyngeal nerve below the inferior ganglion, and perforates the posterior belly of digastric to join the facial nerve near the stylomastoid foramen.

BRANCHES OF DISTRIBUTION

These are tympanic, carotid, pharyngeal, muscular, tonsillar and lingual.

Tympanic nerve – The tympanic nerve leaves the inferior ganglion, ascends to the tympanic cavity through the inferior tympanic canaliculus and divides into branches that contribute to the tympanic plexus. The lesser petrosal nerve is derived from the tympanic plexus.

Carotid branch – The carotid branch is often double. It arises just below the jugular foramen and descends on the internal carotid artery to the wall of the carotid sinus and to the carotid body. The nerve contains primary afferent fibres from chemoreceptors in the carotid body and from the baroreceptors lying in the carotid sinus wall. It may communicate with the inferior ganglion of the vagus, or with one of its branches, and with a sympathetic branch from the superior cervical ganglion.

Pharyngeal branches – The pharyngeal branches are three or four filaments which unite with the pharyngeal branch of the vagus and the laryngopharyngeal branches of the sympathetic trunk to form the pharyngeal plexus near the middle pharyngeal constrictor. They constitute the route by which the glossopharyngeal nerve supplies sensory fibres to the mucosa of the pharynx.

Muscular branch – The muscular branch supplies stylopharyngeus.

Tonsillar, lingual and inferior petrosal branches – The tonsillar, lingual and inferior petrosal branches are described on pages 623, 588, and 237 respectively.

LESIONS OF THE GLOSSOPHARYNGEAL NERVE

Damage to the glossopharyngeal nerve rarely occurs without involvement of other lower cranial nerves. Transient or sustained hypertension may follow surgical section of the nerve, reflecting involvement of the carotid branch. Isolated lesions of the glossopharyngeal nerve lead to loss of sensation over the ipsilateral soft palate, fauces, pharynx and posterior third of the tongue, although this is difficult to assess clinically and requires galvanic stimulation. The palatal and pharyngeal (gag) reflexes are reduced or absent and salivary secretion from the parotid gland may also be reduced. Weakness of stylopharyngeus cannot be tested individually. Glossopharyngeal neuralgia consists of episodic brief but severe pain, often precipitated by swallowing, and experienced in the throat, behind the angle of the jaw and within the ear. Superior jugular bulb thromboses (e.g. in otitis media) and jugular foramen syndrome (associated with nasopharyngeal carcinoma and a glomus tumour) may cause lesions of the adjacent glossopharyngeal, vagus and accessory nerves, with associated weakness in the muscles supplied (in the pharynx and larynx).

VAGUS NERVE

The vagus is a large mixed nerve. It has a more extensive course and distribution than any other cranial nerve, and traverses the neck, thorax and abdomen (**Figs 31.14**, **31.16**, **19.3**, **19.7**, **31.23**). Its central connections are described in Chapter19).

The vagus exits the skull through the jugular foramen accompanied by the accessory nerve, with which it shares an arachnoid and a dural sheath. Both nerves lie anterior to a fibrous septum that separates them from the glossopharyngeal nerve. The vagus descends vertically in the neck in the carotid sheath, between the internal jugular vein and the internal carotid artery, to the upper border of the thyroid cartilage, and then passes between the vein and the common carotid artery to the root of the neck. Its relationships in this part of its course are therefore similar to those described for these structures. Its further course differs on the two sides. The right vagus descends posterior to the internal jugular vein to cross the first part of the subclavian artery and enter the thorax. The left vagus enters the thorax between the left common carotid and subclavian arteries and behind the left brachiocephalic vein.

After emerging from the jugular foramen, the vagus bears two marked enlargements, a small, round, superior ganglion and a larger inferior ganglion (**Fig. 31.23**).

SUPERIOR (JUGULAR) GANGLION
The superior ganglion is greyish, spherical and c.4 mm in diameter. It is connected to the cranial root of the accessory nerve, the inferior glossopharyngeal ganglion, and the sympathetic trunk, the latter by a filament from the superior cervical ganglion. The significance of these connections is not entirely clear, but the first probably contains aberrant motor fibres from the nucleus ambiguus which issue in the accessory nerve, to be distributed to the palatal, pharyngeal, laryngeal and upper oesophageal musculature via the vagus.

INFERIOR (NODOSE) GANGLION
The inferior or nodose ganglion is larger than the superior ganglion, and is elongated and cylindrical in shape with a length of c.25 mm and a maximum breadth of 5 mm. It is connected with the hypoglossal nerve, the loop between the first and second cervical spinal nerves, and with the superior cervical sympathetic ganglion. Just above the ganglion the cranial accessory blends with the vagus nerve, its fibres being distributed mainly in pharyngeal and recurrent laryngeal vagal branches. Most visceral afferent fibres have their cell bodies in the nodose ganglion.

Both vagal ganglia are exclusively sensory, and contain somatic, special visceral and general visceral afferent neurones. The superior ganglion is chiefly somatic, and most of its neurones enter the auricular nerve, whilst neurones in the inferior ganglion are concerned with visceral sensation from the heart, larynx, lungs and the alimentary tract from the pharynx to the transverse colon. Some fibres transmit impulses from taste endings in the vallecula and epiglottis. Large afferent fibres are derived from muscle spindles in the laryngeal muscles. Vagal sensory neurones in the nodose ganglion may show some somatotopic organization. Both ganglia are traversed by parasympathetic, and perhaps some sympathetic fibres, but there is no evidence that vagal parasympathetic components relay in the inferior ganglion. Preganglionic motor fibres from the dorsal vagal nucleus and the special visceral efferents from the nucleus ambiguus, which descend to the inferior vagal ganglion, commonly form a visible band, skirting the ganglion in some mammals. These larger fibres probably provide motor innervation to the larynx in the recurrent laryngeal nerve, together with some contribution to the superior laryngeal nerve supplying cricothyroid.

BRANCHES IN THE NECK
The branches of the vagus in the neck are the meningeal, auricular, pharyngeal, carotid body, superior and recurrent laryngeal nerves and cardiac branches.

Meningeal branch(es) – Meningeal branches appear to start from the superior vagal ganglion and pass through the jugular foramen to be distributed to the dura mater in the posterior cranial fossa.

Auricular branch – The auricular branch arises from the superior vagal ganglion and is joined by a branch from the inferior ganglion of the glossopharyngeal nerve. It passes behind the internal jugular vein and enters the mastoid canaliculus on the lateral wall of the jugular fossa. Traversing the temporal bone, it crosses the facial canal c.4 mm above the stylomastoid foramen and here supplies an ascending branch to the facial nerve. Fibres of the nervus intermedius may pass to the auricular branch at this point, which may explain the cutaneous vesiculation in the auricle that sometimes accompanies geniculate herpes. The auricular branch then traverses the tympanomastoid fissure, and divides into two rami. One ramus joins the posterior auricular nerve and the other is distributed to the skin of part of the ear and to the external acoustic meatus.

Pharyngeal branch – The pharyngeal branch of the vagus is the main motor nerve of the pharynx. It emerges from the upper part of the inferior vagal ganglion and consists chiefly of filaments from the cranial accessory nerve. It passes between the external and internal carotid arteries to the upper border of the middle pharyngeal constrictor, and divides into numerous filaments which join rami of the sympathetic trunk and glossopharyngeal nerve to form a pharyngeal plexus. A minute filament, the ramus lingualis vagi, joins the hypoglossal nerve as it curves round the occipital artery.

Branches to the carotid body – Branches to the carotid body are variable in number. They may arise from the inferior ganglion or travel in the pharyngeal branch, and sometimes in the superior laryngeal nerve. They form a plexus with the glossopharyngeal rami and branches of the cervical sympathetic trunk.

Superior laryngeal nerve – The superior laryngeal nerve is larger than the pharyngeal branch, and issues from the middle of the inferior vagal ganglion. It receives a branch from the superior cervical sympathetic ganglion and descends alongside the pharynx, at first posterior, then medial, to the internal carotid artery, and divides into the internal and external laryngeal nerves.

The internal laryngeal nerve is sensory to the laryngeal mucosa down to the level of the vocal folds. It also carries afferent fibres from the laryngeal neuromuscular spindles and other stretch receptors. It descends to the thyrohyoid membrane, pierces it above the superior laryngeal artery and divides into an upper and lower branch. The upper branch is horizontal and supplies the mucosa of the pharynx, the epiglottis, vallecula and laryngeal vestibule. The lower branch descends in the medial wall of the piriform recess, supplies the aryepiglottic fold, the mucosa on the back of the arytenoid cartilage and one or two branches to transverse arytenoid (the latter unite with twigs from the recurrent laryngeal to supply the same muscle). The internal laryngeal nerve ends by piercing the inferior pharyngeal constrictor to unite with an ascending branch from the recurrent laryngeal nerve. As it ascends in the neck it supplies branches, more numerous on the left, to the mucosa and tunica muscularis of the oesophagus and trachea and to the inferior constrictor.

The external laryngeal nerve, smaller than the internal, descends behind sternohyoid with the superior thyroid artery, but on a deeper plane. It lies first on the inferior pharyngeal constrictor, then pierces it to curve round the inferior thyroid tubercle and reach cricothyroid, which it supplies. The nerve also gives branches to the pharyngeal plexus and the inferior constrictor. Behind the common carotid artery, the external laryngeal nerve communicates with the superior cardiac nerve and superior cervical sympathetic ganglion.

Recurrent laryngeal nerve – The recurrent laryngeal nerve differs, in origin and course, on the two sides. On the right it arises from the vagus anterior to the first part of the subclavian artery, and curves backwards below and then behind it to ascend obliquely to the side of the trachea behind the common carotid artery. Near the lower pole of the lateral lobe of the thyroid gland it is closely related to the inferior thyroid artery, and crosses either in front of, behind, or between, its branches. On the left, the nerve arises from the vagus on the left of the aortic arch, curves below it immediately behind the attachment of the ligamentum arteriosum to the concavity of the aortic arch (**Fig. 30.31**) and ascends to the side of the trachea. As the recurrent laryngeal nerve curves round the subclavian artery, or the aortic arch, it gives cardiac filaments to the deep cardiac plexus. On both sides the recurrent laryngeal nerve ascends in or near a groove between the trachea and oesophagus. It is closely related to the medial surface of the thyroid gland before it passes under the lower border of the inferior constrictor, and it enters the larynx behind the articulation of the inferior thyroid cornu with the cricoid cartilage. The recurrent laryngeal nerve supplies all laryngeal muscles, except the cricothyroid, and it communicates with the internal laryngeal nerve, supplying sensory filaments to the laryngeal mucosa below the vocal folds. It also carries afferent fibres from laryngeal stretch receptors. The recurrent laryngeal nerve is described further with the larynx (p. 644).

ACCESSORY NERVE (Figs 31.20, 31.21, 31.23)

The accessory nerve is conventionally described as a single entity, even though its two components, which join for a relatively short part of its course, are of quite separate origin.

CRANIAL ROOT

The cranial root of the accessory nerve is smaller than the spinal root. It exits the skull through the jugular foramen, and unites for a short distance with the spinal root. It is also connected to the superior vagal ganglion. After traversing the foramen, the cranial root separates from the spinal part and immediately joins the vagus nerve superior to the inferior vagal ganglion. Those of its fibres that are distributed in the pharyngeal branches of the vagus are derived from the nucleus ambiguus, and probably innervate the pharyngeal and palatal muscles except tensor veli palatini. Other fibres enter the recurrent laryngeal nerve to supply the adductor muscles of the vocal cords, thyroarytenoid and lateral cricoarytenoid.

SPINAL ROOT

The spinal root arises from an elongated nucleus of motor cells situated in the lateral aspect of the ventral horn which extends from the junction of the spinal cord and medulla to the sixth cervical segment (**Fig. 31.20**). Some rootlets emerge directly, others turn cranially before exiting. Their line of exit is irregular rather than linear, and the spinal root usually passes through the first cervical dorsal root ganglion. The rootlets form a trunk which ascends between the ligamentum denticulatum and the dorsal roots of the spinal nerves and enters the skull via the foramen magnum, behind the vertebral artery. It then turns upwards and passes laterally to reach the jugular foramen, which it traverses in a common dural sheath with the vagus, but separated from that nerve by a fold of arachnoid mater. As the spinal root exits the jugular foramen it runs posterolaterally and passes either medial or lateral to the internal jugular vein. Occasionally it passes through the vein. The nerve then crosses the transverse process of the atlas and is itself crossed by the occipital artery. It descends obliquely, medial to the styloid process, stylohyoid and the posterior belly of the digastric. Running with the superior sternocleidomastoid branch of the occipital artery, it reaches the upper part of sternocleidomastoid and enters its deep surface, to form an anastomosis with fibres from C2 alone, C3 alone, or C2 and C3, the ansa of Maubrac. The nerve occasionally terminates in the muscle. More commonly it emerges a little above the midpoint of the posterior border of sternocleidomastoid, generally above the emergence of the great auricular nerve (usually within 2 cm of it) and between 4–6 cm from the tip of the mastoid process. However, the point of emergence is very variable. It crosses the posterior triangle on levator scapulae (**Fig. 31.21**), separated from it by the prevertebral layer of deep cervical fascia and adipose tissue. Here the nerve is relatively superficial and related to the superficial cervical lymph nodes. About 3–5 cm above the clavicle it passes behind the anterior border of trapezius, often dividing to form a plexus on its deep surface which receives contributions from C3 and C4, or C4 alone. It then enters the deep surface of the muscle.

The cervical course of the nerve follows a line from the lower anterior part of the tragus to the tip of the transverse process of the atlas and then across the sternocleidomastoid and the posterior triangle to a point on the anterior border of the trapezius 3–5 cm above the clavicle.

Conventionally, the spinal root is thought to provide the sole motor supply to sternocleidomastoid, and the second and third cervical nerves are believed to carry proprioceptive fibres from it. The supranuclear pathway of fibres destined for sternocleidomastoid is not simple: fibres may undergo a double decussation in the brainstem and/or there may be a bilateral projection to the muscle from each hemisphere.

The motor supply to the upper and middle portions of trapezius is primarily from the spinal accessory nerve. However, the lower two-thirds of the muscle, in c.75% of subjects, receives an innervation from the cervical plexus. On the basis of the incomplete denervation of the muscle that sometimes occurs following sacrifice of both the accessory nerve and the cervical plexus, it has been suggested that the trapezius receives a partial motor supply from other sources, possibly via thoracic

roots. In addition to their motor contribution, C3 and 4 carry proprioceptive fibres from trapezius. In c.25% of subjects the spinal accessory nerve receives no fibres from the cervical plexus.

Sensory ganglia have been described along the course of the spinal root.

LESIONS AFFECTING THE ACCESSORY NERVE

Lesions of the accessory nerve may occur centrally; at its exit from the skull; in the neck. The supranuclear fibres which influence motor neurones innervating sternocleidomastoid decussate twice, therefore a lesion of the pyramidal system above the pons produces weakness of the ipsilateral sternocleidomastoid and contralateral trapezius. Episodic contraction of sternocleidomastoid and trapezius, often accompanied by contraction of other muscle groups, e.g. splenius capitis, occurs in spasmodic torticollis, a focal dystonia. In jugular foramen syndrome, caused by pathologies including nasopharyngeal carcinoma or a glomus tumour, lesions of the glossopharyngeal, vagus and accessory nerves coexist. The accessory nerve can be injured more distally in the neck by trauma or by surgical exploration in the posterior triangle. If the accessory nerve is sacrificed as part of a radical neck dissection, and the innervation of trapezius is lost, the patient develops intractable neuralgia due to traction on the brachial plexus caused by the unsupported weight of the shoulder and arm.

HYPOGLOSSAL NERVE (Figs 31.2, 31.14, 31.16, 31.21)

The hypoglossal nerve is motor to all the muscles of the tongue, except palatoglossus. The hypoglossal rootlets run laterally behind the vertebral artery, collected into two bundles which perforate the dura mater separately opposite the hypoglossal canal in the occipital bone, and unite after traversing it. The canal is sometimes divided by a spicule of bone. The nerve emerges from the canal in a plane medial to the internal jugular vein, internal carotid artery, ninth, tenth and eleventh cranial nerves, and passes inferolaterally behind the internal carotid artery and glossopharyngeal and vagus nerves to the interval between the artery and the internal jugular vein. Here it makes a half-spiral turn round the inferior vagal ganglion, and is united with it by connective tissue. It then descends almost vertically between the vessels and anterior to the vagus to a point level with the angle of the mandible, becoming superficial below the posterior belly of digastric and emerging between the internal jugular vein and internal carotid artery. It loops round the inferior sternocleidomastoid branch of the occipital artery, crosses lateral to both internal and external carotid arteries and the loop of the lingual artery a little above the tip of the greater cornu of the hyoid, and is itself crossed by the facial vein. Its course is described further on page 588.

COMMUNICATIONS

The hypoglossal nerve communicates with the sympathetic trunk, vagus, first and second cervical nerves and lingual nerve. Near the atlas it is joined by branches from the superior cervical sympathetic ganglion and by a filament from the loop between the first and second cervical nerves which leaves the hypoglossal as the upper root of the ansa cervicalis (**Fig. 31.2**). The vagal connections occur close to the skull, and numerous filaments pass between the hypoglossal nerve and the inferior vagal ganglion in the connective tissue uniting them. As the hypoglossal nerve curves round the occipital artery it receives the ramus lingualis vagi from the pharyngeal plexus. Near the anterior border of hyoglossus it is connected with the lingual nerve by many filaments which ascend on the muscle.

BRANCHES OF DISTRIBUTION

The branches of distribution of the hypoglossal nerve are meningeal, descending, thyrohyoid and muscular nerves.

Meningeal branches – Meningeal branches leave the nerve in the hypoglossal canal and return through it to supply the diploë of the occipital bone, the dural walls of the occipital and inferior petrosal sinuses and much of the floor of the anterior wall of the posterior cranial fossa, probably through pathways other than that of the hypoglossal nerve, e.g. upper cervical spinal nerves.

Descending branch – The descending branch (descendens hypoglossi) contains fibres from the first cervical spinal nerve. It leaves the hypoglossal nerve when it curves around the occipital artery, and runs down on the carotid sheath. It provides a branch to the superior belly of omohyoid before joining with the descendens cervicalis to form the ansa cervicalis (**Fig. 31.2**).

Nerves to thyrohyoid and geniohyoid – The nerves to thyrohyoid and geniohyoid arise near the posterior border of hyoglossus. They represent the remaining fibres from the first cervical spinal nerves.

LESIONS OF THE HYPOGLOSSAL NERVE

The hypoglossal nerve may be damaged during neck dissection. Complete hypoglossal division causes unilateral lingual paralysis and eventual hemiatrophy; the protruded tongue deviates to the paralysed side, and, on retraction, the wasted and paralysed side rises higher than the unaffected side. The larynx may deviate towards the active side in swallowing, due to unilateral paralysis of the hyoid depressors associated with loss of the first cervical spinal nerve which runs with the hypoglossal nerve. If paralysis is bilateral, the tongue is motionless. Taste and tactile sensibility are unaffected but articulation is slow and swallowing very difficult.

Cervical sympathetic trunk (Figs 31.6, 31.7)

The cervical sympathetic trunk lies on the prevertebral fascia behind the carotid sheath and contains three interconnected ganglia, the superior, middle and inferior (stellate or cervicothoracic). However there may occasionally be two or four ganglia. The cervical sympathetic ganglia send grey rami communicantes to all the cervical spinal nerves but receive no white rami communicantes from them. Their spinal preganglionic fibres emerge in the white rami communicantes of the upper five thoracic spinal nerves (mainly the upper three), and ascend in the sympathetic trunk to synapse in the cervical ganglia. In their course, the grey rami communicantes may pierce longus capitis or scalenus anterior.

SUPERIOR CERVICAL GANGLION

The superior cervical ganglion is the largest of the three ganglia. It lies on the transverse processes of the second and third cervical vertebrae and is probably formed from four fused ganglia judging by its grey rami to C1–4. The internal carotid artery within the carotid sheath is anterior, and longus capitis is posterior (**Fig. 31.6**). The lower end of the ganglion is united by a connecting trunk to the middle cervical ganglion. Postganglionic branches are distributed in the internal carotid nerve, which ascends with the internal carotid artery into the carotid canal to enter the cranial cavity, and in lateral, medial and anterior branches. They supply vasoconstrictor and sudomotor nerves to the face and neck, dilator pupillae and smooth muscle in the eyelids and orbitalis.

Lateral branches – The lateral branches are grey rami communicantes to the upper four cervical spinal nerves and to some of the cranial nerves. Branches pass to the inferior vagal ganglion, the hypoglossal nerve, the superior jugular bulb and associated jugular glomus or glomera, and to the meninges in the posterior cranial fossa. Another branch, the jugular nerve, ascends to the cranial base and divides into two; one part joins the inferior glossopharyngeal ganglion and the other joins the superior vagal ganglion.

Medial branches – The medial branches of the superior cervical ganglion are the laryngopharyngeal and cardiac. The laryngopharyngeal branches supply the carotid body and pass to the side of the pharynx, joining glossopharyngeal and vagal rami to form the pharyngeal plexus. A cardiac branch arises by two or more filaments from the lower part of the superior cervical ganglion and occasionally receives a twig from the trunk between the superior and middle cervical ganglia. It is thought to contain only efferent fibres, the preganglionic outflow being from the upper thoracic segments of the spinal cord, and to be devoid of pain fibres from the heart. It descends behind the common carotid artery, in front of longus colli, and crosses anterior to the inferior thyroid artery and recurrent laryngeal nerve. The courses on the two sides then differ. The right cardiac branch usually passes behind, but sometimes in front

of, the subclavian artery and runs posterolateral to the brachiocephalic trunk to join the deep (dorsal) part of the cardiac plexus behind the aortic arch. It has other sympathetic connections. About midneck it receives filaments from the external laryngeal nerve. Inferiorly, one or two vagal cardiac branches join it. As it enters the thorax it is joined by a filament from the recurrent laryngeal nerve. Filaments from the nerve also communicate with the thyroid branches of the middle cervical ganglion. The left cardiac branch, in the thorax, is anterior to the left common carotid artery and crosses in front of the left side of the aortic arch to reach the superficial (ventral) part of the cardiac plexus. Sometimes it descends on the right of the aorta to end in the deep (dorsal) part of the cardiac plexus. It communicates with the cardiac branches of the middle and inferior cervical sympathetic ganglia and sometimes with the inferior cervical cardiac branches of the left vagus, and branches from these mixed nerves form a plexus on the ascending aorta.

Anterior branches – The anterior branches of the superior cervical ganglion ramify on the common and external carotid arteries and the branches of the external carotid, and form a delicate plexus around each in which small ganglia are occasionally found. The plexus around the facial artery supplies a filament to the submandibular ganglion; the plexus on the middle meningeal artery sends one ramus to the otic ganglion and another, the external petrosal nerve, to the facial ganglion. Many of the fibres coursing along the external carotid and its branches ultimately leave them to travel to facial sweat glands via branches of the trigeminal nerve.

MIDDLE CERVICAL GANGLION (Figs 31.24, 31.25)

The middle cervical ganglion is the smallest of the three, and is occasionally absent, in which case it may be replaced by minute ganglia in the sympathetic trunk or may be fused with the superior ganglion. It is usually found at the level of the sixth cervical vertebra, anterior or just superior to the inferior thyroid artery, or it may adjoin the inferior cervical ganglion. It probably represents a coalescence of the ganglia of the fifth and sixth cervical segments, judging by its postganglionic rami, which join the fifth and sixth cervical spinal nerves (but sometimes also the fourth and seventh). It is connected to the inferior cervical ganglion by two or more very variable cords. The posterior cord usually splits to enclose the vertebral artery, while the anterior cord loops down anterior to, and then below, the first part of the subclavian artery, medial to the origin of its internal thoracic branch, and supplies rami to it. This loop is the ansa subclavia and is frequently multiple, lies closely in contact with the cervical pleura and typically connects with the phrenic nerve, and sometimes with the vagus.

The middle cervical ganglion gives off thyroid and cardiac branches. The thyroid branches accompany the inferior thyroid artery to the

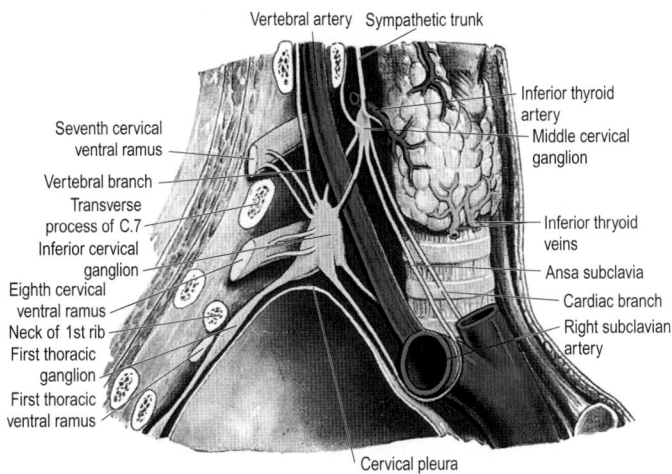

Fig. 31.24 The middle and inferior cervical ganglia of the right side, viewed from the right. Note the proximity of the inferior cervical and first thoracic ganglia, which often fuse to form a cervicothoracic (stellate) ganglion.

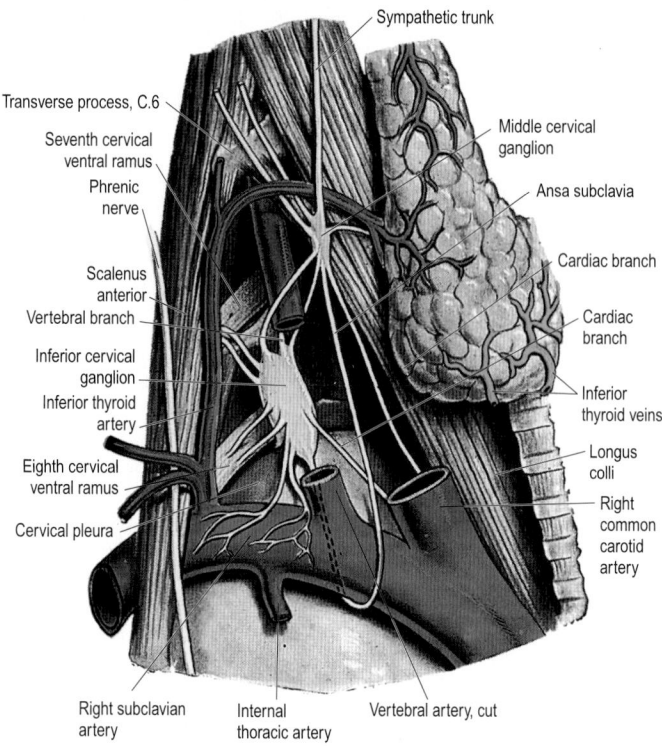

Sympathetic trunk

Transverse process, C.6

Seventh cervical
ventral ramus

Phrenic
nerve

Scalenus
anterior

Vertebral branch

Inferior cervical
ganglion

Inferior thyroid
artery

Eighth cervical
ventral ramus

Cervical pleura

Middle cervical
ganglion

Ansa subclavia

Cardiac branch

Cardiac
branch

Inferior
thyroid veins

Longus
colli

Right
common
carotid
artery

Right subclavian
artery

Internal
thoracic artery

Vertebral artery, cut

Fig. 31.25 The middle and inferior cervical ganglia of the right side, anterior view. Part of the vertebral artery has been excised to show the inferior cervical ganglion.

thyroid gland. They communicate with the superior cardiac, external laryngeal and recurrent laryngeal nerves, and send branches to the parathyroid glands. Fibres to both glands are largely vasomotor but some reach the secretory cells. The cardiac branch, the largest sympathetic cardiac nerve, either arises from the ganglion itself or more often from the sympathetic trunk cranial or caudal to it. On the right side it descends behind the common carotid artery, in front of or behind the subclavian artery, to the trachea where it receives a few filaments from the recurrent laryngeal nerve before joining the right half of the deep (dorsal) part of the cardiac plexus. In the neck, it connects with the superior cardiac and recurrent laryngeal nerves. On the left side the cardiac nerve enters the thorax between the left common carotid and subclavian arteries to join the left half of the deep (dorsal) part of the cardiac plexus. Fine branches from the middle cervical ganglion also pass to the trachea and oesophagus.

INFERIOR (OR CERVICOTHORACIC/STELLATE) GANGLION
(Figs 31.24, 31.25)

The inferior cervical ganglion (cervicothoracic/stellate) is irregular in shape and much larger than the middle cervical ganglion. It is probably formed by a fusion of the lower two cervical and first thoracic segmental ganglia, sometimes including the second and even third and fourth thoracic ganglia. The first thoracic ganglion may be separate, leaving an inferior cervical ganglion above it. The sympathetic trunk turns backwards at the junction of the neck and thorax and so the long axis of the cervicothoracic ganglion becomes almost anteroposterior. The ganglion lies on or just lateral to the lateral border of longus colli between the base of the seventh cervical transverse process and the neck of the first rib (which are both posterior to it). The vertebral vessels are anterior, and the ganglion is separated from the posterior aspect of the cervical pleura inferiorly by the suprapleural membrane. The costocervical trunk of the subclavian artery branches near the lower pole of the ganglion, and the superior intercostal artery is lateral.

A small vertebral ganglion may be present on the sympathetic trunk anterior or anteromedial to the origin of the vertebral artery and directly above the subclavian artery. When present, it may provide the ansa subclavia and is also joined to the inferior cervical ganglion by fibres enclosing the vertebral artery. It is usually regarded as a detached part

of the middle cervical or inferior cervical ganglion. Like the middle cervical ganglion it may supply grey rami communicantes to the fourth and fifth cervical spinal nerves. The inferior cervical ganglion sends grey rami communicantes to the seventh and eighth cervical and first thoracic spinal nerves, and gives off a cardiac branch, branches to nearby vessels and sometimes a branch to the vagus nerve.

The grey rami communicantes to the seventh cervical spinal nerve vary from one to five (two being the usual number). A third often ascends medial to the vertebral artery in front of the seventh cervical transverse process. It connects with the seventh cervical nerve, and sends a filament upwards through the sixth cervical transverse foramen in company with the vertebral vessels to join the sixth cervical spinal nerve as it emerges from the intervertebral foramen. An inconstant ramus may traverse the seventh cervical transverse foramen. Grey rami to the eighth cervical spinal nerve vary from three to six in number.

The cardiac branch descends behind the subclavian artery and along the front of the trachea to the deep cardiac plexus. Behind the artery it connects with the recurrent laryngeal nerve and the cardiac branch of the middle cervical ganglion (the latter is often replaced by fine branches of the inferior cervical ganglion and ansa subclavia).

The branches to blood vessels form plexuses on the subclavian artery and its branches. The subclavian supply is derived from the inferior cervical ganglion and ansa subclavia, and typically extends to the first part of the axillary artery, although a few fibres may extend further. An extension of the subclavian plexus to the internal thoracic artery may be joined by a branch of the phrenic nerve. The vertebral plexus is derived mainly from a large branch of the inferior cervical ganglion that ascends behind the vertebral artery to the sixth transverse foramen. Here it is reinforced by branches of the vertebral ganglion or the cervical sympathetic trunk that pass cranially on the ventral aspect of the artery. Deep rami communicantes from this plexus join the ventral rami of the upper five or six cervical spinal nerves. The plexus, which contains some neuronal cell bodies, continues into the skull along the vertebral and basilar arteries and their branches as far as the posterior cerebral artery, where it meets a plexus from the internal carotid artery. The plexus on the inferior thyroid artery reaches the thyroid gland, and connects with the recurrent and external laryngeal nerves, the cardiac branch of the superior cervical ganglion, and the common carotid plexus.

HORNER'S SYNDROME (Fig. 31.26)
Any condition or injury that destroys the sympathetic trunk ascending from the thorax through the neck into the face results in Horner's syndrome, characterized by a drooping eyelid (ptosis), sunken globe (enophthalmos), narrow palpebral fissure, contracted pupil (meiosis), vasodilatation and lack of thermal sweating (anhydrosis) on the affected side. This occurs classically when a bronchial carcinoma invades the sympathetic trunk. It also occurs as a complication of cervical sympathectomy or a radical neck dissection.

VISCERA

The main viscera to be found in the neck are the submandibular salivary glands, the thyroid and parathyroid glands and the upper components of the respiratory and alimentary systems.

Submandibular salivary gland

Each submandibular salivary gland is situated behind and below the ramus of the mandible, in the region of the submandibular triangle, between the anterior and posterior bellies of digastric. The gland is described in detail on page 602.

Thyroid gland (Fig. 31.27)

The thyroid gland, brownish-red and highly vascular, is placed anteriorly in the lower neck, level with the fifth cervical to the first thoracic vertebrae. It is ensheathed by the pretracheal layer of deep cervical fascia and consists of right and left lobes connected by a narrow, median isthmus. Its weight is usually c.25 g, but this varies. The gland is slightly heavier in females, and enlarges during menstruation and pregnancy. Estimation of the size of the thyroid gland is clinically important in the

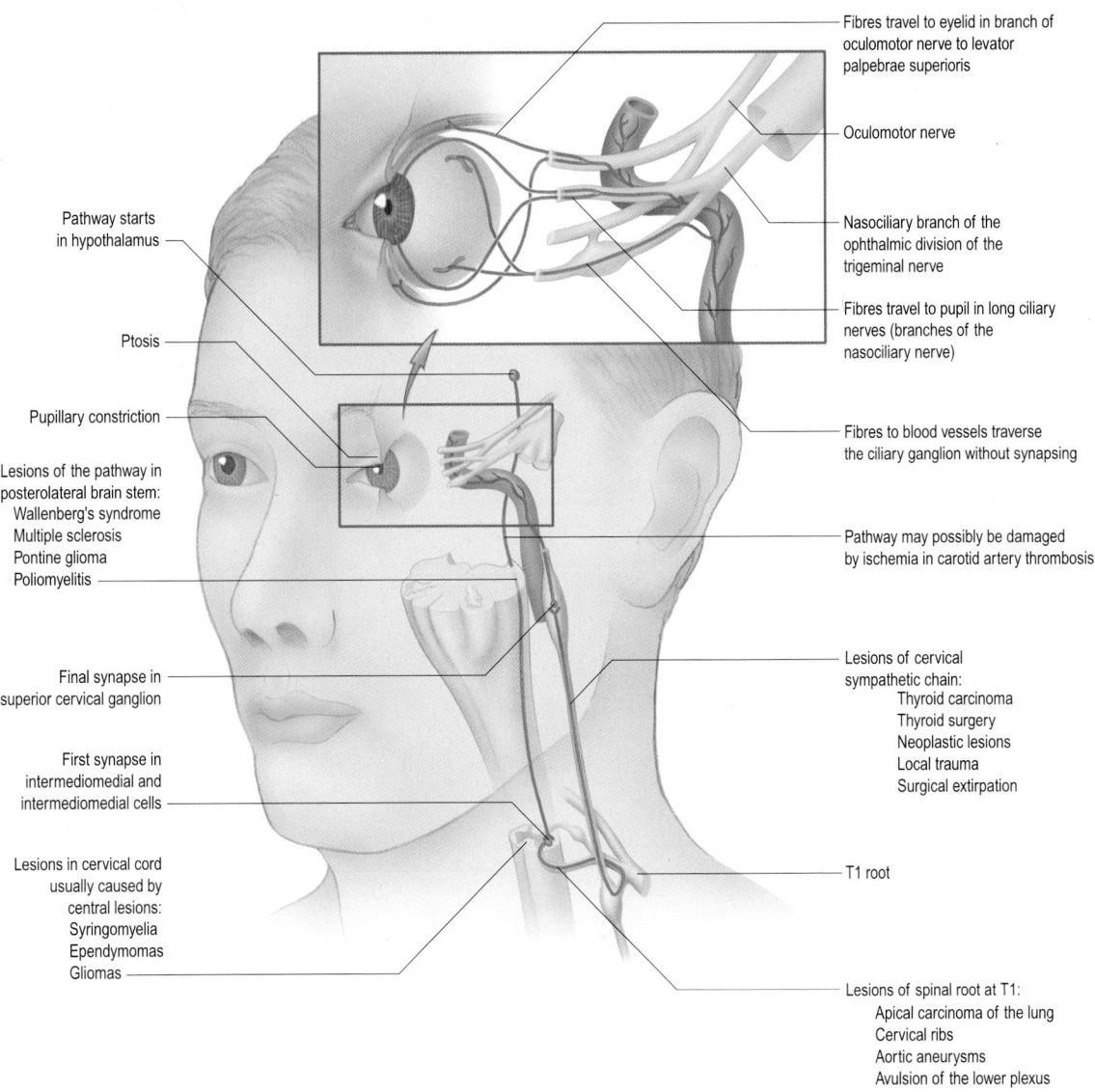

Fibres travel to eyelid in branch of
oculomotor nerve to levator
palpebrae superioris

Oculomotor nerve

Nasociliary branch of the
ophthalmic division of the
trigeminal nerve

Fibres travel to pupil in long ciliary
nerves (branches of the
nasociliary nerve)

Fibres to blood vessels traverse
the ciliary ganglion without synapsing

Pathway may possibly be damaged
by ischemia in carotid artery thrombosis

Lesions of cervical
sympathetic chain:
Thyroid carcinoma
Thyroid surgery
Neoplastic lesions
Local trauma
Surgical extirpation

T1 root

Lesions of spinal root at T1:
Apical carcinoma of the lung
Cervical ribs
Aortic aneurysms
Avulsion of the lower plexus

Pathway starts
in hypothalamus

Ptosis

Pupillary constriction

Lesions of the pathway in
posterolateral brain stem:
Wallenberg's syndrome
Multiple sclerosis
Pontine glioma
Poliomyelitis

Final synapse in
superior cervical ganglion

First synapse in
intermediomedial and
intermediomedial cells

Lesions in cervical cord
usually caused by
central lesions:
Syringomyelia
Ependymomas
Gliomas

Fig. 31.26 Horner's syndrome.

evaluation and management of thyroid disorders and can be achieved non-invasively by means of diagnostic ultrasound. No significant difference in thyroid gland volume has been observed between males and females from 8 months to 15 years.

The lobes of the thyroid gland are approximately conical. Their ascending apices diverge laterally to the level of the oblique lines on the laminae of the thyroid cartilage, and their bases are level with the fourth or fifth tracheal cartilages. Each lobe is c.5 cm long, its greatest transverse and anteroposterior extents being c.3 cm and 2 cm respectively. The posteromedial aspects of the lobes are attached to the side of the cricoid cartilage by a lateral thyroid ligament.

The isthmus connects the lower parts of the two lobes, although occasionally it may be absent. It measures c.1.25 cm transversely and vertically, and is usually anterior to the second and third tracheal cartilages, though often higher or sometimes lower because its site and size vary greatly.

A conical pyramidal lobe often ascends towards the hyoid bone from the isthmus or the adjacent part of either lobe (more often the left). It is occasionally detached or in two or more parts. A fibrous or fibromuscular band, the levator of the thyroid gland, musculus levator glandulae thyroideae, sometimes descends from the body of the hyoid to the isthmus or pyramidal lobe. Small detached masses of thyroid tissue may occur above the lobes or isthmus as accessory thyroid glands. Vestiges of the thyroglossal duct may persist between the isthmus and the foramen caecum of the tongue, sometimes as accessory nodules or cysts of thyroid tissue near the midline or even in the tongue.

SURFACES AND RELATIONS (Fig. 31.15)

The convex lateral (superficial) surface is covered by sternothyroid, whose attachment to the oblique thyroid line prevents the upper pole of the gland from extending on to thyrohyoid. More anteriorly lie sternohyoid and the superior belly of omohyoid, overlapped inferiorly by the anterior border of sternocleidomastoid. The medial surface of the gland is adapted to the larynx and trachea, contacting at its superior pole the inferior pharyngeal constrictor and the posterior part of cricothyroid, which separate it from the posterior part of the thyroid lamina and the side of the cricoid cartilage. The external laryngeal nerve is medial to this part of the gland as it passes to supply cricothyroid. Inferiorly, the trachea and, more posteriorly, the recurrent laryngeal nerve and oesophagus (which is closer on the left) are medial relations. The posterolateral surface of the thyroid gland is close to the carotid sheath, and overlaps the common carotid artery. The thin anterior border of the gland, near the anterior branch of the superior thyroid artery, slants down medially. The rounded posterior border is related below to the inferior thyroid artery and its anastomosis with the posterior branch of the superior thyroid artery. The parathyroid glands are usually related to this border. The lower end of the posterior border on the left side lies near the thoracic duct. The isthmus is covered by sternothyroid, from which it is separated by pretracheal fascia. More superficially it is covered by sternohyoid, the anterior jugular veins, fascia and skin. The superior thyroid arteries anastomose along its upper border and the inferior thyroid veins leave the gland at its lower border.

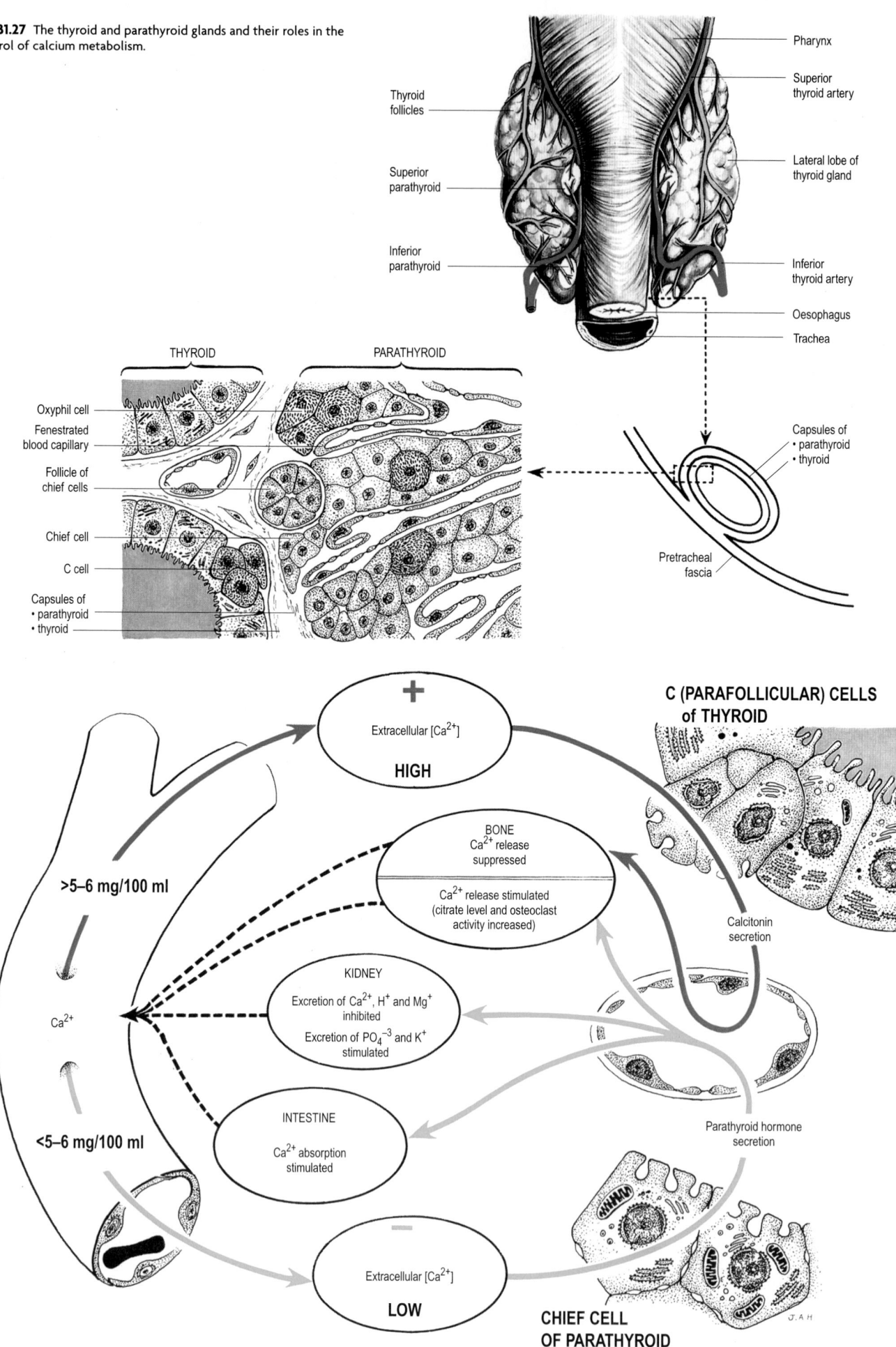

Fig. 31.27 The thyroid and parathyroid glands and their roles in the control of calcium metabolism.

Pharynx

Superior thyroid artery

Lateral lobe of thyroid gland

Inferior thyroid artery

Oesophagus

Trachea

Thyroid follicles

Superior parathyroid

Inferior parathyroid

Capsules of
• parathyroid
• thyroid

Pretracheal fascia

THYROID

PARATHYROID

Oxyphil cell

Fenestrated blood capillary

Follicle of chief cells

Chief cell

C cell

Capsules of
• parathyroid
• thyroid

+

Extracellular [Ca^{2+}]

HIGH

C (PARAFOLLICULAR) CELLS of THYROID

BONE
Ca^{2+} release suppressed

Ca^{2+} release stimulated (citrate level and osteoclast activity increased)

>5–6 mg/100 ml

Calcitonin secretion

KIDNEY

Excretion of Ca^{2+}, H^{+} and Mg^{+} inhibited

Excretion of PO$_4^{-3}$ and K^{+} stimulated

Ca^{2+}

INTESTINE

Ca^{2+} absorption stimulated

Parathyroid hormone secretion

<5–6 mg/100 ml

–

Extracellular [Ca^{2+}]

LOW

CHIEF CELL OF PARATHYROID

J. A H

VASCULAR SUPPLY AND LYMPHATIC DRAINAGE
(Figs 31.15, 31.25, 31.27)

The thyroid gland is supplied by the superior and inferior thyroid arteries and sometimes by an arteria thyroidea ima from the brachiocephalic trunk or aortic arch. The arteries are large and their branches anastomose frequently on and in the gland, both ipsilaterally and contralaterally. The superior thyroid artery pierces the thyroid fascia and then divides into anterior and posterior branches. The anterior branch supplies the anterior surface of the gland, the posterior branch supplies the lateral and medial surfaces. The superior thyroid artery is closely related to the external laryngeal nerve. The inferior thyroid artery approaches the base of the thyroid gland and divides into superior (ascending) and inferior thyroid branches which supply the inferior and posterior surfaces of the gland. The superior branch also supplies the parathyroid glands. The relationship between the inferior thyroid artery and the recurrent laryngeal nerve has clinical importance.

The venous drainage of the thyroid gland is usually via superior, middle, and inferior thyroid veins. The superior thyroid vein emerges from the upper part of the gland and runs with the superior thyroid artery towards the carotid sheath. It drains into the internal jugular vein. The middle thyroid vein collects blood from the lower part of the gland. It emerges from the lateral surface of the gland and drains into the internal jugular vein. The inferior thyroid vein forms a plexus with the vein on the opposite side. This plexus is located below the thyroid gland and in front of the trachea. From the plexus, the left vein descends into the thorax to terminate at the left brachiocephalic vein. The right inferior thyroid vein drains into the right brachiocephalic vein. Alternatively, there may be a common trunk draining into the left brachiocephalic vein.

Thyroid lymphatic vessels communicate with the tracheal plexus, and pass to the prelaryngeal nodes just above the thyroid isthmus and to the pretracheal and paratracheal nodes; some may also drain into the brachiocephalic nodes related to the thymus in the superior mediastinum. Laterally the gland is drained by vessels lying along the superior thyroid veins to the deep cervical nodes. Thyroid lymphatics may drain directly, with no intervening node, to the thoracic duct.

INNERVATION

The thyroid gland receives its innervation from the superior, middle and inferior cervical sympathetic ganglia.

IMAGING

The follicular nature of the thyroid gland is not resolved by current imaging techniques and thus presents a homogeneous texture on cross-sectional imaging (US, CT, MRI). Its superficial location makes the thyroid an ideal organ for sonographic examination (**Fig. 31.28**). The thyroid gland is highly vascular and demonstrates intense contrast enhancement and increased signal on T_2-weighted MRI (**Fig. 31.29**). Radionuclide imaging of the thyroid may be performed with technetium (Tc^{99m}) pertechnetate. This readily available radionuclide is trapped by the thyroid in the same way as iodine, but is not organified. It yields morphological information and will reveal the presence of ectopic thyroid tissue. Functional data can be obtained with the use of ^{131}iodine which is trapped and organified.

MICROSTRUCTURE

The thyroid gland has a thin capsule of connective tissue, which extends into the glandular parenchyma and divides each lobe into irregularly shaped and sized lobules. The functional units of the thyroid are follicles, which are spherical and cyst-like, between 0.02 and 0.9 mm in diameter, and consist of a central colloid core surrounded by a single-layered epithelium resting on a basal lamina (**Fig. 31.30**). Colloid consists almost entirely of an iodinated glycoprotein, iodothyroglobulin. This is the inactive, stored form of the active thyroid hormones, tri-iodothyronine (T_3) and tetraiodothyronine or thyroxine (T_4), and is produced by the follicular epithelial cells. Sufficient iodothyroglobulin is stored extracellularly within follicles to regulate the metabolic activity of the body for up to three months. Follicles are surrounded by a delicate connective tissue stroma, containing dense plexuses of fenestrated capillaries, extensive lymphatic networks and sympathetic nerve fibres which supply the arterioles and capillaries. Some nerve fibres end close to the follicular epithelial cells.

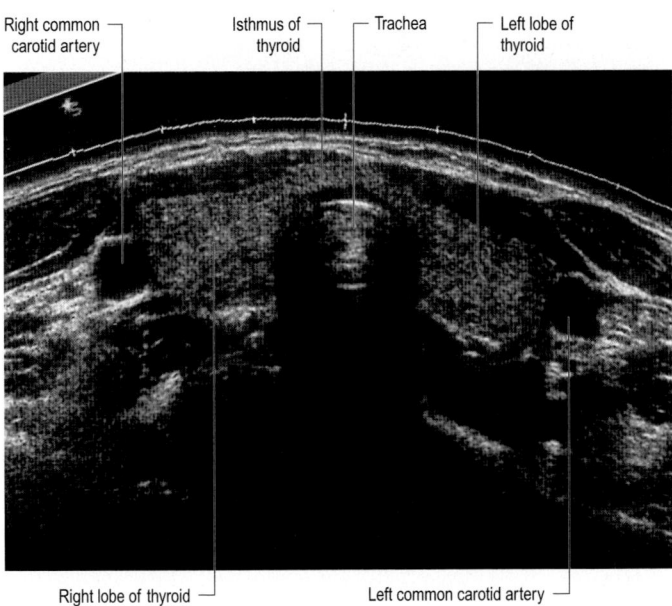

Fig. 31.28 Thyroid sonogram.

Labels: Right common carotid artery — Isthmus of thyroid — Trachea — Left lobe of thyroid — Right lobe of thyroid — Left common carotid artery

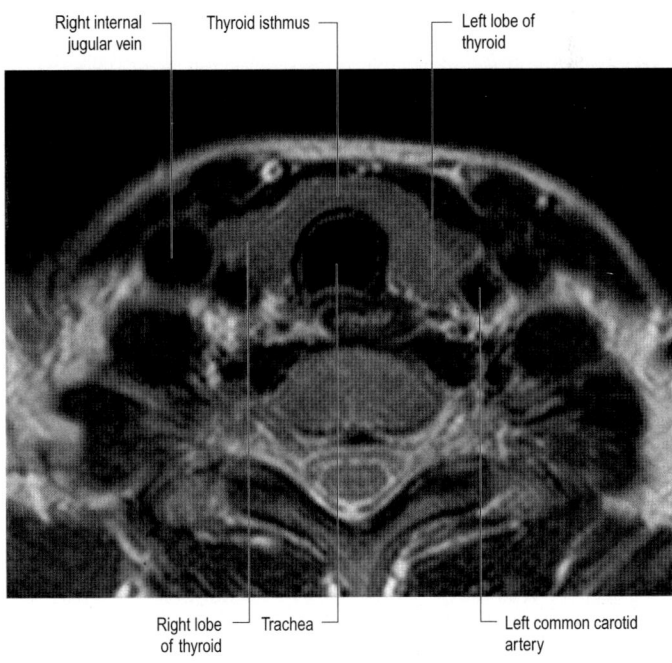

Fig. 31.29 T_2-weighted MRI demonstrating high vascularity of the thyroid gland.

Labels: Right internal jugular vein — Thyroid isthmus — Left lobe of thyroid — Right lobe of thyroid — Trachea — Left common carotid artery

Follicular cells – Follicular cells vary from squamous or low cuboidal to columnar, depending on their level of activity, which is controlled mainly by circulating hypophyseal thyroid-stimulating hormone (TSH, thyrotropin). Resting follicles are large, lined by squamous or low cuboidal epithelium with abundant luminal colloid. Active follicular cells are highly polarized functionally. Synthesis and exocytosis of thyroglobulin occurs at the apices of the cells, and thyroglobulin endocytosis (from stored colloid), lysosomal degradation and liberation of thyroid hormones (T_3 and T_4) occur basally. Follicles showing differing levels of activity may co-exist. The secretion of TSH leads to endocytosis of colloidal droplets at the luminal epithelium (**Fig. 31.30**). Prolonged high levels of circulating TSH induce follicular cell hypertrophy, with progressive resorption of colloid and increased stromal vascularity. Apical microvilli are short in resting cells but elongate and often branch on stimulation by TSH, which also provokes extension of cytoplasmic processes into the luminal colloid. The

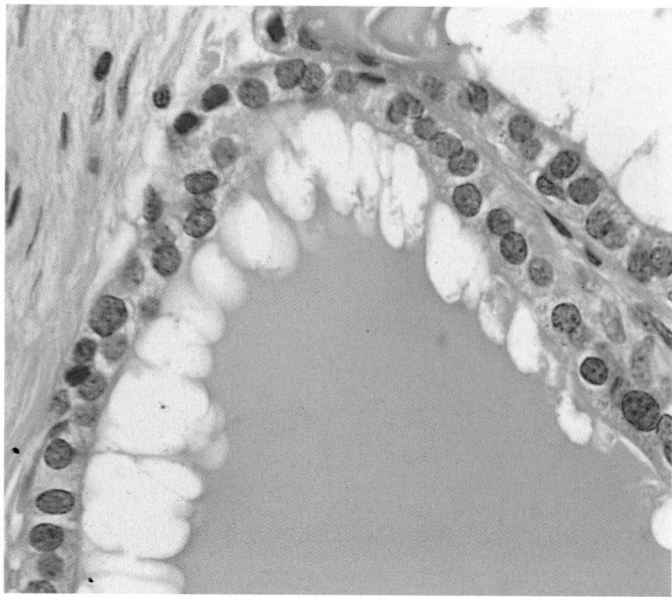

Fig. 31.30 A section through parts of two adjacent thyroid follicles, showing the follicular epithelium enclosing a colloid-filled lumen. Pale cavities in the otherwise homogeneous, eosinophilic colloid are sites of thyroglobulin resorption. Calcitonin-secreting C cells are present but not readily identifiable in routine preparations. A capillary network surrounds the follicles within connective tissue septa. (By permission from Stevens A, Lowe JS 1996 Human Histology, 2nd edn. London: Mosby.)

processes fuse around portions of the colloid and take it into the cell. After colloid endocytosis, lysosomes migrate towards the lumen to fuse with the intracellular droplets of colloid, forming secondary lysosomes. During this period the cytoplasmic colloid gradually disappears as lysosomal acid proteases degrade the iodinated thyroglobulin, releasing the thyroid hormones T_3 and T_4, which pass basally for release, leaving the gland mainly via the blood capillaries and lymphatics.

C cells – Thyroid parenchyma also contains C (clear) cells, so-called from their pale-staining cytoplasm, which is more pronounced in some species than in the human thyroid. They belong to the amine precursor uptake and decarboxylation (APUD) system of dispersed neuroendocrine cells (p. 180), and produce the peptide hormone calcitonin (thyrocalcitonin) which lowers blood calcium by inhibiting bone resorption and calcium recovery from renal tubule ultrafiltrate. C cells populate the middle third of each lateral lobe of the thyroid and are typically found scattered within thyroid follicles, inside the basal lamina but not reaching the follicle lumen: they are occasionally seen in clusters in the interfollicular stroma (which is why they are also called parafollicular cells).

THYROIDECTOMY

Apart from variable enlargement during menstruation and pregnancy, any thyroid swelling is a goitre, which may press on related structures. Symptoms are most commonly due to pressure on the trachea or on the recurrent laryngeal nerves, and there may also be venous engorgement. If thyroidectomy is undertaken, care must be taken when tying off the superior and inferior thyroid arteries to avoid damage to adjacent nerves. The external laryngeal nerve runs close to the superior thyroid artery and the recurrent laryngeal nerve runs close to the inferior thyroid artery. Partial thyroidectomy is often necessary in hyperthyroidism and thyroid enlargement: the posterior parts of both lobes are left intact to preserve the parathyroid glands.

Parathyroid glands (Fig. 31.27)

The parathyroid glands are small, yellowish-brown, ovoid or lentiform structures, usually lying between the posterior lobar borders of the thyroid gland and its capsule. They are commonly c.6 mm long, 3–4 mm across, and 1–2 mm from back to front, each weighing about 50 mg. Usually there are two on each side, superior and inferior. However,

there may be only three or many minute parathyroid islands scattered in connective tissue near the usual sites. Normally the inferior parathyroids migrate only to the inferior thyroid poles, but they may descend with the thymus into the thorax or not descend at all, remaining above their normal level near the carotid bifurcation. To help identification, the anastomotic connection between the superior and inferior thyroid arteries along the posterior border of the thyroid gland usually passes very close to the parathyroids.

The superior parathyroid glands are more constant in location than the inferior and are usually to be found midway along the posterior borders of the thyroid gland, although they may be higher. The inferior pair are more variably situated (related to their embryological development – see p. 617) and may be within the fascial thyroid sheath, below the inferior thyroid arteries and near the inferior lobar poles; or outside the sheath, immediately above an inferior thyroid artery; or in the thyroid gland near its inferior pole. These variations are surgically important. A tumour of the inferior parathyroid situated within the fascial thyroid sheath may descend along the inferior thyroid veins anterior to the trachea into the superior mediastinum, whereas if it is outside the sheath it may extend posteroinferiorly behind the oesophagus into the posterior mediastinum. The superior parathyroids are usually dorsal, the inferior parathyroids ventral, to the recurrent laryngeal nerves.

The parathyroid glands are very flattened in cross-section and are not normally visible by current imaging methods, including scintigraphy.

VASCULAR SUPPLY AND LYMPHATIC DRAINAGE

The parathyroid glands have a rich blood supply from the inferior thyroid arteries or from anastomoses between the superior and inferior vessels. Approximately one-third of human parathyroid glands have two or more parathyroid arteries. Lymph vessels are numerous and associated with those of the thyroid and thymus glands.

INNERVATION

The nerve supply is sympathetic, either direct from the superior or middle cervical ganglia or via a plexus in the fascia on the posterior lobar aspects. Parathyroid activity is controlled by variations in blood calcium level: it is inhibited by a rise and stimulated by a fall. The nerves are believed to be vasomotor but not secretomotor.

Microstructure (Figs 31.27, 31.31)

Each parathyroid gland has a thin connective tissue capsule with intraglandular septa but lacks distinct lobules. The parathyroids synthesize

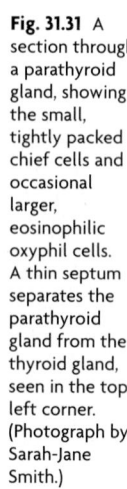

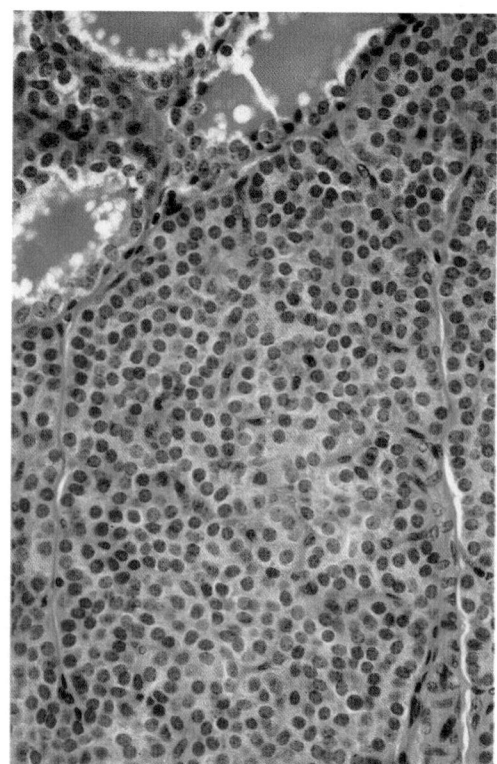

Fig. 31.31 A section through a parathyroid gland, showing the small, tightly packed chief cells and occasional larger, eosinophilic oxyphil cells. A thin septum separates the parathyroid gland from the thyroid gland, seen in the top left corner. (Photograph by Sarah-Jane Smith.)

and secrete parathyroid hormone (PTH, parathormone), a single-chain polypeptide of 84 amino-acid residues concerned with the control of the level and distribution of calcium and phosphorus. In childhood, the gland consists of wide, irregular, interconnecting columns of chief or principal cells separated by a dense plexus of fenestrated sinusoidal capillaries. After puberty, adipose tissue accumulates in the stroma and typically accounts for about one third of the adult tissue mass, increasing further with age.

Chief cells differ ultrastructurally according to their level of activity: active chief cells have large Golgi complexes with numerous vesicles and small membrane-bound granules. Glycogen granules are most abundant in inactive cells, which have few of the cytoplasmic features of synthetic or secretory activity, and appear histologically as 'clear' cells. In normal human parathyroid glands, inactive chief cells outnumber active cells in a ratio of 3–5:1. In contrast to the thyroid, where the activities of adjacent follicular cells are coordinated, individual chief cells of the parathyroid glands go through cycles of secretory activity and rest independently, according to serum calcium levels.

A second cell type, the oxyphil (eosinophil) cell, appears just before puberty and increases in number with age. Oxyphil cells are larger than chief cells and contain more cytoplasm, which stains deeply with eosin. Their nuclei are smaller and more darkly staining than those of chief cells, and their cytoplasm is unusually rich in mitochondria. The functional significance of oxyphil cells and their relationship to chief cells are uncertain.

Oesophagus – cervical portion (Fig. 31.13)

The oesophagus is a muscular tube c.25 cm long, connecting the pharynx to the stomach. It begins in the neck, level with the lower border of the cricoid cartilage and the sixth cervical vertebra. It descends largely anterior to the vertebral column into the superior mediastinum in the thorax. Generally vertical and median, it inclines to the left as far as the root of the neck, and also bends in an anteroposterior plane to follow the cervical curvature of the vertebral column.

Relations – The trachea lies anterior to the oesophagus, attached to it by loose connective tissue. The vertebral column, longus colli and prevertebral layer of deep cervical fascia are posterior, and the common carotid artery and posterior part of the thyroid gland are lateral on each side. In the lower neck, where the oesophagus deviates to the left, it becomes closer to the left carotid sheath and thyroid gland than it is on the right. The thoracic duct ascends for a short distance along its left side. The recurrent laryngeal nerves ascend on each side in or near the groove between the trachea and the oesophagus.

Vascular supply and lymphatic drainage – The cervical part of the oesophagus is mainly supplied by branches from the inferior thyroid arteries. The oesophageal veins drain into the brachiocephalic veins,

and lymphatic vessels pass to retropharyngeal, paratracheal, or deep cervical lymph nodes.

Innervation – The cervical part of the oesophagus is innervated by the recurrent laryngeal nerves and by the sympathetic plexus around the inferior thyroid artery.

Trachea – cervical portion (Fig. 31.15)

The trachea is a tube c.10–11 cm long, formed of cartilage and fibromuscular membrane. It descends from the larynx, and extends from the level of the sixth cervical vertebra to the upper border of the fifth thoracic vertebra. It lies approximately in the sagittal plane but its point of bifurcation is usually a little to the right. The trachea is flexible and can rapidly alter in length. It is flattened posteriorly so that in transverse section it is shaped, with some individual variation, like a letter D. Its external transverse diameter is c.2 cm in adult males, and 1.5 cm in adult females. The lumen in live adults is c.1.2 cm in transverse diameter. In children the trachea is smaller, more deeply placed and more mobile. Tracheal diameter does not exceed 3 mm in the first postnatal year: during later childhood its diameter in millimetres is about equal to age in years.

Relations – The relationships of the trachea to other cervical structures is of clinical significance: tracheostomy is not an uncommon clinical procedure. Anteriorly the cervical part of the trachea is crossed by skin and by the superficial and deep fasciae. It is also crossed by the jugular arch and overlapped by sternohyoid and sternothyroid. The second to fourth tracheal cartilages are crossed by the isthmus of the thyroid gland, above which an anastomotic artery connects the bilateral superior thyroid arteries. Below and in front are the pretracheal fascia, inferior thyroid veins, thymic remnants and the arteria thyroidea ima (when it exists). In children the brachiocephalic artery crosses obliquely in front of the trachea at or a little above the upper border of the manubrium. The left brachiocephalic vein may also rise a little above this level. The oesophagus lies posterior to the trachea, and separates it from the vertebral column. The paired lobes of the thyroid gland, which descend to the fifth or sixth tracheal cartilage, and the common carotid and inferior thyroid arteries, all lie lateral to the trachea. The recurrent laryngeal nerves ascend on each side, in or near the grooves between the sides of the trachea and oesophagus.

Vascular supply and lymphatic drainage – The cervical part of the trachea is mainly supplied by branches from the inferior thyroid arteries. The tracheal veins drain into the bracheocephalic veins via the inferior thyroid plexus, and lymphatic vessels drain into the pretracheal and paratracheal nodes.

Innervation – The trachea is innervated by branches from the vagi, recurrent laryngeal nerves and sympathetic trunks.

REFERENCES

Berkovitz BKB, Kirsch C, Moxham BJ, Alusi G, Cheeseman T 2002 Interactive Head and Neck. London: Primal Pictures.

Cady B, Rossi RL (eds) 1991 Surgery of the Thyroid and Parathyroid Glands. Philadelphia: Saunders.

Crile G 1906 Excision of cancer of the head and neck with special reference to the plan of dissection based on one hundred and thirty two operations. J Am Med Assoc 47: 1780–6.
Seminal paper which considers the surgical anatomy of radical neck dissection.

Froes LB, De Tolosa EMC, Camargo RDC, Pompeu E, Liberti EA 1999 Blood supply to the human sternocleidomastoid muscle by the sternocleidomastoid branch of the occipital artery. Clin Anat 12: 412–6.

Ger R, Evans JT 1993 Tracheostomy: an anatomico-clinical review. Clin Anat 6: 337–41.

Kapandji IA 1975 The Physiology of Joints. Ediburgh: Churchill Livingstone.

Lingeman RE 1998 Surgical anatomy. In: Cummings CW et al (eds) Otolaryngology, Head and Neck Surgery, vol.2. 3rd edition. St Louis: Mosby: 1673–85.

Lucas GDA, Laudanna A, Chopard RP, Raffaelli E Jr 1994 Anatomy of the lesser occipital nerve in relation to cervicogenic headache. Clin Anat 7: 90–6.

Matthers LH Jr, Smith DW, Frankel L 1992 Anatomical considerations in placement of central venous catheters. Clin Anat 5: 89–106.

Robbins KT 1998 Neck dissection. In: Cummings CW et al (eds) Otolaryngology, Head and Neck Surgery, vol. 2. 3rd edition. St Louis: Mosby: 1787–1819.
Considers the relationships of anatomical structures of the neck with reference to radical neck dissection.

Shah JP, Patel SJ 2003 Cervical lymph nodes. In: Head and Neck Surgery and Oncology, 3rd edn. Edinburgh: Mosby: 353–94.

Wilson-Pauwels L, Akesson EJ, Stewart PA 1998 Cranial Nerves: Anatomy and Clinical Comments. Toronto: Decker.

Nose, nasal cavity, paranasal sinuses and pterygopalatine fossa

Chapter

32

The first part of the upper respiratory tract consists of paired nasal cavities divided from each other sagittally by the nasal septum and housed in a bony and cartilaginous framework that extends anteriorly as the external nose. The two halves of the nasal cavity open onto the face through the nares, and are continuous posteriorly with the nasopharynx through the posterior nasal apertures or choanae. The cavity is divisible into three regions, the nasal vestibule anteriorly, the chemosensory olfactory area posterosuperiorly and the respiratory region between them which constitutes the majority of the nasal cavity. The anterior nasal vestibule narrows posteriorly to form the nasal valve (the narrowest portion of the nasal airway). A series of air-filled expansions, the paranasal sinuses, lie within either the lateral walls of the nasal cavities, or in communication with them in adjacent bones. The nasal apparatus serves to warm, humidify, and to some extent filter, particles from the inhaled air, and the olfactory epithelium senses and discriminates between airborne chemicals and mediates the sense of olfaction.

SKIN OF THE EXTERNAL NOSE

The skin covering the nose is thin and loosely connected to the underlying structures. Over the apex and alae it is thicker and more adherent and bears numerous large sebaceous glands: their orifices are usually very distinct.

Vascular supply, lymphatic drainage and innervation of the external nose – The skin of the nose receives its blood supply from branches of the facial, ophthalmic and infraorbital arteries. The alae and lower part of the nasal septum are supplied by lateral nasal and septal branches of the facial artery The dorsal nasal branch of the ophthalmic artery and the infraorbital branch of the maxillary artery supply the lateral aspects and the dorsum of the nose. The venous networks draining the external nose do not run parallel to the arteries. Instead, they correspond to arteriovenous territories of the face: thus, the frontomedian region of

the face, including the nose, drains to the facial vein, and the orbitopalpebral area of the face, including the root of the nose, drains to the ophthalmic veins. The connections of the veins of the nose, upper lip and cheek with the drainage area of the ophthalmic veins are clinically significant. Lymph drainage is primarily to the submandibular group of nodes. Lymph draining from the root of the nose drains to superficial parotid nodes.

The nasal muscles are innervated mainly from the buccal branches of the facial nerve. The nasal skin is innervated by the infratrochlear and external nasal branches of the nasociliary nerve, and from the nasal branch of the infraorbital nerve.

SKELETON OF THE NOSE

BONY SKELETON OF THE EXTERNAL NOSE

The supporting framework is composed of bone and fibro- or elastic cartilages. The bony framework supporting the upper part of the nose consists of the nasal bones, the frontal processes of the maxillae and the nasal process of the frontal bones (**Figs 32.1, 32.2**). The cartilaginous framework consists of the median quadrilateral septal cartilage and the paired upper lateral and major and minor alar nasal cartilages (**Fig. 32.3**), which are connected to each other and to nearby bones by the continuity between the perichondrium and periosteum. The strut formed by the medial crura of the alar cartilages and the overlying skin which lies between the tip of the nose and the philtrum of the upper lip is termed the columella. It is connected to the nasal septum posteriorly by the membranous septum which lacks the central cartilaginous component seen more posteriorly.

Congenital nasal deformities can occur, for example a complete absence of the external nose, with only one aperture existing, or else suppression or malformation on one side e.g. atresia or failed perforation of the choanal plate (the embryonic barrier between the nasopharynx and the posterior nasal cavity).

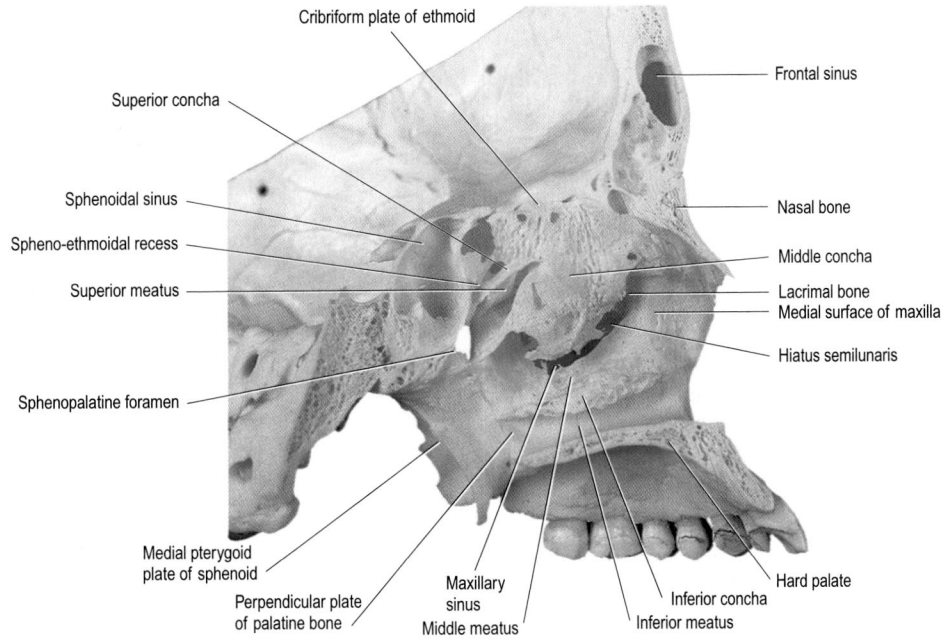

Fig. 32.1 Osteology of lateral wall of the nose. (By permission from Berkovitz BKB, Moxham BJ 1994 Color Atlas of the Skull. London: Mosby.)

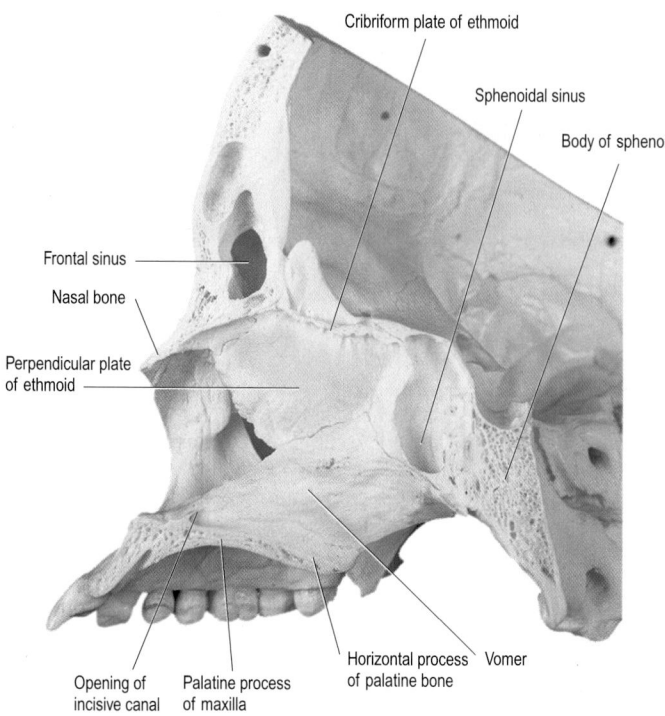

Fig. 32.2 Osteology of medial wall (septum) of the nose. (By permission from Berkovitz BKB, Moxham BJ 1994 Color Atlas of the Skull. London: Mosby.)

Nasal fractures

Trauma to the midface may cause fractures of the bony skeleton ranging from simple displaced fractures of the nasal bones to complex fractures of the midfacial skeleton. The upper dentition may be mobilized as a result of a fracture through the maxilla just above the tooth roots. The fracture line may also run through the ethmoidal air cells resulting in mobility of the whole midface below the orbits. The zygomatic bone may also be depressed by blunt trauma causing damage to the adjacent maxillary nerve and loss of contour of the cheek as the support of the zygomatic process and the lateral margin of the orbit is lost. Direct compressive injury to the contents of the orbit may result in a so called 'blow out' fracture in which the orbital contents prolapse through the disrupted inferior or medial walls of the orbits, often resulting in entrapment of the extra ocular muscles and restriction of eye movements.

CARTILAGINOUS SKELETON OF THE EXTERNAL NOSE (Fig. 32.3)

Septal cartilage

Almost quadrilateral in side view, the septal cartilage is sandwiched between two layers of mucoperichondrium and lies often eccentrically between the anterior parts of the nasal cavity. The anterosuperior margin is connected above to the posterior border of the internasal suture. The middle part is continuous with the upper lateral cartilages, and the lowest part is attached to these cartilages by perichondrial extensions. The anteroinferior border is connected on each side with the medial crurae of the major alar cartilage. The posterosuperior border joins the perpendicular plate of the ethmoid, while the posteroinferior border is attached to the vomer and to the nasal crest and anterior nasal spine of the maxilla. The septal cartilage may extend back (especially in children) as a narrow sphenoidal process for some distance between the vomer and the perpendicular plate of the ethmoid. The anteroinferior part of the nasal septum between the nares is devoid of cartilage and is called the membranous septum. It is continuous with the columnella anteriorly.

Lateral (superior) nasal cartilage

The lateral nasal cartilage is triangular, its anterior margin being thicker than the posterior. The upper part is continuous with the septal cartilage, but anteroinferiorly it may be separated from it by a narrow fissure. The superior margin of the lateral nasal cartilage is attached to the nasal bone and frontal process of the maxilla, while the inferior margin is connected by fibrous tissue to the lateral crus of the major alar cartilage.

Major alar cartilage

The major alar cartilage is a thin flexible plate lying below the upper lateral cartilage, and curved acutely around the anterior part of its naris. The medial part, the narrow medial crus (septal process), is loosely connected by fibrous tissue to its contralateral fellow and to the anteroinferior part of the septal cartilage, thus forming part of the septum mobile nasi. The lateral crus lies lateral to the naris and runs superolaterally away from the margin of the nasal ala. The upper border of the lateral crus of the major alar cartilage is attached by fibrous tissue to the lower border of the lateral nasal cartilage. Its lateral border is connected to the frontal process of the maxilla by a tough fibrous membrane containing three or four minor cartilages of the ala. The junction between the lateral crura of the major alar and the lateral cartilages is variable. The two edges may abut or overlap; the lateral crus is then the more lateral at the junction. The lateral crus of the major alar cartilage is shorter than the lateral margin of the naris and runs away from the margin of the ala nasi. The lateral part of the margin of the ala nasi is fibroadipose tissue covered by skin. In front, the angulations or 'domes' between the medial and lateral crurae of the major alar cartilages are separated by a notch palpable at the tip of the nose.

NASAL CAVITY

The nasal cavity is an irregular space between the roof of the mouth and the cranial base, divided by a vertical osseocartilaginous septum that is approximately median in position. The bony septum reaches the posterior limit of the cavity, which leads into the nasopharynx through a pair of posterior nasal apertures, or choanae, lying above the posterior hard palatal border (**Fig. 27.1**) The medial border of the choanae is formed by the posterior edge of the vomer, and its posteroinferior boundary by the horizontal plate of the palatine bone with the nasal crest of the palatine bone. Lateral to the ala of the vomer the choanae are bounded superiorly by the vaginal processes of the pterygoid processes above, and by the perpendicular plates of the palatine bones laterally. The size of each choana is not usually affected by deviations of the nasal septum.

The cavity is wider below than above, and widest and vertically deepest in its central region. It communicates with the frontal, ethmoidal, maxillary and sphenoidal paranasal sinuses. The posterior nasal apertures are oval openings separated by the posterior border of the vomer, each being limited below by the horizontal plate of the palatine bone, above by the sphenoid and laterally by the medial pterygoid plate. In the adult each is c.2.5 cm in vertical height and 1.3 cm transversely. The vomerovaginal and palatovaginal canals are found in the roof of this region.

Each half of the nasal cavity has a roof, floor, lateral and medial (septal) walls.

Roof

The roof (**Figs 32.1, 32.2**) is horizontal in its central part but slopes downwards in front and behind. The anterior slope is formed by the nasal spine of the frontal bones and by the nasal bones, which contribute to the external nose. The central horizontal region is formed by the cribriform plate of the ethmoid bone which separates the nasal cavity from the floor of the anterior cranial fossa. The cribriform plate contains a separate anterior foramen for the anterior ethmoidal nerve and vessels, and numerous small perforations which transmit the olfactory nerves. The posterior slope is formed by the anterior aspect of the body of the sphenoid – interrupted on each side by an opening of a sphenoidal sinus – and the sphenoidal conchae or superior conchae. The alae of the vomer and the sphenoidal processes of the palatine bones lie below.

Floor (Fig. 32.1)

The floor of the nasal cavity is smooth, concave transversely, and slopes up from anterior to posterior apertures. It constitutes the upper surface of the hard palate. Anteriorly, the palatine processes of the maxillae and, behind them, the horizontal plates of the palatine bones articulate in the midline and with each other. The nasal floor is therefore crossed at the junction of its middle and posterior thirds by the palatomaxillary suture. Anteriorly, near the septum, a small infundibular opening in the nasal floor leads into the incisive canals that descend to the incisive fossa: the opening is marked by a slight depression in the mucosa.

The floor of the nose may be deficient as a result of congenital clefting of the hard and/or soft palate.

Labels in figure:
Cribriform plate of ethmoid
Sphenoidal sinus
Body of sphenoid
Frontal sinus
Nasal bone
Perpendicular plate of ethmoid
Opening of incisive canal
Palatine process of maxilla
Horizontal process of palatine bone
Vomer

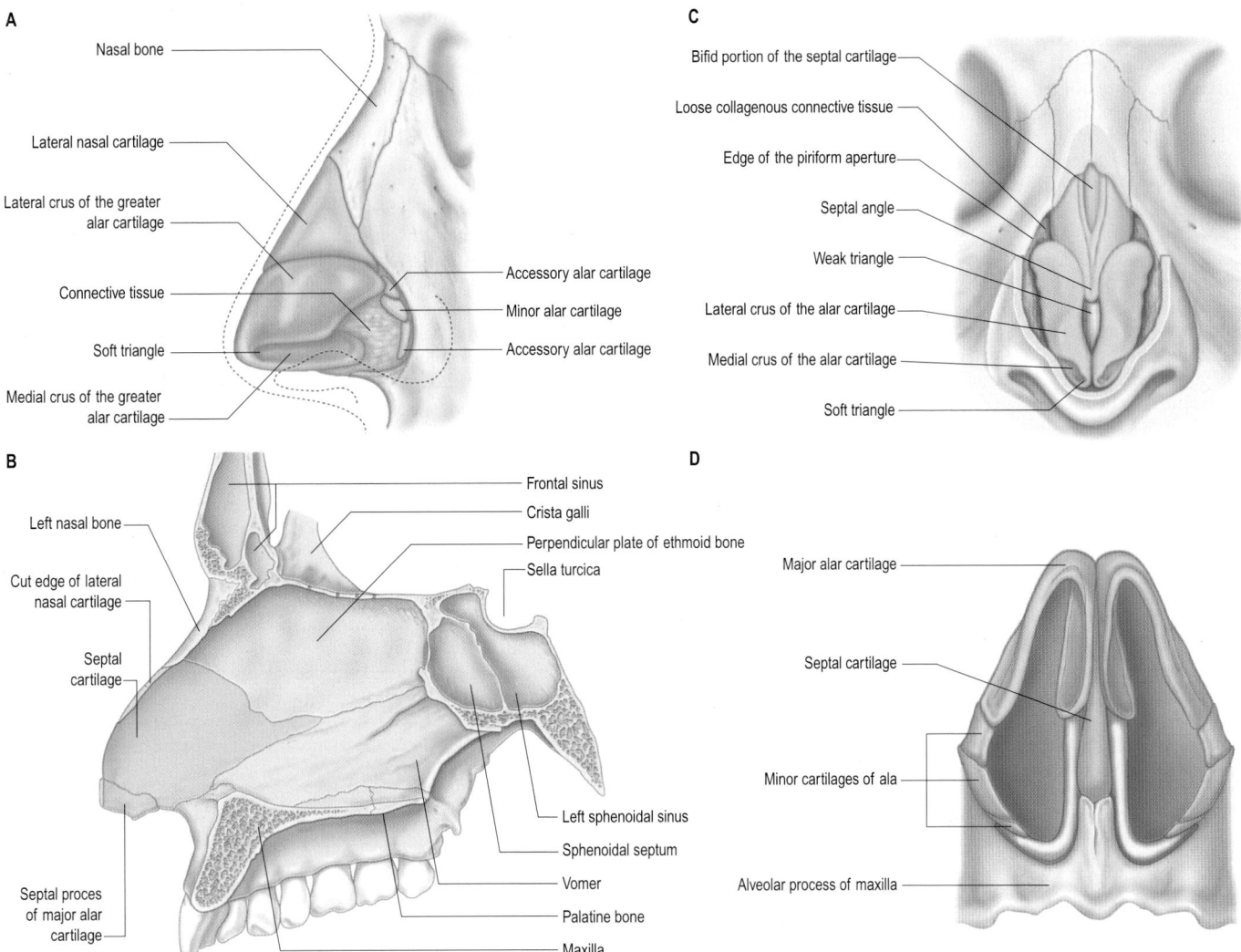

Fig. 32.3 The bone and cartilages of the nose. **A**, lateral view; **B**, nasal septum; **C**, frontal view; **D**, inferior view.

Medial wall (Fig. 32.2)

The medial wall of the nasal cavity is the nasal septum. Relatively featureless, it lies between the roof and floor and is a thin sheet of bone with a wide anterior deficiency occupied by the septal cartilage. Ridges or spurs of bone sometimes project from the septum on either side. The bony part is formed primarily by the vomer and the perpendicular plate of the ethmoid. The vomer extends from the body of the sphenoid to the hard palate, forming the posteroinferior septum (including the posterior border). The surface contains grooves related to the nasopalatine nerves and accompanying vessels. The perpendicular plate of the ethmoid forms the anterosuperior part of the bony nasal septum and is continuous above with its cribriform plate. The nasal septum is often deviated – more usually to the left – and particularly affects the perpendicular plate of the ethmoid. Other bones make minor contributions to the septum at the upper and lower limits of the medial wall. The nasal bones and the nasal spine of the frontal bones are anterosuperior, the rostrum and crest of the sphenoid bone are posterosuperior, and the nasal crests of the maxillary and palatine bones are inferior. Above the incisive canals, at the lower edge of the septal cartilage, there is sometimes a depression pointing downwards and forwards: it occupies the position of the nasopalatine canal which connected the nasal and buccal cavities in early fetal life. A minute orifice may be seen leading back into a blind tubule, 2–6 mm long, on each side of the septum near this recess. The tubules house the vomeronasal organ, a paired accessory olfactory organ similar to the olfactory epithelium in amphibians and reptiles, but believed to be vestigial in man. Posteriorly the mucoperiosteum of the septum may be thickened by a cushion of very vascular tissue.

The nasal septum may be displaced by injury or by some congenital defect, and sometimes the deviation may be so great as to bring the septum and one lateral wall into contact, causing complete unilateral nasal obstruction.

Lateral wall (Fig. 32.1)

The lateral wall of the nasal cavity contains three projections of variable size called the inferior, middle and superior nasal conchae or turbinates. It is formed largely by the maxilla and its anterior and posterior fontanelles (bony deficiencies in the medial wall of the maxilla obliterated to varying degrees by fibrous tissue) anteroinferiorly; by the perpendicular plate of the palatine bone posteriorly; and superiorly by the labyrinth of the ethmoid bone which separates the nasal cavity from the orbit. The nasal conchae curve generally inferomedially, each roofing a groove, or meatus, open to the nasal cavity. The middle conchae may also curve inferolaterally or be expanded by an enclosed air cell to form a so called 'concha bullosa'. The opening associated with the maxillary sinus, the maxillary hiatus, appears as a wide defect in the nasal surface of the isolated maxilla. However, in the articulated state in life, the hiatus is greatly reduced in size by neighbouring bones. Thus it is covered by the maxillary process of the inferior concha below, by the uncinate process of the ethmoid bone above, by the perpendicular plate of the palatine bone behind, and by small parts of ethmoidal labyrinth and lacrimal bone anterosuperiorly (**Fig. 32.1**).

Inferior concha or turbinate

The inferior concha is a thin, curved, independent bone which articulates with the nasal surface of the maxilla and the perpendicular plate of the palatine bone. The free lower border is gently curved and the subjacent inferior meatus reaches the nasal floor. The inferior meatus is the largest meatus, and it extends along almost all of the lateral nasal wall. It is deepest at the junction of its anterior and middle thirds, where the inferior opening of the nasolacrimal canal appears. The nasolacrimal canal is formed by the articulations between the lacrimal groove of the maxilla and the descending process of the lacrimal bone and the lacrimal process of the inferior nasal concha. During postnatal development, the ostium of the nasolacrimal duct moves upwards and is increasingly arched over by the inferior concha.

Middle concha or turbinate

The middle concha is a medial process of the ethmoidal labyrinth, and extends back to articulate with the perpendicular plate of the palatine bone. The middle concha itself may be pneumatized (conchal sinus). The region beneath it is the middle meatus, which is deeper in front than behind, lies below and lateral to the middle concha and continues anteriorly into a shallow fossa above the vestibule, termed the atrium of the middle meatus. Lateral to the atrium an ill-defined curved ridge, the agger nasi, slopes downwards and forwards from the upper end of the anterior free border of the middle concha. The agger nasi is better developed in the newborn than in adults. The middle concha must be displaced to display the lateral wall of the middle meatus fully. The main features of this wall are a rounded elevation, the bulla ethmoidalis and, below it and extending up in front of it, a curved cleft, the hiatus semilunaris (**Figs 32.1, 32.4**). The bulla ethmoidalis is formed by the expansion of the middle ethmoidal sinuses, which open on or just above it. Its size varies according to that of the contained sinuses. The hiatus semilunaris opens laterally into a curved channel, the ethmoidal infundibulum, into which the anterior ethmoidal sinuses open. In at least 50% of subjects the openings of the ethmoidal sinuses are continuous with the opening of the frontonasal duct which drains the frontal sinus. Alternately, the infundibulum may end blindly in front in one or more anterior ethmoidal sinuses (infundibular sinuses) and the frontonasal duct then opens more medially directly into the anterior end of the middle meatus. The opening of the maxillary sinus lies below the bulla, usually hidden by the flange-like lower edge of the uncinate process. This opening is near the roof of the sinus and is therefore unfavourable for drainage. The coordinated beating of the cilia of the mucociliary clearance system of the maxillary sinus is directed towards it. An accessory opening of the maxillary sinus through the posterior fontanelle of the medial wall of the maxillary sinus frequently exists inferoposterior to the hiatus.

Superior concha or turbinate (Fig. 32.1)

The superior concha is a medial process of the ethmoidal labyrinth and presents as a small curved lamina, posterosuperior to the middle concha. It roofs the superior meatus and is the shortest and shallowest of the three conchae. Above the superior concha, the sphenoidal sinus

opens into a triangular sphenoethmoidal recess which separates the superior concha and anterior aspect of the body of the sphenoid. Occasionally a fourth concha, the highest or supreme nasal concha, appears on the lateral wall of this recess: the passage immediately below it is called the supreme nasal meatus, and it sometimes displays an opening of the posterior ethmoidal sinus. The superior meatus is a short oblique passage extending about halfway along the upper border of the middle concha. The posterior ethmoidal sinuses open, via a variable number of apertures, into its anterior part.

The sphenopalatine foramen (**Fig. 32.1**) can be approached through the middle meatus. Clinically it is posterior to the middle meatus and transmits the sphenopalatine artery and nasopalatine and superior nasal nerves from the pterygopalatine fossa. It is bounded above by the body and concha of the sphenoid, below by the superior border of the perpendicular plate of the palatine bone, and in front and behind by the orbital and sphenoidal processes of the palatine bone.

Nasal obstruction

Variations in the anatomy of the structures of the lateral nasal wall, e.g. oversized bulla ethmoidalis air cells, paradoxically curved middle conchae, concha bullosae of the middle concha, or so called 'compensatory hypertrophy' of the inferior concha into a congenital concavity of the nasal septum, may all cause nasal obstruction or impaired sinus ventilation and drainage. Conchae are often excised to open the airway. They may also be 'out-fractured' to lateralize them and improve the airway. The degree of congestion with blood and hence swelling of the vascular mucoperiosteum of the conchae varies cyclically every few hours and may be interfered with by allergy or infection, both of which will cause swelling and inflammation of the conchal mucous membranes. These mucous membranes may be shrunk with vasoconstrictor medication, excised surgically or burned to cause scarring so as to restrict swelling.

SOFT TISSUE

SOFT TISSUE FEATURES OF EXTERNAL NOSE

Externally the nose is pyramidal in shape, its upper angle or root being continuous with the forehead, and its free tip forming the apex. Two ellipsoidal apertures, the external nares or nostrils, are inferior and separated by the nasal septum and columnella. The external nares are narrower in front, and usually measure 1.5–2 cm anteroposteriorly and 0.5–1 cm transversely. By their union in the median plane, the lateral surfaces of the nose form the dorsum nasi, the shape of which varies greatly between individuals. The upper part of the external nose is kept patent by the nasal bones and the frontal processes of the maxillae. Below this the nasal cartilages form the walls of the external nose. The lateral surfaces end below in the rounded alae nasi.

SOFT TISSUE FEATURES OF THE INTERNAL NASAL CAVITY AND SINUS MUCOSA

Nasal vestibule

The nasal vestibule is a slightly expanded anterior part of the air passage just inside the naris. It is bounded laterally by the ala and lateral part of the major alar cartilage, and medially by the medial crus or septal process of this cartilage. The vestibule extends as a small recess towards the apex of the nose. Its lumen is lined with skin, the inferior region bearing sebaceous and sweat glands, and coarse hairs (vibrissae) curving towards the naris and helping to arrest the passage of particles in inspired air. In males, after middle age, these hairs increase considerably in size. The vestibule is limited above and behind by a curved ridge, the limen nasi or nasal valve, corresponding to the lower margin of the upper lateral cartilage anteriorly and the pyriform nasal aperture posteroinferiorly. At this demarcation, the skin of the vestibule is continuous with the nasal mucosa.

Nasal mucosa and respiratory epithelium

The lining of the anterior part of the nasal cavity and vestibule is continuous with the skin, and consists of keratinized stratified squamous epithelium overlying a connective tissue lamina propria. Further posteriorly, at the limen nasi, this grades into a mucosa lined at first by non-keratinizing stratified squamous epithelium, then by pseudostratified ciliated (respiratory) epithelium with numerous goblet cells (p. 31,

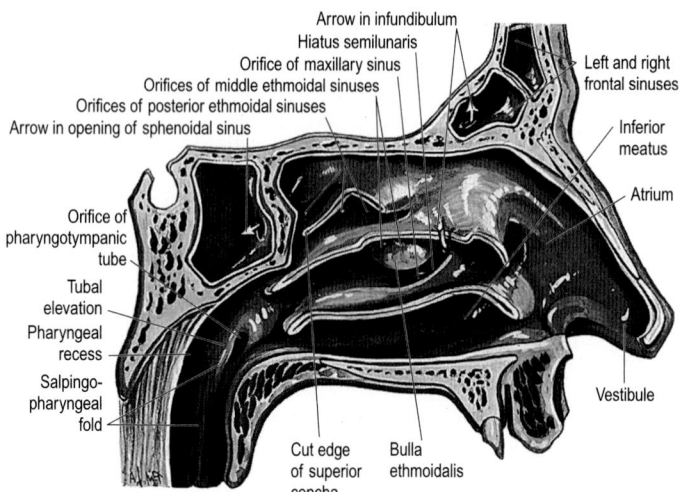

Fig. 32.4 Lateral wall of the left nasal cavity; the conchae have been partially removed. (By permission from Ellis H, Feldman S 1997 Anatomy for Anaesthetists, 7th edn. Oxford: Blackwell.)

Fig. 3.6). Respiratory epithelium forms most of the surface of the nasal cavity, and so covers the conchae, meatuses, floor and roof, except where the olfactory epithelium is present. In some areas, cells of the respiratory epithelium may be low columnar or cuboidal, and the proportion of ciliated to non-ciliated cells is variable.

The nasal mucosa has numerous underlying seromucous glands within its lamina propria, which makes the surface sticky so that particles in the inspired air are deposited on the surface. It is adherent to the periosteum or perichondrium of the neighbouring skeletal structures. The mucosa is continuous with the nasopharyngeal mucosa through the posterior nasal apertures, the conjunctiva through the nasolacrimal duct and lacrimal canaliculi, and the mucosae of the sphenoidal, ethmoidal, frontal and maxillary sinuses through their openings into the meatuses. The epithelium in the sinuses is thinner and has fewer goblet cells than elsewhere. Subepithelial glands are sparse: their combined secretions are directed towards the nasal cavity by ciliary action.

The mucosa is thickest and most vascular over the conchae, especially at their extremities, and also on the nasal septum, but is very thin in the meatuses, on the floor and in the sinuses. Its thickness reduces the volume of the nasal cavity and its apertures significantly. The lamina propria contains cavernous vascular tissue with large venous sinusoids. Local vascular changes, controlled by the vasomotor autonomic innervation and possibly by endocrine stimuli, alter the thickness and contours of the mucosal surfaces, and this is visible as a swelling or shrinkage of the nasal lining. These changes produce periodic alterations in the rate of airflow through the nasal passages, alternating between nares, which may serve to protect their mucosae from desiccation. The conchae add greatly to the surface area of the nasal cavity which increases the turbulence of inhaled air, and may improve olfaction by slowing the passage of air past the olfactory area. Humidification and warming of the inhaled air are also augmented by the increased mucosal area and turbulence.

The mucous film is continually moved by ciliary action backwards into the nasopharynx at a rate of c.6 mm per minute. Palatal movements transfer the mucus and its entrapped particles to the oropharynx for swallowing, but some also enters the nasal vestibule anteriorly. The secretions of the nasal mucosa contain the bacteriocides lysozyme and lactoferrin, and also secretory immunoglobulins (IgA).

Respiratory epithelium extends through the apertures of the paranasal sinuses to line them, and is closely bound to the underlying periosteum in the walls of the sinuses to form a combined mucoperiosteum.

Olfactory epithelium

The peripheral receptors for olfactory sensation are located bilaterally in areas of sensory epithelium lining the posterodorsal parts of the nasal cavities. The sensory epithelium occupies an area of c.5 cm^2 covering the posterior upper parts of the lateral nasal wall, including the back of the superior concha, the sphenoethmoidal recess, the upper part of the perpendicular plate of the ethmoid and the roof of the nose arching between the septum and lateral wall, including the underside of the cribriform plate. This area is pigmented yellowish brown in contrast to the pinker colour of the respiratory mucosa.

Microstructure of the olfactory mucosa

The olfactory mucosa consists of a pseudostratified olfactory epithelium, derived from the embryonic olfactory placodes (p. 245). It contains sensory receptor neurones, and its underlying lamina propria contains their axons, which lie within numerous olfactory nerve fascicles, and subepithelial olfactory glands (of Bowman). The glands secrete a predominantly serous fluid through ducts which open onto the epithelial surface. Their secretions form a thin fluid layer in which sensory cilia and the microvilli of sustentacular cells are embedded.

Olfactory epithelium – The olfactory epithelium (**Figs 32.5, 32.6**) is considerably thicker (up to 100 μm) than the respiratory epithelium. It contains olfactory receptor neurones, sustentacular cells and two classes of basal cell, horizontal basal cells (closest to the basal lamina) and globose basal cells (**Fig. 32.7**). The nuclei of these various cells occupy specific zones within the epithelial thickness. Most superficially is a layer of sustentacular cell nuclei; beneath this, and occupying much of the epithelial thickness, are several tiers of receptor cell bodies and nuclei. Basal cells lie between this zone and the basal lamina underlying the epithelium.

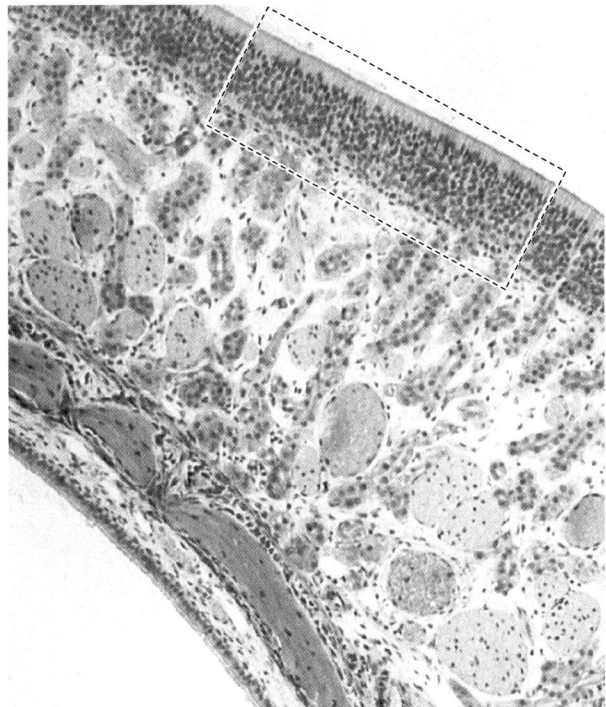

Fig. 32.5 Low power micrograph of the olfactory mucosa covering the superior concha. The olfactory epithelium is shown overlying a lamina propria containing cavernous vascular tissue and olfactory glands (of Bowman). Bundles of olfactory axons (fila olfactoria) pass through the mucosa towards the cribriform plate. A thinner respiratory epithelium covers the lower surface, shown here beneath the bone of the concha. (By permission from Kierszenbaum AL 2002 Histology and Cell Biology. St Louis: Mosby.)

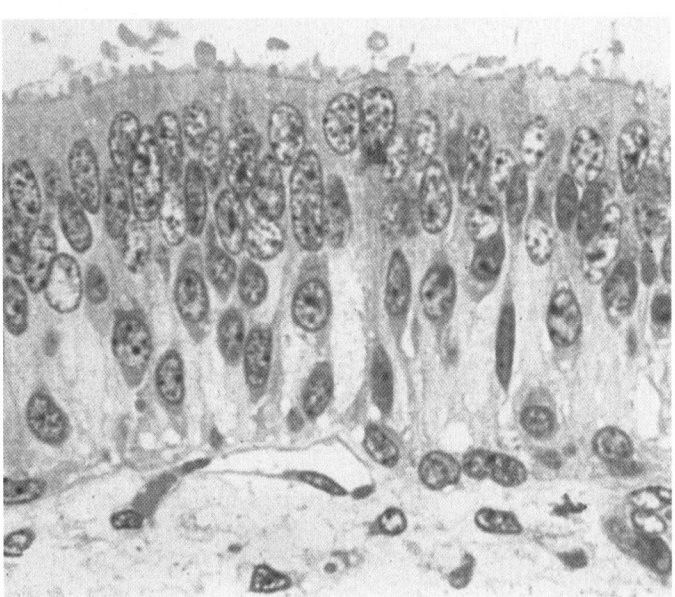

Fig. 32.6 High power micrograph of the olfactory mucosa from an 18-week fetus, showing the nuclei of basal cells, olfactory neurones and sustentacular cells. The olfactory neuronal endings (knobs or vesicles) can be seen projecting from the free surface. (By permission from Stevens A, Lowe JS 1996 Human Histology, 2nd edn. London: Mosby.)

Olfactory receptor neurones – Olfactory receptor neurones are bipolar cells. They have a cell body and nucleus located in the middle zone of the epithelium, a single unbranched apical dendrite c.2 μm across which extends to the epithelial surface, and a basally directed unmyelinated axon c.0.2 μm in diameter, which passes out of the epithelium. Each dendrite projects into the overlying secretory fluid as an expanded

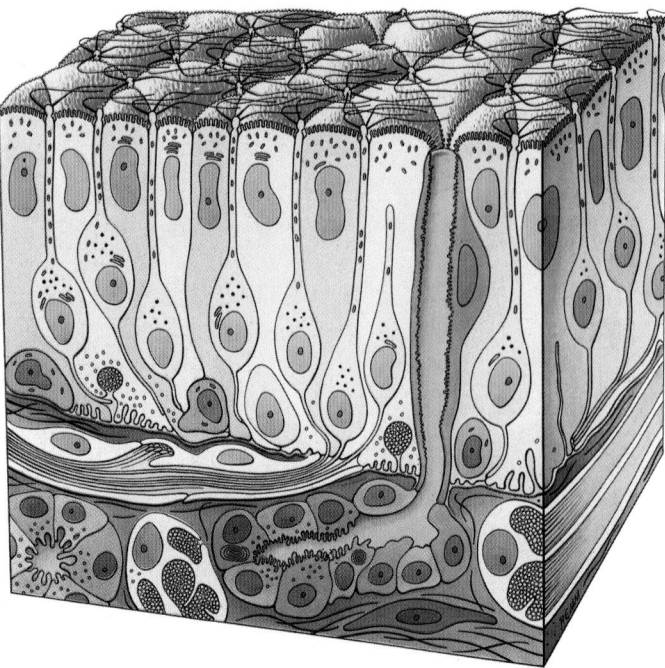

Fig. 32.7 The chief cytological features of the olfactory epithelium. Receptor cells (yellow) are situated among columnar sustentacular cells. The axons of the receptor cells emerge from the epithelium in bundles enclosed by ensheathing glial cells. Rounded globose basal cells (brown) and flattened horizontal basal cells (not shown) lie on the basal lamina and the subepithelial glands (of Bowman) open on to the surface via their intraepithelial ducts (green). At the surface are cilia of the receptor cells and microvilli of the supporting cells.

cylindrical olfactory ending (rod, knob or vesicle). Groups of up to 20 cilia radiate from the circumference of each ending and extend for long distances parallel to the epithelial surface. Internally, the short proximal part of each cilium has the '9 + 2' pattern of microtubules typical of motile cilia (p. 19), while the longer distal trailing end contains only the central pair of microtubules. The cilia lack dynein arms on the peripheral microtubule doublets and are thought to be non-motile, serving to project a large area of sensory surface for the efficient detection of odorants. Individual receptor neurones express receptors for a single (or very few) odorant molecules. Although neurones with the same receptor specificity are randomly distributed within anatomical zones of the epithelium, all project to the same target dendritic field (glomeruli) of the olfactory bulb, and there is a considerable degree of convergence. Specific odours activate a unique spectrum of receptors which in turn activate restricted groups of glomeruli and their second order neurones.

The axons form small intraepithelial fascicles among the processes of sustentacular and basal cells. The fascicles penetrate the basal lamina, and are immediately ensheathed by olfactory ensheathing cells. Groups of up to 50 fascicles join to form larger olfactory nerve rootlets which pass through the cribriform plate to enter the olfactory bulb, there synapsing in glomeruli with secondary sensory neurones, principally mitral cells and, to a lesser extent, smaller tufted cells.

Sustentacular cells – Sustentacular, or supporting, cells (**Fig. 32.7**) are columnar cells that separate and partially ensheathe the olfactory receptors. Their large nuclei form a layer superficial to the receptor nuclei. They send numerous long, irregular microvilli into the secretory fluid layer covering the surface of the epithelium, where they lie among the long trailing ends of olfactory receptor cilia. At their bases, facing the basal lamina, they have expanded end-feet containing numerous lamellated dense bodies resembling neuronal lipofuscin granules. These are remains of secondary lysosomes formed as a result of phagocytic activity, and are largely responsible for the pigmentation of the olfactory area. The granules gradually accumulate with age, and because these cells are long-lived, pigmentation also increases in intensity with age. Cells are linked by desmosomes near the epithelial surface, which gives mechanical coherence to the epithelium, and by

tight junctions between the sustentacular cells and olfactory receptors at the level of the epithelial surface, which provides a protective barrier.

Basal cells – There are two types of basal cell; horizontal basal cells and globose basal cells. Horizontal basal cells are flattened against the basal lamina, and have condensed nuclei and darkly staining cytoplasm containing numerous intermediate filaments of the cytokeratin family, inserted into desmosomes contacting surrounding sustentacular cells. In contrast, globose cells are rounded or elliptical in shape, with a pale, euchromatic nucleus, and a pale cytoplasm. They form a distinct zone spaced slightly from the basal surface of the epithelium. Mitoses are found within this zone because globose basal cells are the immediate source of new olfactory receptor neurones.

Olfactory ensheathing (glial) cells – Olfactory ensheathing cells share properties with astrocytes and non-myelinating Schwann cells, but they possess distinctive features that indicate they are a separate class of glia. Developmentally they are derived from the olfactory placode rather than neural crest. They ensheath olfactory axons in a unique manner throughout their entire course, and accompany them into the central nervous tissue of the olfactory bulb, where they contribute to the glia limitans.

Olfactory glands – The olfactory (Bowman's) glands (**Fig. 32.7**) are branched tubuloalveolar structures that lie beneath the olfactory epithelium and secrete onto the epithelial surface through narrow, vertical ducts. Their secretions, which include defensive substances, lysozyme, lactoferrin, IgA and sulphated proteoglycans, bathe the dendritic endings and cilia of the olfactory receptors. The fluid acts as a solvent for odorant molecules, allowing their diffusion to the sensory receptors. The glands also secrete odorant-binding proteins into the fluid, which increase the efficiency of odour detection.

Turnover of olfactory receptor neurones – Receptor neurones are lost and replaced throughout life. Individual receptor cells have a variable lifespan, averaging 1–3 months. Stem cells situated near the base of the epithelium undergo periodic mitotic division throughout life, giving rise to new olfactory receptor cells which then grow a dendrite to the olfactory surface and an axon to the olfactory bulb. The cell bodies of these new receptor neurones gradually move apically until they reach the region just below the supporting cell nuclei. When they degenerate, dead cells are either shed from the epithelium or are phagocytosed by sustentacular cells. The rate of receptor cell loss and replacement increases after exposure to damaging stimuli, but their capacity to turnover declines slowly with age, and this contributes to diminishing olfactory sensory function in old age.

Vomeronasal organ

Vomeronasal organs are important in sexual behaviour in several species, where they are especially concerned with detecting pheromones, however the organ is considered to be non-functional in adult humans. Putative sensory cells are replaced by non-sensory epithelium if the organ persists into postnatal life.

VASCULAR SUPPLY AND LYMPHATIC DRAINAGE OF THE NASAL CAVITY

Many of the vessels and nerves supplying the nasal cavities arise within the pterygopalatine fossa and these origins are described on page 578.

ARTERIES

These arise as branches of the ophthalmic, maxillary and facial arteries which run to supply different territories within the walls, floor and roof of the nose (**Fig. 32.8**). They ramify to form anastomotic plexuses within and deep to the nasal mucosa. Anastomoses also occur between some larger arterial branches. The anterior and posterior ethmoidal branches of the ophthalmic artery supply the ethmoidal and frontal sinuses and the roof of the nose (including the septum). The sphenopalatine branch of the maxillary artery supplies the mucosa of the conchae, meatuses and posteroinferior part of the nasal septum, i.e. it is the principal vessel supplying the nasal mucosa. The greater palatine branch of the maxillary artery supplies the region of the inferior meatus. Its terminal part ascends through the incisive canal to anastomose on the septum with branches

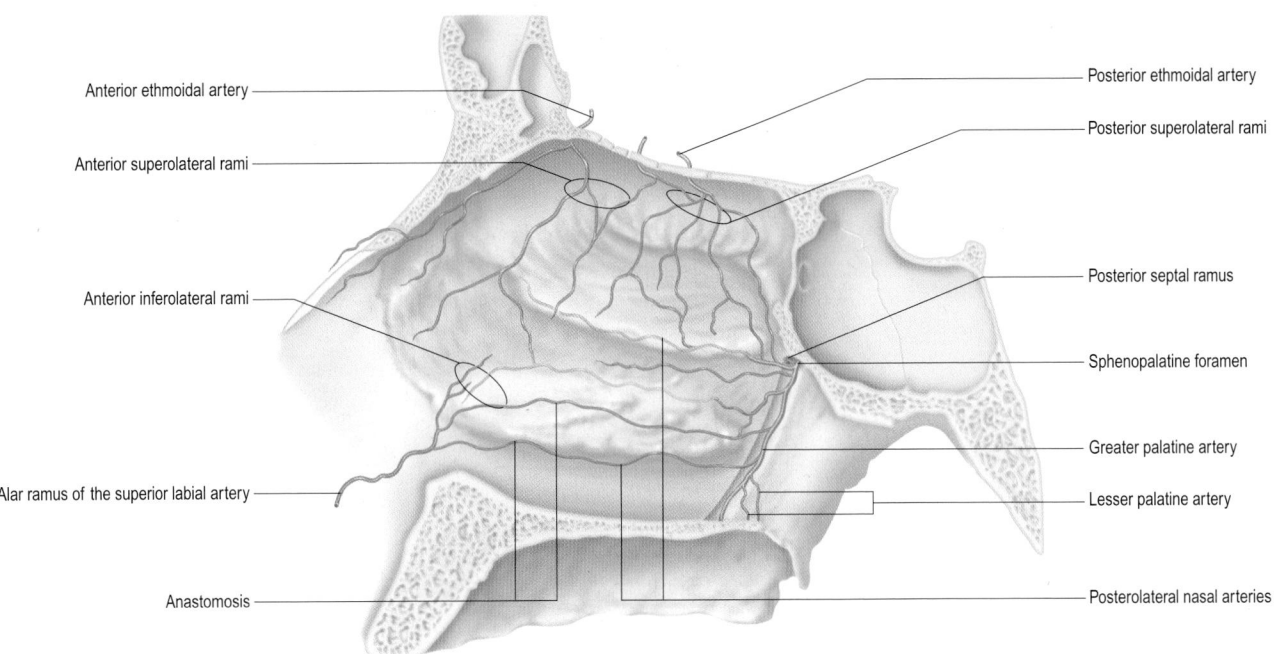

Fig. 32.8 Arteries of the lateral wall of the nose.

of the sphenopalatine and anterior ethmoidal arteries and with the septal branch of the superior labial artery. This septal region (Little's area) is a common site of bleeding from the nose. The infraorbital artery and the superior, anterior, and posterior alveolar branches of the maxillary artery supply the mucosa of the maxillary sinus. The pharyngeal branch of the maxillary artery supplies the sphenoidal sinus.

VEINS

These form a rich submucosal cavernous plexus that is especially dense in the posterior part of the septum and in the middle and inferior conchae. Numerous arteriovenous anastomoses are present in the deep layer of the mucosa and around the mucosal glands. The cavernous conchal plexuses resemble those in erectile tissue: the nasal cavity is susceptible to blockage should they become engorged. Veins from the posterior part of the nose generally pass to the sphenopalatine vein that runs back through the sphenopalatine foramen to drain into the pterygoid venous plexus. The anterior part of the nose is drained mainly through veins accompanying the anterior ethmoidal arteries, and these veins subsequently pass into the ophthalmic or facial veins. A few veins pass through the cribriform plate to connect with those on the orbital surface of the frontal lobes of the brain. When the foramen caecum is patent, it transmits a vein from the nasal cavity to the superior sagittal sinus.

LYMPHATIC DRAINAGE

Lymph vessels from the anterior region of the nasal cavity pass superficially to join those of the external nasal skin, which end in the submandibular nodes. The rest of the nasal cavity, paranasal sinuses, nasopharynx and pharyngeal end of the pharyngotympanic tube all drain to the upper deep cervical nodes, directly or through the retropharyngeal nodes. The posterior nasal floor probably drains to the parotid nodes.

INNERVATION OF THE NASAL CAVITY

Special sensation related to olfaction is associated with the olfactory nerves. General sensation to the nasal mucosa is related to branches from the ophthalmic and maxillary divisions of the trigeminal nerves. The general sensations mediated are touch, pain and temperature. The trigeminal fibres close to, and within, the epithelial layer are also sensitive to noxious chemicals, e.g. ammonia and sulphur dioxide. These latter stimuli may therefore be perceived by the trigeminal nerve even when the olfactory nerves have been damaged. In addition,

autonomic nerves from the pterygopalatine ganglion innervate mucous glands and control cyclical and reactive vasomotor activity.

NERVES OF ORDINARY SENSATION (Figs 32.9, 32.10)

These are all derived from the maxillary nerve, with an additional contribution from the nasociliary branch of the ophthalmic nerve. The anterior ethmoidal branch of the nasociliary nerve leaves the cranial cavity through a small slit near the crista galli and enters the roof of the nasal cavity. Here it runs in a groove on the inner surface of the nasal bone, and supplies the roof of the nasal cavity. It gives off a lateral internal branch to supply the anterior part of the lateral wall and a medial internal branch to the anterior and upper parts of the septum, before emerging at the inferior margin of the nasal bone as the external nasal nerve to supply the skin of the external nose to the nasal tip. The infraorbital nerve supplies the nasal vestibule; the anterior superior alveolar nerve supplies part of the septum, the floor near the anterior nasal spine and the anterior part of the lateral wall as high as the opening of the maxillary sinus; the lateral posterior superior nasal and the posterior inferior nasal branches of the greater palatine nerve together supply the posterior three-quarters of the lateral wall, roof and floor; the medial posterior superior nasal nerves and the nasopalatine nerve supply the inferior part of the nasal septum; branches from the nerve of the pterygoid canal supply the upper and posterior part of the roof and septum.

Autonomic nerves accompany the sensory innervation. Sympathetic postganglionic vasomotor fibres are distributed to the nasal blood vessels, and postganglionic parasympathetic fibres from the pterygopalatine ganglion provide the secretomotor supply to the nasal glands.

OLFACTORY NERVES (Figs 32.9, 32.10)

The olfactory nerves serving the sense of smell have their cells of origin in the olfactory mucosa covering the superior nasal concha, the upper part of the vertical portion of the middle concha and the opposite part of the nasal septum. The axons, which are unmyelinated, originate as the central or deep processes of the olfactory neurones, and collect into bundles that cross in various directions, forming a plexiform network in the mucosa. These bundles finally form c.20 branches that traverse the cribriform plate in lateral and medial groups and end in the glomeruli of the olfactory bulb. Each branch has a sheath consisting of dura mater and pia-arachnoid, the former continuing into the nasal periosteum, the latter into the connective tissue sheaths surrounding the nerve bundles: this arrangement may favour the spread of infection into the cranial cavity from the nasal cavity.

Labels on figure:
Anterior ethmoidal artery
Anterior superolateral rami
Anterior inferolateral rami
Alar ramus of the superior labial artery
Anastomosis
Posterior ethmoidal artery
Posterior superolateral rami
Posterior septal ramus
Sphenopalatine foramen
Greater palatine artery
Lesser palatine artery
Posterolateral nasal arteries

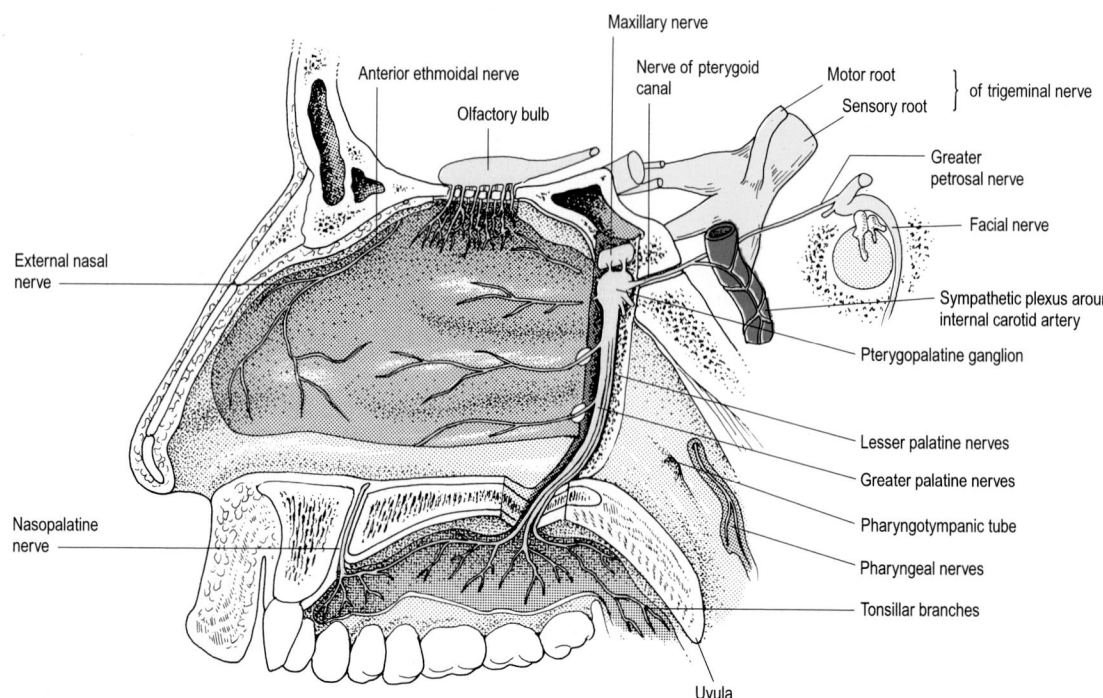

Fig. 32.9 The sensory innervation of the lateral wall of the nasal cavity, hard and soft palates, and nasopharynx. Secretomotor fibres to mucous glands are distributed in branches from the pterygopalatine ganglion.

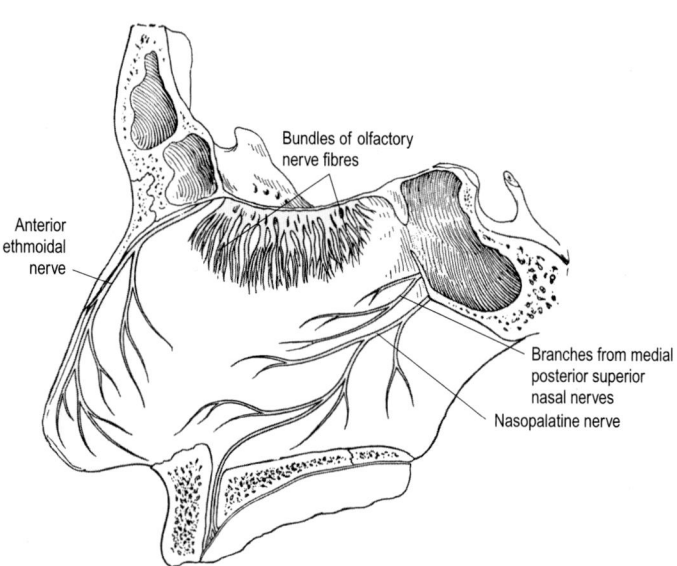

Fig. 32.10 Bundles of olfactory nerve fibres and nerves associated with the septum (left side).

In severe injuries involving the anterior cranial fossa, the olfactory bulb may be separated from the olfactory nerves or the nerves may be torn, producing anosmia, loss of olfaction. Fractures may involve the meninges, admitting cerebrospinal fluid (CSF) into the nose resulting in cerebrospinal rhinorrhoea. Such injuries also open up avenues for infection from the nasal cavity.

VISCERA: PARANASAL SINUSES

The paranasal sinuses are the frontal, ethmoidal, sphenoidal and maxillary sinuses, housed within the bones of the same name. The ethmoidal sinuses differ from the others in being formed of small multiple cavities, divisible into anterior, middle and posterior groups. All sinuses open into the lateral wall of the nasal cavity by small apertures that allow the equilibration of air and movement of mucus. The detailed position of these apertures, and the precise form and sizes of the sinuses, vary enormously between individuals. Their mucosa is continuous with that of the nasal cavity – a feature unfortunately favouring the spread of infections – and is similar histologically, although thinner, less vascular and less adherent to bone. Mucus is secreted by glands within their mucosa and is swept through their apertures into the nose by cilia. Cilia are not uniformly distributed but are always present near the apertures of the sinuses. The mucociliary escalator is the normal mechanism for clearing the sinuses and maintaining aeration and forms the theoretical basis of functional endoscopic sinus surgery (FESS).

Most sinuses are rudimentary or absent at birth, but enlarge appreciably during the eruption of the permanent teeth and after puberty, markedly altering the size and shape of the face at these times.

The functions of the sinuses remain speculative. They clearly add some resonance to the voice, and also allow the enlargement of local areas of the skull whilst minimizing a corresponding increase in bony mass. It is likely that such growth-related changes serve to strengthen particular regions, e.g. the alveolar process of the maxilla when the secondary dentition erupts, but they may also function in contouring the head to provide visual signals indicating the individual's status in a social context (e.g. gender, sexual maturity and group identity).

IMAGING OF THE PARANASAL SINUSES

On standard radiological images, normal sinuses are radiolucent, whereas when they are diseased they show varying degrees of opacity. In lateral views, the extent of the frontal sinus both upwards into the frontal bone and back into the orbital roof can be assessed. The ethmoidal sinuses are seen to extend back from the frontal process of the maxilla as far as the sphenoidal sinus, which is clearly visible below and in front of the hypophyseal fossa, although the two sphenoidal sinuses appear superimposed, and the individual sphenoidal sinuses are seen better from above.

The maxillary sinus is clearly seen in a lateral view, lying below the orbit, and its relationship to the roots of the teeth is obvious. In posteroanterior views of the skull, most of the sinuses are visible. The frontal sinuses appear above the nasal cavity and the medial part of the orbits. Their asymmetry, vertical extent and the position of their septa can be assessed. The ethmoidal sinuses are superimposed on each other and on the sphenoidal sinuses in this view, lying between the orbits below the cribriform plate. The sphenoidal sinuses are obscured in this view. Each maxillary sinus is a pyramidal radiolucent area below the orbit and lateral to the lower part of the nasal cavity, extending inferiorly into the alveolar process of the maxilla. The frontal, maxillary and ethmoidal sinuses are particularly well demonstrated in occipitomental views. The introduction of imaging techniques such as CT has provided infinitely clearer images of the air sinuses and this has significantly aided diagnosis (**Figs 32.11, 32.12, 32.13**).

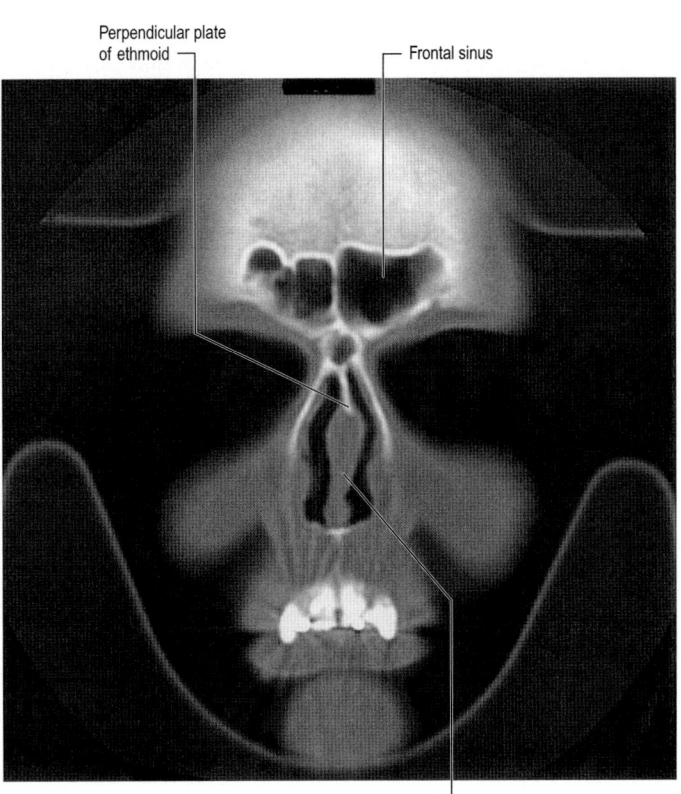

Perpendicular plate of ethmoid — Frontal sinus

Septal cartilage

Fig. 32.11 Coronal CT scan showing frontal sinus. (By kind permission from Dr N Drage.)

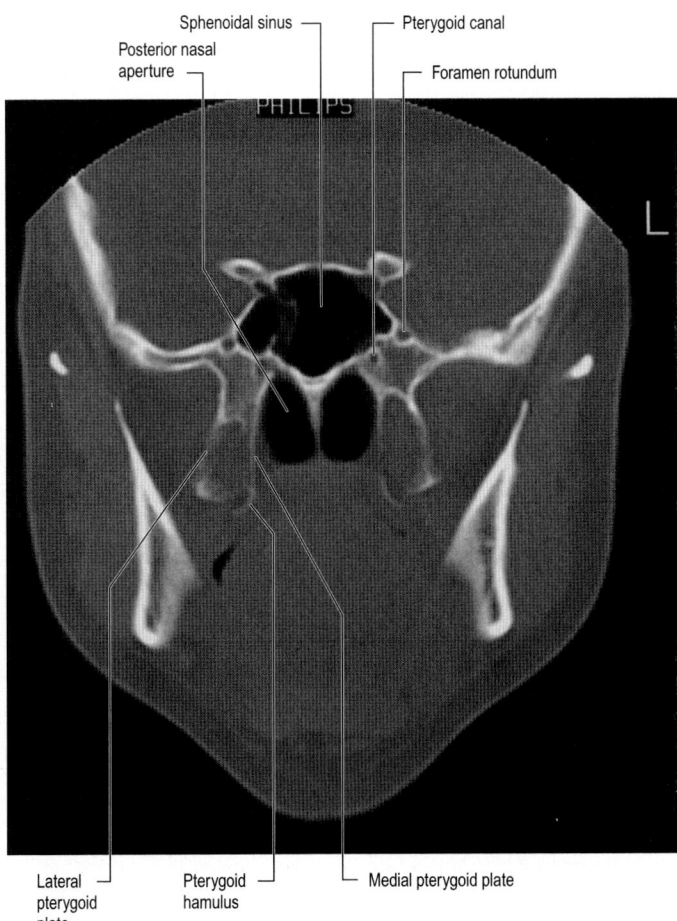

Sphenoidal sinus — Pterygoid canal
Posterior nasal aperture — Foramen rotundum

PHILIPS

L

Lateral pterygoid plate — Pterygoid hamulus — Medial pterygoid plate

Fig. 32.12 Coronal CT scan showing sphenoidal air sinus. (By kind permission from Dr N Drage.)

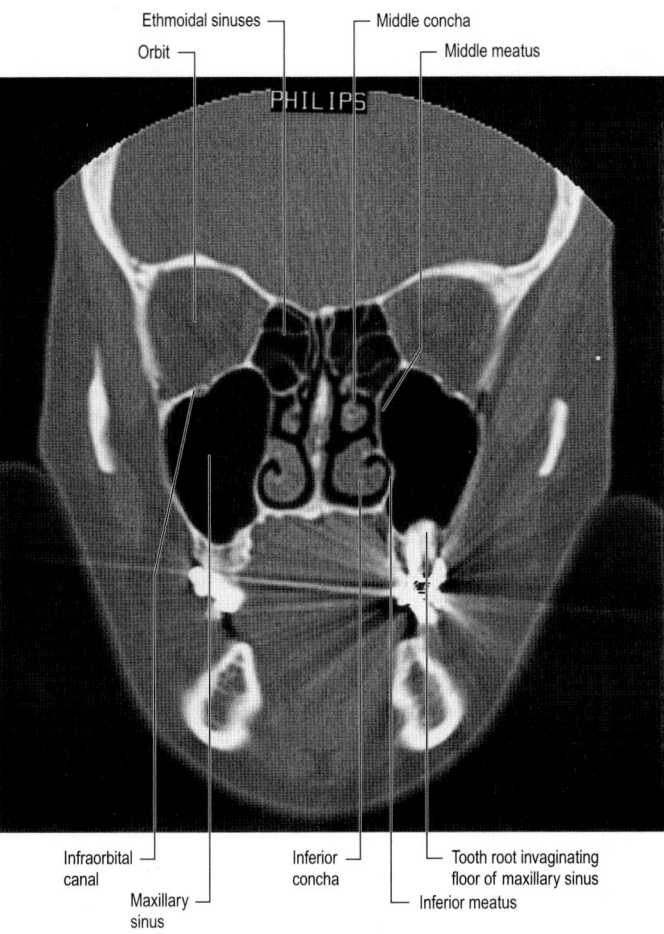

Ethmoidal sinuses — Middle concha
Orbit — Middle meatus

PHILIPS

Infraorbital canal — Inferior concha — Tooth root invaginating floor of maxillary sinus
Maxillary sinus — Inferior meatus

Fig. 32.13 Coronal CT scan showing ethmoidal and maxillary sinuses. (By kind permission from Dr N Drage.)

FRONTAL SINUS (Figs 32.8, 32.10)

The paired frontal sinuses, situated posterior to the superciliary arches, lie between the outer and inner tables of the frontal bone. Each usually underlies a triangular area on the surface, its angles formed by the nasion, a point 3 cm above the nasion and the junction of the medial third and lateral two-thirds of the supraorbital margin. The two sinuses are rarely symmetrical, the septum between them usually deviating from the median plane. Their average dimensions are: height 3.2 cm; breadth 2.6 cm; depth 1.8 cm. Each extends upwards above the medial part of the eyebrow and back into the medial part of the roof of the orbit. The frontal sinus is sometimes divided into a number of communicating recesses by incomplete bony septa. Rarely, one or both sinuses may be absent, and racial differences have been reported. The prominence of the superciliary arches is no indication of the presence or size of the frontal sinuses. The part of the sinus extending upwards in the frontal bone may be small and the orbital part large, or vice versa. Sometimes one sinus may overlap in front of the other. A sinus may extend posteriorly as far as the lesser wing of the sphenoid bone but does not invade it. The morphology of the frontal sinus may be specific enough to allow identification of individuals from radiological evidence for forensic purposes.

The aperture of each frontal sinus usually opens into the anterior part of the corresponding middle meatus by the ethmoidal infundibulum as a hiatus or, more often, as a more elongated frontonasal duct. It may also open medial to the hiatus semilunaris. Rudimentary or absent at birth, the frontal sinuses are generally well developed between the seventh and eighth years, but reach full size only after puberty. They are more prominent in males, giving the forehead an obliquity contrasting with the vertical or convex profile typical of children and females. However, the shape and size of the frontal sinus is highly variable and may be hypoplastic or even absent. In the presence of a persistent metopic suture, the frontal sinuses develop separately on either side of the suture, which can be helpful in excluding frontal fractures.

Vascular supply and innervation – The arterial supply of the frontal sinuses is from the supraorbital and anterior ethmoidal arteries. The veins drain into the anastomotic vein in the supraorbital notch connecting the supraorbital and superior ophthalmic veins. Lymphatic drainage is to the submandibular nodes. The sinuses are innervated by branches from the supraorbital branch of the ophthalmic nerve.

SPHENOIDAL SINUS (Figs 27.13A, 32.8, 32.12, 32.14)

The paired sphenoidal sinuses lie posterior to the upper part of the nasal cavity, within the body of the sphenoid bone. As the sphenoidal septum often deviates from the midline, the sinuses are often unequal in size. They also vary in size and may be further subdivided by accessory septa, especially in the region of former synchondroses. Occasionally one overlaps the other above and, rarely, they intercommunicate. One or both may approach closely to the optic canal or even partly encircle it. The bone overlying the optic nerves and the internal carotid arteries which lie in the lateral wall of the sinus may be dehiscent. The sinuses have average dimensions of: vertical height 2 cm; transverse breadth 1.8 cm; anteroposterior depth 2.1 cm. The degree of pneumatization is highly variable. In nearly 50% they extend into the greater and lesser wing of the sphenoid or the pterygoid process, and may also invade the basilar part of the occipital bone. Gaps in their osseous walls may occasionally leave their mucosa in contact with the overlying dura mater. Bony ridges, produced by the internal carotid artery or pterygoid canal, may project into the sinuses from their lateral walls and floor respectively. A posterior ethmoidal sinus may extend posterosuperior to the relatively smaller sphenoidal sinuses.

The sphenoidal sinuses are related above to the optic chiasma and hypophysis cerebri and on each side to the internal carotid artery and cavernous sinus (**Fig 32.14**). If the sinuses are small, they lie anterior to the hypophysis cerebri. The anterior midline septum often becomes deviated to one side posteriorly and identification of this septation is important prior to trans-sphenoidal surgery.

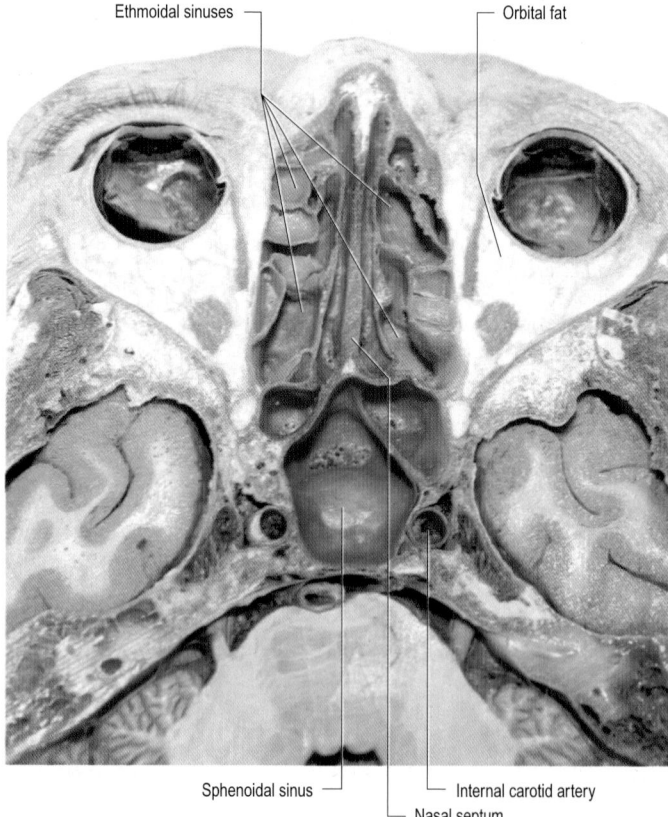

Ethmoidal sinuses — — Orbital fat

Sphenoidal sinus — — Internal carotid artery
— Nasal septum

Fig. 32.14 Horizontal section of head showing ethmoidal and sphenoidal sinuses. (By permission from Berkovitz BKB, Moxham BJ 2002 Head and Neck Anatomy. London: Martin Dunitz.)

The aperture of each sphenoidal sinus opens into the corresponding sphenoethmoidal recess high on the anterior wall of the sinus. At birth the sinuses are minute cavities, and their main development occurs after puberty.

Vascular supply and innervation – The arterial supply of the sphenoidal sinus is via the posterior ethmoidal branch of the ophthalmic artery and nasal branch of the sphenopalatine artery. Venous drainage is through the posterior ethmoidal vein draining into the superior ophthalmic vein. Lymph drainage is to the retropharyngeal nodes. The sensory nerve supply arises from the posterior ethmoidal nerves, while parasympathetic secretomotor fibres are derived from orbital branches of the pterygopalatine ganglion.

ETHMOIDAL SINUSES (Figs 27.19C, 32.13, 32.14)

Ethmoidal sinuses are small, thin-walled cavities in the ethmoidal labyrinth, completed by the frontal, maxillary, lacrimal, sphenoid and palatine bones. They range from 3 large to 18 small sinuses on each side, and their openings into the nasal cavity are also very variable in position. They lie between the upper part of the nasal cavity and the orbit, separated from the latter by the paper-thin lamina papyracea or orbital plate of the ethmoid (a poor barrier to infection that may therefore spread into the orbit). Pneumatization may extend into the middle concha in 4–12% of individuals and into the body and wings of the sphenoid bone lateral to the sphenoid sinus.

Although traditionally divided into anterior, middle and posterior ethmoidal air cells, the ethmoidal sinuses are now commonly considered by clinicians as consisting of anterior and posterior groups on each side, the middle ethmoidal air cells being incorporated into the anterior group. The groups are separated from each other by the basal lamella of the middle concha which may be indented by cells from either group so that it forms a rather tortuous barrier between the two groups. They are, however, distinguished by their sites of communication with the nasal cavity. In each group the sinuses are only partially separated by incomplete bony septa. The ethmoidal sinuses, though small, are of clinical importance at birth because they are susceptible to inflammation. They grow rapidly between 6 and 8 years and after puberty.

Anterior group

Peri-infundibular sinuses (anterior ethmoidal air cells) – There are up to 11 anterior ethmoidal air cells and they open into the ethmoidal infundibulum or the frontonasal duct by one or more orifices. The most anterior group, the agger nasi cells, invaginate beneath the ridge of the same name on the lateral wall of the nasal cavity anteriorly, and are medial relations of the lacrimal sac and duct. Larger anterior and middle cells may develop medially beneath the orbital floor and are known as Haller's cells, and the most anterior supraorbital ethmoidal sinus cells may encroach on the frontal sinus.

Bullar sinuses (middle ethmoidal air cells) – There are usually less than three middle ethmoidal air cells. They open into the middle meatus by one or more orifices on or above the ethmoidal bulla.

Posterior group

The posterior group of ethmoidal air cells vary in number from 1 to 7, and usually open by a single orifice into the superior meatus, although one may open into the supreme meatus when present, and one or more into the sphenoidal sinus. The posterior group lies very close to the optic canal and optic nerve.

Vascular supply and innervation

The ethmoidal sinuses receive their arterial supply from nasal branches of the sphenopalatine artery and the anterior and posterior ethmoidal branches of the ophthalmic artery. Venous drainage is by the corresponding veins. The lymphatics of the anterior group drain to the submandibular nodes, and those of the posterior group to the retropharyngeal nodes. The sensory innervation is from the anterior and posterior ethmoidal branches of the ophthalmic nerve, and the orbital branch of the pterygopalatine ganglion supplies parasympathetic secretomotor fibres.

MAXILLARY SINUS (Figs 27.25C, 32.13, 32.15)

The maxillary sinus is the largest of the paranasal sinuses and is situated in the body of the maxilla. It is pyramidal in shape and its thin walls

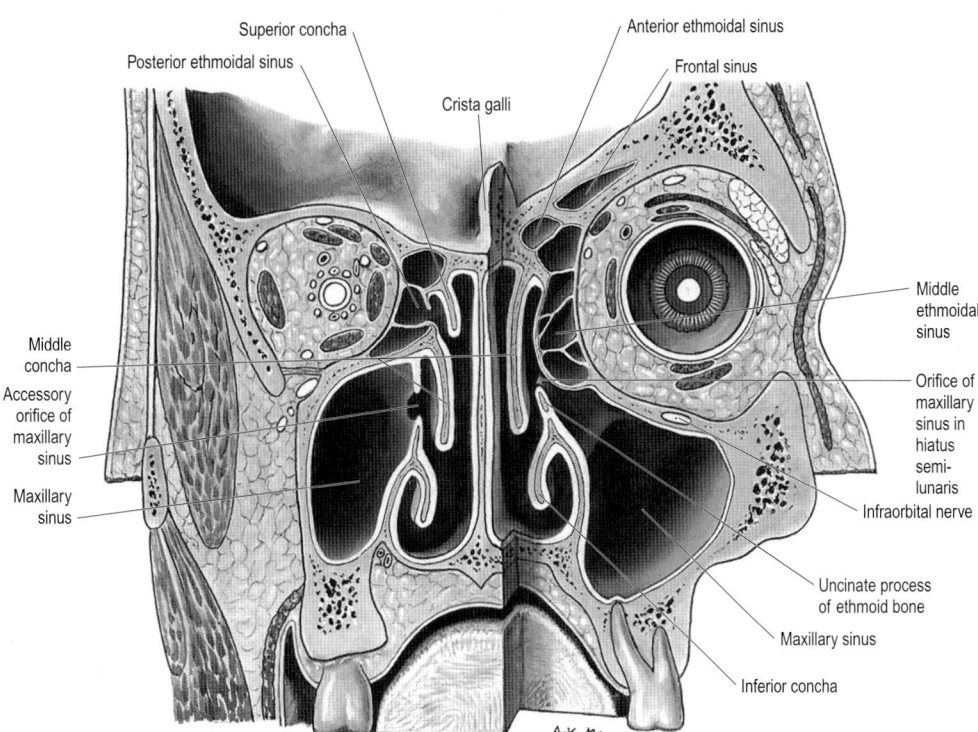

Fig. 32.15 A coronal section through the nasal cavity, viewed from the posterior aspect. On the right side the plane of the section is more anterior. The normal orifice of the maxillary sinus is shown on the right side and a not uncommon accessory orifice on the left side.

correspond to the orbital (roof), alveolar (floor), facial (anterior) and infratemporal (posterior) aspects of the maxilla. Its lateral, truncated apex extends into the zygomatic process, and sometimes even extends into the zygomatic bone forming the zygomatic recess which produces the V-shaped shadows over the antra on a lateral radiograph. Its base is medial and provides much of the lateral wall of the nasal cavity. Its posterior wall contains alveolar canals that may produce ridges in the sinus and that also conduct posterior superior alveolar vessels and nerves to molar teeth. The floor of the sinus is formed by the alveolar process and it often lies below the nasal floor. It is related to the roots of the teeth, especially the second premolar and first molar. However, as the size of the sinus varies, it may extend anteriorly to incorporate the first premolar, and sometimes even the canine, and posteriorly to the third molar tooth. Defects in the bone overlying the roots are not uncommon. The infraorbital canal forms a ridge in the roof of the sinus, and exhibits dehiscences in c.14% of cases. It gives off a fine canal (canalis sinuosus) containing the anterior superior alveolar nerve and vessels that groove the anterior wall. The maxillary sinus may be incompletely divided by septa, complete septa being present only very rarely. The bony medial wall of the sinus is deficient posterosuperiorly at the maxillary hiatus. This large opening is partially closed by the inferior concha and the uncinate process of the ethmoid bone, forming an ostium and anterior and posterior fontanelles. The ostium opens into the middle meatus, usually via the middle part of the hiatus semilunaris: it lies in the angle between the roof and the medial wall and forms the focus of the directional beating of the cilia of the sinus mucoperiosteum. The fontanelles are covered only by periosteum and mucosa and may contain accessory ostia which may be visible on axial CT. All of the openings are nearer the roof than the floor of the sinus which means that the natural drainage of the maxillary sinus is reliant on an intact mucociliary clearance system. Gravitational drainage may be affected by puncture in the lateral wall of the inferior nasal meatus, which is nearer the level of the floor of the sinus. This is useful in disorders of mucociliary clearance such as cystic fibrosis.

Because of the extreme thinness of the sinus walls, a tumour may push up the orbital floor and displace the eyeball; project into the nasal cavity, causing nasal obstruction and bleeding; protrude onto the cheek, causing swelling and numbness when the infraorbital nerve is damaged; spread back into the infratemporal fossa, causing restriction of mouth opening due to pterygoid muscle damage and pain; or spread down into the mouth, loosening teeth and causing malocclusion of the teeth. Extraction of molar teeth may damage the floor, and impact may fracture its walls. Hypoplasia of one maxillary antrum is present in up to 10% of the population, and results in increased density on the plain films.

Osteomeatal complex – The term osteomeatal complex, or osteomeatal unit, refers to the maxillary sinus ostium, ethmoid infundibulum, hiatus semilunaris and frontal recess. It is the final common pathway for drainage of secretions from the maxillary, frontal, anterior and middle ethmoid sinuses into the middle meatus, and obstruction plays a pivotal role in the development and persistence of sinusitis. Coronal high resolution CT (HRCT) reveals these structures in exquisite detail, and is the imaging modality of choice.

Vascular supply and innervation – The arterial supply of the maxillary sinus is derived mainly from the maxillary artery via anterior, middle and superior posterior alveolar branches, and infraorbital and greater palatine arteries. Veins corresponding to the arteries drain into the facial vein or pterygoid venous plexus. Lymph drainage is to the submandibular nodes. The nerve supply is derived from the maxillary nerve via the infraorbital and anterior, middle and posterior superior alveolar nerves.

For further details concerning the dimensions of the various air sinuses and the size and positions of their openings the reader is referred to Lang (1989).

SPREAD OF INFECTION TO CRANIAL CAVITY

Suppuration in the paranasal sinuses occurs frequently. The state of health of the paranasal sinuses is dependent on the state of health of the 'prechambers' through which the sinuses exchange air with the nasal airway and drain mucus. The middle meatus and hiatus semilunaris act as the prechamber for the anterior ethmoidal, frontal and maxillary sinuses, the osteomeatal complex, and can be readily examined with a fibreoptic endoscope. The superior meatus and sphenoethmoidal recess acts as the prechamber for the posterior ethmoidal and sphenoidal sinuses. Obstruction of these prechambers by swollen mucous membranes, polyps or tumours interferes with the ventilation of the sinuses and arrests mucus clearance, which in turn causes overgrowth of bacteria or viruses and consequent sinusitis. Endoscopic examination will show infected mucus draining from the anterior sinus group from the osteomeatal complex onto the superomedial surface of the inferior concha into the pharynx anterior to the pharyngotympanic tubal orifice whilst mucus from the posterior group will drain into the pharynx above and behind the tubal orifice. Maxillary sinus infection may also spread from the infected teeth.

PTERYGOPALATINE FOSSA

OSTEOLOGY OF THE PTERYGOPALATINE FOSSA

The pterygopalatine fossa is a small pyramidal space below the apex of the orbit on the lateral side of the skull. The posterior boundary is the root of the pterygoid process and adjoining anterior surface of the greater wing of the sphenoid, and the anterior boundary is the supero-medial part of the infratemporal surface of the maxilla. The perpendicular plate of the palatine bone, with its orbital and sphenoidal processes forms the medial boundary, and the pterygomaxillary fissure is the lateral boundary. The fossa communicates with the nasal cavity via the sphenopalatine foramen, the orbit via the medial end of the inferior orbital fissure, and the infratemporal fossa via the pterygomaxillary fissure. The latter lies between the back of the maxilla and the pterygoid process of the sphenoid and transmits the maxillary artery. There are two openings in the posterior wall of the pterygopalatine fossa, namely the foramen rotundum, which transmits the maxillary nerve, and the pterygoid canal, which transmits the nerve of the pterygoid canal. When the anterior aspect of the pterygoid plate is examined in a disarticulated sphenoid, it will be seen that the foramen rotundum lies above and lateral to the pterygoid canal (**Fig. 27.13**).

CONTENTS OF THE PTERYGOPALATINE FOSSA

The main contents of the pterygopalatine fossa are the maxillary nerve and many of its branches, the pterygopalatine ganglion and the terminal (third) part of the maxillary artery.

Maxillary nerve (Figs 41.25, 30.6)

The maxillary division of the trigeminal nerve is wholly sensory. It leaves the skull via the foramen rotundum, which leads directly into the posterior wall of the pterygopalatine fossa. Crossing the upper part of the pterygopalatine fossa, the nerve gives off two large ganglionic branches which contain fibres destined for the nose, palate and pharynx, and these pass through the pterygopalatine ganglion without synapsing. It then inclines sharply laterally on the posterior surface of the orbital process of the palatine bone and on the upper part of the posterior surface of the maxilla in the inferior orbital fissure (which is continuous posteriorly with the pterygopalatine fossa): it lies outside the orbital periosteum, and gives off its zygomatic, and then posterior superior alveolar branches. About halfway between the orbital apex and the orbital rim the maxillary nerve turns medially to enter the infraorbital canal as the infraorbital nerve. The subsequent course of the maxillary nerve is described on page 513.

The maxillary nerve gives off many of its branches in the pterygopalatine fossa. They can be subdivided into those that come directly from the nerve, and those that are associated with the pterygopalatine parasympathetic ganglion. Named branches from the main trunk are meningeal, ganglionic, zygomatic, posterior, middle and anterior superior alveolar and infraorbital nerves. Named branches from the pterygopalatine ganglion are orbital, nasopalatine, posterior superior nasal, greater (anterior) palatine, lesser (posterior) palatine and pharyngeal.

Meningeal nerve

The meningeal branch of the maxillary nerve arises within the middle cranial fossa and runs with the middle meningeal vessels. It contributes to the innervation of the dura mater.

Ganglionic branches

There are usually two ganglionic branches that connect the maxillary nerve to the pterygopalatine ganglion.

Zygomatic nerve

The zygomatic branch of the maxillary nerve leaves the pterygopalatine fossa through the inferior orbital fissure together with the maxillary nerve. Its subsequent course is described on page 513.

Posterior superior alveolar nerve

The posterior superior alveolar nerve leaves the maxillary nerve in the pterygopalatine fossa. Its subsequent course and distribution is described in detail on page 601.

Infraorbital nerve

The infraorbital nerve can be regarded as the terminal branch of the maxillary nerve. It leaves the pterygopalatine fossa to enter the orbit at the inferior orbital fissure, and its subsequent course and distribution are described on page 513.

Pterygopalatine ganglion

The pterygopalatine ganglion is the largest of the peripheral parasympathetic ganglia. It is placed deeply in the pterygopalatine fossa, near the sphenopalatine foramen, and anterior to the pterygoid canal and foramen rotundum. It is flattened, reddish-grey in colour, and lies just below the maxillary nerve as it crosses the pterygopalatine fossa. The majority of the 'branches' of the ganglion are connected with it morphologically, but not functionally, because they are primarily sensory branches of the maxillary nerve. Thus they pass through the ganglion without synapsing, and enter the maxillary nerve through its ganglionic branches, but they convey some parasympathetic fibres to the palatine, pharyngeal and nasal mucous glands.

Preganglionic parasympathetic fibres destined for the pterygopalatine ganglion run initially in the greater petrosal branch of the facial nerve, and then in the nerve of the pterygoid canal (Vidian nerve), after the greater petrosal unites with the deep petrosal nerve. The nerve of the pterygoid canal enters the ganglion posteriorly. Postganglionic parasympathetic fibres leave the ganglion and join the maxillary nerve via a ganglionic branch, then travel via the zygomatic and zygomaticotemporal branches of the maxillary nerve to the lacrimal gland (see **Fig. 30.6A**). Preganglionic secretomotor fibres of uncertain origin also travel in the nerve of the pterygoid canal. They synapse in the pterygopalatine ganglion, and postganglionic fibres are distributed to palatine, pharyngeal and nasal mucous glands via palatine and nasal branches of the maxillary nerve (**Fig. 32.9**).

Postganglionic sympathetic fibres pass through the ganglion without synapsing and supply blood vessels and orbitalis. They arise in the superior cervical ganglion and travel via the internal carotid plexus and deep petrosal nerve to enter the pterygopalatine ganglion within the nerve of the pterygoid canal.

General sensory fibres destined for distribution via orbital, nasopalatine, superior alveolar, palatine and pharyngeal branches of the maxillary division of the trigeminal nerve run through the ganglion without synapsing.

Orbital branches

Fine orbital branches enter the orbit through the inferior orbital fissure and supply orbital periosteum. Some fibres also pass through the posterior ethmoidal foramen to supply the sphenoidal and ethmoidal sinuses. The orbital branches probably join branches of the internal carotid nerve to form a 'retro-orbital' plexus from which orbital structures such as the lacrimal gland and orbitalis receive an autonomic innervation.

Nasopalatine nerve (Fig. 32.9)

The nasopalatine nerve leaves the pterygopalatine fossa through the sphenopalatine foramen and enters the nasal cavity. It passes across the cavity to the back of the nasal septum, runs downwards and forwards on the septum in a groove in the vomer, and then turns down through the incisive fossa in the anterior part of the hard palate to enter the roof of the mouth. When an anterior and a posterior incisive foramen exist in this fossa, the left nasopalatine nerve passes through the anterior foramen, and the right nerve passes through the posterior foramen. The nasopalatine nerve supplies the lower part of the nasal septum and the anterior part of the hard palate, where it communicates with the greater palatine nerve.

Posterior superior nasal nerves (lateral and medial)

The posterior superior alveolar nerves enter the back of the nasal cavity through the sphenopalatine foramen. Lateral posterior superior nasal nerves (c.6) innervate the mucosa lining the posterior part of the superior and middle nasal conchae and the posterior ethmoidal sinuses. Two or three medial posterior superior nasal nerves cross the nasal roof below the opening of the sphenoidal sinus to supply the mucosa of the posterior part of the roof and of the nasal septum.

Palatine nerves (greater and lesser)

The greater and lesser palatine nerves pass downwards from the pterygopalatine ganglion through the greater palatine canal. The greater palatine nerve descends through the greater palatine canal, emerges on the hard palate from the greater palatine foramen and runs forwards in a groove on the inferior surface of the bony palate almost to the incisor teeth. It supplies the gingivae, mucosa and glands of the hard palate and also communicates with the terminal filaments of the nasopalatine nerve. In the greater palatine canal it gives off posterior inferior nasal branches that emerge through the perpendicular plate of the palatine bone and ramify over the inferior nasal concha and walls of the middle and inferior meatuses. As it leaves the greater palatine canal, it gives off branches which are distributed to both surfaces of the adjacent part of the soft palate.

The lesser (middle and posterior) palatine nerves are much smaller than the greater palatine nerve. They descend through the greater palatine canal, from which they diverge low down to emerge through the lesser palatine foramina in the tubercle or pyramidal process of the palatine bone. They innervate the uvula, tonsil and soft palate.

Fibres conveying taste impulses from the palate probably pass via the palatine nerves to the pterygopalatine ganglion. They pass through the ganglion without synapsing, and leave via the greater petrosal nerve. Their cell bodies are located in the facial ganglion and their central processes pass via the sensory root of the facial nerve (nervus inter-medius) to the gustatory nucleus in the nucleus of the tractus solitarius.

Pharyngeal nerve (Fig. 32.9)

The pharyngeal branch of the maxillary nerve leaves the pterygopalatine ganglion posteriorly. It passes through the palatovaginal canal with the pharyngeal branch of the maxillary artery and supplies the mucosa of the nasopharynx behind the pharyngotympanic tube.

Vascular supply

Maxillary artery

The maxillary artery passes through the pterygomaxillary fissure from the infratemporal fossa into the pterygopalatine fossa, where it terminates as the third part of the maxillary artery. This part of the artery gives branches which accompany branches of the maxillary nerve (including those associated with the pterygopalatine ganglion).

Posterior superior alveolar artery – The posterior superior alveolar artery arises from the maxillary artery within the pterygopalatine fossa and runs through the pterygomaxillary fissure onto the maxillary tuberosity. It gives off branches which penetrate the bone here to supply the maxillary molar and premolar teeth and the maxillary air sinus, and other branches that supply the buccal mucosa. Occasionally the posterior superior alveolar artery arises from the infraorbital artery.

Infraorbital artery – The infraorbital artery enters the orbit through the inferior orbital fissure. It runs on the floor of the orbit in the infraorbital groove and infraorbital canal and emerges onto the face at the infraorbital foramen to supply the lower eyelid, part of the cheek, the side of the external nose, and the upper lip. While within the infra-orbital canal it gives off the anterior superior alveolar artery which runs downwards to supply the anterior teeth and the anterior part of the maxillary sinus.

Artery of the pterygoid canal – The artery of the pterygoid canal passes through the pterygoid canal and supplies part of the pharyngotympanic tube, tympanic cavity, and the upper part of the pharynx.

Pharyngeal artery – The pharyngeal branch of the maxillary artery passes through the palatovaginal canal, accompanying the nerve of the same name, and is distributed to the mucosa of the nasal roof, nasopharynx, sphenoidal air sinus and pharyngotympanic tube.

Greater (descending) palatine artery – The greater palatine artery leaves the pterygopalatine fossa through the greater (anterior) palatine canal, within which it gives off two or three lesser palatine arteries. The greater palatine artery supplies the inferior meatus of the nose, then passes onto the roof of the hard palate at the greater palatine foramen and runs forwards to supply the hard palate and the palatal gingivae of the maxillary teeth. It gives off a branch that runs up into the incisive canal to anastomose with the sphenopalatine artery, and so contribute to the arterial supply of the nasal septum. The lesser palatine arteries emerge onto the palate through the lesser (posterior) palatine foramen, or foramina, and supply the soft palate.

Sphenopalatine artery – The sphenopalatine branch of the maxillary artery passes through the sphenopalatine foramen and enters the nasal cavity posterior to the superior meatus. From here its posterior lateral nasal branches ramify over the conchae and meatuses, anastomosing with the ethmoidal arteries and nasal branches of the greater palatine artery to supply the frontal, maxillary, ethmoidal and sphenoidal air sinuses. The sphenopalatine artery next crosses anteriorly on the inferior surface of the sphenoid and ends on the nasal septum in a series of posterior septal branches which anastomose with the ethmoidal arteries. A branch descends on the vomer to the incisive canal to anastomose with the greater palatine artery and the septal branch of the superior labial artery.

Nose bleeds

The vast majority of nose bleeds, particularly in children, occur as a result of digital trauma to the anastomosis of arterioles and veins in Little's area (Kiesselbach's plexus), on the nasal septum just inside the nasal vestibule. In older patients brisker bleeding may occur as a result of the spontaneous rupture of arteries further back in the nose. These may be controlled by applying pressure with a nasal pack but where this fails knowledge of the pattern of arterial blood supply to the nasal cavity permits interruption of the appropriate blood supply by ligation or embolization of the feeding vessel. The sphenopalatine artery may be ligated as it enters the nose under endoscopic visualization. The ethmoidal arteries may be exposed within the orbit and ligated to arrest bleeding high up in the nasal cavity. The maxillary artery may be exposed surgically behind the posterior wall of the maxillary sinus and ligated. Alternatively it may be identified radiologically, by instilling a radio-opaque dye, allowing it to be blocked by releasing objects into the artery to embolize and block the bleeding vessel.

Veins of the pterygopalatine fossa

The veins of the pterygopalatine fossa are small and variable. The most consistent is the sphenopalatine vein which drains the posterior aspect of the nose, then passes into the pterygopalatine fossa through the sphenopalatine foramen and ultimately drains into the pterygoid venous plexus via the pterygomaxillary fissure. The inferior ophthalmic vein passes to the pterygoid venous plexus through the inferior orbital fissure.

REFERENCES

Doig TN, McDonald SW, McGregor OA 1998 Possible routes of spread of carcinoma of the maxillary sinus to the oral cavity. Clin Anat 11: 149–56.

Emanuel JM 1998 Epistaxis. In: Cummings CW et al (eds) Otolaryngology Head and Neck Surgery, vol. 2. 3rd edition. St Louis: Mosby: 852–65.
Describes the blood supply to the nose and the surgical approaches to control epistaxis.

Lang J 1989 Clinical Anatomy of the Nose, Nasal Cavity and Paranasal Sinuses. Stuttgart: Thième.

McGowan DA, Baxter PW, James J 1993 The Maxillary Sinus. Oxford: Wright.

Navarro JAC 1997 The Nasal Cavity and Paranasal Sinuses: Surgical Anatomy. Berlin: Springer.

Stammberger H, Kennedy DW (eds) 1995 Paranasal sinuses: anatomic terminology and nomenclature. Ann Otol Rhinol Laryngol (suppl 167) 104(10) Part 2: 7–16.

Traxler H, Windisch A, Geyerhofer U, Surd R, Solar P, Firbas W 1999 Arterial blood supply of the maxillary sinus. Clin Anat 12: 417–21.

Oral cavity

The mouth or oral cavity extends from the lips and cheeks externally to the anterior pillars of the fauces internally, where it continues into the oropharynx. The mouth can be subdivided into the vestibule external to the teeth and the oral cavity proper internal to the teeth. The palate forms the roof of the mouth and separates the oral and nasal cavities. The floor of the mouth is formed by the mylohyoid muscles and is occupied mainly by the tongue. The lateral walls of the mouth are defined by the cheeks and retromolar regions. Three pairs of major salivary glands (parotid, submandibular and sublingual) and numerous minor salivary glands (labial, buccal, palatal, lingual) open into the mouth. The muscles in the oral cavity are associated with the lips, cheeks, floor of the mouth and tongue. The muscles of the lips and cheeks are described with the face on page 504. The muscles of the soft palate are described with the pharynx on page 627.

The mouth is concerned primarily with the ingestion and mastication of food, which is mainly the function of the teeth. The mouth is also associated with phonation and ventilation, but these are secondary functions.

CHEEKS

The external features of the cheeks are described on page 497. Internally, the mucosa of the cheek is tightly adherent to buccinator and is thus stretched when the mouth is opened and wrinkled when closed. Ectopic sebaceous glands may be evident as yellow patches (Fordyce's spots). Their numbers increase in puberty and in later life.

Few structural landmarks are visible. The parotid duct drains into the cheek opposite the maxillary second molar tooth at a small parotid papilla. A hyperkeratinized line (the linea alba) may be seen at a position related to the occlusal plane of the teeth. In the retromolar region, a fold of mucosa which contains the pterygomandibular raphe extends from the upper to the lower alveolus. The entrance to the pterygomandibular space (which contains the lingual and inferior alveolar nerves) lies lateral to this fold and medial to the ridge produced by the anterior border of the ramus of the mandible. This is the site for injection for an inferior alveolar nerve block.

Vascular supply and innervation – The cheek receives its arterial blood supply principally from the buccal branch of the maxillary artery, and is innervated by cutaneous branches of the maxillary division of the trigeminal nerve, via the zygomaticofacial and infraorbital nerves, and by the buccal branch of the mandibular division of the trigeminal nerve.

LIPS

The external features of the lips are described on page 497. The central part of the lips contain orbicularis oris. Internally, the labial mucosa is smooth and shiny and shows small elevations caused by underlying mucous glands.

The position and activity of the lips are important in controlling the degree of protrusion of the incisors. With normal (competent) lips, the tips of the maxillary incisors lie below the upper border of the lower lip, and this arrangement helps to maintain the 'normal' inclination of the incisors. When the lips are incompetent, the maxillary incisors may not be so controlled and the lower lip may even lie behind them, thus producing an exaggerated proclination of these teeth. A tight, or over-active, lip musculature may be associated with retroclined maxillary incisors.

Vascular supply and innervation – The lips are mainly supplied by the superior and inferior labial branches of the facial artery. The upper lip is innervated by superior labial branches of the infraorbital nerve and the lower lip is innervated by the mental branch of the mandibular division of the trigeminal.

ORAL VESTIBULE

The oral vestibule is a slit-like space between the lips or cheeks on one side and the teeth on the other. When the teeth occlude, the vestibule is a closed space that only communicates with the oral cavity proper in the retromolar regions behind the last molar tooth on each side. Where the mucosa that covers the alveolus of the jaw is reflected onto the lips and cheeks, a trough or sulcus is formed which is called the fornix vestibuli. A variable number of sickle-shaped folds containing loose connective tissue run across the fornix vestibuli. In the midline these are the upper and lower labial frena (or frenula). Other folds may traverse the fornix near the canines or premolars. The folds in the lower fornix are said to be more pronounced than those in the upper fornix (**Fig. 33.1**).

The upper labial frenum is normally attached well below the alveolar crest. A large frenum with an attachment near the crest may be associated with a midline gap (diastema) between the maxillary first incisors. This can be corrected by simple surgical removal of the frenum, as it contains no structures of clinical importance. Prominent frena may also influence the stability of dentures.

ORAL MUCOSA

The oral mucosa is continuous with the skin at the labial margins and with the pharyngeal mucosa at the oropharyngeal isthmus. It varies in structure, function and appearance in different regions of the oral cavity and is traditionally divided into lining, masticatory and specialized mucosae.

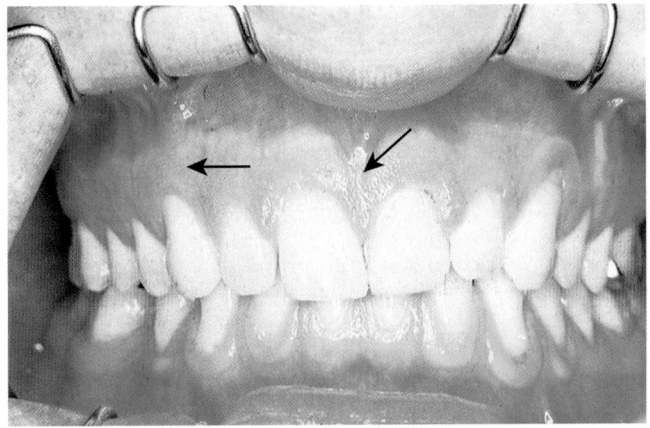

Fig. 33.1 Anterior view of the dentition in centric occlusion, with the lips retracted. Note the pale pink, stippled gingivae and the red, shiny, smooth alveolar mucosa. The degree of overbite is rather pronounced and the gingiva and its epithelial attachment have receded onto the root of the upper left canine. Note frena (arrows).

LINING MUCOSA

The lining mucosa is red in colour, and covers the soft palate, ventral surface of the tongue, floor of the mouth, alveolar processes excluding the gingivae and the internal surfaces of the lips and cheeks. It has a non-keratinized stratified squamous epithelium which overlies a loosely fibrous lamina propria, and the submucosa contains some fat deposits and collections of minor mucous salivary glands. The oral mucosa covering the alveolar bone – which supports the roots of the teeth – and the necks (cervical region) of the teeth is divided into two main components. That portion lining the lower part of the alveolus is loosely attached to the periosteum via a diffuse submucosa and is termed the alveolar mucosa. It is delineated from the masticatory gingival mucosa, which covers the upper part of the alveolar bone and the necks of the teeth, by a well-defined junction, the mucogingival junction. The alveolar mucosa appears dark red, the gingival appears pale pink. These colour differences relate to differences in the type of keratinization and the proximity to the surface of underlying small blood vessels which may sometimes be seen coursing beneath the alveolar mucosa.

MASTICATORY MUCOSA AND THE GINGIVAE

Masticatory mucosa, i.e. mucosa that is subjected to masticatory stress, is bound firmly to underlying bone or to the necks of the teeth, and forms a mucoperiosteum in the gingivae and palatine raphe. Gingival, palatal and dorsal lingual mucosae are keratinized or parakeratinized.

The gingivae may be further subdivided into the attached gingivae and the free gingivae. Attached gingivae are firmly bound to the periosteum of the alveolus and to the teeth, whereas free gingivae, which constitute c.1 mm margin of the gingivae, lie unattached around the cervical region of each tooth. The free gingival groove between the free and attached gingivae corresponds roughly to the floor of the gingival sulcus which separates the inner surface of the attached gingivae from the enamel. The interdental papilla is that part of the gingivae which fills the space between adjacent teeth. The surface of the attached gingivae is characteristically stippled, although there is considerable inter-individual variation in the degree of stippling, and variation according to age, sex and the health of the gingivae. The free gingivae are not stippled. A mucogingival line delineates the attached gingivae on the lingual surface of the lower jaw from the alveolar mucosa towards the floor of the mouth. There is no corresponding obvious division between the attached gingivae and the remainder of the palatal mucosa because this whole surface is orthokeratinized masticatory mucosa, which is pink.

A submucosa is absent from the gingivae and the midline palatine raphe, but is present over the rest of the hard palate. Posterolaterally it is thick where it contains mucous salivary glands and the greater palatine nerves and vessels, and it is anchored to the periosteum of the maxillae and palatine bones by collagenous septa.

VASCULAR SUPPLY AND LYMPHATIC DRAINAGE

The gingival tissues derive their blood supply from the maxillary and lingual arteries. The buccal gingivae around the maxillary cheek teeth are supplied by gingival and perforating branches from the posterior superior alveolar artery and by the buccal branch of the maxillary artery. The labial gingivae of anterior teeth are supplied by labial branches of the infraorbital artery and by perforating branches of the anterior superior alveolar artery. The palatal gingivae are supplied primarily by branches of the greater palatine artery.

The buccal gingivae associated with the mandibular cheek teeth are supplied by the buccal branch of the maxillary artery and by perforating branches from the inferior alveolar artery. The labial gingivae around the anterior teeth are supplied by the mental artery and by perforating branches of the incisive artery. The lingual gingivae are supplied by perforating branches from the inferior alveolar artery and by its lingual branch, and by the main lingual artery, a branch of the external carotid artery.

No accurate description is available concerning the venous drainage of the gingivae, although it may be assumed that buccal, lingual, greater palatine and nasopalatine veins are involved. These veins run into the pterygoid plexuses (apart from the lingual veins, which pass directly into the internal jugular veins).

The lymph vessels of the labial and buccal gingivae of the maxillary and mandibular teeth unite to drain into the submandibular nodes, though in the labial region of the mandibular incisors they may drain into the submental lymph nodes. The lingual and palatal gingivae drain into the jugulodigastric group of nodes, either directly or indirectly through the submandibular nodes.

Table 33.1 Nerve supply to the teeth and gingivae

	Nasopalatine nerve	Greater palatine nerve		Palatal gingivae
Maxilla	Anterior superior alveolar nerve	Middle superior alveolar nerve	Posterior superior alveolar nerve	Teeth
	Infraorbital nerve	Posterior superior alveolar nerve and buccal nerve		Buccal gingivae
	1 2 3	4 5 6	7 8	Tooth position
	Mental nerve	Buccal nerve and perforating branches of inferior alveolar nerve		Buccal gingivae
Mandible	Incisive nerve	Inferior alveolar nerve		Teeth
	Lingual nerve and perforating branches of inferior alveolar nerve			Lingual gingivae

(By permission from Berkovitz BKB, Holland GR, Moxham BJ 2002 Oral Anatomy, Embryology and Histology, 3rd edn. Edinburgh: Mosby.)

INNERVATION (Table 33.1)

The nerves supplying the gingivae in the upper jaw come from the maxillary nerve via its greater palatine, nasopalatine and anterior, middle and posterior superior alveolar branches. Surgical division of the nasopalatine nerve causes no obvious sensory deficit in the anterior part of the palate, which suggests that the territory of the greater palatine nerve reaches as far forwards as the gingivae lingual to the incisor teeth. The mandibular nerve innervates the gingivae in the lower jaw by its inferior alveolar, lingual and buccal branches.

SPECIALIZED ORAL MUCOSA

The specialized mucosa which covers the anterior two-thirds of the dorsum of the tongue is described on page 584.

OROPHARYNGEAL ISTHMUS (Fig. 33.2)

The oropharyngeal isthmus lies between the soft palate and the dorsum of the tongue, and is bounded on both sides by the palatoglossal arches. Each palatoglossal arch runs downwards, laterally and forwards, from the soft palate to the side of the tongue and consists of palatoglossus and its covering mucous membrane. The approximation of the arches shuts off the mouth from the oropharynx, and is essential to deglutition (p. 630).

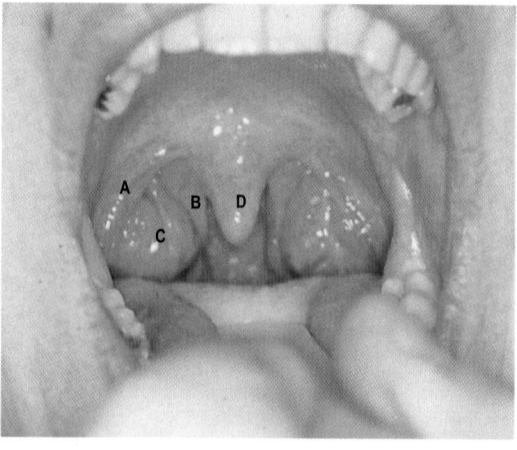

Fig. 33.2 Back of the mouth showing the soft palate and oropharyngeal isthmus. A, palatoglossal fold; B, palatopharyngeal fold; C, palatine tonsil; D, uvula. (By permission from Berkovitz BKB, Holland GR, Moxham BJ 2002 Oral Anatomy, Embryology and Histology, 3rd edn. Edinburgh: Mosby.)

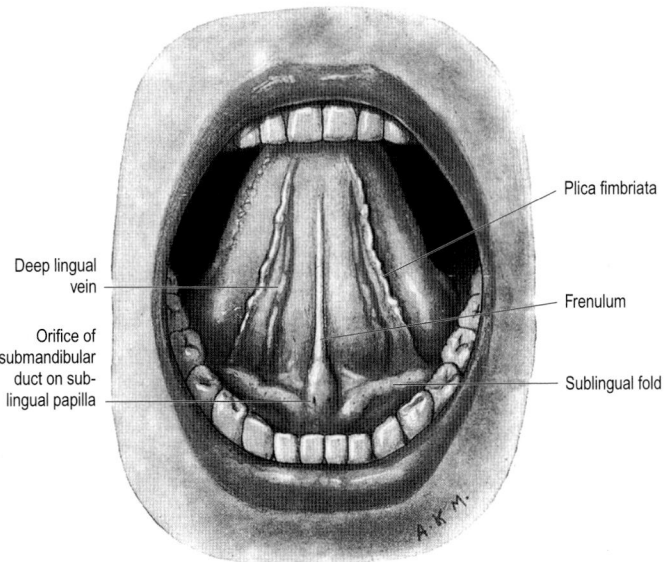

Fig. 33.3 Cavity of the mouth. The tip of the tongue is turned upwards.

Deep lingual vein

Orifice of submandibular duct on sub-lingual papilla

Plica fimbriata

Frenulum

Sublingual fold

FLOOR OF THE MOUTH (Fig. 33.3)

The floor of the mouth is a small horseshoe-shaped region situated beneath the movable part of the tongue and above the muscular diaphragm formed by the mylohyoid muscles. A fold of tissue, the lingual frenum, extends onto the inferior surface of the tongue from near the base of the tongue. It occasionally extends across the floor of the mouth to be attached onto the mandibular alveolus. The submandibular salivary ducts open into the mouth at the sublingual papilla, which is a large centrally positioned protuberance at the base of the tongue.

The sublingual folds lie on either side of the sublingual papilla and cover the underlying submandibular ducts and sublingual salivary glands. The blood supply of the floor of the mouth is described with the blood supply of the tongue (p. 587). The main muscle forming the floor of the mouth is mylohyoid. Immediately above it is geniohyoid.

MYLOHYOID (Fig. 31.10)

Mylohyoid lies superior to the anterior belly of digastric and, with its contralateral fellow, forms a muscular floor for the oral cavity. It is a flat, triangular sheet attached to the whole length of the mylohyoid line of the mandible. The posterior fibres pass medially and slightly downwards to the front of the body of the hyoid bone near its lower border. The middle and anterior fibres from each side decussate in a median fibrous raphe that stretches from the symphysis menti to the hyoid bone. The median raphe is sometimes absent, in which case the two muscles form a continuous sheet, or it may be fused with the anterior belly of digastric. In about one-third of subjects there is a hiatus in the muscle through which a process of the sublingual gland protrudes.

Relations – The inferior (external) surface is related to platysma, anterior belly of digastric, the superficial part of the submandibular gland, the facial and submental vessels, and the mylohyoid vessels and nerve. The superior (internal) surface is related to geniohyoid, part of hyoglossus and styloglossus, the hypoglossal and lingual nerves, the submandibular ganglion, the sublingual gland, the deep part of the submandibular gland and its duct, the lingual and sublingual vessels and, posteriorly, the mucous membrane of the mouth.

Vascular supply – Mylohyoid receives its arterial supply from the sublingual branch of the lingual artery, the maxillary artery, via the mylohyoid branch of the inferior alveolar artery, and the submental branch of the facial artery.

Innervation – Mylohyoid is supplied by the mylohyoid branch of the inferior alveolar nerve.

Actions – Mylohyoid elevates the floor of the mouth in the first stage of deglutition. It may also elevate the hyoid bone or depress the mandible.

GENIOHYOID (Fig. 33.6)

Geniohyoid is a narrow muscle which lies above the medial part of mylohyoid. It arises from the inferior mental spine (genial tubercle) on the back of the symphysis menti, and runs backwards and slightly downwards to attach to the anterior surface of the body of the hyoid bone. The paired muscles are contiguous and may occasionally fuse with each other or with genioglossus.

Vascular supply – The blood supply to geniohyoid is derived from the lingual artery (sublingual branch).

Innervation – Geniohyoid is supplied by the first cervical spinal nerve, through the hypoglossal nerve.

Actions – Geniohyoid elevates the hyoid bone and draws it forwards, and therefore acts partly as an antagonist to stylohyoid. When the hyoid bone is fixed, geniohyoid depresses the mandible.

PALATE

The palate forms the roof of the mouth and is divisible into two regions, namely, the hard palate in front and soft palate behind.

SOFT PALATE

The soft palate is described with the pharynx on page 623.

HARD PALATE (Fig. 33.13A)

The hard palate is formed by the palatine processes of the maxillae and the horizontal plates of the palatine bones. The hard palate is bounded in front and at the sides by the tooth-bearing alveolus of the upper jaw and is continuous posteriorly with the soft palate. It is covered by a thick mucosa bound tightly to the underlying periosteum. In its more lateral regions it also possesses a submucosa containing the main neurovascular bundle. The mucosa is covered by keratinized stratified squamous epithelium which shows regional variations and may be ortho- or parakeratinized.

The periphery of the hard palate consists of gingivae. A narrow ridge, the palatine raphe, devoid of submucosa, runs anteroposteriorly in the midline. An oval prominence, the incisive papilla, lies at the anterior extremity of the raphe and covers the incisive fossa at the oral opening of the incisive canal. It also marks the position of the fetal nasopalatine canal. Irregular transverse ridges or rugae, each containing a core of dense connective tissue, radiate outwards from the palatine raphe in the anterior half of the hard palate: their pattern is unique.

The submucosa in the posterior half of the hard palate contains minor salivary glands of the mucous type. These secrete through numerous small ducts, although bilaterally a larger duct collecting from many of these glands often opens at the paired palatine foveae. These depressions, sometimes a few millimetres deep, flank the midline raphe at the posterior border of the hard palate. They provide a useful landmark for the extent of an upper denture. The upper surface of the hard palate is the floor of the nasal cavity and is covered by ciliated respiratory epithelium.

Vascular supply and lymphatic drainage of the hard palate – The palate derives its blood supply principally from the greater palatine artery, a branch of the third part of the maxillary artery. The greater palatine artery descends with its accompanying nerve in the palatine canal, where it gives off two or three lesser palatine arteries which are transmitted through lesser palatine canals to supply the soft palate and tonsil, and anastomose with the ascending palatine branch of the facial artery. The greater palatine artery emerges on to the oral surface of the palate at the greater palatine foramen and runs in a curved groove near the alveolar border of the hard palate to the incisive canal. It ascends this canal and anastomoses with septal branches of the nasopalatine artery to supply the gingivae, palatine glands and mucous membrane.

The veins of the hard palate accompany the arteries and drain largely to the pterygoid plexus.

Innervation of the hard palate (Fig. 32.9) – The sensory nerves of the hard palate are the greater palatine and nasopalatine branches of the maxillary nerve, which all pass through the pterygopalatine ganglion (p. 579) The greater palatine nerve descends through the greater palatine canal, emerges on the hard palate from the greater palatine foramen, runs forwards in a groove on the inferior surface of the bony palate almost to the incisor teeth and supplies the gums and the mucosa and glands of the hard palate. It also communicates with the terminal filaments of the nasopalatine nerve. As it leaves the greater palatine canal, it supplies palatine branches to both surfaces of the soft palate. The lesser (middle and posterior) palatine nerves, which are much smaller, descend through the greater palatine canal and emerge through the lesser palatine foramina in the tubercle of the palatine bone to supply the uvula, tonsil and soft palate. The nasopalatine nerves enter the palate at the incisive foramen and are branches of the maxillary nerve which pass through the pterygopalatine ganglion to supply the anterior part of the hard palate behind the incisor teeth.

Fibres conveying taste impulses from the palate probably pass via the palatine nerves to the pterygopalatine ganglion, and travel through it without synapsing to join the nerve of the pterygoid canal and the greater petrosal nerve to the facial ganglion, where their cell bodies are situated. The central processes of these neurones traverse the sensory root of the facial nerve (nervus intermedius) to pass to the gustatory nucleus in the nucleus of the tractus solitarius. Parasympathetic postganglionic secretomotor fibres from the pterygopalatine ganglion run with the nerves to supply the palatine mucous glands.

TONGUE

The tongue is a highly muscular organ of deglutition, taste and speech. It is partly oral and partly pharyngeal in position, and is attached by its muscles to the hyoid bone, mandible, styloid processes, soft palate and the pharyngeal wall. It has a root, an apex, a curved dorsum and an inferior surface. Its mucosa is normally pink and moist, and is attached closely to the underlying muscles. The dorsal mucosa is covered by numerous papillae, some of which bear taste buds. Intrinsic muscle fibres are arranged in a complex interlacing pattern of longitudinal, transverse, vertical and horizontal fasciculi and this allows great mobility. Fasciculi are separated by a variable amount of adipose tissue which increases posteriorly. The root of the tongue is attached to the hyoid bone and mandible, and between them it is in contact inferiorly with geniohyoid and mylohyoid. The dorsum (posterosuperior surface) is generally convex in all directions at rest. It is divided by a V-shaped sulcus terminalis into an anterior, oral (presulcal) part which faces upwards, and a posterior, pharyngeal (postsulcal) part which faces posteriorly. The anterior part forms about two-thirds of the length of the tongue. The two limbs of the sulcus terminalis run anterolaterally to the palatoglossal arches from a median depression, the foramen caecum, which marks the site of the upper end of the embryonic thyroid diverticulum. The oral and pharyngeal parts of the tongue differ in their mucosa, innervation and developmental origins.

ORAL (PRESULCAL) PART (Figs 33.4, 33.5)

The presulcal part of the tongue is located in the floor of the oral cavity. It has an apex touching the incisor teeth, a margin in contact with the gums and teeth, and a superior surface (dorsum) related to the hard and soft palates. On each side, in front of the palatoglossal arch, there are four or five vertical folds, the foliate papillae, which represent vestiges of larger papillae found in many other mammals. The dorsal mucosa has a longitudinal median sulcus and is covered by filiform, fungiform and circumvallate papillae. The mucosa on the inferior (ventral) surface is smooth, purplish and reflected onto the oral floor and gums: it is connected to the oral floor anteriorly by the lingual frenulum. The deep lingual vein, which is visible, lies lateral to the frenulum on either side. The plica fimbriata, a fringed mucosal ridge directed anteromedially towards the apex of the tongue, lies lateral to the vein. This part of the tongue develops from the lingual swellings of the mandibular arch and from the tuberculum impar.

PHARYNGEAL (POSTSULCAL) PART (Fig. 33.4)

The postsulcal part of the tongue constitutes its base and lies posterior to the palatoglossal arches. Although it forms the anterior wall of the oropharynx, it is described here for convenience. Its mucosa is reflected laterally onto the palatine tonsils and pharyngeal wall, and posteriorly onto the epiglottis by a median and two lateral glossoepiglottic folds

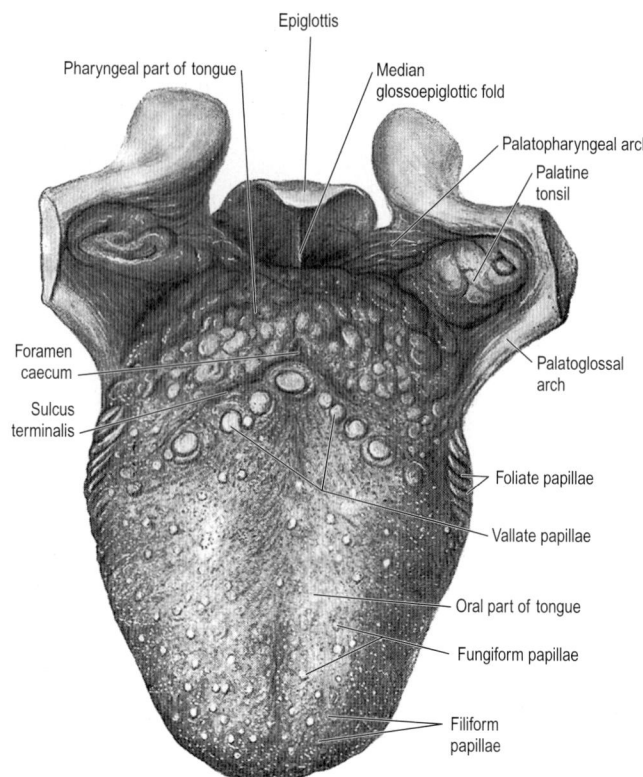

Fig. 33.4 Dorsum of the tongue, with adjoining palatoglossal and palatopharyngeal arches, and epiglottis. The palatine tonsils lie in the tonsillar recesses on either side.

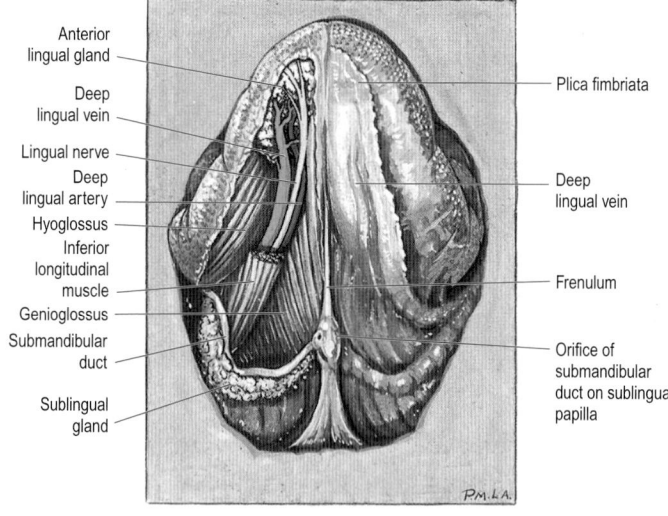

Fig. 33.5 Dissection of the inferior surface of the tongue, also showing the sublingual glands and submandibular duct openings. On the right side the mucous membrane has been removed and the inferior longitudinal muscle has been divided and partially resected.

which surround two depressions or valleculae. The pharyngeal part of the tongue is devoid of papillae, and exhibits low elevations. There are underlying lymphoid nodules which are embedded in the submucosa and collectively termed the lingual tonsil. The ducts of small seromucous glands open on the apices of these elevations. The postsulcal part of the tongue develops from the hypobranchial eminence. On the rare occasions that the thyroid gland fails to migrate away from the tongue during development it remains in the postsulcal part of the tongue as a functioning lingual thyroid gland.

MUSCLES OF THE TONGUE

The tongue is divided by a median fibrous septum, attached to the body of the hyoid bone. There are extrinsic and intrinsic muscles in each half, the former extending outside the tongue and moving it bodily, the latter wholly within it and altering its shape. The extrinsic musculature consists of four pairs of muscles namely genioglossus, hyoglossus, styloglossus (and chondroglossus) and palatoglossus. The intrinsic muscles are the bilateral superior and inferior longitudinal, the transverse and the vertical.

Genioglossus (Fig. 33.6)

Genioglossus is triangular in sagittal section, lying near and parallel to the midline. It arises from a short tendon attached to the superior genial tubercle behind the mandibular symphysis, above the origin of geniohyoid. From this point it fans out backwards and upwards. The inferior fibres of genioglossus are attached by a thin aponeurosis to the upper anterior surface of the hyoid body near the midline (a few fasciculi passing between hyoglossus and chondroglossus to blend with the middle constrictor of the pharynx). Intermediate fibres pass backwards into the posterior part of the tongue, and superior fibres ascend forwards to enter the whole length of the ventral surface of the tongue from root to apex, intermingling with the intrinsic muscles. The muscles of opposite sides are separated posteriorly by the lingual septum. Anteriorly they are variably blended by decussation of fasciculi across the midline. The attachment of the genioglossi to the genial tubercles prevents the tongue from sinking back and obstructing respiration, therefore anaesthetists pull the mandible forward to obtain the full benefit of this connection.

Vascular supply – Genioglossus is supplied by the sublingual branch of the lingual artery and the submental branch of the facial artery.

Innervation – Genioglossus is innervated by the hypoglossal nerve.

Actions – Genioglossus brings about the forward traction of the tongue to protrude its apex from the mouth. Acting bilaterally, the two muscles depress the central part of the tongue, making it concave from side to side. Acting unilaterally, the tongue diverges to the opposite side.

Hyoglossus (Fig. 33.6)

Hyoglossus is thin and quadrilateral, and arises from the whole length of the greater cornu and the front of the body of the hyoid bone. It passes vertically up to enter the side of the tongue between styloglossus laterally and the inferior longitudinal muscle medially. Fibres arising from the body of the hyoid overlap those from the greater cornu.

Relations – Hyoglossus is related at its superficial surface to the digastric tendon, stylohyoid, styloglossus and mylohyoid, the lingual nerve and submandibular ganglion, the sublingual gland, the deep part of the submandibular gland and duct, the hypoglossal nerve and the deep lingual vein. By its deep surface it is related to the stylohyoid ligament, genioglossus, the middle constrictor and the inferior longitudinal muscle of the tongue, and the glossopharyngeal nerve. Posteroinferiorly it is separated from the middle constrictor by the lingual artery. This part of the muscle is in the lateral wall of the pharynx, below the palatine tonsil. Passing deep to the posterior border of hyoglossus are, in

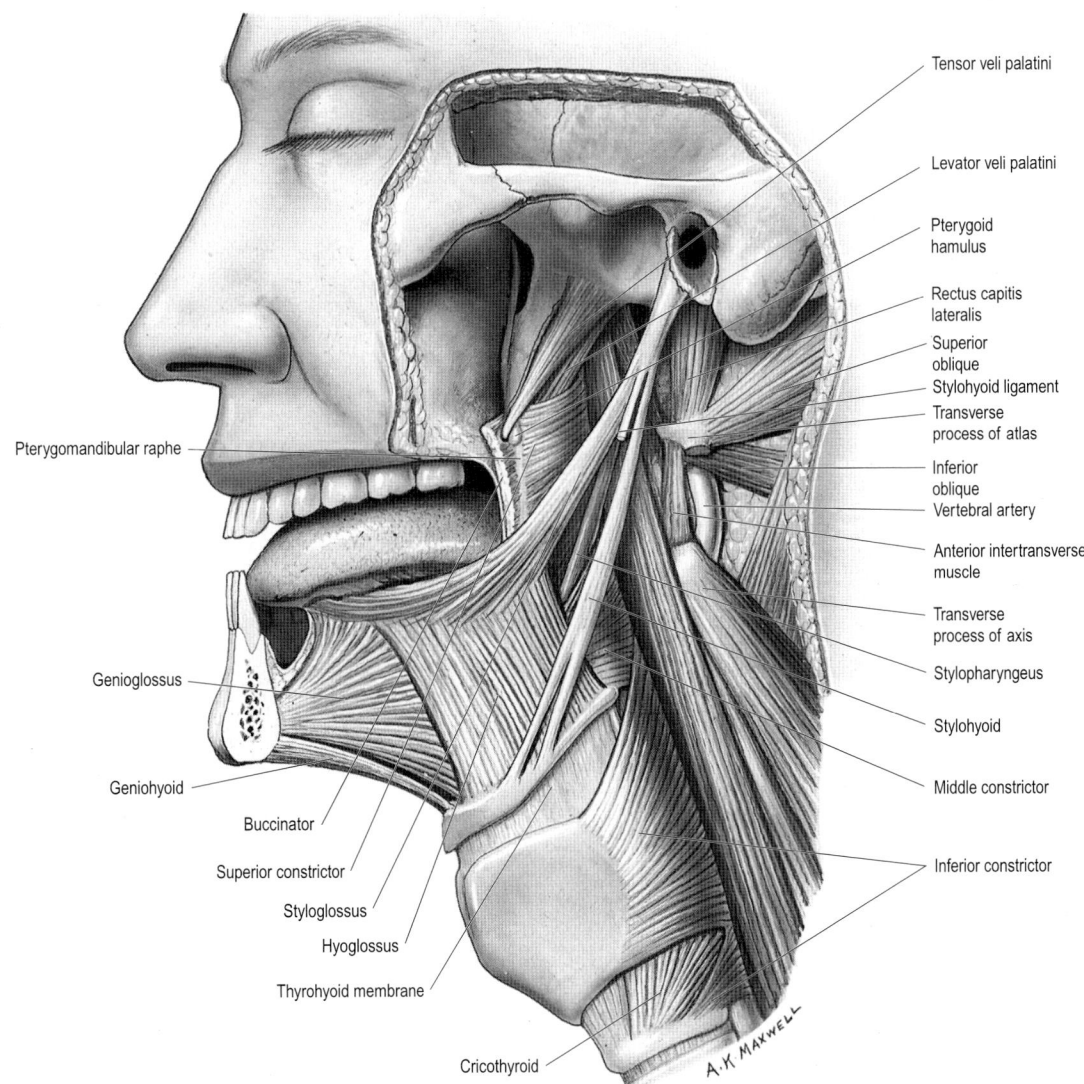

Tensor veli palatini
Levator veli palatini
Pterygoid hamulus
Rectus capitis lateralis
Superior oblique
Stylohyoid ligament
Transverse process of atlas
Inferior oblique
Vertebral artery
Anterior intertransverse muscle
Transverse process of axis
Stylopharyngeus
Stylohyoid
Middle constrictor
Inferior constrictor

Pterygomandibular raphe

Genioglossus
Geniohyoid
Buccinator
Superior constrictor
Styloglossus
Hyoglossus
Thyrohyoid membrane
Cricothyroid

Fig. 33.6 Dissection showing the muscles of the tongue and pharynx. Note that palatoglossus is not shown here, but is depicted in **Fig. 35.3**.

A.K. MAXWELL

descending order: the glossopharyngeal nerve, stylohyoid ligament and lingual artery.

Vascular supply – Hyoglossus is supplied by the sublingual branch of the lingual artery and the submental branch of the facial artery.

Innervation – Hyoglossus is innervated by the hypoglossal nerve.

Action – Hyoglossus depresses the tongue.

Chondroglossus

Sometimes described as a part of hyoglossus, this muscle is separated from it by some fibres of genioglossus, which pass to the side of the pharynx. It is c.2 cm long, arising from the medial side and base of the lesser cornu and the adjoining part of the body of the hyoid. It ascends to merge into the intrinsic musculature between the hyoglossus and genioglossus muscles. A small slip occasionally springs from the cartilago triticea and enters the tongue with the posterior fibres of the hyoglossus muscle.

Vascular supply, innervation and action – These are similar to those described for hyoglossus.

Styloglossus (Fig. 33.6)

Styloglossus is the shortest and smallest of the three styloid muscles. It arises from the anterolateral aspect of the styloid process near its apex, and from the styloid end of the stylomandibular ligament. Passing downwards and forwards, it divides at the side of the tongue into a longitudinal part, which enters the tongue dorsolaterally to blend with the inferior longitudinal muscle in front of hyoglossus, and an oblique part, overlapping hyoglossus and decussating with it.

Vascular supply – Styloglossus is supplied by the sublingual branch of the lingual artery.

Innervation – Styloglossus is innervated by the hypoglossal nerve.

Action – Styloglossus draws the tongue up and backwards.

Stylohyoid ligament (Fig. 33.6)

The stylohyoid ligament is a fibrous cord which extends from the tip of the styloid process to the lesser cornu of the hyoid bone. It gives attachment to some fibres of styloglossus and the middle constrictor of the pharynx and is closely related to the lateral wall of the oropharynx.

Below it is overlapped by hyoglossus. The ligament is derived embryologically from the second branchial arch. It may be partially calcified.

Palatoglossus

Palatoglossus is closely associated with the soft palate in function and innervation, and is described with the other palatal muscles (p. 628).

Intrinsic muscles (Fig. 33.7)

Superior longitudinal

The superior longitudinal muscle constitutes a thin stratum of oblique and longitudinal fibres lying beneath the mucosa of the dorsum of the tongue. It extends forwards from the submucous fibrous tissue near the epiglottis and from the median lingual septum to the lingual margins. Some fibres are inserted into the mucous membrane.

Inferior longitudinal

The inferior longitudinal muscle is a narrow band of muscle close to the inferior lingual surface between genioglossus and hyoglossus. It extends from the root of the tongue to the apex. Some of its posterior fibres are connected to the body of the hyoid bone. Anteriorly it blends with styloglossus.

Transverse

The transverse muscles pass laterally from the median fibrous septum to the submucous fibrous tissue at the lingual margin, blending with palatopharyngeus.

Vertical

The vertical muscles extend from the dorsal to the ventral aspects of the tongue in the anterior borders.

Vascular supply

The intrinsic muscles are supplied by the lingual artery.

Innervation

All intrinsic lingual muscles are innervated by the hypoglossal nerve.

Actions

The intrinsic muscles alter the shape of the tongue. Thus, contraction of the superior and inferior longitudinal muscles tend to shorten the tongue, but the former also turns the apex and sides upwards to make the dorsum concave, while the latter pulls the apex down to make the dorsum convex. The transverse muscle narrows and elongates the tongue

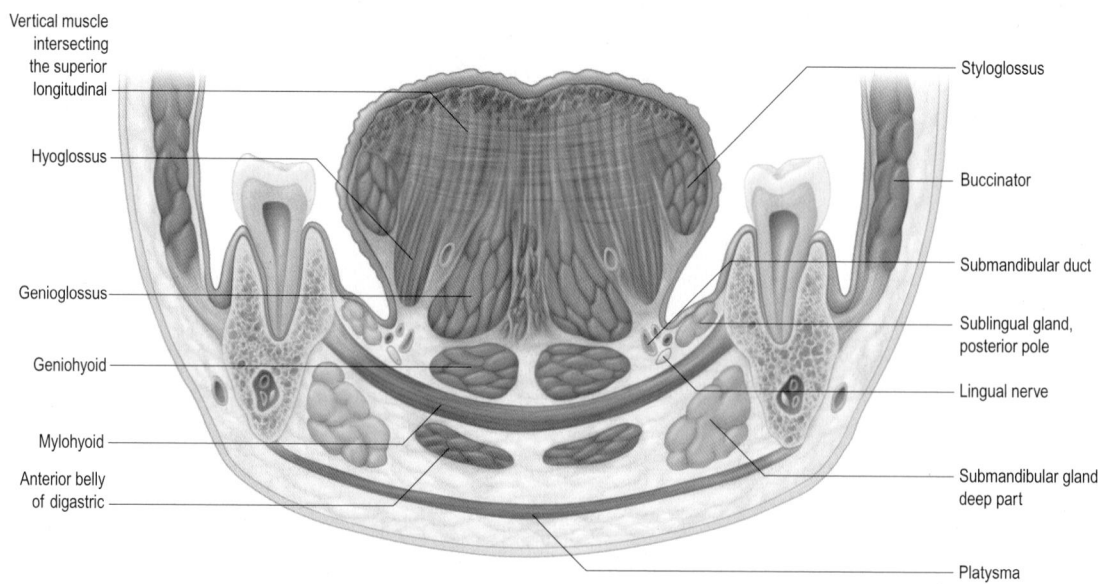

Labels (left, top to bottom): Vertical muscle intersecting the superior longitudinal; Hyoglossus; Genioglossus; Geniohyoid; Mylohyoid; Anterior belly of digastric

Labels (right, top to bottom): Styloglossus; Buccinator; Submandibular duct; Sublingual gland, posterior pole; Lingual nerve; Submandibular gland, deep part; Platysma

Fig. 33.7 Cross-section through the tongue, the mouth and the body of the mandible opposite the first molar tooth.

while the vertical muscle makes it flatter and wider. Acting alone or in pairs and in endless combination, the intrinsic muscles give the tongue precise and highly varied mobility, important not only in alimentary function but also in speech.

VASCULAR SUPPLY AND LYMPHATIC DRAINAGE OF THE TONGUE

Lingual artery (Fig. 33.8)

The tongue and the floor of the mouth are supplied chiefly by the lingual artery, which arises from the anterior surface of the external carotid artery (**Figs 31.7, 31.16, 31.14**). It passes between hyoglossus and the middle constrictor of the pharynx to reach the floor of the mouth accompanied by the lingual veins and the glossopharyngeal nerve. At the anterior border of hyoglossus, the lingual artery bends sharply upwards. It is covered by the mucosa of the tongue and lies between genioglossus medially and the inferior longitudinal muscle laterally. Near the tip of the tongue it anastomoses with its contralateral fellow. The branches of the lingual artery form a rich anastomotic network, which supplies the musculature of the tongue, and a very dense submucosal plexus. Named branches of the lingual artery in the floor of the mouth are the dorsal lingual, sublingual and deep lingual arteries.

Dorsal lingual arteries

The dorsal lingual arteries are usually two or three small vessels. They arise medial to hyoglossus and ascend to the posterior part of the dorsum of the tongue. The vessels supply its mucous membrane, and the palatoglossal arch, tonsil, soft palate and epiglottis. They anastomose with their contralateral fellows.

Sublingual artery

The sublingual artery arises at the anterior margin of hyoglossus. It passes forward between genioglossus and mylohyoid to the sublingual gland, and supplies the gland, mylohyoid and the buccal and gingival mucous membranes. One branch pierces mylohyoid and joins the submental branches of the facial artery. Another branch courses through the mandibular gingivae to anastomose with its contralateral fellow. A single artery arises from this anastomosis and enters a small foramen (lingual foramen) on the mandible, situated in the midline on the posterior aspect of the symphysis immediately above the genial tubercles.

Deep lingual artery

The deep lingual artery is the terminal part of the lingual artery and is found on the inferior surface of the tongue near the lingual frenum.

In addition to the lingual artery, the tonsillar and ascending palatine branches of the facial and ascending pharyngeal arteries also supply tissue in the root of the tongue. In the region of the valleculae, epiglottic branches of the superior laryngeal artery anastomose with the inferior dorsal branches of the lingual artery.

Lingual veins

The veins draining the tongue follow two routes. Dorsal lingual veins drain the dorsum and sides of the tongue, join the lingual veins accompanying the lingual artery between hyoglossus and genioglossus, and empty into the internal jugular vein near the greater cornu of the hyoid bone. The deep lingual vein begins near the tip of the tongue and runs back just beneath the mucous membrane on the inferior surface of the tongue. It joins a sublingual vein from the sublingual salivary gland near the anterior border of hyoglossus and forms the vena comitans nervi hypoglossi, which run back with the hypoglossal nerve between mylohyoid and hyoglossus to join the facial, internal jugular or lingual vein.

Lymphatic drainage (Fig. 33.9)

The mucosa of the pharyngeal part of the dorsal surface of the tongue contains many lymphoid follicles aggregated into dome-shaped groups, the lingual tonsils. Each group is arranged around a central deep crypt, or invagination, which opens onto the surface epithelium. The ducts of mucous glands open into the bases of the crypts. Small isolated follicles also occur beneath the lingual mucosa. The lymphatic drainage of the tongue can be divided into three main regions, namely marginal, central and dorsal. The anterior region of the tongue drains into marginal and central vessels, and the posterior part of the tongue behind the circumvallate papillae drains into the dorsal lymph vessels. The more central regions may drain bilaterally.

Marginal vessels

Marginal vessels from the apex of the tongue and the lingual frenulum area descend under the mucosa to widely distributed nodes. Some vessels pierce mylohyoid as it contacts the mandibular periosteum to enter either the submental or anterior or middle submandibular nodes, or else to pass anterior to the hyoid bone to the jugulo-omohyoid node. Vessels arising in the plexus on one side may cross under the frenulum to end in contralateral nodes. Efferent vessels of median submental nodes pass bilaterally. Some vessels pass inferior to the sublingual gland and accompany the companion vein of the hypoglossal nerve to end in jugulodigastric nodes. One vessel often descends further to reach the jugulo-omohyoid node, and passes either superficial or deep to the intermediate tendon of digastric.

Vessels from the lateral margin of the tongue cross the sublingual gland, pierce mylohyoid and end in the submandibular nodes. Others

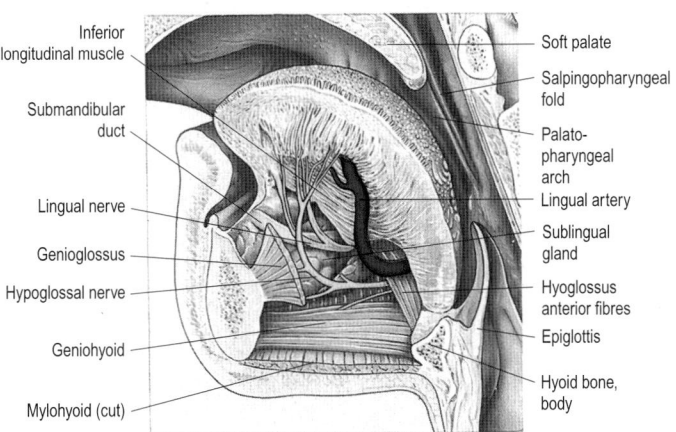

Fig. 33.8 Dissection of the right half of the tongue from the medial side, exposing the end of the second part and the beginning of the third part of the left lingual artery and adjoining structures, in an edentulous subject.

Labels (Fig. 33.8):
Inferior longitudinal muscle
Submandibular duct
Lingual nerve
Genioglossus
Hypoglossal nerve
Geniohyoid
Mylohyoid (cut)
Soft palate
Salpingopharyngeal fold
Palato-pharyngeal arch
Lingual artery
Sublingual gland
Hyoglossus anterior fibres
Epiglottis
Hyoid bone, body

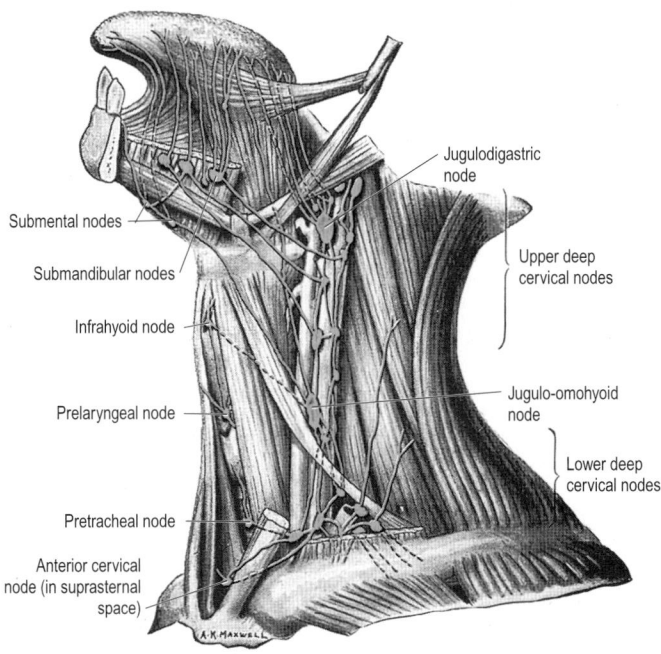

Fig. 33.9 Lymphatic drainage of the tongue. Removal of the sternocleidomastoid has exposed the whole chain of deep cervical lymph nodes. (From The lymphatics of the tongue with particular reference to the removal of lymphatic glands in cancer of the tongue, Jamieson JK, Dobson JF, 8: 80–87, 1920, © British Journal of Surgery Ltd. Reproduced with permission. Permission is granted by John Wiley and Sons Ltd on behalf of the BJSS Ltd.)

Labels (Fig. 33.9):
Submental nodes
Submandibular nodes
Infrahyoid node
Prelaryngeal node
Pretracheal node
Anterior cervical node (in suprasternal space)
Jugulodigastric node
Upper deep cervical nodes
Jugulo-omohyoid node
Lower deep cervical nodes

end in the jugulodigastric or jugulo-omohyoid nodes. Vessels from the posterior part of the lingual margin traverse the pharyngeal wall to the jugulodigastric lymph nodes.

Central vessels

The regions of the lingual surface draining into the marginal or central vessels are not distinct. Central lymphatic vessels ascend between the fibres of the two genioglossi; most pass between the muscles and diverge to the right or left to follow the lingual veins to the deep cervical nodes, especially the jugulodigastric and jugulo-omohyoid nodes. Some pierce mylohyoid to enter the submandibular nodes.

Dorsal vessels

Vessels draining the postsulcal region and the circumvallate papillae run posteroinferiorly. Those near the median plane may pass bilaterally. They turn laterally, join the marginal vessels and all pierce the pharyngeal wall, passing around the external carotid arteries to reach the jugulodigastric and jugulo-omohyoid lymph nodes. One vessel may descend posterior to the hyoid bone, perforating the thyrohyoid membrane to end in the jugulo-omohyoid node.

INNERVATION OF THE TONGUE

The muscles of the tongue, with the exception of palatoglossus, are supplied by the hypoglossal nerve. Palatoglossus is supplied via the pharyngeal plexus (p. 630). The pathways for proprioception associated with the tongue musculature are unknown, but presumably may involve the lingual, glossopharyngeal or hypoglossal nerves, and the cervical spinal nerves which communicate with the hypoglossal nerve.

The sensory innervation of the tongue reflects its embryological development. The nerve of general sensation to the presulcal part is the lingual nerve, which also carries taste sensation derived from the chorda tympani branch of the facial nerve. The nerve supplying both general and taste sensation to the postsulcal part is the glossopharyngeal nerve. An additional area in the region of the valleculae is supplied by the internal laryngeal branch of the vagus nerve.

Lingual nerve (Fig. 30.7)

The lingual nerve is sensory to the mucosa of the floor of the mouth, mandibular lingual gingivae and mucosa of the presulcal part of the tongue (excluding the circumvallate papillae). It also carries postganglionic parasympathetic fibres from the submandibular ganglion to the sublingual and anterior lingual glands.

The lingual nerve arises from the posterior trunk of the mandibular nerve in the infratemporal fossa (Figs 30.6, 30.7, 30.4, 30.8) where it is joined by the chorda tympani branch of the facial nerve and often by a branch of the inferior alveolar nerve. It then passes below the mandibular attachment of the superior pharyngeal constrictor and pterygomandibular raphe, closely applied to the periosteum of the medial surface of the mandible, until it lies opposite the distal (posterior) root of the third molar tooth, where it is covered only by the gingival mucoperiosteum. At this point it usually lies 2–3 mm below the alveolar crest and c.0.6 mm from the bone, but it sometimes lies above the alveolar crest. It next passes medial to the mandibular attachment of mylohyoid, which carries it progressively away from the mandible, and separates it from the alveolar bone covering the mesial root of the third molar tooth, and then passes downward and forward on the deep surface of mylohyoid to cross the lingual sulcus beneath the mucosa. In this position it lies on the deep portion of the submandibular gland. It passes below the submandibular duct which crosses it from medial to lateral, and curves upward, forward and medially to enter the tongue. Within the tongue the lingual nerve lies first on styloglossus and then the lateral surface of hyoglossus and genioglossus, before dividing into terminal branches that supply the overlying lingual mucosa. The lingual nerve is connected to the submandibular ganglion (Fig. 30.8) by two or three branches, and also forms connecting loops with twigs of the hypoglossal nerve at the anterior margin of hyoglossus.

The lingual nerve is at risk during surgical removal of (impacted) lower third molars, and after such operations up to 10% of patients may have symptoms of nerve damage, although these are usually temporary. The nerve is also at risk during operations to remove the submandibular salivary gland, because the duct must be dissected from the lingual nerve during these operations.

Glossopharyngeal nerve

The glossopharyngeal nerve is distributed to the postsulcal part of the tongue and the circumvallate papillae. It communicates with the lingual nerve. The course of the glossopharyngeal nerve in the neck is described on page 555.

Hypoglossal nerve (Fig. 31.21)

The course of the hypoglossal nerve in the neck is described on page 558. After crossing the loop of the lingual artery a little above the tip of the greater cornu of the hyoid, it inclines upwards and forwards on hyoglossus, passing deep to stylohyoid, the tendon of digastric and the posterior border of mylohyoid. Between mylohyoid and hyoglossus the hypoglossal nerve lies below the deep part of the submandibular gland, the submandibular duct and the lingual nerve, with which it communicates. It then passes onto the lateral aspect of genioglossus, continuing forwards in its substance as far as the tip of the tongue. It distributes fibres to styloglossus, hyoglossus and genioglossus and to the intrinsic muscles of the tongue.

The special sensory innervation of the tongue

The sense of taste is dependent on scattered groups of sensory cells, the taste buds, which occur in the oral cavity and pharynx and are particularly plentiful on the lingual papillae of the dorsal lingual mucosa.

Dorsal lingual mucosa

The dorsal mucosa is somewhat thicker than the ventral and lateral mucosae, is directly adherent to underlying muscular tissue with no discernible submucosa, and covered by numerous papillae. The dorsal epithelium consists of a superficial stratified squamous epithelium, which varies from non-keratinized, stratified squamous epithelium posteriorly, to fully keratinized epithelium overlying the filiform papillae more anteriorly. These features probably reflect the fact that the apex of the tongue is subject to greater dehydration than the posterior and ventral parts and is subject to more abrasion during mastication. The underlying lamina propria is a dense fibrous connective tissue, with numerous elastic fibres, and is continuous with similar tissue extending between the lingual muscle fasciculi. It contains numerous vessels and nerves from which the papillae are supplied, and also large lymph plexuses and lingual glands.

Lingual papillae – Lingual papillae are projections of the mucosa covering the dorsal surface of the tongue (Fig. 33.4). They are limited to the presulcal part of the tongue, produce its characteristic roughness and increase the area of contact between the tongue and the contents of the mouth. There are four principal types, named filiform, fungiform, foliate and circumvallate papillae, and all except the filiform papillae bear taste buds. Papillae are more visible in the living when the tongue is dry.

Filiform papillae (Fig. 33.10) – Filiform papillae are minute, conical or cylindrical projections which cover most of the presulcal dorsal area, and are arranged in diagonal rows that extend anterolaterally, parallel with the sulcus terminalis, except at the lingual apex where they are transverse. They have irregular cores of connective tissue and their epithelium, which is keratinized, may split into whitish fine secondary processes. They appear to function to increase the friction between the tongue and food, and facilitate the movement of particles by the tongue within the oral cavity.

Fungiform papillae (Fig. 33.10) – Fungiform papillae occur mainly on the lingual margin but also irregularly on the dorsal surface, where they may occasionally be numerous. They differ from filiform papillae because they are larger, rounded and deep red in colour, this last reflecting their thin, non-keratinized epithelium and highly vascular connective tissue core. Each usually bears one or more taste buds on its apical surface.

Foliate papillae – Foliate papillae lie bilaterally in two zones at the sides of the tongue near the sulcus terminalis, each formed by a series of red, leaf-like mucosal ridges, covered by a non-keratinized epithelium. They bear numerous taste buds.

Circumvallate papillae (Figs 33.11, 33.12) – Circumvallate papillae are large cylindrical structures, varying in number from 8 to 12, which form a V-shaped row immediately in front of the sulcus terminalis on the dorsal surface of the tongue. Each papilla, 1–2 mm in diameter, is surrounded

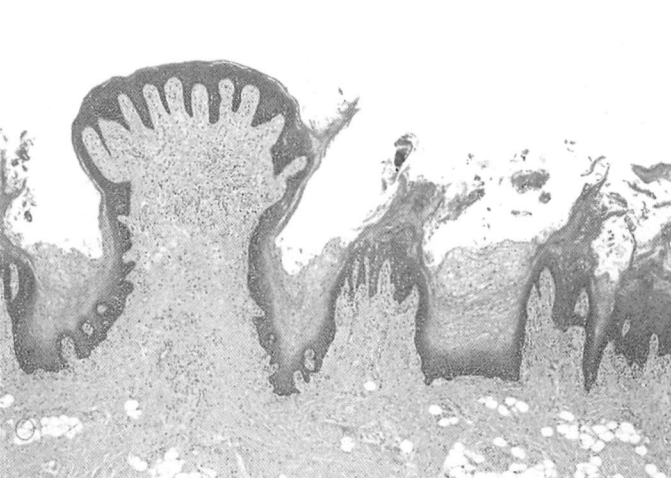

Fig. 33.10 Dorsal surface of the anterior tongue showing non-keratinized fungiform (left) and two keratinized filiform papillae (centre and right) with non-keratinized regions between. (By permission from Young B, Heath JW 2000 Wheater's Functional Histology. Edinburgh: Churchill Livingstone.)

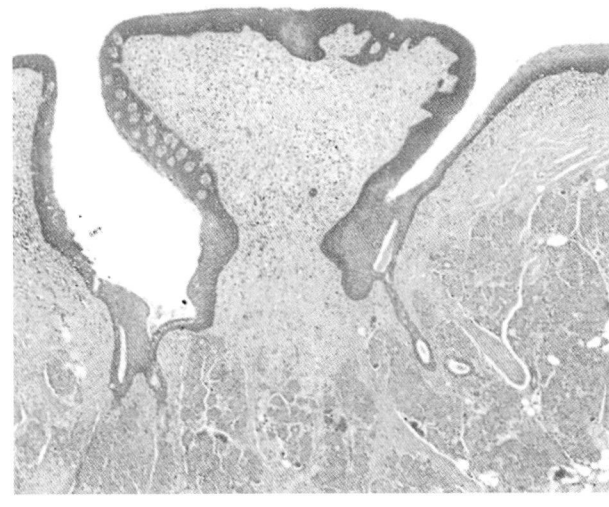

Fig. 33.11 Section through a circumvallate papilla. Serous glands (of von Ebner) empty via ducts into the base of the trench and numerous taste buds are contained within the stratified epithelium of the papillary wall (pale structures on the inner wall of the cleft, left side). (By permission from Young B, Heath JW 2000 Wheater's Functional Histology. Edinburgh: Churchill Livingstone.)

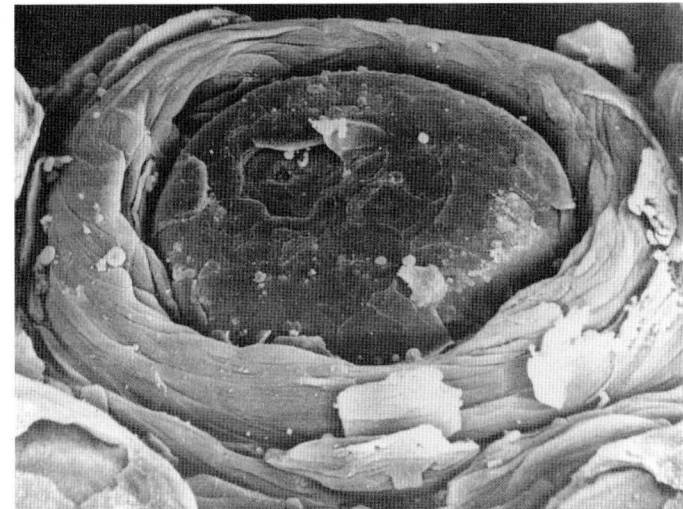

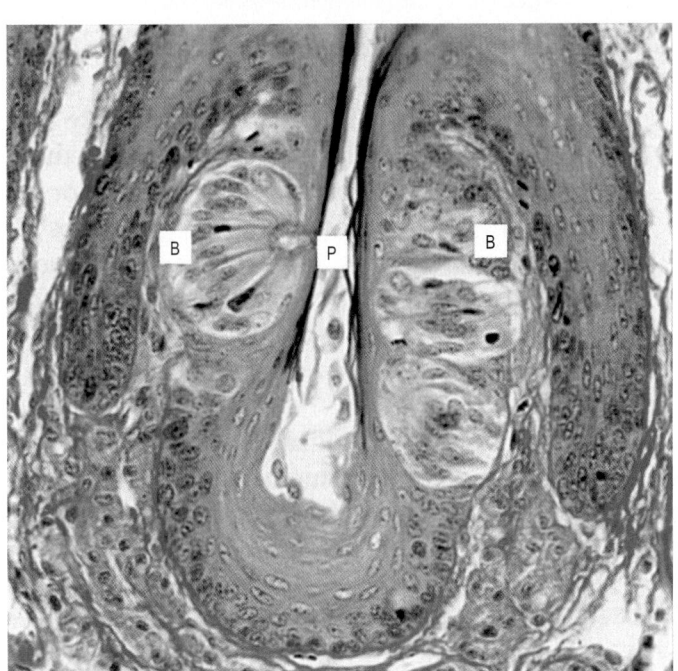

Fig. 33.12 Circumvallate papilla. **A,** Scanning electron micrograph showing a circumvallate papilla surrounded by a trench. **B,** Section of circumvallate papilla showing pale barrel-shaped taste buds (B) in its walls. P, apical pore. (A, by kind permission from S Franey and by permission from Berkovitz BKB, Holland GR, Moxham BJ 2002 Oral Anatomy, Embryology and Histology, 3rd edn. Edinburgh: Mosby; B, by permission from Dr JB Kerr, Monash University, from Kerr JB 1999 Atlas of Functional Histology. London: Mosby.)

by a slight circular mucosal elevation (vallum or wall) which is separated from the papilla by a circular sulcus. The papilla is narrower at its base than its apex and the entire structure is generally covered with non-keratinized stratified squamous epithelium. Numerous taste buds are scattered in both walls of the sulcus, and small serous glands (of von Ebner) open into the sulcal base.

Taste buds

Taste buds are microscopic barrel-shaped epithelial structures which contain chemosensory cells in synaptic contact with the terminals of gustatory nerves. They are numerous on all types of lingual papillae (except filiform papillae) particularly on their lateral aspects. Taste buds are not restricted to the papillae, and are scattered over almost the entire dorsal and lateral surfaces of the tongue and, rarely, on the epiglottis and lingual aspect of the soft palate. Each taste bud is linked by synapses at its base to one of three cranial nerves which carry taste, i.e. the facial, glossopharyngeal or vagus. They share some physiological features with neurones, for example action potential generation and synaptic transmission, and are therefore often referred to as paraneurones.

There is considerable individual variation in the distribution of taste buds in humans. They are most abundant on the posterior parts of the tongue, especially around the walls of the circumvallate papillae and their surrounding sulci, where there is an average of c.250 taste buds for each of the 8–12 papillae. Over 1000 taste buds are distributed over the sides of the tongue, particularly over the more posterior folds of the two foliate papillae, whereas they are rare, and sometimes even absent, on fungiform papillae (c.3 per papilla). Taste buds have been described on the fetal epiglottis and soft palate but most disappear from these sites during postnatal development.

Microstructure of taste buds – Each taste bud is a barrel-shaped cluster of 50–150 fusiform cells which lies within an oval cavity in the epithelium and converges apically on a gustatory pore, a 2 μm wide opening on the mucosal surface. The whole structure is about 70 μm in height by 40 μm across and is separated by a basal lamina from the underlying lamina propria. A small fasciculus of afferent nerve fibres penetrates the basal lamina and spirals around the sensory cells. Chemical substances dissolved in the oral saliva diffuse through the gustatory pores of the taste buds to reach the taste receptor cell membranes, where they cause membrane depolarization.

Innervation of taste buds – Individual nerve fibres branch to give a complex distribution of taste bud innervation. Each fibre may have many terminals, which may spread to innervate widely separated taste buds or may innervate more than one sensory cell in each bud. Conversely, individual buds may receive the terminals of several different nerve fibres. These convergent and divergent patterns of innervation may be of considerable functional importance.

The gustatory nerve for the anterior part of the tongue, excluding the circumvallate papillae, is the chorda tympani, which travels via the lingual nerve. In most individuals, taste fibres run in the chorda tympani to cell bodies in the facial ganglion, but occasionally they diverge to the otic ganglion, which they reach via the greater petrosal nerve. Taste buds in the inferior surface of the soft palate are supplied mainly by the facial nerve, through the greater petrosal nerve, pterygopalatine ganglion and lesser palatine nerve: they may also be supplied by the glossopharyngeal nerve. Taste buds in the circumvallate papillae, postsulcal part of the tongue and in the palatoglossal arches and the oropharynx are innervated by the glossopharyngeal nerve, and those in the extreme pharyngeal part of the tongue and epiglottis receive fibres from the internal laryngeal branch of the vagus.

Each taste bud receives two distinct classes of fibre: one branches in the periphery of the bud to form a perigemmal plexus, the other forms an intragemmal plexus within the bud itself which innervates the bases of the receptor cells. The perigemmal fibres contain various neuropeptides including calcitonin gene-related peptide (CGRP) and substance P, and appear to represent free sensory endings. Intragemmal fibres branch within the taste bud and each forms a series of synapses.

Taste discrimination – Gustatory receptors detect four main categories of taste sensation, classified as salty, sweet, sour and bitter; other taste qualities have been suggested, including metallic, and umami (Japanese: taste typified by monosodium glutamate). Although it is commonly stated that particular areas of the tongue are specialized to detect these different tastes, evidence indicates that all areas of the tongue are responsive to all taste stimuli. Each afferent nerve fibre is connected to widely separated taste buds and may respond to several different chemical stimuli. Some respond to all four classic categories, others to fewer or only one. Within a particular class of tastes, receptors are also differentially sensitive to a wide range of similar chemicals. Moreover, taste buds alone are able to detect only a rather restricted range of chemical substances in aqueous solution. It is difficult to separate the perceptions of taste and smell, because the oral and nasal cavities are continuous. Indeed, much of what is perceived as taste is the result of airborne odorants from the oral cavity which pass through the nasopharynx to the olfactory area above it.

Perceived sensations of taste are the results of the processing (presumably central) of a complex pattern of responses from particular areas of the tongue.

Autonomic innervation of the tongue

The parasympathetic innervation of the various glands of the tongue is from the chorda tympani branch of the facial nerve which synapses in the submandibular ganglion: postganglionic branches are distributed to the lingual mucosa via the lingual nerve. The postganglionic sympathetic supply to lingual glands and vessels arises from the carotid plexus and enters the tongue through plexuses around the lingual arteries. Isolated nerve cells, perhaps postganglionic parasympathetic neurones, have been reported in the postsulcal region: presumably they innervate glandular tissue and vascular smooth muscle.

TEETH

INTRODUCTION AND TERMINOLOGY

Humans have two generations of teeth: the deciduous (primary) dentition and the permanent (secondary) dentition. Teeth first erupt into the mouth at about 6 months after birth and all the deciduous teeth have erupted by 3 years of age. The first permanent teeth appear by 6 years, and thence the deciduous teeth are exfoliated one by one to be replaced by their permanent successors. A complete permanent dentition is present when the third molars erupt at or around the age of 18–21 years. In the complete deciduous dentition there are 20 teeth, 5 in each jaw quadrant. In the complete permanent dentition there are 32 teeth, 8 in each jaw quadrant.

There are three basic tooth forms in both dentitions: incisiform, caniniform and molariform. Incisiform teeth (incisors) are cutting teeth, and have thin, blade-like crowns. Caniniform teeth (canines) are piercing or tearing teeth, and have a single, stout, pointed, cone-shaped crown. Molariform teeth (molars and premolars) are grinding teeth and possess a number of cusps on an otherwise flattened biting surface. Premolars are bicuspid teeth that are restricted to the permanent dentition and replace the deciduous molars.

The tooth-bearing region of the jaws can be divided into four quadrants, the right and left maxillary and mandibular quadrants. A tooth may thus be identified according to the quadrant in which it is located (e.g. a right maxillary tooth or a left mandibular tooth). In both the deciduous and permanent dentitions, the incisors may be distinguished according to their relationship to the midline. Thus, the incisor nearest the midline is the central (first) incisor and the incisor that is more laterally positioned is termed the lateral (second) incisor. The permanent premolars and the permanent and deciduous molars can also be distinguished according to their mesiodistal relationships. The molar most mesially positioned is designated the first molar, and the one behind it is the second molar. In the permanent dentition, the tooth most distally positioned is the third molar. The mesial premolar is the first premolar, and the premolar behind it is the second premolar.

The terminology used to indicate tooth surfaces is shown in **Fig. 33.13**. The aspect of teeth adjacent to the lips or cheeks is termed labial or buccal, that adjacent to the tongue being lingual (or palatal in the maxilla). Labial and lingual surfaces of an incisor meet medially at a mesial surface and laterally at a distal surface, terms which are also used to describe the equivalent surfaces of premolar and molar (postcanine) teeth. On account of the curvature of the dental arch, mesial surfaces of postcanine teeth are directed anteriorly and distal surfaces are directed posteriorly. Thus, the point of contact between the central incisors is the datum point for mesial and distal. The biting or occlusal surfaces of postcanine teeth are tuberculated by cusps which are separated by fissures forming a pattern characteristic of each tooth. The biting surface of an incisor is the incisal edge.

TOOTH MORPHOLOGY (Figs 33.13, 33.14)

There are two incisors, a central and a lateral, in each half jaw or quadrant. In labial view, the crowns are trapezoid, the maxillary incisors (particularly the central) are larger than the mandibular. The biting or incisal edges initially have three tubercles or mamelons, which are rapidly removed by wear. In mesial or distal view their labial profiles are convex while their lingual surfaces are concavo-convex (the convexity near the cervical margin is caused by a low ridge or cingulum, which is prominent only on upper incisors). The roots of incisors are single and rounded in maxillary teeth, but flattened mesiodistally in mandibular teeth. The upper lateral incisor may be congenitally absent or may have a reduced form (peg-shaped lateral incisor).

Behind each lateral incisor is a canine tooth with a single cusp (hence the American term cuspid) instead of an incisal edge. The maxillary canine is stouter and more pointed than the mandibular canine. The canine root, which is the longest of any tooth, produces a bulge (canine eminence) on the alveolar bone externally, particularly in the upper jaw. Although canines usually have single roots, that of the lower may sometimes be bifid.

Distal to the canines are two premolars, each with a buccal and lingual cusp (hence the term bicuspid). The occlusal surfaces of the maxillary premolars are oval (the long axis is buccopalatal) and a mesiodistal fissure separates the two cusps. In buccal view, premolars resemble the canines but are smaller. The maxillary first premolar usually has two roots (one buccal, one palatal) but may have one, and very rarely three, roots (two buccal and one palatal). The maxillary second premolar usually has one root. The occlusal surfaces of the mandibular premolars are more circular or more square than those of the upper premolars. The buccal cusp of the mandibular first premolar towers above the lingual cusp to which it is connected by a ridge separating the mesial and distal occlusal pits. In the mandibular second premolar a mesiodistal fissure usually separates a buccal from two smaller lingual cusps. Each lower premolar has one root, but very rarely the root of the first is bifid. Lower second premolars fail to develop in about 2% of individuals.

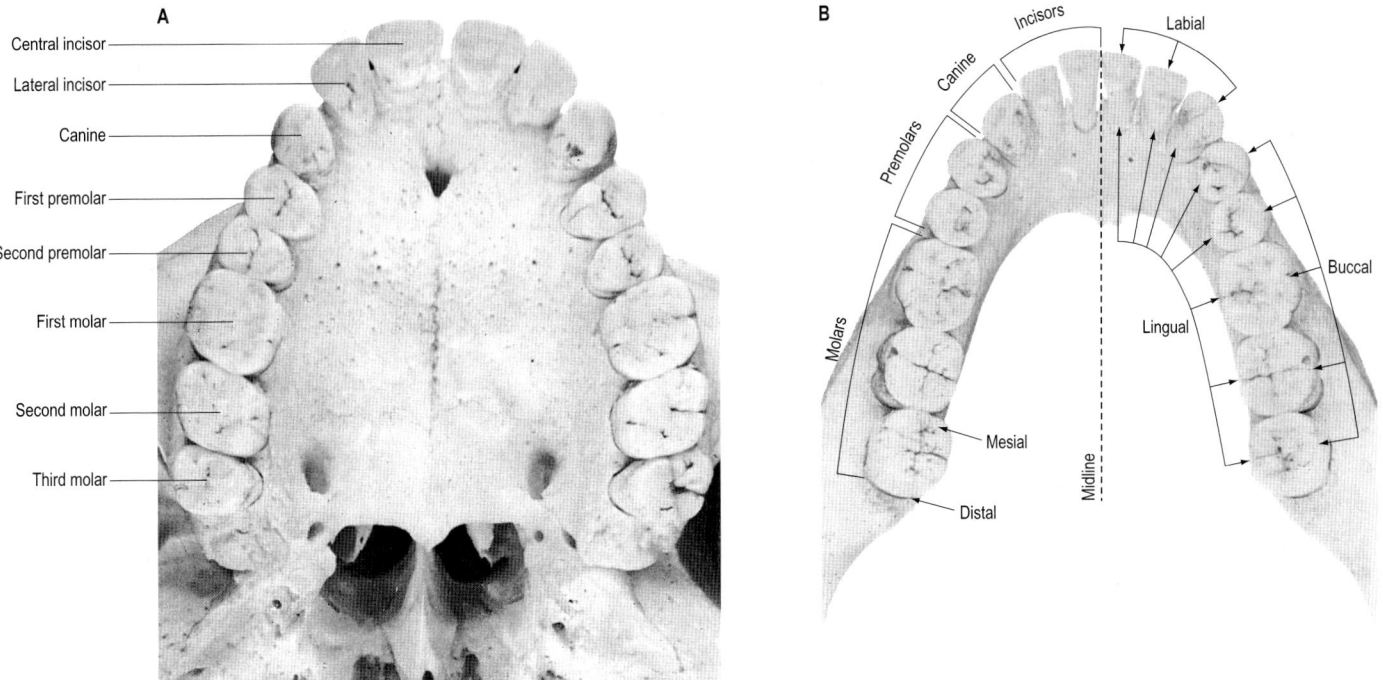

Fig. 33.13 **A**, The permanent teeth of the upper dental arch: occlusal aspect. **B**, The permanent teeth of the lower dental arch: occlusal aspect. **C**, Terminology employed for the identification of teeth according to their location in the lower jaw. The same terminology is employed for the teeth in the upper jaw.

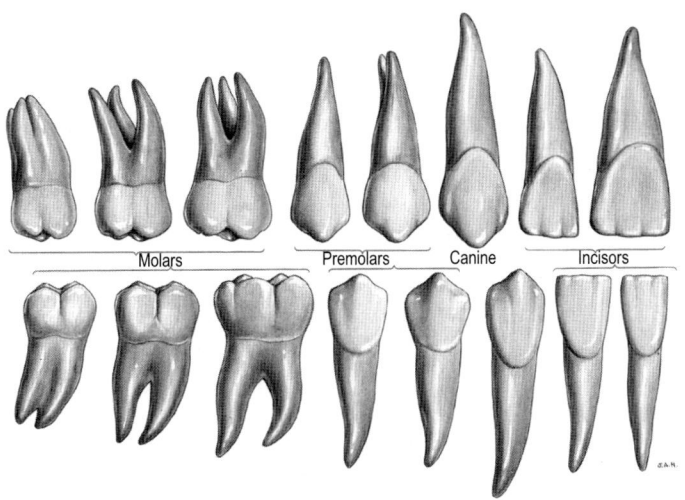

Fig. 33.14 The permanent upper and lower teeth of the right side: labial and buccal surfaces.

Posterior to the premolars are three molars whose size decreases distally. Each has a large rhomboid (upper jaw) or rectangular (lower jaw) occlusal surface with four or five cusps. The maxillary first molar has a cusp at each corner of its occlusal surface and the mesiopalatal cusp is connected to the distobuccal by an oblique ridge. A smaller cusplet or tubercle (cusplet of Carabelli) usually appears on the mesiopalatal cusp (most commonly in Caucasian races). The tooth has three widely separated roots, two buccal and one palatal. The smaller maxillary second molar has a reduced or occasionally absent distopalatal cusp. Its three roots show varying degrees of fusion. The maxillary third molar, the smallest, is very variable in form. It usually has three cusps (the distopalatal being absent) and commonly the three roots are fused.

The mandibular first molar has three buccal and two lingual cusps on its rectangular occlusal surface, the smallest cusp being distal. The cusps of this tooth are all separated by fissures. It has two widely separated roots, one mesial and one distal. The smaller mandibular second molar is like the first, but has only four cusps (it lacks the distal cusp of the first molar) and its two roots are closer together. The mandibular third molar is smaller still and, like the upper third molar, is variable in form. Its crown may resemble that of the lower first or second molar and its roots are frequently fused. As it erupts antero-superiorly, the third molar is often impacted against the second molar, which produces food packing and inflammation, both indications for surgical removal. The maxillary third molar erupts posteroinferiorly and is rarely impacted. One or more third molars (upper or lower) fail to develop in up to 30% of individuals.

Impacted mandibular third molars

In many subjects there is a disproportion between the size of the teeth and the size of the jaws such that there is insufficient space for all the teeth to erupt. As the third mandibular molar teeth (the wisdom teeth) are the last to erupt they are often impeded in their eruption and either become impacted against the distal aspect of the second molar or remain unerupted deeply within the jaw bone. If the tooth is completely covered by bone and mucosa it is very unlikely to cause any symptoms, and the subject remains unaware of their presence unless the teeth are seen on a routine dental radiograph. Very rarely the surrounding dental follicle may undergo cystic degeneration which can 'hollow out' the jaw, usually the mandible, to a considerable degree. The developing cyst may displace the tooth as it expands and the tooth may end up as far away as the condylar neck or coronoid process.

More commonly, the erupting wisdom tooth erupts partially before impacting against the distal aspect of the second molar. When this occurs, symptoms are common due to recurrent soft tissue infection around the partially erupted tooth. This condition is known as pericoronitis and if the infecting organism is virulent, the infection may rapidly spread into the adjacent tissue spaces as described elsewhere. It is for this reason that so many wisdom teeth are removed in adolescents and young adults. The surgery itself requires considerable skill as the lingual nerve passes across the surface of the periosteum lingually, separated from the tooth only by a cortical plate of bone no thicker than an egg shell. Damage to this nerve results in altered sensation to the ipsilateral side of the tongue. The root apices of the impacted tooth often lie immediately above the inferior alveolar canal, and removal of the tooth can result in damage to the underlying nerve and artery. Maxillary third molars are only rarely impacted.

Deciduous teeth (Figs 33.15, 33.16)

The incisors, canine and premolars of the permanent dentition replace two deciduous incisors, a deciduous canine and two deciduous molars in each jaw quadrant. The deciduous incisors and canine are shaped

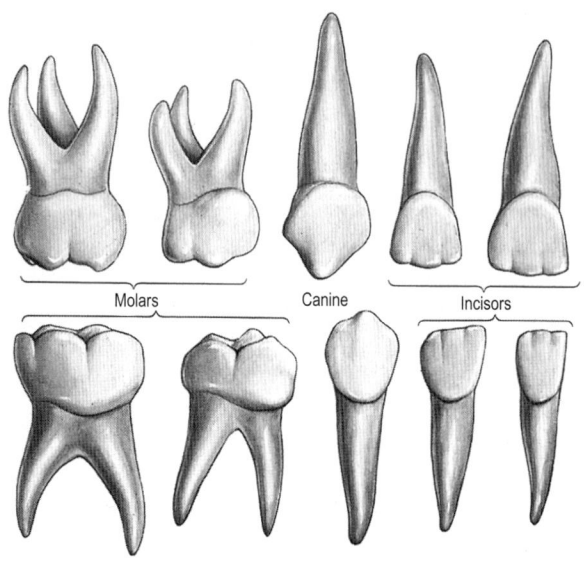

Molars   Canine   Incisors

Fig. 33.15 The deciduous upper and lower teeth of the right side: labial and buccal surfaces.

A

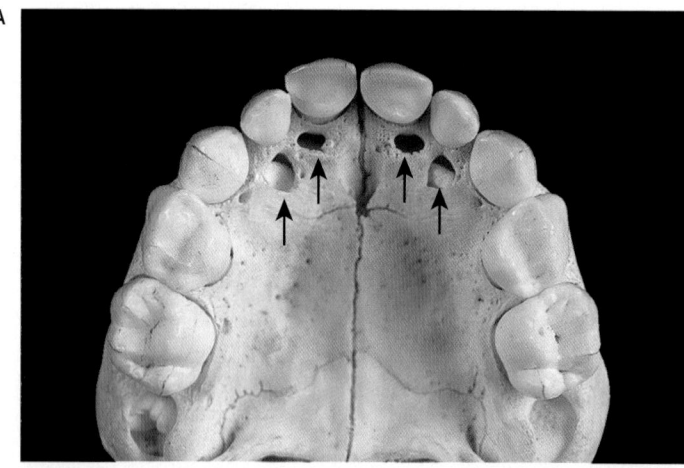

B

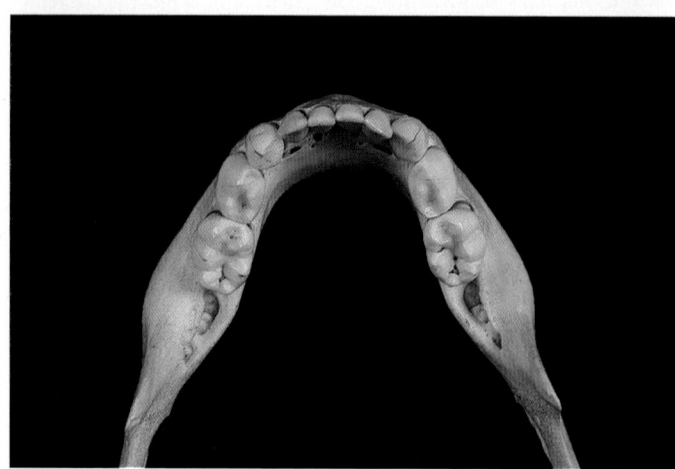

Fig. 33.16 A, The upper deciduous dentition (note the channels (arrows) leading to the developing permanent teeth). **B,** The lower deciduous dentition. (By permission from Berkovitz BKB, Moxham BJ 1994 Color Atlas of the Skull. London: Mosby.)

like their successors but are smaller and whiter and become extremely worn in older children. The deciduous second molars resemble permanent molars rather than their successors, the premolars. Each second deciduous molar has a crown which is almost identical to that of the posteriorly adjacent first permanent molar. The upper first deciduous molar has a triangular occlusal surface (its rounded 'apex' is palatal) and a fissure separates a double buccal cusp from the palatal cusp. The lower first deciduous molar is long and narrow, and its two buccal cusps are separated from its two lingual cusps by a zigzagging mesiodistal fissure. Like permanent molars, upper deciduous molars have three roots and lower deciduous molars have two roots. These roots diverge more than those of permanent teeth because each developing premolar tooth crown is accommodated directly under the crown of its deciduous predecessor. The roots of deciduous teeth are progressively resorbed by osteoclast-like cells (odontoclasts) prior to being shed.

Eruption of teeth (Fig. 33.17)

Information on the sequence of development and eruption of teeth into the oral cavity is important in clinical practice and also in forensic medicine and archaeology. The tabulated data provided in **Table 33.2** are largely based on European-derived populations and there is evidence of ethnic variation. When a permanent tooth erupts, about two-thirds of the root is formed and it takes about another three years for the root to be completed. For deciduous teeth, root completion is more rapid (**Table 33.2**). The developmental stages of initial calcification and crown completion are less affected by environmental influences than eruption, the timing of which may be modified by several factors such as early tooth loss and severe malnutrition.

Figure 33.18 shows the panoramic appearance of the dentition seen with orthopantomograms at the time of birth, 3, $6\frac{1}{2}$, 10 and 16 years of age.

Dental alignment and occlusion

It is possible to bring the jaws together so that the teeth meet or occlude in many positions. When opposing occlusal surfaces meet with maximal 'intercuspation' (i.e. maximum contact), the teeth are said to be in centric occlusion (**Fig. 33.19**). In this position the lower teeth are normally opposed symmetrically and lingually with respect to the upper. Some important features of centric occlusion in a normal (idealized) dentition may be noted. Each lower postcanine tooth is slightly in front of its upper equivalent and the lower canine occludes in front of the upper. Buccal cusps of the lower postcanine teeth lie between the buccal and palatal cusps of the upper teeth. Thus, the lower postcanine teeth are slightly lingual and mesial to their upper equivalents. Lower incisors bite against the palatal surfaces of upper incisors, the latter normally obscuring about one-third of the crowns of the lower. This vertical overlap of incisors in centric occlusion is the overbite. The extent to which upper incisors are anterior to lowers is termed the overjet. In the most habitual jaw position, the resting posture, the teeth are slightly apart, the gap between them being the free-way space or interocclusal clearance. During mastication, especially with lateral jaw movements, the food is comminuted, which facilitates the early stages of digestion.

The ideal occlusion is a rather subjective concept. If there is an ideal occlusion, it can only presently be defined in broad functional terms. Therefore, the occlusion can be considered 'ideal' when the teeth are aligned such that the masticatory loads are within physiological range and act through the long axes of as many teeth in the arch as possible; mastication involves alternating bilateral jaw movements (and not habitual, unilateral biting preferences as a result of adaptation to occlusal interference); lateral jaw movements occur without undue mechanical interference; in the rest position of the jaw, the gap between teeth (the freeway space) is correct for the individual concerned; the tooth alignment is aesthetically pleasing to its possessor.

Variations from the ideal occlusion may be termed malocclusions (although these could be regarded as normal for they are more commonly found in the population: c.75% of the population in the USA have some degree of occlusal 'disharmony'). However, the majority of malocclusions should be regarded as anatomical variations rather than abnormalities for they are rarely involved in masticatory dysfunction or pain, although they may be aesthetically displeasing.

Variations in tooth number, size and form

The incidence of variation in number and form, which is often related to race, is rare in deciduous teeth but not uncommon in the permanent

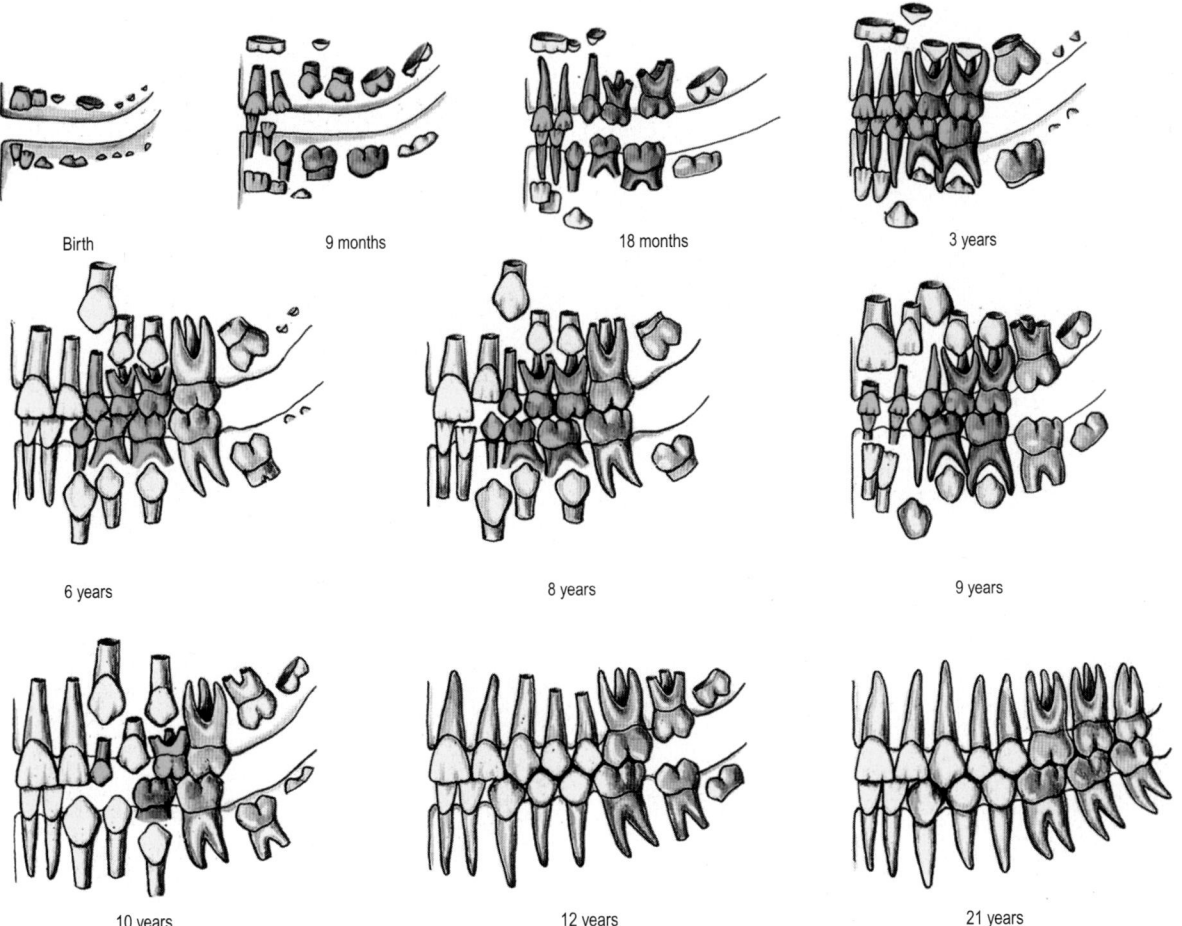

Birth   9 months   18 months   3 years

6 years   8 years   9 years

10 years   12 years   21 years

Fig. 33.17 Development of the deciduous (blue) and permanent (yellow) teeth. (Modified with permission from Schour I, Massler M 1941 The development of the human dentition. J Am Dent Assoc 28: 1153–1160.)

Table 33.2 Chronology of the human dentition

Dentition	Tooth	First evidence of calcification (weeks *in utero* for deciduous teeth)	Crown completed (months)	Eruptiom (months)	Root completed (years)
Deciduous upper	i1	14	$1\frac{1}{2}$	10 (8–12)	$1\frac{1}{2}$
	i2	16	$2\frac{1}{2}$	11 (9–13)	2
	C	17	9	19 (16–22)	$3\frac{1}{4}$
	m1	$15\frac{1}{2}$	6	16 (13–19)	$2\frac{1}{2}$
	m2	19	11	29 (25–33)	3
Deciduous lower	i1	14	$2\frac{1}{2}$	8 (6–10)	$1\frac{1}{2}$
	i2	16	3	13 (10–16)	$1\frac{1}{2}$
	C	17	9	20 (17–23)	$3\frac{1}{4}$
	m1	$15\frac{1}{2}$	$5\frac{1}{2}$	16 (14–18)	$2\frac{1}{4}$
	m2	18	10	27 (23–31)	3
Permanent upper	I1	3–4 months	4–5 yrs	7–8 yrs	10
	I2	10–12 months	4–5 yrs	8–9 yrs	11
	C	4–5 months	6–7 yrs	11–12 yrs	13–15
	P1	$1\frac{1}{2}$–$1\frac{3}{4}$ yrs	5–6 yrs	10–11 yrs	12–13
	P2	2–$2\frac{1}{4}$ yrs	6–7 yrs	10–12 yrs	12–14
	M1	at birth	$2\frac{1}{2}$–3 yrs	6–7 yrs	9–10
	M2	$2\frac{1}{2}$–3 yrs	7–8 yrs	12–13 yrs	14–16
	M3	7–9 yrs	12–16 yrs	17–21 yrs	18–25
Permanent lower	I1	3–4 months	4–5 yrs	6–7 yrs	9
	I2	3–4 months	4–5 yrs	7–8 yrs	10
	C	4–5 months	6–7 yrs	9–10 yrs	12–14
	P1	$1\frac{3}{4}$–2 yrs	5–6 yrs	10–12 yrs	12–13
	P2	$2\frac{1}{4}$–$2\frac{1}{2}$ yrs	6–7 yrs	1–12 yrs	13–14
	M1	at birth	$2\frac{1}{2}$–3 yrs	6–7 yrs	9–10
	M2	$2\frac{1}{2}$–3 yrs	7–8 yrs	11–13 yrs	14–15
	M3	8–10 yrs	12–16 yrs	17–21 yrs	18–25

(Modified with permission from Ash MM 1993 Dental Anatomy, Physiology and Occlusion. Philadelphia: WB Saunders.)

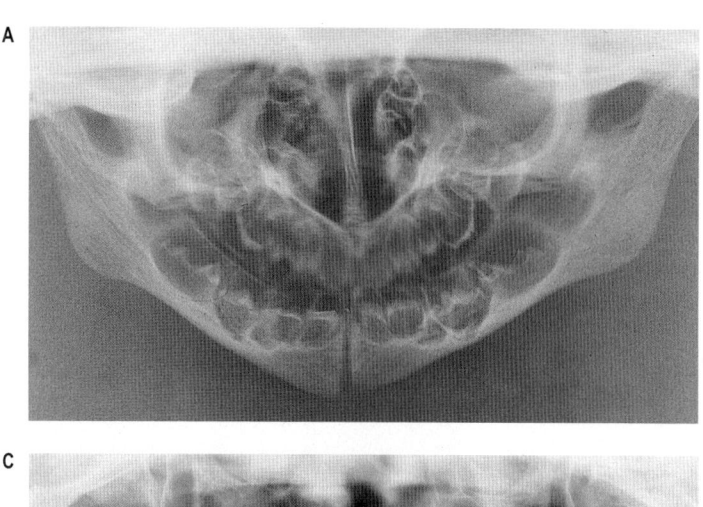

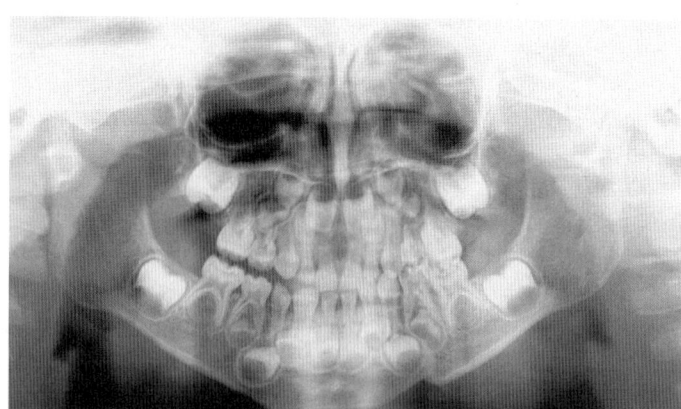

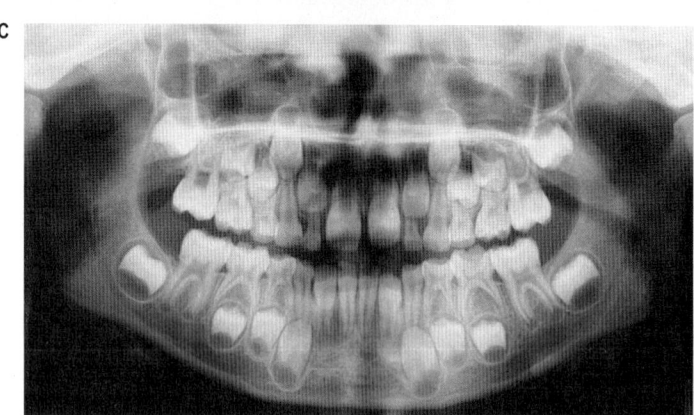

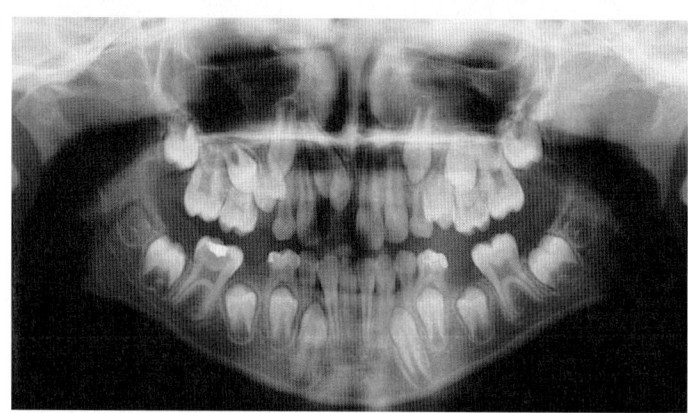

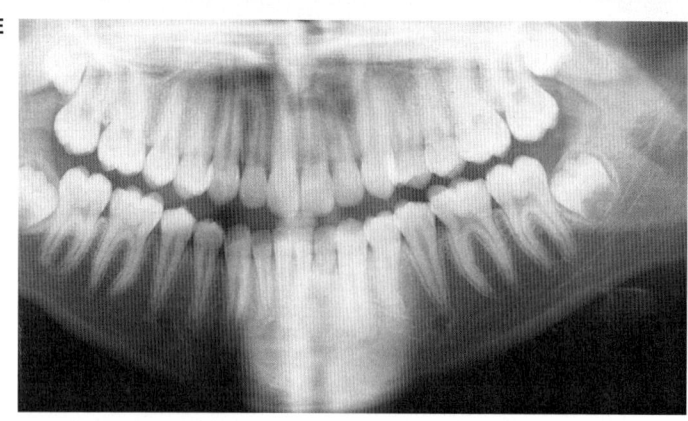

Fig. 33.18 Orthopantomogram of the dentition at birth. **B**, Orthopantomogram of the dentition at 2½ years. **C**, Orthopantomogram of the dentition at 6½ years. **D**, Orthopantomogram of the dentition at 10 years. **E**, Orthopantomogram of the dentition at 16 years. (**B–F**, by permission from Berkovitz BKB, Holland GR, Moxham BJ 2002 Oral Anatomy, Embryology and Histology, 3rd edn. Edinburgh: Mosby; **D–F**, also by kind permission from Eric Whaites.)

dentition. One or more teeth may fail to develop, a condition known as hypodontia. Conversely, additional or supernumerary teeth may form, producing hyperdontia. The third permanent molar is the most frequently missing tooth: in one study one or more third molars failed to form in 32% of Chinese, 24% of English Caucasians and 2.5% of West Africans. In declining order of incidence, other missing teeth are maxillary lateral incisors, maxillary or mandibular second premolars, mandibular central incisors and maxillary first premolars.

Hyperdontia affects the maxillary arch much more commonly than the mandibular dentition. The extra teeth are usually situated on the palatal aspect of the permanent incisors or distal to the molars. More rarely, additional premolars develop. Although supernumerary teeth in the incisor region are often small with simple conical crowns, they may impede the eruption of the permanent incisors. A supernumerary tooth situated between the central incisors is known as a mesiodens. Teeth may be unusually large (macrodontia) or small (microdontia). For example, the crowns of maxillary central incisors may be abnormally wide mesiodistally; in contrast, a common variant of the maxillary lateral incisor has a small, peg-shaped crown. Epidemiological studies reveal that hyperdontia tends to be associated with macrodontia and hypodontia with microdontia, the most severely affected individuals representing the extremes of a continuum of variation. Together with family studies, this indicates that the causation is multifactorial, combining polygenic and environmental influences.

Some variations in the form of teeth, being characteristic of race, are of anthropological and forensic interest. Mongoloid dentitions tend to have shovel-shaped maxillary incisors with enlarged palatal marginal ridges. The additional cusp of Carabelli is commonly found on the mesiopalatal aspect of maxillary first permanent or second deciduous molars in Caucasian but rarely in Mongoloid dentitions. In African races the mandibular second permanent molar often has five rather than four cusps.

GENERAL ARRANGEMENT OF DENTAL TISSUES (Figs 33.20, 33.21, 33.22)
A tooth (**Fig. 33.20**) consists of a crown, covered by very hard translucent enamel and a root covered by yellowish bone-like cementum. These meet at the neck or cervical margin. A longitudinal ground section (**Fig. 32.21**) reveals that the body of a tooth is mostly dentine (ivory) with an enamel covering up to about 2 mm thick, while the cementum is much thinner. The dentine surrounds a central pulp cavity, expanded at its coronal end into a pulp chamber and narrowed in the root as a pulp canal, opening at or near its tip by an apical foramen, occasionally multiple. The pulp is a connective tissue, continuous with the peridontal ligament via the apical foramen. It contains vessels for the support of the dentine and sensory nerves.

The root is surrounded by alveolar bone, its cementum separated from the osseous socket (alveolus) by the connective tissue of the periodontal ligament, c.0.2 mm thick (**Fig. 33.23**). Coarse bundles of

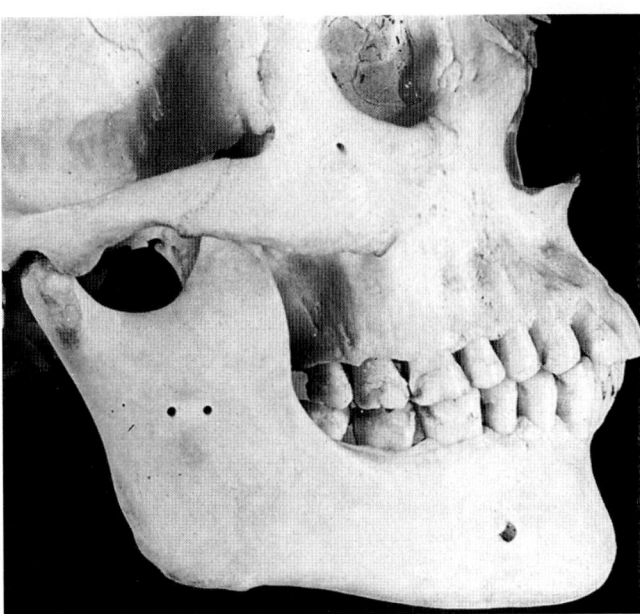

Fig. 33.19 Lateral view of the dentition in centric occlusion.

collagen fibres, embedded at one end in cementum, cross the periodontal ligament to enter the osseous alveolar wall. Near the cervical margin, the tooth, periodontal ligament and adjacent bone are covered by the gingiva. On its internal surface the gingiva is attached to the tooth surface by the junctional epithelium, a zone of profound clinical importance because just above it is a slight recess, the gingival sulcus. As the sulcus is not necessarily self-cleansing, dental plaque may accumulate in it and this predisposes to periodontal disease.

Enamel

Enamel is an extremely hard and rigid material which covers the crowns of teeth. It is a heavily mineralized cell secretion, containing 95–96% by weight crystalline apatites (88% by volume) and less than 1% organic matrix. The organic matrix comprises mainly unique enamel proteins, amelogenins and non-amelogenins such as enamelins, tuftelins. Although comprising a very small percentage of the weight and volume of enamel, the organic matrix permeates the whole of enamel. As its formative cells are lost from the surface during tooth eruption, enamel is incapable of further growth. Repair is limited to the remineralization of minute carious lesions.

Enamel reaches a maximum thickness of 2.5 mm over cusps and thins at the cervical margins. It is composed of closely packed enamel prisms or rods. In longitudinal section, enamel prisms extend from close to the enamel–dentine junction to within c.20 μm of the surface, where they are generally replaced by prismless (non-prismatic, aprismatic)

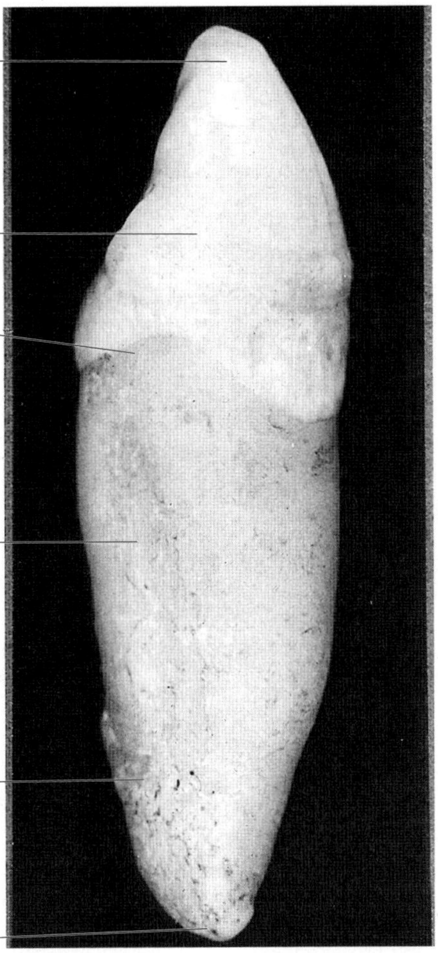

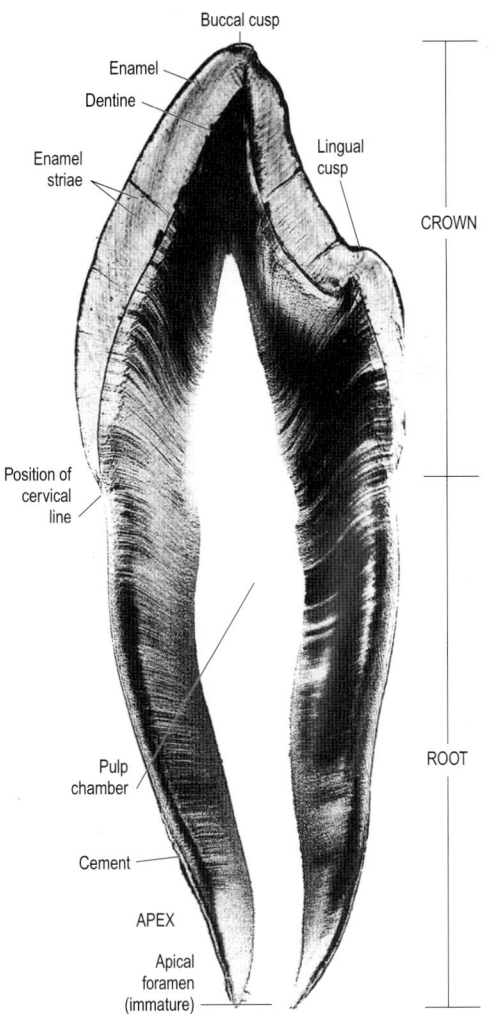

Fig. 33.20 An extracted upper right canine tooth viewed from its mesial aspect, showing its principal parts. Note the root covered by cement (partially removed), and the curved cervical margin, convex towards the cusp of the tooth.

Fig. 33.21 A ground section of a young (permanent) lower first premolar tooth sectioned in the buccolingual longitudinal plane, photographed with transmitted light. The enamel striae are incremental lines of enamel growth (compare with **Fig. 33.31**). Within the dentine the lines of the dentinal tubules are visible, forming S-shaped curves in the apical region but straighter in the root.

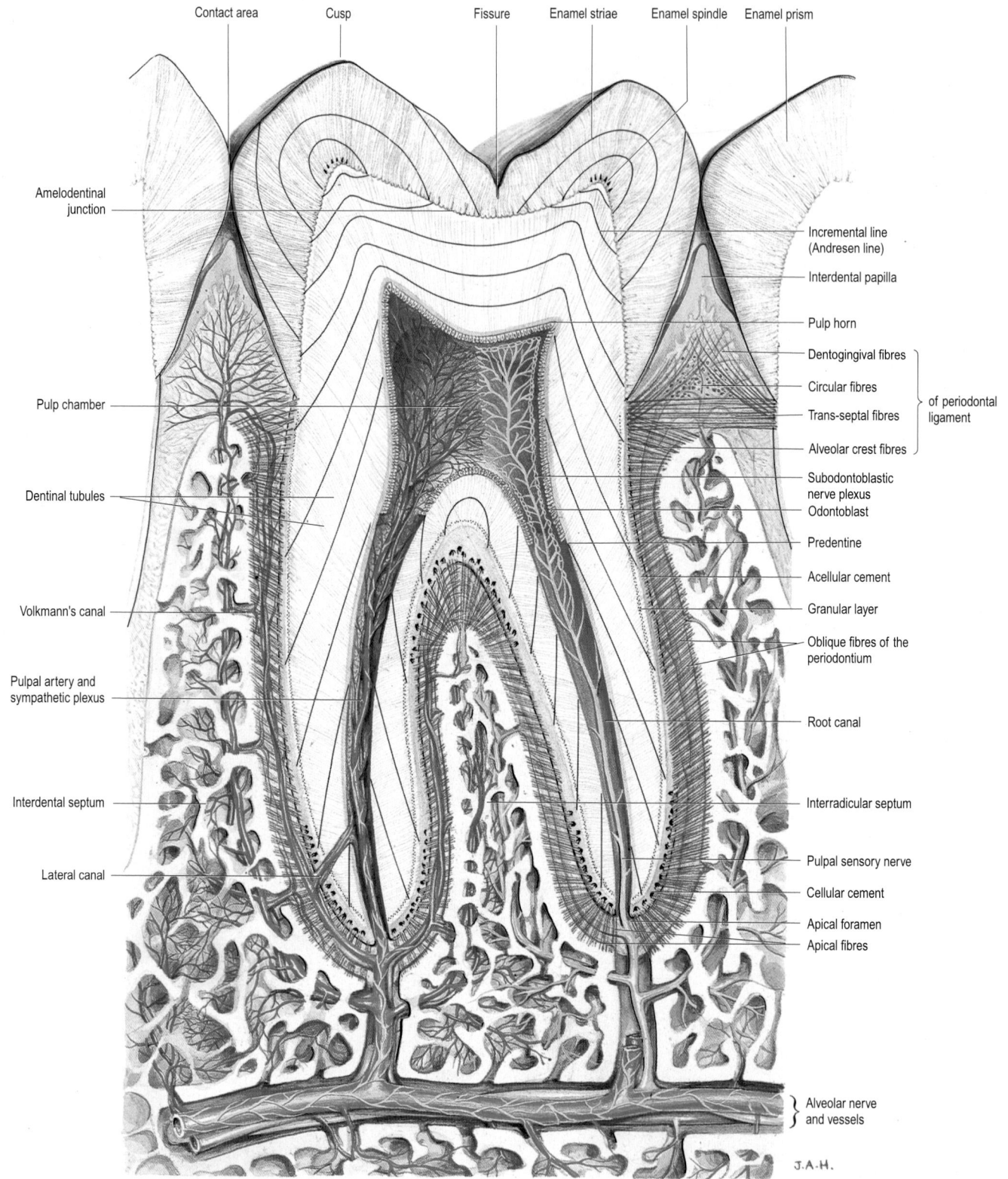

Contact area · Cusp · Fissure · Enamel striae · Enamel spindle · Enamel prism

Amelodentinal junction

Incremental line (Andresen line)

Interdental papilla

Pulp horn

Dentogingival fibres
Circular fibres
Trans-septal fibres
Alveolar crest fibres } of periodontal ligament

Pulp chamber

Subodontoblastic nerve plexus
Odontoblast

Dentinal tubules

Predentine

Acellular cement

Volkmann's canal

Granular layer

Oblique fibres of the periodontium

Pulpal artery and sympathetic plexus

Root canal

Interdental septum

Interradicular septum

Lateral canal

Pulpal sensory nerve

Cellular cement

Apical foramen
Apical fibres

Alveolar nerve and vessels

J.A.H.

Fig. 33.22 Longitudinal section of a tooth and its environs.

enamel (**Fig. 33.24**). In cross-section the prisms are mainly horse-shoe shaped and are arranged in rows that are staggered such that the tails of the prisms in one row lie between the heads of the prism in the row above (prism pattern 3) (**Fig. 33.25**) and the tails are directed rootwards. The appearance of prism boundaries results from sudden changes in crystallite orientation. Prisms have a diameter of c.5 μm, and are packed with flattened hexagonal hydroxyapatite crystals, far larger than those found in the other collagenous-based mineralized tissues.

Two types of incremental lines are visible in enamel, short-term and long-term. At intervals of c.4 μm along its length, each prism is crossed

by a line, probably reflecting diurnal swelling and shrinking in diameter during its growth. This short-term daily growth line is known as a cross striation (**Fig. 33.26**). The longer term incremental lines pass from the enamel–dentine junction obliquely to the surface, where they end in shallow furrows, perikymata, visible on newly erupted teeth. Each line, known as an enamel stria, represents a period of 7–8 days enamel growth (**Fig. 33.27**). A prominent striation, the neonatal line, is formed in teeth whose mineralization spans birth (see above). Neonatal lines are present in the enamel and dentine of teeth mineralizing at the time of birth (all the deciduous teeth and the first permanent molars (see

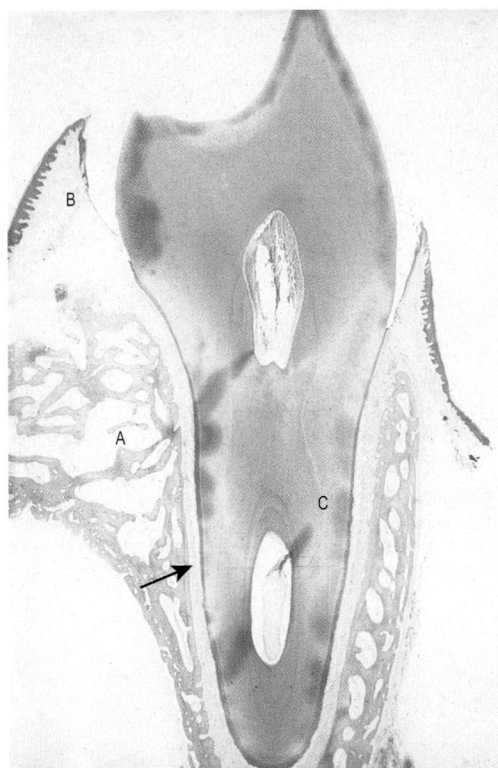

Fig. 33.23 Demineralized section of a tooth with its root attached to the surrounding bone by the periodontal ligament. A, Alveolar bone; C, root of tooth lined by cementum; arrow, peridontal space. (By kind permission from Dr D Lunt.)

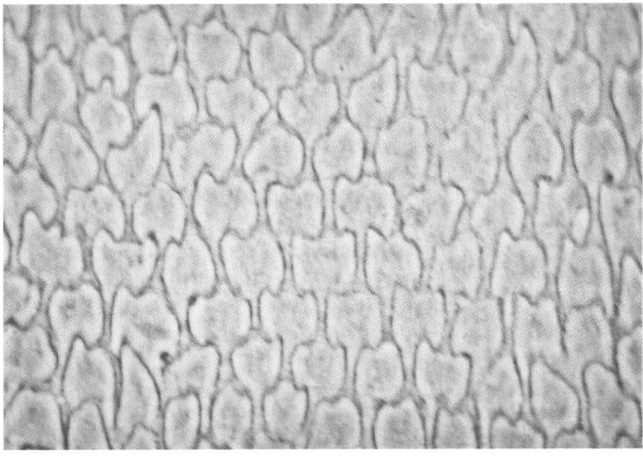

Fig. 33.25 Ground cross-section of enamel showing cross-sectional keyhole (fish scale) appearance of enamel prisms (pattern 3). (By permission from Berkovitz BKB, Holland GR, Moxham BJ 2002 Oral Anatomy, Embryology and Histology, 3rd edn. Edinburgh: Mosby.)

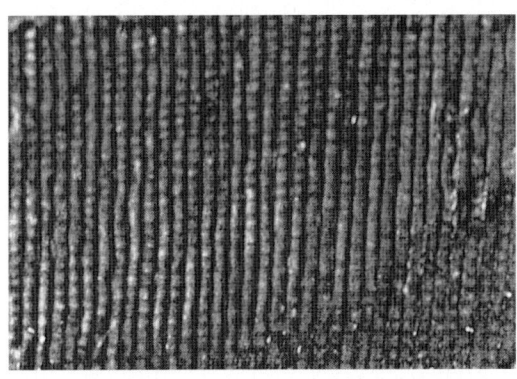

Fig. 33.26 Ground longitudinal section of enamel viewed with phase contrast showing prisms (vertical lines) and cross-striations (horizontal lines). (By permission from Berkovitz BKB, Holland GR, Moxham BJ 2002 Oral Anatomy, Embryology and Histology, 3rd edn. Edinburgh: Mosby.)

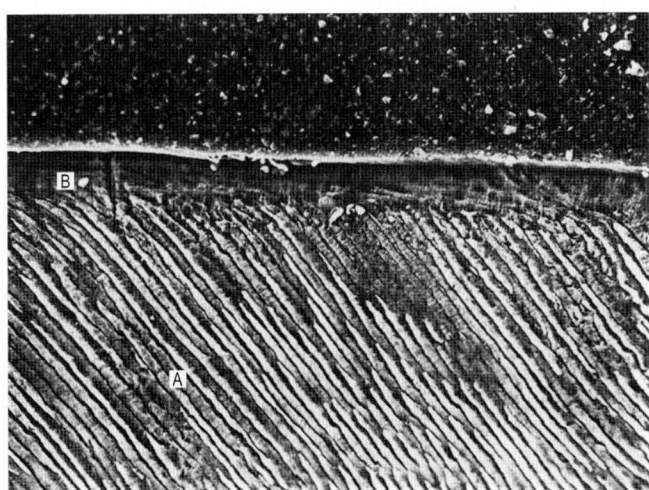

Fig. 33.24 SEM of acid-etched outer enamel (A) showing enamel prisms, each c.5 μm wide. A layer of prismless enamel (B) is evident on the surface. (By kind permission from Professor D Whittaker.)

Fig. 33.13) and are therefore of forensic importance, indicating that an infant has survived for a few days after birth. They reflect a disturbance in mineralization during the first few days after birth.

Dentine

Dentine is a yellowish avascular tissue which forms the bulk of a tooth. It is a tough and compliant composite material, with a mineral content of c.70% dry weight (largely crystalline hydroxyapatite with some calcium carbonate) and 20% organic matrix (type I collagen, glycosaminoglycans and phosphoproteins). Its conspicuous feature is

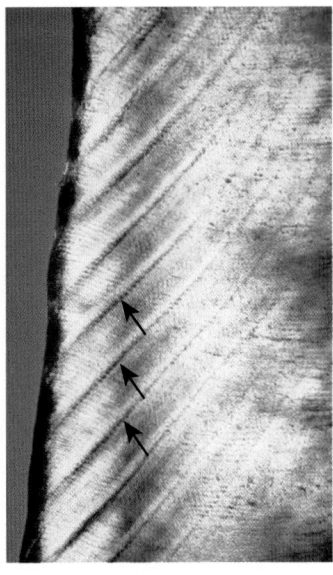

Fig. 33.27 Ground longitudinal section of enamel showing enamel striae (arrows). Viewed between crossed polarizing filters. (By kind permission from Dr AD Beynon.)

the regular pattern of microscopic dentinal tubules, c.3 μm in diameter, which extend from the pulpal surface to the enamel–dentine junction. The tubules show lateral and terminal branching near the enamel–dentine junction (**Fig. 33.28**) and may project a short distance into the enamel (enamel spindles). Each tubule encloses a single cytoplasmic process of an odontoblast whose cell body lies in a pseudostratified layer which lines the pulpal surface. Processes are believed to extend the full thickness of dentine in newly erupted teeth, but in older teeth they may be partly withdrawn and occupy only the pulpal third, while the outer regions contain probably only extracellular fluid. The diameter of the dentine tubule is narrowed by deposition of peritubular dentine. This is different from normal dentine (intertubular dentine) because it is more highly mineralized and lacks a collagenous matrix. Peritubular dentine can therefore be identified by microradiography (**Fig. 33.29**). In time, it may completely fill the tubule, a process which gives rise to translucent dentine and which commences in the apical region of the root.

The outermost zone (10–20 μm) of dentine differs in the crown and the root. In the crown it is referred to as mantle dentine and differs in the orientation of its collagen fibres. In the root, the peripheral zone presents a granular layer – with less overall mineral – beyond which is a hyaline layer which lacks a tubular structure and may function to produce a good bond between the cementum and dentine.

Dentine is formed slowly throughout life, and so there is always an unmineralized zone of predentine at the surface of the mineralized dentine, adjacent to the odontoblast layer at the periphery of the pulp. Biochemical changes within the mineralizing matrix mean that predentine stains differently to the matrix of the mineralized dentine. The predentine–dentine border is generally scalloped, because dentine mineralizes both linearly and as microscopic spherical aggregates of crystals (calcospherites). Dentine, like enamel, is deposited incrementally, and exhibits both short- and long-term incremental lines. Long-term lines are known as Andresen lines and are c.20 μm apart: they represent increments of about 6–10 days (**Fig. 33.30**). Daily incremental lines (von Ebner lines) are c.4 μm apart. Where mineralization spans birth (i.e. all deciduous teeth and usually the first permanent molars) a neonatal line is formed in dentine similar to that which is seen in enamel, and it signals the abrupt change in both environment and nutrition which occurs at birth.

Primary dentine formation proceeds at a steady but declining rate as first the crown and then the root is completed. This slow and intermittent deposition of dentine (regular secondary dentine) continues throughout life and further reduces the size of the pulp chamber. The presence of the odontoblast process means that dentine is a vital tissue. It responds to adverse external stimuli – such as rapidly advancing caries, excessive wear or tooth breakage – by forming poorly mineralized dead tracts, in which the odontoblasts of the affected region die and the tubules remain empty (tertiary dentine). A dead tract may be sealed from the pulp by a thin zone of sclerosed dentine and the deposition of irregular (tertiary) dentine by newly differentiated pulp cells (**Fig. 33.31**).

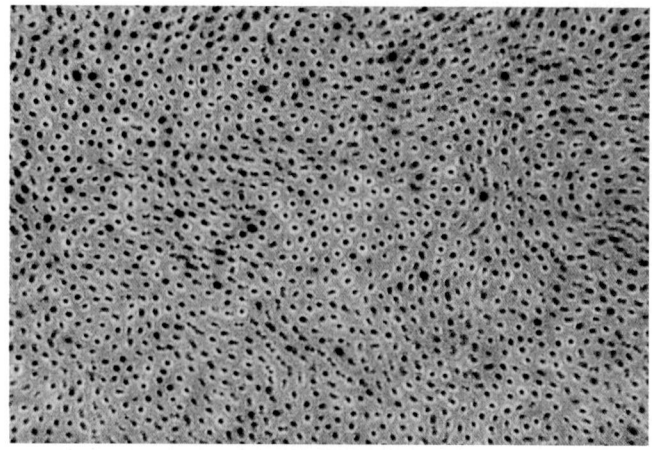

Fig. 33.29 Microradiograph of transversely sectioned dentinal tubules surrounded by a more radiopaque and therefore more mineralized zone of peritubular dentine. (By permission from Berkovitz BKB, Holland GR, Moxham BJ 2002 Oral Anatomy, Embryology and Histology, 3rd edn. Edinburgh: Mosby.)

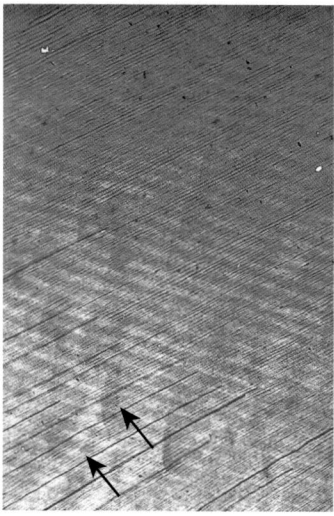

Fig. 33.30 Ground longitudinal section of dentine viewed in polarized light showing alternate light and dark bands representing long-period incremental lines (Andresen lines). The bands are approximately orientated at right angles to the direction of the dentinal tubules (arrows). (By permission from Berkovitz BKB, Holland GR, Moxham BJ 2002 Oral Anatomy, Embryology and Histology, 3rd edn. Edinburgh: Mosby.)

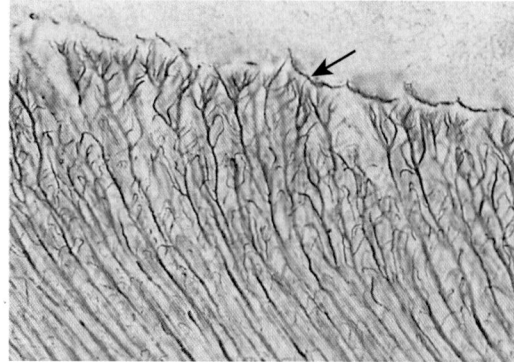

Fig. 33.28 Ground longitudinal section of dentine showing branching of dentine tubules near the enamel–dentine junction (arrow). (By permission from Berkovitz BKB, Holland GR, Moxham BJ 2002 Oral Anatomy, Embryology and Histology, 3rd edn. Edinburgh: Mosby.)

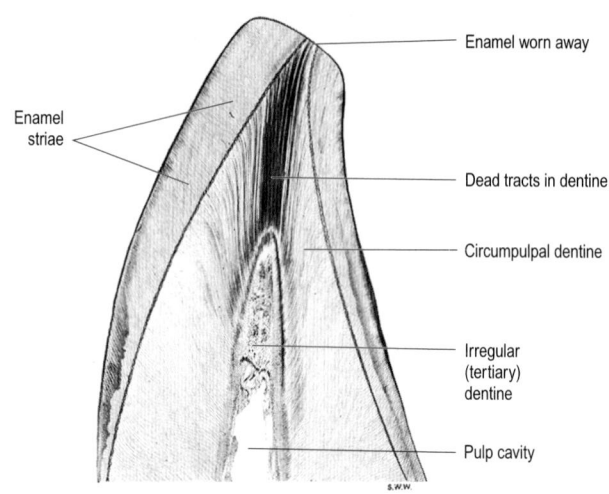

Enamel worn away

Enamel striae

Dead tracts in dentine

Circumpulpal dentine

Irregular (tertiary) dentine

Pulp cavity

Fig. 33.31 Longitudinal ground section of an incisor tooth.

Dental pulp

Dental pulp provides the nutritive support for the synthetic activity of the odontoblast layer. It is a well-vascularized, loose connective tissue, enclosed by dentine and continuous with the periodontal ligament via apical and accessory foramina. Several thin-walled arterioles enter by the apical foramen and run longitudinally within the pulp to an extensive subodontoblastic plexus. Blood flow rate per unit volume of tissue is greater in the pulp than in other oral tissues, and tissue fluid pressures within the pulp appear to be unusually high.

As well as typical connective tissue cells, pulp uniquely contains the cell bodies of odontoblasts whose long processes occupy the dentinal tubules. Pulp also has dendritic antigen-presenting cells. Approximately 60% of pulpal collagen is type I, and the bulk of the remainder is type III. As dentine deposition increases with age, the pulp recedes until the whole of the crown may be removed without accessing the pulp.

Dental pulp is extensively innervated by unmyelinated postganglionic vasoconstrictor sympathetic nerve fibres from the superior cervical ganglion, which enter with the arterioles, and by myelinated (Aδ) and unmyelinated (C) sensory nerve fibres from the trigeminal ganglion, which traverse the pulp longitudinally and ramify as a plexus (Raschkow's plexus) beneath the odontoblast layer (**Fig. 33.22**). Here, any myelinated nerve fibres lose their myelin sheaths and continue into the odontoblast layer, and some enter the dentinal tubules, especially the region beneath the cusps. Stimulation of dentine, whether by thermal, mechanical or osmotic means, evokes a pain response. Pulp nerves release numerous neuropeptides.

Cementum

Cementum is a bone-like tissue which covers the dental roots, and is c.50% by weight mineralized (mainly hydroxyapatite crystals). However, unlike bone, cementum is avascular and lacks nerves. The cementum generally overlaps the enamel slightly, although it may meet it end on. Occasionally, the two tissues may fail to meet, in which case dentine is exposed in the mouth. If the exposed dentinal tubules remain patent then the teeth may be sensitive to stimuli such as cold water. In older teeth, the root may become exposed in the mouth as a consequence of occlusal drift and gingival recession, and cementum is often abraded away by incorrect tooth brushing and dentine exposed.

Like bone, cementum is perforated by Sharpey's fibres, which represent the attachment bundles of collagen fibres in the periodontal ligament (extrinsic fibres). New layers of cementum, which are deposited incrementally throughout life to compensate for tooth movements, incorporate new Sharpey's fibres. Incremental lines are irregularly spaced. The first cement to be formed is thin (up to 200 μm), acellular and contains only extrinsic fibres. Cementum formed later towards the root apex is produced more rapidly and contains cementocytes lying in lacunae joined by canaliculi. The latter are mainly directed towards their source of nutrients from the periodontal ligament. This cementum contains both extrinsic fibres derived from the periodontal ligament and intrinsic fibres of cementoblastic origin which lie parallel to the surface. Varying arrangements of layering between cellular and acellular cement occur. With increasing age, cellular cement may reach a thickness of a millimetre or more around the apices and at the branching of the roots, where it compensates for the loss of enamel by attrition. Cementum is not remodelled but small areas of resorption with evidence of repair may be seen.

Forensic anatomy of teeth

In forensic medicine, dental evidence is valuable in identification of individuals, especially following mass disasters; estimation of age at death of skeletonized remains; establishing guilt in cases of criminal injury by biting.

If teeth have been restored, extracted or replaced by a denture, an individual will have a virtually unique dentition which may have been recorded by the dentist in the form of charts, radiographs or plaster casts. Teeth are the most indestructible bodily structures and can provide an identification when trauma or fire has rendered the face unrecognizable. Moreover, the chronology of crown development, eruption and root formation can be used to estimate age until the third molar is completed at about 21 years. The method is even applicable to the fetus because the weight of mineralized tissue in teeth is closely related to age from about 22 weeks' gestation until birth. The time taken for a crown to form can be calculated from ground sections with considerable accuracy by counting the number of daily cross striations from the neonatal line. For permanent teeth, the time taken for the crown to form can be calculated by counting the number of the enamel striae. The age of adult teeth can be estimated from factors such as wear of the crown, reduction in size of the pulp and increase in thickness of cement in the apical half of the root. However, probably the most useful single characteristic is the amount of translucent dentine in the root, which is proportional to age. Such estimations are within 5–7 years of the chronological age and likely to be closer to the true age than those derived from skeletal changes.

Periodontal ligament

The principal functions of the periodontal ligament are to support the teeth, generate the force of tooth eruption and provide sensory information about tooth position and forces to facilitate reflex jaw activity. The periodontal ligament is a dense fibrous connective tissue c.0.2 mm wide which contains cells associated with the development and maintenance of alveolar bone (osteoblasts and osteoclasts) and of cementum (cementoblasts and odontoclasts). It also contains a network of epithelial cells (epithelial cell rests) which are embryological remnants of an epithelial root sheath. They have no evident function but may give rise to dental cysts.

The majority of collagen fibres of the periodontal ligament are arranged as variously oriented dense fibre bundles that connect alveolar bone and cementum and which may help to resist movement in specific directions (**Fig. 33.32**). About 80% of the collagen in the periodontal ligament is type I, most of the remainder is type III. The rate of turnover of collagen is probably the highest of any site in the body, for reasons which are as yet unclear. A very small volume of fibres are oxytalan fibres.

The periodontal ligament has a rich nerve and blood supply. The nerves are both autonomic (for the vasculature) and sensory (for pain and proprioception). The majority of proprioceptive nerve endings appear to be Ruffini-like endings (p. 62). The blood vessels tend to lie towards the bone side of the periodontal ligament and the capillaries are fenestrated. Tissue fluid pressures appear to be high.

Alveolar bone

That part of the maxilla or mandible which supports and protects the teeth is known as alveolar bone. An arbitrary boundary at the level of the root apices of the teeth separates the alveolar processes from the body of the mandible or the maxilla (**Fig. 33.33**). Like bone in other sites, alveolar bone functions as a mineralized supporting tissue, gives attachment to muscles, provides a framework for bone marrow and acts

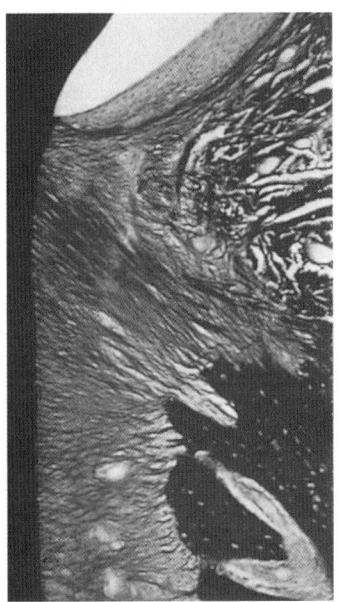

Fig. 33.32 Decalcified longitudinal section of a tooth showing groups of periodontal ligament fibres (the alveolar crest fibres and the horizontal fibres) in the region of the alveolar crest. van Gieson stain. (By permission from Berkovitz BKB, Holland GR, Moxham BJ 2002 Oral Anatomy, Embryology and Histology, 3rd edn. Edinburgh: Mosby.)

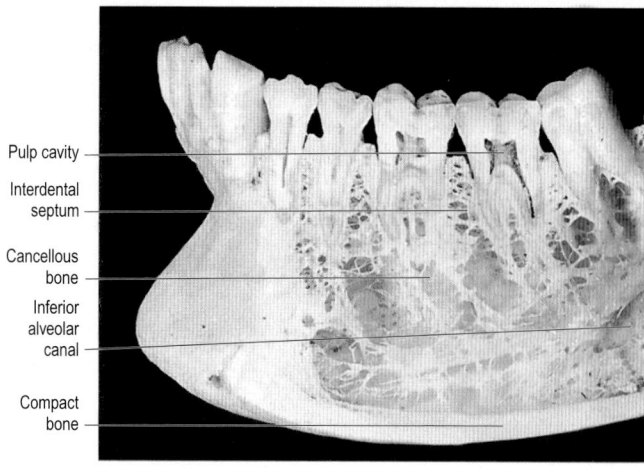

Pulp cavity

Interdental septum

Cancellous bone

Inferior alveolar canal

Compact bone

Fig. 33.33 Anterior part of the left side of the mandible, with the superficial bone removed on the buccal side to show the roots of a number of teeth, some of which have also been sectioned vertically. Note the cortical plate of compact bone lining the sockets of the teeth (the lamina dura of radiographs: see **Fig. 33.35**), and the flat table of bone surmounting the interdental bone septa. In this specimen the inferior alveolar canal is widely separated from the roots of the teeth, a variable condition.

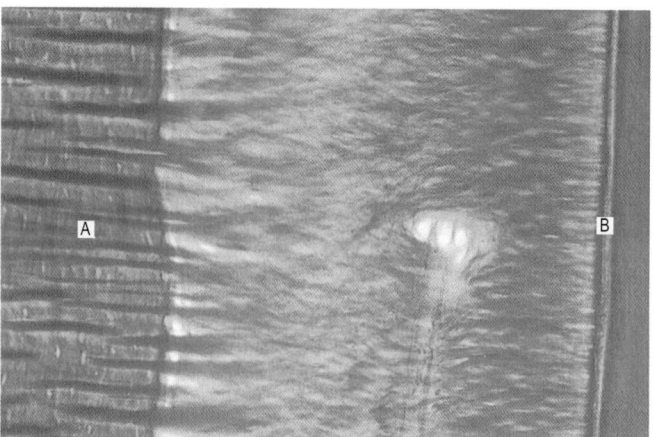

Fig. 33.34 Decalcified section of a root of a tooth showing Sharpey's fibres from the periodontal ligament entering alveolar bone (**A**). The Sharpey's fibres in bone are seen to be thicker, but less numerous, than those entering the cementum (**B**) on the tooth surface. van Gieson stain. (By permission from Berkovitz BKB, Holland GR, Moxham BJ 2002 Oral Anatomy, Embryology and Histology, 3rd edn. Edinburgh: Mosby.)

as a reservoir for ions, especially calcium. It is dependent on the presence of teeth for its development and maintenance, and requires functional stimuli to maintain bone mass. Where teeth are congenitally absent, as for example in anodontia, it is poorly developed, and it atrophies after tooth extraction.

The alveolar tooth-bearing portion of the jaws consists of outer and inner alveolar plates. The individual sockets are separated by plates of bone termed the interdental septa, while the roots of multi-rooted teeth are divided by interradicular septa septas. The compact layer of bone which lines the tooth socket has been called either the cribriform plate, on account of its content of vascular (Volkmann's) canals which pass from the alveolar bone into the periodontal ligament, or bundle bone, because numerous bundles of Sharpey's fibres pass into it from the periodontal ligament (**Fig. 33.34**).

In clinical radiographs, the bone lining the alveolus commonly appears as a continuous dense white line about 0.5–1 mm thick, the lamina dura (**Fig. 33.35**). However, this appearance gives a misleading impression of the density of alveolar bone: the X-ray beam passes tangentially through the socket wall, and so the radio-opacity of the lamina dura is an indication of the quantity of bone the beam has passed through, rather than the degree of mineralization of the bone. Superimposition also obscures the Volkmann's canals. Chronic infections of the dental pulp spread into the periodontal ligament, which leads to resorption of the lamina dura around the root apex. The presence of a continuous lamina dura around the apex of a tooth therefore usually indicates a healthy apical region (except in acute infections where resorption of bone has not yet begun).

On the labial and buccal aspects of upper teeth, the two cortical plates usually fuse, and there is very little trabecular bone between them, except where the buccal bone thickens over the molar teeth near the root of the zygomatic arch. It is easier and more convenient to extract upper teeth by fracturing the buccal than the palatal plate. Anteriorly in the lower jaw, labial and lingual plates are thin, but in the molar region the buccal plate is thickened as the external oblique line. Near the lower third molar, the lingual bone is much thinner than the buccal and it is mechanically easier to remove this tooth, when impacted, via the lingual plate, although it is important to realize that the lingual nerve is here exposed to damage.

VASCULAR SUPPLY AND LYMPHATIC DRAINAGE OF THE TEETH AND SUPPORTING STRUCTURES

Arterial supply of the teeth

The main arteries to the teeth and their supporting structures are derived from the maxillary artery, a terminal branch of the external carotid artery. The upper teeth are supplied by branches from the superior

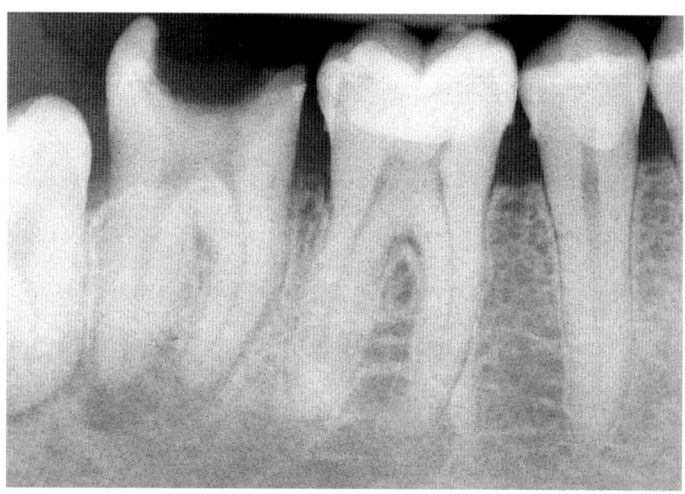

Fig. 33.35 Bite-wing radiograph of teeth and surrounding bone. Note the different radiopacities of enamel and dentine. In a healthy tooth, such as the first molar illustrated here, the lamina dura is complete and appears as a radiopaque line. In the case of the adjacent second molar tooth in which the bulk of the crown has been lost due to dental caries, an abscess has formed at the base of the tooth and as a result the lamina dura has lost its continuity. (By kind permission from Ms Nadine White.)

alveolar arteries and the lower teeth by branches from the inferior alveolar arteries.

Superior alveolar arteries

The upper jaw is supplied by posterior, middle and anterior superior alveolar (dental) arteries. The posterior superior alveolar artery usually arises from the third part of the maxillary artery in the pterygopalatine fossa. It descends on the infratemporal surface of the maxilla, and divides to give branches that enter the alveolar canals to supply molar and premolar teeth, adjacent bone and the maxillary sinus, and other branches that continue over the alveolar process to supply the gingivae. The middle and anterior superior alveolar arteries are branches from the infraorbital artery.

The infraorbital artery often arises with the posterior superior alveolar artery. It enters the orbit posteriorly through the inferior orbital fissure and runs in the infraorbital groove and canal with the infraorbital nerve. When the small middle superior alveolar artery is present it runs down the lateral wall of the maxillary sinus and forms anastomotic arcades with the anterior and posterior vessels, terminating near the canine tooth. The anterior superior alveolar artery curves through the canalis sinuosus to supply the upper incisor and canine teeth and the mucous membrane in the maxillary sinus. The canalis sinuosus swerves laterally from the infraorbital canal and inferomedially below it in the wall of the maxillary sinus, following the rim of the anterior nasal aperture, between the alveoli of canine and incisor teeth and the nasal cavity. It ends near the nasal septum where its terminal branch emerges. The canal may be up to 55 mm long.

Inferior alveolar artery

The inferior alveolar (dental) artery, a branch of the maxillary artery, descends in the infratemporal fossa posterior to the inferior alveolar nerve. Here, it lies between bone laterally and the sphenomandibular ligament medially. Before entering the mandibular foramen it gives off a mylohyoid branch, which pierces the sphenomandibular ligament to descend with the mylohyoid nerve in its groove on the inner surface of the ramus of the mandible (Fig. 30.7). The mylohyoid artery ramifies superficially on the muscle and anastomoses with the submental branch of the facial artery. The inferior alveolar artery then traverses the mandibular canal with the inferior alveolar nerve to supply the mandibular molars and premolars and divides into the incisive and mental branches near the first premolar.

The incisive branch continues below the incisor teeth (which it supplies) to the midline, where it anastomoses with its fellow, although few anastomotic vessels cross the midline. In the canal the arteries supply the mandible, tooth sockets and teeth via branches which enter the minute hole at the apex of each root to supply the pulp. The mental artery leaves the mental foramen and supplies the chin and anastomoses with the submental and inferior labial arteries. Near its origin the inferior alveolar artery has a lingual branch, which descends with the lingual nerve to supply the lingual mucous membrane. The pattern of branching of the inferior alveolar artery reflects that of the nerves of the same name.

Arterial supply of periodontal ligaments

The periodontal ligaments supporting the teeth are supplied by dental branches of alveolar arteries. One branch enters the alveolus apically and sends two or three small rami into the dental pulp through the apical foramen, and other rami into the periodontal ligament. Interdental arteries ascend in the interdental septa, sending branches at right angles into the periodontal ligament, and terminate by communicating with gingival vessels that also supply the cervical part of the ligament. The periodontal ligament therefore receives its blood from three sources: from the apical region; ascending interdental arteries; descending vessels from the gingivae. These vessels anastomose with each other, which means that when the pulp of a tooth is removed during endodontic treatment, the attachment tissues of the tooth remain vital.

Venous drainage of the teeth

Veins accompanying the superior alveolar arteries drain the upper jaw and teeth anteriorly into the facial vein, or posteriorly into the pterygoid venous plexus. Veins from the lower jaw and teeth collect either into larger vessels in the interdental septa or into plexuses around the root apices and thence into several inferior alveolar veins. Some of these veins drain through the mental foramen to the facial vein, others drain via the mandibular foramen to the pterygoid venous plexus.

Lymphatic drainage of the teeth

The lymph vessels from the teeth usually run directly into the ipsilateral submandibular lymph nodes. Lymph from the mandibular incisors, however, drains into the submental lymph nodes. Occasionally, lymph from the molars may pass directly into the jugulodigastric group of nodes.

INNERVATION OF THE TEETH (Fig. 33.36)

The regional supply to the teeth and gingivae is shown in **Table 33.1**. The teeth in the upper jaw are supplied by the superior alveolar nerves while those in the lower jaw are supplied by the inferior alveolar nerve.

Superior alveolar nerves

The teeth in the upper jaw are supplied by the three superior alveolar (dental) nerves (Fig. 30.6). These arise from the maxillary nerve in the pterygopalatine fossa or in the infraorbital groove and canal. The posterior superior alveolar (dental) nerve leaves the maxillary nerve in

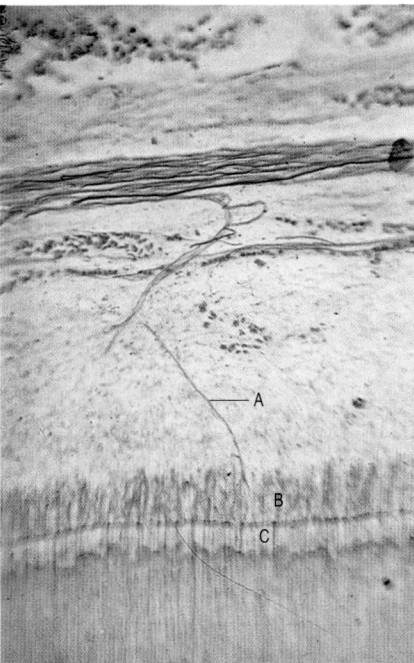

Fig. 33.36 Longitudinal demineralized section of a tooth stained with a silver impregnation technique. Note the horizontal nerve trunk (top) within the pulp, with fine nerve fibres, one of which (A) passes between the odontoblasts (B) lining the surface of the predentine (C).

the pterygopalatine fossa and runs anteroinferiorly to pierce the infratemporal surface of the maxilla, descending under the mucosa of the maxillary sinus. After supplying the lining of the sinus the nerve divides into small branches which link up as the molar part of the superior alveolar plexus, supplying twigs to the molar teeth. It also supplies a branch to the upper gingivae and the adjoining part of the cheek.

The middle superior alveolar (dental) nerve arises from the infraorbital nerve as it runs in the infraorbital groove, and runs downwards and forwards in the lateral wall of the maxillary sinus. It ends in small branches which link up with the superior dental plexus, supplying small rami to the upper premolar teeth. This nerve is variable, and it may be duplicated or triplicated or absent.

The anterior superior alveolar (dental) nerve leaves the lateral side of the infraorbital nerve near the midpoint of its canal and traverses the canalis sinuosus in the anterior wall of the maxillary sinus. It curves first under the infraorbital foramen, then passes medially towards the nose and finally turns downwards and divides into branches to supply the incisor and canine teeth. It assists in the formation of the superior dental plexus and it gives off a nasal branch, which passes through a minute canal in the lateral wall of the inferior meatus to supply the mucous membrane of the anterior area of the lateral wall as high as the opening of the maxillary sinus, and the floor of the nasal cavity. It communicates with the nasal branches of the pterygopalatine ganglion and finally emerges near the root of the anterior nasal spine to supply the adjoining part of the nasal septum.

Inferior alveolar (dental) nerve (Figs 30.4–30.7, 30.6)

The course of the inferior alveolar nerve in the infratemoral fossa is described on page 523. Just before entering the mandibular canal the inferior alveolar nerve gives off a small mylohyoid branch which pierces the sphenomandibular ligament and enters a shallow groove on the medial surface of the mandible following a course roughly parallel to its parent nerve. It passes below the origin of mylohyoid to lie on the superficial surface of the muscle, between it and the anterior belly of digastric, both of which it supplies. It gives a few filaments to supply the skin over the point of the chin.

In the mandibular canal, the inferior alveolar nerve runs downward and forward, generally below the apices of the teeth until below the first and second premolars where it divides into terminal incisive and mental branches. The incisive branch continues forward in a bony canal or in a plexiform arrangement, giving off branches to the first premolar, canine and incisor teeth, and the associated labial gingivae. The lower central incisor teeth receive a bilateral innervation, fibres probably crossing the midline within the periosteum to re-enter the bone via numerous canals in the labial cortical plate.

The mental nerve passes upward, backward and outward to emerge from the mandible via the mental foramen between and just below the apices of the premolar teeth (**Fig. 30.6**). It immediately divides into three branches, two of which pass upward and forward to form an incisor plexus labial to the teeth, supplying the gingiva (and probably the periosteum). From this plexus and the dental branches, fibres turn downwards and then lingually to emerge on the lingual surface of the mandible on the posterior aspect of the symphysis or opposite the premolar teeth, probably communicating with the lingual or mylohyoid nerve. The third branch of the mental nerve passes through the intermingled fibres of depressor anguli oris and platysma to supply the skin of the lower lip and chin. Branches of the mental nerve also communicate with terminal filaments of the mandibular branch of the facial nerve.

Variations in the fascicular organization of the inferior alveolar nerve are clinically important when extracting impacted third molars. It may appear as a single bundle lying a few millimetres below the roots of the teeth, or it may lie much lower, and almost reach the lower border of the bone, so that it gives off a variable number of large rami which pass anterosuperiorly towards the roots before dividing to supply the teeth and interdental septa. Only rarely is it plexiform. The nerve may lie on the lingual or buccal side of the mandible (slightly more commonly on the buccal side). Even when the third molar tooth is in a normal position, the nerve may be so intimately related to it that it grooves its root. Exceptionally the nerve may be similarly related to the second molar.

Nerves may pass from the substance of temporalis to enter the mandible through the retromolar fossa, where they communicate with branches of the inferior alveolar nerve. Foramina occur in c.10% of retromolar fossae and infiltration in this region can abolish sensation which occasionally remains after an inferior alveolar nerve block. Similarly, branches from the buccal, mylohyoid and lingual nerves may enter the mandible and provide additional routes of sensory transmission from the teeth. Thus, even when the inferior alveolar nerve has been anaesthetized correctly, pain may still be experienced by a patient when undergoing dental cavity preparation.

Pain sensation in teeth

The teeth are supplied by nociceptors that generate pain sensation of a very high order. The mechanism underlying this sensitivity is of considerable clinical significance and is controversial. Currently, the most widely accepted view is that fluid movements through the dentine tubules stimulate nerve endings at the periphery of the dental pulp (hydrodynamic hypothesis).

Local analgesia

It is technically possible to achieve profound regional anaesthesia by depositing local anaesthetic solution adjacent to the trigeminal nerve trunks or their branches within the infratemporal fossa (p. 523). These injections can either be performed transorally – posterior superior alveolar nerve block, maxillary nerve block, inferior alveolar nerve block, lingual nerve block and mandibular nerve block – or more rarely by an external route through the skin of the face – maxillary nerve block, inferior alveolar nerve block and mandibular nerve block.

In the case of the mandible, the anterior teeth can be anaesthetized by simple diffusion techniques as the bone is relatively thin. However, this is not adequate for the cheek teeth due to the increased thickness of the bone. In this case, the inferior alveolar nerve has to be anaesthetized before it enters the inferior alveolar canal. The needle has to be placed within the pterygomandibular space to achieve a successful inferior alveolar nerve block. The lingual nerve is also usually blocked as it lies close to the inferior alveolar nerve. Because of the other structures within the infratemporal fossa it is vitally important that the operator has a detailed knowledge of the anatomy in this region to understand, and therefore try to avoid, the complications that may arise. Any damage to blood vessels in the infratemporal fossa, generally the pterygoid venous plexus, can lead to haematoma formation. In extreme cases, bleeding can track through the inferior orbital fissure resulting in a retrobulbar haematoma, which can result in loss of visual acuity or blindness. Intravascular injection of local anaesthetic solution (which usually contains adrenaline (epinephrine)) can have profound systemic effects and for this reason an aspirating syringe is always used to check that the needle has not entered a vessel prior to injection. If the needle is placed too medially it may enter medial pterygoid, while if directed too laterally it

may penetrate temporalis. In either case, there will be lack of anaesthesia followed later by trismus. If the needle is placed too deeply, anaesthetic solution may cause a temporary Bell's palsy due to loss of conduction from the facial nerve in the region of the parotid gland. Finally, if the needle is not sterile, infection of the pterygomandibular space may ensue, which could spread to other important tissue spaces (p. 525). Diffusion of anaesthetic solution through the inferior orbital fissure could give temporary orbital symptoms such as paralysis of lateral rectus due to anaesthesia of the abducens nerve.

THE SALIVARY GLANDS

Salivary glands are compound, tubuloacinar exocrine glands (p. 34) whose ducts open into the oral cavity. They secrete saliva, a fluid which lubricates food to assist deglutition, moistens the buccal mucosa, which is important for speech, and provides an aqueous solvent necessary for taste and a fluid seal for sucking and suckling. They also secrete digestive enzymes, e.g. salivary amylase and antimicrobial agents e.g. IgA, lysozyme and lactoferrin, into saliva. Conditions where there is a significant decrease in the production of saliva (xerostomia) may result in periodontal inflammation and dental caries. An illustration of the position of the major salivary glands and their ducts is shown in **Fig. 33.37**.

The major salivary glands are the paired parotid, submandibular and sublingual glands. In addition, there are numerous minor salivary glands scattered throughout the oral mucosa and submucosa.

Approximately 0.5 litres of saliva is secreted per day. Salivary flow rates are c.0.3 ml/min when unstimulated, and rise to 1.5–2 ml/min when stimulated. Flow rate is negligible during sleep. In the unstimulated state, the parotid gland contributes c.20%, the submandibular gland c.65%, and the sublingual and minor salivary glands c.15% of the daily output of saliva. When stimulated, the parotid contribution rises to 50%.

Parotid gland (Fig. 33.37)

The parotid gland is the largest salivary gland. It is almost entirely serous. The parotid duct runs through the cheek and drains into the mouth opposite the maxillary second permanent molar tooth. The parotid gland is situated in front of the external ear and is described in detail in relation to the face (p. 515).

Submandibular salivary gland (Fig. 33.37)

The submandibular gland is irregular in shape and about the size of a walnut. It consists of a larger superficial and a smaller deep part, continuous with each other around the posterior border of mylohyoid. It is a seromucous (but predominantly serous) gland.

SUPERFICIAL PART OF THE SUBMANDIBULAR GLAND

The superficial part of the gland is situated in the digastric triangle where it reaches forward to the anterior belly of digastric and back to the stylomandibular ligament, by which it is separated from the parotid gland. Above, it extends medial to the body of the mandible. Below, it usually overlaps the intermediate tendon of digastric and the insertion of stylohyoid. This part of the submandibular gland presents inferior, lateral and medial surfaces, and is partially enclosed between two layers of deep cervical fascia that extend from the greater cornu of the hyoid bone. The superficial layer is attached to the lower border of the mandible and covers the inferior surface of the gland. The deep layer is attached to the mylohyoid line on the medial surface of the mandible and covers the medial surface of the gland.

The inferior surface, covered by skin, platysma and deep fascia, is crossed by the facial vein and the cervical branch of the facial nerve. Near the mandible the submandibular lymph nodes are in contact with the gland and some may be embedded within it.

The lateral surface is related to the submandibular fossa on the medial surface of the body of the mandible and the mandibular attachment of medial pterygoid. The facial artery grooves its posterosuperior part, lies at first deep to the gland and then emerges between its lateral surface and the mandibular attachment of the medial pterygoid to reach the lower border of the mandible.

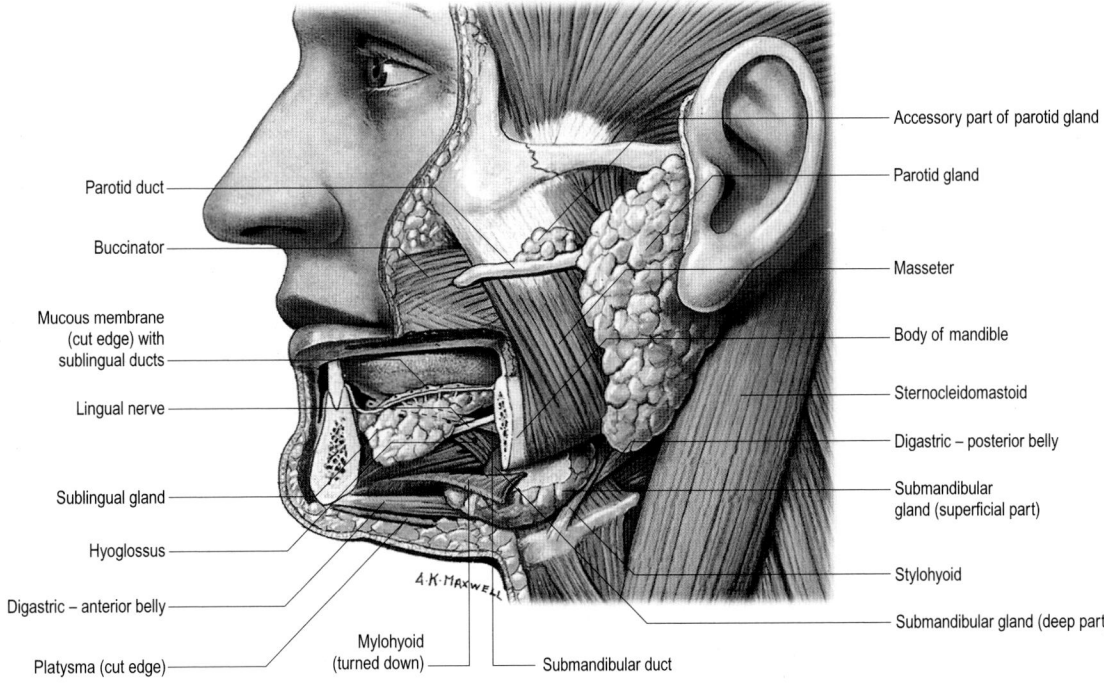

Parotid duct

Buccinator

Mucous membrane
(cut edge) with
sublingual ducts

Lingual nerve

Sublingual gland

Hyoglossus

Digastric – anterior belly

Platysma (cut edge)

Mylohyoid
(turned down)

Submandibular duct

Accessory part of parotid gland

Parotid gland

Masseter

Body of mandible

Sternocleidomastoid

Digastric – posterior belly

Submandibular
gland (superficial part)

Stylohyoid

Submandibular gland (deep part)

A.K.MAXWELL

Fig. 33.37 The salivary glands of the left side. The cranial region of the superficial part of the submandibular gland has been excised and the cut mylohyoid has been turned down to expose a portion of the deep part of the gland.

The medial surface is related anteriorly to mylohyoid, from which it is separated by the mylohyoid nerve and vessels and branches of the submental vessels. More posteriorly, it is related to styloglossus, the stylohyoid ligament and the glossopharyngeal nerve, which separate it from the pharynx. In its intermediate part the medial surface is related to hyoglossus, from which it is separated by styloglossus, the lingual nerve, submandibular ganglion, hypoglossal nerve and deep lingual vein (sequentially from above down). Below, the medial surface is related to the stylohyoid muscle and the posterior belly of digastric.

DEEP PART OF THE SUBMANDIBULAR GLAND

The deep part of the gland extends forwards to the posterior end of the sublingual gland. It lies between mylohyoid inferolaterally, hyoglossus and styloglossus medially, the lingual nerve superiorly, and the hypoglossal nerve and deep lingual vein inferiorly.

VASCULAR SUPPLY AND LYMPHATIC DRAINAGE

The arteries supplying the gland are branches of the facial and lingual arteries. The lymph vessels drain into the deep cervical group of lymph nodes (particularly the jugulo-omohyoid node), interrupted by the submandibular nodes.

INNERVATION

The secretomotor supply to the submandibular gland is derived from the submandibular ganglion. This is a small, fusiform body which lies on the upper part of hyoglossus. There are additional ganglion cells in the hilum of the gland. Like the ciliary, pterygopalatine and otic ganglia, the submandibular is a peripheral parasympathetic ganglion. It is superior to the deep part of the submandibular gland and inferior to the lingual nerve, and is suspended from the latter by anterior and posterior filaments (**Fig. 30.6**). Though related to the lingual nerve, the ganglion is connected functionally with the facial nerve and its chorda tympani branch.

As with the other cranial parasympathetic ganglia, there are three roots associated with the submandibular ganglion (**Fig. 30.8**). The motor, parasympathetic root is the posterior filament which connects it to the lingual nerve. This conveys preganglionic fibres from the superior salivatory nucleus which travel in the facial, chorda tympani and lingual nerves to the ganglion, where they synapse. The postganglionic fibres are secretomotor to the submandibular and sublingual salivary glands. Some fibres may also reach the parotid gland. The sympathetic root is derived from the plexus on the facial artery. It consists of postganglionic fibres from the superior cervical ganglion which traverse the submandibular ganglion without synapsing. They are vasomotor to the blood vessels of the submandibular and sublingual glands. Five or six branches from the ganglion supply the submandibular gland and its

duct. Other fibres pass through the anterior filament that connects the submandibular gland to the lingual nerve and are carried to the sublingual and anterior lingual glands. Sensory fibres are derived from the lingual nerve.

SUBMANDIBULAR DUCT

The submandibular duct is c.5 cm long and has a thinner wall than the parotid duct. It begins from numerous tributaries in the superficial part of the gland and emerges from the medial surface of this part of the gland behind the posterior border of mylohyoid. It traverses the deep part of the gland, passes at first up and slightly back for c.5 mm, and then forwards between mylohyoid and hyoglossus. It next passes between the sublingual gland and genioglossus to open in the floor of the mouth on the summit of the sublingual papilla at the side of the frenulum of the tongue (**Fig. 33.3**). It lies between the lingual and hypoglossal nerves on hyoglossus, but, at the anterior border of the muscle, it is crossed laterally by the lingual nerve, terminal branches of which ascend on its medial side. As the duct traverses the deep part of the gland it receives small tributaries draining this part of the gland.

Like the parotid gland, the duct system of the submandibular gland can be visualized by sialography (**Fig. 33.38**).

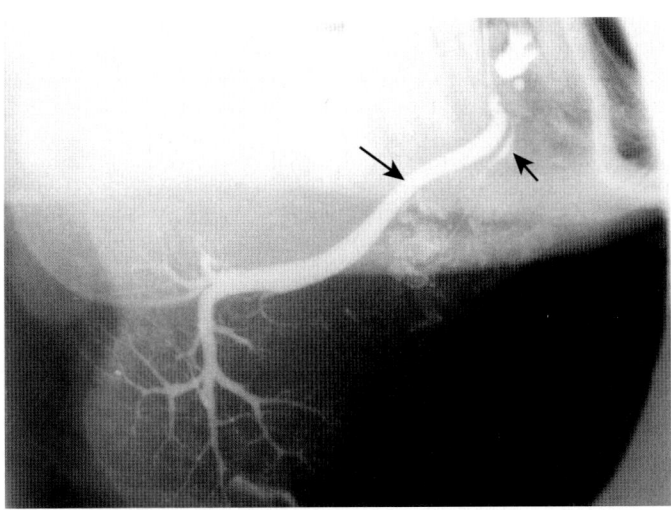

Fig. 33.38 Sialogram showing a normal submandibular duct (large arrow). Unusually, a sublingual duct is also evident (small arrow). (By kind permission from Dr N Drage.)

Sublingual salivary gland (Fig. 33.37)

The sublingual gland is the smallest of the main salivary glands: each gland is narrow, flat, shaped like an almond, and weighs c.4 g. The sublingual gland lies on mylohyoid, and is covered by the mucosa of the floor of the mouth, which is raised as a sublingual fold (Fig. 33.3). The anterior end of the contralateral sublingual gland lies in front, and the deep part of the submandibular gland lies behind. The mandible above the anterior part of the mylohyoid line, the sublingual fossa, is lateral, and genioglossus is medial, separated from the gland by the lingual nerve and submandibular duct.

The sublingual glands are seromucous, but predominantly mucous.

VASCULAR SUPPLY, INNERVATION AND LYMPHATIC DRAINAGE

The arterial supply is from the sublingual branch of the lingual artery and the submental branch of the facial artery. Innervation is via the submandibular ganglion. Lymphatic drainage is to the submental nodes.

SUBLINGUAL DUCTS

The sublingual gland has 8–20 excretory ducts. Smaller sublingual ducts open, usually separately, from the posterior part of the gland onto the summit of the sublingual fold (a few sometimes open into the submandibular duct). Small rami from the anterior part of the gland sometimes form a major sublingual duct (Bartholin's duct), which opens with, or near to, the orifice of the submandibular duct. This duct may be visualized occasionally in a submandibular sialogram (Fig. 33.38).

Ranula

If the ducts draining any salivary gland become obstructed, the gland itself is at risk of developing a retention cyst where the retained secretions dilate the gland itself rather like a balloon. This phenomenon is seen mostly in the minor salivary glands which line the lips and oral cavity. Trauma such as persistent lip biting results in scarring of the overlying oral mucosa and obstruction of the small drainage duct. When trauma occurs in the floor of the mouth and obstructs the drainage duct/s of the sublingual gland, the resulting retention cyst is known as a ranula. (Ranula is the Latin name for a frog and is used here because the tense cystic swelling is said to resemble the throat of a croaking frog.)

A ranula usually presents as a large tense bluish swelling anteriorly in the floor of the mouth just to one side of the midline, which often displaces the tongue. Occasionally the developing retention cyst herniates through a midline dehiscence where the two mylohyoid muscles fail to meet in the midline anteriorly, and then the ranula may present as a submental swelling or as a combined submental and floor of mouth swelling. The treatment of a ranula is excision of the sublingual gland responsible.

Minor salivary glands

The minor salivary glands of the mouth include the labial, buccal, palatoglossal, palatal and lingual glands. The labial and buccal glands contain both mucous and serous elements. The palatoglossal glands are mucous glands and are located around the pharyngeal isthmus. The palatal glands are mucous glands and occur in both the soft and hard palates. The anterior and posterior lingual glands are mainly mucous. The anterior glands are embedded within muscle near the ventral surface of the tongue and open by means of four or five ducts near the lingual frenum and the posterior glands are located in the root of the tongue. The deep posterior lingual glands are predominantly serous. Serous glands (of Von Ebner) occur around the circumvallate papillae, their secretion is watery, and they probably assist in gustation by spreading taste stimuli over the taste buds and then washing them away.

Microstructure of the salivary glands

Salivary glands have numerous lobes composed of smaller lobules separated by dense connective tissue which is continuous with the capsule of the gland, and contains excretory (collecting) ducts, blood vessels, lymph vessels, nerve fibres and small ganglia. Each lobule has a single duct, whose branches terminate at dilated secretory 'endpieces', which are tubular or acinar in shape (Fig. 33.39). Their primary secretion is modified as it flows through intercalated, striated and excretory ducts into one or more main ducts which discharge saliva into the oral cavity. They contain a variable amount of intralobular adipose tissue: adipocytes are particularly numerous in the parotid gland.

The secretory 'endpieces' of the human parotid gland are almost exclusively serous acini (Fig. 33.40): mucous tubules or acini are rare. In the submandibular gland, secretory units are predominantly serous acini, with some mucous tubules and acini (Fig. 33.41). Mucous tubules are often associated with groups of serous cells at their blind ends, appearing as crescent-shaped serous demilunes in routine histological preparations. However this appears to be a fixation artefact, as tissue prepared by rapid freezing methods lacks serous demilunes and the serous secretory cells align with mucous cells around a common lumen. In the sublingual gland mucous tubules and acini predominate (Fig. 33.42), but serous cells also occur, as acini or as serous demilunes.

Serous cells are approximately pyramidal in shape. Their nuclei vary in shape and position, but are more rounded and situated less basally than in mucous cells. Apically, the cytoplasm is filled by proteinaceous secretory (zymogen) granules with high amylase activity. Additionally, serous cells secrete kallikrein, lactoferrin and lysozyme, an antibacterial enzyme whose synthesis has been localized in particular to the serous demilunes of the submandibular and sublingual glands, and which is important in the defence against oral pathogens. In the human parotid and submandibular glands, zymogen granules also show a positive periodic acid-Schiff staining reaction, which indicates the presence of polysaccharides, and some texts refer to these cells as seromucous. Mucous cells are cylindrical and have flattened, basal nuclei. Their apical cytoplasm is typically packed with large, pale-staining and electron-translucent secretory droplets.

DUCTS

Intercalated, striated (both intralobular) and extralobular collecting ducts lead consecutively from the secretory endpieces. The lining cells of intercalated ducts are flat nearest the secretory endpiece, but become cuboidal. They function primarily as a conduit for saliva but, together with the striated ducts, may also modify its content of electrolytes and secrete immunoglobulin A. Striated ducts (Fig. 33.40) are lined by a low columnar epithelium and are so-called because their lining cells have characteristic basal striations. The latter are regions of highly infolded basal plasma membrane, between which lie columns of vertically aligned mitochondria. The nuclei are consequently displaced by the basal striations from a typical ductal basal position to a central or even apical location. Infolding of the basal plasma membrane, and local abundance of mitochondria, are typical features of epithelial cells which actively transport electrolytes. Here, the cells transport potassium and bicarbonate into saliva: they produce a hypotonic saliva by reabsorbing sodium and chloride ions in excess of water. Striated ducts modify electrolyte composition and secrete immunoglobulin A, lysozyme and kallikrein. Immunoglobulin A is produced by subepithelial plasma cells and transported transcytotically across the epithelial barrier to be secreted, once it has been dimerized by epithelial secretory component, into the saliva. This is also a function of serous acinar cells and other secretory epithelia, notably the lactating breast (Chapter 58). The intralobular ductal system of the sublingual gland is less well-developed than that of the parotid and submandibular glands.

Collecting ducts are metabolically relatively inert conduits which run within interlobular connective tissue septa in the glands. They transport saliva to the main duct which opens onto the mucosal surface of the buccal cavity. The lining epithelium of collecting ducts varies. It may be pseudostratified columnar, stratified cuboidal or columnar in the larger ducts, and has a distinct basal layer. It becomes a stratified squamous epithelium near the buccal orifice.

MYOEPITHELIAL CELLS

Myoepithelial cells (Fig. 33.39) are contractile cells associated with secretory endpieces and with much of the ductal system. They lie between the basal lamina and the epithelial cells proper. They extend numerous cytoplasmic processes around serous acini and are often termed basket cells. Myoepithelial cells associated with ducts are more fusiform in shape, and are aligned along the length of the duct. Their cytoplasm contains abundant actin microfilaments which mediate contraction under the control of both sympathetic and parasympathetic stimulation. The outflow of saliva is thus accelerated through reduction in the luminal volume of secretory endpieces and ducts, contributing to the secretory pressure.

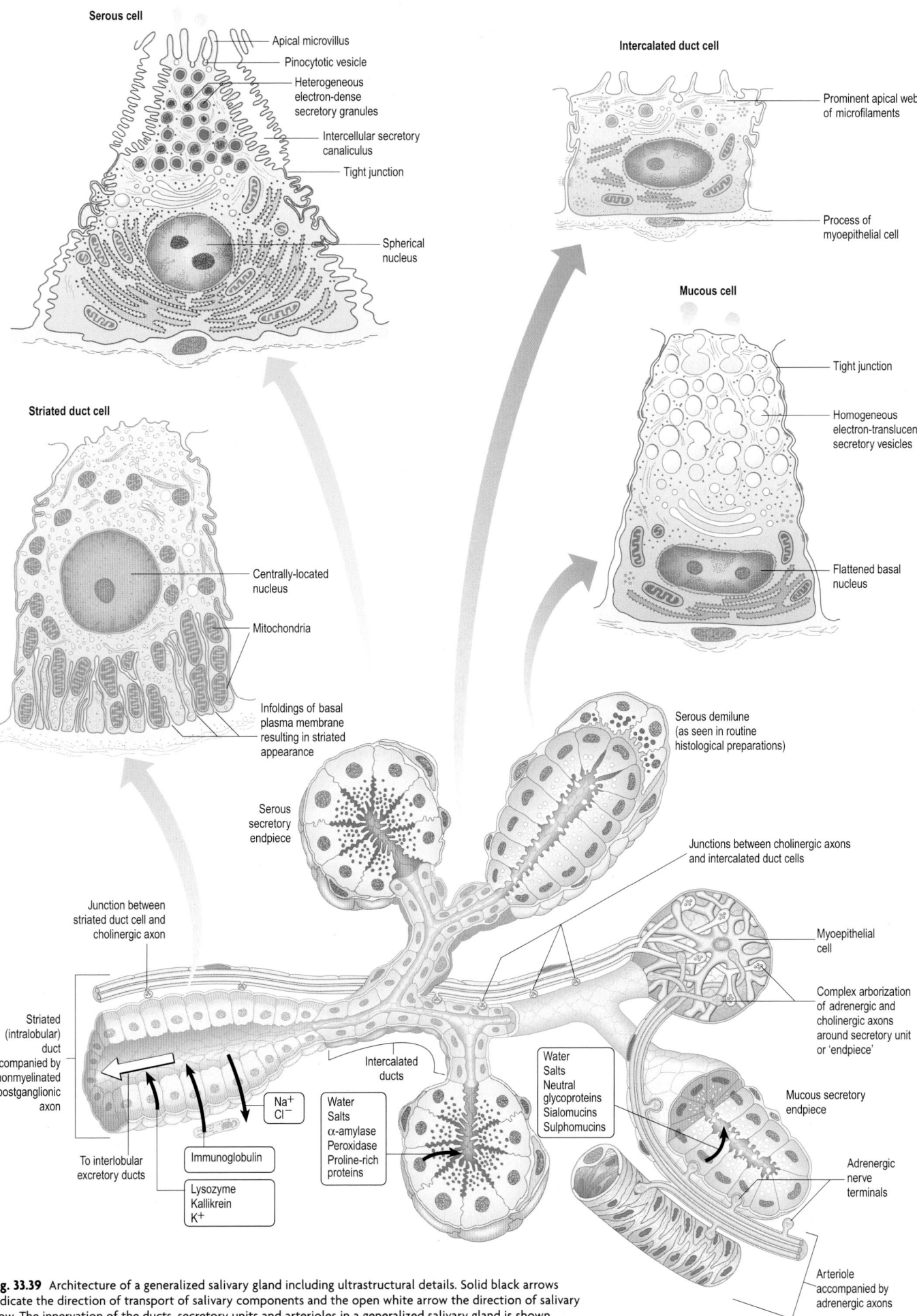

Fig. 33.39 Architecture of a generalized salivary gland including ultrastructural details. Solid black arrows indicate the direction of transport of salivary components and the open white arrow the direction of salivary flow. The innervation of the ducts, secretory units and arterioles in a generalized salivary gland is shown.

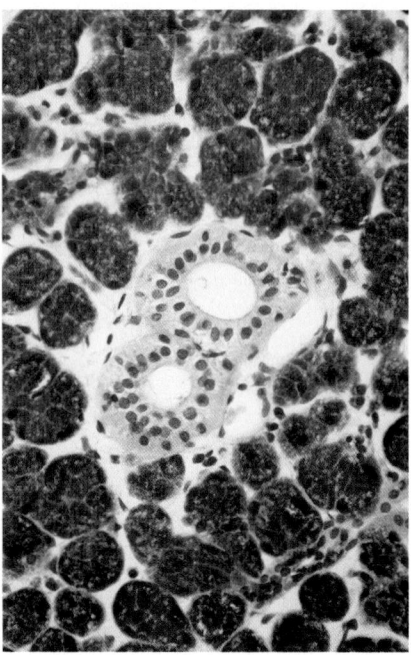

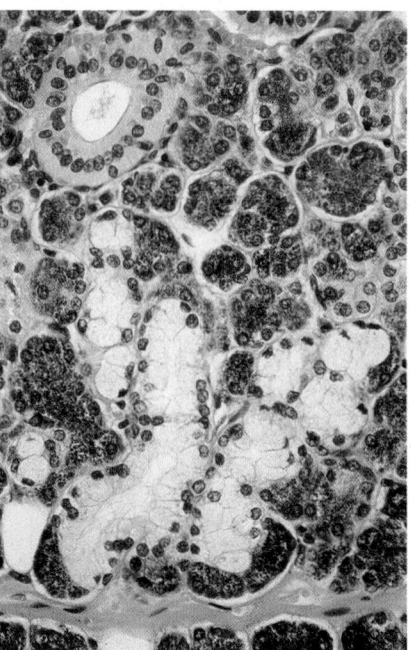

Fig. 33.40 A section through the parotid gland, with deeply stained secretory acini surrounding two striated ducts in transverse section, accompanied by small venules. An intercalated duct is seen in longitudinal section in the bottom right hand corner. (Photograph by Sarah-Jane Smith.)

Fig. 33.41 The mixed secretory units of the submandibular gland. Deeply stained serous acini (above) surround a striated duct (top left). Below are pale-staining mucous tubules, some with serous demilunes. Caps of serous cells appear, artifactually, to form crescentic extensions to the tubule, as seen at the bottom of the field. (Photograph by Sarah-Jane Smith.)

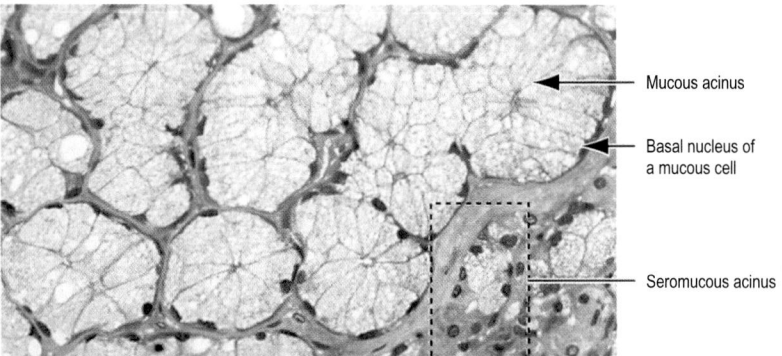

Mucous acinus

Basal nucleus of a mucous cell

Seromucous acinus

Fig. 33.42 Mucous acini in the sublingual gland. Secretory cells are filled with pale-staining mucinogen-containing vesicles and nuclei are displaced basally. (By permission from Kierszenbaum AL 2002 Histology and Cell Biology. St Louis: Mosby.)

CONTROL OF SALIVARY GLAND ACTIVITY

The observed wide and rapid variation in the composition, quantity and rate of salivary secretion in response to various stimuli suggests an elaborate control mechanism. Secretion may be continuous, but at a low resting level, and may also occur spontaneously. It is mainly a response to the drying of the oral and pharyngeal mucosae. A rapid increase can be superimposed on the resting level, e.g. during mastication or when stimulated by the autonomic innervation. The controlled variation in the activity of the many types of salivary effector cells (serous, seromucous and mucous secretory cells, myoepithelial cells, epithelial cells of all the ductal elements and the smooth muscle of local blood vessels) affects the quantity and quality of saliva. There is no clear evidence that circulating hormones evoke secretion directly at physiological levels, but they may alter the response of glandular cells to neural stimuli.

The control of salivation depends on reflex nerve impulses. The afferent inputs to the reflex arc pass to brain stem salivatory centres, especially from taste and mechanoreceptors in the mouth. A variety of other sensory modalities in and around the mouth are also involved, e.g. smell, for certain aspects of submandibular secretion in man. The afferent input is integrated centrally by the salivatory centres, which are themselves influenced by higher centres. The latter may provide facilitatory or inhibitory influences, which presumably explains why the mouth becomes dry under stress. The efferent drive to the glands passes via parasympathetic and sympathetic outputs from the centres. Relatively little is known about the connections of the preganglionic

parasympathetic neurones in the salivatory centres, and virtually nothing is known about either the central location of the sympathetic preganglionic neurones, or the output pathways. No peripheral inhibitory mechanisms exist in the glands.

The typical pattern of innervation is shown in **Fig. 33.39**, but details vary in different glands, and with age. Only the more constant features are illustrated and described here. Cholinergic nerves often accompany ducts and arborize freely around secretory endpieces, but adrenergic nerves usually enter glands along arteries and ramify with them. The main secretomotor nerves are predominantly non-myelinated axons: the few myelinated axons that have been seen are presumably either preganglionic efferent or visceral afferent. Within the glands the nerve fibres intermingle, such that cholinergic and adrenergic axons often lie in adjacent invaginations of one Schwann cell. Secretion and vasoconstriction are mediated via separate sympathetic axons. A single parasympathetic axon may, through serial en passant terminals, induce vasodilatation, secretion and myoepithelial contraction.

Secretory endpieces are usually the most densely innervated structures in the gland: individual cells often have both cholinergic and adrenergic innervation. Secretion of water and electrolytes, which creates the foundation for the volume of saliva secreted, is the outcome of a complex set of processes which is largely induced by parasympathetic impulses. Secretion of protein is an ongoing constitutive process wherever it occurs. The regulated exocytosis of pre-packaged proteins, which is the principle source of protein secretion into saliva, depends on the relative levels of activity in sympathetic and parasympathetic fibres.

The ductal elements of salivary glands can markedly modify the composition of saliva. They are less densely innervated than secretory endpieces but their activity is also under neural control. Adrenal aldosterone promotes resorption of sodium and release of potassium into saliva by striated ductal cells, as it does in kidney tubules. Myoepithelial contraction is stimulated mainly by adrenergic innervation, but there may be an additional role for cholinergic axons.

TISSUE SPACES AROUND THE JAWS (Fig. 33.43)

The dissemination of infection in soft tissues is influenced by the natural barriers presented by bone, muscle and fascia. However, the tissue spaces around the jaws are primarily defined by muscles, principally mylohyoid, buccinator, masseter, medial pterygoid, superior constrictor and orbicularis oris. None of these 'spaces' is actually empty and they should merely be regarded as potential spaces that are normally occupied by loose connective tissue. It is only when inflammatory products destroy the loose connective tissue that a definable space is produced.

The spaces are paired except for the submental, sublingual and palatal spaces.

POTENTIAL TISSUE SPACES AROUND THE LOWER JAW (Fig. 33.43)

The important potential tissue spaces of the lower jaw are the submental; submandibular; sublingual; buccal; submasseteric; parotid; pterygomandibular; peripharyngeal and peritonsillar spaces.

The submental and submandibular spaces are located below the inferior border of the mandible beneath mylohyoid, in the suprahyoid region of the neck. The submental space lies beneath the chin in the midline, between the mylohyoid muscles and the investing layer of deep cervical fascia. It is bounded laterally by the two anterior bellies of the digastric muscles. The submental space communicates posteriorly with the two submandibular spaces. The submandibular space is situated between the anterior and posterior bellies of the digastric muscle and communicates with the sublingual space around the posterior free border of mylohyoid. The sublingual space lies in the floor of the mouth, above the mylohyoid muscles, and is continuous across the midline: it communicates with the submandibular spaces over the posterior free borders of the mylohyoid muscles.

The remaining tissue spaces are illustrated in **Fig. 33.43B**. The buccal space is located in the cheek, on the lateral side of buccinator. The submasseteric spaces are a series of spaces between the lateral surface of the ramus of the mandible and masseter: they are formed because the fibres of masseter have multiple insertions onto most of the lateral surface of the ramus. The pterygomandibular space lies between the medial surface of the ramus of the mandible and medial pterygoid, and the parotid space lies behind the ramus of the mandible, in and around the parotid gland. The parapharyngeal space is bounded by the superior constrictor of the pharynx and the medial surface of medial pterygoid. It is restricted to the infratemporal region of the head and the suprahyoid region of the neck and communicates with the retropharyngeal space, which itself extends into the retrovisceral space in the lower part of the neck (the tissue spaces of the neck are described on p. 542 and of the pharynx on p. 626). The peritonsillar space lies around the palatine tonsil between the pillars of the fauces, and is part of the intrapharyngeal space. It is bounded by the medial surface of the superior constrictor of the pharynx and its mucosa.

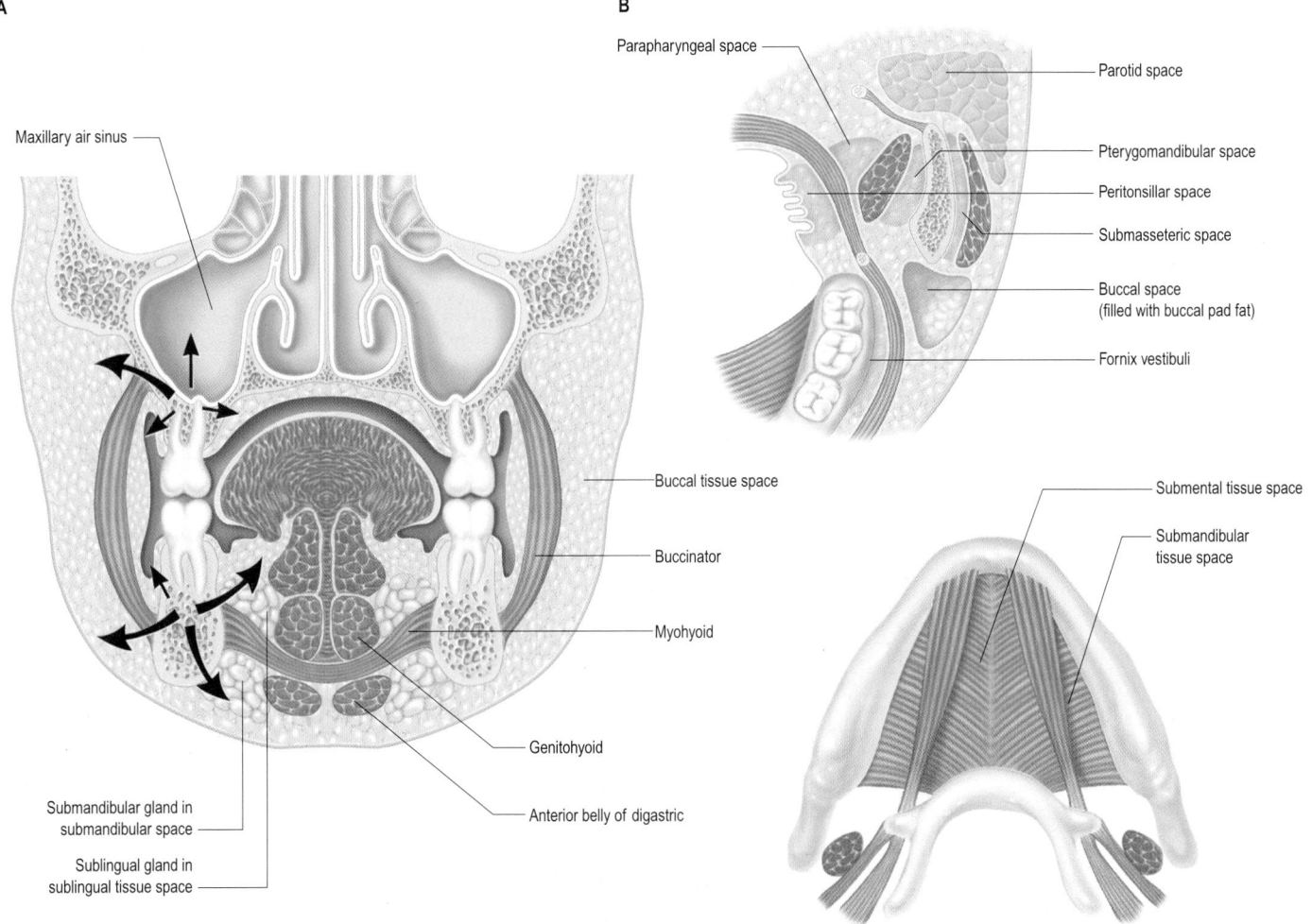

A

B

Maxillary air sinus

Parapharyngeal space

Parotid space

Pterygomandibular space

Peritonsillar space

Submasseteric space

Buccal space
(filled with buccal pad fat)

Fornix vestibuli

Buccal tissue space

Buccinator

Myohyoid

Submental tissue space

Submandibular
tissue space

Genitohyoid

Submandibular gland in
submandibular space

Sublingual gland in
sublingual tissue space

Anterior belly of digastric

Fig. 33.43 Potential tissue spaces around the jaws. **A**, Coronal section showing the sublingual and submandibular spaces in the floor of the mouth and the possible routes for the spread of infections from periapical dental abscesses (left). **B**, Horizontal section through the mandibular molar region showing the associated tissue spaces. **C**, Inferior view of the floor of the mouth (suprahyoid region of the neck) showing the position of the submandibular and sublingual tissue spaces. (**B** and **C**, by permission from Berkovitz BKB, Moxham BJ 2002 Head and Neck Anatomy. London: Martin Dunitz.)

POTENTIAL TISSUE SPACES AROUND THE UPPER JAW

The tissue spaces of the upper jaw are usually associated with spread of infection from the teeth. They are the canine (infraorbital), palatal and infratemporal spaces. The canine (infraorbital) space associated with the canine fossa lies between the levator labii superioris and zygomaticus muscles. The palatal space is not truly a tissue space in the hard palate, as the mucosa there is firmly bound to the periosteum. However, inflammation can strip away some of this periosteum to produce a well-circumscribed abscess. The infratemporal space is the upper extremity of the pterygomandibular space. It is closely related to the maxillary tuberosity and therefore the upper molars.

DENTAL ABSCESS (Fig. 33.43)

Abscesses developing in relation to the apices of roots ultimately penetrate the surrounding bone where it is thinnest. The position of the resultant swelling in the soft tissues is largely determined by the relationship between muscle attachments and the sinus (the path taken by the infected material) in the bone. Thus, in the lower incisor region, because the labial bone is thin, abscesses generally appear as a swelling in the labial sulcus, above the attachment of mentalis. The abscess may open below mentalis, when it will point beneath the chin. If an abscess from a lower postcanine tooth opens below the attachment of buccinator, the swelling is in the neck; if it opens above, the swelling is in the buccal sulcus. If an abscess opens lingually above mylohyoid, the swelling is in the lingual sulcus; if it is below, the swelling is in the neck. Third molar abscesses tend to track into the neck rather than the mouth, because mylohyoid ascends posteriorly.

Apart from canine teeth, which have long roots, abscesses on upper teeth usually open buccally below, rather than above, the attachment of buccinator. Because its root apex is occasionally curved towards the palate, abscesses of the upper lateral incisors may track into the palatal submucosa. Abscesses of upper canines often open facially just below the orbit. Here the swelling may obstruct drainage in the angular part of the facial vein which has no valves, and it is therefore possible for infected material to travel via the angular and ophthalmic veins into the cavernous sinus. Abscesses on the palatal roots of upper molars usually open on the palate.

The superficial lamina of deep cervical fascia opposes the spread of abscesses towards the surface, and pus beneath it tends to migrate laterally. If the pus is in the anterior triangle, it may find its way into the mediastinum, anterior to the pretracheal lamina, but because the fascia here is so thin it more often approaches the surface and 'points' above the sternum. Pus behind the prevertebral lamina may extend laterally and point in the posterior triangle, or it may perforate the lamina and the buccopharyngeal fascia to bulge into the pharynx as a retropharyngeal abscess.

Upper second premolars and first and second molars are related to the maxillary sinus. When this is large, the root apices of these teeth may be separated from its cavity solely by the lining mucosa. Sinus infections may stimulate the nerves entering the teeth, simulating toothache. Upper first premolars and third molars may be closely related to the maxillary sinus. With loss of teeth, alveolar bone is extensively resorbed. Thus in the edentulous mandible the mental nerve, originally inferior to premolar roots, may lie near the crest of the bone. In the edentulous maxilla, the sinus may enlarge to approach the oral surface of the bone. Occasional bony prominences termed the torus mandibularis, torus maxillaris and torus palatinus, may lie lingual to the lower premolars or molars, the upper molars. They in the midline of the palate and may need surgical removal before satisfactory dentures can be fitted.

Severe systemic infections during the time the teeth are developing may lead to faults in enamel, which are visible as horizontal lines (cf. Harris's growth lines).

Development of the face and neck

FACE

Facial development starts during the 4th postovulatory week and is completed at about 18 years of age. Although the most obvious changes in morphology occur up to stage 23 (8 weeks) of development, significant changes in the proportion of the face occur at puberty. The growth and fusion of five main prominences or processes form the face: the midline frontonasal process and bilateral maxillary and mandibular processes from the first pharyngeal arch. Several cell lines are associated with facial development. They are embryonic surface ectoderm, which covers all of the outer, and much of the inner, surfaces of the frontonasal, maxillary and mandibular processes; neural crest from the diencephalic and mesencephalic regions of the neural tube migrates to form the mesenchyme of the frontonasal process, while that from the rostral hindbrain (rhombomeres 1 and 2) migrates to the maxillary and mandibular processes; angiogenic mesenchyme, which develops in and extends from the original aortic arch arteries; paraxial mesenchyme, which provides all the skeletal muscle within the face; prechordal mesenchyme, which gives rise to the extraocular muscles of the eye (Chapter 43); neural plate, from which the afferent components of the cranial nerves extend, the efferent components being provided by neural crest and placodes (Chapter 26).

The diencephalic and mesencephalic neural crest mesenchyme proliferates and migrates rostrally and laterally between the ectoderm and prosen-cephalon to form the frontonasal process (**Fig. 34.1**). Migration begins well before neural tube closure and is completed afterwards. The olfactory placodes within the surface ectoderm remain connected to the neural tube, causing the migrating crest to stream and accumulate around them so that they appear to be displaced to the bottom of olfactory pits. The elevations formed around the pits during stages 14 and 15 are termed medial and lateral nasal processes. By stage 16 the medial processes have moved closer together and project caudally beyond the lateral processes. Internally, the medial processes project into the roof of the stomodeum to form the premaxillary fields. The frontonasal process gives rise to the forehead, nose, philtrum of the upper lip, premaxilla and upper incisor teeth. The surface facial contri-bution of the frontonasal process, which extends over the supraorbital and glabellar regions, includes the upper eyelid and conjunctiva and the external aspects of the nose. Internally the epithelial contribution includes the nasal vestibule, the nasal mucosa of the conchae and paranasal sinuses and the olfactory epithelium (see p. 610).

The mandibular processes approach each other and fuse in the midline superior to the pericardial bulge at stage 12. Viewed from its ventral aspect, the maxillary process a somewhat triangular elevation which arises from the cranial aspect of the dorsal region of each mandibular process from stage 14. Each maxillary process grows in a ventral direction and fuses with the lateral nasal process, although the two are initially separated by a nasomaxillary groove (naso-optic furrow) (**Fig. 34.1**). As the opposed margins of the lateral nasal and maxillary processes grow together they establish continuity between the side of the future nose and the cheek (**Fig. 34.1**). The ectoderm along the boundary between them does not entirely disappear. It gives rise to a solid cellular rod, which at first develops as a linear surface elevation, the nasolacrimal ridge, and then sinks into the mesenchyme. Its caudal end proliferates to connect with the caudal part of the lateral nasal wall, while its cranial extremity later connects with the developing con-junctival sac. The solid rod becomes canalized to form the nasolacrimal duct (**Fig. 34.2B**). The maxillary processes thus give rise to part of the cheek, maxilla, zygoma, lateral portions of the upper lip, hard and soft portions of the secondary palate.

The surface facial contribution of the maxillary process extends from the supratragic point to the lateral angles of eye and mouth, includes the lower eyelid and conjunctiva, and follows the paranasal line of the nasolacrimal duct, finally including a controversial amount of the upper lip. Internally the epithelial contribution includes upper and lower surfaces of the palate, the lining of the maxillary sinus which opens into the nasal cavity, the buccal epithelium lining the upper lip and gums, the invagination of the parotid salivary gland, and the upper teeth from the molars to the canines. The mandibular process gives rise to part of the cheek and the mandible. Fusion between the adjacent surfaces of the mandibular and maxillary processes progressively reduces the relatively wide primitive mouth (stomodeal fissure). At the

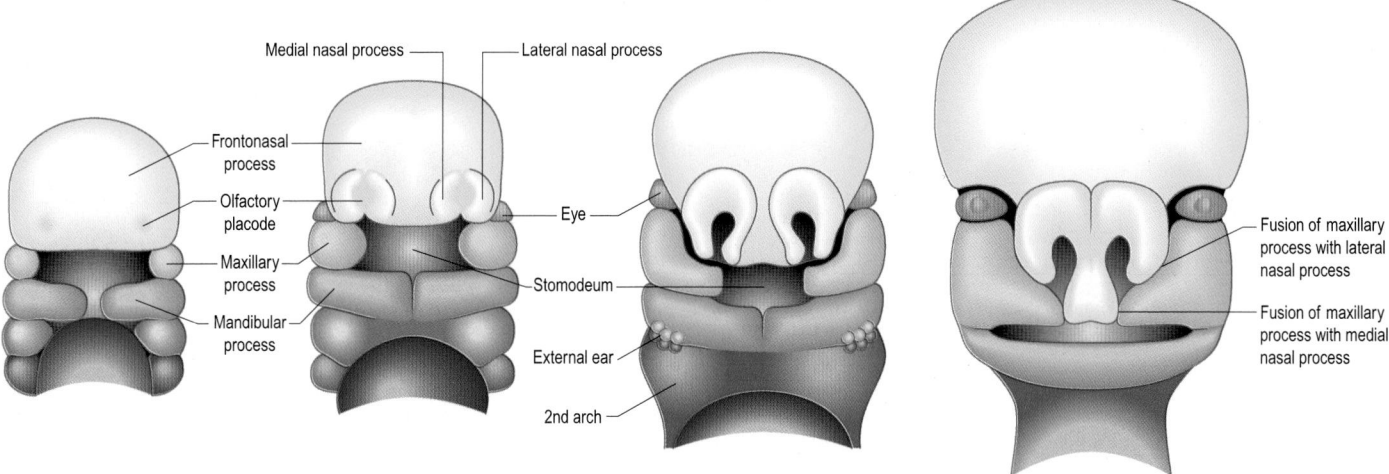

Fig. 34.1 The contribution of the first arch and frontonasal process to the development of the face.

Medial nasal process — Lateral nasal process

Frontonasal process

Olfactory placode

Maxillary process

Mandibular process

Eye

Stomodeum

External ear

2nd arch

Fusion of maxillary process with lateral nasal process

Fusion of maxillary process with medial nasal process

A

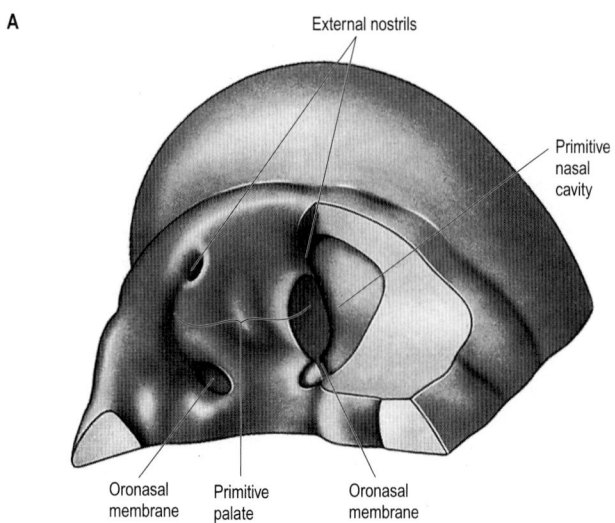

External nostrils

Primitive nasal cavity

Oronasal membrane

Primitive palate

Oronasal membrane

B

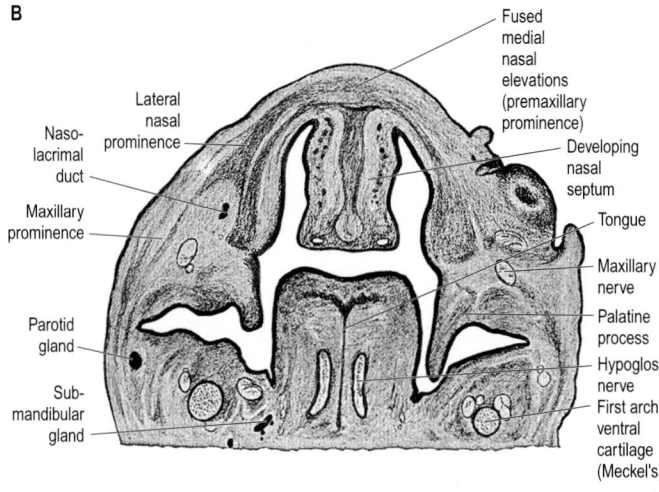

Naso-lacrimal duct

Lateral nasal prominence

Maxillary prominence

Parotid gland

Sub-mandibular gland

Fused medial nasal elevations (premaxillary prominence)

Developing nasal septum

Tongue

Maxillary nerve

Palatine process

Hypoglossal nerve

First arch ventral cartilage (Meckel's)

C

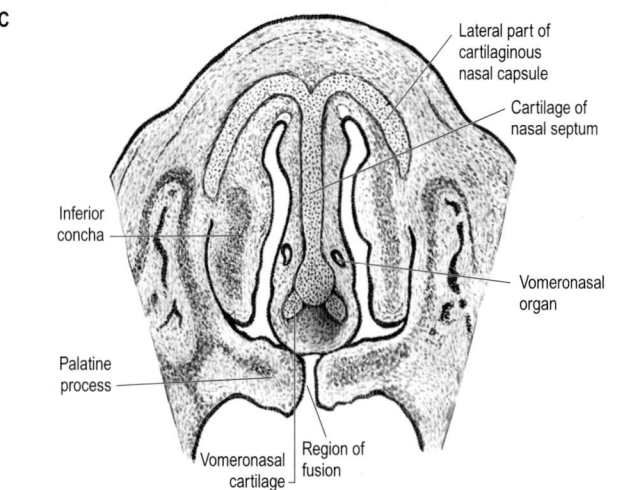

Inferior concha

Palatine process

Vomeronasal cartilage

Region of fusion

Lateral part of cartilaginous nasal capsule

Cartilage of nasal septum

Vomeronasal organ

Fig. 34.2 A, Primitive palate of a human embryo in the seventh week. The figure shows the anterior part of the roof of the mouth; large parts of the left lateral nasal prominence and the left maxillary prominence have been removed to expose the left primitive nasal cavity. **B**, Oblique coronal section through the head of a human embryo 23 mm long. The nasal cavities communicate freely with the cavity of the mouth. **C**, Coronal section through the nasal cavity of a human embryo 28 mm long. (**A**, from a model by K Peter; **C**, after Kollman.)

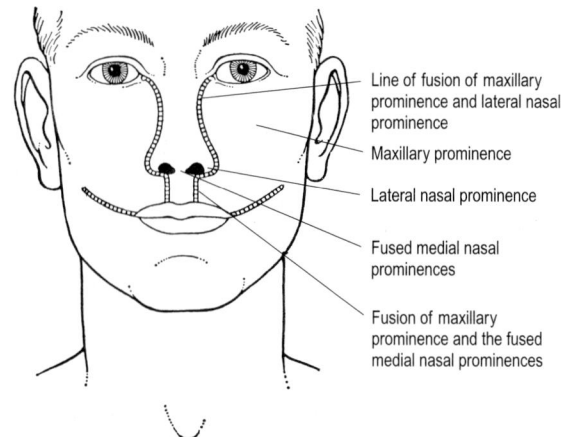

Line of fusion of maxillary prominence and lateral nasal prominence

Maxillary prominence

Lateral nasal prominence

Fused medial nasal prominences

Fusion of maxillary prominence and the fused medial nasal prominences

Fig. 34.3 The parts of the adult face which are derived from the nasal elevations, and the maxillary and mandibular prominences.

roughly triangular: the apex includes the tragus, the upper border extends to the lateral angle of the mouth and the free border of lower lip, and its lower border curves to follow the principal submandibular flexure line of the neck. Internally the mandibular epithelial surface includes the buccal lining of the lower lip and gums, the invagination of the submandibular salivary gland, all the lower teeth and the epithelial surface of the anterior two-thirds of the tongue.

NASAL CAVITY

The apex of the maxillary process extends beyond the lateral nasal process, and crosses the caudal end of the olfactory pit to meet and fuse with the premaxillary elevation that develops at the extremity of the frontonasal process. This closes off the lower or caudal edge of the olfactory pit, and the upper part of the opening is thus defined as the primitive external naris. The growth of the surrounding mesenchyme leads to a deepening of the pit to become a primitive nasal cavity, or nasal sac, the epithelial wall of which is contiguous with the epithelium of the stomodeal roof. The area of contact becomes more extensive as growth continues, and ultimately forms a thin layer, the oronasal membrane (**Fig. 34.2A**), which later disappears. Thereafter, the primitive nasal cavity communicates with the stomodeum through a primitive internal naris (choana), which at this stage is still situated well forward (ventrally) in the stomodeal roof. The nasal cavity thus acquires a floor through the fusion of the nasal and maxillary processes. At this stage the two external nares are still widely separated by an area derived from the frontonasal process, however, this separation is progressively reduced by the fusion of the premaxillary mesenchyme from the two sides. The primitive nasal cavities remain separated but become much more extensive with time. The nasal septum gradually extends backwards and downwards, and fuses with the maxillary palatal shelves to leave a free edge that reaches as far as the attachment of Rathke's pouch to the roof of the buccal cavity. On each side of the nasal septum, in a ventral or anterior position just above the primitive palate, placodal ectoderm is invaginated to form a pair of small diverticula which extend dorsally and cranially into the septum. These are the vomeronasal organs (**Fig. 34.2C**), auxiliary olfactory organs whose openings are close to the junction between the two premaxillae and the maxillae. They appear to be rudimentary in humans. A number of elevations appear on the lateral wall of each nasal cavity, which will develop into the superior, middle and inferior conchae. The paranasal sinuses appear in late fetal and early postnatal life as diverticula which gradually invade the frontal, ethmoid and sphenoid bones. These sinuses and the nasolacrimal duct, which is formed at the line of fusion of the maxillary and lateral nasal processes, all terminate in the lateral wall of the nasal cavity.

OLFACTORY EPITHELIUM

The olfactory nerve fibre bundles (fila olfactoria) develop from a proortion of the placodal cells which line the olfactory pits (p. 610). The

same time, the epithelial and connective tissues of the cheek enlarge. This proceeds from the para-otic region to the angle of the definitive oral fissure. The external ectoderm over the mandibular process becomes the skin of the face (**Fig. 34.3**), and it also takes part in the formation of the tragus of the auricle. Its surface facial contribution is

cells proliferate and give rise to olfactory receptor cells whose central processes are the axons of the olfactory nerve which grow into the overlying olfactory bulbs. The earliest pioneer neurites are devoid of glial ensheathment and cross a mesenchyme-filled gap between the placode and the superjacent brain. Olfactory axons subsequently become enclosed in the cytoplasmic processes of specialized ensheathing cells derived from the rostral neural crest. Within the olfactory bulb, the terminals of the olfactory axons ramify to establish rudimentary olfactory glomeruli. The remaining placodal cells, probably amplified by rostral neural crest cells, differentiate into columnar supporting (sustentacular) cells, rounded basal cells and, by invagination, the flattened duct-lining and polyhedral acinar cells of the glands of Bowman. Basal infiltration by lymphocytes is a relatively late event.

PHARYNGOTYMPANIC TUBE

The ventral end of the first pouch becomes obliterated, but its dorsal end persists and deepens as the head enlarges. It remains close to the ectoderm of the dorsal end of the first cleft and, together with the adjoining lateral part of the pharynx and dorsal part of the second pharyngeal pouch, constitutes the tubotympanic recess. The recess forms the tympanic cavity, the pharyngotympanic tube and their extensions. The dorsal end of the third arch is also considered to take part in the formation of the floor of the pharyngotympanic tube.

ADENOID AND TUBAL TONSILS

A number of focal proliferations of endoderm become invaded by lymphoid tissue. The adenoid or pharyngeal tonsil develops in the posterior midline of the nasopharynx, and the tubal tonsil develops close to the pharyngeal opening of the pharyngotympanic tube (p. 647).

BUCCAL CAVITY

The buccal cavity develops mainly from ventral growth of the upper pharyngeal arches. The rostral growth of the embryo and the formation of the head fold cause the pericardial area and buccopharyngeal membrane to come to lie on the ventral surface of the embryo (p. 198). Further expansion of the forebrain dorsally, and bulging of the pericardium ventrally, together with enlargement of the facial processes laterally, means that the buccopharyngeal membrane becomes depressed at the base of a hollow, the stomodeum or primitive buccal cavity (Figs 34.1, 34.4). At the end of the fourth week (stage 12) the buccopharyngeal membrane breaks down so that communication is established between the stomodeum and cranial end of the foregut (future naso- and oropharynx respectively). No vestige of the membrane is evident in the adult, and this embryonic communication should not be confused with the permanent oropharyngeal isthmus.

The pharyngeal arches grow in a ventral direction and lie progressively between the stomodeum and pericardium. With the fusion of the mandibular processes and the development of the maxillary processes (Fig. 34.1), the opening of the stomodeum assumes a pentagonal form, bounded cranially by the frontonasal process, caudally by the mandibular processes and laterally by the maxillary processes (Figs 34.1, 34.4). The inward growth and fusion of the maxillary palatine processes (Fig. 34.2) divides the stomodeum into a nasal and a buccal part. A shallow groove appears along the free margins of the prominences that bound the mouth cavity, and the ectoderm in its floor thickens and invades the underlying mesenchyme which divides into a medial dental lamina and a lateral vestibular lamina. The central cells of the latter degenerate and the furrow deepens. It is now termed the labiogingival groove or sulcus. The inner wall of the groove contributes to the formation of the alveolar processes of the maxillae and the mandible and their gingivae, while its outer wall forms the lips and cheeks.

Ectoderm/mesenchymal interactions produce structures in the wall of the oral cavity (mucous glands, salivary glands, teeth and taste buds), non-keratinized buccal epithelium, and the keratinized layer of skin.

The site of the original buccopharyngeal membrane may be visualized in the older fetus and adult as a zone posterior to the palatoglossal arch which passes from the junction of the anterior two-thirds and posterior one-third of the tongue to the roof of the nasopharynx, just anterior to the entrance to the auditory tube, and then on to the sella turcica, which contains the ectodermally derived adenohypophysis. The thyroid gland and the auditory tubes are the most anterior endodermal

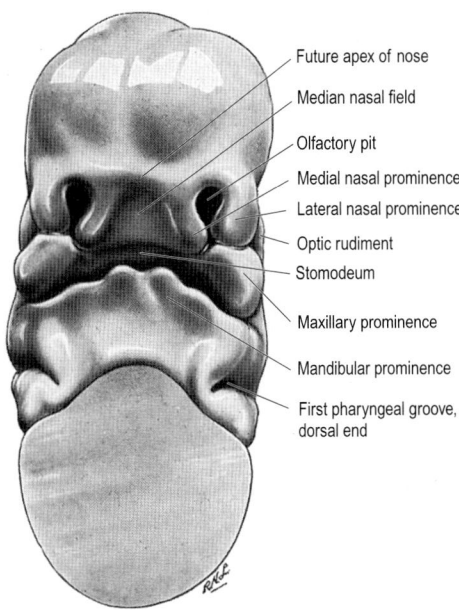

Fig. 34.4 The head of a human embryo in the sixth week: ventral aspect. (From a model by K Peter.)

- Future apex of nose
- Median nasal field
- Olfactory pit
- Medial nasal prominence
- Lateral nasal prominence
- Optic rudiment
- Stomodeum
- Maxillary prominence
- Mandibular prominence
- First pharyngeal groove, dorsal end

derivatives from the upper part of the primitive foregut which arise posterior to the zone. All first arch structures innervated by the trigeminal nerve are anterior to this zone, and permit investigation by touch from the tongue or digits without concern. Structures immediately posterior to the palatoglossal arch are innervated by the third arch nerve, the glossopharyngeal, and inappropriate touch is associated with initiation of the gag reflex.

In the neonate the oral cavity is only potential with the mouth closed. Three spaces are formed in the oral cavity during suckling. There is a median space between the tongue and hard palate which bifurcates posteriorly to produce channels on each side of the approximated soft palate and epiglottis. Two lateral spaces, the lateral arcuate cavities, are formed between the tongue medially and the cheeks laterally: the upper and lower gums situated in these spaces do not touch during suckling. Each cheek is supported by a mass of subcutaneous fat, the suctorial pad, which lies between buccinator and masseter. The larynx is elevated so that its opening is directed into the nasopharynx – i.e. above the level of the spaces – as fluid passes to the pharynx during suckling. This ensures that babies can breathe while suckling. It was thought for many years that neonates preferentially breathe through the nose, resorting to mouth breathing only if the nasal passage is obstructed. Studies have shown that full-term infants are able to establish oral breathing in the presence of nasal occlusion of a mean duration of 7.8 seconds.

PALATE

Once the primitive nasal cavities have been defined the ventral part of the roof of the oral cavity can be regarded as the primitive palate (median palatine prominence; Fig. 34.2A). It is formed by the premaxillary regions and maxillary processes which become confluent and establish continuity with the primitive nasal septum. As the head grows in size, the region of mesenchyme between the forebrain and oral cavity increases greatly by cellular proliferation, and the nasal cavities deepen and extend towards the forebrain. At the same time, they also extend dorsally from the primitive choanae as two deep, narrow grooves in the oral roof (Figs 34.2, 34.5) which are separated by a partition. The grooves and the partition deepen together, and the latter becomes the nasal septum, continuous rostrally with the primitive nasal septum (Fig. 34.2B). The broad dorsocaudal border of the nasal septum is at first in contact with the dorsum of the developing tongue (Fig. 34.2B), and the right and left nasal cavities communicate freely with the mouth except ventrally where the nasal floor has already been established by the primitive palate.

During stage 17 (41 days) the internal aspects of the maxillary prominences produce palatine processes (shelves), which grow caudally and contribute to the development of the linguogingival sulci.

They are separated from each other by the tongue. A coronal section through the head at stage 20 shows the maxillary palatine processes contiguous with the sides of the tongue and bent into a vertical position on each side of it (Figs 34.2B, 34.5). With further growth, the mandibular region and the tongue are carried forwards, ventrally, and the lingual tip passes round to the caudal surface of the primitive palate. At stage 23 (56–57 days) the palatine processes rapidly elevate, and assume a horizontal position which allows them to grow towards each other and thus to fuse (Figs 34.2C, 34.5): this process occurs from before backwards. The change of position, which occurs very rapidly, is caused by region-specific synthesis and accumulation of hyaluronan within the extracellular matrix of the palatal process mesenchyme. Hyaluronan binds more than 1000 times its own weight of water, causing swelling and expansion of the palatal shelves. The process is aided by the alignment of collagen fibrils and palatal mesenchymal cells in the shelves – the latter contract in response to acetylcholine and serotonin, which they secrete, thus regulating the elevation of the shelves – and by the epithelium, which restrains the swelling. Once these forces are in concert and exceed the resistance factors, the palatal shelves will mechanically elevate. This occurs during a period of continuous growth in head height but almost no growth in head width. This latter factor is important, because if palatal shelf elevation is delayed so that it occurs during a period of growth in facial width, the unfused processes are unable to touch physically and cleft palate may result. Other factors affecting palatal closure are the growth in length of the first arch cartilage, which allows the tongue to lower into the developing mandible; and the change in position of the maxilla relative to the anterior cranial base. This is maintained at about 84° during weeks 9 and 10, and has the effect of lifting the head and upper jaw upwards from the mandible which facilitates withdrawal of the tongue from between the palatal shelves and creates space for them to elevate. Mouth opening, tongue protrusion and hiccup movements have also

been noted at this time, and it may be that these movements and their associated pressure changes assist palatal shelf elevation (Ferguson 1990). Generally, in female embryos palatal shelf elevation occurs 7 days later than in males, and congenital cleft palate is more common in female embryos. After elevation, the palatine processes grow medially along the inferior borders of the primitive choanae, and unite with them, and with the margins of the median palatine prominence, except over a small area in the midline where a nasopalatine canal maintains connection between the nasal and oral cavities for some time and marks the future position of the incisive fossa. The plates which form the early (primitive) palate are sometimes known as median palatine processes, the maxillary contributions being then named the lateral palatine processes.

As the medial borders of the maxillary palatine processes fuse with each other and with the free border of the nasal septum, the nasal and oral cavities are progressively separated and the tongue is excluded from the nasal cavity. The nasal cavities extend dorsally until the choanae reach their final position. Slightly later the dorsomedial extremities of the palatine processes, which extend dorsally beyond the choanae, fuse together rostrocaudally to form the future epithelia and connective tissues of the soft palate (Fig. 34.2C). There is a later upgrowth of myogenic mesenchyme from the third and other pharyngeal arches into the palate and around the caudal margins of the auditory tube, along a line corresponding to the definitive palatopharyngeal arches. In the neonate the hard palate is only slightly arched, and it is usually corrugated by five or six irregular transverse folds (rugae) which assist gripping of the nipple when suckling. The epiglottis is high and makes direct contact with the soft palate.

TEETH AND GUMS
Fusion of the mandibular prominences forms the early lower oral margin, and the oral margin is completed by the fusion of the fronto-

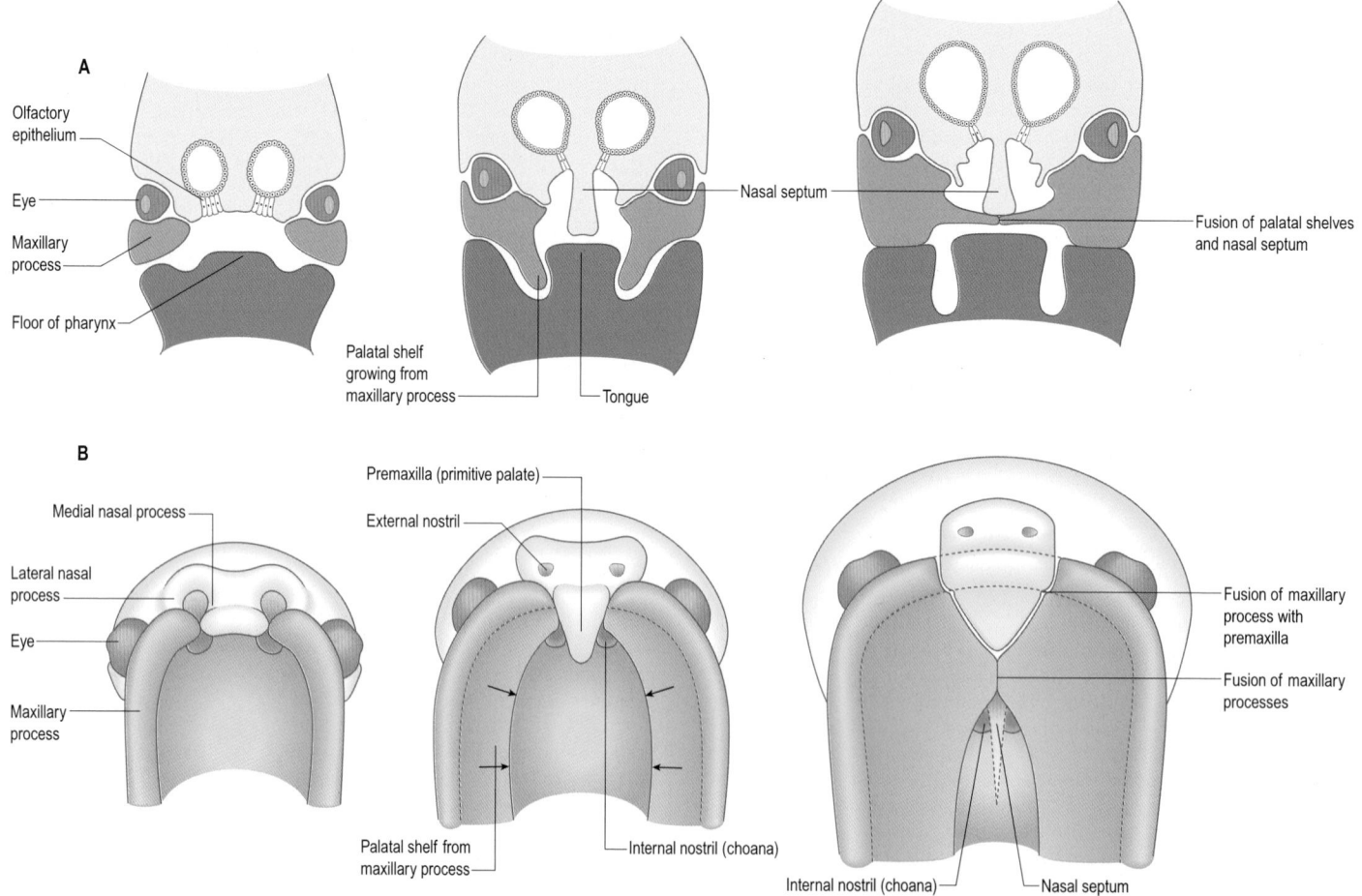

Fig. 34.5 A, Coronal sections through developing head showing formation, elevation and fusion of the palatal processes and the nasal septum. B, View of the roof of the mouth showing fusion of the premaxilla and the maxillary palatal shelves.

nasal process with the maxillary prominences. At this stage there is no distinction between the lips and gums. The lower gingivae form as mesenchymal swellings which are separated from the lip by a labio-gingival sulcus and from the tongue by a linguogingival sulcus. The upper gingivae are similarly separated from the lip by a labiogingival sulcus; however, they remain at the border of the palate. The surfaces of the gingivae differentiate into an oral mucosa that is contiguous with the mucosa lining the lips and cheeks. A series of proliferative epithelial loci signal the site of future tooth development along the ridges of each gum.

Teeth form from a series of epithelial/mesenchymal interactions along the dental lamina (**Fig. 34.6**). In 27 mm embryos individual dental laminae expand into ectodermal (dental) sacs surrounded by vascular mesenchyme. The ectoderm proliferates to form an enamel organ which surrounds a local portion of first arch neural crest mesenchyme, the dental papilla: collectively this unit constitutes a tooth bud or germ. The enamel organ initially forms a cap over the dental papilla and then later it expands into a bell shape.

The inner layer is tightly adherent to the dental papilla and separated from the outer layer by accumulated glycosaminoglycans. The inner cells of the enamel organ differentiate into ameloblasts, and the underlying mesenchymal cells into odontoblasts. Deposition of extracellular matrix onto the adjoining basal lamina produces the tooth. The neural crest dental papilla mesenchyme specifies the type of tooth produced, i.e. incisor or molar; however, the mandibular epithelium is essential and specific for the development of teeth. Recombination of mandibular epithelium and second arch mesenchyme results in tooth development, but second arch epithelium and mandibular mesenchyme does not.

Both the deciduous and permanent teeth develop in the same manner. The permanent teeth develop in accessional positions from the lingual aspects of the existing tooth germs. The tooth germs for the 12 permanent molar teeth develop from posterior extensions of the dental laminae on each side of both jaws. Calcification begins in both deciduous and permanent teeth before birth. The deciduous teeth have well-developed crowns by full term, whereas the permanent teeth remain as tooth buds.

SALIVARY GLANDS

The salivary glands arise bilaterally as a result of epithelial/mesenchymal interactions between the ectodermal epithelial lining of the buccal cavity and the subjacent neural crest mesenchyme. The parotid gland can be recognized in human embryos at stage 15 as an elongated furrow running dorsally from the angle of the mouth between the mandibular and maxillary prominences. The groove, which is converted into a tube, loses its connection with the epithelium of the mouth, except at its ventral end, and grows dorsally into the substance of the cheek. The tube persists as the parotid duct and its blind end proliferates in the local mesenchyme to form the gland. Subsequently the size of the oral fissure is reduced by partial fusion between the maxillary and mandibular prominences and the duct opens thereafter on the inside of the cheek at some distance from the angle of the mouth. In the neonate the parotid gland is rounded and lies between masseter and the ear. During infancy and early childhood, the growing gland covers the parotid duct.

The submandibular gland is identifiable in 13 mm human embryos as an epithelial outgrowth into the mesenchyme from the floor of the linguogingival groove. It increases rapidly in size, and gives off numerous branching processes which later acquire lumina. At first the connection of the submandibular outgrowth with the floor of the mouth lies at the side of the tongue, but the edges of the groove in which it opens come together, from behind forwards, and form the tubular part of the submandibular duct. As a result, the orifice of the duct is shifted forwards till it is below the tip of the tongue, close to the median plane.

The sublingual gland arises in 20 mm embryos as a number of small epithelial thickenings in the linguogingival groove and on the lateral side of the groove: the groove later closes to form the submandibular duct. Each thickening canalizes separately, and so many of the multiple sublingual ducts open separately on the summit of the sublingual fold, while others join the submandibular duct. The topography of the submandibular and sublingual glands is the same as in the adult.

TONGUE

A small median elevation, the tuberculum impar or median tongue bud, appears in the floor of the pharynx before the pharyngeal arches

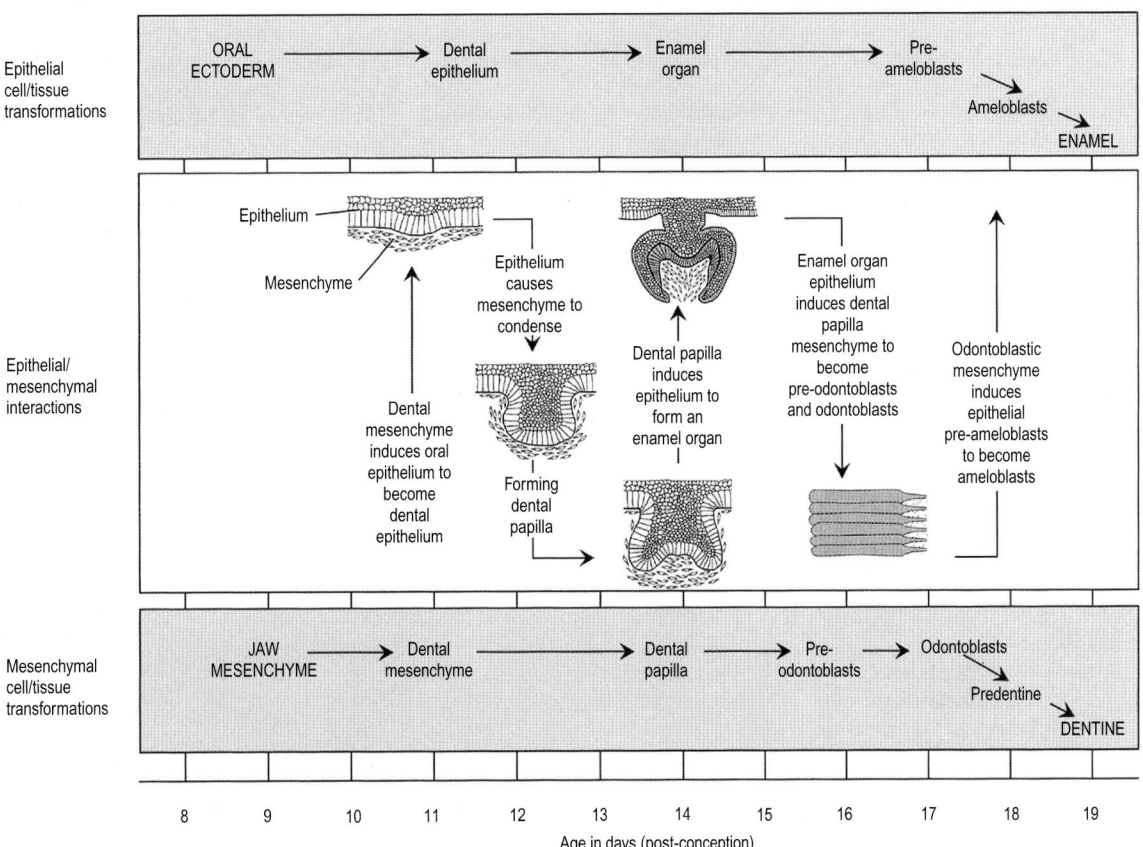

Fig. 34.6 Reciprocal tissue interaction in mammalian tooth development. The sequence of epithelial/mesenchymal interactions involved in the development of teeth in the embryonic mouse. (From a model by K Peter.)

meet ventrally, and it subsequently becomes incorporated in the anterior part of the tongue. A little later two oval mandibular or lingual swellings appear on the inner aspect of the mandibular processes. They meet each other in front, and caudally they converge on the tuberculum impar, with which they fuse (**Fig. 34.7**). A sulcus forms along the ventral and lateral margins of this elevation and deepens, internal to the future alveolar process of the mandible, to form the linguogingival groove, while the elevation constitutes the anterior or buccal (presulcal) part of the tongue. Caudal to the tuberculum impar, a second median elevation, the hypobranchial eminence (copula of His), forms in the floor of the pharynx, and the ventral ends of the fourth, third and, later, second, pharyngeal arches converge into it. A transverse groove separates its caudal part to delineate the epiglottis. Ventrally it approaches the presulcal tongue rudiment, and spreads in the form of a V, to form the posterior or pharyngeal part of the tongue. During this sequence of events, the third arch elements grow over and bury the elements of the second arch, thereby excluding it from the tongue. The mucous membrane of the pharyngeal part of the tongue therefore receives its sensory supply from the glossopharyngeal nerve, which is the nerve of the third arch. In the adult, the union of the anterior and posterior parts of the tongue approximately corresponds to the angulated sulcus terminalis, which has its apex at the foramen caecum, a blind depression produced at the time of fusion of the constituent parts of the tongue, but also marking the site of ingrowth of the median rudiment of the thyroid gland.

The tongue initially consists of a mass of mesenchyme covered on its surface by first arch ectoderm and third arch endoderm. During the second month it is invaded by occipital myotomes which migrate from the lateral aspects of the myelencephalon. They pass ventrally round the pharynx to reach its floor accompanied by the hypoglossal nerve.

The composite character of the tongue is revealed by its sensory innervation. The anterior, buccal part is innervated by the lingual nerve, derived from the post-trematic nerve of the first arch (mandibular nerve) and by the chorda tympani, which is often held to be the pretrematic nerve to the first arch. The posterior, pharyngeal part of the tongue is innervated by the glossopharyngeal, the nerve of the third arch, and the root of the tongue, near the epiglottis, is innervated by the vagus.

The sulcus terminalis cannot be distinguished earlier than the 52 mm stage according to some observers. The vallate papillae appear at about the same time, and increase in number until the 170 mm stage. Serial reconstructions suggest that the territory of the glossopharyngeal nerve extends considerably beyond these papillae. Lymphoid tissue similar to the palatine tonsils usually develops on the surface of the posterior part of the tongue, and is called the lingual tonsil.

In the neonate, the tongue is short and broad, and its entire surface lies within the oral cavity (**Fig. 11.5**). The posterior third of the tongue descends into the neck during the first postnatal year, and by the fourth or fifth year the tongue forms part of the anterior wall of the pharynx.

TONSILS

The palatine tonsils develop from the ventral parts of the second pharyngeal pouches (**Fig. 34.8**). The endoderm lining these pouches grows into the surrounding mesenchyme as a number of solid buds, which are excavated by degeneration and shedding of their central cells, forming tonsillar fossae and crypts. Lymphoid cells accumulate around the crypts and become grouped as lymphoid follicles. A slit-like intra-tonsillar cleft extends into the upper part of the tonsil and is possibly a remnant of the second pharyngeal pouch.

The paired palatine tonsils are situated slightly higher in the tonsillar fossae in the neonate than in the adult. Each descends in position during the second and third postnatal year, but definitive lymph nodes appear after birth. The palatine tonsils begin to atrophy from the fifth year and involution is often complete by puberty.

ANOMALIES OF FACIAL DEVELOPMENT

Congenital malformations produced by arrest of development and/or failure of fusion of components in the formation of the face and palate are not uncommon and variations in the degree of severity of the anomaly produced are seen. Failure of local fusion of one maxillary process with the corresponding premaxillary region, leading to a persistent fissure between the philtrum and lateral part of the upper lip on that side, is called a cleft lip. If the palatal shelves fail to fuse across the midline and with the nasal septum a cleft palate is produced. Failure of fusion of the maxillary process with its adjacent lateral nasal process will lead to a cleft face. The further growth of the face during the fetal period has received little attention, although this period is by no means characterized entirely by incremental growth. It is during fetal life that human facial proportions develop (**Fig. 34.9**). The facial and cranial parts display different patterns of growth, though each influences the other.

Cleft lip

A lack of normal nasolabial muscle attachments is a consequence of uni- or bilateral cleft lip. This results in functional abnormalities that lead to underlying skeletal malformations. The three functional groups of superficial facial muscles – nasolabial (transverse nasalis, levator labii superioris and levator labii superioris alequae nasi), bilabial (orbicularis oris) and labiomental (depressor anguli oris) – are all displaced inferiorly. The absence of the correct insertion of the transverse muscles of the nose and of orbicularis oris on the medial aspect of the cleft onto the tissues around the anterior nasal spine and nasal septum and, most importantly, to the contralateral muscles, is responsible for the deviation of the anterior border of the nasal septum to the non-cleft side. A further consequence is the underdevelopment of the incisor-bearing part of the maxilla. These abnormalities in turn influence the mucocutaneous tissues, which results in the displacement of the skin of the nostril to the upper part of the lip, retraction of the

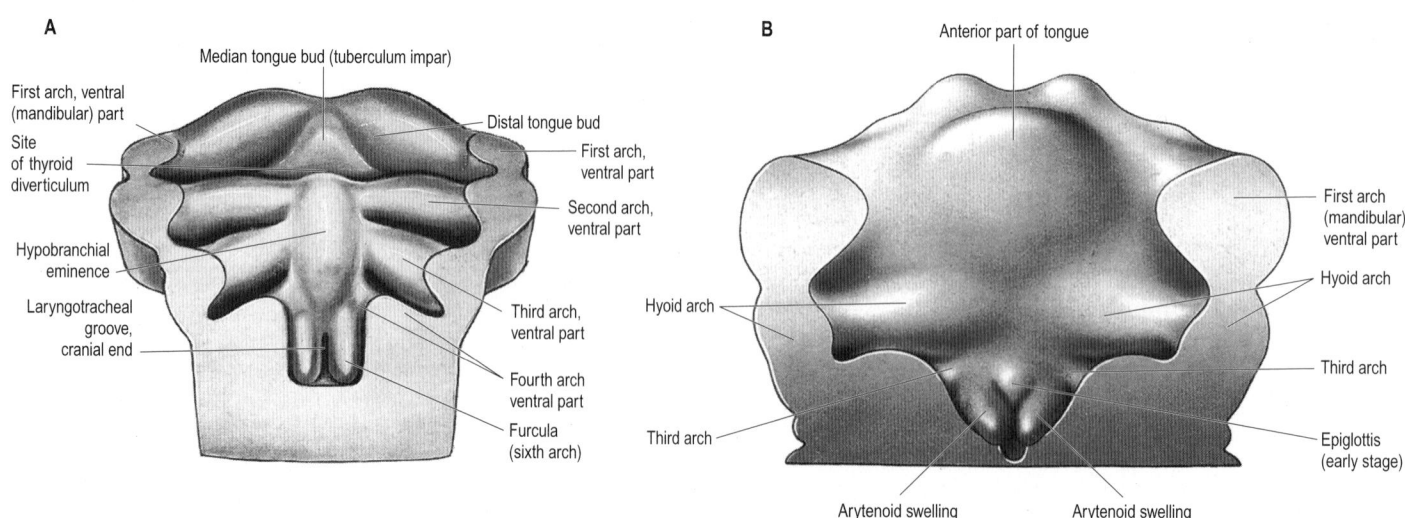

Fig. 34.7 A, The floor of the pharynx of a human embryo at the beginning of the sixth week. **B**, The floor of the pharynx of a human embryo, about 6 weeks old. (From a model by K Peter.)

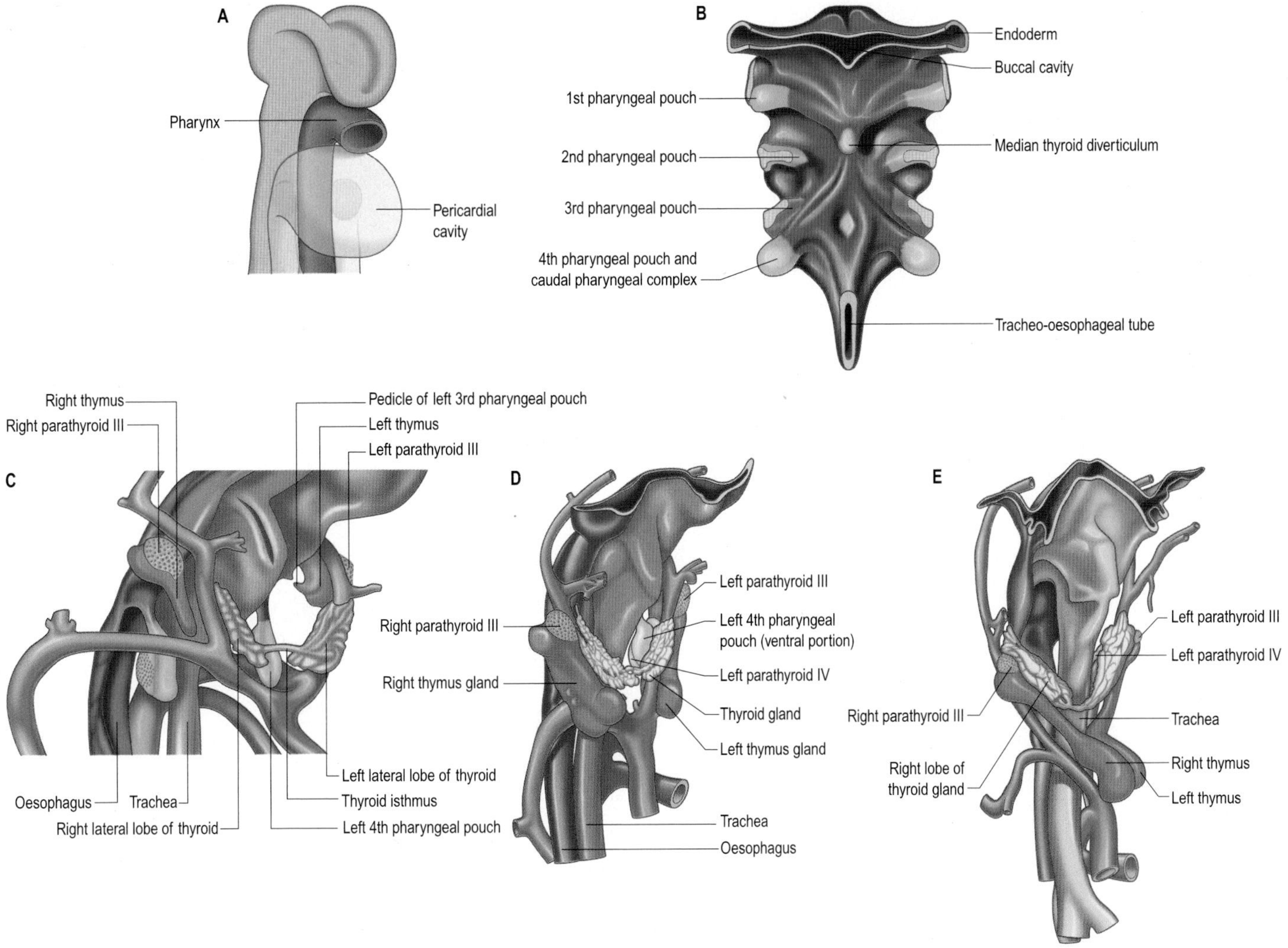

A

Pharynx

Pericardial cavity

B

Endoderm

Buccal cavity

1st pharyngeal pouch

Median thyroid diverticulum

2nd pharyngeal pouch

3rd pharyngeal pouch

4th pharyngeal pouch and caudal pharyngeal complex

Tracheo-oesophageal tube

C

Right thymus
Right parathyroid III

Pedicle of left 3rd pharyngeal pouch
Left thymus
Left parathyroid III

Oesophagus   Trachea

Right lateral lobe of thyroid

Left lateral lobe of thyroid

Thyroid isthmus

Left 4th pharyngeal pouch

D

Right parathyroid III

Right thymus gland

Left parathyroid III

Left 4th pharyngeal pouch (ventral portion)

Left parathyroid IV

Thyroid gland

Left thymus gland

Trachea

Oesophagus

E

Right parathyroid III

Right lobe of thyroid gland

Left parathyroid III

Left parathyroid IV

Trachea

Right thymus

Left thymus

Fig. 34.8 A, Primitive pharynx situated between neural tube and pericardial cavity. **B**, Ventral aspect of the endoderm of the pharynx showing three pharyngeal pouches. The areas of contact of the pharyngeal endoderm with the surface ectoderm are shown as flattened surfaces. **C**, Ventral and dorsal diverticuli of the third and fourth pharyngeal pouches and midline thyroid gland at 6 weeks. **D**, Thymus, thyroid and parathyroid glands at 7 weeks. **E**, Thymus, thyroid and parathyroid glands at 7.5 weeks. (Redrawn by permission from Hamilton WJ, Boyd JD, Mossman HW 1962 Human Embryology: Prenatal Development of Form and Function. Cambridge: W Heffer & Sons.)

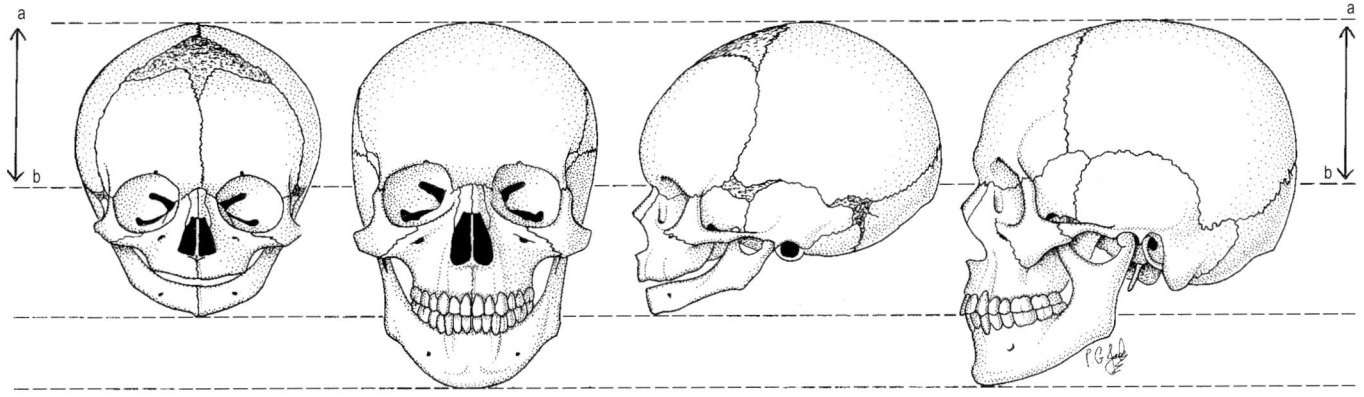

Fig. 34.9 Much of the postnatal growth of the skull is concerned with development of the viscerocranium. This diagram shows that with the height of the cranial vault expressed as similar in newborn and adult skulls (lines a - - - b) the facial skeleton increases particularly during childhood and puberty.

labial skin and abnormalities of the soft tissues on either side of the mucocutaneous junction (**Fig. 34.10A,B**).

As a consequence of the inadequate muscular support, the skin of the nasal floor, the nasal sill, the vestibule and the base of the columella – the lowest, mobile, part of the septal cartilage – drift inferiorly and lie in the region normally occupied by the upper lip. The skin of the lip on both sides of the cleft has an abnormal dome-like appearance because the underlying orbicularis oris is not continuous across the cleft but remains bunched up in the lip. The cartilages of the nose on the side of the cleft adopt a characteristic twisted appearance. The base is more inferiorly positioned, the cartilage is flattened and distended and the cartilaginous nasal septum is deviated to the non-cleft side. These

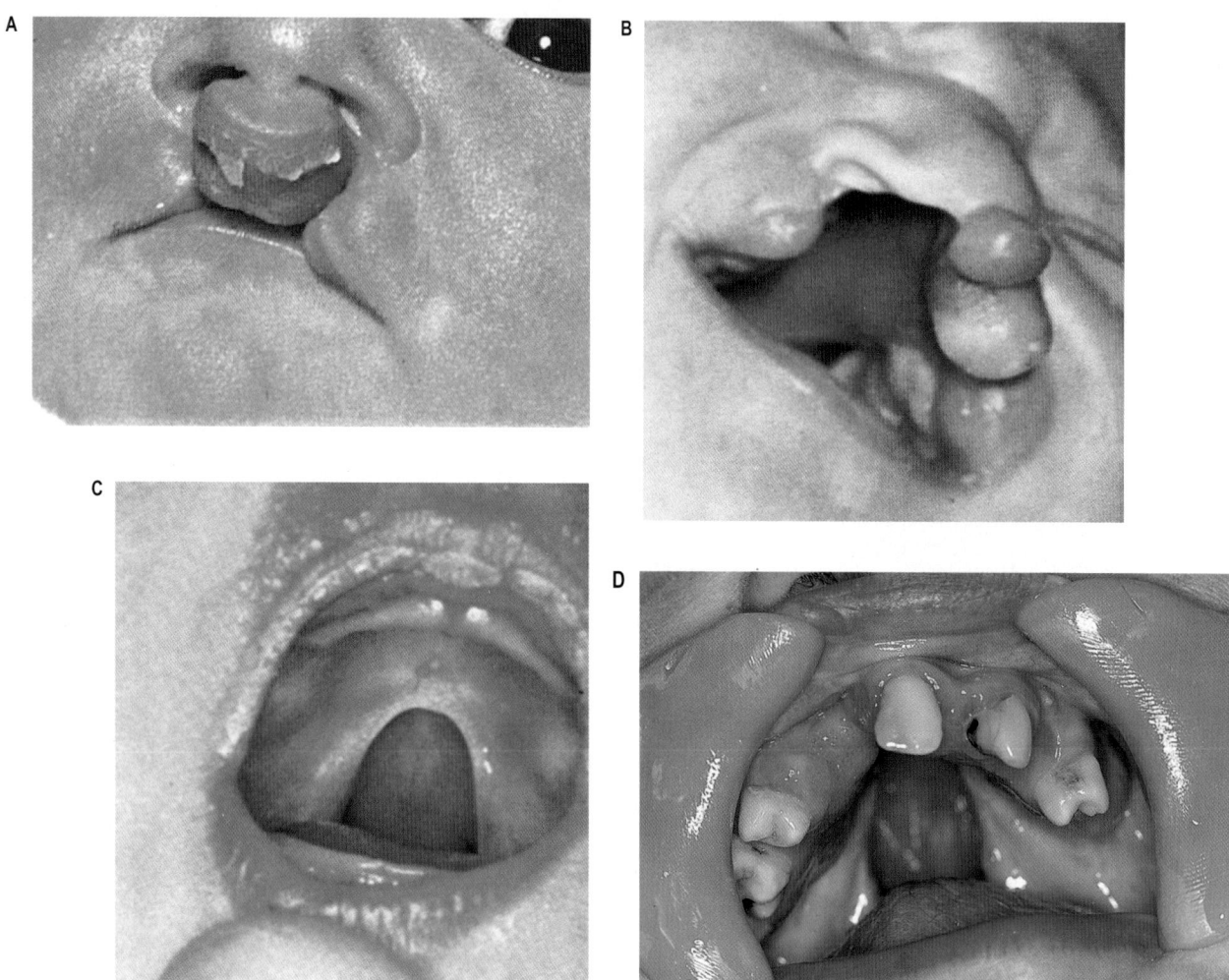

Fig. 34.10 Unrepaired clefts of lip and palate. **A**, Bilateral cleft lip. **B**, Bilateral cleft lip and cleft palate. **C**, Cleft palate. **D**, Cleft lip and palate. (**A–C**, by permission from O'Doherty NJ 1975 Atlas of the Newborn. 5 Congenital Abnormality. London: Pharma Books. **D**, by kind permission from Dr BAW Brown and by permission from Berkovitz BKB, Holland GR, Moxham BJ 2002 Oral Anatomy, Embryology and Histology, 3rd edn. Edinburgh: Mosby.)

deformities are the direct result of abnormal muscle attachments that alter the functional matrix. The underlying maxilla is also affected. The greater segment is displaced toward the non-cleft side and the minor segment toward the cleft side. Again this is due to insufficient stimulation by normally functioning overlying musculature.

The cleft in the lip is normally closed postnatally between the age of 5 and 6 months. Several techniques have been described for lip closure, and they differ most obviously in the description of the details of the skin incisions. The underlying principle is to restore the muscle insertions to their normal position so that functional extracellular matrix can influence the subsequent growth and development. Each of the three muscle groups – nasolabial, bilabial and labiomental – must be separately identified and reattached. Provided this is achieved, subsequent growth and development should proceed normally. The previously displaced maxillary segments will spontaneously correct their position: bone grafting may be undertaken at the age of 9–10 years.

Cleft palate

Many varieties of cleft palate have been observed (**Fig. 34.10C,D**). The commonest type is unilateral, where only one side of the nasal cavity is in communication with the mouth and the extent of the cleft is variable. In the mildest forms, only the soft palate, and sometimes just the uvula, is cleft. Very rarely, palatopharyngeal incompetence is due to muscle hypoplasia, particularly of the musculus uvulae, and a submucous cleft may be revealed clinically as a V-shaped notch in the midline of the soft palate during function. Such examples of arrested development may be associated with disturbances in embryonic nutrition during the second and the third months of gestation and the

grosser varieties, where there is protrusion of the premaxillary region, with associated forwards extension of the nasal septum, are usually coupled with malformations in other regions of the body.

The timing of surgical closure of a cleft palate is critical. All surgical techniques for palatal closure involve raising and mobilizing flaps from adjacent structures. This inevitably results in the formation of scar tissue which subsequently inhibits growth and development of the palate and upper jaw. Many techniques use flaps raised from the vomer to close the nasal layer and lateral palatal flaps based posteriorly on the greater palatine arteries. Unfortunately the use of vomerine flaps results in a reduction of vertical growth of the maxilla whereas the mobilization of palatal mucoperiosteal flaps results in a reduction of transverse growth. For these reasons, palatal closure is delayed for as long as possible. However, if such surgery is delayed beyond 18 months of age, when the infant first begins to develop speech sounds, the child might never develop normal speech. Whatever technique is used to close a cleft palate, it is important to re-establish normal muscle function by approximating the palatoglossus and tensor palatini muscles in the midline whilst avoiding scarring as much as possible (Markus et al 1993).

Cleft face

Facial cleft is a rare malformation which follows failure of fusion between the maxillary process and the lateral nasal process. Here the nasolacrimal duct persists as an open furrow, a condition which is usually associated with ipsilateral cleft lip. The palatine processes may fail to fuse with each other and the nasal septum to variable degrees. In its severest form fusion is wholly lacking, and this produces a wide fissure between the palatine processes through which the nasal septum is visible. On each side the premaxillary parts of the palate are separated from the maxillary palatine processes by clefts which are continuous ventrally with bilateral clefts in the upper lip. In such cases the philtrum is a separate entity that is continuous cranially and dorsally with the nasal septum. The floor of the nasal cavity is deficient throughout its extent and the choanae are incomplete.

Midline anomalies such as median cleft lip (true hare lip), cleft nose and cleft lower jaw are rarely encountered. More common are minor degrees of cleft chin and micrognathia.

NECK

PARATHYROID GLAND

The parathyroid glands develop from interactions between the third and fourth pharyngeal pouch endoderm and local cranial (vagal) neural crest mesenchyme. The third pharyngeal pouch has dorsal and ventral sites of proliferation (**Fig. 34.8**). Bilaterally, the epithelium on the dorsal aspect of the pouch and in the region of its duct-like connection with the cavity of the pharynx becomes differentiated as the primordium of the inferior parathyroid glands (parathyroid III). Although the connection between the pouches and the pharynx is soon lost, the connection between the dorsal parathyroids III and the ventral thymic rudiments persists for some time, and the former passes caudally with the developing thymus. The superior parathyroid glands (parathyroid IV) develop from the dorsal recess of the fourth pharyngeal pouches. They come into relation with, and appear to be anchored by, the lateral lobes of the thyroid gland and thus remain cranial to the parathyroid glands derived from the third pouches. The cardiac neural crest mesenchyme provides the connective tissue elements whereas invading angiogenic mesenchyme gives rise to the vasculature which includes fenestrated capillaries and lymphatics. In the neonate the parathyroid glands are as variable in size and position as they are in the adult. They double in size between birth and puberty. Parathyroid hormone is produced from the 12th week of development.

THYMUS

The thymus gland is formed from the ventral part of the third pharyngeal pouch on each side (**Fig. 34.8**). It cannot be recognized prior to the differentiation of the inferior parathyroid glands at stage 16, but thereafter it is represented by two elongated diverticula which soon become solid cellular masses and grow caudally into the surrounding cardiac (vagal) neural crest mesenchyme. Ventral to the aortic sac the two thymic rudiments meet but do not fuse, and they are subsequently united by connective tissue only. The connection with the third pouch is soon lost, but the stalk may persist for some time as a solid, cellular cord.

As the thymus proliferates and descends the local cardiac (vagal) neural crest mesenchyme controls the pattern and development of the gland. Defective development of cardiac neural crest which affects the heart and peripheral neural ganglia also results in thymic deficiencies as seen in the DiGeorge and Pierre Robin syndromes. Crest mesenchyme forms connective tissue septa which produce the lobulated architecture of the gland. Angiogenic mesenchyme, including lymphoid stem cells, invades this local mesenchyme and by 10 weeks, over 95% of the cells in the gland belong to the T cell lineage, with a few developing erythroblasts and B lymphocytes. Hassall's corpuscles are also present. By 12 weeks, the mesenchymal septa, blood vessels and nerves have reached the newly differentiating medulla, which allows the entry of macrophage lineage precursors. Macrophages and interdigitating cells are first seen at 14 weeks. Granulopoiesis occurs in the perivascular spaces. By 17 weeks, the thymus appears fully differentiated, and after this time it produces the main type of thymocyte that is present throughout life (designated TdT+).

Thymic tissue may also develop from the ventral recess of the fourth pharyngeal pouch in a proportion of embryos, when it is usually found close to the thyroid gland in close association with the superior parathyroid gland. An ectodermal contribution to the thymus, probably of placodal origin, occurs in some mammals but a similar contribution in man is conjectural.

CAUDAL PHARYNGEAL COMPLEX

The most caudal endodermal invaginations of the pharynx are the fourth pharyngeal pouch, elements of the transitory fifth pharyngeal pouch and the ultimobranchial body (**Fig. 34.8**). Collectively these diverticuli are termed the caudal pharyngeal complex, and they are connected to the pharynx via the pharyngobranchial duct. They are surrounded by cardiac (vagal) neural crest and by the tissues of the developing thyroid gland. The cells of the ultimobranchial body, the lowest of the pharyngeal pouches, become incorporated into the lateral thyroid lobes, and give rise to the 'C' or parafollicular cells of the thyroid gland. C-cell hyperplasia is associated with medullary carcinoma, and has been reported within the neck in what are presumed to be remnants of the ultimobranchial body.

THYROID GLAND

The thyroid gland is a midline derivative of the pharynx. It is first identifiable in embryos of c.20 somites as a median thickening of endoderm lying in the floor of the pharynx between the first and second pharyngeal pouches and immediately dorsal to the aortic sac. This area is later invaginated to form a median diverticulum which appears late in the fourth week in the furrow immediately caudal to the median tongue bud (**Fig. 34.8**). It grows caudally as a tubular duct. The tip of the duct bifurcates and the tissue mass subsequently divides into a series of double cellular plates, from which the isthmus and the lateral lobes of the thyroid gland are developed. The primary thyroid follicles differentiate by reorganization and proliferation of the cells of these plates. Secondary follicles subsequently arise by budding and subdivision. These primary and secondary endodermal cells are the progenitors of the follicular parenchyma proper. The parafollicular or C cells of the thyroid gland are derived from the ultimobranchial body.

The original diverticulum, its bifurcation and generations of follicles invade the cardiac neural crest mesenchyme. The latter gives rise to the connective tissue capsule, interlobular septa and perifollicular investments which carry the main neurovascular and lymphatic supply to the gland.

The median diverticulum is connected to the pharynx by the thyroglossal duct. The site of its initial connection with the endodermal floor of the mouth is marked by the foramen caecum, whence it extends caudally in the midline ventral to the primordium of the hyoid bone (behind which it later forms a recurrent loop). The distal part of the duct may differentiate into the pyramidal lobe and levator muscle – or suspensory fibrous band – of the thyroid. The remainder becomes fragmented and disappears, although the lingual part is often identifiable until late in fetal life. Occasionally parts of the midline thyroglossal duct persist and may occur in lingual, suprahyoid, retrohyoid, or infrahyoid positions. They may form aberrant masses of thyroid tissue, cysts, fistulae or sinuses, usually in the midline. A lingual thyroid situated at the junction of the buccal and pharyngeal parts of the tongue is not uncommon, but nodules of glandular tissue may also be found other than in the midline, e.g. laterally placed posterior to sternocleidomastoid, and, on occasion, below the level of the thyroid isthmus.

The thyroid gland is relatively large in the neonate (**Fig. 11.4**), where it has a long narrow isthmus connecting lobes which do not yet contact the upper part of the trachea. The gland attains half the adult size by 2 years postnatally. Colloid is present in the gland from 3 months' gestation and thyroxin is present by 4.5 months' gestation.

VASCULAR SUPPLY OF THE FACE, SCALP AND NECK

ARTERIAL SUPPLY

The arteries supplying the face, scalp and neck arise from the early aortic arch arteries (p. 1042) which develop in a craniocaudal sequence. The first and second aortic arch arteries supply embryonic structures which are dwindling in size as the lower arches are established. When the first and second aortic arch arteries begin to regress, the supply to the corresponding arches is derived from a transient ventral pharyngeal artery, which grows from the aortic sac. It terminates by dividing into mandibular and maxillary branches. Later the stapedial artery develops from the dorsal stem of the second arch artery. It passes through the condensed mesenchymal site of the future ring of the stapes to anastomose with the cranial end of the ventral pharyngeal artery and so annexes its terminal distribution. The fully developed stapedial artery possesses three branches, mandibular, maxillary and supraorbital, which follow the divisions of the trigeminal nerve (**Fig. 34.11**). The mandibular and maxillary branches diverge from a common stem.

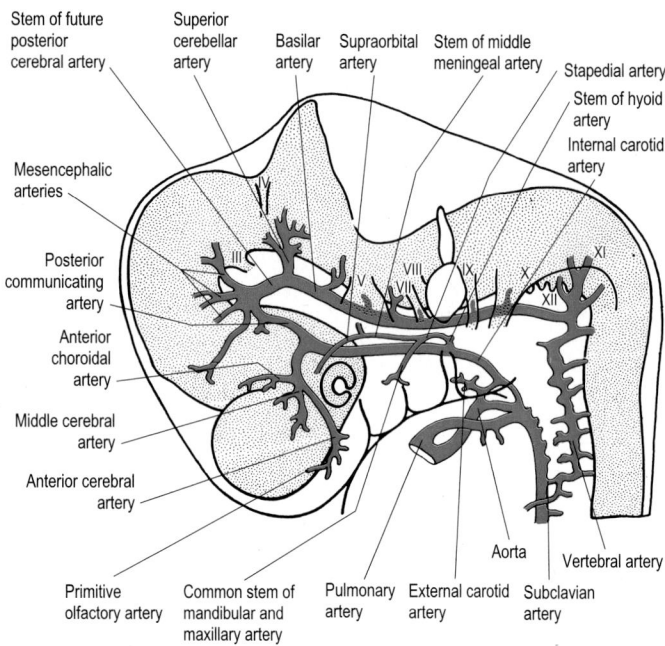

Fig. 34.11 The origins of the main cranial arteries. (After Padget DH 1948 The development of cranial arteries in the human embryo. Contrib Embryol Carnegie Inst Washington 32: 205–261, by permission.)

When the external carotid artery emerges from the base of the third arch it incorporates the stem of the ventral pharyngeal artery, and its maxillary branch communicates with the common trunk of origin of the maxillary and mandibular branches of the stapedial artery and annexes these vessels. The proximal part of the common trunk persists as the root of the middle meningeal artery. More distally the meningeal artery is derived from the proximal part of the supraorbital artery. The maxillary branch becomes the infraorbital artery and the mandibular branch forms the inferior alveolar artery.

When the definitive ophthalmic artery differentiates as a branch from the terminal part of the internal carotid artery, it communicates with the supraorbital branch of the stapedial artery which distally becomes the lacrimal artery. The latter retains an anastomotic connection with the middle meningeal artery. The dorsal stem of the original second arch artery remains as one or more caroticotympanic branches of the internal carotid artery.

VENOUS DRAINAGE

The primary vessels consist of a close-meshed capillary plexus drained on each side by the precardinal vein, which is at first continuous cranially with a transitory primordial hindbrain channel that lies on the neural tube medial to the cranial nerve roots. This is soon replaced by the primary head vein which runs caudally from the medial side of the trigeminal ganglion, lateral to the facial and vestibulocochlear nerves and the otocyst, then medial to the vagus nerve, to become continuous with the precardinal vein. A lateral anastomosis subsequently brings it lateral to the vagus nerve.

The ventral pharyngeal vein drains the mandibular and hyoid arches into the common cardinal vein. As the neck elongates, its termination is transferred to the cranial part of the precardinal vein which later becomes the internal jugular vein. The ventral pharyngeal vein receives tributaries from the face and tongue and becomes the linguofacial vein. As the face develops, the primitive maxillary vein extends its drainage into the territories of supply of the ophthalmic and mandibular divisions of the trigeminal nerve, including the pterygoid and temporal muscles, and it anastomoses with the linguofacial vein over the lower jaw. This anastomosis becomes the facial vein which receives a strong retromandibular vein from the temporal region, and drains through the linguofacial vein into the internal jugular. The stem of the linguofacial vein is now the lower part of the facial vein, whilst the dwindling connection of the facial with the primitive maxillary becomes the deep facial vein. The external jugular vein develops from a tributary of the cephalic vein from the tissues of the neck and anastomoses secondarily with the anterior facial vein. At this stage the cephalic vein forms a venous ring around the clavicle by which it is connected with the caudal part of the precardinal vein. The deep segment of the venous ring forms the subclavian vein and receives the definitive external jugular vein. The superficial segment of the venous ring dwindles, but may persist in adult life.

REFERENCES

Ferguson MWF 1991 The orofacial region. In: Wigglesworth JS, Singer DB (eds) Textbook of Fetal and Perinatal Pathology, Chapter 22. Oxford: Blackwell Scientific.

Markus AF, Smith WP, Delaire J 1993 Primary closure of cleft palate: a functional approach. Br J Oral Maxillofac Surg 31: 71–7.

Pharynx

The pharynx is a 12–14 cm long musculomembranous tube shaped like an inverted cone. It extends from the cranial base to the lower border of the cricoid cartilage (the level of the sixth cervical vertebra), where it becomes continuous with the oesophagus. The width of the pharynx varies constantly because it is dependent on muscle tone, especially of the constrictors: at rest the pharyngo-oesophageal junction is closed as a result of tonic closure of the cricopharyngeal sphincter, and during sleep muscle tone is low and the dimensions of the pharynx are markedly decreased (which may give rise to snoring and sleep apnoea). The pharynx is limited above by the posterior part of the body of the sphenoid and the basilar part of the occipital bone, and it is continuous with the oesophagus below. Behind, it is separated from the cervical part of the vertebral column and the prevertebral fascia that covers longus colli and capitis by loose connective tissue in the prevertebral space.

The muscles of the pharynx are the three constrictors and the three elevators. The constrictors may be thought of as three overlapping cones which arise from structures at the sides of the head and neck and pass posteriorly to insert into a midline fibrous band, the pharyngeal raphe. The arterial supply to the pharynx is derived from branches of the external carotid artery, particularly the ascending pharyngeal artery, but also from the ascending palatine and tonsillar branches of the facial artery; the maxillary artery (greater palatine, pharyngeal and artery of the pterygoid canal), and from dorsal lingual branches of the lingual artery. The pharyngeal veins begin in a plexus external to the pharynx, receive meningeal veins and a vein from the pterygoid canal, and usually end in the internal jugular vein. Lymphatic vessels from the pharynx and cervical oesophagus pass to the deep cervical nodes, either directly or through the retropharyngeal or paratracheal nodes. The motor and sensory innervation is principally via branches of the pharyngeal plexus.

The pharynx lies behind, and communicates with, the nasal, oral and laryngeal cavities via the nasopharynx, oropharynx and laryngopharynx respectively (**Fig. 35.1**). Its lining mucosa is continuous with that lining the pharyngotympanic tubes, nasal cavity, mouth and larynx.

NASOPHARYNX

BOUNDARIES
The nasopharynx lies above the soft palate and behind the posterior nares, which allow free respiratory passage between the nasal cavities and the nasopharynx (**Figs 35.1, 35.2**). The nasal septum separates the two posterior nares, each of which measures c.25 mm vertically and 12 mm transversely. Just within these openings lie the posterior ends of the inferior and middle nasal conchae. The walls of the nasopharynx are rigid (except for the soft palate) and its cavity is therefore never obliterated, unlike the cavities of the oro- and laryngopharynx. The nasal and oral parts of the pharynx communicate through the pharyngeal isthmus which lies between the posterior border of the soft palate and the posterior pharyngeal wall. Elevation of the soft palate and constriction of the palatopharyngeal sphincter close the isthmus during swallowing. The nasopharynx has a roof, a posterior wall, two lateral walls and a floor.

The roof and posterior wall form a continuous concave slope that leads down from the nasal septum to the oropharynx. It is bounded above by mucosa overlying the posterior part of the body of the sphenoid, and further back by the basilar part of the occipital bone as far as the pharyngeal tubercle. Further down, the mucosa overlies the pharyngobasilar fascia and the upper fibres of the superior constrictor, and behind these, the anterior arch of the atlas. A lymphoid mass, the

adenoid, lies in the mucosa of the upper part of the roof and posterior wall in the midline.

The lateral walls of the nasopharynx display a number of important surface features. On either side each receives the opening of the pharyngotympanic tube (also termed the auditory or Eustachian tube), situated 10–12 mm behind and a little below the level of the posterior end of the inferior nasal concha (**Fig. 35.1**). The tubal aperture is approximately triangular in shape, and is bounded above and behind by the tubal elevation which consists of mucosa overlying the protruding pharyngeal end of the cartilage of the pharyngotympanic tube. A vertical mucosal fold, the salpingopharyngeal fold, descends from the tubal elevation behind the aperture (**Fig. 35.1**) and covers salpingopharyngeus in the wall of the pharynx (**Fig. 35.3**), and a smaller salpingopalatine fold extends from the anterosuperior angle of the tubal elevation to the soft palate in front of the aperture. As levator veli palatini enters the soft palate it produces an elevation of the mucosa immediately below the tubal opening (**Fig 35.3**). A small mass of lymphoid tissue, the tubal tonsil, lies in the mucosa immediately behind the opening of the pharyngotympanic tube. Further behind the tubal elevation there is a variable depression in the lateral wall, the pharyngeal recess (fossa of Rosenmüller). The floor of the nasopharynx is formed by the upper surface of the soft palate.

MICROSTRUCTURE OF NON-TONSILLAR NASOPHARYNX
The nasopharyngeal epithelium anteriorly is ciliated, pseudostratified respiratory in type (p. 31, **Fig. 3.6**), with goblet cells. The ducts of mucosal and submucosal seromucous glands open onto its surface. Posteriorly the respiratory epithelium changes to non-keratinized stratified squamous epithelium which continues into the oropharynx and laryngopharynx. The transitional zone between the two types of epithelium consists of columnar epithelium with short microvilli instead of cilia. Superiorly this zone meets the nasal septum, laterally it crosses the orifice of the pharyngotympanic tube, and it passes posteriorly at the union of the soft palate and the lateral wall. There are numerous mucous glands around the tubal orifices.

INNERVATION
Much of the mucosa of the nasopharynx behind the pharyngotympanic tube is supplied by the pharyngeal branch of the pterygopalatine ganglion which traverses the palatovaginal canal with a pharyngeal branch of the maxillary artery. The maxillary nerve is thought to transmit the principal sensory supply from the pharyngotympanic tube and middle ear cavity, presumably through its pharyngeal branch.

ADENOID OR NASOPHARYNGEAL TONSIL (Fig. 35.4)
The adenoid, or nasopharyngeal tonsil, is a median mass of mucosa-associated lymphoid tissue (MALT, p. 77) situated in the roof and posterior wall of the nasopharynx. At its maximal size (during the early years of life) it is shaped like a truncated pyramid, often with a vertically oriented median cleft, so that its apex points towards the nasal septum and its base at the junction of the roof and posterior wall of the nasopharynx.

The free surface of the nasopharyngeal tonsil is marked by folds that radiate forwards and laterally from a median blind recess, the pharyngeal bursa (bursa of Luschka), which extends backwards and up. The recess marks the rostral end of the embryological notochord. The number and position of the folds and of the deep fissures which separate them vary. A median fold may pass forwards from the pharyngeal bursa

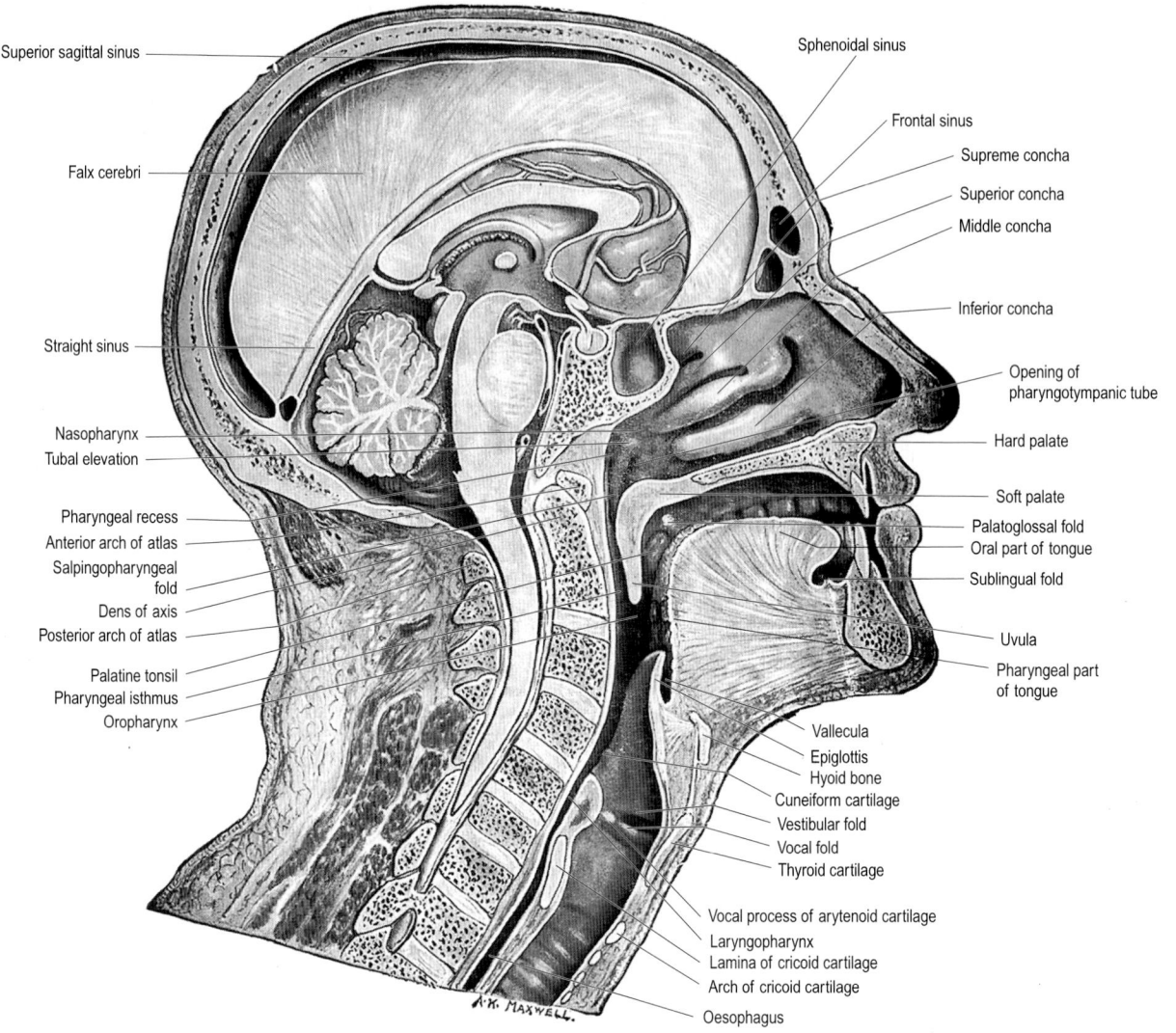

Fig. 35.1 Median sagittal section through the head and neck. Where it passes through the brain, the section passes slightly to the right of the median plane but, below the base of the skull, including the nasal cavity, it passes slightly to the left of the median plane.

towards the nasal septum, or instead a fissure may extend forwards from the bursa, dividing the nasopharyngeal tonsil into two distinct halves which reflect its paired developmental origins (**Fig 35.4**).

The prenatal origins and growth of the nasopharyngeal tonsil are described on pages 611 and 647. After birth it initially grows rapidly, but usually undergoes a degree of involution and atrophy from the age of 8–10 years (although hypoplasia may still occur in adults up to the seventh decade). Relative to the volume of the nasopharynx, the size of the tonsil is largest at 5 years, which may account for the frequency of nasal breathing problems in preschool children, and the incidence of adenoidectomy in this age group.

Vascular supply and lymphatic drainage
The arterial supply of the nasopharyngeal tonsil is derived from the ascending pharyngeal and ascending palatine arteries, the tonsillar branches of the facial artery, the pharyngeal branch of the maxillary artery and the artery of the pterygoid canal. In addition, a nutrient or emissary vessel to the neighbouring bone, the basisphenoid artery, which is a branch of the inferior hypophysial arteries, supplies the bed of the nasopharyngeal tonsil and is a possible cause of persistent post-adenoidectomy haemorrhage in some patients.

Numerous communicating veins drain the nasopharyngeal tonsil into the internal submucous and external pharyngeal venous plexuses. They emerge from the deep lateral surface of the tonsil and join the external palatine (paratonsillar) veins (**Fig. 35.6**), and pierce the superior constrictor either to join the pharyngeal venous plexus, or to unite to

form a single vessel that enters the facial or internal jugular vein. They may also connect with the pterygoid venous plexus.

Microstructure of the nasopharyngeal tonsil (Fig. 35.5)
The adenoid is covered laterally and inferiorly mainly by ciliated respiratory epithelium which contains scattered small patches of non-keratinized stratified squamous epithelium. Its superior surface is separated from the periosteum of the sphenoid and occipital bones by a connective tissue hemicapsule to which the fibrous framework of the tonsil is anchored. The latter consists of a mesh of collagen type III (reticular) fibres which supports a lymphoid parenchyma similar to that in the palatine tonsil.

The nasopharyngeal epithelium lines a series of mucosal folds around which the lymphoid parenchyma is organized into follicles and extrafollicular areas. Internally, the tonsil is subdivided into four to six lobes by connective tissue septa, which arise from the hemicapsule and penetrate the lymphoid parenchyma. Seromucous glands lie within the connective tissue, and their ducts extend through the parenchyma to reach the nasopharyngeal surface.

Functions of the nasopharyngeal tonsil
The nasopharyngeal tonsil forms part of the circumpharyngeal lymphoid ring (Waldeyer's ring), and therefore presumably contributes to the defence of the upper respiratory tract. The territories served by its lymphocytes are uncertain, but may include the nasal cavities, nasopharynx, pharyngotympanic tubes and the middle and inner ears.

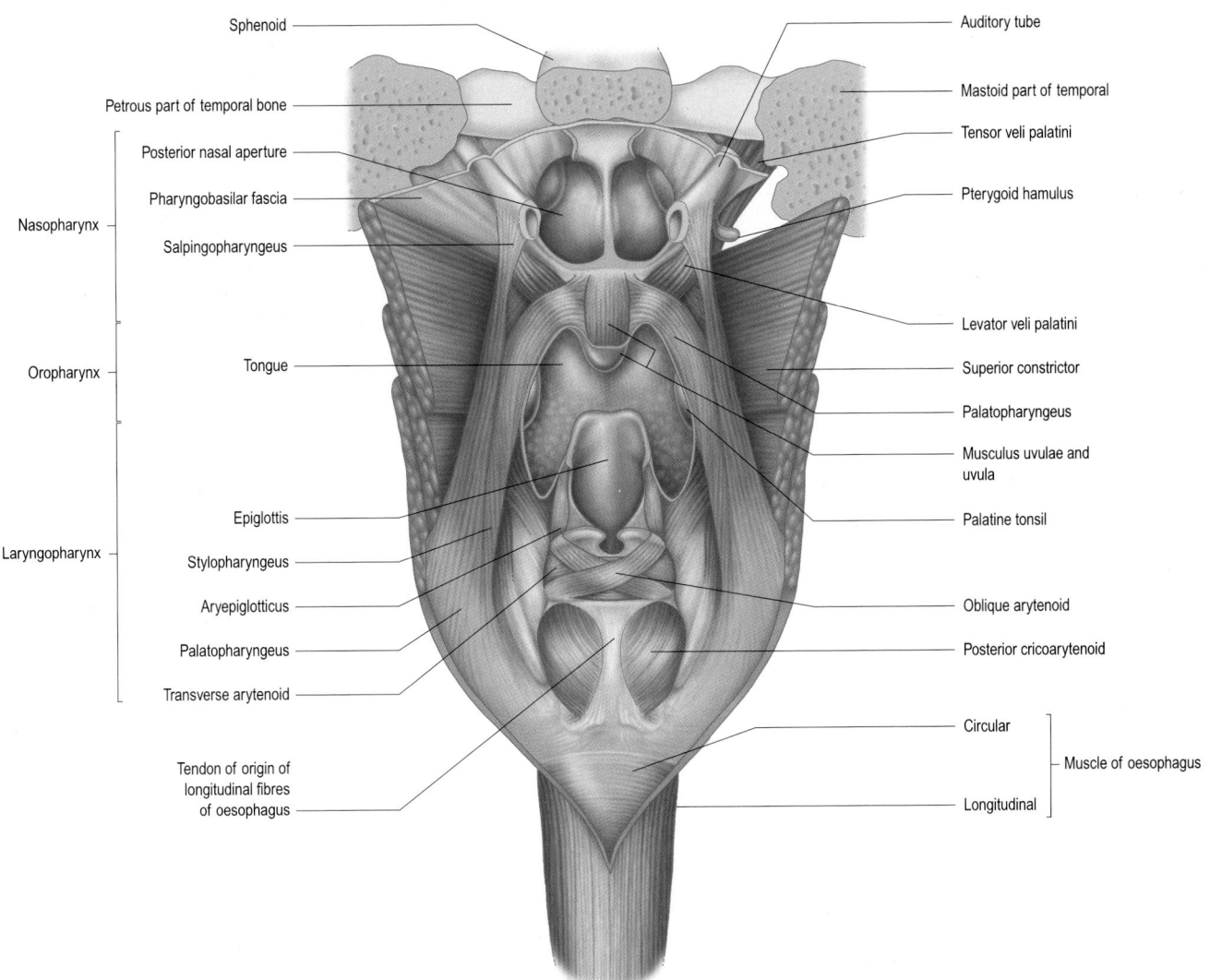

Fig. 35.2 The pharyngeal musculature, exposed from the posterior aspect.

Sphenoid
Petrous part of temporal bone
Posterior nasal aperture
Pharyngobasilar fascia
Salpingopharyngeus
Nasopharynx
Oropharynx
Tongue
Laryngopharynx
Epiglottis
Stylopharyngeus
Aryepiglotticus
Palatopharyngeus
Transverse arytenoid
Tendon of origin of longitudinal fibres of oesophagus

Auditory tube
Mastoid part of temporal
Tensor veli palatini
Pterygoid hamulus
Levator veli palatini
Superior constrictor
Palatopharyngeus
Musculus uvulae and uvula
Palatine tonsil
Oblique arytenoid
Posterior cricoarytenoid
Circular
Longitudinal
Muscle of oesophagus

Adenoidectomy

Surgical removal of the adenoids is commonly performed to clear naso-pharyngeal obstruction and as part of the treatment of chronic secretory otitis media. A variety of methods are employed including suction diathermy, suction microdebridement and most commonly blind curettage. When using the latter it is important to avoid hyperextension of the cervical spine as this throws the arch of the atlas into prominence and may result in damage to the prevertebral fascia and anterior spinal ligaments, with resultant infection and cervical instability. Extreme lateral curettage can result in damage to the tubal orifice and excessive bleeding because the vasculature is denser laterally.

Pharyngotympanic tube (Fig. 38.4)

The pharyngotympanic tube connects the tympanic cavity to the naso-pharynx and allows the passage of air between these spaces in order to equalize the air pressure on both aspects of the tympanic membrane. It is c.36 mm long and descends anteromedially from the tympanic cavity to the nasopharynx at an angle of c.45° with the sagittal plane and 30° with the horizontal (these angles increase with age and elongation of the skull base). It is formed partly by cartilage and fibrous tissue and partly by bone.

The cartilaginous part, c.24 mm long, is formed by a triangular plate of cartilage, the greater part being in the posteromedial wall of the tube.

Its apex is attached by fibrous tissue to the circumference of the jagged rim of the bony part of the tube and its base is directly under the mucosa of the lateral nasopharyngeal wall, forming a tubal elevation behind the pharyngeal orifice of the tube (**Fig. 35.1**). The upper part of the cartilage is bent laterally and downwards, producing a broad medial lamina and narrow lateral lamina. In transverse section it is hook-like and incomplete below and laterally, where the canal is composed of fibrous tissue. The cartilage is fixed to the cranial base in the groove between the petrous part of the temporal bone and the greater wing of the sphenoid, and ends near the root of the medial pterygoid plate. The cartilaginous and bony parts of the tube are not in the same plane, the former descending a little more steeply than the latter. The diameter of the tube is greatest at the pharyngeal orifice, least at the junction of the two parts (the isthmus) and increases again towards the tympanic cavity.

The bony part, c.12 mm long, is oblong in transverse section, with its greater dimension in the horizontal plane. It starts from the anterior tympanic wall and gradually narrows to end at the junction of the squamous and petrous parts of the temporal bone, where it has a jagged margin for the attachment of the cartilaginous part. The carotid canal lies medially.

The mucosa of the pharyngotympanic tube is continuous with the nasopharyngeal and tympanic mucosae. It is lined by a ciliated columnar

Cartilage of
pharyngotympanic tube

Pterygomandibular
raphe

Sphenoidal
sinus

Frontal
sinus

Nasopharyngeal tonsil

Tensor veli palatini

Levator veli palatini

Ascending palatine artery

Salpingopharyngeus

Palatoglossus

Styloglossus

Superior constrictor

Stylopharyngeus

Palatopharyngeus

Stylohyoid ligament

Glossopharyngeal
nerve

Inferior
constrictor

Middle
constrictor

Mucous membrane
of pharynx

Epiglottis

Fig. 35.3 Median sagittal section of the head, showing a dissection of the interior of the pharynx, after the removal of the mucous membrane. The bodies of the cervical vertebrae have been removed and the cut posterior wall of the pharynx then retracted dorsolaterally. Palatopharyngeus is reflected dorsally to show the cranial fibres of the inferior constrictor; the dorsum of the tongue is pulled ventrally to display a part of styloglossus in the angular interval between the mandibular and the lingual fibres of origin of the superior constrictor.

Fig. 35.4 Appearance of a nasopharyngeal tonsil following adenoidectomy by curettage. Rostral surface is to the left; surface folds radiate forward from a median recess (arrowhead). In this example, the impression left by contact with the left Eustachian cushion is evident laterally (arrow). **B**, Transnasal endoscopic view of adenoid. 1, adenoid (in posterior naris); 2, inferior concha (posterior view); 3, posterior end of nasal septum. (**A**, specimen provided by Professor MJ Gleeson, ENT Department, GKT School of Medicine, London.) (**B**, by kind permission from Mr Simon A Hickey.)

A
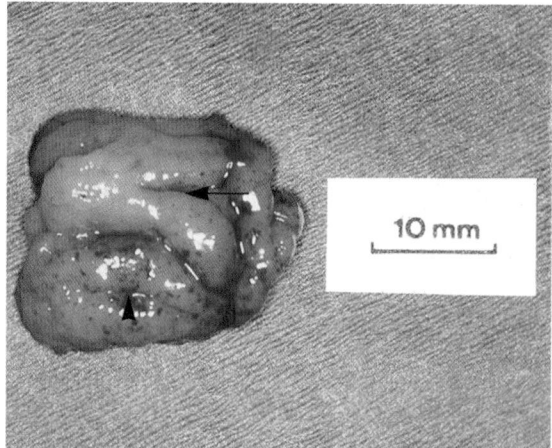

B
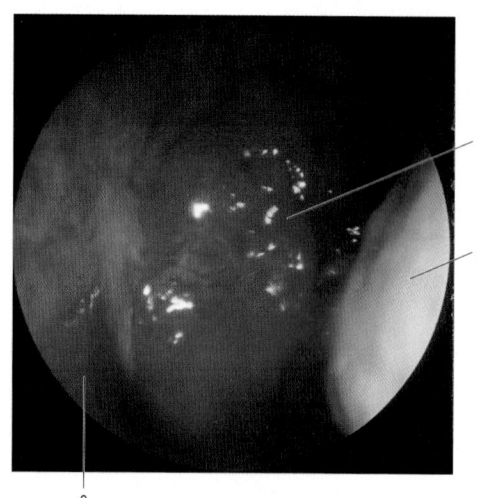

epithelium and is thin in the osseous part but thickened by mucous glands in the cartilaginous part. Near the pharyngeal orifice there is a variable, but sometimes considerable, lymphoid mass, the tubal tonsil.

At birth the pharyngotympanic tube is about half its adult length, it is more horizontal and its bony part is relatively shorter but much wider. The pharyngeal orifice is a narrow slit, level with the palate and without a tubal elevation.

Relations – Salpingopharyngeus is attached to the inferior part of the cartilaginous tube near its pharyngeal opening. Posteromedially are the petrous part of the temporal bone and levator veli palatini, which arises partly from the medial lamina of the tube. Anterolaterally tensor veli palatini separates the tube from the otic ganglion, the mandibular nerve and its branches, the chorda tympani nerve and the middle meningeal artery. Some fibres of tensor veli palatini are attached to the lateral lamina of the cartilage and to the fibrous part, and these fibres are sometimes referred to as dilator tubae. The pharyngotympanic tube

is opened during deglutition but the mechanism is uncertain. Dilator tubae, aided by salpingopharyngeus, may be responsible. Levator veli palatini elevates the cartilaginous part of the pharyngotympanic tube, and so might allow passive opening by releasing tension on the cartilage.

Vascular supply – Arteries to the pharyngotympanic tube arise from the ascending pharyngeal and middle meningeal arteries and from the artery of the pterygoid canal. The veins of the pharyngotympanic tube usually drain to the pterygoid venous plexus.

OROPHARYNX

BOUNDARIES (Figs 35.1, 35.2)
The oropharynx extends from the soft palate to the upper border of the epiglottis (**Fig. 35.1**). It opens into the mouth through the oropharyngeal isthmus, demarcated by the palatoglossal arch, and faces

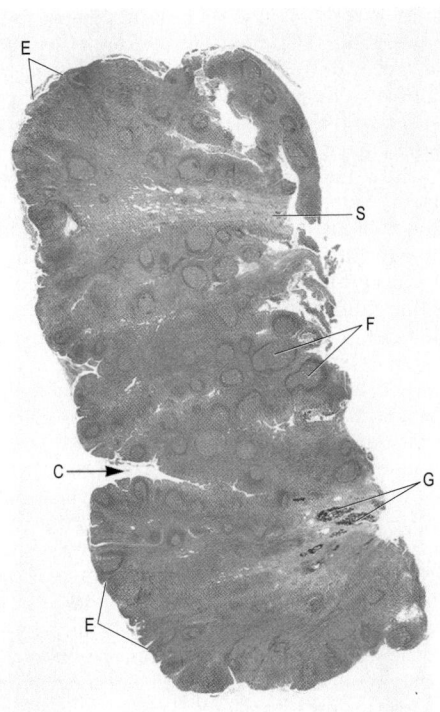

Fig. 35.5 Transverse section of a nasopharyngeal tonsil. Numerous lymphoid follicles (F) are covered on their nasopharyngeal surface by respiratory epithelium (E) with folds and deep crypts (C). Seromucous glands (G) and connective tissue septa (S) penetrate the lymphoid tissue. (Provided by N Kirkpatrick, Division of Anatomy and Cell Biology, GKT School of Medicine, London; photograph by Sarah-Jane Smith.)

the pharyngeal aspect of the tongue. Its lateral wall consists of the palatopharyngeal arch and palatine tonsil (**Fig. 33.2**). Posteriorly, it is level with the body of the second, and upper part of the third, cervical vertebrae (**Fig. 35.1**).

SOFT PALATE

The soft palate is a mobile flap suspended from the posterior border of the hard palate, sloping down and back between the oral and nasal parts of the pharynx. (**Fig. 35.1**). The boundary between the hard and soft palate is readily palpable and may be distinguished by a change in colour, the soft palate being a darker red with a yellowish tint. The soft palate is a thick fold of mucosa enclosing an aponeurosis, muscular tissue, vessels, nerves, lymphoid tissue and mucous glands. In most individuals two small pits, the fovea palatini, one on each side of the midline, may be seen: they represent the orifices of ducts from some of the minor mucous glands of the palate. In its usual relaxed and pendant position, the anterior (oral) surface of the soft palate is concave, and has a median raphe. The posterior aspect is convex and continuous with the nasal floor, the anterosuperior border is attached to the posterior margin of the hard palate, and the sides blend with the pharyngeal wall. The inferior border is free, and hangs between the mouth and pharynx. A median conical process, the uvula, projects downwards from its posterior border (**Fig. 33.2**). Taste buds also occur on the oral aspect of the soft palate.

The anterior third of the soft palate contains little muscle and consists mainly of the palatine aponeurosis. This region is less mobile and more horizontal than the rest of the soft palate and is the chief area acted upon by tensor veli palatini.

A small bony prominence, produced by the pterygoid hamulus, can be felt just behind and medial to each upper alveolar process, in the lateral part of the anterior region of the soft palate. The pterygo-mandibular raphe – a tendinous band between buccinator and the superior constrictor – passes downwards and outwards from the hamulus to the posterior end of the mylohyoid line. When the mouth is opened wide, this raphe raises a fold of mucosa that marks internally the posterior boundary of the cheek, and is an important landmark for an inferior alveolar nerve block.

Palatine aponeurosis

A thin, fibrous, palatine aponeurosis strengthens the soft palate, and is composed of the expanded tendons of the tensor veli palatini muscles. It is attached to the posterior border and inferior surface of the hard palate behind any palatine crests, and extends medially from behind the greater palatine foramina. It is thick in the anterior two-thirds of the soft palate but very thin further back. Near the midline it encloses the musculus uvulae. All the other palatine muscles are attached to the aponeurosis.

Pillars of fauces (Fig. 33.2)

The lateral wall of the oropharynx presents two prominent folds, the pillars of the fauces. The anterior fold, or palatoglossal arch, runs from the soft palate to the side of the tongue and contains palatoglossus. The posterior fold, or palatopharyngeal arch, projects more medially and passes from the soft palate to merge with the lateral wall of the pharynx. It contains palatopharyngeus. A triangular tonsillar fossa (tonsillar sinus) lies on each side of the oropharynx between the diverging palato-pharyngeal and palatoglossal arches, and contains the palatine tonsil.

Vascular supply

The arterial supply of the soft palate is usually derived from the ascending palatine branch of the facial artery. Sometimes this is replaced or supplemented by a branch of the ascending pharyngeal artery which descends forwards between the superior border of the superior constrictor and levator veli palatini, and accompanies the latter to the soft palate. The veins of the soft palate usually drain to the pterygoid venous plexus.

Innervation

The secretomotor supply to most of the mucosa of the soft palate travels via the lesser palatine nerve in postganglionic branches from the pterygopalatine ganglion. The lesser palatine nerve also contains sensory fibres including those supplying taste buds in the oral surface of the soft palate, which travel through the pterygopalatine ganglion without synapsing to access the greater petrosal nerve (a branch of the facial nerve). Postganglionic secretomotor parasympathetic fibres may pass to the posterior parts of the soft palate from the otic ganglion (which receives preganglionic fibres via the lesser petrosal branch of the glossopharyngeal nerve).

Gag reflex

The gag reflex is discussed on page 233.

Uvulopalatopharyngoplasty

The pharyngeal airway is kept patent in the patient who is awake by the combined dilating action of genioglossus, tensor veli palatini, geniohyoid and stylohyoid, which act to counter the negative pressure generated in the lumen of the pharynx during inspiration. The tone in the muscles is reduced during sleep, but is also affected by alcohol and other sedatives, hypothyroidism and a variety of neurological disorders. If the dilator muscle tone is insufficient, the walls of the pharynx may become apposed. Intermittent pharyngeal obstruction may cause snoring, and complete obstruction may cause apnoea, hypoxia and hypercarbia which lead to arousal and sleep disturbance.

Surgical techniques involving reduction in the length of the soft palate, removal of the tonsils and plicating of the tonsillar pillars can be used to raise the intrinsic dilating tone in the pharyngeal wall and to reduce the bulk of (and to stiffen) the soft palate. This will reduce the tendency of the soft palate to vibrate and generate noise during periods of incipient collapse of the pharynx. An alternative treatment is to deliver air to the pharynx at above atmospheric pressure via a closely fitting facemask, thus inflating the pharynx and countering its tendency to collapse.

PALATINE TONSIL (Figs 35.6, 35.7)

The right and left palatine tonsils form part of the circumpharyngeal lymphoid ring. Each tonsil is an ovoid mass of lymphoid tissue situated in the lateral wall of the oropharynx. Size varies according to age, individuality and pathological status (tonsils may be hypertrophied and/or inflamed). It is therefore difficult to define the normal appearance of the palatine tonsil. For the first 5 or 6 years of life the tonsils increase rapidly in size. They usually reach a maximum at puberty when they average 20–25 mm in vertical, and 10–15 mm in transverse, diameters,

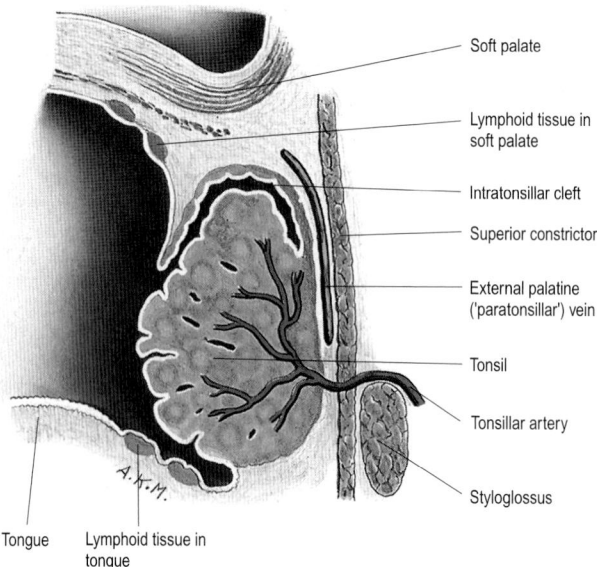

Fig. 35.6 Coronal section through the left palatine tonsil.

and they project conspicuously into the oropharynx. Tonsillar involution begins at puberty, when the reactive lymphoid tissue begins to atrophy, and by old age only a little tonsillar lymphoid tissue remains.

The long axis of the tonsil is directed from above, downwards and backwards. Its medial, free, surface usually presents a pitted appearance. The pits, 10–20 in number, lead into a system of blind-ending, often highly branching, crypts which extend through the whole thickness of the tonsil and almost reach the connective tissue hemicapsule. In a healthy tonsil the openings of the crypts are fissure-like and the walls of the crypt lumina are collapsed so that they are in contact with each other. The human tonsil is polycryptic. The branching crypt system reaches its maximum size and complexity during childhood. The mouth of a deep intratonsillar cleft (recessus palatinus), opens in the upper part of the medial surface of the tonsil (**Fig. 35.6**). It often erroneously

called the supratonsillar fossa, and yet it is not situated above the tonsil but within its substance. The mouth of the cleft is semilunar, curving parallel to the convex dorsum of the tongue in the parasagittal plane. The upper wall of the recess contains lymphoid tissue which extends into the soft palate as the pars palatina of the palatine tonsil. After the age of 5 years this embedded part of the tonsil diminishes in size. From the age of 14, there is a tendency for the whole tonsil to involute, and for the tonsillar bed to flatten out. During young adult life a mucosal fold termed the plica triangularis stretches back from the palatoglossal arch down to the tongue. It is infiltrated by lymphoid tissue and frequently represents the most prominent (anteroinferior) portion of the tonsil. It rarely persists into middle age.

The lateral or deep surface of the tonsil spreads downwards, upwards and forwards. Inferiorly, it invades the dorsum of the tongue, superiorly, the soft palate, and, anteriorly, it may extend for some distance under the palatoglossal arch. This deep, lateral aspect is covered by a layer of fibrous tissue, the tonsillar hemicapsule, separable with ease for most of its extent from the underlying muscular walls of the pharynx which is formed here by the superior constrictor, with styloglossus on its lateral side (**Fig. 35.6**). Anteroinferiorly the hemicapsule adheres to the side of the tongue and to palatoglossus and palatopharyngeus. In this region the tonsillar artery, a branch of the facial, pierces the superior constrictor to enter the tonsil, accompanied by venae comitantes. An important and sometimes large vein, the external palatine or paratonsillar vein, descends from the soft palate lateral to the tonsillar hemicapsule before piercing the pharyngeal wall (**Fig. 35.6**). Haemorrhage from this vessel from the upper angle of the tonsillar fossa may complicate tonsillectomy. The muscular wall of the tonsillar fossa separates the tonsil from the ascending palatine artery, and, occasionally, from the tortuous facial artery itself, which may lie near the pharyngeal wall at the lower tonsillar level. The internal carotid artery lies c.25 mm behind and lateral to the tonsil.

Microstructure of the palatine tonsil

Each tonsil is a mass of lymphoid tissue associated with the oropharyngeal mucosa and fixed in its position, unlike most other examples of mucosa-associated lymphoid tissue (p. 77). It is covered on its oropharyngeal aspect by non-keratinized stratified squamous epithelium. The whole of the tonsil is supported internally by a delicate meshwork of fine collagen type III (reticulin) fibres which are condensed in places to form more robust connective tissue septa that also contain elastin. These septa partition the tonsillar parenchyma, and merge at their ends

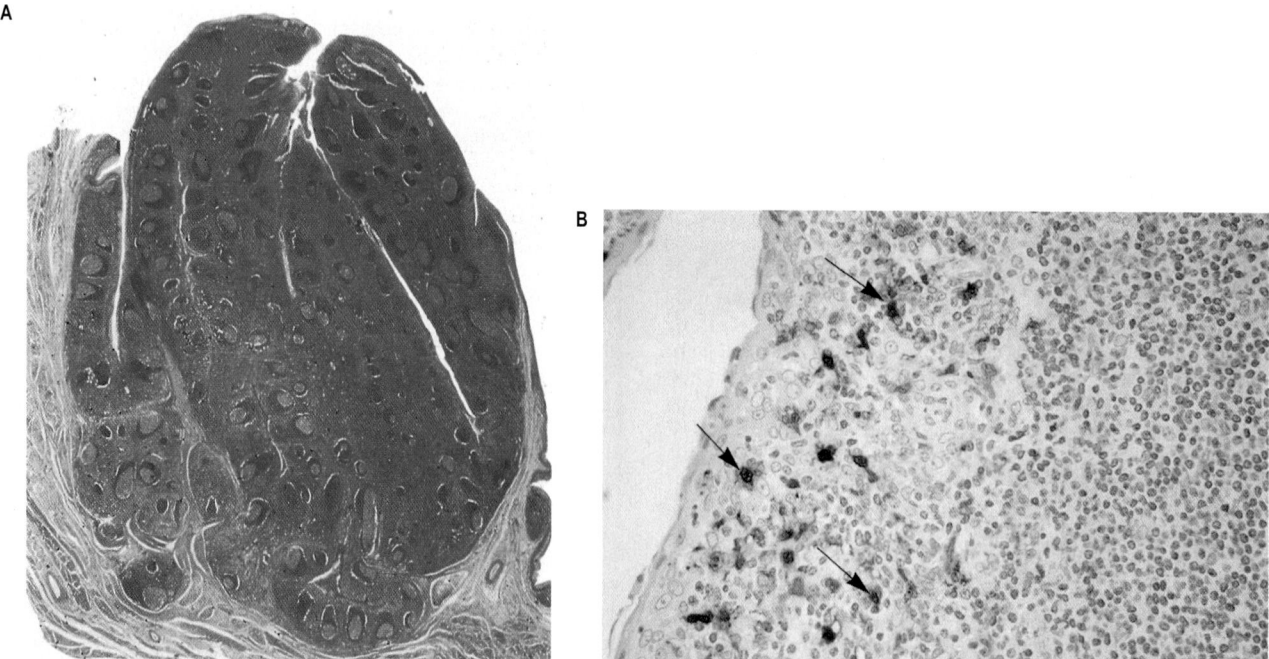

Fig. 35.7 A, Transverse section through a whole palatine tonsil, showing many secondary follicles, oropharyngeal surface epithelium and the connective tissue hemicapsule. **B,** Reticulated epithelium from a crypt of a palatine tonsil, immunostained to show numerous interdigitating cells and macrophages. Note the close contacts between these cells and infiltrating lymphocytes (arrows). (**A**, by permission from Young B, Heath JW 2000 Wheater's Functional Histology. Edinburgh: Churchill Livingstone.) (**B**, provided by M Perry, Division of Anatomy and Cell Biology, GKT School of Medicine, London.)

with the dense irregular fibrous hemicapsule on the deep aspect of the tonsil and with the lamina propria on the pharyngeal surface. Blood vessels, lymphatics and nerves branch or join within the connective tissue condensations. The hemicapsule forms its lateral boundary with the oropharyngeal wall, and with the mucosa which covers its highly invaginated free surface (**Fig. 35.7**).

The 10–20 crypts formed by invagination of the free surface mucosa are narrow tubular epithelial diverticula which often branch within the tonsil and frequently are packed with plugs of shed epithelial cells, lymphocytes and bacteria, which may calcify. The epithelium lining the crypts is mostly similar to that of the oropharyngeal surface, i.e. stratified squamous, but there are also patches of reticulated epithelium, which is much thinner. This has a complex structure which is of great importance in the immunological function of the tonsil.

Reticulated epithelium – Reticulated epithelium lacks the orderly laminar structure of stratified squamous epithelium. Its base is deeply invaginated in a complex manner so that the epithelial cells, with their slender branched cytoplasmic processes, provide a coarse mesh to accommodate the infiltrating lymphocytes and macrophages. The basal lamina of this epithelium is discontinuous. Although the oropharyngeal surface is unbroken, the epithelium may become exceedingly thin in places, so that only a tenuous cytoplasmic layer separates the pharyngeal lumen from the underlying lymphocytes. Epithelial cells are held together by small desmosomes, anchored into bundles of keratin filaments. Interdigitating dendritic cells (antigen-presenting cells, APCs) (p. 80) are also present. The intimate association of epithelial cells and lymphocytes facilitates the direct transport of antigen from the external environment to the tonsillar lymphoid cells, i.e. reticulated epithelial cells are functionally similar to the microfold (M) cells of the gut. The total surface area of the reticulated epithelium is very large because of the complex branched nature of the tonsillar crypts, and has been estimated at $295 \, cm^2$ for an average palatine tonsil. Lymph nodes elsewhere depend on indirect antigen delivery through afferent lymphatic vessels (p. 75), but these are absent from the tonsil (although it is drained by efferent lymphatics).

Tonsillar lymphoid tissue – There are four lymphoid compartments in the palatine tonsils. Lymphoid follicles, many with germinal centres (p. 74), are arranged in rows roughly parallel to neighbouring connective tissue septa. Their size and cellular content varies in proportion to the immunological activity of the tonsil. The mantle zones of the follicles, each with closely packed small lymphocytes, form a dense cap, always situated on the side of the follicle nearest to the mucosal surface. These cells are the products of B-lymphocyte proliferation within the germinal centres. Extrafollicular, or T-lymphocyte areas contain a specialized microvasculature including high endothelial venules (HEVs) (p. 143), through which circulating lymphocytes enter the tonsillar parenchyma. The lymphoid tissue of the reticulated crypt epithelium contains predominantly IgG- and IgA-producing B lymphocytes (including some mature plasma cells), T lymphocytes and antigen-presenting cells, APCs (p. 80). There are numerous capillary loops in this subsurface region.

Vascular supply and lymphatic drainage

The arterial blood supply to the palatine tonsil is derived from branches of the external carotid artery. The principal artery is the tonsillar artery, which is a branch of the facial, or sometimes the ascending palatine, artery. It ascends between medial pterygoid and styloglossus, perforates the superior constrictor at the upper border of styloglossus (**Fig. 35.6**) and ramifies in the tonsil and posterior lingual musculature. Additional small tonsillar branches may be derived from the ascending pharyngeal artery; the dorsal lingual branches of the lingual artery (supplying the lower part of the palatine tonsil); the greater palatine branch of the maxillary artery (supplying the upper part of the tonsil), and the ascending palatine branch of the facial artery. Arteries enter the deep surface of the tonsil, branch within the connective tissue septa, narrow to become arterioles and then give off capillary loops into the follicles, interfollicular areas and the cavities within the base of the reticulated epithelium. The capillaries rejoin to form venules, many with high endothelium, and the veins return within the septal tissues to the hemicapsule as tributaries of the pharyngeal drainage. The tonsillar artery and its venae comitantes often lie within the palatoglossal fold, and may haemorrhage if this fold is damaged during surgery.

Unlike lymph nodes, the tonsils do not possess afferent lymphatics or lymph sinuses. Instead, dense plexuses of fine lymphatic vessels surround each follicle and form efferent lymphatics which pass towards the hemicapsule, pierce the superior constrictor and drain to the upper deep cervical lymph nodes directly (especially the jugulodigastric nodes) or indirectly through the retropharyngeal lymph nodes. The former are typically enlarged in tonsillitis, when they project beyond the anterior border of sternocleidomastoid and are palpable superficially 1–2 cm below the angle of the mandible: when enlarged, they represent the most common swelling in the neck.

Innervation

The palatine tonsil region receives its nerve supply through tonsillar branches of the maxillary nerve and the glossopharyngeal nerve. The maxillary nerve fibres pass through, but do not synapse in, the pterygopalatine ganglion, and are distributed through the lesser palatine nerves. The latter, together with the tonsillar branches of the glossopharyngeal nerve, form a plexus around the tonsil. From this plexus (the circulus tonsillaris), nerve fibres are also distributed to the soft palate and the region of the oropharyngeal isthmus. The tympanic branch of the glossopharyngeal nerve supplies the mucous membrane lining the tympanic cavity. Infection, malignancy and postoperative inflammation of the tonsil and tonsil fossa may therefore be accompanied by pain referred to the ear.

Tonsillectomy

Surgical removal of the pharyngeal tonsils is commonly performed to prevent recurrent acute tonsillitis or to treat airway obstruction by hypertrophied or inflamed palatine tonsils. Occasionally the tonsil may be removed to treat an acute peritonsillar abscess, which is a collection of pus between the superior constrictor and the tonsillar hemicapsule. Many methods have been employed, the commonest being dissection in the plane of the fibrous hemicapsule followed by ligation or electrocautery to the vessels divided during the dissection. The nerve supply to the tonsil is so diffuse that tonsillectomy under local anaesthesia is performed successfully by local infiltration rather than by blocking the main nerves. Surgical access to the glossopharyngeal nerve may be achieved by separating the fibres of superior constrictor.

Waldeyer's ring

Waldeyer's ring is a circumpharyngeal ring of mucosa-associated lymphoid tissue which surrounds the openings into the digestive and respiratory tracts. It is made up anteroinferiorly by the lingual tonsil, laterally by the palatine and tubal tonsils, and posterosuperiorly by the nasopharyngeal tonsil and smaller collections of lymphoid tissue in the inter-tonsillar intervals.

LARYNGOPHARYNX

BOUNDARIES (Figs 35.1, 35.2)

The laryngopharynx (known clinically as the hypopharynx) extends from the superior border of the epiglottis, where it is delineated from the oropharynx by the lateral glossoepiglottic folds, to the inferior border of the cricoid cartilage, where it becomes continuous with the oesophagus. The laryngeal inlet lies in its incomplete anterior wall, and the posterior surfaces of the arytenoid and cricoid cartilages lie below this opening.

Piriform fossa

A small piriform fossa lies on each side of the laryngeal inlet, bounded medially by the aryepiglottic fold and laterally by the thyroid cartilage and thyrohyoid membrane. Branches of the internal laryngeal nerve lie beneath its mucous membrane. At rest, the laryngopharynx extends posteriorly from the lower part of the third cervical vertebral body to the upper part of the sixth. During deglutition it may be elevated considerably by the hyoid elevators.

Inlet of larynx (Fig. 35.2)

The obliquely-sloping inlet of the larynx lies in the anterior part of the laryngopharynx. This inlet is bounded above by the epiglottis, below by the arytenoid cartilages of the larynx, and laterally by the aryepiglottic folds. Below the inlet, the anterior wall of the laryngopharynx is formed by the posterior surface of the cricoid cartilage.

PHARYNGEAL FASCIA

The two named layers of fascia in the pharynx are the pharyngobasilar and the buccopharyngeal fascia. The fibrous layer that supports the pharyngeal mucosa is thickened above the superior constrictor to form the pharyngobasilar fascia (**Fig. 35.8**). It is attached to the basilar part of the occipital bone and the petrous part of the temporal bone medial to the pharyngotympanic tube, and to the posterior border of the medial pterygoid plate and pterygomandibular raphe. Inferiorly, it diminishes in thickness, but is strengthened posteriorly by a fibrous band attached to the pharyngeal tubercle of the occipital bone which descends as the median pharyngeal raphe of the constrictors. This fibrous layer is really the epimysial covering of the muscles and their aponeurotic attachment to the base of the skull. The thinner external part of the epimysium is the buccopharyngeal fascia, which covers the superior constrictor and passes forwards over the pterygomandibular raphe to cover buccinator.

PHARYNGEAL TISSUE SPACES

Pharyngeal tissue spaces can be subdivided into peripharyngeal and intrapharyngeal spaces. The anterior part of the peripharyngeal space is formed by the submandibular and submental spaces, posteriorly by the retropharyngeal space and laterally by the parapharyngeal spaces. The retropharyngeal space is an area of loose connective tissue which lies behind the pharynx and anterior to the prevertebral fascia, and extends upwards to the base of the skull and downwards to the retrovisceral space in the infrahyoid part of the neck. Each parapharyngeal space passes laterally around the pharynx and is continuous with the retropharyngeal space. However, unlike the retropharyngeal space, it is a space which is restricted to the suprahyoid region. It is bounded medially by the pharynx; laterally by the pterygoid muscles – here it is part of the infratemporal fossa – and the sheath of the parotid gland; superiorly by the base of the skull; and is limited inferiorly by suprahyoid structures, particularly the sheath of the submandibular gland. An intrapharyngeal space potentially exits between the inner surface of the constrictor muscles and the pharyngeal mucosa. Infections in this space are either restricted locally or spread through the pharynx into the retropharyngeal or parapharyngeal spaces. The peritonsillar space is an important part of the intrapharyngeal space: it lies around the palatine tonsil between the pillars of the fauces. Infections in the intratonsillar space usually spread up or down the intrapharyngeal space, or through the pharynx into the parapharyngeal space.

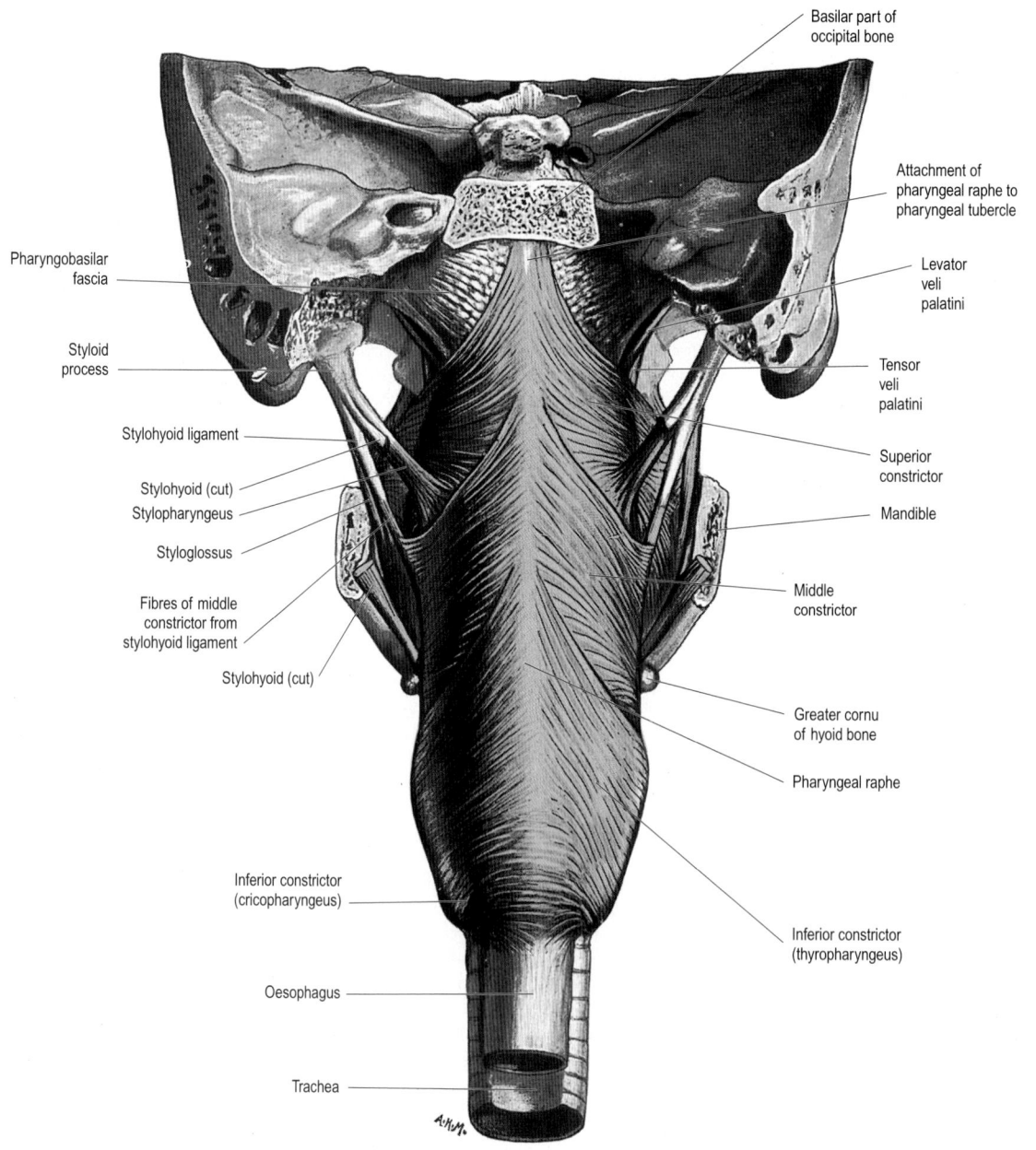

Fig. 35.8 Muscles of the pharynx: posterior view. (From Schaefer EA, Symington J, Bryce TH (eds) 1915 Quain's Anatomy, 11th edn. London: Longmans, Green, with permission from Pearson Education.)

SPREAD OF INFECTION

Infection which spreads into the parapharyngeal space will produce pain, and trismus. There may be swelling in the oropharynx extending up to the uvula, displacing it to the contralateral side, and dysphagia. Posterior spread from the parapharyngeal space into the retropharyngeal space will produce bulging of the posterior pharyngeal wall, dyspnoea and nuchal rigidity. Involvement of the carotid sheath may produce symptoms due to thrombosis of the internal jugular vein and cranial nerve symptoms involving the IX–XII nerves. If the infection continues to spread unchecked, mediastinitis will ensue. A virulent infection in the retropharyngeal space may spread through the prevertebral fascia into the underlying prevertebral space. Infection in this tissue space may descend into the thorax and even below the diaphragm and results in chest pain, severe dyspnoea and retrosternal discomfort.

Pharyngeal infection from mucosally associated lymph tissues such as the palatine tonsil, or as a result of a penetrating injury (e.g. from an ingested foreign body), may result in the spread of infection into the tissue spaces of the neck adjacent to the pharynx. This is an extremely dangerous situation since there is potential for rapid spread throughout the neck and, more dangerously, to the superior mediastinum to cause overwhelming life-threatening infection.

PARAPHARYNGEAL SPACE TUMOURS

Tumours may develop a priori in the parapharyngeal tissue space and remain asymptomatic for some time. When they do present it may be with a diffuse pattern of symptoms, which are often the result of effects of compression on the lower cranial nerves, e.g. dysarthria, resulting from impairment of tongue movements secondary to hypoglossal nerve damage; dysphagia, with overspill and aspiration of ingested material into the airway, resulting from loss of sensory information from the distribution of the pharyngeal plexus nerves, the vagus and cranial accessory; motor dysfunction of the pharynx and larynx resulting from loss of motor innervation via the pharyngeal plexus, and the recurrent laryngeal branch of the vagus to the intrinsic muscles of the larynx.

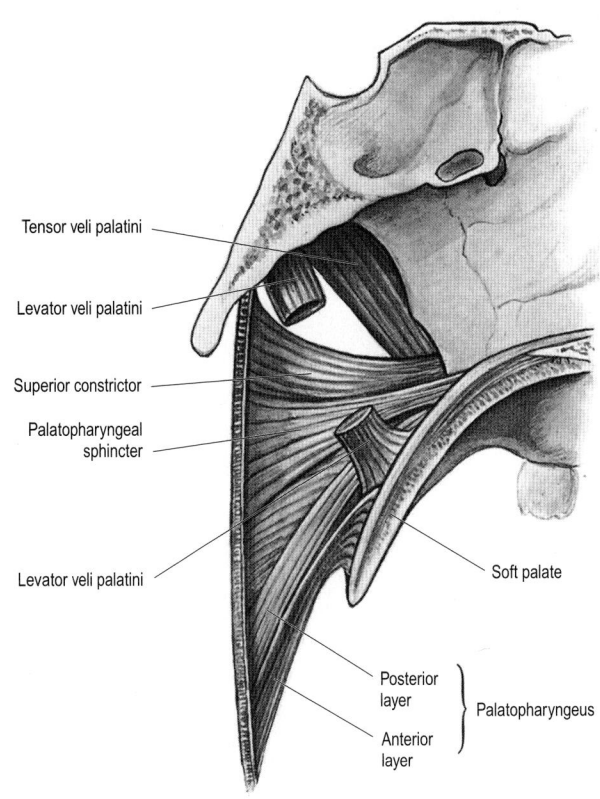

Fig. 35.9 Muscles of the left half of the soft palate and adjoining part of the pharyngeal wall in sagittal section. Part of levator veli palatini is cut sagittally. (Based on a dissection by the late James Whillis, Department of Anatomy, GKT School of Medicine, London.)

MUSCLES OF SOFT PALATE AND PHARYNX

The muscles of the palate and pharynx are levator veli palatini, tensor veli palatini, palatoglossus, palatopharyngeus, musculus uvulae, the superior, middle, and inferior constrictors, salpingopharyngeus and stylopharyngeus. With the exception of tensor veli palatini, which is supplied by the motor branch of the mandibular division of the trigeminal through the nerve to medial pterygoid, and stylopharyngeus, which is supplied by the glossopharyngeal nerve, the muscles are supplied by the cranial part of the accessory nerve via the pharyngeal plexus.

LEVATOR VELI PALATINI (Fig. 35.3, 35.8, 35.9, 35.10)

Levator veli palatini arises by a small tendon from a rough area on the inferior surface of the petrous part of the temporal bone, in front of the lower opening of the carotid canal. Additional fibres arise from the inferior aspect of the cartilaginous part of the pharyngotympanic tube and from the vaginal process of the tympanic bone. At its origin the muscle is inferior rather than medial to the pharyngotympanic tube and only crosses medial to it at the level of the medial pterygoid plate. It passes medial to the upper margin of the superior constrictor and in front of salpingopharyngeus. Its fibres spread in the medial third of the soft palate between the two strands of palatopharyngeus to attach to the upper surface of the palatine aponeurosis as far as the midline, where they interlace with those of the contralateral muscle. Thus the two levator muscles form a sling above and just behind the palatine aponeurosis.

Vascular supply – The blood supply of levator veli palatini is derived from the ascending palatine branch of the facial artery and the greater palatine branch of the maxillary artery.

Innervation – Levator veli palatini is innervated from the cranial part of the accessory nerve via the pharyngeal plexus.

Actions – The primary role of the levator veli palatini muscles is to elevate the almost vertical posterior part of the soft palate and pull it

slightly backwards. During swallowing, the soft palate is at the same time made rigid by the contraction of the tensor veli palatini muscles and touches the posterior wall of the pharynx, thus separating the naso-pharynx from the oropharynx. By additionally pulling on the lateral walls of the nasopharynx posteriorly and medially, the muscles also narrow that space. Levator veli palatini has little or no effect on the pharyngotympanic tube, although it might allow passive opening.

TENSOR VELI PALATINI (Figs 33.6, 35.8, 35.10)

Tensor veli palatini arises from the scaphoid fossa of the pterygoid process and posteriorly from the medial aspect of the spine of the sphenoid bone. Between these two sites it is attached to the antero-lateral membranous wall of the pharyngotympanic tube (including its narrow isthmus where the cartilaginous medial two-thirds meets the bony lateral one-third). Some fibres may be continuous with those of tensor tympani. Inferiorly, the fibres converge on a delicate tendon that turns medially around the pterygoid hamulus to pass through the attachment of buccinator to the palatine aponeurosis and the osseous surface behind the palatine crest on the horizontal plate of the palatine bone. There is a small bursa between the tendon and the pterygoid hamulus.

The muscle is thin and triangular and lies lateral to the medial pterygoid plate, pharyngotympanic tube and levator veli palatini. Its lateral surface contacts the upper and anterior part of medial pterygoid, the mandibular, auriculotemporal and chorda tympani nerves, the otic ganglion and the middle meningeal artery.

Vascular supply – The blood supply of tensor veli palatini is derived from the ascending palatine branch of the facial artery and the greater palatine branch of the maxillary artery.

Innervation – The motor innervation of tensor veli palatini is derived from the mandibular nerve via the nerve to medial pterygoid, and reflects the development of the muscle from the first branchial arch.

Actions – Acting together the tensor veli palatini muscles tauten the soft palate, principally its anterior part, and depress it by flattening its arch.

627

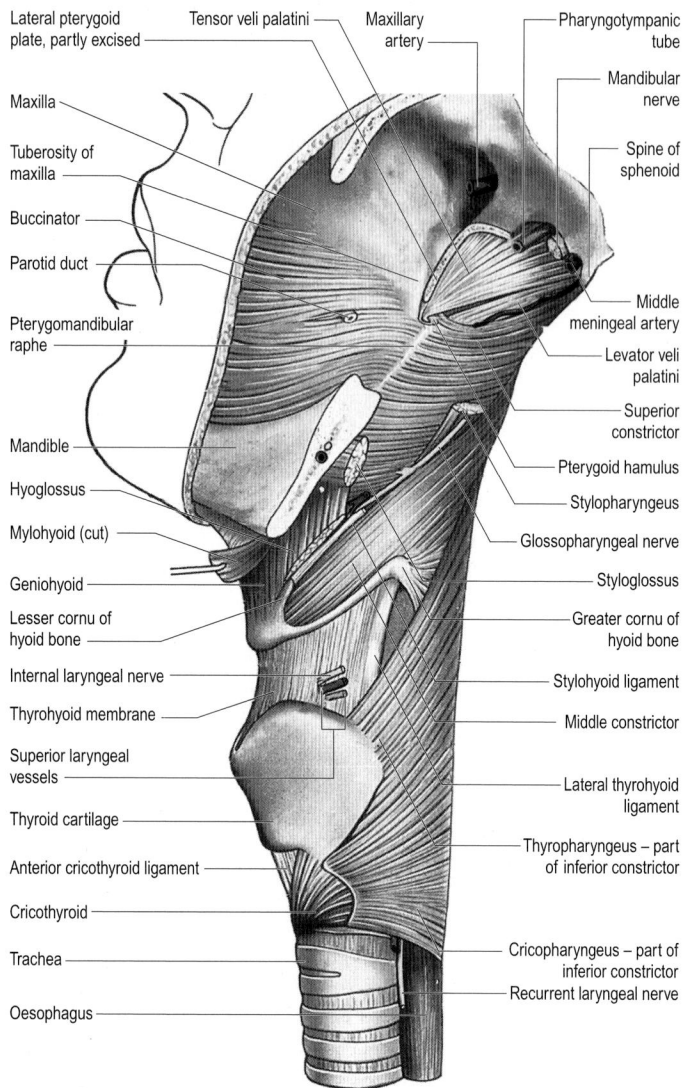

Lateral pterygoid plate, partly excised
Tensor veli palatini
Maxillary artery
Pharyngotympanic tube
Maxilla
Mandibular nerve
Tuberosity of maxilla
Spine of sphenoid
Buccinator
Parotid duct
Middle meningeal artery
Pterygomandibular raphe
Levator veli palatini
Superior constrictor
Mandible
Pterygoid hamulus
Hyoglossus
Stylopharyngeus
Mylohyoid (cut)
Glossopharyngeal nerve
Geniohyoid
Styloglossus
Lesser cornu of hyoid bone
Greater cornu of hyoid bone
Internal laryngeal nerve
Stylohyoid ligament
Thyrohyoid membrane
Middle constrictor
Superior laryngeal vessels
Thyroid cartilage
Lateral thyrohyoid ligament
Anterior cricothyroid ligament
Thyropharyngeus – part of inferior constrictor
Cricothyroid
Trachea
Cricopharyngeus – part of inferior constrictor
Oesophagus
Recurrent laryngeal nerve

Fig. 35.10 Muscles of the pharynx.

Acting unilaterally, the muscle pulls the soft palate to one side. Although contraction of both muscles will slightly depress the anterior part of the soft palate, it is often assumed that the increased rigidity aids palato-pharyngeal closure. However, it is now believed that a primary role of the tensor is to open the pharyngotympanic tube, for example during deglutition and yawning. In this way the muscle equalizes air pressure between the middle ear and nasopharynx.

MUSCULUS UVULAE (Fig. 35.2)

Musculus uvulae arises from the posterior nasal spine of the palatine bone and the superior surface of the palatine aponeurosis, and lies between the two laminae of the aponeurosis. It runs posteriorly above the sling formed by levator veli palatini and inserts beneath the mucosa of the uvula. The two sides of the muscle are united along most of its length.

Vascular supply – The blood supply of musculus uvulae is derived from the ascending palatine branch of the facial artery and the descending palatine branch of the maxillary artery.

Innervation – The nerve supply to musculus uvulae is derived from the cranial part of the accessory nerve via the pharyngeal plexus.

Actions – By retracting the uvular mass and thickening the middle third of the soft palate, musculus uvulae aids levator veli palatini in palato-pharyngeal closure. The two muscles run at right angles to each other and their contraction raises a 'levator eminence' which helps seals off the nasopharynx.

PALATOGLOSSUS (Fig. 35.3)

Palatoglossus is narrower at its middle than at its ends. Together with its overlying mucosa it forms the palatoglossal arch or fold (see **Fig. 33.2**). It arises from the oral surface of the palatine aponeurosis where it is continuous with its fellow. It extends forwards, downwards and laterally in front of the palatine tonsil to the side of the tongue. Some of its fibres spread over the dorsum of the tongue, others pass deeply into its substance to intermingle with fibres of the intrinsic transverse muscle.

Vascular supply – Palatoglossus receives its blood supply from the ascending palatine branch of the facial artery and from the ascending pharyngeal artery.

Innervation – Palatoglossus is supplied by the cranial part of the accessory nerve via the pharyngeal plexus, and is therefore unlike all the other muscles of the tongue, which are supplied by the hypoglossal nerve.

Actions – Palatoglossus elevates the root of the tongue and approxi-mates the palatoglossal arch to its contralateral fellow, thus shutting off the oral cavity from the oropharynx.

PALATOPHARYNGEUS (Figs 35.3, 35.9)

Palatopharyngeus and its overlying mucosa form the palatopharyngeal arch (see **Fig. 33.2**). Within the soft palate palatopharyngeus is com-posed of two fasciculi which are attached to the upper surface of the palatine aponeurosis; they lie in the same plane but are separated from each other by levator veli palatini. The thicker anterior fasciculus arises from the posterior border of the hard palate as well as the palatine aponeurosis, where some fibres interdigitate across the midline. The posterior fasciculus is in contact with the mucosa of the pharyngeal aspect of the palate, and joins the posterior band of the contralateral muscle in the midline. The two layers unite at the posterolateral border of the soft palate, and are joined by fibres of salpingopharyngeus. Passing laterally and downwards behind the tonsil, palatopharyngeus descends posteromedial to and in close contact with stylopharyngeus, to be attached with it to the posterior border of the thyroid cartilage. Some fibres end on the side of the pharynx, attached to pharyngeal fibrous tissue and others cross the midline posteriorly, decussating with those of the contralateral muscle. Palatopharyngeus thus forms an incomplete internal longitudinal muscular layer in the wall of the pharynx.

Passavant's muscle (palatopharyngeal sphincter) – The existence of Passavant's muscle remains controversial. It has been described as a part of the superior constrictor and palatopharyngeus muscles. An alter-native view holds that it is a distinct palatine muscle that arises from the anterior and lateral parts of the upper surface of the palatine aponeurosis, lies lateral to levator veli palatini, blends internally with the upper border of the superior constrictor and encircles the pharynx as a sphincter-like muscle (**Fig. 35.9**). Whatever its origin, when it contracts, it forms a ridge (Passavant's ridge) when the soft palate is elevated. The change from columnar, ciliated, 'respiratory' epithelium to stratified, squamous epithelium that takes place on the superior aspect of the soft palate occurs along the line of attachment of the palatopharyngeal sphincter to the palate. The muscle is hypertrophied in cases of complete cleft palate.

Vascular supply – Palatopharyngeus receives its arterial supply from the ascending palatine branch of the facial artery, the greater palatine branch of the maxillary artery and the pharyngeal branch of the ascending pharyngeal artery.

Innervation – Palatopharyngeus is innervated by the cranial part of the accessory nerve via the pharyngeal plexus.

Actions – Acting together, the palatopharyngei pull the pharynx up, forwards and medially, and thus shorten it during swallowing. They also approximate the palatopharyngeal arches and draw them forwards.

SUPERIOR CONSTRICTOR (Figs 33.6, 35.6, 35.8, 35.9, 35.10)

The superior constrictor is a quadrilateral sheet of muscle and is thinner than the other two constrictors. It is attached anteriorly to the pterygoid hamulus (and sometimes to the adjoining posterior margin of the medial pterygoid plate), the posterior border of the pterygomandibular raphe, the posterior end of the mylohyoid line of the mandible, and, by a few fibres, to the side of the tongue. The fibres curve back into a median pharyngeal raphe which is attached superiorly to the pharyngeal tubercle on the basilar part of the occipital bone

Relations – The upper border of the superior constrictor is separated from the cranial base by a crescentic interval which contains levator veli palatini, the pharyngotympanic tube and an upward projection of pharyngobasilar fascia. The lower border is separated from the middle constrictor by stylopharyngeus and the glossopharyngeal nerve (**Fig. 35.10**). Anteriorly the pterygomandibular raphe separates the superior constrictor from buccinator, and posteriorly the superior constrictor lies on the prevertebral muscles and fascia, from which it is separated by the retropharyngeal space. The ascending pharyngeal artery, pharyngeal venous plexus, glossopharyngeal and lingual nerves, styloglossus, middle constrictor, medial pterygoid, stylopharyngeus, and the stylohyoid ligament all lie laterally, and palatopharyngeus, the tonsillar capsule and the pharyngobasilar fascia lie internally.

Vascular supply – The arterial supply of the superior constrictor is derived mainly from the pharyngeal branch of the ascending pharyngeal artery and the tonsillar branch of the facial artery.

Innervation – The superior constrictor is innervated by the cranial part of the accessory nerve from the pharyngeal plexus.

Actions – The superior constrictor constricts the upper part of the pharynx.

MIDDLE CONSTRICTOR (Figs 33.6, 35.3, 35.8, 35.10)
The middle constrictor is a fan-shaped sheet attached anteriorly to the lesser cornu of the hyoid and the lower part of the stylohyoid ligament (the chondropharyngeal part of the muscle), and to the whole of the upper border of the greater cornu of the hyoid (the ceratopharyngeal part). The lower fibres descend deep to the inferior constrictor to reach the lower end of the pharynx, the middle fibres pass transversely and the superior fibres ascend and overlap the superior constrictor. All fibres insert posteriorly into the median pharyngeal raphe.

Relations – The glossopharyngeal nerve and stylopharyngeus pass through a small gap between the middle and superior constrictors, and the internal laryngeal nerve and the laryngeal branch of the superior thyroid artery pass between the middle and inferior constrictors. The prevertebral fascia and longus colli and longus capitis are posterior, the superior constrictor, stylopharyngeus and palatopharyngeus are internal, and the carotid vessels, pharyngeal plexus of nerves and some lymph nodes are lateral. Near its hyoid attachment, the middle constrictor lies deep to hyoglossus, from which it is separated by the lingual artery.

Vascular supply – The arterial supply of the middle constrictor is derived mainly from the pharyngeal branch of the ascending pharyngeal artery and the tonsillar branch of the facial artery.

Innervation – The middle constrictor is innervated by the cranial part of the accessory nerve from the pharyngeal plexus.

Actions – The middle constrictor constricts the middle part of the pharynx during swallowing.

INFERIOR CONSTRICTOR (Figs 33.6, 35.3, 35.8, 35.10)
The inferior constrictor is the thickest of the three constrictor muscles, and is usually described in two parts, cricopharyngeus and thyropharyngeus. Cricopharyngeus arises from the side of the cricoid cartilage between the attachment of cricothyroid and the articular facet for the inferior thyroid cornu. Thyropharyngeus arises from the oblique line of the thyroid lamina, a strip of the lamina behind this, and by a small slip from the inferior cornu. Some additional fibres arise from a tendinous cord that loops over cricothyroid. Both cricopharyngeus and thyropharyngeus spread posteromedially to join the contralateral muscle. Thyropharyngeus is inserted into the median pharyngeal raphe and its upper fibres ascend obliquely to overlap the middle constrictor, how-

ever cricopharyngeus blends with the circular oesophageal fibres around the narrowest part of the pharynx.

Relations – The buccopharyngeal fascia is external, the prevertebral fascia and muscles are posterior, the thyroid gland, common carotid artery and sternothyroid are lateral, and the middle constrictor, stylopharyngeus, palatopharyngeus and the fibrous lamina are internal. The internal laryngeal nerve and laryngeal branch of the superior thyroid artery reach the thyrohyoid membrane by passing between the inferior and middle constrictors. The external laryngeal nerve descends on the superficial surface of the muscle, just behind its thyroid attachment, and pierces its lower part. The recurrent laryngeal nerve and the laryngeal branch of the inferior thyroid artery ascend deep to its lower border to enter the larynx.

Vascular supply – The arterial supply of the inferior constrictor is derived mainly from the pharyngeal branch of the ascending pharyngeal artery and the muscular branches of the inferior thyroid artery.

Innervation – Both parts of the inferior constrictor are supplied by the cranial part of the accessory nerve from the pharyngeal plexus. Cricopharyngeus is also supplied by the recurrent laryngeal nerve and the external branch of the superior laryngeal nerve.

Actions – Thyropharyngeus constricts the lower part of the pharynx. Cricopharyngeus acts as a sphincter at the junction of the laryngopharynx and the oesophagus.

Hypopharyngeal diverticula (Fig. 35.11)
The pharyngeal mucosa that lies between cricopharyngeus and thyropharyngeus is relatively unsupported by pharyngeal muscles and is called the dehiscence of Killian. A delay in the relaxation of cricopharyngeus, which can occur when the swallowing mechanism becomes discoordinated, generates a zone of elevated pressure adjacent to the mucosa in the dehiscence. The result is the development of a pulsion diverticulum (a pouch of prolapsing mucosa), which breaches the thin muscle wall adjacent to the sixth cervical vertebra and expands, usually a little to the left side, into the parapharyngeal potential space. This may trap portions (or all) of the passing food bolus, resulting in regurgitation of old food, aspiration pneumonia, halitosis and weight loss. Treatment may involve open excision or inversion of the pouch to prevent it filling, coupled with division of the circular fibres of cricopharyngeus, to prevent the build-up of pressure in the region and recurrence of the pouch.

SALPINGOPHARYNGEUS (Fig. 35.3)
Salpingopharyngeus arises from the inferior part of the cartilage of the pharyngotympanic tube near its pharyngeal opening and passes downwards within the salpingopharyngeal fold to blend with palatopharyngeus.

Vascular supply – Salpingopharyngeus receives its arterial supply from the ascending palatine branch of the facial artery, the greater palatine branch of the maxillary artery and the pharyngeal branch of the ascending pharyngeal artery.

Innervation – Salpinopharyngeus is innervated through the cranial part of the accessory nerve from the pharyngeal plexus.

Actions – Salpingopharyngeus elevates the pharynx, and may also assist tensor veli palatini to open the cartilaginous end of the pharyngotympanic tube during swallowing.

STYLOPHARYNGEUS (Figs 33.6, 35.3, 35.8)
Stylopharyngeus is a long slender muscle, cylindrical above and flat below. It arises from the medial side of the base of the styloid process, descends along the side of the pharynx and passes between the superior and middle constrictors to spread out beneath the mucous membrane. Some fibres merge into the constrictors and the lateral glossoepiglottic fold, while others join fibres of palatopharyngeus and are attached to the posterior border of the thyroid cartilage. The glossopharyngeal nerve curves round the posterior border and the lateral side of stylopharyngeus, and passes between the superior and middle constrictors to reach the tongue.

A

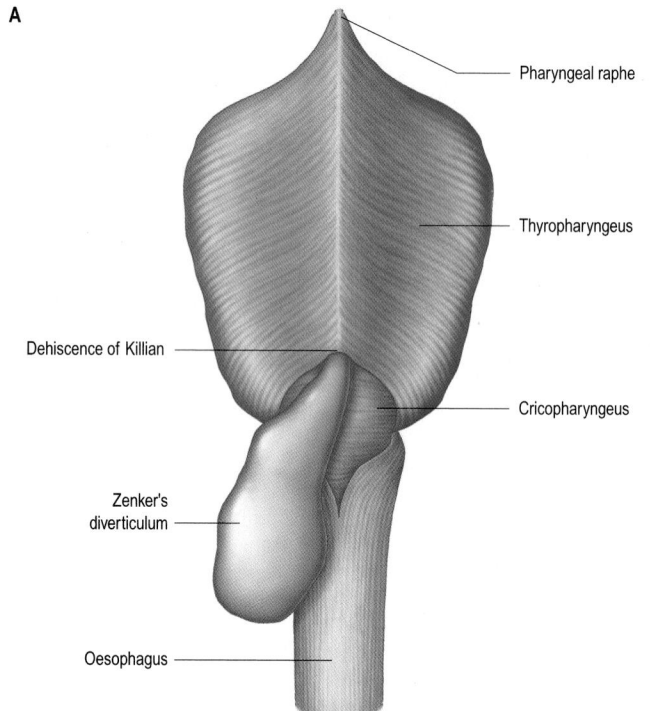

Pharyngeal raphe

Thyropharyngeus

Dehiscence of Killian

Cricopharyngeus

Zenker's
diverticulum

Oesophagus

B

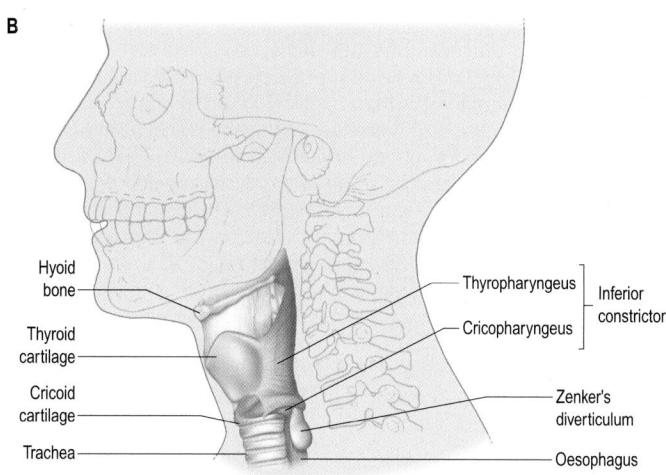

Hyoid
bone

Thyropharyngeus ⎤
Cricopharyngeus ⎦ Inferior constrictor

Thyroid
cartilage

Cricoid
cartilage

Zenker's
diverticulum

Trachea

Oesophagus

Fig. 35.11 Hypopharyngeal diverticulae. Posterior (**A**) and lateral (**B**) views showing Zenker's diverticulum arising from the dehiscence of Killian between cricopharyngeus and thyropharyngeus.

Vascular supply – Stylopharyngeus receives its arterial supply from the pharyngeal branch of the ascending pharyngeal artery.

Innervation – Stylopharyngeus is innervated by the glossopharyngeal nerve.

Actions – Stylopharyngeus elevates the pharynx and larynx.

PHARYNGEAL PLEXUS

Almost all of the nerve supply to the pharynx, whether motor or sensory, is derived from the pharyngeal plexus which lies on the external surface of the pharynx, especially on the middle constrictor. The plexus is formed by the pharyngeal branches of the glossopharyngeal and vagus nerves with contributions from the superior cervical sympathetic ganglion. Mixed nerves leave the plexus and ascend or descend external to the superior and inferior constrictors before branching within the muscular layer and mucosa.

The muscles of the pharynx – with the exception of stylopharyngeus, which is supplied by the glossopharyngeal nerve – are supplied from

the pharyngeal plexus by the pharyngeal branch of the vagus. This branch emerges from the upper part of the inferior vagal ganglion and consists chiefly of filaments from the cranial accessory nerve. It passes between the external and internal carotid arteries to reach the upper border of the middle pharyngeal constrictor. It gives off a minute filament, the ramus lingualis vagi, which joins the hypoglossal nerve as it curves round the occipital artery. The inferior constrictor also receives contributions from the external and recurrent laryngeal nerves.

ANATOMY OF SWALLOWING (DEGLUTITION)

Swallowing is initiated reflexly when food or liquid stimulates sensory nerves in the oropharynx. In man, c.600 swallows are reputed to occur in each 24-hour period, but of these, only some 150 relate to feeding. The remaining swallows, which occur less frequently at night, are unconscious 'empty' swallows that appear to relate primarily to the clearance of saliva from the mouth. However, swallowing in the adult human has traditionally been studied in relation to food swallowing (solid or liquid) carried out on command. Such swallows have been divided into three phases, usually described as the first or oral, the second or pharyngeal and the third or oesophageal, phases. Over the years, the exact dividing line between the first and second phases has changed slightly, and is defined primarily by convention.

ORAL PHASE

The oral phase is traditionally described as a voluntary action in which a bolus of food is moved from the oral cavity up to or through the fauces. Transport of the bolus through the mouth is accomplished by first forming a shallow midline gutter along the tongue to accommodate the bolus, and then by elevating the tongue and the floor of that midline gutter from before backwards. The gutter is probably formed by the co-contraction of the styloglossi and the genioglossi. At this stage a posterior oral seal exists which is associated with elevation of the posterior tongue. Emptying of the longitudinal gutter may involve contraction of hyoglossus and some intrinsic lingual muscles but there is a simultaneous elevation of the anterior and mid tongue, the hyoid bone and the floor of the mouth, which is produced by co-contraction of muscles such as mylohyoid, geniohyoid and stylohyoid. Elevation is accompanied by a relaxation of the posterior oral seal and a forward movement of the posterior tongue which is followed by bilateral contraction of the palatoglossi. The overall effect is of a cam-like action of the tongue which sweeps or squeezes the bolus towards the fauces where the pharyngeal aperture is initially increased and then closed.

PHARYNGEAL PHASE

The pharyngeal stage is considered to be reflex and involves the pharynx changing from being an air channel (between the posterior nares and laryngeal inlet) to being a food channel (from the fauces to the upper end of the oesophagus). This complex action requires a brief cessation of respiratory movements and closure of the airway at two levels. At the upper level, a seal is produced by activation of the superior pharyngeal constrictor and contraction of a subset of palatopharyngeal fibres forming a variable, ridge-like, structure (Passavant's ridge) to which the soft palate is elevated. From an evolutionary perspective, the ridge represents the remnant of a sphincter which formed around a larynx which was situated higher in the neck: a high laryngeal position, by comparison with the human adult, is the norm in other mammals and in the human infant. Interestingly, the pharyngeal ridge becomes hypertrophic in an infant with a cleft palate, presumably in an attempt to produce a seal to the nasal airway. At the lower level, in the normal adult, the seal of the airway at the laryngeal inlet is produced by closure of the glottis. The inlet is further protected by raising and tipping the laryngeal inlet forward under the bulge of the posterior tongue and by the flexing of the epiglottis over the laryngeal inlet as the bolus passes over it.

In this second stage, the three pharyngeal constrictor muscles undergo a sequential contraction which is usually interpreted as the driving force which propels the bolus towards the oesophagus. However, recent evidence that the head of the bolus moves faster than the wave of pharyngeal contraction suggests that, at least in some situations, the kinetic energy imparted to the bolus as it is expelled from the mouth into the pharynx may be sufficient to carry it through the pharynx. The function of sequential contraction of the pharyngeal constrictor muscles may then be to facilitate subsequent pharyngeal clearance.

OESOPHAGEAL PHASE

The third or oesophageal stage involves the relaxation of cricopharyngeus (the upper oesophageal sphincter) to allow the bolus to enter the oesophagus. Once in the oesophagus, the bolus is propelled by sequential waves of contractions of the oesophageal musculature down to the lower oesophageal sphincter, which opens momentarily to allow the bolus to enter the stomach.

CENTRAL PATTERN GENERATION

The patterning and timing of striated muscle contraction in the first, second and in the early part of the third, stages of swallowing are generated at a brain stem level in a network of neural circuits which form a central pattern generator (CPG). In contrast, the patterns of activation in the smooth muscle of the lower part of the oesophagus are generated locally in intramural plexi driven by vagal autonomics.

The CPG is activated by nerve impulses travelling via descending pathways from the motor cortex, and ascending pathways from peripheral sensory nerves, particularly the superior laryngeal nerve, which innervates the valleculae, epiglottis and part of the larynx. Within the CPG, the nucleus of the tractus solitarius receives the descending and peripheral afferent influences. Motor neurones collectively innervate pharyngeal striated muscle and bilaterally represent the outflow from the CPG.

SWALLOWING IN THE NEONATE (Fig. 35.12)

The functional and anatomical differences between the human neonate and the adult suggest that the classical description of the divisions of a swallow should not be applied uncritically to all aspects of swallowing in the human infant. In the adult, the tip of the epiglottis is significantly lower than the inferior edge of the soft palate. In the neonate, the epiglottis may extend above the soft palate so that the laryngeal airway is in direct continuity with the posterior nares, and a potential space is formed between the soft palate above, the epiglottis behind and the tongue anteroinferiorly. In other mammals with an oropharyngeal anatomy similar to that of the human infant, up to 14 cycles of tongue movement or oral phases cause the accumulation of food in this space. Subsequent emptying of the space is a single event followed by movement of the bolus down the oesophagus. The ratio of accumulation cycles to swallow events in the human neonate is c.1.5:1, which is lower than in other mammals, but still implies some temporary accumulation. In the case of a liquid bolus, accumulated material may be passed laterally to the epiglottis through the piriform fossae rather than over the flexed epiglottis, although it is not known whether this happens in the human infant.

The change towards the adult anatomy and co-ordination of the phases of swallowing starts a few months after birth. Differential growth in length of the human pharynx causes the larynx to take up its low adult position and the epiglottis to lose contact with the soft palate. The adult anatomy does not allow any significant accumulation of food to

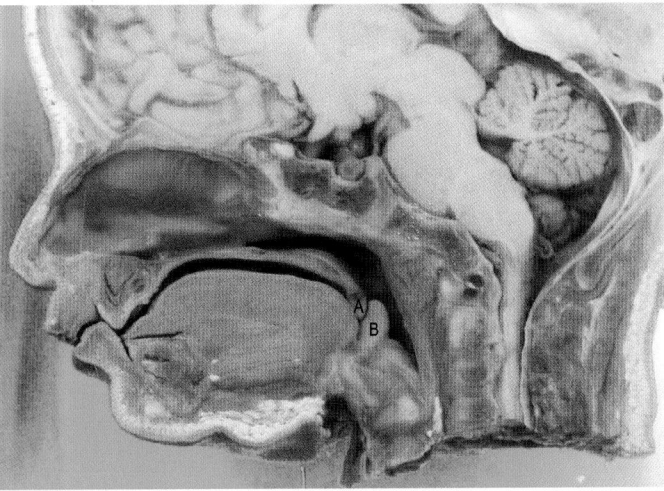

Fig. 35.12 Sagittal section of the head of a neonate. Note the relatively high position of the larynx, the opening being at the level of the soft palate (A). B, epiglottis. (By permission from Berkovitz BKB, Holland GR, Moxham BJ 2002 Oral Anatomy, Embryology and Histology, 3rd edn. Edinburgh: Mosby.)

occur immediately anterior to the epiglottis so that the transport of food through the fauces has to bear a 1:1 relationship to pharyngeal and oesophageal transit.

PHARYNGOSTOMY AND EPIGLOTTOPEXY

Loss of control of the pharyngeal phase of swallowing, e.g. due to neurological disease or ablative head and neck surgery, may result in aspiration of food, especially fluids, leading to pneumonia. This problem may be addressed surgically by pharyngostomy or epiglottopexy. In pharyngostomy, a fine bore feeding tube is passed into the lower oesophagus or stomach via the nose or anterior abdominal wall. Alternatively, a tube may be passed through the cervical skin, fascia and platysma directly into the piriform fossa. This is achieved by passing a curved forcep into the piriform fossa and pushing it laterally, displacing the contents of the carotid sheath and tenting up the platysma and cervical skin from the inside. By cutting down on to the forcep it is possible to grasp the feeding tube and pull it into the piriform fossa prior to feeding it on into the oesophagus. The tract formed by such a puncture epithelializes and may be used for long term alimentation. In epiglottopexy, the neck and the pharynx are opened to expose the laryngeal inlet, the aryepiglottic folds are denuded of mucosa to encourage their adhesion, and the epiglottis is sutured down to the aryepiglottic folds to shield the laryngeal inlet. The resultant compromise of the airway can be offset by the creation of an alternative airway via a tracheostomy. The pharyngeal wall and cervical skin are reconstituted by suturing.

REFERENCES

Bluestone CD 1998 Anatomy and physiology of the Eustachian tube. In: Cummings CW et al (eds) Otolaryngology Head and Neck Surgery. 3rd edition. St Louis: Mosby: 3003–25.

Freelander E 1992 Blood supply of the human levator and tensor veli palatini muscles. Clin Anat 5: 34–44.

Graney DO, Retruzzelli GJ, Myers EW 1998 Anatomy. In: Cummings CW et al (eds) Otolaryngology Head and Neck Surgery. 3rd edition. St Louis: Mosby: 1327–48.
Provides a concise account of the anatomy of the pharynx, highlighting features of clinical relevance.

Sade J (ed) 1989 Basic Aspects of the Eustachian Tube and Middle Ear Disease. Geneva: Kugler and Ghedini.

Thexton A 1998 Some aspects of swallowing. In: Harris M, Edgar M, Meghji S (eds) Clinical Oral Science. Oxford: Wright: 150–66.

Thexton AJ, Crompton AW 1998 The control of swallowing. In: Linden RWA (ed) The Scientific Basis of Eating. Taste and Smell, Salivation, Mastication and Swallowing and their Dysfunctions. Frontiers of Oral Biology Series, vol 9. Basel: Karger: 168–222.

Wood-Jones I 1940 The nature of the soft palate. J Anat 77: 147–70.
Describes the structure of the soft palate and its movements during swallowing.

Larynx

The larynx is an air passage, a sphincter and an organ of phonation. It extends from the tongue to the trachea. It projects ventrally between the great vessels of the neck and is covered anteriorly by skin, fasciae and the hyoid depressor muscles (**Fig. 31.21**) Above, it opens into the laryngopharynx and forms its anterior wall while below it continues into the trachea (**Figs 35.1, 35.2**). It is mobile on deglutition. At rest it lies opposite the third to sixth cervical vertebrae in adult males, although it is somewhat higher in children and adult females. In infants between 6 and 12 months, the tip of the epiglottis (the highest part of the larynx) is a little above the junction of the dens and body of the axis vertebra. Until puberty the male and female larynges are similar in size. After puberty, the male larynx enlarges considerably in comparison with that of the female: all the cartilages increase in size, the thyroid cartilage projects in the anterior midline of the neck, and its sagittal diameter nearly doubles. The male thyroid cartilage continues to increase in size until 40 years of age, after which no further growth occurs. The average measurements of the larynx in European adults are:

	In males	In females
Length	44 mm	36 mm
Transverse diameter	43 mm	41 mm
Sagittal diameter	36 mm	26 mm

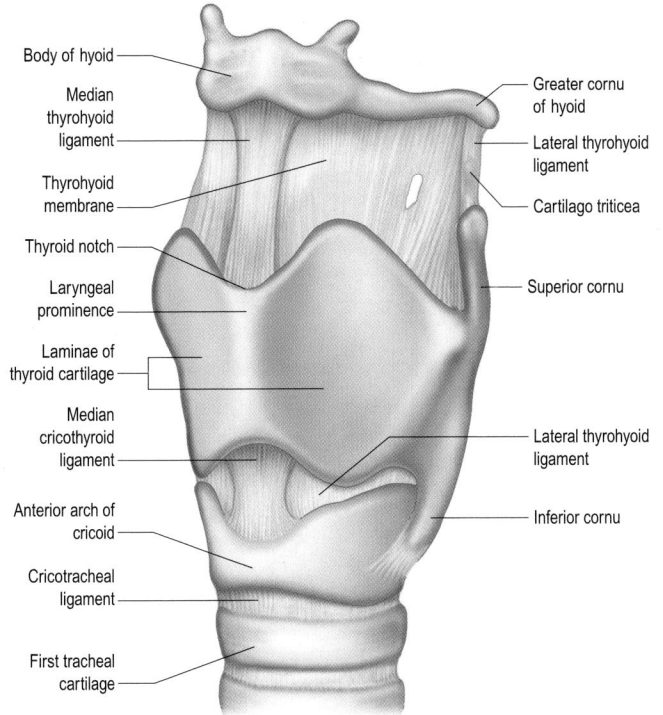

Fig. 36.1 Anterolateral view of the laryngeal cartilages and ligaments.

SKELETON OF THE LARYNX (Figs 36.1, 36.2, 36.3, 36.4)

The skeletal framework of the larynx is formed by a series of cartilages interconnected by ligaments and fibrous membranes, and moved by a number of muscles. The hyoid bone is attached to the larynx: it is usually regarded as a separate structure with distinctive functional roles, and is described on page 541. The laryngeal cartilages are the single cricoid, thyroid and epiglottic cartilages, and the paired arytenoid, cuneiform, corniculate and tritiate cartilages.

In relation to the surface anatomy of the larynx, the levels of the laryngeal cartilages worth noting are: C3 (level of body of hyoid and its greater cornu); C3–4 junction (level of upper border of thyroid cartilage and bifurcation of common carotid artery); C4–5 junction (level of thyroid cartilage); C6 (level of cricoid cartilage).

The corniculate, cuneiform, tritiate and epiglottic cartilages and the apices of the arytenoid are composed of elastic fibrocartilage, with little tendency to calcify. The thyroid, cricoid and the greater part of the arytenoid cartilages consist of hyaline cartilage and may undergo mottled calcification as age advances, commencing about the twenty-fifth year in the thyroid cartilage and somewhat later in the cricoid and arytenoids. By the sixty-fifth year these cartilages commonly appear patchily dense in radiographs.

EPIGLOTTIS (Figs 36.3, 36.4, 36.5)
The epiglottis is a thin leaf-like plate of elastic fibrocartilage, which projects obliquely upwards behind the tongue and hyoid body, and in front of the laryngeal inlet. Its free end, which is broad and round, and occasionally notched in the midline, is directed upwards. Its attached part, or stalk (petiolus), is long and narrow and is connected by the elastic thyroepiglottic ligament to the back of the laryngeal prominence of the thyroid cartilage just below the thyroid notch (**Fig. 36.5**). Its sides are attached to the arytenoid cartilages by aryepiglottic folds (which contain the aryepiglottic muscle). Its free upper anterior surface is covered

by mucosa (the epithelium is non-keratinized stratified squamous), which is reflected onto the pharyngeal aspect of the tongue and the lateral pharyngeal walls as a median glossoepiglottic, and two lateral glossoepiglottic, folds. There is a depression, the vallecula, on each side of the median fold. The lower part of its anterior surface, behind the hyoid bone and thyrohyoid membrane, is connected to the upper border of the hyoid by an elastic hyoepiglottic ligament (**Fig. 36.5**), and separated from the thyrohyoid membrane by adipose tissue, which constitutes the clinically important pre-epiglottic space. The smooth posterior surface is transversely concave and vertically concavo-convex, and is covered by ciliated respiratory mucosa: its lower projecting part is called the tubercle. The cartilage is posteriorly pitted by small mucous glands (**Fig. 36.4**). It is perforated by branches of the internal laryngeal nerve and fibrous tissue, which means that the posterior, i.e. laryngeal, surface of the epiglottis is in continuity through these perforations with the pre-epiglottic space.

Functions of the epiglottis (See also p. 630.)
During deglutition the hyoid bone moves upwards and forwards, and the epiglottis is bent posteriorly as a result of pressure from the base of the tongue and contraction of the aryepiglottic muscles. The food bolus slips over its anterior surface as it bends back over the laryngeal inlet. The bolus then splits to pass into the piriform fossae, which constitute the lateral food passages. The epiglottis is not essential to swallowing, which occurs with minimal aspiration even if the epiglottis is destroyed by disease, nor is it essential for respiration or phonation.

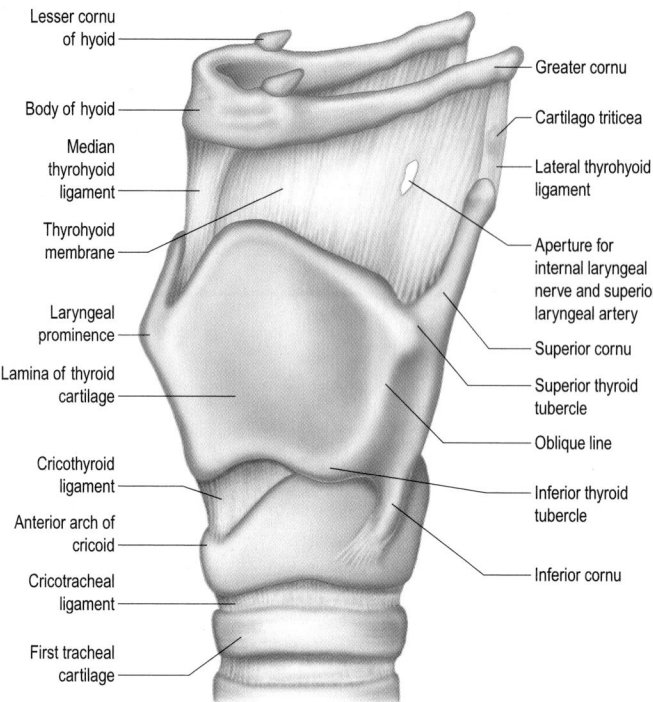

Fig. 36.2 Lateral view of the laryngeal cartilages and ligaments.

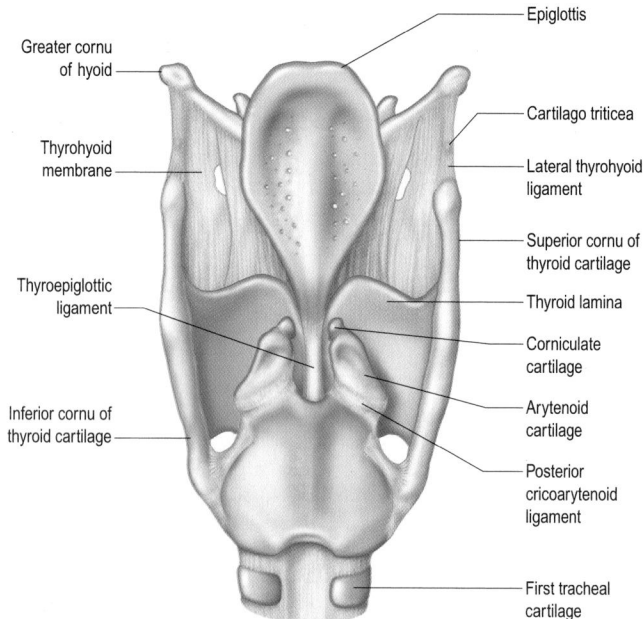

Fig. 36.3 Posterior view of the laryngeal cartilages and ligaments.

THYROID CARTILAGE (Figs 36.1, 36.2, 36.3, 36.4)

The thyroid cartilage is the largest of the laryngeal cartilages. It consists of two quadrilateral laminae whose anterior borders fuse along their inferior two-thirds at a median angle, forming the subcutaneous laryngeal prominence ('Adam's apple'). This projection is most distinct at its upper end, and is well marked in men but scarcely visible in women. Above, the laminae are separated by a V-shaped superior thyroid notch or incisure. Posteriorly the laminae diverge, and their posterior borders are prolonged as slender horns, the superior and inferior cornua. A shallow ridge, the oblique line, curves downwards and forwards on the external surface of each lamina: it runs from the superior thyroid tubercle lying a little anterior to the root of the superior cornu, to the inferior thyroid tubercle on the inferior border of the lamina. Sterno-

thyroid, thyrohyoid, and thyropharyngeus (part of the inferior pharyngeal constrictor) are attached to this line (**Fig. 36.6**).

The internal surface of the lamina is smooth. Above and behind, it is slightly concave and covered by mucosa. The thyroepiglottic ligament, the paired vestibular and vocal ligaments, and the thyroarytenoid, thyroepiglottic and vocalis muscles are all attached to the inner surface of the cartilage, in the angle between the laminae. The superior border of each lamina is concave behind and convex in front, and the thyrohyoid membrane is attached along this edge (**Figs 36.1, 36.2, 36.3**). The inferior border of each lamina is concave behind and nearly straight in front, and the two parts are separated by the inferior thyroid tubercle (**Fig. 36.2**). Anteriorly, the thyroid cartilage is connected to the cricoid cartilage by the anterior (median) cricothyroid ligament, which is a thickened portion of the cricothyroid membrane.

The anterior border of each thyroid lamina fuses with its partner at an angle of c.90° in men and c.120° in women. The shallower angle in men is associated with the larger laryngeal prominence, the greater length of the vocal cords, and the resultant deeper pitch of the voice. The posterior border is thick and rounded and receives fibres of stylopharyngeus and palatopharyngeus. The superior cornu, which is long and narrow, curves upwards, backwards and medially, and ends in a conical apex to which the lateral thyrohyoid ligament is attached. The inferior cornu is short and thick, and curves down and slightly anteromedially. On the medial surface of its lower end there is a small oval facet for articulation with the side of the cricoid cartilage: it is usually only well-defined in c.20% of cases.

A narrow, rhomboidal, flexible strip, the intrathyroid cartilage, lies between the two laminae, and is joined to them by fibrous tissue, during infancy.

CRICOID CARTILAGE (Fig. 36.4)

The cricoid cartilage is attached below to the trachea, and articulates with the thyroid cartilage and the two arytenoid cartilages by synovial joints. It forms a complete ring around the airway, the only laryngeal cartilage to do so (**Fig. 36.4**). It is smaller, but thicker and stronger, than the thyroid cartilage, and has a narrow curved anterior arch, and a broad, flatter posterior lamina.

Cricoid arch

The cricoid arch is vertically narrow in front (5–7 mm in height), and widens posteriorly towards the lamina. Cricothyroid is attached to the external aspect of its front and sides, and cricopharyngeus (part of the inferior pharyngeal constrictor) is attached behind cricothyroid. The arch is palpable below the laryngeal prominence, from which it is separated by a depression containing the resilient cricovocal membrane.

Cricoid lamina

The cricoid lamina is approximately quadrilateral in outline, and 2–3 cm in vertical dimension. It bears a posterior median vertical ridge. The two fasciculi of the longitudinal layer of oesophageal muscle fibres (muscularis externa) are attached by a tendon to the upper part of the ridge. Posterior cricoarytenoid attaches to a shallow depression on either side of the ridge.

A discernible circular synovial facet, facing posterolaterally, sometimes marks the junction of the lamina and arch: it indicates the site where the cricoid articulates with the inferior thyroid cornu. The inferior border of the cricoid is horizontal, and joined to the first tracheal cartilage by the cricotracheal ligament (**Fig. 36.1**). The superior border runs obliquely up and back, and gives attachment anteriorly to the thick median part of the cricothyroid membrane, and laterally to the membranous parts of the cricothyroid membrane (**Fig. 36.1**) and lateral cricoarytenoid. The posterosuperior aspect of the lamina presents a shallow median notch, on each side of which is a smooth, oval, convex facet, directed upwards and laterally, for articulation with the base of an arytenoid cartilage.

The internal surface of the cricoid cartilage is smooth and lined by mucosa.

Subglottic stenosis

Congenital malformation of the cricoid cartilage may result in severe narrowing of the subglottic airway and respiratory obstruction. A similar situation may result from trauma and scarring following prolonged endotracheal intubation for the purposes of ventilation of premature babies on intensive care units.

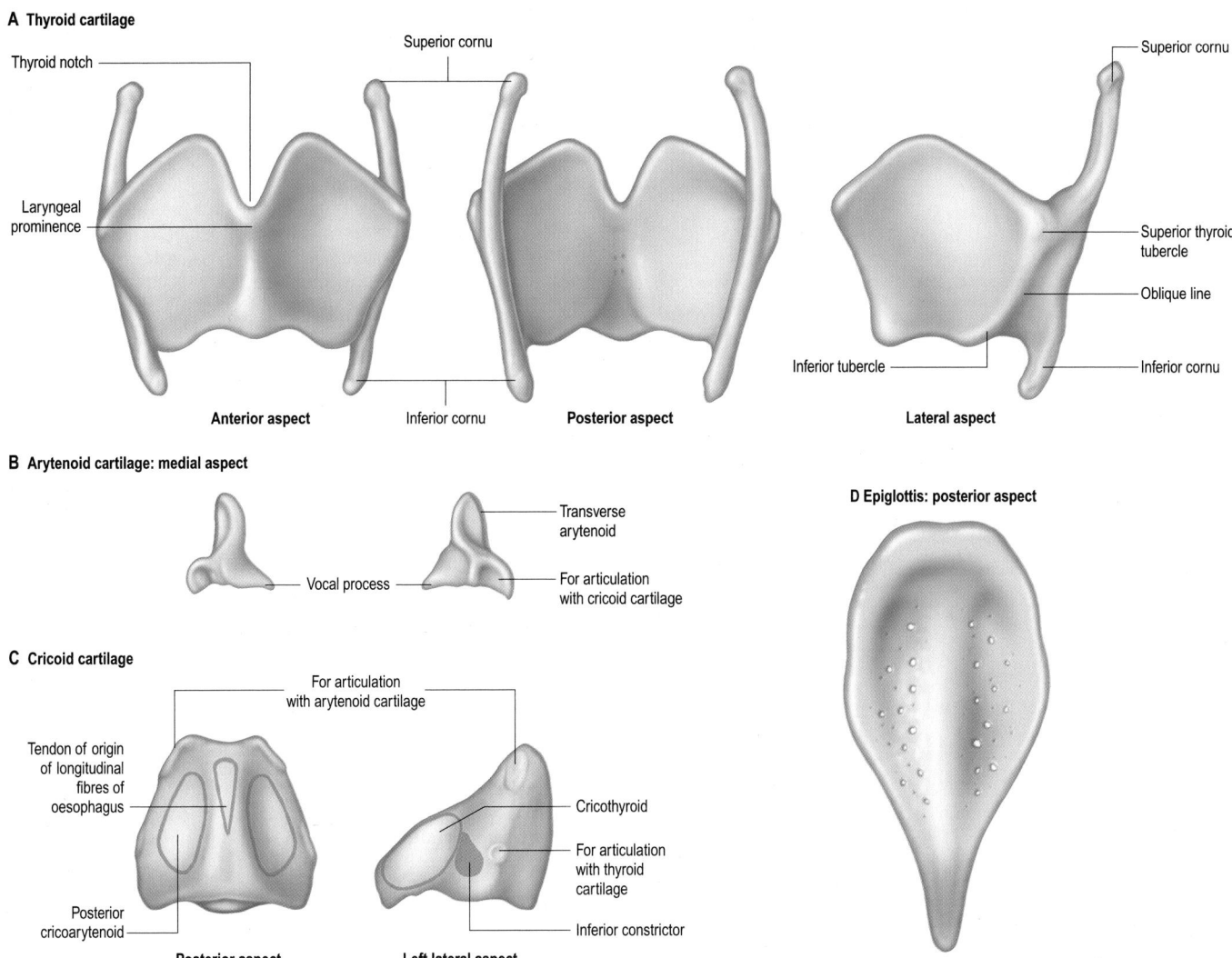

A Thyroid cartilage

Thyroid notch

Superior cornu

Laryngeal prominence

Anterior aspect

Inferior cornu

Posterior aspect

Superior cornu

Superior thyroid tubercle

Oblique line

Inferior tubercle

Inferior cornu

Lateral aspect

B Arytenoid cartilage: medial aspect

Transverse arytenoid

Vocal process

For articulation with cricoid cartilage

D Epiglottis: posterior aspect

C Cricoid cartilage

For articulation with arytenoid cartilage

Tendon of origin of longitudinal fibres of oesophagus

Cricothyroid

For articulation with thyroid cartilage

Posterior cricoarytenoid

Inferior constrictor

Posterior aspect

Left lateral aspect

Fig. 36.4 Cartilages of the larynx: thyroid (**A**), arytenoid (**B**), cricoid (**C**), epiglottis (**D**). The attachments of the vestibular ligaments (above) and the vocal ligaments (below) are shown in **A**, posterior aspect. Note the pitted surface of the epiglottis (**D**).

ARYTENOID CARTILAGE (Figs 36.3, 36.4)

The paired arytenoid cartilages articulate with the lateral parts of the superior border of the cricoid lamina. Each is pyramidal, and has three surfaces, two processes, a base and an apex. The posterior surface, which is triangular, smooth and concave, is covered by transverse arytenoid. The anterolateral surface is convex and rough, and bears, near the apex of the cartilage, an elevation from which a crest curves back, down and then forwards to the vocal process. The lower part of this crest separates two depressions (foveae). The upper is triangular, and the vestibular ligament is attached to it. The lower is oblong, and vocalis and lateral cricoarytenoid are attached to it. The medial surface is narrow, smooth, and flat. It is covered by mucosa and its lower edge forms the lateral boundary of the intercartilaginous part of the rima glottidis. The base is concave, with a smooth surface for articulation with the lateral part of the upper border of the cricoid lamina. Its round, prominent lateral angle, or muscular process, projects backwards and laterally: it gives attachment to posterior cricoarytenoid behind, and lateral cricoarytenoid in front. The vocal ligament is attached to its pointed anterior angle (the vocal process), which projects horizontally forward. The apex curves backwards and medially and articulates with the corniculate cartilage.

CORNICULATE CARTILAGES (Figs 36.3, 36.5)

The corniculate cartilages are two conical nodules of elastic fibrocartilage which articulate with the apices of the arytenoid cartilages, prolonging them posteromedially. They lie in the posterior parts of the aryepiglottic mucosal folds, and are sometimes fused with the arytenoid cartilages.

CUNEIFORM CARTILAGES (Fig. 36.5)

The cuneiform cartilages are two small elongated, club-like nodules of elastic fibrocartilage, one in each aryepiglottic fold anterosuperior to the corniculate cartilages and are visible as whitish elevations through the mucosa.

TRITIATE CARTILAGES (CARTILAGO TRITICEA) (Fig. 36.3)

The tritiate cartilages are two small nodules of elastic cartilage which are situated one on either side above the larynx within the posterior free edge of the thyrohyoid membrane, about halfway between the superior cornu of the thyroid cartilage and the tip of the greater cornua of the hyoid bone. Their functions are unknown, although they may serve to strengthen this connection.

Calcification of laryngeal cartilages

The thyroid, cricoid, and most of the arytenoid, cartilages consist of hyaline cartilage, and may therefore become calcified. This process normally starts at about 18 years of age. Initially it involves the lower and posterior part of the thyroid cartilage, and it subsequently spreads to involve the remaining cartilages. Calcification of the arytenoid cartilage starts at the base. The degree and frequency of calcification of the thyroid and cricoid cartilages appear to be less in females. There is some evidence to suggest that a predilection for tumour invasion may be enhanced by calcification of the laryngeal cartilages.

The tip and upper portion of the vocal process of the arytenoid cartilage consists of non-calcifying, elastic cartilage. This may have

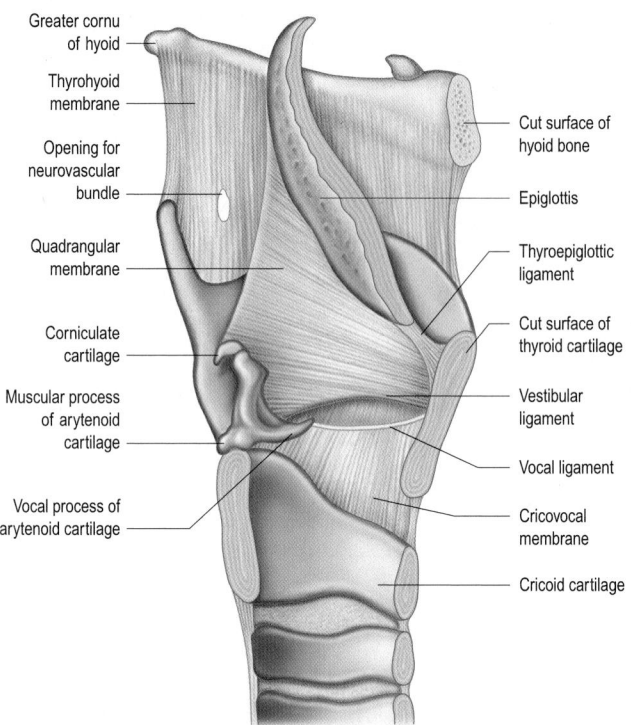

Greater cornu of hyoid

Thyrohyoid membrane

Opening for neurovascular bundle

Quadrangular membrane

Corniculate cartilage

Muscular process of arytenoid cartilage

Vocal process of arytenoid cartilage

Cut surface of hyoid bone

Epiglottis

Thyroepiglottic ligament

Cut surface of thyroid cartilage

Vestibular ligament

Vocal ligament

Cricovocal membrane

Cricoid cartilage

Fig. 36.5 Sagittal section of the left side of the larynx showing laryngeal membranes.

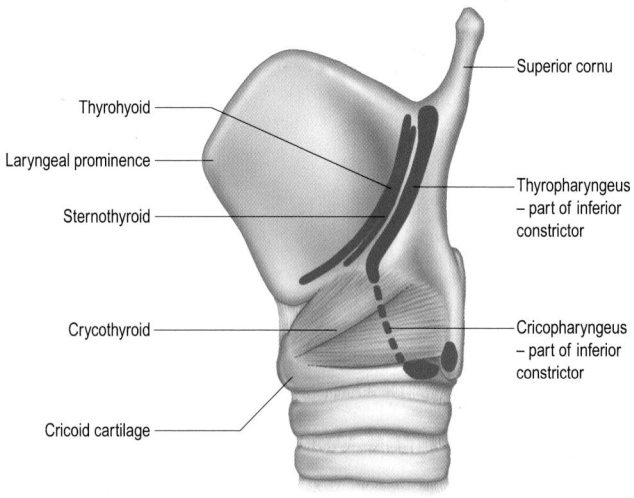

Thyrohyoid

Laryngeal prominence

Sternothyroid

Crycothyroid

Cricoid cartilage

Superior cornu

Thyropharyngeus – part of inferior constrictor

Cricopharyngeus – part of inferior constrictor

Fig. 36.6 Lateral view of the articulated thyroid and cricoid cartilage, showing the position of the muscular attachments (blue lines) and cricothyroid fibres.

considerable functional significance: the vocal process may bend at the elastic cartilage during adduction and abduction, and the two arytenoid cartilages will contact mainly at their 'elastic' superior portions during adduction.

JOINTS

CRICOTHYROID JOINT
The joints between the inferior cornua of the thyroid cartilage and the sides of the cricoid cartilage are synovial. Each is enveloped by a capsular ligament strengthened posteriorly by fibrous bands (**Figs 36.2, 36.3**). Both capsule and ligaments are rich in elastin fibres. The cricoid rotates

on the inferior cornua around a transverse axis which passes transversely through both cricothyroid joints, and, to a limited extent, it also glides in different directions on the thyroid cornua.

CRICOARYTENOID JOINT
A pair of synovial joints exists between the facets on the lateral parts of the upper border of the lamina of the cricoid cartilage and the bases of the arytenoids. Each joint is enclosed by a capsular ligament and strengthened by a ligament that, although traditionally called the posterior cricoarytenoid ligament, is largely medial in position.

The cricoarytenoid joints permit the arytenoids to rotate about an oblique axis (dorso-medio-cranial to ventro-latero-caudal), by which each vocal process swings laterally or medially, thereby increasing or decreasing the width of the rima glottidis. They also permit a gliding movement, by which the arytenoids approach or recede from one another, the direction and slope of their articular surfaces imposing a forward and downward movement on lateral gliding. The movements of gliding and rotation are associated, i.e. medial gliding occurs with medial rotation and lateral gliding with lateral rotation. The posterior cricoarytenoid ligaments limit forward movements of the arytenoid cartilages on the cricoid cartilage. It has been suggested that the 'rest' position of the cricoarytenoid ligament is a major determinant of the position of a denervated vocal cord.

ARYTENOCORNICULATE JOINTS
Synovial or cartilaginous joints link the arytenoid and corniculate cartilages.

INNERVATION OF THE CRICOTHYROID, CRICOARYTENOID AND ARYTENOCORNICULATE JOINTS
The cricothyroid, cricoarytenoid and arytenocorniculate joints are innervated chiefly by branches of the recurrent laryngeal nerves, which arise independently or from branches of the nerve to the laryngeal muscles. Numerous lamellated (Pacinian) corpuscles, Ruffini corpuscles and free nerve endings occur in the capsules of the laryngeal joints.

SOFT TISSUES

The skeletal framework of the larynx is interconnected by ligaments and fibrous membranes, of which the thyrohyoid, cricothyroid, quadrangular and cricovocal membranes are the most significant. The thyrohyoid membrane is external to the larynx, whereas the paired quadrangular and cricovocal membranes are internal. All the membranes are composed of fibroelastic tissue. The named ligaments are the median (anterior) cricothyroid ligament, the hyoepiglottic and thyroepiglottic ligaments and the cricotracheal ligament.

EXTRINSIC LIGAMENTS AND MEMBRANES

Thyrohyoid membrane
The thyrohyoid membrane is a broad, fibroelastic layer, attached below to the superior border of the thyroid cartilage lamina and the front of its superior cornua, and above to the superior margin of the body and greater cornua of the hyoid (**Figs 36.1, 36.2, 36.3**). It thus ascends behind the concave posterior surface of the hyoid, separated from its body by a bursa which facilitates the ascent of the larynx during swallowing. Its thicker part is the median thyrohyoid ligament. The more lateral, thinner, parts are pierced by the superior laryngeal vessels and internal laryngeal nerves (**Fig. 36.2**). Externally it is in contact with thyrohyoid and omohyoid and the body of the hyoid bone. Its inner surface is related to the epiglottis and the piriform fossae of the pharynx. The round, cord-like, elastic lateral thyrohyoid ligaments form the posterior borders of the thyrohyoid membrane, and connect the tips of the superior thyroid cornua to the posterior ends of the greater hyoid cornua (**Fig. 36.2**).

Hyo- and thyroepiglottic ligaments
The epiglottis is attached to the hyoid bone and thyroid cartilage by the extrinsic hyoepiglottic and intrinsic thyroepiglottic ligaments respectively.

Cricotracheal ligament
The cricotracheal ligament unites the lower cricoid border to the first tracheal cartilage, and is thus continuous with the perichondrium of the trachea (**Fig. 36.1**).

INTRINSIC LIGAMENTS AND MEMBRANES (Figs 36.5, 36.7)

The fibroelastic membrane of the larynx lies within the cartilaginous skeleton of the larynx, beneath the laryngeal mucosa. It is interrupted on both sides of the larynx by a horizontal cleft between the vestibular and vocal ligaments. Its upper part, the quadrangular membrane, extends between the arytenoid cartilages and the sides of the epiglottis. Its lower part forms the cricovocal membrane, which connects the thyroid, cricoid and arytenoid cartilages.

Quadrangular membrane

Each quadrangular membrane passes from the lateral margin of the epiglottis to the arytenoid cartilage on its own side. It is often poorly defined. The upper and lower borders of the membrane are free. The upper border slopes posteriorly to form the aryepiglottic ligament, which constitutes the central component of the aryepiglottic fold. It is less defined in its upper portion. Posteriorly it passes through the fascial plane of the oesophageal suspensory ligament, and helps to form a median corniculopharyngeal ligament which extends into the sub-mucosa adjacent to the cricoid cartilage. This ligament may exert vertical traction. The lower border forms the vestibular fold. The cuneiform cartilages lie within the aryepiglottic folds.

Cricothyroid ligament and cricovocal membrane

The cricothyroid ligament is composed mainly of elastic tissue. It consists of two parts: an anterior part, the anterior (median) cricothyroid ligament, and a lateral part, the cricovocal membrane.

Cricothyroid membrane and anterior (median) cricothyroid ligament – The cricothyroid membrane passes upwards from the upper border of the cricoid cartilage to the lower border of the thyroid cartilage. Anteriorly, it is thickened to form the anterior (median) cricothyroid ligament, which is broader below and narrower above.

Cricovocal membrane – This membrane is sometimes called the conus elasticus or the lateral cricothyroid ligament; such terminology ignores the fact that the cricovocal membrane is attached to the arytenoid cartilage as well as to the thyroid cartilage, and that it shows a thickened ligament only where it becomes the vocal ligament.

The cricovocal membrane is thinner than the anterior cricothyroid ligament. It arises beneath the cricothyroid membrane from the inner surface of the cricoid cartilage, near its lower margin. It passes upwards beneath the lower border of the thyroid cartilage and is attached anteriorly to the inner surface of the angle of the thyroid cartilage (just

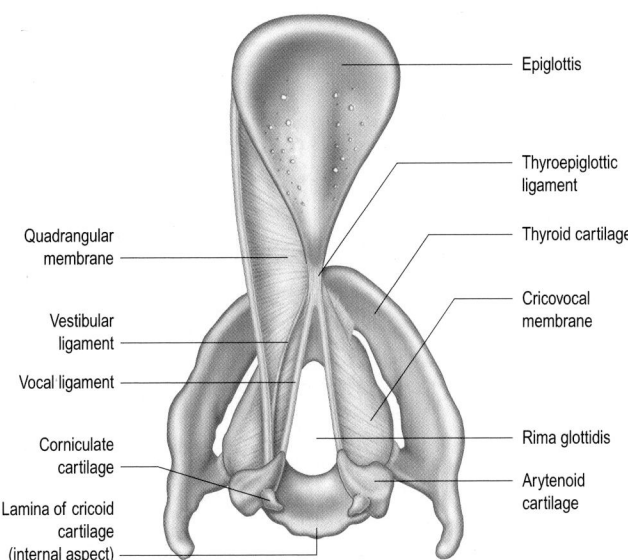

Fig. 36.7 Superior view of laryngeal cartilages together with cricothyroid, quadrangular, and related ligaments and membranes.

below its midpoint) and posteriorly to the tip of the vocal process of the arytenoid cartilage. Between these attachments, the upper edge of the cricovocal membrane is free, horizontally aligned and thickened to form the vocal ligament, which underlines the mucosa-covered vocal cord. The cricovocal membrane is covered internally by mucosa and externally by lateral cricoarytenoid and thyroarytenoid.

MICROSTRUCTURE OF THE LARYNX

The laryngeal mucosa is continuous with that of the pharynx above and the trachea below. It lines the entire inner surface of the larynx including the ventricle and saccule and is thickened over the vestibular folds where it is the chief component. Over the vocal cords it is thinner, and is firmly attached to the underlying vocal ligaments. It is loosely adherent to the anterior surface of the epiglottis, but firmly attached to its anterior surface and the floor of the valleculae. On the aryepiglottic folds it is reinforced by a considerable amount of fibrous connective tissue, and adheres closely to the laryngeal surfaces of the cuneiform and arytenoid cartilages.

The laryngeal epithelium is mainly a ciliated, pseudostratified respiratory epithelium where it covers the inner aspects of the larynx, including the posterior surface of the epiglottis, and it provides a ciliary clearance mechanism shared with most of the respiratory tract (Chapter 62). However, the vocal cords are covered by non-keratinized, stratified squamous epithelium, an important variation which protects the tissue from the effects of the considerable mechanical stresses acting on the surfaces of the vocal cords. The exterior surfaces of the larynx which merge with the laryngopharynx and oropharynx (including the anterior surface of the epiglottis), are subject to the abrasive effects of swallowed food, and are also covered by non-keratinized stratified squamous epithelium.

The laryngeal mucosa has numerous mucous glands, especially over the epiglottis, where they pit the cartilage, and along the margins of the aryepiglottic folds anterior to the arytenoid cartilages, where they are known as the arytenoid glands. Many large glands in the saccules of the larynx secrete periodically over the vocal cords during phonation. The free edges of these folds are devoid of glands and their stratified epithelium is vulnerable to drying and requires the secretions of neighbouring glands. Hoarseness due to excessive speaking is due to partial temporary failure of this secretion. Taste buds, like those in the tongue (p. 588), occur on the posterior epiglottic surface, aryepiglottic folds and less often in other laryngeal regions.

LARYNGEAL CAVITY (Figs 36.8, 36.9)

The laryngeal cavity space extends from the laryngeal inlet (from the pharynx) down to the lower border of the cricoid cartilage, where it continues into the trachea. It is partially divided into upper and lower parts by paired upper and lower mucosal folds which project into its lumen. There is a middle part between the two sets of folds. The upper folds are the vestibular (ventricular or false vocal) folds, and the median aperture which they guard is the rima vestibuli. The lower pair are the (true) vocal cords, and the fissure between the latter is the rima glottidis or glottis. The vocal cords are the primary source of phonation, whereas the vestibular folds normally do not contribute directly to sound production. The clinical term supraglottis refers to that part of the larynx which lies above the glottis. It includes the laryngeal ventricle, vestibular folds, the laryngeal surface of the epiglottis, arytenoid cartilages and the laryngeal aspects of the aryepiglottic folds.

SUPRAGLOTTIS (UPPER PART)

The upper part of the laryngeal cavity contains the laryngeal inlet or aditus, the aryepiglottic fold and the laryngeal ventricle.

Laryngeal inlet or aditus

The upper part of the laryngeal cavity is entered by the laryngeal inlet or 'aditus laryngis', which is the aperture between the larynx and pharynx. This faces backwards and somewhat upwards, because the anterior wall of the larynx is much longer than the posterior (and slopes downwards and forwards in its upper part because of the oblique inclination of the epiglottis). The inlet is bounded anteriorly by the upper edge of the epiglottis, posteriorly by the transverse mucosal fold between the two

Labels on figure:
Epiglottis
Thyroepiglottic ligament
Thyroid cartilage
Cricovocal membrane
Rima glottidis
Arytenoid cartilage
Quadrangular membrane
Vestibular ligament
Vocal ligament
Corniculate cartilage
Lamina of cricoid cartilage (internal aspect)

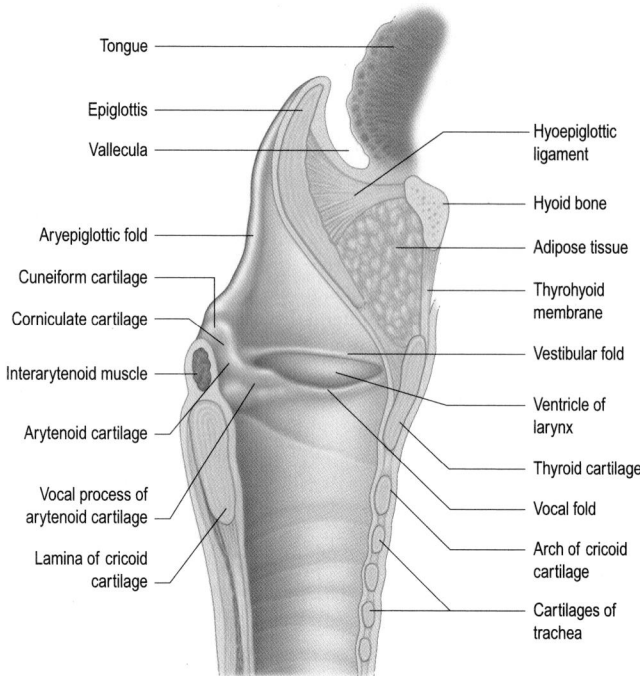

Fig. 36.8 Sagittal section showing the interior aspect of the left half of the larynx.

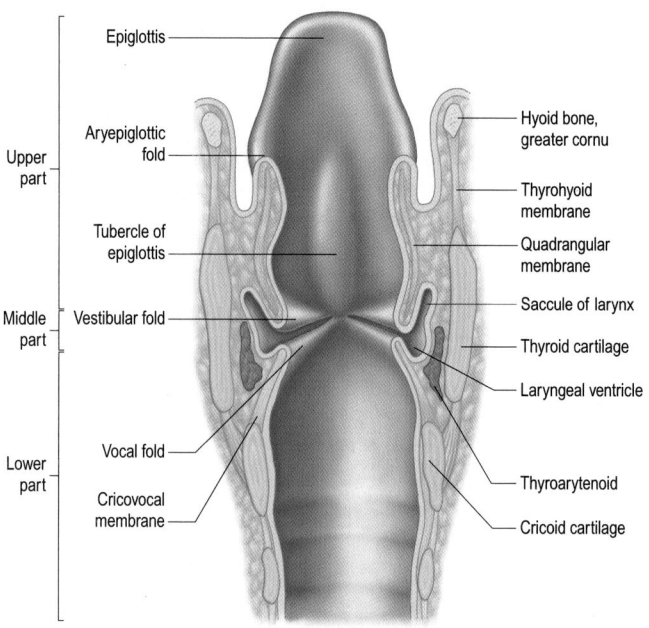

Fig. 36.9 Coronal section through the larynx and the cranial end of the trachea: posterior aspect.

arytenoids (posterior commissure), and on each side by the edge of a mucosal ridge, the aryepiglottic fold, which runs between the side of the epiglottis and the apex of the arytenoid cartilage. The midline groove between the two corniculate tubercles is termed the interarytenoid notch.

Aryepiglottic fold
The aryepiglottic fold contains ligamentous and muscular fibres. The ligamentous fibres represent the free upper border of the quadrangular membrane (**Figs 36.5, 36.7**). The muscle fibres are continuations of the oblique arytenoids. The posterior part of the aryepiglottic fold has two

oval swellings, one above and in front, the other behind and below. These swellings mark the positions of the underlying cuneiform and corniculate cartilages respectively. They are separated by a shallow vertical furrow which is continuous below with the opening of the laryngeal ventricle.

Laryngeal introitus
This clinical term denotes the space between the laryngeal inlet and vestibular folds. It is wide above, narrow below and higher anteriorly than posteriorly. Its anterior wall is formed by the posterior surface of the epiglottis, the lower part of which (the epiglottic tubercle) bulges backwards a little. Its lateral walls, which are higher in front and shallow behind, are the medial surfaces of the aryepiglottic folds. Its posterior wall is the interarytenoid mucosa, above the ventricular folds.

MIDDLE PART
The middle part of the laryngeal cavity is the smallest, and extends from the rima vestibuli above to the rima glottidis below. On each side it contains the vestibular folds, the ventricle and the saccule of the larynx.

Vestibular folds and ligaments
The narrow vestibular ligament represents the thickened lower border of the quadrangular membrane (**Fig. 36.7**). It is fixed in front to the thyroid angle below the epiglottic cartilage and behind to the antero-lateral surface of the arytenoid cartilage above its vocal process. With its covering of mucosa, it is termed the vestibular (ventricular or false vocal) fold (**Figs 36.8, 36.9**). The presence of a loose vascular mucosa lends the vestibular folds a pink appearance *in vivo*, as they lie above and lateral to, the vocal cords.

Ventricle (sinus) of larynx
On each side of the larynx, a slit between the vestibular and vocal cords opens into a fusiform recess called the laryngeal ventricle (**Figs 36.8, 36.9**). The ventricle extends upwards into the laryngeal wall lateral to the vestibular fold.

Saccule of larynx
The ventricle of the larynx opens into the saccule of the larynx (**Fig. 36.9**), a pouch which ascends forwards from the ventricle, between the vestibular fold and thyroid cartilage, and occasionally reaches the upper border of the cartilage. It is conical, and curves slightly backwards; 60–70 mucous glands, sited in the submucosa, open onto its luminal surface. The orifice of the saccule is guarded by a delicate fold of mucosa, the ventriculosaccular fold.

The saccule has a fibrous capsule. This is continuous below with the vestibular ligament, and is covered medially by a few muscular fasciculi from the apex of the arytenoid cartilage, which pass forwards between the saccule and vestibular mucosa into the aryepiglottic fold. Laterally the saccule is separated from the thyroid cartilage by the thyroepiglottic muscle, which compresses the saccule, expressing its secretion onto the vocal cords, which lack glands, to lubricate and protect them against desiccation and infection. Saccules occasionally protrude through the thyrohyoid membrane.

Laryngocoele
The laryngeal ventricle may on occasion become pathologically enlarged due to obstruction of the ventricular aditus by inflammation, by scarring or by a tumour. As the sealed cavity of the ventricle contains the laryngeal saccule, an expanding mucus-filled cyst is formed. This cyst (laryngocoele) may expand into the paraglottic space and extend superiorly to expand the aryepiglottic fold and reach the vallecula (internal laryngocoele). Acute respiratory obstruction may result especially if the contents of the cyst become infected. The cyst may also expand through the thyrohyoid membrane at the point of entry of the internal laryngeal neurovascular bundle to present as a lump in the neck overlying the thyrohyoid membrane (external laryngocoele).

Vocal cords (folds) and ligaments
The free thickened upper edge of the cricovocal membrane forms the vocal ligaments (**Fig. 36.7**). It stretches back on either side from the midlevel of the thyroid angle to the vocal processes of the arytenoids. When covered by mucosa, it is termed the vocal fold or vocal cord (cord

is the preferred clinical term) (**Figs 36.8, 36.9**). The vocal cords form the anterolateral edges of the rima glottidis and are concerned with sound production. The mucosa overlying the vocal ligament is thin and lies directly on the vocal ligament, and so the vocal cord appears pearly white *in vivo*. It is loosely attached to the ligaments: oedema fluid readily collects in this potential space in disease. Known as Reinke's space, it extends along the length of the free margin of the vocal ligament and a little way onto the superior surface of the cord. The site where the vocal cords meet anteriorly is known as the anterior commissure. Fibres of the vocal ligament here pass through the thyroid cartilage to blend with the overlying perichondrium, forming Broyles' ligament. The latter contains blood vessels and lymphatics and is therefore a potential route for the escape of malignant tumours from the larynx. Each vocal ligament is composed of a band of yellow elastic tissue related laterally to vocalis.

Reinke's oedema

The mucous membrane is loosely attached throughout the larynx and can accommodate considerable swelling which may compromise the airway in acute infections. At the edge of the true vocal cords the mucosal covering is tightly bound to the underlying ligament so that oedema fluid does not pass between the upper and lower compartments of the vocal cord mucosa. Any tissue swelling above the vocal cord exaggerates the potential space deep to the mucosa (Reinke's space), causing accumulation of extracellular fluid and flabby swelling of the vocal cords (Reinke's oedema). Smoking and vocal abuse may initiate such changes.

Vocal cord nodules

Aberrant muscle balance during phonation may cause initial contact during vocal cord apposition to occur at a point at the junction of the anterior third and the posterior two-thirds of the vocal ligament. Excessive trauma at this point, for example when singing with poor technique or forcing the voice may produce subepithelial haemorrhage or bruising, and subsequent pathological changes such as subepithelial scarring ('singer's nodes' or 'clergyman's nodes').

Rima glottidis

The rima glottidis or glottis is the fissure between the vocal cords anteriorly and the arytenoid cartilages posteriorly (**Fig. 36.10**). It is bounded behind by the mucosa passing between the arytenoid cartilages at the level of the vocal cords. The rima glottidis is customarily divided into two regions: an anterior intermembranous part, which makes up about three-fifths of its anteroposterior length and is formed by the underlying vocal ligament, and a posterior intercartilaginous part which is formed by the vocal processes of the arytenoid cartilages. The average sagittal diameter of the glottis in adult males is 23 mm and in adult females 17 mm. It is the narrowest part of the larynx. Its width and shape vary with the movements of the vocal cords and arytenoid cartilages during respiration and phonation.

SUBGLOTTIS (LOWER PART)

The lower part of the laryngeal cavity, or the subglottis, extends from the vocal cords to the lower border of the cricoid. In transverse section it is elliptical above and wider and circular below, and is continuous with the trachea. Its walls are lined by respiratory mucosa, and supported by the cricothyroid ligament above and the cricoid cartilage below.

LARYNGOSCOPIC EXAMINATION (Fig. 36.12)

The laryngeal inlet, the structures around it and the cavity of the larynx can all be inspected using fibreoptic endoscopy, either through the mouth (**Fig. 36.11A**) or nasopharynx (**Fig. 36.11B**). The epiglottis is seen foreshortened, but its tubercle is visible. From the epiglottic margins the aryepiglottic folds can be traced posteromedially and the cuneiform and corniculate elevations recognized. The pink vestibular folds and pearly white vocal cords are visible and, when the rima glottidis is wide open, the anterior arch of the cricoid cartilage, the tracheal mucosa and cartilages may be seen. The piriform fossae can also be inspected.

LARYNGEAL OBSTRUCTION AND TRAUMA

Large foreign bodies may obstruct the laryngeal inlet or rima glottidis and suffocation may ensue, while smaller ones can enter the trachea or bronchi, or lodge in the laryngeal ventricle and cause reflex closure of the glottis with consequent suffocation. Inflammation of the upper larynx, e.g. secondary to infection or the effects of smoke inhalation,

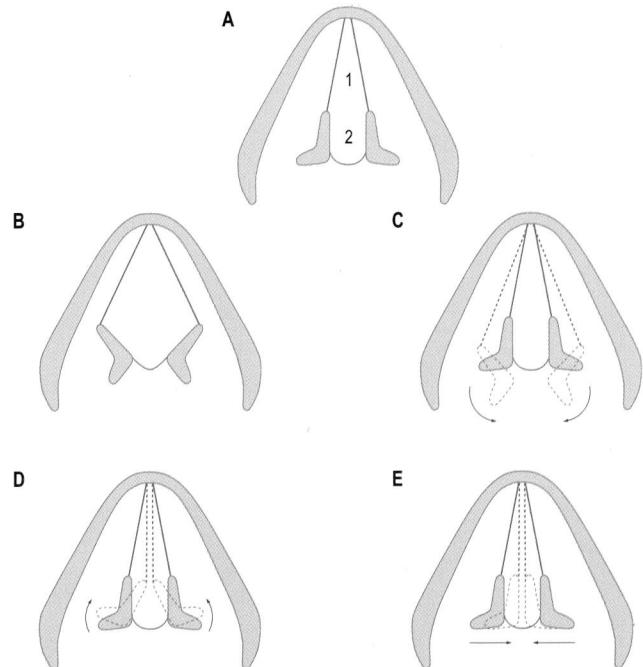

Fig. 36.10 Different positions of the vocal cords and arytenoid cartilages. **A**, Position of rest in quiet respiration. The intermembranous part of the rima glottidis is triangular and the intercartilaginous part is rectangular in shape. Key: 1, intermembranous part of glottis; 2, intercartilagenous part of glottis. **B**, Forced inspiration. Both parts of the rima glottidis are triangular in shape. **C**, Abduction of the vocal cords. The arrows indicate the lines of pull of the posterior cricoarytenoid muscles. The abducted vocal cords and the abducted, retracted and laterally rotated arytenoid cartilages are shown in dotted outline. Both parts of the rima glottidis are triangular. **D**, Adduction of the vocal cords. The arrows indicate the lines of pull of the lateral cricoarytenoid muscles. The adducted vocal cords and the medially rotated arytenoid cartilages are shown in dotted outlines. **E**, Closure of the rima glottidis. The arrows indicate the line of pull of the transverse arytenoid muscle. Both the vocal cords and the arytenoid cartilages are adducted (dotted lines), but there is no rotation of the latter.

may swell the mucosa by effusion of fluid into the abundant, loose submucous tissue (oedema of the supraglottis). The effusion does not involve or extend below the vocal cords, because the mucosa adheres directly to the vocal ligaments without the intervention of submucous tissue.

Laryngotomy below the vocal cords through the cricothyroid ligament or tracheotomy may be necessary to restore a free airway. The mucosa of the upper larynx is highly sensitive, and contact with foreign bodies excites immediate coughing.

Suicidal wounds are usually made through the thyrohyoid membrane, damaging the epiglottis, superior thyroid vessels, external and internal carotid arteries and internal jugular veins. Less frequently they are above the hyoid with damage to the lingual muscles and lingual and facial vessels.

THE INFANT LARYNX

The infant larynx differs markedly from the adult larynx. Its cavity is short and funnel-shaped, and is about one-third the size of the adult, although it is proportionately larger, and this has two main consequences. First, its lumen is disproportionately narrower than the adult, and second, it lies higher in the neck than the adult larynx. At rest the upper border of the epiglottis is at the level of the second or third cervical vertebra, and when the larynx is elevated it reaches the level of the first cervical vertebra. This high position is associated with the ability of the infant to use its nasal airway to breathe while suckling. The epiglottis is X-shaped, with a furled petiole, and the laryngeal cartilages are softer and more pliable than the adult larynx (which may predispose to airway collapse in inspiration, which leads to the clinical picture of laryngomalacia). The thyroid cartilage is shorter and broader than in the adult and lies closer to the hyoid bone in the neonate. This

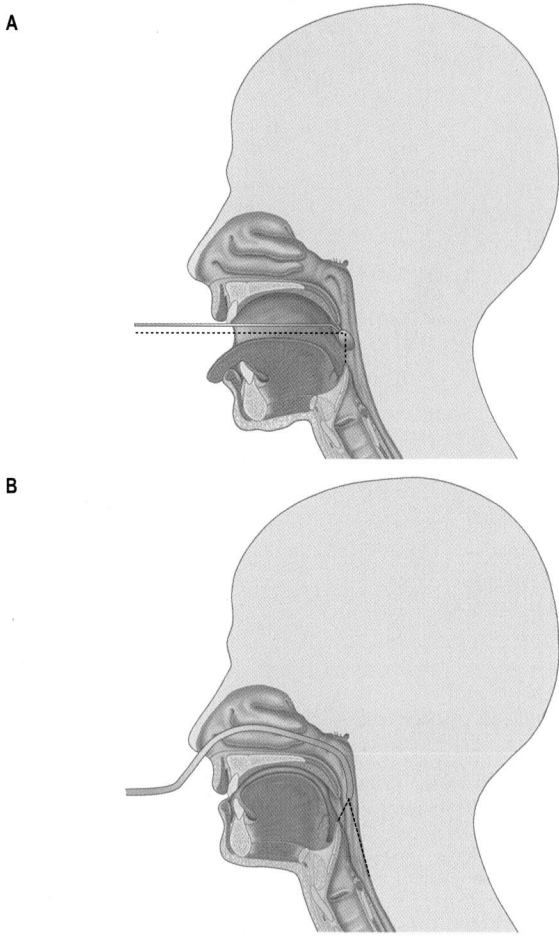

A

B

Fig. 36.11 Laryngoscopic approaches. **A** shows the oral and **B** the nasopharyngeal approaches to the visualization of the larynx.

the infant larynx: it measures 3.5 mm in diameter in neonates. Swelling at this point rapidly results in severe respiratory obstruction. Unlike the adult, the neonatal subglottic cavity extends posteriorly as well as inferiorly, which is important to consider when passing an endotracheal tube. The ventricle of the larynx is small, whereas the saccule of the larynx is often considerably larger than it is in adult life.

By about the third year, sexual differences become apparent in the larynx. It is larger in boys, but the angle between the thyroid laminae is more pronounced in girls. At puberty these changes increase, and there is greater enlargement of the male larynx.

THE PARALUMENAL SPACES

A number of potential spaces or compartments can be identified in and around the larynx. The three most commonly considered are the pre-epiglottic, the paraglottic and the subglottic spaces. They are not closed compartments and their existence does not preclude the spread of tumours. Knowledge of the anatomy of these spaces, and the potential pathways of spread of tumours from them, has significantly influenced the surgical approach to disease in this region.

THE PRE-EPIGLOTTIC SPACE

The pre-epiglottic space might be expected to lie anterior to the epiglottis, but in reality, it also extends beyond the lateral margins of the epiglottis, which gives it the form of a horse-shoe. It is primarily filled with adipose tissue and appears to contain no lymph nodes.

Its upper boundary is formed by the weak hyoepiglottic membrane, which is strengthened medially as the median hyoepiglottic ligament. Its anterior boundary is the thyrohyoid membrane, which is strengthened medially as the median thyrohyoid ligament. Its lower boundary is the thyroepiglottic ligament, which is continuous laterally with the quadrangular membrane behind. Its upper lateral border is the greater cornu of the hyoid bone. Inferolaterally, the pre-epiglottic space is in continuity with the paraglottic space and it is often invaded from the latter by the laryngeal saccule. It is also in continuity with the mucosa of the laryngeal surface of the epiglottis via multiple perforations in the cartilage of the epiglottis. It is through these perforations that malignancies of the laryngeal surface of the epiglottis may invade the fat and areolar tissue of the pre-epiglottic space.

THE PARAGLOTTIC SPACE

The paraglottic space is a region of adipose tissue which contains the internal laryngeal nerve, the laryngeal ventricle and part, or all, of the laryngeal saccule. It is bounded laterally by the thyroid cartilage and thyrohyoid membrane. Superomedially, it is usually continuous with the pre-epiglottic space, although it may be partitioned from it by a fibrous septum. The cricovocal membrane lies inferomedially, and the mucosa of the piriform fossa lies posteriorly. The lower border of the thyroid cartilage is inferior. Anteroinferiorly, there are deficiencies in the paramedian gap at the side of the anterior cricothyroid ligament,

means that the thyrohyoid ligament is relatively short. Neither the superior notch nor the laryngeal prominence are as marked as they are in the adult. The cricoid cartilage is the same shape as in the adult. The vocal cords are 4–4.5 mm long, which is relatively shorter than in either childhood or the adult.

The mucosa of the supraglottis is more loosely attached than it is in the adult larynx and it exhibits multiple submucosal glands. Inflammation of the supraglottis will therefore rapidly result in gross oedema. The mucosa is also lax in the subglottis, which is the narrowest part of

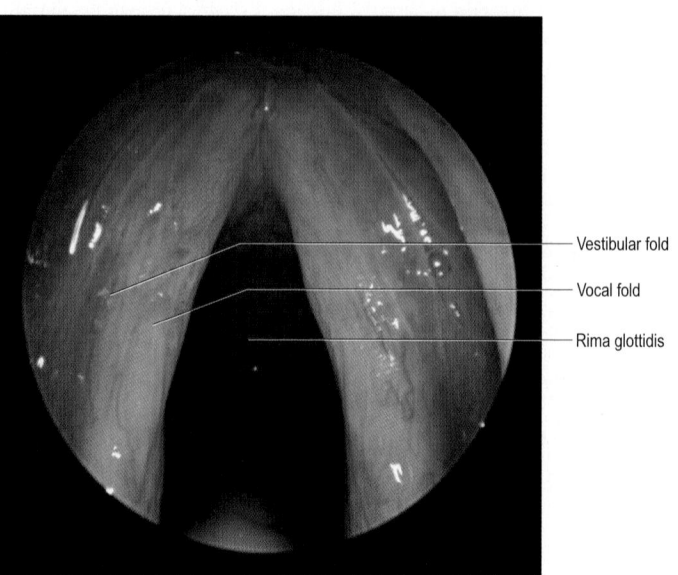

Vestibular fold

Vocal fold

Rima glottidis

Fig. 36.12 Laryngeal folds viewed in abduction, as seen through a laryngoscope. (By permission from Berkovitz BKB, Moxham BJ 2002 Head and Neck Anatomy. London: Martin Dunitz.)

and posteroinferiorly adipose tissue extends towards the cricothyroid joint. Some authorities exclude thyroarytenoid from the paraglottic space.

Supraglottic tumours may spread into the paraglottic space and reach the subglottis, or extend beyond the limits of the larynx. Ventricular tumours may obstruct mucous outflow from the saccule and cause its expansion within the paraglottic space to form a secondary laryngocoele: the tumour itself may also spread transglottically, and thereby fix the vocal cord either by invasion of the cricoarytenoid joint or by damaging the recurrent laryngeal nerve. Fixation of the vocal cord is a good indicator of a tumour within the paraglottic space. The proximity of the mucosa at the piriform fossa makes its removal in surgery mandatory for such disease.

THE SUBGLOTTIC SPACE

The subglottic space is bounded laterally by the cricovocal membrane, medially by the mucosa of the subglottic region and above by the undersurface of Broyle's ligament in the midline. It is continuous below with the inner surface of the cricoid cartilage and its mucosa.

MUSCLES

The muscles of the larynx may be divided into extrinsic and intrinsic groups. The extrinsic muscles connect the larynx to neighbouring structures and are responsible for moving it vertically during phonation and swallowing. They include the infrahyoid strap muscles, i.e. thyrohyoid, sternothyroid and sternohyoid, and the inferior constrictor muscle of the pharynx. Two of the three elevator muscles of the pharynx, i.e. stylo- and palatopharyngeus, are also connected directly to the thyroid cartilage, mainly to the posterior aspect of the thyroid lamina and cornu.

The role of the extrinsic muscles during respiration appears variable. Thus, the larynx has been seen to rise, descend or barely move, during inspiration. The extrinsic muscles can affect the tone and pitch of the voice by raising or lowering the larynx, and geniohyoid elevates and anteriorly displaces the larynx, particularly during deglutition.

The intrinsic muscles are the cricothyroid, posterior and lateral cricoarytenoid, transverse and oblique arytenoid, aryepiglotticus, thyroarytenoid and its subsidiary part, vocalis, and thyroepiglotticus: all are confined to the larynx in their attachments, and all but the transverse arytenoid are paired. Whereas most of the intrinsic muscles lie internally, under cover of the thyroid cartilage or the mucosa, the cricothyroids appear on the outer aspect of the larynx.

The intrinsic laryngeal muscles may be placed in three groups according to their main actions. The posterior and lateral cricoarytenoids and oblique and transverse arytenoids vary the dimensions of the rima glottidis. The cricothyroids, posterior cricoarytenoids, thyroarytenoids and vocales regulate the tension of the vocal ligaments. The oblique arytenoids, aryepiglottic and thyroepiglottic muscles modify the laryngeal inlet. Bilateral pairs of muscles usually act in concert with each other.

Neuromuscular spindles have been found in all human laryngeal muscles, the maximum number (23) being found in the transverse arytenoid. The control of phonation requires very considerable neuromuscular co-ordination, and effective proprioception would appear to be essential to this capacity. The mass of muscle related to adduction far outweighs that related to abduction. In this context, it is of interest to note that histological examination of normal larynges revealed evidence of some degenerative changes in the posterior cricoarytenoid muscle, the single muscle associated with abduction, but none in the remaining muscles.

INTRINSIC MUSCLES

Oblique arytenoid and the aryepiglottic muscle

The oblique arytenoids lie superficial to the transverse arytenoid, and are sometimes considered to be part of it. They cross each other obliquely at the back of the larynx, each extending from the back of the muscular process of one arytenoid cartilage to the apex of the opposite one. Some fibres continue laterally round the arytenoid apex into the aryepiglottic fold, forming the aryepiglottic muscle (**Fig. 36.13**).

Vascular supply – Oblique arytenoid receives its blood supply from the laryngeal branches of the superior and inferior thyroid arteries.

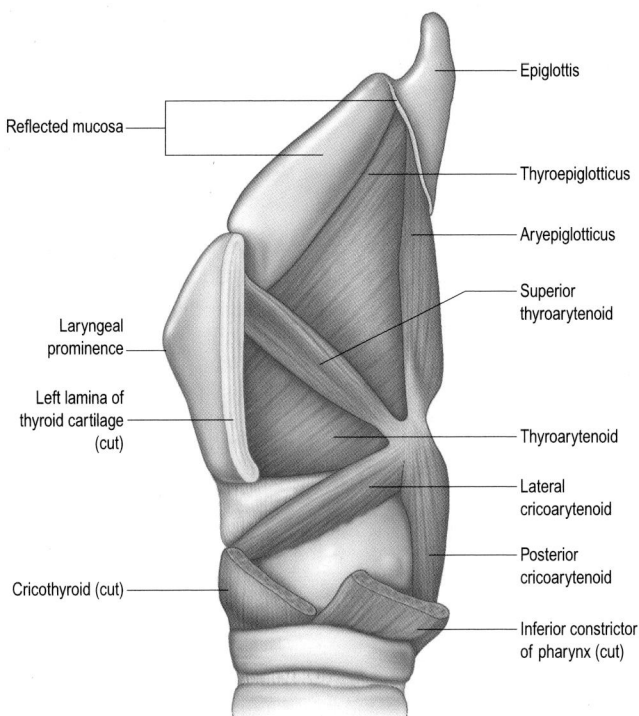

Fig. 36.13 The muscles of the larynx (most of the left lamina of the thyroid cartilage has been removed): left lateral aspect.

Labels (clockwise): Epiglottis; Thyroepiglotticus; Aryepiglotticus; Superior thyroarytenoid; Thyroarytenoid; Lateral cricoarytenoid; Posterior cricoarytenoid; Inferior constrictor of pharynx (cut); Cricothyroid (cut); Left lamina of thyroid cartilage (cut); Laryngeal prominence; Reflected mucosa

Innervation – Oblique arytenoid is innervated by the recurrent laryngeal nerve.

Actions – The oblique arytenoids and aryepiglottic muscles act as a sphincter of the laryngeal inlet by adducting the aryepiglottic folds, and approximating the arytenoid cartilages to the tubercle of the epiglottis. Their poor development limits their capacity to act as a sphincter of the inlet.

Transverse (inter) arytenoid (Fig. 35.2)

Transverse arytenoid is a single, unpaired muscle which bridges the gap at the back of the larynx between the two arytenoid cartilages and fills their posterior concave surfaces. It is attached to the back of the muscular process and adjacent lateral border of both arytenoids.

Vascular supply – Transverse arytenoid receives its blood supply from the laryngeal branches of the superior and inferior thyroid arteries.

Innervation – Transverse arytenoid is innervated by the recurrent laryngeal nerves. It also receives branches from the internal laryngeal nerve, although there is debate as to whether these branches contain any distinct motor input. The nerves form a dense, but highly variable, plexus.

Actions – Transverse arytenoid pulls the arytenoid cartilages towards each other, closing the posterior, intercartilaginous, part of the rima glottidis (**Fig. 36.10E**). This action is accomplished by drawing the arytenoids upwards along the sloping shoulders of the cricoid lamina, without rotation.

Posterior cricoarytenoid (Fig. 35.2)

Posterior cricoarytenoid arises from the posterior surface of the cricoid lamina (**Fig. 36.4**). Its fibres ascend laterally and converge to insert on the back of the muscular process of the ipsilateral arytenoid cartilage. The highest fibres run almost horizontally, the middle obliquely, and the lowest are almost vertical: some reach the anterolateral surface of the arytenoid cartilage. An additional strip of muscle, ceratocricoid, is occasionally seen in relation to the lower border of posterior crico-arytenoid, arising from the cricoid cartilage and inserting on to the posterior aspect of the inferior horn of the thyroid cartilage.

Vascular supply – Posterior cricoarytenoid receives its blood supply from the laryngeal branches of the superior and inferior thyroid arteries.

Innervation – Posterior cricoarytenoid is innervated by the recurrent laryngeal branch of the vagus.

Actions – The posterior cricoarytenoids are the only laryngeal muscles which open the glottis, rotating the arytenoid cartilages laterally around an axis passing through the cricoarytenoid joints, and thus separating the vocal processes and the attached vocal cords (**Fig. 36.10C**). They also pull the arytenoids backwards, assisting the cricothyroids to tense the vocal cords. The most lateral fibres draw the arytenoid cartilages laterally, and so the rima glottidis becomes triangular when the posterior cricoarytenoid muscles contract.

Lateral cricoarytenoid

Lateral cricoarytenoid is attached anteriorly to the upper border of the cricoid arch. It ascends obliquely backwards to be attached to the front of the muscular process of the ipsilateral arytenoid cartilage (**Fig. 36.13**).

Vascular supply – Lateral cricoarytenoid receives its blood supply from the laryngeal branches of the superior and inferior thyroid arteries.

Innervation – Lateral cricoarytenoid is innervated by the recurrent laryngeal nerve via a single branch which forms a homogeneous nerve plexus located in the middle of the muscle. This suggests that lateral cricoarytenoid acts as a single unit, unlike the other intrinsic muscles of the larynx.

Actions – Lateral cricoarytenoid rotates the arytenoid cartilage in a direction opposite to that of posterior cricoarytenoid, and so closes the rima glottidis (**Fig. 36.10D**).

Cricothyroid (Fig. 36.6)

Cricothyroid is attached anteriorly to the external aspect of the arch of the cricoid cartilage. Its fibres pass backwards and diverge into two groups, a lower 'oblique' part which slants backwards and laterally to the anterior border of the inferior cornu of the thyroid; and a superior 'straight' part which ascends more steeply backwards to the posterior part of the lower border of the thyroid lamina. The medial borders of the paired cricothyroids are separated anteriorly by a triangular gap which is occupied by the anterior cricothyroid ligament.

Vascular supply – Cricothyroid is supplied by the cricothyroid artery, a branch of the superior thyroid artery, which crosses high on the cricothyroid ligament to communicate with its contralateral fellow.

Innervation – Unlike the other intrinsic muscles of the larynx, cricothyroid is innervated not by the recurrent laryngeal nerve, but by the external branch of the superior laryngeal nerve.

Actions – The cricothyroids stretch the vocal ligaments by tilting the thyroid cartilage forwards and downwards on the cricoid. Because the arytenoid cartilages are anchored to the cricoid lamina, the sagittally directed rotation of the thyroid cartilage increases the distance between their vocal processes and the anterior angle of the thyroid, and so lengthens, and affects tension in, the vocal ligaments.

Thyroarytenoid and vocalis (Figs 36.9, 36.13)

Thyroarytenoid is a broad, thin muscle, lying lateral to the vocal cord, cricovocal membrane, laryngeal ventricle and saccule. It is attached anteriorly to the lower half of the angle of the thyroid cartilage, and to the cricothyroid ligament. Its fibres pass backwards, laterally and upwards to the anterolateral surface of the arytenoid cartilage. Its lower and deeper fibres form a band which, in a coronal section, appears as a triangular bundle, and is attached to the lateral surface of the vocal process and to the inferior impression on the anterolateral surface of the arytenoid cartilage. This bundle, the vocalis muscle, is parallel with and just lateral to the vocal ligament. It is said to be thicker behind than

in front, because many deeper fibres start from the vocal ligament and so do not extend to the thyroid cartilage. Others consider that all its fibres loop and intertwine as they pass from the thyroid to the arytenoid cartilage. A few fibres extend along the wall of the ventricle from the lateral margin of the arytenoid cartilage to the side of the epiglottis. The superior thyroarytenoid, a small muscle which is not always present, lies on the lateral surface of the main mass of the thyroarytenoid, and extends obliquely from the thyroid angle to the muscular process of the arytenoid cartilage (**Fig. 36.13**).

Vascular supply – Thyroarytenoid receives its arterial blood supply from the laryngeal branches of the superior and inferior thyroid arteries.

Innervation – All parts of thyroarytenoid are supplied by the recurrent laryngeal nerve. It also receives a communicating branch from the external laryngeal nerve, although it is not clear whether such branches carry motor or sensory fibres.

Actions – The thyroarytenoids draw the arytenoid cartilages towards the thyroid cartilage, thereby shortening and relaxing the vocal ligaments. At the same time, they rotate the arytenoids medially to approximate the vocal cords. In addition, they can rotate the arytenoid cartilages medially and so aid closure of the rima glottidis. Relaxation of the posterior parts of the vocal ligaments by the vocalis muscles, combined with tension in the anterior parts of the ligaments, is responsible for raising the pitch of the voice. Vocalis can change the timbre of the voice by affecting the mass of the vocal cords.

Thyroepiglotticus

Many of the fibres of thyroarytenoid are prolonged into the aryepiglottic fold, where some terminate, and others continue to the epiglottic margin as the thyroepiglottic muscle (**Fig. 36.13**). The thyroepiglottics can widen the inlet of the larynx by their action on the aryepiglottic folds.

VASCULAR SUPPLY AND LYMPHATIC DRAINAGE (Fig. 36.14)

The blood supply of the larynx is derived mainly from the superior and inferior laryngeal arteries. Rich anastomoses exist between the corresponding contralateral laryngeal arteries and between the ipsilateral laryngeal arteries. The superior laryngeal arteries supply the greater part of the tissues of the larynx, from the epiglottis down to the level of

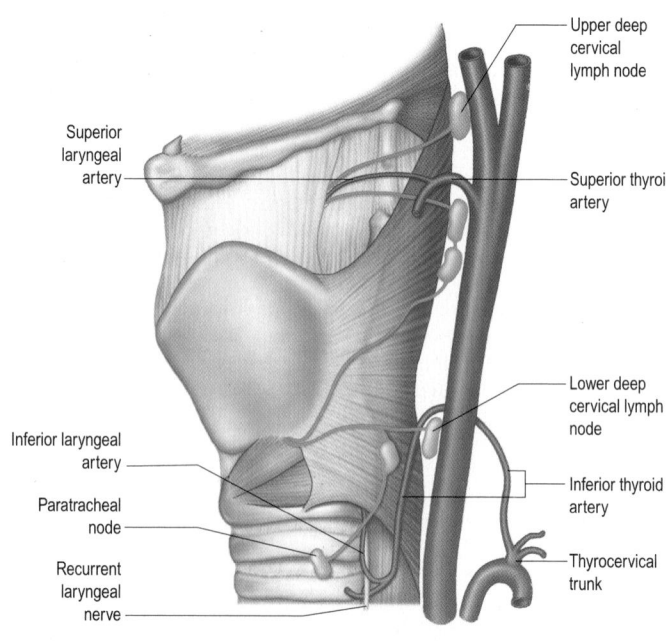

Fig. 36.14 Arterial supply and lymphatic drainage of the larynx. (Adapted from Oxford Textbook of Functional Anatomy, Vol 3 Head and Neck, MacKinnon P, Morris J (eds), 1990. By permission of Oxford University Press.)

the vocal cords, including the majority of the laryngeal musculature. The inferior laryngeal artery supplies the region around cricothyroid, while its posterior laryngeal branch supplies the tissue around posterior cricoarytenoid.

SUPERIOR LARYNGEAL ARTERY

The superior laryngeal artery is normally derived from the superior thyroid artery, a branch of the external carotid artery, as this artery passes down towards the upper pole of the thyroid gland. However, in c.15% of cases, it arises directly from the external carotid artery between the origins of the superior thyroid and lingual arteries. The superior laryngeal artery runs down towards the larynx, with the internal branch of the superior laryngeal nerve lying above it. It enters the larynx by penetrating the thyrohyoid membrane and divides into a number of branches which supply the larynx from the tip of the epiglottis down to the inferior margin of thyroarytenoid. It supplies the larynx, and anastomoses with its fellow and the inferior laryngeal branch of the inferior thyroid artery.

The cricothyroid artery arises from the superior thyroid artery and may contribute to the supply of the larynx. It follows a variable course either superficial or deep to sternothyroid. If superficial, it may be accompanied by branches of the ansa cervicalis, and if deep, it may be related to the external laryngeal nerve. It can anastomose with the artery of the opposite side and with the laryngeal arteries.

INFERIOR LARYNGEAL ARTERY

The inferior laryngeal artery is smaller than the superior laryngeal artery. It is a branch of the inferior thyroid artery, which arises from the thyrocervical trunk of the subclavian artery. It ascends on the trachea with the recurrent laryngeal nerve, enters the larynx at the lower border of the inferior constrictor, just behind the cricothyroid articulation, and supplies the laryngeal muscles and mucosa. It anastomoses with its contralateral fellow, and with the superior laryngeal branch of the superior thyroid artery.

A posterior laryngeal artery of variable size has been described as a regular feature that arises as an internal branch of the inferior thyroid artery.

SUPERIOR AND INFERIOR LARYNGEAL VEINS

Venous return from the larynx occurs via superior and inferior laryngeal veins which run parallel to the laryngeal arteries. They are tributaries of the superior and inferior thyroid veins respectively. The superior thyroid vein drains into the internal jugular vein and the inferior thyroid vein usually into the left brachiocephalic vein.

LYMPHATIC DRAINAGE (Fig. 36.14)

The lymph vessels draining the supraglottic part of the larynx above the vocal cords accompany the superior laryngeal artery, pierce the thyrohyoid membrane, and end in the upper deep cervical lymph nodes, often bilaterally. The supraglottic lymphatics also communicate with those at the base of the tongue. The vocal cords with their firmly bound mucosa and paucity of lymphatics provide a clear demarcation between the upper and lower areas of the larynx. Below the vocal cords, some of the lymph vessels pass through the cricovocal membrane to reach the prelaryngeal (Delphian) and/or pretracheal lymph nodes. Others run with the inferior laryngeal artery to join the lower deep cervical nodes.

Spread of supra- and subglottic tumours

The upper deep cervical lymph nodes act as pathways of spread for malignant tumours of the supraglottic larynx: up to 40% of these tumours will have undergone such spread at the time of clinical presentation. The glottis is very poorly endowed with lymphatic vessels, which means that 95% of malignant tumours confined to the glottis will present with a change in voice or airway obstruction but will not show signs of spread to adjacent lymph nodes at presentation. Tumours of the subglottic larynx will often spread to the paratracheal lymph node chain prior to clinical presentation. However, the presenting symptoms may be voice change and airway obstruction rather than a mass in the neck, because the paratracheal lymph nodes occupy a deep seated position in the root of the neck and so their enlargement may remain occult.

INNERVATION (Fig. 36.15)

The larynx is innervated by the internal and external branches of the superior laryngeal nerve, the recurrent laryngeal nerve and sympathetic nerves. The internal laryngeal nerve is sensory, the external laryngeal nerve is motor, and the recurrent laryngeal nerve is mixed. The internal laryngeal nerve is sensory down to the vocal cords, the recurrent laryngeal nerve is sensory below the vocal cords, and there is overlap between the territories innervated by the two nerves at the vocal cords. All the intrinsic muscles of the larynx are supplied by the recurrent laryngeal nerve except for cricothyroid, which is supplied by the external laryngeal nerve.

The detailed course of the vagus in the neck is described on page 556.

SUPERIOR LARYNGEAL NERVE

The superior laryngeal nerve arises from the middle of the inferior vagal ganglion, and in its course receives one or more communications from the superior cervical sympathetic ganglion: most frequently, the connection is with the external laryngeal nerve. The superior laryngeal nerve divides into two branches, a smaller external and a larger internal branch, c.1.5 cm below the ganglion: rarely both branches may arise from the ganglion.

Internal laryngeal nerve

The internal laryngeal nerve passes forwards c.7 mm before piercing the thyrohyoid membrane, usually at a higher level than the superior thyroid artery. It splits into superior, middle and inferior branches on entering the larynx. The superior branch supplies the mucosa of the piriform fossa. The large middle branch is distributed to the mucosa of the ventricle, specifically the quadrangular membrane, and therefore probably conveys the afferent component of the cough reflex. The inferior ramus is mainly distributed to the mucosa of the ventricle and subglottic cavity. On the medial wall of the piriform fossa, descending branches give twigs to the interarytenoid muscle and share communicating branches with the recurrent laryngeal nerve. The precise nature and function of these communicating nerves have yet to be determined.

External laryngeal nerve

The external laryngeal nerve continues downwards and forwards on the lateral surface of the inferior constrictor to which it contributes some small branches. In c.30% of cases, the nerve is located within the fibres of the constrictor muscle. It passes beneath the attachment of sternothyroid to the oblique line of the thyroid cartilage and supplies cricothyroid. A communicating nerve continues from the posterior

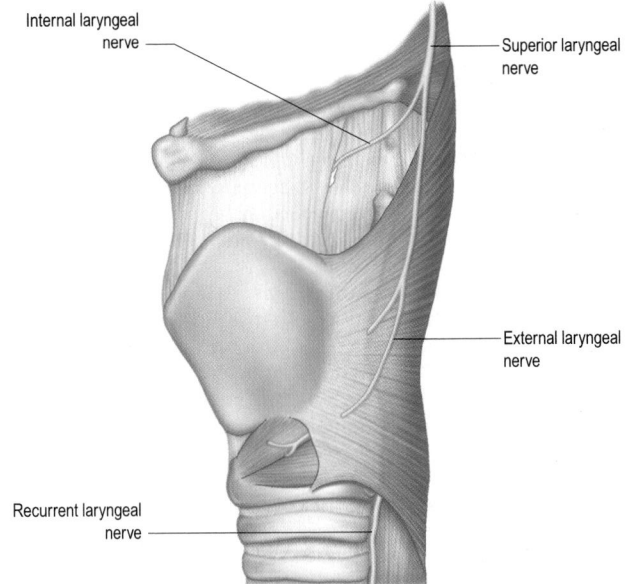

Fig. 36.15 Nerve supply to the larynx. (Adapted from Oxford Textbook of Functional Anatomy, Vol 3 Head and Neck, MacKinnon P, Morris J (eds), 1990. By permission of Oxford University Press.)

surface of cricothyroid, crosses the piriform fossa and enters thyro-arytenoid where it anastomoses with branches from the recurrent laryngeal nerve. It has been suggested that these communicating branches may provide both additional motor components to thyroarytenoid and sensory fibres to the mucosa in the region of the subglottis.

The close relationship of the external laryngeal nerve to the superior thyroid artery puts the nerve at potential risk when the artery is clamped during thyroid lobectomy. The external laryngeal nerve is potentially at risk where it is either particularly close to the artery (in c.20% of cases), or where, instead of crossing the superior thyroid vessels c.1 cm or more above the superior pole of the gland, it actually passes below this point (in c.20% of cases).

RECURRENT LARYNGEAL NERVE

The upper part of the recurrent laryngeal nerve has a close but variable relationship to the inferior thyroid artery: it may pass in front of, behind, or parallel to, the artery. The nerve enters the larynx either by passing deep to (in two-thirds of cases) or between (in one-third of cases) the fibres of cricopharyngeus at its attachment to the lateral aspect of the cricoid cartilage. It supplies cricopharyngeus as it passes. At this point, the nerve is in intimate proximity to the posteromedial aspect of the thyroid gland. The main trunk divides into two or more branches, usually below the lower border of the inferior constrictor, although branching may occur higher up. The anterior branch is mainly motor and sometimes called the inferior laryngeal nerve, and the posterior branch is mainly sensory. The inferior laryngeal nerve passes posterior to the cricothyroid joint and its ligament. In this region, more often than not it may be covered by fibres of posterior cricoarytenoid.

The first ramus of the main motor branch of the recurrent laryngeal nerve innervates posterior cricoarytenoid. It continues and innervates interarytenoid and then lateral cricoarytenoid, before it terminates in thyroarytenoid. Communications exist between the superior laryngeal nerve and its branches and the recurrent laryngeal nerve, and a communicating branch reaches the superior laryngeal nerve via the ansa Galeni.

The recurrent laryngeal nerve does not always lie in a protected position in the tracheo-oesophageal groove, but may be slightly anterior to it (more often on the right), and it may be markedly lateral to the trachea at the level of the lower part of the thyroid gland. On the right the nerve is as often anterior to, or posterior to, or intermingled with, the terminal branches of the inferior thyroid artery. On the left the nerve is usually posterior to the artery, though occasionally anterior to it. The nerve may supply extralaryngeal branches to the larynx, which arise before it passes behind the inferior thyroid cornu.

Outside its capsule the thyroid gland has a distinct covering of pretracheal fascia which splits into two layers at the posterior border of the gland (p. 542). One layer covers the entire medial surface of its lobe and, at or just above the isthmus, has a conspicuous thickening, the lateral ligament of the thyroid gland, which attaches the gland to the trachea and the lower part of the cricoid cartilage. The other layer is posterior; it passes behind the oesophagus and pharynx and is attached to the prevertebral fascia (p. 542). In this way, a compartment is formed on each side, lateral to the trachea and oesophagus, and the recurrent laryngeal nerve and terminal parts of the inferior thyroid artery lie in the fat of this compartment. The nerve may be lateral or medial to the lateral ligament of the thyroid gland, or sometimes may be embedded in it.

An unusual anomaly that is of relevance to laryngeal pathology and surgery is the so-called 'non-recurrent' laryngeal nerve. In this condition, which has a frequency of between 0.3–1%, only the right side is affected and it is always associated with an abnormal origin of the right subclavian artery from the aortic arch on the left side. The right recurrent laryngeal nerve arises directly from the vagus nerve trunk high up in the neck and enters the larynx close to the inferior pole of the thyroid gland. If unrecognized, it may be susceptible to injury during surgery, as well as potentially being compressed by small tumours of the thyroid gland.

AUTONOMIC SUPPLY TO THE LARYNX

Parasympathetic, secretomotor fibres run with both the superior and recurrent laryngeal nerves to mucous glands throughout the larynx. Postganglionic sympathetic fibres run to the larynx with its blood supply, and have their origin in the superior and middle cervical ganglia.

VAGAL NERVE LESIONS AND RECURRENT LARYNGEAL NERVE PARALYSIS

Unilateral complete palsy of the recurrent laryngeal nerve (more commonly on the left side due to its increased length) leads to isolated paralysis of all the laryngeal muscles on the affected side with the exception of cricothyroid (supplied by the external laryngeal nerve). The patient may be asymptomatic or have a hoarse, breathy voice. The hoarseness may be permanent or may become less severe with time as the opposite cord develops the ability to hyperadduct and appose the paralysed cord and thus close the glottis during phonation and coughing.

Clinically, the position of the vocal cord in the acute phase after section of the recurrent laryngeal nerve is very variable. Stridor is more common after bilateral lesions but by no means the rule; indeed the cords may be sufficiently abducted for there to be little problem with airway obstruction, although the voice is always weaker in this situation. With chronic lesions the cords lie more widely separated, which leads to a weakened voice but a more secure upper airway. Variation in the position of paralysed vocal cords in more chronic lesions is probably more related to the degree of associated atrophy and fibrosis of paraglottic muscles than to the relative degrees of weakness and denervation of the apposing adductor and abductor muscle groups.

For many years conventional wisdom was that movements of abduction were affected more than those of adduction when the recurrent laryngeal nerve was partially lesioned (Semon's law). However, it is now recognized that it is difficult to predict the effect that partial lesions of the recurrent laryngeal nerve will have on vocal cord position. Modern studies of human recurrent laryngeal nerve anatomy show that the fibres are randomly arranged in the nerve, which probably contributes to the difficulty in regaining co-ordinated vocal cord movement despite careful microsurgical re-anastomosis of a nerve that has been cut, e.g. after trauma or during laryngeal transplantation.

Involvement of the superior laryngeal nerve in addition to the recurrent laryngeal nerve suggests a lesion proximal to the inferior (nodose) ganglion. This results in paralysis of all laryngeal musculature (including cricothyroid). The affected cord is paralysed and lies in the so-called 'cadaveric' position halfway between abduction and adduction. If the lesion is unilateral the voice is weak and hoarse, but if it is bilateral phonation is almost absent, the vocal pitch cannot be altered and the cough is weak and ineffective.

There is debate as to the effect of lesions of the external laryngeal nerve. Complete section is most likely during the ligation of the vessels forming the vascular pedicle of the thyroid gland during thyroid lobectomy. This often but not always causes a weakening of the voice and mild hoarseness, and sometimes the effect is not really noticeable. Bilateral lesions produce these effects more often than not.

ANATOMY OF SPEECH

During its evolution, the larynx has developed a complex musculo-skeletal structure and refined mechanism of neuromuscular control. These mechanisms allow the larynx to modify the expiratory stream to produce highly complex patterns of sound of varying loudness, frequency and duration, in addition to its sphincteric functions for the protection and control of respiratory activities. The ability to execute these complex movements depends largely on the cerebral hemispheres in which specific parts are involved in the motor aspects of language, such as speech and writing, and sensory manifestations of language, including reading and understanding the spoken word.

SPEECH PRODUCTION

The production of any sound requires a source of energy: for the human voice this is the momentum of the expired air. Structures which can vibrate are also required to produce noise (phonation) in the majority of speech sounds in English. A series of resonators that can interrupt, dampen or amplify certain sound frequencies modify the exhaled airstream into its final form (articulation).

During speech, it is necessary to exert a force sufficient to produce a pressure in the order of 7 cm H_2O beneath the vocal cords (subglottal pressure) to make them vibrate. The subglottal pressure can be increased up to 60 cm H_2O in loud speech or singing. Variations in subglottal pressure mainly affect the loudness but can also influence the pitch of the voice. Vibration of air in the vocal tract superior to the larynx is due primarily to the activity of the vocal cords. Resonance in the larynx above the vocal cords and in the pharynx, mouth and nasal cavity selectively amplifies or dampens certain harmonics. Interruption of airflow through the resonators by articulatory organs, (the lips, tongue, teeth and soft palate), modifies the egressive airstream to produce distinct units of speech (phonemes).

MUSCULAR CONTROL OF THE AIRSTREAM

The expiratory force used in speech is produced by the controlled relaxation of the respiratory muscles to counteract passive elastic recoil of the lungs and thoracic wall. After a rapid inspiration, the intercostal muscles are relaxed slowly to prolong the expiratory phase of respiration as long as the desired utterance. The internal intercostal muscles contract towards the end of the utterance to maintain subglottal pressure as lung air volume nears its resting expiratory level. These muscles also make small contractions to vary the expiratory force and hence the loudness of individual words or phrases for emphasis. The anterior abdominal muscles which are used in prolonged and forced expiration, and in some subjects at the end of quiet respiration, may be involved in speech, especially in singing, shouting and in attempts to speak without the pause necessary for inspiration. Contrary to popular belief, the diaphragm plays little part in regulation of expiratory force. Unlike the intercostal muscles, the diaphragmatic musculature is sparsely supplied with muscle spindles, and therefore control of the diaphragm is poorly regulated: minute changes can be effected more successfully using the intercostal and anterior abdominal muscles.

The pulmonic airstream is the source of energy in normal speech. However, after removal of the larynx, e.g. following laryngeal cancer, patients can be taught to swallow air, store it in a segment of the oesophagus and use it as the energy source (oesophageal speech). Speech in these circumstances tends to have a belching quality and may be badly phrased. Laryngectomy patients always produce phrases that are shorter than normal, and so prostheses incorporating valves and surgical shunts are often inserted to provide a larger egressive airstream by diverting air from the respiratory tract into the oesophagus.

PHONATION

The default position of the rima glottidis is open to maintain patency of the airway during respiration. In quiet respiration, the anterior intermembranous part of the rima glottidis is triangular when viewed from above (see **Fig. 36.10**). Its apex is anterior and its base posterior, and it is represented by an imaginary line c.8 mm long connecting the anterior ends of the arytenoid vocal processes. The intercartilaginous part between the medial surfaces of the arytenoids is rectangular as the two vocal processes lie parallel to each other. During forced respiration, the rima glottidis is widened and the vocal cords are fully abducted to increase the airway. The arytenoid cartilages rotate laterally, and this moves their vocal processes apart, and converts the rima glottidis into a diamond shape in which both intermembranous and intercartilaginous parts are triangular. The greatest width of the rima glottidis is at the point of the attachments of the vocal cords to the vocal processes.

Phonation is necessary for all vowels and a number of consonants in spoken English. Preparatory to phonation, both the intermembranous and intercartilaginous parts of the glottis are adducted, reducing the space between the vocal cords to a linear chink. This position of the vocal cords is achieved by adduction and medial rotation of the arytenoids at the cricoarytenoid joints. Contraction of the lateral cricoarytenoids produces rotatory movements and the transverse arytenoids bring about gliding. The mucous membrane covering the interarytenoid muscles, the interarytenoid fold, intrudes into the larynx when these muscles adduct the arytenoids, and so aids closure of the intercartilaginous part of the rima glottidis. The vocal cords are also tensed, an essential prerequisite for vibration. If sufficient subglottal pressure is generated below the vocal cords after closure and tensing of the glottis, they will be forced apart. The fall in pressure due to their separation and the continued adductor muscle activity result in closure of the glottis. Closure is assisted by the suction effect of the fall in pressure (the Bernoulli effect). During the rapid opening and closing of the glottis, the vocal cords exhibit longitudinal and transverse waves due to their structure. These add harmonics to the fundamental frequency of the tone produced.

The fundamental frequency of the human voice is determined by the resting length of the vocal cords. It varies with age and sex. The frequency range of human speech is from 60–500 Hz with an average of c.120 Hz in males, 200 Hz in females and 270 Hz in children. Variations in frequency (pitch changes) during an utterance are determined by the complex interrelationships between length, tension and thickness of the vocal cords. It must be emphasized that one of these variables cannot be altered without affecting the other two parameters to some extent. Gross changes to the vocal cords demonstrate the effects of these variables. Inflamed and swollen vocal cords are much thicker than normal and result in a hoarse voice. At puberty, growth of the thyroid cartilage in males lengthens the vocal cords and lowers the fundamental frequency: the voice 'breaks' as a result. During panic, the vocal cords may be tensed, which means that the cry for help is a high-pitched squeak.

Pitch is altered by increasing length. At first sight this may seem counterintuitive, but, as the vocal cords are lengthened, there will be a consequent thinning and change in tension. Although an analogy is often drawn between the vocal cords and vibrating strings, a better analogy is a rubber band: if a rubber band is lengthened, the tension will increase, but the thickness will decrease. The vocal cords may be lengthened by up to 50% of their resting length. It is likely that the initial pitch setting is achieved by action of the cricothyroids, and that fine adjustments can then be made using the vocalis muscles. Paralysis of both cricothyroids, which is usually associated with damage to the origins of the superior laryngeal nerve in the vagal nuclei in brainstem stroke, results in permanent hoarseness and inability to vary the pitch of the voice. It is important to remember that once the vocal cords are set in motion they will deviate from their original setting as they vibrate. Auditory feedback of the sounds produced is used to make minute compensatory adjustments to length, tension and thickness to maintain a constant pitch.

Any lengthening of the vocal cords tends to thin them. The thickness can be increased by the vocalis part of thyroarytenoid. Because of its attachment to the vocal ligament, vocalis shortens and relaxes the vocal cords while increasing their thickness. Changes in tension of the vocal cords are produced by the same muscles that change their length, namely cricothyroid, posterior cricoarytenoid and vocalis, probably acting isometrically. In whispering, the intermembranous glottis is closed, but the intercartilaginous part remains widely patent, so that air escapes freely and phonation ceases.

FREQUENCY CHARACTERISTICS OF SPEECH

The sound produced by the mechanism described above is not a pure tone because several harmonics at multiples of the fundamental frequency will also be generated. Harmonics give a note of a particular frequency its defining characteristics. An 'A' played on an oboe or violin is immediately recognizable because of the different harmonics generated by the design of the instrument. In the human vocal tract, the fundamental frequency and its harmonics are transmitted to the column of air which extends from the vocal cords to the exterior, mainly through the mouth. A significant air stream also passes through the nasal cavities during articulation of the nasal consonants /m/, /n/ and /E/ ('ŋg'), as in 'mincing' (/mNnsNE/), when the soft palate is depressed to allow air into the nasopharynx. The supraglottal tract acts as a selective resonator but unlike, for example, an organ pipe, it is variable in length, shape and volume. These parameters may be altered by the muscles of the pharynx, soft palate, fauces, tongue, cheeks and lips. The relative positions of the upper and lower teeth, which are determined by the degree of opening and protrusion or retraction of the mandible, also have an effect. In addition, the tension of the walls of the column can be altered, especially in the pharynx. The result is that the fundamental frequency (pitch) and harmonics produced by the passage of air through the glottis are modified by changes in the supraglottal tract. Harmonics may be amplified, or dampened. The fundamental frequency and its associated harmonics may also be raised or lowered by appropriate elevation or depression of the hyoid bone and the larynx as a unit by the selective actions of the extrinsic laryngeal musculature, namely, the inferior pharyngeal constrictor, the infrahyoid and suprahyoid muscles. Effectively, these movements shorten or lengthen the resonating column, and to some extent also alter the geometry of the walls of the air passages. Analysis of the human voice shows that it has a very similar pattern of harmonics for all fundamental frequencies, determined by the vocal tract acting as a selective filter and resonator. This is necessary for the maintenance of a constant quality of voice without which intelligibility would be lost. For example, recorded speech played back without its harmonics is completely unintelligible. Each human voice is unique and recognizable as belonging to a particular person because of its special characteristics. Indeed, it has been suggested that the unique frequency spectrum of each individual voice could be used for personal identification.

ARTICULATION

During articulation the egressive airstream is given a rapidly changing specific quality by the articulatory organs, the tongue, palate, teeth, lips and nasal cavity. The discipline of phonetics primarily deals with the way in which speech sounds are produced, and consequently with the analysis of the mode of production of phonemes by the vocal apparatus. In order to analyse the way in which the articulators are used in different speech sounds, words are broken down into units called phonemes, which are defined as the minimal sequential contrastive units used in any language.

The human vocal tract can produce many more phonemes than are employed in any one language. Not all languages have the same phonemes. Even within the same language, the phonemes can vary in different parts of the same country and in other countries where that language is also spoken. Anyone who has tried to learn a foreign language knows how difficult it can be to reproduce phonemes that are not used in their native speech because such phonemes require unfamiliar positioning of the speech organs. A native speaker of any language can quickly recognize the origins of anyone attempting to use their language as a second language. The second language speaker will usually speak it with an accent characteristic of their own first language because they are using the familiar configurations of their vocal tract for each phoneme instead of the correct positioning.

PRODUCTION OF VOWELS

All vowel sounds require phonation by vibration of the vocal cords. Each vowel sound has its own characteristic higher harmonics (frequency spectrum) because the pharyngeal and oral cavities act as selective resonators to amplify or dampen different harmonics. These frequencies are always higher multiples of the fundamental frequencies and are called formants.

The sounds of the different vowels are determined by the shape and size of the mouth, and the positions of the tongue and lips are the most important variables. The tongue may be placed high or low (close and open vowels), or further forwards or back (front and back vowels) and the lips may be rounded or spread.

PRODUCTION OF CONSONANTS

Consonants may be defined as speech sounds that are determined by the closure or narrowing of some part of the vocal tract to stop or perturb the airflow. If a consonant is sounded without vibration of the vocal cords, it is defined as unvoiced, while if phonation is a component, it is voiced. There are many pairs of unvoiced and voiced consonants formed by using exactly the same parts of the speech organs, for example (with the voiceless consonant first in each case) /p/ and /b/, /t/ and /d/, /k/ and /g/, /f/ and /v/. Probably the most graphical example is /s/ and /z/. If the larynx is loosely palpated while making a sustained unvoiced 'ssssss' sound, no vibration is felt but if the 'ssssss' is commuted into a prolonged voiced 'zzzzzz' then vibration in the larynx should be readily detectable. The position of the tongue and other articulators is exactly the same for both /s/ and /z/, only the presence or absence of phonation making a difference between them.

Consonants are further classified according to the parts of the speech organs involved, i.e. lips, tongue, teeth and palate, and their positions. For example, /p/ and /b/ are bilabial, the upper and lower lips being approximated to produce them; whereas /f/ and /v/ are labiodental, the lower lip being raised to contact the upper incisor teeth. For the purposes of phonetic analysis, the articulatory organs can be subdivided into a number of regions. For example, the tongue is divided into the tip, anterior edge, the front part of the dorsum, the centre and back parts of the remaining dorsum, and a most posterior part (the root). In some cases, these bear no obvious relationship to the anatomical parts of the tongue but they are useful in describing the part of the dorsum of the tongue contacting other areas of the mouth.

Consonants may be further subclassified by their mechanism of production. A plosive is defined as a consonant requiring sudden explosive release of air e.g. /p/ and /b/. A fricative is a rustling of the breath due to friction as the air column passes through a considerable narrowing of the oral cavity. During articulation of /f/ and /v/, for example, the lower lip is approximated to the upper teeth, without complete closure. An affricate is defined as a plosive followed by a fricative as /ch/ in chain; the 'ch' component is phonetically a plosive /t/ followed by fricative /sh/. A full phonetic description of the phoneme /b/ is a voiced bilabial plosive.

REFERENCES

Berkovitz BKB, Moxham BJ, Hickey S 2000 The anatomy of the larynx. In: Ferlito A (ed) Diseases of the Larynx. London: Chapman and Hall: 25–44.

Durham FC, Harrison TS 1962 The surgical anatomy of the superior laryngeal nerve. Surg Gynecol Obstet 118: 33–44.

Erkki A, Pitkanen R, Suominen H 1987 Observations on the structure and the biomechanics of the cricothyroid articulation. Acta Otolaryngol (Stockh) 103: 117–26.

Friedman M, Toriumi DM, Grybauskas V, Katz A 1986 Nonrecurrent laryngeal nerves and their clinical significance. Laryngoscope 96: 87–90.

Kirchner JA, Carter D 1987 Intralaryngeal barriers to the spread of cancer. Acta Otolaryngol (Stockh) 103: 503–13

Munir Turk L, Hogg DA 1993 Age changes in the human laryngeal cartilages. Clin Anat 6: 154–62.
Provides data concerning the distribution of areas of calcification that occur with age within the cartilages of the larynx.

Pracy R 1983 The infant larynx. J Laryngol Otol 97: 933–47.
Draws attention to features that differ from the adult condition and that may have clinical significance.

Reidenbach MM 1995 Normal topography of the conus elasticus. Anatomical bases for the spread of laryngeal cancer. Surg Radiol Anat 17: 107–11.

Reidenbach MM 1996a The periepiglottic space: topographic relations and histological organisation. J Anat 188: 173–82.

Reidenbach MM 1996b The paraglottic space and transglottic cancer: anatomic considerations. Clin Anat 9: 244–51.

Reidenbach MM 1998 Subglottic region: normal topography and possible clinical implications. Clin Anat 11:9–21.
The four papers by Reidenbach are based on serial reconstruction of sections derived from plastinated material.

Sato I, Shimada K 1995 Arborization of the inferior laryngeal nerve and internal nerve on the posterior surface of the larynx. Clin Anat 8: 379–87.
Discusses the possible clinical significance of connections between the inferior (recurrent) laryngeal nerve and the internal laryngeal nerve.

Welsh LW, Welsh JJ, Rizzo TA 1983 Laryngeal spaces and lymphatics: current anatomic concepts. Ann Otol Rhinol Laryngol Suppl 105: 19–31.
Describes the 'tissue spaces' and lymphatic drainage of the larynx and their importance in determining the route of spread of tumours.

Development of the pharynx, larynx and oesophagus

PHARYNX

Pharyngeal endoderm is in contact with and develops from, mesenchyme and epithelia from neural crest, paraxial mesenchyme of the somitomeres, somites, lateral plate mesenchyme (which at this level is unsplit), cleft ectoderm, general endothelium and the outflow tract of the heart. The mechanism of formation of the pharynx, which is complex, is known to be intimately related to the development of the viscerocranium (Chapter 26) and laryngeal cartilages (Chapters 26, 37): it is likely that some of the processes are regulated by *Hox* gene expression (**Fig. 26.5**).

The distal foregut, and the midgut and hindgut consist of a serous or adventitial layer, a layer of splanchnopleuric mesenchyme – which is derived from the splanchnopleuric coelomic epithelium – and an inner endodermal epithelium. In contrast, the proximal foregut contains a mixture of striated muscle in the upper pharynx, which blends with the smooth muscle of the gut wall within the territory of middle third of the oesophagus. A novel mesenchymal population which develops in a rostrocaudal and lateromedial sequence has been identified at the interface between the endoderm and the paraxial mesenchyme of the somitomeres and occipital somites. It starts as a sparse layer, becomes denser prior to the formation of endothelial networks, and ultimately forms a fenestrated mesenchymal monolayer between developing blood vessels and the endoderm. Later it expands between the notochord and the roof of the foregut, and may participate in the formation of pharyngeal and oesophageal smooth muscle and connective tissues.

NASOPHARYNX

The nasopharynx represents the most rostral portion of the original stomodeum derived from endoderm. The dorsal part of the ectodermal aspect of the first (maxillomandibular) arch contributes to the formation of the lateral wall of the nasopharynx in front of the orifice of the pharyngotympanic tube. This region is the zone of transition of ectoderm to endoderm which passes from the junction of the anterior two-thirds and posterior one-third of the tongue to the developing sella turcica in the sphenoid bone.

OROPHARYNX

The development of the palate subdivides the primitive pharynx so that the original arches and pouches are widely separated. The site of the second arch is partly indicated by the palatoglossal arch; however, the forward growth of the third arch obliterates the middle portion of the second arch and separates its dorsal and ventral ends. The second pharyngeal pouch is represented by the intra-tonsillar cleft, around which the tonsil develops. The third arch forms the lateral glossoepiglottic fold. The ventral ends of the fourth arches fuse with the caudal part of the hypobranchial eminence and so contribute to the formation of the epiglottis. The adjoining portion becomes connected to the arytenoid swelling and may be identified in the aryepiglottic fold.

LARYNGOPHARYNX

After the caudal part of the hypobranchial eminence has separated from the pharyngeal (posterior) part of the tongue (**Figs 26.2, 34.7**), it is in continuity with two linear ridges which appear in the ventral wall of the pharynx. Together these structures form an inverted U, sometimes regarded as an independent formation, the furcula (of His). The ridges have been identified as the sixth arches, and are placed very obliquely owing to the shortness of the pharyngeal floor compared with the greater extent of the roof. They are carried downwards on the ventral wall of the foregut and bound the median laryngotracheal groove, from which the lower part of the larynx, the trachea, bronchi and lungs are developed.

LYMPHOID TISSUE IN THE PHARYNX

The pharyngeal endoderm gives rise to a series of lymphoid organs, namely, the adenoid (pharyngeal tonsil), lateral pharyngeal lymphoid bands, tubal tonsil, lingual tonsils and palatine tonsils, and the thymus (p. 617).

NEONATAL PHARYNX

In the neonate the pharynx is one-third of the relative length in the adult. The nasopharynx is a narrow tube which curves gradually to join the oropharynx without any sharp junctional demarcation. An oblique angle is formed at this junction by 5 years of age and in the adult the nasopharynx and oropharynx join at almost a right angle.

LARYNX

The larynx is probably formed from the lower two pharyngeal arches, although the exact contribution of the sixth arch is still not clear. It lies at the cranial end of the laryngotracheal groove, where it is bounded laterally by the ventral ends of the sixth arches and ventrally by the caudal part of the hypobranchial eminence (**Figs 34.7A&B, 26.2**). Paired arytenoid swellings appear in the ventral ends of the sixth arches, one on each side of the cranial end of the groove. As they enlarge they approximate to each other and to the caudal part of the hypobranchial eminence where the epiglottis develops. The opening into the larynx, at first a vertical slit, is converted into a T-shaped cleft by the enlargement of the arytenoid swellings. The vertical limb of the T lies between the two swellings and its horizontal limb lies between them and the epiglottis. The arytenoid swellings differentiate into the arytenoid and corniculate cartilages (**Fig. 26.7**), and the ridges that join them to the epiglottis become the definitive aryepiglottic folds within which the cuneiform cartilages differentiate from the epiglottis. The thyroid cartilage develops from the ventral ends of the cartilages of the fourth, or fourth and fifth, pharyngeal arches. The cartilage appears as two lateral plates, each chondrified from two centres and united in the midventral line by a fibrous membrane within which an additional centre of chondrification develops. The cricoid cartilage arises from two cartilaginous centres, which soon unite ventrally, gradually extend and ultimately fuse on the dorsal surface of the tube as the cricoid lamina (p. 634).

OESOPHAGUS

An anterior midline lung bud diverticulum first appears at stage 12. By stage 14 the cells of the splanchnopleuric mesenchyme that surrounds the developing trachea and oesophagus are sufficiently diverged in their inductive ability to promote the characteristics of the two different tubes. During stage 17 the oesophageal epithelium is surrounded by a wide submucosal zone and muscular coats can be distinguished. The oesophagus can be distinguished from the stomach at stage 13 (embryo 5 mm). It elongates during successive stages and its absolute length increases more rapidly than that of the embryo as a whole. The oesophagus is invested by splanchnopleuric mesenchyme cranially posterior to the developing trachea, and more caudally between the developing lungs and pericardioperitoneal canals posterior to the pericardium. Caudal to the pericardium, the pregastric segment of the oesophagus acquires a short thick dorsal meso-oesophagus from splanchnopleuric mesenchyme, and a short ventral mesogastrium from the cranial stratum of the mesenchyme of the septum transversum (Ch. 90). The oesophagus has a limited relationship to primary coelomic epithelium. However, it is related to secondary extensions from the primary coelom via the para-oesophageal right and left pneumatoenteric recesses (**Fig. 90.7**), the oblique sinus of the pericardium, and, in the lower thorax, to the mediastinal pleura.

By stage 15 (week 5), the mucosa consists of two layers of cells: their proliferation never occludes the lumen. The mucosa is lined with a ciliated epithelium at 10 weeks, and a stratified squamous epithelium at the end of the 5th month. Occasional patches of ciliated epithelium have been described at birth. Circular muscle can be seen at stage 15, but longitudinal muscle has not been identified until stage 21. Neuroblasts can be demonstrated at relatively early developmental stages, thus myenteric plexuses display cholinesterase activity by 9.5 weeks and

ganglion cells differentiate by 13 weeks. The oesophagus may be capable of peristalsis in the first trimester.

At birth the oesophagus extends 8–10 cm from the cricoid cartilage to the gastric cardiac orifice. It commences and ends 1–2 vertebrae higher than in the adult, and extends from between the fourth to the sixth cervical vertebrae to the level of the ninth thoracic vertebra. Its average diameter is 5 mm and it possesses the constrictions seen in the adult. The narrowest constriction is at its junction with the pharynx, where the inferior pharyngeal constrictor functions to constrict the lumen, and in this region it may be traumatized with instruments or catheters. Peristalsis along the oesophagus and at the lower oesophageal sphincter is immature at birth, which probably accounts for the frequent regurgitation of food that occurs in the newborn period. The pressure at the lower oesophageal sphincter approaches that of the adult at 36 weeks of age.

External and middle ear

The ear can be subdivided into the external, middle and internal ear, all of which are associated with, or lie within, the temporal bone on the lateral aspect of the skull. Each ear is a distance receptor for the collection, conduction, modification, amplification and analysis of complex waves of sound. It also contains the receptors for hearing and balance.

EXTERNAL EAR

The external ear consists of the auricle, or pinna, and the external acoustic meatus. The auricle projects from the side of the head to collect sound waves, and the meatus leads inwards from the auricle to conduct vibrations to the tympanic membrane. These structures do not act merely as a simple ear-trumpet: they are the first of a series of stimulus modifiers in the auditory apparatus.

Skin

The skin of the auricle continues into the external acoustic meatus and covers the external surface of the tympanic membrane. It is thin, has no dermal papillae, and is closely adherent to the cartilaginous and osseous parts of the tube. Inflammation here is therefore very painful. The thick subcutaneous tissue of the cartilaginous part of the meatus contains numerous ceruminous glands which secrete ear wax, or cerumen. Their coiled tubular structure resembles that of sweat glands. The secretory cells are columnar when active, but cuboidal when quiescent. They are covered externally by myoepithelial cells. Ducts open either on to the epithelial surface or into the nearby sebaceous gland of a hair follicle. Cerumen prevents the maceration of meatal skin by trapped water. Overproduction or accumulation of wax may completely block the meatus or obstruct the vibration of the tympanic membrane. Although ceruminous glands and hair follicles are largely limited to the cartilaginous meatus, a few small glands and fine hairs also occur in the roof of the lateral part of the osseous meatus. The warm humid environment of the relatively enclosed meatal air aids the mechanical responses of the tympanic membrane.

Auricle (pinna) (Fig. 38.1)

The lateral surface of the auricle is irregularly concave, faces slightly forwards and displays numerous eminences and depressions. Its prominent curved rim, or helix, usually bears posterosuperiorly a small auricular tubercle, which is quite pronounced around the sixth month of intrauterine life. The antihelix is a curved prominence, parallel and anterior to the posterior part of the helix: it divides above into two crura which flank a depressed triangular fossa. The curved depression between the helix and antihelix is the scaphoid fossa. The antihelix encircles the deep, capacious concha of the auricle, which is incompletely divided by the crus or anterior end of the helix. The conchal area above this, the cymba conchae, overlies the suprameatal triangle of the temporal bone, which can be felt through it, and which overlies the mastoid antrum. The tragus is a small curved flap below the crus of the helix and in front of the concha: it projects posteriorly, partly overlapping the meatal orifice. The antitragus is a small tubercle opposite the tragus and separated from it by the intertragic incisure or notch. Below it is the lobule, composed of fibrous and adipose tissues. It is soft, unlike the majority of the auricle which is supported by elastic cartilage and is firm. The cranial surface of the auricle presents elevations which correspond to the depressions on its lateral surface, and after which they are named (e.g. eminentia conchae, eminentia fossae triangularis).

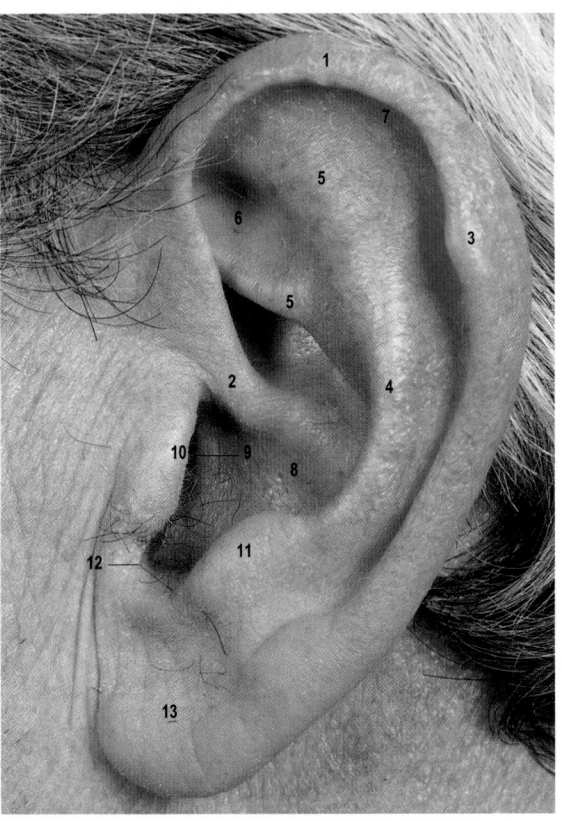

1. Helix.   2. Crus of helix.   3. Auricular tubercle.   4. Antihelix.   5. Crura of antihelix.
6. Triangular fossa.   7. Scaphoid fossa.   8. Concha of auricle.   9. External acoustic meatus.
10. Tragus.   11. Antitragus.   12. Intertragic notch.   13. Lobule of auricle.

Fig. 38.1 Lateral surface of auricle. (By permission from Berkovitz BKB, Moxham BJ 2002 Head and Neck Anatomy. London: Martin Dunitz.)

Cryptotia – Cryptotia or 'pocket ear' is an abnormality of the auricle where the upper part of the auricle is buried beneath the temporal skin. It is fairly easily mobilized into a more normal position surgically, and the posterior surface of the pinna is covered with skin from the post-auricular temporal skin.

Stahl's deformity – Stahl's deformity is a congenital deformity of the auricle where the helix is flattened and the upper crus of the antihelix is duplicated, which produces a ridge of cartilage running from the antihelix to the rim of the helix. This causes a pointing of the ear and a reversal of the normal concavity of the scaphoid fossa. It is easily corrected in the first 6 weeks of life by the application of external moulds, but thereafter the cartilage may be too stiff and a formal surgical correction may be necessary.

Pre-auricular sinus – The auricular tubercles, the embryological precursors of the auricle, arise around the dorsal end of the embryonic first branchial cleft from the first and second branchial arches. They fuse to form the auricle and surround the dorsal end of the first branchial cleft from which the external acoustic meatus arises. Sinuses and cysts are often found just anterior to the root of the helix, near to the point of fusion of the tubercles derived from the first branchial arch and those derived from the second branchial arch. There is debate as to whether the abnormalities are epithelial inclusions between the tubercles or remnants of the first branchial cleft. The sinuses may be simple pits or complex branching sinuses, and they occasionally extend deeply towards the external acoustic meatus so that they lie close to the facial nerve. Clinically they may become chronically infected and require surgical excision: this may be technically demanding surgery given the close proximity to the facial nerve.

CARTILAGINOUS FRAMEWORK OF THE AURICLE

The auricle is a single thin plate of elastic fibrocartilage covered by skin, its surface moulded by eminences and depressions (**Fig. 38.2**). It is connected to the surrounding parts by ligaments and muscles, and is continuous with the cartilage of the external acoustic meatus. There is no cartilage in the lobule or between the tragus and the crus of the helix, where the gap is filled by dense fibrous tissue. Anteriorly, where the helix curves upwards, there is a small cartilaginous projection, the spine of the helix. Its other extremity is prolonged inferiorly as the tail of the helix and it is separated from the antihelix by the fissura anti-tragohelicina. The cranial aspect of the cartilage bears the eminentia conchae and eminentia scaphae, which correspond to the depressions on the lateral surface. The two eminences are separated by a transverse furrow, the sulcus antihelicis transversus, which corresponds to the inferior crus of the antihelix on the lateral surface. The eminentia conchae is crossed by an oblique ridge, the ponticulus, for the attachment of auricularis posterior. There are two fissures in the auricular cartilage, one behind the crus helicis and another in the tragus.

LIGAMENTS OF THE AURICLE

There are two sets of ligaments associated with the auricle. Extrinsic ligaments connect the auricle with the temporal bone, and intrinsic ligaments connect individual auricular cartilages. There are two extrinsic ligaments, anterior and posterior. The anterior ligament extends from the tragus and the spine of the helix to the root of the zygomatic process of the temporal bone. The posterior ligament passes from the posterior surface of the concha to the lateral surface of the mastoid process. The chief intrinsic ligaments are first, a strong fibrous band which passes from the tragus to the helix completing the meatus anteriorly and forming part of the boundary of the concha; and second, a band which passes between the antihelix and the tail of the helix. Less prominent bands also exist on the cranial aspect of the auricle.

AURICULAR MUSCLES

Extrinsic auricular muscles connect the auricle to the skull and scalp and move the auricle as a whole, and intrinsic auricular muscles connect the different parts of the auricle.

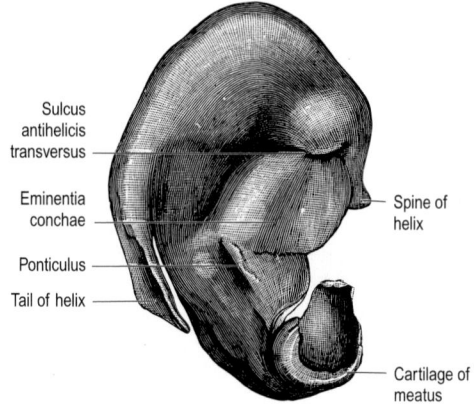

Sulcus
antihelicis
transversus

Eminentia
conchae

Ponticulus

Tail of helix

Spine of
helix

Cartilage of
meatus

Fig. 38.2 The cranial surface of the left auricular cartilage.

EXTRINSIC MUSCLES
The extrinsic auricular muscles are the auriculares anterior, superior and posterior. The auricularis anterior, the smallest of the three, is a thin fan of pale fibres, which arises from the lateral edge of the epicranial aponeurosis: its fibres converge to insert into the spine of the helix. The auricularis superior, the largest of the three, is also thin and fan-shaped and converges from the epicranial aponeurosis via a thin, flat tendon to attach to the upper part of the cranial surface of the auricle. The auricularis posterior consists of two or three fleshy fasciculi which arise by short aponeurotic fibres from the mastoid part of the temporal bone and insert into the ponticulus on the eminentia conchae.

Vascular supply – The arterial supply of the extrinsic auricular muscles is derived mainly from the posterior auricular artery.

Innervation – Auriculares anterior and superior are supplied by temporal branches of the facial nerve and auricularis posterior is supplied by the posterior auricular branch of the facial nerve.

Actions – In man these muscles have very little obvious effect. Auricularis anterior draws the auricle forwards and upwards; auricularis superior elevates the auricle slightly; auricularis posterior draws the auricle back. Despite the paucity of auricular movement, auditory stimuli may evoke patterned responses from these small muscles and electromyography can detect the 'crossed acoustic response' which is elicited by this means in investigative clinical neurology.

INTRINSIC MUSCLES
The intrinsic auricular muscles are helicis major and minor, tragicus, antitragicus, transversus auriculae and obliquus auriculae. Helicis major is a narrow vertical band on the anterior margin of the helix, which passes from its spine to its anterior border, where the helix is about to curve back. Helicis minor is an oblique fasciculus, which covers the crus helicis. Tragicus is a short, flattened, vertical band on the lateral aspect of the tragus. Antitragicus passes from the outer part of the antitragus to the tail of the helix and the antihelix. Transversus auriculae, on the cranial aspect of the auricle, consists of scattered fibres, partly ten-dinous, partly muscular, which extend between the eminentia conchae and the eminentia scaphae. Obliquus auriculae, also on the cranial aspect of the auricle, consists of a few fibres which extend from the upper and posterior parts of the eminentia conchae to the eminentia scaphae.

Vascular supply – The intrinsic auricular muscles are supplied by branches of the posterior auricular and superficial temporal arteries.

Innervation – The intrinsic auricular muscles on the lateral aspect of the auricle are innervated by the temporal branches of the facial nerve, and those on the cranial aspect of the auricle are innervated by the posterior auricular branch of the facial nerve.

Actions – The intrinsic muscles modify auricular shape minimally, if at all, in most human ears. However, rare individuals can modify the shape and position of their external ears.

VASCULAR SUPPLY AND LYMPHATIC DRAINAGE

Arteries – The posterior auricular branch of the external carotid artery supplies three or four branches to the cranial surface of the auricle: twigs from these arteries reach the lateral surface, some through fissures in the cartilage, others round the margin of the helix. The posterior auricular artery ascends between the parotid gland and the styloid process to the groove between the auricular cartilage and mastoid process. The auricle is also supplied by anterior auricular branches of the superficial temporal artery, which are distributed to its lateral surface, and by a branch from the occipital artery.

Veins – Auricular veins correspond to the arteries of the auricle. Arterio-venous anastomoses are numerous in the skin of the auricle and are thought to important in the regulation of core temperature.

Lymphatic drainage – Auricular lymphatics drain into the parotid lymph nodes, especially the node in front of the tragus; the upper deep cervical lymph nodes; and the mastoid lymph nodes.

INNERVATION

The sensory innervation of the auricle is complex and not fully determined. This is perhaps because the external ear represents an area where skin originally derived from a branchial region meets skin originally derived from a postbranchial region. The sensory nerves involved are: the great auricular nerve, which supplies most of the cranial surface and the posterior part of the lateral surface (helix, antihelix, lobule); the lesser occipital nerve, which supplies the upper part of the cranial surface; the auricular branch of the vagus, which supplies the concavity of the concha and posterior part of the eminentia; the auriculotemporal nerve, which supplies the tragus, crus of the helix and the adjacent part of the helix; and the facial nerve, which together with the auricular branch of the vagus probably supplies small areas on both aspects of the auricle, in the depression of the concha, and over its eminence. The details of the cutaneous innervation derived from the facial nerve require further clarification. It is possible that, as the auricular branch of the vagus traverses the temporal bone and crosses the facial canal c.4 mm above the stylomastoid foramen, it contributes an ascending branch to the facial nerve, which carries it to the pinna.

External acoustic meatus (Figs 38.3, 38.4)

The external acoustic meatus extends from the concha to the tympanic membrane. Its length is c.2.5 cm from the floor of the concha and c.4 cm from the tragus. It has two structurally different parts; the lateral third is cartilaginous and the medial two-thirds is osseous. It forms an S-shaped curve, directed at first medially, anteriorly and slightly up (pars externa), then posteromedially and up (pars media) and lastly anteromedially and slightly down (pars interna). It is oval in section, its greatest diameter is obliquely inclined posteroinferiorly at the external orifice, but is nearly horizontal at its medial end. There are two constrictions, one near the medial end of the cartilaginous part, the other, the isthmus, in the osseous part c.2 cm from the bottom of the concha. The tympanic membrane, which closes its medial end, is obliquely set and consequently the floor and the anterior wall of the meatus are longer than its roof and posterior wall.

The lateral, cartilaginous part is c.8 mm long. It is continuous with the auricular cartilage and attached by fibrous tissue to the circumference of the osseous part. This meatal cartilage is deficient posterosuperiorly, and the gap is occupied by a sheet of collagen. Two or three deep fissures exist in its anterior part – the fissures of Santorini.

The osseous part is c.16 mm long, and is narrower than the cartilaginous part. It is directed anteromedially and slightly downwards, with a slight posterosuperior convexity. Its medial end is smaller than the lateral end and it terminates obliquely. The anterior wall projects medially c.4 mm beyond the posterior and is marked, except above, by

a narrow tympanic sulcus, to which the perimeter of the tympanic membrane is attached. Its lateral end is dilated and mostly rough for the attachment of the meatal cartilage. The anterior, inferior, and most of the posterior, parts of the osseous meatus are formed by the tympanic element of the temporal bone, which in the fetus is only a tympanic ring. The posterosuperior region is formed by the squamous part of the temporal bone.

Relations of the meatus – The condylar process of the mandible lies anterior to the meatus and is partially separated from the cartilaginous part by a small portion of the parotid gland. A blow on the chin may cause the condyle to break into the meatus. The middle cranial fossa lies above the osseous meatus and the mastoid air cells are posterior to it, separated from the meatus only by a thin layer of bone. Its deepest part is situated below the epitympanic recess, and is anteroinferior to the mastoid antrum: the lamina of bone which separates it from the antrum is only 1–2 mm thick and provides the 'transmeatal approach' of aural surgery.

Vasculature and lymphatic drainage – The arterial supply of the external acoustic meatus is derived from the posterior auricular artery, the deep auricular branch of the maxillary artery and the auricular branches of the superficial temporal artery. Associated veins drain into the external jugular and maxillary veins and the pterygoid plexus. The lymphatics drain into those associated with the pinna.

Innervation – The sensory innervation of the external acoustic meatus is derived from the auriculotemporal branch of the mandibular nerve – which supplies the anterior and superior walls – and the auricular branch of the vagus – which supplies the posterior and inferior walls. The facial nerve may also contribute via its communication with the vagus nerve.

EXTERNAL SURGICAL APPROACHES TO THE MIDDLE EAR

Surgical access to the middle ear can be achieved via a variety of routes. Provided the external acoustic meatus is wide enough, the tympanic membrane can be elevated by incising the skin of the bony meatus circumferentially and then peeling the deep segment off the bone until the fibrous anulus of the tympanic membrane is visualized. This can then be elevated from the tympanic groove and the middle ear mucosa incised to allow the tympanic membrane to be reflected forwards. This approach, called the permeatal or tympanotomy approach, is used for stapedectomy, and limited middle ear work such as tympanic neurectomy for drooling.

If the external acoustic meatus is too narrow to allow adequate visualization of the middle ear, or if access is required to the mastoid aditus and antrum, it is necessary to displace the superficial soft tissues.

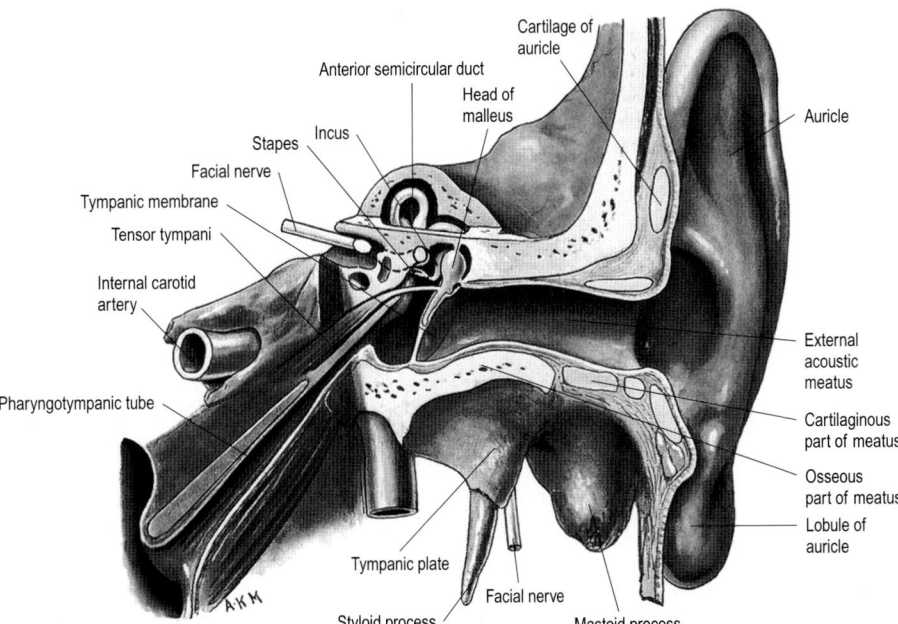

Fig. 38.3 The external and middle regions of the left ear: anterior aspect.

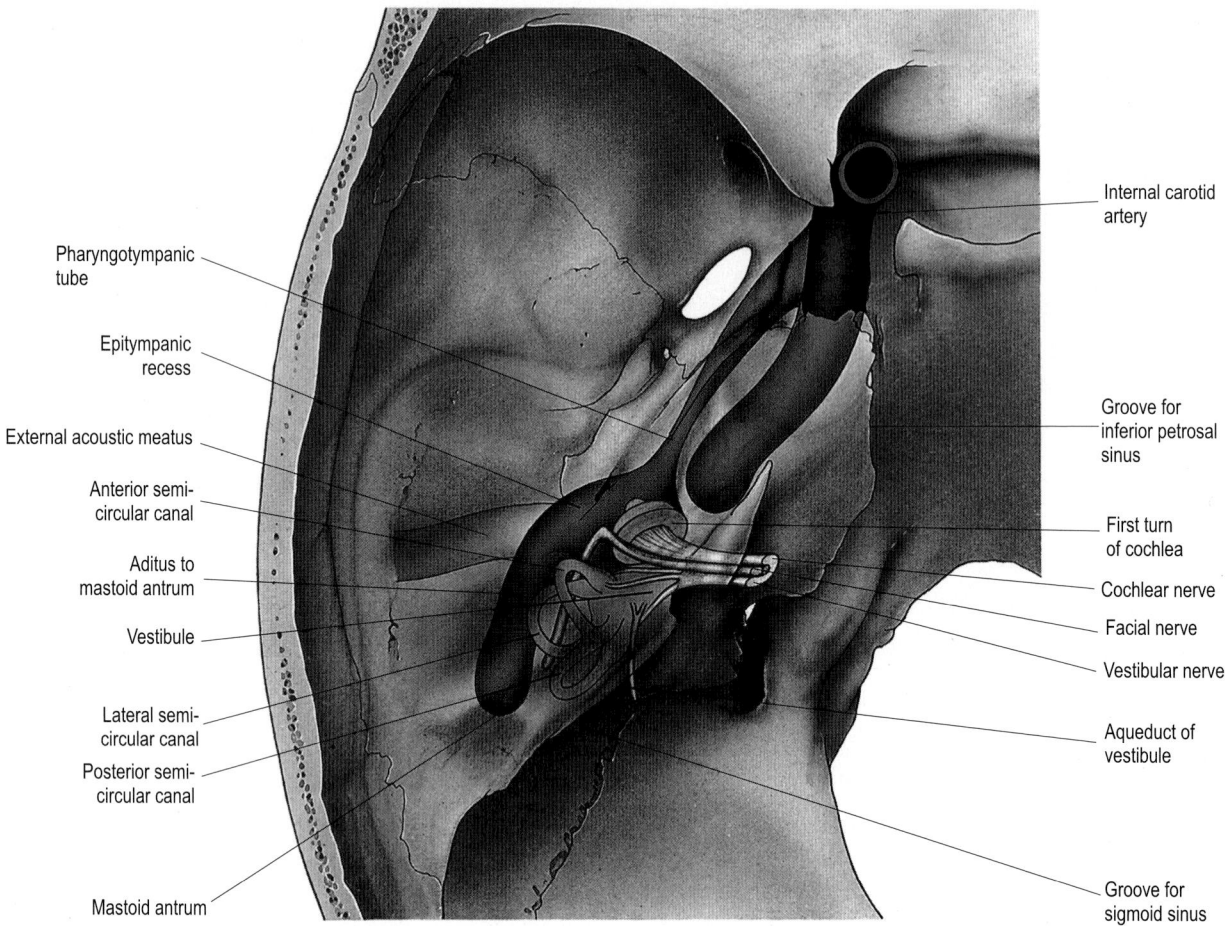

Pharyngotympanic tube

Epitympanic recess

External acoustic meatus

Anterior semi-circular canal

Aditus to mastoid antrum

Vestibule

Lateral semi-circular canal

Posterior semi-circular canal

Mastoid antrum

Internal carotid artery

Groove for inferior petrosal sinus

First turn of cochlea

Cochlear nerve

Facial nerve

Vestibular nerve

Aqueduct of vestibule

Groove for sigmoid sinus

Fig. 38.4 The left auditory apparatus as if viewed through a semi-transparent temporal bone. Compare with Fig. 38.9. Note the bend (genu) in the facial nerve at the site of the geniculate ganglion.

There are two main external approaches to the middle ear: the endaural approach and the postauricular approach.

The endaural approach involves making an incision in the notch between the tragus and the helix. This is carried down to expose the lower margin of temporalis – which can be used to harvest a strong fascial graft for reconstruction – and the bone of the bony external acoustic meatus. The cartilaginous meatus is separated from the bony meatus and reflected laterally as a conchomeatal flap. The bony meatus can then be widened by drilling away bone, so that access to the middle ear and the mastoid antrum and air sinuses is achieved without damaging the ossicular chain or the facial nerve.

The postauricular approach involves making an incision in the post-auricular skin down to temporalis and the periosteum of the mastoid process, dividing the posterior auricular muscles on the way. Grafts can be harvested from the temporalis fascia. The periosteum is incised and elevated to expose the bony external acoustic meatus from behind. The skin over the junction of the bony and cartilaginous meatus is incised so as to allow the cartilage of the auricle and meatus to be swung forward on its blood supply and so expose the bony meatus and mastoid process. Access can then be gained by drilling and elevating a tympanomeatal skin flap as described for the endaural approach.

MIDDLE EAR

The essential function of the middle ear is to transfer energy efficiently from relatively weak vibrations in the elastic, compressible air in the external acoustic meatus, to the incompressible fluid around the delicate receptors in the cochlea. Mechanical coupling between the two systems must match their resistance to deformation or 'flow', i.e. their impedance, as closely as possible. Thus aerial waves of low amplitude and low force per unit area arrive at the tympanic membrane, which has

15–20 times the area of the stapedial footplate in contact with peri-lymph in the inner ear. In this manner, the force per unit area generated by the footplate is increased by a similar amount, while the amplitude of vibration is almost unchanged.

Protective mechanisms are incorporated into the design of the tympanic cavity. These include: the presence of the pharyngotympanic tube to equalize pressure on both sides of the delicate tympanic membrane; the shape of the articulations between the ossicles; and the reflex contractions of stapedius and tensor tympani in response to sounds of fairly high intensity, which prevent damage due to sudden or excessive excursions of the ossicles.

The tympanic cavity or middle ear (**Figs 38.5, 38.6, 38.7**) is an irregular, laterally compressed space in the petrous part of the temporal bone. It is lined with mucous membrane and filled with air, which reaches it from the nasopharynx via the pharyngotympanic tube. It contains three small bones, the malleus, incus and stapes, which collectively are called the auditory ossicles. They form an articulated chain connecting the lateral and medial walls of the cavity, and transmit the vibrations of the tympanic membrane across the cavity to the cochlea.

The space within the middle ear can be subdivided into the tympanic cavity proper, opposite the tympanic membrane, and an epitympanic recess (the attic), above the level of the membrane, which contains the upper half of the malleus and most of the incus. Including the recess, the vertical and anteroposterior diameters of the cavity are each c.15 mm; the transverse diameter is c.6 mm superiorly and 4 mm inferiorly, but opposite the umbo it is only 2 mm. The cavity is bounded laterally by the tympanic membrane and medially by the lateral wall of the internal ear. It communicates posteriorly with the mastoid antrum and with the mastoid air cells. Anteriorly it communicates with the nasopharynx via the pharyngotympanic tube (**Figs 38.3, 38.4**).

The tympanic cavity and mastoid antrum, auditory ossicles and structures of the internal ear are all almost fully developed at birth and

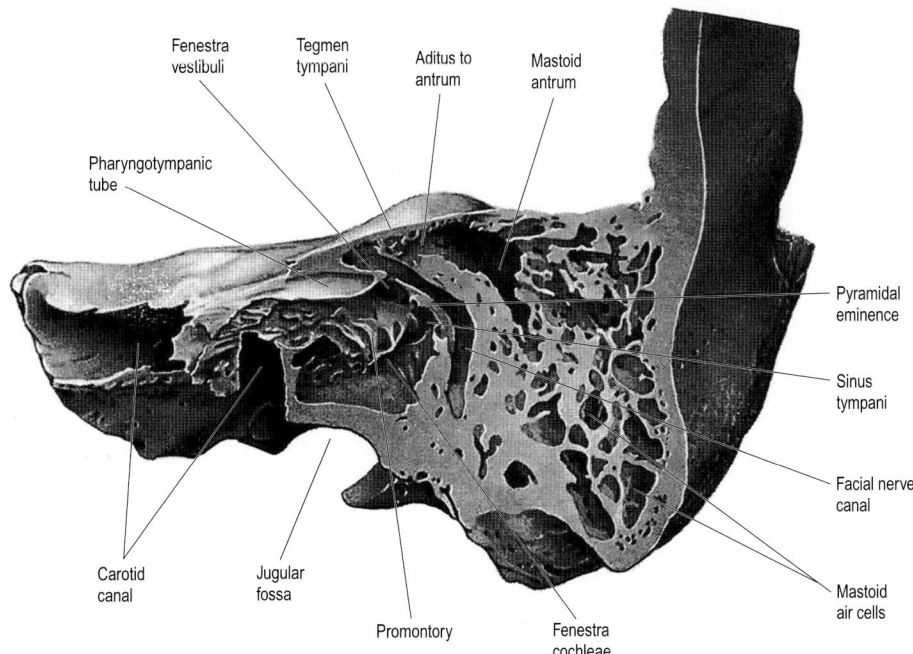

Fig. 38.5 Oblique section through the left temporal bone, showing the medial wall of the middle ear. Compare with Fig. 38.9.

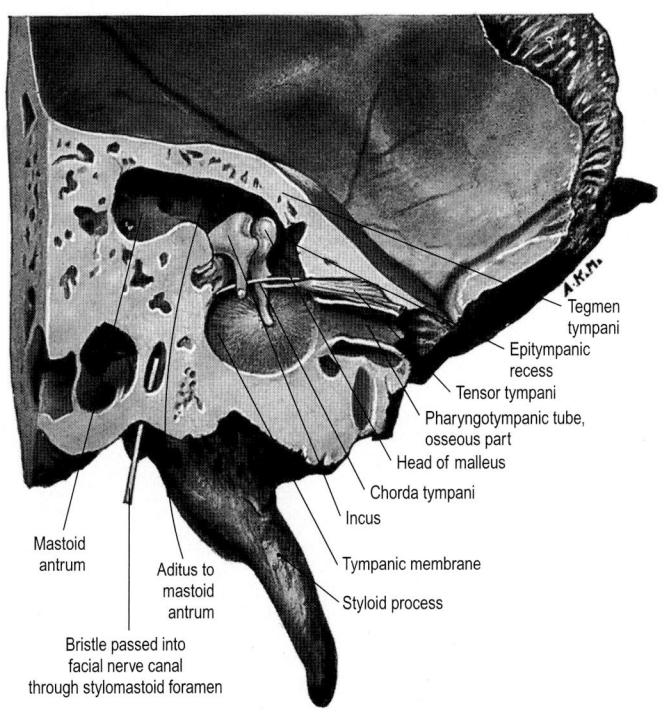

Fig. 38.6 Oblique vertical section through the left temporal bone, to show roof and lateral wall of the middle ear and the mastoid antrum.

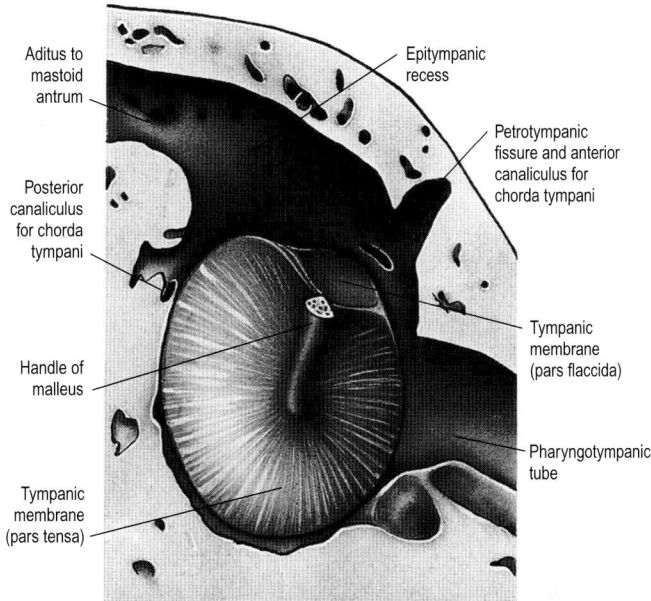

Fig. 38.7 The lateral wall of the left tympanic cavity.

subsequently alter little. In fetuses the cavity contains a gelatinous tissue which has practically disappeared by birth, when it is filled by a fluid which is absorbed when air enters via the pharyngotympanic tube.

The tympanic cavity is a common site of infection, which usually spreads to it from the nose and pharynx along the pharyngotympanic tube.

Boundaries of tympanic cavity

ROOF OF TYMPANIC CAVITY (Fig. 38.6)

A thin plate of compact bone, the tegmen tympani, separates the cranial and tympanic cavities, and forms much of the anterior surface of the petrous temporal bone. The tegmen tympani is prolonged posteriorly as the roof the mastoid antrum and anteriorly it covers the canal for tensor tympani. In youth, the unossified petrosquamosal suture may allow the spread of infection from the tympanic cavity to the meninges. In adults, veins from the tympanic cavity traverse this suture to reach the superior petrosal or petrosquamous sinus and thus may also transmit infection to these structures.

Longitudinal fractures of the middle cranial fossa almost always involve the tympanic roof, accompanied by the rupture of the tympanic membrane or a fractured roof of the osseous external acoustic meatus. Such injuries usually cause bleeding from the ear, with escape of cerebrospinal fluid if the dura mater has been torn.

FLOOR OF TYMPANIC CAVITY

The floor of the tympanic cavity is a narrow, thin, convex plate of bone which separates the cavity from the superior bulb of the internal jugular vein. The bone may be patchily deficient, in which case the tympanic cavity and the vein are separated only by mucous membrane and fibrous tissue. Alternatively, the floor is sometimes thick and may contain some accessory mastoid air cells. A small aperture for the tympanic branch of the glossopharyngeal nerve lies near the medial wall.

LATERAL WALL OF TYMPANIC CAVITY (Figs 38.6, 38.7)

The lateral wall consists mainly of the tympanic membrane, but also contains the ring of bone to which the membrane is attached . There is a deficiency or notch in the upper part of this ring, close to which are the small openings of the anterior and posterior canaliculi for the chorda tympani and the petrotympanic fissure.

The posterior canaliculus for the chorda tympani is situated in the angle between the posterior and lateral walls of the tympanic cavity just behind the tympanic membrane, and level with the upper end of the handle of the malleus. It leads into a minute canal that descends in front of the facial canal and ends in it c.6 mm above the stylomastoid foramen. The canaliculus transmits the chorda tympani and a branch of the stylomastoid artery to the tympanic cavity.

The petrotympanic fissure opens just above and in front of the ring of bone to which the tympanic membrane is attached. It is a mere slit c.2 mm in length, and contains the anterior process and anterior ligament of the malleus. It transmits the anterior tympanic branch of the maxillary artery to the tympanic cavity.

The anterior canaliculus for the chorda tympani opens at the medial end of the petrotympanic fissure: the chorda tympani leaves the tympanic cavity through this canaliculus.

TYMPANIC MEMBRANE (Figs 38.6, 38.7, 38.8, 38.12)

The tympanic membrane separates the tympanic cavity from the external acoustic meatus. It is thin, semi-transparent, and almost oval, though somewhat broader above than below. It lies obliquely, at an angle of c.55° with the meatal floor. Its longest, anteroinferior diameter is from 9 to 10 mm and its shortest is from 8 to 9 mm. Most of its circumference is a thickened fibrocartilaginous ring or anulus which is attached to the tympanic sulcus at the medial end of the meatus. This sulcus is deficient superiorly. Two bands, the anterior and posterior malleolar folds, pass from the ends of the notch to the lateral process of the malleus. The small triangular part of the membrane, the pars flaccida, lies above these folds and is lax and thin. The major part of the tympanic membrane, the pars tensa, is taut. The handle of the malleus is firmly attached to the internal surface of the tympanic membrane as far as its centre, which projects towards the tympanic cavity. The inner surface of the membrane is thus convex and the point of greatest convexity is termed the umbo. Although the membrane as a whole is convex on its inner surface, its radiating fibres are curved with their concavities directed inwards.

MICROSTRUCTURE

Histologically, the tympanic membrane is composed of three strata: an outer cuticular layer, an intermediate fibrous layer and an inner mucous layer. The cuticular stratum is continuous with the thin skin of the meatus. It is keratinized, stratified squamous in type, devoid of dermal papillae and hairless. Its subepithelial tissue is vascularized and may develop a few peripheral papillae. Ultrastructurally, it is c.10 cells thick and has two zones, a superficial layer of non-nucleated squames, and a deep zone which resembles the epidermal stratum spinosum. There are numerous desmosomes between cells, the deepest of which lie on a continuous basal lamina, but lack epithelial pegs and hemidesmosomes. The cells of this stratum have a propensity for lateral migration and differentiation not shared with any other stratified squamous epithelia in the body.

The fibrous stratum consists of an external layer of radiating fibres which diverge from the handle of the malleus, and a deep layer of circular fibres, which are plentiful peripherally, but sparse and scattered centrally. Ultrastructurally the filaments are c.10 nm in diameter, and are linked at 25 nm intervals. They have a distinctive amino acid composition, and may consist of a protein peculiar to the tympanic membrane. Small groups of collagen fibrils appear at 11 weeks *in utero*, interspersed with small bundles of elastin microfibrils. Older specimens contain more typically cross-banded collagen fibrils and an amorphous elastin component. The fibrous stratum is replaced by loose connective tissue in the pars flaccida.

The mucous stratum is a part of the mucosa of the tympanic cavity, and is thickest near the upper part of the membrane. It consists of a single layer of very flat cells, with overlapping interdigitating boundaries.

A

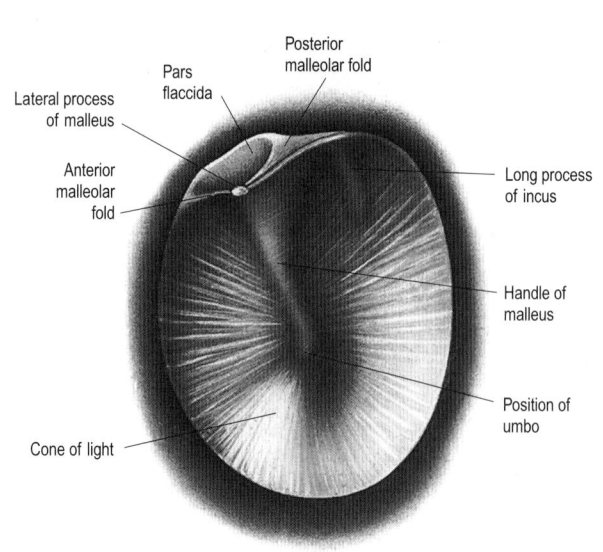

B

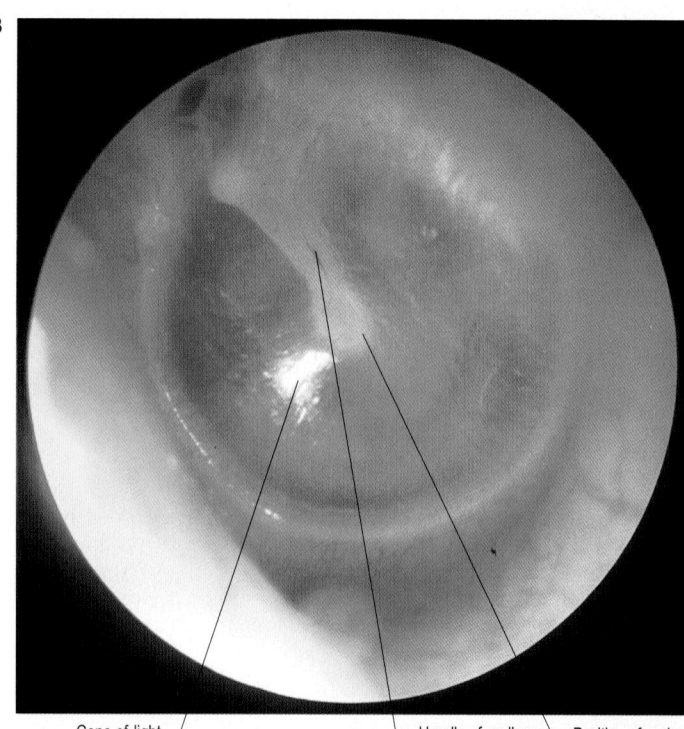

Cone of light ⌐   ⌐ Handle of malleus ⌐ Position of umbo

Fig. 38.8 Left tympanic membrane. **A**, External aspect as seen through a speculum. Note that a bright cone of light is seen in the anteroinferior quadrant of the membrane when it is illuminated. **B**, Viewed in auroscope. (**B**, by kind permission from Mr Simon A Hickey.)

There are desmosomes and tight junctions between adjacent cells. Their cytoplasm contains only a few organelles: the luminal surfaces of these apparently metabolically inert cells have a few irregular microvilli and are covered by an amorphous electron-dense material. Ciliated columnar cells are absent.

INNERVATION OF THE TYMPANIC MEMBRANE

The tympanic membrane is mainly innervated by the auriculotemporal nerve, and appears to perceive only pain. There is a minor, inconstant, overlapping sensory supply from the seventh, ninth and tenth cranial nerves. The auricular branch of the vagus arises from the superior vagal ganglion and is joined soon after by a ramus from the inferior ganglion of the glossopharyngeal nerve. It passes behind the internal jugular vein and enters the mastoid canaliculus on the lateral wall of the jugular fossa. It traverses the temporal bone and crosses the facial canal c.4 mm above the stylomastoid foramen. At this point it supplies an ascending branch to the facial nerve. Fibres of the nervus intermedius may pass to the auricular branch of the vagus here, which may explain the cutaneous vesiculation that sometimes accompanies geniculate herpes. The auricular branch then traverses the tympanomastoid fissure, and divides into two rami. One joins the posterior auricular nerve. The other branch is distributed to the skin of part of the cranial surface of the auricle, the posterior wall and floor of the external acoustic meatus, and to the adjoining part of the outer surface of the tympanic membrane. The auricular branch therefore contains somatic afferent nerve fibres, which probably terminate in the spinal trigeminal nucleus. Stimulation of the vagus nerve – as in syringing the ear – can have a reflex reaction on heart rate.

PHARYNGOTYMPANIC TUBE BLOCKAGE IN CHILDREN

The pharyngotympanic tube serves to ventilate the middle ear, exchanging nasopharyngeal air with the air in the middle ear which has been altered in its composition as a result of transmucosal gas exchange with the haemoglobin in the blood vessels of the mucosa. It also carries mucus from the middle ear cleft to the nasopharynx as a result of ciliary transport. In children the pharyngotympanic tube is relatively narrow and is prone to obstruction as a result of mucosal swelling following infection and allergy. Obstruction of the tube results in a relative vacuum being created in the middle ear secondary to transmucosal gas exchange, and this in turn promotes mucosal secretion and the formation of a middle ear effusion. Because of the collapsibility of the pharyngotympanic tube, the vacuum thus created can overcome the distending effect of the muscles of the tube and 'lock' the tube shut. The resultant persistent middle ear effusion can cause hearing loss by splinting the tympanic membrane and impeding its vibration. It can also provide an ideal environment for the proliferation of bacteria with the result that an acute otitis media may develop. It is possible to relieve the vacuum and unlock the tube, and then remove the effusion by myringotomy, i.e. surgically creating a hole in the tympanic membrane. This hole will generally heal rapidly and it is common practice to insert a flanged ventilation tube – a grommet or tympanostomy tube – to keep the hole open. Migration of the outer squamous layer of the tympanic membrane eventually displaces the tube and the myringotomy heals.

OTITIS MEDIA

Acute otitis media usually arises as a result of ascent of infection from the nasopharynx via the pharyngotympanic tube to the middle ear cleft. From there it may extend to the mastoid aditus and antrum. Swelling secondary to the infection may result in the closure of both exits from the middle ear, i.e. the pharyngotympanic tube and the aditus, with subsequent accumulation of pus under pressure, which causes lateral bulging and inflammation of the tympanic membrane. The latter may burst releasing mucopurulent discharge into the external acoustic meatus, which results in a release of the pressure in the middle ear and a diminution in the levels of pain. After a brief period the discharge dries up, and for the most part the resultant perforation of the tympanic membrane heals. Normal ventilation and drainage of mucus from the middle ear is restored once the swelling in the pharyngotympanic tube resolves. On occasion the process will fail to produce a perforation of the tympanic membrane and the inflammatory exudates will not drain. The immune defence system sterilizes the exudates of organisms, resulting in a sterile mucoid effusion – secretory otitis media – that may cause protracted deafness because its relatively incompressible nature prevents free vibration of the tympanic membrane.

MYRINGOPLASTY

Where pathological perforation of the tympanic membrane occurs and fails to heal there may be hearing impairment and a tendency to infection as a result of contamination with organisms from the external acoustic meatus. This may cause a chronic suppurative discharge. Myringoplasty is a surgical procedure that uses a connective tissue scaffold or graft to support healing of the perforation. The commonest technique involves the elevation of the tympanic anulus and the placement of a piece of fibrous connective tissue, e.g. part of the fibrous deep fascia which invests the lateral surface of temporalis or the perichondrium of the tragal cartilage, onto the undersurface of the tympanic membrane to close the perforation. The healed edges of the perforation are stripped of epithelium to encourage healing and scar formation. The fibrous tissue supports the healing tympanic membrane and may in part be incorporated into the repair. Once the perforation is healed, the vibratory function of the tympanic membrane is usually restored to normal.

MEDIAL WALL OF TYMPANIC CAVITY (Figs 38.5, 38.9)

The medial wall of the tympanic cavity is also the lateral boundary of the internal ear. Its features are the promontory, fenestra vestibuli (oval window), fenestra cochleae (round window) and the facial prominence.

The promontory is a rounded prominence furrowed by small grooves which lodge the nerves of the tympanic plexus. It lies over the lateral projection of the basal turn of the cochlea. A minute spicule of bone frequently connects the promontory to the pyramidal eminence of the posterior wall. The apex of the cochlea lies near the medial wall of the tympanic cavity, anterior to the promontory. A depression behind the promontory, the sinus tympani, indicates the position of the ampulla of the posterior semicircular canal.

The fenestra vestibuli (fenestra ovalis) is a kidney-shaped opening situated above and behind the promontory, and leading from the tympanic cavity to the vestibule of the inner ear. Its long diameter is horizontal and its convex border is directed upwards. It is occupied by the base of the stapes, the circumference of which is attached to the margin of the fenestra by an anular ligament.

The fenestra cochlea (fenestra rotunda) is situated below and a little behind the fenestra vestibuli, from which it is separated by the posterior part of the promontory. It lies completely under the overhanging edge of the promontory in a deep hollow or niche, and is placed very obliquely. In dried specimens it opens anterosuperiorly from the tympanic cavity into the scala tympani of the cochlea. In life, it is closed by the secondary tympanic membrane, which is somewhat concave towards the tympanic cavity and convex towards the cochlea, the membrane being bent so that its posterosuperior one-third forms an angle with its anteroinferior two-thirds. The membrane has three layers: an external layer which is derived from the tympanic mucosa; an internal layer from the cochlear lining membrane; and an intermediate, fibrous layer.

The prominence of the facial nerve canal indicates the position of the upper part of the bony canal which contains the facial nerve. This canal crosses the medial tympanic wall, just above the fenestra vestibuli, and then curves down into the posterior wall of the cavity. Its lateral wall may be partly deficient.

POSTERIOR WALL OF TYMPANIC CAVITY
(Figs 38.5, 38.6, 38.7, 38.9)

The posterior wall of the tympanic cavity is wider above than below. Its main features are the aditus to the mastoid antrum, the pyramid, and the fossa incudis.

The aditus to the mastoid antrum is a large irregular aperture which leads back from the epitympanic recess into the upper part of the mastoid antrum. A rounded eminence on the medial wall of the aditus, above and behind the prominence of the facial nerve canal, corresponds with the position of the lateral semicircular canal.

The pyramidal eminence is situated just behind the fenestra vestibuli and in front of the vertical part of the facial nerve canal. It is hollow and contains stapedius. Its summit projects towards the fenestra vestibuli and is pierced by a small aperture which transits the tendon of stapedius. The cavity in the pyramidal eminence is prolonged down and back in front of the facial nerve canal, and communicates with the latter

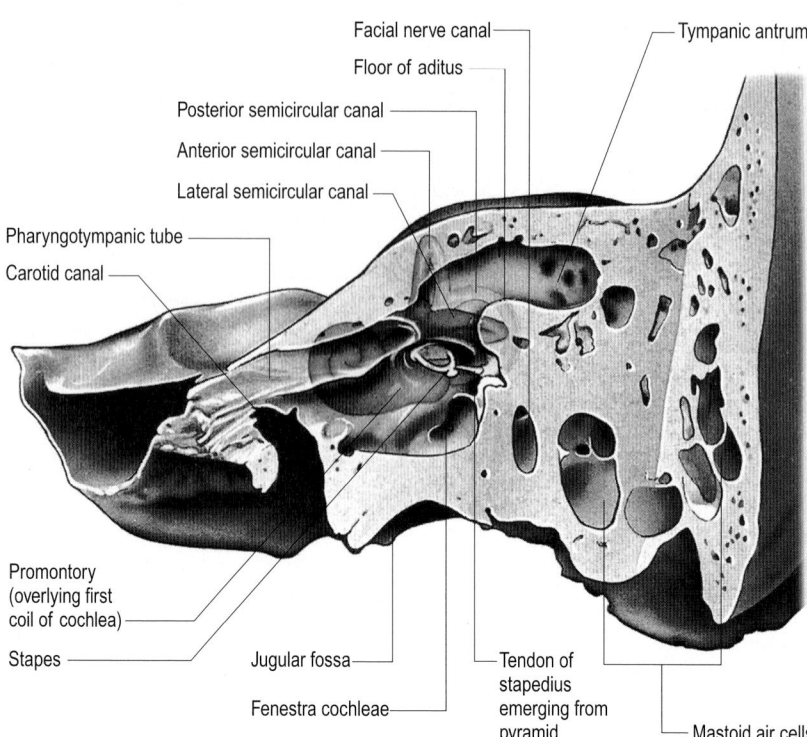

Facial nerve canal
Floor of aditus
Posterior semicircular canal
Anterior semicircular canal
Lateral semicircular canal
Pharyngotympanic tube
Carotid canal
Tympanic antrum
Promontory (overlying first coil of cochlea)
Stapes
Jugular fossa
Fenestra cochleae
Tendon of stapedius emerging from pyramid
Mastoid air cells

Fig. 38.9 Oblique section through the left temporal bone, to show the medial wall of the middle ear. The cochlea and the semicircular canals are in blue. Note the relationship of the first coil of the cochlea to the promontory and the closeness of the facial nerve canal and the lateral semicircular canal to the medial wall of the aditus.

by an aperture through which a small branch of the facial nerve passes to stapedius.

The fossa incudis is a small depression in the lower and posterior part of the epitympanic recess. It contains the short process of the incus, which is fixed to the fossa by ligamentous fibres.

MASTOID ANTRUM (Figs 38.4, 38.5, 38.6, 38.7, 38.9)

The mastoid antrum is an air sinus in the petrous part of the temporal bone. Its topographical relations are of considerable surgical importance. In the upper part of its anterior wall is an opening, the aditus to the mastoid antrum, which leads back from the epitympanic recess. The lateral semicircular canal lies medial to the aditus. The medial wall of the antrum is related to the posterior semicircular canal (**Fig. 38.9**). The sigmoid sinus is posterior, and may be separated from the antrum by mastoid air cells. The roof is formed by the tegmen tympani, and lies below the middle cranial fossa and temporal lobe of the brain. The floor has several openings which communicate with the mastoid air cells. Anteroinferior is the descending part of the facial nerve canal. The lateral wall of the antrum, which offers the usual surgical approach to the cavity, is formed by the postmeatal process of the squamous part of the temporal bone. This is only 2 mm thick at birth but increases at a rate of c.1 mm a year, to attain a final thickness of 12–15 mm. In adults, the lateral wall of the antrum corresponds to the suprameatal triangle on the outer surface of the skull, which is palpable through the cymba conchae. The superior side of the suprameatal triangle, the supramastoid crest, is level with the floor of the middle cranial fossa. The anteroinferior side, which forms the posterosuperior margin of the external acoustic meatus, indicates approximately the position of the descending part of the facial nerve canal. The posterior side, formed by a posterior vertical tangent to the posterior margin of the external acoustic meatus, is just anterior to the sigmoid sinus.

The adult capacity of the mastoid antrum is variable, but on average is c.1 ml and its general diameter c.10 mm. Unlike other air sinuses, it is present at birth, and is indeed then almost adult in size, although it is at a higher level relative to the external acoustic meatus than in adults. In the very young, the thinness of the lateral antral wall and the absence of the mastoid process, means that the stylomastoid foramen and emerging facial nerve are very superficially situated.

MASTOID AIR CELLS (Figs 38.5, 38.9)

The mastoid air cells vary considerably in number, form and size. Usually they interconnect and are lined by a mucosa with squamous non-ciliated epithelium, continuous with that in the mastoid antrum and tympanic cavity. They may fill the mastoid process, even to its tip, and some may be separated from the sigmoid sinus and posterior cranial fossa only by extremely thin bone, which is occasionally deficient. Some may lie superficial to, or even behind the sigmoid sinus and others may occur in the posterior wall of the descending part of the facial nerve canal. Those in the squamous part of the temporal bone may be separated from deeper cells in the petrous part by a plate of bone in the line of the squamomastoid suture (Korner's septum). Sometimes they extend very little into the mastoid process, in which case the process consists largely of dense bone or trabecular bone containing bone marrow. Varieties of the mastoid process occur. The three types most commonly described are pneumatized, with many air cells; sclerotic, with few or none; and mixed, which contains both air cells and bone marrow.

Mastoid air cells may extend beyond the mastoid process into the squamous part of the temporal bone above the supramastoid crest; into the posterior root of the zygomatic process of the temporal bone; into the osseous roof of the external acoustic meatus just below the middle cranial fossa; and into the floor of the tympanic cavity very close to the superior jugular bulb. Rarely, a few may excavate the jugular process of the occipital bone. An important group may extend medially into the petrous part of the temporal bone, even to its apex, related to the pharyngotympanic tube, carotid canal, labyrinth and abducens nerve. However some investigators maintain that these are not continuous with the mastoid cells, but grow independently from the tympanic cavity. The extensions of the mastoid air cells described above are pathologically important since infection may spread to the structures around them. Though the mastoid process antrum is well-developed at birth, the mastoid air cells are merely minute antral diverticula at this stage. As the mastoid develops in the second year, the cells gradually extend into it and by the fourth year they are well formed, although their greatest growth occurs at puberty. In c.20% of skulls the mastoid process has no air cells at all.

Innervation – The mastoid air cells are innervated by a meningeal branch of the mandibular nerve.

MASTOIDITIS

Mastoiditis occurs as a result of the spread of a bacterial infection from the tympanic cavity via the aditus to the mastoid antrum and associated mastoid air cells. This dangerous condition may spread from the antrum to surrounding structures and cause life-threatening infection. In particular the infection may spread through the tegmen tympani to the dura mater of the middle cranial fossa, to cause an extradural collection.

This in turn may cause necrosis of the adjacent dura mater and infection may spread to form a subdural empyema in the subarachnoid space, or an abscess in the substance of the adjacent temporal lobe. Bacterial meningitis may also develop. Similar spread may be seen into the posterior cranial fossa. In both sites the infection may prove fatal.

Infection may spread laterally through the cortical bone of the lateral aspect of the mastoid process to form a subperiosteal postauricular abscess (Bezold's abscess), or through the cortical bone of the mastoid tip of the mastoid process to the attachment of the posterior belly of digastric and sternocleidomastoid, which stimulates painful muscular contraction and torticollis.

ANTERIOR WALL OF TYMPANIC CAVITY (Figs 38.3, 38.6)

The inferior, larger area of the anterior wall is narrowed by the approximation of the medial and lateral walls of the cavity. It is a thin lamina and forms the posterior wall of the carotid canal. It is perforated by the superior and inferior caroticotympanic nerves and the tympanic branch or branches of the internal carotid. The canals for tensor tympani, and the osseous part of the pharyngotympanic tube open above it. The canal for tensor tympani is superior to that for the pharyngotympanic tube. Both canals incline downwards and anteromedially to open in the angle between the squamous and petrous parts of the temporal bone, and are separated by a thin, osseous septum. The canal for tensor tympani and the bony septum runs posterolaterally on the medial tympanic wall, and ends immediately above the fenestra vestibuli. Here, the posterior end of the septum is curved laterally to form a pulley, the processus trochleariformis (cochleariformis). The tendon of tensor tympani turns laterally over the pulley before attaching to the upper part of the handle of the malleus.

Auditory ossicles (Fig. 38.10)

A chain of three mobile ossicles, the malleus, incus and stapes, transfers sound waves across the tympanic cavity from the tympanic membrane to the fenestra vestibuli. The malleus is attached to the tympanic membrane and the base of the stapes is attached to the rim of the fenestra vestibuli. The incus is suspended between them, and articulates with both bones.

MALLEUS (Figs 38.3, 38.6, 38.7, 38.10)

The malleus is the largest of the ossicles, and is shaped somewhat like a mallet. It is 8–9 mm long and has a head, neck, handle (manubrium) and anterior and lateral processes. The head is the large upper end of the bone and is situated in the epitympanic recess. It is ovoid in shape. It articulates posteriorly with the incus, and is covered elsewhere by mucosa. The cartilaginous articular facet for the incus is narrowed near its middle and consists of a larger upper part and a smaller lower part, orientated almost at right angles to each other. Opposite the constriction the lower margin of the facet projects in the form of a process, the spur of the malleus. The neck is the narrowed part below the head and inferior to this is an enlargement from which the processes project.

The handle of the malleus is connected by its lateral margin with the tympanic membrane (**Figs 38.6, 38.7, 38.8**). It is directed downwards, medially and backwards. It decreases in size towards its free end, which is curved slightly forwards and is flattened transversely. Near the upper end of its medial surface there is a slight projection to which the tendon of tensor tympani is attached. The anterior process is a delicate bony spicule, directed forwards from the enlargement below the neck. It is connected to the petrotympanic fissure by ligamentous fibres. In fetal life this is the longest process of the malleus and is continuous in front with Meckel's cartilage. The lateral process is a conical projection from the root of the handle of the malleus. It is directed laterally and is attached to the upper part of the tympanic membrane and, via the anterior and posterior malleolar folds, to the sides of the notch in the upper part of the tympanic sulcus (**Fig. 38.8**).

Ossification – The cartilaginous precursor of the malleus originates as part of the dorsal end of Meckel's cartilage. With the exception of its anterior process, the malleus ossifies from a single endochondral centre which appears near the future neck of the bone in the fourth month *in*

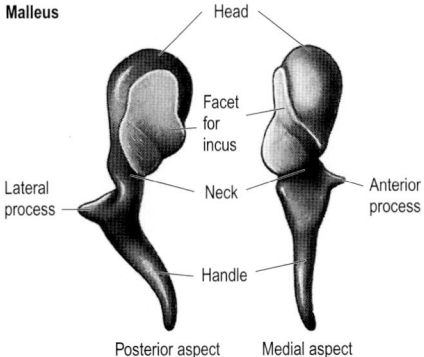

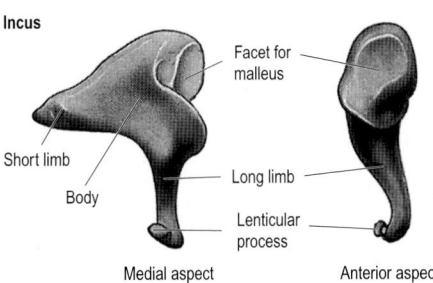

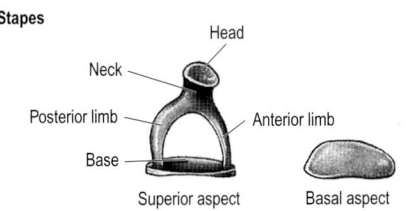

Fig. 38.10 The left ear ossicles.

utero. The anterior process ossifies separately in dense connective tissue and joins the rest of the bone at about the sixth month of fetal life.

INCUS (Figs 38.3, 38.6, 38.7, 38.10)

The incus is shaped less like an anvil – from which it is named – than a premolar tooth, with its two diverging roots. It has a body and two processes. The body is somewhat cubical but laterally compressed. On its anterior surface it has a saddle-shaped facet for articulation with the head of the malleus. The long process, rather more than half the length of the handle of the malleus, descends almost vertically, behind and parallel to the handle. Its lower end bends medially and ends in a rounded lenticular process, the medial surface of which is covered with cartilage and articulates with the head of the stapes. The short process, somewhat conical, projects backwards and is attached by ligamentous fibres to the fossa incudis in the lower and posterior part of the epitympanic recess.

Ossification – The incus has a cartilaginous precursor continuous with the dorsal extremity of Meckel's cartilage. Ossification often spreads from a single centre in the upper part of its long process in the fourth fetal month; the lenticular process may have a separate centre.

STAPES (Figs 38.3, 38.9, 38.10)

The stapes is also known as the stirrup. It has a head, neck, two limbs and a base. The head (caput) is directed laterally and has a small cartilaginous facet for the lenticular process of the incus. The neck is the constricted part supporting the head, and the tendon of stapedius is attached to its posterior surface. The limbs (crura) diverge from the neck and are connected at their ends by a flattened oval plate, the base, which forms the footplate of the stapes. The base is attached to the

657

margin of the fenestra vestibuli by a ring of fibres (the anular ligament). The anterior limb is shorter and less curved than the posterior.

Ossification – The stapes is preformed in the perforated dorsal moiety of the hyoid arch cartilage of the fetus. Ossification starts from a single endochondral centre, which appears in the base in the fourth fetal month and then gradually spreads through the limbs of the stapes to reach the head.

At birth the auditory ossicles have reached an advanced state of maturity.

LIGAMENTS OF AUDITORY OSSICLES

The ossicles are connected to the tympanic walls by ligaments. There are three for the malleus and one each for the incus and stapes. Some of these are mere mucosal folds which carry blood vessels and nerves to and from the ossicles and their articulations, and others contain a central, strong band of collagen fibres.

The anterior ligament of the malleus stretches from the neck of the malleus, just above the anterior process, to the anterior wall of the tympanic cavity near the petrotympanic fissure. Some of its collagen fibres traverse this fissure to reach the spine of the sphenoid, and others continue into the sphenomandibular ligament. The latter, like the anterior malleolar ligament, is derived from the perichondrial sheath of Meckel's cartilage. The anterior malleolar ligament may contain muscle fibres, called laxator tympani or musculus externus mallei. The lateral ligament of the malleus is a triangular band which stretches from the posterior part of the border of the tympanic incisure to the head of the malleus. The superior ligament of the malleus connects the head of the malleus to the roof of the epitympanic recess.

The posterior ligament of the incus connects the end of its short process to the fossa incudis. The superior ligament of the incus is little more than a mucosal fold passing from the body of the incus to the roof of the epitympanic recess.

The vestibular surface and rim of the stapedial base are covered with hyaline cartilage. The cartilage encircling the base is attached to the margin of the fenestra vestibuli by a ring of elastic fibres, the anular ligament of the base of the stapes. The posterior part of this ligament is much narrower than the anterior part: it acts as a kind of hinge on which the stapedial base moves when stapedius contracts and during acoustic oscillation.

ARTICULATION OF AUDITORY OSSICLES

The articulations are typical synovial joints. The incudomalleolar joint is saddle shaped. The incudostapedial joint is a ball and socket articulation. Their articular surfaces are covered with articular cartilage, and each joint is enveloped by a capsule rich in elastic tissue and lined by synovial membrane.

MOVEMENTS OF THE AUDITORY OSSICLES

The handle of the malleus faithfully follows all movements of the tympanic membrane. The malleus and incus rotate together around an axis which runs from the short process and posterior ligament of the incus to the anterior ligament of the malleus. When the tympanic membrane and handle of the malleus move inwards (medially), the long process of the incus moves in the same direction and pushes the stapedial base towards the labyrinth and the perilymph contained within the labyrinth. The movement of the perilymph causes a compensatory outward bulging of the secondary tympanic membrane – which closes the fenestra cochleae. These events are reversed when the tympanic membrane moves outwards. However, if its movement is considerable, the incus does not follow the full outward excursion of the malleus, and merely glides on it at the incudomalleolar joint, thus preventing a dislocation of the base of the stapes from the fenestra vestibuli. When the handle of the malleus is carried medially, the spur at the lower margin of the head of the malleus locks the incudomalleolar joint, and this necessitates an inward movement of the long process of the incus. The joint is unlocked again when the handle of the malleus is carried outwards. The three bones together act as a bent lever so that the stapedial base does not move in the fenestra vestibuli like a piston, but rocks on a fulcrum at its anteroinferior border, where the anular ligament is thick. The rocking movement around a vertical axis, which is like a swinging door, is said to occur only at moderate intensities of sound. With loud, low-pitched sounds, the axis becomes horizontal, and the upper and lower margins of the stapedial base oscillate in opposite directions around this central axis, thus preventing excessive displacement of the perilymph.

OTOSCLEROSIS AND STAPEDECTOMY

Otosclerosis is a hereditary localized disease of bone derived from the embryonic otic capsule in which lamellar bone is replaced by woven bone of greater thickness and vascularity. The position of the focus of new bone determines its effect on the function of the ear. Where it occurs around the footplate of the stapes it may fix the footplate to the margin of the oval window and prevent it moving. This prevents the passage of vibrations of the tympanic membrane passing through the ossicular chain to the inner ear, which results in clinical hearing loss. Complete deafness does not result, because vibrations can still pass directly to the cochlea via the bones of the skull – albeit in a markedly less efficient manner.

Stapedectomy is a surgical procedure designed to bypass the fixation of the stapes footplate caused by otosclerosis. The tympanic membrane is temporarily elevated for access to the middle ear and, under microscopic control, the incudostapedial joint is disarticulated using microinstruments. The limbs of the stapes and stapedius are then divided, usually with microscissors or a laser, and the superstructure of the stapes removed. A small hole is then made in the fixed footplate of the stapes using a microdrill or laser to expose the fluids of the inner ear. A small graft of connective tissue, usually fat or derived from vein, is used to seal the hole with a flexible membrane. A small piston usually made of plastic and wire is crimped onto the long process of the incus and placed in the perforation in the stapes footplate. The tympanic membrane is then returned. The connection between the tympanic membrane and the inner ear is thus reconstituted and hearing restored.

Muscles of tympanic cavity

TENSOR TYMPANI (Figs 38.3, 38.6)

Tensor tympani is a long slender muscle which occupies the bony canal above the osseous part of the pharyngotympanic tube, from which it is separated by a thin bony septum. It arises from the cartilaginous part of the pharyngotympanic tube and the adjoining region of the greater wing of the sphenoid, as well as from its own canal. It passes back within its canal, and ends in a slim tendon which bends laterally round the pulley-like processus trochleariformis and finally attaches to the handle of the malleus, near its root.

Vascular supply – Tensor tympani receives its arterial blood supply from the superior tympanic branch of the middle meningeal artery.

Innervation – Tensor tympani is innervated by a branch of the nerve to medial pterygoid – a ramus of the mandibular nerve – which traverses the otic ganglion without interruption to reach the muscle.

Actions – Tensor tympani draws the handle of the malleus medially, and so tenses the tympanic membrane and helps to damp sound vibrations: its action also pushes the base of the stapes more tightly into the fenestra vestibuli.

STAPEDIUS

Stapedius arises from the wall of a conical cavity in the pyramidal eminence on the posterior wall of the tympanic cavity, and from its continuation anterior to the descending part of the facial nerve canal. Its minute tendon emerges from the orifice at the apex of the pyramid and passes forwards to attach to the posterior surface of the neck of the stapes (**Fig. 38.9**). The muscle is of an asymmetrical bipennate form, and contains numerous small motor units, each of only six to nine muscle fibres. A few neuromuscular spindles exist near the myotendinous junction.

Vascular supply – Stapedius receives its arterial blood supply from branches of the posterior auricular, anterior tympanic and middle meningeal arteries.

Innervation – Stapedius is supplied by a branch of the facial nerve which is given off in the facial canal.

Actions – Stapedius helps to damp down excessive sound vibrations. It opposes the action of tensor tympani that pushes the stapes more tightly into the fenestra vestibuli. Paralysis of stapedius results in hyperacusis.

Stapedial and tensor tympani reflex (p. 342) – When noises are loud, and immediately before speaking, a reflex contraction of stapedius and tensor tympani occurs which helps to damp down the movement of the ossicular chain before vibrations reach the internal ear. The afferent pathways involve the auditory component of the eighth cranial nerve, and higher centres prior to speech. The efferent pathway involves the facial nerve (stapedius) and the mandibular nerve (tensor tympani).

Tympanic mucosa

The mucosa of the tympanic cavity is continuous with that of the pharynx, via the pharyngotympanic tube. It covers the ossicles, muscles and nerves in the cavity, and forms the inner layer of the tympanic membrane and the outer layer of the secondary tympanic membrane. It also spreads into the mastoid antrum and air cells. It forms several vascular folds which extend from the tympanic walls to the ossicles: one descends from the roof of the cavity to the head of the malleus and the upper margin of the body of the incus and a second surrounds stapedius. Other folds invest the chorda tympani nerve and tensor tympani. The folds separate off saccular recesses which give the interior of the tympanic cavity a somewhat honeycombed appearance. The superior recess of the tympanic membrane lies between the neck of the malleus and the pars flaccida. The anterior and posterior recesses of the tympanic membrane, formed by the mucosa around the chorda tympani, lie anterior and posterior respectively to the handle of the malleus. The tympanic mucosa is pale, thin and slightly vascular. It has a ciliated columnar epithelium, except over the posterior part of the medial wall, the posterior wall, and often parts of the tympanic membrane and the auditory ossicles, where the cells are flatter and non-ciliated. Near the pharyngotympanic tube, goblet cells are numerous; otherwise there are no mucous glands. The mastoid antrum and air cells are lined by flat, non-ciliated epithelium. The epithelium is closely attached to periosteum, and forms a mucoperiosteum. It has surfactant on its surface.

CHOLESTEATOMA

Cholesteatoma is the name given to keratinizing squamous epithelium within the middle ear. There is debate as to how such epithelium comes to be in the middle ear. Theories include development from embryological cell rests, metaplasia from inflamed mucoperiosteum, and aberrant migration of squamous epithelium either through a perforation in the tympanic membrane – usually in the pars flaccida or posterosuperior pars tensa – or within an area of tympanic membrane atelectasis where the tympanic membrane becomes adherent to the medial wall of the tympanic cavity. It is likely that all of these may occur at some time. A feature of cholesteatoma that is poorly understood is its ability to erode bone, through activating osteoclasts. This allows the epithelium to proliferate and invade, destroying the temporal bone and carrying infection to the soft tissues. Thus, cholesteatoma can cause: deafness through damage to the ossicles and inner ear; problems with balance through damage to the vestibule and semicircular canals; facial palsy through ischaemia and necrosis of the facial nerve; and intracranial sepsis. Treatment involves microsurgical dissection of the invading sac of epithelium with preservation of these delicate structures wherever possible.

Vascular supply and lymphatic drainage of the tympanic cavity

A number of arteries supply the walls and contents of the tympanic cavity. Three, namely the deep auricular, anterior tympanic and stylomastoid arteries, are larger than the others.

The deep auricular branch of the first part of the maxillary artery often arises with the anterior tympanic artery. It ascends in the parotid gland behind the temporomandibular joint, pierces the cartilaginous or osseous wall of the external acoustic meatus and supplies its cuticular lining, the exterior of the tympanic membrane and the temporomandibular joint.

The anterior tympanic branch of the first part of the maxillary artery ascends behind the temporomandibular joint and enters the tympanic cavity through the petrotympanic fissure. It ramifies on the interior of the tympanic membrane, and forms a vascular circle around it with the posterior tympanic branch of the stylomastoid artery. It also anastomoses with twigs of the artery of the pterygoid canal and caroticotympanic branches of the internal carotid artery in the mucosa of the tympanic cavity.

The stylomastoid branch of the occipital or posterior auricular arteries supplies the posterior part of the tympanic cavity and mastoid air cells. It also enters the stylomastoid foramen to supply the facial nerve and semicircular canals. In the young, its posterior tympanic branch forms a circular anastomosis with the anterior tympanic artery.

The smaller arteries supplying the tympanic cavity include: the petrosal branch of the middle meningeal artery, which enters through the hiatus for the greater petrosal nerve; the superior tympanic branch of the middle meningeal artery, which traverses the canal for tensor tympani; an inferior tympanic branch from the ascending pharyngeal artery, which traverses the tympanic canaliculus – together with the tympanic branch of the glossopharyngeal nerve – to supply the medial wall of the tympanic cavity; a branch from the artery of the pterygoid canal, which accompanies the pharyngotympanic tube; and a tympanic branch or branches from the internal carotid artery, which is given off in the carotid canal and perforates the thin anterior wall of the tympanic cavity.

The mastoid air cells and dura mater are also supplied by a mastoid branch from the occipital artery. This is small in size and sometimes absent. When present, it enters the cranial cavity via the mastoid foramen near the occipitomastoid suture.

In early fetal life a stapedial artery traverses the stapes.

The veins from the tympanic cavity terminate in the pterygoid venous plexus and the superior petrosal sinus. A small group of veins runs medially from the mucosa of the mastoid antrum through the arch formed by the anterior semicircular canal, and emerges onto the posterior surface of the petrous temporal bone at the subarcuate fossa. These veins drain into the superior petrosal sinus and are the remains of the large subarcuate veins of childhood. They represent a potential route for the spread of infection from the mastoid antrum to the meninges.

Lymphatic vessels of the tympanic and antral mucosae drain to the parotid or upper deep cervical lymph nodes. Vessels of the tympanic end of the pharyngotympanic tube probably end in the deep cervical nodes.

Innervation of the tympanic cavity

TYMPANIC PLEXUS

The nerves that constitute the tympanic plexus ramify on the surface of the promontory on the medial wall of the tympanic cavity. They are derived from the tympanic branch of the glossopharyngeal nerve (**Fig. 38.11**) and the caroticotympanic nerves. The former arises from the inferior ganglion of the glossopharyngeal nerve, and reaches the tympanic cavity via the tympanic canaliculus for the tympanic nerve. The superior and inferior caroticotympanic nerves are postganglionic sympathetic fibres which are derived from the carotid sympathetic plexus. They traverse the wall of the carotid canal to join the plexus.

The tympanic plexus supplies branches to the mucosa of the tympanic cavity, pharyngotympanic tube and mastoid air cells. It sends a branch to the greater petrosal nerve via an opening anterior to the fenestra vestibuli. The lesser petrosal nerve, which may be regarded as the continuation of the tympanic branch of the glossopharyngeal nerve, traverses the tympanic plexus. It occupies a small canal below that for tensor tympani. It runs past, and receives a connecting branch from, the geniculate ganglion of the facial nerve. The lesser petrosal nerve emerges from the anterior surface of the temporal bone via a small opening lateral to the hiatus for the greater petrosal nerve and then traverses the foramen ovale or the small canaliculus innominatus to join the otic ganglion (**Fig. 38.11**). Postganglionic secretomotor fibres leave this ganglion in the auriculotemporal nerve to supply the parotid gland.

FACIAL NERVE (Fig. 38.11)

The facial nerve enters the temporal bone through the internal acoustic meatus accompanied by the vestibulocochlear nerve. At this point the

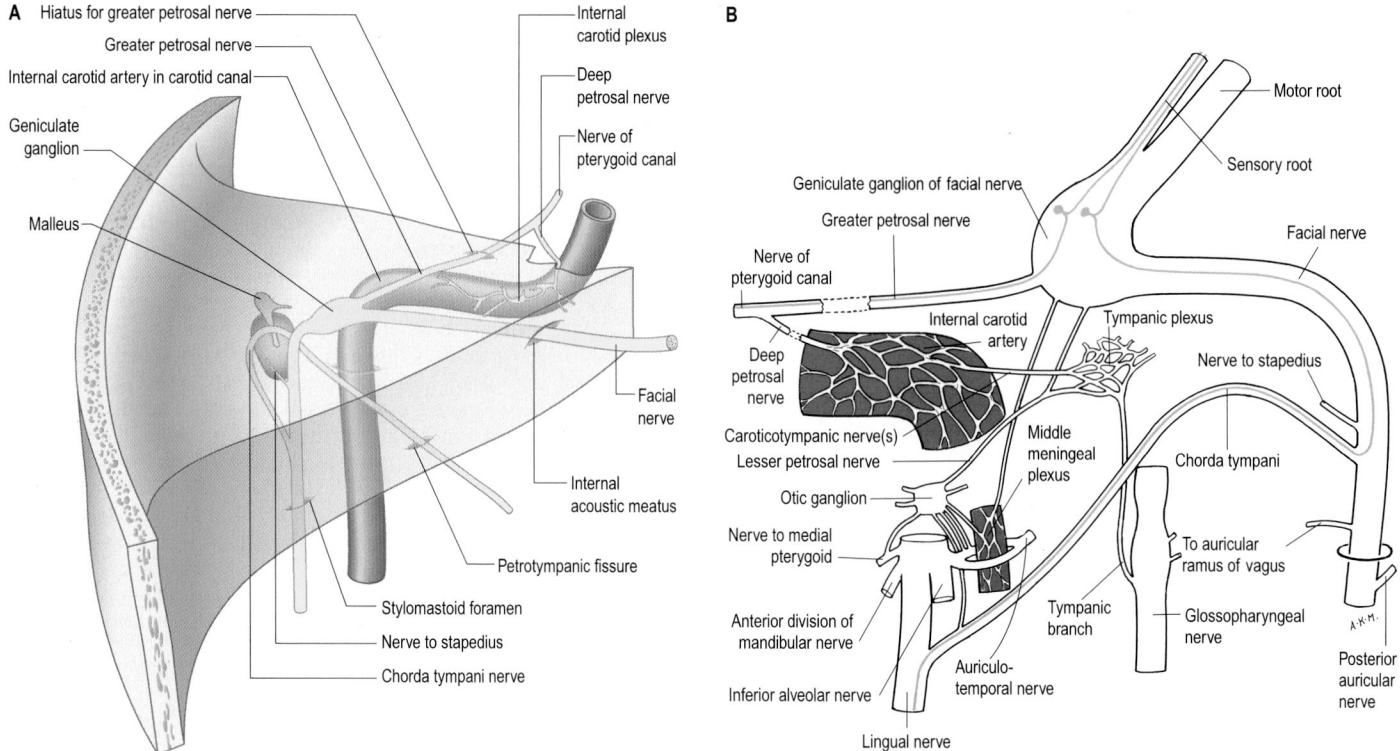

A

Hiatus for greater petrosal nerve
Greater petrosal nerve
Internal carotid artery in carotid canal
Geniculate ganglion
Malleus
Internal carotid plexus
Deep petrosal nerve
Nerve of pterygoid canal
Facial nerve
Internal acoustic meatus
Petrotympanic fissure
Stylomastoid foramen
Nerve to stapedius
Chorda tympani nerve

B

Motor root
Sensory root
Geniculate ganglion of facial nerve
Greater petrosal nerve
Facial nerve
Nerve of pterygoid canal
Deep petrosal nerve
Internal carotid artery
Tympanic plexus
Nerve to stapedius
Caroticotympanic nerve(s)
Lesser petrosal nerve
Middle meningeal plexus
Chorda tympani
Otic ganglion
Nerve to medial pterygoid
Anterior division of mandibular nerve
Inferior alveolar nerve
Tympanic branch
Auriculo-temporal nerve
Lingual nerve
To auricular ramus of vagus
Glossopharyngeal nerve
Tympanic membrane
Posterior auricular nerve

Fig. 38.11 The facial nerve. **A**, Course of the facial nerve and its branches through the temporal bone; the vestibulocochlear nerve has been omitted. **B**, A plan of the intrapetrous section of the facial nerve, its branches and communications. The course of the taste fibres from the mucous membrane of the palate and from the anterior presulcal part of the tongue is represented by the blue lines. (**A**, by permission from Hall-Craggs ECB 1986 Anatomy as a Basis for Clinical Medicine, 2nd edn. Baltimore: Urban and Schwarzenberg.)

motor root, which supplies the muscles of the face, and the nervus intermedius, which contains sensory fibres concerned with the perception of taste and parasympathetic (secretomotor) fibres to various glands, are separate components. They merge within the meatus. At the end of the meatus, the facial nerve enters its own canal, the facial canal, which runs across the medial wall and down the posterior wall of the tympanic cavity to the stylomastoid foramen (**Fig. 38.9**). As the nerve enters the facial canal, there is a bend which contains the geniculate ganglion (**Figs 38.4, 38.11**).

The branches which arise from the facial nerve within the temporal bone can be divided into those which come from the geniculate ganglion and those which arise within the facial canal.

The main branch from the geniculate ganglion is the greater (superficial) petrosal nerve. It is a branch of the nervus intermedius. The greater petrosal nerve passes anteriorly, receives a branch from the tympanic plexus and traverses a hiatus on the anterior surface of the petrous part of the temporal bone. It enters the middle cranial fossa and runs forwards in a groove on the bone above the lesser petrosal nerve. It passes beneath the trigeminal ganglion to reach the foramen lacerum. Here it is joined by the deep petrosal nerve from the internal carotid sympathetic plexus, to become the nerve of the pterygoid canal (Vidian's nerve). The greater petrosal nerve contains parasympathetic fibres destined for the pterygopalatine ganglion, and taste fibres from the palate.

The nerve to stapedius arises from the facial nerve in the facial nerve canal behind the pyramidal eminence of the posterior wall of the tympanic cavity. It passes forwards through a small canal to reach the muscle.

The chorda tympani (**Fig. 38.12**, **Fig. 30.7**) leaves the facial nerve c.6 mm above the stylomastoid foramen and runs anterosuperiorly in a canal to enter the tympanic cavity via the posterior canaliculus. It then curves anteriorly in the substance of the tympanic membrane between its mucous and fibrous layers (**Fig. 38.6**), crosses medial to the upper part of the handle of the malleus to the anterior wall, where it enters the

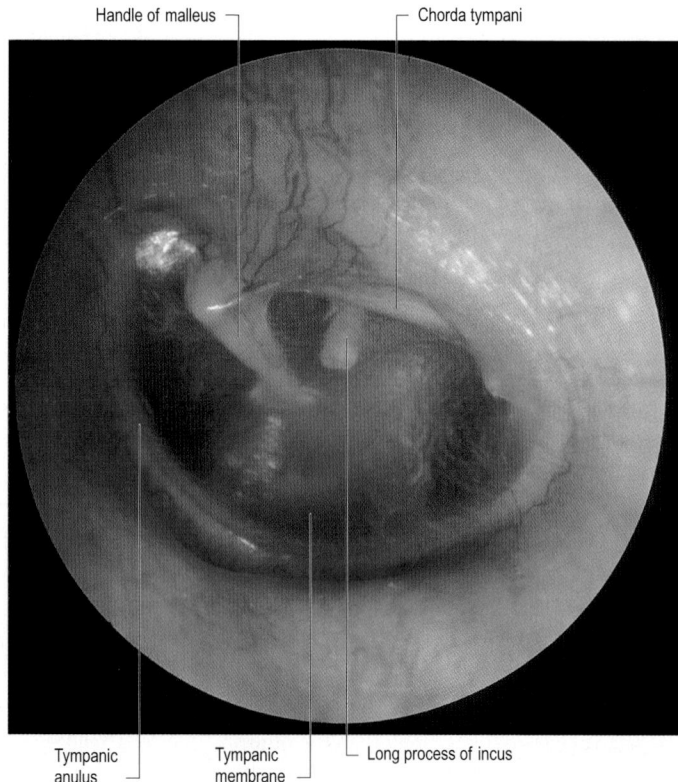

Handle of malleus
Chorda tympani
Tympanic anulus
Tympanic membrane
Long process of incus

Fig. 38.12 Chorda tympani nerve crossing the tympanic membrane. (By kind permission from Mr Simon A Hickey.)

anterior canaliculus (**Fig. 38.7**) It exits the skull at the petrotympanic fissure and its further course is described on page 525. It contains parasympathetic fibres which supply the submandibular and sublingual salivary glands via the submandibular ganglion (**Fig. 30.8**) and taste fibres from the anterior two-thirds of the tongue.

The geniculate ganglion also communicates with the lesser petrosal nerve.

BELL'S PALSY

Bell's palsy is the name given to a lower motor neurone palsy of the facial nerve which occurs spontaneously and without obvious cause. It is characterized by a flaccid paralysis of the ipsilateral muscles of facial expression; decreased lacrimation in the ipsilateral eye (which is controlled by neurones in the greater petrosal nerve); and hyperacusis or decreased tolerance of loud noises in the ipsilateral ear due to paralysis of stapedius. Its cause remains the subject of speculation, but recent MRI studies suggest that it may be the result of viral neuronitis either in the bony first part of the facial canal (labyrinthine segment) at the apex of the internal auditory canal, or in the adjacent brain stem. In the majority of cases spontaneous full recovery occurs after a few weeks.

DEHISCENCES OF FACIAL NERVE CANAL

The facial nerve may be somewhat variable in its anatomical course through the temporal bone. It may split into two or three strands, or pass a few millimetres posteriorly to its second bend, before it turns inferiorly posterior to the fossa incudis – a position where it is particularly vulnerable during surgical exploration of the mastoid antrum. It may be dehiscent, particularly in its second part, when it occasionally overhangs the stapes, or run inferior to the stapes superstructure, a position which renders it vulnerable during surgery to the stapes. The motor fibres to the face may be carried through the chorda tympani, which is then enlarged. When this occurs, the distal facial nerve dwindles to a fibrous strand in a narrowed stylomastoid foramen. In chronic bone disease in the tympanic cavity, the facial nerve may be exposed in its canal. Inflammation may lead to facial paralysis of the infranuclear or lower motor neurone type.

REFERENCES

Anderson SD 1976 The intratympanic muscles. In: Scientific Foundations of Otolaryngology. Hinchcliffe R (ed) Heinemann, London. pp 257–280.

Anson BJ, Donaldson JA 1976 The Surgical Anatomy of the Temporal Bone and Ear. Saunders, Philadelphia.

Baily CM 1997 Surgical anatomy of the skull base. In: Scott Brown's Otolaryngology. Sixth ed. Vol 1. Kerr GA (ed). Butterworth Heinemann, London. Chapter 15. pp. 1–15.

Bluestone C, Klein J 2002 Otitis media, atelectasis and Eustachian tube dysfunction. In: Pediatric Otolaryngology. Bluestone CD, Stool SE (eds) 4th edition. Vol. 1. Saunders, Philadelphia. pp 474–686.

Couter RT 1980 A Colour Atlas of Temporal Bone Surgical Anatomy. Wolfe Medical, London.

Glassock (III) ME, Shambaugh GE 1990 Surgery of the Ear. 4th edition. Saunders, Philadelphia.

Grey P 1995 The clinical significance of the communicating branches of the somatic sensory supply of the middle and external ear. J Laryngol Otol 109: 1141–1145.

Honjo I 1988 Eustachian Tube and Middle Ear Diseases. Springer-Verlag, Berlin.

Phelps PD, Lloyd GAS 1990 Diagnostic Imaging of the Ear. 2nd edition. Springer-Verlag, Berlin.

Wright A 1997 Anatomy and ultrastructure of the human ear. In: Scott Brown's Otolaryngology. Sixth ed. Vol 1. Kerr GA (ed). Butterworth Heinemann, London. Chapter 1. pp. 1–50.

Inner ear

The inner ear contains the organ of hearing, the cochlea, and the organs of balance, the utricle, saccule and semicircular canals. It consists of the bony (osseous) labyrinth, a series of interlinked cavities in the petrous temporal bone, and the membranous labyrinth of interconnected membranous sacs and ducts that lie within the bony labyrinth. The gap between the internal wall of the bony labyrinth and the external surface of the membranous labyrinth is filled with perilymph, a clear fluid with an ionic composition similar to that of other extracellular fluids, i.e. low in potassium ions and high in sodium and calcium. The membranous labyrinth contains endolymph, a fluid with an ionic composition more like that of cytosol, i.e. high in potassium ions and low in sodium and calcium. Moreover, the endolymphatic compartment is c.80 mV more positive than the perilymphatic compartment. These differences in ionic composition and potential are essential to the primary function of the inner ear, because they provide the driving force for mechano-transduction, the process by which sensory hair cells convert the vibrations set up in the inner ear fluids by sound or head movements into electrical signals that are transmitted via the vestibulocochlear nerve to the vestibular and cochlear nuclei in the brain stem.

BONE

TEMPORAL BONE: INTERNAL ACOUSTIC MEATUS

The internal acoustic meatus is separated from the internal ear at its lateral fundus by a vertical plate divided unequally by a transverse crest (**Fig. 39.1**). The canal for the facial nerve passes above and anterior to the crest. Posterior to the crest, the superior vestibular area contains openings for nerves to the utricle and anterior and lateral semicircular ducts. Below the crest, an anterior cochlear area contains a spiral of small holes, the tractus spiralis foraminosus, which encircles the central cochlear canal. Behind this, the inferior vestibular area contains openings for saccular nerves, and most posteroinferior, a single hole (foramen singulare) admits the nerve to the posterior semicircular duct.

LABYRINTH

Bony labyrinth

The bony labyrinth consists of the vestibule, semicircular canals and cochlea, which are all cavities lined by periosteum; they contain the membranous labyrinth (**Figs 38.4, 38.9, 39.2, 39.3, 39.4**). The bony labyrinth consists of bone that is more dense and harder than other parts of the petrous bone, and it is therefore possible, particularly in young skulls, to dissect it out from the petrous temporal bone.

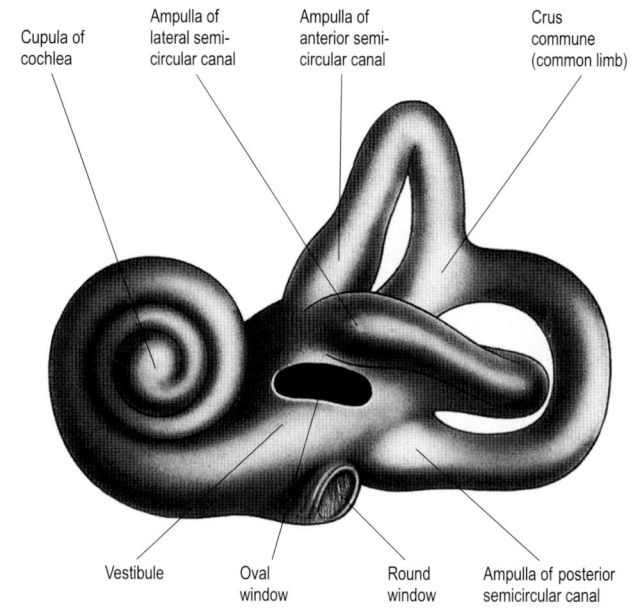

Fig. 39.2 The left bony labyrinth: lateral aspect.

Labels: Cupula of cochlea; Ampulla of lateral semi-circular canal; Ampulla of anterior semi-circular canal; Crus commune (common limb); Vestibule; Oval window; Round window; Ampulla of posterior semicircular canal

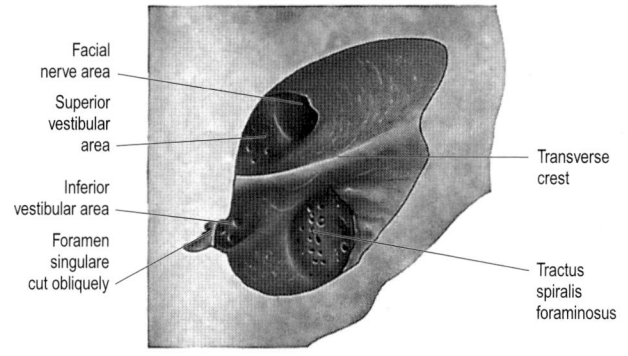

Fig. 39.1 The fundus of the left internal acoustic meatus, exposed by a section through the petrous part of the left temporal bone nearly parallel to the line of its superior border.

Labels: Facial nerve area; Superior vestibular area; Inferior vestibular area; Foramen singulare cut obliquely; Transverse crest; Tractus spiralis foraminosus

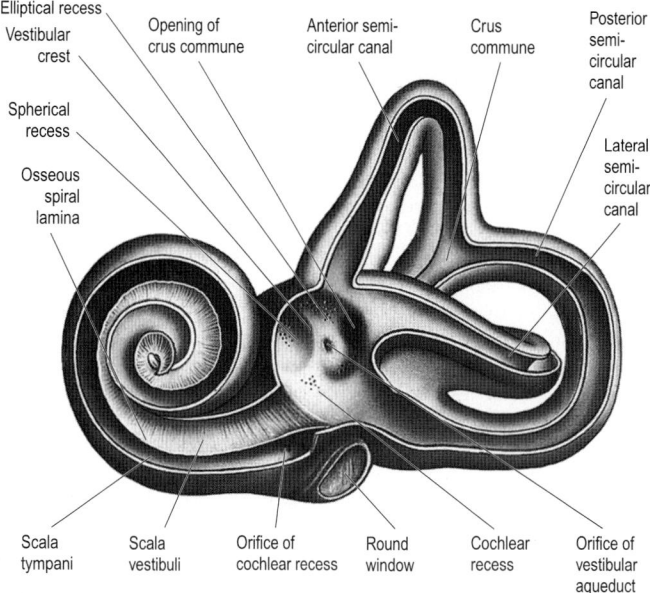

Fig. 39.3 The interior of the left bony labyrinth.

Labels: Elliptical recess; Vestibular crest; Spherical recess; Osseous spiral lamina; Opening of crus commune; Anterior semicircular canal; Crus commune; Posterior semicircular canal; Lateral semicircular canal; Scala tympani; Scala vestibuli; Orifice of cochlear recess; Round window; Cochlear recess; Orifice of vestibular aqueduct

663

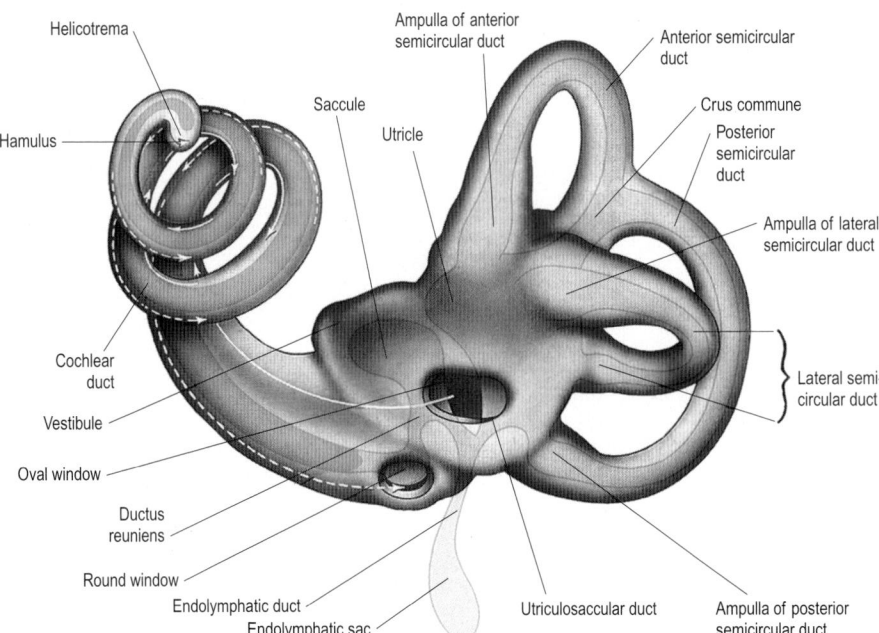

Helicotrema

Ampulla of anterior
semicircular duct

Anterior semicircular
duct

Saccule

Crus commune

Hamulus

Utricle

Posterior
semicircular
duct

Ampulla of lateral
semicircular duct

Cochlear
duct

Vestibule

Lateral semi-
circular duct

Oval window

Ductus
reuniens

Round window

Endolymphatic duct

Endolymphatic sac

Utriculosaccular duct

Ampulla of posterior
semicircular duct

Fig. 39.4 The membranous labyrinth (blue) projected onto the bony labyrinth. The arrows indicate the direction of pressure waves in the cochlea.

Vestibule

The vestibule is the central part of the bony labyrinth and lies medial to the tympanic cavity, posterior to the cochlea and anterior to the semicircular canals (**Figs 38.4, 39.2**). It is somewhat ovoid in shape but flattened transversely, and measures c.5 mm from front to back and vertically, and c.3 mm across. In its lateral wall is the opening of the oval window (fenestra vestibuli) into which the base of the stapes inserts, and to which the base of the stapes is attached by an anular ligament (**Fig. 38.9**). Anteriorly, on the medial wall, is a small spherical recess that contains the saccule; it is perforated by several minute holes, the macula cribrosa media, which transmit fine branches of the vestibular nerve to the saccule (**Figs 39.3, 39.4**). Behind the recess is an oblique vestibular crest, the anterior end of which forms the vestibular pyramid. This crest divides below to enclose a small depression, the cochlear recess, which is perforated by vestibulocochlear fascicles as they pass to the vestibular end of the cochlear duct. Posterosuperior to the vestibular crest, in the roof and medial wall of the vestibule, is the elliptical recess (**Fig. 39.3**), which contains the utricle. The pyramid and adjoining part of the elliptical recess are perforated by a number of holes, the macula cribrosa superior. The holes in the pyramid transmit the nerves to the utricle and those in the recess transmit the nerves to the ampullae of the superior and lateral semicircular canals (**Fig. 38.4, Fig. 39.3**). The region of the pyramid and elliptical recess corresponds to the superior vestibular area in the internal acoustic meatus (**Fig. 39.1**). The vestibular aqueduct opens below the elliptical recess. It reaches the posterior surface of the petrous bone and contains one or more small veins and part of the membranous labyrinth, the endolymphatic duct (**Fig. 39.4**). In the posterior part of the vestibule are the five openings of the semicircular canals; in its anterior wall is an elliptical opening that leads into the scala vestibuli of the cochlea.

Semicircular canals

The three semicircular canals, superior (anterior), posterior and lateral (horizontal), are located posterosuperior to the vestibule (**Figs 38.4, 38.9, 39.2, 39.3, 39.4**). They are compressed from side to side and each forms approximately two-thirds of a circle. They are unequal in length, but similar in diameter along their lengths, except where they bear a terminal swelling, an ampulla, which is almost twice the diameter of the canal.

The superior (anterior) semicircular canal is 15–20 mm long. It is vertical in orientation and lies transverse to the long axis of the petrous temporal bone under the anterior surface of its arcuate eminence. The eminence may not accurately coincide with this semicircular canal, but may instead be adapted to the occipitotemporal sulcus on the inferior surface of the temporal lobe of the brain. The ampulla at the anterior end of the canal opens into the upper and lateral part of the vestibule. Its other end unites with the upper end of the posterior canal to form

the crus commune (common limb), which is c.4 mm long, and opens into the medial part of the vestibule.

The posterior semicircular canal is also vertical but curves backwards almost parallel with the posterior surface of the petrous bone. It is 18–22 mm long and its ampulla opens low in the vestibule, below the cochlear recess where the macula cribrosa inferior transmits nerves to it. Its upper end joins the crus commune.

The lateral (horizontal) canal is 12–15 mm long and its arch runs horizontally backwards and laterally. Its anterior ampulla opens into the upper and lateral angle of the vestibule, above the oval window and just below the ampulla of the superior canal; its posterior end opens below the opening of the crus commune.

The two lateral semicircular canals of the two ears are often described as being in the same plane and the anterior canal of one side as being almost parallel with the opposite posterior canal. However, measurements of the angular relations of the planes of the semicircular osseous canals in 10 human skulls led Blanks et al (1975) to suggest that the planes of the three ipsilateral canals are not completely perpendicular to each other. The angles were measured as: horizontal/anterior 111.76 ± 7.55°, anterior/posterior 86.16 ± 4.72°, posterior/horizontal 95.75 ± 4.66°. The planes of similarly orientated canals of the two sides also showed some departure from being parallel: left anterior/right posterior 24.50 ± 7.19°, left posterior/right anterior 23.73 ± 6.71°, left horizontal/right horizontal 19.82 ± 14.93°. The same observers (Curthoys et al 1977) also measured the dimensions and radii of the canals. The means for the radii of the osseous canals were found to be as follows: horizontal 3.25 mm, anterior 3.74 mm, posterior 3.79 mm. The diameters of the osseous canals are c.1 mm (minor axis) and 1.4 mm (major axis). The membranous ducts within them are much smaller, but are also elliptical in transverse section, and have major and minor axes of 0.23 and 0.46 mm (**Fig. 39.5**). Representative means for ampullary dimensions are as follows: length 1.94 mm, height 1.55 mm. Phylogenetic studies suggest that the arc sizes of the semicircular canals in humans and other primates may be functionally linked to sensory control of body movements. The angulation and dimensions of the canals may be related to locomotor behaviour and possibly to agility, or more specifically to the frequency spectra of natural head movements (see review by Spoor & Zonneveld, 1998).

Cochlea

The cochlea (from the Greek *cochlos* for snail) is the most anterior part of the labyrinth, lying in front of the vestibule (**Figs 38.4, 38.9, 39.2, 39.3, 39.4, 39.6**). It is c.5 mm from base to apex, and 9 mm across its base. Its apex, or cupula, points towards the anterosuperior area of the medial wall of the tympanic cavity (**Figs 38.4, 39.6**). Its base faces the bottom of the internal acoustic meatus and is perforated by numerous apertures for the cochlear nerve. The cochlea has a conical central bony

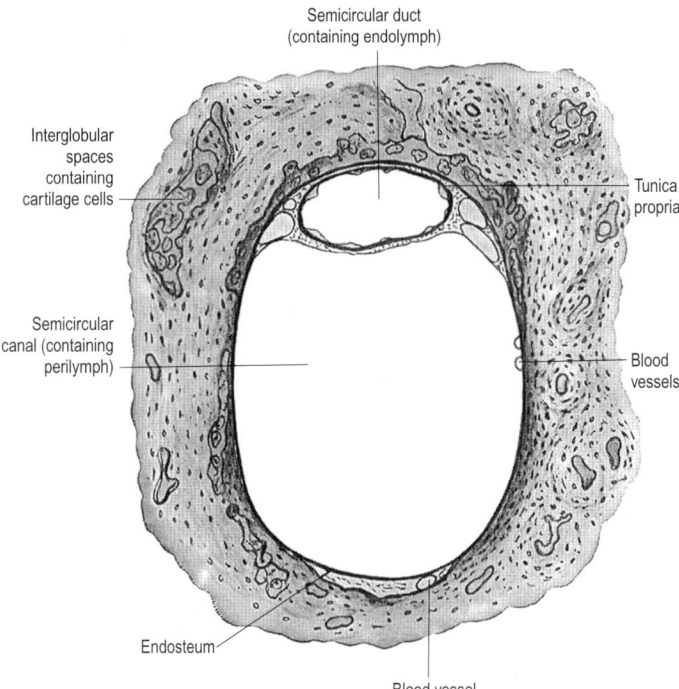

Fig. **39.5** Transverse section through the left posterior semicircular canal and duct of an adult man. (After JK Milne Dickie.)

narrow slit, the helicotrema (**Fig. 39.4**). Two elastic membranes form the upper and lower bounds of the scala media. One is Reissner's membrane, the thin vestibular membrane that separates the scala media from the scala vestibuli. The other is the basilar membrane, which forms the partition between the scala media and the scala tympani. The organ of Corti, the sensory epithelium responsible for hearing, sits on the inner surface of the basilar membrane (p. 671). At the base of the scala vestibuli is the oval window (fenestra vestibuli), which leads onto the vestibular cavity but is sealed by the footplate of the stapes. The scala tympani is separated from the tympanic cavity by the secondary tympanic membrane at the round window (fenestra cochleae). The central cochlear core, the modiolus, has a broad base near the lateral end of the internal acoustic meatus, where it corresponds to the spiral tract (tractus spiralis foraminosus) (**Fig. 39.6**). There are several openings in this area for the fascicles of the cochlear nerve: those for the first $1^1/_2$ turns run through the small holes of the spiral tract, and those for the apical turn run through the hole that forms the centre of the tract. Canals from the spiral tract go through the modiolus and open in a spiral sequence into the base of the osseous spiral lamina. Here the small canals enlarge and fuse to form Rosenthal's canal, a spiral canal in the modiolus which follows the course of the osseous spiral lamina and contains the spiral ganglion (**Fig. 39.7**). The main tract continues through the centre of the modiolus to the cochlear apex.

The osseous cochlear canal spirals for about $2^3/_4$ turns around the modiolus and is c.35 mm long. At its first turn, the canal bulges towards the tympanic cavity where it underlies the promontory. At the base of the cochlea, the canal is c.3 mm in diameter but it becomes progressively reduced in diameter as it spirals apically to end at the cupula. In addition to the round and oval windows, which are the two main openings at it base, the canal has a third smaller opening for the cochlear aqueduct or canaliculus. The latter is a minute funnel-shaped canal that runs to the inferior surface of the petrous temporal bone; it transmits a small vein to the inferior petrosal sinus and connects the subarachnoid space to the scala tympani.

The osseous or primary spiral lamina is a ledge that projects from the modiolus into the osseous canal like the thread of a screw (**Fig. 39.7**). It is attached to the inner edge of the basilar membrane and ends in a hook-shaped hamulus at the cochlear apex, partly bounding the helicotrema (**Fig. 39.4**), which is an opening connecting the scala tympani and scala vestibuli. From Rosenthal's canal, many tiny canals, the habenula perforata, radiate through the osseous lamina to its rim;

core, the modiolus, and a spiral canal runs around it. A delicate osseous spiral lamina (or ledge) projects from the modiolus, partially dividing the canal (**Fig. 39.7**). Within this bony spiral lies the membranous cochlear duct, attached to the modiolus at one edge and to the outer cochlear wall by its other edge. There are therefore three longitudinal channels within the cochlea. The middle canal (the cochlear duct or scala media) is blind, and ends at the apex of the cochlea; its flanking channels communicate with each other at the modiolar apex at a

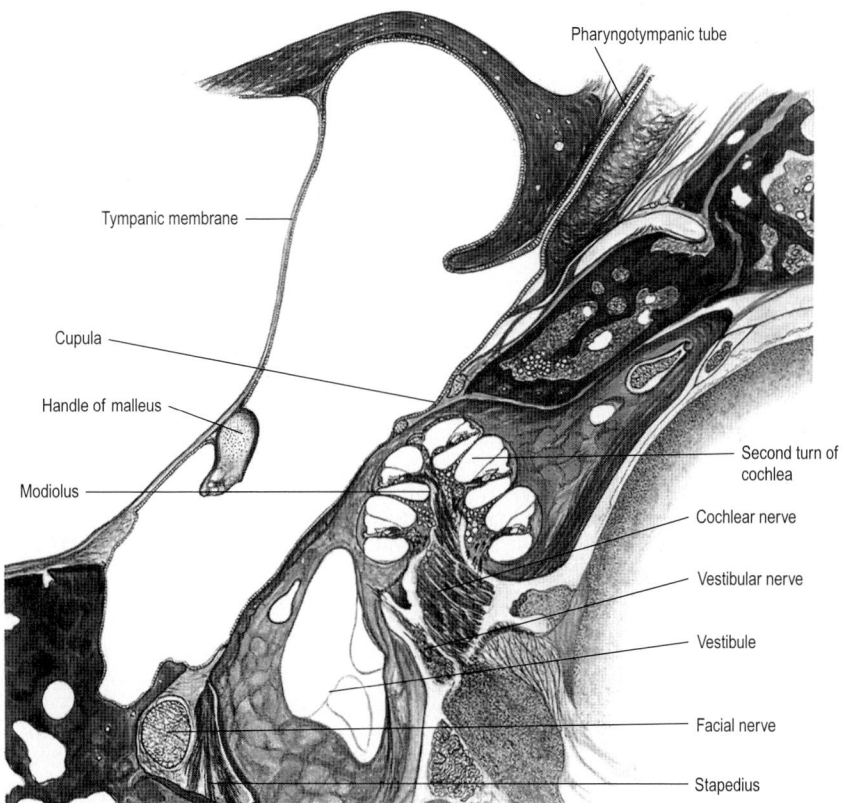

Fig. **39.6** Horizontal section through the left temporal bone. (Drawn from a section prepared at the Ferens Institute and lent by the late J Kirk.)

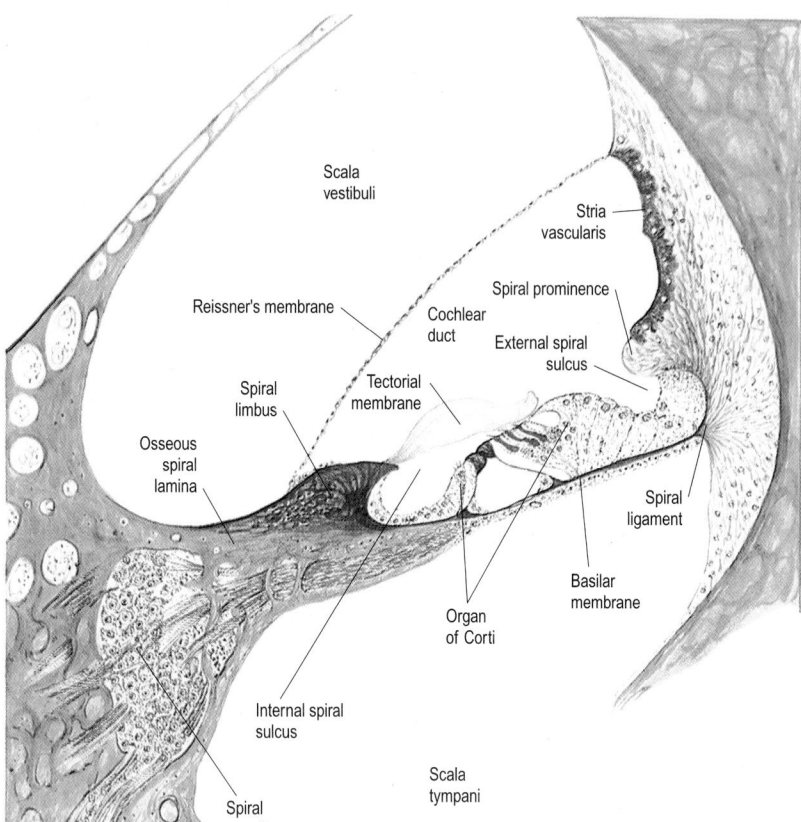

Scala
vestibuli

Stria
vascularis

Spiral prominence

Reissner's membrane

Cochlear
duct

External spiral
sulcus

Spiral
limbus

Tectorial
membrane

Osseous
spiral
lamina

Spiral
ligament

Basilar
membrane

Organ
of Corti

Internal spiral
sulcus

Scala
tympani

Spiral
ganglion

M.CLARK

Fig. 39.7 Section through the second turn of the cochlea seen in
Fig. 39.6. The modiolus is to the left. Mallory's stain.

they carry fascicles of the cochlear nerve to the organ of Corti (**Fig. 39.8**).
A secondary spiral lamina projects inwards from the outer cochlear wall
towards the osseous spiral lamina and is attached to the outer edge of
the basilar membrane. It is most prominent in the lower part of the first
turn: the gap between the two laminae increases progressively towards
the cochlear apex, which means that the basilar membrane is wider at
the apex of the cochlea than at the base.

Microstructure of the bony labyrinth
The wall of the bony labyrinth is lined by fibroblast-like perilymphatic
cells and extracellular fibres (**Fig. 39.5**). The morphology of the cells
varies in different parts of the labyrinth. Where the perilymphatic space
is narrow, as in the cochlear aqueduct, the cells are reticular or stellate

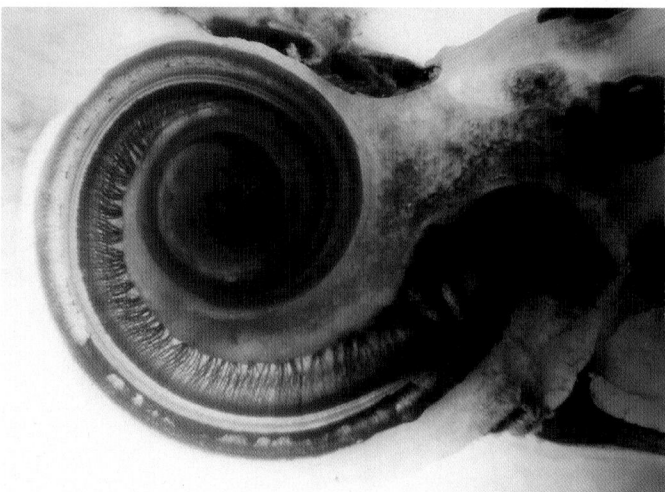

Fig. 39.8 Whole-mount preparation of the organ of Corti from a human
cochlea, stained with osmium to show the distribution of tissues, including the
myelinated axons. (Provided by H Felix, M Gleeson and L-G Johnsson, ENT
Department, University of Zurich and GKT School of Medicine, London.)

in form, and give off sheet-like cytoplasmic extensions that cross the
space. Where the space is wider, as in the scalae vestibuli and tympani
of the cochlea and much of the vestibule, the perilymphatic cells on the
periosteum and the external surface of the membranous labyrinth are
extremely flat, and resemble a squamous epithelium. Elsewhere, on
parts of the perilymphatic surface of the basilar membrane, the cells are
cuboidal. Bundles of collagen fibres are closely related to the periosteal
and labyrinthine aspects of these cells.

Composition of inner ear fluids
The space between the bony and membranous labyrinths is filled
with perilymph (**Figs 39.4, 39.5**). The membranous labyrinth is filled
with endolymph, a fluid produced by the marginal cells of the stria
vascularis and the dark cells of the vestibule (see review by Wangemann
& Schacht 1996) (**Figs 39.7, 39.9**). Whatever their relative contributions, endolymph probably circulates in the labyrinth; it enters the
endolymphatic sac, where it is transferred into the adjacent vascular
plexus via the specialized epithelium of the sac. Pinocytotic removal of
fluid may also occur in other labyrinthine regions.

Perilymph was initially considered to be an ultrafiltrate of plasma
because of its low protein content. However, it more closely resembles
cerebrospinal fluid in ionic composition, particularly in the scala
tympani. Its composition is not precisely the same in both cochlear
scalae: concentrations of potassium, glucose, amino acids and proteins
are greater in the scala vestibuli. This has led to the suggestion that
perilymph in the scala vestibuli is derived from plasma via the endothelial boundary of the cochlear blood vessels, whereas the perilymph
in the scala tympani contains some cerebrospinal fluid derived from
the subarachnoid spaces via the cochlear canaliculus. However, the lack
of significant bulk flow suggests that perilymph homeostasis is predominantly locally regulated. Perilymph contains approximately
5 mM K^+, 150 mM Na^+, 120 mM Cl^- and 1.5 mM Ca^{2+}. Endolymph
contains greater K^+ (150 mM) and Cl^- (130 mM) concentrations and
lower Na^+ (2 mM) and Ca^{2+} (20 µM) concentrations than perilymph.
The major differences in ionic composition between the two fluids
are important for the function of the inner ear. Displacements of the
stereociliary bundles of the sensory cells activate relatively non-specific
cationic channels in the stereociliary tips, which allows an influx of
cations, particularly K^+ and Ca^{2+}, from the endolymph. Hair cells also
possess K^+ channels activated by membrane voltage or intracellular Ca^{2+}

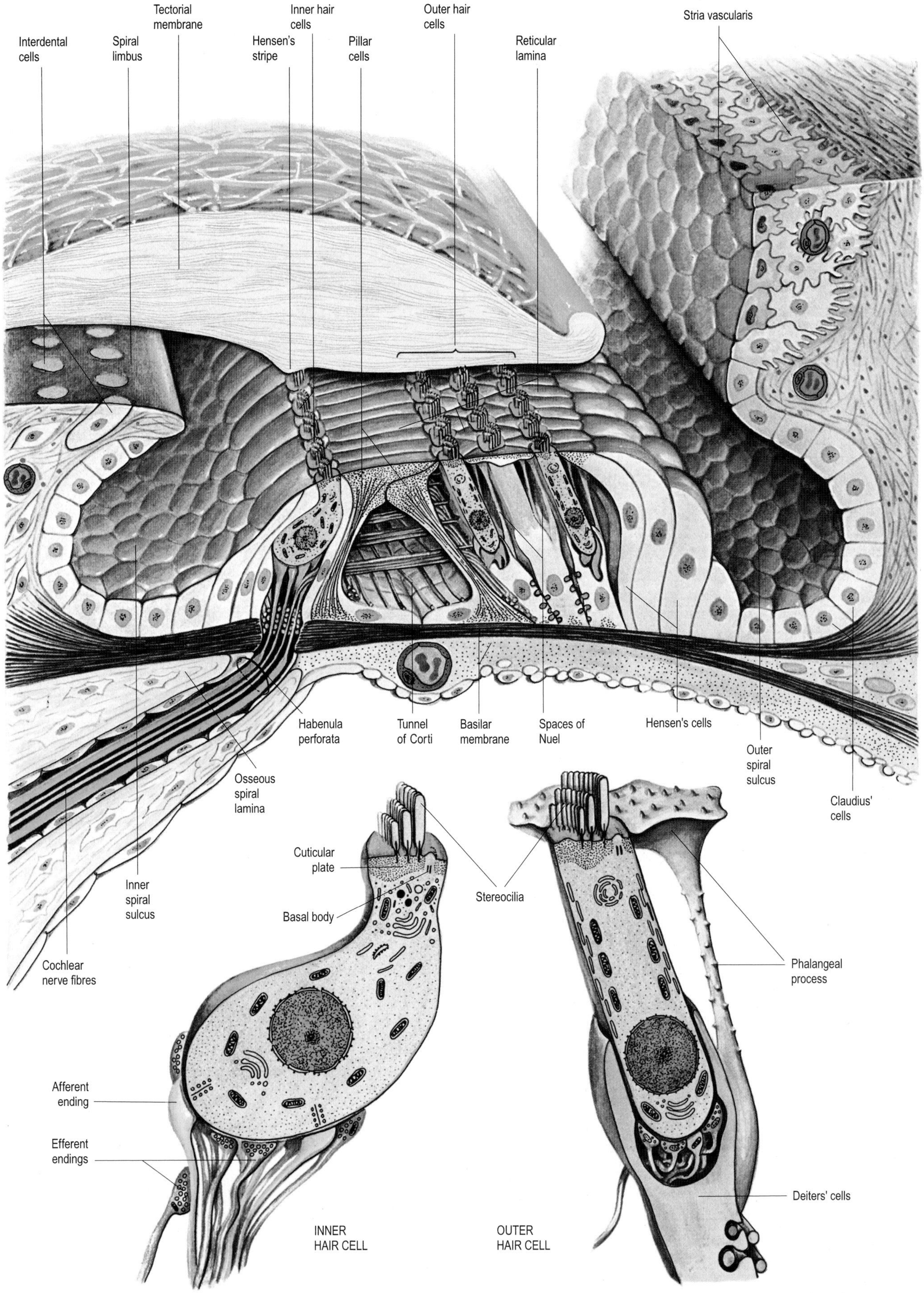

Fig. 39.9 Structure of the cochlear organ of Corti and stria vascularis, showing the arrangement of the various types of cell and their overall innervation. The organization of the inner and outer hair cells and their synaptic connections are depicted below. Afferent nerve terminals are coloured green and efferent fibres purple.

concentrations, and these allow efflux of K^+ into the perilymph which bathes their basal and lateral membranes. In addition, synaptic transmission at the base and sides of hair cells depends on the influx of Ca^{2+} from the perilymph through voltage-dependent calcium channels in order to release neurotransmitter.

Membranous labyrinth

The membranous labyrinth is separated from the periosteum by a space that contains perilymph and a web-like network of fine blood vessels (**Figs 39.4, 39.5**). It can be divided into two major regions, the vestibular apparatus and the cochlear duct.

The vestibular apparatus consists of three membranous semicircular canals which communicate with the utricle, a membranous sac leading into a smaller chamber, the saccule, via the utriculosaccular duct. This Y-shaped duct has a side branch to the endolymphatic duct, which passes to the endolymphatic sac, a small but functionally important expansion situated under the dura of the petrous temporal bone. From the saccule, a narrow canal, the ductus reuniens, leads to the base of the cochlear duct. These various ducts and sacs form a closed system of inter-communicating channels. Endolymph is resorbed into the cerebrospinal fluid from the endolymphatic sac, which therefore provides the site for the drainage of endolymph for the entire membranous labyrinth.

The terminal fibres of the vestibular nerve are connected to five distinct areas of specialized sensory epithelium (two maculae and three crests) in the walls of the membranous labyrinth. Maculae are flat plaques of sensory hair cells surrounded by supporting cells, and are found in the utricle and saccule. The crests are ridges bearing sensory hair cells and supporting cells. They are found in the walls of the ampullae near the utricular openings of the three semicircular canals, one for each canal.

Utricle

The utricle is the larger of the two major vestibular sacs. It is an irregular, oblong, dilated sac that occupies the posterosuperior region of the vestibule (**Fig. 39.4**), and contacts the elliptical recess (where it is a blind-ended pouch) and the area inferior to it.

The macula of the utricle (or utriculus) is a specialized area of neurosensory epithelium lining the membranous wall, and is the largest of the vestibular sensory areas (**Fig. 39.10**). It is triangular or heart-shaped

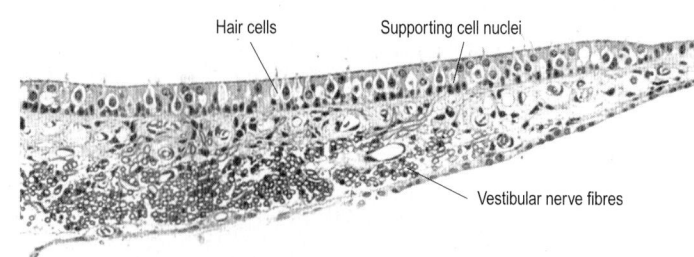

Fig. 39.10 Section of the utricular macula from a guinea pig, showing the relative positions of the hair cells and supporting cell nuclei. Semi-thin resin section, toluidine blue stain. (The inner ear is extremely vulnerable to hypoxia and situated in one of the hardest bones in the body, which means that well-fixed human tissue is rarely obtained for histology. Guinea pigs are one of the most frequently used animal models of human hearing and their inner ear ultrastructure is very similar.) (Provided by RM Walsh, DN Furness and CM Hackney, MacKay Institute of Communication and Neuroscience, Keele University.)

in surface view and lies horizontally with its long axis orientated anteroposteriorly and its sharp angle pointing posteriorly (**Fig. 39.11**). It is flat except at the anterior edge, where it is gently folded in on itself, and it measures c.2.8 mm long by 2.2 mm wide. The mature form of the macula is reached early in development, but in the adult a bulge is often present on the anterolateral border; there is sometimes an indentation at the anteromedial border. The epithelial surface is covered by the otolithic membrane (statoconial membrane), a gelatinous structure in which many small crystals, the otoconia (otoliths, statoliths), are embedded. A curved ridge, the 'snowdrift line', runs along the length of the otolithic membrane. It corresponds to a narrow crescent of underlying sensory epithelium termed the striola, c.0.13 μm wide. The density of sensory hair cells in this strip of epithelium is c.20% less than in the rest of the macula. The striola is convex laterally and runs from the medial aspect of the anterior margin in a posterior direction towards, but not reaching, the posterior pole. The part of the macula medial to the striola is called the pars interna and is slightly larger than the pars externa, which is lateral to it. The significance of this area is that the sensory cells are functionally and anatomically polarized towards it (**Fig. 39.11**). The macula in each utricle is approximately horizontal

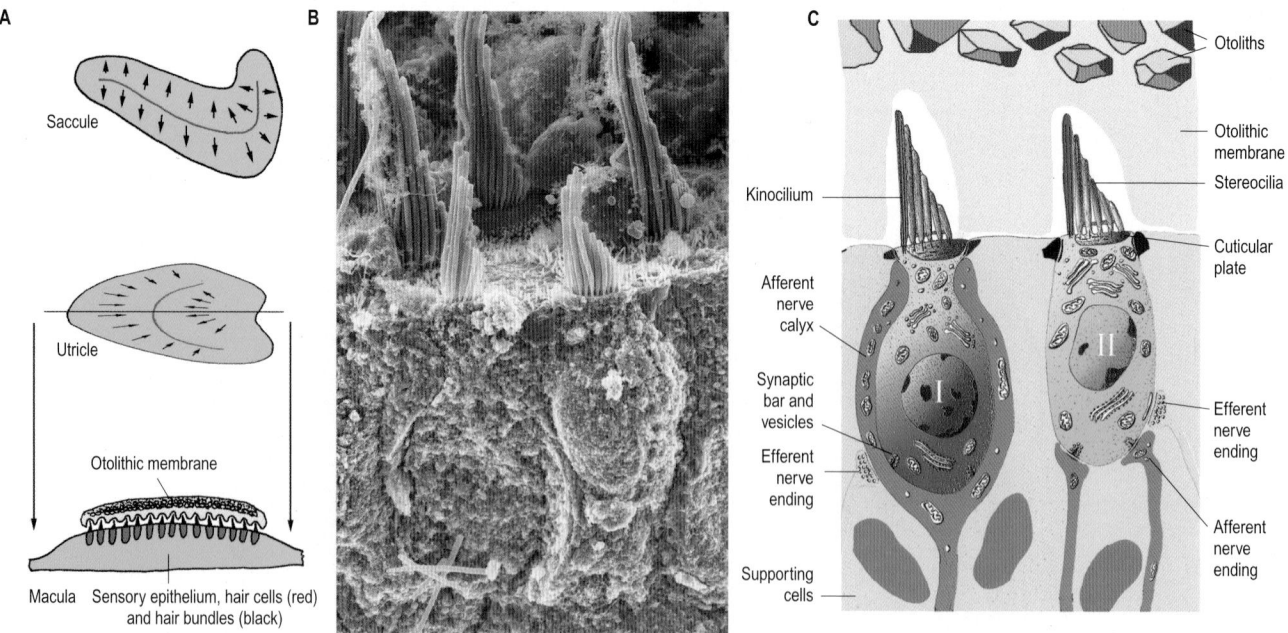

Fig. 39.11 A, Morphological organization of the saccular and utricular maculae and the relationship of their hair cells to the otolithic membrane. The utricular macula has been tilted in the plane of the page to emphasize that it lies horizontally, whereas the saccular macula lies vertically when the head is in an upright position. Note the different shapes of the maculae, the position of the striola as indicated by a curved line in each case, and the different orientations of their stereociliary bundles. The arrows indicate the excitatory direction of deflection. **B**, Scanning electron micrograph of a fracture of a utricular macula (guinea pig) showing a Type I hair cell (left) and a Type II hair cell (right). **C**, The differing innervation patterns of the two types of hair cell. (Provided by DN Furness, MacKay Institute of Communication and Neuroscience, Keele University.)

when the head is in its normal position. Linear acceleration of the head in any horizontal plane will result in the otolithic membrane lagging behind the movement of the membranous labyrinth as a result of the inertia produced by its mass. The membrane thus maximally stimulates one group of hair cells by deflecting their bundles towards the striola whilst inhibiting others by deflecting their bundles away from it. Hence each horizontal movement of the head will produce a specific pattern of firing in the utricular efferents.

Saccule

The saccule (or sacculus) is a slightly elongated, globular sac lying in the spherical recess near the opening of the scala vestibuli of the cochlea (**Fig. 39.11**). As already noted, it is connected to the utricle and endolymphatic duct by the utriculosaccular duct, and to the cochlea by the ductus reuniens, which leaves inferiorly to open into the base of the cochlear duct (**Fig. 39.4**).

The saccular macula is an almost elliptical structure, 2.6 mm long and 1.2 mm at its widest point. Its long axis is orientated antero-posteriorly but, in contrast to the utricular macula, the saccular macula lies in a vertical plane on the wall of the saccule. Its elliptical shape is very slightly distorted by a small anterosuperior bulge. Like the utricular macula, it is covered by an otolithic (statoconial) membrane and possesses a striola, c.0.13 mm wide, which extends along its long axis as an S-shaped strip about which the sensory cells are functionally and anatomically polarized (**Fig. 39.11**). The part of the macula above the striola is termed the pars interna, and that below it, the pars externa. The operation of the saccule is similar to that of the utricle. However, because of its vertical orientation, the saccule is particularly sensitive to linear acceleration of the head in the vertical plane, and is therefore a major gravitational sensor when the head is in an upright position. It is also particularly sensitive to movement along the anteroposterior axis.

Semicircular canals

The lateral, superior and posterior semicircular ducts follow the course of their osseous canals. Throughout most of their length they are securely attached, by much of their circumference, to the osseous walls (p. 462). They are approximately one-quarter of the diameter of their osseous canals (**Fig. 39.5**). The medial ends of the superior and posterior canals fuse to form a single common duct, the crus commune, before entering the utricle. The lateral end of each canal is dilated to form an ampulla, which lies within the ampulla of the osseous canal. The short segment of duct between the ampullae and utricle is the crus ampullaris.

The membranous wall of each ampulla contains a transverse elevation (septum transversum) on the central region of which is a sensory area, the ampullary crest (crista). This is a saddle-shaped ridge that lies transversely across the duct. It is broadly concave on its free edge along most of its length and has a concave gutter (planum semilunatum) at either end between the ridge and the duct wall. Sectioned across the ridge, the crests of the lateral and anterior semicircular canals have smoothly rounded corners; the posterior crest is more angular. A vertical plate of gelatinous extracellular material, the cupula, is attached along the free edge of the crest (**Fig. 39.12**). It projects far into the lumen of the ampulla, so that movements of endolymph within the duct readily deflect the cupula and therefore also the stereocilia of the sensory cells that are inserted into its base. The three semicircular canals thus detect angular accelerations during tilting or turning movements of the head in any direction.

Microstructure of the vestibular system

The maculae and crests detect the orientation of the head with respect to gravity and changes in head movement by means of the mechano-sensitive hair cells that are interspersed among the non-sensory supporting cells in their sensory epithelia. These hair cells are in contact with afferent and efferent endings of vestibular nerve fibres by synapses at their base. The entire epithelium lies on a bed of thick, fibrous connective tissue containing myelinated vestibular nerve fibres and blood vessels. The axons lose their myelin sheaths as they perforate the basal lamina of the sensory epithelium. There are two types of sensory hair cell in the vestibular system, Type I and Type II.

Type I vestibular sensory cells measure c.25 μm in length, with a free surface of 6–7 μm in diameter. The basal part of the cell does not reach the basal lamina of the epithelium. Each cell is typically bottle-shaped, with a narrow neck and a rather broad, rounded basal portion contain-

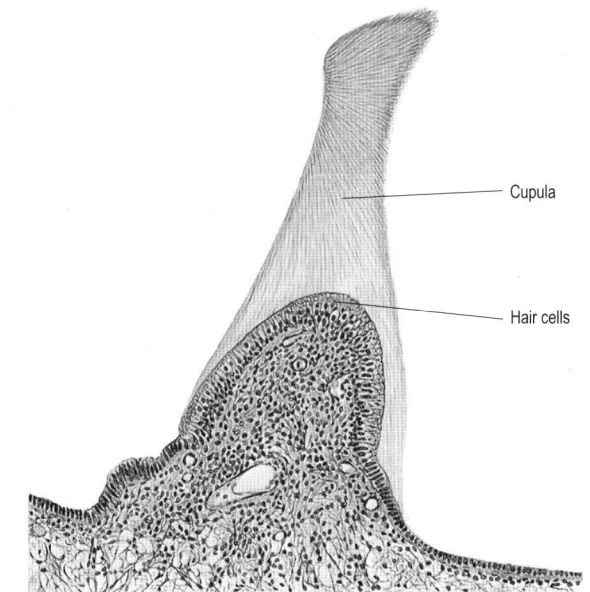

Cupula

Hair cells

Fig. 39.12 Section of an ampullary crest from a 6-month-old human fetus. (Drawn from a section prepared at the Ferens Institute and lent by EW Walls, Professor Emeritus, University College London.)

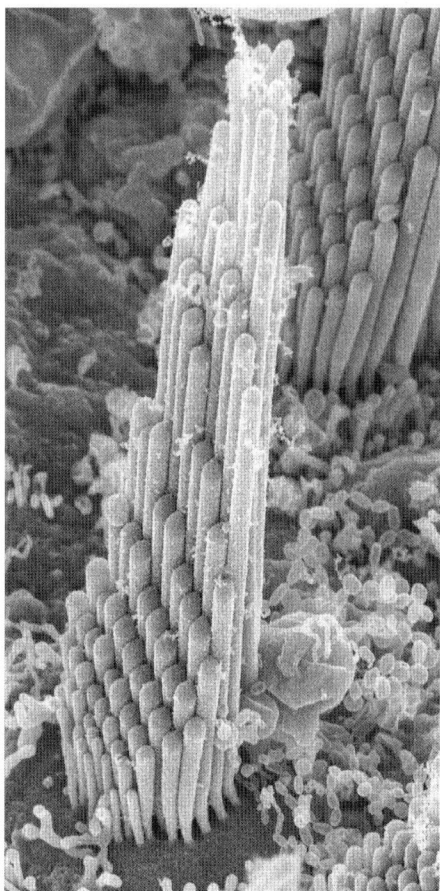

Fig. 39.13 Scanning electron micrograph of a stereociliary bundle from the utricle (guinea pig). The stereocilia are arranged in rows of increasing height towards the tallest element, the kinocilium. Deflection in the direction of the kinocilium results in depolarization of the hair cell. (Provided by DN Furness, MacKay Institute of Communication and Neuroscience, Keele University.)

ing the nucleus (**Fig 39.9, 39.11**). The apical surface is characterized by 30–50 stereocilia (large, regular microvilli c.0.25 μm across) and a single kinocilium (with the typical '9 + 2' arrangement of microtubules characteristic of true cilia). The kinocilium is considerably longer than the stereocilia, and may attain 40 μm, whereas the stereocilia are of graded lengths. They are characteristically arranged in regular rows behind the kinocilium in descending order of height, the longest being next to the kinocilium (**Fig. 39.13**). The kinocilium emerges basally from a typical basal body, with a centriole immediately beneath it. Close to the inner surface of their basal two-thirds, every cell contains numerous synaptic ribbons with associated synaptic vesicles. The post-synaptic surface of an afferent nerve ending encloses the greater part of the sensory cell body in the form of a cup (chalice or calyx) (**Fig. 39.9**). Efferent nerve fibres make synapses with the external surface of the calyx, rather than directly with the sensory cell.

There is much greater variation in the sizes of Type II sensory cells (**Fig. 39.14**). Some are up to 45 μm long, and almost span the entire thickness of the sensory epithelium, whereas others are shorter than Type I cells. They are mostly cylindrical, but otherwise resemble Type I cells in their contents and the presence of an apical kinocilium and stereocilia. However, their kinocilia and stereocilia tend to be shorter and less variable in length. The most striking difference between Type I and II cells is their efferent nerve terminals: Type II cells receive several efferent nerve boutons containing a mixture of small clear and dense-core vesicles around their bases. Afferent endings are small expansions rather than chalices.

Each sensory cell is structurally and functionally polarized (**Fig. 39.13**). Deflection of the hair bundle towards the kinocilium results in depolarization of the hair cell, and increases the rate of neurotransmitter release from its base. Deflection away from the kinocilium hyperpolarizes the hair cell and reduces the release of neurotransmitter. The hair cells have specific orientations within each sensory organ (**Fig. 39.13**). In the maculae, they are arranged symmetrically on either side of the striola. In the utricle, the kinocilia are positioned on the side of the sensory cell nearest to the striola. In the saccule, they are furthest from it. In the ampullary crests, the cells are orientated with their rows of stereocilia at right angles to the long axis of the semicircular duct. In the lateral crest the kinocilia are on the side towards the utricle, whereas in the anterior and posterior crests they are away from it. These different arrangements are important functionally, because any given acceleration of the head maximally depolarizes one group of hair cells and maximally inhibits a complementary set, thus providing a unique representation of the magnitude and orientation of any movement (for further details, see Furness 2002).

The Type I and II sensory cells are set within a matrix of supporting cells that reach from the base of the epithelium to its surface, and form rosettes round the sensory cells, as seen in surface view. Although their form is irregular, they can easily be recognized by the position of their nuclei, which tend to lie below the level of sensory cell nuclei and just above the basal lamina (**Fig. 39.10**). The apices of the supporting cells are attached by tight junctions to neighbouring cells to produce the reticular lamina, a composite layer which forms a plate that is relatively impermeable to cations other than via the mechanosensitive transduction channels of the hair cells.

The otolithic membrane is a layer of extracellular material with a complex structure. It can be divided into two strata. The external layer is composed of otoliths or otoconia, which are barrel-shaped crystals of calcium carbonate with angular ends, up to 30 μm long, and heterogeneous in distribution (**Figs 39.9, 39.10, 39.11, 39.13**). They are attached to a more basal gelatinous layer into which the stereocilia and kinocilia of the sensory cells are inserted. The gelatinous material consists largely of glycosaminoglycans associated with fibrous protein.

Epley's manoeuvre

Benign paroxysmal positional vertigo is a condition in which a sensation of rotation with associated nystagmus is induced by adopting a particular position (with the abnormal ear dependent). It is believed that calcium carbonate crystals from the otoliths become freed from their hair cells and, in certain positions, drop into the ampulla of the posterior semicircular canal, possibly becoming adherent to the cupula and rendering it gravity-sensitive. In certain positions the alignment of the axis of the posterior semicircular canal with gravity results in the

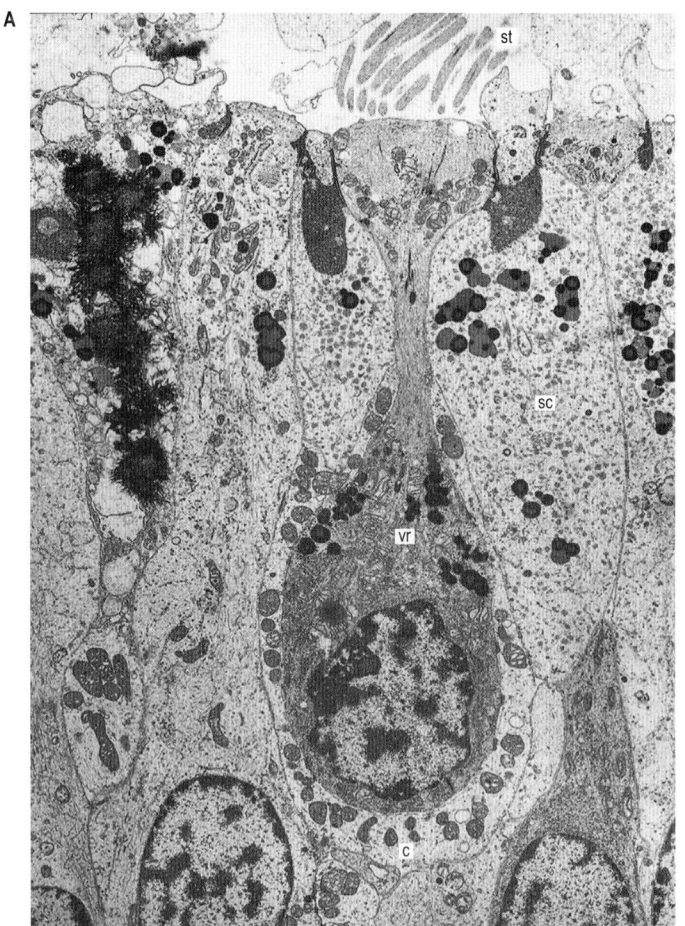

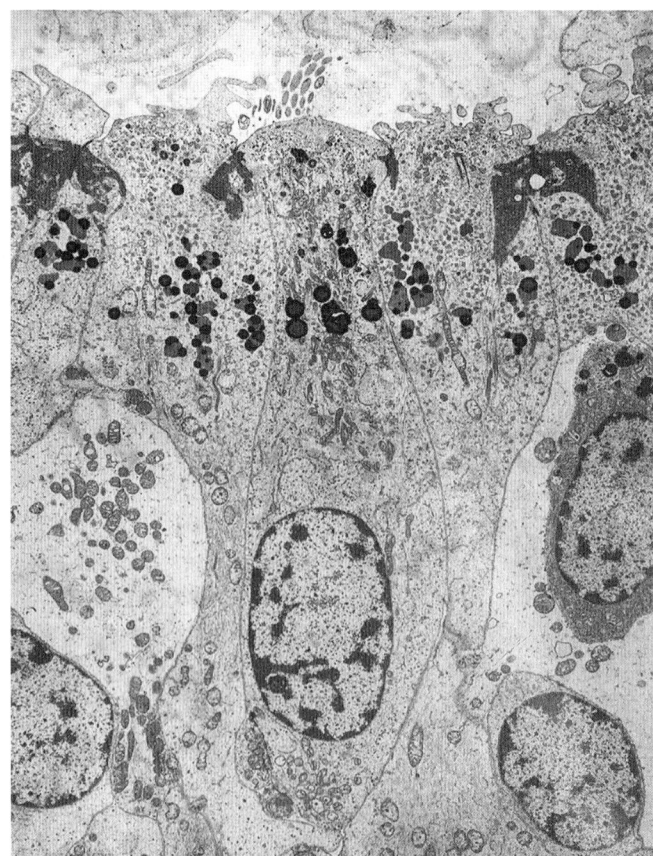

Fig. 39.14 **A**, Transmission electron micrograph of human Type I vestibular hair cell (vr) bearing an apical group of stereocilia (st) seen in a vertical section through the macula. Note that the hair cell is bottle-shaped, and that much of it is enclosed in the calyceal ending (c) of an afferent nerve terminal. Abbreviation: sc, supporting cells. **B**, Transmission electron micrograph of human Type II vestibular hair cell: a bouton-type afferent nerve terminal is in contact with the basal part. (Provided by H Felix, M Gleeson and L-G Johnsson, ENT Department, University of Zurich and GKT School of Medicine, London.)

displacement of the cupula and the activation of the vestibulo-ocular reflex, resulting in compensatory nystagmoid eye movements in response to apparent head movements.

Epley's canalith repositioning procedure relies on the adoption of a series of body postures designed to allow the aberrant crystals (or canaliths) to float out of the posterior semicircular canal and to stick to the wall of the vestibule. Cure rates in excess of 80% have been recorded and the procedures have largely superseded surgical procedures designed to denervate the ampulla of the posterior semicircular canal (cingular neurectomy) or obliterate the canal completely.

Endolymphatic duct and sac

The endolymphatic duct runs in the osseous vestibular aqueduct and becomes dilated distally to form the endolymphatic sac. This is a structure of variable size, which may extend through an aperture on the posterior surface of the petrous bone to end between the two layers of the dura on the posterior surface of the petrous temporal bone near the sigmoid sinus (**Fig. 39.4**). The surface cells throughout the entire endolymphatic duct resemble those lining the non-specialized parts of the membranous labyrinth, and consist of squamous or low cuboidal epithelium. The epithelial lining and subepithelial connective tissue become more complex where the duct dilates to form the endo-lymphatic sac. An intermediate or rugose segment and a distal sac can be distinguished. In the intermediate segment, the epithelium consists of light and dark cylindrical cells. Light cells are regular in form, and have numerous long surface microvilli with endocytic invaginations between them and large clear vesicles in their apical region. In contrast, dark cells are wedge-shaped, and have a narrow base, few apical microvilli and dense, fibrillar cytoplasm.

The endolymphatic sac has important roles in the maintenance of vestibular function. Endolymph produced elsewhere in the labyrinth is absorbed in this region, probably mainly by the light cells. Damage to the sac, or blockage of its connection to the rest of the labyrinth, causes endolymph to accumulate; this produces hydrops, which affects both vestibular and cochlear function. The epithelium is also permeable to leukocytes, including macrophages which can remove cellular debris from the endolymph, and to various cells of the immune system that contribute antibodies to this fluid.

A unique positive electrical potential exists in the endolymphatic spaces, varying from +77 mV in the cochlear duct near the stria vascularis to c.+44 mV in the utricle. This is additional to the normal resting potentials of the receptor cells, so that there is a very considerable potential difference across their membranes. This undoubtedly contributes to the extreme sensitivity to mechanical deformation of the labyrinthine sensory receptors.

Cochlear duct

The cochlear duct is a spiral tube that runs within the bony cochlea (**Figs 39.4, 39.6, 39.7, 39.8**). The osseous spiral lamina projects for part of the distance between the modiolus and the outer wall of the cochlea and is attached to the inner edge of the basilar membrane. The endosteum of the outer wall is thickened to form a spiral cochlear ligament, which projects inwards as a triangular basal crest attached to the outer rim of the basilar membrane. Immediately above this is a concavity, the external spiral sulcus (sulcus spiralis externus), above which the thick, highly vascular periosteum projects as a spiral promi-nence. Above the prominence is a specialized, thick epithelial layer, the stria vascularis. A second, thinner vestibular membrane, Reissner's membrane, extends from the thickened endosteum on the osseous spiral lamina to the outer wall of the cochlea, where it is attached above the stria. Reissner's membrane consists of two layers of squamous epithelial cells separated by a basal lamina. The side facing the scala vestibuli bears flattened perilymphatic cells, with tight junctions between them, creating a diffusion barrier. The endolymphatic side is lined by squamous epithelial cells; these are also joined by tight junctions and are involved in ion transport. The canal thus enclosed between the scala tympani and the scala vestibuli is the cochlear duct (**Fig. 39.7**). It is triangular in cross-section throughout the length of the cochlea. Its closed upper end, the lagaena, is attached to the cupula. The lower end of the duct turns medially, narrowing into the ductus reuniens, and connects with the saccule (**Fig. 39.4**).

The organ of Corti, the sensory epithelium of the cochlea, sits upon the basilar membrane. The apices of the sensory hair cells and support-ing cells it contains are joined by tight junctions to form the reticular lamina. The diffusion barriers which line the cochlear duct ensure that the apices of the sensory hair cells are bathed by endolymph, whereas their lateral and basal regions are bathed in perilymph.

The stria vascularis lies on the outer wall of the cochlear duct, above the spiral eminence (**Fig. 39.7**). It has a special stratified epithelium containing a dense intraepithelial capillary plexus and three cell types: superficial marginal, dark or chromophil cells; intermediate light, or chromophobe cells; and basal cells. The endolymphatic surface consists only of the apices of marginal cells. The intermediate and basal cells lie deeper within the stria and send cytoplasmic processes towards the surface, between the deeper parts of the marginal cells. The long descending cytoplasmic processes of the marginal dark cells and the ascending processes of the intermediate and basal cells envelop the intraepithelial capillaries. The stria vascularis is involved in ion transport, and it helps to produce the unusual ionic composition of endolymph. It is the source of the large positive endocochlear electrical potential, maintenance of which is directly dependent upon adequate oxygenation of the epithelial cells, which is provided by the intraepithelial capillary plexus.

The osseous spiral lamina consists of two plates of bone, between which are canals for the cochlear nerve filaments. On the upper plate, the periosteum is thickened to form the spiral limbus (limbus laminae spiralis) (**Fig. 39.7**). It ends externally in the internal spiral sulcus, which in section is shaped like a C. Its upper part, the overhanging limbic edge, is the vestibular labium and the lower tapering part is the tympanic labium which is perforated by small holes (the habenula perforata) for branches of the cochlear nerve (**Fig. 39.8**). The upper surface of the vestibular labium is crossed at right angles by furrows, separated by numerous elevations, the auditory teeth (dentes acustici) (**Fig. 39.9**). The limbus is covered by a layer that appears superficially to be squamous epithelium; however, only the cells over the 'teeth' are flat, and those in the furrows are flask-shaped interdental cells. The epithelium is continuous with the epithelium in the internal spiral sulcus and on the inferior surface of Reissner's membrane. During development the interdental cells secrete some of the material that forms the tectorial membrane.

Basilar membrane

The basilar membrane stretches from the tympanic lip of the osseous spiral lamina to the basal crest of the spiral ligament (**Figs 39.7, 39.9**). It consists of two zones. The thin zona arcuata stretches from the spiral limbus to the bases of the outer pillar cells and supports the organ of Corti. It is composed of compact bundles of small (8–10 nm diameter) collagenous filaments, mainly radial in orientation. The outer thicker zona pectinata starts beneath the bases of the outer pillar cells and is attached to the crista basilaris. The basilar membrane is trilaminar in the zona pectinata, but the upper and lower layers fuse at its attachment to the crista basilaris. The length of the basilar membrane is c.35 mm; its width increases from 0.21 mm basally to 0.36 mm at its apex, accompanied by corresponding narrowing of the osseous spiral lamina and a decrease in the thickness of the basal crest. The lower or tympanic surface of the basilar membrane is covered by a layer of vascular con-nective tissue and elongated perilymphatic cells. One vessel, the spiral vessel (vas spirale), is larger; it lies immediately below the tunnel of Corti.

Organ of Corti

The organ of Corti consists of a series of epithelial structures that lie on the zona arcuata of the basilar membrane (**Figs 39.7, 39.9, 39.15, 39.16**). The more central of these structures are two rows of cells, the internal and external pillar cells. The bases of the pillar cells are expanded, and rest contiguously on the basilar membrane, but their rod-like cell bodies are widely separated. The two rows incline towards each other and come into contact again at the heads of the pillars, enclosing between them and the basilar membrane the tunnel of Corti, which has a triangular cross-section (**Fig. 39.9**). Internal to the inner pillar cells is a single row of inner hair cells. External to the outer pillar cells are three or four rows of outer hair cells. The bases of the outer hair cells are cupped by supporting cells called Deiters' cells, except for a gap where cochlear axons synapse with them. The apical ends of the hair cells and apical processes of the supporting cells form a regular mosaic called the reticular lamina, which is covered by the tectorial membrane, a gel-like structure projecting from the spiral limbus. A narrow gap separates the tectorial membrane from the reticular lamina except

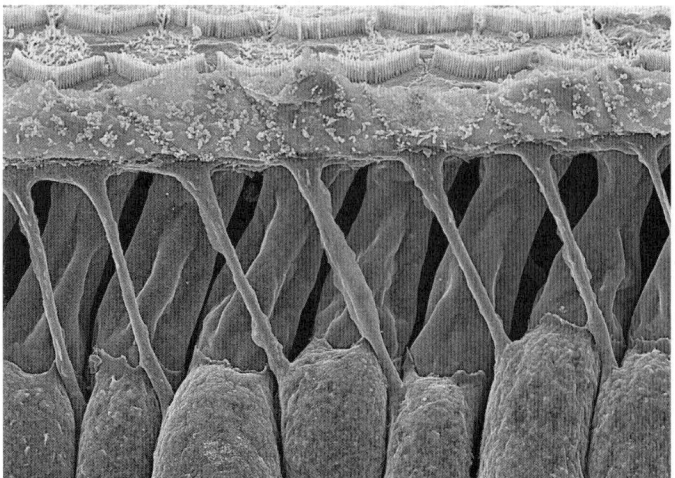

Fig. 39.15 Scanning electron micrograph of a portion of the organ of Corti (guinea pig) dissected to expose the outer row of outer hair cells and their attendant Deiters' cells with narrow phalangeal processes. The stereociliary bundles of two rows of outer hair cells are visible above the reticular lamina. (Provided by DN Furness, MacKay Institute of Communication and Neuroscience, Keele University.)

There are almost 6000 internal pillar cells. Their bases rest on the basilar membrane near the tympanic lip of the internal spiral sulcus, and their bodies form an angle of c.60° with the basilar membrane. Their heads resemble the proximal end of the ulna, with deep concavities for the heads of the outer pillar cells, which they overhang. There are almost 4000 external pillar cells. They are longer and more oblique than the internal pillar cells, and form an angle of c.40° with the basilar membrane. Their heads fit into the concavities on the heads of the inner pillar cells and project externally as thin processes that contact the processes of the Deiters' cells. The distances between the bases of the internal and external pillar cells increase from the cochlear base to its apex, whereas the angles they make with the basilar membrane diminish.

Cochlear hair cells are the sensory transducers of the cochlea: collectively they detect the amplitude and frequency of the sound waves that enter the cochlea (**Fig. 39.9**). All cochlear hair cells have a common pattern of organization. They are elongated cells with a group of modified apical microvilli or stereocilia (which contain parallel arrays of actin filaments) and a group of synaptic contacts with cochlear axons at their rounded bases (**Figs 39.16, 39.17, 39.18**). The inner hair cells form a single row along the inner edge of inner pillar cells (and the spiral tunnel), whereas the outer hair cells are arranged in three or, in some regions of the human cochlea, in four or even five rows, interspersed with supporting cells (**Fig. 39.16**). These two groups have distinctive roles in sound reception; the differences in their detailed structure reflect this functional divergence. There are c.3500 inner hair cells and c.12,000 outer hair cells. The two sets of hair cells lean towards each other apically at about the same angles as the neighbouring inner and outer pillar cells. The geometric arrangement of these cells is very precise, and this pattern is closely related to the sensory performance of the cochlea.

The inner hair cells are pear-shaped and slightly curved; the narrower end is directed towards the surface of the organ of Corti and the wider basal end is positioned some distance above the inner end of the basilar membrane (**Fig. 39.9**). The inner hair cells are surrounded by inner border cells and by inner phalangeal cells, which are attached externally to the heads of the inner pillar cells. The flat apical surface of each inner hair cell is elliptical when viewed from above, its long axis directed in the direction of the row of hair cells (**Fig. 39.17**). The breadth of the apex exceeds that of the inner pillar cells, so that each inner hair cell is related to more than one inner pillar cell. The apex bears 50–60 stereocilia, arranged in several ranks of progressively ascending height, the tallest on the strial side. The tips of the shorter rows are connected diagonally to the sides of the adjacent taller stereocilia by thin filaments called tip links; each stereocilium is also connected to all its neighbours

where the apical stereocilia of the outer hair cells project to make contact with it.

In addition to the tunnel of Corti, other intercommunicating spaces, the spaces of Nuel, surround the outer hair cells. This entire intercommunicating complex of spaces of Nuel and tunnel of Corti is filled with perilymph, which diffuses through the matrix of the basilar membrane. The fluid in these spaces is also sometimes called the cortilymph; it is possible that minor alterations in perilymphatic composition occur within it, because it is exposed to the activities of synaptic endings and specialized excitable cells.

Each pillar cell has a base or crus, an elongated scapus (rod) and an upper end or caput (head) (**Fig. 39.9**); each crus and caput are in contact, but the scapi are separated by the tunnel of Corti. Electron microscopy shows many microtubules, 30 nm in diameter, arranged in linked parallel bundles of 2000 or more in the scapus, originating in the crus and diverging above the scapus to terminate in the head region. The nucleus is situated in the foot-like expansion resting on the basal lamina.

A
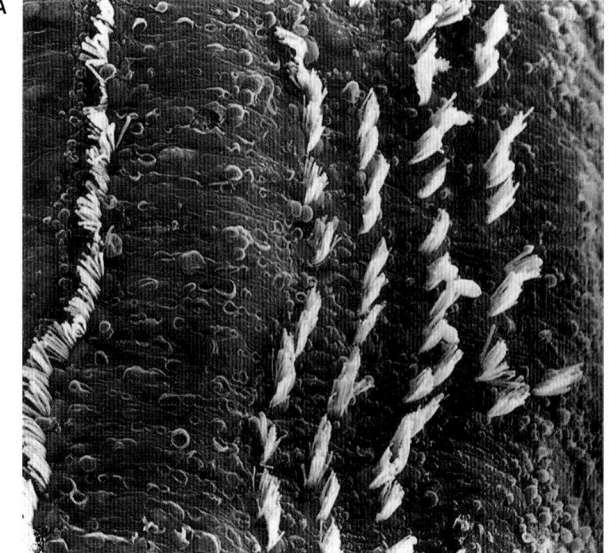

B
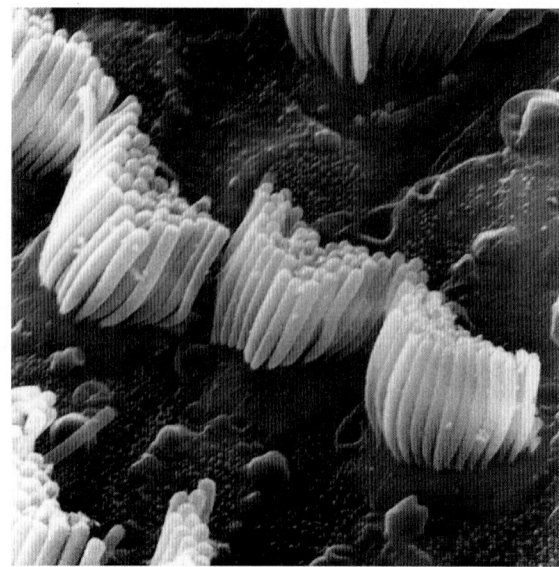

Fig. 39.16 Scanning electron micrographs of the surface of an organ of Corti from a human cochlea. **A,** Low-power view showing a single row of inner hair cells (left) and three rows of outer hair cells, with additional rows in places. **B,** Higher magnification of stereociliary bundles of outer hair cells. (Provided by H Felix, M Gleeson and L-G Johnsson, ENT Department, University of Zurich and GKT School of Medicine, London.)

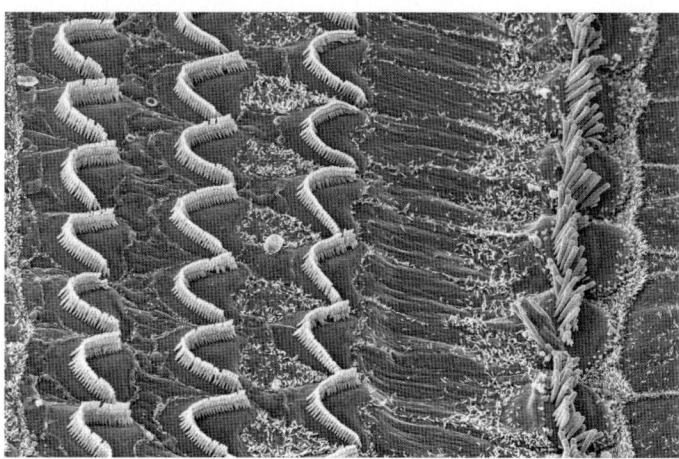

Fig. 39.17 Scanning electron micrograph of the surface of the organ of Corti, the reticular lamina (guinea pig). Three rows of V-shaped stereociliary bundles can be seen protruding from the apices of the outer hair cells. They are separated from the single row of inner hair cells (which have relatively linear stereociliary bundles) by the apices of the inner pillar cells. (Provided by DN Furness, MacKay Institute of Communication and Neuroscience, Keele University.)

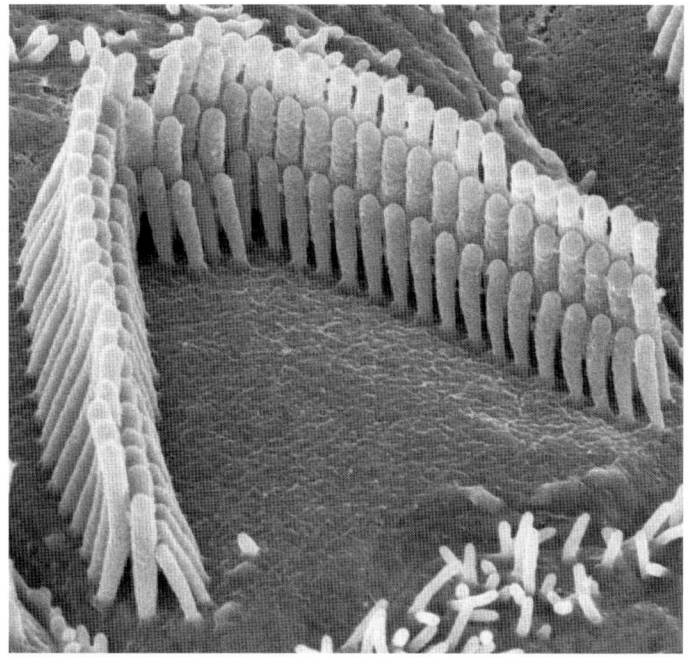

Fig. 39.18 Scanning electron micrograph of stereociliary bundle of one outer hair cell (guinea pig) showing three rows of stereocilia increasing in height. Deflection of the stereocilia in the direction of the tallest row results in depolarization of the hair cell. Microvilli can be seen on the surface of Deiters' cells (front right). (Provided by DN Furness, MacKay Institute of Communication and Neuroscience, Keele University.)

by lateral links. The length of a stereociliary row varies along the length of the cochlea, being longest at the apex and shortest at its base. The stereociliary bases insert into a transverse lamina of dense fibrillar material, the cuticular plate, which lies immediately beneath the apical surface of each inner hair cell. The cuticular plate includes a small aperture containing a basal body. During development, a kinocilium containing microtubules is anchored here, a condition which persists in vestibular hair cells.

At its base, each inner hair cell forms ten or more synaptic contacts with afferent endings, each being marked by a presynaptic structure similar to the ribbon synapses (see Fig. 4.8C) of the retina. Occasionally, an efferent synapse makes direct contact with a hair cell base, but these are usually presynaptic to the terminal expansions of afferent endings, rather than to the hair cell itself.

Outer hair cells are long cylindrical cells which are nearly twice as tall as the inner hair cells (**Figs 39.9, 39.11, 39.16**). There is a gradation of length: the outermost row is longest in any one cochlear region, and those of the cochlear apex are taller than those of the base. They are surrounded by the apical or phalangeal processes of the Deiters' cells or, on the internal side of the inner row, by the heads of the outer pillar cells. The stereocilia, which may number up to 100 per cell, are arranged in three rows of graded heights; the longest is on the outer side. The rows are arranged in the form of a V or W depending on cochlear region, the points of the angles directed externally. The stereocilia are also graded in length according to cochlear region: those of the cochlear base are shortest. Like those of inner hair cells, the stereocilia possess tip links and other filamentous connections with their neighbours, and are inserted at their narrow bases into a cuticular plate. The tallest stereocilia are embedded in shallow impressions on the underside of the tectorial membrane.

The rounded nucleus is positioned near the base of the cell. Below the nucleus are a few ribbon-like synapses associated with afferent endings of the cochlear nerve. The latter are fewer in number and smaller than the cluster of efferent boutons that contact the base of the cell. The neurotransmitter at the afferent synapse in both inner and outer hair cells is probably glutamate, whereas that of the efferent endings is acetylcholine, although other neurotransmitters or neuromodulators have been demonstrated.

Deiters' or phalangeal cells lie between the rows of outer hair cells. Their expanded bases lie on the basilar membrane and their apical ends partially envelop the bases of the outer hair cells (**Fig. 39.9, 39.15**). Each has a finger-like (phalangeal) process that extends diagonally upwards between the hair cells to the reticular membrane, where it forms a plate-like expansion that fills the gaps between hair cell apices.

Five or six rows of columnar supporting cells or external limiting cells, such as Hensen's cells and Claudius' cells lie external to the Deiters' cells (**Fig. 39.9**).

The apices of the hair cells and supporting cells that form the reticular lamina are linked by tight junctions, desmosomes and extensive gap junctions which couple them electrically (**Fig. 39.9**). This arrangement is significant for two reasons. The reticular lamina creates a highly impermeable barrier to the passage of ions other than via the mechano-transducer channels in the stereociliary membranes. It also forms a rigid support between the apices of the hair cells, coupling them mechanically to the movements of the underlying basilar membrane, which causes lateral shearing movements between the stereocilia and the overlying tectorial membrane. If there is hair cell loss as a result of trauma such as excessive noise or ototoxic drugs, the supporting cells expand rapidly to fill the gap, disturbing the regular pattern of the reticular lamina (phalangeal scars), but restoring its function.

Tectorial membrane

The tectorial membrane overlies the sulcus spiralis internus and organ of Corti and is a stiff, gelatinous plate (**Figs 39.7, 39.9**). It contains collagen types II, V and IX, interspersed with glycoproteins (tectorins), which contribute approximately half of the total protein.

In transverse section, the tectorial membrane has a characteristic shape. The underside is nearly flat and the upper surface is convex, and it is thin on the modiolar side where it is attached to the vestibular labium of the spiral limbus. Its outer part forms a thickened ridge, over-hanging the edge of the reticular lamina. The lower surface is relatively smooth, except where the stereocilia of the outer hair cells are embedded in the membrane, leaving a pattern of W- or V-shaped impressions, an S-shaped ridge called Hensen's stripe, which projects towards the stereocilia of the inner hair cells. The interdental cells of the spiral limbus are believed to secrete the membrane.

VASCULAR SUPPLY

ARTERIES

The inner ear is principally supplied by the labyrinthine artery. The stylomastoid branch of either the occipital artery or the posterior auricular artery also supplies the semicircular canals.

Labyrinthine artery – The labyrinthine artery arises from the basilar artery, or sometimes from the anterior inferior cerebellar artery. It divides at the bottom of the internal auditory meatus into cochlear and vestibular branches. The cochlear branch divides into 12–14 twigs, which traverse the canals in the modiolus and are distributed as a capillary plexus to the spiral lamina, basilar membrane, stria vascularis and other cochlear structures. Vestibular arterial branches supply the utricle, saccule and semicircular ducts.

VEINS

The veins draining the vestibule and semicircular canals accompany the arteries. They receive the cochlear veins at the base of the modiolus, and form the labyrinthine vein, which ends in the posterior part of the superior petrosal sinus or in the transverse sinus. A small vessel from the basal cochlear turn traverses the cochlear canaliculus to join the internal jugular vein. For details of the microvasculature of the cochlea of man and other mammals, see Axelsson (1988).

INNERVATION

VESTIBULOCOCHLEAR NERVE (Fig. 39.19)

The vestibulocochlear nerve emerges from the pontocerebellar angle. It courses through the posterior cranial fossa to enter the petrous temporal bone via the internal acoustic meatus, where it divides into an anterior trunk, the cochlear nerve, and a posterior trunk, the vestibular nerve. Both contain the centrally directed axons of bipolar neurones, the cell bodies of which are situated close to their peripheral terminals, together with a smaller number of efferent fibres that arise from brain stem neurones and terminate on cochlear and vestibular sensory cells.

In audiological practice, it is important to distinguish between intra-temporal and intracranial lesions. It is relevant to note therefore that this surgical distinction does not correlate with the precise anatomical description of peripheral and central portions of the auditory and vestibular systems. Clinically, the term 'peripheral auditory lesion' is used to describe lesions peripheral to the spiral ganglion, and the term 'peripheral vestibular disturbance' includes lesions of the vestibular ganglion and the entire vestibular nerve. Furthermore, the intratemporal portion of the vestibulocochlear nerve in humans consists of two histologically distinct portions: a central glial zone adjacent to the brain stem, and a peripheral or non-glial zone. In the glial zone the axons are supported by central neuroglia, whereas in the non-glial zone they are ensheathed by Schwann cells. The non-glial zone extends into the cerebellopontine angle medial to the internal acoustic meatus in more than 50% of human vestibulocochlear nerves.

The central pathways of the vestibular and cochlear nerves are described in Chapter 24 (pp. 436, 436).

Intratemporal vestibular nerve

The maculae and crests are innervated by dendrites of bipolar neurones in the vestibular (Scarpa's) ganglion situated in the trunk of the nerve within the lateral end of the internal auditory meatus (**Fig. 39.20**).

The peripheral processes of the ganglion cells are aggregated into definable nerves, each with a specific distribution (**Fig. 39.1**). The main nerve divides at and within the ganglion into superior and inferior divisions, which are connected by an isthmus. The superior division, the larger of the two, passes through the small holes in the superior vestibular area to supply the ampullary crests of the lateral and anterior semicircular canals via the lateral and anterior ampullary nerves, respectively. A secondary branch of the lateral ampullary nerve supplies the macula of the utricle; however, the greater part of the utricular macula is innervated by the utricular nerve, which is a separate branch of the superior division. Another branch of the superior division, Voit's nerve, supplies part of the saccule.

The inferior division of the vestibular nerve passes through small holes in the inferior vestibular area to supply the remainder of the saccule and the posterior ampullary crest via saccular and singular branches, respectively; the latter passes through the foramen singulare. Occasionally, a very small supplementary or accessory branch innervates the posterior crest; it is probably a vestigial remnant of the crista neglecta, an additional area of sensory epithelium found in some other mammals but seldom in man.

Afferent and efferent cochlear fibres are also present in the inferior division of the vestibular nerve, but leave at the anastomosis of Oort to join the main cochlear nerve (see review by Warr 1992). Another anastomosis, the vestibulofacial anastomosis, is situated more centrally between the facial and vestibular nerves, and is the point at which fibres

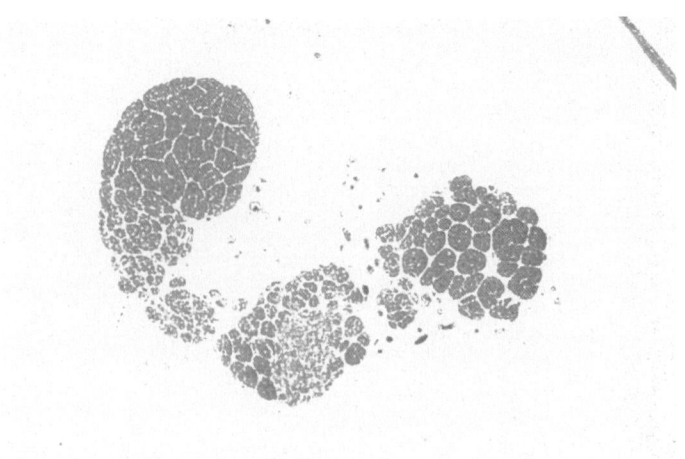

Fig. 39.19 Human vestibulocochlear nerve, in transverse section. On the left, the cochlear nerve (seen as a comma-shaped profile) abuts the inferior division of the vestibular nerve (right). The singular nerve is a separate fascicle between the superior and inferior divisions of the vestibular nerve. (Provided by H Felix, M Gleeson and L-G Johnsson, ENT Department, University of Zurich and GKT School of Medicine, London.)

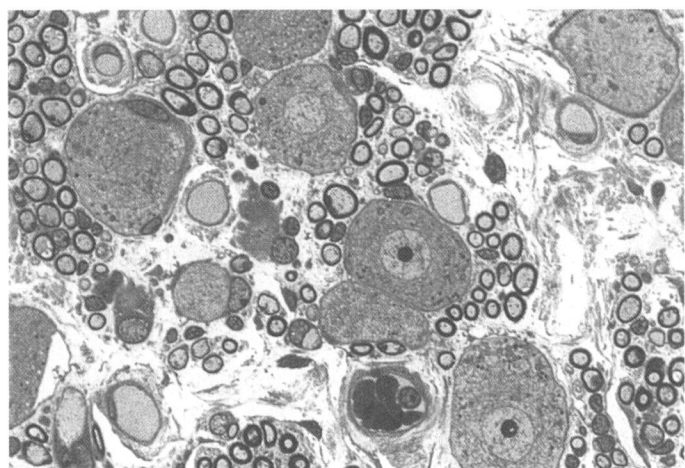

Fig. 39.20 A portion of a human vestibular ganglion, showing neuronal perikarya, myelinated axons and small blood vessels. Toluidine blue stained resin section. (Provided by H Felix, M Gleeson and L-G Johnsson, ENT Department, University of Zurich and GKT School of Medicine, London.)

originating in the intermediate nerve pass from the vestibular nerve to the main trunk of the facial nerve.

There are approximately 20,000 fibres in the vestibular nerve, of which 12,000 travel in the superior division and 8000 travel in the inferior division. The distribution of fibre diameters is bimodal, with peaks at 4 μm and 6.5 μm. The smaller fibres go mainly to the Type II hair cells and the larger fibres tend to supply the Type I hair cells. In addition to the afferents, efferent and autonomic fibres have been identified. Efferent fibres synapse exclusively with the afferent calyceal terminals around Type I cells and usually with the afferent boutons on Type II cells, although a few are in direct contact with the cell bodies of Type II cells. The autonomic fibres do not contact vestibular sensory cells, but terminate beneath the sensory epithelia. Two distinct sympathetic components have been identified in the vestibular ganglion: a perivascular adrenergic system derived from the stellate ganglion, and a blood vessel-independent system derived from the superior cervical ganglion.

Vestibular ganglion – The cell bodies of the bipolar neurones that contribute to the vestibular nerve vary considerably in size: their circumferences range from 45 to 160 μm (Felix et al 1987). No topographically ordered distribution relating to size has been found. The cell bodies are notable for their abundant granular endoplasmic reticulum, which in places forms Nissl bodies, and prominent Golgi complexes (**Fig. 39.20**). They are covered by a thin layer of satellite cells and are often arranged in pairs, closely abutting each other so that only a thin layer of endoneurium separates the adjacent coverings of satellite cells. This arrangement has led to speculation that ganglion cells may affect each other directly by electrotonic spread (ephaptic transmission: see Felix et al 1987) (**Fig. 39.20**).

Anatomy of balance and posture

The vestibular system provides precise information about the orientation of the head in three-dimensional space and its rate and direction of movement. It consists of two otolithic organs, the utricle and the saccule, which detect linear acceleration due to gravitational pull and the direction of other linear accelerations, and three semicircular canals, which detect angular accelerations and hence head rotations. The vestibular labyrinths on each side of the head are arranged symmetrically with respect to each other, so ensuring that any movement of the head will result in a unique pattern of nerve input to the brain. The stereocilia in the apical hair bundles of the mechanosensitive hair cells in each of these organs are embedded in an overlying accessory gel-like structure, the otolithic membrane (in the utricle and the saccule) and the cupula (in the semicircular canals). Their apical surfaces are bathed in endolymph: tight junctional complexes between the apices of the hair cells and their adjacent supporting cells separate the endolymph from the perilymph that bathes their basolateral surfaces. Deflection of the stereocilia (caused by displacements of their overlying accessory membranes by fluid movements in the membranous labyrinth) produces either an increased or decreased rate of opening of the mechanotransduction channels at their tips, depending on whether they are deflected towards or away from the tallest row. This in turn results in signals travelling along the vestibular portion of the vestibulocochlear nerve to the brain for comparison with visual and somatosensory signals, which also signal the position of the head in space (for a more detailed account, see Furness 2002).

Intratemporal cochlear nerve

The cochlear nerve connects the organ of Corti to the cochlear and related nuclei of the brain stem. The cochlear nerve lies inferior to the facial nerve throughout the internal acoustic meatus. It becomes intimately associated with the superior and inferior divisions of the vestibular nerve, which are situated in the posterior compartment of the canal, and leaves the internal acoustic meatus in a common fascicle (**Fig. 39.6**).

There are approximately 30–40 000 nerve fibres in the human cochlear nerve (for review, see Nadol 1988). Their fibre diameter distribution is unimodal, and ranges from 1 to 11 μm, with a peak at 4–5 μm. Functionally, the nerve contains both afferent and efferent somatic fibres, together with adrenergic postganglionic sympathetic fibres from the cervical sympathetic system.

Afferent cochlear innervation

The afferent fibres are myelinated axons with bipolar cell bodies that lie in the spiral ganglion in the modiolus (**Fig. 39.21**). There are two types of ganglion cell: most (90–95%) are large Type I cells, the remainder are smaller Type II cells (see reviews by Nadol 1988, Eybalin 1993). Type I cells contain a prominent spherical nucleus, abundant ribosomes and many mitochondria; in many mammals (although possibly not in humans) they are surrounded by myelin sheaths. In contrast, Type II cells are smaller, always unmyelinated, and have a lobulated nucleus. The cytoplasm of Type II cells is enriched with neurofilaments, but has fewer mitochondria and ribosomes than Type I cells.

Each inner hair cell is in synaptic contact with the unbranched peripheral processes of approximately 10 Type I ganglion cells. The processes of Type II ganglion cells diverge within the organ of Corti and innervate more than 10 outer hair cells. The peripheral and central processes of Type I ganglion cells are relatively large in diameter and are myelinated, whereas those of Type II are smaller and unmyelinated. The peripheral processes of both types of cell radiate from the modiolus into the osseous spiral lamina, where the Type I axons lose their myelin sheaths before entering the organ of Corti through the habenula perforata.

Three distinct groupings of afferent fibres have been identified: inner radial, basilar and outer spiral fibres (**Fig. 39.22**).

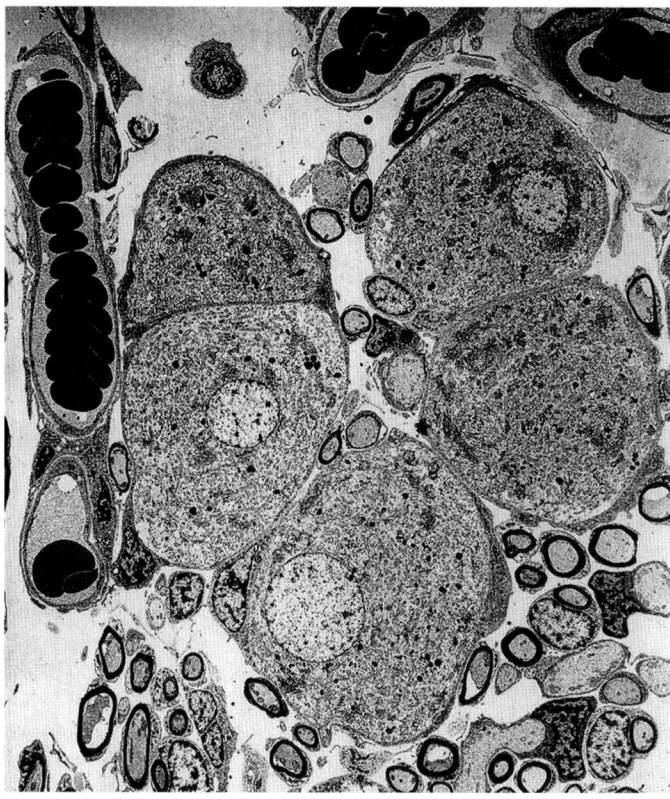

Fig. 39.21 Transmission electron micrograph showing several Type II ganglion cells and nerve fibres in a human spiral ganglion. Note the absence of myelin from the surrounding sheaths of the ganglion cells. (Provided by H Felix, M Gleeson and L-G Johnsson, ENT Department, University of Zurich and GKT School of Medicine, London.)

Inner radial fibres – The inner radial fibre group consists of the majority of afferent fibres. They run directly in a radial direction to the inner hair cells, each of which receives endings from several of these fibres.

Basilar fibres – Basilar fibres are afferent to the outer hair cells and take an independent spiral course, turning towards the cochlear apex near the bases of the inner hair cells. They run for a distance of about five pillar cells before turning radially again and crossing the floor of the tunnel of Corti, often diagonally, to form part of the outer spiral bundle.

Outer spiral bundles – The afferent fibres of the bundles of the outer spiral group course towards the basal part of the cochlea, continually branching off en route to supply several outer hair cells. The outer spiral bundles also contain efferent fibres (see below).

Efferent cochlear fibres

The efferent nerve fibres in the cochlear nerve are derived from the olivocochlear system (see reviews by Warr 1992, Guinan 1996). Within the modiolus, the efferent fibres form the intraganglionic spiral bundle, which may be one or more discrete groups of fibres situated at the periphery of the spiral ganglion (**Fig. 39.22**). There are two main groups of olivocochlear efferents: lateral and medial. The lateral efferents come from small neurones in and near the lateral superior olivary nucleus and arise mainly, but not exclusively, ipsilaterally. They are organized into inner spiral fibres that run in the inner spiral bundle before terminating on the afferent axons that supply the inner hair cells. The medial efferents originate from larger neurones in the vicinity of the medial superior olivary nucleus, and the majority arise contralaterally. They are myelinated and cross the tunnel of Corti to synapse with the outer hair cells mainly by direct contact with their bases, although a few synapse with the afferent terminals. The efferent innervation of the outer hair cells decreases along the organ of Corti from cochlear base to apex, and from the first (inner) row to the third. The efferents use acetylcholine, γ-aminobutyric acid (GABA), or both as their neurotransmitter. They may also contain other neurotransmitters and neuromodulators.

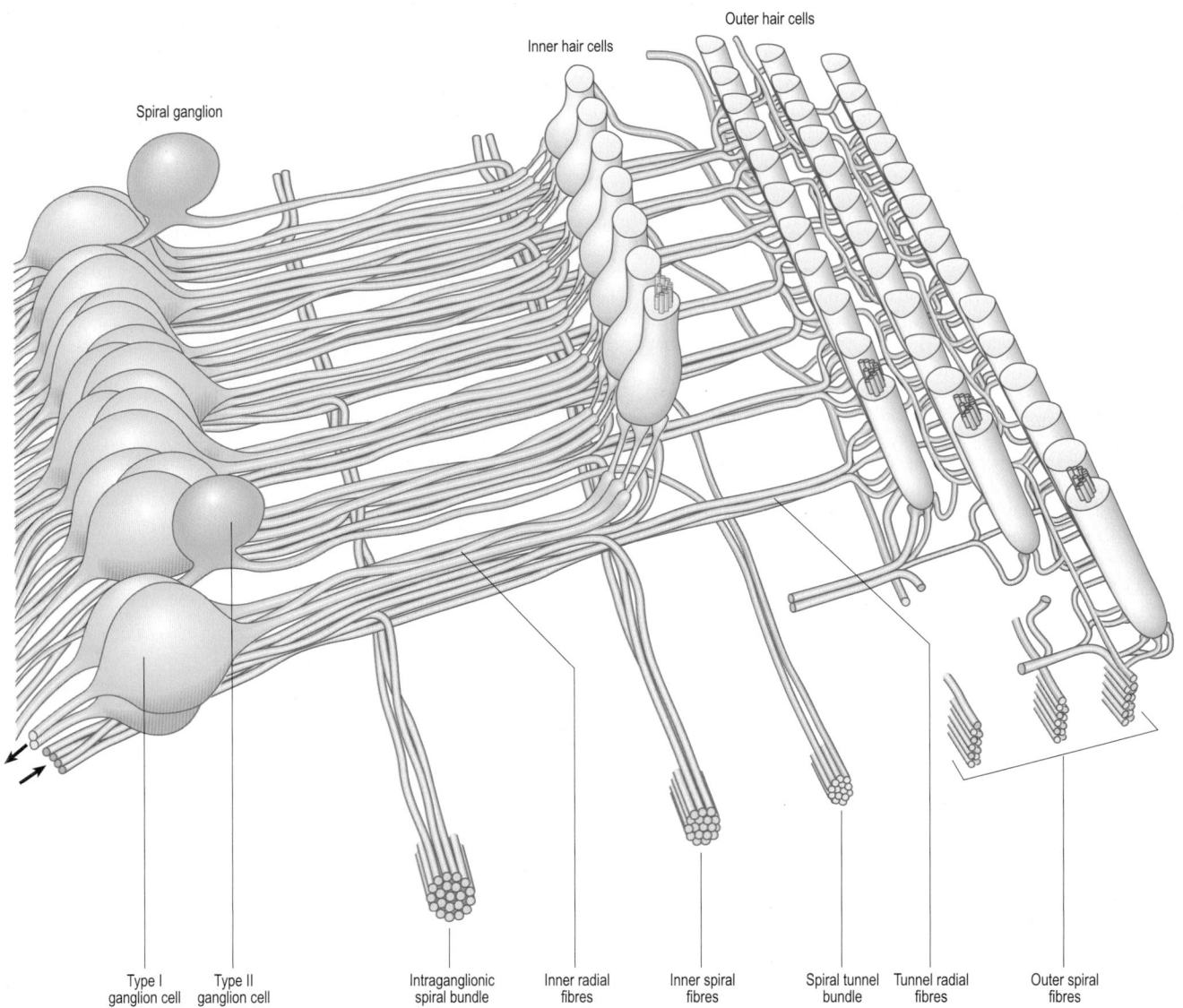

Spiral ganglion

Inner hair cells

Outer hair cells

| Type I
ganglion cell | Type II
ganglion cell | Intraganglionic
spiral bundle | Inner radial
fibres | Inner spiral
fibres | Spiral tunnel
bundle | Tunnel radial
fibres | Outer spiral
fibres |

Fig. 39.22 The innervation of the organ of Corti. The ganglion cells that give rise to the sensory nerve fibres include those related to the inner hair cells (dark green) and others innervating the outer hair cells (light green). Efferent fibres are depicted in purple. There is a great contrast between the convergent afferent innervation of the inner hair cells (c.10 fibres to each cell) and the divergent supply of the outer hair cells (one afferent fibre to c.10 cells). This illustration is a simplified view of the complex innervation of the organ of Corti (see the text for further details).

Activity of the medial efferents inhibits cochlear responses to sound: the strength of the activity grows slowly with increasing sound level. They are believed to modulate the micromechanics of the cochlea by altering the mechanical responses of the outer hair cells, thus changing their contribution to frequency sensitivity and selectivity. The lateral efferents related to the inner hair cells also respond to sound. They appear to modify transmission through their postsynaptic action on inner hair cell afferents. The cholinergic fibres may excite the radial fibres, whilst those containing GABA may inhibit them, although their role is less well understood than that of the medial efferents (see review by Guinan 1996).

Autonomic cochlear innervation

Autonomic nerve endings appear to be entirely sympathetic. Two adrenergic systems have been described within the cochlea: a perivascular plexus derived from the stellate ganglion and a blood vessel-independent system derived from the superior cervical ganglion. Both systems travel with the afferent and efferent cochlear fibres and seem to be restricted to regions away from the organ of Corti. The sympathetic nervous system may cause primary and secondary effects in the cochlea by remotely altering the metabolism of various cell types and by influencing the blood vessels and nerve fibres with which it makes contact.

Anatomy of auditory reception

Sounds waves entering the external ear are converted into electrical signals in the cochlear nerve by the peripheral auditory system (**Fig. 39.23**). Vibrations in the air column in the external acoustic meatus cause a comparable set of vibrations in the tympanic membrane and auditory ossicles. The chain of ossicles acts as a lever which increases the force per unit area at the round window by 1.2 times, whilst the reduction in size of the round window compared with the tympanic membrane increases the force per unit area of the oscillating surface a further 17 times. This overcomes the inertia of the cochlear fluids and produces in them pressure waves that are conducted almost instantaneously to all parts of the basilar membrane. The latter varies continuously in width, mass and stiffness from the basal to the apical end of the cochlea. Each part of the basilar membrane vibrates, but only the region tuned to a specific frequency will respond maximally to a pure tone entering the ear. A wave of mechanical motion, the travelling wave, is propagated along the basilar membrane to the position where it responds maximally and then dies away again. With increasing frequency, the locus of maximum amplitude moves progressively from the apical to the basal end of the cochlea. The pattern of vibrations in the basilar membrane thus varies with the intensity and frequency of the acoustic waves reaching the perilymph. Because of the arrangement of the hair cells on the basilar membrane, these oscillations generate

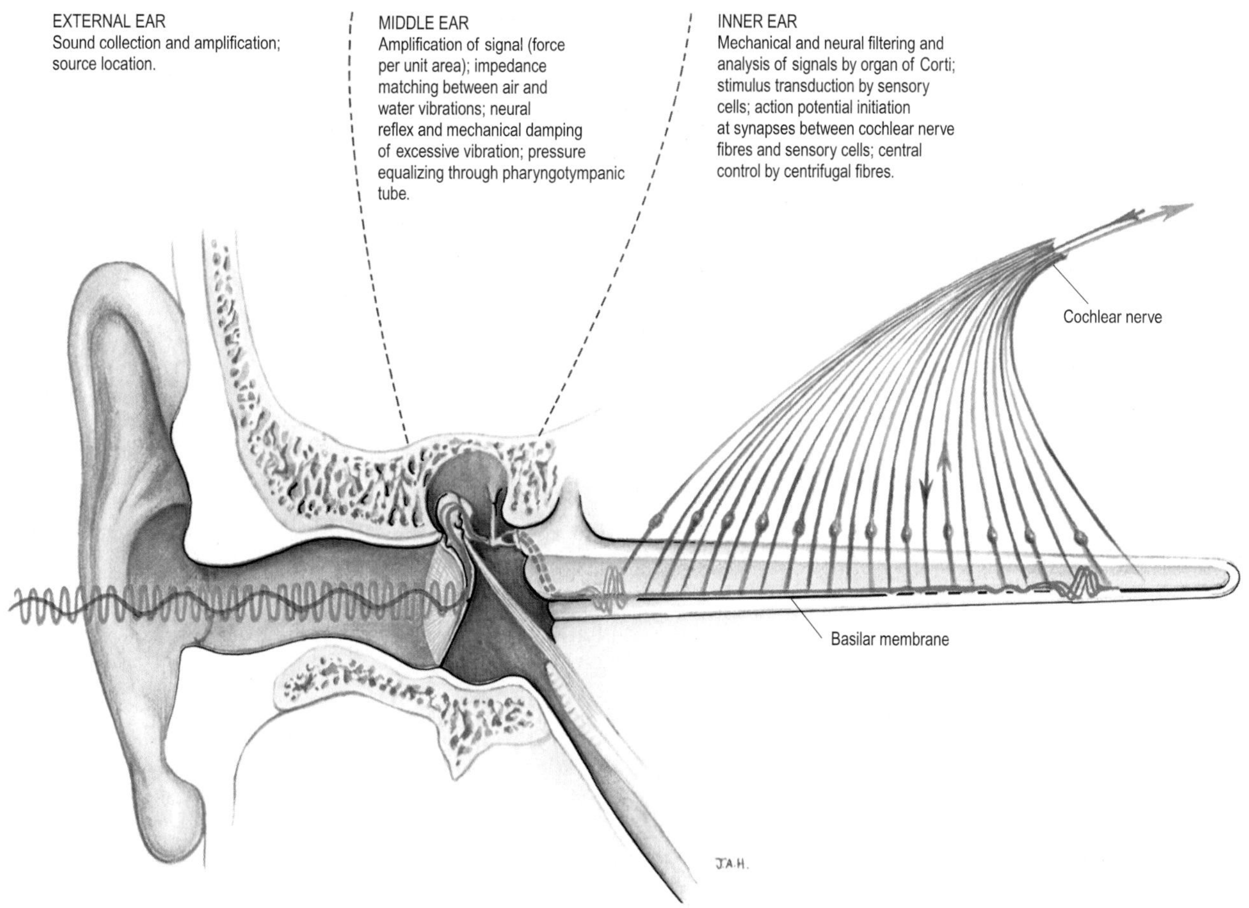

EXTERNAL EAR
Sound collection and amplification;
source location.

MIDDLE EAR
Amplification of signal (force
per unit area); impedance
matching between air and
water vibrations; neural
reflex and mechanical damping
of excessive vibration; pressure
equalizing through pharyngotympanic
tube.

INNER EAR
Mechanical and neural filtering and
analysis of signals by organ of Corti;
stimulus transduction by sensory
cells; action potential initiation
at synapses between cochlear nerve
fibres and sensory cells; central
control by centrifugal fibres.

Cochlear nerve

Basilar membrane

J'A·H.

Fig. 39.23 The principal activities of the peripheral auditory apparatus. For clarity, the cochlea is depicted as though it had been uncoiled. The points of maximal stimulation of the basilar membrane by high frequency (blue) and low frequency (red) vibrations, together with their transmission pathways through the external and middle ear, are also indicated.

a largely transverse shearing force between the outer hair cells and the overlying tectorial membrane (in which the apices of the hair cell stereocilia are embedded). This movement depends on the mechanical properties of the entire organ of Corti, including its cytoskeleton, which stiffens this structure. The inner hair cell stereocilia, which probably do not touch the tectorial membrane although they come very close to it, are likely to be stimulated by local movements of the endolymph. Displacement of the stereociliary bundle of a hair cell opens mechanotransducer channels near the tips of its stereocilia, and this allows potassium and calcium ions from the endolymph to enter the hair cell (see overview by Fettiplace 2002). This induces a depolarizing receptor potential and the release of neurotransmitter onto the cochlear afferents at the base of the cell. In this way a specific group of auditory axons is activated at the position of maximal basilar membrane vibration.

The mechanical behaviour of the basilar membrane is responsible for a rather broad discrimination between different frequencies (passive tuning, see overview by Ashmore 2002), but fine frequency discrimination in the cochlea appears to be related to physiological differences between the hair cells. Individual tuning of hair cells may result from differences in shape, stereociliary length, or possibly variations in the molecular composition of sensory membranes, and may have a role in cochlear amplification (active tuning).

The activity of the outer hair cells appears to play an important part in regulating inner hair cell sensitivity at specific frequencies. Outer hair cells can change length when stimulated electrically at frequencies of many thousands of cycles per second. The rapidity of these changes in length indicates a novel type of motile mechanism, which is believed to depend on conformational changes in proteins located in the plasma membrane of the cells. When the membrane potential of the outer hair cells changes, they generate forces along their axes. When the mechanotransducer channels open, they are thought to oppose the viscous forces which tend to damp down the vibration of the cochlear partition, and

adjust the mechanics of the organ of Corti on a cycle-by-cycle basis. Alternatively they may alter the mechanics of the partition more slowly under the influence of the efferent pathway.

At a particular frequency, an increase in the intensity of stimulus is signalled by an increase in the rate of discharge in individual cochlear axons. At greater intensities it is signalled by the number of activated cochlear axons (recruitment).

The respective roles of the two groups of hair cells have been much debated, particularly since differences in their innervation and physiological behaviour have become apparent. Because of their rich afferent supply, inner hair cells are believed to be the major source of auditory signals in the cochlear nerve. Some evidence for this view is based on the finding that animals treated with antibiotics that are specifically toxic to outer hair cells are still able to hear, but their sensitivity and frequency discrimination is impaired.

Some electrical responses of the cochlea can be recorded with extracellular electrodes. The most significant is the endolymphatic potential, a steady potential recordable between the cochlear duct and the scala tympani, which is caused by the different ionic compositions of their fluids. As the resting potential of hair cells is c.70 mV (negative inside) and the endolymphatic potential is positive in the cochlear duct, the total transmembrane potential across the apices of hair cells is 150 mV. This is a greater resting potential than is found anywhere else in the body, and provides the driving force for mechanotransduction and for the cochlear amplifier.

Under stimulation by sound, a rapid oscillatory cochlear microphonic potential can be recorded. It matches the frequency of the stimulus and movements of the basilar membrane precisely, and appears to depend on fluctuations in the conductance of hair cell membranes, probably of the outer hair cells. At the same time, an extracellular summating potential develops, a steady direct current shift related to the (intracellular) receptor potentials of the hair cells. Cochlear nerve fibres then

677

begin to respond with action potentials, which are also recordable from the cochlea. Intracellular recording of auditory responses from inner hair cells has confirmed that these cells resemble other receptors: their steady receptor potentials are related in size to the amplitude of the acoustic stimulus. At the same time, afferent axons are stimulated by synaptic action at the bases of the inner hair cells. They fire more rapidly as the vibration of the basilar membrane increases in amplitude, up to a threshold that depends on the sensitivity of the specific nerve fibre involved. Each inner hair cell is contacted by axons with response thresholds that range from 0 decibels sound pressure level (dB SPL), the approximate threshold of human hearing, to those which respond to intensities in excess of 100 dB SPL; the loudest sound tolerable is around 120 dB SPL. Each axon responds most sensitively to the frequency represented by its particular cochlear location, its characteristic frequency (**Fig. 39.23**).

Deafness

Two causes of deafness are usually distinguished: conductive hearing loss and sensorineural hearing loss.

Conductive hearing loss may result from trauma to the external or middle ears, blockage of the external auditory meatus, or disruption of the tympanic membrane (e.g. by intense sounds or extreme pressure changes). It may also result from chronic inflammation of the tympanic membrane (e.g. by a cholesteatoma, which may also damage the ossicles); from an infection of the middle ear (otitis media with effusion), which produces a fluid build-up in the normally air-filled middle ear and so impedes the movements of the ossicles; or from otosclerosis, an inappropriate thickening of bone around the footplate of the stapes.

Sensorineural hearing loss refers to loss or damage of the sensory hair cells or their innervation. The sensory cells of the inner ear are particularly vulnerable to mechanical trauma produced by high intensity noise and to changes in their physiological environment caused by infection or hypoxia. Changes in their ionic environment rapidly lead to degenerative processes that result in hair cell loss, often by apoptosis, and produce either hearing loss or vestibular dysfunction. These changes can be induced by drugs such as the aminoglycoside antibiotics, some diuretics, and certain anticancer drugs. A decrease in cochlear sensitivity, presbyacusis, almost invariably occurs with age: hair cells at the high frequency end of the cochlea tend to be lost first. Ménière's disease is a distressing disorder of the inner ear characterized by episodes of hearing loss, tinnitus and vertigo. Histological examination of an affected ear reveals endolymphatic hydrops (swelling of the endolymphatic spaces), suggesting poor drainage of the endolymph via the endolymphatic sac.

SURGICAL APPROACHES TO THE INNER EAR

The inner ear may be approached surgically from various directions. The promontory that overlies the basal turn of the cochlea and the oval window may be opened via the middle ear (after elevating the tympanic membrane). The lateral semicircular canal may be opened via the aditus (after widening the bony external acoustic meatus and removing the incus). The arcuate eminence may be opened to give access to the superior semicircular canal via the floor of the middle cranial fossa. The posterior semicircular canal may be opened deep to the mastoid segment of the Fallopian canal via the mastoid process (after drilling away the overlying air cells). All of these approaches are usually reserved for destructive operations on the labyrinth to treat intractable vertigo.

The round window niche and its membrane may be approached via a posterior tympanotomy. In this procedure, the mastoid air cells are removed to allow access to the bony triangle bounded above by the fossa of incus, superficially by the chorda tympani, and deeply by the descending portion of the facial nerve. This bone is drilled away carefully to expose the facial recess of the tympanic cavity and the round window niche. Using this access, the stimulating electrode of a multichannel intracochlear implant can be passed into the scala tympani of the cochlea so that it lies against the spiral lamina and can stimulate the adjacent fibres of the cochlear nerve.

The endolymphatic sac may be approached after exenteration of the mastoid air cells by elevating the cortical bone of the anterolateral wall of the posterior cranial fossa, anterior to the sigmoid venous sinus and posterior to the posterior semicircular canal (below a line extended from the axis of the lateral semicircular canal). Access to the sac is required in some operations that aim to control vertigo secondary to Ménière's disease.

The internal acoustic meatus may be approached, at a cost to hearing, by drilling away the entire bony labyrinth via the posterior cranial fossa (after craniectomy in the occipital region and retraction of the cerebellum), or via the middle cranial fossa (after a temporal craniotomy and retraction of the dura of the middle fossa and the temporal lobe). These approaches are usually used to access tumours of the cerebellopontine angle and internal acoustic meatus.

REFERENCES

Ashmore J 2002 The mechanics of hearing. In: Roberts D (ed) Signals and Perception: The Fundamentals of Human Sensation. Basingstoke and New York: Palgrave Macmillan: 3–16.

Axelsson A 1988 Comparative anatomy of cochlear blood vessels. Am J Otolaryngol 9: 278–90.

Blanks RH, Curthoys IS, Markham CH 1975 Planar relationships of the semicircular canals in man. Acta Otolaryngol 80: 185–96.

Curthoys IS, Blanks RH, Markham CH 1977 Semicircular canal radii of curvature (R) in cat, guinea pig and man. J Morphol 115: 1–15.

Eybalin M 1993 Neurotransmitters and neuromodulators of the mammalian cochlea. Physiol Rev 73: 309–73.

Felix H, Hoffman V, Wright A, Gleeson MJ 1987 Ultrastructural findings on human Scarpa's ganglion. Acta Otolaryngol Suppl 436: 85–92.

Fettiplace R 2002 The transformation of sound stimuli into electrical signals. In: Roberts D (ed) Signals and Perception: The Fundamentals of Human Sensation. Basingstoke and New York: Palgrave Macmillan: 17–28.

Furness DN 2002 The vestibular system. In: Roberts D (ed) Signals and Perception: The Fundamentals of Human Sensation. Basingstoke and New York: Palgrave Macmillan: 77–90.

Guinan J Jr 1996 Physiology of olivocochlear efferents. In: Dallos P, Popper AN, Fay RR (eds) The Cochlea. New York: Springer Verlag: 435–502.
Comprehensive description of the efferent innervation of the cochlea and its function

Nadol JB 1988 Comparative anatomy of the cochlea and auditory nerve in mammals. Hear Res 34: 253–66.

Spoor F, Zonneveld F 1998 Comparative review of the human bony labyrinth. Am J Phys Anthropol Suppl 27: 211–51.

Wangemann P, Schacht J 1996 Homeostatic mechanisms in the cochlea. In: Dallos P, Popper AN, Fay RR (eds) The Cochlea. New York: Springer Verlag: 130–5.
Reviews what is known about inner ear fluids (perilymph and endolymph), how they are produced and what their functional significance might be.

Warr WB 1992 Organization of olivocochlear efferent systems in mammals. In: Webster DB, Popper AN, Fay RR (eds) Mammalian Auditory Pathway: Neuroanatomy. New York: Springer Verlag: 410–48.

Development of the ear

INNER EAR

The rudiments of the internal ears appear shortly after those of the eyes as two patches of thickened surface epithelium, the otic placodes, lateral to the hindbrain. The early otic epithelium, which is derived from the otic placode, initiates and then suppresses chondrogenesis in the surrounding periotic mesenchyme. Sonic hedgehog protein, fibroblast growth factors and transforming growth factor beta have all been shown to be active in the early stages of otic capsule development in the mouse (Frenz et al 1994).

Each otic placode invaginates as an otic pit while at the same time giving cells to the statoacoustic (vestibulocochlear) ganglion (**Fig. 14.2**). The mouth of the pit then closes to form an otocyst (auditory or otic vesicle) (**Fig. 40.1**). The otocyst is initially piriform, but a vertical infolding of its wall progressively marks off a tubular diverticulum on the medial side, which differentiates into the ductus and saccus endolymphaticus. The latter both communicate via the ductus with the remainder of the vesicle, the utriculosaccular chamber, which is placed laterally. Three compressed diverticula emerge as disc-like evaginations from the dorsal part of this chamber. The central parts of their walls coalesce and disappear and their peripheral portions persist as the semicircular ducts. The anterior duct is completed first, and the lateral last. A medially directed evagination arises from the ventral part of the utriculosaccular chamber and coils progressively as the cochlear duct. Its proximal extremity becomes constricted and forms the ductus reuniens.

The central part of the chamber now represents the membranous vestibule, which becomes divided into a small ventral saccule and a larger utricle. This is achieved mainly by horizontal infolding that extends from the lateral wall of the vestibule towards the opening of the ductus endolymphaticus until only a narrow utriculosaccular duct remains between saccule and utricle. The duct becomes acutely bent on itself: its apex is continuous with the ductus endolymphaticus. During this period the membranous labyrinth rotates so that its long axis, which was originally vertical, becomes more or less horizontal.

Cells derived from the otocyst not only contribute placodal cells to the vestibulocochlear ganglion, but also differentiate into specialized paraneuronal hair cells of the utricle, saccule, ampullae of the semicircular ducts, and organ of Corti; various specialized sustentacular cells and the unique epithelia of the stria vascularis and endolymphatic sac, and cells from which the general epithelial lining of the membranous labyrinth develops.

The periotic mesenchyme surrounding the various parts of the epithelial labyrinth is converted into a cartilaginous otic capsule which ossifies to form most of the bony labyrinth of the internal ear apart from the modiolus and osseous spiral lamina. For a time the cartilaginous capsule is incomplete which means that the cochlear, vestibular and facial ganglia are exposed in the gap between its canicular and cochlear parts. They are soon covered by an outgrowth of cartilage, and the facial nerve becomes enclosed by a growth of cartilage from the cochlear to the canalicular part of the capsule. Perilymphatic spaces develop in the embryonic connective tissue between the cartilaginous capsule and the epithelial wall of the labyrinth. The rudiment of the periotic cistern or vestibular perilymphatic space can be seen in an embryo of from 30–40 mm in length in the reticulum between the saccule and the fenestra vestibuli. The scala tympani develops opposite the fenestra cochleae and is followed later by the scala vestibuli. The two scalae gradually extend along each side of the ductus cochlearis, and when they reach the tip of the ductus a communication, the helicotrema, opens between them. The modiolus and the osseous spiral lamina of the cochlea are not preformed in cartilage but ossify directly from connective tissue.

The rudiment of the eighth nerve appears in the fourth week as the vestibulocochlear ganglion, which lies between the otocyst and the wall of the hindbrain. At first it is fused with the ganglion of the facial nerve (acousticofacial ganglion) but later the two separate. The cells of the vestibulocochlear ganglion are mainly derived from the placodal ectoderm. The ganglion divides into vestibular and cochlear parts, each associated with the corresponding division of the eighth nerve. Ganglionic neurones, which remain bipolar throughout life, are unusual in that many of their somata become enveloped in thin myelin sheaths. Their peripheral processes provide the afferent innervation of the labyrinthine hair cells, which also become associated with the outgrowing axons of the olivocochlear bundle – from cells of the superior olivary complexes in the pons.

MIDDLE EAR (TYMPANIC CAVITY) AND PHARYNGOTYMPANIC TUBE

The pharyngotympanic tube and tympanic cavity are extensions of the early pharynx and develop from a hollow, the tubotympanic recess. This lies between the first and third pharyngeal arches, and has a floor which consists of the second arch and its limiting pouches. The forward growth of the third arch causes the inner part of the recess to narrow to form the tubal region, and also excludes the inner part of the second arch from this portion of the floor. The more lateral part of the recess develops into the tympanic cavity and its floor forms the lateral wall of the tympanic cavity up to approximately the level at which the chorda tympani branches off from the facial nerve. The lateral wall of the tympanic cavity contains first and second arch elements. The first arch territory is limited to that part in front of the anterior process of the malleus, and the second arch forms the outer wall behind this and also turns on to the posterior wall to include the tympanohyal region.

The tubotympanic recess at first lies inferolateral to the cartilaginous otic capsule, but as the capsule enlarges the spatial relationship alters and the tympanic cavity becomes anterolateral. A cartilaginous process grows from the lateral part of the capsule to form the tegmen tympani and it curves caudally to form the lateral wall of the pharyngotympanic tube. In this way, the tympanic cavity and the proximal part of the pharyngotympanic tube become included in the petrous region of the temporal bone. During the sixth or seventh month the mastoid antrum appears as a dorsal expansion of the tympanic cavity.

The malleus develops from the dorsal end of the ventral mandibular (Meckel's) cartilage and the incus from the dorsal cartilage of the first arch (p. 450), which is probably homologous to the quadrate bone of birds and reptiles. The stapes stems mainly from the dorsal end of the cartilage of the second (hyoid) arch, first as a ring (anulus stapes) encircling the small stapedial artery (p. 617). The primordium of the stapedius muscle appears close to the artery and facial nerve at the end of the second month, and at almost the same time the tensor tympani begins to appear near the extremity of the tubotympanic recess. At first the ossicles are embedded in the mesenchymal roof of the tympanic cavity, later they become covered by the mucosa of the middle ear cavity which becomes air filled after birth.

EXTERNAL EAR

The external acoustic meatus develops from the dorsal end of the hyomandibular or first pharyngeal groove. Close to its dorsal extremity this groove extends inwards as a funnel-shaped primary meatus from which the cartilaginous part and a small area of the roof of the osseous

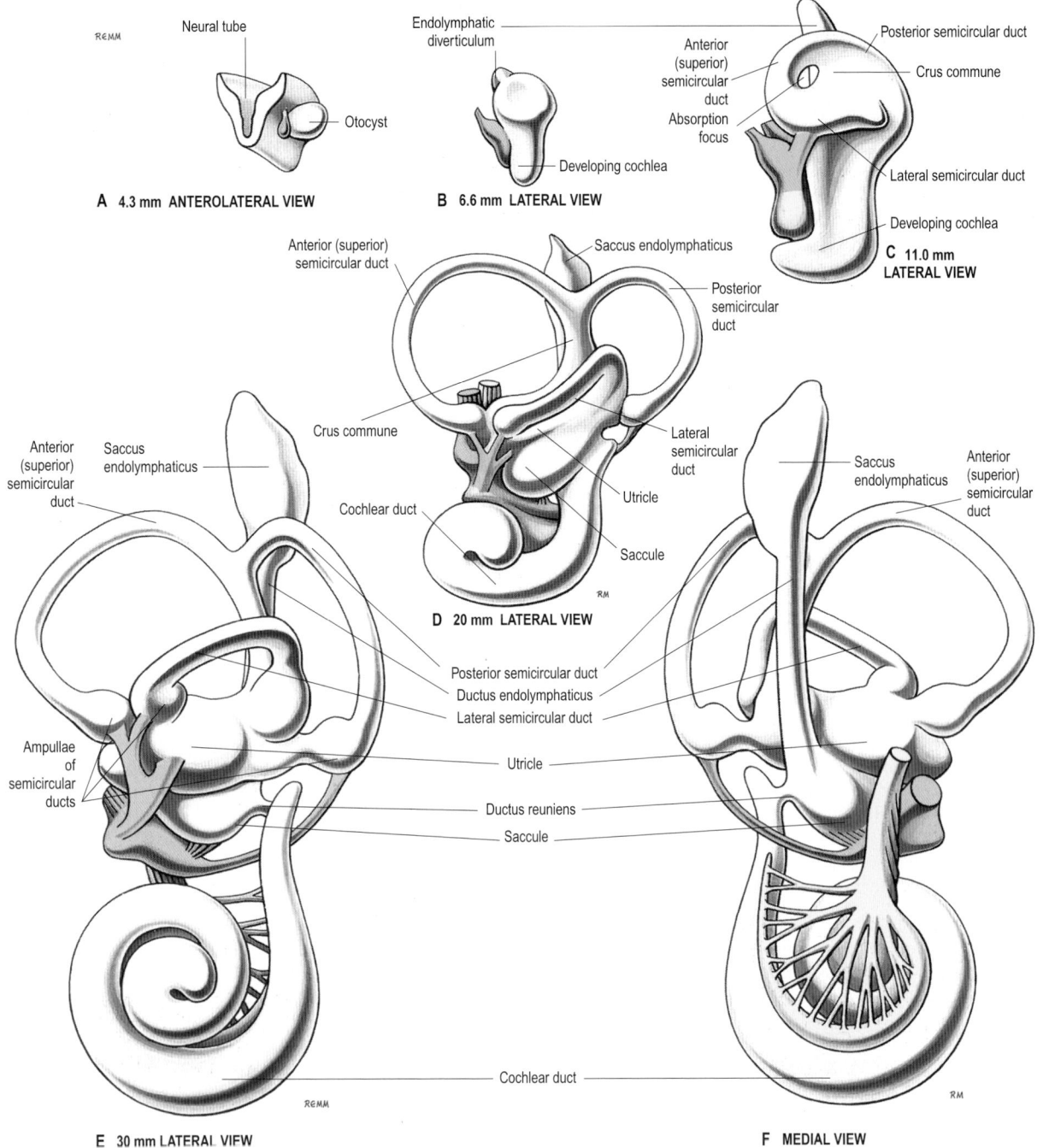

Fig. 40.1 A–F The stages in the development of the membranous labyrinth from the otocyst, at the embryonic stages and viewed from the aspects indicated. Note also the relationship of the vestibular (orange) and cochlear (yellow) parts of the vestibulocochlear nerve.

meatus are developed. A solid epidermal plug extends inwards from the tube along the floor of the tubotympanic recess, and the cells in the centre of the plug subsequently degenerate to produce the inner part of the meatus (secondary meatus). The epidermal stratum of the tympanic membrane is formed from the deepest ectodermal cells of the epidermal plug, and the fibrous stratum is formed from the mesenchyme between the meatal plate and the endodermal floor of the tubotympanic recess.

The development of the auricle is initiated by the appearance of six hillocks which form round the margins of the dorsal portion of the hyomandibular groove at the 4 mm stage. Of the six, three are on the caudal edge of the mandibular arch and three on the cranial edge of

the hyoid arch. These hillocks appear from stage 15. They tend to be less obvious prior to that stage and, of those on the mandibular arch only the most ventral, which subsequently forms the tragus, can be identified throughout earlier stages. The rest of the auricle is formed in the mesenchyme of the hyoid arch, which extends forwards round the dorsal end of the remains of the hyomandibular groove, forming a keel-like elevation which is the forerunner of the helix. The contribution made by the mandibular arch to the auricle is greatest at the end of the second month, and it becomes relatively reduced as growth continues until eventually the area of skin supplied by the mandibular nerve extends little above the tragus. The lobule is the last part of the auricle to develop.

REFERENCE

Frenz DA, Liu W, Williams JD, Hatcher V, Galinovic-Schwartz V, Flanders KC, Van de Water TR 1994 Induction of chondrogenesis: requirement for synergistic interaction of basic fibroblast growth factor and transforming growth factor-beta. Development 120: 415–24.

The orbit and its contents

EYELIDS (Fig. 41.1)

The eyelids (palpebrae) are two thin moveable folds which cover the anterior surface of the eye. They protect the eye, by their closure, from trauma or from excessive light. The act of blinking maintains a thin film of tears over the cornea.

The upper eyelid is larger and more mobile than the lower eyelid, and contains an elevator muscle, levator palpebrae superioris. When the eyelids are open, the upper lid just overlaps the upper part of the cornea, whereas the lower lid lies just below the cornea. An elliptical space, the palpebral fissure, is left between their margins. When the eyelids are closed, the upper lid moves down to cover the whole of the cornea.

The eyelids are covered by skin externally and by conjunctiva internally. The skin of the eyelids is thin and almost translucent. The supporting framework of each eyelid is formed by dense fibrous tissue arranged as a tarsal plate and an orbital septum attaching the plate to the orbital margin. The main muscle within the eyelids is orbicularis oculi.

Each lid margin exhibits a small elevation, the lacrimal papilla, approximately one-sixth of the way along from the medial canthus of the eye. There is a small opening, the punctum lacrimale, in the centre of the papilla. The margin of the eyelid lateral to the lacrimal papilla bears the eyelashes and is termed the ciliary part of the eyelid. The margin of the eyelid medial to the lacrimal papilla lacks eyelashes and is termed the lacrimal part of the eyelid.

The lid margin for both the upper and lower eyelids exhibits a 'grey line' which corresponds to the mucocutaneous junction. The eyelashes lie in front of this line, and the openings of the tarsal glands (meibomian glands) lie behind it. The tarsal glands are seen as a series of parallel, faint yellow lines arranged perpendicular to the lid margins when the eyelids are everted.

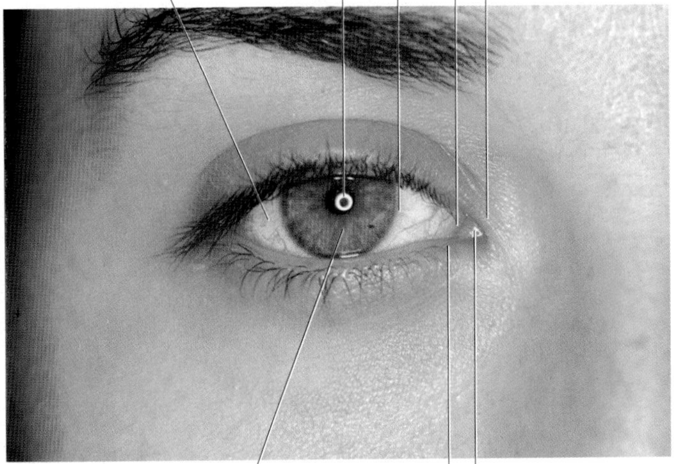

Eyelashes are short, thick, curved hairs, arranged in double or triple rows. The upper, which are more numerous and longer, curve upwards, while those in the lower lid curve down so that upper and lower lashes do not interlace when the lids are closed.

The medial and lateral angles of the eye are referred to as the medial (inner) and lateral (outer) canthi. The lateral canthus is relatively featureless. The medial canthus is c.2 mm lower than the lateral canthus: this distance is increased in some asiatic groups. It is separated from the eyeball by a small triangular space, the lacrimal lake (lacus lacrimalis), in which a small, reddish body called the lacrimal caruncle is situated. The caruncle contains sebaceous and sweat glands, and sometimes accessory lacrimal glands. It represents an area of modified skin containing some fine hairs, and is mounted on the plica semilunaris, a fold of conjunctiva which is believed by some to be a vestige of the nictitating membrane of other animals. In oriental Asians, a semilunar fold of skin termed the epicanthus passes from the medial end of the upper eyelid to the lower eyelid and obscures the caruncle.

The lower eyelid can be everted to reveal its conjunctiva up to the point where it is reflected from the eyelid onto the sclera, i.e. at the inferior fornix. The upper eyelid is less easily everted.

The eyelids are demarcated from the adjacent facial skin by the superior and inferior palpebral furrows. Additional furrows appear with age just beyond the inferior orbital margins, e.g. a nasojugal furrow medially and a malar furrow laterally.

STRUCTURE OF EYELIDS

From its facial surface inwards each eyelid consists of skin, subcutaneous connective tissue, fibres of the palpebral part of orbicularis oculi, submuscular connective tissue, the tarsus with its tarsal glands and orbital septum, and palpebral conjunctiva. The upper lid also contains the aponeurosis of levator palpebrae superioris (**Fig. 41.2**). The skin is extremely thin and is continuous at the palpebral margins with the conjunctiva. The subcutaneous connective tissue is very delicate, seldom contains any adipose tissue and lacks elastic fibres.

The palpebral fibre bundles of orbicularis oculi are thin and pale and run parallel with the palpebral fissure. Deep to them is the submuscular connective tissue, a loose fibrous layer which in the upper lid is continuous with the subaponeurotic layer of the scalp. Effusions of blood or pus at this level can therefore pass down from the scalp into the upper eyelid. The main nerves lie in the submuscular layer, which means that local anaesthetics should be injected deep to orbicularis oculi.

CONJUNCTIVA (Fig. 41.2)

The conjunctiva is a transparent mucous membrane which covers the internal palpebral surfaces and is reflected over the sclera, where its epithelium becomes continuous with that of the cornea.

The palpebral conjunctiva is very vascular, and has a dense subepithelial layer of capillaries. It contains mucosa-associated lymphoid tissue (MALT – Chapter 5) especially at the orbital edges of the tarsi to which it is closely adherent. At the free palpebral margins the conjunctiva is continuous with the skin, the lining epithelium of the ducts of the tarsal glands, and with the lacrimal canaliculi and lacrimal sac (p. 685). There is therefore continuity with the naso-lacrimal duct and nasal mucosa which is important in the spread of infection. The line of reflection of the conjunctiva from the lids to the eyeball, the conjunctival fornix, is subdivided into superior and inferior fornices. The ducts of the lacrimal gland open into the lateral part

Sclerocorneal junction
(limbus) ┐   ┌ Plica semilunaris
Sclera ┐   Pupil ┐ │   ┌ Medial canthus

Iris ┘   Lacrimal papilla ┘   └ Lacrimal caruncle

Fig. 41.1 The eyelids and eyeball. (By permission from Berkovitz BKB, Moxham BJ 2002 Head and Neck Anatomy. London: Martin Dunitz.)

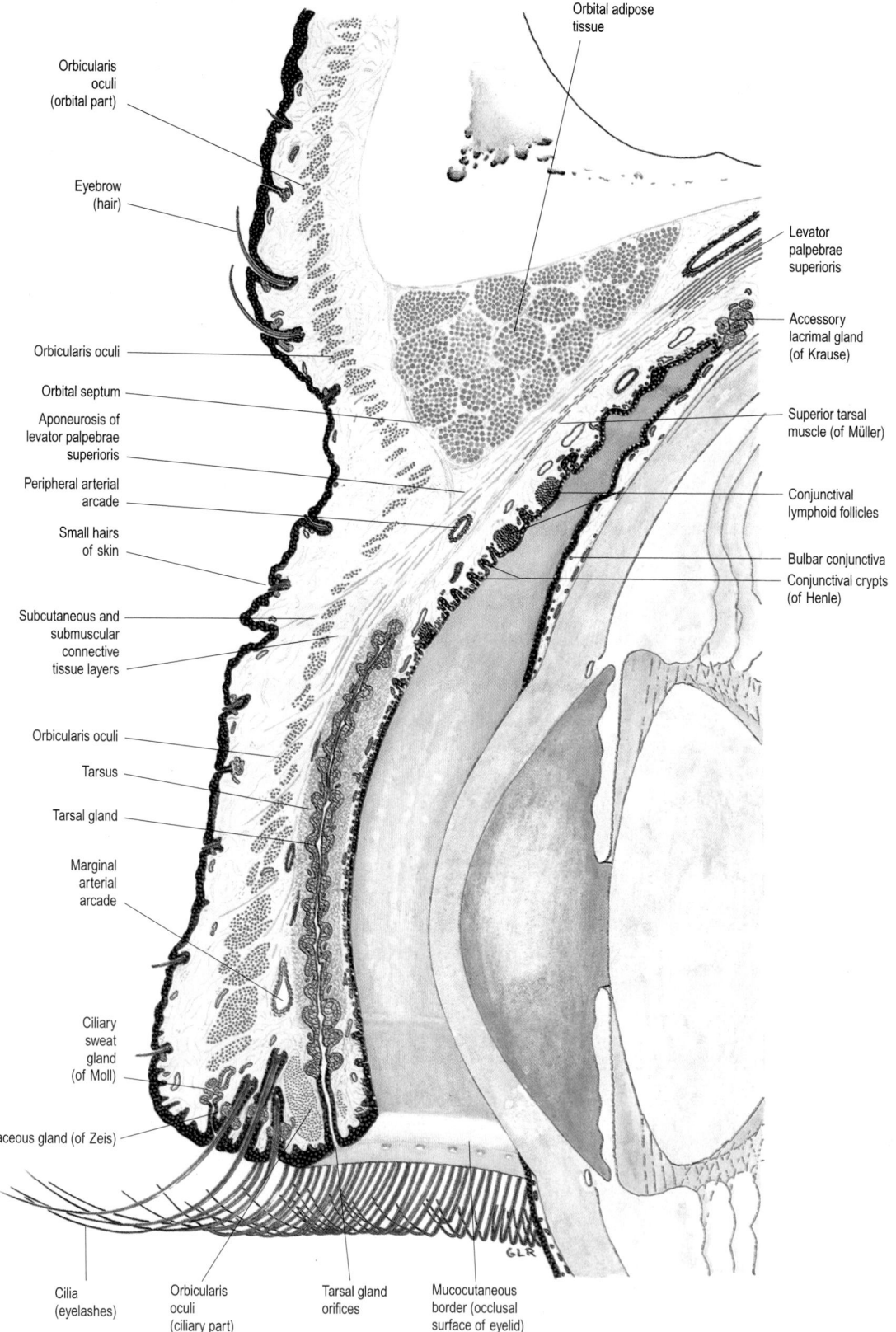

Orbital adipose
tissue

Orbicularis
oculi
(orbital part)

Eyebrow
(hair)

Levator
palpebrae
superioris

Accessory
lacrimal gland
(of Krause)

Orbicularis oculi

Orbital septum

Aponeurosis of
levator palpebrae
superioris

Peripheral arterial
arcade

Small hairs
of skin

Superior tarsal
muscle (of Müller)

Conjunctival
lymphoid follicles

Bulbar conjunctiva

Conjunctival crypts
(of Henle)

Subcutaneous and
submuscular
connective
tissue layers

Orbicularis oculi

Tarsus

Tarsal gland

Marginal
arterial
arcade

Ciliary
sweat
gland
(of Moll)

Sebaceous gland (of Zeis)

Cilia
(eyelashes)

Orbicularis
oculi
(ciliary part)

Tarsal gland
orifices

Mucocutaneous
border (occlusal
surface of eyelid)

Fig. 41.2 The upper eyelid and anterior segment of the eye: sagittal section. (Provided by the late Gordon L Ruskell, Department of Optometry and Visual Science, The City University, London.)

of the superior fornix (**Fig. 41.3**). The bulbar conjunctiva is loosely connected to the eyeball over the exposed sclera, is thin and transparent, and is only slightly vascular.

The epithelium of the palpebral conjunctiva at the margin of the lids is non-keratinized stratified squamous, 10–12 cells thick. About 2 mm from each margin there is often a subtarsal groove in which foreign bodies frequently lodge: here the epithelium has two or three layers, and consists of columnar and flat surface cells. These persist throughout

most of the palpebral conjunctiva. Near the fornices in the orbital conjunctiva the cells are taller, and a trilaminar conjunctival epithelium covers much of the anterior, exposed surface of the sclera. It thickens closer to the corneoscleral junction and then changes to stratified squamous epithelium typical of the cornea. Mucous-secreting goblet cells are scattered in the conjunctival epithelium. They are most frequent on each side of the fornix, but absent from the exposed surfaces of the bulbar conjunctiva and the corneoscleral junction.

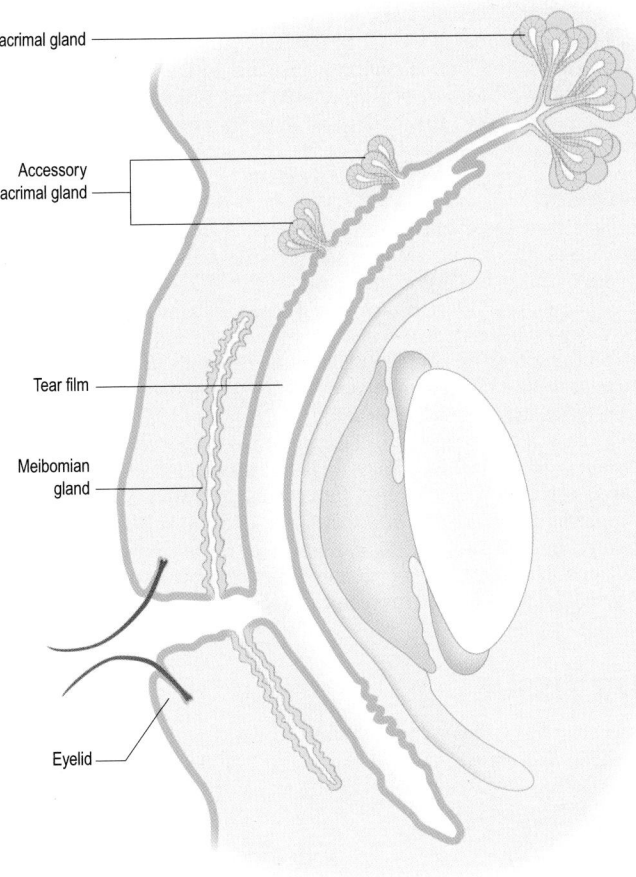

Lacrimal gland

Accessory
lacrimal gland

Tear film

Meibomian
gland

Eyelid

Fig. 41.3 The orbital glands responsible for the secretion of the tear film.

TARSAL PLATES

The two tarsi (**Fig. 41.2**) are thin, elongated, crescent-shaped plates of firm, dense fibrous tissue c.2.5 cm long. There is one in each eyelid to provide support and determine eyelid form. Each tarsal plate is convex forwards, and conforms to the configuration of the anterior surface of the eye. The free ciliary border is straight and adjacent to the eyelash follicles. The orbital, border is convex and attached to the orbital septum.

The superior tarsus, the larger of the two, is semi-oval, c.10 mm in height centrally. Its inferior edge is parallel to, and c.2 mm from, the lid margin. The deepest fibres of the aponeurosis of levator palpebrae superioris are attached to its anterior surface, and the fibrous extension of the superior tarsal muscle is attached to its upper margin (**Fig. 41.4**). The smaller inferior tarsus is narrower, and c.4 mm in vertical height.

The tarsal plates are connected to the margins of the orbit by the orbital septum and by the medial and lateral palpebral (canthal) ligaments. The medial palpebral ligament passes from the medial ends of the two tarsal plates to the anterior lacrimal crest and the frontal process of the maxilla. It splits at its insertion into the tarsal plates to surround the lacrimal canaliculi, and lies in front of the nasolacrimal sac and the orbital septum. The lateral palpebral ligament is relatively poorly developed. It passes from the lateral ends of the tarsal plates to a small tubercle on the zygomatic bone within the orbital margin and is more deeply situated than the medial palpebral ligament. It lies beneath the orbital septum and the lateral palpebral raphe of orbicularis oculi.

Each tarsal plate is associated with a thin lamina of smooth muscle. Opposite the equator of the eye the superior tarsal muscle passes from the inferior face of levator palpebrae superioris to a fibrous extension which projects to the upper margin of the superior tarsus. There is a corresponding but less prominent inferior tarsal muscle in the lower eyelid which unites the inferior tarsus to the anterior expansion of the fused fascial sheath of inferior rectus and inferior oblique. The smooth muscles assist in the elevation of the upper, and depression of the lower, eyelids. They may adjust the size of the aperture of the open eye according to mood and other factors.

Tarsal glands (**Figs 41.2, 41.3**) are modified sebaceous glands embedded in the tarsi, and may be visible through the conjunctiva when the eyelids are everted. They are yellow and arranged in a single row of c.25 in the upper lid, and fewer in the lower lid. They occupy the full tarsal height, and are therefore longer centrally where the tarsi are higher. Each gland consists of a straight tube with many lateral diverticula, and

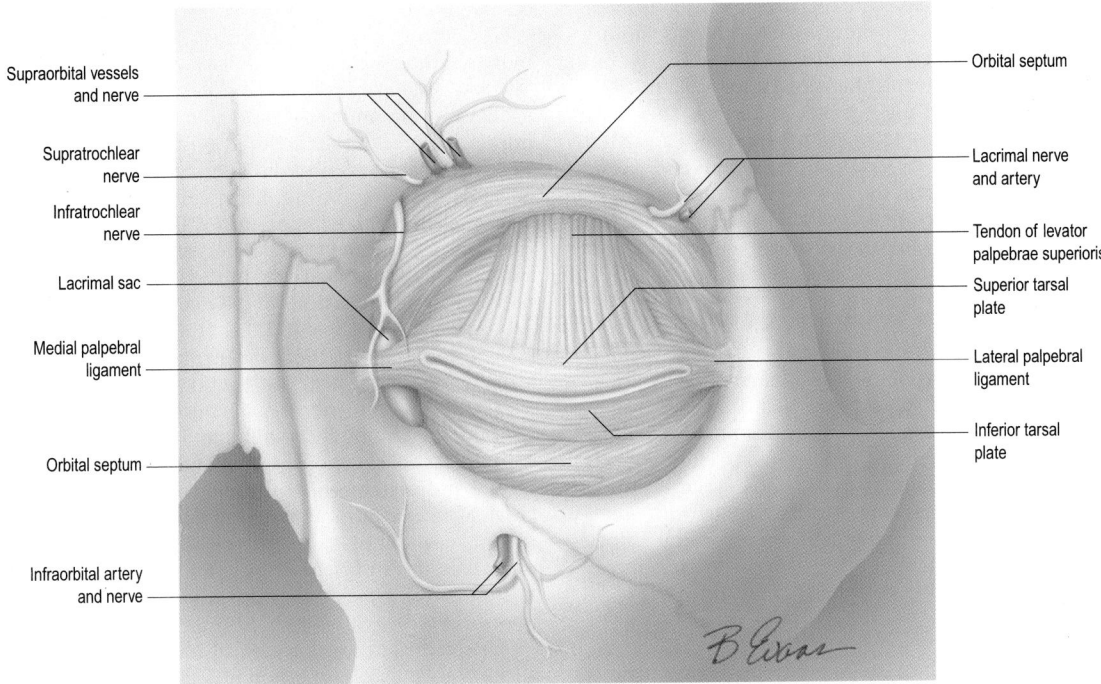

Supraorbital vessels
and nerve

Supratrochlear
nerve

Infratrochlear
nerve

Lacrimal sac

Medial palpebral
ligament

Orbital septum

Infraorbital artery
and nerve

Orbital septum

Lacrimal nerve
and artery

Tendon of levator
palpebrae superioris

Superior tarsal
plate

Lateral palpebral
ligament

Inferior tarsal
plate

Fig. 41.4 The tarsi, their ligaments and the orbital septum: anterior aspect.

opens by a minute orifice on the free palpebral margin. It is enclosed by a basement membrane, and is lined at its orifice by stratified epithelium and elsewhere by a layer of polyhedral cells. The oily secretion of the tarsal glands spreads over the margins of the eyelids, and so an oily layer is drawn over the tear film as the palpebral fissure opens after a blink, reducing evaporation and contributing to tear film stability. The presence of the oily, hydrophobic secretions of tarsal glands along the margins of the eyelids also inhibits the spillage of tears onto the face.

ORBITAL SEPTUM

The orbital septum (**Fig. 41.4**) is a weak membranous sheet which is attached to the orbital rim where it becomes continuous with the periosteum. It passes inwards into each eyelid and blends with the tarsal plates, and, in the upper eyelid, with the superficial lamella of levator palpebrae superioris. The orbital septum is thickest laterally, where it lies in front of the lateral palpebral ligament. It passes behind the medial palpebral ligament and nasolacrimal sac, but in front of the pulley of superior oblique. The orbital septum is pierced above by levator palpebrae superioris and below by the ligament from inferior rectus. The lacrimal, supratrochlear, infratrochlear and supraorbital nerves and vessels pass through the septum from the orbit on the way to the face and scalp.

VASCULAR SUPPLY AND LYMPHATIC DRAINAGE

The eyelids are supplied by the lateral and medial palpebral arteries, both of which have superior and inferior branches which anastomose to form arcades: the superior arteries supply the upper eyelid, and the inferior arteries supply the lower eyelid. The lateral palpebral arteries, usually two, are given off by the lacrimal branch of the ophthalmic artery. The medial palpebral arteries arise directly from the ophthalmic artery below the trochlea, and descend behind the nasolacrimal sac to enter the eyelids, where each bifurcates. Their branches course laterally along the tarsal edges to form superior and inferior arcades which are completed by anastomoses with branches of the supraorbital and zygomatico-orbital arteries (superior arch) and the lateral palpebral artery (both arches). The inferior arch links with the facial artery to supply the mucosa of the nasolacrimal duct. The eyelids are also supplied by branches of the infraorbital, facial, transverse facial and superficial temporal arteries.

The veins which drain the eyelids are larger and more numerous than the arteries. They pass either superficially to veins on the face and forehead, or deeply to the ophthalmic veins within the orbit. Bulbar conjunctival veins pass to the orbital surfaces of the rectal muscles and join the superior or inferior ophthalmic vein.

The lymph vessels which drain the eyelids and conjunctiva commence in a superficial plexus beneath the skin, and in a deep plexus in front of and behind the tarsi. These plexuses communicate with one another and medial and lateral sets of vessels arise from them. The lymph vessels of the lateral set drain the whole thickness of the lateral part of the upper and lower lids and all the ocular conjunctiva. They pass laterally from the lateral commissure to end in the superficial and deep parotid lymph nodes and also in the deep parotid lymph nodes. The lymph vessels of the medial set drain the skin over the medial part of the upper eyelid, the whole thickness of the medial half of the lower lid, and the caruncula lacrimalia. They follow the course of the facial vein and end in the submandibular group of lymph nodes.

INNERVATION (Fig. 41.4)

The cutaneous innervation of the eyelids comes from both the ophthalmic and maxillary divisions of the trigeminal nerve. The upper eyelid is supplied mainly by the supraorbital branch of the frontal nerve. Additional contributions come from the lacrimal nerve, the supratrochlear branch of the frontal nerve, and the infratrochlear branch of the nasociliary nerve. The nerve supply to the lower eyelid is principally from the infraorbital branch of the maxillary nerve, with small contributions from the lacrimal and infratrochlear nerves. The bulbar conjunctiva is supplied by the ophthalmic division of the trigeminal nerve. Autonomic fibres are probably vasomotor in function.

ECTROPION

Ectropion describes the rolling out of the lower eyelid so that it is no longer in contact with the cornea. It is most commonly a senile development but there are also cicatricial and paralytic forms. It causes overspill of tear fluid (epiphora), instability of the tear film, and chronic conjunc-

tivitis resulting from exposure. If the condition persists, the conjunctiva may become dry, thickened and unsightly; in severe cases, drying of the cornea may cause loss of vision. In the senile form ectropion is caused by reduced tension in orbicularis oculi, and in the paralytic form it occurs because orbicularis oculi is unable to contract as a consequence of facial nerve palsy. The condition may warrant treatment by full thickness shortening of the lid.

ENTROPION

Entropion describes the inversion of the eyelids and is largely a problem of later years (the involutional or senile form). Other forms are caused by spasm of the orbicularis oculi (spastic form); by cicatricial contraction of the palpebral conjunctiva, or as a congenital disorder. Connective tissue changes associated with age relax the tension in the lower eyelid in involutional entropion. The tarsal plate becomes thinned, atrophic and unstable, and its attachments to inferior rectus slacken, causing the lid to turn inwards. The lashes abrade the cornea (trichiasis) producing discomfort and in severe untreated cases the cornea becomes inflamed and there is loss of transparency. Spastic entropion is due to an acute spasm of orbicularis oculi, often induced by irritation of the eye, and may be an additional factor in involutional entropion. The tarsal plates of the eyelids stop short of the margins, which are therefore less firm, but they contain the ciliary or marginal part of orbicularis oculi, which may be responsible for the inversion in spastic entropion.

SOFT TISSUE

Certain named regions of soft connective tissue within the orbit have anatomical and clinical significance. These include the orbital septum, canthal ligaments, fascial sheath of the eye, suspensory ligament, periosteum and orbital fat.

ORBITAL SEPTUM

This is described on page 683.

FASCIAL SHEATH OF THE EYEBALL (Fig. 41.5)

A thin fascial membrane, the vagina bulbi (fascia bulbi or Tenon's capsule), envelops the eyeball from the optic nerve to the corneoscleral junction, separates it from the orbital fat, and forms a socket. Its ocular aspect is loosely attached to the sclera by delicate bands of episcleral connective tissue. Posteriorly, the fascia is traversed by ciliary vessels and nerves. It fuses with the sclera and with the sheath of the optic nerve around its entrance to the eyeball. Attachment to the sclera is strongest in this position and again anteriorly, just behind the corneoscleral junction at the limbus.

The fascial sheath is perforated by the tendons of the extraocular muscles and is reflected on to each as a tubular sheath, the muscular fascia. The sheath of superior oblique reaches the fibrous trochlea (pulley) of the muscle. The sheaths of the four recti muscles are very thick anteriorly but are reduced posteriorly to a delicate perimysium. Just before they blend with the vagina bulbi, the thick sheaths of adjacent recti become confluent and form a fascial ring. Expansions from the sheaths are important for the attachments they make. Those from the medial and lateral rectus muscles are triangular and strong, and are attached respectively to the lacrimal and zygomatic bones. As they may limit the actions of the two recti, they are termed the medial and lateral check ligaments (**Figs 41.5, 41.6**). Other extraocular muscles have less substantial check ligaments: the capacity of any of them to actually limit movement has been questioned.

The sheath of inferior rectus is thickened on its underside and blends with the sheath of inferior oblique. These two, in turn, are continuous with the fascial ring noted earlier and therefore with the sheaths of the medial and lateral recti. As the latter are attached to the orbital walls by check ligaments, a continuous fascial band, the suspensory ligament of the eye, is slung like a hammock below the eye. The suspensory ligament provides sufficient support for the eye such that, even when the maxilla forming the floor of the orbit is removed, the eye will retain its position.

The thickened fused sheath of inferior rectus and inferior oblique also has an anterior expansion into the lower eyelid, where, augmented by some fibres of orbicularis oculi (the inferior tarsal muscle), it attaches to the inferior tarsus. Contraction of inferior rectus in downward gaze therefore also draws the lid downward. The sheath of levator palpebrae

A

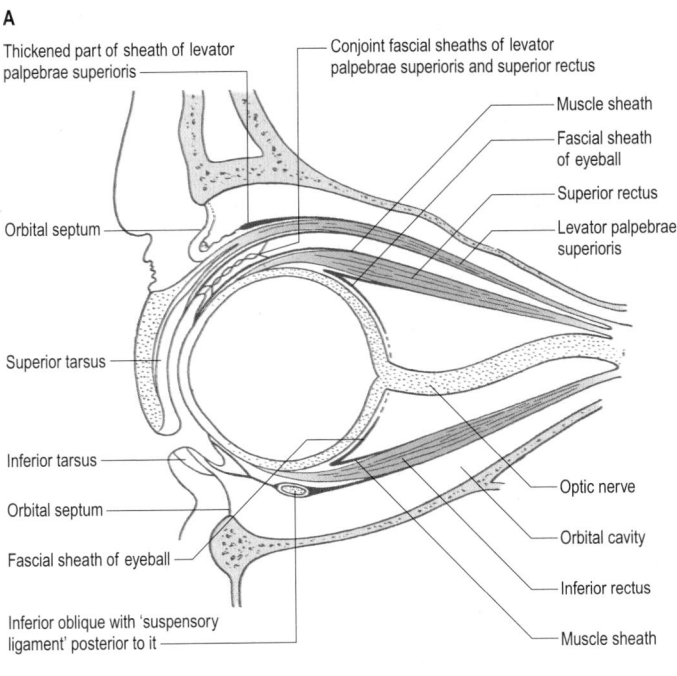

Thickened part of sheath of levator palpebrae superioris

Conjoint fascial sheaths of levator palpebrae superioris and superior rectus

Muscle sheath

Fascial sheath of eyeball

Superior rectus

Levator palpebrae superioris

Orbital septum

Superior tarsus

Inferior tarsus

Orbital septum

Fascial sheath of eyeball

Inferior oblique with 'suspensory ligament' posterior to it

Optic nerve

Orbital cavity

Inferior rectus

Muscle sheath

B

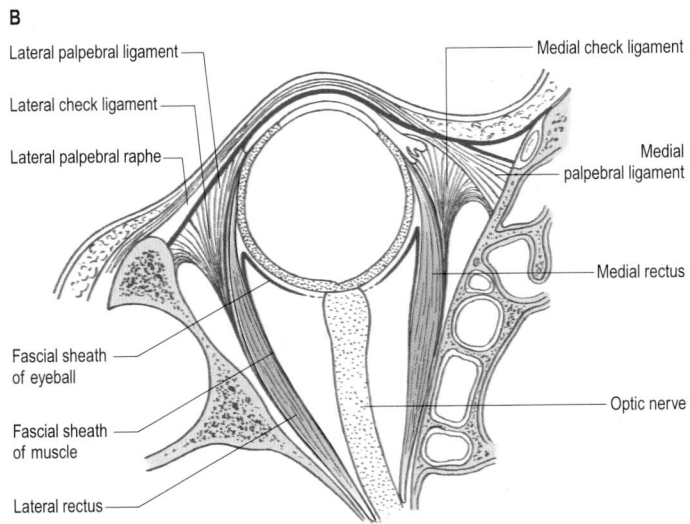

Lateral palpebral ligament

Lateral check ligament

Lateral palpebral raphe

Medial check ligament

Medial palpebral ligament

Medial rectus

Fascial sheath of eyeball

Fascial sheath of muscle

Lateral rectus

Optic nerve

Fig. 41.5 A, The orbital fascia in sagittal section. **B**, Scheme of the orbital fascia in horizontal section. (After Whitnall SE 1932 Anatomy of the Human Orbit, 2nd edn. London: Oxford University Press. By permission of Oxford University Press.)

superioris also thickens anteriorly, and just behind the aponeurosis it fuses inferiorly with the sheath of superior rectus. It extends forward between the two muscles and attaches to the upper fornix of the conjunctiva.

Other extensions of the fascial sheath of the eye pass medially and laterally and attach to the orbital walls, forming the transverse ligament of the eye. This structure is of uncertain significance, but presumably plays a part in drawing the fornix upwards in gaze elevation and it may act as a fulcrum for levator movements. Other numerous finer fasciae form radial septa which extend from the vagina bulbi and the muscle sheaths to the periosteum of the orbit, and so provide compartments for orbital fat. The orbital septum is the most anteriorly placed. Many of the fasciae contain smooth muscle cells. The ocular and orbital fasciae are arranged to assist in the location of the eye within the orbit without obstructing the activities of the extraocular muscles, except possibly in the extremes of rotation. They also prevent the gross displacement of orbital fat, for this could interfere with the accurate positioning of the two eyes in binocular vision.

The periosteum of the orbit is only loosely attached to bone. Behind, it is united with the dura mater of the optic nerve and in front

it is continuous with the periosteum of the orbital margin, where it gives off a stratum contributing to the orbital septum. It also attaches to the trochlea, and, as the lacrimal fascia, forms the roof and lateral wall of the sulcus for the nasolacrimal sac (p. 687).

ORBITAL FAT (Fig. 41.7)

The spaces between the main structures of the orbit are occupied by orbital fat. This is particularly the case between the optic nerve and the cone of muscles (*see* **Fig. 41.8**). The fat helps to stabilize the position of the eyeball and acts as a socket within which the eyeball can rotate. Conditions resulting in an increased overall volume of orbital fat, e.g. hyperthyroidism, may thrust the eyeball forwards (exophthalmos).

NASOLACRIMAL APPARATUS (Figs 41.3, 41.9)

The nasolacrimal apparatus consists of the lacrimal gland, which secretes a complex fluid (tears) and whose excretory ducts convey fluid to the surface of the eye; the paired lacrimal canaliculi; the lacrimal sac, and the nasolacrimal duct, by which the fluid is collected and conveyed into the nasal cavity.

LACRIMAL GLAND

The lacrimal gland consists of an orbital part and a palpebral part. They are continuous posterolaterally around the concave lateral edge of the aponeurosis of levator palpebrae superioris.

The orbital part, about the size and shape of an almond, lodges in the lacrimal fossa on the medial aspect of the zygomatic process of the frontal bone, just within the orbital margin. It lies above levator palpebrae superioris and, laterally, above lateral rectus. Its lower surface is connected to the sheath of levator palpebrae superioris and its upper surface is connected to the orbital periosteum. Its anterior border is in contact with the orbital septum and its posterior border is attached to the orbital fat.

The palpebral part, about one-third the size of the orbital part is subdivided into two or three lobules and extends below the aponeurosis of levator palpebrae superioris into the lateral part of the upper lid, where it is attached to the superior conjunctival fornix. It is visible through the conjunctiva when the lid is everted.

The ducts of the lacrimal gland, about six in number, open into the superior fornix. Those from the orbital part (four or five) penetrate the aponeurosis of levator palpebrae superioris to join those from the palpebral part. Excision of the palpebral part is therefore functionally equivalent to the total removal of the gland.

Many small accessory lacrimal glands occur in or near the fornix. They are more numerous in the upper eyelid. Their presence may explain why the conjunctiva does not dry up after extirpation of the main lacrimal gland.

Vascular supply – The lacrimal gland receives its arterial blood supply from the lacrimal branch of the ophthalmic artery. It may also receive blood from the infraorbital artery. Venous drainage is into the superior ophthalmic vein.

Innervation – The lacrimal gland is innervated by secretomotor parasympathetic fibres from the pterygopalatine ganglion which may reach the gland via zygomatic and lacrimal branches of the maxillary nerve or pass directly to the gland. Preganglionic parasympathetic fibres travel to the ganglion in the greater petrosal nerve, which arises from the facial nerve at the geniculate ganglion.

Microstructure – The lacrimal gland is lobulated and tubuloacinar in form (p. 34). Its secretory units are acini (**Fig. 41.10**) and resemble those of the salivary glands. The secretion is a watery fluid with an electrolyte content similar to that of plasma and contains, amongst other components, a bacteriocidal enzyme, lysozyme. Other components of tears include the proteins lactoferrin, IgA, and tear-specific pre-albumen, as well as some major serum proteins (IgM, IgG, transferrin and serum albumen). It has been suggested that there are two types of secretion from the orbital glands, basic and reflex. The former is a constant slow baseline secretion, and the latter occurs in response to stimulation, e.g.

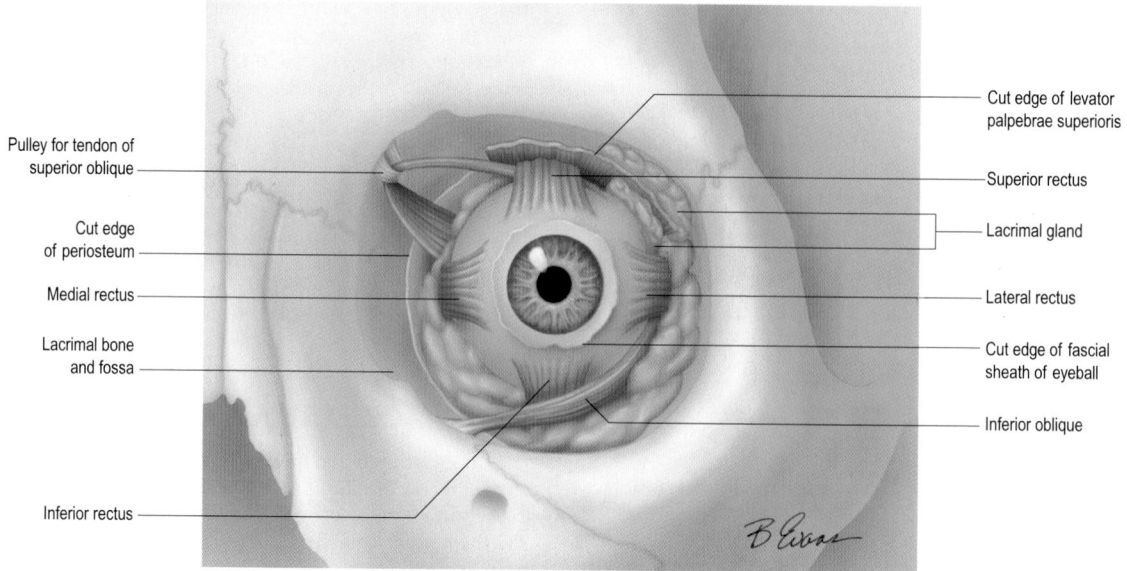

Fig. 41.6 The eye viewed anteriorly showing the extraocular muscles.

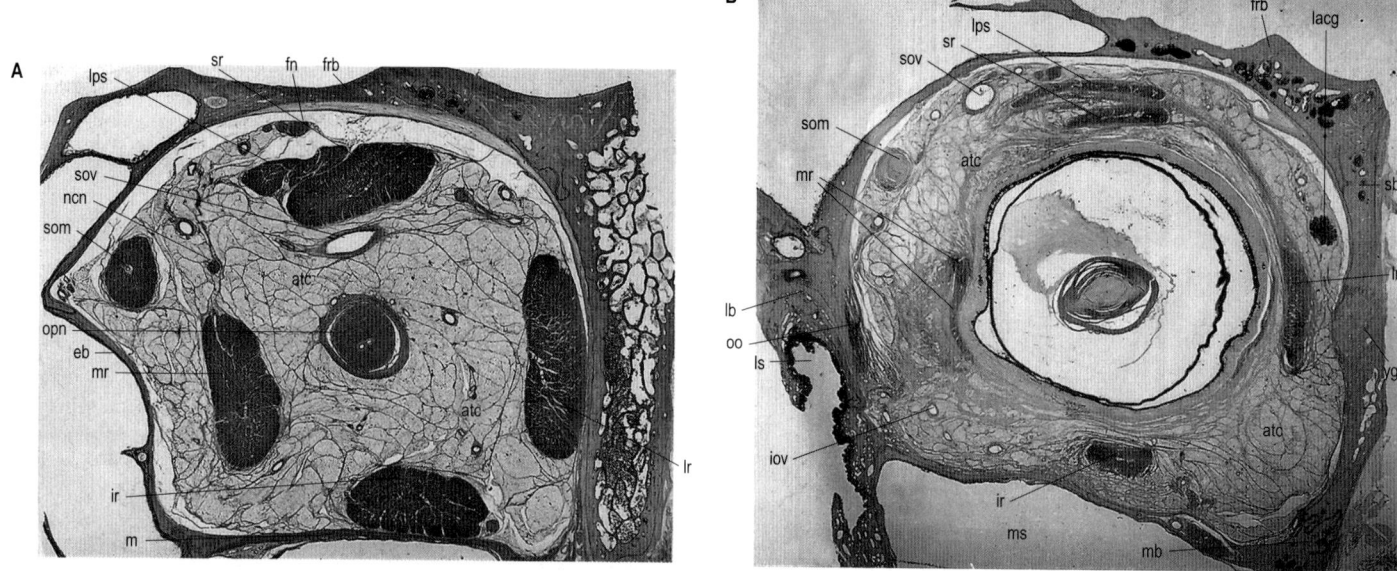

Fig. 41.7 Two coronal sections through the left orbit (viewed from in front: right is lateral) cut through planes passing (**A**) 5 mm behind the posterior pole of the globe of the eye, and (**B**) 4.6 mm in front of its posterior pole (the lens which is visible, has been displaced backwards. atc, adipose tissue compartments; eb, ethmoid bone; fn, frontal nerve; frb, frontal bone; iov, inferior ophthalmic vein; ir, inferior rectus; lb, lacrimal bone; lacg, lacrimal gland; lr, lateral rectus; ls, nasolacrimal sac; m, maxilla (bone); ms, maxillary sinus; mr, medial rectus; ncn, nasociliary nerve; oo, orbicularis oculi; opn, optic nerve; sb, sphenoid bone; lps, levator palpebrae superioris; som, superior oblique; sov, superior ophthalmic vein; sr, superior rectus; zyg, zygomatic bone. (By permission from Kornneef 1977.)

neural stimulation. The content of the tears varies considerably in the non-stimulated and stimulated states.

LACRIMAL CANALICULI (Figs 41.1, 41.9, 41.11)

There is one lacrimal canaliculus in each lid, c.10 mm long. Each commences at a puncta lacrimalia. The superior canaliculus, smaller and shorter than the inferior, at first ascends, and then bends at an acute angle, and passes medially and downwards to reach the nasolacrimal sac. The inferior canaliculus first descends and turns almost horizontally to the sac. At their angles the canaliculi are dilated into ampullae. The mucosa lining the ducts has a non-keratinized stratified squamous epithelium lying on a basement membrane, outside which is a lamina propria rich in elastic fibres (the ducts are therefore easily dilated when probed), and a layer of skeletal muscle fibres continuous with the lacrimal part of orbicularis oculi. At the base of each lacrimal papilla the muscle fibres are circularly arranged in the form of a sphincter.

NASOLACRIMAL SAC Figs 41.9, 41.11)

The lacrimal sac is the closed upper end of the nasolacrimal duct. It is c.12 mm long and lies in a fossa adjacent to the lacrimal groove in the anterior part of the medial wall of the orbit. The sac is bounded in front by the anterior lacrimal crest of the maxilla and behind by the posterior lacrimal crest of the lacrimal bone. Its closed upper end is laterally flattened and its lower part is rounded and merges into the duct. The lacrimal canaliculi open into its lateral wall near its upper end.

A layer of lacrimal fascia, continuous with the orbital periosteum, passes between the lacrimal crest of the maxilla and the lacrimal bone, and forms a roof and lateral wall to the lacrimal fossa. There is

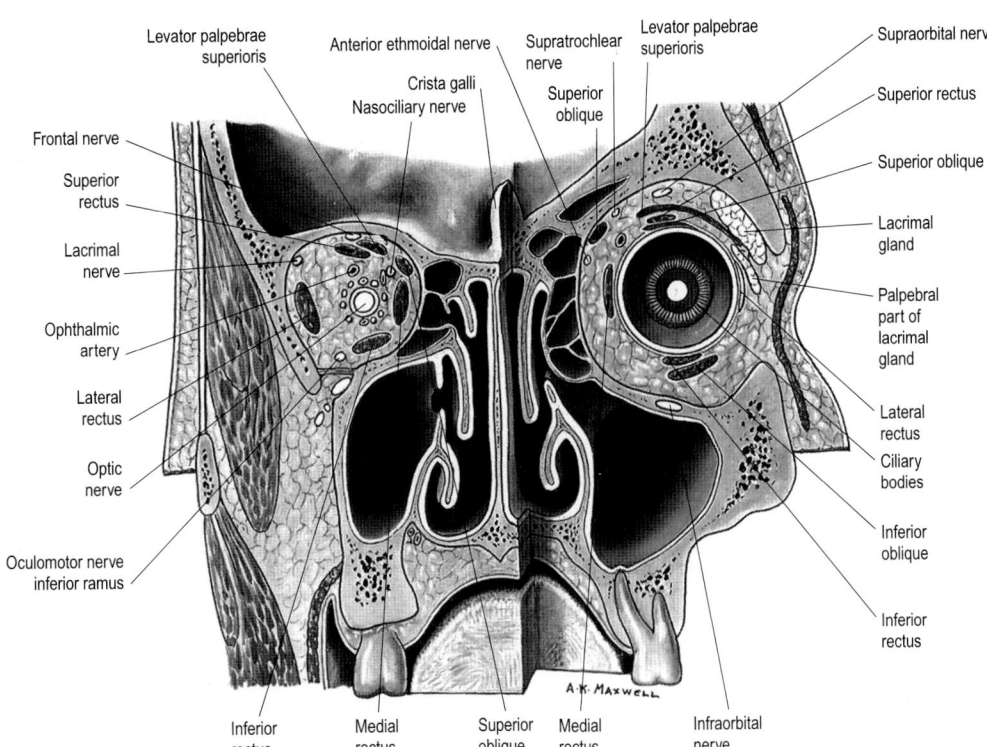

Fig. 41.8 Coronal sections through the two orbits: posterior aspect. On the left side the plane of the section is more posterior and passes behind the eyeball.

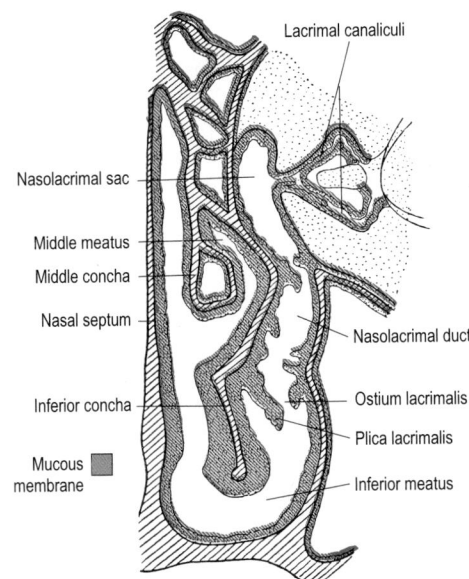

Fig. 41.9 Coronal section through the left half of the nasal cavity (anterior aspect) to show the relation of the lacrimal passages to the maxillary and ethmoidal sinuses and the inferior nasal concha. The mucous membrane is coloured. (After Whitnall SE 1932 Anatomy of the Human Orbit, 2nd edn. London: Oxford University Press. By permission of Oxford University Press.)

a plexus of minute veins between the fascia and the nasolacrimal sac. The fascia separates the sac from the medial palpebral ligament in front and the lacrimal part of orbicularis oculi behind. The lower half of the lacrimal fossa is related medially to the anterior part of the middle meatus, and the upper half to the anterior ethmoidal sinuses. The nasolacrimal sac has a fibroelastic wall. It is lined internally by mucosa which is continuous with the conjunctiva through the lacrimal canaliculi, and with the nasal mucosa through the nasolacrimal duct.

NASOLACRIMAL DUCT (Figs 41.9, 41.11)

The nasolacrimal duct is c.18 mm long, and descends from the lacrimal sac to open anteriorly in the inferior meatus of the nose at an expanded orifice. A fold of mucosa (plica lacrimalis) forms an imperfect valve just above its opening (ostium lacrimalis). The duct runs down an osseous

canal formed by the maxilla, lacrimal bone and inferior nasal concha (**Fig. 41.12**). It is narrowest in the middle and is directed downwards, backwards and a little laterally. The mucosa of the nasolacrimal sac and the nasolacrimal duct has a bilaminar columnar epithelium, which is ciliated in places. Around the duct there is a rich plexus of veins forming erectile tissue: engorgement of these veins may obstruct the duct.

ANATOMY OF TEARS

Lacrimal fluid enters the conjunctival sac at its superolateral angle and, by capillarity and blinking, is carried across the eye to the lacus lacrimalis, mainly between the lower palpebral margin and the eyeball. From the lacus it enters the lacrimal canaliculi. Contraction of orbicularis oculi presses the puncta lacrimalia more firmly into the lacus and capillary attraction draws the secretion into the lacrimal sac. Sudden dilatation of the sac, produced by the lacrimal part of orbicularis oculi during blinking, probably aids this. Normally the tarsal secretions prevent the tears from overflowing the lid margins and also cover the capillary film of fluid on the cornea and sclera with a film of oil, which delays evaporation.

Tear film

The tear film, i.e. the interface between the external environment and the ocular surface has a number of functions. It forms a smooth refracting surface over the corneal surface; lubricates the eyelids; maintains an optimal environment for the epithelia of the cornea and conjunctiva; dilutes and washes away noxious substances; provides an antibacterial system for the ocular surface; serves as an entry pathway for polymorphonuclear leukocytes. The film consists of three layers. The outer layer is a lipid layer c.0.1 μm thick. It floats on an intermediate, aqueous layer, c.7 μm thick, which contains electrolytes, water, IgA and proteins, many of them antibacterial enzymes. The inner layer is mucous which covers the cornea and conjunctiva. Each layer of the tear film is secreted by a different set of orbital glands. The mucous layer is secreted by goblet cells, and it may also contain glycoproteins (possibly mucins) secreted by the stratified squamous epithelial cells of the cornea and conjunctiva. The aqueous layer is secreted by the main and accessory lacrimal glands (**Fig. 41.3**), and may receive a contribution from the corneal epithelial cells. The lipid layer is secreted by the tarsal glands.

LACRIMATION REFLEX (Fig. 41.13)

The lacrimation reflex is stimulated by irritation of the conjunctiva and cornea. The afferent limb of the reflex involves branches of the

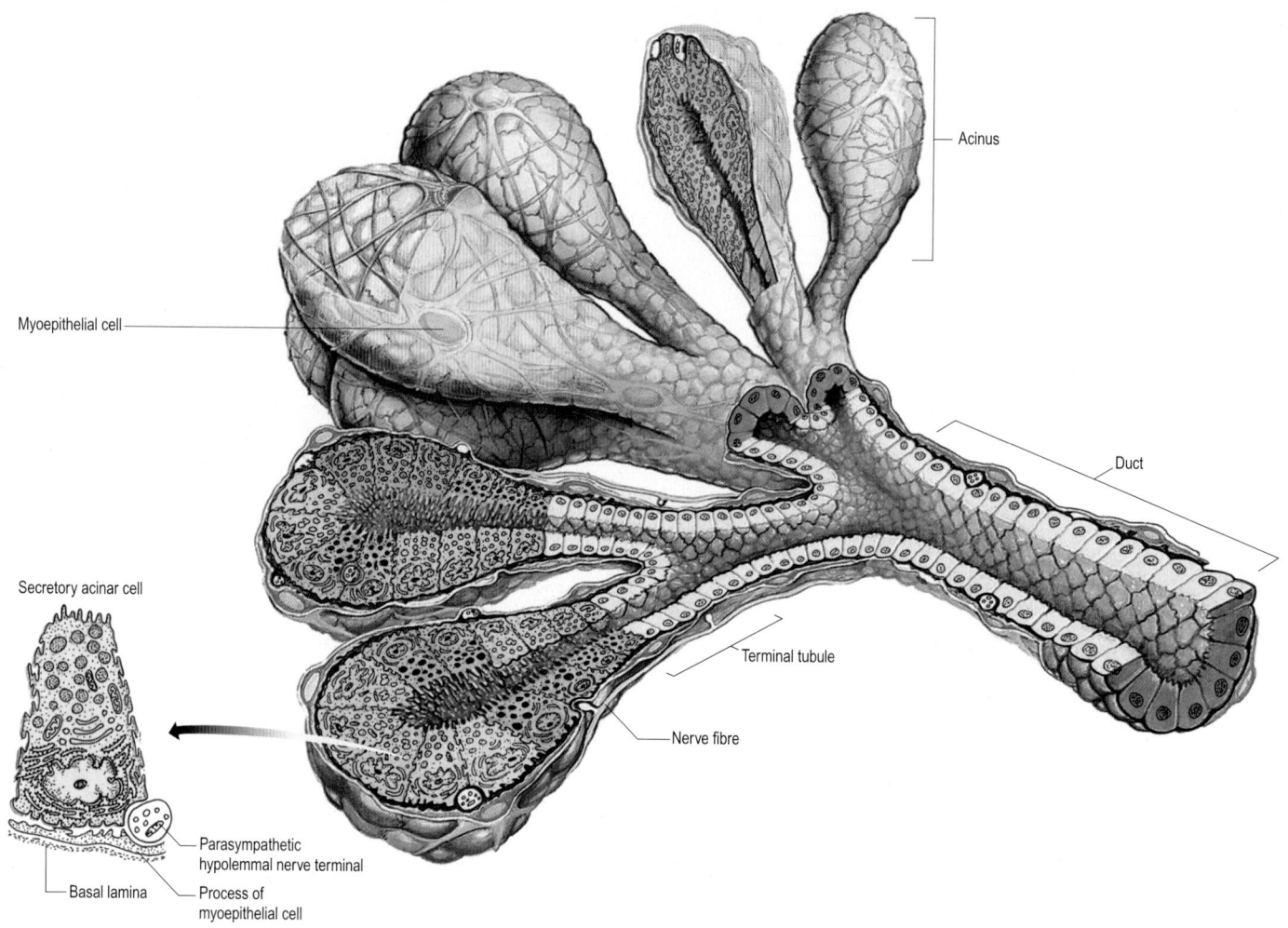

Myoepithelial cell

Acinus

Duct

Secretory acinar cell

Terminal tubule

Nerve fibre

Parasympathetic
hypolemmal nerve terminal

Basal lamina —— Process of
myoepithelial cell

Fig. 41.10 Organization of the secretory units in the lacrimal gland.

ophthalmic nerve, with an additional contribution from the infraorbital nerve if the conjunctiva of the lower eyelid is involved. Impulses enter the brain and spread by interneurones to activate parasympathetic neurones in the superior salivatory centre (associated with the facial nerve) and sympathetic neurones in the upper thoracic spinal cord. The efferent pathway to the lacrimal gland involves the greater petrosal nerve, which carries parasympathetic preganglionic secretomotor fibres, and the deep petrosal nerve, which carries postganglionic sympathetic fibres: the parasympathetic fibres relay in the pterygopalatine ganglion, the sympathetic fibres pass through without synapsing. Lacrimation may also occur in response to emotional triggers.

BONY ORBIT (Figs 41.14, 41.15, 41.16)

The upper part of the facial skeleton contains two orbital cavities. Each cavity is pyramidal, and has a base at the orbital opening and a long, posteromedially directed axis. The major structures which occupy the orbit are the eye and optic nerve; the extraocular muscles; the oculomotor, trochlear and abducent nerves; the ophthalmic and maxillary divisions of the trigeminal nerve; the ciliary parasympathetic ganglion; the ophthalmic vessels and the nasolacrimal apparatus. All of these are contained within, and supported by, a considerable quantity of orbital fat.

Each orbit has a roof, floor, medial and lateral walls, a base and apex.

Roof of the orbit (superior wall)

The roof of the orbit is formed chiefly by the thin orbital plate of the frontal bone. It is gently concave on its orbital aspect, which separates the orbital contents and the brain in the anterior cranial fossa. Antero-

medially it contains the frontal sinus and it displays a small trochlear fovea or spine where the trochlea (pulley) for superior oblique is attached. Anterolaterally there is a shallow lacrimal fossa which houses the orbital part of the lacrimal gland. The common tendinous ring of the four recti is attached to the bone near the superior, medial and lower margins of the orbital opening of the optic canal. Posteriorly, the roof of the orbit includes a part of the inferior aspect of the lesser wing of the sphenoid. The suture between these bones is almost horizontal. The optic canal lies between the roots of the lesser wing, and is bounded medially by the body of the sphenoid.

Medial wall of the orbit (Fig. 41.16)

The medial wall of the orbit is extremely thin except posteriorly. It curves inferolaterally into the floor of the orbit. The vertical lacrimal groove which houses the nasolacrimal sac lies anteriorly: it opens below into the inferior meatus of the lateral wall of the nasal cavity via the nasolacrimal canal. The floor of the groove separates the orbital and nasal cavities anteriorly, but more posteriorly the ethmoidal sinuses intervene. The medial wall is limited in front by the anterior lacrimal crest on the frontal process of the maxilla, to which orbicularis oculi and lacrimal fascia are attached. The maxillolacrimal suture lies behind the lacrimal crest in the floor of the lacrimal groove. The upper opening of the nasolacrimal groove is completed laterally by the lacrimal hamulus, which curves anteromedially to the lower part of the anterior lacrimal crest. The lacrimal part of orbicularis oculi and lacrimal fascia are attached to the posterior lacrimal crest of the lacrimal groove, which is mostly formed by the lacrimal bone, and they bridge the groove. Posteriorly the orbital surface of the lacrimal bone is flat, and it articulates by a vertical suture with the orbital plate of the ethmoid labyrinth. The frontolacrimal and lacrimal maxillary sutures limit the medial wall in front.

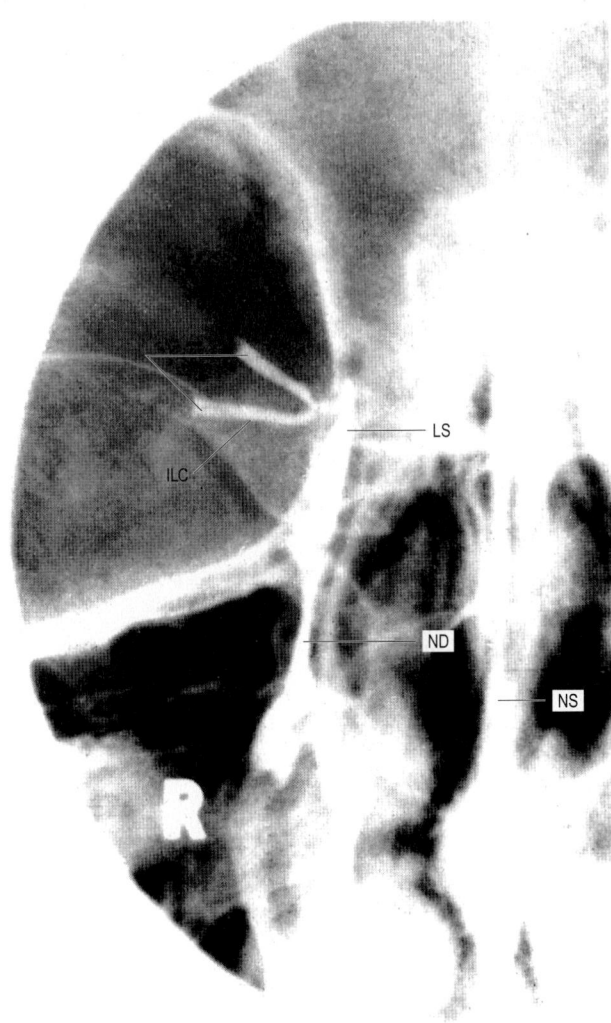

Fig. 41.11 Radiograph of the lacrimal drainage pathway, demonstrated by the injection of radio-opaque tracer into the lacrimal duct. PL, puncta lacrimalia; ILC, inferior lacrimal canaliculus; LS, lacrimal sac; ND, nasolacrimal duct; NS, nasal septum. (Provided by TD Hawkins, Addenbrooke's Hospital, Cambridge; photograph by Sarah-Jane Smith.)

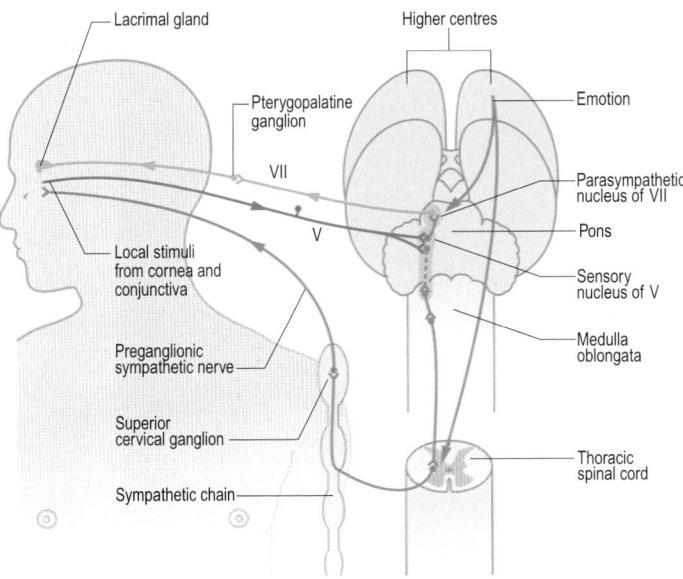

Fig. 41.13 Lacrimation reflex. (Redrawn from MacKinnon P, Morris J 1990 Oxford Textbook of Functional Anatomy, Vol 3. Head and Neck. Oxford: Oxford University Press.. By permission of Oxford University Press.)

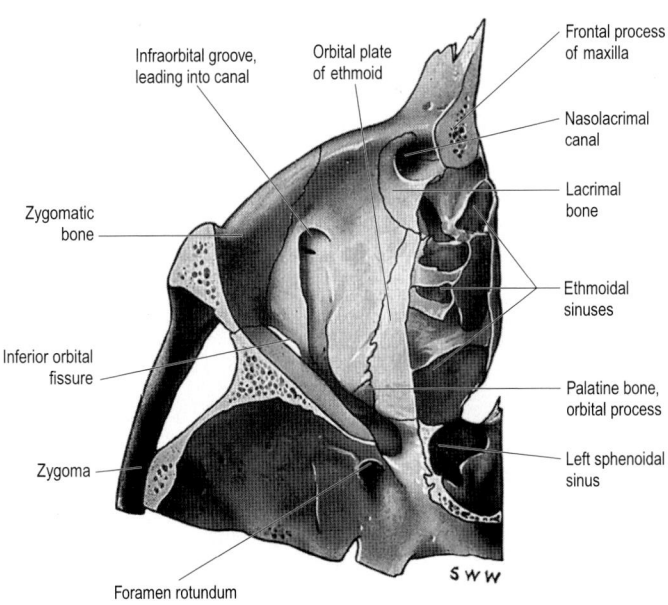

Fig. 41.14 Horizontal section through the left orbit and nasal cavity viewed from above.

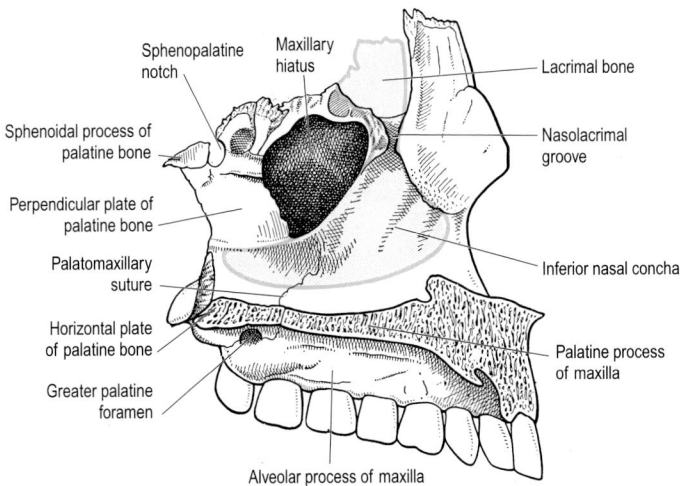

Fig. 41.12 The medial wall of the nasolacrimal canal is formed by the maxilla and the articulation of the descending process of the lacrimal bone with the lacrimal process of the inferior nasal concha.

The orbital plate of the ethmoid bone contributes most to the remainder of the medial wall. It is almost rectangular, and very thin, and forms the lateral walls of the ethmoidal sinuses. Above, it articulates with the medial edge of the orbital plate of the frontal bone at a suture which is interrupted by anterior and posterior ethmoidal foramina. The posterior foramen may be absent; occasionally there is a middle ethmoidal foramen. The anterior ethmoidal canal transmits its vessels and nerves into the anterior cranial fossa and also to the anterior nasal mucosa at the lateral edge of the cribriform plate. Below, the orbital plate of the ethmoid articulates with the medial edge of the orbital surface of the maxilla and posteriorly with the orbital process of the palatine bone. Posteriorly, it articulates with the body of the sphenoid, which forms the medial wall of the orbit posteriorly, separated from the orbital roof by the optic canal.

Floor of the orbit (inferior wall) (Figs 41.14, 41.15, 41.16)
The floor of the orbit is mostly formed by the maxilla and, antero-laterally, by the zygomatic bone. Posteromedially the small triangular orbital process of the palatine bone joins the medial wall.

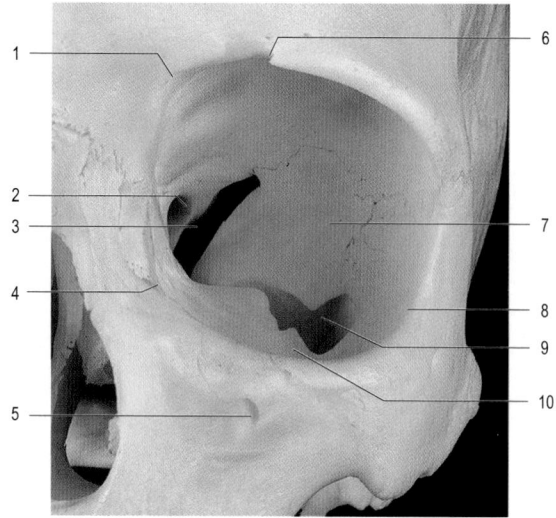

1. Frontal notch.
2. Optic canal.
3. Superior orbital fissure.
4. Opening of nasolacrimal canal.
5. Infraorbital foramen.
6. Supraorbital notch.
7. Orbital surface of greater wing of sphenoid.
8. Orbital surface of zygomatic bone.
9. Inferior orbital fissure.
10. Infraorbital groove.

Fig. 41.15 Lateral wall of left orbit. (By permission from Berkovitz BKB, Moxham BJ 1989 A Colour Atlas of the Skull. London: Mosby-Wolfe.)

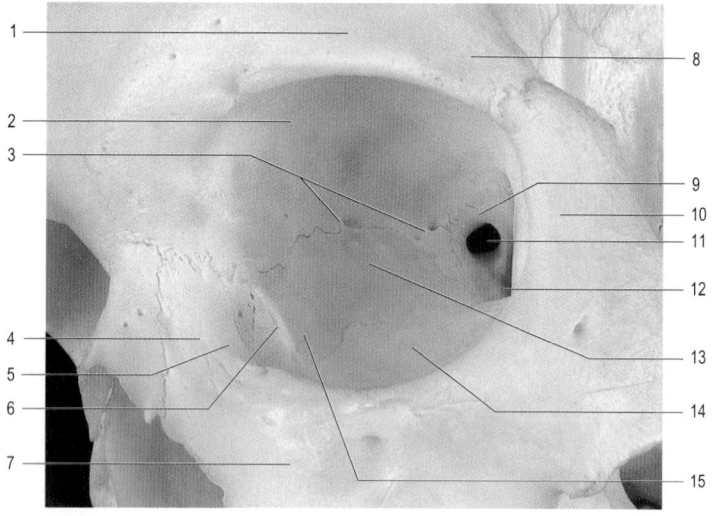

1. Frontal bone.
2. Orbital part of frontal bone.
3. Anterior and posterior ethmoidal foramina.
4. Anterior lacrimal crest of maxilla.
5. Fossa for nasolacrimal sac.
6. Posterior lacrimal crest.
7. Maxilla.
8. Zygomatic process of frontal bone.
9. Lesser wing of sphenoid.
10. Zygomatic bone.
11. Optic canal.
12. Body of sphenoid.
13. Orbital plate of ethmoid.
14. Orbital surface of maxilla.
15. Lacrimal bone.

Fig. 41.16 Medial wall of left orbit. (By permission from Berkovitz BKB, Moxham BJ 1989 A Colour Atlas of the Skull. London: Mosby-Wolfe.)

The floor is thin and largely roofs the maxillary sinus. Not quite horizontal, it ascends a little laterally. Anteriorly it curves into the lateral wall. Posteriorly it is separated from the lateral wall by the inferior orbital fissure, which connects the orbit posteriorly to the pterygopalatine fossa, and more anteriorly to the infratemporal fossa. The medial lip is notched by the infraorbital groove. The latter passes forwards and sinks into the floor to become the infraorbital canal which opens on the face at the infraorbital foramen. Infraorbital groove, canal and foramen contain the infraorbital nerve and vessels. The infraorbital foramen is sometimes double (even multiple), accessory foramina are usually smaller and recorded at incidences of 2–18% in various populations.

Lateral wall of the orbit (Fig. 41.15)

The lateral wall is formed by the orbital surface of the greater wing of the sphenoid posteriorly and by the frontal process of the zygomatic bone anteriorly. The bones meet at the sphenozygomatic suture. The zygomatic surface contains the openings of minute canals for the zygomaticofacial and zygomaticotemporal nerves, the former near the junction of the floor and lateral wall, the latter at a slightly higher level, sometimes near the suture.

The lateral wall is the thickest wall of the orbit, especially posteriorly where it separates the orbit from the middle cranial fossa. Anteriorly the lateral wall separates the orbit and the infratemporal fossa. The lateral wall and roof are continuous anteriorly but are separated posteriorly by the superior orbital fissure. This lies between the greater wing (below) and lesser wing (above) of the sphenoid, and communicates with the middle cranial fossa. It tapers laterally but widens at its medial end, its long axis descending posteromedially. Where the fissure begins to widen, its inferolateral edges shows a projection, often a spine, for the lateral attachment of the common tendinous ring. An infraorbital sulcus which runs from the superolateral end of the superior orbital fissure towards the orbital floor, has been described, sometimes associated with an anastomosis between the middle meningeal and infraorbital arteries.

Apex of the orbit

The apex of the orbit lies near the medial end of the superior orbital fissure and contains the optic canal.

ORBITAL FISSURES AND OPTIC CANAL

The superior and inferior orbital fissures and the optic canal open into the orbit and transmit important nerves and vessels.

Superior orbital fissure

The superior orbital fissure connects the cranial cavity with the orbit. It is bounded medially by the body of the sphenoid, above by the lesser wing of the sphenoid, below by the medial margin of the orbital surface of the greater wing, and laterally, between the greater and lesser wings of the sphenoid, by the frontal bone. It transmits the oculomotor, trochlear and abducens nerves, branches of the ophthalmic nerve and the ophthalmic veins.

Inferior orbital fissure (Fig. 41.14)

The inferior orbital fissure is bounded above by the greater wing of the sphenoid, below by the maxilla and the orbital process of the palatine bone, and laterally by the zygomatic bone or zygomaticomaxillary suture. The maxilla and sphenoid often meet at the anterior end of the fissure, and exclude the zygomatic bone. The inferior orbital fissure connects the orbit with the pterygopalatine and infratemporal fossae. It transmits the infraorbital and zygomatic branches of the maxillary nerve and accompanying vessels; orbital rami from the pterygopalatine ganglion; and a connection between the inferior ophthalmic vein and pterygoid venous plexus. Anteromedially, lateral to the lacrimal hamulus, a small maxillary depression may mark the attachment of inferior oblique.

Optic canal

The lesser wing of the sphenoid is connected to the body of the sphenoid by a thin, flat anterior root and a thick, triangular posterior root. The optic canal lies between these roots and connects the orbit to the middle cranial fossa. It contains the optic nerve and ophthalmic artery.

Common tendinous ring (Fig. 41.17)

Many important structures pass through the superior orbital fissure and optic foramen at the apex of the orbit. Their disposition is best understood by referring to the origin of the four recti muscles from a fibrous ring called the common tendinous ring. This ring surrounds the optic canal and encloses part of the superior orbital fissure. Since the optic nerve and ophthalmic artery enter the orbit via the optic canal, they lie within the ring. The superior and inferior divisions of the oculomotor nerve, nasociliary branch of the ophthalmic nerve, and abducens nerve also enter the orbit within the common tendinous ring, but via the superior orbital fissure. The trochlear nerve, and the frontal and lacrimal branches of the ophthalmic nerve enter the orbit through the superior orbital fissure but lie outside the common tendinous ring. Structures entering the orbit through the inferior orbital fissure obviously lie outside the common tendinous ring.

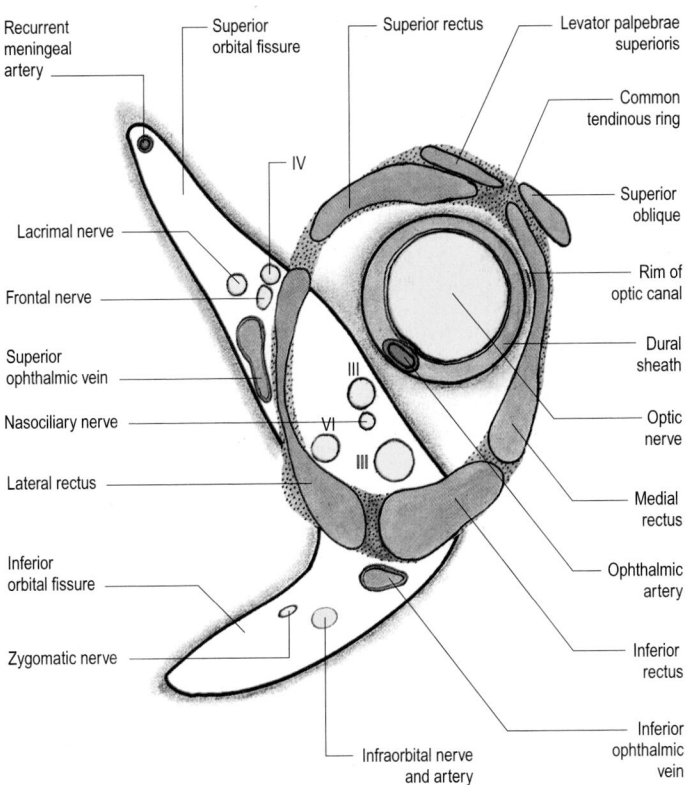

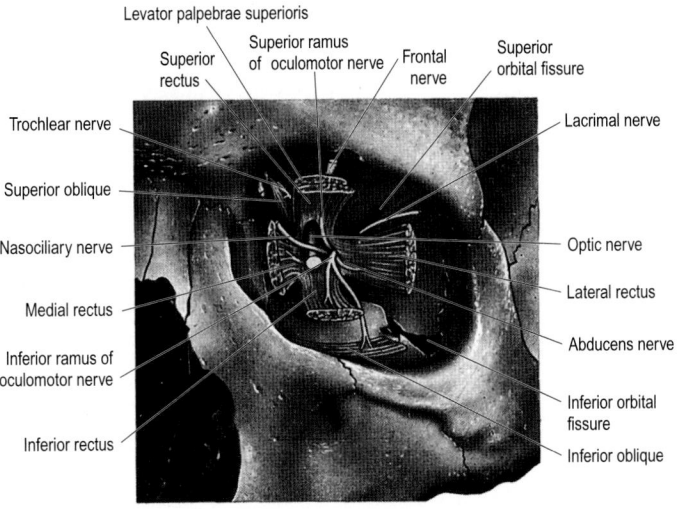

Fig. 41.17 The common tendinous ring with its muscle origins superimposed, and the relative positions of the nerves entering the orbital cavity through the superior orbital fissure and optic canal. Note that the attachments of levator palpebrae superioris and superior oblique lie external to the common tendinous ring but are attached to it. The ophthalmic veins frequently pass through the ring. The recurrent meningeal artery, a branch of the ophthalmic artery, is often conducted from the orbit to the cranial cavity through its own foramen. (Based mainly on the data of Whitnall SE 1932 Anatomy of the Human Orbit, 2nd edn. London: Oxford University Press, and Koornneef (1977). Provided by the late Gordon L Ruskell, Department of Optometry and Visual Science, The City University, London.)

Fig. 41.18 A dissection of the left orbit, viewed from in front, to show the origins of the orbital muscles and the relative positions of the nerves of the orbit.

EXTRAOCULAR MUSCLES

There are seven extraocular or extrinsic muscles associated with the eye. Levator palpebrae superioris is an elevator of the upper eyelid, while the other six, i.e. four recti (superior, inferior, medial and lateral), and two obliqui (superior and inferior), are capable of moving the eye in almost any direction.

LEVATOR PALPEBRAE SUPERIORIS (Figs 41.4, 41.8, 41.17, 41.18)

Levator palpebrae superioris is a thin, triangular muscle which arises from the inferior aspect of the lesser wing of the sphenoid, above and in front of the optic canal, and separated from it by the attachment of superior rectus. It has a short narrow tendon at its posterior attachment, and broadens gradually, then more sharply as it passes anteriorly above the eyeball. The muscle ends in front in a wide aponeurosis. Some of its tendinous fibres pass straight into the upper eyelid to attach to the anterior surface of the tarsus, while the rest radiate and pierce orbicularis oculi to pass to the skin of the upper eyelid.

The connective tissue coats of the adjoining surfaces of levator palpebrae superioris and superior rectus are fused. Where the two muscles separate to reach their anterior attachments, the fascia between them forms a thick mass to which the superior conjunctival fornix is attached: this is usually described as an additional attachment of levator palpebrae superioris. Traced laterally, the aponeurosis of the levator passes between the orbital and palpebral parts of the lacrimal gland to a tubercle (Whitnall's tubercle) on the zygomatic bone, just within the orbital margin. Traced medially, it loses its tendinous nature as it passes closely over the reflected tendon of superior oblique, and continues on to the medial palpebral ligament as loose strands of connective tissue.

Vascular supply – Levator palpebrae superioris receives its arterial supply both directly from the ophthalmic artery and indirectly from its supra-orbital branch.

Innervation – Levator palpebrae superioris is supplied by a branch of the superior division of the oculomotor nerve which enters the inferior surface of the muscle. Sympathetic fibres to the smooth muscle component of levator palpebrae superioris are derived from the plexus surrounding the internal carotid artery. These nerve fibres may join the oculomotor nerve in the cavernous sinus and pass forward in its superior branch.

Actions – Levator palpebrae superioris elevates the upper eyelid. During this process the lateral and medial parts of its aponeurosis are stretched and thus limit its action: the elevation is also said to be checked by the orbital septum. 'Check' mechanisms abound in the orbit, but there is little direct evidence that connective tissue structures thus implicated do function in this manner. Elevation of the eyelid is opposed by the palpebral part of orbicularis oculi. Levator palpebrae superioris is linked to superior rectus by a check ligament, thus there is elevation of the upper eyelid when the gaze of the eye is directed upwards.

The position of the eyelids depends on reciprocal tone in orbicularis oculi and levator palpebrae superioris, and on the degree of ocular protrusion. In the opened position the margin of the inferior eyelid usually crosses the eyeball level with the lower edge of the circumference of the iris, the upper eyelid covering about half of the width of the upper part of the iris. The eyes are closed by movements of both lids, produced by the contraction of the palpebral part of orbicularis oculi and relaxation of levator palpebrae superioris. In looking upwards, the levator contracts and the upper lid follows the ocular movement. At the same time, the eyebrows are also usually raised by the frontal parts of occipitofrontalis to diminish their overhang. The lower lid lags behind ocular movement, so that more sclera is exposed below the cornea and the lid is bulged a little by the lower part of the elevated eye. When the eye is depressed both lids move, the upper retains its normal relation to the eyeball and still covers about a quarter of the iris. The lower lid is depressed because the extension of the thickened fascia of rectus inferior and obliquus inferior pull on its tarsus as the former contracts.

The palpebral fissures are widened in states of fear or excitement by contraction of the smooth muscle of the superior and inferior tarsal muscles, as a result of increased sympathetic activity. Lesions of the sympathetic supply result in drooping of the upper eyelid (ptosis), as seen in Horner's syndrome.

THE FOUR RECTI (Figs 41.18, 41.19, 41.20)

The four recti are approximately strap-shaped; each has a thickened middle part which thins gradually to a tendon. They are attached posteriorly to a common tendinous ring around the superior, medial

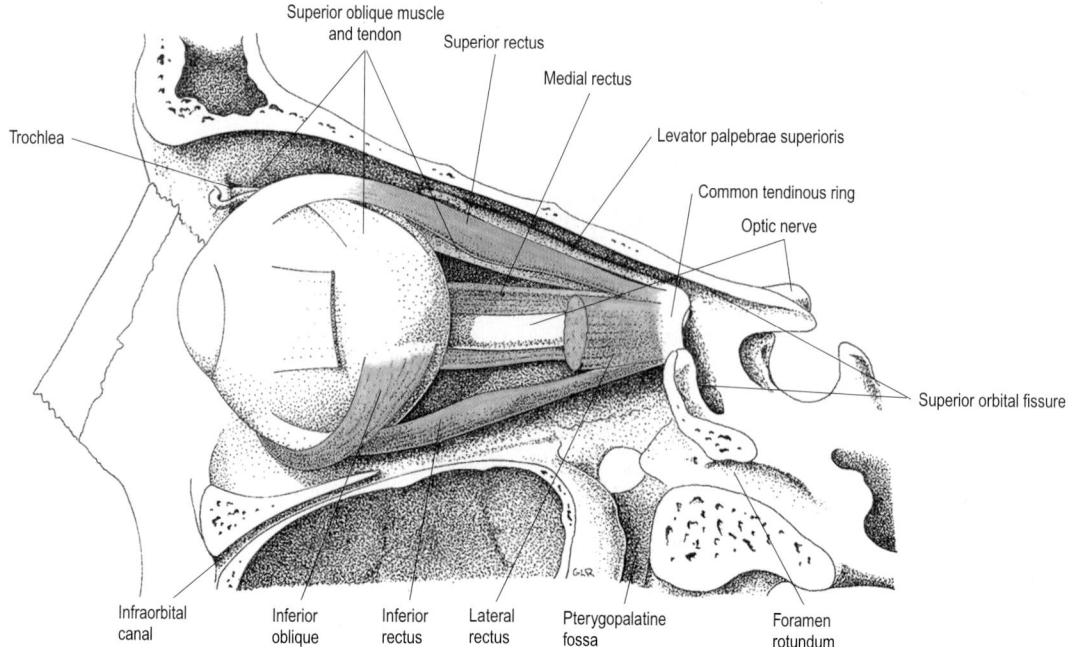

Fig. 41.19 The muscles of the left orbit, lateral view. (Provided by the late Gordon L Ruskell, Department of Optometry and Visual Science, The City University, London.)

and inferior margins of the optic canal (**Fig. 41.17**). This continues laterally across the inferior and medial parts of the superior orbital fissure and is attached to a tubercle or spine on the margin of the greater wing of the sphenoid. The tendon is closely adherent to the dural sheath of the optic nerve medially and to the surrounding periosteum. Inferior rectus, part of medial rectus and the lower fibres of lateral rectus are attached to the lower part of the ring and superior rectus, part of medial rectus and the upper fibres of lateral rectus are attached to the upper part. A second small tendinous slip of lateral rectus is attached to the orbital surface of the greater wing of the sphenoid, lateral to the common tendinous ring. The relationship of structures associated with the common tendinous ring is described on page 690.

Each rectus muscle passes forwards, in the position implied by its name, to be attached anteriorly by a tendinous expansion into the sclera, posterior to the margin of the cornea.

Superior rectus

Superior rectus is slightly larger than the other recti muscles. It arises from the upper part of the common tendinous ring, above and lateral to the optic canal. Some fibres also arise from the dural sheath of the optic nerve. The fibres pass forwards and laterally (at an angle of c.25° to the median plane of the eye in the primary position) to insert into the upper part of the sclera c.8 mm from the limbus. The insertion is slightly oblique, the medial margin more anterior than the lateral margin.

Vascular supply – Superior rectus receives its arterial supply both directly from the ophthalmic artery and indirectly from its supraorbital branch.

Innervation – Superior rectus is supplied by the superior division of the oculomotor nerve which enters the inferior surface of the muscle.

Actions – Superior rectus moves the eye so that the cornea is directed upwards (elevation) and medially (adduction). To obtain upward movement alone, the muscle must function with inferior oblique. Superior rectus also causes intorsion of the eye (i.e. medial rotation). Because a check ligament extends from the muscle to levator palpebrae superioris, elevation of the cornea also results in elevation of the upper eyelid. For more detailed discussion of its actions, see page 694.

Inferior rectus

Inferior rectus arises from the common tendinous ring, below the optic canal. It runs along the orbital floor in a similar direction to superior rectus (i.e. forwards and laterally) and inserts obliquely into the sclera below the cornea, c.6.5 mm from the limbus.

Vascular supply – Inferior rectus receives its arterial supply from the ophthalmic artery and from the infraorbital branch of the maxillary artery.

Innervation – Inferior rectus is innervated by a branch of the inferior division of the oculomotor nerve which enters the superior surface of the muscle.

Actions – The principal activity of inferior rectus is to move the eye so that the cornea is directed downwards (depression). Inferior rectus also causes the cornea to deviate medially. To obtain downward movement alone, inferior rectus must function with superior oblique. Inferior rectus is responsible for extorsion of the eye (i.e. lateral rotation). A ligament passes from the muscle to the inferior tarsal plate of the eyelid, and this causes the lower eyelid to be depressed when inferior rectus contracts. For more detailed discussion of its actions, see page 694.

Medial rectus

Medial rectus is slightly shorter than the other recti muscles, but is said to be the strongest. It arises from the medial part of the common tendinous ring, and also from the dural sheath of the optic nerve, and passes horizontally forwards along the medial wall of the orbit, below superior oblique. Medial rectus inserts into the medial surface of the sclera, c.5.5 mm from the limbus and slightly anterior to the other recti muscles.

Vascular supply – Medial rectus receives its arterial supply from the ophthalmic artery.

Innervation – Medial rectus is supplied by a branch from the inferior division of the oculomotor nerve which enters the lateral surface of the muscle.

Actions – Medial rectus moves the eye so that the cornea is directed medially (adducted). The two medial recti muscles acting together are responsible for convergence. For more detailed discussion of its actions, see page 694.

Lateral rectus

Lateral rectus arises from the lateral part of the common tendinous ring and bridges the superior orbital fissure. Some fibres also arise from a spine on the greater wing of the sphenoid. The muscle passes horizontally forward along the lateral wall of the orbit to insert into the lateral surface of the sclera, c.7 mm from the limbus.

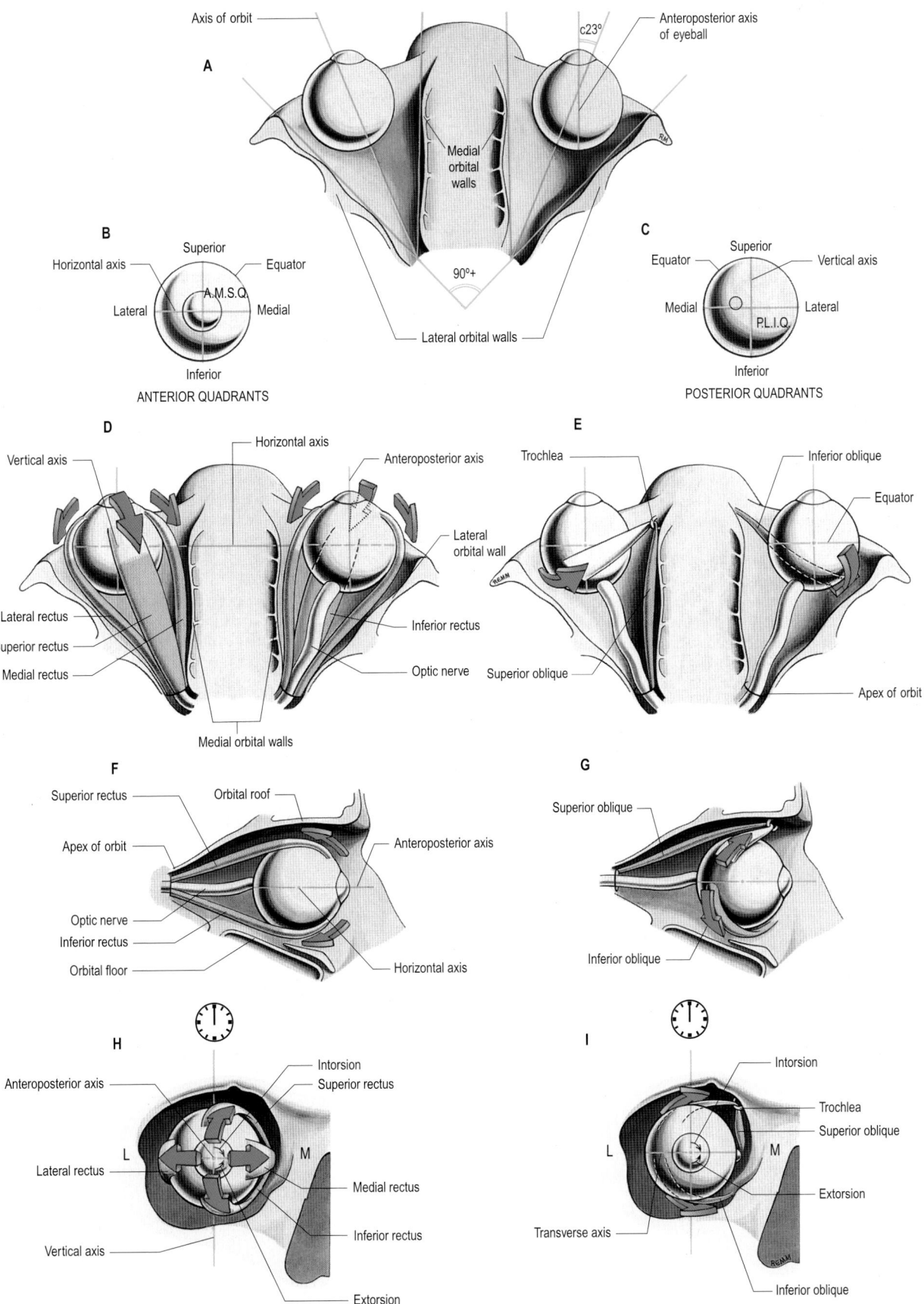

Fig. 41.20 The geometrical basis of ocular movements. **A**, The relationship between the orbital and ocular axes, with the eyes in the primary position, where the visual axes are parallel. **B** and **C**, The ocular globe in anterior and posterior views to show conventional geometry. A.M.S.Q., anterior medial superior quadrant; P.L.I.Q., posterior lateral inferior quadrant. **D**, The orbits from above showing the medial and lateral recti and the superior rectus (left) and the inferior rectus (right), indicating turning moments primarily around the vertical axis. **E**, Superior (left) and inferior (right) oblique muscles showing turning moments primarily around the vertical and also anteroposterior axes. **F**, Lateral view to show the actions of the superior and inferior recti around the horizontal axis. **G**, Lateral view to show the action of the superior and inferior oblique muscles around the anteroposterior axis. **H**, Anterior view to show the medial rotational movement of the superior and inferior recti around the vertical axis. Conventionally the 12 o'clock position indicated is said to be intorted (superior rectus) or extorted (inferior rectus) as indicated by the small arrows on the cornea. **I**, Anterior view to show the torsional effects of the superior oblique (intorsion) and inferior oblique (extorsion) around the anteroposterior axis, as indicated by the small arrows on the cornea.

Vascular supply – Lateral rectus receives its arterial supply from the ophthalmic artery directly and/or from its lacrimal branch.

Innervation – Lateral rectus receives its nerve supply from the abducens nerve by branches which enter the medial surface of the muscle.

Actions – Lateral rectus moves the eye so that the cornea is directed laterally (abducted). For more detailed discussion of its actions, see page 694.

SUPERIOR OBLIQUE (Figs 41.6, 41.8, 41.17, 41.18, 41.19)
Superior oblique is a fusiform muscle which arises from the body of the sphenoid superomedial to the optic canal and the tendinous attachment of the superior rectus. It passes forwards to end in a round tendon which plays through a fibrocartilaginous loop, the trochlea, attached to the trochlear fossa of the frontal bone. Tendon and trochlea are separated by a delicate synovial sheath. Having passed through the trochlea, the tendon descends posterolaterally and inferior to superior rectus, and is attached to the sclera in the superolateral part of the posterior quadrant behind the equator, between the superior and lateral recti.

Vascular supply – Superior oblique receives its arterial supply directly from the ophthalmic artery and indirectly from its supraorbital branch.

Innervation – Superior oblique is supplied by the trochlear nerve which enters the superior surface of the muscle.

Actions – Because of its insertion into the posterior part of the eyeball, contraction of superior oblique elevates the back of the eye, which results in depression of the cornea (particularly with the eye in the adducted position). Superior oblique moves the eye laterally and also causes intorsion. For more detailed discussion of its actions, see page 694.

INFERIOR OBLIQUE (Figs 41.6, 41.18, 41.19)
Inferior oblique is a thin, narrow muscle near the anterior margin of the floor of the orbit. It arises from the orbital surface of the maxilla lateral to the nasolacrimal groove and ascends posterolaterally, at first between inferior rectus and the orbital floor, and then between the eyeball and lateral rectus. It is inserted into the lateral part of the sclera behind the equator of the eyeball, in the inferolateral part of the posterior quadrant between the inferior and lateral recti, near to, but slightly posterior to, the attachment of superior oblique. The muscle broadens and thins, and, in contrast to the other extraocular muscles, it has a barely discernible tendon at its scleral attachment.

Vascular supply – Inferior oblique receives its arterial supply from the ophthalmic artery and from the infraorbital branch of the maxillary artery.

Innervation – Inferior oblique is innervated by a branch of the inferior division of the oculomotor nerve which enters the orbital surface of the muscle.

Actions – Because of its insertion into the posterior part of the eye, contraction of inferior oblique depresses the back of the eye, which results in elevation of the cornea (particularly in the adducted position). The muscle moves the eye laterally and also causes extorsion. For more detailed discussion of its actions, see page 694.

MINOR MUSCLES OF THE EYELIDS
Several smooth muscles are associated with the orbit, although they are not directly attached to the eyeball. Orbitalis, the orbital muscle of Müller, lies at the back of the orbit and spans the infraorbital fissure. Its functions are uncertain, but its contraction may possibly produce a slight forward protrusion of the eyeball. The superior and inferior tarsal muscles are small muscle laminae inserted into the upper and lower eyelids. They are described in more detail with the tarsal plates (p. 683).

Since they are composed of smooth muscles, all three minor muscles receive a sympathetic innervation from the superior cervical ganglion via the internal carotid plexus. They are affected by dysfunction of the sympathetic innervation, e.g. in Horner's syndrome, which means that the upper eyelid droops (ptosis).

MOVEMENTS OF THE EYES
Ocular movements are frequently accompanied by movements of the head, which can be likened to the coarse adjustment of an optical instrument, whereas the finer adjustments are made by the ocular musculature.

Actions of extraocular muscles (Figs 41.20, 41.21)
Levator palpebrae superioris elevates the upper lid, and its antagonist is the palpebral part of orbicularis oculi. The degree of elevation of the lid, which, apart from blinking, is maintained for long periods during waking hours, is a compromise between ensuring an adequate exposure of the optical media and controlling the amount of incident light. In very bright sunshine, the latter can be reduced by lowering the upper lid, and so limiting glare. Electrically, the levator discharges steadily for a given fixation, but with increasing rates with upward lid position, and relaxes during closure of the palpebral fissure. The role of the superior tarsal muscle is less clear. Its tonus is related to sympathetic nerve activity, since ptosis is a consequence of impairment of the sympathetic nerve supply to the head.

The six extraocular muscles all rotate the eyeball in directions dependent upon the geometrical relation between their osseous and global attachments (**Fig. 41.20A,D,E**): these are altered by the ocular movements themselves. For convenience each muscle is considered in isolation. However, it is essential to appreciate that any movement of an eyeball alters the tension and/or length in all six muscles. Because they form more obvious groupings as antagonists or synergists, it is useful to consider the four recti and two obliques as separate groups, remembering always that they act in concert. It has been suggested that the extrinsic ocular muscles collectively position the eyeball in the orbital cavity and prevent anteroposterior movements of the eyeball, other than a slight retraction during blinks, because the recti exert a posterior traction while the obliques pull the eyeball to some degree anteriorly. They may be assisted by various 'check ligaments' (p. 684). A simplified description of the actions of the extraocular muscles is summarized in **Fig. 41.21**.

Of the four recti, the medial and lateral exert comparatively straightforward forces on the eyeball. Being approximately horizontal, when the visual axis is in its primary position, directed to the horizon, they rotate the eye medially (adduction) or laterally (abduction) about an imaginary vertical axis (**Fig. 41.20D**). They are antagonists. The visual axis can be swept through a horizontal arc by reciprocal adjustment of their lengths. When, as is usual, both eyes are involved, the four medial

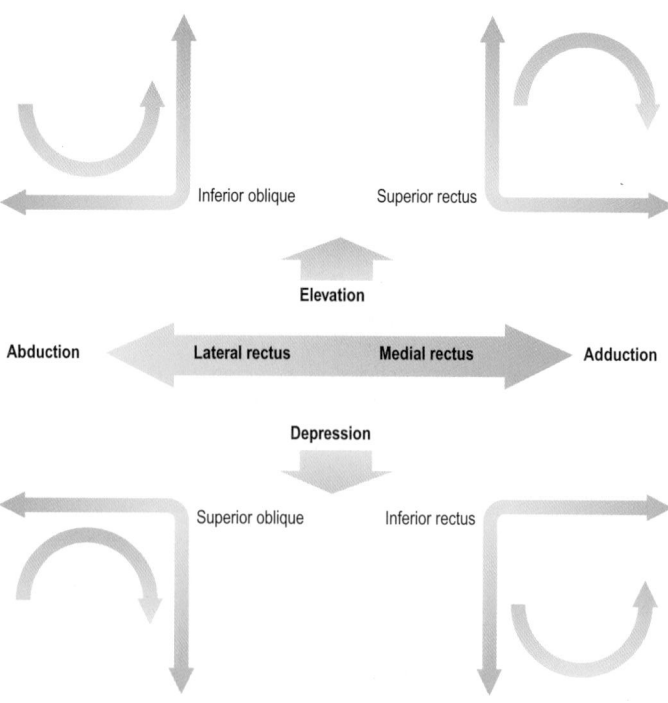

Fig. 41.21 Simplified summary of the actions of the extraocular muscles.

and lateral recti can either adjust both visual axes in a conjugate movement from point to point at infinity, their axes remaining parallel, or they can converge or diverge the axes to or from nearer or more distant objects of attention in the visual field.

The medial and lateral recti do not rotate the eye around its transverse axis and so cannot elevate or depress the visual axes as gaze is transferred from nearer to more distant objects or the reverse. This movement requires the superior and inferior recti (aided by the two oblique muscles). It must be remembered that the orbital axis does not correspond with the visual axis in its primary position but diverges from it at an angle of c.23° (the value varies between individuals, and depends on the angle between the orbital axes and the median plane) (Fig. 41.20A). Thus the simple rotation caused by an isolated superior rectus, analysed with reference to the three hypothetical ocular axes, appears more complex, being primarily elevation (transverse axis), and secondarily a less powerful medial rotation (vertical axis) and slight intorsion (anteroposterior axis) in which the midpoint of the upper rim of the cornea (often referred to as '12 o'clock') is rotated medially towards the nose. These actions, compounded as a single, simple rotation, are easily appreciated when it is seen that the direction of traction of superior rectus runs in a posteromedial direction from its attachment in front, which is anterior to the equator and superior to the cornea, to its osseous attachment near the orbital apex (Fig. 41.20D,H).

Inferior rectus pulls in a similar direction to superior rectus, but rotates the visual axis downwards about the transverse axis. It rotates the eye medially on a vertical axis but its action around the anteroposterior axis extorts the eye, i.e. rotates it so that the corneal '12 o'clock' point turns laterally. The combined, equal contractions of the superior and inferior recti therefore rotate the eyeball medially, since their effects around the transverse and anteroposterior axes are opposed. In binocular movements they assist the medial recti in converging the visual axes, and by reciprocal adjustment they can elevate or depress the visual axes. As the eyeball is rotated laterally, the lines of traction of the superior and inferior recti approach the plane of the anteroposterior ocular axis (Fig. 41.20H), and so their rotational effects about this and the vertical ocular axis diminish. In abduction to c.23°, they become almost purely an elevator and depressor respectively of the visual axis.

Superior oblique acts on the eye from the trochlea, and, since the attachment of inferior oblique is for practical purposes vertically below this, both muscles approach the eyeball at the same angle, being attached in approximately similar positions in the superior and inferior posterolateral ocular quadrants (Fig. 41.20I). Superior oblique elevates the posterior aspect of the eyeball, and inferior oblique depresses it, which means that the former rotates the visual axis downwards and the latter rotates it upwards, and both movements occur around the transverse axis. When the eye is in the primary position, the obliquity of both muscles means that they pull in a direction posterior to the vertical axis and both therefore rotate the eye laterally around this axis. With regard to the anteroposterior axis, in isolation, superior oblique intorts the eye and inferior oblique extorts it. Like the superior and inferior recti, therefore, the two obliques have a common turning movement around the vertical axis but they are opposed forces in respect of the other two. Acting in concert they could therefore assist the lateral rectus in abducting the visual axis, as in divergence of the eyes in transferring attention from near to far. Again, like the superior and inferior recti, the directions of traction of the oblique muscles also vary with ocular position, such that they become more nearly a pure elevator and a depressor as the eye is adducted.

Ocular rotations are for the most part under voluntary control, whereas torsional movements cannot be voluntarily initiated. When the head is tilted in a frontal plane, reflex torsions occur. Any small lapse in the concerted adjustment of both eyes produces diplopia.

Movements that shift or stabilize gaze

The role of eye movements is to bring the image of objects of visual interest onto the fovea of the retina and to hold the image steady in order to achieve and maintain the highest level of visual acuity. Several types of eye movement are required to ensure that these conditions are met. Moreover, the movements of both eyes must be near perfectly matched to achieve the benefits of binocularity. Both volitional and reflexive movements are involved and may be so classified. Alternatively, they may be grouped into those movements that shift gaze as visual interest changes, and those that stabilize gaze by maintaining a steady image on the retina. They have distinct characteristics, and are

generated by different neural mechanisms in response to different stimuli, but share a common final motor pathway. Movements that shift gaze are of three types, saccades, vergence, and vestibular-generated rapid changes in fixation.

In so-called 'fixation' of a focus of attention, whether uniocular or binocular, the visual axis is not 'fixed' in a perfectly steady manner but undergoes minute, but observable flicking (of a few minutes or even seconds of arc) across the true line of fixation. These microsaccades are rapid and surprisingly complex. When interest changes to another feature of the visual scene, the eyes execute a fast or saccadic movement to take up fixation. If the required rotation is small the saccade is accurate, whereas small supplementary corrective saccades are needed if the shift is substantial. In addition to visually evoked saccades, they may occur in response to other extroreceptive stimuli, e.g. auditory, tactile, or centrally evoked. They may be volitional or reflex. As an example of the latter, in reading a line of print the eyes make three or four jerky saccades rather than following the line smoothly: the line is usefully imaged only when the eye is stationary, consequently little of the line is seen by the centre of the fovea. The term saccade, a French word of obscure origin meaning a 'jerk on the reins', was introduced by Dodge in 1903 for the swings of fixation observed in subjects reading a line of print. In general, reaction times and movements are measured in microseconds; amplitude varies from seconds of arc to many degrees, with an accuracy of 0.2° or better, and the velocity of a large saccade may reach 500° per second. The speed of saccades is assured by an initial contraction of the appropriate muscles which is slightly excessive. The necessary deceleration when the target is fixated is apparently largely dependent on the viscoelasticity of the extraocular muscles and orbital soft tissues, and not on antagonistic muscular activity.

Vergence is a relatively slow movement permitting maintenance of single binocular vision of close objects. The eyes converge towards the midline between the two eyes to achieve imagery of the object on both foveas. The view of the object at the two eyes is not quite the same and the disparity is used to assess depth. Additionally the pupils constrict and the eyes accommodate to achieve sharp focused images. These three activities constitute the near reflex.

The vestibular apparatus induces a variety of reflex eye movements to compensate for the potentially disruptive effects on vision caused by head and body movement. Receptors of the semicircular canals respond to active or passive rotational (angular) accelerations of the head. When the body makes substantial rotational movements a vestibulo-ocular reflex generates a cycle of responses involving both the shifting and stabilizing of gaze. Body rotation is matched by counter-rotation of the eyes so that gaze direction is unaltered and clear vision is maintained. Physical constraint limits the rotation to 30° or less and is followed by a rapid saccadic movement of the eyes, a physiological nystagmus, to another object in the visual scene and the cycle is repeated. Consequently vision is clear throughout most of the cycle while the image is stationary, but at the cost of no useful vision during the brief periods of the saccades. The reflex is efficient and rapid. Such speed could not be generated by the visual system which is slow relative to the short latency of vestibular receptors.

Other vestibular generated reflexes, which induce compensatory eye movements to stabilize gaze, are activated during brief head movements. When the head is sharply rotated in any direction, the eyeball rotates by an equal amount in the opposite direction as a consequence of the stimulation of semicircular canal cristae (angular acceleration), and gaze is undisturbed. Brief rotational movements are commonly combined with translational (linear acceleration) movements monitored by otolith organs. For example, a linear displacement occurs in walking as the head bobs vertically with each stride, and a rotational displacement occurs as the head rolls, invoking otolith and canal responses respectively to stabilize the retinal image. Head perturbations induced by the vibrations of, for example, an idling bus engine, may generate a vertical linear displacement alone. Vestibular disease incurring the loss of the rapid, fine compensatory eye movements in locomotion destabilizes the retinal image, blurs vision and may render locomotion intolerable.

The otoliths also respond to the pull of gravity, generating static vestibulo-ocular reflexes associated with head tilt. When static otolith orientation is changed, e.g. when the head is tilted upwards or downwards, the eyes counter-rotate to maintain fixation of the horizontal meridian. Lateral tilt towards a shoulder generates a torsional counter-rotation of the eyes, a movement which cannot be made voluntarily.

The torsional tilt reflex, equal and opposite in direction by the two eyes, is fully compensatory over 40° or so in afoveate animals, but in man it is vestigial: it is fractionally compensatory and varies in extent between individuals. Because the foveal image is unaffected by torsional movements, the subject is unaware of any visual penalty.

Pursuit eye movements are used to track a moving object of visual interest, maintaining the image approximately on the fovea. They are usually preceded by a saccade to capture the image but, unlike saccades, they are slow and motivated by vision. If the angular shift required to track the moving object is large or is moving swiftly, the initial saccade is frequently inaccurate and one or more small corrective saccades are made before tracking begins. Because the stimulus is visual, the pursuit system response is subject to a relatively long latency (c.100 msec): the limitation in performance this imposes may be offset by a predictive capacity when object movement follows a regular pattern, and the eye movements adjust in anticipation to speed and direction.

The optokinetic response is another visually mediated reflex which stabilizes retinal imagery during rotational movement. As the visual scene changes the eyes follow, holding the retinal image steady until the eyes shift rapidly in the opposite direction to another area of the visual scene. The full field of vision, rather than small objects within it, is the stimulus, and the alternating slow and fast phases of movement generated describes optokinetic nystagmus. This reflex functions in collaboration with the rotational vestibulo-ocular reflex. In sustained rotations of the body, the vestibulo-ocular reflex fades because of the mechanical arrangements of the semicircular canals. In darkness the reflex, which is initially compensatory, loses velocity, and after c.45 seconds the eyeballs become stationary. With a visual input, the reflex is sustained by the optokinetic response. Because the reflex is already initiated, the relative delay of visual input is overcome. The integration of the two systems is served by an accessory optic system projection to the vestibular nuclei via the inferior olive and cerebellum. The usual method of evoking optokinetic nystagmus in the laboratory or clinic is to present a horizontally moving pattern of vertical black-on-white stripes while the head of the subject is held stationary.

Saccadic activity is almost ever-present in human vision. Thus both visual axes are endlessly and rapidly transferred to new points of interest in any part of the total visual field. Binocular gaze is very frequently made to travel routes of the most variable complexity in examining objects of some extent in the field, and both visual axes must be maintained with sufficient accuracy to avoid diplopia. Binocular movements involving convergence are markedly slower than conjugate movements, which presumably reflects the greater complexity of neural control that these movements require (and the speed of contraction of ciliaris must be a factor). Most human visual activity concerns targets of regard near enough to demand convergence and hence a neuronal intermediation of greater flexibility. Since the prime purpose is the clear perception of a 'target', it is not surprising that the visual input is itself utilized in continuous feedback to achieve the correct aiming of visual axes.

Continual movements of the eyeball appear to be essential for vision to occur. Retinal and more central neural networks appear to be designed primarily to detect transient events such as movements rather than static, maintained stimuli. Indeed, images which are essentially static, such as those due to retinal blood vessels, are not detectable unless the shadows they cast on photoreceptors are made to move, e.g. by shifting narrow-angle illumination with an ophthalmoscope.

The central control of conjugate gaze is discussed in Section 2.

VASCULAR SUPPLY AND LYMPHATIC DRAINAGE

ARTERIES WITHIN THE ORBIT

The main vessel supplying orbital structures is the ophthalmic artery. Its terminal branches anastomose on the face and scalp with those of the facial, maxillary and superficial temporal arteries, thereby establishing connections between the external and internal carotid arteries. In addition to the ophthalmic artery, the infraorbital branch of the maxillary artery, and possibly the recurrent meningeal artery, supply orbital structures.

Ophthalmic artery (Fig. 41.22)

The ophthalmic artery leaves the internal carotid artery as it quits the cavernous sinus medial to the anterior clinoid process. It enters the orbit

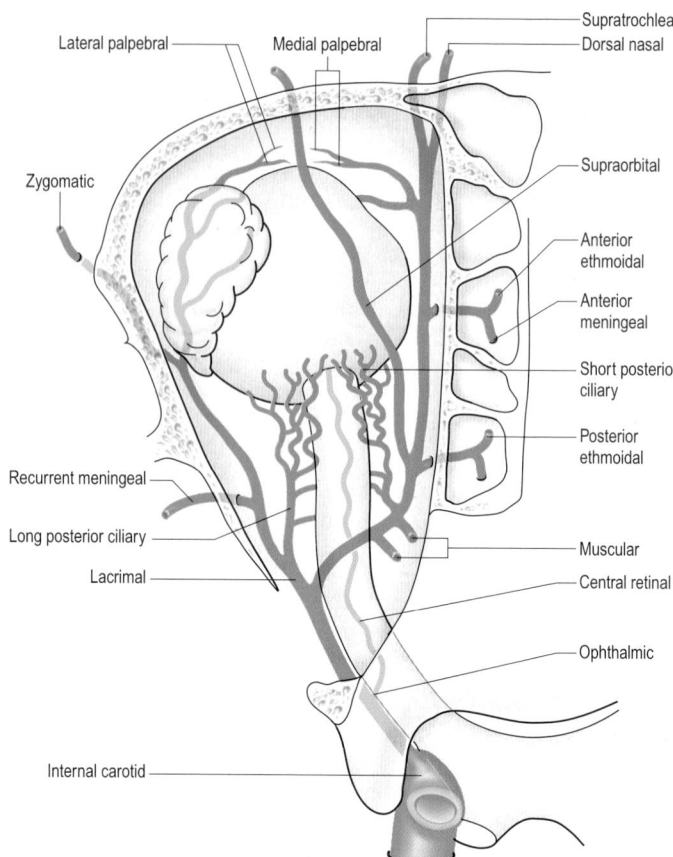

Fig. 41.22 Distribution of the branches of the ophthalmic artery viewed from above. The artery has several anastomoses with branches of the external carotid artery, e.g. the middle meningeal with the recurrent meningeal, the facial (angular) with the frontal or dorsal nasal, the superficial temporal with the supraorbital (inconstant). (By permission from MacKinnon P, Morris J 1990 Oxford Textbook of Functional Anatomy, Vol 3. Head and Neck. Oxford: Oxford University Press. By permission of Oxford University Press.)

by the optic canal, inferolateral to the optic nerve. For a short distance it is then lateral to the optic nerve and medial to the oculomotor and abducens nerves, the ciliary ganglion and lateral rectus. It crosses between the optic nerve and superior rectus to reach the medial wall of the orbit, running between superior oblique and medial rectus. At the medial end of the upper eyelid, it divides into supratrochlear and dorsal nasal branches. As it crosses the optic nerve with the nasociliary nerve, it is separated from the frontal nerve by superior rectus and levator palpebrae superioris. Its terminal branch accompanies the infratrochlear nerve. In c.15% of subjects the ophthalmic artery crosses below the optic nerve. It has the following branches: central artery of the retina, lacrimal artery, muscular branches, ciliary arteries, supraorbital artery, posterior ethmoidal artery, anterior ethmoidal artery, meningeal branch, medial palpebral arteries, supratrochlear artery, dorsal nasal artery. Many of the branches of the ophthalmic artery accompany sensory nerves of the same name and have a similar distribution.

Central artery of the retina

The small central artery of the retina is the first branch. It begins below the optic nerve and for a short distance it lies in the dural sheath of the nerve. It enters the inferomedial surface of the nerve c.1.25 cm behind the eye, and runs to the retina along its axis. Its further distribution is described on page 716.

Muscular branches

Muscular branches frequently spring from a common trunk to form superior and inferior groups, most of which accompany branches of the oculomotor nerve. The inferior, more constant, contains most of the anterior ciliary arteries. Other muscular vessels branch from the lacrimal and supraorbital arteries or from the trunk of the ophthalmic artery.

Ciliary arteries

There are three groups of ciliary arteries: long and short posterior, and anterior. Long posterior ciliary arteries, usually two, pierce the sclera near the optic nerve, pass anteriorly along the horizontal meridian and join the greater arterial circle in the iris. About seven short posterior ciliary arteries pass close to the optic nerve to reach the eyeball where they divide into 15–20 branches. They pierce the sclera around the optic nerve to supply the choroid, and anastomose with twigs of the central retinal artery at the optic disc. Anterior ciliary arteries arise from muscular branches of the ophthalmic artery. They reach the eyeball on the tendons of the recti, form a circumcorneal subconjunctival vascular zone, and pierce the sclera near the sclerocorneal junction to end in the greater arterial circle of the iris.

Lacrimal artery

The lacrimal artery is a large branch which usually leaves the ophthalmic artery near its exit from the optic canal, although it occasionally arises before the ophthalmic artery enters the orbit. It accompanies the lacrimal nerve along the upper border of lateral rectus, supplies and traverses the lacrimal gland, and ends in the eyelids and conjunctiva as the lateral palpebral arteries. The latter run medially in the upper and lower lids and anastomose with the medial palpebral arteries. The lacrimal artery gives off one or two zygomatic branches. One reaches the temporal fossa via the zygomaticotemporal foramen, and anastomoses with the deep temporal arteries. The other reaches the cheek by the zygomaticofacial foramen, and anastomoses with transverse facial and zygomatico-orbital arteries. A recurrent meningeal branch, usually small, passes back via the lateral part of the superior orbital fissure to anastomose with a middle meningeal branch: it is sometimes large, replacing the lacrimal artery, and becomes a greater contributor to the orbital blood supply.

Supraorbital artery

The supraorbital artery leaves the ophthalmic artery where it crosses the optic nerve, ascends medial to superior rectus and levator palpebrae superioris, meets the supraorbital nerve and runs with it between the periosteum and levator palpebrae superioris to the supraorbital foramen (or notch). It passes through the foramen and divides into superficial and deep branches which supply the skin, muscles and frontal periosteum, and anastomose with the supratrochlear artery, and the frontal branch of the superficial temporal artery and its contralateral fellow. It supplies superior rectus and levator palpebrae superioris, and sends a branch across the trochlea to the medial canthus. At the supraorbital margin it often sends a branch to the diploe of the frontal bone and may also supply the mucoperiosteum in the frontal sinus.

Posterior ethmoidal artery

The posterior ethmoidal artery runs through the posterior ethmoidal canal and supplies the posterior ethmoidal air sinuses. It enters the cranium, sends a meningeal branch to the dura mater and nasal branches which descend into the nasal cavity via the cribriform plate, and anastomoses with branches of the sphenopalatine artery.

Anterior ethmoidal artery

The anterior ethmoidal artery passes with its accompanying nerve through the anterior ethmoidal canal to supply ethmoidal and frontal air sinuses. Entering the cranium, it gives off a meningeal branch to the dura mater and nasal branches which descend into the nasal cavity with the anterior ethmoidal nerve. It runs in a groove on the deep surface of the nasal bone to supply the lateral nasal wall and septum. A terminal branch appears on the nose between the nasal bone and the upper nasal cartilage.

Meningeal branch

A meningeal branch, usually small, passes back through the superior orbital fissure to the middle cranial fossa, and anastomoses with the middle and accessory meningeal arteries. It is sometimes large when it becomes a major contributor to the orbital blood supply.

Medial palpebral arteries

The medial palpebral arteries are described on page 510.

Supratrochlear artery

The supratrochlear artery is a terminal branch of the ophthalmic artery. It leaves the orbit superomedially with the supratrochlear nerve, ascends

on the forehead to supply the skin, muscles and pericranium, and anastomoses with the supraorbital artery and with its contralateral fellow.

Dorsal nasal artery

The dorsal nasal artery is the other terminal branch of the ophthalmic artery, and emerges from the orbit between the trochlea and medial palpebral ligament. It gives a branch to the upper part of the nasolacrimal sac and then divides into two branches. One branch joins the terminal part of the facial artery, and the other runs along the dorsum of the nose, supplies its outer surface and anastomoses with its contralateral fellow and the lateral nasal branch of the facial artery.

Infraorbital branch of the maxillary artery

The infraorbital branch of the maxillary artery enters the orbit through the posterior part of the inferior orbital fissure. It passes along the infra-orbital groove of the maxilla in the floor of the orbit before entering the infraorbital canal, and comes out onto the face through the infraorbital foramen. Whilst in the infraorbital groove, it gives off branches which supply inferior rectus and inferior oblique, the nasolacrimal sac and, inconstantly, the lacrimal gland.

VEINS WITHIN THE ORBIT

The veins draining the orbit are the superior and inferior ophthalmic veins and the infraorbital vein. The veins of the eyeball mainly drain into the vortex veins.

Superior and inferior ophthalmic veins (Figs 41.7, 41.17, 41.23)

The superior and inferior ophthalmic veins link the facial and intra-cranial veins. They are devoid of valves. The superior ophthalmic vein forms posteromedial to the upper eyelid from two tributaries which connect anteriorly with the facial and supraorbital veins. It runs with the ophthalmic artery, lying between the optic nerve and superior rectus, and receives the corresponding tributaries, the two superior vortex veins of the eyeball, and the central vein of the retina. The central vein of the retina sometimes drains directly into the cavernous sinus, although it still gives a communicating branch to the superior ophthalmic vein. The superior ophthalmic vein may also receive the inferior ophthalmic vein. It traverses the superior orbital fissure usually above the common tendinous ring of the recti muscles and ends in the cavernous sinus.

The inferior ophthalmic vein begins in a network near the anterior region of the orbital floor and medial wall. It runs backwards on inferior rectus and across the inferior orbital fissure, and then either joins the superior ophthalmic vein or passes through the superior orbital fissure – within or below the common tendinous ring of the recti muscles – to drain directly into the cavernous sinus. The inferior ophthalmic vein receives tributaries from inferior rectus and inferior oblique, the nasolacrimal sac and the eyelids. It also receives the two inferior vortex veins of the eyeball. The inferior ophthalmic vein communicates with

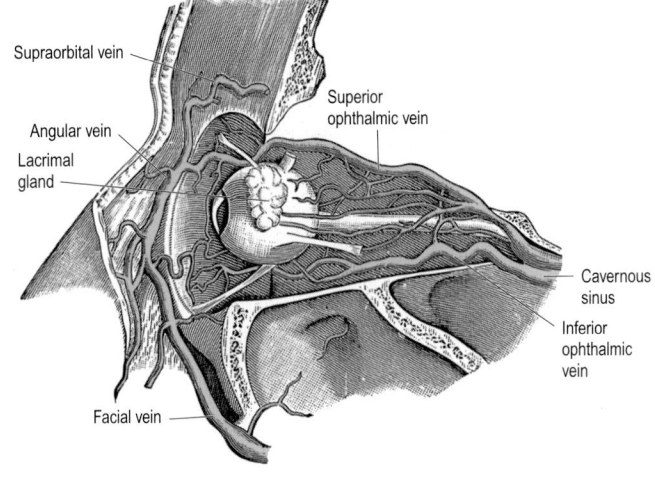

Fig. 41.23 The veins of the left orbit: lateral aspect. Note that the eyeball is shown at c.50% of real size, relative to the orbit, to reveal the veins.

the pterygoid venous plexus by a branch which passes through the inferior orbital fissure. It may also communicate with the facial vein across the inferior margin of the orbit.

The infraorbital vein

The infraorbital vein runs with the infraorbital nerve and artery in the floor of the orbit, and passes backwards through the inferior orbital fissure into the pterygoid venous plexus. It drains structures in the floor of the orbit and communicates with the inferior ophthalmic vein. The infraorbital vein may communicate with the facial vein on the face.

Central retinal vein

The central retinal vein first traverses the optic nerve, and receives branches which drain the optic nerve, including a central vein which drains forwards. It then leaves the nerve to pursue a short course in the subarachnoid space before entering the cavernous sinus or the superior ophthalmic vein.

LYMPHATIC DRAINAGE

Lymphatic vessels other than those draining the conjunctiva have not been identified.

INNERVATION

Somatic and autonomic motor and somatic sensory nerves are found in the orbit. The motor nerves are the oculomotor, trochlear and abducens nerves, and they supply the extraocular muscles. Parasympathetic fibres from the oculomotor nerve (via the ciliary ganglion) supply sphincter pupillae and ciliaris, and from the facial nerve (via the pterygopalatine ganglion) supply the lacrimal gland and choroid. Sympathetic fibres supply dilator pupillae. Both sympathetic and parasympathetic nerves supply the arteries. The sensory nerves within the orbit are the optic, ophthalmic and maxillary nerves, although the maxillary nerve and most ophthalmic branches only pass through the orbit to supply the face and jaws.

OCULOMOTOR NERVE (Figs 41.17, 41.18, 41.24)

The oculomotor nerve is the third cranial nerve. It is the main source of innervation to the extraocular muscles and also contains parasympathetic fibres which relay in the ciliary ganglion.

The oculomotor nerve emerges at the midbrain, on the medial side of the crus of the cerebral peduncle. It passes along the lateral dural wall

of the cavernous sinus where it divides into superior and inferior divisions which run beneath the trochlear and ophthalmic nerves. The two divisions of the oculomotor nerve enter the orbit through the superior orbital fissure, within the common tendinous ring of the recti muscles, separated by the nasociliary branch of the ophthalmic nerve.

The superior division of the oculomotor nerve passes above the optic nerve to enter the inferior (ocular) surface of superior rectus. It supplies this muscle and gives off a branch which runs to supply levator palpebrae superioris. The inferior division of the oculomotor nerve divides into three branches, medial, central and lateral. The medial branch passes beneath the optic nerve to enter the lateral (ocular) surface of medial rectus. The central branch runs downwards and forwards to enter the superior (ocular) surface of inferior rectus. The lateral branch travels forwards on the lateral side of inferior rectus to enter the orbital surface of inferior oblique. The lateral branch also communicates with the ciliary ganglion to distribute parasympathetic fibres to sphincter pupillae and ciliaris.

TROCHLEAR NERVE (Fig. 41.24)

The trochlear nerve is the fourth cranial nerve and is the only cranial nerve which emerges from the dorsal surface of the brain. It passes from the midbrain onto the lateral surface of the crus of the cerebral peduncle and runs through the lateral dural wall of the cavernous sinus. It then crosses the oculomotor nerve and enters the orbit through the superior orbital fissure, above the common tendinous ring of the recti muscles and levator palpebrae superioris, and medial to the frontal and lacrimal nerves. The trochlear nerve travels but a short distance to enter the superior (orbital) surface of superior oblique, which is its sole target.

ABDUCENS NERVE (Figs 41.24, 41.25)

The abducens nerve is the sixth cranial nerve, and emerges from the brain stem between the pons and the medulla oblongata. It is related to the cavernous sinus, but unlike the oculomotor, trochlear, ophthalmic and maxillary nerves, which merely invaginate the lateral dural wall, it passes through the sinus itself, lying lateral to the internal carotid artery. The abducens nerve enters the orbit through the superior orbital fissure, within the common tendinous ring of the recti muscles (**Fig. 41.17**), at first below, and then between, the two divisions of the oculomotor nerve and lateral to the nasociliary nerve. It passes forwards to enter the medial (ocular) surface of lateral rectus, which is its sole target.

OPHTHALMIC NERVE

The ophthalmic nerve, a division of the trigeminal nerve, travels through the orbit to supply targets that are primarily in the upper part of the face. It arises from the trigeminal ganglion in the middle cranial fossa and passes forwards along the lateral dural wall of the cavernous sinus. It gives off three main branches, the lacrimal, frontal and nasociliary nerves, just before it reaches the superior orbital fissure.

Lacrimal nerve (Figs 41.18, 41.24, 41.25)

The lacrimal nerve enters the orbit through the superior orbital fissure, above the common tendinous ring of the recti muscles, and lateral to the frontal and trochlear nerves. It passes forwards along the lateral wall of the orbit on the superior border of lateral rectus, and travels through the lacrimal gland and the orbital septum to supply conjunctiva and skin covering the lateral part of the upper eyelid. The lacrimal nerve communicates with the zygomatic branch of the maxillary nerve, and so parasympathetic fibres associated with the pterygopalatine ganglion might be conveyed to the lacrimal gland.

Frontal nerve (Figs 41.18, 41.24, 41.25)

The frontal nerve is the largest branch of the ophthalmic nerve. It enters the orbit through the superior orbital fissure, above the common tendinous ring of the recti muscles, and lies between the lacrimal nerve laterally and the trochlear nerve medially. It passes forwards on levator palpebrae superioris, towards the rim of the orbit: about halfway along this course it divides into the supraorbital and supratrochlear nerves.

The supraorbital nerve is the larger of the terminal branches of the frontal nerve. It continues forwards along levator palpebrae superioris and leaves the orbit through the supraorbital notch or foramen to emerge onto the forehead. The supraorbital nerve supplies the mucous

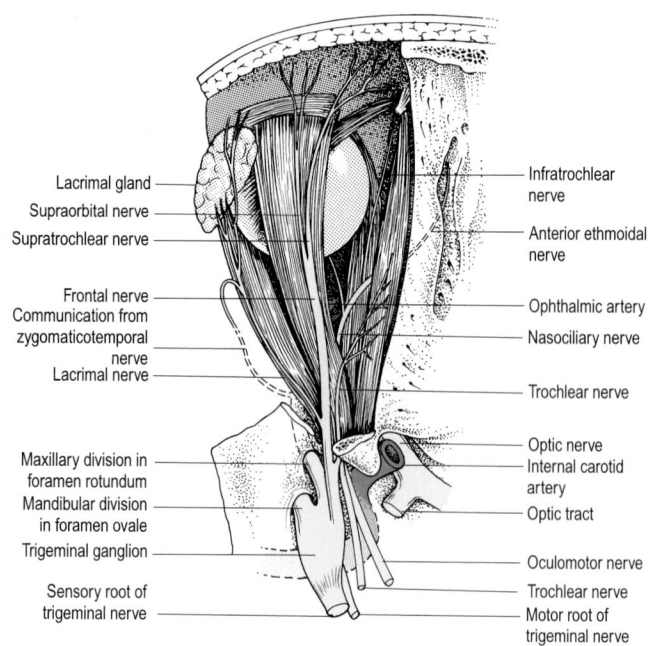

Lacrimal gland
Supraorbital nerve
Supratrochlear nerve

Frontal nerve
Communication from zygomaticotemporal nerve
Lacrimal nerve

Maxillary division in foramen rotundum
Mandibular division in foramen ovale
Trigeminal ganglion

Sensory root of trigeminal nerve

Infratrochlear nerve

Anterior ethmoidal nerve

Ophthalmic artery
Nasociliary nerve

Trochlear nerve

Optic nerve
Internal carotid artery
Optic tract

Oculomotor nerve
Trochlear nerve
Motor root of trigeminal nerve

Fig. 41.24 The nerves of the left orbit: superior aspect.

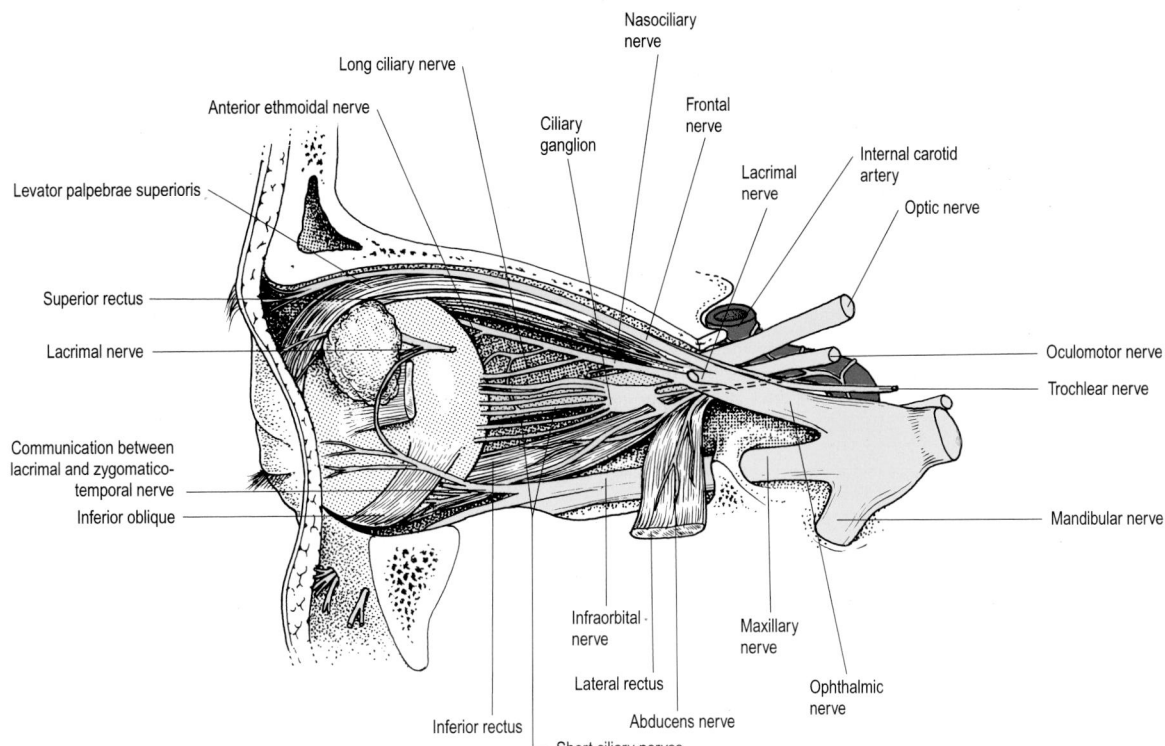

Fig. 41.25 The nerves of the left orbit and the ciliary ganglion: lateral aspect.

Labels on figure: Nasociliary nerve; Long ciliary nerve; Anterior ethmoidal nerve; Ciliary ganglion; Frontal nerve; Internal carotid artery; Levator palpebrae superioris; Lacrimal nerve; Optic nerve; Superior rectus; Lacrimal nerve; Oculomotor nerve; Trochlear nerve; Communication between lacrimal and zygomatico-temporal nerve; Inferior oblique; Mandibular nerve; Infraorbital nerve; Maxillary nerve; Lateral rectus; Ophthalmic nerve; Inferior rectus; Abducens nerve; Short ciliary nerves

membrane which lines the frontal sinus, skin and conjunctiva covering the upper eyelid, and skin over the forehead and scalp. The post-ganglionic sympathetic fibres which innervate the sweat glands of the supraorbital area probably travel in the supraorbital nerve, having entered the ophthalmic nerve through its communication with the abducens nerve within the cavernous sinus.

The supratrochlear nerve runs medially above the pulley for superior oblique. It gives a descending branch to the infratrochlear nerve and ascends onto the forehead through the frontal notch to supply skin and conjunctiva covering the upper eyelid, and skin over the forehead.

Nasociliary nerve (Figs 41.18, 41.24, 41.25)

The nasociliary nerve is intermediate in size between the frontal and lacrimal nerves, and is more deeply placed in the orbit, which it enters through the common tendinous ring, lying between the two rami of the oculomotor nerve. It crosses the optic nerve with the ophthalmic artery and runs obliquely below superior rectus and superior oblique to reach the medial orbital wall. Here, as the anterior ethmoidal nerve, it passes through the anterior ethmoidal foramen and canal and enters the cranial cavity. It runs forwards in a groove on the upper surface of the cribriform plate beneath the dura mater and descends through a slit lateral to the crista galli into the nasal cavity, where it occupies a groove on the internal surface of the nasal bone and gives off two internal nasal branches (p. 573). The medial internal nasal nerve supplies the anterior septal mucosa, and the lateral internal nasal nerve supplies the anterior part of the lateral nasal wall. The anterior ethmoidal nerve emerges, as the external nasal nerve (p. 512), at the lower border of the nasal bone, and descends under the transverse part of nasalis to supply the skin of the nasal ala, apex and vestibule.

The nasociliary nerve has connections with the ciliary ganglion and has long ciliary, infratrochlear and posterior ethmoidal branches.

The ramus communicans to the ciliary ganglion usually branches from the nerve as it enters the orbit lateral to the optic nerve. It is sometimes joined by a filament from the internal carotid sympathetic plexus or from the superior ramus of the oculomotor nerve as it enters the posterosuperior angle of the ganglion.

Two or three long ciliary nerves branch from the nasociliary nerve as it crosses the optic nerve (**Fig. 41.25**). They accompany the short ciliary nerves and pierce the sclera near the attachment of the optic nerve. Running forwards between sclera and choroid, they supply the ciliary body, iris and cornea and are said to contain postganglionic sympathetic fibres for the dilator pupillae from neurones in the superior cervical

ganglion. An alternative pathway for the supply of the dilator pupillae is via the sympathetic root associated with the ciliary ganglion.

The posterior ethmoidal nerve leaves the orbit by the posterior ethmoidal foramen and supplies the ethmoidal and sphenoidal sinuses.

MAXILLARY NERVE

The maxillary nerve is a sensory division of the trigeminal nerve. Most of the branches from the maxillary nerve arise in the pterygopalatine fossa. It gives rise to the zygomatic and infraorbital nerves that pass into the orbit through the inferior orbital fissure and two others that pass through the pterygopalatine ganglion without synapsing and are distributed to the nose, palate and pharynx.

Zygomatic nerve

The zygomatic nerve is located close to the base of the lateral wall of the orbit. It soon divides into two branches, the zygomaticotemporal and the zygomaticofacial nerves, which run for only a short distance in the orbit before passing onto the face through the lateral wall of the orbit. They may either enter separate canals within the zygomatic bone or the zygomatic nerve itself may enter the bone before dividing.

The zygomaticotemporal nerve exits the zygomatic bone on its medial surface, and pierces the temporal fascia to supply the skin over the temple. It also gives a branch to the lacrimal nerve which may carry parasympathetic fibres to the lacrimal gland (**Figs 41.25, 30.6**).

The zygomaticofacial nerve leaves the zygomatic bone on its lateral surface to supply skin overlying the prominence of the cheek.

Infraorbital nerve (Fig. 41.25)

The infraorbital nerve initially lies in the infraorbital groove on the floor of the orbit. As it approaches the rim of the orbit it runs into the infraorbital canal through which it passes to emerge onto the face at the infraorbital foramen. The infraorbital nerve supplies the skin of the lower eyelid, possibly the conjunctiva, and skin over the upper jaw, and also provides the middle and anterior superior alveolar nerves.

Orbital branches of pterygopalatine ganglion

Several rami orbitales arise dorsally from the pterygopalatine ganglion and enter the orbit through the inferior orbital fissure. Branches leave the orbit through the posterior ethmoidal air sinus. There is strong experimental evidence from studies of animals including monkeys that postganglionic parasympathetic branches pass directly to the lacrimal gland, ophthalmic artery and choroid.

OPTIC NERVE (Figs 41.17, 41.18)

The optic nerve is the second cranial nerve. It arises from the optic chiasma on the floor of the diencephalon and enters the orbit through the optic canal, accompanied by the ophthalmic artery. It changes its shape from being flattened at the chiasma to rounded as it passes through the optic canal. In the orbit it passes forwards, laterally and downwards, and pierces the sclera at the lamina cribrosa, slightly medial to the posterior pole. It has a somewhat tortuous course within the orbit to allow for movements of the eyeball. It is surrounded by extensions of the three layers of meninges.

The optic nerve has important relationships with other orbital structures. As it leaves the optic canal, it lies superomedial to the ophthalmic artery, and is separated from lateral rectus by the oculomotor, nasociliary and abducens nerves, and sometimes by the ophthalmic veins. The optic nerve is closely related to the origins of the four recti muscles, whereas more anteriorly, where the muscles diverge, it is separated from them by a substantial amount of orbital fat. Just beyond the optic canal, the ophthalmic artery and the nasociliary nerve cross the optic nerve to reach the medial wall of the orbit. The central artery of the retina enters the substance of the optic nerve about halfway along its length. Near the back of the eye, it becomes surrounded by long and short ciliary nerves and vessels.

CILIARY GANGLION (Figs 41.25, 41.26)

The ciliary ganglion is a parasympathetic ganglion which is concerned functionally with the motor innervation of certain intraocular muscles. It is a small, flat, reddish-grey swelling, 1–2 mm in diameter, connected to the nasociliary nerve, and located near the apex of the orbit in loose fat c.1 cm in front of the medial end of the superior orbital fissure. It lies between the optic nerve and lateral rectus, usually lateral to the ophthalmic artery. Its neurones, which are multipolar, are larger than in typical autonomic ganglia; a very small number of more typical neurones are also present.

Its connections or roots enter or leave it posteriorly. Eight to ten delicate filaments, termed the short ciliary nerves, emerge anteriorly from the ganglion arranged in two or three bundles, the lower being larger. They run forwards sinuously with the ciliary arteries, above and below the optic nerve, and divide into 15–20 branches that pierce the sclera around the optic nerve and run in small grooves on the internal scleral surface. They convey parasympathetic, sympathetic and sensory fibres between the eyeball and the ciliary ganglion: only the parasympathetic fibres synapse in the ganglion.

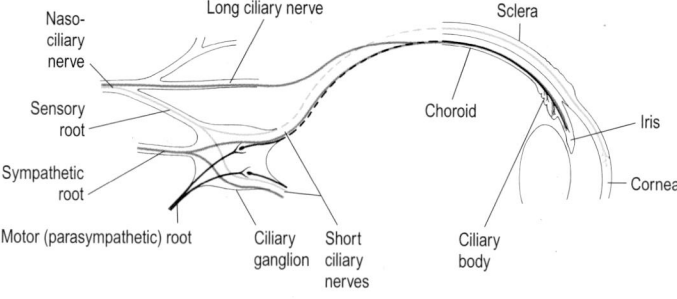

Fig. 41.26 The ciliary ganglion, with its roots and branches of distribution. Red, sympathetic fibres; heavy black, parasympathetic fibres; blue, sensory (cerebrospinal) fibres. Alternative pathways are given for the sympathetic fibres.

The parasympathetic root, derived from the branch of the oculomotor nerve to the inferior oblique, consists of preganglionic fibres from the Edinger–Westphal nucleus, which relay in the ganglion. Postganglionic fibres travel in the short ciliary nerves to the sphincter pupillae and ciliaris. More than 95% of these fibres supply ciliaris, which is much the larger muscle in volume.

The sympathetic root contains fibres from the plexus around the internal carotid artery within the cavernous sinus. These postganglionic fibres, derived from the superior cervical ganglion, form a fine branch which enters the orbit through the superior orbital fissure inside the common tendinous ring of the recti muscles. The fibres either pass directly to the ganglion, or join the nasociliary nerve and travel to the ganglion in its sensory root. Either way, they traverse the ganglion without synapsing to emerge into the short ciliary nerves. They are distributed to the blood vessels of the eyeball. Sympathetic fibres innervating dilator pupillae may sometimes travel via the short ciliary nerves (rather than the more usual route via the ophthalmic, nasociliary and long ciliary nerves).

The sensory fibres which pass through the ciliary ganglion are derived from the nasociliary nerve. They enter the short ciliary nerves and carry sensation from the cornea, the ciliary body and the iris.

REFERENCES

Hayreh SS 1942 The ophthalmic artery. III Branches. Br J Ophthalmol 46: 212–46.

Jones LT 1964 The anatomy of the upper eyelid and its relation to ptosis surgery. Am J Ophthalmol 57: 943–59.

Knop E, Knop N 2002 A functional unit for ocular surface immune defence formed by the lacrimal gland, conjunctiva and lacrimal drainage system. Adv Exp Med Biol 506B: 635–44.

Koornneef L 1977 Spatial Aspects of Orbital Musculo-fibrous Tissue in Man. Amsterdam: Swestsa Zeitlinger.

Leigh RJ, Zee DS 1999 The Neurology of Eye Movement. 3rd edition. Oxford: Oxford University Press.

Ruskell GL 1975 Nerve terminals and epithelial cell variety in the human lacrimal gland. Cell Tiss Res 138: 121–36.

The eye

The eyeball, the peripheral organ of vision, is situated in a skeletal cavity, the orbit, the walls of which help to protect it from injury. The orbit also has a more fundamental role in the visual process itself, in providing a rigid support and direction to the eye and in forming the sites of attachment for its external muscles. This setting permits the accurate positioning of the visual axis under neuromuscular control, and determines the spatial relationship between the two eyes – essential for binocular vision and conjugate eye movements.

The eyeball is embedded in orbital fat, separated from it by a thin fascial sheath (Chapter 41). It is composed of the segments of two spheres of different radii. The anterior segment, part of the smaller sphere, is transparent and forms c.7% of the surface of the whole globe. It is more prominent than the posterior segment, which is part of a larger sphere and opaque, and forms the remainder of the globe. The anterior segment is bounded by the cornea and the lens, and is incompletely subdivided into anterior and posterior chambers by the iris. These chambers are continuous through the pupil. The anterior chamber is slightly overlapped by the sclera peripherally. The angle between the iris and cornea therefore forms an annulus of greater diameter than the limbus, the junction between the sclera and cornea. The difference between these two varies from 1 to 2 mm, the angle being deeper above and below than at the sides of the eyeball. The posterior chamber lies between the posterior surface of the iris and the anterior aspect of the lens and its supporting ligament, the zonule, and is triangular in section. The apex of the triangle is the point where the iris touches the lens, and the base, or zonular region, extends among the collagenous bundles of the zonule, sometimes even into a retrozonular space between the zonule and the vitreous humour in the posterior segment of the eyeball. The posterior segment consists of the parts of the eye posterior to the zonule and lens.

The anterior pole is the centre of the anterior (corneal) curvature, and the posterior pole is the centre of its posterior (scleral) curvature; a line joining these two points forms the optic axis. (By the same convention, the eye has an equator, equidistant between the poles: any circumferential line joining the poles is a meridian.) The optic axes of the two eyes, in their primary position, are parallel and do not correspond with the orbital axes, which diverge anterolaterally at a marked angle to each other (Chapter 41). The optic nerves follow the orbital axes and are therefore not parallel; each enters its eye c.3 mm medial (nasal) to the posterior pole. The ocular vertical diameter (23.5 mm) is rather less than the transverse and anteroposterior diameters (24 mm); the anteroposterior diameter at birth is c.17.5 mm and at puberty 20–21 mm; it may vary considerably in myopia (c.29 mm) and in hypermetropia (c.20 mm). In females all diameters are on average slightly less than in the male.

OCULAR FIBROUS TISSUE

The eye has three layers enclosing its contents. From the outer surface these are a fibrous layer, which consists of the sclera behind and the cornea in front; a vascular, pigmented layer which consists of (from behind forwards) the choroid, ciliary body and iris, collectively termed the uveal tract; and a neural layer, known as the retina.

The fibrous layer of the eyeball (Fig. 42.1) has an opaque posterior sclera and a transparent anterior cornea. Together these form the protective enclosing capsule of the eye, a semi-elastic structure which when made turgid by intraocular pressure, determines with great precision the optical geometry of the visual apparatus. The sclera also provides attachments for the extraocular muscles which rotate the eye, its smooth external surface rotating easily on the adjacent tissues of the orbit. The cornea admits light, refracts it towards a retinal focus, and plays an important role in the image-processing mechanism.

Sclera (Fig. 42.1)

The sclera, so named from its relatively hard consistency, is a dense layer. When distended by intraocular pressure it maintains the shape of the eyeball. It is thickest (c.1.1 mm) posteriorly, near the optic nerve entry point, and is thinnest (0.4 mm) at the equator and at the attachments of the recti (Chapter 41). Its external surface is covered by a delicate episcleral lamina of loose fibrous tissue which contains sparse blood vessels and is in contact with the inner surface of the fascial sheath of the eyeball.

The anterior part is covered by conjunctiva which is reflected onto it from the deep surfaces of the eyelids. The scleral internal surface is attached to the choroid by a delicate fibrous layer, the suprachoroid lamina, which contains numerous fibroblasts and melanocytes. Anteriorly, it is attached to the ciliary body by the lamina supraciliaris. Posteriorly, the sclera is pierced by the optic nerve and is continuous with the fibrous nerve sheath and hence with the dura mater. The sclera has the appearance of a perforated plate, the lamina cribrosa sclerae, where the nerve pierces it (Fig. 42.2): the optic nerve fascicles pass through these minute orifices. The central retinal artery and vein pass through a larger, central aperture. Numerous small apertures transmit the ciliary vessels and nerves through the sclera close to the perimeter of the cribriform plate. Just behind the equator four larger apertures transmit the venae vorticosae. The lamina cribrosa is the weakest part of the sclera and bulges outwards in the condition of a cupped disc when intraocular pressure is raised chronically as in glaucoma.

Anteriorly, the sclera is directly continuous with the cornea at the corneoscleral junction or limbus (Fig. 42.3). Near the internal surface of the sclera there is an annular endothelial canal, the sinus venosus sclerae (canal of Schlemm), at this junction. In section, the canal appears as an oval cleft, whose outer wall grooves the sclera. Posteriorly, the cleft extends as far as a rim of scleral tissue, the scleral spur, which in section forms a triangle with its apex directed forwards. The sinus may be double or multiple in part of its course. Its inner wall, adjoining the aqueous chamber, consists of loose trabecular tissue continuous anteriorly with the posterior limiting lamina and endothelium of the cornea. There are spaces among its fibres through which aqueous humour filters from the anterior chamber to the sinus, draining peripherally to the anterior ciliary veins. Most of the fibres of the trabecular tissue mentioned above are attached to the anterior, external aspect of the scleral spur. Of the remainder, most are continuous with meridional fibres of the ciliary muscle, some of which attach to the posterior internal aspect of the scleral spur. The iridocorneal angle of the anterior chamber is bordered anteriorly by trabecular tissue and the scleral spur, and posteriorly by the periphery of the iris.

The sclera is composed of dense collagenous tissue mixed with occasional elastic fibres and interspersed with flat fibroblasts. Collagen forms 75% of the dry scleral weight, a factor which is important in the regulation of intraocular pressure. Fibre bundles are arranged circumferentially around the optic disc, and around the orifices of the lamina cribrosa. Elsewhere on the external surface of the sclera, fibres are arranged mostly in a reticular manner. The fibres of the tendons of the recti muscles intersect scleral fibres at right angles at their attachments, and then interlace deeper in the sclera. Collagen fibres of the scleral spur are orientated circularly, and there is an increased incidence of

701

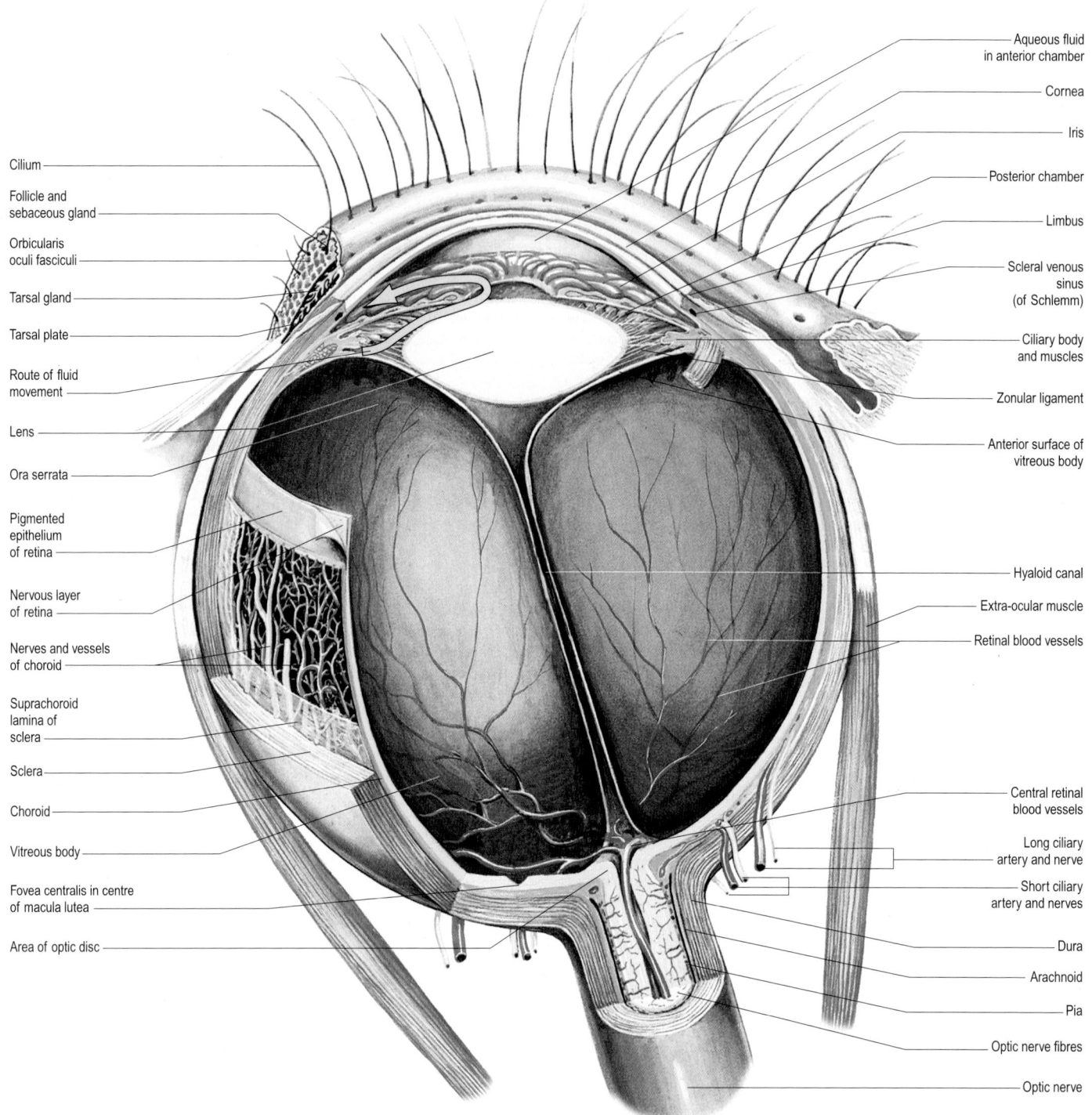

Cilium

Follicle and sebaceous gland

Orbicularis oculi fasciculi

Tarsal gland

Tarsal plate

Route of fluid movement

Lens

Ora serrata

Pigmented epithelium of retina

Nervous layer of retina

Nerves and vessels of choroid

Suprachoroid lamina of sclera

Sclera

Choroid

Vitreous body

Fovea centralis in centre of macula lutea

Area of optic disc

Aqueous fluid in anterior chamber

Cornea

Iris

Posterior chamber

Limbus

Scleral venous sinus (of Schlemm)

Ciliary body and muscles

Zonular ligament

Anterior surface of vitreous body

Hyaloid canal

Extra-ocular muscle

Retinal blood vessels

Central retinal blood vessels

Long ciliary artery and nerve

Short ciliary artery and nerves

Dura

Arachnoid

Pia

Optic nerve fibres

Optic nerve

Fig. 42.1 The organization of the eye, viewed from above. In this illustration the left eye and part of the lower eyelid are depicted in horizontal section and also cut away to show internal structure.

elastic fibres here. Scleral vessels are few and mainly disposed in the episcleral lamina, especially close to the limbus. The sclera provides passage for nerves of the cornea and vascular autonomic nerves, but its own innervation is sparse.

Cornea (Figs 42.3, 42.4, 42.5)

The cornea is the anterior, projecting, transparent part of the external tunic. Its tear film cover is the major site of refraction of light which enters the eye. Convex anteriorly, it projects from the sclera as a dome-shaped elevation forming c.7% of the external tunic area. Its curvature changes very little after the first year or so of life. Since it is more

curved (radius (r) = 6.8–8.5 mm, averaging 7.8 mm) than the sclera (r = 11.5 mm), a slight sulcus sclerae marks the corneoscleral junction. Corneal thickness is c.0.7 mm close to the corneoscleral junction, and 0.5–0.6 mm at its centre. Viewed from in front, the corneal perimeter is slightly elliptical, and its transverse diameter is a little greater than its vertical. Its posterior perimeter is circular and is more extensive than the anterior surface in its vertical axis, because in section the corneoscleral junction is slightly oblique above and below. The corneal diameter is c.11.7 mm on its posterior aspect; anteriorly it is 11.7 mm horizontally and 10.6 mm vertically. Of the total 60 dioptres refractive power of the eye, the cornea provides c.40 dioptres.

Microscopically, the cornea consists of five layers arranged antero-posteriorly as follows: corneal epithelium, which is continuous with the

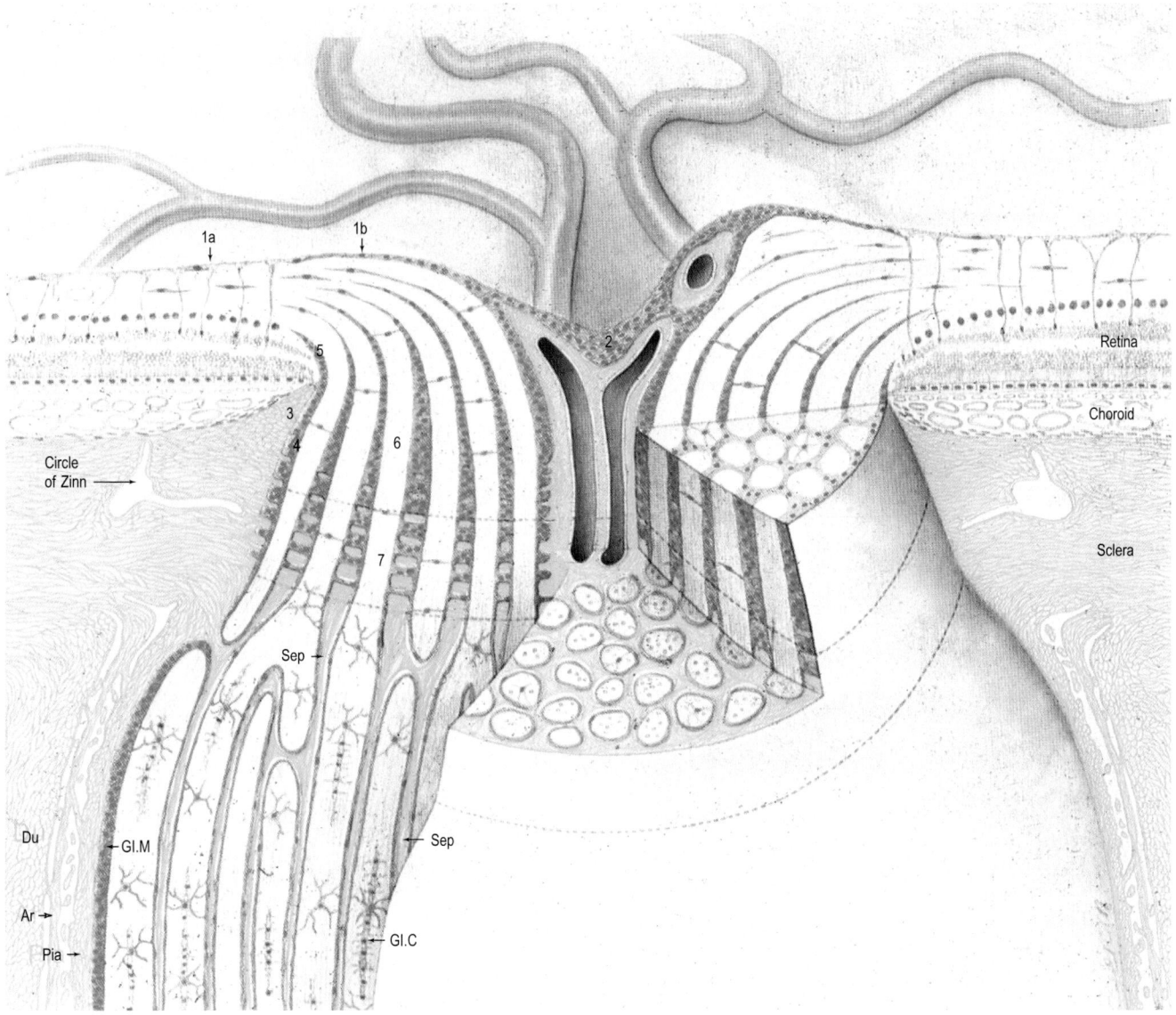

Fig. 42.2 Exit of the human optic nerve from the eyeball, showing the distribution of collagenous (blue) and neuroglial (magenta) tissues. Sep, septa of collagenous connective tissue carried into the nerve from the pia mater and dividing the nerve fibres into numerous fascicles; Gl.M, astroglial membrane separating nerve fibres from connective tissue; Gl.C, astrocytes and oligodendrocytes among the fibres in their fascicles; Du, Ar, Pia, dura, arachnoid and pia maters respectively. (1a) is the internal limiting membrane of the retina, which is continuous with an astroglial membrane (of Elschnig) covering the optic disc (1b). An accumulation of astrocytes forms a central meniscus of Kuhnt in the centre of the disc (2). The anterior or so-called 'choroidal part' of the lamina cribrosa (6) is separated from the choroid by a spur of collagenous tissue (3). The 'border tissue of Jacoby' (4), which is largely astroglia, frequently extends beyond the choroid (5) to separate much of the retina from the 'retinal part' of the optic nerve head. The posterior part of the lamina cribrosa (7) contains collagenous tissue derived from the optic nerve septa and fenestrated sheets of collagen fibres continuous with those of the sclera. (By permission from Anderson DR, Hoyt W 1969 Ultrastructure of intraorbital portion of human and monkey optic nerve. Arch Ophthalmol 82: 506–530.)

conjunctival epithelium; anterior limiting lamina; substantia propria; posterior limiting lamina; endothelium.

CORNEAL EPITHELIUM

The corneal epithelium covers the anterior surface of the cornea and generally has five layers of cells. The deepest are columnar with flat bases and rounded apices, and large rounded or oval nuclei. Cells in the second layer are polyhedral and resemble those in the epidermal stratum spinosum. In the more superficial layers the cells become progressively flatter. However, unlike the cells of the epidermis, they contain flat nuclei, are not normally keratinized, and present a smooth, optically perfect surface. At the corneoscleral junction (limbus) the corneal epithelium merges with the limbal conjunctival epithelium, which thickens (up to 12 cells) and soon loses the regular surface of the cornea. It is of clinical significance that the cornea does not appear to possess epithelial stem cells. Cell replacement depends on the centripetal migration (from the edges of the cornea) of cells which are the progeny of mitotic limbal stem cells.

ANTERIOR LIMITING LAMINA

The anterior limiting lamina lies behind the corneal epithelium. It contains a dense mass of collagen fibrils set in a matrix similar to that of the substantia propria. The lamina is 12 μm thick and is readily distinguishable from the substantia propria because it contains no fibroblasts. It appears amorphous by light microscopy.

SUBSTANTIA PROPRIA OR STROMA

The substantia propria or stroma forms the bulk of the cornea. It is a compact and transparent layer, composed of 200–250 sequential lamellae, each made up of fine parallel collagen fibrils mainly of type I collagen. Flat dendritic interconnecting fibroblasts form a coarse mesh between the lamellae. Alternate lamellae are typically orientated at large angles to each other (**Fig. 42.5**). Each lamella is c.2 μm thick and of variable breadth (10–250 μm, or, rarely, more). All fibrils in a given lamella have similar diameters, and are smaller in anterior lamellae than more posteriorly (a range of 21–65 nm). The dimensions of the fibrils

703

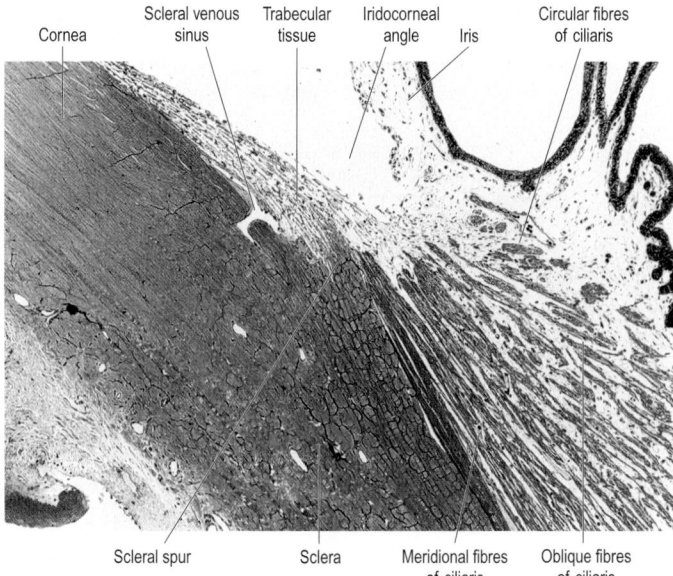

Fig. 42.3 Meridional section through the iridocorneal angle. The conjunctiva (left) was damaged in preparation. (Provided by the late Gordon L Ruskell, Department of Optometry and Visual Science, The City University, London.)

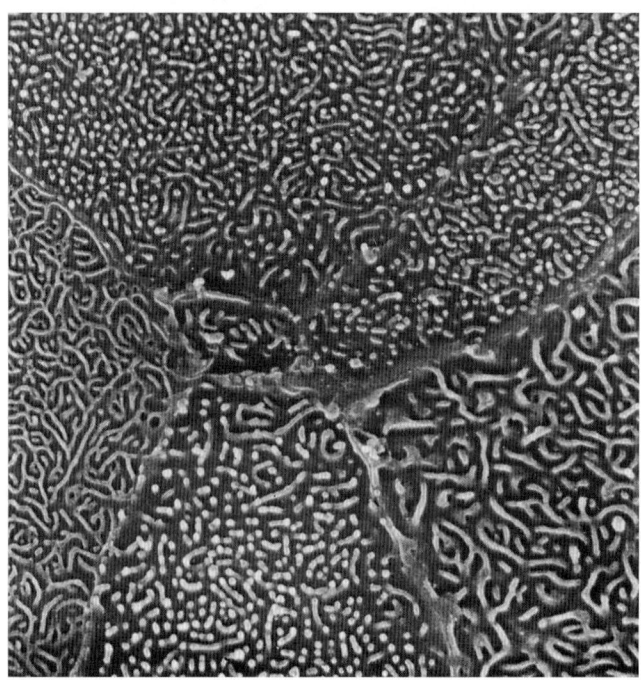

Fig. 42.4 Normal human corneal epithelial cells. Parts of the outlines of several cells are visible; in the upper and lower cells, microvilli predominate but some microplicae are seen. The cells at the right of the field display predominantly microplicae, with only a few microvilli. (From Pfister RR, Burstein NL 1977 The normal and abnormal human corneal epithelial surface. Invest Ophthalmol Vis Sci 16: 614–622. By permission from the Association for Research in Vision and Ophthalmology.)

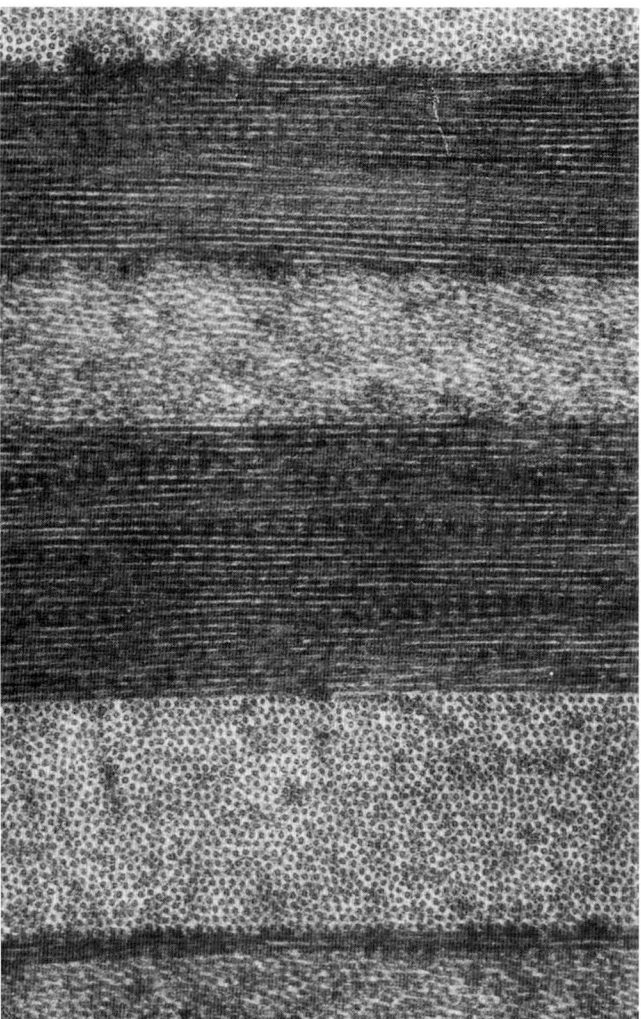

Fig. 42.5 Substantia propria of the human cornea; note the geometric precision of the alternation in direction of adjacent layers of collagen fibres. (By kind permission from John Marshall, Institute of Ophthalmology, London.)

are much smaller than the wavelength of light: this feature, and the regularity of their spacing, are the principal factors which determine stromal transparency (Hogan et al 1971).

POSTERIOR LIMITING LAMINA

The posterior limiting lamina covers the substantia propria posteriorly. It is thin and apparently homogeneous, and is regarded as the basement membrane of the endothelium. It is known to grow throughout life. It is 5 μm thick at birth, and may increase to 17 μm by the ninth

decade. At the limbus of the cornea it disperses into the fibres of trabecular tissue which adjoin the inner wall of the scleral venous sinus.

Aqueous humour drains from the eye through the iridocorneal angle (the 'filtration angle' in clinical terminology; Figs 42.3, 42.6). The trabecular spaces are interconnected, and it is believed that there is no impediment to flow from the anterior chamber to the inner wall of the sinus. The wall of the sinus is constructed of a continuous single thin endothelial layer. Passage of aqueous humour to the sinus probably occurs via giant pinocytotic vacuoles, which form on the inner face of the endothelium and discharge into the sinus at the outer face, and through intercellular clefts. Aqueous humour then passes through a plexus of fine intrascleral vessels which connect the sinus with anterior ciliary veins. Normally the sinus does not contain blood: pressure gradients prevent the reflux of blood even though the channels between the sinus and veins have no valves. In venous congestion, blood may enter the sinus, however, the continuous endothelial outer wall of the trabeculae prevents further reflux.

ENDOTHELIUM

The corneal endothelium covers the posterior surface of the cornea and lines the spaces of the iridocorneal angle. It is a layer of polygonal, flattened cells: there are prominent interdigitations between adjacent cells.

VASCULAR SUPPLY

The cornea contains neither blood nor lymphatic vessels: the capillaries of the conjunctiva and sclera end in loops near its periphery.

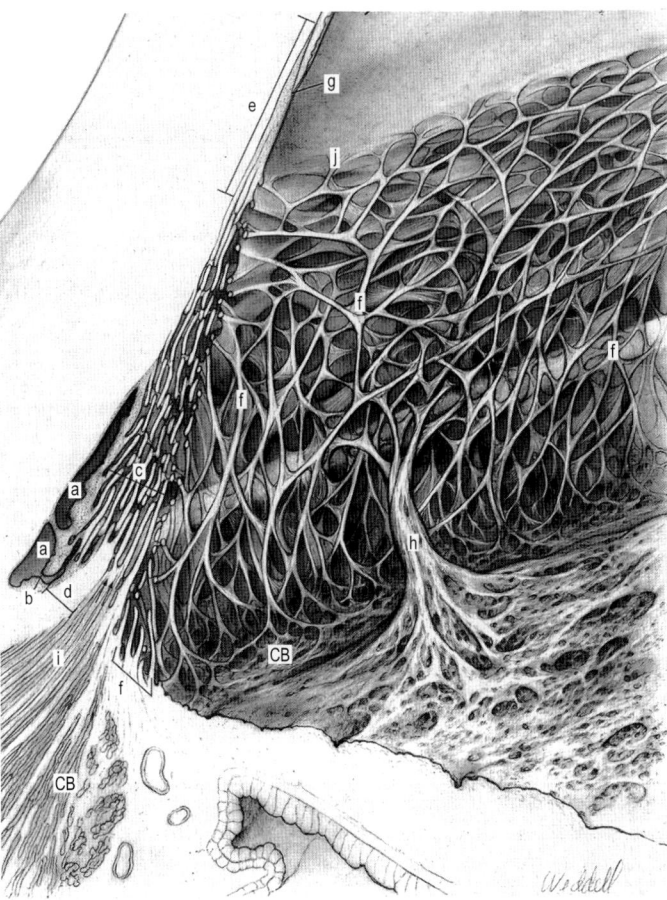

Fig. 42.6 The iridocorneal angle and adjoining structures, showing the proximity of the scleral venous sinus (a) to the pectinate ligaments (f). The trabecular meshwork of the latter is partly uveal, being continuous with the iris (h) and ciliary body (CB) and muscle (i). Anterior to the scleral spur (d), scleral trabecular tissue (c) is even closer to the scleral venous sinus. Aqueous fluid percolates through this trabecular region, reaching the lumen of the sinus through small apertures (b). The pectinate ligament diminishes as it approaches the corneal limbus (e) and in this junctional zone the posterior limiting membrane (of Descemet) also terminates (g). The endothelium of the anterior chamber (posterior corneal epithelium) is continuous with the endothelium of the trabeculae (j) at the limbus.
(By permission from Hogan MJ, Alvarado JA, Weddell JE 1971 Histology of the Human Eye. Philadelphia: WB Saunders.)

INNERVATION

The cornea is well innervated by numerous branches of the ophthalmic nerve which either form an annular plexus around the periphery of the cornea, or pass directly from the sclera and enter the substantia propria radially as 70–80 small groups of fibres. Upon entering the cornea, the few myelinated nerves lose their myelin sheaths. The nerves ramify throughout the corneal matrix in a delicate reticulum, and their terminal filaments form an intricate subepithelial plexus. Fine varicose axons from this plexus cross the anterior limiting membrane and form an intraepithelial plexus. There are no specialized end organs, the epithelial nerve fibres are devoid of Schwann cells, and they do not arborize.

OCULAR VASCULAR TUNIC

The vascular tunic, or uveal tract, consists of the choroid, ciliary body and iris, which collectively form a continuous structure. The choroid covers the internal scleral surface, and extends forwards to the ora serrata. The ciliary body continues forward from the choroid to the circumference of the iris, which is a circular diaphragm behind the cornea and in front of the lens. It presents an almost central aperture, the pupil.

Choroid (Figs 42.1, 42.7)

The choroid is a thin, highly vascular, dark brown tissue which lines almost five-sixths of the eye posteriorly. It is pierced behind by the optic

nerve where it is firmly adherent to the sclera. Elsewhere its external surface is loosely connected to the sclera by the suprachoroid layer (lamina fusca). Internally it is firmly attached to the pigmented layer of the retina, and at the optic disc it is continuous with the pia-arachnoid tissues around the optic nerve.

Structurally, the choroid consists largely of a dense capillary plexus. The blood flow through the choroid is high, a feature probably associated with an intraocular pressure of 15–20 mmHg, which means that a venous pressure above 20 mmHg is required to maintain circulation. The cooling effect of the choroidal circulation on the retina may be important. Externally, the suprachoroid layer, c.30 μm thick, is composed of delicate non-vascular lamellae, each one a network of fine collagen and elastic fibres, and stellate cells which contain dark brown granules. Ganglionic neurones and neural plexuses are present in the connective tissue.

The choroid proper lies internal to the suprachoroid layer, which is partly scleral tissue, and consists of a number of layers. Although descriptions of these vary, the following are generally recognized: an external vascular layer of small arteries and veins, loose connective tissue and scattered pigment cells; a capillary layer; a thin, apparently structureless, basal layer.

The vascular layer is sometimes subdivided on the basis of blood vessel calibre, which naturally decreases towards the capillary layer. It also contains the terminal branches of short posterior ciliary arteries (**Fig. 42.1**) which extend meridionally from their entry through the sclera near the optic disc. The veins are larger, and converge spirally onto four, or very occasionally more, principal vorticose veins. These pierce the sclera behind the equator to reach tributaries of the ophthalmic veins. The capillary layer is separated from the retina only by the thin basal layer of the choroid, and provides nutrition to the retina. It consists of a close meshwork of large vessels: the meshes widen slightly towards the ciliary body. The basal layer appears as a glassy, homogeneous layer (lamina vitrea), only 2–4 μm thick, under the light microscope. It consists largely of an elastic fibre mesh. Its function is uncertain, but is thought to be related to the passage of fluid and solutes from the choroidal capillaries to the retina. It is derived from both the retina and the choroid. In advancing years, lipid may be deposited in this membrane, which impairs the exchange of gases, nutrients and metabolites between the choroidal blood and the outer layers of the retina, and causes degenerative disease in the photoreceptor layer of the neural retina.

The choroidal pigment cells limit the passage of light through the sclera to the retina. More importantly, they may absorb light traversing the retina beyond the receptors, so preventing internal reflection within the vitreous body. The vessels of the choroid have a rich autonomic vasomotor supply, however, the sensory supply is at most very poor.

Ciliary body (Figs 42.8, 42.9)

The ciliary body is directly continuous with the choroid behind, and with the iris in front. While all of these regions of the uveal tract share certain various features, they also exhibit regional differences related to variations in their function. The ciliary body is concerned with the suspension of the lens and with accommodation, and it contains an accumulation of muscle fibres which cause it to bulge internally. It is also the major source of aqueous fluid for the anterior segment of the eye, which its anterior aspect faces. Posteriorly it is contiguous with the vitreous humour, and it probably secretes some of the glycosaminoglycans (GAGs) of the vitreous body. The anterior and the long ciliary arteries meet in the ciliary body (**Fig. 42.7**), and so it is a highly vascular region. The major nerves to all the anterior tissues of the eyeball pass through the ciliary body.

Externally, the ciliary body may be represented by a line which extends from c.1.5 mm posterior to the limbus of the cornea (corresponding also to the scleral spur) to a line c.7.5–8 mm posterior to this on the temporal side, and 6.5–7 mm on the nasal side. The ciliary body is thus slightly eccentric. It projects posteriorly from the scleral spur, which is its attachment, with a meridional width varying from 5.5 to 6.5 mm. Internally, it exhibits a posteriorly crenated or scalloped periphery, the ora serrata, where it is continuous with the choroid and retina. Anteriorly, it is confluent with the periphery of the iris, and externally bounds the iridocorneal angle of the anterior chamber.

Melanin in the deeper layer of its epithelium renders the ciliary body brown. It has an anterior plicated part, the corona ciliaris (pars plicata),

Fig. 42.7 **Fig. 42.7** The vascular arrangements of the uveal tract. The long posterior ciliary arteries, one of which is visible (A), branch at the ora serrata (b) and feed the capillaries of the anterior part of the choroid. Short posterior ciliary arteries (C) divide rapidly to form the posterior part of the choriocapillaris. Anterior ciliary arteries (D) send recurrent branches to the choriocapillaris (e) and anterior rami to the major arterial circle (f). Branches from the circle extend into the iris (g) and to the limbus. Branches of the short posterior ciliary arteries (C) form an anastomotic circle (h) (of Zinn) round the optic disc, and twigs (i) from this join an arterial network on the optic nerve. The vorticose veins (J) are formed by the junctions (k) of suprachoroidal tributaries (l). Smaller tributaries are also shown (m, n). The veins draining the scleral venous sinus (o) join anterior ciliary veins and vorticose tributaries. (By permission from Hogan MJ, Alvarado JA, Weddell JE 1971 Histology of the Human Eye. Philadelphia: WB Saunders.)

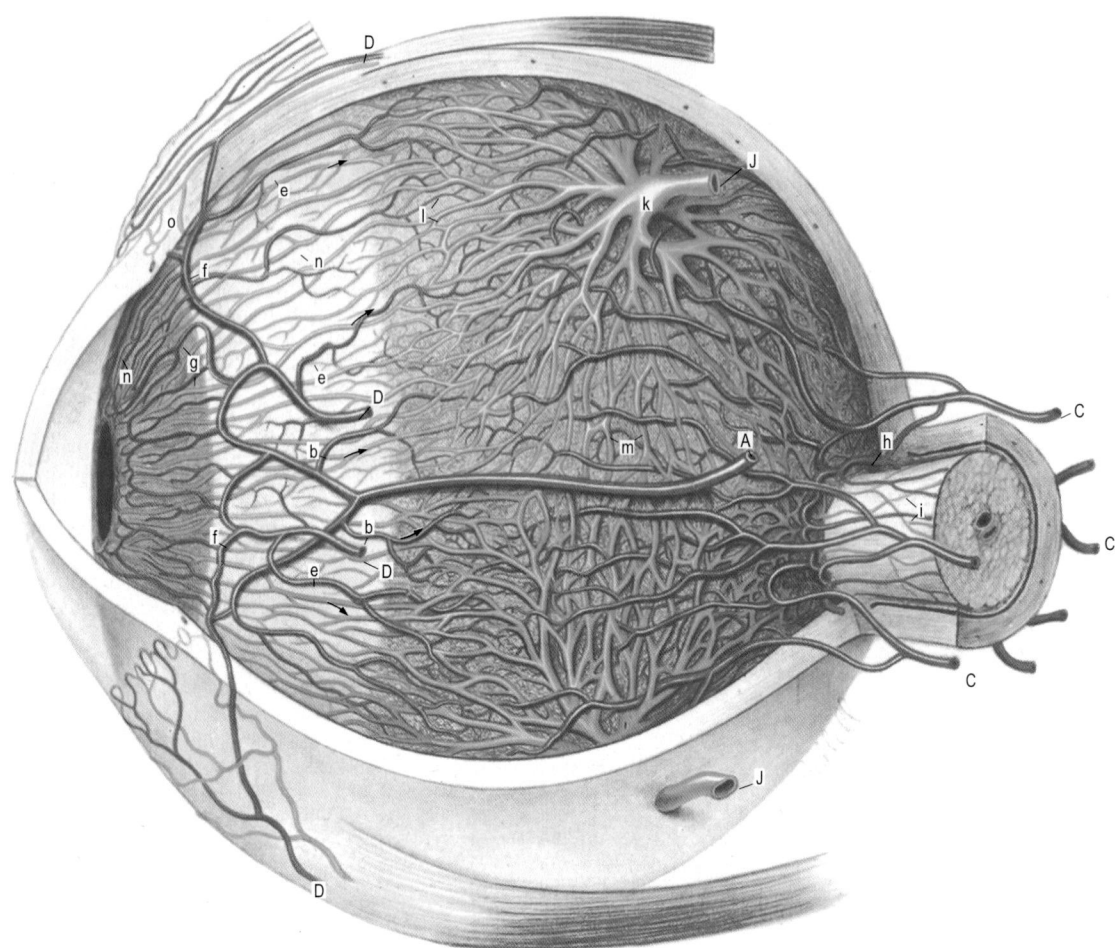

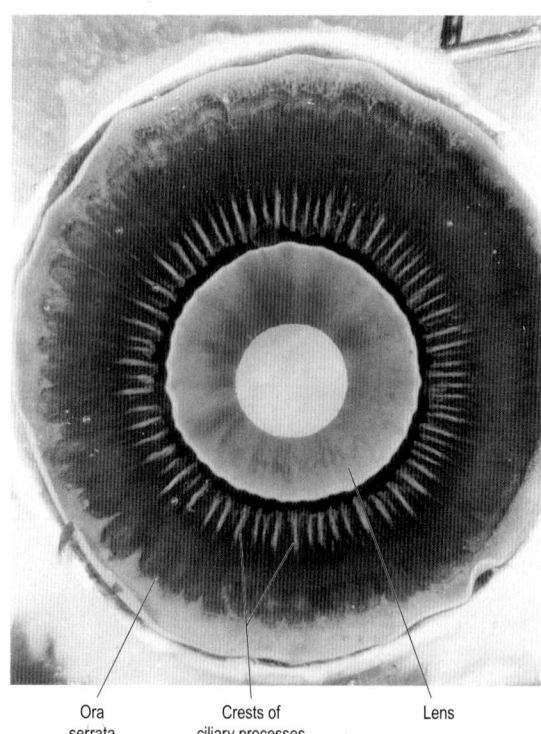

Ora serrata   Crests of ciliary processes   Lens

Fig. 42.8 The posterior aspect of the anterior half of the eyeball showing the termination of the neural retina at the ora serrata and the ciliary body. The definition of the serrations is less clear temporally (right). Note the lighter crests of the ciliary processes and the greater width of the ciliary body temporally. The lens has retained sufficient transparency to reveal the iris border and its crenated perimeter is due to tension imposed by the attached suspensory ligaments (unseen). (Provided by the late Gordon L Ruskell, Department of Optometry and Visual Science, The City University, London.)

which surrounds the base of the iris. Posterior to this is a smooth, annular orbiculus ciliaris (pars plana, ciliary ring). The orbiculus forms more than half of the meridional width of the ciliary body, and is 3.5–4 mm across. Its peripheral rim is the ora serrata, at which the optical or sensory part of the retina is suddenly reduced to two layers of epithelial cells, which extend over the whole ciliary body as the pars ciliaris retinae, and beyond this extend to the posterior surface of the iris. The corona ciliaris, a smaller annular region within the orbiculus, is ridged meridionally by 70–80 ciliary processes radiating from the base of the iris. A minor ridge, or ciliary plica, lies in the valley between most of the processes. The crests of the processes are less pigmented, and this gives them the appearance of white (or light) striae, from which the name ciliary is derived. Fibres of the zonule (the suspensory ligament of the lens) extend into the valleys. They pass beyond the ciliary processes to fuse with the basal lamina of the superficial epithelial layer of the orbiculus ciliaris. Their sites of attachment are marked by striae which pass back from the valleys of the corona, across the orbiculus, almost as far as the apices of the dentate processes of the ora serrata (**Fig. 42.9**).

CILIARY EPITHELIUM

The ciliary epithelium is bilaminar, and consists of two layers of simple epithelium which are derived embryonically from the two layers of the optic cup. The superficial layer consists of columnar cells over the orbiculus, and cuboidal cells over the ciliary processes: it becomes irregular and more flattened between the processes. These cells contain little or no pigment and are the sole anterior continuation of the neural retina. The pigment epithelium of the retina is continuous with the deeper layer of the ciliary epithelium, where the cells are approximately cuboidal and are loaded with pigment. The two layers are normally firmly united, but fluid may separate them pathologically. The pigment layer is united to the stroma of the ciliary body by its basal lamina, which continues back into the basal lamina of the choroid (**Fig. 42.10**). A basal lamina covers the free surface of the bilayer and is continuous with the internal limiting membrane of the retina. This arrangement

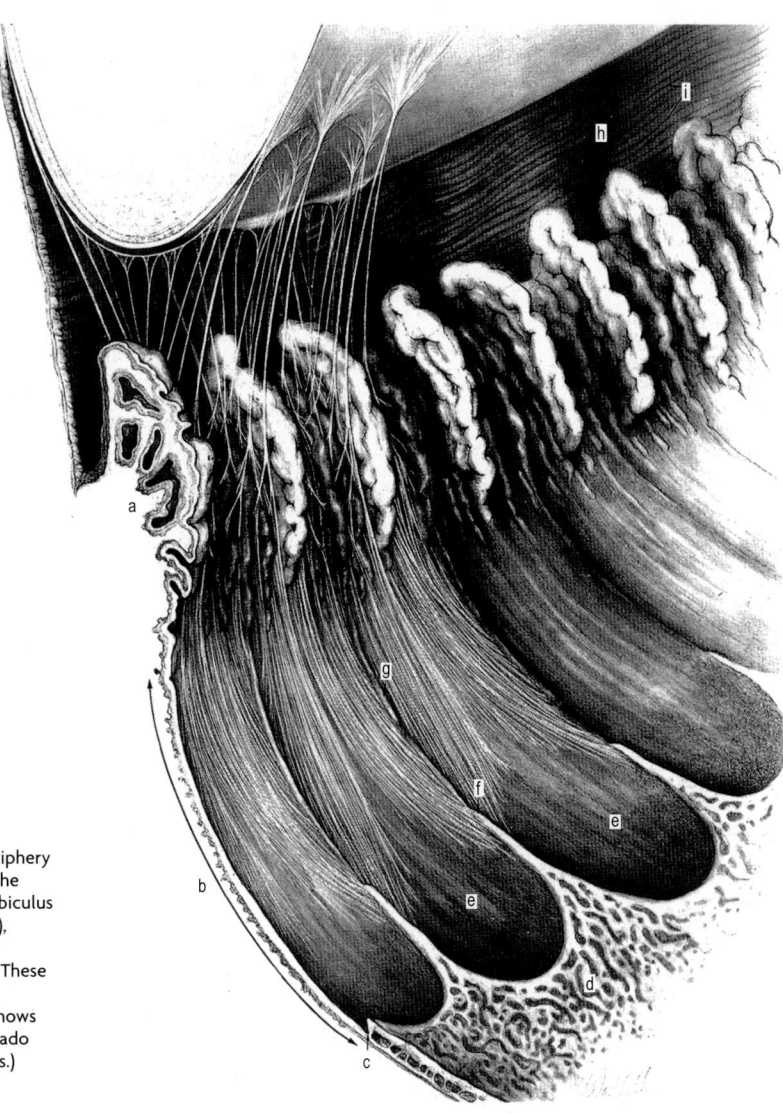

Fig. 42.9 The ciliary region seen from the ocular interior. Above is the periphery of the lens, attached by the fibres of the zonule (suspensory ligament) to the processes of the corona ciliaris (pars plicata) of the ciliary body (a). The orbiculus ciliaris or pars plana ciliaris (b) has a scalloped boundary, the ora serrata (c), which separates it from the retina (d). Flanking the 'bays' (e) of this are the dentate processes (f), with which linear ridges or striae (g) are continuous. These striae extend forwards between the main ciliary processes, providing an attachment for the longer zonular fibres. The posterior aspect of the iris shows radial (h) and circumferential (i) sulci. (By permission from Hogan MJ, Alvarado JA, Weddell JE 1971 Histology of the Human Eye. Philadelphia: WB Saunders.)

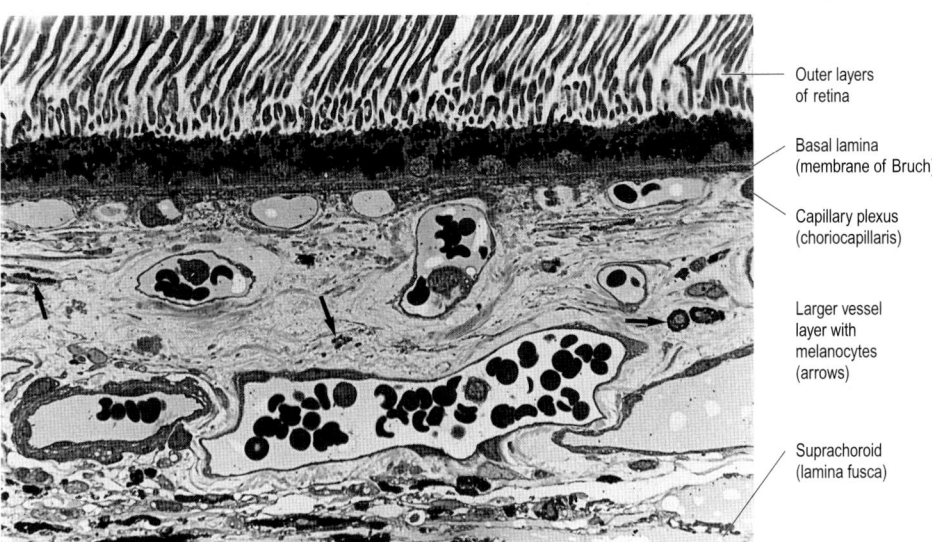

Outer layers
of retina

Basal lamina
(membrane of Bruch)

Capillary plexus
(choriocapillaris)

Larger vessel
layer with
melanocytes
(arrows)

Suprachoroid
(lamina fusca)

Fig. 42.10 Transverse section through the choroid. (Provided by the late Gordon L Ruskell, Department of Optometry and Visual Science, The City University, London.)

is a consequence of the invagination of the optic cup during development.

CILIARY STROMA

The ciliary stroma is composed largely of loose bundles of collagen, which form a considerable mass between the ciliary muscle and over-lying processes, and extend into both of them. This inner layer of connective tissue contains numerous larger branches of the ciliary vessels. A dense reticulum of large capillaries is concentrated in the ciliary processes. Anteriorly, near the periphery of the iris, is the major arterial circle (**Fig. 42.7**), which is formed chiefly by long posterior ciliary branches of the ophthalmic artery. These enter the eye some distance behind the ocular equator and pass between the choroid and sclera to

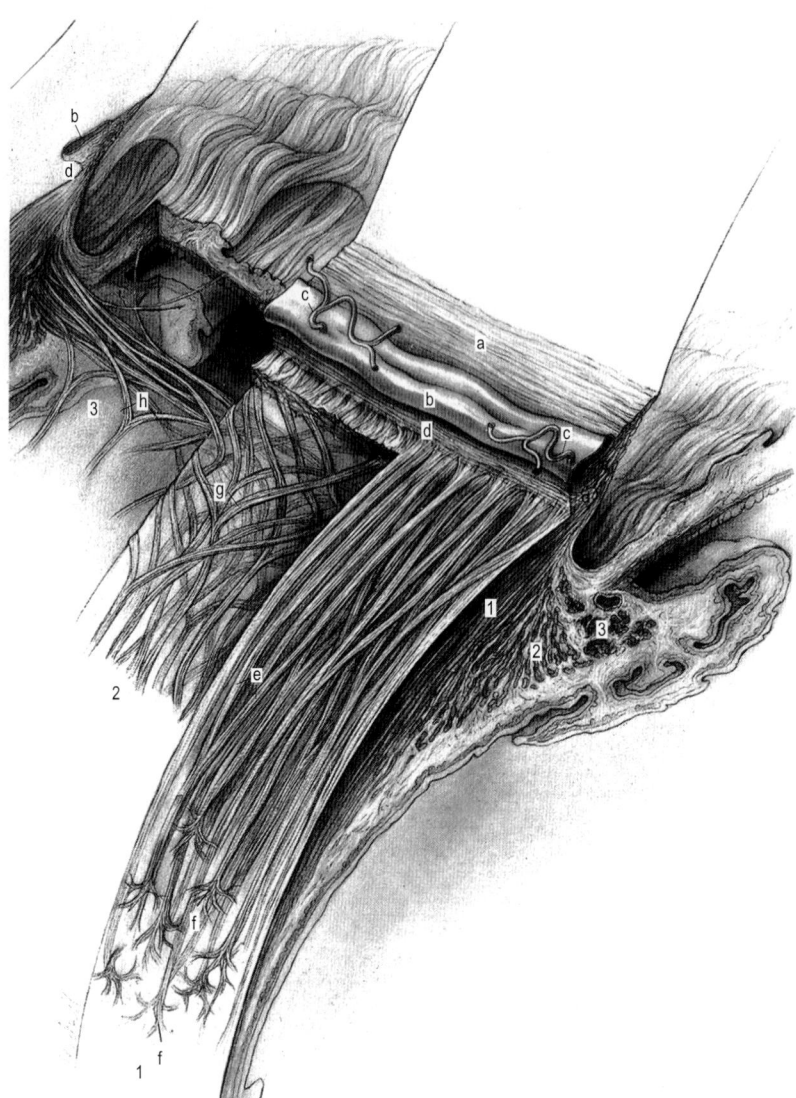

Fig. 42.11 The ciliary muscle and its components. The meridional or longitudinal (1), radial or oblique (2), and circular or sphincteric (3) layers of muscle fibres are displayed by successive removal towards the ocular interior. The cornea and sclera have been removed, leaving the pectinate ligament (a), the scleral venous sinus (b), collecting venules (c) and scleral spur (d). The meridional fibres often display acutely angled junctions (e) and terminate in epichoroidal stars (f). The radial fibres meet at obtuse angles (g) and similar junctions, at even wider angles (h), occur in the circular stratum of the ciliaris. (By permission from Hogan MJ, Alvarado JA, Weddell JE 1971 Histology of the Human Eye. Philadelphia: WB Saunders.)

the ciliary body. Ciliary veins, also draining the iris, pass posteriorly to join the vorticose veins of the choroid.

CILIARY MUSCLE (Fig. 42.11)

The ciliary muscle is a small annular mass of smooth muscle. Descriptions of the muscle generally recognize three main parts: meridional, radial or oblique, and circular or sphincteric. Most, perhaps almost all, ciliary muscle fibres are attached to the scleral spur. The outermost fibres are meridional or longitudinal, and pass posteriorly into the stroma of the choroid. The innermost fibres swerve acutely from the spur to run circumferentially as a sphincteric element near the periphery of the lens. Obliquely interconnecting radial fibres run between these two muscular strata, frequently forming an interweaving lattice.

Myelinated and non-myelinated nerve fibres abound in the ciliary muscle and ciliary body. The former are postganglionic parasympathetic fibres from the ciliary ganglion which stimulate the ciliary muscle to contract. Sympathetic fibres are sparse: they have a very limited capacity to relax the muscle. On contraction the muscle is displaced radially towards the optic axis. All parts of the muscle act in concert, and tension on the zonular ligaments is relaxed which frees the lens to assume its accommodated shape.

Iris (Fig. 42.12)

The iris is an adjustable diaphragm around a central aperture (slightly medial to true centre), the pupil, which controls the amount of light entering the eye (**Fig. 42.1**). Pupillary diameter varies from 1 to at least 8 mm, and has an even wider range under the influence of drugs. This gives an aperture range in excess of f20–f2.5, and a ratio of 32:1 for the amount of light permitted to enter the eye. While this is not enough to save the retina from the effects of intense illumination, it moderates the great range of luminosity encountered in ordinary use, and preserves useful vision under highly variable conditions. (The pupillary diameters noted above and the average iridial diameter of c.12 mm are estimated through the cornea, which introduces a magnification factor of c.12%.) Pupillary constriction and dilatation are self-explanatory terms, for which miosis and mydriasis are used clinically, though they are more properly reserved for the extreme limits of contraction and dilatation. Loewenstein and Loewenfeld (1970) should be consulted for further information.

Though the iris is named after the rainbow, its range of colour extends only from light blue to very dark brown. The colour often varies between the two eyes and even within the same iris (**Fig. 42.12**). It is a product of the combined effect of the iridial connective tissue and the pigment cells which selectively absorb and reflect different frequencies of light energy. Pigment is necessary to confine light transmission to the pupil and central lens, where optical aberrations are least. The concentration of melanocytes is the main factor which determines the hue of the iris. The distribution of pigment is often irregular, and this produces a flecked appearance. When pigment is largely absent, other than in the epithelial layers, which is the condition at birth, the colour is light blue.

The iris is not a flat diaphragm because the lens causes it to bulge a little. This means that it is more accurately described as a shallow cone, truncated by the pupillary aperture. It is sited between the cornea and lens and immersed in aqueous fluid. It therefore partially divides the anterior segment into an anterior chamber, enclosed by the cornea and iris (which meet at the iridocorneal angle), and a confusingly termed posterior chamber, which lies between the iris and the lens.

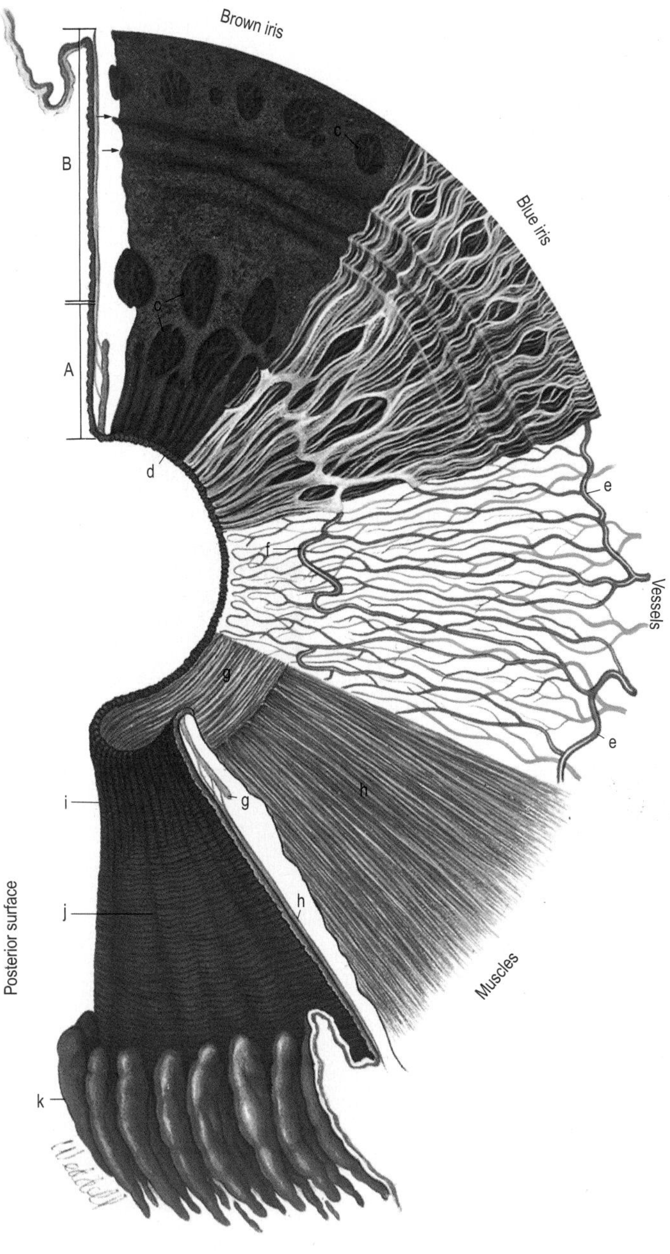

Fig. 42.12 Composite view of the surfaces and internal strata of the iris. In a clockwise direction from above, the pupillary (**A**) and ciliary (**B**) zones are shown in successive segments. The first (brown iris) shows the anterior border layer and the openings of crypts (c). In the second segment (blue iris), the layer is much less prominent and the trabeculae of the stroma are more visible. The third segment shows the iridial vessels, including the major arterial circle (e) and the incomplete minor arterial circle (f). The fourth segment shows the muscle stratum, including the sphincter (g) and dilator (h) of the pupil. The everted 'pupillary ruff' of the epithelium on the posterior aspect of the iris (d) appears in all segments. The final segment, folded over for pictorial purposes, depicts this aspect of the iris, showing radial folds (i and j) and the adjoining ciliary processes (k). (By permission from Hogan MJ, Alvarado JA, Weddell JE 1971 Histology of the Human Eye. Philadelphia: WB Saunders.)

MICROSTRUCTURE

The stroma of the iris is formed of fibroblasts, melanocytes and loose collagenous matrix. The intercellular spaces appear to communicate freely with the anterior chamber, and interchange of fluid between the two may assist the considerable changes in thickness which occur during contraction and relaxation of the iris. There is no elastic tissue.

The anterior surface of the iris does not possess a distinct epithelium, but is a modified superficial layer of the general stroma of the iris, formed mainly by an increased number of fibroblasts and melanocytes. At the periphery it blends with the pectinate ligament and the trabecular connective tissue of the iridocorneal angle (Hogan et al 1971), and at

the pupillary rim it meets the epithelium of the posterior surface of the iris. This stroma contains the regional vessels and nerves. An aggregation of smooth muscle cells near the pupillary rim forms an annular contractile sphincter pupillae. The epithelial surface covering the iris posteriorly is a continuation of the bilaminar epithelium of the ciliary body formed from the two layers of the optic cup. The pupil, through which this epithelium curves for a short distance on to the anterior surface as the pigment ruff or 'border', therefore corresponds to the opening of the optic cup.

The deeper of the two epithelial layers is confusingly termed the anterior epithelium, although it lies posterior to the stroma. Its cells are pigmented, as are those of the same layer in the ciliary epithelium. They give rise to the dilator pupillae, which like the sphincter has an unusual embryological origin, from the neural ectoderm of the optic cup which interacts with the local neural crest. Superficial (posterior) to this layer is a stratum of heavily pigmented cells, the so-called posterior epithelium, which is continuous with the internal non-pigmented, retinal, layer of the ciliary epithelium. The surface bears numerous delicate radial ridges at its free surface which facilitate the movement of aqueous humour from the posterior to the anterior chamber.

MUSCLES OF THE IRIS

The muscles of the iris are sphincter and dilator pupillae.

SPHINCTER PUPILLAE

Sphincter pupillae is a flat annulus of smooth muscle c.0.75 mm wide and 0.15 mm thick. Its densely packed fusiform muscle cells are often arranged in small bundles, as in the ciliary muscle, and pass circumferentially around the pupil (**Fig. 42.12**). Collagenous connective tissue lies in front of and behind the muscle fibres and is very dense posteriorly, where it binds the sphincter to the pupillary end of the dilator muscle. It is attached to the epithelial layer at the pupil margin. Small axons, mostly non-myelinated, ramify in the connective tissue between bundles.

DILATOR PUPILLAE

Dilator pupillae is a thin layer which lies immediately anterior to the epithelium of the posterior surface of the iris. Its 'fibres' are the muscular processes of the anterior layer of this epithelium, whose cells are therefore myoepithelial. Myofilaments are present in both parts of these cells, but are more abundant in the fusiform basal muscular processes, which are c.4 μm thick, 7 μm wide and 60 μm in length. They form a layer some 3–5 elements thick through most of the iris, from its periphery to the outer perimeter of the sphincter, which it slightly overlaps. Here the dilator thins out, and sends spurs to blend with the sphincter. Unlike the apical parts of the myoepithelial cells, these have a basal lamina and are joined by gap junctions like those between the sphincteric muscle cells. Non-myelinated nerve axons pass between, and terminate on, their muscular processes.

VASCULAR SUPPLY OF THE IRIS (Figs 42.7, 42.12)

The iris receives its blood supply from the long posterior and anterior ciliary arteries (**Fig. 42.7**). Both long ciliary arteries, on reaching the attached margin of the iris, divide into an upper and a lower branch. The branches anastomose with the corresponding contralateral arteries, and the anterior ciliary arteries, to form a vascular circle, the circulus arteriosus major. Vessels converge from this circle to the free margin of the iris, where they anastomose to form an incomplete circulus arteriosus minor: there is a view that these vessels are venous. The smaller arteries and veins are very similar in their structure and also share some peculiarities. They are often slightly helical, which may allow them to adapt to changes in iridial shape as the pupil varies in size. All of the vessels, including the capillaries, have a non-fenestrated endothelium and a prominent, often thick, basal lamina. There is no elastic lamina in the arteries or veins, and there are few smooth muscle cells, especially in the veins. Connective tissue in the tunica media is loose, whereas the adventitia is remarkably dense and collagenous, so that it appears to form almost a separate tube. The loose stratum of the media has been regarded as a lymph space, but this is improbable; it is c.7 μm in width, and contains a matrix which is probably derived from the endothelial basal lamina (Hogan et al 1971).

INNERVATION OF THE IRIS

The iris is innervated largely by branches of the long ciliary rami of the nasociliary nerve and of the short ciliary rami of the ciliary ganglion (p. 700). The latter provide parasympathetic postganglionic myelinated axons which innervate the sphincter pupillae. They lose their myelin well before entering the muscle. The dilator is supplied with non-myelinated postganglionic fibres from the superior sympathetic ganglion; their routes are less well established. The internal carotid sympathetic plexus is said to send a branch via the ciliary ganglion, which reaches the eye in the short ciliary nerves: other fibres may travel in the long ciliary nerves. Both the sphincter and the dilator may have a double autonomic supply. An additional small fraction of dilator and sphincter muscle nerve endings have been identified as parasympathetic and sympathetic respectively in experimental animal studies, including those on primates. Although ganglion cells have been noted in the iris, almost all nerve fibres are probably postganglionic. They form a plexus around the periphery of the iris, from which small nerves and fibres extend to the two muscles, to vessels, and to the anterior border layer. Some fibres may be afferent and some are vasomotor: it is difficult to identify afferent nerve endings in the iris and ciliary body or to distinguish them from efferent autonomic endings.

PUPILLARY MEMBRANE

In the fetus, the pupil is closed by a thin, vascular pupillary membrane. Its vessels are derived partly from those of the iridial margin, and partly from those of the lens capsule. They end in loops near the centre of the membrane, which is avascular. At about the sixth month of gestation, absorption of the membrane begins, from the centre towards the periphery, until at birth when only scattered fragments remain. Exceptionally the pupillary membrane may persist and interfere with vision.

RETINA (Figs 42.13, 42.14, 42.15)

The retina is the sensory neural layer of the eyeball. It is a most complex structure and should be considered as a special area of the brain, from which it is derived by outgrowth from the diencephalon (Chapter 14). It is dedicated to the detection and early analysis of visual information and is an integrated part of the much larger apparatus of visual analysis present in the thalamus, cortex and other areas of the central nervous system (Section 2).

The retina lies between the choroid externally and the vitreous body internally. It is thin, being thickest (0.56 mm) near the optic disc, diminishing to 0.1 mm anterior to the equator, and continuing at this thickness to the ora serrata. It also thins locally at the fovea of the macula. The retina is continuous with the optic nerve at the optic disc. Anteriorly, at the ora serrata (p. 705), a thin, non-neural prolongation of the retina extends forwards over the ciliary processes and iris as the ciliary and iridial parts of the retina respectively: they consist of pigmented and columnar epithelial layers only. The optic part of the retina extends from the optic disc to the ora serrata. It is soft, translucent

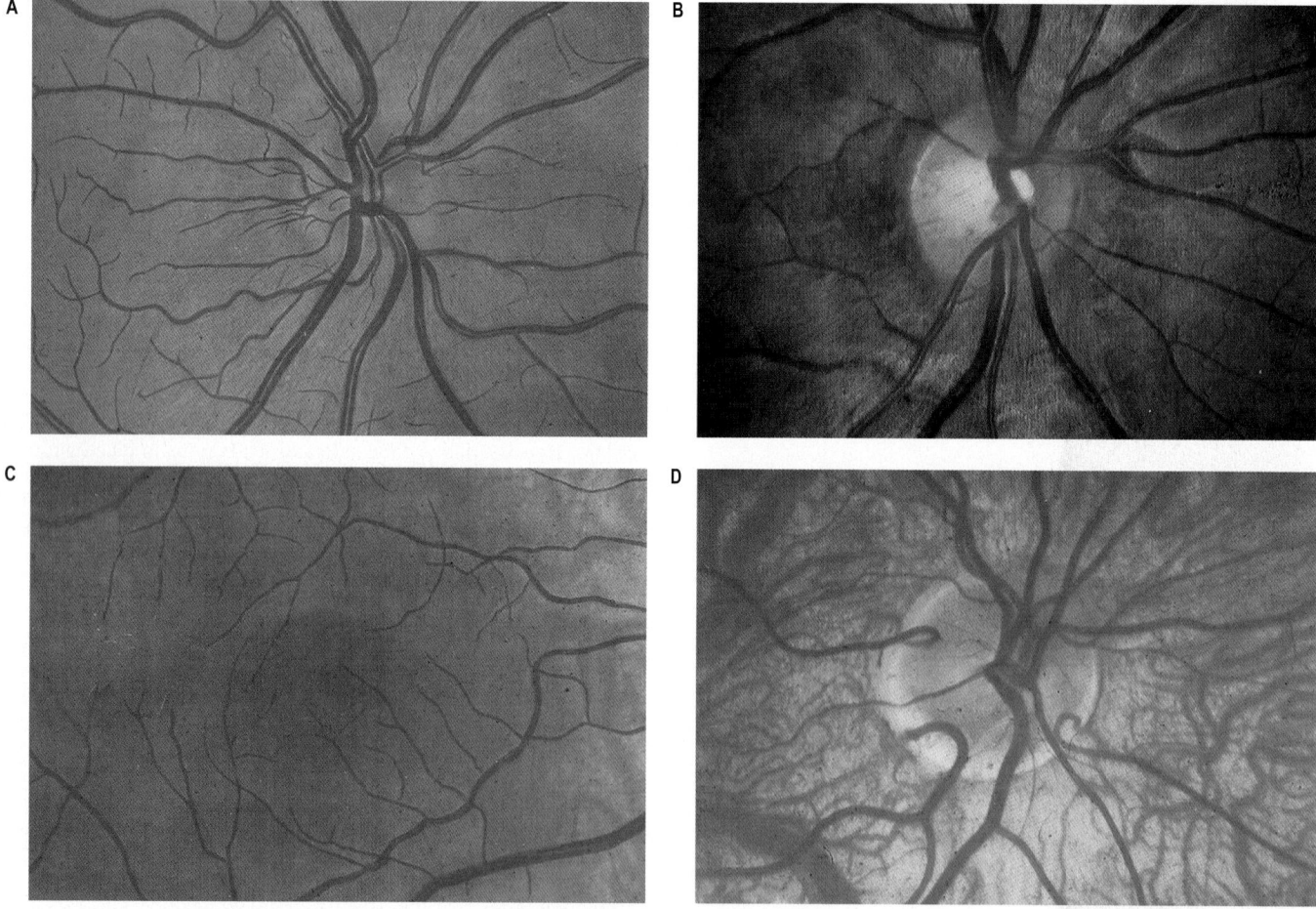

Fig. 42.13 Ophthalmoscopic photographs of the right human retina. **A**, Note dichotomous branching of vessels, arteries being brighter red and showing a more pronounced 'reflex' to light, as a pale stria along their length. The veins are also larger in calibre; more of them cross arteries superficially than is usual. The optic disc, around the entry of the vessels, is a light pink, with a surrounding zone of heavier pigmentation. Compare with **Fig. 42.14A** from the same Caucasian adult. **B**, Appearances in a heavily pigmented individual (African-origin adult), with a paler optic disc than in A. Note accentuation of the edge of the disc by retinal and choroidal pigmentation. The arteries cross the veins superficially in this retina. **C**, Normal macula of a young Caucasian subject. The vessels radiate from the centrally placed fovea. The macular branches of the central retinal artery are approaching from the right. The macula is largely free of vessels of macroscopic size, but the capillaries here form a particularly close network, except at the fovea. **D**, The region of the optic disc in an eye with poorly developed pigmentation. Three cilioretinal arteries are curving round the edge of the disc (two on the left, one on the right). Between the two cilioretinal arteries a single macular artery is apparent. Due to the depressed pigmentation choroidal vessels are also visible, especially veins; and on the left of the photograph two large vorticose venous tributaries can be seen.

and purple in the fresh, unbleached state, because of the presence of rhodopsin (visual purple), but soon becomes opaque and bleached when exposed to light.

Near the centre of the retina there is a region 5–6 mm in diameter, which contains the macula lutea (**Fig. 42.14C,D**), an elliptical yellowish area, c.2 mm horizontally and 1 mm vertically. Its colour is due to the presence of xanthophyll derivatives. The macula lutea contains a central depression, the fovea centralis or foveola, with a diameter of c.0.4 mm, where visual resolution is highest (**Fig. 42.15**). Here, all elements except pigment epithelium cone photoreceptors are displaced laterally. The

minute size of the foveola is the reason why the visual axes must be directed with great accuracy in order to achieve the most discriminative vision.

About 3 mm medial (nasal) and 1 mm superior to the foveola, the optic nerve becomes continuous with the retina at the optic disc ('blind spot'). It is c.1.5 mm in diameter. The name 'optic papilla', often applied to the disc, is a misnomer, since almost all of a normal disc is level with the retina. Centrally it contains a shallow depression, where it is pierced by the central retinal vessels (**Figs 42.1**, **42.13**, **42.14A,B**). The disc is devoid of photoreceptors and is therefore insensitive to light.

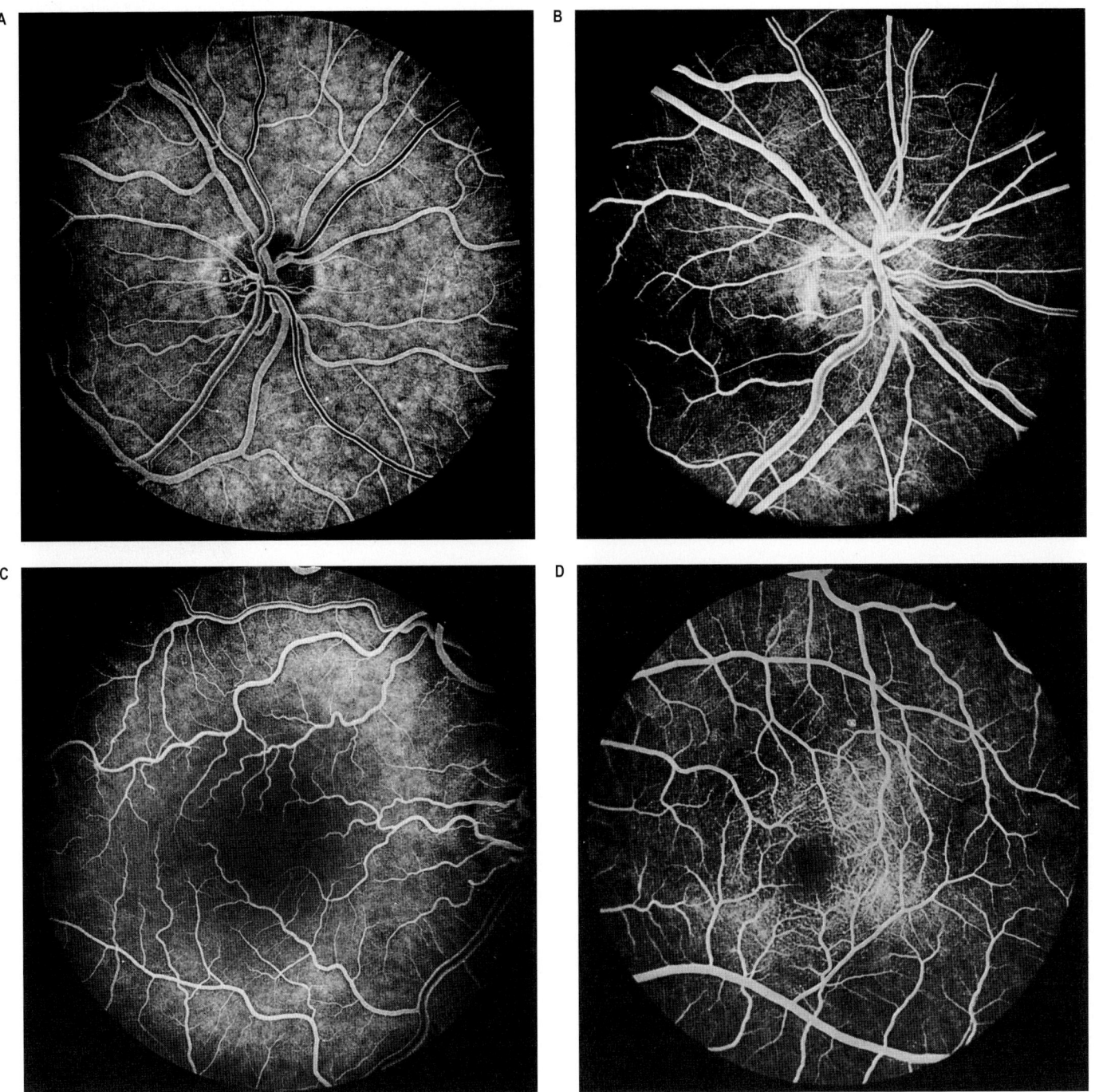

Fig. 42.14 Fluorescence angiograms of the retina. These are produced by photography with a fundus camera at known periods of time following introduction of fluorescein into the circulation. **A**, Angiogram of the same retina as that appearing in **Fig. 42.13A** taken in 'mid-venous' phase. The arteries display an even fluorescence, but the veins appear striped, due to laminar flow. This appearance is the reverse of and not to be compared with the arterial 'reflex' which is seen in **Fig. 42.13A**. The background mottling is due to fluorescence from the choroidal vessels. **B**, Angiogram of the left optic disc, showing the major arteries and veins and also their smaller branches. Note particularly the radial pattern in the retinal capillaries. The laminar flow in the veins is less obvious than in **Fig. 42.13A**. **C**, Angiogram showing the macular region of a right eye. The main macular vessels are approaching from the right. The subject was an elderly person with considerable macular pigmentation, which masks fluorescence from the choroidal circulation. Compare with: **D**, Angiogram of the macula of a young subject (left eye) showing the macular capillaries in detail. Note the central avascular fovea. Compare with C.

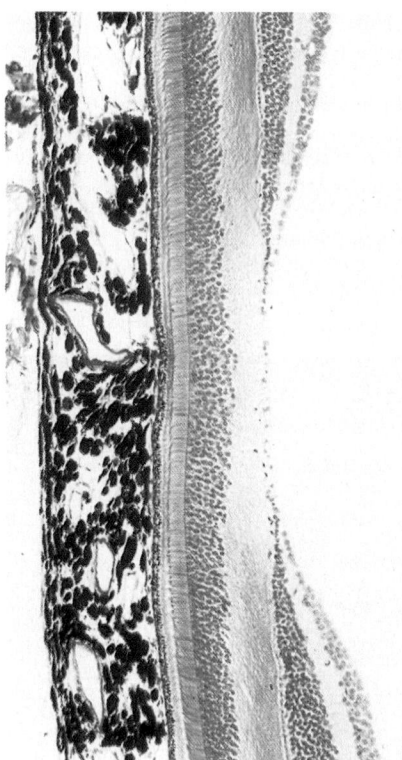

Fig. 42.15 Section through the fovea centralis. (By permission from Young B, Heath JW 2000 Wheater's Functional Histology. Edinburgh: Churchill Livingstone.)

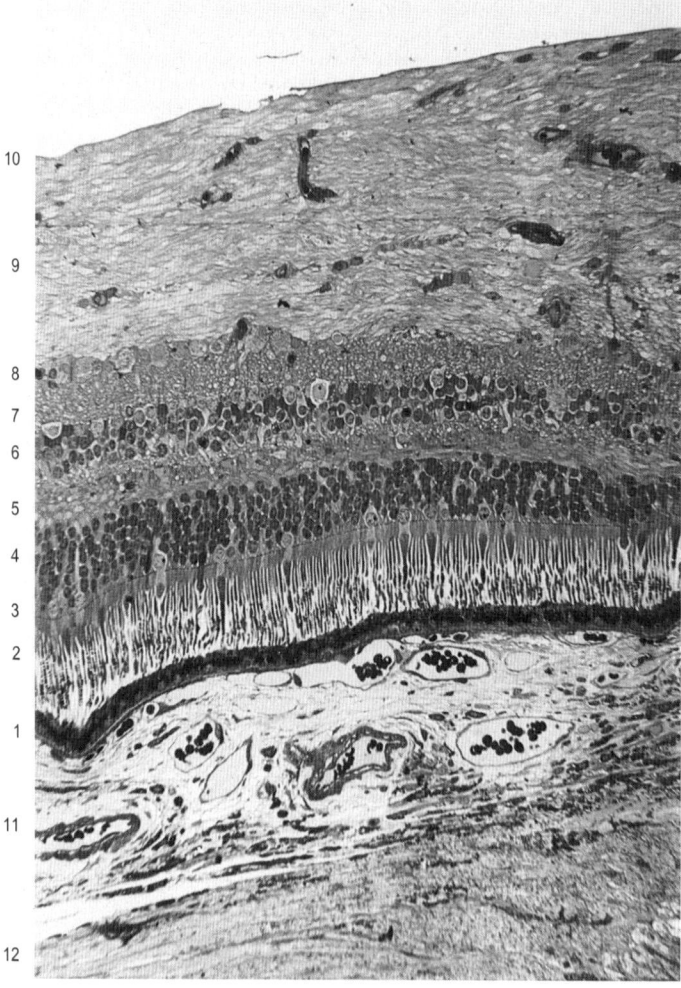

1. Pigment epithelial layer.
2. Rod and cone layer.
3. External limiting membrane.
4. Outer nuclear layer.
5. Outer plexiform layer.
6. Inner nuclear layer.
7. Inner plexiform layer.
8. Ganglion cell layer.
9. Nerve fibre layer.
10. Internal limiting membrane.
11. Choroid.
12. Sclera.

Fig. 42.16 The retina of a 60-year-old male. The section was made close to the optic nerve head explaining the thickened nerve fibre layer. (Provided by the late Gordon L Ruskell, Department of Optometry and Visual Science, The City University, London.)

By ophthalmoscopy it is normally pink but it is much paler than the retina, and may be grey or almost white. In optic atrophy the capillary vessels disappear and the disc is then white.

MICROSTRUCTURE

The retina is derived from the two layers of the invaginated optic vesicle (p. 245); the outer layer becomes the layer of pigment cells, the inner layer develops into a complex multilaminar structure of sensory and neural cells. Anteriorly, sensory and neural cells are absent from the retina as it approaches the ora serrata and merges into the ciliary body and iris (p. 705).

The neural retina contains a variety of cell types. They include the photoreceptors (rod and cone cells), their first order neurones (bipolar cells) and the somata and axons of the second order neurones (ganglion cells); and two major classes of interneurones, the horizontal and amacrine cells. The retina also contains neuroglial elements and a rich vascular system, chiefly of capillaries. It is backed by specialized pigment epithelial cells.

LAYERS OF THE RETINA (Fig. 42.16)

The retina is organized into layers or zones where distinctive components of its cells are clustered together or in register to form continuous strata. These layers extend uninterrupted throughout the photoreceptive retina except at the exit point of the optic nerve fibres at the optic disc, although certain layers are much reduced at the foveola where the photoreceptive elements predominate. The names given to the different layers reflect in part the components present within them, and also their position in the thickness of the retina. Conventionally, those structures furthest from the vitreous (i.e. towards the choroid) are designated as outer or external, and those towards the vitreous are inner or internal.

Customarily, ten retinal layers are distinguished (**Fig. 42.17**), beginning at the choroidal edge and passing towards the vitreous. These are: retinal pigment epithelium; layer of rods and cones (outer segments and inner segments); external limiting membrane; outer nuclear layer; outer plexiform layer (OPL); inner nuclear layer (INL); inner plexiform layer (IPL); ganglion cell layer; nerve fibre layer; internal limiting membrane. Some of these are subdivisible into substrata, and an innermost plexiform layer between layers 8 and 9 has also been demonstrated.

Rod and cone cells reach radially inwards from the rod and cone lamina through the outer nuclear layer, where they have their nuclei, to the outer plexiform layer in which they synapse with bipolar and horizontal cells. Bipolar cells possess dendrites in the outer plexiform layer, cell bodies and nuclei in the inner nuclear layer, and axons in the inner plexiform layer where they synapse with ganglion cell and amacrine cell dendrites. Horizontal cells have their dendrites and axons in the outer plexiform layer and their nuclei in the inner nuclear layer, while ganglion cells have their dendrites in the inner plexiform layer, their cell bodies in the ganglion cell layer, and their axons in the layer of nerve fibres (and within the optic nerve). Amacrine cell dendrites are mainly in the inner plexiform layer, although some (interplexiform cells) extend into the outer plexiform layer; amacrine cell dendrites are either situated in the inner nuclear layer or in the outer part of the ganglionic layer (displaced amacrines). Pigment cells lie behind the retina, and several types of retinal glial cell are distributed in distinctive locations among its different layers.

The composition of the different retinal layers is as follows:

Layer 1: Pigment epithelium – This is a simple low cuboidal epithelium which forms the back of the retina, and, therefore forms the boundary with the choroid, from which it is separated by a thick composite basal lamina.

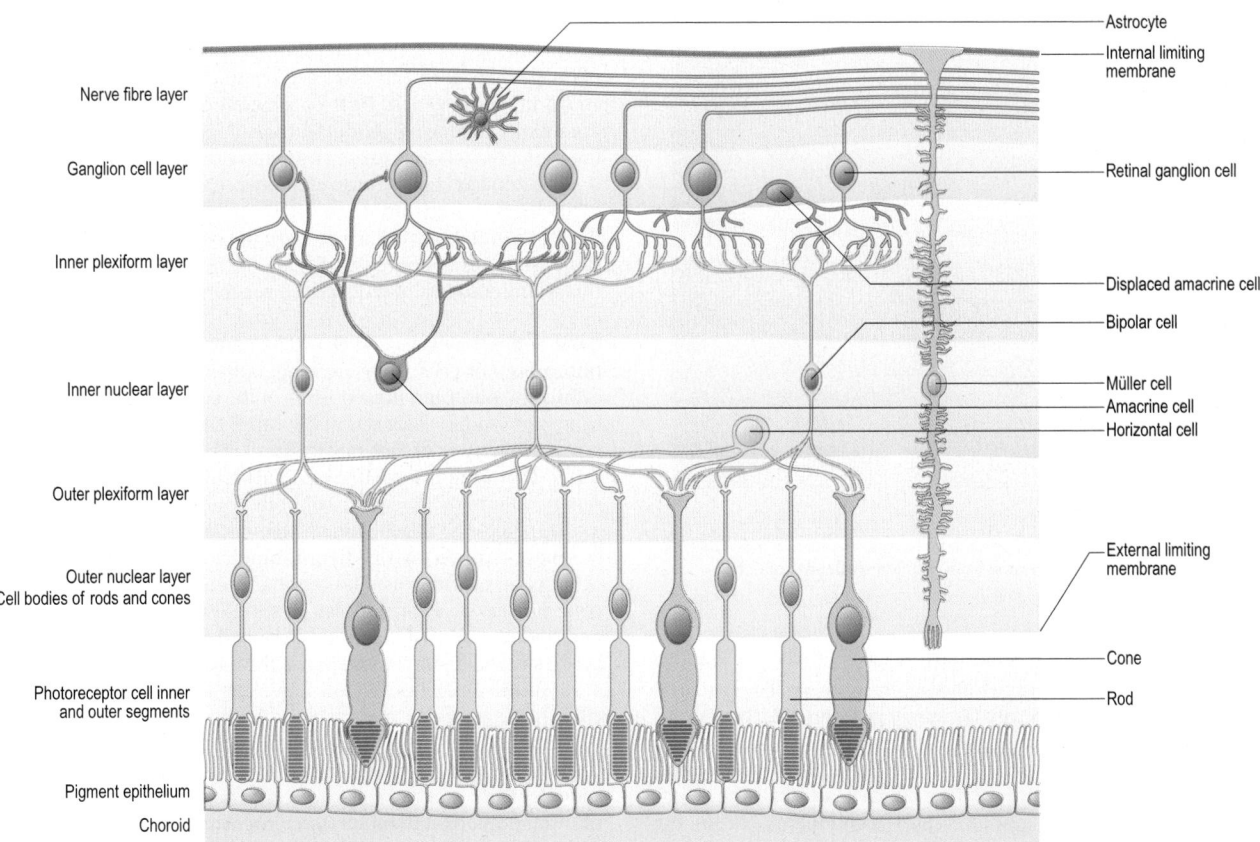

Nerve fibre layer

Ganglion cell layer

Inner plexiform layer

Inner nuclear layer

Outer plexiform layer

Outer nuclear layer
Cell bodies of rods and cones

Photoreceptor cell inner
and outer segments

Pigment epithelium
Choroid

Astrocyte
Internal limiting
membrane

Retinal ganglion cell

Displaced amacrine cell
Bipolar cell

Müller cell
Amacrine cell
Horizontal cell

External limiting
membrane

Cone

Rod

Fig. 42.17 The layered arrangement of neuronal cell bodies in the retina and the interconnections of their processes in the intervening plexiform layers. Also shown are the two principal types of neuroglial cell in the retina; microglia are also present but not shown.

Layer 2: Rod and cone cell processes – This contains the photoreceptive outer segments and the outer part of the inner segments of rod and cone cells.

Layer 3: External limiting membrane – This layer appears as a distinct line by light microscopy. It consists of a zone of intercellular junctions of the zonula adherens type (p. 7) between the processes of radial glial cells and photoreceptor processes.

Layer 4: Outer nuclear layer – This consists of several tiers of rod and cone cell bodies and their nuclei, the cone nuclei lying outermost. Mingled with these are the outer and inner fibres from the same cell bodies, directed outward to the bases of inner segments, and inwards towards the outer plexiform layer.

Layer 5: Outer plexiform layer – This is a region of complex synaptic arrangements between the processes of the cells whose cell bodies lie in the adjacent layers. The outer plexiform layer contains the synaptic processes of rod and cone cells, bipolar cells, horizontal cells, and some interplexiform cells (which in this account are grouped with the amacrines).

Layer 6: Inner nuclear layer – This is composed of three nuclear strata. Horizontal cell nuclei form the outermost zone, then in sequence inwards, the nuclei and cell bodies of bipolar cells, radial glial cells, and the outer set of amacrine cells, including the interplexiform cells whose dendrites cross this layer.

Layer 7: Inner plexiform layer – This is divisible into three layers depending on the types of contact occurring. The outer or 'OFF' layer contains synapses between 'OFF' bipolar cells, ganglion cells and some amacrines; a middle or 'ON' layer contains synapses between the axons of 'ON' bipolars and the dendrites of ganglion cells and displaced amacrines; and an inner 'rod' layer contains synapses between rod bipolars and displaced amacrines. (Refer to Wässle & Boycott 1991 for an explanation of the 'OFF' and 'ON' cell designations.)

Layer 8: Ganglion cell layer – This layer contains the nuclei of the displaced amacrine cells. Its inner regions consist of the cell bodies, nuclei and initial segments of retinal ganglion cells of various classes.

Layer 9: Nerve fibre layer – This contains the unmyelinated axons of retinal ganglion cells. It forms a zone of variable thickness over the inner retinal surface, and is the only component of the retina at the point where the fibres pass into the nerve at the optic disc. The inner aspect of this layer contains the nuclei and processes of astrocytes which, together with radial glial cells, ensheath the nerve fibres. Between the nerve fibre layer and the ganglion cells there is another narrow innermost plexiform layer where neuronal processes make synaptic contact with the axon hillocks and initial segments of ganglion cells.

Layer 10: Internal limiting membrane – This is a glial boundary between the retina and the vitreous body. It is formed by the end feet of radial glial cells and astrocytes, and is separated from the vitreous body by a basal lamina.

CELLS OF THE RETINA

Retinal pigment epithelial cells – The retinal pigment epithelial cells are low cuboidal cells which form a single continuous layer extending from the periphery of the optic disc to the ora serrata, and continue from there into the ciliary epithelium (p. 705). They are flat in radial section, hexagonal or pentagonal in surface view and number about 4–6 million in the human retina. Their cytoplasm contains numerous melanin granules (**Fig. 42.18**). Apically (towards the rods and cones), the cells bear long (5–7 μm) microvilli which contact or project between the outer ends of rod and cone processes. The tips of rod outer segments are deeply inserted into invaginations in the apical membrane. The attachments are unsupported by junctional complexes and are broken in the clinical condition of retinal detachment arising from trauma or disease processes.

Pigment epithelial cells play a major role in the turnover of rod and cone photoreceptive components. Their cytoplasm contains the

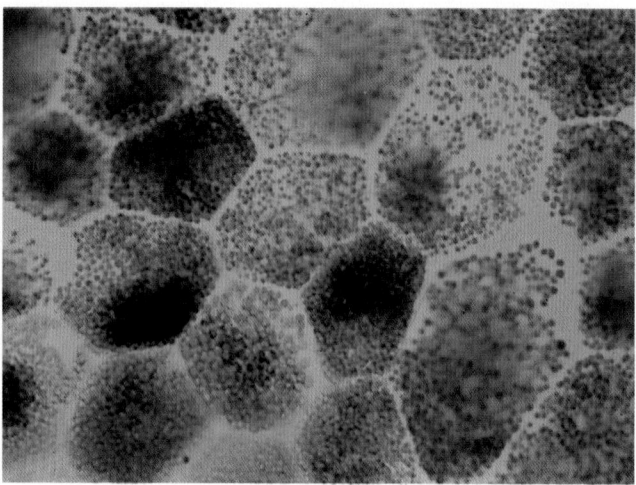

Fig. 42.18 Unstained retinal pigment epithelium from a 40-year-old individual, seen in surface view. (By kind permission from John Marshall, Institute of Ophthalmology, London.)

phagocytosed ends of rods and cones undergoing lysosomal destruction. The final products of this process are lipofuscin granules, which accumulate in these cells and add to their granular appearance. The failure of some part of this process may cause progressive loss of retinal function and eventual blindness, e.g. when enzyme deficiencies cause the build-up of shed, but undegraded, photoreceptor components within the retina.

The epithelium also acts as an anti-reflection device and prevents the light bouncing back into the photoreceptive layer with consequent loss of image sharpness. This process is complex, because the energy absorbed could be dissipated as heat or generate free radicals, which are both potentially damaging products. Indeed, very intense light may damage the pigment cells and cause epithelial breakdown.

The zone of tight junctions between the pigment cells allows the epithelium to function as an important blood–retinal barrier between the retina and the vascular system of the choroid. These guard the special ionic environment of the retina, and inhibit the entry of leukocytes into this immunologically sequestered compartment of the eye.

Cone and rod cells (Fig. 42.19) – The cone and rod cells are the retinal photoreceptor cells. They are long, radially orientated structures with a cylindrical photoreceptive portion at the end nearest the pigment epithelium and synaptic contacts at the other end, within the outer plexiform layer. Both types of cell have a similar organization, although details differ. From the external (choroidal) end inwards, the cells consist of outer and inner segments, a cell body containing the nucleus, and either a cone pedicle or a rod spherule (depending on cell type); this is an area of synaptic contact with adjacent bipolar and horizontal cells and with other cone or rod cells. The outer and inner segments together form a cone process or a rod process (it should be noted that the terms cone and rod are also often loosely applied to the whole cell); the cone process is wider, but tapers (hence the name), whereas the rod processes are cylindrical. The outer and inner segments are connected by a short cilium.

Cone cells are chiefly responsible for high spatial resolution and colour vision in good lighting conditions (photopic vision). Rod cells provide high monochromatic sensitivity to a much wider range of illumination down to much lower intensities (scotopic vision), although with relatively low spatial discrimination because of their different

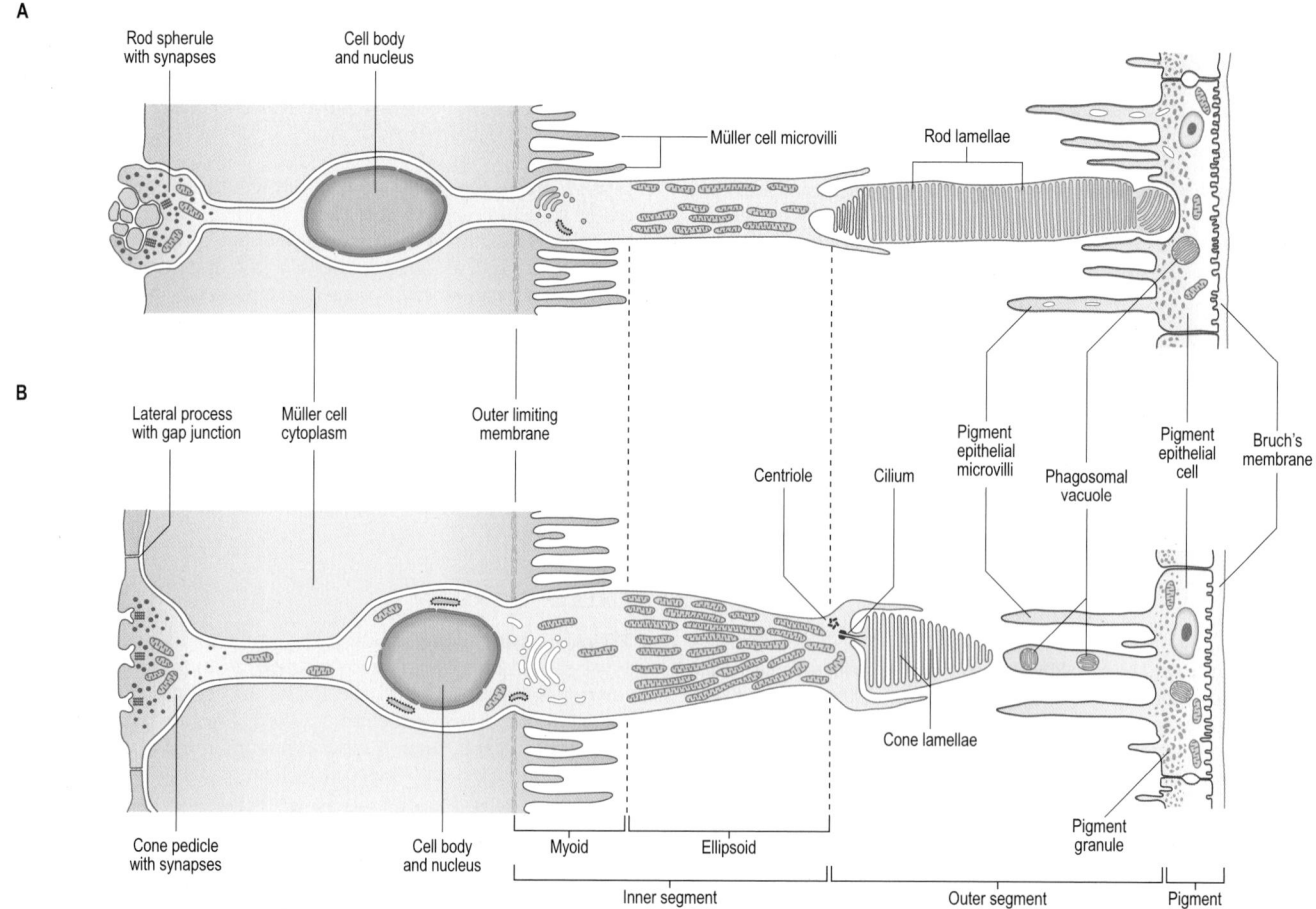

Fig. 42.19 The major features of (**A**) a retinal rod cell and (**B**) a retinal cone cell. Note that the relative size of the pigment epithelial cells has been exaggerated for illustrative purposes.

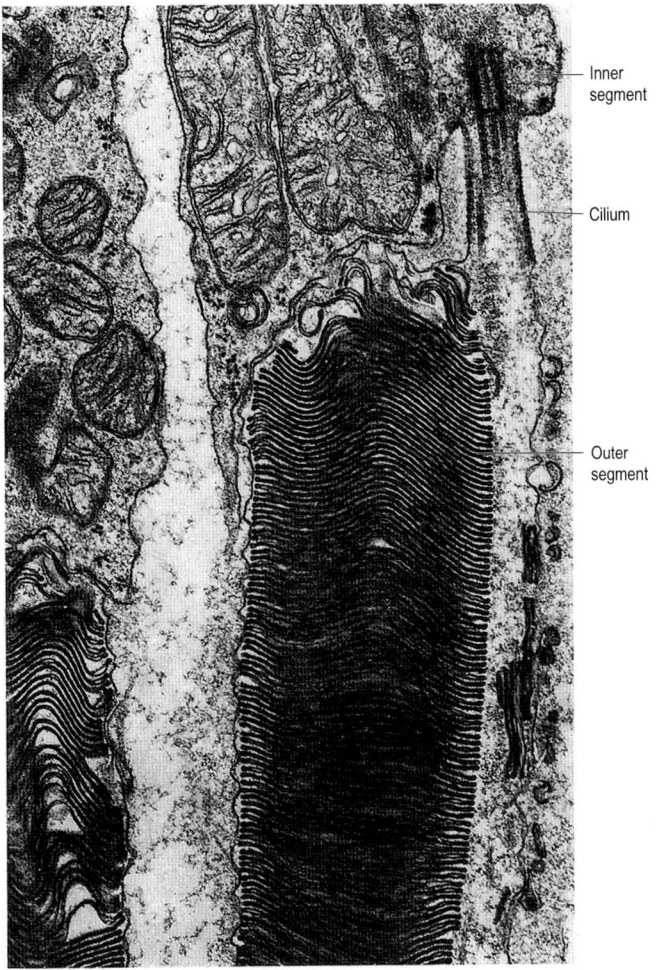

Inner segment

Cilium

Outer segment

Fig. 42.20 Section of a human retinal rod showing the junction between the inner and outer segments. (By kind permission from G Vrenson and B Willekens, Ophthalmic Research Institute of Amsterdam.)

neural connections. Cone cells are of three types, red, green and blue, according to their maximum spectral sensitivities. They are highly concentrated in the centre of the retina (the fovea) where visual acuity is greatest, but they populate the whole retina, intermingled with rods, as far as its neural edge. Rods are excluded from the fovea. The total number of rods in the human retina has been estimated at 110–125 million, and of cones at 63–68 million (Österberg 1935).

The outer segments of rods contain the photoreceptive protein rhodopsin (visual purple). Related photosensitive pigments with different absorption properties are present in cones. Photoreceptive pigments are incorporated into flattened membranous discs which form as deep infoldings of the plasma membrane and stack together within the photoreceptor outer segments (**Fig. 42.20**). They bud off as free discs within the outer segment of rods, where their turnover is rapid. New discs are generated at the proximal end closest to the soma, and shed at the distal end embedded in the pigment epithelium, where they are phagocytosed. Turnover appears to be less rapid in cones, where the discs retain continuity with the plasma membrane, and a more random insertion of disc components may occur. Cones are much narrower at the fovea where they closely resemble rods in size.

Bipolar cells (Fig. 42.17) – Bipolar cells are radially orientated neurones, each with one or more dendrites which synapse with cones or rods and horizontal cells and interplexiform cells in the outer plexiform layer. Their somata are located in the inner nuclear layer, and axonal branches given off in the inner plexiform layer synapse with dendrites of ganglion cells or amacrine cells (**Fig. 42.17**). Cone bipolars are of three major types, namely midget, blue cone or diffuse, according to their connectivity and size. As their name implies, midget cone bipolars are small cells, each one a part of a single, one-to-one, channel from cone to

ganglion cell; they are thought to mediate high spatial resolution. Blue cones have similar connectivity and selectively form part of a short wavelength mediating channel. The larger diffuse cone bipolars are connected to up to ten cones and are thought to signal luminosity rather than colour. Rod bipolars receive direct photoreceptive inputs from many rods and relate to ganglion cells indirectly via a synapse with amacrine cells.

Horizontal cells (Fig. 42.17) – Horizontal cells are inhibitory interneurones whose dendrites and axons extend within the outer plexiform layer, making synaptic contacts with the bases of cones and rods, and, via gap junctions at the tips of their dendrites, with each other. Their cell bodies lie in the outer part of the inner nuclear layer. Because of their interactions with photoreceptor cells and bipolar cells, horizontal cells create inhibitory surrounds. When illumination of a photoreceptor cluster with a point of light causes depolarization of synaptically connected 'ON' bipolars at its bright centre, horizontal cell dendrites cause inhibition at the edge of the illuminated area, thus sharpening contrast and maximizing spatial resolution.

Amacrine cells (Fig. 42.17) – Amacrine cells lack typical axons but their dendrites function as axons and dendrites, and make both incoming and outgoing synapses. Each neurone has a cell body either in the inner nuclear layer; near its boundary with the inner plexiform layer; or on the outer aspect of the ganglion cell layer, when they are known as displaced amacrine neurones. The processes of amacrine neurones make scattered chemical synaptic contacts with the axons of bipolar cells; dendrites (and possibly axons) of ganglion cells; and the processes of other amacrine cells. They also receive numerous synapses from bipolar cells. Some amacrine cells form electrical synapses with bipolar cells.

There are several classes of amacrine cell which variously serve a number of important functions in vision. One class (amacrine II cells) transmits signals from rod bipolars on to ganglion cells and is therefore an essential element in the rod pathway. Others appear to be important modulators of photoreceptive signals, and serve to adjust or maintain relative colour and luminosity inputs under changing light conditions, e.g. at different times of day. They are probably responsible for some of the complex forms of image analysis known to occur within the retina, e.g. directional movement detection.

Ganglion cells (Fig. 42.17) – Ganglion cells are the final common pathway neurones of the retina. Their dendrites are synaptically connected with processes of bipolar and amacrine neurones in the inner plexiform layer, and their axons likewise with neurones in the CNS. Their axons form the layer of nerve fibres on the inner surface of the retina. They turn tangentially to the optic disc, through which they leave the eye as fibres of the optic nerve, and the axons are subsequently distributed to various parts of the brain including the lateral geniculate nucleus, pretectal area and superior colliculus of the midbrain, the thalamic pulvinar and the accessory optic system.

Ganglion cell bodies form a single stratum in most of the retina, but become progressively more numerous near the macula. They are ranked in about 10 rows in the macular area, and their number diminishes again towards the fovea, from which they are almost totally excluded. Ganglion cells are multipolar neurones, varying from 10–30 μm or more in diameter. Their dendrites vary in number and branching patterns, and usually emerge opposite the axon. Numbers of ganglion cells in the human macular area reach 38,000/mm²: they are more numerous in the nasal retina than the temporal, and in the superior retina compared with the inferior, although numbers vary considerably in different eyes. In total, each human retina has c.10^6 ganglion cells, each of which receives signals from large numbers of photoreceptor cells.

Nerve fibre layer – In the nerve fibre layer, axons of ganglion cells converge on to the optic disc from the whole retina. They converge in a simple radial pattern from the medial (nasal) half of the retina. However, the macular area, inferolateral to the optic disc, complicates the course of the lateral (temporal) axons. Axons from the macula form a papillomacular fasciculus which passes almost straight to the disc. The more temporal fibres, which are more peripheral, swerve circumferentially above and below the macula to reach the disc.

Axons of ganglion cells are almost always non-myelinated within the retina, which is an optical advantage because myelin is refractile. They are surrounded by the processes of radial glial cells and retinal astrocytes. A few small myelinated fibres may occur, but in general myelin sheaths usually only commence as the axons enter the optic disc to become the optic nerve.

Retinal glial cells

Retinal glial cells are of three types, radial (Müller) cells, astrocytes and microglia. Radial glial cells form the predominant glial element of most of the retina. Retinal astrocytes are largely confined to the ganglion cell and nerve fibre layers. Microglial cells are scattered throughout the neural part of the retina in small numbers (**Fig. 42.17**).

Radial glial cells span the entire thickness of the neural retina. They ensheath and separate the various photoreceptive and neural cells except at synaptic sites. They form the outer boundary of the retinal tissue at the level of the inner rod and cone segments, and the inner boundary at the internal limiting membrane. Their nuclei lie within the inner nuclear layer, and from this region a single thick fibre ascends radially, giving off complex lateral lamellae which branch among the processes of the outer plexiform layer. Apically the central process terminates in a surface from which microvilli project into the space between the rod and cone processes. Just beneath this area the radial glial cells form a line of dense zonulae adherentes with each other and with receptor inner segments, and so form the external limiting membrane. On the inner aspect of the retina, the main radial glial cell process expands in a terminal foot plate which contacts those of neighbouring radial glial cells and astrocytes and attaches to the internal limiting membrane. Like other neuroglia (Chapter 4), radial glia also contact blood vessels, especially capillaries, and their basal laminae fuse with those of the vascular smooth muscle in the media of larger vessels or of the endothelia lining capillaries. These extensive neuroglial cells form much of the total retinal volume, and almost totally fill the extracellular space between neural elements. Their functions appear to be similar to those of astrocytes, i.e. maintenance of the stability of the retinal extracellular environment by ionic transport; uptake of neurotransmitter; removal of debris; storage of glycogen; electrical insulation of receptors and neurones; mechanical support of the neural retina.

The cell bodies of retinal astrocytes lie between the layer of nerve fibres and the internal limiting membrane, whilst their processes branch to form sheaths around ganglion cell axons. They are present only in regions of the retina that are vascularized, and are therefore absent from the fovea. Astrocytes contribute substantially to the glia limitans which surrounds the capillaries. Retinal microglia are scattered mainly within the inner plexiform layer. Their radiating branched processes spread mainly parallel to the retinal plane, and this gives them a star-like appearance when viewed microscopically from the surface of the retina. They can act as phagocytes, and their number increases in the injured retina.

Internal limiting membrane – The expanded end-feet of radial glial cells and astrocytes are separated from the vitreous body by a complex, rather thick (0.5 μm) internal limiting membrane which is continuous with the internal limiting membrane of the ciliary body. The delicate collagen fibrils of the vitreous body blend with the glial basal lamina. The internal limiting membrane is involved in fluid exchange between the vitreous and the retina and, perhaps through the latter, with the choroid. It has various other functions including anchorage of retinal glial cells, and inhibition of cell migration into the vitreous body.

Modifications in the macular area – All the retinal layers are modified in the macular area, and to a marked degree in the fovea, which is largely devoid of rod cells or processes. Approximately 2500 close-packed, elongated, very narrow cone cells lie in the floor of the fovea (foveola), an arrangement which favours photopic vision, and the high degree of spatial discrimination typical of foveal vision.

The general displacement of the outer nuclear layer to the foveal periphery means that the internal processes of the photoreceptors are stretched out tangentially in the external plexiform layer, and consequently there are no cone pedicles or rod spherules in the central fovea and foveola. The inner nuclear layer is also displaced to the edge of the foveal depression, and the internal plexiform, ganglionic and nerve fibre layers are almost absent from the whole fovea. Therefore, even on the foveal wall, the retina is thinner and more transparent than elsewhere. Capillaries reach the foveal margin, but they only invade the ganglionic layer at its circumference, so that the fovea is normally devoid of all blood vessels.

OPTIC DISC AND RETINAL BLOOD VESSELS

The retina is placed between two sets of arteries and veins, the ciliary vessels of the choroid, and the branches of the central retinal vessels. It depends on both circulations, since neither is sufficient independently to maintain full visual activity in the retina. The choroidal circulation is described on page 716, and the orbital and intraneural parts of the central retinal vessels are described on page 705. The central retinal vessels enter and leave the retina at the optic disc, which will be described before the vessels are considered.

Optic disc (Figs 42.1, 42.2, 42.13, 42.14)

The optic disc is the region where retinal tissues meet the neural and glial elements of the optic nerve and the connective tissues of the sclera and meninges. It is the exit point for the optic nerve fibres, and a point of entry and exit for the retinal circulation. It is the only site where anastomoses occur with other arteries (the posterior ciliary arteries). It is visible, by ophthalmoscopy , and is a region of much clinical importance, since it is here that the central vessels can be inspected directly: the only vessels so accessible in the whole body. Oedema of the disc (papilloedema) may be the first sign of raised intracranial pressure, which is transmitted into the subarachnoid space around the optic nerve and compresses the central retinal vein where it crosses the space.

The optic disc is superomedial to the posterior pole of the eye, and so lies away from the visual axis. It is round or oval, usually c.1.6 mm in transverse diameter and 1.8 mm in vertical diameter, and its appearance is very variable (for details see Jonas et al 1988). In light-skinned subjects, the general retinal hue is a bright terracotta-red, with which the pale pink of the disc contrasts sharply; its central part is usually even paler and may be light grey. These differences are due in part to the degree of vascularization of the two regions, which is much less at the optic disc, and also to the total absence of choroidal or retinal pigment cells, since the retina is represented in the disc by little more than the internal limiting membrane. In subjects with strongly melanized skins, both retina and disc are darker (**Fig. 42.13B**). The optic disc does not project at all in many eyes, and rarely does it project sufficiently to justify the term papilla. It is usually a little elevated on its lateral side, where the papillomacular nerve fibres turn into the optic nerve. There is usually a slight depression where the retinal vessels traverse its centre.

RETINAL VASCULAR SUPPLY

The central retinal artery enters the optic nerve as a branch of the ophthalmic artery, c.1.2 cm behind the eyeball. It travels in the optic nerve to its head, where its fascicles traverse the lamina cribrosa. At this level, which is usually not visible to ophthalmoscopy, the central artery divides into two equal branches, superior and inferior. After a few millimetres, these divide into superior and inferior nasal, and superior and inferior temporal, branches. Each of these four supplies its own 'quadrant' of the retina, although each territory is much more than a quadrant, since the branches ramify as far as the ora serrata. Corresponding retinal veins unite to form the central retinal vein. However, the courses of the venous and arterial vessels do not correspond exactly, and arteries often cross veins, usually lying superficial to them. In severe hypertension the arteries may press on the veins and cause visible dilations distal to these crossings. Arterial pulsation is not visible by routine ophthalmoscopy without higher magnification.

The branching of the artery is usually dichotomous, and equal rami diverge at angles of 45–60°. Smaller branches may leave singly and at right angles. Arteries and veins ramify in the nerve fibre layer, near the internal limiting membrane, which accounts for their clarity when seen through an ophthalmoscope (**Figs 42.13, 42.14A,B**). Arterioles pass deeper into the retina and may penetrate to the internal nuclear lamina, from which venules return to larger superficial veins. The question of whether or not the dense capillary bed is diffusely organized or layered is unsettled. Some lamination has been identified, most noticeably at the interface between the inner nuclear and outer plexiform layers. The structure of the blood vessels resembles that of vessels elsewhere, except that the internal elastic lamina is absent from the arteries, and muscle cells may appear in their adventitia. Capillaries have a non-fenestrated endothelium.

Microcirculatory studies of the human retina in flat preparations, stained after trypsin digestion, have revealed many details of the capillary arrangement. It resembles that seen in renal glomeruli, i.e. a network of capillaries which connect individual arterioles and venules which are themselves devoid of anastomoses and arteriovenous shunts. Thus the territories of the arteries which supply a particular quadrant do not overlap, nor do the branches within a quadrant anastomose with each other. In consequence, a blockage in a retinal artery causes loss of vision in the corresponding part of the visual field. The only exception to this end-arterial pattern is in the vicinity of the optic disc. Here, the posterior ciliary arteries enter the eye near the disc (**Figs 42.1, 42.7**), and their rami not only supply the adjacent choroid, but also form an anastomotic circle in the sclera around the head of the optic nerve (**Fig. 42.2**). Branches from this ring join the pial arteries of the nerve, and small cilioretinal arteries from any arteries in this region may enter the eye and contribute to the retinal vasculature (**Fig. 42.13D**). Similarly, small retinociliary veins may sometimes also be present.

Retinal capillaries do not pass towards the external surface of the retina beyond the inner nuclear lamina. They show regional differences in density, and are especially numerous in the macula, but absent from the central fovea. They become less numerous in the peripheral retina and are altogether absent from a zone c.1.5 mm wide which adjoins the ora serrata. Within the optic nerve, the central artery is innervated by sympathetic and parasympathetic fibres: the nerve supply does not extend to the retina.

OCULAR REFRACTIVE MEDIA

The components of the eye that transmit and refract light are the cornea, the aqueous humour, the lens and the vitreous body. Of these, only the refracting power of the lens can be varied. The cornea is described on page 702.

Aqueous humour

To satisfy the requirements of vision the eye has its own circulatory system. Aqueous humour is secreted into the posterior chamber by the non-pigmented epithelium of the ciliary processes. It passes into the anterior chamber through the pupil and drains to the scleral venous sinus at the iridocorneal angle through the spaces of the trabecular tissue. It is responsible for maintaining the metabolism of the avascular transparent media, vitreous, lens and cornea, and it also maintains and regulates the relatively high intraocular pressure (c.17 mmHg), and hence the constancy of the ocular dimensions of the eyeball, via the balance between production and drainage. Depth of the anterior chamber may be assessed using slit-lamp biomicroscopy, and the filtration angle may be viewed directly by gonioscopy. Any interference with its drainage into the sinus increases intraocular pressure leading to the condition of glaucoma.

GLAUCOMA

The characteristic physical sign of glaucoma is increased intraocular pressure, which is usually caused by obstruction of aqueous humour drainage at the iridocorneal angle (filtration angle). Increased formation of aqueous humour, or raised pressure in the veins draining the canal of Schlemm, are less commonly responsible. Although some drainage normally also occurs through uveoscleral channels, this alternative pathway cannot compensate adequately if the angle is blocked. Sustained raised pressure leads to defects in the visual field, and subsequently to blindness, either because of direct mechanical damage (particularly at the optic nerve head), or impairment of the blood supply, or both.

Glaucoma may be either primary or secondary to a specific anomaly or disease of the eye.

Secondary glaucoma

A variety of conditions may lead to secondary glaucoma: the following are the most common. Inflammatory glaucoma causes an increased pressure because the drainage channels become clogged by a turbid aqueous humour and by inflammatory exudates. As a later consequence of inflammation, exudates may form annular posterior synechiae, and these may attach the iris to the lens and prevent aqueous flow from the posterior to the anterior chamber. The root of the iris may attach to the cornea and block the angle: this may occur after perforation of the cornea, as a consequence of trauma or postoperatively, or following damage to the lens. Infantile glaucoma (buphthalmos) is an obstructive

type which is usually the result of a failure in the development of the tissues of the iridocorneal angle.

Primary glaucoma

The two distinct types of primary glaucoma are primary closed-angle and primary open-angle glaucoma. They differ in their clinical course and symptomatology. The closed-angle type characteristically affects hypermetropic eyes with a shallow anterior chamber where the angle is narrowed by the proximity of the root of the iris to the cornea. These features arise because the hypermetropic eye is generally small and the angle is likely to be narrowed further by the normal growth of the lens which presses the iris forward; lens development could explain the preponderance of the condition in the fifth and sixth decades, mostly in women. Attacks of raised pressure are usually sudden and subacute, and there is transient reduced vision and corneal oedema, followed later by persistent pressure instability. Without treatment, this ultimately leads to acute, painful congestive attacks and to permanent loss of vision.

Primary open-angle glaucoma is the commonest type, and the least readily diagnosed; there are no overt structural changes in the anterior segment of the eye. The disease is practically symptomless and slowly progressive, usually over several years. The outcome is similar to that of the other forms of glaucoma in that there is permanent congestion and blindness. Cellular changes in the trabecular meshwork reduce the facility of aqueous drainage, and this causes raised intraocular pressure, although the increment may not be maintained throughout the day. In the later stages a reduction in the visual field may be noticed.

Lens (Fig. 42.1, 42.21)

The lens is a transparent, encapsulated, biconvex body, which lies between the iris and the vitreous body. Posteriorly, the lens contacts the hyaloid fossa (p. 719) of the vitreous body. Anteriorly, it forms a ring of contact with the free border of the iris, but further away from the axis of the lens the gap between the two increases to form the posterior chamber of the eye (p. 708). The lens is encircled by the ciliary processes, and is attached to them by the zonular fibres which issue mainly from the pars plana of the ciliary body. Collectively, the fibres form the zonule which holds the lens in place and transmits the forces which stretch the lens (except in visual accommodation).

The lens has a characteristic shape (**Fig. 42.1**). Its anterior convexity is less steep, and has a greater radius of curvature, than the posterior, which has a more parabolic shape. The central points of these surfaces are the anterior and posterior poles; a line connecting these is the axis of the lens. The marginal circumference of the lens is its equator. In fetuses the lens is nearly spherical, has a slight reddish tinge, and is soft, such that it breaks up on application of the slightest pressure. A hyaloid artery from the central retinal artery traverses the vitreous body to the posterior pole of the lens, whence its branches spread as a plexus. This covers the posterior surface and is continuous round the capsular circumference with the vessels of the pupillary membrane and iris.

In infants and adults the lens is avascular, colourless and transparent, but still quite soft in texture. In old age, the anterior surface becomes a little more curved, which pushes the iris forward slightly. It becomes less clear, with an amber tinge, and its nucleus is denser. In cataract, the lens gradually becomes opaque, causing blindness.

The dimensions of the lens are optically and clinically important, but they change with age as a consequence of continuous growth. Its equatorial diameter at birth is 6.5 mm, increasing rapidly at first, then more slowly to 9.0 mm at 15 years of age, and even more gradually to reach 9.5 mm in the ninth decade. Its axial dimension increases from 3.5–4.0 mm at birth to 4.75–5.0 mm at age 95. The radii of curvature reduce throughout life; the anterior surface shows the greater change as the lens thickens (Brown 1974). Average adult radii of the anterior and posterior surfaces are 10 mm and 6 mm respectively; the reduction during accommodation occurs mainly at the anterior surface.

MICROSTRUCTURE OF THE LENS

The lens is derived from embryonic ectoderm (p. 198) and consists almost entirely of large numbers of stiff, very elongated, prismatic cells known as lens fibres, which are tightly packed together in a highly organized manner (**Fig. 42.22**). The anterior surface of the lens, as far as the equator, is covered by a layer of lens cells. The whole is surrounded

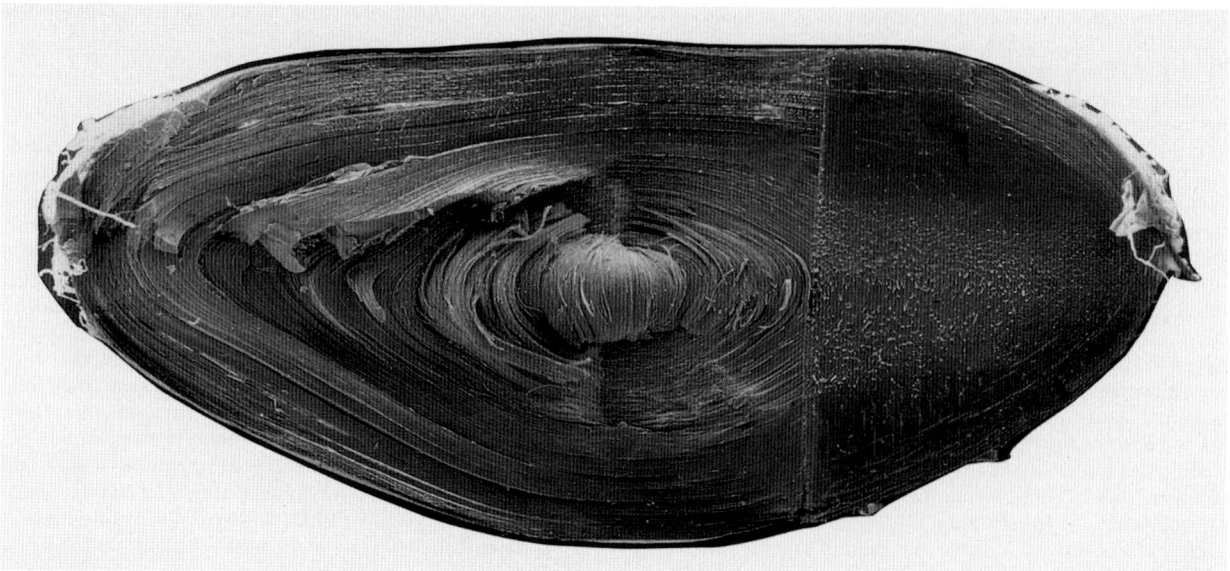

Fig. 42.21 An adult human lens, fractured across to reveal its lamellar structure. Note that the small central part with a different fibre orientation may represent the embryonic nucleus; the adult nucleus cannot be distinguished from the cortex. The more steeply curved surface (below) is posterior. The different texture of the lens in the right part of this picture is caused by cutting prior to the fracture procedure. (Reprinted from Experimental Eye Research, Vrensen et al, Membrane architecture as a function of lens maturation. 54: 433–446, 1992, with permission from Elsevier.)

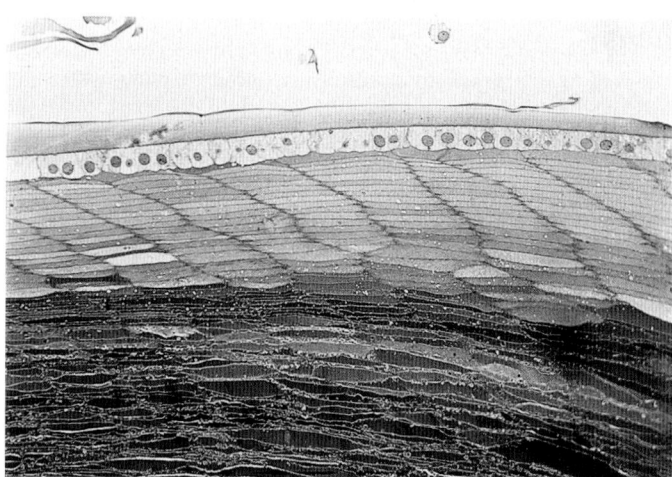

Fig. 42.22 Section through the anterior layers of the lens. The thin capsule covers the single row of epithelial cells and the lens substance is composed of regularly stacked younger fibres and more densely stained and complex deeper fibres. (Provided by the late Gordon L Ruskell, Department of Optometry and Visual Science, The City University, London.)

by the lens capsule. The lens is avascular and devoid of nerve fibres or other structures which might affect its transparency. Its surface forms a very effective barrier against invasion by cells or elements of the immune system, and so creates an immunologically sequestered environment.

LENS FIBRES

Each lens fibre is up to 12 mm long, depending on age and position in the lens (related to their time of formation). Fibres near the surface at the equator are nucleated, and the nuclei form a short S-shaped bow which extends inwards from the surface, reflecting their sequence of formation from the superficial layer of anterior epithelial cells. The deeper fibres lose their nuclei. In cross-section, individual fibres are flattened hexagons measuring c.10 μm by 2 μm. They are tightly packed, and adjacent fibres are firmly adherent and interlocked by innumerable junctions of various kinds, resembling ball-and-socket or tongue-and-groove joints, or close-fitting angular processes. Lens fibres are also in contact through desmosomes and numerous gap junctions.

The cells contain crystallins, proteins which are responsible for the transparency and refractile properties, and for much of the elasticity, of the lens. At least two varieties coexist, α and β. They occur in very high concentrations, and form up to 60% of the lens fibre mass. Variations in their concentration in different parts of the lens give rise to regional differences in refractive index, and these correct for spherical and chromatic aberrations which might otherwise occur in a homogeneous lens.

Variations in lens fibre structure and composition make it possible to distinguish a softer cortical zone and a firmer central part, the nucleus (**Fig. 42.21**). Where sheaves of lens fibres contact each other at their ends, faint sutural lines are formed, which radiate out from the poles towards the equator (**Fig. 42.23**). In fetuses, the sutures on the anterior surface of the lens form a triradiate pattern (**Fig. 42.23A**), centred on the anterior pole and resembling the limbs of an upright letter Y; posteriorly, a similar, though inverted, sutural configuration is present. In adults, the sutures increase in number and complexity as a consequence of lens growth and other changes in the arrangement of lens fibres (**Fig. 42.23B**). The sutures represent the lines of linearly registered interlocking junctions between terminating lens fibres. If an extracted lens is hardened with fixatives and then broken open, the arrangement of lens fibres produces a striking, onion-like appearance, the fibres splitting into a series of concentric lamellae of varying thicknesses (**Fig. 42.21**).

All lens fibres cross the equator (or the plane passing through it) where they are generated, and terminate on both an anterior and a posterior suture. Because of the curious growth pattern of the lens, fibres which start near the central axis of the lens anteriorly, terminate posteriorly on a suture near the periphery, and vice versa.

ANTERIOR LENS CELLS

Anterior lens cells form a transparent layer of simple cuboidal epithelium over the anterior surface of the lens (**Fig. 42.22**). They divide and migrate to the equator where they transform into lens fibres. In surface view, anterior lens cells are polygonal. They are c.15 μm across and slightly less in height, while in the central area they may be flattened to 6 μm. They are tall and thin towards the equator, and mitosis is more frequent. Near the equator of the lens, they differentiate, i.e. they synthesize the characteristic lens fibre proteins, and undergo extreme elongation. As other cells follow suit, the earlier cells come to occupy a deeper position in the lens; they lose their nuclei as new recruits are added to the lens fibre population.

Lens capsule

The lens capsule is a thick basement membrane which covers the outer surface of the lens (**Fig. 42.22**) and the anterior lens cell layer. It is thickest anteriorly (c.10 μm), becomes thinner posteriorly and consists of various classes of collagen fibre (I, III and IV), as well as a range of

A

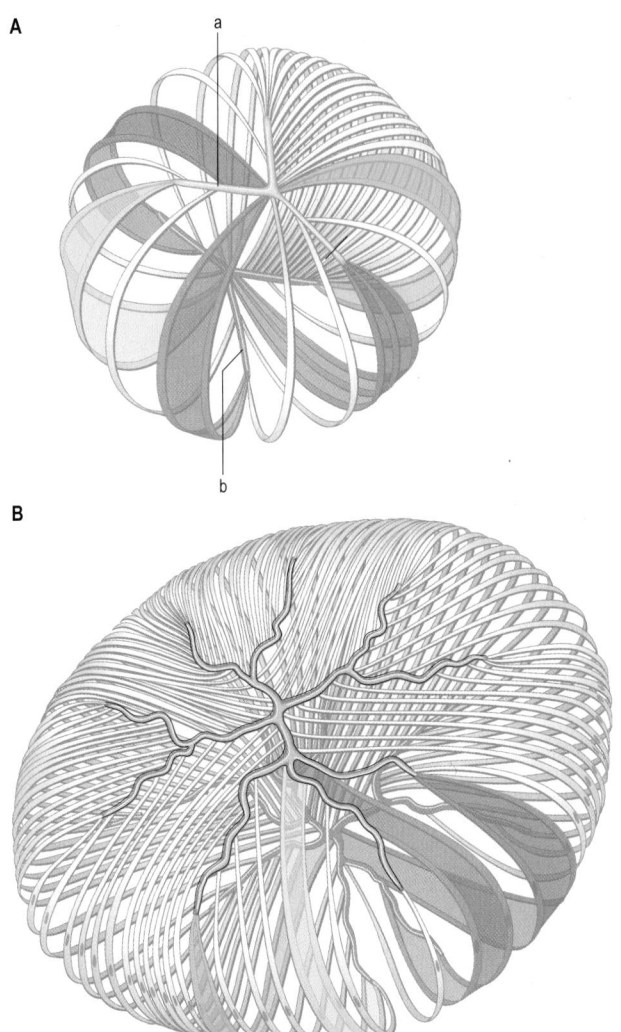

B

Fig. 42.23 The structure of the fetal (**A**) and adult (**B**) human lens, showing the major details of arrangement of the lens cells or fibres. The anterior (a) and posterior (b) triradiate sutures are shown in the fetal lens. Fibres pass from the apex of an arm of one suture to the angle between two arms at the opposite pole, as shown in the coloured segments. Intermediate fibres show the same reciprocal behaviour. The suture pattern becomes much more complex as successive strata are added to the exterior of the growing lens, and the original arms of each triradiate suture show secondary and tertiary dichotomous branchings. (By permission from Hogan MJ, Alvarado JA, Weddell JE 1971 Histology of the Human Eye. Philadelphia: WB Saunders.)

glycosaminoglycans and glycoproteins, e.g. fibronectin and laminin. It is probably derived from the anterior lens cells and their fetal precursors. The capsule is elastic: during lens flattening it can stretch up to about 60% in circumference without tearing. Zonular fibres are inserted into the capsule in the region of the equator. They are composed of thin (4–7 nm) fibrils with hollow centres, and resemble fibrils associated with elastic connective tissue fibres. They possess some elasticity, although this decreases with age.

LENS REFRACTION

The dioptric power of the lens is much less than that of the cornea. All ocular optical media have a refractive index close to that of water, but the corneal surface is in contact with air and most of the 60 dioptres of the refractive power of the eye are affected here. The value of the lens is its ability to vary its dioptric power, which is dependent upon its capacity to change shape. It has a greater refractive index than the adjacent media, varying from 1.386 at its periphery to 1.406 at its core, and contributes c.17 dioptres to the total of the relaxed eye. Its range in dioptric power permits a further 12 dioptres in youth, but the available dioptric range decreases with age, being halved at 40 years and reduced to 1 dioptre or less at 60. Most young children show minor refractive errors modifying towards emmetropia in preschool and later years.

For further information on physiological optics consult Bennett and Rabetts (1989).

DISORDERS OF REFRACTION

In a relaxed eye, when the refracting structures are so related to its length that the retina receives a focused image of a distant object it is said to be emmetropic. A majority of eyes are emmetropic or nearly so and this state is maintained throughout life including the early years when growth demands a fine adjustment between cornea, lens power and eye length. But a large minority, have errors of refraction or ametropia that takes three different forms. These are: myopia, when the eye is too long for its refractive power; hyperopia, when it is too short; and astigmatism, when the refractive power of the eye is not the same in different meridians. Astigmatism usually occurs together with myopia and hyperopia. In myopia the image falls in front of the retina and if accommodation is attempted, blurring of the image is increased, however the myope has the advantage that close objects at an appropriate distance are conjugate to the retina and are therefore seen clearly. In hyperopia the image falls on an imaginary point behind the retina but the hyperope has the advantage that with accommodation, increasing the power of the eye, the image can be brought to a focus. This requires effort, perhaps sufficient to cause symptoms of asthenopia. No adjustments can be made to correct for astigmatism but the condition may induce an unrewarding effort to seek the best focus and again give rise to symptoms. There is a hereditable factor in ametropia and a relationship with the demands of close work in the young is widely accepted. These errors of refraction are amenable to correction using spectacle or contact lenses or less commonly by various forms of refractive surgery.

There is a moderate deviation from emmetropia in the neonate including 1–3 dioptres of astigmatism in 50% and slight hyperopia. This is reduced after a year and mostly eliminated by school age when emmetropia predominates. Surveys show that in later years, mean hyperopia increases a fraction and myopia reduces.

During the fifth decade the ability to change the power of the lens diminishes to an extent that neither the corrected ametrope nor the emmetrope is able to focus near objects clearly and reading spectacles become necessary. The disability increases gradually until the ability to accommodate is completely lost in the seventh decade. This condition, presbyopia, is treated using reading lenses. It is offset to a very limited extent by the reduction of the pupil aperture with age. This increases depth of focus, but at the cost of creating the further problem of requiring greater illumination.

Other errors of refraction are the concomitants of eye disease, especially those which affect the cornea. Corneal curvature may be sufficiently altered as a residual defect of past disease to cause irregular astigmatism. This can be corrected conservatively only by using contact lenses which in effect provide a substitute for the irregular anterior corneal surface. In keratoconus, the cornea is thinned and steepened centrally, which distorts the refracting surface of the cornea to an extent that spectacle correction may not improve vision. Again contact lenses provide adequate treatment and in a large majority of cases keratoplasty does not become necessary. A dislocated lens, e.g. in Marfan's syndrome, disrupts the refractive status of the eye, and may not be amenable to spectacle correction.

Vitreous body

The vitreous body fills the vitreous chamber, and occupies about four-fifths of the eyeball. It is hollowed in front as a deep concavity, the hyaloid fossa, which is adapted to the lens. It is colourless, consisting of c.99% water, but not entirely structureless. At its perimeter it has a gel-like consistency (100–300 μm thick) and is firmly attached to the surrounding structures of the eye; nearer the centre it has a more liquid zone. Hyaluronan, in the form of long glycosaminoglycan chains, fills the whole vitreous. In addition, the peripheral gel or cortex contains a random loose network of type II collagen fibrils which are occasionally grouped into fibres. The cortex also contains scattered cells, the hyalocytes, which possess the characteristics of mononuclear phagocytes. They are responsible for the production of hyaluronan. Whilst they are normally in a resting state, they have the capacity to be actively phagocytic in inflammatory conditions. Hyalocytes are not present in the cortex bordering the lens. The liquid vitreous is absent at birth, appears first at 4 or 5 years, and increases to occupy half the vitreous

719

space by the seventh decade. The cortex is most dense at the pars plana of the ciliary body adjacent to the ora serrata, where attachment is strongest, and this is often referred to as the base of the vitreous. Here the vitreous is thickened into a mass of radial (zonular) fibres which form the suspensory ligament of the lens.

A narrow hyaloid canal (**Fig. 42.1**) runs from the optic nerve head to the central posterior surface of the lens. In the fetus this contains the hyaloid artery which normally disappears about 6 weeks before birth. It persists as a very delicate fibrous structure and is of no functional importance.

REFERENCES

Bennett AG, Rabbets RB 1989 Clinical Visual Optics, 2nd edn. London: Butterworth-Heinemann
   A detailed account of human ocular media in relation to physiological optics.
Brown NP 1974 The change in lens curvature with age. Exp Eye Res 19: 175–183
Hogan MJ, Alvarado JA, Weddell JE 1971 Histology of the Human Eye. Philadelphia: Saunders
Jonas JB, Gusek GC, Naumann GO 1988 Optic disc, cup and neuroretinal rim size, configuration and correlations in normal eyes. Invest Ophthalmol Vis Sci 29: 1151–1158
   A clinical template of a normal range.

Loewenstein O, Loewenfeld IE 1969 The pupil. In: Davson H (ed) The eye, vol. 3, New York: Academic Press
Osternerg GA 1935 Topography of the layers of the rods and cones in the human retina. Acta Ophthalmol Suppl 6
Wässle H, Boycott BB 1991 Functional architecture of the mammalian retina. Physiol Rev 71: 447–480
   Unitary cell responses of the various retinal neurones and their connectivity.

Development of the eye

The development of the eye involves a series of interactions between neighbouring tissues in the head. These are the neurectoderm of the forebrain, which forms the sensory retina and accessory pigmented structures; the surface ectoderm, which forms the lens and cornea, and the intervening neural crest mesenchyme, which contributes to the fibrous coats of the eye. These interactions lead to the development of the potential to form optic vesicles throughout a broad anterior domain of neurectoderm. Subsequent interactions between mesenchyme and neurectoderm subdivide this region into bilateral domains at the future sites of the eyes. The parallel process of lens determination appears to depend on a brief period of inductive influence which spreads through the surface ectoderm from the rostral neural plate and elicits a lens-forming area of the head. Reciprocal interactions which are necessary for the complete development of both tissues take place as the optic vesicle forms and contacts the potential lens ectoderm (Saha et al 1992). Vascular tissue of the developing eye may form by local angiogenesis or vasculogenesis of angiogenetic mesenchyme. (Accounts of the development of the eye are given in O'Rahilly 1966 and 1983.)

EMBRYONIC COMPONENTS OF THE EYE

The first morphological sign of eye development is a thickening of the diencephalic neural folds at 22 days postovulation, when the embryo has 7–8 somites. This optic primordium extends on both sides of the neural plate and crosses the midline at the primordium chiasmatis. A slight transverse indentation, the optic sulcus, appears in the inner surface of the optic primordium on each side of the brain. During the period when the rostral neuropore closes, at about 24 days, the walls of the forebrain at the optic sulcus begin to evaginate, projecting laterally towards the surface ectoderm so that, by 25 days, the optic vesicles are formed. The lumen of each vesicle is continuous with that of the forebrain. Cells delaminate from the walls of the optic vesicle and, probably joined by head mesenchyme and cells derived from the mesencephalic neural crest, invest the vesicle in a sheath of mesenchyme. By 28 days, regional differentiation is apparent in each of the source tissues of the eye. The optic vesicle is visibly differentiated into its three primary parts. Thus, a thick-walled region marks the future optic stalk at the junction with the diencephalon; laterally, the tissue which will become the sensory retina forms a flat disc of thickened epithelium in close contact with the surface ectoderm; and the thin-walled part of the vesicle which lies between these regions will later form the pigmented layer of the retina. The area of surface ectoderm that is closely apposed to the optic vesicle also thickens to form the lens placode. The mesenchymal sheath of the vesicle begins to show signs of angiogenesis. Between 32 and 33 days postovulation, the lens placode and optic vesicle undergo coordinated morphogenesis. The lens placode invaginates, forming a pit which pinches off from the surface ectoderm to form the lens vesicle. The surface ectoderm reforms a continuous layer which will become the corneal epithelium. The lateral part of the optic vesicle also invaginates to form a cup, the inner layer of which – facing the lens vesicle – will become the sensory retina, and the outer layer becomes the pigmented retinal epithelium. As a result of these folding movements, what were the apical (luminal) surfaces of the two layers of the cup now face one another across a much reduced lumen, the intraretinal space. The pigmented layer becomes attached to the mesenchymal sheath, but the junction between the pigmented and sensory layers is less firm and is the site of pathological detachment of the retina. The two layers are continuous at the lip of the cup which, at the end of the third month,

grows round the front of the lens and forms the pigmented iris. Between the base of the cup and the brain, the narrow part of the optic vesicle forms the optic stalk. The anteroventral surface of the vesicle and distal part of the stalk are also infolded, forming a wide groove – the choroid fissure – through which mesenchyme extends with an associated artery, the hyaloid artery. As growth proceeds, the fissure closes, and the artery is included in the distal part of the stalk. Failure of the optic fissure to close is a rare anomaly that is always accompanied by a corresponding deficiency in the choroid and iris (congenital coloboma).

DIFFERENTIATION OF THE FUNCTIONAL COMPONENTS OF THE EYE

The developments just described bring the embryonic components of the eye into the spatial relationships necessary for the passage, focusing, and sensing of light. The next phase of development involves further patterning and cell-type differentiation in order to develop the specialized structures of the adult organ.

The optic cup becomes patterned, from the base to the rim, into regions with distinct functions (**Fig. 43.1**). The external stratum remains as a rather thin layer of cells which begin to acquire pigmented melanosomes and form the pigmented epithelium of the retina around 36 days. In a parallel process, which had already begun before invagination, the cells of the inner layer of the cup proliferate to form a thick epithelium. The inner layer forms neural tissue over the base and sides of the cup and non-neural tissue around the lip. The non-neural epithelium is further differentiated into the components of the prospective iris at the rim, and the ciliary body a little further back adjacent to the neural area. The development of this pattern is reflected in regional differences in the expression of various genes which encode transcriptional regulators and which are therefore likely to play key roles in controlling and coordinating development. Each of these genes is expressed prior to overt cell-type differentiation. For example, *PAX6* is expressed in the prospective ciliary and iris regions of the optic cup. Individuals heterozygous for mutations in *PAX6* lack an iris, which suggests a causal role for this gene in the development of the iris. The genes expressed in the eye are also active at a variety of other specific sites in the embryo, and this may, in part, account for the co-involvement of the eye and other organs in syndromes which result from single genetic lesions.

DEVELOPING NEURAL RETINA

This comprises an outer nuclear zone and an inner marginal zone which is devoid of nuclei. Around 36 days the cells of the nuclear zone invade the marginal zone, and by 44 days the nervous stratum of the retina consists of inner and outer neuroblastic layers. The inner neuroblastic layer gives rise to the ganglion cells, the amacrine cells and the somata of the 'fibrous' sustentacular cells (of Muller); the outer neuroblastic layer is the source of the horizontal and rod-and-cone bipolar neurones and probably the rod-and-cone cells, which first appear in the central part of the retina. By the eighth month all the named layers of the retina can be identified. However, the retinal photoreceptor cells continue to form after birth, generating an array of increasing resolution and sensitivity.

The divergent differentiation of the pigmented and sensory layers of the retina depends on interactions mediated by diffusible molecules. For example, soluble factors from the retina elicit the polarized distribution

A

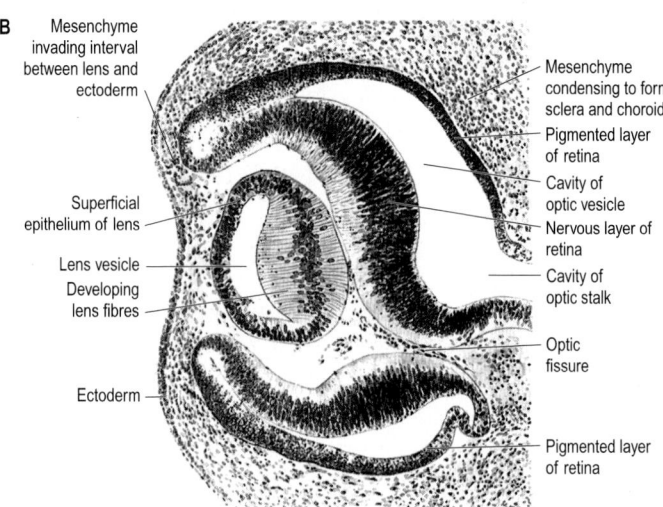

B

Mesenchyme
invading interval
between lens and
ectoderm

Mesenchyme
condensing to form
sclera and choroid

Pigmented layer
of retina

Cavity of
optic vesicle

Superficial
epithelium of lens

Nervous layer of
retina

Lens vesicle

Developing
lens fibres

Cavity of
optic stalk

Optic
fissure

Ectoderm

Pigmented layer
of retina

C

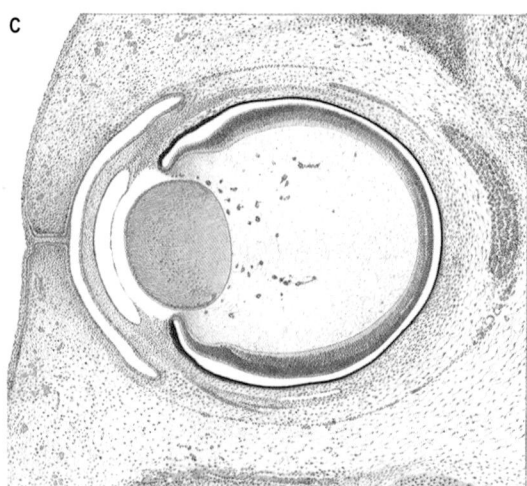

Fig. 43.1 A–C, Section through the developing eyes of human embryos.
A, 8 mm CR length. The thick nervous and the thinner pigmented layers of the
retina and the developing lens are shown. Stained with haematoxylin and eosin.
B, 13.2 mm CR length. **C,** 40 mm CR length. Note the layers of the retina,
developing lens, pupillary membrane, cornea, conjunctival sac, anterior and
posterior aqueous chambers, the developing vitreous body, and condensing
circumoptic mesenchyme and the fused eyelids. Stained with haematoxylin and
eosin. (**A**, from material loaned by Professor RJ Harrison; **B**, by permission from
Streeter GL 1948 Developmental horizons in human embryos. Contrib Embryol
Carnegie Inst Washington 32: 133–203.)

of plasma membrane proteins and the formation of tight junctions
in the pigmented epithelium. Neural retinal differentiation appears
to be mediated by fibroblast growth factors. However, the pigmented
epithelium retains the potential to become neural retina and will do so
if the embryonic retina is wounded.

OPTIC NERVE

The optic nerve develops from the optic stalk. The centre of the optic
cup, where the optic fissure is deepest, will later form the optic disc. Here
the neural retina is continuous with the corresponding invaginated cell
layer of the optic stalk; consequently the developing nerve fibres of the
ganglion cells pass directly into the wall of the stalk and convert it into
the optic nerve. The fibres of the optic nerve begin to acquire their
myelin sheaths shortly before birth, but the process is not completed
until some time later. The optic chiasma is formed by the meeting and
partial decussation of the fibres of the two optic nerves in the ventral
part of the lamina terminalis at the junction of the telencephalon with
the diencephalon in the floor of the third ventricle. Beyond the chiasma,
the fibres are continued backwards as the optic tracts, and pass principally
to the lateral geniculate bodies and to the superior tectum.

CILIARY BODY

The ciliary body is a compound structure. Its epithelial components are
the region of the inner layer of the retina between the iris and the neural
retina and the adjacent outer layer of pigmented epithelium. The cells
here differentiate in close association with the surrounding mesenchyme to form highly vascularized folds that secrete fluid into the globe
of the eye. The inner surface of the ciliary body also forms the site of
attachment of the lens, while the outer layer is associated with smooth
muscle derived from mesenchymal cells in the choroid lying between
the anterior scleral condensation and the pigmented ciliary epithelium.

IRIS

The iris develops from the tip of the optic cup where the two layers
remain thin and are associated with vascularized, muscular connective
tissue. The muscles of the sphincter and dilator pupillae are unusual in
being of neurectodermal origin, and develop from the cells of the pupillary part of the optic cup. The mature colour of the iris develops after
birth and is dependent on the relative contributions of the pigmented
epithelium on the posterior surface of the iris and the chromatophore
cells in the mesenchymal stroma of the iris. If only epithelial pigment
is present, the eye appears blue, whereas if there is an additional contribution from the chromatophores, the eye appears brown.

LENS

The lens develops from the lens vesicle (**Fig. 43.1A**). Initially this is
a ball of actively proliferating epithelium which encloses a clump of
disintegrating cells, but by 37 days there is a discernible difference
between the thin anterior (i.e. outward facing) epithelium and the
thickened posterior epithelium. Cells of the posterior wall lengthen and
fill the vesicle (**Fig. 43.1B,C**) and reduce the original cavity to a slit by
about 44 days. The posterior cells become filled with a very high concentration of proteins (crystallins) which render them transparent. They
also become densely packed within the lens as primary lens fibres. Cells
at the equatorial region of the lens elongate and contribute secondary
lens fibres to the body of the lens in a process which continues into
adult life, sustained by continued proliferation of cells in the anterior
epithelium. The polarity and growth of the lens appear to depend on
the differential distribution of soluble factors which promote either cell
division or lens fibre differentiation and are present in the anterior
chamber and vitreous humour respectively.

The developing lens is surrounded by a vascular mesenchymal
condensation, the vascular capsule, the anterior part of which is named
the pupillary membrane. The posterior part of the capsule is supplied
by branches from the hyaloid artery, and the anterior part is supplied by
branches from the anterior ciliary arteries. During the fourth month,
the hyaloid artery gives off retinal branches. By the sixth month all of
the vessels have atrophied except the hyaloid artery. The latter becomes
occluded during the eighth month of intrauterine life, although its
proximal part persists in the adult as the central artery of the retina.
Atrophy of the hyaloid vasculature and of the pupillary membrane
appears to be an active process of programmed tissue remodelling
which is macrophage-dependent. The hyaloid canal, which carries the
vessels through the vitreous, persists after the vessels have become
occluded. In the newly born child it extends more or less horizontally
from the optic disc to the posterior aspect of the lens but when the adult
eye is examined with a slit-lamp it can be seen to follow an undulating
course, sagging downwards as it passes forwards to the lens. With the
loss of its blood vessels the vascular capsule disappears and the lens
becomes dependent for its nutrition on diffusion via the aqueous and

vitreous humours. The lens remains enclosed in the lens capsule, a thickened basal lamina derived from the lens epithelium. Sometimes the pupillary membrane persists at birth, which gives rise to congenital atresia of the pupil.

VITREOUS BODY

The vitreous body develops between the lens and the optic cup as a transparent, avascular gel of extracellular substance. The precise derivation of the vitreous remains controversial. The lens rudiment and the optic vesicle are at first in contact, but they draw apart after closure of the lens vesicle and formation of the optic cup, and remain connected by a network of delicate cytoplasmic processes. This network, derived partly from cells of the lens and partly from those of the retina, is the primitive vitreous body. At first these cytoplasmic processes are connected to the whole of the neuroretinal area of the cup, but later they become limited to the ciliary region where, by a process of condensation, they form the basis of the suspensory ligaments of the ciliary zonule. The vascular mesenchyme which enters the cup through the choroidal fissure and around the equator of the lens associates locally with this reticular tissue and thus contributes to the formation of the vitreous body.

AQUEOUS CHAMBER

The aqueous chamber of the eye develops in the space between the surface ectoderm and the lens that is invaded by mesenchymal cells of neural crest origin. The chamber initially appears as a cleft in this mesenchymal tissue. The mesenchyme superficial to the cleft forms the substantia propria of the cornea, and that deep to the cleft forms the mesenchymal stroma of the iris and the pupillary membrane. Tangentially, this early cleft extends as far as the iridocorneal angle where communications are established with the sinus venosus sclerae. When the pupillary membrane disappears the cavity continues to form between the iris and the lens capsule as far as the zonular suspensory fibres. In this way the aqueous chamber is divided by the iris into anterior and posterior chambers, which communicate through the pupil. The walls of these chambers furnish both the sites of production of and the channels for circulation and reabsorption of the aqueous humour.

CORNEA

The cornea is induced in front of the anterior chamber by the lens and optic cup. The corneal epithelium is formed from surface ectoderm and the epithelium of the anterior chamber is formed from mesenchyme. A regular array of collagen fibres is established between these two layers and these serve to reduce scattering of light entering the eye.

CHOROID AND SCLERA

The choroid and sclera differentiate as inner, vascular, and outer, fibrous, layers from the mesenchyme that surrounds the optic cup. The blood vessels of the choroid develop from the fifteenth week and include the vasculature of the ciliary body. The choroid is continuous with the internal sheath of the optic nerve which is pia-arachnoid mater, and the sclera is continuous with the outer sheath of the optic nerve, and thus with the dura mater.

DIFFERENTIATION OF STRUCTURES AROUND THE EYE

EXTRAOCULAR MUSCLES

The extrinsic ocular muscles derive from prechordal mesenchyme which ingresses at the primitive node very early in development. The prechordal

cells lie at the rostral tip of the notochordal process and remain mesenchymal after the notochordal process becomes epithelial and gains a basal lamina (**Fig. 26.5**). The prechordal mesenchyme migrates laterally towards the paraxial mesenchyme. Although this is a singular origin for muscle, the early myogenic properties of these cells have been demonstrated experimentally; moreover, if transplanted into limb buds, the cells are able to develop into muscle tissue (Wachtler & Jacob 1986).

Early embryos develop bilateral premandibular, intermediate and caudal cavities in the head – previously described as preotic somites. The walls of the premandibular head cavities are lined by flat or cylindrical cells which do not exhibit the characteristics of a germinal epithelium. As the oculomotor nerve grows down to the level of the head cavity, a condensation of premuscle cells appears at its ventrolateral side which later subdivides into the blastemata of the different muscles that are supplied by the nerve. Similar events occur with respect to the intermediate head cavity (trochlear nerve and superior oblique), and the caudal head cavity (abducens nerve and lateral rectus) (**Fig. 26.5**).

There is no doubt that the head cavities are formed by a mesenchymal/epithelial shift similar to that seen in the somites. However, the epithelial plate of the somite is a germinal centre which produces postmitotic myoblasts destined for epaxial regions, and migratory premitotic myoblasts destined for the limbs and body wall. The head cavities may serve a similar purpose if a mesenchyme/epithelial shift is part of a maturation process for putative myoblasts. However, it may not need to provide a centre for cell replication because premitotic myoblasts differentiated directly from the prechordal mesenchyme may form the premuscular masses.

EYELIDS

The eyelids are formed as small cutaneous folds of surface ectoderm and neural crest mesenchyme (**Fig. 43.1C**). During the middle of the third month their edges come together and unite over the cornea to enclose the conjunctival sac, and they usually remain united until about the end of the sixth month. When the eyelids open, the conjunctiva which lines their inner surfaces and covers the white (scleral) region of the eye fuses with the corneal epithelium. The eyelashes and the lining cells of the tarsal (meibomian), ciliary and other glands which open onto the margins of the eyelids are all derived from the tarsal plate. Orbicularis oculi develops from skeletal myoblasts which invade the eyelids from the second pharyngeal arch. Levator palpebrae superioris develops from the prechordal mesenchyme and is attached to the upper eyelid by tendons derived from the neural crest. Smooth muscle also develops within the eyelids.

LACRIMAL APPARATUS

The epithelium of the alveoli and ducts of the lacrimal gland arise as a series of tubular buds from the ectoderm of the superior conjunctival fornix. These buds are arranged in two groups: one forms the gland proper and the other forms its palpebral process (de la Cuadra-Blanco et al 2003). The lacrimal sac and nasolacrimal duct are derived from ectoderm in the nasomaxillary groove between the lateral nasal process and the maxillary process of the developing face (p. 609). This thickens to form a solid cord of cells, the nasolacrimal ridge, which sinks into the mesenchyme. During the third month the cord becomes canalized to form the nasolacrimal duct. The lacrimal canaliculi arise as buds from the cranial extremity of the cord which establish openings (puncta lacrimalia) on the margins of the lids. The inferior canaliculus isolates a small part of the lower eyelid to form the lacrimal caruncle and plica semilunaris.

REFERENCES

de la Cuadra-Blanco C, Peces-Peña MD, Mèrida-Velasco JR 2003 Morphogenesis of the human lacrimal gland. J Anat 203: 531–6.

O'Rahilly R 1966 The early development of the eye in staged human embryos. Contrib Embryol Carnegie Inst 38: 1.

O'Rahilly R 1983 The timing and sequence of events in the development of the human eye and ear during the embryonic period proper. Anat Embryol 168: 87–99.

Saha MS, Servetnick M, Grainger RM 1992 Vertebrate eye development. Curr Opin Genet Dev 2: 582–8.
Reviews the interactions involved in eye development and discusses genes responsible for development of the eye.

Wachtler F, Jacob M 1986 Origin and development of the cranial skeletal muscles. Bibl Anat 29: 24–46.

BACK AND MACROSCOPIC ANATOMY OF SPINAL CORD

Editors:

Andrew Williams *(Lead Editor)*

Richard LM Newell *(Editor)*

Patricia Collins *(Embryology, Growth and Development)*

Critical reviewers:

Michael A Adams *(biomechanics)*, **Paul Cartwright** *(chapter 44)*, **Alison McGregor** *(biomechanics)*

Surface anatomy of the back

Most clinical disorders of the back present as low back pain with or without associated lower limb pain, so historically most attention has been paid to the anatomy of the lower (lumbosacral) back. In this chapter, the term 'the back' will include the whole of the posterior aspect of the trunk and of the neck. The whole of this region has great clinical importance but its anatomy has often been neglected. Recent understanding of the detailed topography of the bony and soft-tissue elements of the lower back owes much to the work of Bogduk (1997).

The soft tissues of the back of the trunk and neck include the skin and subcutaneous fat, the underlying fascial layers, and the musculature. The deep, 'true' or epaxial muscles lie within compartments in their own fascial 'skeleton'. The bony framework to which the muscles and fasciae attach includes not only elements of the axial skeleton, i.e. the

vertebral column and occiput, but also elements of the pectoral and pelvic girdles as well as the ribs. The occiput is described on p. 463, the scapula on p. 819, the ribs on p. 955 and the pelvis on p. 1421.

SKELETAL LANDMARKS (Figs 44.1, 44.2, 44.3)

VERTEBRAL SPINES

In the midline a median furrow runs from the external occipital protuberance above to the natal cleft below. The furrow is most shallow in the lower cervical region and is deepest in the midlumbar zone. Inferiorly, it widens out into a flattened, triangular area, the apex of which lies at the start of the natal cleft and corresponds to the third

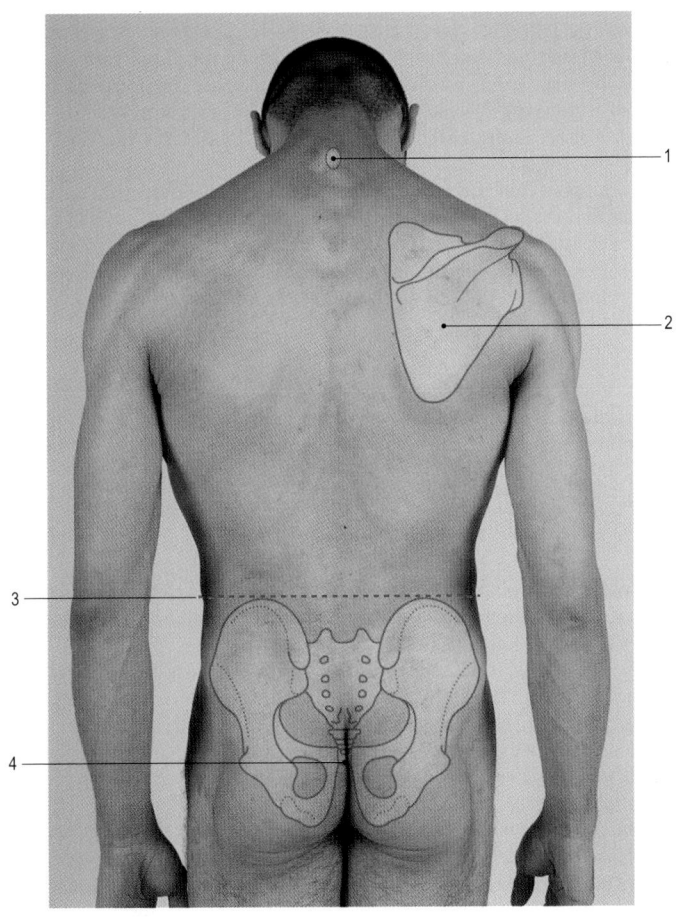

1. Medial border of scapula.
2. Spine of scapula.
3. Supracristal plane.
4. Position of sacral hiatus.

Fig. 44.1 Back view of trunk. (Photograph by Sarah-Jane Smith.)

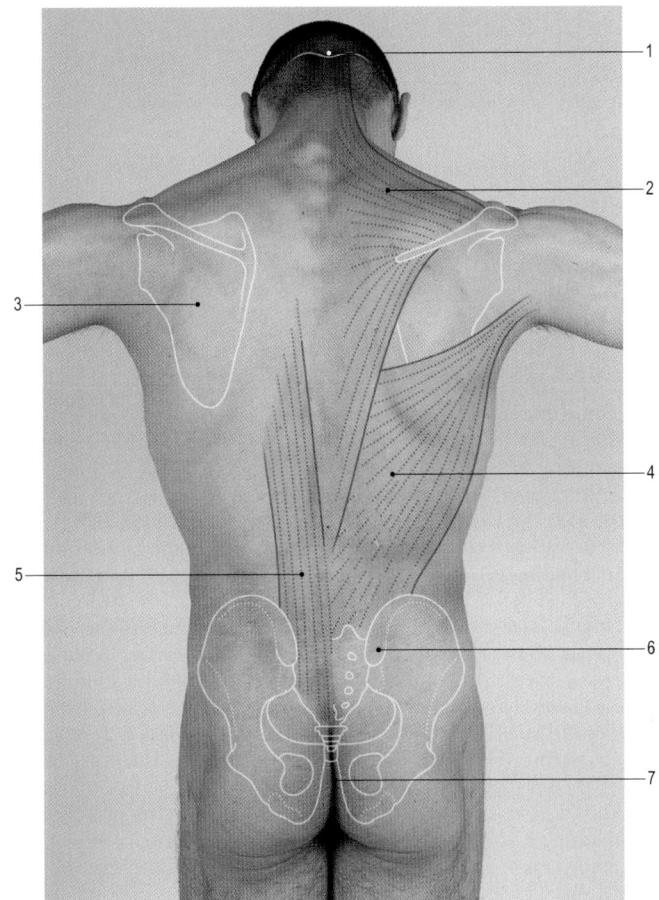

1. External occipital protuberance.
2. Trapezius.
3. Inferior angle of scapula.
4. Latissimus dorsi.
5. Erector spinae.
6. Posterior superior iliac spine underlying sacral dimple.
7. Natal cleft.

Fig. 44.2 Back view of trunk, arms abducted. (Photograph by Sarah-Jane Smith.)

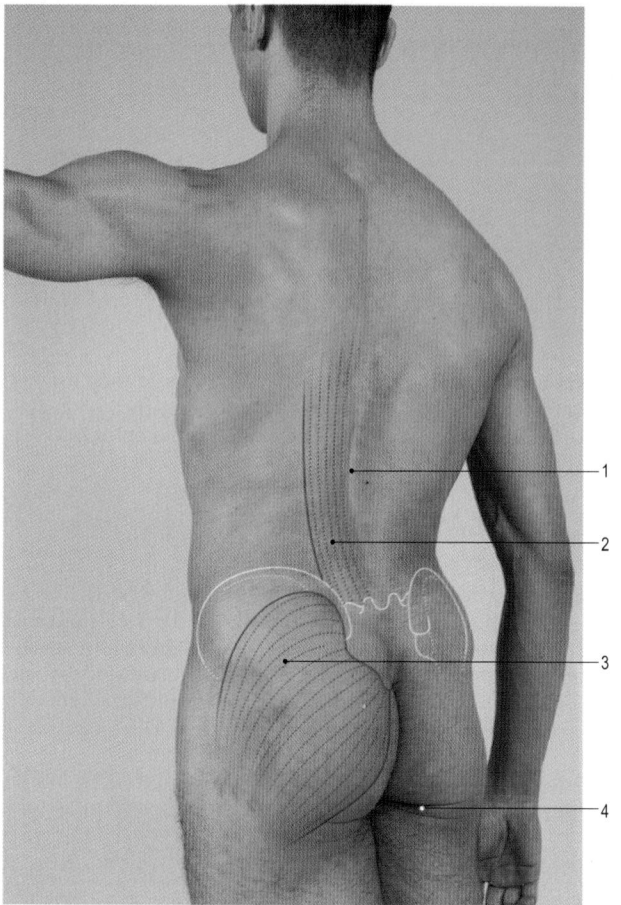

1. Median furrow.
2. Lateral border of erector spinae.
3. Gluteus maximus.
4. Gluteal fold.

Fig. 44.3 Back of trunk, oblique view. (Photograph by Sarah-Jane Smith.)

Table 44.1 Vertebral spines as landmarks for the viscera

Spine	Viscera
C5	Cricoid cartilage, start of oesophagus
C7	Apex of lung
T3	Aorta reaches spine. Tracheal bifurcation
T4	Aortic arch ends. Upper border of heart
T8	Lower border of heart. Central tendon of diaphragm.
T10	Lower border of lung. Cardia of stomach. Upper border of kidney
T12	Lowest level of pleura. Pylorus
L1	Hilum of kidney. Renal arteries. Superior mesenteric artery
L2	Spinal cord terminates. Pancreas. Duodenojejunal flexure
L3	Lower border of kidney
L4	Bifurcation of aorta
L5	Inferior vena cava begins

opposite the inferior part of its own body. The body of the fourth lumbar vertebra is level with the summits of the iliac crests, so the fourth lumbar spine overlies the L4/5 interspace (a point useful in lumbar puncture). The second sacral spine is level with the posterior superior iliac spines. Sacral and coccygeal landmarks are described below (p. 728).

Note that when the subject lies in the lateral position (on the side), the median soft-tissue furrow may not coincide with the median plane, especially in the lumbar region in the obese. Careful palpation may be necessary to identify the spines, a point which is of particular importance during lumbar or epidural puncture in this position.

Spinal levels of viscera
The palpable vertebral spines can be used as landmarks for the levels of the viscera. Some of the more important are shown in **Table 44.1** (minor differences between the two sides are ignored).

SCAPULAR LANDMARKS
The shape of the back in the upper thoracic region is determined largely by the scapula and the muscles which attach to it, especially trapezius. The relative prominence of the scapula and its muscles depends upon the state of contraction of the latter. Bony scapular landmarks are most evident when the arms hang by the sides.

The scapula overlies the second to seventh ribs. Its superior angle is palpable beneath trapezius, and its inferior angle is just covered by latissimus dorsi. These angles are joined by the medial border of the scapula which runs vertically. The scapular spine runs subcutaneously and is easily palpable from its root medially to the acromion process laterally.

The root of the spine of the scapula lies opposite the third thoracic spine and the inferior angle lies opposite the seventh thoracic spine when the arm is by the side.

POSTERIOR PELVIC AND SACROCOCCYGEAL BONY LANDMARKS
At the lower part of the back the iliac crest can be palpated throughout its whole length, and can be traced backwards and upwards from the anterior superior iliac spine to its highest point, and then downwards and medially to the posterior superior iliac spine, which is overlain by a dimple in the skin. A line joining these sacral dimples passes through the second sacral spine and the body of the second sacral vertebra, and is a useful landmark for the lower end of the adult dural sac. There may also be a less prominent pair of dimples at the level of the L4/5

sacral spine. Palpation of the median furrow reveals the sagittal curves of the spine: the cervical curve is convex forwards (lordosis) and extends from the first cervical to the second thoracic vertebra; the thoracic curvature is concave forwards (kyphosis) and extends from the second to the twelfth thoracic vertebra; the lumbar curvature is convex forwards and extends from the twelfth thoracic vertebra to the lumbosacral prominence. The external occipital protuberance is subcutaneous and can be felt and often seen, and it can be palpated without difficulty when it is approached from below. The inion is the point situated on this protuberance in the median plane. The tips of the spines of the cervical vertebrae are obscured by the overlying ligamentum nuchae. The tubercle on the posterior arch of the atlas is impalpable; the first bony prominence which is encountered when the finger is drawn downwards in the midline from the external occipital protuberance is the spine of the second cervical vertebra. The ligamentum nuchae terminates inferiorly at the spine of the seventh cervical vertebra, which is the highest, and sometimes the only, visible projection in this region (vertebra prominens). Immediately below this the spine of the first thoracic vertebra is palpable; it is usually more prominent than the seventh cervical vertebra. The spine of the second thoracic vertebra can also often be felt. The third thoracic spinous process is level with the spine of the scapula, and the seventh with the inferior scapular angle when the arm is by the side. The identification of the remaining thoracic spines is not easy, even in a thin subject when the trunk is fully flexed, because of the manner in which they overlap one another in the midthoracic region. In the upper and lower thoracic regions, the tips of the thoracic spines lie opposite the upper part of the body of the immediately subjacent vertebra. In the midthoracic region, they lie opposite the lower part of the vertebra below. The tip of the spine of each lumbar vertebra can usually be palpated without difficulty, especially if the trunk is flexed. Each lies

intervertebral disc. The posterior superior iliac spine lies over the centre of the sacroiliac joint. The supracrestal plane joins the highest points of the iliac crest on each side. It passes through the body of the fourth lumbar vertebra and has been used as a clinical landmark when performing a lumbar puncture (p. 730) though difficulty in its definition reduces its reliability in this procedure (Broadbent et al 2000). The tip of the coccyx can be felt deeply near the centre of the natal cleft. As the examining finger passes cranially, the sacral cornua can be felt on either side: these demarcate the sacral hiatus, and form the landmark for performing a caudal anaesthetic block.

MUSCULOTENDINOUS LANDMARKS
(Figs 44.1, 44.2, 44.3)

In the upper and middle cervical region the median furrow lies between the cylindrical prominences formed mainly by the semispinalis muscles, which are accentuated by neck extension against resistance. In the thoracic and lumbar regions, a broad elevation produced by the erector spinae muscle group extends for about one hand's breadth on either side of the median furrow and is present between the iliac crest and the twelfth rib. The lateral border of this elevation then crosses the ribs at their angles, passing medially as it ascends. The muscle group can be demonstrated by extending the back against resistance.

Trapezius is a flat, triangular muscle which covers the back of the neck and shoulder. Together, the two trapezius muscles resemble a trapezium or quadrilateral in which two of the angles correspond to the shoulders, a third to the occipital protuberance and the fourth to the spine of the twelfth thoracic vertebra. The two muscles cover the back of the neck and shoulders like a monk's cowl, hence the ancient name of the trapezius was musculus cucullaris. The upper part of trapezius is demonstrated by elevation of the shoulders, or by extension and lateral flexion of the neck, against resistance. The lower fibres are best seen when the subject pushes both hands hard against a wall with the elbows extended. The anterosuperior border of the muscle forms the posterior boundary of the posterior triangle of the neck and can be seen in muscular subjects, especially during elevation of the shoulder against resistance.

In a well-muscled subject the outline of latissimus dorsi can easily be traced, particularly if the arm is adducted against resistance. The triangle of auscultation lies between the upper border of latissimus dorsi, the lower lateral border of trapezius and the medial border of the scapula.

The lumbar triangle, one of the sites of the rare primary lumbar hernia, lies inferiorly, between the lowermost outer border of latissimus dorsi, the posterior free border of the external oblique, and the iliac crest.

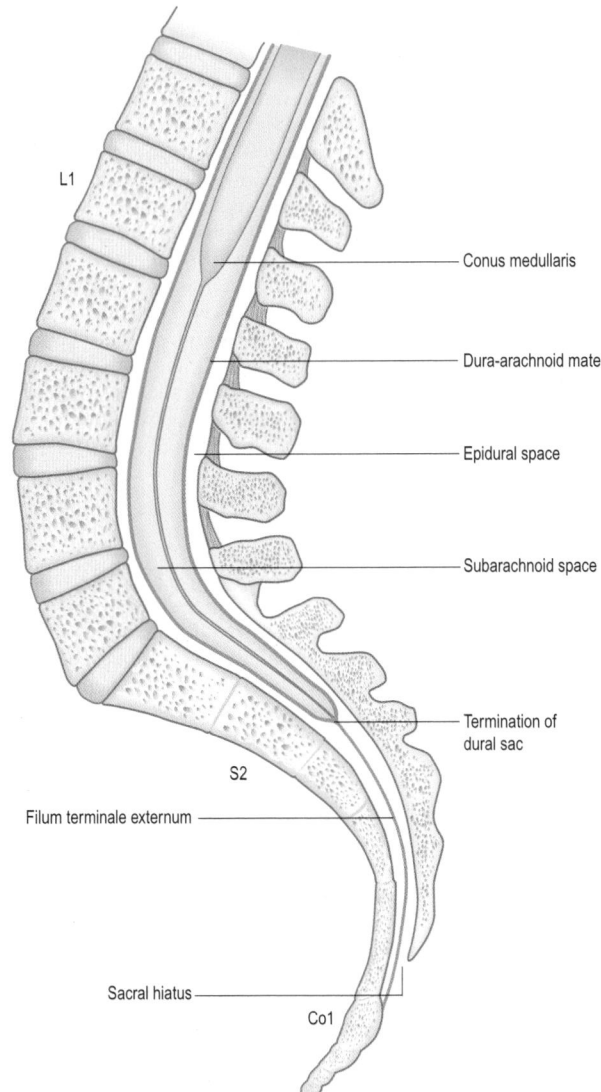

Fig. 44.4 Contents of the vertebral canal in the lumbosacral region. Adapted from Mackintosh RR 1951 Lumbar Puncture and Spinal Analgesia. Edinburgh: E&S Livingstone. (Modified with permission from Mackintosh RR 1951 Lumbar Puncture and Spinal Analgesia. Edinburgh: E&S Livingstone.)

SPINAL CORD AND ITS COVERINGS (Fig. 44.4)

The surface relationships of the spinal cord and its coverings are of great clinical importance throughout life.

During development the vertebral column elongates more rapidly than the spinal cord, which leads to an increasing discrepancy between the anatomical level of spinal cord segments and their corresponding vertebrae. At stage 23 the vertebral column and spinal cord are the same length, and the cord ends at the last coccygeal vertebra: this arrangement continues until the third fetal month. At birth the spinal cord terminates at the lower border of the second lumbar vertebra, and may sometimes reach the third lumbar vertebra. In the adult, the spinal cord is said to terminate at the level of the disc between the first and second lumbar vertebral bodies, which lies a little above the level of the elbow joint when the arm is by the side, and also lies approximately in the transpyloric plane (p. 1099). However, there is considerable variation in the level at which the spinal cord ends. It may end below this level in as many as 40% of subjects, or opposite the body of either the first or second lumbar vertebra: very occasionally it ends opposite the twelfth thoracic or even the third lumbar vertebra.

In estimating the vertebral levels of cord segments in the adult, a useful approximation is that in the cervical region the tip of a vertebral spinous process corresponds to the succeeding cord segment (i.e. the sixth cervical spine is opposite the seventh spinal segment); at upper thoracic levels the tip of a vertebral spine corresponds to the cord two segments lower (i.e. the fourth spine is level with the sixth segment), and in the lower thoracic region there is a difference of three segments (i.e. the tenth thoracic spine is level with the first lumbar segment). The eleventh thoracic spine overlies the third lumbar segment and the twelfth is opposite the first sacral segment. In making this estimate by palpation of the vertebral spines, the relationship of the individual spines to their vertebral bodies should be remembered (p. 727).

The dural sac (theca), and thus the subarachnoid space and its contained cerebrospinal fluid (CSF), usually extends to the level of the second segment of the sacrum. This corresponds to the line joining the sacral dimples located in the skin over the posterior superior iliac spines. Occasionally the dural sac ends as high as the fifth lumbar vertebra, and very rarely it may extend to the third part of the sacrum, in which case it is occasionally possible to enter the subarachnoid space inadvertently during the course of a sacral nerve block.

UNDERLYING VISCERA

The posterior surface markings of the abdominal viscera are described on page 1098.

729

CLINICAL EXAMINATION

Clinical examination of the back of the trunk and neck best follows the order of inspection, palpation and movement. The examination will be determined by the circumstances of presentation and by the history, and may include musculoskeletal, neurological and vascular observations. Information relevant to the neurological and vascular examination of the skin and material relating to spinal movements and deeper innervation are found below. Palpation of the region involves careful assessment of the bony and musculotendinous landmarks described above, looking in particular for asymmetry, deformity and tenderness. Note that, apart from the spines, most of the bony elements of the vertebrae and almost all of the intervertebral joints are not palpable from behind. In regions of lordosis (sagittal plane curves of the spine with anterior convexity, i.e. midcervical and mid- and lower lumbar), parts of the vertebral column can often be palpated anteriorly with care in well-relaxed, thin subjects.

CLINICAL PROCEDURES

ACCESS TO CEREBROSPINAL FLUID

The safest approach to the cerebrospinal fluid (CSF) is to enter the lumbar cistern of the subarachnoid space in the midline, well below the level at which the spinal cord normally terminates (see p. 729). The fine needle employed is unlikely to damage the mobile nerve roots of the cauda equina. This procedure is called lumbar puncture. It is also possible to access the CSF by midline puncture of the cerebello-medullary cistern (cisterna magna) (Chapter 16): this is cisternal puncture.

LUMBAR PUNCTURE: ADULT

Lumbar puncture in the adult may be performed with the patient either sitting or lying on the side on a firm flat surface. In each position, the lumbar spine must be flexed as far as possible, in order to separate the vertebral spines maximally and expose the ligamentum flavum in the interlaminar window (Fig. 44.5). A line is then taken between the highest points of the iliac crests: this line intersects the vertebral column just above the palpable spine of L4. With the spines now identified, the skin is anaesthetised and a needle is inserted between the spines of L3 and L4 (or L4 and L5). Exact identification of the level by palpation is difficult (Broadbent et al 2000). The soft tissues which the needle will ultimately traverse should also be anaesthetised, though care should be taken lest the injection of an excessive amount of local anaesthetic compromise appreciation of the structures being traversed. These include the subcutaneous fat, and supraspinous and interspinous ligaments down to the ligamentum flavum itself. The lumbar puncture needle may then be inserted in the midline or just to one side, and angled in the horizontal and sagittal planes sufficiently to pierce the ligamentum flavum in or very near the midline (Fig. 44.6). There is then a slight loss of resistance as the needle enters the epidural space, and careful advancement will next pierce the dura and arachnoid to release CSF.

LUMBAR PUNCTURE: NEONATE AND INFANT

At full term (40 weeks) the spinal cord usually terminates somewhat lower than the adult level, sometimes reaching the body of L3. The supracristal plane intersects the vertebral column slightly higher (L3–4). By the second postnatal month the level of cord termination has usually reached its permanent position level with the body of the first lumbar vertebra. The lower end of the subarachnoid spine is found at sacral levels 1 or 2. These differences must be borne in mind when identifying the landmarks before undertaking lumbar puncture in the neonate and infant.

A lumbar puncture is performed by placing the baby in a position, either lying or 'sitting', which gives maximum convex curvature to the lumbar spine. A needle with trocar is inserted into the back between the spines of the third and fourth lumbar vertebrae and into the subarachnoid space below the level of the conus medullaris. The space between L3 and L4 is approximately level with the iliac crests and it is usual to insert the needle and trocar into the intervertebral space immediately above or below the iliac crests.

CISTERNAL PUNCTURE

In cisternal puncture, the cisterna magna (Chapter 16) is entered by midline puncture through the posterior atlanto-occipital membrane.

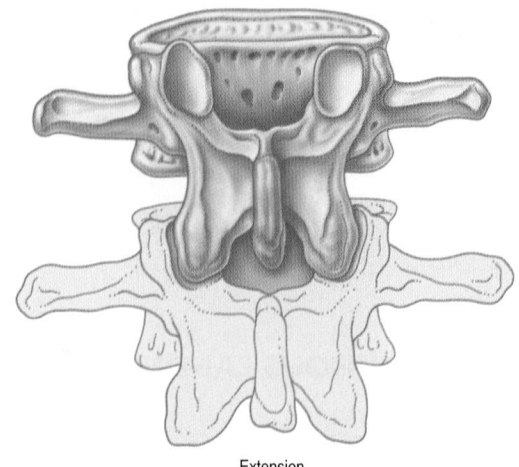

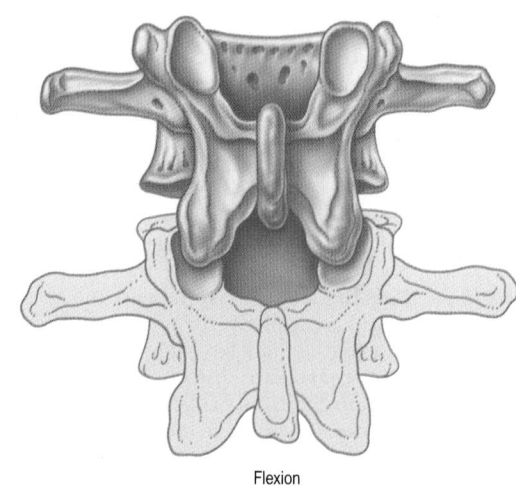

Extension

Flexion

Fig. 44.5 The lumbar interlaminar window in extension and flexion.

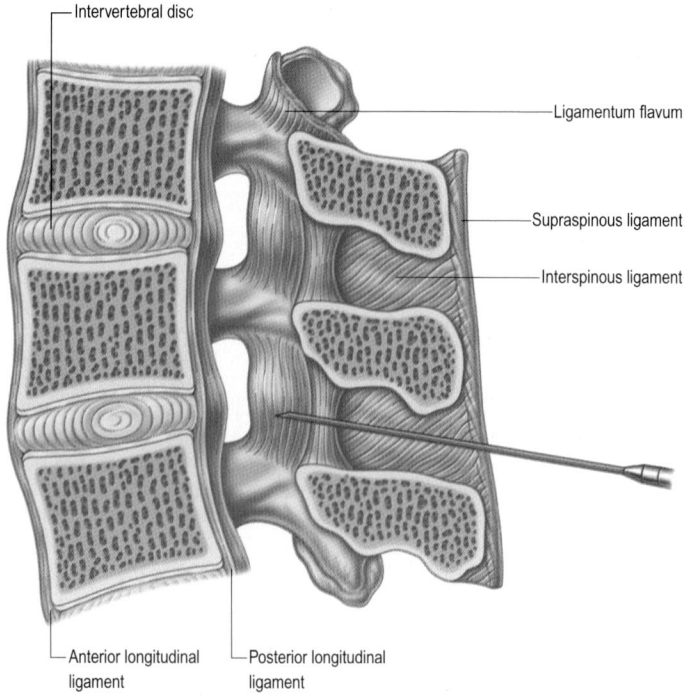

Intervertebral disc

Ligamentum flavum

Supraspinous ligament

Interspinous ligament

Anterior longitudinal ligament

Posterior longitudinal ligament

Fig. 44.6 The position of the needle in lumbar puncture.

Further details of this difficult specialist technique are beyond the scope of this book.

ACCESS TO THE EPIDURAL SPACE

The epidural 'space' lies between the spinal dura and the wall of the vertebral canal (p. 778). It contains epidural fat and a venous plexus. Access to this space, usually in the lumbar region, is required for the administration of anaesthetic and analgesic drugs, and for endoscopy. The caudal route is used mainly for analgesic injections.

Lumbar epidural

For access to the lumbar epidural space, the approach is as for lumbar puncture. The intention in epidural injection is to avoid dural puncture, so it is best to enter the epidural space in the midline posteriorly, where the depth of the space is greatest. Techniques for entering the epidural space rely on the appreciation of loss of resistance to injection of the chosen medium (usually air or saline) as the space is entered. There is very little distance between the ligamentum flavum and the underlying dura on either side of the median plane.

Caudal epidural

The route of access to the caudal epidural space is via the sacral hiatus. The space is thus entered below the level of termination of the dural sac (S2). With the patient in the lateral position or lying prone over a pelvic pillow, the sacral hiatus is identified by palpation of the sacral cornua (p. 749) (**Fig. 44.7**). These are felt at the upper end of the natal cleft c.5 cm above the tip of the coccyx. Alternatively, the sacral hiatus may be identified by constructing an equilateral triangle based on a line joining the posterior superior iliac spines: the inferior apex of this triangle overlies the hiatus. After local anaesthetic infiltration, a needle is introduced at 45° to the skin, to penetrate the posterior sacrococcygeal ligament and enter the sacral canal. Once the canal is entered, the hub of the needle is lowered so that the needle may pass along the canal (**Fig. 44.8**). If the needle is angled too obliquely it will strike bone; if it is placed too superficially it will lie outside the canal. The latter mal-position can be confirmed by careful injection of air while palpating the skin over the lower sacrum.

Thoracic and cervical epidurals

It is possible to access the epidural space at thoracic and cervical levels, but the specialist techniques required are outside the scope of this book. The principles are the same as those for lumbar epidurals, but the special anatomy of the vertebral spines at the other levels requires the angle of approach to be modified.

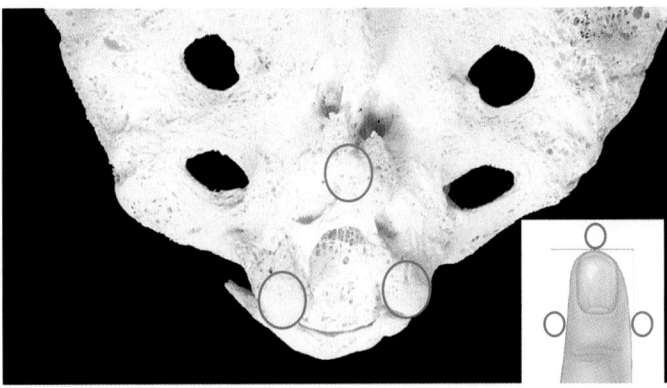

Fig. 44.7 Palpation of the sacral cornua for caudal epidural injection. With permission from Ellis H, Feldman SA 1997 Anatomy for Anaesthetists, 7th edn. Oxford: Blackwell Science. (By permission from Ellis H, Feldman S 1997 Anatomy for Anaesthetists, 7th edn. Oxford: Blackwell Science.)

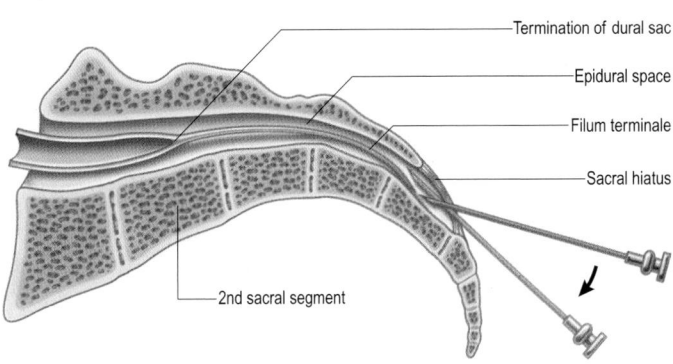

Fig. 44.8 Position of the needle in caudal epidural injection.

REFERENCES

Bogduk N 1997 Clinical Anatomy of the Lumbar Spine and Sacrum, 3rd edn. Edinburgh: Churchill Livingstone.

Broadbent CR, Maxwell WE, Ferrie R, Wilson DJ, Gawne-Cain M, Russell R 2000 Ability of anaesthetists to identify a marked lumbar interspace. Anaesthesia 55: 1122–6.

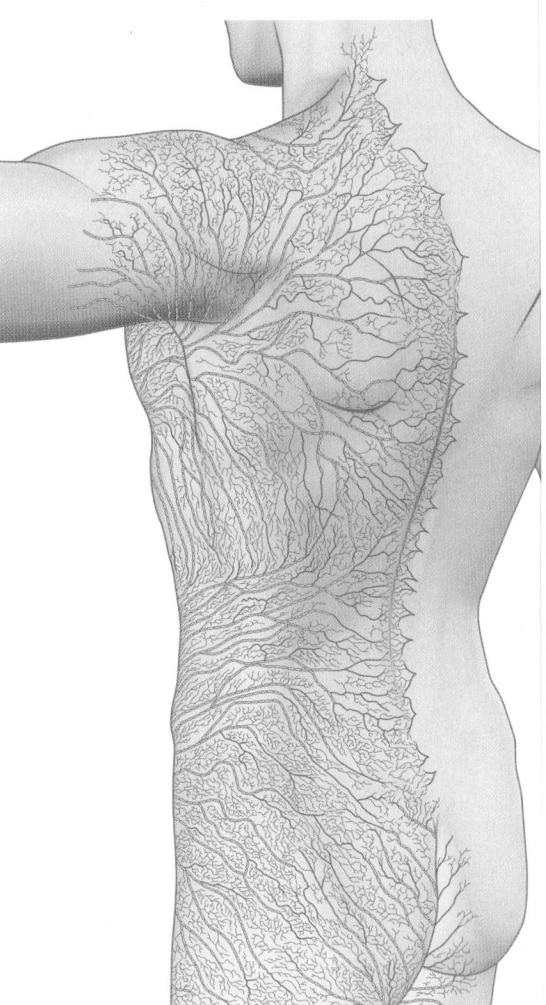

Fig. 45.5 Cutaneous lymphatics on the dorsum of the trunk. (By permission from Romanes GJ (ed) 1964 Cunningham's Textbook of Anatomy, 10th edn. London: Oxford University Press.)

with varying orientation of the constituent collagen fibres [...] the biomechanical function of the fascia. The posterior [...] layers of the thoracolumbar fascia and the vertebral colum[...] form an osteofascial compartment which encloses the ere[...] muscle group. The attachments of the fascia, especially thos[...] it continuity with the abdominal wall musculature, give it a[...] role in lifting, though the exact details of this role remain c[...] The fascia may also play an important role in load transfer [...] trunk and the limbs: its tension is affected by the actions [...] dorsi, gluteus maximus, and the hamstrings. An erector spin[...] ment syndrome may be one cause of low back pain.

DEEP CERVICAL FASCIA

The investing layer of the deep cervical fascia forms the de[...] the posterior aspect of the neck. It attaches in the midline to [...] occipital protuberance, the ligamentum nuchae and the s[...] seventh cervical vertebra, and splits to enclose trapezius o[...] Inferiorly the posterior part of the investing layer att[...] trapezius to the spine and acromion of the scapula.

VERTEBRAL COLUMN (Figs 45.7, 45.8)

The vertebral column is a curved linkage of individua[...] vertebrae. A continuous series of vertebral foramina runs [...] articulated vertebrae posterior to their bodies, and collectively [...] the vertebral canal, which transmits and protects the spin[...] nerve roots, their coverings and vasculature. A series of p[...]

The back

SKIN

The skin of the back of the trunk is thick and highly protective, but has low discriminatory sensation. The superficial fascia is thick and fatty in most areas of the back. Its attachment to the deeper fascial layers is strong in the midline, especially in the neck, but becomes weaker more laterally. The skin of the back of the neck is thicker than that of the front of the neck, but thinner than that of the back of the trunk. The quantity, texture and distribution of hair vary with sex, race and the individual, though well-defined hair tracts have been delineated (**Fig. 45.1**).

Lines of skin tension (p. 173) run horizontally in the cervical and lumbosacral regions but form segments of two adjacent circles in the thoracic region (**Fig. 45.2**).

CUTANEOUS INNERVATION AND DERMATOMES (Figs 46.14, 45.3)

The skin of the back of the neck and trunk is innervated by the dorsal (posterior primary) rami of the spinal nerves (**Fig. 46.14**) where dorsal rami are covered in detail. In the cervical and upper thoracic regions (down to T6) skin is supplied by the medial branches of these rami, while in the lower thoracic, lumbar and sacral regions it is supplied by the lateral branches. The total area supplied by these dorsal rami is shown in **Fig. 46.14**. The spinal nerves involved include C2 to C5, T2 to L3, S2 to S4, and Co1. The pattern of their dermatomes is shown in **Fig. 45.3**. There is about half a segment of overlap between these cutaneous 'strips': the strips supplied by the dorsal rami do not correspond exactly to those served by ventral rami, and differ slightly in both width and position.

CUTANEOUS VASCULAR SUPPLY AND LYMPHATIC DRAINAGE
(Figs 45.4, 45.5)

The skin of the back of the trunk receives its arterial blood supply mainly from musculocutaneous branches of posterior intercostal, lumbar and lateral sacral arteries, which all accompany the cutaneous branches of

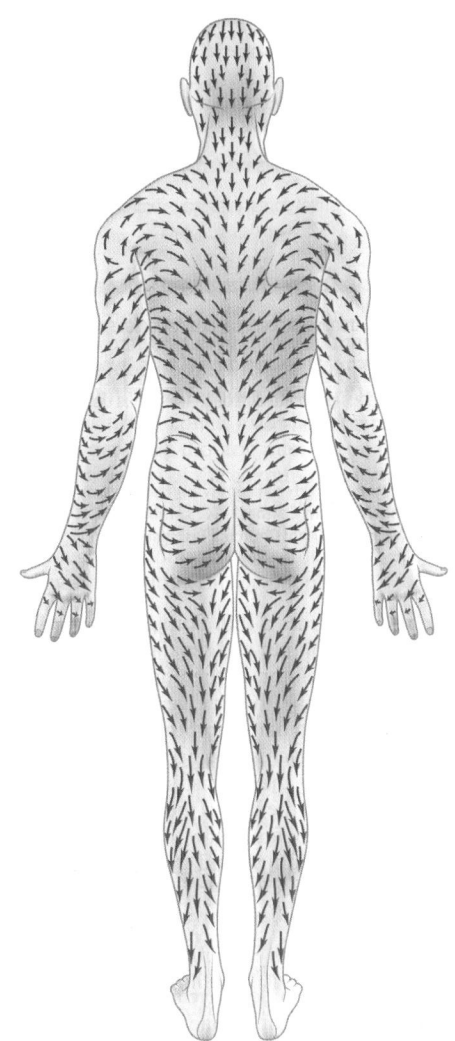

Fig. 45.1 Hair tracts on the dorsal surface of the body. (By permission from Wood Jones F (ed) 1949 Buchanan's Manual of Anatomy, 8th edn. London: Baillière Tindall and Cox.)

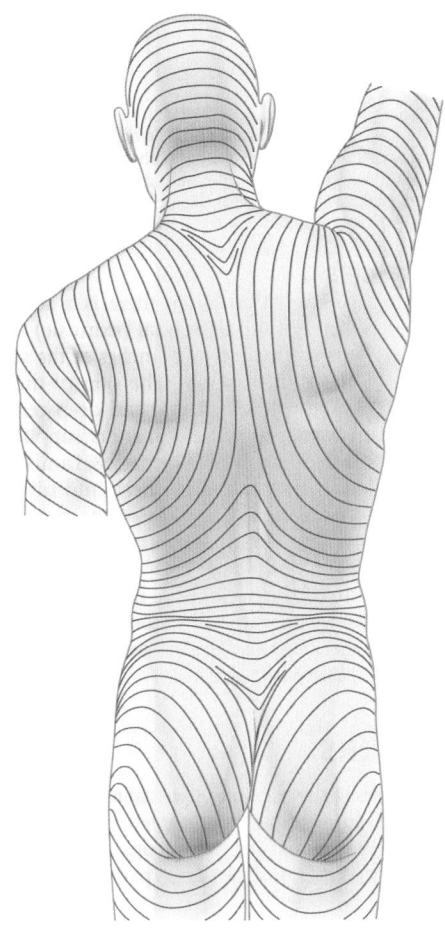

Fig. 45.2 Lines of skin tension on the dorsum of the trunk and head. (From Kriassl CL, Plast Reconstruct Surg 8: 1–28, 1951. By permission from Lippincott Williams and Wilkins.)

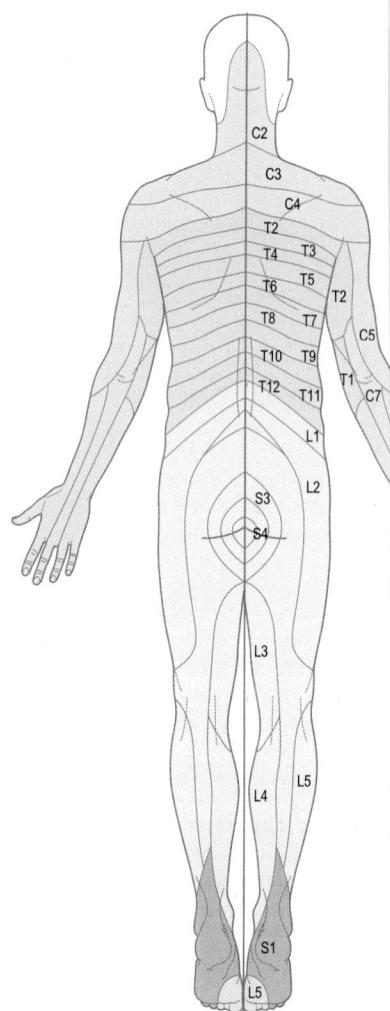

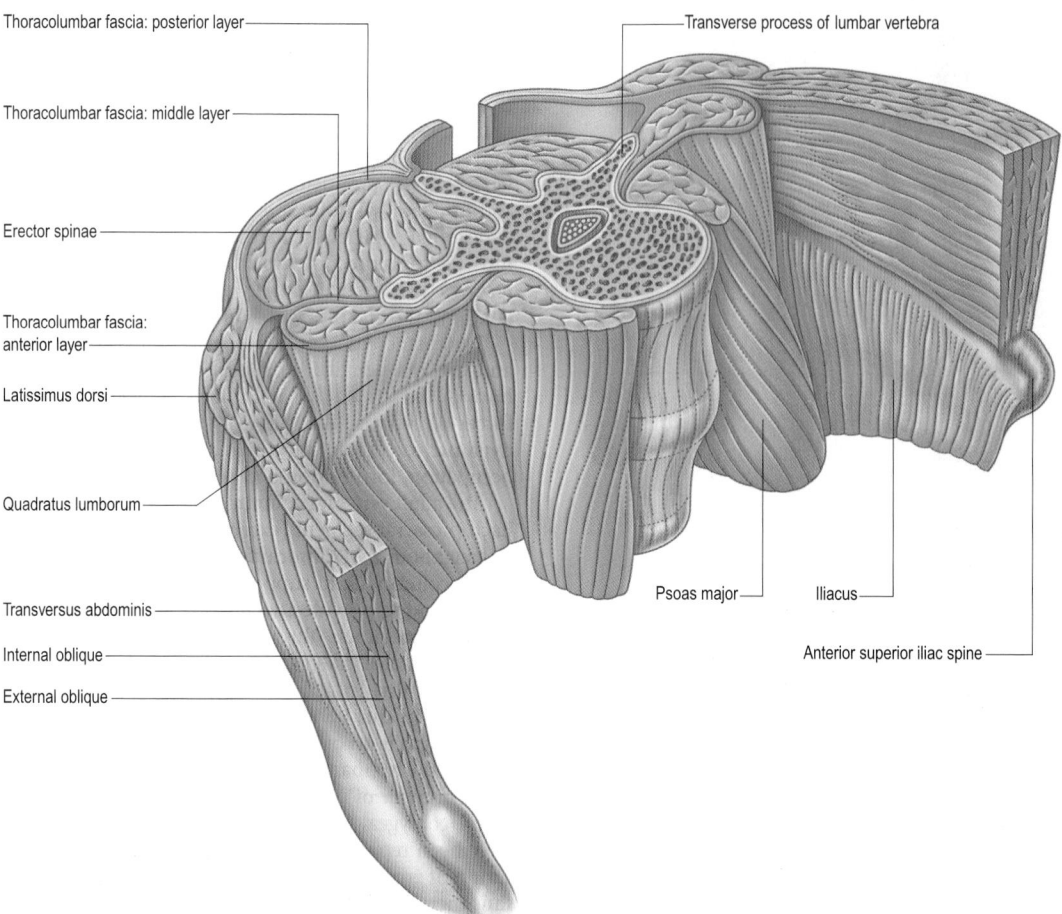

Fig. 45.3 Dermatomes on the dorsal surface of th shows the regular arrangement of dermatomes in the embryo. (Adapted with permission from Moff Anatomy, 2nd edn. Oxford: Blackwell Scientific.)

Fig. 45.6 Muscles and fasciae of the posterior abdominal wall. (By permission from Kiss F, Szentagothai J 1964 Atlas of Human Anatomy. Oxford: Pergamon Press.)

their respective dorsal rami. In addition, dominant vascular pedicles of the superfici The skin over the scapula is supplied by bra dorsal scapular and subscapular arteries. T neck is supplied mainly from the occipital The superficial cervical or transverse cervica the lower part of the back of the neck (Cor

Veins drain the skin of the back of the occipital and deep cervical veins. The skin drains into the azygos system, via tributaries and lumbar veins.

Lymph from the skin of the back of the lateral deep cervical and axillary nodes. Fr drainage is to the posterior (subscapular) lateral superficial inguinal nodes.

FASCIAL LAYERS

The main fascial layers in the axial and para neck are the thoracolumbar fascia, the de continuous prevertebral plane. The latter c endothoracic, retroperitoneal and posterior

THORACOLUMBAR FASCIA (Figs 45.6, 68.1, The thoracolumbar (lumbodorsal) fascia c the back and the trunk. Above, it passes ar superior and is continuous with the supe

cervical fascia on the back of the neck. I

Structural defects of the posterior bony elements

Deformity and bony deficiency may occur at several sites within the posterior elements. The laminae may be wholly or partially absent, or the spinous process alone may be affected, even without overlying soft tissue signs (spina bifida occulta). A defect may occur in the part of the lamina between the superior and inferior articular processes (pars inter-articularis): this condition is spondylolysis, and may be developmental or result from acute or fatigue fracture. If such defects are bilateral, the column becomes unstable at that level, and forward displacement of that part of the column above (cranial to) the defects may occur: this is spondylolisthesis. Abnormality of the laminar bone, or degenerative changes in the facet joints, may also lead to similar displacement in the absence of pars defects. The deformity of the vertebral canal resulting from severe spondylolisthesis may lead to neural damage. Much more rarely, bony defects may occur elsewhere in the posterior elements, e.g. in the pedicles.

Detailed anatomical relations of all aspects of the vertebral column at the various levels are best appreciated by the study of horizontal (axial) sections and images (**Figs 45.35D** and **45.54**).

CURVATURES

Embryonic and fetal curvatures

The embryonic body appears flexed. It has primary thoracic and pelvic curves which are convex dorsally. Functional muscle development leads to the early appearance of secondary cervical and lumbar spinal curvatures in the sagittal plane. The cervical curvature appears at the end of the embryonic period, and reflects the development of function in the muscles responsible for head extension, an important component of the 'grasp reflex'. Radiographic examination of human fetuses aged from 8 to 23 weeks shows that the secondary cervical curvature is almost always present. Lumbar flattening has also been identified as early as the eighth week. Ultrasound investigations support the role of move-

ment in the development of these curvatures. The early appearance of the secondary curves is probably accentuated by postnatal muscular and nervous system development at a time when the vertebral column is highly flexible and is capable of assuming almost any curvature.

Neonatal curvatures

In the neonate the vertebral column has no fixed curvatures (**Figs 11.5, 11.6**). It is particularly flexible and if dissected free from the body it can easily be bent (flexed or extended) into a perfect half circle. A slight sacral curvature can be seen which develops as the sacral vertebrae ossify and fuse. The thoracic part of the column is the first to develop a relatively fixed curvature, which is concave anteriorly. An infant can support its head at c.3 or 4 months, sit upright at c.9 months, and will commence walking between 12 and 15 months. These functional changes exert a major influence on the development of the secondary curvatures in the vertebral column and changes in the proportional size of the vertebrae, in particular in the lumbar region. The secondary lumbar curvature becomes important in maintaining the centre of gravity of the trunk over the legs when walking starts, and thus changes in body proportions exert a major influence on the subsequent shape of curvatures in the vertebral column.

Adult curvatures

In adults, the cervical curve is a lordosis (convex forwards), and the least marked. It extends from the atlas to the second thoracic vertebra, with its apex between the fourth and fifth cervical vertebrae. Sexual dimorphism has been described in the cervical curvatures. The thoracic curve is a kyphosis (convex dorsally). It extends between the second and the eleventh and twelfth thoracic vertebrae, and its apex lies between the sixth and ninth thoracic vertebrae. This curvature is caused by the increased posterior depth of the thoracic vertebral bodies. The lumbar curve is also a lordosis. It has a greater magnitude in females and extends from the twelfth thoracic vertebra to the lumbosacral angle:

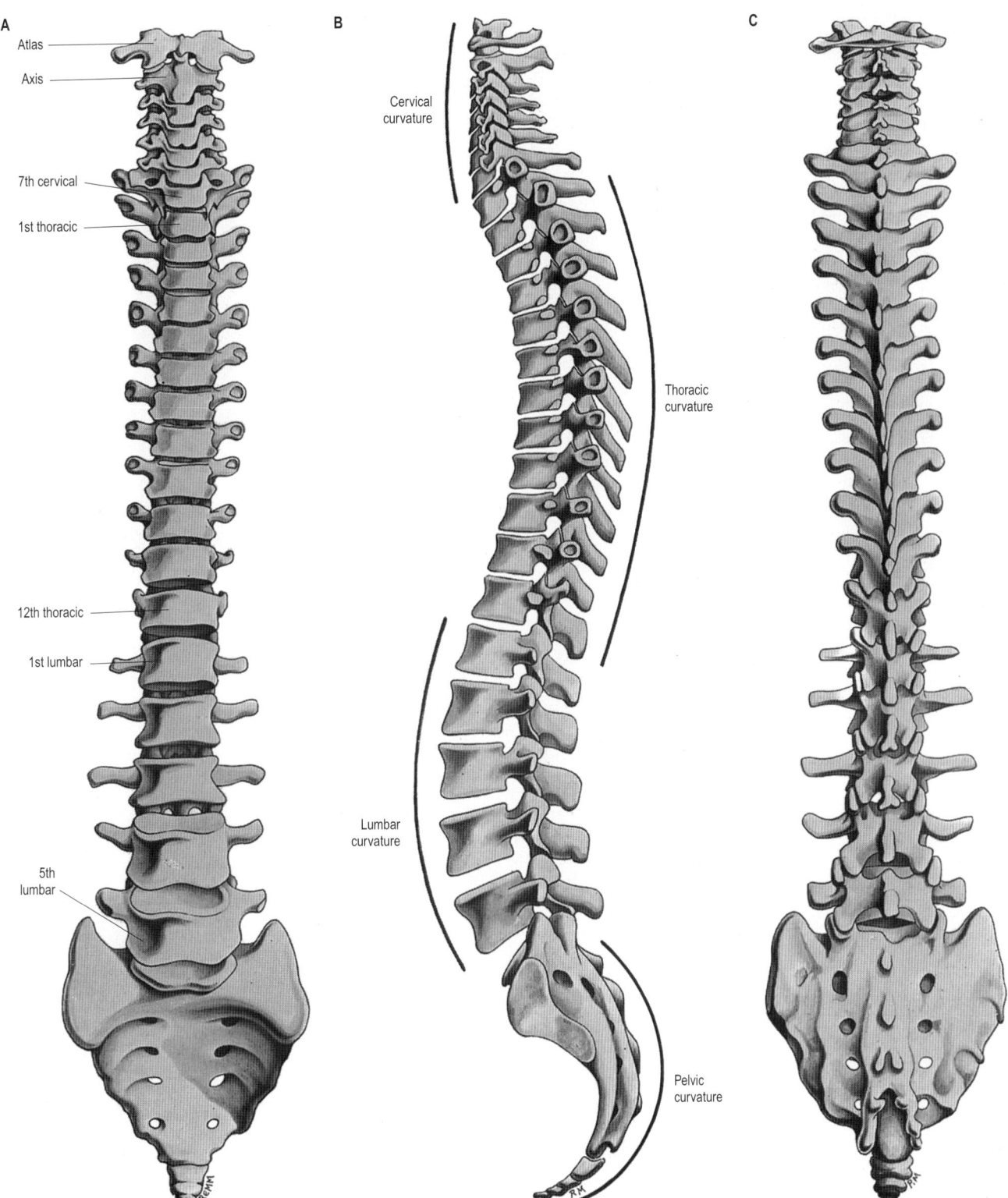

Fig. 45.7 The vertebral column: **A**, anterior aspect; **B**, lateral aspect; **C**, posterior aspect.

there is an increased convexity of the last three segments as a result of the greater anterior depth of the intervertebral discs and some posterior wedging of the vertebral bodies. Its apex is at the level of the third lumbar vertebra. The pelvic curve is concave anteroinferiorly and involves the sacrum and coccygeal vertebrae. It extends from the lumbosacral junction to the apex of the coccyx.

The presence of these curvatures means that the cross-sectional profile of the trunk changes with spinal level. The anteroposterior diameter of the thorax is much greater than that of the lower abdomen. In the normal vertebral column there are well-marked curvatures in the sagittal plane and no lateral curvatures other than in the upper thoracic region, where there is often a slight lateral curvature, convex to the right in right-handed persons, and to the left in the left-handed. Compensatory lateral curvature may also develop to cope with pelvic obliquity such as that imposed by inequality of leg length. The sagittal curvatures are present in the cervical, thoracic, lumbar and pelvic regions (**Fig. 45.7**). These curvatures have developed with rounding of the thorax and pelvis as an adaptation to bipedal gait.

VERTEBRAL COLUMN IN THE ELDERLY

In older people, age-related changes in the structure of bone lead to broadening and loss of height of the vertebral bodies. These changes are

737

A

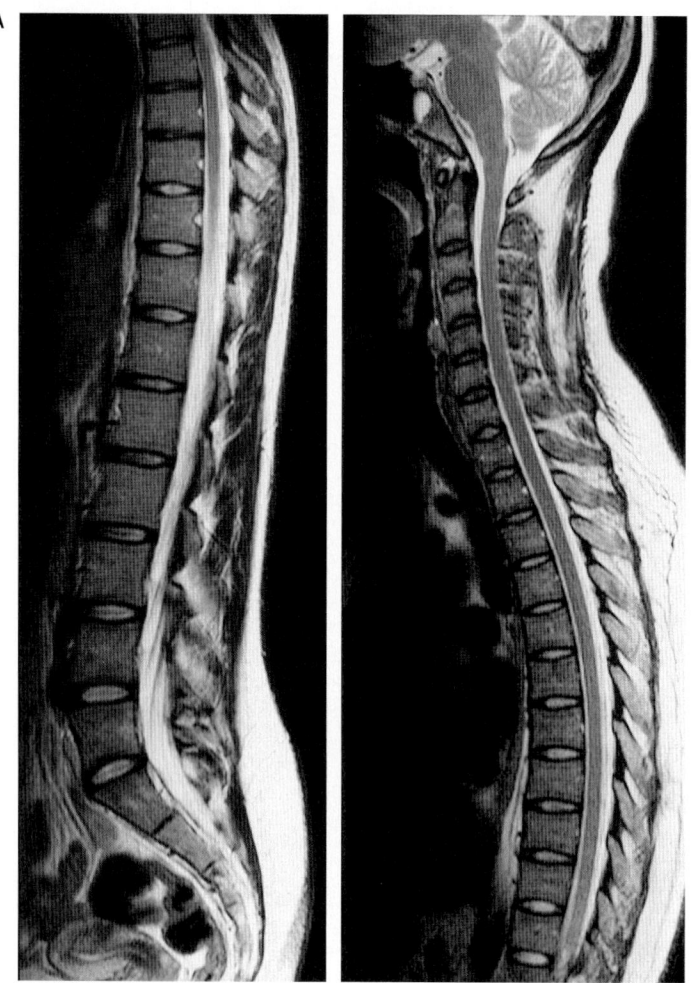

Fig. 45.8 A, Sagittal MRI of thoracolumbosacral spine. **B**, Sagittal MRI of cervicothoracic spine. (By kind permission from Dr Justin Lee, Chelsea and Westminster Hospital, London.)

B

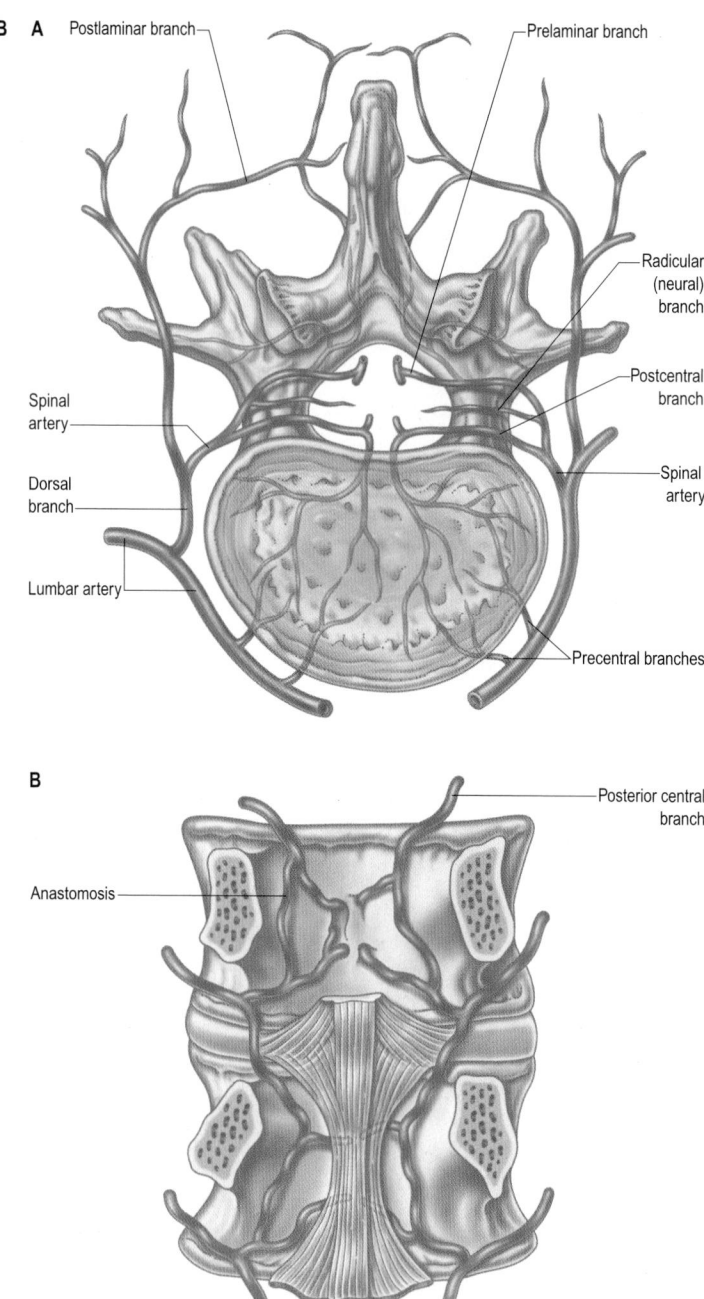

Fig. 45.9 Arterial supply to the vertebrae and the contents of the vertebral canal. **A**, Branching pattern of lumbar segmental arteries. **B**, Arterial anastomoses between postcentral branches of spinal arteries within the vertebral canal.

more severe in females. The bony changes in the vertebral column are accompanied by changes in the collagen content of the discs and by decline in the activity of the spinal muscles. This leads to progressive decline in vertebral column mobility, particularly in the lumbar spine. The development of a 'dowager's hump' in the midthoracic region in females, caused by age-related osteoporosis, increases the thoracic kyphosis and cervical lordosis. Overall, these changes in the vertebral column lead directly to loss of total height in the individual.

In mid-lumbar vertebrae the width of the body increases with age. In men there is a relative decrease of posterior to anterior body height, while in both sexes anterior height decreases relative to width. Twomey et al (1983) observed a reduction in bone density of lumbar vertebral bodies with age, principally as a result of a reduction in transverse trabeculae (more marked in females as a result of postmenopausal osteoporosis), which was associated with increased diameter and increasing concavity in their juxtadiscal surfaces (end-plates).

Other changes affect the vertebral bodies. Osteophytes (bony spurs) may form from the compact cortical bone on the anterior and lateral surfaces of the bodies. Although individual variations occur, these changes appear in most individuals from c.20 years onwards. They are most common on the anterior aspect of the body, and never involve the ring epiphysis. Osteophytic spurs are frequently asymptomatic, but may result in diminished movements within the spine.

VASCULAR SUPPLY AND LYMPHATIC DRAINAGE
(See also Crock 1996.)

Arteries (Fig. 45.9)
The vertebral column, its contents and its associated soft-tissues, all receive their arterial supply from derivatives of dorsal branches of

the embryonic intersegmental somatic arteries (Ch. 61 and **Fig. 61.24**). The named artery concerned depends on the level of the column. These intersegmental vessels persist in the thoracic and lumbar regions as the posterior intercostal and lumbar arteries. In the cervical and sacral regions, longitudinal anastomoses between the intersegmental vessels persist as longitudinal vessels which themselves give spinal branches to the vertebral column. In the neck the postcostal anastomosis becomes most of the vertebral artery, while the post-transverse anastomosis forms most of the deep cervical artery. The ascending cervical artery and the lateral sacral artery are persistent parts of the precostal anastomosis.

In the thorax and abdomen the primitive arterial pattern is retained by the paired branches of the descending aorta which supply the vertebral column (**45.9A**). On each side, the main trunk of the artery (posterior intercostal or lumbar (p. 1119) passes around the vertebral body, giving off primary periosteal and equatorial branches to the body, and then a major dorsal branch. The dorsal branch gives off a spinal

A

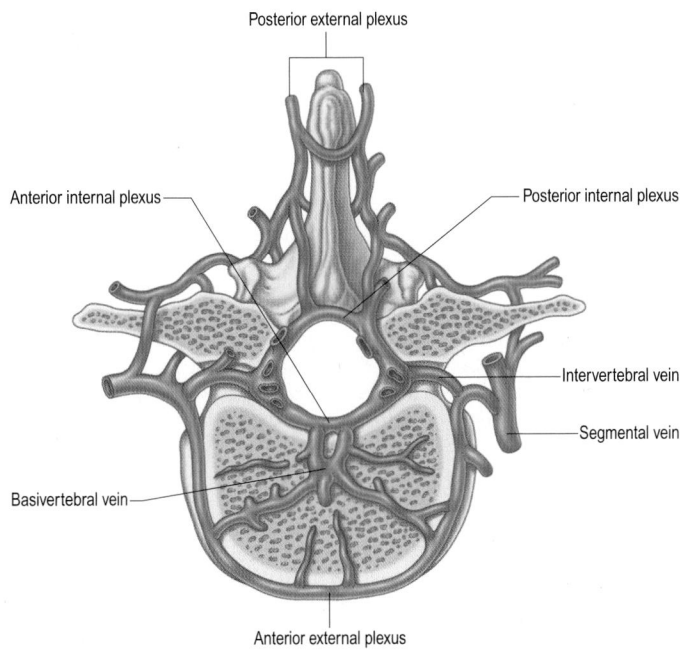

Anterior internal
vertebral (epidural)
venous plexus

Posterior internal
vertebral (epidural)
venous plexus

Anterior external
vertebral venous plexus

Posterior external
vertebral venous plexus

Basivertebral vein

Intervertebral vein

branch which enters the intervertebral foramen, before itself supplying
the facet joints, the posterior surfaces of the laminae and the overlying
muscles and skin. There is free anastomosis between these dorsal
articular and soft-tissue branches, extending over several segments
(Crock & Yoshizawa 1976; Boelderl et al 2002). At cervical and sacral
levels the longitudinally running arteries described above have direct
spinal branches. The spinal branches are the main arteries of supply to
all bony elements of the vertebrae and to the dura and epidural tissues,
and also contribute to the supply of the spinal cord and nerve roots via
radicular branches (p. 784). As they enter the vertebral canal the spinal
arteries divide into postcentral, prelaminar and radicular branches.
The postcentral branches, which are the main nutrient arteries to the
vertebral bodies and to the periphery of the intervertebral discs,
anastomose beneath the posterior longitudinal ligament with their
fellows above and below as well as across the midline (**Fig. 45.9A,B**).
This anastomosis also supplies the anterior epidural tissues and dura.
The majority of the vertebral arch, the posterior epidural tissues and
dura and the ligamentum flavum are supplied by the prelaminar
branches and their anastomotic plexus on the posterior wall of the
vertebral canal.

Veins (Fig. 45.10)

Veins of the vertebral column form intricate plexuses along the entire
column, external and internal to the vertebral canal. Both groups are
devoid of valves, anastomose freely with each other, and join the intervertebral veins. Interconnections are widely established between these
plexuses and longitudinal veins early in fetal life. When development
is complete, the plexuses drain into the caval and azygos/ascending
lumbar systems via named veins which accompany the arteries described
above.

The veins also communicate with cranial dural venous sinuses and
with the deep veins of the neck and pelvis. The venous complexes
associated with the vertebral column can dilate considerably, and can
form alternative routes of venous return in patients with major venous
obstruction in the neck, chest or abdomen. The absence of valves allows

B

Posterior external plexus

Anterior internal plexus

Posterior internal plexus

Intervertebral vein

Segmental vein

Basivertebral vein

Anterior external plexus

Fig. 45.10 A, B Venous drainage of the vertebral column.

pathways for the wide and sometimes paradoxical spread of malignant
disease and sepsis. Pressure changes in the body cavities are transmitted
to these venous plexuses and thus to the CSF, though the cord itself may
be protected from such congestion by valves in the small veins which
drain from the cord into the internal vertebral plexus.

External vertebral venous plexuses

The external vertebral venous plexuses are anterior and posterior. They anastomose freely, and are most developed in the cervical region. Anterior external plexuses are anterior to the vertebral bodies, communicate with basivertebral and intervertebral veins, and receive tributaries from vertebral bodies. Posterior external plexuses lie posterior to the vertebral laminae and around spines, transverse and articular processes. They anastomose with the internal plexuses and join the vertebral, posterior intercostal and lumbar veins.

Internal vertebral venous plexuses

The internal vertebral venous plexuses occur between the dura mater and vertebrae, and receive tributaries from the bones, red bone marrow and spinal cord. They form a denser network than the external plexuses and are arranged vertically as four interconnecting longitudinal vessels, two anterior and two posterior.

The anterior internal plexuses are large plexiform veins on the posterior surfaces of the vertebral bodies and intervertebral discs. They flank the posterior longitudinal ligament, beneath which they are connected by transverse branches into which the large basivertebral veins open. The posterior internal plexuses, on each side in front of the vertebral arches and ligamenta flava, anastomose with the posterior external plexuses via veins which pass through and between the ligaments. The internal plexuses interconnect by venous rings near each vertebra. Around the foramen magnum they form a dense network connecting with vertebral veins, occipital and sigmoid sinuses, the basilar plexus, the venous plexus of the hypoglossal canal, and the condylar emissary veins.

Basivertebral veins

The basivertebral veins emerge from the posterior foramina of the vertebral bodies. They are large and tortuous channels in bone, like those in the cranial diploë. The basivertebral veins also drain into the anterior external vertebral plexuses through small openings in the vertebral bodies. Posteriorly they form one or two short trunks which open into the transverse branches and unite anterior internal vertebral plexuses. They enlarge in advanced age.

Intervertebral veins

The intervertebral veins accompany the spinal nerves through intervertebral foramina, draining the spinal cord and internal and external vertebral plexuses, and ending in the vertebral, posterior intercostal, lumbar and lateral sacral veins. Upper posterior intercostal veins may drain into the caval system via brachiocephalic veins, whereas the lower intercostals drain into the azygos system. Lumbar veins are joined longitudinally in front of the transverse processes by the ascending lumbar veins, in which they may terminate. Alternatively, they may proceed around the vertebral bodies to drain into the inferior vena cava. Whether the basivertebral or intervertebral veins contain effective valves is uncertain but experimental evidence strongly suggests that their blood flow can be reversed (Batson 1957). This may explain how pelvic neoplasms, e.g. carcinoma of the prostate, may metastasize in vertebral bodies: the cells spread into the internal vertebral plexuses via their connections with the pelvic veins when blood flow is temporarily reversed by raised intra-abdominal pressure or postural alterations.

Lymphatic drainage

Little is known in detail about the lymphatic drainage of the vertebral column and its associated soft tissues. In general, deep lymphatic vessels tend to follow the arteries. The cervical vertebral column drains to deep cervical nodes, the thoracic to (posterior) intercostal nodes, and the lumbar column to lateral aortic and retro-aortic nodes. The pelvic part of the column drains to lateral sacral and internal iliac nodes.

INNERVATION

Innervation of the vertebral column and its associated soft tissues has been studied in greatest detail in the lumbar region. The account given here relies particularly on the work of Bogduk, to whose textbook on the lumbosacral spine (Bogduk 1997) the interested reader is referred. See also the work of Groen et al (1990).

Innervation is derived from the spinal nerves where they branch, in and just beyond the intervertebral foramina. There is also an important input from the sympathetic system via grey rami communicantes or directly from thoracic sympathetic ganglia. The branches of the spinal nerve concerned are the dorsal ramus and the recurrent meningeal or sinuvertebral nerves (usually more than one at each level) (p. 782 and also **Fig. 46.11**). The dorsal ramus branches to supply the facet joints, periosteum of the posterior bony elements, overlying muscles and skin. The exact origin and branching pattern of the sinuvertebral nerves is controversial, but they may be best considered to be recurrent branches of the ventral rami. They receive the sympathetic input described above, then re-enter the intervertebral foramina to supply the structures forming the walls of the vertebral canal as well as the dura and epidural soft tissues. Their subsequent course is described on page 782.

VERTEBRAE: GENERAL FEATURES

A typical vertebra has a ventral body, a dorsal vertebral (neural) arch, extended by lever-like processes, and a vertebral foramen, which is occupied in life by the spinal cord, meninges and their vessels (**Fig. 45.11**).

Opposed surfaces of adjacent bodies are bound together by intervertebral discs of fibrocartilage. The complete column of bodies and discs forms the strong but flexible central axis of the body and supports the full weight of the head and trunk. It also transmits even greater forces generated by muscles attached to it directly or indirectly. The foramina form a vertebral canal for the spinal cord, and between adjoining neural arches, near their junctions with vertebral bodies, intervertebral foramina transmit mixed spinal nerves, smaller recurrent nerves and blood and lymphatic vessels.

The cylindroid vertebral body varies in size, shape and proportions in different regions of the vertebral column. Its superior and inferior (discal) surfaces vary in shape from approximately flat (but not parallel) to sellar, with a raised peripheral smooth zone formed from an 'anular' epiphyseal disc within which the surface is rough. These differences in texture reflect variations in the early structure of intervertebral discs. In the horizontal plane the profiles of most bodies are convex anteriorly, but concave posteriorly where they complete the vertebral foramen. Most sagittal profiles are concave anteriorly but flat posteriorly. Small vascular foramina appear on the front and sides, and posteriorly there are small arterial foramina and a large irregular orifice (sometimes double) for the exit of basivertebral veins (**Fig. 45.12**). The adult vertebral body is not coextensive with the developmental centrum but includes, posterolaterally, parts of the neural arch.

Viewed anteriorly there is a cephalocaudal increase in vertebral body width from the second cervical to the third lumbar vertebra, which is associated with an increased load-bearing function. The increase is linear in the neck but not in the thoracic and lumbar regions. There is some variation in size of the last two lumbar bodies, but thereafter width diminishes rapidly to the coccygeal apex. In the two lowest lumbar vertebrae there is an inverse relation between the areas of the

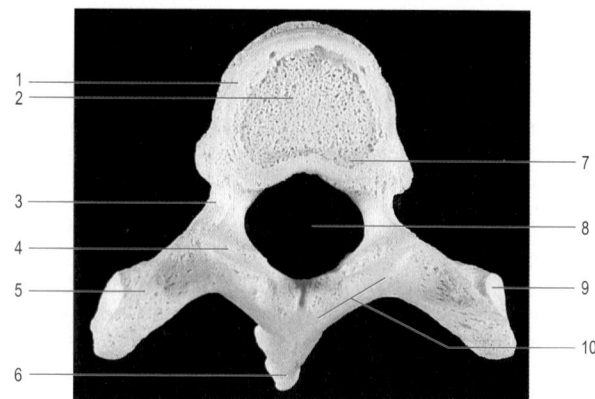

1. Bone derived from anular epiphysis.   2. Vertebral body – bone derived from centrum.
3. Pedicle.   4. Superior articular facet.   5. Transverse process.   6. Spinous process.
7. Vertebral body – bone derived from neural arch.   8. Vertebral foramen.
9. Costal facet.   10. Lamina.

Fig. 45.11 Fourth thoracic vertebra, superior aspect. (Photograph by Sarah-Jane Smith.)

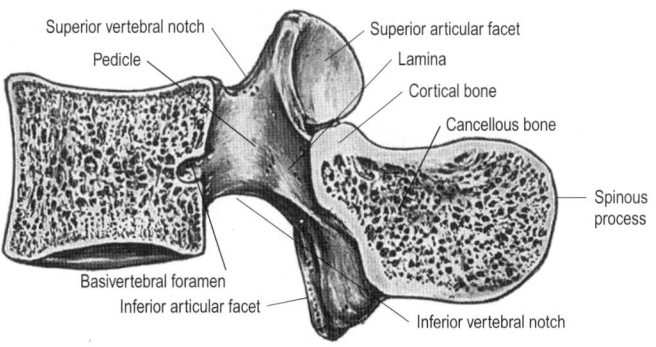

Fig. 45.12 Median sagittal section through a lumbar vertebra.

upper and lower surfaces of the bodies and the size of the pedicles and transverse processes.

On each side the vertebral arch has a vertically narrower ventral part, the pedicle, and a broader lamina dorsally. Paired transverse, superior and inferior articular processes project from their junctions. There is a median dorsal spinous process.

Pedicles are short, thick, rounded dorsal projections from the superior part of the body at the junction of its lateral and dorsal surfaces: the concavity formed by the curved superior border of the pedicle is shallower than the inferior one (**Fig. 45.12**). When vertebrae articulate by the intervertebral disc and facet joints, these adjacent vertebral notches contribute to an intervertebral foramen. The complete perimeter of an intervertebral foramen consists of the notches, the dorsolateral aspects of parts of adjacent vertebral bodies and the intervening disc, and the capsule of the synovial facet joint.

The laminae are directly continuous with the pedicles. They are vertically flattened and curve dorsomedially to complete, with the base of the spinous process, a vertebral foramen.

Lateral to the spinous processes, vertebral grooves contain the deep dorsal muscles. At cervical and lumbar levels these grooves are shallow and mainly formed by laminae. In the thoracic region they are deeper, broader and formed by the laminae and transverse processes. The laminae are broad for the first thoracic vertebra, narrow for the second to seventh, broaden again from the eighth to eleventh, but become narrow thereafter down to the third lumbar vertebra.

The spinous process (vertebral spine) projects dorsally and often caudally from the junction of the laminae. Spines vary considerably in size, shape and direction. They lie approximately in the median plane and project posteriorly, although in some individuals a minor deflection of the processes to one side may be seen. The spines act as levers for muscles which control posture and active movements (flexion/extension, lateral flexion and rotation) of the vertebral column.

The paired superior and inferior articular processes (zygapophyses) arise from the vertebral arch at the pediculolaminar junctions. The superior processes project cranially, bearing dorsal facets which may also have a lateral or medial inclination, depending on level. Inferior processes run caudally with articular facets directed ventrally, again with a medial or lateral inclination which depends on vertebral level. Articular processes of adjoining vertebrae thus contribute to the synovial zygapophyseal or facet joints (p. 757), and form part of the posterior boundaries of the intervertebral foramina. These joints permit limited movement between vertebrae: mobility varies considerably with vertebral level.

Transverse processes project laterally from the pediculolaminar junctions as levers for muscles and ligaments, particularly those concerned in rotation and lateral flexion. In the cervical region, the transverse processes are anterior to the articular processes, lateral to the pedicles and between the intervertebral foramina. In the thoracic region, they are posterior to the pedicles, considerably behind those of the cervical and lumbar regions. In the lumbar region, the transverse processes are anterior to the articular processes, but posterior to the intervertebral foramina. There is considerable regional variation in the structure and length of the transverse processes. In the cervical region, the transverse process of the atlas is long and broad, which allows the rotator muscles maximum mechanical advantage. Breadth varies little

from the second to the sixth cervical vertebra, but increases in the seventh. In thoracic vertebrae, the first is widest, and breadth decreases to the twelfth, where the transverse elements are usually vestigial. The transverse processes become broader in the upper three lumbar vertebrae, and diminish in the fourth and fifth. The transverse process of the fifth lumbar vertebra is the most robust. It arises directly from the body and pedicle to allow for force transmission to the pelvis through the iliolumbar ligament.

The thoracic transverse processes articulate with ribs, but at other levels the mature transverse process is a composite of 'true' transverse process and an incorporated costal element. Costal elements develop as basic parts of neural arches in mammalian embryos, but become independent only as thoracic ribs. Elsewhere they remain less developed and fuse with the 'transverse process' of descriptive anatomy (**Fig. 47.7**).

Vertebrae are internally trabecular, and have an external shell of compact bone perforated by vascular foramina (**Fig. 45.12**). The shell is thin on the superior and inferior body surfaces but thicker in the arch and its processes. The trabecular interior contains red bone marrow and one or two large ventrodorsal canals which contain the basivertebral veins.

Sexual dimorphism in vertebrae has received little attention, but Taylor and Twomey (1984) have described radiological differences in adolescent humans and have reported that female vertebral bodies have a lower ratio of width to depth. Vertebral body diameter has also been used as a basis for sex prediction in the analysis of skeletal material (MacLaughlin & Oldale 1992).

VERTEBRAL CANAL (Fig. 45.13)

The vertebral canal extends from the foramen magnum to the sacral hiatus, and follows the vertebral curves. In the cervical and lumbar regions, which exhibit free mobility, it is large and triangular, but in the thoracic region, where movement is less, it is small and circular. These differences are matched by variations in the diameter of the spinal cord and its enlargements. In the lumbar region, the vertebral canal decreases gradually in size between L1 and L5, with a greater relative width in the female.

For clinical purposes it is useful to consider the vertebral canal as having three zones. These are a central zone, between the medial margins of the facet joints, and two lateral zones, beneath the facet joints and entering the intervertebral foramina. Each lateral zone, which passes into and just beyond the intravertebral foramen, can be further subdivided into subarticular (lateral recess), foraminal and extraforaminal regions (Macnab & McCulloch 1990). The lateral zone thus described forms the canal of the spinal nerve (the radicular or 'root' canal). The central zone of the canal is a little narrower than the radiological interpedicular distance if the lateral recess is considered to be part of the radicular canal rather than part of the central zone.

Spinal stenosis

Narrowing (stenosis) of the vertebral canal may occur at single or multiple spinal levels, and mainly affects the lumbar and cervical regions. Stenosis may affect the central canal and the 'root canals' either together or separately. There is a developmental form of the condition which mainly affects the central canal, but more commonly the stenosis is degenerative, and results from intervertebral disc narrowing and osteoarthritic changes in the facet joints. This latter combination is more likely to narrow the intervertebral foramen and the 'root canal', even though the sectional profile of the vertebral canal in affected lumbar vertebrae typically changes from the shape of a bell to that of a trefoil. The lumbosacral intervertebral foramen, which is normally the smallest in the region, is particularly liable to such stenosis.

Severe spinal stenosis may compress the spinal cord and compromise its arterial supply. More localized 'root canal' stenosis will present with the clinical features of spinal nerve compression, but without the tension signs which characterize the stretching of nerve roots over a prolapsed disc. Ischaemia of the nerves and roots may be more responsible for the damage than is the actual physical compression of the neural tissue.

INTERVERTEBRAL FORAMINA (See also p. 735 and p. 782.)

Intervertebral foramina are the principal routes of entry and exit to and from the vertebral canal, and are closely related to the main intervertebral articulations. (Minor routes occur between the median, often

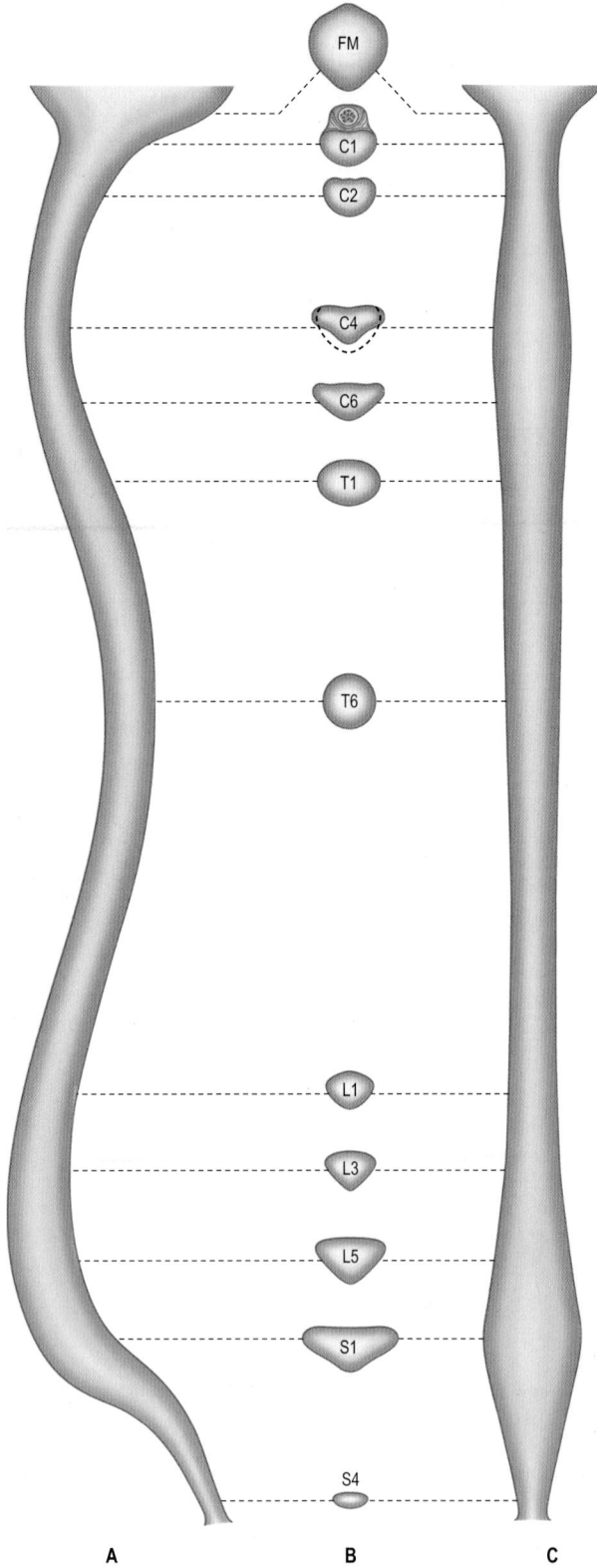

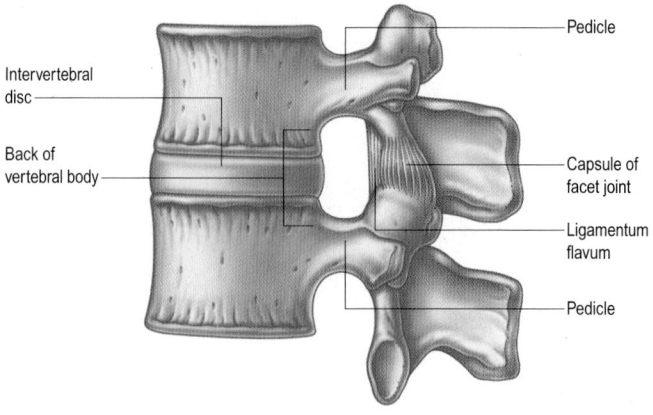

Fig. 45.14 The boundaries of an intervertebral foramen.

Fig. 45.13 The vertebral canal in section: **A**, sagittal; **B**, transverse (axial); **C**, coronal.

The boundaries of a generalized intervertebral foramen (**Fig. 45.14**) are anteriorly, from above downwards, the posterolateral aspect of the superior vertebral body, the posterolateral aspect of the intervertebral symphysis (including the disc), and a small (variable) posterolateral part of the body of the inferior vertebra; superiorly, the compact bone of the deep arched inferior vertebral notch of the vertebra above; inferiorly, the compact bone of the shallow superior vertebral notch of the vertebra below; and posteriorly a part of the ventral aspect of the fibrous capsule of the facet synovial joint. Cervical intervertebral foramina are distinct in having superior and inferior vertebral notches of almost equal depth which, in accord with the direction of the pedicles, face anterolaterally. External to them, and oriented in the same direction, is a transverse process. The thoracic and lumbar intervertebral foramina face laterally and their transverse processes are posterior. In addition, the anteroinferior boundaries of the first to tenth thoracic foramina are formed by the articulations of the head of a rib and the capsules of double synovial joints (with the demifacets on adjacent vertebrae and the intra-articular ligament between the costocapitular ridge and the intervertebral symphysis). Lumbar foramina lie between the two principal lines of vertebral attachment of psoas major. The walls of each foramen are covered throughout by fibrous tissue which is in turn periosteal (though the presence of a true periosteum lining the vertebral canal is controversial [Newell 1999]), perichondrial, annular and capsular. The more lateral parts of the foramina may be crossed at a variable level by narrow fibrous bands, the transforaminal ligaments. The true foramen is the foraminal region of the canal of the spinal nerve (the radicular or 'root' canal). A foramen contains a segmental mixed spinal nerve and its sheaths, from two to four recurrent meningeal (sinuvertebral) nerves, variable numbers of spinal arteries, and plexiform venous connections between the internal and external vertebral venous plexuses. These structures, particularly the nerves, may be affected by trauma or one of the many disorders which may affect tissues bordering the foramen. In particular, nerve compression and irritation may be caused by intervertebral disc prolapse, or by bony entrapment as the size of the foramen decreases as a result of facet joint osteoarthritis, osteophyte formation or disc degeneration, all of which may lead to lateral or foraminal spinal stenosis.

CERVICAL VERTEBRAE (Figs 45.8B, 45.15, 45.16)

The cervical vertebrae are the smallest of the moveable vertebrae, and are characterized by a foramen in each transverse process. The first, second and seventh have special features and will be considered separately. The third, fourth and fifth cervical are almost identical, and the sixth, while typical in its general features, has minor distinguishing differences.

TYPICAL CERVICAL VERTEBRA (Figs 45.17, 45.18)
A typical cervical vertebra has a small, relatively broad vertebral body. The pedicles project posterolaterally and the longer laminae posteromedially, enclosing a large, roughly triangular vertebral foramen; the vertebral canal here accommodates the cervical enlargement of the

partly fused, margins of the ligamenta flava.) The same general arrangement applies throughout the vertebral column, between the axis and sacrum, although there are some quantitative and structural regional variations. Because of their construction, contents and susceptibilities to multiple disorders, the intervertebral foramina are loci of great biomechanical, functional and clinical significance. The specializations cranial to the axis and at sacral levels are described with the individual bones and articulations.

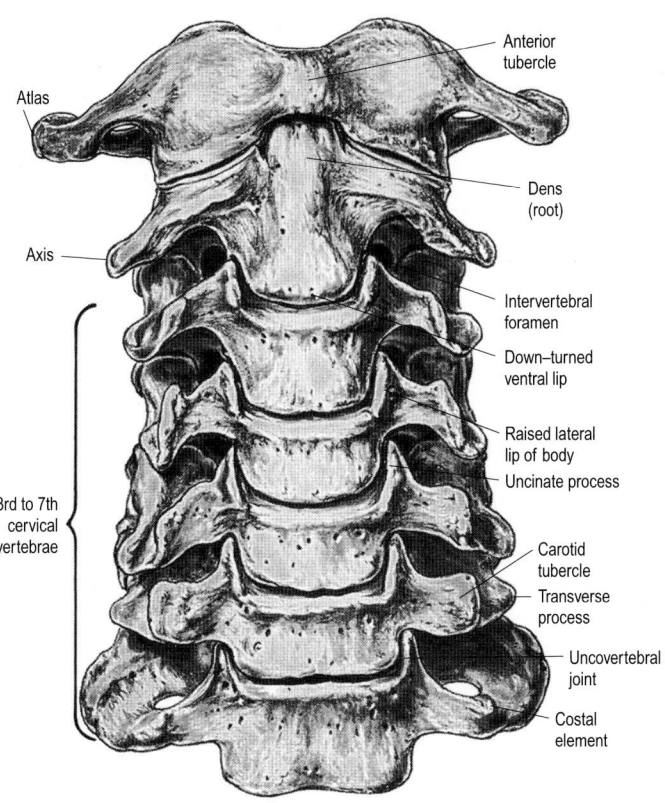

Fig. 45.15 The cervical vertebrae (anterior aspect).

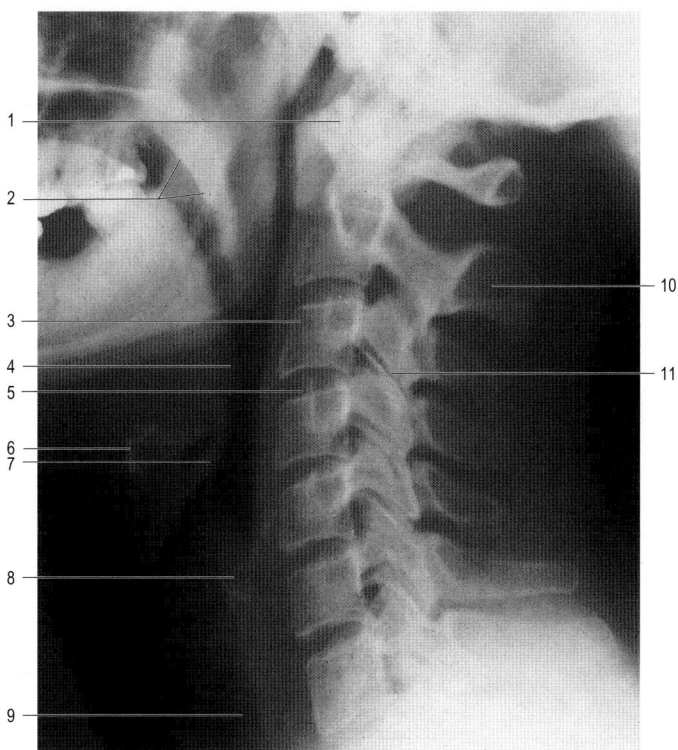

1. Anterior tubercle of the atlas. 2. Soft palate. 3. Characteristic cervical body.
4. Pharyngeal part of the tongue. 5. Intervertebral disc. 6. Body of the hyoid bone.
7. Epiglottis. 8. Thyroid cartilage which is undergoing calcification. 9. Air in trachea.
10. Spinous process of the axis. 11. Zygapophyseal joint.

Fig. 45.16 Lateral radiograph of the neck. The cervical curve of the vertebral column is well shown. (Provided by Shaun Gallagher, GKT School of Medicine, London; photograph by Sarah-Jane Smith.)

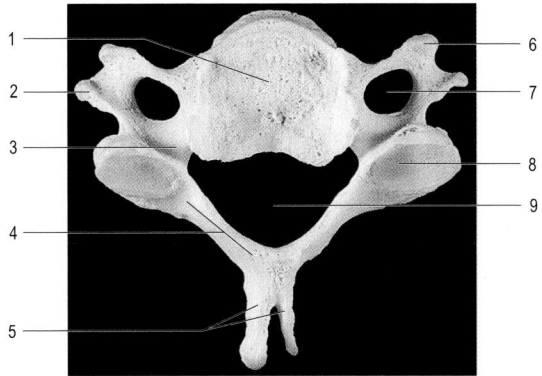

1. Body. 2. Posterior tubercle of transverse process. 3. Pedicle. 4. Lamina.
5. Bifid spinous process. 6. Anterior tubercle of transverse process. 7. Foramen transversarium.
8. Superior articular facet. 9. Vertebral foramen.

Fig. 45.17 Fourth cervical vertebra, superior aspect. (Photograph by Sarah-Jane Smith.)

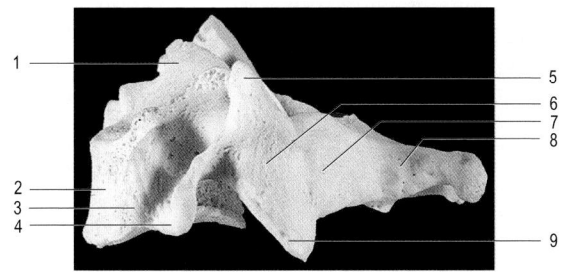

1. Uncinate process. 2. Body. 3. Anterior tubercle of transverse process.
4. Posterior tubercle of transverse process. 5. Superior articular process. 6. Lateral mass.
7. Lamina. 8. Spinous process. 9. Inferior articular process.

Fig. 45.18 Fourth cervical vertebra, lateral aspect. (Photograph by Sarah-Jane Smith.)

spinal cord. The pedicles attach midway between the discal surfaces of the vertebral body, so the superior and inferior vertebral notches are of similar depth. The laminae are thin and slightly curved, with a thin superior and slightly thicker inferior border. The spinous process ('spine') is short and bifid, with two tubercles which are often unequal in size. The junction between lamina and pedicle bulges laterally between the superior and inferior articular processes to form, when articulated, an articular pillar ('lateral mass') on each side. The transverse process is morphologically composite around the foramen transversarium. Its dorsal and ventral bars terminate laterally as corresponding tubercles. The tubercles are connected, lateral to the foramen, by the costal (or intertubercular) lamella: these three elements represent morphologically the capitellum, tubercle and neck of a cervical costal element (p. 795). The attachment of the dorsal bar to the pediculolaminar junction

represents the morphological transverse process and the attachment of the ventral bar to the ventral body represents the capitellar process.

The vertebral body has a convex anterior surface. The discal margin gives attachment to the anterior longitudinal ligament. The posterior surface is flat or minimally concave, and its discal margins give attachment to the posterior longitudinal ligament. The central area displays several vascular foramina, of which two are commonly relatively larger. These are the basivertebral foramina which transmit basivertebral veins to the anterior internal vertebral veins. The superior discal surface is saddle-shaped, formed by flange-like lips which arise from most of the lateral circumference of the upper margin of the vertebral body; these are sometimes referred to as uncinate or neurocentral lips or processes. The inferior discal surface is also concave: the convexity is produced mainly by a broad projection from the anterior margin which partly

743

overlaps the anterior surface of the intervertebral disc. The discal surfaces of cervical vertebrae are so shaped in order to restrict both lateral and anteroposterior gliding movements during articulation. The paired ligamenta flava extend from the superior border of each lamina below to the roughened inferior half of the anterior surfaces of the lamina above. The superior part of the anterior surface of each lamina is smooth, like the immediately adjacent surfaces of the pedicles, which are usually in direct contact with the dura mater and cervical root sheaths to which they may become loosely attached. The spinous process of the sixth cervical vertebra is larger, and is often not bifid.

The superior articular facets, flat and ovoid, are directed supero-posteriorly, whereas the corresponding inferior facets are directed mainly anteriorly, and lie nearer the coronal plane than the superior facets. The dorsal rami of the cervical spinal nerves curve posteriorly, close to the anterolateral aspects of the lateral masses, and may actually lie in shallow grooves, especially on the third and fourth pair. The dorsal root ganglion of each cervical spinal nerve lies between the superior and inferior vertebral notches of adjacent vertebrae. The large anterior ramus passes posterior to the vertebral artery, which lies on the concave upper surface of the costal lamella: the concavity of the lamellae increases from the fourth to the sixth vertebra. The fourth to sixth anterior tubercles are elongated and rough for muscle attachment. The sixth is the longest, the carotid tubercle of Chassaignac. The carotid artery can be forcibly compressed in the groove formed by the vertebral bodies and the larger anterior tubercles, especially the sixth. The posterior tubercles are rounded and more laterally placed than the anterior, and all but the sixth are also more caudal; the sixth is at about the same level as the anterior.

Muscle attachments – The ligamentum nuchae and numerous deep extensors, including semispinalis thoracis and cervicis, multifidus, spinales and interspinales, are all attached to the spinous processes. Tendinous slips of scalenus anterior, longus capitis and longus colli are attached to the fourth to sixth anterior tubercles. Splenius, longissimus and iliocostalis cervicis, levator scapulae and scalenus posterior and medius are all attached to the posterior tubercles. Shallow anterolateral depressions on the anterior surface of the body lodge the vertical parts of the longus colli.

Ossification – Cervical vertebrae ossify according to the standard vertebral pattern described on page 792. Incomplete segmentation ('block vertebra') is common in the cervical spine and most commonly involves the axis and third cervical vertebra.

C1, THE ATLAS (Fig. 45.19)

The atlas, the first cervical vertebra, supports the head. It is unique in that it fails to incorporate a centrum, whose expected position is occupied by the dens, a cranial protuberance from the axis. The atlas consists of two lateral masses connected by a short anterior and a longer

posterior arch. The transverse ligament retains the dens against the anterior arch.

The transverse ligament divides the vertebral canal into two compartments. The anterior third (approximately) of the canal is occupied by the dens. The posterior compartment is occupied by the spinal cord and its coverings, and the cord itself takes up about half of this space (i.e. the cord, like the dens, occupies one third of the canal).

The anterior arch is slightly convex anteriorly, and carries a roughened anterior tubercle to which is attached the anterior longitudinal ligament (which is cord-like at this level). Its upper and lower borders provide attachment for the anterior atlanto-occipital membrane and diverging lateral parts of the anterior longitudinal ligament. The posterior surface of the anterior arch carries a concave, almost circular, facet for the dens.

The lateral masses are ovoid, their long axes converging anteriorly. Each bears a kidney-shaped superior articular facet for the respective occipital condyle, which is sometimes completely divided into a larger anterior and a smaller posterior part (Lang 1986). The inferior articular facet of the lateral mass is almost circular and is flat or slightly concave. It is orientated more obliquely to the transverse plane than the superior facet, and faces more medially and very slightly backwards. On the medial surface of each lateral mass is a roughened area which bears vascular foramina and a tubercle for attachment of the transverse ligament. In adults the distance between these tubercles is shorter than the transverse ligament itself, with a mean value of c.16 mm.

The posterior arch forms three-fifths of the circumference of the atlantal ring. The superior surface bears a wide groove for the vertebral artery and venous plexus immediately behind, and is variably overhung by the lateral mass; the first cervical nerve intervenes. The flange-like superior border gives attachment to the posterior atlanto-axial membrane, and the flatter inferior border to the highest pair of ligamenta flava. The posterior tubercle is a rudimentary spinous process, roughened for attachment of the ligamentum nuchae.

The transverse processes are longer than those of all cervical vertebrae except the seventh (**Fig. 45.15**). They act as strong levers for the muscles which make fine adjustments to keep the head balanced. Maximum atlantal width varies from 74–95 mm in males and 65–76 mm in females, and this affords a useful criterion for assessing sex in human remains. The apex of the transverse process, which is usually broad, flat and palpable between the mastoid process and ramus of the mandible, is homologous with the posterior tubercle of typical cervical vertebrae: the remaining part of the transverse process consists of the costal lamella. A small anterior tubercle is sometimes visible on the anterior aspect of the lateral mass. The costal lamella is sometimes deficient, which leaves the foramen transversarium open anteriorly.

Muscle attachments – The superior oblique parts of longus colli are attached on each side of the anterior tubercle. The anterior surface of the lateral mass gives attachment to rectus capitis anterior. Rectus capitis posterior minor is attached just lateral to the posterior tubercle. Rectus capitis lateralis is attached to the transverse process superiorly, and obliquus capitis superior is located more posteriorly. Obliquus capitis inferior is attached laterally on the apex, below which are slips of levator scapulae, splenius cervicis and scalenus medius.

Ossification – The atlas is commonly ossified from three centres (**Fig. 45.20**). One appears in each lateral mass at about the seventh week, gradually extending into the posterior arch where they unite between the third and fourth years, usually directly but occasionally through a separate centre. At birth, the anterior arch is fibrocartilaginous, and a separate centre appears about the end of the first year. This unites with the lateral masses between the sixth and eighth year, the lines of union extending across anterior parts of the superior articular facets. Occasionally the anterior arch is formed by the extension and ultimate union of centres in the lateral masses and sometimes from two lateral centres in the arch itself.

The central part of the posterior arch may be absent and replaced by fibrous tissue. Frequently bony spurs arise from the anterior and posterior margins of the groove for the vertebral artery. These are sometimes referred to as ponticles, and they occasionally convert the groove into a foramen. More often the foramen is incomplete superiorly. Rarely the atlas may be wholly or partially assimilated into (fused with) the occiput.

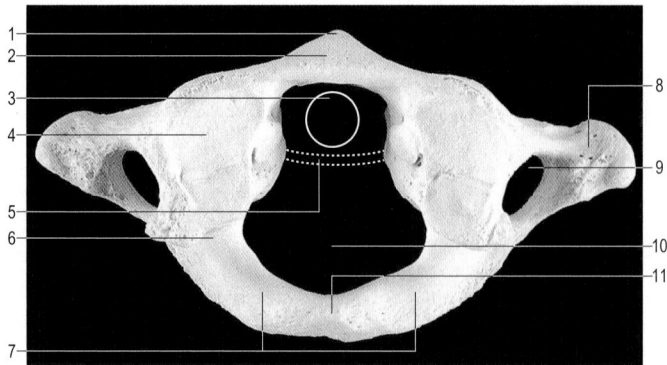

1. Anterior tubercle. 2. Anterior arch. 3. Outline of dens.
4. Superior articular facet, on lateral mass (bipartite facet in this specimen).
5. Outline of transverse ligament. 6. Groove for vertebral artery and C1
(beneath bony overhang from lateral mass here). 7. Posterior arch. 8. Transverse process.
9. Foramen transversarium. 10. Vertebral foramen. 11. Posterior tubercle.

Fig. 45.19 First cervical vertebra (atlas), superior aspect. (Photograph by Sarah-Jane Smith.)

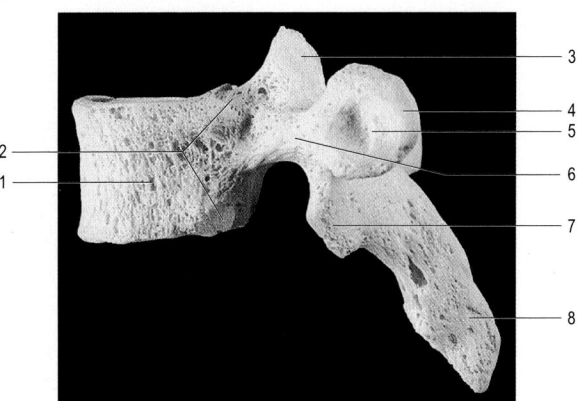

1. Body. 2. Costocapitular demifacets. 3. Superior articular facet. 4. Transverse process.
5. Costotubercular facet. 6. Pedicle. 7. Inferior articular process. 8. Spinous process.

Fig. 45.24 Fourth thoracic vertebra, lateral aspect. (Photograph by Sarah-Jane Smith.)

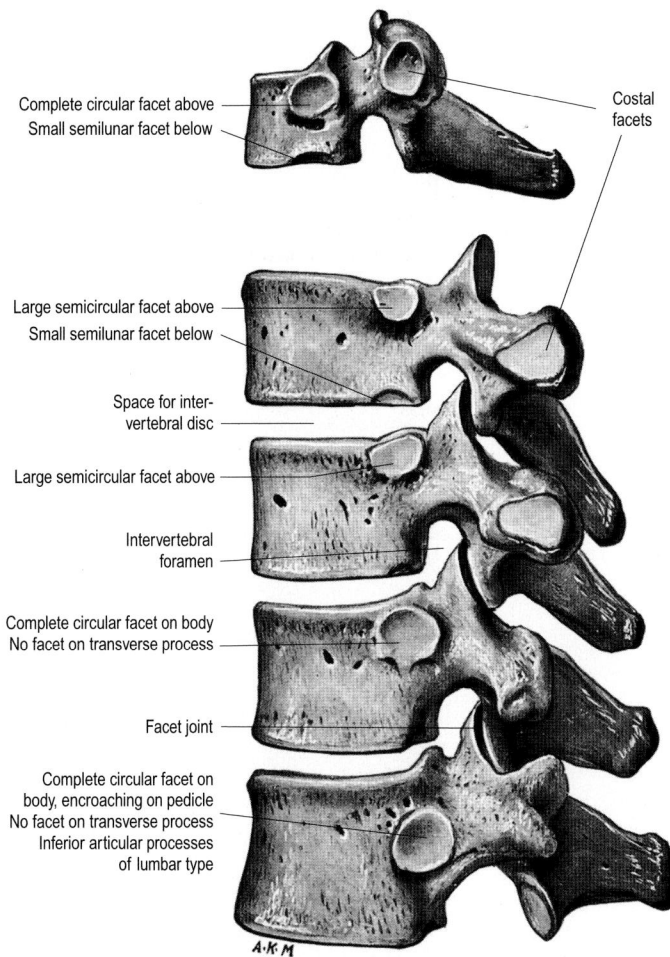

Complete circular facet above
Small semilunar facet below

Costal facets

Large semicircular facet above
Small semilunar facet below

Space for inter-vertebral disc

Large semicircular facet above

Intervertebral foramen

Complete circular facet on body
No facet on transverse process

Facet joint

Complete circular facet on body, encroaching on pedicle
No facet on transverse process
Inferior articular processes of lumbar type

A·K·M

Fig. 45.25 The first, ninth, tenth, eleventh and twelfth thoracic vertebrae, lateral aspect.

but change little transversely. These four, in transverse section, are asymmetrical, their left sides being flattened by pressure of the thoracic aorta. The rest increase more rapidly in all measurements, so that the twelfth body resembles that of a typical lumbar vertebra. These modifications may contribute to the greater range of flexion–extension seen at the cervical and lumbar ends of the thoracic vertebral column.

The anterior and posterior longitudinal ligaments are attached to the borders of the bodies, and around the margins of the costal facets

there are the capsular and radiate ligaments of the costovertebral joints. Thoracic pedicles show a successive caudal increase in thickness. The superior vertebral notch is recognizable only in the first thoracic vertebra, whereas the inferior notch is deep in all. Ligamenta flava are attached at the upper borders and lower anterior surfaces of the laminae.

Thoracic transverse processes shorten in caudal succession. In the upper five or six vertebrae the costal facets are concave and face antero-laterally, and at lower levels the facets are flatter and face superolaterally and slightly forwards. The costotransverse ligament is attached to the anterior surface medial to the facet; the lateral costotransverse ligament is attached to its tuberculated apex and the superior costotransverse ligament is attached to its lower border.

Thoracic spines overlap from the fifth to the eighth vertebra, whose spine is the longest and most oblique. Supraspinous and interspinous ligaments are attached to the spines.

A change in orientation of articular processes from thoracic to lumbar type usually occurs at the eleventh thoracic vertebra, but sometimes at the twelfth or tenth. In the transitional vertebra the superior articular processes are thoracic, and face posterolaterally, while the inferior are transversely convex and face anterolaterally. The transitional vertebra marks the site of a sudden change of mobility from predominantly rotational to predominantly flexion–extension.

Muscle attachments – Longus colli arises from the upper three thoracic vertebral bodies, lateral to the anterior longitudinal ligament, and psoas major and minor arise from the sides of the twelfth near its lower border. Upper and lower borders of the transverse processes provide attachment for the intertransverse muscles or their fibrous vestiges. The posterior surfaces of the transverse processes provide attachment for the deep dorsal muscles, and levator costae is attached posteriorly on the apex. Trapezius, rhomboid major and minor, latissimus dorsi, serratus posterior superior and inferior and many deep dorsal muscles are attached to the spines. Rotatores attach to the posterior aspects of the laminae.

Ossification – Thoracic vertebrae all ossify according to the standard vertebral pattern described on page 792.

T1 (Fig. 45.25)
The first thoracic vertebra resembles a cervical vertebra in its body, both in shape and in the distinctive posterolateral 'lipping' which forms the anterior border of the superior vertebral notch. There are circular superior costal facets for articulation with the whole facet on the head of the first rib. The smaller, semilunar inferior facets articulate with a demifacet on the head of the second rib. The upper costal facet is often incomplete, in which case the first rib articulates with the seventh cervical vertebra and the intervening disc. A small, deep depression often occurs below the facet. The long, thick spine is horizontal and commonly as prominent as that of the seventh cervical vertebra.

T9 (Fig. 45.25)
The ninth thoracic vertebra is otherwise typical, but it often fails to articulate with the tenth ribs, in which case the inferior demifacets are absent.

T10 (Fig. 45.25)
The tenth thoracic vertebra only articulates with the tenth pair of ribs, so that superior facets only appear on the body. These are usually large and semilunar, or oval when the tenth ribs fail to articulate with the ninth vertebra and intervening disc. The transverse process may or may not bear a facet for the tenth rib tubercle.

T11 (Fig. 45.25)
The eleventh thoracic vertebra articulates only with the heads of the eleventh ribs. The circular costal facets are close to the upper border of the body and extend onto the pedicles. The small transverse processes lack articular facets. The eleventh and twelfth thoracic spinous processes are triangular, with blunt apices, a horizontal lower and an oblique upper border.

T12 (Fig. 45.25)
The twelfth thoracic vertebra articulates with the heads of the twelfth ribs by circular facets somewhat below the upper border, spreading on to the pedicles. The body is large and the vertebra has some lumbar

features. The transverse process is replaced by three small tubercles: the superior is largest, projects upwards and corresponds to a lumbar mammillary process, though it does not lie as close to the superior articular process; the lateral tubercle is the homologue of a transverse process; the inferior is the homologue of a lumbar accessory process. The superior and inferior processes are surprisingly long in some specimens.

LUMBAR VERTEBRAE (Figs 45.26, 45.27, 45.28, 45.29)

LUMBAR VERTEBRAE IN GENERAL

The five lumbar vertebrae are distinguished by their large size and absence of costal facets and transverse foramina. The body is wider transversely, and normally is deeper in front. The vertebral foramen is triangular, larger than at thoracic levels but smaller than at cervical levels. The pedicles are short. The spinous process is almost horizontal, quadrangular and thickened along its posterior and inferior borders. The superior articular processes bear vertical concave articular facets facing posteromedially, with a rough mammillary process on their posterior borders. The inferior articular processes have vertical convex articular facets which face anterolaterally. The transverse processes are thin and long, except on the more substantial fifth pair. A small accessory process marks the posteroinferior aspect of the root of each transverse process. The accessory and mammillary processes are linked by a fine

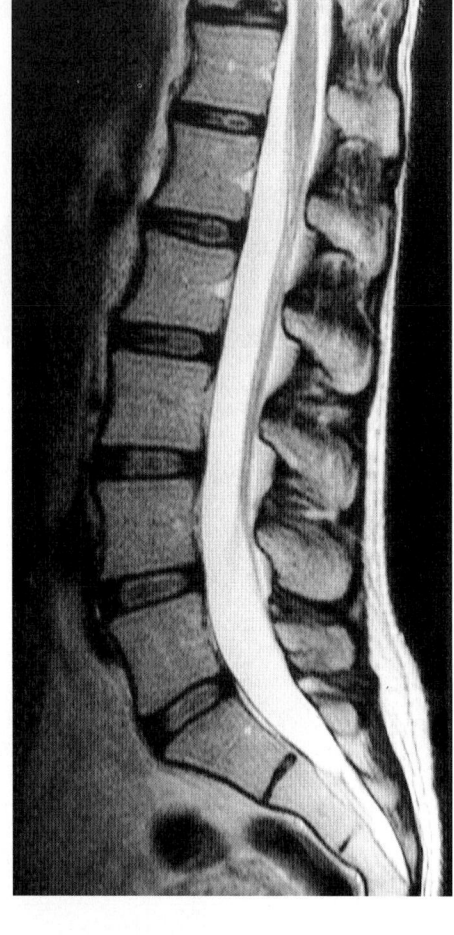

Fig. 45.28 Median sagittal MRI lumbar spine. (By kind permission from Dr Justin Lee, Chelsea and Westminster Hospital, London.)

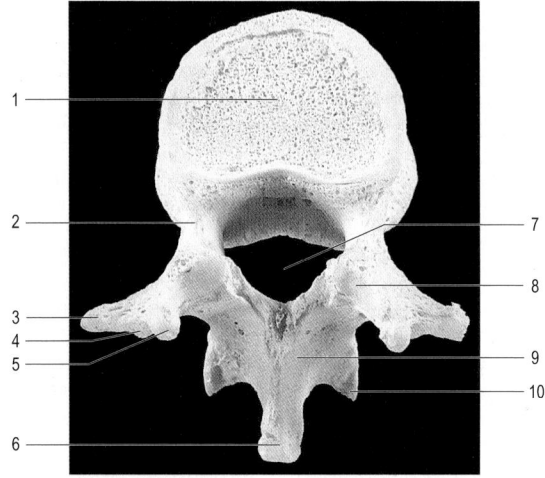

1. Body. 2. Pedicle. 3. Transverse process. 4. Accessory process.
5. Mammillary process. 6. Spinous process. 7. Vertebral foramen.
8. Superior articular facet. 9. Lamina. 10. Inferior articular facet.

Fig. 45.26 First lumbar vertebra, superior aspect. (Photograph by Sarah-Jane Smith.)

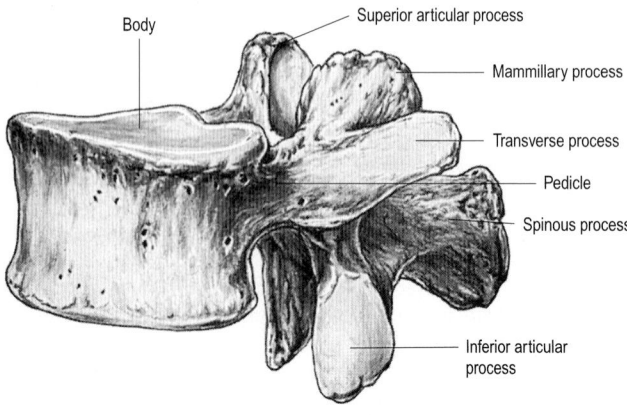

Body
Superior articular process
Mammillary process
Transverse process
Pedicle
Spinous process
Inferior articular process

Fig. 45.27 Lumbar vertebra, lateral aspect.

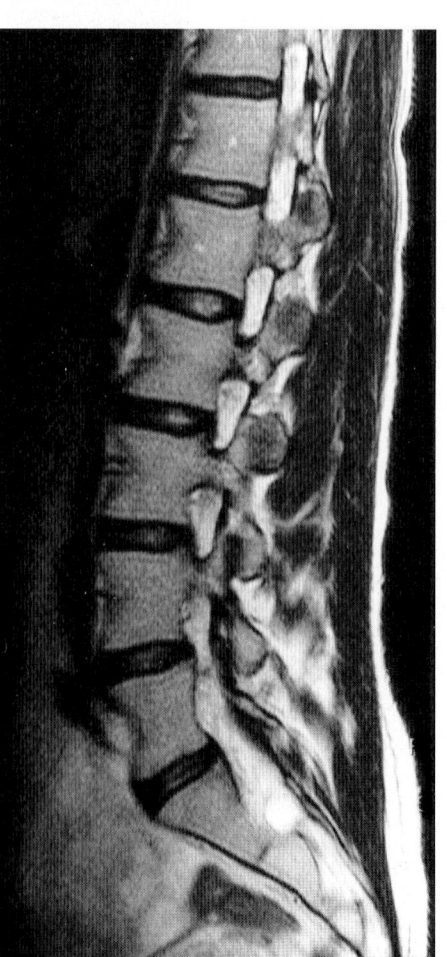

Fig. 45.29 Paramedian sagittal MRI lumbar spine, showing intervertebral foramina. (By kind permission from Dr Justin Lee, Chelsea and Westminster Hospital, London.)

ligament, the mammillo-accessory ligament, which is sometimes ossified, and beneath which runs the medial branch of the dorsal primary ramus of the spinal nerve.

Strong paired pedicles arise posterolaterally from each body near its upper border. Superior vertebral notches are shallow and the inferior ones are deep. The laminae are broad and short, but do not overlap as much as those of the thoracic vertebrae. The fifth spine is the smallest, and its apex is often rounded and down-turned. Upper lumbar superior articular processes are further apart than inferior ones, but the difference is slight in the fourth and negligible in the fifth. The articular facets are reciprocally concave (superior) and convex (inferior), which allows flexion, extension, lateral bending and some degree of rotation. There are sex differences in the angle of inclination and depth of curvature of the articular facets. The facets are sometimes asymmetrical. Transverse processes, except the fifth, are anteroposteriorly compressed and project posterolaterally. The lower border of the fifth transverse process is angulated, passes laterally and then superolaterally to a blunt tip, and the whole process presents a greater upward inclination than the fourth. The angle on the inferior border may represent the tip of the costal element and the lateral end the tip of the true transverse process. The lumbar transverse processes increase in length from first to third and then shorten. The fifth pair incline both upwards and posterolaterally. The costal element is incorporated in the mature transverse process.

The first lumbar vertebral foramen contains the conus medullaris of the spinal cord, while lower foramina contain the cauda equina and spinal meninges. Variation occurs in the sagittal and coronal dimensions of the lumbar vertebral canal, both within and between normal populations.

Muscle and fascial attachments (See also p. 734.) – Upper and lower borders of lumbar bodies give attachment to the anterior and posterior longitudinal ligaments (p. 754). The upper bodies (three on the right, two on the left) give attachments to the crura of the diaphragm lateral to the anterior longitudinal ligament. Posterolaterally, psoas major is attached to the upper and lower margins of all the lumbar bodies, and between them, tendinous arches carry its attachments across their concave sides (**Fig. 2.1**). The posterior lamella of the thoracolumbar fascia, erectores spinae, spinales thoracis, multifidi, interspinal muscles and ligaments, and supraspinous ligaments are all attached to spinous processes. All lumbar transverse processes present a vertical ridge on the anterior surface, nearer the tip, which marks the attachment of the anterior layer of the thoracolumbar fascia, and separates the surface into medial and lateral areas for psoas major and quadratus lumborum respectively. The middle layer of the fascia is attached to the apices of the transverse processes; the medial and lateral arcuate ligaments attach to the apices of the first pair, and the iliolumbar ligament attaches to the apices of the fifth pair. Posteriorly the transverse processes are covered by deep dorsal muscles, and fibres of longissimus thoracis are attached to them and to their accessory processes. The ventral lateral intertransverse muscles are attached to their upper and lower borders, while the dorsal attach cranially to the accessory process and caudally to the upper border of the transverse process. The mammillary process, homologous with the superior tubercle of the twelfth thoracic vertebra, gives attachment to multifidus and the medial intertransverse muscle. The latter also attaches to the accessory process, which is sometimes difficult to identify.

Ossification (Fig. 45.20) – Lumbar vertebrae ossify according to the standard vertebral pattern described on page 792, but also have two additional centres for the mammillary processes. A pair of scale-like epiphyses usually appear on the tips of the costal elements of the fifth lumbar vertebra.

L5 (Fig. 45.30)

The fifth lumbar vertebra has a massive transverse process which is continuous with the whole of the pedicle and encroaching on the body. The body is usually the largest and markedly deeper anteriorly, so contributing to the lumbosacral angle.

Segmentation anomalies (sacralization) are considered below with the sacrum. The costal element of the first lumbar vertebra may form a short lumbar rib, which articulates with the transverse process, but not usually with the body, of the vertebra.

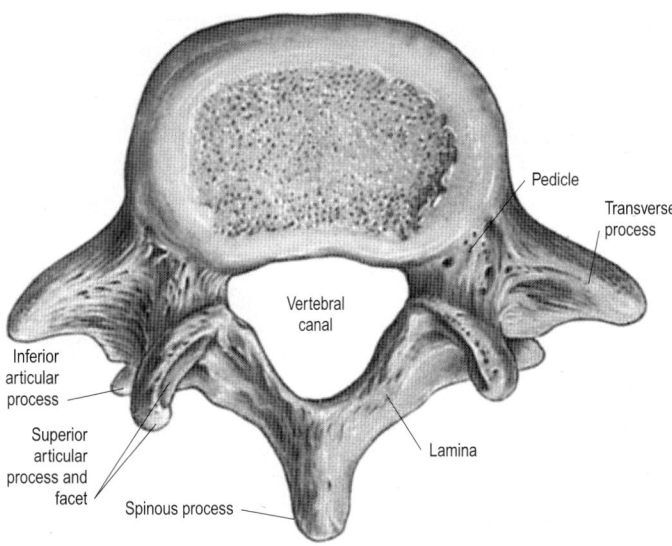

Fig. 45.30 Fifth lumbar vertebra, superior aspect.

Labels: Pedicle; Transverse process; Vertebral canal; Inferior articular process; Superior articular process and facet; Spinous process; Lamina

SACRUM (Figs 45.31, 45.32, 45.33, 45.34, 45.35)

The sacrum is a large, triangular fusion of five vertebrae and forms the posterosuperior wall of the pelvic cavity, wedged between the two innominate bones. Its blunted, caudal apex articulates with the coccyx and its superior, wide base with the fifth lumbar vertebra at the lumbosacral angle. It is set obliquely and curved longitudinally, its dorsal surface is convex, and the pelvic surface is concave. This ventral curvature increases pelvic capacity. Between base and apex are dorsal, pelvic and lateral surfaces and a sacral canal. In childhood, individual sacral vertebrae are connected by cartilage, and the adult bone retains many vertebral features. The sacrum consists of trabecular bone enveloped by a shell of compact bone of varying thickness.

Base – The base is the upper surface of the first sacral vertebra, the least modified from the typical vertebral plan. The body is large and wider transversely, and its anterior projecting edge is the sacral promontory. The vertebral foramen is triangular, its pedicles are short and diverge posterolaterally. The laminae are oblique, inclining down postero-medially to meet at a spinous tubercle. The superior articular processes project cranially, with concave articular facets directed posteromedially to articulate with the inferior articular processes of the fifth lumbar vertebra. The posterior part of each process projects backwards and its lateral aspect bears a rough area homologous with a lumbar mammillary process.

The transverse process is much modified as a broad, sloping mass which projects laterally from the body, pedicle and superior articular process. It is formed by the fusion of the transverse process and the costal element to each other and to the rest of the vertebra, and forms the upper surface of the sacral lateral mass or ala.

Terminal fibres of the anterior and posterior longitudinal ligaments are attached to the ventral and dorsal surfaces of the first sacral body. Its upper laminar borders receive the lowest pair of ligamenta flava. The ala is smooth superiorly, concave medially and rough laterally, and covered almost entirely by psoas major. The smooth area is grooved obliquely by the lumbosacral trunk. The rough area is for the lower band of the iliolumbar ligament, which lies lateral to the fifth lumbar spinal nerve and to the anterior sacroiliac ligament.

Pelvic surface – The anteroinferior pelvic surface is vertically and transversely concave, but the second sacral body may produce a convexity. Four pairs of pelvic sacral foramina communicate with the sacral canal through intervertebral foramina, and transmit ventral rami of the upper four sacral spinal nerves. The large area between the right and left foramina, which is formed by the flat pelvic aspects of the sacral bodies, bears evidence of their fusion at four transverse ridges. The longitudinal bars between the foramina are costal elements, which fuse to the vertebrae. Lateral to the foramina the costal elements unite. Posteriorly

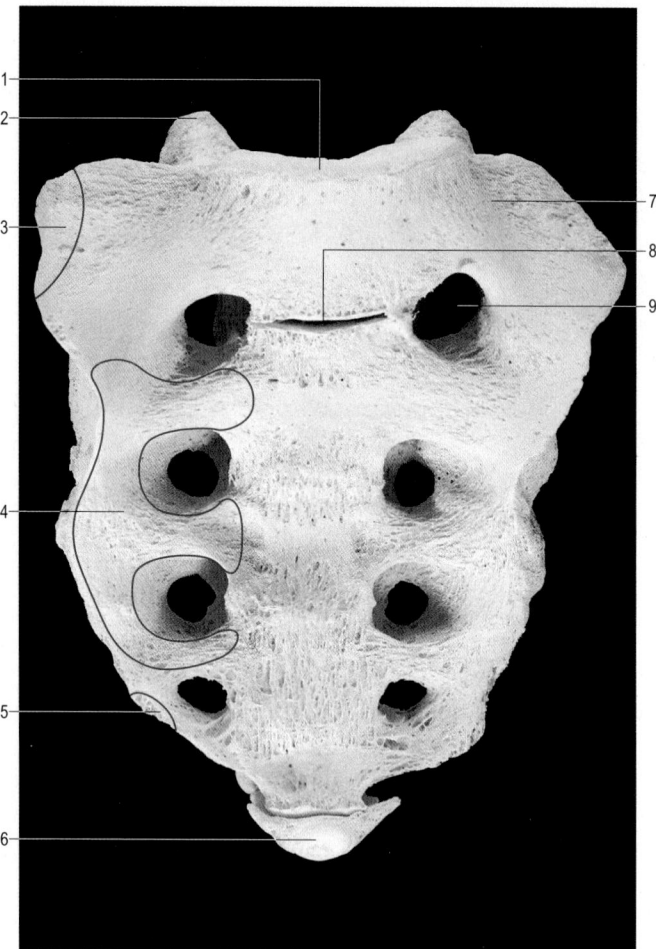

1. Upper border of body of S1 (sacral promontory). **2.** Superior articular process of S1.
3. Attachment of iliacus. **4.** Attachment of piriformis. **5.** Attachment of coccygeus. **6.** Coccyx.
7. Ala. **8.** Incompletely fused S1–2 intervertebral joint. **9.** First pelvic sacral foramen.

Fig. 45.31 Sacrum, anterior (pelvic) surface. (Photograph by Sarah-Jane Smith.)

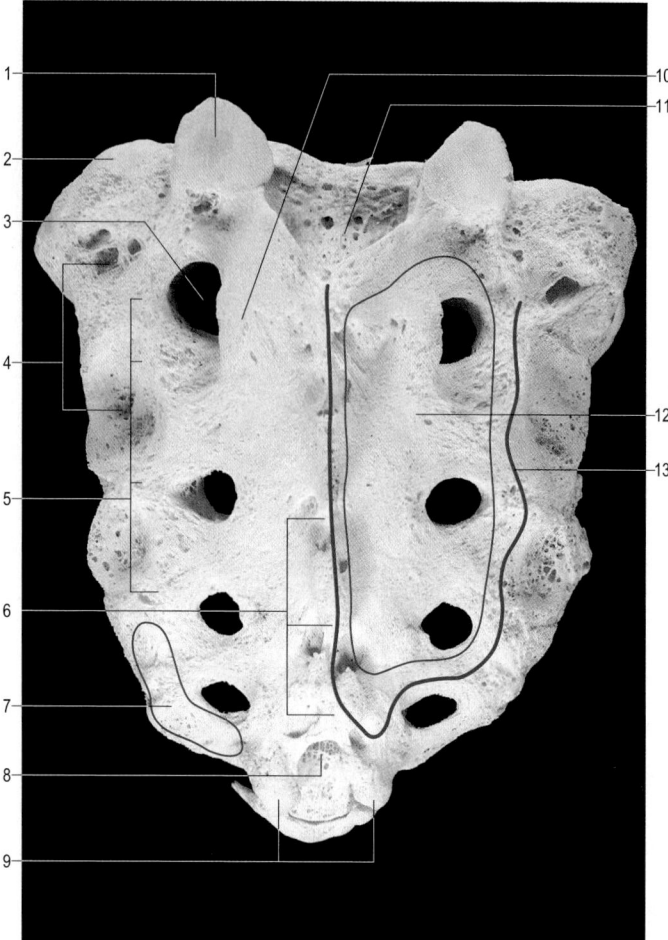

1. Superior articular facet of S1. **2.** Ala. **3.** First dorsal sacral foramen.
4. Attachments of interosseous sacroiliac ligaments. **5.** Lateral crest and transverse tubercles.
6. Median crest and spinous processes. **7.** Attachment of gluteus maximus. **8.** Sacral hiatus.
9. Cornua. **10.** Intermediate crest and articular tubercle (inferior articular process).
11. Posterior surface of body of S1 forming anterior wall of sacral canal.
12. Area of attachment of multifidus (bounded by thin line).
13. Attachment of erector spinae aponeurosis (thick line).

Fig. 45.32 Sacrum, posterior (dorsal) surface. (Photograph by Sarah-Jane Smith.)

they unite with the transverse processes to form the lateral part of the sacrum, which expands basally as the ala.

The first three sacral ventral rami emerge from the pelvic sacral foramina and pass anterior to piriformis. The sympathetic trunks descend in contact with bone, medial to the foramina, as do the median sacral vessels in the midline. Lateral to the foramina, lateral sacral vessels are related to bone. Ventral surfaces of the first, second, and part of the third sacral bodies are covered by parietal peritoneum and crossed obliquely, left of the midline, by the attachment of the sigmoid mesocolon. The rectum is in contact with the pelvic surfaces of the third to fifth sacral vertebrae and with the bifurcation of the superior rectal artery between the rectum and third sacral vertebra.

Dorsal surface – The posterosuperior aspect of the dorsal surface bears a raised, interrupted, median sacral crest with four (sometimes three) spinous tubercles which represent fused sacral spines. Below the fourth (or third) tubercle there is an arched sacral hiatus in the posterior wall of the sacral canal. This hiatus is produced by the failure of the laminae of the fifth sacral vertebra to meet in the median plane, and as a result the posterior surface of the body of that vertebra is exposed on the dorsal surface of the sacrum. Flanking the median crest, the posterior surface is formed by fused laminae, and lateral to this are four pairs of dorsal sacral foramina. Like the pelvic foramina, they lead into the sacral canal through intervertebral foramina, and each transmits the dorsal ramus of a sacral spinal nerve. Medial to the foramina, and vertically below each articular process of the first sacral vertebra, is a row of four small tubercles, which collectively constitute the intermediate sacral crest. These are sometimes termed articular tubercles, and represent fused contiguous articular processes. The inferior articular

processes of the fifth sacral vertebra are free and project downwards at the sides of the sacral hiatus as sacral cornua, connected to coccygeal cornua by intercornual ligaments. The interrupted roughened crest to the lateral side of the dorsal sacral foramina is the lateral sacral crest which is formed by fused transverse processes, whose apices appear as a row of transverse tubercles.

The upper three sacral spinal dorsal rami pierce multifidus as they emerge via dorsal foramina.

Lateral surface – The lateral surface is a fusion of transverse processes and costal elements. It is wide above, and rapidly narrows in its lower part. The broad upper part bears an auricular surface for articulation with the ilium, and the area posterior to this is rough and deeply pitted by the attachment of ligaments. The auricular surface, borne by costal elements, is like an inverted letter L. The shorter, cranial limb is restricted to the first sacral vertebra; the caudal limb descends to the middle of the third. Beyond this the lateral surface is non-articular and reduced in breadth. Caudally it curves medially to the body of the fifth sacral vertebra at the inferior lateral angle, beyond which the surface becomes a thin lateral border. A variable accessory sacral articular facet sometimes occurs, posterior to the auricular surface.

The auricular surface is covered by hyaline cartilage, and formed entirely by costal elements. It shows cranial and caudal elevations and an intermediate depression, behind which a third elevation is visible in the elderly. The surface becomes more corrugated with age. The rough area behind the auricular surface shows two or three marked depressions

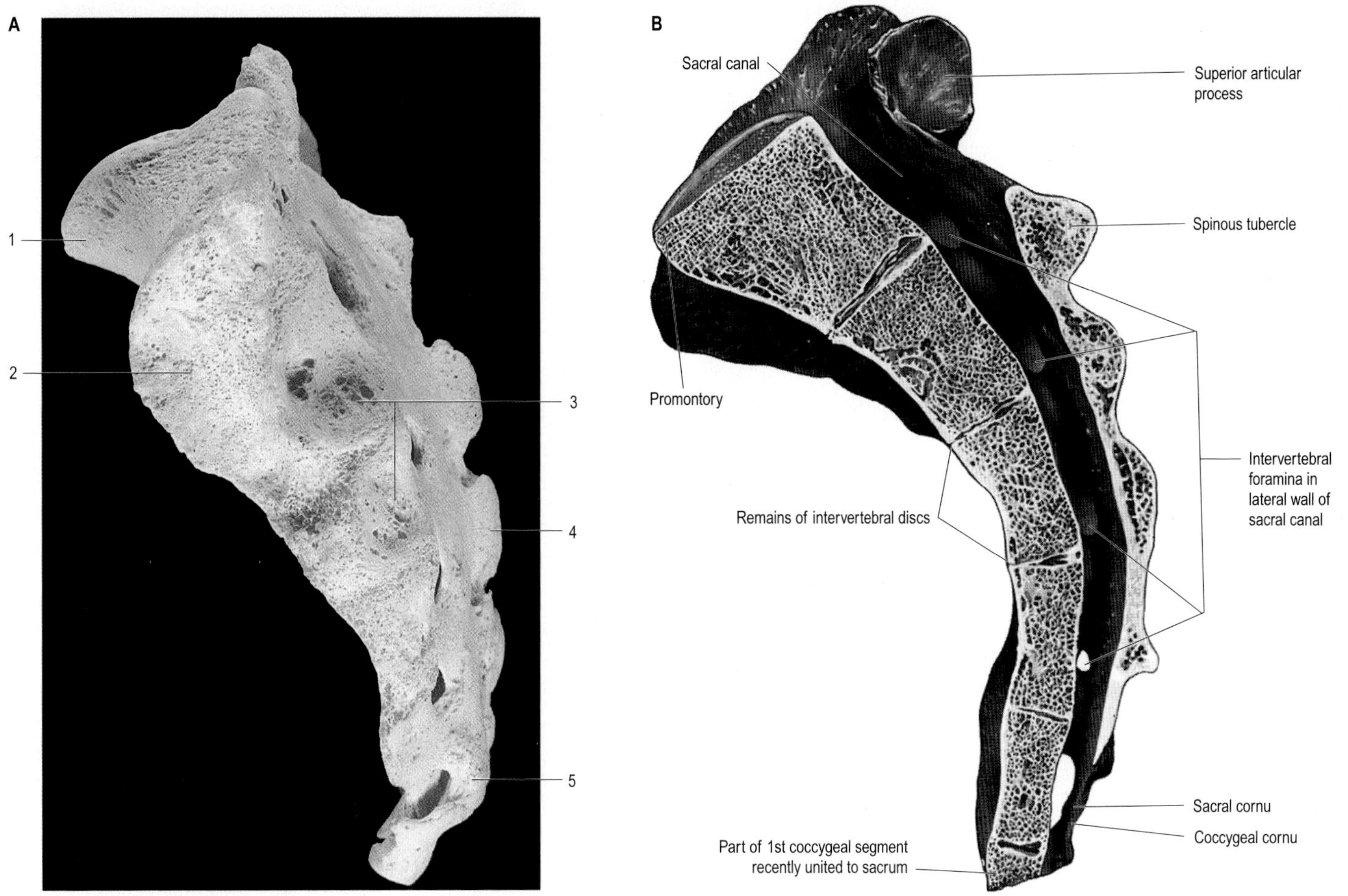

A

B

Sacral canal

Superior articular process

Promontory

Spinous tubercle

Remains of intervertebral discs

Intervertebral foramina in lateral wall of sacral canal

Part of 1st coccygeal segment recently united to sacrum

Sacral cornu

Coccygeal cornu

1. Promontory. 2. Auricular (articular) surface. 3. Attachments of interosseous sacroiliac ligaments. 4. Spinous process. 5. Sacral cornu (left).

Fig. 45.33 **A**, Sacrum, lateral aspect. **B**, Median sagittal section through the sacrum. (**A**, photograph by Sarah-Jane Smith.)

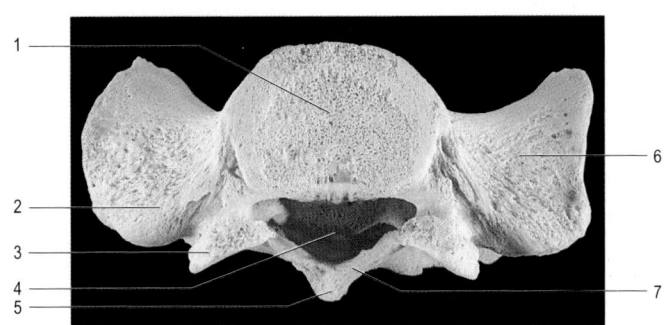

1. Body of S1. 2. Posterosuperior ala (transverse process element).
3. Superior articular process. 4. Sacral canal. 5. Spinous process of S1.
6. Anterosuperior ala (costal element). 7. Lamina.

Fig. 45.34 Sacrum, superior aspect (base). (Photograph by Sarah-Jane Smith.)

for the attachment of strong interosseous sacroiliac ligaments. Below the auricular surface the sacrotuberous and sacrospinous ligaments are attached between gluteus maximus dorsally and coccygeus ventrally.

Apex – The apex is the inferior aspect of the fifth sacral vertebral body, and bears an oval facet for articulation with the coccyx.

Sacral canal (Fig. 45.33B) – The sacral canal is formed by sacral vertebral foramina, and is triangular in section. Its upper opening, seen on the basal surface, appears to be set obliquely. The inclination of the sacrum means that it is directed cranially in the standing position. Each lateral

wall presents four intervertebral foramina, through which the canal is continuous with pelvic and dorsal sacral foramina. Its caudal opening is the sacral hiatus. The canal contains the cauda equina and the filum terminale, and the spinal meninges. Opposite the middle of the sacrum, the subarachnoid and subdural spaces close: the lower sacral spinal roots and filum terminale pierce the arachnoid and dura mater at that level. The filum terminale emerges below the sacral hiatus and passes downwards across the dorsal surface of the fifth sacral vertebra and sacrococcygeal joint to reach the coccyx. The fifth sacral spinal nerves also emerge through the hiatus medial to the sacral cornua, and groove the lateral aspects of the fifth sacral vertebra.

Muscle attachments – The pelvic surface gives attachment to piriformis in its second to fourth segments, to iliacus superolaterally, and to coccygeus inferolaterally. The dorsal surface gives attachment to the aponeurosis of erector spinae along a U-shaped area of spinous and transverse tubercles, covering multifidus which occupies the enclosed area (**Fig. 45.34**). On the lateral border below the auricular surface, gluteus maximus is attached dorsal and coccygeus is attached ventral to the sacrotuberous and sacrospinous ligaments.

Ossification (Fig. 45.36) – The sacrum resembles typical vertebrae in the ossification of its segments. Primary centres for the centrum and each half vertebral arch appear between the tenth and twentieth weeks. Primary centres for the costal elements of the upper three or more segments appear superolateral to the pelvic sacral foramina, between the sixth and eighth prenatal months. Each costal element unites with its half vertebral arch between the second and fifth years, and the conjoined element so formed unites anteriorly with the centrum and posteriorly with its opposite fellow at about the eighth year. Thereafter the upper and lower surfaces of each sacral body are covered by an

A

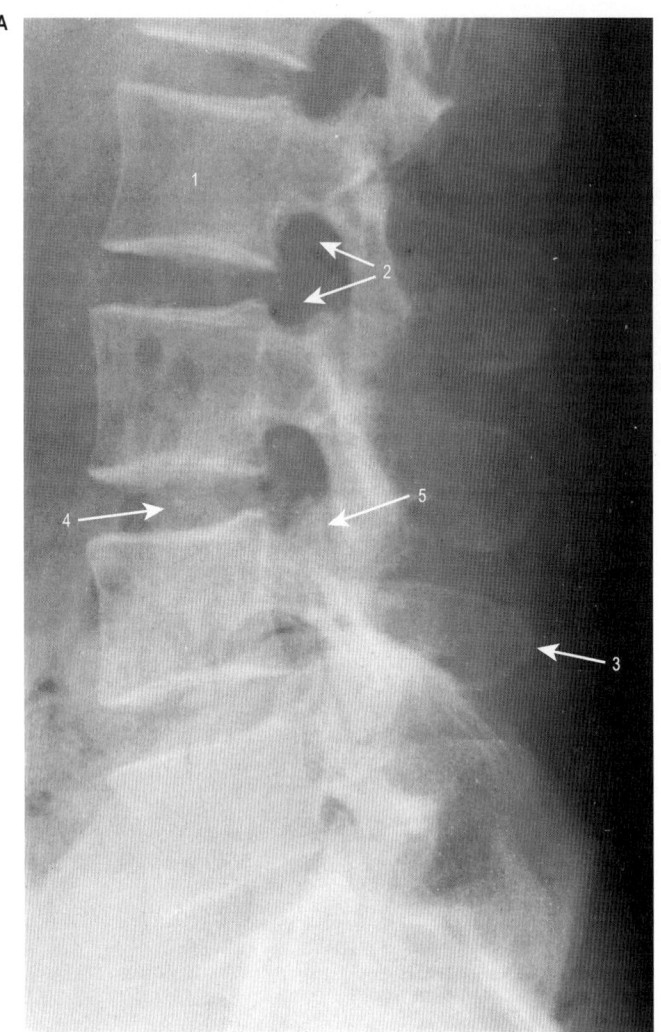

1. Lumbar vertebral body. 2. Intervertebral foramen. 3. Spinous process.
4. Site of intervertebral disc. 5. Synovial joint between articular processes.

B

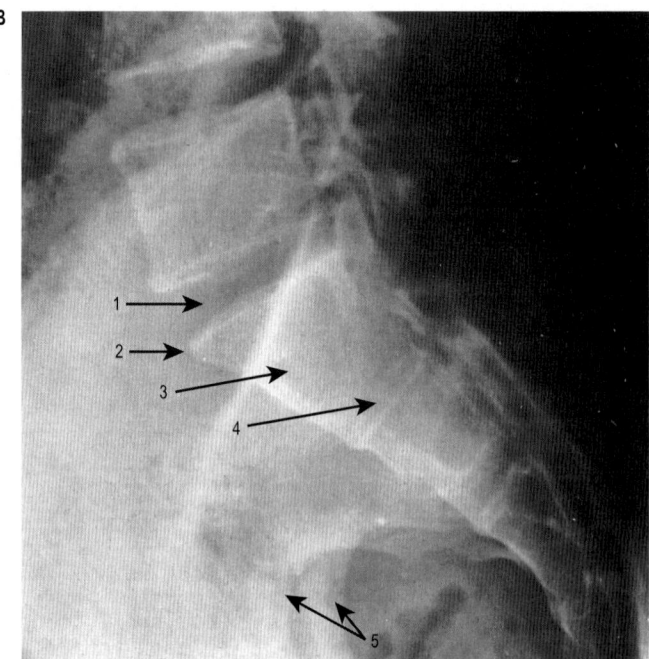

1. Site of lumbosacral disc. 2. Sacral promontory. 3. First sacral segment.
4. Remains of sacral intervertebral disc. 5. Profiles of greater sciatic notches.

C

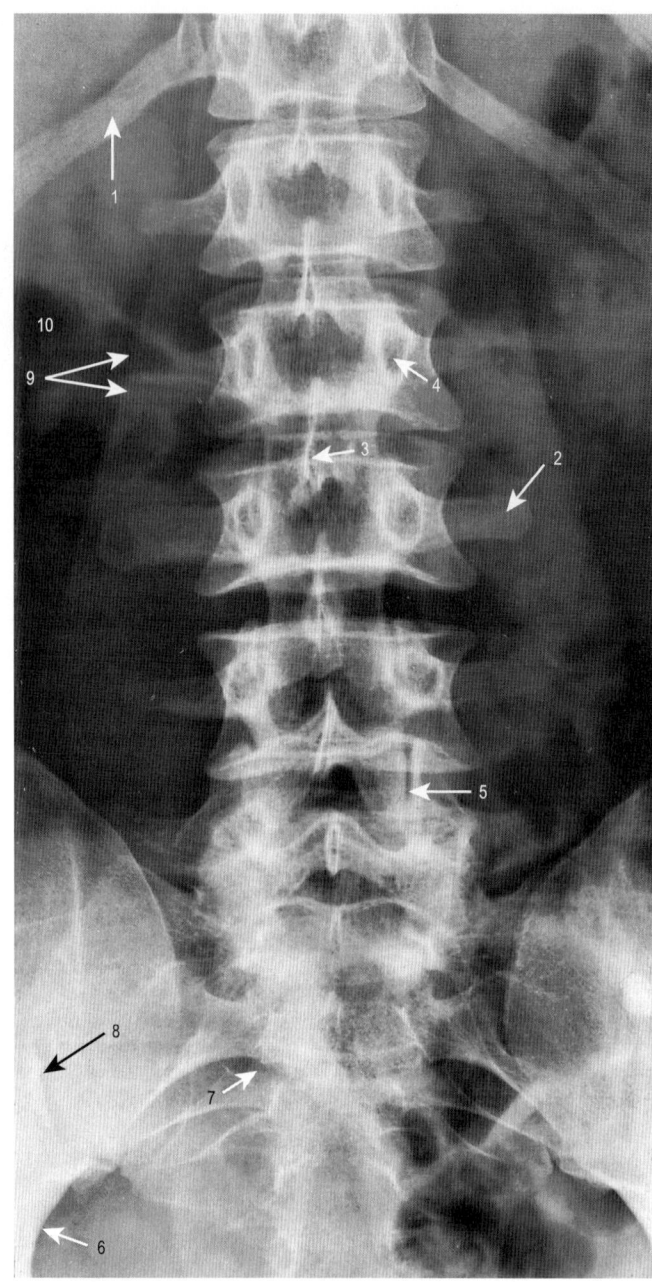

1. Twelfth rib. 2. Transverse process. 3. Spinous process (2nd lumbar).
4. Pedicle (2nd lumbar). 5. Joint between articular processes (4th and 5th lumbar).
6. Pelvic brim. 7. Anterior sacral foramen. 8. Sacroiliac joint.
9. Lateral border of psoas major. 10. Gas in colon.

Fig. 45.35 **A** and **B**, Lateral radiographs of lumbosacral vertebral column in an adult male aged 26 years. **C**, Anteroposterior radiograph of lumbosacral vertebral column in a young adult male aged 22 years. (Provided by Shaun Gallagher, GKT School of Medicine, London; photographs by Sarah-Jane Smith.)

D

R   L

1

2

3

4

5

6

7

8

1. Inferior vena cava.
2. Psoas major.
3. Facet synovial joint between L4 and 5.
4. Erector spinae muscle mass.
5. Bifurcation of aorta.
6. Fourth lumbar vertebral body.
7. Thecal sac.
8. Spinous process.

Fig. 45.35 (*Cont'd*) **D**, High resolution computed tomogram through posterior abdominal wall at the level of the body of the fourth lumbar vertebra, showing zygapophyseal joints between fourth and fifth lumbar vertebrae.

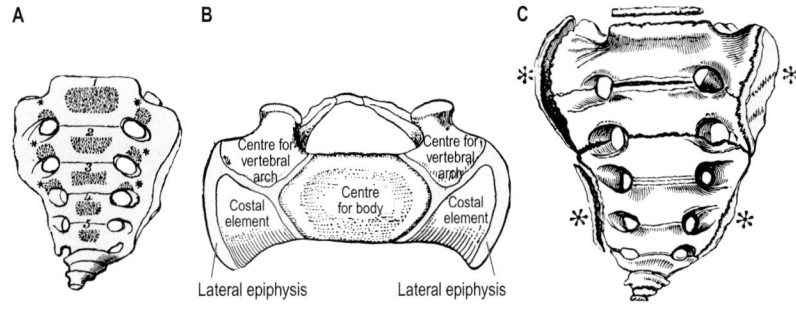

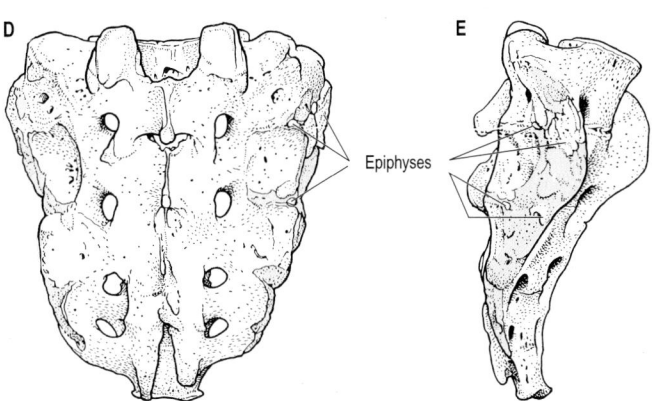

Fig. 45.36 Ossification of the sacrum and coccyx. **A**, At birth. **B**, The base of the sacrum of a child about four years old. **C**, At the twenty-fifth year: epiphyseal plates for each lateral surface are marked by asterisks. **D**, **E**, The epiphyses of the costal and transverse process of the sacrum at the eighteenth year.

753

epiphyseal plate of hyaline cartilage which is separated from its neighbour by the fibrocartilaginous precursor of an intervertebral disc. Laterally, successive conjoined vertebral arches and costal elements are separated by hyaline cartilage; a cartilaginous epiphysis, sometimes divided into upper and lower parts, develops on each auricular and adjacent lateral surface. Soon after puberty the fused vertebral arches and costal elements of adjacent vertebrae begin to coalesce from below upwards. At the same time individual epiphyseal centres develop for the upper and lower surfaces of bodies, spinous tubercles, transverse tubercles and costal elements.

The costal epiphyseal centres appear at the lateral extremities of the hyaline cartilages between adjacent costal elements; two anterior and two posterior centres appear in each of the intervals between the first, second and third sacral vertebrae. Ossification spreads from these into the auricular epiphyseal plates. One costal epiphyseal centre, placed anteriorly, occurs in each remaining interval and from them ossification spreads to the epiphyseal plate covering the lower part of the lateral surface of the sacrum. Sacral bodies unite at their adjacent margins after the twentieth year, but the central and greater part of each intervertebral disc remains unossified up to or beyond middle life.

Variants – The sacrum may contain six vertebrae, by development of an additional sacral element or by incorporation of the fifth lumbar or first coccygeal vertebrae. Inclusion of the fifth lumbar vertebra (sacralization) is usually incomplete and limited to one side. In the most minor degree of the abnormality a fifth lumbar transverse process is large and articulates, sometimes by a synovial joint, with the sacrum at the posterolateral angle of its base. Reduction of sacral constituents is less common but lumbarization of the first sacral vertebra does occur: it remains partially or completely separate. The bodies of the first two sacral vertebrae may remain unfused when the lateral masses are fused. The dorsal wall of the sacral canal may be variably deficient, due to imperfect development of laminae and spines. Orientation of the superior sacral articular facets displays wide variation, as does the sagittal curvature of the sacrum. Asymmetry (facet tropism) of the superior facets alters the relation between the planes of the two lumbosacral facet joints.

Sex differences in sacra – Sex differences in sacra are described on page 1428.

COCCYX (Fig. 45.37)

The coccyx is a small triangular bone often asymmetrical in shape. It usually consists of four fused rudimentary vertebrae: the number varies from three to five, the first is sometimes separate. The bone is directed downwards and ventrally from the sacral apex: its pelvic surface is tilted upwards and forwards, its dorsum downwards and backwards. Orientation varies with mobility and between individuals.

The base or upper surface of the first coccygeal vertebral body has an oval, articular facet for the sacral apex. Posterolateral to this, two coccygeal cornua project upwards to articulate with sacral cornua: they are homologues of the pedicles and superior articular processes of other vertebrae. A rudimentary transverse process projects superolaterally from each side of the first coccygeal body and may articulate or fuse with the inferolateral sacral angle, completing the fifth sacral foramina.

The second to fourth coccygeal vertebrae diminish in size and are usually mere fused nodules. They represent rudimentary vertebral bodies, though the second may show traces of transverse processes and pedicles.

The gap between the fifth sacral body and the articulating cornua represents, on each side, an intervertebral foramen which transmits the fifth sacral spinal nerve. The dorsal ramus descends behind the rudimentary transverse process, and the ventral ramus passes anterolaterally between the transverse process and sacrum.

Muscle and ligament attachments – The lateral parts of the pelvic surface, including the rudimentary transverse processes, give attachment to the levatores ani and coccygei. The anterior sacrococcygeal ligament is attached to the front of the first and sometimes second coccygeal vertebral bodies (**Fig. 111.11**). The cornua give attachment to the intercornual ligaments. The lateral sacrococcygeal ligament connects the transverse process to the inferolateral sacral angle. Gluteus maximus is attached to the dorsal surface, and both levator ani and sphincter ani externus are attached to the tip of the bone. The median area gives attachment to the deep and superficial posterior sacrococcygeal ligaments, the superficial descending from the margins of the sacral hiatus and sometimes closing the sacral canal. The filum terminale, which is situated between the two ligaments, blends with them on the dorsum of the first coccygeal vertebra.

Ossification – Each coccygeal segment is ossified from one primary centre. A centre in the first segment appears about birth and its cornua may soon ossify from separate centres. Remaining segments ossify at wide intervals up to the twentieth year or later. Segments slowly unite: union between the first and second is frequently delayed until 30 years. The coccyx often fuses with the sacrum in later decades, especially in females.

LIGAMENTS OF THE VERTEBRAL COLUMN

LIGAMENTUM NUCHAE (Fig. 45.38)
The ligamentum nuchae is a bilaminar fibroelastic intermuscular septum which is often considered homologous with, but structurally distinct from, the supraspinous and interspinous ligaments in the neck. Its dense bilateral fibroelastic laminae are separated by a tenuous layer of areolar tissue and the laminae are blended at its posterior free border. This border is superficial and extends from the external occipital protuberance to the spine of C7. The fibroelastic laminae are attached to the median part of the external occipital crest, the posterior tubercle of C1 and the medial aspects of the bifid spines of cervical vertebrae, as a septum for the bilateral attachment of cervical muscles and their sheaths. There is also a midline attachment to the posterior spinal dura at atlanto-occipital and atlanto-axial levels (Dean & Mitchell 2002). In bipeds the ligamentum nuchae is the reduced representative of a much thicker, complex elastic ligament which in quadrupeds aids suspension of the head and controls its flexion.

ANTERIOR LONGITUDINAL LIGAMENT (Fig. 45.41B)
The anterior longitudinal ligament is a strong band extending along the anterior surfaces of the vertebral bodies. It is broader caudally, and thicker and narrower in thoracic than in cervical and lumbar regions. It

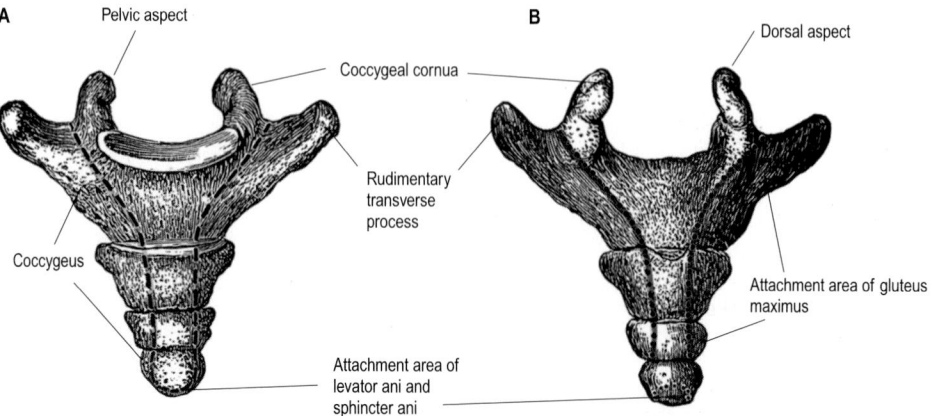

Fig. 45.37 The coccyx. **A**, Anterior (pelvic) aspect. **B**, Posterior (dorsal) aspect.

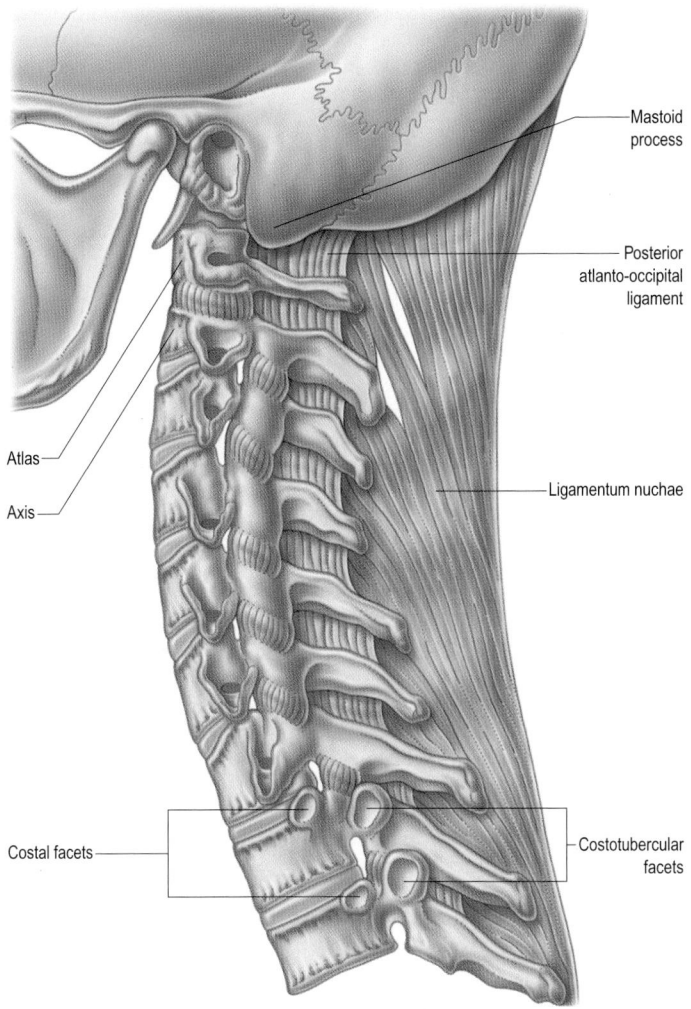

Fig. 45.38 The ligamentum nuchae. (By permission from Kiss F, Szentagothai J 1964 Atlas of Human Anatomy. Oxford: Pergamon Press.)

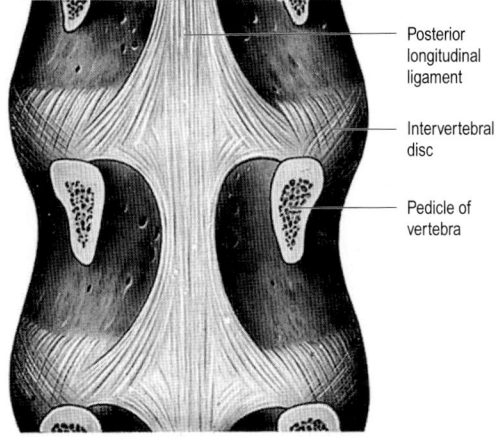

Fig. 45.39 The posterior longitudinal ligament in the lumbar region.

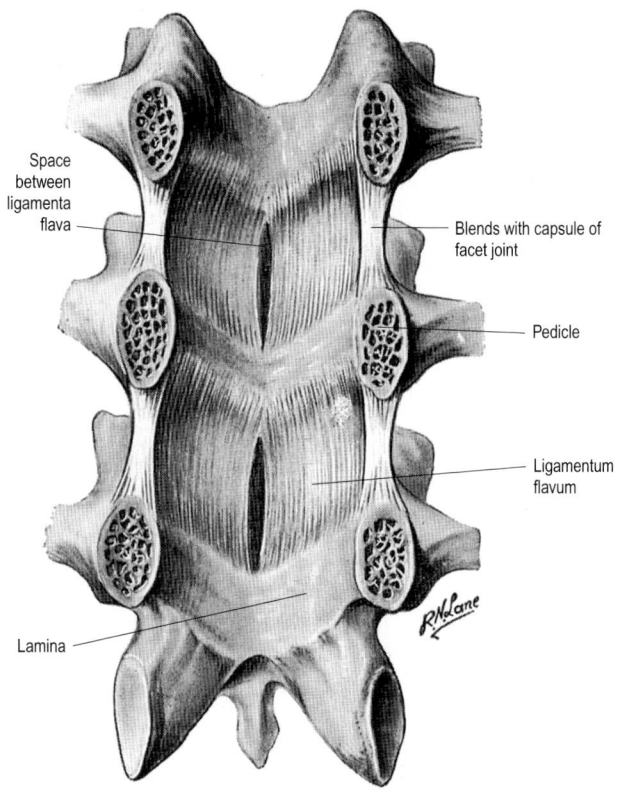

Fig. 45.40 Ligamenta flava (anterior aspect) in the lumbar region.

is also relatively thicker and narrower opposite vertebral bodies than at the levels of intervertebral symphyses. It extends from the basilar part of the occipital bone to the anterior tubercle of C1 and the front of the body of C2, then continues caudally to the front of the upper sacrum. Its longitudinal fibres are strongly adherent to the intervertebral discs, hyaline cartilage end-plates and margins of adjacent vertebral bodies, and are loosely attached at intermediate levels of the bodies, where the ligament fills their anterior concavities, flattening the vertebral profile. At these various levels ligamentous fibres blend with the subjacent periosteum, perichondrium and periphery of the annulus fibrosus. The anterior longitudinal ligament has several layers. The most superficial fibres are the longest and extend over three or four vertebrae, the intermediate extend between two or three, and the deepest from one body to the next. Laterally, short fibres connect adjacent vertebrae.

POSTERIOR LONGITUDINAL LIGAMENT (Fig. 45.39)

The posterior longitudinal ligament lies on the posterior surfaces of the vertebral bodies in the vertebral canal, attached between the body of C2 and the sacrum, and continuous with the membrana tectoria above (p. 761). Its smooth glistening fibres, attached to intervertebral discs, hyaline cartilage end-plates and adjacent margins of vertebral bodies, are separated between attachments by basivertebral veins and the venous rami which drain them into anterior internal vertebral plexuses. At cervical and upper thoracic levels the ligament is broad and of uniform width, but in lower thoracic and lumbar regions it is denticulated, narrow over vertebral bodies and broad over discs. Its superficial fibres bridge three or four vertebrae, while deeper fibres extend between adjacent vertebrae as perivertebral ligaments, which are close to and, in adults, fused with, the annulus fibrosus of the intervertebral disc. The layers are more distinct in the immediate postnatal years.

LIGAMENTA FLAVA (Figs 45.39, 45.40)

The ligamenta flava connect laminae of adjacent vertebrae in the vertebral canal. Their attachments extend from facet joint capsules to the point where laminae fuse to form spines. Here their posterior margins meet and are partially united; the intervals between them admit veins which connect the internal and posterior external vertebral venous plexuses. Their predominant tissue is yellow elastic tissue, whose almost perpendicular fibres descend from the lower anterior surface of one lamina to the posterior surface and upper margin of the lamina below. The anterior surface of the ligaments is covered by a fine, continuous smooth lining membrane (Newell 1999). The ligaments are thin, broad and long in the cervical region, thicker in the thoracic and thickest at lumbar levels. They arrest separation of the laminae in spinal flexion, preventing abrupt limitation, and also assist restoration to an erect posture after flexion, perhaps protecting discs from injury.

755

INTERSPINOUS LIGAMENTS (Fig. 45.41B)

Interspinous ligaments are thin, almost membranous and connect adjoining spines, their attachments extending from the root to the apex of each. They meet the ligamenta flava in front and the supraspinous ligament behind. The ligaments are narrow and elongated in the thoracic region, broader, thicker and quadrilateral at lumbar levels, and poorly developed in the neck. Some observers designate all cervical interspinous fibres as part of the ligamentum nuchae, while others regard them as distinct structures. Their fibres run obliquely posterosuperiorly from the upper border of one spine to the lower border of that immediately above.

SUPRASPINOUS LIGAMENT (Fig. 45.41B)

The supraspinous ligament is a strong fibrous cord which connects the tips of spinous process from C7 to the sacrum. It is thicker and broader at lumbar levels, where it is intimately blended with neighbouring fascia, though only lightly attached to the spines of L3–5. The most superficial fibres extend over three or four vertebrae, the deeper span two or three, while the deepest connect adjacent spines and are continuous with interspinous ligaments. Between the spine of C7 and the external occipital protuberance the supraspinous ligament is expanded as the ligamentum nuchae.

INTERTRANSVERSE LIGAMENTS

Intertransverse ligaments run between adjacent transverse processes. At cervical levels they consist of a few, irregular fibres which are largely replaced by intertransverse muscles; in the thoracic region they are cords intimately blended with adjacent muscles; in the lumbar region they are thin and membranous.

LIGAMENTOUS INSTABILITY

Damage to the ligaments controlling stability of the column may occur in the absence of evident bony pathology. This is particularly prevalent in inflammatory disease of the upper cervical spine, where rheumatoid arthritis may weaken or destroy the ligaments on which atlanto-axial stability depends (p. 759). The transverse ligament is stronger than the dens, which usually fractures before the ligament ruptures. The alar ligaments are weaker, and combined head flexion and rotation may avulse one or both alar ligaments: rupture of one side results in an increase of about a third in the range of rotation to the opposite side. Pathological softening of the transverse and adjacent ligaments or of the lateral atlanto-axial joints results in atlanto-axial subluxation, which may cause spinal cord injury. Ligamentous damage may also occur in spinal injuries, particularly at cervical levels.

Developmental laxity of ligaments may also lead to problems with instability, especially if there is an episode of trauma: this combination is probably responsible for atlanto-axial rotational instability. Laxity of cervical spinal ligaments may be a normal variant in children, and lead to diagnostic difficulties. In radiographs of the upper cervical spine in children aged less than 8, a deceptive appearance of subluxation ('pseudosubluxation') may result from a combination of ligamentous laxity and facet orientation. This usually occurs between C2 and C3, but may occasionally be seen at C3/4. Clinical and other radiological features should facilitate the correct diagnosis.

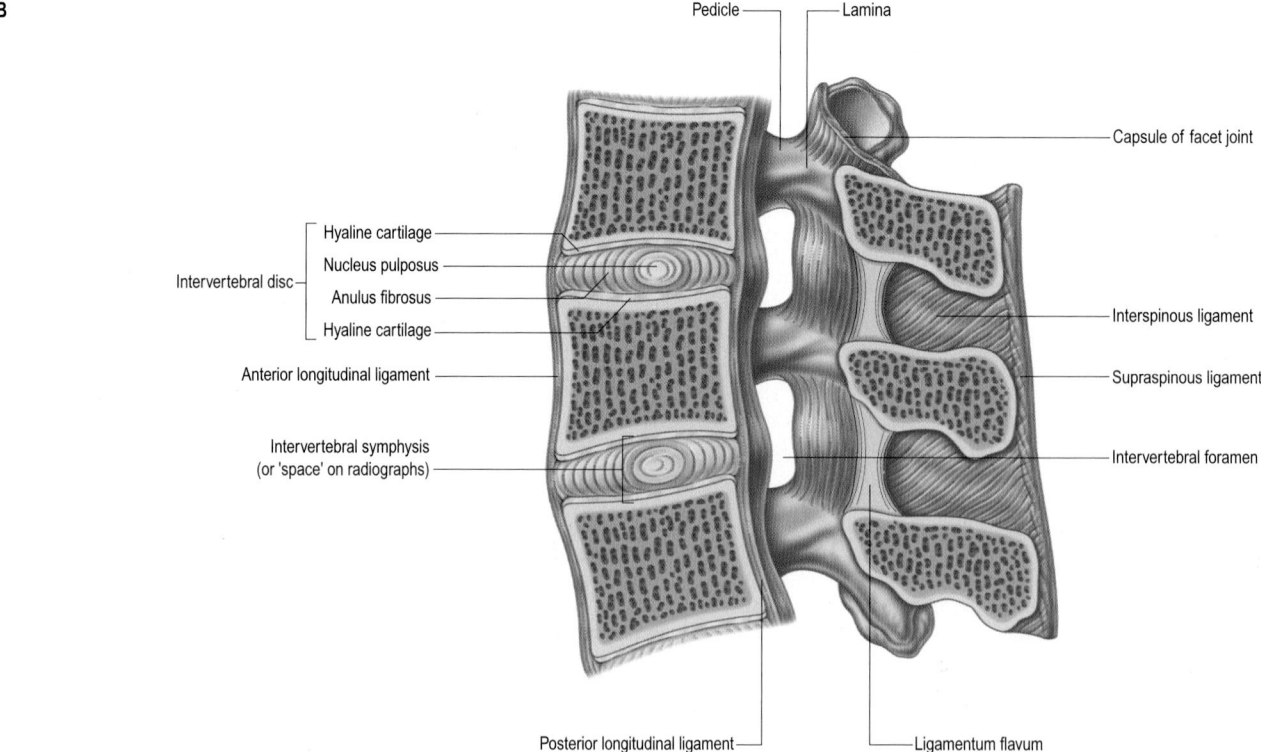

A

Anulus fibrosus

Nucleus pulposus

Laminae of fibro-cartilage

Vertebral body

B

Pedicle — Lamina

Capsule of facet joint

Hyaline cartilage

Nucleus pulposus

Intervertebral disc

Anulus fibrosus

Hyaline cartilage

Interspinous ligament

Anterior longitudinal ligament

Supraspinous ligament

Intervertebral symphysis (or 'space' on radiographs)

Intervertebral foramen

Posterior longitudinal ligament

Ligamentum flavum

Fig. 45.41 A, Schematic representation of the main structural features of an intervertebral disc. For clarity the number of fibrocartilaginous laminae has been greatly reduced. Note alternating obliquity of collagen fascicles in adjacent laminae (after Inoue). **B**, Median sagittal section through upper lumbar vertebral column showing discs and ligaments. (**A**, after Inoue H 1973 Three-dimensional observation of collagen framework of intervertebral discs in rats, dogs and humans. Arch Histol Jpn 36: 39–56.)

JOINTS

All vertebrae from C2 to S1 articulate by secondary cartilaginous joints (symphyses) between their bodies, synovial joints between their articular processes, and fibrous joints between their laminae, transverse and spinous processes. In the cervical region, from C3 to C7, there are also laterally placed articulations between the uncinate or neurocentral processes (p. 742) of the inferior vertebral body and the bevelled lateral border of the superior body at each level. These small joints, the unco-vertebral or neurocentral joints of Luschka, have a synovial element, with articular cartilage and a partial capsule.

INTERVERTEBRAL JOINTS

Joints between the vertebral bodies

Joints between vertebral bodies are symphyses. Typical vertebral bodies are united by anterior and posterior longitudinal ligaments and by fibro-cartilaginous intervertebral discs between sheets of hyaline cartilage (vertebral end-plates). The ligaments are described on pages 735 and 754.

Articulating surfaces: intervertebral discs (Fig. 45.41A)

The intervertebral discs are the chief bonds between the adjacent surfaces of vertebral bodies from C2 to the sacrum. Except at the sites of the uncovertebral (neurocentral) joints of Luschka, disc outlines correspond with the adjacent bodies. Their thickness varies in different regions and within individual discs. Each disc consists of an outer lamellated anulus fibrosus and an inner nucleus pulposus. In cervical and lumbar regions the discs are thicker anteriorly, contributing to the anterior convexity of the vertebral column. In the thoracic region they are nearly uniform, and the anterior concavity is largely due to the vertebral bodies.

Discs are thinnest in the upper thoracic region and thickest in the lumbar region. They adhere to thin layers of cartilage on the superior and inferior vertebral surfaces, the vertebral end-plates. The latter do not reach the periphery of the vertebral bodies but are encircled by ring apophyses (p. 735). The end-plates contain both hyaline cartilage and fibrocartilage. The fibrocartilaginous component lies nearer to the disc, and is sometimes considered not to be part of the end-plate itself. The fibrocartilaginous components of the end-plates above and below the nucleus pulposus, together with the innermost lamellae of the anulus fibrosus, form a flattened sphere of collagen which surrounds and encloses the nucleus (**Fig. 45.42**). The overall proportion of fibrocartilage in the end-plate increases with age. While all discs are attached to the anterior and posterior longitudinal ligaments, discs in the thoracic region are additionally tied laterally, by intra-articular ligaments, to the heads of ribs articulating with adjacent vertebrae. Intervertebral discs form about a quarter of the length of the postaxial vertebral column: cervical and lumbar regions make a greater contribution than the thoracic and are thus more pliant.

Anulus fibrosus – The anulus fibrosus has a narrow outer collagenous zone and a wider inner fibrocartilaginous zone. Its lamellae, which are convex peripherally when seen in vertical section, are incomplete collars. The internal vertical concavity of the lamellae conforms to the surface profile of the nucleus pulposus. In all quadrants of the anulus, about half the lamellae are incomplete; the proportion increases in the posterolateral region. The exact nature of the interlamellar substance remains in some doubt. Posteriorly, lamellae join in a complex manner. Fibres in the rest of each lamella are parallel and run obliquely between vertebrae at about 65° to the vertical. Fibres in successive lamellae cross each other obliquely in opposite directions, thus limiting rotation. The obliquity of fibres in deeper zones varies in different lamellae. Posterior fibres may sometimes be predominantly vertical, which possibly pre-disposes them to herniation.

This standard description of the anulus may not apply at all spinal levels: a recent cadaveric study indicates that the anulus is usually incomplete posteriorly in adult cervical discs (Mercer & Bogduk 1999).

Nucleus pulposus – The nucleus pulposus is better developed in cervical and lumbar regions and lies between the centre of the disc and its posterior surface. At birth it is large, soft, gelatinous and composed of mucoid material. It contains a few multinucleated notochordal cells and is invaded by cells and collagen fibres from the inner zone of the adjacent anulus fibrosus. Notochordal cells disappear in the first decade, and the mucoid material is gradually replaced by fibrocartilage, derived mainly from the anulus fibrosus and the plates of hyaline cartilage adjoining the vertebral bodies. The nucleus pulposus becomes less differentiated from the remainder of the disc as age progresses, and gradually becomes less hydrated and increasingly fibrous. The type II collagen of the nucleus becomes more like the type I of the anulus as its fibril diameter increases. The quantity of aggregated proteoglycans in the nucleus decreases, while the keratan sulphate/chondroitin sulphate ratio increases. As increased cross-linking occurs between collagen and the proteoglycans the discs lose their water-binding capacity, become stiffer and more liable to injury. Contrary to what was previously thought, it has now been shown that lumbar discs do not decrease in overall height as a part of normal ageing. The anulus gradually loses height as its radial bulge increases, but the nucleus retains height and may increase in convexity as it increasingly indents the end-plate. Loss of trunk height with age results from a decrease in vertebral body depth (Bogduk 1997). When the disc is not loaded, pressure in the nucleus pulposus is low at all ages.

For a review of the structure and function of the human inter-vertebral disc see Adams et al (2002).

Ligaments

The ligaments associated with the joints between the vertebral bodies are described on pages 735 and 754.

Vascular supply (See also p. 735.)

Small offshoots of spinal branches of arteries supplying the vertebral column form an anastomosis on the outer surface of the anulus fibrosus and supply its most peripheral fibres. Normal discs are other-wise avascular and are dependent for their nutrition on diffusion from vertebral bone beneath adjacent end-plates and from the peripheral anulus. Vascular and avascular parts differ in their reaction to injury. Venous drainage is via the external and internal vertebral venous plexuses to the intervertebral veins and thence to the larger named veins which drain the vertebral column. Lymphatic drainage of the vertebral column is briefly considered above. Nothing specific is known about the lymphatic drainage of the disc.

Innervation

The nerve supply of intervertebral discs has been studied in detail in the lumbar region. The outer third of the anulus is innervated by the sinuvertebral nerves: the anterior anulus is supplied by the sympathetic (grey rami) component rather than by the mixed nerve. In damaged and degenerate discs the nerves may penetrate more centrally into the disc substance. The sinuvertebral nerves are condensations within exten-sive nerve plexuses which lie on the posterior longitudinal ligament. Similar plexuses have been demonstrated anteriorly, covering the anterior longitudinal ligament, and laterally in the fetus. Each sinuvertebral nerve supplies both the disc at the level of its spinal nerve of origin and the disc one level above.

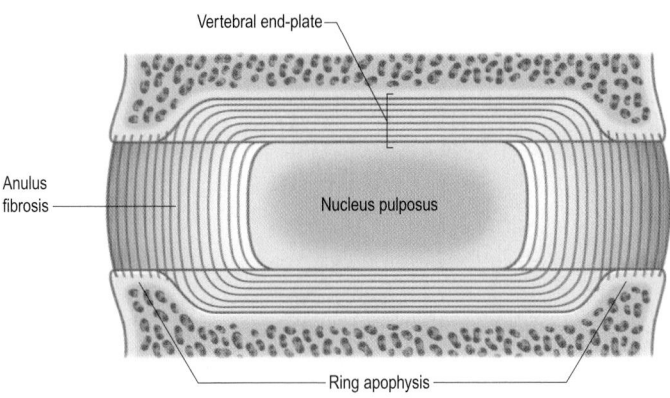

Fig. 45.42 Structure of the vertebral end plate: the collagen fibres of the inner two-thirds of the anulus fibrosus sweep around into the vertebral end plate and form its fibrocartilaginous component. The peripheral fibres of the anulus are anchored into the bone of the ring apophysis. (By permission from Bogduk N 1997 Clinical Anatomy of the Lumbar Spine and Sacrum, 3rd edn. Edinburgh: Churchill Livingstone.)

Relations and 'at risk' structures

Posterior, lateral and anterior relations of the intervertebral disc are important in the planning of interventional investigative and therapeutic procedures ranging from discography to open disc surgery. The postero-lateral surface of the disc forms the anterior boundary of the inter-vertebral foramen on each side (p. 757), and so is closely related to the spinal nerve and its accompanying vessels. More centrally the disc is related posteriorly to the dura mater covering the spinal cord and the cauda equina. Anterior relations of the discs vary considerably with vertebral level, but important 'at risk' structures include the pharynx and oesophagus, the descending aorta and the inferior vena cava. Laterally, relations change with level, but the parietal pleura in the thorax, and the sympathetic trunk and psoas muscles in the lumbar region, are important examples.

Prolapsed intervertebral disc

A prolapsed intervertebral disc most commonly affects the 20–55 year age group, and is most often seen at the L4/5 and lumbosacral levels. It may also affect the cervical discs, particularly at C5/6 and C6/7. The thoracic discs are rarely affected. Acute tearing or chronic degeneration of the posterior lamellae of the anulus fibrosus allows deformation and herniation of the softer nucleus pulposus. The disc most often prolapses just lateral to the posterior longitudinal ligament and can compress one or two spinal nerves unilaterally (**Fig. 45.43**). Much less commonly, the prolapse is central, in the midline posteriorly. The compression of neural structures may then be bilateral, affecting the cord itself or the whole cauda equina. If the damaged anulus ruptures completely, some of the nuclear tissue may escape into the vertebral and 'root' canals. This sequestrated material may migrate within the canals and cause nerve compression at spinal levels distant from that of the disc rupture. The disc material itself may have an irritative effect on the spinal nerve.

Regarding the anatomy of the vertebral canal and intervertebral foramen in relation to disc prolapse, it is important to understand that one or both of two spinal nerves and their roots may be affected by a single prolapse, depending upon the exact site of the prolapse in the horizontal plane. At the level of each disc and foramen, there are two spinal nerves (and their roots) to consider: these are the exiting nerve and the traversing nerve (Macnab & McCulloch 1990) (**Fig. 45.44**). The nerve usually affected at lumbar levels is the traversing nerve, which crosses the back of the disc on its way to become the exiting nerve at the level below. Thus a lumbosacral (i.e. L5/S1) disc prolapse usually compresses the S1 nerve. However, a prolapse may affect the exiting nerve at its own level. This is especially likely if the prolapse is in the extra-foraminal zone of the 'root' canal (p. 735), the so-called 'far lateral' prolapse. At cervical levels, because the roots and nerve leave the vertebral canal almost horizontally, the prolapse usually affects the exiting nerve. This nerve will still bear the number of the vertebra below the affected disc, because cervical nerves exit the canal above the pedicle of their numerically corresponding vertebra. Neurological presentation will include signs and symptoms of spinal nerve damage at the affected level. Thus pain and sensory loss will be dermatomal in distribution. Sensory changes usually precede motor loss.

Internal disruption of a lumbar intervertebral disc is more common than disc prolapse, and is now an increasingly recognized cause of back pain. Typically, the nucleus is decompressed and the inner lamellae of the anulus appear to collapse into it.

For more detail on disc pathology and its consequences, see Adams et al (2002).

Facet (zygapophyseal) joints

Joints between the vertebral articular processes (zygapophyses) are synovial. They are termed zygapophyseal joints, or in more common clinical usage, facet joints. For a detailed description of these joints, see Bogduk (1997).

Articulating surfaces

Facet joints are of the simple (cervical and thoracic) or complex (lumbar) synovial variety: the articulating surfaces are covered in hyaline cartilage and are carried on mutually adapted articular processes. The size and shape of these processes vary with spinal level and are described with the individual vertebrae.

Fibrous capsule

The fibrous capsule is thin and loose and attached peripherally to the articular facets of adjacent articular processes. The capsules are longer

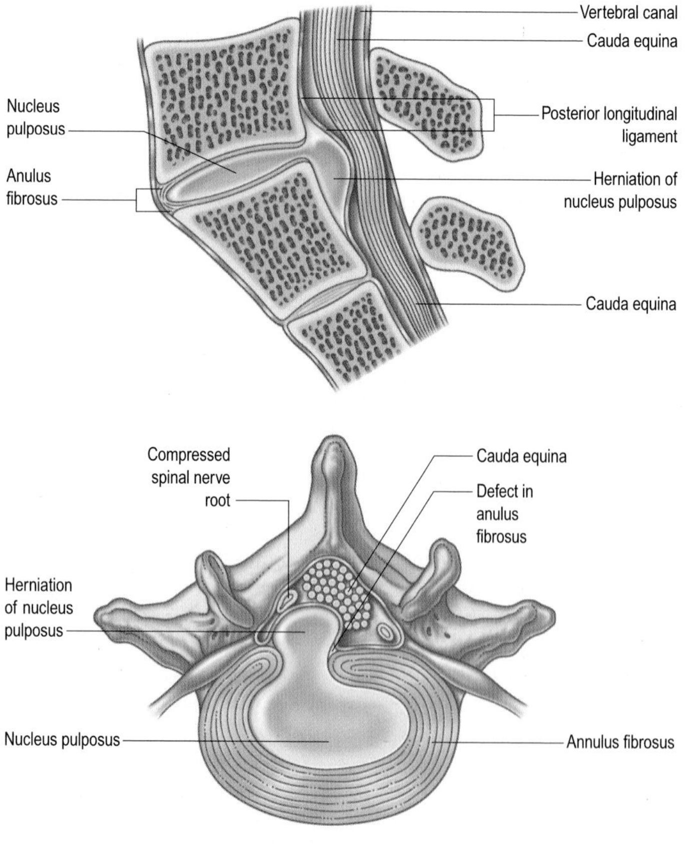

Fig. 45.43 Posterolateral disc prolapse. (By permission from Moore K, Agur AMR 2002 Essential Clinical Anatomy, 2nd edn. Philadelphia: Lippincott Williams and Wilkins.)

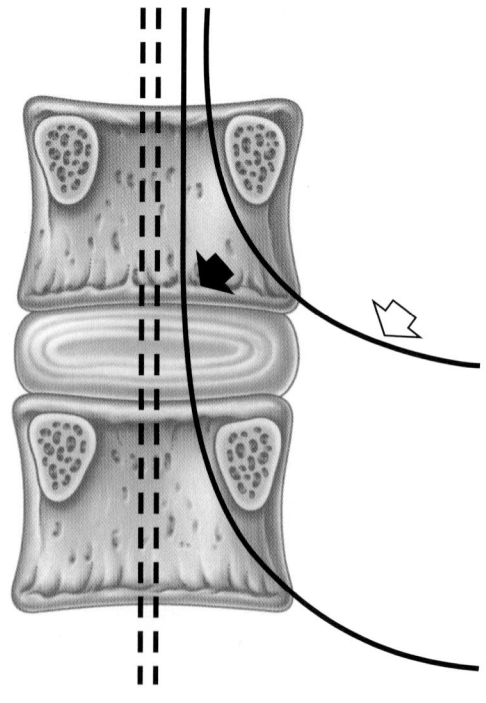

Fig. 45.44 Exiting and traversing nerve roots. The upper root (open arrow) is the exiting root at this level: the lower (arrow) is the traversing root here, which becomes the exiting root at the level below. The dotted roots are traversing roots of the lower segment.

and looser in the cervical region. According to Bogduk, the anterior fibrous capsule is replaced entirely by the ligamentum flavum in the lumbar spine.

Intracapsular structures – Bogduk describes two types of intra-articular structure in lumbar facet joints, namely subcapsular fat and 'meniscoid' structures. The latter structures may be collagenous, fibroadipose or purely adipose, and project into the crevices between non-congruent articular surfaces. They resemble inclusions seen in the small joints of the hand; their function is conjectural.

Ligaments
Ligaments which work in conjunction with, and modify the function of, the facet joints throughout the vertebral column are described on page 735.

Synovial membrane
The synovium attaches around the periphery of the articular cartilages and lines the fibrous capsule. In the lumbar region it is reflected over the intracapsular structures described above.

Vascular supply
Arterial anastomoses around the facet joints are formed from posterior spinal branches of those arteries which supply the vertebral column. Venous drainage is via the external and internal posterior vertebral venous plexuses to the intervertebral veins and thence to the larger named veins which drain the vertebral column. Lymphatic drainage follows the principles described for the vertebral column.

Innervation
The facet joints are copiously innervated by medial branches of the dorsal primary rami of the spinal nerves, which give articular branches to the joints above and below them.

Relations and 'at risk' structures
Anteriorly the capsules of the facet joints form the posterior boundaries of the intervertebral foramina (p. 741). Posteriorly and laterally the joints are related to the deep muscles of the back, some of whose fibres attach to the capsules. The joints also lie in close relation to the medial branches of the dorsal rami of the spinal nerves and to their accompanying arteries and veins. Damage to the medial branches of the dorsal rami may denervate the deep back muscles. Access to the facet joints and their related nerves may be required in the diagnosis and treatment of spinal pain.

Lumbar articular tropism
In the lumbar region, asymmetrical orientation of the facet joints occurs in about one fifth of the population. Such facet tropism does not predispose to degenerative disc disease.

CRANIOVERTEBRAL JOINTS (Figs 45.45, 45.46, 45.47, 45.48)
The articulation between the cranium and vertebral column is specialized to provide a wider range of movement than in the rest of the axial skeleton. It consists of the occipital condyles, and the atlas and axis, and functions like a universal joint which permits horizontal and vertical scanning movements of the head and is adapted for eye–head co-ordination.

Atlanto-occipital joints
The atlas articulates with the occipital bone of the skull by a pair of synovial joints. The bones are connected by articular capsules and by the anterior and posterior atlanto-occipital membranes.

Articulating surfaces
Each joint consists of two reciprocally curved articular surfaces, one on the occipital condyle and the other on the lateral mass of the atlas. The atlantal facets are concave and tilted medially.

Fibrous capsules
The fibrous capsules surround the occipital condyles and superior atlantal articular facets. They are thicker posteriorly and laterally, where the capsule is sometimes deficient, and may communicate with the joint cavity between the dens and the transverse ligament of the atlas.

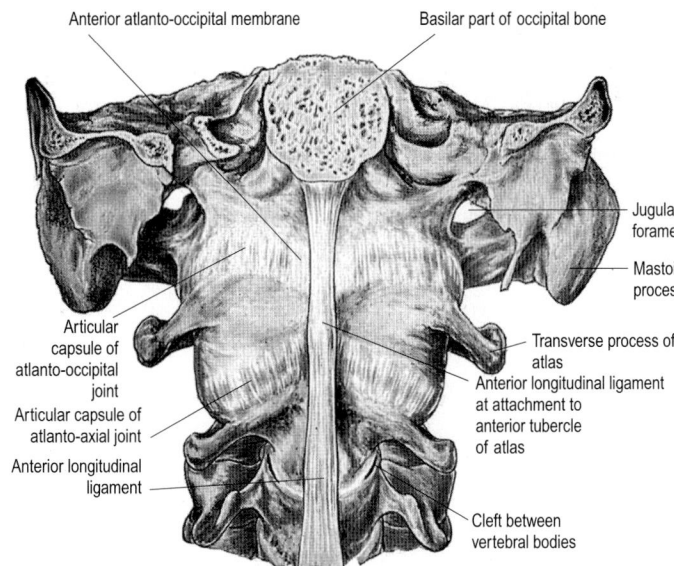

Fig. 45.45 Atlanto-occipital and atlanto-axial joints: anterior aspect. On each side a small cleft has been opened between the lateral part of the upper surface of the body of the third cervical vertebra and the bevelled, inferior surface of the body of the axis.

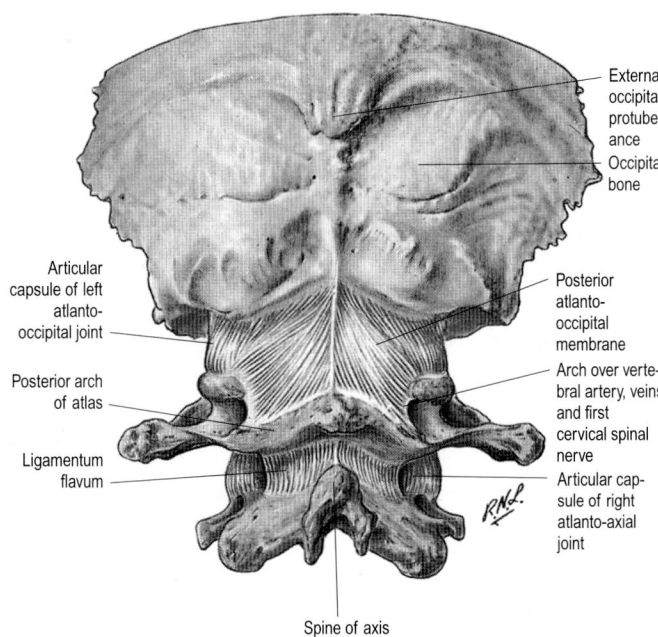

Fig. 45.46 Atlanto-occipital and atlanto-axial joints: posterior aspect.

Ligaments

The anterior atlanto-occipital membrane – The anterior atlanto-occipital membrane is a broad, dense fibrous structure which connects the anterior margin of the foramen magnum to the upper border of the anterior arch of the atlas. Laterally, it blends with the capsular ligaments, and medially it is strengthened by a median cord, which is the anterior longitudinal ligament stretching between the basilar occipital bone and anterior atlantal tubercle.

The posterior atlanto-occipital membrane – The posterior atlanto-occipital membrane is broad, but relatively thin, and connects the posterior margin of the foramen magnum to the upper border of the posterior atlantal arch, blending laterally with the joint capsules. It arches over the grooves for the vertebral arteries, venous plexuses and

759

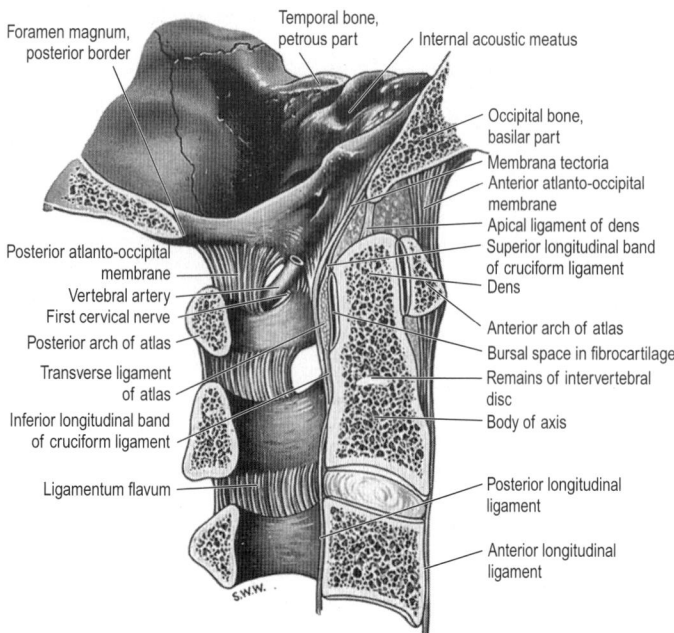

Fig. 45.47 Median sagittal section through the occipital bone and first to third cervical vertebrae.

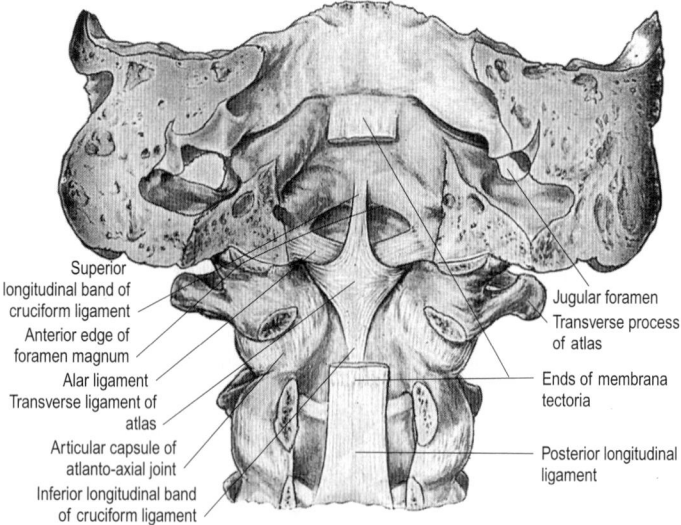

Fig. 45.48 Posterior aspect of the atlanto-occipital and atlanto-axial joints. The posterior part of the occipital bone and the laminae of the cervical vertebrae have been removed and the atlanto-occipital joint cavities opened.

first cervical nerve. The ligamentous border of the arch is sometimes ossified. The ligaments connecting the axis and the occipital bone are also functionally involved (p. 760).

Synovial membrane

The synovial cavities of one or both joints may communicate with that of the posterior component of the median atlanto-axial joint.

Vascular supply

The arterial supply of this region is derived from an anastomosis between branches of the deep cervical, occipital and vertebral arteries.

Innervation

The joints are innervated by branches of the dorsal primary rami of the first and second cervical spinal nerves. The medial branches of these rami often communicate with each other and with the third cervical nerve to form the posterior cervical plexus.

Factors maintaining stability (See also pp. 735, 760 and 768.)
Factors maintaining stability include the fibrous capsules, the atlanto-occipital membranes, the shape of the articular surfaces, the ligaments connecting the axis and the occipital bone, the ligamentum nuchae and the posterior neck muscles. The suboccipital muscles play an important proprioceptive and postural role.

Movements and muscles

The long axes of the joints run anteromedially. Taken together with their articular curvatures, this means that the joints act as one around both transverse and anteroposterior axes of movement, but not about a vertical axis. The main movement is flexion (about 18° in young subjects), with a few degrees of lateral flexion and rotation.

The following muscles produce these movements. For flexion: longus capitis and rectus capitis anterior; for extension: recti capitis posteriores major and minor, obliquus capitis superior, semispinalis capitis, splenius capitis and trapezius (cervical part); for lateral flexion: rectus capitis lateralis, semispinalis capitis, splenius capitis, sternocleidomastoid and trapezius (cervical part); and for rotation: obliquus capitis superior, rectus capitis posterior minor, splenius capitis and sternocleidomastoid.

Relations and 'at risk' structures

Posteriorly the joints are closely related to the vertebral arteries as they pass from the foramina transversaria into the foramen magnum. The dorsal primary ramus of the first cervical nerve and rectus capitis posterior major lie posteromedially. Rectus capitis anterior lies anteriorly.

Atlanto-axial joints

The atlas articulates with the axis at three synovial joints. These are a pair between the lateral masses and a median complex between the dens of the axis and the anterior arch and transverse ligament of the atlas.

Articulating surfaces

The articular surfaces of the joints between the lateral masses are often classified as planar. The bony articular surfaces are more complex in shape and are usually reciprocally concave in the coronal plane; the medial parts are somewhat convex in the sagittal plane (especially that of the axis). The cartilaginous articular surfaces are usually less concave. The median joint is a pivot between the dens and a ring formed by the anterior arch and transverse ligament of the atlas. A vertically ovoid facet on the anterior dens articulates with a facet on the posterior aspect of the anterior atlantal arch.

Fibrous capsules

The fibrous capsules for the lateral joints are attached to the articular margins and are thin and loose. Each has a posteromedial accessory ligament attached below to the axial body near the base of its dens, and above to the lateral atlantal mass near the transverse ligament. The fibrous capsule for the median joint is also relatively weak and loose, especially superiorly.

Ligaments

Anteriorly, the vertebral bodies are connected by the anterior longitudinal ligament: here a strong, thickened band attaches above to the lower border of the anterior tubercle of the anterior arch of the atlas and below to the front of the axial body. Posteriorly the vertebral bodies are joined by the ligamenta flava which are attached to the lower border of the atlantal arch above, and to the upper borders of the axial laminae. At this level these ligaments form a thin membrane, pierced laterally by the second cervical nerves.

The transverse atlantal and cruciform ligaments – The transverse atlantal ligament is a broad, strong band which arches across the atlantal ring behind the dens: its length varies about a mean of 20 mm. It is attached laterally to a small but prominent tubercle on the medial side of each atlantal lateral mass, and broadens medially where it is covered anteriorly by a thin layer of articular cartilage. It consists almost entirely of collagen fibres, which, in the central part of the ligament, cross one another at an angle to form an interlacing mesh. From its upper margin a strong median longitudinal band arises which inserts into the basilar part of the occipital bone between the apical ligament of the dens and membrana tectoria, and from its inferior surface a weaker and less consistent longitudinal band passes to the posterior surface of the axis. These transverse and longitudinal components together constitute the cruciform ligament. The transverse ligament divides the ring of the atlas into unequal parts (**Fig. 45.19**). The posterior two-thirds surrounds the spinal cord and meninges, the anterior third contains the dens, which it retains in position even when all other ligaments are divided.

Ligaments connecting axis and occipital bone – Ligaments connecting axis and occipital bone consist of the membrana tectoria, the paired alar ligaments, the median apical ligament, and the longitudinal components of the cruciform ligament.

Membrana tectoria – Inside the vertebral canal, the membrana tectoria is a broad strong band representing the upward continuation of the posterior longitudinal ligament (p. 754). Its superficial and deep laminae are both attached to the posterior surface of the axial body. The superficial lamina expands as it ascends to the upper surface of the basilar occipital bone, and attaches above the foramen magnum, where it blends with the cranial dura mater. The deep lamina consists of a strong median band which ascends to the foramen magnum, and two lateral bands which pass to, and blend with, the capsules of the atlanto-occipital joints as they reach the foramen magnum. The membrane is separated from the cruciform ligament of the atlas by a thin layer of loose areolar tissue, and sometimes by a bursa.

Alar ligaments – The alar ligaments are thick cords c.11 mm long, which pass horizontally and laterally from the longitudinally ovoid flattenings on the posterolateral aspect of the apex of the dens to the roughened areas on the medial side of the occipital condyles. In most individuals there is also an anteroinferior band, c.3 mm long, which inserts into the lateral mass of the atlas in front of the transverse ligament. Fibres occasionally pass from the dens to the anterior arch of the atlas. In addition, in c.10% of cases a continuous transverse band of fibres, the transverse occipital ligament, passes between the occipital condyles immediately above the transverse ligament. The ligaments consist mainly of collagen fibres arranged in parallel. The main function of the alar ligaments is now considered to be limitation of atlanto-axial rotation, the left becoming taut on rotation to the right and vice versa. The slightly upward movement of the axis during rotation helps permit a wider range of movement by reducing tension in the alar ligaments, and in the capsules and accessory ligaments of the lateral atlanto-occipital joint.

The apical ligament of the dens – The apical ligament of the dens fans out from the apex of the dens into the anterior margin of the foramen magnum between the alar ligaments, and represents the cranial continuation of the notochord and its sheath. It is separated for most of its extent from the anterior atlanto-occipital membrane and cruciform ligament by pads of fatty tissue, though it blends with their attachments at the foramen magnum, and with the alar ligaments at the apex of the dens.

The ligamentum nuchae and the anterior longitudinal ligament also connect cervical vertebrae with the cranium (p. 754).

Synovial membrane

The synovial membranes of the lateral joints have no special features. The median joint has two synovial cavities which sometimes communicate. The synovial cavity of the posterior component of the median joint complex is larger, lying between the horizontally orientated ovoid facet, on the posterior surface of the dens and the cartilaginous anterior surface of the transverse ligament: communication often exists with one or both of the atlanto-occipital joint cavities.

Vascular supply

The arterial supply of this region is derived from an anastomosis between branches of the deep cervical, occipital and vertebral arteries.

Innervation

The joints are innervated by branches of the dorsal primary rami of the first and second cervical spinal nerves. The medial branches of these rami often communicate with each other and with the third cervical nerve to form the posterior cervical plexus.

Factors maintaining stability (See also pp. 735, and 768.)

The most important factors maintaining stability are the ligaments, of which the transverse atlantal ligament is the strongest. The alar liga-

ments are weaker. Other ligaments connecting the axis and the occipital bone, the fibrous capsules, the ligamentum nuchae and the posterior neck muscles also contribute. The suboccipital muscles play an important proprioceptive and postural role.

Movements and muscles

Movement is simultaneous at all three joints, and consists almost exclusively of rotation around the axis. The shape of the articular surfaces is such that, when rotation occurs, the axis ascends slightly into the atlantal ring, limiting stretch on the lateral atlanto-axial joint capsules. Rotation is limited mainly by the alar ligaments, with a minor contribution from the accessory atlanto-axial ligament. The normal range of atlanto-axial rotation is about 40°.

The muscles producing atlanto-axial rotation act on the cranium, transverse processes of the atlas and spinous process of the axis. They are mainly obliquus capitis inferior, rectus capitis posterior major and splenius capitis of one side, and the contralateral sternocleidomastoid.

Relations and 'at risk' structures

The most important 'at risk' relation is the spinal cord, lying posterior to the median atlanto-axial joint. Anteriorly the atlanto-axial articulations, capsules and ligaments are separated from the buccopharyngeal fascia and superior constrictor by the longus capitis and longus colli, the prevertebral fascia and the retropharyngeal potential space.

LUMBOSACRAL JUNCTION

Articulations between the fifth lumbar and first sacral vertebrae resemble those between other vertebrae. The bodies are united by a symphysis which includes a large intervertebral disc. The latter is deeper anteriorly at the lumbosacral angle. The synovial facet joints are separated by a wider interval than those above. Segmentation (transitional) anomalies affecting the lumbosacral junction are described on page 749.

Articulating surfaces

The reciprocally curved surfaces of the facet joints show considerable individual variation in alignment and shape. Asymmetry (facet tropism) is not unusual.

Ligaments

Iliolumbar ligament (Figs 111.11, 45.49) – The fifth lumbar vertebra is attached to the ilium and sacrum by the iliolumbar ligament, which has several distinct parts. It is attached to the tip and anteroinferior aspect of the fifth lumbar transverse process, and sometimes has a weak attachment to the fourth transverse process. It radiates laterally and is attached to the pelvis by two main bands. A lower band passes from the inferior aspect of the fifth lumbar transverse process and the body of the fifth lumbar vertebra across the anterior sacroiliac ligament to reach the posterior margin of the iliac fossa. An upper band, which is part of the attachment of quadratus lumborum, passes to the iliac crest anterior to the sacroiliac joint, and is continuous above with the anterior layer of the thoracolumbar fascia (p. 734). The lower ligament has a more vertical component which reaches the posterior iliopectineal line: this component is a lateral relation of the L5 ventral ramus. A posterior component of the iliolumbar ligament passes behind quadratus lumborum to attach to the ilium.

In neonates and children the iliolumbar 'ligament' is muscular: the muscle is gradually replaced by ligament up to the fifth decade of life.

Other ligaments concerned with this joint are described on page 735.

Vascular supply

The vascular supply of the lumbosacral junction is derived mainly from the iliolumbar and superior lateral sacral arteries.

Innervation

The lumbosacral junction is innervated by branches derived from the fourth and fifth lumbar spinal nerves: the pattern of distribution is as described on page 735.

Relations and 'at risk' structures

The lumbosacral disc is related anteriorly to the common iliac veins, the median sacral vessels, and the superior hypogastric plexus of nerves. The sympathetic trunks cross it anterolaterally, while the obturator

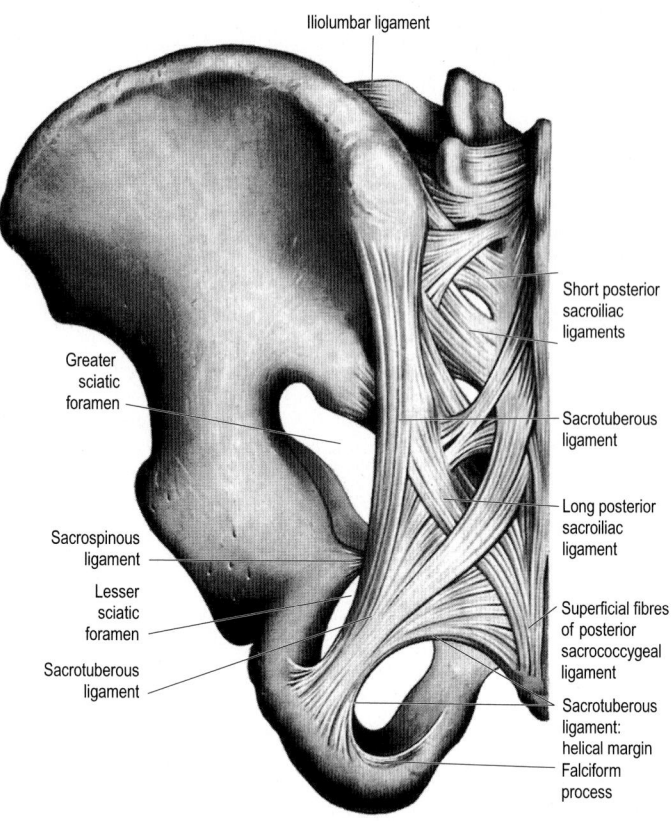

Iliolumbar ligament

Greater
sciatic
foramen

Sacrospinous
ligament

Lesser
sciatic
foramen

Sacrotuberous
ligament

Short posterior
sacroiliac
ligaments

Sacrotuberous
ligament

Long posterior
sacroiliac
ligament

Superficial fibres
of posterior
sacrococcygeal
ligament

Sacrotuberous
ligament:
helical margin
Falciform
process

Fig. 45.49 Joints and ligaments on the posterior aspect of the left half of the pelvis and the fifth lumbar vertebra.

nerves and lumbosacral trunks pass close laterally. The relations of the lumbosacral facet joints are similar to those of the lumbar facet joints described above (p. 759).

SACROCOCCYGEAL JUNCTION
The sacrococcygeal joint is usually a symphysis between the sacral apex and coccygeal base, united by a thin fibrocartilaginous disc which is somewhat thicker in front and behind than laterally. Its surfaces carry hyaline cartilage which varies from thin veils to small islands. Occasionally the coccyx is more mobile and the joint is synovial.

Ligaments

Anterior sacrococcygeal ligament (Fig. 111.11) – The anterior sacrococcygeal ligament consists of irregular fibres which descend on the pelvic surfaces of both sacrum and coccyx: it is attached like the anterior longitudinal ligament.

Superior posterior sacrococcygeal ligament – The superior posterior sacrococcygeal ligament is flat and passes from the margin of the sacral hiatus to the dorsal coccygeal surface (**Fig. 45.49**), roofing the lower sacral canal.

Deep dorsal sacrococcygeal ligament – The deep dorsal sacrococcygeal ligament passes from the back of the fifth sacral vertebral body to the dorsum of the coccyx and corresponds to the posterior longitudinal ligament.

Lateral sacrococcygeal ligaments – The lateral sacrococcygeal ligaments are bilateral, and connect the coccygeal transverse processes to the infero-lateral sacral angles, completing foramina for the fifth sacral spinal nerves.

Intercornual ligaments – The intercornual ligaments connect sacral and coccygeal cornua on each side. A fasciculus also connects the sacral cornua to the coccygeal transverse processes.

Vascular supply
The arterial supply of the sacrococcygeal junction is derived from the inferior lateral sacral and median sacral arteries.

Innervation
The innervation of the sacrococcygeal junction is derived from the lower two sacral and the coccygeal nerves.

INTERCOCCYGEAL JOINTS
In the young the intercoccygeal joints are symphyses, with thin discs of fibrocartilage between coccygeal segments. Segments are also connected by extensions of the anterior and posterior sacrococcygeal ligaments. In adult males all segments unite comparatively early, but in females union is later. In advanced age the sacrococcygeal joint becomes obliterated. Occasionally the joint between the first and second segments is synovial. The apex of the terminal segment is connected to overlying skin by white fibrous tissue.

MUSCLES (Figs 45.50, 45.58)

The musculature of the back is arranged in a series of layers, of which only the deeper are true, intrinsic, back muscles. These true back muscles are characterized by their position and by their innervation by branches of the posterior (dorsal) rami of the spinal nerves. Those below the neck lie deep to posterior layer of the thoracolumbar fascia. In the lumbar region, where the layers of the thoracolumbar fascia are well-defined, they occupy the compartment between its posterior and middle layers (p. 734).

Lying superficial to the true, intrinsic muscles are the extrinsic, 'immigrant' muscles. The most superficial of these run between the upper limb and the axial skeleton, and consist of trapezius, latissimus dorsi, levator scapulae and the rhomboid muscles. Beneath this layer lie the serratus posterior group, superior and inferior, which are variably developed but usually thin, muscles, whose function may be respiratory or possibly proprioceptive. All the extrinsic muscles are innervated by anterior (ventral) rami.

Trapezius, latissimus dorsi, levator scapulae, rhomboid major and rhomboideus minor are described on pages 836–838; serratus posterior muscles are described on page 963.

The muscles of the posterior abdominal wall are described on page 1115.

The intrinsic muscles also have superficial and deep layers. The more superficial layers contain the splenius muscles in the neck and upper thorax, and the erector spinae group in the trunk as a whole. The deeper layers include the transversospinal group, which is itself layered into semispinalis, multifidus and the rotatores, and the suboccipital muscles. Deepest of all lie the interspinal and intertransverse muscles. The latter group are not all innervated by dorsal rami: lumbar intertransversarii mediales, thoracic intertransversarii and medial parts of cervical posterior intertransversarii are so innervated, but the others are supplied by ventral rami and are thus not true muscles of the back.

VASCULAR SUPPLY
The deep muscles of the back receive their blood supply from the following arteries: vertebral artery; deep cervical artery; superficial and deep descending branches of the occipital artery; deep branch of the transverse cervical artery, when present; superior intercostal artery via dorsal branches of the upper two posterior intercostal arteries; posterior intercostal arteries of the lower nine spaces via dorsal branches; dorsal branches of the subcostal arteries; dorsal branches of the lumbar arteries; dorsal branch of arteria lumbalis ima; dorsal branches of the lateral sacral arteries.

The detailed pattern of the arterial supply of the deep muscles of the back has been described by Michel Salmon (Taylor & Razaboni 1994). These muscles are supplied by dorsal branches of the posterior intercostal and lumbar arteries. In the thoracic and upper lumbar regions, where the components of the erector spinae run in well-defined longitudinal columns, arterial trunks from these branches run in the sulci between the columns and between the erector spinae and multifidus, giving off branches to supply the muscles. In the lumbar region, where

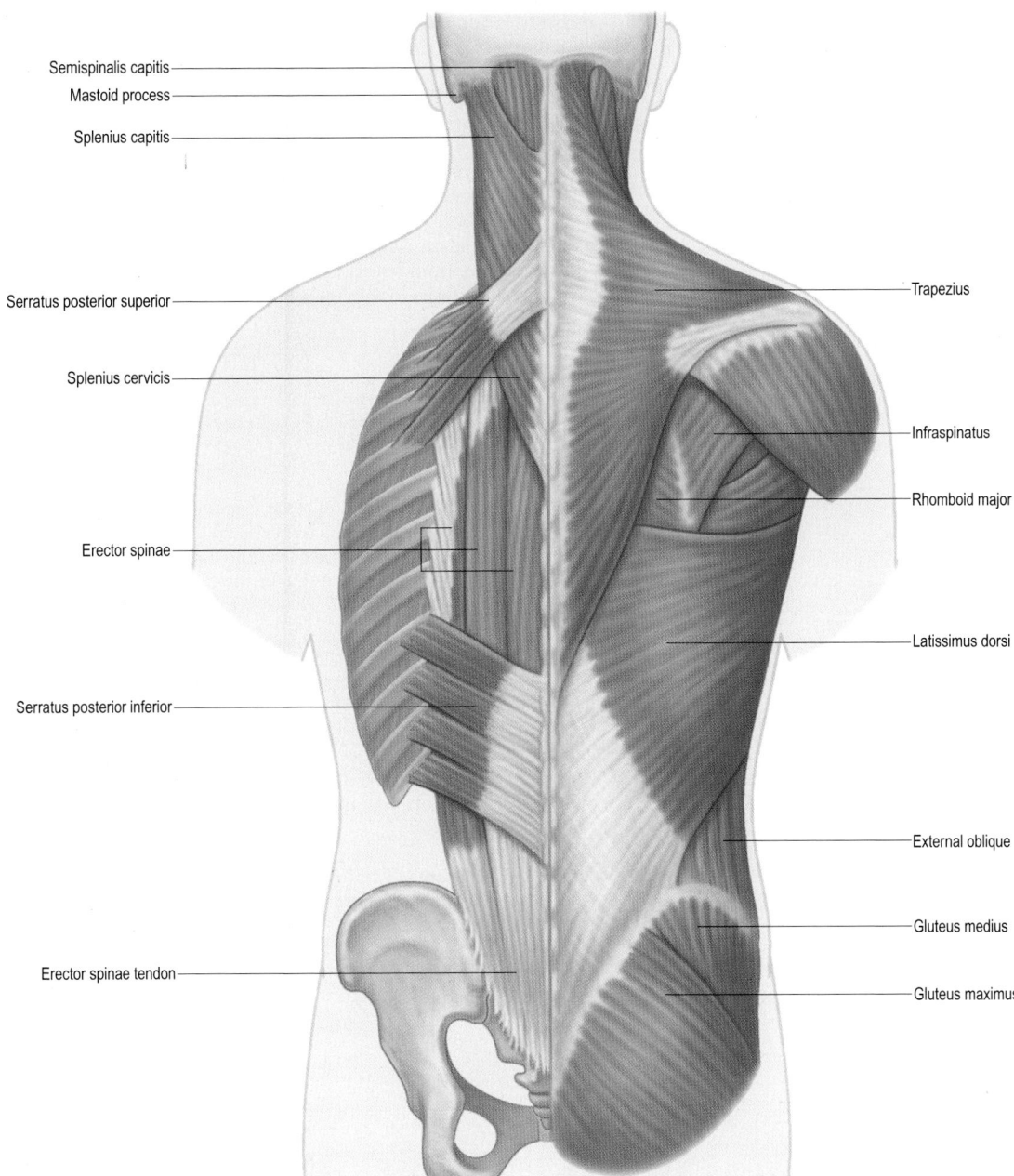

Semispinalis capitis

Mastoid process

Splenius capitis

Serratus posterior superior

Splenius cervicis

Erector spinae

Serratus posterior inferior

Erector spinae tendon

Trapezius

Infraspinatus

Rhomboid major

Latissimus dorsi

External oblique

Gluteus medius

Gluteus maximus

Fig. 45.50 Superficial (extrinsic) muscles of the back.

the erector spinae is more of a common muscle mass, this vascular pattern is less regular.

SPLENIUS CAPITIS

Attachments – Splenius capitis arises from the dorsal edge of the lower half of the ligamentum nuchae, the spines of the seventh cervical and upper three or four thoracic vertebrae, and their supraspinous ligaments. The muscle passes upwards and laterally to be attached to the mastoid process and the rough surface on the occipital bone just below the lateral third of the superior nuchal line.

Relations – The upper part of splenius capitis lies beneath sterno-cleidomastoid and the remainder lies deep to serratus posterior superior, the rhomboids and trapezius. Between sternocleidomastoid and trapezius it forms part of the floor of the posterior triangle of the neck, above and behind levator scapulae. Deep to splenius lie the upper parts of the erector spinae complex and the semispinalis cervicis.

Vascular supply – See page 762.

Innervation – Splenius capitis is innervated by medial branches of the dorsal rami of the middle cervical spinal nerves.

Actions – The action of splenius capitis is described under splenius cervicis.

SPLENIUS CERVICIS

Attachments – Splenius cervicis is attached to the spines of the third to the sixth thoracic vertebrae. It ascends to the posterior tubercles of the transverse processes of the upper two or three cervical vertebrae, immediately anterior to the attachment of levator scapulae. The splenii may be absent or vary in their vertebral attachments. Accessory slips also occur.

Relations – Splenius cervicis lies deep to serratus posterior superior, the rhomboids and trapezius. Its deep relations include the upper parts of the erector spinae complex and the lower semispinalis muscles.

Vascular supply – See page 762.

Innervation – Splenius cervicis is innervated by the medial branches of the dorsal rami of the lower cervical and upper thoracic spinal nerves.

Actions – Acting together, the splenii of the two sides draw the head directly backwards. Acting separately, they draw the head to one side, and rotate it slightly, turning the face to the same side. Each is therefore synergistic with the contralateral sternocleidomastoid.

ERECTOR SPINAE (Figs 45.53, 45.54, 68.1, 68.2, 68.3)

The erector spinae (sacrospinalis) muscle complex lies on either side of the vertebral column. It forms a large musculotendinous mass, which varies in size and composition at different levels. In the sacral and lower lumbar regions it narrows and becomes increasingly strong and tendinous as it approaches its attachments. In the upper lumbar region it expands to form a thick fleshy mass which divides into three columns which are, from lateral to mid-line, iliocostalis, longissimus and spinalis. The columns may be subdivided as follows:

Iliocostalis	Longissimus	Spinalis
Iliocostalis lumborum	Longissimus thoracis	Spinalis thoracis
Iliocostalis thoracis	Longissimus cervicis	Spinalis cervicis
Iliocostalis cervicis	Longissimus capitis	Spinalis capitis

The main muscle mass can readily be felt in the lumbar region in the living subject. Its lateral border is flanked by a visible groove (**Fig. 44.3**), which ascends over the back of the thorax, traversing the ribs at their angles and running first laterally, then vertically, and finally medially until it is obscured by the scapula.

Attachments – Erector spinae arises from the anterior surface of a broad, thick tendon or aponeurosis, which is attached in the midline to the median sacral crest, the spines of the lumbar and the eleventh and twelfth thoracic vertebrae, their supraspinous ligaments, and laterally to the medial aspect of the posterior iliac crest and to the lateral sacral crest, where it blends with the sacrotuberous and dorsal sacroiliac ligaments. Some of its fibres are continuous with gluteus maximus and multifidus.

Iliocostalis – Iliocostalis lumborum is attached, by flattened tendons, to the inferior borders of the angles of the lower six or seven ribs.

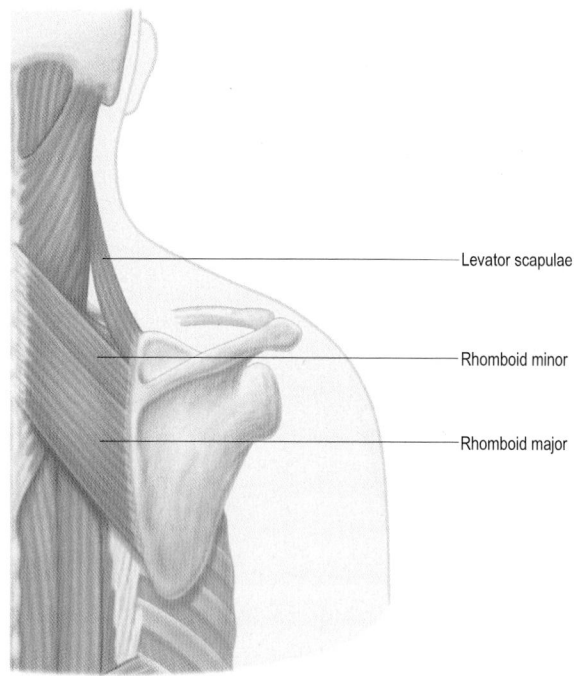

Levator scapulae

Rhomboid minor

Rhomboid major

Fig. 45.51 Rhomboid muscles.

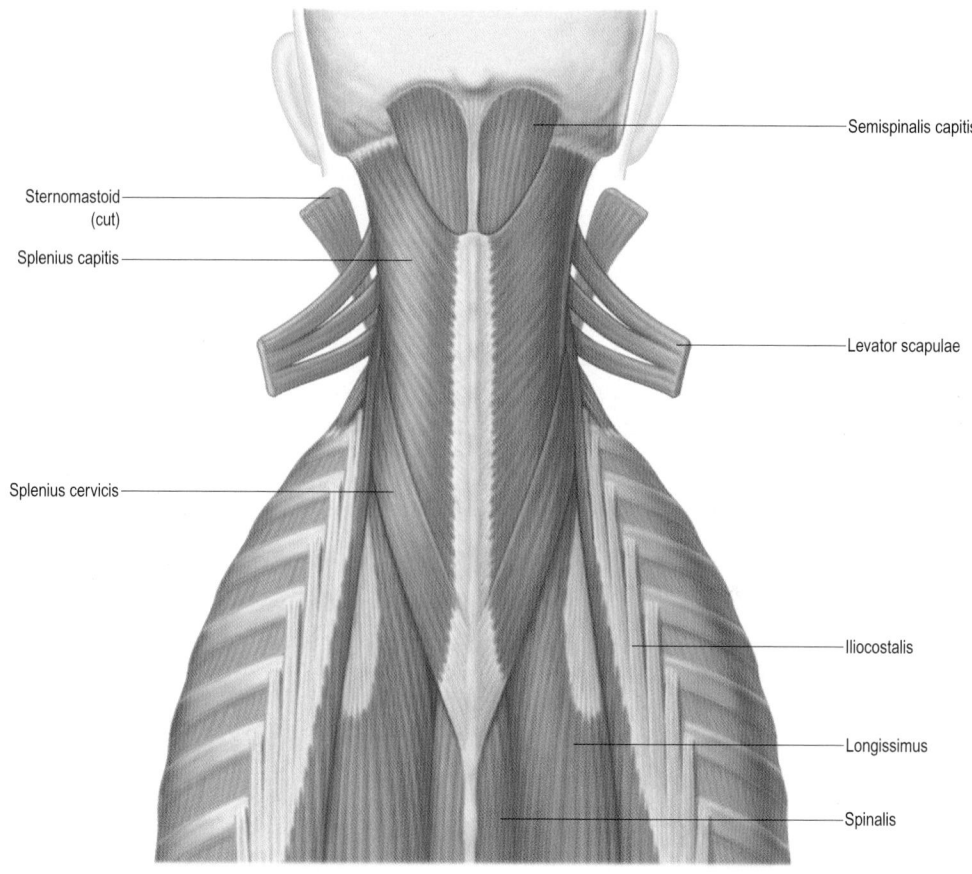

Sternomastoid (cut)

Splenius capitis

Splenius cervicis

Semispinalis capitis

Levator scapulae

Iliocostalis

Longissimus

Spinalis

Fig. 45.52 Splenius cervicis and splenius capitis.

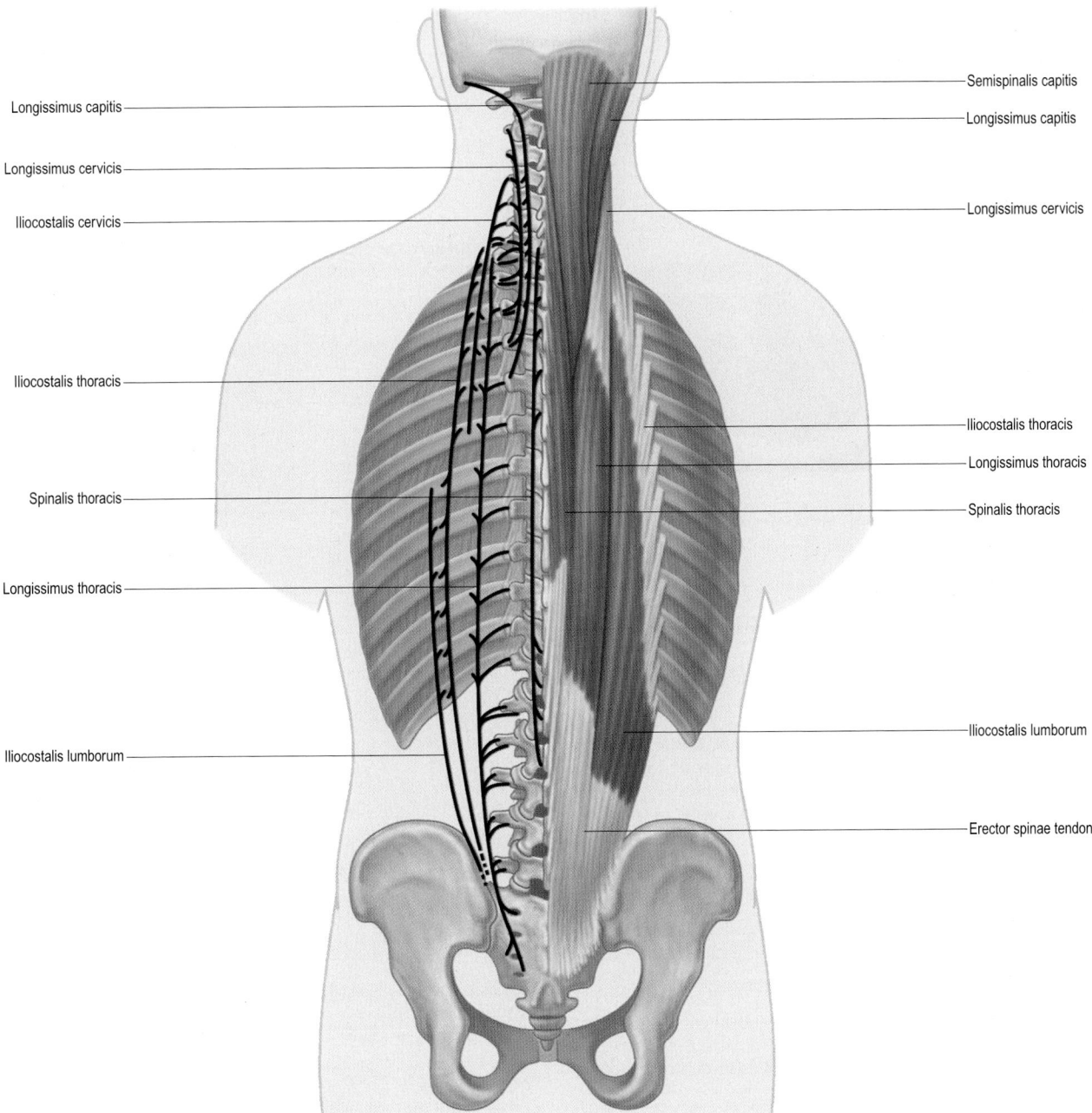

Fig. 45.53 Erector spinae muscle group.

Iliocostalis thoracis attaches below to the upper borders of the angles of the lower six ribs medial to the tendons of insertion of iliocostalis lumborum, and above to the superior borders of the angles of the upper six ribs and the back of the transverse process of the seventh cervical vertebra.

Iliocostalis cervicis attaches below to the angles of the third to the sixth ribs, medial to the tendons of insertion of iliocostalis thoracis, and above to the posterior tubercles of the transverse processes of the fourth, fifth and sixth cervical vertebrae.

Longissimus – Longissimus thoracis is the largest of the continuations of the erector spinae. In the lumbar region, where it blends with iliocostalis lumborum, some of its fibres are attached to the whole length of the posterior surfaces of the transverse processes and the accessory processes of the lumbar vertebrae, and to the middle layer of the thoracolumbar fascia. In the thoracic region it is attached, by rounded tendons, to the tips of the transverse processes of all the thoracic vertebrae, and by fleshy slips to the lower nine or ten ribs between their tubercles and angles.

Longissimus cervicis lies medial to longissimus thoracis. It is attached by long thin tendons to the transverse processes of the upper four or five thoracic vertebrae, and again by tendons to the posterior tubercles of the transverse processes of the second to the sixth cervical vertebrae.

Longissimus capitis lies between longissimus cervicis and semi-spinalis capitis. It is attached below by tendons to the transverse processes of the upper four or five thoracic vertebrae and the articular processes of the lower three or four cervical vertebrae and above to the posterior margin of the mastoid process, deep to splenius capitis and sternocleidomastoid. It is usually traversed by a tendinous intersection near its upper end.

Spinalis – Spinalis thoracis, the medial continuation of erector spinae, is barely separable as a distinct muscle. It lies medial to longissimus thoracis, and blends intimately with it. It is attached below by three or four tendons to the eleventh and twelfth thoracic and the first and second lumbar vertebral spines: these unite in a small muscle which is attached above by separate tendons to the spines of the upper thoracic vertebrae (the number varies from four to eight). It blends closely with semispinalis thoracis, which lies anterior to it.

Spinalis cervicis, when it is present, is attached to the lower part of the ligamentum nuchae and the spine of the seventh cervical vertebra (and sometimes to the first and second thoracic vertebrae), and to the

765

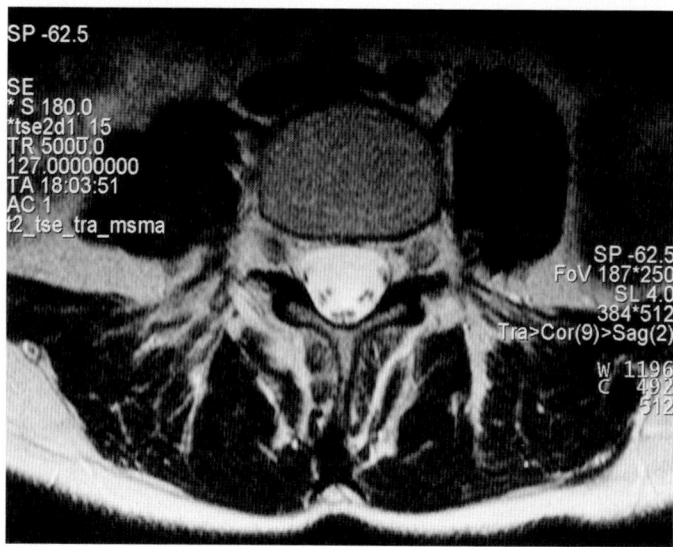

Fig. 45.54 Axial MRI of lumbar spine showing erector spinae.

spine of the axis. Occasionally it is also attached to the spines of the two vertebrae immediately below it.

Spinalis capitis usually blends to some extent with semispinalis capitis (see below), but can be separate.

Relations – Erector spinae is covered in the lumbar and thoracic regions by the thoracolumbar fascia (p. 734), and by serratus posterior inferior below and the rhomboids and splenii above. In the lumbar region it lies in the compartment between the posterior and middle layers of the thoracolumbar fascia.

Vascular supply – See page 762.

Innervation – Erector spinae is innervated by lateral and intermediate branches of the dorsal rami of the lower cervical, thoracic and lumbar spinal nerves.

Actions – Erector spinae as a group extends and laterally flexes the vertebral column when acting against gravity. It contracts eccentrically to control the movement as the column is flexed forwards or laterally with the aid of gravity.

Contraction of the erectores spinae extends the trunk, a movement controlled largely by opposing activity of the abdominal muscle complex (rectus abdominus and the oblique abdominals). Flexion of the trunk is initiated by flexor muscles such as rectus abdominis: as the centre of gravity moves forward control is transferred to the erectores spinae which then contract eccentrically. When the trunk is fully flexed the erectores spinae are relaxed and electromyographically quiet: in this position, flexion may be limited by passive forces generated by tension in the thoracolumbar fascia and in the spinal ligaments and by resistance to deformation of the intervertebral discs. Electromyographic activity in the erector spinae group is greater when work is carried out on a low surface from a standing position. Lateral flexion is controlled by the contralateral erector spinae, with input from the oblique muscles.

Longissimus capitis extends the head and turns the face to the ipsilateral side.

TRANSVERSOSPINALIS

The transversospinalis muscular group consists of the following muscles:

Semispinalis thoracis	Multifidus	Rotatores thoracis
Semispinalis cervicis		Rotatores cervicis
Semispinalis capitis		Rotatores lumborum

These muscles run obliquely upwards and medially from transverse processes to adjacent, and sometimes more distant, spinous processes.

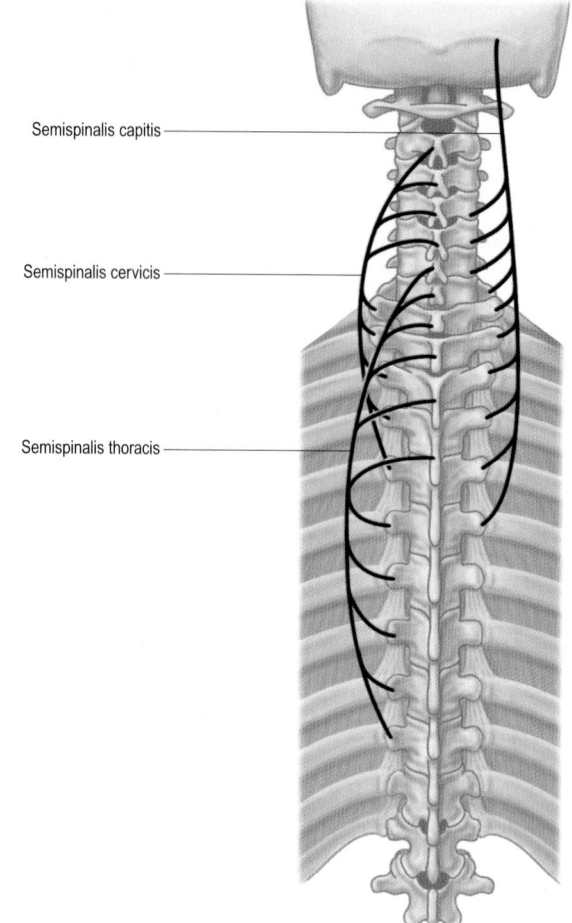

Semispinalis capitis

Semispinalis cervicis

Semispinalis thoracis

Fig. 45.55 Attachments of semispinalis.

Bogduk and his co-workers believe that, in the lumbar region at least, multifidus should be considered to run downwards and laterally (Macintosh et al 1986).

Semispinalis (Fig. 45.55) – Semispinalis thoracis consists of thin, fleshy fasciculi interposed between long tendons. It is attached below by a series of tendons to the transverse processes of the sixth to the tenth thoracic vertebrae, and above, again by tendons, to the spines of the upper four thoracic and lower two cervical vertebrae.

Semispinalis cervicis, a thicker muscle, is attached below by a series of tendinous and fleshy fibres to the transverse processes of the upper five or six thoracic vertebrae, and above to the spines of the second to the fifth cervical vertebrae. The fasciculus connected with the axis is the largest, and is composed chiefly of muscle.

Semispinalis capitis is attached by a series of tendons to the tips of the transverse processes of the upper six or seven thoracic and seventh cervical vertebrae, to the articular processes of the fourth, fifth, and sixth cervical vertebrae and, occasionally, to the spine of the seventh cervical or first thoracic vertebra. The tendons come together in a broad muscle which attaches above to the medial part of the area between the superior and inferior nuchal lines of the occipital bone. The medial part of the muscle, which is usually more or less distinct from the rest, is sometimes called biventer cervicis, because it is traversed by an incomplete tendinous intersection.

Multifidus (Fig. 45.56) – Multifidus consists of a number of fleshy and tendinous fasciculi which lie deep to the foregoing muscles and fill the groove at the side of the spines of the vertebrae from the sacrum to the axis. Its fasciculi attach as follows: most caudally, to the back of the sacrum as low as the fourth sacral foramen, to the posterior superior iliac spine and dorsal sacroiliac ligaments; in the lumbar region, to all the mammillary processes; in the thoracic region, to all the transverse

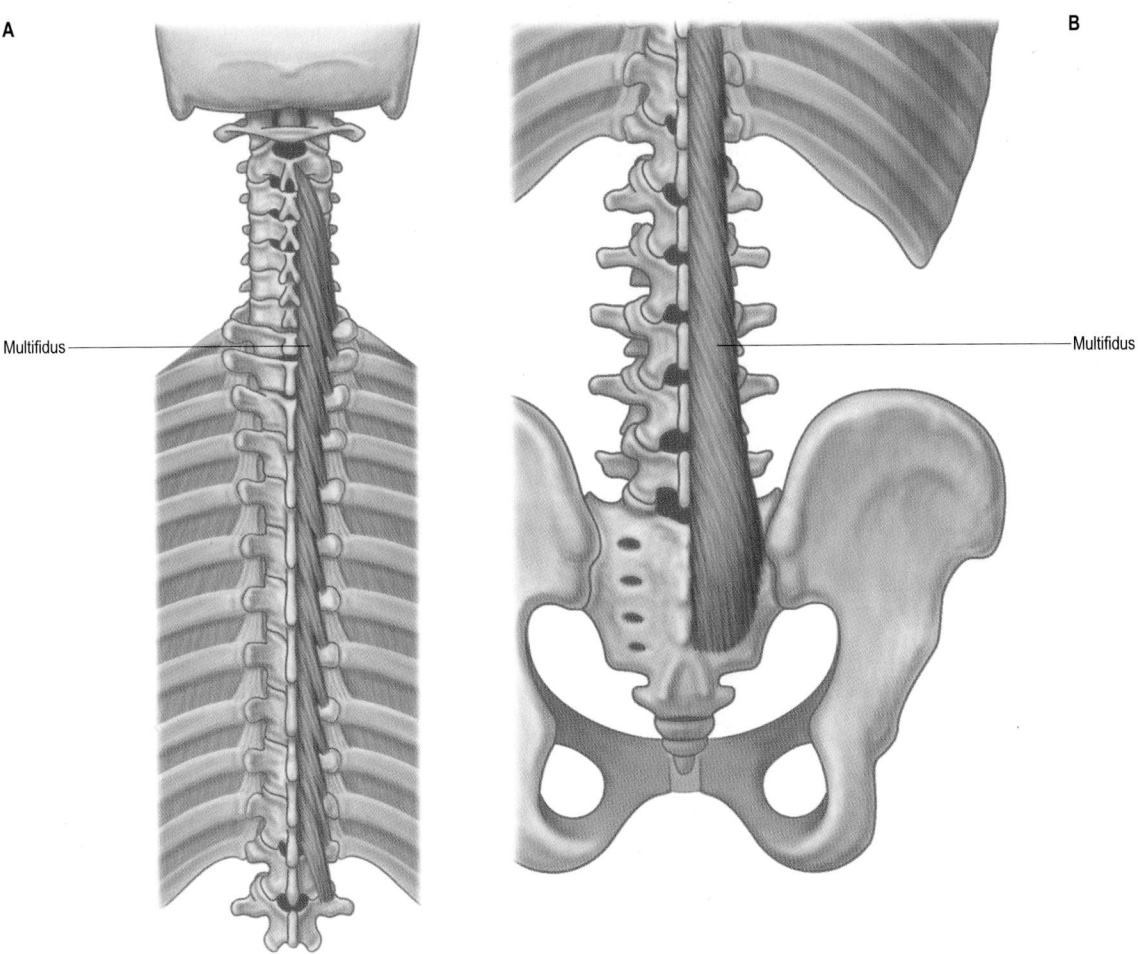

Fig. 45.56 Multifidus. **A**, cervicothoracic. **B**, lumbosacral parts.

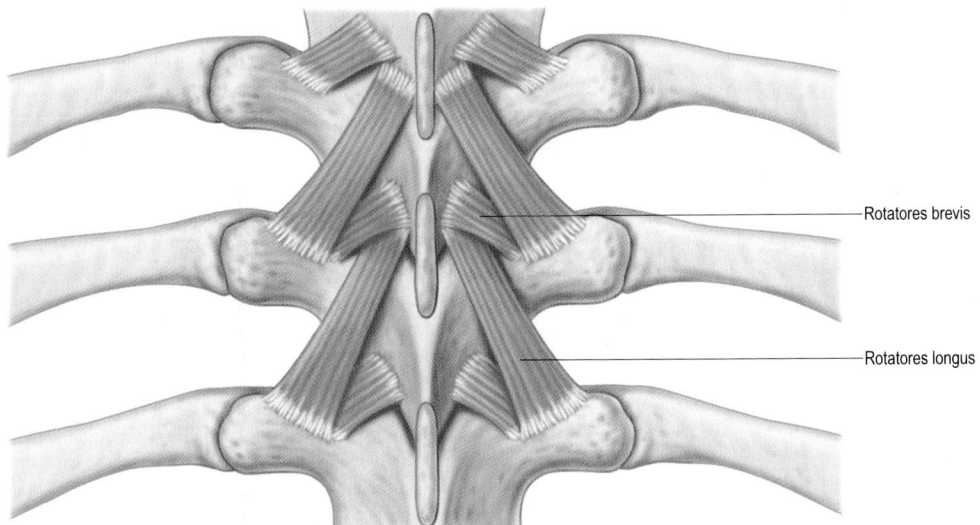

Fig. 45.57 Rotatores (thoracic region). (By permission from Benninghoff, Anatomie, 15th edition © Urban and Schwarzenberg, 1994.)

processes; in the cervical region, to the articular processes of the lower four vertebrae. In the lumbar region a few fibres may attach to the tendon (aponeurosis) of the erector spinae, and to the capsules of the facet joints. Each fasciculus is attached to the spinous process of one of the vertebrae above. Some fasciculi attach to the base of the spinous process, while others reach its tip. The fasciculi vary in length. Thus the most superficial connect one vertebra to the third or fourth above, those next in depth connect one vertebra to the second or third above, and

the deepest connect adjacent vertebrae. For further detail of the structure of this muscle, see Kalimo et al (1989).

Rotatores (Fig. 45.57) – Rotatores thoracis consists of eleven pairs of small roughly quadrilateral muscles. Each connects the upper and posterior part of the transverse process of one vertebra to the lower border and lateral surface of the lamina of the vertebra immediately above. Some fibres may extend to the base of the spinous process of the vertebra above (rotatores longi). The first is found between the first and second thoracic vertebrae, and the last between the eleventh and twelfth thoracic vertebrae. One or more may be absent from the upper or lower ends of the series.

Rotatores cervicis and lumborum are represented only by irregular and variable muscle bundles, whose attachments are similar to those of rotatores thoracis.

Relations – The transversospinalis group lie deep to erector spinae, except in the neck where semispinalis lies mainly deep to splenius and trapezius. A small section of semispinalis capitis may lie even more superficially, forming the uppermost part of the floor of the posterior triangle of the neck. In the lumbosacral region multifidus lies immediately deep to the erector spinae tendon (aponeurosis). The components of transversospinalis themselves lie in three planes, semispinalis is the most superficial and the rotatores are the most deeply placed. Semispinalis is absent in the lumbar and sacral regions, and the rotatores are well represented only in the thoracic region.

Vascular supply – See page 762.

Innervation – All of the transversospinalis group is innervated by dorsal rami of spinal nerves, usually by medial branches.

Actions – Semispinales thoracis and cervicis extend the thoracic and cervical regions of the vertebral column, and rotate them towards the opposite side. Semispinalis capitis extends the head, and turns the face slightly towards the opposite side.

INTERSPINALES

Interspinales are short paired muscular fasciculi attached above and below to the apices of the spines of contiguous vertebrae, one on either side of the interspinous ligament. They are most distinct in the cervical region, where they consist of six pairs, the first between the axis and third vertebra, and the last between the seventh cervical and first thoracic vertebrae. In the thoracic region they occur between the first and second vertebrae (sometimes between the second and third), and the eleventh and twelfth vertebrae. In the lumbar region there are four pairs between the five lumbar vertebrae. A pair is occasionally found between the last thoracic and first lumbar vertebrae, and another between the fifth lumbar vertebra and the sacrum. Sometimes cervical interspinales span more than two vertebrae.

INTERTRANSVERSARII

Intertransversarii are small muscles between the transverse processes of the vertebrae. They are best developed in the cervical region, where they consist of posterior and anterior sets of muscles separated by the ventral rami of spinal nerves. Posterior intertransverse muscles are divisible into medial and lateral slips, which are supplied by the dorsal and ventral rami of the spinal nerves, respectively. Each medial slip, the intertransverse muscle 'proper', is often further subdivided into medial and lateral parts by the passage through it of the dorsal ramus of a spinal nerve. Anterior intertransverse muscles and lateral parts of the posterior muscles connect the costal processes of contiguous vertebrae and medial parts of the posterior muscles connect true transverse processes. There are seven pairs of these muscles, the highest between the atlas and axis, and the lowest between the seventh cervical vertebra and the first thoracic: the anterior muscles between atlas and axis are often absent. In the thoracic region they consist of single muscles, which are present between the transverse processes of only the last three thoracic and first lumbar vertebrae. In the lumbar region they again consist of two sets of muscles. One set, intertransversarii mediales, connects the accessory process of one vertebra with the mammillary process of the next. The other set, intertransversarii laterales, can be divided into ventral and dorsal parts: the ventral parts connect the transverse processes (costal elements) of the lumbar vertebrae, and the dorsal parts connect the accessory processes to the transverse processes of succeeding vertebrae. Both ventral and dorsal lumbar intertransversarii are innervated by ventral primary rami (Bogduk 1997).

Thoracic intertransverse muscles and ligaments are homologous with the medial slips of the 'proper' posterior intertransverse muscles of the cervical region, and levatores costarum (p. 962) are homologous with their lateral slips. The lateral branch of the dorsal ramus of a spinal nerve separates thoracic intertransverse from levator costae. The lumbar

levatores costarum are represented by the medial intertransverse muscles; the lateral intertransverse are homologous with the intercostal muscles. For other views on the homologies and classification of transversospinal musculature consult Sato (1973).

Actions of the short muscles of the back

The short muscles of the back probably function, for the most part, as postural muscles. In effect, the vertebral column consists of a series of short, jointed levers. A mechanical arrangement of this type is unstable under compression and will tend to buckle unless movement at the individual joints is controlled. The short muscles may serve to stabilize adjoining vertebrae, controlling their movement during motion of the vertebral column as a whole, and providing for more effective action of the long erector spinae muscles. In theory, the short muscles are capable of producing extension (multifidus, interspinales), lateral flexion (multifidus, intertransversarii) and rotation (multifidus and rotatores), but their detailed patterns of activity remain unknown. The deep muscles of the back as a whole are certainly involved in the control of posture: they contract intermittently during the swaying movements that take place from an upright position.

SUBOCCIPITAL MUSCLES (Fig. 45.58)

The suboccipital muscles are four small muscles which connect the occipital bone, atlas and axis posteriorly. They lie inferior to the anterior part of the occipital bone, where three of the muscles form the boundaries of the suboccipital triangle. Above and medially lie rectus capitis posterior major; above and laterally, obliquus capitis superior, and below and laterally, obliquus capitis inferior. With the head in the anatomical position the suboccipital triangle lies almost in the horizontal plane.

Rectus capitis posterior major – Rectus capitis posterior major is attached by a pointed tendon to the spine of the axis, becomes broader as it ascends, and is attached to the lateral part of the inferior nuchal line and the occipital bone immediately below it. As the muscles of the two sides pass upwards and laterally, they leave between them a triangular space in which parts of the recti capitis posteriores minores are visible.

Rectus capitis posterior minor – Rectus capitis posterior minor is attached by a narrow pointed tendon to the tubercle on the posterior arch of the atlas. As it ascends it broadens before attaching to the medial part of the inferior nuchal line and to the occipital bone between the inferior nuchal line and the foramen magnum (p. 463). Either muscle may be doubled longitudinally. There may be an attachment to the dura mater.

Obliquus capitis inferior – Obliquus capitis inferior, the larger of the two oblique muscles, passes laterally and slightly upwards from the lateral surface of the spine and the adjacent upper part of the lamina of the axis to the inferoposterior aspect of the transverse process of the atlas.

Obliquus capitis superior – Obliquus capitis superior is attached by tendinous fibres to the upper surface of the transverse process of the atlas. It expands in width as it ascends dorsally, and is attached to the occipital bone between the superior and inferior nuchal lines, lateral to semispinalis capitis and overlapping the insertion of rectus capitis posterior major.

Relations of the suboccipital triangle – Medially the suboccipital triangle is covered by a layer of dense adipose tissue, deep to semispinalis capitis. Laterally it lies under longissimus capitis and sometimes splenius capitis, both of which overlap obliquus capitis superior. The 'floor' of the triangle is formed by the posterior atlanto-occipital membrane and the posterior arch of the atlas. The vertebral artery and the dorsal ramus of the first cervical nerve lie in a groove on the upper surface of the posterior arch of the atlas.

Vascular supply – The suboccipital muscles receive their blood supply from the vertebral artery and deep descending branches of the occipital artery.

Innervation – All the suboccipital muscles are supplied by the dorsal ramus of the first cervical spinal nerve.

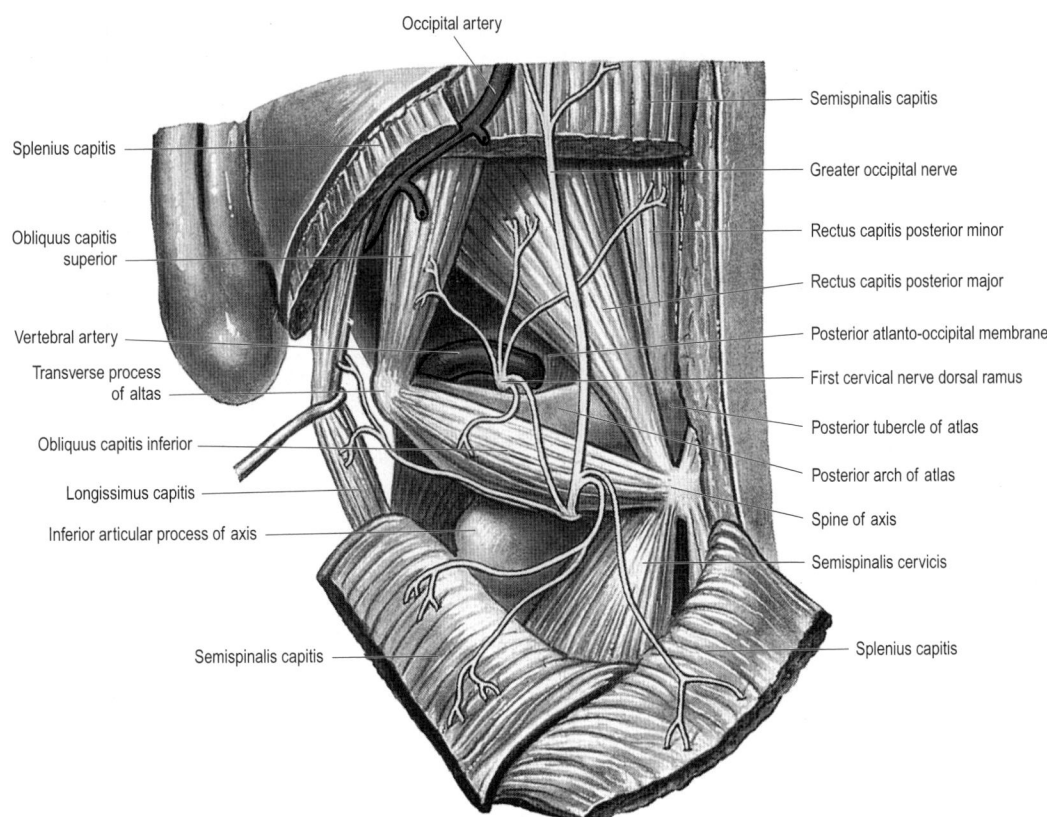

Fig. 45.58 Posterior view of the left suboccipital triangle.

Actions of the suboccipital triangle – The suboccipital muscles are involved in extension of the head at the atlanto-occipital joints and rotation of the head and atlas on the axis. Obliquus capitis superior and the two recti are probably more important as postural muscles than as prime movers, but this is difficult to confirm by direct observation. Rectus capitis posterior major extends the head and, acting with obliquus capitis inferior, rotates the face towards the ipsilateral side. Rectus capitis posterior minor extends the head. Obliquus capitis superior extends the head and laterally flexes it to the ipsilateral side.

MOVEMENTS OF THE VERTEBRAL COLUMN

Spinal movements between individual vertebrae cannot be measured accurately by skin-surface techniques. Only biplanar radiography is good enough for this purpose. The best values for the normal adult lumbar spine are from Pearcy (1984a,b). Movements of the entire lumbar spine can be measured using skin-surface techniques, but such measurements are of limited clinical use because of high inter- and intra- observer variation.

The intervertebral discs are the principal sites of vertebral column movement. At most levels they are also the limiting factor for motion according to their available deformation. Bony deformation in the subchondral bone and articular cartilage may contribute. Regional variations in mobility of the spine depend on the geometry, orientation and properties of the facet joints and related ligamentous complexes. Physiological intervertebral movements usually combine tilting (bending) and gliding (shear), so the instantaneous centre of rotation moves continually during the movement. During flexion and extension of lumbar vertebrae, the centre of rotation usually lies near the centre of the intervertebral discs, close to the end-plate of the inferior vertebra.

The oblique and ovoid articular surfaces of the facet joints ensure that spinal movements in different planes are usually 'coupled' to a certain extent. For example, lateral flexion would cause impingement of the articular surfaces on that side, leading to a posteriorly directed force on the upper vertebra which would act to rotate it about its long axis. Physiologically, coupled movements are variable, and are probably influenced by muscular control. Although movements between individual vertebrae are small, their summation gives a large total range to the vertebral column in flexion, extension, lateral flexion, and axial rotation. Each pair of vertebrae with its interposed disc and ligaments is termed a motion segment or functional spinal unit.

In flexion the anterior longitudinal ligament becomes relaxed as the anterior parts of the intervertebral discs are compressed. At its limit, the posterior longitudinal ligament, ligamenta flava, interspinous and supraspinous ligaments and posterior fibres of intervertebral discs are tensed; interlaminar intervals widen, inferior articular processes glide on superior processes of subjacent vertebrae and their capsules become taut. Tension of extensor muscles is also important in limiting flexion, e.g. when carrying a load on the shoulders. Flexion is effectively absent in the thoracic region. In forward flexion of the lumbar spine, the muscles protect the osteoligamentous spine from injury but the margin of safety can be compromised during repetitive or sustained bending by a failure of the spinal reflexes. Once the muscle protection is lost, flexion injury affects first the interspinous ligaments and then the capsules of the facet joints. The ligamentum flavum has such a high content of elastin that it is always under tension, and can be stretched by 80% without damage. This ligament probably functions to provide a constant smooth lining to the vertebral canal, one which never is overstretched in flexion, and never goes slack in extension.

In extension the opposite events occur, and there is compression of posterior discal fibres. Extension is limited by tension of the anterior longitudinal ligament, anterior discal fibres and approximation of spines and facet joints. It is marked in cervical and lumbar regions, and much less at thoracic levels, partly because of the discs are thinner, but also because of the presence of the ribs and chest musculature. In full extension, the axis of movement passes posterior to the disc, moving forwards as the column straightens and passes into flexion, reaching the centre of the intervertebral disc in full flexion.

In lateral flexion, which is always combined with 'coupled' axial rotation, intervertebral discs are laterally compressed and contralaterally tensed and lengthened, and motion is limited by tension of antagonist muscles and ligaments. Lateral movements occur in all parts of the column but are greatest in cervical and lumbar regions.

Axial rotation involves twisting of vertebrae relative to each other with accompanying torsional deformation of intervening discs. About 70% of cervical rotation occurs at the upper two cervical levels, mainly the atlanto-axial joint. Elsewhere in the column, although movement is slight between individual vertebrae, the range summates to become large for the column as a whole. In the post-cervical column, the effective range of rotation is greatest at the thoracolumbar junction. There is very little rotation in the remainder of the lumbar region.

In the cervical region the upward inclination of the superior articular facets allows free flexion and extension. The latter is usually greater, and is checked above by locking of the posterior edges of the superior facets of C1 in the occipital condylar fossae, and below by slipping of the inferior processes of C7 into grooves inferoposterior to the first thoracic superior articular processes. Flexion stops where the cervical convexity is straightened, checked by apposition of the projecting lower lips of vertebral bodies on subjacent bodies. Cervical lateral flexion and rotation are always coupled, and the superomedial inclination of the superior articular facets imparts rotation during lateral flexion.

Cervical motion can be considered to involve the upper (i.e. the atlanto-occipital and atlanto-axial complexes) and the lower cervical spine (C3–7). Two physiological movements take place at the atlanto-occipital joints, those of flexion–extension and lateral flexion. The atlanto-axial joints allow flexion–extension and rotation. Some studies have suggested that maximum flexion–extension occurs between the occiput and C1; however, Frobin et al (2002) noted between 12.6 and 14.5° at this level, which is less than at some of the other cervical levels. Global cervical flexion ranges from 45 to 58° depending on the method of assessment, age and sex: older subjects and females exhibit less motion (Ordway et al 1997; Trott et al 1996). At an intersegmental level, motion increases from the second cervical level, peaking at the mid cervical level, with 14–17° recorded at C4/5, before reducing at the junction of the cervical and thoracic spine (9.8–11.5° noted at C6/7) (Frobin et al 2002). Global ranges of lateral flexion range from 32 to 47°, again with a gradual reduction in range with age and sex, whilst rotational movements range from 63 to 78°. Intersegmental ranges of motion vary from 4.7 to 6° for lateral flexion to between C2 and C7 and 2–12° for rotation (White & Panjabi 1990).

In the thoracic region, especially superiorly, all movements are limited, reducing interference with respiration. Lack of upward inclination of the superior articular facets prohibits much flexion, and extension is checked by contact of the inferior articular margins with the laminae and of the spines with each other. Thoracic rotation is freer, though limited by the ribs at upper levels. Its axis is in the vertebral bodies in the midthoracic region, and in front of them elsewhere, so that rotation involves some lateral displacement. The direction of articular facets would allow free lateral flexion, but this is limited in the upper thoracic region by the resistance of the ribs and sternum. Rotation is usually combined with slight lateral flexion to the same side.

Movement in the thoracic spine is frequently regionalized to upper, mid- and lower thoracic. In the upper thoracic flexion ranges from 7.8 to 9.5°, increasing to 10–11.4° in the mid-thoracic and 12.5 to 12.8° in the lower thoracic (Willems et al 1996). Extension is more consistent throughout the thoracic spine ranging from 7.1 to 9.7°. Lateral flexion increases as the thoracic spine is descended ranging from 5.6 to 6.2° in the upper thoracic; 7.9 to 8.1° in the mid-thoracic and 11.9 to 13.2° in the lower thoracic. Rotation however, is greatest in the mid-thoracic region being between 11.8 to 15.9° in the upper thoracic; 21.5 to 25.3° in the mid-thoracic; and 8.3 to 11.8° in the lower thoracic.

Lumbar flexion movements are generally greater than extension or lateral flexion. Axial rotation occurs about a centre of rotation in the posterior anulus, and is limited by bony contact in the facet joints after only 1–2° of movement. Functional transition between thoracic and lumbar regions is usually between the eleventh and twelfth thoracic vertebrae (p. 746), where the facet joints usually fit so tightly that slight compression locks them, and prevents all movements but flexion.

During flexion of the lumbar spine there is an unfolding or straightening of the lumbar lordosis. Thus in full flexion the lumbar spine assumes a straight alignment or is curved slightly forwards. Normal ranges of global lumbar flexion range from 58 to 72° in under 40-year-olds and 40 to 60° in the over forties: females exhibit a reduced range compared with males (McGregor et al 1995; Dvořák et al 1995). At an intersegmental level, the L3/4 junction and L4/5 junction exhibit the greatest mobility, c.12 and 13° respectively, whilst at the lowest level L5/S1 there is only 9° and at the upper lumbar levels 8 and 10° respectively (Pearcy et al 1984). Movements into extension are the converse of those seen in flexion. Normal ranges of global extension range from 25 to 30° in under 40-year-olds and 15 to 20° in those over forty. At an intersegmental level, L5/S1 and L1/2 exhibit the greatest mobility at c.5° whilst the remaining levels exhibit less than 5° of extension. Ranges of lateral flexion and rotation in the lumbar spine are

reduced compared to other regions of the spine. Global lateral flexion ranges from 20 to 35°, whilst rotation ranges from 25 to 40°, and again is reduced with age. Assessment of intersegmental rotation and lateral flexion has proven difficult because of the limitations of measurement techniques.

ROLE OF MUSCULATURE

Although muscles will move the spinal column, the majority of muscular activity is involved in providing stability to maintain posture and to provide a firm platform for limb function. Hence the concept of 'core stability' in modern rehabilitation programmes, especially in sports-related problems.

It is important to recognize the way in which the muscles of the back work in conjunction with those of the abdominal wall, particularly the oblique and transversus muscles, and with those of the lower limbs. The erector spinae group and the internal oblique and transversus-abdominis are anatomically and functionally connected by the thoracolumbar fascia which encloses the former, and into which the latter are inserted. This fascia, together with collagenous tissue within the back muscles, plays an important role in resisting forward bending of the trunk, and in manual handling. The fascia is tensioned primarily by flexing the trunk, although this tension may be enhanced slightly by the lateral pull of the abdominal muscles. It is functionally advantageous to generate tension in the fascia and muscle sheaths, because the elastic strain energy stored in these stretched tissues can be used to help bring the trunk to an upright position and so reduce the metabolic cost of the movement (Adams et al 2002). The thoracolumbar fascia may also have an important function in transferring load between the trunk and the lower limbs: tension in the fascia can be increased by the actions of gluteus maximus and the hamstrings as well as by trunk flexion.

Muscles producing vertebral movements

The spinal column is moved both directly by muscles attached to it, and indirectly by muscles attached to other bones. Gravity always plays a part. Flexion is effected by longus capitis and longus colli, scaleni, sternocleidomastoid and rectus abdominis of both sides, aided in the lumbar region by the abdominal obliques; extension is achieved by the erector spinae complex and the transversospinalis group, splenius, semispinalis capitis and trapezius of both sides, together with the sub-occipital muscles; lateral flexion by longissimus and iliocostocervicalis, oblique abdominal muscles and flexors on the side of lateral flexion, quadratus lumborum; and lastly, rotation by sternocleidomastoid, splenius cervicis, oblique abdominal muscles, rotatores and multifidus.

FACTORS INVOLVED IN STABILITY

The vertebral column is remarkable in that it combines mobility, stability and load-bearing capacity and also protects its contained neural structures, irrespective of its position. Much of the stability of the vertebral column depends on dynamic muscular control. However there are bony and ligamentous 'static' stabilizers. There is considerable variation between segments of the column regarding stability and mobility: the most mobile levels are the least stable. The latter are those in which the ratio of intervertebral disc height to vertebral body height is highest.

Stability may be compromised by damage to any of the structures involved. Trauma may affect any vertebral region. Levels of specialized mobility (e.g. atlanto-axial joint) and junctions of mobile and relatively fixed regions (e.g. cervicothoracic, thoracolumbar) are particularly vulnerable to severe structural damage, which is often accompanied by spinal cord and nerve injury. Injuries of the vertebral column may be purely soft-tissue (ligaments, joint capsules and muscles) or may affect bony structures. Pure ligamentous/capsular injuries leading to instability may be particularly difficult to diagnose in the absence of gross radiological signs. In the cervical spine, subluxation and dislocation of the facet joints commonly occur without bony injury because of the orientation of the articular facets.

Chronic infections of many types (e.g. tuberculosis) may involve the vertebrae and lead to their deformity and collapse, affect their mechanical properties and compromise their neuroprotective function. Acute infections, spreading locally or via the bloodstream, may lead to the collection of pus within the vertebral canal causing spinal cord compression (epidural abscess).

The integrity of the vertebrae may also be affected by malignant disease, most commonly metastatic. Vertebrae have a copious blood supply throughout life, and many of the common cancers (e.g. breast, bronchus) spread via the arterial system. Cancers of the haemopoietic system (e.g. multiple myeloma) also commonly affect the vertebrae. Prostatic carcinoma has a predilection to metastasize to the vertebral column, often using the venous (Batson's plexus) rather than the arterial route. Metastatic deposits may occur within the epidural space, compressing the contents of the dural sac at multiple levels.

Systemic inflammatory diseases may cause both deformity and instability of the vertebral column. Rheumatoid arthritis inflames facet joints and weakens ligaments, leading to instability, especially in the cervical spine. Ankylosing spondylitis and other seronegative arthritides affect joints and ligamentous attachments (entheses), leading to ectopic ossification of collagenous structures, fusion (ankylosis) of interbody and facet joints, and loss of the normal spinal curvatures. Widespread new bone formation at and around the joints of the column occurs in DISH (diffuse idiopathic skeletal hyperostosis). Such conditions would seem to increase stability of the column, at the expense of its mobility and function, but an ankylosed spine is very liable to fracture which carries an associated risk of neural damage.

Full stability and load-bearing capacity both require intact vertebral bodies and intervertebral discs. Earlier views regarding the relative importance of the disc–body complex and the posterior elements have proved somewhat simplistic. Clinical observation led to the 'three-column concept' of spinal stability (Denis 1983), in which the column was divided into three longitudinal parts rather than two. The anterior column is formed by the anterior longitudinal ligament, the anterior half of the vertebral body and the anterior anulus fibrosus. The middle column is made up of the posterior longitudinal ligament, the posterior half of the vertebral body and pedicles and the posterior anulus fibrosus. The posterior column consists of the neural arch and facet joints and the posterior ligamentous complex. Failure of any column can lead to some instability: the status of the middle column is the most important. The more columns affected, the worse the instability. An injury to two columns is usually unstable.

The intervertebral discs, by elastic deformability, permit tilting and axial rotation between vertebral bodies, and also help to reduce vertical accelerations of the head. The main shock-absorbing mechanism of the column stems from the spinal curves, which increase and decrease slightly during locomotion against the restraining tension of the trunk muscles. It is the elastic strain energy in the stretched tendons of the muscle which actually does the shock absorbing.

Both body height and spinal stability are subject to a marked diurnal variation. Body height is affected by changes from recumbency to the upright posture. These diurnal variations appear to be due to changes which occur within the cervical, thoracic and lumbar regions of the spine. Investigations using stereophotogrammetry have demonstrated that 40% of diurnal changes occur in the thoracic spine, affecting the degree of kyphosis, and a further 40% in the lumbar spine, without affecting the lordosis. (Wing et al 1992). The greatest change in vertebral column length is found in adolescents and young adults. The height loss occurs within 3 hours of rising in the morning, with the overall loss being c.15 mm.

Although the curvatures within the vertebral column contribute to the changes in height, changes within the intervertebral disc contribute both to observed height loss and to variation in stability. Magnetic resonance imaging investigations reveal a dynamic movement of fluid into and out of an intervertebral disc and adjacent vertebral body over a 24-hour period, which is related to body position. In the early morning, the discs are swollen with water, the intervertebral ligaments and the anulus fibrosus are taut, and the intrinsic bending stiffness and stability of the osteoligamentous spine are relatively high. After several hours of normal activity, the discs lose c.20% of their water and height which makes the ligaments slack and greatly reduces the bending stiffness of the spine. Relatively more of the stability of the spine must then be provided by the musculature.

This diurnal expulsion of water from intervertebral discs also affects the distribution of compressive loading in the spine. As the day progresses, the hydrostatic pressure in the nucleus pulposus falls, and stress concentrations arise in the anulus fibrosus and facet joints.

All ligaments of the column, as well as the facet joint capsules, are important in the maintenance of stability. The anterior longitudinal ligament is very strong, and resists translational displacement (shear) of

the vertebrae as well as extension. All the ligaments of the posterior complex resist flexion and rotation, and their integrity determines the range of movements allowed. These ligaments can support the whole column when the muscles are inactive, e.g. in quiet standing. At the limit of lumbar flexion the column is supported mainly by the thoracolumbar fascia and by collagenous tissue within the electrically silent muscles of the back.

Movements are both determined and constrained by the shape and orientation of the facet joints, whose articular surfaces stabilize the column primarily by resisting horizontal gliding (shear) movements and axial rotation. In the most mobile regions the joint surfaces are flatter and more horizontally placed, as will become apparent if a typical cervical facet joint is compared with a typical lumbar joint.

Certain regions of the vertebral column are further stabilized by additional, extraspinal factors. The thoracic spine is stabilized by its position as an integral part of the thoracic cage and by its strong ligamentous linkages with the ribs. The sacrum is effectively a virtually fixed integral element of the bony pelvis.

The contribution to stability conferred by the musculature has in the past been grossly underrated. The whole vertebral column is stabilized by the 'guy-rope' or staying effect of the long muscles which attach it to the girdles, the head and the appendicular skeleton, especially erector spinae, which controls global posture and movement. The small and deep muscles of the back are best able to resist shear movements between vertebrae because only they have sufficient angulation to the long axis of the vertebral column to do this effectively. These deep muscles can also fine-tune intervertebral movements.

For most back problems in clinical practice, especially chronic low back pain, enhancing muscle strength, stamina, and coordination with the many other muscle groups which contribute to stability, e.g. pelvic girdle muscles, is the most appropriate and effective therapeutic avenue. Only a minority of cases benefit from surgery. Furthermore, neglecting the musculature may explain the relatively high failure rates from surgery.

Injury to the vertebral column may result from several different mechanisms: flexion, extension, distraction, rotation, shear and compression. Some of these mechanisms, often flexion, axial rotation and compression, commonly occur together.

POSTURE AND ERGONOMICS

Posture is a descriptive term for the relative position of the body segments during rest or activity. The maintenance of good posture is a compromise between minimizing the load on the spine and minimizing the muscle work required.

The well-balanced erect body has a line of gravity which extends from the level of the external auditory meatus, through the dens of the axis just anterior to the body of the second thoracic vertebra, through the centre of the body of the twelfth thoracic vertebra, and through the rear of the body of the fifth lumbar vertebra to lie anterior to the sacrum. The position of the line of gravity may move anteriorly with locomotion, and may vary between individuals.

The normal curvature of the cervical spine is a lordosis. However, as a result of pain, injury or poor ergonomics, this curve can become exaggerated to give a 'protruding chin' stance, i.e. hyperlordosis in the lower cervical spine with a kyphosis in the upper cervical spine. This can result in shortness and over-activity of the neck extensor muscle group, and elongation and under-activity of the neck flexor group.

The thoracic spine is held convex posteriorly, and this posture primarily results from the structure of the underlying vertebrae. However, this curve or kyphosis can become exaggerated to give the impression of a rounded back. Poor posture and ergonomics can lead to this exaggerated curvature but other important causes include tuberculosis, a wedge or compression fracture of a vertebral body, Scheuermann's osteochondritis, ankylosing spondylitis, osteoporosis, and metastatic carcinoma.

The lumbar spine is held in a lordosis. The degree of this lordosis is determined by the lumbosacral angle and is normally 30–45°. The muscles responsible for this posture include erector spinae, rectus abdominus, the internal and external obliques, psoas major, iliacus, the gluteal and hamstring muscles. The lordosis can be increased (as a result of weak abdominal muscles and tight hamstring muscles), decreased, flattened (common in people either with acute or chronic low back pain), or reversed.

A common postural deviation seen throughout the spine is scoliosis or lateral curvature of the spine. It can be structural, compensatory or protective. In structural scoliosis, the lateral curvature is associated with vertebral rotation, and both the curve and the rotation become more accentuated on forward flexion. Such a scoliosis is common in adolescent girls and its cause is unknown. It may also be secondary to an underlying disorder, e.g. muscular dystrophy, spinal muscular atrophy or spina bifida. A compensatory scoliosis occurs when the pelvis is tilted laterally, e.g. as a result of unequal leg length or of a fixed abduction or adduction deformity at the hip joint. Usually there is no intrinsic abnormality of the spine itself and the scoliosis disappears when the pelvic tilt is corrected. A sciatic or antalgic scoliosis is a temporary deformity produced by the protective action of muscles in certain painful conditions of the spine.

Ergonomics has been defined as 'the way humans work', and it permits an appreciation of the effects of tasks and the work environment on underlying postural biomechanics. Nachemson (1975) showed that discs were loaded maximally in sitting and in lifting in a forward leaning position, so sitting posture and lifting have received considerable ergonomic attention.

In sitting the goal has been to determine the seat type and reclining angle associated with lowest disc pressure and the least paraspinal muscle activity. When sitting with the hips and knees flexed to 90° the pelvis rotates posteriorly, flattening the lumbar lordosis and consequently increasing the load on the intervertebral discs. Thus it is now advised that in sitting the angle between trunk and thigh should be between 105 and 135°, with the sacrum tilted at 16° and the fourth and fifth lumbar vertebrae supported.

In lifting heavy weights there is considerable initial compression of lumbar intervertebral discs, and large increases in thoracic and intra-abdominal pressure. The compressive force acting on the spine is shared between the vertebral bodies and the neural arch. In the lumbar spine, the neural arch typically resists 20% of this force once the disc height has been reduced by diurnal fluid expulsion, and when the spine is positioned upright. However, age-related narrowing of the disc can cause more than 50% of the compressive force to be resisted by the neural arch, which may explain why osteoarthritis of the facet joints commonly follows disc degeneration.

When lifting, manual handling advisors emphasize the importance of leg lifting as opposed to back lifting. Loads should also be kept close to the body to reduce the lever arm of the load. The use of deep inspiration to raise intra-abdominal pressure while lifting has also been advised, as this is believed to offer further support to the lumbar spine. The spine is at risk when lifting is combined with twisting, lateral bending, and asymmetric postures. However, heavy lifting remains one of the key work related risk factors for the spine together with whole body vibration, prolonged sitting, twisting and bending.

REFERENCES

Adams MA, Bogduk N, Burton K, Dolan P 2002 The Biomechanics of Back Pain. Edinburgh: Churchill Livingstone.
A comprehensive and detailed source of information on the functional anatomy, tissue biology and biomechanics of the lumbar spine.

Batson OV 1957 The vertebral vein system. Am J Roentgenol 78: 195–212.
A pioneering study of the venous plexuses of the vertebral column which has become the standard of reference in its field.

Boelderl A, Daniaux H, Kathrein A, Maurer H 2002 Danger of damaging the medial branches of the posterior rami of spinal nerves during a dorsomedian approach to the spine. Clin Anat 15: 77–81.
Detailed descriptions of the vascular supply and innervation of the posterior elements of the thoracolumbar spine and the overlying muscles.

Bogduk N 1997 Clinical Anatomy of the Lumbar Spine and Sacrum, 3rd edn. Edinburgh: Churchill Livingstone.
The most thorough text currently available on the topographical and functional anatomy of the lumbosacral spine, with over 800 references. The book incorporates biomechanical and physiological information which is related to the clinical problem of low back pain.

Cormack GC, Lamberty BGH 1994 Arterial Anatomy of Skin Flaps, 2nd edn. Edinburgh: Churchill Livingstone.
A comprehensive plastic surgical textbook in which the cutaneous arterial supply is described in detail.

Crock HV 1996 Atlas of Vascular Anatomy of the Skeleton and Spinal Cord. London: Martin Dunitz.

Crock HV, Yoshizawa H 1976 The blood supply of the lumbar vertebral column. Clin Orthop 115: 6–21.

Dean NA, Mitchell BS 2002 Anatomic relation between the nuchal ligament (ligamentum nuchae) and the spinal dura mater in the craniocervical region. Clin Anat 15: 182–5.
Describes continuity in the midline between the spinal dura and the ligamentum nuchae in human cadavers.

Denis F 1983 The three column spine and its significance in the classification of acute thoracolumbar spinal injuries. Spine 8: 817–31.
Seminal paper for the understanding and classification of spinal instability.

Dvorák J, Vajda EG, Grob D, Panjabi MM 1995 Normal motion of the lumbar spine related to age and gender. Eur Spine J 4: 18–23.

Frobin W, Leivseth G, Biggeman M, Brinckmann P 2002 Sagittal plane segmental motion of the cervical spine. A new precision measurement protocol and normal motion data of healthy adults. Clin Biomech 17: 21–31.

Groen G, Baljet B, Drukker J 1990 The nerves and nerve plexuses of the human vertebral column. Amer J Anat 188: 282–96.
An acetylcholinesterase whole-mount study of human fetal material giving detail of the perivertebral nerve plexuses and of the sinuvertebral nerves.

Kalimo H, Rantanen J, Viljanen T, Einola S 1989 Lumbar muscles: structure and function. Ann Med 21: 353–9.
A source of detailed information, particularly on the anatomy of multifidus.

Lang J 1986 Craniocervical region, osteology and articulations. Neuro Orthop 1: 67–92.

Macintosh JE, Valencia F, Bogduk N, Munro RR 1986 The morphology of the lumbar multifidus muscles. Clin Biomech 1: 196–204.

Macnab I, McCulloch J 1990 Backache, 2nd edn, Baltimore: Williams and Wilkins. Chapter 1.
The functional anatomy of the lumbar spine, described as a basis for the clinical management of low back pain.

MacLaughlin SM, Oldale KNM 1992 Vertebral body diameters and sex prediction. Ann Hum Biol 19: 285–93.
Describes the archaeological and forensic examination of skeletal material.

McGregor AH, McCarthy ID, Hughes SPF 1995 Motion characteristics of the lumbar spine in the normal population. Spine 20: 22: 2421–8.

Mercer S, Bogduk N 1999 The ligaments and anulus fibrosus of human adult cervical intervertebral discs. Spine 24: 619–28.
A human cadaveric microdissection study showing that the cervical anulus fibrosus is an anterior crescent rather than a uniformly circumferential structure.

Nachemson A 1975 Towards a better understanding of low-back pain: a review of the mechanics of the lumbar disc. Rheumatol Rehab 14: 129–43.

Newell RLM 1999 The spinal epidural space. Clin Anat 12: 375–9.
Review of the morphological, developmental and topographical aspects of the spinal epidural space.

Ordway NR, Seymour R, Donelson RG, Hojnowski L, Lee E, Edwards T 1997 Cervical sagittal range of motion using three methods. Spine 22: 501–508.

Pearcy M, Protek I, Shepherd J 1984a Three-dimensional X-ray analysis of normal movement in the lumbar spine. Spine 9: 294–7.

Pearcy M, Tibrewal SB 1984b Axial rotation and lateral bending in the normal lumbar spine Spine 9: 582–7.

Sato T 1973 A new classification of the transverso-spinalis system. Proc Jap Acad 49: 51–6.
An alternative view of a controversial aspect of true back muscle homology.

Taylor GI, Razaboni RM (eds) 1994 Michel Salmon: Anatomic Studies, Book 1. Arteries of the Muscles of the Extremities and Trunk. St Louis: Quality Medical Publishing.
A translated, updated and edited version of a classic French text first published in 1933. Now a major source-book in plastic surgery.

Taylor JR, Twomey LT 1984 Sexual dimorphism in human vertebral shape. J Anat 138: 281–6.
Anthropometric and radiological studies of children and adolescents.

Trott PH, Pearcy MJ, Ruston SA, Fulton I, Brien C 1996 Three-dimensional analysis of active cervical motion: the effect of age and gender. Clin Biomech 11: 201–206.

Twomey L, Taylor J, Furniss B 1983 Age changes in the bone density and structure of the lumbar vertebral column. J Anat 136: 15–25.

White AA, Panjabi MM 1990 Clinical Biomechanics of the Spine, 2nd edn. Philadelphia: JB Lippincott.

Willems JM, Jull GA, Ng JK-F 1996 An in vivo study of the primary and coupled rotations of the thoracic spine. Clin Biomech 11: 311–16.

Wing P, Tsang I, Gagnon F, Susak L, Gagnon R 1992 Diurnal changes in the profile shape and range of motion of the back. Spine 17: 761–5.

SECTION

4

Chapter

45

Macroscopic anatomy of the spinal cord and spinal nerves

This chapter deals with the gross anatomy of the structures which lie within the vertebral canal and its extensions through the intervertebral foramina, the spinal nerve or radicular ('root') canals. The spinal cord, its blood vessels and nerve roots lie within a meningeal sheath, the theca, which occupies the central zone of the vertebral canal and extends from the foramen magnum, where it is in continuity with the meningeal coverings of the brain, to the level of the second sacral vertebra in the adult. Distal to this level the dura extends as a fine cord, the filum terminale externum, which fuses with the posterior periosteum of the first coccygeal segment. Tubular prolongations of the dural sheath extend around the spinal roots and nerves into the lateral zones of the vertebral canal and out into the 'root' canals, eventually fusing with the epineurium of the spinal nerves. Between the theca and the walls of the vertebral canal is the epidural (spinal extradural) space (p. 778), which is loosely filled with fat, connective tissue containing small arteries and lymphatics, and an important venous plexus. Three-dimensional appreciation of the anatomy of the spinal theca and its surroundings is essential for the efficient management of spinal pain and of spinal injuries, tumours and infections. Equally significant clinically is the anatomy of the often precarious blood supply of the spinal cord and its associated structures. The increasing application and refinement of diagnostic imaging and endoscopic procedures lend a new importance to topographical detail here.

SPINAL CORD (MEDULLA) (Figs 46.1, 46.2, 46.3, 46.4, 46.5, 46.6)

The spinal cord is an elongated, approximately cylindrical part of the CNS, occupying the superior two-thirds of the vertebral canal. Its average length in European males is 45 cm, its weight c.30 g. (For dimensional data consult Barson & Sands 1977.) It extends from the upper border of the atlas to the junction between the first and second lumbar vertebrae: this lower level varies, and there is some correlation with the length of the trunk, especially in females. The termination may be as high as the caudal third of the twelfth thoracic vertebra or as low as the disc between the second and third lumbar vertebra, and its position rises slightly in vertebral flexion. The spinal cord is enclosed in the dura, arachnoid and pia mater, separated from each other by the subdural and subarachnoid spaces respectively. The former is a potential space, while the latter contains cerebrospinal fluid (CSF). The cord is continuous cranially with the medulla oblongata, and narrows caudally to the conus medullaris, from whose apex a connective tissue filament, the filum terminale, descends to the dorsum of the first coccygeal vertebral segment. The spinal cord varies in transverse width, gradually tapering craniocaudally, except at the levels of the enlargements. It is not cylindrical, being wider transversely at all levels, especially in the cervical segments.

The cervical enlargement is the source of the large spinal nerves which supply the upper limbs. It extends from the third cervical to the second thoracic segments, its maximum circumference (c.38 mm) is in the sixth cervical segment. (A spinal cord segment provides the attachment of the rootlets of a pair of spinal nerves.)

The lumbar enlargement corresponds to the innervation of the lower limbs, and extends from the first lumbar to the third sacral segments, the equivalent vertebral levels being the ninth to twelfth thoracic vertebrae. The greatest circumference (c.35 mm) is near the lower part of the body of the twelfth thoracic vertebra, below which it rapidly dwindles into the conus medullaris.

Fissures and sulci extend along most of the external surface. An anterior median fissure and a posterior median sulcus and septum

almost completely separate the cord into right and left halves, but they are joined by a commissural band of nervous tissue which contains a central canal.

The anterior median fissure extends along the whole ventral surface with an average depth of 3 mm, although it is deeper at caudal levels. It contains a reticulum of pia mater. Dorsal to it is the anterior white commissure. Perforating branches of the spinal vessels pass from the fissure to the commissure to supply the central spinal region. The posterior median sulcus is shallower, and from it a posterior median septum of neuroglia penetrates more than halfway into the cord, almost to the central canal. The septum varies in anteroposterior extent from 4 to 6 mm, and diminishes caudally as the canal becomes more dorsally placed and the cord contracts.

A posterolateral sulcus exists from 1.5 to 2.5 mm lateral to each side of the posterior median sulcus. Dorsal roots (strictly rootlets) of spinal

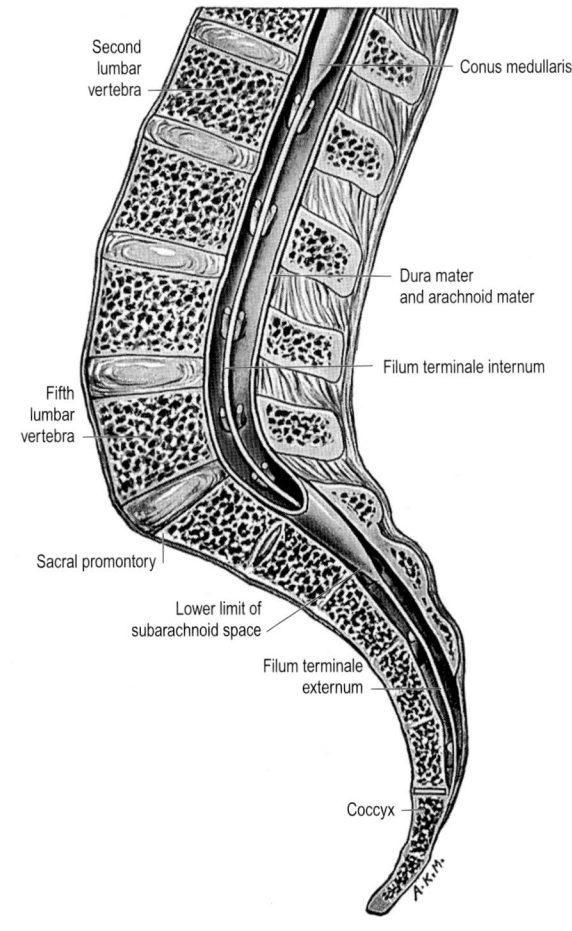

Fig. 46.1 Median sagittal section of the lumbosacral part of the vertebral column to show the conus medullaris and filum terminale. The section has opened up the subarachnoid space as far as the first sacral vertebra. Note the difference in levels between the inferior limits of the spinal cord and meninges. Note that there are two inaccuracies in this figure retained from an earlier edition: the epidural space is not shown; the fibres of interspinous ligaments should slope dorsocranially.

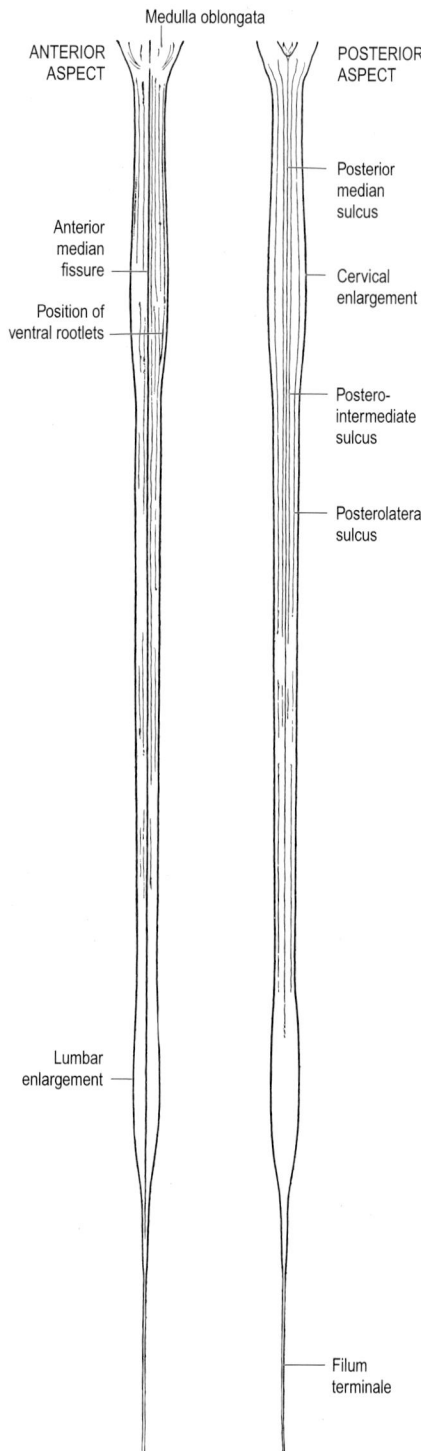

Medulla oblongata

ANTERIOR
ASPECT

POSTERIOR
ASPECT

Posterior
median
sulcus

Anterior
median
fissure

Cervical
enlargement

Position of
ventral rootlets

Postero-
intermediate
sulcus

Posterolateral
sulcus

Lumbar
enlargement

Filum
terminale

Fig. 46.2 The main features of the spinal cord.

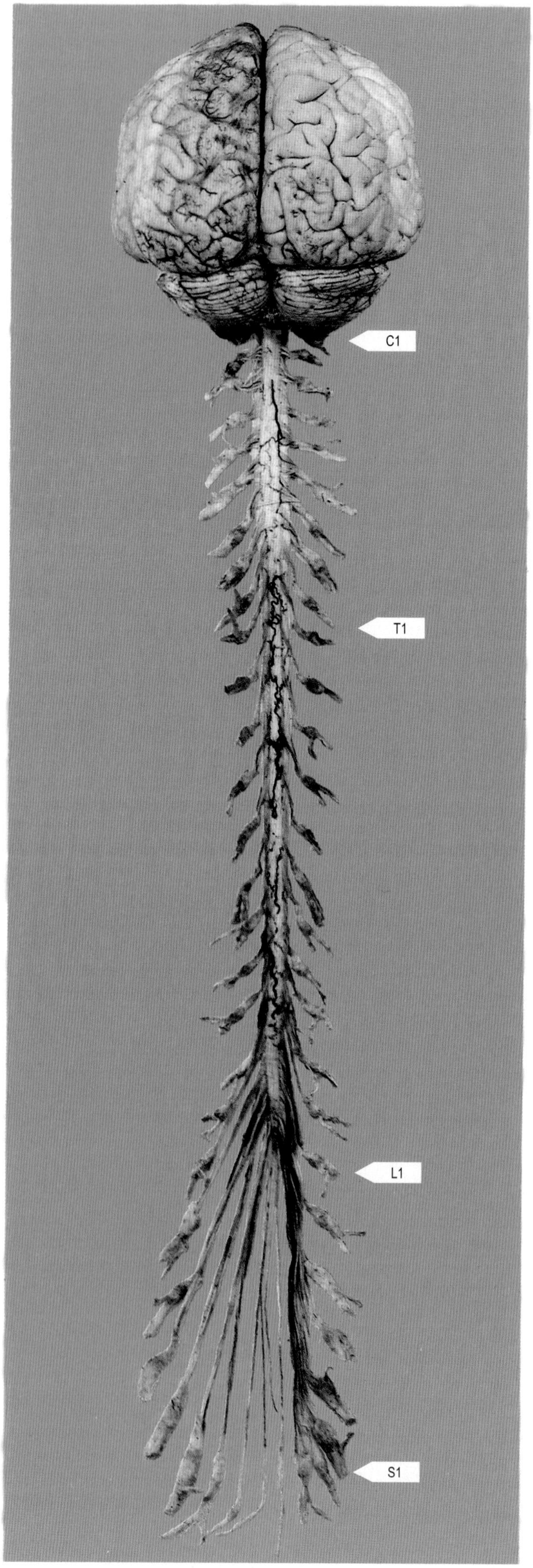

Fig. 46.3 (*Right*) Brain and spinal cord with attached spinal nerve roots and dorsal root ganglia, photographed from the dorsal aspect. Note the fusiform cervical and lumbar enlargements of the cord, and the changing obliquity of the spinal nerve roots as the cord is descended. The cauda equina is undisturbed on the right but has been spread out on the left to show its individual components. (Dissection by MCE Hutchinson, GKT School of Medicine; photograph by Kevin Fitzpatrick on behalf of GKT School of Medicine, London.)

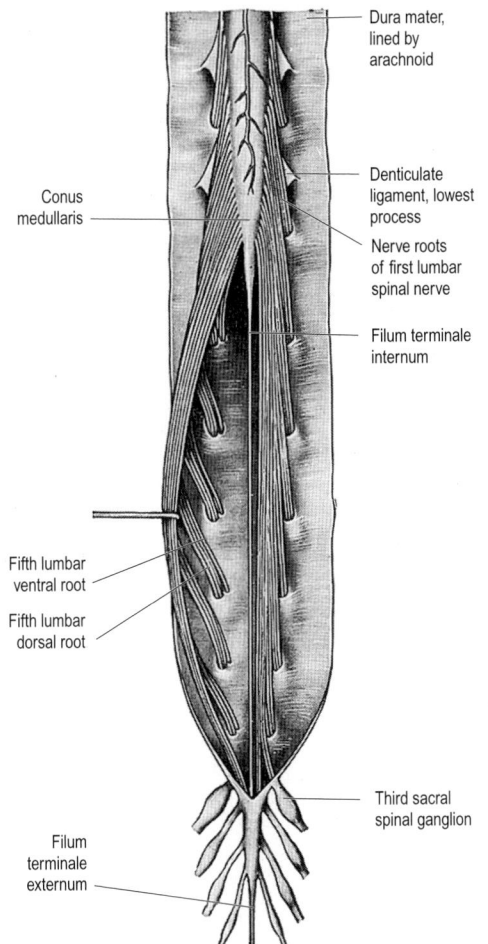

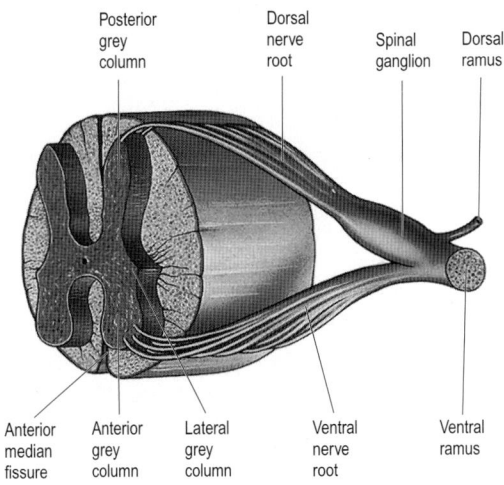

Fig. 46.6 Diagram of a spinal cord segment showing mode of formation of a typical spinal nerve and the gross relationships of the grey and white matter. Note dorsal nerve rootlets in a single linear row, ventral rootlets in three or more rows.

Fig. 46.4 Lower end of spinal cord, filum terminale and cauda equina exposed from behind. The dura mater and the arachnoid have been opened and spread out.

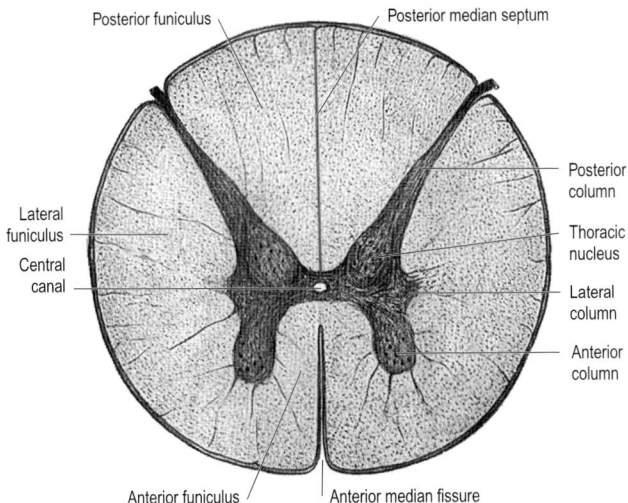

Fig. 46.5 Transverse section of the spinal cord at a mid-thoracic level.

fissure is the anterolateral funiculus. This is subdivided into anterior and lateral funiculi by ventral spinal roots which pass through its substance to issue from the surface of the cord. The anterior funiculus is medial to, and includes, the emerging ventral roots, whilst the lateral funiculus lies between the roots and the posterolateral sulcus. In upper cervical segments, nerve rootlets emerge through each lateral funiculus to form the spinal accessory nerve which ascends in the vertebral canal lateral to the spinal cord and enters the posterior cranial fossa via the foramen magnum (**Fig. 46.7**).

The filum terminale, a filament of connective tissue c.20 cm long, descends from the apex of the conus medullaris. Its upper 15 cm, the filum terminale internum, is continued within extensions of the dural and arachnoid meninges and reaches the caudal border of the second sacral vertebra. Its final 5 cm, the filum terminale externum, fuses with the investing dura mater, and then descends to the dorsum of the first coccygeal vertebral segment. The filum is continuous above with the spinal pia mater. A few strands of nerve fibres which probably represent roots of rudimentary second and third coccygeal spinal nerves adhere to its upper part. The central canal is continued into the filum for 5–6 mm. A capacious part of the subarachnoid space surrounds the filum terminale internum, and is the site of election for access to the CSF (lumbar puncture).

DORSAL AND VENTRAL ROOTS

(Fig. 46.6)(*See also* p. 781.)

The paired dorsal and ventral roots of the spinal nerves are continuous with the spinal cord. They cross the subarachnoid space and traverse the dura mater separately, uniting in or close to their intervertebral foramina to form the (mixed) spinal nerves. Since the spinal cord is shorter than the vertebral column, the more caudal spinal roots descend for varying distances around and beyond the cord to reach their corresponding foramina. In so doing they form, mostly distal to the apex of the cord, a divergent sheaf of spinal nerve roots, the cauda equina, which is gathered round the filum terminale in the spinal theca (*see also* p. 781).

Ventral spinal roots contain efferent somatic and, at some levels, efferent sympathetic, nerve fibres which emerge from their spinal sources. There are also afferent nerve fibres in these roots. The rootlets comprising each ventral root emerge from the anterolateral sulcus over an elongated vertical elliptical area. Dorsal spinal roots bear ovoid swellings, the spinal ganglia, one on each root proximal to its junction with a corresponding ventral root in an intervertebral foramen. Each root fans out into six to eight rootlets before entering the cord in a vertical row in the posterolateral sulcus. Dorsal roots are usually said to contain only afferent axons (both somatic and visceral) from unipolar neurones in spinal root ganglia, but they may also contain a small number (3%) of efferent fibres and autonomic vasodilator fibres.

nerves enter the cord along the sulcus. The white substance between the posterior median and posterolateral sulcus on each side is the posterior funiculus. In cervical and upper thoracic segments a longitudinal postero-intermediate sulcus marks a septum dividing each posterior funiculus into two large tracts: the fasciculus gracilis (medial) and fasciculus cuneatus (lateral). Between the posterolateral sulcus and anterior median

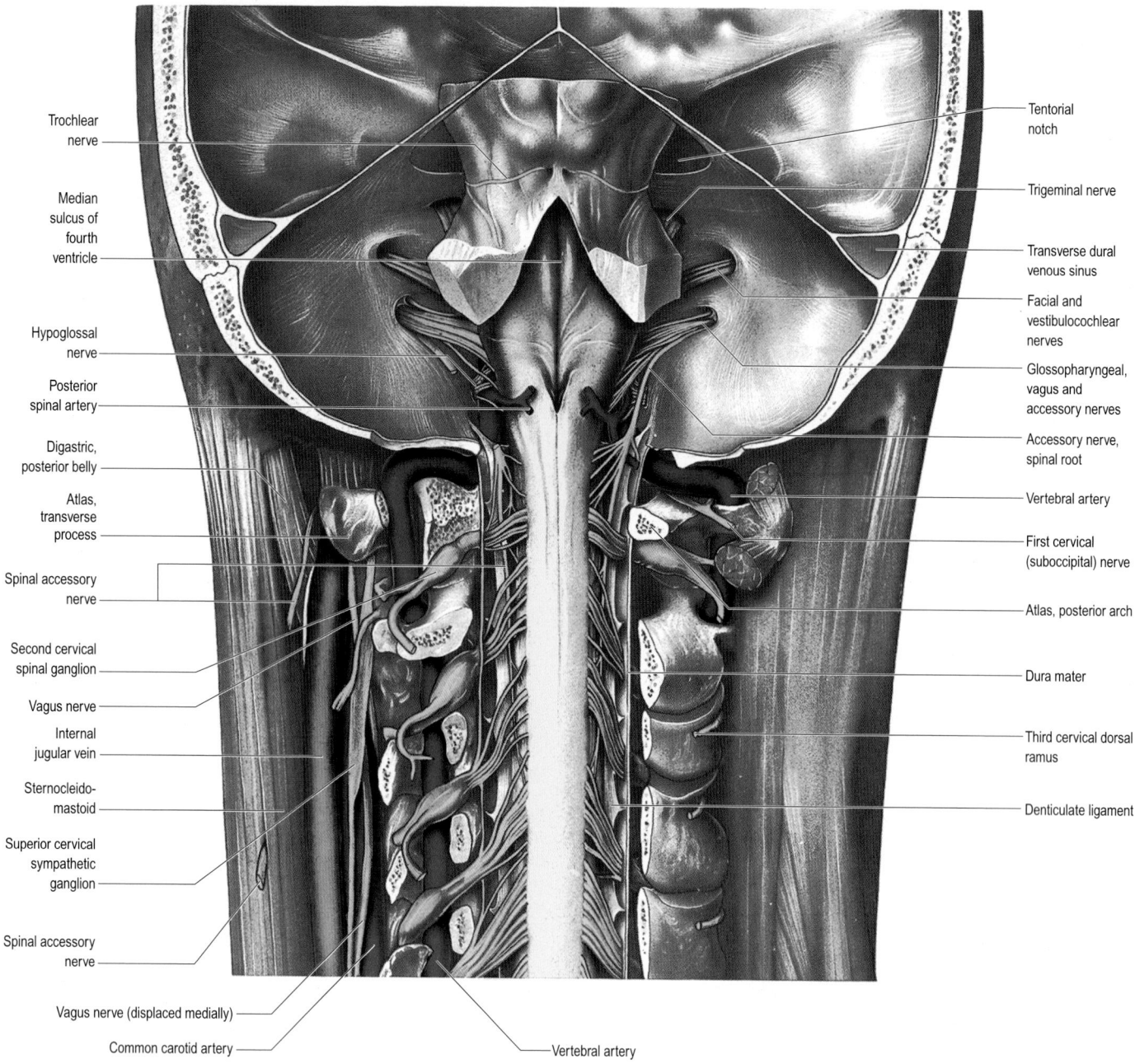

Trochlear
nerve

Median
sulcus of
fourth
ventricle

Hypoglossal
nerve

Posterior
spinal artery

Digastric,
posterior belly

Atlas,
transverse
process

Spinal accessory
nerve

Second cervical
spinal ganglion

Vagus nerve

Internal
jugular vein

Sternocleido-
mastoid

Superior cervical
sympathetic
ganglion

Spinal accessory
nerve

Vagus nerve (displaced medially)

Common carotid artery

Tentorial
notch

Trigeminal nerve

Transverse dural
venous sinus

Facial and
vestibulocochlear
nerves

Glossopharyngeal,
vagus and
accessory nerves

Accessory nerve,
spinal root

Vertebral artery

First cervical
(suboccipital) nerve

Atlas, posterior arch

Dura mater

Third cervical dorsal
ramus

Denticulate ligament

Vertebral artery

Fig. 46.7 Dissection showing the brain stem and upper five cervical spinal segments after removal of large portions of the occipital and parietal bones and the cerebellum together with the roof of the fourth ventricle. On the left, the foramina transversaria of the atlas and of the third, fourth and fifth cervical vertebrae have been opened to expose the vertebral artery. On the right, the posterior arch of the atlas and the laminae of the succeeding cervical vertebrae have been removed.

Each ganglionic neurone has a single short stem which divides into a medial branch which enters the spinal cord via a dorsal root, and a lateral branch which passes peripherally to a sensory end organ. The central branch is an axon while the peripheral one is an elongated dendrite (but when traversing a peripheral nerve is, in general structural terms, indistinguishable from an axon). The region of spinal cord associated with the emergence of a pair of nerves is a spinal segment, but there is no actual surface indication of segmentation. Moreover, the deep neural sources or destinations of radicular fibres may lie far beyond the confines of the 'segment' so defined.

MENINGES

DURA MATER
The single layer of dura which lines the cranial cavity divides into two layers as it passes downwards through the foramen magnum, although it is still a single layer as it forms the anterior and posterior atlanto-

occipital membranes. Within the vertebral column, it has been suggested that the outer endosteal layer becomes the periosteum of the vertebral canal, which is separated from the spinal dura mater by an extradural (epidural) space (see below). This interpretation, which would make the epidural space 'intradural', is not generally agreed (see Newell 1999). The spinal dura mater forms a tube whose upper end is attached to the edge of the foramen magnum and to the posterior surfaces of the second and third cervical vertebral bodies, and also by fibrous bands to the posterior longitudinal ligament, especially towards the caudal end of the vertebral canal. The dural tube narrows at the lower border of the second sacral vertebra. It invests the thin spinal filum terminale, descends to the back of the coccyx, and blends with the periosteum. For details of the meningeal coverings of the spinal roots and nerves see page 782.

Epidural space (Fig. 46.8)
The epidural space lies between the spinal dura mater and the tissues which line the vertebral canal. It is closed above by fusion of the spinal dura with the edge of the foramen magnum, and below by the posterior

sacrococcygeal ligament which closes the sacral hiatus. It contains loosely packed connective tissue, fat, a venous plexus, small arterial branches, lymphatics and fine fibrous bands which connect the theca with the lining tissue of the vertebral canal. These bands, the meningovertebral ligaments, are best developed anteriorly and laterally. Similar bands tether the nerve root sheaths or 'sleeves' within their canals. There is also a midline attachment from the posterior spinal dura to the ligamentum nuchae at atlanto-occipital and atlanto-axial levels (Dean & Mitchell 2002). The venous plexus consists of longitudinally arranged chains of vessels, connected by circumdural venous 'rings'. The anteriorly placed vessels receive the basivertebral veins.

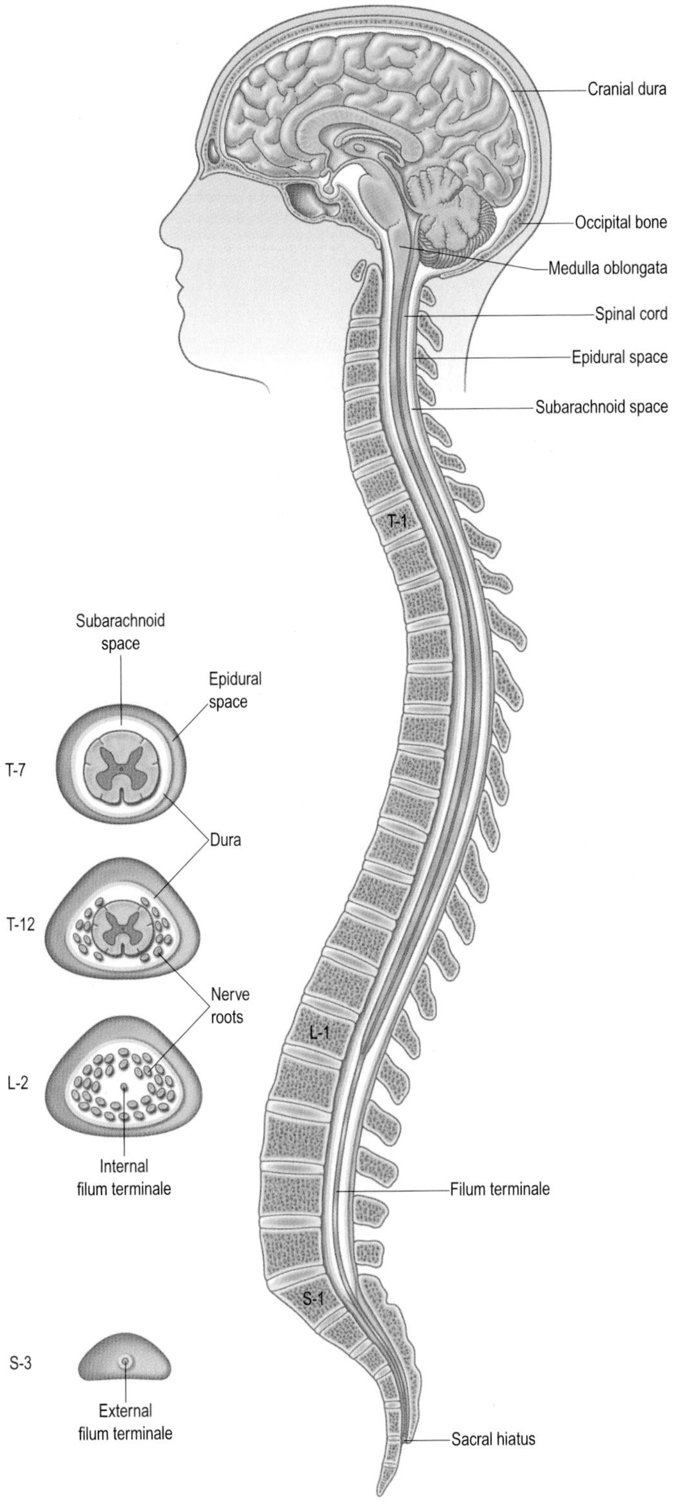

The shape of the space within each spinal segment is not uniform, though the segmental pattern is metamerically repeated. It is difficult to define the true shape of the 'space', because it changes with the introduction of fluid or as a result of preservation techniques. In the lumbar region, the dura mater is apposed to the walls of the vertebral canal anteriorly and attached by connective tissue in a manner that permits displacement of the dural sac during movement and venous engorgement. Adipose tissue is present posteriorly in recesses between the ligamentum flavum and the dura. The connective tissue extends for a short distance through the intervertebral foramina along the sheaths of the spinal nerves. Like the main thecal sac, the root sheaths are partially tethered to the walls of the foramina by fine meningovertebral ligaments. Contrast media and other fluids injected into the epidural space at the sacral level can spread up to the cranial base. Local anaesthetics injected near the spinal nerves, just outside the intervertebral foramina, may spread up or down the epidural space to affect the adjacent spinal nerves or may pass to the opposite side. The paravertebral spaces of each side communicate via the epidural space, particularly at lumbar levels.

For a review of the morphology of the epidural space, see Newell (1999).

Subdural space

The subdural space is a potential space in the normal spine because the arachnoid and dura are closely apposed (Haines et al 1993). It does not connect with the subarachnoid space, but continues for a short distance along the cranial and spinal nerves. Accidental subdural catheterization may occur during extradural injections. Injection of fluid into the subdural space may either damage the cord by direct toxic effects or by compression of the vasculature.

ARACHNOID MATER (Figs 46.9, 46.10)

The arachnoid mater which surrounds the spinal cord is continuous with the cranial arachnoid mater. It is closely applied to the deep aspect of the dura mater. At sites where vessels and nerves enter or leave the subarachnoid space, the arachnoid mater is reflected on to the surface

Fig. 46.8 The epidural space. Adapted with permission from Rosse C & Gaddum-Rosse P 1997. Hollinshead's Textbook of Anatomy 5th edn. Philadelphia: Lippincott-Raven, Fig. 13–3.

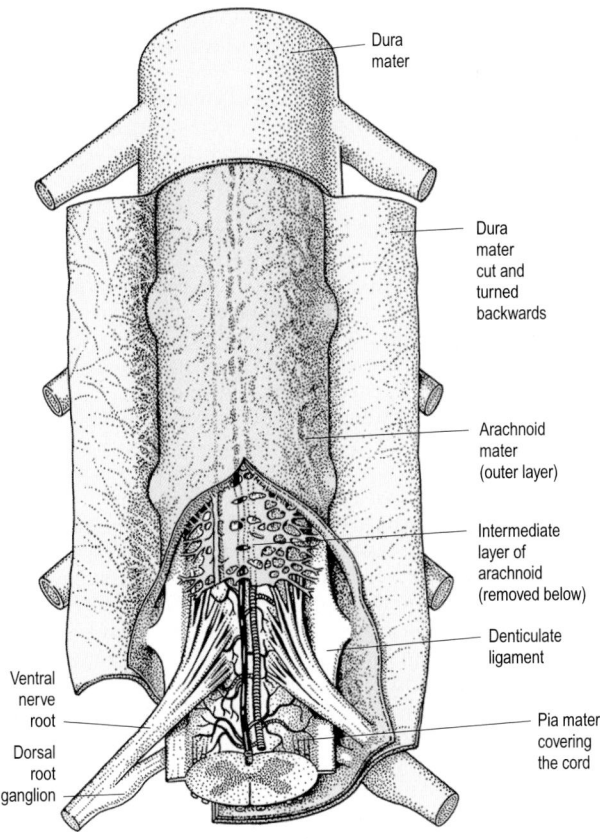

Fig. 46.9 Part of the spinal cord exposed from the anterior aspect to show meningeal coverings.

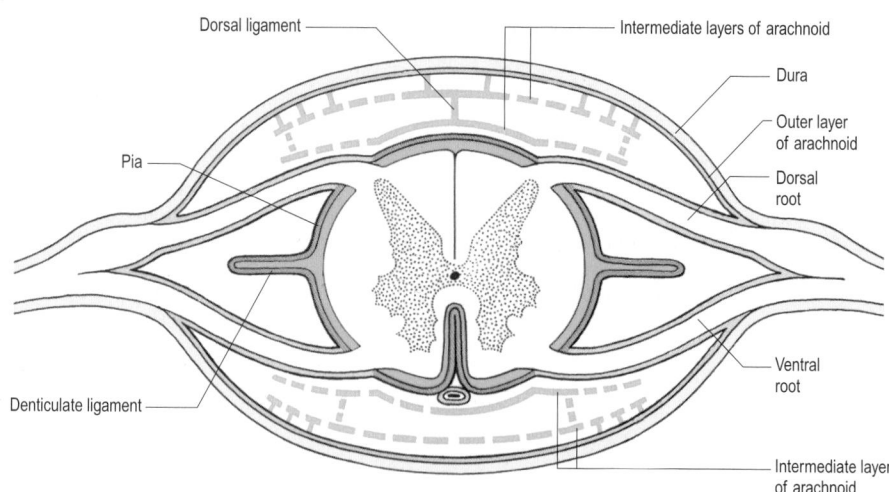

Fig. 46.10 Transverse section through the spinal cord and meninges to show the relationships between the meninges and ligaments with the spinal cord and roots: dura mater (yellow), outer layer of arachnoid mater (pale blue), intermediate layer of arachnoid mater (dark blue), pia mater (pink), subpial connective tissue (green).

of these structures and forms a thin coating of leptomeningeal cells over the surface of both vessels and nerves. Thus a subarachnoid angle is formed as nerves pass through the dura into the intervertebral foramina. At this point, the layers of leptomeninges fuse and become continuous with the perineurium. The epineurium is in continuity with the dura. Such an arrangement seals the subarachnoid space so that particulate matter does not pass directly from the subarachnoid space into nerves. The existence of a pathway of lymphatic drainage from the CSF is controversial.

PIA MATER (Figs 46.9, 46.10)

The spinal pia mater closely invests the surface of the spinal cord and passes into the anterior median fissure. As in the cranial region, there is a subpial 'space', however over the surface of the spinal cord the subpial collagenous layer is thicker than in the cerebral region, and it is continuous with the collagenous core of the ligamentum denticulatum.

The ligamentum denticulatum is a flat, fibrous sheet which lies on each side of the spinal cord between the ventral and dorsal spinal roots. Its medial border is continuous with the subpial connective tissue of the cord and its lateral border forms a series of triangular processes, the apices of which are fixed at intervals to the dura mater. There are usually 21 processes on each side. The first crosses behind the vertebral artery where it is attached to the dura mater, and is separated by the artery from the first cervical ventral root. Its site of attachment to the dura mater is above the rim of the foramen magnum, just behind the hypoglossal nerve: the spinal accessory nerve ascends on its posterior aspect (**Fig. 46.7**). The last of the dentate ligaments lies between the exiting twelfth thoracic and first lumbar spinal nerves and is a narrow, oblique band which descends laterally from the conus medullaris. Changes in the form and position of the dentate ligaments during spinal movements have been demonstrated by cine-radiography.

Beyond the conus medullaris, the pia mater continues as a coating of the filum terminale.

INTERMEDIATE LAYER (Fig 46.10)

In addition to the well-defined coats of arachnoid and pia mater, the cord is also surrounded by an extensive intermediate layer of leptomeninges. This layer is concentrated in the dorsal and ventral regions and forms a highly perforated, almost lace-like structure which is focally compacted to form the dorsal, dorsolateral and ventral ligaments of the spinal cord. Dorsally, the intermediate layer is adherent to the deep aspect of the arachnoid mater and forms a discontinuous series of dorsal ligaments which attach the spinal cord to the arachnoid. The dorsolateral ligaments are more delicate and fenestrated, and they extend from the dorsal roots to the parietal arachnoid. As the intermediate layer spreads laterally over the dorsal surface of the dorsal roots, it becomes increasingly perforated and eventually disappears. A similar arrangement is seen over the ventral aspect of the spinal cord, but the intermediate layer is less substantial.

The intermediate layer is structurally similar to the trabeculae which cross the cranial subarachnoid space, in that a collagenous core is coated by leptomeningeal cells. The intermediate layers of leptomeninges around

the spinal cord may act as a baffle within the subarachnoid space to dampen waves of CSF in the spinal column. Inflammation within the spinal subarachnoid space may result in extensive fibrosis within the intermediate layer and the complications of chronic arachnoiditis.

CEREBROSPINAL FLUID (CSF)

The cerebrospinal fluid is described in detail on page 292. Though there is free communication between the spinal and cerebral subarachnoid spaces, the mode of circulation of the spinal CSF remains uncertain. Spinal arachnoid granulations have been described.

SPINAL NERVES

In those body segments which largely retain a metameric (segmental) structure, e.g. the thoracic region, spinal nerves show a common plan (**Fig. 46.11**). The dorsal, epaxial, ramus passes back lateral to the articular processes and divides into medial and lateral branches which penetrate the deeper muscles of the back: both branches innervate the adjacent muscles and supply a band of skin from the posterior median line to the scapular line (p. 782). The ventral, hypaxial, ramus is connected to a corresponding sympathetic ganglion by white and grey rami communicantes. It innervates the prevertebral muscles and curves round in the body wall to supply the lateral muscles of the trunk. Near

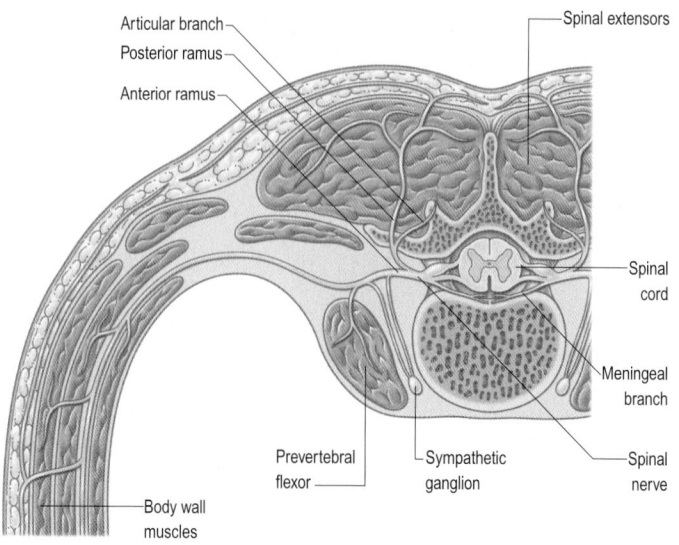

Fig. 46.11 Formation and branching pattern of a typical spinal nerve.

the midaxillary line it gives off a lateral branch which pierces the muscles and divides into anterior and posterior cutaneous branches. The main nerve advances in the body wall, where it supplies the ventral muscles and terminates in branches to the skin.

Spinal nerves are united ventral and dorsal spinal roots, attached in series to the sides of the spinal cord. The term spinal nerve strictly applies only to the short segment after union of the roots and before branching occurs. This segment, the spinal nerve proper, lies in the intervertebral foramen: in clinical practice it is often loosely termed the 'nerve root'. There are 31 pairs of spinal nerves: 8 cervical, 12 thoracic, 5 lumbar, 5 sacral, 1 coccygeal. The abbreviations C, T, L, S and Co, with appropriate numerals, are commonly applied to individual nerves. The nerves emerge through intervertebral foramina. At thoracic, lumbar, sacral and coccygeal levels the numbered nerve exits the vertebral canal by passing below the pedicle of the corresponding vertebra, e.g. L4 nerve exits the intervertebral foramen between L4 and L5. However, in the cervical region, nerves C1–7 pass above their corresponding vertebrae. C1 leaves the vertebral canal between the occipital bone and atlas and hence is often termed the suboccipital nerve. The last pair of cervical nerves does not have a correspondingly numbered vertebra and C8 passes between the seventh cervical and first thoracic vertebrae. Each nerve is continuous with the spinal cord by ventral and dorsal roots; the latter each bears a spinal ganglion ('dorsal root ganglion').

SPINAL ROOTS AND GANGLIA

Ventral (anterior) roots
Ventral roots contain axons of neurones in the anterior and lateral spinal grey columns. Each emerges as a series of rootlets in two or three irregular rows in an area c.3 mm in horizontal width.

Dorsal (posterior) roots
Dorsal roots contain centripetal processes of neurones sited in the spinal ganglia. Each consists of medial and lateral fascicles which both diverge into rootlets which enter along the posterolateral sulcus. The rootlets of adjacent dorsal roots are often connected by oblique filaments, especially in the lower cervical and lumbosacral regions.

Little is known of the detail of the regions of entry and emergence of afferent and efferent rootlets in humans, but these zones of transition between the central and peripheral nervous systems have been extensively described in rodents (Fraher 2000) (see also p. 65).

Appearance and orientation of roots at each spinal level
The size and direction of spinal nerve roots vary. The upper four cervical roots are small, the lower four are large. Cervical dorsal roots have a thickness ratio to the ventral roots of 3:1, which is greater than in other regions. The first dorsal root is an exception, being smaller than the ventral and it is occasionally absent. The conventional view is that the first and second cervical spinal roots are short, running almost horizontally to their exits from the vertebral canal, and that from the third to the eighth cervical levels the roots slope obliquely down. Obliquity and length increase successively, although the distance between spinal attachment and vertebral exit never exceeds the height of one vertebra. An alternative view (Kubik & Müntener 1969) states that upper cervical roots descend, the fifth is horizontal, the sixth to eighth ascend, the first two thoracic roots are horizontal, the next three ascend, the sixth is horizontal and the rest descend. This view is based on the observation that the cervicothoracic part of the spinal cord grows more in length than other parts.

Thoracic roots, except the first, are small, and the dorsal root only slightly exceeds the ventral in thickness. They increase successively in length. In the lower thoracic region, the roots descend in contact with the spinal cord for at least two vertebrae before emerging from the vertebral canal.

Lower lumbar and upper sacral roots are the largest, and their rootlets are the most numerous. Coccygeal roots are the smallest. Kubik & Müntener (1969) confirm that lumbar, sacral and coccygeal roots descend with increasing obliquity to their exits. The spinal cord ends near the lower border of the first lumbar vertebra, and so the lengths of successive roots rapidly increase: the consequent collection of roots is the cauda equina (**Fig. 46.3**). The largest roots, and hence the largest spinal nerves, are continuous with the spinal cervical and lumbar swellings and innervate the upper and lower limbs.

Spinal ganglia (dorsal root ganglia)
Spinal ganglia are large groups of neurones on the dorsal spinal roots. Each is oval and reddish; its size is related to that of its root. A ganglion is bifid medially where the two fascicles of the dorsal root emerge to enter the cord. Ganglia are usually sited in the intervertebral foramina, immediately lateral to the perforation of the dura mater by the roots (**Fig. 46.4**). However, the first and second cervical ganglia lie on the vertebral arches of the atlas and axis, the sacral lies inside the vertebral canal, and the coccygeal ganglion usually lies within the dura mater. The first cervical ganglion may be absent. Small aberrant ganglia sometimes occur on the upper cervical dorsal roots between the spinal ganglia and the cord.

SPINAL NERVES PROPER (Figs 46.11, 46.12)
Immediately distal to the spinal ganglia, ventral and dorsal roots unite to form spinal nerves. These very soon divide into dorsal and ventral rami, both of which receive fibres from both roots. At all levels above the sacral, this division occurs within the intervertebral foramen. Division of the sacral spinal nerves occurs within the sacral vertebral canal, and the dorsal and ventral rami exit separately through posterior and anterior sacral foramina at each level. Spinal nerves trifurcate at some cervical and thoracic levels, and the third branch is called a ramus intermedius. At or distal to its origin each ventral ramus gives off recurrent meningeal (sinuvertebral) branches and receives a grey ramus communicans from the corresponding sympathetic ganglion. The thoracic and first and second lumbar ventral rami each contributes a white ramus communicans to the corresponding sympathetic ganglia. The second, third and fourth sacral nerves also supply visceral branches, unconnected with sympathetic ganglia, which carry a parasympathetic outflow direct to the pelvic plexuses.

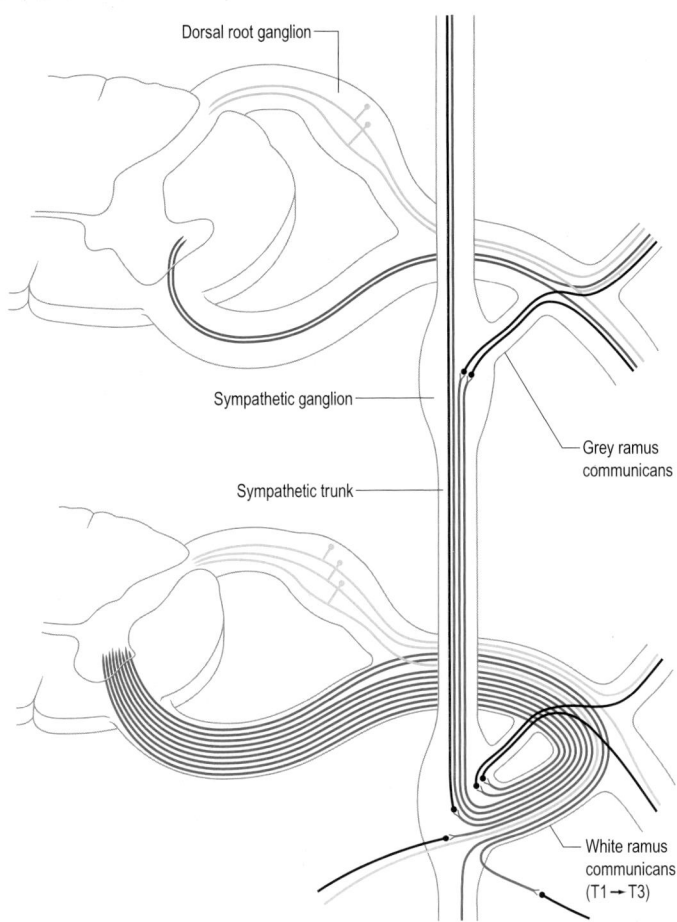

Dorsal root ganglion

Sympathetic ganglion

Sympathetic trunk

Grey ramus communicans

White ramus communicans (T1 → T3)

Fig. 46.12 The constitution of a typical spinal nerve. In the upper part of the diagram the spinal nerve roots show the somatic components, in the lower part the visceral components. Red: somatic efferent and preganglionic sympathetic fibres; blue: somatic and visceral afferent fibres; black: postganglionic sympathetic fibres.

Cervical spinal nerves enlarge from the first to the sixth nerve. The seventh and eighth cervical and the first thoracic nerve are similar in size to the sixth cervical nerve. The remaining thoracic nerves are relatively small. Lumbar nerves are large, increasing in size from the first to the fifth. The first sacral is the largest spinal nerve, thereafter the sacral nerves decrease in size. The coccygeal nerves are the smallest spinal nerves.

Meningeal branches

The recurrent meningeal or sinuvertebral nerves number two to four filaments on each side, and occur at all vertebral levels. Each receives one or more rami from a nearby grey ramus communicans or directly from a thoracic sympathetic ganglion, and most then pursue a recurrent (often perivascular) course into the vertebral canal through the intervertebral foramen ventral to the dorsal root ganglion. Here these mixed sensory and sympathetic nerves divide into transverse, ascending and descending branches which are distributed to the dura mater, the walls of blood vessels, the periosteum, ligaments and intervertebral discs in the anterolateral region of the vertebral canal. Fine meningeal branches occasionally pass dorsal to reach the spinal ganglia to innervate the dorsal dura, periosteum and ligaments, and others pass ventrally to the posterior longitudinal ligament. Ascending branches of the upper three cervical meningeal nerves are large and distributed to the dura mater in the posterior cranial fossa. Meningeal nerves are important in relation to the referred pain which is characteristic of many spinal disorders and in occipital headache.

Coverings and relations of the spinal roots and nerves in the radicular canal (Figs 46.9, 46.10, 46.13)

Tubular prolongations of the spinal dura mater, closely lined by the arachnoid, extend around the spinal roots and nerves as they pass through the lateral zone of the vertebral canal and through the intervertebral foramina. These prolongations, the spinal nerve sheaths ('root sheaths'), gradually lengthen as the spinal roots become increasingly oblique. Each individual dorsal and ventral root runs in the subarachnoid space with its own covering of pia mater. Each root pierces the dura

separately, taking a sleeve of arachnoid with it, before joining within the dural prolongation just distal to the spinal ganglion. The dural sheaths of the spinal nerves fuse with the epineurium, within or slightly beyond the intervertebral foramina. The arachnoid prolongations within the sheaths do not extend as far distally as their dural coverings, but the subarachnoid space and its contained CSF extend sufficiently distally to form a radiologically demonstrable 'root sleeve' for each nerve. Shortening or obstruction of this sleeve seen on the radiculogram indicates compression of the spinal nerve. At the cervical level, where the nerves are short and the vertebral movement is greatest, the dural sheaths are tethered to the periosteum of the adjacent transverse processes. In the lumbosacral region there is less tethering of the dura to the periosteum, though there may be an attachment posteriorly to the facet joint capsule.

In the radicular ('root') canal and intervertebral foramen, the spinal nerve is related to the spinal artery of that level and its radicular branch, and to a small plexus of veins. At the outer end of the foramen the nerve may lie above or below transforaminal ligaments.

The size of the spinal nerve and its associated structures within the intervertebral foramen is not in direct relation to the size of the foramen. At lumbar levels, though L5 is the largest nerve, its foramen is smaller than those of L1–4, which renders this nerve particularly liable to compression.

Functional components of spinal nerves

Each typical spinal nerve contains somatic and visceral (autonomic) fibres.

Somatic components

Somatic components are efferent and afferent. Somatic efferent fibres which innervate skeletal muscles are axons of α, β and γ neurones in the spinal anterior grey column. Somatic afferent fibres convey impulses into the CNS from receptors in the skin, subcutaneous tissue, muscles, tendons, fasciae and joints: they are peripheral processes of unipolar neurones in the spinal ganglia.

Visceral components

Visceral components are also afferent and efferent, and belong to the autonomic nervous system. They include sympathetic or parasympathetic fibres at different spinal levels. Preganglionic visceral efferent sympathetic fibres are axons of neurones in the spinal lateral grey column in the thoracic and upper two or three lumbar segments: they join the sympathetic trunk along corresponding white rami communicantes and synapse with postganglionic neurones distributed to non-striated muscle or glands. The preganglionic visceral efferent parasympathetic fibres are axons of neurones in the spinal lateral grey column of the second to fourth sacral segments: they leave the ventral rami of corresponding sacral nerves and synapse in pelvic ganglia. The postganglionic axons are distributed mainly to muscle or glands in the walls of the pelvic viscera. Visceral afferent fibres have cell bodies in the spinal ganglia. Their peripheral processes pass through white rami communicantes and, without synapsing, through one or more sympathetic ganglia to end in viscera. Some visceral afferent fibres may enter the spinal cord in the ventral roots.

Central processes of ganglionic unipolar neurones enter the spinal cord by posterior roots and synapse on somatic or sympathetic efferent neurones, usually through interneurones, completing reflex paths. Alternatively, they may synapse with other neurones in the spinal or brain stem grey matter which give origin to a variety of ascending tracts.

Variations of spinal roots and nerves

The courses of spinal roots and nerves in relation to the thecal sac and vertebral and radicular canals may be aberrant. An individual intervertebral foramen may contain a duplicated sheath, nerve and roots, which will then be absent at an adjacent level. Abnormal communications between roots may occur within the vertebral canal. These anomalies have been described and classified for the lumbosacral spine by Neidre & Macnab (1983).

Rami of the spinal nerves

Ventral (anterior primary) rami supply the limbs and the anterolateral aspects of the trunk, and in general are larger than the dorsal rami. Thoracic ventral rami run independently and retain a largely segmental distribution. Cervical, lumbar and sacral ventral rami connect near their

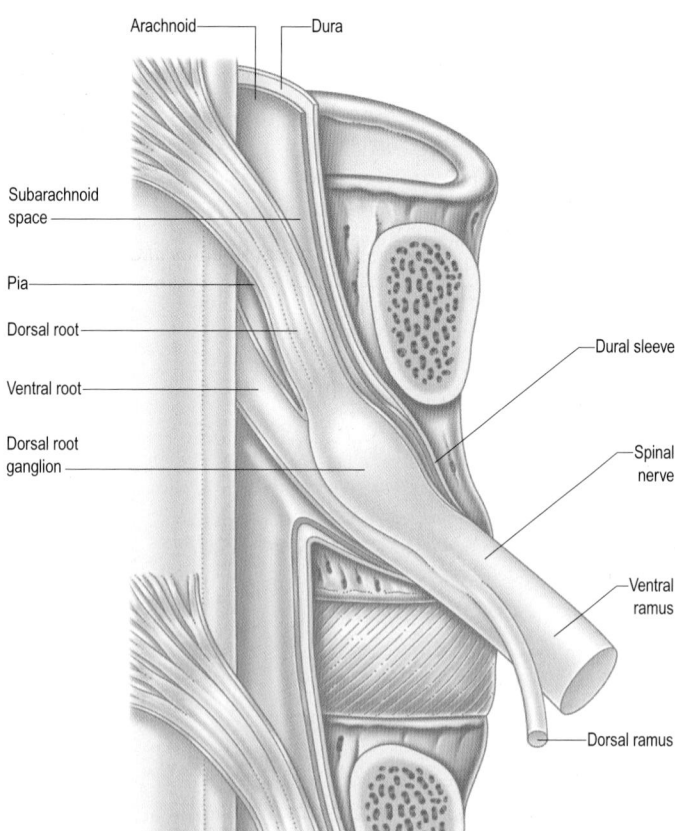

Fig. 46.13 A lumbar spinal nerve and its roots and meningeal coverings.

Arachnoid — Dura

Subarachnoid space

Pia

Dorsal root

Ventral root

Dorsal root ganglion

Dural sleeve

Spinal nerve

Ventral ramus

Dorsal ramus

origins to form plexuses. Dorsal rami do not join these plexuses. The ventral rami are described in the appropriate regional Sections.

Dorsal (posterior primary) rami of spinal nerves are usually smaller than the ventral rami and are directed posteriorly. Retaining a segmental distribution, all, except for the first cervical, fourth and fifth sacral and the coccygeal, divide into medial and lateral branches which supply the muscles and skin of the posterior regions of the neck and trunk (**Fig. 46.14**).

Cervical dorsal spinal rami
Each cervical spinal dorsal ramus, except the first, divides into medial and lateral branches which all innervate muscles. In general only medial branches of the second to fourth, and usually the fifth, supply the skin. Except for the first and second, each dorsal ramus passes back medial to a posterior intertransverse muscle, curving round the articular process into the interval between semispinalis capitis and semispinalis cervicis.

First cervical dorsal ramus (suboccipital nerve) (Fig. 54.58) – The first cervical dorsal ramus, the suboccipital nerve, is larger than the ventral. It emerges superior to the posterior arch of the atlas and inferior to the vertebral artery and enters the suboccipital triangle to supply rectus capitis posterior major and minor, obliquus capitis superior and inferior,

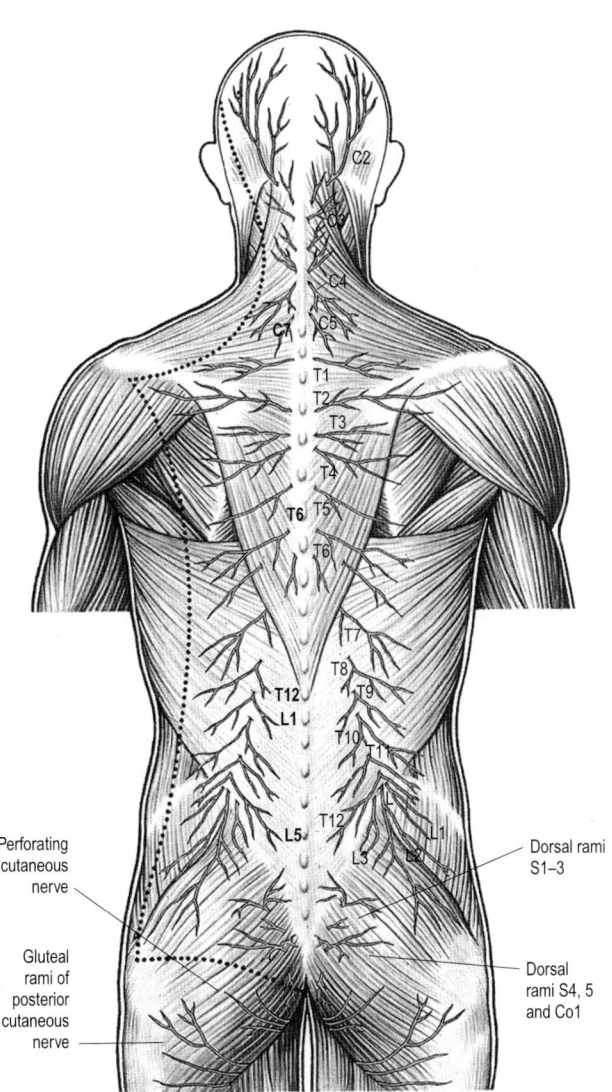

Fig. 46.14 Cutaneous distribution of the dorsal rami of the spinal nerves. The nerves are shown lying on the superficial muscles; on the left side the limit of the skin area supplied by these nerves is indicated by the dotted line. The nerves are numbered on the right side; the spines of the seventh cervical, sixth and twelfth thoracic, and first and fifth lumbar vertebrae are labelled in bold on the left side.

and semispinalis capitis. A filament from the branch to the inferior oblique joins the second dorsal ramus. The suboccipital nerve occasionally has a cutaneous branch which accompanies the occipital artery to the scalp, and connects with the greater and lesser occipital nerves. It may also communicate with the accessory nerve.

Second cervical dorsal ramus (Figs 54.58, 29.9B) – The second cervical dorsal ramus is slightly larger than the ventral and all the other cervical dorsal rami. It emerges between the posterior arch of the atlas and the lamina of the axis, below inferior oblique, which it supplies. It receives a connection from the first cervical dorsal ramus and divides into a large medial and smaller lateral branch. The medial branch, termed the greater occipital nerve, ascends between inferior oblique and semispinalis capitis, pierces the latter and trapezius near their occipital attachments, and is joined by a filament from the medial branch of the third dorsal ramus. It ascends with the occipital artery, divides into branches which connect with the lesser occipital nerve, and supplies the skin of the scalp as far forward as the vertex. It supplies semispinalis capitis and, occasionally, the back of the auricle. The lateral branch supplies splenius capitis, longissimus capitis and semispinalis capitis, and is often joined by the corresponding third cervical branch.

Greater occipital neuralgia – Greater occipital neuralgia is a syndrome of pain and paraesthesiae felt in the distribution of the greater occipital nerve. It is usually due to an entrapment neuropathy of the nerve as it pierces the attachment of the neck extensors to the occiput. A similar syndrome may be caused by upper facet joint arthritis involving the second cervical root.

Third cervical dorsal ramus – The third cervical dorsal ramus is intermediate in size between the second and fourth. It courses back round the articular pillar of the third cervical vertebra, medial to the posterior intertransverse muscle, and divides into medial and lateral branches. Its medial branch runs between spinalis capitis and semispinalis cervicis, and pierces the splenius and trapezius to end in the skin. Deep to trapezius it gives rise to a branch, the third occipital nerve, which pierces trapezius to end in the skin of the lower occipital region, medial to the greater occipital nerve and connected to it. The lateral branch often joins a branch of the second cervical dorsal ramus. The dorsal ramus of the suboccipital nerve and medial branches of the dorsal rami of the second and third cervical nerves are sometimes joined by loops to form the posterior cervical plexus.

Dorsal rami of the lower five cervical nerves – The dorsal rami of the lower five cervical nerves curve back round the vertebral articular pillars and divide into medial and lateral branches. Medial branches of the fourth and fifth run between semispinalis cervicis and semispinalis capitis, reach the vertebral spines and pierce splenius and trapezius to end in the skin. The fifth medial branch may not reach the skin. The medial branches of the lowest three cervical nerves are small and end in semispinalis cervicis, semispinalis capitis, multifidus and interspinales. The lateral branches supply iliocostalis cervicis, longissimus cervicis and longissimus capitis.

Thoracic dorsal spinal rami
Thoracic dorsal rami pass backwards close to the vertebral facet joints to divide into medial and lateral branches. Each medial branch emerges between a joint and the medial edges of the superior costotransverse ligament and intertransverse muscle. Each lateral branch runs in the interval between the ligament and the muscle before inclining posteriorly on the medial side of levator costae.

Medial branches of the upper six thoracic dorsal rami pass between and supply the semispinalis thoracis and multifidus, then pierce the rhomboids and trapezius, and reach the skin near the vertebral spines.

Medial branches of the lower six thoracic dorsal rami mainly supply multifidus and longissimus thoracis and occasionally the skin in the median region. Lateral branches increase inferiorly in size, and run through, or deep to, longissimus thoracis to the interval between it and iliocostalis cervicis, supplying these muscles and the levatores costarum. The lower five or six also have cutaneous branches, and pierce serratus posterior inferior and latissimus dorsi in line with the costal angles. Some upper thoracic lateral branches supply the skin. The twelfth thoracic lateral branch sends a filament medially along the iliac crest, then passes down to the anterior gluteal skin. Medial cutaneous branches of the thoracic dorsal rami descend close to the vertebral spines before reaching the skin; lateral branches descend across as many as four ribs before becoming superficial. The branch of the twelfth thoracic reaches the skin a little above the iliac crest.

Lumbar dorsal spinal rami

Lumbar dorsal rami pass back medial to the medial intertransverse muscles, and divide into medial and lateral branches.

Medial branches run near the vertebral articular processes to end in the multifidus. They are related to the bone between the accessory and mammillary processes and may groove it, crossing a distinct notch or even a foramen. Lateral branches supply the erector spinae. In addition, the upper three rami give rise to cutaneous nerves which pierce the aponeurosis of latissimus dorsi at the lateral border of the erector spinae and cross the iliac crest posteriorly to reach the gluteal skin, some reaching as far as the level of the greater trochanter.

Sacral dorsal spinal rami

Sacral dorsal rami are small, diminishing downwards, and other than the fifth, all emerge though the dorsal sacral foramina. The upper three are covered at their exit by multifidus, and divide into medial and lateral branches. Medial branches are small and end in multifidus. Lateral branches join together and with lateral branches of the last lumbar and fourth sacral dorsal rami to form loops dorsal to the sacrum. Branches from these loops run dorsal to the sacrotuberous ligament and form a second series of loops under gluteus maximus. From these, two or three gluteal branches pierce gluteus maximus (along a line from the posterior superior iliac spine to the coccygeal apex) to supply the posterior gluteal skin.

The dorsal rami of the fourth and fifth sacral nerves are small and lie below multifidus. They unite with each other and with the coccygeal dorsal ramus to form loops dorsal to the sacrum: filaments from these supply the skin over the coccyx.

Coccygeal dorsal spinal ramus

The coccygeal dorsal spinal ramus does not divide into medial and lateral branches. Its connections and distribution are noted above.

VASCULAR SUPPLY OF SPINAL CORD, ROOTS AND NERVES

Arteries (Fig. 46.15) (See Crock 1996.)

The spinal cord, its roots and nerves are supplied with blood by both longitudinal and segmental vessels. Three major longitudinal vessels, a single anterior and two posterior spinal arteries (each of which is sometimes doubled to pass on either side of the dorsal rootlets), originate intracranially from the vertebral artery and terminate in a plexus around the conus medullaris. The anterior spinal artery forms from the fused anterior spinal branches of the vertebral artery, and descends in the anterior median fissure of the cord. Each posterior spinal artery originates either directly from the ipsilateral vertebral artery or from its posterior inferior cerebellar branch, and descends in a posterolateral sulcus of the cord. The segmental arteries are derived in craniocaudal sequence from spinal branches of the vertebral, deep cervical, intercostal and lumbar arteries. These vessels enter the vertebral canal through the intervertebral foramina and anastomose with branches of the longitudinal vessels to form a pial plexus on the surface of the cord. The segmental spinal arteries send anterior and posterior radicular branches to the spinal cord along the ventral and dorsal roots. Most anterior radicular arteries are small, and end in the ventral nerve roots or in the pial plexus of the cord. The small posterior radicular arteries also supply the dorsal root ganglia: branches enter at both ganglionic poles to be distributed around ganglion cells and nerve fibres.

Segmental medullary feeder arteries

Some radicular arteries, mainly situated in the lower cervical, lower thoracic and upper lumbar regions, are large enough to reach the anterior median sulcus where they divide into slender ascending and large descending branches. These are the anterior medullary feeder arteries (Dommisse 1975). They anastomose with the anterior spinal arteries to form a single or partly double longitudinal vessel of uneven calibre along the anterior median sulcus. The largest anterior medullary feeder, the great anterior segmental medullary artery of Adamkiewicz, varies in level, arising from a spinal branch of either one of the lower posterior

intercostal arteries (T9–11), or of the subcostal artery (T12), or less frequently of the upper lumbar arteries (L1 and L2). It most often arises on the left side (Carmichael & Gloviczki 1999). Reaching the spinal cord, it sends a branch to the anterior spinal artery below and another to anastomose with the ramus of the posterior spinal artery which lies anterior to the dorsal roots. It may be the main supply to the lower two-thirds of the cord. Central branches of the anterior spinal artery enter the anterior median fissure, and then turn right or left to supply the ventral grey column, the base of the dorsal grey column, including the dorsal nucleus, and the adjacent white matter (**Fig. 46.16**).

Each posterior spinal artery contributes to a pair of longitudinal anastomotic channels, anterior and posterior to the dorsal spinal roots. These are reinforced by posterior medullary feeders from the posterior radicular arteries. The latter are variable in number and size, but smaller, more numerous and more evenly distributed than the anterior medullary feeders. The anterior channel is joined by a ramus from the descending branch of the great anterior segmental medullary artery of Adamkiewicz. In all longitudinal spinal arteries the width of the lumen is uneven, and complete interruptions may occur. At the conus medullaris they communicate by anastomotic loops. Anastomoses other than those between the pial or peripheral spinal arterial branches may be important, e.g. a posterior spinal series of anastomoses between rami of the dorsal divisions of segmental arteries near the spinous processes.

Intramedullary arteries

The central branches of the anterior spinal artery supply about two-thirds of the cross-sectional area of the cord. The rest of the dorsal grey and white columns and peripheral parts of the lateral and ventral white columns are supplied by numerous small radial vessels which branch from posterior spinal arteries and the pial plexus. In a micro-angiographic study of the human cervical spinal cord, up to six anterior, and eight posterior, radicular spinal arteries were described, and up to eight central branches arose from each centimetre of the anterior spinal artery (Turnbull et al 1966).

Spinal cord ischaemia

The spinal cord can rely neither for its transverse nor for its longitudinal blood supply entirely on the longitudinal arteries. The anterior longitudinal artery and the intramedullary arteries are functional end-arteries, although overlap of territories of supply has been described. Damage to the anterior longitudinal artery can result in loss of function of the anterior two-thirds of the cord. The longitudinal arteries cannot supply the whole length of the cord, and the input of the segmental medullary feeder vessels is essential. This is especially true of the artery of Adamkiewicz (great anterior segmental medullary artery), which may effectively carry the major supply for the lower cord. The midthoracic cord, distant from the main anterior medullary feeders, is particularly liable to become ischaemic after periods of hypotension.

Veins (Fig. 46.17)

The venous drainage of the spinal cord follows a similar pattern to that of its arterial supply (Gillilan 1970). Intramedullary veins within the substance of the cord drain into a plexus of surface veins, the coronal plexus. There are six tortuous longitudinal channels within this plexus, one in each of the anterior and posterior median fissures, and four others which run on either side of the ventral and dorsal nerve roots. Only the anterior median vein, which drains the central grey matter, is consistently complete. These vessels connect freely. They drain superiorly into the cerebellar veins and cranial sinuses, and segmentally mainly into medullary veins. These segmental veins drain into the intervertebral veins and thence into the external vertebral venous plexuses, the caval and azygos systems.

Segmental veins

Anterior and posterior medullary veins run along some of the ventral and dorsal roots. They are larger than radicular veins, and drain the cord but not the roots themselves. Like the medullary feeder arteries, they are largest in the cervical and lumbar regions of the cord, but do not necessarily occur in the same segments as the medullary feeders. Anterior and posterior great medullary veins may arise in the lower thoracic or upper lumbar cord segments. There are 8–14 anterior medullary veins. Posterior medullary veins are more numerous.

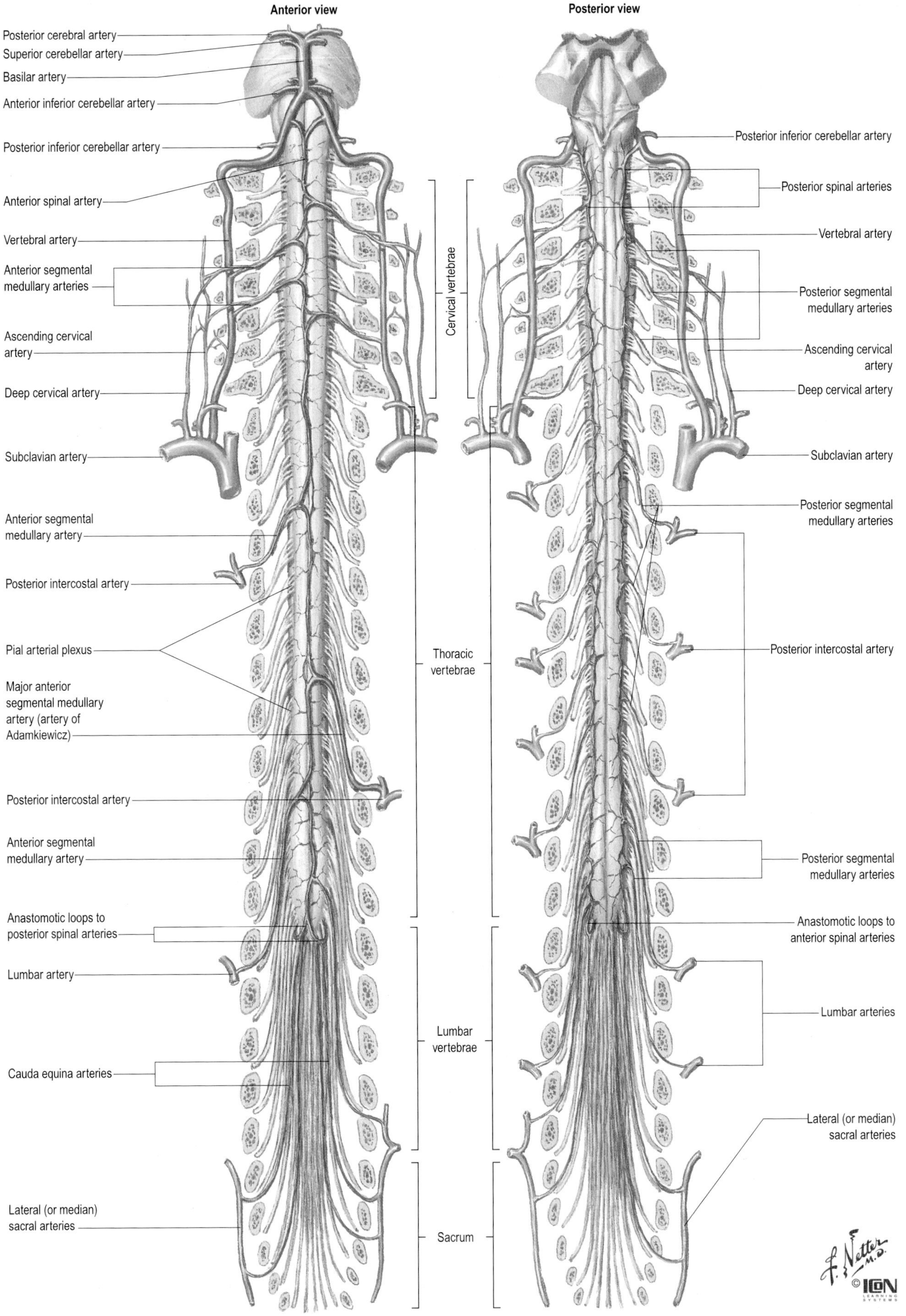

Anterior view

Posterior view

Posterior cerebral artery

Superior cerebellar artery

Basilar artery

Anterior inferior cerebellar artery

Posterior inferior cerebellar artery

Anterior spinal artery

Vertebral artery

Anterior segmental
medullary arteries

Ascending cervical
artery

Deep cervical artery

Subclavian artery

Anterior segmental
medullary artery

Posterior intercostal artery

Pial arterial plexus

Major anterior
segmental medullary
artery (artery of
Adamkiewicz)

Posterior intercostal artery

Anterior segmental
medullary artery

Anastomotic loops to
posterior spinal arteries

Lumbar artery

Cauda equina arteries

Lateral (or median)
sacral arteries

Cervical vertebrae

Thoracic
vertebrae

Lumbar
vertebrae

Sacrum

Posterior inferior cerebellar artery

Posterior spinal arteries

Vertebral artery

Posterior segmental
medullary arteries

Ascending cervical
artery

Deep cervical artery

Subclavian artery

Posterior segmental
medullary arteries

Posterior intercostal artery

Posterior segmental
medullary arteries

Anastomotic loops to
anterior spinal arteries

Lumbar arteries

Lateral (or median)
sacral arteries

Fig. 46.15 Arteries of the spinal cord. (Netter Illustrations used with permission from Icon Learning Systems, a division of MediMedia USA, Inc. All rights reserved.)

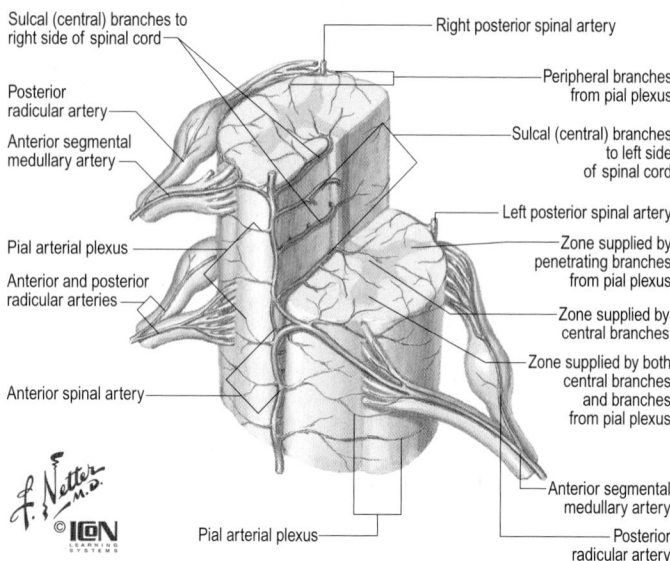

Fig. 46.16 Arterial disposition within the spinal cord. (Netter Illustrations used with permission from Icon Learning Systems, a division of MediMedia USA, Inc. All rights reserved.)

Very small anterior and posterior radicular veins occur in most spinal segments, accompanying and draining the ventral and dorsal roots and some of the cord at the points of entry and exit of the rootlets. They usually drain into the intervertebral veins.

SPINAL CORD INJURY AND VERTEBRAL COLUMN INJURY

In the assessment of a patient with spinal injury and neurological damage, it is important to remember that the level of cord and root injury will not coincide with that of the skeletal damage to the vertebral column.

In estimating the vertebral levels of cord segments in the adult, a useful approximation is that in the cervical region the tip of a vertebral spinous process corresponds to the succeeding cord segment (i.e. the sixth cervical spine is opposite the seventh spinal segment); at upper

thoracic levels the tip of a vertebral spine corresponds to the cord two segments lower (i.e. the fourth spine is level with the sixth segment), and in the lower thoracic region there is a difference of three segments (i.e. the tenth thoracic spine is level with the first lumbar segment). The eleventh thoracic spine overlies the third lumbar segment and the twelfth is opposite the first sacral segment. In making this estimate by palpation of the vertebral spines, the relationship of the individual spines to their vertebral bodies should be remembered (p. 727).

Complete division above the fourth cervical segment causes respiratory failure because of the loss of activity in the phrenic and intercostal nerves. Lesions between C5 and T1 paralyse all four limbs (quadriplegia), the effects in the upper limbs varying with the site of injury: at the fifth cervical segment paralysis is complete; at the sixth, each arm is positioned in abduction and lateral rotation, with the elbow flexed and the forearm supinated, due to unopposed activity in the deltoid, supraspinatus, rhomboid and brachial flexors (all supplied by the fifth cervical spinal nerves). In lower cervical lesions upper limb paralysis is less marked. Lesions of the first thoracic segment paralyse small muscles in the hand and damage the sympathetic outflow, resulting in contraction of the pupil, recession of the eyeball, narrowing of the palpebral fissure and loss of sweating in the face and neck (Horner's syndrome). However, sensation is retained in areas innervated by segments above the lesion, thus cutaneous sensation is retained in the neck and chest down to the second intercostal space, because this area is innervated by the supraclavicular nerves (C3 and C4). At thoracic levels, division of the cord paralyses the trunk, below the segmental level of the lesion, and both lower limbs (paraplegia). The first sacral neural segment is approximately level with the thoracolumbar vertebral junction: injury, which commonly occurs here, paralyses the urinary bladder, the rectum and muscles supplied by the sacral segments, and cutaneous sensibility is lost in the perineum, buttocks, the back of the thighs and the legs and soles of the feet. The roots of lumbar nerves descending to join the cauda equina may be damaged at this level, causing complete paralysis of both lower limbs. Lesions below the first lumbar vertebra may divide or damage the cauda equina, but severe nerve damage is uncommon and is usually confined to the spinal roots at the level of the trauma. Neurological symptoms may also occur as a result of interference with the spinal blood supply, particularly in the lower thoracic and upper lumbar segments.

SPINAL CORD INJURY WITHOUT RADIOLOGICAL ABNORMALITY: 'SCIWORA'

The spinal cord may be damaged without radiological evidence of skeletal injury in some injuries to the vertebral column. This is particularly liable to occur if the vertebral canal is abnormally narrowed, usually by osteoarthritic changes. In the elderly patient there may in

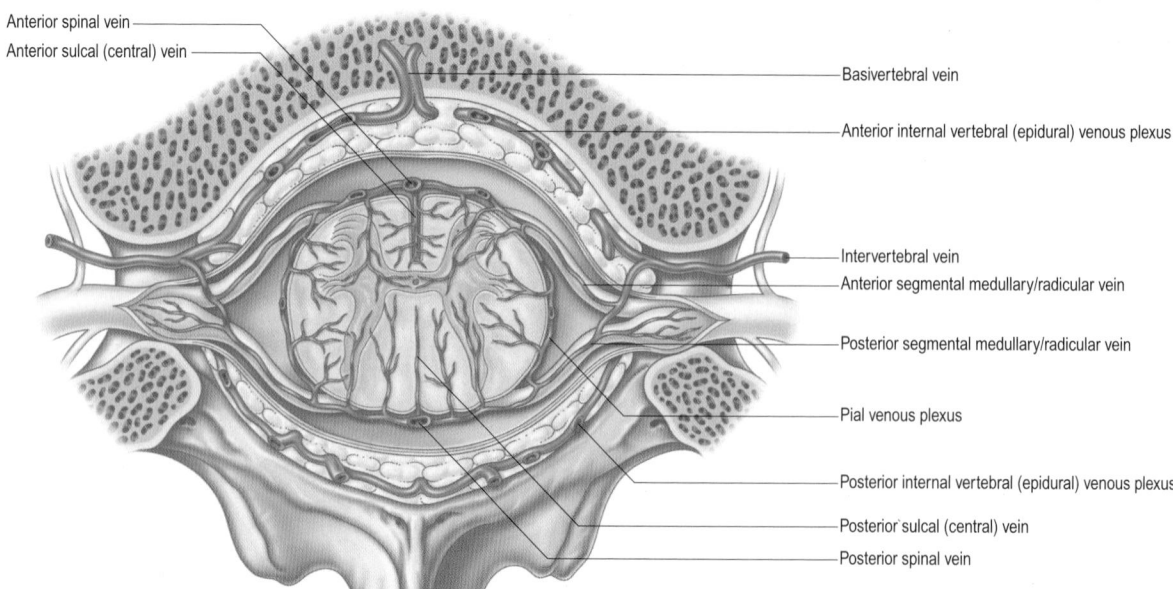

Fig. 46.17 Venous disposition within the spinal cord.

addition be occlusive arterial disease, directly compromising an already precarious blood supply to the cord (p. 784). This type of injury not uncommonly occurs in hyperextension injuries of the cervical spine in this age group. The cause of the damage may be direct injury to neural tissue by osteophytes or by an infolded ligamentum flavum, or direct or indirect injury to the vasculature of the cord. For cervical spinal injury, several cord syndromes have been described, relating the clinical picture to the anatomy of the neurological lesion within the cord. The commonest of these is central cord syndrome, which usually results from hyperextension injury to an osteoarthritic neck, in which the major injury is to the central grey matter. This gives a greater motor loss in the upper than in the lower limbs, with variable sensory loss. In anterior cord syndrome, which may occur in flexion–compression injuries of the neck, the damage occurs in the area of supply of the anterior spinal artery, sparing the posterior columns. Here the motor loss is usually proportionately greater in the lower than in the upper limbs, while sensory loss is less of a problem.

LESIONS OF THE SPINAL ROOTS, NERVES AND GANGLIA

The spinal roots, nerves and ganglia may be damaged in the vertebral and 'root' canals and at the intervertebral foramina (p. 741). Neurofibromas may occur on the roots and nerves in the 'root' canals, and as they enlarge become dumb-bell in shape with both an intra- and an extraspinal component in continuity. The clinical picture may thus include paradoxical features as this asymmetrical space-occupying lesion grows.

Root compression usually presents acutely with pain which may be severe. The pain, paraesthesiae and numbness occur in a dermatomal distribution. It may be difficult to demonstrate sensory loss on the trunk, because of the overlap of the dermatomes. Severe traction injuries of the upper limbs may cause avulsion of spinal roots from the cord in the cervical region.

THE ANATOMY OF PAIN OF SPINAL ORIGIN (See also p. 316.)

In the diagnosis and description of pain of spinal origin it is particularly important to distinguish anatomically between radicular ('nerve root') pain, referred pain and radiating pain. The second and third terms are often used imprecisely and their meanings are confused.

Radicular pain occurs in spinal nerve (dermatomal) distribution, is well localized and results from involvement of the spinal nerve in the pathological process, e.g. when it is compressed by a disc prolapse.

Referred pain is not strictly 'of spinal origin'. The source of the pain is usually a visceral structure whose afferent innervation shares an interneuronal pool in the posterior horn of the spinal cord with the somatic structure in which the pain is felt. The pain may be felt in a dermatome; however, the pain-producing lesion is not in the spinal nerve.

Radiating pain does not adopt any particular anatomical distribution. It is often vaguely localized and is described by the patient using the whole of the hand to indicate the affected area. The extent of its area of distribution often relates directly to the severity of the pain. Spinal pain of this type commonly radiates around the hip and down into the thigh.

LESIONS OF THE CONUS AND CAUDA EQUINA

Lesions of the conus and cauda equina, e.g. tumours, cause bilateral deficit, often with pain in the back extending into the sacral segments and to the legs. Loss of bladder and erectile function can be early features. There are lower motor neurone signs in the legs with fasciculation and muscle atrophy. Sensory loss usually involves the perineal or 'saddle area' as well as involving other lumbar and sacral dermatomes. There may be congenital abnormalities, e.g. spina bifida, lipomata or dystematomyelia, and the conus may extend below the lower border of L1, often with a tethered filum terminale. Extramedullary lesions include prolapsed intervertebral discs. A midline (central) disc protrusion in the lumbar region may present with involvement of only the sacral segments.

REFERENCES

Barson AJ, Sands J 1977 Regional and segmental characteristics of the human adult spinal cord. J Anat 123: 797–803.

Bogduk N 1997 Clinical Anatomy of the Lumbar Spine and Sacrum, 3rd edn. Edinburgh: Churchill Livingstone.

Carmichael SW, Gloviczki P 1999 Anatomy of the blood supply to the spinal cord: the artery of Adamkiewicz revisited. Perspect Vasc Surg 12: 113–22.

Crock HV 1996 An Atlas of Vascular Anatomy of the Skeleton and Spinal Cord. London: Martin Dunitz.

Dean NA, Mitchell BS 2002 Anatomic relation between the nuchal ligament (ligamentum nuchae) and the spinal dura mater in the craniocervical region. Clin Anat 15: 182–5.

Dommisse GF 1975 The Arteries and Veins of the Human Spinal Cord From Birth. Edinburgh: Churchill Livingstone.

Fraher JP 2000 The transitional zone and CNS regeneration. J Anat 196: 137–58.

Gillilan LA 1970 Veins of the spinal cord. Anatomic details; suggested clinical applications. Neurology 20: 860–8.

Haines DE, Harkey HL, Al-Mefty O 1993 The 'subdural' space: a new look at an outdated concept. Neurosurgery 32: 111–20.
Proposes the view that the subdural 'space' is a pathological cleavage plane rather than a normal anatomical element

Kubik S, Müntener M 1969 Zur Topographie der spinalen Nervenwurzeln. II Der Einfuss des Wachstums des Duralsackes, sowie der Krümmagen und der Bewegungen der spinalen Nervenwurzeln. Acta Anat 74: 149–68.
An alternative view of the obliquity of the cervicothoracic spinal nerve roots based on observations of differential cord growth

Neidre A, Macnab I 1983 Anomalies of the lumbosacral nerve roots. Spine 8: 294–9.

Newell RLM 1999 The spinal epidural space. Clin Anat 12: 375–9.

Turnbull IM, Brieg A, Hassler O 1966 Blood supply of cervical spinal cord in man. A microangiographic cadaver study. J Neurosurg 24: 951–65.

Development of the vertebral column

Vertebrae and their alternating intervertebral discs are one of the main manifestations of body segmentation or metamerism. A chain of segments arranged in sequence allows the overall structure to bend when it is moved by the associated muscles. The original body segments, the somites, provide the embryonic cell populations for bone and muscle. The vertebrae form between the early body segments by the recombination of portions of the somites on the craniocaudal axis, and the muscles attach to adjacent vertebrae. The axial skeleton, the vertebral column and associated muscles, are formed by the paraxial mesenchyme which is found lateral to the neural tube and notochord in the early embryo. Each vertebra develops from bilateral origins to form a midline centrum, two lateral arches, bearing transverse processes, which develop lateral and dorsal to the spinal cord, and a midline fused dorsal portion with a spinous process. Individual vertebrae may be distinguished by modifications of these component parts. The intervertebral discs develop from the same origins as the centra, and are composed of outer dense fibrous tissue surrounding a softer central zone.

SEGMENTATION OF PARAXIAL MESENCHYME

Epiblast cells which ingress through the lateral aspect of the primitive node and the rostral primitive streak (Chapter 10) become committed to a somitic lineage (**Fig. 10.15**). After passing through the streak the cells retain contact with both the epiblast and hypoblast basal laminae as they migrate and for some time after reaching their destination. The cells form populations of paraxial mesenchyme on each side of the notochord, termed presomitic or unsegmented mesenchyme. Somites will form from cultured presomitic mesenchyme with or without the presence of neural tube tissue or primitive node tissue. As well as specifying somitic lineage, the position of ingression of the epiblast informs the specific destination of the cells. Thus those cells which ingress through the lateral portion of Hensen's node form the medial halves of the somites, whereas those ingressing through the primitive streak c.200 μm caudal to the node produce the lateral halves of the somites. The two somite halves do not appear to intermingle.

The segmentation of the paraxial presomitic mesenchyme occurs as a sequential process along the craniocaudal axis. In amniote embryos a pair of somites is formed every 90 minutes until the full number is obtained. The molecular pathway for this synchronous segmentation has been termed the segmentation clock. It has been identified as a conserved process in vertebrates from fish to mammals, and is based on the rhythmic production of mRNAs for the transcription of genes related to Notch, a large transmembrane receptor, and a number of trans-membrane ligands.

Intrinsically coordinated pulses of mRNA expression appear as a wave within the presomitic mesenchyme as each somite forms. As new cells enter the paraxial mesenchyme caudally they begin phases of up-regulation of the cycling genes followed by downregulation of these genes. During each cycle the most cranial presomitic mesenchyme will segment to form the next somite.

Experimental evidence (from chick embryos) shows that newly formed paraxial mesenchyme cells undergo 12 such cycles before they finally form a somite (Pourquie & Kusumi 2001). Thus from ingression through the primitive streak to segmentation into a somite takes c.18 hours. As the somite number varies between vertebrate species it is likely that the rate of somite formation also varies. Indeed those vertebrates with elongated bodies and many somites appear to form somites more rapidly than those with shorter bodies, a finding which supports the concept that somite number is controlled in part by species-specific cyclical properties of the presomitic mesenchyme (Richardson et al 1998).

The final determination of somitic boundary formation has not yet been fully elucidated, but seems to require a periodic repression of the Notch pathway genes. The caudal presomitic mesenchyme cells are thought to be maintained in an immature state by their production of FGF8. The cells become competent for segmentation when FGF8 levels drop below a certain threshold. They would then be in close apposition to cells that have segmented (i.e. the next cranial somite).

This area of research is moving rapidly. A detailed critique of the conceptual models of segmentation is given by Stern & Vasiliauskas (2000). An overview of the processes involved in the development of the paraxial mesenchyme, based on the work of Christ et al (2000), is shown in **Fig. 47.1**.

SOMITOGENESIS

Following segmentation, and once the somite boundaries have been defined, the cells within the somite undergo somitogenesis, a process in which five main stages can be identified (**Figs 47.2, 47.3**). These are compaction, formation of the spherical epithelial somite surrounding free somitocoele cells, epithelial/mesenchymal transition of the ventral and ventromedial walls of the somite to form the sclerotome, bilateral migration of the ventromedial mesenchyme populations towards the notochord to form the perinotochordal sheath and of similar cells around the neural tube as the sclerotome, and formation of the epithelial plate of the somite, also termed the dermomyotome, from the remaining somitic epithelium.

After the onset of neurulation the paraxial mesenchyme caudal to the otic vesicle undergoes segmentation in a craniocaudal progression and forms discrete clusters of mesenchyme cells: this stage is termed compaction and denotes the start of somitogenesis.

The Golgi apparatus, and actin and α-actinin are all located in the apical region of the epithelial somite cells; cilia develop on the free surface. The cells are joined by tight junctions (a variety of cell adhesion molecules has been demonstrated in epithelial somites). The basal surface rests on a basal lamina which contains collagen, laminin, fibronectin and cytotactin. Processes from the somite cells pass through this basal lamina to contact the basal laminae of the neural tube and notochord. Dorsoventral patterning of the putative vertebral column is dependent on the interaction of SHH from the notochord/floor plate with BMP4 from the roof plate and overlying ectoderm.

The epithelial somite undergoes rapid development. The cells of the ventromedial wall undergo an epithelial/mesenchyme transformation and break apart. The newly formed mesenchymal cells, which are collectively termed the sclerotome, proliferate and migrate medially towards the notochord. Initially they provide an axial cell population (now termed the perinotochordal sheath); they subsequently provide lateral sclerotomal populations which will give rise to the bones, joints and ligaments of the vertebral column. The remaining cells of the somite are now termed the epithelial plate of the somite (or dermomyotome). This epithelium is proliferative. It produces the cell lines which will give rise to (nearly) all the striated muscles of the body (see also p. 723). Three separate myogenic lines can be identified. First, cells produced along the craniomedial edge of the epithelial plate elongate from the cranial to the caudal edge on the underside of the basal lamina of the plate. They are collectively termed the myotome and will give rise to the skeletal muscle dorsal to the vertebrae, the epaxial musculature (p. 797). (The term 'myotome' was used previously to describe all the muscle

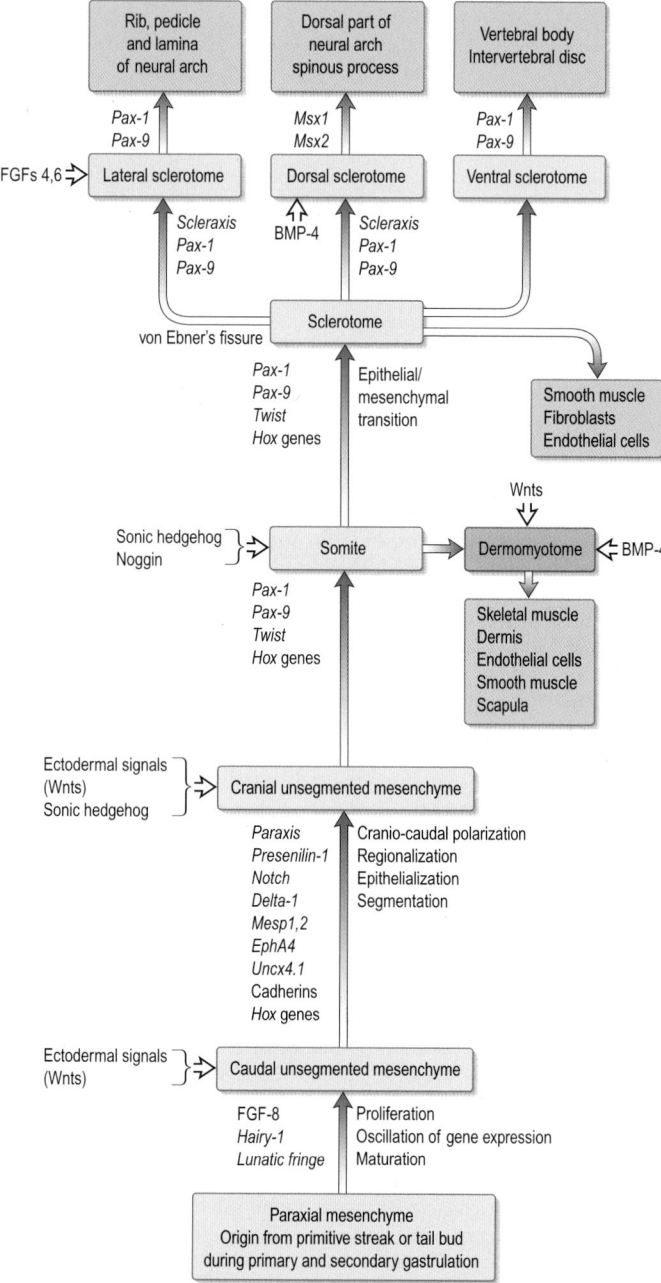

Fig. 47.1 Processes in the development of the paraxial mesenchyme in the avian embryo. Signals are indicated by open arrows; genes are printed in italics. (Redrawn with permission from Christ B, Huang R, Wilting J. The development of the avian vertebral column. Anat Embryol 202: 179–194, 2000, Springer.)

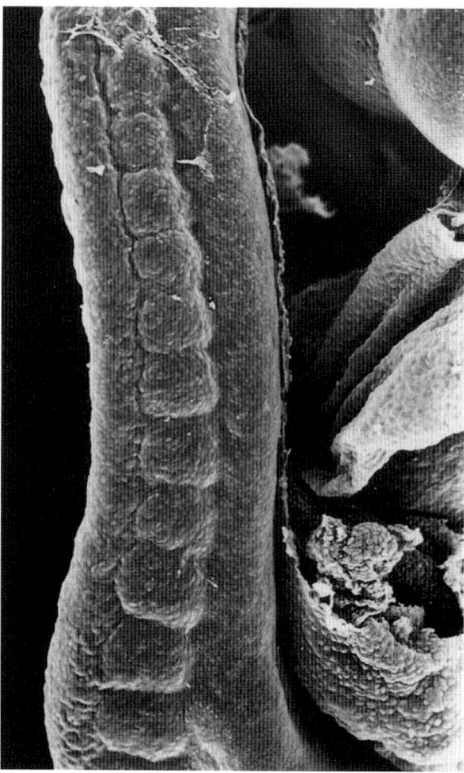

Fig. 47.2 Scanning electron micrograph of a lateral view of an embryo showing the somites. The cranial somites are at the lower border and the more caudal somites are at the upper border. A change in size of the cranially more advanced somites is apparent. (Photograph by P Collins; printed by S Cox, Electron Microscopy Unit, Southampton General Hospital.)

distribution than the segmental portion of skin usually implied by the term dermatome. The concept that an embryological dermatome, derived from the somite, produces all of the dermis of the skin is therefore outdated.

The regularity of somite formation provides criteria for staging embryos. The staging scheme proposed by Ordahl (1993) will be used in the following account of relative somite development. Ordahl noted that morphogenetic events occur in successive somites at approximately the same rate. The somite most recently formed from the unsegmented mesenchyme is designated as stage I, the next most recent as stage II, etc. After the embryo forms an additional somite, the ages of the previously formed somites increase by one Roman numeral. According to this scheme, compaction occurs at stage I; epithelialization at stages II to III; formation of mesenchymal sclerotome cells from stage V; myotome formation at stage VI; early migration of the ventrolateral lip of the epithelial plate, and production of myotome cells are still occurring at stage X.

DEVELOPMENT OF SCLEROTOMES

Sclerotomal populations form from the ventromedial border of the epithelial somite. An intrasegmental boundary (fissure or cleft, sometimes termed von Ebner's fissure) appears within the sclerotome, dividing it into loosely packed cranial and densely packed caudal halves; this boundary is initially filled with extracellular matrix and a few cells. The epithelial plate, and later the dermomyotome, spans the two half-sclerotomes. The bilateral sclerotomal cell populations migrate towards the notochord and surround it to form the perinotochordal sheath. They undergo a matrix-mediated interaction with the notochord, differentiating chondrogenetically to form the cartilaginous precursor of the vertebral centrum. The perinotochordal sheath transiently expresses type II collagen, and this is believed to initiate type II collagen expression, and thereafter a chondrogenic fate, in those mesenchyme cells which contact it. Each vertebra is formed by the combination of much of the caudal half of one bilateral pair of sclerotomes with much of the cranial half of the next caudal pair of sclerotomes. Their fusion around the notochord produces the blastemal centrum of the vertebra (**Figs 47.4,**

forming cells of the somite. However, it is now usually restricted to cells which are derived from the craniomedial edge.) Second, after initiation of the myotome, cells produced from the ventrolateral edge of the epithelial plate, opposite the limb bud, migrate into the developing limb and give rise to its skeletal muscle. Cells produced from this portion of the occipital somites migrate anteriorly to give rise to the intrinsic muscles of the tongue (p. 614). The remaining epithelial plate and underlying myotome cells grow into the flank region of the body. The epithelial plate is still proliferating at the beginning of this stage. Later the epithelial plate cells revert to mesenchyme, and processes from contiguous somites fuse to form a unified premuscular mass which gives rise to the ventrolateral muscles of the body wall (p. 797).

It was thought that the somite gave rise to segmental portions of the dermis of the skin as well as bone and muscle. However, it is now clear that the epithelial plate of the somite continues to provide a significant source of myogenic precursor cells as it elongates into the body wall. The somitic contribution to the skin from the epithelial plate is limited to the dermis over the epaxial muscles alone, which is a much smaller

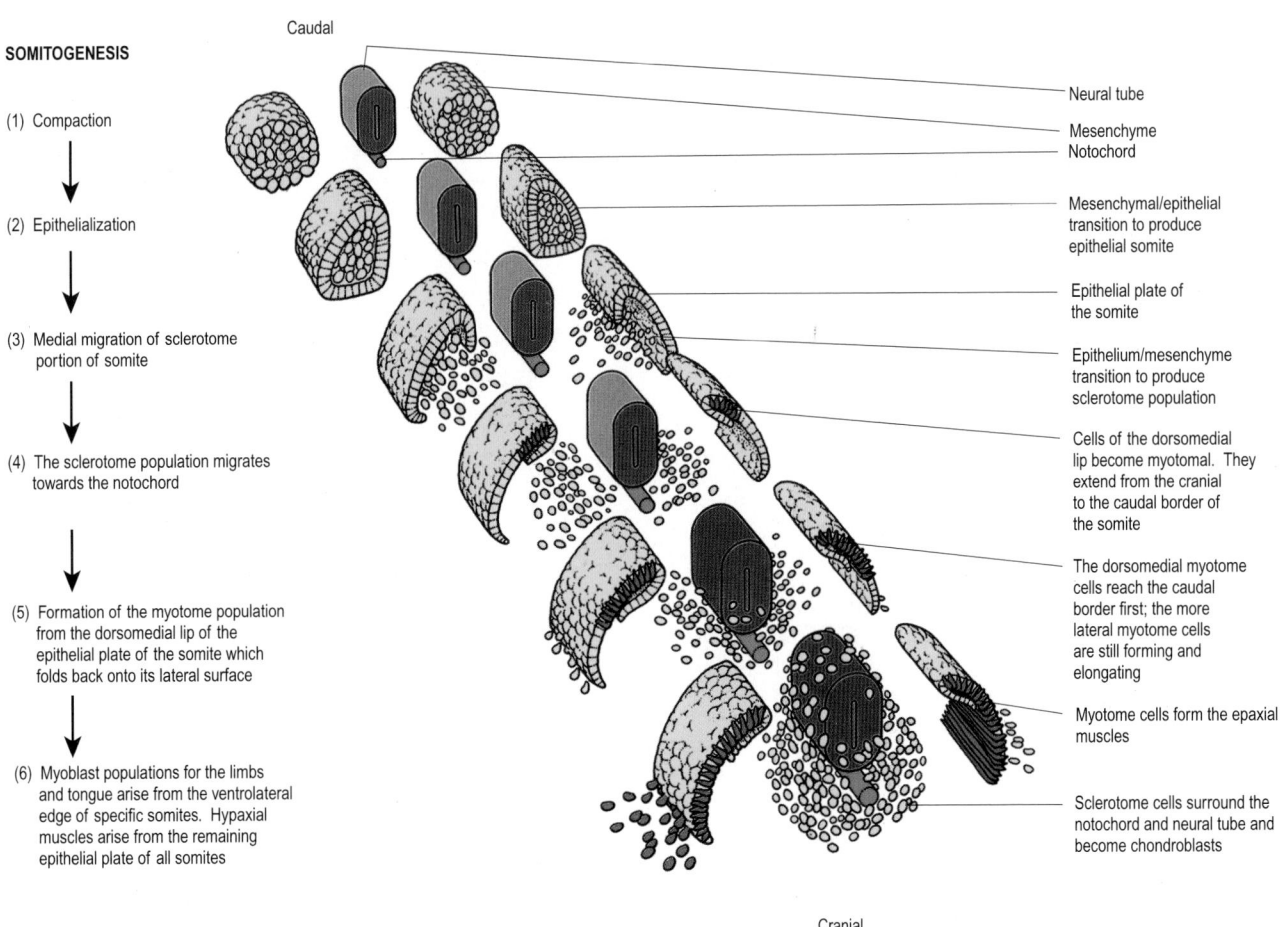

SOMITOGENESIS

(1) Compaction

(2) Epithelialization

(3) Medial migration of sclerotome portion of somite

(4) The sclerotome population migrates towards the notochord

(5) Formation of the myotome population from the dorsomedial lip of the epithelial plate of the somite which folds back onto its lateral surface

(6) Myoblast populations for the limbs and tongue arise from the ventrolateral edge of specific somites. Hypaxial muscles arise from the remaining epithelial plate of all somites

Caudal

Neural tube
Mesenchyme
Notochord

Mesenchymal/epithelial transition to produce epithelial somite

Epithelial plate of the somite

Epithelium/mesenchyme transition to produce sclerotome population

Cells of the dorsomedial lip become myotomal. They extend from the cranial to the caudal border of the somite

The dorsomedial myotome cells reach the caudal border first; the more lateral myotome cells are still forming and elongating

Myotome cells form the epaxial muscles

Sclerotome cells surround the notochord and neural tube and become chondroblasts

Cranial

Fig. 47.3 The stages of somitogenesis. Development proceeds in a craniocaudal progression. The more cranially placed somites (at the lower right of the figure) are further developed than those caudally placed (at the upper left of the figure). The stages in somitogenesis are given on the left of the figure; more detailed information is given on the right.

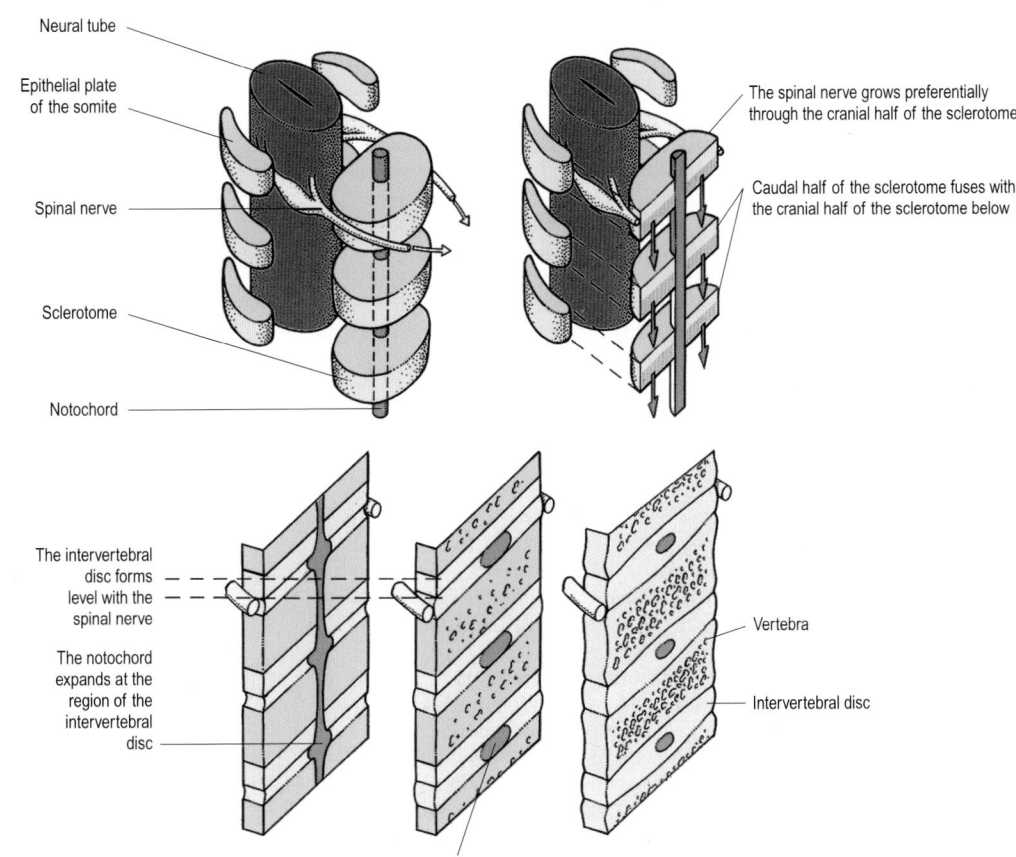

Neural tube

Epithelial plate of the somite

Spinal nerve

Sclerotome

Notochord

The spinal nerve grows preferentially through the cranial half of the sclerotome

Caudal half of the sclerotome fuses with the cranial half of the sclerotome below

The intervertebral disc forms level with the spinal nerve

The notochord expands at the region of the intervertebral disc

Vertebra

Intervertebral disc

Nucleus pulposus

Fig. 47.4 Formation of vertebrae and intervertebral discs from the mesenchymal sclerotomes. Each vertebra is formed from the cranial half of one bilateral pair of sclerotomes and the caudal half of the next pair of sclerotomes. The spinal nerves preferentially migrate through the cranial portion of the sclerotomes. (Redrawn from Tuchmann-Duplessis H, Haegel P 1972 Illustrated Human Embryology, Vol 2 Organogenesis. London: Chapman and Hall.)

47.5). The mesenchyme adjoining the intrasegmental sclerotomic fissure now increases greatly in density to form a well-defined perichordal disc which intervenes between the centra of two adjacent vertebrae and is the future anulus fibrosus of the intervertebral symphysis ('disc') (see below).

The basic pattern of a typical vertebra is initiated by this recombination of caudal and cranial sclerotome halves (**Fig. 47.6**), followed by differential growth and sculpturing of the sclerotomal mesenchyme which encases the notochord and neural tube. The centrum encloses the notochord and lies ventral to the neural tube. Condensation of the sclerotomal mesenchyme around the notochord and right and left neural processes can be seen in stage 15 human embryos. The neural processes extend from the dorsolateral angles of the centrum and curve to enclose the neural tube. The neural arch consists of paired bilateral pedicles (ventrolaterally) and laminae (dorsolaterally) which coalesce in the midline dorsal to the neural tube to form the spinous process. On each side three further processes project cranially, caudally and laterally from the junction of the pedicle and laminae. The cranial and caudal projections are the blastemal articular processes (zygapophyses) which become contiguous with reciprocal processes of adjacent vertebrae; their junctional zones mark the future zygapophyseal or facet joints. The lateral projections are the true vertebral transverse processes. Bilateral costal processes (ribs) grow anterolaterally from the ventral part of the pedicles (i.e. near the centrum), from the neighbouring perichordal disc, and, at most thoracic levels, with accessions from the next adjacent caudal pedicles. The costal processes expand to meet the tips of the transverse processes. The definitive vertebral body is compound, and is formed from a median centrum (derived from the cells of the perinotochordal sheath), and bilaterally from the expanded pedicle ends (derived from the migrating sclerotomal populations). These portions of the vertebral body fuse at the neurocentral synchondroses.

The segmental nature of the vertebrae is promoted by the notochord, which induces the ventral elements of the vertebrae and represses dorsal structures, e.g. the spinous processes. Excision of the notochord in early embryos results in fusion of the centra and formation of a cartilaginous plate ventral to the neural tube. Dorsal segmentation is influenced by the spinal ganglia: experimental removal of the ganglia results in fusion of the neural arches and the formation of a uniform cartilaginous plate dorsal to the neural tube.

Intervertebral discs

Vertebral centra are derived from caudal and cranial sclerotomal halves. An intervertebral disc is formed from the free somitocoele cells within the epithelial somite which migrate with the caudal sclerotomal cells. The sclerotomal mesenchyme which forms the centra of the vertebrae replaces the notochordal tissue which it surrounds. In contrast, the notochord expands between the developing vertebrae as localized aggregates of cells and matrix which form the nucleus pulposus of the intervertebral disc (**Figs 47.4, 47.7**). The intermediate part of each perichordal disc, which forms the anulus fibrosus, surrounds the nucleus pulposus and differentiates into an external laminated fibrous zone and an internal cuff (which lies next to the nucleus pulposus). The inner zone contributes to the growth of the outer. Near the end of the second month of embryonic life it begins to merge with the notochordal tissue, and is ultimately converted into fibrocartilage. After the sixth month of fetal life, notochordal cells in the nucleus pulposus degenerate, and are replaced by cells from the internal zone of the anulus fibrosus. This degeneration continues until the second decade of life, by which time all the notochordal cells have disappeared. In the adult, notochordal vestiges are limited, at the most, to non-cellular matrix.

The original sclerotomes are coextensive with the individual metameric body segments: each sclerotomic fissure, perichordal disc, and maturing intervertebral disc lie opposite the centre of each fundamental body segment. It therefore follows that the discs correspond in level to (i.e. form the anterior boundary of) the intervertebral foramina and their associated mixed spinal nerves, ganglia, vessels and sheaths. Posteriorly, the foramina are bounded by the capsules of the synovial facet joints; the rims of the vertebral notches of adjacent vertebrae lie cranially and caudally. Thus all the structures listed (and other associated ones) are often designated segmental, whereas vertebral bodies are designated intersegmental because of their mode of development.

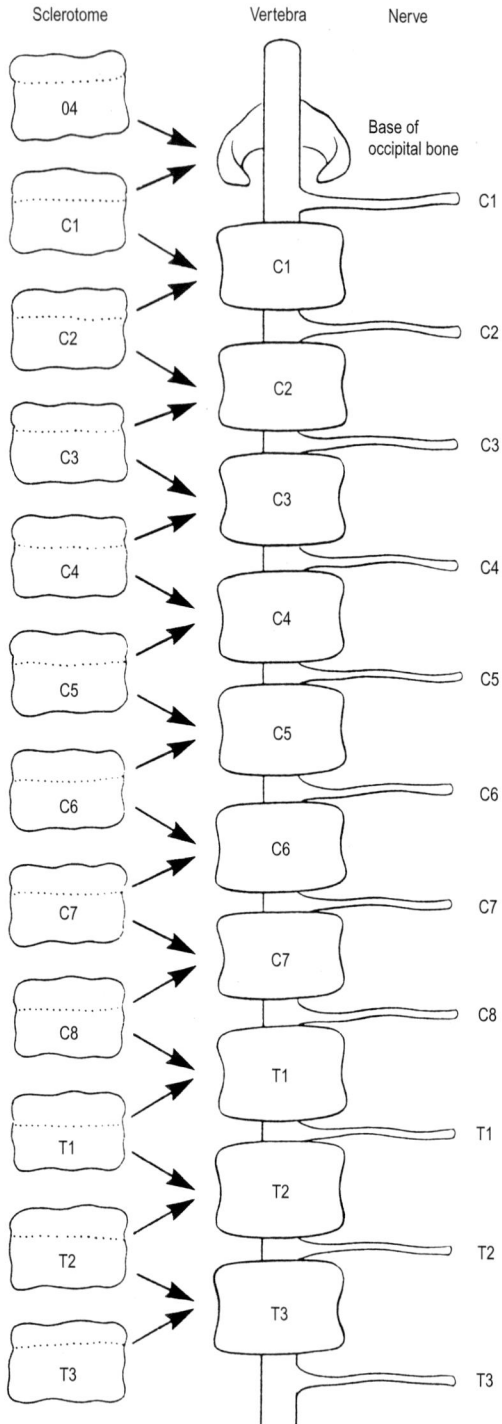

Fig. 47.5 Contribution of the somites to the vertebrae. Each somite induces a ventral root to grow out from the spinal cord. When the sclerotomes recombine the cranial half of the first cervical sclerotome fuses with the occipital sclerotome above contributing to the occipital bone of the skull. The cervical nerves beginning with C1 exit above the corresponding vertebra. Nerve C8 exits below the last cervical vertebra (C7). After this level nerves arise below their vertebrae. (By permission from Larsen WJ 1997 Human Embryology, 2nd edn. Edinburgh: Churchill Livingstone.)

(For further discussion of resegmentation theories, the reader is directed to Muller & O'Rahilly 1986; Brand-Saberi & Christ 2000; Huang et al 2000; Stern & Vasiliauskas 2000.)

Development of vertebrae

The initial movements of sclerotomal cells round the neural tube and the expression of type II collagen signals the blastemal stage of vertebral

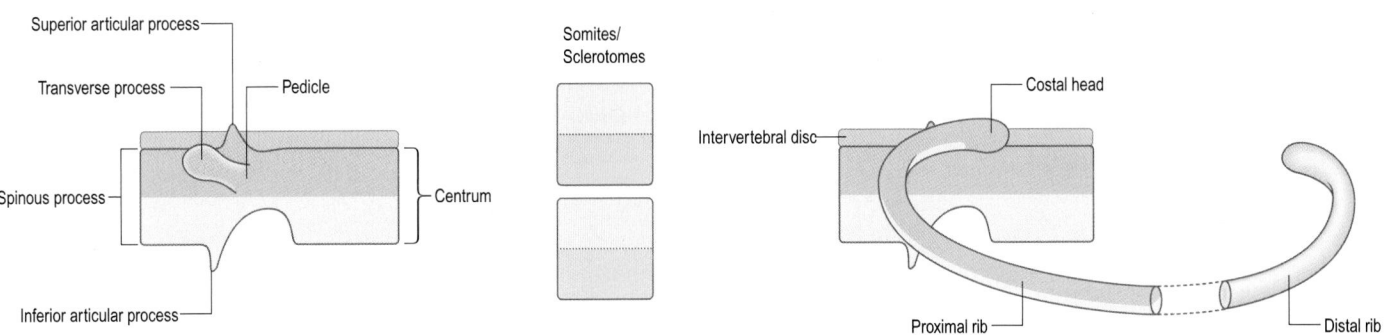

Fig. 47.6 Contribution of two adjacent somites to one vertebra and rib. The intervertebral disc and the costal head are derived from somitocoele cells from one somite which migrate with the caudal half of the sclerotome. The proximal rib is formed from caudal and cranial somite halves with no mixing of cells; in the distal rib there is more mixing of cranial and caudal cells as segmentation diminishes in the ventral body wall. (Redrawn with permission from Christ B, Huang R, Wilting J. The development of the avian vertebral column. Anat Embryol 202: 179–194, 2000, Springer.)

development (**Fig. 47.7**). Chondrification begins at stage 17, initiating the cartilaginous stage. Each centrum chondrifies from one cartilage anlage. Each half of a neural arch is chondrified from a centre, starting in its base and extending dorsally into the laminae and ventrally into the pedicles, to meet, expand and blend with the centrum. By stage 23 there are 33 or 34 cartilaginous vertebrae (**Fig. 11.6**), but the spinous processes have not yet developed, so the overall appearance is of total spina bifida occulta. Fusion of the spines does not occur until the fourth month. The transverse and articular processes are chondrified in continuity with the neural arches. Intervening zones of mesenchyme which do not become cartilage mark the sites of the facet joints and the complex of costovertebral joints, within which synovial cavities later appear.

A typical vertebra is ossified from three primary centres, one in each half vertebral arch and one in the centrum (**Fig. 45.20**). Centres in arches appear at the roots of the transverse processes, and ossification spreads backwards into laminae and spines, forwards into pedicles and postero-lateral parts of the body, laterally into transverse processes and upwards and downwards into articular processes. Classically centres in vertebral arches are said to appear first in upper cervical vertebrae in the ninth to tenth week, and then in successively lower vertebrae, reaching lower lumbar levels in the twelfth week. However, in a radiographic study of unsexed human fetuses (Bagnall et al 1977), a pattern was noted which differed from such a simple craniocaudal sequence. A regular cervical progression was not observed. Centres first appeared in the lower cervical/upper thoracic region, quickly followed by others in the upper cervical region. After a short interval a third group appeared in the lower thoracolumbar region and remaining centres then appeared, spreading regularly and rapidly in craniocaudal directions.

The major part of the body, the centrum, ossifies from a primary centre dorsal to the notochord. Centra are occasionally ossified from bilateral centres which may fail to unite. Suppression of one of these produces a cuneiform vertebra (hemivertebra), which is one cause of lateral spinal curvature (scoliosis). At birth (**Fig. 11.6**) and during early postnatal years the centrum is connected to each half neural arch by a synchondrosis or neurocentral joint. In thoracic vertebrae costal facets on the bodies are posterior to neurocentral joints.

During the first year the arches unite behind, first in the lumbar region and then throughout the thoracic and cervical regions. In upper typical cervical vertebrae, centra unite with arches about the third year, but in lower lumbar vertebrae, union is not complete until the sixth. The upper and lower surfaces of bodies and apices of transverse and spinous processes are cartilaginous until puberty, at which time five secondary centres appear, one in the apex of each transverse and spinous process and two annular epiphyses ('ring apophyses') for the circumferential parts of the upper and lower surfaces of the body. Costal articular facets are extensions of these anular epiphyses. They fuse with the rest of the bone at c.25 years. There are two secondary centres in bifid cervical spinous processes. Exceptions to this pattern of ossification are described in the appropriate subsections in Chapter 45.

Vertebrae are specified as to region very early in development. If a group of thoracic somites is transplanted to the cervical region, ribs will still develop. It is the sclerotome which is restricted: the myotome will produce muscle characteristic of the new location.

OCCIPITOCERVICAL JUNCTION

In humans, the junction between the head and neck (termed occipito-cervical, craniovertebral or spinomedullary) corresponds to the boundary between the 4th and 5th somites (Muller & O'Rahilly 1994). It can first be determined at stage 12 by the observation of hypoglossal nerve rootlets (**Fig. 47.8**). At stages 14 and 15 the junction is seen between the hypoglossal rootlets and the 1st spinal ganglion. The exact position of this boundary is controversial. Wilting et al (1995) suggest that in human embryos the boundary may be between the 5th and 6th somites and that previous studies were based on older embryos in which the transitory 1st somite had already disappeared. In avian embryos, where all embryonic stages may be obtained experimentally, the occipitocervical boundary has been determined as the 5th–6th somite boundary.

The first occipital somite disappears early and the caudal three fuse to form the basiocciput. Occipital sclerotomes 3 and 4 are the most distinct at stage 14, by which time the first three sclerotomes have fused. Vertebrae are formed from the 5th somite caudally: the first cervical vertebra is formed by the caudal half of occipital somite 4 and the cranial half of cervical somite 1 (**Fig. 47.5**). This shift of somite number and vertebral number accounts for the production of seven cervical vertebrae from eight cervical somites.

The segmental pattern present in the cervical somites can be seen rostrally in the developing skull base, where mesenchymal condensations equivalent to the centra of occipital somites 2, 3 and 4 are apparent. The hypoglossal rootlets pass through the less dense portion of occipital sclerotome 4, accompanied by the hypoglossal artery. Occipital sclerotome 4 forms an incomplete centrum axially and exoccipital elements laterally, which are regarded as corresponding to neural arches. They form the rim of the foramen magnum. The occipital condyles develop from the 1st cervical somite (as also happens in the chick).

In the occipitocervical junctional region the centra formed from sclerotomes 5, 6 and 7 have a different fate from those more caudally placed. The lateral portions of these sclerotomes generally develop similarly to those of lower ones. In a study of occipitocervical segmentation in human embryos, Muller and O'Rahilly designated the three complete rostral centra which develop in the atlanto-axial region X, Y and Z (**Figs 47.9, 47.10**; Muller & O'Rahilly 1986). They noted that the height of the XYZ complex is equal to that of three centra elsewhere. X is on the level of sclerotome 5, and Y and Z are in line with sclerotome 6 and with the less dense portion of sclerotome 7. During stage 17 a temporary intervertebral disc appears peripherally between Y and Z. It begins to disappear in stage 21, although remains may be found in the adult. No disc develops between X and Y.

The origin of the anterior arch of the atlas is unclear. It is evident at stages 21–23 at the level of X or sometimes between X and Y. The posterior arch of the atlas arises from the dense area of sclerotome 5 at the level of X. The XYZ complex belongs to the axis, which means that the atlas does not incorporate a part of the central column (Muller & O'Rahilly 1994).

The posterior arch of the axis arises from the dense area of sclerotome 6 and is at the level of Y and Z, particularly Z. XYZ correspond to the

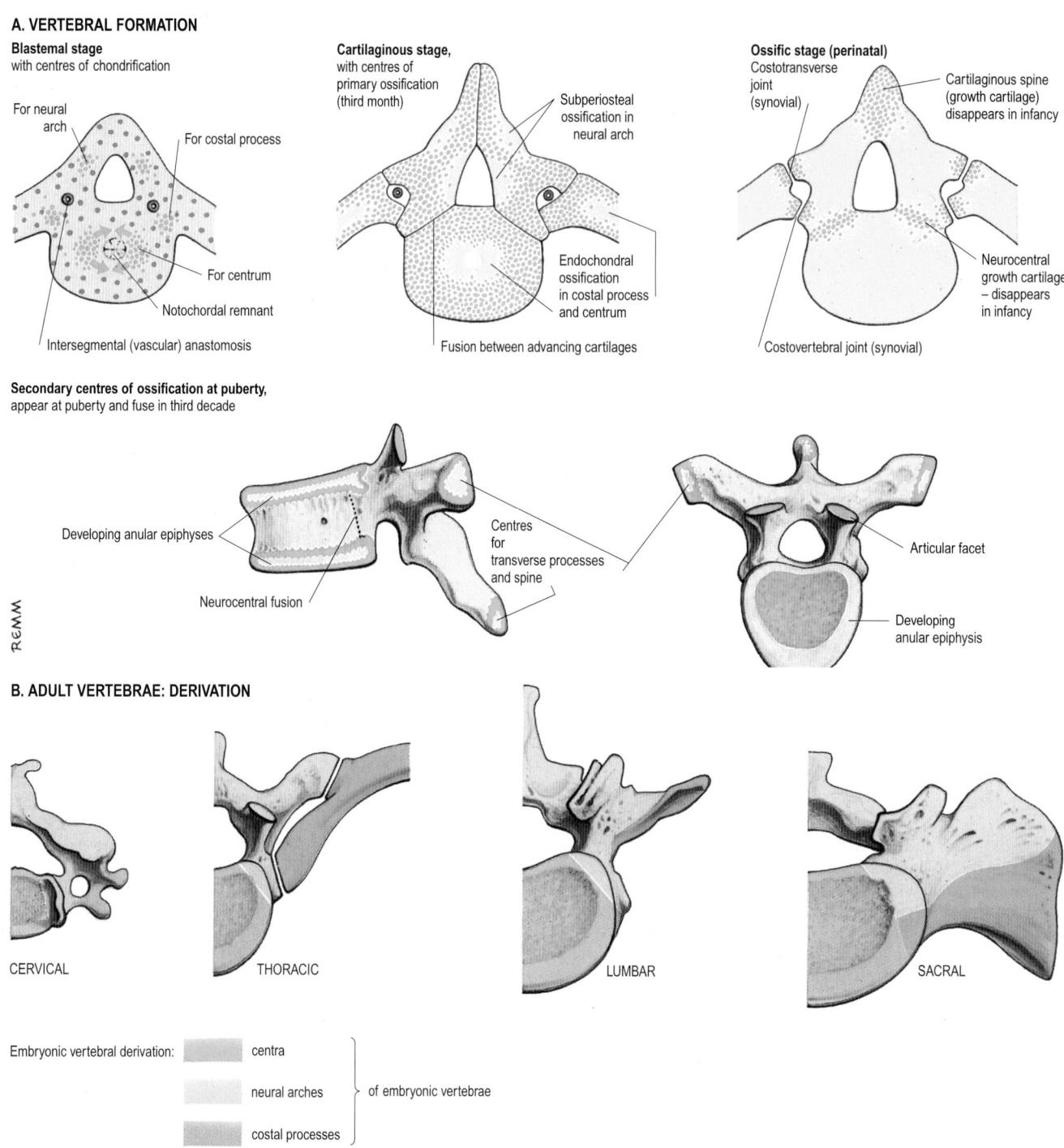

A. VERTEBRAL FORMATION

Blastemal stage
with centres of chondrification

For neural arch

For costal process

For centrum

Notochordal remnant

Intersegmental (vascular) anastomosis

Cartilaginous stage,
with centres of
primary ossification
(third month)

Subperiosteal ossification in neural arch

Endochondral ossification in costal process and centrum

Fusion between advancing cartilages

Ossific stage (perinatal)
Costotransverse joint (synovial)

Cartilaginous spine (growth cartilage) disappears in infancy

Neurocentral growth cartilage – disappears in infancy

Costovertebral joint (synovial)

Secondary centres of ossification at puberty,
appear at puberty and fuse in third decade

Developing anular epiphyses

Neurocentral fusion

Centres for transverse processes and spine

Articular facet

Developing anular epiphysis

B. ADULT VERTEBRAE: DERIVATION

CERVICAL

THORACIC

LUMBAR

SACRAL

Embryonic vertebral derivation:

centra

neural arches — of embryonic vertebrae

costal processes

Fig. 47.7 Vertebral development through blastemal, cartilaginous and pre- and postnatal ossificatory stages. Bottom row indicates principal morphological parts of adult vertebrae. **A**, Vertebral development through blastemal, cartilaginous and pre- and postnatal ossificatory stages. **B**, Derivation of principal morphological parts of adult vertebrae.

three parts of the median column of the axis, where X represents the tip of the dens, Y represents the base of the dens and Z represents the centrum of the axis. The latter differs from other cervical vertebrae in that it is thicker and square-shaped.

The development of the cervical spine, particularly the upper cervical vertebrae, is closely related to the development of the basiocciput and exocciput: anomalous development will affect both regions. Anomalies of the occiput are associated with decreased skull base height; the dens lies at or above the level of the foramen magnum; a distinctive margin of the foramen magnum lies above the bottom of the posterior fossa; and the posterior arch of the atlas is at the same level as the foramen magnum. The last three structural defects are collectively termed basilar invagination. Malfusions of the caudal portion of occipital sclerotome 4 and the cranial portion of cervical sclerotome 1 may produce defects

of the occipital condyles. Disassociated occipital condyles are called a proatlas, because in lower vertebrates the cranial half of the first cervical sclerotome forms a separate bone between the occipital bone and the atlas.

Decreased skull base height and diminished volume in the posterior fossa are structural anomalies associated with the Arnold–Chiari malformation. Although this is considered clinically to be a neurological defect, in that the medulla oblongata, and sometimes the cerebellar tonsils, project through the foramen magnum, there is good evidence that the underlying cause is a series of abnormalities of the occipitocervical junction. When the volume of the brain in the posterior cranial fossa and the volume of the fossa (delineated by bone and the tentorium cerebelli) were compared in controls and Arnold–Chiari cases, no significant difference was found between brain volume in the two groups,

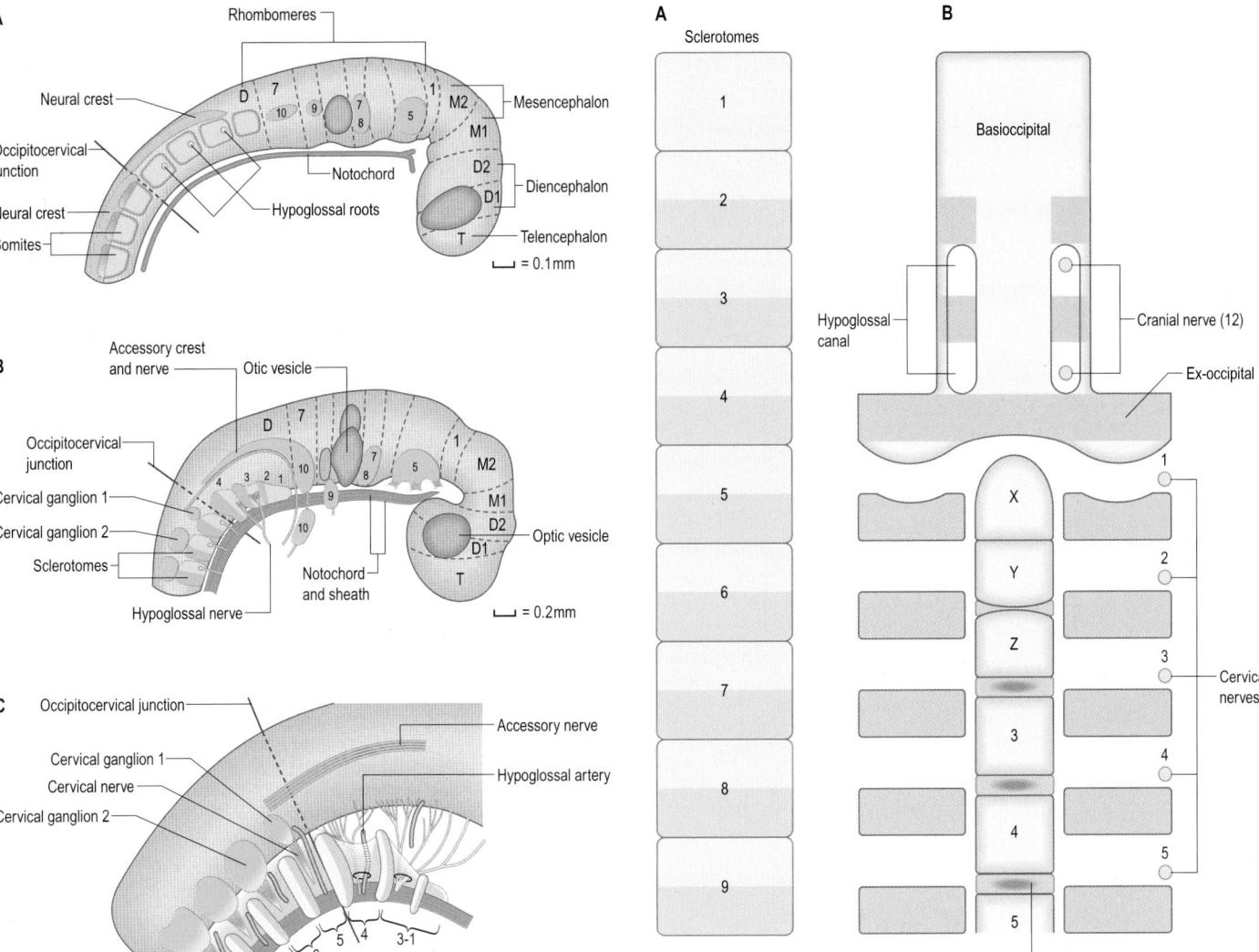

Fig. 47.8 Reconstructions of the occipitocervical region of human embryos. **A**, Stage 12: occipital somites innervated by hypoglossal fibres (small circles). Three cervical somites are shown. The crest derived ganglia of cranial nerves 5, 7, 8, 9 and 10 are shown in green. Neural crest associated with the occipital somites is hypoglossal and perhaps accessory (also shown in green). **B**, Stage 14: the somites have transformed into sclerotomes and moved ventrally. The less dense cranial and dense caudal parts of the sclerotomes and occipital sclerotomes 1–4 are indicated. Hypoglossal fibres and cervical ventral rami migrate through the less dense parts of the sclerotomes. The occipital neural crest is now seen to be mostly accessory. The cervical crest is subdivided into spinal ganglia. A perinotochordal sheath can be seen extending rostrally to the termination of the notochord. **C**, Stage 15: the dense parts of sclerotomes 1–8 are shown. Intersegmental arteries are visible in the less dense areas of the sclerotomes, as are the spinal nerve fibres. In all diagrams the occipitocervical junction is indicated by the asterisks and line. (After Muller F, O'Rahilly R 1994 Occipitocervical segmentation in staged human embryos. J Anat 185: 251–258. Permission by Blackwell Publishing.)

Fig. 47.9 The relationship between the centra and neural arches of the vertebrae and the related spinal ganglia and nerves. Scheme of the details of the early development of the occipitocervical region. **A**, The column of sclerotomes from occipital somite 1. **B**, Dorsal view of the developing vertebrae with the centra in the middle and the bilateral components of the neural processes laterally. X, Y and Z are three centra which will produce the tip of the dens of the axis (X), the base of the dens of the axis (Y) and the centrum of the axis (Z). An intervertebral disc appears temporarily between Y and Z during stage 17. No disc develops between X and Y. The occipital condyles are derived from the first cervical sclerotome. (After Muller F, O'Rahilly R 1994 Occipitocervical segmentation in staged human embryos. J Anat 185: 251–258. Permission by Blackwell Publishing.)

though the basiocciput, exocciput and supraocciput were significantly smaller in affected individuals (Nishikawa et al 1997). In patients with the Arnold–Chiari malformation, proatlas remnants and atlas assimilation are found. The sagittal canal diameter of the foramen magnum is critical: patients become symptomatic when this is less than 19 mm (Menezes 1995). Secondary skull base and cervical spine deformations, e.g. foramen magnum and cervical canal enlargement, may develop in association with the Arnold–Chiari malformation.

Most defects of the atlas do not contribute to abnormal occipitocervical anomalies and are not associated with basilar invagination.

Abnormalities of the axis are usually concerned with fusion of the dens with the centrum of the second cervical sclerotomes. Using the classification of the three complete centra which develop in the atlantoaxial region as X, Y and Z (Muller & O'Rahilly 1986), failure of fusion of X with the YZ complex produces an ossiculum terminale, a dissociated apical odontoid epiphysis. Failure of fusion of the XY complex with Z at the dentocentral synchondrosis, or maintenance of the transitory intervertebral disc at this point, produces an os odontoideum, thought to be induced by excessive movement at the time of ossification of the dens (Crockard & Stevens 1995). Hypoplasia and aplasia of the X and Y centra, and aplasia of the Z centrum, will all lead to reduced size of the dens. There are widely differing views about whether this will lead to atlanto-axial instability.

C3–7, THIRD TO SEVENTH CERVICAL VERTEBRAE

In cervical vertebrae 3–7 (**Fig. 47.7**) the transverse process is dorsomedial to the foramen transversarium. The costal process, corresponding to the head, neck and tubercle of a rib, limits the foramen ventrolaterally and dorsolaterally. The distal parts of these cervical costal processes do not normally develop; they do so occasionally in the case of the seventh cervical vertebra, and may even develop costovertebral joints. These cervical ribs may reach the sternum.

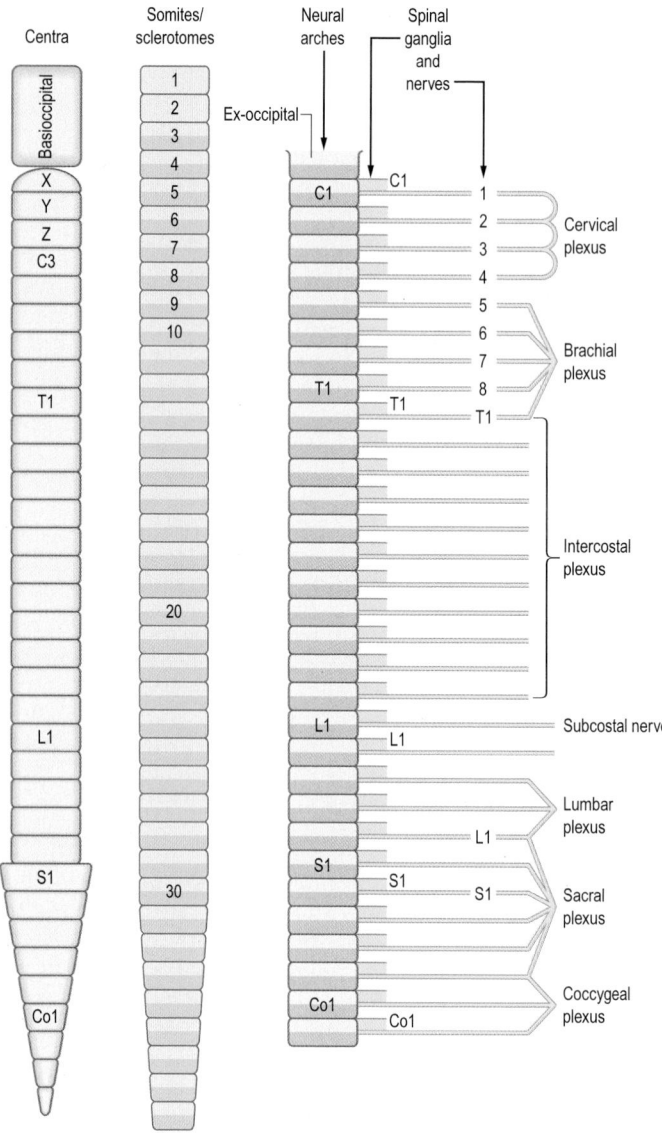

Fig. 47.10 The relationship between the centra and neural arches of the vertebrae with the related spinal ganglia and nerves. Cells of the somites from 1 to c.27 are derived from the primitive streak. Somite 31 illustrates the level of final closure of the caudal neuropore. All neural and somitic tissue caudal to that is derived from secondary neurulation. An intervertebral disc appears temporarily between Y and Z during stage 17. No disc develops between X and Y. The occipital condyles are derived from the first cervical sclerotome. (After Muller F, O'Rahilly R 1994 Occipitocervical segmentation in staged human embryos. J Anat 185: 251–258. Permission by Blackwell Publishing.)

The seventh cervical vertebra is transitional in shape between cervical and thoracic vertebrae. The laminae are longer than other cervical vertebrae in the neonate and lie almost perpendicular to the basal plane; the inferior articular facets are more upright, and resemble those of thoracic vertebrae; and, in the lateral view, the superior articular facets extend transversely to the top of the transverse processes.

Anomalies of the lower cervical vertebrae are generally caused by inappropriate cervical vertebral fusion: collectively this is termed Klippel–Feil syndrome. This term includes all congenital fusions of the cervical spine, from two segments to the entire cervical spine. Affected individuals have a low posterior hairline, short neck and limitations of head and neck movement. Scoliosis and/or kyphosis is common.

THORACIC VERTEBRAE

At stage 23 the neural processes of thoracic vertebrae are short, slightly bifurcated and joined by collagenous fibres. The transverse process is prominent. The three facets for articulation with the ribs at the costo-vertebral and costotransverse joints are present. The thoracic neuro-

central and posterior synchondroses are not fused in the neonate: the posterior synchondroses close within 2 to 3 months of postnatal development and the neurocentral synchondroses are open until 5 to 6 years of age.

In general, the thoracic spine develops ahead of the cervical and lumbar spine. However, towards the end of the second month, ossification begins in the cartilaginous vertebrae in a craniocaudal progression.

RIBS

Ribs usually develop in association with the thoracic vertebrae. Occasionally they can arise from the seventh cervical and first lumbar vertebrae.

The costal processes attain their maximum length as the ribs in the thoracic region. Each rib originates from the caudal half of one sclerotome and the cranial half of the next subjacent sclerotome (**Fig. 47.6**). The head of the rib develops from somitocoele cells from one somite, which migrate with the caudal half of the sclerotome. The proximal portion of the rib forms from both caudal and cranial sclerotomal halves; there is no mixing of cells from these origins. The distal portion of the rib forms from caudal and cranial sclerotomal halves; these cells mix as the rib extends into the ventral body wall and segmentation diminishes.

The ribs arise anterolaterally from the ventral part of the pedicles, and form bilateral costal processes which expand to meet the tips of the transverse processes. As they elongate laterally and ventrally they come to lie between the myotomic muscle plates. In the thorax (**Fig. 47.7**) the costal processes grow laterally to form a series of precartilaginous ribs. The transverse processes grow laterally behind the vertebral ends of the costal processes, at first connected by mesenchyme which later becomes differentiated into the ligaments and other tissues of the costotransverse joints. The capitular costovertebral joints are similarly formed from mesenchyme between the proximal end of the costal processes and the perichordal disc, and the adjacent parts of two (sometimes one) vertebral bodies, which are derived from the neural arch. Ribs 1–7 (vertebrosternal) curve round the body wall to reach the developing sternal plates. Ribs 8–10 (vertebrochondral) are progressively more oblique and shorter, only reaching the costal cartilage of the rib above, and contributing to the costal margin. Ribs 11 and 12 are free (floating), and have cone-shaped terminal cartilages to which muscles become attached (p. 955).

LUMBAR VERTEBRAE

The costal processes do not develop distally in lumbar vertebrae (**Fig. 47.7**). Their proximal parts become the 'transverse processes', while the morphologically true transverse processes may be represented by the accessory processes of the vertebrae. Occasionally, movable ribs may develop in association with the first lumbar vertebra.

Lumbar intervertebral discs are thicker than thoracic discs. By stage 23 the annulus fibrosus can be seen in the peripheral part, and internally the notochordal cells are expanding to form the nucleus pulposus.

SACRUM

Sacral vertebrae have lower centra and are narrower overall from side to side than their thoracic and lumbar counterparts. Each sacral vertebra is composed of a centrum and bilateral neural processes. The contribution of the costal processes to sacral development was examined by O'Rahilly et al (1990). These authors divided the neurocentral junctional area into two parts, anterolateral or alar, and posterolateral. They found the alar element in sacral vertebra 1 to be novel, since it was absent in lumbar vertebra 5. There is support for this view if the course of the dorsal rami of the spinal nerves is used to distinguish the costal elements ventrally from the transverse elements dorsally. The alar elements of the sacral vertebrae are ventral to the sacral dorsal rami, and both costal and transverse portions are posterolateral. The alar element of S1 and S2 forms the auricular surface of the sacrum. At stage 23 the cartilaginous sacral vertebrae have joined and the outline of the future bone can be recognized. Individual pedicles and laminae are very small and can be detected in S3–5.

Ossification of the vertebral column proceeds in a craniocaudal direction. After 16 weeks it has progressed to L5. Ossification of each additional vertebra occurs over a period of 2–3 weeks; S2 is ossified by 22 weeks.

Very rarely significant malformation of the sacral or lumbosacral vertebrae may develop, often in association with a maternal history of diabetes. When there is sacral agenesis, motor paralysis is profound below the affected vertebral level, whereas the sensory disturbance does not relate to the vertebral level so clearly and sensation may be present down to the knees. Bladder involvement is a consistent feature.

Spina bifida

Spina bifida is the generic term for a range of discrete defects of neurulation and subsequent vertebral formation. The spectrum of neural tube and vertebral defects includes a range of open neural tube defects: craniorachischisis (non-fusion of the entire neural tube and no vertebral arch development); anencephaly (non-fusion of the rostral portion of the neural tube with no calvarial or occipital development); and myelocoele (non-fusion of caudal portions of the neural tube and local failure of vertebral arch development)(see **Fig. 14.8**).

Spina bifida cystica occurs where the meninges have developed adjacent to or over the defective neural tissue. Local accumulation of CSF may push a defective neural plaque or spinal cord superficial to the level of the vertebrae forming a meningomyelocoele. Alternatively, a meningeal sac may protrude in the midline if one or two spinous processes are absent; this condition is a meningocoele. In both cases the meningeal sac may be covered with skin or skin may be contiguous with the edges of a neural plaque.

Prior to antenatal diagnosis of spina bifida by ultrasonography, most live births with spina bifida cystica had meningomyelocoele. Meningomyelocoele occurs in thoracolumbar, lumbar or lumbosacral regions. Sacral lesions are less common. The vertebral lesion usually extends cranially further than the neural lesion, showing deformities of the vertebral bodies and laminae. Vertebrae may be wedge shaped or hemivertebrae and ribs may be fused or absent. Concomitant kyphosis at birth is associated with a worse prognosis. Prenatal diagnosis of meningomyelocoele and termination of affected fetuses has led to a significant decrease in the incidence of live births with this condition.

Up to 10% of spina bifida cystica cases are meningocoele. This lesion may occur in cervical and upper thoracic levels or in lower lumbar and sacral levels: the latter are most common. In its mildest form no neurological abnormality occurs with this condition.

Spina bifida occulta affects about 5% of the population. Affected individuals have bifid spinous processes often at the lumbosacral junction. A very small proportion of those with this condition have a naevus, dimple or tuft of hair over the lesion.

TETHERING OF THE CORD AND DIASTEMATOMYELIA

The greatest change of vertebral length occurs within the last 6 months of intrauterine life. When there is any degree of spina bifida, the upward migration of the spinal cord which normally occurs within the vertebral canal during growth is limited, and the cord is said to be tethered. Neurological deficits caused by this condition in neonates become apparent soon after birth, although some individuals show symptoms later in life, especially degrees of urinary dysfunction.

Very rarely, tethering symptoms may be associated with abnormal development of the vertebral centra, e.g. when a midline cartilaginous or osseous spicule or a fibrous septum projects into the vertebral canal. These obstacles may split the spinal cord or intraspinal nerve roots into two columns, a condition termed diastematomyelia. Usually patients with this condition have a cutaneous abnormality, such as a dimple, pigmented naevi or patch of hair, along their back at the level of the tethering.

DEVELOPMENT OF DERMOMYOTOMES

The dorsal half of the somite, the dermomyotome, gives rise to all the skeletal muscle in the trunk. The medial dermomyotome produces the epaxial muscles and the lateral portion produces the muscles of the tongue, limbs and of the ventrolateral body wall. Muscles in the head arise from the unsegmented paraxial mesenchyme rostral to the occipital somites (p. 453).

Myogenic determination factors, MyoD, myogenin, Myf 5 and herculin/MRF 4 can first be detected in the medial half of the somite as early as stage II, several hours prior to the onset of myotome formation. Cells of the epithelial plate are mainly orientated perpendicular to the back, but they have different orientations according to their positions: they are transversely orientated along the dorsomedial edge and longitudinally orientated within the cranial edge of the epithelial plate (**Figs 47.2, 47.3**).

Myotome cells originate from longitudinally orientated cells at the cranial edge of the epithelial plate. Individual cells, which are originally produced and anchored at the craniomedial corner of the epithelial plate, send processes to the caudal edge of the plate where they form a second anchor point. In this way, myotome formation continues caudally along the dorsomedial edge and laterally along the cranial edge, and each mononucleated myotome cell becomes very elongated perpendicular to the cells of the epithelial plate. Development of subsequent cells imparts a triangular shape to the early myotome. The growing myotome first reaches the caudal somite border on the medial side and later the ventrolateral edge. When the vertebral bodies form, the future intervertebral fissure divides the sclerotome into rostral and caudal halves. The myotome fibres span the intervertebral joints and foramina, which means that the muscles which are derived from the myotome are positioned to move adjacent vertebrae relative to each other.

EPAXIAL MUSCLE: DORSAL TRUNK MUSCLES

Myotome cells are all postmitotic embryonic myoblasts: later in development they fuse to form syncytia which form the epaxial musculature. The presence of the neural tube is required for normal myoblast development. There is evidence to suggest that interactions between precursor myotome cells and the medial neural crest cells, which are commencing their migration at this time, may also be important. The epaxial muscles are innervated by the dorsal ramus of each spinal nerve (p. 782).

At much later stages satellite cells enter the myotome. Interestingly the development of endo-, peri- and epimysium in relation to the epaxial muscles has not been addressed.

HYPAXIAL MUSCLE: VENTROLATERAL TRUNK MUSCLES

The ventrolateral trunk muscles are formed from the epithelial plate of the somite. After production of the myotome and the precursor myogenic cells of the limb, the remaining epithelial plate and attached myotome grows into the flank somatopleuric mesenchyme. At this stage the epithelial plate is still proliferating and producing myogenic precursor cells. The epithelial plate has a leading edge or process from which single cells or clusters of cells migrate in a ventral direction. It may be that these epithelial plate cells, which are in a more immature state of differentiation, act as pioneer cells for further cell movement. The previously segmented processes from adjacent epithelial plates form a unified premuscular mass. Both postmitotic myoblast cells and mitotic plate cells can be seen in the body wall; they may represent early and later forming myoblasts which will form heterokaryotic myotubes.

The premuscular mass subdivides into abdominal muscle blastemata for the external and internal oblique muscles, transversus abdominis and rectus abdominis. At this time the number of somatopleural fibroblasts situated within the muscle-forming zone increases, and myotubes can be first seen. There is a subsequent ventral shift of the already separated muscle blastemata within the growing abdominal wall as they attain their definitive positions. Muscle differentiation continues and muscular connective tissue, tendons and aponeuroses develop.

OTHER STRUCTURES DERIVED FROM THE SOMITES

Dermal precursors undergo an epithelial/mesenchyme transformation from the dermomyotome and migrate dorsally toward the ectoderm over the dorsal region of the embryo. Their transformation seems to be controlled by factors from the neural tube. There is a sharp boundary between dermis which is somite-derived and that which is derived from the splachnopleuric mesenchyme of the lateral plate (which covers the limbs, part of the lateral and all of the ventral body wall).

Smooth muscle cells within and around the developing somites and endothelial cell precursors are now considered to arise from somitic cells. All compartments of the epithelial somite, including the somitocoele cells, give rise to angioblasts (Brand-Saberi & Christ 2000).

REFERENCES

Bagnall KM, Harris PF, Jones PRM 1977 A radiographic study of the human spine II. The sequence of development of ossification centres in the vertebral column. J Anat 124: 791–802.

Brand-Saberi B, Christ B 2000 Evolution and development of distinct cell lineages derived from somites. Current Topics in Developmental Biology Vol 47. New York: Academic Press.

Christ B, Huang R, Wilting J 2000 The development of the avian vertebral column. Anat Embryol 202: 179–94.

Crockard HA, Stevens JM 1995 Craniovertebral junction anomalies in inherited disorders: part of the syndrome or caused by the disorder? Eur J Pediatr 154: 504–12.

Gumpel-Pinot M 1984 Muscle and skeleton of limbs and body wall. In: Le Douarin N, McLaren A (eds) Chimeras in Developmental Biology. London: Academic Press: 281–310.

Huang R, Zhi Q, Brand-Saberi B, Christ B 2000 New experimental evidence for somite resegmentation. Anat Embryol 202: 195–200.

Menezes AH 1995 Primary craniovertebral anomalies and the hindbrain herniation syndrome (Chiari 1); database analysis. Pediatr Neurosurg 23: 260–9.

Muller F, O'Rahilly R 1986 Somitic–vertebral correlation and vertebral levels in the human embryo. Am J Anat 177: 3–19.

Muller F, O'Rahilly R 1994 Occipitocervical segmentation in staged human embryos. J Anat 185: 251–8.

Nishikawa M, Sakamoto H, Hakuba A, Nakanishi N, Inoue Y 1997 Pathogenesis of Chiari malformations: a morphometric study of the posterior cranial fossa. J Neurosurg 86: 40–7.

O'Rahilly R, Muller F, Meyer DB 1990 The human vertebral column at the end of the embryonic period proper. 4. The sacrococcygeal region. J Anat 168: 95–111.

Ordahl CP 1993 Myogenic lineages within the developing somite. In: Bernfield M (ed.) Molecular Basis of Morphogenesis. New York: Wiley Liss: 165–76.

Pourquie O, Kusumi K 2001 When body segmentation goes wrong. Clin Genet 60: 409–16.

Richardson MK, Allen SP, Wright GM, Raynaud A, Hanken J 1998 Somite number and vertebrate evolution. Development 125: 151–60.

Stern CD, Vasiliauskas D 2000 Segmentation: a view from the border. Current Topics in Developmental Biology, Vol 47. New York: Academic Press. *Presents three different models of somite formation in the context of recent molecular data.*

Wilting J, Ebensperger C, Müller TS, Kosecki H, Wallin J, Christ B 1995 *Pax-1* in the development of the cervico-occipital transitional zone. Anat Embryol 192: 221–227.

PECTORAL GIRDLE AND UPPER LIMB

Editors:

David Johnson and Harold Ellis *(Lead Editors)*

Patricia Collins *(Embryology, Growth and Development)*

David Johnson and Harold Ellis *(Editors)*

With specialist contributions on clinical and functional anatomy by

Vivien Lees *(chapter 53)*

Critical reviewers:

Paul Cartwright *(chapter 48)*, **Steve Corbett** *(49 & 51)*, **David Woods** *(49 & 51)*

General organization and surface anatomy of the upper limb

This chapter is divided into two sections. The first is an overview of the general organization of the upper limb, with particular emphasis on the distribution of the major blood vessels and lymphatic channels, and of the branches of the brachial plexus: it is intended to complement the detailed regional anatomy described in Chapters 49 to 53. The second section describes the surface anatomy of the upper limb.

SKIN, FASCIA AND SOFT TISSUES

The skin of the anterior aspect of the upper arm and forearm differs from that of the posterior aspect in that it is thinner and hairless. The palmar skin is thick and hairless: firm attachments to the underlying palmar fascia reflect its role in gripping and shock absorption. The dorsal skin of the hand is much thinner, lax and mobile, and this allows the extensor tendons to glide underneath the subcutaneous tissue.

The direction in which skin tension is greatest varies regionally in the upper limb as in other areas of the body. Skin tension lines that follow the furrows formed when the skin is relaxed are known as 'relaxed skin tension lines' (p. 173) and can act as a guide in planning elective incisions.

The superficial fascia is a layer of subcutaneous fatty tissue. Its thickness depends on the degree of obesity of the subject: measurement of the thickness of the subcutaneous tissue of the posterior upper arm is used as an indicator of obesity. There is less subcutaneous tissue in the palm of the hand than on the dorsum of the hand.

The depth of deep fascia varies according to the stresses to which it is subjected in the different areas of the limb. It is a thin but quite obvious layer in the upper arm, where intermuscular septa pass to the medial and lateral sides of the humerus and separate the upper arm muscles into anterior and posterior groups within their respective compartments. In addition, each muscle also lies within its own delicate fascial sheath, an arrangement that allows individual muscles to glide upon each other.

At the elbow the deep fascia condenses anteriorly as the tough bicipital aponeurosis. In the forearm it is relatively thin and is attached along the subcutaneous border of the ulna. Intermuscular septa divide the forearm into three compartments, anterior (flexors), posterior (extensors) and the mobile wad compartment for brachioradialis and extensor carpi radialis longus and brevis.

At the wrist the deep fascia becomes condensed anteriorly and posteriorly as the flexor and extensor retinacula respectively. Further condensation occurs in the palm of the hand, where the palmar aponeurosis is reinforced by the insertion of the tendon of palmaris longus, and in the flexor tendon sheaths and fascial system associated with the digits.

BONES AND JOINTS

The bones of the upper limb are the clavicle, scapula, humerus, radius and ulna (connected for a large portion of their length by an interosseous membrane) and the bones of the hand, i.e. the carpals, metacarpals and phalanges (**Figs 48.1, 48.2**).

The shoulder girdle is extremely mobile because reciprocal movements at the sternoclavicular and glenohumeral joints enable 180° abduction of the upper limb. Movement occurs in all three planes at the glenohumeral joint.

The elbow joint is a hinge joint. It incorporates the superior (proximal) radio-ulnar joint within its capsule. The proximal and distal radio-ulnar joints permit pronation and supination of the forearm – a unique feature of the primate upper limb.

The range of movement at the condyloid wrist joint, between the distal ends of the radius and ulna and the proximal carpal bones, is supplemented by gliding movements between the carpal bones. The saddle-shaped first metacarpal joint, between the trapezium and the base of the first metacarpal, is unique to the primate forelimb and permits opposition of the thumb. The hand is clenched by flexion at the metacarpophalangeal joints, supplemented by gliding movements of the fourth and fifth carpometacarpal joints. In grasping, the thumb is of equal value to the remaining four digits: loss of the thumb is almost as disabling as loss of all of the other digits.

MUSCLES

Posterior and anterior muscle groups connect the pectoral girdle to the axial skeleton; the only bony connection is at the sternoclavicular joint. The posterior muscles are trapezius, levator scapulae and the rhomboid muscles: their actions include raising the shoulder and drawing the scapula medially. The anterior muscles are pectoralis minor, serratus anterior, and subclavius. Serratus anterior and trapezius together rotate the scapula in abduction of the arm.

Latissimus dorsi (posteriorly) and pectoralis major (anteriorly) run from the axial skeleton to the humerus. They are both powerful adductors and medial rotators of the shoulder, and latissimus dorsi is also a powerful extensor.

A large group of muscles arise from the shoulder girdle and pass to the humerus. They are the four muscles of the rotator cuff (subscapularis, supraspinatus, infraspinatus and teres minor), teres major, deltoid, the clavicular origin of pectoralis major, biceps brachii, coracobrachialis and the long head of triceps.

The muscles of the upper arm can be divided into an anterior group of elbow flexors (biceps, brachialis and coracobrachialis) and a posterior group of elbow extensors (triceps and anconeus). Biceps brachii is also a powerful supinator of the radio-ulnar joints.

The extensor muscles of the wrist and fingers, together with brachioradialis and a slip of origin of supinator, arise from the lateral epicondyle of the humerus. The principal head of pronator teres, the carpal flexor muscles, palmaris longus and, at a deeper level, the main origin of flexor digitorum superficialis, all arise from the medial epicondyle of the humerus. More deeply, flexor pollicis longus, flexor digitorum profundus and pronator quadratus arise from the anterior aspects of the shafts of the radius and ulna and the intervening interosseous membrane. Abductor pollicis longus, extensors pollicis longus and brevis and extensor indicis all arise from the posterior aspects of these bones and the intervening interosseous membrane.

The small (intrinsic) muscles of the hand consist of a thenar and a hypothenar group, and the muscles of the palm, which are the anterior and posterior interossei and the lumbricals. These muscles are all concerned with the intricate movements of the digits.

VASCULAR SUPPLY AND LYMPHATIC DRAINAGE

ARTERIAL SUPPLY (Fig. 48.3)

The blood supply to the skin of the upper limb comes from a combination of direct cutaneous, fasciocutaneous and musculocutaneous vessels (**Fig. 8.20**). **Figure 48.4** provides an overview of the anatomical territories of the cutaneous vessels.

The axial artery to the upper limb is the subclavian artery: it becomes the axillary artery after crossing the lateral edge of the first rib, and the

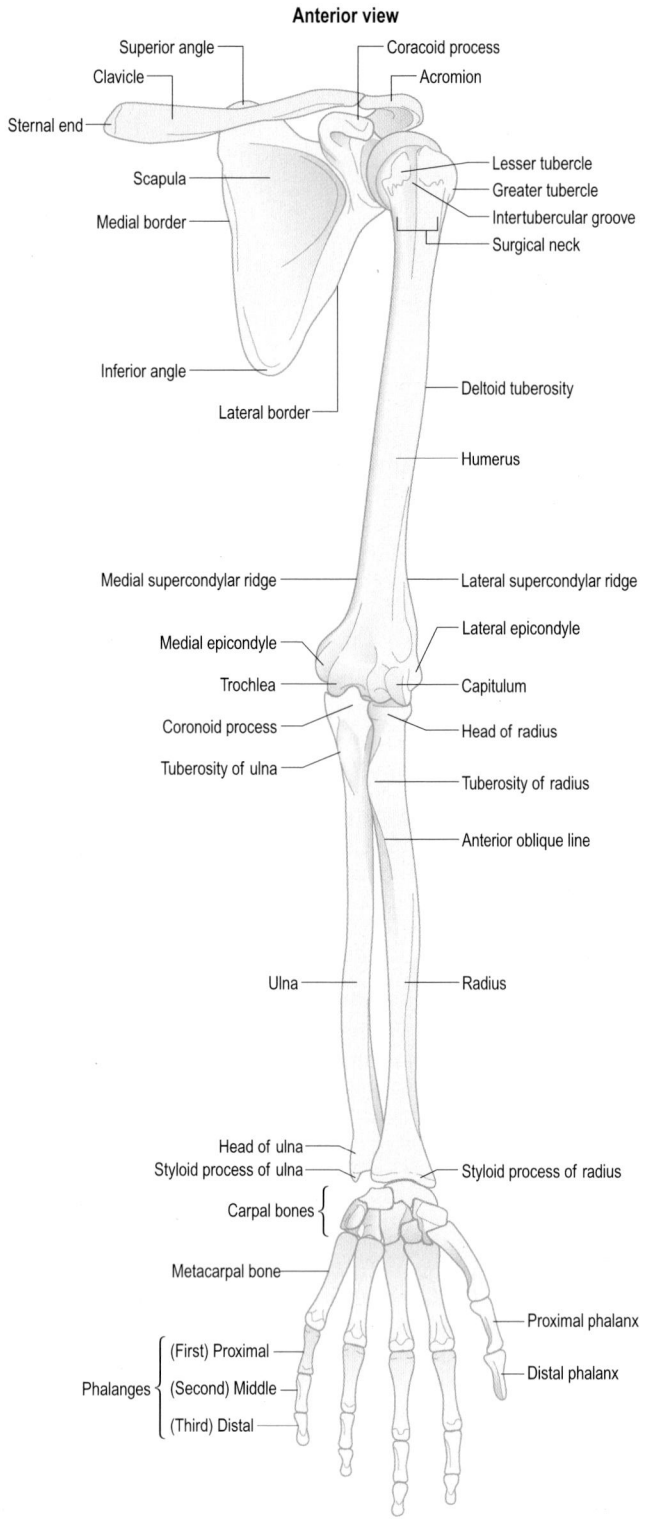

Anterior view

Superior angle — Clavicle — Sternal end — Scapula — Medial border — Inferior angle — Lateral border — Coracoid process — Acromion — Lesser tubercle — Greater tubercle — Intertubercular groove — Surgical neck — Deltoid tuberosity — Humerus — Medial supercondylar ridge — Lateral supercondylar ridge — Medial epicondyle — Lateral epicondyle — Trochlea — Capitulum — Coronoid process — Head of radius — Tuberosity of ulna — Tuberosity of radius — Anterior oblique line — Ulna — Radius — Head of ulna — Styloid process of ulna — Styloid process of radius — Carpal bones — Metacarpal bone — Proximal phalanx — Distal phalanx — Phalanges { (First) Proximal — (Second) Middle — (Third) Distal }

Fig. 48.1 Overview of the bones of the left pectoral girdle and upper limb: anterior view.

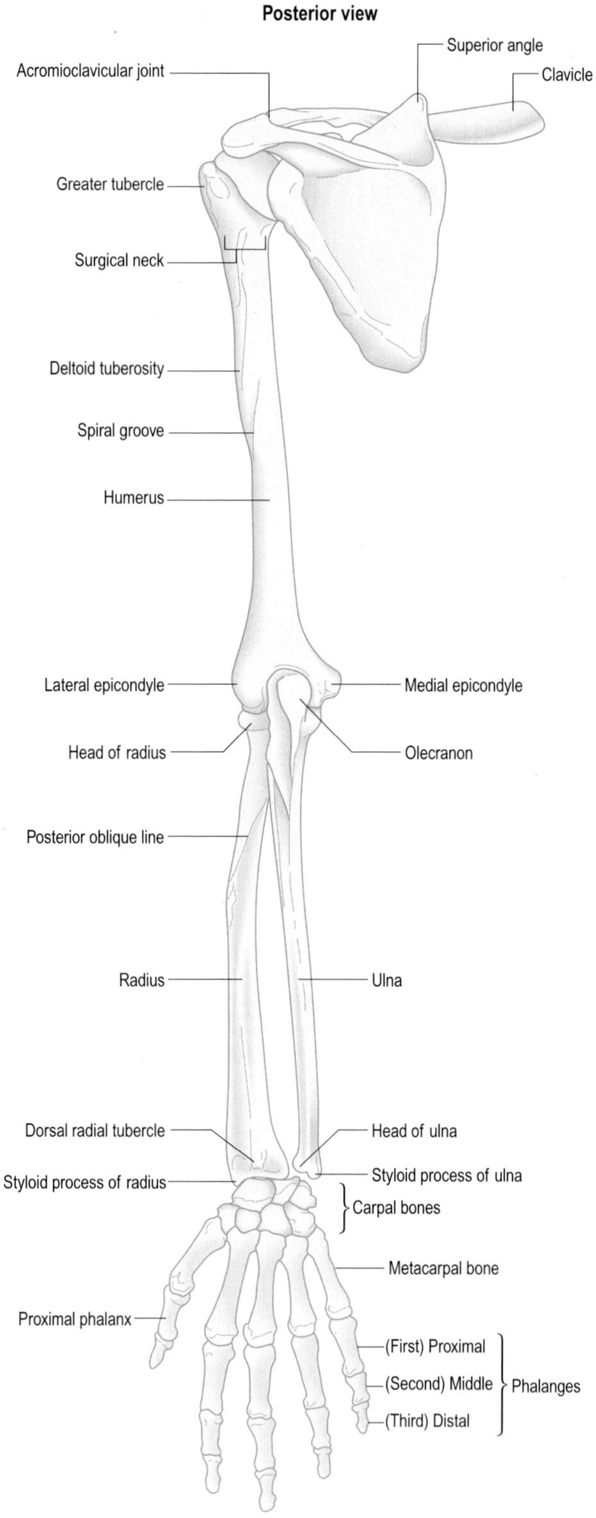

Posterior view

Acromioclavicular joint — Superior angle — Clavicle — Greater tubercle — Surgical neck — Deltoid tuberosity — Spiral groove — Humerus — Lateral epicondyle — Medial epicondyle — Head of radius — Olecranon — Posterior oblique line — Radius — Ulna — Dorsal radial tubercle — Head of ulna — Styloid process of radius — Styloid process of ulna — Carpal bones — Metacarpal bone — Proximal phalanx — Phalanges { (First) Proximal — (Second) Middle — (Third) Distal }

Fig. 48.2 Overview of the bones of the left pectoral girdle and upper limb: posterior view.

axillary artery becomes the brachial artery as it crosses the distal edge of the posterior axillary fold, i.e. at the lower border of teres major. At first, the brachial artery lies on the medial side of the upper arm, in the flexor compartment. It then inclines laterally until it lies anterior to the elbow joint. Just distal to the elbow, it divides into the radial and ulnar arteries, both of which remain in, and supply, the flexor compartment. The ulnar artery quickly gives rise to the common interosseous artery, which divides into anterior and posterior interosseous arteries: these vessels travel towards the wrist on either side of the interosseous membrane (the anterior interosseous artery lying directly on the membrane

and the posterior interosseous artery separated from it by the deep extensor muscles).

The muscles and other components of the extensor aspect are supplied by the profunda brachii artery in the upper arm, and by the posterior interosseous artery in the forearm. The hand is supplied by rich, and somewhat variable, anastomoses between branches of the radial and ulnar arteries, principally on the palmar aspect.

Each upper limb joint is supplied by an extensive anastomosis of arteries fed by descending vessels that arise proximal to the joint and ascending recurrent branches that arise distal to the joint.

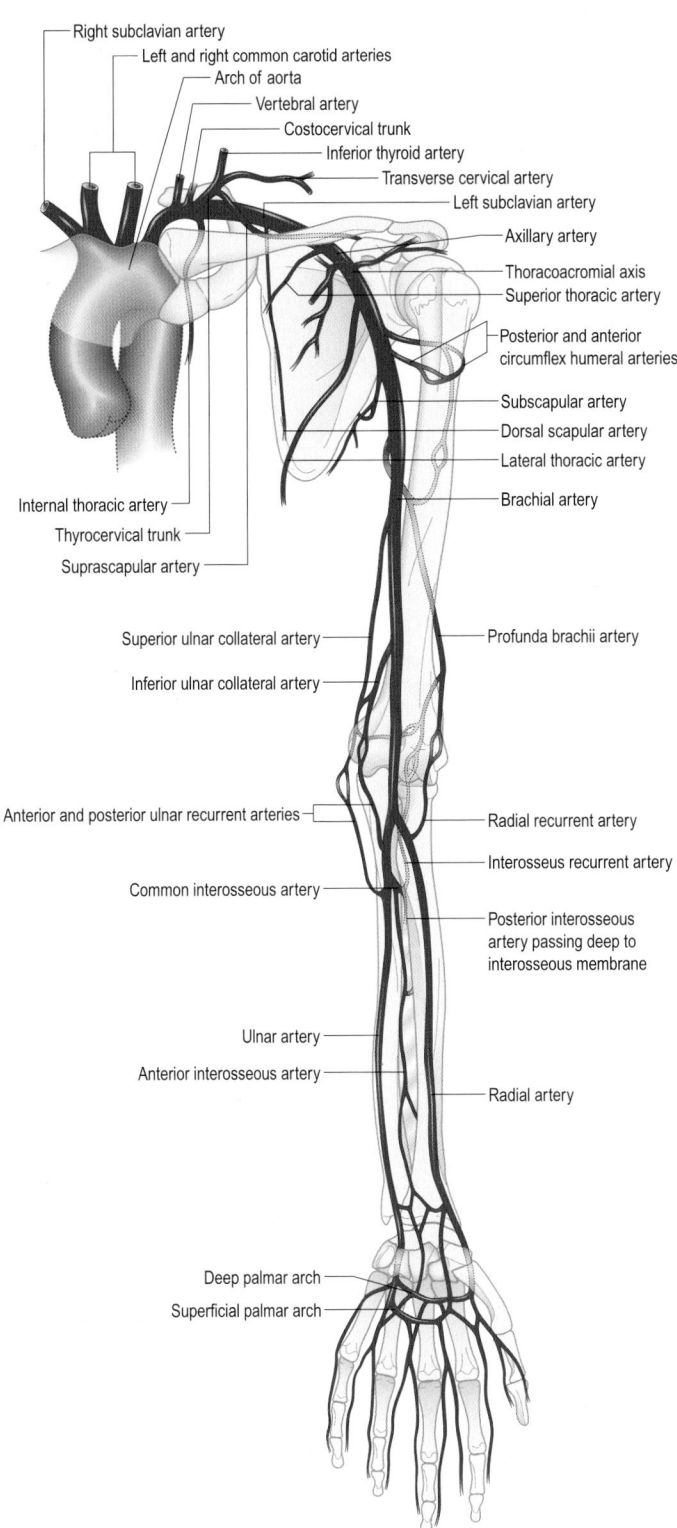

Fig. 48.3 Overview of arteries of the left upper limb.

Right subclavian artery
Left and right common carotid arteries
Arch of aorta
Vertebral artery
Costocervical trunk
Inferior thyroid artery
Transverse cervical artery
Left subclavian artery
Axillary artery
Thoracoacromial axis
Superior thoracic artery
Posterior and anterior circumflex humeral arteries
Subscapular artery
Dorsal scapular artery
Lateral thoracic artery
Brachial artery

Internal thoracic artery
Thyrocervical trunk
Suprascapular artery

Superior ulnar collateral artery
Profunda brachii artery

Inferior ulnar collateral artery

Anterior and posterior ulnar recurrent arteries
Radial recurrent artery
Interosseus recurrent artery

Common interosseous artery

Posterior interosseous artery passing deep to interosseous membrane

Ulnar artery
Anterior interosseous artery

Radial artery

Deep palmar arch
Superficial palmar arch

VENOUS DRAINAGE

The venous drainage of the upper limb is composed of superficial and deep groups of vessels.

The superficial group starts as an irregular dorsal arch on the back of the hand. The pattern of these veins is variable. The cephalic vein begins at the radial extremity of the arch. It ascends along the lateral aspect of the arm within the superficial fascia and then pierces the deep fascia to enter the axillary vein just distal to the clavicle (**Fig. 48.5**).

The basilic vein drains the ulnar end of the arch. It passes along the medial aspect of the forearm, pierces the deep fascia at the elbow and joins the venae comitantes of the brachial artery to form the axillary vein. In front of the elbow, the prominent median cubital vein links the cephalic and basilic veins. It receives a number of tributaries from the front of the forearm and gives off the deep median vein, which pierces the fascial roof of the antecubital fossa to join the venae comitantes of the brachial artery.

The deep veins accompany the arteries, usually as venae comitantes: they become the axillary and then the subclavian vein. They drain the tissues beneath the deep fascia of the upper limb and are connected to the superficial system by perforating veins.

LYMPH NODES AND DRAINAGE

Lymphatic drainage of superficial tissues

Superficial lymphatic vessels begin in cutaneous plexuses. In the hand, the palmar plexus is denser than the dorsal plexus. Digital plexuses drain along the digital borders to their webs; here they join the distal palmar vessels, which pass back to the dorsal aspect of the hand. The proximal palm drains towards the carpus, medially by vessels that run along its ulnar border, and laterally to join vessels draining the thumb. Several vessels from the central palmar plexus form a trunk that winds round the second metacarpal bone to join the dorsal vessels draining the index finger and thumb.

In the forearm and arm, superficial vessels run with the superficial veins. Collecting vessels from the hand pass into the forearm on all carpal aspects. Dorsal vessels, after running proximally in parallel, curve successively round the borders of the limb to join the ventral vessels. Anterior carpal vessels run through the forearm parallel with the median vein of the forearm to the cubital region. They subsequently follow the medial border of biceps brachii then pierce the deep fascia at the anterior axillary fold to end in the lateral axillary lymph nodes (**Fig. 48.6**).

Lymph vessels that lie laterally in the forearm follow the cephalic vein to the level of the deltoid tendon, where most incline medially to reach the lateral axillary nodes; a few continue with the vein and drain into the infraclavicular nodes. They receive vessels that curve round the lateral border from the dorsal aspect of the limb. Vessels lying medially in the forearm follow the basilic vein. Proximal to the elbow some end in supratrochlear lymph nodes whose efferents, together with the medial vessels that have bypassed them, pierce the deep fascia with the basilic vein and end in the lateral axillary nodes or deep lymphatic vessels. They are joined by vessels that curve round the medial border of the limb.

Collecting vessels from the deltoid region pass round the anterior and posterior axillary fold to end in the axillary nodes. The scapular skin drains either to subscapular axillary nodes or by channels following the transverse cervical vessels to the inferior deep cervical nodes.

Lymphatic drainage of deep tissues

Deep lymph vessels follow the main neurovascular bundles (radial, ulnar, interosseous and brachial) to the lateral axillary nodes. They are less numerous than the superficial vessels and communicate with them at intervals. A few lymph nodes occur along the vessels. Scapular muscles drain mainly to the subscapular axillary nodes, and pectoral muscles to the pectoral, central and apical nodes (**Fig. 48.6**).

INNERVATION

AUTONOMIC INNERVATION

The autonomic supply to the limbs is exclusively sympathetic. The preganglionic sympathetic inflow to the upper limb is derived from neurones in the lateral horn of the upper thoracic spinal segments T2–6(7). Fibres pass in white rami communicantes to the thoracic sympathetic chain and synapse in the stellate and second thoracic ganglia. Postganglionic fibres to the skin are distributed via cutaneous branches of the brachial plexus. The blood vessels to the upper limb receive their sympathetic supply via adjacent peripheral nerves, thus the median nerve supplies postganglionic sympathetic fibres to the brachial artery and the palmar arches, and the ulnar nerve supplies the ulnar artery.

OVERVIEW OF THE BRACHIAL PLEXUS (Figs 48.7, 49.30)

The brachial plexus is a union of the ventral rami of the lower four cervical nerves and the greater part of the first thoracic ventral ramus. The fourth ramus usually gives a branch to the fifth, and the first

A

Posterior

Anterior

B

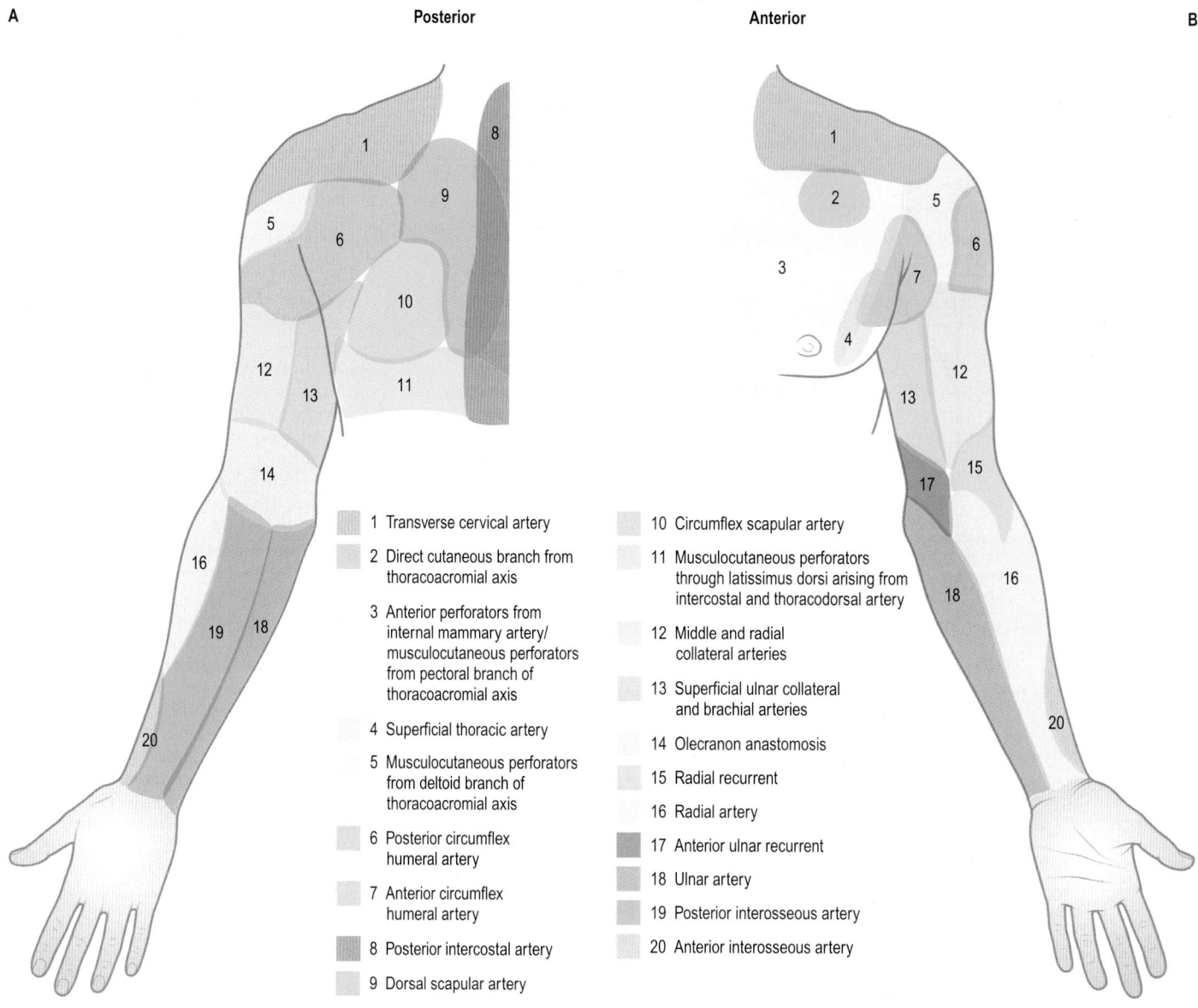

1 Transverse cervical artery

2 Direct cutaneous branch from thoracoacromial axis

3 Anterior perforators from internal mammary artery/ musculocutaneous perforators from pectoral branch of thoracoacromial axis

4 Superficial thoracic artery

5 Musculocutaneous perforators from deltoid branch of thoracoacromial axis

6 Posterior circumflex humeral artery

7 Anterior circumflex humeral artery

8 Posterior intercostal artery

9 Dorsal scapular artery

10 Circumflex scapular artery

11 Musculocutaneous perforators through latissimus dorsi arising from intercostal and thoracodorsal artery

12 Middle and radial collateral arteries

13 Superficial ulnar collateral and brachial arteries

14 Olecranon anastomosis

15 Radial recurrent

16 Radial artery

17 Anterior ulnar recurrent

18 Ulnar artery

19 Posterior interosseous artery

20 Anterior interosseous artery

Fig. 48.4 The anatomical territories served by the cutaneous blood supply to the upper limb.

thoracic frequently receives one from the second. These ventral rami are the roots of the plexus and are almost equal in size but variable in their mode of junction. Contributions to the plexus by C4 and T2 vary. When the branch from C4 is large, that from T2 is frequently absent and the branch from T1 is reduced, forming a 'prefixed' type of plexus. If the branch from C4 is small or absent, the contribution from C5 is reduced but that from T1 is larger and there is always a contribution from T2: this arrangement constitutes a 'postfixed' type of plexus.

Close to their exit from the intervertebral foramina, the fifth and sixth cervical ventral rami receive grey rami communicantes from the middle cervical sympathetic ganglion, and the seventh and eighth receive grey rami from the cervicothoracic ganglion. The first thoracic ventral ramus receives a grey ramus from, and contributes a white ramus to, the cervicothoracic ganglion.

The most common arrangement of the brachial plexus is as follows: the fifth and sixth rami unite at the lateral border of scalenus medius as the upper trunk; the eighth cervical and first thoracic rami join behind scalenus anterior as the lower trunk; the seventh cervical ramus becomes the middle trunk. The three trunks incline laterally, and either just above or behind the clavicle each bifurcates into anterior and posterior divisions. The anterior divisions of the upper and middle trunks form a lateral cord that lies lateral to the axillary artery. The anterior division of the lower trunk descends at first behind and then medial to the

axillary artery and forms the medial cord, which often receives a branch from the seventh cervical ramus. Posterior divisions of all three trunks form the posterior cord, which is at first above and then behind the axillary artery. The posterior division of the lower trunk is much smaller than the others and contains few, if any, fibres from the first thoracic ramus. It is frequently derived from the eighth cervical ramus before the trunk is formed.

OVERVIEW OF THE PRINCIPAL NERVES

Axillary nerve (C5, 6)

The axillary nerve is a branch of the posterior cord of the brachial plexus. It winds posteriorly around the neck of the humerus together with the circumflex humeral vessels and supplies deltoid and teres minor and an area of skin over the deltoid region (**Fig. 48.8**).

Radial nerve (C5–8, T1) (Fig. 48.9)

The radial nerve is the continuation of the posterior cord of the brachial plexus. In the upper arm it lies in the spiral groove of the humerus where it is accompanied by the profunda brachii artery and its venal comitantes. It enters the posterior (extensor) compartment and supplies triceps, then re-enters the anterior compartment of the arm by piercing the lateral intermuscular septum. At the level of the lateral epicondyle

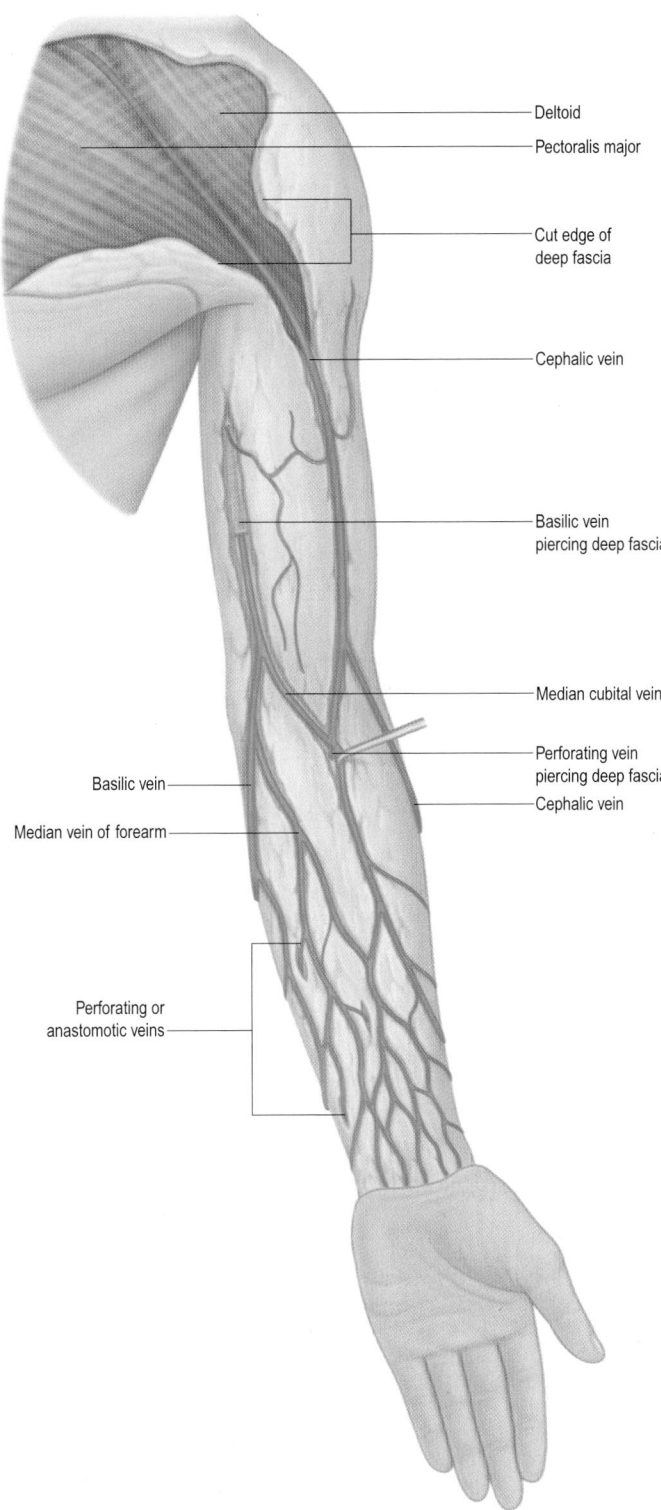

Deltoid

Pectoralis major

Cut edge of
deep fascia

Cephalic vein

Basilic vein
piercing deep fascia

Median cubital vein

Perforating vein
piercing deep fascia

Cephalic vein

Basilic vein

Median vein of forearm

Perforating or
anastomotic veins

Fig. 48.5 Overview of superficial veins of the left upper limb.

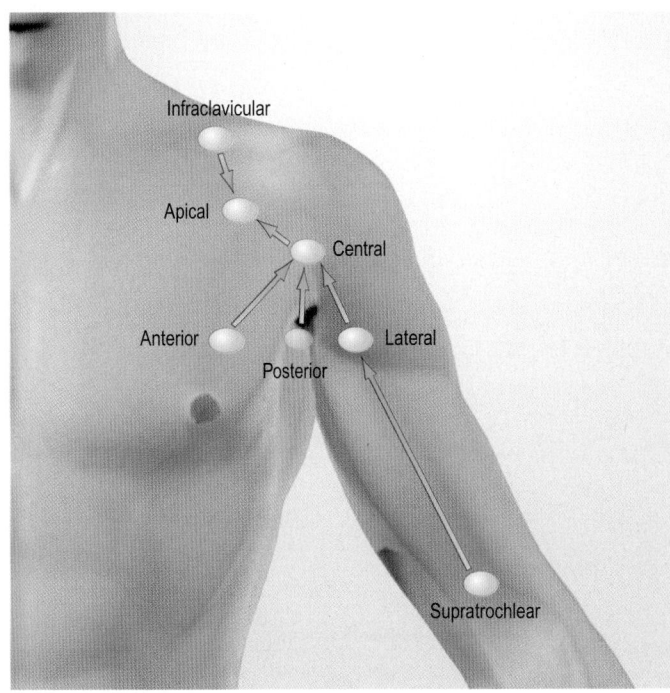

Infraclavicular

Apical

Central

Anterior

Posterior

Lateral

Supratrochlear

Fig. 48.6 Lymph nodes of the left upper limb.

it and biceps and brachialis, and then continues into the forearm as the lateral cutaneous nerve of the forearm (**Fig. 48.10**).

Median nerve (C6–8, T1) (Fig. 48.11)

The median nerve is formed by the union of the terminal branch of the lateral and medial cords of the brachial plexus. It has no branches in the upper arm. It enters the forearm between the two heads of pronator teres and gives off the anterior interosseous nerve, which supplies all the flexor muscles of the forearm apart from flexor carpi ulnaris and the ulnar half of flexor digitorum profundus. The median nerve itself passes deep to the flexor retinaculum at the wrist. On entering the palm, it gives off motor branches to the thenar muscles and the radial two lumbricals and cutaneous branches to the palmar aspect of the thumb, index and middle fingers and the radial half of the ring finger.

Ulnar nerve (C7, C8, T1) (Fig. 48.12)

The ulnar nerve is the continuation of the medial cord of the brachial plexus. Like the median nerve, it has no branches in the upper arm. It enters the posterior compartment of the upper arm midway down its length by piercing the medial intermuscular septum and passes behind the medial epicondyle of the humerus to enter the forearm. It passes to the wrist deep to flexor carpi ulnaris, giving branches to this muscle and to the ulnar half of flexor digitorum profundus. Just proximal to the wrist it gives off a dorsal cutaneous branch that supplies the skin over the dorsal aspect of the little finger and the ulnar half of the ring finger. The ulnar nerve crosses into the palm superficial to the flexor retinaculum in Guyon's canal. It divides into a motor branch, which supplies the hypothenar muscles, the intrinsics (apart from the radial two lumbricals) and adductor pollicis, and cutaneous branches, which supply the skin of the palmar aspect of the little finger and ulnar half of the ring finger.

SURFACE ANATOMY

SURFACE FEATURES AND MARKINGS (Figs 48.13, 48.14, 48.15, 48.16, 48.17, 48.18)

Skin, fascia and soft tissues

Palmar skin is marked by a number of creases, but they are of little value as points of reference. Transverse skin creases cross the palmar aspects of the fingers in three situations. The most proximal crease is placed at the junction of the digit with the palm and lies nearly 2 cm

it gives off the posterior interosseous nerve, which passes between the two heads of supinator and enters the extensor compartment of the forearm. The posterior interosseous nerve supplies these muscles. The radial nerve itself continues into the forearm in the anterior compartment deep to brachioradialis. It terminates by supplying the skin over the posterior aspect of the thumb, index, middle and radial half of the ring finger.

Musculocutaneous nerve (C5–7)

The musculocutaneous nerve is formed from the continuation of the lateral cord of the brachial plexus. It pierces coracobrachialis, supplies

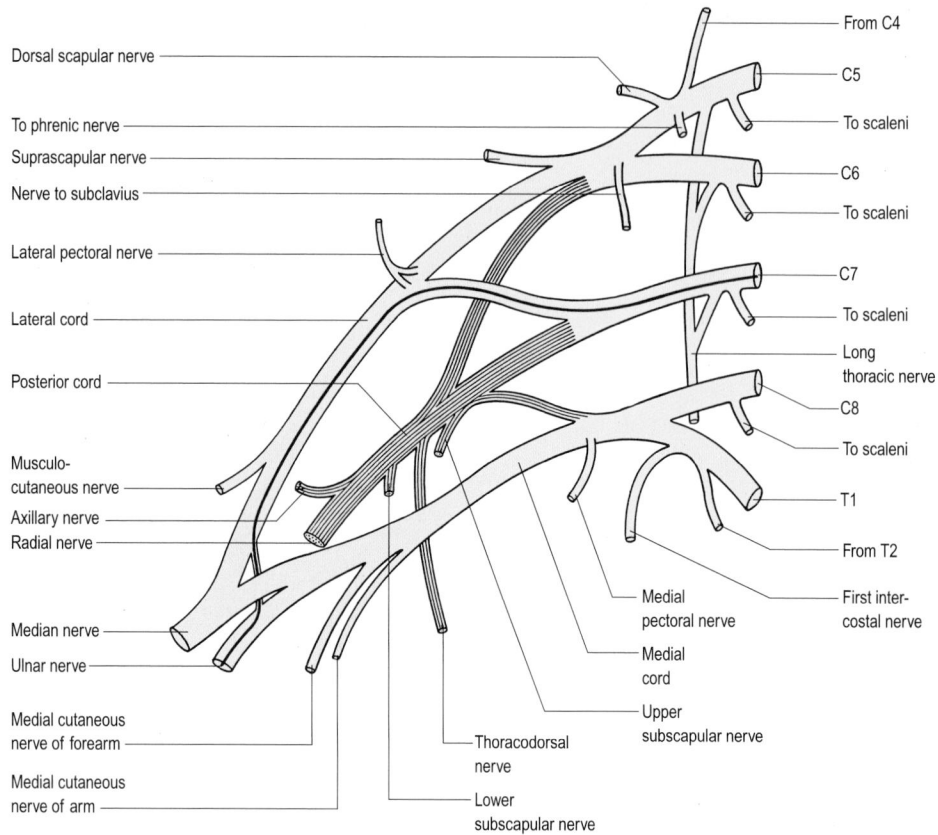

Fig. 48.7 A plan of the brachial plexus. The posterior division of the trunks and their derivatives are shaded; the fibres from C7 that enter the ulnar nerve are shown as a heavy black line. Letters and numbers C4–8 and T1, T2 indicate the ventral rami of these cervical and thoracic spinal nerves.

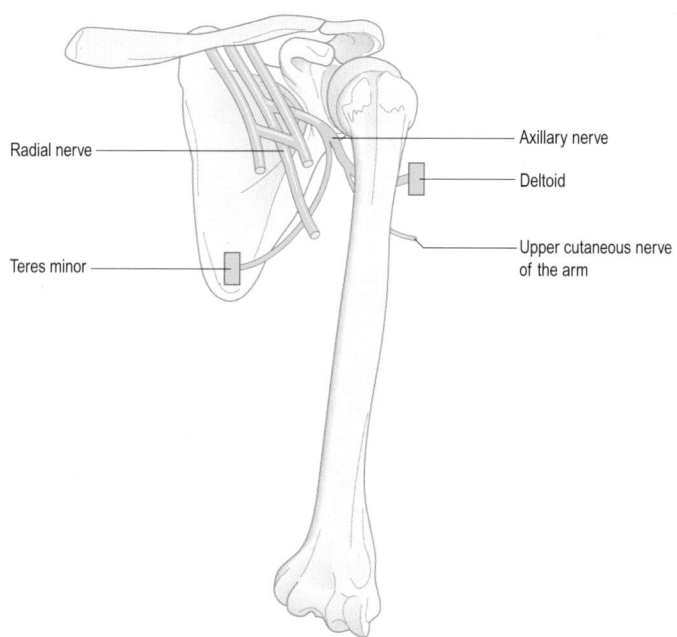

Fig. 48.8 Motor and sensory branches of the axillary nerve. (From Aids to the Examination of the Peripheral Nervous System. 2000. 4th edition. London: Saunders. With permission of Guarantors of Brain.)

of the hamate. Its proximal border may be indicated by a curved line, concave upwards, that joins the tubercle of the scaphoid to the pisiform. Flexion of the wrist produces a number of transverse skin creases (usually two or three) at the wrist. The dominant crease, which is distal, overlies the proximal edge of the flexor retinaculum; the carpal tunnel lies distal to this crease, under the palmar skin.

Bones and joints

The clavicle is both visible and palpable throughout its course. Its outline can be traced from the expanded sternal end, which forms the lateral boundary of the suprasternal notch, to the flattened acromial extremity. The line of the acromioclavicular joint is palpable as a distinct 'step' in an anteroposterior plane. The acromion can be traced from the acromioclavicular joint to its tip, and then backwards across the top of the shoulder until it meets the crest of the spine of the scapula at the prominent acromial angle. From this point, the spine of the scapula can be palpated as it passes medially from the acromial angle to the medial (vertebral) border of the scapula, where it lies opposite the spine of the third thoracic vertebra. The spine is subcutaneous and is easily visible in a thin subject.

The medial border of the scapula is hidden in its upper part by trapezius, but below the spine it can be palpated as it passes downwards to the inferior angle. Although covered by teres major and latissimus dorsi, the inferior angle can easily be felt when it is approached from below, and it can be seen to move laterally and forwards around the chest wall when the arm is raised above the head. The inferior angle of the scapula is at the level of the spine of the seventh thoracic vertebra and overlies the seventh rib. When a thoracotomy is being performed, it is a convenient landmark from which the ribs can be counted along the lateral chest wall.

A small depression can be seen inferior to the clavicle at the junction of its convex medial and concave lateral portions. This is the infraclavicular fossa (or deltopectoral triangle) and it intervenes between the surface elevations produced by the clavicular origins of pectoralis major and the deltoid. The apex of the coracoid process lies 2.5 cm below the clavicle immediately to the lateral side of this fossa, under cover of the

distal to the metacarpophalangeal joint; the intermediate crease lies opposite the proximal interphalangeal joint; and the distal crease is placed just proximal to the distal interphalangeal joint.

The flexor retinaculum may be outlined by defining its bony attachments. Its distal border, concave downwards, may be indicated on the surface by a curved line that joins the crest of the trapezium to the hook

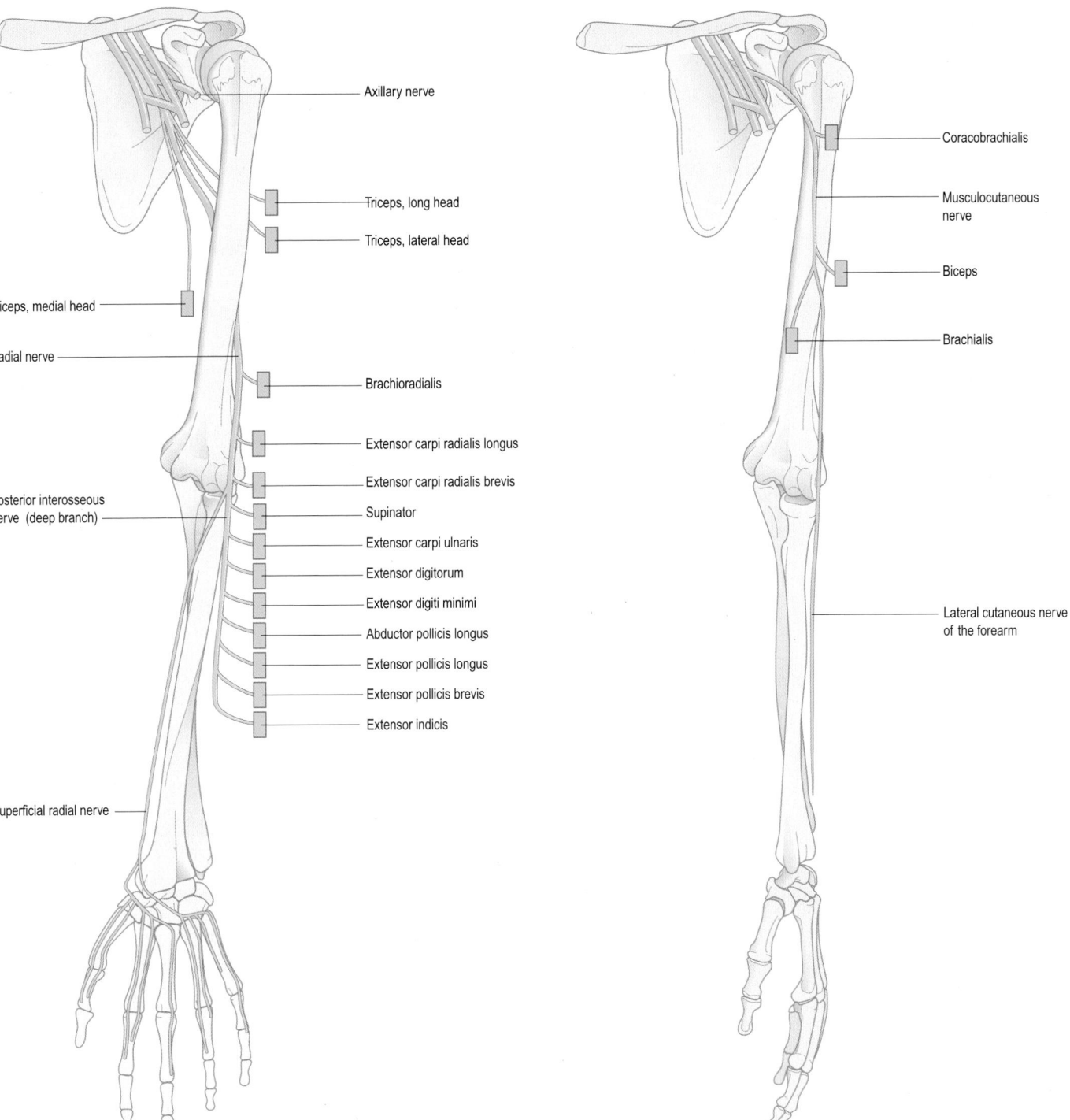

Fig. 48.9 Motor and sensory branches of the radial nerve. Variation exists in a cutaneous innervation of the dorsal aspects of the digits. Here the radial nerve is shown to supply all five digits. The dorsum of the ring and little fingers is frequently innervated by the dorsal branch of the ulnar nerve. (From Aids to the Examination of the Peripheral Nervous System. 2000. 4th edition. London: Saunders. With permission of Guarantors of Brain.)

Fig. 48.10 Motor and sensory branches of the musculocutaneous nerve. (From Aids to the Examination of the Peripheral Nervous System. 2000. 4th edition. London: Saunders. With permission of Guarantors of Brain.)

anterior fibres of deltoid. If the examining finger is passed laterally from the coracoid process, the lesser tubercle of the humerus will be felt below the tip of the acromion on deep pressure through deltoid. This bony prominence slips away from the examining finger when the humerus is rotated laterally or medially. The greater tubercle of the humerus is the most lateral bony point in the shoulder region and projects laterally below and in front of the acromial angle. It can also be felt to move on rotation of the humerus. When the arm is abducted, the head of the humerus can be palpated on deep pressure in the apex of the axilla.

The shaft of the humerus can only be felt indistinctly through its course because its outline is obscured by covering muscles. Distally, the

medial epicondyle of the humerus is a conspicuous landmark and is easily felt, particularly when the elbow is flexed; proximally it can be traced upwards into the medial supracondylar ridge. The ulnar nerve can be rolled from side to side posterior to the base of the medial epicondyle. The lateral epicondyle is not so prominent, but its posterior surface is easily palpated and its lateral margin can be traced upwards into the lateral supracondylar ridge on deep pressure. Inspection of the posterior aspect of the extended elbow reveals a well-marked depression to the lateral side of the midline. This is bounded laterally by the fleshy elevation formed by the superficial group of forearm extensor muscles and medially by the lateral side of the olecranon. The floor of this depression contains, in its upper part, the posterior surface of the lateral epicondyle and, in its lower part, the head of the radius. Although the latter is covered by the anular ligament, it can be felt to rotate when the

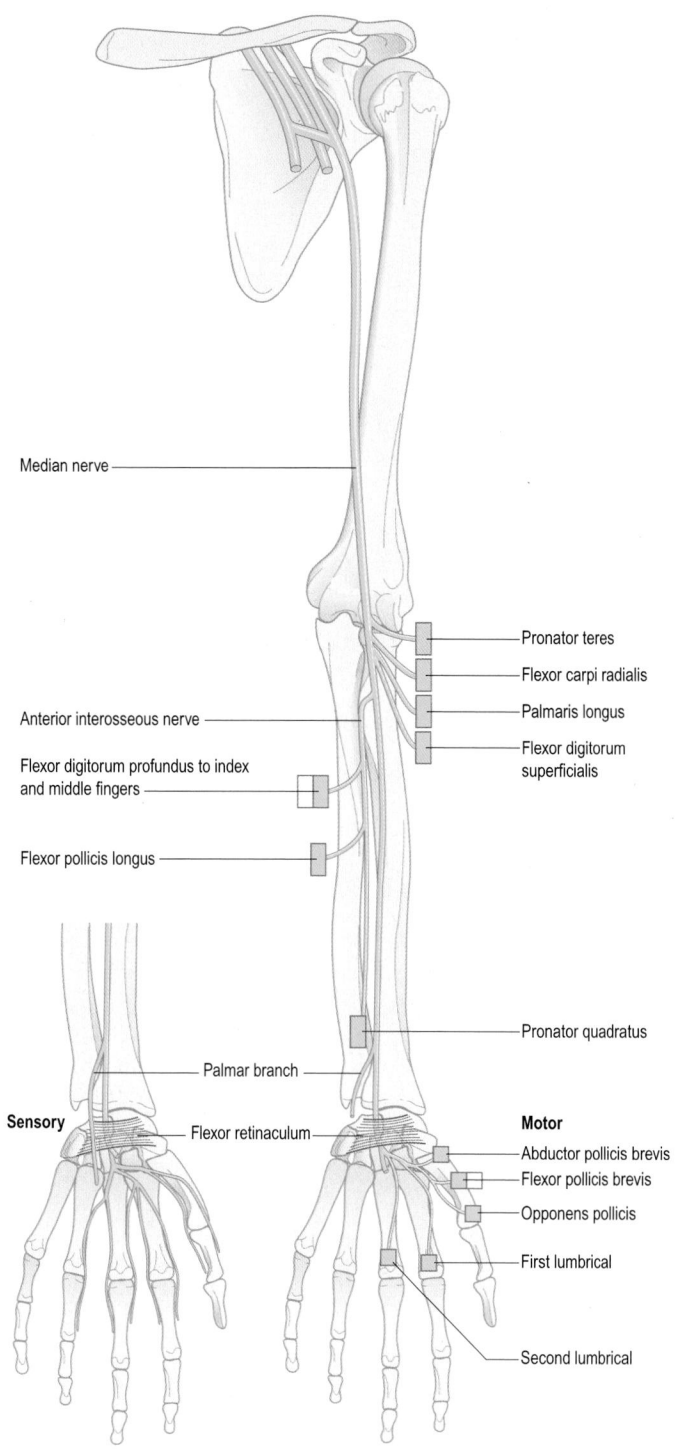

Fig. 48.11 Motor and sensory branches of the median nerve. Flexor digitorum profundus to ring and little fingers are supplied by the ulnar nerve. Flexor pollicis brevis may be supplied by both median nerve and ulnar nerve. (From Aids to the Examination of the Peripheral Nervous System. 2000. 4th edition. London: Saunders. With permission of Guarantors of Brain.)

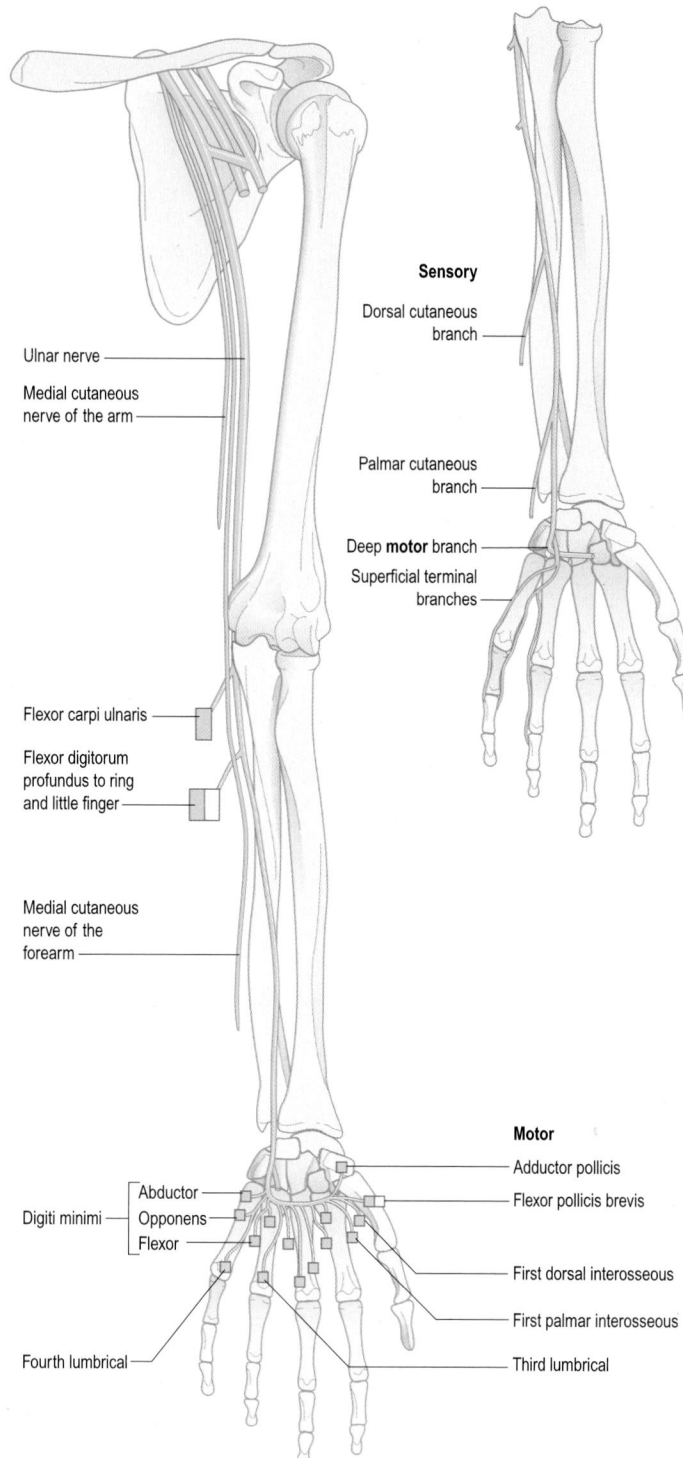

Fig. 48.12 Motor and sensory branches of the ulnar nerve together with the medial cutaneous nerve of the arm and the forearm. Flexor digitorum profundus to index and middle fingers are supplied by the median nerve. Flexor pollicis brevis may be supplied by both median nerve and ulnar nerve. (From Aids to the Examination of the Peripheral Nervous System. 2000. 4th edition. London: Saunders. With permission of Guarantors of Brain.)

forearm is pronated and supinated. Between the lateral epicondyle and the radial head, the humero-radial part of the elbow joint can be felt as a distinct transverse depression.

When the elbow is extended, the apex of the olecranon can be felt and seen to lie in a line level with the two epicondyles. When the elbow is flexed, the apex of the olecranon descends and the three bony points then form the angles of a triangle. This relationship is lost in dislocation of the elbow. The posterior surface of the olecranon is subcutaneous and tapers from above downwards. It can be felt with ease immediately below the apex.

The level of the elbow joint is situated 2 cm below a line joining the two epicondyles. It slopes downwards and medially from its lateral extremity, and this obliquity produces the 'carrying angle'. When the

elbow is fully extended and the forearm and hand are in supination ('the anatomical position'), the carrying angle is c.165° in the female and 175° in the male. It disappears on full flexion of the elbow, when the shafts of the ulna and humerus come to lie in the same plane, and is also obscured in full pronation of the forearm.

The posterior border of the ulna is subcutaneous throughout its whole extent, from the subcutaneous surface of the olecranon superiorly to the styloid process below. Its position corresponds to the longitudinal furrow that can be seen on the posterior aspect of the forearm when the elbow is fully flexed, which separates the flexor group of muscles from the extensors. In contrast, the shaft of the radius can only be felt indistinctly because of its covering of muscles. The rounded head of the ulna forms a surface elevation on the medial part of the posterior aspect of the wrist when the hand is pronated. The styloid process of the ulna projects distally from the posteromedial aspect of the head.

The expanded lower end of the radius forms a slight surface elevation on the lateral side of the wrist and can be traced downwards into the styloid process of the radius. The posterior aspect of the lower end of the radius is partly obscured by the extensor tendons but can be palpated without difficulty. It presents a tubercle (of Lister), which is grooved on its ulnar aspect by the tendon of extensor pollicis longus. The tubercle lies in line with the cleft between the index and the middle fingers.

The wrist joint is easily identified between the carpus and the distal ends of the radius and ulna on flexion and extension of the wrist, even though it is covered by tendons. The line of the wrist joint corresponds to a line, convex upwards, that joins the styloid process of the radius to that of the ulna. It is delineated by the proximal of the two transverse anterior wrist skin creases.

Four of the bones of the carpus can be palpated and identified. The pisiform forms an elevation that can be both seen and felt on the palmar aspect of the wrist at the base of the hypothenar eminence. It can be moved over the articular surface of the triquetrum when the wrist is passively flexed. The hook of the hamate lies 2.5 cm distal to the pisiform and is in line with the ulnar border of the ring finger. It can be felt by deep pressure in this situation, and here the superficial division of the ulnar nerve can be rolled from side to side over the tip of the hook. The tubercle of the scaphoid is situated at the base of the thenar eminence. In many subjects it forms a small visible elevation. Immediately distal to it, but covered by the muscles of the thenar eminence, the crest of the trapezium can be identified on deep pressure. The scaphoid and trapezium can also be palpated in the 'anatomical snuffbox'.

The heads of the metacarpal bones form the prominence of the knuckles, that of the middle finger being the most prominent. Their convex palmar aspects can be felt on deep pressure over the front of the metacarpophalangeal joints and can be gripped between the finger and the thumb. Deep pressure over the distal aspect of the head of the metacarpal bone reveals the base of the corresponding proximal phalanx; the line of the metacarpophalangeal joint can be detected on the dorsum of the hand as the fingers are flexed and extended. The dorsal aspects of the shafts of the metacarpal bones of the fingers and thumb and of the trapezium can be felt rather indistinctly, since they are obscured by the extensor tendons. The interphalangeal joints can be felt on the dorsal aspect of the flexed finger, just distal to the prominences caused by the heads of the proximal and middle phalanges.

Muscles

Deltoid may be delineated when the arm is abducted against resistance, and its tendon can be identified about half-way down the lateral aspect of the humerus. Its anterior border can be traced upwards and medially from the anterior aspect of the humerus, across the tendon of pectoralis major, to form the lateral boundary of the infraclavicular fossa. The posterior border runs upwards and medially from the posterior aspect of the deltoid tendon and reaches the crest of the spine of the scapula

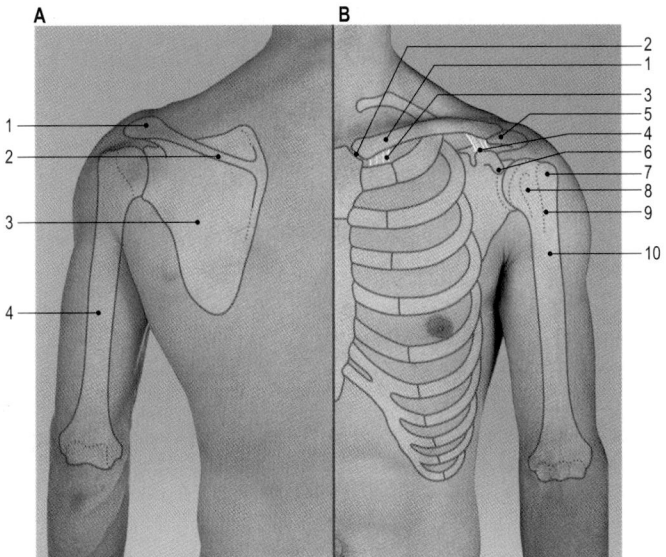

PART A: **1.** Acromion. **2.** Spine of scapula. **3.** Scapula. **4.** Humerus.

PART B: **1.** Clavicle. **2.** Sternoclavicular joint. **3.** Costoclavicular ligament. **4.** Coracoclavicular ligaments. **5.** Acromion. **6.** Coracoid process. **7.** Greater tubercle (tuberosity). **8.** Lesser tubercle (tuberosity). **9.** Bicipital groove. **10.** Humerus.

Fig. 48.13 Posterior (A) and anterior (B) views of the shoulder region. (By permission from Lumley JSP 2002 Surface Anatomy, 3rd edn. Edinburgh: Churchill Livingstone.)

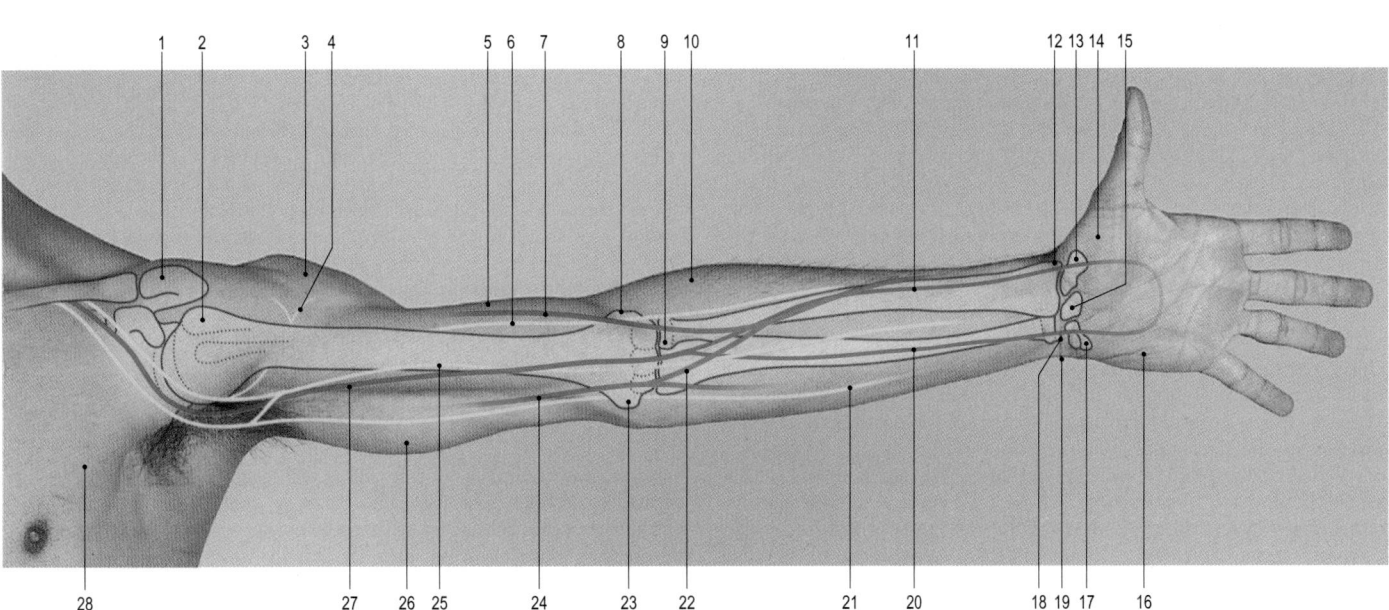

1. Acromion. **2.** Greater tubercle (tuberosity). **3.** Deltoid. **4.** Axillary nerve. **5.** Biceps brachii. **6.** Radial nerve. **7.** Cephalic vein. **8.** Lateral epicondyle. **9.** Head of radius. **10.** Brachioradialis. **11.** Radial artery. **12.** Styloid process of radius. **13.** Scaphoid. **14.** Thenar eminence. **15.** Lunate. **16.** Hypothenar eminence. **17.** Triquetrum. **18.** Styloid process of ulna. **19.** Proximal wrist crease. **20.** Ulnar artery. **21.** Ulnar nerve. **22.** Median cubital vein. **23.** Median epicondyle. **24.** Basilic vein. **25.** Median nerve. **26.** Triceps. **27.** Brachial artery. **28.** Pectoralis major.

Fig. 48.14 Anterior view of the arm abducted at the shoulder. (Photograph by Sarah-Jane Smith.)

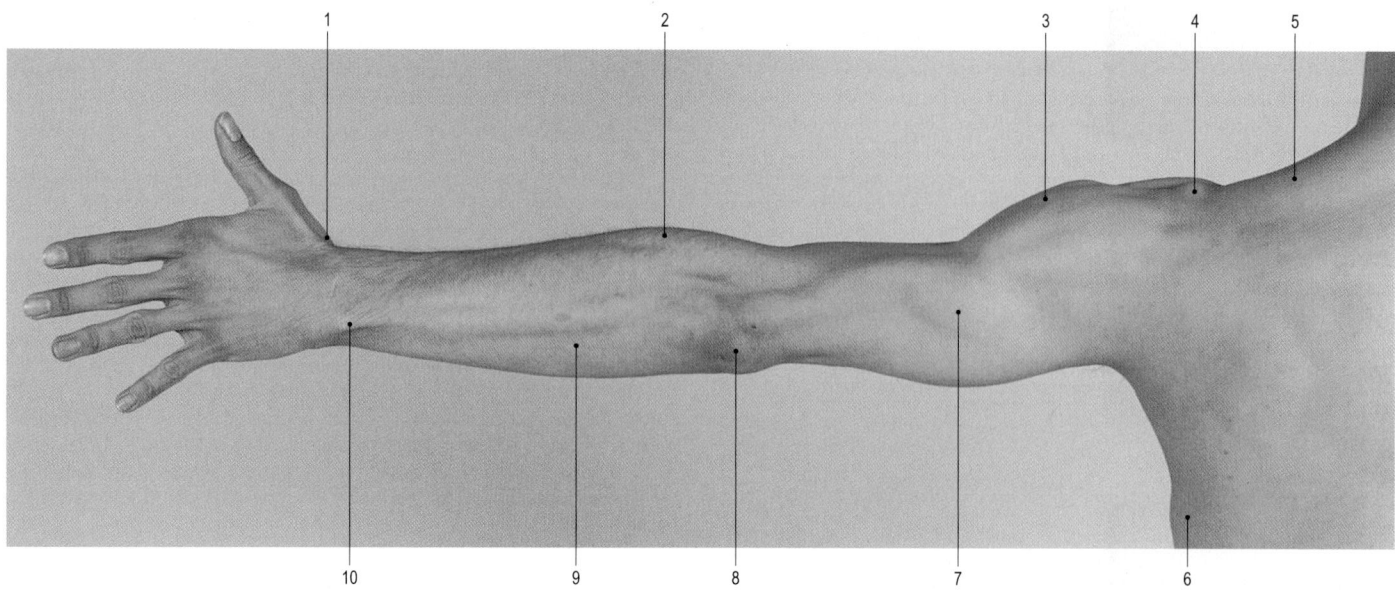

1. Anatomical snuffbox. **2.** Brachioradialis. **3.** Deltoid. **4.** Acromion. **5.** Trapezius. **6.** Latissimus dorsi. **7.** Triceps. **8.** Olecranon process. **9.** Common extensor muscle group.
10. Extensor carpi ulnaris

Fig. 48.15 Posterior view of the arm abducted at the shoulder. (Photograph by Sarah-Jane Smith.)

near its medial end. The normal rounded contour of the shoulder is produced by deltoid, which spreads out over the lateral aspect of the greater tubercle of the humerus. In dislocation of the shoulder, the greater tubercle is displaced medially, deltoid descends vertically to its humeral attachment, and the normal rounded contour of the shoulder is lost.

The rounded lower border of pectoralis major forms the anterior axillary fold. It is rendered more conspicuous when the abducted arm is adducted against resistance, e.g. when the hand is placed on the hip and pressed firmly against the trunk. When the arm is flexed to a right angle against resistance, the clavicular head of the muscle can be felt and seen to contract. When the flexed arm is extended against resistance, the clavicular head becomes relaxed but the sternocostal head stands out in relief.

The posterior fold of the axilla, produced by latissimus dorsi and the underlying teres major, reaches a lower level on the humerus than the anterior fold. Both latissimus dorsi and teres major participate in adduction of the arm: when the abducted arm is adducted against resistance, the posterior fold of the axilla is accentuated and the lateral border of latissimus dorsi can be traced downwards to its attachment to the iliac crest. When the arm is raised above the head, the lower five or six serrations of serratus anterior can be seen on the lateral aspect of the chest; they pass downwards and forwards to interdigitate with the serrations of external oblique. When serratus anterior is paralysed following injury to its nerve, the medial border, and especially the lower angle of the scapula, stand out prominently to produce a characteristic 'winged' appearance that can be accentuated by asking the patient to press both hands against a wall.

The belly of biceps produces a conspicuous elevation on the anterior aspect of the arm. It diminishes above, where it is covered by pectoralis major, and below, where it is replaced by its tendon just above the elbow joint. Shallow furrows indicate its medial and lateral borders. When the elbow is flexed against resistance, biceps becomes still more obvious, and the bicipital tendon can be held between finger and thumb and traced down into the cubital fossa. With the arm held in this position, the sharp upper margin of the bicipital aponeurosis can be traced downwards and medially over the elevation produced by the superficial group of forearm flexor muscles. Coracobrachialis emerges from the lateral wall of the axilla and forms a rounded ridge on the upper part of the medial side of biceps.

Posteriorly, the lateral head of triceps forms an elevation medial and parallel to the posterior border of deltoid and is thrown into prominence when the elbow is extended against resistance. On its medial side, the fleshy mass produced by the long head of triceps disappears above under cover of deltoid.

Brachioradialis is the most superficial of the muscles on the lateral side of the forearm. When the elbow is flexed in the semi-prone position against resistance brachioradialis stands out as a prominent ridge extending upwards beyond the level of the elbow joint on the lateral side of the arm.

Proximal to the wrist crease, the prominent tendon of flexor carpi radialis can be seen and palpated when the wrist is flexed; the radial artery lies on its lateral side. By palpating lateral to flexor carpi radialis, 3 or 4 cm proximal to the wrist crease, it is possible to feel flexor pollicis longus: bending and straightening the thumb will confirm that the examining finger is in the correct place. The area on the ulnar side of flexor carpi radialis is packed most densely with functionally important structures. The median nerve lies very close to the skin surface and is therefore often injured in lacerations. It is covered by palmaris longus, when that muscle is present (best confirmed by pinching thumb and ring finger together, when the muscle will be seen to stand out). When palmaris longus is absent, only a thin covering of subcutaneous fat and deep fascia separates skin and nerve. The four tendons of flexor digitorum superficialis lie deep to the median nerve: the tendons for the middle and ring fingers lie in front of those for the index and little fingers as they pass deep to the flexor retinaculum and can be felt, and usually seen, to move on flexion of the fingers. Deeper still are the tendons of flexor digitorum profundus. The large and robust tendon of flexor carpi ulnaris is easily palpated on the ulnar side of the front of the wrist; the ulnar nerve, artery and venae comitantes lie in the shelter of its radial edge. Any sharp injury powerful enough to cut through this strong tendon usually has enough energy left to cut the nerve and vessel.

When the thumb is fully extended, a depression known as the anatomical snuffbox is seen on the lateral aspect of the wrist, immediately distal to the radial styloid process (**Fig. 48.18**). Palpating distally from the styloid process, three structures are usually encountered: the convex ovoid proximal articular surface of the scaphoid (best felt during alternate ulnar and radial deviation at the wrist); less distinctly, the radial aspect of the trapezium; and the expanded base of the first metacarpal (best felt during circumduction of the thumb). When clinically assessing wrist stability throughout the range of wrist movements, the scaphoid may be effectively compressed (bidigitally, between index finger and thumb) along its oblique long axis between tubercle and articular surface. The trapezium may be similarly compressed between its crest and radial aspect.

The cephalic vein can be seen in the proximal roof of the snuffbox, and the pulsation of the radial artery can be felt in its depth. The snuffbox is bounded on the radial side by the tendons of abductor pollicis longus laterally and extensor pollicis brevis medially; these tendons lie close to each other. The tendon of extensor pollicis longus

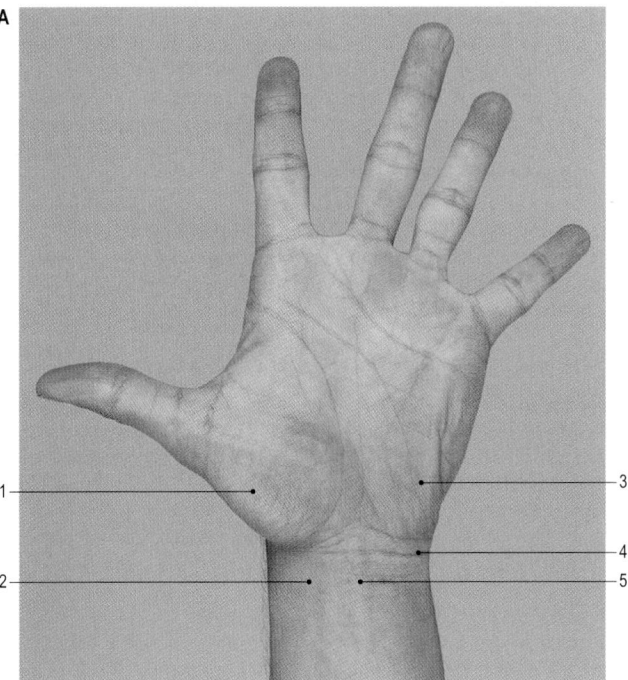

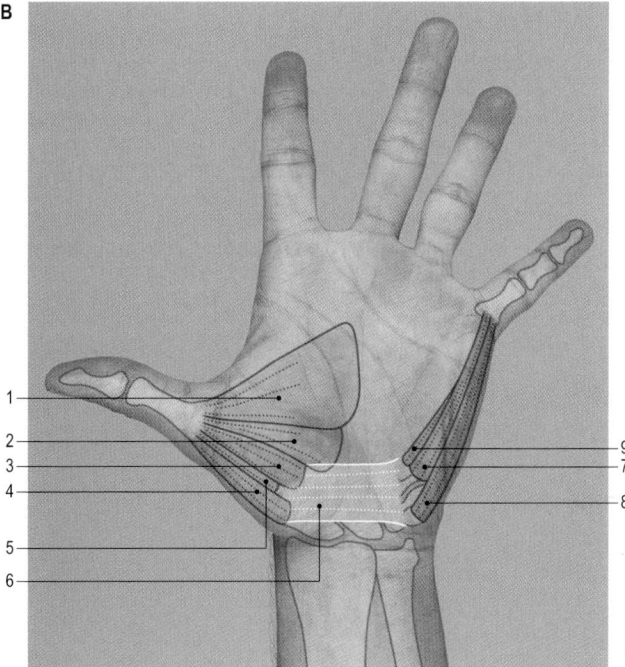

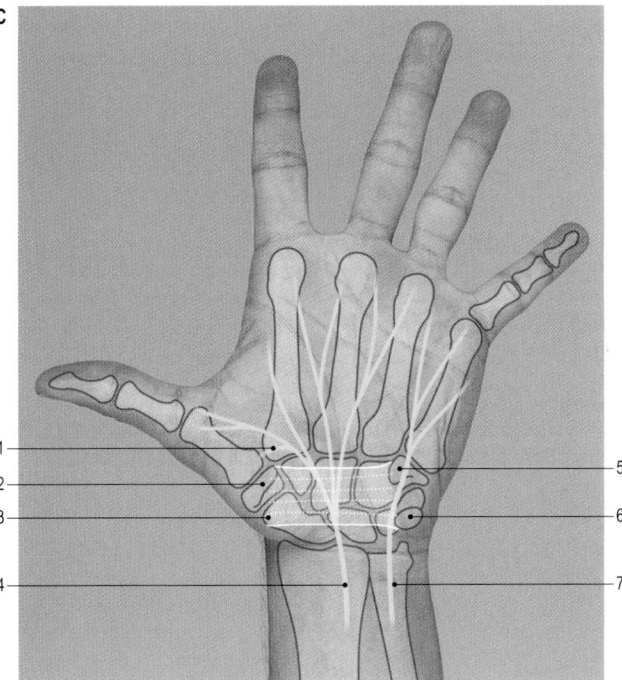

PART A:
1. Thenar eminence.
2. Tendon of flexor carpi radialis.
3. Hypothenar eminence.
4. Proximal skin crease of the wrist.
5. Tendon of palmaris longus

PART B:
1. Adductor pollicis transverse head.
2. Adductor pollicis oblique head.
3. Flexor pollicis brevis.
4. Abductor pollicis brevis.
5. Opponens pollicis.
6. Flexor retinaculum.
7. Flexor digiti minimi.
8. Abductor digiti minimi.
9. Opponens digiti minimi.

PART C:
1. Recurrent branch of median nerve.
2. Ridge of trapezium.
3. Scaphoid tubercle.
4. Median nerve.
5. Hook of hamate.
6. Pisiform bone.
7. Ulnar nerve.

Fig. 48.16 Volar surface of the distal forearm and hand. (Photograph by Sarah-Jane Smith.)

lies on the ulnar side of the snuffbox: it stands out conspicuously in full extension of the thumb, and can be seen to extend to the base of the distal phalanx of the thumb. If a finger is run along this tendon proximally, the superficial radial nerve can be rolled from side to side as it crosses the tendon.

The tendons of the radial extensors of the wrist can be identified on the back of the carpus when the fist is alternately clenched and relaxed. The tendons of extensor digitorum can readily be seen on the back of the hand when the fingers are fully extended. When the wrist is extended and deviated to the ulnar side, the tendon of extensor carpi ulnaris may be felt distal to the ulnar styloid as it crosses the wrist. The lateral part of the dorsal aspect of the hand between the index finger and thumb shows a fleshy elevation caused by the first dorsal interosseous: it becomes more conspicuous when the index finger is abducted against resistance. The corresponding anterior aspect of the first web space is formed by adductor pollicis.

The thenar eminence is a fleshy elevation produced by abductor and flexor pollicis brevis, which overlie opponens pollicis. On the medial side of the palm the hypothenar eminence is formed by the corresponding muscles of the little finger but is not so prominent. The medial border of the hand is formed by the medial aspect of the hypothenar eminence. The lateral border of the hand is formed by the dorsal aspect of the metacarpal bone of the thumb, which can be palpated throughout its extent.

Arteries

By applying pressure laterally against the shaft of the humerus, the pulsation of the brachial artery can be felt in the furrow along the medial side of biceps and, more superiorly, in the depression posterior to coracobrachialis. In its lower part, the artery can be felt adjacent and posteromedial to the tendon of biceps before it disappears deep to the bicipital aponeurosis. Note that the brachial artery lies medial to the humerus in its upper part, but then lies directly in front of the distal end of the shaft of the bone. The proximity of the artery to a bone against which it can be compressed makes this the favoured site for non-invasive measurement of blood pressure. The median nerve is intimately related to the brachial artery throughout its course in the arm. It is at first lateral to the artery, then half-way along the arm the nerve crosses the artery, usually passing in front of it, and descends on its medial side into the cubital fossa.

The ulnar artery begins in the midline of the forearm opposite the neck of the radius. In the upper, and deepest, part of its course through the forearm it can be represented by a line which passes downwards and medially across the elevation produced by the superficial flexor muscles of the forearm to reach the radial side of the ulnar nerve at the junction of the upper one-third with the lower two-thirds of the forearm. In the rest of its course, the ulnar artery lies along the radial side of the ulnar nerve.

The radial artery begins opposite the neck of the radius on the medial side of the tendon of biceps. It runs downwards and radially through the forearm to the wrist, where it crosses the anterior margin of the expanded lower end of the radius, passes posteriorly, deep to the tendons of abductor pollicis longus and extensor pollicis brevis, and enters the anatomical snuffbox where its pulsation can be felt. The upper part of its course can be represented by a line that passes deep to the medial part of the elevation produced by brachioradialis on the anterior aspect of the forearm.

The superficial palmar arch is indicated by a horizontal line c.4 cm long at the level of the fully extended and partially abducted thumb. The deep palmar arch is indicated by a horizontal line c.4 cm long from a point just distal to the hook of the hamate, and is c.1 cm proximal to the superficial arch.

Pulses/palpation/arterial gases

Brachial pulse – The pulsation of the brachial artery can be felt in the furrow along the medial side of biceps and, more superiorly, in the depression posterior to coracobrachialis, by applying pressure laterally against the shaft of the humerus. In its lower part, the artery can be felt adjacent and posteromedial to the tendon of biceps before it disappears deep to the bicipital aponeurosis. This is a useful site at which to pass an arterial catheter for coronary angiography or cardiac catheterization.

Radial pulse – The radial pulse is most easily felt on the ventral aspect of the wrist in the interval between the tendon of flexor carpi radialis medially and the lower lateral aspect of the radius. This is the most accessible pulse for palpation under normal clinical circumstances.

Ulnar pulse – The pulse of the ulnar artery is usually palpable on deep pressure radial to the tendon of flexor carpi ulnaris at the wrist.

Sites for arterial cannulation – The most useful and commonly used site for cannulation of an artery (for blood pressure monitoring and arterial blood sampling) in the upper limb is the radial artery at the wrist. The presence of the palmar arches, which supply a collateral circulation to the hand, means that thrombosis at this site will not normally jeopardize the circulation of the hand.

The deep branch of the ulnar artery supplies the intrinsic muscles of the thumb via the deep palmar anastomosis. Cannulation should be avoided, therefore, if the ulnar artery has previously been damaged. An adequate collateral circulation is demonstrated by Allen's test.

Allen's test – Allen's test examines the patency of the radial and ulnar arteries at the wrist and so determines whether each individual artery is sufficient to maintain the arterial supply to the hand in isolation. Both

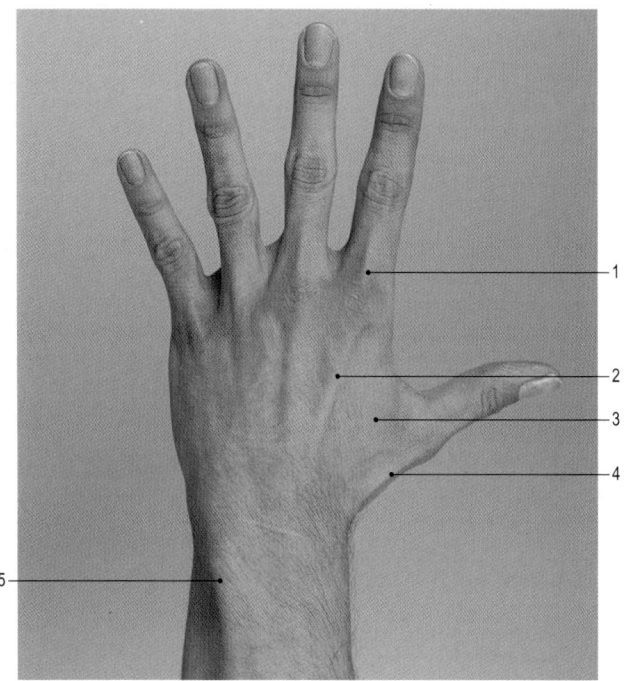

1. Extensor expansion of finger.   2. Tendon of extensor digitorum to index finger.
3. First dorsal interosseous.   4. Tendon of extensor pollicis longus.
5. Tendon of extensor carpi ulnaris.

Fig. 48.17 Dorsal surface of the distal forearm and hand. (Photograph by Sarah-Jane Smith.)

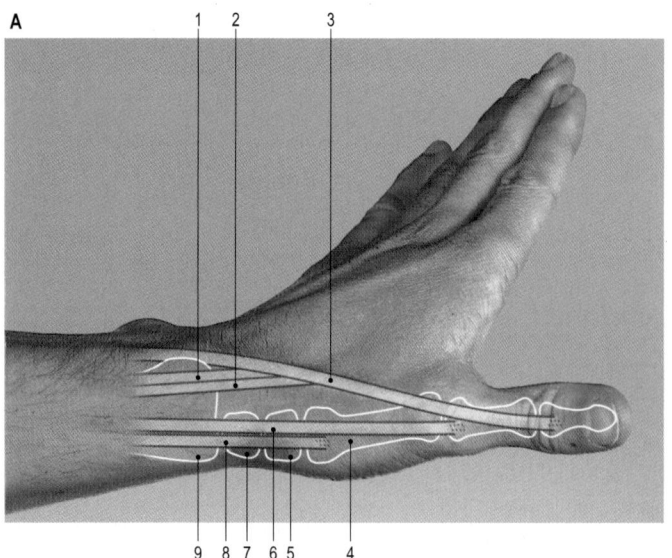

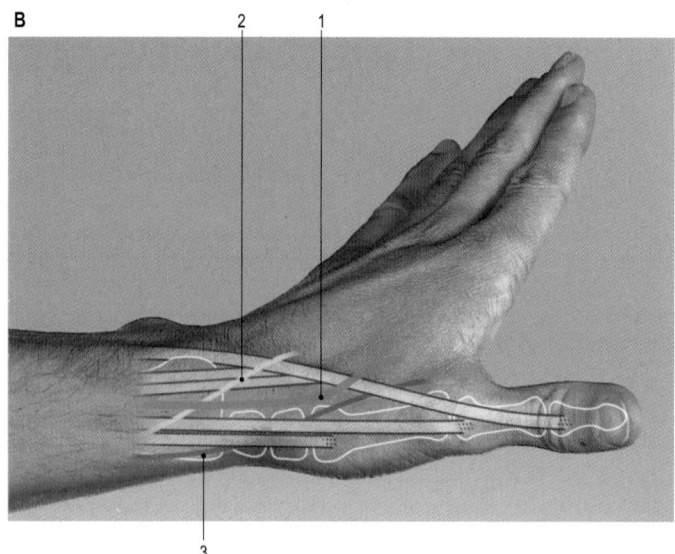

PART A: **1.** Tendon of extensor carpi radialis brevis.   **2.** Tendon of extensor carpi radialis longus.   **3.** Tendon of extensor pollicis longus.   **4.** First metacarpal.   **5.** Trapezium.
   6. Tendon of extensor pollicis brevis.   **7.** Scaphoid.   **8.** Tendon of abductor pollicis longus.   **9.** Radial styloid.
PART B: **1.** Cephalic vein.   **2.** Radial nerve.   **3.** Radial artery.

Fig. 48.18 Radial aspect of the distal forearm and wrist to show the anatomical snuffbox. (By permission from Lumley JSP 2002 Surface Anatomy, 3rd edn. Edinburgh: Churchill Livingstone.)

the radial and ulnar arteries are compressed by the examiner's index and middle fingers of both hands. The forearm is then elevated and the hand exsanguinated by clenching the fist. The hand is then opened while continuing the arterial compression. The palm of the hand appears pale unless there is an anomalous arterial supply, e.g. from a persistent median artery. The brisk return of a normal pink colour to the palmar skin following removal of digital pressure from one of the arteries suggests that that artery is patent and capable of perfusing the hand adequately in isolation. If the palmar skin remains pale, it must be assumed that there is either a distal obstruction to the artery or that this artery cannot adequately perfuse the hand in isolation. The test is then repeated with release of digital pressure on the other artery.

Veins

At the wrist the cephalic vein is situated over the dorsolateral aspect of the lower end of the radius just proximal to the anatomical snuffbox. This is one of the few constantly sited peripheral veins. In the upper arm, the cephalic vein lies in the deltopectoral groove between deltoid and pectoralis major, and then ascends to the infraclavicular fossa, where it pierces the clavipectoral fascia to enter the axillary vein.

The median cubital and basilic veins may be identified in the cubital fossa. They are frequently covered by fat, especially in the female, which makes them difficult to see; however, they are usually palpable, especially if the venous return is occluded proximally by a tourniquet. The median cubital vein usually arises from the cephalic vein c.2.5 cm distal to the lateral epicondyle of the humerus and runs upwards and medially to join the basilic vein 2.5 cm above the transverse crease of the elbow. The median vein of the forearm drains the venous plexuses on the palmar surface of the hand. It ascends on the front of the forearm and usually ends in either the basilic vein or the median cubital vein: sometimes it divides just distal to the elbow into two branches, one of which joins the basilic vein and the other the cephalic vein.

The bicipital aponeurosis is crossed by the median cubital vein, which runs medially and proximally from the cephalic vein to join the basilic vein. It may be distended into prominence by applying gentle constriction to the upper arm.

Venepuncture (elbow)

Median cubital vein – Blood sampling, blood transfusion and intravenous injection are commonly carried out near the elbow or more distally in the forearm: the largest vein is usually the median cubital. The cubital veins are also used for cardiac catheterization.

A high bifurcation of the brachial artery may occur in c.1% of cases. This may produce an anomalous superficial ulnar artery that descends superficial to the common origin of the forearm flexor muscles. When this occurs, the ulnar artery, although deep to the deep fascia, may lie subcutaneously, either at the elbow or in the upper forearm. It is this anomalous ulnar artery, superficial to the bicipital aponeurosis and immediately deep to the median cubital vein, that is at greatest risk of intra-arterial puncture when the median cubital vein is selected for intravenous injection.

The cephalic vein may be accessed where it lies superficial to the distal end of the radius in the anatomical snuffbox. This site has many advantages for placing an indwelling cannula when a lengthy period is contemplated: the position of the arm, forearm and hand are all optimal for this purpose.

Lymph nodes

Outlying supratrochlear nodes (in reality supra-epicondylar nodes) lie next to the basilic vein. If enlarged, they may be palpated along the line of the vein a few centimetres above the elbow joint.

Nerves

The trunks of the brachial plexus lie in the posterior triangle of the neck in the angle between the clavicle and lower posterior border of sternocleidomastoid, where they are palpable through the skin, platysma and deep fascia.

The initial course of the radial nerve may be indicated on the posterior aspect of the arm. It passes laterally from the start of the brachial artery to the junction of the upper and middle thirds of a line between the lateral epicondyle and deltoid tuberosity, and then continues anteriorly as far as the lateral epicondyle, a finger's breadth to the lateral side of the tendon of biceps. From here its course in the forearm can be mapped

out along a line descending vertically to a point on the dorsum of the wrist midway between the head of the ulna and the dorsal tubercle of the radius. The point at which the posterior interosseous nerve winds round the upper end of the radius may be indicated by placing the index finger of the contralateral hand on the dorsal aspect of the head of the radius, and aligning the middle and ring fingers below the index finger. The ring finger then lies over the posterior interosseous nerve. This is an important surgical landmark in making an incision for exposure and removal of a fractured head of radius: the incision should not extend more than a finger's breadth below the head of the radius. The terminal branches of the superficial radial nerve can be palpated in the region of the anatomical snuffbox as they pass over the tendon of extensor pollicis longus.

The median nerve is intimately related to the brachial artery throughout its course in the upper arm. Its course can be marked on the surface by a line from the medial side of the brachial artery in the cubital fossa along the midline of the forearm to the wrist.

The ulnar nerve can be palpated and rolled by the examining fingers as it passes posterior to the medial epicondyle of the humerus. In the forearm its course corresponds to a line drawn from the base of the posterior aspect of the medial epicondyle of the humerus to the radial side of the pisiform and across the hook of the hamate. Deep pressure at these bony landmarks will produce paraesthesia. In the lower part of the forearm the line of the nerve lies along the radial side of the tendon of flexor carpi ulnaris medial to the ulnar artery and its venae comitantes.

Dermatomes (Fig. 48.19)

Our knowledge of the extent of individual dermatomes, especially in the limbs, is largely based on clinical evidence. The dermatomes of the upper limb arise from spinal nerves C5–8 and T1: C7 supplies the central part of the hand. Considerable overlap exists between adjacent dermatomes innervated by nerves derived from consecutive spinal cord segments.

Myotomes

Each spinal nerve originally supplies the musculature derived from its own myotome. Where myotomal derivatives remain entities, they retain their original segmental supply. When derivatives from adjoining myotomes fuse, the resulting muscles do not always retain a nerve supply from each corresponding spinal nerve. Since muscles develop *in situ* in the mesodermal cores of the developing limbs, it is impossible to identify their original segments by a developmental study. Most limb muscles are innervated by neurones from more than one segment of the spinal cord. **Tables 48.1** to **48.4** summarize the predominant segmental origin of the nerve supply for each of the upper limb muscles and for movements taking place at the joints of the upper limb: damage to these segments or to their motor roots results in maximum paralysis.

Reflexes

Biceps jerk (C5, 6) – The elbow is flexed to a right angle and slightly pronated. A finger is placed on the biceps tendon and struck with a percussion hammer: this should elicit flexion and slight supination of the forearm.

Triceps jerk (C6–8) – The arm is supported at the wrist and flexed to a right angle. Triceps is struck with a percussion hammer just proximal to the olecranon: this should elicit extension of the elbow.

Radial jerk (C7, 8) – The radial jerk is a periosteal, not a tendon, reflex. The elbow is flexed to a right angle and the forearm placed in the mid position. The radial styloid is struck with the percussion hammer. This elicits contraction of brachioradialis, which causes flexion of the elbow.

CLINICAL PROCEDURES

NERVE BLOCKS

Brachial plexus block

There are three common approaches to achieve anaesthetic blockade of the brachial plexus – the interscalene, supraclavicular and axillary routes.

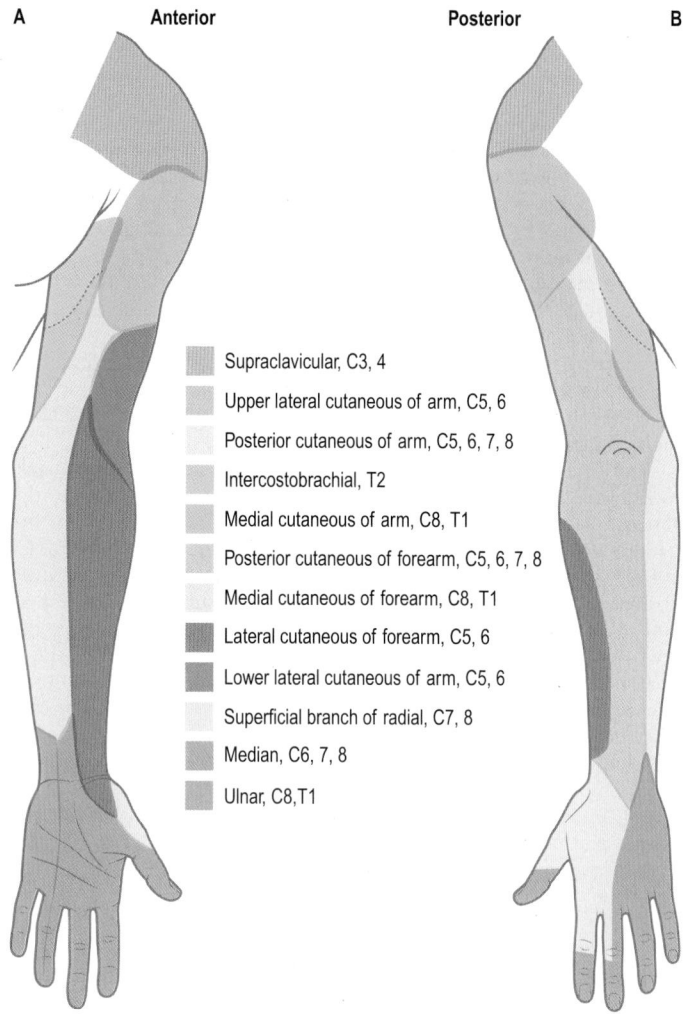

A   Anterior   Posterior   B

Supraclavicular, C3, 4

Upper lateral cutaneous of arm, C5, 6

Posterior cutaneous of arm, C5, 6, 7, 8

Intercostobrachial, T2

Medial cutaneous of arm, C8, T1

Posterior cutaneous of forearm, C5, 6, 7, 8

Medial cutaneous of forearm, C8, T1

Lateral cutaneous of forearm, C5, 6

Lower lateral cutaneous of arm, C5, 6

Superficial branch of radial, C7, 8

Median, C6, 7, 8

Ulnar, C8, T1

Fig. 48.19 The arrangement of dermatomes and cutaneous nerves of the left upper limb. **A**, Viewed from the anterior aspect. The heavy black line represents the ventral axial line: overlap across it is minimal. In marked contrast, overlap is considerable across the interrupted lines. **B**, Viewed from the posterior aspect. The heavy black line represents the dorsal axial line: overlap across this line is minimal. Overlap is considerable across the interrupted lines.

The interscalene route requires identification of the interscalene groove. The patient is asked to sniff, an action that involves the scalene muscles as accessory muscles of respiration. A needle is inserted perpendicular to the skin and enters the interscalene groove. Paraesthesia may be elicited, and local anaesthetic solution is injected. There is a risk that some local anaesthetic may move in a retrograde direction and reach the cervical epidural space. The proximal nature of the block means that there is almost always some involvement of the phrenic nerve, and sympathetic block (as evidenced by a Horner's syndrome) is universal.

The supraclavicular route places local anaesthetic solution in the plane occupied by the trunks of the brachial plexus as they emerge between scalenus anterior and medius on the first rib, immediately posterior to the third part of the subclavian artery. The site of injection is 2 cm above the midpoint of the clavicle. The needle is directed backwards, inwards and downwards to make contact with the upper surface of the first rib. During this procedure the patient will usually complain of paraesthesia down the arm, which indicates that the needle is correctly placed. Preliminary aspiration ensures that a major vessel has not been punctured. If the first rib is missed, there is the risk of producing a pneumothorax. There is often a transient Horner's syndrome, caused by diffusion of the local anaesthetic towards the stellate ganglion.

The axillary approach blocks the nerves as they group around the axillary artery.

Wrist blocks

Useful anaesthesia of the palm of the hand (except for the lateral surface of the thumb base) can be achieved by blockade of the ulnar and median nerves at the wrist. The ulnar nerve may be blocked via a needle inserted lateral to the tendon of flexor carpi ulnaris at the wrist. The median nerve may be blocked via a needle inserted at the midline between the tendons of palmaris longus and flexor carpi radialis at the level of the proximal wrist crease.

The radial nerve, which supplies the dorsal skin of the hand, may be blocked by injecting local anaesthetic around the subcutaneous dorso-radial border of the wrist, where branches of the nerve can be rolled over the tendon of extensor pollicis longus.

Digital nerve block

The digital nerves lie on either side of the flexor sheath in a plane immediately anterior to the phalanx. The needle should be inserted, therefore, on either side of the base of the digit just anterior to the anterolateral margin of the phalanx. A common alternative approach to blocking the digital nerves is via a dorsal skin approach: the needle is inserted through the dorsal skin on either side of the base of the proximal phalanx and advanced towards the volar location of the digital nerves while continually infusing the local anaesthetic agent. This is thought to be less painful than the volar approach because the dorsal skin is less sensitive than the volar skin.

DETERMINATION OF LOCATION OF A LESION

In clinical practice it is only necessary to test a relatively small number of muscles in order to determine the location of a lesion. For example, abduction of the arm might test shoulder abduction, a C5 root lesion, the axillary nerve or deltoid.

Any muscle to be tested must satisfy a number of criteria. It should be visible, so that wasting or fasciculation can be observed and the muscle consistency with contraction can be felt. It should have an isolated action, so that its function can be tested separately. It should help to differentiate between lesions at different levels in the neuraxis and in the peripheral nerve, or between peripheral nerves. It should be tested in such a way that normal can be differentiated from abnormal, so that slight weakness can be detected early with reliability. Some preference should be given to muscles with an easily elicited reflex.

Table 48.4 gives a list of movements and muscles chosen according to these criteria. For example, with an upper motor neurone lesion, shoulder abduction, elbow extension, wrist and finger extension and finger abduction are weaker than their opposing movements. Since this weakness may be more distal than proximal or *vice versa*, normal shoulder abduction and finger abduction excludes an upper motor neurone weakness of the arm. Some muscles are difficult to test but are included for special reasons. For example, the strength of brachioradialis is difficult to assess but it can be seen and felt, it is mostly innervated by the C6 root, and it has an easily elicited reflex.

To determine the root level of a lesion, it is necessary to know an appropriate muscle to test for each root, preferably with an easily elicited reflex.

Knowledge of the sequence in which motor branches leave a peripheral nerve to innervate specific muscles is very helpful in locating the level of the lesion. For example, with radial nerve lesions, if triceps is involved, then the lesion must be high in the axilla. If, as is usual, triceps is spared but brachioradialis, wrist extensors, finger extensors and the superficial radial nerve are all involved, then the lesion is in the arm where the radial nerve is vulnerable to pressure against the humerus. If wrist extension is normal and the superficial radial nerve is not involved but finger extension is weak, then the lesion involves the posterior interosseous branch of the radial nerve.

Table 48.1 Movements, muscles and segmental innervation in the upper limb

Joint	Movement	Muscle	Innervation	C3	C4	C5	C6	C7	C8	T1
SCAPULA	ELEVATION	Upper trapezius	Spinal accessory n.							
		Levator scapulae	Dorsal scapular n.							
	DEPRESSION	Lower trapezius	Spinal accessory n.							
	RETRACTION	Middle trapezius	Spinal accessory n.							
		Rhomboids	Dorsal scapular n.							
SHOULDER	PROTRACTION	Serratus anterior	Long thoracic n.							
	FLEXION	Anterior deltoid	Axillary n.							
		Pectoralis major (clavicular head)	Medial & lateral pectoral nn.							
		Pectoralis major (sternocostal head)	Medial & lateral pectoral nn.							
		Coracobrachialis	Musculocutaneous n.							
	EXTENSION	Posterior deltoid	Axillary n.							
		Infraspinatus	Suprascapular n.							
		Teres minor	Axillary n.							
		Teres major	Lower subscapular n.							
		Latissimus dorsi	Thoracodorsal n.							
	VERTICAL ABDUCTION	Middle deltoid	Axillary n.							
		Supraspinatus	Suprascapular n.							
	VERTICAL ADDUCTION	Pectoralis major (sternocostal head)	Medial & lateral pectoral nn.							
		Latissimus dorsi	Thoracodorsal n.							
		Coracobrachialis	Musculocutaneous n.							
	HORIZONTAL ABDUCTION	Posterior deltoid	Axillary n.							
	HORIZONTAL ADDUCTION	Pectoralis major (clavicular head)	Medial & lateral pectoral nn.							
		Pectoralis minor	Medial & lateral pectoral nn.							
		Anterior deltoid	Axillary n.							
	MEDIAL ROTATION	Subscapularis:								
		Teres major	Brachial plexus							
		Latissimus dorsi	Thoracodorsal n.							
		Anterior deltoid	Axillary n.							
	LATERAL ROTATION	Infraspinatus	Suprascapular n.							
		Teres minor	Axillary n.							
		Posterior deltoid	Axillary n.							
ELBOW	FLEXION	Biceps brachii	Musculocutaneous n.							
		Brachialis	Musculocutaneous & radial nn.							
		Brachioradialis	Radial n.							
	EXTENSION	Triceps	Radial n.							
	SUPINATION	Biceps brachii	Musculocutaneous n.							
		Supinator	Posterior interosseous n.							
	PRONATION	Pronator quadratus	Anterior interosseous n.							
		Pronator teres	Median n.							
WRIST	FLEXION	Flexor carpi radialis	Median n.							
		Palmaris longus	Median n.							
		Flexor carpi ulnaris	Ulnar n.							
	EXTENSION	Extensor carpi radialis longus	Radial n.							
		Extensor carpi radialis brevis	Posterior interosseous n.							
		Extensor carpi ulnaris	Posterior interosseous n.							
	ABDUCTION	Extensor carpi radialis longus	Radial n.							
		Extensor carpi radialis brevis	Posterior interosseous n.							
		Flexor carpi radialis	Median n.							
	ADDUCTION	Extensor carpi ulnaris	Posterior interosseous n.							
		Flexor carpi ulnaris	Ulnar n.							
FINGERS	FLEXION (MP/PIP Joints)	Flexor digitorum superficialis	Median n.							
	FLEXION (DIP Joints)	Flexor digitorum profundus (lateral)	Anterior interosseous n.							
		Flexor digitorum profundus (medial)	Ulnar n.							
		Dorsal interossei	Ulnar n.							
		Palmar interossei	Ulnar n.							
	FLEXION (MP Joint)	Flexor digiti minimi brevis	Ulnar n.							
	EXTENSION (MP/PIP/DIP Joints)	Extensor digitorum	Posterior interosseous n.							
		Extensor indicis	Posterior interosseous n.							
	EXTENSION (MP/PIP/DIP Joints)	Flexor digiti minimi	Posterior interosseous n.							
	EXTENSION (PIP/DIP Joints)	Lumbricals I & II	usu. Median n.							
		Lumbricals III & IV	usu. Ulnar n.							
	ABDUCTION	Dorsal interossei	Ulnar n.							
	ABDUCTION (thumb fixed)	Abductor pollicis brevis	Median n.							
	ABDUCTION	Abductor digiti minimi	Ulnar n.							
	ADDUCTION	Palmar interossei	Ulnar n.							
	OPPOSITION	Opponens digiti minimi	Ulnar n.							
THUMB	FLEXION (IP Joint)	Flexor pollicis longus	Anterior interosseous n.							
	FLEXION/ROTATION (MP Joint)	Flexor pollicis brevis	Median n. and/or ulnar n.							
	EXTENSION (MP Joint)	Extensor pollicis brevis	Posterior interosseous n.							
	EXTENSION (IP Joint)	Extensor pollicis longus	Posterior interosseous n.							
	ABDUCTION	Abductor pollicis longus	Posterior interosseous n.							
	ABDUCTION/ROTATION	Abductor pollicis brevis	Median n.							
	ADDUCTION/ROTATION	Adductor pollicis	Ulnar n.							
	ADDUCTION/FLEXION (MP Joint)	Palmar interosseous I	Ulnar n.							
	OPPOSITION	Opponens pollicis	Median n. and ulnar n.							

Table 48.2 Segmental innervation of the muscles of the upper limb

C3, 4	Trapezius, levator scapulae
C5	Rhomboids, deltoids, supraspinatus, infraspinatus, teres minor, biceps
C6	Serratus anterior, latissimus dorsi, subscapularis, teres major, pectoralis major (clavicular head), biceps, coracobrachialis, brachialis, brachioradialis, supinator, extensor carpi radialis longus
C7	Serratus anterior, latissimus dorsi, pectoralis major (sternal head), pectoralis minor, triceps, pronator teres, flexor carpi radialis, flexor digitorum superficialis, extensor carpi radialis longus, extensor carpi radialis brevis, extensor digitorum, extensor digiti minimi
C8	Pectoralis major (sternal head), pectoralis minor, triceps, flexor digitorum superficialis, flexor digitorum profundus, flexor pollicis longus, pronator quadratus, flexor carpi ulnaris, extensor carpi ulnaris, abductor pollicis longus, extensor pollicis longus, extensor pollicis brevis, extensor indicis, abductor pollicis brevis, flexor pollicis brevis, opponens pollicis
T1	Flexor digitorum profundus, intrinsic muscles of the hand (except abductor pollicis brevis, flexor pollicis brevis, opponens pollicis)

Table 48.3 Segmental innervation of joint movements of the upper limb

Shoulder	Abductors and lateral rotators	C5
	Abductors and medial rotators	C6–8
Elbow	Flexors	C5, 6
	Extensors	C7, 8
Forearm	Supinators	C6
	Pronators	C7, 8
Wrist	Flexors and extensors	C6, 7
Digits	Long flexors and extensors	C7, 8
Hand	Intrinsic muscles	C8, T1

Table 48.1 complements the mainly topographical description of muscles in Chapters 49–53 by bringing together information about the innervation and functions of muscles in the upper limb. To achieve this, some simplification has been necessary. **Movements**. At the central nervous level of control, muscles are not recognized as individual actuators but as components of movement. Muscles may contribute to several types of movement, acting variously as prime movers, antagonists, fixators or synergists. For example, in the movement of the scapula around the thorax, serratus anterior acts as an antagonist of trapezius, but in the forward rotation of the scapula the two muscles combine as prime movers. Moreover, a muscle that crosses two joints can produce more than one movement. Even a muscle that acts across one joint can produce a combination of movements, such as flexion with medial rotation, or extension with adduction. Some muscles have therefore been included in more than one place in the table, but even these listings are not exhaustive. **Nerve roots**. The spinal roots listed as contributing to the innervation of the muscles vary in different texts: this is a reflection of the often unreliable nature of the information available. The most positive identifications have been obtained by electrically stimulating spinal roots and recording the evoked electro-

myographic activity in the muscles. This is, however, a laborious process and data of this quality are in limited supply. Much of the information in the table is based on neurological experience gained in examining the effects of lesions, and some of it is far from new. **Major and minor contributions**. Spinal roots have been given the same shading when they innervate a muscle to a similar extent or when differences in their contribution have not been described. Heavy shading has been used to indicate roots from which there is known to be a dominant contribution. From a clinical viewpoint, some of these roots may be regarded as innervating the muscle almost exclusively: for example, deltoid by C5, brachioradialis by C6, and triceps by C7. Minor contributions have nevertheless been retained in the table in order to increase its utility in other contexts, such as electromyography and comparative anatomy. **Clinical testing**. For diagnostic purposes, it is neither necessary nor possible to test every muscle, and the experienced neurologist can cover every clinical possibility with a much shorter list. Red has been used to highlight those muscles or movements that have diagnostic value. The emphasis in this table is on the differentiation of lesions at different root levels. Other lists may be developed to differentiate lesions at the level of the root, plexus or peripheral nerve, at different sites along the length of a nerve, or between different peripheral nerves. The preferred criteria for including a given muscle in such a list are that it is visible and palpable; that its action is isolated or can be isolated by the examiner; that it is innervated by one peripheral nerve or (predominantly) one root; that it has a clinically elicitable reflex; and that it is useful in differentiating between different nerves, roots or levels of lesion.

Table 48.4 Movements and muscles tested to determine the location of a lesion in the upper limb

Arm movement	Muscle	Upper motor neurone	Root	Relflex	Nerve
Shoulder abduction	Deltoid	++	C5		Axillary
Elbow flexion	Biceps		C5/6	+	Musculocutaneous
	Brachioradialis		C6	+	Radial
Elbow extension	Triceps	+	C7	+	Radial
Radial wrist extensor	Extensor carpi radialis longus	+	C6		Radial
Finger extensors	Extensor digitorum	+	C7	(+)	Posterior interosseous
Finger flexors	Felxor pollicis longus + flexor digitorum profundus Index		C8	+	Anterior interosseous
	Flexor digitorum profundus Ring & little				Ulnar
Finger abduction	First dorsal interosseous	++	T1		Ulnar
	Abductor pollicis brevis		T1		Median

*The muscles listed in the column Upper motor neurone are those which are preferentially affected in upper motor neurone lesions. The root level is the principal supply to a muscle.

Pectoral girdle, shoulder region and axilla

SKIN AND SOFT TISSUE

SKIN

Cutaneous vascular supply

The area over the lateral end of the clavicle is supplied by the supra-clavicular artery which pierces the deep fascia superior to the clavicle and anterior to trapezius (**Fig. 50.1**). In the majority of cases this artery arises from the superficial cervical/transverse cervical artery, but it occasionally arises from the suprascapular artery. The area over the deltoid is supplied by the anterior and posterior circumflex humeral arteries. The deltoid branch of the thoraco-acromial axis contributes to the blood supply of the anterior aspect of the shoulder via musculocutaneous perforators through deltoid. For details of the cutaneous supply to the anterior, lateral and posterior chest wall see page 951.

Cutaneous innervation

The segmental supply is described in Chapter 48, page 813. The cutaneous supply to the shoulder region comes from the supraclavicular nerves (p. 555) (**Fig. 48.18**). The floor of the axilla together with part of the upper medial aspect of the arm is supplied by the intercostobrachial nerve (lateral branch of the second intercostal nerve). Occasionally the lateral branch of the third intercostal nerve contributes to the supply of skin in the floor of the axilla. The upper lateral cutaneous nerve of the arm supplies the skin over the inferolateral part of the shoulder.

SOFT TISSUE

Deep fascia

Fascia over deltoid – The deep fascia over deltoid sends numerous septa between its fasciculi and is continuous with the pectoral fascia in front and the thick and strong infraspinous fascia behind. Above it is attached to the clavicle, acromion and crest of the scapular spine; below it is continuous with the brachial fascia.

Subscapular fascia – The subscapular fascia is a thin aponeurosis attached to the entire circumference of the subscapular fossa; subscapularis itself is partly attached to its deep surface.

Supraspinous fascia – The supraspinous fascia completes the osseo-fibrous compartment in which supraspinatus is attached. It is thick medially, but thinner laterally under the coraco-acromial ligament. It is attached to the scapula around the boundaries of the attachment of supraspinatus.

Infraspinous fascia – The infraspinous fascia covers infraspinatus and is attached to the margins of the infraspinous fossa. The fascia is continuous with the deltoid fascia along the overlapping posterior border of deltoid.

Pectoral and axillary fascia – The pectoral fascia is a thin lamina which covers pectoralis major and extends between its fasciculi. It is attached medially to the sternum, above to the clavicle and is continuous infero-laterally with the fascia of the shoulder, axilla and thorax. Although thin over pectoralis major, it is thicker between this muscle and latissimus dorsi, and forms the floor of the axilla as the axillary fascia. The latter divides at the lateral margin of latissimus dorsi into two layers, which ensheathe the muscle and are attached behind to the spines of the thoracic vertebrae. As the fascia leaves the lower edge of pectoralis major to cross the axilla, a layer ascends under cover of the muscle and

splits to envelop pectoralis minor: it becomes the clavipectoral fascia at the upper edge of pectoralis minor. The hollow of the armpit is produced mainly by the action of this fascia in tethering the skin to the floor of the axilla, and it is sometimes referred to as the suspensory ligament of the axilla. The axillary fascia is pierced by the tail of the breast (Ch. 58).

Clavipectoral fascia – The clavipectoral fascia is a strong fibrous sheet behind the clavicular part of pectoralis major. It fills the gap between pectoralis minor and subclavius, and covers the axillary vessels and nerves. It splits around subclavius and is attached to the clavicle both anterior and posterior to the groove for subclavius. The posterior layer fuses with the deep cervical fascia which connects omohyoid to the clavicle and with the sheath of the axillary vessels. Medially it blends with the fascia over the first two intercostal spaces and is attached to the first rib, medial to subclavius. Laterally, it is thick and dense, and is attached to the coracoid process, blending with the coracoclavicular ligament. Between the first rib and coracoid process the fascia often thickens to form a band, the costocoracoid ligament. Below this the fascia becomes thin, splits around pectoralis minor and descends to blend with the axillary fascia and laterally with the fascia over the short head of biceps. The cephalic vein, thoraco-acromial artery and vein, and lateral pectoral nerve pass through the fascia.

Spread of infection

When axillary suppuration occurs the local fascial arrangement affects the spread of pus. Suppuration may be superficial or deep to the clavipectoral fascia, either between the pectoral muscles or behind pectoralis minor. In the former, an abscess would appear at the edge of the anterior axillary fold or the groove between deltoid and pectoralis major; in the latter, pus would tend to surround vessels and nerves and ascend into the neck, the direction of least resistance. Pus may also track along vessels into the arm. When an axillary abscess is incised, the knife should enter the axillary 'base', midway between the anterior and posterior margins and near the thoracic side to avoid the lateral thoracic, subscapular and axillary vessels on the anterior, posterior and lateral walls respectively.

BONE

CLAVICLE

The clavicle lies almost horizontally at the root of the neck and is subcutaneous throughout its whole extent (**Fig. 49.1**). It acts as a prop which braces back the shoulder and enables the limb to swing clear of the trunk and transmits part of the weight of the limb to the axial skeleton. The lateral or acromial end of the bone is flattened and articulates with the medial side of the acromion, whereas the medial or sternal end is enlarged and articulates with the clavicular notch of the manubrium sterni and first costal cartilage. The shaft is gently curved and in shape resembles the italic letter *f*, being convex forwards in its medial two-thirds and concave forwards in its lateral third. The inferior aspect of the intermediate third is grooved in its long axis. The clavicle is trabecular internally, with a shell of much thicker compact bone in its shaft. Although elongated, the clavicle is unlike typical long bones in that it usually has no medullary cavity.

The female clavicle is shorter, thinner, less curved and smoother, and its acromial end is carried lower than the sternal in comparison with the male. In males the acromial end is on a level with, or slightly higher than, the sternal end when the arm is pendent. Midshaft circumference

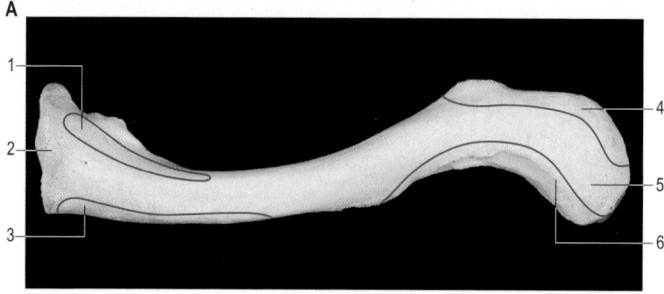

1. Sternocleidomastoid (clavicular head). 2. Sternal end. 3. Pectoralis major. 4. Trapezius. 5. Acromial end. 6. Deltoid.

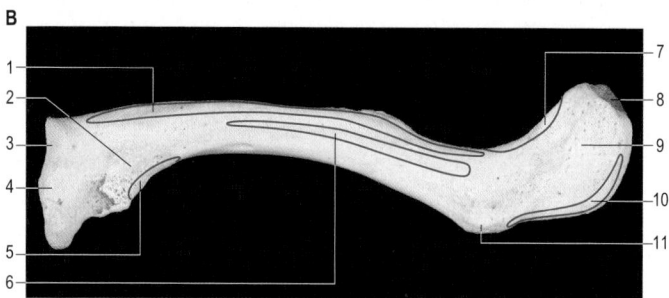

1. Pectoralis major. 2. For costoclavicular ligament. 3. For first costal cartilage. 4. For sternum. 5. Sternohyoid. 6. Subclavius. 7. Deltoid. 8. For acromion. 9. Trapezoid line. 10. Trapezius. 11. Conoid tubercle.

Fig. 49.1 A, Superior view of left clavicle **B,** Inferior view of left clavicle. (Photographs by Sarah-Jane Smith.)

is the most reliable single indicator of sex: a combination of this measurement with weight and length yields better results. The clavicle is thicker and more curved in manual workers, and its ridges for muscular attachment are better marked.

Lateral third

The lateral third of the clavicle is flattened and has a superior and an inferior surface, limited by an anterior and a posterior border. The anterior border is concave, thin and roughened and may be marked by a small deltoid tubercle.

The posterior border, also roughened by muscular attachments, is convex backwards. The superior surface is roughened near its margins but is smooth centrally, where it can be felt through the skin. The inferior surface presents two obvious markings. Close to the posterior border, at the junction of the lateral fourth with the rest of the bone, there is a prominent conoid tubercle which gives attachment to the conoid part of the coracoclavicular ligament. A narrow, roughened strip, the trapezoid line, runs forwards and laterally from the lateral side of this tubercle, almost as far as the acromial end (**Fig. 49.1B**). The trapezoid part of the coracoclavicular ligament is attached to it. A small oval articular facet, for articulation with the medial aspect of the acromion, faces laterally and slightly downwards at the lateral end of the shaft.

Subclavius lies in a groove on the inferior surface (**Fig. 49.1B**). The clavipectoral fascia is attached to the edges of the groove; the posterior edge of the groove runs to the conoid tubercle, where fascia and conoid ligament merge. Lateral to the groove there is a laterally inclined nutrient foramen. Deltoid (anterior) and trapezius (posterior) are attached to the lateral third of the shaft: both muscles reach the superior surface. The coracoclavicular ligament, which is attached to the conoid tubercle and trapezoid line (**Fig. 49.1A**), transmits the weight of the upper limb to the clavicle, counteracted by trapezius which supports its lateral part. From the conoid tubercle this weight is transmitted through the medial two-thirds of the shaft to the axial skeleton.

The clavicle is often fractured, commonly by indirect forces, as a result of a violent impact to the hand or shoulder. The break is usually at the junction of the lateral and intermediate thirds, where the curvature changes, for this is the weakest part of the bone. A fracture medial to the conoid tubercle interrupts weight transmission from the arm to the

axial skeleton. The resulting deformity is caused by the weight of the arm, which acts on the lateral fragment through the coracoclavicular ligament and draws it downwards. The medial fragment, as a rule, is a little displaced.

Medial two-thirds

The medial two-thirds of the shaft of the clavicle is cylindrical or prismoid in form and possesses four surfaces, but the inferior surface is often reduced to a mere ridge. The anterior surface is roughened over most of its extent but it is smooth and rounded at its lateral end, where it forms the upper boundary of the infraclavicular fossa. The upper surface is roughened in its medial part and smooth at its lateral end. The posterior surface is smooth and featureless. The inferior surface is marked, near the sternal end, by a roughened oval impression, which is often depressed below the surface. Its margins give attachment to the costoclavicular ligament, which connects the clavicle to the upper surface of the first rib and its cartilage. Rarely, this area is smooth or raised to form an eminence which may articulate with the upper surface of the first rib by means of a synovial joint. There is a groove in the long axis of the bone in the lateral half of the posterior surface.

The medial two-thirds provide attachment, anteriorly, for the clavicular head of pectoralis major: the area is usually clearly indicated on the bone. The clavicular head of sternocleidomastoid is attached to the medial half of the superior surface, but the marking on the bone is not very conspicuous. The smooth, posterior surface is devoid of muscular attachments except at its lower part immediately adjoining the sternal end, where the lateral fibres of sternohyoid are attached. Medially, this surface is related to the lower end of the internal jugular vein (from which it is separated by sternohyoid), the termination of the subclavian vein, and the start of the brachiocephalic vein. More laterally, it arches in front of the trunks of the brachial plexus and the third part of the subclavian artery. The suprascapular vessels are related to the upper part of this surface. The inferior surface gives insertion to subclavius in the subclavian groove: the clavipectoral fascia, which encloses subclavius, is attached to the edges of the groove. The posterior lip of the groove runs into the conoid tubercle and carries the fascia into continuity with the conoid ligament. A nutrient foramen is found in the lateral end of the groove, running in a lateral direction: the nutrient artery is derived from the suprascapular artery. The impression for the costoclavicular ligament is very variable in its character.

Sternal end

The sternal end of the clavicle is directed medially, and a little downwards and forwards, to articulate with the clavicular notch of the manubrium sterni. The sternal surface, usually irregular and pitted, is quadrangular (sometimes triangular). Its uppermost part is slightly roughened for attachment of the interclavicular ligament, sternoclavicular capsule and articular disc. Elsewhere the surface is smooth and articular and it extends onto the inferior surface for a short distance, where it articulates with the first costal cartilage. The sternal end of the clavicle projects upwards beyond the manubrium sterni and can be felt without difficulty and usually seen (a prominent clinical landmark), in the lateral wall of the jugular fossa.

Ossification

The clavicle begins to ossify before any other bone in the body, and is ossified from three centres. The shaft of the bone is ossified in condensed mesenchyme from two primary centres, medial and lateral, which appear between the fifth and sixth weeks of intrauterine life, and fuse about the forty-fifth day. Cartilage then develops at both ends of the clavicle. The medial cartilaginous mass contributes more to growth in length than does the lateral mass: the two centres of ossification meet between the middle and lateral thirds of the clavicle. A secondary centre for the sternal end appears in late teens, or even early twenties, usually 2 years earlier in females (**Fig. 49.2**). Fusion is probably rapid but reliable data are lacking. An acromial secondary centre sometimes develops at c.18 to 20 years, but this epiphysis is always small and rudimentary and rapidly joins the shaft.

The clavicle does not ossify exclusively by intramembranous ossification. In 14 mm embryos the clavicle is a band of condensed mesenchyme between the acromion and apex of the first rib, which is continuous with the sternal rudiment. Medial and lateral zones of early cartilage transformation ('precartilage') occur within this band, and intramembranous centres of ossification appear, and soon fuse, in the

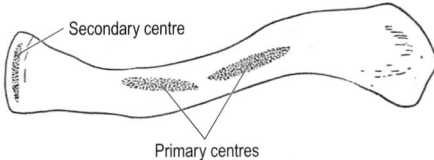

Fig. 49.2 Diagram showing the three constant centres of ossification of the clavicle.

mesenchyme between them. Sternal and acromial zones soon become true cartilage into which ossification extends from the shaft. Length increases by interstitial growth of these terminal cartilages; the latter develop zones of hypertrophy, calcification and advancing endochondral ossification like other growth cartilages. Diameter increases by sub-perichondral deposition in the extremities and subperiosteal deposition in the shaft. Epiphyses are endochondral and probably fuse in the same way as they do in long bones. Defects of ossification in the clavicle and those cranial bones which ossify by intramembranous ossification occasionally coincide e.g. in cleidocranial dysostosis.

SCAPULA

The scapula is a large, flat, triangular bone which lies on the postero-lateral aspect of the chest wall, covering parts of the second to seventh ribs (**Figs 49.3, 49.4, 49.5, 49.6**). It has costal and dorsal surfaces, superior, lateral and medial borders, inferior, superior and lateral angles, and three processes, the spine, its continuation the acromion and the

coracoid process. The lateral angle is truncated and bears the glenoid cavity for articulation with the head of the humerus. This part of the bone may be regarded as the head, and it is connected to the plate-like body by an inconspicuous neck. The long axis of the scapula is nearly vertical and the relatively featureless costal surface can easily be distinguished from the dorsal surface, which is interrupted by the shelf-like projection of the spine (**Fig. 49.3**). The bone is very much thickened in the immediate neighbourhood of the lateral border, which runs from the inferior angle below, to the glenoid cavity above. The main processes, and thicker parts of the scapula, contain trabecular bone; the rest consists of a thin layer of compact bone. The central supraspinous fossa and the greater part of the infraspinous fossa are thin and even translucent; occasionally the bone in them is deficient, and the gaps are filled by fibrous tissue.

The inferior angle lies over the seventh rib, or over the seventh intercostal space. It can be felt through the skin and the muscles which cover it and, when the arm is raised above the head, it can be seen to pass forwards round the chest wall. The superior angle is placed at the junction of the superior and medial borders, and is obscured by the muscles which cover it. The lateral angle is truncated and broadened. It constitutes the head of the bone. On its free surface it bears the glenoid cavity for articulation with the head of the humerus in the shoulder joint. Very gently hollowed out, the glenoid forms a poor socket for the humeral head. It is narrow above and wider below, and is pear-shaped in outline. Immediately above the glenoid cavity a small roughened area encroaches on the root of the coracoid process and is termed the supraglenoid tubercle. The neck of the scapula is the constriction

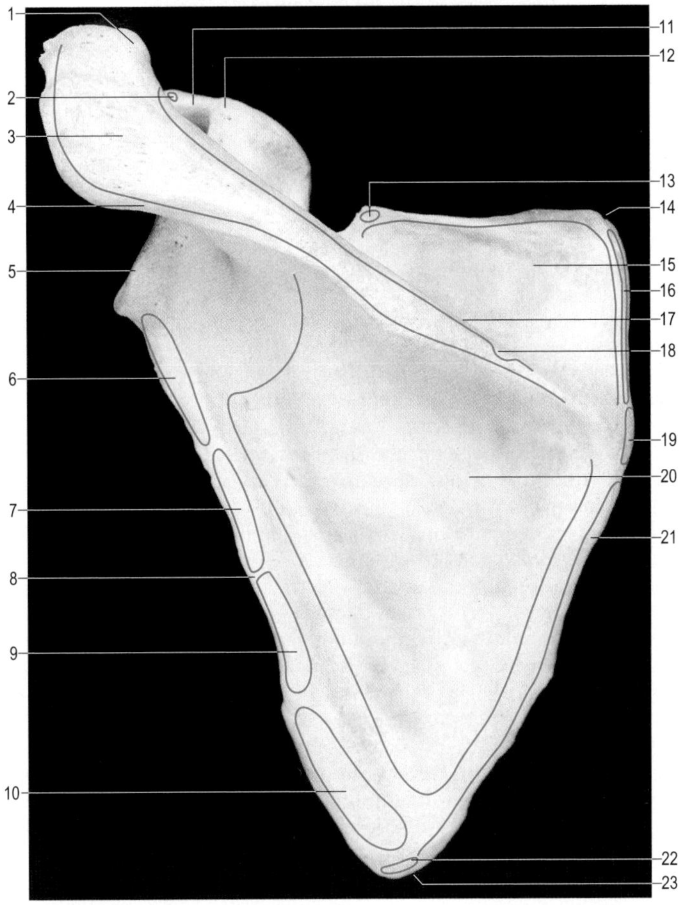

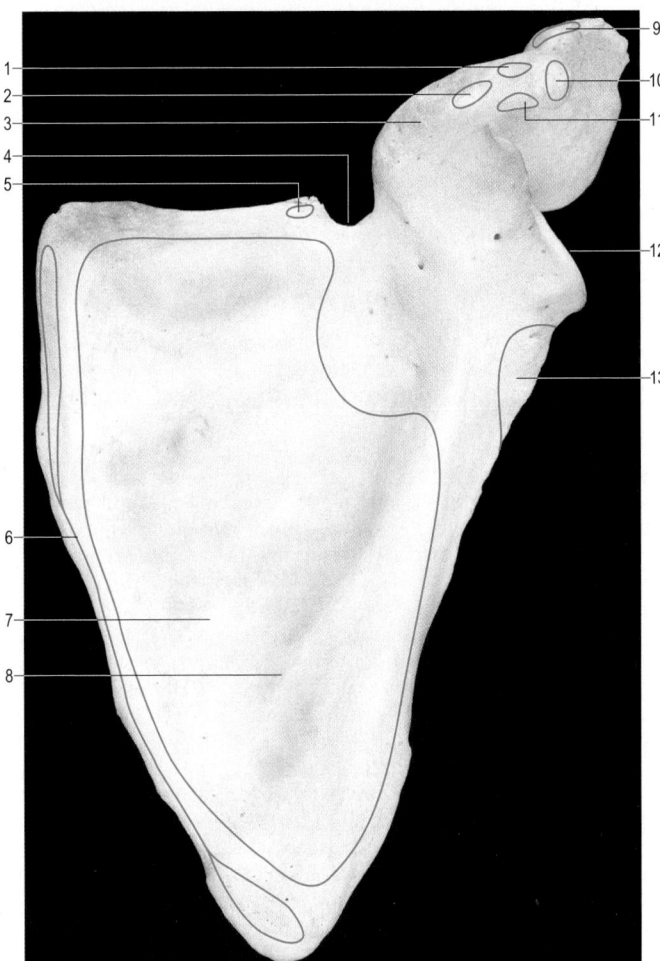

1. Clavicular facet. 2. Biceps (short head). 3. Acromion. 4. Deltoid. 5. Glenoid fossa.
6. Triceps brachii (long head). 7 and 9. Teres minor. 8. Groove for circumflex scapular artery.
10. Teres major. 11. Conoid tubercle. 12. Coracoid process. 13. Omohyoid (inferior belly).
14. Superior angle. 15. Supraspinatus. 16. Levator scapulae. 17. Spine. 18. Trapezius.
19. Rhomboid minor. 20. Infraspinatus. 21. Rhomboid major. 22. Latissimus dorsi.
23. Inferior angle.

Fig. 49.3 Posterior aspect of left scapula. (Photograph by Sarah-Jane Smith.)

1. Trapezoid ligament attachment. 2. Conoid ligament attachment. 3. Acromion process.
4. Suprascapular notch. 5. Omohyoid (inferior belly). 6. Serratus anterior.
7. Subscapularis. 8. Ridge for intermuscular tendon of subscapularis. 9. Deltoid.
10. Biceps (short head) and coracobrachialis. 11. Pectoralis minor. 12. Glenoid fossa.
13. Triceps (long head).

Fig. 49.4 Anterior aspect of left scapula. (Photograph by Sarah-Jane Smith.)

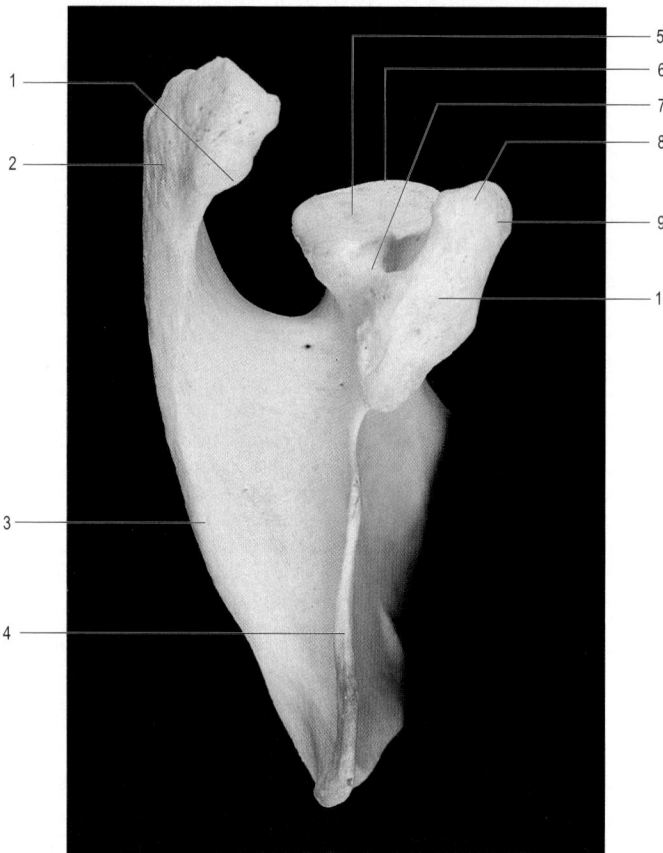

1. Facet for clavicle. 2. Acromial process. 3. Spine. 4. Superior border. 5. Head.
6. Glenoid fossa. 7. Neck. 8. Conoid tubercle (for conoid ligament). 9. Coracoid process.
10. Trapezoid ligament attachment.

Fig. 49.5 Superior aspect of left scapula. (Photograph by Sarah-Jane Smith.)

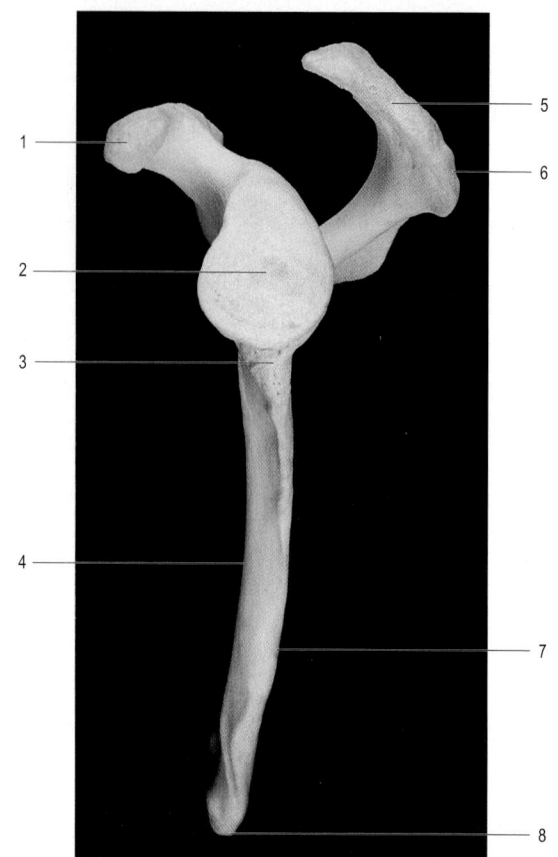

1. Coracoid process. 2. Glenoid fossa. 3. Infraglenoid tubercle for long head of triceps.
4. Ventral surface. 5. Acromion. 6. Acromial angle. 7. Lateral border. 8. Inferior angle.

Fig. 49.6 Lateral aspect of left scapula. (Photograph by Sarah-Jane Smith.)

immediately adjoining the head. It can be identified most easily on its inferior and dorsal aspects. Ventrally, it can be regarded as extending between the infraglenoid tubercle and the anterior margin of the suprascapular notch.

Costal surface (Fig. 49.4)
The costal surface, which is directed medially and forwards when the arm is by the side, is slightly hollowed out, especially in its upper part. Near the lateral border there is a longitudinal rounded ridge, prominent near the neck, but less so below, which is separated from the lateral border by a narrow grooved area.

Subscapularis arises from nearly the whole of the costal surface, including the grooved area immediately adjoining the lateral border, but excluding the area next to the neck of the bone. Small intramuscular tendons are attached to the roughened ridges which subdivide this surface incompletely into a number of smooth areas. The anterior aspect of the neck is separated from subscapularis by a bursal protrusion of the synovial membrane of the shoulder joint (subscapular 'bursa'). The lower five or six digitations of serratus anterior are attached to an oval area near the inferior angle. The remainder of the muscle is inserted into a narrow strip along the ventral aspect of the medial border, which is wider above, where it receives the large first digitation. The longitudinal thickening of the bone near the lateral border provides a lever of the necessary strength to withstand the pull of serratus anterior on the inferior angle during lateral scapular rotation, when the glenoid cavity is turned to face more directly upwards as the arm is raised from the side and carried above the head against gravity.

Dorsal surface (Fig. 49.3)
The dorsal surface is divided by the shelf-like spine of the scapula into a small upper and a large lower area, which are confluent at the spinoglenoid notch between the lateral border of the spine and the dorsal aspect of the neck.

Supraspinatus is attached to the medial two-thirds of the supraspinous fossa on the dorsal surface: the fascia which covers the muscle is attached to the margins of the fossa. Teres major is attached to the upper two-thirds of a flattened strip which adjoins the lateral border. The strip is grooved near its upper end by the circumflex scapular vessels, which pass between teres major and the bone as they enter the infraspinous fossa. The lower limit of the attachment of teres minor is indicated by an oblique ridge, which runs from the lateral border to the neighbourhood of the inferior angle and cuts off a somewhat oval area where teres major is attached. The dorsal aspect of the inferior angle may give origin to a small slip which joins the deep surface of latissimus dorsi. The infraspinous fossa is hollowed out laterally but is convex medially. Infraspinatus is attached to the infraspinous fossa, with the exception of an area near the neck of the bone. The strong infraspinatus fascia passes onto teres minor and teres major, and sends fascial partitions between them which reach the bone along the ridges which mark the limits of their attachments.

Superior border
The superior border, thin and sharp, is the shortest. At its anterolateral end it is separated from the root of the coracoid process by the suprascapular notch (**Fig. 49.5**). Near the suprascapular notch it gives origin to the inferior belly of omohyoid. The notch is bridged by the superior transverse ligament which is attached laterally to the root of the coracoid process and medially to the limit of the notch. The ligament is sometimes ossified. The foramen, thus completed, transmits the suprascapular nerve to the supraspinous fossa, whereas the suprascapular vessels pass backwards above the ligament.

Lateral border
The lateral border of the scapula forms a clearly defined, sharp, roughened ridge, which runs sinuously from the inferior angle to the glenoid cavity. At its upper end it widens into a rough, somewhat triangular area, which is termed the infraglenoid tubercle (**Fig. 49.6**).

The lateral border separates the attachments of subscapularis and teres minor and major. These muscles project beyond the bone and, with latissimus dorsi, cover it so completely that it cannot be felt through the skin. The long head of triceps is attached to the infraglenoid tubercle.

The grooved part of the costal surface, the narrow flat lateral strip of the dorsal surface and the adjacent thickened ridge (**Fig. 49.6**), are often included in the 'lateral border' during clinical examination.

Medial border

The medial border of the scapula extends from the inferior to the superior angle. In its lower two-thirds this border can easily be felt through the skin, but its upper third is more deeply placed and cannot be palpated. It is thin and often angled opposite the root of the spine. Levator scapulae is attached to a narrow strip, extending from the superior angle to the root of the spine, and rhomboid minor is attached below this, opposite the root of the spine. Rhomboid major is attached to the remainder of the border.

Scapular angles

The inferior angle overlies the seventh rib or intercostal space. Palpable through the skin and covering muscles, it is also visible as it advances round the thoracic wall when the arm is raised. It is covered on its dorsal aspect by the upper border of latissimus dorsi, a small slip from which is frequently attached to the inferior angle. The superior angle, at the junction of the superior and medial borders, is obscured by the upper part of trapezius. The lateral angle, truncated and broad, bears the glenoid cavity which articulates with the head of the humerus at the glenohumeral joint. It provides a shallow, and limited, socket for the humeral head. Its outline is piriform, narrower above (**Fig. 49.6**). The glenohumeral ligaments are attached to its anterior margin. When the arm is by the side, the cavity is directed forwards, laterally and slightly upwards. When the arm is raised above the head it is directed almost straight upwards. Just above it a small rough supraglenoid tubercle encroaches on the root of the coracoid process. The anatomical neck, the constriction adjoining the rim of the glenoid cavity, is most distinct at its inferior and dorsal aspects. Anteriorly and posteriorly it extends between the infraglenoid and supraglenoid tubercles, passing lateral to the root of the coracoid process. The long head of biceps brachii is attached to the supraglenoid tubercle, and the long head of triceps brachii is attached to the infraglenoid tubercle.

Spine of the scapula

The spine of the scapula forms a shelf-like projection on the upper part of the dorsal surface of the bone, and is triangular in shape (**Fig. 49.3**). Its lateral border is free, thick and rounded and helps to bound the spinoglenoid notch, which lies between it and the dorsal surface of the neck of the bone. Its anterior border joins the dorsal surface of the scapula along a line which runs laterally and slightly upwards from the junction of the upper and middle thirds of the medial border. The plate-like body of the bone is bent along this line, which accounts for the concavity of the upper part of the costal surface. The dorsal border is the crest of the spine, and is subcutaneous throughout nearly its whole extent. At its medial end the crest expands into a smooth, triangular area. Elsewhere the upper and lower edges and the surface of the crest are roughened for muscular attachments. The upper surface of the spine widens as it is traced laterally, and is slightly hollowed out. Together with the upper area of the dorsal surface of the bone, the upper surface of the spine forms the supraspinous fossa. The lower surface is overhung by the crest at its medial, narrow end, but is gently convex in its wider, lateral portion. Together with the lower area of the dorsal surface of the bone, the lower surface of the spine forms the infraspinous fossa, which communicates with the supraspinous fossa through the spinoglenoid notch.

Supra- and infraspinatus are attached to the upper and lower surfaces of the spine of the scapula, respectively. The flattened triangular area at its root lies opposite the spine of the third thoracic vertebra and is covered by the tendon of trapezius; a bursa intervenes to enable the tendon to play over this part of the bone. The posterior fibres of deltoid are attached to the lower border of the crest. The middle fibres of trapezius are attached to the upper border of the crest, and the lowest fibres of trapezius terminate in a flat triangular tendon which glides over the smooth area at the base of the spine and inserts into a rough prominence, erroneously called the deltoid tubercle, on the dorsal or subcutaneous aspect of the spine near its medial end.

Acromion

The acromion projects forwards, almost at right angles, from the lateral end of the spine, with which it is continuous. The lower border of the crest of the spine becomes continuous with the lateral border of the acromion at the acromial angle, which forms a subcutaneous, bony landmark. The medial border of the acromion is short and is marked anteriorly by a small, oval facet, directed upwards and medially, for articulation with the lateral end of the clavicle. The lateral border, tip and upper surface of the acromion can all be felt through the skin without difficulty. There may be an accessory articular facet on the inferior surface of the acromion.

The acromion is subcutaneous over its dorsal surface, being covered only by the skin and superficial fascia. The lateral border, which is thick and irregular, and the tip of the process, as far round as the clavicular facet, give origin to the middle fibres of deltoid. The medial aspect of the tip gives attachment, below deltoid, to the lateral end of the coraco-acromial ligament. The articular capsule of the acromioclavicular joint is attached around the margins of the clavicular facet. Behind the facet, the medial border of the acromion gives insertion to the horizontal fibres of trapezius. The inferior aspect of the acromion is relatively smooth, and together with the coraco-acromial ligament and the coracoid process forms a protective arch over the shoulder joint. The tendon of supraspinatus passes below the overhanging acromion and is separated from it and from deltoid by the subacromial bursa.

Coracoid process (Figs 49.4, 49.5)

The coracoid process arises from the upper border of the head of the scapula and is bent sharply so as to project forwards and slightly laterally. When the arm is by the side, the coracoid process points almost straight forwards and its slightly enlarged tip can be felt through the skin, although it is covered by the anterior fibres of deltoid. It lies c.2.5 cm below the junction of the lateral fourth of the clavicle with the rest of the bone. The supraglenoid tubercle marks the root of the coracoid process where it adjoins the upper part of the glenoid cavity. There is another impression on the dorsal aspect of the coracoid process at the point where it changes direction: it gives attachment to the conoid part of the coracoclavicular ligament.

The coracoid process lies below the clavicle at the junction of the lateral fourth with the rest of the bone and is connected to its under surface by the coracoclavicular ligament. It is covered by the anterior fibres of deltoid and can be identified only on deep pressure through the lateral border of the infraclavicular fossa. The attachment of the conoid part of the ligament has already been considered: the trapezoid part is attached to the upper aspect of the horizontal part of the process. Pectoralis minor is attached to the superior aspect of the coracoid process. The wider, medial end of the coraco-acromial ligament and, below that, the coracohumeral ligament, are attached to the lateral border. Coracobrachialis is attached to the medial side of the tip of the process, and the short head of biceps is attached to the lateral side of the tip. The inferior aspect of the process is smooth and helps to complete the coraco-acromial arch.

Ligaments

The main scapular ligaments are the coracoacromial and superior transverse scapular; there may also be a weaker, variable inferior transverse scapular (spinoglenoid) ligament (see **Fig. 49.4**).

Coracoacromial ligament – The coracoacromial ligament is a strong triangular band between the coracoid process and acromion. It is attached apically to the acromion anterior to its clavicular articular surface and by its base along the whole lateral border of the coracoid. Together with the coracoid process and acromion it completes an arch above the humeral head. It may be composed of two strong marginal bands with a thinner centre; when pectoralis minor is inserted into the humeral capsule instead of the coracoid process, which happens occasionally, its tendon passes between the bands. The subacromial bursa facilitates movement between the coracoacromial arch and the subjacent supraspinatus and shoulder joint, functioning as a secondary synovial articulation.

Superior transverse scapular (suprascapular) ligament – The superior transverse scapular (suprascapular) ligament converts the scapular notch into a foramen: it is sometimes ossified. A flat fasciculus, it narrows towards its attachments to the base of the coracoid process and medial

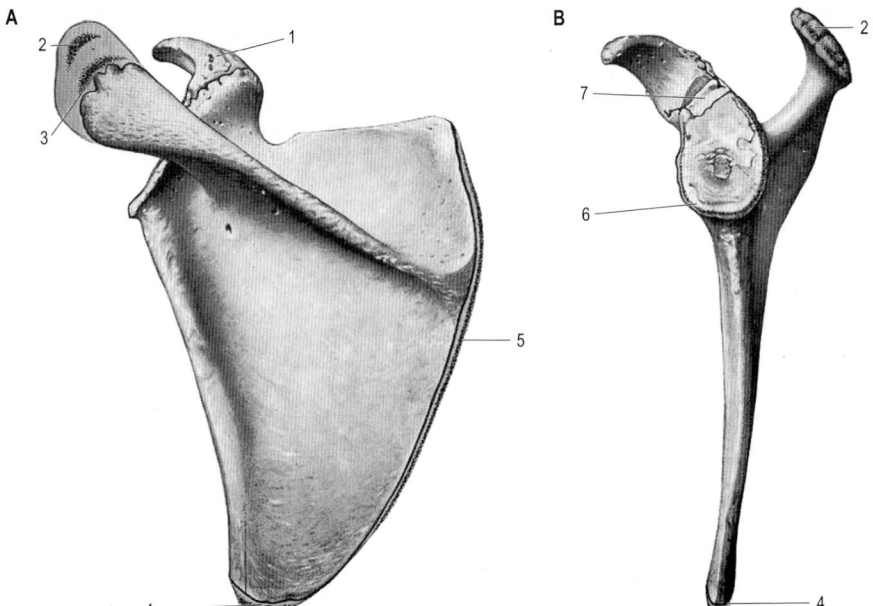

A

B

1. Coracoid centre.   2. Distal acromial centre.   3. Proximal acromial centre.
4. Centre at inferior angle.   5. Centre for medial border.   6. Glenoid centre.
7. Subcoracoid centre.

Fig. 49.7 Ossification of the scapula. **A**, Dorsal aspect;
B, Lateral aspect.

side of the scapular notch. The suprascapular nerve traverses the foramen and the suprascapular vessels cross above the ligament.

Inferior transverse scapular (spinoglenoid) ligament – When present, the inferior transverse scapular ligament is a membranous ligament which may stretch from the lateral border of the spine of the scapula to the glenoid margin. It forms an arch over the suprascapular nerve and vessels entering the infraspinous fossa.

Ossification

The cartilaginous scapula is ossified from eight or more centres: one in the body, two each in the coracoid process and the acromion, one each in the medial border, inferior angle and lower part of the rim of the glenoid cavity (**Fig. 49.7**). The centre for the body appears in the eighth intrauterine week. Ossification begins in the middle of the coracoid process in the first year or in a small proportion of individuals before birth and the process joins the rest of the bone about the fifteenth year. At or soon after puberty centres of ossification occur in the rest of the coracoid process (subcoracoid centre), in the rim of the lower part of the glenoid cavity, frequently at the tip of the coracoid process, in the acromion, in the inferior angle and contiguous part of the medial border and in the medial border. A variable area of the upper part of the glenoid cavity, usually the upper third, is ossified from the subcoracoid centre; it unites with the rest of the bone in the fourteenth year in the female and the seventeenth year in the male. A horseshoe-shaped epiphysis appears for the rim of the lower part of the glenoid cavity; thicker at its peripheral than at its central margin, it converts the flat glenoid cavity of the child into the gently concave fossa of the adult. The base of the acromion is formed by an extension from the spine; the rest of the acromion is ossified from two centres which unite and then join the extension from the spine. The various epiphyses of the scapula have all joined the bone by about the twentieth year.

HUMERUS

The humerus, the longest and largest bone in the upper limb, has expanded ends and a shaft (**Figs 49.8, 49.9, 49.10**). The rounded head occupies the proximal and medial part of the upper end of the bone and forms an enarthrodial articulation with the glenoid cavity of the scapula. The lesser tubercle projects from the front of the shaft, close to the head, and is limited on its lateral side by a well-marked groove. The distal end, loosely termed 'condylar', is adapted to the forearm bones at the elbow joint.

The capsular ligament of the elbow joint is attached anteriorly to the upper limits of the radial and coronoid fossae, so that both these bony depressions are intracapsular and therefore lined with synovial membrane. Medially it is attached to the medial non-articular aspect of the projecting lip of the trochlea and to the root of the medial epicondyle. Posteriorly it ascends to, or almost to, the upper margin of the olecranon fossa, which is therefore intracapsular and covered with synovial membrane. Laterally it skirts the lateral borders of the trochlea and capitulum, lying medial to the lateral epicondyle.

With the arm by the side, the medial epicondyle lies on a plane which is posterior to that of the lateral epicondyle, so that the humerus *appears* to be rotated medially. In this position the head of the humerus is directed almost equally backwards and medially, and the posterior surface of the shaft faces posterolaterally. Since the glenoid fossa of the scapula faces anterolaterally, the humerus is not rotated medially relative to the scapula in this position of rest, but it is so rotated relative to the conventional anatomical position. This position of the bone must be remembered when movements of the arm and forearm are considered.

Proximal end

The proximal end of the humerus consists of the head, anatomical neck and the greater and lesser tubercles. It joins the shaft at an ill-defined 'surgical neck', which is closely related on its medial side to the axillary nerve and posterior humeral circumflex artery (**Fig. 49.9A,B**).

Head (Fig. 49.9A,B) – The head of the humerus forms rather less than half a spheroid; in sectional profile it is spheroidal (strictly ovoidal). Its smooth articular surface is covered with hyaline cartilage, which is thicker centrally. When the arm is at rest by the side, it is directed medially, backwards and upwards to articulate with the glenoid cavity of the scapula. The humeral articular surface is much more extensive than the glenoid cavity, and only a portion of it is in contact with the cavity in any one position of the arm.

Anatomical neck – The anatomical neck of the humerus immediately adjoins the margin of the head and forms a slight constriction, which is least apparent in the neighbourhood of the greater tubercle, and superiorly, and for some distance anteriorly and posteriorly: it indicates the line of capsular attachment of the shoulder joint (**Fig. 49.9A,B**), other than at the intertuberous sulcus, where the long tendon of biceps emerges. Medially, the capsular attachment diverges from the anatomical neck and descends 1 cm or more onto the shaft.

Lesser tubercle – The lesser tubercle is anterior to and just beyond the anatomical neck. It has a smooth, muscular impression on its upper part palpable through the thickness of deltoid 3 cm below the acromial apex. The bony prominence slips away from the examining finger when the humerus is rotated. The lateral edge of the lesser tubercle is sharp and forms the medial border of the intertuberous sulcus. Subscapularis is attached to the lesser tubercle (**Fig. 49.8A**), and the transverse ligament of the shoulder joint is attached to the lateral margin.

Greater tubercle – The greater tubercle is the most lateral part of the proximal end of the humerus. It projects beyond the lateral border of

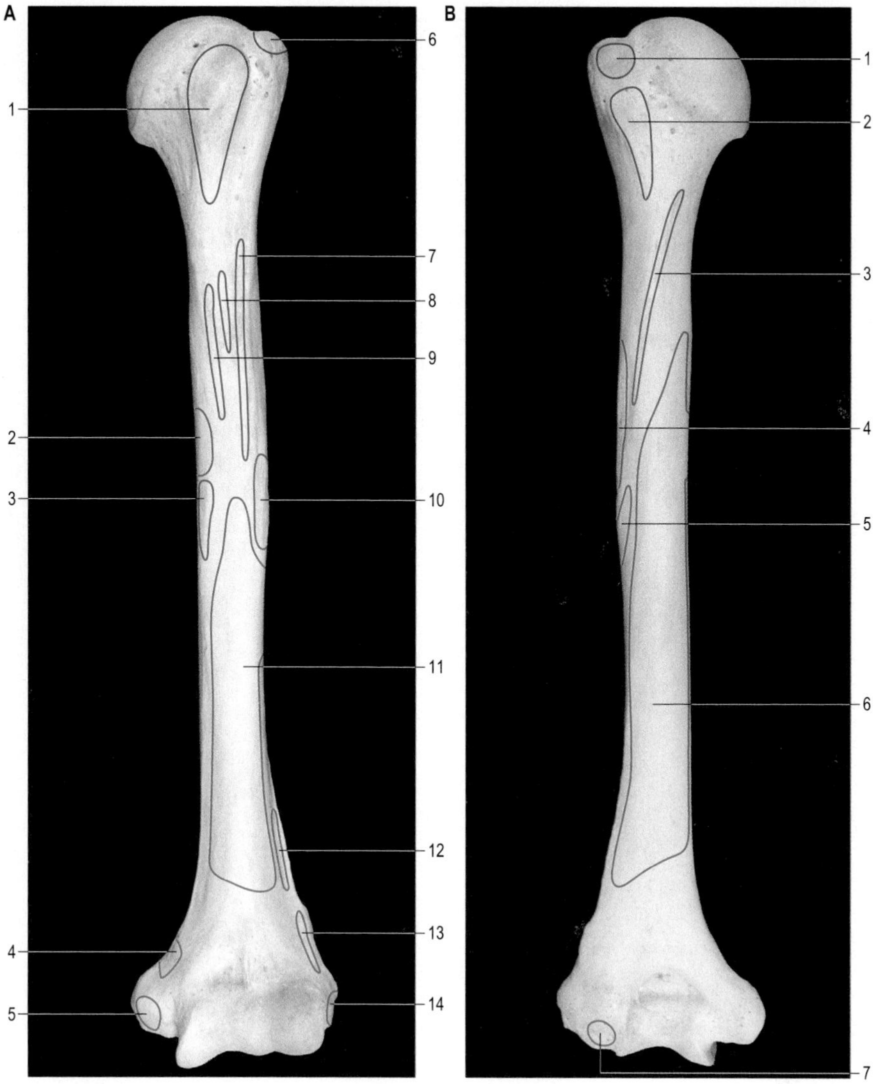

A   B

Part A:
1. Subscapularis.
2. Triceps (medial head).
3. Coracobrachialis.
4. Pronator teres (humeral head).
5. Common flexor origin.
6. Supraspinatus.
7. Pectoralis major.
8. Lastissimus dorsi.
9. Teres major.
10. Deltoid.
11. Brachialis.
12. Brachioradialis.
13. Extensor carpi radialis longus.
14. Common extensor origin.

Part B:
1. Infraspinatus.
2. Teres minor.
3. Triceps (lateral head).
4. Deltoid.
5. Brachialis.
6. Triceps (medial head).
7. Anconeus.

Fig. 49.8 A, Anterior aspect of left humerus. **B**, Posterior aspect of left humerus. (Photographs by Sarah-Jane Smith.)

the acromion. Its posterosuperior aspect, near the anatomical neck, bears three smooth flattened impressions for the attachment of supraspinatus (uppermost), infraspinatus (middle) and teres minor (lowest and placed on the posterior surface of the tubercle) (**Figs 49.8A,B**). The attachments of subscapularis and teres minor are not confined to their respective tubercles, but extend for varying distances on to the adjacent metaphysis. The projecting lateral surface of the tubercle presents numerous vascular foramina and is covered by the thick, fleshy deltoid, which produces the normal rounded contour of the shoulder. A part of the subacromial bursa may cover the upper part of this area and separate it from deltoid.

The intertuberous sulcus (bicipital groove) lies between the tubercles. It contains the long tendon of biceps, its synovial sheath, and an ascending branch from the anterior circumflex humeral artery. The rough lateral lip of the groove is marked by the bilaminar tendon of pectoralis major, its floor by the tendon of latissimus dorsi and its medial lip by the tendon of teres major; the attachment of pectoralis major extends beyond that of teres major, that of latissimus dorsi is least extensive.

Shaft

The shaft of the humerus is almost cylindrical in its proximal half but is triangular on section in its distal half, which is compressed in an anteroposterior direction. It can be identified when the arm is grasped firmly, but its outline is obscured by the strong muscles which surround it. It has three surfaces and three borders – which are not everywhere equally obvious.

Anterior border – The anterior border starts on the front of the greater tubercle and runs downwards almost to the lower end of the bone. Its proximal third forms the lateral lip of the intertuberous sulcus and is

roughened for muscular attachments. The succeeding portion is also roughened and forms the anterior limit of the deltoid tubercle; the lower half of the border is smooth and rounded.

Lateral border – The lateral border is conspicuous at the lower end of the bone, where its sharp edge is roughened along its anterior aspect. In its middle and upper thirds the border is barely discernible, but in a well-marked bone it can be traced upwards to the posterior surface of the greater tubercle. About its middle, the border is interrupted by a wide, shallow groove (radial or spiral groove), which crosses the bone obliquely, passing downwards and forwards from its posterior to its anterior surface.

Medial border – The medial border, although rounded, can be identified without difficulty in the lower half of the shaft, where it becomes the medial supracondylar ridge. A little above its middle it is marked by a V-shaped roughened area which is termed the deltoid tubercle. The limbs of the V are broad; behind the posterior limb the groove for the radial nerve runs downwards and fades away on the lower part of the surface. Proximal to the deltoid tubercle the medial border is indistinct until it reappears as the medial lip of the intertuberous sulcus, where it is again rough and reaches the lesser tubercle.

Surfaces – The anterolateral surface is bounded by the anterior and lateral borders and is smooth and featureless in its upper part, which is covered by deltoid. About, or a little above, the middle of this surface, deltoid is inserted into the deltoid tubercle; further distally the surface gives origin to the lateral fibres of brachialis, which extend upwards into the floor of the lower end of the groove for the radial nerve (**Fig. 49.8A,B**). Brachioradialis is attached to the proximal two-thirds of the roughened anterior aspect of the lateral supracondylar

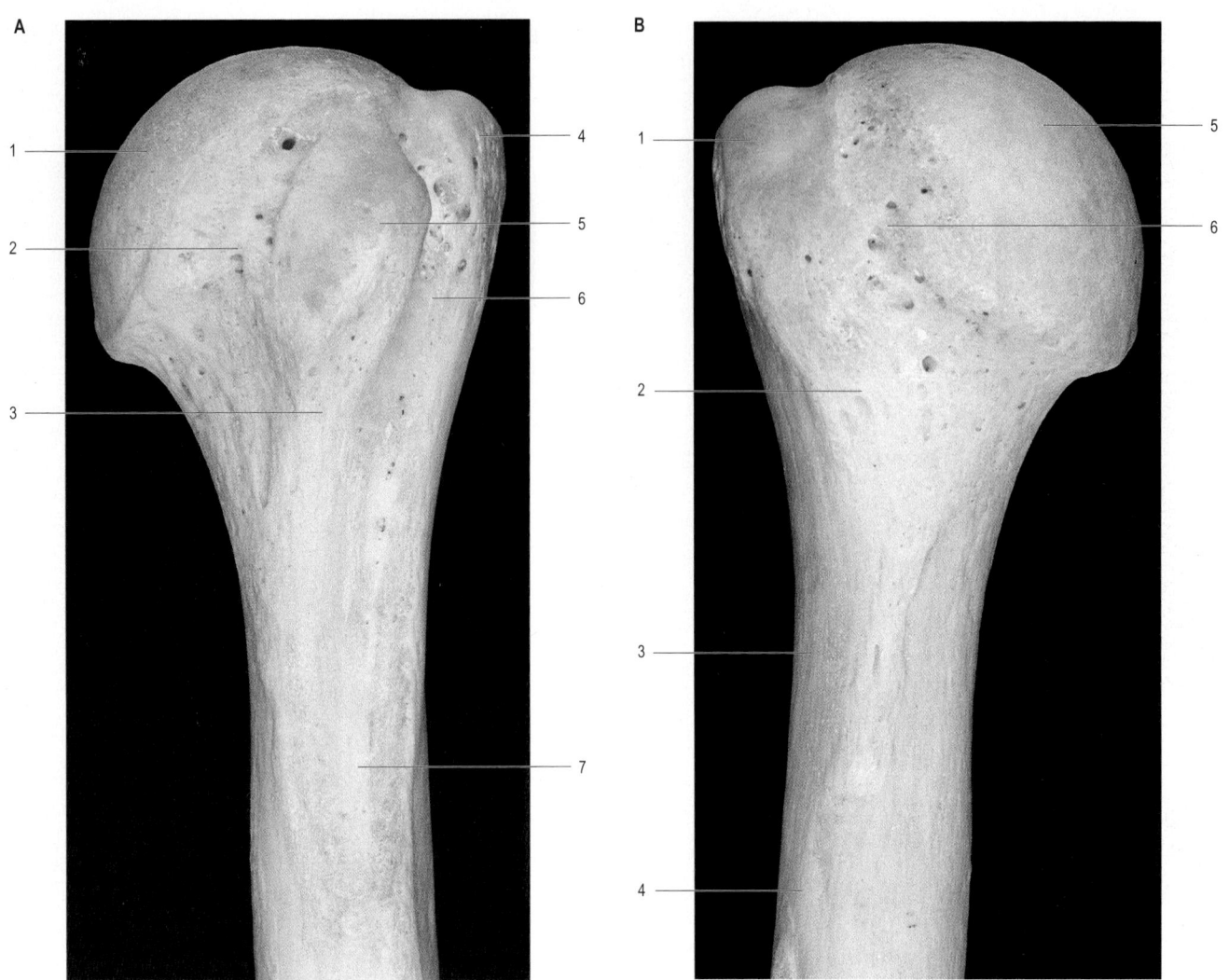

A

B

Part A: **1.** Head. **2.** Anatomical neck. **3.** Surgical neck. **4.** Greater tubercle. **5.** Lesser tubercle. **6.** Intertuberous sulcus. **7.** Shaft.
Part B: **1.** Greater tubercle. **2.** Surgical neck. **3.** Shaft. **4.** Radial groove. **5.** Head. **6.** Anatomical neck.

Fig. 49.9 A, Anterior aspect of proximal end of left humerus. **B**, Posterior aspect of proximal end of left humerus. (Photographs by Sarah-Jane Smith.)

ridge, and extensor carpi radialis longus is attached to its distal third. Behind these muscles, the ridge gives attachment to the lateral intermuscular septum of the arm.

The anteromedial surface is bounded by the anterior and medial borders. Rather less than its upper third forms the rough floor of the intertuberous sulcus; the rest of the surface is smooth. Distal to the intertuberous sulcus a small area of the anteromedial surface is devoid of muscular attachment, but its lower half is occupied by the medial part of brachialis (**Fig. 49.8A**). Coracobrachialis is attached to a roughened strip on the middle of the medial border. The humeral head of pronator teres is attached to a narrow area close to the lowest part of the medial supracondylar ridge, and the ridge itself gives attachment to the medial intermuscular septum of the arm.

A little below its midpoint, the nutrient foramen, which is directed downwards, opens close to the medial border. A hook-shaped process of bone, the supracondylar process, from 2 to 20 mm in length, occasionally projects from the anteromedial surface of the shaft, c.5 cm proximal to the medial epicondyle. It is curved downwards and forwards, and its pointed apex is connected to the medial border, just above the epicondyle, by a fibrous band to which part of pronator teres is attached. The foramen completed by this fibrous band usually transmits the median nerve and brachial artery, but sometimes encloses only the nerve, or the nerve plus the ulnar artery (in cases of high division of the brachial artery). A groove which lodges the artery and nerve usually exists behind the process, and may protect the nerve and artery from compression by muscles.

The posterior surface, between the medial and lateral borders, is the most extensive surface. It is occupied mostly by the medial head of triceps. A ridge, sometimes rough, descends obliquely and laterally across its proximal third, and gives attachment to the lateral head of triceps. Above triceps, the axillary nerve and the posterior circumflex humeral vessels wind round this aspect of the bone under cover of deltoid. Below and medial to the attachment of the lateral head of triceps, a shallow groove which contains the radial nerve and the profunda brachii vessels, runs downwards and laterally to gain the anterolateral surface of the shaft. The area for the origin of the fleshy medial head of triceps includes a very large part of the posterior surface of the bone. It covers an elongated triangular area, the apex of which is placed on the medial part of the posterior surface above the level of the lower limit of the insertion of teres major. The area widens below and covers the whole surface almost down to the lower end of the bone.

Fractures of the humeral shaft – Fractures of the humerus are comparatively common and may occur at almost any level. The humerus is fractured by muscular action probably more frequently than any other long bone: usually the shaft is broken below the attachment of deltoid. The radial nerve may be injured in its groove or may very rarely become involved later in the growth of callus. Fractures at the proximal end of the humerus may rarely damage the axillary nerve, but fractures of the medial epicondyle are often complicated by damage to the ulnar nerve. Supracondylar fractures are relatively common in children. Here, the end of the proximal fragment can sometimes injure the brachial artery

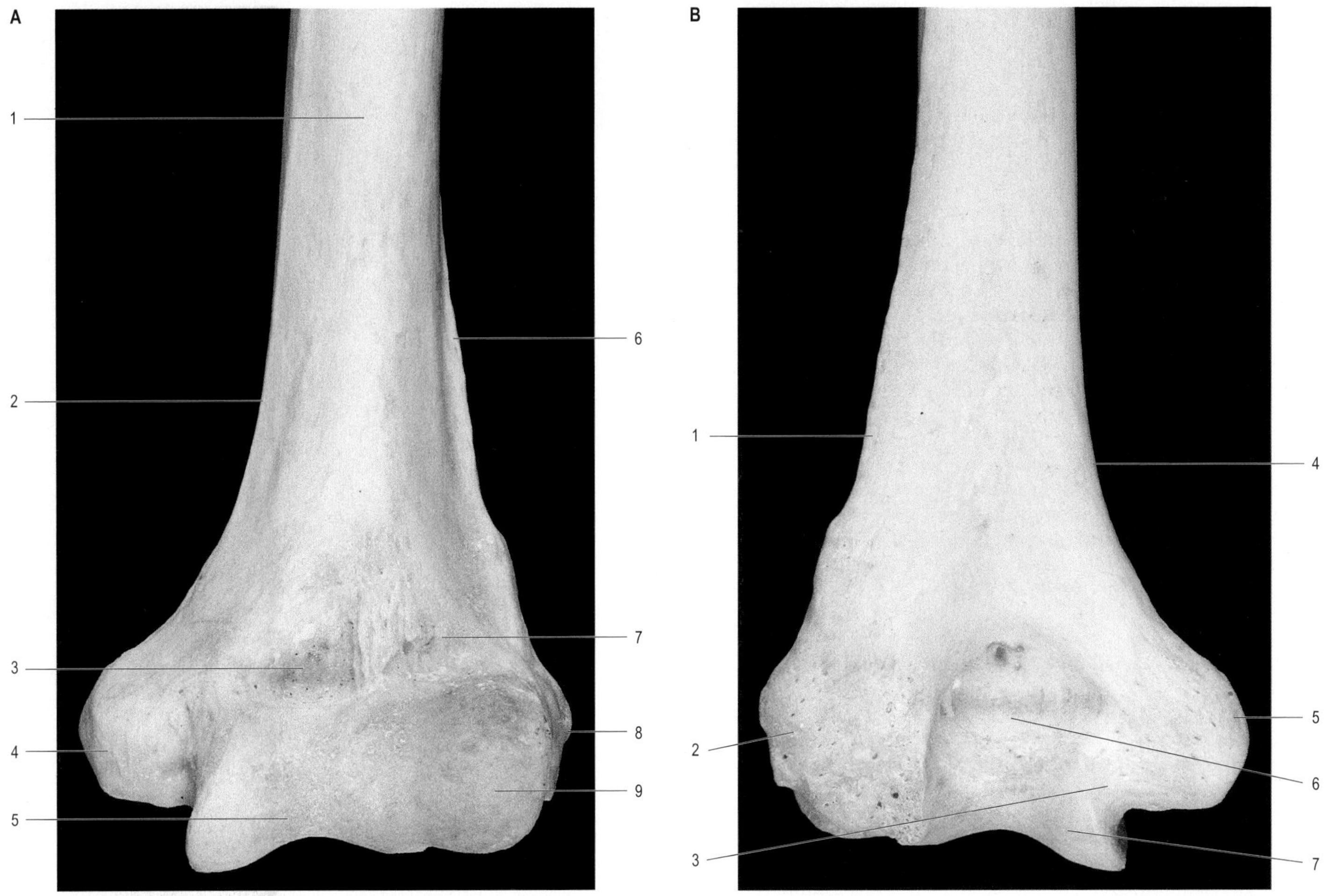

A

B

Part A: **1.** Shaft. **2.** Medial supracondylar ridge. **3.** Coronoid fossa. **4.** Medial epicondyle. **5.** Trochlea. **6.** Lateral supracondylar ridge. **7.** Radial fossa. **8.** Lateral epicondyle. **9.** Capitulum.
Part B: **1.** Lateral supracondylar ridge. **2.** Lateral epicondyle. **3.** Sulcus for ulnar nerve. **4.** Medial supracondylar ridge. **5.** Medial epicondyle. **6.** Olecranon fossa. **7.** Trochlea.

Fig. 49.10 A, Anterior aspect of distal end of left humerus. **B**, Posterior aspect of distal end of left humerus. (Photographs by Sarah-Jane Smith.)

or median nerve. In adults, non-union is commoner in the humerus than in any other bone except the tibia.

Distal end (Figs 49.10A,B, 49.11)

The distal end of the humerus is a modified condyle: it is wider transversely and has articular and non-articular parts. The articular part is curved forwards, so that its anterior and posterior surfaces lie in front of the corresponding surfaces of the shaft. It articulates with the radius and the ulna at the elbow joint, and is divided by a faint groove into a lateral capitulum, and a medial trochlea.

The capitulum is a rounded, convex projection, considerably less than half a sphere, which covers the anterior and inferior surfaces of the lateral part of the condyle of the humerus but does not extend onto its posterior surface. It articulates with the discoid head of the radius, which lies in contact with its inferior surface in full extension of the elbow but slides onto its anterior surface during flexion.

The groove of the trochlea winds backwards and laterally as it is traced from the anterior to the posterior surface of the bone, and it is wider, deeper and more symmetrical posteriorly. Anteriorly, the medial flange of the pulley is much longer than the lateral, and the surface adjoining its projecting medial margin is convex to accommodate itself to the medial part of the upper surface of the coronoid process of the ulna. These asymmetries entail varying angulation between the humeral and ulnar axes, together with some conjunct rotation.

The non-articular part of the condyle includes the medial and lateral epicondyles, olecranon and coronoid and radial fossae.

Trochlea – The trochlea is a pulley-shaped surface, which covers the anterior, inferior and posterior surfaces of the condyle of the humerus medially. It articulates with the trochlear notch of the ulna. On its

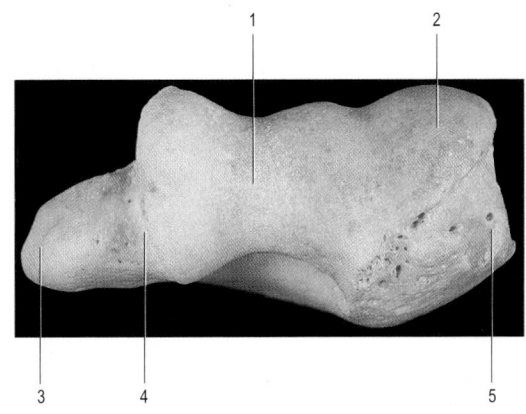

1. Trochlea. **2.** Capitulum. **3.** Medial epicondyle. **4.** Sulcus for ulnar nerve.
5. Lateral epicondyle.

Fig. 49.11 Inferior aspect of distal end of left humerus. (Photograph by Sarah-Jane Smith.)

lateral side it is separated from the capitulum by a faint groove; its medial margin projects downwards beyond the rest of the bone. When the elbow is extended the inferior and posterior aspects of the trochlea are in contact with the ulna, but, as the joint is flexed, the trochlear notch slides on to the anterior aspect and the posterior aspect is then left uncovered. The downward projection of the medial edge of the trochlea is the principal factor in determining the angulation between

825

the long axis of the humerus and the long axis of the supinated forearm when the elbow is extended.

Medial epicondyle – The medial border of the humerus ends by turning slightly backwards as the medial epicondyle, which forms a conspicuous, blunt projection on the medial side of the condyle. It is subcutaneous and usually visible, especially in passive flexion of the elbow. Its posterior surface is smooth and is crossed by the ulnar nerve, which lies in a shallow sulcus as it enters the forearm. In this situation the nerve can be felt and rolled against the bone, and if it is jarred against the epicondyle, characteristic tingling sensations result. The lower part of the anterior surface of the medial epicondyle is marked by the attachment of the superficial group of forearm flexors. They arise from the epiphysis for the epicondyle, but are entirely extracapsular.

Lateral epicondyle – The lateral border of the humerus terminates at the lateral epicondyle, and its lower portion constitutes the lateral supracondylar ridge. The lateral epicondyle occupies the lateral part of the non-articular portion of the condyle, but does not project beyond the lateral supracondylar ridge. It turns slightly forwards, unlike the medial epicondyle, which turns slightly backwards. Its lateral and anterior surfaces show a well-marked impression for the superficial group of the extensor muscles of the forearm (**Fig. 49.8B**), which arise from the lateral side of the lower humeral epiphysis, and, like the flexors, are situated outside the articular capsule. The posterior surface, which is very slightly convex, is easily felt in a depression visible behind the extended elbow. A small area on the posterior surface gives origin to anconeus.

Olecranon, coronoid and radial fossae – There is a deep hollow, the olecranon fossa, on the posterior surface of the condyle, immediately above the trochlea. It lodges the tip of the olecranon of the ulna when the elbow is extended. The floor of the fossa is always thin and may be partially deficient. A similar but smaller hollow lies immediately above the trochlea on the anterior surface of the condyle and is termed the coronoid fossa. It accommodates the anterior margin of the coronoid process of the ulna during flexion of the elbow. A very slight depression lies above the capitulum on the lateral side of the coronoid fossa. It is termed the radial fossa, since it is related to the margin of the head of the radius in full flexion of the elbow.

Ossification

The humerus is ossified from eight centres, in the shaft, head, greater and lesser tubercles, capitulum with the lateral part of the trochlea, the medial part of the trochlea, and one for each epicondyle (**Fig. 49.12**). The centre for the shaft appears near its middle in the eighth week of intrauterine life, and gradually extends towards the ends. Before birth (20%), or in the first six months afterwards, ossification begins in the head, during the first year in females and second year in males in the greater tubercle, and about the fifth in the lesser tubercle. The existence of a centre in the lesser tubercle is often questioned, perhaps because it is often obscured in the usual anteroposterior radiological views (**Fig. 49.13**).

By the sixth year the centres for the head and tubercles have joined to form a single large epiphysis, which is hollowed out on its inferior

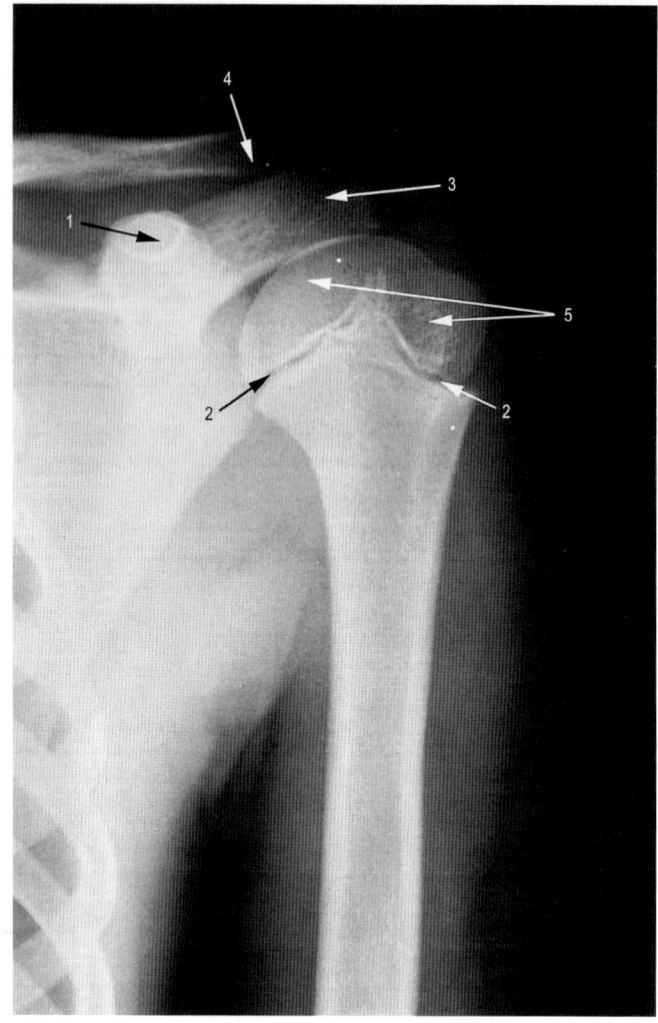

1. Coracoid process. 2. Growth plate of cartilage at upper end of humeral metaphysis.
3. Acromion. 4. Lateral end of clavicle, not yet completely ossified.
5. Proximal humeral epiphysis.

Fig. 49.13 Anteroposterior radiograph of the left shoulder in a boy aged 11. Note the conical junction of the humeral epiphysis with the diaphysis.

surface to adapt it to the somewhat conical upper end of the metaphysis. It fuses with the shaft of the humerus about the twentieth year in males, two years earlier in females. The lower end is ossified as follows. During the first year ossification begins in the capitulum and extends medially to form the chief part of the articular surface; the centre for the medial part of the trochlea appears in the ninth year in females and tenth year in males.

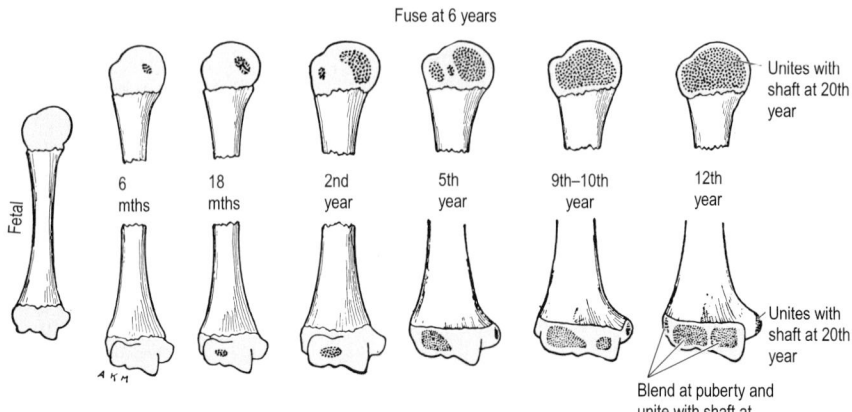

Fuse at 6 years

Fetal | 6 mths | 18 mths | 2nd year | 5th year | 9th–10th year | 12th year

Unites with shaft at 20th year

Unites with shaft at 20th year

Blend at puberty and unite with shaft at 14–16 years

Fig. 49.12 The stages in ossification of the humerus (not to scale).

Ossification begins in the medial epicondyle in the fourth year in females, sixth in males, and in the lateral epicondyle about the twelfth year. The centres for the lateral epicondyle, capitulum and trochlea fuse around puberty and the composite epiphysis unites with the shaft in the fourteenth year in females, sixteenth in males. The centre for the medial epicondyle forms a separate epiphysis, which is entirely extra-capsular and is placed on the posteromedial aspect of the epicondyle. It is separated from the rest of the lower epiphysis by a downgrowth from the shaft, with which it unites about the twentieth year.

Amputation of the humerus in youth

The proximal epiphysis joins the humeral shaft later than the distal, which means that growth in length is mainly attributable to growth from the proximal epiphysial plate. After amputation through the arm in youth, the humerus continues to grow and its lower end progressively moulds the surrounding soft tissues so that the stump becomes conical.

JOINTS

STERNOCLAVICULAR JOINT

The sternoclavicular joint is a synovial sellar joint.

Articulating surfaces

The articulating surfaces are the sternal end of the clavicle and the clavicular notch of the sternum, together with the adjacent superior surface of the first costal cartilage (**Fig. 49.14**). The larger clavicular articular surface is covered by fibrocartilage, which is thicker than the fibrocartilaginous lamina on the sternum. The joint is convex vertically but slightly concave anteroposteriorly, and is therefore sellar; the clavicular notch of the sternum is reciprocally curved, but the two surfaces are not fully congruent. An articular disc completely divides the joint.

Fibrous capsule

The capsule is thickened in front and behind, but above, and especially below, it is little more than loose areolar tissue.

Ligaments

Anterior sternoclavicular ligament – The anterior sternoclavicular liga-ment is broad and attached above to the anterosuperior aspect of the sternal end of the clavicle. It passes inferomedially to the upper anterior aspect of the manubrium, spreading onto the first costal cartilage.

Posterior sternoclavicular ligament – The posterior sternoclavicular ligament is a weaker band posterior to the joint. It descends infero-medially from the back of the sternal end of the clavicle to the back of the upper manubrium.

Interclavicular ligament – The interclavicular ligament is continuous above with deep cervical fascia, and unites the superior aspect of the sternal ends of both clavicles; some fibres are attached to the superior manubrial margin.

Costoclavicular ligament – The costoclavicular ligament is like an inverted cone, but short and flattened. It has anterior and posterior laminae which are attached to the upper surface of the first rib and costal cartilage, and ascends to the margins of an impression on the inferior clavicular surface at its medial end. Fibres of the anterior lamina ascend laterally and those of the posterior lamina (which are shorter) ascend medially (**Fig. 49.14**); they fuse laterally and merge medially with the capsule.

Articular disc

The articular disc is flat and almost circular, between the sternal and clavicular surfaces. It is attached above to the posterosuperior border of the articular surface of the clavicle, below to the first costal cartilage near its sternal junction, and by the rest of its circumference to the capsule. It is thicker peripherally, especially in its superoposterior part and a smaller inferomedial one. The capsule around the former is more lax: movements between the clavicle and the disc are more extensive than those between the disc and sternum. The sellar shape of the articular surfaces permits movement in approximately anteroposterior and vertical planes, and some rotation about the long axis of the clavicle. Close-packing probably coincides with maximum posterior rotation associated with full scapular rotation. Some anteroposterior translation also occurs.

Vascular supply

The sternoclavicular joint is supplied by branches from the internal thoracic and suprascapular arteries.

Innervation

The sternoclavicular joint is innervated by branches from the anterior supraclavicular nerve and the nerve to subclavius.

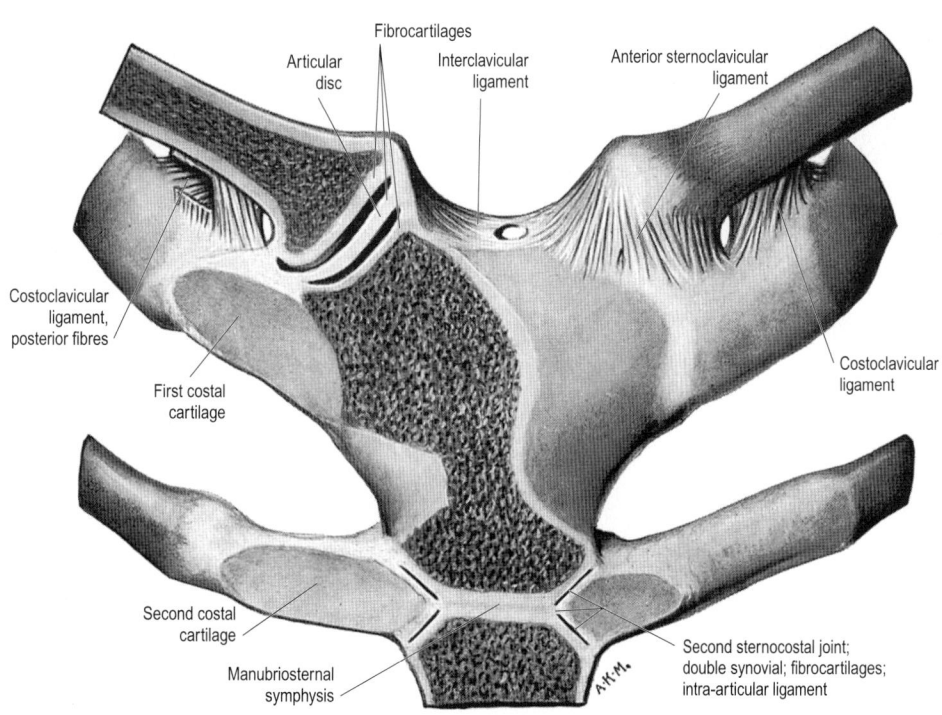

Fig. 49.14 Sternoclavicular joints: anterior aspect; left joint intact and right in coronal section.

Factors maintaining stability

The strength of the sternoclavicular joint depends on its associated ligaments, and especially on its disc. These factors, and the usual transmission of forces along the clavicle, make dislocation rare and fracture far more common.

ACROMIOCLAVICULAR JOINT

The acromioclavicular joint is a synovial plane joint.

Articulating surfaces

The acromioclavicular joint lies between the acromial end of the clavicle and the medial acromial margin (**Fig. 49.15**). It is approximately plane, but either surface may be slightly convex, the other reciprocally concave. Both are covered by fibrocartilage; the clavicular surface is a narrow, oval area which faces inferolaterally and overlaps a corresponding facet on the medial acromial border. The long axis is anteroposterior.

Fibrous capsule

The capsule completely surrounds the articular margins and is strengthened above by the acromioclavicular ligament. The capsule is lined by synovial membrane.

Ligaments

Acromioclavicular ligament – The acromioclavicular ligament is quadrilateral. It extends between the upper aspects of the lateral end of the clavicle and the adjoining acromion. Its parallel fibres interlace with the aponeuroses of trapezius and deltoid.

Articular disc – The articular disc often occurs in the upper part of the joint, partially separating the articular surfaces: occasionally it completely divides the joint.

Coracoclavicular ligament (Fig. 49.16) – The coracoclavicular ligament connects the clavicle and the coracoid process of the scapula. Though separate from the acromioclavicular joint, it is a most efficient accessory ligament, and maintains the apposition of the clavicle to the acromion. Its trapezoid and conoid parts, usually separated by fat or, frequently, a

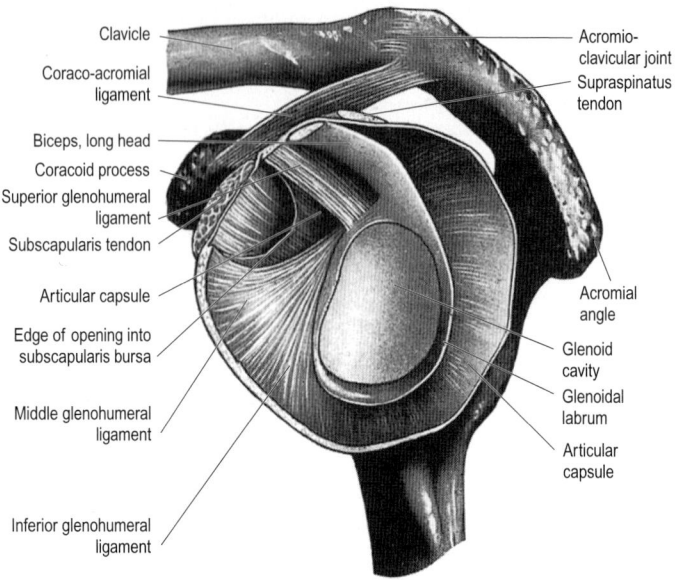

Fig. 49.15 Interior of the left shoulder joint: anterolateral aspect.

A

B

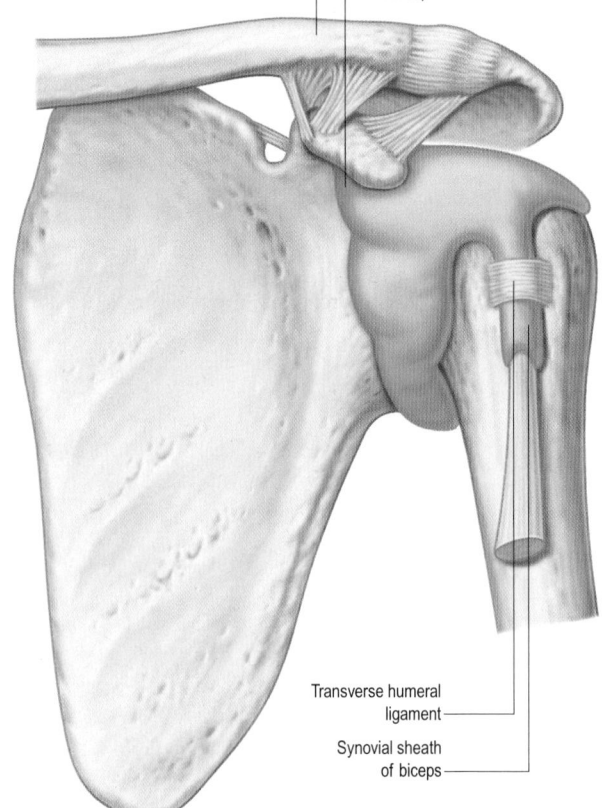

Fig. 49.16 **A**, The anterior aspect of the left shoulder. **B**, A deeper view of the anterior aspect than in (A), showing the bursae and acromioclavicular ligaments.

C

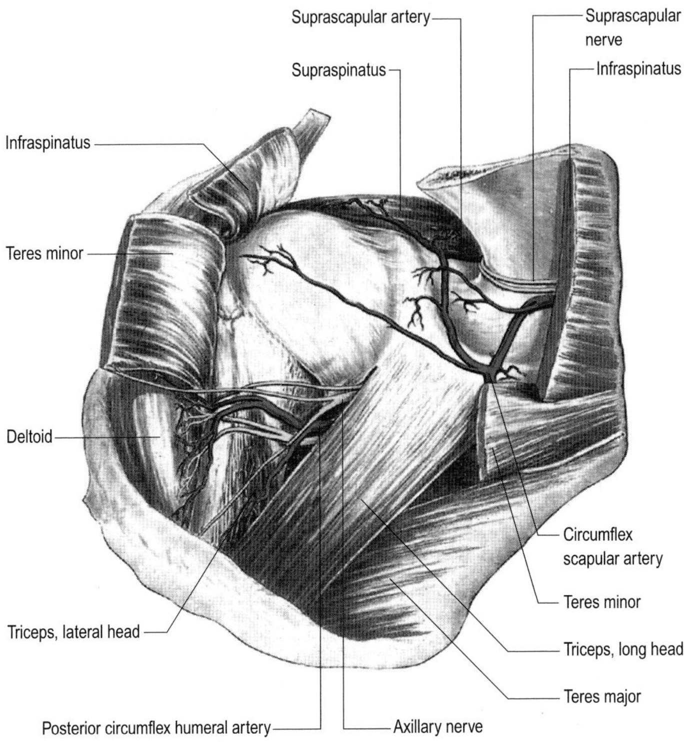

Suprascapular artery

Suprascapular nerve

Supraspinatus

Infraspinatus

Infraspinatus

Teres minor

Deltoid

Circumflex scapular artery

Teres minor

Triceps, long head

Teres major

Triceps, lateral head

Posterior circumflex humeral artery

Axillary nerve

Fig. 49.16 (*Cont'd*) **C**, Posterior aspect of the left shoulder joint with the acromion removed. Parts of infraspinatus and teres minor have been excised and their tendons turned forwards.

bursa, connect the medial horizontal part of the coracoid process and lateral end of the subclavian groove of the clavicle; these adjacent areas may even be covered by cartilage to form a coracoclavicular joint.

Trapezoid part – The trapezoid part is anterolateral and is broad, thin and quadrilateral, ascending slightly from the upper coracoid surface to the trapezoid line on the inferior clavicular surface. It is almost horizontal, its anterior border is free, and its posterior border is joined to the conoid part, forming an angle which projects backwards.

Conoid part – The conoid part is posteromedial and is a dense, almost vertical triangular band. Its base is attached to the conoid tubercle of the clavicle and its inferior apex is attached posteromedially to the root of the coracoid process in front of the scapular notch.

Vascular supply
The acromioclavicular joint receives its arterial supply from branches from the suprascapular and thoracoacromial arteries.

Innervation
The acromioclavicular joint is innervated by branches from the suprascapular and lateral pectoral nerves.

Factors maintaining stability
The coracoclavicular ligament stabilizes the acromioclavicular joint. In acromioclavicular dislocation, the ligament is torn and the scapula falls away from the clavicle. Dislocation readily recurs because of the flatness and orientation of the joint surfaces.

Movements
Movements at the joint are like those of the sternoclavicular joint. These are passive, i.e. no muscle directly moves the joint, but muscles which move the scapula indirectly move the clavicle. Axial rotation of the clavicle is c.30°, the two joints together therefore, permit c.60° of scapular rotation. Angulation with the scapula occurs in any direction.

MOVEMENTS OF THE PECTORAL (SHOULDER) GIRDLE
Clavicular movements at the sternoclavicular and acromioclavicular joints are inevitably associated with movements of the scapula, and these are usually accompanied by movements of the humerus. The acromioclavicular joint allows anteroposterior gliding and rotation of the acromion, and hence the scapula, on the clavicle: scapular range is increased by movements at the sternoclavicular joint.

In all scapular movements, it is assumed that subclavius probably steadies the clavicle by drawing it medially and downwards, although its inaccessibility for electromyographic analysis makes its role uncertain. Scapular movements on the thoracic wall are facilitated by areolar tissue between subscapularis, serratus anterior and the chest wall. With the arm by the side, the normal posture of the shoulder girdle relative to the trunk involves moderate activity in trapezius and serratus anterior, and this increases when the limb is loaded.

The following account should be read together with the description of movements of the glenohumeral joint.

Elevation and depression – Scapular elevation and depression, as in 'shrugging the shoulders', do not necessarily imply movement at the shoulder joint. In elevation, slight angulation or swing occurs at the acromioclavicular joint. The sternal end of the clavicle, rotating about an anteroposterior axis through the bone above the medial attachment of the costoclavicular ligament, slides down over the articular disc (translation). This is checked by antagonist muscles and tension in the costoclavicular ligament and lower capsule. It is produced by the upper part of trapezius and levator scapulae, and since these tend to rotate the scapula in opposite directions, pure elevation can occur. In depression, slight angulation occurs at the acromioclavicular joint, and the clavicle slides up on the disc at the sternoclavicular joint. The movements are checked by antagonist muscles, the interclavicular and sternoclavicular ligaments and the articular disc. Usually gravity alone is sufficient: when necessary, the lowest part of serratus anterior and pectoralis minor are active depressors.

Protraction and retraction – Protraction (forward movement) round the thoracic wall occurs in pushing, thrusting and reaching movements, usually with some lateral rotation. The acromion advances over the clavicular facet to the limit, and the shoulder is simultaneously advanced by forward movement of the lateral end of the clavicle and posterior translation of its sternal end over the sternal facet, carrying the disc with it. Antagonist muscles, together with the anterior sternoclavicular ligament and posterior lamina of the costoclavicular ligament, check backward slide of the sternal end. Serratus anterior and pectoralis minor are prime movers and maintain continuous apposition of the scapula, especially its medial border, in smooth gliding on the thoracic wall. The upper part of latissimus dorsi also acts like a strap across the inferior scapular angle in protraction and lateral rotation.

In scapular retraction, i.e. bracing back the shoulders, these movements are reversed and checked at the sternoclavicular joint by the posterior sternoclavicular ligament and anterior lamina of the costoclavicular ligament. Trapezius and the rhomboids are prime movers, but gravity may also produce retraction when the weight of the trunk is taken by the arms in leaning forwards, which is to a degree controlled by protractive musculature.

When force is applied at the end of an outstretched arm, e.g. in a fall on the hand, pressure transmitted to the glenoid fossa tends to drive the sloping acromial facet below the acromial end of the clavicle. It also tenses the trapezoid ligament, which resists the displacement.

Lateral and medial rotation – Lateral rotation of the scapula increases the range of humeral elevation by turning the glenoid cavity to face almost directly up, e.g. raising an arm above the head. This movement is always associated with some humeral elevation and with protraction of the scapula. Scapular rotation requires movement at both sternoclavicular and acromioclavicular joints: the sternoclavicular joint permits elevation of the lateral end of the clavicle, a movement which is almost complete when the arm is abducted to 90°. The acromioclavicular joint moves in the first 30° of abduction, when the conoid ligament becomes taut, and is subsequently accompanied by clavicular rotation at the sternoclavicular joint around the longitudinal axis of the bone. The medial end is depressed further as the lateral end continues to rise. Some acromioclavicular movement also occurs in the final stages of humeral abduction. Trapezius (upper part) and serratus anterior (lower part) are prime movers.

Medial rotation is usually effected by gravity: gradual active lengthening of trapezius and serratus anterior is sufficient to control it. When more force is needed, levator scapulae, the rhomboids and, in the initial stages, pectoralis minor, are prime movers in returning the scapula to a position of rest.

Muscles which are antagonists in one movement may combine as prime movers in another. Movements, not muscles, are represented in cerebral motor areas. Muscles are not grouped unalterably in nervous control but can be variably combined as demands dictate. Thus serratus anterior and trapezius are opposed in scapular movement round the thorax, but combine as prime movers in lateral rotation of the scapula.

Glenohumeral (shoulder) joint

The glenohumeral joint is a synovial multiaxial spheroidal joint between the roughly hemispherical head of the humerus and the shallow glenoid fossa of the scapula (**Fig. 49.17**). Notable for its relative lack of bony constraint, the joint possesses three degrees of freedom. Its static and dynamic stability depends on the surrounding muscular and soft tissue envelope more than on its shape and ligaments: effective function is achieved by a complex interaction between the articular and soft tissue restraints.

Articulating surfaces

The articular surfaces are reciprocally curved and are really ovoids. (Here, as in the hip, where ovoid surfaces are almost spherical they are often termed spheroidal.) The area of the humeral convexity exceeds that of the glenoid concavity such that only a small portion opposes the glenoid in any position (**Fig. 49.18**). The remaining capitular articular surface is in contact with the capsule, so that contact on the glenoid

fossa is much more uniformly distributed over its entire articular surface. The radius of curvature of the glenoid fossa in the coronal plane is greater than that of the humeral head, and is deepened by a fibro-cartilaginous rim, the glenoid labrum (**Figs 49.15, 49.19**). Both articular surfaces are covered by hyaline cartilage, which is thickest centrally and thinner peripherally over the humerus, and the reverse in the glenoid cavity. In most positions, their curvatures are not fully congruent, and the joint is loose-packed. Close packing (full congruence) is reached with the humerus abducted and laterally rotated (**Figs 49.20, 6.62**).

Glenoid labrum

The glenoid labrum is a fibrocartilaginous rim around the glenoid fossa. Triangular in section, its base is attached to the margin of the fossa, and its thin margin projects as a continuation of the curve of the glenoid. It blends above with two fasciculi from the long tendon of biceps. The labrum deepens the cavity, may protect the bone, and probably assists lubrication. Its attachment is sometimes partly deficient anterosuperiorly, in which case synovial membrane may protrude through the gaps.

Fibrous capsule

A fibrous capsule envelops the joint (**Figs 49.16, 49.18**). It is attached medially to the glenoid margin outside the glenoid labrum, and encroaches on the coracoid process to include the attachment of the long head of biceps. Laterally, it is attached to the anatomical neck of the humerus, i.e. near the articular margin, except inferomedially, where it descends more than 1 cm on the humeral shaft. It is so lax that the bones can be distracted for 2 or 3 cm, which accords with the very wide range of movement possible at the glenohumeral joint. However, such unnatural separation requires relaxation of the upper capsule by abduction.

The fibrous capsule is supported by the tendons of supraspinatus (above), infraspinatus and teres minor (behind), subscapularis (in front)

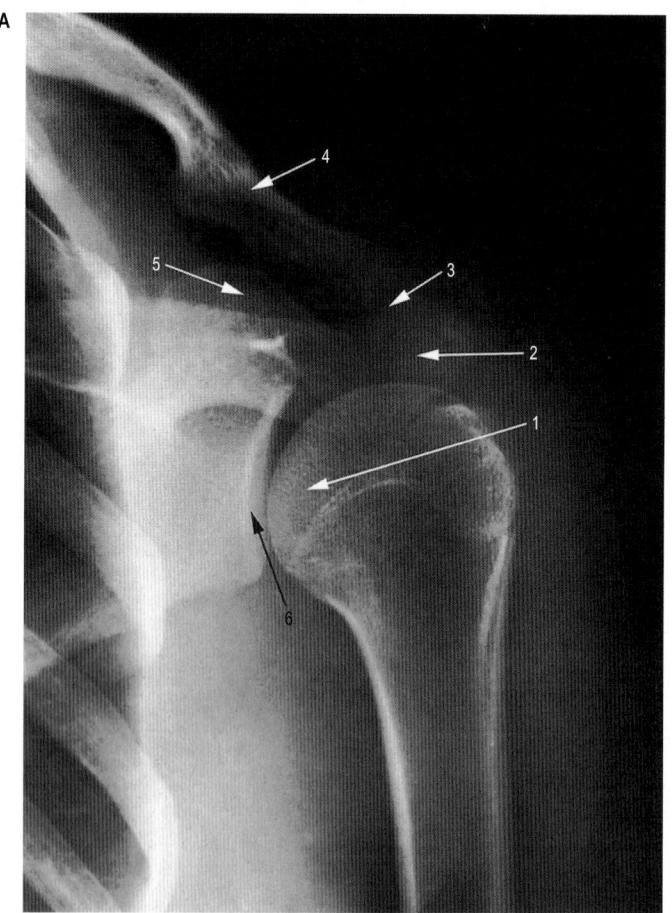
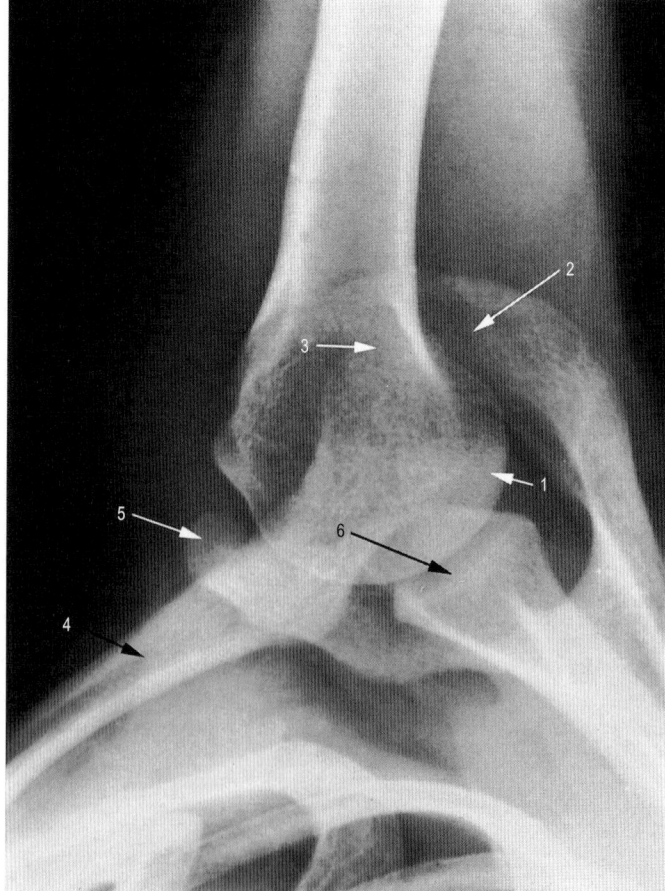

1. Head of humerus.   **2.** Acromion.   **3.** Acromioclavicular joint.   **4.** Clavicle.   **5.** Coracoid process.   **6.** Glenoid (osseous, subchondral) articular surface.

Fig. 49.17 Radiograph of shoulder in a young female of 18 years in anteroposterior view (**A**) and axillary view with the arm abducted (**B**).

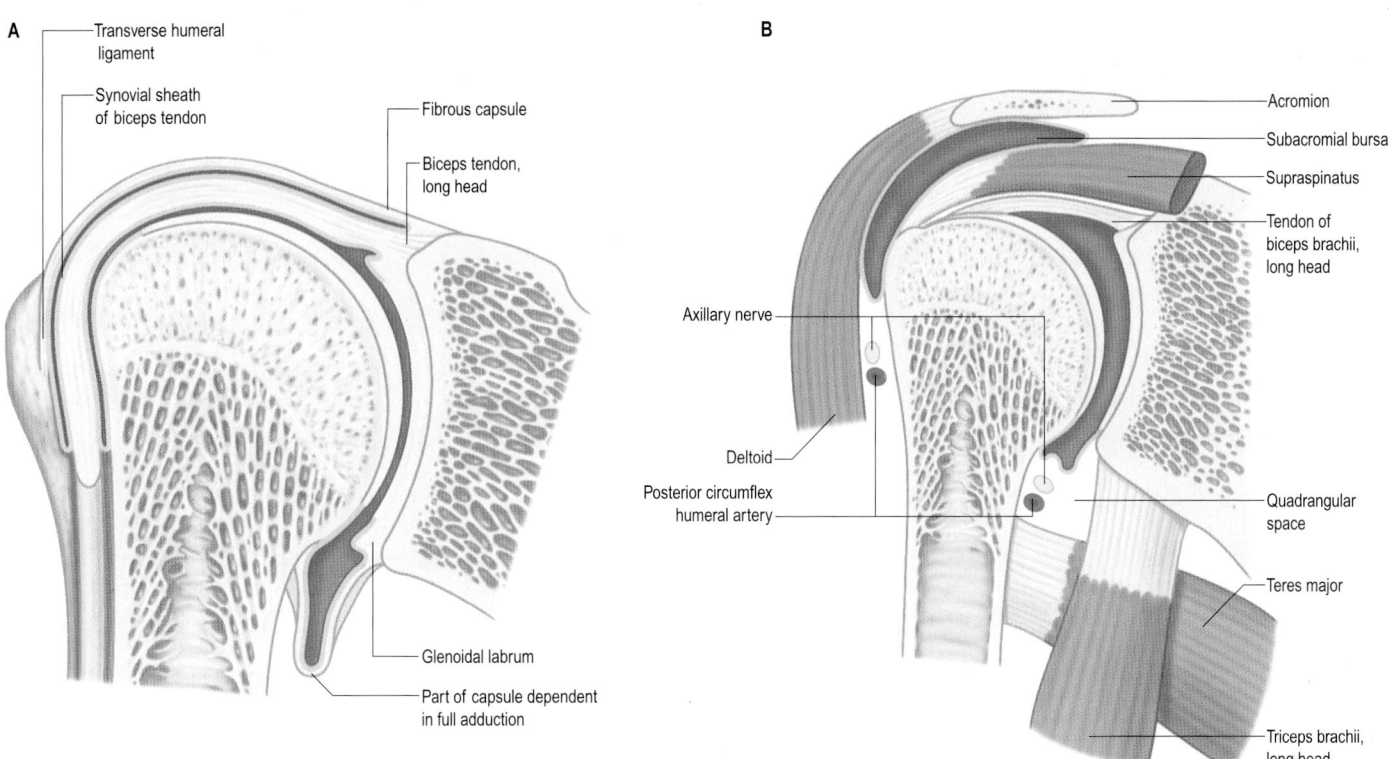

Fig. 49.18 A, B, Coronal section through the left shoulder joint viewed from the posterior aspect A, anteriorly placed coronal section to show tendon of biceps, long head B, posteriorly placed coronal section to show subacromial bursa and contents of quadrangular space. (**B**, by permission from Agur AMR, Lee MJ (eds) 1999 Grant's Atlas of Anatomy, 10th edn. Philadelphia: Lippincott Williams and Wilkins.)

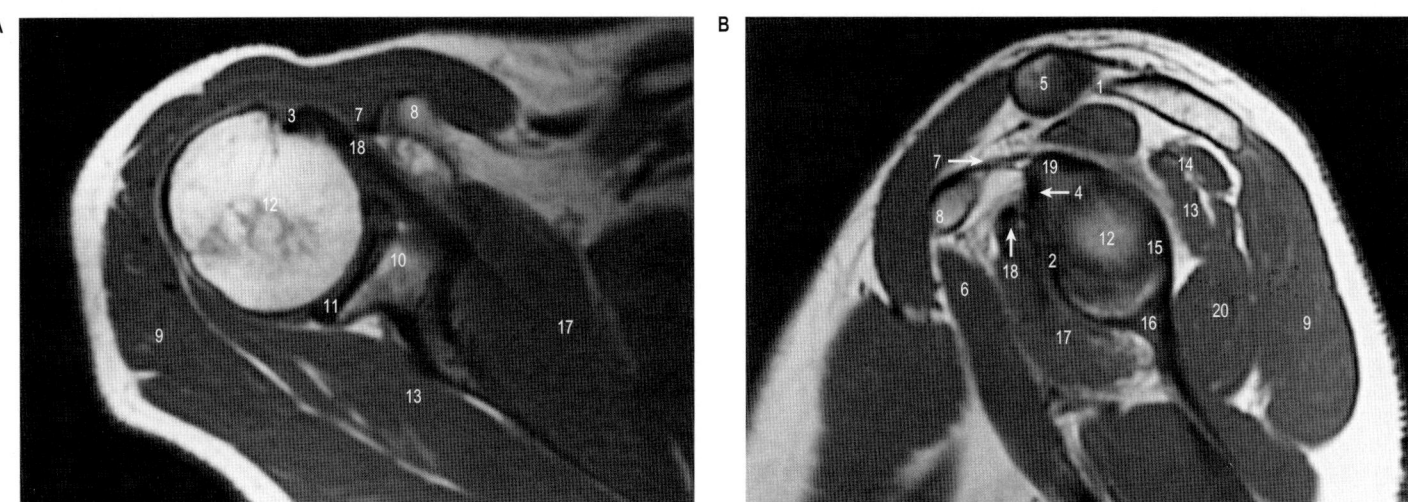

1. Acromioclavicular joint. 2. Anterior labrum. 3. Biceps brachii tendon. 4. Biceps brachii tendon – long head. 5. Clavicle. 6. Coracobrachialis muscle. 7. Coracohumeral ligament.
8. Coracoid process. 9. Deltoid muscle. 10. Glenoid. 11. Glenoid labrum. 12. Head of humerus. 13. Infraspinatus muscle. 14. Infraspinatus tendon. 15. Posterior labrum. 16. Scapula.
17. Subscapularis muscle. 18. Subscapularis tendon. 19. Superior labrum. 20. Teres minor muscle.

Fig. 49.19 MRI of shoulder. **A,** Axial image. **B,** Sagittal oblique section. (By permission from Weir J, Abrahams PH 2003 Imaging Atlas of Human Anatomy, 3rd edn, London: Mosby, and contributions from Anna-Maria Belli, Margaret Hourihan, Naill Moore and Philip Owen.)

and by the long head of triceps (below). All but triceps blend with the capsule as the rotator cuff, which reinforces the capsule and actively supports it unless the muscles are fully relaxed. Triceps is separated from the capsule by the axillary nerve and posterior circumflex humeral vessels as they pass back from the axilla (**Fig. 49.16**). The capsule is least supported inferiorly, and subjected to the greatest strain in full abduction, when it is stretched tightly across the humeral head. It is strengthened anteriorly by extensions from the tendons of pectoralis major and teres major.

There are usually two or three openings in the capsule: below the coracoid process, connecting the joint to a bursa behind the tendon of subscapularis (anterior); between the humeral tubercles, transmitting the long tendon of biceps and its synovial sheath; connecting the joint to a bursa under the tendon of infraspinatus (posterior and inconstant).

Ligaments

Glenohumeral ligaments – Three glenohumeral ligaments, best visible from within the joint, reinforce the capsule anteriorly (**Fig. 49.15**). They do not act as traditional ligaments (which carry a pure tensile force along their length), and become taut at varying positions of abduction and humeral rotation. Moreover, they do not have the strength

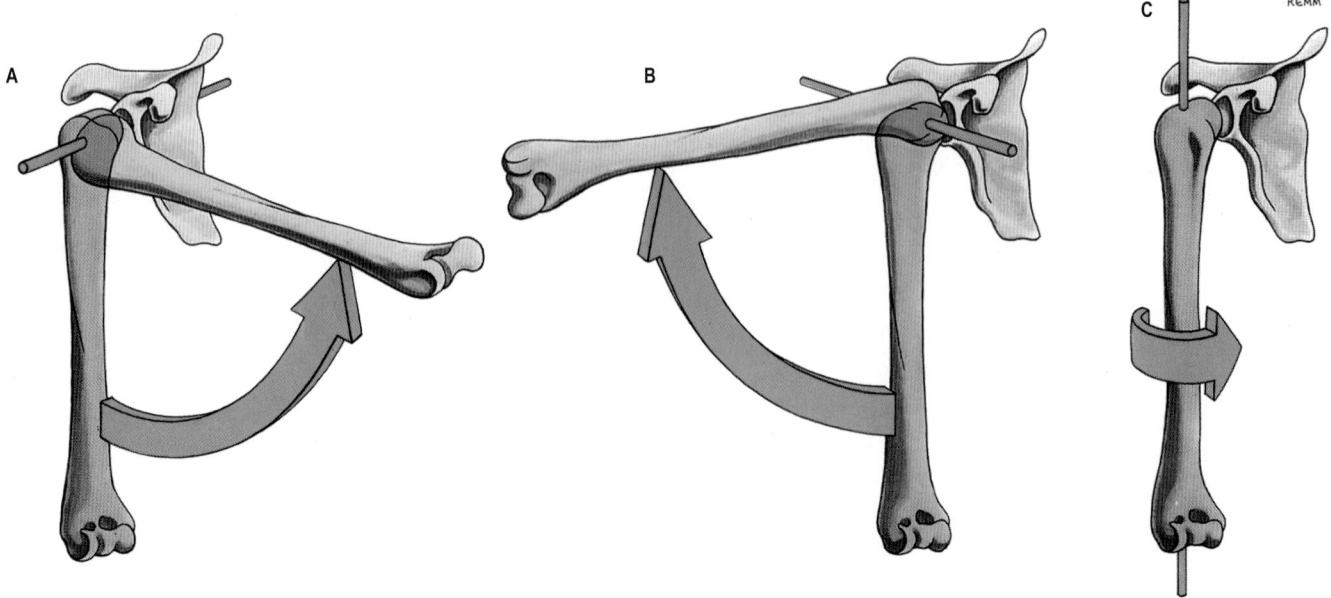

Fig. 49.20 The three mutually perpendicular axes around which the principal movements of flexion–extension (**A**), abduction–adduction (**B**) and medial and lateral rotation (**C**) occur at the shoulder. The axes are referred to the plane of the scapula and not to the coronal and sagittal planes of the erect body as a whole. An infinite variety of additional movements may occur at such a joint, involving intermediate planes, and there may be movement combinations or sequences. However, these can always be resolved mathematically into components related to the three axes illustrated.

characteristics of the ligaments at the knee. The superior glenohumeral ligament passes from the supraglenoid tubercle, just anterior to the origin of the long head of biceps, to the humerus near the proximal tip of the lesser tubercle on the medial ridge of the intertuberous groove. It forms an anterior cover around the long head of biceps, and is part of the rotator interval. Together with the coracohumeral ligament it is an important stabilizer in the inferior direction (the coracohumeral ligament is more robust than the superior glenohumeral ligament). The middle glenohumeral ligament arises from a wide attachment below the superior glenohumeral ligament, along the anterior glenoid margin as far as the inferior third of the rim, and passes obliquely infero-laterally, enlarging as it does, to attach to the lesser tubercle deep to the tendon of subscapularis, with which it blends. The width and thickness of this ligament may be as much as 2 cm and 4 mm respectively. It provides anterior stability at 45° and 60° abduction. The thicker and longer inferior glenohumeral ligament complex is a hammock-like structure with anchor points on the anterior and posterior sides of the glenoid. It arises from the anterior, middle and posterior margins of the glenoid labrum, below the epiphyseal line, and passes anteroinferiorly to the inferior and medial aspects of the neck of the humerus. The anterior, superior edge of the inferior ligament is thickened as the superior band, and the diffuse thickening of the anterior part of the capsule to which it is attached is known as the axillary pouch. The anterior band of the inferior glenohumeral ligament is thought to be the primary anterior stabilizer of the glenohumeral joint. (For further details consult Burkart & Debski 2002.)

Coracohumeral ligament – The coracohumeral ligament is attached to the dorsolateral base of the coracoid process and extends as two bands, which blend with the capsule, to the greater and lesser tubercles (**Fig. 49.16**). Portions of the coracohumeral ligament form a tunnel for the biceps tendon on the anterior side of the joint. The rotator interval, the region of the capsule between the anterior border of suraspinatus and the superior border of subscapularis, is reinforced by the coracohumeral ligament. It also blends inferiorly with the superior glenohumeral ligament.

Transverse humeral ligament – The transverse humeral ligament is a broad band which passes between the humeral tubercles, and is attached superior to the epiphyseal line (**Fig. 49.16**). It converts the intertuberous sulcus into a canal, and acts as a retinaculum for the long tendon of biceps.

Synovial membrane
The synovial membrane lines the capsule and covers parts of the anatomical neck. The long tendon of biceps traverses the joint in a synovial sheath which continues into the intertuberous sulcus as far as the surgical neck of the humerus (**Figs 49.16, 49.18**).

Bursae
Many bursae adjoin the shoulder joint. They are usually found between the tendon of subscapularis and the capsule, communicating with the joint between the superior and middle glenohumeral ligaments; on the superior acromial aspect; between the coracoid process and capsule; between teres major and the long head of triceps: anterior and posterior to the tendon of latissimus dorsi. The subacromial bursa, between deltoid and the capsule, does not communicate with the joint cavity but is prolonged under the acromion and coracoacromial ligament, and between them and supraspinatus: it appears to be attached, together with the subdeltoid fascia, to the acromion. Bursae sometimes occur behind coracobrachialis and between the tendon of infraspinatus and the capsule, occasionally opening into the joint.

Vascular supply
The glenohumeral joint is supplied by branches from the anterior and posterior circumflex humeral, suprascapular and circumflex scapular vessels.

Innervation
The glenohumeral joint is innervated mainly from the posterior cord of the brachial plexus. The capsule is supplied by the suprascapular nerve (posterior and superior parts), axillary nerve (anteroinferior) and the lateral pectoral nerve (anterosuperior).

Factors maintaining stability
The articulation between the relatively large humeral head and the shallow glenoid fossa allow a wide range of movement at the expense of providing an unstable bony complex. The joint capsule is strong but lax. A variety of additional factors help to increase the stability of the joint. The glenoid labrum deepens the concavity of the articulating glenoid. The coracoacromial arch (coracoid, acromion and coraco-acromial ligament) prevents upward dislocation of the humerus. The tendons of subscapularis, supraspinatus, infraspinatus and teres minor fuse with the lateral part of the joint capsule to form the 'rotator cuff'.

These short muscles collectively produce a compressive force during active glenohumeral movements which maintains congruent contact between the head of the humerus and the glenoid fossa, helps to resist skid, and checks excessive translation. The rotator cuff also provides strong lateral stability and prevents this part of the lax capsule from being nipped during joint movements. The long head of biceps offers additional superior support. The long head of triceps offers inferior support which is particularly important when the shoulder is abducted. However, the glenohumeral joint is least stabile inferiorly when the shoulder is fully abducted.

Movements at the shoulder (glenohumeral) joint

The shoulder is capable of any combination of swing and spin over a very wide range. Laxity of the capsule, and a humeral head which is large relative to a shallow glenoid fossa, afford a wider range of movement than at any other joint. Flexion–extension, abduction–adduction, circumduction and medial and lateral rotation all occur at the shoulder.

In analysis of shoulder movements it is preferable to refer humeral movement to the scapula, rather than to conventional anatomical planes (**Fig. 49.21**). When the arm hangs at rest the glenoid fossa faces almost equally forwards and laterally, and the humeral capitular and scapular (topographical) axes correspond, although the humerus, relative to the anatomical position, is medially rotated. Flexion carries the arm antero-medially on an axis through the humeral head orthogonal to the glenoid fossa at its centre. Abduction and adduction occur in a vertical plane orthogonal to that of flexion–extension; the axis is horizontal, through the humeral head, parallel with the glenoid plane. Pure abduction raises the arm anterolaterally in the plane of the scapula. However, when referred to the trunk, flexion and extension occur in the paramedian plane, and abduction and adduction in the coronal plane. In this sense, raising the arm vertically from flexion or raising it from abduction are both accompanied by humeral rotation in opposite directions. Whether 'scapular' or any other plane of abduction is described, these are selections from an infinite series. In scapular abduction points on the humeral surface pursue vertical cords but in rotation they are horizontal. In 'pure' flexion–extension, in a plane orthogonal to the scapula the axis of movement, and the notional 'mechanical axis', are regarded as projected from the centre of the glenoid cavity.

Glenohumeral abduction is c.90°, but angles up to 120° have been reported. Some 60° further abduction occurs at the sterno- and acromioclavicular articulations. Contralateral vertebral flexion also aids in bringing the arm to the vertical. During active elevation, movements at the glenohumeral and acromioclavicular joints are simultaneous, except in the initial few degrees, when most, often all, movement is glenohumeral. For every 15° of elevation, glenohumeral movement is said to be 10° and scapular movement 5°. During the initial stages of abduction, subscapularis, infraspinatus and teres minor counteract the strong upward component of pull of deltoid, which would otherwise cause the humeral head to slide up; the additive turning moments exerted by deltoid and supraspinatus about the shoulder joint can then abduct the arm.

In flexion, the humerus swings at right angles to the scapular plane and scapular rotation cannot increase the elevation (120°) obtainable in full flexion. If the fully flexed humerus is also abducted, elevation increases pro rata until, when the humerus reaches the scapular plane, i.e. when true abduction is reached, 180° of elevation becomes possible. In medial or lateral rotation, the humerus revolves about one-quarter of a circle around a vertical axis; the range is greatest when the arm is pendent, and least when it is vertical. When assessing the rotational range at the glenohumeral joint, the forearm should be flexed to a right angle at the elbow: this will prevent the effects of superadded pronation or supination in the pendent limb. In circumduction, which is a succession of the foregoing movements, the distal end of the humerus describes the base of a cone, its apex at the humeral head. This gleno-humeral movement can be much increased by scapular movements, e.g. in acts of slinging objects with force.

The peculiar relation of the long head of biceps to the shoulder joint may serve several purposes. By its connection with both the shoulder and elbow, the muscle harmonizes their actions as an elastic ligament during all their movements. It helps to prevent the humeral head impinging on the acromion when deltoid contracts and to steady it in movements of the arm. In paralysis of supraspinatus it may also help initiate abduction of the arm, particularly when the humerus is laterally rotated.

Muscles producing movements

The muscles which produce movements at the glenohumeral joint are principally deltoid, pectoralis major, latissimus dorsi and teres major. These long muscles all converge on the humerus, acting at mechanical advantage on a joint which, as a result of glenoid shallowness and capsular laxity, is relatively unstable. The long muscles are counteracted by the rotator cuff, a group of short muscles (subscapularis, supra-spinatus, infraspinatus and teres minor) which are attached nearer to the joint, and which centre the head of the humerus in the glenoid fossa through the midrange of motion, when the capsuloligamentous structures are lax.

Flexion: pectoralis major (clavicular part), deltoid (anterior fibres) and coracobrachialis assisted by biceps. The sternocostal part of pectoralis major is a major force in flexion forwards to the coronal plane from full extension.

Extension: deltoid (posterior fibres) and teres major, from the dependent position. When the fully flexed arm is extended against resistance, latissimus dorsi and the sternocostal part of pectoralis major act powerfully until the arm reaches the coronal plane.

Abduction: deltoid. Initially its effect is mainly upward and, unless opposed, this would displace the humerus upwards. Subscapularis, infraspinatus and teres minor exert downward traction and so apply an opposing force: together with deltoid they constitute a 'couple' to produce abduction in the scapular plane. Supraspinatus assists in effecting and maintaining this movement, but its precise role is controversial.

Medial rotation: pectoralis major, deltoid (anterior fibres), latissimus dorsi, teres major and, with the arm pendent, subscapularis.

Lateral rotation: infraspinatus, deltoid (posterior fibres) and teres minor. Lateral rotation is important for clearance of the greater tubercle and its associated tissues as it passes under the coracoacromial arch, as well as for relaxation of the capsular ligamentous constraints.

Rotator cuff impingement syndrome

The subacromial space is defined by the humeral head inferiorly, and the anterior edge and inferior surface of the anterior third of the acromion, coracoacromial ligament and acromioclavicular joint superiorly. It is occupied by the supraspinatus tendon, subacromial bursa, tendon of the long head of biceps brachii, and the capsule of the shoulder joint. Rotator cuff impingement syndrome is a painful disorder caused by severe or chronic impingement of the rotator cuff tendons under the coracoacromial arch (Michiner et al 2003). The cuff normally impinges against the coracoacromial arch when the humerus is abducted, flexed and internally rotated. This is known as the impingement position. The supraspinatus tendon is anatomically affected most by the impingement, which interestingly also coincides with an area of reduced vascularity in this tendon. Severe impingement can be caused by osteoarthritic thickening of the coracoacromial arch; inflammation of the cuff from disorders such as rheumatoid arthritis; and prolonged overuse in the impingement position, e.g. in cleaning windows, which, when associated with a tendinopathy from age-related degenerative changes within the tendon, can lead to subsequent partial or complete tears of the cuff. Clinically, this condition causes tenderness over the anterior portion of the acromion, and pain which typically occurs on abducting the shoulder between 60° and 120° (the painful arc).

Glenohumeral joint dislocations

The glenohumeral joint is the most frequently dislocated joint in the body. It is most unstable inferiorly. The vast majority of dislocations are anterior and occur when the arm is forced into abduction, external rotation and extension. Clinically, a dislocated shoulder loses its normal contour, and the acromion process, rather than the greater tubercle, becomes the most lateral bony structure. The axillary nerve and artery may be injured during dislocation, and this can lead to inability to abduct the shoulder together with an area of anaesthesia over the distal part of the muscle, as well as ischaemic changes in the limb. Posterior dislocation is rare and typically occurs when violent movements produce marked internal rotation and adduction, e.g. in epileptic seizures or electric shock.

MUSCLES

PECTORALIS MAJOR

Attachments – Pectoralis major (**Fig. 49.21**) is a thick, fan-shaped muscle. It arises from the anterior surface of the sternal half of the

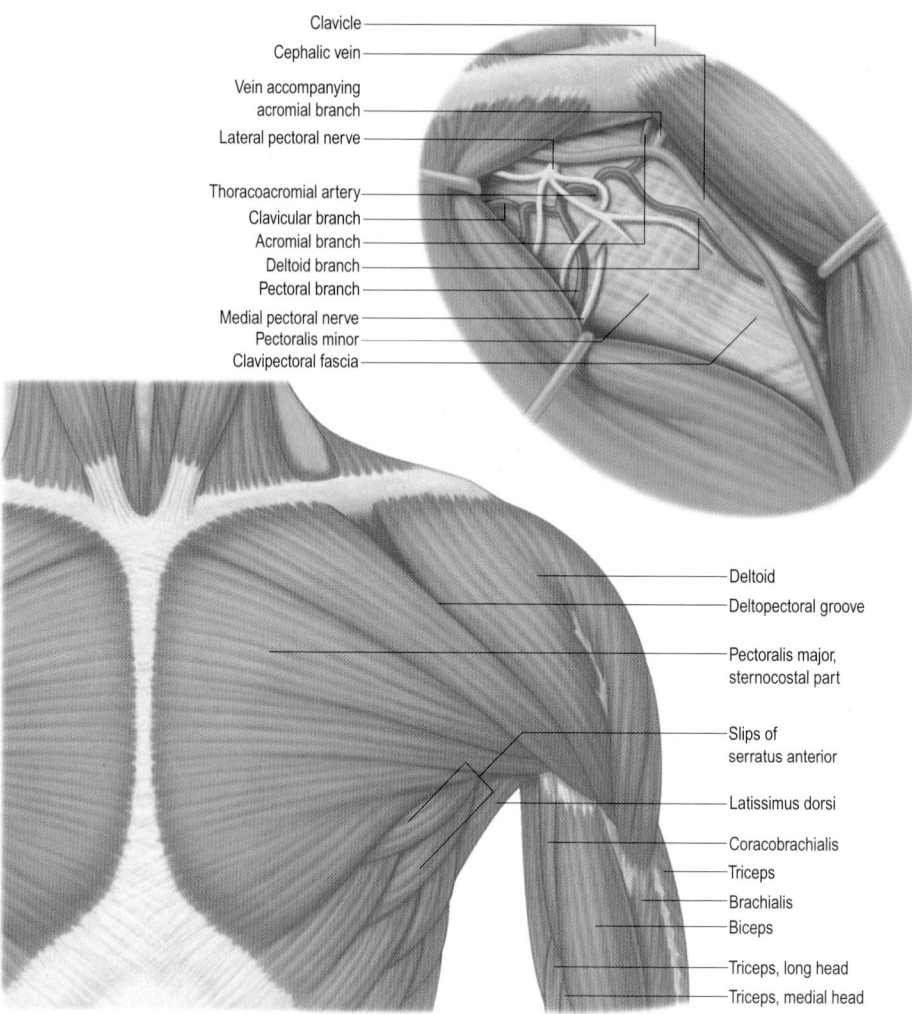

Fig. 49.21 Superficial muscles of the front of the chest and left upper arm, showing thoracoacromial axis.

clavicle; half the breadth of the anterior surface of the sternum down to the level of the sixth or seventh costal cartilage; the first to the seventh costal cartilages (first and seventh often omitted); the sternal end of the sixth rib; and the aponeurosis of external oblique. The clavicular fibres are usually separated from the sternal fibres by a slight cleft. The muscle converges to a flat tendon, c.5 cm across, which is attached to the lateral lip of the intertuberous sulcus of the humerus. The tendon is bilaminar. The thicker anterior lamina is formed by fibres from the manubrium, which are joined superficially by clavicular fibres and deeply by fibres from the sternal margin and the second to fifth costal cartilages. Clavicular fibres may be prolonged into the deltoid tendon. The posterior lamina receives fibres from the sixth (and often seventh) costal cartilages, sixth rib, sternum, and aponeurosis of the external oblique. Costal fibres join the lamina without twisting. Fibres from the sternum and aponeurosis curve around the lower border, turning successively behind those above them, which means that this part of the muscle is twisted so that the fibres that are lowest at their medial origin are highest at their insertion on the humerus. The posterior lamina reaches higher on the humerus than the anterior, and gives off an expansion which covers the intertuberous sulcus and blends with the capsular ligament of the shoulder joint. An expansion from the deepest part of the lamina lines the intertuberous sulcus at its linear insertion; from its lower border another expansion descends into the deep fascia of the upper arm.

The rounded lower border of the muscle forms the anterior axillary fold, and becomes conspicuous in abduction against resistance.

Variants – The abdominal slip from the aponeurosis of the external oblique is sometimes absent. The number of costal attachments and the extent to which the clavicular and costal parts are separated vary. Right and left muscles may decussate across the sternum. A superficial vertical slip, or slips, may ascend from the lower costal cartilages and rectus sheath to blend with sternocleidomastoid or to attach to the upper sternum or costal cartilages. This is sternalis (rectus sternalis). The muscle may be partially or completely absent.

Relations – Skin, superficial fascia, platysma, anterior and middle supraclavicular nerves, breast, and deep fascia are all anterior. The sternum, ribs and costal cartilages, clavipectoral fascia, subclavius, pectoralis minor, serratus anterior, external intercostal muscles and membranes are all posterior. Pectoralis major forms the superficial layer of the anterior axillary wall, and hence lies anterior to the axillary vessels and nerves and the upper parts of biceps and coracobrachialis. Its upper border is separated from deltoid by the infraclavicular fossa, which contains the cephalic vein and deltoid branch of the thoraco-acromial artery. Its lower border forms the anterior axillary fold. Pectoralis major is separated from latissimus dorsi on the medial axillary wall, but the two muscles converge as they approach the lateral axillary wall: the floor of the intertubercular sulcus lies between their attachments.

Vascular supply – Pectoralis major is supplied by one dominant vascular pedicle from the pectoral branch of the thoraco-acromial axis, supplemented by several smaller secondary segmental vessels from the deltoid and clavicular branches of the thoraco-acromial axis, and perforating branches of the internal thoracic arteries and superior and lateral thoracic arteries.

The presence of a dominant vascular pedicle (together with its musculocutaneous perforators) means that a musculocutaneous flap in this region can be surgically raised solely on the pectoral branch (the pectoralis major musculocutaneous flap). This flap can be used to reconstruct areas of missing tissue following head and neck cancer resections.

Innervation – Pectoralis major is supplied through the medial and lateral pectoral nerves. Fibres for the clavicular part are from C5 and 6; those for the sternocostal part are from C6, 7, 8, and T1.

Action – The two parts of the muscle can act separately or together. The whole muscle assists adduction and medial rotation of the humerus against resistance. It swings the extended arm forwards and medially, its clavicular part acting with the anterior fibres of deltoid and coraco-brachialis: the sternocostal part is relaxed. The opposite movement is usually aided by gravity. When it is resisted, the sternocostal part acts together with latissimus dorsi, teres major and the posterior fibres of deltoid: the clavicular part is relaxed. With the raised arms fixed, e.g. gripping a branch, the same combination of muscles draws the trunk up and forwards. Pectoralis major is active in deep inspiration. Electro-myography suggests that the clavicular part acts alone in medial rotation.

Clinical anatomy: testing – To test the clavicular head, the abducted arm is flexed against resistance. To test the sternocostal head, the arm is adducted against resistance.

Poland syndrome – Poland syndrome is a rare congenital anomaly where there is hypoplasia of the thoracic chest wall muscles and ipsilateral hypoplasia of the arm and hand. It occurs in c.1:50,000 live births. The major clinical features are that the sternocostal head of pectoralis major and all of pectoralis minor are absent. In addition, there may be hypoplasia of latissimus dorsi, serratus anterior, external oblique, supraspinatus, infraspinatus, deltoid and the intercostal muscles, and hypoplasia of the hemithorax and ribs. There may be ipsilateral breast hypoplasia and absent nipple-areolar-complex (Ch. 59).

Hypoplasia affecting the arm ranges from syndactyly to symbrachydactyly and ectrodactyly. The second, third and fourth fingers are the most affected; the wrist, forearm, upper arm and scapula are variably involved.

The aetiology is unclear. It has been suggested that the condition is caused by disruption of the arterial blood supply to the subclavian vessels during the sixth and seventh week of embryonic life, or by disruption of lateral plate mesoderm 2–4 weeks after fertilization.

PECTORALIS MINOR

Attachments – Pectoralis minor is a thin, triangular muscle lying posterior (deep) to pectoralis major (**Fig. 49.22**). It arises from the upper margins and outer surfaces of the third to fifth ribs (frequently second to fourth), near their cartilages, and from the fascia over the adjoining external intercostal muscles. Its fibres ascend laterally under cover of pectoralis major, converging in a flat tendon which is attached to the medial border and upper surface of the coracoid process of the scapula. Part or all of the tendon may cross the coracoid process into the coraco-acromial ligament, or even beyond to the coracohumeral ligament, thereby gaining attachment to the humerus.

Variants – Slips of the muscle are sometimes separated and vary in number and level. In rare cases, one passes from the first rib to the coracoid (pectoralis minimus). The costal attachments can be 2nd to 5th ribs; 3rd to 5th; 2nd to 4th; 3rd to 4th. The muscle can be present or absent when the pectoralis major is absent.

Relations – Pectoralis major, the lateral pectoral nerve and pectoral branches of the thoraco-acromial artery are anterior. The ribs, external intercostals, serratus anterior, the axilla, axillary vessels, lymphatics and brachial plexus are all posterior. The upper border of pectoralis minor is separated from the clavicle by a triangular gap which is filled by the clavipectoral fascia, behind which are the axillary vessels, lymphatics and nerves. The lateral thoracic artery follows the lower border of the muscle. The medial pectoral nerves pierce and partly supply the muscle.

Vascular supply – Pectoralis minor is supplied by pectoral and deltoid branches of the thoraco-acromial and superior and lateral thoracic arteries.

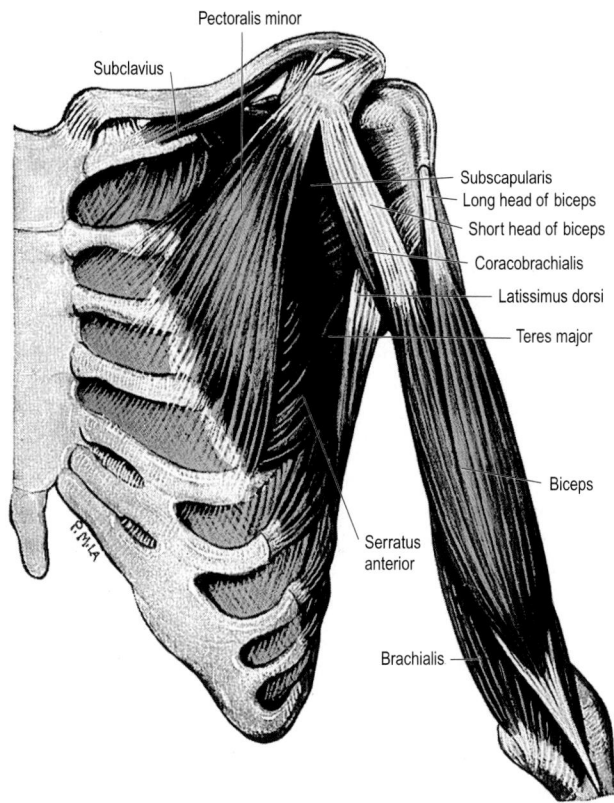

Fig. 49.22 Deep muscles of the front of the chest and left arm.

Innervation – Pectoralis minor is innervated by branches of the medial and lateral pectoral nerves, C5, 6, 7, 8 and T1.

Action – Pectoralis minor assists serratus anterior in drawing the scapula forwards around the chest wall. With levator scapulae and the rhomboids it rotates the scapula, depressing the point of the shoulder. Both pectoral muscles are electromyographically quiescent in normal inspiration, but are active in forced inspiration.

SUBCLAVIUS

Attachments – Subclavius is a small, triangular muscle tucked between the clavicle and the first rib (**Fig. 49.22**). It arises from the junction of the first rib and its costal cartilage by a thick tendon, prolonged at its inferior margin and anterior to the costoclavicular ligament. It passes upwards and laterally to a groove on the under surface of the middle third of the clavicle, where it is attached by muscular fibres.

Subclavius may be attached to the coracoid process or the upper border of the scapula as well as, or instead of, the clavicle.

Relations – Posteriorly subclavius is separated from the first rib by the subclavian vessels and brachial plexus, and anteriorly it is separated from pectoralis major by the anterior lamina of the clavipectoral fascia.

Vascular supply – Subclavius is supplied by the clavicular branch of the thoraco-acromial artery and the suprascapular artery.

Innervation – Subclavius is supplied by the subclavian branch of the brachial plexus, which contains fibres from C5 and 6.

Action – Subclavius probably pulls the point of the shoulder down and forwards and braces the clavicle against the articular disc of the sterno-clavicular joint: however it is inaccessible to palpation, and difficult to investigate by electromyography. It 'protects' the subclavian vessels in fractures of the clavicle, which rarely involve these vessels.

TRAPEZIUS

Attachments – Trapezius is a flat, triangular muscle which extends over the back of the neck and upper thorax (**Fig. 57.19**). The paired trapezius muscles form a diamond shape, from which the name is derived: the lateral angles occur at the shoulder tips, the superior angle at the occipital protuberance and superior nuchal lines, and the inferior angle at the spine of the twelfth thoracic vertebra. On either side, the muscle is attached to the medial third of the superior nuchal line, external occipital protuberance, ligamentum nuchae, and apices of the spinous processes and their supraspinous ligaments from C7 to T12. Superior fibres descend, inferior fibres ascend, and the fibres between them proceed horizontally: all converge laterally on the shoulder. The superior fibres are attached to the posterior border of the lateral third of the clavicle; the middle fibres to the medial acromial margin and superior lip of the crest of the scapular spine; and the inferior fibres pass into an aponeurosis which glides over a smooth triangular surface at the medial end of the scapular spine and is attached to a tubercle at its lateral apex. The occipital attachment is by a fibrous lamina, which is also adherent to the skin. The spinal attachment is by a broad triangular aponeurosis from the sixth cervical to the third thoracic vertebrae, and by short tendinous fibres below this.

Variants – The clavicular attachment of trapezius varies in extent, sometimes reaching mid-clavicle, and occasionally blending with sterno-cleidomastoid. The vertebral attachment sometimes stops at the eighth thoracic spine. The occipital attachment may be absent. Cervical and dorsal parts are occasionally separate.

Vascular supply – The upper third of trapezius is supplied by a transverse muscular branch which arises from the occipital artery at the level of the mastoid process. It enters the muscle on its deep surface and gives off several musculocutaneous perforators to the overlying skin.

The middle portion of trapezius, together with an area of overlying skin, is supplied by the superficial cervical artery or by a superficial branch of the transverse cervical artery, via musculocutaneous perforators.

The lower third of trapezius is supplied by a muscular branch from the dorsal scapular artery, passing medial to the medial border of the scapula. It reaches the deep surface of the muscle either by piercing the rhomboids or by passing between rhomboid major and minor at the level of the base of the spine of the scapula. It anastomoses with the medial and lateral perforating branches of the posterior intercostal arteries.

The presence of these three discrete vascular pedicles means that musculocutaneous flaps can be surgically raised based on these individual arteries and their accompanying venae comitantes. These flaps can be used for reconstructing areas in the posterior head and neck.

Innervation – Trapezius is innervated by the spinal part of the accessory nerve. Sensory (proprioceptive) branches are derived from the ventral rami of C3 and C4.

Action – Trapezius cooperates with other muscles in steadying the scapula, controlling it during movements of the arm, and maintaining the level and poise of the shoulder. Electromyographic activity is minimal in the unloaded arm, and heavy loads can be suspended with a small contribution from the upper part. Acting with levator scapulae, the upper fibres elevate the scapula and with it the point of the shoulder; acting with serratus anterior, trapezius rotates the scapula forward so that the arm can be raised above the head; and acting with the rhomboids, it retracts the scapula, bracing back the shoulder. With the shoulder fixed, trapezius may bend the head and neck backwards and laterally. Trapezius, levator scapulae, rhomboids and serratus anterior combine in producing a variety of scapular rotations (p. 829).

Clinical anatomy: testing – Trapezius is palpated while the shoulder is shrugged against resistance.

DELTOID

Attachments – Deltoid is a thick, curved triangle of muscle. It arises from the anterior border and superior surface of the lateral third of the clavicle, the lateral margin and superior surface of the acromion, and

the lower edge of the crest of the scapular spine (other than its smooth medial triangular surface) (**Figs 57.19, 49.21**). The fibres converge inferiorly to a short, substantial tendon which is attached to the deltoid tubercle on the lateral aspect of the midshaft of the humerus. Anterior and posterior fibres converge directly to this tendon. The intermediate part is multipennate: four intramuscular septa descend from the acromion to interdigitate with three septa ascending from the deltoid tubercle. The septa are connected by short muscle fibres, which provide powerful traction. The fasciculi are large, producing a coarse longitudinal striation. The muscle surrounds the glenohumeral articulation on all sides except inferomedially, lending the shoulder its rounded profile. In contraction its borders are easily seen and felt. The tendon gives off an expansion into the brachial deep fascia which may reach the forearm.

Variants – Deltoid may fuse with pectoralis major or may receive additional slips from trapezius, the infraspinous fascia or the lateral scapular border.

Relations – The skin, superficial and deep fasciae, platysma, lateral supraclavicular and upper lateral brachial cutaneous nerves are all superficial. The coracoid process, coraco-acromial ligament, subacromial bursa, tendons of pectoralis minor, coracobrachialis, both heads of biceps, pectoralis major, subscapularis, supraspinatus, infraspinatus, teres minor, long and lateral heads of triceps, the circumflex humeral vessels, axillary nerve, and the surgical neck and upper shaft of the humerus, including both tubercles, all lie deep to deltoid. The anterior border of the muscle is separated proximally from pectoralis major by the infraclavicular fossa, which contains the cephalic vein and deltoid branches of the thoraco-acromial artery. Distally, the muscles are in contact, and their tendons are usually united. The posterior border overlies infraspinatus and triceps.

Vascular supply – Deltoid is supplied by acromial and deltoid branches of the thoraco-acromial artery; the anterior and posterior circumflex humeral arteries; subscapular artery; and the deltoid branch of profunda brachii.

Innervation – Deltoid is innervated by the axillary nerve, C5 and 6.

Action – Different parts of the muscle can act independently as well as together. Anterior fibres assist pectoralis major in drawing the arm forwards and rotating it medially. Posterior fibres act with latissimus dorsi and teres major in drawing the arm backwards and rotating it laterally. The multipennate acromial part of deltoid is a strong abductor: aided by supraspinatus it abducts the arm until the joint capsule is tense below. Movement takes place in the plane of the body of the scapula, which is the only way that scapular rotation can be fully effective in raising the arm above the head. In true abduction (**Fig. 49.21B**), acromial fibres contract strongly, while clavicular and posterior fibres prevent departure from the plane of motion. In the early stages of abduction, traction by the deltoid is upward, but the humeral head is prevented from translating upward by the synergistic downward pull of subscapularis, infraspinatus and teres minor. Electromyography suggests that deltoid contributes little to medial or lateral rotation but confirms that it takes part in most other shoulder movements. It may also aid supraspinatus in resisting the downward drag of a loaded arm. A common action of the deltoid is arm-swinging while walking.

Clinical anatomy: testing – Deltoid can be seen and felt to contract when the arm is abducted against resistance.

LEVATOR SCAPULAE

Attachments – Levator scapulae is a slender muscle attached by tendinous slips to the transverse processes of the atlas and axis, and to the posterior tubercles of the transverse processes of the third and fourth cervical vertebrae (**Figs 31.11, 57.19**). It descends diagonally to approach the medial scapular border between its superior angle and the triangular smooth surface at the medial end of the scapular spine.

Variants – Levator scapulae varies considerably in its vertebral attachments and the extent to which it separates into slips. There may be accessory attachments to the mastoid process, occipital bone, first or second rib, scaleni, trapezius, and serratus muscles.

Vascular supply – Levator scapulae receives its arterial supply mainly from the transverse cervical and ascending cervical arteries. The vertebral extremity of the muscle is supplied by branches from the vertebral artery.

Innervation – Levator scapulae is innervated directly by branches of the third and fourth cervical spinal nerves, and from the fifth cervical nerve via the dorsal scapular nerve.

Action – The levator scapulae and the rhomboids assist other scapular muscles in controlling the position and movement of the scapula. Acting with trapezius, rhomboids retract the scapula, bracing back the shoulder; with levator scapulae and pectoralis minor they rotate the scapula, depressing the point of the shoulder. With the cervical vertebral column fixed, levator scapulae acts with trapezius to elevate the scapula or to sustain a weight carried on the shoulder; with the shoulder fixed, the muscle inclines the neck to the same side.

LATISSIMUS DORSI

Attachments – Latissimus dorsi is a large, flat, triangular muscle which sweeps over the lumbar region and lower thorax and converges to a narrow tendon (**Fig. 57.19**). It arises by tendinous fibres from the spines of the lower six thoracic vertebrae anterior to trapezius; from the posterior layer of thoracolumbar fascia, by which it is attached to the spines and supraspinous ligaments of the lumbar and sacral vertebrae; and from the posterior part of the iliac crest. It also springs by muscular fibres from the posterior part (outer lip) of the iliac crest lateral to erector spinae, and by fleshy slips from the three or four lower ribs, interdigitating with external oblique (**Fig. 67.8**). From this extensive attachment, fibres pass laterally with different degrees of obliquity (the upper fibres are nearly horizontal, the middle oblique, and the lower almost vertical) to form a sheet c.12 or 13 mm thick that overlaps the inferior scapular angle. The muscle curves around the inferolateral border of teres major to gain its anterior surface. Here it ends as a flattened tendon, c.7 cm long, in front of the tendon of teres major. It is attached to the floor of the intertuberous sulcus of the humerus, with an expansion to the deep fascia. The attachment extends higher on the humerus than that of teres major. As the muscle curves round teres major, the fasciculi rotate around each other, so that fibres that originate lowest at the midline insert highest on the humerus, and fibres that originate highest at the midline insert lowest on the humerus. A bursa sometimes occurs between the muscle and the inferior scapular angle. The tendons of latissimus dorsi and teres major are united at their lower borders: they are separated by a bursa near their humeral attachments.

Latissimus dorsi and teres major together form the posterior axillary fold. When the arm is adducted against resistance, this fold is accentuated, and the whole inferolateral border of latissimus dorsi can then be traced to its attachment to the iliac crest.

The lower, lateral margin of the muscle is usually separated from the posterior border of external oblique by the lumbar triangle; the base of this small triangle is the iliac crest and its floor the internal oblique (**Fig. 57.19**). It should not be confused with the triangle of auscultation, which is medial to the scapula, and is bounded above by the trapezius, below by latissimus dorsi and laterally by the medial border of the scapula; part of rhomboid major is exposed in the triangle. If the scapulae are drawn forwards, by folding the arms across the chest, and the trunk is bent forwards, parts of the sixth and seventh ribs and the interspace between them (overlying the apex of the lower pulmonary lobe) become subcutaneous.

Variants – Latissimus dorsi commonly receives some additional fibres from the scapula as it crosses the inferior scapular angle. A muscular axillary arch, 7–10 cm in length and 5–15 mm in breadth, may sometimes be present: it crosses from the edge of latissimus dorsi, midway in the posterior fold, over the front of the axillary vessels and nerves to join the tendons of pectoralis major, coracobrachialis or the fascia over the biceps. The vertebral and costal attachments of latissimus dorsi may be reduced or, in rare cases, increased. A fibrous slip usually passes from the tendon, near its humeral insertion, to the long head of triceps.

Vascular supply –Latissimus dorsi is supplied by a single dominant vascular pedicle, the thoracodorsal artery, itself a continuation of the subscapular artery (p. 844). The thoracodorsal artery (and its accompany-ing venae comitantes) enters the muscle at a single neurovascular hilum on its costal surface, 6–12 cm from the subscapular artery and 1–4 cm medial to the lateral border of the muscle. The artery gives off one to three large branches to serratus anterior before dividing at, or even before, the hilum to supply latissimus dorsi itself. The basic pattern of branching is a bifurcation into lateral and medial branches. The larger lateral branch follows a course parallel to, and 1–4 cm from, the upper border of the muscle; the smaller branch diverges at an angle of 45° and travels medially. In a small number of cases the artery trifurcates: this usually yields a small recurrent branch which returns to supply the proximal part of the muscle, but in some cases it provides a third major branch which supplies the distal part of the muscle. Occasionally the lateral branch gives off a further collateral to serratus anterior. The major branches give off 5–9 longitudinal branches which travel distally, parallel with the muscle fibres. Musculocutaneous perforators arising from these vessels supply the overlying skin.

In addition to the dominant vascular pedicle, latissimus dorsi is supplied distally by several smaller secondary segmental vascular pedicles. These are dorsal perforating arteries derived from the 9th, 10th and 11th posterior intercostal and 1st, 2nd and 3rd lumbar arteries, and they all enter the muscle on its deep surface. They anastomose within the muscle with branches of the thoracodorsal artery.

The blood supply of latissimus dorsi is particularly important because of its applications in plastic and reconstructive surgery. The presence of the dominant vascular pedicle provides the anatomical basis for raising the muscle either alone, or together with an overlying paddle of skin in the form of a musculocutaneous flap based solely on the thoracodorsal artery and its accompanying venae comitantes. These flaps can be used in a pedicle fashion, e.g. in reconstructing a breast following a mastectomy, or used as free tissue transfer to cover large areas of tissue loss anywhere in the body.

Innervation – Latissimus dorsi is supplied by the thoracodorsal nerve, from the posterior cord of the brachial plexus, C6, 7 and 8. This nerve runs in the neurovascular pedicle and divides c.1.3 cm proximal to the point of bifurcation or trifurcation of the thoracodorsal artery. The pattern of branching follows that of the artery closely, and the neural and vascular branches travel together.

Action – Latissimus dorsi is active in adduction, extension and especially in medial rotation of the humerus. Humeral adduction and extension are most powerful when the initial position of the arm is one of partial abduction, flexion or a combination of the two. With the sternocostal part of pectoralis major and teres major it adducts the raised arm against resistance. It assists backward swinging of the arm, as in walking and many athletic pursuits. When the arms are raised above the head, as in climbing, it pulls the trunk upwards and forwards. It takes part in all violent expiratory efforts, such as coughing or sneezing: this is readily confirmed by palpation. Electromyography suggests that it aids deep inspiration, but it is also active towards the end of forcible expiration, e.g. when blowing a sustained note on a musical instrument. When the arm is elevated, the stretched fibres of latissimus dorsi press on the inferior scapular angle, keeping it in contact with the chest wall. Despite this range of actions, surgical transposition of the muscle does not produce any serious restriction of normal activity.

Clinical anatomy: testing – Latissimus dorsi is palpated when the abducted arm is adducted against resistance and can be felt to contract during coughing.

SERRATUS ANTERIOR

Attachments – Serratus anterior is a large muscular sheet which curves around the thorax. It arises from an extensive costal attachment and inserts on the scapula (**Figs 57.19, 49.21, 49.22**). Fleshy digitations spring anteriorly from the outer surfaces and superior borders of the upper eight, nine or even ten ribs, and from fasciae which cover the intervening intercostals. They lie on a long, slightly curved, line which passes inferolaterally across the thorax. The first digitations springs from the first and second ribs and intercostal fascia, the others from a single rib, and the lower four interdigitate with the upper five slips of external oblique. The muscle follows the contour of the chest wall closely. It passes ventral to the scapula and reaches the medial border of the scapula in the following way. The first digitation encloses, and is attached to, a triangular area of both the costal and dorsal surfaces of the superior scapular angle. The next two or three digitations form a triangular sheet which is attached to the costal surface along almost its entire medial border. The lower four or five digitations converge to be attached by musculotendinous fibres to a triangular impression on the costal surface of the inferior angle: they enclose the inferior angle and are also attached to a smaller triangular part of its dorsal surface near its tip.

Variants – Digitations may be absent, particularly the first and eighth, and sometimes also the intermediate part. Serratus anterior may be partly fused with levator scapulae, adjacent external intercostals or external oblique.

Vascular supply – Serratus anterior is supplied by superior and lateral thoracic arteries, and branches from the thoracodorsal artery before (occasionally after) it divides in latissimus dorsi.

Innervation – Serratus anterior is innervated by the long thoracic nerve, C5, 6 and 7, which descends on the external surface of the muscle.

Action – With pectoralis minor, serratus anterior protracts (draws forward) the scapula, as a prime mover in all reaching and pushing movements. The upper part, with levator scapulae and upper fibres of trapezius, suspends the scapula, but slight activity is sufficient to support the unloaded arm. The heavier insertion lower down pulls the inferior scapular angle forwards around the thorax, assisting trapezius in upward rotation of the bone, an action that is essential to raising the arm above the head. In the initial stages of abduction, serratus anterior helps other muscles to fix the scapula, so that deltoid acts effectively on the humerus, and not the scapula. While deltoid is raising the arm to a right angle with the scapula, serratus anterior and trapezius are simultaneously rotating the scapula: the combination allows the arm to be raised to the vertical. To effect this upward rotation of the scapula, forward pull on the inferior angle by the lower digitations of serratus anterior is coupled with an upward and medial pull on the lateral end of the clavicle and acromion by the upper fibres of trapezius, and a downward pull on the base of the scapular spine by the lower fibres of trapezius. Conversely, slow downward scapular rotation assisted by gravity is achieved by controlled lengthening of these muscles. More powerful downward rotation requires balanced contraction of the upper fibres of serratus anterior, levator scapulae, rhomboids, pectoralis minor and the middle part of trapezius. When weights are carried in front of the body, serratus anterior prevents backward rotation of the scapula. Electromyography shows that serratus anterior is not active in normal human respiration. This may not apply to laboured respiration, e.g. when asthmatics and athletes may be observed to fix the scapula by grasping a rail or other support.

Clinical anatomy: testing – The muscular digitations of serratus anterior can be seen and felt when the outstretched hand pushes against resistance.

When serratus anterior is paralysed, the medial border of the scapula, and especially its lower angle, stand out prominently. The arm cannot be raised fully. Pushing is ineffective, indeed attempts to do so produce further projection, known as 'winging' of the scapula.

RHOMBOID MAJOR

Attachments – Rhomboid major is a quadrilateral sheet of muscle which arises by tendinous fibres from the spines and supraspinous ligaments of the second to fifth thoracic vertebrae, and descends laterally to the medial border of the scapula between the root of the spine and the inferior angle (**Fig. 57.19**). Most of its fibres usually end in a tendinous band between these two points, joined to the medial border by a thin membrane. Occasionally this is incomplete, in which case some muscular fibres are attached directly into the scapula. The attachments of rhomboid major – and also those of rhomboid minor, levator scapulae and serratus anterior – can be more extensive, with 'folds' or extensions passing to both dorsal and costal aspects of the scapula adjacent to its medial margin.

Vascular supply, innervation, action and clinical anatomy: testing – All described with rhomboid minor.

RHOMBOID MINOR

Attachments – Rhomboid minor is a small, cylindrical muscle which runs from the lower ligamentum nuchae and the spines of the seventh cervical and first thoracic vertebrae to the base of a smooth triangular surface at the medial end of the spine of the scapula (**Fig. 57.19**). Here, dorsal and ventral layers enclose the inferior border of levator scapulae. The dorsal layer of rhomboid minor is attached to the rim of the triangular surface, dorsolateral to and below levator scapulae. The ventral layer is strong and wide, extending 2–3 cm medial to and below levator scapulae; here the fasciae of rhomboid minor and serratus anterior are tightly fused. Rhomboid minor is usually separate from rhomboid major, but the muscles overlap and are occasionally united.

Variants – There is some variability in the vertebral and scapular attachments of rhomboids major and minor. A slip of muscle may extend from the upper border of rhomboid minor to reach the occipital bone (rhomboid occipitalis).

Vascular supply of the rhomboids – Rhomboids major and minor are supplied by the dorsal scapular artery or deep branch of the transverse cervical artery and by dorsal perforating branches from the upper five or six posterior intercostal arteries.

Innervation of the rhomboids – Rhomboids major and minor are innervated by a branch of the dorsal scapular nerve, C4, 5.

Action of the rhomboids – Both rhomboid major and minor retract the medial border of the scapula superiorly and medially. They are used in squaring the shoulders.

Clinical anatomy: testing of the rhomboids – Rhomboids major and minor can be palpated deep to trapezius on bracing the shoulder back against resistance.

SUPRASPINATUS

Attachments – Supraspinatus arises from the medial two-thirds of the supraspinous fossa and from the supraspinous fascia (**Fig. 49.23**). The fibres converge, under the acromion, into a tendon which crosses above the shoulder joint and is attached to the highest facet of the greater tubercle of the humerus. The tendon blends into the articular capsule and may give a slip to the tendon of pectoralis major. Fibrocartilage has been described at the tendinous insertion, as in other tendons attached to epiphyseal bone.

Vascular supply – Supraspinatus is supplied by the suprascapular and dorsal scapular arteries.

Innervation – Supraspinatus is innervated by the suprascapular nerve, C5 and 6.

Action – Supraspinatus initiates abduction of the shoulder and assists deltoid in abduction thereafter. As part of the rotator cuff, it helps to stabilize the head of the humerus in the glenoid fossa during movements of the glenohumeral joint. With the arm dependent, even when moderately loaded, supraspinatus and tension in the upper capsule prevent downward displacement of the humerus.

Clinical anatomy: testing – Supraspinatus can be palpated deep to trapezius when the arm is abducted at the shoulder joint against resistance.

The tendon of supraspinatus is separated from the coraco-acromial ligament, acromion and deltoid by the large subacromial bursa; when this is inflamed, abduction of the shoulder joint is painful. The tendon is the most frequently ruptured element of the musculotendinous cuff around the shoulder joint.

INFRASPINATUS

Attachments – Infraspinatus is a thick triangular muscle which occupies most of the infraspinous fossa (**Fig. 49.23**). It arises by muscular fibres from the medial two-thirds of the fossa, by tendinous fibres from ridges on its surface and from the deep surface of the infraspinous fascia, which separates it from teres major and minor. Its fibres converge to a

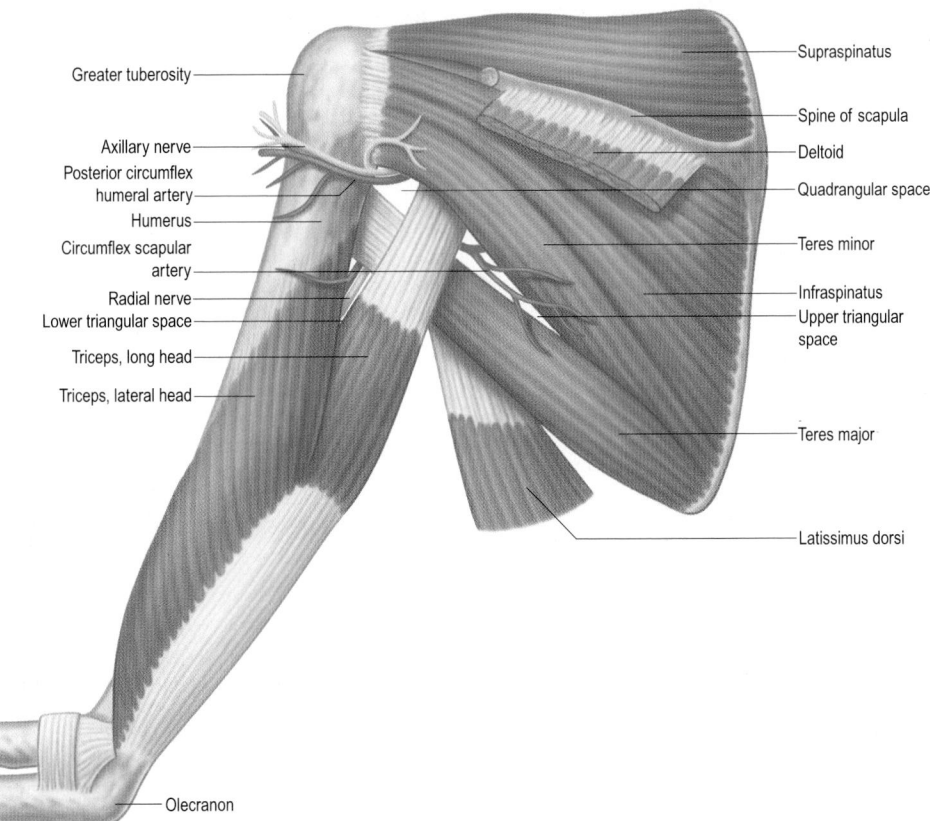

Greater tuberosity

Axillary nerve
Posterior circumflex
humeral artery
Humerus
Circumflex scapular
artery
Radial nerve
Lower triangular space
Triceps, long head
Triceps, lateral head

Olecranon

Supraspinatus
Spine of scapula
Deltoid
Quadrangular space
Teres minor
Infraspinatus
Upper triangular
space
Teres major
Latissimus dorsi

Fig. 49.23 The dorsal scapular muscles and triceps of the left side. The spine of the scapula has been divided near its lateral end and the acromion has been removed together with a large part of deltoid. The humerus is laterally rotated and the forearm pronated.

tendon which glides under the lateral border of the spine of the scapula, and then passes across the posterior aspect of the capsule of the shoulder joint to be attached to the middle facet on the greater tubercle of the humerus. The tendon is sometimes separated from the capsule by a bursa, which may communicate with the joint cavity. Infraspinatus is sometimes fused with teres minor.

Vascular supply – Infraspinatus is supplied by the suprascapular and circumflex scapular arteries.

Innervation – Infraspinatus is innervated by the suprascapular nerve, C5 and 6.

Action – Infraspinatus is a lateral rotator of the humerus. Together with supraspinatus, subscapularis and teres minor, it helps to stabilize the head of the humerus in the glenoid fossa during shoulder movements (p. 830).

SUBSCAPULARIS

Attachments – Subscapularis is a bulky, triangular muscle which fills the subscapular fossa (**Fig. 49.22**). In its medial two-thirds, the fibres are attached to the periosteum of the costal surface of the scapula. Other fibres arise from tendinous intramuscular septa, which are attached to ridges on the bone, and from the aponeurosis which covers the muscle and separates it from teres major and the long head of triceps. The fibres converge laterally into a broad tendon which is attached to the lesser tubercle of the humerus and the front of the articular capsule. The tendon is separated from the neck of the scapula by the large subscapular bursa, which communicates with the shoulder joint.

Variation is unusual. A separate slip may pass from the medial border of the scapula to the glenohumeral capsule or to the periosteum medial to the intertuberous sulcus of the humerus.

Relations – Subscapularis forms much of the posterior axillary wall. Its anterior surface is apposed inferomedially to serratus anterior, and

superolaterally to coracobrachialis and biceps, the axillary vessels, brachial plexus and subscapular vessels and nerves. Its posterior surface is attached to the scapula and glenohumeral capsule. Its lower border contacts teres major and latissimus dorsi.

Vascular supply – Subscapularis is supplied by small branches from the suprascapular, axillary and subscapular arteries.

Innervation – Subscapularis is innervated by the upper and lower subscapular nerves, C5, 6.

Action – Subscapularis is a medial rotator of the humerus. Together with supraspinatus, infraspinatus and teres minor, it helps to stabilize the head of the humerus in the glenoid fossa during shoulder movements (p. 830).

TERES MAJOR

Attachments – Teres major is a thick, flat muscle which arises from the oval area on the dorsal surface of the inferior scapular angle, and from the fibrous septa interposed between the muscle and teres minor and infraspinatus (**Fig. 49.23**). Its fibres ascend laterally and end in a flat tendon, c.5 cm long, which is attached to the medial lip of the intertuberous sulcus of the humerus. The tendon lies behind that of latissimus dorsi, from which it is separated by a bursa; the tendons are united along their lower borders for a short distance.

Variants – Teres major may be fused with the scapular part of latissimus dorsi, and it may send a slip to join the long head of triceps or the brachial fascia.

Vascular supply – Teres major is supplied by the thoracodorsal branch of the subscapular artery on its way to latissimus dorsi and by the posterior circumflex humeral artery.

Innervation – Teres major is innervated by the lower subscapular nerve, C5, 6 and 7.

Action – Despite its name, teres major has a nerve supply and action that is distinct from teres minor. Teres major draws the humerus backwards and rotates it medially. Electromyographic studies are equivocal about its major role in movement, but its involvement as a contributor to static posture and arm-swinging is not contested.

Clinical anatomy: testing – Teres major can be palpated posterior to the posterior axillary fold during adduction of the humerus against resistance.

TERES MINOR

Attachments – Teres minor is a narrow elongated muscle. It arises from the upper two-thirds of a flattened strip on the dorsal surface of the scapula adjoining its lateral border, and from two aponeurotic laminae which separate it from infraspinatus and teres major (**Fig. 49.23**). It runs upwards and laterally. The upper fibres end in a tendon attached to the lowest facet on the greater tubercle of the humerus. The lower fibres are attached directly into the humerus distal to this facet and above the origin of the lateral head of triceps. The tendon passes across, and blends with, the lower posterior surface of the capsule of the shoulder joint.

Teres minor may be fused with infraspinatus.

Vascular supply – Teres minor is supplied by the circumflex scapular artery, which pierces the origin of the muscle as it turns upward in the infraspinous fossa, and by the posterior circumflex humeral artery.

Innervation – Teres minor is innervated by the axillary nerve, C5 and 6.

Action – Teres minor acts as a lateral rotator and weak adductor of the humerus. Together with supraspinatus, infraspinatus and subscapularis, it helps stabilize to the head of the humerus in the glenoid fossa during shoulder movements. (p. 830).

THE QUADRANGULAR AND TRIANGULAR SPACES

Anteriorly, the quadrangular space is bounded by subscapularis, the capsule of the shoulder joint and teres minor above, teres major below, the long head of triceps medially, and the surgical neck of the humerus laterally. Posteriorly, the quadrangular space is bounded above by teres minor. The axillary nerve and the posterior circumflex artery and vein pass through the space (**Fig. 49.23**).

There are two triangular spaces (**Fig. 49.23**). The upper triangular space is bounded above by subscapularis anteriorly, teres minor posteriorly, teres major below, and the long head of triceps laterally. The circumflex scapular artery passes through this space. The lower triangular space (triangular interval) is bounded above by subscapularis anteriorly and teres major posteriorly; the long head of triceps medially and the humerus laterally. The radial nerve and the profunda brachii vessels pass through this space.

AXILLA

BOUNDARIES

The axilla is a pyramidal region between the upper thoracic wall and the arm (**Figs 49.24, 49.25**). Its blunt apex continues into the root of the neck (cervico-axillary canal) between the external border of the first rib, superior border of the scapula, posterior surface of the clavicle and the medial aspect of the coracoid process. Its base, which is virtual, can be imagined as facing downwards: it is broad at the chest and narrow at the arm, and corresponds to the skin and a thick layer of axillary fascia

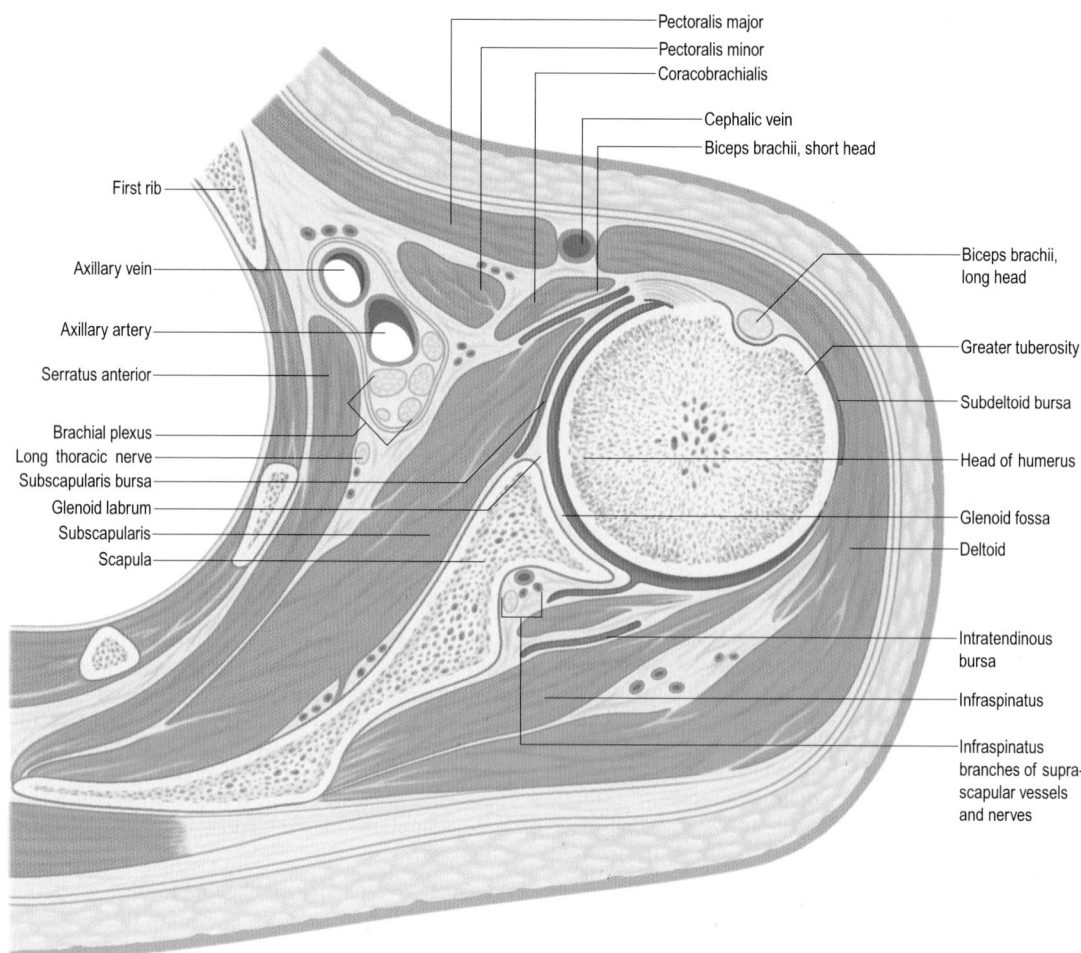

Fig. 49.24 Transverse section through left shoulder joint and axilla, viewed from below. (By permission from Agur AMR, Lee MJ (eds) 1999 Grant's Atlas of Anatomy, 10th edn. Philadelphia: Lippincott Williams and Wilkins.)

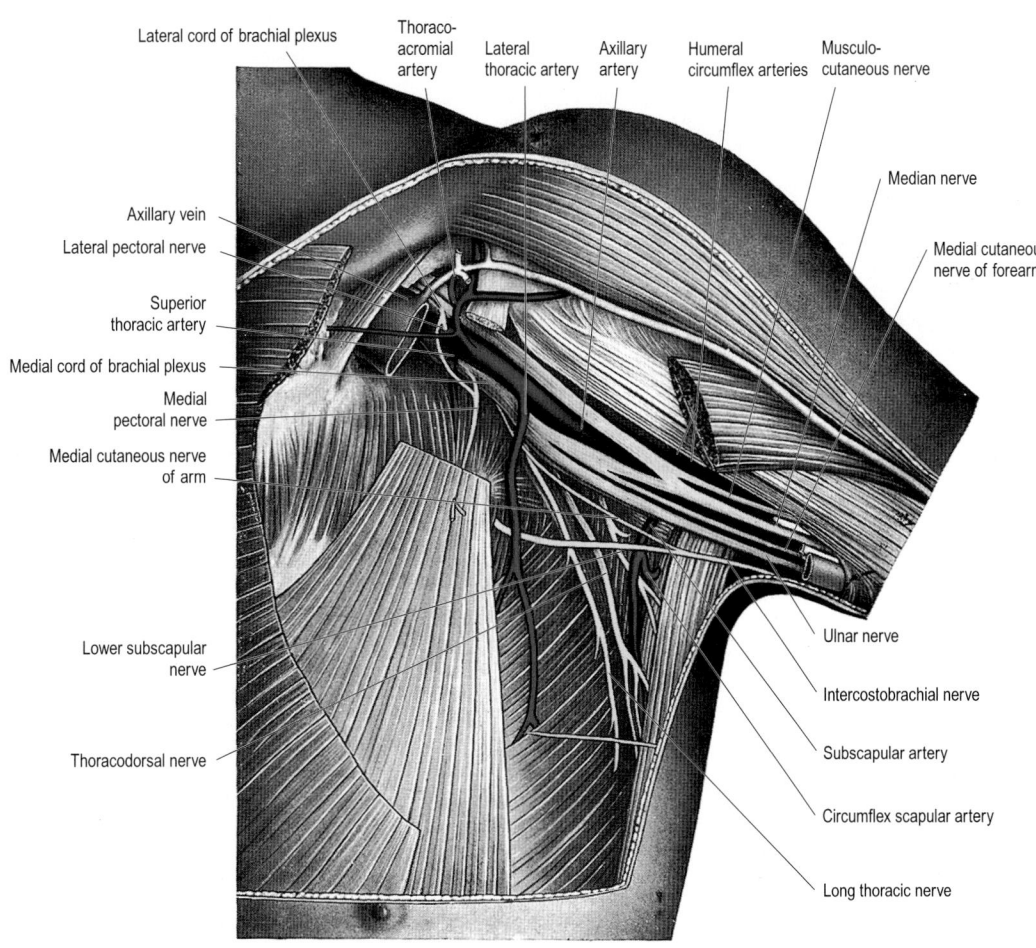

Fig. 49.25 The left axillary artery and its branches. The pectoralis major and part of the pectoralis minor have been removed. Prominent but unlabelled features are the medial and lateral roots of the median nerve.

Labels on figure:
Lateral cord of brachial plexus
Thoraco-acromial artery
Lateral thoracic artery
Axillary artery
Humeral circumflex arteries
Musculo-cutaneous nerve
Median nerve
Medial cutaneous nerve of forearm
Axillary vein
Lateral pectoral nerve
Superior thoracic artery
Medial cord of brachial plexus
Medial pectoral nerve
Medial cutaneous nerve of arm
Lower subscapular nerve
Thoracodorsal nerve
Ulnar nerve
Intercostobrachial nerve
Subscapular artery
Circumflex scapular artery
Long thoracic nerve

between the inferior borders of pectoralis major (anterior) and latissimus dorsi (posterior). It is convex upwards, conforming to the concavity of the armpit.

The anterior wall is formed by pectorales major and minor, the former covering the whole wall, the latter its intermediate part. The interval between the upper border of pectoralis minor and clavicle is occupied by the clavipectoral fascia. The posterior wall is formed by subscapularis above, and teres major and latissimus dorsi below. The medial 'wall' is convex laterally and is composed of the first four ribs and their associated intercostal muscles, together with the upper part of serratus anterior. The anterior and posterior walls converge laterally: the 'wall' is narrow and consists of the humeral intertuberous sulcus. The lateral angle lodges coracobrachialis and biceps.

CONTENTS

The axilla contains the axillary vessels, the infraclavicular part of the brachial plexus and its branches, lateral branches of some intercostal nerves, many lymph nodes and vessels, loose adipose areolar tissue and, in many instances, the 'axillary tail' of the breast. The axillary vessels and brachial plexus run from the apex to the base along the lateral wall, nearer to the anterior wall: the axillary vein is anteromedial to the artery. The obliquity of the upper ribs means that the neurovascular bundle, after it emerges from behind the clavicle, crosses the first intercostal space: its relations are therefore different at upper and lower levels. Thoracic branches of the axillary artery are in contact with the pectoral muscles; the lateral thoracic artery reaches the thoracic wall along the lateral margin of pectoralis minor. Subscapular vessels descend on the posterior wall at the lower margin of subscapularis. The subscapular and thoracodorsal nerves cross the anterior surface of latissimus dorsi at different inclinations. Circumflex scapular vessels wind round the lateral border of the scapula; posterior circumflex humeral vessels and the axillary nerve curve back and laterally around the surgical neck of the humerus.

No large vessel lies on the medial 'wall', which is crossed proximally only by small branches of the superior thoracic artery. The long thoracic

nerve descends on serratus anterior and the intercostobrachial nerve perforates the upper anterior part of this wall, crossing the axilla to its lateral 'wall'.

VASCULAR SUPPLY AND LYMPHATIC DRAINAGE

ARTERIES

Suprascapular artery (Figs 31.8, 49.26)

The suprascapular artery usually arises from the thyrocervical trunk of the subclavian artery, although it may arise from the third part of the subclavian artery. It first descends laterally across scalenus anterior and the phrenic nerve, posterior to the internal jugular vein and sternocleidomastoid, then crosses anterior to the subclavian artery and brachial plexus, posterior and parallel with the clavicle and subclavius and the inferior belly of omohyoid, to reach the superior border of the scapula. Here it passes above (sometimes under) the superior transverse ligament, separating it from the suprascapular nerve, and enters the supraspinous fossa (**Fig. 49.26**), where it lies on the bone, and supplies supraspinatus. It descends behind the scapular neck, and passes through the great scapular notch deep to the inferior transverse ligament to gain the deep surface of infraspinatus, where it anastomoses with the circumflex scapular and deep branch of the transverse cervical artery. Its muscular branches supply sternocleidomastoid, subclavius and infraspinatus. It also gives off a suprasternal branch which crosses the sternal end of the clavicle to supply the skin of the upper thorax, and an acromial branch which pierces trapezius to supply the skin over the shoulder. This last branch anastomoses with the thoraco-acromial and posterior circumflex humeral arteries.

As the suprascapular artery passes over the superior transverse ligament, it gives off a branch which enters the subscapular fossa beneath subscapularis and anastomoses with the subscapular artery and the deep branch of the transverse cervical artery. It also supplies the acromioclavicular and glenohumeral joints, the clavicle and the scapula.

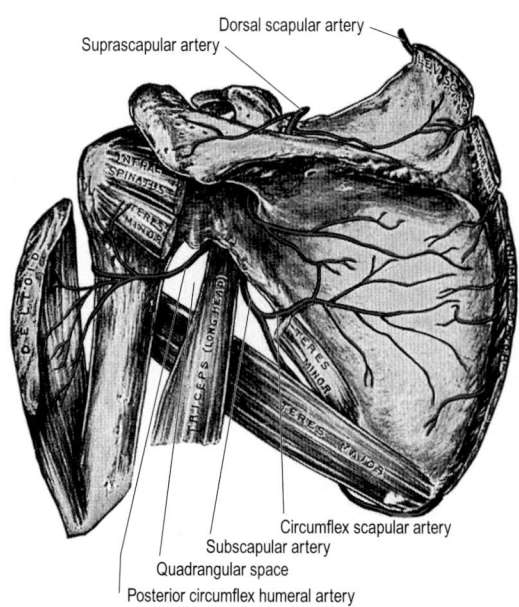

Fig. 49.26 The scapular anastomosis of the left side.

Dorsal scapular artery

In the majority of cases, the dorsal scapular artery arises from the third, or less often the second, part of the subclavian artery. It passes laterally through the trunks of the brachial plexus in front of scalenus medius and then deep to levator scapulae to reach the superior scapular angle. Here it descends with the dorsal scapular nerve under the rhomboids along the medial border of the scapula to the inferior angle (**Figs 31.8, 49.26**). It supplies the rhomboids, latissimus dorsi and the inferior portion of trapezius. It supplies the skin over the inferomedial aspect of trapezius via musculocutaneous perforators. It anastomoses with the suprascapular and subscapular and with posterior branches of some posterior intercostal arteries. It sends a small branch to scalenus anterior: sometimes this arises directly from the subclavian artery.

Variants – About a third of the superficial cervical and dorsal scapular arteries arise in common from the thyrocervical trunk as a transverse cervical artery, together with a superficial and a deep branch (superficial cervical and dorsal scapular arteries respectively). In this case the dorsal scapular artery arises near the superior border of the scapula: it passes laterally, anterior to the brachial plexus and then posterior to levator scapulae. (**Fig. 49.27**).

Supraclavicular artery

This small vessel arises from either the transverse cervical or superficial cervical artery. It pierces the deep fascia just superior to the clavicle and anterior to trapezius and supplies an area of skin over the lateral end of the clavicle.

Axillary artery

The axillary artery, a continuation of the subclavian artery, begins at the outer border of the first rib, and ends nominally at the inferior border of teres major where it becomes the brachial artery (**Fig. 49.28**). Its direction varies with the position of the limb: it is almost straight when the arm is raised at right angles, concave upwards when the arm is elevated above this, and convex upwards and laterally when the arm is by the side. At first deep, it subsequently becomes superficial, when it is covered only by the skin and fasciae. Pectoralis minor crosses it and so divides it into three parts which are proximal, posterior and distal to the muscle.

Relations of the first part

The skin, superficial fascia, platysma, supraclavicular nerves, deep fascia, clavicular fibres of pectoralis major and the clavipectoral fascia, lateral pectoral nerve and the loop of communication between the lateral and medial pectoral nerves, and the thoraco-acromial and cephalic veins are all anterior. The first intercostal space and external intercostal, first and second digitations of serratus anterior, long thoracic and medial pectoral nerves and the medial cord of the brachial plexus are all posterior. The posterior cord of the brachial plexus is lateral and the axillary vein is anteromedial. The first part is enclosed with the axillary vein and brachial plexus in a fibrous axillary sheath, which is continuous with the prevertebral layer of the deep cervical fascia.

Relations of the second part

The skin, superficial and deep fascia, and pectorales major and minor are all anterior. The posterior cord of the brachial plexus and the areolar tissue between it and subscapularis are posterior. The axillary vein is medial, separated from the artery by the medial cord of the brachial plexus and the medial pectoral nerve. The lateral cord of the brachial plexus is lateral, separating the artery from coracobrachialis. The cords

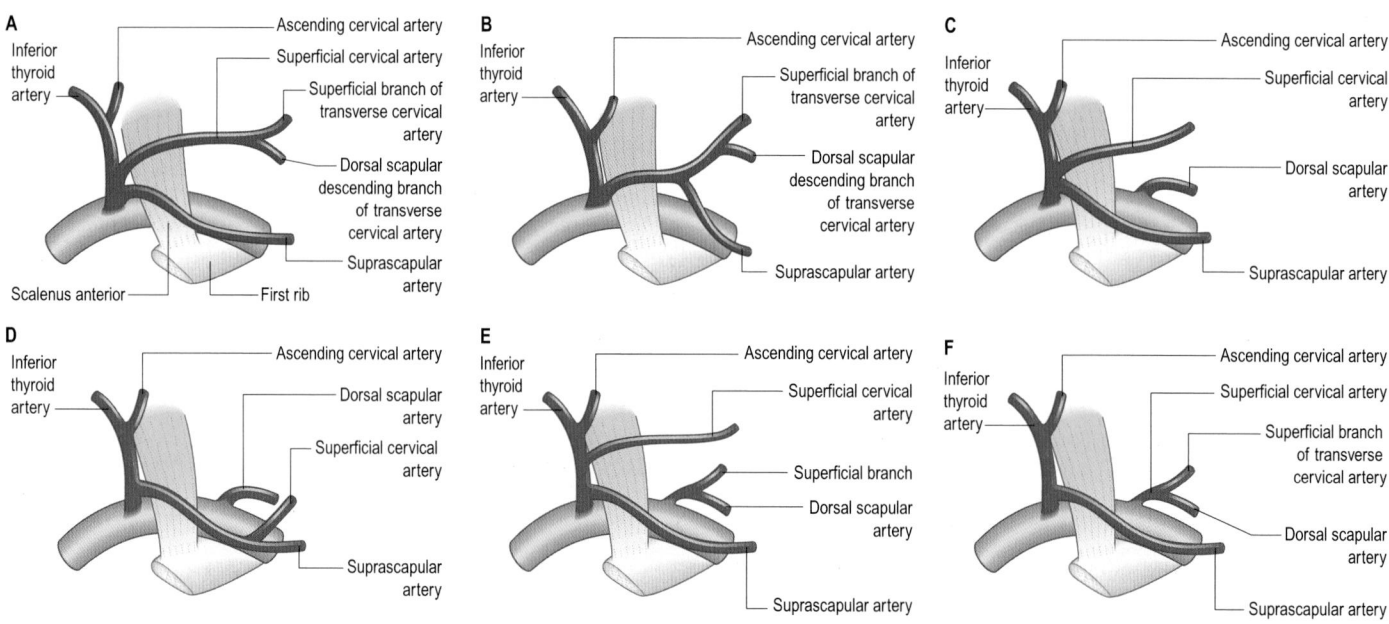

Fig. 49.27 Variations in origin and branches of the thyrocervical trunk. The superficial cervical artery is the distinct vessel arising from the thyrocervical trunk (C and E) or from the suprascapular artery (D), which supplies the territory of the superficial branch of the (absent) transverse cervical artery. (By permission from Cormack GC, Lamberty BGH 1994 The Arterial Anatomy of Skin Flaps, 2nd edn. Edinburgh: Churchill Livingstone.)

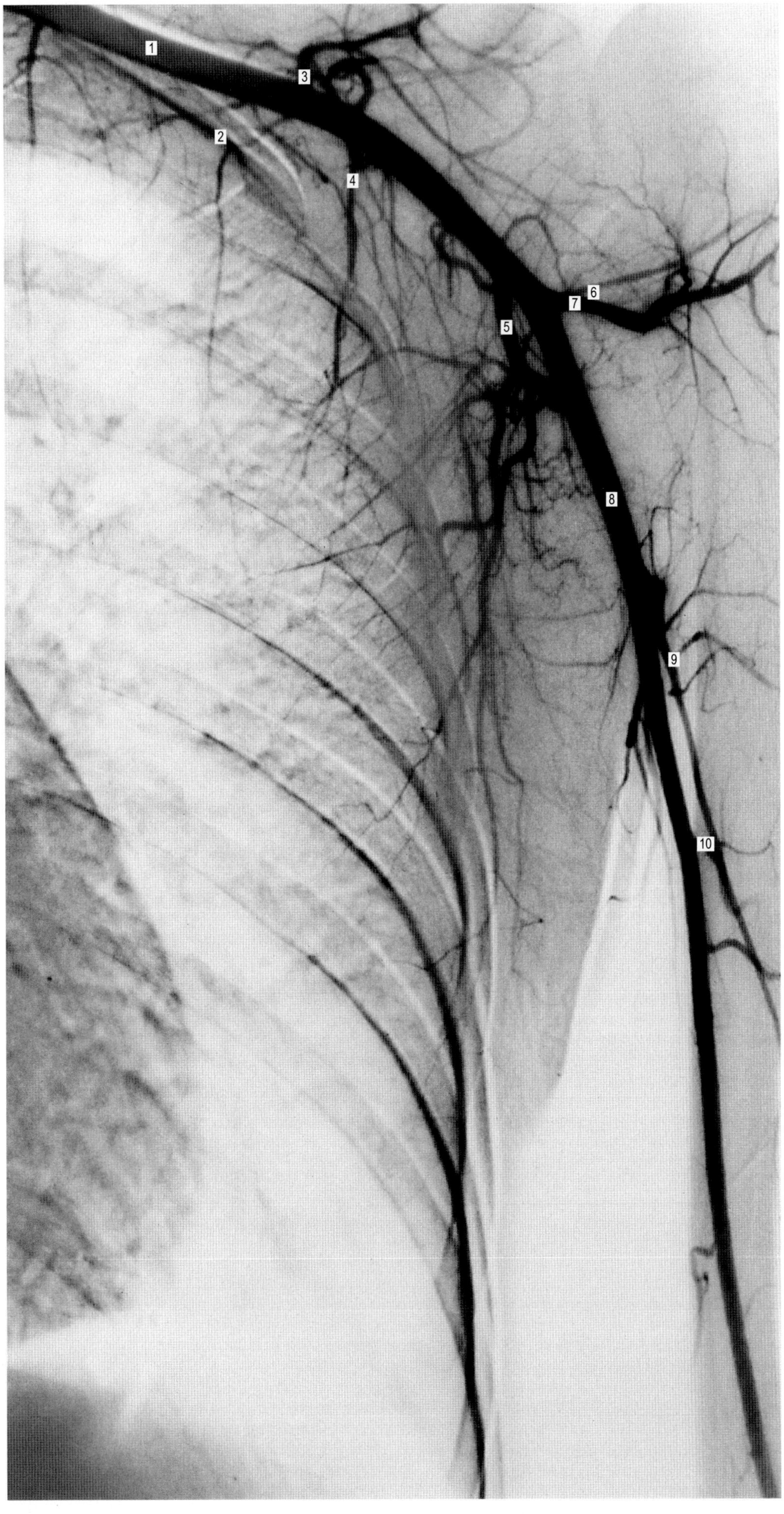

1. Axillary artery.
2. Superior thoracic artery.
3. Thoracoacromial artery.
4. Lateral thoracic artery.
5. Subscapular artery.
6. Anterior circumflex humeral artery.
7. Posterior circumflex humeral artery.
8. Brachial artery.
9. Profunda brachii artery.
10. Muscular branches of brachial artery.

Fig. 49.28 Left axillary arteriogram.
(By permission from Weir J, Abrahams PH
2003 Imaging Atlas of Human Anatomy,
3rd edn, London: Mosby, and
contributions from Anna-Maria Belli,
Margaret Hourihan, Naill Moore and
Philip Owen.)

of the brachial plexus thus surround the second part on three sides, with the dispositions implied by their names, and separate it from the vein and adjacent muscles.

Relations of the third part

Pectoralis major, and, distal to the muscle, skin and fasciae, are anterior. The lower part of subscapularis and the tendons of latissimus dorsi and teres major are posterior. Coracobrachialis is lateral and the axillary vein is medial. Branches of the brachial plexus are arranged as follows: laterally, the lateral root and then trunk of the median nerve and, for a short distance, the musculocutaneous nerve; medially, the medial cutaneous nerve of the forearm between the axillary artery and vein anteriorly, and the ulnar nerve between these vessels posteriorly; anteriorly, the medial root of the median nerve; posteriorly, the radial and axillary nerves, the latter only to the distal border of subscapularis.

Branches

The branches of the axillary artery are superior thoracic, thoraco-acromial, lateral thoracic, subscapular, anterior and posterior circumflex humeral.

Superior thoracic artery (Fig. 49.25) – The superior thoracic artery is a small vessel which arises from the first part of the axillary artery near the lower border of subclavius: it is sometimes arises from the thoraco-acromial artery. It runs anteromedially above the medial border of pectoralis minor, then passes between it and pectoralis major to gain the thoracic wall. It supplies these muscles and the thoracic wall, and anastomoses with the internal thoracic and upper intercostal arteries.

Thoraco-acromial (acromio-thoracic) artery (Figs 31.8, 49.21, 49.25, 49.28) – The thoraco-acromial artery is a short branch which arises from the second part of the axillary artery. It is at first overlapped by pectoralis minor; skirting its medial border. It pierces the clavipectoral fascia and divides into pectoral, acromial, clavicular and deltoid branches, which supply the anterior portion of deltoid, pectoralis major and minor and an area of skin over the clavipectoral fascia.

Pectoral branch – The pectoral branch is the largest branch. It descends between the pectoral muscles, gives a branch to pectoralis minor, and then continues on the deep surface of pectoralis major. It enters the muscle and anastomoses with the intercostal branches of the internal thoracic and lateral thoracic arteries. It gives off perforating branches to the breast, and musculocutaneous perforators to the skin over pectoralis major.

Acromial branch – The acromial branch crosses the coracoid process under deltoid, which it supplies, pierces the muscle and ends on the acromion. It anastomoses with branches of the suprascapular artery, the deltoid branch of the thoraco-acromial artery and the posterior circumflex humeral arteries.

Clavicular branch – The clavicular branch ascends medially between the clavicular part of pectoralis major and the clavipectoral fascia. It supplies the sternoclavicular joint and subclavius.

Deltoid branch – The deltoid branch often arises with the acromial branch. It crosses pectoralis minor to accompany the cephalic vein between pectoralis major and deltoid, and supplies both muscles.

Lateral thoracic artery (Fig. 49.25) – The lateral thoracic artery arises from the second part of the axillary artery. Following the lateral border of pectoralis minor, it passes to the deep surface of pectoralis major as far distally as the fifth intercostal space. It supplies serratus anterior and the pectoral muscles, the axillary lymph nodes and subscapularis. It anastomoses with the internal thoracic, subscapular, and intercostal arteries and with the pectoral branch of the thoraco-acromial artery. In females it is large and has lateral mammary branches, which curve round the lateral border of pectoralis major to the breast. In both males and females, it gives off cutaneous branches which pass around the lateral border of pectoralis major to supply the skin in this region.

Subscapular artery (Figs 49.25, 49.26) – The subscapular artery is the largest branch of the axillary artery. It usually arises from the third part of the axillary artery at the distal (inferior) border of subscapularis,

which it follows to the inferior scapular angle, where it anastomoses with the lateral thoracic and intercostal arteries and the deep branch of the transverse cervical artery. It supplies adjacent muscles and the thoracic wall. It is accompanied distally by the nerve to latissimus dorsi. Approximately 4 cm from its origin the subscapular artery divides into the circumflex scapular and thoracodorsal arteries.

Circumflex scapular artery – The circumflex scapular artery (**Fig. 49.28**), the larger of the two terminal branches of the subscapular artery, curves backwards around the lateral border of the scapula, traversing a triangular space between subscapularis above and teres major below and the long head of the triceps laterally (p. 840). It enters the infraspinous fossa under teres minor and then divides. One branch (infrascapular) enters the subscapular fossa deep to subscapularis, and anastomoses with the suprascapular and dorsal scapular arteries (or deep branch of the transverse cervical artery). The other branch continues along the lateral border of the scapula between teres major and minor and, dorsal to the inferior angle, anastomoses with the dorsal scapular artery. Small branches supply the posterior part of deltoid and the long head of triceps, and anastomose with an ascending branch of the profunda brachii artery.

Two significant cutaneous branches arise from the circumflex scapular artery as it emerges through the upper triangular space. The superior, or horizontal, branch is a direct cutaneous artery which passes medially at the level of the deep fascia parallel with the spine of the scapula: it supplies a band of skin overlying the spine of the scapula. The lower branch (parascapular branch) is also a direct cutaneous vessel which passes in an inferomedial direction, again at the level of the deep fascia, and supplies an area of skin overlying the lateral border of the scapula. Both these cutaneous vessels provide the anatomical basis of skin flaps which can be surgically raised in this region (scapular flap based on the horizontal branch and parascapular flap based on the lower, parascapular branch) to reconstruct areas of missing tissue elsewhere in the body.

Thoracodorsal artery – The other terminal branch of the subscapular artery, the thoracodorsal artery, follows the lateral margin of the scapula, posterior to the lateral thoracic artery, between latissimus dorsi and serratus anterior. Before entering the deep surface of latissimus dorsi, it supplies teres major and the intercostals and sends one or two branches to serratus anterior. It enters latissimus dorsi muscle with the thoracodorsal nerve: this constitutes the principle neurovascular pedicle to the muscle. It provides numerous musculocutaneous perforators which supply the skin over the superior part of latissimus dorsi. The intramuscular portion of the artery anastomoses with intercostal arteries and lumbar perforating arteries.

Anterior circumflex humeral artery – The anterior circumflex humeral artery arises from the lateral side of the axillary artery at the distal border of subscapularis. It runs horizontally behind coracobrachialis and the short head of biceps, anterior to the surgical neck of the humerus. Reaching the intertuberous sulcus, it sends an ascending branch to supply the humeral head and shoulder joint. It continues laterally under the long head of biceps and deltoid, and anastomoses with the posterior circumflex humeral artery.

Posterior circumflex humeral artery (Fig. 49.26, 49.29)
The posterior circumflex humeral artery is larger than the anterior. It branches from the third part of the axillary artery at the distal border of subscapularis and runs backwards with the axillary nerve through a quadrangular space which is bounded by subscapularis, the capsule of the shoulder joint and teres minor above, teres major below, the long head of triceps medially, and the surgical neck of the humerus laterally (p. 840). It curves round the humeral neck and supplies the shoulder joint, deltoid, teres major and minor, and long and lateral heads of triceps. It gives off a descending branch which anastomoses with the deltoid branch of the profunda brachii artery and with the anterior circumflex humeral and acromial branches of the suprascapular and thoraco-acromial arteries.

Variants

Branches vary considerably; an alar thoracic, often from the second part, may supply fat and lymph nodes in the axilla. The lateral thoracic artery may be absent when it is replaced by lateral perforating branches

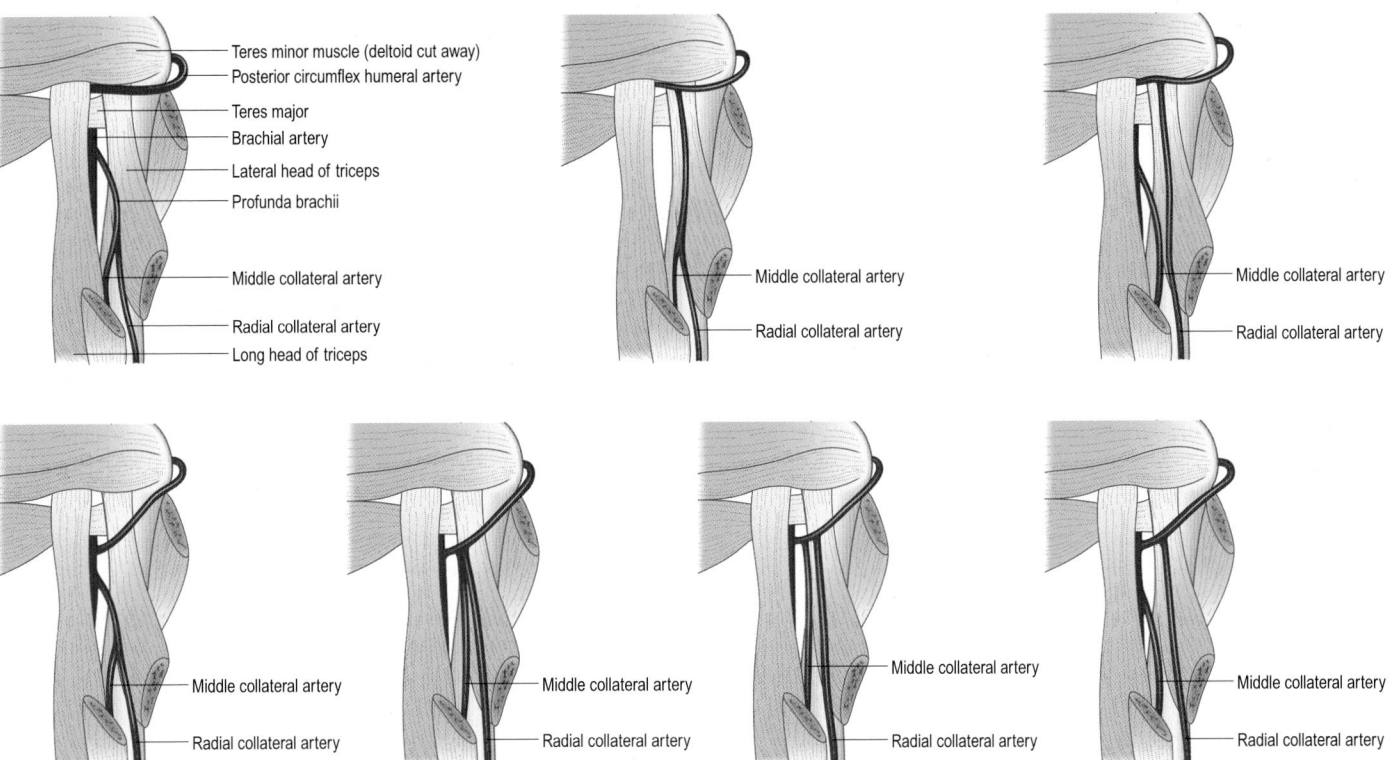

Fig. 49.29 Variation in origin and course of the posterior circumflex humeral artery. The axillary artery, shown in red outline, runs anterior to the radial nerve.
(By permission from Cormack GC, Lamberty BGH 1994 The Arterial Anatomy of Skin Flaps, 2nd edn. Edinburgh: Churchill Livingstone.)

of the intercostal arteries. It may become, or give off, a direct cutaneous vessel (named the superficial thoracic artery by some sources) which supplies the skin over the lateral border of pectoralis major. In up to 30% of cases, the subscapular artery can arise from a common trunk with the posterior circumflex humeral artery. Occasionally the subscapular, circumflex humeral and profunda brachii arteries arise in common, in which case, branches of the brachial plexus surround this common vessel instead of the axillary artery. The posterior circumflex humeral artery may arise from the profunda brachii artery, and pass back below teres major instead of passing through the quadrangular space. Sometimes the axillary divides into radial and ulnar arteries (anomalous 'high division'), and is occasionally the source of the anterior interosseous artery.

VEINS

Axillary vein

The axillary vein is the continuation of the basilic vein. It begins at the lower border of teres major, and ascends to the outer border of the first rib, where it becomes the subclavian vein. It is joined by the brachial vein near subscapularis, and by the cephalic vein near its costal end; other tributaries follow the axillary arterial branches. It lies medial to the axillary artery, which it partly overlaps. The medial pectoral nerve, medial cord of the brachial plexus, ulnar nerve and medial cutaneous nerve of the forearm lie between the artery and the vein. The medial cutaneous nerve of the arm is medial to the vein; the lateral group of axillary lymph nodes is posteromedial. There are a pair of valves near its distal end, and valves also occur near the ends of the cephalic and subscapular veins.

Subclavian vein (Fig. 31.8)

The subclavian vein is a continuation of the axillary vein. It extends from the outer border of the first rib to the medial border of scalenus anterior, where it joins the internal jugular to form the brachiocephalic vein. The clavicle and subclavius are anterior, and the subclavian artery is posterosuperior, separated by scalenus anterior and the phrenic nerve. The first rib and pleura are inferior. The vein usually has a pair of valves c.2 cm from its end. Its tributaries are the external jugular, dorsal scapular and (sometimes) anterior jugular veins, and occasionally a

small branch from the cephalic vein which ascends anterior to the clavicle. At its junction with the internal jugular vein, the left subclavian receives the thoracic duct: the right subclavian vein receives the right lymphatic duct.

AXILLARY LYMPH NODES

There are between 20 to 30 axillary nodes, which may be divided into five not wholly distinct groups, namely, lateral, anterior (pectoral), posterior (subscapular), central and apical (**Figs 58.4, 48.6**). Four of the groups are intermediary, and only the apical group is terminal. Collectively they drain the entire upper limb, breast and trunk above the umbilicus.

The lateral group of four to six nodes is posteromedial to the axillary vein, its afferents drain the whole limb except the vessels accompanying the cephalic vein (**Figs 58.4, 48.6**). Efferent vessels pass partly to the central and apical axillary groups, and partly to the inferior deep cervical nodes. The anterior group of four or five nodes spreads along the inferior border of pectoralis minor near the lateral thoracic vessels. Their afferents drain the skin and muscles of the supra-umbilical antero-lateral body wall and breast, and efferents pass partly to the central and partly to the apical axillary nodes. The posterior group of six or seven nodes lie on the inferior margin of the posterior axillary wall, along the subscapular vessels. Their afferents drain the skin and superficial muscles of the inferior posterior region of the neck and the dorsal aspect of the trunk down to the iliac crest, and efferents pass to the apical and central axillary nodes. A central group of three or four large nodes embedded in axillary fat receives afferents from all preceding groups, and their efferents drain to the apical nodes. An apical group of six to twelve nodes is partly posterior to the superior part of pectoralis minor and partly above its superior border, extending to the apex of the axilla medial to the axillary vein. The only direct territorial afferents are those which accompany the cephalic vein or some which drain the upper peripheral region of the breast: the group drains all the other axillary nodes. Their efferents unite as the subclavian trunk and drain directly to the jugulosubclavian venous junction, or the subclavian vein, or jugular lymphatic trunk or (occasionally) to a right lymphatic duct; the left trunk usually ends in the thoracic duct. A few efferents from apical nodes usually reach the inferior deep cervical nodes.

One or two infraclavicular nodes appear beside the cephalic vein, in the groove between pectoralis major and deltoid, just inferior to the clavicle. Their efferents pass through the clavipectoral fascia to the apical axillary nodes. Occasionally some pass anterior to the clavicle to the inferior deep cervical (supraclavicular) nodes.

INNERVATION: BRACHIAL PLEXUS

For an overview of the brachial plexus see page 803 and **Figure 48.7**.

In the axilla, the lateral and posterior cords of the brachial plexus are lateral to the first part of the axillary artery, and the medial cord is behind it. The cords surround the second part of the artery: their names indicate their relationship. In the lower axilla the cords divide into nerves which supply the upper limb (**Fig. 49.30**). Except for the medial root of the median nerve, these nerves are related to the third part of the artery as their cords are to the second, i.e. branches of the lateral cord are lateral, of the medial cord, medial, and of the posterior cord, posterior, to the artery.

Branches of the brachial plexus may be described as supraclavicular and infraclavicular.

SUPRACLAVICULAR BRANCHES

Supraclavicular branches arise from roots or from trunks:

From roots	1. Nerves to scaleni and longus colli	C5, 6, 7, 8
	2. Branch to phrenic nerve	C5
	3. Dorsal scapular nerve	C5
	4. Long thoracic nerve	C5, 6 (7)
From trunks	1. Nerve to subclavius	C5, 6
	2. Suprascapular nerve	C5, 6

Branches to the scaleni and longus colli arise from the lower cervical ventral rami near their exit from the intervertebral foramina. The phrenic nerve is joined by a branch from the fifth cervical ramus anterior to scalenus anterior.

Dorsal scapular nerve

The dorsal scapular nerve comes from the fifth cervical ventral ramus, pierces scalenus medius, passes behind levator scapulae, which it occasionally supplies, and runs with the deep branch of the dorsal scapular artery to the rhomboids, which it supplies.

Long thoracic nerve (Fig. 49.31)

The long thoracic nerve is usually formed by roots from the fifth to the seventh cervical rami, although the last ramus may be absent. The upper two roots pierce scalenus medius obliquely, uniting in or lateral to it. The nerve descends dorsal to the brachial plexus and the first part of the axillary artery and crosses the superior border of serratus anterior to reach its lateral surface. It may be joined by the root from C7, which emerges between scalenus anterior and scalenus medius, and descends on the lateral surface of medius. The nerve continues downwards to the lower border of serratus anterior, and supplies branches to each of its digitations.

The long thoracic nerve is the most common nerve to be affected by neuralgic amyotrophy. Winging of the scapula may be the only clinical manifestation: it is best demonstrated by asking the patient to push against resistance with the arm extended at the elbow and flexed to 90° at the shoulder.

Nerve to subclavius

The nerve to subclavius is small and arises near the junction of the fifth and sixth cervical ventral rami. It descends anterior to the plexus and

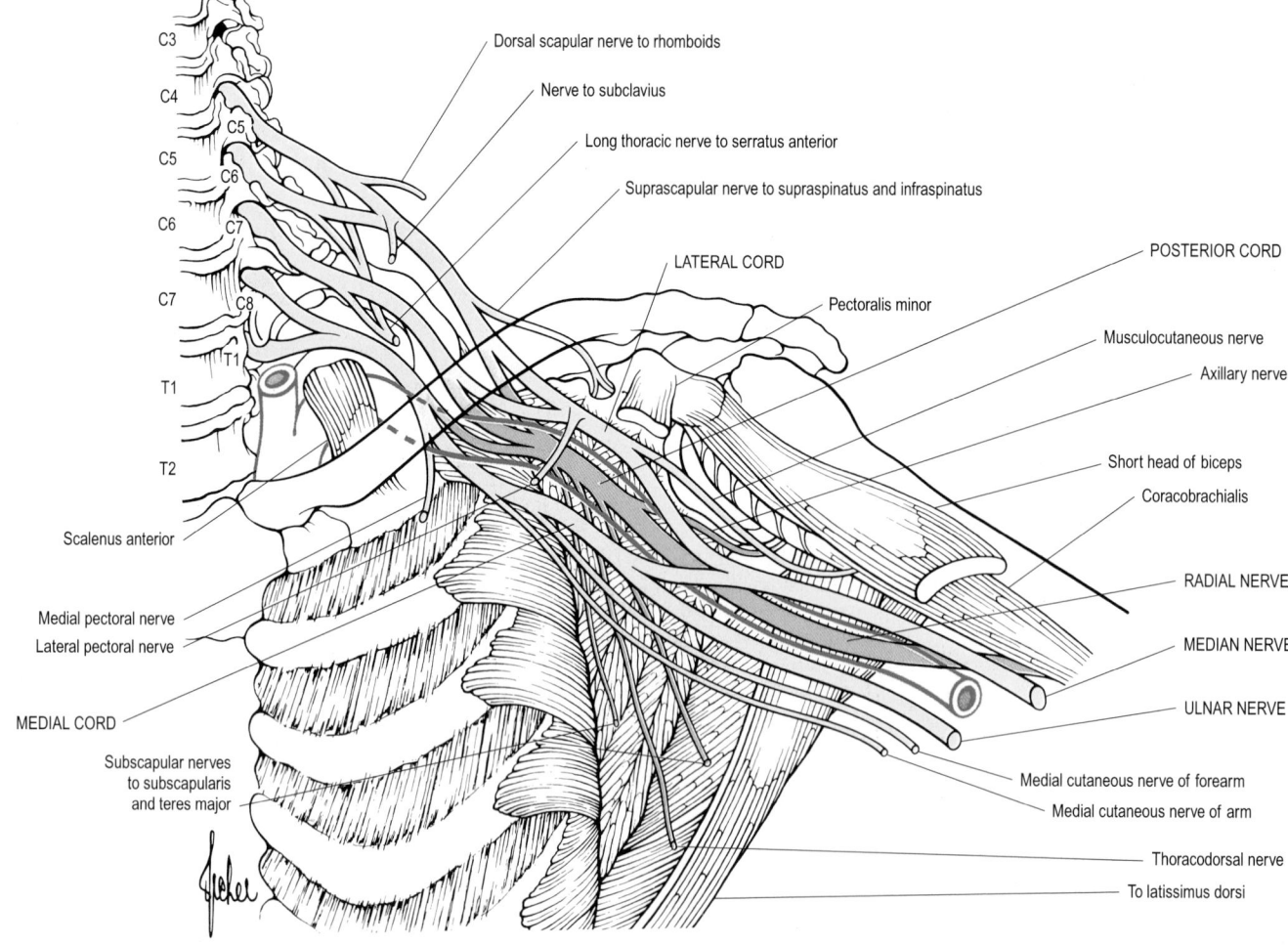

Fig. 49.30 Diagram of the brachial plexus, its branches and the muscles which they supply. The axillary artery, shown in red outline, runs anterior to the radial nerve. (By permission from Aids to the Examination of the Peripheral Nervous System. 2000. 4th edition. London: Saunders.)

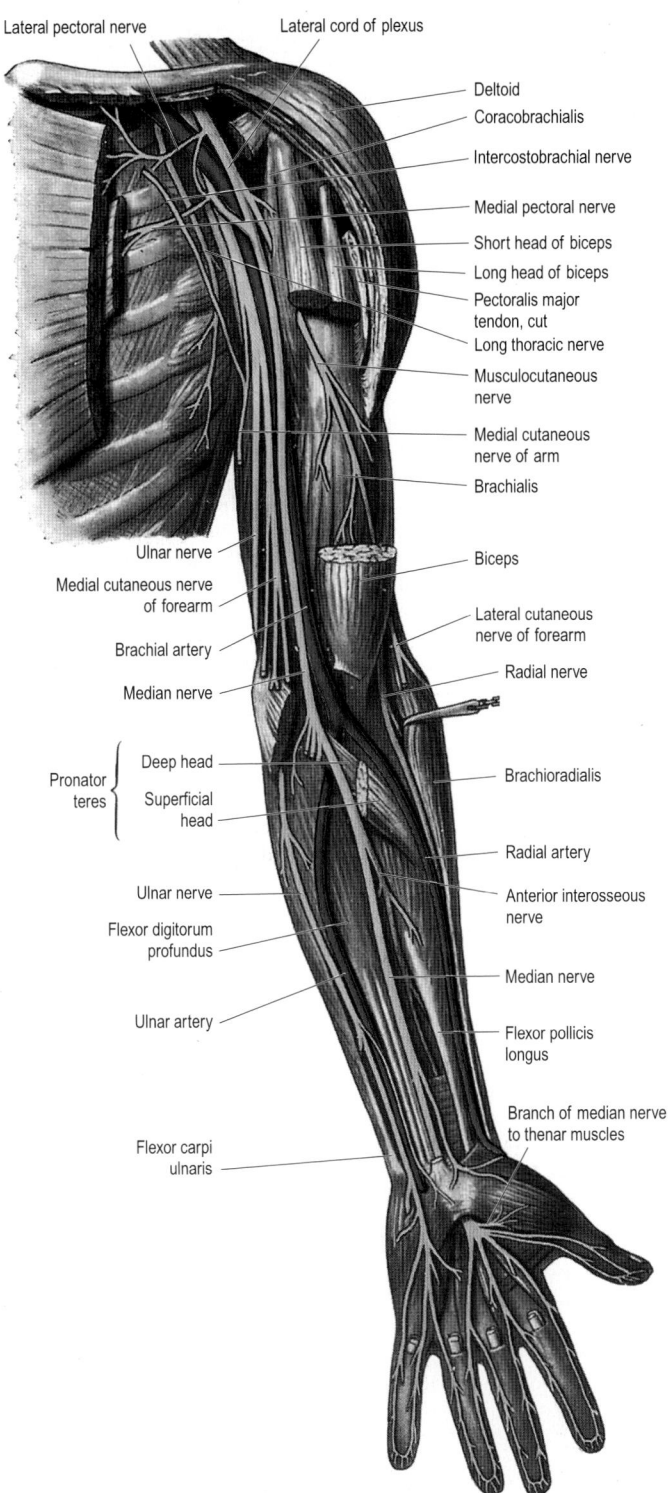

Fig. 49.31 The nerves of the left upper limb, dissected from the anterior aspect.

Labels on figure:
Lateral pectoral nerve
Lateral cord of plexus
Deltoid
Coracobrachialis
Intercostobrachial nerve
Medial pectoral nerve
Short head of biceps
Long head of biceps
Pectoralis major tendon, cut
Long thoracic nerve
Musculocutaneous nerve
Medial cutaneous nerve of arm
Brachialis
Biceps
Ulnar nerve
Medial cutaneous nerve of forearm
Lateral cutaneous nerve of forearm
Brachial artery
Radial nerve
Median nerve
Pronator teres { Deep head, Superficial head }
Brachioradialis
Radial artery
Ulnar nerve
Anterior interosseous nerve
Flexor digitorum profundus
Median nerve
Ulnar artery
Flexor pollicis longus
Flexor carpi ulnaris
Branch of median nerve to thenar muscles

pierces deltoid close to the tip of the acromion and supplies the skin of the proximal third of the arm within the territory of the axillary nerve.

Lesions of the suprascapular nerve – The commonest cause involving the suprascapular nerve is neuralgic amyotrophy. An entrapment neuropathy may occur in the scapular notch or the nerve may be damaged by trauma to the scapula and shoulder. There is pain in the shoulder and wasting and weakness of supraspinatus and infraspinatus.

INFRACLAVICULAR BRANCHES
Infraclavicular branches come from the cords, but their axons may be traced back to the spinal nerves detailed in the box.

Lateral cord	Lateral pectoral	C5, 6, 7
	Musculocutaneous	C5, 6 7
	Lateral root of median	C(5), 6, 7
Medial cord	Medial pectoral	C8, T1
	Medial cutaneous of forearm	C8, T1
	Medial cutaneous of arm	C8, T1
	Ulnar	C(7), 8, T1
	Medial root of median	C8, T1
Posterior cord	Upper subscapular	C5, 6
	Thoracodorsal	C6, 7,8
	Lower subscapular	C5, 6
	Axillary	C5, 6
	Radial	C5, 6, 7, 8, (T1)

Lateral pectoral nerve (Fig. 49.31)
The lateral pectoral nerve is larger than the medial, and may arise from the anterior divisions of the upper and middle trunks, or by a single root from the lateral cord. Its axons are from the fifth to seventh cervical rami. It crosses anterior to the axillary artery and vein, pierces the clavipectoral fascia and supplies the deep surface of pectoralis major. It sends a branch to the medial pectoral nerve, forming a loop in front of the first part of the axillary artery (**Fig. 49.31**), to supply some fibres to pectoralis minor.

Medial pectoral nerve
The medial pectoral nerve is derived from the eighth cervical and first thoracic ventral rami and branches from the medial cord while the latter lies posterior to the axillary artery. It curves forwards between the axillary artery and vein. Anterior to the artery it joins a ramus of the lateral pectoral nerve, and enters the deep surface of pectoralis minor, which it supplies. Two or three branches pierce pectoralis minor and others may pass round its inferior border to end in pectoralis major.

Upper (superior) subscapular nerve
The superior subscapular nerve is smaller than the inferior. It arises from the posterior cord (C5 and 6), enters subscapularis at a high level, and is frequently double.

Lower (inferior) subscapular nerve
The inferior subscapular nerve arises from the posterior cord (C5 and 6). It supplies the lower part of subscapularis, and ends in teres major, which is sometimes supplied by a separate branch.

Thoracodorsal nerve
The thoracodorsal nerve arises from the posterior cord (C6 to 8) between the subscapular nerves. It accompanies the subscapular artery along the posterior axillary wall and supplies latissimus dorsi, reaching its distal border.

Axillary nerve (Fig. 49.23)
The axillary nerve arises from the posterior cord (C5, 6). It is at first lateral to the radial nerve, posterior to the axillary artery and anterior to subscapularis. At the lower border of subscapularis it curves back inferior to the humeroscapular articular capsule and, with the posterior circumflex humeral vessels, traverses a quadrangular space bounded above by subscapularis (anterior) and teres minor (posterior), below by teres major, medially by the long head of triceps, and laterally by the surgical neck of the humerus. It divides in the space into anterior and posterior branches. The anterior branch curves round the neck of the humerus

the third part of the subclavian artery and is usually connected to the phrenic nerve. It passes above the subclavian vein to supply subclavius.

Suprascapular nerve (Fig. 31.8)
The suprascapular nerve is a large branch of the superior trunk. It runs laterally, deep to trapezius and omohyoid and enters the supraspinous fossa through the suprascapular notch inferior to the superior transverse scapular ligament. It runs deep to supraspinatus and curves round the lateral border of the spine of the scapula with the suprascapular artery to reach the infraspinous fossa, where it gives two branches to supraspinatus and articular rami to the shoulder and acromioclavicular joints. The suprascapular nerve rarely has a cutaneous branch. When present, it

with the posterior circumflex humeral vessels, deep to deltoid. It reaches the anterior border of the muscle and supplies it, and gives off a few small cutaneous branches which pierce deltoid and ramify in the skin over its lower part. The posterior branch courses medially and posteriorly along the attachment of the lateral head of triceps, inferior to the glenoid rim. It usually lies medial to the anterior branch in the quadrangular space. It gives off the nerve to teres minor and the upper lateral cutaneous nerve of the arm at the lateral edge of the origin of the long head of triceps. The nerve to teres minor enters the muscle on its inferior surface. The posterior branch frequently supplies the posterior aspect of deltoid, usually via a separate branch from the main stem, occasionally from the superior lateral cutaneous nerve of the arm. However, the posterior part of deltoid has a more consistent supply from the anterior branch of the axillary nerve, which should be remembered when performing a posterior deltoid-splitting approach to the shoulder. The upper lateral cutaneous nerve of the arm pierces the deep fascia at the medial border of the posterior aspect of deltoid and supplies the skin over the lower part of deltoid and the upper part of the long head of triceps. The posterior branch is intimately related to the inferior aspects of the glenoid and shoulder joint capsule, which may place it at particular risk during capsular plication or thermal shrinkage procedures (Ball et al 2003). There is often an enlargement or pseudoganglion on the branch to teres minor. The axillary trunk supplies a branch to the shoulder joint below subscapularis.

Lesions of the axillary nerve – The commonest causes of axillary nerve lesions are trauma (dislocation of the shoulder, fracture of the surgical neck of the humerus), and neuralgic amyotrophy. There is wasting and weakness of deltoid, which is usually clinically evident, and a patch of sensory loss on the outer aspect of the arm. This can be differentiated from a C5 root lesion by finding normal function in the distribution of the suprascapular nerve.

Musculocutaneous nerve (Fig. 49.31)

The musculocutaneous nerve arises from the lateral cord (C5–7), opposite the lower border of pectoralis minor. It pierces coracobrachialis and descends laterally between biceps and brachialis to the lateral side of the arm. Just below the elbow it pierces the deep fascia lateral to the tendon of biceps, and continues as the lateral cutaneous nerve of the forearm. A line drawn from the lateral side of the third part of the axillary artery across coracobrachialis and biceps to the lateral side of the biceps tendon is a surface projection for the nerve (but this varies according to its point of entry into coracobrachialis). It supplies coracobrachialis, both heads of biceps and most of brachialis. The branch to coracobrachialis is given off before the musculocutaneous nerve enters the muscle: its fibres are from the seventh cervical ramus and may branch directly from the lateral cord. Branches to biceps and brachialis leave after the musculocutaneous has pierced coracobrachialis: the branch to brachialis also supplies the elbow joint. The musculocutaneous nerve supplies a small branch to the humerus, which enters the shaft with the nutrient artery.

Lesions of the musculocutaneous nerve – An isolated lesion of the musculocutaneous nerve is rare, but may occur in injuries to the upper arm and shoulder, e.g. fracture of the humerus, and in patients with neuralgic amyotrophy. There is marked weakness of elbow flexion, because biceps brachii and much of brachialis are paralysed, and sensory impairment on the extensor aspect of the forearm in the distribution of the lateral cutaneous nerve of the forearm. Pain and paraesthesiae may be aggravated by elbow extension.

Medial cutaneous nerve of arm

The medial cutaneous nerve of the arm is the smallest and most medial branch of the brachial plexus, and arises from the medial cord (C8, T1). It crosses the axilla, either anterior or posterior to the axillary vein, then passes medial to the axillary vein, communicates with the intercostobrachial nerve, and descends medial to the brachial artery and basilic vein. It pierces the deep fascia at the midpoint of the upper arm to supply the skin over the medial aspect of the distal third of the upper arm.

Medial cutaneous nerve of forearm

The medial cutaneous nerve of the forearm arises from the medial cord (C8, T1). It is described further on pages 858 and 887.

Median nerve

The median nerve has two roots from the lateral (C5, 6, 7) and medial (C8, T1) cords, which embrace the third part of the axillary artery, and unite anterior or lateral to it (**Fig. 49.31**). Some fibres from C7 often leave the lateral root in the lower part of the axilla and pass distomedially posterior to the medial root, and usually anterior to the axillary artery, to join the ulnar nerve. They may branch from the seventh cervical ventral ramus. Clinically they are believed to be mainly motor and to supply flexor carpi ulnaris. If the lateral root is small, the musculocutaneous nerve (C5, 6, 7) connects with the median nerve in the arm.

Ulnar nerve

The ulnar nerve arises from the medial cord (C8, T1) but often receives fibres from the ventral ramus of C7 (**Fig. 49.31**). It runs distally through the axilla medial to the axillary artery, between it and the vein. It is described further on page 857.

Radial nerve

The radial nerve is the largest branch of the brachial plexus. It arises from the posterior cord (C5, 6, 7, 8, (T1)) (**Fig. 49.23**), and descends behind the third part of the axillary artery and the upper part of the brachial artery, anterior to subscapularis and the tendons of latissimus dorsi and teres major. With the arteria profunda brachii it inclines dorsally, and passes through the triangular space below the lower border of teres major, between the long head of triceps and the humerus. It is described further on page 857.

BRACHIAL PLEXUS LESIONS

Lesions of the brachial plexus commonly affect either the upper part of the plexus, i.e. C5 and C6 roots and the upper trunk, or the lower part of the plexus, i.e. C8 and T1 roots and the lower trunk. Lesions affecting the upper part are usually traumatic, whereas those affecting the lower part may be caused by trauma but may also be produced by malignant infiltration or a thoracic outlet syndrome. Severe trauma may affect the whole plexus.

Upper plexus palsies

Downward traction of an infant's arm during birth, or, in adults, a severe fall on the side of the head and the shoulder, forcing the two apart, as frequently occurs in a motor cycle injury, may tear the roots of C5 and C6. This will result in paralysis of deltoid, the short muscles of the shoulder, and of brachialis and biceps. The last two are both elbow flexors, and biceps is also a powerful supinator of the superior radio-ulnar joint. The arm therefore hangs by the side, with the forearm pronated and the palm facing backwards, like a waiter hinting for a tip (Erb–Duchenne paralysis). There is sensory loss over the lateral aspect of the upper arm.

Lower plexus palsies

Upward traction on the arm, e.g. in a forcible breech delivery, may tear the lowest root, T1, which provides the segmental supply to the intrinsic muscles of the hand. The hand assumes a clawed appearance reflecting the unopposed action of the long flexors and extensors of the fingers (Klumpke's paralysis). There is sensory loss along the medial aspect of the forearm and there is often an associated Horner's syndrome (ptosis and constriction of the pupil) which occurs as a result of traction on the cervical sympathetic chain.

Malignant infiltration of the brachial plexus may result from extension of an apical lung carcinoma (Pancoast tumour) or from metastatic spread, often from carcinoma of the breast. There is slowly progressive weakness which usually starts in the small muscles of the hand (T1) and spreads to involve the finger flexors (C8). This is usually a painful condition, and the pain may be severe. There is sensory loss on the medial aspect of the forearm (T1) extending into the medial side of the hand and to the little finger (C8). A Horner's syndrome may occur if there is involvement of the cervical sympathetic ganglia. A similar syndrome may occur following radiotherapy for breast carcinoma, but this is usually painless. Thoracic surgery involving a sternal split may cause traction on the brachial plexus and usually affects the lower part of the plexus.

The lower trunk of the brachial plexus (C8, T1), together with the subclavian artery, may be angulated over a cervical rib (thoracic outlet syndrome). Patients may present with vascular symptoms as a result of kinking of the subclavian artery (this is more likely to occur with large bony ribs), or they may present with neurological deficit (this is more likely in patients with small rudimentary ribs which extend into a fibrous band which joins the first rib anteriorly). Cervical ribs are quite common and are rarely associated with symptoms. There is a slow insidious onset of wasting of the small muscles of the hand, which often starts on the lateral side with involvement of the thenar eminence and first dorsal interosseous. There is pain and paraesthesiae in the medial aspect of the forearm extending to the little finger, and this is often aggravated by carrying shopping or suitcases. A bruit may be heard over the subclavian artery, and the radial pulse may be easily obliterated by movements of the arm, particularly with the arm extended and abducted at the shoulder.

REFERENCES

Ball CM, Steger T, Galatz LM, Yamaguchi K 2003 The posterior branch of the axillary nerve: an anatomic study. J Bone Joint Surg 85: 1497–1501.

Burkart AC, Debski RE 2002 Anatomy and function of the glenohumeral ligaments in anterior shoulder instability. Clin Orthopaed Related Res 400: 32–39.

Michener LA, McClure PW, Karduna AR 2003 Anatomical and biomechanical mechanisms of subacromial impingement syndrome. Clin Biomech 18: 369–79.

Taylor GI, Razaboni RM (eds) 1994 Michael Salmon: Anatomic Studies. Book 1, Arteries of the Muscles of the Extremities and the Trunk. Book 2, Arterial anastomotic pathways of the extremities. St Louis: Quality Medical Publishing. *Contains the translated work of Dr Michel Salmon and describes the blood supply to muscle as well as the anastomotic pathways in the limbs.*

Upper arm

SKIN AND SOFT TISSUE

CUTANEOUS VASCULAR SUPPLY

The blood supply to the skin of the upper arm can be divided into three regions with separate supply; the deltoid region, supplied by musculo-cutaneous perforators, and the medial and lateral regions, supplied by fasciocutaneous perforators (Cormack & Lamberty 1994; Salmon 1994) (**Figs 50.1, 50.2, 50.3**).

The deltoid region is supplied by the posterior circumflex humeral artery (p. 844) via musculocutaneous perforators. After the posterior circumflex humeral artery passes through the quadrangular space (p. 840) it gives off a descending branch, which runs down to the deltoid insertion and the overlying skin, and an ascending branch which passes superiorly towards the acromion, pierces the edge of deltoid and the deep fascia to fan out and supply the overlying skin.

The medial side of the upper arm is supplied by five or six fascio-cutaneous perforators which arise from the brachial artery, the superior ulnar collateral artery and, if present, the single artery to biceps. These perforators pass along the medial intermuscular septum to spread out in the deep fascia and anastomose with perforating vessels superiorly and inferiorly and from the lateral side. There are virtually no musculo-cutaneous perforators through biceps or triceps.

The lateral side of the upper arm below deltoid is supplied by perforating vessels from the middle collateral and radial collateral arteries (the terminating bifurcation of the profunda brachii). The middle collateral artery sends perforators to the skin via the lateral inter-muscular septum between brachioradialis and triceps, while the radial collateral artery gives off cutaneous perforators via the intermuscular septum between brachialis and brachioradialis. These cutaneous vessels anastomose with those from the medial side.

CUTANEOUS INNERVATION

The skin of the shoulder region is supplied by the supraclavicular nerves from the cervical plexus. The floor of the axilla and upper medial surface of the arm is supplied by the lateral branch of the second intercostal nerve (the intercostobrachial nerve). The lower aspect of the medial side of the upper arm is supplied by the medial cutaneous nerve of the arm. The lateral aspect of the upper arm is supplied by the upper lateral cutaneous nerve (a branch of the axillary nerve) and the lower lateral cutaneous nerve (a branch of the radial nerve). The posterior aspect is supplied by the posterior cutaneous nerve of the arm, a branch of the radial nerve (**Figs 45.3, 48.18**).

SOFT TISSUE

Brachial fascia

Brachial fascia, the deep fascia of the upper arm, is continuous with the fascia covering deltoid and pectoralis major: it forms a thin, loose sheath for muscles of the upper arm, and sends septa between them. It is thin over biceps, but thicker over triceps and the humeral epicondyles, and is strengthened by fibrous aponeuroses from pectoralis major and

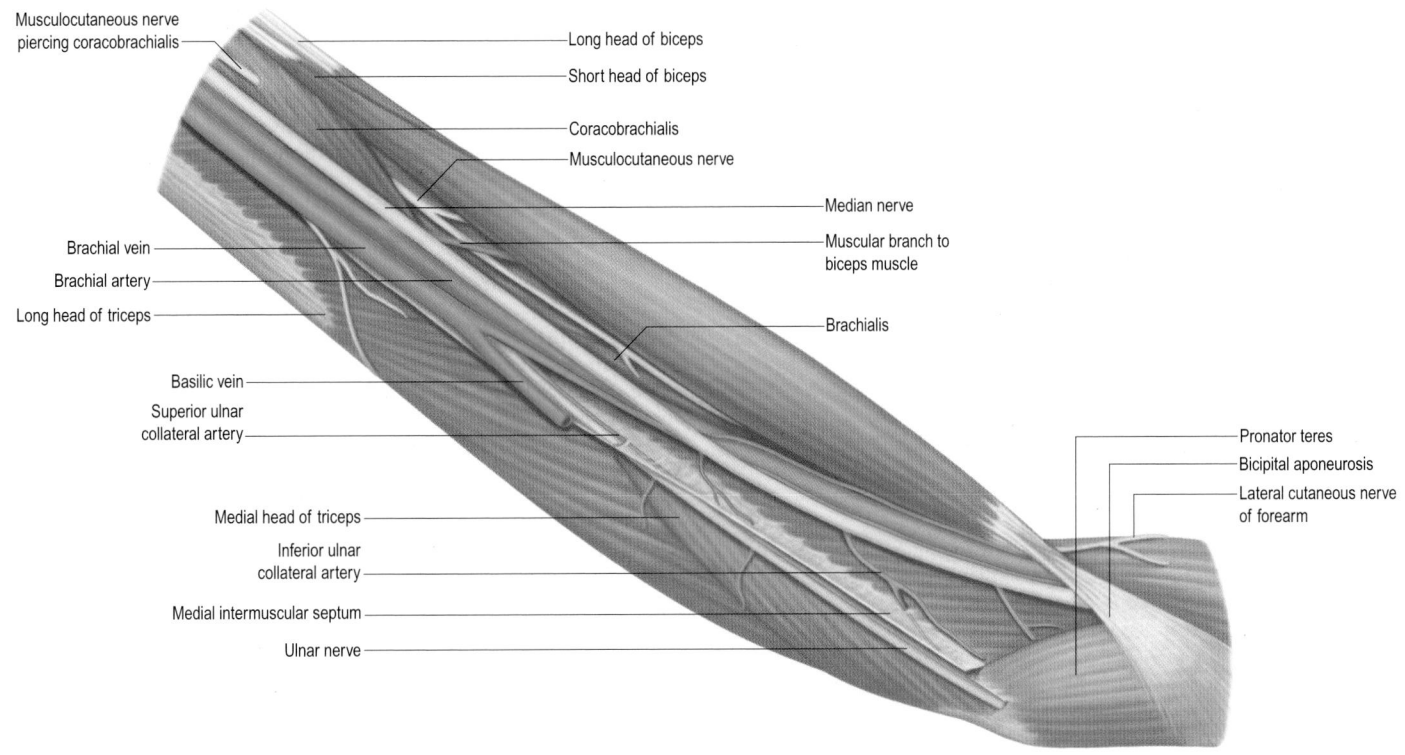

Fig. 50.1 Muscles, vessels and nerves of the left upper arm viewed from the medial aspect.

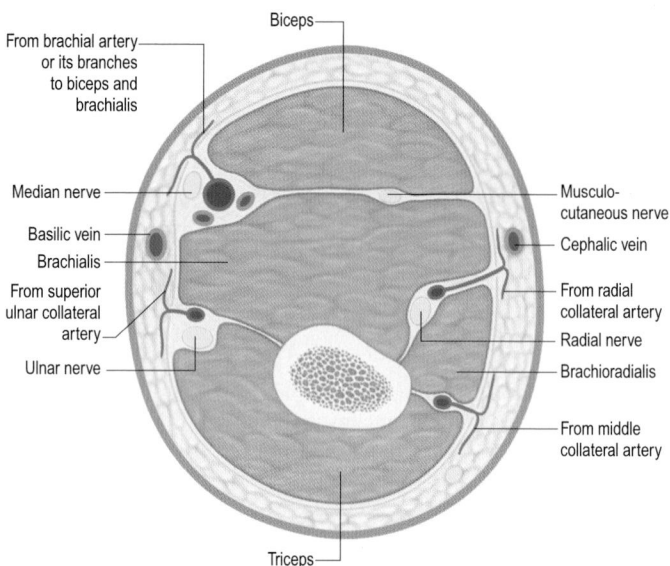

Fig. 50.2 Transverse section through the upper arm to show the location of fasciocutaneous perforators lying on the superficial aspect of the deep fascia. (Adapted and redrawn with permission from Cormack GC, Lamberty BGH 1994 The Arterial Anatomy of Skin Flaps, 2nd edn. Edinburgh: Churchill Livingstone.)

latissimus dorsi medially and from deltoid laterally. Strong medial and lateral intermuscular septa extend from it on each side.

The lateral intermuscular septum extends distally from the lateral lip of the intertubercular sulcus of the humerus along the lateral supracondylar ridge to the lateral epicondyle, and blends with the tendon of deltoid. It gives attachment to triceps behind, and brachialis, brachioradialis and extensor carpi radialis longus in front. It is perforated near the junction of its upper and middle thirds by the radial nerve and the radial collateral branch of the profunda brachii artery. The thicker medial intermuscular septum extends from the medial lip of the intertubercular sulcus, distal to teres major, along the medial supracondylar ridge to the medial epicondyle, and blends with the tendon of coracobrachialis. It gives attachment to triceps behind, and brachialis in front. It is perforated by the ulnar nerve, superior ulnar collateral artery, and the posterior branch of the inferior ulnar collateral artery. At the elbow, the brachial fascia is attached to the epicondyles of the humerus and the olecranon of the ulna, and is continuous with the antebrachial fascia. Medially, just below the middle of the upper arm, it is traversed by the basilic vein and lymphatic vessels and, at various levels, branches of the brachial cutaneous nerves.

Together, the lateral and medial intermuscular septa of the upper arm divide the upper arm into anterior and posterior compartments.

MUSCLES

The muscles of the upper arm are coracobrachialis, which acts only on the shoulder joint; biceps and triceps, which cross both shoulder and elbow joints; and brachialis, which acts only at the elbow joint (**Figs 50.1, 50.3, 50.4**).

ANTERIOR COMPARTMENT

Coracobrachialis

Attachments – Coracobrachialis arises from the apex of the coracoid process, together with the tendon of the short head of biceps, and also by muscular fibres from the proximal 10 cm of this tendon; it ends on an impression, 3–5 cm in length, midway along the medial border of the humeral shaft between the attachments of triceps and brachialis (**Figs 49.22, 50.5**). Accessory slips may be attached to the lesser tubercle, medial epicondyle or medial intermuscular septum.

Relations – Coracobrachialis forms an inconspicuous rounded ridge on the upper medial side of the arm; pulsation of the brachial artery can be felt and often seen in the depression behind it. The muscle is perforated

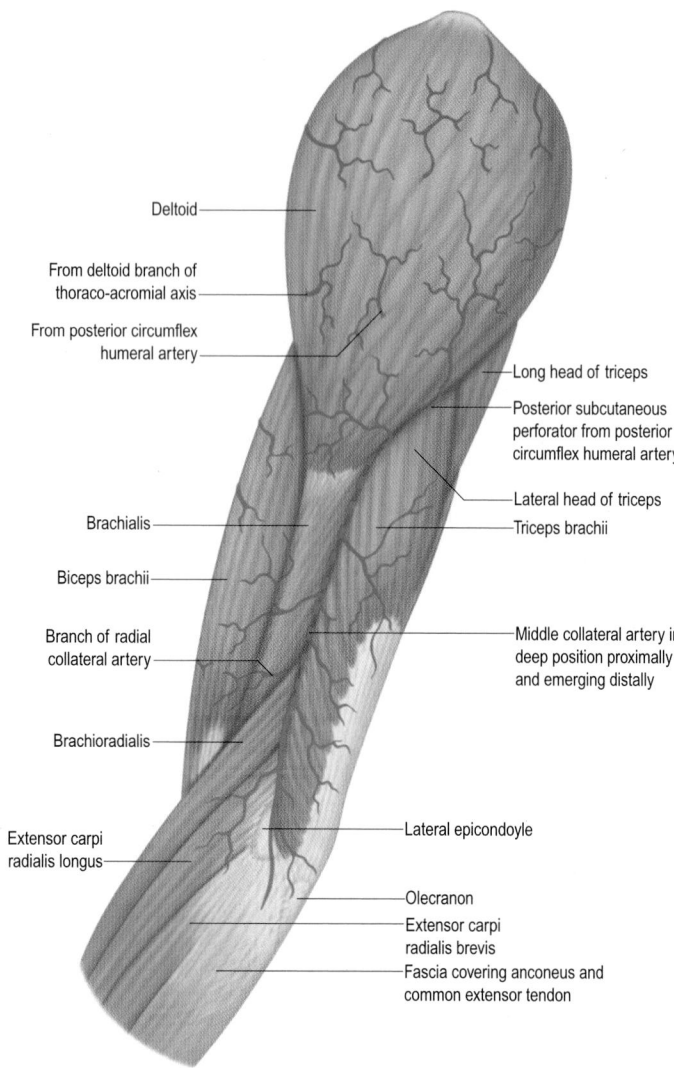

Fig. 50.3 Muscles of the left upper arm viewed from the lateral aspect showing fasciocutaneous and musculocutaneous perforating vessels.

by the musculocutaneous nerve. Anteriorly it is related to pectoralis major above and, at its humeral insertion, to the brachial vessels and median nerve, which cross it. The tendons of subscapularis, latissimus dorsi, and teres major, the medial head of triceps, the humerus and the anterior circumflex humeral vessels all lie posterior. The axillary artery (third part) and proximal parts of the median and musculocutaneous nerves lie medial. Biceps and brachialis lie lateral.

Vascular supply – One or more branches from the axillary artery pass deep to the lateral root of the median nerve, and the musculocutaneous nerve, to reach the deep surface of the muscle. Branches from the anterior circumflex humeral artery also supply the deep surface of the muscle. The accompanying artery of the musculocutaneous nerve sends a recurrent branch to the coracoid attachment and gives off a series of branches to the muscle during its intramuscular course. Accessory branches from the thoracoacromial artery provide additional supply to the superficial part of coracobrachialis.

Innervation – Coracobrachialis is innervated by the musculocutaneous nerve, C5, 6 and 7.

Actions – Coracobrachialis flexes the arm forward and medially, especially from a position of brachial extension. In abduction it acts with anterior fibres of deltoid to resist departure from the plane of motion.

Clinical anatomy: testing – Coracobrachialis can be tested by palpating its fibres during shoulder flexion against resistance.

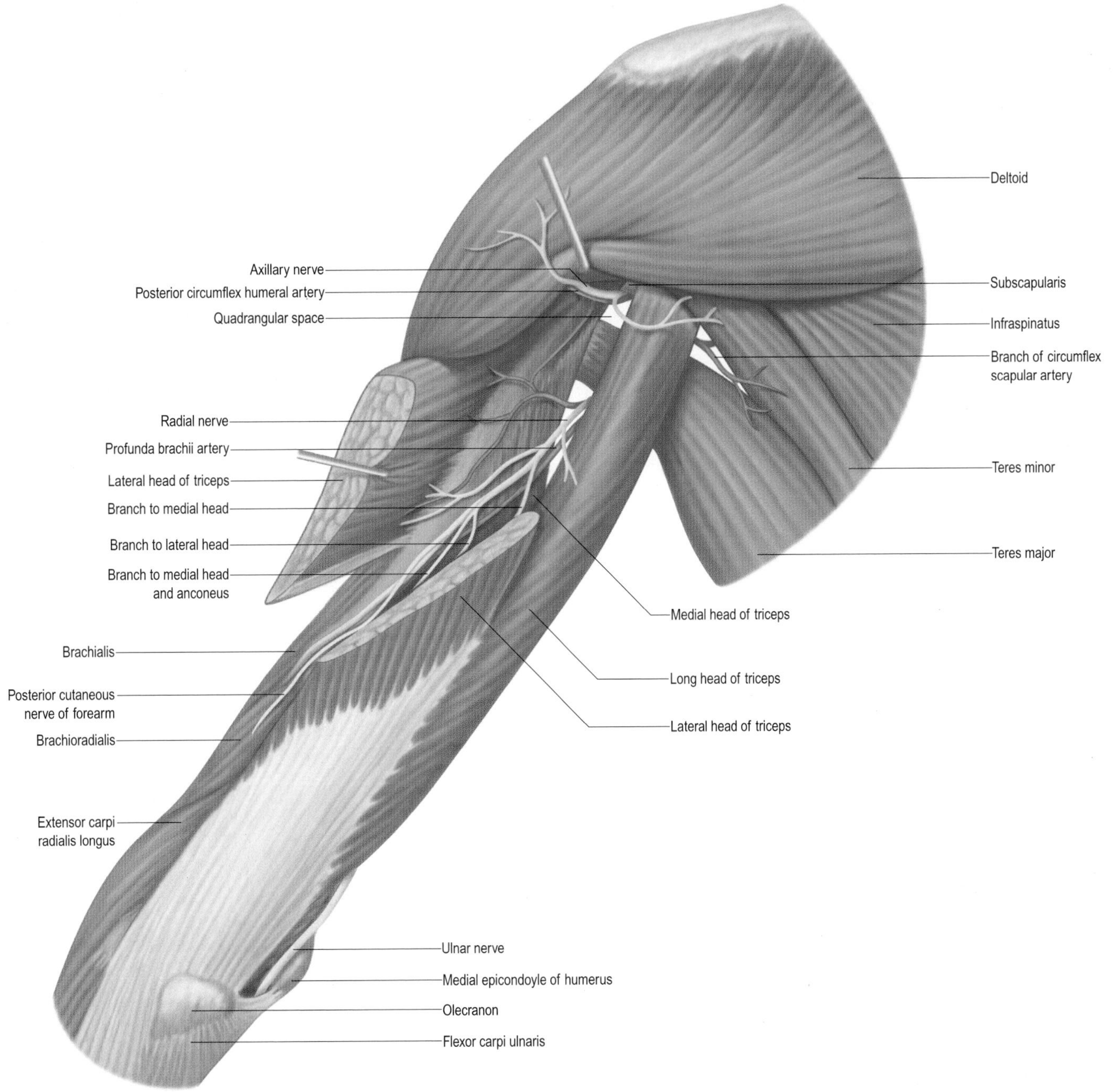

Fig. 50.4 Muscles, vessels and nerves of the left upper arm viewed from the posterior aspect.

Biceps brachii

Attachments – Biceps brachii derives its name from its two proximally attached parts or 'heads' (**Figs 49.22, 50.1, 50.5, 50.6, 50.7**). The short head arises by a thick flattened tendon from the coracoid apex, together with coracobrachialis. The long head starts within the capsule of the shoulder joint as a long narrow tendon, running from the supraglenoid tubercle of the scapula at the apex of the glenoidal cavity, where it is continuous with the glenoidal labrum (p. 830). The tendon of the long head, enclosed in a double tubular sheath (an extension of the synovial membrane of the joint capsule), arches over the humeral head, emerges from the joint behind the transverse humeral ligament, and descends in the intertubercular sulcus, where it is retained by the transverse humeral ligament and a fibrous expansion from the tendon of pectoralis major. The two tendons lead into elongated bellies that, although closely applied, can be separated to within 7 cm or so of the elbow joint. At this joint they end in a flattened tendon, which is attached to the rough posterior area of the radial tuberosity; a bursa separates the tendon from the smooth anterior area of the tuberosity. As it approaches the radius, the tendon spirals, its anterior surface becoming lateral before

being applied to the tuberosity. The tendon has a broad medial expansion, the bicipital aponeurosis, which descends medially across the brachial artery to fuse with deep fascia over the origins of the flexor muscles of the forearm (**Fig. 50.8**). The tendon can be split without difficulty as far as the tuberosity, whence it can be confirmed that its anterior and posterior layers receive fibres from the short and long heads, respectively.

In 10% of cases, a third head arises from the superomedial part of brachialis and is attached to the bicipital aponeurosis and medial side of the tendon of insertion. It usually lies behind the brachial artery, but it may consist of two slips, which descend in front of and behind the artery. Less often, other slips may spring from the lateral aspect of the humerus or intertubercular sulcus.

Relations – Biceps is overlapped proximally by pectoralis major and deltoid; distally it is covered only by fasciae and skin, and it forms a conspicuous elevation on the front of the arm. Its long head passes through the shoulder joint; its short head is anterior to the joint. Distally it lies anterior to brachialis, the musculocutaneous nerve and supinator. Its medial border touches coracobrachialis, and overlaps the

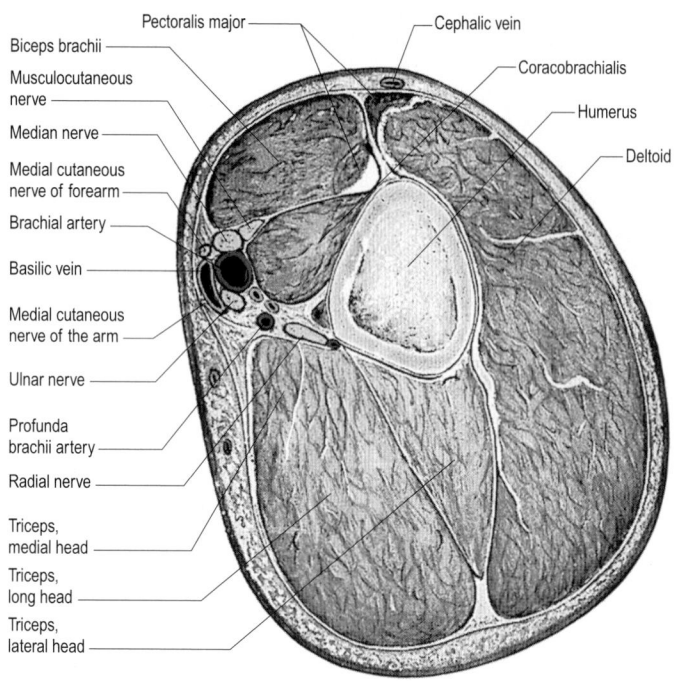

Fig. 50.5 Transverse section through the left arm at the junction of the proximal and middle thirds of the humerus: distal aspect.

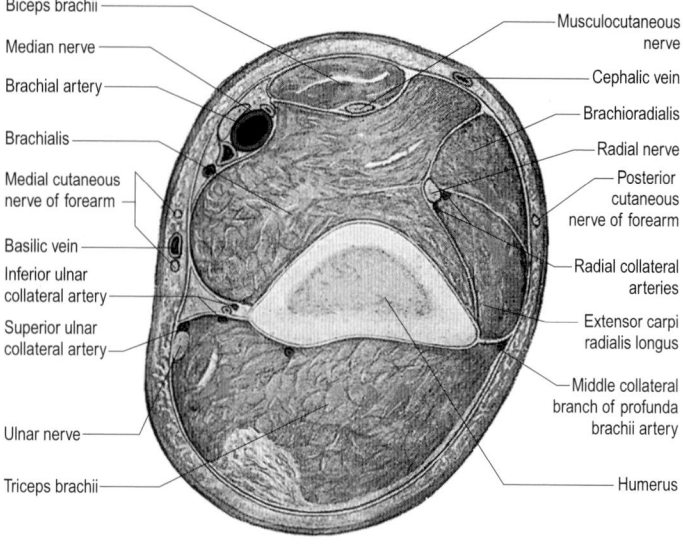

Fig. 50.7 Transverse section through the left arm 2 cm above the medial epicondyle of the humerus: distal aspect.

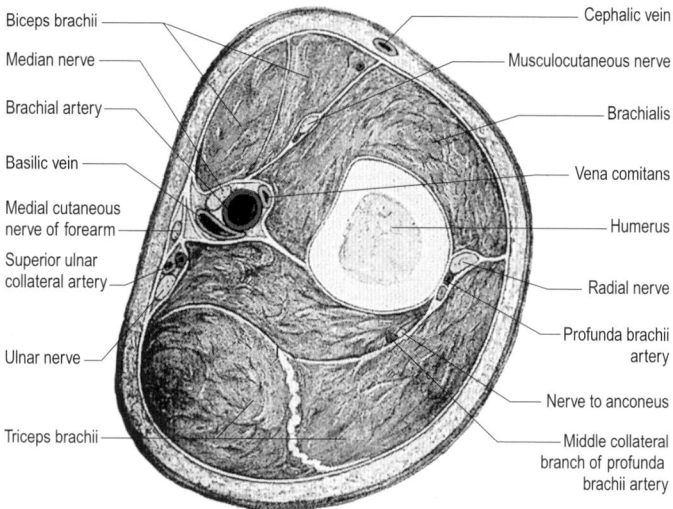

Fig. 50.6 Transverse section through the left arm a little below the middle of the shaft of the humerus: distal aspect.

brachial vessels and median nerve; its lateral border is related to deltoid and brachioradialis.

Vascular supply – Biceps brachii is typically supplied by up to eight vessels originating from the brachial artery in the middle third of the arm. These vessels pass laterally, posterior to the median nerve and divide into ascending and descending branches just before reaching the deep surface of the muscle. Smaller branches arise from the anterior circumflex humeral artery and the deltoid branch of the acromial division of the thoracoacromial axis.

There is great variation in the arterial supply to the muscle. The main arterial supply may originate from the superior or inferior ulnar collateral artery, subscapular artery, axillary artery, ulnar or radial arteries in cases of proximal bifurcation of the brachial artery, or the profunda brachii artery.

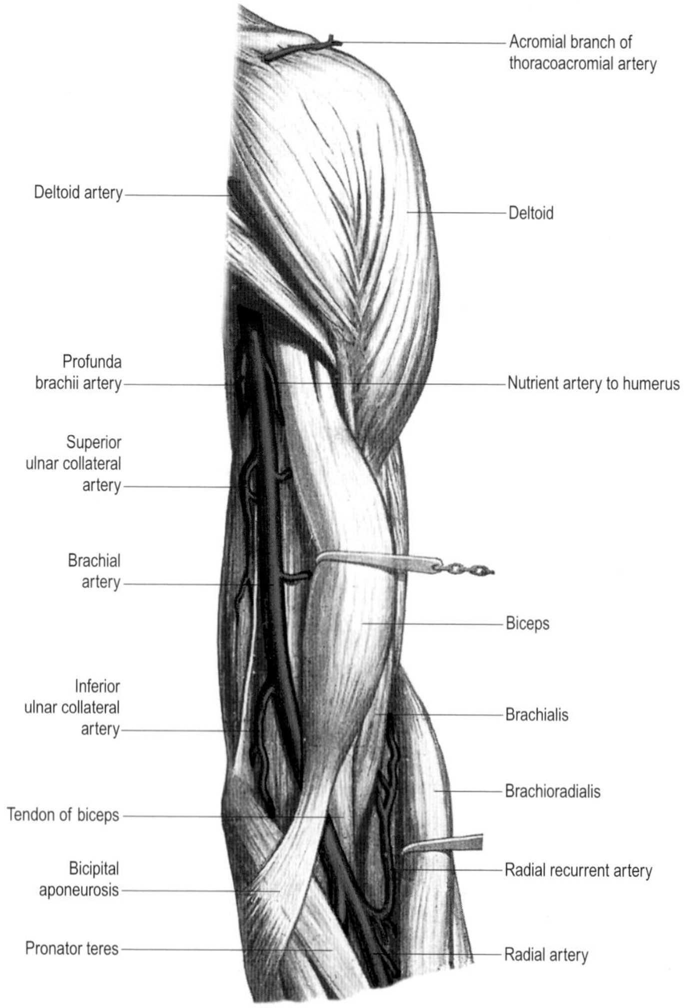

Fig. 50.8 The left brachial artery and its branches.

Innervation – Biceps brachii is innervated by the musculocutaneous nerve, C5 and 6, with separate branches passing to each belly.

Actions – Biceps brachii is a powerful supinator, especially in rapid or resisted movements. It flexes the elbow, most effectively with the forearm supinated, and acts to a slight extent as a flexor of the shoulder joint. It is attached, via the bicipital aponeurosis, to the posterior border of the ulna, the distal end of which is drawn medially in supination. The long head helps to check upward translation of the humeral head during contraction of deltoid. When the elbow is flexed against resistance, the tendon of insertion and bicipital aponeurosis become conspicuous.

Lowering the hand under the influence of gravity by extension at the elbow calls for controlled lengthening of biceps. This is an example of a habitual movement in which muscle tension increases despite increasing length. As the hand descends and the elbow extends, the vertical through the centre of gravity of the forearm is carried further from the fulcrum of movement; the turning moment exerted by the load therefore increases and must be matched by an increase in the moment exerted by the muscle.

Clinical anatomy: testing – With the forearm supinated, biceps brachii can be tested by palpating its fibres during elbow flexion against resistance.

Brachialis

Attachments – Brachialis arises from the lower half of the front of the humerus, starting on either side of the insertion of deltoid, and extending distally to within 2.5 cm of the cubital articular surface (**Figs 49.22, 50.1, 50.6, 50.7**). It also arises from the intermuscular septa, more from the medial than the lateral, since it is separated distally from the lateral intermuscular septum by brachioradialis and extensor carpi radialis longus. Its fibres converge to a thick, broad tendon which is attached to the ulnar tuberosity and to a rough impression on the anterior aspect of the coronoid process.

Brachialis may be divided into two or more parts. It may be fused with brachioradialis, pronator teres or biceps. In some cases it sends a tendinous slip to the radius or bicipital aponeurosis.

Relations – Anterior are biceps, the brachial vessels, musculocutaneous and median nerves. Posterior are the humerus and capsule of the elbow joint. Medial are pronator teres, and the medial intermuscular septum, which separates it from triceps and the ulnar nerve. Lateral are the radial nerve, radial recurrent and radial collateral arteries, brachioradialis and extensor carpi radialis longus.

Vascular supply – The blood supply to brachialis typically consists of two main arteries (superior and inferior) supplemented by a system of accessory arteries. The superior main artery originates from the brachial artery distal to the site of origin of the superior ulnar collateral artery and travels laterally to enter the anterior surface of the upper third of the muscle. The inferior main artery originates either from the superior ulnar collateral artery or directly from the brachial artery and enters the mid-portion of the muscle. The accessory arteries are small, variable in number, origin and course. They can arise from the brachial artery, the superior and inferior ulnar collateral arteries, or the profunda brachii artery.

Innervation – Brachialis is innervated by the musculocutaneous nerve (C5 and 6), and radial nerve (C7) to a small lateral part of the muscle.

Action – Brachialis is a flexor of the elbow joint with the forearm either prone or supine, whether or not the movement is resisted.

Clinical anatomy: testing – Brachialis can be tested by palpating its fibres during elbow flexion against resistance.

POSTERIOR COMPARTMENT

Triceps

Attachments – Triceps fills most of the extensor compartment of the upper arm (**Figs 49.23, 50.4, 50.5, 50.6, 50.7**). It arises by three heads (long, lateral and medial), from which it takes its name.

The long head arises by a flattened tendon from the infraglenoid tubercle of the scapula, blending above with the glenohumeral capsule. Its muscular fibres descend medial to the lateral head and superficial to the medial head, and join them to form a common tendon.

The lateral head arises by a flattened tendon from a narrow, linear, oblique ridge on the posterior surface of the humeral shaft, and from the lateral intermuscular septum. The origin on the humerus ascends with varying obliquity from its lateral border above the radial groove and behind the deltoid tuberosity to the surgical neck medial to the insertion of teres minor. These fibres also converge to the common tendon.

The medial head, which is overlapped posteriorly by the lateral and long heads, has a particularly extensive origin, from the entire posterior surface of the humeral shaft, below the radial groove from the insertion of teres major to within 2.5 cm of the trochlea, from the medial border of the humerus; the medial intermuscular septum and the lower part of the lateral intermuscular septum. Some muscular fibres reach the olecranon directly, the rest converge to the common tendon.

The tendon of triceps begins near the middle of the muscle. It has two laminae, one superficial in the lower half of the muscle, the other in its substance. After receiving the muscle fibres, the two layers unite above the elbow and are attached, for the most part, to the upper surface of the olecranon. On the lateral side a band of fibres continues down over anconeus to blend with antebrachial fascia.

Relations – The long head descends between teres minor and major, dividing the wedge-shaped interval between them and the humerus into triangular and quadrangular parts (**Fig. 49.23**). The triangular space contains the circumflex scapular vessels; it is bounded above by teres minor, below by teres major, laterally by the long head of triceps. The quadrangular space transmits the posterior circumflex humeral vessels and the axillary nerve; it is bounded above by subscapularis, teres minor and the articular capsule, below by teres major, medially by the long head of triceps, and laterally by the humerus.

The lateral head of triceps forms an elevation, parallel and medial to the posterior border of the deltoid; it stands out prominently when the elbow is actively extended. The mass which lies medial to it, and disappears under the deltoid, is the long head.

Vascular supply – The blood supply to triceps is mainly from the profunda brachii artery and the superior ulnar collateral artery, with an accessory supply from the posterior circumflex humeral artery. The medial head of triceps is supplied on its anterior surface by two or three branches from the superior ulnar collateral artery. The posterior surface is supplied by a large proximal branch from the profunda which passes medially in front of the radial nerve. The long head of triceps is supplied on its anterior surface by two arteries, one arising from the axillary artery in front of the tendon of latissimus dorsi and the other arising from either the brachial artery or the superior ulnar collateral. The posterior surface receives a recurrent branch from the posterior circumflex humeral artery immediately after traversing the quadrangular space. The lateral surface receives a number of small branches from the profunda brachii in its distal portion. The lateral head of the triceps is primarily supplied by branches of the profunda brachii, with an additional supply from a branch of the posterior circumflex humeral artery.

Innervation – Triceps is innervated by the radial nerve, C6, 7 and 8, with separate branches for each head.

Action – Triceps is the major extensor of the forearm at the elbow joint. The medial head is active in all forms of extension. The lateral and long heads are minimally active except in extension against resistance, as in thrusting or pushing or supporting body weight on the hands with the elbows semiflexed. When the flexed arm is extended at the shoulder joint, the long head may assist in drawing back and adducting the humerus to the thorax. The long head supports the lower part of the capsule of the shoulder joint, especially when the arm is raised. Articularis cubiti probably draws up the posterior part of the capsule of the elbow joint during extension of the forearm. In forceful supination of the semiflexed forearm, involving contraction of both supinator and biceps brachii, the triceps contracts synergistically to maintain the semiflexed position.

Clinical anatomy: testing – The muscle can be tested by palpating its fibres during elbow extension against resistance.

Anconeus
Anconeus is described on page 880.

VASCULAR SUPPLY AND LYMPHATIC DRAINAGE

ARTERIES

Brachial artery
The brachial artery, a continuation of the axillary, begins at the distal (inferior) border of the tendon of teres major and ends about a centimetre distal to the elbow joint (at the level of the neck of the radius) by dividing into radial and ulnar arteries (**Figs 50.1, 50.8, 50.9**). At first it is medial to the humerus, but gradually spirals anterior to it until it lies midway between the humeral epicondyles. Its pulsation can be felt throughout.

Relations
The brachial artery is wholly superficial, covered anteriorly only by skin and superficial and deep fasciae. The bicipital aponeurosis crosses it anteriorly at the elbow, separating it from the median cubital vein; the median nerve crosses it lateromedially near the distal attachment of coracobrachialis. Posterior are the long head of triceps, separated by the radial nerve and profunda brachii artery, and then successively by the medial head of triceps, the attachment of coracobrachialis and brachialis. Proximally the median nerve and coracobrachialis lie laterally while distally the biceps and the muscles overlap the artery. Proximally the medial cutaneous nerve of the forearm and ulnar nerve lie medially, while distally the median nerve and basilic vein lie. With the artery are two venae comitantes, connected by transverse and oblique branches.

At the elbow the brachial artery sinks deeply into the triangular intermuscular cubital fossa (p. 859).

Variants
The brachial artery, with the median nerve, may diverge from the medial border of the biceps, descending towards the medial humeral epicondyle, usually behind a supracondylar process from which a fibrous arch crosses the artery, and which then runs behind or through pronator teres to the elbow. Occasionally the artery divides proximally into two trunks which reunite. Frequently it divides more proximally than usual into radial, ulnar and common interosseous arteries. Most often the radial branches arise proximally, leaving a common trunk for the ulnar and common interosseous; sometimes the ulnar arises proximally, the radial and common interosseous forming the other division; the common interosseous may also arise proximally. Sometimes slender vasa aberrantia connect the brachial to the axillary artery or to one of the forearm arteries, usually the radial. The brachial artery may be crossed by muscular or tendinous slips from coracobrachialis, biceps, brachialis or pronator teres. Rarely the median nerve crosses behind, and not in front of, the brachial artery near the insertion of coracobrachialis.

Branches
These are profunda brachii, nutrient, superior, middle and inferior ulnar collateral, deltoid, muscular, radial and ulnar arteries.

Profunda brachii artery (Figs 50.4, 50.5, 50.8, 50.9) – The profunda brachii is a large branch from the posteromedial aspect of the brachial artery, distal to teres major. It follows the radial nerve closely, at first posteriorly between the long and medial heads of triceps, then in the spiral groove covered by the lateral head of triceps. It supplies muscular branches, the nutrient artery of the humerus, and finally divides into terminal radial and middle collateral branches (**Fig. 50.9**). The radial collateral branch pierces the lateral intermuscular septum to reach the anterior aspect of the epicondyle of the humerus in the groove between brachioradialis and brachialis, and takes part in the anastomosis around the elbow. The middle collateral branch runs posterior to the septum and epicondyle.

The profunda brachii can originate from a common origin with the posterior circumflex humeral artery, from the axillary artery proximal to the tendon of latissimus dorsi or from the distal portion of the axillary artery.

Middle collateral (posterior descending) branch – The middle collateral artery is the larger terminal vessel. It arises posterior to the humerus and descends down the posterior surface of the lateral intermuscular septum to the elbow (**Figs 50.6, 50.9**). Proximally, the artery lies between brachialis (anteriorly) and the lateral head of triceps (posteriorly) while distally it lies between brachioradialis (anteriorly) and the lateral head of triceps (posteriorly). It may pierce the deep fascia and become cutaneous or remain deep to the fascia until anastomosing with the interosseous recurrent artery behind the lateral epicondyle; it gives off about five small fasciocutaneous perforators and often has a small branch that accompanies the nerve to anconeus.

This artery and its fasciocutaneous perforators provide the anatomical basis to allow a skin flap (the lateral arm flap) to be surgically raised (either pedicled or by free tissue transfer) for reconstructing areas of tissue missing elsewhere in the body.

Radial collateral (anterior descending) branch – The radial collateral artery is the continuation of the profunda (**Figs 50.7, 50.9**). It accompanies the radial nerve through the lateral intermuscular septum, descending between brachialis and brachioradialis anterior to the lateral epicondyle, anastomosing with the radial recurrent artery. It supplies brachialis, brachioradialis, the radial nerve and a few fasciocutaneous perforators.

Nutrient artery of humerus – The nutrient artery of the humerus arises near the mid-level of the upper arm, and enters the nutrient canal near the attachment of coracobrachialis, posterior to the deltoid tuberosity; it is directed distally.

Superior ulnar collateral artery (Figs 50.6, 50.7, 50.8, 50.9) – The superior ulnar collateral artery arises a little distal to the mid-level of the upper arm, usually from the brachial artery, but often as a branch from the profunda brachii. It accompanies the ulnar nerve, piercing the medial intermuscular septum to descend in the posterior compartment and supply the medial head of triceps. It passes between the medial epicondyle and olecranon, ending deep to flexor carpi ulnaris by anastomosing with the posterior ulnar recurrent and inferior collateral arteries. A branch sometimes passes anterior to the medial epicondyle and anastomoses with the anterior ulnar recurrent artery.

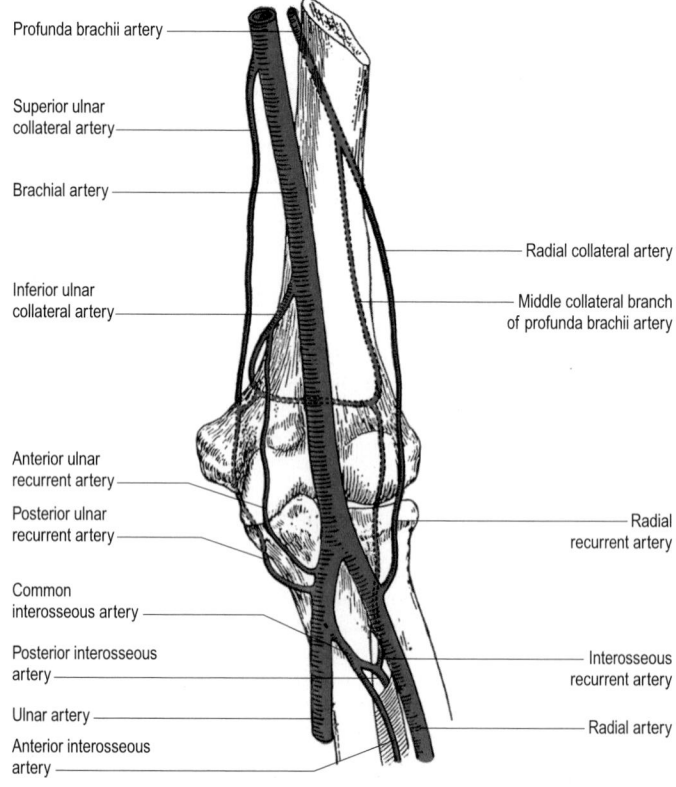

Fig. 50.9 The arterial anastomoses around the left elbow joint viewed from the anterior aspect.

Profunda brachii artery

Superior ulnar collateral artery

Brachial artery

Inferior ulnar collateral artery

Anterior ulnar recurrent artery

Posterior ulnar recurrent artery

Common interosseous artery

Posterior interosseous artery

Ulnar artery

Anterior interosseous artery

Radial collateral artery

Middle collateral branch of profunda brachii artery

Radial recurrent artery

Interosseous recurrent artery

Radial artery

Middle ulnar collateral artery – If present, the middle ulnar collateral artery arises from the brachial artery between the superior and inferior ulnar collaterals. It passes anterior to the medial epicondyle and anastomoses with the anterior ulnar recurrent artery. It supplies triceps and sends small fasciocutaneous perforators to the skin.

Inferior ulnar collateral (supratrochlear) artery (Figs 50.7, 50.8, 50.9, 52.15) – The inferior ulnar collateral artery begins c.5 cm proximal to the elbow, passes medially between the median nerve and brachialis and, piercing the medial intermuscular septum, curls round the humerus between the triceps and bone. It forms, by its junction with the middle collateral branch of the profunda brachii artery, an arch proximal to the olecranon fossa. As it lies on brachialis it gives off branches which descend anterior to the medial epicondyle to anastomose with the anterior ulnar recurrent artery. Behind the epicondyle a branch anastomoses with the superior ulnar collateral and posterior ulnar recurrent arteries.

Muscular branches – Muscular branches are distributed to the coraco-brachialis, biceps and brachialis.

Deltoid (ascending) branch – The deltoid branch ascends between the lateral and long heads of triceps, and anastomoses with a descending branch of the posterior humeral circumflex artery.

Radial and ulnar arteries – The radial and ulnar arteries are described in detail on page 863.

VEINS

Brachial veins
The brachial veins flank the brachial artery, as venae comitantes with tributaries similar to the arterial branches; near the lower margin of subscapularis they join the axillary vein. The medial branch, however, often joins the basilic before it becomes the axillary.

These deep veins have numerous anastomoses with each other and with the superficial veins.

Superficial veins (Fig. 48.5)
The cephalic vein ascends in front of the elbow superficial to a groove between the brachioradialis and biceps, crosses superficial to the lateral cutaneous nerve of the forearm, ascends lateral to biceps and between pectoralis major and deltoid, where it adjoins the deltoid branch of the thoracoacromial artery. Entering the infraclavicular fossa to pass behind the clavicular head of pectoralis major, it pierces the clavipectoral fascia, crosses the axillary artery and joins the axillary vein just below clavicular level. It may connect with the external jugular by a branch anterior to the clavicle. Sometimes the median cubital vein is large, transferring most blood from the cephalic to the basilic vein; the proximal cephalic vein is then absent or much diminished.

LYMPHATIC DRAINAGE
Lymphatics follow the usual pattern in that superficial lymphatics follow the veins; deep lymphatics follow the arteries.

For details of supratrochlear nodes see page 864.
For details of infraclavicular nodes see page 846.

INNERVATION

MEDIAN NERVE (Figs 50.1, 49.31)
The median nerve enters the arm lateral to the brachial artery. Near the insertion of coracobrachialis it crosses in front of (rarely behind) the artery, descending medial to it to the cubital fossa where it is posterior to the bicipital aponeurosis and anterior to brachialis, separated by the latter from the elbow joint.

It gives off vascular branches to the brachial artery and usually a branch to pronator teres, a variable distance proximal to the elbow joint.

MUSCULOCUTANEOUS NERVE
The musculocutaneous nerve is the nerve of the anterior compartment of the arm (Fig. 49.31). It gives a branch to the shoulder joint and then passes through coracobrachialis, which it supplies, emerging to pass between biceps and brachialis. It sends branches to both these muscles.

In the cubital fossa it lies at the lateral margin of the biceps tendon where it continues as the lateral cutaneous nerve of the forearm.

The musculocutaneous nerve has frequent variations. It may run behind coracobrachialis or adhere for some distance to the median nerve and pass behind biceps. Some fibres of the median nerve may run in the musculocutaneous nerve, leaving it to join their proper trunk; less frequently the reverse occurs, and the median nerve sends a branch to the musculocutaneous. Occasionally it supplies pronator teres and may replace radial branches to the dorsal surface of the thumb.

ULNAR NERVE (Figs 50.1, 49.31)
The ulnar nerve gives no branches in the arm. It runs distally through the axilla medial to the axillary artery and between it and the vein, continuing distally medial to the brachial artery as far as the midarm. Here it pierces the medial intermuscular septum, inclining medially as it descends anterior to the medial head of triceps to the interval between the medial epicondyle and the olecranon, with the superior ulnar collateral artery.

RADIAL NERVE (Figs 50.4, 49.31)
The radial nerve descends behind the third part of the axillary artery and the upper part of the brachial artery, anterior to subscapularis and the tendons of latissimus dorsi and teres major. With the profunda brachii artery it inclines dorsally, passing through the triangular space (p. 833) below the lower border of teres major, between the long head of triceps and the humerus. Here it supplies the long head of triceps, and gives rise to the posterior cutaneous nerve of the arm which supplies the skin along the posterior surface of the upper arm. It then spirals obliquely across the back of the humerus, lying posterior to the uppermost fibres of the medial head of triceps which separate the nerve from the bone in the first part of the spiral groove. Here it gives off a muscular branch to the lateral head of triceps and a branch which passes through the medial head of triceps to anconeus. On reaching the lateral side of the humerus it pierces the lateral intermuscular septum to enter the anterior compartment; it then descends deep in a furrow between brachialis and proximally brachioradialis, then more distally extensor carpi radialis longus. Anterior to the lateral epicondyle it divides into superficial and deep terminal rami.

The branches of the radial nerve in the upper arm are: muscular, cutaneous, articular and superficial terminal and posterior interosseous.

Muscular branches
Muscular branches supply triceps, anconeus, brachioradialis, extensor carpi radialis longus and brachialis in medial, posterior and lateral groups. Medial muscular branches arise from the radial nerve on the medial side of the arm. They supply the medial and long heads of triceps; the branch to the medial head is a long, slender filament which, lying close to the ulnar nerve as far as the distal third of the arm, is often termed the ulnar collateral nerve. A large posterior muscular branch arises from the nerve as it lies in the humeral groove. It divides to supply the medial and lateral heads of triceps and anconeus, that for the latter being a long nerve which descends in the medial head of triceps and partially supplies it; it is accompanied by the middle collateral branch of the profunda brachii artery and passes behind the elbow joint to end in anconeus. Lateral muscular branches arise in front of the lateral intermuscular septum; they supply the lateral part of brachialis, brachioradialis and extensor carpi radialis longus.

Cutaneous branches
Cutaneous branches are the posterior and lower lateral cutaneous nerves of the arm and the posterior cutaneous nerve of the forearm (**Fig. 48.18**).

Lower lateral cutaneous nerve of the arm
The lower lateral cutaneous nerve of the arm perforates the lateral head of triceps distal to the deltoid tuberosity, passes to the front of the elbow close to the cephalic vein and supplies the skin of the lateral part of the lower half of the arm.

Posterior cutaneous nerve of the arm
The small posterior cutaneous nerve of the arm arises in the axilla and passes medially to supply the skin on the dorsal surface of the arm nearly as far as the olecranon. It crosses posterior to and communicates with the intercostobrachial nerve.

Posterior cutaneous nerve of the forearm

The posterior cutaneous nerve of the forearm arises with the lower lateral cutaneous nerve of the arm. Perforating the lateral head of triceps, it descends first lateral in the arm, then along the dorsum of the forearm to the wrist, supplying the skin in its course and joining, near its end, with dorsal branches of the lateral cutaneous nerve of the forearm.

Articular branches to elbow joint

See page 859.

Lesions of the radial nerve in the upper arm

Lesions of the radial nerve at its origin from the posterior cord in the axilla may be caused by pressure from a long crutch (crutch palsy). Triceps is only involved when lesions occur at this level and is usually spared in the more common lesions of the radial nerve in the arm as it lies alongside the spiral groove, where the nerve is commonly affected by fractures of the humerus. Compression of the nerve against the humerus occurs if the arm is rested on a sharp edge such as the back of a chair ('Saturday night palsy'). Both these injuries cause weakness of brachioradialis with wasting and loss of the reflex. There is both wrist and finger drop due to weakness of wrist and finger extensors, as well as weakness of extensor pollicis longus and abductor pollicis longus. There may be sensory impairment or paraesthesiae in the distribution of the superficial radial nerve. However, nerve overlap means that only a small area of anaesthesia usually occurs on the dorsum of the hand between the first and second metacarpal bones.

Medial cutaneous nerve of arm

The medial cutaneous nerve of arm supplies the skin of the medial aspect of the arm (**Figs 48.18, 49.31**). It is the smallest branch of the brachial plexus, and arises from the medial cord and contains fibres from the eighth cervical and first thoracic ventral rami. It traverses the axilla, crossing anterior or posterior to the axillary vein, to which it is then medial, and communicating with the intercostobrachial nerve; it descends medial to the brachial artery and basilic vein (**Fig. 49.31**) to a point midway in the upper arm, where it pierces the deep fascia to supply a medial area in the distal third of the arm, extending on to its anterior and posterior aspects. Rami reach the skin anterior to the medial epicondyle, and over the olecranon. It connects with the posterior branch of the medial cutaneous nerve of the forearm. Sometimes the medial cutaneous nerve of the arm and the intercostobrachial nerve are connected in a plexiform manner in the axilla. The intercostobrachial nerve may be large and reinforced by part of the lateral cutaneous branch of the third intercostal nerve. It then replaces the medial cutaneous nerve of the arm and receives a connection representing the latter from the brachial plexus (occasionally this connection is absent).

Medial cutaneous nerve of forearm (Fig. 49.31)

The medial cutaneous nerve of forearm comes from the medial cord. It is derived from the eighth cervical and first thoracic ventral rami. At first it is between the axillary artery and vein and gives off a ramus which pierces the deep fascia to supply the skin over the biceps, almost to the elbow. The nerve descends medial to the brachial artery, pierces the deep fascia with the basilic vein midway in the arm and divides into anterior and posterior branches. The larger, anterior branch usually passes in front of, occasionally behind, the median cubital vein, descending anteromedial in the forearm to supply the skin as far as the wrist and connecting with the palmar cutaneous branch of the ulnar nerve. The posterior branch descends obliquely medial to the basilic vein, anterior to the medial epicondyle, and curves round to the back of the forearm, descending on its medial border to the wrist, supplying the skin. It connects with the medial cutaneous nerve of the arm, the posterior cutaneous nerve of the forearm, and the dorsal branch of the ulnar.

REFERENCES

Cormack GC, Lamberty BGH 1994 The Arterial Anatomy of Skin Flaps. Edinburgh: Churchill Livingstone.

Salmon M 1994 Anatomic studies. In: Taylor GI, Razaboni RM (eds) Book 1: Arteries of the Muscles of the Extremities and the Trunk. Book 2: Arterial Anastomotic Pathways of the Extremities. New York: Quality Medical Publishing.

Elbow

SKIN AND SOFT TISSUE

SKIN

Cutaneous vascular supply (Fig. 48.4)
The skin overlying the cubital fossa receives its blood supply on its anterolateral side by small perforating vessels from the radial collateral artery, together with some small musculocutaneous perforators from the radial recurrent artery which traverse brachioradialis. On the antero-medial side, skin is supplied by small branches from the anastomosis between the inferior ulnar collateral artery and the anterior ulnar recurrent artery and by small branches from the brachial artery.

A plexus of anastomosing vessels covers the posterior aspect of the elbow region. On the medial side, the plexus is supplied by small branches from the superior and inferior ulnar collateral arteries and the posterior ulnar recurrent artery. The lateral side is supplied from the middle collateral artery and the posterior interosseous recurrent artery.

Cutaneous innervation (Fig. 48.18)
The skin of the cubital fossa and the epicondylar regions is innervated by the medial and lateral cutaneous nerves of the forearm. A small proximal area on the lateral aspect is supplied by the distal part of the lower lateral cutaneous nerve of the arm. The skin over the olecranon region is innervated by the distal branches of the posterior cutaneous nerve of the arm, together with proximal branches of the posterior cutaneous nerve of the forearm.

SOFT TISSUE: CUBITAL FOSSA
The cubital fossa forms a triangular depression in the middle of the upper part of the anterior aspect of the forearm (**Fig. 51.1**). The superior border of the fossa is an imaginary line, which joins the two epicondyles of the humerus. The fleshy elevation which constitutes its medial border is formed by the lateral margin of pronator teres and the elevation which forms the lateral border is the medial edge of brachioradialis. The roof of the fossa is formed by the deep fascia of the forearm, reinforced by the bicipital aponeurosis on the medial aspect. The median cubital vein lies on this deep fascia crossed superficially (or sometimes deeply) by the medial cutaneous nerve of the forearm. Brachialis and supinator form the floor of the fossa.

From medial to lateral, the fossa contains the median nerve, the terminal part of the brachial artery and accompanying veins together with the start of the radial and ulnar arteries, the tendon of biceps and the radial nerve just under cover of brachioradialis.

JOINTS

The humerus articulates with both the radius and the ulna at the elbow joint. The radius and ulna articulate by synovial superior (proximal) and inferior (distal) radio-ulnar joints and by an intermediate interosseous membrane and ligament, which constitute a non-synovial middle radio-ulnar union.

ELBOW JOINT
The elbow joint is a synovial joint. Its complexity is increased by continuity with the superior radio-ulnar joint. It includes two articulations (**Figs 51.2, 51.3**). These are the humero-ulnar, between the trochlea of the humerus and the ulnar trochlear notch, and the humero-radial, between the capitulum of the humerus and the radial head.

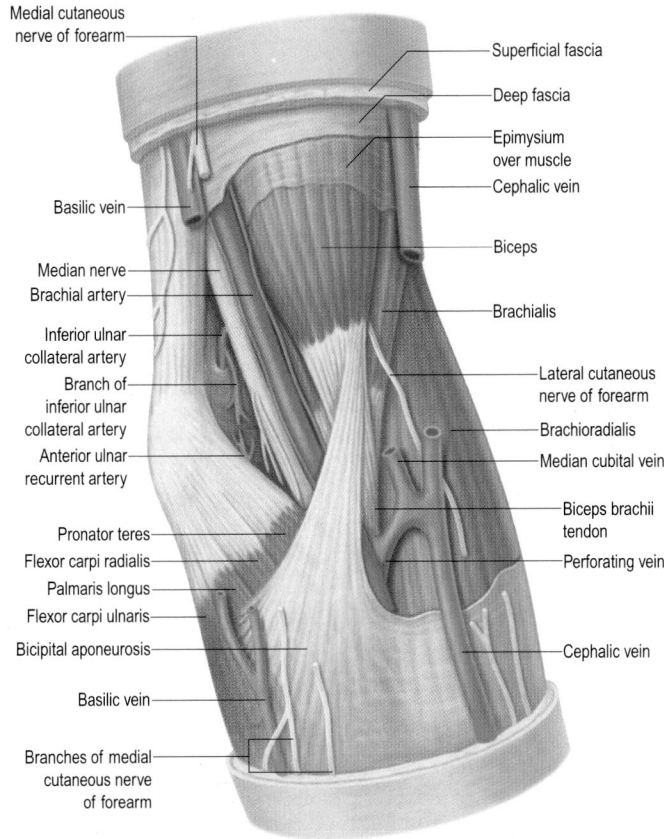

Fig. 51.1 Anterior aspect of the left elbow, showing superficial structures. Compare with **Fig. 51.9**.

Articulating surfaces – The articular surfaces are the humeral trochlea and capitulum, and the ulnar trochlear notch and radial head. The trochlea is not a simple pulley because its medial flange exceeds its lateral, thus projecting to a lower level. This means that the plane of the joint, c.2 cm distal to the inter-epicondylar line, is tilted inferomedially; the trochlea is also widest posteriorly and here its lateral edge is sharp. The trochlear notch is not wholly congruent with it: in full extension the medial part of its upper half is not in contact with the trochlea and a corresponding lateral strip loses contact in flexion. The trochlea has an asymmetrical sellar surface, largely concave transversely, convex antero-posteriorly: sections show that these profiles are compounded spirals. Swing is therefore accompanied (as in all hinge joints) by screwing and conjunct rotation. The olecranon and coronoid parts of the trochlear notch are usually separated by a rough strip, devoid of articular cartilage and covered by fibroadipose tissue and synovial membrane. The capitulum and the radial head are reciprocally curved; closest contact occurs with a semiflexed radius in midpronation. The rim of the head, which is more prominent medially, fits the groove between humeral capitulum and trochlea.

859

A

B

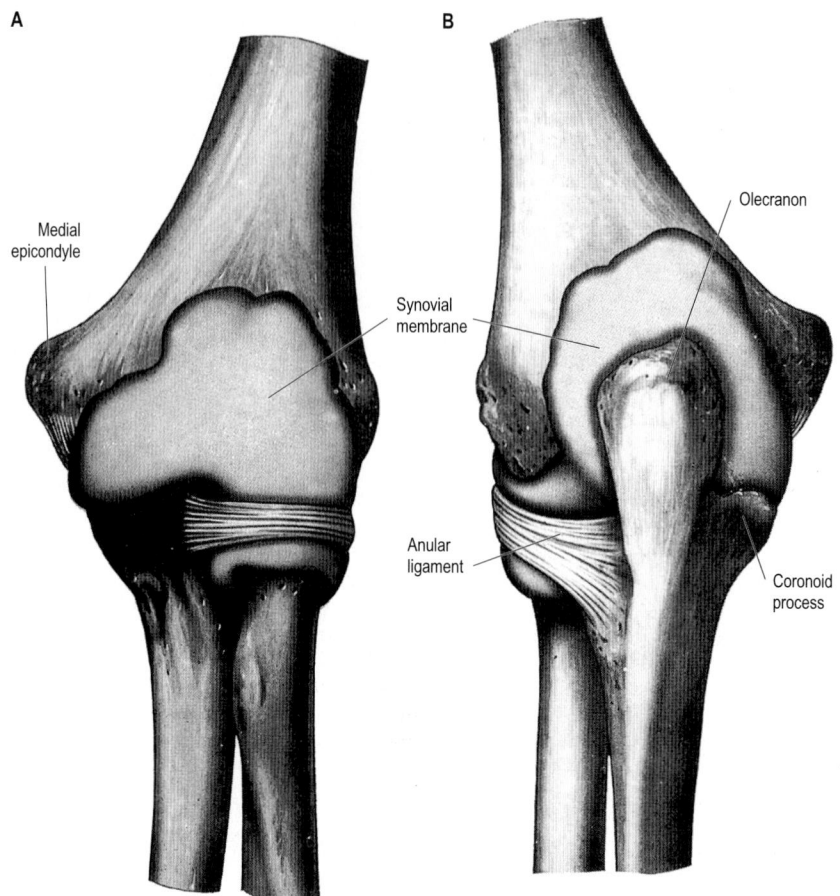

Medial epicondyle

Olecranon

Synovial membrane

Anular ligament

Coronoid process

Fig. 51.2 A, Synovial cavity of the left elbow joint, partially distended: anterior aspect. The fibrous capsule of the elbow joint has been removed but the thick part of the anular ligament has been left *in situ*. Note that the synovial membrane (blue) descends below the lower border of the anular ligament. **B**, Synovial cavity of the left elbow joint, partially distended: posterior aspect of the specimen represented in A. In A and B a small part of the ulnar (medial) collateral ligament may be seen. (Drawn from a specimen prepared by JCB Grant.)

Since the humero-ulnar and humeroradial articulations form a largely uniaxial joint, the ligaments are capsular and ulnar and radial collateral.

Fibrous capsule – The fibrous capsule (**Figs 51.4, 51.5**) is broad and thin anteriorly. It is attached proximally to the front of the medial epicondyle and humerus above the coronoid and radial fossae, and distally to the edge of the ulnar coronoid process and anular ligament, and is continuous at its sides with the ulnar and radial collateral ligaments. Anteriorly it receives numerous fibres from brachialis. Posteriorly the capsule is thin and attached to the humerus behind its capitulum and near its lateral trochlear margin, to all but the lower part of the edge of the olecranon fossa, and to the back of the medial epicondyle. Inferomedially it reaches the superior and lateral margins of the olecranon and is laterally continuous with the superior radio-ulnar capsule deep to the anular ligament. It is related posteriorly to the tendon of triceps and to anconeus.

Ligaments

Ulnar collateral ligament – This is a triangular band, consisting of thick anterior, posterior and inferior parts united by a thin region (**Fig. 51.5A**). The strongest and stiffest anterior part is attached by its apex to the front of the medial epicondyle and by its broad distal base to a proximal tubercle on the medial coronoid margin. The posterior part, also triangular, is attached low on the back of the medial epicondyle and to the medial margin of the olecranon. Between these two bands intermediate fibres descend from the medial epicondyle to an inferior, oblique band, often weak, between the olecranon and coronoid processes. This converts a depression on the medial margin of the trochlear notch into a foramen, through which the intracapsular fat pad is continuous with extracapsular fat medial to the joint. The anterior band is taut throughout most of the range of flexion, while the posterior band becomes taut between half and full flexion.

The ulnar collateral ligament is related to triceps, flexor carpi ulnaris and the ulnar nerve. Along it, anteriorly, the attachment of flexor

digitorum superficialis extends from the medial epicondyle to the medial coronoid border.

Radial collateral ligament – This is attached low on the lateral epicondyle and to the anular ligament (**Fig. 51.5B**). Some of its posterior fibres cross the ligament to the proximal end of the supinator crest of the ulna. It is intimately blended with attachments of supinator and extensor carpi radialis brevis. It is taut throughout most of the range of flexion.

Synovial membrane (Figs 51.2, 51.4) – This extends from the humeral articular margins, lines the coronoid, radial and olecranon fossae, the flat medial trochlear surface, the deep surface of the capsule and the lower part of the anular ligament. Projecting between the radius and ulna from behind is a crescentic synovial fold, which partly divides the joint into humero-radial and humero-ulnar parts. Irregularly triangular, it contains extra synovial fat (**Fig. 51.6**). Between the capsule and synovial membrane are three other pads of fat: the largest, at the olecranon fossa, is pressed into the fossa by triceps during flexion; the other two, at the coronoid and radial fossae, are pressed in by brachialis during extension. They are all slightly displaced in contrary movements. Smaller synovial-covered tags of fat project into the joint near constrictions flanking the trochlear notch, and cover small non-articular areas of bone.

A small bursa, the olecranon bursa, lies between the elbow joint capsule and the insertion of triceps tendon. Pressure and friction can lead to inflammation and enlargement of this bursa.

Vascular supply and lymphatic drainage – Articular arteries are derived from the numerous periarticular anastomoses (**Fig. 50.9**).

Innervation – Articular nerves are mainly from branches of the musculocutaneous and radial nerves, but the ulnar, median, and sometimes anterior interosseous nerves also contribute. The musculocutaneous branch is from the nerve to brachialis and innervates an anterior part of the capsule; branches of the radial supply posterior and anterolateral

A

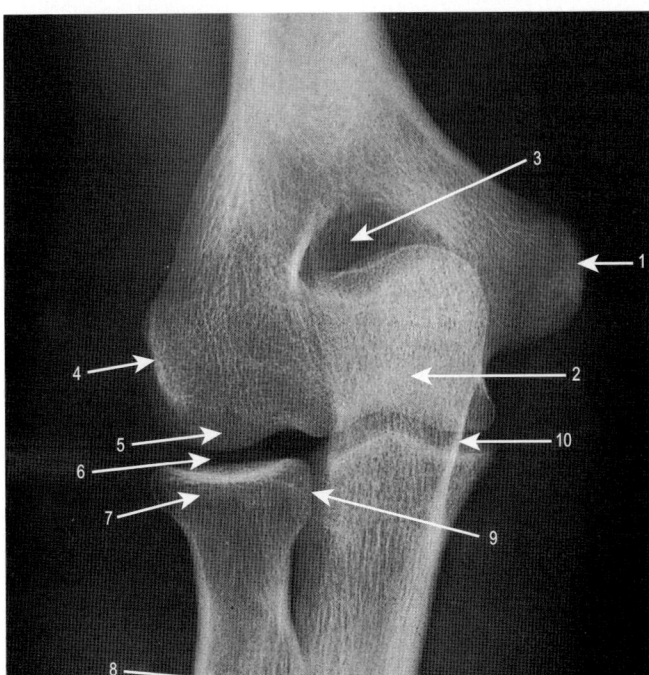

B

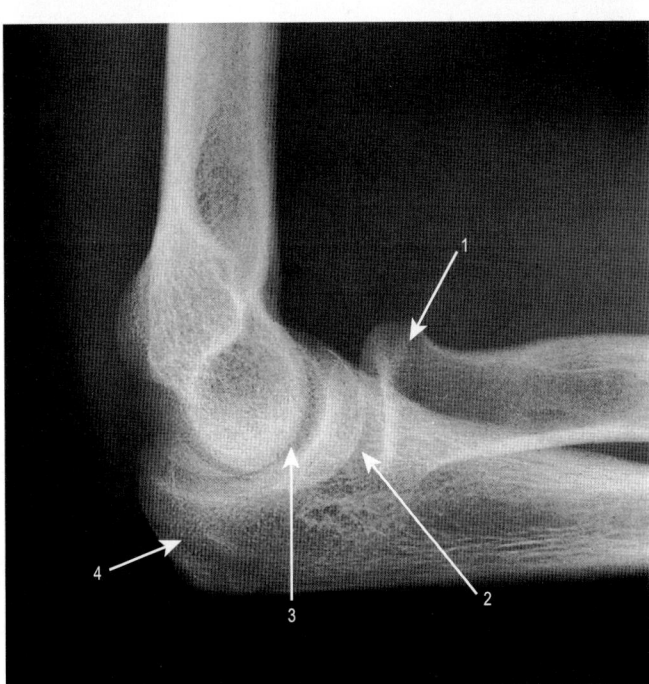

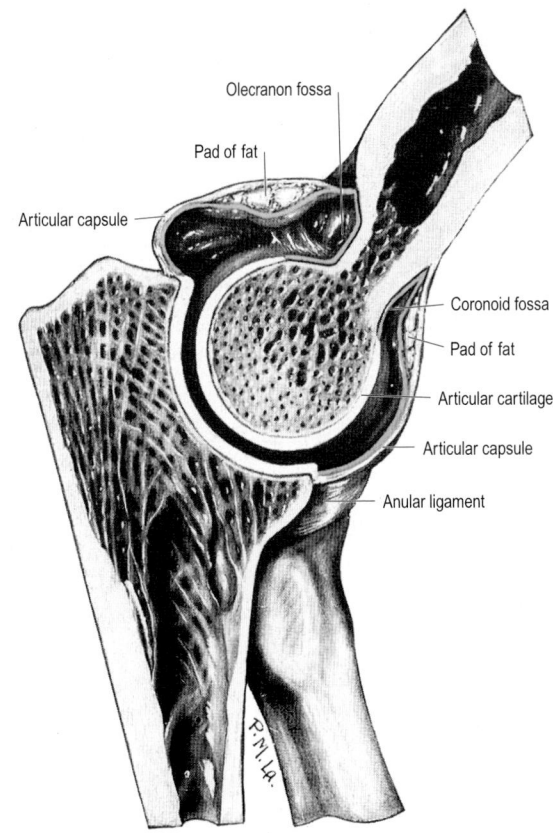

Fig. 51.4 Sagittal section through the left elbow joint: medial aspect. The synovial membrane is shown in blue.

Part A: **1.** Medial humeral epicondyle. **2.** Shadow of olecranon superimposed on trochlea.
3. Olecranon fossa. **4.** Lateral epicondyle. **5.** Capitulum.
6. Humero-radial joint. **7.** Head of radius. **8.** Radial tuberosity.
9. Radial head articulating with radial notch of ulna. **10.** Humero-ulnar joint.
Part B: **1.** Head of radius. **2.** Profile of capitulum. **3.** Profile of trochlea. **4.** Olecranon.

Fig. 51.3 Anteroposterior (A) and lateral (B) radiographs of an adult elbow joint. The joint is semiflexed in B.

regions and come from the nerve to anconeus and the ulnar collateral branch to the medial head of triceps. The ulnar nerve supplies the ulnar collateral ligament behind the medial epicondyle. These articular nerves accompany blood vessels supplying the synovial membrane, fat pads and epiphyses; they presumably contain vasomotor fibres as well as afferent fibres serving pain and proprioception.

Movements – Being a uniaxial joint, the elbow allows flexion and extension, the ulna moving on the trochlea, and the radial head on the capitulum. However, ulnar flexion–extension is not a pure swing but is accompanied by slight conjunct rotation, the ulna being slightly pronated in extension, supinated in flexion. Since the capitulum is smaller than the radial facet, the head of the radius can be felt at the back of the joint in full extension, which is limited by tension in the capsule and muscles anterior to the joint (extension being the close-packed position) and the entry of the tip of the olecranon into the olecranon fossa. Flexion is limited chiefly by apposition of soft parts: in full flexion the rim of the radial head and the tip of the ulnar coronoid process enter the radial and coronoid fossae of the humerus respectively.

When the forearm is fully extended and supinated, it diverges laterally forming with the upper arm a 'carrying angle' of c.163°; its ulnar border cannot contact the lateral surface of the thigh. The 'carrying angle' is caused partly by projection of the medial trochlear edge c.6 mm beyond its lateral edge and partly by the obliquity of the superior articular surface of the coronoid, which is not orthogonal to the shaft of the ulna. Tilt of the humeral and ulnar articular surfaces is approximately equal, hence the carrying angle disappears in full flexion, the two bones reaching the same plane. When the adducted arm is flexed the little finger meets the clavicle, because of the position of the resting humerus; when the humerus is rotated laterally, the hand reaches the front of the shoulder. The carrying angle is also masked by pronation of the extended forearm, which brings the upper arm, semipronated forearm and hand into line, increasing manual precision in full extension of the elbow or during extension.

Accessory movements – These are limited to slight ulnar screwing, abduction and adduction, and anteroposterior translation of the radial head on the humeral capitulum. In translation the radial head moves on the ulnar radial notch and the anular ligaments are slewed backwards and forwards, more so when the elbow is semiflexed.

Muscles producing movement – Flexion: brachialis, biceps and brachioradialis. In slow flexion or its maintenance against gravity, brachialis and biceps are principally involved, even for light loads. With increasing speed, activity in brachioradialis is increasingly prominent; its

861

A

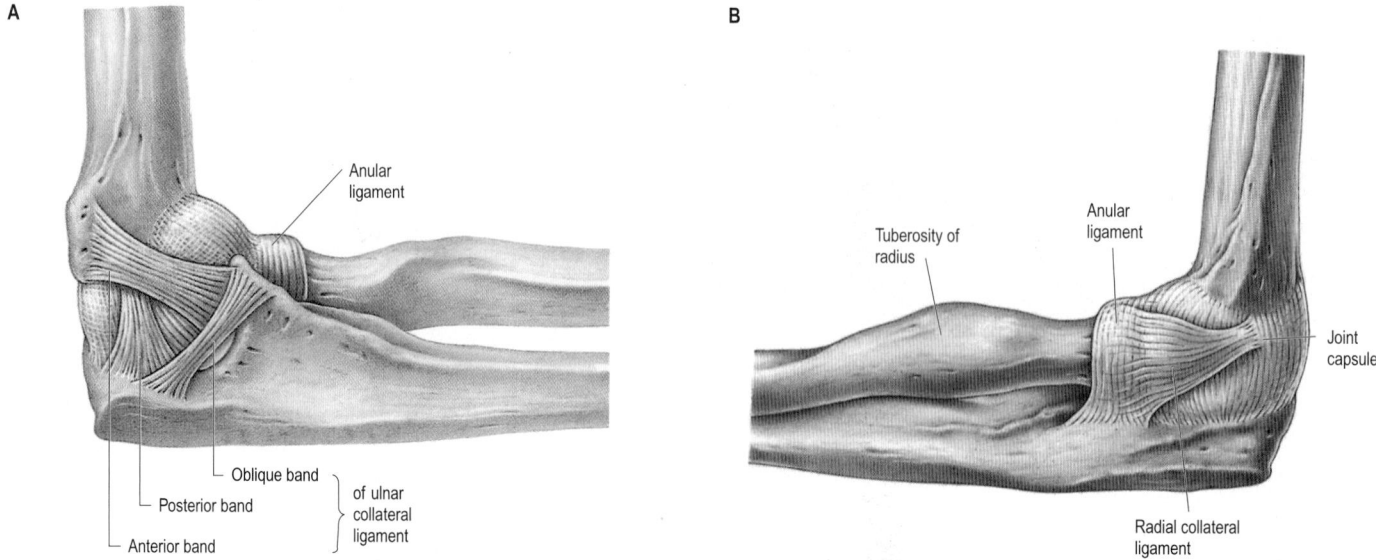

B

Fig. 51.5 The left elbow joint. **A**, Medial aspect; **B**, lateral aspect.

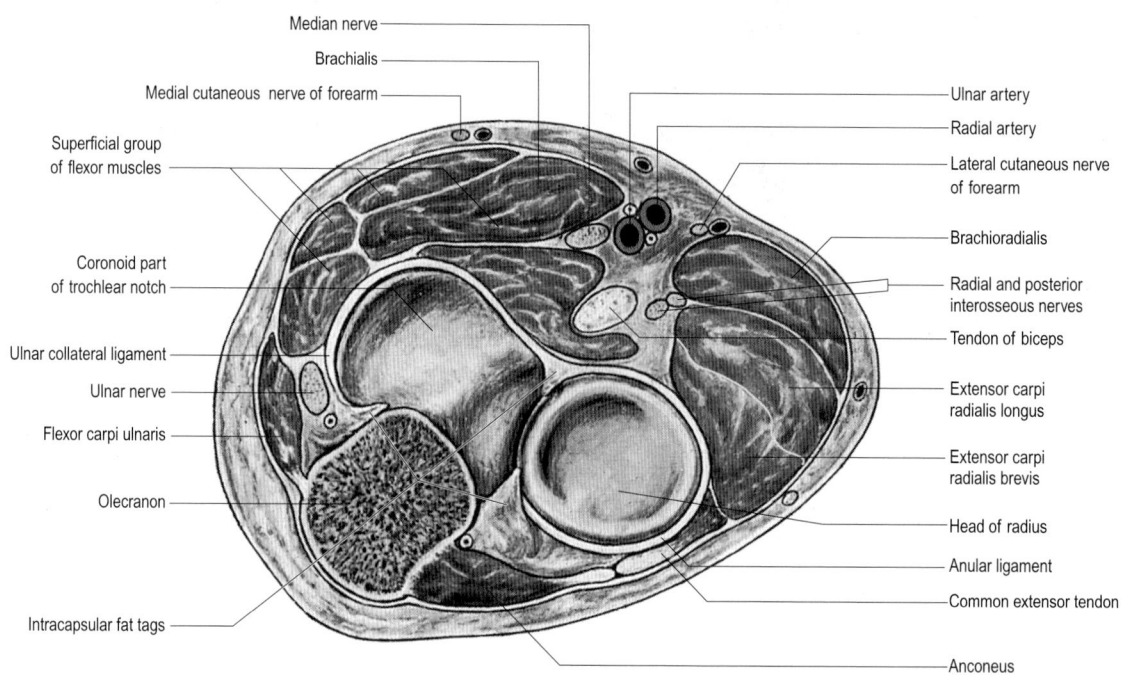

Fig. 51.6 Transverse section of the left elbow joint to show the relations of the joint: distal aspect. Note the intracapsular fat 'tags' with meniscoid transverse sectional profiles.

attachments determine that it acts most effectively in midpronation. Against resistance, pronator teres and flexor carpi radialis may also act.

Extension: triceps, anconeus and gravity. In rapid extension brachio-radialis may be active.

Relations – Muscles related to the joint are: (anteriorly) brachialis, (posteriorly) triceps and anconeus, (laterally) supinator and the common extensor tendon, and (medially) the common flexor tendon and flexor carpi ulnaris.

PROXIMAL (SUPERIOR) RADIOULNAR JOINT

The proximal radioulnar joint is a uniaxial pivot joint.

Articulating surfaces – The articulating surfaces are between the circumference of the radial head and the fibro-osseous ring made by the ulnar radial notch and anular ligament.

Fibrous capsule – The capsule is continuous with that of the elbow joint and is attached to the anular ligament.

Ligaments

Anular ligament – This is a strong band, which encircles the radial head, holding it against the radial notch of the ulna. Forming about four-fifths of the ring, it is attached to the anterior margin of the notch, broadens posteriorly and may divide into several bands. It is attached to a rough ridge at or behind the posterior margin of the notch; diverging bands may also reach the lateral margin of the trochlear notch above and proximal end of the supinator crest below (**Fig. 51.7**). The proximal anular border blends with the elbow joint capsule, except posteriorly where the capsule passes deep to the ligament to reach the posterior and inferior margins of the radial notch. From the distal anular border a few fibres pass over reflected synovial membrane to attach loosely on the radial neck. The external surface of the anular ligament blends with

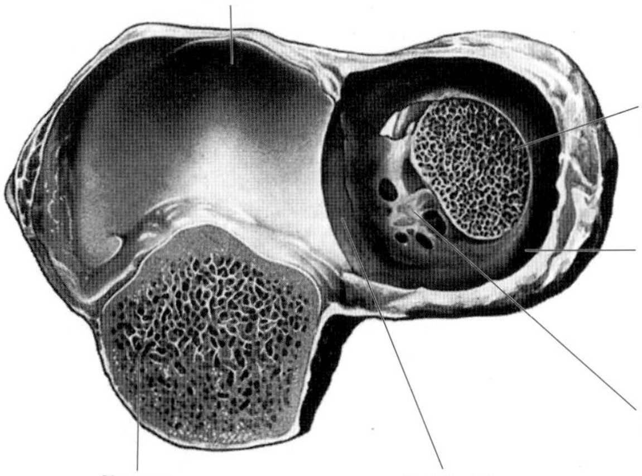

Fig. 51.7 Distal socket of the proximal radioulnar joint. The radial neck has been transected and its head withdrawn. The socket consists of the chondrified aspect of the anular ligament, the articular cartilage of the radial notch of the ulna and the lax almost retiform quadrate ligament. Section of the base of the olecranon reveals, anteriorly, the sellar articular surface of the coronoid part of the trochlear notch (humero-ulnar joint).

the radial collateral ligament and provides an attachment for part of supinator. Posterior to it are anconeus and the interosseous recurrent artery. Internally the ligament is thinly covered by cartilage where it is in contact with the radial head; distally it is covered by synovial membrane, reflected up onto the radial neck.

Quadrate ligament – This thin, fibrous ligament stretches between the neck of the radius and the upper part of the supinator fossa of the ulnar and covers the synovial membrane on the distal surface of the joint (**Fig. 51.7**). It maintains constant tension throughout pronation and supination.

Synovial membrane – The synovial membrane is continuous with that of the elbow joint so that the proximal radio-ulnar joint and elbow joint form one continuous synovial cavity. It is attached to the articular margins and lines the capsule and anular ligament. It is prevented from herniation between the anterior and posterior free edges of the anular ligament by the quadrate ligament.

Vascular supply – Articular arteries are derived from the numerous peri-articular anastomoses (**Fig. 50.9**).

Innervation – Superior radio-ulnar joint is innervated by small branches from the musculocutaneous, median, radial and ulnar nerves.

Factors maintaining stability (Figs 51.5, 51.7) – The prime stabilizing factor is the anular ligament which encircles the radial head and holds it against the radial notch of the ulna.

Movements and muscles producing movement – See the description of the distal radioulnar joint pp. 863, 901.

Injuries around the elbow
Posterior dislocation of the elbow joint with ulnar abduction is often complicated by fracture of the coronoid process as it impinges against the trochlea of the humerus. The normal triangular relationship between the olecranon and the two humeral epicondyles is disrupted. The brachial artery and/or median and ulnar nerves can occasionally be damaged in these injuries. The strength of the collateral ligaments is such that the medial epicondyle is frequently torn off in lateral dislocations.

Subluxation of the radial head through the anular ligament arising from a sudden jerk on the arm is a relatively common injury in young children (known as 'pulled elbow'). This is because the anular ligament has vertical sides in children compared with more funnel-shaped sides in adults. Reduction involves forcefully supinating and flexing the elbow which snaps the ligament back into place.

Supracondylar distal humeral fractures are usually seen in children following a fall on the outstretched hand. The distal fragment in usually displaced posteriorly. The jagged end of the proximal fragment can sometimes injure the brachial artery or the median nerve.

DISTAL (INFERIOR) RADIOULNAR JOINT
Movements at the radioulnar joint complex pronate and supinate the hand. The distal radioulnar joint and the movements which occur during supination and pronation are described on page 901.

VASCULAR SUPPLY AND LYMPHATIC DRAINAGE

ARTERIES

Brachial artery
The brachial artery is central and divides near the neck of the radius into its terminal branches, namely the radial and ulnar arteries (**Figs 51.1, 51.8, 51.9**). The skin, superficial fascia and median cubital vein are anterior, separated by the bicipital aponeurosis. Posteriorly, brachialis separates it from the elbow joint. The median nerve is medial proximally but is separated from the ulnar artery by the ulnar head of pronator teres. Lateral are the tendon of biceps and the radial nerve, the latter concealed between supinator and brachioradialis.

Radial artery
The radial artery passes deep to brachioradialis and gives off the radial recurrent artery before continuing into the forearm (**Figs 51.1, 51.9**).

Radial recurrent artery (Figs 50.9, 51.9, 51.10) – The radial recurrent artery arises just distal to the elbow, passing between superficial and deep branches of the radial nerve to ascend behind brachioradialis, anterior to supinator and brachialis. It supplies these muscles and the elbow joint, anastomosing with the radial collateral branch of the profunda brachii.

Ulnar artery
The ulnar artery gives off the anterior and then the posterior ulnar recurrent arteries before passing deep to pronator teres to continue its course in the forearm (**Figs 51.1, 51.9**). In the forearm, the posterior interosseous artery (a branch of the ulnar artery via the common interosseous artery), gives rise to the posterior interosseous recurrent artery which passes proximally to supply the elbow region.

The common interosseous, anterior interosseous and posterior interosseous arteries, and muscular branches of the ulnar artery, are described in Chapter 52 (p. 882).

Anterior ulnar recurrent artery (Figs 50.9, 51.10) – The anterior ulnar recurrent artery arises just distal to the elbow, ascends between brachialis and pronator teres, supplies them and anastomoses with the inferior ulnar collateral artery anterior to the medial epicondyle.

Posterior ulnar recurrent artery (Figs 50.9, 51.10) – The posterior ulnar recurrent artery arises distal to the anterior ulnar recurrent, and passes dorsomedially between flexores digitorum profundus and superficialis, ascending behind the medial epicondyle; between this and the olecranon, it is deep to flexor carpi ulnaris, ascending between its heads with the ulnar nerve. It supplies adjacent muscles, nerve, bone and elbow joint, and anastomoses with the ulnar collateral and interosseous recurrent arteries (**Fig. 50.9**).

Posterior interosseous recurrent artery – The posterior interosseous recurrent artery is a branch of the posterior interosseous artery. It passes proximally through supinator to lie deep to anconeous posterior to the lateral epicondyle. It gives off branches which take part in the anastomotic cutaneous plexus around the olecranon.

VEINS
The deep and superficial veins supplying the elbow and related structures are described on pages 885 and 885.

863

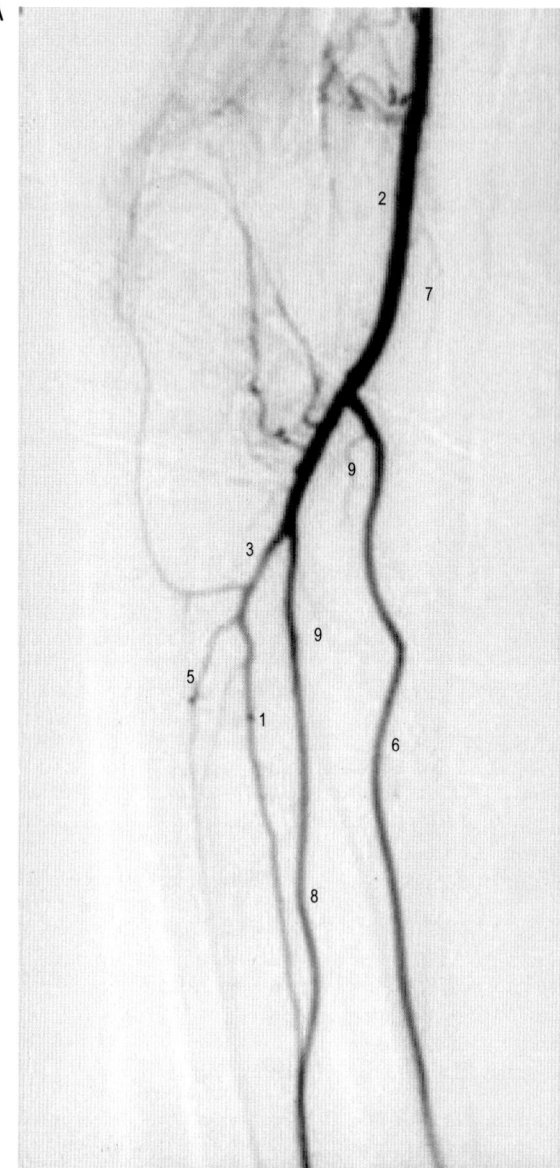

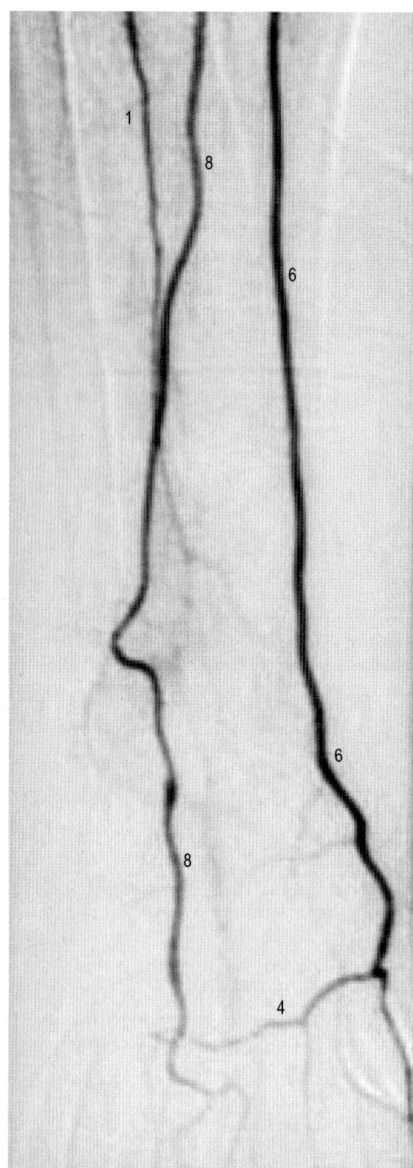

1. Anterior interosseous artery.
2. Brachial artery.
3. Common interosseous artery.
4. Deep palmar arch.
5. Posterior interosseous artery.
6. Radial artery.
7. Radial recurrent artery
   (just visible due to poor contrast filling).
8. Ulnar artery.
9. Ulnar recurrent artery.

Fig. 51.8 A, Arteriogram showing division of left brachial artery into radial and ulnar arteries. **B,** Arteriogram showing arteries of the forearm. (By permission from Weir J, Abrahams PH 2003 Imaging Atlas of Human Anatomy, 3rd edn, London: Mosby, and contributions from Anna-Maria Belli, Margaret Hourihan, Naill Moore and Philip Owen.)

LYMPHATIC DRAINAGE: SUPRATROCHLEAR NODES

One or two supratrochlear nodes are superficial to the deep fascia proximal to the medial epicondyle and medial to the basilic vein; their efferents accompany the vein to join the deep lymph vessels.

Small isolated nodes sometimes occur along the radial, ulnar and interosseous vessels, in the cubital fossa near the bifurcation of the brachial artery, or in the arm medial to the brachial vessels.

INNERVATION

MEDIAN NERVE

In the cubital fossa the median nerve lies medial to the brachial artery, deep to the bicipital aponeurosis and anterior to brachioradialis (**Figs 51.1, 51.9**).

Pronator syndrome

This is an uncommon entrapment neuropathy of the median nerve occurring in the elbow region. Entrapment can occur typically at four sites. The first occurs at the site of the ligament of Struthers. This ligament represents an anatomical variant and when present connects a small supracondyloid spur of bone to an accessory origin of pronator teres. The median nerve can be compressed as it passes under this ligament. The nerve may also be trapped as it passes deep to the bicipital aponeurosis; the aponeurotic edge of the deep head of pronator teres

muscle; or the tendinous aponeurotic arch forming the proximal free edge of the radial attachment of flexor digitorum superficialis.

The syndrome presents with pain on the volar aspect of the distal arm and proximal forearm. The symptoms may be aggravated by flexing the elbow against resistance, pronating the forearm against resistance, or flexion of superficialis to the middle finger against resistance, depending on the precise cause of the entrapment. If the anterior interosseous nerve is also compressed there is weakness of all the muscles innervated by the median nerve, including abductor pollicis brevis and the long finger flexors, and sensory impairment on the palm of the hand.

The treatment is exploration of the nerve and surgical decompression.

MUSCULOCUTANEOUS NERVE

In the cubital fossa the musculocutaneous nerve lies at the lateral margin of the biceps tendon where it continues on as the lateral cutaneous nerve of the forearm.

ULNAR NERVE

At the elbow the ulnar nerve is in a groove on the dorsum of the epicondyle. It enters the forearm between the two heads of flexor carpi ulnaris superficial to the posterior and oblique parts of the ulnar collateral ligament (**Figs 51.9, 51.11, 51.12**).

Articular branches

Articular branches to the elbow joint issue from the ulnar nerve between the medial epicondyle and olecranon.

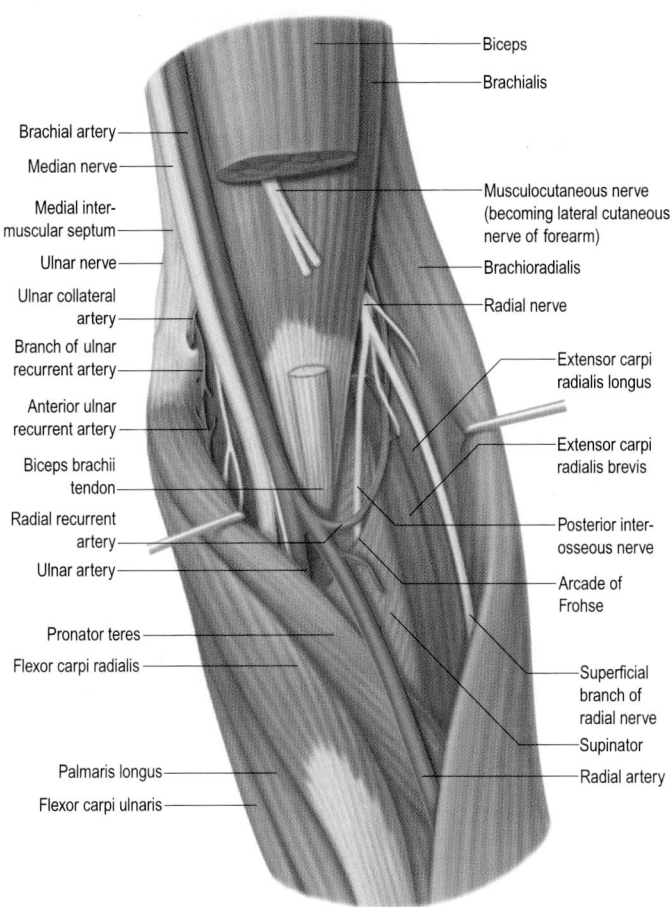

Fig. 51.9 Anterior aspect of the left elbow showing deep structures. Compare with **Fig. 51.1**.

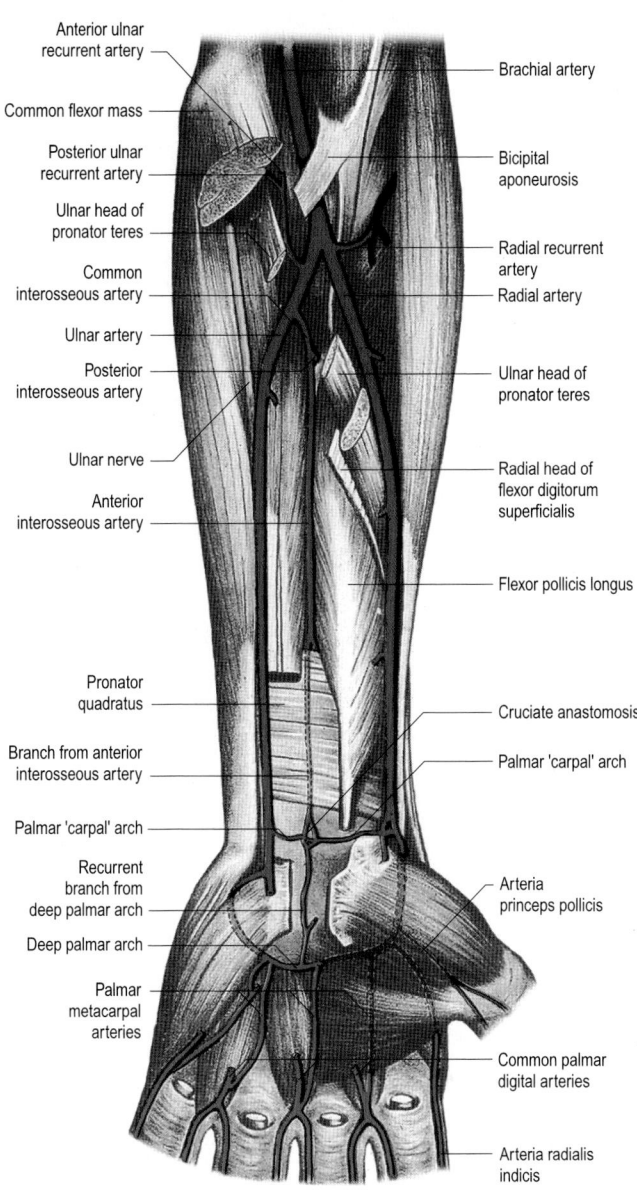

Fig. 51.10 The arteries of the left forearm: deep dissection. The palmar carpal arch lies across forearm bones.

Cubital tunnel syndrome

Typically the ulnar nerve can be compressed in the tunnel formed by the tendinous arch connecting the two heads of flexor carpi ulnaris at their humeral and ulnar attachments. Other local causes of compression and neuritis at this site include trauma, compression by the medial head of the triceps, osteophytes, recurrent subluxation of the nerve across the medial epicondyle of the humerus and abnormal muscular variants such as the anconeus epitrochlearis.

The symptoms are pain at the medial aspect of the proximal forearm together with paraesthesia and numbness of the little finger and ulnar half of the ring finger and the ulnar side of the dorsum of the hand. These symptoms are typically worse on forced elbow flexion. There may also be associated weakness of the muscles of the forearm and the intrinsic muscles of the hand innervated by the ulnar nerve. Interestingly, flexor carpi ulnaris and profundus to the ring and little fingers are frequently spared, presumably because the fascicles supplying these muscles are located on the deep aspect of the nerve. Clawing of the hand is therefore unusual in this syndrome.

Surgical treatment involves decompression of the tunnel by division of the aponeurosis of flexor carpi ulnaris with or without subsequent anterior transposition of the ulnar nerve.

Ulnar nerve division at the elbow

The ulnar nerve is in a vulnerable position as it lies between the median epicondyle and the olecranon: it lies on bone covered only by a thin layer of skin. It is easily damaged if the ulnar groove is shallow and the nerve may become more prominent than the medial epicondyle or the olecranon when the elbow is fully flexed.

Division of the nerve at the elbow paralyses flexor carpi ulnaris, flexor digitorum profundus to the ring and little fingers and all the intrinsic muscles of the hand (apart from the radial two lumbricals). The clawing of the hand is less intense than occurs after division of the ulnar nerve at the wrist, reflecting the imbalance in action between the long flexors and extensors to the ring and little fingers when digit flexion is produced only by superficialis. In addition there is sensory loss over the little finger and the ulnar half of the ring finger.

RADIAL NERVE

The radial nerve at the elbow lies deep in a groove between brachialis and brachioradialis proximally and extensor carpi radialis distally. It divides into the superficial terminal branch and the posterior interosseous nerve just anterior to the lateral epicondyle (**Fig. 51.9**).

Articular branches are distributed to the elbow joint.

MEDIAL AND POSTERIOR CUTANEOUS NERVES OF THE FOREARM

The medial cutaneous nerve is described on pages 858 and 887, and the posterior cutaneous nerve is described on pages 858 and 887.

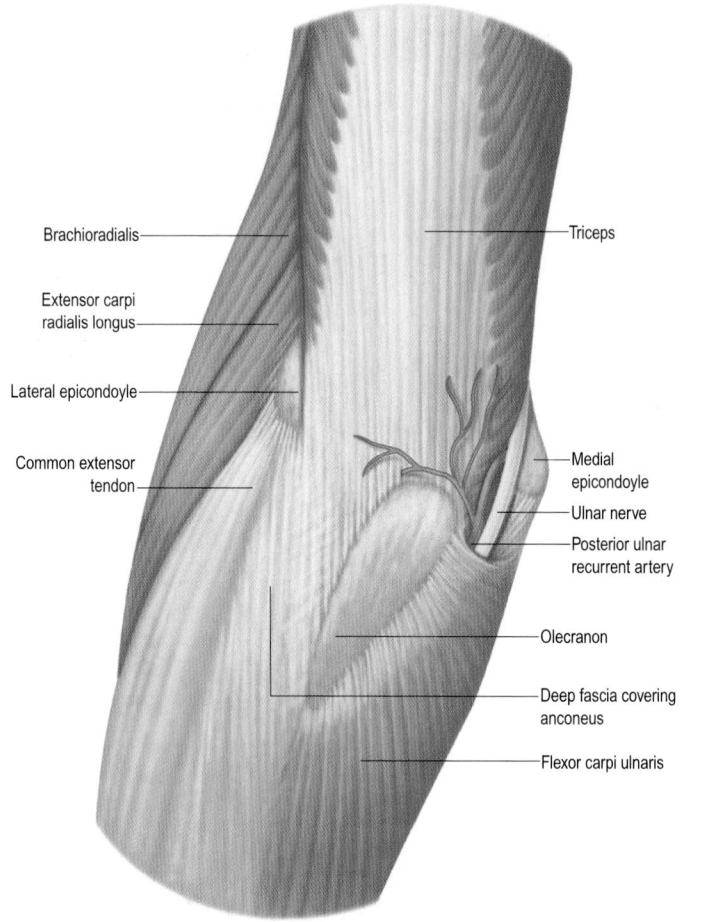

Fig. 51.11 Posterior aspect of the left elbow showing superficial structures.

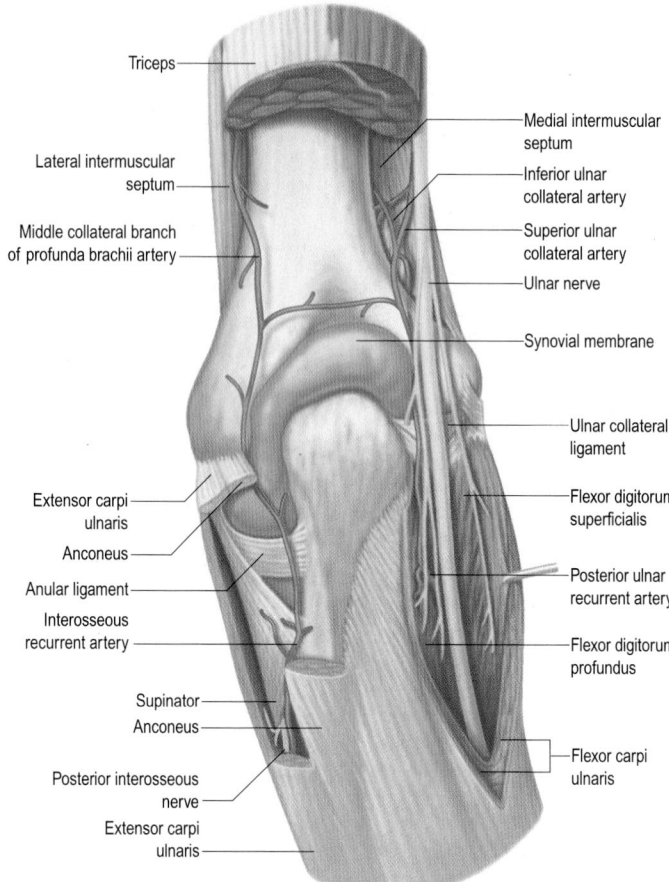

Fig. 51.12 Posterior aspect of the left elbow region showing deep structures.

REFERENCE

Green DP (ed) 1982 Operative Hand Surgery. New York/London: Churchill Livingstone.

Forearm

Chapter

52

SKIN

CUTANEOUS VASCULAR SUPPLY

Fasciocutaneous perforators from the radial artery supply the lateral two-thirds of the anterior surface of the forearm, the lateral (radial) border and the posterior one-quarter of the forearm (except in the distal third) (**Fig. 48.4**). These perforators pass in the intermuscular fascia between brachioradialis and flexor carpi radialis and between flexor carpi radialis and flexor digitorum superficialis (**Figs 52.1, 52.2**). Within the territory of the radial artery is the area of the largest fasciocutaneous perforator,

which has recently been named the inferior cubital artery. It extends from the distal apex of the antecubital fossa to midway down the forearm. Fasciocutaneous perforators from the ulnar artery supply an anatomical area which extends from the cubital fossa to the wrist, and from the medial (ulnar) third of the anterior aspect of the forearm around the medial border to the medial one-quarter of the posterior surface of the forearm (**Figs 52.1, 52.2, 48.4**).

Very small musculocutaneous perforators pass through brachioradialis and flexor carpi ulnaris. The contribution from these is far less than that of the fasciocutaneous perforators.

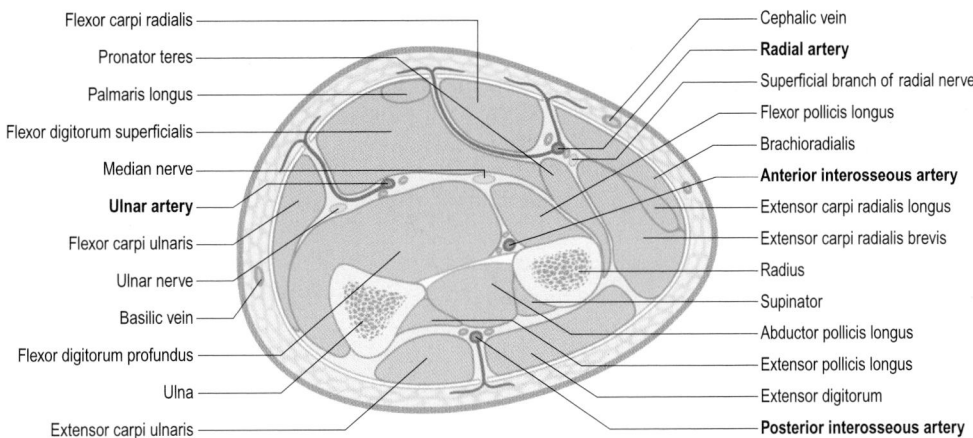

Fig. 52.1 Schematic transverse section through the mid-forearm to demonstrate the location of the principal fasciocutaneous perforators. (By permission from Cormack GC, Lamberty BGH 1994 The Arterial Anatomy of Skin Flaps, 2nd edn. Edinburgh: Churchill Livingstone.)

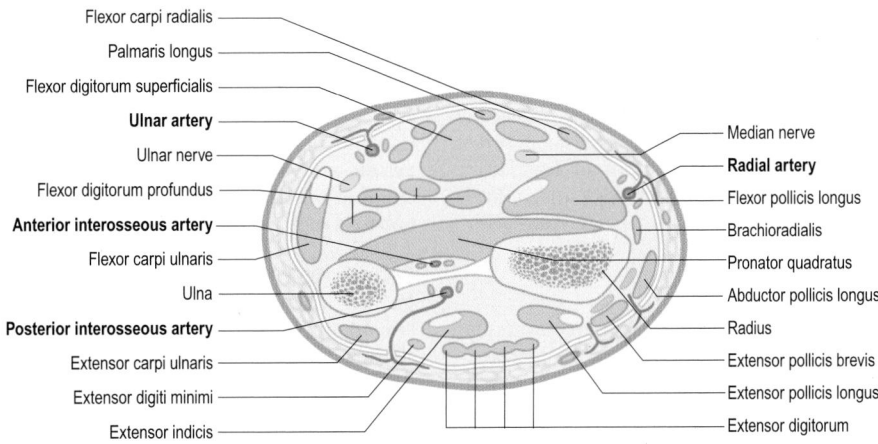

Fig. 52.2 Schematic transverse section through the distal forearm to demonstrate the location of the principal fasciocutaneous perforators. The terminal branches of the anterior interosseous artery pass through the interosseous membrane to reach the posterior compartment where they emerge around extensor pollicis brevis and abductor pollicis longus. (By permission from Cormack GC, Lamberty BGH 1994 The Arterial Anatomy of Skin Flaps, 2nd edn. Edinburgh: Churchill Livingstone.)

The distal third of the lateral (radial) aspect of the forearm is supplied by the terminal perforating branches of the anterior interosseous artery (**Fig. 48.4**).

The central half of the posterior surface of the forearm, from the lateral edge of extensor digitorum, just below the lateral epicondyle of the humerus, to the wrist, is supplied by fasciocutaneous perforators which arise from the posterior interosseous artery. They reach the skin by passing along the intermuscular fascia between extensor carpi ulnaris and extensor digit minimi (**Figs 52.1, 52.2, 48.4**).

For a detailed account of the cutaneous blood supply to the forearm see Cormack & Lamberty (1994) and the translated works of Salmon (1994).

CUTANEOUS INNERVATION (Fig. 48.18)

The anterior aspect of the forearm is supplied by the anterior branches of the medial and lateral cutaneous nerves of the forearm. The medial and lateral regions of the posterior aspect of the forearm are supplied by the posterior branches of the medial and lateral cutaneous nerves of the forearm respectively. The central part of the posterior aspect of the forearm is supplied by the posterior cutaneous nerve of the forearm.

SOFT TISSUE

INTEROSSEOUS MEMBRANE

The radial and ulnar shafts are connected by syndesmoses – an oblique cord and an interosseous membrane.

Oblique cord (Fig. 52.3)

The oblique cord is a small inconstant flat fascial band on the deep head of supinator. It extends from the lateral side of the ulnar tuberosity to the radius a little distal to its tuberosity. Its fibres are at right angles to those in the interosseous membrane. Its functional significance is dubious.

Interosseous membrane (Figs 52.3, 52.13)

The interosseous membrane is a broad, thin, collagenous sheet. Its fibres slant distomedially between the radial and ulnar interosseous borders, and its distal part is attached to the posterior division of the radial border. Two or three posterior bands occasionally descend distolaterally across the other fibres. The membrane is deficient proximally, starting c.2 or 3 cm distal to the radial tuberosity, and broader at midlevel. An oval aperture near its distal margin conducts the anterior interosseous vessels to the back of the forearm, and the posterior interosseous vessels pass through a gap between its proximal border and the oblique cord.

The membrane provides attachments for the deep forearm muscles and connects the radius and ulna. Its fibres appear to transmit forces which act proximally from the hand to the radius, thence to the ulna and humerus. However the hand is usually pronated when subject to these forces, and the membrane is relaxed in complete pronation and supination: the interosseous membrane is only tense when the hand is midway between prone and supine positions. Moreover, the radius can transmit substantial forces directly to the humerus. Anteriorly, in its proximal three-quarters, the membrane is related laterally to flexor pollicis longus and medially to flexor digitorum profundus, and between them to the anterior interosseous vessels and nerve. In its distal quarter it is related to pronator quadratus. Its posterior relations are supinator, abductor pollicis longus, extensors pollicis brevis, longus and indicis and, near the carpus, the anterior interosseous artery and posterior interosseous nerve.

COMPARTMENTS OF THE FOREARM

The antebrachial fascia (deep fascia of the forearm), which is continuous above with the brachial fascia, is a dense general sheath for muscles, collectively and individually, in this region. It is attached to the olecranon and posterior border of the ulna. From its deep surface septa pass between muscles, providing partial attachment for them, and some of these septa reach bone. Muscles also arise from its internal aspect, especially in the upper forearm. This deep fascia, together with the interosseous membrane and fibrous intermuscular septa, divide the forearm into a number of compartments. These are the superficial and deep flexor (anterior) compartments, the extensor (posterior compartment) and a proximolateral compartment known as the mobile wad (encompassing brachioradialis and extensors carpi radialis longus and

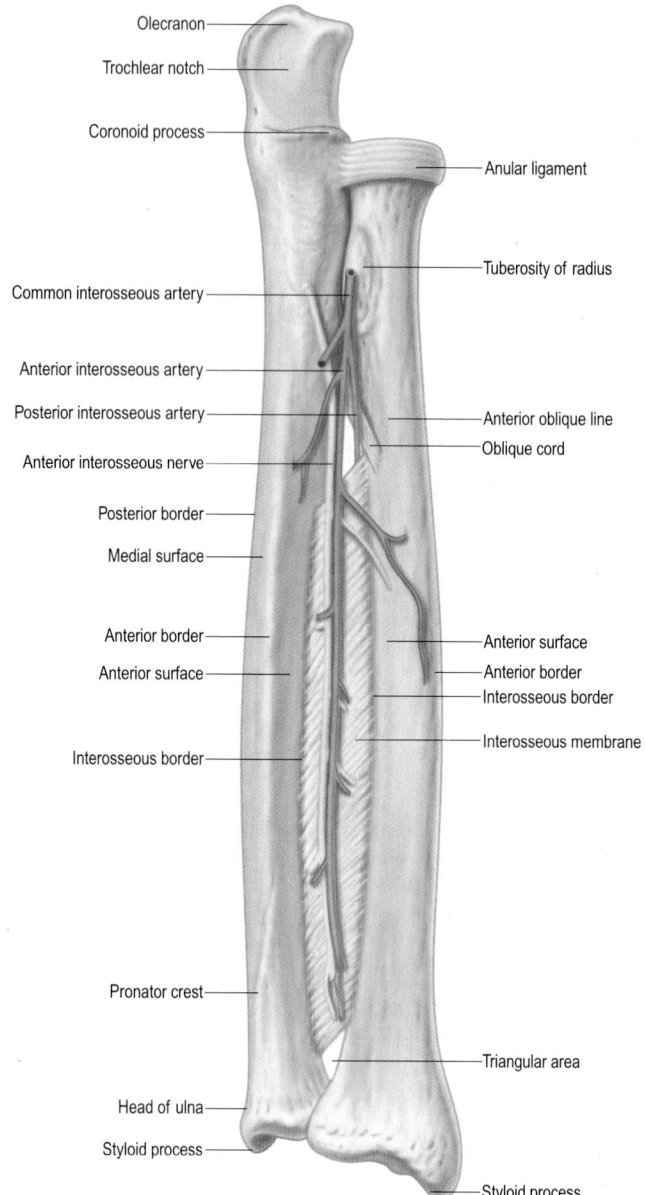

Fig. 52.3 Interosseous membrane and oblique cord of the forearm: anterior aspect. Membrane and cord are syndesmoses.

brevis) (**Fig. 52.4**). The fascia is much thicker posteriorly and in the lower forearm. It is strengthened above by tendinous fibres from biceps and triceps. Near the wrist, two localized thickenings, the flexor and extensor retinacula, retain the digital tendons in position (p. 913). Vessels and nerves pass through apertures in the fascia. One large aperture anterior to the elbow transmits a venous communication between superficial and deep veins.

Compartment syndrome

The deep fascia in the forearm has limited elasticity and consequently any accumulation of fluid within this space (e.g. from haemorrhage, swelling from trauma, burns) can lead to increased tension in the compartment. If this pressure is high enough (c.35 mmHg), tissue perfusion pressure will be compromised and this will lead to a compartment syndrome where ischaemia and necrosis of the tissues ensues. Once muscle becomes infarcted the damage is irreversible: muscle fibres become contracted and replaced by inelastic fibrous tissue (termed Volkmann's ischaemic contracture). The symptoms and signs associated with compartment syndrome are pain (particularly on passive stretching of the compartmental muscles), weakness of the compartment muscles, tenseness of the compartment, paraesthesia and hyperaesthesia. The pulse can still be normal in compartment syndrome, because systolic

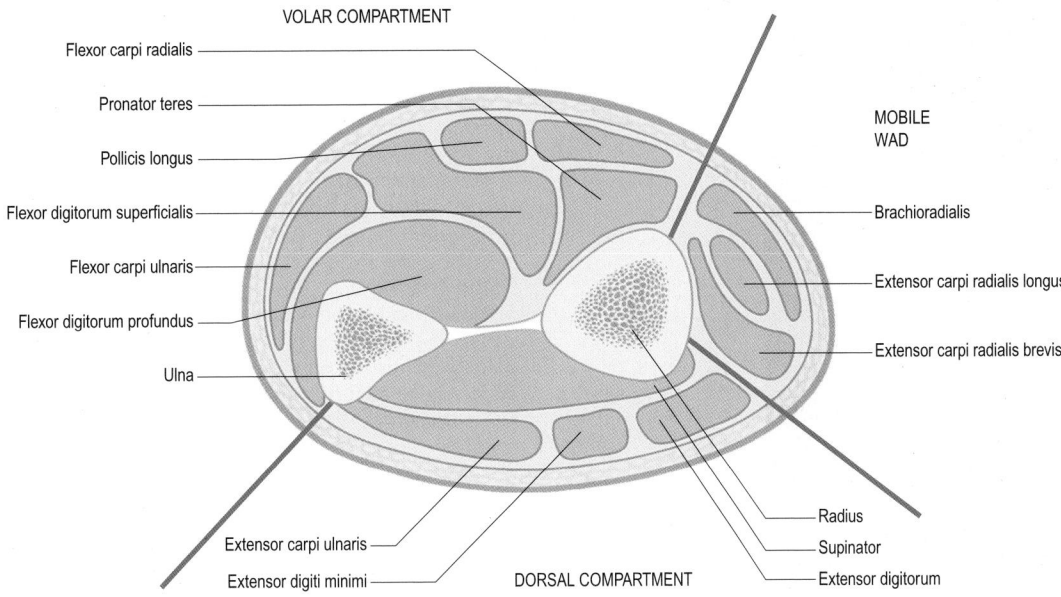

Fig. 52.4 Compartments of the forearm. Cross-section through the upper third of the forearm.

blood pressure is well above the critical closing pressure of vessels which supply the tissues within the compartment.

Compartment syndromes can occur at various sites in the body, but more commonly affect the anterior compartment of the forearm, the intrinsic muscles of the hand, and the lower leg. The identification of a compartment syndrome requires urgent surgical decompression. Here, both the skin and deep fascia are incised throughout the whole length of the compartment to relieve the pressure.

BONE

RADIUS (Figs 52.5, 52.6, 52.7)

The radius is the lateral bone of the forearm. It has expanded proximal and distal ends; the distal is much the broader. The shaft widens rapidly towards its distal end, is convex laterally and concave anteriorly in its distal part.

Proximal end

The proximal end includes a head, neck and tuberosity. The head is discoid, its proximal surface a shallow cup for the humeral capitulum. Its smooth articular periphery is vertically deepest medially, where it contacts the ulnar radial notch. Its posterior surface is palpable in a small depression on the lateral side of the back of the extended elbow. The neck is the constriction distal to the head, which overhangs it, especially on the lateral side. The tuberosity is distal to the medial part of the neck; posteriorly it is rough, but anteriorly it is usually smooth.

Shaft

The shaft has a lateral convexity, and is triangular in section (**Figs 52.3, 52.13**). The interosseous border is sharp, except for two areas: proximally, near the tuberosity; and distally, where the interosseous border is the posterior margin of a small, elongated, triangular area, proximal to the ulnar notch. These two areas form the so-called medial surface. The interosseous membrane is attached to its distal three-fourths, and connects the radius to the ulna. The anterior border is obvious at both ends, but rounded and indefinite between them. It descends laterally from the anterolateral part of the tuberosity as the anterior oblique line, which distally becomes a sharp, palpable crest along the lateral margin of the anterior surface. The posterior border is well defined only in its middle third: proximally it ascends medially towards the posteroinferior part of the tuberosity, and distally it is merely a rounded ridge. The anterior surface, between anterior and

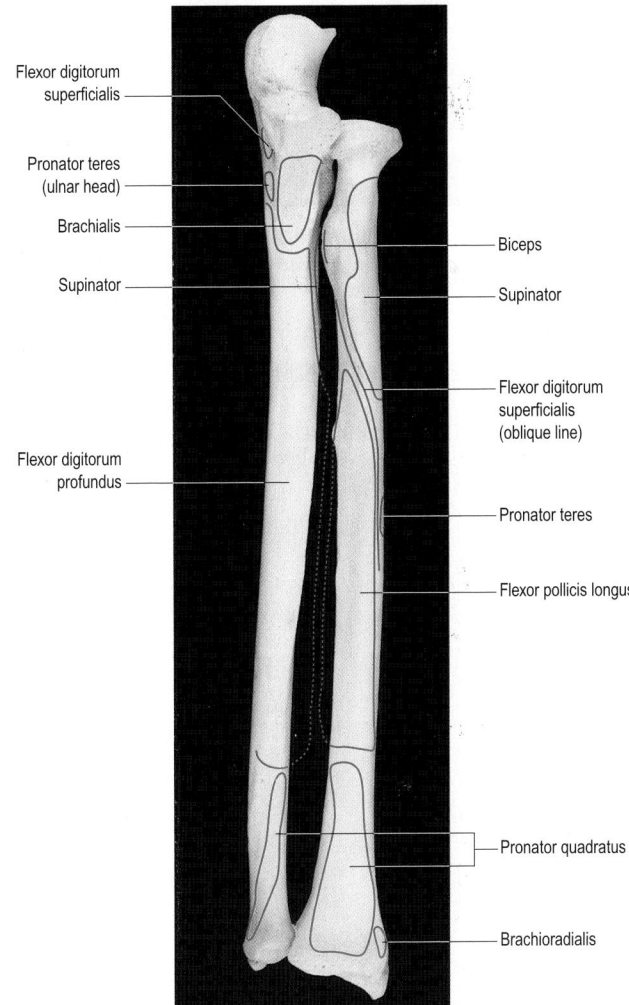

Fig. 52.5 Articulated radius and ulna: anterior view showing muscle attachments. Note that the hatched lines denote extension of muscular attachments onto the interosseous membrane. (Photograph by Sarah-Jane Smith.)

869

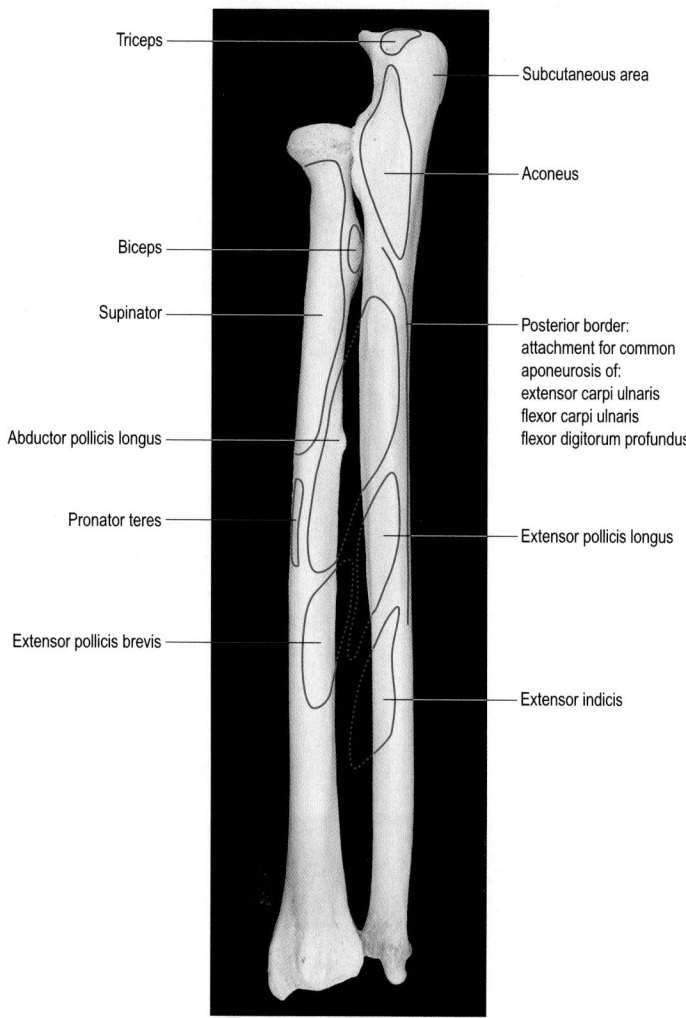

Fig. 52.6 Articulated radius and ulna: posterior view showing muscle attachments. (Photograph by Sarah-Jane Smith.)

interosseous borders, is concave transversely and shows a distal forward curvature. Near its midpoint there is a proximally directed nutrient foramen and canal. The posterior surface, between interosseous and posterior borders, is largely flat but may be slightly hollow in the proximal area. The lateral surface is gently convex. Proximally, due to the obliquity of the anterior and posterior borders, it encroaches on the anterior and posterior aspects and is here slightly rough. A finely irregular oval area occurs near the midshaft, and beyond it the surface is smooth.

Distal end (Fig. 52.8)

The distal end is the widest part. It is four-sided in section. The lateral surface is slightly rough, projecting distally as a styloid process which is palpable when tendons around it are slack. The smooth carpal articular surface is divided by a ridge into medial and lateral areas. The medial is quadrangular, whereas the lateral is triangular and curves on to the styloid process. The anterior surface is a thick, prominent ridge, palpable even through overlying tendons, 2 cm proximal to the thenar eminence. The medial surface is the ulnar notch, which is smooth and antero-posteriorly concave for articulation with the head of the ulna. The posterior surface displays a palpable dorsal tubercle (Lister's tubercle), which is limited medially by an oblique groove and is in line with the cleft between the index and middle fingers. Lateral to the tubercle there is a wide, shallow groove, divided by a faint vertical ridge.

Muscle, ligament and articular attachments

The proximal articular surface of the radial head and its circumference are covered by hyaline cartilage. The upper rim (margin) fits the groove between the capitulum and trochlea and enters the radial fossa in flexion. The articular circumference articulates with the ulnar radial notch and annular ligament, within which it rotates in pronation and supination. The radial neck is enclosed by the narrower distal part of the ligament, from which it is separated by a synovial protrusion from the superior radio-ulnar joint. The posterior area of the tuberosity is marked by the biceps tendon, which is separated from a smooth anterior area by a bursa. The oblique cord is attached just distal to the bursa.

The thin, wide radial head of flexor digitorum superficialis is attached proximally on the anterior border. The lateral edge of the extensor retinaculum is attached to its conspicuous distal part. A small, triangular area proximal to the ulnar notch gives attachment to the deepest part of pronator quadratus.

The proximal two-thirds of the anterior surface provides an extensive area for attachment of flexor pollicis longus, which conceals the

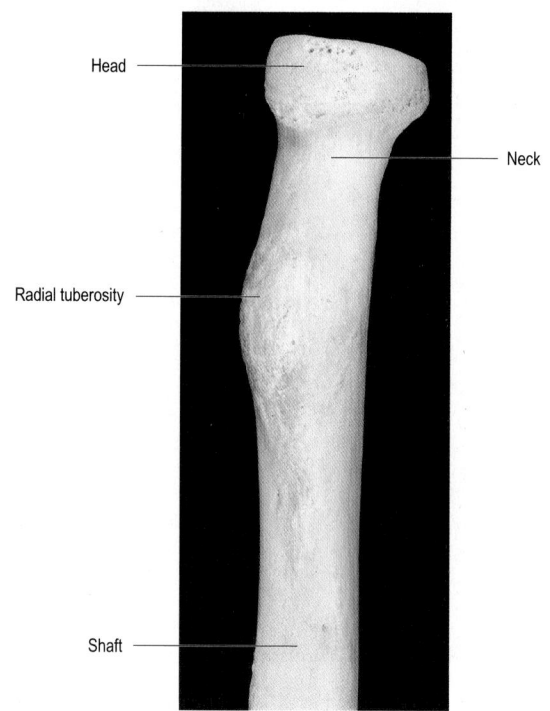

Fig. 52.7 Proximal end of radius. (Photograph by Sarah-Jane Smith.)

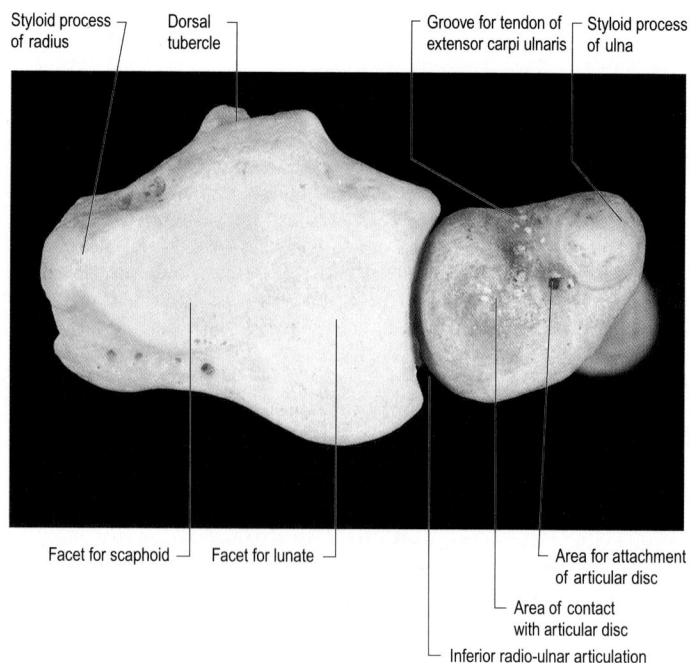

Fig. 52.8 Distal radius and ulna. (Photograph by Sarah-Jane Smith.)

nutrient foramen. Pronator quadratus is attached to the distal quarter, and pronator teres is attached to a rough area near the midpoint of its lateral surface, at its maximal curvature. Proximally, the lateral surface widens into a long V-shaped area for supinator (**Figs 52.5, 52.6**). Distal to pronator teres, the lateral surface is covered by tendons of the radial extensors. On the posterior surface, abductor pollicis longus is attached proximally and, more distally, extensor pollicis brevis. The remaining surface is devoid of attachments and covered by the long and short extensors of the thumb.

The radial styloid process projects beyond that of the ulna, its apex concealed by the tendons of abductor pollicis longus and extensor pollicis brevis. The lateral radiocarpal ligament is attached to its tip. The lateral surface, near the styloid process, receives the attachment of brachioradialis and is crossed obliquely, downwards and forwards, by the tendons of abductor pollicis longus and extensor pollicis brevis. The terminal ridge on the anterior surface of the lower end is an attachment for the palmar radiocarpal ligament. The base of the triangular articular disc of the inferior radio-ulnar joint is attached to a smooth ridge distal to the ulnar notch. From the latter, a narrow protrusion of synovial membrane extends proximally anterior to the lower end of the interosseous membrane (p. 868). The lateral part of the carpal articular surface articulates with the scaphoid, and the medial part with the lateral part of the lunate. In full adduction, the proximal surface of the lunate is wholly in contact with the radius.

The radial dorsal tubercle receives a slip from the extensor retinaculum and is grooved medially by the tendon of extensor pollicis longus. The wide groove lateral to the tubercle contains the tendons of extensor carpi radialis longus laterally, and extensor carpi radialis brevis medially, together with their synovial sheaths. Medially the dorsal surface is grooved by the tendons of extensor digitorum, which are separated from the bone by the tendons of extensor indicis and the posterior interosseous nerve. The dorsal radiocarpal ligament is attached to the distal margin of this surface.

Vascular supply

There are multiple metaphyseal nutrient foramina that transmit branches of the radial, ulnar, anterior and posterior interosseous arteries. Typically, there is one nutrient diaphyseal foramina located on the anterior surface of the bone and directed proximally toward the elbow. There is also a network of small fascioperiosteal and musculoperiosteal vessels which arise from the compartmental vessels and reach the bone via septal and muscular attachments.

The dorsal metaphyseal supply of the distal radius is of particular importance to reconstructive hand surgeons because of its potential use in raising vascularized pedicled bone grafts (**Fig. 52.9**). Consistent branches connecting the anterior interosseous artery proximally to the dorsal carpal arch distally pass through the fourth and fifth extensor compartments of the wrist and provide metaphyseal nutrient arteries. Intercompartmental vessels send nutrient arteries to the radius through the retinaculum between the first and second dorsal compartments, and the second and third dorsal compartments. These vessels originate from the radial artery and anterior interosseous arteries respectively, and anastomose with the dorsal carpal arch. For an anatomical description detailing the practical application of such pedicled bone grafts see Sheetz et al (1995).

Ossification

The radius ossifies from three centres. One appears centrally in the shaft in the eighth week of fetal life, and the others appear in each end (**Figs 52.10, 52.11**). Ossification begins in the distal epiphysis towards the end of the first postnatal year, and in the proximal epiphysis during the fourth year in females, and fifth in males. The proximal epiphysis fuses in the fourteenth year in females, seventeenth in males, and the distal in the seventeenth and nineteenth years respectively. A fourth centre sometimes appears in the tuberosity at about the fourteenth or fifteenth year.

ULNA (Figs 52.5, 52.6)

The ulna is medial to the radius in the supinated forearm. Its proximal end is a massive hook which is concave forwards (**Fig. 52.12**). The lateral border of the shaft is a sharp interosseous crest. The bone diminishes progressively from its proximal mass throughout almost its whole length, but at its distal end expands into a small rounded head

and styloid process. The shaft is triangular in section but has no appreciable double curve. In its whole length it is slightly convex posteriorly. Mediolaterally, its profile is sinuous. The proximal half has a slight laterally concave curvature, and the distal half a medially concave curvature.

Proximal end

The proximal end has large olecranon and coronoid processes and trochlear and radial notches which articulate with the humerus and radius (**Fig. 52.12**). The olecranon is more proximal and is bent forwards at its summit like a beak, which enters the humeral olecranon fossa in extension. Its posterior surface is smooth, triangular and subcutaneous, and its proximal border underlies the 'point' of the elbow. In extension it can be felt near a line joining the humeral epicondyles, but in flexion it descends, so that the three osseous points form an isosceles triangle. Its anterior, articular surface forms the proximal area of the trochlear notch. Its base is slightly constricted where it joins the shaft and is the narrowest part of the proximal ulna. The coronoid process projects anteriorly distal to the olecranon. Its proximal aspect forms the distal part of the trochlear notch. On the lateral surface, distal to the trochlear notch, there is a shallow, smooth, oval radial notch which articulates with the radial head. Distal to the radial notch the surface is hollow to accommodate the radial tuberosity during pronation and supination. The anterior surface of the coronoid is triangular. Its distal part is the tuberosity of the ulna. Its medial border is sharp and bears a small tubercle proximally.

The trochlear notch articulates with the trochlea of the humerus. It is constricted at the junction of the olecranon and coronoid processes, where their articular surfaces may be separated by a narrow rough non-articular strip. A smooth ridge, adapted to the groove on the humeral trochlea, divides the notch into medial and lateral parts. The medial fits into the trochlear flange. The radial notch, an oval or oblong proximal depression on the lateral aspect of the coronoid process, articulates with the periphery of the radial head, and is separated from the trochlear notch by a smooth ridge (**Fig. 52.12**).

Shaft

The shaft is triangular in section in its proximal three-fourths, but distally is almost cylindrical (**Figs 52.5, 52.6**). It has anterior, posterior and medial surfaces and interosseous, posterior and anterior borders (**Fig. 52.13**). The interosseous border is a conspicuous lateral crest in its middle two-fourths. Proximally it becomes the supinator crest, which is continuous with the posterior border of a depression distal to the radial notch. Distally, it disappears. The rounded anterior border starts medial to the ulnar tuberosity, descends backwards, and is usually traceable to the base of the styloid process. The posterior border, also rounded, descends from the apex of the posterior aspect of the olecranon, and curves laterally to reach the styloid process. It is palpable throughout its length in a longitudinal furrow which is most obvious when the elbow is fully flexed.

The anterior surface, between the interosseous and anterior borders, is longitudinally grooved, sometimes deeply (**Fig. 52.5**). Proximal to its midpoint there is a nutrient foramen, which is directed proximally and contains a branch of the anterior interosseous artery. Distally, it is crossed obliquely by a rough, variable prominence, descending from the interosseous to the anterior border. The medial surface, between the anterior and posterior borders, is transversely convex and smooth. The posterior surface, between the posterior and interosseous borders, is divided into three areas (**Fig. 52.6**). The most proximal is limited by a sometimes faint oblique line ascending laterally from the junction of the middle and upper thirds of the posterior border to the posterior end of the radial notch. The region distal to this line is divided into a larger medial and narrower lateral strip by a vertical ridge, usually distinct only in its proximal three-fourths.

Distal end

The distal end is slightly expanded and has a head and styloid process. The head is visible in pronation on the posteromedial carpal aspect, and can be gripped when the supinated hand is flexed. Its lateral convex articular surface fits the radial ulnar notch. Its smooth distal surface (**Fig. 52.8**) is separated from the carpus by an articular disc, the apex of which is attached to a rough area between the articular surface and styloid process. The latter, a short, round, posterolateral projection of the distal end of the ulna, is palpable (most readily in supination)

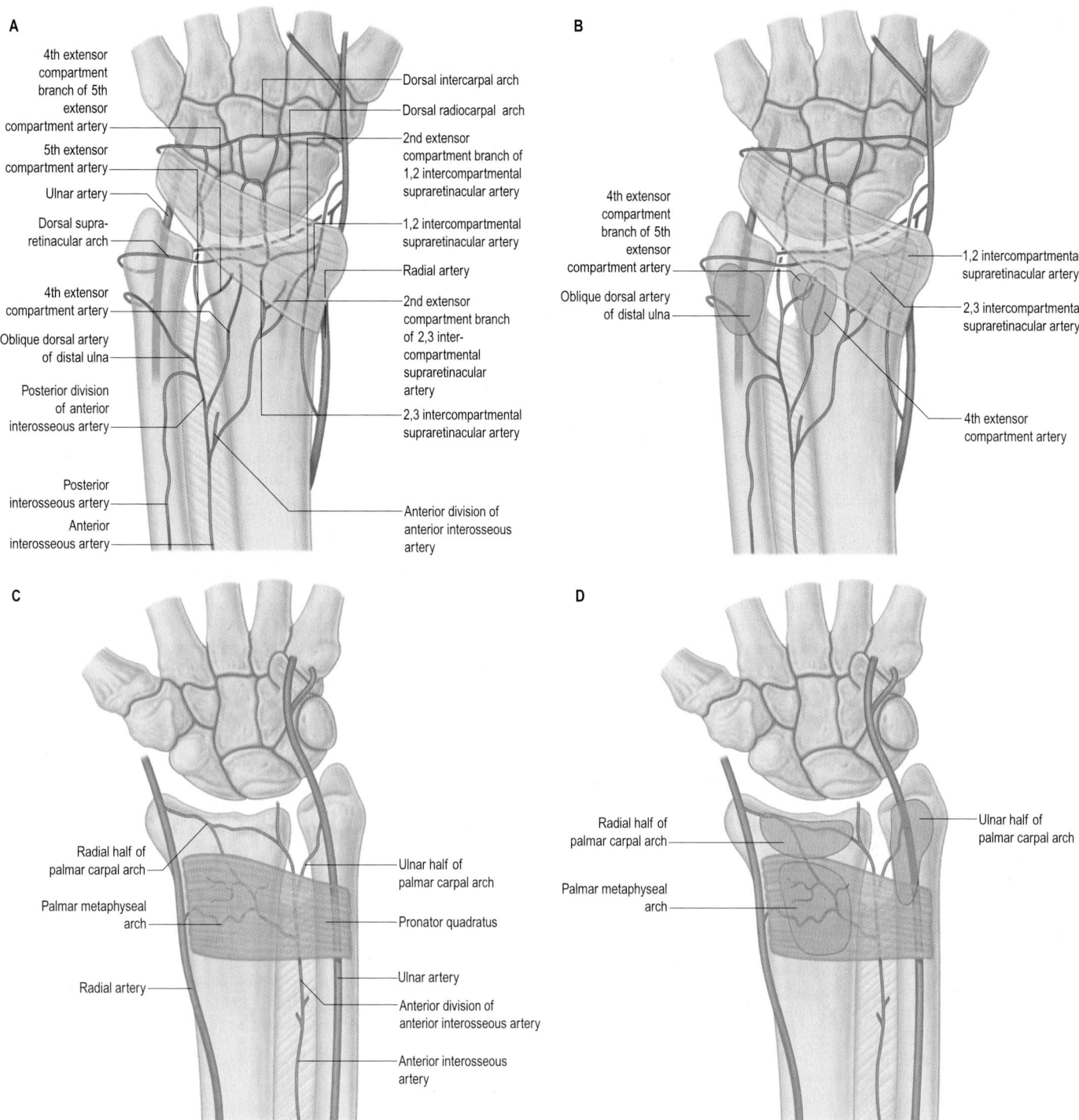

A

4th extensor compartment branch of 5th extensor compartment artery

5th extensor compartment artery

Ulnar artery

Dorsal supra-retinacular arch

4th extensor compartment artery

Oblique dorsal artery of distal ulna

Posterior division of anterior interosseous artery

Posterior interosseous artery

Anterior interosseous artery

Dorsal intercarpal arch

Dorsal radiocarpal arch

2nd extensor compartment branch of 1,2 intercompartmental supraretinacular artery

1,2 intercompartmental supraretinacular artery

Radial artery

2nd extensor compartment branch of 2,3 inter-compartmental supraretinacular artery

2,3 intercompartmental supraretinacular artery

Anterior division of anterior interosseous artery

B

4th extensor compartment branch of 5th extensor compartment artery

Oblique dorsal artery of distal ulna

1,2 intercompartmental supraretinacular artery

2,3 intercompartmental supraretinacular artery

4th extensor compartment artery

C

Radial half of palmar carpal arch

Palmar metaphyseal arch

Radial artery

Ulnar half of palmar carpal arch

Pronator quadratus

Ulnar artery

Anterior division of anterior interosseous artery

Anterior interosseous artery

D

Radial half of palmar carpal arch

Palmar metaphyseal arch

Ulnar half of palmar carpal arch

Fig. 52.9 A, B, Extraosseous arterial supply to the dorsal distal radius and ulna. **C, D**, Extraosseous arterial supply to the palmar distal radius and ulna. The shaded regions demonstrate where the nutrient vessels from the labelled arteries penetrate bone. (Adapted from Sheetz KK, Bishop AT, Berger RA. The arterial blood supply of the distal radius and ulna and its potential use in vascularized pedicled bone grafts; 20(6): 902–914, 1995, with permission from The American Society for Surgery of the Hand.)

c.1 cm proximal to the plane of the radial styloid. A posterior vertical groove is present between the head and styloid process.

Muscle, ligament and articular attachments (Figs 52.5, 52.6)

Anteriorly, the capsule of the elbow joint is attached to the proximal olecranon surface. The tendon of triceps is attached to its rough posterior two-thirds: the capsule and tendon can be separated by a bursa. The medial surface of the olecranon is marked proximally by the attachment of the posterior and oblique bands of the ulnar collateral ligament and the ulnar part of flexor carpi ulnaris. The smooth area distal to this is the most proximal attachment of flexor digitorum profundus. Anconeus is attached to the lateral olecranon surface and the adjoining posterior surface of the ulnar shaft as far as its oblique line. The posterior

surface of the ulna is separated from the skin by a subcutaneous bursa.

Brachialis is attached to the anterior surface of the coronoid process, including the ulnar tuberosity. The oblique and anterior bands of the ulnar collateral ligament and the distal part of the humero-ulnar slip of flexor digitorum superficialis are attached to a small tubercle at the proximal end of the medial border. Distal to this the margin provides attachment for the ulnar part of pronator teres. An ulnar part of flexor pollicis longus may be attached to the lateral or, more rarely, the medial border of the coronoid process. Fibres of flexor digitorum profundus are attached to its medial surface. The annular ligament is attached to the anterior rim of the radial notch and posteriorly to a ridge at or just behind the posterior margin of the notch. The depressed area distal to the notch is limited behind by the supinator crest, and both provide attachment for supinator.

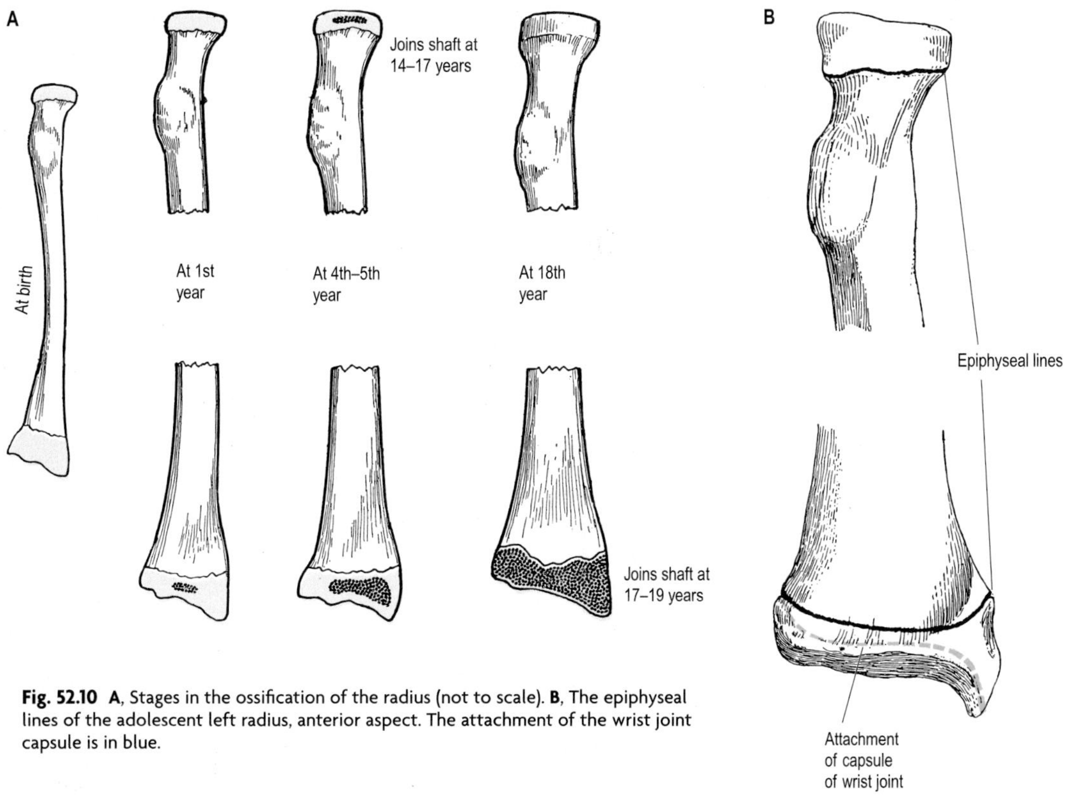

Fig. 52.10 A, Stages in the ossification of the radius (not to scale). **B**, The epiphyseal lines of the adolescent left radius, anterior aspect. The attachment of the wrist joint capsule is in blue.

The olecranon area of the trochlear notch is usually divided into three areas. The most medial faces anteromedially, and is grooved to fit the medial flange of the humeral trochlea, with which it makes increasing contact during flexion. A flat intermediate area fits the lateral flange, and the most lateral area, a narrow strip, abuts the trochlea in extension. The articular surface is narrower than the base of the olecranon: non-articular parts are related to the synovial processes. The coronoid area of the trochlear notch is also divided, and its medial and lateral areas correspond to medial and intermediate areas of the olecranon. The medial is more hollow, and conforms to the convex medial trochlear flange. The medial and anterior parts of the capsular ligament are attached to its medial and anterior borders.

The deep fascia of the forearm is attached to the subcutaneous posterior border. This border also provides an attachment for the aponeurosis of flexor digitorum profundus in its proximal three-quarters, for flexor carpi ulnaris in its proximal half, and for extensor carpi ulnaris in its middle third. These three muscles connect with the posterior border through a common blended aponeurosis. The interosseous membrane is attached to the interosseous border, except proximally.

Flexor digitorum profundus is attached to the proximal three-fourths of the anterior border and medial surface, attaching medial to the coronoid process and olecranon. The rough strip across the distal fourth of the anterior surface provides part of the bony attachment for pronator quadratus. Anconeus is attached to the posterior surface proximal to the oblique line and lateral to the olecranon. The narrow strip between the interosseous border and vertical ridge gives rise to the attachment of three deep muscles: abductor pollicis longus arises from the proximal fourth, extensor pollicis longus arises from the succeeding fourth (sometimes a ridge is interposed between them), and extensor indicis is attached to the third quarter. The broad strip medial to the vertical ridge is covered by extensor carpi ulnaris, whose tendon grooves the posterior aspect of the distal end of the ulna. The ulnar collateral ligament is attached to the apex of the styloid process.

Vascular supply

Multiple metaphyseal nutrient foramina transmit branches of the radial, ulnar, anterior and posterior interosseous arteries (**Fig. 52.9**). These vessels give off a number of smaller segmental branches. Usually one, but occasionally two, major nutrient diaphyseal foramina are located on the anterior surface of the bone, directed proximally toward the elbow. A network of small fascioperiosteal and musculoperiosteal branches

given off from the compartmental vessels reach the bone via septal and muscular attachments.

Ossification

The ulna ossifies from four main centres, one each in the shaft and distal end and two in the olecranon (**Fig. 52.14**). Ossification begins in the midshaft about the eighth fetal week, and extends rapidly. In the fifth (females) and sixth (males) years, a centre appears in the distal end, and extends into the styloid process. The distal olecranon is ossified as an extension from the shaft, the remainder from two centres, one for the proximal trochlear surface, and the other for a thin scale-like proximal epiphysis on its summit. The latter appears in the ninth year in females, eleventh in males. The whole proximal epiphysis has joined the shaft by the fourteenth year in females, sixteenth in males. The distal epiphysis unites with the shaft in the seventeenth year in females, eighteenth in males.

MUSCLES

ANTERIOR COMPARTMENT

The anterior compartment contains the flexor muscles of the forearm which are arranged in superficial and deep groups. Chronic tendonitis of the common flexor tendon origin produces medial epicondylitis of the elbow, leading to pain and tenderness. It is a frequent complaint among golfers. A detailed account of the architectural properties of the muscles of the arm and forearm is given by Leiber et al (1992).

Superficial flexor compartment

Muscles of the superficial flexor compartment arise from the medial epicondyle of the humerus by a common tendon. They are pronator teres, flexor carpi radialis, palmaris longus, flexor digitorum superficialis, and flexor carpi ulnaris (**Fig. 52.15**). They have additional attachments to the antebrachial fascia near the elbow and to the septa that pass from this fascia between individual muscles.

Pronator teres

Attachments – Pronator teres has humeral and ulna attachments (**Figs 52.5, 52.15**). The humeral head, the larger and more superficial of the two, arises just proximal to the medial epicondyle, from the common tendon of origin of the flexor muscles, from the intermuscular septum

873

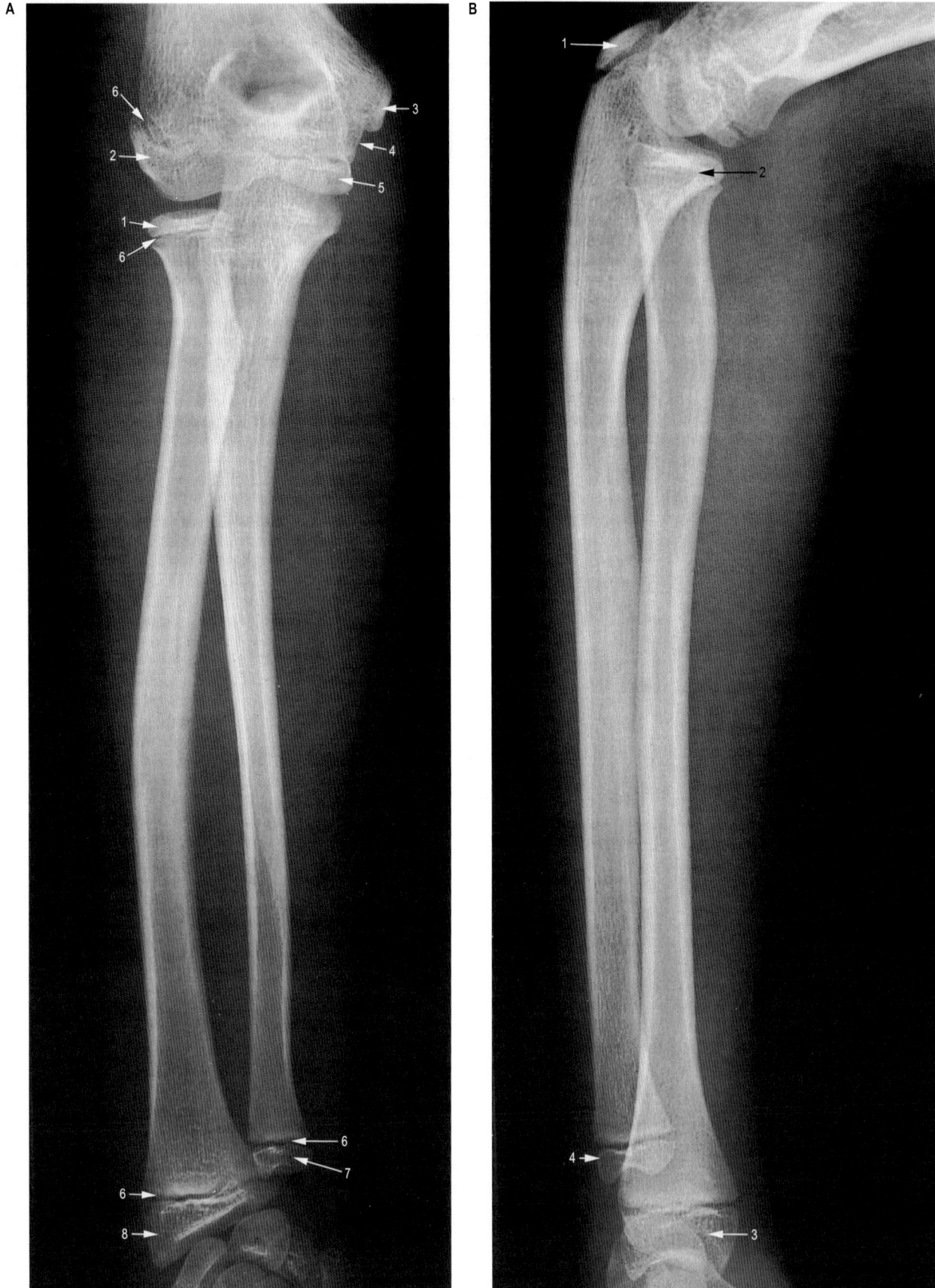

A

B

Part A: 1. Proximal radial epiphysis.   2. Conjoined epiphyses of capitulum and lateral epicondyle.   3. Epiphysis of medial epicondyle.   4. Diaphysial bone.   5. Trochlear epiphysis.
6. Cartilaginous growth plates.   7. Distal ulnar epiphysis.   8. Distal radial epiphysis.
Part B: 1. Olecranon.   2. Proximal radial.   3. Distal radial.   4. Distal ulna.

Fig. 52.11 A, Anteroposterior radiograph of the forearm of a girl aged 11. **B**, Lateral radiograph of forearm of a girl of 11 years, semiflexed at the elbow. Note the epiphyses and adjacent radiotranslucent growth cartilages.

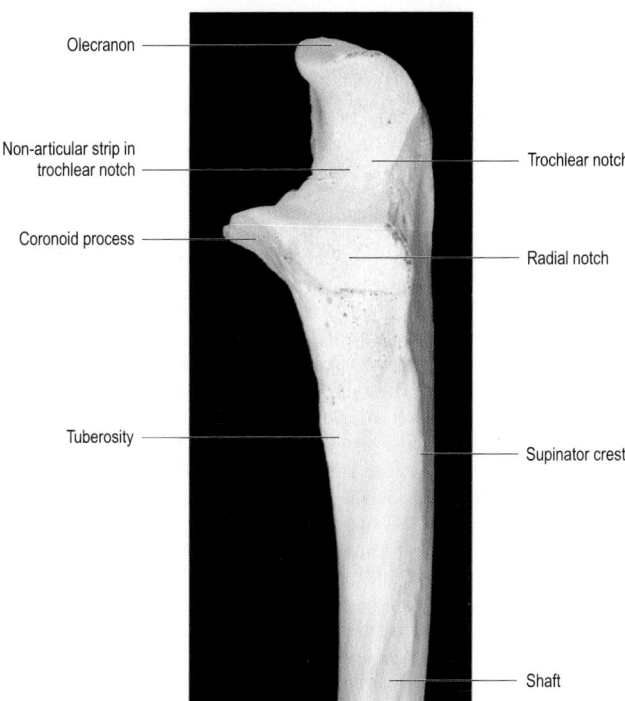

Olecranon

Non-articular strip in
trochlear notch

Coronoid process

Tuberosity

Trochlear notch

Radial notch

Supinator crest

Shaft

Fig. 52.12 Proximal end of ulna: lateral view. (Photograph by Sarah-Jane Smith.)

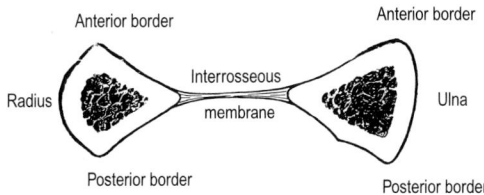

Anterior border

Anterior border

Radius

Interrosseous
membrane

Ulna

Posterior border

Posterior border

Fig. 52.13 Transverse section of the left radius and ulna showing attachment of interosseous membrane. Viewed from proximal aspect.

between it and flexor carpi radialis, and from antebrachial fascia. The smaller ulnar head springs from the medial side of the coronoid process of the ulna, distal to the attachment of flexor digitorum superficialis, and joins the humeral head at an acute angle. The muscle passes obliquely across the forearm to end in a flat tendon that is attached to a rough area midway along the lateral surface of the radial shaft at the 'summit' of its lateral curve. The coronoid attachment may be absent. Accessory slips may arise from a supracondylar process of the humerus, if it is present, or from biceps, brachialis or the medial intermuscular septum.

Relations – The median nerve usually enters the forearm between the two heads of pronator teres, and is separated from the ulnar artery by the ulnar head. The lateral border of pronator teres is the medial limit of the cubital fossa, the triangular hollow anterior to the elbow joint.

Vascular supply – The humeral head of pronator teres is supplied by the inferior ulnar collateral artery and the anterior ulnar recurrent artery. The ulnar head is supplied by the common interosseous artery. The mid portion of the muscle belly is supplied by direct branches from the ulnar artery, while the attachment to the radius is supplied by the radial artery.

Innervation – Pronator teres is innervated by the median nerve, C6 and 7.

Action – Pronator teres rotates the radius on the ulna (pronation of the forearm), turning the palm medially so that it faces backwards. It acts with pronator quadratus (which is always active in pronation) only in rapid or forcible pronation. Like all of the muscles which arise from the medial epicondyle, pronator teres acts as a weak flexor of the elbow joint.

Clinical anatomy: testing – Pronator teres is tested by palpating its contracting fibres during pronation against resistance.

Flexor carpi radialis

Attachments – Flexor carpi radialis lies medial to pronator teres, and arises from the medial epicondyle via the common flexor tendon, from the antebrachial fascia and from adjacent intermuscular septa (**Fig. 52.15**). Its fusiform belly ends, rather more than halfway to the wrist, in a long tendon which passes within a synovial sheath through a lateral canal, formed by the flexor retinaculum above and a groove on

A

Joins
at
14th–16th
year

At birth

5th–6th
year

9th–11th
year

16th
year

Joins shaft
at 17th–18th year

Fig. 52.14 **A**, Stages in the ossification of the ulna. The diagram is simplified in relation to the ossification of the olecranon epiphysis, which is said to have two centres. **B**, The epiphyseal lines of the adolescent left ulna, lateral aspect. The attachment of the joint capsules is in blue.

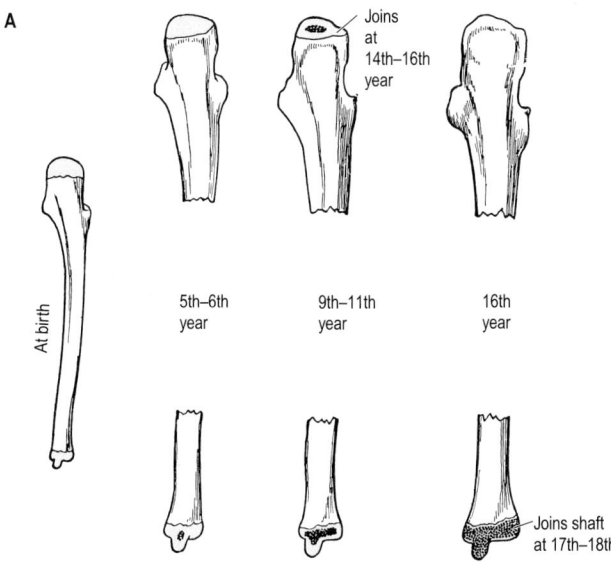

B

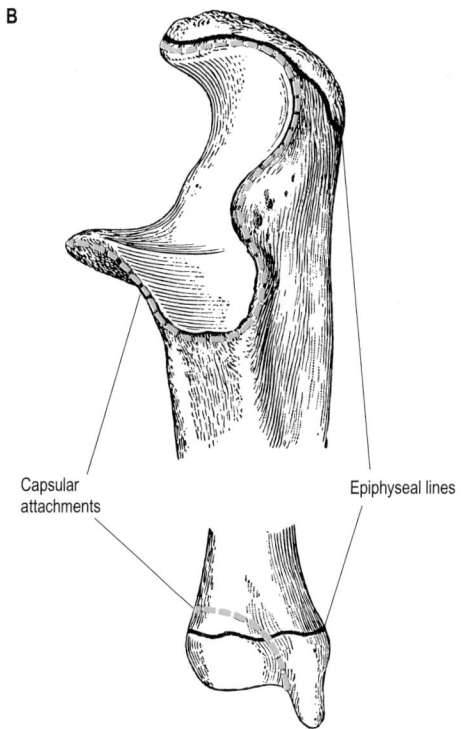

Capsular
attachments

Epiphyseal lines

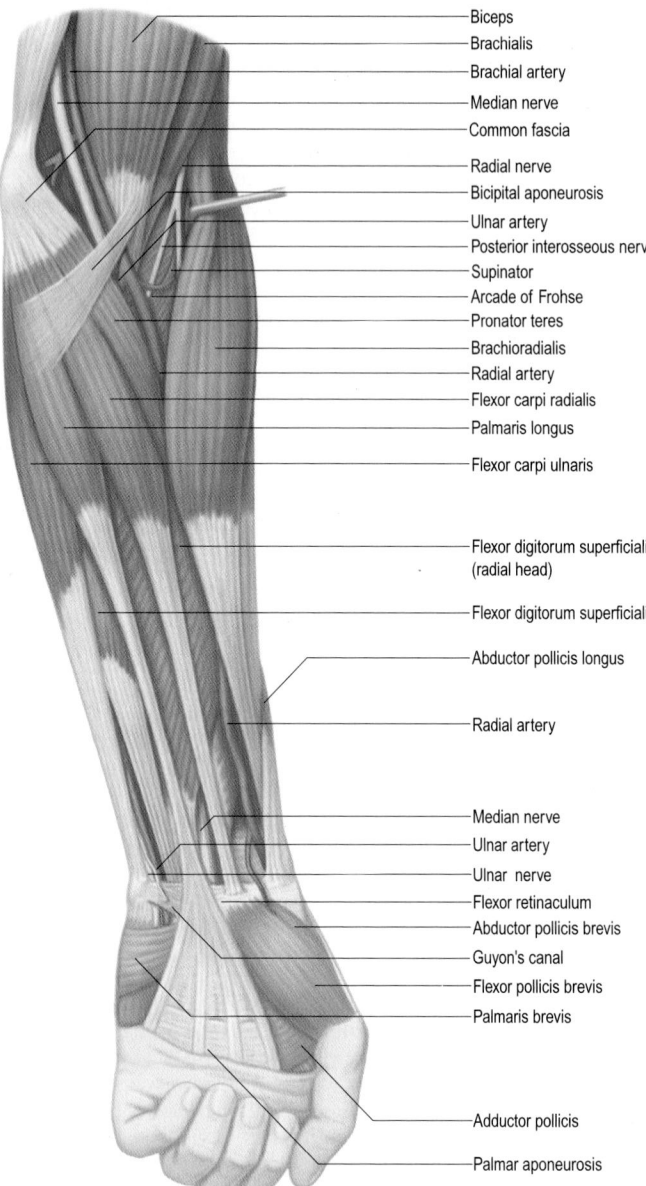

Biceps
Brachialis
Brachial artery
Median nerve
Common fascia
Radial nerve
Bicipital aponeurosis
Ulnar artery
Posterior interosseous nerve
Supinator
Arcade of Frohse
Pronator teres
Brachioradialis
Radial artery
Flexor carpi radialis
Palmaris longus
Flexor carpi ulnaris

Flexor digitorum superficialis
(radial head)

Flexor digitorum superficialis

Abductor pollicis longus

Radial artery

Median nerve
Ulnar artery
Ulnar nerve
Flexor retinaculum
Abductor pollicis brevis
Guyon's canal
Flexor pollicis brevis
Palmaris brevis

Adductor pollicis

Palmar aponeurosis

Fig. 52.15 The superficial flexor muscles of the left forearm.

the trapezium beneath. It inserts on the palmar surface of the base of the second metacarpal, sending a slip to the third metacarpal. These distal attachments are hidden by the oblique head of adductor pollicis. The muscle rarely may be absent. It may have accessory slips from the biceps tendon, bicipital aponeurosis, coronoid process or radius. Distally it may also be attached to the flexor retinaculum, trapezium or fourth metacarpal.

Relations – In the lower part of the forearm the radial artery lies between the tendon of flexor carpi radialis and that of brachioradialis. The surface groove for the radial pulse is well known to all physicians.

Vascular supply – Flexor carpi radialis is supplied by a single dominant proximal pedicle and several distal minor pedicles. The dominant pedicle is formed by a branch which arises from either the anterior or posterior ulnar recurrent artery. The latter passes deep to pronator teres to enter the deep surface of flexor carpi radialis, whereupon it divides into a small ascending branch and a larger descending branch. The distal minor pedicles amount to six to eight branches from the radial artery which enter the muscle on the anterolateral side.

Innervation – Flexor carpi radialis is innervated by the median nerve, C6 and 7.

Action – Acting with flexor carpi ulnaris, and sometimes flexor digitorum superficialis, flexor carpi radialis flexes the wrist, and helps radial extensors of the wrist in abducting the hand.

Clinical anatomy: testing – Flexor carpi radialis is tested by palpating its contracting fibres during flexion of the wrist against resistance.

Flexor digitorum superficialis

Attachments – Flexor digitorum superficialis (sublimis) lies deep to the preceding muscles (**Fig. 52.15**). It is the largest of the superficial flexors, and arises by two heads. The humero-ulnar head arises from the medial epicondyle of the humerus via the common tendon; the anterior band of the ulnar collateral ligament; adjacent intermuscular septa, and from the medial side of the coronoid process proximal to the ulnar origin of pronator teres. The radial head, a thin sheet of muscle, arises from the anterior radial border extending from the radial tuberosity to the insertion of pronator teres. The median nerve and ulnar artery descend between the heads. The muscle usually separates into two strata, directed to digits 2–5. The superficial stratum, joined laterally by the radial head, divides into two tendons for the middle and ring finger. The deep stratum gives off a muscular slip to join the superficial fibres directed to the ring finger, and then ends in two tendons for the index and little finger. As the tendons pass behind the flexor retinaculum they are arranged in pairs: the superficial pair pass to the middle and ring fingers, the deep to the index and little finger. Distal to the carpal tunnel the four tendons diverge. Each passes towards a finger superficial to the corresponding flexor digitorum profundus tendon. The two tendons for each finger enter the digital flexor sheath (which starts over the metacarpophalangeal joint) in this relationship. The superficialis tendon then splits into two bundles which pass around the profundus to lie posteriorly. They subsequently reunite and insert into the anterior surface of the middle phalanx (p. 913). Some fibres interchange from one bundle to another.

An intermediate tendon is always found in the central branching area of the muscle belly and is an important landmark in deep dissection: it can initially be confused with the median nerve. The radial head of flexor digitorum superficialis may be absent and the muscular slip from the deep stratum may provide most or all of the fibres acting on the index finger. The fibres associated with the little finger may be absent, when they are replaced by a separate slip from the ulna, flexor retinaculum or palmar fascia. Variations occur in the arrangement of the tendons.

Relations – The median nerve and ulnar artery descend between the heads of flexor digitorum superficialis.

Vascular supply – The humeral head of flexor digitorum superficialis is supplied by the anterior ulnar recurrent artery. The main part of the muscle is supplied on its anterior surface by three or four branches from both the ulnar and radial arteries. The posterior surface is supplied by the ulnar artery and median artery, and the lateral surface by additional branches from the radial artery.

Innervation – Flexor digitorum superficialis is innervated by the median nerve, C8 and T1.

Action – Flexor digitorum superficialis is potentially a flexor of all the joints over which it passes, i.e. proximal interphalangeal, metacarpophalangeal and wrist joints. Its precise action depends on which other muscles are acting. It has independent muscle slips to all four fingers, unlike flexor digitorum profundus, which has a muscle group common to the middle, ring and little fingers. It is therefore able to flex the proximal interphalangeal joints individually.

Clinical anatomy: testing – The independent action of flexor digitorum superficialis for a particular finger is tested by flexing that digit while holding the three other fingers in full extension. This eliminates any simultaneous contraction of the flexor digitorum profundus which might flex the digit.

Palmaris longus

Attachments – Palmaris longus (**Fig. 52.15**) is a slender, fusiform muscle medial to flexor carpi radialis. It springs from the medial epicondyle by the common tendon, and from adjacent intermuscular septa and deep fascia. It converges on a long tendon, which passes anterior (superficial) to the flexor retinaculum. A few fibres leave the tendon and interweave with the transverse fibres of the retinaculum, but most of the tendon passes distally. As the tendon crosses the retinaculum it broadens out to become a flat sheet which becomes incorporated into the palmar aponeurosis (p. 891). Palmaris longus is often absent on one or both sides.

Relations – The median nerve at the wrist lies partly under the cover of the tendon of palmaris longus, and partly between the tendons of palmaris longus and flexor carpi radialis.

Vascular supply – The muscle belly of palmaris longus is supplied by a small branch from the anterior ulnar recurrent artery. A small contribution is sometimes made by the median artery, if this is well developed.

Innervation – Palmaris longus is innervated by the median nerve, C7 and 8.

Action – It has been suggested that palmaris longus is a phylogenetically degenerate metacarpophalangeal joint flexor. Although consideration of the line of action would suggest that it plays a role in carpal flexion, its main function appears to be as an anchor for the skin and fascia of the hand, in resisting horizontal shearing forces in a distal direction, (e.g. as in holding a golf club), which would tend to deglove the skin of the palm.

Clinical anatomy: testing – If the wrist is flexed against resistance, the taut tendon of palmaris longus will be seen in the midline of the flexor wrist crease as the tendon passes superficial to the flexor retinaculum. It helps to oppose the thumb to the middle fingertip at the same time as the wrist if flexed.

Flexor carpi ulnaris

Attachments – Flexor carpi ulnaris is the most medial of the superficial forearm flexors (**Fig. 52.15**). It arises by two heads, humeral and ulnar, connected by a tendinous arch. The small humeral head arises from the medial epicondyle via the common tendon. The ulnar head has an extensive origin from the medial margin of the olecranon and proximal two-thirds of the posterior border of the ulna, an aponeurosis (which it shares with extensor carpi ulnaris and flexor digitorum profundus), and from the intermuscular septum between it and flexor digitorum superficialis. Occasionally there is a slip from the coronoid process. A thick tendon forms along its anterolateral border in its distal half. The tendon is attached to the pisiform, and thence prolonged to the hamate and fifth metacarpal by pisohamate and pisometacarpal ligaments. The attachment to the flexor retinaculum and the fourth or fifth metacarpal bones is sometimes substantial.

Relations – The ulnar nerve and posterior ulnar recurrent artery pass under the tendinous arch between the humeral and ulnar heads of flexor carpi ulnaris. Ulnar vessels and nerve lie lateral to the tendon of insertion.

Vascular supply – The main arterial supply of flexor carpi ulnaris is derived from three pedicles. The proximal pedicle arises from a branch of the posterior ulnar recurrent artery as it passes between the humeral and ulnar heads. The middle and distal pedicles arise from the ulnar artery and enter the muscle at the junction of the upper and middle thirds, and the musculotendinous junctions, respectively. Flexor carpi ulnaris also receives a small supply near its origin which arises from the inferior ulnar collateral artery.

Innervation – Flexor carpi ulnaris is innervated by the ulnar nerve, C7 and 8 and T1.

Action – Acting with flexor carpi radialis, flexor carpi ulnaris flexes the wrist. Acting with extensor carpi ulnaris, it adducts (ulnar deviates) the hand.

Clinical anatomy: testing – Flexor carpi ulnaris is tested by palpating its fibres while the wrist is flexed against resistance. A more positive test is to palpate the tendon while the patient abducts the little finger against resistance. FCV synergistically contracts to stabilize the pisiform, giving abducted digiti minimi a stable origin.

Deep flexor compartment

The muscles of the deep flexor compartment are flexor digitorum profundus, flexor pollicis longus and pronator quadratus.

Flexor digitorum profundus

Attachments – Flexor digitorum profundus arises deep to the superficial flexors from about the upper three-quarters of the anterior and medial surfaces of the ulna (**Fig. 52.16**). It embraces the attachment of brachialis above and extends distally almost to pronator quadratus. It also arises from a depression on the medial side of the coronoid process, the upper three-quarters of the posterior ulnar border (by an aponeurosis which it shares with flexor and extensor carpi ulnaris), and the anterior surface of the ulnar half of the interosseous membrane. The muscle ends in four tendons, which run initially posterior (deep) to the tendons of flexor digitorum superficialis and the flexor retinaculum. The part of the flexor digitorum profundus muscle which acts on the index finger is usually distinct throughout. The tendons for the other fingers are interconnected by areolar tissue and tendinous slips as far as the palm. Anterior to their proximal phalanges, the tendons pass through the tendons of flexor digitorum superficialis to insert on the palmar surfaces of the bases of the distal phalanges. The tendons of the profundus undergo fascicular rearrangement as they pass through those of superficialis.

Flexor digitorum profundus may be joined by accessory slips from the radius (which act on the index finger), flexor superficialis, flexor pollicis longus, the medial epicondyle or the coronoid process.

Relations – Flexor digitorum profundus forms most of the surface elevation medial to the palpable posterior ulnar border. In the palm, the lumbrical muscles are attached to its tendons (p. 920).

Vascular supply – The origin of flexor digitorum profundus is supplied by the inferior ulnar collateral and ulnar recurrent arteries. The proximal part of is supplied by one or two branches from either the ulnar or common interosseous arteries. The distal part is supplied by a series of branches from the ulnar artery, the anterior interosseous artery and the median artery.

Innervation – The medial part of flexor digitorum profundus, i.e. the muscle bellies to the little and ring fingers, is innervated by the ulnar nerve. The lateral part, i.e. the muscle bellies to the middle and index fingers, is innervated by the anterior interosseous branch of the median nerve, C8 and T1.

Action – Flexor digitorum profundus is capable of flexing any or all of the joints over which it passes. It therefore has a role in coordinated finger flexion, but it is the only muscle capable of flexing the distal interphalangeal joints. The index finger tendon is usually capable of independent function, whereas the other three work together. Electromyographically flexor digitorum profundus acts alone in gentle digital flexion and is reinforced by superficialis for greater force and/or velocity.

Clinical anatomy: testing – Flexor digitorum profundus is tested by flexing the distal interphalangeal joint while holding the proximal interphalangeal joint in extension.

Flexor pollicis longus

Attachments – Flexor pollicis longus is lateral to flexor digitorum profundus (**Fig. 52.16**). It arises from the grooved anterior surface of the radius, and extends from below its tuberosity to the upper attachment of pronator quadratus. It also arises from the adjacent interosseous membrane, and frequently by a variable slip from the lateral, or more rarely medial, border of the coronoid process, or from the medial epicondyle of the humerus. The muscle ends in a flattened tendon, which passes behind the flexor retinaculum, between opponens pollicis and the oblique head of adductor pollicis, to enter a synovial sheath. It inserts on the palmar surface of the base of the distal phalanx of the thumb.

Flexor pollicis longus is sometimes connected to flexor digitorum superficialis, or profundus, or pronator teres. The interosseous attachment, and indeed the whole muscle, may be absent. Anomalous tendon slips from the flexor pollicis longus to the flexor digitorum profundus are common.

Relations – The anterior interosseous nerve and vessels descend on the interosseous membrane between flexor pollicis longus and flexor digitorum profundus.

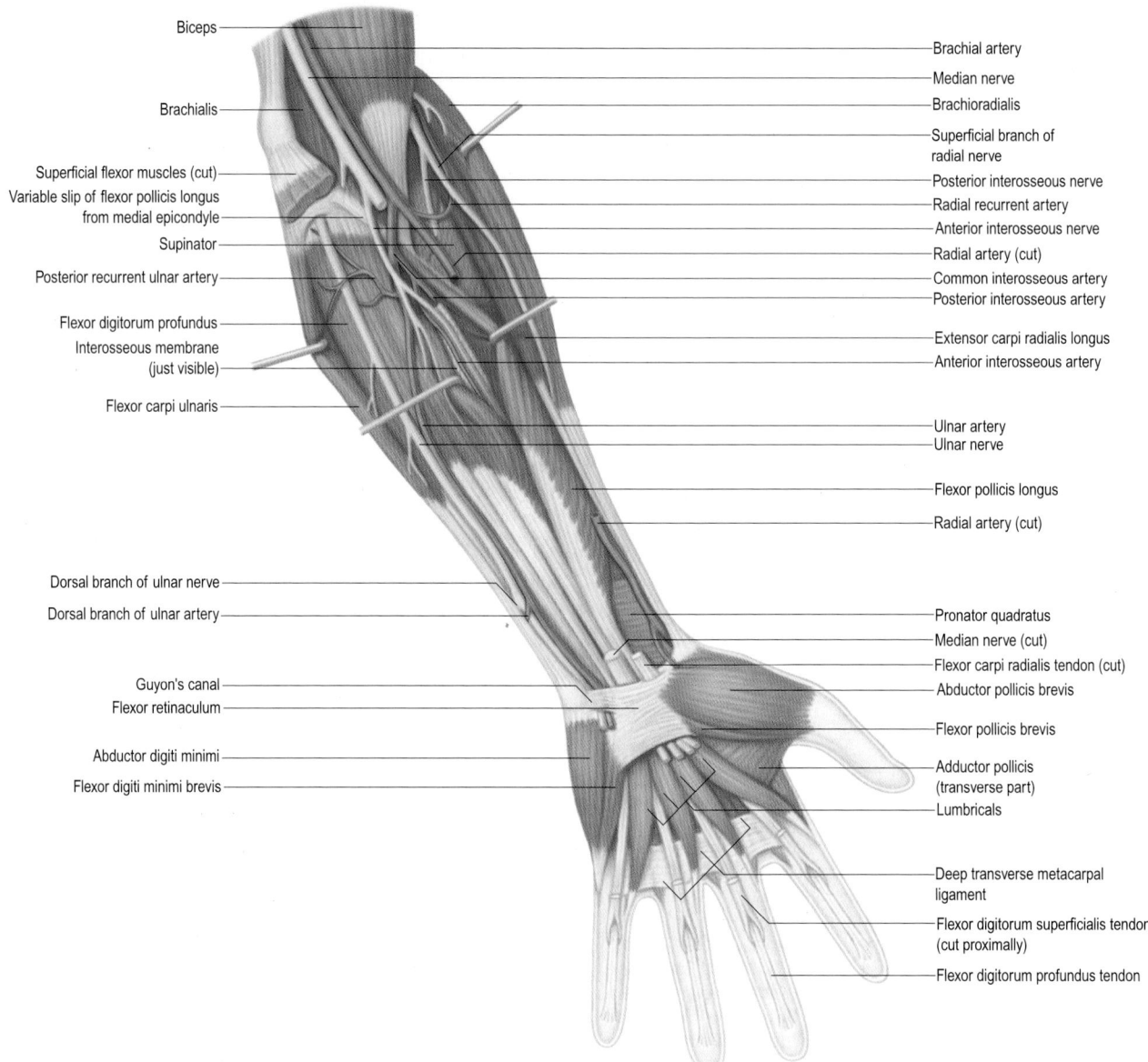

Biceps

Brachialis

Superficial flexor muscles (cut)

Variable slip of flexor pollicis longus from medial epicondyle

Supinator

Posterior recurrent ulnar artery

Flexor digitorum profundus

Interosseous membrane (just visible)

Flexor carpi ulnaris

Dorsal branch of ulnar nerve

Dorsal branch of ulnar artery

Guyon's canal

Flexor retinaculum

Abductor digiti minimi

Flexor digiti minimi brevis

Brachial artery

Median nerve

Brachioradialis

Superficial branch of radial nerve

Posterior interosseous nerve

Radial recurrent artery

Anterior interosseous nerve

Radial artery (cut)

Common interosseous artery

Posterior interosseous artery

Extensor carpi radialis longus

Anterior interosseous artery

Ulnar artery

Ulnar nerve

Flexor pollicis longus

Radial artery (cut)

Pronator quadratus

Median nerve (cut)

Flexor carpi radialis tendon (cut)

Abductor pollicis brevis

Flexor pollicis brevis

Adductor pollicis (transverse part)

Lumbricals

Deep transverse metacarpal ligament

Flexor digitorum superficialis tendon (cut proximally)

Flexor digitorum profundus tendon

Fig. 52.16 The deep flexor muscles of the left forearm.

Vascular supply – The medial half of flexor pollicis longus is supplied by the anterior interosseous artery, while the lateral half is supplied by branches of the radial artery. The median artery may contribute if it is well developed.

Innervation – Flexor pollicis longus is innervated by the anterior interosseous branch of the median nerve, C7 and 8.

Action – Flexor pollicis longus flexes the phalanges of the thumb and the carpometacarpal joint of the thumb, especially if the more distal joints are stiff or fused.

Clinical anatomy: testing – Flexor pollicis longus is tested by flexing the interphalangeal joint of the thumb against resistance.

Pronator quadratus

Attachments – Pronator quadratus is a flat, quadrilateral muscle which extends across the front of the distal parts of the radius and ulna (**Fig. 52.16**). It arises from the oblique ridge on the anterior surface of the shaft of the ulna, the medial part of this surface, and a strong aponeurosis which covers the medial third of the muscle. The fibres pass laterally and slightly downwards to the distal quarter of the anterior border and surface of the shaft of the radius. Deeper fibres insert into the triangular area above the ulnar notch of the radius.

Vascular supply – Pronator quadratus receives its main arterial supply from the anterior interosseous artery as it passes through the interosseous membrane.

Innervation – Pronator quadratus is innervated by anterior interosseous branch of the median nerve, C7 and 8.

Action – Pronator quadratus is the principal pronator of the forearm, and is assisted by pronator teres only in rapid or forceful pronation. The deeper fibres oppose separation of the distal ends of the radius and ulna when upward thrusts are transmitted through the carpus.

Clinical anatomy: testing – Pronator quadratus is tested by pronation of the forearm against resistance while the wrist finger flexors are relaxed. The simultaneous contraction of pronator teres makes it difficult to test the independent action of pronator quadratus.

POSTERIOR COMPARTMENT

The posterior compartment contains the extensor muscles of the forearm and brachioradialis and supinator. Chronic tendonitis of the common extensor tendon origin produces lateral epicondylitis of the elbow leading to pain and tenderness. It is a frequent complaint among tennis players.

Superficial extensor compartment

Brachioradialis

Attachments – Brachioradialis is the most superficial muscle along the radial side of the forearm, and forms the lateral border of the cubital fossa (**Fig. 52.17**). It arises from the proximal two-thirds of the lateral supracondylar ridge of the humerus and the anterior surface of the lateral intermuscular septum. The muscle fibres end above mid-forearm level in a flat tendon which inserts on the lateral side of the distal end of the radius, usually just proximal to its styloid process. Occasionally this attachment may be much more proximal.

The muscle is often fused proximally with brachialis. Its tendon may divide into two or three separately attached slips. In rare instances it is double or absent.

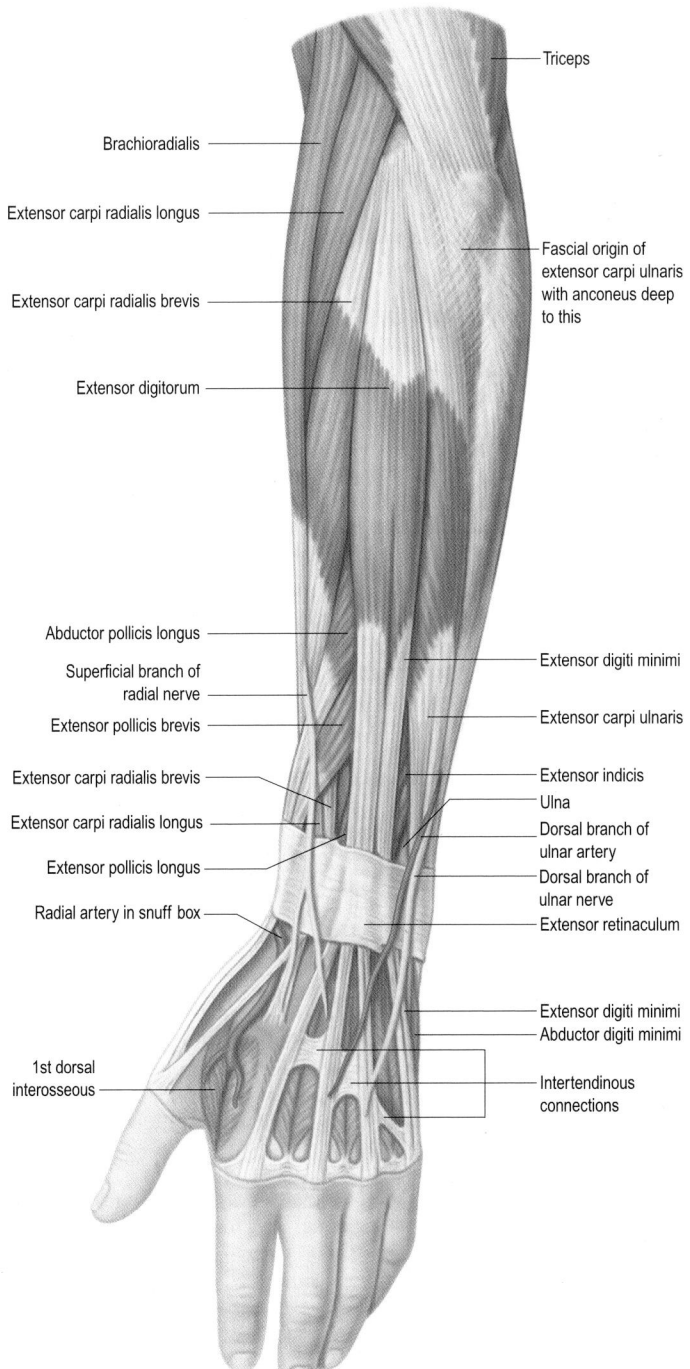

Triceps

Brachioradialis

Extensor carpi radialis longus

Extensor carpi radialis brevis

Extensor digitorum

Fascial origin of extensor carpi ulnaris with anconeus deep to this

Abductor pollicis longus

Superficial branch of radial nerve

Extensor pollicis brevis

Extensor carpi radialis brevis

Extensor carpi radialis longus

Extensor pollicis longus

Radial artery in snuff box

1st dorsal interosseous

Extensor digiti minimi

Extensor carpi ulnaris

Extensor indicis

Ulna

Dorsal branch of ulnar artery

Dorsal branch of ulnar nerve

Extensor retinaculum

Extensor digiti minimi

Abductor digiti minimi

Intertendinous connections

Fig. 52.17 The superficial extensor muscles of the left forearm.

Relations – The radial nerve and the anastomosis between the profunda brachii artery and the radial recurrent artery lie between the lateral intermuscular septum and brachialis. The tendon is crossed near its distal termination by the tendons of abductor pollicis longus and extensor pollicis brevis. The radial artery is on its ulnar (medial) side.

Vascular supply – Brachioradialis is supplied by branches of the radial recurrent artery which pierce the posteromedial surface of the muscle. It also receives branches from the radial collateral branch of the profunda brachii and directly from the radial artery in the distal part of the muscle.

Innervation – Brachioradialis is innervated by the radial nerve, C5 and 6.

Action – Brachioradialis is a flexor of the elbow (despite being supplied by an 'extensor' nerve). It acts most effectively with the forearm in mid-pronation. It is minimally active in slow, easy flexions, or with the forearm supine, but generates a powerful burst of activity in both flexion and extension when movement is rapid. Under these conditions it develops a pronounced transarticular component of its force which helps to stabilize the elbow joint by balancing the centrifugal force of rapid swings in either direction.

Clinical anatomy: testing – Brachioradialis can be seen and felt when the semi-pronated forearm is flexed against resistance.

Extensor carpi radialis longus

Attachments – Extensor carpi radialis longus arises mainly from the distal third of the lateral supracondylar ridge of the humerus and the front of the lateral intermuscular septum. Some fibres come from the common tendon of origin of the forearm extensors. The belly ends at the junction of the proximal and middle thirds of the forearm in a flat tendon which runs along the lateral surface of the radius, deep to abductor pollicis longus and extensor pollicis brevis. The tendon then passes under the extensor retinaculum, where it lies in a groove on the back of the radius just behind the styloid process. It inserts on the radial side of the dorsal surface of the base of the second metacarpal, and may send slips to the first or third metacarpal bones. It contributes to the intermetacarpal ligaments.

Relations – Extensor carpi radialis longus (**Fig. 52.17**) is partly over-lapped by brachioradialis.

Vascular supply – Extensor carpi radialis longus receives its principal arterial supply from a single branch from the radial recurrent artery. Addition blood supply comes from branches from the radial collateral branch of the profunda brachii and directly from the radial artery in the distal part of the muscle.

Innervation – Extensor carpi radialis longus is innervated by the radial nerve, C6 and 7.

Action – Extensor carpi radialis longus acts as an extensor and abductor of the wrist and midcarpal joints. It acts in synergism with the finger flexors when making a fist.

Clinical anatomy: testing – The muscle belly and tendon of extensor carpi radialis longus can be palpated when the wrist is extended and abducted against resistance with the forearm pronated.

Extensor carpi radialis brevis

Attachments – Extensor carpi radialis brevis arises from the lateral epicondyle of the humerus by a tendon of origin which it shares with other forearm extensors, the radial collateral ligament of the elbow joint, a strong aponeurosis which covers its surface, and adjacent intermuscular septa. Its belly ends at about mid-forearm in a flat tendon which closely accompanies that of the longer carpal extensor to the wrist. The tendon passes under the extensor retinaculum and is attached to the dorsal surface of the base of the third metacarpal on its radial side, distal to its styloid process, and on adjoining parts of the second metacarpal base.

The tendons of both extensor carpi radialis longus and brevis may split into slips, which are variably attached to the second and third metacarpal bones. The muscles themselves may be united or may exchange muscular slips.

Relations – Extensor carpi radialis brevis is shorter than extensor carpi radialis longus and is covered by it (**Fig. 52.17**). The tendon passes deep to abductor pollicis longus and extensor pollicis brevis, then under the extensor retinaculum, where it lies in a shallow groove on the back of the radius, medial to the tendon of extensor carpi radialis longus, and separated from it by a low ridge. These two tendons share a common synovial sheath.

Vascular supply – Extensor carpi radialis brevis receives its arterial supply principally from two pedicles. One is a single branch from the radial recurrent artery, and the other is a branch of the radial artery which arises about one third of the way down the forearm. There is an additional blood supply proximally from branches from the radial collateral branch of the profunda brachii.

Innervation – Extensor carpi radialis brevis is innervated by the posterior interosseous nerve, C7 and 8.

Action – Extensor carpi radialis brevis acts with extensor carpi radialis longus as an extensor and abductor of the wrist and midcarpal joints. It acts in synergism with the finger flexors when making a fist.

Clinical anatomy: testing – The muscle belly and tendon of extensor carpi radialis brevis can be palpated when the wrist is extended and abducted against resistance with the forearm pronated.

Extensor digitorum

Attachments – Extensor digitorum arises from the lateral epicondyle of the humerus via the common extensor tendon, the adjacent intermuscular septa and the antebrachial fascia (**Fig. 52.17**). It divides distally into four tendons, which pass, in a common synovial sheath with the tendon of extensor indicis, through a tunnel under the extensor retinaculum. The tendons diverge on the dorsum of the hand, one to each finger. The tendon to the index finger is accompanied by extensor indicis, which lies ulnar (medial) to it. On the dorsum of the hand, adjacent tendons are linked by three variable intertendinous connections (juncturae tendinae), which are inclined distally and radially. The digital attachments enter a fibrous expansion on the dorsum of the proximal phalanges to which lumbrical, interosseous and digital extensor tendons all contribute.

The tendons of extensor digitorum may be variably deficient. More commonly, they are doubled or even tripled in one or more digits, most often the index finger or the middle finger. Occasionally a slip of tendon passes to the thumb. The arrangement of the intertendinous connections on the dorsum of the hand is highly variable. The medial connection is strong and pulls the tendon of the little finger towards that of the ring finger, whereas the connection between the middle two tendons is weak and may be absent.

Relations – The extensor tendon to the index finger lies radial (lateral) to the tendon of extensor indicis. The extensor tendon to the little finger lies radial (lateral) to the tendon of extensor digiti minimi.

Vascular supply – The proximal third of extensor digitorum is supplied by branches from the radial recurrent artery, and the distal two-thirds are supplied by branches from the posterior interosseous artery. The very distal portion is supplied by a perforating branch from the anterior interosseous artery which passes through the interosseous membrane.

Innervation – Extensor digitorum is innervated by the posterior interosseous nerve, C7 and 8.

Action – Extensor digitorum can extend any or all of the joints over which it passes, i.e. wrist, metacarpophalangeal, proximal and distal interphalangeal joints (the latter two via the extensor expansion of the digits). When acting on the metacarpophalangeal joints, extensor digitorum tends to spread the digits apart, an action that is due principally to the different axes of the individual joints imposed by the transverse arch of the hand. This is a 'trick' movement used by patients with interosseous muscle paralysis. The function of the intertendinous bands is not clear, but they may affect independent extension of digits.

Testing – The tendons of extensor digitorum can be readily felt, and usually seen, when the fingers are extended against resistance and the forearm is pronated.

Extensor digiti minimi

Attachments – Extensor digiti minimi is a slender muscle medial to, and usually connected with, extensor digitorum (**Fig. 52.17**). It arises from the common extensor tendon by a thin tendinous slip and adjacent intermuscular septa. It frequently has an additional origin from the antebrachial fascia. Its long tendon slides in a separate compartment of the extensor retinaculum just behind the inferior radio-ulnar joint. Distal to the retinaculum, the tendon typically splits into two, and the lateral slip is joined by a tendon from extensor digitorum. All three tendons are attached to the dorsal digital expansion of the fifth digit, and there may be a slip to the fourth digit.

Extensor digiti minimi is rarely absent, but sometimes it is fused with extensor digitorum.

Relations – The tendon of extensor digiti minimi lies ulnar (medial) to the common extensor tendon to the little finger.

Vascular supply – Extensor digiti minimi is supplied by branches from the radial recurrent and posterior interosseous arteries, and by terminal branches from the anterior interosseous artery after it has pierced the interosseous membrane.

Innervation – Extensor digiti minimi is innervated by the posterior interosseous nerve, C7 and 8.

Action – Extensor digiti minimi can extend any of the joints of the little finger, or contribute to wrist extension. It permits extension of the little finger independently of the other digits even in extremes of ulnar or radial wrist deviation.

Clinical anatomy: testing – Extensor digiti minimi is tested by extending the little finger while holding the remaining fingers flexed at the metacarpophalangeal joints. This eliminates any simultaneous contraction of extensor digitorum.

Extensor carpi ulnaris

Attachments – Extensor carpi ulnaris arises from the lateral epicondyle via the common extensor tendon, the posterior border of the ulna (by an aponeurosis shared with flexor carpi ulnaris and flexor digitorum profundus), and overlying fascia (**Fig. 52.17**). It ends in a tendon that slides in a groove between the head and the styloid process of the ulna, in a separate compartment of the extensor retinaculum, and is ultimately attached to a tubercle on the medial side of the fifth metacarpal base.

Vascular supply – Proximally extensor carpi ulnaris receives branches from the radial recurrent artery. Distally, it is supplied by several branches from the posterior interosseous artery.

Innervation – Extensor carpi ulnaris is innervated by the posterior interosseous nerve, C7 and 8.

Action – Together with extensors carpi radialis longus and brevis, extensor carpi ulnaris acts synergistically with the digital flexors to extend and to fix the wrist when objects are being gripped or when the fist is clenched. Observation shows that it is impossible to grip strongly unless the wrist is extended. Acting with flexor carpi ulnaris, extensor carpi ulnaris adducts the hand.

Clinical anatomy: testing – If the wrist is extended and adducted against resistance, and the forearm is pronated and the fingers are extended, extensor carpi ulnaris can be felt lateral to the groove that overlies the posterior subcutaneous border of the ulna.

Anconeus

Attachments – Anconeus is a small, triangular muscle posterior to the elbow joint and is partially blended with triceps (**Figs 52.15, 52.17**). Anconeus arises by a separate tendon from the posterior surface of the lateral epicondyle of the humerus. Its fibres diverge medially towards the ulna, covering the posterior aspect of the annular ligament, and are attached to the lateral aspect of the olecranon and proximal quarter of the posterior surface of the shaft of the ulna.

The extent to which anconeus fuses with triceps or extensor carpi ulnaris is variable.

Vascular supply – Anconeus is supplied by branches from the posterior interosseous recurrent artery. A small number of musculocutaneous perforators reach the skin overlying the muscle.

Innervation – Anconeus is innervated by the radial nerve, C6, 7 and 8.

Action – Anconeus assists triceps in extending the elbow joint. Its major function is not clear, but it may be the control of ulnar abduction in pronation, which is necessary if the forearm is to turn over the hand without translating it medially. In this way a tool can be revolved 'on the spot' or it can be swept through an arc.

Deep extensor compartment

The five deep forearm extensor muscles are abductor pollicis longus, extensor pollicis longus and extensor pollicis brevis (which all act on the thumb), extensor indicis and supinator (**Fig. 52.18**). Apart from supinator, all are attached proximally only to the forearm bones.

Abductor pollicis longus

Attachments – Abductor pollicis longus arises from the posterior surface of the shaft of the ulna distal to anconeus, the adjoining interosseous membrane, and the middle third of the posterior surface of the radius distal to the attachment of supinator (**Fig. 52.18**). It descends laterally, becoming superficial in the distal forearm, where it is visible as an

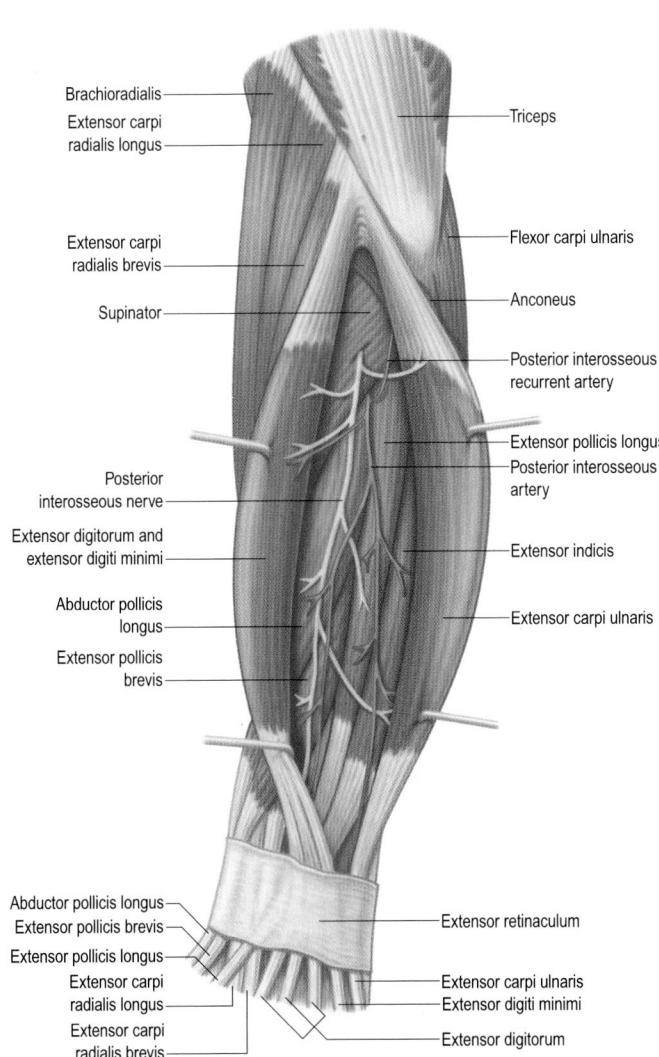

Brachioradialis
Extensor carpi radialis longus
Extensor carpi radialis brevis
Supinator
Posterior interosseous nerve
Extensor digitorum and extensor digiti minimi
Abductor pollicis longus
Extensor pollicis brevis

Triceps
Flexor carpi ulnaris
Anconeus
Posterior interosseous recurrent artery
Extensor pollicis longus
Posterior interosseous artery
Extensor indicis
Extensor carpi ulnaris

Abductor pollicis longus
Extensor pollicis brevis
Extensor pollicis longus
Extensor carpi radialis longus
Extensor carpi radialis brevis

Extensor retinaculum
Extensor carpi ulnaris
Extensor digiti minimi
Extensor digitorum

Fig. 52.18 The deep extensor muscles of the left forearm.

oblique elevation (**Fig. 52.17**). The muscle fibres end in a tendon just proximal to the wrist. The tendon runs in a groove on the lateral side of the distal end of the radius accompanied by the tendon of extensor pollicis brevis. It usually splits into two slips, one of which is attached to the radial side of the first metacarpal base, and the other is attached to the trapezium. Slips from the tendon may continue into opponens pollicis or abductor pollicis brevis. Occasionally the muscle itself may be wholly or partially divided.

Vascular supply – Abductor pollicis longus is supplied proximally by a lateral branch from the posterior interosseous artery. Distally it is supplied on the medial side by a perforating branch from the anterior interosseous artery.

Innervation – Abductor pollicis longus is innervated by the posterior interosseous nerve, C7 and 8.

Action – Abductor pollicis longus abducts the wrist joint. Acting with abductor pollicis brevis it aids abduction of the thumb radially (i.e. in the plane of the palm). Acting with the pollicial extensors it extends the thumb at its carpometacarpal joint. The tendon may also stabilize the trapezium upon which the first metacarpal can move.

Clinical anatomy: testing – The tendon of abductor pollicis longus can be seen and felt at the radial aspect of the anatomical snuff box when the thumb and wrist are abducted against resistance at the carpometacarpal joint.

Extensor pollicis longus

Attachments – Extensor pollicis longus is larger than extensor pollicis brevis, whose proximal attachment it partly covers (**Figs 52.17, 52.18**). It arises from the lateral part of the middle third of the posterior surface of the shaft of the ulna below abductor pollicis longus, and the adjacent interosseous membrane. The tendon passes through a separate compartment of the extensor retinaculum in a narrow, oblique groove on the back of the distal end of the radius. It turns around a bony fulcrum, Lister's tubercle, which changes its line of pull from that of the forearm to that of the thumb, and is attached to the base of the distal phalanx of the thumb. The sides of the tendon are joined on the dorsum of the proximal phalanx by expansions from the tendon of abductor pollicis brevis laterally, and from the first palmar interosseous and adductor pollicis medially.

Relations – After passing around Lister's tubercle, the tendon of extensor pollicis longus crosses the tendons of extensor carpi radialis brevis and longus obliquely (**Fig. 52.17**). When the thumb is fully extended the tendon is separated from extensor pollicis brevis by a triangular depression or fossa, the so-called 'anatomical snuff-box'. Bony structures can be felt in the floor of this fossa by deep palpation. In proximal to distal order they are the radial styloid, the smooth convex articular surface of the scaphoid, the trapezium, and the base of the first metacarpal. The latter are more easily felt during metacarpal movement, while the scaphoid is more easily felt during adduction and abduction of the hand.

Vascular supply – Extensor pollicis longus is supplied on its superficial surface by branches from the posterior interosseous artery, and on its deep surface by perforating branches from the anterior interosseous artery.

Innervation – Extensor pollicis longus is innervated by the posterior interosseous nerve, C7 and 8.

Action – Extensor pollicis longus extends the distal phalanx of the thumb. Acting in association with extensor pollicis brevis and abductor pollicis longus, it extends the proximal phalanx and the metacarpal. In continued action, as a consequence of the obliquity of its tendon, extensor pollicis longus adducts the extended thumb and rotates it laterally.

Clinical anatomy: testing – The tendon of extensor pollicis longus can be palpated at the ulnar border of the anatomical snuff-box when the thumb is extended at the interphalangeal joint against resistance. When the thumb is opposed and adducted, abductor pollicis brevis can extend the interphalangeal joint of the thumb, mimicking the action of extensor pollicis longus.

Extensor pollicis brevis

Attachments – Extensor pollicis brevis arises from the posterior surface of the radius distal to abductor pollicis longus, and from the adjacent interosseous membrane (**Figs 52.17, 52.18**). The tendon is inserted into the base of the proximal phalanx of the thumb, and commonly has an additional attachment to the base of the distal phalanx, usually through a fasciculus which joins the tendon of extensor pollicis longus. Extensor pollicis brevis may be absent or fused completely with abductor pollicis longus.

Relations – Extensor pollicis brevis is ulnar (medial) to, and closely connected with, abductor pollicis longus (**Figs 52.17, 52.18**). In the distal forearm, the two muscles emerge between extensor carpi radialis brevis and extensor digitorum, and pass obliquely across the tendons of the radial extensors of the wrist. They cover the distal part of brachioradialis, and pass through the most lateral compartment of the extensor retinaculum in a single synovial sheath, sharing a groove in the distal radius. Ultimately they cross, superficial to the radial styloid process and radial artery, to reach the dorsolateral base of the proximal phalanx of the thumb.

Vascular supply – Extensor pollicis brevis is supplied from branches from the posterior interosseous artery together with perforating branches from the anterior interosseous artery.

Innervation – Extensor pollicis brevis is innervated by the posterior interosseous nerve, C7 and 8.

Action – Extensor pollicis brevis extends the proximal phalanx and metacarpal of the thumb.

Clinical anatomy: testing – The tendon of extensor pollicis brevis can be felt at the radial border of the anatomical snuff-box, lying medial to the tendon of abductor pollicis longus, when the metacarpophalangeal joint of the thumb is extended against resistance.

Extensor indicis

Attachments – Extensor indicis is a narrow, elongated muscle which lies medial and parallel to extensor pollicis longus (**Fig. 52.18**). It arises from the posterior surface of the ulna distal to extensor pollicis longus, and the adjacent interosseous membrane. Its tendon passes under the extensor retinaculum in a common compartment with the tendons of extensor digitorum. Opposite the head of the second metacarpal it joins the ulnar side of the tendon of extensor digitorum which serves the index finger.

Extensor indicis occasionally sends accessory slips to the extensor tendons of other digits. Rarely its tendon may be interrupted on the dorsum of the hand by an additional muscle belly (extensor indicis brevis manus).

Relations – The tendon of extensor indicis lies on the ulnar aspect of the extensor digitorum tendon to the index finger on the dorsum of the hand.

Vascular supply – Extensor indicis is supplied on its superficial surface by branches from the posterior interosseous artery, and on its deep surface by perforating branches from the anterior interosseous artery.

Innervation – Extensor indicis is innervated by the posterior interosseous nerve, C7 and 8.

Action – Extensor indicis helps to extend the index finger and the wrist. It permits extension of the index finger independently of the other digits, even in extremes of ulnar or radial wrist deviation.

Clinical anatomy: testing – Extensor indicis is tested by extending the index finger while holding the remaining fingers flexed at the metacarpophalangeal joints. This eliminates the effects of any simultaneous contraction of extensor digitorum.

Supinator

Attachments – Supinator surrounds the proximal third of the radius and has superficial and deep layers (**Figs 52.18, 52.19**). The two parts

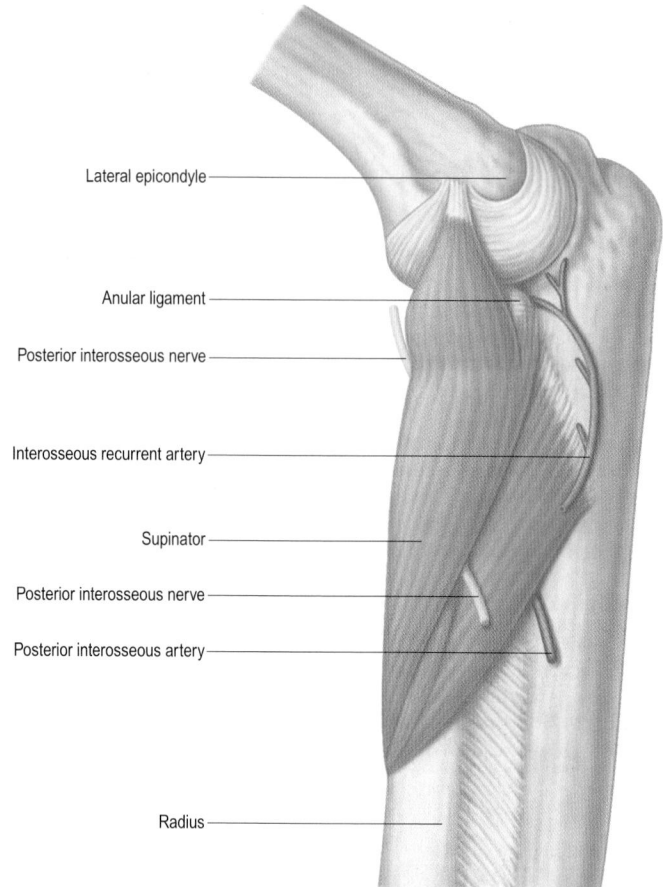

Fig. 52.19 The left supinator muscle: posterolateral aspect.

Lateral epicondyle

Anular ligament

Posterior interosseous nerve

Interosseous recurrent artery

Supinator

Posterior interosseous nerve

Posterior interosseous artery

Radius

arise together, the superficial by tendinous, and the deep by muscular fibres, from the lateral epicondyle of the humerus; the radial collateral ligament of the elbow joint and the anular ligament of the superior radio-ulnar joint; the supinator crest of the ulna and the posterior part of the triangular depression in front of it; and an aponeurosis which covers the muscle. Supinator is attached distally to the lateral surface of the proximal third of the radius, down to the insertion of pronator teres. The radial attachment extends on to the anterior and posterior surfaces between the anterior oblique line and the fainter posterior oblique 'ridge' (**Fig. 52.6**).

Supinator is subject to frequent variation, and small parts of the muscle have acquired individual names, e.g. lateral and medial tensors of the annular ligament.

Relations – The posterior interosseous nerve enters the forearm by passing between the superficial and deep heads of supinator.

Vascular supply – The superficial part of supinator is supplied by branches from the radial recurrent artery. The deep part of supinator is supplied by branches from the posterior interosseous artery and the posterior interosseous recurrent artery.

Innervation – Supinator is innervated by the posterior interosseous nerve, C6 and 7 as it traverses the muscle.

Action – Supinator rotates the radius so as to bring the palm to face anteriorly. It acts alone in slow, unopposed supination, and together with biceps brachii in fast or forceful supination. An object which may potentially be heavy is often picked up with the forearm initially pronated. The more powerful supinators lift the object against gravity, and rotation is often combined with increasing elbow flexion to bring the object towards the eyes.

Clinical anatomy: testing – Supinator is too deep to be palpated and independent testing is difficult. Biceps is inactive on supination with the elbow fully extended, therefore this must be produced by supination alone and can be used to test its function.

VASCULAR SUPPLY AND LYMPHATIC DRAINAGE

ARTERIES

Radial artery (Figs 52.1, 52.2, 52.15, 52.16, 52.19, 52.20)

The radial artery is smaller than the ulnar artery, yet appears a more direct continuation of the brachial artery. It normally starts c.1 cm distal to the flexion crease of the elbow. It descends along the lateral side of the forearm, accompanied by paired venae comitantes, from the medial side of the neck of the radius to the wrist, where it is palpable between flexor carpi radialis medially and the salient anterior border of the radius. The artery is medial to the radial shaft proximally, and anterior to it distally. Proximally it is overlapped anteriorly by the belly of brachioradialis, but elsewhere in its course it is covered only by the skin, and superficial and deep fasciae. Its posterior relations in the forearm are successively the tendon of biceps, supinator, the distal attachment of pronator teres, the radial head of flexor digitorum superficialis, flexor pollicis longus, pronator quadratus and the lower end of the radius (where its pulsation is most accessible). Brachioradialis is lateral to the artery throughout its length. Pronator teres is medial to the proximal part of the artery and the tendon of flexor carpi radialis is medial to the distal portion. The superficial radial nerve lies lateral to the middle third of the radial artery: multiple branches from the artery supply the nerve throughout its length.

The radial artery may occasionally arise from the continuation of a superficial brachial artery, or as a high proximal division of an otherwise normal brachial artery. It can give rise to the common interosseous artery.

The course and distribution of the radial artery in the wrist and hand are described on page 928.

Branches in the forearm

Radial recurrent artery – The radial recurrent artery is discussed in Chapter 51, page 863.

Cutaneous branches – Cutaneous branches emerge between brachioradialis and pronator teres in the proximal third of the forearm. The largest perforator, which is also the largest in the forearm, has been named the inferior cubital artery. It reaches the deep fascia by passing superficially between brachioradialis and pronator teres in the apex of the antecubital fossa. It lies lateral to the tendon of biceps, emerging between the median cubital vein and its communicating branch to the venae comitantes of the radial artery. In the distal two-thirds of the forearm, the cutaneous perforators emerge through the fascia between brachioradialis and flexor carpi radialis and between flexor carpi radialis and flexor digitorum superficialis and fan out at the level of the deep fascia (**Fig. 52.2**). These vessels anastomose with their counterparts from the ulnar artery and the posterior interosseous artery.

The fasciocutaneous branches provide the anatomical basis for raising a skin flap containing the whole width of forearm skin, either pedicled or as a free flap, based on the radial artery and its venae comitantes. Known as the radial forearm fasciocutaneous flap, it is used for reconstructing areas of missing tissue elsewhere in the body. It is possible to incorporate the lateral aspect of the radius with the flap because a few fascioperiosteal branches supply this part of the bone.

Muscular branches – Muscular branches are distributed to the muscles on the radial side of the forearm.

Ulnar artery (Figs 52.1, 52.2, 52.15, 52.16, 52.20, 52.21)

The ulnar artery is the larger terminal branch of the brachial artery. It starts 1 cm distal to the flexion crease of the elbow and reaches the medial side of the forearm midway between elbow and wrist. In the forearm the artery initially lies on brachialis and deep to pronator teres, flexor carpi radialis, palmaris longus and flexor digitorum superficialis. It subsequently lies on flexor digitorum profundus, between flexor carpi ulnaris and flexor digitorum superficialis, and is covered by the skin, superficial and deep fasciae. The median nerve is a medial relation for c.2.5 cm distal to the elbow, and then crosses the artery, from which it is separated by the ulnar head of pronator teres. The ulnar nerve lies medial to the distal two-thirds of the artery, which supplies the nerve throughout its length. The palmar cutaneous branch of the ulnar nerve descends along the ulnar artery to reach the hand. The ulnar artery crosses the flexor retinaculum lateral to the ulnar nerve and pisiform bone to enter the hand.

The ulnar artery is accompanied throughout its length by venae comitantes.

The ulnar artery may arise proximal to the elbow, usually from the brachial artery, when it usually lies superficial to the forearm flexors under the deep fascia: only rarely is it subcutaneous. When this occurs, the brachial artery supplies the common interosseous and the ulnar recurrent arteries.

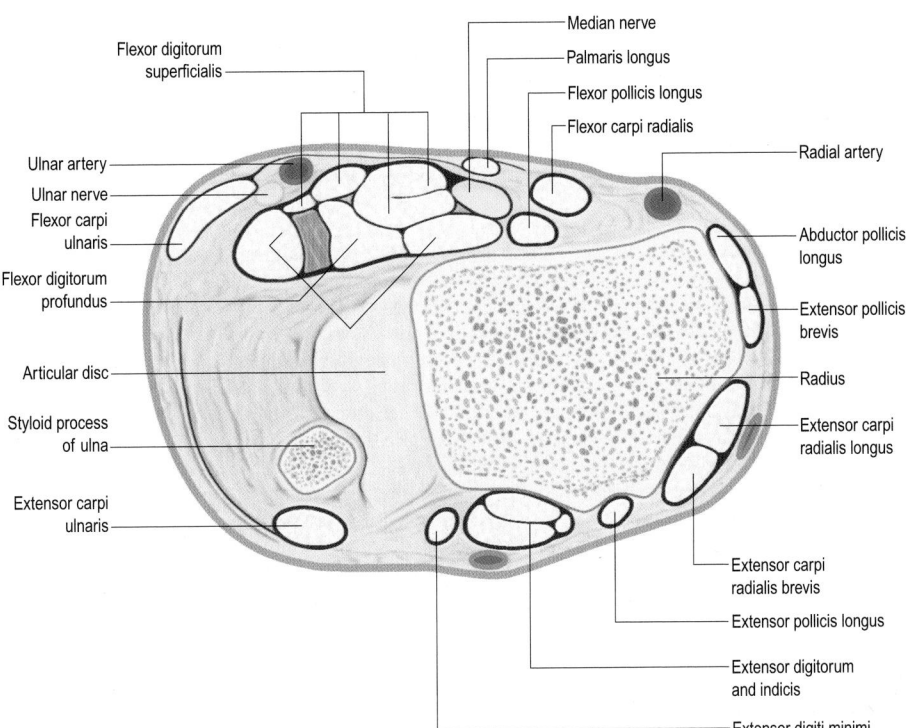

Flexor digitorum superficialis
Median nerve
Palmaris longus
Flexor pollicis longus
Flexor carpi radialis
Radial artery
Ulnar artery
Ulnar nerve
Flexor carpi ulnaris
Flexor digitorum profundus
Abductor pollicis longus
Extensor pollicis brevis
Radius
Articular disc
Extensor carpi radialis longus
Styloid process of ulna
Extensor carpi ulnaris
Extensor carpi radialis brevis
Extensor pollicis longus
Extensor digitorum and indicis
Extensor digiti minimi

Fig. 52.20 Transverse section through the left forearm, passing through the distal end of the radius and the styloid process of the ulna, with the hand and forearm in full supination: distal (inferior) aspect.

883

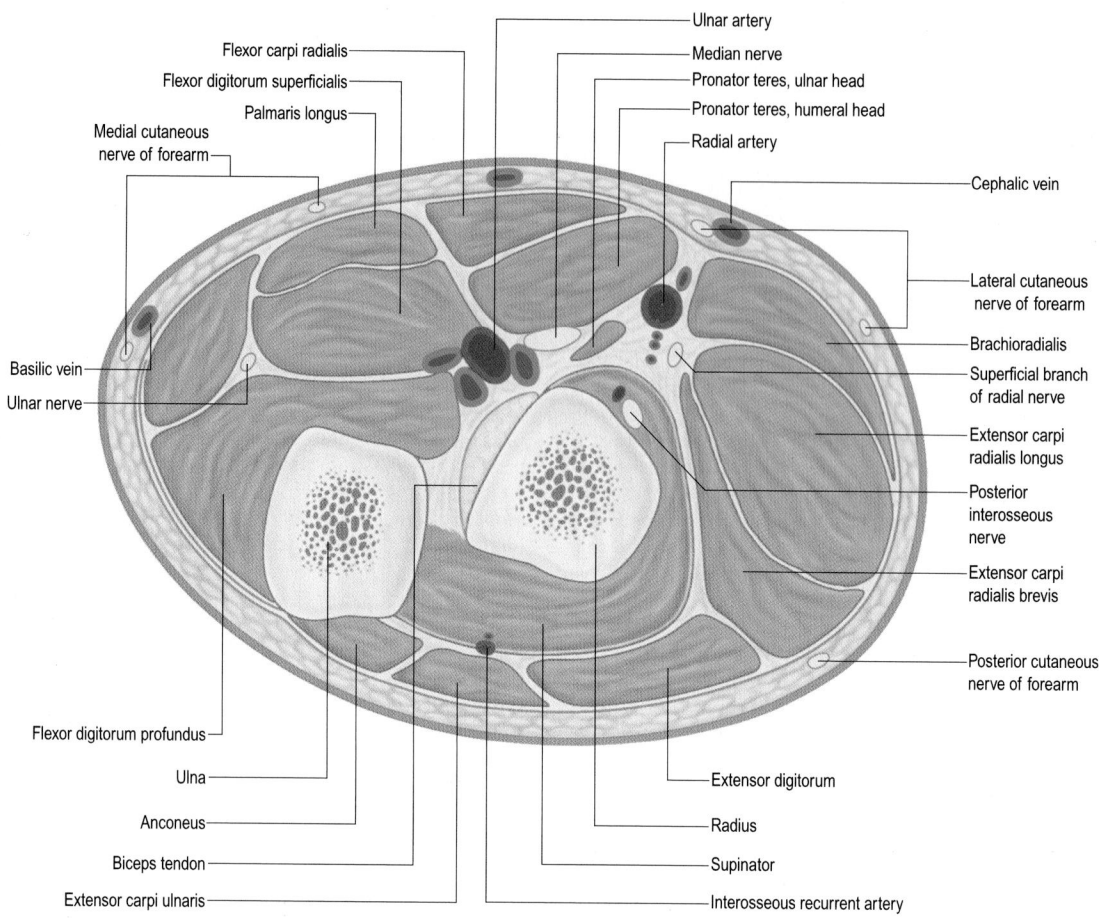

Fig. 52.21 Transverse section through the left forearm at the level of the radial tuberosity: proximal aspect.

The course and distribution of the ulnar artery in the wrist and hand are described on page 929.

Branches in the forearm

Anterior and posterior ulnar recurrent arteries – The anterior and posterior ulnar recurrent arteries are described in Chapter 51, page 863.

Common interosseous artery (Fig. 52.16) – The common interosseous artery is a short branch of the ulnar artery. It arises just distal to the radial tuberosity and passes back to the proximal border of the interosseous membrane, where it divides into the anterior and posterior interosseous arteries. Occasionally, the common interosseous artery is a branch of the radial artery.

Anterior interosseous artery (Fig. 50.9) – The anterior interosseous artery descends on the anterior aspect of the interosseous membrane with the anterior interosseous branch of the median nerve. It is overlapped by contiguous sides of flexor digitorum profundus and flexor pollicis longus. Shortly after its origin, it usually gives off a slender median artery. This accompanies and supplies the median nerve as far as the palm, where it may join the superficial palmar arch or end as one or two palmar digital arteries. (The median artery can also arise from the ulnar or the common interosseous artery.)

Muscular and nutrient branches from the anterior interosseous artery pierce the interosseous membrane to supply deep extensor muscles and the radius and ulna respectively. A branch descends deep to pronator quadratus before piercing the interosseous membrane to join the anterior 'carpal' arch.

The anterior interosseous artery proper leaves the anterior compartment by piercing the interosseous membrane proximal to pronator quadratus. It anastomoses with the posterior interosseous artery in the posterior compartment of the forearm, and travels through a tunnel under the extensor retinaculum with the tendons of the digital extensors

before joining the dorsal carpal arch. Three small cutaneous perforating branches supply the skin over the lower lateral border of the forearm.

Posterior interosseous artery (Figs 52.2, 52.18, 52.22) – The posterior interosseous artery is usually smaller than the anterior. It passes dorsally between the oblique cord and proximal border of the interosseous membrane and then between supinator and abductor pollicis longus. It descends deep in the groove between extensor carpi ulnaris and the extensor digiti minimi part of extensor digitorum. While in the groove it gives rise to multiple muscular branches which supply these muscles and fasciocutaneous perforators which travel in the intermuscular septum between extensor carpi ulnaris and extensor digiti minimi. These fasciocutaneous vessels provide the anatomical basis for raising a dorsal forearm skin flap, which is usually pedicled, based on the posterior interosseous artery and its venae comitantes. Known as the posterior interosseous artery flap, it is used for reconstructing areas of missing tissue in the forearm and proximal part of the hand.

The posterior interosseous artery accompanies the deep branch of the radial nerve (posterior interosseous nerve) on abductor pollicis longus. Distally it anastomoses with the terminal part of the anterior interosseous artery and the dorsal carpal arch.

Sometimes the posterior interosseous artery disappears halfway down the forearm, in which case the anterior interosseous artery pierces the interosseous membrane more proximally to anastomose with it. Rarely no anastomosis occurs between the anterior and the posterior interosseous arteries.

Posterior interosseous recurrent artery – The posterior interosseous recurrent artery leaves the posterior interosseous artery near its origin and ascends between the lateral epicondyle and olecranon, either on or through supinator, and deep to anconeus. It anastomoses with the middle collateral branch of the arteria profunda brachii, posterior ulnar recurrent and ulnar collateral arteries. Occasionally the artery is absent.

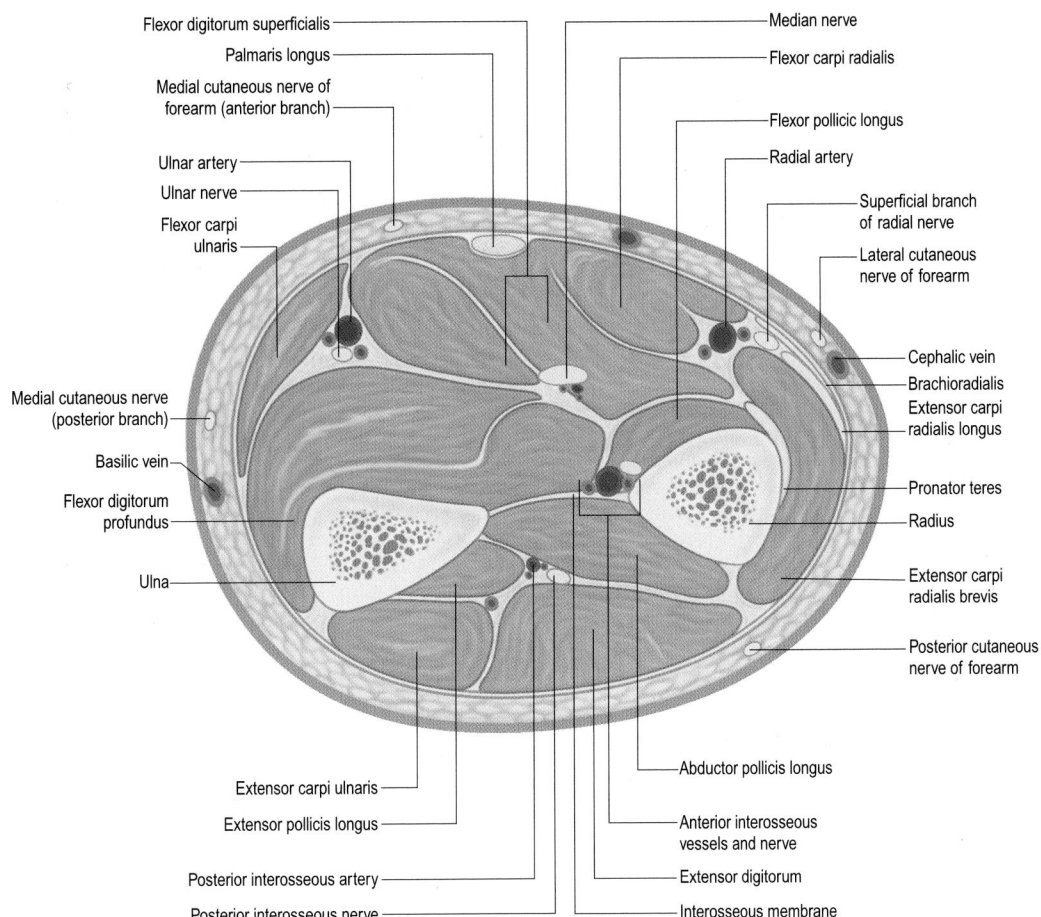

Flexor digitorum superficialis
Palmaris longus
Medial cutaneous nerve of forearm (anterior branch)
Ulnar artery
Ulnar nerve
Flexor carpi ulnaris
Medial cutaneous nerve (posterior branch)
Basilic vein
Flexor digitorum profundus
Ulna
Extensor carpi ulnaris
Extensor pollicis longus
Posterior interosseous artery
Posterior interosseous nerve

Median nerve
Flexor carpi radialis
Flexor pollicic longus
Radial artery
Superficial branch of radial nerve
Lateral cutaneous nerve of forearm
Cephalic vein
Brachioradialis
Extensor carpi radialis longus
Pronator teres
Radius
Extensor carpi radialis brevis
Posterior cutaneous nerve of forearm
Abductor pollicis longus
Anterior interosseous vessels and nerve
Extensor digitorum
Interosseous membrane

Fig. 52.22 Transverse section through the middle of the left forearm: distal aspect.

Cutaneous branches – The cutaneous perforators of the ulnar artery reach the skin by passing along the fascial septum between flexor carpi ulnaris and flexor digitorum superficialis throughout the length of the forearm. A constant dorso-ulnar perforator vessel is given off distally c.2–5 cm proximal to the pisiform and it accompanies the dorsal cutaneous branch of the ulnar nerve. The vessel emerges between flexor carpi ulnaris and extensor carpi ulnaris. A few small musculocutaneous perforators reach the skin via flexor carpi ulnaris and anastomose with their counterparts derived from the radial and the posterior interosseous arteries.

Muscular branches – Muscular branches arise directly from the main vessel and are distributed to the muscles on the ulnar side of the forearm.

VEINS

Deep veins
The venae comitantes running with the radial and ulnar arteries drain the deep and superficial palmar venous arches respectively. They unite near the elbow as paired brachial veins. The radial veins are smaller, and receive the deep dorsal veins of the hand. The ulnar veins drain the deep palmar venous arch, and connect with superficial veins near the wrist. Near the elbow they receive the venae comitantes of the anterior and posterior interosseous arteries, and a large branch connects them to the median cubital vein.

Superficial veins

Cephalic vein (Fig. 48.5)
The cephalic vein usually forms over the 'anatomical snuff-box' from the radial end of the dorsal venous plexus. It curves proximally around the radial side of the forearm to gain its ventral aspect, and receives veins from both aspects of the forearm. Distal to the elbow a branch, the median cubital vein, diverges proximomedially to reach the basilic vein. The median cubital vein is joined by a branch from the deep veins.

The further course of the cephalic vein is described in the arm on page 857.

Accessory cephalic vein – The accessory cephalic vein may arise either in a dorsal forearm plexus or from the ulnar side of the dorsal venous network in the hand. It joins the cephalic vein distal to the elbow. A large oblique vein often connects the basilic and cephalic veins dorsally in the forearm.

Basilic vein (Fig. 48.5)
The basilic vein starts medially in the dorsal venous network of the hand. It ascends posteromedially in the forearm, inclining forwards to the anterior surface distal to the elbow, where it is joined by the median cubital vein. It then ascends superficial to and between biceps and pronator teres, and is crossed by filaments of the medial cutaneous nerve of the forearm which pass both superficial and deep to the vein.

The course of the basilic vein in the arm is described on p. 857.

Median vein (Fig. 48.5)
The median vein of the forearm drains the superficial palmar venous plexus and ascends through the anterior part of the forearm to join either the basilic or median cubital vein. It may divide distal to the elbow to join both veins.

INNERVATION

MEDIAN NERVE (Figs 52.15, 52.16, 52.20, 52.21, 52.22)
The median nerve usually enters the forearm between the heads of pronator teres. (Occasionally the nerve passes posterior to both heads of pronator teres, or it may pass through the humeral head). It crosses to the lateral side of the ulnar artery, from which it is separated by the deep head of pronator teres. It passes behind a tendinous bridge between the humero-ulnar and radial heads of the flexor digitorum superficialis,

and descends through the forearm posterior and adherent to flexor digitorum superficialis and anterior to flexor digitorum profundus. About 5 cm proximal to the flexor retinaculum it emerges from behind the lateral edge of flexor digitorum superficialis, and becomes superficial just proximal to the wrist. Here it lies between the tendons of flexor digitorum superficialis and flexor carpi radialis, projecting laterally from beneath the tendon of palmaris longus (**Fig. 52.20**). It then passes deep to the flexor retinaculum into the palm. In the forearm the median nerve is accompanied by the median branch of the anterior interosseous artery.

The course and distribution of the median nerve in the wrist and hand is described on page 931.

Martin–Gruber connection

Multiple communicating branches between the median nerve (and sometimes the anterior interosseous nerve) arise proximally and pass medially between flexors digitorum superficialis and profundus, deep to the ulnar artery, and join the ulnar nerve. This motor fibre communication (commonly referred to as the Martin–Gruber connection) is estimated to be present in 17% of individuals. It results in a median nerve innervation of a variable number of intrinsic muscles of the hand (Leibovic & Hastings 1992), and presumably explains why isolated ulnar and median nerve lesions can sometimes be unpredictable in terms of the pattern of intrinsic muscle paralysis.

Branches in the forearm

Anterior interosseous nerve

The anterior interosseous nerve branches posteriorly from the median nerve between the two heads of pronator teres, just distal to the origin of its branches to the superficial forearm flexors and proximal to the point at which the median nerve passes under the tendinous arch of flexor digitorum superficialis. With the anterior interosseous artery it descends anterior to the interosseous membrane, between and deep to flexor pollicis longus and flexor digitorum profundus. It supplies flexor pollicis longus and the lateral part of flexor digitorum profundus (which sends tendons to the index and middle finger). Terminally, the anterior interosseous nerve lies posterior to pronator quadratus, which it supplies via its deep surface. It also supplies articular branches to the distal radio-ulnar, radiocarpal and carpal joints.

Anterior interosseous nerve syndrome – The anterior interosseous nerve may be affected with the median nerve or by itself in any of the causes of pronator syndrome (p. 864). Median nerve compression is typically caused by pressure from fascial bands on the deep head of the pronator teres or the tendinous radial attachment of flexor digitorum superficialis. Anterior interosseous nerve palsy may be due to external pressure, a form of 'Saturday night palsy', and sometimes by tight grip in association with pronation without obvious cause. It may be a manifestation of neuralgic amyotrophy and tends to resolve spontaneously over several months. A variety of aberrant muscles, e.g. an accessory head of flexor pollicis longus, palmaris profundus, or flexor carpi radialis brevis, have all been described as causing entrapment neuropathy of the anterior interosseous nerve.

An anterior interosseous nerve palsy causes weakness of pinch grip due to involvement of flexor pollicis longus and flexor digitorum profundus to the index finger. Innervation of flexor digitorum profundus to the middle finger is rather variable, and therefore this muscle may or may not be weak. The branches to these three muscles may arise separately from the median nerve, so that isolated weakness of the terminal phalanx to the thumb or index finger may occur. Pronator quadratus is also involved but is not clinically significant. Anterior interosseous nerve palsy can be distinguished from pronator syndrome because there are no sensory symptoms. The treatment is exploration of the nerve and surgical decompression.

Muscular branches

Muscular branches are given off near the elbow to all the superficial flexor muscles except flexor carpi ulnaris, i.e. to pronator teres, flexor carpi radialis, palmaris longus and flexor digitorum superficialis. The branch to the part of flexor digitorum superficialis which serves the index finger is given off near mid-forearm and may be derived from the anterior interosseous nerve.

Other branches

Articular branches, arising at or just distal to the elbow joint, supply the joint and the proximal radio-ulnar joint. The palmar cutaneous branch is described in Chapter 53, page 931.

ULNAR NERVE (Figs 52.16, 52.20, 52.21, 52.22)

The ulnar nerve descends on the medial side of the forearm, lying on flexor digitorum profundus. Proximally it is covered by flexor carpi ulnaris: its distal half lies lateral to the muscle and is covered only by skin and fasciae. In the upper third of the forearm, the nerve is distant from the ulnar artery, but more distally it comes to lie close to the medial side of the artery. About 5 cm proximal to the wrist it gives off a dorsal branch which continues distally into the hand, anterior to the flexor retinaculum on the lateral side of the pisiform and posteromedial to the ulnar artery. It passes deep to the superficial part of the retinaculum (in Guyon's canal) with the artery and divides into superficial and deep terminal branches.

The course and distribution of the ulnar nerve in the hand is described on page 932.

Muscular branches

There are usually two muscular branches. They begin near the elbow and supply flexor carpi ulnaris and the medial half of flexor digitorum profundus.

Palmar cutaneous branch

The palmar cutaneous branch arises about mid-forearm. It descends on the ulnar artery, which it supplies, and then perforates the deep fascia to end in the palmar skin, after communicating with the palmar branch of the median nerve. It sometimes supplies palmaris brevis.

Dorsal branch

The dorsal branch of the ulnar nerve is described on page 932.

RADIAL NERVE (Figs 52.19, 52.20, 52.22)

There is some variation in the level at which branches of the radial nerve arise from the main trunk in different subjects. Branches to extensor carpi radialis brevis and supinator may arise from the main trunk of the radial nerve or from the proximal part of the posterior interosseous nerve, but almost invariably above the arcade of Frohse.

Radial tunnel syndrome

Radial tunnel syndrome is an entrapment neuropathy of the radial nerve near the elbow, where four structures can potentially cause compression of the nerve. These are fibrous bands (which can tether the radial nerve to the radiohumeral joint); the sharp tendinous medial border of extensor carpi radialis brevis; a leash of vessels from the radial recurrent artery as it passes to supply brachioradialis and extensor carpi radialis longus; the arcade of Frohse, which is the free aponeurotic proximal edge of the superficial part of supinator (see **Fig. 51.9**).

Usually the only presenting symptom is pain over the extensor mass just distal to the elbow. There is no sensory disturbance or motor loss, but there is frequently tenderness along the course of the radial nerve over the radial head. The pain is exacerbated when the elbow is extended and the wrist is passively flexed and pronated, or extended and supinated against resistance. Extension of the middle finger against resistance when the elbow in fully extended also may lead to increased pain. These manoeuvres tighten the anatomical structures which cause compression.

Superficial terminal branch

The superficial terminal branch descends from the lateral epicondyle anterolaterally in the proximal two-thirds of the forearm, initially lying on supinator, lateral to the radial artery and behind brachioradialis. In the middle third of the forearm it lies behind brachioradialis, close to the lateral side of the artery, and is successively anterior to pronator teres, the radial head of flexor digitorum superficialis and flexor pollicis longus. It leaves the artery c.7 cm proximal to the wrist and passes deep to the tendon of brachioradialis. It curves round the lateral side of the radius as it descends, pierces the deep fascia and divides into five, sometimes four, dorsal digital nerves. On the dorsum of the hand it usually communicates with the posterior and lateral cutaneous nerves of the forearm.

As the nerve crosses the lateral aspect of the radius it is superficial and relatively unprotected: it is easily compressed here by tight bracelets, watch straps and handcuffs.

Radial sensory nerve entrapment (Wartenberg's disease)
Entrapment of the superficial radial nerve can occur as it emerges from beneath the edge of the brachioradialis tendon c.6 cm proximal to the radial styloid. The condition is frequently associated with previous trauma in this region. The symptoms are pain and paraesthesia over the radial aspect of the dorsum of the wrist and hand.

Posterior interosseous nerve (Fig. 52.21)
The posterior interosseous nerve is the deep terminal branch of the radial nerve. It reaches the back of the forearm by passing round the lateral aspect of the radius between the two heads of supinator. It supplies extensor carpi radialis brevis and supinator before entering supinator: as it passes through the muscle it supplies it with additional branches. The branch to extensor carpi radialis brevis may arise from the beginning of the superficial branch of the radial nerve. As it emerges from supinator posteriorly, the posterior interosseous nerve gives off three short branches to extensor digitorum, extensor digiti minimi and extensor carpi ulnaris, and two longer branches, a medial to extensor pollicis longus and extensor indicis, and a lateral which supplies abductor pollicis longus and extensor pollicis brevis. The nerve at first lies between the superficial and deep extensor muscles, but at the distal border of extensor pollicis brevis it passes deep to extensor pollicis longus and, diminished to a fine thread, descends on the interosseous membrane to the dorsum of the carpus. Here it presents a flattened and somewhat expanded termination or 'pseudoganglion', from which filaments supply the carpal ligaments and articulations. Articular branches from the posterior interosseous nerve supply carpal, distal radio-ulnar and some intercarpal and intermetacarpal joints. Digital branches supply the metacarpophalangeal and proximal interphalangeal joints.

The distal portion of the nerve lies in a separate fascial sheath in the radial, deep aspect of the fourth dorsal compartment of the extensor retinaculum of the wrist, where it is located deep to extensor digitorum and extensor indicis. This portion of the nerve can be used as a donor nerve for grafting segmental digital nerve defects, as there is no clinically discernible donor site deficit.

Posterior interosseous nerve palsy
There are many causes of posterior interosseous nerve palsy. These include trauma and inflammatory swellings, as well as entrapment at the same anatomical sites that can cause radial tunnel syndrome. Pain is similar in nature to that of radial tunnel syndrome and is later accompanied by weakness and paralysis. When fully developed, there is inability to extend the fingers at the metacarpophalangeal joints, weakness of thumb extension and abduction. There is weakness and radial deviation of wrist extension because extensor carpi ulnaris is usually affected, while the radial wrist extensors and brachioradialis are normal (because their nerve supply is given off proximal to the origin of the posterior interosseous nerve). There are no sensory disturbances, because the superficial radial nerve arises above this level.

MEDIAL CUTANEOUS NERVE OF THE FOREARM (Fig. 48.18)
The medial cutaneous nerve of the forearm has already divided into anterior and posterior branches before it enters the forearm. The larger anterior branch usually passes in front of, occasionally behind, the median cubital vein, and descends anteromedially in the forearm to supply the skin as far as the wrist. It curves round to the back of the forearm, descending on its medial border to the wrist, supplying the skin. It connects with the medial cutaneous nerve of the arm, the posterior cutaneous nerve of the forearm, and the dorsal branch of the ulnar nerve.

LATERAL CUTANEOUS NERVE OF THE FOREARM (Figs 48.18, 48.10)
The lateral cutaneous nerve of the forearm is a direct continuation of the musculocutaneous nerve as it lies lateral to the biceps tendon in the antecubital fossa. It passes deep to the cephalic vein, descending along the radial border of the forearm to the wrist. It supplies the skin of the anterolateral surface of the forearm and connects with the posterior cutaneous nerve of the forearm and the terminal branch of the radial nerve by branches which pass around its radial border. Its trunk gives rise to a slender recurrent branch which extends along the cephalic vein as far as the middle third of the upper arm, distributing filaments to the skin over the distal third of the anterolateral surface of the upper arm close to the vein. At the wrist joint the lateral cutaneous nerve of the forearm is anterior to the radial artery. Some filaments pierce the deep fascia and accompany the artery to the dorsum of the carpus. The nerve then passes to the base of the thenar eminence, where it ends in cutaneous rami. It has branches which connect with the terminal branch of the radial nerve and the palmar cutaneous branch of the median nerve.

POSTERIOR CUTANEOUS NERVE OF THE FOREARM
The posterior cutaneous nerve of the forearm passes along the dorsum of the forearm to the wrist. It supplies the skin along its course and near its end joins the dorsal branches of the lateral cutaneous nerve of the forearm (**Fig. 48.18**).

REFERENCES

Cormack GC, Lamberty BGH 1994 The Arterial Anatomy of Skin Flaps. Edinburgh: Churchill Livingstone.

Salmon M. 1994 Anatomic studies. In: Taylor GI, Razaboni RM (eds) Book 1. Arteries of the Muscles of the Extremities and the Trunk. Book 2 Arterial Anastomotic Pathways of the Extremities. St Louis, MO: Quality Medical Publishing.
  Contains the translated work of Dr Michel Salmon concerning the blood supply to muscle as well as the anastomotic pathways in the limbs.

Sheetz KK, Bishop AT, Berger RA 1995 The arterial blood supply of the distal radius and ulna and its potential use in vascularized pedicled bone grafts. J Hand Surg 20A: 902–914.

Leiber RL, Jacobson MD, Fazeli BM, Abrams RA, Botte MJ. Architecture of selected muscles of the arm and forearm: anatomy and implications for tendon transfer. J Hand Surg 1992; 17A: 787–98.

Tan ST, Smith PJ. Anomalous extensor muscles of the hand: a review. J Hand Surg 1999; 24A: 449–55.

Leibovic SJ, Hastings II H. Martin–Gruber revisited. J Hand Surg 1992; 17A: 47–53.
  Examines the literature on reported connections between the median and ulnar nerves in the forearm and classifies these connections.

Wrist and hand

53

SKIN

DORSAL SKIN VERSUS PALMAR SKIN

The skin over the dorsum of the hand is thin and mobile and this allows for flexion at the metacarpophalangeal and interphalangeal joints. The dorsal skin is frequently hirsute over the dorsal aspect of the proximal phalanges and the ulnar aspect of the dorsum of the hand. In comparison, the palm is adapted for padding and anchorage. The palmar skin and the skin over the volar surface of the digits is thick and hairless, and has a well-defined stratum lucidum, a higher density of nerve endings, and eccrine sweat glands, but no sebaceous glands.

SKIN CREASES AND FINGERPRINTS (Fig. 53.1)

Flexure lines commonly crease the skin across the flexor surfaces of the wrist and hand (**Fig. 53.1**). Though not all directly over their function-ally related subjacent skeletal joints, they are produced by adhesion of the skin to subjacent deep fascia and are sites of folding of the skin during movement. These flexures are useful landmarks. Less regular, but quite prominent, crease-line complexes are centred over the dorsal (extensor) aspects of the radiocarpal, carpal, metacarpophalangeal and interphalangeal joints. They are mainly transverse but display varying curvatures. During flexion the dorsal skin is stretched and the lines

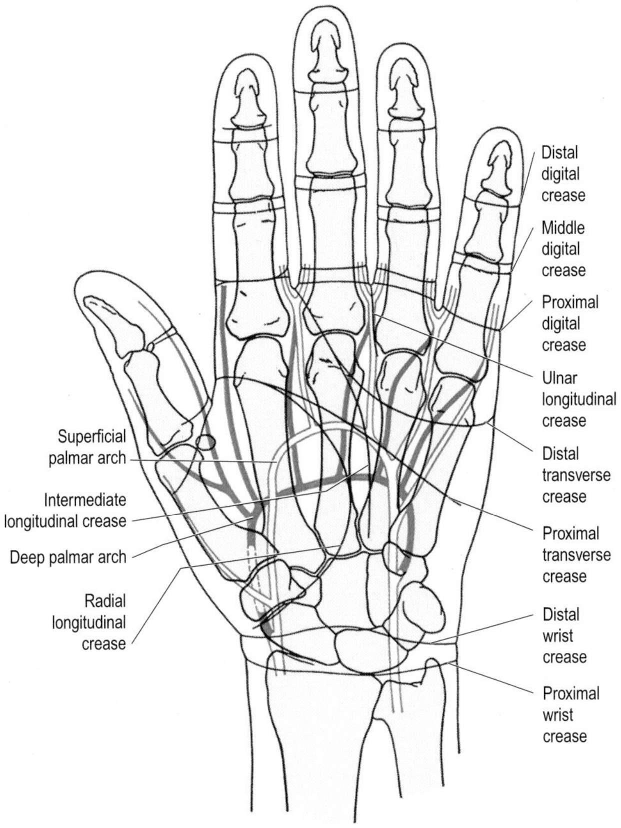

become less prominent (but can still be identified). During extension the now redundant skin becomes increasingly puckered and the lines are finally maximally prominent. (For a general review of 'skin lines' see p. 173.)

Near the junction of the carpus and forearm there are usually three anterior transverse lines. The proximal marks the proximal limit of the flexor synovial sheaths, an intermediate line overlies the wrist joint, and a distal line is at the proximal border of the flexor retinaculum.

In the palm a curved radial longitudinal line encircles the thenar eminence, ending at the radial (lateral) margin of the palm. Several less constant longitudinal lines lie medial and roughly parallel to it. Proximal and distal transverse lines ascend medially across the palm. The proximal line begins at the distal end of the radial longitudinal line and runs obliquely to the middle of the hypothenar eminence across the shafts of the metacarpals. The distal line begins at or near the cleft between the index and middle finger and crosses the palm with a proximal convexity over the second to fourth metacarpal heads, near the proximal ends of the fibrous flexor sheaths.

The second to fifth digits show proximal, middle and distal sets of transverse lines. The proximal, often double, are at the digital roots, c.2 cm distal to the metacarpophalangeal joints. The middle are typically double: the proximal line lies directly over the proximal interphalangeal joint. The distal lines are usually single, and lie proximal to the distal interphalangeal joints: their levels are sometimes marked by a fainter, more distal line. The free pollicial base is partly encircled by a line which starts on the radial side and crosses distally over the metacarpophalangeal joint to end between the thumb and index finger level with the base of the proximal pollicial phalanx. There is a second, shorter crease c.1 cm distal to this line. There are two lines comparable to the middle digital lines in other digits opposite the interphalangeal joint of the thumb. (*See also* p. 174.)

CUTANEOUS VASCULAR SUPPLY (Fig. 53.2)

The skin of the volar aspect of the wrist is supplied directly by cutaneous branches from the superficial palmar branch of the radial artery, the ulnar artery and occasionally the median artery if it is large enough. The skin over the thenar eminence is supplied by small perforating branches from the superficial palmar branch of the radial artery and the princeps pollicis. The skin over the hypothenar eminence is supplied by per-forating branches from the ulnar artery, some of which pass through palmaris brevis. The remainder of the palm is supplied by small perforating branches from the common palmar digital arteries which pierce the palmar aponeurosis, and small branches from the radialis indicis artery. The blood supply to the volar aspect of the digital skin comes from small branches from each digital artery. At the level of the distal phalanx the two digital arteries typically form an H-shaped anastomosis from which cutaneous perforators fan out within the pulp. Deep digital veins accompanying the digital arteries are usually very small and frequently absent. More commonly, superficial palmar veins tend to pass dorsally and drain into the larger superficial dorsal venous system.

The skin of the dorsal aspect of the wrist is supplied by branches from a plexus overlying the extensor retinaculum. Branches from the radial artery, including its dorsal carpal branch, dorsal carpal branch of the ulnar artery, and anterior and posterior interosseous arteries all contribute to this plexus. The blood supply to the dorsum of the hand arises from longitudinal rows of four or five tiny branches from each of the dorsal metacarpal arteries, which usually arise either from the radial artery directly or the dorsal carpal arch. At the level of the neck of the

Fig. 53.1 Relation of the skin flexure lines and palmar arterial arches to the bones of the left hand.

Distal digital crease

Middle digital crease

Proximal digital crease

Ulnar longitudinal crease

Distal transverse crease

Proximal transverse crease

Distal wrist crease

Proximal wrist crease

Superficial palmar arch

Intermediate longitudinal crease

Deep palmar arch

Radial longitudinal crease

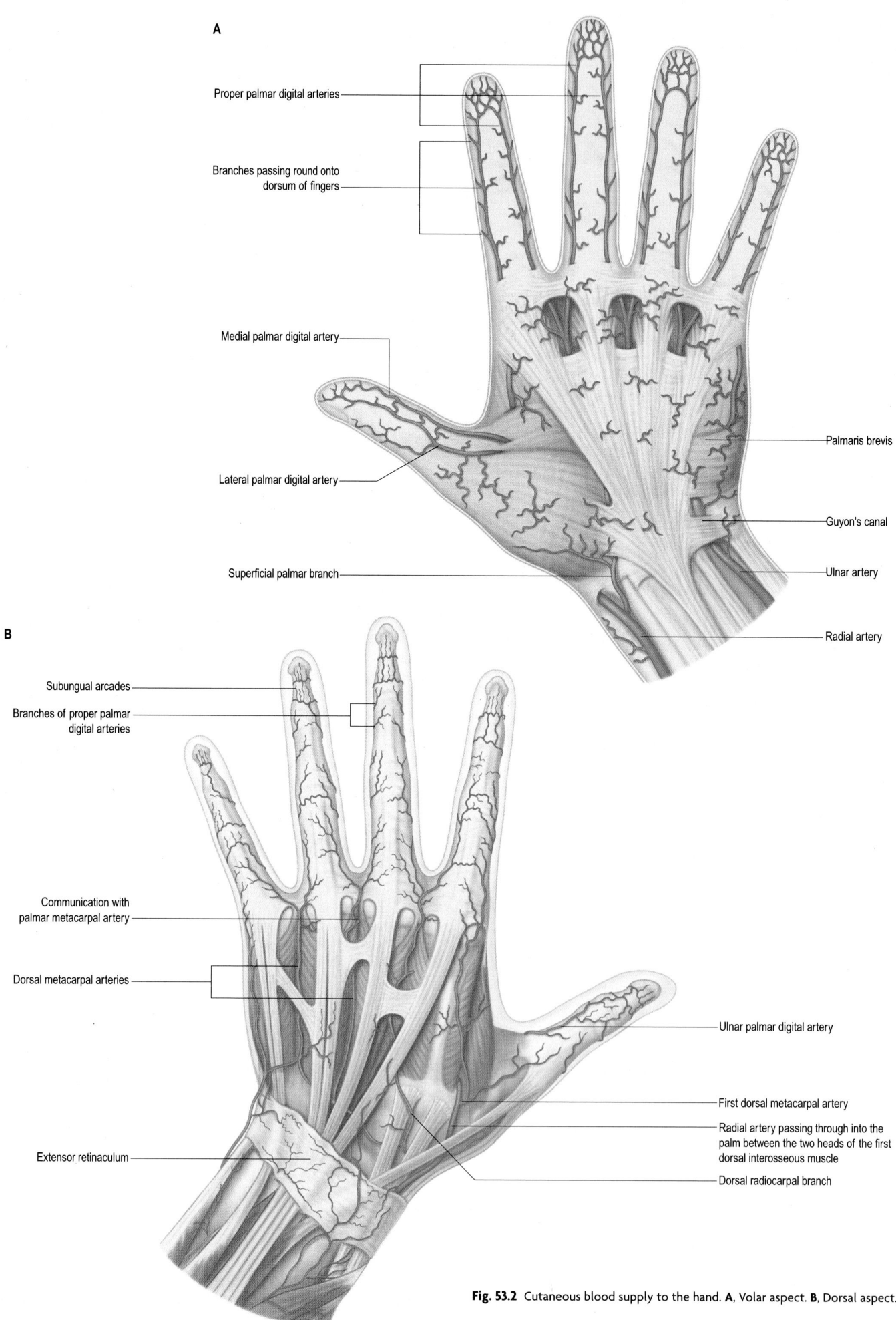

A

Proper palmar digital arteries

Branches passing round onto dorsum of fingers

Medial palmar digital artery

Lateral palmar digital artery

Superficial palmar branch

Palmaris brevis

Guyon's canal

Ulnar artery

Radial artery

B

Subungual arcades

Branches of proper palmar digital arteries

Communication with palmar metacarpal artery

Dorsal metacarpal arteries

Extensor retinaculum

Ulnar palmar digital artery

First dorsal metacarpal artery

Radial artery passing through into the palm between the two heads of the first dorsal interosseous muscle

Dorsal radiocarpal branch

Fig. 53.2 Cutaneous blood supply to the hand. **A**, Volar aspect. **B**, Dorsal aspect.

metacarpals, where the second, third and fourth dorsal metacarpal arteries communicate with branches from the corresponding common palmar digital arteries, a large cutaneous perforating branch passes proximally to supply an area of skin as far as the dorsal aspect of the wrist.

The blood supply to the dorsum of the fingers comes proximally from the terminal branches of the dorsal metacarpal arteries – supplying a region as far distally as the proximal interphalangeal joint – as well as from dorsal branches of the palmar digital arteries which are given off at each phalangeal level. At the level of the distal phalanx the cutaneous supply comes from three dorsal arcades: a superficial arcade over the base of the distal phalanx, and two distal subungual arcades. The skin of the dorsum of the thumb is supplied by longitudinal axial branches of the princeps pollicis and dorsal branches from the palmar digital arteries.

CUTANEOUS INNERVATION (Fig. 53.3)

The skin of the volar aspect of the wrist is innervated by the terminal branches of the lateral and medial cutaneous nerves of the forearm. The skin of the palm is innervated by the palmar branches of the ulnar nerve and the palmar branch of the median nerve. The skin of the volar aspect of the thumb, index, middle and radial aspect of the ring fingers is supplied by cutaneous branches of the median nerve, while that of the little finger and ulnar side of the ring finger is supplied by the ulnar nerve.

The cutaneous innervation of the radial aspect of the dorsum of the wrist and hand, as well as the dorsal aspect of the radial three and a half digits as far distally as the nail bed, arises from the terminal branches of the radial nerve, the dorsal digital nerves. Between two and five dorsal digital nerves supply each digit. The cutaneous innervation of the ulnar aspect of the dorsum of the wrist and hand, and the dorsal aspect of the ulnar one and a half digits as far distally as the nail bed, arises from the dorsal branch of the ulnar nerve, again ending as dorsal digital nerves. The skin of the dorsum of the middle and distal phalanges is also supplied by dorsal branches of the palmar digital nerves.

NAIL APPARATUS

The nail apparatus consists of the nail plate, proximal and lateral nail folds, nail matrix, nail bed and hyponychium. It is described on page 167.

SOFT TISSUE

PALMAR FASCIAL COMPLEX

The palmar fascia is a three-dimensional ligamentous system composed of longitudinal, transverse and vertical fibres (**Fig. 53.4**).

LONGITUDINAL FIBRE SYSTEM

The longitudinal fibres represent the phylogenetically degenerated metacarpophalangeal joint flexor. They run proximally from the palmaris longus tendon or the flexor retinaculum of the wrist across the whole width of the central third of the palm, producing four well-defined longitudinal bundles to the index, middle, ring and little fingers. A less well-defined bundle passes to the thumb. Distal to the transverse fibres of the palmar aponeurosis the longitudinal fibres pass in three layers (McGrouther 1982). The most superficial longitudinal fibres (layer 1) are inserted superficially into the skin of the distal palm between the distal palmar crease and the proximal digital crease. Some superficial fibres pass distally into the palmar midline of the digit. Deeper longitudinal fibres (layer 2) pass deep to the natatory ligament and neurovascular bundles into the apex of the web space skin and into the fingers themselves where they are continuous with Cleland's ligaments and the lateral digital sheet. These are known as the spiral bands of Gosset. Deeper still, the longitudinal fibres in layer 3 perforate the deep transverse metacarpal ligament to pass around the sides of the metacarpophalangeal joint and attach to the metacarpal bone and proximal phalanx, and extensor tendon.

TRANSVERSE FIBRE SYSTEM

The transverse fibre system consists of the natatory ligament (also known as superficial transverse metacarpal ligament), the transverse fibres of the palmar aponeurosis (also known as fibres of Skoog), and the transverse metacarpal ligament (also known as the deep transverse metacarpal ligament).

Natatory ligament (superficial transverse metacarpal ligament)

The fibres of the natatory ligament (superficial transverse metacarpal ligament) cross the apex of the web skin and extend into the digit to blend with the lateral digital sheet, thus limiting the spreading of the skin of the distal palm and the separation of the adjacent fingers. The natatory ligament in the first web is called the distal commissural ligament.

Transverse fibres of the palmar aponeurosis

The transverse fibres of the palmar aponeurosis (fibres of Skoog) lie more proximally than the natatory fibres and represent the deepest layer of the palmar fascia. They lie proximal to the distal palmar crease in a band c.2 cm wide, and connect the anterior fibres of the flexor tendon sheaths with one another and to the fasciae over the thenar and hypothenar muscles groups. The extension to the first ray is called the proximal commissural ligament.

Transverse metacarpal ligament

The strong transverse fibres of the transverse metacarpal ligament are deep to the palmar aponeurosis and flexor sheaths. They connect the metacarpal heads of the index to little fingers by their attachment with the volar plates.

VERTICAL FIBRE SYSTEM

The vertical fibres are more delicate, and pass from the dermis, between the longitudinal and transverse fibres, to the fibrous flexor sheaths and the metacarpal bones. They are concentrated on either side of the palmar skin creases as well as the thenar and hypothenar eminences.

A series of vertical septa lie deep to the transverse fibres of the palmar aponeurosis, and connect it to the underlying deep transverse ligament. They provide compartments which contain the flexor tendons and the lumbricals and neurovascular bundles.

DUPUYTREN'S DISEASE

Dupuytren's disease (contracture) is a progressive condition of uncertain aetiology resulting from fibrous contracture of the palmar aponeurosis where the little and ring fingers are especially affected. Longitudinal thickening in the palm produces cords and thickened nodules which can progress to flexion deformities of the metacarpophalangeal and proximal interphalangeal joints of the affected fingers. The palmar aponeurosis only extends as far as the sides of the middle phalanx, therefore the distal interphalangeal joint is uncommonly involved. Indeed, in advanced cases, the distal interphalangeal joint can be hyperextended as the distal phalanx is pushed backwards against the palm.

The pattern of fascial involvement in this condition can be complex. For example, the normal anatomical position of the digital nerves and arteries may be distorted because they are often displaced medially. Since surgical treatment involves excising the affected area of palmar fascia, the digital nerves and arteries may be at risk in this procedure.

A similar contracture may affect the plantar fascia in the sole of the foot.

DIGITAL FASCIAL COMPLEX (Fig. 53.4)

The superficial fascia within the finger is fibrofatty in the palmar and dorsal aspects, but more sheet-like laterally, where it is termed the lateral digital sheet. Within the core of the finger the fascia is thickened in areas, forming the flexor sheath, Cleland's, Grayson's and Landsmeer's ligaments. The flexor sheath is discussed in detail on page 913. Cleland's ligaments extend from the sides of the phalanges, pass dorsal to the neurovascular bundles and insert into the lateral digital sheet. Grayson's ligaments are more delicate, may even be discontinuous and pass from the lateral sides of the phalanges volar to the neurovascular bundles to insert into the lateral digital sheet. Landsmeer's ligaments are inconsistent anatomical structures made up of transverse and oblique retinacular ligaments (see **Fig. 53.43**). The transverse retinacular ligament passes from the A3 pulley of the fibrous flexor sheath at the level of the proximal interphalangeal joint to the lateral border of the lateral extensor band. The oblique retinacular ligament lies deep to the transverse retinacular ligament. It originates from the lateral aspect of the proximal phalanx and flexor sheath (A2 pulley) and passes volar to the axis of rotation of

A

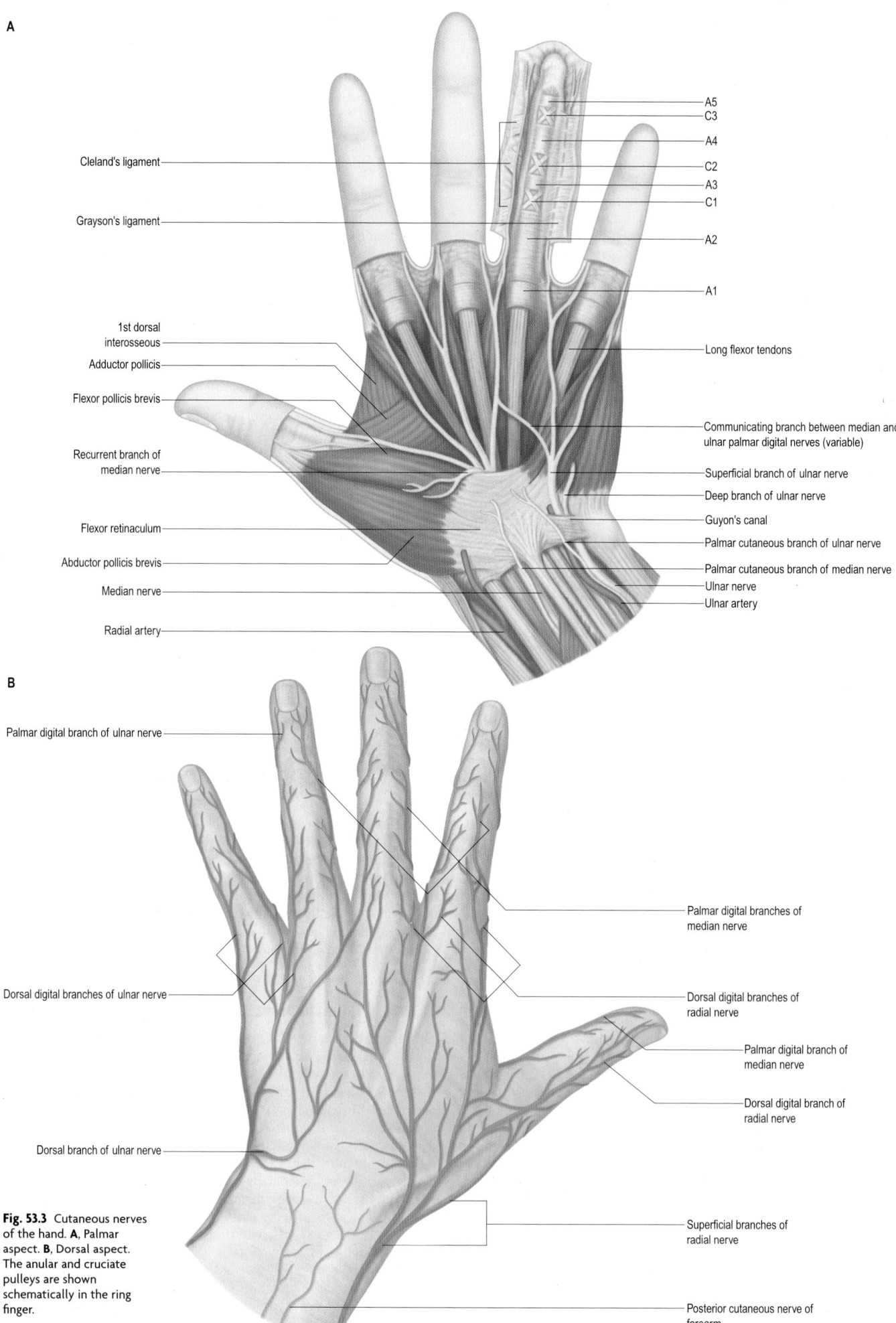

Cleland's ligament

Grayson's ligament

1st dorsal interosseous

Adductor pollicis

Flexor pollicis brevis

Recurrent branch of median nerve

Flexor retinaculum

Abductor pollicis brevis

Median nerve

Radial artery

A5
C3
A4
C2
A3
C1
A2
A1

Long flexor tendons

Communicating branch between median and ulnar palmar digital nerves (variable)

Superficial branch of ulnar nerve

Deep branch of ulnar nerve

Guyon's canal

Palmar cutaneous branch of ulnar nerve

Palmar cutaneous branch of median nerve

Ulnar nerve

Ulnar artery

B

Palmar digital branch of ulnar nerve

Dorsal digital branches of ulnar nerve

Dorsal branch of ulnar nerve

Palmar digital branches of median nerve

Dorsal digital branches of radial nerve

Palmar digital branch of median nerve

Dorsal digital branch of radial nerve

Superficial branches of radial nerve

Posterior cutaneous nerve of forearm

Fig. 53.3 Cutaneous nerves of the hand. **A**, Palmar aspect. **B**, Dorsal aspect. The anular and cruciate pulleys are shown schematically in the ring finger.

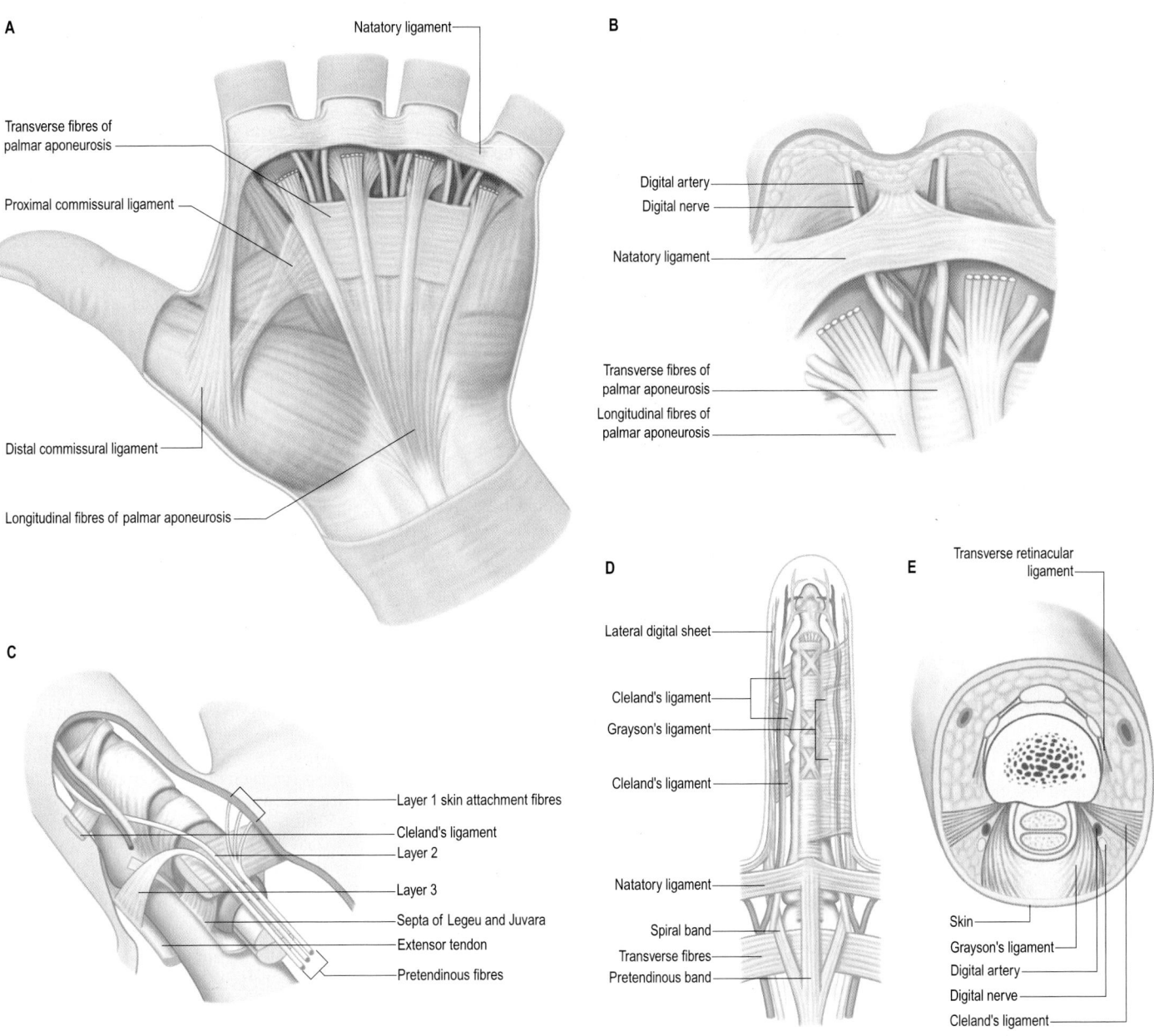

Fig. 53.4 Palmar aponeurosis and distal fascial complex. **A**, Schematic diagram of the palmar fascia. **B**, More detailed view of structures at the web space. **C**, Fate of the distal longitudinal fibres. **D**, **E**, Normal digital fascia.

the proximal interphalangeal joint in a dorsal and distal direction to insert into the terminal extensor tendon.

FUNCTIONS OF THE FASCIA OF THE HAND

The fascial continuum of the hand performs a number of different, but inter-related, functions. It channels and lubricates structures in transit between the forearm and the digits; transmits loads; anchors the skin; protects underlying vessels; and provides a framework for muscle attachments.

Channelling of structures in transit between forearm and digits

The vertical septa act as spacers between the tendons and neurovascular bundles of the individual digital rays.

Where tendons change direction around a concave surface the channels are thickened. They perform a retinacular role, forming sheaths with specialized pulleys to prevent the tendon springing away from the underlying skeleton (see flexor tendon sheaths, p. 913).

Transmission of loads

At points where compressive loading is applied to the hand, such as the finger pulp and palm, loculi of fat act as shock absorbers. The loculi

are contained within defined fibrous boundaries, which means that the shape, but not the volume, of each loculus can change. The compliance or deformability of the boundaries determines the amount of shock absorption. Local 'turgor' (deformability) and blood volume are measures of this anatomical property.

The palm also contains much larger fibrous compartments between skin and skeleton which transmit muscles, tendons and other structures. The honeycomb pattern of these compartments constitutes the palmar shock absorption system. The soft padded parts of the hand are able to conform to the contours of objects which are grasped, and this permits better interpretation of sensation and better grip.

The hand must also resist tensile loading. Tendons and ligaments are particularly suitable for resisting such forces but many other parts of the fascial continuum, e.g. the anchorage system of the palm, also play a major role in resisting 'pulling' forces.

Anchorage

Skin is retained by fascial ligaments which allow the hand to flex while retaining the skin in position. Skin folds at palmar and digital creases possess few deep-anchoring fibres. However, the skin on either side of the crease lines contains deep anchorage ligaments, and these allow the unanchored skin between them to fold in a repetitive pattern. The palmar creases have been described as skin 'joints'. Fascial anchors may be vertical (perpendicular to the palm), e.g. in the midpalm where scattered vertical fibres run from the dermis down into the depths of the hand; horizontal (in the plane of the palm); or oblique to the skin surface.

The insertion of the longitudinal (pretendinous) fibres of the palmar aponeurosis is an example of a well-developed horizontal anchorage system. The most superficial longitudinal fibres insert into the dermis of the distal palm. This arrangement resists horizontal shearing force in gripping tasks, e.g. holding a golf club, where it prevents distal skin slippage or degloving of the palm on striking the golf ball. The characteristic blisters on the palms of those unaccustomed to such sports map out the sites of the skin anchorage points. This anchorage system can be demonstrated by flexing the palm until the skin of the distal palm folds loosely. An attempt to pull the loose skin distally will reveal the anchoring longitudinal fibres of the palmar aponeurosis.

Oblique anchors occur in the fingers where Cleland's ligaments tether the skin of the proximal and middle segments of the digits to the region of the proximal interphalangeal joints.

Binding

Transversely orientated fascial structures help to maintain the transverse arch of the hand by 'binding' the underlying skeletal structures or the tendon sheaths.

Limiting or tethering

Joint motion is limited not only by joint ligamentous action, but also in some cases by skin tightness. Skin in the interdigital webs is generally reinforced by fascial ligamentous fibres which run just beneath the dermis in a direction which resists stretch. They are well developed in the thumb web.

Lubrication

There are many other gliding planes, e.g. between periosteum and the extensor apparatus, and between the latter and the skin, on the dorsum of the digits. The flexor tendon sheaths possess low friction and are lubricated by synovial fluid.

Vascular protection and pumping action

The blood vessels of the palm are surrounded by a cuff of tough fascia or by a fatty pad. When the hand is compressed, as in gripping, these relatively incompressible fascial structures function as a venous pumping mechanism to assist return of blood from the limb. In contrast, large capacitance veins on the dorsum of the hand lie in gliding skin, surrounded by loose areolar tissue, which allows venous dilatation.

Framework for muscle attachments

Many of the small muscles of the hand are attached to the fascial skeleton, at least in part, e.g. abductor pollicis brevis, palmaris longus. The fascial framework can be visualized as a harness by which muscles can act on the underlying skeleton. For example, the metacarpophalangeal joint is moved by a ring of fascial and ligamentous structures which surround the joint and to which tendons are attached.

DIGITAL AND PALMAR SPACES

There are many potential spaces within the hand, often with ill-defined margins.

The nail fold is a 'U-shaped' space made up of the eponychium and the lateral nail fold. The apical spaces at the tip of the finger are formed by the fibrous attachments of the distal phalanx to the tip of the digital pulp skin. The digital pulp spaces are confined compartments bounded by the digital creases which overlie the joints, and are attached to the underlying pulleys. The synovial flexor tendon sheaths are described on page 913. The web space is bounded distally by the skin and natatory ligament, by the deep transverse metacarpal ligament posteriorly, and by the deep attachments of the palmar fascia, together with their lateral attachments to the tendon sheaths proximally. The deep palmar space is a complex three-dimensional space limited proximally by the carpal tunnel. It lies deep to the palmar aponeurosis, between the radial and ulnar condensations of vertical fibres which connect the palmar aponeurosis to the thenar and hypothenar eminences. Partitions which pass deeply from the longitudinal bands of the palmar aponeurosis form eight narrow compartments: four contain the digital flexor

tendons and four contain the lumbricals and the neurovascular bundles.

INFECTIONS OF THE HAND

The spaces of the hand limit the spread of infection. Infections in the digit can occur in the nail fold (paronychia), the apical spaces at the very tip of the finger, the distal pulps (a felon) and the flexor sheaths. Anatomically, because the flexor synovial sheath of the thumb and the little finger are continuous throughout the palm, they have the potential to spread infection to the palm and so communicate with other sheaths within the carpal tunnel. Pus can certainly spread proximally within flexor tendon sheaths, but from a clinical point of view it is as disastrous in those digits whose sheaths do not communicate with the carpal tunnel sheaths (index, middle, ring) as it is in those that do (thumb, little finger). It is preferable, therefore, to know the structures rather than the potential spaces between them. Deep infections in the palm are usually not confined to any particular space.

BONE

The skeleton of the hand consists of the carpus, metacarpus and the phalanges. In the following description, proximal and distal are used in preference to superior and inferior, and palmar and dorsal, rather than anterior and posterior.

CARPAL BONES (Figs 53.5, 53.6)

The carpus contains eight bones in proximal and distal rows of four. In radial (lateral) to ulnar (medial) order, the scaphoid, lunate, triquetrum and pisiform make up the proximal row, and the trapezium, trapezoid, capitate and hamate make up the distal row. The pisiform articulates with the palmar surface of the triquetrum, and is thus separated from the other carpal bones, all of which articulate with their neighbours. The other three proximal bones form an arch which is proximally convex, and which articulates with the radius and articular disc of the distal radio-ulnar joint. The concavity of the arch is a distal recess embracing, proximally, the projecting aspects of the capitate and hamate. The two rows of carpal bones are thus mutually and firmly adapted without any loss of movement.

The dorsal carpal surface is convex. The palmar surface forms a deeply concave carpal groove, accentuated by the palmar projection of the radial (lateral) and ulnar (medial) borders. The ulnar projection is formed by the pisiform and the hamulus (hook), an unciform palmar process of the hamate. The pisiform is at the proximal border of the hypothenar eminence, on the ulnar side of the palm, and it is easily felt in front of the triquetrum. The hamulus is concave in a radial direction, its tip is palpable 2.5 cm distal to the pisiform, in line with the radial border of the ring finger. The superficial division of the ulnar nerve can be rolled on it. The radial border of the carpal groove is formed by the tubercles of the scaphoid and trapezium. The former is distal on the anterior scaphoid surface and palpable (sometimes also visible) as a small medial knob at the proximal border of the palmar thenar eminence, radial to the tendon of flexor carpi radialis. The tubercle of the trapezium is a vertically rounded ridge on the anterior surface of the bone, slightly hollow medially and just distal and radial to the scaphoid tubercle: it is difficult to palpate. (Both the scaphoid and trapezium may be grasped individually, and moved passively, by firm pressure between an opposed index finger and thumb applied to the palmar surface and 'anatomical snuff-box' simultaneously.) The carpal groove is made into an osseofibrous carpal tunnel by a fibrous retinaculum attached to its margins. The tunnel carries flexor tendons and the median nerve into the hand. The retinaculum strengthens the carpus and augments flexor efficiency. Radiocarpal, intercarpal and carpometacarpal ligaments are attached to the palmar and dorsal surfaces of all of the carpal bones, except the triquetrum and pisiform.

INDIVIDUAL CARPAL BONES

Scaphoid

The scaphoid is the largest element in the proximal carpal row (**Fig. 53.7**). It has a long axis which is distal, radial and slightly palmar in direction. A round tubercle on the distolateral part of its palmar surface is directed anterolaterally (**Fig. 53.6**, left), and provides an attachment for the flexor retinaculum and abductor pollicis brevis: it is crossed by

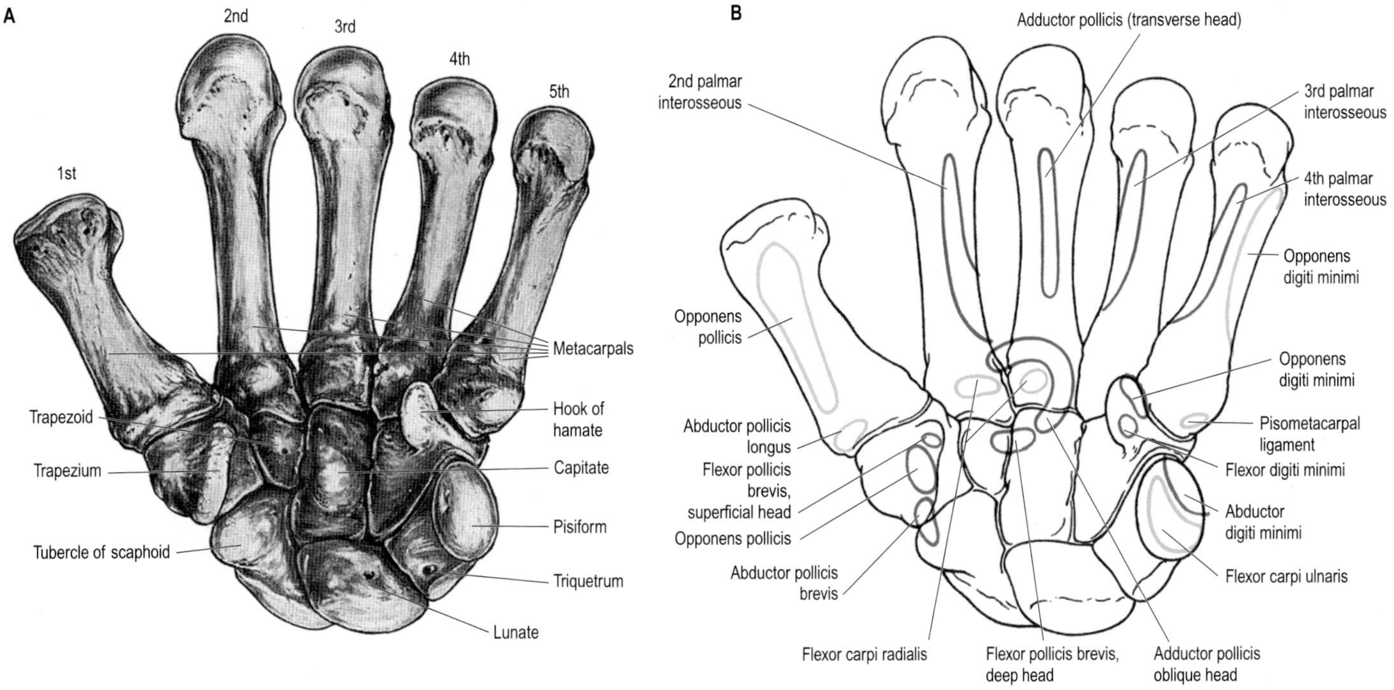

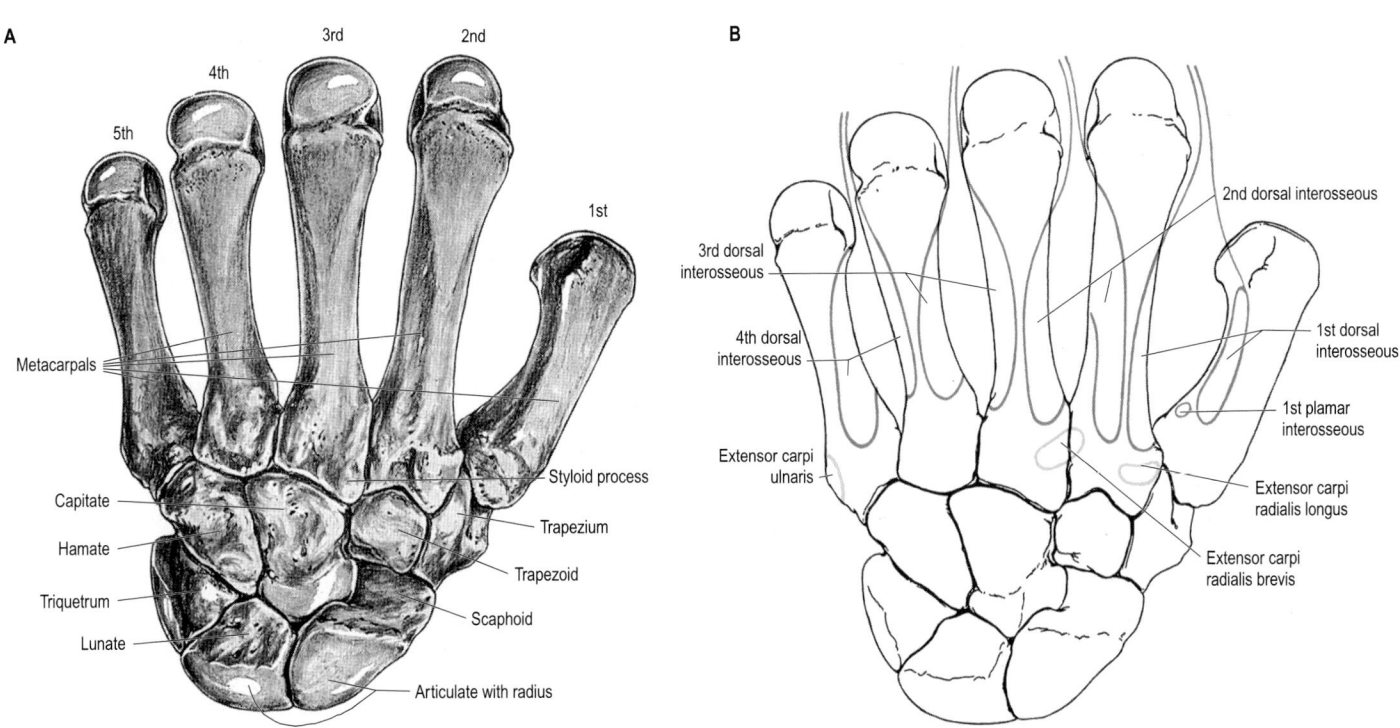

A

2nd 3rd 4th 5th

1st

Trapezoid

Trapezium

Tubercle of scaphoid

Metacarpals

Hook of hamate

Capitate

Pisiform

Triquetrum

Lunate

B

Adductor pollicis (transverse head)

2nd palmar interosseous

3rd palmar interosseous

4th palmar interosseous

Opponens digiti minimi

Opponens pollicis

Opponens digiti minimi

Abductor pollicis longus

Flexor pollicis brevis, superficial head

Opponens pollicis

Abductor pollicis brevis

Pisometacarpal ligament

Flexor digiti minimi

Abductor digiti minimi

Flexor carpi ulnaris

Flexor carpi radialis

Flexor pollicis brevis, deep head

Adductor pollicis oblique head

Fig. 53.5 Palmar aspect of the carpal and metacarpal bones of the left hand. Muscle attachments, except for the dorsal interossei, are shown on the line drawing on the right.

A

3rd 2nd

4th

5th

1st

Metacarpals

Capitate

Hamate

Triquetrum

Lunate

Styloid process

Trapezium

Trapezoid

Scaphoid

Articulate with radius

B

2nd dorsal interosseous

3rd dorsal interosseous

4th dorsal interosseous

1st dorsal interosseous

1st plamar interosseous

Extensor carpi ulnaris

Extensor carpi radialis longus

Extensor carpi radialis brevis

Fig. 53.6 Dorsal aspect of the carpal and metacarpal bones of the left hand. Muscle attachments are shown on the line drawing on the right.

the tendon of flexor carpi radialis. The rough dorsal surface is slightly grooved, narrower than the palmar, and pierced by small nutrient foramina, which are often restricted to the distal half (13%). The radial collateral ligament is attached to the lateral surface, which is also narrow and rough. The remaining surfaces are all articular. The radial (proximal) surface is convex, proximal and directed proximolaterally; the lunate surface is flat, semilunar, and faces medially; the capitate surface is large, concave and distal, and directed distomedially. The surface for the trapezium and trapezoid is continuous, convex and distal.

Scaphoid bone fractures – The scaphoid is the most frequently fractured carpal bone, typically as a result of a fall onto an outstretched hand. The fracture usually crosses the long axis of the bone. Fractures of its proximal part or its 'waist' may fail to unite because the proximal fragment has lost its blood supply: avascular necrosis of the proximal fragment is then inevitable.

Lunate

The lunate is approximately semilunar and articulates between the scaphoid and triquetrum in the proximal carpal row (**Fig. 53.8**). Its rough

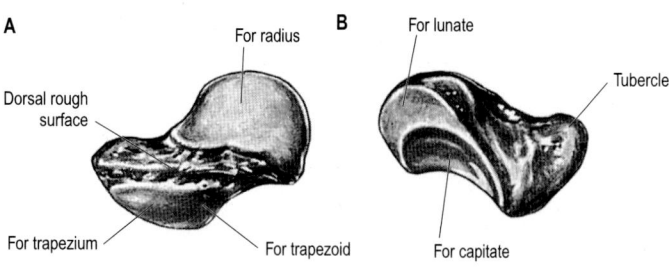

Fig. 53.7 The left scaphoid: **A**, dorsal, **B**, palmar aspects.

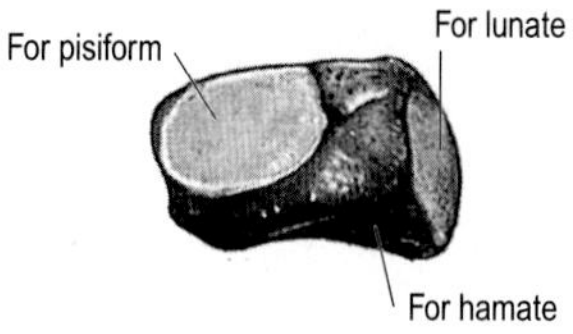

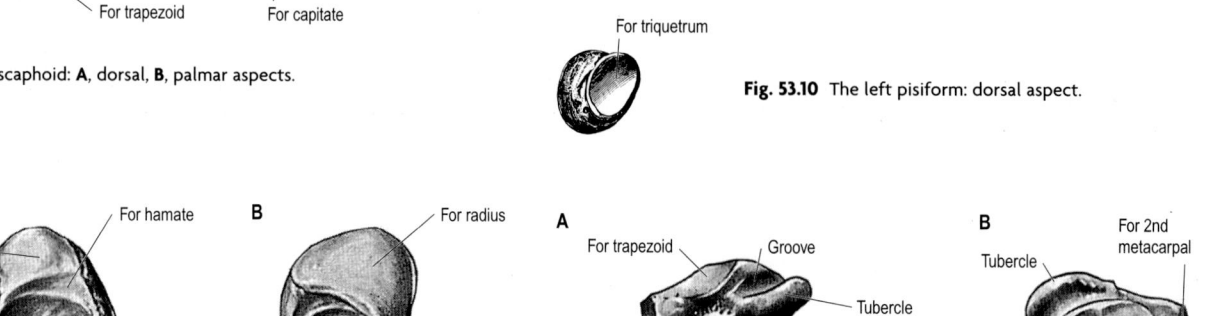

Fig. 53.9 The left triquetrum: palmar aspect.

Fig. 53.10 The left pisiform: dorsal aspect.

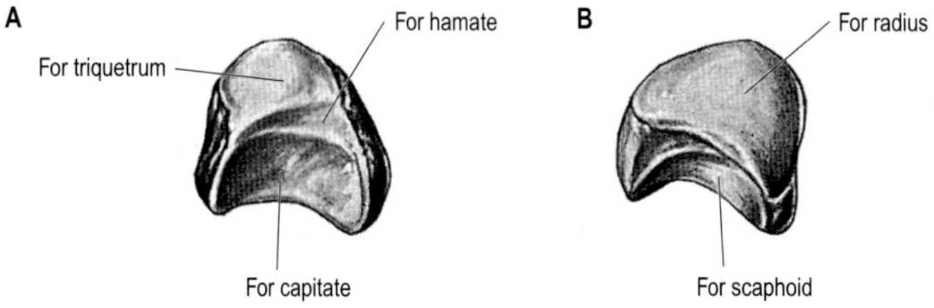

Fig. 53.8 The left lunate: **A**, distomedial; **B**, proximolateral aspects.

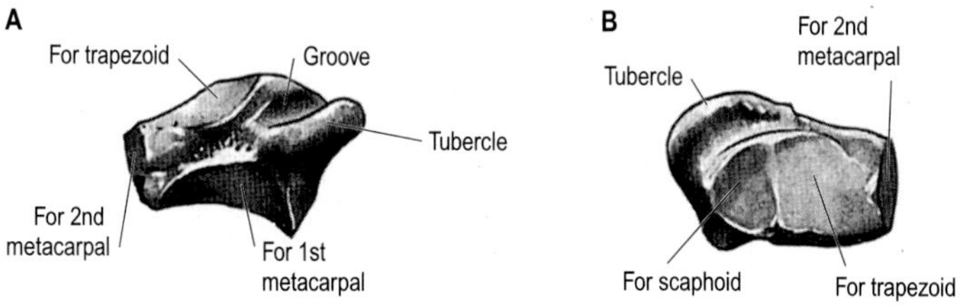

Fig. 53.11 The left trapezium: **A**, palmar; **B**, proximomedial aspects.

palmar surface, almost triangular, is larger and wider than the rough dorsal surface. Its smooth convex proximal surface articulates with the radius and the articular disc of the distal radio-ulnar joint. Its narrow lateral surface bears a flat semilunar facet for the scaphoid. The medial surface, almost square, articulates with the triquetrum and is separated from the distal surface by a curved ridge, usually somewhat concave for articulation with the edge of the hamate in adduction (**Fig. 53.8A**). The distal surface is deeply concave to fit the medial part of the head of the capitate.

Triquetrum

The triquetrum is somewhat pyramidal and bears an oval isolated facet for articulation with the pisiform on its distal palmar surface (**Fig. 53.9**). Its medial and dorsal surfaces are confluent, and marked distally by the attachment of the ulnar collateral ligament, but smooth proximally to receive the articular disc of the distal radio-ulnar joint in full adduction. The hamate surface, lateral and distal, is concavoconvex, broad proximally, narrow distally. The lunate surface, almost square, is proximal and lateral.

Pisiform

The pisiform is shaped like a pea, with a distolateral long axis (**Fig. 53.10**). It bears a dorsal flat articular facet for the triquetrum. The tendon of flexor carpi ulnaris and the distal continuations of the tendon, the pisometacarpal and pisohamate ligaments, are all attached to the palmar non-articular area, which surrounds and projects distal to the articular surface. The pisiform therefore has attributes of a sesamoid bone.

Trapezium

The trapezium has a tubercle and groove on its rough palmar surface (**Fig. 53.11**). The groove, which is medial, contains the tendon of flexor carpi radialis, and two layers of the flexor retinaculum are attached to its margins (**Fig. 53.12**) (p. 913). The tubercle is obscured by the thenar muscles which are attached to it (opponens pollicis, flexor pollicis brevis and abductor pollicis brevis) (**Fig. 53.5B**). The elongated, rough dorsal surface is related to the radial artery. The large lateral surface is rough for attachment of the radial collateral ligament and capsular ligament of the thumb carpometacarpal joint. A large sellar surface faces distolaterally and articulates with the base of the first metacarpal. Most distally it projects between the bases of the first and second metacarpal bones and carries a small, quadrilateral, distomedially directed facet which articulates with the base of the second metacarpal. The large medial surface is gently concave for articulation with the trapezoid. The proximal surface is a small, slightly concave facet for

articulation with the scaphoid. Its ridge, or 'summit', fits the concavity of the first metacarpal base, and extends in a palmar and lateral direction, at an angle of c.60° with the plane of the second and third metacarpals. Abduction and adduction occur in the plane of the ridge, which is shorter than the corresponding metacarpal groove. Their contours vary reciprocally: they are more curved near the second metacarpal base, whereas the radius of curvature is longer further away from this site. The two surfaces are not completely congruent, and the area of close contact probably moves towards the palm in adduction and dorsally in abduction. While the axis of flexion/extension passes through the trapezium, that for adduction/abduction is in the metacarpal base. Flexion is accompanied by medial rotation, and extension by lateral rotation (p. 910).

Trapezoid

The trapezoid is small and irregular. It has a rough palmar surface which is narrower and smaller than its rough dorsal surface: the former invades the lateral aspect (**Fig. 53.13**). The distal surface, which articulates with the grooved base of the second metacarpal, is triangular, convex transversely and concave at right angles to this. The medial surface articulates by a concave facet with the distal part of the capitate, the lateral surface articulates with the trapezium, and the proximal surface articulates with the scaphoid.

Capitate

The capitate is the central and largest carpal bone. It articulates with the base of the third metacarpal via its triangular distal concavoconvex surface (**Fig. 53.14**). Its lateral border is a concave strip for articulation with the medial side of the base of the second metacarpal. Its dorso-medial angle usually bears a facet for articulation with the base of the fourth metacarpal. The head projects into the concavity formed by the lunate and scaphoid: the proximal surface articulates with the lunate, and the lateral surface with the scaphoid. The facets for the scaphoid and trapezoid, though usually continuous on the distolateral surface, may be separated by a rough interval. The medial surface bears a large facet for articulation with the hamate, which is deeper proximally where it is partly non-articular. Palmar and dorsal surfaces are roughened for carpal ligaments, the dorsal being the larger.

Hamate

The hamate is cuneiform and bears an unciform hamulus (hook) which projects from the distal part of its rough palmar surface. The hamulus is curved with a lateral concavity and its tip inclines laterally, contributing to the medial wall of the carpal tunnel (**Fig. 53.15**). The

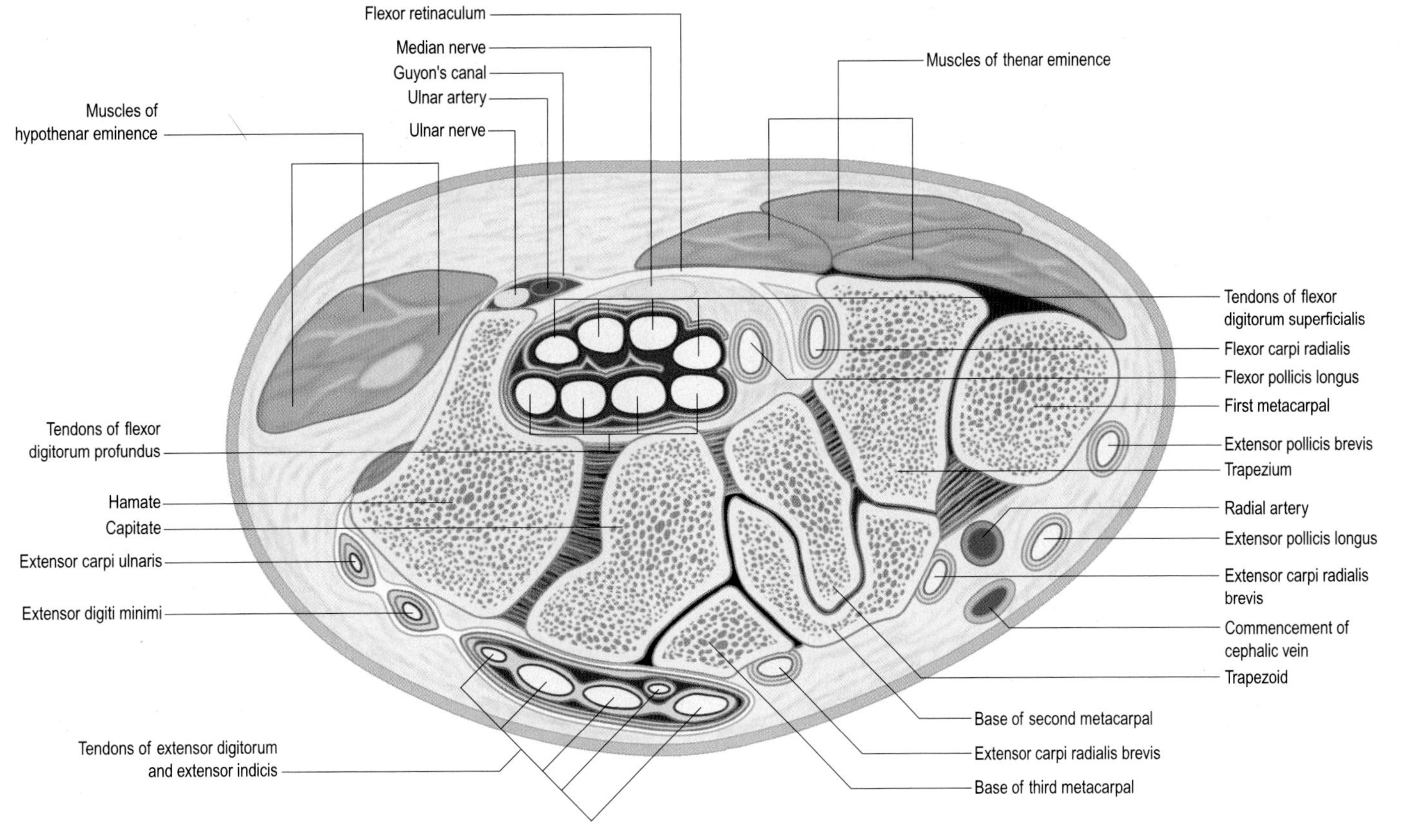

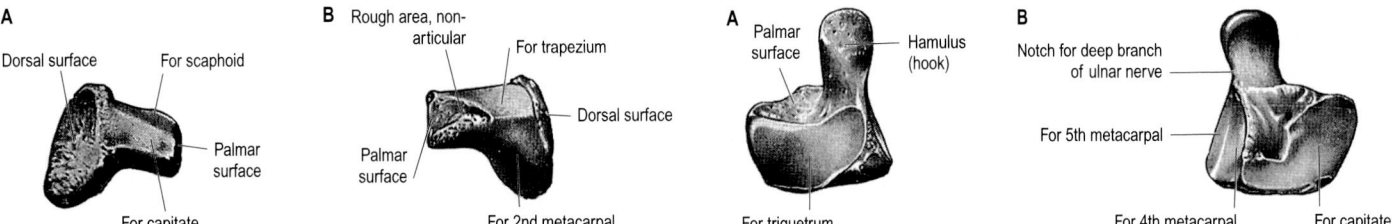

Muscles of hypothenar eminence

Flexor retinaculum
Median nerve
Guyon's canal
Ulnar artery
Ulnar nerve

Muscles of thenar eminence

Tendons of flexor digitorum superficialis
Flexor carpi radialis
Flexor pollicis longus
First metacarpal
Extensor pollicis brevis
Trapezium
Radial artery
Extensor pollicis longus
Extensor carpi radialis brevis
Commencement of cephalic vein
Trapezoid

Tendons of flexor digitorum profundus
Hamate
Capitate
Extensor carpi ulnaris
Extensor digiti minimi

Tendons of extensor digitorum and extensor indicis

Base of second metacarpal
Extensor carpi radialis brevis
Base of third metacarpal

Fig. 53.12 Transverse section through the left wrist, showing the tendons and their synovial sheaths: distal aspect. The section is slightly oblique and passes through the distal row of the carpus and the bases of the first, second and third metacarpal bones. Note that the carpometacarpal joint of the thumb is separate from the joint between the trapezium and the base of the second metacarpal bone.

A
Dorsal surface
For scaphoid
Palmar surface
For capitate

B Rough area, non-articular
For trapezium
Dorsal surface
Palmar surface
For 2nd metacarpal

Fig. 53.13 The left trapezoid: **A**, proximomedial; **B**, distolateral aspects.

A
Palmar surface
Hamulus (hook)
For triquetrum

B
Notch for deep branch of ulnar nerve
For 5th metacarpal
For 4th metacarpal
For capitate

Fig. 53.15 The left hamate: **A**, medial; **B**, lateral aspects.

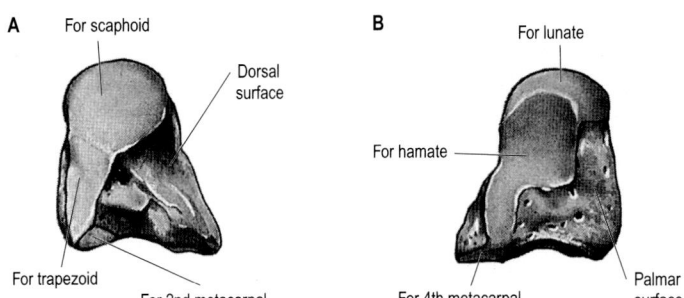

A
For scaphoid
Dorsal surface
For trapezoid
For 2nd metacarpal

B
For lunate
For hamate
For 4th metacarpal
Palmar surface

Fig. 53.14 The left capitate: **A**, lateral; **B**, medial aspects.

flexor retinaculum is attached to the apex of the hamulus. Distally, on the hamular base, a slight transverse groove may be in contact with the terminal deep branch of the ulnar nerve. The remaining palmar surface, like the dorsal, is roughened for attachment of ligaments. A faint ridge divides the distal surface into a smaller lateral facet which articulates with the base of the fourth metacarpal base, and a medial facet for articulation with the base of the fifth. The proximal surface, the thin margin of the wedge, usually bears a narrow facet which contacts the lunate in adduction. The medial surface is a broad strip, convex proximally, concave distally, which articulates with the triquetrum: distally a narrow medial strip is non-articular. The lateral surface articulates with the capitate by a facet covering all but its distal palmar angle.

OSSIFICATION (Figs 53.16, 53.17, 53.18, 53.19, 53.20)
Carpal bones are cartilaginous at birth, although ossification may have started in the capitate and hamate. Each carpal bone is ossified from

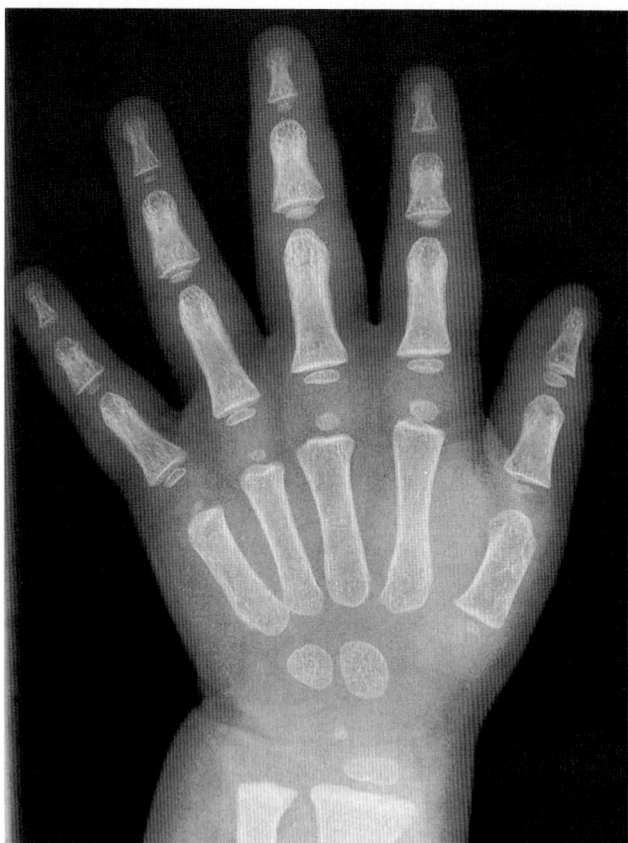

Fig. 53.16 Radiograph of a hand at $2\frac{1}{2}$ years (male), dorsopalmar projection. Note early stages of ossification in the epiphyses at the proximal ends of the phalanges and first metacarpal; at the distal ends of the remaining metacarpals and radius; in the capitate, hamate and lunate. Typically, the centre for the lunate is preceded by the centre for the triquetrum. Compare with **Figs 53.17** and **53.18**.

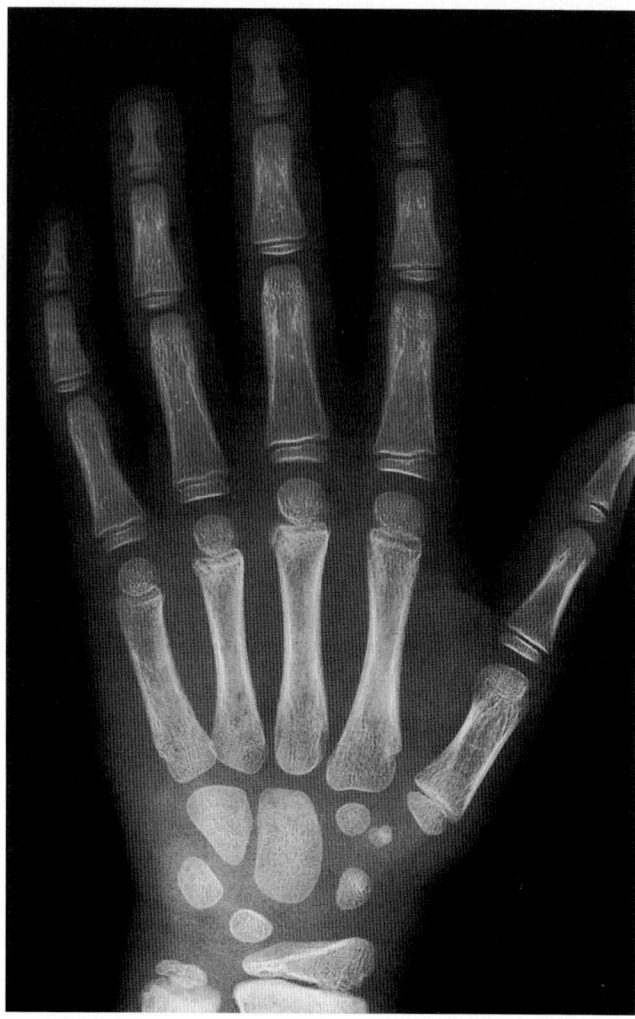

Fig. 53.17 Radiograph of a hand at $6\frac{1}{2}$ years (male), dorsopalmar projection. Note the more advanced state of the centres of ossification which were already visible in **Fig. 53.16**, and the appearance of additional centres in the distal ulnar epiphysis and in the triquetrum, scaphoid, trapezium and trapezoid.

one centre, capitate first, and pisiform last: the order in the others varies. The capitate begins to ossify in the second month, the hamate at the end of the third month, the triquetrum in the third year, the lunate, scaphoid, trapezium and trapezoid in the fourth year in females and fifth year in males. The pisiform begins to ossify in the ninth or tenth year in females, and the twelfth in males. The order varies according to sex, nutrition and, possibly, race Occasionally an os centrale occurs between the scaphoid, trapezoid and capitate bones: during the second prenatal month it is a cartilaginous nodule which usually fuses with the scaphoid. Occasionally, lunate and triquetral elements may fuse. Other fusions and accessory ossicles have also been described.

METACARPALS

The metacarpus consists of five metacarpal bones, conventionally numbered in radio-ulnar order. These are miniature long bones, with a distal head, shaft and expanded base. The rounded heads articulate with the proximal phalanges. Their articular surfaces are convex, although less so transversely, and extend further on the palmar surfaces, especially at their margins. The knuckles are produced by the metacarpal heads. The metacarpal bases articulate with the distal carpal row and with each other, except the first and second. The shafts have longitudinally concave palmar surfaces, which form hollows for the palmar muscles. Their dorsal surfaces bear a distal triangular area, which is continued proximally as a round ridge. These flat areas are palpable proximal to the knuckles.

The medial four metacarpals are sometimes described as parallel; strictly speaking, they diverge somewhat, and radiate gently proximodistally. However, the first metacarpal, relative to the others, is more anterior and rotated medially on its axis through 90°, so that its morphologically dorsal surface is lateral, its radial border palmar, its palmar surface medial, and its ulnar border dorsal. Hence the thumb flexes medially across the palm and can be rotated into opposition with

each finger. Opposition depends on medial rotation and is the prime factor in manual dexterity: when an object is grasped, fingers and thumb encircle it from opposite sides, greatly increasing the power and skill of the grip.

INDIVIDUAL METACARPAL BONES

First metacarpal (Fig. 53.21)

The first metacarpal is short and thick. Its dorsal (lateral) surface can be felt to face laterally; its long axis diverges distolaterally from its neighbour. The shaft is flattened, dorsally broad and transversely convex. The palmar (medial) surface is longitudinally concave and divided by a ridge into a larger lateral (anterior) and smaller medial (posterior) part. Opponens pollicis is attached to the radial border and adjoining palmar surface; the first dorsal interosseous muscle (radial head) is attached to its ulnar border and adjacent palmar surface. The base is concavoconvex and articulates with the trapezium. Abductor pollicis longus is attached on its lateral (palmar) side, the first palmar interosseous muscle to its ulnar side. The head is less convex than in other metacarpals and is transversely broad. Sesamoid bones glide on radial and ulnar articular eminences on its palmar aspect.

Second metacarpal (Fig. 53.22)

The second metacarpal has the longest shaft and largest base. The latter is grooved in a dorsopalmar direction for articulation with the trapezoid. Medial to the groove a deep ridge articulates with the capitate; laterally, nearer the dorsal surface of the base, there is a quadrilateral facet for articulation with the trapezium, and just dorsal to this facet a rough

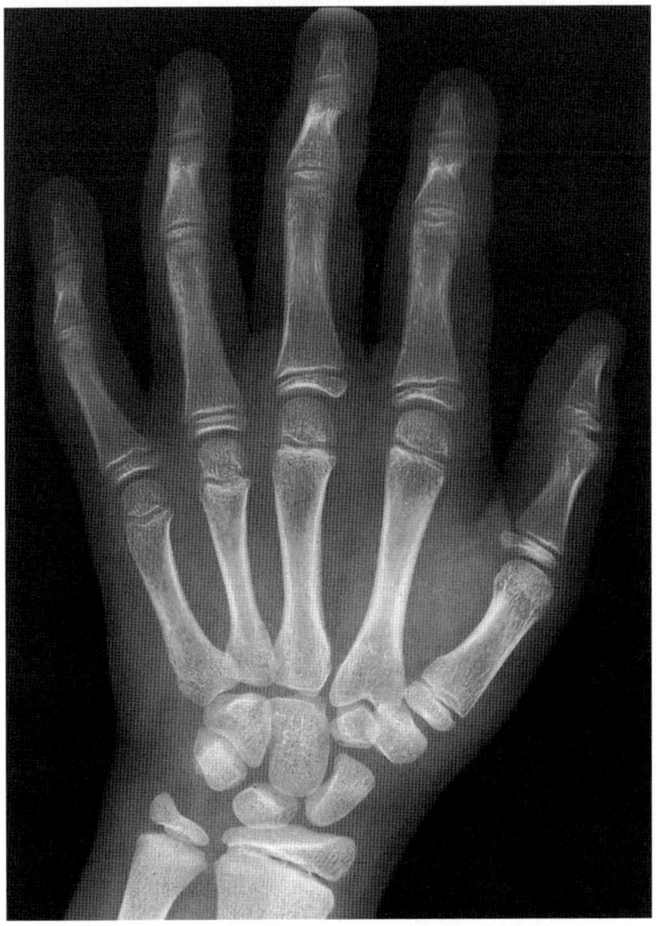

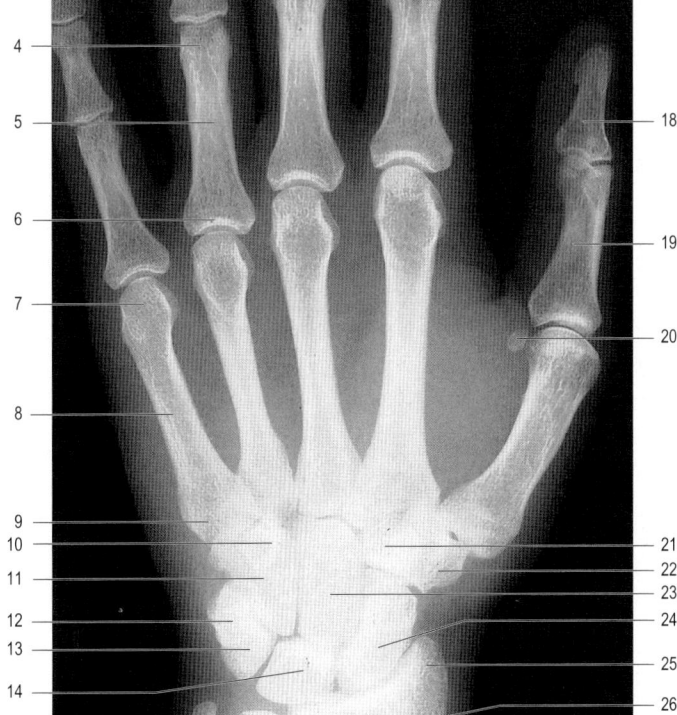

Fig. 53.18 Radiograph of a hand at 11 years (female), dorsopalmar projection. Note the maturing shapes of all the ossifications previously seen in **Figs 53.16** and **53.17**, with the addition of the pisiform.

1. Head of middle phalanx of middle finger.   2. Shaft of middle phalanx of middle finger.
3. Base of middle phalanx of middle finger.   4. Head of proximal phalanx of ring finger.
5. Shaft of proximal phalanx of ring finger.   6. Base of proximal phalanx of ring finger.
7. Head of fifth metacarpal.   8. Shaft of fifth metacarpal.   9. Base of fifth metacarpal.
10. Hook of hamate.   11. Hamate.   12. Pisiform.   13. Triquetrum.   14. Lunate.
15. Styloid process of ulna.   16. Head of ulna.   17. Distal phalanx of index finger.
18. Distal phalanx of thumb.   19. Proximal phalanx of thumb.   20. Sesamoid bone.
21. Trapezoid.   22. Trapezium.   23. Capitate.   24. Scaphoid.   25. Styloid process of radius.
26. Ulnar (sigmoid) notch of radius.   27. Radius.

Fig. 53.19 Radiograph of adult hand for comparison (male of 19 years), dorsopalmar projection. Note additional ossification in the sesamoid bones of the thumb. (By permission from Weir J, Abrahams PH 2003 Imaging Atlas of Human Anatomy, 3rd edn, London: Mosby, and contributions from Anna-Maria Belli, Margaret Hourihan, Naill Moore and Philip Owen.)

impression marks the attachment of extensor carpi radialis longus. On the palmar surface a small tubercle or ridge receives flexor carpi radialis. The medial side of the base articulates with that of the third metacarpal by a long facet, centrally narrowed. The shaft is prismatic in section and longitudinally curved, convex dorsally, concave towards the palm. Its dorsal surface is distally broad but proximally narrows to a ridge which is covered by extensor tendons of the index finger. Its converging borders begin at the tubercles, one on each side of its head for the attachment of collateral ligaments. Proximally the lateral surface inclines dorsally for the ulnar head of the first dorsal interosseous. The medial surface inclines similarly, and is divided by a faint ridge into a palmar strip for attachment of the second palmar interosseous, and a dorsal strip for attachment of the radial head of the second dorsal interosseous.

Third metacarpal (Fig. 53.23)
The third metacarpal has a short styloid process, projecting proximally from the radial side of the dorsal surface. Its base articulates with the capitate by a facet anteriorly convex but dorsally concave where it invades the styloid process on the lateral aspect of its base. A strip-like facet, constricted centrally, articulates with the bases of the second metacarpal (laterally) and the fourth metacarpal (medially), the latter by two oval facets. The palmar facet may be absent; less frequently the facets are connected proximally by a narrow bridge. The palmar surface of the base receives a slip from the tendon of flexor carpi radialis; extensor carpi radialis brevis is attached to its dorsal surface, beyond the styloid process. The shaft resembles that of the second metacarpal. The ulnar head of the second dorsal interosseous is attached to its lateral surface; the radial head of the third dorsal interosseous is attached to its medial surface, and the transverse head of adductor pollicis is attached to the intervening palmar ridge in its distal two-thirds. Its dorsal surface is covered by the extensor tendon.

Fourth metacarpal (Fig. 53.24)
The fourth metacarpal is shorter and thinner than the second and third. On its base it displays two lateral oval facets for articulation with the base of the third metacarpal; the dorsal is usually larger and proximally in contact with the capitate. A single medial elongated facet is for articulation with the base of the fifth metacarpal. The quadrangular proximal surface articulates with the hamate, and is anteriorly convex, dorsally concave. The shaft is like the second, but a faint ridge on its lateral surface separates the attachments of the third palmar interosseous and the ulnar head of the third dorsal interosseous. The radial head of the fourth dorsal interosseous is attached to the medial surface.

Fifth metacarpal (Fig. 53.25)
The fifth metacarpal differs in its medial basal surface, which is non-articular and bears a tubercle for extensor carpi ulnaris. The lateral basal surface is a facet, transversely concave, convex from palm to dorsum, for articulation with the hamate. A lateral strip articulates with the base of

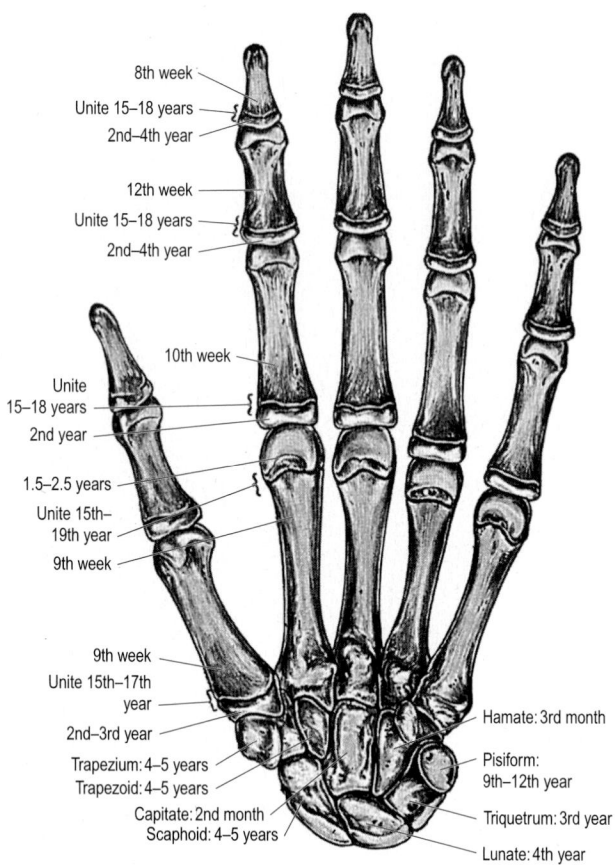

Fig. 53.20 The bones of the hand of a child, indicating the general plan of ossification.

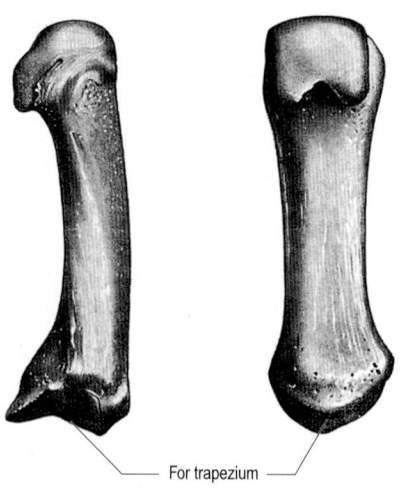

Fig. 53.21 The first left metacarpal bone: palmar and lateral aspects.

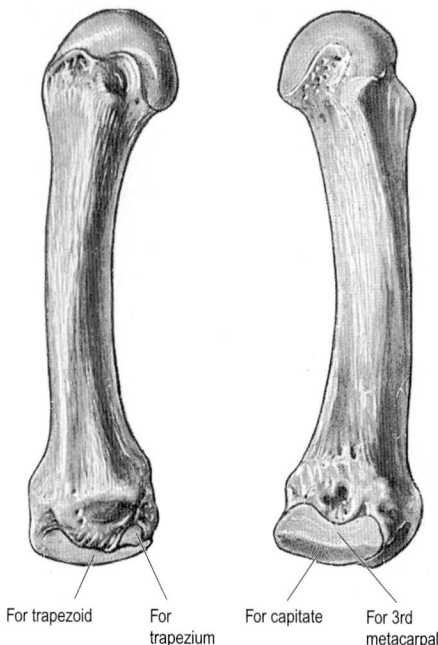

Fig. 53.22 The left second metacarpal bone: dorsolateral and medial aspects.

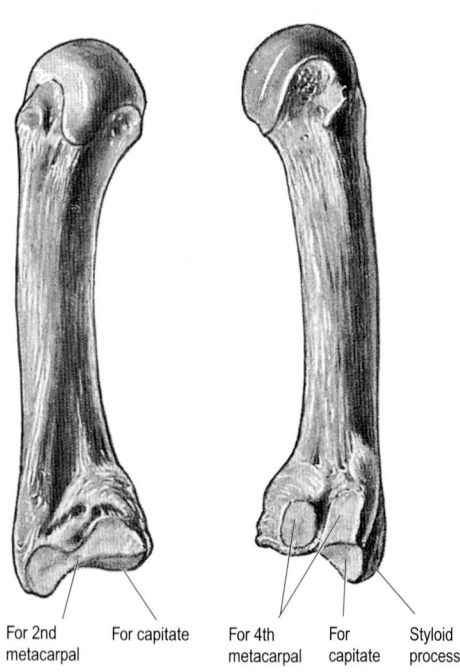

Fig. 53.23 The left third metacarpal bone: lateral and medial aspects.

the fourth metacarpal. The shaft bears a triangular dorsal area which almost reaches the base; the lateral surface inclines dorsally only at its proximal end. Opponens digiti minimi is attached to the medial surface. The lateral surface is divided by a ridge, which is sometimes sharp, into a palmar strip for the attachment of the fourth palmar interosseous and a dorsal strip for the ulnar part of the fourth dorsal interosseous.

OSSIFICATION (Figs 53.16, 53.17, 53.18, 53.19)
Each metacarpal ossifies from a primary centre for the shaft and a secondary centre which is in the base of the first metacarpal and in the heads of the other four. Ossification begins in the midshaft about the ninth week. Centres for the second to fifth metacarpal heads appear in

that order in the second year in females, and between $1\frac{1}{2}$ to $2\frac{1}{2}$ years in males. They unite with the shafts about the fifteenth or sixteenth year in females, eighteenth or nineteenth in males. The first metacarpal base begins to ossify late in the second year in females, early in the third year in males, uniting before the fifteenth year in females and seventeenth in males. Sometimes the styloid process of the third metacarpal is a separate ossicle. (The thumb metacarpal ossifies like a phalanx.) Some authorities therefore consider that the thumb skeleton consists of three phalanges. Others believe that the distal phalanx represents fused middle and distal phalanges, a condition occasionally observed in the fifth toe. When the thumb has three phalanges, the metacarpal has a distal and a proximal epiphysis. It occasionally bifurcates distally. When it does,

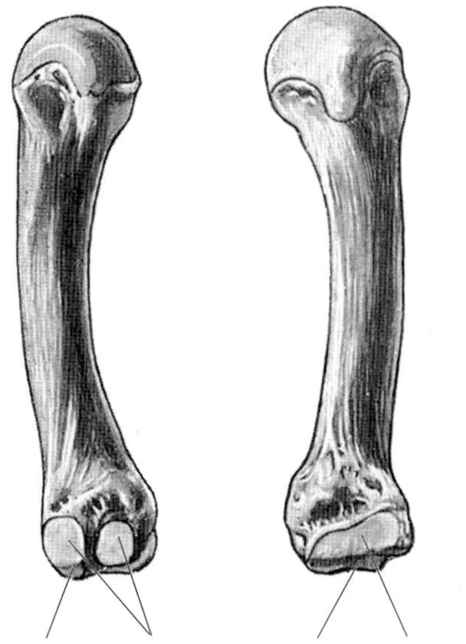

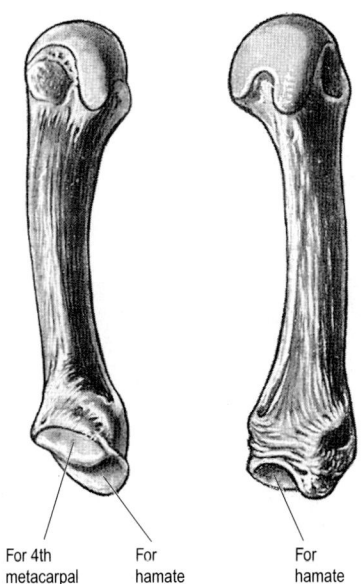

Fig. 53.24 The left fourth metacarpal bone: lateral and medial aspects.

For
capitate   For 3rd   For   For 5th
matacarpal   hamate   metacarpal

For 4th   For   For
metacarpal   hamate   hamate

Fig. 53.25 The left fifth metacarpal bone: lateral and medial aspects.

the medial branch has no distal epiphysis and bears two phalanges, while the lateral branch shows a distal epiphysis, and three phalanges. The existence of only a distal metacarpal epiphysis may be associated with a greater range of movement at the metacarpophalangeal joint. In the thumb, the carpometacarpal joint has the wider range, and the first metacarpal has a basal epiphysis. A distal epiphysis may appear in the first, and a proximal epiphysis in the second, metacarpal.

PHALANGES

There are 14 phalanges, three in each finger, two in the thumb. Each has a head, shaft and proximal base. The shaft tapers distally, its dorsal surface transversely convex. The palmar surface is transversely flat but gently concave anteriorly in its long axis. The bases of the proximal phalanges carry concave, oval facets adapted to the metacarpal heads. Their own heads are smoothly grooved like pulleys and encroach more on to the palmar surfaces. The bases of the middle phalanges carry two concave facets separated by a smooth ridge, conforming to the heads of

the proximal phalanges. The bases of the distal phalanges are adapted to the pulley-like heads of the middle phalanges. The heads of the distal phalanges are non-articular and carry a rough, crescentic palmar tuberosity to which the pulps of the fingertips are attached.

Articular ligaments and numerous muscles are attached to the phalanges. A corresponding tendon of flexor digitorum profundus and, on its dorsal surface, extensor digitorum, are attached to the base of each distal phalanx on its palmar surface. A tendon of flexor digitorum superficialis and its fibrous sheath are attached to the sides of a middle phalanx, and a part of extensor digitorum is attached to the base dorsally. A fibrous flexor sheath is attached to the sides of a proximal phalanx, part of the corresponding dorsal interosseous is attached to its base laterally, and another dorsal interosseous is attached medially.

The phalanges of the little finger and the thumb differ. Abductor and flexor digiti minimi are attached to the medial side of the base of the proximal phalanx of the little finger. The tendon of extensor pollicis brevis and the oblique head of adductor pollicis (dorsally), and the oblique and transverse heads of adductor pollicis, sometimes conjoined with the first palmar interosseous (medially), are attached to the base of the proximal pollicial phalanx.

The margins of the proximal pollicial phalanx are not sharp, because the fibrous sheath is less strongly developed than it is in the other digits.

OSSIFICATION (Figs 53.16, 53.17, 53.18, 53.19, 53.20)

Phalanges are ossified from a primary centre for the shaft and a proximal epiphyseal centre. Ossification begins prenatally in shafts as follows: distal phalanges in the eighth or ninth week, proximal phalanges in the tenth, middle phalanges in the eleventh week or later. Epiphyseal centres appear in proximal phalanges early in the second year (females), and later in the same year (males); and in middle and distal phalanges in the second year (females), or third or fourth year (males). All epiphyses unite about the fifteenth to sixteenth year in females, and seventeenth to eighteenth year in males.

JOINTS

DISTAL RADIO-ULNAR JOINT

The distal radio-ulnar joint is a uniaxial pivot joint.

Articulating surfaces – The articulating surfaces are between the convex distal head of the ulna and the concave ulnar notch of the radius. These surfaces are connected by an articular disc.

Fibrous capsule – The fibrous capsule is thicker anteriorly and posteriorly. The proximal part of the capsule is lax.

Articular disc – The articular disc is fibrocartilaginous (collagen with few elastic fibres in the young) and is triangular, binding the distal ends of the ulna and radius. Its periphery is thicker, its centre sometimes perforated. The disc is attached by a blunt, thick apex to a depression between the ulnar styloid process and distal articular surface, and by its wider thin base to the prominent edge between the ulnar notch and carpal articular surface of the radius. Its margins are united to adjacent carpal ligaments, its surfaces are smooth and concave: the proximal articulates with the ulnar head, the distal is part of the radiocarpal joint, and articulates with the lunate and, when the hand is adducted, the triquetrum. The disc shows age-related degeneration, becoming thinned and ultimately perforated in about half the subjects over the age of 60.

Synovial membrane – The capsule is lined by synovial membrane which projects proximally between the radius and ulna as a recessus sacciformis in front of the distal part of the interosseous membrane.

Vascular supply and lymphatic drainage – The arterial supply to the distal radio-ulnar joint and disc is mainly derived from the palmar and dorsal branches of the anterior interosseous artery, reinforced by the posterior interosseous and ulnar arteries.

Innervation – The distal radio-ulnar joint is innervated by branches of the anterior and posterior interosseous nerves.

Movements – Movements at the radio-ulnar joint complex pronate and supinate the hand. In pronation the radius, carrying the hand, turns anteromedially and obliquely across the ulna, its proximal end remains lateral, its distal becomes medial. During this action the interosseous membrane becomes spiralled. In supination the radius returns to a position lateral and parallel to the ulna and the interosseous membrane becomes unspiralled. The hand can be turned through 140–150°: with the elbow extended, this can be increased to nearly 360° by humeral rotation and scapular movements. Power is greater in supination, a fact which has affected the design of nuts, bolts and screws, which are tightened by supination in right-handed subjects. Moreover, supination is an antigravity movement with a pendent upper arm and semiflexed forearm; in seizing objects for examination or manipulation, pronation is merely a preliminary and is aided by gravity.

Forearm rotation occurs between the articulation of the head of the ulna and sigmoid notch distally, and the head of the radius and the radial notch of the ulna proximally. These distal and proximal radio-ulnar joints are pivot-type synovial joints: they act as a pair permitting stable rotary motion (pronation 61–66°, supination 70–77°). During rotation, the radius moves around the ulnar head. The axis for pronation and supination is often represented as a line through the centre of the radial head (proximal) and the ulnar attachment of the articular disc (distal). More correctly this is the axis of movement of the radius relative to the ulna and it does not remain stationary. The radial head rotates in the fibro-osseous ring: its distal lower end and articular disc swing round the ulnar head. During rotation of the radial head its proximal surface spins on the humeral capitulum. As the forearm moves from full pronation into supination the ulna translocates laterally by 9–10 mm, such that the axis of rotation shifts but still passes through the ulnar head. In addition the sigmoid notch changes its contact position with the ulnar head, lying dorsal proximal in pronation and volar distal in supination. The distal end of the ulna is not stationary during these movements; it moves a variable amount along a curved course, posterolaterally in pronation, anteromedially in supination. The axis of movement, as defined above, is therefore displaced laterally in pronation, medially in supination. Hence the axis for supination and pronation of the whole forearm and hand passes between the bones at both the superior and distal radio-ulnar joints when ulnar movement is marked, but through the centres of the radial head and ulnar styloid when it is minimal. The axis may be prolonged through any digit, depending on the medial or lateral displacement of the distal end of the ulna. The hand will rotate further than the forearm because of the sliding–rotatory movement which occurs between the carpal bones and the bases of the metacarpals and, to a very minor degree, at the radio-carpal joint.

Accessory movements – Accessory movements include anterior and posterior translation of the radial head on the ulnar radial notch, and of the ulnar head likewise on the radial ulnar notch.

MUSCLES PRODUCING MOVEMENT
The muscles producing movements at the distal radio-ulnar joint are as follows.

Pronation – Pronator quadratus, aided in rapid movement and against resistance by pronator teres. Gravity also assists.

Supination – Supinator, in slow unresisted movement and extension, assisted by biceps in fast movements in flexion, especially when resisted.

Electromyographic studies have not confirmed activity in brachio-radialis during pronation and supination.

RADIOCARPAL (WRIST) JOINT (Figs 53.26, 53.27)

Articulating surfaces – The radiocarpal joint is a synovial biaxial and ellipsoid joint formed by articulation of the distal end of the radius and the triangular articular disc with the scaphoid, lunate and triquetrum. In the neutral position of the wrist, only the scaphoid and lunate are in contact with the radius and articular disc: the triquetrum comes into apposition with the disc only in full adduction of the wrist joint. The radial articular surface and distal discal surface form an almost elliptical, concave surface with a transverse long axis. The radial surface is bisected by a low ridge into two concavities. A similar ridge usually appears between the medial radial concavity and the concave distal discal surface.

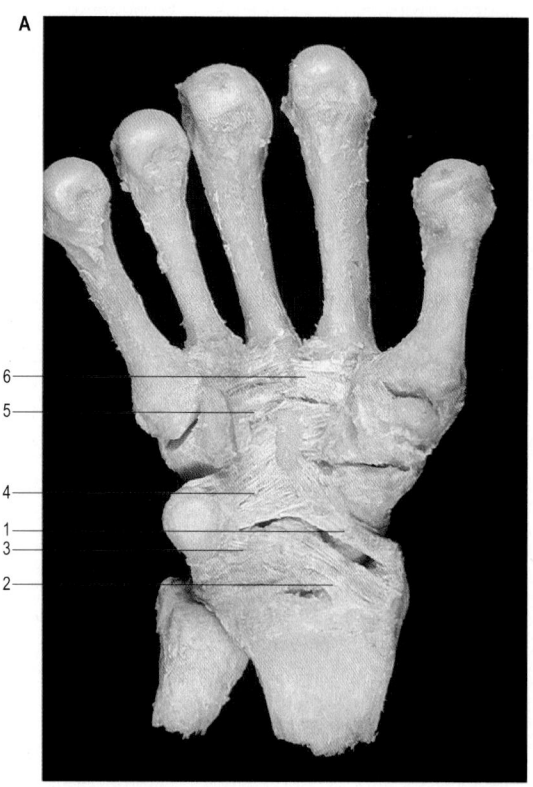 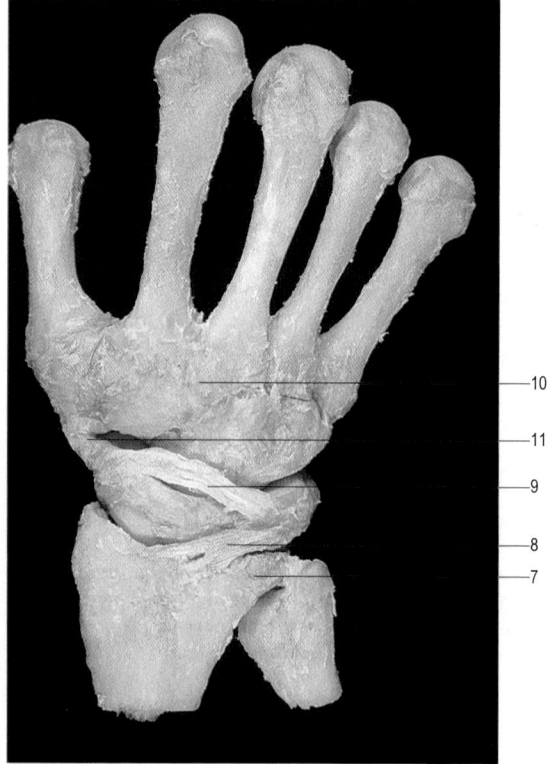

PART A: **1.** Radioscaphocapitate ligament.   **2.** Long radiolunate ligament.   **3.** Palmar lunotriquetral interosseous ligament.   **4.** Palmar triquetrohamate and triquetrocapitate ligaments.
     5/6. Palmar distal row interosseous ligaments.
PART B: **7.** Dorsal radio-ulnar ligament.   **8.** Dorsal radiolunotriquetral ligament.   **9.** Dorsal intercarpal ligament.   **10.** Dorsal distal row interosseous ligament.   **11.** Scaphotrapeziotrapezoidal ligament.

Fig. 53.26 Anatomic dissection of the major extrinsic and intrinsic wrist ligaments. **A**, Palmar view. **B**, Dorsal view. (By permission from Kirk Watson H, Weinzweig J (eds) 2001 The Wrist. Philadelphia: Lippincott Williams and Williams.)

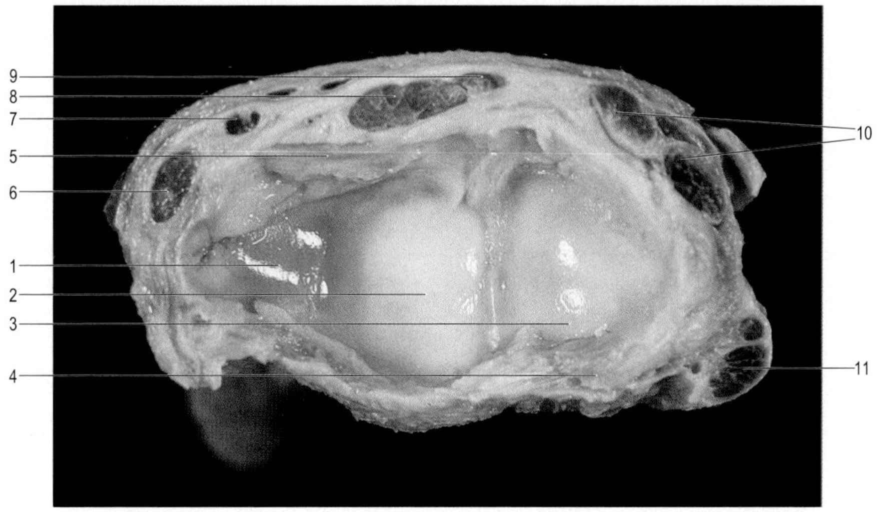

1. Triangular fibrocartilage.   **2.** Lunate fossa.   **3.** Scaphoid fossa.   **4.** Palmar radiocarpal ligament.   **5.** Dorsal radiolunotriquetral ligament.   **6.** Extensor carpi ulnaris tendon (sixth extensor compartment).
7. Extensor digiti minimi (fifth compartment).   **8.** Extensor digitorum and extensor indicis (fourth compartment).   **9.** Extensor pollicis longus (third compartment).
10. Extensor carpi radialis brevis and longus (second compartment).   **11.** Extensor pollicis brevis and abductor pollicis longus (first compartment).

Fig. 53.27 Distal articular surface of the radius. (By permission from Kirk Watson H, Weinzweig J (eds) 2001 The Wrist. Philadelphia: Lippincott Williams and Williams.)

The proximal articular surfaces of the scaphoid, lunate and triquetrum, and their interosseous ligaments, form a smooth convex surface which is received into the proximal concavity.

Fibrous capsule – The fibrous capsule is lined by synovial membrane which is usually separate from that of the distal radio-ulnar and intercarpal joints. A protruding prestyloid recess (recessus sacciformis), anterior to the articular disc, is present and ascends close to the styloid process. The recess is bounded distally by a fibrocartilaginous meniscus, which projects from the ulnar collateral ligament between the tip of the ulnar styloid process and the triquetrum; both are clothed with hyaline articular cartilage. The meniscus may ossify. The capsule is strengthened by palmar radiocarpal and ulnocarpal, dorsal radiocarpal and radial and ulnar collateral ligaments.

Synovial membrane – The synovial membrane lines the fibrous capsule.

Vascular supply – The radiocarpal joint is supplied by branches of the anterior interosseous artery, anterior and posterior carpal branches of the radial and ulnar arteries, palmar and dorsal metacarpal arteries and recurrent rami of the deep palmar arch.

Innervation – The radiocarpal joint is innervated by the anterior and posterior interosseous nerves.

Muscles producing movement – Movements accompany those of the intercarpal and midcarpal joints and are described on page 903. The close-packed position is in full extension.

CARPAL JOINTS

The intercarpal joints interconnect the carpal bones. They may be summarized as joints between the proximal row of carpal bones, between the distal row of carpal bones, and a complex joint between the rows, the midcarpal joint.

Carpal bones are connected by an extensive array of ligaments, not all of which are specifically named. The flexor retinaculum is an accessory intercarpal ligament. Articular surfaces are either sellar, ellipsoid or spheroidal.

JOINTS OF THE PROXIMAL CARPAL ROW

Joints of the proximal carpal row are between the scaphoid, lunate and triquetrum. In addition, the pisiform articulates with the palmar surface of the triquetrum at a small, oval, almost flat, synovial pisotriquetral joint.

A thin capsule surrounds the joint. The synovial cavity is usually separate but may communicate with that of the radiocarpal joint.

JOINTS OF THE DISTAL CARPAL ROW

Joints of the distal carpal row are between the trapezium, trapezoid, capitate and hamate. There is virtually no movement at these joints.

MIDCARPAL JOINT

The midcarpal joint, between the scaphoid, lunate and triquetrum (proximally) and trapezium, trapezoid, capitate and hamate (distally) is a compound articulation which may be divided descriptively into medial and lateral parts. Throughout most of the medial compartment the convexity formed by the head of the capitate and hamate articulates with a reciprocal concavity formed by the scaphoid, lunate and much of the triquetrum. However, most medially the curvatures are reversed, forming a compound sellar joint. In the lateral compartment the trapezium and trapezoid articulate with the scaphoid, forming a second compound articulation, often said to be plane, but which is also sellar.

Carpal synovial membrane – The carpal synovial membrane is most extensive, and lines an irregular articular cavity. Its proximal part is between the distal surfaces of the scaphoid, lunate and triquetrum and the proximal surfaces of the second carpal row. It has proximal prolongations between the scaphoid and lunate, and lunate and triquetrum, and three distal prolongations between the four bones of the second row. The absence of an interosseous ligament means that the prolongation between the trapezium and trapezoid and/or between the trapezoid and capitate is often continuous with corresponding carpometacarpal joints, variably from the second to the fifth, or often the second and third only. In the latter case, the joint between the hamate and fourth and fifth metacarpal bones has a separate synovial membrane and the carpometacarpal interosseous ligament is interposed. Synovial cavities of carpometacarpal joints are prolonged slightly between the metacarpal bases. The synovial joint between the pisiform and triquetrum is usually isolated.

Vascular supply – The carpal joints are supplied by the posterior carpal branches of the radial and ulnar arteries and by the anterior interosseous artery.

Innervation – Precise details about innervation of the carpal joints are lacking. They appear to be innervated by small branches from the deep terminal branch of the ulnar nerve, the anterior interosseous branch of the median nerve, and the posterior interosseous branch of the radial nerve.

WRIST LIGAMENTS

Wrist ligaments situated between the fibrous and synovial layers of the wrist joint are termed intracapsular, while those lying superficial to the fibrous layer are extracapsular. Almost all ligaments of the wrist actually lie within the joint capsule and the only exceptions are the flexor and extensor retinaculae and the pisotriquetral ligament. The intracapsular ligaments appear to blend one into another and the edges of the ligaments may not be distinct or discrete.

The ligaments are further classified into extrinsic and intrinsic named ligaments. In addition there are superficial and deep parts to some of the extrinsic ligaments: the latter are identifiable at wrist arthroscopy, the former are not.

It is important to appreciate that the wrist ligaments are named from proximal to distal and from radial to ulnar. Thus a ligament passing between the capitate, scaphoid and radius is called the radio-scaphocapitate ligament.

Extrinsic ligaments

Extrinsic ligaments connect the carpus with the forearm bones. The extrinsic ligaments as a group tend to be longer than the intrinsic ligaments. They are approximately one-third as strong but easier to repair following rupture.

Extrinsic palmar carpal ligaments

When the synovial lining of the carpal tunnel is dissected away, two V-shaped ligamentous bands are visible with their apices lying distally (**Fig. 53.26A**). The limbs of the 'V' take origin from the radius and ulna respectively: the apex of one 'V' attaches to the distal row and that of the second 'V' to the proximal row.

Radioscaphocapitate ligament – The radioscaphocapitate ligament originates from the radial styloid and the palmar lip of the radius. It courses distally and is then described by some authors as having three parts. The first is the most radial and inserts onto the lateral aspect of the waist of the scaphoid (radial collateral ligament). The second continues as part of the distal 'V' and inserts onto the distal pole of the scaphoid. The third passes over the proximal pole of the scaphoid towards the midcarpus and blends with the fibres originating from the ulnar side – part of the triangular fibrocartilage complex – to form the arcuate ligament over the palmar aspect of the capitate. A few of the fibres of the radioscaphocapitate ligament attach to the body of the capitate. There is a discrete interval between the inferior margin of this ligament and the palmar horn of the lunate which is known as the space of Poirier.

Long radiolunate ligament – The long radiolunate ligament takes origin adjacent to the radioscaphocapitate ligament on the palmar lip of the radius. It passes over and supports the proximal pole of the scaphoid before inserting into the palmar horn of the lunate. This ligament is discrete from the radioscaphocapitate ligament and the visible separation is known as the interligamentous sulcus (continuous with the space of Poirier).

Radioscapholunate (ligament of Testut) – Histological studies have shown the radioscapholunate ligament is not a true ligament because it contains neurovascular structures which supply the scapholunate interosseous membrane and is covered by a thick synovial lining. However it a visible landmark inside the wrist joint when undertaking wrist arthroscopy.

Short radiolunate ligament – The short radiolunate ligament is part of the proximal 'V'. It arises from the palmar lip of the lunate fossa of the radius and passes directly to the palmar horn of the lunate. To the ulnar side its fibres blend with those of the palmar triangular fibrocartilage complex as these also pass to their insertion on the lunate. This ligament contributes to the stability of the lunate.

Ulnolunate ligament – The ulnolunate ligament originates from the palmar aspect of the ulna adjacent to the short radiolunate ligament and inserts onto the palmar horn of the lunate. Part of this fibre complex arches radially and blends with part of the radioscaphocapitate complex, forming the arcuate ligament.

Ulnotriquetral (ulnar collateral) ligament – The ulnotriquetral ligament arises from the palmar aspect of the ulna and inserts into the medial aspect of the triquetrum. It continues distally to a further attachment to the medial aspect of the hamate. It is generally thought that the ulnolunate and ulnotriquetral ligaments take some origin from the marginal ligament of the TFCC as well.

Extrinsic dorsal carpal ligaments

The dorsal wrist ligaments are comparatively thin. They are reinforced by the floor and septa of the fibrous tunnels for the six dorsal compartments. The extrinsic dorsal carpal ligaments and the intrinsic dorsal intercarpal ligaments have a 'Z-shaped' configuration (**Fig. 53.26B**). The pattern and shape of these ligaments is utilized in one surgical approach to the dorsum of the wrist joint where incisions are oriented parallel with the ligaments: this reduces scarring and restriction of subsequent motion caused by the arthrotomy.

Dorsal radiolunotriquetral ligament – The dorsal radiolunotriquetral ligament is a true intracapsular ligament. It is the only extrinsic ligament on the dorsum of the carpus and has superficial and deep components. The superficial part connects the radius and triquetrum, and the deep part connects the radius, lunate and triquetrum. The two components are inseparable. The wide superficial component arises from the dorsal margin of the distal radius and courses ulnarly to insert on the dorsal edge of the triquetrum. The deep component takes a narrower origin from the ulnar aspect of the distal dorsal radius and passes in an ulnar direction to attach to part of the lunotriquetral articulation and the intrinsic lunotriquetral ligament.

Intrinsic ligaments

Intrinsic ligaments of the wrist are attached to carpal bones. They are stronger and shorter than extrinsic ligaments and are connected with the extrinsic ligament complexes by interdigitating fibres. Rupture of one or more intrinsic ligaments frequently leads to a clinical instability of the carpus. The intrinsic ligaments are subdivided into ligaments which connect the carpal bones of the proximal and distal rows respectively and those which connect the rows by crossing over the midcarpal joint.

Proximal row interosseous ligaments – The scapholunate and lunotriquetral ligaments are clinically and biomechanically important structures. In the sagittal plane they have an approximately horseshoe-shape configuration with palmar, midcarpal and dorsal components (**Fig. 53.28**). The scapholunate ligament contains short transverse fibres connecting the dorsal aspect of the respective bones and more obliquely oriented fibres connecting the palmar aspect. The functional significance of this arrangement is that the tighter dorsal component of the ligament acts as a hinge facilitating flexion and extension of the scaphoid: these movements are important to carpal mechanics. The ligament continues on its midcarpal section as an interosseous membrane. The lunotriquetral ligament has similar dorsal, midcarpal interosseous and palmar components, but the fibres of the dorsal and palmar components are similarly rather than differentially oriented, which precludes the same pattern of preferential movement as occurs between the lunate and scaphoid. The interosseous membranes of the scapholunate and lunotriquetral ligaments separate the midcarpal from the radiocarpal joint spaces. Dye injected into one of these joint spaces which leaks to the other denotes a tear of one of these ligaments.

Distal row interosseous ligaments – The distal row interosseous ligaments are powerful ligaments between the capitate, hamate, trapezium and trapezoid, with an important stabilizing function for the distal carpal row. They have superficial and deep components. Unlike the ligaments of the proximal row, these are seldom torn.

Palmar midcarpal ligaments – Anterolaterally lies the fan-shaped palmar scaphocapitate–trapezoid ligament which originates from the scaphoid tuberosity and is thought to be an important stabilizer of the scaphoid. This ligament may be subdivided into two parts known as the scapho-trapeziotrapezoidal ligament (having the attachments as its name suggests) and a more ulnar component known as the scaphocapitate ligament. The triquetrohamate and triquetrocapitate ligaments lie towards the ulnar side of the carpus. Together these palmar midcarpal ligaments contribute to the arcuate ligament (**Fig. 53.26A**).

Dorsal midcarpal ligaments – The dorsal intercarpal ligament assists in stabilization of the proximal carpal row. It arises from the trapezoid and distal pole of scaphoid, and passes across the dorsal horn of the lunate to be attached to the triquetrum. The ligament forms the floor of the fourth and fifth extensor compartments. On the radial side is the lateral scaphotrapeziotrapezoidal ligament which acts as a stabilizer of the scaphoid and trapezium.

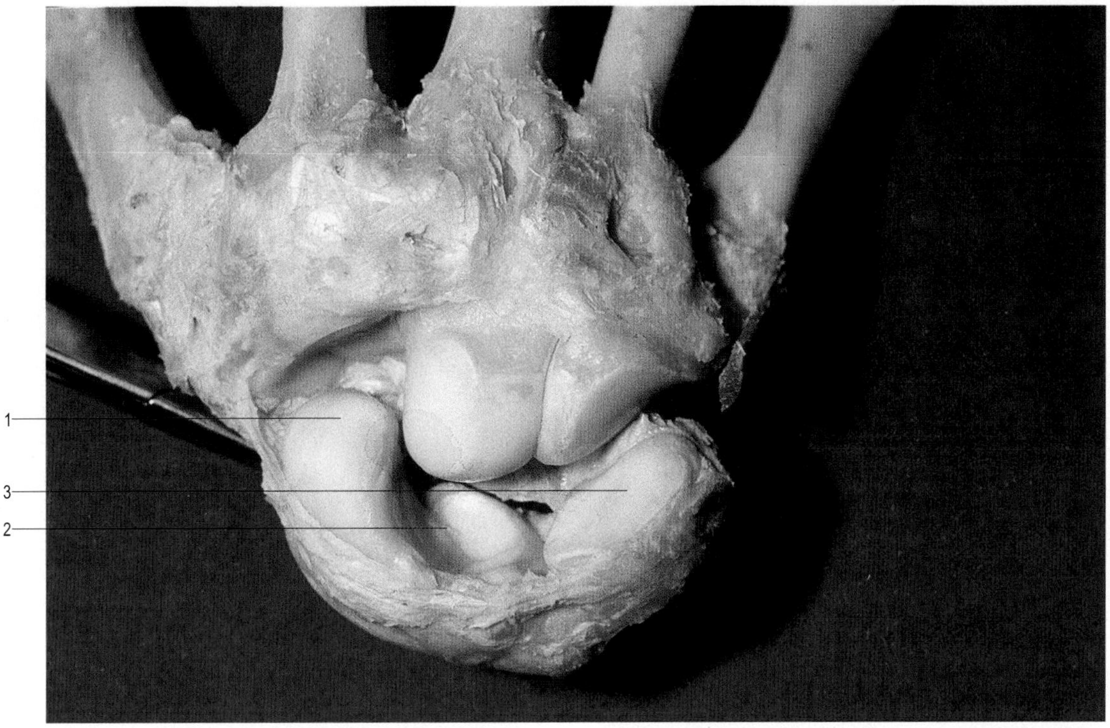

Fig. 53.28 Open view of the midcarpal joint, viewed from the dorsum. (By Kirk Watson H, Weinzweig J (eds) 2001 The Wrist. Philadelphia: Lippincott Williams and Williams.) Three articular structures are evident: 1. scaphoid–trapezium–trapezoid (proximal condyle–distal glenoid); 2. lunate–scaphoid–capitate (distal condyle–proximal glenoid); 3. triquetrum–hamate (helicoidal-shaped).

Distal radio-ulnar ligaments

The triangular fibrocartilage complex (TFCC) is a ligamentous and carti-laginous structure which suspends the distal radius and ulnar carpus from the distal ulna (**Fig. 53.27**). By definition, it is made up of the cartilaginous disc, the meniscus homologue (an embryological remnant of the 'ulnar' wrist that is only occasionally present), volar and dorsal distal radio-ulnar ligaments, ulnar collateral ligament, floor of extensor carpi ulnaris subsheath, ulnolunate and ulnotriquetral ligaments. The triangular fibrocartilage proper (TFC) is a biconcave body composed of chondroid fibrocartilage. It extends across the dome of the ulnar head and varies between 2 and 5 mm in thickness.

From its distal aspect, the TFCC resembles a hammock supporting the ulnar carpus with the disc proper as the base of the hammock. From the proximal side, the TFCC appears in the shape of a fan extending from the fovea of the ulna along either side of the sigmoid notch. This fan-shaped structure is divided into dorsal, central and palmar portions where the central portion is the triangular fibrocartilage and the peripheral margins are thick lamellar collagen, structurally adapted to tensile loading and known as the distal (palmar and dorsal) radio-ulnar ligaments. In keeping with other extrinsic ligaments of the wrist joint proper there are thought to be superficial and deep components of the distal radio-ulnar ligaments which act as a functional couple stabilizing the rotation of the ulnar head on the sigmoid notch of the radius.

Stability of the distal radio-ulnar joint during forearm rotation is conferred by the triangular fibrocartilage complex (TFCC), dorsal and volar distal radio-ulnar ligaments, interosseous membrane and sub-sheath of the extensor carpi ulnaris tendon (floor of sixth dorsal extensor compartment).

COORDINATED MOVEMENTS AND LOAD-BEARING AT THE WRIST JOINT

WRIST MOVEMENTS

The movements at the radiocarpal and intercarpal joints are considered together since they are both involved in all movements as well as being acted upon by the same muscles. Active movements are flexion (c.85°), extension (c.85°), adduction (ulnar deviation) (c.45°), abduction (radial deviation) (c.15°) and circumduction.

The range of flexion is greater at the radiocarpal joint, while in extension there is more movement at the midcarpal joint (**Fig. 53.29**). Hence the proximal surfaces extend further posteriorly on the lunate and scaphoid bones. These movements are limited chiefly by antagonistic muscles, and therefore the range of flexion is perceptibly diminished when the fingers are flexed, due to increased tension in the extensors. Only when the joints are forced to the limits of flexion or extension are the dorsal or palmar ligaments fully stretched (but see below).

Adduction of the hand is considerably greater than abduction, perhaps due to the more proximal site of the ulnar styloid process. Most adduction occurs at the radiocarpal joint. The lunate articulates with both the radius and articular disc when the hand is in the midposition, but in adduction it articulates solely with the radius, and the triquetrum now comes into contact with the articular disc (**Fig. 53.30A**). Much of the proximal articular surface of the scaphoid becomes subcapsular beneath the radial collateral ligament and forms a smooth, convex, palpable prominence in the floor of the 'anatomical snuff-box'.

Abduction from the neutral position occurs at the midcarpal joint, the proximal carpal row not moving. Radiographs of abducted hands show that the capitate rotates round an anteroposterior axis so that its head passes medially and the hamate conforms to this: the distance between the lunate and the apex of the hamate is increased (**Fig. 53.30B**). The scaphoid rotates around a transverse axis, and its proximal articular surface moves away from the capsule to articulate solely with the radius. Movements are limited by antagonistic muscles and, at extremes, by the carpal collateral ligaments.

Circumduction of the hand is not rotatory, but involves successive flexion, adduction, extension and abduction or vice versa.

Muscles producing movements

Flexion – Flexors carpi radialis and ulnaris and palmaris longus, assisted by flexors digitorum superficialis and profundus and flexor pollicis longus.

Extension – Extensors carpi radialis longus, brevis and ulnaris, assisted by extensors digitorum, digiti minimi, indicis and pollicis longus.

Adduction – Flexor and extensor carpi ulnaris.

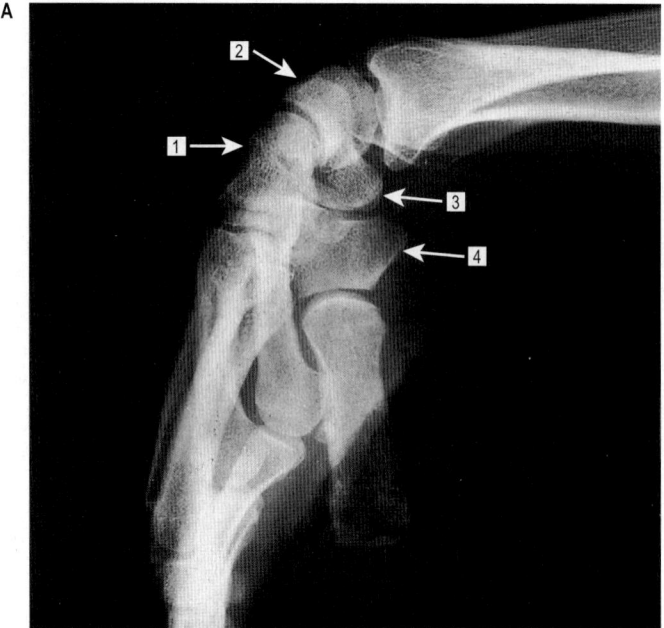

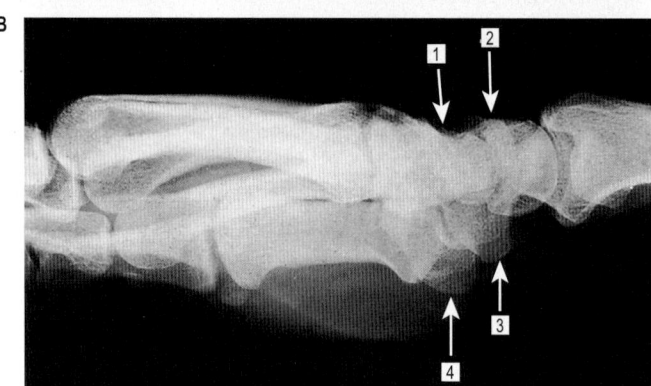

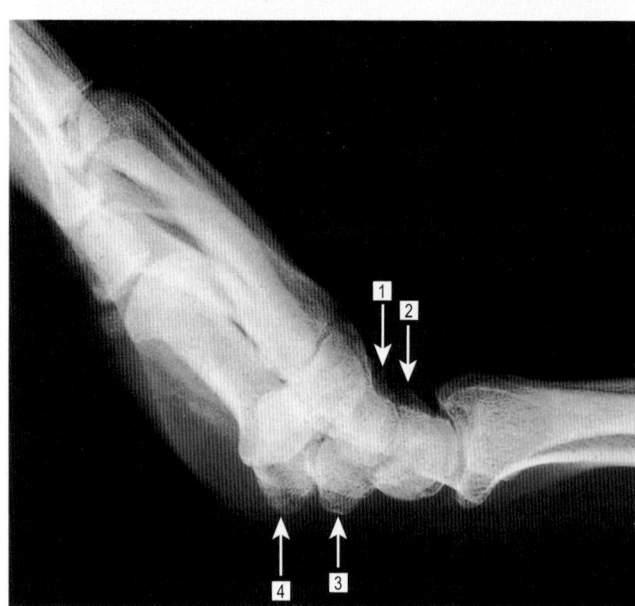

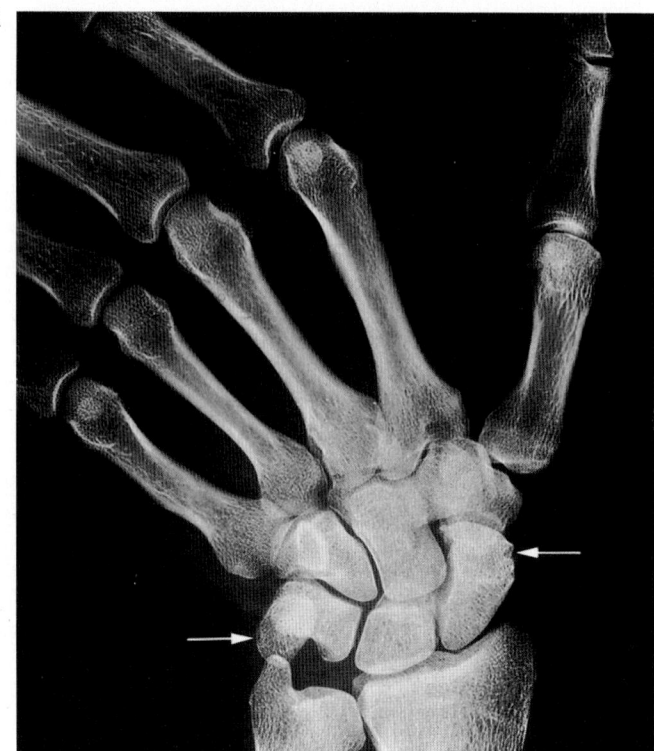

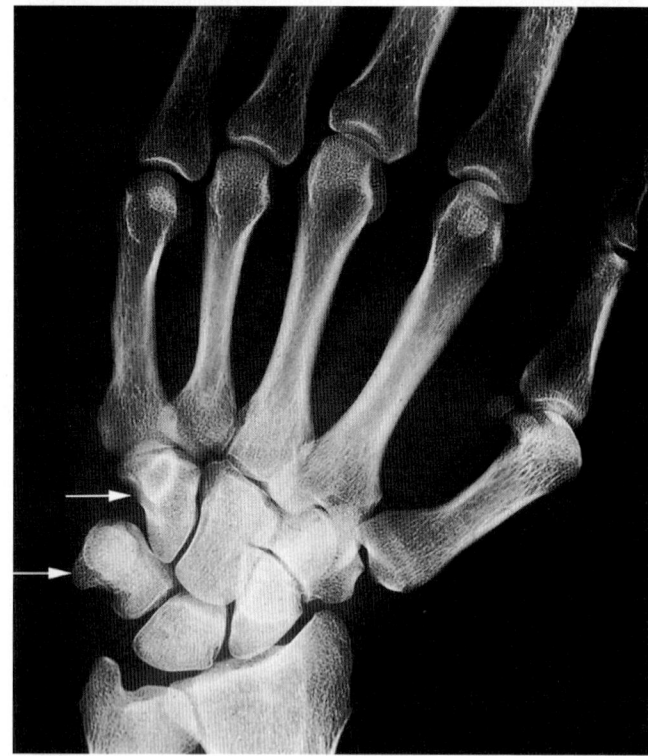

Fig. 53.29 A, Radiograph of the hand and wrist in full flexion: lateral aspect. The arrows point to (1) capitate; (2) lunate; (3) tubercle of the scaphoid; (4) tubercle of the trapezium. Compare with B, and note the relative positions of the capitate and lunate, and the lunate and radius. **B**, Radiograph of the hand and wrist: lateral aspect. The long axes of the third metacarpal, capitate and lunate are, approximately, in line with the long axis of the radius. The arrows point to the same structures as in A. Note the relative positions of the capitate and lunate, and the lunate and radius. **C**, Radiograph of the hand and wrist in full extension: lateral aspect. The arrows point to the same structures as in A. Compare with B and note the alterations in the relative positions of the capitate and lunate, and the lunate and the radius.

Fig. 53.30 A, Radiograph of the hand in full adduction (ulnar deviation), dorsopalmar projection. The arrows point to the scaphoid on the radial side and to the pisiform on the ulnar side. Note that the shadow of the pisiform bone overlaps the shadow of the tip of the styloid process of the ulna. Compare with B and observe that the movements occur at both the radiocarpal and intercarpal joints. **B**, Radiograph of the same hand in full abduction (radial deviation). The arrows point to the hamate and pisiform. Compare with A and note that: (1) the scaphoid and lunate have passed medially (ulnarly) so that the latter articulates to a large extent with the articular disc of the distal radio-ulnar joint; (2) the pisiform is now widely separated from the styloid process of the ulna; (3) the scaphoid, having rotated round a transverse axis, is much foreshortened; (4) the apex of the hamate has been thrust away from the lunate by the rotation of the capitate around an anteroposterior axis; (5) a gap has opened up between the distal portions of the hamate and triquetrum; and (6) the long axes of the capitate and lunate are now almost in the same straight line.

Abduction – Flexor carpi radialis, extensors carpi radialis longus and brevis, with abductor pollicis longus and extensor pollicis brevis.

Integrated model of wrist movement (carpal kinematics)

The proximal row (scaphoid, lunate and triquetrum) is an intercalated segment: no tendons insert onto the bones of the row (**Fig. 53.31**). It is inherently unstable and controlled by specific retaining and gliding ligaments. Its relative position is determined by the spatial configurations of the radius, triangular fibrocartilage complex (TFCC) and ulna on one side, and the rigid distal carpal row on the other. The proximal carpal row is subject to two opposing moments: the scaphoid straddles the proximal and distal rows and tends to rotate the proximal row into flexion under axial load and radial deviation. At the same time there is a force tending to extend the proximal row which is initiated by the distal row and transmitted via the midcarpal ligaments to the triquetrum (**Fig. 53.32**). Stability of the midcarpal joint is thus ensured during both movement and loading.

The distal carpal row (trapezium, trapezoid, capitate and hamate) can be regarded as one rigid structure tightly bound together. The scaphoid bridges the proximal and distal carpal rows and provides a functional couple between the two.

The carpus was originally thought to move simply as proximal and distal rows (row or rigid body theory). According to this view, during the composite movement of wrist flexion and extension, approximately two-thirds of movement occurred at the radiocarpal joint and one-third at the midcarpal joint. The carpus was later judged to move in lateral central and medial columns more than it did in rows, and the radius–lunate–capitate was described as a three-bar linkage system (column theory). This theory was modified to incorporate the specific stabilizing role of the scaphoid as it bridges the proximal and distal rows. A further theory proposed that the bones were linked by their ligaments in a ring configuration, so that any breakage of the key links leads to instability (ring theory). Most recently the 'four unit' theory suggests that the distal carpal row moves as a single unit, and the

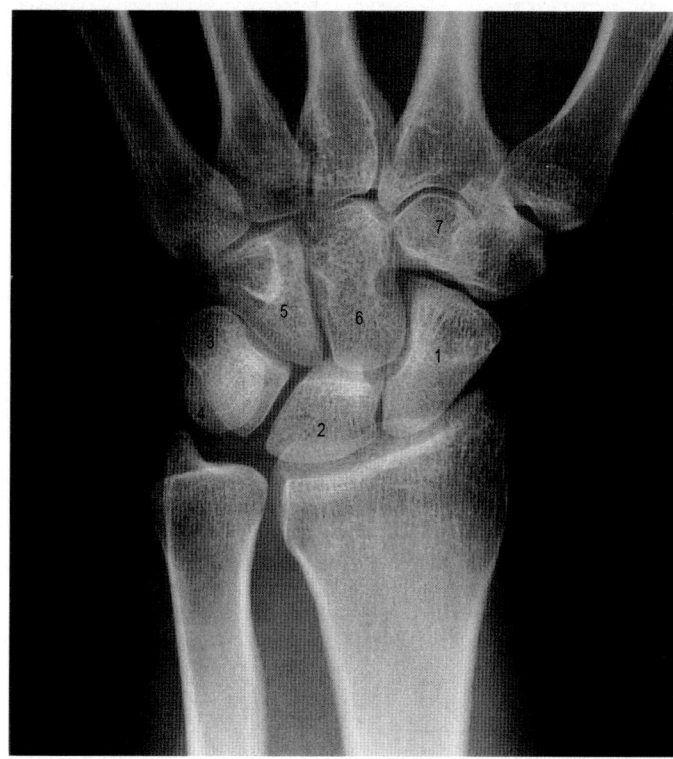

1. Scaphoid. 2. Lunate. 3. Triquetrum. 4. Pisiform. 5. Hamate. 6. Capitate.
7. Trapezoid. 8. Trapezium.

Fig. 53.31 Posteroanterior radiograph of wrist demonstrating the individual carpal bones.

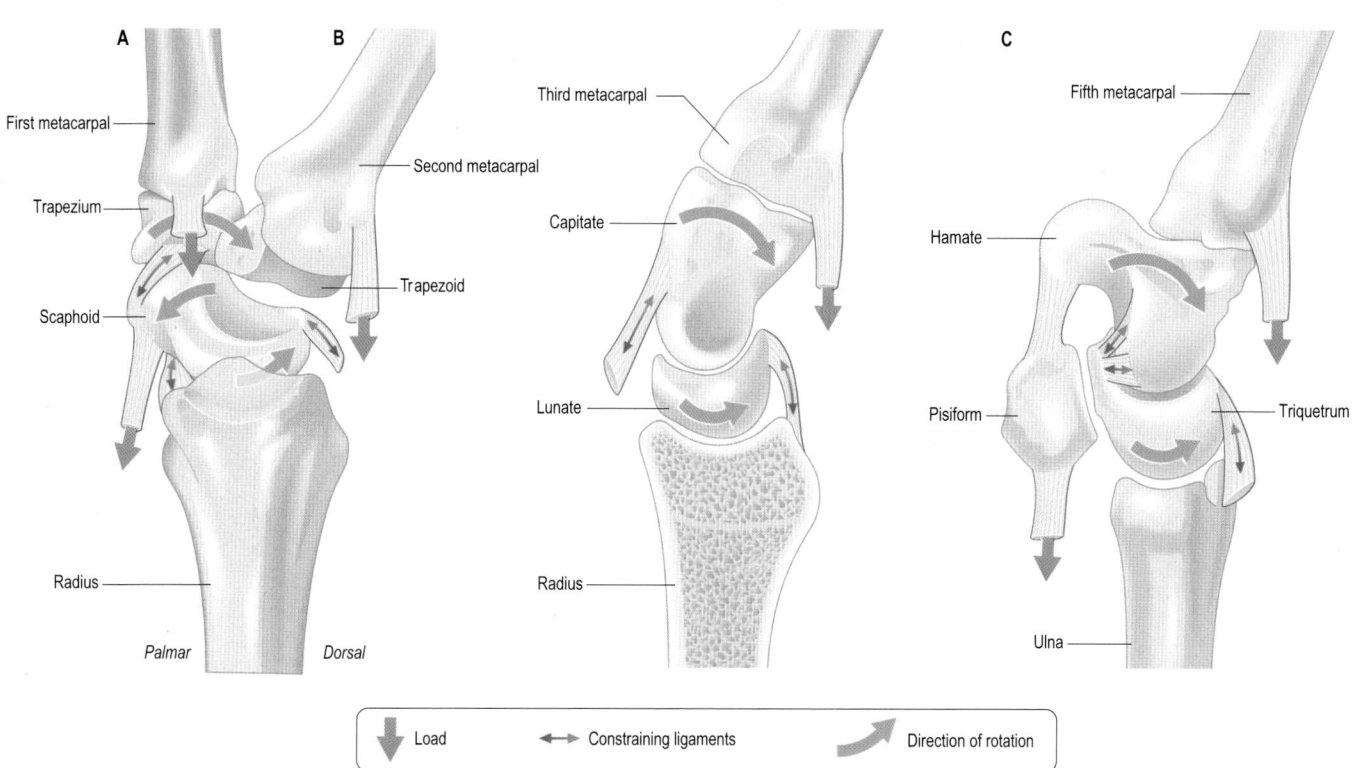

Fig. 53.32 The balance of rotatory moments occurring during axial loading are explained in this series of line diagrams representing sagittal sections of the wrist. In this representation the white arrows show the tendency for movement of the individual carpal bones and the black arrows show the tension developed in the restraining ligaments. **A**, The scaphoid tends to move into flexion with axial loading and is simultaneously constrained palmarly by the scaphotrapeziotrapezoidal ligaments and dorsally by the scapholunate ligament. **B**, The lunate tends to follow the scaphoid restrained only by the dorsal radiolunate ligament. **C**, The triquetrum tends to flex along with the two other bones of the proximal carpal row and is constrained palmarly by the triquetrohamate and triquetrocapitate ligaments and dorsally by the radiotriquetral ligament. Redrawn with permission from Büchler U 1996 Wrist instability. London: Martin Dunitz. (By permission from Wrist Instability, Büchler U, 1996. London: Martin Dunitz.)

scaphoid, lunate and triquetrum move in complex but characteristic relationships which are dependent on the given movement (**Fig. 53.33**). Clinical observation provides some support for each of these theories.

Carpometacarpal joints (CMCJs)

(See also p. 910.)

The first CMCJ or basal joint of the thumb is a modified saddle joint permitting opposition of the thumb and conferring the ability to hold and manipulate objects. The actions of 'pinch' grip, 'tripod' pinch and 'chuck' grip are specifically facilitated. Significant forces pass across and compress this joint as compared to the remaining CMCJs. The second to fifth CMCJs exhibit an increasing range of movement progressing from the radial to the ulnar sides. Thus there is little mobility at the base of the index ray but considerable mobility at the base of the small finger ray, which facilitates 'cupping' of the palm of the hand. Compressive forces between the metacarpals and the distal carpal row are estimated to be upwards of ten times the forces at the tips of the fingers during 'pinch' or 'chuck' grip.

Triangular fibrocartilage complex (TFCC)

The TFCC stabilizes the ulnocarpal and radio-ulnar joints, transmits and distributes load from the carpus to the ulna and facilitates complex movements at the wrist (**Fig. 53.34**).

WRIST LOADING

Axial loading refers to load or force applied along a line parallel to the long bones of the arm and therefore corresponds to power grip manoeuvres, e.g. clenching the fist. In the normal activities of daily living, loading is usually multiplanar with a combination of vectors of force, e.g. grasping an object and then lifting it against gravity with the elbow flexed would engender transverse and axial loading with respect to the long axis of the forearm.

Force transmission

Radiocarpal joint

The articulation of the carpus with the radius (radiocarpal) and ulna (ulnocarpal) can be described in terms of specific fossae, i.e. the scaphoid and lunate fossae of the radius and the facet formed by the distal aspect of the TFCC. The scaphoid fossa contributes 43%, the lunate fossa 46%, and the TFCC 11%, of the total area of this articulating surface. Under physiological conditions, the contact area between this surface and the proximal carpal row is of the order of 20% of the whole. It varies consistently with position: greater contact is seen in forearm supination, radial deviation and dorsiflexion of the wrist, and lesser contact in forearm pronation, ulnar deviation and palmar flexion of the wrist. Further increase in contact area is seen with axial loading. Maximum contact areas are recorded at 40%. Force across the joint also varies with

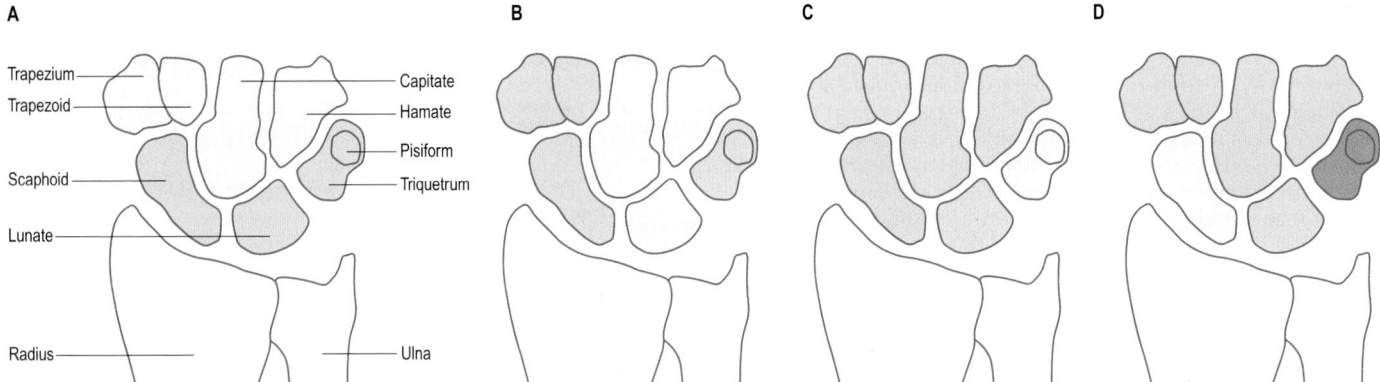

Fig. 53.33 Different theories of carpal mechanics. **A**, Row or rigid body theory; **B**, central column theory of Navarro; **C**, ring theory of Taleisnik; **D**, four-unit concept of Viegas.

In image A, the labels are: Trapezium, Trapezoid, Scaphoid, Lunate, Radius (left side); Capitate, Hamate, Pisiform, Triquetrum, Ulna (right side).

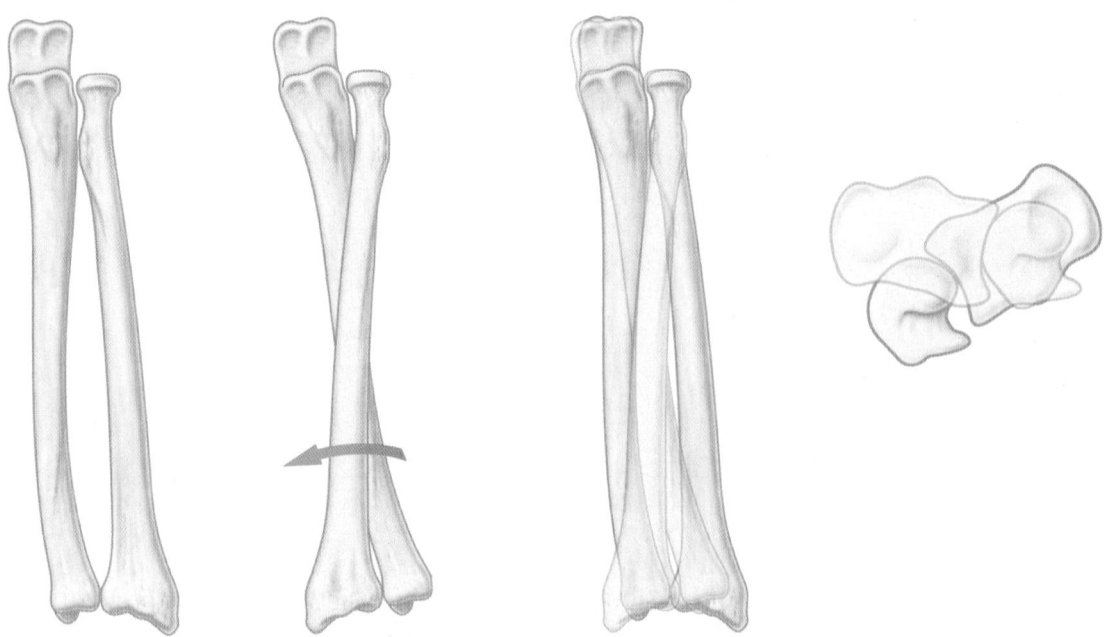

Fig. 53.34 Representation of the manner in which the radius moves around the ulna during forearm rotation. The curvature of the shaft of the radius is important in facilitating this movement. The axis of forearm rotation passes through the head of the ulna and varies slightly in position through the range of rotation.

the position of the forearm and the degree of wrist flexion. For a given load in wrist neutral position, 50% of force passes across the scaphoid fossa, 35% through the lunate fossa, and 15% across the TFCC. With a power grip there is slight ulnar deviation, and the proportion of force passing across the scaphoid and lunate fossae reverses.

Midcarpal joint

With the wrist in neutral position, c.50–60% of a given load is transmitted from the distal row through the capitate to the scaphoid and lunate. Up to 30% of the load is transmitted via the scaphotrapeziotrapezoid joint, and up to 20% via the hamate–triquetral joint.

Distal radio-ulnar joint (DRUJ)

Static axial loading of the wrist increases the contact areas of the joint surfaces of the distal radio-ulnar joint, DRUJ. Force transmitted across the DRUJ also increases with axial loading and varies with position of forearm rotation. It is maximal at 60° supination, when the ulnar head lies most directly under the ulnar-sided carpus, and least in full pronation. It has been shown that with the wrist in neutral position, 70–80% of axial load passes down the radius and 20–30% down the ulna. The proportion of force passing down the ulna varies with increasing load, and changes with position of the hand and carpus relative to the forearm bones. The interosseous membrane between the radius and ulna plays a role in distributing load in the forearm. Distal radio-ulnar joint loading also depends on relative radial and ulnar lengths, ie ulnar negative, neutral or positive variance.

SPECIFIC ACTIONS

Power grip

There is a predictable pathway of force transmission during axial loading of the hand such as occurs in power grip. During this action the wrist is positioned in mid-dorsiflexion and the object is tightly gripped. Force is transmitted from the hand and wrist via the radiocarpal joint and TFCC to both bones of the forearm, through the elbow joint to

the humerus, and thence via the glenohumeral joint to the pectoral girdle. Dynamic muscle action accounts for transmission of a large part of the force, and a smaller proportion is transmitted through the osseoligamentous structures. The distribution of force between the radius and ulna varies dynamically. It depends on the absolute value of load, degree of forearm rotation, and position of the carpus relative to the forearm.

Hammer action

The action exemplified by hammering, where the wrist alternates between the dorsoradial and the palmar–ulnar position, is an important movement. The reciprocal movement is more constrained and awkward to perform. The former movement is important in a wide variety of activities of daily living. In primates this movement is needed (along with forearm rotation at the distal radio-ulnar joint) for brachiation.

It is believed that load distributes dynamically as the position of the carpus moves relative to the forearm and there are consequent changes in the relative position of the carpal bones.

WRIST INSTABILITY

During evolution the upper limb has developed to facilitate prehension, i.e. the placing of the hand in three-dimensional space. However, mobility of the hand on the forearm has evolved at the expense of stability. A wrist is said to be kinetically unstable when it cannot bear physiological loads without giving way or causing injury. A wrist is kinematically unstable when it exhibits sudden changes in carpal alignment, i.e. during a specific movement there is a 'clunk' as one or more of the carpal bones moves abnormally with respect to the others. Stability of the various joints such that the bones maintain normal anatomical relations with respect to each other throughout the normal range of motion is essential for physiological load-bearing.

Carpal instability is produced by rupture or attenuation of intrinsic and extrinsic carpal ligaments and may be detected either clinically or evidenced on radiographs as malalignment of the carpal bones (**Fig. 53.35**).

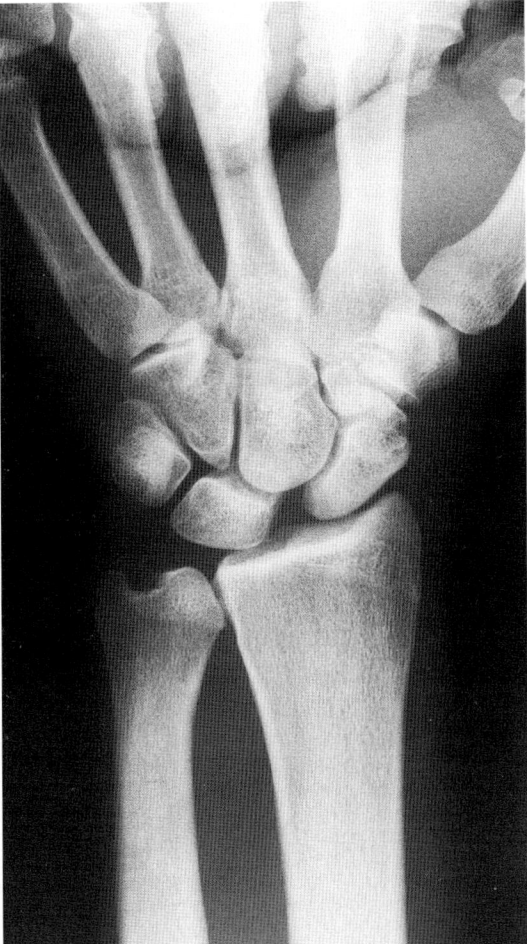
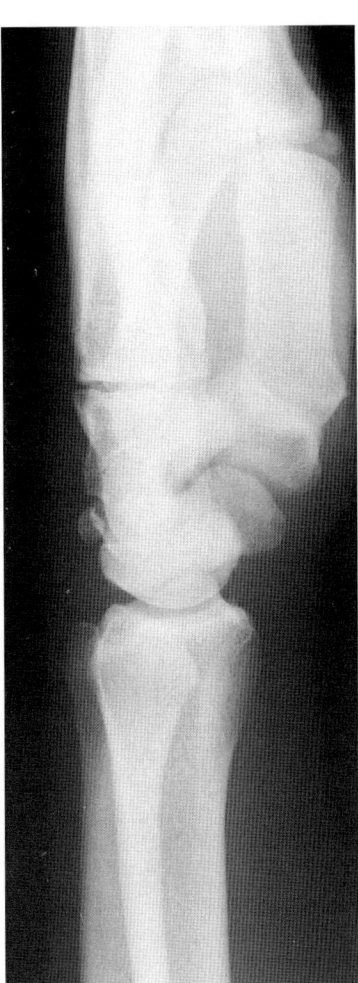

Fig. 53.35 Scapholunate dissociation shown in posteroanterior power grip view (A) and lateral view (B). Scapholunate dissociation shown in anteroposterior power grip view B. Dissociation between the scaphoid and lunate as shown here leads to collapse of the scaphoid into flexion and the lunate into extension (dorsal intercalated segment instability, or DISI) thus removing the inbuilt tension across the proximal row. This causes the increased scapholunate angle to 90 degrees in Fig. 53.35B.

CARPOMETACARPAL JOINTS

CARPOMETACARPAL JOINT OF THE THUMB

Articulating surfaces – The carpometacarpal joint of the thumb is a sellar (saddle) joint between the first metacarpal base and trapezium. It enjoys wide mobility due to its extensive articular surfaces and their topology.

Ligaments – The first metacarpal and trapezium are connected by lateral, anterior and posterior ligaments and a fibrous capsule. The broad lateral ligament runs from the lateral surface of the trapezium to the radial side of the metacarpal base. The palmar and dorsal ligaments are oblique bands which converge to the ulnar side of the metacarpal base from the palmar and dorsal surfaces of the trapezium respectively.

Synovial membrane – The synovial membrane lines the joint capsule and is separate from it.

Vascular supply – The carpometacarpal joint of the thumb receives its blood supply from the radial artery and its first dorsal metacarpal branch.

Innervation – The carpometacarpal joint of the thumb is innervated by articular twigs from the posterior interosseous nerve.

Joint movements – (See also p. 923.)

Except at initiation, flexion is accompanied by medial rotation; conversely, medial rotation involves flexion. Linkage of movements is due largely to the shape of the articular surfaces (which impose some conjunct rotation), and to the obliquity of the dorsal ligament (which, when taut, anchors the ulnar side of the metacarpal base while its radial side continues to move). Contraction of flexor pollicis brevis, assisted by opponens pollicis, thus produces medial rotation with flexion; combined with abduction this brings the thumb pulp into contact with the pulps of the slightly flexed fingers, a movement termed opposition. (The flexed fingers have varying degrees of lateral metacarpophalangeal rotation, which is minimal in the index, but maximal in minimus.) Conversely, full extension of the thumb metacarpal entails slight lateral rotation, attributable to the sellar form of the joint and to the action of the palmar ligament (which is similar to that of the dorsal ligament in flexion).

Muscles producing movements – The muscles producing movements at the carpometacarpal joint of the thumb are as follows.

Flexion – Flexor pollicis brevis and opponens pollicis, aided by flexor pollicis longus when the other joints of the thumb are flexed. Flexion entails medial rotation.

Extension – Abductor pollicis longus and extensors pollicis brevis and longus. In full extension extensor pollicis longus, owing to its oblique pull and the disposition of the palmar ligament, rotates the thumb laterally and draws it dorsally, i.e. slightly adducts it.

Abduction – Abductors pollicis brevis and longus. When abduction is maximal the digit and metacarpal are not in line, and the thumb is abducted at both metacarpophalangeal and carpometacarpal joints.

Adduction – Adductor pollicis alone.

Opposition – Opponens pollicis and flexor brevis pollicis simultaneously flex and medially rotate the abducted thumb. Interpulpal pressure, or that generated by digital grasping, is increased by adductor pollicis and flexor pollicis longus.

Circumduction – Extensors, abductors, flexors and adductors acting consecutively in this, or reverse, order.

SECOND TO FIFTH CARPOMETACARPAL JOINTS

The second to fifth carpometacarpal joints are synovial ellipsoid joints between the carpus and second to fifth metacarpals. Although widely classed as plane, they have curved articular surfaces which are often of complex sellar shape. The bones are united by articular capsules, and dorsal, palmar and interosseous ligaments.

Ligaments – The dorsal ligaments are the strongest, and connect the dorsal surfaces of the carpal and metacarpal bones. The second metacarpal has two ligaments, from the trapezium and trapezoid; the third has two, from the trapezoid and capitate; the fourth has two, from the capitate and hamate; the fifth has a single band from the hamate, which is continuous with a similar palmar ligament, forming an incomplete capsule.

The palmar ligaments are similar, except that the third metacarpal has three: a lateral from the trapezium, superficial to the tendon sheath of flexor carpi radialis, an intermediate from the capitate, and a medial from the hamate.

The interosseous ligaments consist of two short, thick, fibrous bands. They are limited to one part of the carpometacarpal articulation and connect contiguous distal margins of the capitate and hamate with adjacent surfaces of the third and fourth metacarpal bones. They may be united proximally.

Synovial membranes – The synovial membranes are often continuous with those of the intercarpal joints. Occasionally, the joint between the hamate and fourth and fifth metacarpal bones has a separate synovial cavity, bounded laterally by the medial interosseous ligament and its extensions to the palmar and dorsal parts of the capsule.

Vascular supply – The second to fifth carpometacarpal joints are supplied by the posterior carpal branches of the radial and ulnar arteries, by twigs from the anterior interosseous artery, and from the palmar digital arteries.

Innervation – The second to fifth carpometacarpal joints are innervated by the deep terminal branches of the ulnar nerve, the anterior interosseous branch of the median nerve, and the posterior interosseous branch of the radial nerve.

Muscles producing movements – Slight gliding movements are effected by the long flexor and extensor muscles of the digits.

INTERMETACARPAL JOINTS

Articulating surfaces – The second to fifth metacarpal bases articulate reciprocally by small cartilage-covered facets connected by dorsal, palmar and interosseous ligaments.

Fibrous capsule – The intermetacarpal joints have fibrous capsules.

Ligaments – The dorsal and palmar ligaments pass transversely from bone to bone. The interosseous ligaments connect contiguous surfaces just distal to their articular facets.

Synovial membranes – The synovial membranes are continuous with those of the carpometacarpal articulations.

Movements at the carpometacarpal and intermetacarpal joints – Movements at the carpometacarpal and intermetacarpal articulations are limited to slight gliding, sufficient to permit some flexion–extension and adjunct rotation: ranges vary in different joints. They are partly accessory movements occurring when the palm is 'cupped', as in grasping an object. Active movements also occur and are familiar, e.g. to the pianist or violinist. The fifth metacarpal is most movable and the second and third are the least mobile. These variations are easily demonstrated by opposing each digit to the thumb over the palmar centre. About two-thirds of the movements are pollicial, as described above, but during opposition to minimus, the latter is flexed, abducted and laterally rotated, accounting for the remaining third of the movement. These actions occur at both the carpometacarpal and metacarpophalangeal joints. The close-packed position probably coincides with carpal extension, as in gripping. Further accessory movements are spiral twisting of the whole metacarpus on the carpus.

Muscles producing movements – Movements at carpometacarpal and intermetacarpal joints are effected by the flexors and extensors of the second to fifth digits.

METACARPOPHALANGEAL JOINTS

The metacarpophalangeal joints are usually considered ellipsoid. However, the metacarpal heads are adapted to shallow concavities on the phalangeal bases: they are not regularly convex but partially divided on their palmar aspects and thus almost bicondylar (**Fig. 53.36**).

Fibrous capsule – The metacarpophalangeal joints all have fibrous capsules.

Ligaments – Each metacarpophalangeal joint has a palmar and two collateral ligaments.

Palmar ligaments – The palmar (volar plates) ligaments are unusual. They are thick, dense and fibrocartilaginous, and sited between, and connected to, the collateral ligaments. They are attached loosely to the metacarpals but firmly to the phalangeal bases. Their palmar aspects are blended with the deep transverse palmar ligaments and are grooved for the flexor tendons, whose fibrous sheaths connect with the sides of the grooves. Their deep surfaces increase articular areas for the metacarpal heads.

Deep transverse metacarpal ligaments – The deep transverse metacarpal ligaments are three short, wide, flat bands which connect the palmar ligaments of the second to fifth metacarpophalangeal joints. They are related anteriorly to the lumbricals and digital vessels and nerves, and posteriorly to the interossei. Bands from the digital slips of the central palmar aponeurosis join their palmar surfaces. On both sides of the third and fourth metacarpophalangeal joints, but only the ulnar side of the second and radial side of the fifth, transverse bands of the dorsal digital expansions join the deep transverse metacarpal ligaments. The lumbricals and the phalangeal attachments of the dorsal interossei lie anterior to this band, and the remaining attachments of dorsal interossei and palmar interossei are posterior to it (*see* **Fig. 53.43**).

Collateral ligaments – The collateral ligaments are strong, round cords which flank the joints. Each is attached to the posterior tubercle and adjacent pit on the side of its metacarpal head, and each passes distoanteriorly to the side of the anterior aspect of its phalangeal base (**Fig. 53.36**).

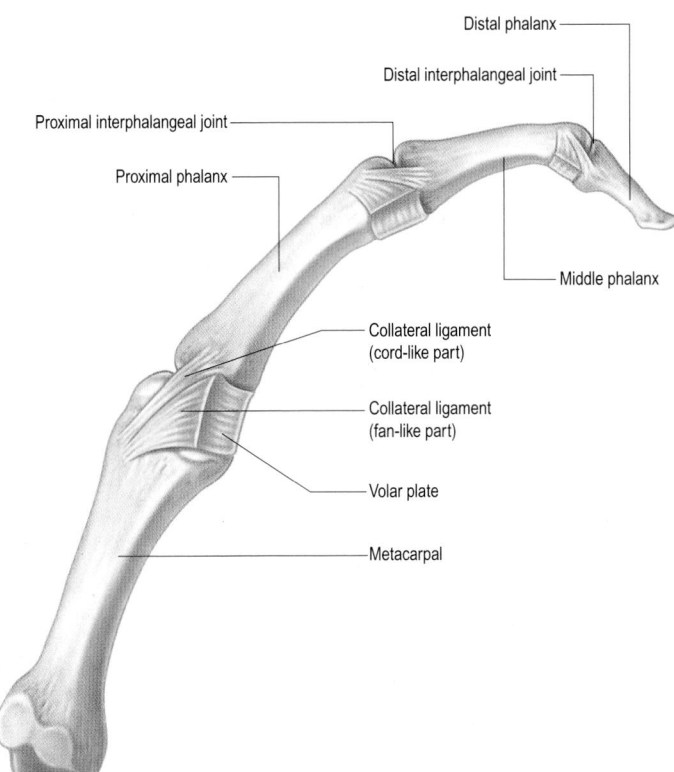

Proximal interphalangeal joint

Proximal phalanx

Distal phalanx

Distal interphalangeal joint

Middle phalanx

Collateral ligament
(cord-like part)

Collateral ligament
(fan-like part)

Volar plate

Metacarpal

Fig. 53.36 Metacarpophalangeal and digital joints of the left third finger: medial aspect.

Synovial membrane – The metacarpophalangeal joints are lined by a synovial membrane.

Vascular supply – The metacarpophalangeal joints receive their blood supply from the dorsal and palmar metacarpal arteries, the arteria princeps pollicis, and the arteria radialis indicis.

Innervation – The metacarpophalangeal joints are innervated by twigs from the palmar digital branches of the median nerve, the deep terminal branch of the ulnar nerve, and the posterior interosseous nerve.

Joint movements – Flexion, extension, adduction, abduction, circumduction and limited rotation all take place at the metacarpophalangeal joints. Rotation cannot occur in isolation, but may accompany flexion–extension. This may be initiated voluntarily in the free hand (e.g. each finger flexing and rotating to place its tip near the palmar centre); the range of rotation is frequently increased as a result of the resistance of a grasped object. Flexion is almost 90°, whereas extension is only a few degrees: both movements are limited mostly by antagonistic muscles. Flexion is often terminated by the resistance offered by a grasped object. The metacarpophalangeal joint of the thumb has a flexion–extension range of c.60°, which is almost entirely flexion. Other movements are adduction–abduction (maximal range 25°), which invariably accompanies the corresponding carpometacarpal movements and increases their combined range, and slight conjunct rotation, but greater adjunct rotation, which accompanies flexion–extension. Of the second to fifth metacarpophalangeal joints, the second is most mobile in adduction–abduction (c.30°), followed by the fifth, fourth, and third.

Accessory movements – Accessory movements are further rotation (most marked in the thumb), anteroposterior and lateral translation of a phalanx or metacarpal, and distraction.

Muscles producing movements – The muscles producing movements at the metacarpophalangeal joints are as follows.

Flexion – Flexors digitorum superficialis and profundus, assisted by the lumbricals and interossei and, in the minimus, flexor digiti minimi brevis. In the thumb, flexors pollicis longus and brevis and the first palmar interosseous. Slight lateral rotation accompanies digital flexion of digits 3–5. Flexion of the index finger may be accompanied by minimal lateral rotation or no rotation: a small degree of medial rotation is frequently observed.

Extension – Extensor digitorum, assisted in the second and fifth digits by extensor indicis and extensor digiti minimi respectively. In the thumb, extensors pollicis longus and brevis.

Adduction – In extended fingers, palmar interossei; the long flexors are predominant during flexion. In the thumb, limited metacarpophalangeal adduction is possible and may be attributable to adductor pollicis and the first palmar interosseous.

Abduction – In extended fingers, dorsal interossei assisted by the long extensors (except in the middle finger), and abductor digiti minimi in the little finger. In the thumb, abductor pollicis brevis (which also contributes to opposition). When the fingers are flexed at the IP joints, active abduction is impossible: if the long digital flexors are inactive, passive abduction is free. Inability to abduct actively in this position may be due to shortening of the dorsal interossei and abductor digiti minimi by flexion. However the altered line of pull of the interossei relative to the axis of movement is probably the determining factor: in digital extension the axis of lateral movements is anteroposterior, whereas in flexion it is proximodistal, and the line of pull of the interossei is then nearly parallel to the axis.

Gamekeeper's thumb – The ulnar collateral ligament of the metacarpophalangeal joint of the thumb can be avulsed from its distal attachment to the base of the proximal phalanx by a combination of forced extension and radial deviation of the joint. The injury was reported to occur in gamekeepers while breaking the necks of game, but can occur following simple falls onto the outstretched hand, especially in skiers who have the straps of ski poles wrapped around their thumbs.

The ulnar collateral ligament is normally covered by the aponeurotic insertion of the adductor pollicis tendon. Following avulsion, the proximal end can become superficially displaced around the proximal free edge of the aponeurotic insertion of the adductor. This soft tissue interposition prevents the ends of the avulsed ligament from healing. If left untreated, a firm palpable inflammatory swelling occurs, known as the 'Stener lesion'. Surgical repair requires division of the aponeurotic insertion of adductor pollicis, followed by bony reattachment of the avulsed ligament and repair of the aponeurosis.

INTERPHALANGEAL JOINTS

The interphalangeal joints are uniaxial hinge joints (**Fig. 53.36**).

Fibrous capsule – Each interphalangeal joint has a fibrous capsule.

Ligaments – Each interphalangeal joint has a palmar ligament (also known as the volar plate) and two collateral ligaments. The long extensor tendons take the place of the dorsal capsular ligaments. Extensions from the extensor expansion, each collateral ligament and the palmar ligament pass into the joint cavity. They provide a significant increase to the articular surface area of the phalangeal base and their deformable nature improves joint congruence.

Palmar ligament (volar plate) – The volar plate constitutes the floor of the interphalangeal joint. In the proximal interphalangeal joint, the distal end of the volar plate is thickened laterally where it is firmly attached to the base of the middle phalanx at the position of the true collateral ligament attachment. Centrally, it is more delicate and blends with the volar periosteum of the middle phalanx. Proximally, the volar plate is also very delicate in its central portion, but it is thickened laterally to form the so-called check rein ligaments which attach to the periosteum of the proximal phalanx just within the walls of the A2 pulley component of the fibrous flexor sheath. Nutrient branches of the digital arteries pass underneath these check ligaments to reach the vinculae (**Fig. 53.37**). A detailed account of the anatomy of the volar plate can be found in Bowers et al (1980).

Collateral ligaments – The collateral ligaments pass from the lateral aspect of the head of one phalanx to the volar aspect of the base of the adjacent phalanx. An accessory component to the collateral ligament arises in continuity with the main ligament and passes in a volar direction to attach to the volar plate.

Synovial membrane – Each interphalangeal joint has a synovial lining.

Vascular supply – The interphalangeal joints are supplied by branches from the palmar digital arteries.

Innervation – The interphalangeal joints are innervated by the palmar digital branches of the median nerve (to the thumb, index, middle and ring fingers), and the ulnar nerve (to the ring and little fingers).

Factors maintaining stability – Stability is conferred by the articular contours of the joint surfaces and the collateral ligaments. The flexor and extensor tendons and retinacular ligaments provide secondary stabilization. Stability against hyperextension of the proximal interphalangeal joint is enhanced by the three-dimensional box arrangement that is produced by the collateral ligament–volar plate complex.

Joint movements – Movements (active) at the interphalangeal joints are flexion and extension, and are greater in range at the proximal joints. Flexion is considerable, whereas extension is limited by tension of the digital flexors and terminated by tension in the palmar ligaments and conarticular compression. Full extension is the close-packed position, which is assumed whenever the fingers are used as props to transmit body weight or powerful thrust. In contrast, the fully clenched fist may also be used for this purpose. Flexion and extension are accompanied by slight conjunct rotation: during flexion this turns the digital pulps slightly laterally, i.e. to face the opposed thumb, and an opposite rotation occurs during extension.

Accessory movements – Accessory movements are limited rotation, abduction, adduction and anteroposterior translation. They permit the

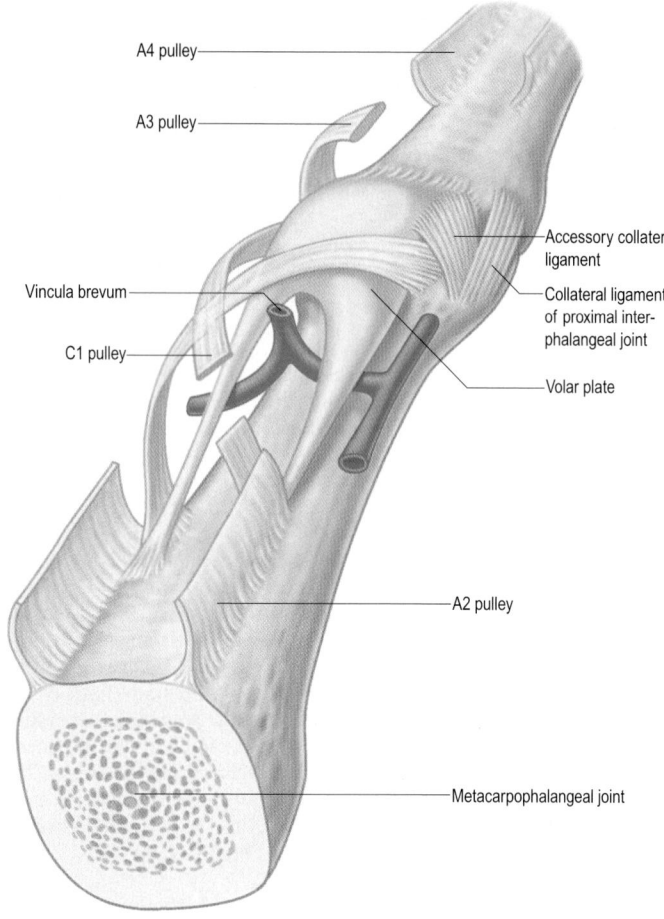

Fig. 53.37 Anatomy of the proximal interphalangeal joint volar plate.

fingers to adapt to the shapes of gripped objects and help to protect against stresses and strains.

Muscles producing movements – The muscles producing movements at the interphalangeal joints are as follows.

Flexion – At proximal interphalangeal joints, flexors digitorum superficialis and profundus; at distal interphalangeal joints, flexor digitorum profundus; at the thumb interphalangeal joint, flexor pollicis longus.

Extension – Extensors digitorum, digiti minimi and pollicis longus, in association with abductor pollicis longus and extensor pollicis brevis. Extension occurs simultaneously in both joints in digits 2–5.

Simultaneous flexion at the metacarpophalangeal joints and extension at the interphalangeal joints of a digit are essential for the fine movements of writing, drawing, threading a needle, etc. The lumbricals and interossei have long been accepted as not only primary agents in flexing the metacarpophalangeal joints but also in extending the interphalangeal joints via their attachments to the dorsal digital expansions.

Mallet finger – Mallet finger is a traumatic rupture, avulsion fracture or laceration of the terminal slip of the extensor tendon to the terminal phalanx of the finger. It can result from forced flexion of the distal phalanx of the fully extended finger and is a well-known injury in cricketers. The patient is unable actively to extend the terminal phalanx although the distal interphalangeal joint can be extended passively.

Swan neck deformity – Swan neck deformity involves hyperextension of the proximal interphalangeal joint together with distal interphalangeal joint flexion. It is caused by a relative overactivity of the extensors acting at the proximal interphalangeal joint compared with the flexors. It arises as a result of intrinsic muscle spasm, long standing mallet finger or dysfunction of flexor digitorum superficialis and can only occur if there is also same laxity of the volar plate.

Boutonnière deformity – Boutonnière deformity is a flexion deformity of the proximal interphalangeal joint following either division or laxity in the central slip of the extensor tendon, which normally inserts into the base of the middle phalanx. An essential feaure is hyper extension at the distal interphalangeal joint. It usually occurs as a result of either trauma or rheumatoid arthritis which cause the lateral bands of the extensor tendon to migrate in a volar direction and the head of the proximal phalanx to migrate dorsally. Initially the deformity is passively correctable. With time, the soft tissues around the joint contract and a fixed deformity results.

MUSCLE

EXTRINSIC LONG FLEXORS AND EXTENSORS

The extrinsic long flexors and extensors are described on page 873.

FLEXOR RETINACULUM (Fig. 53.12)

The flexor retinaculum is a strong, fibrous band which crosses the front of the carpus and converts its anterior concavity into the carpal tunnel. The latter transmits the flexor tendons of the digits and the median nerve. The retinaculum is short and broad, c.2.5–3 cm both transversely and proximodistally. It is attached medially to the pisiform and the hook of the hamate. Laterally, it splits into superficial and deep laminae. The superficial lamina is attached to the tubercles of the scaphoid and trapezium. The deep lamina is attached to the medial lip of the groove on the trapezium. Together with this groove, the two laminae form a tunnel, lined by a synovial sheath, which contains the tendon of flexor carpi radialis. The retinaculum is crossed superficially by the ulnar vessels and nerve – immediately radial to the pisiform – and by the palmar cutaneous branches of the median and ulnar nerves. A slender

band of fascia, the superficial part of the flexor retinaculum, bridges over the ulnar neurovascular bundle and attaches to the radial side of the pisiform, forming a tunnel (Guyon's canal) which is an occasional site of ulnar nerve entrapment. The tendons of palmaris longus and flexor carpi ulnaris are partly attached to the anterior surface of the retinaculum. Distally some of the intrinsic muscles of the thumb and little finger are attached to the retinaculum.

LONG FLEXOR TENDON APPARATUS

Flexor tendon sheaths

The fibrous sheaths of the flexor tendons are specialized parts of the palmar fascial continuum. Each finger has an osseoaponeurotic tunnel which extends from midpalm to the distal phalanx. The thumb has a tunnel for flexor pollicis longus which extends from the metacarpal to the distal phalanx. The proximal border is to some extent a matter of definition, because the transverse fibres of the palmar aponeurosis may be considered to be a part of the pulley system. The sheath consists of arcuate fibres which arch anteriorly over bone, tendons (where the sheath is required to be stiff), and the centres of joints (where a bucket-handle of arcuate fibres is a mechanically favourable arrangement). In contrast, where the sheath is required to fold to permit joint flexion, it consists of cruciate fibres. These fibrous sheaths are lined by a thin synovial membrane which provides a sealed lubrication system containing synovial fluid. The synovial membrane extends from the distal phalanx to midpalm in the case of the index, middle and ring fingers, and further proximally in the case of the little finger (**Fig. 53.38**). The sheaths around the thumb and little finger are continuous with the flexor sheaths in front of the wrist. The parietal synovial membrane is reflected onto the surface of the flexor tendon, forming a visceral synovium.

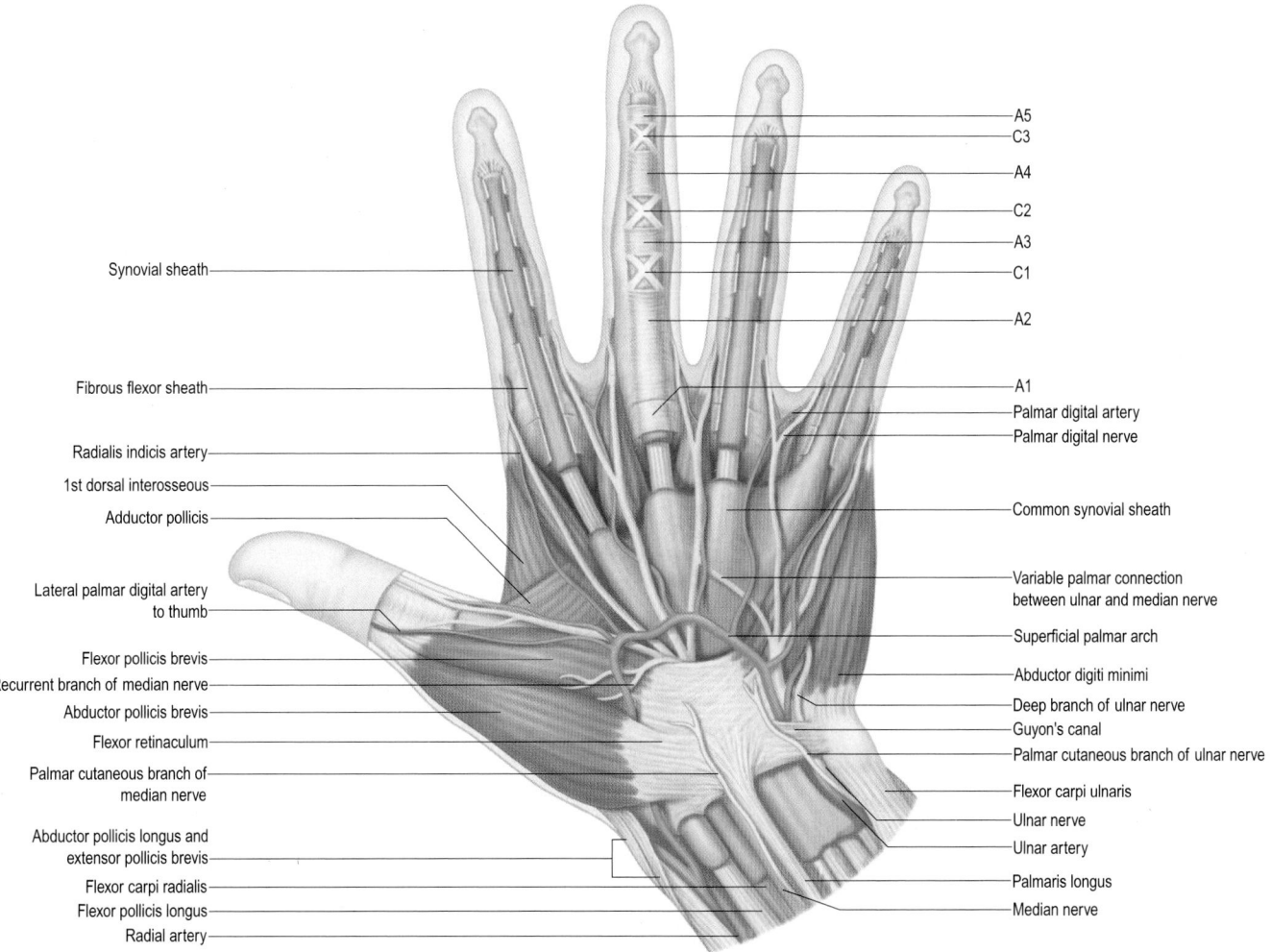

Synovial sheath —
Fibrous flexor sheath —
Radialis indicis artery —
1st dorsal interosseous —
Adductor pollicis —
Lateral palmar digital artery to thumb —
Flexor pollicis brevis —
Recurrent branch of median nerve —
Abductor pollicis brevis —
Flexor retinaculum —
Palmar cutaneous branch of median nerve —
Abductor pollicis longus and extensor pollicis brevis —
Flexor carpi radialis —
Flexor pollicis longus —
Radial artery —

— A5
— C3
— A4
— C2
— A3
— C1
— A2
— A1
— Palmar digital artery
— Palmar digital nerve
— Common synovial sheath
— Variable palmar connection between ulnar and median nerve
— Superficial palmar arch
— Abductor digiti minimi
— Deep branch of ulnar nerve
— Guyon's canal
— Palmar cutaneous branch of ulnar nerve
— Flexor carpi ulnaris
— Ulnar nerve
— Ulnar artery
— Palmaris longus
— Median nerve

Fig. 53.38 Synovial sheaths of the tendons on the flexor aspect of the left wrist and hand. Where they are exposed, the synovial sheaths are shown in blue.

A standard nomenclature for the anular and cruciform pulleys that make up the sheath has been adopted by the American Society for Surgery of the Hand: the letters A and C respectively are used (Doyle & Blythe 1975).

The usual pattern is as follows (**Fig. 53.39**). The A1 pulley is situated anterior to the palmar cartilaginous plate of the metacarpophalangeal joint and may extend over the proximal part of the proximal phalanx. The A2 overlies the middle third of the proximal phalanx. It is the strongest pulley and arises from well-defined longitudinal ridges on the palmar aspect of the phalanx. Its distal edge is well developed. A pouch or recess of synovium extends superficial to the free edge of the pulley fibres so that the free edge forms a lip protruding into the synovial space. A3 is a narrow pulley lying palmar to the proximal interphalangeal joint. A4 overlies the middle third of the middle phalanx, and A5 overlies the distal interphalangeal joint. The cruciate fibres are numbered in a slightly different manner. C0 is palmar to the metacarpophalangeal joint. There are two cruciate zones, C1 and C2, at the proximal interphalangeal joint and they lie just proximal and distal respectively to A3. At the distal interphalangeal joint there is one pronounced cruciate system, C3, which lies between A4 and A5. Variations occur frequently. During flexion, the cruciate fibres become orientated more transversely in the digits and the edges of adjacent anular pulleys approximate so that they form, in full flexion, a continuous tunnel of transversely orientated fibres. Surgically the most important pulleys which prevent bowstringing of the flexor tendons are the A2 and A4 pulleys.

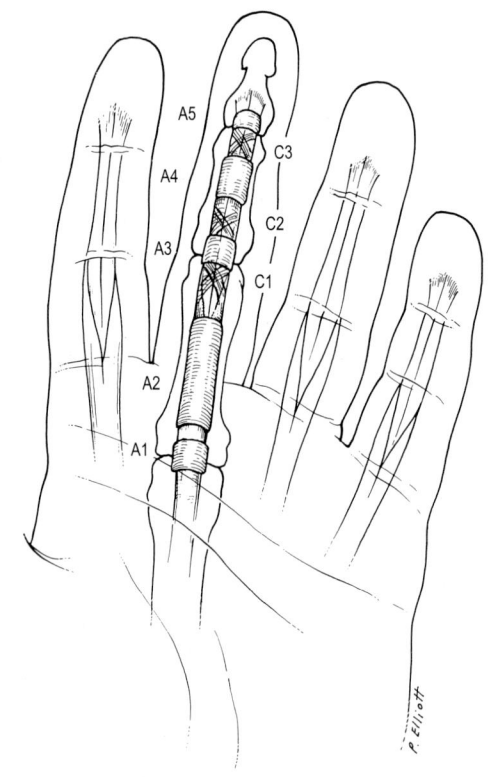

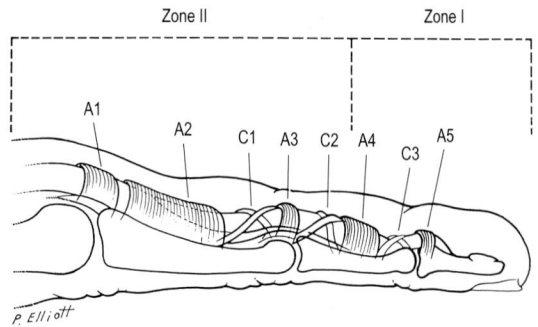

Fig. 53.39 Arrangement of the anular and cruciate pulleys of the flexor tendon sheath. **A**, Palmar aspect of left hand; **B**, lateral view.

The pulley arrangement in the thumb is different from that in the other digits. There are three constant pulleys – two anular and one oblique (**Fig. 53.40**). The A1 pulley is located at the metacarpophalangeal joint. The oblique pulley is located over the mid-portion of the proximal phalanx, and its fibres pass from the ulnar aspect proximally to the radial aspect dorsally. The A2 pulley is thinner than the A1 pulley and is situated just proximal to the interphalangeal joint. The oblique pulley is the most important pulley in the thumb for maintaining the action of flexor pollicis longus.

Synovial sheaths of the carpal flexor tendons
Two synovial sheaths envelop the flexor tendons as they traverse the carpal tunnel, one for the flexores digitorum superficialis and profundus, the other for flexor pollicis longus (**Fig. 53.12**). These sheaths extend into the forearm for c2.5 cm proximal to the flexor retinaculum, and occasionally communicate with each other deep to it. The sheath of the flexores digitorum tendons reaches about halfway along the metacarpal bones, where it ends in blind diverticula around the tendons to the index, middle and ring fingers (**Fig. 53.38**). It is prolonged around the tendons to the little finger and is usually continuous with their digital synovial sheath. A transverse section through the carpus shows that the tendons are invaginated into the sheath from the lateral side (**Fig. 53.12**). The parietal layer lines the flexor retinaculum and the floor of the carpal tunnel. It is reflected laterally as the visceral layer over the tendons of flexor digitorum superficialis ventrally and flexor digitorum profundus dorsally. Medially a recess formed by the visceral layer of the sheath insinuates between the two groups of tendons and passes laterally for a variable distance. The sheath of flexor pollicis longus, which is usually separate, is continued along the thumb as far as the insertion of the tendon.

Vincula
The phenomenon of tendon gliding within a fibrous sheath requires a very specialized arrangement of the vascular supply. Folds of synovial membrane (containing a loose plexus of fascial fibres) carry blood vessels to the tendons at certain defined points (**Fig. 53.41**). These folds, vincula tendinum, are of two kinds. Vincula brevia, of which there are two in each finger, are attached to the deep surfaces of the tendons near to their insertions. There is thus one vinculum brevium attaching flexor digitorum profundus to the region of the distal interphalangeal joint, and a more proximal vinculum deep to flexor digitorum superficialis at the proximal interphalangeal joint. Vincula longa are filiform: usually two are attached to each superficial tendon, one to each deep tendon.

Trigger finger
Trigger finger is a stenosing tenovaginitis which affects the fibrous flexor sheaths of the fingers or thumb within the palm. The affected sheath thickens and entraps the contained tendons, which become constricted at the site of entrapment and bulge distal to it, to produce a distinct nodule in the palm of the hand. The finger now snaps as the tendon nodule passes through the constriction on flexing the finger. The corresponding extensor muscle is insufficiently powerful to extend the affected finger. The patient does this passively, accompanied by a painful snap. Treatment frequently requires surgical division of the A1 pulley of the flexor sheath to relieve the stricture.

EXTENSOR RETINACULUM (Fig. 53.42)
The extensor retinaculum is a strong, fibrous band which extends obliquely across the back of the wrist. It is attached laterally to the anterior border of the radius, medially to the triquetral and pisiform bones, and, in passing across the wrist, to the ridges on the dorsal aspect of the distal end of the radius. It prevents bowstringing of the tendons across the wrist joint.

Synovial sheaths of the carpal extensor tendons
Six tunnels deep to the extensor retinaculum transmit the extensor tendons, each contains a synovial sheath (**Fig. 53.42**).

The tendons of abductor pollicis longus and extensor pollicis brevis lie in a tunnel on the lateral side of the styloid process of the radius. Occasionally there may be a separate synovial sheath for each, or the tendon of the abductor may be double. The tendons of extensores carpi radiales longus and brevis lie behind the styloid process. The tendon of extensor pollicis longus lies on the medial side of the dorsal tubercle of

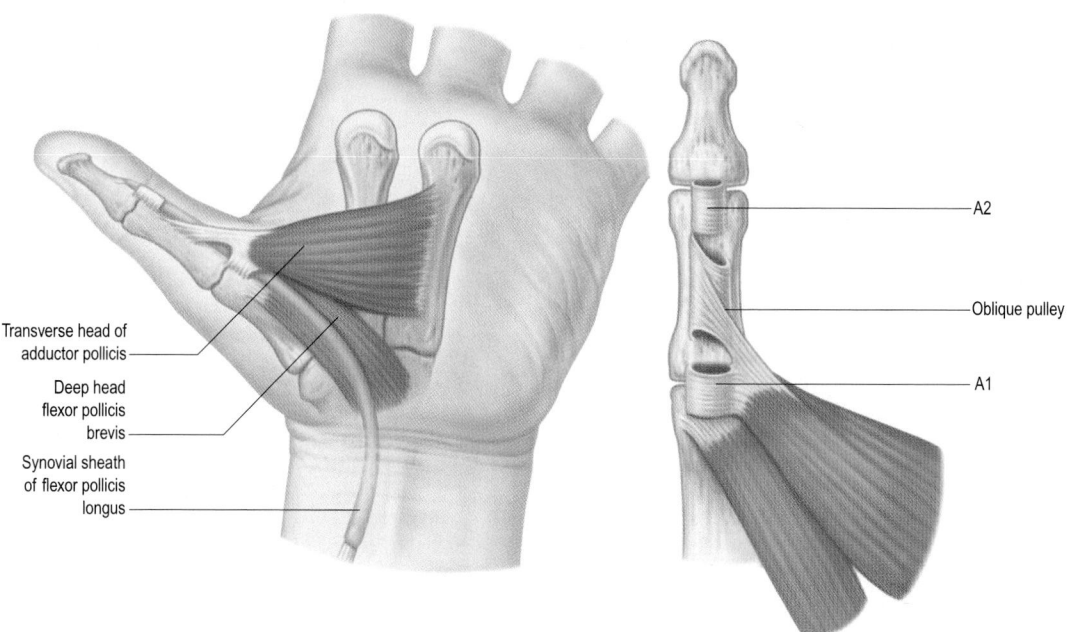

Transverse head of
adductor pollicis

Deep head
flexor pollicis
brevis

Synovial sheath
of flexor pollicis
longus

A2

Oblique pulley

A1

Fig. 53.40 Flexor sheath of the left thumb showing the anular and oblique pulleys. (From Doyle JR, Blythe WF 1977 Anatomy of the flexor tendon sheath and pulleys of the thumb. J Hand Surg 2: 149–151. With permission from the American Society for Surgery of the Hand.)

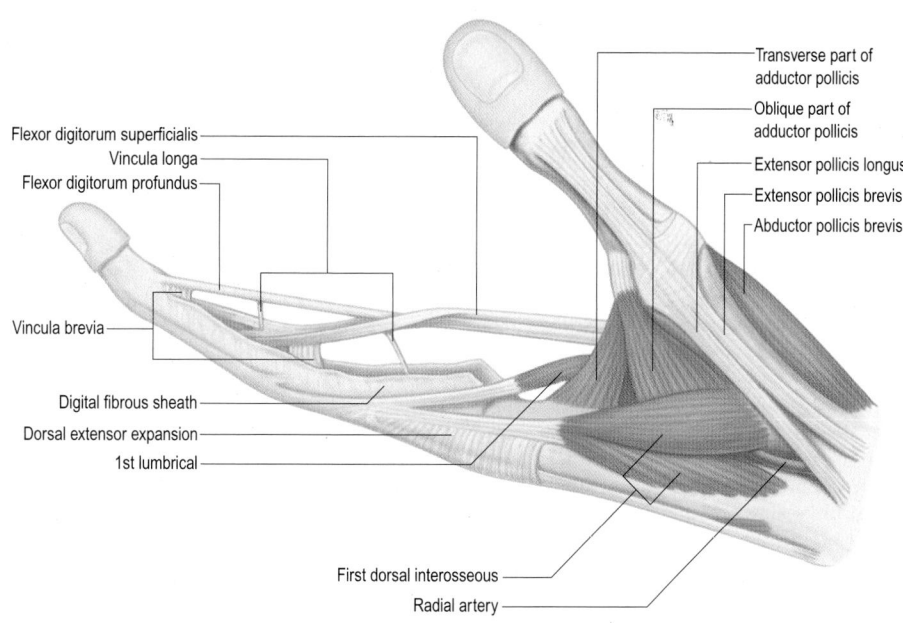

Flexor digitorum superficialis
Vincula longa
Flexor digitorum profundus

Transverse part of
adductor pollicis
Oblique part of
adductor pollicis
Extensor pollicis longus
Extensor pollicis brevis
Abductor pollicis brevis

Vincula brevia

Digital fibrous sheath
Dorsal extensor expansion
1st lumbrical

First dorsal interosseous
Radial artery

Fig. 53.41 Lateral part of the left hand showing the tendons and vincula tendinum of the index finger and the muscles in the first intermetacarpal space.

the radius and the tendons of extensor digitorum and extensor indicis lie in a tunnel on the medial side of the tubercle. The tendon of extensor digiti minimi lies opposite the interval between the radius and ulna, and the tendon of extensor carpi ulnaris lies between the head and the styloid process of the ulna.

The tendon sheaths of abductor pollicis longus, extensores pollicis brevis and longus, extensores carpi radiales and extensor carpi ulnaris stop immediately proximal to the bases of the metacarpal bones; those of extensor digitorum, extensor indicis and extensor digiti minimi are sometimes prolonged a little more distally along the metacarpus.

De Quervain's tenovaginitis

De Quervain's tenovaginitis is a stenosing tenovaginitis of unknown aetiology which occurs at the level of the radial styloid. It involves the common extensor sheath containing the tendons of abductor pollicis longus and extensor pollicis brevis. There is palpable thickening of the tendon sheath with painful limitation of extension of the thumb. Treat-

ment frequently requires division of the thickened sheath, care being taken to avoid the adjacent superficial radial nerve. Division of the sheath produces no functional impairment.

EXTENSOR TENDON APPARATUS

(See also p. 922.)

The extensor digitorum tendons emerge through the fourth dorsal compartment onto the dorsum of the hand, where they are joined together distally by a varying pattern of oblique interconnections, the juncturae tendinae. These typically pass in a distal direction from middle finger to index finger and from ring finger to middle and little fingers. Proximal lacerations to the middle finger extensor tendon may result in only partial loss of extension because of these tendinous interconnections.

At the level of the metacarpophalangeal joint, each extensor tendon is held in a central position over the dorsum of the joint by a flat fibrous

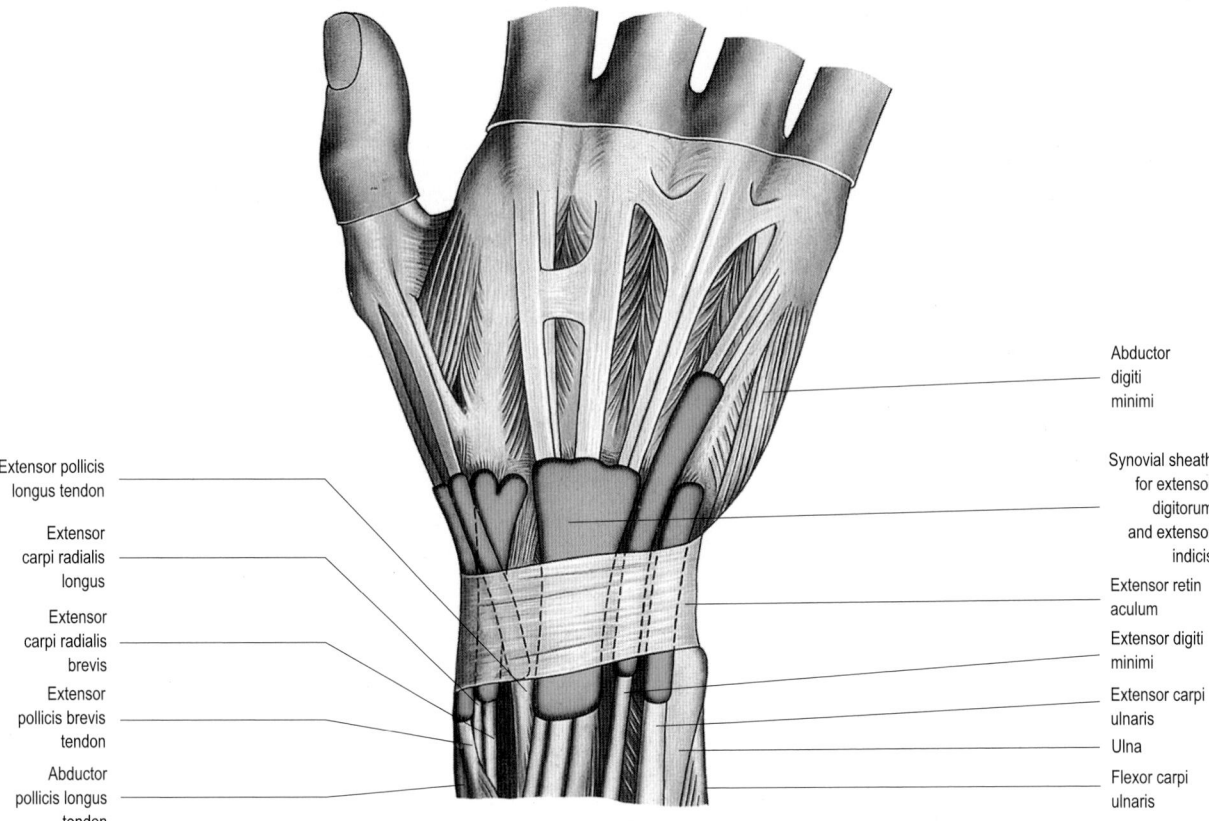

Extensor pollicis
longus tendon

Extensor
carpi radialis
longus

Extensor
carpi radialis
brevis

Extensor
pollicis brevis
tendon

Abductor
pollicis longus
tendon

Abductor
digiti
minimi

Synovial sheath
for extensor
digitorum
and extensor
indicis

Extensor retin
aculum

Extensor digiti
minimi

Extensor carpi
ulnaris

Ulna

Flexor carpi
ulnaris

Fig. 53.42 A simplified representation of the synovial sheaths of the tendons on the extensor aspect of the right wrist (preparation by Professor J C B Grant). The synovial sheaths are shown in blue, but they have not been coloured where they lie deep to the extensor retinaculum. In this situation, and where one sheath lies deep to another, the margins of the sheaths are indicated by broken lines.

extensor expansion (**Fig. 53.43**). The expansion extends onto the dorsum of the proximal phalanx of each digit. It forms a movable hood, which moves distally when the metacarpophalangeal joint is flexed, and proximally when it is extended (in which position it is most closely applied to the joint).

Each extensor tendon blends with the extensor expansion along its central axis, and is separated from the metacarpophalangeal joint by a small bursa. The expansion is triangular in shape, with its base proximal. It receives the conjoined tendons of the intrinsic muscles. The expansion is almost translucent between its margins and the extensor digitorum tendon. Transverse fibres (the sagittal bands) pass to the volar plate and transverse metacarpal ligaments. They separate the phalangeal attachment of the dorsal interosseus from the rest of the muscle, and the palmar interosseus from the lumbrical muscle. Injuries to the sagittal bands can lead to subluxation of the extensor tendon.

The margins of the extensor expansions are thickened on the radial side by the tendons of lumbrical and interosseous muscles and on the ulnar side by the tendon of an interosseous alone or, in the case of the fifth digit, by abductor digiti minimi. In clinical practice these attachments of the intrinsic muscles are referred to as 'wing tendons'. Proximal and distal 'wings' can be identified in the fingers usually on both sides of each expansion. The attachments of the interossei to these wings has led some to classify these muscles as 'distal' and 'proximal', in place of the more usual 'palmar' and 'dorsal'.

The interossei tendons join the extensor expansion at the level of the proximal portion of the proximal phalanx, while the lumbrical tendons join the extensor mechanism further distally at the mid-portion of the proximal phalanx. Their line of pull is proximal to the axis of rotation at the metacarpophalangeal joint, but dorsal to the axis of rotation at the proximal interphalangeal joint. The extensor mechanism trifurcates into a central slip and two lateral bands just proximal to the proximal interphalangeal joint. The central slip receives a contribution from the lumbrical and interosseous tendons via the lateral bands. Similarly, some fibres from the central region pass to each lateral band, producing a criss-cross arrangement of fibres. The central slip attaches to the base of the middle phalanx, while the lateral bands continue distally and

eventually fuse together and insert into the distal phalanx. The tension in the central slip and the lateral bands varies as the finger moves between flexion and extension and plays a crucial role in coordinating synchronous activity between the proximal and distal interphalangeal joints.

The transverse and oblique retinacular ligaments of Landsmeer connect the fibrous flexor sheath to the extensor apparatus. The transverse retinacular ligament passes from the A3 pulley of the fibrous flexor sheath at the level of the proximal interphalangeal joint to the lateral border of the lateral extensor band. The oblique retinacular ligament lies deep to the transverse retinacular ligament. It originates from the lateral aspect of the proximal phalanx and flexor sheath (A2 pulley) and passes volar to the axis of rotation of the proximal interphalangeal joint but in a dorsal and distal direction to insert into the terminal extensor tendon.

INTRINSIC MUSCLES OF THE HAND

The intrinsic muscles of the hand are organized into three groups plus a superficial muscle. Flexor pollicis brevis, abductor pollicis brevis, opponens pollicis and adductor pollicis all act on the thumb and are known collectively as the thenar muscles. Abductor digiti minimi, flexor digiti minimi brevis and opponens digiti minimi all act on the little finger and are known collectively as hypothenar muscles. Interossei and lumbricals act on the fingers. Palmaris brevis is a superficial muscle which lies beneath the ulnar palmar skin.

FLEXOR POLLICIS BREVIS

Attachments – Flexor pollicis brevis lies medial to abductor pollicis brevis (**Fig. 53.44**). It has superficial and deep parts. The superficial head arises from the distal border of the flexor retinaculum and the distal part of the tubercle of the trapezium, and passes along the radial side of the tendon of flexor pollicis longus. It is attached, by a tendon containing a sesamoid bone, to the radial side of the base of the proximal phalanx of the thumb. The deep part arises from the trapezoid

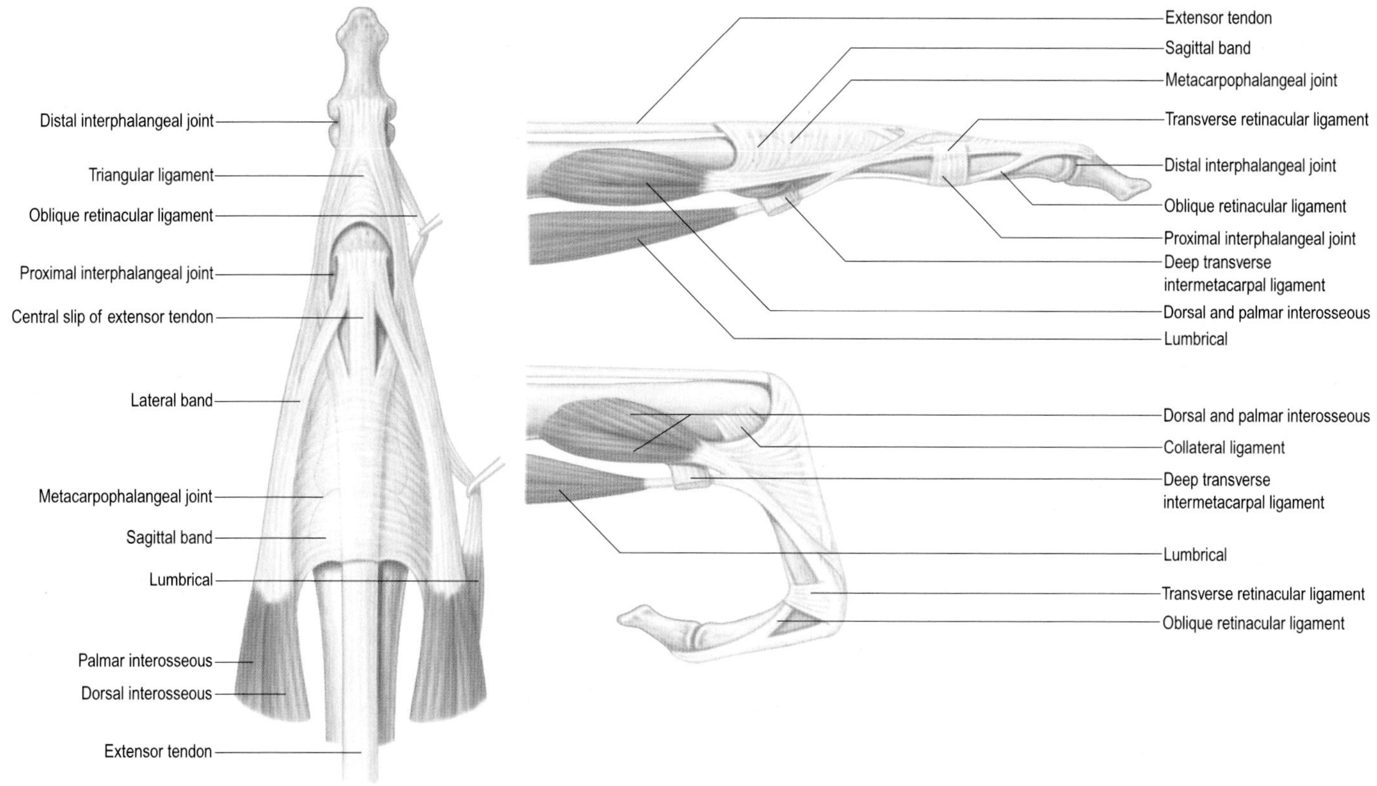

Distal interphalangeal joint

Triangular ligament

Oblique retinacular ligament

Proximal interphalangeal joint

Central slip of extensor tendon

Lateral band

Metacarpophalangeal joint

Sagittal band

Lumbrical

Palmar interosseous

Dorsal interosseous

Extensor tendon

Extensor tendon

Sagittal band

Metacarpophalangeal joint

Transverse retinacular ligament

Distal interphalangeal joint

Oblique retinacular ligament

Proximal interphalangeal joint

Deep transverse intermetacarpal ligament

Dorsal and palmar interosseous

Lumbrical

Dorsal and palmar interosseous

Collateral ligament

Deep transverse intermetacarpal ligament

Lumbrical

Transverse retinacular ligament

Oblique retinacular ligament

Fig. 53.43 Extensor mechanism of the finger. **A**, Dorsal view; **B**, lateral view; **C**, lateral view in flexion.

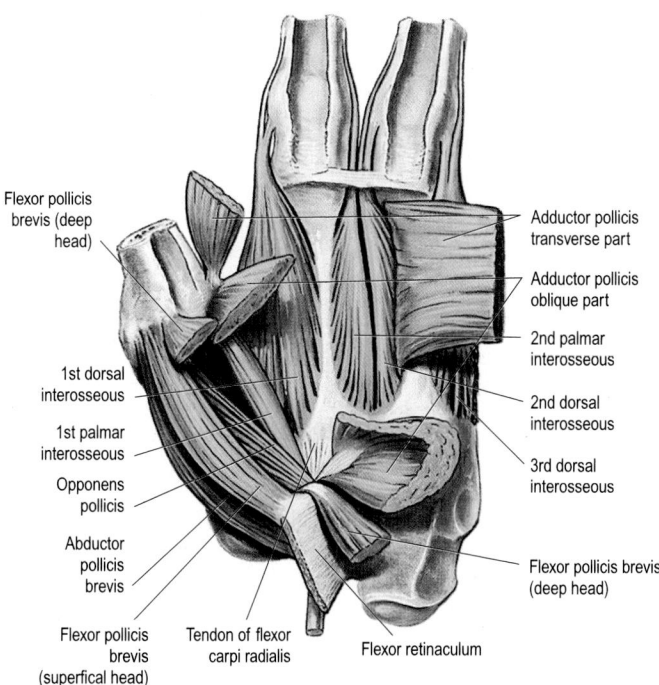

Flexor pollicis brevis (deep head)

1st dorsal interosseous

1st palmar interosseous

Opponens pollicis

Abductor pollicis brevis

Flexor pollicis brevis (superficial head)

Tendon of flexor carpi radialis

Adductor pollicis transverse part

Adductor pollicis oblique part

2nd palmar interosseous

2nd dorsal interosseous

3rd dorsal interosseous

Flexor pollicis brevis (deep head)

Flexor retinaculum

Fig. 53.44 Dissection of the left thenar eminence and palm over the two lateral intermetacarpal spaces. Adductor pollicis and the 'deep head' of flexor pollicis brevis, have been transected.

and capitate bones and from the palmar ligaments of the distal row of carpal bones, and passes deep to the tendon of flexor pollicis longus. It unites with the superficial head on the sesamoid bone and base of the first phalanx.

The superficial head is frequently blended with opponens pollicis. The deep head varies considerably in size and may even be absent.

Relations – Flexor pollicis brevis lies superficial in the thenar eminence and is distal to abductor pollicis brevis. It is crossed by the motor branch of the median nerve.

Vascular supply – Flexor pollicis brevis is supplied by the superficial palmar branch of the radial artery, and branches from the princeps pollicis artery and radialis indicis artery.

Innervation – The superficial head of flexor pollicis brevis is usually innervated by the lateral terminal branch (motor branch) of the median nerve. The deep head is usually innervated by the deep branch of the ulnar nerve, C8 and T1. Some variation is common.

Action – Flexor pollicis brevis flexes the metacarpophalangeal joint.

Testing – Flexor pollicis brevis is palpated in the thenar eminence whilst the subject flexes the metacarpophalangeal joint of the thumb, keeping the interphalangeal joint fully extended.

ABDUCTOR POLLICIS BREVIS

Attachments – Abductor pollicis brevis is a thin, subcutaneous muscle in the proximolateral part of the thenar eminence (**Fig. 53.44**). It arises mainly from flexor retinaculum: a few fibres spring from the tubercles of the scaphoid bone and trapezium, and from the tendon of abductor pollicis longus. Its medial fibres are attached by a thin, flat tendon to the radial side of the base of the proximal phalanx of the thumb. Its lateral fibres join the dorsal digital expansion of the thumb. The muscle may receive accessory slips from the long and short extensors of the thumb, opponens pollicis, or the styloid process of the radius.

Relations – Abductor pollicis brevis lies proximomedial to flexor pollicis brevis in the superficial part of the thenar eminence.

Vascular supply – Abductor pollicis brevis is supplied by the superficial palmar branch of the radial artery, and often by an independent branch directly from the radial artery lying on the radial aspect of thumb.

Innervation – Abductor pollicis brevis is innervated by the lateral terminal branch (motor branch) of the median nerve, C8 and T1. Note that this is the only muscle of the thenar eminence which is constantly supplied by the median nerve.

Action – Abductor pollicis brevis draws the thumb ventrally in a plane at right angles to the palm of the hand (abduction).

Testing – The hand is placed with its dorsum on the table. The subject's thumb is placed so that the nail is in a plane at right angles to the palm of the hand. The subject is instructed to touch with his thumb an object held vertically above the thumb. This is a highly specific test for a median nerve lesion.

OPPONENS POLLICIS

Attachments – Opponens pollicis lies deep to abductor pollicis brevis (**Fig. 53.44**). It arises from the tubercle of the trapezium and flexor retinaculum, and is attached to the whole length of the lateral border, and the adjoining lateral half of the palmar surface of the metacarpal bone of the thumb.

Relations – Opponens pollicis lies deep between the other two muscles of the thenar eminence and is only revealed when they are retracted.

Vascular supply – Opponens pollicis is supplied by the superficial palmar branch of the radial artery, and by branches from the first palmar metacarpal artery (when present), princeps pollicis artery, radialis indicis artery and the deep palmar arch.

Innervation – Opponens pollicis is innervated by the lateral terminal branch of the median nerve, C8 and T1, and commonly by a branch of the deep terminal branch of the ulnar nerve.

Action – Opponens pollicis flexes the metacarpal bone of the thumb.

Testing – The subject tries, against resistance, to touch the tip of the little finger with the thumb. The key observation is whether or not the thumb can be strongly adducted without flexing the IP joint.

ADDUCTOR POLLICIS

Attachments – Adductor pollicis arises by oblique and transverse heads (**Fig. 53.44**). The oblique head is attached to the capitate bone, the bases of the second and third metacarpal bones, the palmar ligaments of the carpus and the sheath of the tendon of flexor carpi radialis. Most of the fibres converge into a tendon (which contains a sesamoid bone), which unites with the tendon of the transverse head, and is attached to the ulnar side of the base of the proximal phalanx of the thumb. The deepest fibres may pass into the medial side of the dorsal digital expansion of the thumb. On the lateral side of the oblique head a considerable fasciculus passes deep to the tendon of flexor pollicis longus to join flexor pollicis brevis; this has been described as the 'deep head' of flexor pollicis brevis. The transverse head is the deepest of the pollicial muscles. It is triangular, and arises from the distal two-thirds of the palmar surface of the third metacarpal. The fibres converge to be attached, with the oblique head and the first palmar interosseous, to the base of the proximal phalanx of the thumb. The two parts of the adductor vary in relative size and degree of connection.

Relations – The deep palmar arch and the deep branch of the ulnar nerve pass between the two heads of the muscle (**Fig. 53.45**). Anteriorly adductor pollicis is crossed by the flexor tendons of the index finger and their sheath, and the first lumbrical, and is overlapped by flexor pollicis brevis. Posteriorly it abuts against the first dorsal interosseous muscle: together these muscles form the mass of the first web space of the hand.

Vascular supply – Adductor pollicis is supplied by the arteria princeps pollicis and the arteria radialis indicis (which are sometimes combined as the first palmar metacarpal artery) and by branches from the deep palmar arch.

Innervation – Adductor pollicis is innervated by the deep branch of the ulnar nerve, C8 and T1.

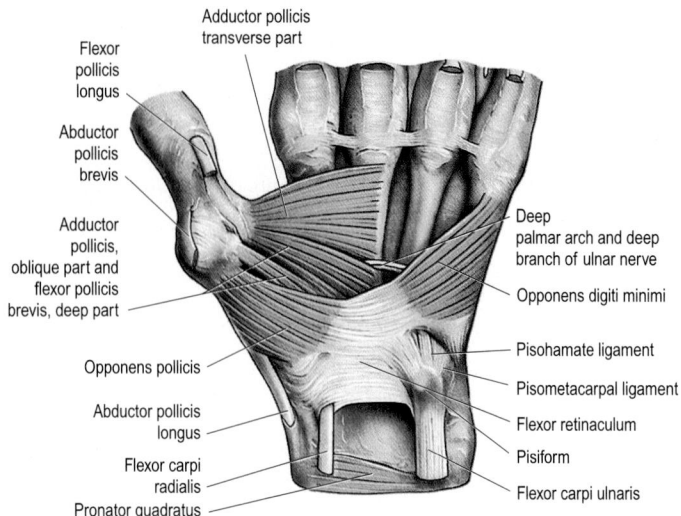

Fig. 53.45 Deep dissection of the left palm, showing opponens pollicis and opponens digiti minimi and the two parts of adductor pollicis, including the 'deep head' of flexor pollicis brevis. The superficial thenar and hypothenar muscles and palmaris longus have been removed.

Action – Adductor pollicis approximates the thumb to the palm of the hand. It acts to greatest advantage when the abducted, rotated and flexed thumb is opposed to the fingers in gripping.

Testing – With the thumb lying along the palmar aspect of the index finger, and with its nail in a plane at right angles to the palm, the subject is asked to retain a strip of paper between the thumb and palm against resistance.

ABDUCTOR DIGITI MINIMI

Attachments – Abductor digiti minimi arises from the pisiform bone, the tendon of flexor carpi ulnaris and the pisohamate ligament (**Fig. 53.42**). It ends in a flat tendon which divides into two slips. One is attached to the ulnar side of the base of the proximal phalanx of the little finger, and the other to the ulnar border of the dorsal digital expansion of extensor digiti minimi.

The muscle may have two or three slips and may be fused with flexor digiti minimi brevis. An additional slip may arise from flexor retinaculum, antebrachial fascia, or tendons of palmaris longus or flexor carpi ulnaris. It may be partly attached to the fifth metacarpal by a slip from the pisiform.

Relations – Abductor digiti minimi lies along the ulnar border of flexor digit minimi brevis and overlies opponens digiti minimi.

Vascular supply – Abductor digiti minimi is supplied by the deep palmar branch of the ulnar artery, branches from the ulnar end of the superficial palmar arch and the palmar digital artery for the medial border of the little finger.

Innervation – Abductor digiti minimi is innervated by the deep branch of the ulnar nerve, C8 and T1.

Action – Abductor digiti minimi abducts the little finger away from the fourth, e.g. in the habitual spreading of the digits when they are extended. Abduction is also possible when digits 2–4 are tightly adducted in flexion or extension.

Testing – Abductor digiti minimi is tested by abducting the little finger against resistance.

FLEXOR DIGITI MINIMI BREVIS

Attachments – Flexor digiti minimi brevis arises from the convex surface of the hook of the hamate and the palmar surface of the flexor retinaculum. It inserts into the ulnar side of the base of the proximal phalanx of the little finger with abductor digiti minimi.

It may be absent, or fused with the abductor, and it may attach to the distal end of the fifth metacarpal by a muscular slip.

Relations – Flexor digiti minimi brevis lies lateral to the abductor (**Fig. 53.46**). Its origin is separated from that of the abductor by the deep branches of the ulnar artery and nerve.

Vascular supply – Flexor digiti minimi brevis is supplied by the deep palmar branch of the ulnar artery, branches from the ulnar end of the superficial palmar arch, and the palmar digital artery for the medial border of the little finger.

Innervation – Flexor digiti minimi brevis is innervated by the deep branch of the ulnar nerve, C8 and T1.

Action – Flexor digiti minimi brevis produces flexion of the little finger at its metacarpophalangeal joint, together with some lateral rotation.

Testing – The subject flexes the metacarpophalangeal joint of the little finger while the examiner maintains the interphalangeal joints in extension.

OPPONENS DIGITI MINIMI

Attachments – Opponens digiti minimi is a triangular muscle, lying under cover of the flexor and abductor (**Figs 53.45, 53.46**). It arises from the convexity of the hook of the hamate, and the contiguous portion of flexor retinaculum. It inserts along the whole length of the ulnar margin of the fifth metacarpal bone, and the adjacent palmar surface.

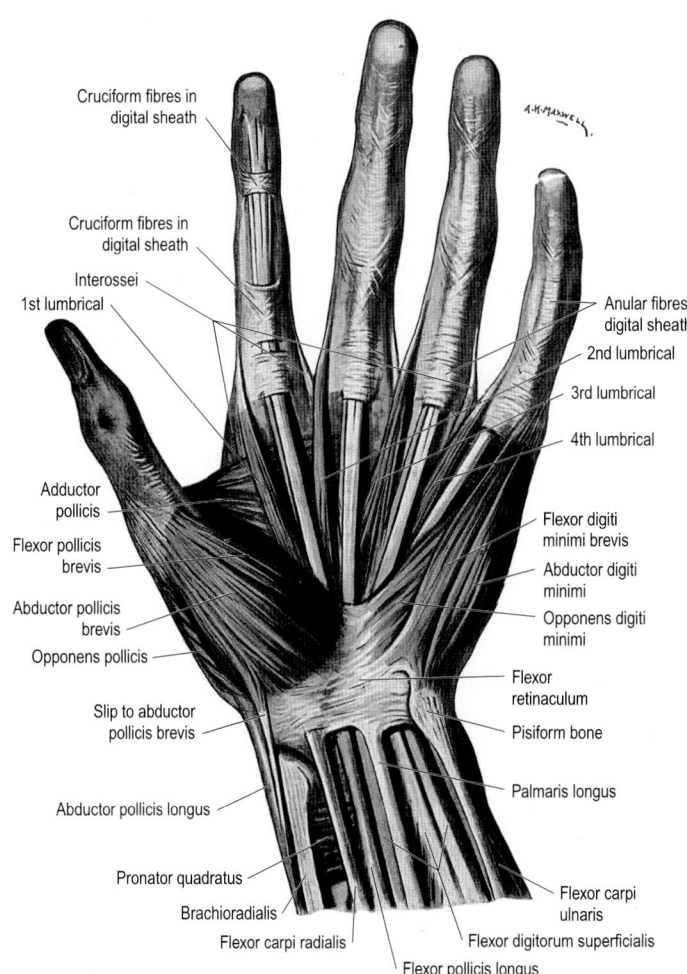

Fig. 53.46 Superficial dissection of muscles of the palm of the left hand.

Cruciform fibres in digital sheath
Cruciform fibres in digital sheath
Interossei
1st lumbrical
Adductor pollicis
Flexor pollicis brevis
Abductor pollicis brevis
Opponens pollicis
Slip to abductor pollicis brevis
Abductor pollicis longus
Pronator quadratus
Brachioradialis
Flexor carpi radialis
Flexor pollicis longus
Anular fibres in digital sheath
2nd lumbrical
3rd lumbrical
4th lumbrical
Flexor digiti minimi brevis
Abductor digiti minimi
Opponens digiti minimi
Flexor retinaculum
Pisiform bone
Palmaris longus
Flexor carpi ulnaris
Flexor digitorum superficialis

The muscle is often divided into two lamellae by the deep branches of the ulnar artery and nerve. It blends to a variable degree with its neighbours.

Relations – Opponens digiti minimi lies on the ulnar margin and adjacent palmar surface of the fifth metacarpal, overlapped by, and often partly fused with, the other two muscles of the hypothenar eminence.

Vascular supply – Opponens digiti minimi is supplied by the deep palmar branch of the ulnar artery, and branches from the medial end of the deep palmar arch.

Innervation – Opponens digiti minimi is innervated by the deep branch of the ulnar nerve, C8 and T1.

Action – Opponens digiti minimi flexes the fifth metacarpal bone, drawing it forwards and rotating it laterally at the carpometacarpal joint: this deepens the hollow of the palm. These actions, together with flexion and some lateral rotation at the metacarpophalangeal and interphalangeal joints, bring the digit into opposition with the thumb.

Testing – The subject is asked to place the tip of the little finger, against resistance, onto the tip of the opposed thumb while the examiner maintains the interphalangeal joints of the little finger in extension.

PALMARIS BREVIS

Attachments – Palmaris brevis is a thin, quadrilateral muscle, lying beneath the skin of the ulnar side of the palm (**Fig. 53.4**). It arises from the flexor retinaculum and the medial border of the central part of the palmar aponeurosis, and is attached to the dermis on the ulnar border of the hand.

Relations – Palmaris brevis is superficial to the ulnar artery and the superficial terminal branch of the ulnar nerve.

Vascular supply – Palmaris brevis is supplied by branches from the ulnar end of the superficial palmar arch.

Innervation – Palmaris brevis is innervated by the superficial branch of the ulnar nerve, C8 and T1.

Action – Palmaris brevis wrinkles the skin on the ulnar side of the palm of the hand and deepens the hollow of the palm by accentuating the hypothenar eminence. In this way it may contribute to the security of the palmar grip.

Testing – Against resistance, the subject touches the tip of the opposed thumb with the tip of the little finger; the skin on the ulnar side of the palm is seen to pucker.

INTEROSSEI

The interossei occupy the intervals between the metacarpal bones, and are divided into a palmar and a dorsal set.

Palmar interossei

Attachments – Palmar interossei are smaller than dorsal interossei and lie on the palmar surfaces of the metacarpal bones rather than between them (**Fig. 53.47**). With the exception of the first, each of the four arises from the entire length of the metacarpal bone of one finger, and passes to the appropriate (adductor) side of the dorsal digital expansion.

The middle finger has no palmar interosseus. The remaining digits have palmar interossei on their aspects which face the middle finger. The first arises from the ulnar side of the palmar surface of the base of the first metacarpal bone. It is inserted into a sesamoid bone on the ulnar side of the proximal phalanx and from there passes to the phalanx and usually also into the dorsal digital expansion. It lies in front of the lateral head of the first dorsal interosseous, and is overlapped anteriorly by the oblique head of adductor pollicis (**Figs 53.44, 53.47**). It is often very rudimentary because the thumb has its own powerful adductor. The second arises from the ulnar side of the second metacarpal bone, and is inserted into the same side of the digital expansion of the index finger. The third arises from the radial side of the fourth metacarpal bone, and is inserted together with the third lumbrical (**Fig. 53.43**). The

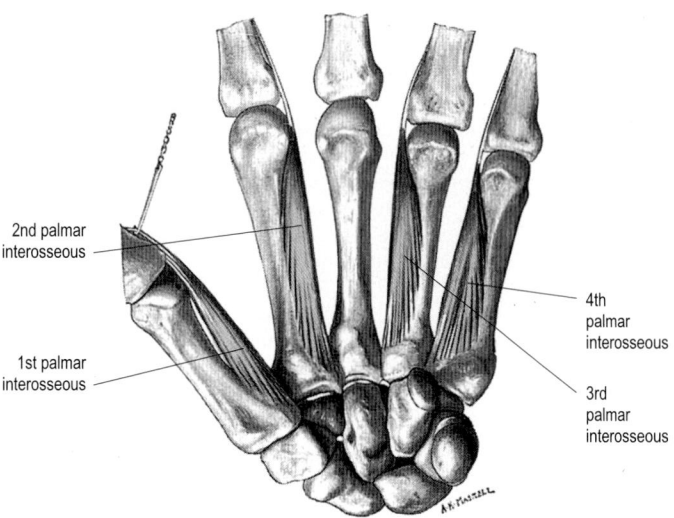

Fig. 53.47 Palmar interossei of the left hand: palmar aspect. Note the first palmar interosseous is often absent or rudimentary because the thumb has its own powerful adductor.

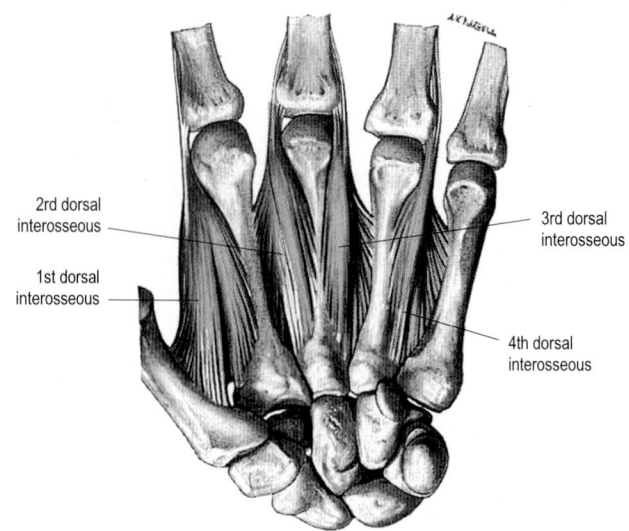

Fig. 53.48 Dorsal interossei of the left hand: palmar aspect.

fourth arises from the radial side of the fifth metacarpal bone, and is attached with the fourth lumbrical and also to the base of the proximal phalanx. The attachment of these muscles to the dorsal digital expansions (**Fig. 53.43**) stabilizes the extensor tendons on the convex heads of the metacarpal bones during flexion and extension at the metacarpophalangeal joints.

The interossei show little variation in their arrangement. They are occasionally reduplicated.

Relations – The first palmar interosseous lies anterior to the lateral head of the first dorsal interosseous. It is overlapped anteriorly by the oblique head of adductor pollicis, which also crosses anterior to the second palmar interosseous. The third and fourth are overlapped by the long flexor tendons of the ring and little finger respectively within their flexor sheaths.

Vascular supply – Palmar interossei are supplied by branches from the deep palmar arch, princeps pollicis artery, radialis indicis artery, palmar metacarpal arteries, proximal and distal perforating arteries and common and proper digital (palmar) arteries.

Innervation – All the interossei are innervated by the deep branch of the ulnar nerve, C8 and T1.

Action – Palmar interossei adduct the fingers to an imaginary longitudinal axis through the centre of the middle finger. Interossei have a considerable cross-sectional area and therefore contribute strongly to metacarpophalangeal joint flexion and interphalangeal extension. When paralysed, as in ulnar nerve paralysis, the grip strength of the hand is severely impaired and the arc of finger motion is abnormal, with a tendency for the fingers to claw. Each interosseous has a considerable ability to rotate the digit at the metacarpophalangeal joint. Generally this is not obvious, because interossei act in pairs, but it may occur where one interosseus is deficient as a result of injury or congenital deformity.

Testing – Adduction of the index, ring and little fingers against resistance. The subject grips a piece of paper between the index and middle fingers with the hand placed flat on the table. The examiner can assess the strength of adduction on trying to pull the paper away. This is a reliable test of ulnar nerve integrity.

Dorsal interossei

Attachments – Dorsal interossei consist of four bipennate muscles, each arising from the adjacent sides of two metacarpal bones, but more extensively from the metacarpal bone of the finger into which the

muscle passes (**Fig. 53.48**). They insert on the bases of the proximal phalanges and separately into the dorsal digital expansions. Between the double origin of each of these muscles there is a narrow triangular interval. The radial artery passes through the first of these intervals, and a perforating branch from the deep palmar arch passes through each of the others. The first and largest muscle is sometimes named abductor indicis. It is attached to the radial side of the proximal phalanx of the index finger and to the capsule of the adjoining metacarpophalangeal joint. The second and third are attached to the radial and ulnar sides of the middle finger, respectively. Whereas the second generally reaches the digital expansion and the proximal phalanx, the third usually extends only to the digital expansion (**Fig. 53.43**). The fourth may be wholly attached to the digital expansion, but it often sends an additional slip to the proximal phalanx.

Relations – The first dorsal interosseous abuts anteriorly with adductor pollicis. The other dorsal interossei occupy the spaces between the second and the fifth metacarpal bones.

Vascular supply – Dorsal interossei are supplied by the dorsal metacarpal arteries (1st–4th), palmar metacarpal arteries (2nd–4th), radial artery (1st); princeps pollicis artery, radialis indicis artery, three perforating branches from the deep palmar arch (proximal perforating arteries), and three distal perforating branches. The tendons are supplied by branches from the common and proper palmar digital arteries and the dorsal digital arteries.

Innervation – All the interossei are innervated by the deep branch of the ulnar nerve, C8 and T1.

Action – Dorsal interossei abduct the fingers from an imaginary longitudinal axis through the centre of the middle finger. *See also* action of palmar interossei.

Testing – Abduction of the index, middle and ring fingers against resistance. Most conveniently, the first dorsal interosseous is tested with the subject's fingers and palm flat upon the table. The subject tries to abduct the index finger against the examiner's resistance. The muscle belly can be felt and seen. This provides a reliable test for the integrity of the ulnar nerve.

LUMBRICALS

Attachments – The lumbricals are four small fasciculi which arise from the tendons of flexor digitorum profundus (**Fig. 53.46**). The first and second arise from the radial sides and palmar surfaces of the tendons of the index and middle fingers respectively. The third arises from the adjacent sides of the tendons of the middle and ring fingers, and the fourth from the adjoining sides of the tendons of the ring and little fingers. Each passes to the radial side of the corresponding finger, and is attached to the lateral margin of the dorsal digital expansion of extensor digitorum which covers the dorsal surface of the finger.

Variations in the attachments of the lumbricals are common. Any of them may be unipennate or bipennate. When bipennate, the two heads arise from adjoining tendons of flexor digitorum profundus, and from the tendon of flexor pollicis longus in the case of the first lumbrical. Accessory lumbrical slips may be attached to an adjacent tendon of flexor digitorum superficialis.

Vascular supply – First and second lumbricals are supplied by the first and second dorsal metacarpal and dorsal digital arteries. Third and fourth lumbricals are supplied by the second and third common palmar digital arteries, and the third and fourth dorsal digital arteries and their anastomoses with the palmar digital arteries.

Innervation – The first and second lumbricals are innervated by the median nerve, C8 and T1, and the third and fourth lumbricals by the deep terminal branch of the ulnar nerve, C8 and T1. The third lumbrical frequently receives a supply from the median nerve. The first and second lumbricals are occasionally innervated by the deep terminal branch of the ulnar nerve.

Action – Lumbricals arise from flexor tendons and insert into the extensor apparatus. Since both attachments are mobile, they have the potential for producing movement at either. The action on the extensor apparatus is easier to understand and consists of extension of both interphalangeal joints in a coordinated manner. The mode of action at the metacarpophalangeal joints is disputed, but if there is a flexor action it is very weak. The effect on the flexor digitorum profundus attachment is to pull the tendon distally. The combined action on both origin and insertion is therefore to alter the posture of the finger to allow more interphalangeal extension. Pinching the index finger against the thumb without a lumbrical would result in a nail-to-nail contact: the addition of the lumbrical increases the interphalangeal joint extension, and results in pulp-to-pulp pinch. Lumbricals contain many muscle spindles and have a long fibre length: it is therefore reasonable to assume that they play a role in proprioception.

Testing – Lumbricals cannot be tested in isolation, but the lumbrical–interosseous muscle complex can readily be examined together. The examiner holds the metacarpophalangeal joint of the index finger in hyperextension. The subject is the instructed to extend the two interphalangeal joints against resistance. This test is repeated seriatim on the middle, ring and little fingers.

COORDINATED MOVEMENTS OF THE HAND

The apparently simple human functions of closing the hand to grasp an object, or opening the palm to release it, are in reality tasks of considerable mechanical complexity, requiring the simultaneous contraction of many individual muscles. The isolated action of a single muscle may be inferred from the positions of its origin and insertion, and the estimated line of action (usually the centre line of the muscle) in relation to the axes of all the joints traversed by the muscle and its tendon. The limb can be regarded as a chain of joints crossed by muscles. If it is known which muscles are active, then the reason why one joint moves and others do not is a matter of simple mechanical relationships.

For example, flexor pollicis longus is considered to have a major role as a flexor of the interphalangeal joint of the thumb. However, the position of its tendon relative to more proximal joints in the limb gives it the potential for producing flexion at the metacarpophalangeal joint and also at the trapeziometacarpal and wrist joints. In the living subject the actual motion that takes place depends on which other muscle groups are acting, and so the potential for movement must be considered for each joint in the chain in turn. Motion at the wrist is generally balanced by wrist extensors. Motion at the trapeziometacarpal joint is balanced by abductor pollicis longus. Flexor pollicis longus will then have an action as a flexor of the metacarpophalangeal and interphalangeal joints only.

The factor that determines whether one or both of two joints will move is the turning moment at each. The greater the perpendicular distance from the line of muscle or tendon pull to the axis of the joint, the stronger is the turning effect of the muscle at the joint, but the smaller the range of joint motion that can be produced. In the case of flexor pollicis longus, the tendon is situated further from the axis of the metacarpophalangeal joint than from the axis of the interphalangeal joint: it will therefore tend to produce flexion preferentially at the metacarpophalangeal joint unless that joint is restrained by extensor pollicis brevis. In this way different postures of the thumb can be produced by the interplay of flexor and extensor forces. These simple guiding principles should provide an understanding of muscle action in the hand that is sufficient for most purposes.

In considering the role of a particular muscle, there is a tendency to concentrate on motion. Indeed, many muscles are named on the basis of the movements that they generate, although others – often those whose actions are the most difficult to interpret – are described according to their morphology or situation. A more important function may be the nature of the force generated. For example, although flexor pollicis longus flexes the thumb (see above), a large range of flexion is actually required in only a few activities, such as certain ripping tasks. In most pinch and manipulative tasks the role of the thumb is to apply isometric force, which it does with such precision that it is possible to pick up an egg and neither crush nor drop it. Thus for much of the time flexor pollicis longus behaves as an extremely sophisticated mechanism for the application of force, in which contraction and proprioception are equally important.

The anatomical position of the hand (palm flat and pointing anteriorly, forearm supinated) is a convenient standard for studying structural relationships. The hand in the relaxed (anaesthetized) position adopts a posture of partial flexion and mid-supination/pronation (the reader can verify this by relaxing completely and observing forearm and hand position).

SPECIAL FUNCTIONS OF THE HAND

CLOSING THE HAND

It is clear that the fingers and palm of the hand flex in gripping, grasping or making a fist, but there are subtle differences in hand posture in these various activities. The basic mechanisms of hand closure will be described before special grips are considered.

As the digits flex, the wrist usually extends (dorsiflexes) at the same time. The involvement of the long digital flexors in this movement will be considered first, followed by an analysis of the role of the wrist.

ROLE OF THE LONG DIGITAL FLEXORS
(See also p. 913.)

Flexor digitorum superficialis acts to flex principally the proximal interphalangeal joints, through its insertions into the middle phalanges. However, in each digit it also has an action on the metacarpophalangeal joint, because the tendon passes anterior to that joint. The muscle has the potential to produce flexion at the wrist for the same reason. The fact that each tendon arises from an individual muscle slip allows the clinician to test one finger at a time. The reader can verify this by attempting to flex each digit individually while using the other hand to keep the distal interphalangeal joints of the remaining fingers in extension. This test is frequently used in clinical practice and is useful for the middle and ring fingers, where flexion of one finger alone must be attributed to flexor digitorum superficialis. The index finger, however, has its own profundus musculotendinous unit and may therefore move independently under the action of this tendon. Many individuals cannot flex the proximal interphalangeal joint of the little finger alone, probably because superficialis is deficient, although most can flex the metacarpophalangeal joint of the little finger using flexor digiti minimi.

Flexor digitorum profundus has similarities to superficialis: because it reaches further (to the distal phalanx), it is the only muscle available for flexion of the distal interphalangeal joint. It also contributes, together with superficialis, to flexion at the proximal interphalangeal and metacarpophalangeal joints. These two long flexors (sometimes called extrinsic flexors, because the muscle bellies are outside the hand) can be considered to act together to flex the finger. However, their action alone would wind up the interphalangeal before the metacarpophalangeal joints and the finger would not move in a normal arc of flexion. This is precisely what happens in an ulnar nerve paralysis, in which the interossei and lumbricals are not functioning. These small (intrinsic) muscles have been described earlier in terms of their individual actions. For their role in coordinated activity it is sufficient to appreciate that their contribution changes the arc produced by the long flexors, increasing flexion at the metacarpophalangeal joint and reducing flexion at the proximal interphalangeal joint. All three joints are then angulated to the same degree and the fingers form a normal arc of flexion.

As the finger flexes, the long extensor tendons (extensor digitorum, extensor indicis and extensor digiti minimi) aid the process by relaxing and allowing the extensor apparatus to glide distally on the dorsum of the phalanges.

ROLE OF THE WRIST
(See also p. 905.)

As the fingers wind up to make a fist, the wrist tends to extend, particularly when force is applied. This extension has a marked effect on the excursion of the long flexor tendons. On its own, digital flexion would require the long tendons to move proximally in their sheaths and the flexor muscles in the forearm would shorten. Dorsiflexion of the wrist tends to produce a lengthening of the same muscles, which in normal use is almost enough to balance the shortening due to finger flexion; the net effect is a very slight shortening (c.1 cm) of the long flexors in the forearm. The wrist can therefore be seen as a mechanism for maximizing force, because it allows the fingers to flex while maintaining the resting length of the extrinsic muscles near to the peak of the force–length curve. It is, of course, possible to wind up the fingers with the wrist held in a neutral position, but the grip is somewhat weaker. With the wrist in full flexion it is not possible to flex the fingers fully.

Flexion of the fingers on gripping tends to result in a distal excursion of the long extensors. However, this tendency is counteracted by dorsiflexion of the wrist. The net effect is a very small proximal excursion of the long extensor tendons on gripping, mirroring the effect on the flexor surface. If the movement of the wrist is exaggerated so that the wrist is a little flexed on opening the hand, and fully dorsiflexed on closing it, the net excursion of long flexors and extensors is zero, i.e. this whole movement sequence can be completed with the forearm flexor and extensor muscles contracting isometrically.

The reader can observe the relationship between digits and wrist by performing the following manoeuvre. The wrist is held in a relaxed, mid-supinated position, with the elbow flexed at 90°. If the forearm is now rotated into pronation, the wrist will fall into flexion and the fingers will automatically extend. If the forearm is rotated into supination, the wrist will extend and the fingers flex. The finger movements compensate for the wrist movements and are entirely automatic; they are made without the need for any excursion of forearm flexor or extensor tendons. This test, the wrist tenodesis test, is a useful way of examining the limb for tendon injury. The pointing finger (which does not move with wrist motion) 'points to' a tendon injury.

Wrist motion is controlled principally by two wrist flexors (flexor carpi radialis and flexor carpi ulnaris) and three extensors (extensors carpi radialis longus and brevis, and extensor carpi ulnaris). Although the radiocarpal joint has some functional similarity to a ball and socket joint, it is possible to conceive of the wrist as a variable hinge joint, the axis of which may be set in a number of inclinations. For example, in using a hammer it is useful to rotate the wrist backwards and forwards about an axis that permits not only wrist flexion but also ulnar deviation. It would be very restricting to have a pure hinge joint with collateral ligaments of fixed length. In this context, the wrist flexors and extensors may be regarded as variable collateral ligaments which allow the joint to be set about a number of different axes.

For movement about major axes, the wrist tendons can be considered to act in pairs:

Wrist flexion: flexor carpi radialis and flexor carpi ulnaris
Wrist extension: extensor carpi radialis longus and brevis, and extensor carpi ulnaris
Ulnar deviation: extensor carpi ulnaris and flexor carpi ulnaris
Radial deviation: flexor carpi radialis, extensor carpi radialis longus and brevis, extensor pollicis brevis and abductor pollicis longus

---

MAKING A TIGHT FIST
It is possible to observe and to palpate the muscle groups that are active in making a tight fist. The flexor compartment of the forearm is contracted tightly and electromyogram evidence confirms that flexor digitorum profundus and flexor digitorum superficialis are active. Flexor carpi ulnaris may be seen and felt to contract strongly. The extensor compartment is tightly contracted and the wrist extensors would certainly be expected to be active. Palpation of the long digital extensors on the back of the wrist will show these to be contracting as well. It seems that when the fingers are held tightly closed, the long digital extensors are unable to move the extensor apparatus: they have acquired a new fixed point on which to act, namely the proximal limit of the extensor apparatus over the metacarpophalangeal joint. They therefore perform the only task available to them and act together as an additional wrist extensor.

In the thumb web, palpation confirms that the first dorsal interosseous is contracting, as are all the other interossei and the thenar and hypothenar muscles. As the firm fist is swung forward in anger the brachioradialis stands out, and at the moment of impact virtually every muscle in the limb is in a state of contraction, with the exception of the lumbricals.

OPENING THE HAND
The hand is opened from its relaxed balanced posture, e.g. when stretching out to reach an object. This motion is made up of extension of the distal interphalangeal, proximal interphalangeal and metacarpophalangeal joints. The hand is provided with an ingenious mechanism that allows this to happen. The laws of mechanics would suggest that one motor would be required for every joint in a chain, together with some sort of controlling mechanism to ensure that the chain of joints moved together in a coordinated fashion. In the hand this is achieved through an extensor apparatus which minimizes the number of motors required for movement by allowing the muscles to act on more than one joint, and by linking different levels in the mechanism so that the arc of motion is controlled.

The tendons of extensor digitorum run distally over the metacarpal heads, forming the major component of the extensor apparatus. Extensor digitorum has no insertion into the proximal phalanx and therefore exerts its extensor action on the metacarpophalangeal joint indirectly through more distal insertions. The first point of insertion is at the base of the middle phalanx (in clinical practice the term central slip has been adopted). Acting at this insertion alone, extensor digitorum can extend both metacarpophalangeal and proximal interphalangeal joints together. The interossei are also active in hand opening, since they will tend to increase extension of the proximal interphalangeal joint. There is therefore a range of possibilities. At one extreme, with no interosseous contribution, the long extensor will exert all of its action at the metacarpophalangeal joint: this leads to full extension, and even hyperextension, while the proximal interphalangeal joint remains flexed (the typical claw hand of ulnar nerve paralysis, or 'intrinsic minus' hand). At the other extreme, when the intrinsics act strongly together with extensor digitorum, the proximal interphalangeal joint will extend completely while the metacarpophalangeal joint remains flexed ('intrinsic plus' hand). Thus the hand possesses in the proximal part of the extensor apparatus a variable mechanism that allows different amounts of relative metacarpophalangeal or proximal interphalangeal joint motion.

In contrast, the more distal part of the extensor apparatus acts as an automatic or fixed mechanism which determines that the two interphalangeal joints, proximal and distal, will move together. The lateral slips of the extensor apparatus arise from extensor digitorum and pass distally on either side of the central slip and thus over the proximal interphalangeal joint. Being further lateral they are nearer the joint axis, because the dorsal surface curves away on each side. A helpful analogy that has been suggested for this arrangement is to consider it as two pulleys of different size on one axle. The central slip can be regarded as a cord that passes over the larger wheel, and each lateral slip as a cord that passes over the smaller wheel. Since these latter pulleys are smaller there is less longitudinal excursion for a given rotation of the wheel, and this allows some of the excursion to be used for another function, namely extension at the distal joint. There is an additional mechanism by which the lateral slips move laterally during flexion of the proximal interphalangeal joint. The effect of this lateral movement is to reduce further the distance between the lateral slips and the joint axis, thereby reducing the amount of excursion at the proximal interphalangeal joint still more and allowing more excursion at the distal joint. When the hand flexes, this mechanical linkage system allows both interphalangeal joints to flex together in a coordinated way.

The extensor expansion also receives contributions from the interossei and lumbricals, which approach the digits from the webs and join the corresponding expansion in the proximal segment of the digit. These small muscles can therefore act on the extensor apparatus at two levels: they can extend the proximal interphalangeal joint through fibres that radiate towards the central slip, and they can act on the distal interphalangeal joint through fibres that join the lateral slip.

Apart from the components of the extensor expansion that are concerned with joint function, the whole structure requires additional anchorage. This must be arranged in such a way that it is not displaced from the underlying skeleton, yet it must not restrict longitudinal movement. These difficult requirements are met by transverse retinacular ligaments at the level of the joints, the transverse ligaments running to relatively fixed attachment points in the region of the joint axis. As the expansion glides backwards and forwards the transverse fibres move like bucket handles. Smooth gliding layers are required under the expansion and retinacular ligaments to allow motion to occur without friction.

One final component of the extensor apparatus provides an additional automatic function. This is a fibrous anchorage system, Landsmeer's oblique retinacular ligament, which anchors the distal expansion to the middle phalanx. The role of the oblique retinacular ligament is controversial (reviewed by Bendz 1985). Some argue it may act in a dynamic tenodesis effect to synchronize the movements of the interphalangeal joints, i.e. it may initiate extension of the distal interphalangeal joint as the proximal interphalangeal joint is extended from a fully flexed position, and relax with proximal interphalangeal joint flexion to allow full distal interphalangeal joint flexion. Others argue that it only becomes taut when the proximal interphalangeal joint is fully extended and the distal interphalangeal joint is flexed, so that it functions as a restraining force to stabilize the fingertip when it is flexed against resistance, e.g. in the hook grip. A further suggestion is that the ligament is merely a secondary lateral stabilizer of the proximal interphalangeal joint and that it acts to centralize the extensor components over the dorsum of the middle phalanx.

MOVEMENTS OF THE THUMB
(See also p. 910.)

An opposable thumb requires a different system of control from the other digits. Since the metacarpal is much more mobile than in the digits, muscles are needed to control the extra freedom of movement.

The thumb does not easily assume the classical anatomical position. Therefore the normal descriptive anatomical terms – anterior, posterior, medial and lateral – do not readily apply. The terms 'palmar, dorsal, ulnar and radial' have been adopted in clinical practice.

The basic active movements are flexion–extension, abduction–adduction, rotation, and circumduction. In the resting position of the first metacarpal, flexion and extension are parallel with the palmar plane, and abduction and adduction occur at right angles to this.

Flexion and extension should be confined to motion at the interphalangeal or metacarpophalangeal joints (**Fig. 53.49A–C**). Palmar abduction (**Fig. 53.49D,E**), in which the first metacarpal moves away from the second at right angles to the plane of the palm, and radial abduction (**Fig. 53.49D,F**), in which the first metacarpal moves away from the second with the thumb in the plane of the palm, occur at the carpometacarpal joint. The opposite of radial abduction is ulnar adduction, or transpalmar adduction, in which the thumb crosses the palm towards its ulnar border. In clinical practice the term adduction is generally used without qualification. Circumduction describes the angular motion of the first metacarpal, solely at the carpometacarpal joint, from a position of maximal radial abduction in the plane of the palm towards the ulnar border of the hand, maintaining the widest possible angle between the first and second metacarpals (**Fig. 53.49G**). Lateral inclinations of the first phalanx maximize the extent of excursion of the circumduction arc. Opposition is a composite position of the thumb achieved by circumduction of the first metacarpal, internal rotation of the thumb ray and maximal extension of the metacarpophalangeal and interphalangeal joints (**Fig. 53.49H**). Retroposition is the opposite to opposition (**Fig. 53.49I**). Flexion adduction is the position of maximal transpalmar adduction of the first metacarpal: the

metacarpophalangeal and interphalangeal joints are flexed and the thumb is in contact with the palm (**Fig. 53.49J**).

Rotary movements occur during circumduction. The simple angular movements described above combine with rotation about the long axis of the metacarpal shaft. In opposition, the shaft must rotate medially into pronation. In retroposition, the thumb must rotate laterally into supination. Axial rotation of the thumb metacarpal is produced by muscle activity (which moves the thumb through its arc of circumduction); the geometry of the articular surfaces of the trapeziometacarpal joint; tensile forces in the ligaments (which combine with forces exerted by the muscles of opposition and retroposition to produce axial rotation). The stability of the first metacarpal is greatest after complete pronation in the position of full opposition, when ligamentary tension, muscular contraction and joint congruence combine to maximal effect.

POSITION OF REST

The hand has a well-recognized position of rest, with the wrist in extension and the digits in some degree of flexion. The precise position of the thumb in the position of rest appears to be rather variable. Typically it is considered as the midpoint between maximal palmar abduction and maximal retroposition. In this position the carpometacarpal joint lies within 20° of radial abduction and 30° of palmar abduction, and from clinical observations it seems that the metacarpophalangeal joint lies within c.40° of flexion and the interphalangeal joint between extension and 10° of flexion.

GRIPS

From the position of rest, the tip of the thumb can approach the radial aspect of the fingers without incurring axial rotation because the palmar and dorsal trapeziometacarpal ligaments remain relaxed (see below).

From different positions of the arc of circumduction, numerous different types of pinch grip are possible (**Fig. 53.50**). In clinical practice these have been classified into two main types: tip pinch and lateral (or key) pinch. Many forces contribute to these configurations.

The thumb is a triarticular system, unlike the finger, which is a biarticular system. The thumb is activated by monoarticular muscles (abductor pollicis longus and opponens pollicis), biarticular muscles (extensor pollicis brevis, adductor pollicis, abductor pollicis brevis and flexor pollicis brevis), and triarticular muscles (extensor pollicis longus and flexor pollicis longus). It appears, however, that even a monoarticular muscle can change posture in all three joints by altering the overall balance of forces, and it is therefore very difficult to attribute function to the individual intrinsic muscles. However, the thumb muscles do seem to provide two broad functions. They control metacarpal positioning (the guy-rope function): this activity is automatically accompanied by rotation. They also control the axial stability of the skeleton of the thumb.

The thumb muscles can be classified into those used for retroposition, opposition and pinch grip.

Retroposition muscles

The muscles that bring about retroposition are extensor pollicis longus, extensor pollicis brevis and abductor pollicis longus. As the thumb moves into retroposition, automatic axial rotation produces supination of the first metacarpal. This is produced by the off-axis action of two parallel, but oppositely directed, forces, one exerted by extensors pollicis longus and brevis and the other by abductor pollicis longus and the anterior oblique carpometacarpal ligament.

Opposition muscles

A succession of activity occurs in the thenar muscles during the movement of opposition. Three subgroups of radial (abductor pollicis longus and extensor pollicis brevis), central (abductor pollicis brevis and opponens pollicis) and ulnar (flexor pollicis brevis) muscles are involved.

These forces act simultaneously but with different intensities, depending on the situation of the thumb. As the thumb moves into opposition there is automatic axial rotation of the first metacarpal shaft to produce pronation. This is produced by the paired action of oppositely directed forces: the opposition muscles provide one force, and the posterior oblique carpometacarpal ligament provides the other.

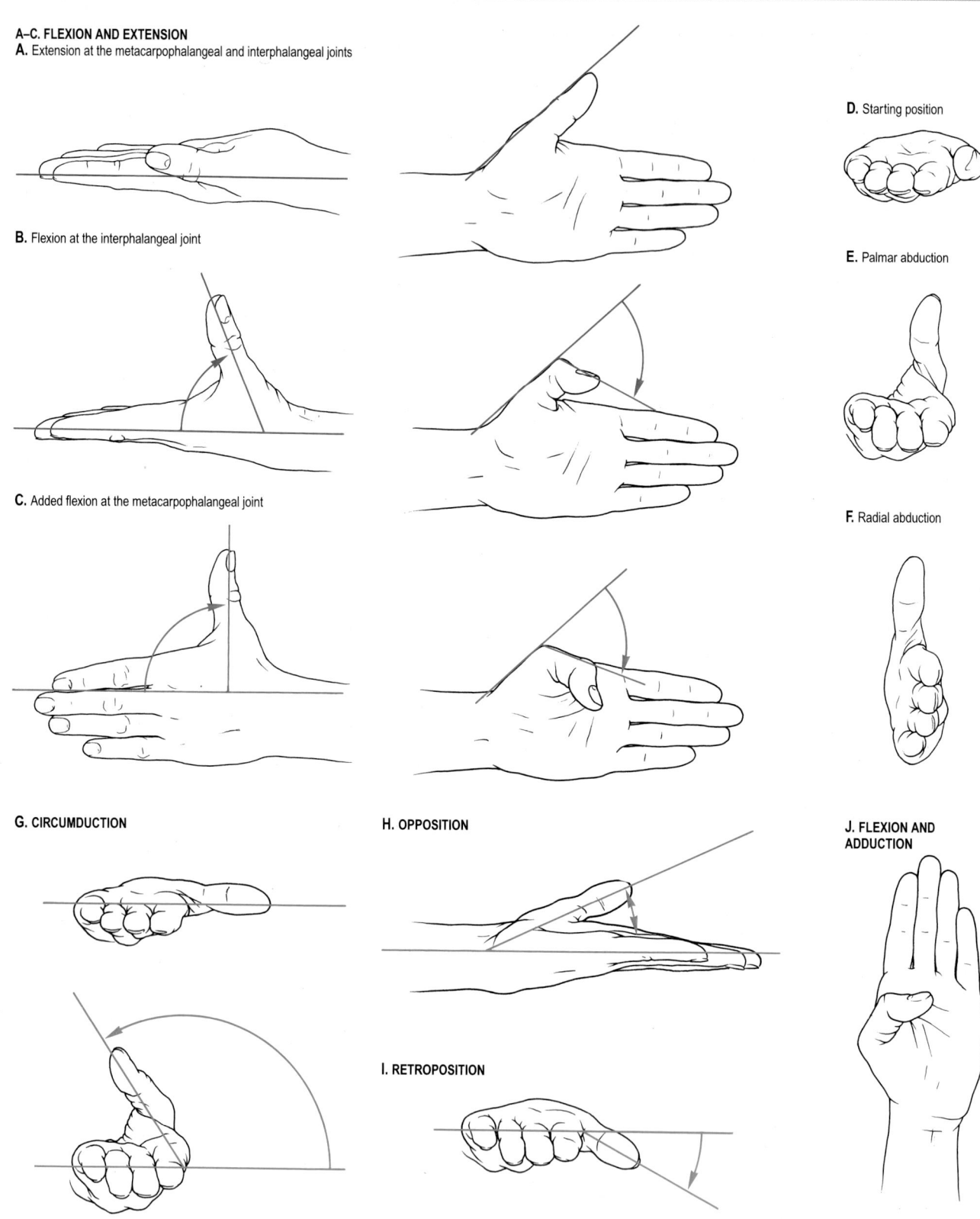

A–C. FLEXION AND EXTENSION
A. Extension at the metacarpophalangeal and interphalangeal joints

B. Flexion at the interphalangeal joint

C. Added flexion at the metacarpophalangeal joint

D. Starting position

E. Palmar abduction

F. Radial abduction

G. CIRCUMDUCTION

H. OPPOSITION

I. RETROPOSITION

J. FLEXION AND ADDUCTION

Fig. 53.49 Movements of the thumb.

Pinch grip muscles

The muscles of pinch grip can be divided into lateral, medial and intermediate subgroups. The lateral subgroup (opposition muscles) moves the first metacarpal into palmar abduction. The metacarpal shaft rotates medially into pronation. Radial angulation at the metacarpophalangeal joint increases the span of the hand. The metacarpophalangeal joint is stabilized principally by extensor pollicis brevis and flexor pollicis brevis. Flexion of the proximal and distal phalanges is controlled.

Muscles of the medial subgroup (abductor pollicis brevis and first dorsal interosseous) produce an approach of the first metacarpal towards the palm. Since they act with the lateral group they have a strong controlling effect on the position and rotation of the first metacarpal. The intermediate subgroup consists simply of flexor pollicis longus, which flexes the interphalangeal or metacarpophalangeal joint, as described earlier. Palpating the thenar eminence during tip and lateral pinch provides some appreciation of the action of the pinch grip muscles.

A
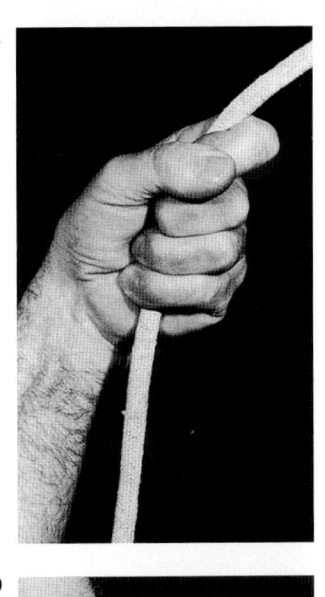

B
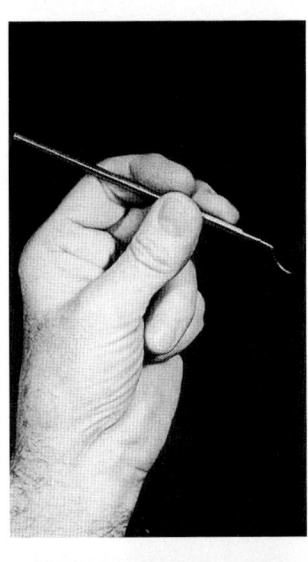

C
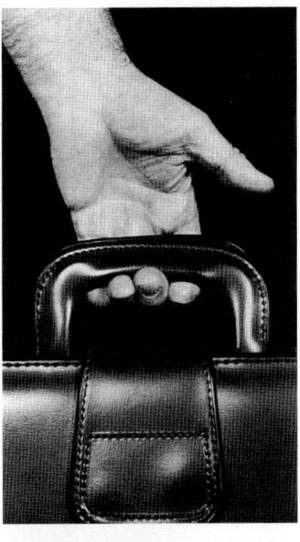

D
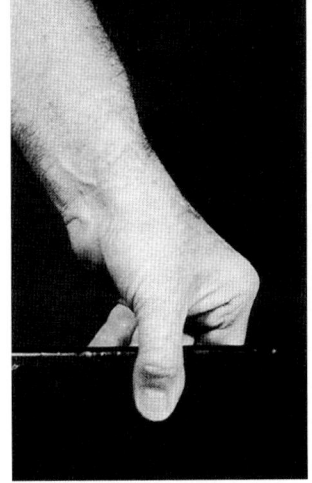

E
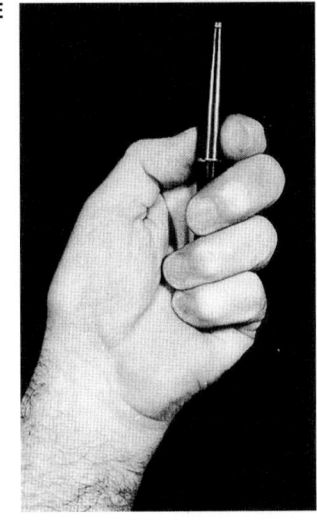

F
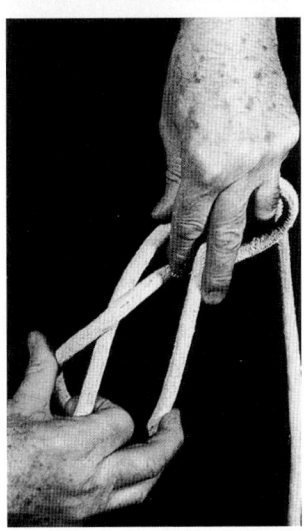

Fig. 53.50 Some of the many varieties of functional posture that may be adopted by the human hand. **A**, In the power grip, the fingers are flexed around an object, with counter pressure from the thumb. Any skill in wielding the object derives from the limb, including the wrist; relative movements of the thumb and fingers are not involved. **B**, The precision grip, which varies considerably with the task, stabilizes the object between the tips of one or more fingers and the thumb. The gross position of the object may be adjusted by movements at the wrist, elbow, or even shoulder, but the most skilled manipulations are carried out by the digits themselves, e.g. in advancing a thread through the eye of a needle. **C**, The hook grip is used to suspend or to pull open objects. The fingers are flexed around the object; the thumb may or may not be involved. It is a grip for the transmission of forces, not for skillful manipulation. **D**, Powerful opposition of the thumb to the radial side of the index finger produces a lateral pinch grip, e.g. to hold a door key; here the object is larger than a key, and all the fingers are involved. **E**, Many activities involve a combination of grips. Here a fountain pen is stabilized in a power grip by flexion of digits 4–5 against the palm, while the index finger and thumb, used in a precision grip, unscrew the cap. **F**, Complex manipulation.

VASCULAR SUPPLY AND LYMPHATIC DRAINAGE

ARTERIES

Anastomoses occur between the radial and ulnar arteries at the wrist (via the palmar and dorsal carpal arches), in the hand (via the superficial and deep palmar arches) and between their digital and metacarpal branches.

RADIAL ARTERY (Fig. 53.51)

At the wrist the radial artery passes on to the dorsal aspect of the carpus between the lateral carpal ligament and the tendons of abductor pollicis longus and extensor pollicis brevis. It crosses the scaphoid bone and trapezium (in the 'anatomical snuff-box'), where again its pulsation is obvious, and as it passes between the heads of the first dorsal interosseous it is crossed by the tendon of extensor pollicis longus. Between the thumb extensors it is crossed by the start of the cephalic vein and the digital branches of the radial nerve which supply the thumb and index finger (**Fig. 53.52**). Occasionally it gives off a distal superficial dorsal branch which crosses the radial extensor tendons at the wrist together with the superficial radial nerve. Filaments of the lateral cutaneous nerve of the forearm run along its distal part as it curves round the carpus.

In the hand the radial artery passes through the first interosseous space between the heads of the first dorsal interosseous and crosses the palm. At first it lies deep to the oblique head of adductor pollicis and then passes between its oblique and transverse heads or through the transverse head. At the fifth metacarpal base it anastomoses with the deep branch of the ulnar artery, completing the deep palmar arch (**Fig. 53.53**).

Palmar carpal branch (Fig. 53.55)

The palmar carpal branch is a small vessel which arises from the radial artery near the distal border of pronator quadratus. It crosses the anterior surface of the distal end of the radius, near the palmar carpal surface, and passes medially to anastomose behind the long flexor tendons with the palmar carpal branch of the ulnar artery. This transverse anastomosis is joined by longitudinal branches from the anterior interosseous artery and recurrent branches from the deep palmar arch, to form a cruciate palmar carpal arch which supplies the carpal articulations and bones by descending branches. (Although so named, this anastomosis is usually sited near the wrist joint on the distal forearm bones.)

Superficial palmar branch (Fig. 53.56)

The superficial palmar branch arises from the radial artery just before it curves round the carpus. It passes through, and occasionally over, the thenar muscles, which it supplies, sometimes anastomosing with the end of the ulnar artery to complete a superficial palmar arch.

Dorsal carpal branch

The dorsal carpal branch arises deep to the thumb extensor tendons. It runs medially across the dorsal carpal surface under them and anastomoses with the ulnar dorsal carpal branch and also with the anterior and posterior interosseous arteries to form a dorsal carpal arch. The carpal arches are both close to bone and supply the distal epiphyseal parts of the radius and ulna. From the dorsal arch three dorsal metacarpal arteries descend on the second to fourth dorsal interossei and bifurcate into the dorsal digital branches to supply the adjacent sides of all four fingers.

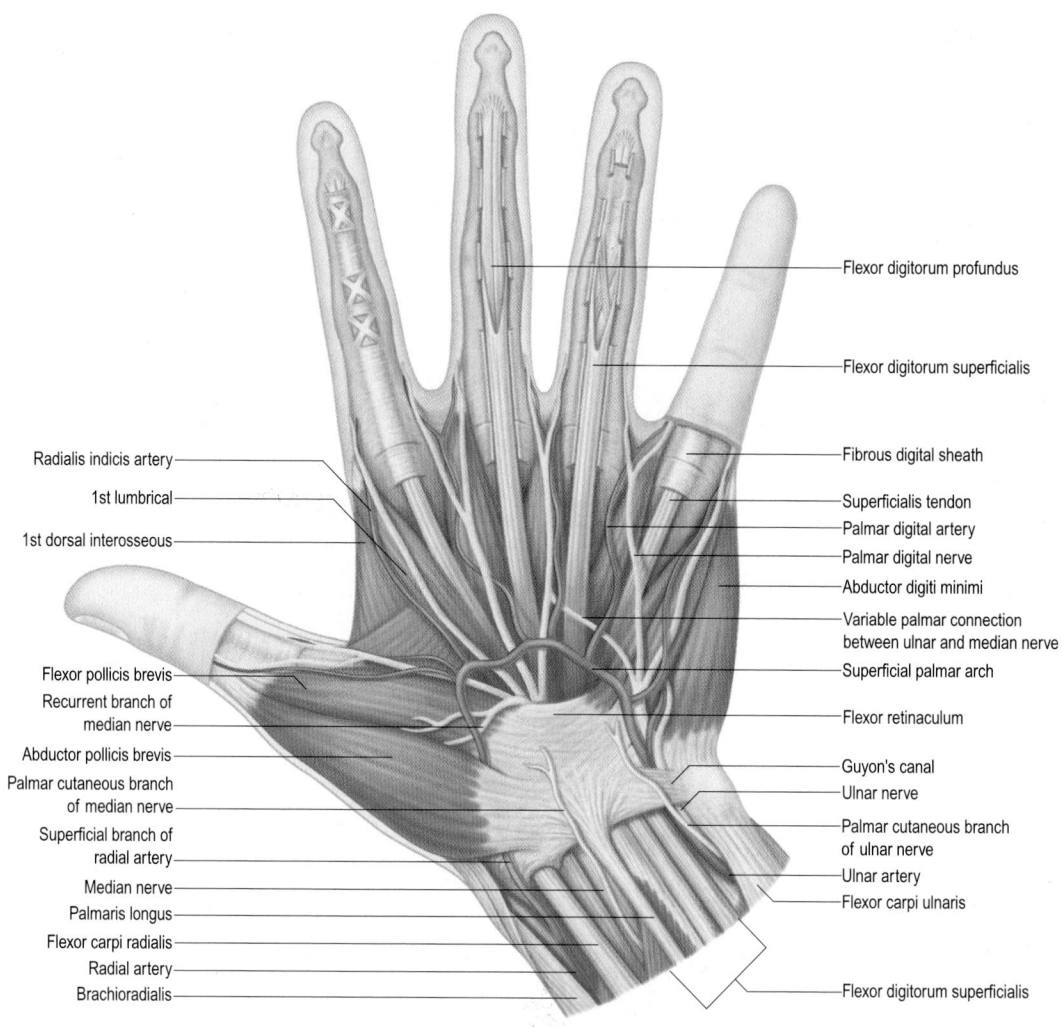

Radialis indicis artery
1st lumbrical
1st dorsal interosseous

Flexor pollicis brevis
Recurrent branch of
median nerve
Abductor pollicis brevis
Palmar cutaneous branch
of median nerve
Superficial branch of
radial artery
Median nerve
Palmaris longus
Flexor carpi radialis
Radial artery
Brachioradialis

Flexor digitorum profundus
Flexor digitorum superficialis
Fibrous digital sheath
Superficialis tendon
Palmar digital artery
Palmar digital nerve
Abductor digiti minimi
Variable palmar connection
between ulnar and median nerve
Superficial palmar arch
Flexor retinaculum
Guyon's canal
Ulnar nerve
Palmar cutaneous branch
of ulnar nerve
Ulnar artery
Flexor carpi ulnaris
Flexor digitorum superficialis

Fig. 53.51 Superficial structures of the left palm and wrist. See also note at Fig. 53.53

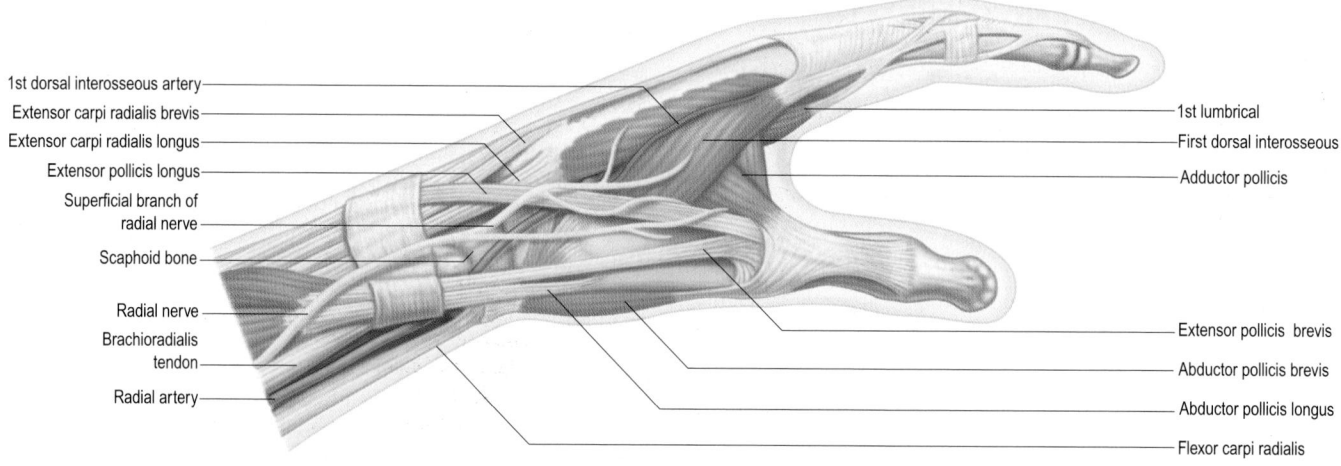

1st dorsal interosseous artery
Extensor carpi radialis brevis
Extensor carpi radialis longus
Extensor pollicis longus
Superficial branch of
radial nerve
Scaphoid bone
Radial nerve
Brachioradialis
tendon
Radial artery

1st lumbrical
First dorsal interosseous
Adductor pollicis

Extensor pollicis brevis
Abductor pollicis brevis
Abductor pollicis longus
Flexor carpi radialis

Fig. 53.52 Lateral view of the left wrist: radial aspect.

First dorsal metacarpal artery (Fig. 53.2)

The first dorsal metacarpal artery arises from the radial artery just before it passes between the heads of the first dorsal interosseous. It divides almost at once into two branches which supply the adjacent sides of the thumb and index finger as far distally as the proximal interphalangeal joint. The radial side of the thumb receives a branch direct from the radial artery proper.

In the majority of cases the first dorsal metacarpal artery follows a fascial course overlying the first dorsal interosseous and parallel to the second metacarpal bone. Occasionally it may follow an intramuscular course. Distally, over the proximal phalanx, it anastomoses with the dorsal branches of the radiopalmar digital artery of the index finger.

In a small number of cases, the first dorsal interosseous artery either arises from, or gives rise to, an ulnodorsal digital artery of the thumb.

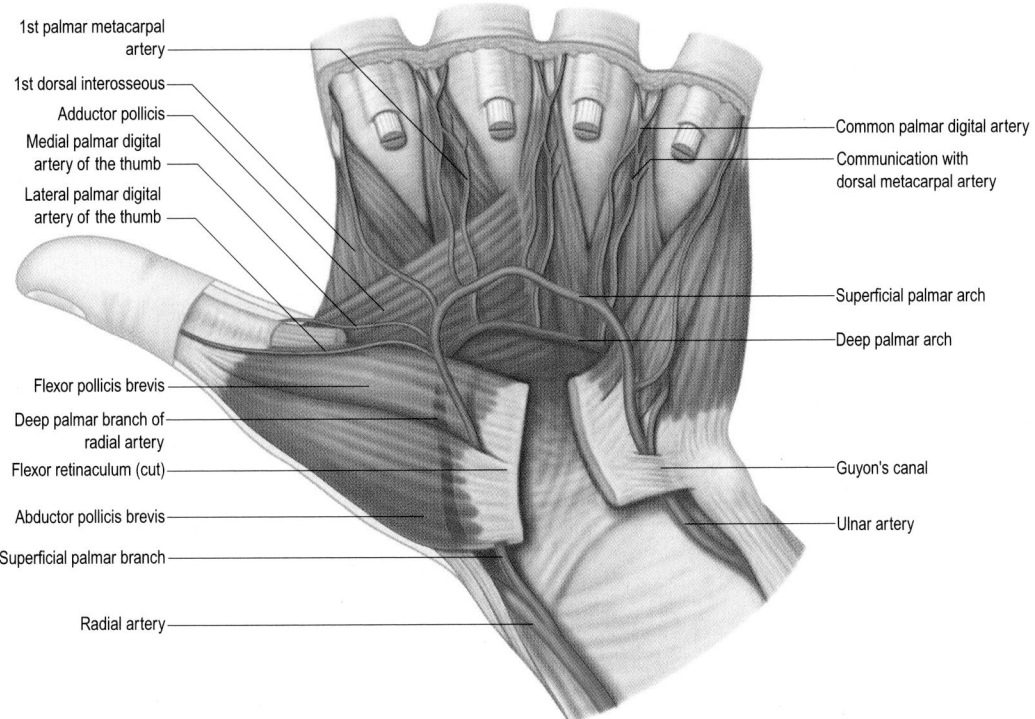

1st palmar metacarpal artery

1st dorsal interosseous

Adductor pollicis

Medial palmar digital artery of the thumb

Lateral palmar digital artery of the thumb

Flexor pollicis brevis

Deep palmar branch of radial artery

Flexor retinaculum (cut)

Abductor pollicis brevis

Superficial palmar branch

Radial artery

Common palmar digital artery

Communication with dorsal metacarpal artery

Superficial palmar arch

Deep palmar arch

Guyon's canal

Ulnar artery

Fig. 53.53 The deep palmar arch and its branches. Note the palmar digital arteries to the thumb have a separate origin from the superficial palmar arch in this specimen; this variation occurs in 20% of cases. There is no princeps pollicis artery in this specimen.

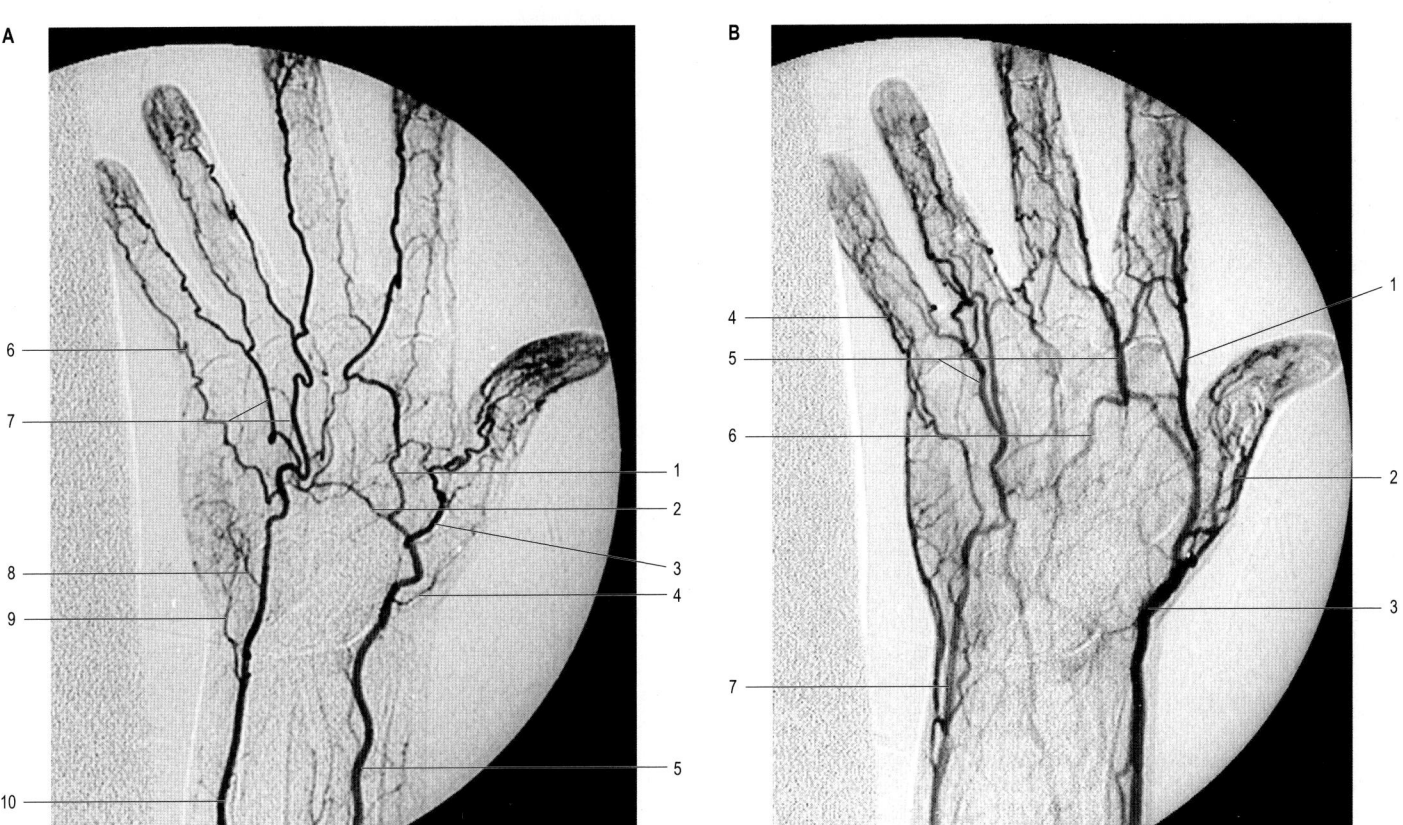

Part A: **1.** Palmar metacarpal artery. **2.** Deep palmar arch. **3.** Princeps pollicis artery. **4.** Artery to radial aspects of thumb. **5.** Radial artery. **6.** Proper palmar digital artery. **7.** Common palmar digital artery. **8.** Palmar carpal branch of ulnar artery. **9.** Deep palmar branch of of ulnar artery. **10.** Ulnar artery.

Part B: **1.** Radialis indicis vein. **2.** Princeps pollicis vein. **3.** Cephalic vein. **4.** Palmar digital vein. **5.** Common palmar digital vein. **6.** Superficial palmar arch. **7.** Basilic vein.

Fig. 53.54 **A,** Digitally subtracted hand arteriogram, dorsopalmar projection. Note that this patient has an incomplete superficial palmar arch. **B,** Venous phase of hand arteriogram. (By permission from Weir J, Abrahams PH 2003 Imaging Atlas of Human Anatomy, 3rd edn, London: Mosby, and contributions from Anna-Maria Belli, Margaret Hourihan, Naill Moore and Philip Owen.)

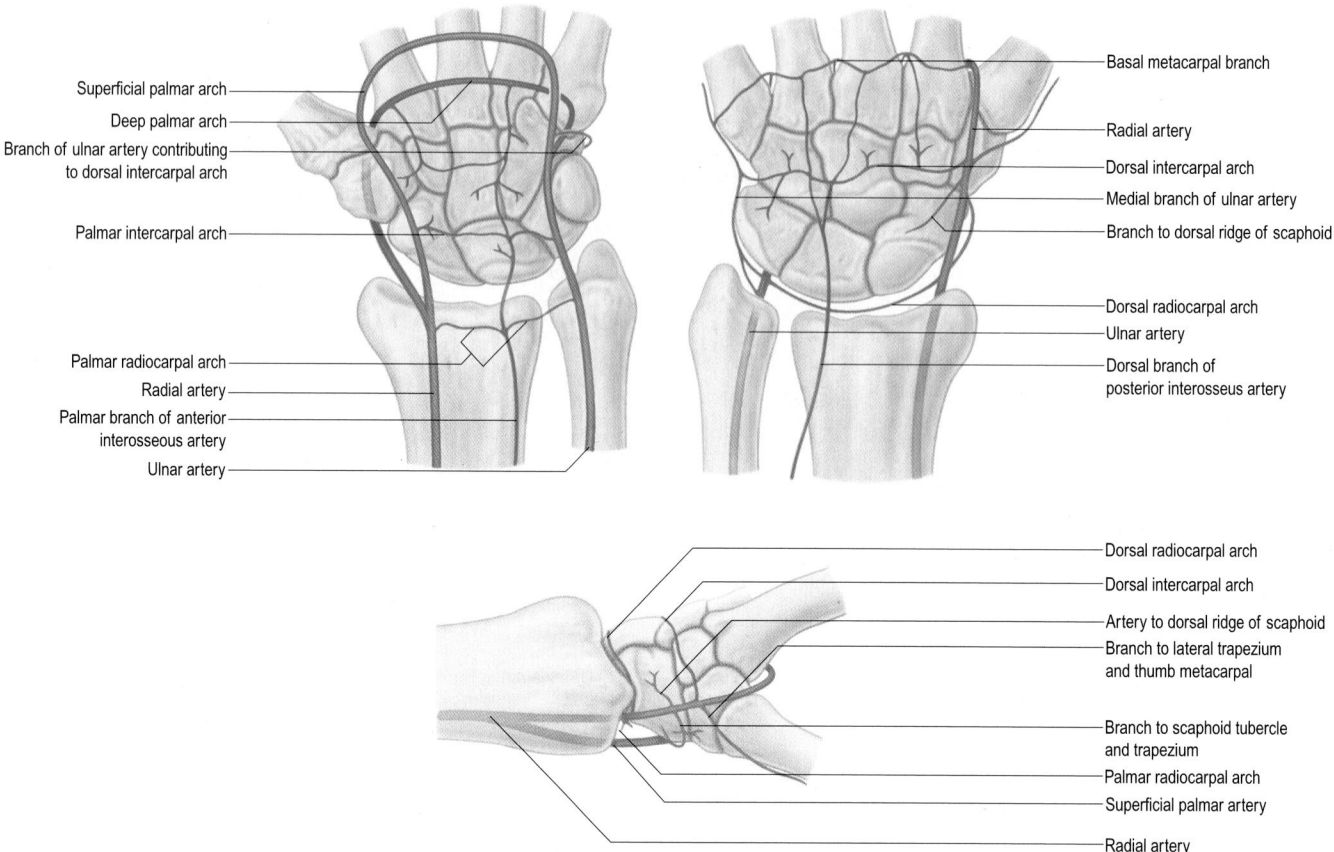

Fig. 53.55 The extraosseous blood supply to the carpus. **A**, Palmar aspect; **B**, dorsal aspect; **C**, lateral aspect viewed from the radial side. (Reprinted from J Hand Surgery, vol 8, Gelberman et al, Arterial anatomy of the human carpus, part 1, 1984, with permission from The American Society for the Surgery of the Hand.)

Occasionally it gives rise to the ulnopalmar digital artery of the thumb, and rarely may give rise to the second dorsal metacarpal artery.

This anatomical arrangement allows a flap of skin over the dorsum of the proximal phalanx of the index finger to be raised on this artery and its accompanying venae comitantes. This is particularly useful under certain circumstances for reconstruction of the thumb following injury.

Second, third and fourth dorsal metacarpal arteries
The second to fourth dorsal metacarpal arteries arise from the dorsal carpal arch. Near their origins they anastomose with the deep palmar arch by proximal perforating arteries and, near their bifurcation, with dorsal perforating branches from the palmar metacarpal arteries which pass between the metacarpal necks. They also anastomose distally at the level of the web spaces with dorsal perforating branches from the palmar digital arteries from the superficial palmar arch. The third and fourth dorsal metacarpal arteries are much smaller than the first and second.

Cutaneous branches from the dorsal metacarpal arteries supply the dorsal skin as far distally as the proximal interphalangeal joint. At the level of the neck of the second, third and fourth metacarpals, a direct cutaneous branch is given off which passes proximally and supplies an area of skin between the two adjacent metacarpals (**Fig. 53.57**).

These anatomical arrangements permit the surgical elevation of flaps of dorsal skin to be based either proximally on the dorsal metacarpal arteries proper, or distally on the direct cutaneous branch. These flaps may be used for reconstructing areas of missing tissue elsewhere in the hand.

Arteria princeps pollicis
The arteria princeps pollicis arises from the radial artery as it turns into the palm to form the deep palmar arch. It descends on the palmar aspect of the first metacarpal under the oblique head of adductor pollicis lateral to the first palmar interosseous. At the base of the proximal phalanx, deep to the tendon of flexor pollicis longus, the artery divides into two branches. It appears between the medial and lateral attachments of the oblique head of adductor pollicis to run along both sides of the thumb. On the palmar surface of its distal phalanx it forms a pollicial arch which supplies the skin and subcutaneous tissue. The arteria princeps pollicis is the usual nutrient of supply to the first metacarpal bone.

Arteria radialis indicis (Fig. 53.55)
The arteria radialis indicis is often a proximal branch of the arteria princeps pollicis. It descends between the first dorsal interosseous and transverse head of adductor pollicis, and along the lateral side of the index finger to its end. It anastomoses with the indicial medial digital artery. At the distal border of the transverse head of adductor pollicis it anastomoses with the arteria princeps pollicis and links with the superficial palmar arch. It may arise from the superficial arch or from the first dorsal metacarpal artery.

The arteria princeps pollicis and radialis indicis may be combined as the first palmar metacarpal artery.

Deep palmar arch
The deep palmar arch is formed by anastomosis of the end of the radial artery with the deep palmar branch of the ulnar artery (**Fig. 53.53**). It crosses the bases of the metacarpal bones and interossei, covered by the oblique head of adductor pollicis, the digital flexor tendons and lumbricals. In its concavity, running laterally, is the deep branch of the ulnar nerve. Rarely the arch is incomplete. There are variations in the size of contribution from the ulnar artery.

Palmar metacarpal artery
The three palmar metacarpal arteries run distally from the convexity of the deep palmar arch on the interossei of the second to fourth spaces, and join the common digital branches of the superficial arch at the digital clefts (**Fig. 53.53**). They supply nutrient branches to the medial four metacarpals.

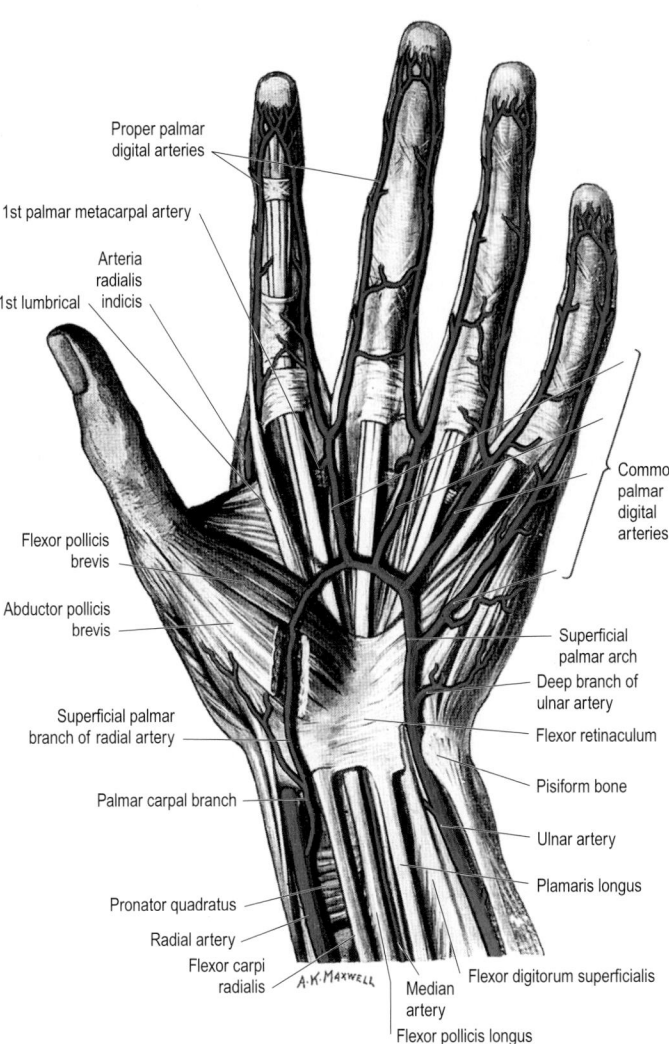

Fig. 53.56 The superficial palmar arch and its branches in the left hand. Part of the abductor pollicis brevis has been excised to expose the superficial palmar branch of the radial artery.

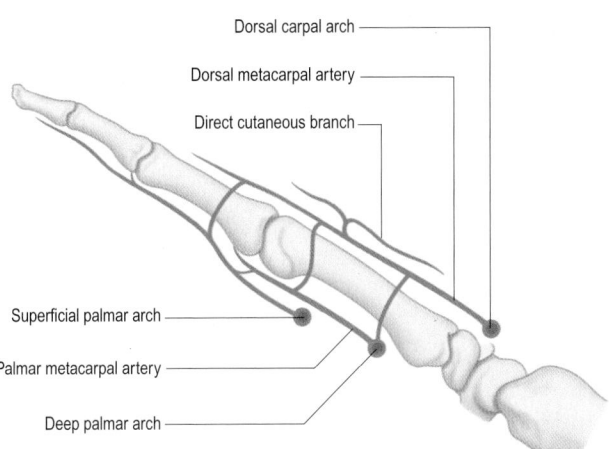

Fig. 53.57 Sagittal view showing communication between the palmar and dorsal metacarpal arteries and the direct cutaneous branch given off the dorsal metacarpal artery c.0.5–1.0 cm proximal to the metacarpophalangeal joint.

Perforating branches

Three perforating branches from the deep palmar arch cross the second to fourth interosseous spaces between the heads of the corresponding dorsal interossei and anastomose with the dorsal metacarpal arteries.

Recurrent branches

Recurrent branches ascend proximally from the deep palmar arch anterior to the carpus to supply the carpal bones and intercarpal articulations. They end in the palmar carpal arch.

ULNAR ARTERY (Figs 53.51, 53.53, 53.56, 53.58)

At the wrist the ulnar artery is covered by skin, fasciae and palmaris brevis. It lies between the superficial and main parts of the flexor retinaculum (p. 913). The ulnar nerve and pisiform are medial.

Dorsal cutaneous branch

A constant dorsoulnar perforator vessel is given off distally. It arises c.2–5 cm proximal to the pisiform and accompanies the dorsal cutaneous branch of the ulnar nerve (p. 884). It emerges between flexor carpi ulnaris and extensor carpi ulnaris. The cutaneous perforator can support a flap of skin on the medial aspect of the distal forearm just proximal to the wrist and is useful in reconstructing areas of missing skin in this region.

Palmar carpal branch

A small palmar carpal branch crosses the distal ulna deep to the tendons of flexor digitorum profundus (**Fig. 53.55**). It anastomoses with a palmar carpal branch of the radial to make a palmar carpal arch.

Dorsal carpal branch

A dorsal carpal branch arises just proximal to the pisiform (**Fig. 53.55**). It curves deep to the tendon of flexor carpi ulnaris to reach the carpal dorsum, which it crosses laterally beneath the extensor tendons. It anastomoses with the radial dorsal carpal branch to complete the dorsal carpal arch. Near its origin it sends a small digital branch along the ulnar side of the fifth metacarpal to supply the medial side of the dorsal surface of the fifth finger.

Deep palmar branch

The deep palmar branch is often double (**Fig. 53.55**). It passes between the abductor and flexor digiti minimi, through or deep to the opponens digiti minimi. It anastomoses with the radial artery, completing the deep palmar arch. The deep palmar branch accompanies the deep branch of the ulnar nerve.

SUPERFICIAL PALMAR ARCH

The superficial palmar arch is an anastomosis fed mainly by the ulnar artery (**Figs 53.2, 53.54, 53.56**). The latter enters the palm with the ulnar nerve, anterior to the flexor retinaculum and lateral to the pisiform. It passes medial to the hook of the hamate, then curves laterally to form an arch, convex distally and level with a transverse line through the distal border of the fully extended pollicial base. About a third of the superficial palmar arches are formed by the ulnar alone; a further third are completed by the superficial palmar branch of the radial artery; and a third by the arteria radialis indicis, a branch of arteria princeps pollicis or the median artery. The superficial palmar arch is covered by palmaris brevis and the palmar aponeurosis and it is superficial to flexor digiti minimi, branches of the median nerve and to the long flexor tendons and lumbricals.

Common and proper palmar digital arteries

Three common palmar digital arteries arise from the convexity of the superficial palmar arch (**Fig. 53.56**). They pass distally on the second to fourth lumbricals, each joined by a corresponding palmar metacarpal artery from the deep palmar arch, and divide into two proper palmar digital arteries. These run along the contiguous sides of all four fingers, dorsal to the digital nerves, between Grayson's and Cleland's ligaments (p. 891), anastomosing in the subcutaneous tissue of the finger tips and near the interphalangeal joints. Each digital artery has two dorsal branches which anastomose with the dorsal digital arteries and supply the soft parts dorsal to the middle and distal phalanges, including the matrices of the nails. The palmar digital artery for the medial side of the little finger leaves the arch under palmaris brevis. Palmar digital arteries supply the metacarpophalangeal and interphalangeal joints and nutrient

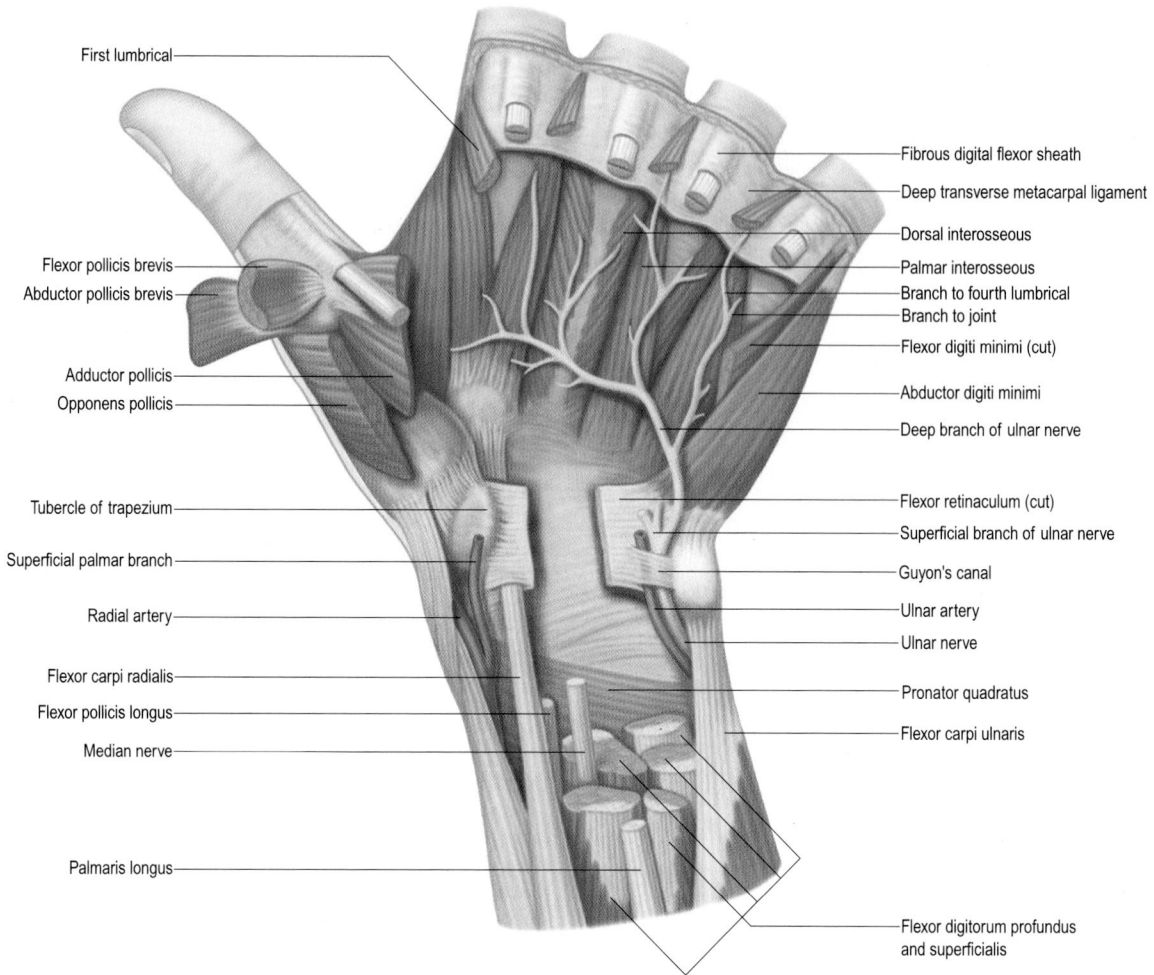

First lumbrical

Flexor pollicis brevis
Abductor pollicis brevis

Adductor pollicis
Opponens pollicis

Tubercle of trapezium

Superficial palmar branch

Radial artery

Flexor carpi radialis
Flexor pollicis longus
Median nerve

Palmaris longus

Fibrous digital flexor sheath
Deep transverse metacarpal ligament
Dorsal interosseous
Palmar interosseous
Branch to fourth lumbrical
Branch to joint
Flexor digiti minimi (cut)
Abductor digiti minimi
Deep branch of ulnar nerve

Flexor retinaculum (cut)
Superficial branch of ulnar nerve
Guyon's canal
Ulnar artery
Ulnar nerve

Pronator quadratus
Flexor carpi ulnaris

Flexor digitorum profundus
and superficialis

Fig. 53.58 Deep structures in the left palm and wrist.

rami to the phalanges. They are the main digital supply, because the dorsal digital arteries are minute.

The origins of the palmar digital arteries of the thumb are quite variable. Both may arise from a single princeps pollicis, or they may arise separately from the superficial palmar arch. The ulnar digital artery may arise from the first dorsal metacarpal artery.

The terminal branches of the digital arteries contribute to a number of vascular arcades which provide a rich vascular supply for the distal elements of each digit (**Fig. 53.59**). Three distal phalangeal dorsal arterial arcades anastomose with each other and with those from the other side of the digit. The superficial arcade occurs at the level of the proximal nailfold and is supplied primarily by a dorsal branch from the palmar digital artery, which is given off at the level of the middle phalanx. The proximal subungual arcade is at the level of the lunula and is supplied by a terminal branch of the digital artery, which passes dorsally. The distal subungual arcade occurs more distally in the nail bed. It is supplied by a dorsal vessel which emerges from the point of confluence of the 'H'-shaped anastomosis between the terminal portions of both digital arteries, and passes from volar to dorsal aspect of the digit under the interosseous ligament which connects the proximal and distal parts of the distal phalanx (**Fig. 53.59**).

Glomus tumours

Glomus tumours are very painful (often tiny and sometimes difficult to identify) tumours of the glomus bodies (small AV anastomoses involved in the regulation of peripheral skin temperature control (**Fig. 7.14**). These typically occur in the proximal nailfold/subungual regions of the finger tips (p. 167) in association with the dorsal digital arterial arcades, although they can occur anywhere. They are diagnosed by exquisite point tenderness over the swelling with reduction of tenderness when the finger is exsanguinated. If the tumour is not visible (as is often the

case) then the best way surgically to explore the dorsal fingertip region to look for the tumour is to incise the lateral nailfold and hyponychium and raise this as a flap along with the underlying periosteum pedicled on the blood supply from the opposite nailfold. The dorsal distal phalangeal digital arterial arcades are then identified from their deep surface and any glomus tumour identified.

VEINS (Fig. 53.4)

SUPERFICIAL VEINS OF THE HAND

Dorsal and palmar digital veins

Dorsal digital veins pass along the sides of the fingers, joined by oblique branches. They unite from the adjacent sides of the digits into three dorsal metacarpal veins (**Fig. 53.60**), which form a dorsal venous network over the metacarpus. This is joined laterally by a dorsal digital vein from the radial side of the index finger and both dorsal digital veins of the thumb, and is prolonged proximally as the cephalic vein. Medially a dorsal digital vein from the ulnar side of minimus joins the network, which ultimately drains proximally into the basilic vein. A vein often connects the central parts of the network to the cephalic vein near the midforearm.

Palmar digital veins connect to their dorsal counterparts by oblique intercapitular veins which pass between metacarpal heads. They also drain to a plexus superficial to the palmar aponeurosis, extending over both thenar and hypothenar regions.

Cephalic vein

The cephalic vein forms over the anatomical snuff-box from the radial extremity of the dorsal venous plexus. It runs proximally over the distal lateral aspect of the radius, where it is easily visible.

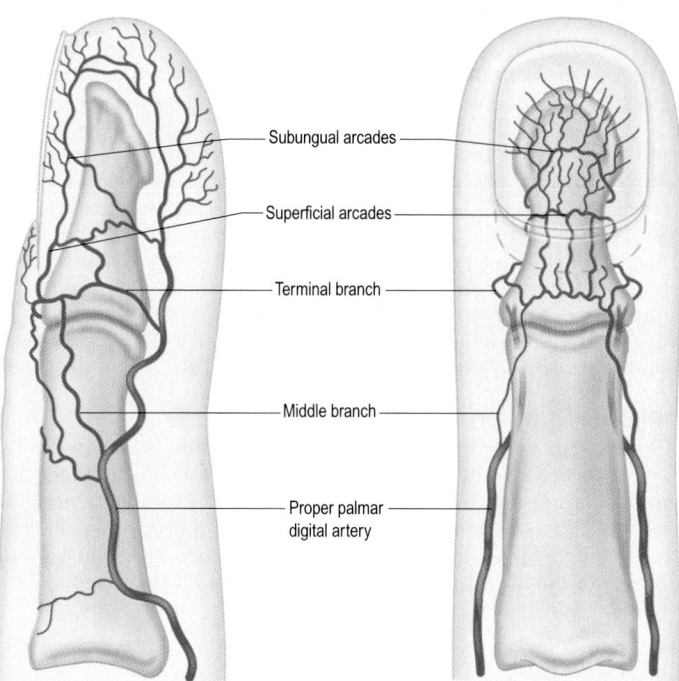

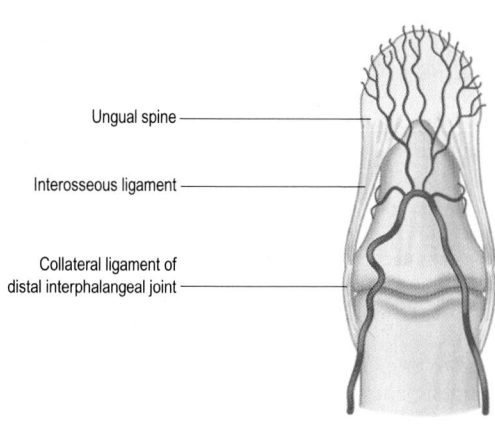

Fig. 53.59 Terminal vascular arcades over the distal phalanx. (By permission from Flint MH 1956 Some observations on the vascular supply of the nail bed and terminal segments of the fingers. BJPS 8: 186–195.)

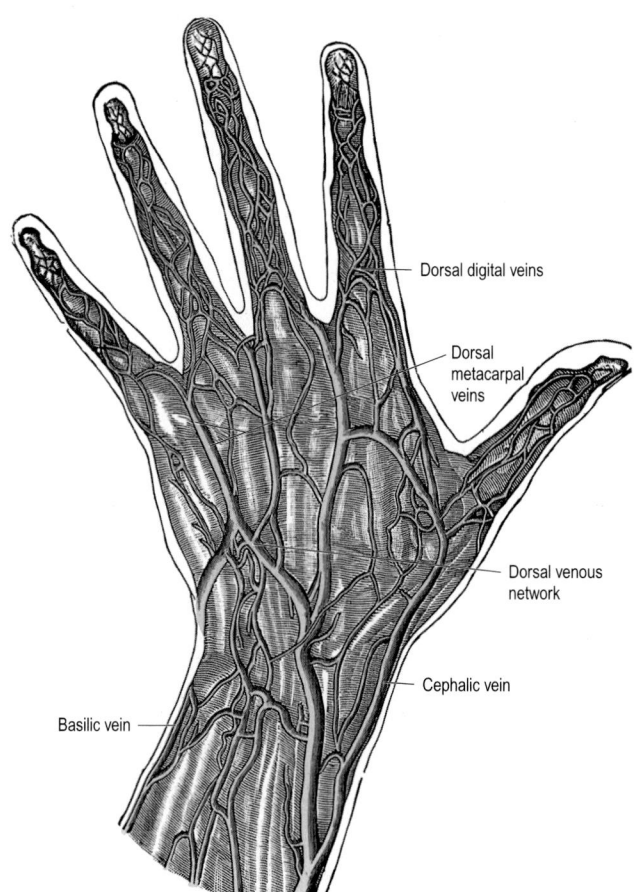

Fig. 53.60 The veins of the dorsum of the hand.

DEEP VEINS OF THE HAND

Superior and deep palmar venous arches

Superficial and deep palmar venous arches accompany their arterial counterparts and receive the corresponding branches. Thus common palmar digital veins join the superficial arch, and palmar metacarpal veins join the deep arch.

Palmar and dorsal metacarpal veins

Deep veins accompanying the dorsal metacarpal arteries receive perforating branches from the palmar metacarpal veins. They end in the radial veins and the dorsal venous network over the metacarpus. This network is joined laterally by a dorsal digital vein from the radial side of the index finger and by both digital veins of the thumb. It is prolonged proximally as the cephalic vein.

INNERVATION

MEDIAN NERVE

The median nerve proximal to the flexor retinaculum is lateral to the tendons of flexor digitorum superficialis and lies between the tendons of flexor carpi radialis and palmaris longus. It passes under the retinaculum in the 'carpal tunnel' (p. 913) where it may be compressed in the carpal tunnel syndrome (see p. 932). Distal to the retinaculum the nerve enlarges and flattens, and usually divides into five or six branches: the mode and level of division are variable.

PALMAR CUTANEOUS BRANCH

The palmar cutaneous branch starts just proximal to flexor retinaculum. It pierces the retinaculum or the deep fascia and divides into lateral branches which supply the thenar skin and connect with the lateral cutaneous nerve of the forearm. Medial branches supply the central palmar skin and connect with the palmar cutaneous branch of the ulnar nerve.

Communicating branches, which may be multiple, often arise in the proximal forearm, sometimes from the anterior interosseous branch. They pass medially between flexores digitorum superficialis and profundus and behind the ulnar artery to join the ulnar nerve. This communication is a factor in explaining anomalous muscular innervation in the hand (see below).

MUSCULAR BRANCH (MOTOR OR RECURRENT BRANCH)

The muscular branch is short and thick, and arises from the lateral side of the nerve; it may be the first palmar branch or a terminal branch which arises level with the digital branches. It runs laterally, just distal to the flexor retinaculum, with a slight recurrent curve beneath the part of the palmar aponeurosis covering the thenar muscles. It turns round the distal border of the retinaculum to lie superficial to flexor pollicis brevis, which it usually supplies, and continues either superficial to the muscle or traverses it. It gives a branch to abductor pollicis brevis, which enters the medial edge of the muscle and then passes deep to it to supply opponens pollicis, entering its medial edge. Its terminal part occasionally gives a branch to the first dorsal interosseous, which may be its sole or partial supply. The muscular branch may arise in the carpal tunnel and pierce the flexor retinaculum, which is a point of surgical importance.

PALMAR DIGITAL BRANCHES

The median nerve usually divides into four or five digital branches. It often divides first into a lateral ramus which provides digital branches to the thumb and the radial side of the index finger, and a medial ramus, which supplies digital branches to adjacent sides of the index, middle and ring fingers. Other modes of termination can occur.

Digital branches are commonly arranged as follows. They pass distally, deep to the superficial palmar arch and its digital vessels, at first anterior to the long flexor tendons. Two proper palmar digital nerves, sometimes from a common stem, pass to the sides of the thumb: the nerve supplying its radial side crosses in front of the tendon of flexor pollicis longus. The proper palmar digital nerve to the lateral side of the index also supplies the first lumbrical. Two common palmar digital nerves pass distally between the long flexor tendons. The lateral divides in the distal palm into two proper palmar digital nerves which traverse adjacent sides of the index and middle finger. The medial divides into two proper palmar digital nerves which supply adjacent sides of the middle and ring fingers. The lateral common digital nerve supplies the second lumbrical, and the medial receives a communicating twig from the common palmar digital branch of the ulnar nerve and may supply the third lumbrical. In the distal part of the palm the digital arteries pass deeply between the divisions of the digital nerves: the nerves lie anterior to the arteries on the sides of the digits. The median nerve usually supplies palmar cutaneous digital branches to the radial three and one-half digits (thumb, index, middle and the lateral side of the ring): sometimes the radial side of the ring finger is supplied by the ulnar nerve. Occasionally, there is a communicating branch between the common digital nerve to the middle and ring fingers (derived from the median nerve) and the common digital nerve to the ring and little fingers (derived from the ulnar nerve). This can explain variations in sensory patterns that do not conform to the classic pattern.

The proper palmar digital nerves pass along the medial side of the index finger, and both sides of the middle and the lateral side of the ring finger. They enter these digits in fat between slips of the palmar aponeurosis (p. 891). Together with the lumbricals and palmar digital arteries, they pass dorsal to the superficial transverse metacarpal ligament (p. 891) and ventral to the deep transverse metacarpal ligament (p. 891). In the digits, the nerves run distally beside the long flexor tendons (outside their fibrous sheaths), level with the anterior phalangeal surfaces and anterior to the digital arteries, between Grayson's and Cleland's ligaments (p. 891). Each nerve gives off several branches to the skin on the front and sides of the digit, where many end in Pacinian corpuscles. It also sends branches to the metacarpophalangeal and interphalangeal joints.

The digital nerves supply the fibrous sheaths of the long flexor tendons, digital arteries (vasomotor) and sweat glands (secretomotor). Distal to the base of the distal phalanx each digital nerve gives off a branch which passes dorsally to the nail bed. The main nerve frequently trifurcates to supply the pulp and skin of the terminal part of the digit. Distal to the base of the proximal phalanx, each proper digital nerve also gives off a dorsal branch to supply the skin over the back of the middle and distal phalanges. The proper palmar digital nerves to the thumb and the lateral side of the index finger emerge with the long flexor tendons from under the lateral edge of the palmar aponeurosis. They are arranged in the digits as described above, but in the thumb small distal branches supply the skin on the back of the distal phalanx only.

OTHER BRANCHES

In addition to the branches of the median nerve described above, variable vasomotor branches supply the radial and ulnar arteries and their branches. Some of the intercarpal, carpometacarpal and intermetacarpal joints are said to be supplied by the median nerve or its anterior interosseous branch: the precise details are uncertain.

CARPAL TUNNEL SYNDROME

Carpal tunnel syndrome is the most common entrapment mononeuropathy. It is caused by compression of the median nerve as it passes through the fibro-osseous tunnel beneath flexor retinaculum. The carpal tunnel may be narrowed by arthritic changes in the wrist joint,

particularly rheumatoid arthritis; soft tissue thickening as may occur in myxoedema and acromegaly; and with oedema and obesity including pregnancy. Usually the condition is idiopathic. Normally the nerve slides smoothly in and out of the carpal tunnel during flexion and extension of the wrist. When the nerve is compressed, additional damage may be produced during these movements. The dominant hand is usually affected first, probably because this hand is used more frequently and more vigorously. Typically, the syndrome produces pain, paraesthesia and numbness in the thumb, index, middle and medial side of the ring finger, which is worse at night and on gripping objects. The palmar branch of the median nerve is spared since it does not pass through the carpal tunnel. With time, the compression leads to wasting and weakness of abductor pollicis brevis. Treatment is usually surgical decompression of the nerve by dividing the flexor retinaculum.

MEDIAN NERVE DIVISION AT THE WRIST

The median nerve is vulnerable to division from lacerations at the wrist. Division leads to paralysis of the lumbricals to the index and middle fingers and the thenar muscles (apart from adductor pollicis), as well as loss of sensation to the thumb, index, middle and radial half of the ring fingers. The radial half of the hand becomes flattened as a result of wasting of the thenar muscles and the adducted posture of the thumb.

ULNAR NERVE

At the wrist, the ulnar nerve passes under the superficial part of the retinaculum (in Guyon's canal) with the ulnar artery and divides into superficial and deep terminal branches.

DORSAL BRANCH

The dorsal branch arises c.5 cm proximal to the wrist. It passes distally and dorsally, deep to flexor carpi ulnaris, perforates the deep fascia, descends along the medial side of the back of the wrist and hand and then divides into two, or often three, dorsal digital nerves. The first supplies the medial side of the little finger, the second, the adjacent sides of the little and ring fingers, while the third, when present, supplies adjoining sides of the ring and middle fingers. The latter may be replaced, wholly or partially, by a branch of the radial nerve, which always communicates with it on the dorsum of the hand (**Fig. 53.4**). In the little finger, the dorsal digital nerves extend only to the base of the distal phalanx, and in the ring finger they extend only to the base of the middle phalanx. The most distal parts of the little finger and of the ulnar side of the ring finger are supplied by dorsal branches of the proper palmar digital branches of the ulnar nerve. The most distal part of the lateral side of the ring finger is supplied by dorsal branches of the proper palmar digital branch of the median nerve.

SUPERFICIAL AND DEEP TERMINAL BRANCHES

Superficial terminal branch

The superficial terminal branch supplies palmaris brevis and the medial palmar skin. It divides into two palmar digital nerves, which can be palpated against the hook of the hamate bone. One supplies the medial side of the little finger, the other (a common palmar digital nerve) sends a twig to the median nerve and divides into two proper digital nerves to supply the adjoining sides of little and ring fingers. The proper digital branches are distributed like those derived from the median nerve.

Deep terminal branch (Fig. 53.58)

The deep terminal branch accompanies the deep branch of the ulnar artery as it passes between abductor digiti minimi and flexor digiti minimi and then perforates the opponens digiti minimi to follow the deep palmar arch dorsal to the flexor tendons. At its origin it supplies the three short muscles of the little finger. As it crosses the hand, it supplies the interossei and the third and fourth lumbricals. It ends by supplying adductor pollicis, the first palmar interosseous and usually flexor pollicis brevis. It sends articular filaments to the wrist joint.

The medial part of flexor digitorum profundus is supplied by the ulnar nerve, as are the third and fourth lumbricals which are connected with the tendons of this part of the muscle. Similarly, the lateral part of flexor digitorum profundus and the first and second lumbricals are supplied by the median nerve. The third lumbrical is often supplied by both nerves. The deep terminal branch is said to give branches to some intercarpal, carpometacarpal and intermetacarpal joints: precise details are uncertain. Vasomotor branches, arising in the forearm and hand, supply the ulnar and palmar arteries.

ULNAR TUNNEL SYNDROME

Ulnar tunnel syndrome is an entrapment neuropathy of the ulnar nerve as it passes through Guyon's canal at the wrist (p. 932). Causes of compression at this site include a ganglion, trauma, and proximity of aberrant or accessory muscles. The symptoms include pain in the hand or forearm and sensory changes in the palmar aspect of the little and ulnar half of the ring fingers, however sensation on the ulnar aspect of the dorsum of the hand is normal. In addition there may be weakness and wasting of the intrinsic muscles of the hand supplied by the ulnar nerve, with clawing posture in extreme cases.

Surgical treatment involves decompression of the nerve by division of the roof of Guyon's canal and removal of the causative lesion, eg. ganglion.

ULNAR NERVE DIVISION AT THE WRIST

Division of the ulnar nerve at the wrist paralyses all the intrinsic muscles of the hand (apart from the radial two lumbricals). The intrinsic muscle action of flexing the metacarpophalangeal joint and extending the interphalangeal joints is therefore lost. The unopposed action of the long extensors and flexors of the fingers cause the hand to assume a clawed appearance with extension of the metacarpophalangeal joints and flexion of the interphalangeal joints. The clawing is less intense in the index and middle fingers because of their intact lumbricals, supplied by the median nerve. For a detailed account of the hand posture adopted in ulnar nerve lesions, see Smith 2002.

There is sensory loss over the little finger and the ulnar half of the ring finger. In comparison to an ulnar nerve division at the elbow, the skin over the ulnar aspect of the dorsum of the hand is spared because the dorsal branch of the ulnar nerve is given off c.5 cm proximal to the wrist joint.

A combined median and ulnar nerve palsy at the wrist results in a full claw hand with thenar and hypothenar flattening, and thumb adduction and flexion. This posture is known as a simian hand because of the similarity to the appearance of the hand of an ape.

RADIAL NERVE

Branches of the superficial branch of the radial nerve reach the hand by curving around the wrist deep to the tendon of brachioradialis. They divide into dorsal digital nerves. On the dorsum of the hand they usually communicate with the posterior and lateral cutaneous nerves of the forearm.

DORSAL DIGITAL NERVES

There are usually four or five small dorsal digital nerves. The first supplies the skin of the radial side of the thumb and the adjoining thenar eminence, and communicates with branches of the lateral cutaneous nerve of the forearm. The second supplies the medial side of the thumb; the third, the lateral side of the index finger; the fourth, the adjoining sides of the index and middle fingers; the fifth communicates with a ramus of the dorsal branch of the ulnar nerve and supplies the adjoining sides of the middle and ring fingers, but is frequently replaced by the dorsal branch of the ulnar nerve. The pollicial digital nerves reach only to the root of the nail, those in the index finger, midway along the middle phalanx, those to the middle and the lateral part of the ring finger may reach no further than the proximal interphalangeal joints. The remaining distal dorsal areas of the skin in these digits are supplied by palmar digital branches of the median and ulnar nerves. The superficial terminal branch of the radial nerve may supply the whole dorsum of the hand.

REFERENCES

An K-N, Berger RA, Cooney WP (eds) 1991 Biomechanics of the Wrist Joint. New York: Springer-Verlag.

Bendz P 1985 The functional significance of the oblique retinacular ligament of Landsmeer. A review and new proposals. J Hand Surg 10: 25–9.

Bowers WH, Wolf JW Jr, Nehil JL, Bittinger S 1980 The proximal interphalangeal joint volar plate. I. An anatomical and biochemical study. J Hand Surg [Am] 5: 79–88.

Cormack GC, Lamberty BGH 1994 The Arterial Anatomy of Skin Flaps, 2nd edn. Edinburgh: Churchill Livingstone.

Doyle JR, Blythe WF 1975 The finger flexor tendon sheath and pulleys: anatomy and reconstruction. AAOS Symposium on Tendon Surgery in the Hand. St Louis: Mosby: 81–8.

Garcia-Elias M 1996 Carpal kinetics. In: Büchler V (ed) Wrist Instability. London: Martin Dunitz, Chapter 2.

Garcia Elias M 2001 Anatomy of the wrist. In: Watson HK, Weinzweig J (ed) The Wrist. Phildephia: Lippincott, Williams & Wilkins.

Green D, Hotchkiss R, Pederson W 1999 Green's Operative Hand Surgery, 4th edn. New York: Churchill Livingstone.

Kauer JMG 1996 The functional anatomy of the carpal joint: the whole and its components. In: Wrist Instability. London: Martin Dunitz.

Kirk Watson H, Weinzweig J 2001 The Wrist. Philadelphia: Lippincott, Williams & Wilkins.

McGrouther D 1982 The microanatomy of Dupuytren's contracture. The Hand 14: 215–36.

Salmon M 1994 Anatomic studies. In: Taylor GI, Razaboni RM (eds) Book 1: Arteries of the muscles of the extremities and the trunk. Book 2: Arterial anastomotic pathways of the extremities. St Louis: Quality Medical Publishing.

Smith PJ 2002 Lister's The Hand. Diagnosis and Indications, 4th edn. Edinburgh: Churchill Livingstone.

Spinner MJB 1984 Kaplan's Functional and Surgical Anatomy of the Hand, 3rd edn. Philadelphia: Lippincott, Williams & Wilkins.

Stanley J, Saffar P 1994 Anatomy. In: Wrist Arthroscopy. London: Martin Dunitz.

Watson HK, Weinzweig J (eds)2001 The Wrist. Philadelphia: Lippincott Williams and Wilkins. In particular the following chapters in this book: Garcia-Elias M, Anatomy of the wrist; and Ryu J, Biomechanics of the wrist.

Development of the limbs

Limb development may be conceptualized as the result of a series of ectodermal–mesenchymal interactions. Such concepts are supported by experimental evidence from amphibian, avian and reptilian species, which demonstrate a remarkable conservation of developmental processes. Chimeric experimentation has further revealed the specific fates of cell populations within the developing limb. The demonstration of conserved homeobox-containing genes in the developing limb is now providing opportunities for reconciling molecular models of development with the results of chimeric experimentation.

The limbs develop via a continual series of complex epithelial/mesenchymal interactions initiated in the lateral body walls. The proliferating somatopleuric mesenchyme forms a ridge externally, ventrolateral to the somites, which extends caudally from the most caudal (sixth) pharyngeal arch, finally tapering towards the tail. Interaction of specialized regions of the somatopleuric mesenchyme with the overlying ectoderm gives rise to local, thickened regions of surface ectoderm and proliferation of the underlying mesenchyme, which specifies the

position of the future limb buds. At the site of each putative limb, the ectoderm forms a longitudinal ridge of high columnar epithelial cells, the apical ectodermal ridge (**Fig. 54.1**).

The apical ectodermal ridge and the underlying specialized somatopleuric mesenchyme are termed the progress zone: this remains at the distal tip of the limb until the digits are formed. The progress zone controls the orientation and progression of limb development and specifies the position of the skeletal elements. The somatopleuric mesenchyme controls the specific developmental fate of the overlying ectoderm and within the limb becomes the skeletal and connective tissue elements. Precursor muscle cells and neurones migrate into the limb somewhat later.

The appendicular skeleton and muscles thus arise from both paraxial mesenchyme (the epithelial somite) and lateral plate mesenchyme (somatopleuric). The upper limb develops in advance of the lower, which is consistent with the craniocaudal progression of development.

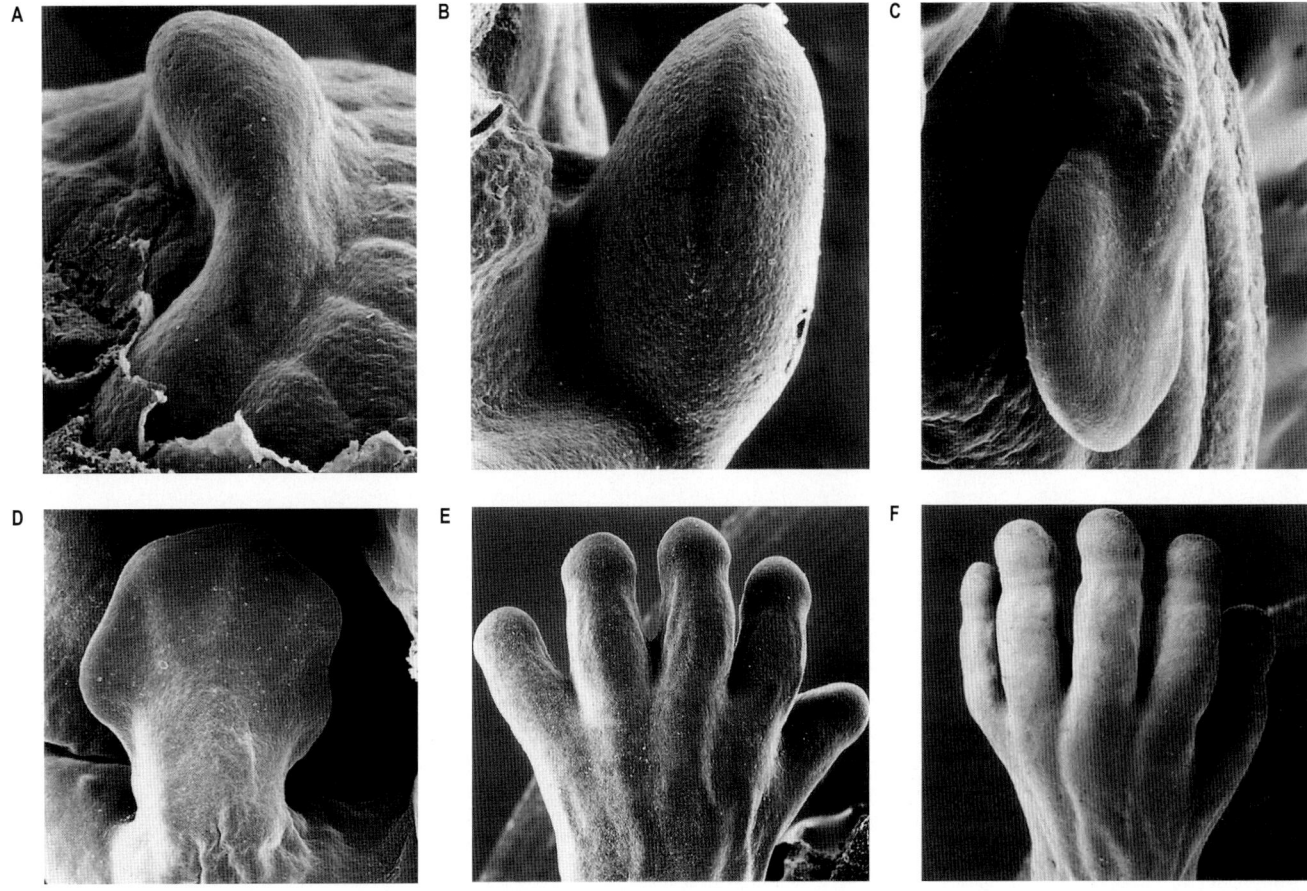

Fig. 54.1 Scanning electron micrographs to show the development of the upper limb. **A**, The earliest limb bud viewed from the postaxial border. **B**, Limb bud viewed from postaxial border; the apical ectodermal ridge can be seen. **C**, Limb bud, ventrolateral view; the shoulder and elbow region are specified and a hand plate has formed. The apical ectodermal ridge is still obvious at the margin of the hand plate. **D**, Digital rays are present in the hand plate and the margin of the plate is becoming notched. **E**, The fingers are nearly separated and proliferations are commencing at the distal end of each digit to form the nail bed. **F**, The fingers each have tactile pads distally, and nail development continues. (Photographs by P Collins; printed by S Cox, Electron Microscopy Unit, Southampton General Hospital.)

AXES OF LIMBS

For descriptive, experimental and conceptual purposes, it has been necessary to define and name various 'axes', borders, surfaces and lines in relation to the developing limb bud (**Fig. 54.2**). An imaginary line from the centre of the elliptical base of the bud, through the centre of its mesenchymal core, to the centre of the apical ectodermal ridge, defines the proximodistal axis of the limb bud (previously known in descriptive embryology simply as the axis). Named in relation to the latter, the cranially placed limb border is the preaxial border, and the caudally placed limb border is the postaxial border. (In tetrapods and birds, the last two are termed anterior and posterior borders, respectively.) Any line that passes through the limb bud from preaxial to postaxial border, orthogonal to the proximodistal axis, constitutes a craniocaudal axis. The dorsal and ventral ectodermal surfaces thus clothe their respective aspects from preaxial to postaxial borders, and any line that passes from dorsal to ventral aspect, orthogonal to both proximodistal and craniocaudal axes, constitutes a dorsoventral axis. It should be noted here that the terms dorsal and ventral axial lines are to be used exclu-sively in relation to developing and definitive patterns of cutaneous innervation of the limbs and their associated levels of the trunk.

The three developmental axes can be identified in the developing limb bud by stage 13 (**Figs 54.2, 54.3**). These are, as noted above, the proximodistal, the dorsoventral and the craniocaudal axes. Each of the three principal axes seem to be specified by different mechanisms. The proximodistal axis is controlled by the progress zone, i.e. the apical ectodermal ridge and subjacent somatopleuric mesenchyme. The cranio-caudal axis is controlled by a small population of mesenchymal cells on the postaxial border of the limb bud, some distance from the apical ectodermal ridge; this mesenchyme is termed the zone of polarizing activity. The dorsoventral axis of the limb appears to be controlled by the ectoderm of the limb

Early differential growth of parts of the limb bud results in two main changes to the originally symmetric axes of the limb. The dorsal aspect of the limb grows faster than the ventral, which causes the limb bud to curve around the body wall. The ventral surface of the limb that is closest to the body wall remains relatively flat, but the dorsal surface bulges into the amniotic cavity. The originally laterally facing apical

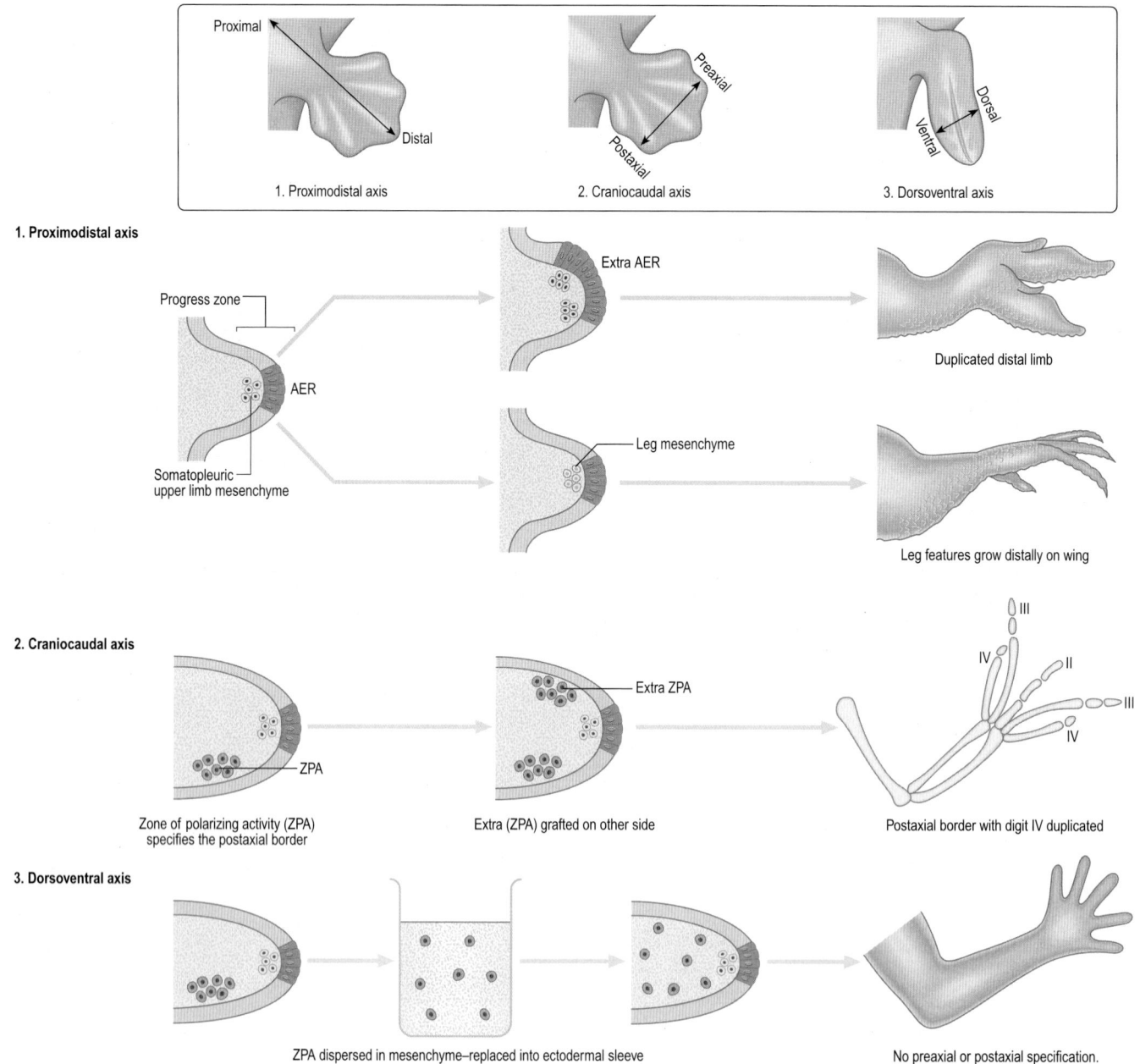

Fig. 54.2 Axes of the developing limb. Abbreviations: AER, apical ectodermal ridge; ZPA, zone of polarizing activity.

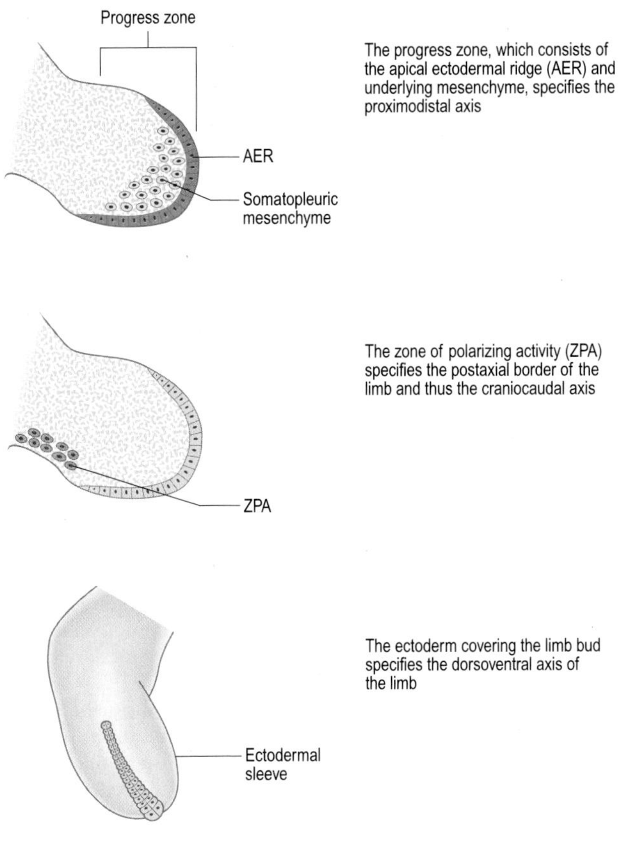

The progress zone, which consists of the apical ectodermal ridge (AER) and underlying mesenchyme, specifies the proximodistal axis

Progress zone

AER

Somatopleuric mesenchyme

The zone of polarizing activity (ZPA) specifies the postaxial border of the limb and thus the craniocaudal axis

ZPA

The ectoderm covering the limb bud specifies the dorsoventral axis of the limb

Ectodermal sleeve

Fig. 54.3 Specification of the axes of the developing limb. The three axes are specified by different interactions. The pattern of development within the limb and the ectodermal specializations are controlled by the limb mesenchyme. The timescale of limb development is controlled by the apical ectodermal ridge (AER). Abbreviation: ZPA, zone of polarizing activity.

mesenchyme beneath the apical ectodermal ridge provides an 'apical ectodermal ridge maintenance factor' essential to the function of the ridge. Temporal information passes from the apical ectodermal ridge to the underlying mesenchyme. A graft of a young limb bud to an older one with the progress zone removed results in duplication of limb elements. Conversely a graft of an old progress zone onto the stump of a younger limb produces a limb with intermediate sections missing. The progress zone behaves independently, as if no communication concerning positional values travels in a proximodistal direction. As cells leave the progress zone, their proximodistal values are specified (**Fig. 54.3**).

In grafting experiments, only whole limb bones develop. Eight states of the progress zone can be described: humerus, ulna-radius, carpals I, carpals II, metacarpals, phalanges I, phalanges II, phalanges III. Each state takes approximately 8 hours. It appears that the progress zone behaves like a clock, the ticks of which are cell-division cycles. The precision with which skeletal growth occurs is often not appreciated. In calculating the growth in left limbs versus right limbs, it may be noted that the length of the left ulna of a limb does not vary by more than 5% of the length of the right.

ZONE OF POLARIZING ACTIVITY

The zone of polarizing activity is a region of somatopleuric mesenchyme on the postaxial limb border posterior to the apical ectodermal ridge. If it is grafted beneath an apical ectodermal ridge, duplication of the limb occurs from that time onwards. If the zone of polarizing activity is grafted onto the preaxial border of the limb, a duplicated distal portion grows, with the orientation reversed (**Fig. 54.3**). The digit closest to the zone of polarizing activity is always digit five; further away from the zone of polarizing activity, digits four, three, two and one develop. This region of mesenchyme is seen as a morphogenetic field. Hox gene expression in the distal limb bud shows a nested arrangement similar to that of Russian dolls: the postaxial border of the limb has all Hox-d genes (d-13, d-12, d-11, d-10 and d-9) expressed; in the next anterior zone, only four genes are expressed (d-12, d-11, d-10 and d-9), and so on until only d-9 is expressed. The five Hox genes can thus specify five different types of digit. Fibroblast growth factors maintain the zone of polarizing activity and Shh gene co-localizes with the zone of polarizing activity.

ECTODERMAL INTERACTION

If the mesenchyme of a limb is removed, dissociated and then repacked into the ectodermal sleeve, a limb will develop that has no anterior–posterior axis, i.e. the zone of polarizing activity has been dispersed. However, the limb does have dorsal and ventral surfaces, which can be identified by the directions of the joints and position and type of hair. Thus the ectoderm specifies the dorsoventral axis.

EARLY SKELETAL ELEMENTS OF THE LIMB

It has been suggested that formation of the cartilaginous elements of a limb is related to the shape of that limb and the conditions necessary for chondrogenesis. There is an antichondrogenic zone beneath the ectoderm of the limb, which prevents chondrogenesis within the dermis and myogenic zones. Foci of chondrogenesis occur in the centre of the limb bud where the cell density is greatest; the production of extracellular matrix by these cells encourages chondrogenic differentiation. In more distal portions of the limb, the limb bud widens, forming first two centres of chondrogenesis then, later, five centres. The apical ectodermal ridge is believed to control the width of the digital plate, which will subsequently reflect this width by the number of digits that develop. Zones that show preprogrammed cell death can be identified on the cranial and caudal, or preaxial and postaxial, borders of the limb at the same time as the zone of polarizing activity. These zones limit the length of the apical ectodermal ridge. (It should be noted that, in the literature relating to work on animal embryos, the preaxial and postaxial borders are termed anterior and posterior borders. Thus the regions in which programmed cell death occurs are termed, in animals, the anterior and posterior necrotic zones.)

If the length of the apical ectodermal ridge becomes reduced, then fewer digits will form (oligodactyly), whereas if the apical ectodermal ridge is not reduced and becomes longer, then more digits will form

ectodermal ridge becomes increasingly directed ventrally. Slightly later, the preaxial border grows faster than the postaxial, resulting in a further shift of the apical ectodermal ridge caudally rather than ventrally. These reorientations in the upper limb form the shoulder, arm and forearm; however, their effects cannot be seen until later.

APICAL ECTODERMAL RIDGE AND PROGRESS ZONE

The outgrowth of a limb bud is controlled by the apical ectodermal ridge (AER) and the underlying somatopleuric mesenchyme. The epithelium seems to control the developmental stage of the limb and the somatopleuric mesenchyme controls the type of limb, interpreting the temporal information from the apical ectodermal ridge in a proximodistal developmental progression. These two tissue arrangements form the progress zone, a region which is believed to be the site where assignments are made to cell populations in the limb. As cells leave the progress zone, their proximal/distal value becomes fixed. Once the mesenchyme has been assigned, it specifies the developmental pattern of the overlying ectoderm.

The fundamental interactions seen in limb development are discussed in Wessells (1977) and in detail in Hinchcliffe and Johnson (1980). The knowledge may be summarized as follows:

The apical ectodermal ridge and underlying mesenchyme provide the orientating influence for limb outgrowth. Removal of the apical ectodermal ridge results in cessation of limb development, whereas insertion of a second apical ectodermal ridge results in two axes of development, and duplication of distal structures from the graft onwards. Replacement of the underlying mesenchyme with any other mesenchyme results in no limb development, as only 'limb' mesenchyme will promote limb bud formation. However, replacement of upper limb mesenchyme with lower limb mesenchyme does support limb growth, but leads to the development of leg structures. In addition, the leg mesenchyme will pass information back to the local ectoderm, causing the appropriate epidermal development. It is presumed that the

(polydactyly). Supernumerary digits may develop on either the pre- or postaxial borders. Other regions of cell death occur between the digits and result in digital separation, but these occur later than the anterior and posterior necrotic zones. The cells between the digits are removed by macrophages. Note that cells in the anterior necrotic zone, posterior necrotic zone and between the digits undergo apoptosis.

The first evidence of bone formation is seen at the mid part of the diaphysis of long bones at 8 weeks. Vascular invasion of the cartilage matrix precedes the formation of a periosteal collar, which extends proximally and distally until it reaches the future epiphyseal level, where a growth plate will be established. By 10 weeks, columns of chondrocytes can be seen at the epiphyseal level of most bones; however, only the lower end of the femur and upper end of the tibia develop ossification centres before birth. The pelvis forms from two hemipelves, which each develop from one cartilaginous focus. Ossification of the pelvis commences with the ilium, which undergoes endochondral ossification (similar to the long bones) at 9.5 weeks.

Further details of the development of cartilage are to be found on page 83; for the development of bone, see page 97.

DEVELOPMENT OF JOINTS

Regions of developing cartilage are easily recognized in the developing limb, because they have widely spaced cells surrounded by matrix. Between the developing skeletal elements, the somatopleuric mesenchyme is more condensed and forms plates of interzonal mesenchyme, which mark the sites of future joints. Their development varies according to the type of joint formed.

In fibrous joints, the interzone is converted into collagen, which is the definitive medium connecting the bones involved. In synchondroses it becomes (growth) cartilage of the modified hyaline type, and in symphyses it is predominantly fibrocartilage, but retains narrow para-osseous laminae of hyaline (growth) cartilage. The interzonal mesenchyme of developing synovial joints becomes trilaminar, as a more tenuous intermediate zone appears between two dense strata next to the cartilaginous ends of the skeletal elements of the region. As the skeletal elements chondrify and in part ossify, the dense strata of the interzonal mesenchyme also become cartilaginous and cavitation of the intermediate zone establishes the cavity or discontinuity of the joint. The loose mesenchyme around the cavity forms the synovial membrane and probably also gives rise to all other intra-articular structures, such as tendons, ligaments, discs and menisci. In joints containing discs or menisci, and in compound articulations, more than one cavity may appear initially, sometimes merging later into a complex single one. As development proceeds, thickenings in the fibrous capsule can be recognized as the specializations peculiar to a particular joint. In some joints, however, such accessions to the fibrous capsule are derived from neighbouring tendons, muscles or cartilaginous elements.

Although the initial stages in the process of cavitation of joints is independent of movements, a full, true joint cavity can form only in the presence of movements.

Generally, the literature suggests that all musculoskeletal elements are in their appropriate positions by 10 weeks. For a review of the literature concerning the chronology of events in human embryonic limbs, consult O'Rahilly and Gardner (1975) and Uhthoff (1990).

EARLY MUSCULATURE OF THE LIMB

It is now well established that all limb muscle precursor cells originate from the somites. These precursor cells are committed at an early stage and can be identified in the lateral halves of the somites. After the mesenchymal sclerotome cells have migrated from the epithelial somite, the remaining dorsolateral portion is termed the epithelial plate of the somite (**Fig. 47.4**). Cells from the cranial edge of this plate form the axial musculature, whereas cells from the ventrolateral edge of those somites opposite limb buds migrate into the limb anlagen. Initially, the cells migrate as single mesenchyme-like cells; later, they migrate in groups. They are surrounded by a non-random, structured network of extracellular fibrils. The migrating cells exhibit at their leading ends filopodia, which are in contact with the extracellular fibrils or with other cells. It is believed that the orientation of the extracellular fibrils may direct the migration of the cells. However, the precursor muscle cells are not competent to produce limb muscles before their migration into the limb, and it is believed that the somito–somatopleural migration is a

time when precursor myogenic cells acquire their responsiveness to the somatopleuric connective tissue.

The proliferation of the limb bud is controlled at the distal tip where the somatopleuric mesenchyme and the overlying ectoderm form the apical ectodermal ridge. The myogenic cells colonize the limb bud in a proximodistal direction only, and never reach the most distal portion of the limb, where there seems to be a distal boundary for the muscle cells. The speed of migration of myogenic cells into the limb is considered to be constant, as the border of invasion seems to lag behind as soon as the rate of elongation of the limb bud becomes more pronounced. Myogenic cells are still indifferent regarding their region-specific determination when they first enter the limb. Myogenic cells from a limb will, if grafted into brachial or pelvic somites, assume the myogenic potentialities of the somites and give rise to normal wing or leg musculature. The muscle cells, unlike the somatopleuric mesenchyme, have no 'limbness'. Further, the muscle pattern developed in the limb reflects the pattern of the skeletal elements: duplication or lack of digits is accompanied by the duplication or lack of the corresponding muscles.

Two subpopulations of myogenic cells can be discerned in the limb bud. In the early buds, there are mainly replicating presumptive myoblasts, considered to be premitotic, whereas in later stages there are also postmitotic myoblasts. It is interesting that the invading myoblasts are still replicating; this may be a prerequisite for the formation of the considerable amount of skeletal muscular tissue that will develop in the limbs.

The first myogenic cells to arrive in the limb form the principal dorsal and ventral premuscular masses. It is believed that all classes of tetrapods begin limb muscle development with these blocks, which produce all the skeletal muscle in the limb. The blocks of premuscle undergo a spatiotemporal sequence of divisions and subdivisions as the limb lengthens, and this leads to the individualization of about 19 muscles in the upper limb and 14 muscles in the lower limb. Small changes in the extracellular environment of myoblasts are believed to induce local fusion of some cells, and thus create a gap that divides the muscle mass into two. In the upper limb, the premuscle masses first divide into three masses, the next division gives rise to the muscles attached to the carpus, and the final division produces the long muscles of the digits. A similar pattern is seen in the lower limb. Thus the patterning of the musculature of the limb is controlled by the somatopleuric mesenchyme.

The axial development of the limb, particularly that controlled by the zone of polarizing activity, also affects the formation of individual muscles from the premuscular mass, as it has been shown experimentally that, if the somatopleuric mesenchyme is dissociated and repacked in an ectodermal sleeve before myoblast migration, the muscle masses remain unsplit.

Each anatomical muscle appears as a composite structure. The muscle cells and myosatellite cells are of somitic origin, and the connective tissue envelopes and the tendons are of somatopleuric origin. The precise way in which the muscles are anchored to the developing bones by the tendons is not clear.

For further development of skeletal muscle, see page 123.

EMBRYONIC MOVEMENTS

Embryonic movements are vital for development of the musculoskeletal system. They have effects on the developing muscle, and are necessary to align trabeculae within bones, and to ensure the correct attachments of the tendons and the appropriate coiling of the constituent collagen fibres within the tendons. Simple movements of an extremity have been observed sporadically as early as the seventh week of gestation. Combined movements of limb, trunk and head commence between 12 and 16 weeks of gestation. Movements of the embryo and fetus encourage normal skin growth and flexibility, in addition to the progressive maturation of the musculoskeletal system.

FETAL MOVEMENTS

Fetal movements have been detected by ultrasonography in the second month of gestation. Fetal movements related to trunk and lower limb movements are perceived consistently by the mother from about 16 weeks' gestation (quickening). Movements of the fetus often involve slow and asymmetric twisting and stretching movements of the trunk and limbs, which resemble athetoid movements. There may also be rapid, repetitive, wide-amplitude limb movements, similar to myoclonus.

By 32 weeks' gestation, symmetric flexor movements are most frequent. By term, the quality of the movements has generally matured to smooth alternating movement of the limbs, with medium speed and intensity. The reduced effect of gravity *in utero* may cause certain fetal movements to appear, on ultrasonography, more fluent than the equivalent movements observed postnatally. The number of spontaneous movements decreases after the thirty-fifth week of gestation, and from this time there is an increase in the duration of fixed postures. This restriction of normal fetal movements in late gestation reflects the degree of compliance of the maternal uterus: there is a slowing of growth at this time.

In addition to promoting normal musculoskeletal development, movements of the fetus encourage skin growth and flexibility indirectly. Fetuses with *in utero* muscular dystrophies, or other conditions that result in small or atrophied muscles, have webs of skin, pterygia, which pass across the flexor aspect of the joints and severely limit movement. Multiple pterygium syndrome is characterized by webbing across the neck, the axillae and antecubital fossae. Usually, the legs are maintained straight and webbing is not seen at the hip and knee. A group of congenital disorders, collectively termed 'multiple congenital contractures', may result from genetic causes, or limitations of embryonic and fetal joint mobility, or be secondary to muscular, connective tissue, skeletal or neurological abnormalities. These conditions may be recognized on prenatal ultrasound examination by the appearance of fixed, immobile limbs in bizarre positions, or by webbing in limb flexures. Specific syndromes, lethal multiple pterygium syndrome, and congenital muscular dystrophy, have been described.

The workload undertaken by the musculoskeletal system before birth is relatively light because the fetus is supported by the amniotic fluid and therefore under essentially weightless conditions. The load on the muscles and bones is generated by the fetus itself, with little gravitational effect. The reduction of gravitational force afforded by the supporting fluid means that all parts of the fetus are subject to relatively equal forces, and that the position assumed by the fetus relative to gravity is of little consequence. This is important, to ensure the normal modelling of fetal bones, especially the skull. Skulls of premature babies may become distorted as a result of the weight of the head on the mattress, despite regular changes in position, and the application of oxygen therapy via a mask attached by a band around the head can cause dysostosis of the occipital bone.

EARLY BLOOD VESSELS IN THE LIMB

ARTERIES

The early limb bud receives blood via intersegmental arteries that contribute to a primitive capillary plexus. At the tip of the limb bud, there is a terminal plexus which is constantly renewed in a distal direction as the limb grows (**Figs 55.1, 116.1**). Later, one main vessel, the axial artery, supplies the limb and the terminal plexus. The terminal plexus is separated from the outer ectodermal sleeve of the limb by an avascular zone of mesenchyme, which contains an extracellular matrix consisting largely of hyaluronic acid. There is experimental evidence that ectodermal/mesenchymal interactions and extracellular matrix components control the initial patterning of blood vessels within the limb. During these early stages of limb development, the proximodistal regions of the limb are patterned by the progress zone beneath the apical ectodermal ridge; later, after the main elements of the limb have developed, the ectoderm and underlying mesenchyme interact to produce the epidermis and dermis. It may be that the early presence of the avascular zone ensures that little interaction of these tissues occurs until a later stage of development, thus preventing premature development of the skin.

The development of the vasculature in the limb precedes the morphological and molecular changes that occur within the limb mesenchyme. The differentiation of cartilage within the limb occurs only after local vascular regression begins, and only in areas with few or no capillaries. Regions of mesenchyme free of capillaries and at high cell density are the sites of chondrogenesis (p. 937). It is not known whether the presence, or lack, of blood vessels affords different local environmental stimuli for mesenchymal cells (by varying the supply of nutrients to the tissue), or whether the local environment is controlled by the diversity of the endothelial cells. Similarly, it is not clear whether inductive factors from the limb mesenchyme cause the changes in the pattern of blood vessels.

VEINS

At the tip of the early limb bud, blood in the terminal capillary plexus returns to the body via a marginal vein that develops along the pre- and postaxial borders of the limb. The marginal vein is separated from the overlying ectoderm by an avascular zone of mesenchyme. As the limb enlarges, the marginal vein can be subdivided into pre- and postaxial veins, which run along their respective borders and which are the precursors of the superficial veins of the limb. Generally, the preaxial (superficial) veins join the deep veins at the proximal joint, and the postaxial (superficial) veins join the deep veins at the distal joint of the limb. Deep veins develop *in situ* alongside the arteries.

REFERENCES

Hinchcliffe JR, Johnson DR 1980 The Development of the Vertebrate Limb. An Approach through Experiment, Genetics, and Evolution. Oxford: Clarendon Press.
Presents the classic experiments on limb development.
Kawakami Y, Tsukui T, Ng JK, Izpisua-Belmonte JC 2003 Insights into the molecular basis of vertebrate forelimb and hindlimb identity. In: Tickle C (ed) Vertebrate Development. Frontiers in Molecular Biology, vol. 41. Oxford: Oxford University Press: 198–213.
Presents the most recently identified genes involved in the control of limb specification.

O'Rahilly R, Gardner E 1975 The timing and sequence of events in the development of the limbs in the human embryo. Anat Embryol 148: 1–23.
Uhthoff HK 1990 The Embryology of the Human Locomotor System. Berlin: Springer-Verlag.
Wessells NK 1977 Tissue Interactions and Development. London: Benjamin/Cummings.
Sets out the main concepts of epithelial–mesenchymal interactions.

Development of the pectoral girdle and upper limb

STAGES OF UPPER LIMB DEVELOPMENT

The upper limb bud is first visible as a ridge along the lateral longitudinal axis of the body wall opposite somites 8–10, at the level of the entrance to the cranial intestinal portal during stage 12. It enlarges, protruding laterally from its elliptical base at the body wall as a flattened plate, with a curved border and an apical ectodermal ridge forming its distal tip. It also has initially equal and relatively flat dorsal and ventral ectodermal surfaces, and a somatopleuric mesenchymal core.

By stage 13 (28 days) the upper limb bud is curved ventrally, and in stage 14 embryos the preaxial border has started to lengthen. At this stage the limb bud is opposite the developing ventricles of the heart. In stage 15, the upper limb can be subdivided into definite regions. The proximal portion of the limb still shows the dorsal bulge and ventral curve: this is the shoulder region and upper arm region. The next distal portion (which was derived from the increase in the length of the preaxial border) can now be identified as the forearm, and the most distal portion is now expanded into a flattened hand plate.

At stage 16, the upper limb appears much more substantial. It is sometimes close to the body wall and sometimes abducted. The hand plate has the first indications of digit rays. By stage 17, the upper limb has an elbow region and digit rays; in advanced members of this stage, the hand plate has a crenated rim indicating the beginning of tissue removal between the digits (**Fig. 54.1**). In stage 18 embryos (44 days), there is further crenation of the hand plate between the digit rays. Changes during stages 19–23 are concerned with growth of the limb and separation of the digits. The hands are now curving over the cardiac region. The distal phalangeal portions of the fingers enlarge at stage 21, forming the nail beds.

Most of the bones in the appendicular skeleton are derived from somatopleuric mesenchyme. Within the upper limb, however, although the clavicle and coracoid portion of the scapula arise from somatopleuric mesenchyme, the body and spine of the scapula are derived from the somites. Prechondroblasts are present in the upper limb at stage 13, and condensations of cartilage can be detected at stage 16, when the humeral anlage can be recognized. Cavitation of the shoulder and elbow joints occurs at 7–8 weeks. By stage 17, when the radius and ulna chondrify, the branched tips of the radial, median and ulnar nerves have migrated to the distal hand plate. The carpal bones chondrify at stage 18, when the hand plate shows notching of the digital rays.

VESSELS IN THE UPPER LIMB

In the upper limb bud, usually only one trunk, the subclavian, persists and it probably represents the lateral branch of the seventh intersegmental artery. Its main continuation (axis artery) to the upper limb (**Fig. 55.1**), later the axillary and brachial arteries, passes into the forearm deep to the flexor muscle mass and terminates as a deep plexus in the developing hand. This vessel ultimately persists as the anterior interosseous artery and the deep palmar arch. A branch from the main trunk passes dorsally between the early radius and ulna as the posterior interosseous artery; a second branch accompanies the median nerve into the hand, where it ends in a superficial capillary plexus. The radial and ulnar arteries are the latest arteries to appear in the forearm; at first the radial artery arises more proximally than the ulnar, crosses in front of the median nerve, and supplies biceps. Later, the radial artery establishes a new connection with the main trunk at or near the level of origin of the ulnar artery and the upper portion of its original stem usually largely disappears. On reaching the hand, the ulnar artery links up with the superficial palmar plexus, from which the superficial palmar

arch is derived, while the median artery commonly loses its distal connections and is reduced to a small vessel. The radial artery passes to the dorsal surface of the hand but, after giving off dorsal digital branches, it traverses the first intermetacarpal space and joins the deep palmar arch.

Anomalies of the forelimb arterial tree are fairly common, probably because they have multiple and plexiform sources, display a temporal succession of emergence of principal arteries, anastomoses and periarticular networks, and some paths that are initially functionally dominant subsequently regress. In general, anomalous patterns may present as: differences in the mode and proximodistal level of branching; the presence of unusual compound arterial segments; aberrant vessels that connect with other principal vessels, arcades or plexuses; vessels that occupy exceptional tissue planes (e.g. superficial fascia instead of the usual subfascial route) or which have unexpected neural, myological or osteoligamentous relationships.

In the upper limb, the preaxial vein becomes the cephalic vein, and drains into the axillary vein at the shoulder. The postaxial vein becomes the basilic vein, which passes deep in the arm to continue as the axillary vein.

NEONATAL UPPER LIMB

In general, the upper limbs are proportionately shorter than they are in the adult. They are long compared with the neonatal trunk and lower limbs, extending to the upper thigh as in the adult; however, the trunk is much shorter in the neonate (**Fig. 11.6**). At birth, the upper limbs are about the same length as the lower limbs, but much more developed. When the proportions of parts of the upper limb are examined, the forearm is longer than the upper arm in the newborn, more so in boys than girls. Only primary centres of ossification are present in the upper limb, apart from a centre in the head of the humerus. The elbow of the newborn cannot achieve full extension, being some 10–15% short; it can flex to 145°. The neonate has a relatively strong grasp within the first few days. The fingernails of the upper limb usually extend to the finger tips or just beyond; they are soft at birth but soon dry, to become quite firm and sharp.

UPPER LIMB ANOMALIES

Approximately 1 in 600 neonates will have a congenital anomaly of the hand or forearm, 30% of which will be bilateral. There is about equal frequency in males and females. It is twice as likely that a limb defect will occur in the upper limb rather than the lower.

A classification of congenital limb malformation uses seven subgroups (Swanson 1976). These describe a clinical picture and do not always relate accurately to the developmental process occurring in the limb. Failure of formation of parts of a limb is caused by developmental arrest affecting the long bones. The second subgroup, failure of differentiation, includes unsuccessful separation of parts, and so includes the range of syndactyly. Groups three to five include limb duplication, overgrowth and undergrowth. Group six includes limb amputations, mainly by adherent amniotic bands, and the last group includes all other generalized skeletal anomalies.

LIMB REDUCTION DEFECTS

These anomalies are categorized as failures of development. The limb reductions seen in infants whose mothers took thalidomide during their

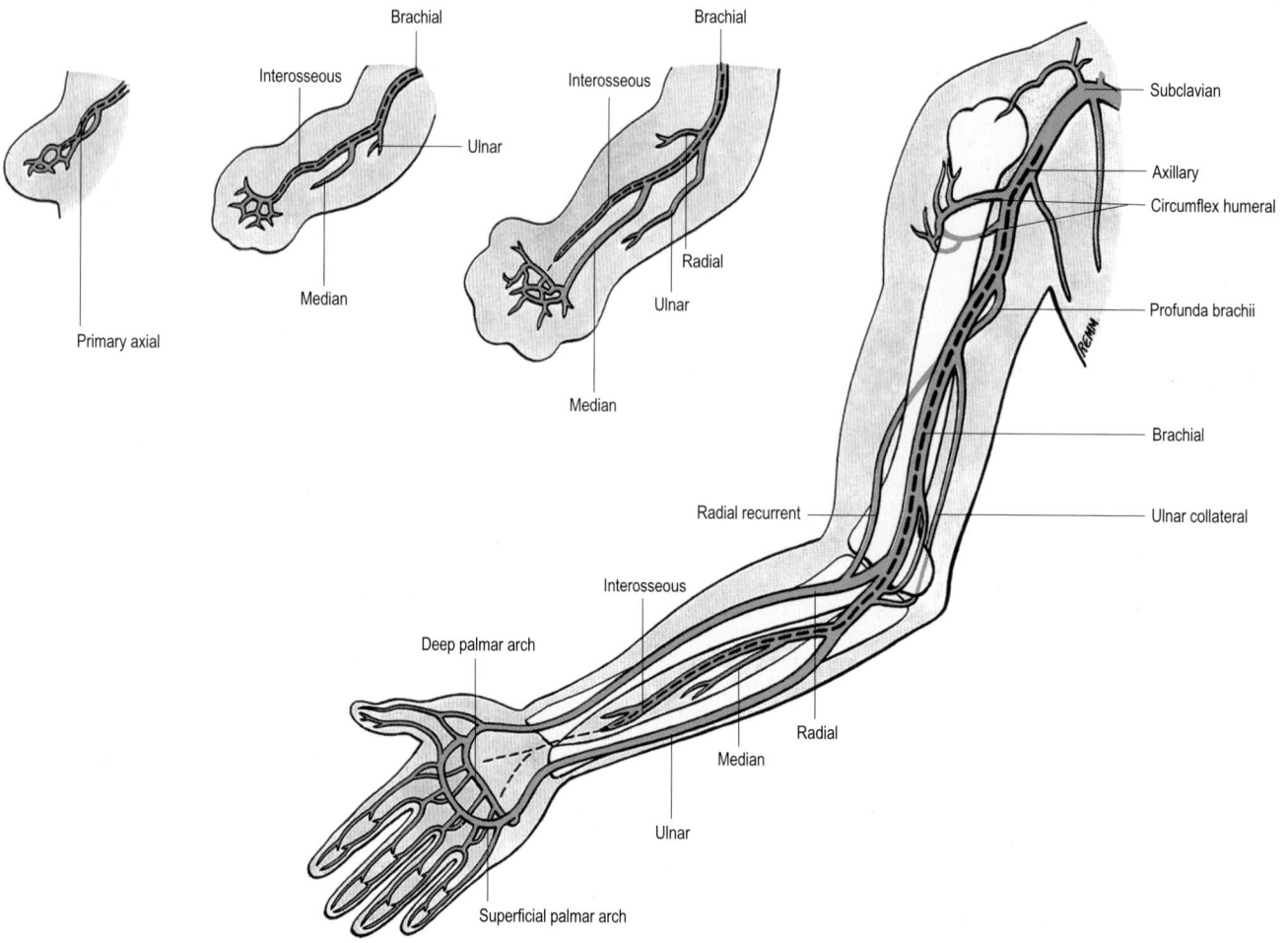

Fig. 55.1 Stages in the development of the arteries of the arm. The original path of the axis artery is indicated by an interrupted line. (After Patten.)

pregnancy seemed to disrupt the apical ectodermal ridge and under-lying progress zone, causing amelia and phocomelia. Proximal segments of the limb were lost with, in some cases, normal distal segments.

In congenital absence of the radius, the ulna is usually shortened and curved towards the radial side. If the thumb is present, it is usually hypoplastic and the first metacarpal is absent.

Inheritance of autosomal dominant genes may cause anomalies of the hand, resulting in absence of the central digit ray of the distal hand plate and subsequent absence of the middle or ring finger and its metacarpals. Extra digits or too few digits can result from alterations in the preaxial (p. 937) and postaxial (p. 937) necrotic zones, producing an extra or missing thumb (preaxial) or little finger (postaxial). The middle digits are not duplicated.

ANOMALIES OF THE DIGITS

Webbing of the fingers is the most common congenital anomaly of the hand, and occurs because of failure to remove cells between the digit rays during stages 19–23, or because of a dominantly inherited disorder.

Clinodactyly is a congenital condition in which the little finger is curved towards the ring finger. It can occur in isolation, or be associated with chromosomal abnormalities like Down's syndrome. Camptodactyly is a congenital condition in which the little finger, sometimes the ring finger, is held in a fixed flexed position. Symphalangism is a rare congenital disorder in which there is fusion of the interphalangeal joints. The affected finger is stiff, with an absence of skin creases of the affected joint. There is minimal joint space, and sometimes the digit is shorter than normal.

REFERENCE

Swanson AB 1976 A classification for congenital limb malformations. J Hand Surg 1: 8–22.

THORAX

Editors:

David Johnson (Lead Editor)

Pallav Shah (Editor)

Patricia Collins (Embryology, Growth and Development)

Caroline Wigley (Microstructure)

Critical reviewers:

Paul Cartwright (chapter 56), **Michael A Gatzoulis** (61), **John Pepper** (60)

Surface anatomy of the thorax

The thoracic skeleton is an osteocartilaginous frame around the principal organs of respiration and circulation (**Fig. 57.3**). It is narrow above, broad below, flattened anteroposteriorly and longer behind. The forward projection of the vertebral bodies means that it is reniform in horizontal section.

Posteriorly, the thorax includes the thoracic vertebrae and the posterior parts of the ribs. The posterolateral curvature of the ribs from their vertebral ends to their angles produces a large groove on both sides of the vertebral column. Anteriorly are the sternum and the anterior parts of the ribs and costal cartilages; this aspect is slightly convex. Laterally, the thorax is convex and formed only by ribs. The ribs and costal cartilages are separated by 11 intercostal spaces, which are occupied by intercostal muscles and membranes, neurovascular bundles and lymphatic channels.

The thoracic inlet is reniform, c.5 cm anteroposteriorly and c.10 cm transversely. Its plane slopes down and forwards, bounded by the first thoracic vertebral body behind, the superior border of the manubrium sterni in front and the first rib on each side. The outlet is limited posteriorly by the twelfth thoracic vertebral body, the twelfth and eleventh ribs laterally, and anteriorly by the tenth to seventh ribs, which ascend to form the infrasternal angle. It is wider transversely and oblique, and slopes down towards the back, and is closed by the diaphragm, which forms a floor to the thoracic cavity.

Thoracic variations in dimensions and proportions are partly individual and also linked to age, sex and race. At birth, the transverse diameter is relatively less than it is in the adult, but adult proportions develop as walking begins. Thoracic capacity is less in females than it is in males, both absolutely and proportionately: the sternum is shorter, the thoracic inlet more oblique, and the suprasternal notch level with the third thoracic vertebra (whereas it is level with the second in males). The upper ribs are more mobile in females, allowing greater upper thoracic expansion.

SURFACE FEATURES

BREAST
In females, the site of the nipple is dependent on the size and shape of the breasts. In the male, the nipple is usually sited in the fourth intercostal space in the midclavicular line. In the young adult of either sex, the nipples are usually positioned 20–23 cm from the suprasternal notch in the midclavicular line and 20–23 cm apart in the horizontal plane.

SKELETAL LANDMARKS (Figs 56.1)
Anteriorly, the clavicle and sternoclavicular joint are not only palpable, but also visible in all but the most obese individuals. The sternum can be felt throughout its length in the midline, but laterally it may be obscured by pectoralis major. The jugular notch at the superior end of the sternum is easily found, and the trachea may be felt deep to it. The cartilaginous rings are usually palpable: by rolling one's finger over the trachea, or by using two fingers within the notch, it is possible to assess whether the trachea is in the midline or deviated to one side. The jugular notch lies at the level of the junction between the second and third thoracic vertebrae. The sternal angle (angle of Louis), is more pronounced in the male than in the female, and is felt at the junction of the manubrium with the body of the sternum. It is a particularly useful landmark because it indicates the medial ends of the second costal cartilages, and is level with the junction of the fourth and fifth thoracic vertebrae. The xiphisternal joint and xiphoid process may be

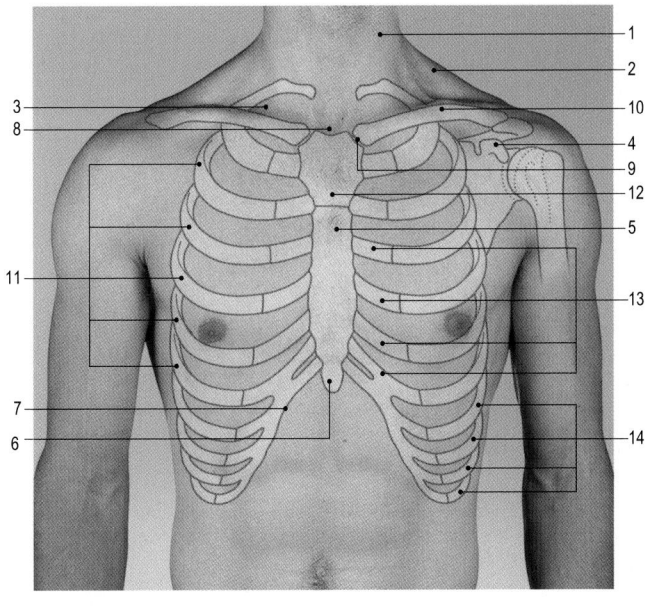

1. Sternocleidomastoid.   2. Trapezius.   3. Supraclavicular fossa.   4. Coracoid process.
5. Body of sternum.   6. Xiphisternum.   7. Costal margin.   8. Suprasternal notch.
9. Sternoclavicular joint.   10. Clavicle.   11. True ribs.   12. Manubrium.
13. Costal cartilages.   14. False ribs.

Fig. 56.1 Frontal view of trunk demonstrating bony and soft tissue structures. (By permission from Lumley JSP 2002 Surface Anatomy, 3rd edn. Edinburgh: Churchill Livingstone.)

felt at the inferior end of the sternum. The joint usually lies at the level of the ninth thoracic vertebra. Lateral to this may be felt the costal margin, formed here by the anterior ends of the seventh costal cartilages. The rest of the costal margin is formed by the fused anterior ends of the eighth, ninth and tenth costal cartilages, whereas posteriorly the free ends of the eleventh and twelfth ribs may be palpable. In thin individuals, it is possible to palpate all the ribs from the first down to the costal margin. However, well-developed musculature or the female breast will obscure the ribs anteriorly and the shaft of the first rib (which lies predominantly behind the clavicle).

Posteriorly (**Fig. 56.2**), the spinous processes of the thoracic vertebrae are easily palpable; the posterior angles of the ribs can be felt lateral to the spinous processes. The surface anatomy of the back and skeletal surface landmarks are described in Chapter 110.

MUSCULOTENDINOUS LANDMARKS
In a muscular subject, pectoralis major, the slips of serratus anterior, and latissimus dorsi, trapezius, external oblique and rectus abdominis are all easily visible (**Figs 56.2, 56.3**). The anterior chest wall of females may be largely obscured by the breasts.

INTRATHORACIC VISCERA (Fig. 56.4; see 56.5)
Anteriorly, the manubriosternal joint (sternal angle) overlies the concavity of the aortic arch and marks the level at which the trachea bifurcates and the azygos vein enters the superior vena cava. The costal cartilages of the second ribs meet the sternum here, and so the joint offers an accurate point at which to start counting ribs. The transverse

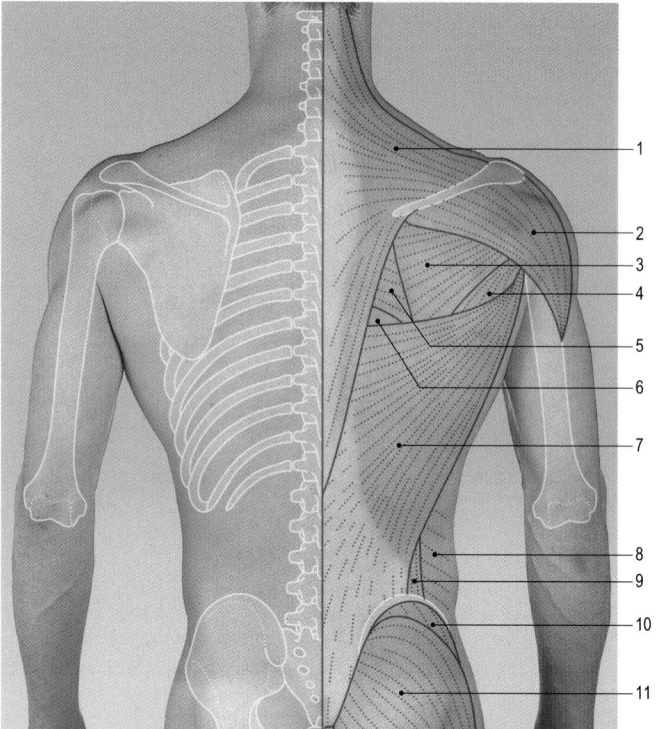

1. Trapezius.   2. Deltoid.   3. Infraspinatus.   4. Teres major.   5. Rhomboid major.
6. Ausculatory triangle.   7. Latissimus dorsi.   8. External oblique.   9. Lumbar triangle.
10. Gluteus medius.   11. Gluteus maximus.

Fig. 56.2 Posterior aspect of the trunk to show surface anatomy, bony and soft tissue structures. (By permission from Lumley JSP 2002 Surface Anatomy, 3rd edn. Edinburgh: Churchill Livingstone.)

thoracic plane, which includes the sternal angle, demarcates the lower border of the superior mediastinum and the point at which the aortic arch receives the ascending aorta (anteriorly) and becomes the descending aorta (posteriorly). At this point the right and left pleurae are in contact with each other; it is therefore a useful starting point when delineating the surface markings of the parietal pleura (see **Fig. 56.5**).

Heart

The surface projections to be described below apply to an average adult. It must be appreciated that they are considerably modified by age, sex, stature and proportions, ventilation and posture. The projections of the position of the valves on the surface are not the best sites for their auscultation (**Fig. 60.10**). The cardiac apex almost corresponds to the apex beat, which is usually visible and always palpable in the fifth intercostal space, slightly medial to midclavicular line, c.9 cm from the midline in average adult males. The apex beat is the most inferolateral point at which a pulsation can be felt; however, the true cardiac apex is a short distance further inferolaterally and does not contact the thoracic wall in systole.

The cardiac sternocostal surface, projected onto the anterior thoracic wall, is a trapezoid (**Figs 56.4, 60.10**). The area of superficial cardiac dullness as mapped out by light percussion is roughly triangular and corresponds to the area of the heart not covered by lung. The borders of the heart, although frequently given as being fixed, are in fact variable and depend largely on the position of the diaphragm and the obesity and build of the patient.

The following borders are usually recognized. The upper border forms a gently sloping line from the second left costal cartilage to the third right costal cartilage. The right border is a gently curved line, convex to the right from the third right to the sixth right costal cartilage, usually 1–2 cm lateral to the sternal edge. The inferior or acute border runs from the sixth right costal cartilage to the apex of the heart, which lies in the fifth left intercostal space approximately in the midclavicular line. The left ('obtuse') border extends superomedially, convex laterally, from the apex to meet the second left costal cartilage c.1 cm from the

left sternal edge. An oblique line joining the sternal end of the third left and sixth right costal cartilages represents the anterior part of the coronary sulcus, which separates the right atrium from the right ventricle (the left atrium lies behind the heart). The left and right borders can be identified by heavy percussion.

The surface projection of the anterior part of the atrioventricular groove is an oblique line that joins the sternal ends of the third left and sixth right costal cartilages and separates the atrial and ventricular areas. Although in different planes, the projections of the cardiac valves are also sited along or close to this line (**Fig. 60.10**).

The pulmonary orifice lies partly behind the superior border of the third left costal cartilage, and partly behind the left third of the sternum. It is represented by a horizontal line, 2.5 cm long, which crosses cartilage and sternum. Parallel lines from the ends of this line, up to the second left costal cartilage, indicate the site of the pulmonary trunk.

The aortic orifice is below and a little right of the pulmonary, and is marked by a line 2.5 cm long running from the medial end of the third left intercostal space downward to the right. Two parallel lines from the ends of this line, slanting up to the right half of the sternal angle, outline the location of the ascending aorta.

The tricuspid valvar orifice is represented by a line, 4 cm long, starting near the midline just below the level of the fourth right costal cartilage, and passing down and slightly to the right. The centre of this line should be level with the middle of the fourth right intercostal space.

The mitral orifice is behind the left half of the sternum opposite the fourth left costal cartilage, and is represented by a line, 3 cm long, descending to the right.

The sites of auscultation for the cardiac valves do not correspond directly to the surface anatomy of the valves, because the intensity of the sounds is influenced by direction of blood flow, which carries the sound with it. Thus convenient sites at which to apply the stethoscope bell or diaphragm are (**Fig. 56.4**): the sternal end of the second left intercostal space (pulmonary area); the sternal end of the second right intercostal space (aortic area); near the cardiac apex (mitral area); over the left lower sternal border, at the level of the fifth intercostal spaces (tricuspid area).

Great vessels

The aortic arch lies predominantly behind the manubrium sterni. Starting at the aortic valve (behind the lower border of third left costal cartilage), the ascending aorta curves forwards, upwards and to the right, to become the aortic arch behind the right half of the manubrium at the level of the second right costal cartilage. It continues to ascend behind the right side of the manubrium sterni, arching over the transthoracic plane and descending such that the aortic knuckle protrudes just to the left of the manubrium sterni in the first intercostal space. The pulmonary trunk and tracheal bifurcation lie within its concavity. The brachiocephalic artery arises approximately behind the centre point of the manubrium and ascends to the right sternoclavicular joint. The superior vena cava descends predominantly behind, but also just to the right of, the right manubrial border and enters the right atrium at the level of the third right costal cartilage. The short right brachiocephalic vein descends almost vertically from behind the medial end of the clavicle just lateral to the right sternoclavicular junction, whereas the much longer left brachiocephalic vein passes almost horizontally behind the superior portion of the manubrium sterni. Both join behind the first right costal cartilage to form the superior vena cava, which descends as a band 2 cm wide along the right sternal margin, reaching the right atrium at the level of the third right costal cartilage.

Lungs and pleurae (Fig. 56.5)

Anteriorly, the apex of the lung is c.2.5 cm above the centre of the medial one-third of the clavicle; posteriorly it lies at the level of the seventh cervical vertebra. The surface markings of the apical dome and costovertebral border of the lung correspond to those of the parietal pleura. The anterolateral surface projection of the lung may be represented by a curved line that crosses the midclavicular line at the level of the sixth rib, and the midaxillary line at the level of the eighth rib. On inspiration, the lower border of the lung moves downwards, from the level of the tenth thoracic vertebra to the level of the twelfth thoracic vertebra (these levels are approximate). In full expiration, the lower border of the lung retreats anteriorly a short distance from the retrosternal costomediastinal recess; laterally, the lower margin of the lung may rise 5 cm above the parietal pleural reflection (the costodiaphragmatic recess).

A

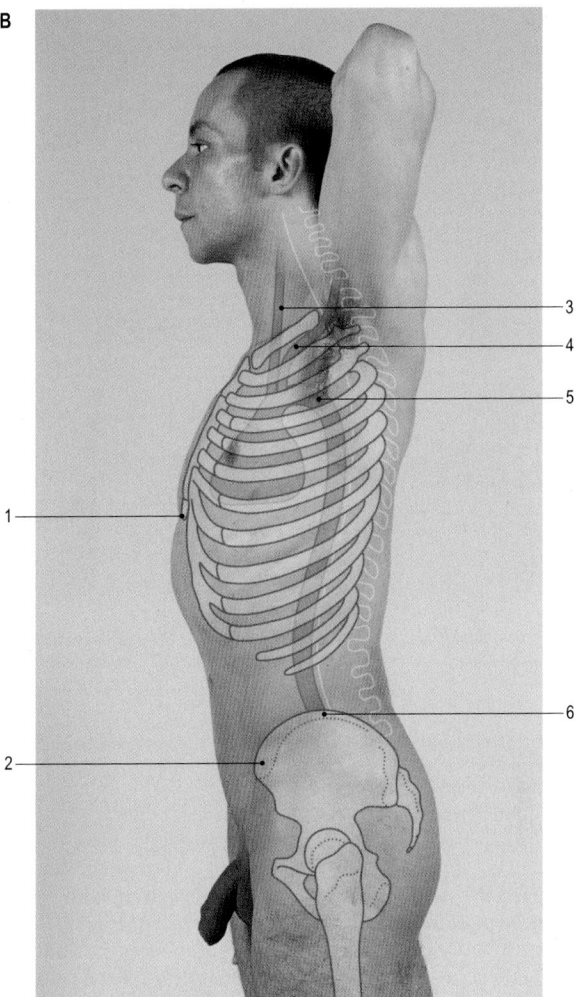

B

Part A: **1.** Infraclavicular fossa. **2.** Anterior axillary fold. **3.** Pectoralis major. **4.** Rectus abdominis. **5.** Linea semilunaris. **6.** External oblique. **7.** Triceps. **8.** Deltoid. **9.** Axilla. **10.** Posterior axillary fold. **11.** Teres major. **12.** Latissimus dorsi. **13.** Serratus anterior. **14.** Inferior costal margin.
Part B: **1.** Xiphoid process. **2.** Anterior superior iliac spine. **3.** Common carotid artery. **4.** Axillary artery. **5.** Aorta. **6.** Iliac crest.

Fig. 56.3 Lateral view of trunk demonstrating bony and soft tissue structures. (Photograph by Sarah-Jane Smith.)

Trachea, bronchi

The trachea originates at the level of the cricoid cartilage (C6), and usually runs in the midline. It is palpable within the suprasternal notch, where it may be felt either by rolling one finger over its convex surface or by defining its lateral extent with two fingers. A shift to one side indicates that the mediastinum has either been pulled over to that side by loss of lung volume, or pushed over, e.g. by a large pneumothorax or pleural effusion. The trachea bifurcates at the level of the sternal angle; the posterior landmark for the bifurcation is the fourth thoracic vertebra.

Fissures

The fissures are depicted in **Fig 56.5A.**

On either side, the upper and lower lobes of the lung are separated by the oblique fissure. This may be marked by a line running from the posterior end of the third rib downwards and forwards to cross the fifth rib in the midaxillary line and then to the sixth costal cartilage at the midclavicular line (7–8 cm lateral to the midline). As a convenient approximation, the oblique fissure follows the medial border of the scapula when the arm is in full abduction. The left oblique fissure is slightly more vertical than the right.

The horizontal fissure, between the middle and upper lobes, lies at the level of the fourth costal cartilage on the right. It starts from the anterior border of the lung and passes posterolaterally to meet the oblique fissure: the horizontal fissure therefore extends from the fifth rib in the midaxillary line to the fourth rib at the right sternal border. The upper and middle lobes lie anterior to the oblique fissure and so

are best examined from the front of the chest, whereas the lower lobes lie posteriorly and should be examined from the back of the chest. The right middle lobe may be projected onto the chest wall as a triangular surface where the three points of the triangle are represented by the fourth rib at the right para-sternal edge, the fifth rib at the midaxillary line, and the sixth rib at the midclavicular line.

Pleural reflections

The pleural reflections are depicted in **56.4 and 56.5A.**

Starting in the midline at the manubriosternal junction, the anterior reflections of the parietal pleura may be traced superiorly along a line that diverges from the midline and extends up and outwards to the apex of the pleural cavity. This point lies 3–4 cm above the anterior end of the first rib, on a level with the posterior end of the rib; its surface marking is c.2.5 cm above the centre of the medial one-third of the clavicle. The parietal pleura is intimately fused with the inner aspect of the thoracic cavity, and it can be followed laterally and inferiorly down the inner aspect of the chest wall to the level of the tenth rib in the midaxillary line. Followed medially, the pleura covers the diaphragm; its position will therefore vary according to the phase of ventilation.

The costodiaphragmatic reflections of the pleurae can be followed anteriorly from the midaxillary line towards the midline. On the right, the pleura crosses the eighth rib in the midclavicular line, passes to the xiphisternum and then ascends to the sternal angle. On the left, the pleura does not reach the midline, but turns superiorly at the anterior end of the sixth rib, 3–5 cm from the midline, and passes up to the level of the fourth costal cartilage. This deviation produces an area between

947

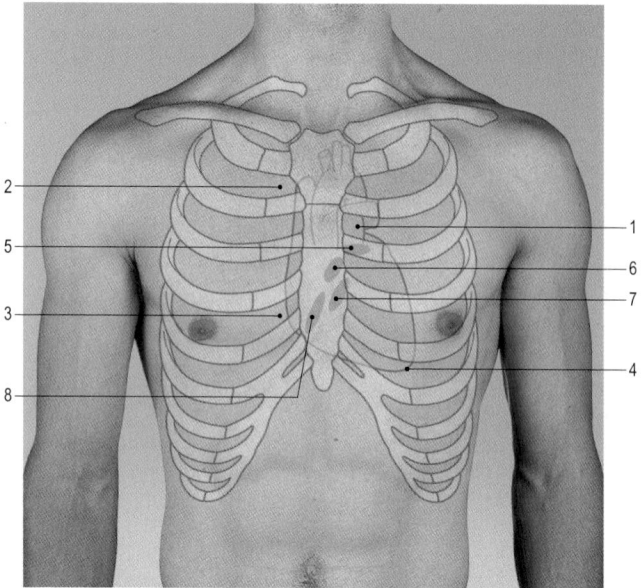

1. Pulmonary valve ausculation.   2. Aortic valve ausculation.   3. Tricuspid valve auscultation.
4. Mitral valve auscultation.   5. Pulmonary valve.   6. Aortic valve.   7. Tricuspid valve.
8. Mitral valve.

Fig. 56.4 Frontal view of trunk demonstrating the surface anatomy of the heart and optimal sites for auscultation.

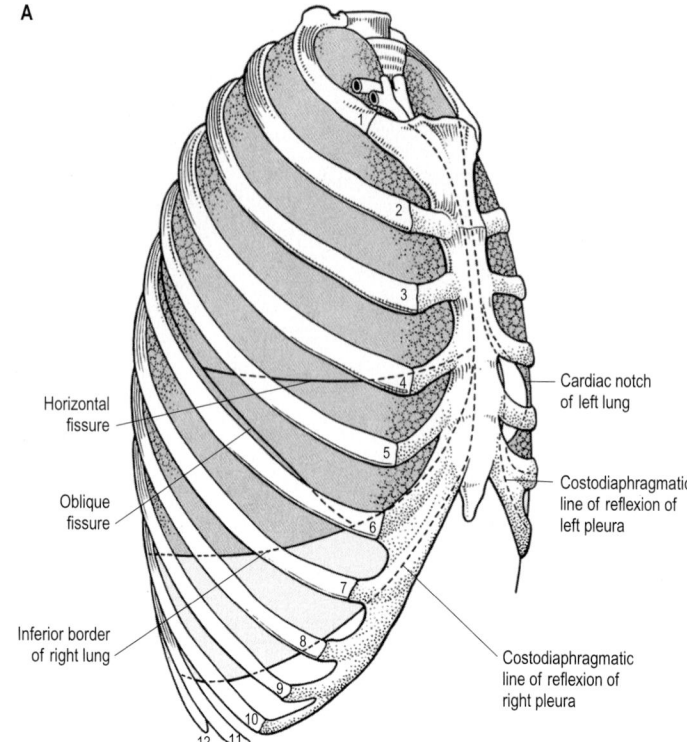

A

Horizontal fissure

Oblique fissure

Inferior border of right lung

Cardiac notch of left lung

Costodiaphragmatic line of reflexion of left pleura

Costodiaphragmatic line of reflexion of right pleura

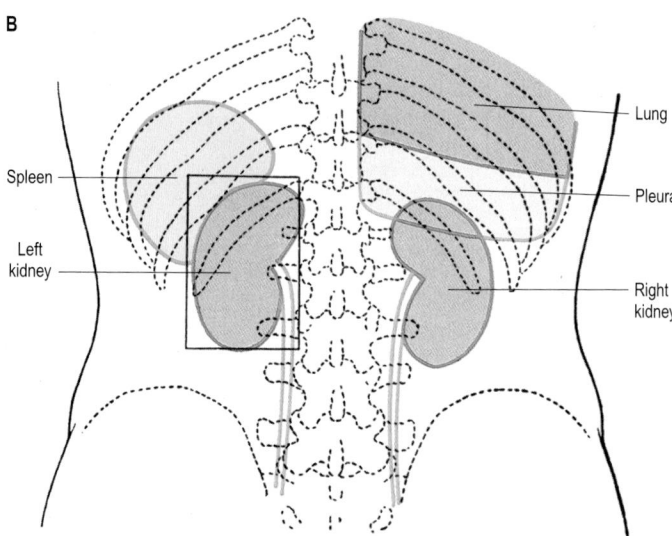

B

Spleen

Left kidney

Lung

Pleura

Right kidney

Fig. 56.5 A, Relation of the pleura and lungs to the chest wall: right lateral aspect. Key: purple, lungs, covered with the pleural sacs; blue, pleural sac, with no underlying lung. **B**, Lower limits of the lung and pleura: posterior view. The lower portions of the lung and the pleura are shown on the right side.

the heart and the sternum that is free of pleura; a needle puncture of the heart may be performed at this site without risk of damaging the pleura. The right and left pleurae meet at the level of the fourth costal cartilage and maintain contact up to the level of the second costal cartilage.

Viewed from the back, the medial edge of the pleura may be followed along a line joining the transverse processes of the second to the twelfth thoracic vertebrae. It extends horizontally laterally, and crosses the twelfth and eleventh ribs to meet the tenth rib in the midaxillary line (**Fig. 56.5**).

CLINICAL PROCEDURES (Fig. 56.6)

CENTRAL VENOUS ACCESS
Central venous cannulation permits monitoring of the central venous pressure and the administration of drugs directly into the central circulation.

Subclavian vein cannulation
Subclavian vein cannulation is performed with the patient supine, the head turned slightly to the opposite side, and the arms placed by the side. The bed is tilted down by c.10° and a small bedroll may be placed between the shoulder blades in order to ensure that the infraclavicular area is more prominent. The skin is cleaned and local anaesthetic injected into the skin c.3 cm lateral to the midpoint of the clavicle. The central venous needle is then inserted from the inferior edge of the clavicle towards the suprasternal notch. The needle is directed so that it passes just below the posterior border of the clavicle; care must be taken to avoid downward direction of the needle, which may cause a pneumothorax. Gentle aspiration of the syringe is performed whilst the needle is being advanced until the subclavian vein is punctured.

Internal jugular vein cannulation
The patient is placed in the supine position with the head turned slightly towards the contralateral side. The key anatomical landmarks are the two inferior heads of sternocleidomastoid, which form two sides of a triangle with the clavicle as its base. The internal jugular vein lies between the two heads of the muscle, slightly lateral and anterior to the common carotid artery. After the skin has been prepared, local anaesthetic is injected around the apex of the triangle. With one hand palpating the carotid artery, the physician inserts a needle at the apex of

the triangle and the tip is directed lateral to the midpoint of the triangle, with a downward angulation of c.30°. From a high internal jugular approach, the needle is inserted at the midpoint of the medial border of sternocleidomastoid and directed towards the ipsilateral nipple with a downward angulation of 30–45°.

When the left internal jugular vein is cannulated, additional care must be taken to avoid the thoracic duct and the cupula of the pleura, which is higher than on the right side, an arrangement which increases the risk of accidental pneumothorax. The left internal jugular vein is often smaller in diameter than the right.

THORACOCENTESIS (PLEURAL ASPIRATION)
Thoracocentesis or pleural aspiration is an essential step in the assessment of pleural effusions. A chest radiograph will confirm the location and extent of the effusion and clinical examination will identify the best

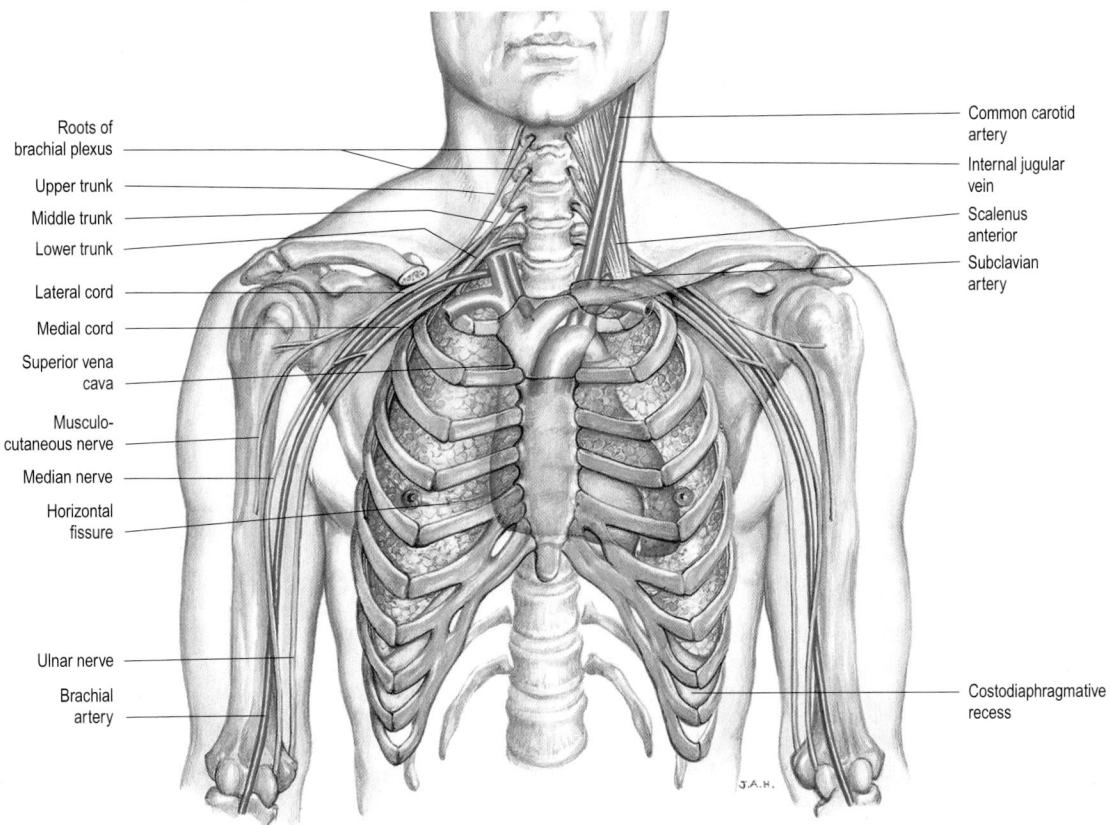

Roots of brachial plexus

Upper trunk

Middle trunk

Lower trunk

Lateral cord

Medial cord

Superior vena cava

Musculo-cutaneous nerve

Median nerve

Horizontal fissure

Ulnar nerve

Brachial artery

Common carotid artery

Internal jugular vein

Scalenus anterior

Subclavian artery

Costodiaphragmative recess

Fig. 56.6 Anterior view of thorax, root of neck and axilla, showing heart, great vessels and brachial plexus.

position for aspiration: the posterior midscapular line is a common site. The skin of the desired interspace is cleaned and anaesthetized, and the aspiration needle is inserted at the lower margin of the interspace. The needle is not inserted in the middle of the interspace because the intercostal vessels run along the middle of the interspace posteriorly, and from the axilla forwards onto the anterior chest wall they are protected only by the lower border of the rib. After appropriate local analgesia has been applied, the needle is carefully advanced in a perpendicular direction in the lower portion of the interspace until it enters the pleural space. More complex or small effusions should be aspirated under ultrasound guidance.

PLACEMENT OF ELECTROCARDIOGRAPH LEADS

The 12-lead electrocardiograph (ECG) provides three-dimensional information on the electrical activity of the heart. The limb leads provide information about the electrical activity in the frontal plane. They are placed on the left and right wrists, and the left foot, with the right foot acting as a neutral grounding point. The chest leads provide information about the electrical activity in the horizontal plane. They are placed as follows: V1, right fourth intercostal space, para-sternal position; V2, left fourth intercostal space, para-sternal position; V3, mid-point of V2 and V4 on the left; V4, fifth intercostal space, midclavicular line on the left; V5, fifth intercostal space, anterior axillary line on the left; V6, fifth intercostal space, midaxillary line on the left.

PERICARDIOCENTESIS

Pericardiocentesis is performed to aspirate a pericardial effusion or, in an emergency, to decompress a cardiac tamponade, where pressure from blood in the pericardial space prevents the heart chambers from filling during the cardiac cycle, and seriously impairs cardiac output.

Pericardial puncture can be performed in either the fifth or sixth left intercostal space near the sternum (to avoid the internal thoracic artery), or at the left costoxiphoid angle. The needle is passed 1–2 cm to the left of the costoxiphoid angle at 45° to the skin, and then up and backwards towards the tip of the scapula until it enters the pericardial sac.

NEEDLE THORACOCENTESIS

Needle thoracocentesis is performed in patients in whom a life-threatening tension pneumothorax is suspected. A needle is inserted into the second intercostal space in the midclavicular line on the side of the tension pneumothorax, with the patient in an upright position. A sudden escape of air is heard when the needle enters the parietal pleura. A chest tube must be inserted after this procedure.

CHEST DRAIN INSERTION

The insertion site for a chest drain is usually the fifth intercostal space, just anterior to the midaxillary line on the affected side. A 2 cm horizontal incision is followed by blunt dissection through the subcutaneous tissues to the top of the rib. The parietal pleura is punctured with the tip of a clamp and a gloved finger inserted into the pleural space to free up any adhesions. The chest drain (thoracostomy tube) is then inserted into the pleural space and attached to an underwater sealed container placed below the level of the lungs: the water level rises and falls in the tube with ventilation.

THORACOTOMY INCISIONS

Posterolateral

A posterolateral incision is most commonly used in thoracic surgery for unilateral pulmonary resections, bullectomy, unilateral lung volume reduction surgery, chest wall resection and oesophageal surgery (Fry 2000). The patient is placed in a lateral decubitus position with adequate support of the elbow, axilla and knee with padding. The standard approach is via an incision from the anterior axillary line which curves c.4 cm below the tip of the scapula and then vertically between the posterior midline and medial edge of the scapula. The incision is usually extended to the level of the spine of scapula. Overall, the incision forms an S-shape in the fifth intercostal space. The sixth or seventh intercostal space is used in oesophageal surgery.

The lower portions of trapezius and latissimus dorsi are divided. Serratus anterior is retracted, and may be divided in a high thoracotomy.

949

The costal muscle and pleura are dissected along the inferior margin of the intercostal space to avoid damaging the neurovascular bundle. A small section of rib is removed at the costovertebral angle to reduce the risk of fracture, particularly in patients older than 40 years. This technique provides good access to the thoracic contents; the main problem is postoperative pain as a consequence of intraoperative musculoskeletal traction.

Anterolateral

Using an anterolateral approach, the patient is placed in the supine position with the arms by the sides. A roll is placed vertically under the back and hips so as to raise the operative side by c.45°. The incision is from the midaxillary line over the fifth intercostal space along the inframammary fold, and curves upwards para-sternally. The pectoral muscles are divided, and subsequent access to the thorax is similar to that used in the posterolateral approach. However, access is limited, and may be improved by dividing costal cartilages.

'Clam shell'

The transverse thoracosternotomy is known as the 'clam shell' incision. It provides excellent exposure to both sides of the chest and is therefore used in bilateral lung transplantation and in lung volume reduction surgery with bilateral lung resections. The patient is placed in the supine position with a roll vertically along the upper thoracic spine. Bilateral anterolateral incisions are made in the inframammary fold and the sternum is transected. This allows the upper portion of the thorax to be displaced upwards with a rib-spreader – hence the name clam shell. The main disadvantage of the clam shell procedure is the need to transect the sternum: even after careful repair with sternal wires, there is a risk of sternal instability.

Sternotomy

Sternotomy is commonly needed in cardiac surgery (p. 1018). The patient is placed in the supine position with both arms extended by the side. A vertical incision is made in the midline from the suprasternal notch to a point just below the xiphoid process. The tissues around the manubrium and the xiphoid process are mobilized. The pectoralis fascia in the midline is incised and the sternum is split and its two edges retracted. The sternum is closed using interosseous wire sutures.

Axillary thoracotomy

The patient is placed in the lateral decubitus position, with arms abducted at 90° and supported on an arm rest. The incision is based along the desired intercostal space, which, for upper thoracic lesions, is the second or third space. Latissimus dorsi is elevated and retracted, whereas serratus anterior is divided in the direction of its fibres. The anterior aspect of serratus anterior is divided to expose the intercostal muscles, which are divided in turn. The overall size in the incision is limited and provides good access to the upper thorax. Postoperative pain is less than with some other approaches, but the long thoracic nerve may be damaged if serratus anterior is divided too posteriorly.

Thoracoscopic access

Occasionally, video-assisted thoracoscopic surgery is required to assess the mediastinum. The thoracoscope is usually introduced via the fifth intercostal space in the midclavicular line, with additional ports at the third and sixth intercostal spaces to assess the anterior mediastinum. To assess the posterior mediastinum, the thoracoscope is inserted into the seventh intercostal space in the midclavicular line.

REFERENCE

Fry WA 2000 Thoracic incisions. In: Shields TW, LoCicero III J, Ponn RB (eds) General Thoracic Surgery, 5th edn. Philadelphia: Lippincott Williams and Wilkins: 367–74.

Chest wall

SKIN

VASCULAR SUPPLY

The skin of the thorax is supplied by a combination of direct cutaneous vessels and musculocutaneous perforators which reach the skin primarily via the intercostal muscles, pectoralis major, latissimus dorsi and trapezius.

Branches from the thoraco-acromial axis, lateral thoracic artery, internal thoracic artery, anterior and posterior intercostal arteries, thoraco-dorsal, transverse cervical/dorsal scapular and circumflex scapular arteries are the major contributing vessels (**Figs 57.1, 57.2, 45.4**).

The anterior aspect of the thoracic skin is supplied by the thoraco-acromial axis, the internal thoracic arteries, perforating branches from the intercostal arteries and branches from the lateral thoracic and superficial thoracic arteries. The thoraco-acromial axis supplies the skin primarily via musculocutaneous perforators from its pectoral branch, which reach the skin through pectoralis major. In addition, direct cutaneous branches arise from the acromial and deltoid branches. The internal thoracic artery sends direct perforating branches to the skin of the upper six intercostal spaces, accompanied by the cutaneous branches of the anterior intercostal nerves. The branches reach the skin after passing through pectoralis major; they travel laterally in the subcutaneous fat as direct cutaneous vessels. The second intercostal perforator is usually the largest.

The lateral aspect of the thoracic skin is supplied by the lateral thoracic, superficial thoracic and lateral cutaneous branches of the intercostal arteries. The lateral thoracic artery gives off direct cutaneous branches to the lateral chest wall, in addition to musculocutaneous branches passing through pectoralis major.

The posterior aspect of the thoracic skin is supplied by the medial and lateral dorsal cutaneous branches of the posterior intercostal arteries (which reach the skin by passing through erector spinae and latissimus dorsi), musculocutaneous perforating branches from the superficial cervical artery and the transverse cervical/dorsal scapular artery (via trapezius), musculocutaneous perforating branches from the thoracodorsal artery and the intercostal arteries (via latissimus dorsi) and direct cutaneous branches from the circumflex scapular artery.

INNERVATION

The skin of the thorax is supplied by cutaneous branches of cervical and thoracic nerves in consecutive, curved zones, the upper almost horizontal and the lower oblique. On the upper ventral thoracic aspect, the third and fourth cervical areas adjoin the first and second thoracic areas (**Fig. 45.3**) because the intervening nerves provide the sensory and motor supply to the upper limb. There is a similar, but less extensive, posterior 'gap': most of the skin of the back of the thorax is supplied by the dorsal rami of the thoracic nerves. The subcostal margin is supplied by the seventh thoracic nerve.

The ventral rami of the first to the eleventh thoracic nerves pass into the intercostal spaces. Each intercostal nerve gives off a lateral cutaneous branch, which arises beyond the angle of the ribs and divides into anterior and posterior branches, and terminates near the sternum in an anterior cutaneous branch.

Branches of the supraclavicular nerve, which originates from the third and fourth cervical nerve roots, supply the skin in the upper pectoral region. Most of the first thoracic nerve joins the brachial plexus: it gives off a small inferior branch, which becomes the first intercostal nerve. The lateral cutaneous branch of the second intercostal nerve supplies the skin of the axilla and is known as the intercostobrachial nerve. The

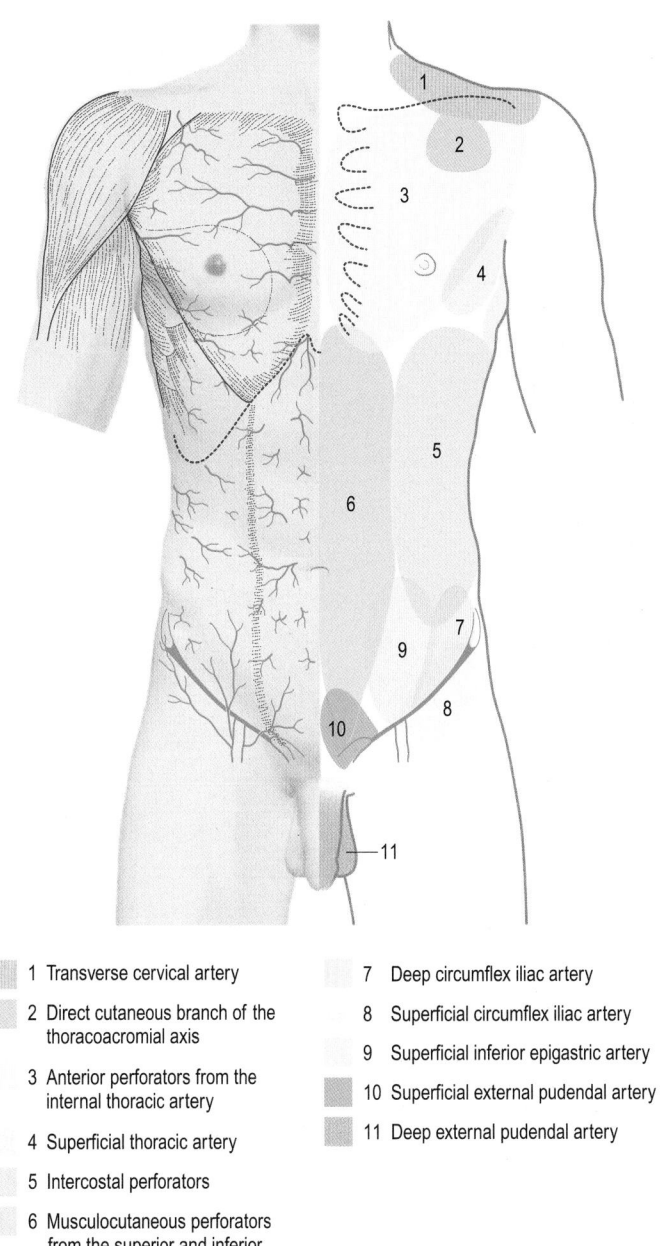

1	Transverse cervical artery
2	Direct cutaneous branch of the thoracoacromial axis
3	Anterior perforators from the internal thoracic artery
4	Superficial thoracic artery
5	Intercostal perforators
6	Musculocutaneous perforators from the superior and inferior deep epigastric arteries
7	Deep circumflex iliac artery
8	Superficial circumflex iliac artery
9	Superficial inferior epigastric artery
10	Superficial external pudendal artery
11	Deep external pudendal artery

Fig. 57.1 Anatomical territories of cutaneous blood vessels on the anterior trunk. (By permission from Cormack GC, Lamberty BGH 1994 The Arterial Anatomy of Skin Flaps, 2nd edn. Edinburgh: Churchill Livingstone.)

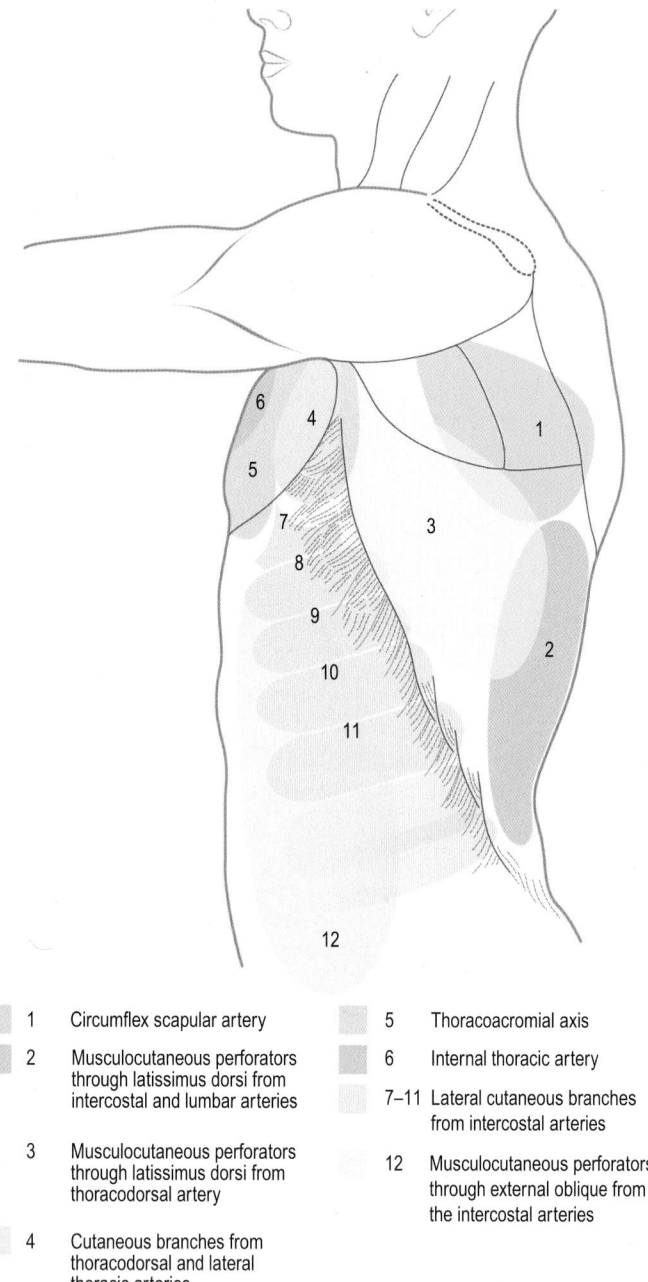

	1	Circumflex scapular artery		5	Thoracoacromial axis
	2	Musculocutaneous perforators through latissimus dorsi from intercostal and lumbar arteries		6	Internal thoracic artery
				7–11	Lateral cutaneous branches from intercostal arteries
	3	Musculocutaneous perforators through latissimus dorsi from thoracodorsal artery		12	Musculocutaneous perforators through external oblique from the intercostal arteries
	4	Cutaneous branches from thoracodorsal and lateral thoracic arteries			

Fig. 57.2 Anatomical territories of cutaneous blood vessels on the lateral trunk. (By permission from Cormack GC, Lamberty BGH 1994 The Arterial Anatomy of Skin Flaps, 2nd edn. Edinburgh: Churchill Livingstone.)

costal margin is supplied by a branch from the seventh thoracic nerve, and the tenth thoracic nerve supplies the skin of the abdomen at the level of the umbilicus. The seventh to eleventh thoracic nerves supply the skin of the thoracic wall as they pass anteriorly and inferiorly; they continue beyond the costal cartilages and supply the skin and subcutaneous tissues of the abdominal wall. The subcostal nerve follows the inferior border of the twelfth rib and supplies the skin of the lower abdominal wall.

SOFT TISSUE

SUPERFICIAL FASCIA
The superficial fascia lies below the skin. It consists primarily of fat and is only loosely attached to the skin, an arrangement that allows some movement of the underlying structures. Small blood vessels and nerves perforate the superficial fascia to supply the skin.

The mammary gland lies within the superficial fascia (Ch. 58).

DEEP FASCIA
The deep fascia is a tough and fibrous membrane; it conserves fluid and allows some movement of structures over one another.

Clavipectoral fascia
The clavipectoral fascia (p. 817) is a sheet of deep fascia that extends between the clavicle and pectoralis minor. It surrounds subclavius and extends medially to the first rib.

BONE AND CARTILAGE (Fig. 57.3)

The thoracic part of the vertebral column consists of 12 vertebrae and their associated intervertebral discs, and is described in detail in Chapter 45 (p. 746).

STERNUM
The sternum (**Figs 57.4, 57.5**) consists of a cranial manubrium (prosternum), an intermediate body (mesosternum), and a caudal xiphoid process (metasternum). Until puberty, the mesosternum consists of four sternebrae; from their costal relations, these appear to be intersegmental. The total length of the sternum is c.17 cm in males, less in females. The ratio between manubrial and mesosternal lengths differs between the sexes. Growth may continue beyond the third decade and possibly throughout life.

In natural stance, the sternum slopes down and slightly forwards. It is convex in front, concave behind, and broadest at the junction with the first costal cartilages. It is narrow at the manubriosternal joint, below which it widens to its articulation with the fifth cartilages, and narrows again below this.

The sternum contains highly vascular trabecular bone enclosed by a compact layer which is thickest in the manubrium between the clavicular notches. Centrally, the bone is lightly constructed, whereas laterally the trabeculae are thicker and wider. The medulla contains haemopoietic (red) bone marrow.

Manubrium of sternum
The manubrium is level with the third and fourth thoracic vertebrae. It is broad and thick above, and narrows to its junction with the body. The anterior surface is smooth, transversely convex and vertically concave, and the posterior surface is concave and smooth. The superior border is thick, and contains a central jugular (suprasternal) notch between two oval fossae, the clavicular notches, which are directed up and posterolaterally for articulation with the sternal ends of the clavicles. Fibres of the interclavicular ligament are attached to the jugular notch. The inferior border, oval and rough, carries a thin layer of cartilage for articulation with the body. The lateral borders are marked above by a depression for the first costal cartilage and below by a small articular demifacet, which articulates with part of the second costal cartilage. The narrow curved edge descends medially between these facets.

Unlike all the other sternocostal joints, the manubriocostal joint (between the manubrium and the first costal cartilage) is an unusual form of synarthrosis.

Body (mesosternum)
The body is level with the fifth to ninth thoracic vertebrae. It is longer, narrower and thinner than the manubrium, and is broadest near its lower end. The anterior surface is nearly flat and faces slightly upwards. It bears three variable transverse ridges, which mark the levels of fusion of its four sternebrae. A sternal foramen, of varying size and form, may occur between the third and fourth sternebrae. The posterior surface, slightly concave, also displays three less distinct transverse lines. The oval upper end articulates with the manubrium at the level of the sternal angle (manubriosternal joint), which lies opposite the inferior border of the fourth vertebral body. The manubriosternal joint is marked by a posterior transverse groove (**Fig. 57.5**) and is palpable anteriorly as a ridge.

The lower end of the manubrium is narrow and continuous with the xiphoid process. On each lateral border, at its superior angle, a small notch articulates with part of the second costal cartilage (**Fig. 57.4**).

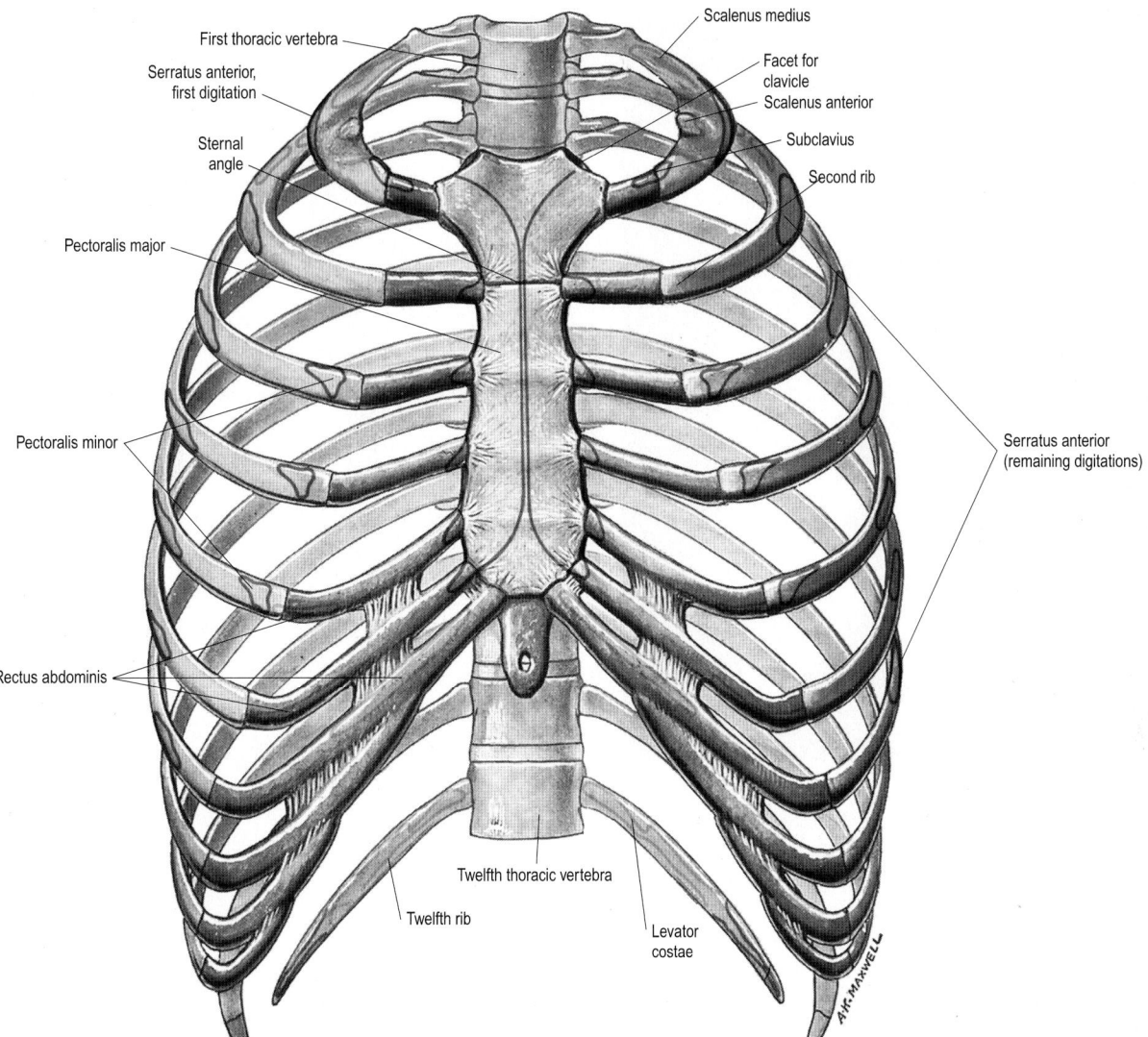

First thoracic vertebra

Serratus anterior,
first digitation

Sternal
angle

Pectoralis major

Pectoralis minor

Rectus abdominis

Scalenus medius

Facet for
clavicle

Scalenus anterior

Subclavius

Second rib

Serratus anterior
(remaining digitations)

Twelfth thoracic vertebra

Twelfth rib

Levator
costae

Fig. 57.3 The skeleton of the thorax: anterior aspect, showing muscle attachments.

Below this, four costal notches articulate with the third to sixth costal cartilages. The inferior angle bears a small facet which, together with the xiphoid process, articulates with the seventh costal cartilage. Between these articular depressions, a series of curved edges diminish in length downwards and form the anterior limits of the intercostal spaces.

Xiphoid process (xiphisternum)

The xiphoid process is in the epigastrium. It is the smallest and most variable sternal element, and may be broad and thin, pointed, bifid, perforated, curved or deflected. The xiphoid is cartilaginous in youth, but more or less ossified in adults. It is continuous with the lower end of the body at the xiphisternal joint. Anterior to its superolateral angles there are demifacets that articulate with parts of the seventh costal cartilages (**Fig. 57.5**).

Pectus excavatum and carinatum

Pectus excavatum occurs to some extent in about 1 in 500 live births. It is a depression of the sternum and costal cartilage that results in a funnel-shaped chest. The lower costal cartilages and the body of the sternum are depressed and there is some asymmetric curving of the ribs posteriorly. There is frequently an abnormal posture with dorsal lordosis, and some patients also develop a scoliosis. The deformity is either found at birth or occurs early in life: more than 85% of affected individuals show signs of the abnormality in the first 12 months of life. The aetiology is unknown, but some cases are associated with conditions such as Marfan's syndrome, in which the connective tissue is abnormal.

Pectus carinatum is the anterior protrusion of the sternum or a pigeon chest. The deformity develops in childhood and in 50% of cases it occurs after the age of 10 years.

Muscle attachments

The sternal ends of pectoralis major and sternocleidomastoid are attached to the anterior surface of the manubrium. Sternothyroid is attached to the posterior surface, opposite the first costal cartilage, and the most medial fibres of sternohyoid are attached above sternothyroid. The articular capsules of the sternocostal joints and sternal fibres of pectoralis major are attached to the anterior surface of the body. Transversus thoracis (sternocostalis) is attached to its posterior surface. The external intercostal membranes are attached to the borders of the body between the costal facets. The most medial fibres of rectus abdominis and the aponeuroses of external and internal oblique are attached to the anterior surface of the xiphoid. The linea alba is attached to its lower end, and the aponeuroses of internal oblique and transversus abdominis are attached to its borders. Slips of the diaphragm are attached to its posterior aspect, and the sternum is here related to the liver.

Vascular supply

The internal thoracic artery provides the main blood supply for the sternum. A sternal network of vessels derived from the internal thoracic arteries provides a network of perforating arteries at the level of each intercostal space. The anterior network is formed by anastomoses between anterior superior and anterior inferior sternal branches and laterosternal and anterosternal arches. It provides branches that go

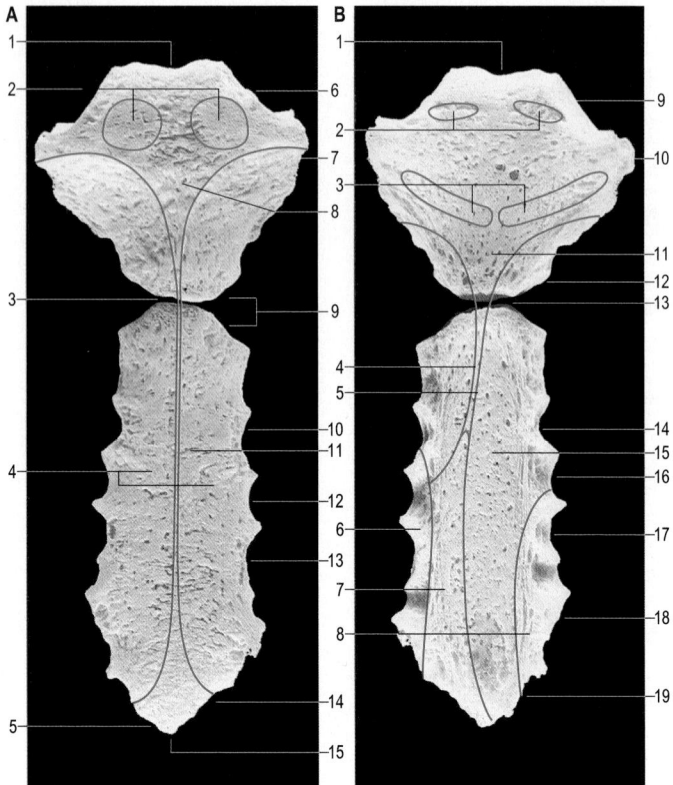

Part A: 1. Jugular notch. **2.** Attachment for sternocleidomastoid.
3. Sternal angle and manubriosternal joint. **4.** Attachment for pectoralis major.
5. Notches for seventh costal cartilage. **6.** Clavicular notch. **7.** Notch for first costal cartilage
8. Manubrium. **9.** Notches for second costal cartilage. **10.** Notches for third costal cartilage.
11. Body of sternum. **12.** Notches for fourth costal cartilage. **13.** Notches for fifth costal cartilage.
14. Notches for sixth costal cartilage. **15.** Xiphisternal joint.

Part B: 1. Jugular notch. **2.** Attachment for sternohyoid. **3.** Attachment for sternothyroid.
4. Edge of area covered by left pleura. **5.** Edge of area covered by right pleura.
6. Attachment for transversus thoracis. **7.** Area in contact with pericardium.
8. Attachment for transversus thoracis. **9.** Clavicular notch. **10.** Notch for costal cartilage.
11. Manubrium. **12.** Notches for second costal cartilage.
13. Sternal angle and manubriosternal joint. **14.** Notches for third costal cartilage.
15. Body of sternum. **16.** Notches for fourth costal cartilage. **17.** Notches for fifth costal cartilage.
18. Notches for sixth costal cartilage. **19.** Notches for seventh costal cartilage.

Fig. 57.4 The sternum. **A**, Anterior aspect. **B**, Posterior aspect. (Photographs by Sarah-Jane Smith.)

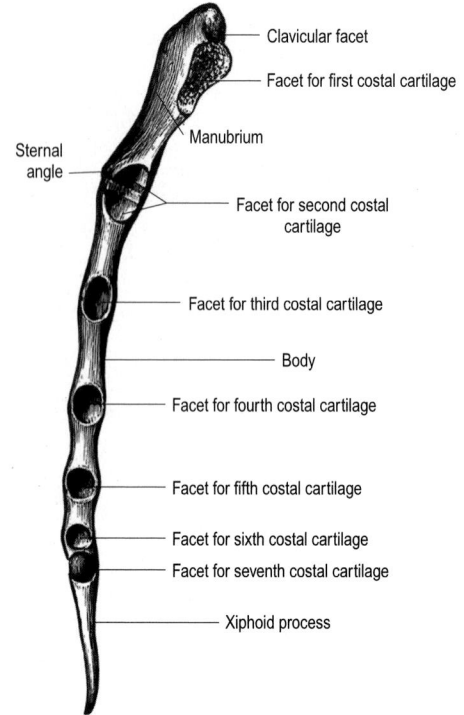

Fig. 57.5 The sternum: lateral aspect.

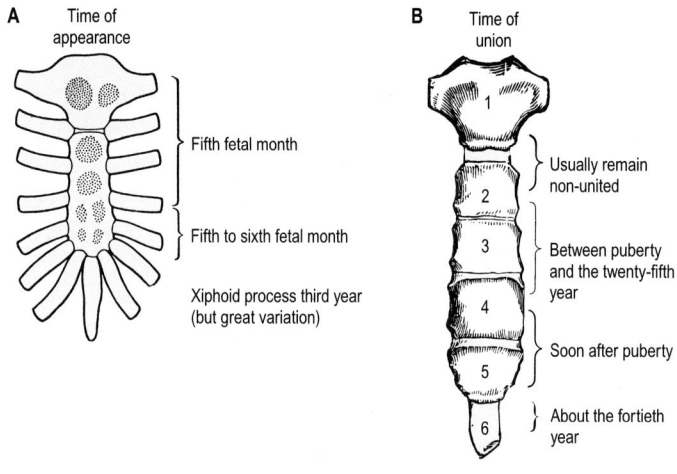

Fig. 57.6 The ossification of the sternum. **A**, Before birth. **B**, At puberty.

directly into the sternum. A similar network of vessels exists posteriorly and is formed by anastomoses between posterior superior and posterior inferior vessels and laterosternal and retrosternal arches. The posterior network is more highly developed than the anterior system; these networks are particularly developed at the level of the fourth and fifth intercostal spaces.

The venous network is less developed and formed mainly by large vessels. The inframedullary network of sinuses form a network in the bone and then drain into the venous system. They are transcortical veins, and drain either into the peripheral sternal networks or into the internal thoracic vein.

Innervation

The manubrium is supplied by the anterior branch of the supraclavicular nerve and the anterior cutaneous branch of the first intercostal nerve, whereas the body of the sternum is supplied largely by anterior branches of the intercostal nerves. The anterior branch of the phrenic nerve runs anteromedially from the diaphragm and supplies the lower portion of the sternum with its contralateral counterpart.

Ossification (Fig. 57.6)

The sternum is formed by fusion of two cartilaginous sternal plates flanking the median plane. The arrangement and number of centres of ossification vary according to the level of completeness and time of fusion of the sternal plates, and to the width of the adult bone. Incomplete fusion leaves a sternal foramen. The manubrium is ossified

from one to three centres appearing in the fifth fetal month. The first and second sternebrae usually ossify from single centres that appear at about the same time. Centres in the third and fourth sternebrae are commonly paired, and appear in the fifth and sixth months, respectively, but one of either pair may be delayed until the seventh or even eighth month. The fourth sternebral centre may be absent. The xiphoid process begins to ossify in the third year or later. In some sterna, all centres are single and median, in others the manubrial centre is single and the sternebral centres are all paired, symmetric or asymmetric. Union between mesosternal centres begins at puberty and proceeds from below upwards: by the age of 25 years they are all united.

Suprasternal ossicles, paired or single, occur in about 7% of sterna. They may fuse to the manubrium or articulate posteriorly at the lateral border of the jugular notch. When well formed, they are pyramidal, and their base is articular. The ossicles are cartilaginous at birth, and ossify during adolescence.

CLAVICLE

The clavicle is described in Chapter 49 (p. 817).

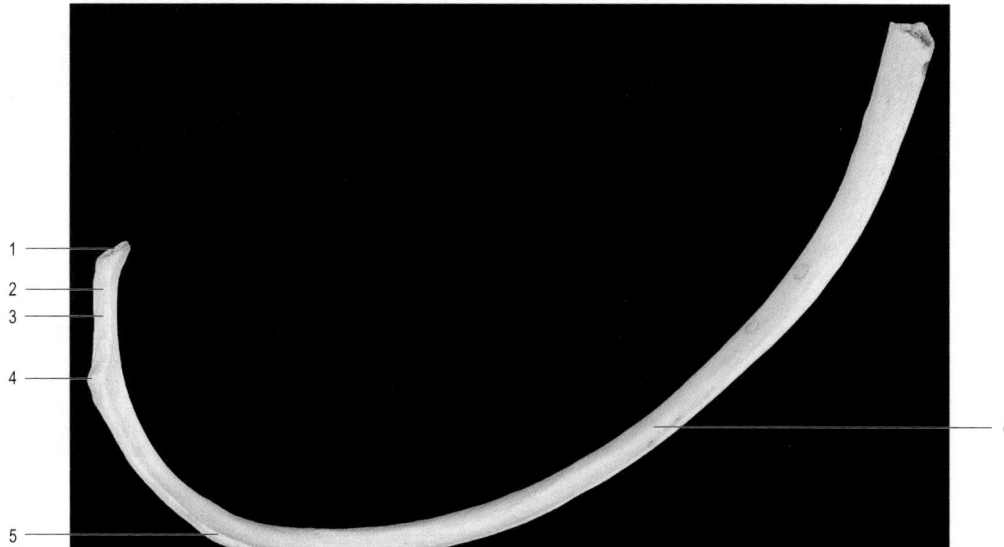

1. Articular facets of head.
2. Crest of head.
3. Neck of rib.
4. Articular facet of tubercle.
5. Angle.
6. Shaft.

Fig. 57.7 A typical rib of the left side: inferior aspect. (Photograph by Sarah-Jane Smith.)

RIB

The ribs are 12 pairs of elastic arches that articulate posteriorly with the vertebral column. They form much of the thoracic skeleton. Their number may be increased by cervical or lumbar ribs or reduced by the absence of the twelfth pair. The first seven pairs are connected to the sternum by costal cartilages, and are referred to as the true ribs (**Fig. 57.4**). The remaining five are the so-called false ribs: the cartilages of the eighth to tenth usually join the superjacent costal cartilage, whereas the eleventh and twelfth ribs, which are free at their anterior ends, are sometimes termed the 'floating' ribs. The tenth rib may also be a floating rib; the incidence varies from 35% to 70% in different races.

The ribs are separated by the intercostal spaces, which are deeper in front and between the upper ribs. The latter are less oblique than the lower ribs; obliquity is maximal at the ninth rib and decreases to the twelfth. Ribs increase in length from the first to seventh, and thereafter diminish to the twelfth. They decrease in breadth downwards; in the upper 10, the greatest breadth is anterior. The first two and last three ribs present special features, whereas the remainder conform to a common plan.

Ribs consist of highly vascular trabecular bone, enclosed in a thin layer of compact bone and containing large amounts of red marrow.

Typical rib

A typical rib has a shaft with anterior and posterior ends (**Figs 57.7, 57.8**). The anterior, costal, end has a small concave depression for the lateral end of its cartilage. The shaft has an external convexity and is grooved internally near its lower border, which is sharp, whereas its upper border is rounded. The posterior, vertebral end has a head, neck and tubercle. The head presents two facets, separated by a transverse crest. The lower and larger facet articulates with the body of the corresponding vertebra, its crest attaching to the intervertebral disc above it. The neck is the flat part beyond the head, anterior to the corresponding transverse process. It is oblique, and faces anterosuperiorly. Its postero-inferior surface is rough and pierced by foramina. Its upper border is the sharp crest of the neck, its lower border rounded. The tubercle, which is more prominent in upper ribs, is posteroexternal at the junction of the neck and shaft and is divided into medial articular and lateral non-articular areas. The articular part bears a small, oval facet for the transverse process of the corresponding vertebra. The non-articular area is roughened by ligaments. The shaft is thin and flat and has external and internal surfaces, and superior and inferior borders. It is curved, bent at the posterior angle (5–6 cm from the tubercle), and twisted about its long axis. The part behind the angle inclines superomedially, and so its external surface is posteroinferior. In front of the angle it faces slightly up. It is convex and smooth, and near the tubercle is crossed by a rough line, directed inferolaterally, towards the posterior angle. The smooth internal surface is marked by a costal groove, bounded below by the inferior border. The superior border of the groove continues behind the lower border of the neck, but terminates anteriorly at the

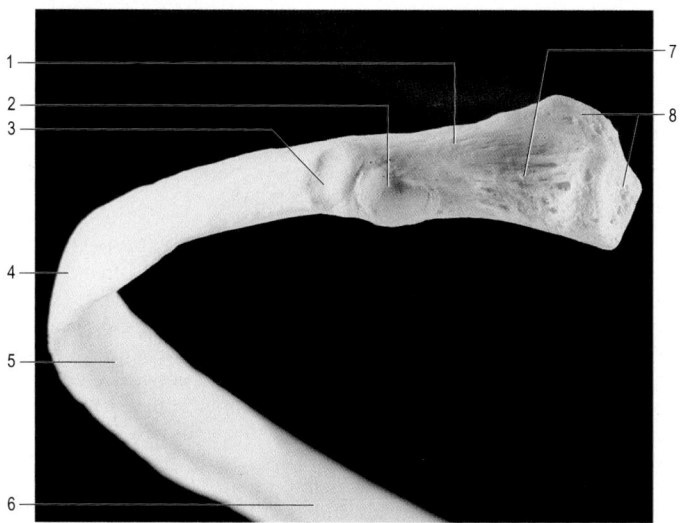

1. Neck of rib. 2. Articular facet of tubercle. 3. Non-articular part of tubercle. 4. Angle. 5. Costal groove. 6. Shaft. 7. Crest of head. 8. Articular facets of head.

Fig. 57.8 A typical rib of the left side: distal end. (Photograph by Sarah-Jane Smith.)

junction of the middle and anterior thirds of the shaft, anterior to which the groove is absent.

Attachments and relations – A radiate ligament is attached along the anterior border of the head and an intra-articular ligament is attached to the crest of the head. The anterior surface of the head is related to costal pleura and, in lower ribs, to the sympathetic trunk. The anterior surface of the neck is divided by a faint transverse ridge for the internal intercostal membrane and is continuous with the inner lip of the superior border of the shaft. The area above the ridge, which is more or less triangular, is separated from the membrane by fatty tissue. The lower, smooth area is covered by costal pleura. The posterior surface of the neck gives attachment to the costotransverse ligament and is pierced by vascular foramina. The superior costotransverse ligament is attached to the crest of the neck, which extends laterally into the outer lip of the superior border of the shaft. The rounded inferior border of the neck continues laterally into the upper border of the costal groove, and gives attachment to the internal intercostal membrane. The articular area of the tubercle in the upper six ribs is convex and faces posteromedially. In the succeeding three or four ribs it is almost flat, and faces down, back and slightly medially. The lateral costotransverse ligament is attached to the non-articular area.

The ridge on the external surface of the shaft (near its posterior angle) gives attachment to an upward continuation of the thoracolumbar fascia and lateral fibres of iliocostalis thoracis. From the second to the tenth ribs, the distance between angle and tubercle increases. Medial to the angle, the external surface gives attachment to a levator costae and is covered by erector spinae. Near the sternal end of this surface an indistinct oblique line, the anterior 'angle', separates the attachments of external oblique and serratus anterior (or latissimus dorsi, in the case of the ninth and tenth ribs). The internal intercostal muscle is attached to the costal groove on the internal surface, and separates the bone and the intercostal neurovascular bundle. At its vertebral end, the groove faces down, its borders in the same plane. The shaft broadens near the posterior angle, and the groove reaches its internal surface. The innermost intercostal is attached to the superior rim of the groove, and this attachment occasionally extends to the anterior quarter of the rib. Posteriorly, the superior rim meets the lower border of the neck. The external intercostal muscle is attached to the sharp inferior costal border. The superior border has two lips posteriorly: an inner and an outer lip. The internal intercostal muscles and the innermost intercostal muscles are attached to the inner lip. The external intercostal muscle is attached to the outer lip.

Vascular supply and innervation – Typical ribs receive their blood supply anteriorly via branches from the internal thoracic artery (first six intercostal spaces) or musculophrenic artery (subsequent spaces), and posteriorly from intercostal arteries derived directly from the aorta. Venous drainage is into the corresponding intercostal vein and then into the azygos system. Typical ribs are innervated segmentally by branches from the corresponding intercostal nerves.

Cervical rib

A cervical rib, the costal element of the seventh cervical vertebra, may be a mere epiphysis on its transverse process, but more often it has a head, neck and tubercle. When a shaft is present, it is of variable length, and extends anterolaterally into the posterior triangle of the neck, where it may end freely or join the first rib or costal cartilage, or even the sternum. A cervical rib may be partly fibrous, but its effects are not related to the size of its osseous part. If it is long enough, its relations are those of a first thoracic rib: the brachial plexus (usually lower trunk) and subclavian vessels are superior and apt to suffer compression in a narrow angle between rib and scalenus anterior. Hence cervical ribs may first be revealed by nervous and vascular symptoms, particularly those caused by pressure on the eighth cervical and first thoracic spinal nerves.

A cervical rib or pleurapophysis may show synostosis or diarthrosis with either the anterior (parapophyseal) or posterior (diapophyseal) 'roots' of the so-called seventh cervical transverse process or, more usually, with both.

First rib

Most acutely curved and usually shortest, the first rib is broad and flat, its surfaces are superior and inferior, and its borders are internal and external (**Fig. 57.9**). It slopes obliquely down and forwards to its sternal end. The obliquity of the first ribs accounts for the appearance of pulmonary and pleural apices in the neck.

The head of the first rib is small and round. It bears an almost circular facet, and articulates with the body of the first thoracic vertebra. The neck is rounded and ascends posterolaterally. The tubercle, wide and prominent, is directed up and backwards; medially an oval facet articulates with the transverse process of the first thoracic vertebra. At the tubercle, the rib is bent, its head turned slightly down, and so the angle and tubercle coincide. The superior surface of the flattened shaft is crossed obliquely by two shallow grooves, separated by a slight ridge, which usually ends at the internal border as a small pointed projection, the scalene tubercle, to which scalenus anterior is attached. The groove anterior to the scalene tubercle forms a bed for the subclavian vein, and the rough area between this and the first costal cartilage gives attachment to the costoclavicular ligament and, more anteriorly, to subclavius. The subclavian artery and (usually) the lower trunk of the brachial plexus pass in the groove behind the tubercle. Behind this, scalenus medius is attached as far as the costal tubercle.

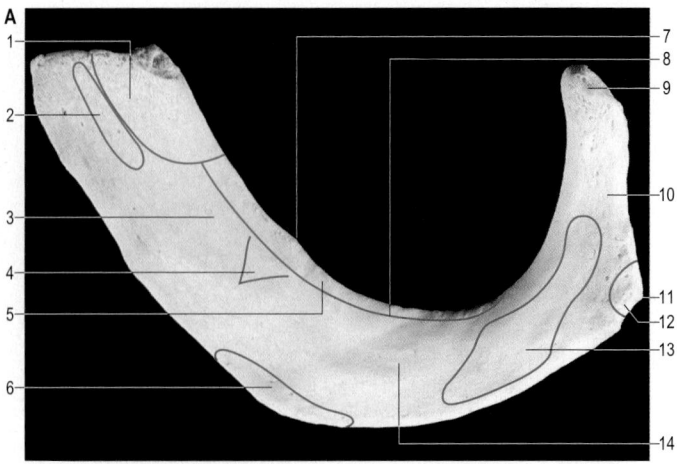

1. Costoclavicular ligament. 2. Attachment of subclavius. 3. Groove for subclavian vein.
4. Scalene anterior. 5. Groove for subclavian artery and first thoracic nerve.
6. Serratus anterior. 7. Scalene tubercle. 8. Suprapleural membrane. 9. Head.
10. Neck. 11. Tubercle. 12. Attachment of lateral costrotransverse ligament.
13. Scalenus medius. 14. Shaft.

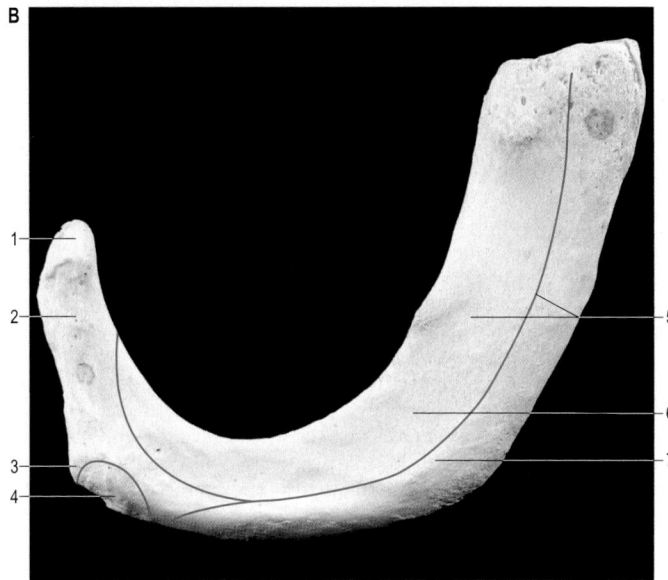

1. Head. 2. Neck. 3. Tubercle. 4. Attachment of lateral costotransverse ligament.
5. Area and edge of area covered by pleura. 6. Shaft.
7. Attachment of intercostal muscles and membranes.

Fig. 57.9 A, Superior and **B**, inferior aspects of the first rib. (Photographs by Sarah-Jane Smith.)

The external border is convex, thick posteriorly and thin anteriorly. It is covered behind by scalenus posterior descending to the second rib. The first digitation of serratus anterior is, in part, attached to it, behind the subclavian (arterial) groove. The internal border is concave and thin, and the scalene tubercle is near its midpoint. The suprapleural membrane, which covers the cervical dome of the pleura, is attached to the internal border.

The inferior surface is smooth. The anterior end is larger than in any other rib.

Vascular supply and innervation – The first rib is supplied by the internal thoracic artery and the superior intercostal artery. Venous drainage is via the intercostal vein. It is innervated by the first intercostal nerve.

Ossification – The first rib has a primary centre for the shaft, and secondary ossification centres for the head of the rib and the tubercle.

Second rib

The second rib is twice the length of the first rib, with a similar curvature. The non-articular area of the tubercle is small. The angle is slight

A

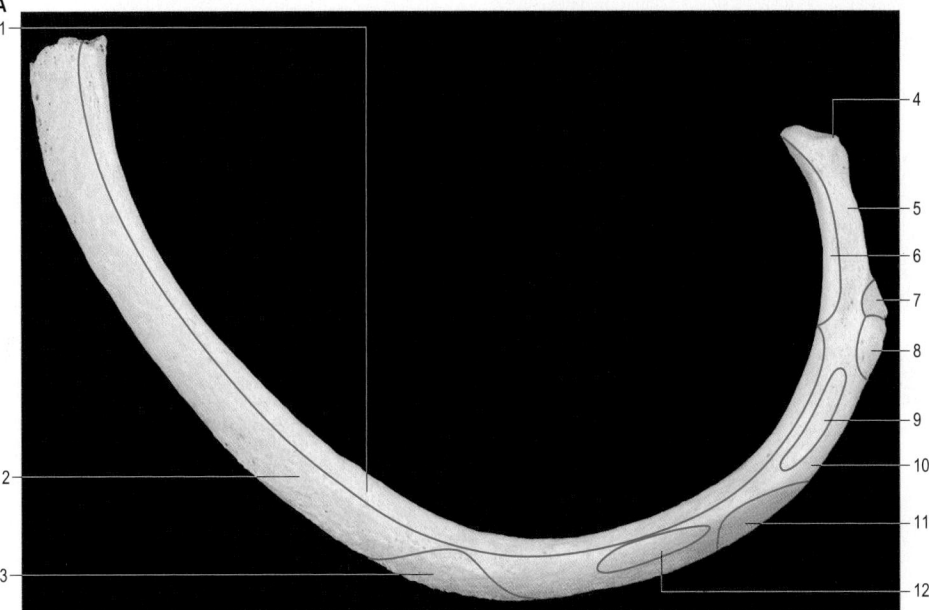

B

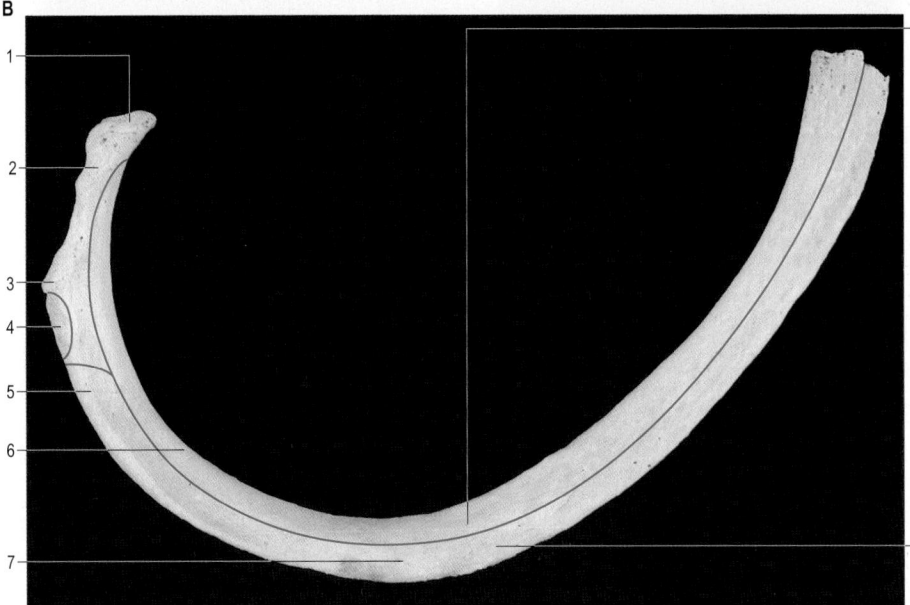

Part A:
1. Attachment of intercostal muscles and membranes.
2. Shaft of rib.
3. Attachment of serratus anterior on serratus anterior tuberosity.
4. Head.
5. Neck.
6. Attachment of superior costotransverse ligament.
7. Tubercle
8. Attachment of lateral costotransverse ligament.
9. Attachment of levator costae.
10. Angle.
11. Attachment of serratus posterior superior.
12. Attachment of scalenus posterior.

Part B:
1. Head.
2. Neck.
3. Tubercle.
4. Attachment of lateral costotransverse ligament.
5. Angle.
6. Costal groove.
7. Shaft.
8. Area covered by pleura.
9. Attachment of intercostal muscles and membranes.

Fig. 57.10 **A**, Superior and **B**, inferior aspects of the second rib. (Photographs by Sarah-Jane Smith.)

and near the tubercle. The shaft is not twisted, but at the tubercle is convex upwards, as in the first rib, but less so. The external surface of the shaft is convex and superolaterally is marked centrally by a rough, muscular impression that continues posteromedially towards the tubercle as a narrow, roughened ridge. The internal surface, smooth and concave, faces inferomedially and there is a short costal groove posteriorly.

The lower parts of the first and second digitations of serratus anterior are attached to a rough prominence that extends from just behind the midpoint of the external surface (**Fig. 57.10**). The distinct lips of the upper border are widely separated behind; scalenus posterior and serratus posterior superior are attached to the outer lip in front of the angle.

Vascular supply and innervation – The blood supply of the second rib is the internal thoracic artery and the superior intercostal artery. Venous drainage is via the superior intercostal vein, which drains into the brachiocephalic vein, and the anterior intercostal veins, which drain into the internal thoracic vein. The bone is innervated by branches of the first intercostal nerve.

Ossification – The second rib is ossified from a primary centre for the shaft, which appears near the angle, late in the second month. The secondary centres for the head and articular and non-articular parts of the tubercle appear about puberty, uniting to the shaft soon after the age of 20 years.

Tenth, eleventh and twelfth ribs

The tenth rib has a single facet on its head that may articulate with the intervertebral disc above, in addition to the upper border of the tenth thoracic vertebra near its pedicle. The ninth and tenth ribs are usually united anteriorly by a fibrous joint. However, the tenth rib may be free, in which case it is pointed like the eleventh and twelfth ribs.

The eleventh and twelfth ribs each have one large, articular facet on the head, but no neck or tubercle. Their pointed anterior ends are tipped with cartilage. The eleventh rib has a slight angle and shallow costal groove. The twelfth rib has neither, is much shorter and slopes cranially at its vertebral end. The internal surfaces of both ribs face slightly upwards, more so in the twelfth.

Numerous muscles and ligaments are attached to the twelfth rib (**Fig. 57.11**). Quadratus lumborum and its anterior covering layer of thoracolumbar fascia are attached to the lower part of its anterior surface in its medial one-half to two-thirds; the upper part is related to the costodiaphragmatic pleural recess. The internal intercostal muscle (medially) and the diaphragm (laterally) are attached at or near the upper border. The lower border gives attachment to the middle lamella

957

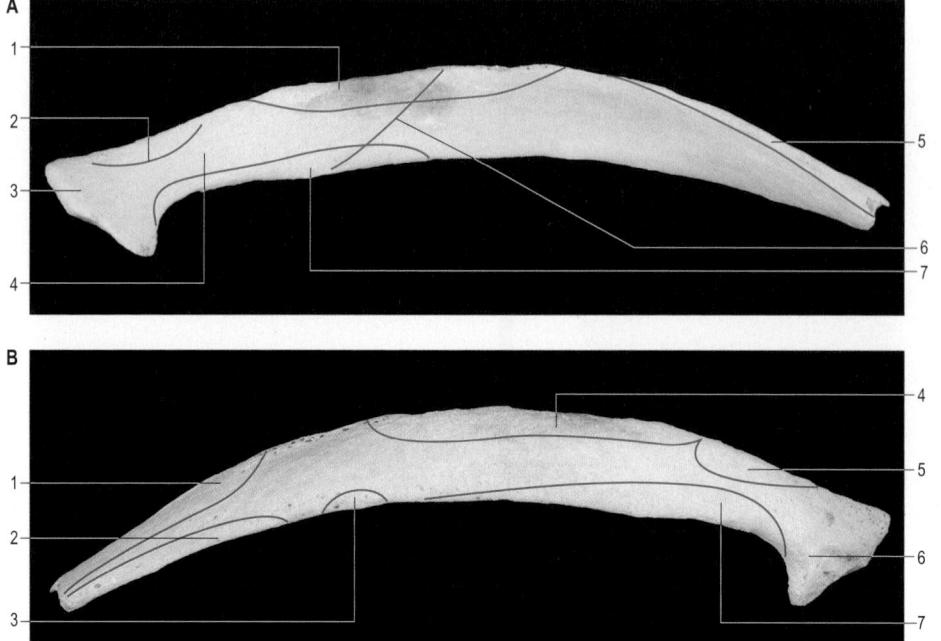

Part A:
1. Attachment of internal intercostal muscle.
2. Attachment of costotransverse ligament.
3. Head.
4. Area covered by pleura.
5. Attachment of diaphragm.
6. Line of pleural reflection.
7. Attachment of quadratus lumborum.

Part B:
1. Attachment of latissimus dorsi.
2. Attachment of external oblique.
3. Serratus posterior inferior.
4. Attachment of external intercostal muscle.
5. Attachment of levator costae.
6. Head.
7. Attachment of erector spinae.

Fig. 57.11 The twelfth rib of the left side.
A, Anterior aspect. **B**, Posterior aspect.
(Photographs by Sarah-Jane Smith.)

of the thoracolumbar fascia and, lateral to quadratus lumborum, to the lateral arcuate ligament and posterior lamella of the thoracolumbar fascia. The lumbocostal ligament is attached posteriorly, close to the head, connecting it to the first lumbar transverse process. The lowest levator costae, longissimus thoracis and iliocostalis are attached to the medial half of the external surface, and serratus posterior inferior, latissimus dorsi and external oblique are attached to its lateral half. The external intercostal muscle is attached along the upper border. These attachments vary: those of the internal intercostal, levator costae and erector spinae merge and those of latissimus dorsi, diaphragm and external oblique may reach the costal cartilage. The lower limit of the pleural sac crosses in front of the rib, approximately at the point where it is crossed by the lateral border of iliocostalis. Its lateral end is usually below the line of costodiaphragmatic pleural reflection and is therefore not covered by pleura.

The tenth rib ossifies from a primary centre in the shaft and secondary centres for the head and articular parts of the tubercle. The eleventh and twelfth ribs, without tubercles, have two centres each.

Vascular supply and innervation – The tenth and eleventh ribs are supplied by the posterior intercostal artery and branches from the musculophrenic artery. The twelfth rib is supplied by the subcostal artery. Venous drainage is via the posterior intercostal and subcostal veins, which in turn drain into the hemiazygos vein. There is additional drainage via the anterior intercostal veins (branches of the musculo-phrenic vein). The tenth and eleventh ribs are innervated by the corresponding intercostal nerve, and the twelfth rib is innervated by the subcostal nerve.

Costal cartilages

Costal cartilages are the persistent, unossified anterior parts of the cartilaginous models in which the ribs develop. They are flat bars of hyaline cartilage that extend from the anterior ends of the ribs, and contribute greatly to thoracic mobility and elasticity (**Fig. 57.12**). The upper seven pairs join the sternum; the eighth to tenth articulate with the lower border of the cartilage above; the lowest two have free, pointed ends in the abdominal wall. They increase in length from the first to the seventh, and then decrease to the twelfth. They diminish in breadth from first to last, like the intercostal spaces. The costal cartilages are broad at their costal continuity and taper as they pass forward. The first and second are of even breadth and the sixth to eighth enlarge where their margins are in contact. The first descends a little, the second is horizontal and the third ascends slightly; the others are angulated and incline up towards the sternum or cartilage above, a little anterior to their ribs.

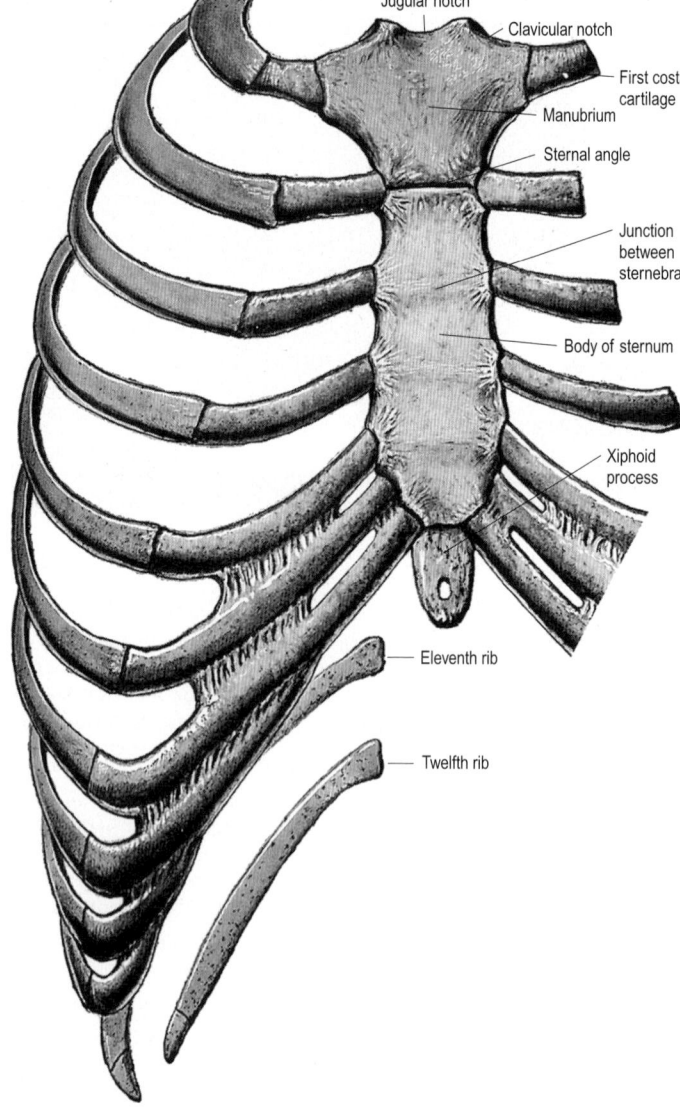

Fig. 57.12 The sternum and costal cartilages: anterior aspect.

Jugular notch
Clavicular notch
First costal cartilage
Manubrium
Sternal angle
Junction between sternebrae
Body of sternum
Xiphoid process
Eleventh rib
Twelfth rib

Each costal cartilage has two surfaces, borders and ends. The anterior surface is convex, facing anterosuperior. The sternoclavicular articular disc, costoclavicular ligament and subclavius are attached to the first cartilage. Pectoralis major is attached to the medial aspect of the first six cartilages. The others are covered by the partial attachments of the anterior abdominal muscles. The posterior surface is concave, and really posteroinferior. Sternothyroid is attached to the first cartilage, transversus thoracis is attached to the second to sixth, and transversus abdominis is attached to the lower six. The internal intercostal muscles and external intercostal membranes are attached to the concave superior and convex inferior borders. The inferior borders of the fifth (sometimes), and sixth to ninth cartilages project at points of greatest convexity. Oblong facets on these projections articulate with facets on slight projections from the superior borders of subjacent cartilages. The lateral end of each cartilage is continuous with its rib. The medial end of the first is continuous with the sternum; those of the six succeeding cartilages are round and articulate with shallow costal notches on the lateral margins of the sternum; those of the eighth to tenth are pointed, each connected with the cartilage above; those of the eleventh and twelfth are pointed and free. With the exception of the synarthrosis between the first rib and sternum, all these articulations are synovial.

In old age the costal cartilages tend to ossify superficially, lose pliability and become brittle.

Rib fractures

Elastic recoil of the ribs, which suspend the sternum, may explain the rarity of sternal fractures. Despite their pliability, the ribs are much more frequently broken: the middle ribs are the most vulnerable. Because traumatic stress is often the result of compression of the thorax, the usual site of fracture is the weakest point of the rib, which is just in front of the angle. Direct impact may fracture a rib anywhere, and the broken ends of bone may be driven inwards, with possible injury to thoracic or upper abdominal viscera.

JOINTS

MANUBRIOSTERNAL JOINT

The manubriosternal joint lies between the manubrium and sternal body, and is usually a symphysis. The bony surfaces are covered by hyaline cartilage and connected by a fibrocartilage, which may ossify in the aged. In more than 30%, the central part of the disc is absorbed and the joint appears synovial. The manubriosternal joint is connected by a fibrous membrane enveloping the entire bone. In occasional individuals older than 30 years, the manubrium is joined to the sternal body by bone, but the intervening cartilage may be only superficially ossified; it is in the aged that this is complete. Early synostosis has been attributed to a persistent synchondrosis in place of a symphysis. In the newborn, union is by collagenous and elastic fibres, without chondrocytes.

Movements – The symphysis permits a small range of angulation between longitudinal axes of the manubrium and body of the sternum, and also limited anteroposterior displacement. A study of these movements in 62 male athletes yielded (standing position) mean values of 162.7° (full inspiration) and 164.7° (full expiration) for the manubriosternal angle. Both movements contribute to respiratory excursions of the sternum.

XIPHISTERNAL JOINT

The joint between the xiphoid process and the body of the sternum process is a symphysis. Usually transformed to a synostosis by the fortieth year, it sometimes remains unchanged even in old age.

STERNOCLAVICULAR JOINT

The sternoclavicular joint is described in Chapter 49 (p. 827).

COSTOVERTEBRAL, STERNOCOSTAL AND INTERCHONDRAL JOINTS

The heads of the ribs articulate with vertebral bodies (costocorporeal joints) and their necks and tubercles articulate with transverse processes (costotransverse joints).

Joints of costal heads

Heads of typical ribs articulate with facets (often termed demifacets) on the margins of adjacent thoracic vertebral bodies and with the inter-

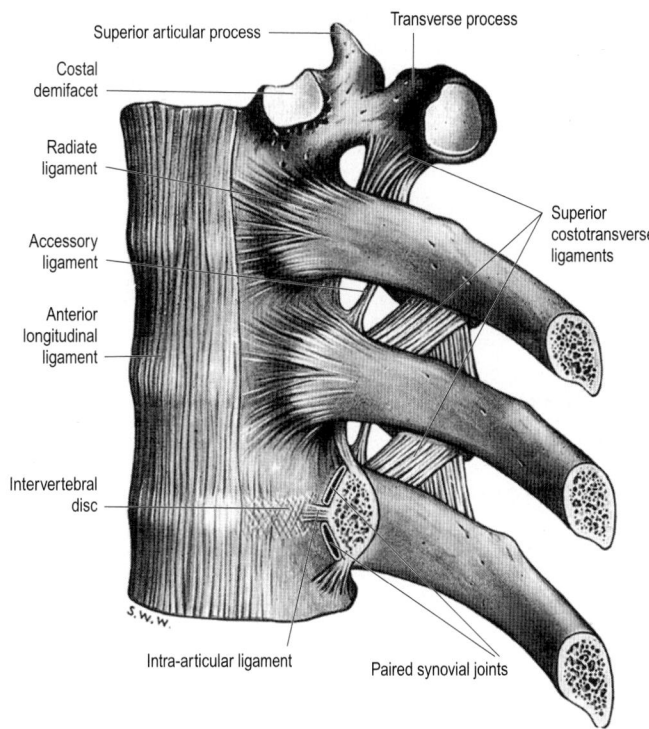

Fig. 57.13 Costovertebral joints: left anterolateral aspect. In the lowest joint shown, most of the radiate ligament and the anterior part of the head of the rib have been excised to show the two joint cavities and the intra-articular ligament between them.

vertebral discs between them (**Fig. 57.13**). The first and tenth to twelfth ribs articulate with a single vertebra by a simple synovial joint. In the others, an intra-articular ligament bisects the joint, producing a double synovial compartment, so the joint is classified as both compound and complex. Often inaccurately described as plane, their articular surfaces are slightly ovoid and the upper and lower synovial articulations are obtusely angled to each other (**Fig. 57.13**). Ligaments are capsular, radiate and intra-articular.

Fibrous capsules – The fibrous capsule connects the costal head to the circumference of the articular surface formed by an intervertebral disc and demifacets of two adjacent vertebrae. Some of their upper fibres traverse their intervertebral foramina to blend with the posterior aspects of intervertebral discs (strictly symphyses). The posterior fibres are continuous with costotransverse ligaments.

Radiate ligaments – Radiate ligaments connect the anterior parts of each costal head to the bodies of two vertebrae and their intervening intervertebral disc. Each is attached to the head just beyond its articular surface. Superior fibres ascend to the vertebral body above, inferior to the body below. Intermediate fibres, shortest and least distinct, are horizontal and attached to the disc. The radiate ligament associated with the first rib is attached to the seventh cervical and first thoracic vertebrae. In the joints of the tenth to twelfth ribs, which articulate with single vertebrae, the radiate ligament is attached to the numbered vertebra and the one above.

Intra-articular ligament – The intra-articular ligament is a short, flat band, attached laterally to the crest between the costal articular facets and medially to the intervertebral disc, dividing the joint. The ligament is absent from the first and tenth to twelfth joints.

Costotransverse joints

The facet of a costal tubercle articulates reciprocally with the transverse process of its corresponding vertebra (**Fig. 57.14**). The eleventh and twelfth ribs lack this articulation. In the upper five or six joints, articular surfaces are reciprocally curved, but below this they are flatter (**Fig. 57.15**). Their ligaments are capsular, costotransverse, superior and lateral

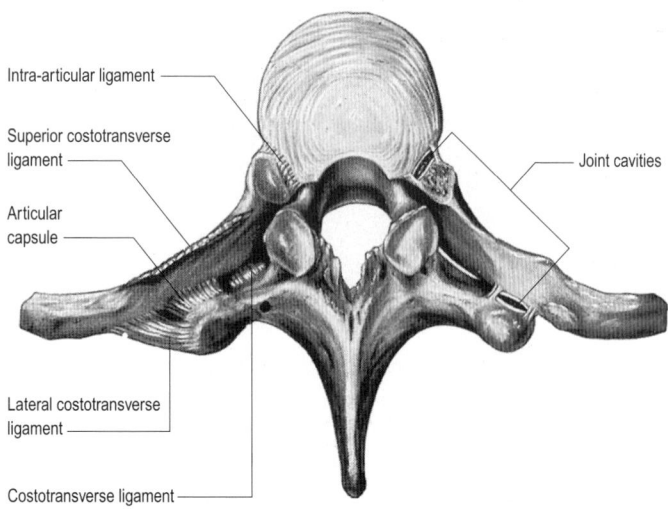

Fig. 57.14 Costovertebral joints: superior aspect. On the left the free demifacet superior to the intra-articular ligament is apparent on the head of the rib. On the right the inferior costovertebral and costotransverse synovial cavities have been opened.

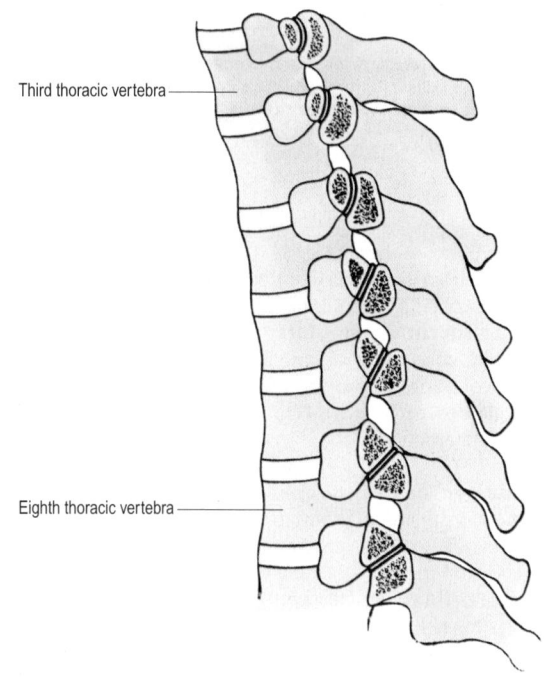

Fig. 57.15 Section through the costotransverse joints from the third to the ninth inclusive. Contrast the concave facets on the upper transverse processes with the less curved facets on the lower transverse processes.

costotransverse and accessory. The fibrous capsule is thin and attached to articular peripheries; it has a synovial lining.

The costotransverse ligament – The costotransverse ligament fills the costotransverse foramen between the rib neck and its adjacent corresponding transverse process. Its numerous short fibres extend back from the posterior rough surface on the neck to the anterior surface of the transverse process. In the eleventh and twelfth ribs it is rudimentary or absent.

The superior costotransverse ligament – The superior costotransverse ligament has an anterior layer attached between the crest of the costal neck and lower aspect of the transverse process above (Fig. 57.13). Laterally, it blends with the internal intercostal membrane and is crossed by the intercostal vessels and nerve. Its posterior layer is attached posteriorly on the costal neck, ascending posteromedially to the transverse process above. Laterally, the posterior layer blends with the external intercostal muscle. The first rib has no such ligament. The shaft of the twelfth rib, near its head, is connected to the base of the first lumbar transverse process by a lumbocostal ligament in series with the superior costotransverse ligaments.

Accessory ligament – An accessory ligament is usually present. It lies medial to the superior costotransverse ligament, and is separated from it by the dorsal ramus of a thoracic spinal nerve and accompanying vessels (Fig. 57.13). These bands are variable in their attachments, but usually pass from a depression medial to a costal tubercle to the inferior articular process immediately above. Some fibres also pass to the base of the transverse process.

The lateral costotransverse ligament – The lateral costotransverse ligament is short, thick and strong. It passes obliquely from the apex of the transverse process to the rough non-articular part of the adjacent costal tubercle. The ligaments of upper ribs ascend from their transverse processes; they are shorter and more oblique than those of the lower ribs, which descend.

Movements at costotransverse joints – Costal heads are so firmly tied to vertebral bodies by radiate and intra-articular ligaments that only slight gliding can occur. Strong ligaments binding costal necks and tubercles to transverse processes also limit movements at costotransverse joints to slight gliding, which is guided by the shape and direction of the articular surfaces (Fig. 57.15). Those on tubercles of the upper six ribs are oval and vertically convex, and fit corresponding concavities on the anterior surfaces of transverse processes, consequently up and down movements of tubercles involve rotation of costal necks about their long axes. Articular surfaces of the seventh to tenth tubercles are almost flat, and face down, medially and backwards; their opposing surfaces are on the upper aspects of transverse processes, and so when these tubercles ascend they also move posteromedially. Both sets of joints move simultaneously and in the same directions. The costal neck therefore moves as if at a single joint in which the two articulations form its ends.

In the upper six ribs, the neck moves slightly up and down but its chief movement is one of rotation about its long axis, which means that downward rotation of its anterior aspect is associated with depression and upward rotation with elevation of the shaft and anterior end of the rib. In the seventh to tenth ribs, the neck ascends posteromedially or descends anterolaterally, increasing or diminishing the infrasternal angle respectively; slight rotation accompanies these movements.

Sternocostal joints

Costal cartilages articulate with small concavities on the lateral sternal borders (chondrosternal articulations, Fig. 57.16). Perichondrium and periosteum are continuous. The first sternocostal joint is an unusual variety of synarthrosis, often inaccurately called a synchondrosis. The second to seventh costal cartilages articulate by synovial joints, although articular cavities are often absent, particularly in the lower joints. Fibrocartilage covers articular surfaces and also unites the costal cartilages and the sternum in those joints where cavities are absent. The seventh costosternal joint may be synovial or 'symphyseal'. Ligaments involved are capsular, radiate sternocostal, intra-articular and costoxiphoid.

Fibrous capsules – Fibrous capsules surround the second to seventh sternocostal joints. They are thin, blended with the sternocostal ligaments and are strengthened above and below by fibres connecting the costal cartilages to the sternum.

Radiate sternocostal ligaments – These are broad, thin bands, which radiate from the front and back of the sternal ends of the costal cartilages of true ribs to corresponding sternal surfaces. Their superficial fibres intermingle with adjacent ligaments above and below, with those of the opposite side and with tendinous fibres of pectoralis major; collectively, these tissues form a thick fibrous membrane around the sternum, more markedly in its lower part.

Intra-articular ligaments – Intra-articular ligaments are constant only between the second costal cartilages and sternum. The ligament associated with the second costal cartilage extends from the costal

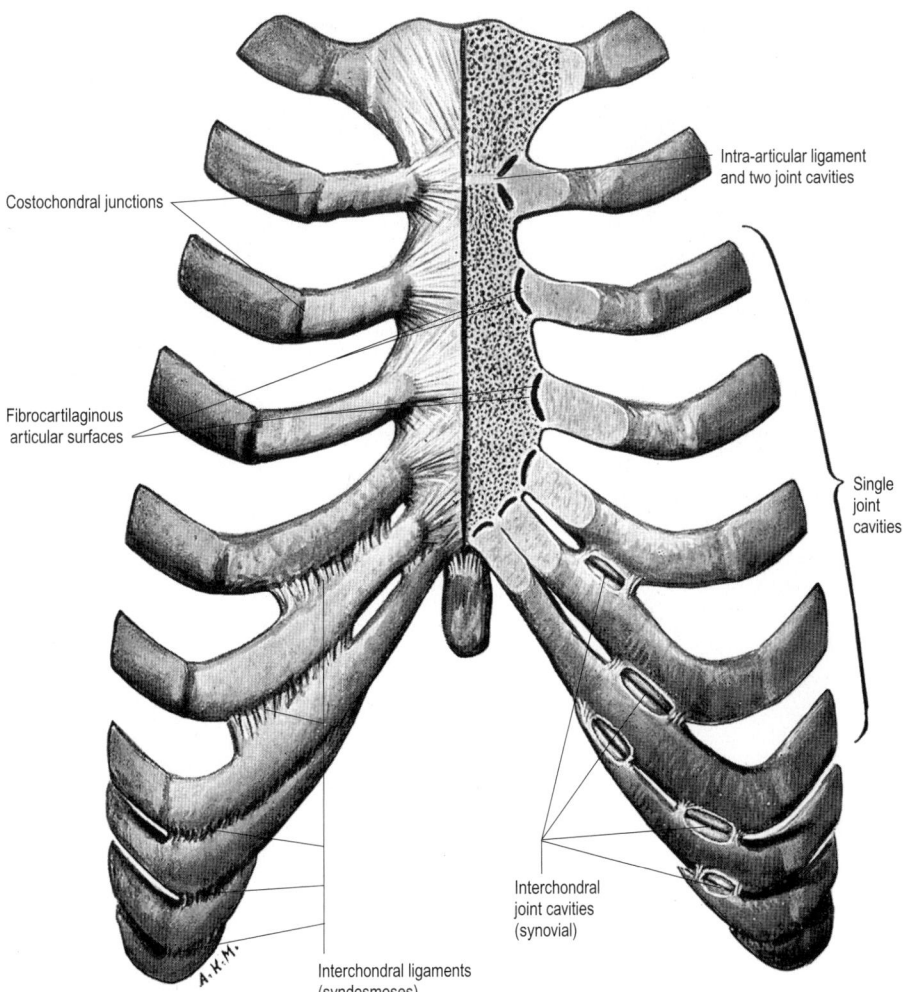

Costochondral junctions

Fibrocartilaginous
articular surfaces

Intra-articular ligament
and two joint cavities

Single
joint
cavities

Interchondral
joint cavities
(synovial)

Interchondral ligaments
(syndesmoses)

A.K.M.

Fig. 57.16 Sternocostal and interchondral joints: anterior aspect.

cartilage to the fibrocartilage uniting the manubrium and sternal body and is therefore intra-articular. Occasionally, the third sternal cartilage is connected with the first and second sternal segments by a similar ligament. Fibrocartilaginous strands may occur in the third and lower joints. Articular cavities may be absent at any age.

Costoxiphoid ligaments – Costoxiphoid ligaments connect the anterior and posterior surfaces of the seventh (and sometimes sixth) costal cartilage to the same surfaces of the xiphoid process. They vary in length and breadth; the posterior is less distinct.

Movements – Slight gliding movements occur at sternocostal joints, sufficient for ventilation.

Interchondral joints

Contiguous borders of the sixth to ninth costal cartilages articulate by apposition of small oblong facets. Each articulation is enclosed in a thin fibrous capsule, lined by synovial membrane with lateral and medial interchondral ligaments (**Fig. 57.16**). Sometimes the fifth cartilage, and more rarely the ninth, articulate at their inferior borders with adjoining cartilages; this connection is more often by ligamentous fibres. Articulation between the ninth and tenth cartilages is never synovial and sometimes absent.

COSTOCHONDRAL JUNCTIONS

Artificially separated from its rib, a costal cartilage has a rounded end that fits a reciprocal depression in the rib. Periosteum and perichondrium are continuous across the costochondral junctions, and the collagen of the osseous and cartilaginous matrices blend. No movement occurs at costochondral junctions.

INTRINSIC CHEST WALL MUSCLES

INTERCOSTALS

The intercostals (**Figs 57.17, 57.18, 67.9, 67.11**) are thin multiple layers of muscular and tendinous fibres that occupy the intercostal spaces. Their names are derived from their spatial relationship, i.e. external, internal and innermost intercostals.

External intercostals

Eleven pairs of external intercostals extend from the tubercles of the ribs, where they blend with the posterior fibres of the superior costotransverse ligaments, almost to the costal cartilages, where each continues forwards to the sternum as an aponeurotic layer called the external intercostal membrane. Each muscle passes from the lower border of one rib to the upper border of the rib below. In the upper two or three spaces, they do not quite reach the ends of the rib, and in the lower two spaces they extend to the free ends of the costal cartilages. The external intercostals are thicker than the internal intercostals. Their fibres are directed obliquely downwards and laterally at the back of the thorax, and downwards, forwards and medially at the front.

Innervation – External intercostals are supplied by the adjacent intercostal nerves.

Action – External intercostals are believed to act with the internal intercostals (p. 1084).

Internal intercostals

Eleven pairs of internal intercostals begin anteriorly at the sternum, in the interspaces between the cartilages of the true ribs, and at the anterior extremities of the cartilages of the 'false' ribs. Their greatest

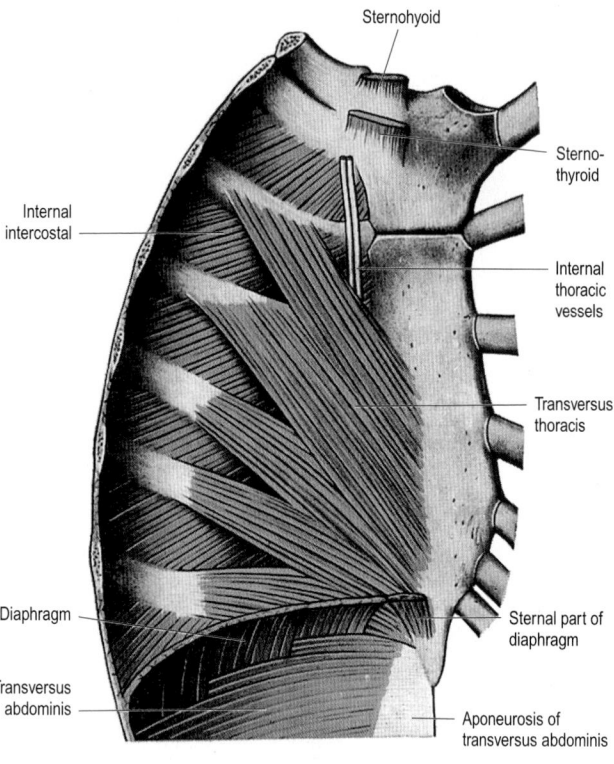

Fig. 57.17 The left transversus thoracis, exposed and viewed from its posterior aspect. Note that the lower border of transversus thoracis is in contact with the upper border of transversus abdominis in the interval between the sternal and costal origins of the diaphragm.

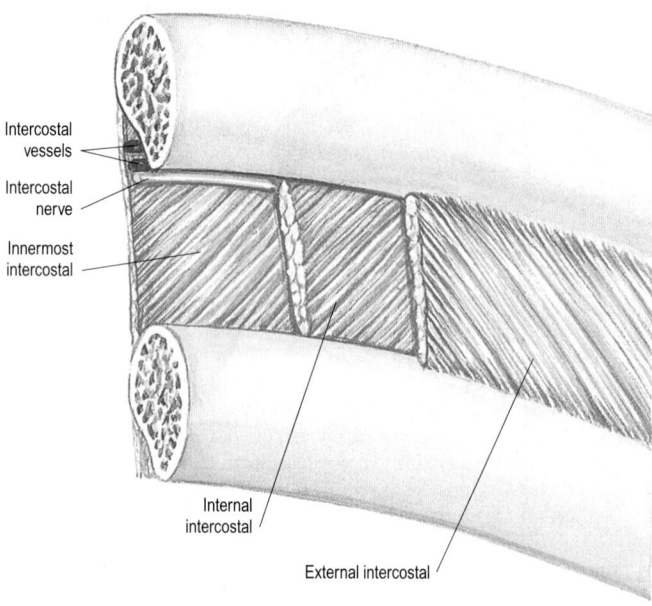

Fig. 57.18 Dissection of part of an intercostal space, showing the position of the intercostal vessels and nerve relative to the intercostal muscles.

thickness lies in this intercartilaginous or parasternal part. They continue back as far as the posterior costal angles, where each is replaced by an aponeurotic layer called the internal intercostal membrane. The latter is continuous posteriorly with the anterior fibres of a superior costo-transverse ligament, and anteriorly with the fascia between the internal and external intercostal muscles. Each muscle descends from the floor of a costal groove and adjacent costal cartilage, and inserts into the upper border of the rib below. Their fibres are directed obliquely, nearly at right angles to those of the external intercostal muscles.

Innervation – Internal intercostals are supplied by the adjacent intercostal nerves.

Action – Internal intercostals are believed to act with the external intercostals (p. 1084).

Innermost intercostals
The innermost intercostals were once regarded as internal laminae of the internal intercostal muscles, and fibres in the two layers do coincide in direction. Each muscle is attached to the internal aspects of two adjoining ribs. They are insignificant, and sometimes absent, at highest thoracic levels, but become progressively more substantial below this, extending through about the middle two quarters of the lower intercostal spaces. Posteriorly the innermost intercostals, in those spaces where they are well developed, may come together with the corresponding subcostales. The innermost intercostals are related internally to the endothoracic fascia and parietal pleura, and externally to the intercostal nerves and vessels.

Innervation – Innermost intercostals are supplied by the adjacent intercostal nerves.

Action – Innermost intercostals are believed to act with the internal intercostals (p. 1084).

SUBCOSTALES
Subcostales consist of muscular and aponeurotic fasciculi, and are usually well developed only in the lower part of the thorax. Each descends from the internal surface of one rib, near its angle, to the internal surface of the second or third rib below. Their fibres run parallel to those of the internal intercostals and, like the innermost intercostals, they lie between the intercostal vessels and nerves and the pleura.

Innervation – Subcostales are supplied by the adjacent intercostal nerves.

Action – Subcostales depress the ribs.

TRANSVERSUS THORACIS
Transversus thoracis (also called the triangularis sternae and sternocostalis) spreads over the internal surface of the anterior thoracic wall (**Fig. 57.17**). It arises from the lower one-third of the posterior surface of the sternum, the xiphoid process and the costal cartilages of the lower three or four true ribs near their sternal ends. Its fibres diverge and ascend laterally as slips that pass into the lower borders and inner surfaces of the costal cartilages of the second, third, fourth, fifth and sixth ribs. The lowest fibres are horizontal, and are contiguous with the highest fibres of transversus abdominis; the intermediate fibres are oblique; the highest are almost vertical. Transversus thoracis varies in its attachments, not only between individuals but even on opposite sides of the same individual. Like the innermost intercostals and subcostales, transversus thoracis separates the intercostal nerves from the pleura.

Innervation – Transversus thoracis is supplied by the adjacent intercostal nerves.

Action – Transversus thoracis draws down the costal cartilages to which it is attached.

LEVATORES COSTARUM
Levatores costarum are strong bundles, twelve on each side, that arise from the tips of the transverse processes of the seventh cervical and first to eleventh thoracic vertebrae. They pass obliquely downwards and laterally, parallel with the posterior borders of the external intercostals. Each is attached to the upper edge and external surface of the rib immediately below the vertebra from which it takes origin, between the tubercle and the angle (levatores costarum breves). Each of the four lower muscles divides into two fasciculi: one is attached as already described, and the other descends to the second rib below its origin (levatores costarum longi).

Innervation – Levatores costarum are supplied by the lateral branches of the dorsal rami of the corresponding thoracic spinal nerves.

Action – Levatores costarum elevate the ribs, but their importance in ventilation is disputed. They are also said to act from their costal attachments as rotators and lateral flexors of the vertebral column.

SERRATUS POSTERIOR

Serratus posterior superior
Serratus posterior superior is a thin, quadrilateral muscle, external to the upper posterior part of the thorax. It arises by a thin aponeurosis from the lower part of the nuchal ligament, the spines of the seventh cervical and upper two or three thoracic vertebrae and their supraspinous ligaments. It descends laterally, and ends in four digitations attached to the upper borders and external surfaces of the second, third, fourth and fifth ribs, just lateral to their angles. It is superficial to the thoracic part of the thoracolumbar fascia and deep to the rhomboids. The number of digitations can vary from three to six, and the muscle may even be absent.

Innervation – Serratus posterior superior is innervated by the second, third, fourth and fifth intercostal nerves.

Action – The attachments of serratus posterior superior clearly indicate that it could elevate the ribs; however, experiments in dogs do not support a ventilatory function. Its role in man is uncertain.

Serratus posterior inferior
Serratus posterior inferior is a thin, irregularly quadrilateral muscle at the junction of the thoracic and lumbar regions (**Fig. 57.19**). It arises from the spines of the lower two thoracic and upper two or three lumbar vertebrae and their supraspinous ligaments by a thin aponeurosis that blends with the lumbar part of the thoracolumbar fascia. It ascends laterally, and its four digitations pass into the inferior borders and outer surfaces of the lower four ribs, a little lateral to their angles. There may be fewer digitations and in rare cases the entire muscle may be absent.

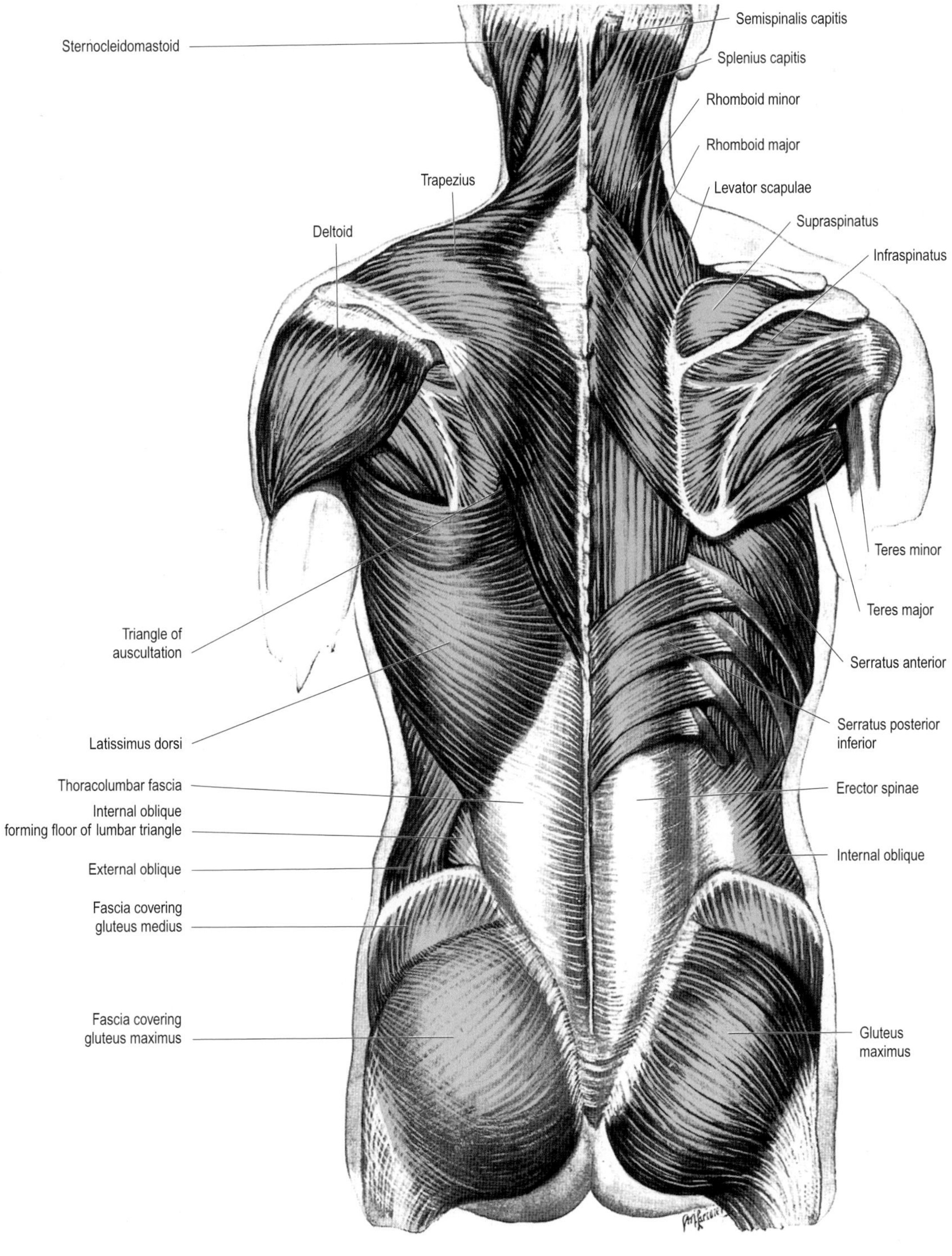

Fig. 57.19 Superficial muscles of the back of the neck and trunk. On the left only the skin, superficial and deep fasciae (other than gluteofemoral) have been removed; on the right, sternocleidomastoid, trapezius, latissimus dorsi, deltoid and external oblique have been dissected away.

Sternocleidomastoid

Trapezius

Deltoid

Triangle of auscultation

Latissimus dorsi

Thoracolumbar fascia

Internal oblique forming floor of lumbar triangle

External oblique

Fascia covering gluteus medius

Fascia covering gluteus maximus

Semispinalis capitis

Splenius capitis

Rhomboid minor

Rhomboid major

Levator scapulae

Supraspinatus

Infraspinatus

Teres minor

Teres major

Serratus anterior

Serratus posterior inferior

Erector spinae

Internal oblique

Gluteus maximus

Innervation – Serratus posterior inferior is innervated by ventral rami of the ninth, tenth, eleventh and twelfth thoracic spinal nerves.

Action – Serratus posterior inferior draws the lower ribs downwards and backwards, although possibly not in ventilation.

MECHANISM OF THORACIC CAGE MOVEMENT

Breathing involves changing the thoracic volume by altering the vertical, transverse and anteroposterior dimension of the thorax (p. 1084). The diaphragm is the key muscle in this process, whereas the intercostal muscles maintain the rigidity of the chest wall. The muscle fibres of the diaphragm descend from their relatively 'high' anterior sternocostal attachments steeply to the central tendon and obliquely to their complex 'low' posterior attachments (**Fig. 64.1**). The central tendon is fixed and hence when the diaphragm contracts it allows the lower rib cage to move inferiorly and anteriorly without any change to the curvature of the diaphragm. The external and internal intercostals, transversus thoracis, subcostales, levatores costarum, serratus posterior superior and serratus posterior inferior can elevate or depress the ribs, and hence can act as accessory muscles of ventilation.

MUSCLES OF THE SCAPULA, AND MUSCLES CONNECTING THE UPPER LIMB WITH THE CHEST WALL AND VERTEBRAE

Trapezius, latissimus dorsi, rhomboid major, rhomboid minor, levator scapulae, pectoralis major, pectoralis minor, subclavius, serratus anterior, deltoid, subscapularis, supraspinatus, infraspinatus, teres minor and teres major are described in detail in Chapter 49 (p. 833).

VASCULAR SUPPLY AND LYMPHATIC DRAINAGE

ARTERIES

Muscles of the thoracic wall receive their blood supply from the internal thoracic artery, either directly or via the musculophrenic artery, the superior intercostal artery, descending thoracic aorta, and the subcostal and superior thoracic (p. 844) arteries. Additional contributions come from vessels that supply proximal muscles of the upper limb, namely, suprascapular, superficial cervical, thoracoacromial, lateral thoracic and subscapular arteries.

The blood supply to the diaphragm is described in Chapter 64 (p. 1081).

Internal thoracic artery

The internal thoracic artery arises inferiorly from the first part of the subclavian artery, c.2 cm above the sternal end of the clavicle, opposite the root of the thyrocervical trunk (**Fig. 57.20**). It descends behind the first six costal cartilages c.1 cm from the lateral sternal border. It divides at the level of the sixth intercostal space into musculophrenic and superior epigastric branches.

Relations – At first, the internal thoracic artery descends anteromedially behind the sternal end of the clavicle, the internal jugular and brachiocephalic veins and the first costal cartilage. As it enters the thorax, the phrenic nerve crosses it obliquely from its lateral side, usually in front. The artery then descends almost vertically to its bifurcation, lying behind pectoralis major, the first six costal cartilages, external intercostal membranes, internal intercostals and terminations of the upper six intercostal nerves. It is separated from the pleura, down to the second or third cartilage, by a strong layer of fascia, and below this by transversus thoracis. The artery is accompanied by a chain of lymph nodes and venae comitantes, which unite at about the third costal cartilage into a single vein medial to the artery. Its intermediate branches are sternal, anterior intercostal and perforating.

Sternal branches – Sternal branches are distributed to transversus thoracis, the periosteum of the posterior sternal surface and the sternal red bone marrow. These branches, together with small branches of the pericardiacophrenic artery, anastomose with branches of the posterior intercostal and bronchial arteries to form a subpleural mediastinal plexus.

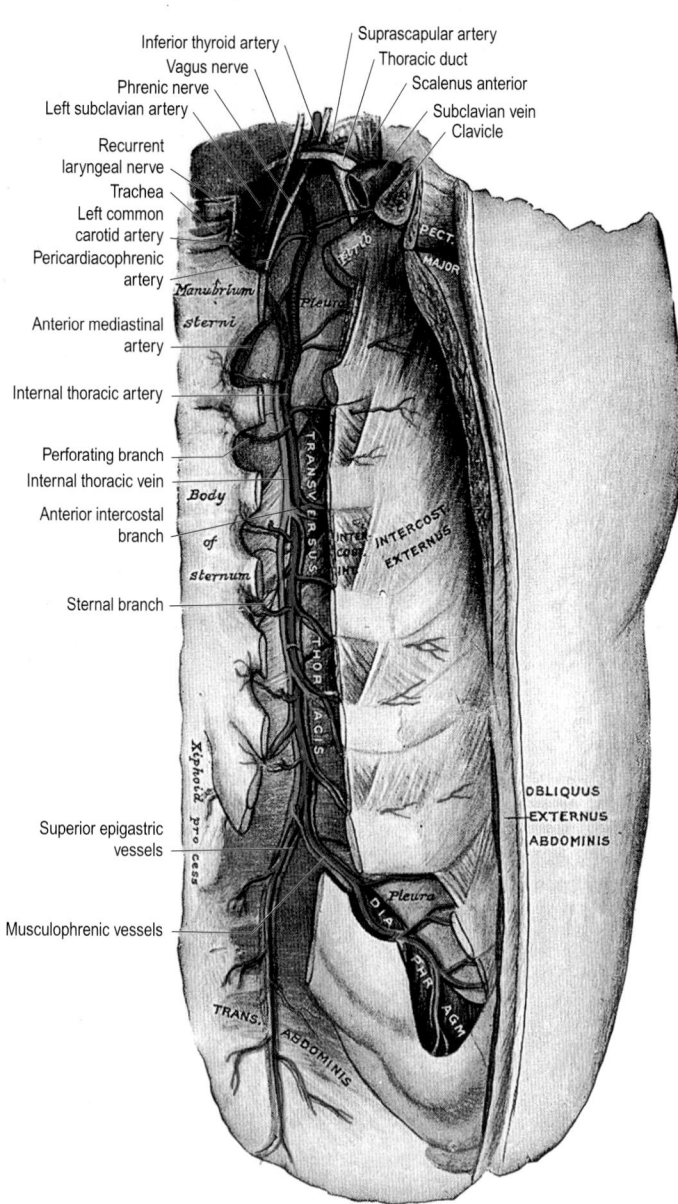

Fig. 57.20 The left internal thoracic artery and vein and their main branches: Anterior view after resection and elevation of the clavicle and removal of the overlying costal cartilages.

Anterior intercostal branches – Anterior intercostal arteries are distributed to the upper six intercostal spaces. They pass laterally along the borders of the space to anastomose with the posterior intercostal arteries (and their collateral branches). Usually, the anterior intercostals arise from the internal thoracic artery as single vessels (sometimes as two separate branches) that soon divide into two branches, one passing to the superior and one to the inferior part of each intercostal space. Occasionally, one branch passes to the space above, and one to the space below. They lie at first between the pleura and the internal intercostals, then between the innermost intercostals and the internal intercostals. They supply the intercostal muscles and send branches through them to the pectoral muscles, breast and skin.

Perforating branches – Perforating branches traverse the upper five or six intercostal spaces with anterior cutaneous branches of the corresponding intercostal nerves. They pierce and supply pectoralis major, and then curve laterally to become direct cutaneous vessels that supply the skin. These cutaneous vessels provide the anatomical basis for surgically raising a skin flap in this region (deltopectoral flap) for reconstructing areas of missing tissue in the head and neck.

The second to fourth branches supply the breast; during lactation they are enlarged.

Musculophrenic artery – The musculophrenic artery passes infero-laterally behind the seventh to ninth costal cartilages, traverses the diaphragm near the ninth, and ends near the last intercostal space. It anastomoses with the inferior phrenic and lower two posterior intercostal arteries and ascending branches of the deep circumflex iliac arteries. Two anterior intercostal arteries branch from it for each of the seventh to ninth intercostal spaces, and are distributed like their counterparts in higher spaces. The musculophrenic artery also supplies the lower part of the pericardium and the abdominal muscles.

Superior intercostal artery

The superior intercostal artery arises from the costocervical trunk. It descends between the pleura and necks of the first and second ribs to anastomose with the third posterior intercostal artery. Crossing the neck of the first rib, it lies medial to the ventral branch of the first thoracic spinal nerve, which it crosses at a lower level, and lateral to the stellate ganglion. In the first space it gives off the first posterior intercostal artery, which is similar in distribution to the lower posterior intercostal arteries. It descends to become the second posterior intercostal artery, usually joining a branch from the third. The artery is not constant, and is more common on the right; when absent, it is replaced by a direct branch from the aorta.

Posterior intercostal arteries (Fig. 57.21)

There are usually nine pairs of posterior intercostal arteries. They arise from the posterior aspect of the descending thoracic aorta and are distributed to the lower nine intercostal spaces. Right posterior intercostal arteries are longer, reflecting the aortic deviation to the left: they cross the vertebral bodies behind the oesophagus, thoracic duct and azygos vein, right lung and pleura. Left posterior intercostal arteries turn backwards on the vertebral bodies in contact with the left lung and pleura; the upper two are crossed by the left superior intercostal vein, and the lower by the hemiazygos and accessory hemiazygos veins. The further course of the arteries is the same on both sides. The sympathetic trunk lies anterior to all of the arteries, and the splanchnic nerves descend in front of the lower arteries.

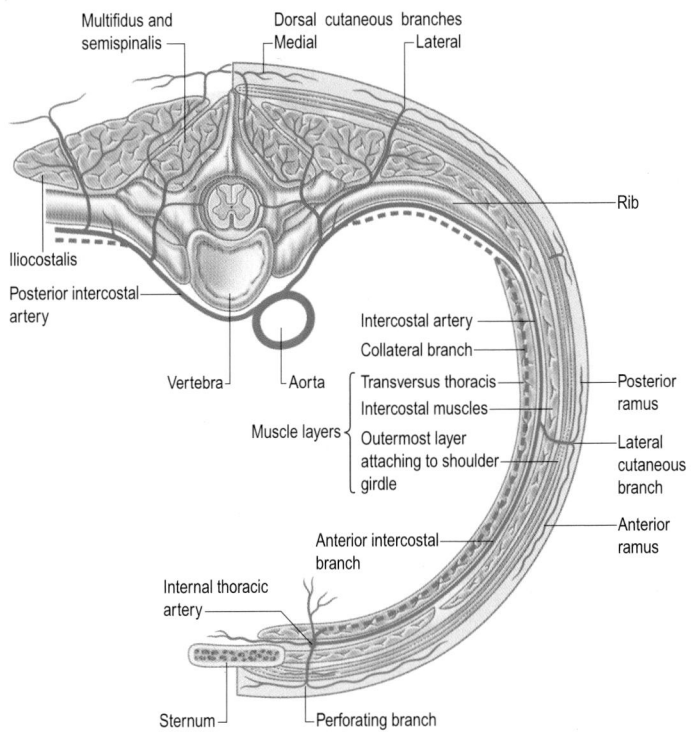

Fig. 57.21 Schematic transverse section through one half of a lower intercostal space to show the branches of a typical intercostal artery. The usual branching arrangement of the dorsal cutaneous branch is shown to the right of the spine and a common variant is shown to the left. (By permission from Cormack GC, Lamberty BGH 1994 The Arterial Anatomy of Skin Flaps, 2nd edn. Edinburgh: Churchill Livingstone.)

Each artery crosses its intercostal space obliquely towards the angle of the rib above and continues forward in its costal groove (**Fig. 30.31**). At first between the pleura and internal intercostal membrane as far as the costal angle, it passes between the internal intercostal and innermost intercostal muscles, anastomosing with an anterior intercostal branch from either the internal thoracic or musculophrenic artery. Each artery has a vein above and a nerve below, except in the upper spaces, where the nerve at first lies above the artery. The third posterior intercostal artery anastomoses with the superior intercostal artery and may provide the major supply to the second space. The lower two arteries continue anteriorly into the abdominal wall, where they anastomose with the subcostal, superior epigastric and lumbar arteries. Each posterior intercostal artery has dorsal, collateral, muscular and cutaneous branches.

Dorsal branch – Each dorsal branch runs dorsally between the necks of adjoining ribs; a vertebral body and superior costotransverse ligament lie medial and lateral, respectively. Each dorsal branch gives off a spinal branch which enters the vertebral canal via the intervertebral foramen and supplies the vertebrae, spinal cord and meninges, and anastomoses with the spinal arteries above and below and with its contralateral fellow. It then divides into a medial and a lateral dorsal musculocutaneous branch (occasionally these arise separately from the posterior intercostal artery rather than from a common trunk). The medial branch crosses a transverse process with the medial dorsal branch of a thoracic spinal nerve to supply spinalis and longissimus thoracis and an area of overlying skin. The lateral branch supplies longissimus thoracis and iliocostalis, and the medial aspects of latissimus dorsi and trapezius, in addition to an area of overlying skin.

Collateral intercostal branch – A collateral intercostal branch arises near the costal angle and descends to the upper border of the subjacent rib, along which it courses to anastomose with an anterior intercostal branch of the internal thoracic or musculophrenic artery.

Muscular branches – Muscular branches supply intercostal and pectoral muscles and serratus anterior. They anastomose with the superior and lateral thoracic branches of the axillary artery. Lateral cutaneous branches accompany the same branches of the thoracic spinal nerves. Mammary branches from the vessels in the second to fourth spaces supply the pectoral muscles, skin and mammary tissue and enlarge during lactation.

Lateral cutaneous branch – The lateral cutaneous branch is given off in the posterior part of the intercostal space and travels anteriorly for a few centimetres with an accompanying vein and the lateral cutaneous branch of the equivalent intercostal nerve. This neurovascular bundle pierces the intercostal muscles and emerges lower down between the interdigitations of serratus anterior and external oblique. It divides into anterior and posterior rami, which contribute to the blood supply of the skin of the lateral trunk; these vessels are less significant in the upper three intercostal spaces.

Unnamed branches – Other unnamed branches supply tissues of the thoracic wall, e.g. costal periosteum, bone and bone marrow of the ribs, tissues of synovial and synarthrodial joints and the parietal pleura.

VEINS

Internal thoracic veins

The internal thoracic veins are venae comitantes to the inferior half of the internal thoracic artery. They have several valves. Near the third costal cartilages, the veins unite and ascend medial to the artery to end in their appropriate brachiocephalic vein (**Figs 57.21, 31.15**). Tributaries correspond to branches of the artery, and include a pericardiacophrenic vein.

Left superior intercostal vein

The left superior intercostal vein drains the second and third (sometimes fourth) left posterior intercostal veins. It ascends obliquely forwards across the left aspect of the aortic arch, lateral to the left vagus and medial to the left phrenic nerve, to open into the left brachiocephalic vein (**Fig. 31.15**). It usually receives the left bronchial veins, sometimes the left pericardiacophrenic vein, and connects inferiorly with the accessory hemiazygos vein.

Posterior intercostal veins

The posterior intercostal veins accompany their arteries in eleven pairs. Approaching the vertebral column, each vein receives a posterior tributary returning blood from the dorsal muscles and skin and vertebral venous plexuses (**Figs 59.2, 60.31**). On both sides, the first posterior intercostal vein ascends anterior to the neck of the first rib, arching forward above the pleural dome to end in the ipsilateral brachiocephalic or vertebral vein. On the right the second, third and often fourth, form a right superior intercostal vein joining the arch of the azygos vein. Veins from the lower spaces drain directly to it. On the left the second and third (sometimes fourth) form a left superior intercostal vein. Veins from the fourth (or fifth) to eighth intercostal spaces end in the accessory hemiazygos vein; veins from the ninth to the eleventh intercostal spaces end in the hemiazygos vein.

Posterior intercostal veins are so called to distinguish them from small anterior intercostal veins, which are tributaries of the internal thoracic and musculophrenic veins.

Azygos and hemiazygos veins

The hemiazygos vein is formed on the left side from the lower three posterior intercostal veins, a common trunk formed by the left ascending lumbar and subcostal veins, and by oesophageal and mediastinal tributaries (p. 1026).

The accessory hemiazygos vein descends to the left of the vertebral column, receiving veins from the fourth (or fifth) to eighth intercostal spaces and sometimes the left bronchial veins. It crosses the seventh thoracic vertebra to join the azygos vein. It sometimes joins the hemiazygos vein, and their common trunk opens into the azygos vein.

Variations of the azygos veins – The azygos veins vary greatly in their mode of origin, course, tributaries, anastomoses and termination. The accessory hemiazygos is the most variable, and may drain into the left brachiocephalic, azygos or hemiazygos vein. The arrangement shown in **Figure 60.32** represents a common pattern. Typically, there is a main 'right-sided' azygos and at least some representative of the hemiazygos veins. The latter vary: one or other may be absent or poorly developed. Very occasionally, independent left and right azygos veins (the early embryonic form) persist, or a single azygos vein may occur in a midline position without hemiazygos tributaries. Retro-aortic transvertebral connections from hemiazygos and accessory hemiazygos veins to the azygos are also extremely variable: there may be from one to at least five, and when either hemiazygos is absent, the relevant intercostal veins cross vertebral bodies and end in the azygos. These transvertebral routes are often very short, because the azygos vein is more commonly anterior to the vertebral column and often passes left of the midline in part of its course.

LYMPHATIC DRAINAGE

Superficial lymphatic vessels of the thoracic wall ramify subcutaneously and converge on the axillary nodes. Those superficial to trapezius and latissimus dorsi unite to form 10 or 12 trunks, which end in the subscapular nodes. Those in the pectoral region, including vessels from the skin covering the periphery of the mammary gland and its subareolar plexus, run back, collecting those superficial to serratus anterior, to reach the pectoral nodes. Vessels near the lateral sternal margin pass between the costal cartilages to the parasternal nodes, but also anastomose across the sternum. A few vessels from the upper pectoral region ascend over the clavicle to the inferior deep cervical nodes. Lymph vessels from deeper tissues of the thoracic walls drain mainly to the parasternal, intercostal and diaphragmatic lymphatic nodes.

Parasternal (internal thoracic) nodes

There are four or five parasternal nodes along each internal thoracic artery, at the anterior ends of the intercostal spaces. They drain afferents from the mammary gland, deeper structures of the supra-umbilical anterior abdominal wall, the superior hepatic surface (through a small group of nodes behind the xiphoid process) and deeper parts of the anterior thoracic wall. Their efferents usually unite with those from the tracheobronchial and brachiocephalic nodes to form the bronchomediastinal trunk. The latter may open, on either side, directly into the jugulo–subclavian junction or into either great vein near the junction or may join the right subclavian trunk or right lymphatic duct, or the thoracic duct on the left.

Intercostal nodes

Intercostal nodes occupy the intercostal spaces near the heads and necks of the ribs. They receive deep lymph vessels from the posterolateral aspects of the chest and the mammary gland, some of which are interrupted by small lateral intercostal nodes. Efferents of nodes in the lower four to seven spaces unite into a trunk that descends to the abdominal confluence of lymph trunks or to the start of the thoracic duct. Efferents of nodes in the left upper spaces end in the thoracic duct; those of the right upper spaces end in one of the right lymph trunks.

Diaphragmatic nodes

Located on the thoracic surface of the diaphragm, these nodes are arranged in anterior, right and left lateral and posterior groups.

The anterior group – This consists of two or three small nodes behind the base of the xiphoid process, draining the convex hepatic surface, and one or two nodes on each side near the junction of the seventh rib and cartilage, which receive anterior lymph vessels from the diaphragm. The anterior group drains to the parasternal nodes.

The lateral groups – These each contain two or three nodes, and lie close to the point where the phrenic nerves enter the diaphragm. On the right, some nodes lie within the fibrous pericardium anterior to the intrathoracic end of the inferior vena cava. Their afferents drain the central diaphragm, those on the right also draining the convex surface of the liver. Their efferents pass to the posterior mediastinal, parasternal and brachiocephalic nodes.

The posterior group – This contains a few nodes on the back of the crura, which are connected with the lateral aortic and posterior mediastinal nodes.

LYMPHATIC DRAINAGE OF DEEPER TISSUES

Collecting vessels of the deeper thoracic tissues include lymphatics that drain the muscles attached to the ribs. Most end in axillary nodes; some from pectoralis major also drain to the parasternal nodes. Intercostal vessels drain the intercostal muscles and parietal pleura: those from the anterior thoracic wall and pleura end in the parasternal nodes, and their posterior counterparts drain to intercostal nodes.

Vessels from the diaphragm form two plexuses, thoracic and abdominal, which anastomose freely, especially in areas covered by pleurae and peritoneum, respectively. The thoracic plexus unites with lymph vessels draining the costal and mediastinal pleura. Its efferents are: anterior, which drain to the anterior diaphragmatic nodes near the junctions of the seventh ribs and cartilages; middle, which drain to nodes on the oesophagus and around the end of the inferior vena cava; posterior, which drain to nodes around the aorta where it leaves the thorax. The abdominal plexus anastomoses with the hepatic lymphatics and peripherally with those of the subperitoneal tissue. Efferents from its right half end in a group of nodes on the inferior phrenic artery, and in others in the right lateral aortic nodes. Those from the left half of the abdominal diaphragmatic plexus pass to the pre-aortic and lateral aortic nodes and to nodes near the terminal oesophagus.

INNERVATION

THORACIC VENTRAL SPINAL RAMI

There are twelve pairs of thoracic ventral rami. The upper eleven lie between the ribs (intercostal nerves), and the twelfth lies below the last rib (subcostal nerve) (**Figs 57.22, 57.23**). Each is connected with the adjoining ganglion of the sympathetic trunk by grey and white rami communicantes; the grey ramus joins the nerve proximal to the point at which the white ramus leaves it. Intercostal nerves are distributed primarily to the thoracic and abdominal walls. The first two nerves supply fibres to the upper limb in addition to their thoracic branches, the next four supply only the thoracic wall, and the lower five supply both thoracic and abdominal walls. The subcostal nerve is distributed to the abdominal wall and the gluteal skin. Communicating branches link the intercostal nerves posteriorly in the intercostal spaces, and the lower five nerves communicate freely in the abdominal wall.

The first to sixth thoracic ventral rami

The first thoracic ventral ramus divides unequally. A large branch ascends across the neck of the first rib, lateral to the superior intercostal

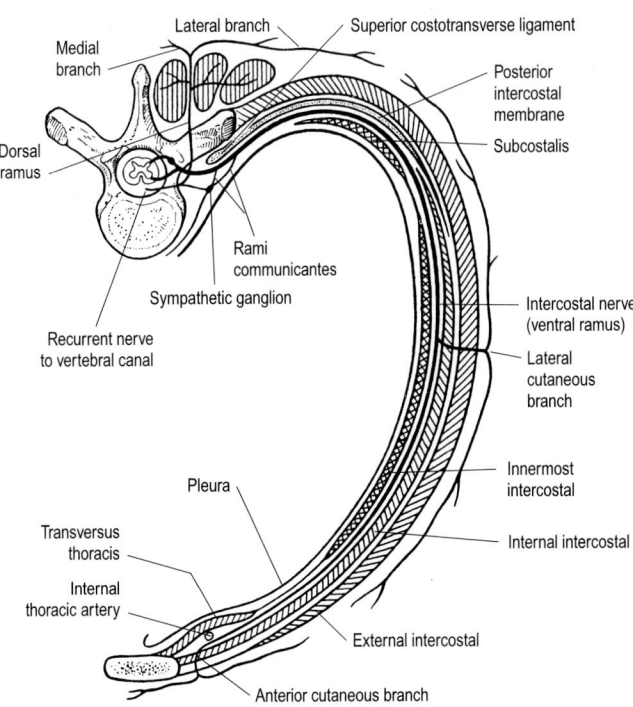

Fig. 57.22 The course of a typical intercostal nerve. The muscular and the collateral branches are not shown.

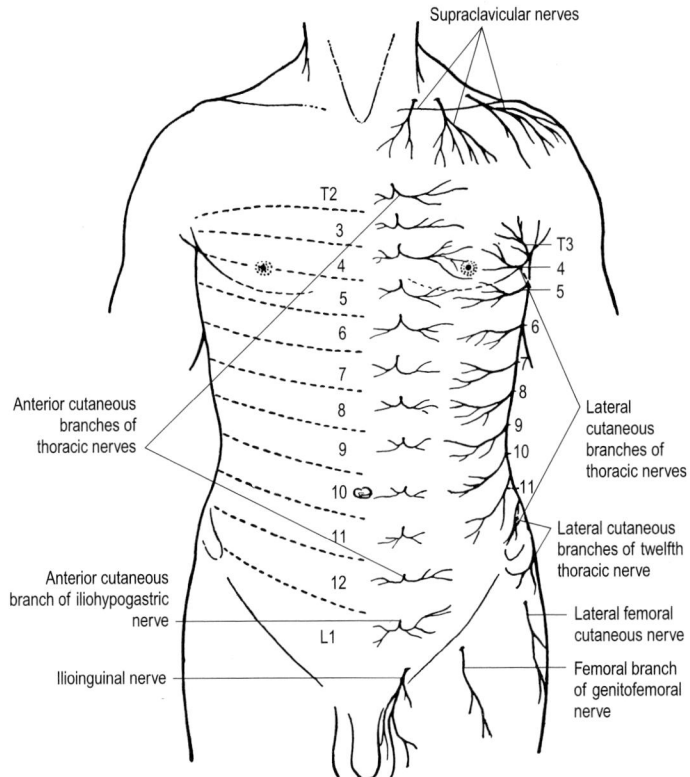

Fig. 57.23 The approximate segmental distribution of the cutaneous nerves on the front of the trunk. The contribution from the first thoracic spinal nerve is not shown and the considerable overlap that occurs between adjacent segments is not indicated.

artery, and enters the brachial plexus. The smaller branch is the first intercostal nerve; it runs in the first intercostal space and ends on the front of the chest as the first anterior cutaneous nerve of the thorax. It gives off a lateral cutaneous branch, which pierces the chest wall in front of serratus anterior and supplies the axillary skin; it may communicate with the intercostobrachial nerve and sometimes joins the medial cutaneous nerve of the arm. The first thoracic ramus often receives a connecting ramus from the second, which ascends in front of the neck of the second rib.

The second to sixth thoracic ventral rami pass forwards in their intercostal spaces below the intercostal vessels. At the back of the chest they lie between the pleura and external intercostal membranes, but in most of their course they run between the internal intercostals and the subcostales and innermost intercostals (**Fig. 57.23**). Near the sternum, they cross anterior to the internal thoracic vessels and transversus thoracis, pierce the internal intercostals, the external intercostal membranes and pectoralis major, and end as the anterior cutaneous nerves of the thorax, which supply the skin on the front of the thorax. The second anterior cutaneous nerve may be connected to the medial supraclavicular nerves of the cervical plexus; twigs from the sixth intercostal nerve supply abdominal skin in the upper part of the infrasternal angle.

Branches – Numerous slender muscular filaments supply the intercostals, serratus posterior superior and transversus thoracis. Anteriorly, some cross the costal cartilages from one intercostal space to another.

Each intercostal nerve gives off a collateral and a lateral cutaneous branch before it reaches the angle of the adjoining ribs. The collateral branch follows the inferior border of its space in the same intermuscular place as the main nerve, which it may rejoin before it is distributed as an additional anterior cutaneous nerve. The lateral cutaneous branch accompanies the main nerve a little way and then pierces the intercostal muscles obliquely. With the exception of the lateral cutaneous branches of the first and second intercostal nerves, each divides into anterior and posterior rami that subsequently pierce serratus anterior. Anterior branches run forwards over the border of pectoralis major to supply the overlying skin; those of the fifth and sixth also supply twigs to a variable number of upper digitations of external oblique. Posterior branches run backwards and supply the skin over the scapula and latissimus dorsi.

The lateral cutaneous branch of the second intercostal nerve is the intercostobrachial nerve (**Fig. 49.31**). It crosses the axilla to gain the medial side of the arm and joins a branch of the medial cutaneous nerve of the arm. It then pierces the deep fascia of the arm, and supplies the skin of the upper half of the posterior and medial parts of the arm, communicating with the posterior cutaneous branch of the radial nerve. Its size is in inverse proportion to the size of the medial cutaneous nerve. A second intercostobrachial nerve often branches off from the anterior part of the third lateral cutaneous nerve and sends filaments to the axilla and the medial side of the arm.

The seventh to eleventh thoracic ventral rami

The ventral rami of the seventh to eleventh thoracic nerves are continued anteriorly from the intercostal spaces into the abdominal wall; their further course is described in Chapter 68.

Lesions of the intercostal nerves

Subluxation of the interchondral joints between the lower costal cartilages may trap the intercostal nerves, causing referred abdominal pain. The dorsal cutaneous branch of an intercostal nerve can become entrapped as it penetrates the fascia of erector spinae. This produces an area of numbness, usually with painful paraesthesiae, which extends from the midline laterally c.10 cm and c.10 cm in length (notalgia paraesthetica). Commonly, the area between the medial edge of the scapula and the spine is affected. The anterior cutaneous branches of the intercostal nerves can become entrapped as they penetrate the fascia of rectus abdominis; this produces an area of numbness on the abdomen, usually with painful paraesthesiae, which extends from the midline laterally 10 or 12 cm (rectus abdominis syndrome).

The twelfth thoracic ventral ramus (subcostal nerve)

The ventral ramus of the twelfth thoracic nerve (subcostal nerve) is larger than the others. It gives a communicating branch to the first lumbar ventral ramus (sometimes termed the dorsolumbar nerve). Like the intercostal nerves, it soon gives off a collateral branch. It accompanies the subcostal vessels along the inferior border of the twelfth rib, passing behind the lateral arcuate ligament and kidney and in front of the upper part of quadratus lumborum. It perforates the aponeurosis of the origin of transversus abdominis and passes forwards between that muscle and internal oblique, to be distributed in the same manner as the lower intercostal nerves. It connects with the iliohypogastric nerve of the lumbar plexus and sends a branch to pyramidalis. The lateral cutaneous branch of the subcostal nerve pierces the internal and external oblique muscles and supplies the lowest slip of the latter. It descends over the iliac crest c.5 cm behind the anterior superior iliac spine (**Fig. 67.3**) and is distributed to the anterior gluteal skin; some filaments reach as low as the greater trochanter of the femur.

THORACIC DORSAL SPINAL RAMI

Thoracic dorsal rami pass backwards close to the vertebral zygapophyseal joints and divide into medial and lateral branches. The medial branch emerges between the joint and the medial edge of the superior costotransverse ligament and intertransverse muscle. The lateral branch runs in the interval between the ligament and the muscle before inclining posteriorly on the medial side of levator costae.

Medial branches of the upper six thoracic dorsal rami pass between and supply semispinalis thoracis and multifidus; they then pierce the rhomboids and trapezius, and reach the skin near the vertebral spines (**Fig. 46.14**). Medial branches of the lower six thoracic dorsal rami are distributed mainly to multifidus and longissimus thoracis; occasionally they give filaments to the skin in the median region. Lateral branches increase in size from above downwards. They run through or deep to longissimus thoracis to the interval between it and iliocostalis cervicis, and supply these muscles and levatores costarum; the lower five or six also give off cutaneous branches, which pierce serratus posterior inferior and latissimus dorsi in line with the costal angles (**Fig. 46.14**). The lateral branches of a variable number of the upper thoracic rami also supply the skin. The lateral branch of the twelfth sends a filament medially along the iliac crest, then passes down to the skin of the anterior part of the gluteal region.

Medial cutaneous branches of the thoracic dorsal rami descend for some distance close to the vertebral spines before reaching the skin. Lateral branches descend for a considerable distance, which may be as much as the breadth of four ribs, before they become superficial; e.g. the branch of the twelfth thoracic reaches the skin only a little way above the iliac crest.

REFERENCE

Kurihara Y, Yakushiji YK, Matsumoto J, Ishikawa T, Hirata K 1999 The ribs: anatomic and radiologic considerations. Radiographics 19: 105–19.
Includes some chest wall and rib cage abnormalities.

Breast

The breasts form a secondary sexual feature of females and are the source of nutrition for the neonate. They are also present in a rudimentary form in males. The breasts are the site of malignant change in as many as one in ten women. For reviews of normal breast structure, consult Ellis et al (1993).

In young adult females, each breast is a rounded eminence lying within the superficial fascia, largely anterior to the upper thorax but spreading laterally to a variable extent (**Fig. 58.1**). Breast shape and size depend upon genetic, racial and dietary factors, and the age, parity and menopausal status of the individual. Breasts may be hemispherical, conical, variably pendulous, piriform or thin and flattened. In the adult female the base of the breast – its attached surface – extends vertically from the second or third to the sixth rib, and from the sternal edge, medially, almost to the midaxillary line laterally in the transverse plane. The superolateral quadrant is prolonged towards the axilla along the inferolateral edge of pectoralis major, from which it projects a little, and may extend through the deep fascia up to the apex of the axilla (the axillary tail).

The breast lies upon the deep pectoral fascia, which in turn overlies pectoralis major and serratus anterior, and inferiorly, external oblique and its aponeurosis as the latter forms the anterior wall of the sheath of rectus abdominis. Between the breast and the deep fascia is loose connective tissue in the 'submammary space'. This allows the breast some degree of movement on the deep pectoral fascia. (Advanced mammary

carcinoma may, by invasion, fix the breast to pectoralis major.) Occasionally, small projections of glandular tissue may pass through the deep fascia into the underlying muscle in normal subjects.

The nipple projects from the centre of the breast anteriorly (**Figs 58.1, 58.2**); its shape varies from conical to flattened, depending on nervous, hormonal, developmental and other factors. Its level in the thorax varies widely, but is at the fourth intercostal space in most young women. In the nulliparous it is pink, light brown or darker, depending on the general melanization of the body. Occasionally the nipple may not evert during prenatal development (p. 973), and it remains permanently retracted and so causes difficulty in suckling.

The areola is a disc of skin, which circles the base of the nipple, varying in colour from pink to dark brown depending on parity and race (**Figs 58.1, 58.2**).

SKIN

The female breast is covered by typical thin skin of the anterior thoracic wall, and bears fine hairs (Chapter 8). Where it covers the nipple, which lacks hairs, and the surrounding areola, the skin is modified. Here, the skin has a convoluted surface, and contains many sweat and sebaceous glands which open directly on to the skin surface. The oily secretion of the sebaceous glands is a protective lubricant during

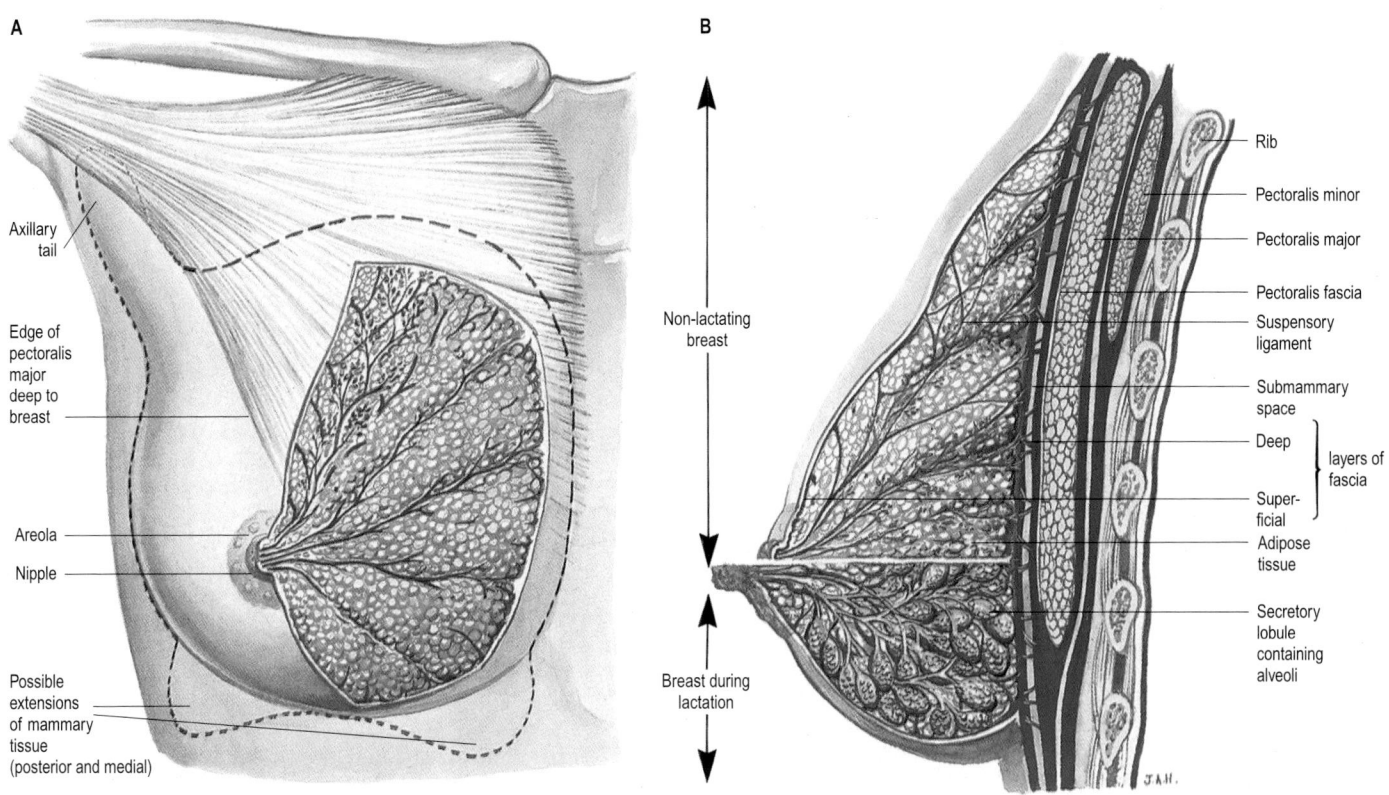

Fig. 58.1 A, The macroscopic structure of the breast. **B**, Changes during lactation.

A

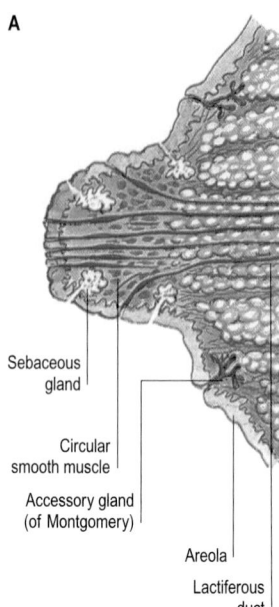

Fig. 58.2 A, Section of the nipple. **B**, Cross-section of the nipple. There is a corrugated layer of stratified squamous keratinized epithelium over the nipple surface; 20 or more lactiferous ducts (L) open onto the surface; sebaceous glands (S) are deep to the epidermis. (**B**, by permission from Dr JB Kerr, Monash University, from Kerr JB 1999 Atlas of Functional Histology. London: Mosby.)

Sebaceous gland

Circular smooth muscle

Accessory gland (of Montgomery)

Areola

Lactiferous duct

B

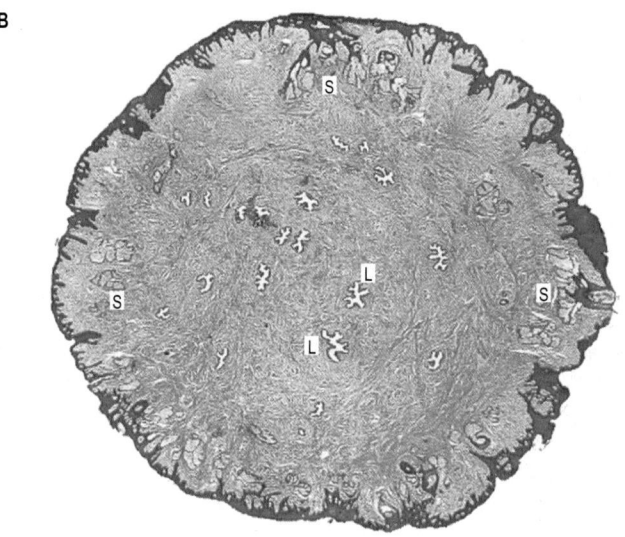

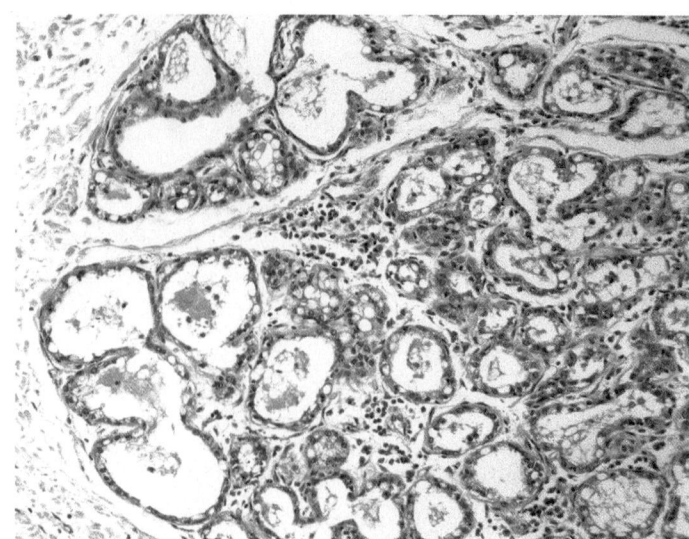

Fig. 58.3 The peripheral part of a lactating breast lobule enclosed by a connective tissue septum (left). The alveoli are distended by milk secretion. Milk protein appears as eosinophilic material in the lumen and milk fat as pale cytoplasmic vacuoles in the flattened alveolar epithelium. Intralobular connective tissue between the alveoli contains a prominent lymphocytic infiltration, including plasma cells secreting IgA. (Photograph by Sarah-Jane Smith.)

lactation. Other areolar glands are intermediate in structure between mammary and sweat glands: they enlarge in pregnancy and lactation as subcutaneous tubercles. Melanocytes are quite numerous in the skin of the nipple and areola, giving them a darker colour than the remainder of the breast. Further darkening of the nipple and areola occurs during the second month of pregnancy, a change that persists to a variable degree.

CUTANEOUS VASCULAR SUPPLY AND LYMPHATIC DRAINAGE

Medially, the skin of the breast is supplied by branches from the anterior intercostal arteries as the vessels pass laterally supplying the intercostal muscles. Laterally the skin is supplied by branches from the lateral thoracic artery, a branch of the axillary artery, and by lateral cutaneous branches of the posterior intercostal arteries. The venous drainage of the areola and surrounding skin is into a circular venous plexus, which drains into the veins, which accompany the corresponding arteries, i.e. the axillary, internal thoracic and intercostal veins. The density of lymphatic drainage channels in the skin is much greater than for the soft tissue of the breast. Lymph drainage is towards the axilla. The lymphatics of the lateral skin of the breast, including the subareolar plexus, pass to the pectoral nodes. Vessels near the sternal edge pass between the costal cartilages to parasternal nodes and also anastomose across the sternum. A few vessels from the upper pectoral region ascend over the clavicle to drain to the inferior deep cervical nodes.

INNERVATION OF THE NIPPLE AND AREOLA

The innervation of the nipple and areola is described on page 972.

SOFT TISSUE

The breasts are composed of lobes, which contain a network of glandular tissue consisting of branching ducts and terminal secretory lobules in a connective tissue stroma. Although the lobes are usually described as discrete territories within the breast, they merge at their edges and do not appear distinct during surgery. The connective tissue stroma which surrounds the lobules is dense and fibrocollagenous, whereas intra-lobular connective tissue has a loose texture, which allows the rapid expansion of secretory tissue during pregnancy (**Figs 58.1, 58.3**). Fibrous condensations of stromal tissue extend from the ducts to the dermis. These are often well developed in the upper part of the breast as suspensory ligaments which assist in supporting the breast tissue. Elsewhere in the normal breast, fibrous tissue surrounds the glandular components and extends to the skin and nipple, assisting in the mechanical coherence of the gland. The interlobar stroma contains variable amounts of adipose tissue, which contributes largely to the increase in breast size at puberty (p. 974).

VASCULAR SUPPLY AND LYMPHATIC DRAINAGE

Arteries

The breasts are supplied by branches of the axillary artery, the internal thoracic artery, and some intercostal arteries. The axillary artery supplies blood from several branches, namely the superior thoracic, the pectoral branches of the thoraco-acromial artery, the lateral thoracic (via branches which curve around the lateral border of pectoralis major to supply the lateral aspect of the breast) and the subscapular artery. The internal thoracic artery supplies perforating branches to the anteromedial part of the breast. The second to fourth anterior intercostal arteries supply perforating branches more laterally in the anterior thorax. The second perforating artery is usually the largest, and supplies the upper region of the breast, and the nipple, areola and adjacent breast tissue.

Veins

There is a circular venous plexus around the areola. From this, and from the glandular tissue, blood drains in veins which accompany the corresponding arteries that supply the breast, i.e. to the axillary, internal thoracic and intercostal veins. Great individual variation may occur. The internal thoracic veins are venae comitantes to the inferior half of the internal thoracic artery and veins unite at the third costal cartilage to ascend medial to the artery, ending in the brachiocephalic vein.

Lymphatic drainage (Fig. 58.4)

The lymphatic drainage of the breast can be very variable. There are communicating lymphatic plexi in the interlobular connective tissue and the walls of the lactiferous ducts and the subareolar region. There is also a plexus of minute vessels on the subjacent deep fascia, but it plays little part in normal lymphatic drainage or in early spread of carcinoma. It offers an alternative route when the usual pathways are obstructed.

Axillary nodes receive more than 75% of the lymph from the breast. There are 20–40 nodes, grouped artificially as pectoral (anterior), subscapular (posterior), central and apical. Surgically, the nodes are described in relation to pectoralis minor. Those lying below pectoralis minor are the low nodes (level 1), those behind the muscle are the middle group (level 2), while the nodes between the upper border of pectoralis minor and the lower border of the clavicle are the upper or apical nodes (level 3). There may be one or two other nodes between pectoralis minor and major. Efferent vessels directly from the breast pass round the anterior axillary border through the axillary fascia to the pectoral lymph nodes; some may pass directly to the subscapular nodes. A few vessels pass from the superior part of the breast to the apical axillary nodes, sometimes interrupted by the infraclavicular nodes or by small, inconstant, interpectoral nodes.

Most of the remainder drains to parasternal nodes from the medial and lateral parts of the breast; they accompany perforating branches of the internal thoracic artery. Lymphatic vessels occasionally follow lateral cutaneous branches of the posterior intercostal arteries to the intercostal nodes. Cutaneous lymphatic drainage is described on page 970.

Efferent vessels drain from the subareolar plexus to the contralateral breast, the internal lymph node chain and the axillary lymph nodes. The internal thoracic chain drains via the mediastinal lymph nodes to the para-aortic lymph nodes, bronchomediastinal trunks, thoracic duct and right thoracic duct and, inferiorly, via the superior and inferior epigastric lymphatic routes to the groin.

Axillary surgery in breast cancer

Axillary lymph node sampling is a standard component of the breast surgery for breast cancer. This is primarily performed because the presence of metastases and axillary lymph nodes has strong prognostic significance and influences adjuvant therapy. However, axillary lymph node dissection can lead to chronic postoperative problems such as pain, reduced mobility of the arm, impaired sensation, lymphoedema and occasionally the development of a seroma. The vessels and nerves have to be carefully identified to preserve the medial pectoral vessels and nerve, long thoracic nerve and the thoracodorsal artery, vein and nerve.

Lymphatic drainage in breast cancer and role of sentinel lymph node biopsy

Lymphatic mapping with sentinel lymph node biopsy has become an important technique in the staging of patients with breast cancer. Radio-labelled colloids are injected into the peri-tumoural tissue and the lymph node site where the radiolabelled tracer accumulates identified (Rubio & Klimberg 2001, Tanis et al 2001). Peri-areolar, subareolar, intraductal, or subcutaneous injection over the primary tumour site are also used. The lymph node where the isotope accumulates is considered to be the node that receives drainage from the primary tumour and is then biopsied to assess lymph node involvement. If there is no evidence

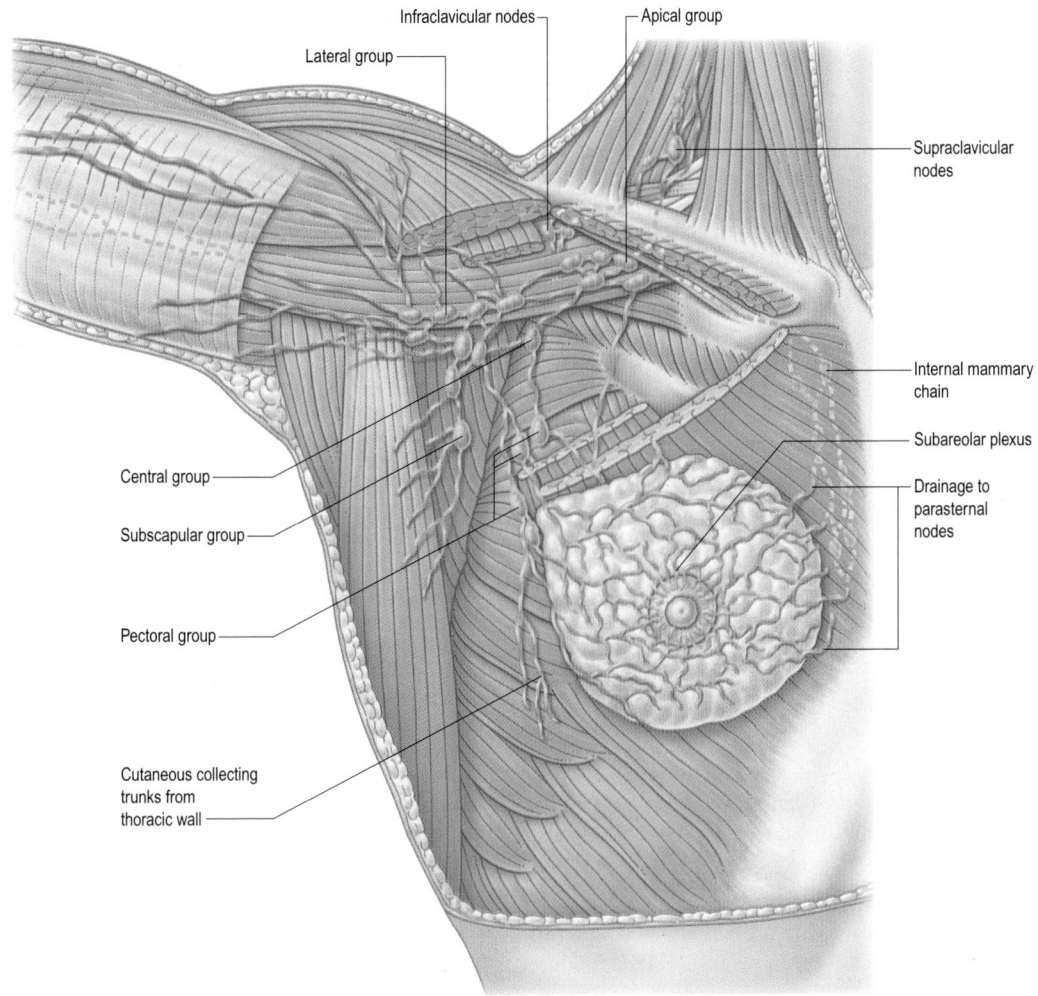

Fig. 58.4 Lymph vessels of the breast and the axillary lymph nodes.

of metastatic involvement then it is unlikely that metastases will be present in the axillary lymph nodes, which are distal to the node that has been biopsied. The accuracy of this technique has been shown to be over 90% in a number of studies. Involvement of the sentinel lymph node is a poor prognostic marker and indicates the need for axillary dissection and clearance. If the biopsy is negative, then the inference is that the other lymph nodes in the axilla will be clear of tumour, and sparing the need to remove these nodes removes the morbidity of an axillary dissection.

INNERVATION

The breast is innervated by anterior and lateral branches of the fourth to sixth intercostal nerves, which carry sensory and sympathetic efferent fibres. The nipple is supplied from the anterior branch of the lateral cutaneous branch of T4 (Yap et al 2002). This forms an extensive plexus within the nipple, and its sensory fibres terminate close to the epithelium as free endings, Meissner corpuscles and Merkel disc endings (p. 59). These are essential in signalling suckling to the central nervous system. Secretory activities of the gland are largely controlled by ovarian and hypophyseal hormones rather than by efferent motor fibres. The areola has fewer sensory endings.

MICROSTRUCTURE

The microstructure of breast tissue varies with age, time in the menstrual cycle, pregnancy and lactation (p. 974). The following description relates to the mature, resting breast. For most of their lengths, the ducts are lined by columnar epithelium (**Fig. 58.5**). In the larger ducts these are two cells thick, but in the smaller ones only a single layer of columnar or cuboidal cells is present. The bases of these cells are in close contact with numerous myoepithelial cells of ectodermal origin, similar to those of certain other glandular epithelia (**Fig. 58.9**). Myoepithelial cells are so numerous that they form a distinct layer surrounding the ducts and presumptive alveoli and give the epithelium a bilayered appearance.

Lactiferous ducts draining each lobe of the breast pass through the nipple and open on to its tip as 15–20 orifices. Near its orifice, each of these ducts is slightly expanded as a lactiferous sinus, which, in the lactating breast, is further dilated by the presence of milk. Each lactiferous duct is therefore connected to a system of ducts and lobules, surrounded by connective tissue stroma, collectively forming a lobe of the mammary gland. Lobules consist of the portions of the glands that have secretory potential. Their structure varies according to hormonal status. In the mature resting breast each lobule consists of a cluster of blind-ended, branched ductules whose termini lack terminal alveoli (acini), which are the sites of milk secretion in the lactating breast. The stratified cuboidal lining is replaced by keratinized stratified squamous epithelium, continuous with the epidermis, close to the openings of the lactiferous ducts on the nipple. Shed squames may sometimes block the duct apertures in the non-pregnant breast.

Internally the nipple is composed mostly of collagenous dense connective tissue and contains numerous elastic fibres which wrinkle the overlying skin. Smooth muscle cells, arranged in a predominantly circular direction, are present in, and just deep to, the nipple. Their contraction, induced by cold or tactile stimuli (e.g. in suckling), causes erection of the nipple and wrinkling of the surrounding areola.

The stroma of the breast, including interlobar adipose tissue, is described on page 970.

BREAST CANCER

Breast cancer is a common disease, particularly in postmenopausal women (see Fentiman 1993). Male breast cancers make up c.1% of all mammary malignancies (p. 974) and may include tissue beyond the areolar boundary.

Breast cancers arise within the epithelia of lobules or ducts. As they increase in size and infiltrate the stroma they often lead to a fibrous tissue reaction. Breast lumps may be classified into those with clinical signs suggesting malignancy, i.e. hard and irregular, skin-tethering, muscle fixation, skin infiltration or oedema (peau d'orange), and those which are mobile and without sinister signs. Investigations include needle aspiration, which will drain cysts, or in the case of a solid lump, obtaining cells for cytological evaluation. Additional investigations include mammography and ultrasonography, which can distinguish

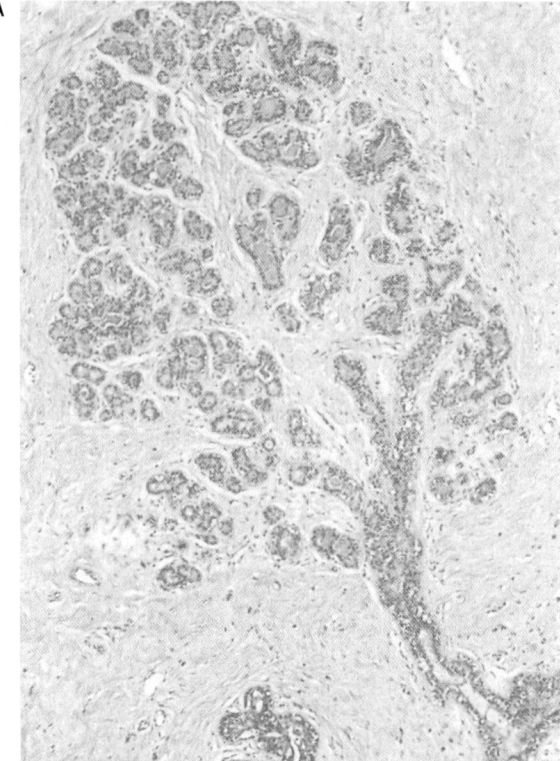

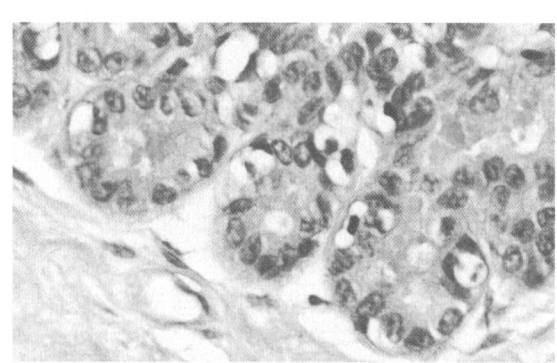

Fig. 58.5 A, A glandular lobule surrounded by collagenous interlobular connective tissue in the mature resting breast. A terminal duct (bottom right) branches extensively to terminate in rudimentary acini, which are shown at higher magnification in the lower panel (**B**). (By permission from Young B, Heath JW 2000 Wheater's Functional Histology. Edinburgh: Churchill Livingstone.)

cysts from solid lumps. A common problem in young women is the fibroadenoma, an overgrowth of a lobule.

If a breast lump has to be removed, incision should be based whenever possible in the relaxed skin tension lines for best cosmetic results, although for women with larger lumps which may be malignant, the incision should be compatible with a possible subsequent mastectomy. Most women with single breast cancers up to 4 cm in diameter are treated by breast conservation rather than mastectomy. This is a combination of surgery (tumour excision and axillary lymph node sampling or clearance) together with external radiotherapy. Patients with larger tumours are treated by modified radical mastectomy with clearance of the axilla and preservation of the nerve to serratus anterior, latissimus dorsi and the lateral and medial pectoral nerves. Failure to preserve the nerve to serratus anterior will result in winging of the scapula and reduced function of the shoulder.

Patients with bloodstained nipple discharge without a palpable lump are treated by duct excision (microdochectomy) carried out through a circumareolar incision. Bloodstained nipple discharge is caused by either an intraduct papilloma, or duct ectasia, and only rarely (5% of cases) is it due to malignancy.

The papillary ducts are radially orientated and incisions should hence also be radial. An obstructed lactiferous duct may distend as a galactocele. Abscesses may occur between the septa in the glandular tissue, subcutaneously near the papilla or between gland and deep fascia anterior to the pectoralis major.

RECONSTRUCTIVE SURGERY FOR BREAST CANCER DISEASE

Breast reconstruction may be performed at the time of mastectomy for breast cancer, or at a later stage (Serletti & Moran 2000). During a mastectomy, skin as well as the glandular breast tissue is removed, and so a reconstructive procedure needs to replace both skin and volume. This can be achieved in a number of ways.

First, the existing skin can be stretched by placing a tissue expander underneath it and gradually inflating the expander until the skin has stretched to the required amount. The expander then acts as an implant.

Second, the skin and volume component of the breast can be replaced by the latissimus dorsi musculocutaneous flap with or without an underlying silicone breast implant. Here latissimus dorsi with an overlying paddle of skin is raised on its dominant vascular pedicle consisting of the thoracodorsal artery and vein which enter the muscle on its deep surface. These vessels send perforating branches through the muscle to the overlying skin. The flap is transferred in an arc from the back to the front of the chest and fashioned to make a new breast. An implant is usually required to provide additional volume replacement, in which case it is placed beneath the flap.

The donor defect on the back is directly sutured and there is minimal coding from the ectopic transfer of latissimus dorsi.

Third, the skin and volume component of the breast can be replaced by a transverse rectus abdominis musculocutaneous flap (TRAM flap). Here a portion of one rectus abdominis and an overlying paddle of skin is raised on either of its two main vascular pedicles. This can be either the superior epigastric artery or the deep inferior epigastric artery. Cutaneous perforators near the level of the umbilicus pass to the skin in two rows (a medial and a lateral row). If the superior epigastric artery is used as the pedicle for the flap then the deep inferior epigastric artery is ligated and the flap is swung on the pedicle and tunnelled up into the chest where it is fashioned into a new breast. If the deep inferior epigastric artery is used as the pedicle then the superficial epigastric artery is divided and the flap is transferred as a free flap and the deep inferior epigastric artery and vein are anastomosed to recipient vessels in either the chest (internal thoracic vessels by removing the third costal cartilage) or the axilla. The advantage of the TRAM flap over the latissimus dorsi flap is that there is sufficient volume to reconstruct even a large breast without the need for an implant. The donor defect in the abdomen is sutured directly. It is possible to dissect a single cutaneous perforator through rectus abdominus to its origin from the deep inferior epigastric artery and so obviate the need to sacrifice this muscle when raising the flap. The flap is then named a DIEP flap (deep inferior epigastric artery perforator flap).

DEVELOPMENT

The epithelial/mesenchymal interactions which will give rise to the glandular tissue of the breast, in both sexes, can first be seen at about the fifth or sixth week, when two ventral bands of thickened ectoderm, the mammary ridges or milklines, extend from the axilla to the inguinal region. Usually invagination of the thoracic mammary bud occurs by day 49, and the remaining mammary line involutes.

The thoracic ectodermal ingrowths branch into 15–20 solid buds of ectoderm which will become the lactiferous ducts and their associated lobes of alveoli in the fully formed gland. These are surrounded by somatopleuric mesenchyme which forms the connective tissue, fat and vasculature and is invaded by the mammary nerves. By proliferation, elongation and further branching the alveoli are formed and the duct system defined. Nipple formation begins at day 56 and primitive ducts (mammary sprouts) develop at 84 days with canalization occurring at about the 150th day. During the last two months of gestation the ducts become canalized and the epidermis at the point of original development of the gland forms a small mammary pit, into which the lactiferous tubules open (**Fig. 58.6**). Perinatally the nipple is formed by mesenchymal proliferation. Should this fail the ducts open into shallow pits, a malformation known as inverted nipple. Rarely, the nipple may not develop (athelia) although this occurs more commonly in accessory breast tissue.

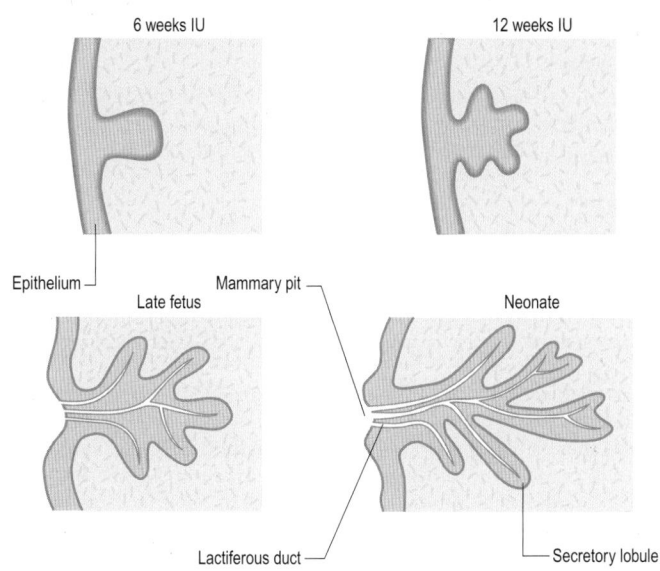

Fig. 58.6 Early development of breast epithelium.

At birth the mammary glands are alike in their stage of development in both sexes; the combination of fetal prolactin and maternal oestrogen may give rise to transient hyperplasia and secretion of 'witch's milk'. In males, thereafter, the mammary glands normally remain undeveloped; in females at puberty, in late pregnancy and during the period of lactation they undergo further, hormone-dependent, developmental changes.

ACCESSORY BREAST TISSUE AND NIPPLES

Polymastia (supernumerary breasts) and polythelia (supernumerary nipples) may develop in males and females anywhere along the length of the mammary ridges (milk lines, **Fig. 58.7**). Conversely breast tissue may not develop at all (amastia) or there may be nipple development but no breast tissue (amazia). Supernumerary breast development is in most cases in the thoracic region (90%), just inferior to the normal breast, but other sites include the axillary (5%) and abdominal regions (5%). Polythelia occurs along the same mammary line but no underlying glandular tissue develops. About 1% of the female population have this condition, however, it is more common in males where the accessory nipple may be mistaken for a mole.

CONGENITAL INVERSION OF NIPPLE

Congenital inversion of the nipples occurs in about 3% of the female population. The condition is bilateral in over 85% of cases and unilateral in about 15%. The majority of the cases are umbilicated (over 75%) where the nipple can be easily pulled down from its depressed position underneath the alveolar surface. The condition is thought to be due to failure of proliferation of the mesenchymal tissue which fails to push the nipple out. The remaining cases are due to invagination of the nipple. Apart from psychological implications, inversion of the nipple may cause recurrent mastitis and difficulty with breast feeding. The abnormality may be corrected surgically.

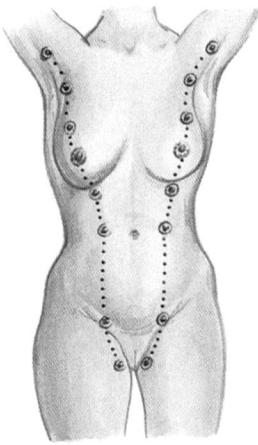

Fig. 58.7 The milk lines.

AGE-RELATED CHANGES IN THE BREAST

PREPUBERTY

The neonatal breast contains lactiferous ducts but no alveoli. Until puberty little branching of the ducts occurs, and slight mammary enlargement is due to the growth of fibrous stroma and fat.

PUBERTY

After puberty in the female, the ducts, stimulated by ovarian oestrogens, develop branches whose ends form solid, spheroidal masses of granular polyhedral cells, the potential alveoli. Oestrogens also promote adipocyte differentiation from mesenchymal cells in the interlobar stroma. Breast enlargement at puberty is largely a consequence of lipid accumulation by these adipocytes.

From puberty onwards, externally recognizable breast development (thelarche) can be divided into five separate phases (**Fig. 58.8**). In Phase I there is elevation of the nipple. In phase II glandular subareolar tissue is present and both nipple and breast project from the chest wall as a single mass. Phase III encompasses increase in diameter and pigmentation of the areola, with proliferation of palpable breast tissue. In phase IV further pigmentation and enlargement in the areola occurs so that the nipple and areola form a secondary mass anterior to the main part of the breast. In phase V a smooth contour to the breast develops.

DURING THE MENSTRUAL CYCLE

Changes occur in the breast tissues in the menstrual cycle. In the follicular phase (days 3–14) the stroma becomes less dense and various changes take place in the ducts. These include the expansion of their lumen, with occasional mitoses but no secretion. In the luteal phase (days 15–28) there is a progressive increase in stromal density and the ducts have an open lumen containing secretion, associated with flattening of epithelial cells. Cell proliferation is maximal on day 26. Thereafter, the ductal system undergoes reduction, and epithelial cell apoptosis is greatest on day 28 of the cycle. These activities may have clinical significance in terms of the most appropriate timing for surgery related to carcinoma of the breast (*see* Fentiman 1993). In addition to these alterations there are changes in blood flow, which are greatest at mid-cycle, and an increase in the water content of the stroma in the second half of the menstrual cycle.

POSTMENOPAUSAL

Progressive atrophy of lobules and ducts occurs after the menopause, with fatty replacement of glandular breast tissue, although a few ducts may remain. The stroma becomes much less cellular and collagenous fibres decrease. The amount of adipose tissue varies widely between individuals, and the breast may return to a condition similar to the pre-pubertal state.

CHANGES ASSOCIATED WITH PREGNANCY AND LACTATION

PREGNANCY

As the output of oestrogen and progesterone produced first by the corpus luteum and later by the placenta rises during pregnancy, the intralobular ductal epithelium proliferates and the number and lengths of their branches therefore increase. Alveoli develop at their termini: with the synthesis and secretion of milk, the alveoli expand as their cells and lumens fill. The myoepithelial cells, which are initially spindle-shaped, become highly branched stellate cells, especially around the alveoli. Adjacent myoepithelial cells intermesh to form a basket-like network around the alveoli and ducts, interposed between the basal lamina and the luminal cells. Their cytoplasm contains actin and myosin filaments and they are contractile.

There is a concomitant reduction in adipose tissue in the stroma. The numbers of lymphocytes, including plasma cells, and eosinophils increase greatly. Blood flow through the breast increases. Secretory activity in the alveolar cells rises progressively in the latter half of pregnancy. In late pregnancy, and for a few days after parturition, their product is different from the later milk and is known as colostrum. This is low in lipid but rich in protein and immunoglobulins, and confers a measure of passive immunity to the neonatal alimentary tract; it also has laxative properties.

Total weight gain of each breast during pregnancy is c.400 g.

LACTATION (Fig. 58.9)

True milk secretion begins a few days after parturition as a result of a reduction in circulating oestrogen and progesterone, a change which appears to stimulate production of prolactin by the anterior hypophysis.

Milk distends the alveoli so that the cells flatten as secretion increases (**Figs 58.1**, **58.3**). The alveolar cell cytoplasm accumulates membrane-bound granules of casein and other milk proteins, and these are released from the apical plasma membrane by membrane fusion (merocrine secretion). Lipid vacuoles are formed directly in the apical cytoplasm as small lipid droplets. They fuse with each other to create large 'milk vacuoles' up to 10 µm across, frequently protruding from the cell surface. These are released as intact lipid droplets with a thin surround of apical plasma membrane and adjacent cytoplasm (apocrine secretion). On hormonal stimulation by oxytocin, myoepithelial cells contract to expel alveolar secretions into the ductal system in readiness for suckling.

After the onset of lactation there is a gradual reduction in the numbers of lymphocytes and eosinophils in the stroma, although plasma cells continue to synthesize IgA for secretion into the milk. Alveolar cells take up IgA synthesized by adjacent plasma cells by endocytosis at their basal surfaces and secrete it apically, as dimers complexed to epithelial secretory component.

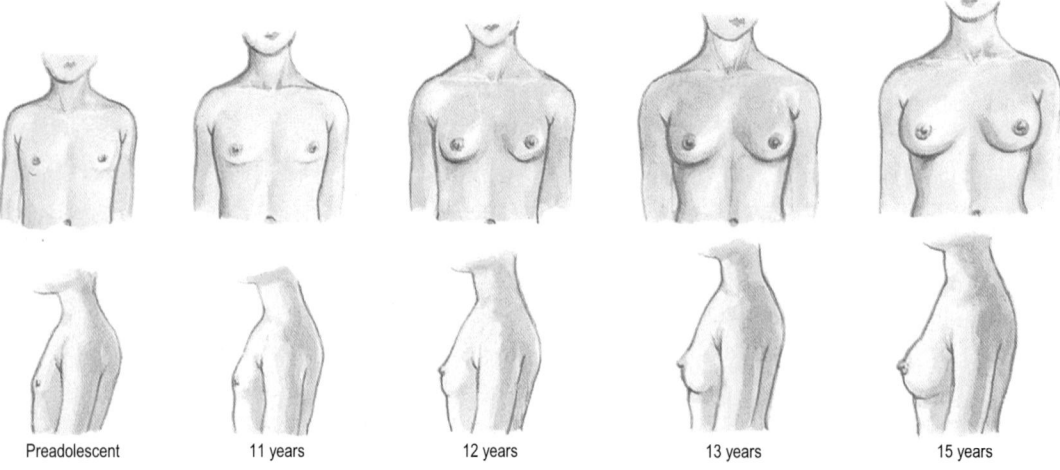

Preadolescent   11 years   12 years   13 years   15 years

Fig. 58.8 Pre and postpubertal development and structure of the female breast demonstrating changes in the contour of the breast.

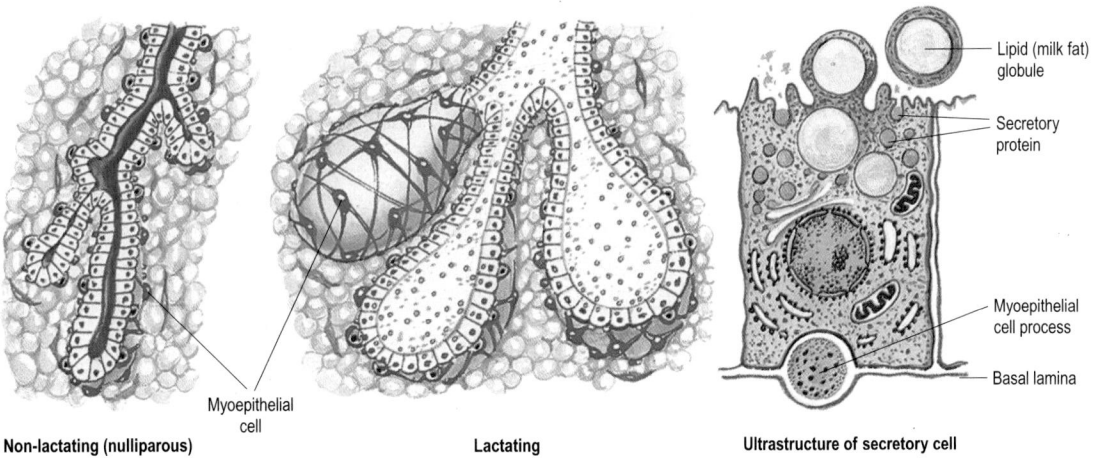

Fig. 58.9 Microstructure of breast epithelium; note that the myoepithelial process is actually about half the relative size shown in the right-hand diagram.

POSTLACTATION

When lactation ceases, which may be after $3^1/_2$ years or longer if frequent suckling is maintained, the secretory tissue undergoes some involution, but the ducts and alveoli never return completely to the pre-pregnant state. Two major processes are responsible for the regression of the alveolar–ductal system: a reduction in epithelial cell size, and a reduction in cell numbers through apoptosis. Gradually the breast tissue reverts to the resting state. If another pregnancy occurs, the resting glandular tissue is reactivated, and the process outlined above recurs. Up to the age of c.50 years, increasing amounts of elastic tissue tend to be laid down around vessels and ducts (elastosis), and also in the stroma, although elastosis does not typically continue thereafter except pathologically.

MALE BREAST

The male breast remains rudimentary throughout life. It is formed of small ducts (without lobules or alveoli) or solid cellular cords and a little supporting fibro-adipose tissue (see Ellis et al 1993). Slight temporary enlargement may occur in the newborn, reflecting the influence of maternal hormones, and again at puberty. The areola is well developed, although limited in area, and the nipple is relatively small. It is usually stated that the ducts do not extend beyond the areola, but glandular tissue can be more extensive.

GYNAECOMASTIA

Gynaecomastia is a benign proliferation of subareolar breast tissue or excessive growth of breast tissue. It is usually bilateral but may be unilateral. It is commonly associated with pain or tenderness, which is thought to be due to accumulation of fluid in the glandular ducts. Histological changes are fibrosis, followed by hyalinization. It is usually due to an imbalance in the ratio of free oestrogens and androgens. Hence it is commonly seen after anti-androgen therapy for conditions such as prostatic cancer, but other drugs such as spironolactone and cimetidine have been implicated.

REFERENCES

Ellis H, Colborn GL, Skandalakis JE 1993 Surgical embryology and anatomy of the breast and its related anatomic structures. Surg Clin North Am 73: 611–32.

Fentiman IS 1993 Detection and treatment of early breast cancer. London: Martin Dunitz.

Rubio IT, Klimberg S 2001 Techniques of sentinel lymph node biopsy. Semin Surg Oncol 20: 214–23.

Serletti JM, Moran SL 2000 Microvascular reconstruction of the breast. Semin Surg Oncol 19: 264–71.

Tanis PJ, Nieweg OE, Valdes Olmos RA, Kroon BB 2001 Anatomy and physiology of lymphatic drainage of the breast from the perspective of sentinel node biopsy. J Am Coll Surg 192(3): 399–409.

Yap LH, Whiten SC, Forster A, Stevenson JH 2002 The anatomical and neuro-physiological basis of the sensate free TRAM and DIEP flaps. Br J Plastic Surg 55: 35–45.

Mediastinum

Strictly speaking, the mediastinum is the partition between the lungs and includes the mediastinal pleura; however, the term is commonly applied to the region between the two pleural sacs. It is bounded anteriorly by the sternum and posteriorly by the thoracic vertebral column (**Figs 59.1, 59.2**), and extends vertically from the thoracic inlet to the diaphragm. For descriptive purposes, it is arbitrarily divided into a superior and an inferior mediastinum, and the latter is subdivided into anterior, middle and posterior parts. The plane of division into superior and inferior mediastina crosses the manubriosternal joint and the lower surface of the fourth thoracic vertebra (**Fig. 59.1**). Detailed accounts of the mediastinal contents are included with descriptions of the respiratory organs (Chapter 63), the heart (Chapter 60) and the oesophagus (p. 986).

SUPERIOR MEDIASTINUM (Figs 59.3, 59.4, 59.5, 59.6, 60.4E,F)

The superior mediastinum lies between the manubrium sterni and the upper four thoracic vertebrae. It is bounded below by the sternal plane, above by the plane of the thoracic inlet and laterally by the mediastinal pleurae. It contains the lower ends of sternohyoid, sternothyroid and longus colli, thymic remnants, internal thoracic arteries and veins, brachiocephalic veins and the upper half of the superior vena cava, the aortic arch, the brachiocephalic, left common carotid and subclavian arteries, the left superior intercostal vein, the vagus, cardiac, phrenic and left recurrent laryngeal nerves, the trachea, oesophagus, the superficial part of the cardiac plexus and the thoracic duct. It also contains the para-

tracheal, brachiocephalic and tracheobronchial lymph nodes associated with their named structures.

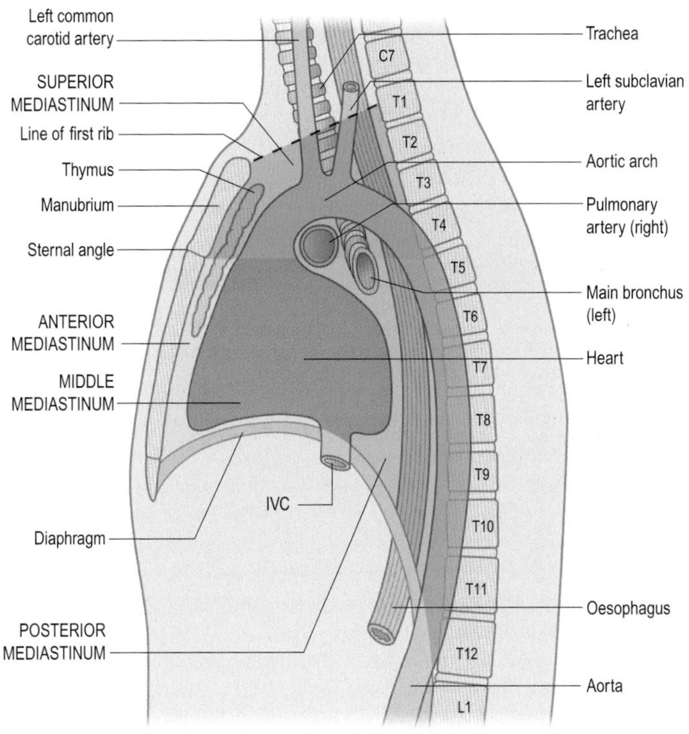

ANTERIOR MEDIASTINUM (Figs 59.7, 59.8, 60.4A,B)

The anterior mediastinum lies between the sternal body and pericardium. It narrows above the fourth costal cartilages, where the pleural sacs come close to each other. It contains loose connective tissue, the sternopericardial ligaments, a few lymph nodes and the mediastinal branches of the internal thoracic artery. It may sometimes contain part of the thymus gland or its degenerated remains (p. 980).

MIDDLE MEDIASTINUM (Figs 59.2, 59.7, 59.8, 60.4A,B)

The middle mediastinum is the broadest part of the inferior mediastinum. It contains the pericardium, heart, ascending aorta, the lower half of the superior vena cava, the terminal azygos vein, tracheal bifurcation and both main bronchi, the pulmonary trunk and the right and left pulmonary arteries, both pulmonary veins, the phrenic nerves, the deep part of the cardiac plexus and the tracheobronchial lymph nodes.

POSTERIOR MEDIASTINUM (Figs 59.2, 59.7, 59.8, 60.4A,B)

The posterior mediastinum is bounded in front by the tracheal bifurcation, pulmonary vessels, pericardium and the posterior part of the upper surface of the diaphragm. Behind, it is bounded by the vertebral column, from the lower border of the fourth to the twelfth thoracic vertebrae, and on each side by the mediastinal pleura. It contains the descending thoracic aorta, the azygos, hemiazygos and accessory azygos veins, the vagus and splanchnic nerves, the oesophagus, thoracic duct and posterior mediastinal lymph nodes.

MEDIASTINAL IMAGING

COMPUTED TOMOGRAPHY AND MAGNETIC RESONANCE IMAGING OF THE MEDIASTINAL SPACES

Computed tomography (CT) scans provide excellent cross-sectional views of the anatomy of the mediastinum (**Figs 59.3, 59.4, 59.5, 59.6, 59.7, 59.8**; compare with **Fig. 59.1**). Intravenous contrast enhancement of the vessels improves the detail of the scan and improves distinction of blood vessels from lymph nodes and soft tissue opacities. Cross-sectional CT scanning is very useful in evaluating the mediastinal spaces, which include the pretracheal space, aortopulmonary window, subcarinal space, right para-tracheal space and posterior tracheal space. These areas are where mediastinal lymph node masses are located and hence of importance in the staging of lung cancer.

The pretracheal space, as seen in cross-section, is bordered by the trachea posteriorly, the superior vena cava and right brachiocephalic vein anteriorly, and the descending aorta and the superior pericardial sinus to the left. The aortopulmonary window is located underneath the aortic arch and above the left pulmonary artery. The trachea forms its medial border and the lungs its lateral border. The right para-tracheal space is in between the lung and the trachea on the anterolateral aspects, whereas the posterior tracheal space is formed between the lung and the posterior lateral aspect of the trachea. The subcarinal space is located below the carina and bounded by the two bronchi. On the right, the azygo-oesophageal recess is located posterior to the subcarinal space and on the left side is the oesophagus. All these areas are in direct continuity with each other and are traversed during cervical mediastinoscopy.

The junctional areas are where the two lungs approach each other. The anterior or prevascular junction is anterior to the great vessels and

Fig. 59.1 The major divisions of the mediastinum (see text for further details). Note that not all mediastinal contents are depicted. IVC, inferior vena cava.

Left common carotid artery — Trachea
SUPERIOR MEDIASTINUM — Left subclavian artery
Line of first rib
Thymus — Aortic arch
Manubrium — Pulmonary artery (right)
Sternal angle
ANTERIOR MEDIASTINUM — Main bronchus (left)
MIDDLE MEDIASTINUM — Heart
IVC
Diaphragm
POSTERIOR MEDIASTINUM — Oesophagus
— Aorta

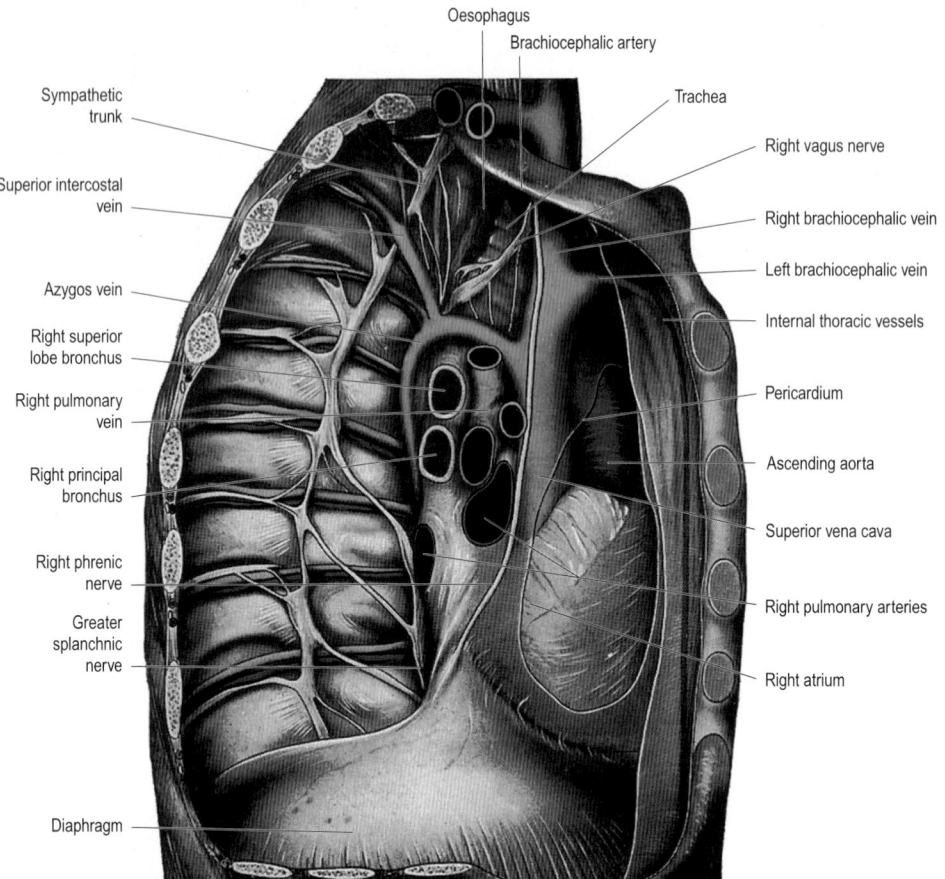

Oesophagus
Brachiocephalic artery
Trachea
Sympathetic trunk
Superior intercostal vein
Azygos vein
Right superior lobe bronchus
Right pulmonary vein
Right principal bronchus
Right phrenic nerve
Greater splanchnic nerve
Diaphragm
Right vagus nerve
Right brachiocephalic vein
Left brachiocephalic vein
Internal thoracic vessels
Pericardium
Ascending aorta
Superior vena cava
Right pulmonary arteries
Right atrium

Fig. 59.2 The mediastinum: right lateral aspect. A part of the pericardial sac has been removed to expose the lateral surface of the right atrium.

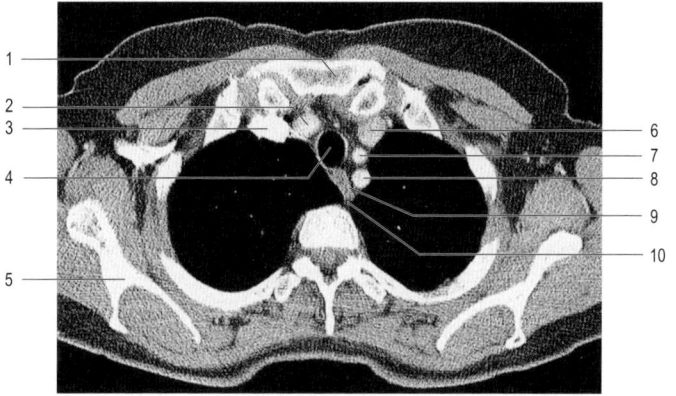

1. Manubrium. 2. Right brachiocephalic artery. 3. Right brachiocephalic vein.
4. Trachea. 5. Scapula. 6. Left brachiocephalic vein. 7. Left common carotid artery.
8. Left subclavian artery. 9. Oesophagus. 10. Posterior junction.

Fig. 59.3 Transverse section of thorax at the level of the junction of the first rib; obtained by computed tomography.

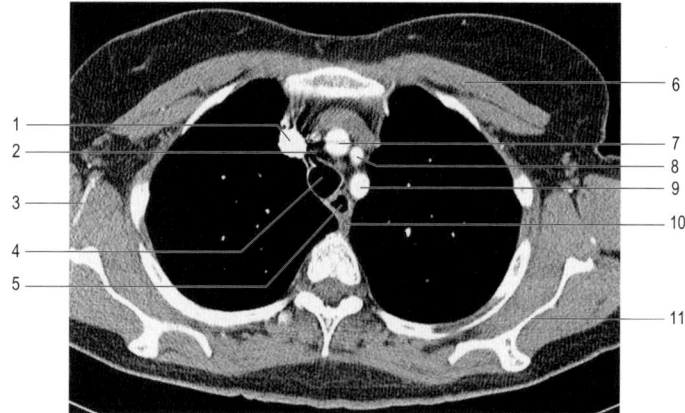

1. Brachiocephalic vein. 2. Pretracheal space. 3. Axillary vein. 4. Trachea. 5. Oesophagus.
6. Pectoralis major. 7. Right brachiocephalic artery. 8. Left common carotid artery.
9. Left subclavian artery. 10. Posterior junction. 11. Scapula.

Fig. 59.4 Transverse section of thorax through the lower portion of the third thoracic vertebra; obtained by computed tomography.

posterior to the chest wall, and between the two lungs. The left brachiocephalic vein, highest mediastinal nodes, thymus and phrenic nerves are located in the anterior junction. The posterior junction is an area posterior to the trachea and is where the lungs lie close to each other. The para-spinal area is a space between the lateral margins of the spine and the lungs. The intercostal vessels and small lymph nodes are located within the para-spinal space. The retrocrural space is between the diaphragmatic crura and the lungs. The structures that pass through it include the aorta, azygos and hemiazygos veins, intercostal arteries and the splanchnic nerves.

NORMAL MEDIASTINAL CONTOURS ON FRONTAL CHEST RADIOGRAPH (Fig. 59.9)

In a standard posteroanterior chest radiograph the X-ray beams pass from back to the front of the chest. The patient is asked to hold their breath in full inspiration and with arms abducted so as to rotate the scapulae and clear the lung fields. In this view (**Fig. 59.9**) the heart and large blood vessels appear as the 'mediastinal shadow'. Forming its left border from above down, are the left subclavian artery, aortic arch ('aortic knuckle'), left auricle and left ventricle. Below the arch, the infundibulum of the right ventricle or the pulmonary trunk may be

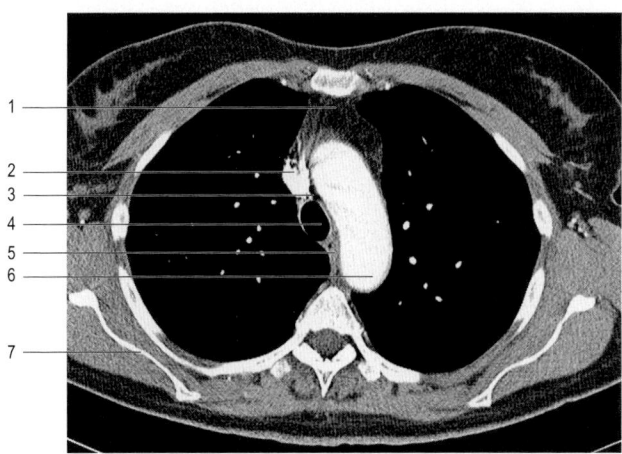

1. Anterior junction. 2. Superior vena cava. 3. Pretracheal space. 4. Trachea.
5. Oesophagus. 6. Arch of aorta. 7. Scapula.

Fig. 59.5 Transverse section of thorax through the middle of the fourth thoracic vertebra and aortic arch; obtained by computed tomography.

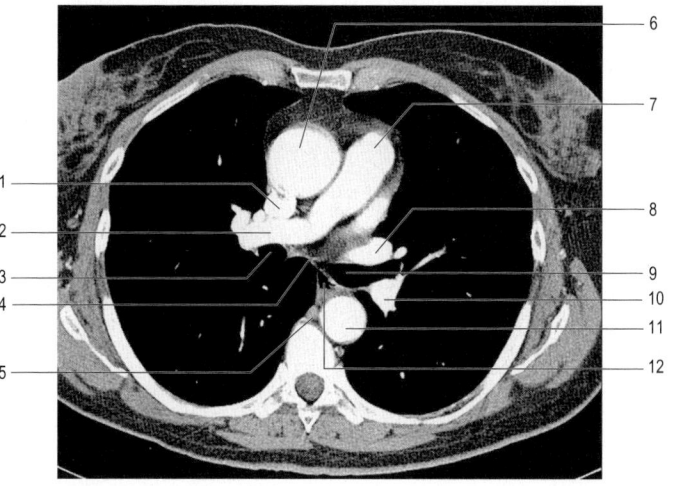

1. Superior vena cava. 2. Right pulmonary artery. 3. Right main bronchus.
4. Subcarinal space. 5. Azygos vein. 6. Ascending aorta. 7. Trunk of pulmonary artery.
8. Superior branch of left pulmonary artery. 9. Left main bronchus.
10. Inferior branch of left pulmonary artery. 11. Descending aorta. 12. Oesophagus.

Fig. 59.7 Transverse section of thorax at the upper border of the sixth thoracic vertebra, below the carina at the level of the pulmonary trunk and the right main pulmonary artery; obtained by computed tomography.

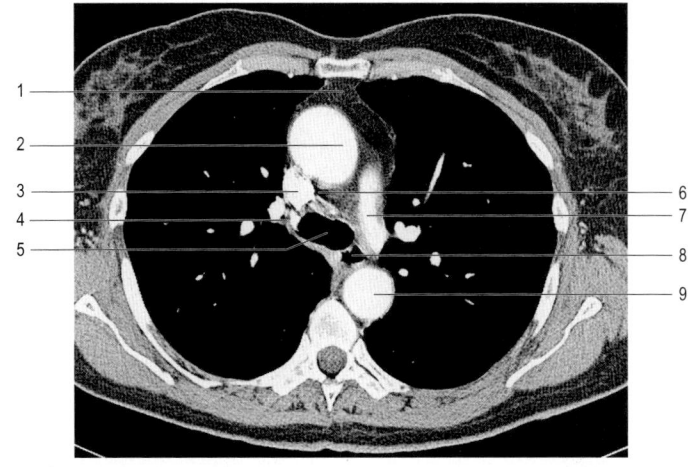

1. Anterior junction. 2. Ascending aorta. 3. Superior vena cava. 4. Right para-tracheal space.
5. Carina (bifurcation of trachea). 6. Superior pericardial recess. 7. Left pulmonary artery.
8. Oesophagus. 9. Descending aorta.

Fig. 59.6 Transverse section of thorax at the level of the lower border of the fourth thoracic vertebra, just at the level of the tracheal bifurcation; obtained by computed tomography.

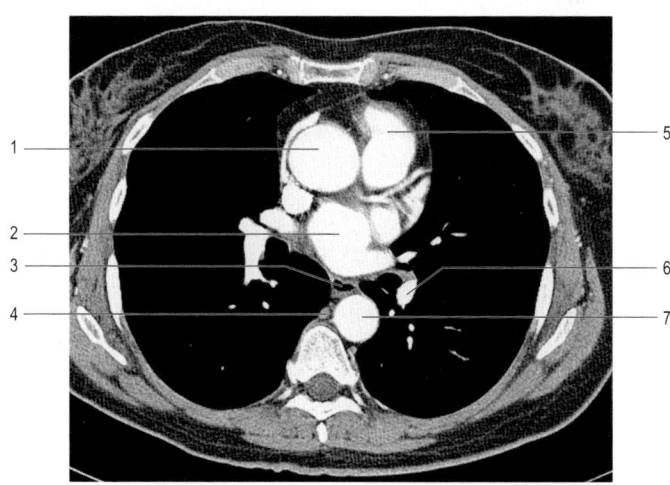

1. Aortic root. 2. Left atrium. 3. Oesophagus. 4. Azygos vein.
5. Right ventricular outflow tract. 6. Left inferior pulmonary vein. 7. Descending aorta.

Fig. 59.8 Transverse section of thorax through the lower portion of the seventh thoracic vertebra, passing through the aortic root; obtained by computed tomography.

recognizable. The descending aorta is visible as a continuous border down to the diaphragm and on some chest radiographs the aortopulmonary stripe, a reflection of the mediastinal pleura, is visible from the aorta to the pulmonary artery. On the right border are the right brachiocephalic vein, superior vena cava, right atrium and thoracic inferior vena cava. A right para-tracheal stripe may be visualized in some chest radiographs. Enlargements or displacements of any of these structures accentuate the normal bulges on the borders of the mediastinal shadow. On both sides, opacities caused by pulmonary vessels associated with the roots of the lungs form hilar shadows. In the upper thorax, the less dense shadow of the trachea is visible in the median plane. The anterior junction is visible in some individuals as the two lungs approximate above the heart. In some patients, the posterior junction line, where the lungs are close together behind the oesophagus, is also visible. The azygo-oesophageal recess is where a portion of the right lung is in contact with the azygos vein and the lateral wall of the

oesophagus; the interface is occasionally seen on a chest radiograph and termed the azygo-oesophageal line. The para-spinal lines are also visible as a line parallel to the right and left margins of the thoracic spine.

NORMAL MEDIASTINAL CONTOURS ON A LATERAL CHEST RADIOGRAPH (Fig. 59.10)

In lateral or oblique views, the cardiac shadow is above the anterior part of the diaphragm. In front of it is the retrosternal space (anterior mediastinum); behind is the retrocardiac space (posterior mediastinum) containing the oesophagus, which can be visualized with a barium swallow (**Fig. 59.11**), and the descending thoracic aorta. Above, the less dense trachea and bronchi are recognizable.

The aortic arch and large vessels produce faint shadows in the superior mediastinum. In this supra-aortic region, the brachiocephalic artery is visible anterior to the trachea. The brachiocephalic veins are

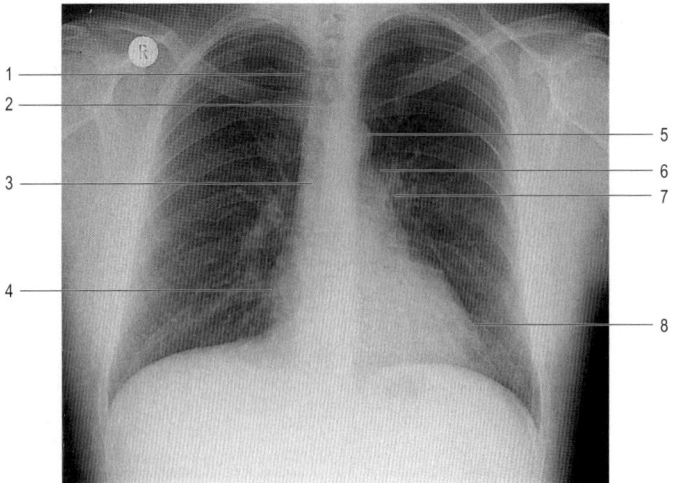

1. Right brachiocephalic vein.   2. Right para-tracheal stripe.   3. Azygo-oesophageal line.
4. Right ventricular border.   5. Aortic arch.   6. Aortopulmonary stripe.   7. Pulmonary artery.
8. Left ventricular border.

Fig. 59.9 Radiograph of chest of adult male: posteroanterior view.

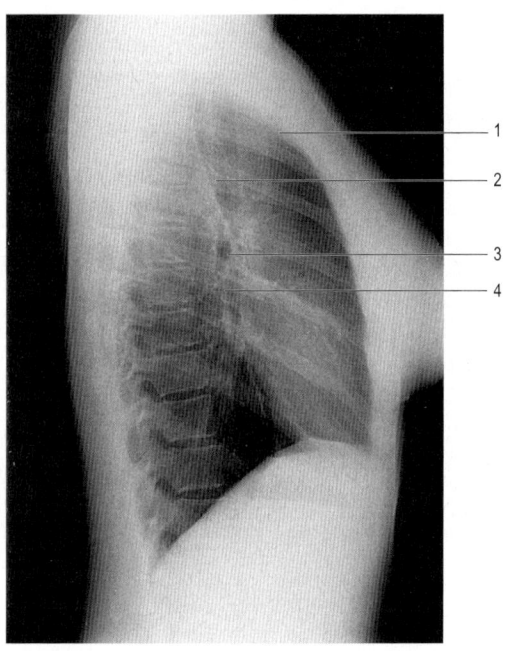

1. Anterior extrapleural line.   2. Posterior tracheal band.   3. Right main bronchus.
4. Bronchus intermedius.

Fig. 59.10 Radiograph of chest of adult female: lateral view.

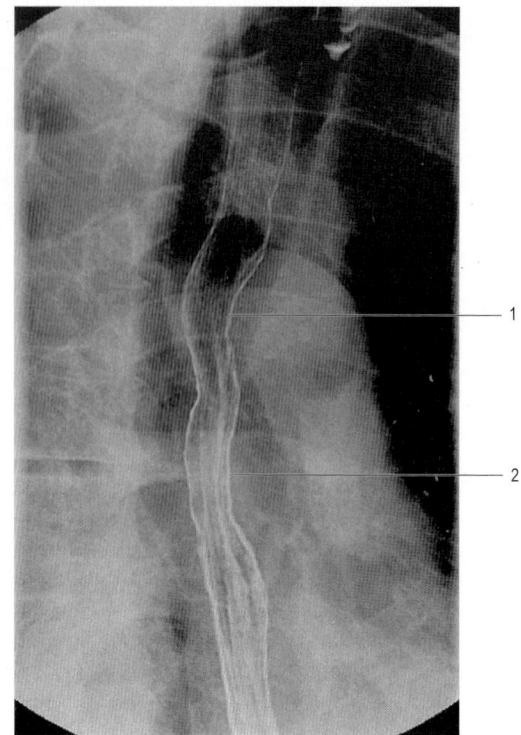

1. Indentation from aortic arch.   2. Indentation from left main bronchus.

Fig. 59.11 Oblique radiograph of the thorax during the oesophageal transit of part of a 'meal' of barium sulphate paste.

visible as an extrapleural bulge directly behind the manubrium. The oesophagus is directly behind the trachea; the posterior tracheal stripe, which is seen in the majority of lateral radiographs, is composed of the anterior oesophageal wall and posterior tracheal wall. The retrosternal line is created by differences in the anterior extent of the right and left lungs and seen as a substernal band in the lower half of the chest. The inferior vena cava is visible in the majority of patients as it drains into the right atrium.

THYMUS (Figs 59.12, 59.13, 59.14, 59.15, 59.16, 59.17)

The thymus is one of the two primary lymphoid organs; the other is the bone marrow. It is responsible for the provision of thymus-processed

lymphocytes (T lymphocytes) to the entire body, and provides a unique microenvironment in which T-cell precursors (thymocytes) undergo development, differentiation and clonal expansion. During this process, the exquisite specificity of T-cell responses is acquired, as is their immune tolerance to the body's own components. These steps involve intimate interactions between thymocytes and other cells (mainly epithelial cells and antigen-presenting cells) and chemical factors in the thymic environment. The thymus is also part of the neuroendocrine axis of the body, and it both influences and is influenced by the products of this axis. Its activity, therefore, varies throughout life under the influence of different physiological states, disease conditions and chemical insults, such as drugs and pollutants.

ANATOMY AND RELATIONS

The appearance of the thymus varies considerably with age. It is largest in the early part of life up to the age of c.15 years, although it persists actively into old age. It is a soft, bilobed organ, and its two parts lie close together side by side, joined in the midline by connective tissue that merges with the capsule of each lobe. The thymus is visible on CT and magnetic resonance imaging (MRI) axial sections just anterior to the aorta and inferior to the brachiocephalic vein. The CT density in younger individuals is homogenous and similar to or greater than that of muscle. With MRI on T_2-weighted images, the signal intensity is similar to or greater than that of fat.

Position and relations

The greater part of the thymus lies in the superior and anterior inferior mediastinum, and the lower border of the thymus reaches the level of the fourth costal cartilages. Superiorly, extensions into the neck are common, reflecting the (bilateral) embryonic origins of the thymus from the third pharyngeal pouch (p. 617). It sometimes reaches the inferior poles of the thyroid gland or even higher. Its shape is largely moulded by the adjacent structures. Inferiorly, the lower end of the right lobe is commonly between the right side of the ascending aorta and the right lung, anterior to the superior cava. Anterior to the gland in the neck are sternohyoid and sternothyroid and fascia; in the thorax the gland is covered anteriorly by the manubrium, the internal thoracic vessels, the upper three costal cartilages, and laterally by the pleura.

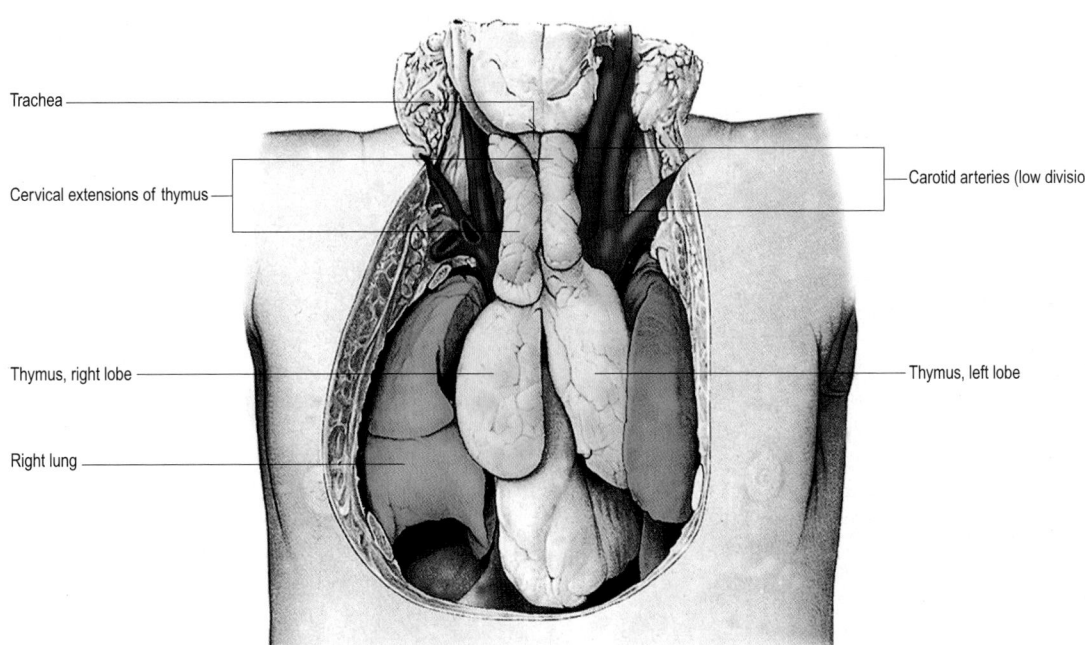

Trachea

Cervical extensions of thymus

Thymus, right lobe

Right lung

Carotid arteries (low division)

Thymus, left lobe

Fig. 59.12 Dissection to display the neonatal thymus.

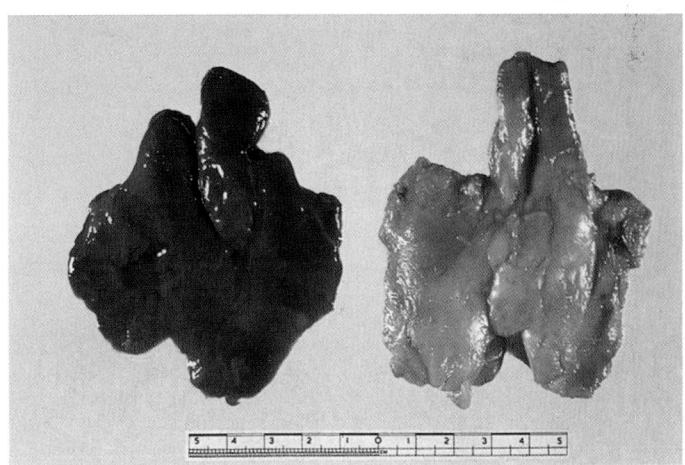

Fig. 59.13 Human thymus from a 9-year-old girl (left) and an 80-year-old man (right). Note the fatty infiltration of the older thymus. (Provided by M Kendall, Department of Physiology, GKT School of Medicine, London.)

Posteriorly, it is in contact with the vessels of the superior mediastinum, especially the left brachiocephalic vein, which may be partly embedded in the gland, and with the upper part of the thoracic trachea and the upper part of the anterior surface of the heart.

Ectopic thymic tissue is sometimes found. Small accessory nodules may occur in the neck. They represent portions that have become detached during their early descent. The thymus may be found even more superiorly as thin strands along this path, reaching the thyroid cartilage or above. Connective tissue marking the line of descent during early development may occasionally run between the thymus and the parathyroids.

VASCULAR SUPPLY AND LYMPHATIC DRAINAGE

Arteries

The thymus is supplied mainly from branches of the internal thoracic and inferior thyroid arteries, which also supply the surrounding mediastinal connective tissue. A branch from the superior thyroid artery is sometimes present. There is no main hilum, but arterial branches pass either directly through the capsule or, more often, into the depths of the interlobar septa before entering the thymus at the junction of the cortex and medulla.

Veins

Thymic veins drain to the left brachiocephalic, internal thoracic and inferior thyroid veins. One or more veins often emerge medially from each lobe of the thymus to form a common trunk opening into the left brachiocephalic vein.

Lymphatic drainage

The thymus has no afferent lymphatics. Efferent lymphatics arise from the medulla and corticomedullary junction and drain through the extravascular spaces in company with the arteries and veins entering and leaving the thymus. Thymic lymphatic vessels end in the brachiocephalic, tracheobronchial and para-sternal nodes. It is not known whether there is perithymic lymphatic drainage.

INNERVATION

The thymus is innervated from the sympathetic chain via the cervicothoracic (stellate) ganglion or from the ansa subclavia and from the vagus. Branches from the phrenic nerve and descending cervical nerve are distributed mainly to the capsule of the thymus. During development, the thymus is innervated by the vagus in the neck before its descent into the thorax. The two lobes are innervated separately through their dorsal, lateral and medial aspects, and rich neural plexuses are formed in the medulla. After its descent, the thymus receives the sympathetic nerves along vascular routes: their terminals branch radially and form a plexus with the vagal fibres at the corticomedullary junction. Innervation is complete by the onset of thymic function. Many of the autonomic nerves are doubtless vasomotor, but many terminal branches also (at least in rodents) leave their perivascular pathways and pass among the cells of the thymus, particularly the medulla, suggesting that they may have other roles. The medulla contains a variety of non-lymphoid cells, including cells positive for vasoactive intestinal polypeptide and acetylcholinesterase, large, non-myoid cells and cells containing oxytocin, vasopressin and neurophysin, of possible neural crest origin. The roles of the nervous system and other neuroendocrine elements in the overall biology of the thymus are little understood.

MICROSTRUCTURE (Figs 59.14, 59.17)

General architecture

It is useful to consider the embryological origins of the thymus in order to understand its cellular organization. The thymus is derived from a number of sources, including epithelial derivatives of the pharyngeal pouches, mesenchyme, haemolymphoid cells and vascular tissue. In section, the thymus can be seen to consist of an outer cortex of densely packed cells mainly of the T-lymphocyte lineage, the thymocytes and an inner medulla, with fewer lymphoid cells.

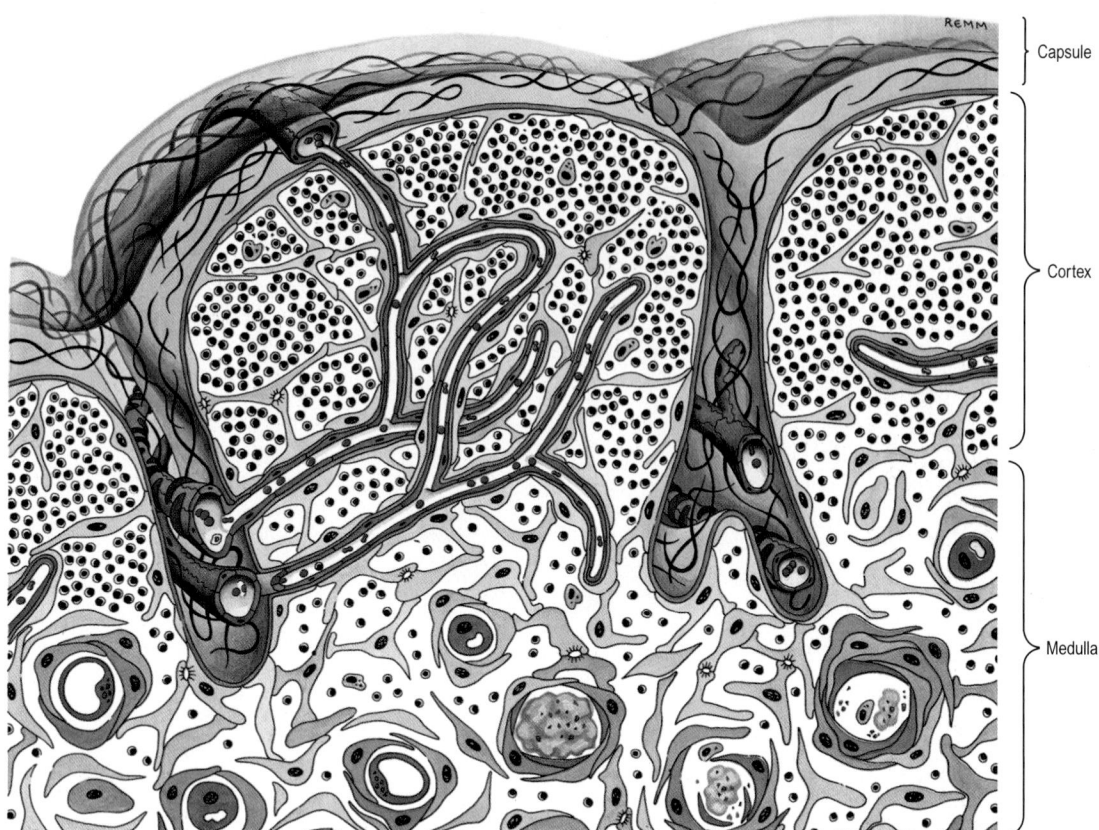

Fig. 59.14 Thymic structure (not drawn to scale). Note the lobular outline, capsule, delicate interlobular septa, cortical lymphocytes, the epithelial cells and the medullary Hassall's corpuscles showing a graded series of increasing maturity. The transcortical circulation is also shown.

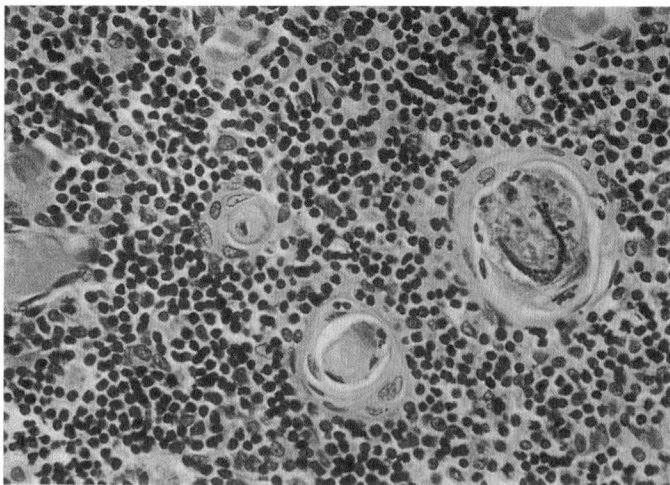

Fig. 59.15 The medulla of a neonatal thymus, showing three concentric Hassall's corpuscles of varying degrees of maturity, surrounded by closely packed lymphocytes and a few epithelial cells with larger nuclei.

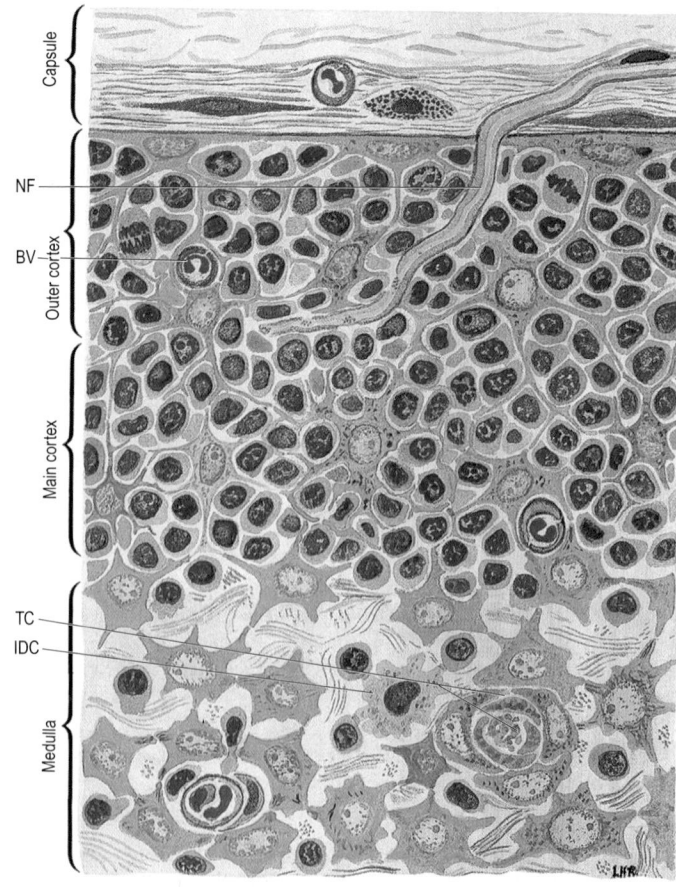

Fig. 59.16 Cellular organization of the thymus showing thymocytes (blue) and epithelial cell framework (green). BV, blood vessel; IDC, interdigitating dendritic cell; NF, nerve fibre; TC, thymic (Hassall's) corpuscle.

Both thymic lobes have a loose fibrous connective tissue capsule, from which septa penetrate to the junction of the cortex and medulla, and partially separate the irregular lobules (Figs 59.14, 59.16), which are each 0.5–2.0 mm in diameter. The connective tissue septa form a route of entry and exit for blood vessels and nerves and carry efferent lymphatics. Most migrant cells enter or leave the thymus by this route. A loose network of interconnected epithelial cells populates the cortex and medulla. In each lobule, the cortex is composed of a superficial outer cortical region (subcapsular cortex), which is a narrow band of cells immediately beneath the capsule, and the main cortex, which is much more extensive. The central medulla of both thymic lobes is continuous from one lobule to the next.

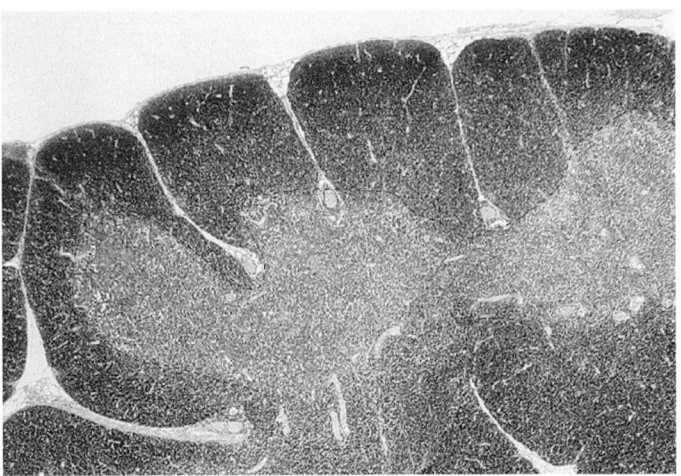

Fig. 59.17 The lobular structure of the thymic cortex (dark blue, resulting from the high density of developing T cells) and shared central medulla. The capsular connective tissue extends into the thymus as septa that divide the cortex into its lobules. (By permission from Kierszenbaum AL 2002 Histology and Cell Biology. St Louis: Mosby.)

Epithelial framework (Figs 59.14, 59.17)

Unlike other lymphoid structures, in which the supportive framework is chiefly collagenous reticular tissue, the thymus contains a network of interconnected epithelial cells supporting lymphoid and other cells. By cell–cell contact and the release of paracrine factors, the epithelial cells create an appropriate microenvironment in which thymic lymphocytes (T cells) develop and mature (p. 80).

Epithelial cells vary in size and shape according to their positions within the thymus. Typically they have pale, oval nuclei, a rather eosinophilic cytoplasm and desmosomal attachments between cells. Intermediate (cytokeratin) filament bundles lie within their cytoplasm. The subcapular cells form a continuous external lining to the thymus beneath its fibrous capsule, and follow its lobulated profile. They ensheath the vessels that pass into it, contributing to the functional blood–thymus barrier. Other cortical epithelial cells extend long processes, with large spaces between them, whereas those of the medulla tend to form more solid cords in addition to the characteristic thymic or Hassall's corpuscles. Although differing in morphology, all the epithelial cells of the thymus share a common origin from pharyngeal endoderm. Lymphocytes lie within the meshes and between the cords formed by these various cells. Large epithelial cells with many associated thymocytes (50 or more) are sometimes called thymic nurse cells.

Hassall's corpuscles are whorls of flattened, concentrically layered medullary epithelial cells, from 30 to 100 μm in diameter, and are characteristic features of the thymic medulla. They start to form before birth and their numbers increase throughout life. Their function is not clear, although they may represent a site for removal of dying apoptotic thymocytes. The centre of the corpuscle is eosinophilic, partly keratinized and often contains cellular debris. Corpuscles with a similar appearance have been described in the palatine tonsil (Ch. 35).

Other non-lymphocytic thymic cells

The thymus also contains cells of the myeloid lineage, fibroblasts and myoid cells. Myeloid lineage cells include monocytes at the corticomedullary junction, mature macrophages throughout, but particularly in the cortex, and interdigitating dendritic (antigen-presenting) cells (p. 81) at the corticomedullary junction and in the medulla. Some dendritic cells are of lymphoid rather than myeloid origin. Fibroblasts are found in the capsule, perivascular spaces and medulla, but are infrequent in the cortex, except in the involuted thymus. Myoid cells, which are relatively rare, are situated mainly in the medulla and at the corticomedullary junction. They are large, rounded cells, and possess a central nucleus surrounded by irregularly arranged bundles of myofilaments. Their functions are unknown, although it has been suggested that their contractions might aid the movement of lymphoid cells across or out of the thymus.

Thymocytes

In the cortex, massive numbers of densely packed small thymocytes (thymic lymphocytes, presumptive T cells) predominate. They occupy the interstices of the epithelial reticulum, which in histological sections they largely obscure, and form c.90% of the total weight of the neonatal thymus. A distinct subcapsular zone is present, housing the thymic stem cells and lymphoblasts undergoing mitotic division. The first stem cells to enter the thymus in the embryo come from the yolk sac and liver during their haemopoietic phases. During later developmental periods, it is probable that all thymic lymphocytes originate in the bone marrow, before passing in the blood stream to the thymus.

Thymocytes undergo mitosis in all cortical zones as the differentiating T cells mature, gradually moving deeper into the cortex. The processes of thymocyte development and maturation to generate T cells depends on the microenvironment provided by epithelial cells, dendritic cells, macrophages and fibroblasts. T cells which fail to recognize self-MHC (histocompatibility) molecules and those which recognize self-antigens (p. 77) die by apoptosis, processes which are necessary for functional immune reactivity and self-tolerance, respectively. Over 95% of cortical thymocytes die within the thymus; the surviving T cells migrate through the walls of venules and efferent lymphatics to enter the circulation and populate secondary lymphoid tissues.

Microcirculation

Vessels in the cortex

The pattern of blood flow differs in the cortex and medulla. Major blood vessels enter the gland at the corticomedullary junction and pass within each lobe, giving off small capillaries to the cortex and larger vessels to the medulla. Most cortical capillaries loop around at different depths in the cortex and join venous vessels at the corticomedullary junction. Some continue through the cortex to join larger veins running in the capsule and so leave the thymus. These smaller capillaries usually have a narrow perivascular space, which sometimes contains pericytes and other cells, but rarely nerves. Sheaths of thymic epithelial cells of the blood–thymus barrier lie between the perivascular space and cortical thymocytes.

Vessels in the medulla

Medullary blood vessels are not so protected by epithelial cells, and those of the corticomedullary junction are only partially ensheathed (usually on their cortical aspect). Medullary vessels are very variable in size, and some may have short lengths of high (cuboidal) endothelium similar to those in lymph nodes and mucosa-associated lymphoid tissue.

Development

The embryology and prenatal development of the thymus are discussed in Chapter 34.

Thymic changes during postnatal life (Fig. 59.18) – At birth, the thymus is most often bilobar. It is 4–6 cm long, 2.5–5 cm wide and 1 cm thick. The thickest part of the gland at birth is not at the superior thoracic aperture, but lies immediately above the base of the heart. During childhood the thymus narrows and lengthens and the cervical portion becomes less noticeable. CT and imaging studies of the thorax have given similar results: the right lobe of the thymus measures c.9 mm and the left c.11 mm in normal children. After the age of 20 years, it decreases to c.5–6 mm in thickness.

The thymus is largest relative to body weight at birth, when its weight is 10–15 g. It rapidly increases to c.20 g, then remains at that weight thereafter. Studies of thymus weight after sudden death have recorded a wide variation at all ages, but the general pattern is that, after the first year of life, when there is an increase, the mean weight is fairly constant at c.20 g until the sixth decade, when a reduction occurs.

Although the weight of the thymus may be fairly constant, it becomes increasingly infiltrated by adipose tissue and so the total amount of active lymphoid tissue becomes progressively smaller. At birth, individual adipocytes may be seen in connective tissue septa, and increased numbers are found within the cortex in the second and third decades. Fatty infiltration is usually complete by the fourth decade, when only the medulla and small patches of associated cortex are spared. This process is independent of obesity.

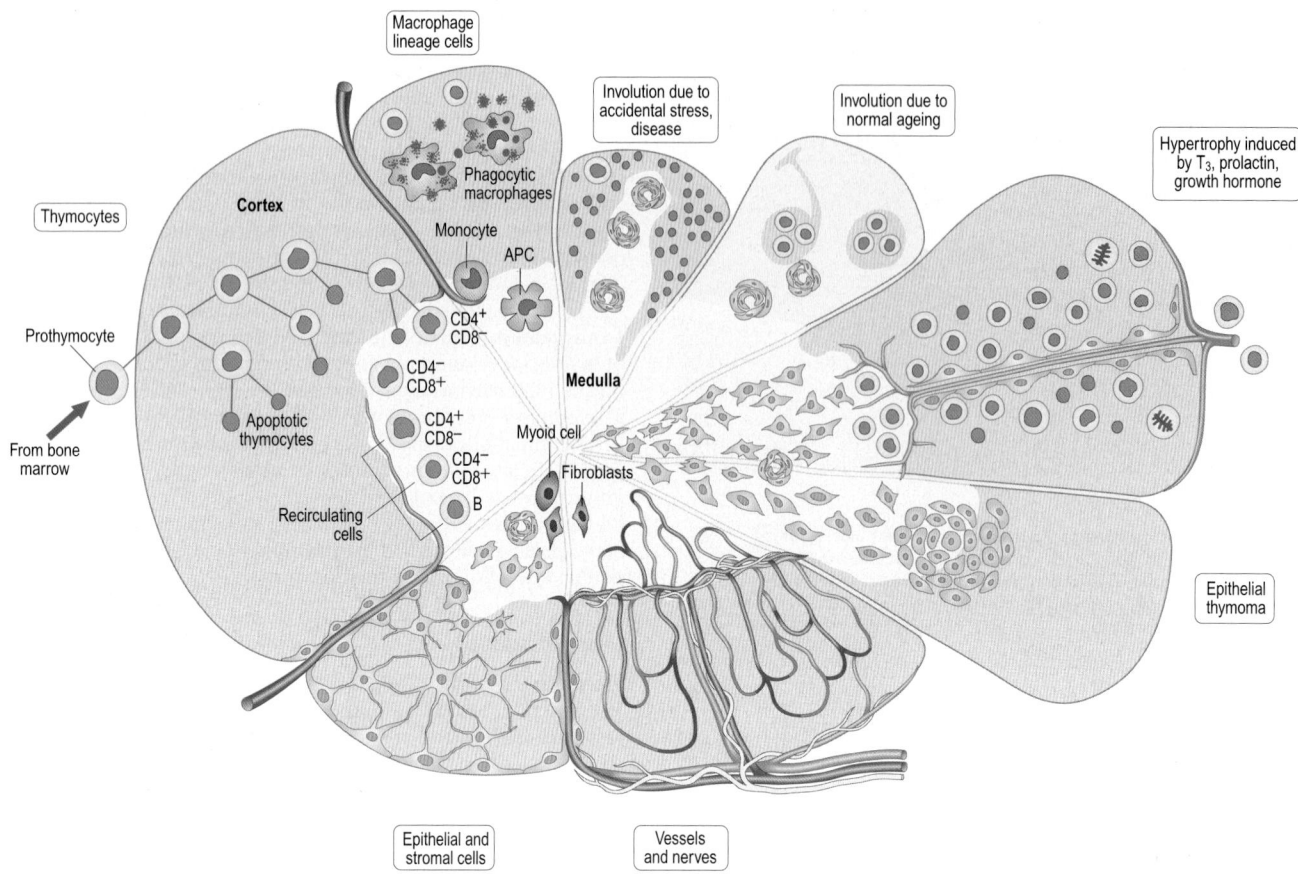

Fig. 59.18 The microscopic organization of the thymus at various stages of life and under different conditions. APC, antigen-presenting cell; T₃, thyroid hormone (tri-iodothyronine).

In children the gland is more pyramidal in shape and firmer than in later life, when its lymphoid content is reduced. In the fresh state it is deep red as a result of its rich vascular supply (**Fig. 59.13**). With age it becomes thinner and greyer, before yellowing as adipose tissue infiltrates the organ, and the amount of lymphoid tissue gradually decreases. Each of the two lobes is partially divided by the ingrowth of shallow septa so that, superficially, the gland appears lobulated. As fatty atrophy proceeds during ageing, this lobulation becomes more distinct. The older thymus can be distinguished from the surrounding mediastinal fat only by the presence of its capsule, although even within greatly atrophied glands there are usually greyer areas around blood vessels, which are formed by persistent lymphoid tissue.

Thymic hormone-secreting cells in the medulla persist throughout life. The reduction in size of the thymus with ageing suggests that the numbers of thymocytes present must be greatly reduced in old age, and this has been found in cultured tissue. However, thymocyte production and differentiation persist throughout life, and T cells from this source continue to populate the peripheral lymphoid tissue, blood and lymph.

Thymomas and myasthenia gravis – Thymic tumours may compress the trachea, oesophagus and large veins in the neck, causing hoarseness, cough, dysphagia and cyanosis. Thymic masses can be accurately assessed according to signal intensity by MRI. Tumours tend to have an inhomogeneous signal intensity. Thymomas may develop in one lobe of the thymus without affecting the other. Many affected patients also have myasthenia gravis and other autoimmune conditions. Myasthenia gravis, a chronic autoimmune disease of adults, presents as a diminution in power of repetitive contraction in certain voluntary muscles. Although there may be more than one condition with these signs, myasthenia gravis is essentially an autoimmune disease in which acetylcholine receptor proteins of neuromuscular junctions are attacked by auto-antibodies. Muscles commonly involved are levator palpebrae superioris (leading to ptosis) and extraocular muscles (leading to diplopia). Other muscles in the face, jaws, neck and limbs may be involved, and in severe cases the ventilatory muscles are compromised. About 10% of Caucasian individuals with myasthenia gravis have a thymoma and 50% have medullary follicular hyperplasia. These are predominantly females younger than 40 years of age who have strong expression of HLA-B8-DR3. Thymectomy in this latter group often results in improvements in their symptoms. In the absence of a thymoma, the onset of myasthenia gravis occurs after 40 years of age in patients with an HLA-B7-DR2 phenotype, except for a group in whom weaknesses are restricted to eye and eyelid movements.

The thymus is essential to the normal development of lymphoid tissues during neonatal and early postnatal life. Thymectomy during this period leads to a progressively fatal condition, with hypoplasia of the peripheral lymphoid organs, wasting and an inability to mount an effective immune response. By puberty, when the main lymphoid tissues are fully developed, thymectomy is less debilitating, but a reduction in effective responses to novel antigens ultimately ensues.

Congenital anomalies of the thymus – Undescended thymus, accessory thymic bodies and rare cysts of the third branchial pouch are of no clinical significance (except where thymectomy is indicated). Patients with thymic agenesis, aplasia and hypoplasia, as in severe combined immune deficiency disease, have reduced lymphocyte numbers, and early death from infection is common. Most cases are familial, with autosomal recessive genes.

In young children a large thymus may press on the trachea, causing attacks of ventilatory stridor.

THORACIC DUCT (Figs 59.19, 59.20, 59.21)

The origin of the thoracic duct is described in Chapters 61 (p. 1051) and 68 (p. 1122).

In adults the thoracic duct, including the confluence of lymph trunks (or the cisterna chyli in the small proportion in whom the latter is saccular) is 38–45 cm in length and extends from the second lumbar

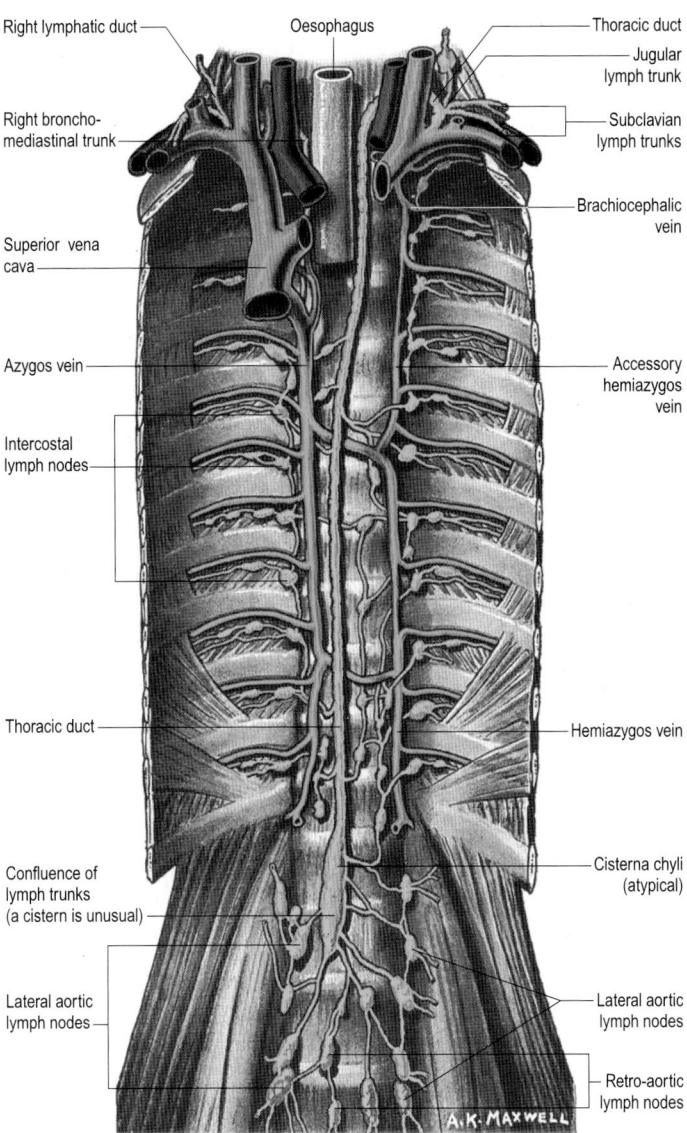

Right lymphatic duct
Oesophagus
Thoracic duct
Jugular lymph trunk
Right broncho-mediastinal trunk
Subclavian lymph trunks
Brachiocephalic vein
Superior vena cava
Azygos vein
Accessory hemiazygos vein
Intercostal lymph nodes
Thoracic duct
Hemiazygos vein
Confluence of lymph trunks (a cistern is unusual)
Cisterna chyli (atypical)
Lateral aortic lymph nodes
Lateral aortic lymph nodes
Retro-aortic lymph nodes

A.K.MAXWELL

Fig. 59.19 The thoracic and right lymphatic ducts. The accessory hemiazygos vein is crossing the median plane lower and the hemiazygos is higher than usual. Note also the comments concerning the more common course of the azygos vein made in **Fig. 60.32**. Two features are also uncommon: there is a single right lymphatic duct (usually two or more trunks open independently), and a simple cisterna chyli is infrequent (it is usually a confluence of lymph trunks of varying morphology).

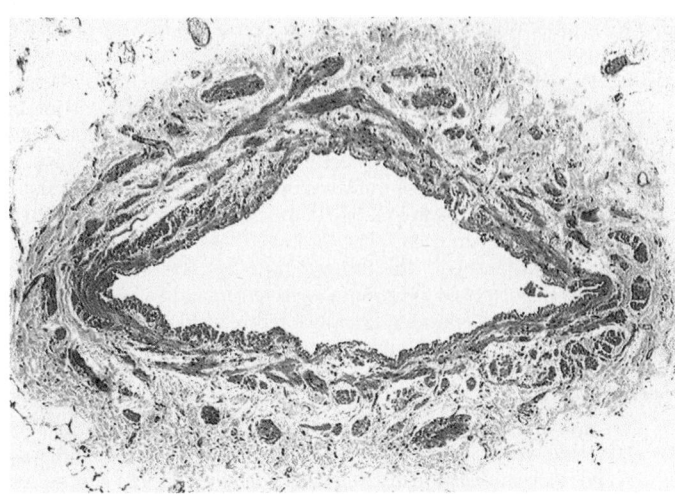

Fig. 59.20 Transverse section of the thoracic duct showing the fibromuscular coat. (Preparation by Millie Harrison, Department of Anatomy, GKT School of Medicine, London.)

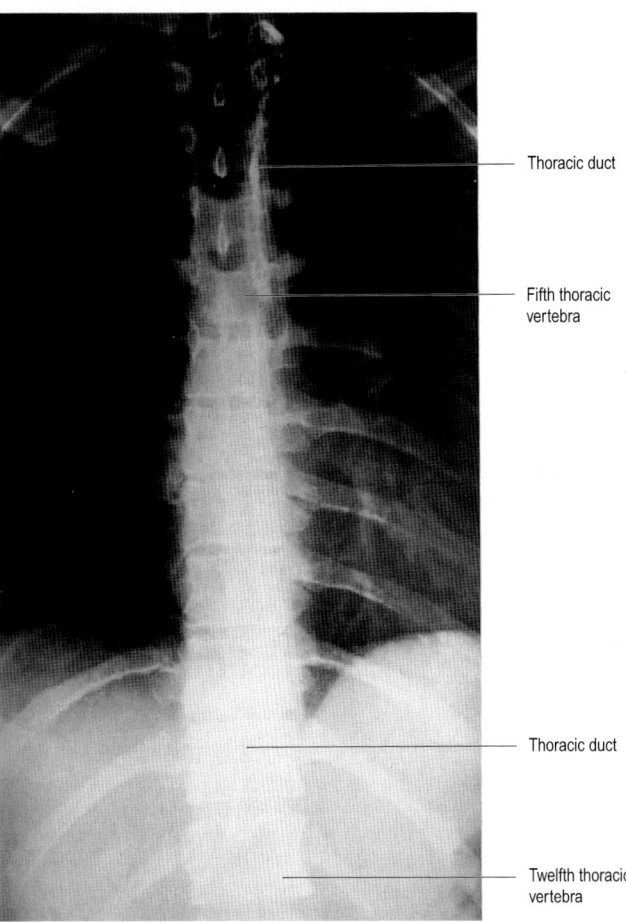

Thoracic duct
Fifth thoracic vertebra
Thoracic duct
Twelfth thoracic vertebra

Fig. 59.21 Lymphangiogram showing the entire length of the thoracic duct, approximately 24 hours after injection of lipiodol into a lymphatic vessel on the dorsum of each foot. The cisterna chyli is not evident. (Provided by GI Verney, Addenbrooke's Hospital, Cambridge; photograph by Sarah-Jane Smith.)

vertebra to the base of the neck. Starting from the superior pole of the confluence near the lower border of the twelfth thoracic vertebra, it traverses the aortic aperture of the diaphragm, then ascends the posterior mediastinum, right of the midline, between the descending thoracic aorta (on its left) and the azygos vein (on its right). The vertebral column (vertebral bodies, symphyses, anterior longitudinal ligament), the right aortic intercostal arteries and terminal segments of the hemiazygos and accessory hemiazygos veins are posterior relations. The diaphragm and oesophagus are anterior; a recess of the right pleural cavity may separate the duct and oesophagus. At the level of the fifth thoracic vertebral body, the duct gradually inclines to the left, enters the superior mediastinum and then ascends to the thoracic inlet along the left border of the oesophagus. In this part of its course the duct is first crossed anteriorly by the aortic arch and then runs posterior to the initial segment of the left subclavian artery, in close contact with the left mediastinal pleura. Passing into the neck, it arches laterally at the level of the transverse process of the seventh cervical vertebra. Its arch rises 3 or 4 cm above the clavicle and curves anterior to the vertebral artery and vein, the left sympathetic trunk, thyrocervical artery or its branches and the left phrenic nerve and medial border of scalenus anterior (but is separated

from the nerve and muscle by the prevertebral fascia). It passes posterior to the left common carotid artery, vagus nerve and internal jugular vein. Finally, the duct descends anterior to the arched cervical first part of the left subclavian artery and ends by opening into the junction of the left subclavian and internal jugular veins. It may also open into either of the great veins, near the junction, or it may divide into a number of smaller vessels before terminating (see below).

985

At its abdominal origin, the thoracic duct is c.5 mm in diameter. It diminishes in calibre at midthoracic levels, then in c.50% of individuals is again slightly dilated before its termination. It is slightly sinuous, constricted at intervals and appears varicose. It may divide in its mid course into two unequal vessels that soon reunite, or into several small branches that form a plexus before continuing as a single duct. At a higher level it occasionally bifurcates, the left branch ending as usual, the right branch diverging to join one of the right lymph trunks or, when present, a right lymphatic duct. The combined vessel usually opens into the right subclavian vein. The thoracic duct has several valves corresponding to sites exposed to pressure. At its termination a bicuspid valve faces into the vein to prevent or reduce reflux of blood. (After death, blood regurgitates freely into the duct, which then looks like a vein.)

TERMINATION

In rare individuals there is no apparent thoracic duct on the left. Several terminal openings are frequent (10–40%, according to different observers). Patterns vary greatly in different studies, but the commonly reported sites of termination are internal jugular vein (36–48%), jugulo-subclavian junction (35%) and subclavian vein (9% and 17%). Termination in the left brachiocephalic vein occurs in c.8%.

TRIBUTARIES

The tributaries of the thoracic duct may be summarized as follows. Bilateral descending thoracic lymph trunks from intercostal lymph nodes of the lower six or seven intercostal spaces of both sides traverse the aortic orifice and join the lateral aspects of the thoracic duct in the abdomen immediately after its origin. Bilateral ascending lumbar lymph trunks from the upper lateral aortic nodes ascend and pierce their corresponding diaphragmatic crus, and then join the thoracic duct at a variable level within the thorax. The upper intercostal trunks drain the intercostal nodes in the upper five or six left intercostal spaces. The mediastinal trunks drain various nodal groups (noted below) and provide paths to the thoracic duct from the convex diaphragmatic aspect of the liver, the diaphragm, the pericardium, heart and oesophagus. The left subclavian trunk usually joins the thoracic duct, but may open independently into the left subclavian vein. The left jugular trunk usually joins the thoracic duct, but may open independently into the left internal jugular vein. The left bronchomediastinal trunk occasionally joins the thoracic duct, but usually has an independent venous opening.

Many of the trunks listed above are described as possessing terminal bicuspid valves, which possibly prevent reflux of lymph.

LYMPHOGRAPHY

The central lymphatic vessels and thoracic duct are narrow and occasionally difficult to delineate anatomically. Anomalies of the thoracic duct may be delineated by dissection into the inguinal lymphatics followed by cannulation and subsequent injection of an oily contrast medium. Cross-sectional CT can then be utilized to obtain better anatomical detail.

DEVELOPMENT

The development of the thoracic duct is described in Chapter 61 (p. 1051).

INJURY DURING OESOPHAGEAL SURGERY

The thoracic duct is vulnerable to damage after thoracic surgery and particularly after oesophageal surgery (Wemyss-Holden et al 2001). The incidence is between 0.2 and 3% and increases with trans-hiatal and thoracoscopic procedures. Thoracic duct laceration is a potentially life-threatening complication: mortality rates are more than 50% with conservative management and as high as 10–16% even after early surgical duct ligation. Rupture of the thoracic duct leads to leakage of chyle, which is rich in lipid, protein and lymphocytes and hence a progressive nutritional and immune deficit occurs. Fortunately, the incidence of true thoracic duct transection is rare, and cases in which there are some postoperative chylous effusions are usually the result of damage to some of the tributaries of the thoracic duct, rather than to the duct itself. These are usually self-limiting and respond to conservative treatment.

The variable course of the thoracic duct, coupled with failure to identify it at surgery, may lead to inadvertent incision or transection of the duct. The greater incidence of injury with trans-hiatal resection may be attributable to shear forces during the mobilization of the distal oesophagus; whereas the limited field of view probably contributes to the greater incidence of thoracic duct injury during thoracoscopic surgery. Injury should be suspected in the postoperative period if there is an enlarging mediastinal shadow on chest radiograph, or there is significant drainage of a cream-coloured liquid from the chest drains or abdominal drains. In cases of uncertainty, an electrophoretic confirmation for the presence of chylomicrons in the pleural fluid is diagnostic.

Conservative management consists of adequate drainage of the chylous fluid, in conjunction with enteral or parenteral nutrition. However, the mortality rate remains high from sepsis with this approach. Early surgical management with thoracic duct ligation above the diaphragm or repair of the laceration is preferable. Repair of the laceration requires preoperative identification of the site of injury, and this is usually achieved with lymphangiography. This involves the subcutaneous injection of an oily contrast media into both feet. Serial chest radiographs are then taken at intervals to identify the site of leakage. However, even during surgical re-exploration, accurate identification of laceration may be difficult. It may be necessary to administer fatty feed enterally, which increases the rate of leakage of chyle from the laceration.

RIGHT LYMPHATIC TRUNK (Fig. 7.14)

The right lymphatic trunk has a variable anatomy, which includes doubling of the duct, left-sided, right or bilateral termination. The plexiform nature of the trunks from which the thoracic duct develops leads to a number of possible abnormalities. The most common is duplication of the duct for a variable part of its course and subsequent merging to form a single duct, which drains into the left internal jugular trunk. Occasionally, the duct has dual terminations in the right and left internal jugular veins, and rarely the duct terminates only into the right internal jugular vein.

MEDIASTINOSCOPY

In cervical mediastinoscopy, a transverse incision is made in the suprasternal notch through the deep cervical fascia after retraction of sternohyoid and sternothyroid. The pretracheal plane is dissected along the anterior surface of the trachea. A space is created between the trachea and the brachiocephalic artery anteriorly down to the level of the carina and along both sides of the trachea and main bronchi. This allows insertion of the endoscope to inspect and biopsy lymph-node masses in the upper para-tracheal (station 2), lower para-tracheal (station 4) and subcarinal nodes in station 7. The superior prevascular part of the anterior mediastinum is more difficult to assess by mediastinoscopy and usually requires an anterior mediastinostomy, with the use of a special retractor with the cervical extended approach. Here the mediastinoscope is inserted retrosternally along the prevascular plane. The nodes at stations 5 and 6 of the mediastinum can be accessed by this technique.

OESOPHAGUS
(Figs 35.1, 35.2, 35.8, 59.22, 71.1)

The oesophagus is a muscular tube c.25 cm (10 in) long, which connects the pharynx to the stomach. It begins in the neck, level with the lower border of the cricoid cartilage and the sixth cervical vertebra. It descends largely anterior to the vertebral column through the superior and posterior mediastina, passes through the diaphragm, level with the tenth thoracic vertebra, and ends at the gastric cardiac orifice level with the eleventh thoracic vertebra. Generally vertical in its course, the oesophagus has two shallow curves. It starts in the median plane, but inclines to the left as far as the root of the neck, gradually returns to the median plane near the fifth thoracic vertebra, and at the seventh thoracic vertebra deviates left again, before it pierces the diaphragm. The oesophagus also bends in an anteroposterior plane to follow the cervical and thoracic curvatures of the vertebral column. It is the narrowest part of the alimentary tract, except for the vermiform appendix, and is constricted at the beginning (15 cm (6 in) from the incisor teeth), where it is crossed by the aortic arch (22.5 cm (9 in) from the incisor teeth), where it is crossed by the left principal bronchus (27.5 cm (11 in) from the incisors) and as it passes through the diaphragm (40 cm (16 in) from the incisors). These measurements are important clinically with regard to the passage of instruments along the oesophagus.

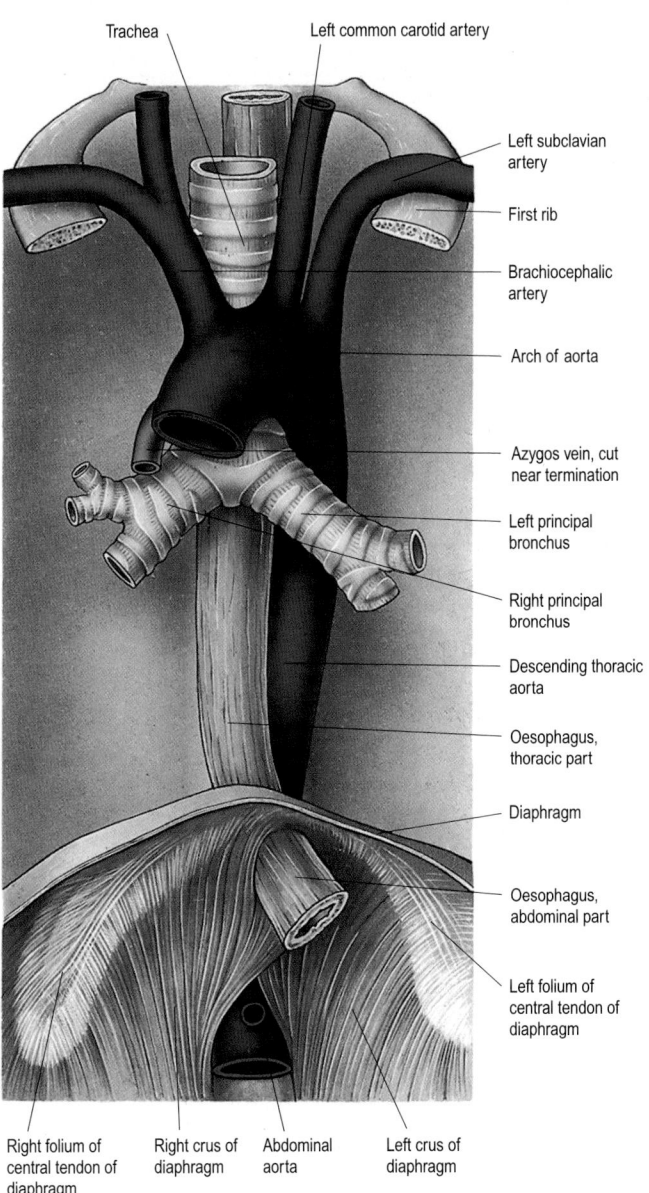

Trachea
Left common carotid artery
Left subclavian artery
First rib
Brachiocephalic artery
Arch of aorta
Azygos vein, cut near termination
Left principal bronchus
Right principal bronchus
Descending thoracic aorta
Oesophagus, thoracic part
Diaphragm
Oesophagus, abdominal part
Left folium of central tendon of diaphragm
Right folium of central tendon of diaphragm
Right crus of diaphragm
Abdominal aorta
Left crus of diaphragm

Fig. 59.22 Dissection to expose the oesophagus in the posterior mediastinum and in the abdomen, and its relation to the trachea and aorta in the thorax.

CERVICAL OESOPHAGUS (Figs 35.1, 35.8)

The cervical oesophagus is posterior to the trachea and attached to it by loose connective tissue. The recurrent laryngeal nerves ascend on each side in or near the groove between the trachea and the oesophagus. Posterior are the vertebral column, longus colli and prevertebral layer of deep cervical fascia. Lateral on each side are the common carotid artery and posterior part of the thyroid gland. In the lower neck, where the oesophagus deviates left, it is closer to the left carotid sheath and thyroid gland than it is on the right. The thoracic duct ascends for a short distance along its left side.

THORACIC OESOPHAGUS (Figs 59.22, 60.4E,F)

The thoracic oesophagus is situated a little to the left in the superior mediastinum between the trachea and the vertebral column. It passes behind and to the right of the aortic arch to descend in the posterior mediastinum along the right side of the descending thoracic aorta. Below, as it inclines left, it crosses anterior to the aorta and enters the abdomen through the diaphragm at the level of the tenth thoracic vertebra. From above downwards the trachea, right pulmonary artery, left principal bronchus, pericardium (separating it from the left atrium) and the diaphragm are anterior. The vertebral column, longus colli, right posterior (aortic) intercostal arteries, thoracic duct, azygos vein and the terminal parts of the hemiazygos and accessory hemiazygos veins

and, near the diaphragm, the aorta, are posterior. A long recess of the right pleural sac lies between the oesophagus (in front) and the azygos vein and vertebral column (behind) in the posterior mediastinum.

In the superior mediastinum, the terminal part of the aortic arch, the left subclavian artery, thoracic duct, the left pleura and the recurrent laryngeal nerve (which ascends in or near the groove between the oesophagus and trachea) are left lateral relations. In the posterior mediastinum, the oesophagus is related to the descending thoracic aorta and left pleura. The right pleura, and the azygos vein that intervenes as it arches forwards above the right principal bronchus to join the superior vena cava, are right lateral relations. Below the pulmonary roots, the vagus nerves descend in contact with the oesophagus, the right chiefly behind and the left in front: they unite to form an oesophageal plexus around it. Low in the posterior mediastinum, the thoracic duct is behind and to the right of the oesophagus. Higher, the thoracic duct is posterior, crossing to the left of the oesophagus at about the level of the fifth thoracic vertebra and then ascending on the left. On the right of the oesophagus, just above the diaphragm, a small serous infracardiac bursa may occur, which represents the detached apex of the right pneumatoenteric recess.

ABDOMINAL OESOPHAGUS (Fig. 71.1)

The abdominal oesophagus emerges from the right diaphragmatic crus, slightly left of the midline and level with the tenth thoracic vertebra, grooving the posterior surface of the left lobe of the liver. It forms a truncated cone, c.1 cm long, curving sharply left, its base continuous with the cardiac orifice of the stomach. Its right side continues smoothly into the lesser curvature, whereas the left is separated from the gastric fundus by the cardiac notch. Covered by peritoneum on its front and left side, it is contained in the upper left part of the lesser omentum. The peritoneum reflected from its posterior surface to the diaphragm is part of the gastrophrenic ligament, through which oesophageal branches of the left gastric vessels reach it. The left crus and left inferior phrenic artery are posterior. The relations of the vagus nerves vary as the oesophagus traverses the diaphragm. Usually, the left vagus is composed of two or three trunks, which are firmly applied to the anterior aspect of the oesophagus. The right vagus is usually single, a thick cord some distance from the posterior aspect of the oesophagus.

VASCULAR SUPPLY AND LYMPHATIC DRAINAGE

Arteries

The cervical oesophagus is supplied by the inferior thyroid artery. The thoracic oesophagus is supplied by bronchial arteries and oesophageal arteries. There are four or five oesophageal arteries, which arise anteriorly from the aorta and descend obliquely to the oesophagus. They form a vascular chain on the oesophagus that anastomoses above with the oesophageal branches of the inferior thyroid arteries and below with ascending branches from the left phrenic and left gastric arteries.

Veins

Blood from the oesophagus drains into a submucous plexus and then into a peri-oesophageal venous plexus. The oesophageal veins originate from this venous plexus. Those from the thoracic oesophagus drain predominantly into the azygos veins and, to a lesser extent, the hemiazygos and intercostal veins. There is some drainage into the bronchial veins. The cervical oesophagus drains into the inferior thyroid vein.

The left gastric vein meets the oesophageal vein at the oesophageal opening in the lesser curvature and then drains into the portal vein.

Oesophageal varices

Cirrhosis or fibrosis of the liver affects the vascular tree within the liver and results in a decrease in hepatic vascular compliance. There is also an increased vascular tone, which may be the result of reduction in endothelial vasodilators such as nitric oxide. The portal resistance increases, leading to the formation of a collateral circulation. There is a concomitant increase in the systemic and splanchnic blood flow. Portosystemic shunting of blood occurs between the short gastric coronary veins and the oesophageal veins. This is primarily attributable to the dilatation of pre-existing embryonic channels. In the normal situation, the circulation is a flow of c.1000 ml/min, with a pressure of c.7 mmHg within the portal circulation. The pressure increases to c.10–12 mmHg in portal hypertension. The resulting varices are formed throughout the gastrointestinal tract (Paquet 2000).

Varices in the distal oesophagus are easily visible at endoscopy, because they are situated superficially in the lamina propria. The blood from the superficial veins drains into a superficial venous plexus and then into a deeper intrinsic venous plexus. Blood then drains into the peri-oesophageal veins via perforating veins. In this region bidirectional flow is possible, and this allows pressure changes during breathing and Valsalva manoeuvres. In portal hypertension, the valves within the perforating vessels become incompetent and hence there is retrograde flow, which causes dilatation of the deep intrinsic veins. The greater pressure within this region predisposes the varices to bleeding.

Treatment is directed towards controlling the formation of collateral circulation and the obliteration of varices that are susceptible to bleeding. This is achieved by para-variceal endoscopic injection of a sclerosant, which causes obliteration of the varices as a result of thrombus formation. Fibrosis is also induced within the mucosa, which reduces the formation of new collateral vessels. An alternative technique is to apply rubber bands in an attempt to ligate the varices. Bleeding from varices is associated with a 25% mortality, reflecting the problems of re-bleeding and development of liver failure.

Lymphatic drainage

The oesophagus has an extensive submucosal lymphatic system. Efferent vessels from the cervical oesophagus drain to the deep cervical nodes either directly or through the para-tracheal nodes. Vessels from the thoracic oesophagus drain to the posterior mediastinal nodes and those from the abdominal oesophagus drain to the left gastric lymph nodes. Some may pass directly to the thoracic duct (p. 984).

INNERVATION

The upper oesophagus is supplied by the branches of the recurrent laryngeal nerve and by postganglionic sympathetic fibres that reach it by travelling along the inferior thyroid arteries. The lower oesophagus is supplied by the oesophageal plexus, a wide-meshed autonomic network that surrounds the oesophagus below the level of the lung roots, and which contains a mixture of parasympathetic and sympathetic fibres.

Motor fibres to the striated and smooth muscle of the oesophageal wall travel in the vagus. Fibres with cell bodies in the nucleus ambiguus travel via the recurrent laryngeal and supply cricopharyngeus and the striated muscle of the upper one-third of the oesophagus. Fibres with cell bodies in the dorsal nucleus pass through the oesophageal plexus and supply the smooth muscle that makes up the lower part of the oesophagus, after local relay in the oesophageal wall. Other branches are given off by the vagus as it travels through the mediastinum, and pass directly to the oesophagus. The vagus also carries secretomotor fibres to mucous glands in the oesophageal mucosa, and sensory fibres to cell bodies in its inferior ganglion.

Vasomotor sympathetic fibres destined for the oesophagus arise from the upper four to six thoracic spinal cord segments. Those from the upper ganglia pass to the middle and inferior cervical ganglia, where they synapse on postganglionic neurones of which the axons innervate the vessels of the cervical and upper thoracic oesophagus. Those from the lower ganglia pass directly to the oesophageal plexus or to the coeliac ganglion (in the greater splanchnic nerve), where they synapse; postganglionic axons innervate the distal oesophagus. Afferent visceral pain fibres travel via the sympathetic fibres to the first four segments of the thoracic spinal cord. As these segments also receive afferents from the heart, it is sometimes difficult to distinguish between oesophageal and cardiac pain.

MICROSTRUCTURE (Figs 59.23, 70.1)

The tissues forming the thoracic oesophageal wall, from lumen outwards, are the mucosa (consisting of epithelium, lamina propria, and muscularis mucosae), submucosa, muscularis externa and adventitia.

Mucosa

The mucosa is thick and, in the living, pink above and pale below. At its lowermost end, at the gastro-oesophageal junction, a jagged boundary line separates the greyish-pink, smooth, oesophageal mucosa from the reddish-pink gastric mucosa, which is covered by minute bulges and depressions (p. 1152). Throughout its length, the oesophageal lumen

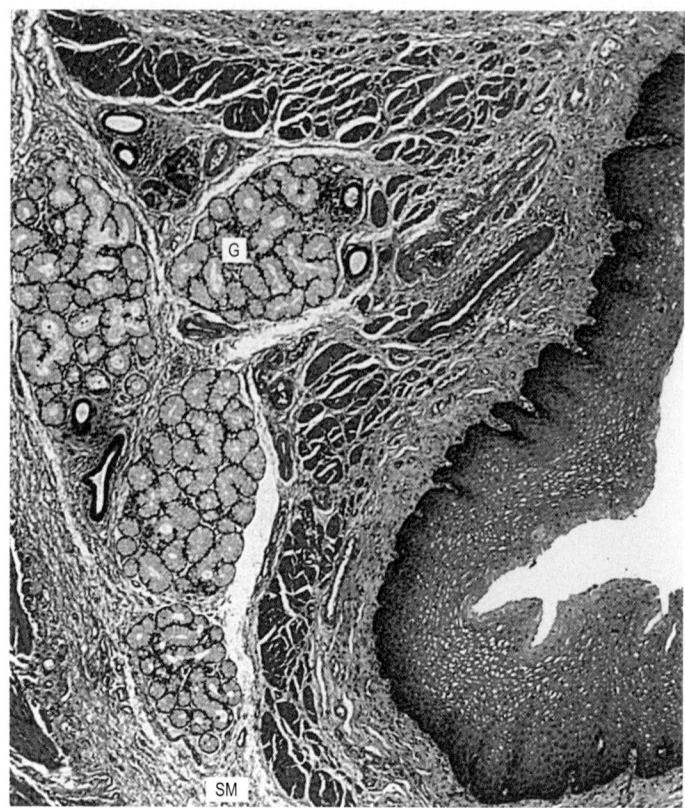

Fig. 59.23 The wall of the oesophagus. A stratified squamous, non-keratinizing epithelium lines the lumen (right), and submucosal glands (G) in the submucosa (SM) secrete mucus that lubricates the passage of food. (By permission from Dr JB Kerr, Monash University, from Kerr JB 1999 Atlas of Functional Histology. London: Mosby.)

is marked by deep longitudinal grooves and ridges, which disappear when the lumen is distended, but obliterate the lumen at all other times.

Epithelium

The epithelium is a non-keratinized, stratified squamous epithelium, continuous with that of the oropharynx. In humans this protective layer is quite thick (300–500 μm) (Fig. 59.23), and is not affected by oesophageal distension. The boundary between the oesophageal epithelium and its lamina propria is distinct but markedly uneven, as tall connective tissue papillae invaginate the epithelial base, assisting in the anchorage of the epithelium to underlying tissues (Fig. 59.23). These papillae are permanent structures, also unaffected by oesophageal distension, and they are rich in blood vessels and nerve fibres. At the base of the epithelium there is a basal lamina, to which epithelial cells are attached by hemidesmosomes, as occurs in the oral mucosa. The oesophageal epithelium is similar to other stratified squamous epithelia (p. 32). It can be divided into a basal, proliferative layer, a parabasal layer of cells undergoing terminal differentiation and a flattened layer of superficial cells or squames, which retain their nuclei. The most superficial strata of cells contain a few keratohyalin granules, in addition to cytokeratin filaments.

The epithelial cell population is constantly renewed by mitosis in the cuboidal basal cells and the deepest of the parabasal cells. As they migrate towards the lumen, they become progressively polygonal and then more flattened, and are eventually desquamated at the epithelial surface. This sequence of events normally takes 2–3 weeks, and is markedly slower than in the stomach and intestine.

The epithelium is an effective protection against mechanical injury during swallowing because of its thickness and the presence of mucus at its surface. However, protection is limited by repeated exposure to the strongly acidic, protease-rich secretions of the stomach, as occurs abnormally during reflux. Normally, the lower oesophageal sphincter prevents reflux, but if reflux does occur, ulceration and fibrosis of the oesophageal wall, accompanied by considerable pain and difficulties in swallowing may ensue. Exposure to acid may also cause oesophageal epithelial metaplasia to a gastric-like mucosa (Barrett's mucosa), or to more overt neoplastic changes.

Langerhans cells – Langerhans cells are present in the oesophageal epithelium. They are immature dendritic cells (p. 82) and resemble those of the epidermis. They perform similar antigen-processing and presenting roles, important in immunostimulation of naive T cells and mucosal defence.

Lamina propria

The oesophageal lamina propria contains scattered groups of lymphoid follicles (mucosa-associated lymphoid tissue, p. 77), which are especially prominent near the gastro-oesophageal junction. Small tubular mucous glands occur in this region, and in the upper part of the oesophagus close to the pharynx.

Muscularis mucosae

The muscularis mucosae is composed of mainly longitudinal smooth muscle, and forms a thin sheet near the epithelium, the contours of which it follows closely. At the pharyngeal end of the oesophagus it may be absent or represented only by sparse, scattered bundles; below this it becomes progressively thicker. The longitudinal orientation of its cells changes to a more plexiform arrangement near the gastro-oesophageal junction.

Submucosa

The submucosa loosely connects the mucosa and the muscularis externa, and penetrates the longitudinal ridges of the oesophageal lumen. It contains larger blood vessels, nerves and mucous glands. Its elastic fibres are also important in the re-closure of the oesophageal lumen after peristaltic dilatation.

Oesophageal glands

Oesophageal glands are small tubulo-acinar glands lying in the submucosa, each group sending a single long duct through the intervening layers of the gut wall to the surface. They are composed mostly of mucous cells, although they also contain serous cells that secrete lysozyme. In the region close to the pharynx, and at the lower end close to the stomach, the glands are simpler in form and restricted to the lamina propria of the mucosa. The mucosal mucous glands of the abdominal oesophagus closely resemble the cardiac glands of the stomach (p. 1152) and are termed oesophageal cardiac glands.

Muscularis externa

The muscularis externa is up to 300 μm thick, and is composed of the outer longitudinal and inner circular layers typical of the intestine. The longitudinal fibres form a continuous coat around almost the entire length of the oesophagus, but posterosuperiorly, 3–4 cm below the cricoid cartilage, they diverge as two fascicles ascending obliquely to the front of the tube. Here, they pass deep to the lower border of the inferior constrictor, and end in a tendon attached to the upper part of the ridge on the back of the cricoid lamina (**Fig. 35.2**). The V-shaped space between these fascicles is filled by circular fibres of the oesophagus, which are thinly covered below by some decussating longitudinal fibres and above by the overlapping inferior constrictor. The longitudinal layer is generally thicker than the circular. Accessory slips of smooth muscle sometimes pass between the oesophagus and left pleura or the root of the left principal bronchus, trachea, pericardium or aorta, and are sometimes considered to fix the oesophagus to these structures. Superiorly, the circular fibres are continuous behind with the inferior pharyngeal constrictor. In front, the uppermost fibres are attached to the lateral margins of the tendon of the two longitudinal fasciculi of the oesophagus. Inferiorly, the circular muscle is continuous in the stomach wall with the oblique layer of its muscle fibres (p. 1152). In the upper one-third of the human oesophagus, the muscularis externa is formed by skeletal muscle. In the middle one-third, smooth muscle fascicles intermingle with striated muscle, and this increases distally such that the lower one-third contains only smooth muscle.

OESOPHAGOSCOPY AND TRANSOESOPHAGEAL ULTRASOUND

The oesophagus can be inspected visually by oesophagoscopy. This may be indicated in patients with persistent oesophageal symptoms such as atypical chest pain, dysphagia, odynophagia (painful swallowing) or symptoms of reflux. The procedure is performed with or without sedation. The endoscope is passed orally under direct vision with the patient in a lateral decubitus position. The endoscope is manoeuvred into the oesophageal inlet and the patient asked to swallow. Once the endoscope passes the oesophageal inlet, it is advanced slowly under direct vision and the mucosa carefully inspected. The mucosa normally appears whitish pink and changes at the lower oesophagus to a reddish mucosa at the squamocolumnar junction (Z line). This is closely related to the diaphragmatic hiatus and displacement by more than 2 cm is indicative of a hiatus hernia. There may be slight extrinsic compression at the level of the aorta and occasionally at the left main stem bronchus.

Endoscopic transoesophageal ultrasound permits assessment of the oesophageal wall and para-oesophageal structures such as lymph nodes. This technique is more sensitive than CT scanning in detecting mediastinal lymph nodes. It allows lymph nodes less than 10 mm in size to be assessed for possible malignant involvement. Normal lymph nodes cannot be easily identified by endoscopic ultrasound, because they have the same sonar characteristics as surrounding tissue. However, normal lymph nodes in the subcarinal position or reactive lymph nodes may occasionally be detected. Hypoechoic or inhomogeneous pattern on ultrasound is considered more suspicious of malignancy. Endoscopic ultrasound-guided fine-needle aspiration allows accurate localization of lymph nodes, but only mediastinal nodes adjacent to the oesophagus can be fully evaluated. Transbronchial fine-needle aspiration is an alternative approach for sampling mediastinal nodes. The choice of lymph nodes to be sampled is based on CT findings.

Oesophageal rupture

The majority of oesophageal ruptures are iatrogenic, and occur during the instrumentation of the oesophagus during endoscopy, endoscopic intervention and nasogastric tube placement. Other causes are traumatic, barotrauma, foreign bodies and oesophageal carcinoma. Barotrauma usually occurs with intense retching and vomiting. It usually causes a longitudinal tear in the posterior wall of the thoracic oesophagus. Overall, c.60% of the perforations are located in the thoracic oesophagus, 25% in the cervical and 15% in the abdominal oesophagus. The perforation in the cervical oesophagus occurs in the posterior wall, where it is at its thinnest. Often this corresponds to an area of mucosa where there is no covering with muscle, which is bordered by the pharyngeal inferior constrictor and cricopharyngeus. Mortality from oesophageal perforations is c.20% and results from mediastinitis and necrotizing infection.

Presenting symptoms include thoracic pain, odynophagia, haematemesis, subacute emphysema, tachycardia and breathlessness. Early diagnosis (within 24 hours) and repair are associated with a better prognosis and a mortality rate of between 10 and 15%, whereas late diagnosis has a much greater mortality rate. For a perforation in the upper two-thirds of the thoracic oesophagus, a right thoracotomy in the fifth and sixth intercostal space is performed. The lower one-third of the oesophagus is approached through a left thoracotomy in the sixth and seventh intercostal space. The perforation is closed in layers after any necrotic tissue has been debrided. Conservative treatment consists of broad-spectrum antibiotics, total parental nutrition and drainage of effusions.

BARIUM STUDIES

A barium swallow with fluoroscopy gives anatomical functional assessment of the oesophagus. A standard examination involves the patient swallowing a barium solution in both the supine and recumbent position. The upright posture fully dilates the oesophagus and is useful in evaluating any constrictions. The narrow tubular lumen of the oesophagus is slightly indented by the aortic arch and the left mainstem bronchus (**Fig. 59.6**). The supine view allows better evaluation of any motor dysfunction. Both spot films and cine loops of fluoroscopy are obtained. The fluoroscopic images demonstrate defective opening of the pharyngeal oesophageal sphincter and the nature of the contractions in the body of the oesophagus. The cardio-oesophageal sphincter can be assessed in achalasia. Other abnormalities such as hiatus hernia, and areas of narrowing or dilatation of the oesophagus may be demonstrated. Mucosal relief images are obtained once the bulk of the contrast media has passed into the stomach, leaving a thin layer of contrast media. This allows demonstration of the mucosa of the oesophagus and reveals abnormalities such as ulcers. Air contrast/air interface images detect more subtle changes that may occur in the mucosa.

CROSS-SECTIONAL IMAGING
Cross-sectional imaging is usually used for the preoperative planning and staging of oesophageal tumours, and is of value in radiotherapy planning.

DEVELOPMENT
The development of the oesophagus is described in Chapter 37 (p. 647).

Tracheo-oesophageal fistula
Tracheo-oesophageal fistula is described in Chapter 65 (p. 1091).

Oesophageal atresia
The majority of cases (92%) of oesophageal atresia occur in conjunction with a tracheo-oesophageal fistula, with an incidence of 1:3000–4000 births. There is a high incidence of associated congenital abnormalities such as cardiac, genitourinary, skeletal and other gastrointestinal anomalies. Prenatal diagnosis is unusual because of the lack of specific ultrasound features. The only prenatal indicators are polyhydramnios and absence of stomach gas, which occurs in c.1% of cases. Other clinical signs are the presence of a pharyngeal pouch on ultrasound. Postnatal clinical features are regurgitation of feeds. Other signs, such as recurrent cough and choking spells, are related to the presence of a tracheo-oesophageal fistula.

Corrective surgery is essential, with postoperative nasogastric feeding. Overall survival is influenced by the presence of associated cardiac anomalies, when survival may be as poor as 44%, compared with 94% in infants who do not have an associated malformation.

OESOPHAGEAL SPHINCTERIC MECHANISMS
Radiological studies show that swallowed food stops momentarily in the gastric end of the oesophagus, before entering the stomach (**Fig. 59.11**), suggesting the presence of a sphincter at this point. In the past there was much controversy as to the reason for this behaviour, as only slight thickening of the muscle coat has been found in humans. There is now ample physiological and clinical evidence that closure depends on two major mechanisms operating at the lower end of the oesophagus. The more important of these is the lower oesophageal sphincter, a specialized zone of circular smooth muscle surrounding the oesophagus at its transit through the diaphragm and for much of its short abdominal course. This region of the oesophagus is maintained under tonic contraction, except during swallowing, when it relaxes briefly to admit ingesta to the stomach, and during vomiting. It is controlled by the intramural plexuses of the enteric nervous system, the neural release of nitric oxide contributing to its relaxation. The second mechanism is a functional external sphincter provided by the crural diaphragm, usually the right crus, which encircles the oesophagus as it passes into the abdomen and is attached to it by the phreno-oesophageal ligament. Radiological, electromyographic and manometric analyses have shown that its muscular fibres contract around the oesophagus during inspiration and when intra-abdominal pressure is increased, thus helping to prevent gastro-oesophageal reflux, even when the lower oesophageal sphincter is inhibited experimentally with atropine. The relative importance of these two agents in the prevention of oesophageal reflux is still being debated; clinically, there is a good correlation of this condition with lower oesophageal sphincter dysfunction in some cases, whereas in others failure of the diaphragmatic component, as seen in hiatus hernia, appears to be a major factor. The anatomical configuration of the gastro-oesophageal orifice may also play some part in these processes (see below).

OESOPHAGEAL DYSMOTILITY
The main disorders of the oesophageal motility are disorders of upper oesophageal sphincter, lower oesophageal sphincter (discussed in detail in the section on upper gastro-oesophageal reflux, p. 1083) and achalasia. Problems with the upper oesophageal sphincter predominantly have a neurological aetiology. Brain stem disease impairs relaxation of crico-pharyngeus, leading to dysphagia of solids and liquids, with a tendency to aspirate. Videofluoroscopy may demonstrate the abnormality.

Achalasia of the cardia is a primary motor disorder of the oesophagus in which there is failure of relaxation of the cardio-oesophageal sphincter and loss of peristalsis in the body of the oesophagus. There is degeneration of neuronal cell bodies in the myenteric nerve plexus. The clinical presentation is dysphagia, regurgitation of undigested food, retrosternal chest pain and occasional weight loss. A simple chest radiograph may show dilatation of the oesophagus and retention of food products. Barium swallow shows a classical bird-beak appearance as a result of failure of relaxation of the lower oesophageal sphincter and an absence of peristalsis. Oesophageal manometry with pressure measurements confirms the diagnosis and demonstrates absent or impaired relaxation of the lower oesophageal sphincter. Treatment consists of pneumatic balloon dilatation during endoscopy or minimal-access surgical myotomy of the cardia. An alternative in frail patients is intra-sphincteric injection of botulinum toxin. The advantages are lower morbidity and mortality, with much lower risk of oesophageal perforation.

Diffuse oesophageal spasm may present with dysphagia and chest pain. It is characterized by abnormal oesophageal contractions on barium swallow and produces simultaneous segmental contractions that obliterate the oesophageal lumen to produce a corkscrew oesophagus. Manometry also demonstrates titanic contractions of the oesophagus. Non-specific oesophageal motility disorder occurs with ageing and is characterized by a decreased incidence of normal or even absent peristalsis after swallowing. This may be accompanied by repetitive contractions and failure of relaxation of the lower oesophageal sphincter. Oesophageal dysmotility also includes oesophageal spasm and disorders caused by scleroderma or other connective tissue diseases in which there is atrophy of smooth muscle and fibrous replacement in the submucosa and lamina propria.

GASTRO-OESOPHAGEAL REFLUX
Gastro-oesophageal reflux is described in Chapter 71 (p. 1144).

HIATUS HERNIA
Hiatus hernia is described in Chapter 64 (p. 1083).

MEDIASTINAL LYMPH NODES (Fig. 59.24)

The mediastinal lymph nodes are now classified into regional lymph node stations for the purposes of staging lung cancer. Involvement of these lymph nodes by cancer cells has important prognostic implications and influences the choice of treatment (Mountain & Dresler 1997). The staging system for lung cancer classifies involvement of hilar lymph nodes as N1, mediastinal lymph nodes as N2 and supraclavicular or scalene nodes as N3. Nodes that are contralateral to the tumour site are also classed as N3 nodes. The mediastinal nodes (N2 nodes) consist of all lymph node stations within the mediastinal pleural reflections.

Station 1: highest mediastinal nodes lie above a horizontal line at the level at which the left brachiocephalic vein crosses the trachea.

Station 2: upper para-tracheal nodes lie below the line of the highest mediastinal nodes and above a line drawn horizontally at the level of the upper border of the aortic arch.

Station 3: prevascular and retro-tracheal nodes lie behind the trachea but in front of the great vessels.

Station 4: lower para-tracheal nodes lie below the upper margin of the aortic arch and down to the upper margin of the corresponding upper lobe bronchus. On the right side, this is the upper margin of the right upper lobe bronchus; the majority of nodes in this area tend to be positioned anterolateral to the trachea. On the left side, the nodes are located below the upper margin of the aortic arch and above the margin of the left upper lobe bronchus. They lie medial to the ligamentum arteriosum and are usually lateral to the trachea.

Station 5: subaortic nodes lie in the aortopulmonary window and are situated lateral to the ligamentum arteriosum or aorta or left pulmonary artery, but proximal to the first division of the left pulmonary artery.

Station 6: para-aortic nodes lie between the upper margin of the aortic arch and lateral to the ascending aorta and aortic arch.

Station 7: subcarinal nodes lie below the carina of the trachea, but are not associated with the lower lobe bronchi.

Station 8: para-oesophageal nodes lie at either side of the oesophagus, well below the level of the subcarinal nodes.

Station 9: pulmonary ligament nodes lie within the pulmonary ligament.

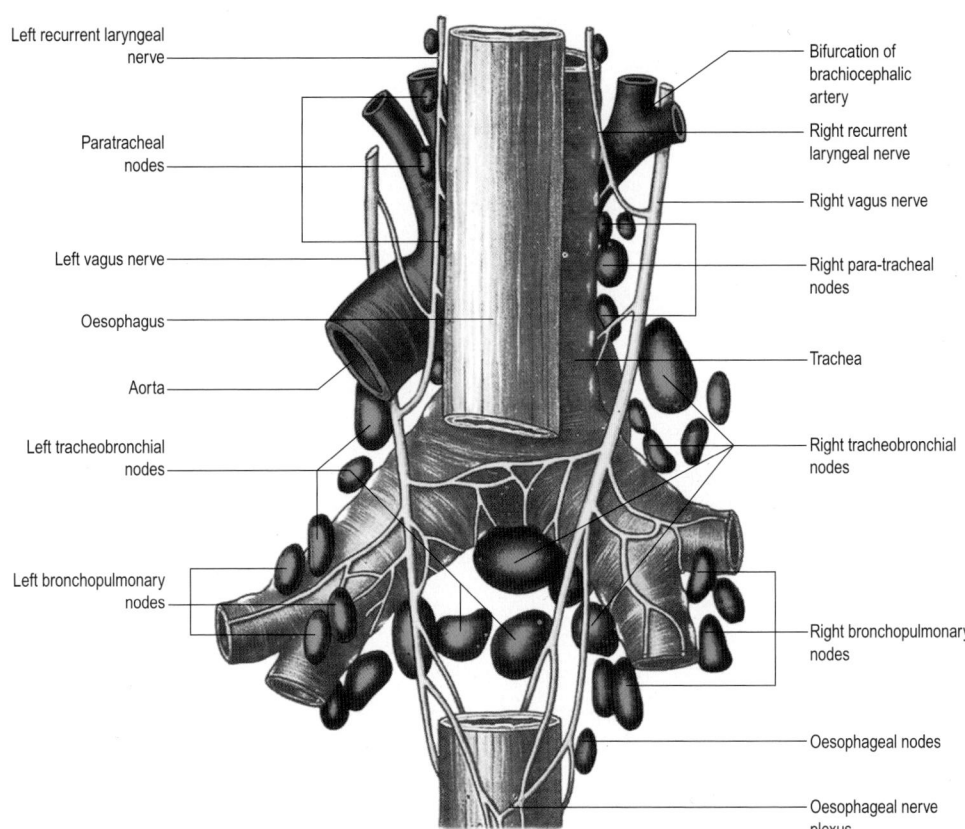

Left recurrent laryngeal nerve

Paratracheal nodes

Left vagus nerve

Oesophagus

Aorta

Left tracheobronchial nodes

Left bronchopulmonary nodes

Bifurcation of brachiocephalic artery

Right recurrent laryngeal nerve

Right vagus nerve

Right para-tracheal nodes

Trachea

Right tracheobronchial nodes

Right bronchopulmonary nodes

Oesophageal nodes

Oesophageal nerve plexus

Fig. 59.24 The lymph nodes of the trachea, bronchi and lungs. Note the large 'carinal' node lodged between the bifurcation of the principal bronchi.

These groups are not sharply demarcated. Pulmonary nodes become continuous with the bronchopulmonary nodes, and they in turn merge with the inferior and superior tracheobronchial nodes, which are continuous with the para-tracheal group. Afferents of tracheobronchial nodes drain the lungs and bronchi, thoracic trachea, heart and some efferents of the posterior mediastinal nodes. Their efferent vessels ascend on the trachea to unite with efferents of the para-sternal and brachiocephalic nodes as the right and left bronchomediastinal trunks. The right trunk may occasionally join a right lymphatic duct or another right-sided lymph trunk and on the left the thoracic duct; however, more often they open independently in or near the ipsilateral jugulo-subclavian junction.

AUTONOMIC NERVOUS SYSTEM

The autonomic nervous system in the thorax consists of a ganglionated sympathetic chain, the vagus nerve and three autonomic plexuses: the cardiac plexus, the oesophageal plexus and the pulmonary plexus (p. 1075).

THORACIC SYMPATHETIC TRUNK (Figs 59.25, 59.26)
The thoracic sympathetic trunk contains ganglia almost equal in number to those of the thoracic spinal nerves (11 in more than 70% of individuals; occasionally 12, rarely 10 or 13). The first thoracic ganglion is usually fused with the inferior cervical ganglion, forming the cervicothoracic ganglion (c.80% of individuals). Rarely, the middle cervical or second thoracic ganglion may be included. The succeeding ganglion is counted as the second in order to make the other ganglia correspond numerically with other segmental structures. Except for the lowest two or three, the thoracic ganglia lie against the costal heads, posterior to the costal pleura. The lowest two or three are lateral to the bodies of the corresponding vertebrae. Caudally, the thoracic sympathetic trunk passes dorsal to the medial arcuate ligament (or through the crus of the diaphragm) to become the lumbar sympathetic trunk. The ganglia are small and interconnected by intervening segments of

the trunk. Two or more rami communicantes, white and grey, connect each ganglion with its corresponding spinal nerve, white rami joining the nerve distal to the grey. Sometimes a grey and a white ramus fuse to form a 'mixed' ramus.

The medial branches from the upper five ganglia are very small, supplying filaments to the thoracic aorta and its branches. On the aorta they form a fine thoracic aortic plexus with filaments from the greater splanchnic nerve. Rami of the second to fifth or sixth ganglia enter the posterior pulmonary plexus. Others, from the second to fifth ganglia, pass to the deep (dorsal) part of the cardiac plexus. Small branches of these pulmonary and cardiac nerves pass to the oesophagus and trachea. The medial branches from the lower seven ganglia are large, supplying the aorta and uniting to form the greater, lesser and lowest splanchnic nerves, the last not always being identifiable.

The greater splanchnic nerve, consisting mainly of myelinated pre-ganglionic efferent and visceral afferent fibres, is formed by branches from the fifth to ninth or tenth thoracic ganglia, but fibres in the upper branches may be traced to the first or second thoracic ganglia. Its roots vary from one to eight, four being the most usual number. It descends obliquely on the vertebral bodies, supplies branches to the descending thoracic aorta and perforates the ipsilateral crus of the diaphragm to end mainly in the coeliac ganglion, but partly in the aorticorenal ganglion and suprarenal (adrenal) gland. A splanchnic ganglion exists on the nerve opposite the eleventh or twelfth thoracic vertebra in a majority of individuals.

The lesser splanchnic nerve, formed by rami of the ninth and tenth (sometimes the tenth and eleventh) thoracic ganglia and the trunk between them, pierces the diaphragm with the greater splanchnic, to join the aorticorenal ganglion.

The lowest (least) splanchnic nerve (or renal nerve) from the lowest thoracic ganglion enters the abdomen with the sympathetic trunk to end in the renal plexus.

The prevalence of the splanchnic nerves, according to seven observers, is as follows: the greater is always present, the lesser is present in 94% (86–100%), and the least is present in 56% (16–98%). A fourth (accessory) splanchnic nerve has been described.

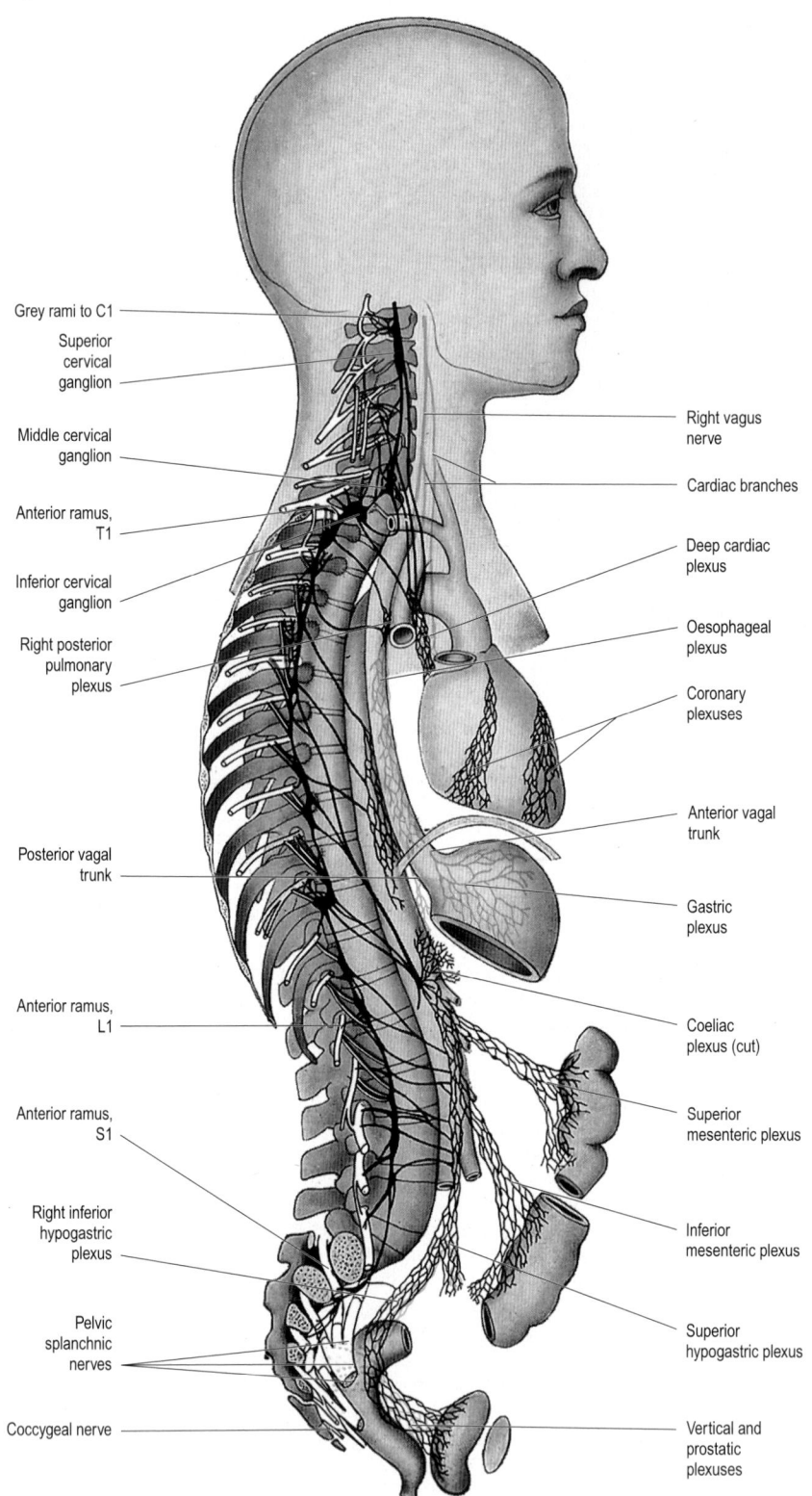

Grey rami to C1

Superior
cervical
ganglion

Middle cervical
ganglion

Anterior ramus,
T1

Inferior cervical
ganglion

Right posterior
pulmonary
plexus

Posterior vagal
trunk

Anterior ramus,
L1

Anterior ramus,
S1

Right inferior
hypogastric
plexus

Pelvic
splanchnic
nerves

Coccygeal nerve

Right vagus
nerve

Cardiac branches

Deep cardiac
plexus

Oesophageal
plexus

Coronary
plexuses

Anterior vagal
trunk

Gastric
plexus

Coeliac
plexus (cut)

Superior
mesenteric plexus

Inferior
mesenteric plexus

Superior
hypogastric plexus

Vertical and
prostatic
plexuses

Fig. 59.25 The right sympathetic trunk and its connections with the thoracic, abdominal and pelvic plexuses. Parasympathetic fibres are blue; sympathetic trunk and branches are black; white rami communicantes are red.

THORACIC VAGUS NERVE AND THORACIC BRANCHES

The vagus nerve contains preganglionic parasympathetic fibres that arise in its dorsal nucleus and travel in the nerve and its pulmonary, cardiac, oesophageal, gastric, intestinal and other branches. Some cardiac parasympathetic fibres may originate from neurones in or near the nucleus ambiguus. The proportion of efferent parasympathetic fibres in the vagus varies at different levels, but is small relative to its sensory and sensorimotor content. Efferent fibres relay in minute ganglia in the visceral walls. The disproportion in the numbers of preganglionic to postganglionic fibres is greater in the vagus than in other cranial nerves. Cardiac branches slow the cardiac cycle, joining the cardiac plexuses and relaying in ganglia distributed freely over both atria in the sub-

epicardial tissue. The terminal fibres are distributed to the atria and the atrioventricular bundle and concentrated around the SA and (to a lesser extent) the atrioventricular nodes. It has been claimed in the past that only through the latter can the vagi influence ventricular muscle, although there is a sparse postganglionic parasympathetic innervation of the ventricles. The smaller branches of the coronary arteries are innervated mainly via the vagus. Larger arteries, with a dual innervation, are chiefly supplied by sympathetic fibres. Pulmonary branches are motor to the circular smooth muscle fibres of the bronchi and bronchioles and are therefore bronchoconstrictor; synaptic relays occur in the ganglia of the pulmonary plexuses. Gastric branches are secretomotor and motor to the smooth muscle of the stomach, with the exception of the pyloric

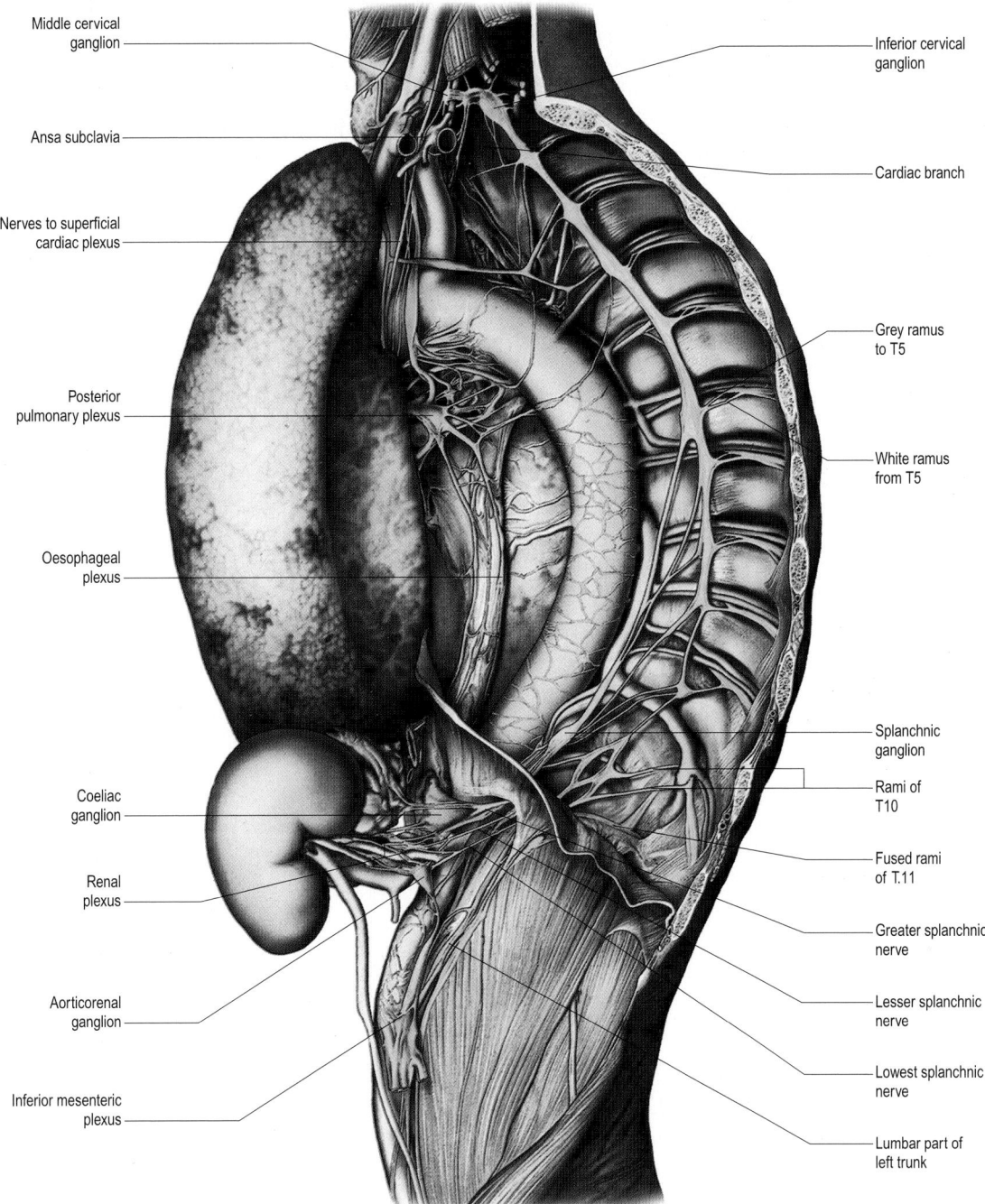

Middle cervical ganglion

Ansa subclavia

Nerves to superficial cardiac plexus

Posterior pulmonary plexus

Oesophageal plexus

Coeliac ganglion

Renal plexus

Aorticorenal ganglion

Inferior mesenteric plexus

Inferior cervical ganglion

Cardiac branch

Grey ramus to T5

White ramus from T5

Splanchnic ganglion

Rami of T10

Fused rami of T.11

Greater splanchnic nerve

Lesser splanchnic nerve

Lowest splanchnic nerve

Lumbar part of left trunk

Fig. 59.26 The thoracic part of the sympathetic system of the left side. Note that the diaphragm has been divided to its posterior attachment and the left lung and the left kidney have been drawn forwards and rotated to the right, to expose the posterior surface of the left kidney and suprarenal gland. (Drawn from a dissection by the late GD Channel, GKT School of Medicine, London.)

sphincter, which they inhibit. Intestinal branches have a corresponding action in the small intestine, caecum, vermiform appendix, ascending colon, right colic flexure and most of the transverse colon; they are secretomotor to the glands, motor to the intestinal muscular coats, but inhibitory to the ileocaecal sphincter. The synaptic relays are situated in the myenteric (Auerbach's) and the submucosal (Meissner's) plexuses.

Course of vagus in mediastinum

The right vagus nerve descends posterior to the internal jugular vein to cross the first part of the subclavian artery to enter the thorax. It descends through the superior mediastinum, at first behind the right brachiocephalic vein, and then to the right of the trachea and postero-medial to the right brachiocephalic vein and superior vena cava. The right pleura and lung are lateral to it above and are separated from it

below by the azygos vein, which arches forwards above the right pulmonary hilum (**Fig. 59.2**). It passes behind the right principal bronchus and lies on the posterior aspect of the right hilum, where it divides into the posterior pulmonary (bronchial) branches. The latter unite with rami from the second to fifth or sixth thoracic sympathetic ganglia to form the right posterior pulmonary plexus. Two or three branches descend from the caudal part of this plexus on the posterior surface of the oesophagus and join a left vagal branch to form the posterior oesophageal plexus. A vagal trunk containing fibres from both right and left vagi leaves the plexus and runs down on the posterior surface of the oesophagus. It enters the abdomen by passing through the diaphragmatic oesophageal opening.

The left vagus enters the thorax between the left common carotid and subclavian arteries and behind the left brachiocephalic vein. It descends through the superior mediastinum and crosses the left side of the aortic arch to pass behind the left pulmonary hilum. Above the aortic arch, it is crossed anterolaterally by the left phrenic nerve and on the arch by the left superior intercostal vein (**Fig. 60.6**). Behind the hilum it divides into the posterior pulmonary (or bronchial) branches, which unite with rami of the second to fourth thoracic sympathetic ganglia to form the left posterior pulmonary plexus. Two or three branches descend anteriorly on the oesophagus and join with a ramus from the right posterior pulmonary plexus to form the anterior oesophageal plexus. A trunk containing fibres from both vagi descends anterior to the oesophagus and enters the abdomen through the oesophageal diaphragmatic opening.

AUTONOMIC PLEXUSES

Pulmonary plexus

The pulmonary plexus is formed from extensions of the cardiac plexus and by vagal and sympathetic branches (p. 1075). The nerve plexus lies anterior and posterior to the other hilar structures of the lungs.

Oesophageal plexus

The oesophageal plexus is described on page 988.

Cardiac plexus

The cardiac plexus is derived from the autonomic nerves and ganglia located in the thorax (**Figs 59.24, 59.25**).

SWALLOWING

The oesophageal phase of swallowing is described in Chapter 35.

VOMITING

The lower oesophageal sphincter relaxes in the initial phase of vomiting. This is coordinated with relaxation of the crural fibres around the oesophagus. Subsequently, there is rapid contraction of the diaphragm and abdominal muscles, with a resultant increase in intra-abdominal pressure.

REFERENCES

Armstrong P 2000 The normal chest. In: Armstrong P, Wilson AG, Dee P, Hansell DM (eds) Imaging of Diseases of the Chest, 3rd edn. London: Mosby: 21–62.

Mountain CF, Dresler CM 1997 Regional lymph node classification for lung cancer staging. Chest 111: 1718–23.

Paquet K-J 2000 Causes and pathomechanisms of oesophageal varices development. Med Sci Monit 6: 915–28.

Spitz L 1996 Esophageal atresia: past, present and future. J Paediatr Surg 31: 19–25.

Wemyss-Holden SA, Launois B, Maddern GJ 2001 Management of thoracic duct injuries after oesophagectomy. Br J Surg 88: 1442–8.

Heart and great vessels

PERICARDIUM

The pericardium contains the heart and the juxtacardiac parts of its great vessels. It consists of two components, the fibrous and the serosal pericardium. The fibrous pericardium is a sac made of tough connective tissue, completely surrounding the heart without being attached to it. This fibrous sac develops by a sequential process of cavitation of the embryonic body wall by expansion of the secondary pleural cavity. Thus its lateral walls are clothed externally by parietal mediastinal pleura. The serosal pericardium consists of two layers of serosal membrane, one inside the other: the inner (visceral) one adheres to the heart and forms its outer covering known as the epicardium, whereas the outer (parietal) one lines the internal surface of the fibrous pericardium. The two serosal surfaces are apposed and separated by a film of fluid. This allows movement of the inner membrane and the heart adhering to it, except at the arterial and venous areas of the pericardium where the two serosal membranes merge. These last constitute two parietovisceral lines of serosal reflexion. The separation of the two membranes of the serosal pericardium creates a narrow space, the pericardial cavity, which provides a complete cleavage between the heart and its surroundings and so allows it some freedom to move and change shape.

FIBROUS AND SEROSAL PERICARDIUM

The fibrous pericardium is compact collagenous fibrous tissue. The serosal pericardium is a single layer of flat cells on a thin subserosal layer of connective tissue, which blends with the fibrous pericardium in the parietal membrane and with the interstitial myocardial tissue in the visceral membrane. On the cardiac side, the subserosal layer contains fat, especially along the ventricular side of the atrioventricular groove, the inferior cardiac border and the interventricular grooves. The main coronary vessels and their larger branches are embedded in this fat; the amount is related to the general extent of body fat and gradually increases with age.

Fibrous pericardium

The fibrous pericardium is roughly conical and clothes the heart. Superiorly, it is continuous exteriorly with the adventitia of the great vessels; inferiorly it is attached to the central tendon of the diaphragm and a small muscular area of its left half. Above, the fibrous pericardium not only blends externally with the great vessels, but is continuous with the pretracheal fascia. Anteriorly, it is also attached to the posterior surface of the sternum by superior and inferior sternopericardial ligaments, although the extent of these 'ligaments' is extremely variable, and the superior one is often undetectable. The pericardium is securely anchored by these connections and maintains the general thoracic position of the heart, serving as the 'cardiac seat belt'.

Anteriorly, the fibrous pericardium is separated from the thoracic wall by the lungs and the pleural coverings. However, in a small area behind the lower left half of the body of the sternum and the sternal ends of left fourth and fifth costal cartilages, the pericardium is in direct contact with the thoracic wall. Until it regresses, the lower end of the thymus is also anterior to the upper pericardium. The principal bronchi, oesophagus, oesophageal plexus, descending thoracic aorta and posterior parts of the mediastinal surface of both lungs are posterior relations. Laterally are the pleural coverings of the mediastinal surface of the lungs. The phrenic nerve, with its accompanying vessels, descends between the fibrous pericardium and mediastinal pleura on each side. Inferiorly, the pericardium is separated by the diaphragm from the liver and fundus of the stomach.

The aorta, superior vena cava, right and left pulmonary arteries and the four pulmonary veins all receive extensions of the fibrous pericardium. The inferior vena cava, which traverses the central tendon, has no such covering.

Serosal pericardium

The serosal pericardium is a closed sac within the fibrous pericardium, and has a visceral and a parietal layer. The visceral layer, or epicardium, covers the heart and great vessels and is reflected into the parietal layer, which lines the internal surface of the fibrous pericardium. The reflections of the serosal layer are arranged as two complex 'tubes': the aorta and pulmonary trunk are enclosed in one, and the superior and inferior venae cavae and the four pulmonary veins in the other. The tube surrounding the veins has the shape of an inverted J (**Figs 60.1, 60.2**). The cul-de-sac within its curve is behind the left atrium and is termed the oblique sinus. The transverse sinus is a passage between the two pericardial 'tubes' (**Fig. 60.1**). It has the aorta and pulmonary trunk in front and the atria and great veins behind. The arrangement of the oblique

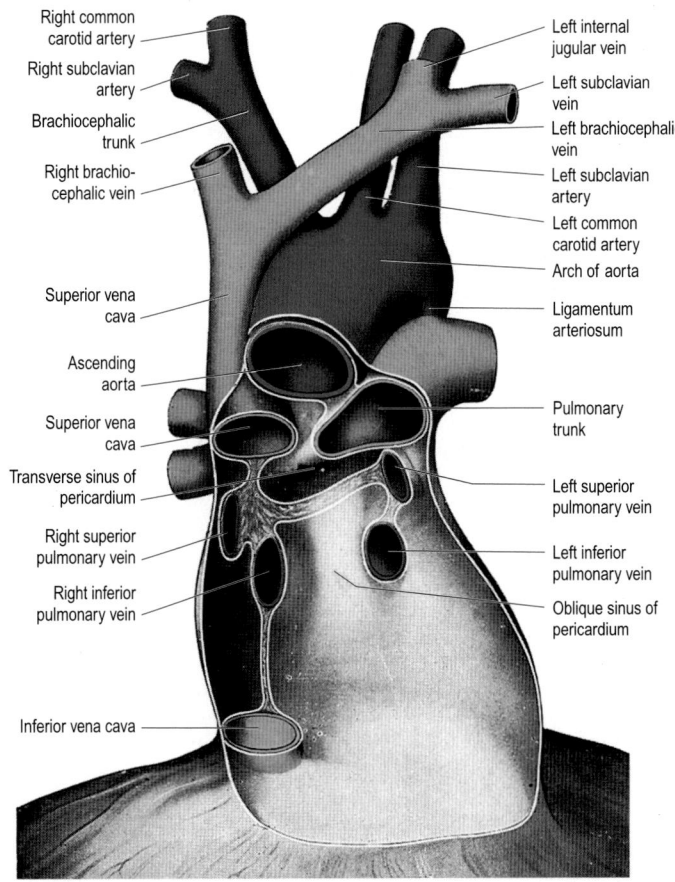

Right common carotid artery
Right subclavian artery
Brachiocephalic trunk
Right brachio-cephalic vein
Superior vena cava
Ascending aorta
Superior vena cava
Transverse sinus of pericardium
Right superior pulmonary vein
Right inferior pulmonary vein
Inferior vena cava

Left internal jugular vein
Left subclavian vein
Left brachiocephalic vein
Left subclavian artery
Left common carotid artery
Arch of aorta
Ligamentum arteriosum
Pulmonary trunk
Left superior pulmonary vein
Left inferior pulmonary vein
Oblique sinus of pericardium

Fig. 60.1 Interior of the serosal pericardial sac after section of the large vessels at their cardiac origin and removal of the heart (seen from the front). *See* text for additional named recesses of the general serosal pericardial cavity and its transverse sinus.

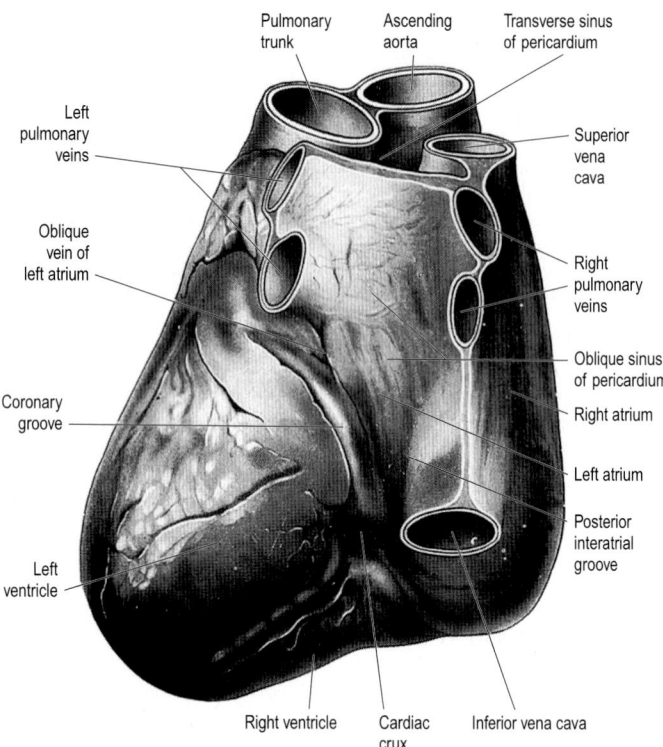

Pulmonary trunk

Ascending aorta

Transverse sinus of pericardium

Left pulmonary veins

Superior vena cava

Oblique vein of left atrium

Right pulmonary veins

Coronary groove

Oblique sinus of pericardium

Right atrium

Left atrium

Posterior interatrial groove

Left ventricle

Right ventricle

Cardiac crux

Inferior vena cava

Fig. 60.2 The base and the diaphragmatic surface of the heart. The serosal pericardium is *in situ* and its cut edge is seen around the great vessels; its disposition is highly schematic (recesses omitted). *See* text for additional details. The cardiac crux results from the confluence of the posterior interatrial groove, the posterior atrioventricular groove and the posterior interventricular groove.

and transverse sinuses, along with that of the main 'principal' cavity, is further affected by the development of complex three-dimensional pericardial recesses between adjacent structures. These recesses can be grouped according to the siting of their orifices or 'mouths'. From the principal pericardial cavity, the postcaval recess projects towards the left behind the atrial termination of the superior vena cava. It is limited above by the right pulmonary artery and below by the upper right pulmonary vein. Its mouth opens superolaterally to the right. The right and left pulmonary venous recesses each project medially and upwards on the back of the left atrium between the superior and inferior pulmonary veins on each side, indenting the side walls of the oblique sinus. The superior aortic recess extends from the transverse sinus. From its mouth, located inferiorly, it ascends posterior to, then to the right of, the ascending aorta and ends at the level of the sternal angle. The inferior aortic recess, also extending from the transverse sinus, is a diverticulum descending from a superiorly located mouth to run between the lower ascending part of the aorta and the right atrium. The left pulmonary recess, with its mouth under the fold of the left vena cava, passes to the left between the inferior aspect of the left pulmonary artery and the upper border of the superior left pulmonary vein. The right pulmonary recess lies between the lower surface of the proximal part of the right pulmonary artery and the upper border of the left atrium.

A triangular fold of serosal pericardium is reflected from the left pulmonary artery to the subjacent upper left pulmonary vein as the fold of the left superior vena cava. It contains a fibrous ligament, a remnant of the obliterated left common cardinal vein (left duct of Cuvier, p. 1033). This ligament descends anterior to the left pulmonary hilum from the upper part of the left superior intercostal vein to the back of the left atrium, where it is continuous with the oblique vein of the left atrium. The left common cardinal vein may persist as a left superior vena cava which then replaces the oblique vein of the left atrium and empties into the coronary sinus. When both common cardinal veins persist as right and left superior venae cavae, the transverse anastomosis between them, which normally forms the left brachiocephalic vein, may be small or absent. When there is a left superior vena cava, it is joined by the left superior intercostal vein.

VASCULAR SUPPLY AND LYMPHATIC DRAINAGE

The arteries of the pericardium are derived from the internal thoracic and musculophrenic arteries and the descending thoracic aorta. The veins are tributaries of the azygos system.

INNERVATION

The pericardium is innervated by the vagus, together with phrenic nerves and the sympathetic trunks. Pericardial pain is typically a sharp severe substernal pain. It may be exacerbated by lying back or on the left side and relieved by leaning forward. It occasionally radiates to the upper border of trapezius.

CARDIAC TAMPONADE

Cardiac tamponade is external compression of the heart usually caused by accumulation of fluid in the pericardial space. This causes compression of the right atrium and reduces venous return, which reduces cardiac output. It may occur after trauma, proximal extension from a dissecting aortic aneurysm or cardiac surgery. Patients develop hypotension and circulatory collapse. Emergency treatment involves first relieving the tamponade by percutaneous pericardial aspiration, followed by surgery to address the underlying cause. Echocardiography can be useful in assessing tamponade and is also useful in guiding percutaneous pericardial aspiration (p. 949). Surgery is via a subxiphoid incision or a left anterior thoracotomy.

HEART

The microstructure of smooth muscle, the cardiovascular and lymphatic systems and cardiac muscle are described in detail in Chapter 7 (pp. 137, 146, 150).

General organization

The heart is a pair of valved muscular pumps combined in a single organ (**Fig. 60.3**). Although the fibromuscular framework and conducting tissues of these pumps are structurally interwoven, each pump (the so-called 'right' and 'left' hearts) is physiologically separate, and is interposed in series at different points in the double circulation. Despite this functional disposition in series, the two pumps are usually described topographically in parallel.

Of the four cardiac chambers, the two atria receive venous blood as weakly contractile reservoirs for final filling of the two ventricles, which then provide the powerful expulsive contraction that forces blood into the main arterial trunks.

The right heart commences at the right atrium, and receives the superior and inferior venae cavae together with the main venous inflow from the heart itself via the coronary sinus. This systemic venous blood traverses the right atrioventricular orifice, guarded by the tricuspid valve, to enter the inlet component of the right ventricle. Contraction of the ventricle, particularly its apical trabecular component, closes the tricuspid valve and, with increasing pressure, ejects the blood through the muscular right ventricular outflow tract into the pulmonary trunk. The blood then flows through the pulmonary vascular bed, which has a relatively low resistance. Changes in pressure, time relations and valvular events are described below. Many structural features of the 'right heart', including its overall geometry, myocardial architecture and the construction and the relative strengths of the tricuspid and pulmonary valves, accord with this low resistance, being associated with comparatively low changes in pressure.

The left heart commences at the left atrium, which receives all the pulmonary inflow of oxygenated blood and some coronary venous inflow. It contracts to fill the left ventricle through the left atrioventricular orifice guarded by its mitral valve. The valve is the entry to the inlet of the left ventricle. Ventricular contraction rapidly increases the pressure in the apical trabecular component, closing the mitral valve and opening the aortic valve, enabling the ventricle to eject via the left ventricular outflow tract into the aortic sinuses and the ascending aorta, and thence to the entire systemic arterial tree, including the coronary arteries. This vast vascular bed presents a high peripheral resistance that, with large metabolic demands (especially the sustained requirements of the cerebral tissues), explains the more massive structural organization of the 'left heart'. The ejection phase of the left ventricle is shorter than that of the right, but its fluctuations in pressure are very much greater.

A

B

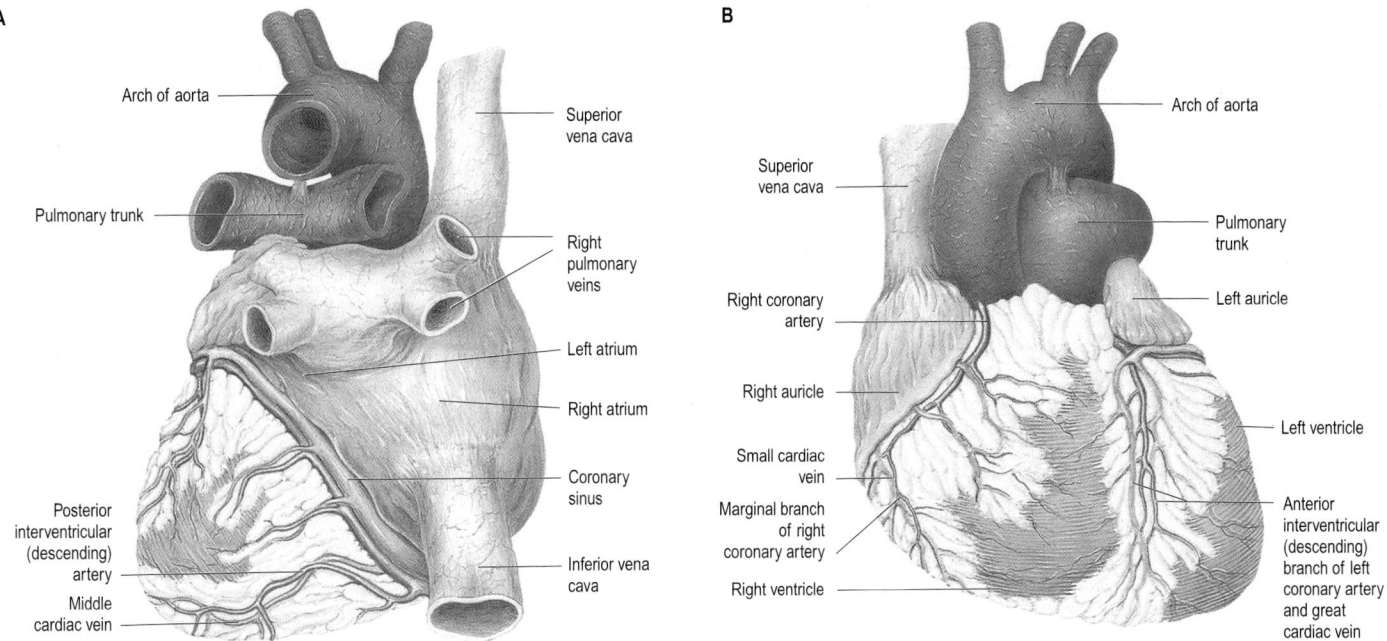

Fig. 60.3 The heart and great vessels. The pulmonary veins carry oxygenated blood, and the pulmonary trunk carries deoxygenated blood.

Because of its contrasting functional demands, the heart is far from a simple pair of (structurally combined) parallel pumps, even though the right and left ventricles must deliver more or less the same volume with each contraction. The heart has a complicated, spiral, three-dimensional organization which is markedly skewed when compared with the planes of the body. Terms such as 'left' and 'right', 'anterior' and 'posterior', 'superior' and 'inferior', therefore, do not always assist the descriptions of cardiac anatomy. Another potential source of confusion is the usual study of isolated whole or dissected hearts, with the subsequent difficulty in relating details to the heart as it is positioned within the body. The following preliminary description emphasizes such difficulties in order to circumvent certain misconceptions, before proceeding to an account of more detailed structure.

The right heart, while forming the right aspect or 'border' (pp. 1000, 1001), follows a gentle curve and covers most of the anterior aspect of the left heart (except for a left-sided strip including the apex). Thus the right heart forms the largest part of the anterior surface, its outflow tract ascending until it terminates on the left side of the outflow tract from the left ventricle. The sites of the tricuspid and pulmonary valves are widely separated and on different planes, the flat cavity of the right ventricle (crescentic in its section) splaying out between them. Conversely, the left heart (except the left-sided strip mentioned above) is largely posterior in position and when viewed from the front is obscured by the chambers of the right heart. The inlet to the left ventricle (containing the mitral valve) is very close to its outlet (the aortic valve), the two being embraced by the wide tract linking inlet and outlet components of the right ventricle. The planes of the left ventricular orifices, although relatively inclined, are more nearly co-planar than those of the right. The left ventricular cavity is narrow and conical, and its tip occupies the cardiac apex. Most of the base of the heart is made up of the left atrium.

CARDIAC SIZE, SHAPE AND EXTERNAL FEATURES

The heart is a hollow, fibromuscular organ of a somewhat conical or pyramidal form, with a base, apex and a series of surfaces and 'borders'. Enclosed in the pericardium (**Figs 60.1, 60.4**), it occupies the middle mediastinum between the lungs and their pleural coverings. It is placed obliquely behind the body of the sternum and the adjoining costal cartilages and ribs. Approximately one-third of the mass lies to the right of the midline.

An average adult heart is c.12 cm from base to apex, 8–9 cm at its broadest transverse diameter and 6 cm anteroposteriorly. Its weight varies from 280 to 340 g (average 300 g) in males and from 230 to 280 g (average 250 g) in females. Cardiac weight is c.0.45% of body weight in males and 0.40% in females. Adult weight is achieved between the ages of 17 and 20 years. The oblique position of the heart may be emphasized by comparing it to a rather deformed pyramid, with the base facing posteriorly and to the right, and the apex anteriorly and to the left. A line from the apex to the approximate centre of the base, projected posterolaterally, emerges near the right midscapular line. Some surfaces of the cardiac 'pyramid' are flat, others more or less convex, these aspects merging along rather ill-defined 'borders'. Precise definition of surfaces and intervening 'borders' is, therefore, difficult. In the account that follows, official nomenclature (*Terminologia Anatomica* 1998) and more generally used terms from clinical practice are given as alternatives. The heart is described as having a base and apex, its surfaces being designated as sternocostal (anterior), diaphragmatic (inferior) and right and left (pulmonary). Its borders are termed upper, inferior ('acute' margin or border) and left ('obtuse' margin or border). Some name the right surface a 'border', despite its extent. One avoidable source of confusion is the use of 'posterior', which can be replaced with the unambiguous term 'diaphragmatic'. If posterior is to be used for a cardiac surface, it should be reserved for the base. (However, compounding this difficulty, there are a number of different usages of the term 'cardiac base'.)

The heart is placed obliquely in the thorax. The atrial and ventricular septal structures are virtually in line, but inclined forwards and to the left at c.45° to a sagittal plane. The planes of the mitral and tricuspid valves, although vertical and not precisely co-planar, are broadly at right angles to the septal plane. The right atrium, therefore, is not only to the right, but also anterior and inferior to the left atrium. It is also partly anterior to the left ventricle, an important atrioventricular septum intervening. The right ventricle forms most of the anterior aspect of the ventricular mass (**Fig. 60.5**), only its inferior end is to the right of the left ventricle, its upper left extremity (pulmonary orifice) is to the left and superior relative to the aortic valve. The left atrium forms most of the posterior aspect of the heart, whereas the left ventricle is only prominent inferiorly, running along the left margin to reach the apex. The atria are essentially right of and posterior to their respective ventricles. These general dispositions are of the greatest importance in planning or interpreting radiographs, scans, angiocardiograms and echocardiograms.

GROOVES ON THE CARDIAC SURFACE

The division of the heart into four chambers produces boundaries that are visible externally as grooves (sulci). Some are deep and obvious and

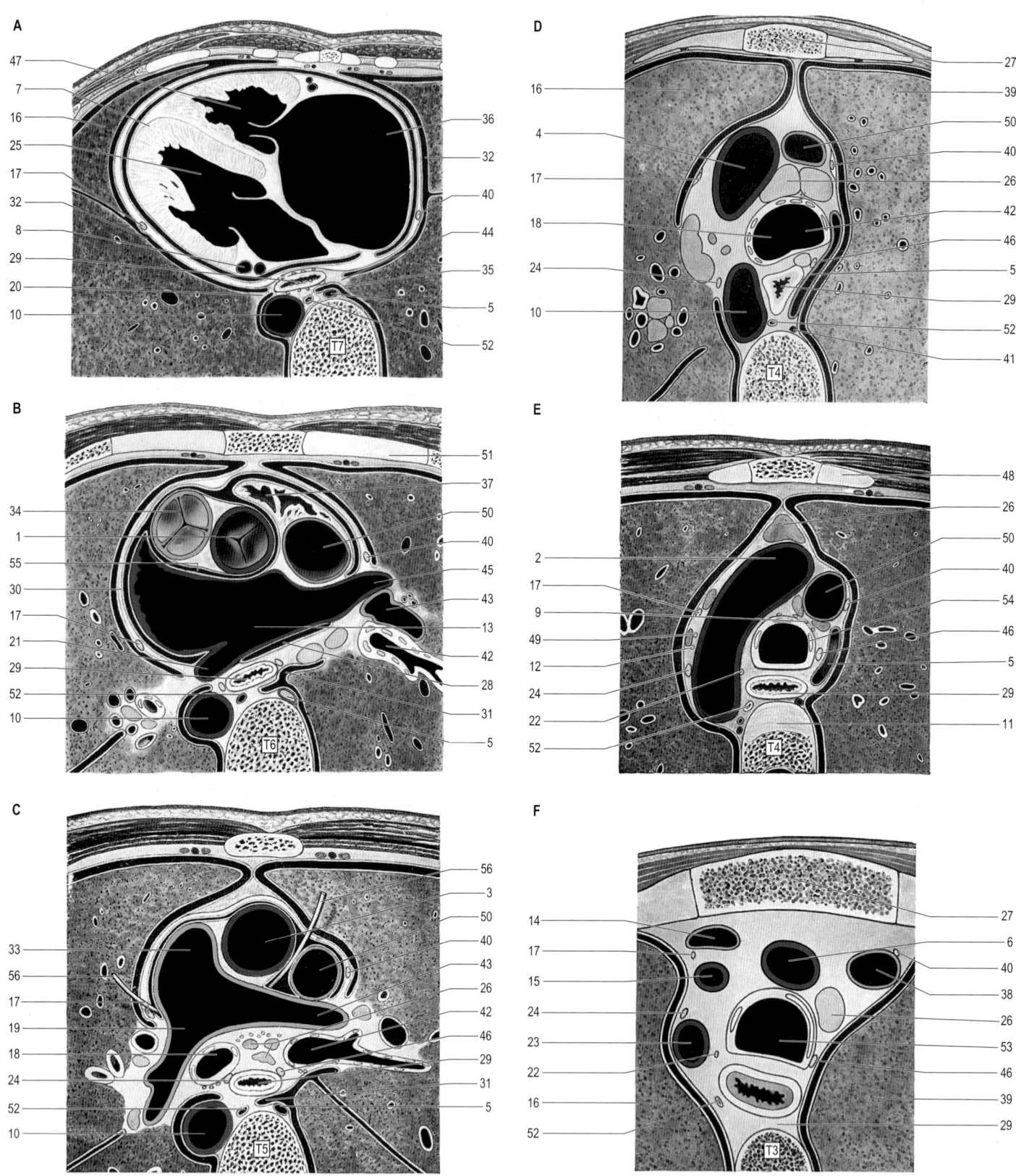

1. Aortic valve. 2. Arch of aorta. 3. Ascending aorta. 4. Ascending aorta near termination. 5. Azygos vein. 6. Brachiocephalic artery. 7. Cardiac apex. 8. Coronary sinus. 9. Deep cardiac plexus. 10. Descending thoracic aorta. 11. Disc between T3 and T4. 12. Inferior cervical branch of left vagus. 13. Left atrium. 14. Left brachiocephalic vein. 15. Left common carotid artery. 16. Left lung. 17. Left phrenic nerve. 18. Left principal bronchus. 19. Left pulmonary artery. 20. Left pulmonary ligament. 21. Left pulmonary vein. 22. Left recurrent laryngeal nerve. 23. Left subclavian artery. 24. Left vagus nerve. 25. Left ventricle. 26. Lymph node. 27. Manubrium of sternum. 28. Oblique sinus. 29. Oesophagus. 30. Pericardium. 31. Pleural recess. 32. Pleural sac. 33. Pulmonary trunk. 34. Pulmonary valve. 35. Recess of right pleural sac. 36. Right atrium. 37. Right auricle. 38. Right brachiocephalic vein. 39. Right lung. 40. Right phrenic nerve. 41. Right posterior intercostal artery. 42. Right principal bronchus. 43. Right pulmonary artery. 44. Right pulmonary ligament. 45. Right pulmonary vein. 46. Right vagus nerve. 47. Right ventricle. 48. Second costal cartilage. 49. Superior cervical cardiac branch of left sympathetic chain. 50. Superior vena cava. 51. Third costal cartilage. 52. Thoracic duct. 53. Trachea. 54. Tracheal bifurcation. 55. Transverse sinus of pericardium. 56. Wire in transverse sinus.

Fig. 60.4 Transverse sections through the mediastinum at six levels, viewed from below. **A**, At the body of T7. Note the general disposition of the cardiac cavities, their intervening septa (c.45° to sagittal and coronal planes) and, orthogonal to this, the plane of the atrioventricular valves. The oesophageal plexus of nerves is clear but not labelled. **B**, At the body of T6. **C**, At the upper border of T5. Note the nerve fibres of the deep cardiac and posterior pulmonary plexuses, and the inferior tracheobronchial and hilar lymph nodes. **D**, At the lower part of the body of T4. **E**, At the upper part of the body of T4. **F**, At the body of T3.

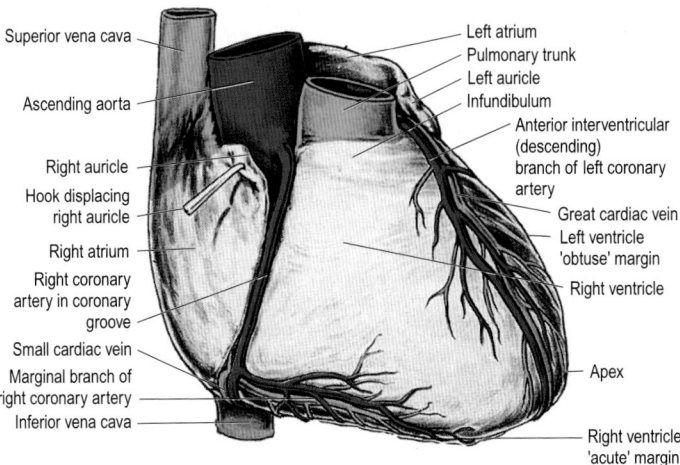

Superior vena cava
Ascending aorta
Right auricle
Hook displacing right auricle
Right atrium
Right coronary artery in coronary groove
Small cardiac vein
Marginal branch of right coronary artery
Inferior vena cava

Left atrium
Pulmonary trunk
Left auricle
Infundibulum
Anterior interventricular (descending) branch of left coronary artery
Great cardiac vein
Left ventricle 'obtuse' margin
Right ventricle
Apex
Right ventricle 'acute' margin

Fig. 60.5 The anterior or sternocostal surface of the heart. The pulmonary trunk is coloured blue because it contains deoxygenated blood.

contain prominent structures. Others are less distinct, even barely perceptible, and are sometimes obscured, in part, by the major structures that cross them. The interatrial groove is a shallow groove separating the two atria. The lateral limits are defined by the borders of the atria. The atrioventricular (coronary) groove (or sulcus) separates the atria from the ventricles. This groove, containing the main trunks of the coronary arteries, is oblique. It descends to the right on the sternocostal surface (**Fig. 60.5**), separating the right atrium (and its auricle) from the oblique right margin of the right ventricle and its infundibulum. Its upper left part is obliterated where it is crossed by the pulmonary trunk and, behind this, the aorta, from which the coronary arteries originate. Continuing to the left, the groove curves around the 'obtuse' margin and descends to the right, separating the atrial base from the diaphragmatic surface of the ventricles (**Fig. 60.2**). This diaphragmatic part of the atrioventricular groove then curves around the 'acute' margin at its lower right end to become confluent with the sternocostal part. Thus the groove passes from high on the left to low on the right, with the diaphragmatic part being a little to the left of the sternocostal. A section that includes the atrioventricular groove is at c.45° to the sagittal plane and at a greater but variable angle to the transverse and coronal planes. It approximately traverses the lines of attachment of the atrioventricular valves and (even less precisely) those of the aortic and pulmonary valves. A line at right angles to the centre of this plane will descend forwards and leftwards to the cardiac apex.

Internally, the ventricles are separated by the septum. The mural margins of the septum correspond to the anterior and inferior (diaphragmatic) interventricular grooves. The anterior groove, seen on the sternocostal cardiac surface, is near and almost parallel to the left ventricular obtuse margin. On the diaphragmatic surface, the groove is closer to the midpoint of the ventricular mass. The interventricular grooves extend from the atrioventricular groove to the apical notch on the acute margin, which is a little to the right of the true cardiac apex.

CARDIAC BASE, APEX, SURFACES AND BORDERS

Posterior aspect of the heart – The true cardiac base is somewhat quadrilateral, with curved lateral extensions. It faces back and to the right, separated from the thoracic vertebrae (fifth to eighth in the recumbent, sixth to ninth in the erect posture) by the pericardium, right pulmonary veins, oesophagus and aorta. It is formed mainly by the left atrium, and only partly by the posterior part of the right atrium (**Fig. 60.2**). It extends superiorly to the bifurcation of the pulmonary trunk and inferiorly to the posterior part of the atrioventricular groove, which contains the coronary sinus and branches of the coronary arteries (pp. 1018, 1014). It is limited to the right and left by the rounded surfaces of the corresponding atria. These are separated by the shallow interatrial groove. The point of junction of the atrioventricular, interatrial and posterior interventricular grooves is termed the crux of the heart (**Fig. 60.2**). Two pulmonary veins on each side open into the left atrial part of the base, whereas the superior and the inferior vena cava

open into the upper and lower parts of the right atrial basal region. The area of the left atrium between the openings of right and left pulmonary veins forms the anterior wall of the oblique pericardial sinus (**Fig. 60.1**). This description of the anatomical base reflects the usual position of the heart in the thorax. Some confusion is produced by other current usages of the term 'base'. It is often applied to the segment of the atrioventricular and ventriculoarterial junctions seen after dissections through the atrioventricular groove. This area is better termed the base of the ventricles. In clinical practice, auscultation in or near the parasternal parts of the second intercostal spaces is often described as occurring at the clinical 'base', to make the contrast with the clinical 'apex'. Such descriptions, while less than perfect anatomically, will almost certainly persist.

Anatomical apex of the heart – This is the apex of the conical left ventricle, which is directed down, forwards and to the left. It is overlapped by the left lung and pleura. The apex is located most commonly behind the fifth left intercostal space, near or a little medial to the midclavicular line.

Anterior, sternocostal surface of the heart– Facing forwards and upwards, the anterior surface has an acute right and a more gradual left convexity (**Figs 60.5, 60.6**). It consists of an atrial area above and to the right, and a ventricular part below and to the left of the atrioventricular groove. The atrial area is occupied almost entirely by the right atrium. The left atrium is largely hidden by the ascending aorta and pulmonary trunk. Only a small part of the left appendage projects forwards to the left of the pulmonary trunk. Of the ventricular region, about one-third is made up by the left and two-thirds by the right ventricle. The site of the septum between them is indicated by the anterior interventricular groove. The sternocostal surface is separated by the pericardium from the body of the sternum, the sternocostal muscles and the third to the sixth costal cartilages. Because of the bulge of the heart to the left, more of this surface is behind the left costal cartilages than behind the right ones. It is also covered by the pleural membranes and by the thin anterior edges of the lungs, except for a triangular area at the cardiac incisure of the left lung. The lungs and their pleural coverings are variable in their degree of overlap of the heart.

Inferior, diaphragmatic surface of the heart – Largely horizontal, the inferior surface of the heart slopes down and forwards a little towards the apex (**Fig. 60.2**). It is formed by the ventricles (chiefly the left) and rests mainly upon the central tendon but also, apically, on a small area of the left muscular part of the diaphragm. It is separated from the anatomical base by the atrioventricular groove and is traversed obliquely by the posterior interventricular groove.

Left surface of the heart – Facing up, back and to the left, the left surface consists almost entirely of the obtuse margin of the left ventricle, but a small part of the left atrium and its auricle contribute superiorly. Convex and widest above, where it is crossed by the atrioventricular groove, it narrows to the cardiac apex. It is separated by the pericardium from the left phrenic nerve and its accompanying vessels, and by the left pleura from the deep concavity of the left lung.

Right surface of the heart – The right surface is rounded and formed by the right atrial wall. It is separated from the mediastinal aspect of the right lung by the pericardium and the pleural coverings. Its convexity merges below into the short intrathoracic part of the inferior vena cava and above into the superior vena cava. The sulcus terminalis (terminal groove) is a prominent landmark between the true atrial and the venous components of the right atrium, curving approximately along the junction of the sternocostal and right surfaces.

Upper border of the heart – This is atrial (mainly the left atrium). Anterior to it are the ascending aorta and the pulmonary trunk (**Fig. 60.1**). At its extremity, the superior vena cava enters the right atrium.

Right border of the heart – Corresponding to the right atrium, the profile of the right border is slightly convex to the right and it approaches the vertical.

Inferior border of the heart – Also known as the acute margin of the heart, the inferior border is sharp, thin and nearly horizontal. It extends

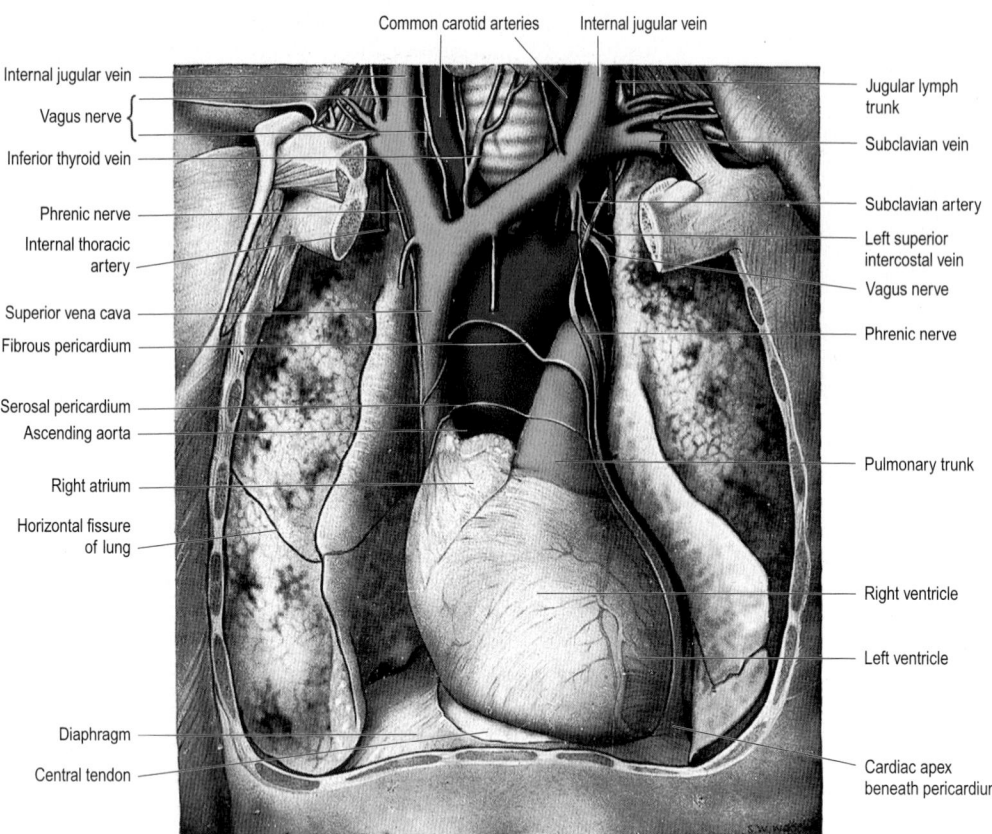

Common carotid arteries

Internal jugular vein

Internal jugular vein

Vagus nerve

Inferior thyroid vein

Phrenic nerve

Internal thoracic artery

Superior vena cava

Fibrous pericardium

Serosal pericardium

Ascending aorta

Right atrium

Horizontal fissure of lung

Diaphragm

Central tendon

Jugular lymph trunk

Subclavian vein

Subclavian artery

Left superior intercostal vein

Vagus nerve

Phrenic nerve

Pulmonary trunk

Right ventricle

Left ventricle

Cardiac apex beneath pericardium

Fig. 60.6 Dissection that displays the heart, the great vessels and the lungs *in situ*. The sternum and the sternal ends of the costal cartilages, together with the parietal pleura on each side, have been excised and the mediastinal pleura and parietal layer of the pericardium over the sternocostal surface of the heart have been removed. The lungs have been displaced to expose the heart and the epicardium dissected off the heart and roots of the great vessels. On the right side, the inferior cardiac branch of the vagus nerve descends between the brachiocephalic artery and the right brachiocephalic vein. On the left side, a communication descends from the left superior intercostal vein and crosses the aortic arch and the left pulmonary artery to become continuous with the oblique vein of the left atrium.

from the lower limit of the right border to the apex and it is formed mainly by the right ventricle, with a small contribution from the left ventricle near the apex.

Left border of the heart – Also known as the obtuse margin, the left border separates the sternocostal and left surfaces. It is round and mainly formed by the left ventricle but, to a slight extent superiorly, is formed by the auricle of the left atrium. It descends obliquely, convex to the left, from the auricle to the cardiac apex.

RIGHT ATRIUM

GENERAL AND EXTERNAL FEATURES

The interatrial septum (or atrial septum) is oblique, so the right atrium is both anterior and to the right of the left atrium (**Figs 60.2, 60.5**), also extending inferior to it. Its walls form the right upper sternocostal surface, the convex right (pulmonary surface) and a little of the right side of the anatomical base. The superior vena cava opens into its dome and the inferior vena cava into its lower posterior part (**Fig. 60.5**). An extensive muscular pouch, the auricle, projects anteriorly to overlap the right side of the ascending aorta. The auricle is a broad, triangular structure and has a wide junction with the true atrial component of the atrium (**Fig. 60.3**). The junction between the venous part (sinus venarum) and the atrium proper is marked externally by a shallow groove, the sulcus terminalis, extending between the right sides of the openings of the two venae cavae. The sulcus terminalis corresponds, internally, to the terminal crest (crista terminalis) which is the site of origin of the extensive pectinate muscles that arise serially at right angles from the crest (**Fig. 60.7**). Posteriorly, the vertical interatrial groove descends to the crux.

Anteriorly, the right atrium is related to the anterior part of the mediastinal surface of the right lung, from which it is separated by pleura and pericardium. Laterally, the atrium is also related to the mediastinal surface of the right lung, but anterior to its hilum and separated from it by the pleura, right phrenic nerve and pericardiacophrenic vessels and pericardium. Posteriorly and to the left (**Fig. 60.2**), the atrial septum and the surrounding infolded atrial walls separate the right from the left atrium (the mural infolding is indicated by an extensive interatrial groove). Posteriorly and to the right are the right pulmonary veins.

Medially are the ascending aorta and, to a lesser extent, the root of the pulmonary trunk and its bifurcation.

INTERIOR SURFACE

The interior surface of the right atrium can be divided into three regions: a smooth-walled venous component posteriorly that leads, anteriorly, to the vestibule of the tricuspid valve and the auricle (**Fig. 60.7**). The wall of the vestibule is smooth, but its junction with the auricle is ridged all around the atrioventricular junction. The smooth-walled part receives the opening of the venae cavae and the coronary sinus. It represents the venous component ('sinus venosus') of the developing heart (p. 1033). The wall of the vestibule has a ridged surface and that of the auricle is trabeculated. Both are derived from the embryonic atrium proper.

The superior and inferior venae cavae open into the venous component. The superior vena cava returns blood from head, neck and upper limb through an orifice that faces inferoanteriorly and has no valve. The inferior vena cava is larger than its superior counterpart and returns blood from the lower part of the body into the lowest part of the atrium near the septum. Anterior to its orifice is a flap-like valve, the Eustachian valve or valve of the inferior vena cava (**Fig. 60.7**). Of varying size, this valve is found along the lateral, or right, margin of the vein. When traced inferiorly, it runs into the sinus septum (see below), where it is contiguous with the valve of the coronary sinus (Thebesius' valve, also known as the Thebesian valve). The lateral part of the Eustachian valve becomes continuous with the lower end of the terminal crest. The valve is a fold of endocardium enclosing a few muscular fibres. It is large during fetal life, when it serves to direct richly oxygenated blood from the placenta through the foramen ovale of the atrial septum into the left atrium. The valve varies markedly in size in postnatal life; it is sometimes cribriform or filamentous but often is absent. A particularly prominent recess, behind the Eustachian valve, is seen posteroinferiorly relative to the ostium of the coronary sinus.

The coronary sinus opens into the venous atrial component between the orifice of the inferior vena cava, the oval fossa and the vestibule of the atrioventricular opening (**Fig. 60.7**). The coronary sinus is often guarded by a thin, semicircular valve that covers the lower part of the orifice (Thebesius' valve). The upper limb of this valve joins with the Eustachian valve and, from this commissure, a tendinous structure runs

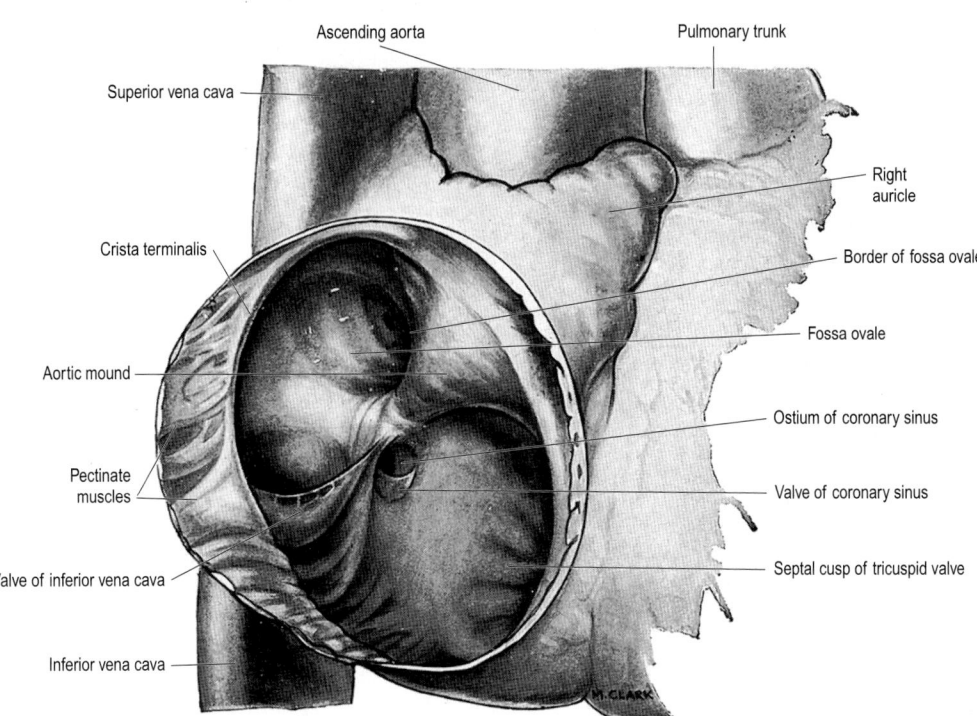

Ascending aorta

Pulmonary trunk

Superior vena cava

Right
auricle

Crista terminalis

Border of fossa ovale

Aortic mound

Fossa ovale

Ostium of coronary sinus

Pectinate
muscles

Valve of coronary sinus

Valve of inferior vena cava

Septal cusp of tricuspid valve

Inferior vena cava

Fig. 60.7 The interior of the right atrium, viewed from the front. The sinu-atrial node is embedded in the anterior wall of the atrium at the upper end of the crista terminalis just below the opening of the superior vena cava. The atrioventricular node is in the interatrial septum, just above and to the left of the opening of the coronary sinus.

into the sinus septum (the septum between the coronary sinus and the fossa ovale). The tendinous structure, called the tendon of Todaro, runs forwards to insert into the central fibrous body. It is one of the landmarks of the triangle of Koch (**Fig. 60.8**). The ostium of the coronary sinus forms a prominent landmark in the right atrium (**Fig. 60.7**). The sinus itself lies within the left atrioventricular groove (**Fig. 60.2**). It is the conduit for return of most of the venous blood from the heart, although some atrial veins drain directly to the right or left atrial chambers. The coronary sinus begins at the point where the oblique vein of the left atrium joins the great cardiac vein. The sinus receives the middle and small cardiac veins close to its junction with the right atrium.

Several small venous ostia, draining the minimal atrial veins, are found scattered around the atrial walls. They return a small fraction of blood from the heart, and are most numerous on the septal aspect. The anterior cardiac veins and, sometimes, the right marginal vein may enter the atrium through larger ostia.

The atrium proper and the auricle are separated from the venous sinus by the crista terminalis. This smooth, muscular ridge begins on the upper part of the septal surface and, passing anterior to the orifice of the superior vena cava, skirts its right margin to reach the right side of the orifice of the inferior vena cava (**Fig. 60.7**). It marks the site of the right venous valve of the embryonic heart (p. 1033), and corresponds externally to the terminal groove. Within the superior part of the groove, lateral to and extending below the orifice of the superior vena cava, is the sinu-atrial node.

The pectinate muscles (musculi pectinati), almost parallel muscular ridges, extend anterolaterally from the terminal crest and reach into the auricle, where they form several trabeculations.

The septal wall presents the fossa ovale, an oval depression above and to the left of the orifice of the inferior vena cava. Its floor is the primary atrial septum, the septum primum. The rim of the fossa is prominent and, although often said to represent the edge of the so-called septum secundum, in reality it is merely the infolded walls of the atrial chambers. It is most distinct above and in front of the fossa, and is usually deficient inferiorly. A small slit is sometimes found at the upper margin of the fossa, ascending beneath the rim to communicate with the left atrium. This represents failure of obliteration of the fetal foramen ovale, which remains patent in up to one-third of all normal hearts.

Anteroinferior in the right atrium is the large, oval vestibule leading to the orifice of the tricuspid valve. A triangular zone (the triangle of Koch, **Fig. 60.8**) is found between the attachment of the septal cusp of the tricuspid valve, the anteromedial margin of the ostium of the coronary sinus, and the round, collagenous, palpable, subendocardial

tendon of Todaro. The triangle is a landmark of particular surgical importance, indicating the site of the atrioventricular node and its atrial connections. Anterosuperior to the insertion of the tendon of Todaro, the septal wall is formed by the atrioventricular component of the membranous septum, intervening between the right atrium and subaortic outlet of the left ventricle (**Fig. 60.8**). The atrial wall bulges anterosuperiorly above the membranous septum. This area is the aortic mound (torus aorticus) and marks the location of the non-coronary sinus of the aorta with its enclosed valvular cusp.

RIGHT VENTRICLE

The right ventricle extends from the right atrioventricular (tricuspid) orifice nearly to the cardiac apex. It then ascends to the left to become the infundibulum, or conus arteriosus, reaching the pulmonary orifice and supporting the cusps of the pulmonary valve. Topographically, the ventricle possesses: an inlet component, supporting and surrounding the tricuspid valve, a coarsely trabeculated apical component, and the muscular outlet or infundibulum, which surrounds the attachments of the cusps of the pulmonary valve.

EXTERNAL FEATURES

The convex anterosuperior surface of the right ventricle makes up a large part of the sternocostal aspect of the heart (**Fig. 60.3**), separated from the thoracic wall only by the pericardium. The left pleura and, to a lesser extent, the anterior margin of the left lung are interposed above and to the left. The inferior surface is flat and is related mainly, with the interposition of the pericardium, to the central tendon and a small adjoining muscular part of the diaphragm. The left and posterior wall is the ventricular septum. This is slightly curved and bulges into the right ventricle so that, in sections across the cardiac axis, the outline of the right ventricle is crescentic. A delicate collagenous band, the tendon of the infundibulum (conus ligament), is believed by some to connect the pulmonary muscular infundibulum posteriorly to the root of the aorta. The wall of the right ventricle is significantly thinner (3–5 mm on average) than that of the left, the ratio usually being c.1:3.

INTERNAL FEATURES

The inlet and outlet components of the ventricle, supporting and surrounding the cusps of the tricuspid and pulmonary valves respectively, are separated in the roof of the ventricle by the prominent supraventricular crest (crista supraventricularis; **Fig. 60.9**). The crest is a thick, muscular, highly arched structure, extending obliquely forwards and to the right from a septal limb high on the interventricular septal wall to

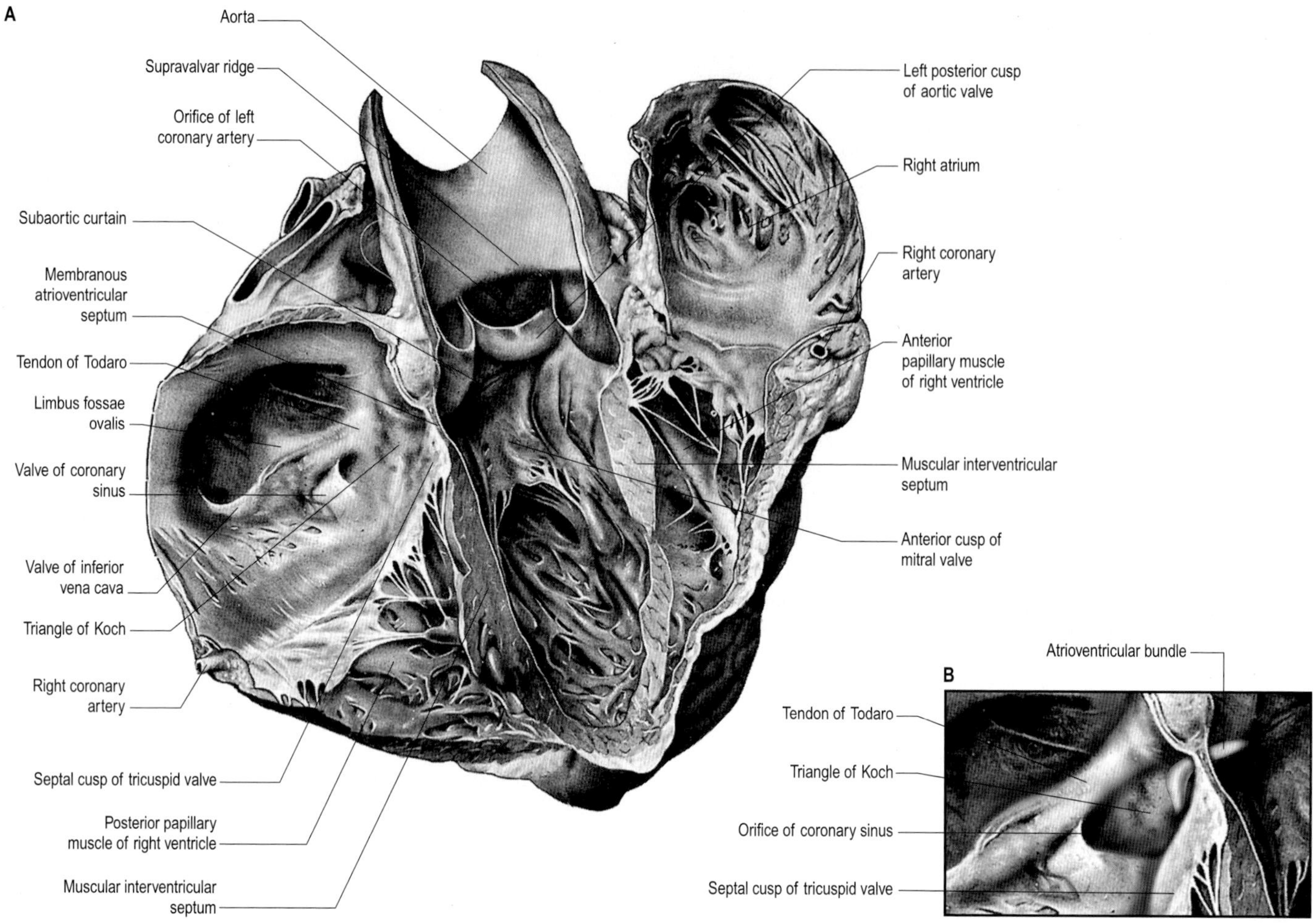

A

Aorta

Supravalvar ridge

Orifice of left
coronary artery

Subaortic curtain

Membranous
atrioventricular
septum

Tendon of Todaro

Limbus fossae
ovalis

Valve of coronary
sinus

Valve of inferior
vena cava

Triangle of Koch

Right coronary
artery

Septal cusp of tricuspid valve

Posterior papillary
muscle of right ventricle

Muscular interventricular
septum

Left posterior cusp
of aortic valve

Right atrium

Right coronary
artery

Anterior
papillary muscle
of right ventricle

Muscular interventricular
septum

Anterior cusp of
mitral valve

B

Atrioventricular bundle

Tendon of Todaro

Triangle of Koch

Orifice of coronary sinus

Septal cusp of tricuspid valve

Fig. 60.8 A, The interior of the heart, revealed by incising it along its right and lower surfaces and excising the pulmonary trunk and infundibulum. The rest of the heart has been turned over to the left. **B**, The triangle of Koch, which is defined by the tendon of Todaro, ostium of the coronary sinus and the septal aspect of the tricuspid valve.

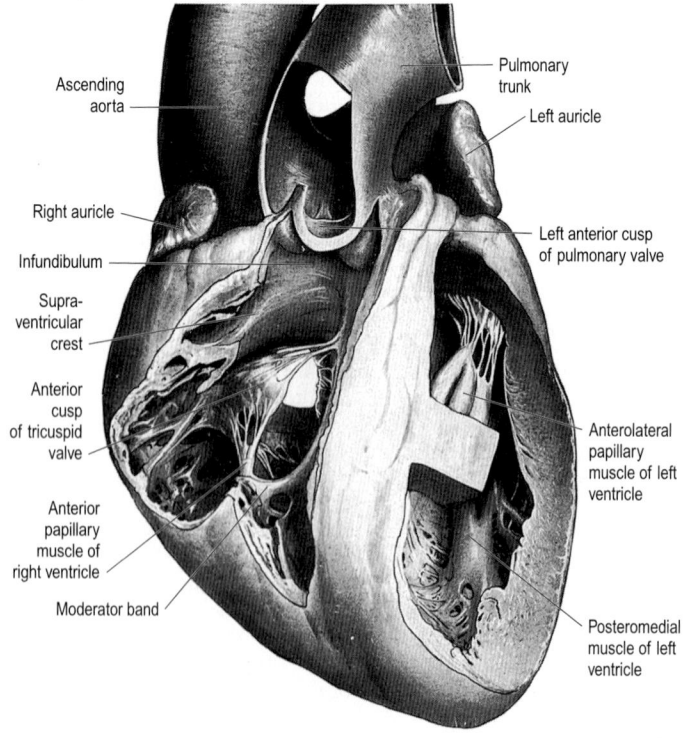

Ascending
aorta

Right auricle

Infundibulum

Supra-
ventricular
crest

Anterior
cusp
of tricuspid
valve

Anterior
papillary
muscle of
right ventricle

Moderator band

Pulmonary
trunk

Left auricle

Left anterior cusp
of pulmonary valve

Anterolateral
papillary
muscle of left
ventricle

Posteromedial
muscle of left
ventricle

Fig. 60.9 A dissection opening the ventricles, viewed from the front.

a mural or parietal limb on the anterolateral right ventricular wall. The posterolateral aspect of the crest provides a principal attachment for the anterosuperior cusp of the tricuspid valve. The septal limb of the crest may be continuous with, or embraced by, the septal limbs of the septomarginal trabecula. The inlet and outlet regions extend apically into and from the prominent coarsely trabeculated component of the ventricle. The inlet component is itself also trabeculated, whereas the outlet component (or infundibulum) has predominantly smooth walls. The trabeculated appearance is caused by a myriad of irregular muscular ridges and protrusions, which are known collectively as trabeculae carneae, and are lined by endocardium. These protrusions and intervening grooves impart great variation in wall thickness. Protrusions vary in extent from mere ridges to trabeculae that are fixed at both ends but free in between. Other conspicuous protrusions are the papillary muscles, which are inserted at one end onto the ventricular wall and are continuous at the other end with collagenous cords, the chordae tendineae, inserted on the free edge and elsewhere on the free aspect of the atrioventricular valves. One protrusion in the right ventricle, the septomarginal trabecula or septal band, is particularly prominent. It reinforces the septal surface where, at the base, it divides into limbs that embrace the supraventricular crest. Towards the apex, it supports the anterior papillary muscle of the tricuspid valve and, from this point, crosses to the parietal wall of the ventricle as the 'moderator band' (this alternative name records an old idea that the septomarginal trabecula prevents overdistension of the ventricle). A further series of prominent trabeculae extend from its anterior surface and run onto the parietal ventricular wall. These are the septoparietal trabeculations. The smooth-walled outflow tract, or infundibulum (conus arteriosus), ascends to the left above the septoparietal trabeculations and below the arch of the supraventricular crest to the pulmonary orifice.

TRICUSPID VALVE

The atrioventricular valvular complex, in both right and left ventricles, consists of the orifice and its associated anulus, the cusps, the supporting chordae tendineae of various types and the papillary muscles.

Harmonious interplay of all these, together with the atrial and ventricular myocardial masses, depends on the conducting tissues and the mechanical cohesion provided by the fibroelastic cardiac skeleton. All parts change substantially in position, shape, angulation and dimensions during a single cardiac cycle.

TRICUSPID VALVULAR ORIFICE

The tricuspid valve orifice is best seen from the atrial aspect and measures 11.4 cm in circumference in males and 10.8 cm in females. It has a clear line of transition from the atrial wall or septum to the lines of attachment of the valvular cusps. Its margins are not precisely in a single plane. It is almost vertical, but at c.45° to the sagittal plane and slightly inclined to the vertical, such that it 'faces' (on its ventricular aspect) anterolaterally to the left and somewhat inferiorly (**Fig. 60.10**). Roughly triangular, its margins are described as anterosuperior, inferior and septal, corresponding to the lines of attachment of the valvular cusps.

The connective tissues around the orifice of the atrioventricular valves separate the atrial and ventricular myocardial masses completely, except at the point of penetration of the atrioventricular bundle, and vary in density and disposition around the valvular circumference. Extending from the right fibrous trigone component of the central fibrous body are a pair of curved, tapered, subendocardial tendons, or 'prongs' (fila coronaria) that partly encircle the circumference. The latter is completed by more tenuous, deformable fibroblastic sulcal areolar tissue. The extent of fibrous tissue also varies with sex and age. Nevertheless, the tissue within the atrioventricular junction around the tricuspid orifice is less robust than similar elements found at the attachments of the mitral

valve. Furthermore, in the tricuspid valve, the topographical 'attachment' of the free valvular cusps does not wholly correspond to the internal level of attachment of the fibrous core of the valve to the junctional atrioventricular connective tissue. It is the line of attachment of the cusp that is best appreciated in the heart when examined grossly, and this feature is also more readily discerned clinically.

TRICUSPID VALVE CUSPS

It is usually possible to distinguish three cusps in the tricuspid valve, hence the name. They are located anterosuperiorly, septally and inferiorly, corresponding to the marginal sectors of the atrioventricular orifice so named. Each is a reduplication of endocardium enclosing a collagenous core, continuous marginally and on its ventricular aspect with diverging fascicles of chordae tendineae (see below) and basally confluent with the anular connective tissue. All cusps of the atrioventricular valves display, passing from the free margin to the inserted margin, rough, clear and basal zones. The rough zone is relatively thick, opaque and uneven on its ventricular aspect where most chordae tendineae are attached. The atrial aspect of the rough zone makes contact with the comparable surface of the adjacent cusps during full closure of the valve. The clear zone is smooth and translucent, receives few chordae tendineae and has a thinner fibrous core. The basal zone, extending c.2–3 mm from the circumferential attachment of the cusps, is thicker, contains more connective tissue and is vascularized and innervated. It contains the insertions of the atrial myocardium.

The anterosuperior cusp is the largest component of the tricuspid valve. It is attached chiefly to the atrioventricular junction on the posterolateral aspect of the supraventricular crest, but extends along its septal limb to the membranous septum, ending at the anteroseptal commissure. One or more notches often indent its free margin. The attachment of the septal cusp passes from the inferoseptal commissure on the posterior ventricular wall across the muscular septum and then angles across the membranous septum to the anteroseptal commissure. The septal cusp defines one of the borders of the triangle of Koch, which aids location of the atrioventricular node, which lies at the apex of the triangle. It ensures that this area can be avoided when the tricuspid valve is operated on (**Fig. 60.8**).

The inferior cusp is wholly mural in attachment and guards the diaphragmatic surface of the atrioventricular junction. Its limits are the inferoseptal and anteroinferior commissures.

CHORDAE TENDINEAE (TENDINOUS CORDS)

The chordae tendineae are fibrous collagenous structures supporting the cusps of the atrioventricular valves. False chordae connect papillary muscles to each other or to the ventricular wall including the septum, or pass directly between points on the wall (or septum, or both); they are irregular in numbers and dimensions in the right ventricle. The true chordae usually arise from small projections on the tips or margins of the apical one-thirds of papillary muscles, but sometimes arise from the bases of papillary muscles or directly from the ventricular walls and the septum. They are attached to various parts of the ventricular aspects or the free margins of the cusps. They have been classified into first-, second- and third-order chordae according to the distance of the attachment from the margins of the cusps; this scheme has little functional or morphological merit.

Fan-shaped chordae have a short stem from which branches radiate to attach to the margins (or the ventricular aspect) of the zones of apposition between cusps and to the ends of adjacent cusps. Rough zone chordae arise from a single stem which usually splits into three components that attach to the free margin, the ventricular aspect of the rough zone and to some intermediate point on the cusp, respectively. Free-edge chordae are single, thread-like and often long, passing from either the apex or the base of a papillary muscle into a marginal attachment, usually near the midpoint of a cusp or one of its scallops. Deep chordae, also long, pass beyond the margins and, branching to various extents, reach the more peripheral rough zone or even the clear zone. Basal chordae are round chordae or flat ribbons, long and slender, or short and muscular. They arise from the smooth or trabeculated ventricular wall and attach to the basal component of a cusp.

PAPILLARY MUSCLES

The two major papillary muscles in the right ventricle are located in anterior and posterior positions. A third, smaller muscle has a medial position together with several smaller, and variable, muscles attached to

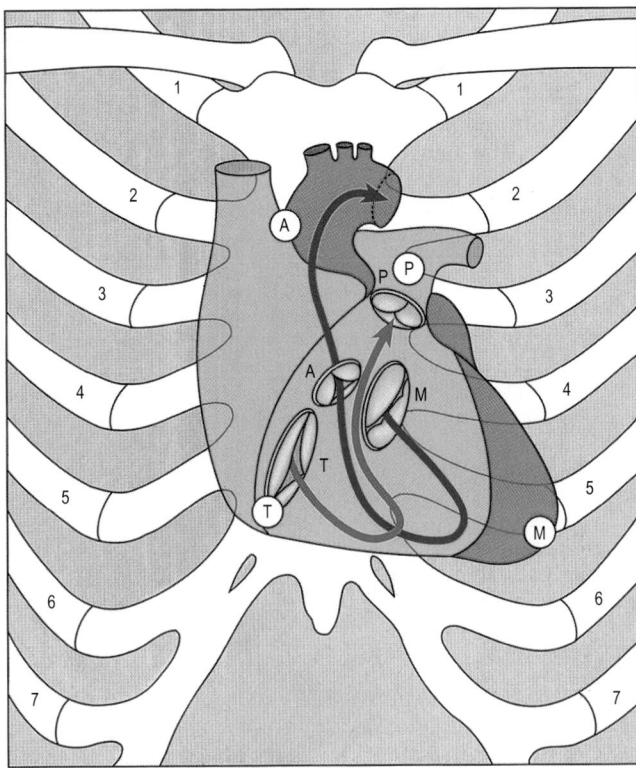

Fig. 60.10 Relation of the sternocostal surface and valves of the heart to the thoracic cage. The right heart is blue, the arrow denoting the inflow and outflow channels of the right ventricle; the left heart is treated similarly in red. The positions, planes and relative sizes of the cardiac valves are shown. The position of the letters, A, P, T and M indicate respectively the aortic, pulmonary, tricuspid and mitral auscultation areas of clinical practice. Note that, for the purpose of illustration, the orifices of the aortic, mitral and tricuspid valves are shown with some separation between them. In reality, the cusps of the three valves are in fibrous continuity (*see* **Fig. 60.12**).

the ventricular septum. The anterior papillary muscle is largest. Its base arises from the right anterolateral ventricular wall below the antero-inferior commissure of the inferior cusp and it also blends with the right end of the septomarginal trabecula. The posterior, or inferior, papillary muscle arises from the myocardium below the inferoseptal commissure. It is frequently bifid or trifid. The septal, or medial, papillary muscle is small but typical, and arises from the posterior septal limb of the septomarginal trabecula. All the major papillary muscles supply chordae to adjacent components of the cusps they support. A feature of the right ventricle is that the septal cusp is tethered by individual chordae tendineae directly to the ventricular septum; such septal insertions are never seen in the left ventricle. When closed, the three cusps fit snugly together, the pattern of the zones of apposition confirming the trifoliate arrangement of the tricuspid valve.

OPENING OF THE TRICUSPID VALVE

Despite its name, the tricuspid valve acts more like a bicuspid valve, because the septal cusp, the smallest of the three cusps, is fixed between the right and left fibrous trigones and the atrial and ventricular septa. The remainder of the tricuspid anulus is muscular. During diastole the right ventricle relaxes, the anulus dilates and the large anterior and posterior cusps move away from the plane of the anulus into the right ventricle. During systole the anulus constricts as the right ventricle contracts, and the two major cusps move like sails to abut a relatively immobile septal cusp and the septum itself.

PULMONARY VALVE

The pulmonary valve, guarding the outflow from the right ventricle, surmounts the infundibulum and is situated at some distance from the other three cardiac valves (**Figs 60.11, 60.12**). Its general plane faces superiorly to the left and slightly posteriorly. It has three semilunar cusps attached by convex edges partly to the infundibular wall of the right ventricle and partly to the origin of the pulmonary trunk. The line of attachments is curved, rising at the periphery of each cusp near their zones of apposition (the commissures) and reaching the sinutubular ridge of the pulmonary trunk (**Fig. 60.13A**). Removal of the cusps shows that the fibrous semilunar attachments enclose three crescents of infundibular musculature within the pulmonary sinuses, whereas three roughly triangular segments of arterial wall are incorporated within the ventricular outflow tract beneath the apex of each commissural attachment (**Fig. 60.13A**). There is, thus, no proper circular 'anulus' supporting the cusps of the valve, and the fibrous semilunar attachment is an essential requisite for snug closure of the nodules and lunules of the cusps (see below) during ventricular diastole. It is difficult to name the cusps and corresponding sinuses of the pulmonary valve and trunk precisely according to the coordinates of the body, because the valvular orifice is obliquely positioned. The official nomenclature (*Terminologia*

Anatomica 1998) refers to an anterior, a posterior and a septal cusp, based on their position in the fetus. The position changes with development and in the adult there are two anterior cusps, right and left, and a posterior one.

Each cusp is a fold of endocardium, with an intervening, and variably developed, fibrous core. The core is substantial along both the free edge and the semilunar attached border, and the latter is particularly thickened at the deepest central part (nadir) of the base of each cusp (thus never forming a simple complete fibrous ring). Central in the free margin of each cusp is a localized thickening of collagen, the nodule of the semilunar 'cusp' (nodule of Arantius). Perforations within the cusps close to the free margin and near the commissures are frequently present, but are of no functional significance. Each semilunar cusp is contained within one of the three sinuses of the pulmonary trunk.

OPENING OF THE PULMONARY VALVE

Except for differences in relations of timing and pressures, opening and closure of the pulmonary valve has much in common with that of the aortic valve (p. 1008; **Fig. 60.14**). During diastole, the pulmonary valve is closed and all three cusps of the valve are tightly apposed. The pulmonary valve is difficult to visualize at echocardiography and usually only the posterior cusp is visible when the valve is closed. Atrial systole may cause a slight posterior movement of the valve cusps. The pulmonary valve opens passively during ventricular systole and then closes rapidly at the end of systole.

LEFT ATRIUM

Although smaller in volume than the right, the left atrium has thicker walls (3 mm on average). Its cavity and walls are formed largely by the proximal parts of the pulmonary veins, which are incorporated into the atrium during development (p. 1033). The only clear derivative of the left part of the embryonic atrium is the auricle, together with the vestibule of the mitral valve. The left atrium is roughly cuboidal and extends behind the right atrium, separated from it by the obliquely positioned septum. Thus the right atrium is in front and anterolateral to the right part of the left atrium. The left part is concealed anteriorly by the initial segments of the pulmonary trunk and aorta: part of the transverse pericardial sinus lies between it and these arterial trunks. Anteroinferiorly, and to the left, it adjoins the base of the left ventricle at the orifice of the mitral valve. Its posterior aspect forms most of the anatomical base of the heart and is approximately quadrangular, receiving the terminations of (usually) two pulmonary veins from each lung. It forms the anterior wall of the oblique pericardial sinus (**Fig. 60.1**). This surface ends at the shallow vertical interatrial groove, which descends to the cardiac crux. The left atrial auricle is constricted at its atrial junction and all the pectinate muscles of the left atrium are contained within it. It is characteristically longer, narrower and more hooked than the right auricle, its margins being more deeply indented. It turns forwards to the left of the pulmonary trunk, overlapping its origin (**Fig. 60.15**). Interiorly, the four pulmonary veins open into the upper posterolateral surfaces of the left atrium, two on each side. Their orifices are smooth and oval, the left pair frequently opening via a common channel. Some minimal cardiac veins return blood directly from the myocardium to the cavity of the left atrium. The left atrial aspect of the septum has a characteristically rough appearance, bounded by a crescentic ridge, concave upwards, which marks the site of the foramen ovale (p. 1033).

LEFT VENTRICLE

GENERAL AND EXTERNAL FEATURES

The left ventricle is constructed in accordance with its role as a powerful pump that sustains pulsatile flow in the high-pressured systemic arteries. Variously described as half-ellipsoid or cone-shaped, it is longer and narrower than the right ventricle, extending from its base in the plane of the atrioventricular groove to the cardiac apex. Its long axis descends forwards and to the left. In transverse section, at right angles to the axis, its cavity is oval or nearly circular, with walls about three times thicker (8–12 mm) than those of the right ventricle. It forms part of the sterno-costal, left and inferior (diaphragmatic) cardiac surfaces. Except where obscured by the aorta and pulmonary trunk, the base of the ventricular cone is superficially separated from the left atrium and atrial auricle by part of the atrioventricular groove; the coronary sinus runs in the posterior aspect of the groove to reach the right atrium (**Fig. 60.2**). The

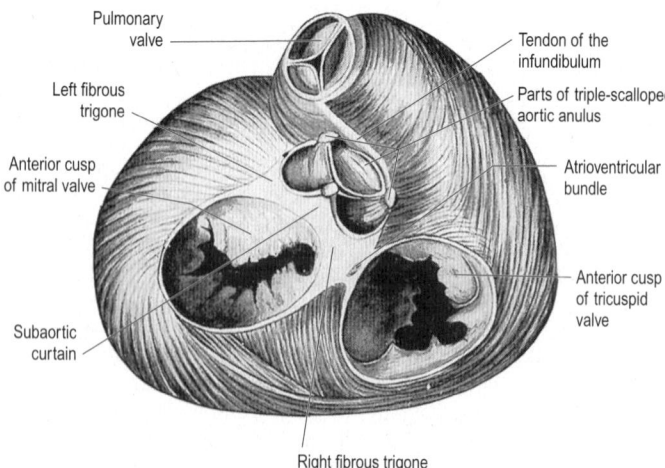

Pulmonary valve
Left fibrous trigone
Anterior cusp of mitral valve
Subaortic curtain
Tendon of the infundibulum
Parts of triple-scalloped aortic anulus
Atrioventricular bundle
Anterior cusp of tricuspid valve
Right fibrous trigone

Fig. 60.11 The base of the ventricles, after removal of the atria and the pericardium. Contrast the planes and positions of aortic and pulmonary valves. Contrast with **Fig. 60.12**. (By permission from Walsmley T 1929 The heart. In: Quain J (ed) Elements of descriptive and practical anatomy. Vol 4, Pt 3. London: Longmans, Green.)

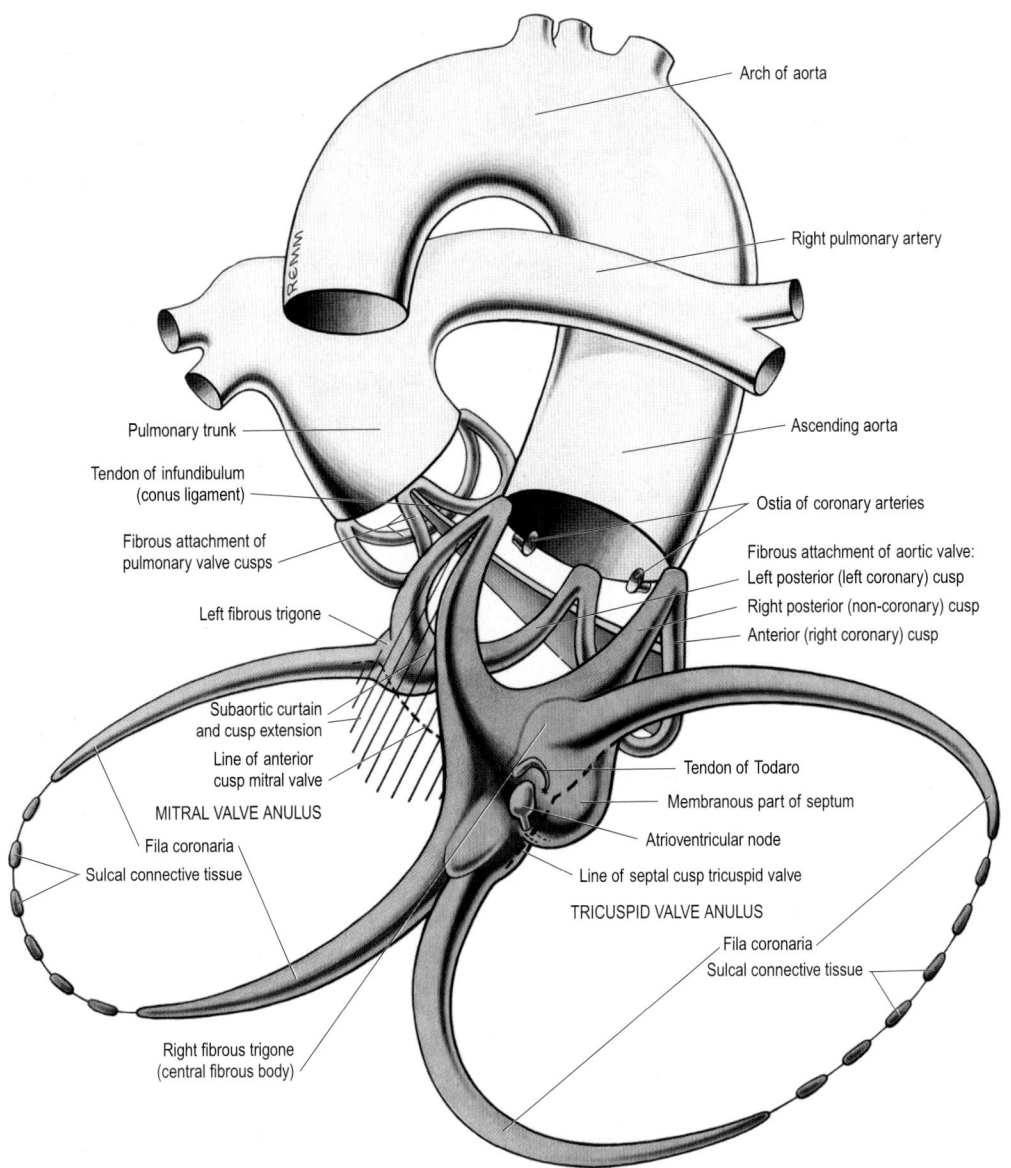

Arch of aorta

Right pulmonary artery

Ascending aorta

Pulmonary trunk

Tendon of infundibulum
(conus ligament)

Fibrous attachment of
pulmonary valve cusps

Left fibrous trigone

Ostia of coronary arteries

Fibrous attachment of aortic valve:
Left posterior (left coronary) cusp
Right posterior (non-coronary) cusp
Anterior (right coronary) cusp

Subaortic curtain
and cusp extension

Line of anterior
cusp mitral valve

MITRAL VALVE ANULUS

Fila coronaria

Sulcal connective tissue

Tendon of Todaro

Membranous part of septum

Atrioventricular node

Line of septal cusp tricuspid valve

TRICUSPID VALVE ANULUS

Fila coronaria

Sulcal connective tissue

Right fibrous trigone
(central fibrous body)

Fig. 60.12 Principal elements of the fibrous skeleton of the heart. For clarity, the view is from the right posterosuperior aspect. Perspective causes the pulmonary anulus to appear smaller than the aortic anulus, whereas in fact the reverse is the case. Consult text for an extended discussion. Key: red, mitral and aortic 'anuli'; blue, tricuspid and pulmonary 'anuli'; green, tendon of the infundibulum. (Copyright from The Royal College of Surgeons of England. Reproduced with permission.)

anterior and posterior interventricular grooves indicate the lines of mural attachment of the ventricular septum and the limits of the left and right ventricular territories. The sternocostal surface of the ventricle curves bluntly into its left surface at the obtuse margin.

INTERNAL FEATURES

The left ventricle has an inlet region, guarded by the mitral valve (ostium venosum), an outlet region, guarded by the aortic valve (ostium arteriosum), and an apical trabecular component. The left atrioventricular orifice admits atrial blood during diastole, flow being towards the cardiac apex. After closure of the mitral cusps, and throughout the ejection phase of systole, blood is expelled from the apex through the aortic orifice. In contrast to the orifices within the right ventricle, those of the left ventricle are in close contact, with fibrous continuity between the cusps of the aortic and mitral valves (the subaortic curtain; **Fig. 60.16**). The inlet and outlet turn sharply round this fibrous curtain (**Fig. 60.11**).

The anterolateral wall is the concavo-convex ventricular septum, a muscular wall the convexity of which is the posteromedial profile of the right ventricle as seen in section. It thus completes the circular outline of the left ventricle. Towards the aortic orifice, the septum becomes the thin, collagenous interventricular component of the membranous septum, an oval or round area below and confluent with the fibrous triangle separating the right and the non-coronary cusps of the aortic valve.

Between the lower limits of the free margins of the cusps of the mitral valve and the apex of the ventricle, the muscular walls are deeply trabeculated. These trabeculae carneae are finer and more intricate than those of the right ventricle, but similar in structure. Trabeculation is

characteristically well developed near the apex, whereas the upper reaches of the septal surface are smooth (**Fig. 60.16**).

HYPERTROPHY OF HEART MUSCLE

In hypertrophic cardiomyopathy, there is an increase in the thickening of the myocardial walls, particularly the interventricular septum, which is disproportionately thickened in comparison with the posterior wall. Echocardiography allows accurate assessment of the thickening and of systolic function. Other features in hypertrophic cardiomyopathy are dynamic left ventricular outflow obstruction, systolic anterior motion of the anterior mitral valve cusp, and midsystolic closure of the aortic valve. A degree of diastolic dysfunction is also present in some cases of hypertrophic cardiomyopathy. Serial short-axis magnetic resonance imaging (MRI) allows accurate measurement of wall thickness and is particularly useful in assessing hypertrophy confined to the apex. Gradient-echo MRI also allows some functional assessment of the hypertrophy. A number of histological changes are observed, including disarray of the cardiac myocytes with replacement fibrosis, and expansion of the collagen component. Treatment is usually medical, except for refractory cases and those in whom the left ventricular outflow tract obstruction has a gradient of greater than 50 mmHg. Ventricular septal myotomy and myectomy are performed in such cases. Two vertical parallel myotomies are performed in the septum c.1 cm apart, followed by a connecting transverse incision. The segment that is isolated is excised, creating a channel between the aortic anulus and the mitral valve cusps.

An athlete's heart may also hypertrophy and may require differentiation from hypertrophic cardiomyopathy. However, in athletes there is

A

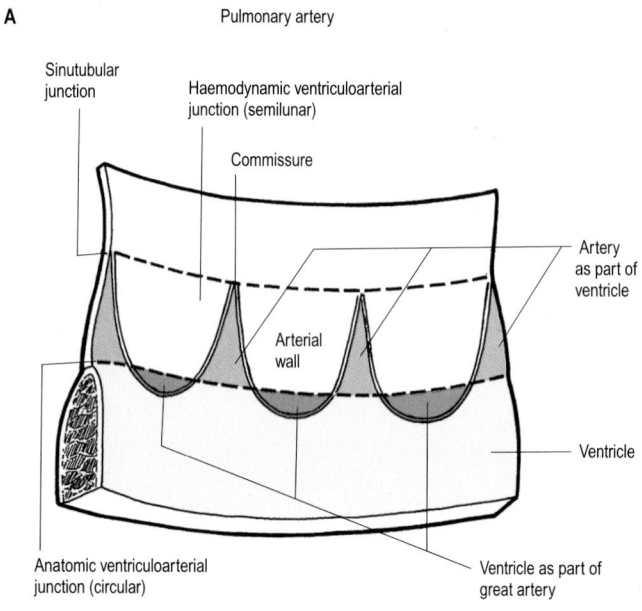

B

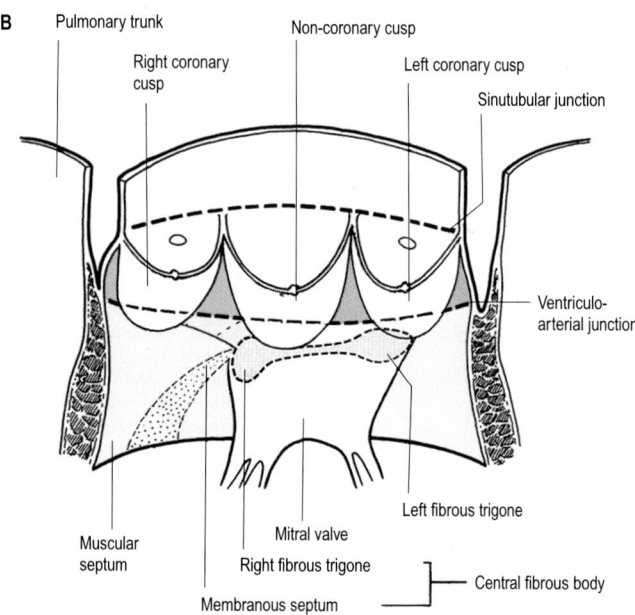

Fig. 60.13 **A**, In this diagram of the aortic root, the cusps have been resected at the attachment to the aortic wall. Note the relation of the cusp insertions and the ventriculo–arterial junction. **B**, The root of the aorta cut open and distended, to show the insertion of the semilunar cusps. The diagram illustrates the structure of the zone of fibrous continuity between the cusps of the aortic valve and the cusps of the mitral valve and their relation with the fibrous trigones. It also shows the semilunar attachment of the cusps (compare with **A**).

uniform hypertrophy, the left ventricle cavity is usually less than 55 mm in size, and the thickness decreases with deconditioning. Hypertrophic cardiomyopathy, in contrast, may show unusual patterns of left ventricular hypertrophy, which is often asymmetric with sharp transitions between segments, left atrial enlargement and bizarre electrocardiographic patterns. Furthermore, there is an autosomal dominant inheritance pattern of abnormalities in genes coding for myocardial proteins associated with hypertrophic cardiomyopathy. Individuals with mutations of the β-MHC (major histocompatibility complex) gene usually develop the classical form of hypertrophy, whereas those with cardiac troponin T gene mutations generally have only mild or clinically undetectable hypertrophy. Rare forms of hypertrophy include localized left ventricular apical hypertrophy as a result of cardiac troponin I mutations, and isolated midcavity hypertrophy caused by cardiac actin and MLC (myosin light chain) gene mutations.

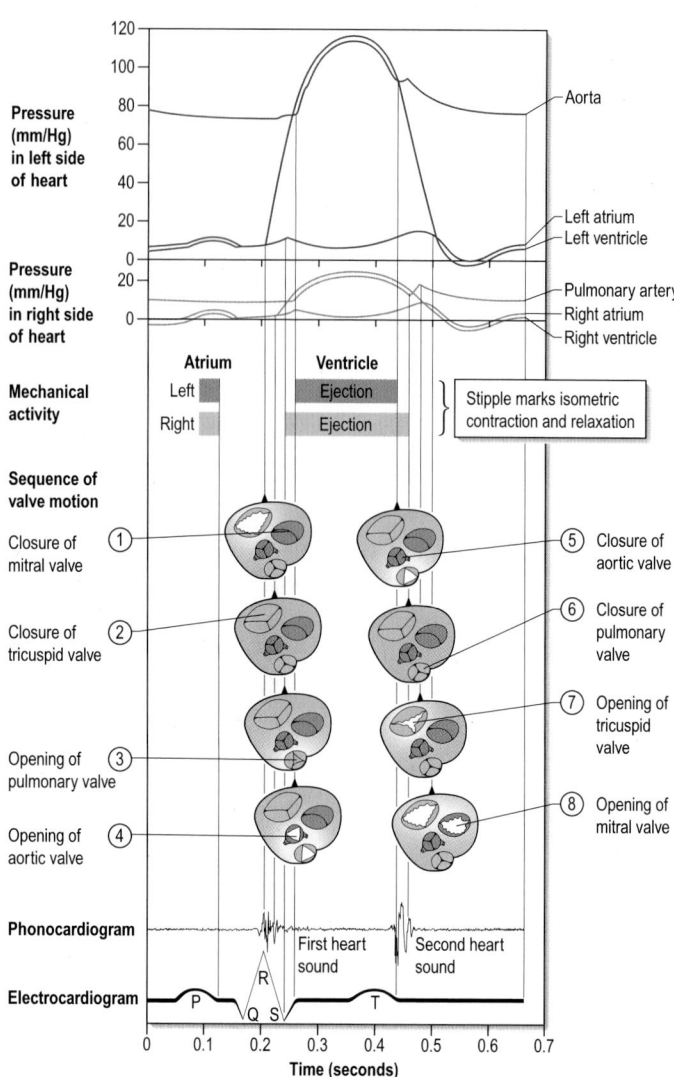

Fig. 60.14 Summary of some of the principal events that occur in the cardiac cycle and which are mentioned at various points throughout the chapter.

MITRAL VALVE

The general comments already made in respect to the tricuspid valve apply equally to the mitral. The valve has an orifice with its supporting anulus, cusps and a variety of chordae tendineae and papillary muscles.

MITRAL VALVULAR ORIFICE

The mitral orifice is a well-defined transitional zone between the atrial wall and the bases of the cusps. It is smaller than the tricuspid orifice (mean circumference is 9.0 cm in males, 7.2 cm in females). The approximately circular orifice is almost vertical in diastole and at 45° to the sagittal plane, but with a slight forward tilt. Its ventricular aspect faces anterolaterally to the left and a little inferiorly towards the left ventricular apex. It is almost co-planar with the tricuspid orifice but posterosuperior to it, whereas it is posteroinferior and slightly to the left of the aortic orifice. The mitral, tricuspid and aortic orifices are intimately connected centrally at the central fibrous body. When the cusps of the mitral valve close, they form a single zone of coaptation, sometimes termed the commissure.

The anulus of the valve is not a simple fibrous ring, but is made up of fibrocollagenous elements of varying consistency from which the fibrous core of the cusps take origin. These variations allow major changes in the shape and dimensions of the anulus at different stages of the cardiac cycle and ensure optimal efficiency in valvular action.

The anulus is strongest at the internal aspects of the left and right fibrous trigones (**Fig. 60.11**). Extending from these structures, the anterior and posterior coronary prongs (which are tapering, fibrous,

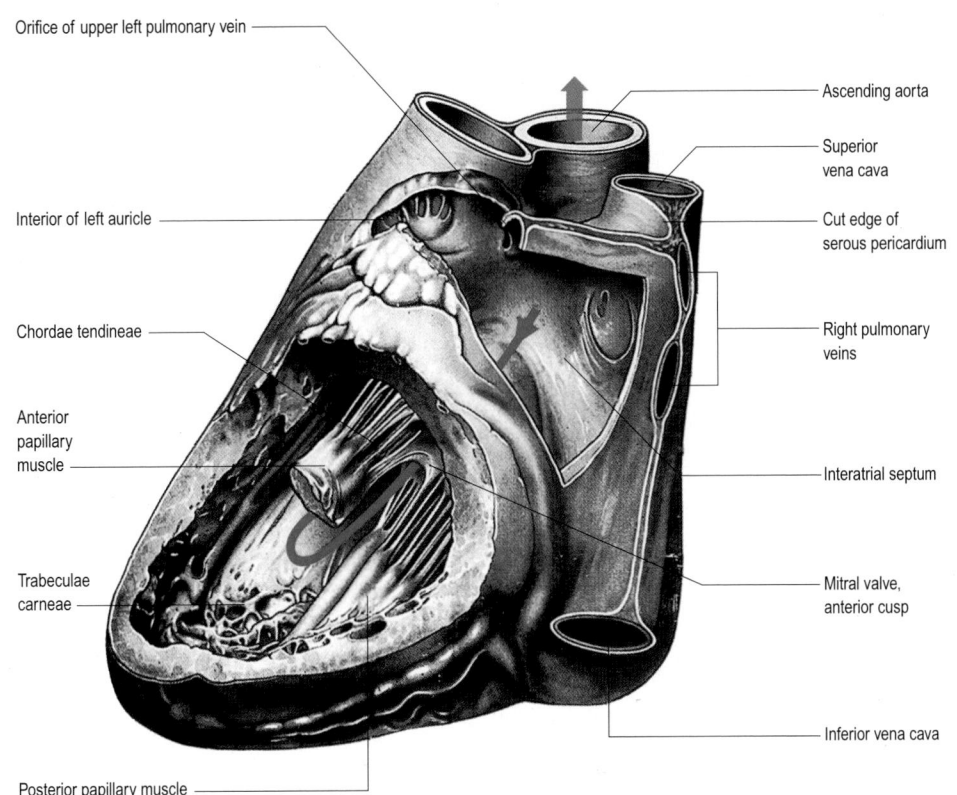

Orifice of upper left pulmonary vein

Interior of left auricle

Chordae tendineae

Anterior
papillary
muscle

Trabeculae
carneae

Posterior papillary muscle

Ascending aorta

Superior
vena cava

Cut edge of
serous pericardium

Right pulmonary
veins

Interatrial septum

Mitral valve,
anterior cusp

Inferior vena cava

Fig. 60.15 Dissection showing the interior of the left side of the heart. The red arrow indicates the course of blood flow from the left atrium through the left ventricle to the aorta.

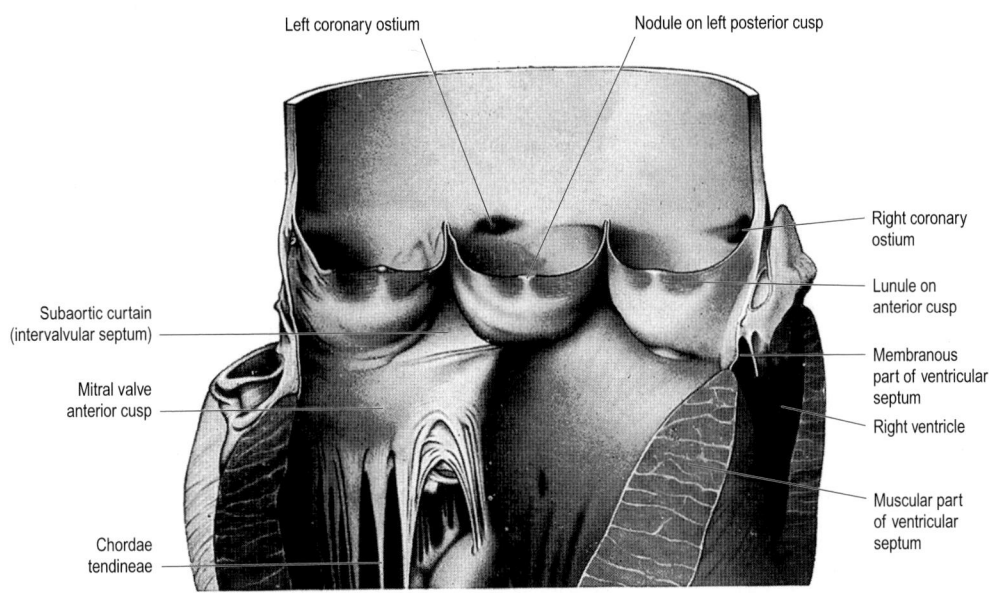

Left coronary ostium

Nodule on left posterior cusp

Subaortic curtain
(intervalvular septum)

Mitral valve
anterior cusp

Chordae
tendineae

Right coronary
ostium

Lunule on
anterior cusp

Membranous
part of ventricular
septum

Right ventricle

Muscular part
of ventricular
septum

Fig. 60.16 The aortic orifice opened from the front to show the cusps of the aortic valves, their nodules, lunules, commissures and the triple-scalloped line of anular attachment. Also shown is the continuity of the subaortic curtain with the mitral anterior cusp (i.e. 'aortic baffle') and the coronary ostia.

subendocardial tendons) partly encircle the orifice at the atrioventricular junction (**Figs 60.11, 60.12**). Between the tips of the prongs, the atrial and ventricular myocardial masses are separated by a more tenuous sheet of deformable fibroelastic connective tissue. Spanning anteriorly between the trigones, the fibrous core of the central part of the anterior aortic cusp of the mitral valve is a continuation of the fibrous subaortic curtain that descends from the adjacent halves of the left and non-coronary cusps of the aortic valve (**Fig. 60.16**).

MITRAL VALVE CUSPS

Since the earliest descriptions, the mitral valvular cusps have been described as paired structures. Hence, the name 'bicuspid valve' is more explicit, although erroneous (the cusps are not cuspid, or 'peaked', in form) and surely less picturesque than the clinical term 'mitral'. Confusion, controversy and difficulties in quantitation have arisen, however, because small accessory cusps are almost always found between the two major cusps. These problems can be resolved if the mitral valve is described as consisting of a continuous veil attached around the

entire circumference of the mitral orifice. Its free edge bears several indentations; two are sufficiently deep and regular to be nominated as the ends of a solitary and oblique zone of apposition, or commissure. It is more usual, however, for these anteromedial and posterolateral extremities to be designated as two independent commissures, each positionally named as indicated. The official names for these cusps, anterior and posterior, although simple, are somewhat misleading because of the obliquity of the valve.

When the valve is laid open, the anterior cusp (aortic, septal, 'greater' or anteromedial) is seen to guard one-third of the circumference of the orifice and to be semicircular or triangular, with few or no marginal indentations. Its fibrous core (lamina fibrosa) is continuous, on the outflow aspect, beyond the margins of the fibrous subaortic curtain, with the right and left fibrous trigones (**Figs 60.8, 60.11, 60.13B**). Between these, it is continuous with the fibrous curtain itself and, beyond the trigones, with the roots of the anular fibrous prongs (**Fig. 60.12**). The cusp has a deep crescentic rough zone, which receives various chordae tendineae. The ridge limiting the outer margin of the rough zone indicates the maximal extent of surface contact with the mural cusp in full closure. A clear zone is seen between the rough zone and the valvular anulus, which is devoid of attachments of chordae, although its fibrous core carries extensions from chordae attached in the rough zone. The anterior cusp has no basal zone, continuing instead into the valvular curtain. Hinging on its anular attachment, and continuous with the subaortic curtain, it is critically placed between the inlet and the outlet of the ventricle. During passive ventricular filling and atrial systole, its smooth atrial surface is important in directing a smooth flow of blood towards the body and apex of the ventricle. After the onset of ventricular systole and closure of the mitral valve, the ventricular aspect of its clear zone merges into the smooth surface of the subaortic curtain which, with the remaining fibrous walls of the subvalvular aortic vestibule, forms the smooth boundaries of the ventricular outlet.

The posterior cusp (mural, ventricular, 'smaller' or posterolateral) usually has two or more minor indentations. Lack of definition of major intervalvular commissures has previously led to disagreement and confusion concerning the territorial extent of this cusp and the possible existence of accessory 'scallops'. Examination of the valve in the closed position, however, shows that the posterior cusp can conveniently be regarded as all the valvular tissue posterior to the anterolateral and posteromedial ends of the major zone of apposition with the aortic cusp. Thus defined, it has a wider attachment to the anulus than does the anterior cusp, guarding two-thirds of the circumferential attachments. Further indentations usually divide the mural cusp into a relatively large middle scallop and smaller anterolateral and posteromedial commissural scallops. Each scallop has a crescentic, opaque rough zone, receiving on its ventricular aspect the attachments of the chordae that define the area of valvular apposition in full closure. From the rough zone to within 2–3 mm of its anular attachment, there is a membranous clear zone devoid of chordae. The basal 2–3 mm is thick and vascular, and receives basal chordae. The ratio of rough to clear zone in the anterior cusp is c.0.6; in the middle scallop of the posterior cusp it is 1.4. Much more of the mural cusp is in apposition with the aortic cusp during closure of the mitral valve.

MITRAL CHORDAE TENDINEAE (TENDINOUS CORDS)
The chordae tendineae resemble those supporting the tricuspid valve. False chordae (trabeculae carneae; **Fig. 60.15**) are also irregularly distributed as in the right ventricle. They occur in about 50% of all human left ventricles, and often cross the subaortic outflow. Many contain extensions from the ventricular conducting tissues. These left ventricular bands can often be identified by cross-sectional echocardiography. Their role, if any, has still to be determined. True chordae of the mitral valve may be divided into intercusp (or commissural) chordae, rough zone chordae, including the special strut chordae, so-called 'cleft' chordae and basal chordae. Most true chordae divide into branches from a single stem soon after their origin from the apical one-third of a papillary muscle, or proceed as single chordae that divide into several branches near their attachment. Basal chordae, in contrast, are solitary structures passing from the ventricular wall to the mural cusp.

There is such marked variation between the arrangement of the chordae in individual normal hearts that any detailed classification loses much of its clinical significance. Suffice it to say that, in the majority of hearts, the chordae support the entire free edges of the valvular cusps, together with varying degrees of their ventricular aspects and bases. There is some evidence to suggest that those valves with unsupported areas of the free edge become prone to prolapse in later life.

PAPILLARY MUSCLES
The two muscles supporting the cusps of the mitral valve also vary in length and breadth and may be bifid. The anterolateral muscle arises from the sternocostal mural myocardium, the posteromedial from the diaphragmatic region. Chordae tendineae arise mostly from the tip and apical one-third of each muscle, but sometimes take origin near their base. The chordae from each papillary muscle diverge and are attached to corresponding areas of closure on both valvular cusps.

OPENING OF THE MITRAL VALVE
At the onset of diastole, opening is passive but rapid, the cusps parting and projecting into the ventricle as left atrial pressure exceeds left ventricular diastolic pressure. Passive ventricular filling proceeds as atrial blood pours to the apex, directed by the pendant aortic cusp of the valve. The cusps begin to float passively together, hinging on their

anular attachments, partially occluding the ventricular inlet. Atrial systole now occurs, jetting blood apically and causing re-opening of the cusps. As maximal filling is achieved, the cusps again float rapidly together. Closure is followed by ventricular systole, which starts in the papillary muscles and continues rapidly as a general contraction of the walls and septum. Coordinated contraction of the papillary muscles increases the tension in the chordae and promotes joining of the corresponding points on opposing cusps, preventing their eversion. With general mural and septal excitation and contraction, left ventricular pressure increases rapidly (**Fig. 60.14**). The cusps 'balloon' towards the atrial cavity and the atrial aspects of the rough zones come into maximal contact. Precise papillary contraction, and increasing tension in the chordae, continue to prevent valvular eversion and maintain valvular competence.

The orifices and the cusps of both atrioventricular valves undergo considerable changes in position, form and area during a cardiac cycle. Both valves move anteriorly and to the left during systole, and reverse their motion in diastole. The mitral valve reduces its orificial (anular) area by as much as 40% in systole. Its shape also changes from circular to crescentic at the height of systole, the anular attachment of its aortic cusp being the concavity of the crescent. The attachment of its mural cusp, although remaining convex, contracts towards the anterior wall of the heart.

AORTIC VALVE

The smooth left ventricular outflow tract, or aortic vestibule, ends at the cusps of the aortic valve. Although stronger in construction, the aortic valve resembles the pulmonary (**Figs 60.13, 60.16, 60.17, 60.18, 60.19**) in possessing three semilunar cusps, supported within the three aortic sinuses of Valsalva. Although the aortic valve, like the pulmonary valve, is often described as possessing an anulus in continuity with the fibrous skeleton, there is no complete collagenous ring supporting the attachments of the cusps. As with the pulmonary valve, the anatomy of the aortic valve is dominated by the fibrous semilunar attachment of the cusps (**Fig. 60.13B**).

AORTIC VALVE CUSPS
The cusps are attached in part to the aortic wall and in part to the supporting ventricular structures. The situation is more complicated than in the pulmonary valve, because parts of the cusps also take origin from the fibrous subaortic curtain, and are continuous with the aortic cusp of the mitral valve (**Fig. 60.16**). This area of continuity is thickened at its two ends to form the right and left fibrous trigones (**Fig. 60.11**). However, as with the pulmonary valve (**Fig. 60.13B**), the semilunar attachments incorporate segments of ventricular tissue within the base of each aortic sinus. These sinuses and cusps are conveniently named as right, left and non-coronary, according to the origins of the coronary arteries (**Fig. 60.13B**). The semilunar attachments also incorporate three triangular areas (trigones) of aortic wall within the apex of the left ventricular outflow tract. As these triangular areas are part of the wall of the aorta rather than of the left ventricle, and are interposed between the bulbous aortic sinuses, they separate the cavity of the left ventricle from the pericardial space. Removal of the trigones in an otherwise intact heart is instructive in demonstrating the relationships of the aortic valve, which can justly be considered as the keystone of the heart. The base of the triangle between the non-coronary and the left coronary cusps is continuous inferiorly with the fibrous aortic–mitral curtain. The apex of this triangle 'points' into the transverse pericardial space. The triangle between right and non-coronary cusps has, as its base, the membranous components of the interventricular septum and thus 'faces' the right ventricle, whereas its apex 'points' towards the transverse pericardial space behind the origin of the right coronary artery. The third triangle, between the two coronary cusps, has its base on the muscular ventricular septum. Its apex 'points' to the plane of space found between the aortic wall and the free-standing sleeve of right ventricular infundibular musculature that supports the cusps of the pulmonary valve. Although the basal attachments of each cusp are thickened and collagenous at their ventricular origins, there is no continuous collagenous skeleton supporting, in circular fashion, all the attachments of the cusps of the aortic valve. Valvular function depends primarily upon the semilunar attachments of the cusps.

The cusps themselves are folds of endocardium with a central fibrous core. With the valve half open, each equals slightly more than a quarter

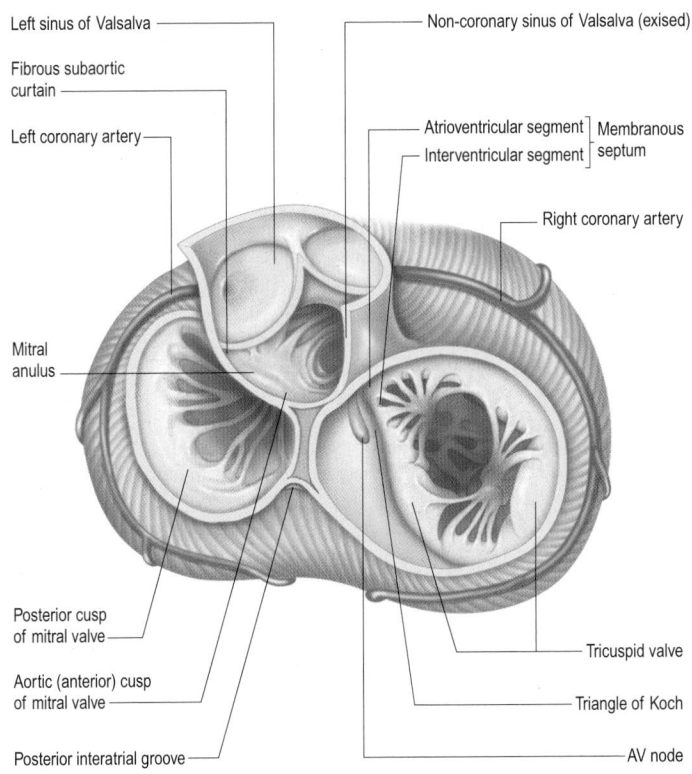

Left sinus of Valsalva

Fibrous subaortic curtain

Left coronary artery

Non-coronary sinus of Valsalva (exised)

Atrioventricular segment ⎤ Membranous
Interventricular segment ⎦ septum

Right coronary artery

Mitral anulus

Posterior cusp of mitral valve

Aortic (anterior) cusp of mitral valve

Posterior interatrial groove

Tricuspid valve

Triangle of Koch

AV node

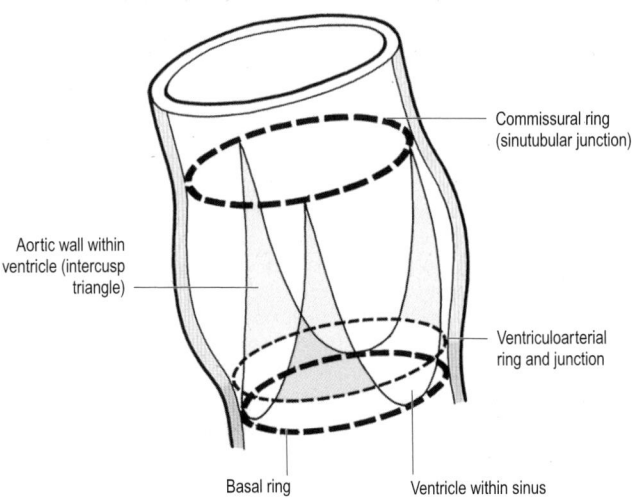

Aortic wall within ventricle (intercusp triangle)

Commissural ring (sinutubular junction)

Ventriculoarterial ring and junction

Basal ring

Ventricle within sinus

Fig. 60.18 Diagram showing how the structure of the aortic root is best conceptualized in terms of a three-pronged coronet. There are at least three rings within this coronet, but none supports the entirety of the attachments of the valvular cusps (see also **Fig. 60.13B**).

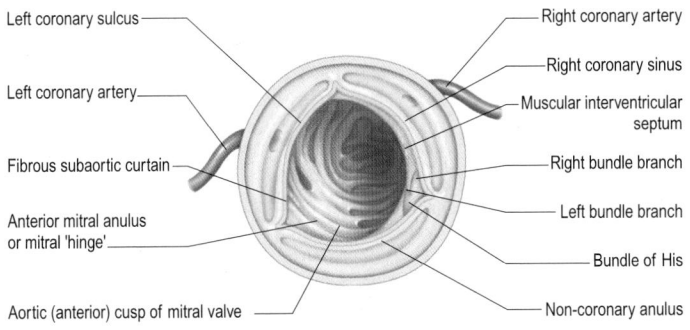

Left coronary sulcus

Left coronary artery

Fibrous subaortic curtain

Anterior mitral anulus or mitral 'hinge'

Aortic (anterior) cusp of mitral valve

Right coronary artery

Right coronary sinus

Muscular interventricular septum

Right bundle branch

Left bundle branch

Bundle of His

Non-coronary anulus

Fig. 60.17 The crucial relation between subaortic outflow tract and ventricular inlet components. The non-coronary sinus of the aorta, with its corresponding aortic valvular cusp, has been removed.

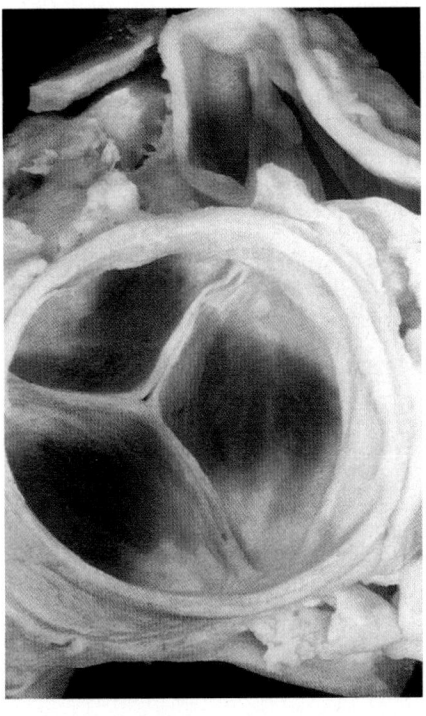

Fig. 60.19 The arterial view of the aortic valve in its closed position shows the snug fit between its component cusps.

of a sphere, an approximate hemisphere being completed by the corresponding sinus. Each cusp has a thick basal border, deeply concave on its aortic aspect, and a horizontal free margin. The latter is only slightly thickened, except at its midpoint, where there is an aggregation of fibrous tissue, the valvular nodule of the semilunar cusp. Flanking each nodule, the fibrous core is tenuous, and forms the lunules of translucent and occasionally fenestrated valvular tissue (**Fig. 60.16**). Fenestrations are of no functional significance. The aortic surface of each cusp is rougher than its ventricular aspect.

Currently, three sets of names are used to describe the aortic cusps. Posterior, right and left refer to presumed fetal positions before full cardiac rotation has occurred. Corresponding terms based on the approximate positions in maturity are anterior, left posterior and right posterior. However, as already indicated, widespread clinical terminology links both cusps and sinuses to the origins of the coronary arteries. Thus the anterior is termed the right coronary cusp, left posterior is left coronary, and right posterior is non-coronary. These clinical terms are preferable because they are simple and unambiguous.

AORTIC SINUSES (OF VALSALVA)
The aortic sinuses are more prominent than those in the pulmonary trunk. The upper limit of each sinus reaches considerably beyond the

level of the free border of the cusp and forms a well-defined complete circumferential sinotubular ridge when viewed from the aortic aspect (**Fig. 60.13B**). Coronary arteries usually open near this ridge within the upper part of the sinus, but are markedly variable in their origin. The walls of the sinuses are largely collagenous near the attachment of the cusps, but the amount of lamellated elastic tissue increases with distance from the zone of attachment. Strands of myocardium may enter this fibroelastic wall. At the mid level of each sinus, its wall is about half the thickness of the supravalvular aortic wall and less than one-quarter of the thickness of the sinotubular ridge. At this level, the mean luminal diameter of the beginning of the aortic root is almost double that of the ascending aorta. These details are functionally significant in the mechanism of valvular motion.

OPENING OF THE AORTIC VALVE
During diastole, the closed aortic valve supports an aortic column of blood at high but slowly diminishing pressure. Each sinus and its cusp form a hemispherical chamber. The three nodules are apposed and the margins and lunular parts of adjacent cusps are tightly apposed on their

ventricular aspects. From the aortic aspect, the closed valve is triradiate, three pairs of closely compressed lunules radiating from their nodules to their peripheral commissural attachments at the sinutubular junction (**Fig. 60.19**). As ventricular systolic pressure increases, it exceeds aortic pressure and the valve is passively opened. The fibrous wall of the sinuses nearest the aortic vestibule is almost inextensible but, in the upper parts of sinuses, the wall is fibroelastic. Under left ventricular ejection pressure, the radius here increases c.16% in systole. Hence the commissures move apart, making the orifice triangular when fully open. The free margins of the cusps then become almost straight lines between peripheral attachments. However, they do not flatten against the sinus walls, even at maximal systolic pressure, which is probably an important factor in subsequent closure. During ejection, most blood enters the ascending aorta, but some enters the sinuses, forming vortices that help to maintain the triangular 'mid position' of the cusp during ventricular systole and probably initiate their approximation with the end of systole. Tight and full closure ensues, with the rapid decrease in ventricular pressure in diastole. Commissures narrow, nodules aggregate and the valve reassumes its triradiate form. Experiments indicate that c.4% of ejected blood regurgitates through a valve with normal sinuses, whereas 23% regurgitates through a valve without them. The normal structure of the aortic sinuses also promotes non-turbulent flow into the coronary arteries.

ECHOCARDIOGRAPHY

The gross anatomy of the heart can be evaluated by two-dimensional echocardiography in the para-sternal, apical, suprasternal and subcostal positions. The standardized planes used are long axis, short axis and four-chamber. Echocardiography allows a detailed assessment of the functional anatomy of the heart. The long-axis view is obtained by placing the ultrasound transducer in the left apicosternal position and provides detailed images of the left ventricle, aorta, left atrium, and mitral and aortic valves (**Fig. 60.20**). Angling the beam towards the right also allows assessment of the right atrium, right ventricle and tricuspid valves. Rotating the transducer by 90° in the clockwise direction produces the short-axis view, which allows assessment of the left ventricle, papillary muscles, chordae tendineae and mitral valves. The four-chamber view demonstrates the ventricles, atria, and mitral and tricuspid valves (**Fig. 60.20**). Rotation of the transducer allows two-chamber views of the heart and more detailed assessment of the aorta and aortic valves.

Connective tissue and fibrous skeleton of the heart

From epicardium to endocardium, and from the orifices of the great veins to the roots of the arterial trunks, the intercellular spaces between contractile and conducting elements are everywhere permeated by connective tissue. The amount varies greatly in arrangement and texture in different locations.

A fine layer of areolar tissue is found beneath the mesothelium of the serosal visceral epicardium over much of the heart. This accumulates subepicardial fat, the amount increasing with age, which becomes concentrated along the acute margin, the atrioventricular and interventricular grooves and their side channels. The coronary vessels and their main branches are embedded in this fat. The endocardium also lies on a fine areolar tissue rich in elastic fibres. Fibrocellular components of these subepicardial and subendocardial layers blend on their mural aspects with the endomysial and perimysial connective tissue on the myocardium. Each cardiac myocyte is invested by a delicate endomysium composed of fine reticular fibres, collagen and elastin fibres embedded in ground substance. This matrix is lacking only at desmosomal and gap junctional contacts of intercalated discs. Similar arrangements apply to myocytes of the ventricular conducting tissues and their extensive contacts with the working myocardium. The connective tissue matrix itself is interconnected laterally to form bundles, strands or sheets of macroscopic proportions showing a complex geometric pattern. The larger myocardial bundles are surrounded by, and attached to, stronger perimysial condensations. The overall pattern is described in terms of struts and weaves.

The myocardial matrix, despite its importance, cannot be dissected grossly. Running at the ventricular base, and intimately related to atrioventricular valves and the aortic orifice, is a complex framework of dense collagen with membranous, tendinous and fibroareolar extensions. The whole is sufficiently distinct to be termed the fibrous skeleton of the heart.

Although it is often stated that all four valves are contained within this skeleton, this is not the case. The cusps of the pulmonary valve are supported on a free-standing sleeve of right ventricular infundibulum which can easily be removed from the heart without disturbing either the fibrous skeleton or the left ventricle. The fibrous skeleton is strongest at the junction of the aortic, mitral and tricuspid valves, the so-called central fibrous body (**Figs 60.11, 60.12**). Two pairs of curved, tapering, collagenous prongs (fila coronaria) extend from the central fibrous body. They are stronger on the left, passing partially around the mitral and tricuspid orifices, which are almost co-planar and incline to face the cardiac apex. The aortic valve, in contrast, faces up, right and slightly forwards. It is anterosuperior and to the right of the mitral orifice. As already described, two of the cusps of the aortic valve are in fibrous continuity with the aortic cusp of the mitral valve. This aortic–mitral or subaortic curtain (**Figs 60.11, 60.13B**) is also an integral part of the fibrous skeleton. The two ends of the curtain are strengthened as the right and left fibrous trigones, which are the strongest part of the skeleton. The right trigone, together with the membranous septum, constitutes the central fibrous body (**Fig. 60.11**). This important structure is penetrated by the mechanism for atrioventricular conduction (the bundle of His,

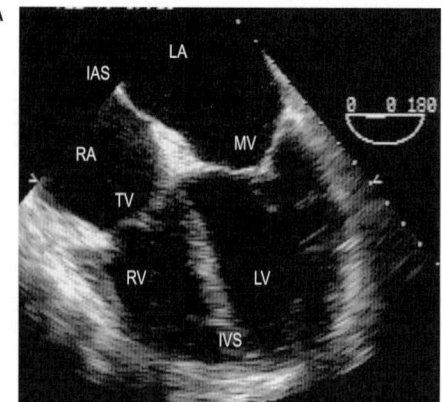 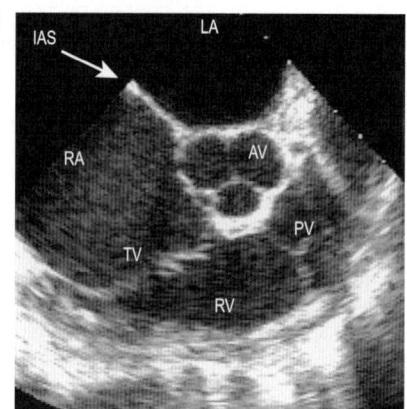 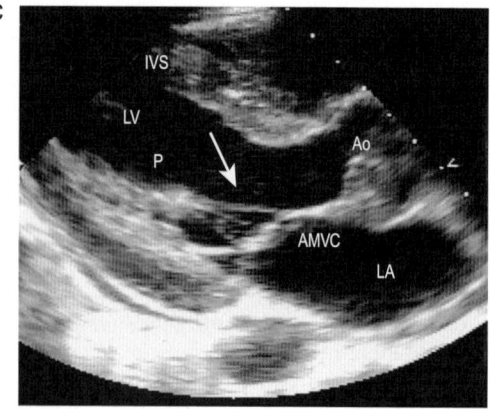

Fig. 60.20 Cardiac anatomy shown by transthoracic echocardiography. **A**, Four-chamber view. IAS, interatrial septum; IVS, interventricular septum; LA, left atrium; LV, left ventricle; MV, mitral valve; RA, right atrium; RV, right ventricle; TV, tricuspid valve. **B**, Short-axis view at aortic valve level. AV, aortic valve (note three cusps); IAS (arrow), interatrial septum; LA, left atrium; PV, pulmonary valve; RA, right atrium; RV, right ventricle; TV, tricuspid valve. **C**, Parasternal long-axis view. AMVC, anterior mitral valve cusp; Ao, aortic outflow; IVS, interventricular septum; LA, left atrium; LV, left ventricle; P, papillary muscle. The arrow shows the chordae tendineae attaching the mitral valve cusps to the papillary muscles. (By kind permission from Dr Sam Kaddoura, Chelsea and Westminster Hospital, London.)

or atrioventricular bundle), whereas the membranous septum is crossed on its right aspect by the attachment of the tricuspid valve, which divides the septum into atrioventricular and interventricular components.

The fibrous skeleton has two functions. It ensures electrophysiological discontinuity between the atrial and ventricular myocardial masses except at the site of penetration of the conducting tissue. It also functions as a stable but deformable base for the attachments of the fibrous cores of the atrioventricular valves.

The aortic root is central within the fibrous skeleton and is often described in terms of an 'anulus' integrated within the fibrous skeleton. As with the pulmonary valve, however, the structure of the aortic root corresponds to the triple fibrous semilunar attachments of its cusps. Within this complex circumferential zone there are three crucially important triangular areas that separate, on the ventricular aspect, the aortic bulbous sinuses that house the valvular cusps. As a whole, these three triangles can be conceptualized in terms of a three-pointed coronet (**Fig. 60.18**) and are known as the subaortic spans. Their triangular apices correspond to the tips of the valvular commissures. Their walls, which are significantly thinner than those of the sinuses, variously consist of collagen or admixed muscle strands and fibroelastic tissue. They form the subvalvular extensions of the aortic vestibule. The interval between the non-coronary and left coronary sinuses is filled with the deformable subaortic curtain. The span between the non-coronary and right coronary sinuses is continuous with the anterior surface of the membranous septum. The third subaortic span, namely that between the two coronary aortic sinuses, is filled with fibroelastic tissue, which separates the extension of the subaortic root from the wall of the free-standing subpulmonary infundibulum. Previously, this was held to be the location of the tendon of the infundibulum (conus ligament). Similar fibrous triangles are found separating the sinuses of the pulmonary trunk, but these are significantly less robust.

The mitral and tricuspid rings (anuli) are not simple and rigid collagenous structures but dynamic, deformable lines of valvular attachment that vary greatly at different peripheral points and change considerably with each phase of the cardiac cycle and with increasing age. The tricuspid attachments are even less robust than those of the mitral valve. At several sites only fibroareolar tissue separates the atrial and ventricular muscular masses.

Congenital cardiac malformations

Congenital malformations of the heart are relatively common, amounting to about one-quarter of all developmental abnormalities. Their incidence is estimated at 8 per 1000 live births, but they are found in up to 2% of stillbirths. Only a small proportion of the anomalies are directly attributable to genetic or environmental factors; the majority are the result of multifactorial events.

ABNORMALITIES OF CARDIAC POSITION

The most severe abnormality of position is an extrathoracic heart, so-called ectopia cordis. The heart usually projects to the surface through the lower thoracic and upper abdominal wall, remaining covered, in most instances, by the fibrous pericardium. There is usually additional herniation of the abdominal contents. Another abnormality of position is a mirror-like reversal in shape and position of the heart, which is found in the right hemithorax with its apex directed to the right instead of the left (dextrocardia). This arrangement may be part of a general mirror-like reversal of great vessels (so-called general 'situs inversus'). More usually, an abnormal location of the heart is found in cases of isomerism, in which both sides of the thorax, including the atrial appendages, retain features of either morphological rightness or leftness. Isomerism is also usually associated with anomalous arrangement of the abdominal organs, right isomerism is associated with absence of the spleen (asplenia) and left isomerism with multiple spleens (polysplenia). The heart can also be abnormally located when the rest of the body is normal. This usually indicates the presence of additional lesions within the heart, but can simply be the consequence of an abnormality of the lungs, and the abnormally located heart is anatomically normal.

More significant congenital abnormalities are usually detected during antenatal ultrasound screening. They may present postnatally with tachypnoea, cyanotic spells, difficulty in feeding or with circulatory collapse. There may be audible murmurs on auscultation. The majority of abnormalities may be detected by echocardiography, but in a few cases cardiac catheterization and measurement of blood oxygen saturation may be required.

ACYANOTIC CARDIAC DEFECTS

Acyanotic heart defects are the result of a left to right intracardiac shunt, which leads to increased work and stress on the heart as a consequence of the pumping of greater volume into the pulmonary circulation. Examples of these defects are simple septal defects (p. 1040) such as atrial or ventricular septal defects. Complex septal defects include complete atrial ventricular septal defects, and a combination of ventricular septal defects with coarctation of the aorta and double-outlet ventricle or interrupted aortic artery. An obstruction of blood flow in the left side of the heart against either the mitral valve or the aortic valve or in the aorta itself also increases the workload of the heart.

Treatment in all cases is directed towards reducing the cardiac output and pulmonary blood flow to normal. Surgical correction is usually required, except with aortic stenosis, for which balloon dilatation is effective.

CYANOTIC CARDIAC DEFECTS

Cyanotic cardiac defects may be attributable to a right to left intracardiac shunt or to a reduction in flow to the pulmonary circulation. They may be caused by simple lesions such as pulmonary stenosis with an atrial right to left shunt. Complex lesions include Fallot's tetralogy, in which there is a ventricular septal defect, right ventricular outlet tract obstruction, right ventricular hypertrophy and an over-riding aorta. Other complex lesions include transposition of the aorta (p. 1049), truncus arteriosus, tricuspid atresia and total anomalous pulmonary venous return. Most of these patients survive because there is a significant blood flow into the pulmonary vasculature via a patent ductus arteriosus.

Conducting tissue
IMPULSE-CONDUCTING TISSUES OF THE HEART

The cells of cardiac muscle differ from those of skeletal muscle in having the inherent ability to contract and relax spontaneously. This myogenic rhythm is shown by small pieces of cardiac tissue, and even isolated myocytes. The underlying mechanism appears to be based on a further specialization of the sarcolemma that permits a slow inward leakage of sodium ions. Ventricular cells contract and relax at a lower frequency than atrial cells, but in the intact heart both are synchronized to a more rapid rhythm, generated by pacemaker tissue and conveyed to them by a system of fibres specialized for conduction. The anatomical arrangement of these tissues is described in the context of the heart. Here, consideration is restricted to the cells that make up the impulse-generating and conducting system. All are modified cardiac cells. Three types may be distinguished morphologically from normal working cardiac cells: P (= pale-staining = primitive = pacemaker) cells, transitional cells and Purkinje fibres.

Although these terms will be used in the following account, it is important to recognize that there is a continuum of morphology between P cells, transitional cells, Purkinje fibres and working cardiac muscle cells.

OVERVIEW OF THE CONDUCTING SYSTEM

Of all the cells in the heart, those of the sinu-atrial node generate the most rapid rhythm, and therefore function as the pacemaker of the heart. The impulse, believed to be generated in the P cells, is transmitted over preferentially conducting pathways to right and left atria and to the atrioventricular node. At the atrioventricular node, the impulse is delayed by c.40 ms. This delay allows the atria to eject their contents fully before contraction of the ventricles begins. It also places an upper limit on the frequency of signals that can be transmitted to the ventricles. Slender transitional cells, closer in morphology to normal cardiac cells, extend from the node into the stem and principal branches of the atrioventricular bundle (of His). Here, they become continuous with cells of more distinctive appearance, the Purkinje fibres. Conduction of the impulse is rapid in the bundle and its branches (c.2–3 metres per second, as opposed to 0.6 metres per second in normal myocardium). The cardiac impulse therefore arrives at the apex of the heart before spreading through the ventricular walls, producing a properly coordinated ventricular ejection.

The human heart beats ceaselessly at c.70 cycles every minute for many decades, maintaining perfusion of pulmonary and systemic tissues. The rate and stroke volume fluctuate in response to prevailing physiological demands. **Fig. 60.14** summarizes the principal events in a cardiac cycle, including: the electrical events recorded in the electro-cardiogram; the mechanical sequences of diastole, atrial systole, isovolumetric contraction, ejection and isovolumetric relaxation in ventricular systole; the acoustic phenomena recorded in the phono-cardiogram; the pressure profiles of right and left hearts and arterial trunks: the sequences of valvular events. Cardiac efficiency depends on precise timing of the operation in interdependent structures. Passive diastolic filling of the atria and ventricles is followed by atrial systole, stimulated by discharge from the sinu-atrial node, which completes ventricular filling. Excitation and contraction of the atria must be synchronous and finish before ventricular contraction. This is effected by a delay in the conduction of excitation from atria to ventricles. There-after, ventricular contraction proceeds in a precise manner. A specialized ventricular conduction system ensures that closure of atrioventricular valves is followed rapidly by a wave of excitation and contraction, which spreads from the ventricular apices towards the outflow tracts and orifices, rapidly accelerating the blood during ejection.

Cardiac contraction originates unequivocally in specialized myocytes, but neural influences are important in adapting the intrinsic cardiac rhythm to functional demands from the entire body. All cardiac myocytes are excitable, and display autonomous rhythmic depolarization and repolarization of the cell membrane, conduction of waves of excitation via gap junctions to adjacent myocytes, and excitation–contraction coupling to their actomyosin complexes. These properties are developed to different degrees in different sites and in different types of myocyte. The rate of depolarization and repolarization is slowest in the ven-tricular myocardium, intermediate in the atrial muscle and fastest in the myocytes of the sinuatrial node. These last over-ride those generating slower rhythms and, in the normal heart, are the locus for the rhythmic initiation of cardiac cycles. Conversely, conduction velocity is slow in nodal myocytes, intermediate in general 'working' cardiac myocytes and fastest in the myocytes of the ventricular conducting system.

The nodes and networks of the so-called specialized myocardial cells constitute the cardiac conducting system (**Figs 60.21, 60.22**). The com-ponents of this system are the sinu-atrial and atrioventricular nodes, the atrioventricular bundle with its left and right bundle branches and the subendocardial plexus of ventricular conducting cells (Purkinje fibres). Within the system, the main pacemaker rhythm of the heart is generated (sinus), is influenced by nerves (sinus and its innervation) and is trans-mitted specifically from atria to ventricles (atrioventricular node and bundle) and, within the ventricles, to all their musculature. The spread of excitation is very rapid, but not instantaneous. Different parts of the ventricles are excited at slightly different times, with important func-tional consequences. Failure of the conducting system will not block cardiac contraction, but the system will become poorly coordinated or uncoordinated. The rhythm will be slower because it originates from a spontaneous (myogenic) activity in the working cardiac myocytes or in a subsidiary pacemaker in a more distal part of the diseased or disrupted conduction system.

There are no specialized internodal and interatrial conducting path-ways. The excitation emanating from the sinuatrial node spreads to the atrial musculature and to the atrioventricular node through ordinary atrial working myocardium. The geometric arrangement of fibres along well-organized atrial muscle bundles, e.g. the terminal crest and the rims of the oval fossa, ensure that conduction is marginally more rapid than elsewhere within the atrium.

SINUATRIAL NODE

The sinuatrial node is an elliptical structure, c.10–20 mm long. It is located at the junction between parts of the right atrium derived from the embryonic venous sinus and the atrium proper (**Figs 60.21A, 60.22**). The node is often covered by a plaque of subepicardial fat, making it visible in some instances to the naked eye. It extends between 1 and 2 cm on the right from the crest of the right auricle and runs postero-

inferiorly into the upper part of the terminal groove. In a small pro-portion of individuals, about 1 in 10, it extends in horseshoe fashion across the crest of the auricle. Nodal tissue does not occupy the full thickness of the right atrial wall from epicardium to endocardium in humans, but rather sits as a wedge of specialized tissue subepicardially within the terminal groove. Its location is marked consistently by a large central artery, which is a branch of either the left circumflex or posterior descending branch of the right coronary artery. Nodal cells are grouped circumferentially around this artery and interwoven into its dense collagenous adventitia. These cells are now considered the 'pacemakers', although the functional implications of this relationship are not fully understood. Many nerve fibres are present, although none appears to terminate on cells. There are no autonomic ganglion cells within the node, although many border it anteriorly and posteriorly. P cells are most abundant in the central region. They are small, empty-looking cells, c.5–10 μm in greatest diameter, with a large central nucleus. Their pale appearance is attributable to the sparsity of organelles: myofibrils are few and irregularly arranged, and there is no proper sarcotubular system and little glycogen. P cells are less abundant in the periphery of the node, where they mix with slender fusiform tran-sitional cells. The latter are part of a heterogeneous group intermediate in appearance between P cells and normal working cardiac cells. They link P cells to other cells.

ATRIOVENTRICULAR NODE

The atrioventricular node is an atrial structure that lies at the root of an extensive tree of conducting tissue reaching the apex of the ventricles, the papillary muscles and other regions of the ventricles (**Fig. 60.22**). The node, with its transitional zones, is located within the atrial com-ponent of the muscular atrioventricular septum. Its anatomical land-marks are the boundaries of the triangle of Koch (p. 1001). These are: inferiorly, the attachment of the septal cusp of the tricuspid valve; basally, the ostium of the coronary sinus; superiorly, the tendon of Todaro (**Fig. 60.21A**). The compact node is a half oval set against the central fibrous body towards the apex of this triangle. Its atrial aspect is convex, and is overlain by atrial myocardium. Its left margin is concave and abuts on the superior aspect of the central fibrous body. Its basal end projects into the atrial muscle and its anteroinferior end enters the central fibrous body to become the penetrating atrioventricular bundle. The node is pervaded by an irregular collagenous reticulum enmeshing the myocytes, but this is less dense than in the sinu-atrial node. Its arterial supply is from a characteristic vessel that originates from the dominant coronary artery at the crux of the heart. The node has a well-formed compact zone made up of interlocking nodal cells, which frequently show stratification. The transitional cell zones are found superficially and posteriorly. The larger component of atrioventricular delay is probably produced in these transitional zones of the node.

Internodal conducting pathways converge on the atrioventricular node. This is similar in general appearance to the sinuatrial node, although the collagenous component is less dense. The majority of cells are of the transitional type, but P cells resembling those of the sinuatrial node are found in a more fibrous central region. Autonomic ganglia are present between the node and the coronary sinus. In both sinu-atrial and atrioventricular nodes, the intercellular contacts between P cells, and between P cells and transitional cells, are much less specialized than the intercalated discs between normal cardiac cells. A sparsity of gap junctions is consistent with the absence from these areas of connexin-43, which is a major protein component of mammalian gap junctions. This probably accounts for the observed difficulty in exciting these cells from adjacent cells. The atrioventricular delay may owe much to this relative inexcitability of the P cells, which appears to disturb the spread of potential in a manner that delays propagation. The narrow diameter of the transitional cells may contribute to the conduction delay.

ATRIOVENTRICULAR BUNDLE

The atrioventricular bundle is the direct continuation of the atrio-ventricular node, becoming oval, quadrangular or triangular in trans-verse sectional profile as it enters the central fibrous body (**Fig. 60.21A**). Traversing the fibrous body, it branches on the crest of the muscular interventricular septum, the branching tract being sandwiched between the muscular and the membranous components of the septum. The

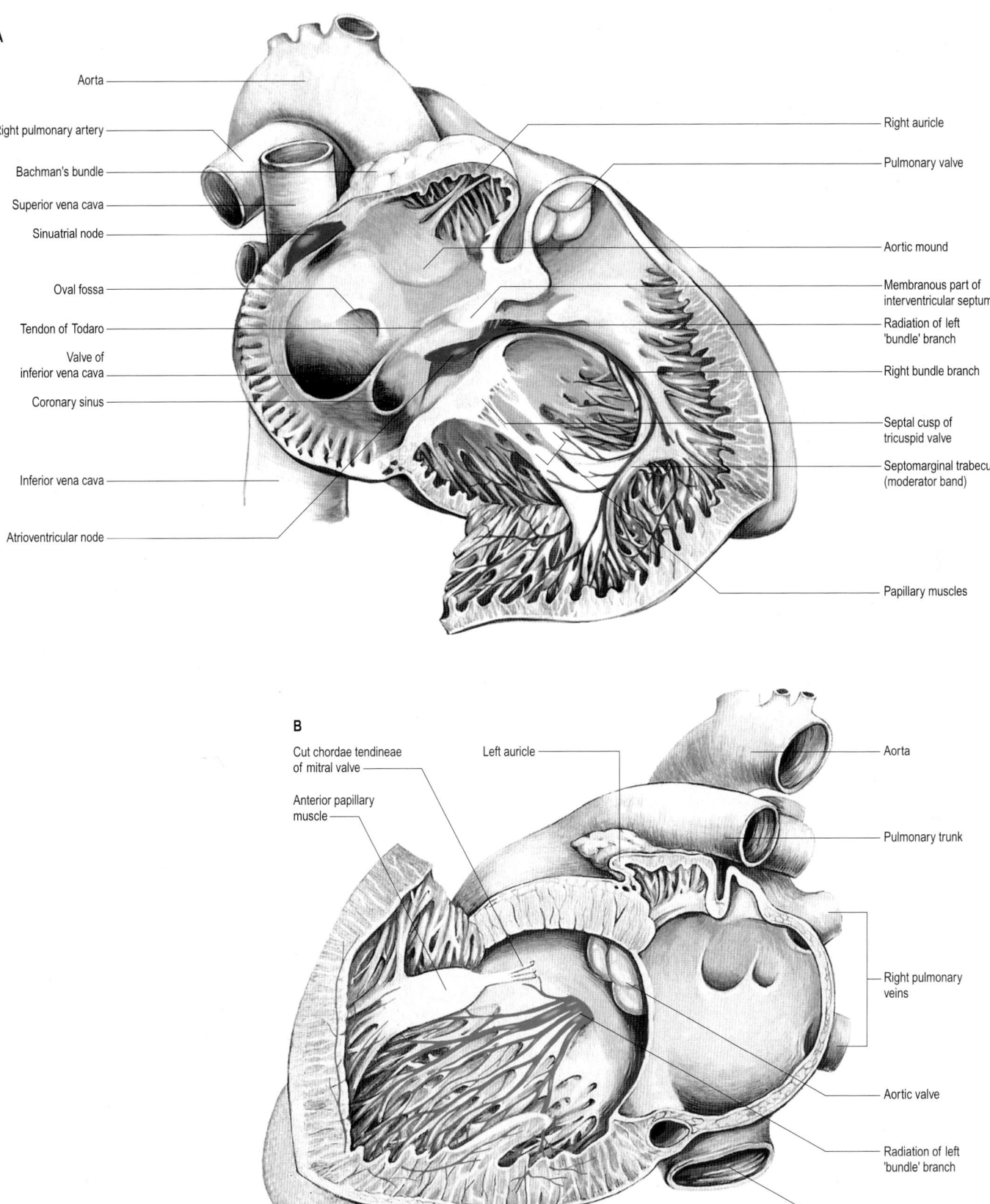

A

Aorta

Right pulmonary artery

Bachman's bundle

Superior vena cava

Sinuatrial node

Oval fossa

Tendon of Todaro

Valve of
inferior vena cava

Coronary sinus

Inferior vena cava

Atrioventricular node

Right auricle

Pulmonary valve

Aortic mound

Membranous part of
interventricular septum

Radiation of left
'bundle' branch

Right bundle branch

Septal cusp of
tricuspid valve

Septomarginal trabecula
(moderator band)

Papillary muscles

B

Cut chordae tendineae
of mitral valve

Anterior papillary
muscle

Left auricle

Aorta

Pulmonary trunk

Right pulmonary
veins

Aortic valve

Radiation of left
'bundle' branch

Inferior vena cava

Fig. 60.21 Diagrams of the conducting tissue of the heart: **A**, right aspect; **B**, left aspect. The elements of the conducting system are shown in red. Note the conducting tissue accompanying fine trabeculae carneae and false chordae. In reality, the radiation of the left bundle branch is directly related to the cusps of the aortic valve.

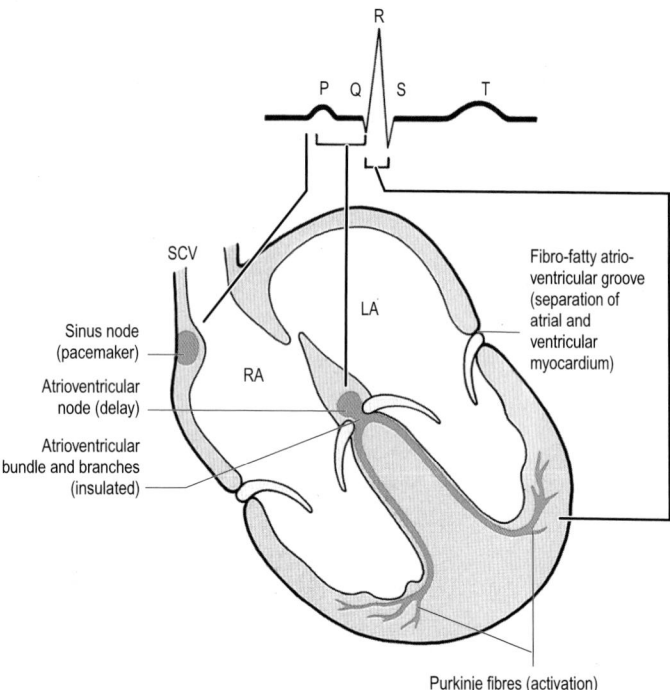

Fig. 60.22 The basic structure of the conducting system, and its relationship with the electrocardiogram. LA, left atrium; RA, right atrium; SCV, superior vena cava.

right branch of the bundle (crus dextrum) is a narrow, discrete round group of fascicles that courses at first within the myocardium and then subendocardially towards the apex of the ventricle, entering the septomarginal trabecula to reach the anterior papillary muscle. It gives few branches to the ventricular walls in its septal course. At the origin of the anterior papillary muscle, it divides profusely into fine subendocardial fascicles that diverge and, first, embrace the papillary muscle, and then recurve subendocardially to be distributed to the remaining ventricular walls. The left branch (crus sinistrum) arises as numerous fine intermingling fascicles that leave the left margin of the branching bundle through much of its course along the crest of the muscular ventricular septum (**Fig. 60.21B**). These fascicles form a flattened sheet down the smooth left ventricular septal surface. The sheet diverges apically and subendocardially across the left aspect of the ventricular septum, separating into anterior, septal and posterior divisions. Fine branches leave the sheets, forming subendocardial networks, which first surround the papillary muscles and then curve back subendocardially to be distributed to all parts of the ventricle.

The principal branches of the bundle are insulated from the surrounding myocardium by sheaths of connective tissue. Functional contacts between ventricular conduction and working myocytes become numerous only in the subendocardial terminal ramifications. Hence, papillary muscles contract first, followed by a wave of excitation and ensuing contraction that travels from the apex of the ventricle to the arterial outflow tract. Because the Purkinje network is subendocardial, muscular excitation proceeds from the endocardial to the epicardial aspect. In the developing heart, it can be shown that the bundle responsible for atrioventricular conduction is a much more extensive structure. Immunohistochemical analysis has revealed that the precursor of the system is a ring of cells that surrounds the inlet and outlet components of the developing ventricular loop (p. 1037). This ring becomes modified after septation of the ventricles, so that it encircles the right atrioventricular orifice and the aortic outlet from the left ventricle. With subsequent growth, only the septal components of this 'figure of eight' persist as the atrioventricular conducting tract. However, remnants of the aortic ring can persist as a 'dead-end tract'.

The Wolff–Parkinson–White syndrome is caused by abnormal small strands of otherwise unremarkable ventricular myocardium, which connect the atrial and ventricular myocardial masses at some point around the atrioventricular junctions. Histologically, they are strands of working myocardium running through the fibroareolar tissue of the atrioventricular groove.

CARDIAC PACING

Temporary pacing wires are usually inserted by cannulation of either the internal jugular vein or the subclavian vein. The subclavian vein approach carries a slightly greater risk of a pneumothorax because of the proximity of the pleural cavity. Other potential risks are brachial plexus injury if the entry site is too posterior, and thoracic duct injury if the left subclavian vein is cannulated. With permanent pacemakers, the most common site at which to locate the device is in a subcutaneous pocket on the anterior chest wall. Access to the heart and the endocardium of the right ventricle and right atrium is gained via the cephalic vein, where it lies in the deltopectoral groove.

CARDIAC CONDUCTION STUDIES

Intracardiac electrocardiography and electrophysiology are used to assess cardiac conduction and rhythm abnormalities. A catheter is inserted via the femoral, subclavian or internal jugular veins using a guidewire technique. Fluoroscopy is used to guide accurate placement of the catheter in the appropriate position. The sites of study are high right atrium (for assessing the atrioventricular bundle and right bundle branch) and the coronary sinus (for evaluating atrioventricular junctional arrhythmias and accessory pathways). The multipolar electrodes provide detailed electroanatomical mapping of the sequence of excitation from the atria, atrioventricular junction and ventricles. The origin of supraventricular arrhythmias, ventricular tachycardias, accessory conduction pathways and re-entrant pathways can be identified and used to guide radiofrequency ablation.

CONGENITAL CONDUCTION ABNORMALITIES

The majority of congenital conduction abnormalities have an anatomical basis for their origin and are the product of either accessory pathways or abnormal morphogenesis within the conducting tissue at any point from the atrioventricular node through the atrioventricular bundle. Some of the abnormalities are caused by tumours such as multifocal Purkinje cell tumours, and benign congenital polycystic tumours of the atrioventricular node.

Vascular supply and lymphatic drainage
CORONARY ARTERIAL SUPPLY

The right and left coronary arteries issue from the ascending aorta in its anterior and left posterior sinuses (**Figs 60.4C, 60.23, 60.24**). The levels of the coronary ostia are variable: they are usually at or above cuspal margins. The two arteries, as indicated by their name, form an oblique inverted crown, in which an anastomotic circle in the atrioventricular groove is connected by marginal and interventricular (descending) loops intersecting at the cardiac apex (**Figs 60.23, 60.24**). This is, of course, only an approximation. The degree of anastomosis varies and is usually insignificant. The main arteries and major branches are usually subepicardial, but those in the atrioventricular and interventricular grooves are often deeply sited, and occasionally hidden by overlapping myocardium or embedded in it.

The term 'dominant' is used to refer to the coronary artery that gives the posterior interventricular (descending) branch (which supplies the posterior part of the ventricular septum and often part of the posterolateral wall of the left ventricle). This is usually the left coronary artery (70%), which is also invariably the larger of the two vessels. Where it is not, the posterior interventricular (descending) branch is either bilateral, issuing from both the right coronary artery and the left circumflex artery, or absent and replaced by a network of smaller vessels given off from both right and left coronary arteries. Anastomoses between right and left coronary arteries are abundant during fetal life, but are much reduced by the end of the first year of life. Anastomoses providing collateral circulation may become prominent in conditions of hypoxia and in coronary artery disease. An additional collateral circulation is provided by small branches from mediastinal, pericardial and bronchial vessels.

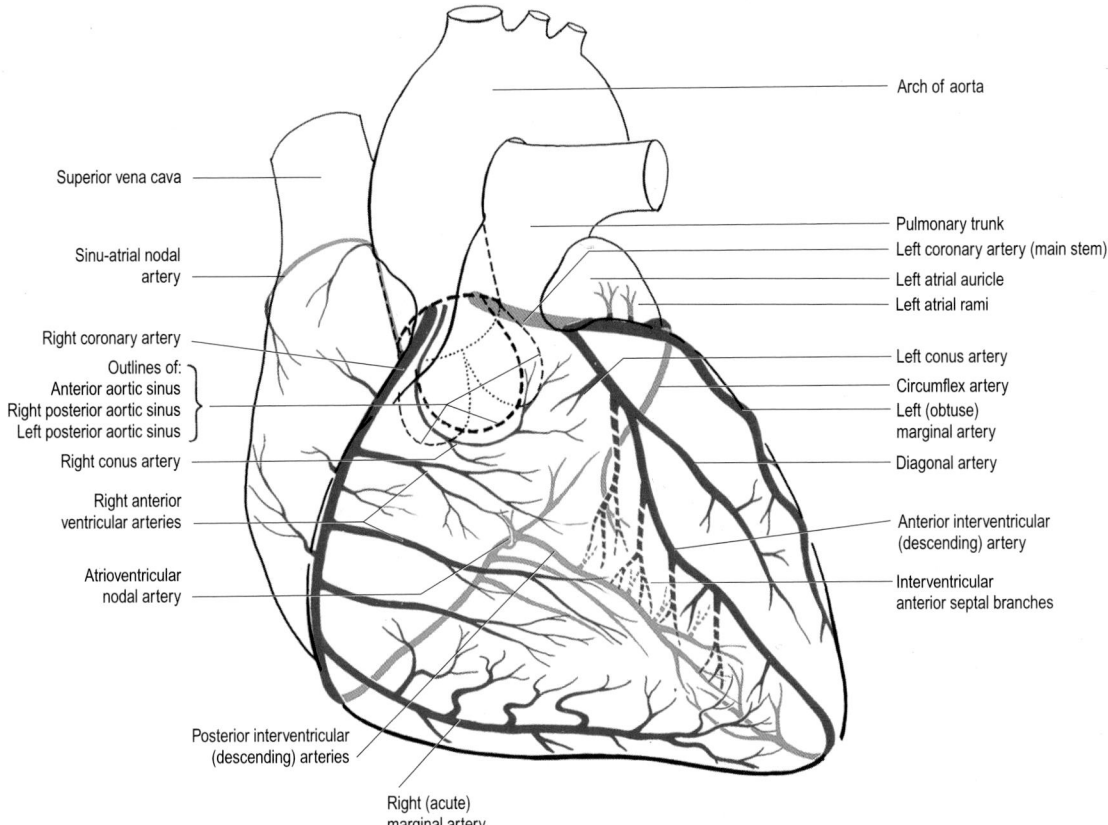

A

Arch of aorta

Superior vena cava

Sinu-atrial nodal artery

Right coronary artery

Outlines of:
Anterior aortic sinus
Right posterior aortic sinus
Left posterior aortic sinus

Right conus artery

Right anterior ventricular arteries

Atrioventricular nodal artery

Pulmonary trunk
Left coronary artery (main stem)
Left atrial auricle
Left atrial rami

Left conus artery
Circumflex artery
Left (obtuse) marginal artery
Diagonal artery

Anterior interventricular (descending) artery

Interventricular anterior septal branches

Posterior interventricular (descending) arteries

Right (acute) marginal artery

B

C

Sinu-atrial artery

Fig. 60.23 Anterior views of the coronary arterial system, with the principal variations. The right coronary arterial tree is shown in magenta, the left in full red. In both cases posterior distribution is shown in a paler shade. **A**, The most common arrangement. **B**, A common variation in the origin of the sinuatrial nodal artery. **C**, An example of left 'dominance' by the left coronary artery, showing also an uncommon origin of the sinu-atrial artery.

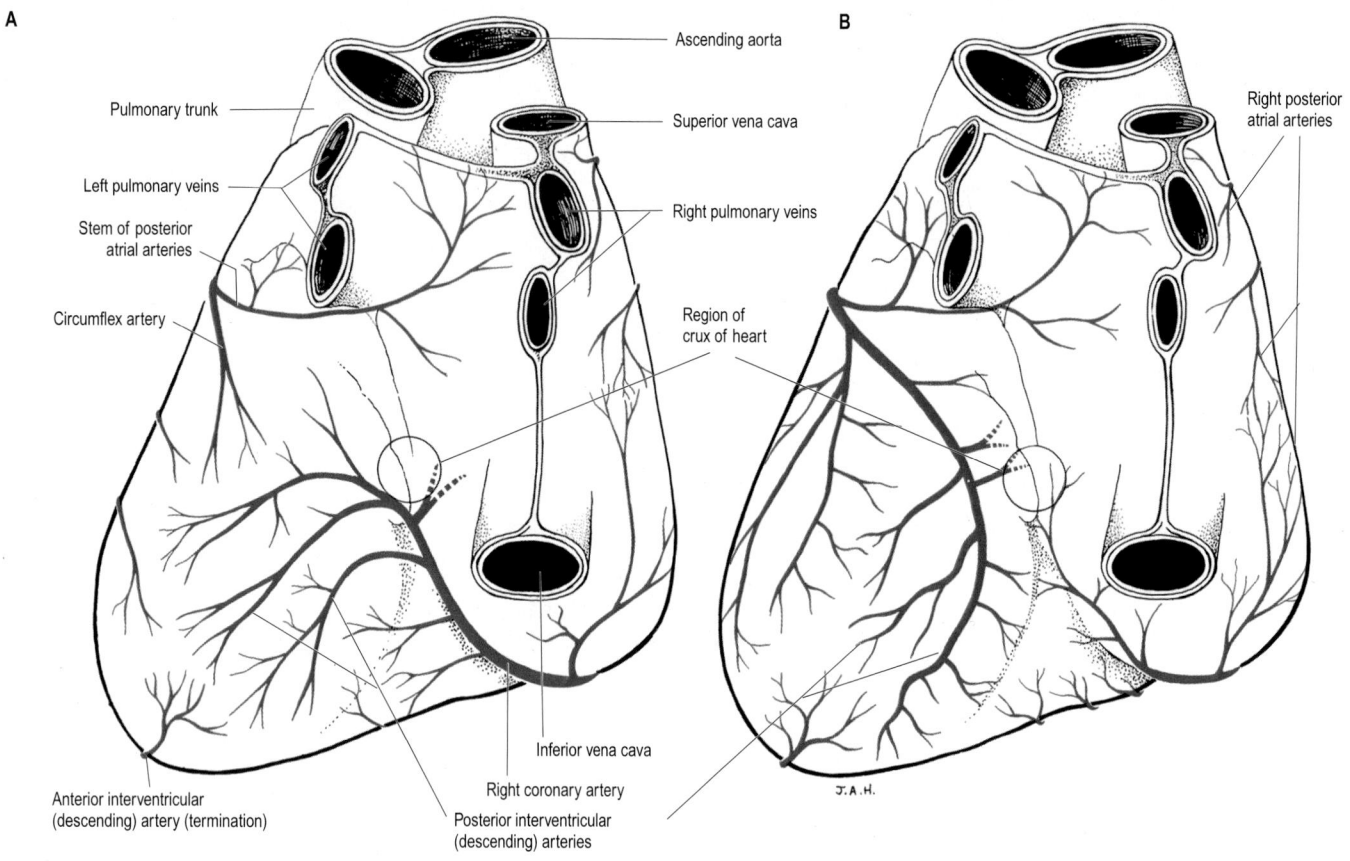

Fig. 60.24 Posteroinferior views of the coronary arterial system. The right coronary arterial tree is shown in magenta, the left in full red. **A**, An example of the more normal distribution in right 'dominance'. **B**, A less common form of left 'dominance'. In these 'posterior' views, the diaphragmatic (inferior) surface of the ventricular part of the heart has been artificially displaced and foreshortening ignored, to clarify the details of the so-called posterior (inferior) distribution of the coronary arteries.

The calibre of coronary arteries, both main stems and larger branches, based on measurements of arterial casts or angiograms, ranges between 1.5 and 5.5 mm for coronary arteries at their origins. The left exceed the right in c.60% of hearts, the right being larger in 17%, and the vessels approximately equal in 23%. The diameters of the coronary arteries may increase up to the thirtieth year.

RIGHT CORONARY ARTERY

The right coronary artery arises from the anterior ('right coronary') aortic sinus: the ostium is below the margin of the cusps in c.10%. The artery is usually single, but as many as four right coronary arteries have been observed. It passes at first anteriorly and slightly to the right between the right auricle and pulmonary trunk, where the sinus usually bulges. It reaches the atrioventricular groove and descends in this almost vertically to the right (acute) cardiac border, curving around it into the posterior part of the groove, where the latter approaches its junction with both interatrial and interventricular grooves, a region appropriately termed the crux of the heart. The artery reaches the crux and ends a little to the left of it, often by anastomosing with the circumflex branch of the left coronary artery. In a minority of individuals, the right coronary artery ends near the right cardiac border (c.10%), or between this and the crux (c.10%); more often (c.20%) it reaches the left border, replacing part of the circumflex artery.

Branches of the right coronary supply the right atrium and ventricle and, variably, parts of the left chambers and atrioventricular septum. The first branch (arising separately from the anterior aortic sinus in 36% of individuals) is the arteria coni arteriosi or conus artery. This is sometimes termed a 'third coronary' artery, but as a similar vessel comes from the left coronary, it is more correctly named the right conus artery. It ramifies anteriorly on the lowest part of the pulmonary conus and upper part of the right ventricle. It commonly anastomoses with a similar left coronary branch to form the 'anulus of Vieussens', a tenuous anastomotic 'circle' around the pulmonary trunk.

The first segment of the right coronary artery (between its origin and the right margin of the heart) gives off anterior atrial and ventricular branches. These vessels diverge widely, approaching a right angle in the case of ventricular arteries, which is in marked contrast to the more acute origins of the left coronary ventricular branches. The anterior ventricular branches, usually two or three, ramify towards the cardiac apex, which they rarely reach unless the right marginal artery is included in this group of branches, as it is by some authors. The right marginal artery is greater in calibre than the other anterior ventricular arteries and long enough to reach the apex in most hearts (93%). When it is very large, the remaining anterior ventricular branches may be reduced to one, or may be absent. Up to three small posterior ventricular branches, commonly two, arise from the second segment of the right coronary artery (between the right border and crux); they supply the diaphragmatic aspect of the right ventricle. Their size is inversely proportional to that of the right marginal artery, which usually extends to the diaphragmatic surface of the heart. As the right coronary approaches the crux, it normally produces one to three posterior interventricular branches (occasionally there are none). One, the posterior interventricular (descending) artery, lies in the interventricular groove. It is usually single (c.70%), and flanked either to the right or left or bilaterally by parallel branches from the right coronary artery. When these flanking vessels exist, branches of the posterior interventricular artery are small and sparse. The posterior interventricular (descending) artery is replaced by a left coronary branch in c.10% of individuals.

Although the atrial branches of the right coronary artery are sometimes described as anterior, lateral (right or marginal) and posterior groups, they are usually small single vessels c.1 mm in diameter. The right anterior and lateral branches are occasionally double, very rarely triple, and mainly supply the right atrium. The posterior branch is usually single and supplies the right and left atria. The artery of the sinuatrial node is an atrial branch, distributed largely to the myocardium of both atria, mainly the right. Its origin is variable: it comes from the circumflex branch of the left coronary in c.35%. However, more commonly it arises from the anterior atrial branch of the right coronary artery, less often from its right lateral part, least often from its posterior atrioventricular part. This 'nodal' artery thus usually passes back in the groove between the right auricular appendage and aorta. Whatever its origin, it usually branches around the base of the superior vena cava, typically as an arterial loop from which small branches supply the right atrium. A large 'ramus cristae terminalis' traverses the sinu-atrial node (**Fig. 60.23**); it would seem more appropriate to name this branch the 'nodal artery', as most of the currently named vessel actually supplies the atria and serves as the 'main atrial branch'.

Septal branches of the right coronary artery are relatively short, and leave the posterior interventricular (descending) branch to supply the posterior interventricular septum. They are numerous, but do not usually reach the apical parts of the septum. The largest posterior septal artery, usually the first, commonly arises from the inverted loop which is said to characterize the right coronary artery at the crux. It supplies the atrioventricular node in 80% of hearts.

Small recurrent atrioventricular branches are given off from the ventricular branches of the right coronary artery as they cross the atrio-ventricular groove; they supply the adjoining atrial myocardium.

LEFT CORONARY ARTERY

The left coronary artery is larger in calibre than the right, and supplies a greater volume of myocardium, including almost all the left ventricle and atrium, except in so-called 'right dominance', in which the right coronary artery partly supplies a posterior region of the left ventricle (**Fig. 60.23**). The left coronary artery usually supplies most of the inter-ventricular septum. It arises from the left posterior (left 'coronary') aortic sinus; the ostium is below the margin of the cusps in c.15%, and may be double, leading into major initial branches, usually the circumflex and anterior interventricular (descending) arteries. Its initial portion, between its ostium and its first branches, varies in length from a few millimetres to a few centimetres. The artery lies between the pulmonary trunk and the left atrial auricle, emerging into the atrioventricular groove, in which it turns left. This part is loosely embedded in sub-epicardial fat and usually has no branches, but may give off a small atrial ramus and, rarely, the sinu-atrial nodal artery.

Reaching the atrioventricular groove, the left coronary divides into two or three main branches: the anterior interventricular (descending) artery is commonly described as its continuation. This artery descends obliquely forward and to the left in the interventricular groove, some-times deeply embedded in or crossed by bridges of myocardial tissue, and by the great cardiac vein and its tributaries. It almost invariably reaches the apex, and terminates there in one-third of specimens. How-ever, more often it turns round the apex into the posterior interventricular groove, and passes one-third to one-half of the way along its length, where it meets the terminal twigs of the posterior interventricular (descending) branches of the right coronary artery.

The anterior interventricular (descending) artery produces right and left anterior ventricular and anterior septal branches, and a variable number of corresponding posterior branches. Anterior right ventricular branches are small and rarely number more than one or two; the right ventricle is supplied almost wholly by the right coronary artery.

From two to nine large left anterior ventricular arteries branch at acute angles from the anterior interventricular (descending) artery and cross the anterior aspect of the left ventricle diagonally; larger terminals reach the rounded (obtuse) left border. One is often large and may arise separately from the left coronary trunk (which then ends by trifur-cation). This left diagonal artery, reported in 33–50% or more indi-viduals, is sometimes duplicated (20%). A small left conus artery frequently leaves the anterior interventricular (descending) artery near its start, and anastomoses on the conus with its counterpart from the right coronary artery and with the vasa vasorum of the pulmonary artery and aorta. The anterior septal branches leave the anterior inter-ventricular (descending) artery almost perpendicularly, and pass back and down in the septum, usually supplying its ventral two-thirds. Small posterior septal branches from the same source supply the posterior one-third of the septum for a variable distance from the cardiac apex.

The circumflex artery, comparable to the anterior interventricular (descending) in calibre, curves left in the atrioventricular groove, continuing round the left cardiac border into the posterior part of the groove and ending left of the crux in most hearts, but sometimes continuing as a posterior interventricular (descending) artery. Proximally, the left atrial auricle usually overlaps it. In c.90%, a large ventricular

branch, the left marginal artery, arises perpendicularly from the circum-flex artery and ramifies over the rounded 'obtuse' margin, supplying much of the adjacent left ventricle, usually to the apex. Smaller anterior and posterior branches of the circumflex artery also supply the left ventricle. Anterior ventricular branches (from one to five, commonly two or three) course parallel to the diagonal artery, when it is present, and replace it when it is absent. Posterior ventricular branches are smaller and fewer; the left ventricle is partly supplied by the posterior interventricular (descending) artery. When this is small or absent, it is accompanied or replaced by an interventricular continuation of the circumflex artery, which is frequently double or triple. The circumflex artery may supply the left atrium via anterior, lateral and posterior atrial branches.

The circumflex artery has inconstant branches. The artery to the sinu-atrial node is a branch in c.35%, usually from the anterior circum-flex segment, less often the circum-marginal. It passes over and supplies the left atrium, encircling the superior vena cava like a right coronary nodal branch. It sends a large branch to (and through) the node, but is predominantly atrial in distribution. The artery to the atrioventricular node, the terminal branch in 20%, arises near the crux, in which case the circumflex usually supplies the posterior interventricular (descending) artery, an example of so-called 'left dominance'. Kugel's anastomotic artery ('arteria anastomotica auricularis magna') has been described as a constant circumflex branch, usually from its anterior part, traversing the interatrial septum (near its ventricular border) to establish direct or indirect anastomosis with the right coronary; its existence has been questioned.

CORONARY DISTRIBUTION

Details of coronary distribution require integration into a concept of total cardiac supply. Most commonly, the right coronary artery supplies all the right ventricle (except a small region right of the anterior inter-ventricular groove), a variable part of the left ventricular diaphragmatic aspect, the posteroinferior one-third of the intraventricular septum, the right atrium and part of the left, and the conducting system as far as the proximal parts of the right and left crura. Left coronary distribution is reciprocal, and includes most of the left ventricle, a narrow strip of right ventricle, the anterior two-thirds of the interventricular septum and most of the left atrium. As noted (**Figs 60.23, 60.24**), variations in the coronary arterial system mainly affect the diaphragmatic aspect of the ventricles; they consist of the relative 'dominance' of supply by the left or the right coronary artery. The term is misleading, as the left artery almost always supplies a greater volume of tissue. In 'right dominance', the posterior interventricular (descending) artery is derived from the right coronary; in 'left dominance' it derives from the left. In the so-called 'balanced' pattern, branches of both arteries run in or near the groove. Less is known of variation in atrial supply because the small vessels involved are not easily preserved in the corrosion casts that are used for analysis. In more than 50% of individuals, the right atrium is supplied only by the right coronary; in the remainder the supply is dual. More than 62% of left atria are largely supplied by the left and c.27% by the right coronary; in each group a small accessory supply from the other coronary artery exists, and 11% are supplied almost equally by both arteries. Sinu-atrial and atrioventricular supplies also vary. Various studies have reported that the right and left coronary arteries supply the sinu-atrial node in 51–65% and 35–45% respec-tively (fewer than 10% of nodes receive a bilateral supply). The atrio-ventricular node is supplied by the right coronary (80–90%) and left coronary arteries (10–20%).

CORONARY ANASTOMOSIS

Anastomoses between branches of coronary arteries, subepicardial or myocardial, and between these arteries and extracardiac vessels are of prime medical importance. Clinical experience suggests that anastomoses cannot rapidly provide collateral routes sufficient to circumvent sudden coronary obstruction, and the coronary circulation is assumed to be end-arterial. Nevertheless, it has long been established that anastomoses do occur, particularly between fine subepicardial branches, and they may increase during individual life. Analyses of coronary radiographs and resin corrosion casts, and the results of radio-opaque perfusion studies, have revealed intra- and intercoronary anastomoses in vessels up to 100–200 μm in calibre. The most frequent sites of extramural anastomoses are the apex, the anterior aspect of the right ventricle, the posterior aspect of the left ventricle, crux, interatrial and interventricular grooves and between the sinuatrial nodal and other atrial vessels. The functional value of such anastomoses must vary, but they appear to become more effective in slowly progressive pathological conditions. Their structure is uncertain: most observations that have been made on corrosion casts suggest that anastomotic vessels are relatively straight in normal hearts, but much coiled in hearts that have been subject to coronary occlusion. Little has been recorded of their microscopic structure; they appear little more than endothelial tubes, without muscles or elastic tissue.

Extracardiac anastomoses may connect various coronary branches with other thoracic vessels via the pericardial arteries and arterial vasa vasorum of vessels that link the heart with systemic and pulmonary circulations. The effectiveness of these connections as collateral routes in coronary occlusion is unpredictable.

Coronary arteriovenous anastomoses and numerous connections between the coronary circulation and cardiac cavities, producing so-called 'myocardial sinusoids' and 'arterioluminal' vessels, have been reported; their importance in coronary disease is uncertain.

CORONARY ARTERY DISEASE

Atherosclerosis is characterized by deposition of lipid and accumulation of macrophages in the intima. Endothelial dysfunction leads to the recruitment of inflammatory cells into the vascular wall and the release of various cytokines and adhesion molecules that propagate the process of atherosclerosis. Lipid accumulation and smooth muscle proliferation lead to the formation of an atheromatous plaque. The formation of the plaque itself may cause stenosis of the coronary arteries, and reduces coronary blood flow (classically on exertion). The plaques are also susceptible to rupture with concomitant thrombus formation, which leads to acute occlusion of one of the coronary arteries and may cause myocardial infarction. Plaques may rupture as a result of fatigue within the fibrous cap, but are also more vulnerable when the lipid content is greater than 40% of the composition of the plaque. Superficial erosion of the plaque may also promote critical thrombus formation.

Assessment of coronary artery disease is possible via a number of radiological techniques, including MRI, positron emission tomography, scintigraphy and ultrasound, and invasively by coronary arteriography (which displays the anatomy and delineates regions of stenosis).

CORONARY ANGIOGRAPHY

Coronary angiography may be performed by introducing a catheter through the femoral, radial or brachial arteries. The femoral artery is punctured with a needle c.3 cm below the inguinal ligament while the leg is held adducted and slightly externally rotated (p. 1450). The exact position is guided by palpation of the femoral arterial pulse, and the needle is inserted at an angle of 45°. After arterial puncture, a fine guidewire is inserted through the needle and fed into the artery. The catheter is then inserted over the guidewire and manipulated via the iliac artery into the aorta, up the aortic arch and located in the ascending aorta. The brachial or radial artery may be used for percutaneous access to the circulation. Once the catheter is located in the ascending aorta, a variety of guidewires (straight tip, left and right curved catheters, and pigtail catheters) are used to enter the coronary vessels for selective arteriography and interventions. Angiography is performed with standard high osmolality contrast medium with cineangiography. In selected patients, new-generation low osmolality contrast medium may also be used. All the coronary arteries are catheterized and evaluated in a variety of views to obtain a full evaluation of the anatomy of the coronary arteries and determine the location and degree of any stenoses. The ostium of the left coronary artery arises from the left sinus and is best viewed in the direct frontal and left anterior oblique directions. The right anterior oblique view is useful in demonstrating the diagonal branches and anterior descending coronary artery. The right coronary artery originates from the right sinus of Valsalva and is usually visualized in the right anterior oblique and left anterior oblique views. Pressure and oxygen saturations can be measured via the catheter. Changes in pressure across valves allow the degree of stenosis to be measured. Coronary blood flow and relative flow reserve can also be calculated. Significant stenosis may be treated initially by balloon angioplasty followed by insertion of stents. The balloon exerts pressure against the plaque in the arterial wall and fractures and splits the plaque. The splinting effect of the plaque and elastic recoil are reduced, resulting in an increase in the arterial lumen. Insertion of a stent reduces the rate of restenosis.

CORONARY REVASCULARIZATION

Atherosclerosis causing greater than 60% stenosis of the terminal diameter of the coronary arteries is likely to cause a significant reduction in myocardial perfusion. Patients with high-grade lesions or left main-stem coronary artery or triple-vessel disease with impaired left ventricular function are usually considered for coronary artery bypass grafting. The common grafts that are used are the saphenous veins and internal thoracic (mammary) arteries. Other grafts that are occasionally used are the radial artery, ulnar artery, gastroepiploic artery and inferior epigastric artery.

The left internal thoracic artery grafts have a greater patency rate than saphenous vein grafts. Approximately 15% of saphenous vein grafts occlude in 1 year and from then on at a rate of 1–2% in the first 6 years and 4% thereafter; 40–50% of saphenous vein grafts have re-occluded by 10 years. In contrast, only about 10% of left internal thoracic artery grafts will have re-occluded at 10 years.

The common surgical approach is via a midline sternotomy. If the internal thoracic artery is used as a donor graft, it is divided distally (maintaining its proximal origin from the thyrocervical trunk) and anastomosed to the coronary artery distal to the stenosis. If saphenous vein grafts are used, they must be anastomosed both proximal and distal to the coronary artery, to bridge the site of the stenosis.

In selected cases, minimally invasive direct coronary artery bypass grafting is performed, but the approach is dependent on the vessel being grafted. The anterior approach is via mini-thoracotomy over the fourth intercostal space underneath the nipple for grafting the mid-left anterior descending and diagonal branches. The anterolateral approach is via an incision in the third intercostal space from the midclavicular line to the anterior axillary line and is used for grafting early marginal branches of the circumflex system. The lateral approach allows grafting of the circumflex vessels via lateral thoracotomy measuring only c.10 cm in size through the fifth or sixth intercostal space. Extrathoracic approaches that are occasionally used include the subxiphoid approach for the distal right coronary artery and posterior descending artery. Port access surgery allows for full re-vascularization with cardiopulmonary bypass, but obviates the need for midline sternotomy.

CARDIAC VEINS

The heart is drained by the coronary sinus and its tributaries, the anterior cardiac veins and the small cardiac veins. The coronary sinus and its tributaries return blood to the right atrium from the entire heart (including its septa) except for the anterior region of the right ventricle and small, variable parts of both atria and left ventricle. The anterior cardiac veins drain an anterior region of the right ventricle and a region around the right cardiac border when the right marginal vein joins this group, ending principally in the right atrium. The small cardiac veins (Thebesius' veins) open into the right atrium and ventricle and, to a lesser extent, the left atrium and sometimes left ventricle.

Variation in cardiac veins – Attempts to categorize variations in cardiac venous circulation into 'types' have not produced any accepted pattern. There are major variations concerning the general directions of drainage. The coronary sinus may receive all the cardiac veins (except the small veins), including the anterior cardiac veins (33%), which may be reduced by diversion of some into the small cardiac vein and then to the coronary sinus (28%). The remainder (39%) represent the 'normal' pattern, as described above.

CORONARY SINUS

The large majority of cardiac veins drain into the wide coronary sinus, c.2 or 3 cm long, lying in the posterior atrioventricular groove between the left atrium and ventricle (Figs 60.2, 60.25). The sinus opens into the right atrium between the opening of the inferior vena cava and the right atrioventricular orifice; the opening is guarded by an endocardial fold (semilunar valve of the coronary sinus; Fig. 60.7). Its tributaries are the great, small and middle cardiac veins, the posterior vein of the left ventricle and the oblique vein of the left atrium; all except the last have valves at their orifices.

Great cardiac vein – The great cardiac vein begins at the cardiac apex, ascends in the anterior interventricular groove to the atrioventricular groove and follows this, passing to the left and posteriorly to enter the coronary sinus at its origin (Fig. 60.25). It receives tributaries from the

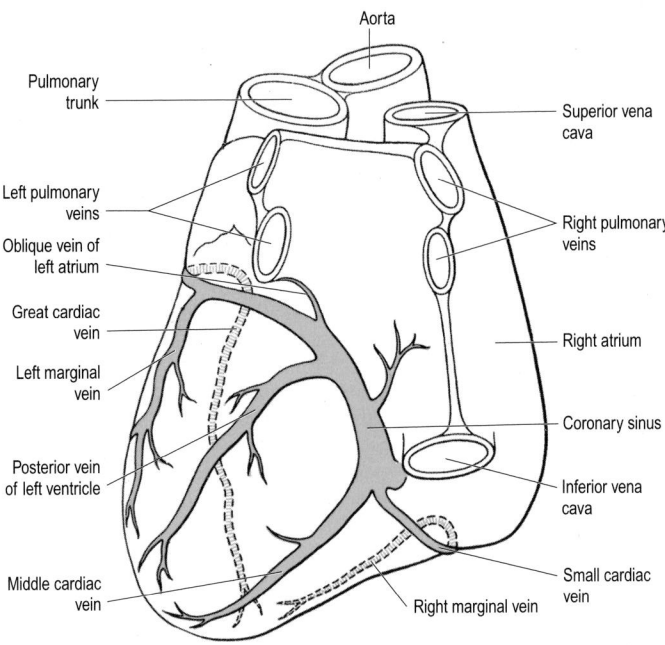

Fig. 60.25 The principal veins of the heart.

left atrium and both ventricles, including the large left marginal vein that ascends the left aspect ('obtuse border') of the heart.

Small cardiac vein – The small cardiac vein lies in the posterior atrio-ventricular groove between the right atrium and ventricle and opens into the coronary sinus near its atrial end (**Fig. 60.25**). It receives blood from the posterior part of the right atrium and ventricle. The right marginal vein passes right, along the inferior cardiac margin ('acute border'). It may join the small cardiac vein in the atrioventricular groove, but more often opens directly into the right atrium.

Middle cardiac vein – The middle cardiac vein (**Fig. 60.25**) begins at the cardiac apex, and runs back in the posterior interventricular groove to end in the coronary sinus near its atrial end.

Posterior vein of the left ventricle – The posterior vein of the left ventricle (**Fig. 60.25**) is found on the diaphragmatic surface of the left ventricle a little to the left of the middle cardiac vein. It usually opens into the centre of the coronary sinus, but sometimes opens into the great cardiac vein.

Oblique vein of the left atrium – The small vessel that is the oblique vein of the left atrium (**Fig. 60.25**) descends obliquely on the back of the left atrium to join the coronary sinus near its end. It is continuous above with the ligament of the left vena cava. The two structures are remnants of the left common cardinal vein.

ANTERIOR CARDIAC VEINS

The anterior cardiac veins drain the anterior part of the right ventricle. Usually two or three, sometimes even five, they ascend in subepicardial tissue to cross the right part of the atrioventricular groove, passing deep or superficial to the right coronary artery. They end in the right atrium, near the groove, separately or in variable combinations. A subendocardial collecting channel, into which all may open, has been described. The right marginal vein courses along the inferior ('acute') cardiac margin, draining adjacent parts of the right ventricle, and usually opens separately into the right atrium. It may join the anterior cardiac veins or, less often, the coronary sinus. Because it is commonly independent, it is often grouped with the small cardiac veins, but it is larger in calibre, being comparable to the anterior cardiac veins or even wider.

SMALL CARDIAC VEINS

The existence of small cardiac veins, opening into all cardiac cavities, has been confirmed, but they are more difficult to demonstrate than larger cardiac vessels. Their numbers and size are highly variable: up to 2 mm in diameter opening into the right atrium and c.0.5 mm into the right ventricle. Numerous small cardiac veins have been identified in the right atrium and ventricle, but they are rare in the left atrium and left ventricle.

CARDIAC VENOUS ANASTOMOSIS

There are widespread anastomoses at all levels of the cardiac venous circulation, on a scale exceeding that of the arteries and amounting to a veritable venous plexus. Not only are adjacent veins often connected, but connections also exist between tributaries of the coronary sinus and those of the anterior cardiac veins. Abundant anastomoses occur at the apex and its anterior and posterior aspects. Like coronary arteries, cardiac veins connect with extracardiac vessels, chiefly the vasa vasorum of the large vessels continuous with the heart.

LYMPHATIC DRAINAGE OF THE HEART

Cardiac lymphatic vessels form subendocardial, myocardial and sub-epicardial plexuses, the first two draining into the third. Efferents from the subepicardial plexuses form the left and right cardiac collecting trunks. Two or three left trunks ascend the anterior interventricular groove, receiving vessels from both ventricles. Reaching the atrioventricular groove, they are joined by a large vessel from the diaphragmatic surface of the left ventricle, which first ascends in the posterior interventricular groove and then turns left along the atrioventricular groove. The vessel formed by this union ascends between the pulmonary artery and the left atrium, usually ending in an inferior tracheobronchial node. The right trunk receives afferents from the right atrium and right border and diaphragmatic surface of the right ventricle. It ascends in the atrio-ventricular groove, near the right coronary artery, and then anterior to the ascending aorta to end in a brachiocephalic node, usually on the left.

Innervation

Initiation of the cardiac cycle is myogenic, originating in the sinu-atrial node. It is harmonized in rate, force and output by autonomic nerves operating on the nodal tissues and their prolongations, on coronary vessels and on the working atrial and ventricular musculature. This supply has both efferent (sympathetic and parasympathetic) and afferent components. All the cardiac branches of the vagus and sympathetic contain both afferent and efferent fibres, except the cardiac branch of the superior cervical sympathetic ganglion, which is purely efferent. The efferent preganglionic cardiac sympathetic fibres arise from neurones in the intermediolateral column of the upper four or five thoracic spinal segments. They pass by white rami communicantes to synapse in the upper thoracic sympathetic ganglia, although many ascend to synapse in the cervical ganglia. Postganglionic fibres from these ganglia form the sympathetic cardiac nerves, which accelerate the heart and dilate the coronary arteries. Of the sympathetic axons from the first four or five thoracic spinal segments, the upper pass to the ascending aorta, pulmonary trunk and ventricles, the lower to the atria.

Efferent cardiac parasympathetic axons from the dorsal vagal nucleus and neurones near the nucleus ambiguus run in vagal cardiac branches to synapse in the cardiac plexuses and atrial walls. These vagal fibres slow the heart and cause constriction of the coronary arteries. In man (like most mammals) intrinsic cardiac neurones are limited to the atria and interatrial septum. They are most numerous in the subepicardial connective tissue near the sinu-atrial and atrioventricular nodes. There is evidence that these intrinsic ganglia are not simple nicotinic relays, but may act as sites for integration of extrinsic nervous inputs and form complex circuits for the local neuronal control of the heart, and perhaps even local reflexes.

CARDIAC PLEXUS

Nearing the heart, the autonomic nerves form a mixed cardiac plexus, usually described in terms of a superficial component inferior to the aortic arch lying between it and the pulmonary trunk, and a deep part between the aortic arch and tracheal bifurcation. The cardiac plexus is

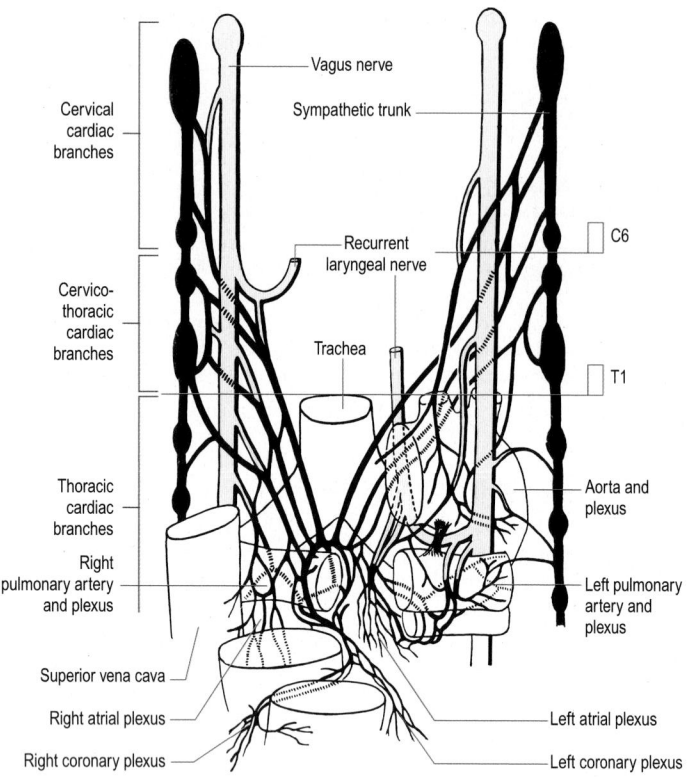

Fig. 60.26 The human cardiac plexus: its source from the cervical parts of the vagus nerves and sympathetic trunks and its extensions, the pulmonary, atrial and coronary plexuses. Note the numerous junctions between sympathetic and parasympathetic (vagal) branches that form the plexus. Concerning the frequent variations, consult Mizeres (1963). (By permission from Mizeres NJ 1963 The cardiac plexus in man. Am J Anat 112: 141–151.)

also described by regional names for its coronary, pulmonary, atrial and aortic extensions (**Fig. 60.26**). These plexuses contain ganglion cells, and ganglion cells are also found in the heart along the distribution of branches of the plexus. They are confined to the atrial tissues, with a preponderance adjacent to the sinu-atrial node. Their axons are considered to be largely, if not exclusively, postganglionic parasympathetic. Cholinergic and adrenergic fibres, arising in or passing through the cardiac plexus, are distributed most profusely to the sinus and atrio-ventricular nodes; there is a much less dense supply to the atrial and ventricular myocardium. Adrenergic fibres supply the coronary arteries and cardiac veins. Rich plexuses of nerves containing cholinesterase, adrenergic transmitters and other peptides, e.g. neuropeptide Y, are found in the subendocardial regions of all chambers and in the cusps of the valves.

Superficial (ventral) part of the cardiac plexus – The superficial (ventral) part of the cardiac plexus lies below the aortic arch and anterior to the right pulmonary artery. It is formed by the cardiac branch of the left superior cervical sympathetic ganglion and the lower of the two cervical cardiac branches of the left vagus. A small cardiac ganglion is usually present in this plexus immediately below the aortic arch, to the right of the ligamentum arteriosum. This part of the cardiac plexus connects with the deep part, the right coronary plexus and the left anterior pulmonary plexus.

Deep (dorsal) part of the cardiac plexus – The deep (dorsal) part of the cardiac plexus is anterior to the tracheal bifurcation, above the point of division of the pulmonary trunk and posterior to the aortic arch. It is formed by the cardiac branches of the cervical and upper thoracic sympathetic ganglia and of the vagus and recurrent laryngeal nerves. The only cardiac nerves which do not join it are those that join the superficial part of the plexus.

Branches from the right half of the deep part of the cardiac plexus pass in front of and behind the right pulmonary artery. Those anterior

to it, the more numerous, supply a few filaments to the right anterior pulmonary plexus and continue on to form part of the right coronary plexus. Those behind the pulmonary artery supply a few filaments to the right atrium and then continue into the left coronary plexus. The left half of the deep part of the cardiac plexus is connected with the superficial, and supplies filaments to the left atrium and left anterior pulmonary plexus. It forms much of the left coronary plexus.

Left coronary plexus – The left coronary plexus is larger than the right, and is formed chiefly by the prolongation of the left half of the deep part of the cardiac plexus and a few fibres from the right. It accompanies the left coronary artery to supply the left atrium and ventricle.

Right coronary plexus – The right coronary plexus is formed from both superficial and deep parts of the cardiac plexus, and accompanies the right coronary artery to supply the right atrium and ventricle.

Atrial plexuses – The atrial plexuses are derivatives of the right and left continuations of the cardiac plexus along the coronary arteries. Their fibres are distributed to the corresponding atria, overlapping those from the coronary plexuses.

MAJOR BLOOD VESSELS

The major blood vessels comprise the pulmonary trunk, the thoracic aorta and its branches, the superior and inferior venae cavae and their tributaries.

Arteries

PULMONARY TRUNK

The pulmonary trunk, or pulmonary artery, conveys deoxygenated blood from the right ventricle to the lungs (**Figs 60.4C,D, 60.27**). About 5 cm in length and 3 cm in diameter, it is the most anterior of the cardiac vessels and arises from the base of the right ventricle (from the pulmonary anulus surmounting the conus arteriosus) above and to the left of the supraventricular crest. It slopes up and back, at first in front of the ascending aorta, then to its left. Below the aortic arch it divides, level with the fifth thoracic vertebra and to the left of the midline, into right and left pulmonary arteries of almost equal size. The pulmonary trunk bifurcation lies below, in front and to the left of the tracheal bifurcation (which is also associated with the inferior tracheobronchial lymph nodes and the deep cardiac nerve plexus). In the fetus, at the level of the bifurcation the pulmonary artery is connected to the aortic arch by the ductus arteriosus, which lies in the same direction as the pulmonary artery.

Relations – The pulmonary artery is entirely within the pericardium, enclosed with the ascending aorta in a common tube of visceral pericardium. The fibrous pericardium gradually disappears within the adventitia of the pulmonary arteries. Anteriorly, it is separated from the sternal end of the left second intercostal space by the pleura, left lung and pericardium. Posterior are the ascending aorta and left coronary artery initially, then the left atrium. The ascending aorta ultimately lies on its right. An auricle and coronary artery lie on each side of its origin. The superficial cardiac plexus is between the pulmonary bifurcation and the aortic arch. The tracheal bifurcation, lymph nodes and nerves are above, bilateral and right.

During fetal life, when blood pressure is similar in the pulmonary artery and the aorta, the structure of the vessels is similar. After birth, the lungs expand and pulmonary arterioles dilate, and so pulmonary vascular resistance decreases, whereas blood flow increases. The systolic pressure in the pulmonary artery consequently decreases and this is accompanied by a structural remodelling of its wall. The elastic material, which originally had a lamellar structure, becomes aggregated into star-shaped units linked to many muscle cells. The amount of muscular tissue grows extensively after birth and exceeds that found in the aorta. The thickness of the wall of the aorta is about twice that of the pulmonary artery.

RIGHT AND LEFT PULMONARY ARTERIES

The pulmonary arteries are described in Chapter 63 (p. 1070).

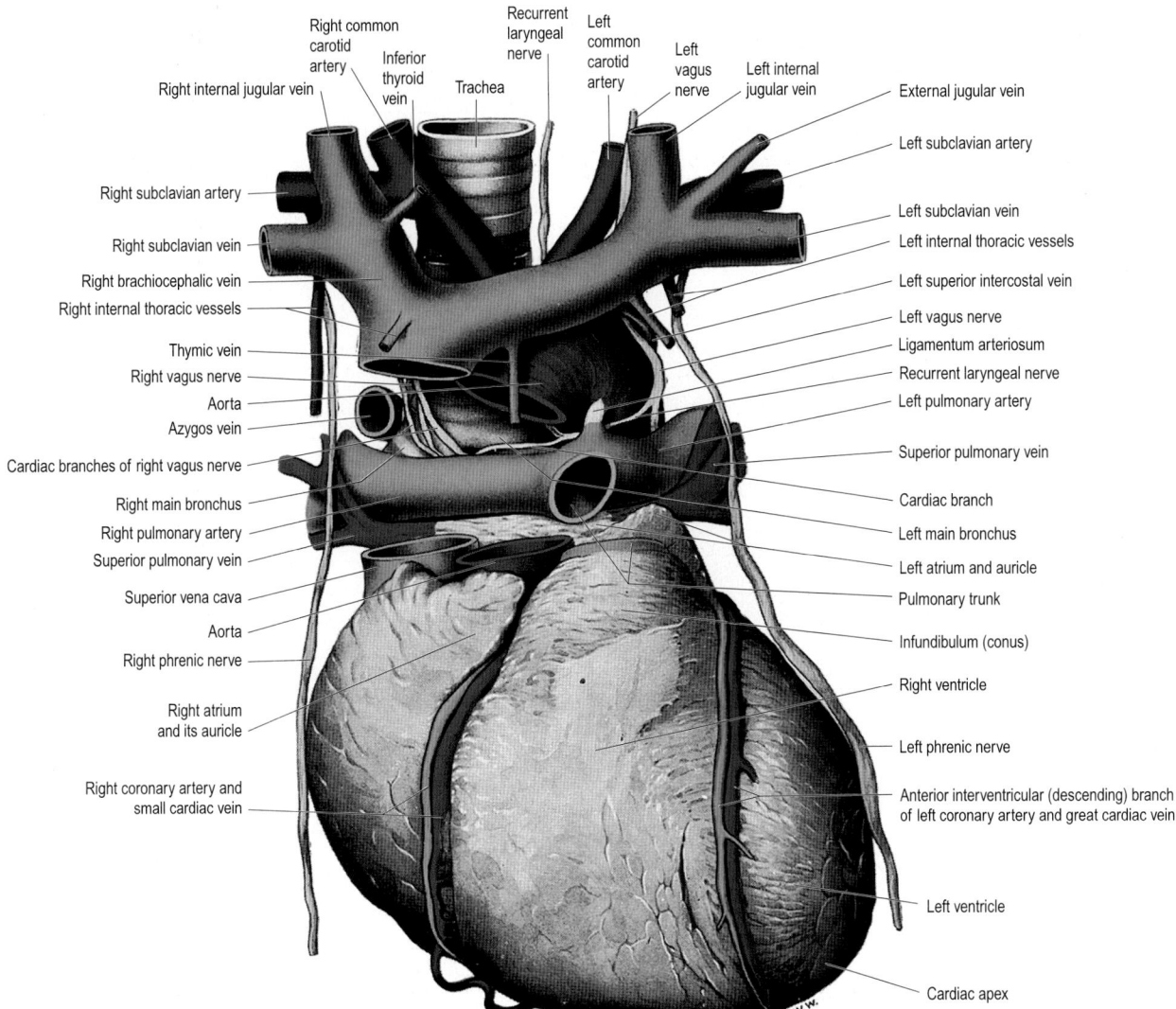

Fig. 60.27 The relations of the pulmonary arteries and primary bronchi seen from the front. Parts of the ascending aorta, pulmonary trunk and superior vena cava have been removed in the dissection.

THORACIC AORTA

ASCENDING AORTA

The ascending aorta (**Figs 60.4C, 60.6, 60.23, 60.24, 60.27**), c.5 cm long, begins at the base of the left ventricle, level with the lower border of the third left costal cartilage; it ascends obliquely, curving forwards and right, behind the left half of the sternum to the level of the upper border of the second left costal cartilage. At its origin, close to the aortic anulus, the sectional profile is larger and not circular because of three almost hemispherical outward bulges (sinuses of Valsalva), one posterior (non-coronary), one left and one right, which correspond to the three cusps of the aortic valve. Distal to the aortic anulus are three aortic sinuses, beyond which the calibre of the vessel is slightly increased by a bulging of its right wall. This aortic bulb gives the vessel an oval section.

Relations – The ascending aorta is within the fibrous pericardium, enclosed in a tube of serosal pericardium with the pulmonary trunk (**Fig. 60.1**). Anterior to its lower part are the infundibulum, the initial segment of the pulmonary trunk and the right auricle. Superiorly, it is separated from the sternum by the pericardium, right pleura, anterior margin of the right lung, loose areolar tissue and the remains of the thymus gland. Posterior are the left atrium, right pulmonary artery and principal bronchus. Right lateral are the superior vena cava and right atrium, the former partly posterior. Left lateral are the left atrium and, at a higher level, the pulmonary trunk. At least two structures, aortico-pulmonary bodies (reminiscent of the carotid arterial chemoreceptors

and baroreceptors), lie between the ascending aorta and the pulmonary trunk. The inferior aorticopulmonary body is near the heart and anterior to the aorta. The middle aorticopulmonary body is near the right side of the ascending aorta.

AORTIC ARCH

The aortic arch continues from the ascending aorta (**Fig. 60.4C,E**). Its origin, slightly to the right, is level with the upper border of the second right sternocostal joint. The arch first ascends diagonally back and to the left over the anterior surface of the trachea, then back across its left side and finally descends to the left of the fourth thoracic vertebral body, continuing as the descending thoracic aorta. It ends level with the sternal end of the second, left costal cartilage. Thus the aortic arch lies wholly in the superior mediastinum. It curves around the hilum of the left lung, and extends upwards to the mid level of the manubrium of the sternum. The shadow of the arch is easily identified in antero-posterior radiographs and its left profile is sometimes called the 'aortic knuckle' (**Figs 60.28, 60.29**). The arch may also be visible in left anterior oblique views enclosing a pale space, 'the aortic window', in which shadows of the pulmonary trunk and its left branch may be discerned. Its diameter at the origin is the same as in the ascending aorta, c.28 mm, but it is reduced to 20 mm at the end, after the issue of its large collateral branches. At the border with the thoracic aorta, a small stricture (aortic isthmus), followed by a dilatation, can be recognized. In fetal life the isthmus lies between the origin of the left subclavian artery and the opening of the ductus arteriosus.

A

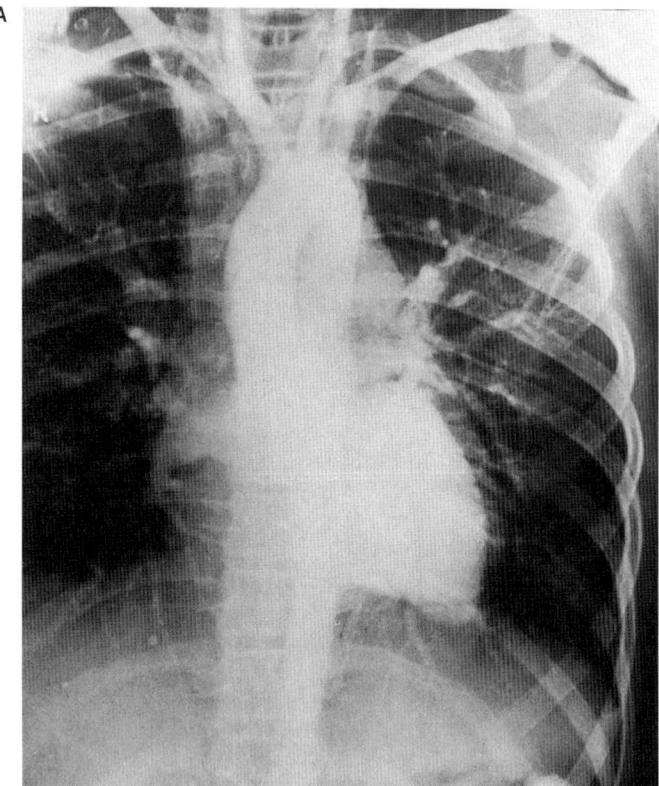

A

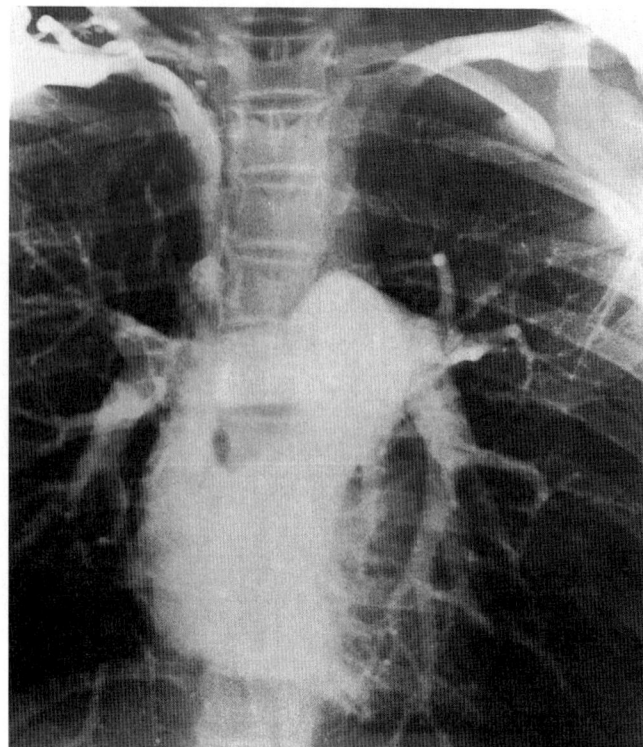

B

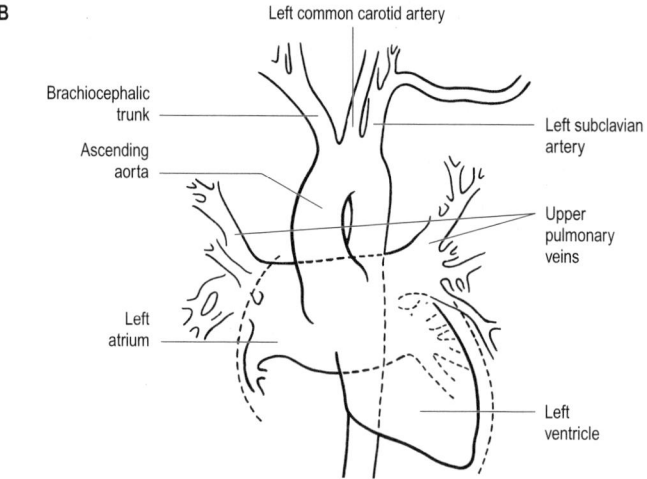

Fig. 60.28 Angiocardiogram showing the left side of the heart in a child of 11 years: anteroposterior view. Note that, because of the great obliquity of the atrial septum, the left atrium extends to the right behind the right atrium, and that, because the arms of the patient are raised above the head, the distal end of the left subclavian artery passes upwards. (Provided by Frances Gardner.)

B

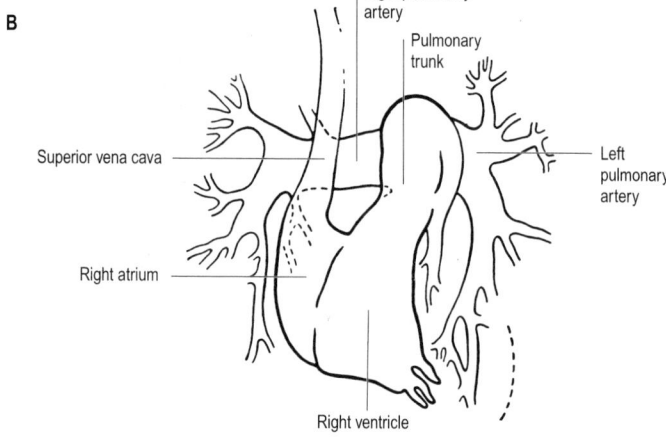

Fig. 60.29 Angiocardiogram showing the right side of the heart in a child of 12 years: anteroposterior view. (Provided by Frances Gardner.)

Relations – Anteriorly and to the left of the aortic arch is the left mediastinal pleura. Deep to the pleura it is crossed, in anteroposterior order by: the left phrenic nerve, left lower cervical cardiac branch of the vagus, left superior cervical cardiac branch of the sympathetic and left vagus. As the left vagus crosses the arch, its recurrent laryngeal branch hooks below the vessel left and behind (developmentally caudal to) the ligamentum arteriosum and then ascends on the right of the arch. The left superior intercostal vein ascends obliquely forwards on the arch, superficial to the left vagus, deep to the left phrenic nerve (**Fig. 60.6**). The left lung and pleura separate all these from the thoracic wall. Posterior and to the right are the trachea and deep cardiac plexus, the left recurrent laryngeal nerve, oesophagus, thoracic duct and vertebral column. Above, the brachiocephalic, left common carotid and left subclavian arteries arise from its convexity, and are crossed anteriorly near their origins by the left brachiocephalic vein. Below are the pulmonary bifurcation, left principal bronchus, ligamentum arteriosum, superficial cardiac plexus and left recurrent laryngeal nerve. Best viewed from the left, the concavity of the aortic arch is the upper curved limit through which structures gain access to or leave the hilum of the left lung.

Variations of the arch and its branches – The summit of the arch is usually about 2.5 cm below the superiosternal border, but may diverge from this. In the infant it is closer to the upper border of the sternum; the same is often the case in old age, because of the dilatation of the vessel. Sometimes the aorta curves over the right pulmonary hilum and descends to the right of the vertebral column. This is usually accompanied by transposition of thoracic and abdominal viscera. Less often, after arching over the right hilum, it passes behind the oesophagus to gain its usual position (this is not accompanied by visceral transposition). The aorta may divide into ascending and descending trunks, the former dividing into three branches to supply the head and upper limbs. Sometimes it divides near its origin, the two branches soon reuniting, and the oesophagus and trachea usually pass through the interval between them.

Branches – Three branches arise from the convex aspect of the arch: the brachiocephalic trunk, left common carotid and left subclavian arteries (**Figs 31.15, 60.6**). They may branch from the beginning of the arch or the upper part of the ascending aorta. The distance between these origins varies, the most frequent being approximation of the left common carotid artery to the brachiocephalic trunk.

Primary branches from the aortic arch may be reduced to one, but more commonly two. The left common carotid may arise from the brachiocephalic trunk (7%). More rarely, the left common carotid and subclavian arteries may arise from a left brachiocephalic trunk, or the right common carotid and right subclavian may arise separately, in which case the latter more often branches from the left end of the arch and passes behind the oesophagus. The left vertebral artery may arise between the left common carotid and the subclavian arteries. Very rarely, external and internal carotid arteries arise separately, the common carotid being absent on one or both sides, or both carotids and one or both vertebral arteries may be separate branches. When a 'right aorta' occurs, the arrangement of its three branches is reversed. The common carotids may have a single trunk. Other arteries may branch from it, most commonly one or both bronchial arteries and the thyroid ima artery.

An analysis of variation in branches from 1000 aortic arches showed the usual pattern in 65%; a left common carotid shared the brachiocephalic trunk in 27% (contrast percentage quoted above) and the four large arteries branched separately in 2.5%. The remaining 5% showed a great variety of patterns, the most common (1.2%) being symmetric right and left brachiocephalic trunks.

COARCTATION OF THE AORTA

The aortic lumen is occasionally partly or completely obliterated, above (preductal or infantile type), opposite or just beyond (postductal or adult type) the entry of the ductus arteriosus. The condition, coarctation of the aorta, is congenital; the ductus arteriosus may remain patent, but rarely compensates, because systemic blood pressure is usually much greater than pulmonary.

In the preductal type, the length of the coarctation is variable and may involve the left subclavian and even the brachiocephalic artery, and there is little scope for the development of an effective collateral circulation to regions distal to the stenosis. Many cases are incompatible with survival for more than a few months and surgical problems are great. However, coarctation may be restricted to a short segment between the brachiocephalic and left subclavian arteries, when pressures in the left arm are lower than in the right; a collateral circulation may develop through branches of the brachiocephalic.

The postductal type of coarctation has been attributed to abnormal extension of the ductal tissue into the aortic wall, stenosing both vessels as the duct contracts after birth. This form can permit many years of normal life, allowing the development of an extensive collateral circulation to the aorta distal to the stenosis. High vascularity of the thoracic wall is important and clinically characteristic; many arteries arising indirectly from the aorta, proximal to the coarctation segment, anastomose with vessels connected with it distal to the block; all of these vessels become greatly enlarged. In the anterior thoracic wall, the thoraco-acromial, lateral thoracic and subscapular arteries from the axillary artery, the suprascapular from the subclavian artery and the first and second posterior intercostal arteries from the costocervical trunk anastomose with other posterior intercostal arteries; the internal thoracic artery and its terminal branches anastomose with the lower posterior intercostal and inferior epigastric arteries. Posterior intercostal arteries are always involved, and enlargement of their dorsal branches may eventually groove ('notch') the inferior margins of the ribs. The radiograph shadow of the enlarged left subclavian artery is also increased. Enlargement of the scapular vessels and anastomoses may lead to widespread interscapular pulsation (easily appreciated with the palm of the hand, and sometimes heard on auscultation).

AORTIC ANEURYSM FORMATION

An aneurysm (abnormal dilatation) may form in any part of the aorta. Degeneration of the medial wall of the aorta and intimal dissection occur in the majority of thoracic aneurysms, particularly affecting the ascending aorta and aortic arch. These are often the result of abnormalities of connective tissue such as occur in Marfan's syndrome, homocystinuria and Ehlers–Danlos syndrome. Descending aortic aneurysms are generally caused by atherosclerosis (90%); the remainder result from mycotic disease or trauma. Some aortic aneurysms are incidental findings on chest X-rays or computed tomography scans. Symptomatic cases present with breathlessness, chest pain, back pain, hoarse voice, cough and haemoptysis. Early diastolic murmurs may be audible on cardiac auscultation and are caused by aortic regurgitation. Repair is carried out in patients with symptoms or fusiform dilatation measuring more than 5 cm in diameter.

AORTIC DISSECTION

Aortic dissection occurs as a result of degeneration of the medial aspect of the aortic wall as a result of ageing, persistent hypertension or in fibrillin diseases such as Marfan's disease. An intimal tear may occur, producing a split into the medial wall, which creates a false lumen. These cases present acutely with severe retrosternal or intrascapular chest pain. Depending on the extent of the dissection, they may be associated with neurological signs, diarrhoea or leg weakness. Extension into the pericardium causes cardiac tamponade (p. 949) and circulatory collapse. Diagnosis is established by echocardiography and on contrast-enhanced computed tomography scans. Surgical repair is essential for ascending aortic or aortic arch dissection.

BRACHIOCEPHALIC ARTERY

The brachiocephalic (innominate) artery, the largest branch of the aortic arch, is 4–5 cm in length (**Figs 31.15, 60.4F, 60.27**). It arises from the convexity of the arch posterior to the centre of the manubrium of sternum, and ascends posterolaterally to the right, at first anterior to the trachea, then on its right. Level with the upper border of the right sternoclavicular joint, it divides into the right common carotid and right subclavian arteries.

Relations – Sternohyoid and sternothyroid, the remains of the thymus, left brachiocephalic and right inferior thyroid veins, crossing its root, and sometimes the right cardiac branches of the vagus, all separate the brachiocephalic artery from the manubrium. Posterior are the trachea below, right pleura above. The right vagus is posterolateral before passing lateral to the trachea. Right lateral are the right brachiocephalic vein, the upper part of the superior vena cava and pleura. Left lateral are the thymic remains, the origin of the left common carotid artery, the inferior thyroid veins and the trachea.

Branches – The brachiocephalic artery usually has only terminal branches, the right common carotid (p. 1025) and right subclavian artery (p. 1025). Occasionally a thyroid ima artery arises from it. This is a small and inconstant artery that ascends on the trachea to the thyroid isthmus, where it ends. It may arise from the aorta, right common carotid, subclavian or internal thoracic arteries. Sometimes a thymic or bronchial branch arises from the brachiocephalic artery.

DESCENDING THORACIC AORTA

The thoracic aorta is the segment of descending aorta confined to the posterior mediastinum (**Fig. 60.30**). It begins level with the lower border of the fourth thoracic vertebra, continuous with the aortic arch, and ends anterior to the lower border of the twelfth thoracic vertebra in the diaphragmatic aortic aperture. At its origin it is left of the vertebral column; as it descends it approaches the midline and at its termination is directly anterior to it.

Relations – Anterior to the descending thoracic aorta, from above down, are the left pulmonary hilum, the pericardium separating it from the left atrium, oesophagus and diaphragm. Posterior are the vertebral column and hemiazygos veins. Right lateral are the azygos and thoracic duct and below, the right pleura and lung. Left lateral are the pleura and lung. The oesophagus, with its plexus of nerves, is right lateral above, but becomes anterior in the lower thorax, and close to the diaphragm it is left anterolateral. To a limited degree, the descending aorta and oesophagus are mutually spiralized.

Surface anatomy – The descending thoracic aorta is projected as a 2.5 cm broad band from the sternal end of the second left costal cartilage to a median position c.2 cm above the transpyloric plane.

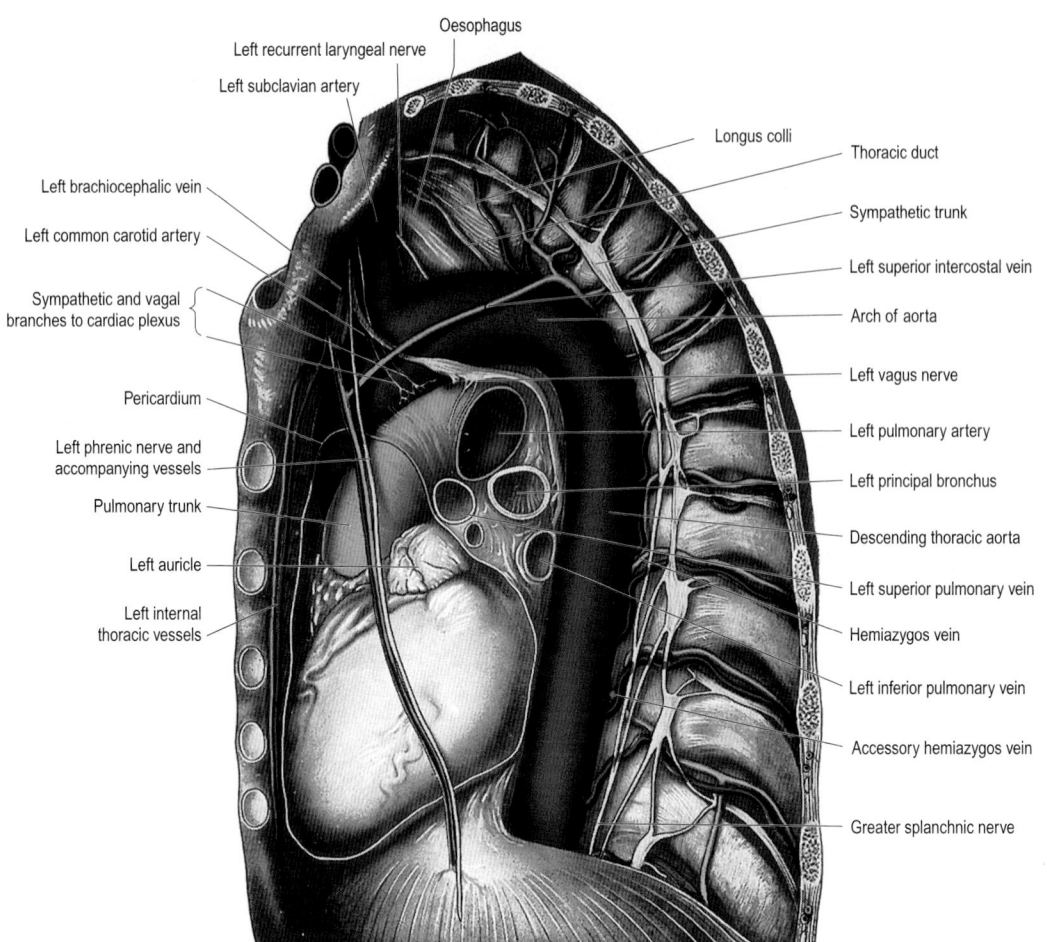

Oesophagus
Left recurrent laryngeal nerve
Left subclavian artery
Left brachiocephalic vein
Left common carotid artery
Sympathetic and vagal branches to cardiac plexus
Pericardium
Left phrenic nerve and accompanying vessels
Pulmonary trunk
Left auricle
Left internal thoracic vessels

Longus colli
Thoracic duct
Sympathetic trunk
Left superior intercostal vein
Arch of aorta
Left vagus nerve
Left pulmonary artery
Left principal bronchus
Descending thoracic aorta
Left superior pulmonary vein
Hemiazygos vein
Left inferior pulmonary vein
Accessory hemiazygos vein
Greater splanchnic nerve

Fig. 60.30 The left aspect of the mediastinum. The left lung and pleura have been removed and an extensive opening has been made into the pericardial sac to expose the heart. Note the oblique orientation of the thoracic inlet, and the forward inclination of longus colli, upper oesophagus and thoracic duct.

Branches

The thoracic aorta provides visceral branches to the pericardium, lungs, bronchi and oesophagus, and parietal branches to the thoracic wall.

Pericardial branches – A few small vessels are distributed to the posterior aspect of the pericardium.

Bronchial arteries – Bronchial arteries vary in number, size and origin. There is usually only one right bronchial artery. This arises either from the third posterior intercostal or upper left bronchial artery, and runs posteriorly on the right bronchus. Its branches supply these structures, in addition to the pulmonary areolar tissue and the bronchopulmonary lymph nodes, pericardium and oesophagus (p. 1077). The left bronchial arteries, usually two, arise from the thoracic aorta, the upper near the fifth thoracic vertebra, the lower below the left bronchus. They run posteriorly to the left bronchus and are distributed as on the right.

Mediastinal branches – Numerous small vessels supply lymph nodes and areolar tissue in the posterior mediastinum.

Phrenic branches – Phrenic branches arise from the lower thoracic aorta and are distributed posteriorly to the superior diaphragmatic surface. They anastomose with the musculophrenic and pericardiacophrenic arteries.

Posterior intercostal arteries – The posterior intercostal arteries and their branches are described in Chapter 57 (p. 965).

Subcostal arteries – Subcostal arteries are the last paired branches of the thoracic aorta, in series with the posterior intercostal arteries, and are below the twelfth ribs. Each runs laterally anterior to the twelfth thoracic vertebral body and posterior to the splanchnic nerves, sympathetic trunk, pleura and diaphragm. The right is also posterior to the thoracic duct and azygos vein, the left is posterior to the accessory hemiazygos vein. Each then enters the abdomen posterior to the lateral arcuate ligament with the twelfth thoracic (subcostal) nerve at the lower border

of the twelfth rib, anterior to quadratus lumborum and posterior to the kidney. The right artery courses posterior to the ascending colon, the left to its descending part. Piercing the aponeurosis of transversus abdominis, each proceeds between this and internal oblique, anastomosing with the superior epigastric, lower posterior intercostal and lumbar arteries. Each has a dorsal branch, distributed like those of the posterior intercostal arteries.

Aberrant artery – A small artery sometimes leaves the thoracic aorta on its right near the right bronchial artery origin. It ascends to the right behind the trachea and oesophagus and may anastomose with the right superior intercostal. It is a vestige of the right dorsal aorta; occasionally it is enlarged as the first part of a right subclavian artery.

AORTIC BODIES

Aortic bodies develop progressively during fetal life. They attain maximum size in the first three postnatal years, when the largest are two brownish bodies c.1 cm long, which flank the abdominal aorta and are usually united anterior to it by a horizontal mass immediately above the inferior mesenteric artery (**Fig. 9.4**). They thus form an inverted crescentic or H-shaped arrangement, intimately related to the intermesenteric and superior hypogastric plexuses. Their constituent cells disperse and atrophy and by 14 years they may have disintegrated completely. When well developed, they consist of masses of polygonal chromaffin cells embedded in wide-meshed capillary plexuses and secreting noradrenaline (norepinephrine). Other small chromaffin bodies are also widespread in the fetus in the abdominal and pelvic prevertebral sympathetic plexuses. They reach a maximum size between the fifth and eighth fetal months, and survive in adults mainly near the coeliac and superior mesenteric arteries and as microscopic collections of cells that persist in the lower parts of the intermesenteric plexus.

AORTIC RUPTURE IN TRAUMA

Aortic rupture resulting from blunt trauma is a life threatening injury. It commonly occurs in road traffic accidents and has a poor survival rate of c.20%. There is usually a transverse tear in the wall of the aorta, which may involve the intima through to the media of the aorta. The pressure within the systemic circulation may itself cause the formation of a false aneurysm. Rupture of the isthmus region of the descending aorta is more common, probably because the isthmus tends to be the junction between the mobile and fixed portions of the aorta. Other sites include the ascending aorta proximal to the origin of the brachiocephalic artery, the aortic arch and the abdominal aorta. Rupture is likely to be the result of a number of factors, including torsion and shear and stretching forces, and is possibly compounded by hydrostatic pressure.

AORTIC ATHEROSCLEROSIS OR CALCIFICATION

Aortic sclerosis or calcification may be implicated in embolic events and strokes. Echocardiography, and particularly transesophageal echocardiography, allows very detailed assessment of the proximal aorta. The extent of turbulent flow appears as signal loss in the ascending aorta using MRI, and can be used to assess any functional narrowing. MRI also allows an accurate assessment of the composition and size of atherosclerotic plaques, which permits assessment of the risk of plaque rupture and thrombus formation.

SUBCLAVIAN ARTERIES

RIGHT SUBCLAVIAN ARTERY

The right subclavian artery arises from the brachiocephalic trunk and is the first branch to be given off the ascending aorta. The right subclavian artery is formed behind the upper border of the right sternoclavicular joint. It ascends above the clavicle superomedial and then posterior to scalenus anterior. It next descends laterally to scalenus anterior, to the outer border of the first rib, where it becomes the axillary artery.

LEFT SUBCLAVIAN ARTERY

In the majority of individuals, the left subclavian artery originates independently from the aortic arch after the origin of the brachiocephalic trunk and left common carotid artery. The left subclavian artery arises from the aortic arch below the left common carotid artery and rises into the neck lateral to the medial border of scalenus anterior, crosses behind this muscle and then descends towards the outer border of the first rib, where it becomes the axillary artery. A common origin exists occasionally between the left subclavian artery and left vertebral artery (2.5%). Rarely, there are bilateral brachiocephalic trunks, which subsequently divide on both sides into common carotid and subclavian arteries (1.2%).

Relations – In the thorax the left subclavian artery is related anteriorly to the left common carotid artery and left brachiocephalic vein, from which it is separated by the left vagus, cardiac and phrenic nerves. More superficially, the anterior pulmonary margin, pleura, sternothyroid and sternohyoid lie between the vessel and the upper left area of the manubrium of sternum. The left side of the oesophagus, the thoracic duct and longus colli are posterior. The left subclavian artery is in contact posterolaterally with the left lung and pleura. The trachea, the left recurrent laryngeal nerve, oesophagus and thoracic duct are medial. Laterally, the artery grooves the mediastinal surface of the left lung and pleura, which also encroach on its anterior and posterior aspects.

COMMON CAROTID ARTERIES

The right and left carotid arteries differ in length and origin. The right carotid is exclusively cervical, and arises from the brachiocephalic trunk behind the right sternoclavicular joint. The left carotid originates directly from the aortic arch immediately posterolateral to the brachiocephalic trunk and therefore has both thoracic and cervical parts.

RIGHT COMMON CAROTID ARTERY

The right common carotid artery and its relations are described in Chapter 31 (p. 543).

LEFT COMMON CAROTID ARTERY

The left common carotid artery (**Figs 31.15, 60.4F**) ascends until level with the left sternoclavicular joint, where it enters the neck. It is 20–25 mm long and it lies at first in front of the trachea, then it inclines to the left. The further course of the artery is described in Chapter 31 (p. 543).

Relations – Sternohyoid and sternothyroid, the anterior parts of the left pleura and lung, the left brachiocephalic vein and the thymic remnants are anterior and separate the left common carotid artery from the manubrium. The trachea, left subclavian artery, left border of the oesophagus, left recurrent laryngeal nerve and thoracic duct are posterior. To the right are the brachiocephalic trunk (below) and the trachea, inferior thyroid veins and thymic remains (above). To the left are the left vagus and phrenic nerves, left pleura and lung.

Veins

SUPERIOR VENA CAVA

The superior vena cava is c.7 cm in length, formed by the junction of the brachiocephalic veins. It returns blood to the heart from the superior half of the body. It begins behind the lower border of the first right costal cartilage near the sternum, descends vertically behind the first and second intercostal spaces, and ends in the upper right atrium behind the third right costal cartilage. Its inferior half is within the fibrous pericardium, which it pierces level with the second costal cartilage. Covered anterolaterally by serous pericardium (from which a retrocaval recess projects), it is slightly convex to the right (**Figs 31.15, 60.4D,E, 60.27, 60.6**). The superior vena cava has no valves.

Relations – The anterior margins of the right lung and pleura are anterior, the pericardium intervening below. These separate the superior vena cava from the internal thoracic artery, first and second intercostal spaces, and second and third costal cartilages. Posteromedial are the trachea and right vagus; the right lung and pleura are posterolateral. The right pulmonary hilum is posterior. Right lateral are the right phrenic nerve and pleura; left lateral are the brachiocephalic artery and ascending aorta, the latter overlapping the superior vena cava.

Variations – The brachiocephalic veins may enter the right atrium separately, the right vein descending like a normal superior vena cava. A left superior vena cava may have a slender connection with the right and then cross the left side of the aortic arch to pass anterior to the left pulmonary hilum before turning to enter the right atrium. It replaces the oblique atrial vein and coronary sinus and receives all the tributaries of the coronary sinus. The left brachiocephalic vein sometimes projects above the manubrium (more frequently in childhood), and crosses the suprasternal fossa in front of the trachea.

Tributaries – Tributaries of the superior vena cava are the azygos vein and small veins from the pericardium and other mediastinal structures.

SUPERIOR VENA CAVAL OBSTRUCTION

Superior vena caval obstruction is characterized by headaches, facial congestion and facial oedema. It is often caused by bronchial carcinoma involving the right upper lobe of the lung or metastatic involvement of the right paratracheal lymph nodes causing circumferential narrowing or complete obstruction of the superior vena cava. This impairs venous drainage of the head, neck and upper arms. This is usually considered to be an oncological emergency and symptoms may be relieved by insertion of a vascular stent or by radiotherapy to the affected region after a tissue diagnosis is established.

INFERIOR VENA CAVA

The inferior vena cava is described in Chapter 68 (p. 1120). The thoracic part is very short, partly inside and partly outside the pericardial sac. The extrapericardial part is separated from the right pleura and lung by the right phrenic nerve. The intrapericardial part is covered, except posteriorly, by inflected serous pericardium. The venous drainage from the tissues below the diaphragm finally ends in the inferior vena cava. The inferior vena cava traverses the diaphragm at the level of the eight and ninth thoracic vertebrae between the right and central tendon of the diaphragm (p. 1081). It then passes through the pericardium and drains into the inferoposterior part of the right atrium.

COLLATERAL VENOUS CHANNELS

In obstruction of the upper inferior vena cava, the azygos and hemiazygos veins and vertebral venous plexuses are the main collateral channels maintaining venous circulation. They connect the superior and inferior venae cavae and communicate with the common iliac vein by the ascending lumbar veins and with many tributaries of the inferior vena cava.

BRACHIOCEPHALIC VEINS

RIGHT BRACHIOCEPHALIC VEIN

About 2.5 cm long, the right brachiocephalic vein begins posterior to the sternal end of the right clavicle, and descends almost vertically to join the left brachiocephalic vein, forming the superior vena cava posterior to the lower border of the first right costal cartilage, near the right sternal border. It is anterolateral to the brachiocephalic artery and right vagus nerve. The right pleura, phrenic nerve and internal thoracic artery are posterior to it above, becoming lateral below (**Fig. 31.15**). Its tributaries are the right vertebral, internal thoracic, inferior thyroid and sometimes the first right posterior intercostal veins.

LEFT BRACHIOCEPHALIC VEIN

Some 6 cm long, the left brachiocephalic vein begins posterior to the sternal end of the left clavicle, anterior to the cervical pleura. It descends obliquely to the right, posterior to the upper half of the manubrium sterni, to the sternal end of the first right costal cartilage, uniting here with the right brachiocephalic vein to form the superior vena cava. It is separated from the left sternoclavicular joint and manubrium by sternohyoid and sternothyroid, the thymus or its remains and areolar tissue; terminally it is overlapped by the right pleura. It crosses anterior to the left internal thoracic, subclavian and common carotid arteries, left phrenic and vagus nerves, trachea and brachiocephalic artery. The aortic arch is inferior to it. Its tributaries are the left vertebral, internal thoracic, inferior thyroid, superior intercostal, sometimes the first left posterior intercostal, thymic and pericardial veins.

AZYGOS VENOUS SYSTEM

AZYGOS VEIN

The azygos vein typically starts from the posterior aspect of the inferior vena cava, at or below the level of the renal veins (**Figs 60.31, 60.32, 31.15**); the origin is not constant. When present, the lumbar azygos ascends anterior to the upper lumbar vertebrae. It may pass behind the right crus of the diaphragm or pierce it, or it may traverse the aortic opening on the right of the cisterna chyli. Anterior to the twelfth thoracic vertebral body, it is joined by a large vessel formed by the right ascending lumbar and right subcostal veins, which passes forward and to the right of the twelfth thoracic vertebra behind the right crus. This common trunk may, in the absence of a lumbar azygos, form the azygos vein itself. Whatever its origin, the azygos vein ascends in the posterior mediastinum to the level of the fourth thoracic vertebra, arching forward above the right pulmonary hilum to end in the superior vena cava, before the latter pierces the pericardium. It is anterior to the lower eight thoracic vertebral bodies, anterior longitudinal ligament and right posterior intercostal arteries. Right lateral are the right greater splanchnic nerve, lung and pleura; left lateral in most of its course are the thoracic duct and aorta and, where it arches forward, the oesophagus, trachea and right vagus. In the lower thorax it is covered anteriorly by a recess of the right pleural sac and oesophagus, emerging from behind the latter to ascend behind the right hilum (**Fig. 59.2**). Because of the closeness of the azygos vein to the right posterolateral aspect of the descending thoracic aorta, aortic pulsations may assist venous return in azygos and hemiazygos veins.

HEMIAZYGOS VEIN

The hemiazygos vein starts on the left, like the azygos. It ascends anterior to the level of the vertebral column to the eighth thoracic level. It crosses the vertebral column posterior to the aorta, oesophagus and

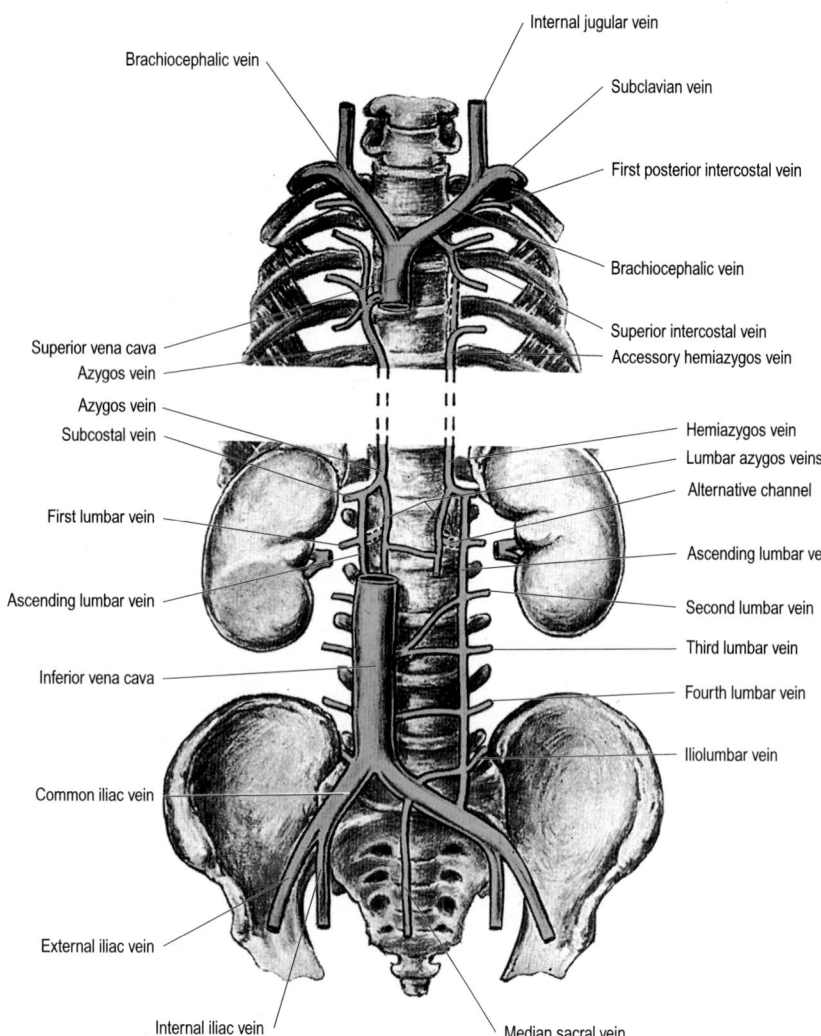

Labels on figure:
Internal jugular vein
Brachiocephalic vein
Subclavian vein
First posterior intercostal vein
Brachiocephalic vein
Superior intercostal vein
Accessory hemiazygos vein
Superior vena cava
Azygos vein
Azygos vein
Subcostal vein
Hemiazygos vein
Lumbar azygos veins
Alternative channel
First lumbar vein
Ascending lumbar vein
Ascending lumbar vein
Second lumbar vein
Third lumbar vein
Inferior vena cava
Fourth lumbar vein
Iliolumbar vein
Common iliac vein
External iliac vein
Internal iliac vein
Median sacral vein

Fig. 60.31 The superior and inferior extremities of the azygos system of veins and their principal associated veins. The intervening parts have been omitted because diagrams are often topographically misleading. Considerable variation occurs in the transthoracic parts of the azygos and hemiazygos veins, in terms of numbers of radicles, levels of transmedian crossing, etc.

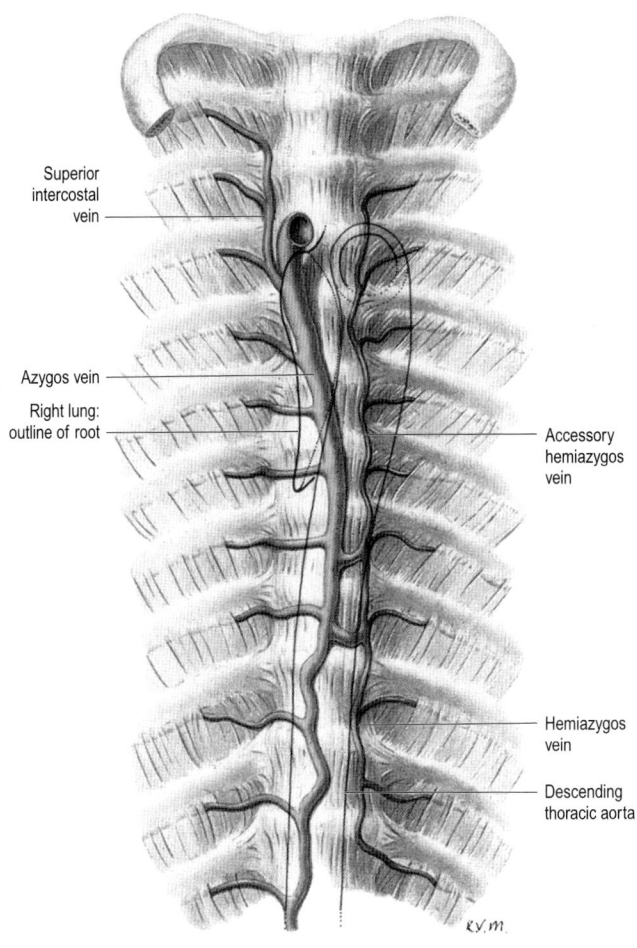

Superior intercostal vein

Azygos vein

Right lung: outline of root

Accessory hemiazygos vein

Hemiazygos vein

Descending thoracic aorta

Fig. 60.32 A frequent (perhaps the most common) course followed by the intrathoracic azygos, hemiazygos and accessory hemiazygos veins. Outlines of the root of the right lung and descending thoracic aorta are included. (Dissection by MCE Hutchinson, GKT School of Medicine, London.)

thoracic duct, to end in the azygos vein. Its tributaries are the lower three posterior intercostal veins, a common trunk formed by the left ascending lumbar and subcostal veins, and oesophageal and mediastinal branches. Its lower end often connects with the left renal vein.

ACCESSORY HEMIAZYGOS VEIN

The accessory hemiazygos vein descends to the left of the vertebral column, receiving veins from the fourth (or fifth) to eighth intercostal spaces and sometimes the left bronchial veins. It crosses the seventh thoracic vertebra to join the azygos vein. It sometimes joins the hemiazygos, and their common trunk opens into the azygos vein.

INTERNAL THORACIC VEINS

The internal thoracic veins are venae comitantes to the inferior half of the internal thoracic artery; they have several valves. Near the third

costal cartilages, the veins unite to ascend medial to the artery, ending in their brachiocephalic vein (**Figs 31.15, 57.21**). Tributaries correspond to branches of the artery and include a pericardiophrenic vein.

INFERIOR THYROID VEINS

The inferior thyroid veins arise in a glandular venous plexus, which also connects with the middle and superior thyroid veins (**Fig. 31.15**). These veins form a pretracheal plexus, from which the left inferior vein descends to join the left brachiocephalic vein, the right descending obliquely across the brachiocephalic artery to the right brachiocephalic vein, at its junction with the superior vena cava. The inferior thyroid veins often open in common into the superior vena cava or left brachiocephalic vein. They drain the oesophageal, tracheal and inferior laryngeal veins and have valves at their terminations.

LEFT SUPERIOR INTERCOSTAL VEIN

The left superior intercostal vein drains the second and third (sometimes fourth) left posterior intercostal veins, ascending obliquely forwards across the left aspect of the aortic arch, lateral to the left vagus, and medial to the left phrenic nerve, to open into the left brachiocephalic vein (**Fig. 31.15**). It usually receives the left bronchial veins, and sometimes the left pericardiacophrenic vein; it connects inferiorly with the accessory hemiazygos vein.

POSTERIOR INTERCOSTAL VEINS

The posterior intercostal veins accompany their arteries in eleven pairs. They are described in Chapter 57 (p. 966).

BRONCHIAL VEINS

Usually two on each side, the bronchial veins drain blood from larger bronchi and from hilar structures. The right bronchial veins join the end of the azygos, the left join the left superior intercostal or hemiazygos vein. Some blood carried to the lungs by bronchial arteries returns via the pulmonary veins.

PULMONARY VEINS

The pulmonary veins (p. 1070) return oxygenated blood to the left atrium. Usually four, two from each lung, and devoid of valves, they originate from capillary networks in the alveolar walls. By repeated junctions, tributary veins finally form a single trunk in each lobe, i.e. three in the right lung, and two in the left. The right middle and superior lobar veins usually join so that two veins, superior and inferior, leave each lung; they perforate the fibrous pericardium and open separately in the posterosuperior aspect of the left atrium (**Figs 60.2, 60.15, 60.21B**). Occasionally the three right lobar veins remain separate. Sometimes the two left pulmonary veins form a single trunk, or they may be augmented by an accessory lobar vein from each lobe which unite to form a third left pulmonary vein.

In the pulmonary hilum, the superior pulmonary vein is anteroinferior to the pulmonary artery, and the inferior is the most inferior hilar structure and also slightly posterior. On the right, the superior pulmonary vein passes posterior to the superior vena cava, the inferior behind the right atrium. On the left both pass anterior to the descending thoracic aorta. In the pericardium, the pulmonary veins are partly covered by serous pericardium. Between the terminations of the right and left veins is, centrally, the oblique pericardial sinus and, laterally, smaller and variable pulmonary venous pericardial recesses that are directed medially and upwards.

REFERENCES

Anderson RH, Ho SY, Becker AE 1983 The surgical anatomy of the conduction tissues. Thorax 38: 408–20.
Federative Committee on Anatomical Terminology 1998 Terminologia Anatomica. Stuttgart: Thieme.

James TN 1993 Congenital disorders of cardiac rhythm and conduction. J Cardiovasc Electrophysiol 4: 702–18.
Mizeres NJ 1963 The cardiac plexus in man. Am J Anat 112: 141–51.

Development of the cardiovascular and lymphatic systems

DEVELOPMENT OF THE HEART

Cells that give rise to the heart

The heart is formed from at least three sources: midline splanchnopleuric coelomic epithelium, angioblastic mesenchyme and neural crest cells. The splanchnopleuric coelomic epithelium is ventral to the foregut endoderm after the head fold stage. The angioblastic mesenchyme is lateral to the cranial intestinal portal. The neural crest cells are derived from the region between the otic vesicle and the caudal limit of somite three. These sources will produce respectively: the myocardium, including the conducting tissue of the heart, and the specific extracellular matrix proteins associated with the developing heart, i.e. the cardiac jelly; the endocardium and cardiac mesenchymal cells that produce the valvular tissue of the heart; and the aorticopulmonary septum and the tunica media of the great vessels.

A novel population of cells has recently been described that contribute to the heart. Ventrally emigrating neural tube cells originate from the ventral part of the rhombencephalon and migrate from the site of attachment of the cranial nerves. Extirpation of ventrally emigrating neural tube cells in animals before their migration from the neural tube results in thin walled ventricles and atria (Ali et al 2003).

Primitive cardiac myocytes can first be seen in stage 9 embryos. During the onset of neurulation and somitogenesis, the intraembryonic coelom forms across the midline, initially above the endoderm, and then as the head fold emerges it undergoes a reversal, so that the future pericardial cavity comes to lie ventral to the endodermal foregut. The splanchnopleuric wall of the pericardial coelom (subjacent to the endoderm) provides a germinal epithelium that produces the cardiac myocytes, and is characterized by the expression of myocardial specific markers such as the cardiac myosin heavy chain. The somatopleuric wall, which is also proliferative, gives rise to cells that contribute mesenchymal populations to the thoracic wall and septum transversum (Figs 10.24, 61.1).

The endocardium develops during stage 9 from a network of mesenchymal cells, the endocardial plexus, between the splanchnopleuric coelomic epithelium of the pericardial cavity and the endoderm. These groups of angioblastic cells are among the earliest intraembryonic vascular precursors to appear. They arise as single cells at the ventrolateral edges of the cranial intestinal portal and subsequently aggregate to form an epithelium, the endocardium, which encloses small cavities. These cells express markers for the endothelial cell lineage. The endocardial lined spaces coalesce in the vicinity of the developing foregut to establish bilateral, hollow tubular structures that become connected (Fig. 61.1), merging to form one endocardial tube that is almost completely surrounded by putative myocardial cells by stage 10. The endocardium is supported by a fine extracellular reticulum that holds it apart from the myocytes. Close to the foregut endoderm, the local mesenchymal cells form the primitive dorsal mesocardium, which may stabilize the developing endothelium and promote the fusion of the bilateral endocardial tubes. The two endocardial tubes fuse across the midline progressively, commencing at the future outflow tract (arterial end) and extending to the inflow tract (venous end). Thus the earliest heart is composed of an inner endocardial epithelial tube that is incompletely surrounded by an outer proliferating myocardial epithelial tube. These tubes are separated widely by an extracellular matrix secreted by the myocardial cells.

Neural crest cells migrate from the developing pharyngeal arches into the outflow tract, where they contribute to the endocardial mesenchyme. Generally these cells are believed to play a role in the spatio-temporal regulation of the development of the outflow septum. A second route for the migration of crest cells into the early heart is via the dorsal mesocardium.

The epicardium is not present at these early stages, although it is sometimes included in descriptions of the myocardium. The epicardial layer proper develops later from septum transversum mesenchyme cells that spread over the myocardial tube. Cells facing the coelomic wall (termed epicardial in many studies) contribute cell lines to the developing heart. It is not clear how these epicardial cells differ from the proliferating coelomic wall that produces the early populations of cardiac myocytes.

EXTRACELLULAR MATRIX AND CARDIAC MESENCHYME

The extracellular matrix of the heart, historically termed cardiac jelly, promotes occlusion of the endocardial tubular lumen during myocardial contraction, thus providing mechanical assistance for the generation of blood flow. It also acts as a site for the deposition of inductive factors from the myocardial cells, which may modify the differentiation of specific endocardial cells. It has been called a gelatinoreticulum, a myoepicardial reticulum (**Fig. 61.1C,D**) and, more recently, the myocardial basement membrane. It is composed of, among other things, hyaluronic acid, hyaluronidase and fibronectin. Inductive signals originating from the myocardial cells cause a subset of endocardial cells lining the atrioventricular canal and the proximal outflow tract to transform into mesenchyme (cardiac mesenchyme), while the endocardial cells in other regions of the heart, e.g. in the ventricle, remain epithelial. When activated by myocardial inductive factors, the endocardial cells lose their cell–cell associations, showing decreased expression of N-CAM (neural cell adhesion molecule) and increased expression of substrate adhesion molecules such as chondroitin sulphate and fibronectin. They undergo cytoskeletal rearrangements necessary for migration, and they express type I procollagen. The transformation of endocardium to mesenchyme may, perhaps, be the only example of a mesenchymal population that is derived from an endothelial lineage. The cells uniquely retain expression of the endothelial marker, QH1. It is believed that the transformation is triggered by an intrinsic clock, because a similar change occurs *in vitro* when atrioventricular endocardium is cultured with myocardium.

Formation of cardiac mesenchyme cells at the atrioventricular canal and the proximal outflow tract is followed by their migration into the myocardial basement membrane. Accumulation of mesenchyme and matrix in these regions produces protrusions, the subendocardial cushions, which bulge into the primary heart tube and support the valve function of the atrioventricular canal and outflow tract.

Formation and twisting of the heart tube

The initial concept of heart development described a number of different segments, termed primitive cardiac cavities, each of which was believed to give rise to a definitive cardiac chamber. Experimental studies have challenged this view and shown that each definitive cardiac chamber is formed by the integration of several primitive cardiac segments.

The first segment of the heart to be formed is the bulbus cordis, the future trabeculated portion of the right ventricle. When this forms the heart tube is straight, and more putative caudal portions of the heart are bilateral structures. The second segment to form is the future trabeculated portion of the left ventricle. The atrioventricular canal is segment three. The proximal inflow tract, the sinuatrial chamber, is then added as segment four and the distal outflow tract, the truncus arteriosus, forms segment five. When all segments are present the heart tube is elongated

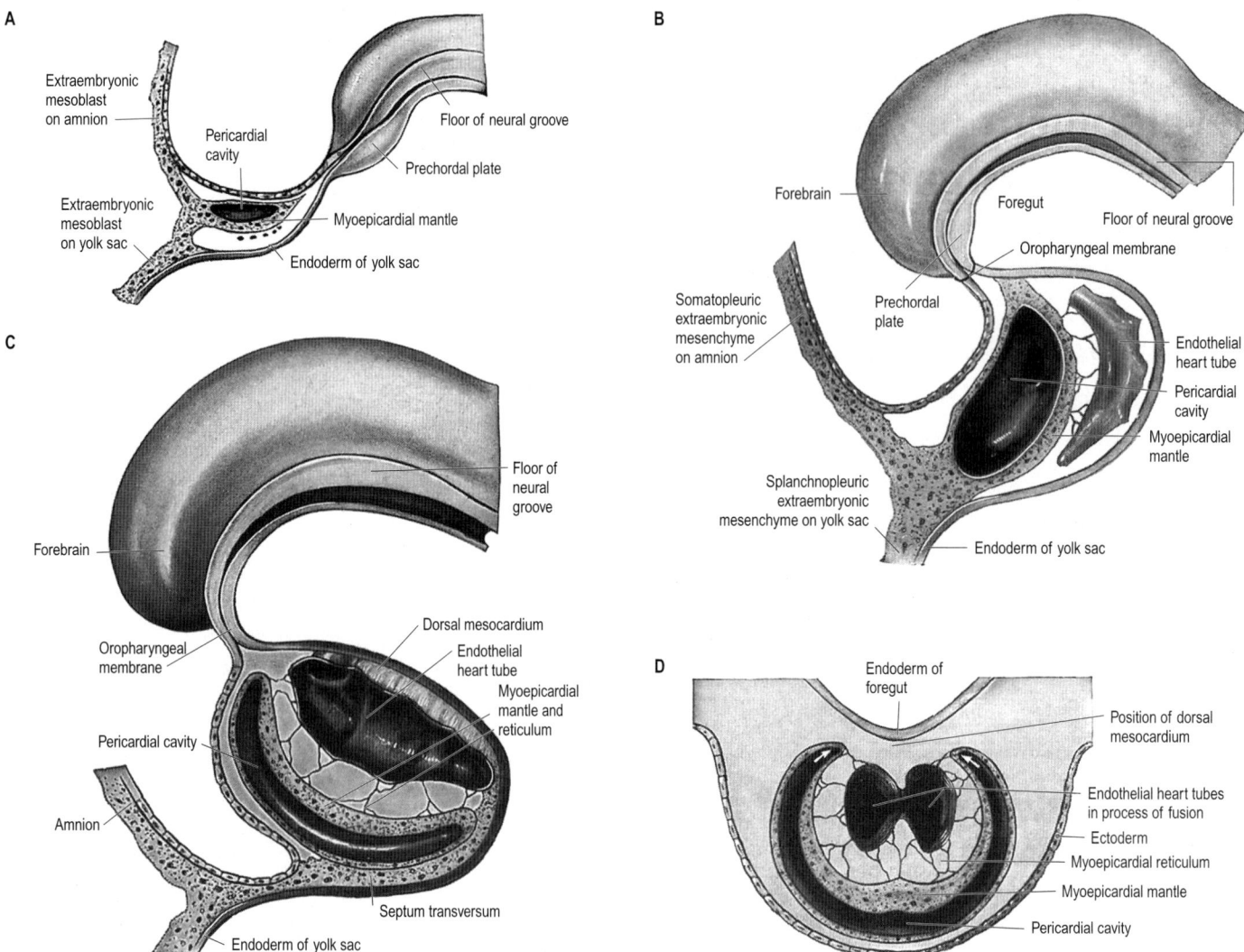

Fig. 61.1 A, Median section through the cranial end of an early human embryo to show the position of the pericardium before the formation of the head fold. A few scattered angioblasts are seen between the cardiogenic plate and the yolk sac; they will ultimately form the endothelial heart tubes. **B**, Median section through the cranial end of a young human embryo, showing the head fold in process of formation and its reversal effect on the position of the pericardium and endothelial heart; also intervening reticulum and myoepicardium. **C**, Median section through the cranial end of a young human embryo, after completion of the head fold and reversal of the pericardium. **D**, Horizontal section through the pericardium and developing heart of the embryo shown in **C**. The arrows indicate the directions in which the dorsolateral recesses of the pericardium deepen so as to define the transient dorsal mesocardium. (**A** and **D**, modified with permission from Davis CL 1923 Description of a human embryo having twenty paired somites. Contrib Embryol Carnegie Inst Washington 15: 1–51.)

sufficiently to form a ventral curve, then a ventral fold, and the entire tube subsequently develops an asymmetric twist (**Fig. 61.2**).

During stage 10, three chambers of the early heart tube can be identified (**Fig. 61.3**). They are atrial, which will give rise to right and left atria; ventricular, which will give rise to the left ventricle; and bulbar, which will give rise to the bulb of the heart, producing the right ventricle proximally. With further growth the distal portion of the bulbar region will extend to produce the truncus arteriosus. (The bulbus cordis and the outflow tract is sometimes subdivided into the conus cordis and truncus arteriosus.)

The endocardium within the myocardial mantle may at this stage consist of two parallel channels interconnected by transverse vessels. Externally two sulci, atrioventricular and bulboventricular (interventricular), are apparent at stage 10.

The atrial region is disposed transversely. On each side, this common atrium is joined caudally by a short venous trunk. These trunks represent the right and left horns of the sinus venosus, sinusal horns. Each receives the union of the corresponding umbilical vein, vitelline radicles and the common cardinal vein (**Fig. 61.3**). Thus, at the earliest stages, the common atrium may justifiably be termed a common sinu-atrial chamber.

Early in stage 10 the ventricular and bulbar parts of the heart tube occupy the midline. Later, the heart tube grows more rapidly and the bulboventricular portion of the tube bulges ventrally and caudally,

forming a U-shaped loop with the bulbus cordis on the right and the ventricle on the left (**Fig. 61.3**). This loop is conspicuous throughout the fourth and fifth weeks of development, and appears as a deep bulboventricular sulcus externally. A corresponding bulboventricular ridge projects internally. The bulbus cordis initially communicates with the dorsal aortae through the first pair of aortic arches. Towards the end of the fourth week, as successive aortic arches develop, the connection between the bulbus cordis and the most caudal pair of aortic arches lengthens to form the conus cordis and truncus arteriosus.

While these bulboventricular changes are occurring, the atrial part of the heart is also affected. The atrioventricular opening moves cranially and to the left, and both parts of the common atrial or sinu-atrial chamber 'rise' or emerge from the mesenchyme of the septum transversum to grow cranially into the pericardial cavity dorsal to the ventricle. As a result of these changes, the atrioventricular canal for a time connects the left part of the atrium to the ventricle, so that venous blood from the right side has to pass through both parts of the atrium.

The heart begins to contract during stage 10, producing an 'ebb and flow' movement of the fluids in the early circulatory system and in the nutritive fluid filling the pericardial cavity, coelomic ducts and exocoelom, on which the embryo is still heavily dependent. The deposition of extracellular matrix between the endocardial channel and the myocardium promotes occlusion of the tubular lumen during contraction. However, it is only after recruitment of cardiac mesenchyme

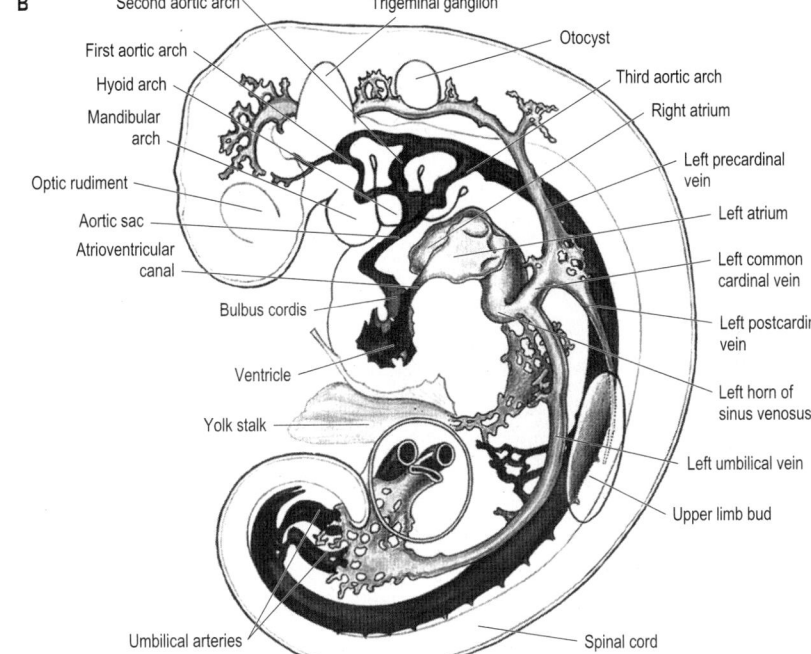

Fig. 61.2 A, The blood vascular system of a human embryo with 14 paired somites: estimated age, 23.5 days; crown–rump length 2.4 mm. The arteries and veins are only in the process of development, so that no true circulation is possible at this stage. Only the endothelial lining of the heart tube is shown. **B,** Profile reconstruction of the blood vascular system of a human embryo having 28 somites; crown–rump length 4 mm; estimated age 26 days. Note: Only the endothelial lining of the heart chambers is shown and, as the muscular wall has been omitted, the pericardial cavity appears much larger than the contained heart. Observe that the atrioventricular canal still connects the left atrium with the single ventricle. (Modified with permission from Streeter GL 1942 Developmental horizons in human embryos. Contrib Embryol Carnegie Inst Washington 30: 211–245.)

into specific inflow and outflow tract positions that directional movement of fluid can occur.

SUBENDOCARDIAL CUSHIONS

Cardiac mesenchyme cells are produced by an epithelial–mesenchymal transformation of a subset of endocardial cells that line the inflow tract at the atrioventricular canal and the outflow tract in the distal bulbus cordis and truncus arteriosus. These cells proliferate between the endocardium and myocardium and, with local accumulation of extracellular matrix molecules, produce protrusions which bulge into the primary heart tube. The early subendocardial cushions thus support the narrowed atrioventricular canal and the outflow tract. Their position corresponds to the future positions of the fibrous skeleton of the heart and the valves.

The atrioventricular cushions are formed from cardiac extracellular matrix (cardiac jelly) and mesenchymally transformed endocardial cells. The cushions bulge into the lumen of the atrioventricular canal and ultimately fuse, forming a wedge of mesenchyme that serves to guide the union of the internal muscular septa. At their time of fusion, the atrioventricular endocardial cushions are large relative to the size of the atrioventricular orifices. They will give rise to the tricuspid and mitral valve boundaries and cusps.

The conotruncal, outflow tract, cushions are formed from cardiac extracellular matrix, mesenchymally transformed endocardial cells and neural crest cells. The cushions of the conus cordis ultimately fuse to form the conal or outlet septum. This divides the conus into a potential outlet for both left and right ventricles. The truncal cushions become the pulmonary and aortic valves.

The aortic sac, which is the connection of the truncus arteriosus to the aortic arch arteries, becomes divided by subendocardial cushions of neural crest origin into the proximal roots of the aorta and pulmonary trunk.

THE DORSAL MESOCARDIUM

As the heart enlarges the early, or primary, dorsal mesocardium that supported the endocardial heart tubes is reinforced by further mesenchyme from the coelomic epithelium. Dorsolateral recesses of the splanchnopleuric pericardial layer adjacent to the myocardium deepen and approach one another (**Fig. 61.1D**). Their apposed walls fuse, completing a broad dorsal attachment between the edge of the myocardium and the parietal pericardium. The persisting stalk of the dorsal mesocardium connects the sinu-atrial chamber with the splanchnopleuric mesenchyme around the developing lung buds and with the septum transversum mesenchyme, which will give rise to the liver. The primary dorsal mesocardium is transient. It breaks down early in the fourth week and establishes a passage across the pericardial cavity, from side to side dorsal to the heart, which persists as the transverse sinus of the pericardium. The removal of the dorsal mesocardium is crucial because it allows the straight heart tube to loop, promoting the development of the bulboventricular sulcus and rearrangement of the myocardial wall at this point.

The significance of the dorsal mesocardium to cardiac and local development has only recently been realized. It is the site of development of the pulmonary veins from persistent dorsal mesocardial endothelial strands, and the region also provides a passageway for the migration of neural crest and other mesenchymal population into the

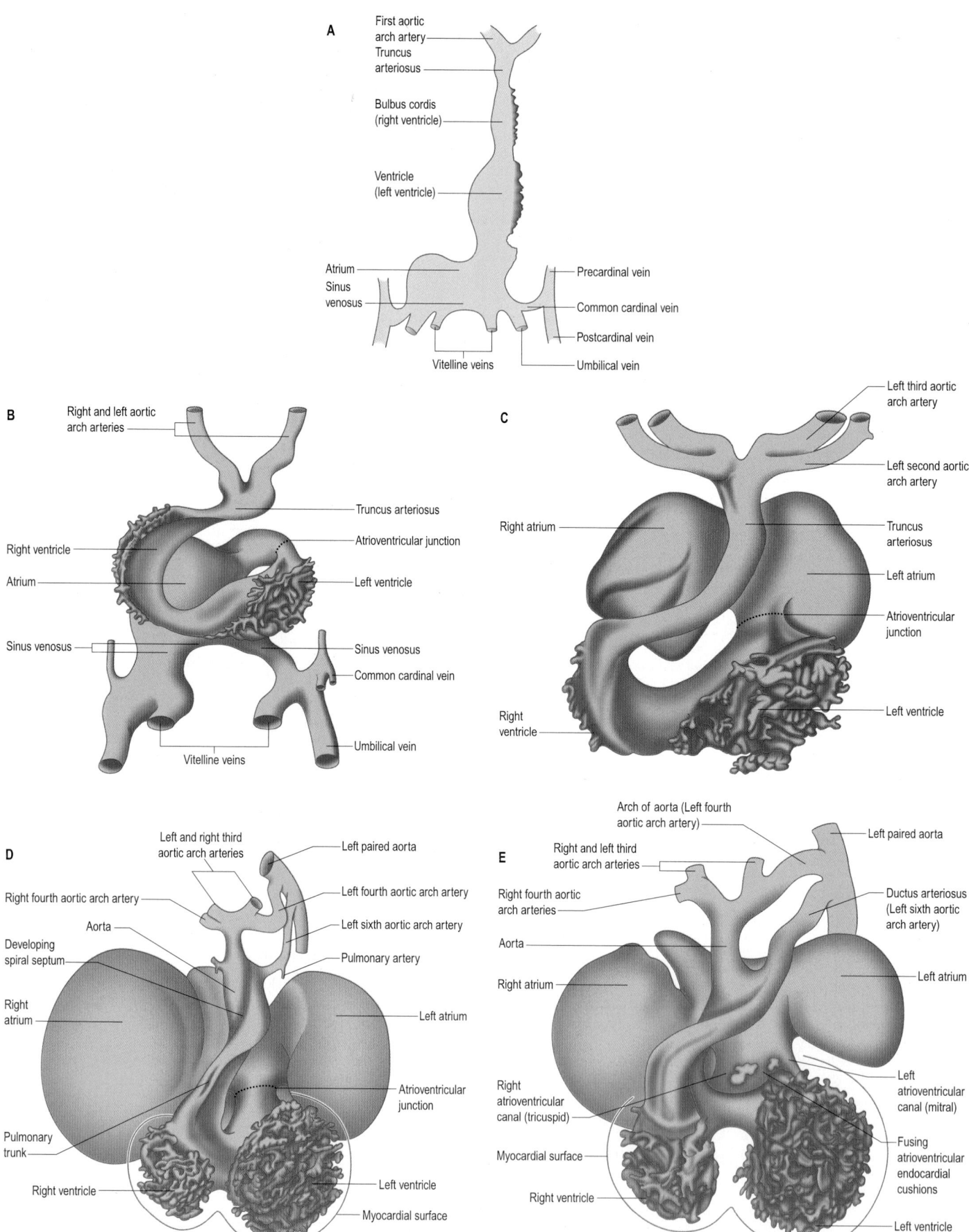

Fig. 61.3 Reconstructions of human heart showing the endocardium. At the left and right ventricles, the endocardium interdigitates with the myocardium and appears trabeculated; elsewhere it is separated from the myocardium by the cardiac extracellular matrix. **A**, Heart tube shown straightened at stage 11. **B**, Heart tube showing normal folding at stage 11. **C**, Heart tube at stage 13. **D**, Heart tube at stage 15. **E**, Heart tube at stage 16. (Modified from O'Rahilly and Muller. Developmental Stages in Human Embryos 1987 Carnegie Institution of Washington. Pub 637.)

inflow region, venous pole, of the heart tube. It is believed that further endothelial to mesenchymal transformations may be taking place here, similar to that in the endocardial cushions, although such dorsal mesocardium derived mesenchyme can be distinguished from endocardial cushion cells immunohistochemically. The subsequent development and the molecular and cellular interactions involved in this intracardiac mesenchymal portion of the dorsal mesocardium, also termed the spina vestibuli, is unclear.

Inflow and outflow regions of the heart

Before septation of the heart, the following chambers can be clearly denoted: the sinus venosus, common atrium, ventricle (now noted as the left ventricle), bulbus cordis (now noted as the right ventricle), the conus cordis and the truncus arteriosus.

DEVELOPMENT OF INFLOW TRACT

SINUS VENOSUS

The sinus venosus is initially a wide channel extending transversely above the cranial intestinal portal in direct communication with the atrial chamber (**Fig. 61.3**). Thus the term sinu-atrial chamber is not inappropriate. On each side the confluence of the umbilical, vitelline and common cardinal veins, which deliver blood into the atrial cavity, produces a dilation, the sinus horn. The early symmetric arrangement of vessels entering the heart (**Fig. 61.24**, p. 1045) is rapidly remodelled and this is reflected in differences between the right and left sinus horns (**Fig. 61.27**). With growth of the liver, the right sinus horn increases rapidly in size at the expense of the left (**Fig. 61.25**, p. 1046). The vitello-umbilical blood flow enters the right horn through a wide but short vessel, the common hepatic vein, which becomes the cranial end of the inferior vena cava. In addition, the right horn receives the right common cardinal vein from the body wall of the right side, and blood from the left common cardinal vein, which passes across the body of the sinus. Later, when transverse connections are established between the cardinal veins, the blood from the body wall of the left side reaches the heart via the veins of the right side. The left common cardinal vein then becomes much reduced in size and forms the oblique vein of the left atrium and the fold of the left caval vein, whereas the left horn and the body of the sinus venosus persist as the coronary sinus. The disposition of some of the main abdominal and intrathoracic veins in the later prenatal months is shown in **Fig. 61.26** (p. 1046).

The right sinual horn opens into the right atrium through its dorsal and caudal walls. The orifice, elongated and often slit-like, is guarded by two muscular folds, the right and left sinu-atrial (venous) valves (valvules) (**Fig. 61.4**). These two valves meet cranially and become continuous with a fold that projects into the atrium from its roof, the septum spurium. Caudally, the valves meet and fuse with the dorsal endocardial cushion of the atrial canal. The cranial part of the right sinu-atrial valve loses its fold-like form, but its position is indicated in the adult heart by the crista terminalis of the right atrium. Its caudal part forms the valve of the coronary sinus and most of the valve of the inferior vena cava. The medial (or left) end of the valve of the inferior vena cava is formed by a small fold continuous with the dorsal wall of the sinus venosus, the sinus septum. The latter intervenes between the orifice of the common hepatic vein and the opening of the body of the sinus. (In the mature heart, see the tendon of Todaro and triangle of Koch, p. 1001).

The left venous valve blends with the right side of the atrial septum and usually no trace of it can be seen in the adult heart.

As the sinu-atrial valves undergo these changes, the right sinus horn becomes incorporated in the right atrium and expands to form its smooth dorsal wall, medial to the crista terminalis. This part of the adult atrium is termed the sinus venarum, the receiving chamber of the large venous orifices. The right half of the primitive atrium forms the internally ridged, more muscular, wall anterior to the crista terminalis and the right auricle.

ATRIA

The common atrium is derived from the cranial part of the sinu-atrial chamber (**Fig. 61.3**). It receives the opening of the sinus venosus dorso-caudally and to the right of the median plane. It communicates ventrally

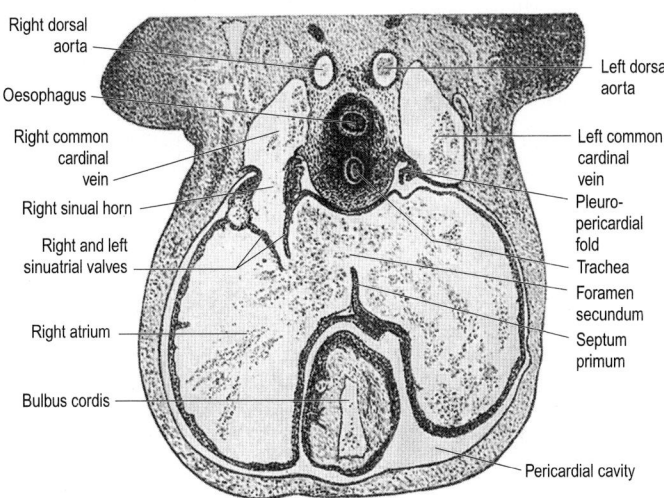

Fig. 61.4 Transverse section of a human embryo, 8 mm long. The atria bulge forwards on each side of the bulbus cordis. The septum primum has broken down in its dorsal region and the two atria communicate through the foramen secundum.

with the ventricle through the atrioventricular canal, which has resumed its median position by the middle of the fifth week, thus permitting both right and left parts of the atrium to communicate with the common ventricular cavity. Dorsal and ventral subendocardial cushions (p. 1031) develop in the walls of the atrioventricular canal between the endothelium and the myoepicardial mantle. These, the atrioventricular endocardial cushions, encroach on the canal and eventually fuse, leaving a relatively small orifice on each side. The fused tissue constitutes the septum intermedium (of His), which separates the two small right and left atrioventricular orifices and canals.

Development of the pulmonary veins

Early in the development of the atrium a single common pulmonary vein, believed to develop from angiogenic cells positioned in the early dorsal mesocardium but in continuity with the endoderm, opens into the caudodorsal wall of the left atrium close to the septum. It is the union of a right and a left pulmonary vein, each formed by two small veins issuing in turn from the developing lung buds. Subsequently, the common trunk and the two veins forming it expand and are incorporated in the left atrium to make up the greater part of its cavity. This expansion usually continues as far as the orifices of the four veins, which thus open separately into the left atrium. However, variations are quite common. The left half of the primitive atrium is progressively restricted to the mature auricle.

SEPTATION OF ATRIA

Internal separation into right and left atria is mainly effected by sequential growth of two septa together with additional, less prominent structures. First, the septum primum grows from the dorsocranial atrial wall as a crescentic fold (**Fig. 61.5A**), separated from the left sinu-atrial valve by the interseptovalvular space. The leading edge of the septum primum is covered by a mesenchymal cap, which is in continuity with the dorsal mesocardium. The ventral horn of the crescentic septum reaches the ventral atrioventricular cushion; the dorsal horn reaches the dorsal cushion. 'Ventral' and 'dorsal' refer to the positions of the cushions after the atrium repositions to lie dorsal to the bulbus cordis. Ventral and caudal to the advancing edge of the septum, the two atria communicate through the foramen primum (= ostium primum) (**Fig. 61.5A**). Free passage of blood from right to left atrium is essential throughout fetal life, as oxygenated blood from the placenta reaches the heart via the inferior vena cava. Therefore, as the foramen primum diminishes, the septum primum breaks down dorsally and a new right–left shunt, through the foramen secundum (= ostium secundum), is formed before the end of the fifth week. The foramen primum is finally occluded by fusion of the edge of the septum primum with the fused atrioventricular cushions in the median plane (**Fig. 61.7**, p. 1034). The foramen secundum enlarges, allowing sufficient free passage of blood

Image labels (Fig. 61.4):
Right dorsal aorta · Oesophagus · Right common cardinal vein · Right sinual horn · Right and left sinuatrial valves · Right atrium · Bulbus cordis · Left dorsal aorta · Left common cardinal vein · Pleuro-pericardial fold · Trachea · Foramen secundum · Septum primum · Pericardial cavity

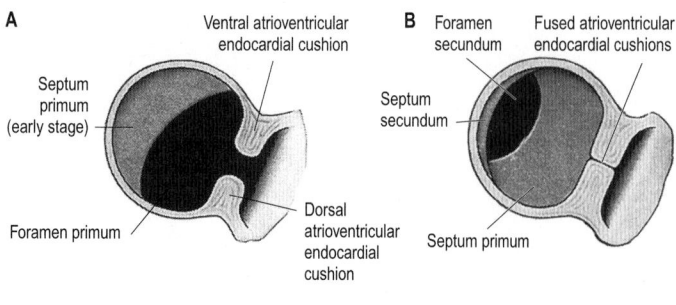

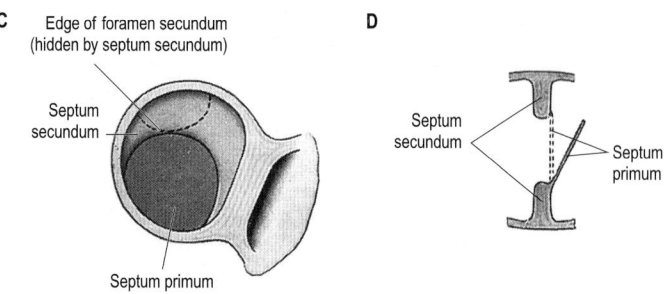

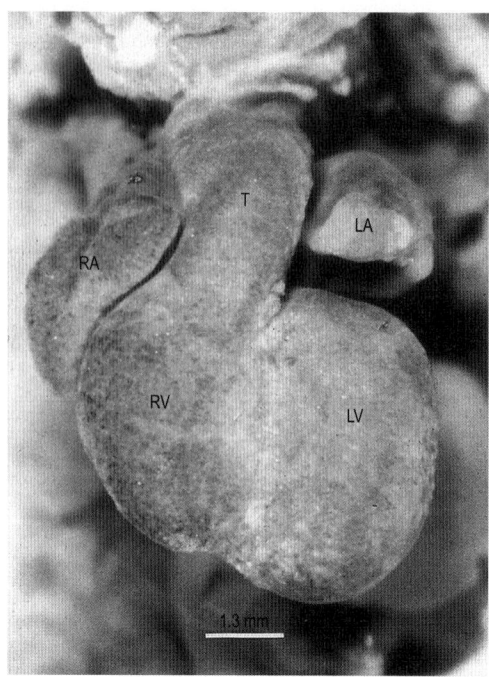

Fig. 61.5 Three representative stages in the development of the atrial septum, viewed from the right side. The heart has been divided in its long axis to the right of its median plane and only the atria and the adjoining part of the ventricular cavity are depicted. **A**, The septum primum has not yet obliterated the original communication between the two atria and the atrioventricular endocardial cushions have not yet fused. **B**, The atrioventricular endocardial cushions have fused with each other and with the septum primum, which has broken down in its dorsal part. The foramen secundum, thus formed, subsequently moves to the position shown in **C**. **C**, The septum secundum has formed and hides the foramen secundum, the margins of which are indicated by the curved, dotted line. **D**, The valve-like character of the foramen secundum. When the pressure in the right atrium exceeds that in the left atrium, blood passes from the right to the left side of the heart, but when the two pressures are equal the septum primum assumes the position indicated by the dotted outline.

Fig. 61.6 Human heart at 32 days (stage 15). Both atria are clearly visible. Abbreviations: LA, left atrium; LV, left ventricle; RA, right atrium; RV, right ventricle; T, truncus arteriosus.

from right to left atrium (**Fig. 61.5**), and it persists throughout intra-uterine life as the interatrial septal complex. At first the foramen secundum is sited craniodorsally in the septum primum, but it becomes modified until it is cranioventral.

Towards the end of the second month, the muscular wall of the atrium becomes invaginated as another crescentic septum on the right side of the septum primum (**Fig. 61.5B,C**). This, the septum secundum, involves more than the entire width of the interseptovalvular space. Thus the dorsal attachments of the septum primum and the left sinu-atrial valve are carried into the interior of the atrium on its left and right surfaces, respectively. The superior and inferior horns of the septum secundum at first grow ventrally. The superior horn grows much more rapidly and fuses first with the septum intermedium. It is then continuous with the sinus septum. The free edge of the septum secundum (crista dividens) is thus at first directed caudoventrally and later caudally alone. It overlaps the foramen secundum (**Fig. 61.1C,D**) and hence the septum primum acts as a flap valve. As the blood pressure is greater in the right atrium than in the left, the blood flows from right to left, but not conversely. The right–left flow occurs through the 'true', but some-what misnamed, foramen ovale. It flows from the right atrium under the crescentic free border of the septum secundum, then through the oblique cleft between the (parted) secondary and primary septal surfaces, and finally enters the left atrium through the foramen secundum.

During the second month, the two atria bulge ventrally, one on each side of the bulbus cordis, which lies in a groove on their ventral surface (**Figs 61.3, 61.6**). These projecting parts of the atria form the auricles of the adult heart.

DEVELOPMENT OF OUTFLOW TRACT

VENTRICLE, BULBUS CORDIS, TRUNCUS ARTERIOSUS

By stage 11, the endocardial walls of the primitive ventricle (left ventricle) and the bulbus cordis (right ventricle) have trabeculated portions, and the interventricular septum is just apparent. The most differentiated

myocardial cells are found close to the cardiac lumen, forming loops and strands that interlock with the endocardium, thus producing the trabeculae (**Fig. 61.3**). During stage 12, the partitioning of left and right circulations is initiated when the ventricular pumps begin to operate in parallel rather than in series, and left and right ventricles begin to contract simultaneously.

Blood enters the bulboventricular cavity through the right and left atrioventricular canals (**Fig. 61.3**) (ventricular inflow tracts) and is ejected through the proximal and distal bulbus (outflow tracts). Blood flow from the future left ventricle passes obliquely to the dorsal part of the bulbus, whereas right ventricular blood has a reverse inclination to the former and is expelled through the ventral part of the bulbus. These inclinations impose a mutually spiral flow on the two streams as they traverse the truncus.

The blood flow through the truncus arteriosus compresses some portions of the vessels wall and not others. The regions with little haemodynamic force accumulate extracellular matrix and also neural crest cells, and bulge into the truncal lumen. Because the blood flow spirals as it passes along the truncus, the position of the matrix accumu-lation also spirals as two ridges. The right ridge passes obliquely onto the ventral and then the left wall, whereas the left ridge extends on to the dorsal wall and then the right wall. The fusion of these ridges forms the spiral aorticopulmonary septum.

SEPTATION OF VENTRICLES

The separation of the two ventricles from each other leaves the right ventricle in communication with the right atrium (inflow tract) and the pulmonary artery (outflow tract), and the left ventricle in communi-cation with the left atrium (inflow tract) and the aorta (outflow tract). It involves a series of complex changes in which three distinct factors contribute to the formation of the adult ventricular septum. These are the muscular ventricular septum, the proximal bulbar septum (continuous with the aorticopulmonary spiral septum) and the atrioventricular endo-cardial cushions.

The appearance of a caudal crescentic ridge in the inside of the heart indicates the separation between the two ventricles. In the trabeculated part of the ventricles there is less extracellular matrix and it is this part of the chambers that expand on each side of the early ventricular septum which remains between them. The inner crest of the septum is the older portion and the deeper parts are added as the ventricular chambers enlarge. The dorsal and ventral horns of the septum grow along the

Fig. 61.7 Two stages in the formation of the adult ventricular septum. **A**, The right and left ventricles communicate with each other. **B**, The interventricular communication has been closed by the fusion of the ventricular septum with the enlarged right extremity of the fused atrioventricular cushions. Note the position of the septum primum relative to the fused atrioventricular cushions and, in **B**, that cushion tissue intervenes between the two ventricles (membranous part of ventricular septum), and also between the right atrium and the left ventricle (atrioventricular septum).

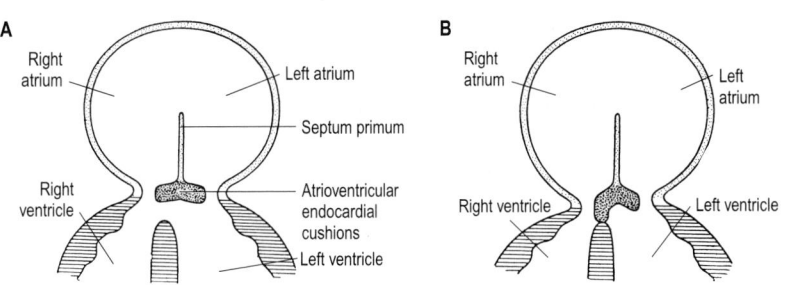

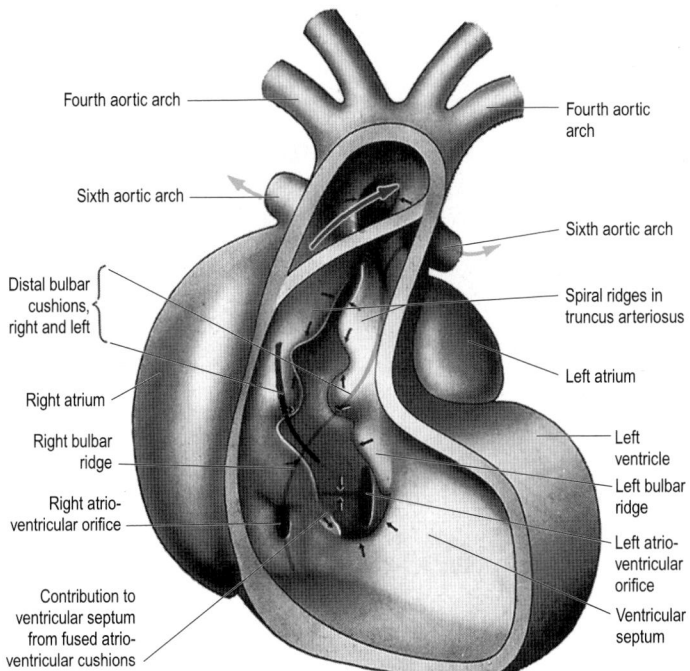

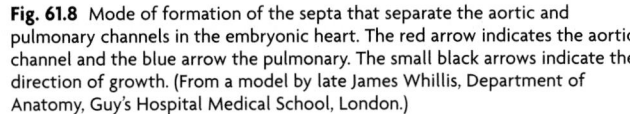

Fig. 61.8 Mode of formation of the septa that separate the aortic and pulmonary channels in the embryonic heart. The red arrow indicates the aortic channel and the blue arrow the pulmonary. The small black arrows indicate the direction of growth. (From a model by late James Whillis, Department of Anatomy, Guy's Hospital Medical School, London.)

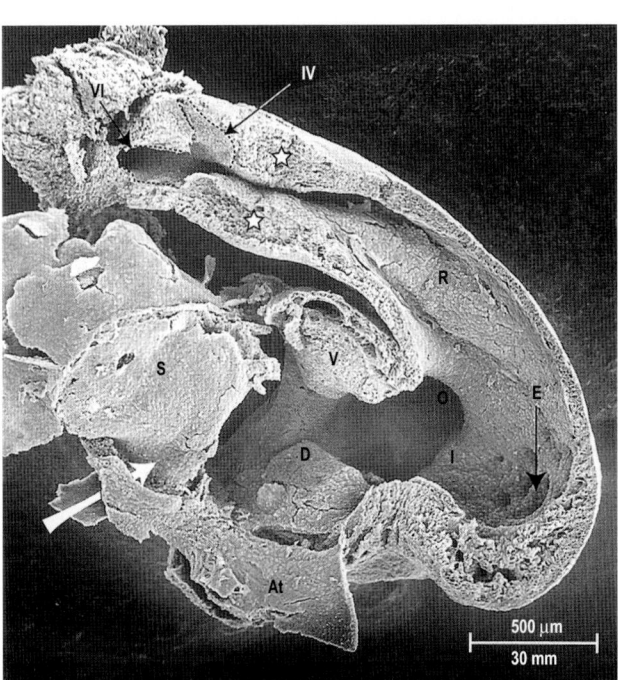

Fig. 61.9 Human heart at 32 days (stage 15). The right lateral wall of the right atrium, right ventricle and the outflow tract have been removed. The septum primum (S) and the developing valve of the sinus venosus (white arrow) are at a distance from the unfused ventral (V) and dorsal (D) atrioventricular cushions. The interventricular foramen (primum) is open (O). Its lower margin is made up by the developing interventricular septum (I). Note the left anterolateral ridge (R) and, at the distal margins of the truncus arteriosus, the valve swellings (☆) of the putative aorta and pulmonary trunk. The swellings are in continuity with the IVth and Vth aortic arches. Abbreviations: At, atrium; E, embryonic trabeculae.

ventricular walls to meet and fuse with the corresponding endocardial cushions of the atrioventricular canal near their right extremities (**Fig. 61.7**). The septum has a free sickle-shaped margin which, with the endocardial cushions, bounds a circular interventricular foramen (sometimes delineated temporally as the interventricular foramen primum) (**Figs 61.8, 61.9**).

At first the bulboventricular junction is marked by a distinct notch on the outside of the heart, and inside by a corresponding bulbo-ventricular ridge. The latter lies between the atrioventricular orifice and the caudal part of the bulb (**Fig. 61.10**) and its absorption is essential for the development of a four-chambered heart. Partly by absorption of the bulboventricular ridge and partly by growth of the atrioventricular region, the right extremity of the atrioventricular canal comes to lie caudal to the orifice of the bulb (**Fig. 61.8**). This alteration in relative positions of the structures concerned occurs while the ventricular septum is forming, paving the way for completion of ventricular partition.

Completion of ventricular septation is achieved by growth of the spiral aorticopulmonary septum back to the proximal bulbar region. The right bulbar ridge grows across the dorsal wall of the bulb and right extremity of the fused atrioventricular endocardial cushions to reach the dorsal horn of the free, crescentic edge of the ventricular septum and obliterates the ventral or cranial part of the right atrioventricular orifice (**Fig. 61.8**). The left bulbar ridge crosses the ventral wall of the bulb to reach the ventral or cranial horn of the ventricular septum. The bulbar ridges fuse and separate the conus arteriosus of the right ventricle from the aortic vestibule. However, the caudal edge of the bulbar septum

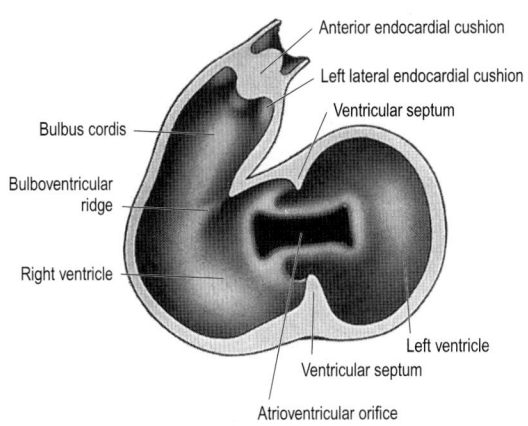

Fig. 61.10 An early stage in the relationships between the atrioventricular opening and ventricles, the cavity of the bulbus cordis and the bulboventricular ridge. The endocardial cushions at the distal end of the bulb are shown in a more differentiated state than they really exhibit at this stage. (After JE Frazer.)

is still separated from the free crescentic edge of the ventricular septum by a diminishing interventricular channel (sometimes termed the interventricular foramen secundum). The latter is closed by growth of tissue from the right extremity of the fused atrioventricular cushions that fuses, on its one aspect with the caudal border of the proximal bulbar septum, and on its other with the margin of the ventricular septum. (A transitory interventricular foramen tertium has been described; it can be seen towards the end of the sixth week of gestation as an orifice 80 μm in its largest diameter.) A dimple less than 40 μm in diameter is left for a brief period of time at the site of closure on the endocardial surface of the left ventricle. The dorsal part of the bulb largely becomes absorbed, but its position is indicated by the dorsal wall of the aortic vestibule, which is mainly formed by tissue extensions from the fused atrioventricular endocardial cushions.

Fibrous skeleton of the heart

The valve complexes of the heart, four in number, arise in two main cardiac zones. These are the mitral and tricuspid complexes, which extend from their inception between the atrioventricular junctions and loci on the interior of the ventricular walls (the inflow tract of the heart) and the aortic and pulmonary valves at the distal bulbotruncal junction (the outflow tract of the heart).

Each commences as an internal endocardial projection of varying form enclosing cardiac mesenchyme (myocardial basement membrane matrix and mesenchymal cells). In some regions the mesenchymatous cells proliferate, transform into fibroblasts and produce a geometrically organized collagenous framework that varies with site and functional demands. Elsewhere, the core is invaded by differentiating cardiac myoblasts.

ATRIOVENTRICULAR VALVES

Initially, the atrial myocardium is continuous with the ventricular myocardium through the myocardium of the atrioventricular canal. The atrioventricular canal is characterized by sulcus tissue on the epicardial side and subendocardial cushion on the endocardial side. As the atrioventricular valves develop, the sulcus and cushion tissues fuse at the ventricular margin of the atrioventricular canal. This disrupts the myocardial continuity at this site.

The atrioventricular valves develop as shelf-like projections from the margins of the atrioventricular orifices, directed as almost complete conical sheets towards the ventricles, their advancing edges continuing, initially as trabecular ridges, deep into the ventricular cavity. With continued differential growth and excavation on their ventricular aspects, each sheet develops two (mitral) and three (tricuspid) marginal indentations, defining the principal valve cusps. Minor marginal indentations (clefts) subdivide some cusps into scallops. Each cusp develops functionally significant regional variations in surface texture. Its core condenses as a collagenous lamina fibrosa. The latter blends, at its atrioventricular base, with the inappropriately named fibroareolar valve 'annulus' – each a part of the complex, functionally crucial, fibrous 'skeleton' of the heart. The anterior cusp of the tricuspid valve and both the anterolateral and posteromedial cusps of the mitral valve appear at about the time when fusion of the atrioventricular cushions and bulbar ridges takes place. Delamination of the septal cusp of the tricuspid valve occurs after closure of the interventricular foramen during the seventh to eighth week of gestation (**Fig. 61.11**).

AORTIC AND PULMONARY VALVES

The aortic and pulmonary valves form in the outflow tract of the heart, from the four endocardial cushions that appear at the distal end of the bulbus cordis in the truncus arteriosus. These cushions become populated by neural crest cells, in addition to endocardial derived mesenchyme. The completion of the distal bulbar septum results in division of each lateral cushion into two. Thus the number of thickenings is increased to six, three associated with the pulmonary orifice, and three with the aortic. These are the rudiments of the aortic and pulmonary valves. Each cushion-derived intrusion grows and is excavated on its truncal aspect to form a semilunar valve cusp. Similar events affect the adjacent truncal or septal wall. Thus the pouches between the valves and the walls of the vessels gradually enlarge and form their related sinuses. The

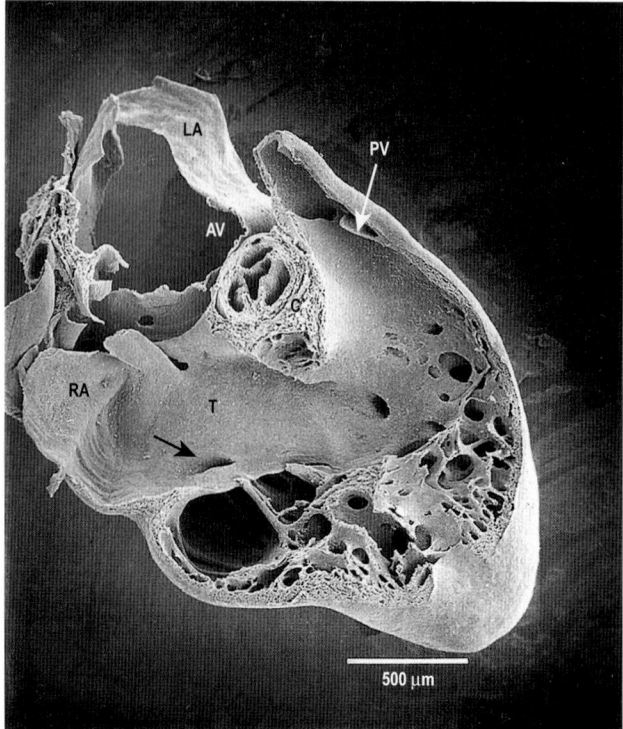

Fig. 61.11 Septal aspect of the right ventricle of a human heart at 8 weeks gestation. Delamination of the septal cusp of the tricuspid valve (T) is taking place. A cleft (black arrow) has appeared, marking the posterior margin of the septal cusp. There are no clefts delineating the anterior margins in the region adjacent to the supraventricular crest (C), and the endocardium is continuous. No tension apparatus is present. Abbreviations: AV, aortic valve; LA, left atrium; PV, pulmonary valve; RA, right atrium.

core of each cusp forms a collagenous lamina fibrosa, delicate and thin in each crescentic lunule, thick and compact in the central nodule, with marginal radiate and basal bands. The latter blend with the complex, scalloped, mural valve ring. Initially, one cusp of the pulmonary valve lies anteriorly and the other two posterolaterally, whereas one cusp of the aortic valve lies posteriorly and the other two anterolaterally. However, a rotation of the heart to the left before birth changes the orientation of the cusps of the pulmonary and aortic valves, and this is reflected in the various schemes for the designation of these cusps in the mature heart.

EMBRYONIC TRABECULAE

During stage 15 (32 days) embryonic trabeculae start to emerge in the apical endocardial region of the primitive ventricles. By stage 17 (42 days) well developed embryonic trabeculae show a typical spatial orientation, creating a number of ventricular sinuses and giving a sponge-like appearance to the internal aspect of both ventricles (**Fig. 61.12**). Definitive trabeculae are first observed about the fortieth day of gestation, appearing initially in the walls of both ventricles at the level of the atrioventricular junction; they develop towards the apex of the heart (**Fig. 61.13**). By 10 weeks' gestation, the trabeculae are fewer and confined to the apical region, where they gradually disappear after a process of simplification, deletion and reabsorption. The remodelling process is accomplished without the intervention of macrophages or inflammatory cells in the immediate interstitium. Mesenchymal tissue surrounding the trabeculae passes between the margins of the valve cusps, indentations, clefts and defined zones of the cusp surface as white, glistening, compacted, collagenous tendinous cords. These converge towards the tip and sides of the single or grouped papillary muscles and blend with their connective tissue framework. The muscles are the ventricular ends of the original embryonic trabeculae and, although they are free throughout their length, their mural ends are confluent with mural ventricular musculature and receive a dense population of its nerves and specialized conducting tissues.

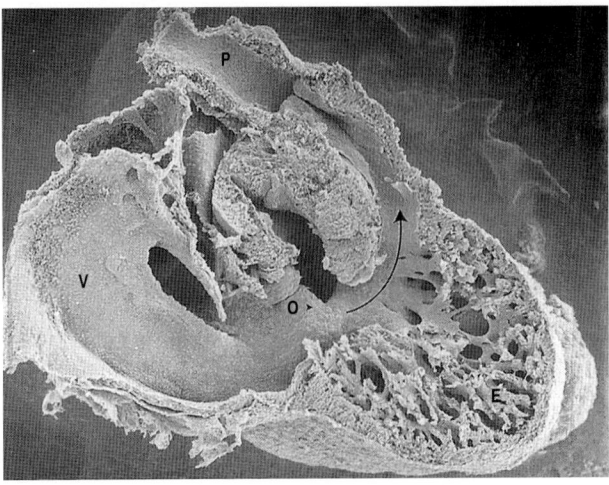

Fig. 61.12 Human heart at 42 days' gestation. The right lateral wall of the right atrium, right ventricle and the outflow tract have been removed. The valve of the sinus venosus (V) is prominent. There is no septal cusp of the tricuspid valve guarding the inlet portion of the right ventricle. The parietal cusp has been removed. The atrioventricular cushions are fused. Note the adjacent right lateral tubercles (O). A small interventricular foramen (secundum, see text) is indicated (small arrowhead). There is a well developed right ventricular outflow tract (curved arrow). Abbreviations: E, embryonic trabeculae; P, pulmonary trunk.

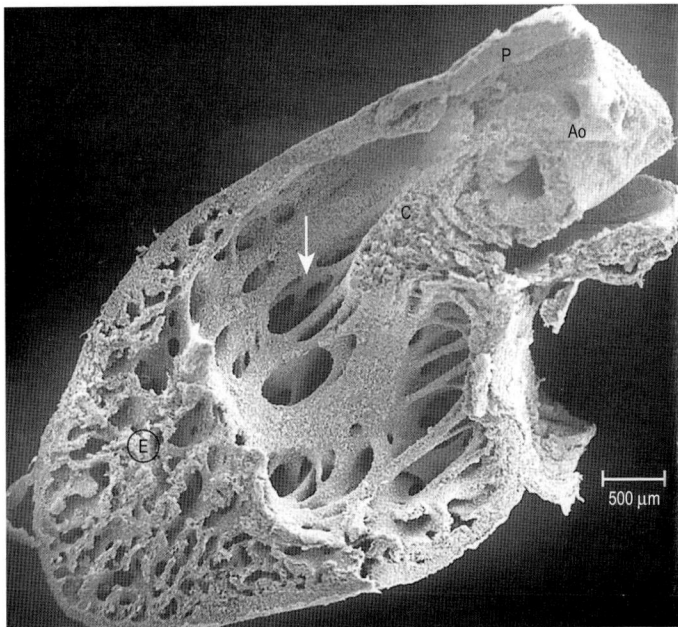

Fig. 61.13 Parietal aspect of the right ventricle at 8 weeks' gestation. The embryonic trabeculae (E) are confined to the lower half of the ventricular wall. An arrow shows the definitive trabeculae. Abbreviations: Ao, aorta; C, supraventricular crest; P, pulmonary trunk.

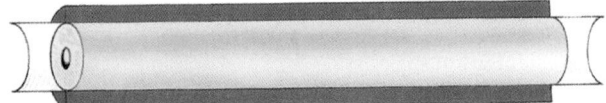

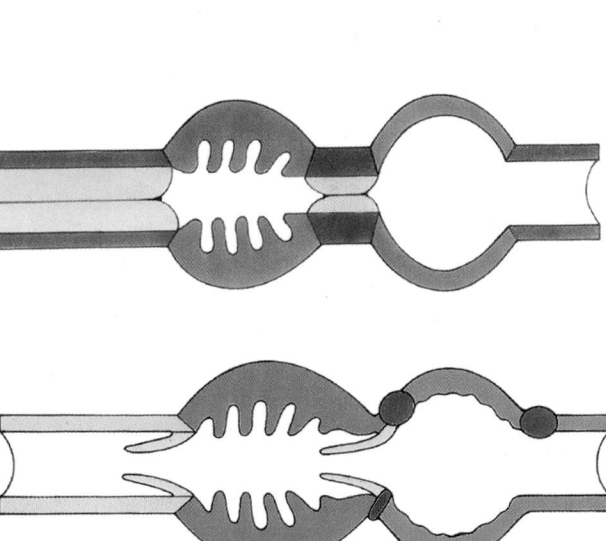

Fig. 61.14 Development of cardiac segments in three 'prototypic' human stages, showing the tubular heart at c.24 days (top) and 38 days (middle) of development, and the adult configuration (bottom). Blood flow is from right to left. Colour key: purple, primary myocardium; blue, atrial working myocardium; red, ventricular working myocardium; yellow, cushion/valvular tissue; green, no longer myocardium.

Heart conducting system

The development of the conducting system has been difficult to elucidate because conventional histological staining methods are unable to identify and delineate conducting tissues from other cardiac components during development. However, recent descriptions of the patterns of expression of a number of markers for the conducting system, e.g. HNK-1, GIN2, neurofilament, connexin-43 and Msx-2 (Hox-8), have brought more clarity to this field.

In the formed heart, two types of myocardium have been distinguished: first, the working myocardium of atria and ventricles, which is specialized in contraction, and second, the conducting system, which is specialized in the coordinated propagation of the impulse over the myocardium. The conducting system consists of the sinu-atrial node, where the impulse is generated; the atrioventricular node, responsible for the delayed transmission of the impulse from the atria to the ventricles; and the atrioventricular bundle and left and right bundle branches, by which the impulse is rapidly spread over the ventricles. This differentiation in the nomenclature between contracting and conducting cardiac myocytes has focused attention on morphological evidence for different cell lineages, yet the embryonic heart has a measurable electrical activity, as seen by electrocardiographic measurements, with no distinct conducting system.

The early heart tube is not segmented and, although a polarity can be observed along its craniocaudal axis, it is in essence a homogeneous tissue (**Fig. 61.14**). Pacemaker activity is seen in the inflow tract from the earliest time. Initially there is a poorly coupled pattern of excitation and contraction, but this rapidly becomes a rhythmic activation pattern. Impulses so generated are slowly propagated, leading to a peristaltoid form of contraction that is characteristic of the tubular heart. Indeed, the slow propagation of the impulse is the predominant functional feature that distinguishes the myocardium of the early heart tube from that of the more advanced stages, leading to its description as primary myocardium. It is suggested that the primary myocardium will give rise to both working myocardium and the conducting system, although there is also some support for the view that these myogenic lineages are separate and arise from different cell lines. Neural crest has been suggested to give rise to the conducting system, in some part due to the expression of HNK-1 and neurofilament in the conducting tissue. However, sinus node activity can be demonstrated before arrival of crest cells in the heart, and the expression of such markers may reflect the ambiguous neural and myocardial properties of the conducting system.

As development proceeds, segments of rapidly conducting atrial and ventricular working myocardium differentiate within the slowly conducting primary myocardium. The resulting heart consists of five segments displaying alternately slow and fast conduction (**Fig. 61.14**). This is also reflected in the alternating concentrations of the major cardiac gap junctional protein, connexin-43, in the consecutive segments and the appearance of an electrocardiographic output. This architecture permits the pumping function of the embryonic heart, although no valves are present. The slowly conducting segments between the atrium and ventricle (atrioventricular canal), and ventricle and great arteries (outflow tract), contain the endocardial cushions, which function as sphincteric valves. The segments persist until one-way valves have been sculpted from the endocardial cushions. The primary myocardium of the outflow tract regresses along with the formation of the semilunar valves and has virtually disappeared around the twelfth week of human development. The primary myocardium of the atrioventricular canal will become incorporated into the atria upon the formation of the atrioventricular valves from the ventricular inlets and the annulus fibrosus between 6 and 12 weeks of development. Some persists as the still slowly conducting atrioventricular node.

It has been believed that rings of cardiac specialized tissue, precursor tissue of the conducting system in the formed heart, are present in the embryonic heart at the sinu-atrial, atrioventricular, bulboventricular (interventricular) and bulbotruncal junctions, as in the 'four ring theory'. However, the primary myocardial, slowly conducting, segments that remain after the formation of the atrial and ventricular segments should not be considered as newly formed rings. The presence of an interventricular ring has been immunohistochemically confirmed. It gives rise to the rapidly conducting ventricular part of the conducting system encompassing the atrioventricular bundle and bundle branches. Thus the conducting system of the formed heart encompasses two distinct functional components: the slowly conducting nodal component, consisting of persisting primary myocardium of the flanking segments, and the rapidly conducting ventricular component, consisting of the atrioventricular bundle and bundle branches.

The concept of cardiac specialized tissue may unintentionally suggest that it is a homogeneous tissue with a single function, and is more specialized than other myocardium. However, it is contradictory to suggest that the nodal tissue that is reminiscent of primary myocardium is more specialized than the well differentiated working myocardium. Since the discovery of the nodes, attempts have been made to identify internodal tracts of specialized atrial cells, but as yet there is no convincing evidence to substantiate the presence of such tracts. Preferential conducting pathways in certain areas of the atrium can be accounted for by regional differences in the histological architecture and geometry of the atrial walls and septum.

With the evolutionary emergence of two ventricles, the development of the ventricular conducting system appears to have become essential to guarantee simultaneous contraction of both ventricles. The development of the ventricular conducting system is therefore obligatorily associated with ventricular septation. In the early human embryo (stage 14, 5 weeks) a myocardial ring can be identified, encircling the foramen between the presumptive left and right ventricles on top and astride the developing ventricular septum (**Fig. 61.15**). At this stage of development the atria are connected to the left ventricle only. The interventricular ring is a ventricular structure which, in the inner curvature of the ring, is also part of the myocardium of the atrioventricular canal. Between stages 16 and 19, as a result of the rightward expansion of the atrioventricular canal during subsequent stages, the right atrium gains access to the right ventricle, and the left ventricle gains access to the subaortic outflow tract, as a result of an apparent leftward expansion of the outflow tract (**Figs 61.16, 61.17**). This entire process can be visualized by the expression of GIN2, one of the neuronal markers of cardiac

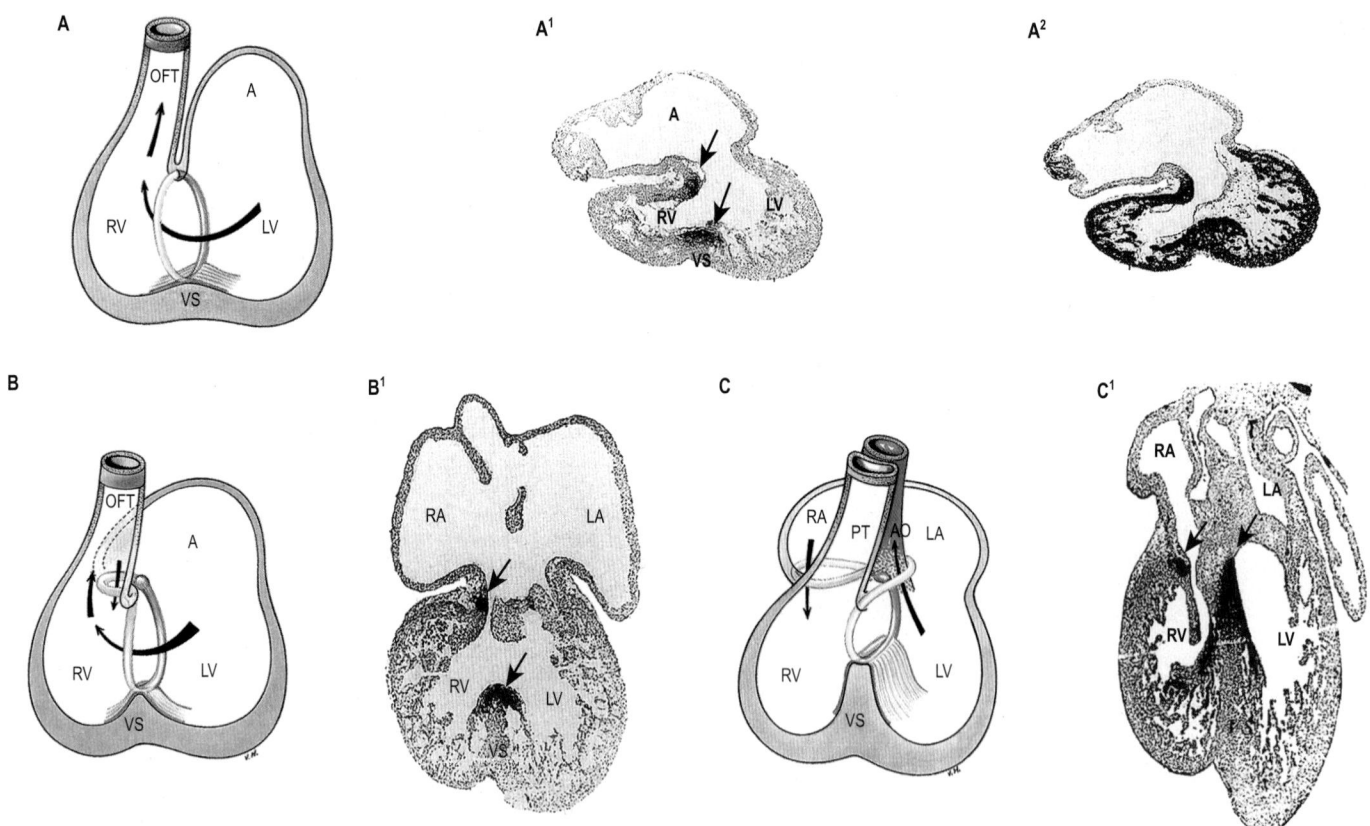

Fig. 61.15 Development of the ventricular conducting system in the human heart. The sequence (**A–C**) shows schematic representations. The red part of the interventricular ring will give rise to the atrioventricular bundle and bundle branches, whereas the yellow part of the interventricular myocardium will not participate in the formation of the adult conducting system. The sequence (**A¹–C¹; A²**) demonstrates immunohistochemical detection of GIN2, a marker for the developing conducting system.
A, At 5 weeks of development (**A¹**), expression of the neural marker is present in the interventricular myocardium, in the right atrioventricular junction and on top of the ventricular septum (arrowed); (**A²**) shows a serial section stained for the presence of ventricular myosin (β-myosin heavy chain), indicating that the neural marker is expressed entirely in the ventricular myocardium.
B, At 6 weeks of development, the atrioventricular canal is expanding towards the right and the original interventricular myocardium becomes part of the right atrioventricular junction. In (**B¹**), expression of GIN2 is clearly present at the right atrioventricular junction and at the top of the ventricular septum (arrowed).
C, At 7 weeks of development, the right atrium has become positioned entirely above the right ventricle and the outflow tract has expanded to the left; the left ventricle has gained access to the aorta. In (**C¹**), expression of GIN2 clearly identifies the right atrioventricular ring; the atrioventricular bundle and the bundle branches can also be identified. Abbreviations: A, embryonic atrium; AO, aorta; LV, embryonic left ventricle; OFT, outflow tract; PT, pulmonary trunk; RV, embryonic right ventricle; VS, developing ventricular septum.

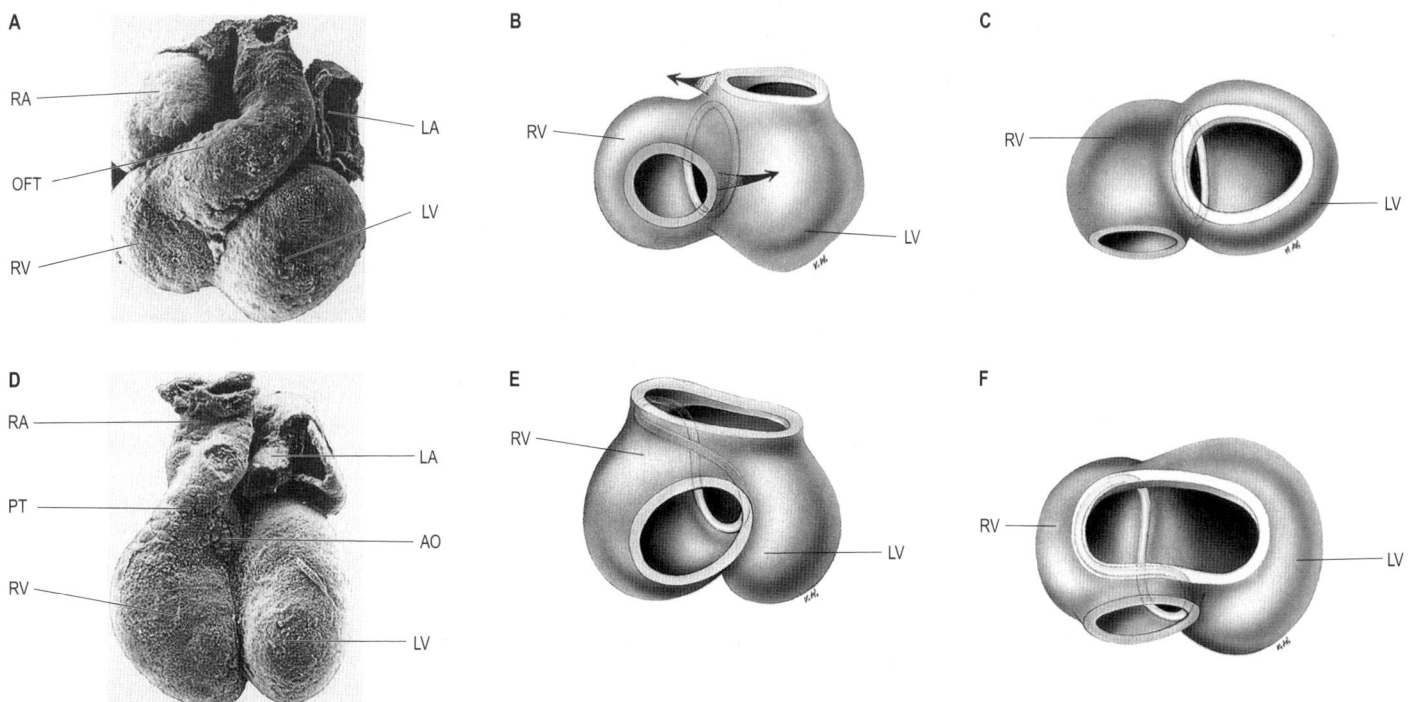

Fig. 61.16 **A**, Scanning electron micrograph of a heart at 5 weeks' development. **B**, Schematic representation of the same heart, with atria and outflow tract removed. The arrows indicate the morphogenetic movements that will occur in the next stage, i.e. rightwards expansion of the atrioventricular canal and apparent leftwards expansion of the outflow tract. **C**, The same scheme as in **B**, but turned 90° to permit an unobstructed view of the atrioventricular canal and of the developing ventricular septum. The atrium (removed in this scheme) would be positioned entirely above the left ventricle. **D**, Scanning electron micrograph of a heart at 7 weeks development. **E**, Schematic representation of the same heart, with atria and outflow tract removed. The atrioventricular canal has expanded towards the right. **F**, The same scheme as in **E**, but turned 90° to permit an unobstructed view in the atrioventricular canal and onto the developing ventricular septum. Note that the embryonic atrium has become positioned above the right and left ventricles. Abbreviations: AO, aorta; LA, left embryonic atrium; LV, left embryonic ventricle; OFT, outflow tract; PT, pulmonary trunk; RA, right embryonic atrium; RV, right embryonic ventricle. (Reprinted from Developmental Biology, Viragh and Challice, Vol 56: 382–396 and 397–411, with permission from Elsevier.)

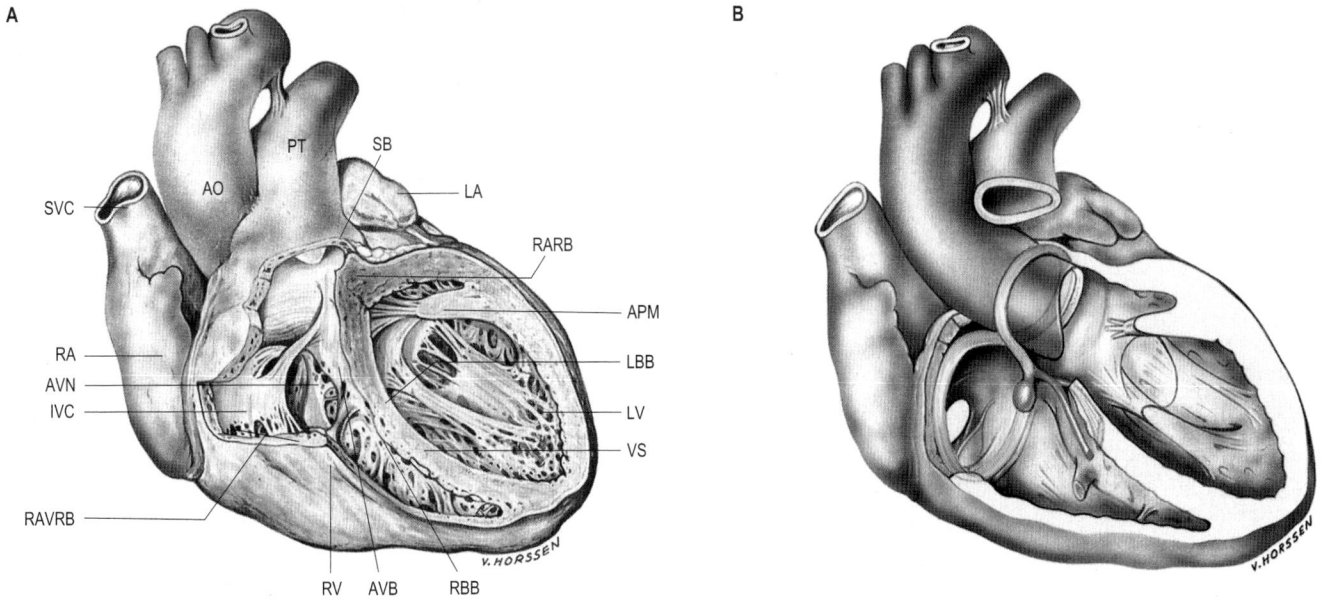

Fig. 61.17 Position of the original interventricular myocardium in the formed heart. **A**, Heart with opened ventricles; **B**, same heart with the pulmonary trunk removed and the position of the original ring indicated. The yellow parts have disappeared. Abbreviations: AO, aorta; APM, anterior papillary muscle; AVB, atrioventricular bundle; AVN, atrioventricular node; IVC, inferior vena cava; LA, left atrium; LBB, left bundle branch; LV, left ventricle; PT, pulmonary trunk; RA, right atrium; RARB, retroaortic root branch; RAVRB, right atrioventricular root bundle; RBB, right bundle branch; RV, right ventricle; SB, septal branch; SVC, superior vena cava; VS, ventricular septum.

myocytes. The atrioventricular bundle develops from the dorsal portion of the interventricular ring and is contiguous with the left and right bundle branches in the top of the ventricular septum. The anterior portion of this ring has been called the septal branch. Also called the 'third branch' of the atrioventricular bundle, it has been described as a 'dead-end track' in some malformed hearts. It is not yet clear whether the GIN2-positive ring contributes to the formation of the atrioventricular node. As a consequence of the rightward expansion of the atrioventricular canal, part of the GIN2-positive ring encircles the right atrioventricular junction and will finally be located in the lower rim of the atrium. This part of the ring is called the right atrioventricular ring bundle and has been demonstrated in fetal human hearts. As a consequence of the apparent leftward expansion of the outflow tract, the GIN2-positive ring becomes positioned at the root and behind the subaortic outflow tract. This part is called the retroaortic branch. The septal branch, retroaortic branch and right atrioventricular ring bundle disappear during normal development in mammals. **Fig. 61.17** represents the entire system in the adult heart.

The fact that the ventricular conducting system originates from a single interventricular ring provides a solid base for understanding the disposition of the conducting system in a number of congenital malformations. The concept accounts particularly well for the morphology and disposition of the atrioventricular node and bundle in hearts with straddling tricuspid valves, with double inlet left ventricles, and with tricuspid atresia. The morphology of the latter heart defect is remarkably similar to the embryonic condition.

Fetal/neonatal heart

At full term the heart is situated midway between the crown of the head and the lower level of the buttocks (**Fig. 11.4**). The anterior surface is formed mainly by the right atrium and right ventricle, as it is in the adult; this surface is usually covered by the thymus, which may extend over the base of the right ventricle. The heart is relatively large at birth and weighs c.20 g (**Figs 61.18, 65.5**); the cardiac output is c.550 ml/min, and the blood pressure 80/46 mmHg. The fetal heart rate is c.150 beats/min near term, at birth it is c.180 beats/min, and it decreases over the neonatal period to 170 beats/min after about 10 min and to 120–140 beats/min from 15 min to 1 hour after birth. Any signs of fetal distress will increase this general basic level. The heart rate decreases further with increasing age: it is normally between 113 and 127 beats/min from 6 months to 1 year, settling to c.100 beats/min by the end of the first year.

Within the atrial septum, the foramen ovale lies at the level of the third intercostal space, with its long axis in the median plane. It is about 4–6 mm in vertical length and 3–4 mm wide (**Fig. 11.4**). It is almost exactly in the coronal plane of the body; thus blood passes from the anteriorly placed right atrium posteriorly and upwards to reach the upper, posterior part of the left atrium After birth, the intra-atrial pressures are equalized and the free edge of the septum primum is therefore kept in contact with the left side of the septum secundum and fusion occurs. The initially free crescentic margin of the septum secundum forms, after fusion, the border of the fossa ovalis, and the septum primum forms the floor of the fossa ovalis of the adult heart.

At all ages the interventricular septum is considered part of the left ventricle. The heart ratio is expressed as the weight of left ventricle and septum: weight of right ventricle. At birth the left ventricle weighs c.25% more than the right. However, the right ventricle has been working against the systemic pressure in the fetus (the pulmonary circulation being not yet active) and there is a preponderance of right ventricular function in the first 2 or 3 months after birth. With the establishment of the pulmonary circulation, the work of the right side of the heart decreases and the left side of the heart, particularly the ventricle, grows rapidly to meet the demands of the active neonate. By the end of the second year, the left weighs twice as much as the right, a condition that continues to middle age. At birth, the average thicknesses of the lateral walls of the ventricles are approximately equal (5 mm). By the end of the third month, the left ventricle is thicker than the right, it becomes twice as thick by the second year, and three times as thick by puberty.

CONGENITAL HEART DEFECTS

Defects of heart development may not come to light until after birth, although many can be observed on ultrasound examination (p. 1011). They may affect the atrial septum, the atrioventricular septum, the ventricular septum or the arterial pole of the developing heart. More complex forms with abnormal septation represent failure, or inappropriate connection, of the atria to the ventricles. They include anomalies such as double inlet ventricle, absence of one atrioventricular connection (tricuspid or mitral atresia) and discordant atrioventricular connections (congenitally corrected transposition).

Congenital cardiac malformations are often multiple and probably occur more frequently in siblings and in children of consanguineous marriages. There is a low correlation, however, among monozygotic twins. Ventricular septal defects are the most common lesions, making up c.20% of all cases, followed by persistent patency of the ductus arteriosus, coarctation, pulmonary stenosis, Fallot's tetralogy, complete transposition, aortic stenosis and hypoplastic left heart syndrome (each of these accounts for between 5 and 10% of all cases).

ATRIAL SEPTAL DEFECTS

A persistent communication between the atrial chambers within the fossa ovalis is common, and results from failure of fusion of the primary atrial septum (the flap valve) with the infolded muscular rims of the fossa. When the flap valve is still able to overlap the rims, the communication is of no functional significance as long as left atrial pressure is greater than right, which is usually the case. In contrast, when the flap valve is smaller than the fossa, or when it is perforate, there is a true atrial septal defect (**Fig. 61.19**).

In normal development, the free edge of the septum primum fuses with the atrioventricular endocardial cushions, permitting subsequent formation of the atrioventricular septum. When this process fails to occur, the entire atrioventricular junction is malformed, and an atrioventricular septal defect is part of the complex anomaly. This defect can be found when the cusps of the atrioventricular valves are fused to the crest of the ventricular septum (**Fig. 61.20**), producing an interatrial communication at the expected site of the atrioventricular septum. This so-called ostium primum defect is correctly classed as an atrioventricular septal defect. Other interatrial communications can be formed in the mouths of the venae cavae, most frequently the superior vena cava, and are usually associated with drainage of the right pulmonary veins into the cavo–atrial junction. Known as sinus venosus defects (**Fig. 61.19**), their essential feature is a bi-atrial connection of the vena cava. An interatrial communication can also occur through the mouth of the coronary sinus when there is a deficiency or absence of the wall that usually separates the sinus from the left atrium.

Atrioventricular septal defects result from failure of fusion of the endocardial atrioventricular cushions, leaving a common atrioventricular orifice and deficiencies of the adjacent septal structures (**Fig. 61.20**). The common orifice is guarded by a basically common valve, with superior and inferior cusps bridging the scooped-out ventricular septum to be tethered in both right and left ventricles. Although the left component of the valve thus formed is often interpreted as a 'cleft mitral valve', in reality it bears no resemblance to the normally structured mitral valve, having three cusps and with the 'cleft' forming the zone of apposition between the left ventricular components of the bridging cusps. The defects show marked variation according to the attachments of the bridging cusps of the common valve to each other, and to the adjacent atrial and ventricular septal structures. Two major subgroups are identified. The more frequent pattern has a common atrioventricular orifice and the potential for shunting through the septal defect at both atrial and ventricular levels (**Fig. 61.20**, middle). The minority of cases have separate right and left atrioventricular orifices, with shunting possible only at atrial level. Although the latter defect is often described as an ostium primum atrial septal defect, it is, in reality, an atrioventricular septal defect.

VENTRICULAR SEPTAL DEFECTS

The most common defect of the ventricular septum is found in the environs of the expected site of the membranous septum in the right wall of the aortic vestibule, below the commissure between the non-coronary and right coronary cusps of the aortic valve (**Fig. 61.21**). The defect is closely related to the septal cusp of the tricuspid valve, but can extend to open into the ventricular outlet beneath the supraventricular crest. It results from incomplete closure of the ventricular septum by its membranous component, and is often associated with over-riding of the crest of the muscular septum by the aortic orifice, along with pulmonary stenosis or atresia and hypertrophy of the right ventricle (Fallot's tetralogy). Rarely, the pulmonary trunk can be normal or even dilated with this combination, giving the so-called Eisenmenger complex. Perimembranous defects, so called because they have the remnant of the membranous septum as part of their perimeter, can also be found with abnormal ventriculo–arterial connections. It is then often the pulmonary trunk that over-rides the muscular septum, giving the so-called Taussig–Bing syndrome. In perimembranous ventricular septal defects, the atrioventricular bundle and its right and left branches are always found along the posteroinferior margin of the defect.

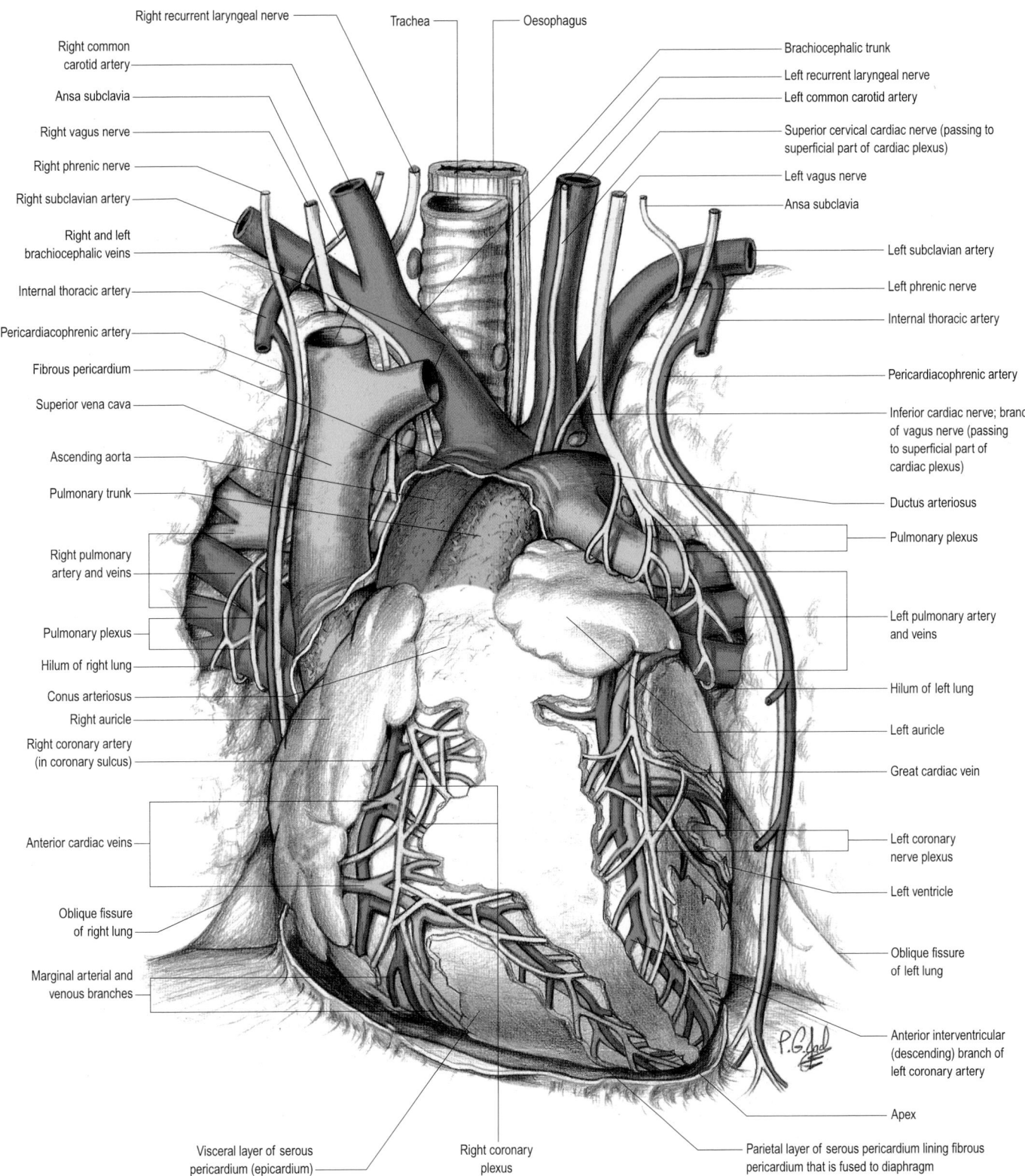

Fig. 61.18 Anterior view of heart and great vessels in a full-term neonate. The lungs have been displaced to expose the heart and the epicardium dissected off the heart and roots of the great vessels. Note that, after birth, blood flow reverses through the ductus arteriosus prior to its closure. (After Crelin ES 1969 Anatomy of the Newborn. Philadelphia: Lea and Febiger.)

Less commonly, a septal defect can be found in the ventricular outflow tracts roofed by the conjoined facing cusps of the aortic and pulmonary valves. Such juxta-arterial defects are doubly committed, in that they open beneath the orifices of both aortic and pulmonary valves. They are the result of failure of formation of both the outlet component of the muscular ventricular septum and the free-standing subpulmonary muscular infundibulum, but with appropriate septation at the ventriculo–arterial junction. They usually have a muscular

posteroinferior rim, which protects the atrioventricular bundle, but can extend to become perimembranous.

The third type of ventricular septal defect occurs within the musculature of the septum. These muscular defects can occur in all parts of the septum, and can be multiple, producing a so-called 'Swiss-cheese' septum.

Defects within the inlet part of the septum are important, because the atrioventricular bundle passes in the upper border. This is in

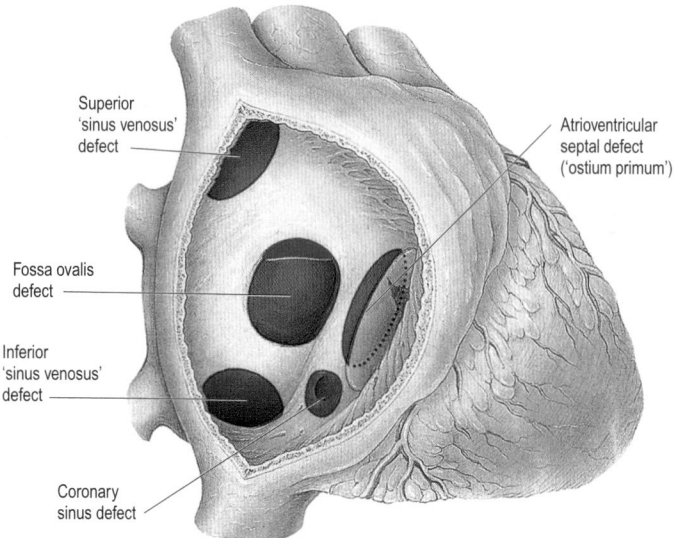

Fig. 61.19 Location of the defects that produce an interatrial communication. Only defects within the fossa ovalis are true atrial septal defects.

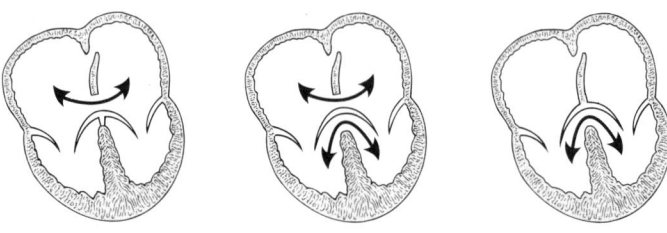

Fig. 61.20 Shunting across an atrioventricular septal defect. This can be atrial (left), ventricular (right) or at both levels (middle), depending on the attachment of the bridging cusps.

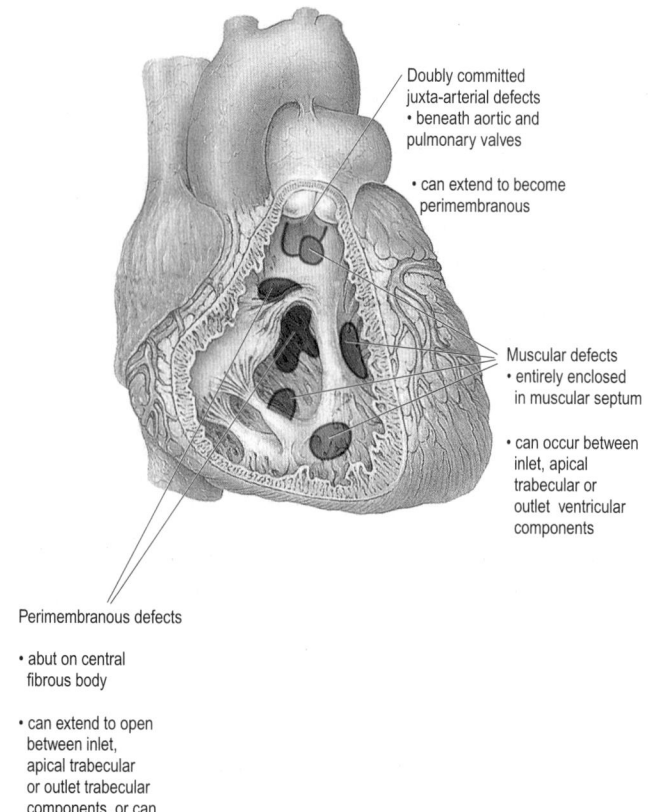

Fig. 61.21 Ventricular septal defects. Depending on the structure of the anatomic borders seen from the right ventricle, these defects can be placed into perimembranous, muscular or doubly committed groups.

contrast to perimembranous defects, which open into the inlet of the right ventricle, where the atrioventricular bundle is posteroinferiorly located.

DEVELOPMENT OF BLOOD VESSELS

All the vascular channels – atrial, venous and lymphatic – are developing at the same time, and are influenced by the same growth factors (p. 209).

Arteries

The first aortic arches run through the mandibular arches, and five additional pairs are developed within the corresponding pharyngeal arches caudal to them so that, in all, six pairs of aortic arches are formed (**Fig. 61.22A**). The fifth arches are atypical and probably transient, at most, in mankind.

EMBRYONIC AORTIC ARCHES (Fig. 61.22)

The embryonic aortic arches, with the exception of the fifth, are developed in a craniocaudal sequence. The more cranial are in process of disappearing before the caudal ones are completed. The first and second embryonic aortic arches are already dwindling by the time the third is established. The first disappears entirely. The dorsal end of the second arch or hyoid artery remains as the stem of the stapedial artery, but the remainder of this arch also disappears (**Fig. 34.11**). The external carotid artery first appears as a sprout, which grows headward from the aortic sac close to the ventral end of the third arch artery. The common carotid arises from an elongation of the adjacent part of the aortic sac,

and the third arch artery becomes the proximal part of the internal carotid artery. The fourth embryonic aortic arch on the right forms the proximal part of the right subclavian artery, whereas the corresponding vessel on the left constitutes the arch of the definitive aorta between the origins of the left common carotid and left subclavian arteries. (It has proved difficult to assess accurately the contributions of the fourth embryonic aortic arches. It has also been claimed that the left fourth aortic arch is subsequently drawn into the descending or ascending, or both, limbs of the definitive aortic arch, and the corresponding vessel of the right contributes to the brachiocephalic artery.)

The identity and status of the fifth embryonic aortic arch artery is uncertain. It is usually incomplete, and may connect the fourth aortic arch or subjacent aortic sac with the dorsal ends of the sixth aortic arch (whereas the other embryonic aortic arches pass between sac and dorsal aorta). The fifth aortic arch eventually disappears on both sides.

From its inception, the sixth embryonic arch vessel is associated with a developing lung bud. Initially each bud is supplied by a capillary plexus from the aortic sac. Later, the plexus connects with the dorsal aorta and the sixth aortic arch is defined as a channel in the vascular connection between sac and dorsal aorta, which continues to supply the developing lung bud. When the aorticopulmonary septum divides the truncus arteriosus into pulmonary trunk and ascending aorta, the sixth aortic arches retain continuity with the former. On the right, the ventral part of the sixth aortic arch persists as the stem of the right pulmonary artery, but its dorsal segment disappears, possibly because of a decreased blood flow resulting from partitioning of the aortic and pulmonary blood streams. On the left side, the ventral part of the sixth aortic arch is absorbed into the pulmonary trunk, whereas its dorsal segment persists as the ductus arteriosus (p. 1053), which is functional during intrauterine life but becomes obliterated after birth, ultimately forming the fibrous ligamentum arteriosum. Postnatal functional closure nears completion within a few weeks, but structural changes continue over many months.

The transformation of the aortic arches described above is conditioned by environmental changes and results largely from changes in

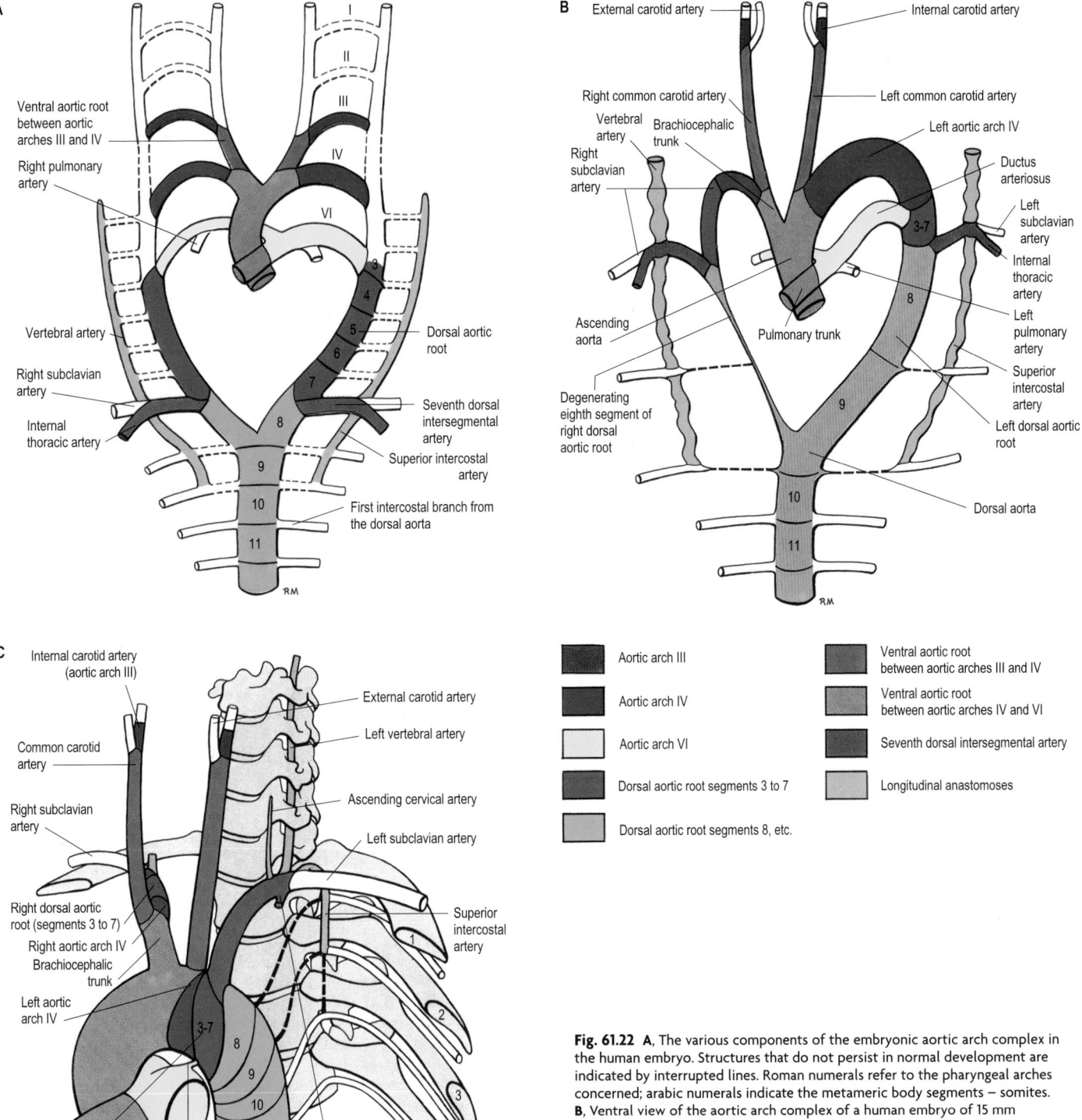

Fig. 61.22 **A**, The various components of the embryonic aortic arch complex in the human embryo. Structures that do not persist in normal development are indicated by interrupted lines. Roman numerals refer to the pharyngeal arches concerned; arabic numerals indicate the metameric body segments – somites. **B**, Ventral view of the aortic arch complex of a human embryo of 15 mm crown–rump length. Note the asymmetry in the pattern that has developed by this stage. Compare with **A** and **C**. **C**, The adult human aorta and its branches, left ventrolateral aspect, showing the position and relative sizes of the definitive contributions from the various embryonic components shown in **A** and **B**. (Based on the work of Barry A 1951 The aortic arch derivatives in the human adult. Anat Rec 111: 221–238, with permission of the author and publisher.)

the pharynx and from the descent of the heart. The entire period of transformation can be divided, both temporally and spatially, into two phases: pharyngeal and postpharyngeal. In the pharyngeal phase, which lasts until about the 12 mm crown–rump length stage (stage 17), the arrangement of the aortic arches resembles that in lower vertebrates. In this phase the course of the blood from the heart to the dorsal aorta follows a succession of different pathways: first arch, first and second arches, second and third arches, third and fourth aortic arches and finally third, fourth and sixth aortic arches. In the postpharyngeal phase, which extends onwards into, and beyond, intrauterine life, the

definitive human pattern and disposition of the vessels is finally established.

DORSAL AORTAE

The dorsal aortae persist on the cranial side of the third aortic arches as continuations of the internal carotid arteries (**Fig. 61.22**). The dorsal aorta between the third and fourth aortic arches, the ductus caroticus, diminishes and finally disappears. From the fourth arch to the origin of the seventh intersegmental artery, the right dorsal aorta becomes part of the right subclavian artery. Caudal to the seventh intersegmental artery, the right dorsal aorta disappears as far as the locus of fusion of thoracic aortae. After disappearance of the left ductus caroticus, the remainder persists to form the descending part of the arch of the aorta. Thence the fused right and left embryonic dorsal aortae persist as the definitive descending thoracic and abdominal aorta. A constriction, the aortic isthmus, is sometimes present in the aorta between the final site of origin of the left subclavian artery and reception of the ductus arteriosus.

In the adult, the right subclavian artery occasionally arises from the arch of the aorta distal to the origin of the left subclavian and then passes upwards and to the right, behind the trachea and oesophagus. This condition is possibly explained by the persistence of the embryonic right dorsal aorta and the obliteration of the fourth aortic arch of the right side.

The heart originally lies ventral to the pharynx, immediately caudal to the stomodeum (**Fig. 61.2A**). With the elongation of the neck and the development of the lungs, it recedes within the thorax and, correspondingly, the vessels are drawn out and the original position of the fourth and sixth aortic arches is greatly modified. Thus on the right the fourth aortic arch recedes only to the thoracic inlet, whereas on the left side it descends into the thorax. The recurrent laryngeal nerves (in contrast to the other arch nerves) originally pass to the larynx caudal to the sixth pair of aortic arches, and are therefore affected by the descent of these structures. Thus in the adult the left nerve hooks round the ligamentum arteriosum within the thorax. On the right, as a result of the disappearance of the fifth and the dorsal part of the sixth aortic arches, the right recurrent laryngeal nerve hooks round the fourth aortic arch, i.e. the start of the right subclavian artery (just above the thoracic inlet).

At first the aortae are the only longitudinal vessels present, for their branches all run at right angles to the long axis of the embryo. Later these transverse arteries become connected, in certain situations, by longitudinal anastomosing channels, which in part persist, forming such arteries as the internal thoracic, the superior and inferior epigastric, the gastroepiploic, etc. Each primitive dorsal aorta gives off ventral splanchnic arteries (paired segmental branches to the digestive tube), lateral splanchnic arteries (paired segmental branches to the mesonephric ridge), somatic arteries (intersegmental branches to the body wall) and a caudal continuation (which passes into the body stalk, the umbilical arteries).

SEGMENTAL EMBRYONIC ARTERIES

VENTRAL SPLANCHNIC ARTERIES

The ventral splanchnic arteries are originally paired vessels distributed to the capillary plexus in the wall of the yolk sac. After fusion of the dorsal aortae, they merge as unpaired trunks that are distributed to the increasingly defined and lengthening primitive digestive tube. Longitudinal anastomotic channels connect these branches along the dorsal and ventral aspects of the tube, forming dorsal and ventral splanchnic anastomoses (**Fig. 61.23**). These vessels obviate the need for so many 'subdiaphragmatic' ventral splanchnic arteries, and these are reduced to three: i.e. the coeliac trunk and superior and inferior mesenteric arteries. As the viscera supplied descend into the abdomen, their origins migrate caudally by differential growth. Thus the origin of the coeliac artery is transferred from the level of the seventh cervical segment to the level of the twelfth thoracic; the superior mesenteric from the second thoracic to the first lumbar; and the inferior mesenteric from the twelfth thoracic to the third lumbar. (Above the diaphragm, however, a variable number of ventral splanchnic arteries persist, usually four or five, supplying the thoracic oesophagus.) The dorsal splanchnic anastomosis persists in the gastroepiploic, pancreaticoduodenal and the primary branches of the colic arteries, whereas the ventral splanchnic anastomosis forms the right and left gastric and the hepatic arteries.

LATERAL SPLANCHNIC ARTERIES

The lateral splanchnic arteries supply, on each side, the mesonephros, metanephros, the testis or ovary and the suprarenal (adrenal) gland. All these structures develop, in whole or in part, from the intermediate mesenchyme of the mesonephric ridge. One testicular or ovarian artery and three suprarenal arteries persist on each side. The phrenic artery branches from the most cranial suprarenal artery, and the renal artery arises from the most caudal. Additional renal arteries are frequently

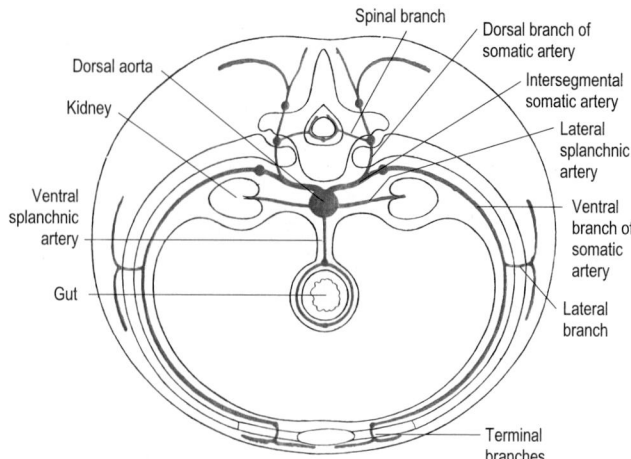

Fig. 61.23 The segmental and intersegmental arteries. Note the positions of the longitudinal anastomoses (small pink dilatations).

present and may be looked on as branches of persistent lateral splanchnic arteries.

SOMATIC ARTERIES

The somatic arteries are intersegmental in position. They persist, almost unchanged, in the thoracic and lumbar regions, as the posterior intercostal, subcostal and lumbar arteries. Each gives off a dorsal ramus, which passes backwards in the intersegmental interval and divides into medial and lateral branches to supply the muscles and superficial tissues of the back (**Fig. 61.23**). It also gives off a spinal branch, which enters the vertebral canal and divides into a series of branches to the tissues constituting the walls and joints of the osteoligamentous canal, and neural branches to the spinal cord and spinal nerve roots. Having produced its dorsal branch, the intersegmental artery runs ventrally in the body wall, gives off a lateral branch and terminates in muscular and cutaneous rami. Before their division, the stems of the somatic arteries, at thoracic and lumbar levels, provide small rami that enter the developing vertebral bodies.

Numerous longitudinal anastomoses link up the intersegmental arteries and their branches (**Fig. 61.23**). On both sides a postcostal anastomosis connects their dorsal branches in the intervals between the necks of ribs and the vertebral transverse processes. This persists in the cervical region where it forms the greater part of the vertebral artery. A post-transverse anastomosis also connects the dorsal branches and forms the greater part of the deep cervical artery. A precostal anastomosis connects intersegmental arteries beyond the origins of their dorsal branches. The ascending cervical and the superior intercostal arteries are persistent parts of this vessel. Near the anterior median line, intersegmental arteries are linked by a ventral somatic anastomosis. Most of these vessels persist bilaterally as the internal thoracic and the superior and inferior epigastric arteries.

UMBILICAL ARTERIES

The umbilical arteries at first are the direct caudal continuation of the primitive dorsal aortae and are present in the body stalk before any vitelline (yolk sac) or visceral branches emerge, indicating the dominance of the allantoic over the vitelline circulation in the human embryo. (On a comparative basis, the umbilical vessels are chorio-allantoic and therefore 'somatovisceral'.) After the fusion of the dorsal aortae, the umbilical arteries arise from their ventrolateral aspects and pass medial to the primary excretory duct to the umbilicus. Later, the proximal part of each umbilical artery is joined by a new vessel that leaves the aorta at its termination and passes lateral to the primary excretory duct. This, possibly the fifth lumbar intersegmental artery, constitutes the dorsal root of the umbilical artery (the original stem, the ventral root). The dorsal root gives off the axial artery of the lower limb, branches to the pelvic viscera and, more proximally, the external iliac artery. The ventral root disappears entirely, the umbilical artery now arising from that part of its dorsal root distal to the external iliac artery, i.e. the internal iliac artery.

Embryonic veins

VISCERAL VESSELS AND SOMATIC VEINS

Often, for convenience and apparent simplicity, the early embryonic veins are segregated into two groups, visceral and somatic. The visceral group contains the derivatives of the vitelline and umbilical veins, and the somatic group includes all remaining veins. It should be noted that embryonic veins, with time, change the principal tissues they drain. Others have some radicles from patently parietal tissues which become confluent with drainage channels that are clearly visceral, and so form a compound vessel.

The arrangement of the early embryonic veins is initially symmetrical. The primitive tubular symmetric heart receives its venous return through the right and left sinual horns which are initially embedded in the mesenchyme of the septum transversum. Each horn receives, most medially, the termination of the principal vitelline vein, more laterally, the umbilical vein and, most laterally, having encircled the pleuroperitoneal canal, the common cardinal vein. This symmetric pattern changes as the heart and gut develop and the cardiac return is diverted to the right side of the heart.

VITELLINE VEINS

The vitelline veins drain capillary plexuses developed in the splanchnopleuric mesenchyme of the secondary yolk sac. With head, tail and lateral fold formation, the upper recesses of the yolk sac are enclosed within the embryo as the splanchnopleuric gut tube, extending from the stomodeal buccopharyngeal membrane to the proctodeal cloacal membrane. Derivatives from all these levels possess a venous drainage, originally vitelline in origin.

The deep aspects of the maxillomandibular facial prominences, retrogingival oral cavity, the pharyngeal walls and their lymphoid and endocrine derivatives, and the cervicothoracic oesophagus, all have drainage channels that connect with the precardinal complex, ultimately returning blood to the heart via the superior vena cava. Laryngeal and tracheobronchial veins also drain to the precardinal complex, whilst

the capillary plexuses, developed in the (splanchnopleuric) walls of the fine terminal respiratory passages and alveoli, converge on pulmonary veins of increasing calibre, finally making secondary connections with the left atrium of the heart, and may be grouped with the vitelline systems. Even the heart itself first differentiates in splanchnopleure that, after head fold formation, forms the dorsal wall of the primitive pericardial cavity (floor of the rostral foregut) and may therefore be considered a highly specialized vitelline vascular derivative. Similarly, at the caudal extremity of the splanchnopleuric gut tube (the future lower rectum and upper anal canal) the vitelline venous drainage makes connections with the internal iliac radicles of the postcardinal complex.

The increasingly extensive remainder of the gut tube, from the gastric terminal segment of the future oesophagus to the upper rectum, is, as elsewhere, clothed with splanchnopleuric mesenchyme permeated by a capillary plexus. The latter drains into an anastomosing network of veins. The net is more dense ventrally and in the central midgut region; for a while, it receives a leash of small veins from the definitive yolk sac that enter the embryo through the umbilicus, embedded in the yolk stalk. Later, in normal development, both stalk and vessels atrophy. Within the splanchnopleuric net, progressing rostrally, longitudinal channels anterolateral to the gut become increasingly well defined as the embryonic abdominal vitelline veins. Entering the septum transversum, the right and left vitelline veins incline slightly, becoming parallel to the lateral aspects of the gut. They establish connections with capillary plexuses in the septal mesenchyme, then continue, finally curving to enter the medial part of the cardiac sinual horn of their corresponding side. The parts of the gut closely related to the presinual segments of the vitelline veins are the future subdiaphragmatic end of the oesophagus, primitive stomach, the superior (first) and descending (second) regions of the duodenum, and the remainder of the duodenal tube.

The principal ascending vitelline veins flanking the sides of the abdominal part of the foregut receive venules from its splanchnopleuric capillaries, and those of the septal mesenchyme. Within these venular nets, enlarged (but still plexiform) anastomoses connect the two vitelline veins (**Fig. 61.24**) (for clarity, these are represented as simple transverse

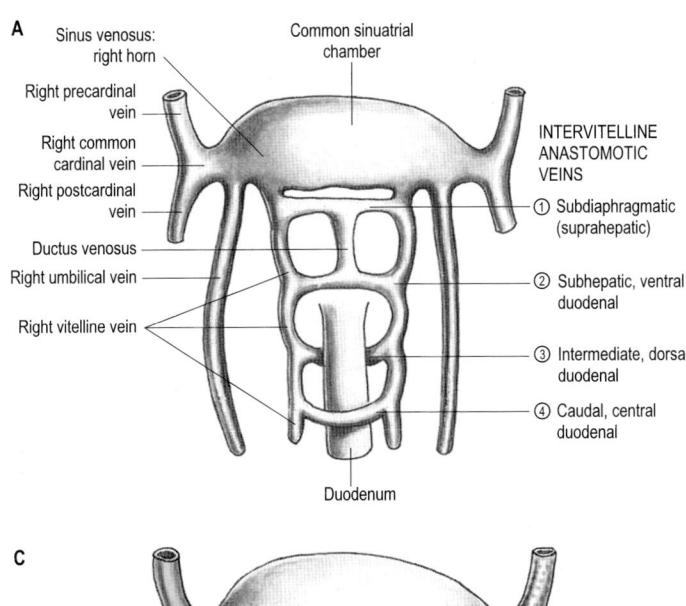

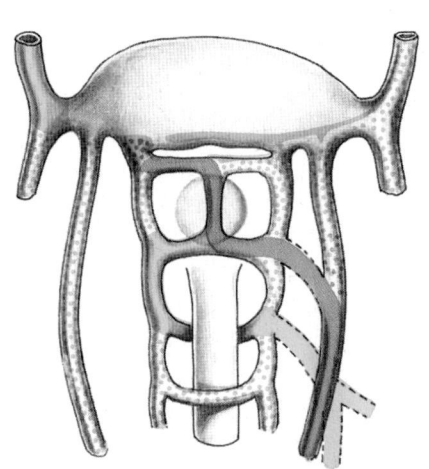

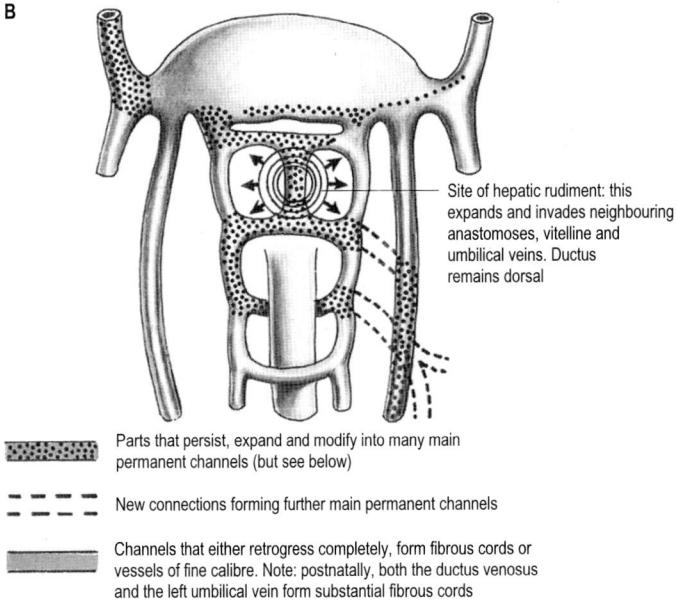

Fig. 61.24 Development of the vitelline, umbilical and terminal cardinal vein complexes: the early symmetric condition. **A**, The topography and nomenclature of the veins forming the right and left sinual horns, the intervitelline anastomoses and the median ductus venosus. **B**, Further details of cardiac development. To assist understanding of later changes, the symmetric pattern is used to indicate which segments persist or retrogress, the sites of formation of new channels and the intimately involved hepatic rudiment. **C**, Simplified representation of the subsequent main flow paths of oxygenated and deoxygenated blood.

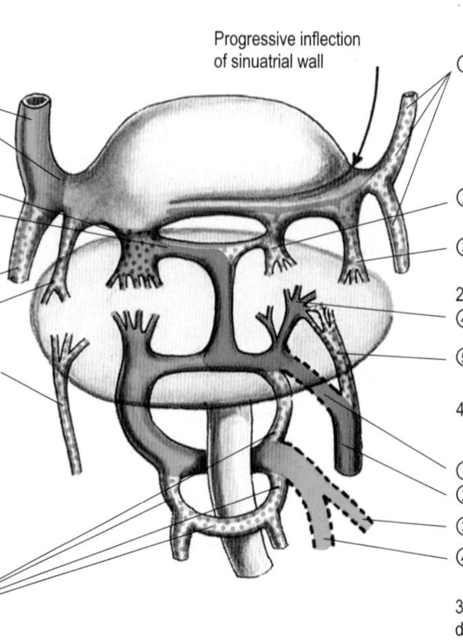

ENLARGING

① Right precardinal and common cardinal veins

② Right hepatocardiac vein (termination of right vitelline vein – future inferior vena cava)

③ Right half of subdiaphragmatic anastomosis

DIMINISHING

① Right postcardinal vein

② Hepatocardiac part of right umbilical vein

③ Hepatic terminal right umbilical vein

Progressive inflection of sinuatrial wall

DIMINISHING

① Left precardinal, common and postcardinal veins

② Hepatocardiac part of left vitelline vein

③ Hepatocardiac part of left umbilical vein

2 + 3 = left venae revehentes

④ Hepatic terminals of left vitelline vein

⑤ Hepatic terminals of left umbilical vein

4 + 5 = left venae advehentes

ENLARGING

① New venous connections

② Left umbilical vein

③ Presumptive splenic vein

④ Presumptive superior mesenteric vein

3 + 4 merge to form root of definitive hepatic portal vein

DIMINISHING

Vitelline vein segments and ventral anastomosis

Fig. 61.25 Development of the vitelline, umbilical and terminal cardinal vein complexes: a mid-stage of asymmetry has been reached between the early symmetric condition (**Fig. 61.24**) and the definitive late prenatal state. Note the definition of the coronary sinus and the central role of the liver; compare homologous left- and right-sided vessels.

channels in the figure). A subdiaphragmatic intervitelline anastomosis develops in the rostral septal mesenchyme, lying a little caudal to the cardiac sinuatrial chamber, connecting the veins near their sinual terminations. (The channel is sometimes termed suprahepatic because of the position of the hepatic primordium; with expansion of the latter it becomes partly intrahepatic.) The presumptive duodenum is crossed by three transverse duodenal intervitelline anastomoses. Their relation to the gut tube alternates so that the most cranial, the subhepatic, is ventral, the intermediate is dorsal and the caudal is ventral. It has become customary to describe the paraduodenal vitelline veins and their associated anastomoses as forming a figure 8. At this early stage when left and right embryonic veins are still symmetric, the cranial duodenal anastomosis becomes connected with the subdiaphragmatic anastomosis by a median longitudinal channel, the primitive median ductus venosus, which is dorsal to the expanding hepatic primordium, but ventral to the gut. The further development of the vitelline veins and anastomoses is, as indicated, closely interlocked, with rapid hepatic expansion and gut changes, and umbilical vein disposition and modification is closely involved.

UMBILICAL VEINS

The umbilical veins form by the convergence of venules draining the splanchnopleure of the extraembryonic allantois. The human endodermal allantois is very small, projecting just into the embryonic end of the connecting stalk, so the latter is regarded as precociously formed allantoic mesenchyme, and the umbilical vessels as allantoic. The peripheral venules drain the mesenchymal cores of the chorionic villous stems and terminal villi (extraembryonic somatopleuric structures). These are the radicles of, usually single, vena umbilicalis impar which traverses the compacting mixed mesenchyme of the umbilical cord to reach the caudal rim of the umbilicus. Here, the single cordal vein divides into primitive right and left umbilical veins. Each curves rostrally in the somatopleuric lateral border of the umbilicus (i.e. where intraembryonic and extraembryonic or amniotic somatopleure are continuous), where it lies lateral to the communication between both the intraembryonic and extraembryonic coeloms. Rostrolateral to the umbilicus, the two umbilical veins reach, enter and traverse the junctional mesenchyme of the septum transversum, to connect with septal capillary plexuses. They then continue to enter their corresponding cardiac sinual horns lateral to the terminations of the vitelline veins. This early symmetric disposition of the vitelline veins and anastomoses, umbilical and common cardinal veins, and locus of the hepatic primordial complex is summarized in **Fig. 61.24**.

CHANGES IN THE VITELLO-UMBILICAL VEINS

Progressive changes in the vitello-umbilical veins are rapid, profound and closely linked with regional modifications in shape and position of the gut, expansion and invasion of venous channels by hepatic tissue,

asymmetry of the heart and cardiac venous return. The principal events are summarized in **Figs 61.24, 61.25** and **61.26**.

From the cranial portion of the early hepatic evagination of the foregut, interconnected sheets and 'cords' of endodermal cells, the presumptive hepatocytes, penetrate the septum transversum mesenchyme. Hepatic mesenchyme is composed of a mixed population of cells with endothelial/angiogenic and connective tissue lineages. Capillary plexuses develop within this mesenchyme and, possibly under the influence of the endodermal hepatic sheets, the plexuses become more profuse by further addition of angioblastic septal mesenchyme, which also forms masses of perivascular intrahepatic haemopoietic tissue. These processes extend along the plexiform connections of the vitelline, and later the umbilical, veins until their intrahepatic (trans-septal) zones themselves become largely plexiform. Initially capillary in nature, they transform into a mass of rather wider, irregular, sinusoidal vessels with a discontinuous endothelium containing many phagocytic cells (p. 1255). The lengths of vitelline veins involved in these processes are the intermediate parts of the segments extending from the subhepatic (cranioventral duodenal) to the suprahepatic (subdiaphragmatic) transverse intervitelline anastomoses, and the corresponding lengths of the umbilical veins. Thus at this early stage the liver sinusoids are perfused by mixed blood reaching them through a series of branching vessels collectively called the venae advehentes, or afferent hepatic veins. They are deoxygenated from the gut splanchnopleure via vitelline vein hepatic terminals and oxygenated from the placenta via hepatic terminals of the umbilical veins. Blood leaves the liver through four venae revehentes (efferent hepatic veins); two on each side reach and open into their respective cardiac sinual horns. This full complement of four hepatocardiac veins is only transient, and becomes reduced to one dominant, rapidly enlarging channel. As detailed below, the originally bilaterally symmetric cardinal vein complexes, both rostral and caudal, develop transverse or oblique anastomoses such that the cardiac venous return is restricted to the definitive right atrium. (The pulmonary veins are the only major ones returning to the left atrium (p. 1033)).

These cardiac and concomitant hepatoenteric changes are accompanied by events in supra-, intra- and subhepatic parts of the vitelloumbilical veins. Some vessels enlarge, persisting as definitive vessels to maturity and, in places, they are joined later by other channels that become defined in already established capillary plexuses. Other vessels retrogress, either disappearing completely or remaining as vestigial tags and, occasionally, vessels of fine calibre. Some vessels of crucial importance in the circulatory patterns of embryonic and fetal life become obliterated postnatally and transformed to substantial fibrous cords. Both right and left umbilical hepatocardiac and the left vitelline hepatocardiac veins continue, for a time, to discharge blood into their sinual horns; however, they begin to retrogress (**Figs 61.24, 61.25**). The right umbilical channel atrophies completely. The left channels also disappear, but their cardiac terminals may, on occasion, be found as conical fibrous tags attached to the inferior wall of the coronary sinus.

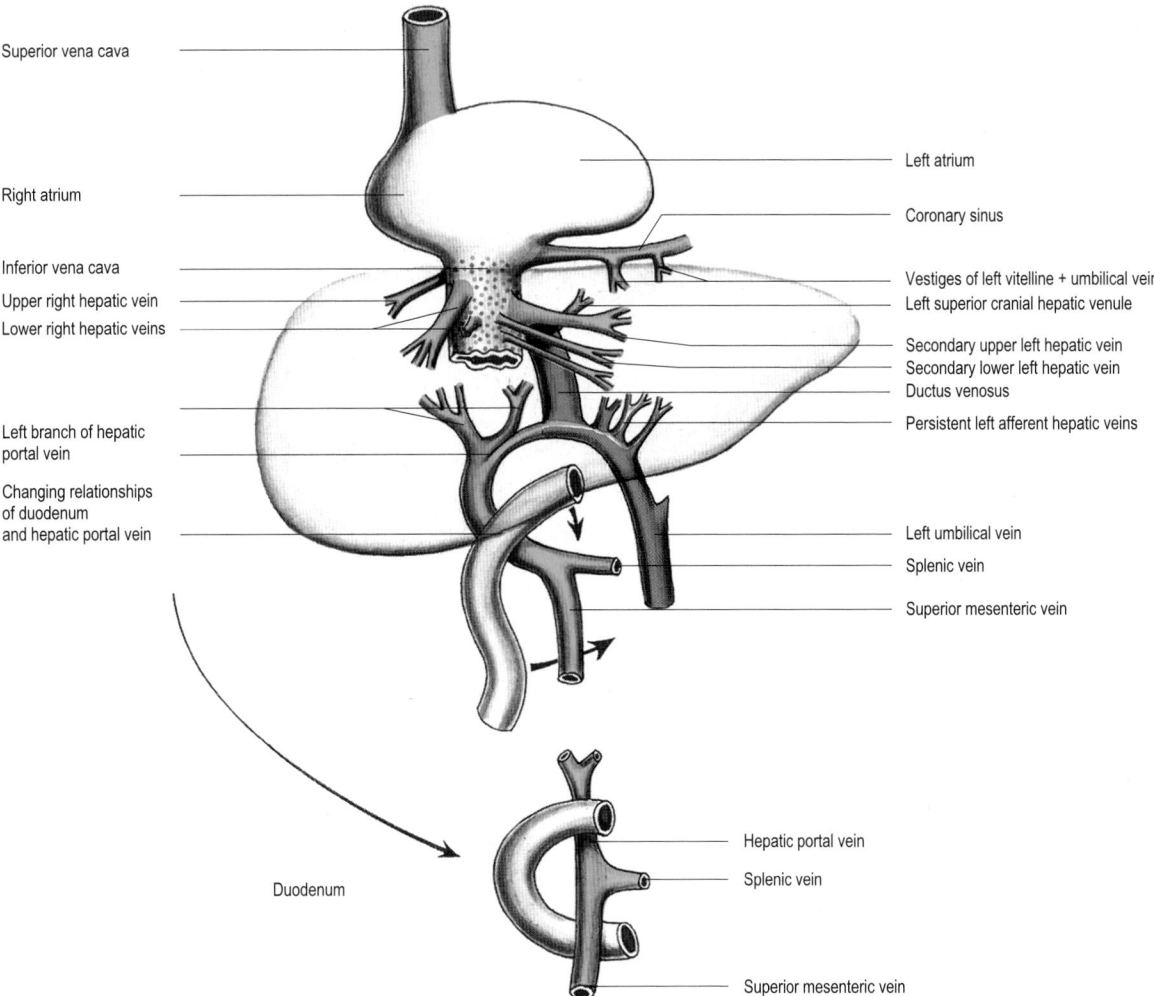

Superior vena cava

Right atrium

Inferior vena cava
Upper right hepatic vein
Lower right hepatic veins

Left branch of hepatic
portal vein

Changing relationships
of duodenum
and hepatic portal vein

Duodenum

Left atrium

Coronary sinus

Vestiges of left vitelline + umbilical veins
Left superior cranial hepatic venule

Secondary upper left hepatic vein
Secondary lower left hepatic vein
Ductus venosus

Persistent left afferent hepatic veins

Left umbilical vein

Splenic vein

Superior mesenteric vein

Hepatic portal vein

Splenic vein

Superior mesenteric vein

Fig. 61.26 The condition of some main upper abdominal and intrathoracic right atrial terminal veins in the later prenatal months. Note the coronary sinus and attached vestiges; the terminations of the superior and inferior venae cavae; the grouped hepatic veins; the convergent formation and hepatic divarication of the hepatic portal vein, and the routes available for return of oxygenated left umbilical venous blood; the changing disposition of the duodenal loop and its relationship to the definitive portal vein; the manner in which the left terminal branch of the latter establishes connections with the ductus venosus and the left umbilical vein. Return of placental blood to the fetal heart is along an (embryologically) complex path; **Figs 61.24** and **61.25** should assist clarification.

The right vitelline hepatocardiac vein continues enlarging and ultimately forms the terminal segment of the inferior vena cava. The latter receives the right efferent hepatic veins and new channels draining the territories of the left efferent hepatic veins. These collectively form the upper and lower groups of right and (secondary) left hepatic veins. The terminal caval segment also shows the orifice of the right half of the intervitelline subdiaphragmatic anastomosis, and a large new connection with the right subcardinal vein.

The hepatic terminals of the right and left duodenal parts of the vitelline veins are destined to form the corresponding branches of the hepatic portal vein, the left branch incorporating the cranial ventral intervitelline anastomosis. With rotation of the gut and formation of the duodenal loop, segments of the original vitelline veins and the caudal transverse anastomosis atrophy (indicated in **Figs 61.24, 61.25, 61.26**), while new splanchnopleuric venous channels, the superior mesenteric and splenic veins, converge and join the left end of the dorsal intermediate anastomosis. The numerous other radicles of the portal vein and its principal branches, including the inferior mesenteric vein, are later formations.

For a period, placental blood returns from the umbilicus via right and left umbilical veins, both discharging through afferent hepatic veins into the hepatic sinusoids, where admixture with vitelline blood occurs. At approximately 7 mm crown–rump length, the right umbilical vein retrogresses completely. The left umbilical vein retains some vessels discharging directly into the sinusoids, but new enlarging connections with the left half of the subhepatic intervitelline anastomosis emerge. The latter is the start of a bypass channel for the majority of the placental

blood, which continues through the median ductus venosus and finally the right half of the subdiaphragmatic anastomosis, to reach the termination of the inferior vena cava. Postnatally these channels are obliterated with the resulting ligamentum teres extending from the umbilicus to the porta hepatis, whence, having established connections with the left branch of the portal vein, it continues as the ligamentum venosum to join an upper left hepatic vein, and terminates in the suprahepatic inferior vena cava.

SOMATIC VENOUS COMPLEXES

The initial venous channels in the early embryo have traditionally been termed cardinal because of their importance at this stage. The cardinal venous complexes (**Fig. 61.27**) are first represented by two large vessels on each side: the precardinal portion is rostral and the postcardinal, caudal, to the heart. The two veins on each side unite to form a short common cardinal vein, which passes ventrally, lateral to the pleuro-pericardial canal, to open into the corresponding horn of the sinus venosus (**Fig. 61.2B**).

The precardinal veins undergo remodelling as the head develops. The postcardinal veins, which in the early embryo drain the body wall, are insufficient channels for venous return from the developing meso-nephros and gonads and for the growing body wall. As the embryo increases in size, they are supplemented by a range of bilateral longitudinal channels that anastomose with the posterior cardinal system and with each other. They are, as follows: subcardinal, supracardinal, azygos line, subcentral and precostal veins.

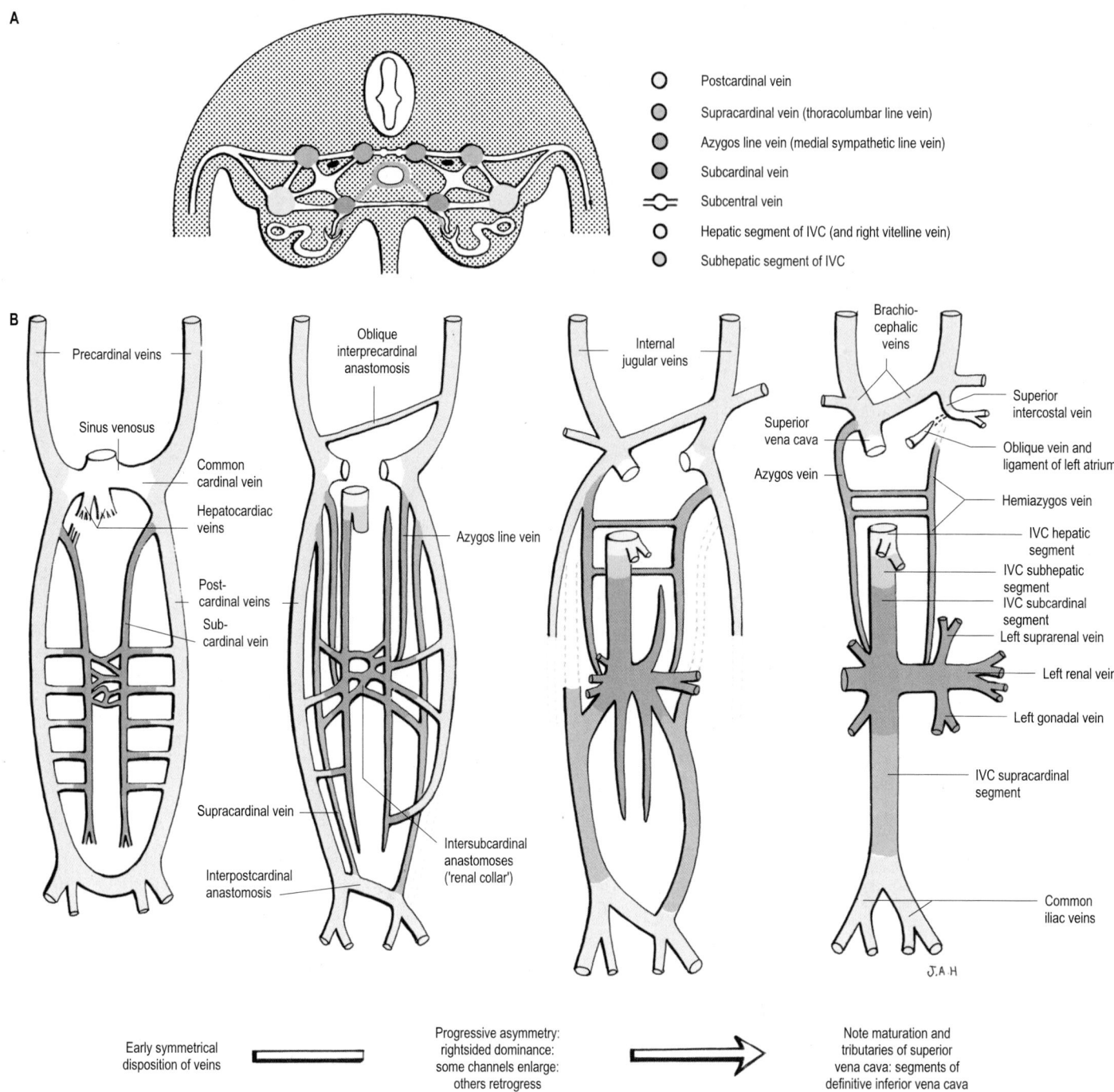

A

- ○ Postcardinal vein
- ◑ Supracardinal vein (thoracolumbar line vein)
- ● Azygos line vein (medial sympathetic line vein)
- ● Subcardinal vein
- ─◯─ Subcentral vein
- ○ Hepatic segment of IVC (and right vitelline vein)
- ○ Subhepatic segment of IVC

B

Precardinal veins
Sinus venosus
Common cardinal vein
Hepatocardiac veins
Post-cardinal veins
Sub-cardinal vein
Supracardinal vein
Interpostcardinal anastomosis

Oblique interprecardinal anastomosis
Azygos line vein
Intersubcardinal anastomoses ('renal collar')

Internal jugular veins
Superior vena cava
Azygos vein

Brachio-cephalic veins
Superior intercostal vein
Oblique vein and ligament of left atrium
Hemiazygos vein
IVC hepatic segment
IVC subhepatic segment
IVC subcardinal segment
Left suprarenal vein
Left renal vein
Left gonadal vein
IVC supracardinal segment
Common iliac veins

J.A.H

Early symmetrical disposition of veins → Progressive asymmetry: rightsided dominance: some channels enlarge: others retrogress ⟹ Note maturation and tributaries of superior vena cava: segments of definitive inferior vena cava

Fig. 61.27 Somatic venous development. **A,** Schematic section through the embryonic trunk. Principal longitudinal veins are colour-coded. Interconnections and intersegmental veins remain uncoloured. **B,** Plan of development of principal somatic veins from the early symmetric state, through states of increasing asymmetry, to the definitive arrangement. Abbreviation: IVC, inferior vena cava. (Modified from Williams PL, Wendell-Smith CP, Treadgold S 1969 Basic Human Embryology, 2nd edn. Philadelphia: Lippincott.)

Subcardinal veins – form in the ventromedial parts of the mesonephric ridges and become connected to the postcardinal veins by a number of vessels traversing the medial part of the ridges. The subcardinal veins assume the drainage of the mesonephros, they intercommunicate by a pre-aortic anastomotic plexus, which later constitutes the part of the left renal vein crossing anterior to the abdominal aorta.

Supracardinal veins – form dorsolateral to the aorta and lateral to the sympathetic trunk. They take over the intersegmental venous drainage from the posterior cardinal vein. This is also referred to as the thoraco-lumbar line or lateral sympathetic line vein.

Azygos line veins – form dorsolateral to the aorta and medial to the sympathetic trunk. This channel, also referred to as the medial sympathetic line vein, gradually takes over the intersegmental venous

drainage from the supracardinal veins. The intersegmental veins now reach their longitudinal channel by passing medial to the autonomic trunk, a relationship that the lumbar and intercostal veins maintain thenceforth. Cranially, the azygos lines join the persistent cranial ends of the posterior cardinal veins.

Subcentral veins – form directly dorsal to the aorta in the interval between the origins of the paired intersegmental arteries. These veins communicate freely with each other and with the azygos line veins, and these connections ultimately form the retro-aortic parts of the left lumbar veins and of the hemiazygos veins.

A precostal or lumbocostal venous line – is recognized by some authorities, anterior to the vertebrocostal element, and posterior to the supracardinal. A possible derivative is the ascending lumbar vein.

The supracardinal veins are, as indicated, lateral to the aorta and sympathetic trunks, which therefore intervene between them and the azygos lines. They communicate caudally with the iliac veins and cranially with the subcardinal veins in the neighbourhood of the pre-aortic intersubcardinal anastomosis. The supracardinal veins also communicate freely with each other through the medium of the azygos lines and the subcentral veins. The most cranial of these connections, together with the supracardinal–subcardinal and the intersubcardinal anastomoses, complete a venous ring around the aorta below the origin of the superior mesenteric artery, termed the 'renal collar'.

The ultimate arrangement of these embryonic abdominal and thoracic longitudinal cardinal veins may be summarized as follows. The terminal part of the left postcardinal vein forms the distal part of the left superior intercostal vein. On the right side, its cranial end persists as the terminal part of the azygos vein. The caudal part of the subcardinal vein is in part incorporated in the testicular or ovarian vein and partly disappears. The cranial end of the right subcardinal vein is incorporated into the inferior vena cava and also forms the right supra-renal vein. The left subcardinal vein, cranial to the intersubcardinal anastomosis, is incorporated into the left suprarenal vein. The renal and testicular or ovarian veins on both sides join the supracardinal–subcardinal anastomosis. On the left side, this is connected directly to the part of the inferior vena cava which is of subcardinal status through an intersubcardinal anastomosis. The right supracardinal vein forms much of the postrenal (caudal) segment of the inferior vena cava. The left supracardinal vein disappears entirely. The right azygos line persists in its thoracic part to form all but the terminal part of the azygos vein. Its lumbar part can usually be identified as a small vessel that leaves the vena azygos on the body of the twelfth thoracic vertebra and descends on the vertebral column, deep to the right crus of the diaphragm, to join the posterior aspect of the inferior vena cava at the upper end of its postrenal segment. The left azygos line forms the hemiazygos veins. The subcentral veins give rise to the retro-aortic parts of the left lumbar veins and of the hemiazygos veins.

SUPERIOR VENA CAVA

The precardinal veins enlarge as the head and brain develop. They are further augmented by the subclavian veins from the upper limb buds, and so become the chief tributaries of the common cardinal veins, which gradually assume an almost vertical position in association with the descent of the heart into the thorax. That part of the original precardinal vein rostral to the subclavian is now the internal jugular vein, and their confluence is the brachiocephalic vein of each side. The right and left common cardinal veins are originally of the same diameter. By the development of a large oblique transverse connection, the left brachio-cephalic vein carries blood across from the left to the right (**Fig. 61.27**). The part of the original right precardinal vein between the junction of the two brachiocephalics and the azygos veins forms the upper part of the superior vena cava; the caudal part of the latter vessel (below the entrance of the azygos vein) is formed by the right common cardinal vein. Caudal to the transverse branching of the left brachiocephalic vein, the left precardinal and left common cardinal veins largely atrophy, the former constituting the terminal part of the left superior intercostal vein, while the latter is represented by the ligament of the left vena cava and the oblique vein of the left atrium (**Fig. 61.27B**). The remainder of the left superior intercostal vein is developed from the cranial end of the postcardinal vein and drains the second, third and, on occasion, the fourth intercostal veins. The oblique vein passes downwards across the back of the left atrium to open into the coronary sinus, which, as already indicated, represents the persistent left horn of the sinus venosus. Right and left superior venae cavae are present in some animals, and occasionally persist in mankind.

INFERIOR VENA CAVA

The inferior vena cava of the adult is a composite vessel. The precise mode of development of its postrenal segment (caudal to the renal vein) is still somewhat uncertain. Its function is initially carried out by the right and left postcardinal veins (**Fig. 61.27**), which receive the venous drainage of the lower limb buds and pelvis and run in the dorsal part of the mesonephric ridges, receiving tributaries from the body wall (intersegmental veins) and from the derivatives of the mesonephroi.

The early postcardinal veins communicate across the midline via an interpostcardinal anastomosis. This remains as an oblique transverse anastomosis between the iliac veins, and becomes the major part of the definitive left common iliac vein. It diverts an increasing volume of blood into the right longitudinal veins, which accounts for the ultimate disappearance of most of those on the left.

The supracardinal veins receive the larger venous drainage of the growing body wall. The right supracardinal vein persists and forms the greater part of the postrenal segment of the inferior vena cava. The continuity of the vessel is maintained by the persistence of the anastomosis between the right supracardinal and the right subcardinal in the renal collar. The left supracardinal disappears, but some of the renal collar formed by the left supracardinal–subcardinal anastomosis persists in the left renal vein. Both supracardinal veins drain cranially into the subcardinal veins. On the right side, the subcardinal vein comes into intimate relationship with the liver. An extension of the vessel takes place in a cranial direction and meets and establishes continuity with a corresponding new formation that is growing caudally from the right vitelline hepatocardiac (common hepatic) vein. In this way, on the right side a more direct route is established to the heart and the prerenal (cranial) segment of the inferior vena. In summary, therefore, the inferior vena cava is formed from below upwards by the confluence of: the common iliac veins; a short segment of the right postcardinal vein; the postcardinal–supracardinal anastomosis; part of the right supracardinal vein; the right supracardinal–subcardinal anastomosis; right subcardinal vein; a new anastomotic channel of double origin, the hepatic segment of the inferior vena cava; and the cardiac termination of the right vitelline hepatocardiac vein (common hepatic vein).

Only the supracardinal part of the inferior vena cava receives intersegmental venous drainage. The postrenal (caudal) segment of the inferior vena cava is on a plane that lies dorsal to the plane of the prerenal (cranial) segment. Thus the right phrenic, suprarenal and renal arteries, which represent persistent mesonephric arteries, pass behind the inferior vena cava, whereas the testicular or ovarian artery, which has a similar developmental origin, passes anterior to it.

In some animals, the right postcardinal vein constitutes a large part of the postrenal segment of the inferior vena cava. In these cases the right ureter, on leaving the kidney, passes medially dorsal to the vessel and then, curving round its medial side, crosses its ventral aspect. Rarely, a similar condition is found in humans, and indicates the persistence of the right postcardinal vein and failure of the right supracardinal to play its normal part in the development of the inferior vena cava.

Abnormal connections of the great arteries and veins

Should the bulbar spiral septum (aorticopulmonary septum, p. 1011) fail to develop at all, or in an incorrect position, a number of outflow anomalies may occur. When no spiral septum develops, a common arterial trunk lesion is present with an undivided arterial channel, guarded by a common arterial valve positioned above and astride the free margin of the muscular ventricular septum (**Fig. 61.28**). There is, therefore, a coexisting juxta-arterial deficiency of the ventricular septum. The right and left pulmonary arteries usually arise via a confluent segment, but can take independent origin from the common arterial trunk, which continues as the ascending aorta. The common valve usually has three cusps, but may have two, four or more. The lesion is almost certainly linked to abnormal migration of cells into the heart from the neural crest.

Complete transposition of the great vessels is the condition in which the aorta arises from the right ventricle and the pulmonary trunk from the left. Better described as showing discordant ventriculo–arterial connections, such hearts can coexist with deficiencies of cardiac septation. They can also be found with discordant connections at the atrioventricular junction (congenitally corrected transposition). The developmental history of discordant connections remains unknown.

Double outlet ventricle exists when the greater parts of both arterial valves are attached within the same ventricle, almost always the right. For circulation to continue, it is then necessary for the ventricular septum to be deficient, although the septal defect can rarely close as a secondary event. The position of the septal defect serves for sub-classification. It is usually beneath the aorta or the pulmonary trunk, but can be doubly committed or even non-committed.

Either the systemic or pulmonary veins can be anomalously connected. The most common systemic anomaly is found when a persistent left

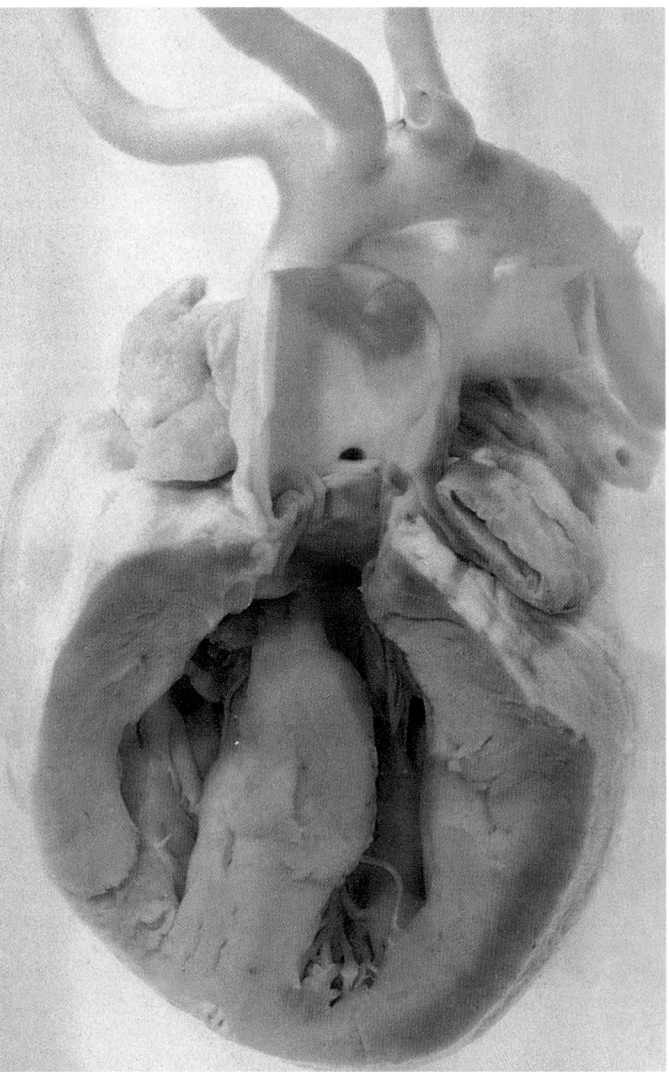

Fig. 61.28 This heart possesses a common arterial trunk, with a common truncal valve over-riding a juxta-arterial deficiency of the ventricular septum, the result of failure of septation of the arterial pole of the developing heart. (By kind permission from Dr Leon M Gerlis.)

superior vena cava drains into the right atrium through the enlarged orifice of the coronary sinus.

More rarely, the left vena cava may connect directly with the superior aspect of the left atrium, usually associated with unroofing of the coronary sinus, so that the orifice of the sinus functions as an interatrial communication. The most common lesion of the inferior vena cava is when its abdominal course is interrupted, with drainage to the heart via the azygos or hemiazygos venous system. This lesion is found most frequently with left isomerism.

The pulmonary veins can be connected to an anomalous site individually or in combination. Totally anomalous connection is of most significance. Usually, the veins form a confluence behind the left atrium that then connects to the superior vena cava, the coronary sinus or the portal venous system after traversing the diaphragm.

A right aortic arch is found most frequently with Fallot's tetralogy or with a common arterial trunk. It can also exist, together with a left arch, in various combinations known as arterial rings, which compress the oesophagus, giving so-called dysphagia lusoria. Persistent patency of the ductus arteriosus must be distinguished from delayed closure. The persistently patent duct can be an obligatory part of the circulation when associated with aortic or pulmonary atresia. Coarctation of the aorta can be found as an isolated lesion when the ductus arteriosus is closed, or with an open duct, when it is more likely to be associated with additional lesions within the heart (p. 1023).

DEVELOPMENT OF LYMPHATIC VESSELS AND TISSUES

There is little recent work on the development of the lymphatic channels, although the cellular components of lymphoid tissue are widely researched. Two theories of lymphatic channel development have been put forward. In one, the earliest lymphatic vessels are believed to arise as offshoots from the endothelium of the veins, as capillary plexuses that later lose their connections with the venous system and become confluent to form lymph sacs. In the other, lymphatic spaces commence as clefts in local angiogenic mesenchyme that take on the characteristics of endothelium. These spaces form capillary plexuses from which certain lymph sacs are derived. The connections of the lymphatic and venous systems are regarded as entirely secondary. The balance of the evidence suggests that all but the earliest lymphatic channels originate independently of the venous system and acquire connections with it only at a later stage. However, it should be appreciated that both venous and lymphatic drainage are part of the circulatory system in the embryo, fetus and adult.

Recent interest in lymphangiogenesis has been stimulated by the identification of novel growth factors, receptors, cell surface proteins and transcription factors in the lymphatic endothelium. These are termed vascular endothelial growth factors (VEGF). Growth factors VEGF-C and VEGF-D, and their cognate receptor tyrosine kinase, VEGF receptor-3, are critical regulators of lymphangiogenesis (Partanen & Paavonen 2001). This tyrosine kinase receptor appears to be abnormally phosphorylated in patients with Milroy disease, an autosomal dominant condition of chromosome 5q that causes lymphoedema, hypoplasia, dilation and tortuosity of lymphatic vessels. The homeobox transcription factor Prox-1 is also proving to be a useful tool in this field. It is strongly expressed in lymphatic endothelium, in addition to other sites. Mice deficient for Prox-1 are practically devoid of lymphatic vessels (Rodregues-Niedenfuhr et al 2001).

In the human embryo, the lymph vessels are derived from six lymph sacs. Two are paired (the jugular and the posterior lymph sacs) and two unpaired (the retroperitoneal and the cisterna chyli). In lower mammals an additional pair (subclavian) is present, but in the human embryo these are merely extensions of the jugular sacs.

The jugular lymph sac is the first to appear, at the junction of the subclavian vein with the precardinal, with later prolongations along the internal and external jugular veins; the posterior lymph sac encircles the left common iliac vein; the retroperitoneal sac appears in the root of the mesentery near the suprarenal glands; and the cisterna chyli appears opposite the third and fourth lumbar vertebrae (**Fig. 61.29**).

From the lymph sacs, the lymph vessels bud out along lines corresponding more or less closely with the course of embryonic blood

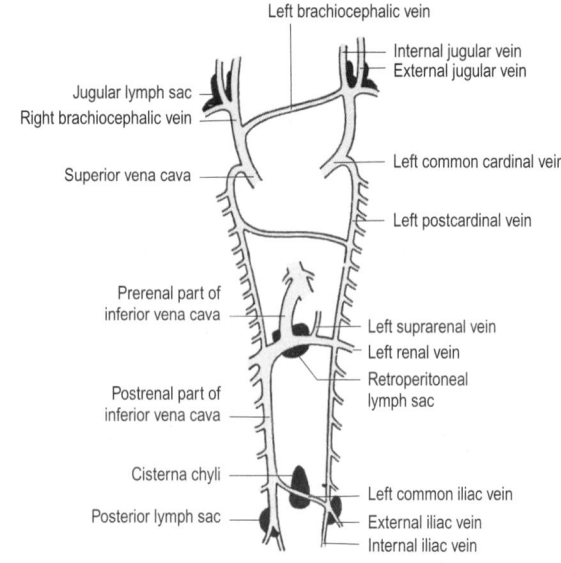

Fig. 61.29 Relative positions of the primary lymph sacs. (After Sabin FR 1912 On the origin of the abdominal lymphatics in mammals from the vena cava and the renal glands. Anat Rec 6: 335–342, by permission from John Wiley.)

vessels, which are most commonly veins, but many arise *de novo* in the mesenchyme and establish connections with existing vessels. In the body wall and wall of the intestine, the deeper plexuses are the first to be developed; by continued growth, the vessels in the superficial layers are gradually formed.

Thoracic duct

The thoracic duct is, phylogenetically, a bilateral structure. In man it comprises the caudal part of the right vessel, a transverse anastomosis and the cranial part of the left vessel. It is believed to be formed from anastomosing outgrowths from the jugular sacs and cisterna chyli. At its connection with the cisterna it is at first double, but the vessels soon join. Numerous valves are laid down in the duct during the fifth month, but many of them disappear before birth. Those that persist are formed in situations where the duct may be subjected to pressure, e.g. where it is crossed by the oesophagus and the aortic arch.

The thoracic duct is the largest single lymph vessel in the body in both neonates and adults. It is about 10–11 cm long in the neonate. The right lymphatic duct, which drains lymph from the right side of the head and neck, is only 2–3 cm long and surrounded by lymph nodes.

Cisterna chyli

All the lymph sacs except the cisterna chyli are, at a later stage, divided by a number of slender connective tissue bridges. Subsequently, they are invaded by lymphocytes and transformed into groups of lymph nodes, the lymph sinuses representing portions of the original cavity of the sac. The caudal part of the cisterna chyli is similarly converted, but its rostral part sometimes persists as a definitive cisterna. In many cases the cisterna chyli is plexiform. The siting of the major groups of lymph nodes follows a similar basic pattern amongst the mammals.

Lymph nodes

Lymphatic vessels can be seen in the embryo in the cervical region from stage 16. Lymph nodes have been identified from week 9. Early lymph sacs become infiltrated by lymphoid cells and the outer portion of the sacs becomes the subcapsular sinus of the lymph node. Morphological differentiation of medullary and cortical compartments has not been observed until the end of week 10 (Tonar et al 2001). At the same time as these early lymph nodes are developing, the nasopharyngeal wall is infiltrated by lymphoid cells that are believed to herald the early development of the tubal and pharyngeal tonsils. The total amount of lymphoid tissue in the form of lymph nodes is considerable in the neonate. Generally, lymphoid tissues increase in amount during childhood because of the growth of nodes already present in the neonate. Definitive follicles with germinal centres are formed during the first postnatal year. The pharyngeal tonsil reaches its maximal development at 6 years; thereafter involution is completed by puberty.

CIRCULATION

Embryonic circulation

The earliest circulatory components are seen with the production of endothelial and early blood cells in the extraembryonic tissues. Angioblastic cells differentiate from extraembryonic mesenchyme in the splanchnopleure of the yolk sac, in the body stalk (containing the allantois), and in the somatopleure of the chorion. At these sites small, spherical groups of cells, termed blood islands, are found early in the third week. The peripheral cells flatten as a vascular endothelium, whereas the central cells transform into primitive red blood corpuscles. Later, contiguous islands merge, forming a continuous network of fine vessels.

Intraembryonic blood vessels are first seen at the endoderm–mesenchyme interface within the lateral splanchnic mesenchyme at the caudolateral margins of the cranial intestinal portal. All mesenchymal tissue apart from notochord and prochordal plate contains angiogenic cells that are capable of differentiating into endothelium or primitive blood cells. Ectodermal tissues do not appear to give rise to angiogenic cells; however, evidence suggests that endodermal tissues are necessary

for endothelial differentiation. Angioblastic competence has been demonstrated among the ventral (splanchnopleuric) mesenchymes with which the endoderm interacts. Embryonic angioblasts are highly invasive, moving in every direction throughout embryonic mesenchyme tissue.

Before the establishment of the circulation, endothelial vessels are formed either by vasculogenesis, whereby new vessels develop *in situ* (e.g. endothelial heart tubes, dorsal aortae, umbilical and early vitelline vessels) or by angiogenesis, whereby vessels develop by sprouting and branching from endothelium of pre-existing vessels (e.g. as seen in most other vessel production).

The ultimate pattern of vessels formed is controlled by the surrounding, non-angiogenic, mesenchyme. Blood vessels become morphologically specific for the organ in which they develop and immunologically specific, expressing organ-specific proteins.

All blood vessels are initially surrounded by a fibronectin-rich matrix that is later incorporated into the basal lamina along with laminin, a particularly early constituent. Several layers of fibronectin-expressing cells can be seen around the larger vessels (e.g. dorsal aortae). The endothelium does not synthesize a basal lamina in those regions where remodelling is active and, similarly, the mesenchyme around such endothelium does not express α-actin, laminin, etc. Appearance of these molecules is indicative of cessation of branching and differentiation of the media. It is not known how differentiation of pericytes and smooth muscle cells is induced.

Major restructuring changes take place during the early development of the circulation. Anastomoses appear and disappear, capillaries fuse and give rise to arteries or veins, and the direction of blood flow may reverse several times. The tunica media of the vessels appears after a stable vascular pattern has formed. The majority of arteries accumulate layers of smooth muscle derived from the surrounding mesenchyme in the tunica media. The embryonic aortic arch arteries of the third, fourth and sixth arches and the dorsal aorta initially contain smooth muscle cells that are not elastogenic and not of cardiac neural crest origin. Two populations of neural crest cells surround these arteries: one that does not express either smooth muscle or elastin antigens, and a second larger population that differentiates into an elastogenic phenotype. This is expressed from the truncus arteriosus to the aortic arch arteries until all of them are elastogenic. At the same time, the original smooth muscle cells disappear along the great vessels to their first branch point. The ductus arteriosus and the pulmonary arteries, however, have a muscular tunica media and not an elastic media like the other arch arteries.

Apart from the aortae, none of the main vessels of the adult arises as a single trunk in the embryo. Along the course of each vessel a capillary network is first laid down and, by selection and enlargement of definite paths in this network, the larger arteries and veins are defined. The branches of main arteries are not always simple modifications of the vessels of a capillary network, but arise as outgrowths from the enlarged stem.

Subsequent to head fold formation, each primitive aorta consists of ventral and dorsal parts that are continuous through the first embryonic aortic arch. The ventral aortae are fused and form a dilated aortic sac. The dorsal aortae run caudally, one on each side of the notochord, but in the fourth week they fuse from about the level of the fourth thoracic to that of the fourth lumbar segment to form a single definitive descending aorta (**Fig. 61.2A**). The dorsal continuation of the primitive dorsal aortae directs blood into an anastomosing network around the allantois. This will form the umbilical arteries. Blood is channelled back to the developing heart from the allantois via umbilical veins, from the primitive yolk sac anastomoses via the vitelline veins, and from the body via pre- and postcardinal veins that join to form the common cardinal veins (**Fig. 61.2B**). Generally, the embryonic circulation is symmetric. Modifications of this early pattern produce a functioning fetal circulation that is able to change rapidly at birth.

In early development, the arteries of the embryo are disproportionately large and their walls consist of little more than a single layer of endothelium. The cardiac orifices are also relatively large and the force of the cardiac contraction is weak. As a result, despite the rapid rate of contraction, the circulation is sluggish, but this is compensated for because the tissues are able to draw nourishment not only from the capillaries but also from the large arteries and the intraembryonic coelomic fluid.

It has been suggested that a site and mechanism for filling the rapidly expanding cardiovascular system with plasma is accomplished by the movement of fluid from the intraembryonic coelom to the veins. Generally, the intraembryonic coelom wall is composed of proliferating cells producing splanchnopleuric and somatopleuric mesenchymal populations. However, the walls of a portion of the pericardioperitoneal canals are thin at the time when the canals surround the hepatocardiac channels (veins). These vessels are situated between the hepatic plexus and the sinus venosus. The hepatocardiac channel on the right side is more developed and on the left it is more plexiform, with only a transitory connection to the sinus venosus. The differentiation of this specific coelomic region occurs just in advance of the expansion and filling of the right and left atria, at about stage 12.

As the heart muscle thickens, compacts and strengthens, the cardiac orifices become both relatively and absolutely reduced in size, the valves increase their efficiency and the large arteries acquire their muscular walls and undergo a relative reduction in size. From this time onwards, the embryo is dependent for its nourishment on the expanding capillary beds and henceforth the function of the larger arteries becomes restricted to that of controllable distribution channels to keep the embryonic tissues constantly and appropriately supplied.

The heart starts to beat early, before the development of the conducting system, and a circulation is established before a competent valvular mechanism has formed. Cardiac output increases in proportion with the weight of the embryo. Cardiac rate increases with development; however, most of the increase in cardiac output results from a geometric increase in stroke volume. When dorsal aortic blood flow is matched to embryonic weight, blood flow remains constant over a more than 150-fold change in mass of the embryo.

Fetal circulation

The pattern of the fetal circulation develops in such a way as to provide for the sudden establishment of the pulmonary circulation at birth while maintaining the persistence of the placental circulation during fetal life. Fetal blood reaches the placenta via two umbilical arteries and returns in early fetal life by two umbilical veins (**Fig. 61.30**). Later, the right one disappears. The persisting left umbilical vein enters the abdomen at the umbilicus and traverses the edge of the falciform ligament to reach the hepatic surface. It then joins the left branch of the portal vein at the hepatic portal. Opposite the junction, a large vessel, the ductus venosus, arises and ascends posterior to the liver to join the left hepatic vein near its termination in the inferior vena cava. (For a detailed developmental account, with illustrations, of the circumhepatic veins see p. 1046.) The portal vein is small in the fetus compared with the size of the umbilical vein. Parts of its left branch, proximal and distal to their junctions, function as branches of the portal vein, carrying oxygenated blood to the right and left parts of the liver. Hence, blood in the left umbilical vein reaches the inferior vena cava by three routes: some enters the liver directly and reaches the vena cava via the hepatic veins; a considerable quantity circulates through the liver with portal venous blood before also entering by the hepatic veins; the remainder is bypassed into the inferior vena cava by the ductus venosus.

Blood from the ductus venosus and hepatic veins mixes in the inferior vena cava with blood from the lower limbs and abdominal wall. It enters the right atrium and, guided by the valve of the inferior vena cava, c.75% passes through the foramen ovale into the left atrium, where it mingles with the limited venous return from the pulmonary veins. The remainder of the blood returning via the inferior vena cava, instead of traversing the foramen ovale, joins blood from the superior vena cava and passes through the right atrium to reach the right ventricle. From the left atrium, blood enters the left ventricle and thence the aorta, by which it is probably distributed almost entirely to the heart, head and upper limbs, so that little reaches the descending aorta. Blood from the head and upper limbs returns via the superior vena cava to the right atrium, flowing through the right atrioventricular orifice along with the small amount returned via the inferior vena cava. From the right ventricle, this blood enters the pulmonary trunk. The fetal lungs are largely inactive, so only a little of the blood from the right ventricle flows through the right and left pulmonary arteries and this returns by the pulmonary veins to the left atrium. The greater part of the outflow through the pulmonary trunk is carried by the ductus arteriosus directly to the aorta, where it mixes with the small quantity of blood passed from the left ventricle into this part of the aorta. The mixture descends the aorta and is partly distributed to the lower limbs and the organs

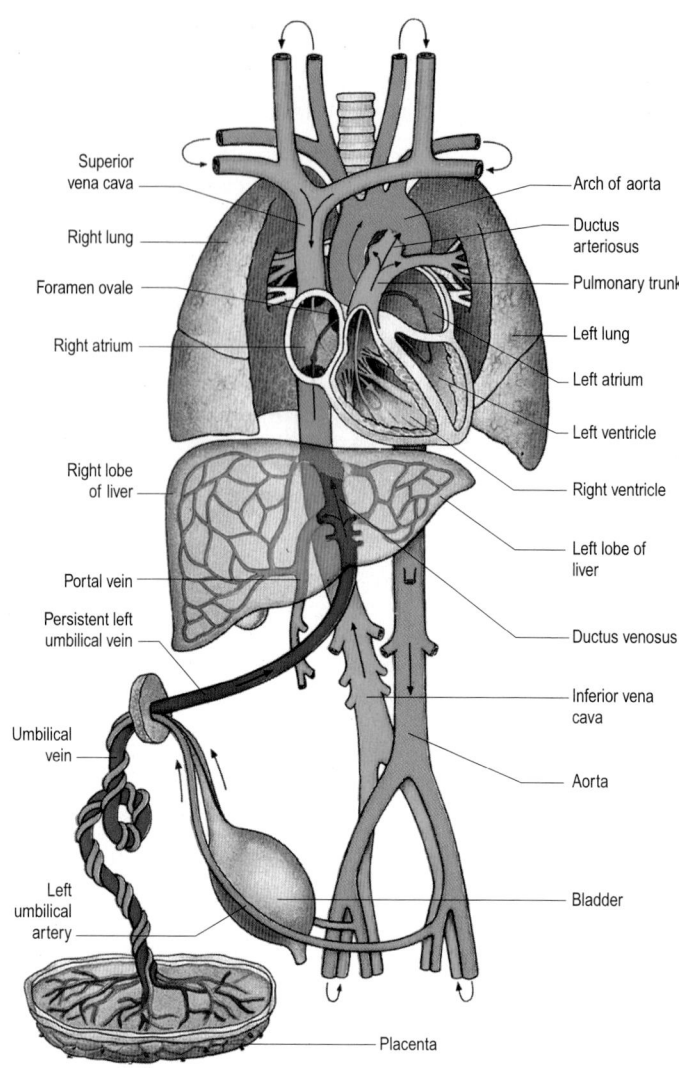

Superior vena cava

Right lung

Foramen ovale

Right atrium

Right lobe of liver

Portal vein

Persistent left umbilical vein

Umbilical vein

Left umbilical artery

Arch of aorta

Ductus arteriosus

Pulmonary trunk

Left lung

Left atrium

Left ventricle

Right ventricle

Left lobe of liver

Ductus venosus

Inferior vena cava

Aorta

Bladder

Placenta

Fig. 61.30 Plan of the fetal circulation. The arrows indicate the direction of blood flow. The placenta is drawn to a greatly reduced scale.

of the abdomen and pelvis. Most is returned via the umbilical arteries to the placenta.

In terms of function, it is the placenta that serves as the organ for fetal nutrition and excretion, receiving deoxygenated fetal blood and returning it oxygenated and detoxified. Most of the blood entering the left atrium comes from the right atrium, because right atrial pressure is much greater than that in the left atrium, and this forces the flap-like valve of the septum primum to the left (**Fig. 61.5D**), allowing passage of blood from the right to the left atrium. The valve of the inferior vena cava is so placed as to direct nearly all the richly oxygenated blood from the umbilical vein to the foramen ovale and left atrium, whereas most of the venous blood from the superior vena cava enters the right ventricle directly through the right atrioventricular orifice. The refreshed placental blood, mixed with blood from the portal vein and inferior vena cava, passes almost directly to the aorta for distribution to the head and upper limbs. In contrast, the blood that reaches the descending aorta through the ductus arteriosus is mostly the blood that has circulated through the head and upper limbs, with only a small amount coming from the pulmonary veins and left atrium. This blood is distributed to the abdomen and lower limbs, but principally returns to the placenta.

Changes in the fetal circulation and occlusion of fetal vessels after birth

At birth, as pulmonary respiration begins, increased amounts of blood from the pulmonary trunk traverse the pulmonary arteries to the lungs and return by the pulmonary veins to the left atrium. Consequently, pressure increases within the left atrium. A decrease in pressure also occurs in the inferior vena cava as a result of reduction of venous return concomitant with occlusion of the umbilical vein and ductus venosus. Atrial pressures become equal and the valvular foramen ovale is closed by apposition, and later fusion, of the septum primum to the rims of the foramen. Contraction of the atrial septal muscle, synchronized with that in the superior vena cava, may assist this closure, which occurs after functional closure of the ductus arteriosus. Although the foramen ovale closes functionally after pulmonary respiration is established, it does not become structurally closed until some time later. It is obliterated in fewer than 3% of infants 2 weeks after birth, but in 87% by 4 months after birth. Sometimes fusion is incomplete (p. 1040), and a potential atrial communication (atrial septal defect) persists throughout life. Almost always this has no functional effect, because the inequality of atrial pressures and the valve-like arrangement of the opening do not favour passage of blood. Soon after birth, a number of fetal vessels occlude, but the majority of vessels do not. This differential constriction suggests that the walls of a population of fetal vessels are different than those of the remaining vessels. In many cases, the tunica media contains populations of smooth muscle, elastic fibres and connective tissue that proliferate before birth. Bradykinin, one of the kinin polypeptide hormones that induce contraction or relaxation of smooth muscle, forms in the blood of the umbilical cord when the temperature of the cord decreases at or shortly after birth. It is also formed and released by granular leukocytes in the lungs of the neonate after exposure to adequate oxygen. Bradykinin is a potent constrictor of the umbilical arteries and veins and the ductus arteriosus, while being at the same time a potent inhibitor of contraction of the pulmonary vessels. It has long been realized that intact endothelium is required for the relaxation response to bradykinin.

DUCTUS ARTERIOSUS

In the fetus, the ductus arteriosus shunts blood from the pulmonary trunk to the arch of the aorta, thus bypassing the lungs (**Figs 61.18, 61.31**). It arises as a direct continuation of the pulmonary trunk, where it divides into right and left pulmonary arteries. It is 8–12 mm long, and joins the aorta at an angle of 30–35° on the left side, anterolaterally, below the origin of the left subclavian artery. The opening of the ductus arteriosus into the aorta is greatly elongated. The diameter of the ductus at its origin from the pulmonary trunk, when distended with blood, is 4–5 mm, which is nearly equal to the diameter of the adjacent ascending aorta (5–6 mm). Both arteries taper to a smaller diameter as they pass inferiorly and the aorta remains slightly larger (4 mm; **Fig. 61.31**). In the neonate, the ductus arteriosus is closely related to the left primary bronchus inferiorly and the thymus gland anteriorly.

The ductus arteriosus is very different from the other great vessels arising from the heart. They develop tunicae mediae that are elastic in nature, whereas the ductus has a muscular morphology. A relationship between the recurrent laryngeal branch of the vagus nerve and the developing ductus arteriosus could account for the histological difference in the ductus. The vagus nerve in the stage 16 embryo is very large in relation to the aortic arch system. The recurrent laryngeal nerve has a greater proportion of connective tissue than other nerves, making it more resistant to stretch. It has been suggested that tension applied by the left recurrent laryngeal nerve as it wraps around the ductus arteriosus could provide a means of support that would permit the ductus to develop as a muscular artery, rather than an elastic artery.

It is essential that the ductus arteriosus remains patent during intra-uterine life. Prostaglandins appear to have a role in maintaining this patency. Fetal and neonatal ductal tissue can produce prostaglandins E_2, I_2 and F_2a, which inhibit the ability of the ductus to contract in response to oxygen.

CLOSURE OF THE DUCTUS ARTERIOSUS

Closure of the ductus arteriosus starts immediately after birth, although blood probably continues to flow intermittently through it for a week or so. This flow is reversed relative to that occurring in the fetal circulation as the consequence of the increase in systemic vascular resistance that results from exclusion of the placental circulation, and the decrease in pulmonary resistance that occurs with expansion of the lungs. Initial constriction at birth has been attributed to increased

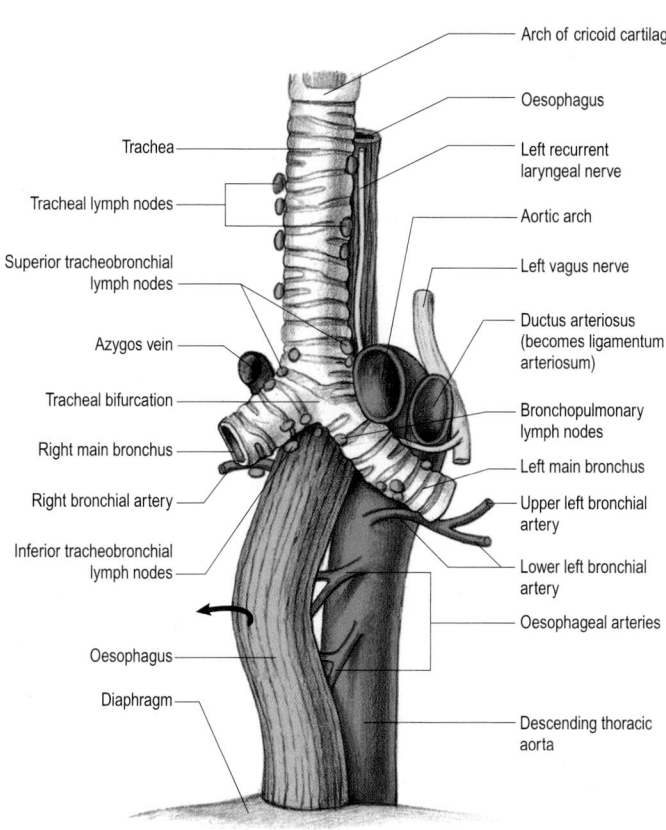

Fig. 61.31 Anterior view with the heart removed to show the relationship between the left primary bronchus, the aortic arch and the ductus arteriosus in a full-term fetus. (After Crelin ES 1969 Anatomy of the Newborn. Philadelphia: Lea and Febiger.)

oxygen tension. A neural factor may also be involved, the muscular wall having afferent and efferent nerve endings and responding to adrenaline (epinephrine) and noradrenaline (nonepinephrine).

The first stage of ductal closure is completed within 10–15 hours and the second stage takes 2–3 weeks. The first stage consists of contraction of the smooth muscle cells and development of subendothelial oedema. Destruction of the endothelium and proliferation of the intima subsequently occurs, leading to permanent closure. Diverse factors have been identified that may promote ductal closure. They include increased oxygen tension; increased plasma catecholamine concentrations, suppression of prostaglandin I_2 production, switching off prostaglandin E receptors, a synergistic role of prostaglandin F_2a and oxygen concentrations and a decrease in plasma adenosine concentration.

After birth, these interrelated events result in the closure of the ductus arteriosus. It has been proposed that the high oxygen tension of the reversed blood flow through the ductus initiates the synthesis of a hydroperoxy fatty acid that suppresses prostacyclin production, thus exposing the ductus to the contractile effects of prostaglandin endoperoxide.

After closure, the duct becomes the ligamentum arteriosum, which connects the left pulmonary artery (near its origin) with the aortic arch.

UMBILICAL VESSELS

UMBILICAL ARTERIES

The umbilical arteries are in direct continuation with the internal iliac arteries (**Fig. 11.4**). Their lumen is c.2–3 mm in diameter at their origin, when distended. This narrows as they approach the umbilicus, where there is a reciprocal thickening of the tunica media, as a result, in particular, of an increase in the number of longitudinal smooth muscle fibres and elastic fibres. Before birth there is a proliferation of connective tissue within the vessel wall. The umbilical vessels constrict in response to handling, stretching, cooling and altered tensions of oxygen and carbon dioxide. Umbilical vessels are muscular, but devoid of a nerve supply in their extra-abdominal course. After the cord is severed the umbilical arteries contract, preventing significant blood loss; thrombi often form in the distal ends of the arteries. The arteries obliterate from their distal ends until, by the end of the second or third month, involution has occurred at the level of the superior vesical arteries. The proximal parts of the obliterated vessels remain as the medial umbilical ligaments.

Umbilical arterial catheterization

Insertion of an umbilical catheter is undertaken to provide direct access to the arterial circulation. Arterial blood can be withdrawn repeatedly for measurement of oxygen and carbon dioxide partial pressures, pH, base excess and many other parameters of blood biochemistry and haematology. The indwelling catheter also enables the continuous measurement of arterial blood pressure.

The catheter is inserted directly into either the cut end or the side of one of the two umbilical arteries in the umbilical cord stump that remains attached to the baby after transection of the umbilical cord at the time of delivery. The catheter tip is then advanced along the length of the umbilical artery, through the internal iliac artery, into the common iliac artery and from there into the aorta. In order to keep the catheter patent, a small volume of fluid is continuously infused through it. It is important that the tip of the catheter should be located well away from arteries branching from the aorta, to avoid potentially harmful perfusion of these arteries with the catheter fluid. Thus umbilical arterial catheter tips are placed in the descending aorta either in a 'high' position, above the coeliac artery but well below the ductus arteriosus, or in a 'low' position, below the renal and inferior mesenteric arteries but above the point where the aorta bifurcates into the two common iliac arteries. The length of catheter to be inserted can be estimated from charts relating the required catheter length to external body measurements, or from birth weight. Positioning of the catheter is assessed by means of radiographs of the abdomen or chest: a 'high' catheter tip should be located in the descending aorta somewhere between the levels of the sixth and ninth thoracic vertebrae (T6–9), while a 'low' catheter tip should be at a level between the third and fourth lumbar vertebrae (L3–4). Relevant anatomical reference points are given in **Table 61.1**.

UMBILICAL VEIN

The umbilical vein in the neonate is 2–3 cm long and 4–5 mm in diameter when distended (**Figs 11.4, 11.5**). It passes from the umbilicus, within the layers of the falciform ligament, superiorly and to the right, to the porta hepatis. Here it gives off several large intrahepatic branches to the liver and then joins the left branch of the portal vein and the ductus venosus. The umbilical vein is thin walled. It possesses a definite internal lamina of elastic fibres at the umbilical ring, but not in its intra-abdominal course. The tunica media contains smooth muscle fibres, collagen and elastic fibres. When the cord is severed, the umbilical vein contracts, but not so vigorously as the arteries. The rapid decrease in pressure in the vein after the cord is clamped means that the elastic tissue at the umbilical ring is sufficient to arrest any retrograde flow along the vessel. Before birth there is a subintimal proliferation of connective tissue around the periphery of the lumen. After birth, the contraction of the collagen fibres in the tunica media and the increased

connective tissue form the ligamentum teres. Obliteration of the vessel occurs from the umbilical ring towards the hepatic end and no thrombi are formed in the obliteration process. For up to 48 hours after birth, the intra-abdominal portion of the umbilical vein can be easily dilated, and in most adults the original lumen of the vein persists through the ligamentum teres and can be dilated to 5–6 mm in diameter.

Ductus venosus

The ductus venosus is a direct continuation of the umbilical vein arising from the left branch of the portal vein, directly opposite the termination of the umbilical vein. The ductus venosus passes for 2–3 cm within the layers of the lesser omentum, in a groove between the left lobe and caudate lobe of the liver. It terminates either in the inferior vena cava, or in the left hepatic vein immediately before it joins the inferior vena cava. The tunica media of the ductus venosus contains circularly arranged smooth muscle fibres, an abundant amount of elastic fibres and some connective tissue. The ductus venosus shuts down by an unknown mechanism. It is already closed in about one-third of newborn infants. Obliteration of this vessel is initiated at the portal vein end and passes to the vena cava. It begins in the second postnatal week and the lumen is completely obliterated by the second or third month after birth. Its fibrous remnant is the ligamentum venosum.

Umbilical vein catheterization

The umbilical vein is catheterized to enable exchange and transfusion of blood, for central venous pressure measurement and, usually in an emergency, for vascular access. The catheter is inserted into the cut end of the umbilical vein and is advanced along the length of the vein, through the ductus venosus and into the inferior vena cava, the tip being placed between the ductus venosus and the right atrium. Positioning of the catheter tip is confirmed radiologically and it should be located just above the diaphragm at a point which is level with the ninth or tenth thoracic vertebrae (T9/T10). As with umbilical arterial catheters, estimation of the required catheter length can be determined from standard charts.

Neonatal arterial and venous vessels

In the neonate, the blood vessels of the trunk, with their associated visceral branches, are relatively larger than those in the limbs, favouring central pooling of blood. Vessels in the periphery are nearly microscopic in the neonate and cannulation poses much more of a problem than in the adult. Large vessels are in the same relative positions as in the adult, but may correspond to different vertebral levels. Thus, although the bifurcation of the common carotid artery into the internal and external carotid arteries occurs at the level of the upper border of the thyroid cartilage, as in the adult, the thyroid cartilage is relatively higher in the neonate neck than in the adult. The renal arteries similarly arise higher, often between T12 and L1 (in the adult they arise at the upper border of L2). The abdominal aorta bifurcates into common iliac arteries at the upper border of L4, rather than at the lower border as in the adult.

CENTRAL VENOUS CATHETERIZATION

Small-bore catheters can be fed into large central veins or into the right atrium via needles or catheters inserted in the peripheral veins. Typically, the median cubital or basilic veins are used in the upper limb and the long saphenous vein at the medial malleolus in the lower limb. The tip of the catheter is sited at the entrance to the right atrium. The required catheter length is assessed from direct measurement of the distance between the point of surface entry in the limb to the right atrium, estimated at midsternal level.

PERIPHERAL ARTERIAL PUNCTURE

It is common practice to insert a small-bore cannula into a peripheral artery in neonates receiving intensive care when either the umbilical artery is not accessible or there are clinical reasons to avoid cannulation of the umbilical vessels. Transillumination can be used to provide an outline of the artery to be cannulated. The peripheral arteries that are most commonly used are the radial artery, just above the anterior surface of the wrist, and the posterior tibial artery, posterior to the medial

Table 61.1 Key anatomical reference points for umbilical arterial catheterization.

Structure	Vertebral level
Ductus	T4–5
Coeliac artery	T12
Superior mesenteric artery	T12–L1
Renal artery	L1
Inferior mesenteric artery	L3
Aortic bifurcation	L4–5

malleolus. The proximity of the ulnar nerve to the ulnar artery increases the risk of nerve damage associated with arterial cannulation of the ulnar artery, and the relatively poor collateral circulation associated with the dorsalis pedis artery means that this artery is used only as a last resort. The brachial artery at the antecubital fossa also has a poor collateral circulation and the median nerve is in close proximity; it is generally considered, therefore, that cannulation of this artery is not justified.

Confirmation that an adequate collateral circulation is present when cannulating the radial artery can be obtained by performing Allen's test, in which both the radial and ulnar arteries are compressed at the wrist after exsanguination of the hand; release of pressure on the ulnar artery while maintaining occlusion of the radial artery should result in reperfusion of the hand if an adequate collateral ulnar arterial supply is present. Alternatively, intact arterial flow can usually be confirmed, particularly in the preterm infant, by direct visualization of the arteries using transillumination. A cold light source is placed on the posterior aspect of the lower forearm and the shadow of the pulsating arteries can be seen on the anterior surface of the forearm.

REFERENCES

Ali MM, Farooqui FA, Sohal GS 2003 Ventrally emigrating neural tube cells contribute to the normal development of heart and great vessels. Vascul Pharmacol 40: 133–40.
Identification of the latest cell line suggested to be involved in heart development.

De la Cruz MV, Markwald RR, Krug EL et al 2001 Living morphogenesis of the ventricles and congenital pathology of their component parts. Cardiol Young 11: 588–600.
Explains the development of a range of cardiac anomalies.

Mjaatvedt CH, Nakaoka T, Moreno-Rodriguez R et al 2001 The outflow tract of the heart is recruited from a novel heart-forming field. Dev Biol 238: 97–109.
Presents experimental evidence establishing the origin of mesenchyme contributing to the heart. Discusses all the cells contributing to heart development.

Moorman AFM, De Jong F, Denyn MMFJ, Lamers WH 1998 Development of the cardiac conduction system. Circ Res 82: 29–644.
The primary ring and its contribution to septation and segmentation of the heart.

Partanen TA, Paavonen K 2001 Lymphatic versus blood vascular endothelial growth factors and receptors in humans. Microsc Res Tech 55: 108–121.
Provides the most up-to-date information on vascular endothelial growth factors in lymphangiogenesis.

Pierpoint MEM, Markwald RR, Lin AE 2000 Genetic aspects of atrioventricular septal defects. Am J Med Genet 97: 289–96.
An overview of transcription factors and signalling molecules involved in atrial septation.

Rodrigues-Niedenfuhr M, Papoutsi M, Christ B et al 2001 Prox-1 is a marker of ectodermal placodes, endodermal compartments, lymphatic endothelium and lymphangioblasts. Anat Embryol (Berl) 204: 399–406.
The distribution of Prox-1 in a range of embryos including human.

Tonar Z, Kocova J, Liska V, Slipkja J 2001 Early development of the jugular lymphatics. Sb Lek 102: 217–25.
Study of human lymphatic vessel and lymph node development.

Wessels A & Markwald RR 2000 Cardiac morphogenesis and dysmorphogenesis. I. Normal development. Methods Mol Biol 136: 239–59.
A general review of cardiac development.

Wessels A, Anderson RH, Markwald RR et al 2000 Atrial development in the human heart: an immunohistochemical study with emphasis on the role of mesenchymal tissues. Anat Rec 259: 288–300.
Detailed information on the dorsal mesocardium and development of the pulmonary veins.

Microstructure of trachea, bronchi and lungs

The trachea, major bronchi and lungs are epithelial–mesenchymal outgrowths of the anterior foregut (Chapter 65), and form tubes which branch dichotomously as they grow. The larger proximal tubes become conducting airways (larynx, trachea, bronchi, bronchioles and terminal bronchioles). The more distal conduits and terminal expansions form the surfaces for respiratory exchange between the atmosphere and adjacent capillaries (respiratory bronchioles, alveolar ducts and sacs and alveoli).

The conducting airways are lined internally by a mucosa (p. 41), and the epithelium lies on a thin connective tissue lamina propria. External to this is a submucosa, also composed of connective tissue, in which are embedded airway smooth muscle, glands, cartilage plates (depending on the level in the respiratory tree), vessels, lymphoid tissue and nerves. Cartilage is present from the trachea to the smallest bronchi but is absent (by definition) from bronchioles.

THE CONDUCTING AIRWAYS

EPITHELIUM (Fig. 62.1)

The epithelia of the trachea, bronchi and bronchioles are in general similar to each other, with graded variations in the numbers of different cell types. The extrapulmonary and larger intrapulmonary passages are lined with respiratory epithelium, which is pseudostratified, predominantly ciliated, and contains interspersed mucus-secreting goblet cells. There are fewer cilia in terminal and respiratory bronchioles, and the cells are reduced in height to low columnar or cuboidal. The epithelium of smaller bronchi and bronchioles is folded into conspicuous longitudinal ridges, which allow for changes in luminal diameter (**Figs 62.1, 62.2, 62.3**). The epithelium in the respiratory bronchioles progressively reduces in height towards the alveoli, and is eventually composed of cuboidal, non-ciliated cells. Respiratory bronchioles have lateral pouches in their walls, which are lined with squamous cells, so providing an accessory respiratory surface.

Six distinct types of epithelial cell have been described in the conducting airways, namely, ciliated columnar, goblet, Clara, basal, brush and neuroendocrine (Jeffery 1990). Lymphocytes and mast cells migrate into the epithelium from the underlying connective tissue.

Ciliated columnar cells – Ciliated columnar cells are the driving force of the mucociliary rejection current (escalator) in the bronchial tree. They vary from low to tall columnar, and each has up to 300 cilia projecting from the apical surface. The cilia extend into a watery fluid secreted by serous cells of the submucosal glands, but their tips are in contact with a more superficial layer of thicker mucus secreted by surface goblet cells and mucous cells in the submucosal glands. The rate of ciliary beating is usually c.12–16 per second, although mechanical stimulation of the epithelial surface, and inflammatory mediators, increase the rate. In addition to tight junctions which seal the apical intercellular space from the airway lumen, the ciliated cells are coupled by gap junctions which allow a change in rate of beating to spread from stimulated cells to their neighbours (probably via calcium) so that their metachronal coordination (p. 19) remains intact.

Goblet cells – Goblet cells are present from the trachea (6000–7000 per mm^2) down to the smaller bronchi, but are normally absent from bronchioles. They contain an apical region full of large secretory vacuoles filled with mucinogen. When the epithelium is irritated, e.g. by tobacco smoke, there is an overall increase in the number of goblet cells, and they also extend into the bronchioles.

Clara cells – Cuboidal non-ciliated cells, with apices which bulge into the lumen. They contain numerous electron-dense secretory granules and many lysosomes. Clara cells produce surfactant lipoprotein and thus share functional similarities with the type II alveolar cell of pulmonary alveoli, although their secretory granules differ in structure and composition. They may also regulate ion transport.

Basal cells – Basal cells are present in parts of the airway which are lined by pseudostratified respiratory epithelium. These small rounded cells are in contact with the basal lamina and are most frequent in the larger conducting passages. Basal cells are mitotic stem cells for other epithelial cell types.

Brush cells – Brush cells are slender, non-ciliated cells with characteristically long, stiff apical microvilli from which they derive their name. Although infrequent, they are present throughout all parts of the conducting airway passages including the respiratory epithelium of the nasopharynx (p. 568). They are in contact with afferent nerve fibres basally and so are considered to have a sensory receptor function.

Neuroendocrine cells – Neuroendocrine cells, also termed dense-core or small granule (Kulchitsky) cells, have a rounded shape, contain numerous small dense-cored vesicles c.150 nm diameter which lie basal to their nuclei, and are found mainly in the basal part of the epithelium. They form part of the dispersed neuroendocrine system of amine precursor uptake and decarboxylation (APUD) cells (p. 180). Neuroendocrine cells are most numerous in fetal lungs. Their number decreases dramatically after birth, although they may proliferate in certain pulmonary diseases. There appears to be little further change in their frequency during adult life.

Lymphocytes – Small lymphocytes, mainly T cells derived from mucosa-associated lymphoid tissue (MALT; p. 77) in the walls of the passages, occur within the epithelium throughout the conducting airway tissues, particularly in the extrapulmonary portion: they are concerned with the immune surveillance of the epithelium. Clusters of lymphocytes sometimes lie beneath non-ciliated epithelial cells of the microfold (M-cell) type (Chapter 72).

Mast cells – Mast cells are present within the basal regions of the epithelium. They resemble connective tissue mast cells, and their cytoplasmic histamine-containing granules are released in response to irritants, including inhaled allergens.

SUBMUCOSAL GLANDS

Tubulo-acinar, seromucous glands are present in the submucosa of the trachea and bronchi and, to a lesser extent, in the larger bronchioles. They contain separate mucous and serous cells, and are an important source of the mucous layer at the surface of the ciliated respiratory epithelium. Their secretions include mucins; the bacteriostatic substances lysozyme and lactoferrin; secretory antibodies (IgA) produced by plasma cells in the submucosal connective tissue; and protease inhibitors (e.g. α_1 antitrypsin) important for neutralizing leukocyte-derived proteases, particularly elastase, in the respiratory tract. The secretory acini and tubules are surrounded by myoepithelial cells, which are innervated by autonomic fibres.

CONNECTIVE TISSUE AND MUSCLE (Figs 62.1, 62.2, 62.3, 62.4)

Broad, longitudinal bands of elastin within the submucosa follow the course of the respiratory tree and connect with the elastin networks

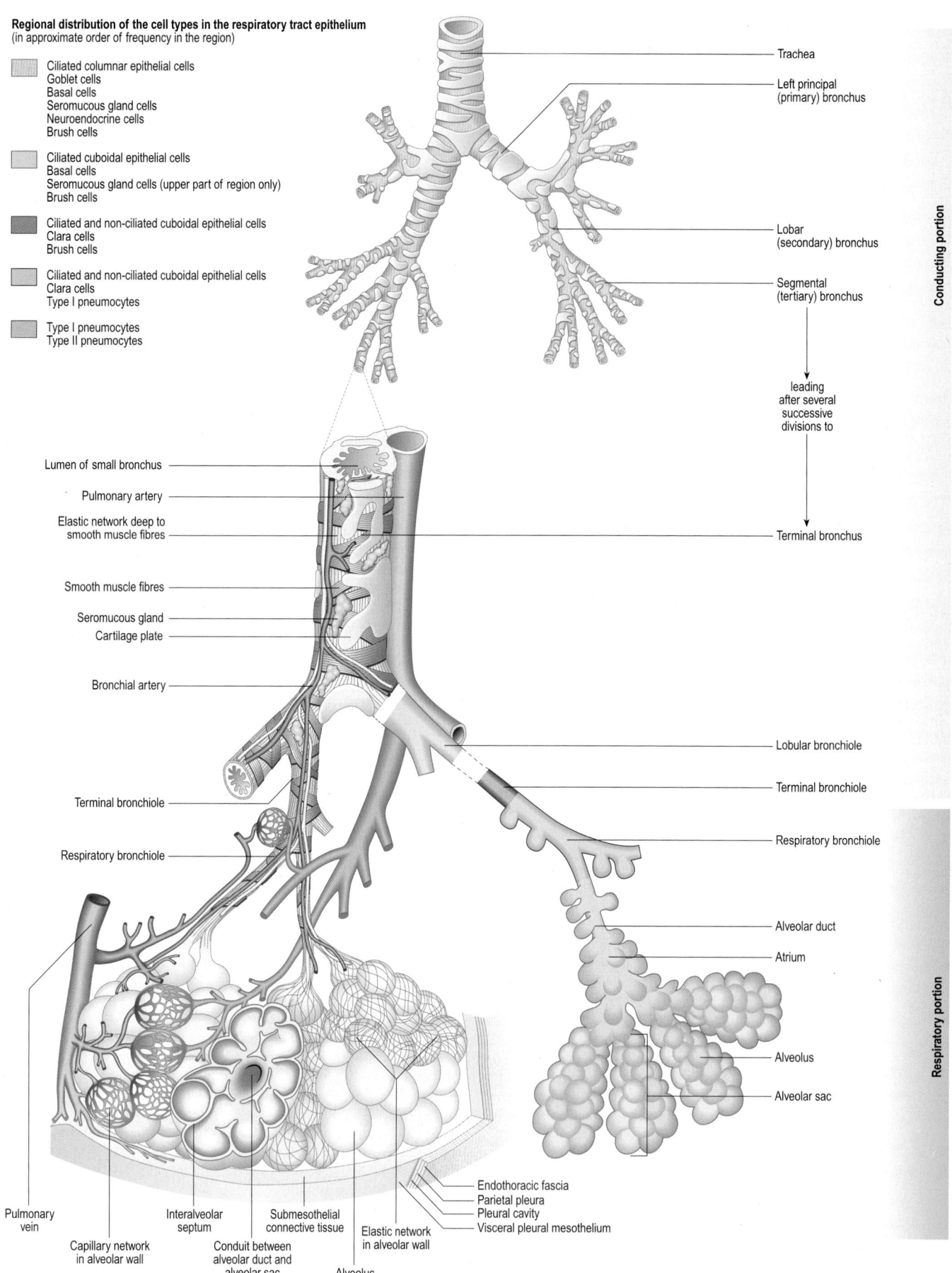

Regional distribution of the cell types in the respiratory tract epithelium
(in approximate order of frequency in the region)

Ciliated columnar epithelial cells
Goblet cells
Basal cells
Seromucous gland cells
Neuroendocrine cells
Brush cells

Ciliated cuboidal epithelial cells
Basal cells
Seromucous gland cells (upper part of region only)
Brush cells

Ciliated and non-ciliated cuboidal epithelial cells
Clara cells
Brush cells

Ciliated and non-ciliated cuboidal epithelial cells
Clara cells
Type I pneumocytes

Type I pneumocytes
Type II pneumocytes

Trachea

Left principal (primary) bronchus

Lobar (secondary) bronchus

Segmental (tertiary) bronchus

leading after several successive divisions to

Terminal bronchus

Conducting portion

Lumen of small bronchus

Pulmonary artery

Elastic network deep to smooth muscle fibres

Smooth muscle fibres

Seromucous gland

Cartilage plate

Bronchial artery

Lobular bronchiole

Terminal bronchiole

Respiratory bronchiole

Terminal bronchiole

Respiratory bronchiole

Alveolar duct

Atrium

Alveolus

Alveolar sac

Respiratory portion

Endothoracic fascia
Parietal pleura
Pleural cavity
Visceral pleural mesothelium

Pulmonary vein

Capillary network in alveolar wall

Interalveolar septum

Conduit between alveolar duct and alveolar sac

Submesothelial connective tissue

Alveolus

Elastic network in alveolar wall

Fig. 62.1 The respiratory tree and its blood supply and drainage, lymphatic drainage and nerve supply. The distribution of the different epithelial cells is shown. Blue = vessels which contain deoxygenated blood; red = vessels which contain oxygenated blood.

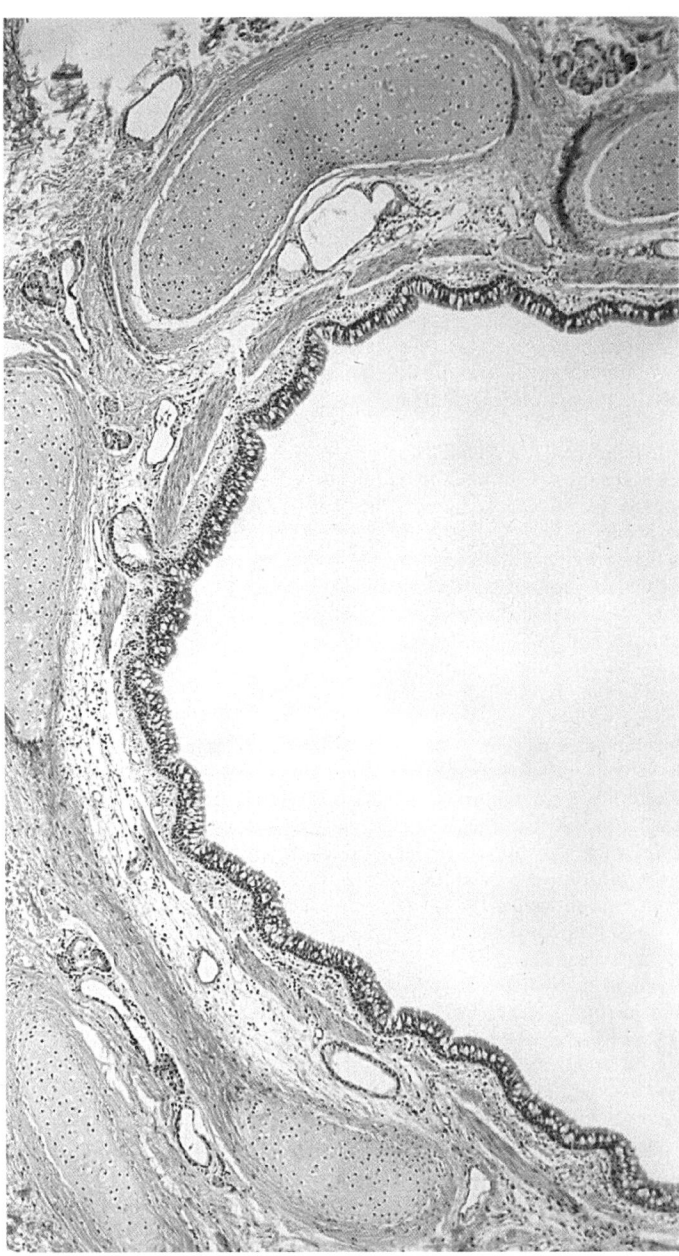

Fig. 62.2 Micrograph of the wall of a bronchus, showing the respiratory epithelial lining, bundles of smooth muscle underlying the mucosa, discontinuous cartilage plates and submucosal seromucous glands. (By permission from Kierszenbaum AL 2002 Histology and Cell Biology. St Louis: Mosby.)

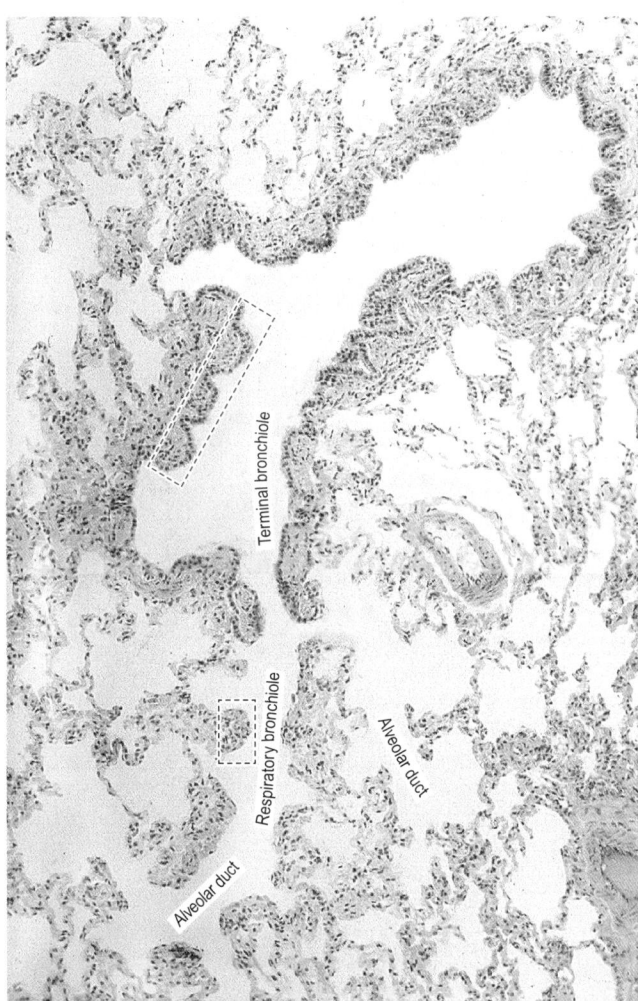

Fig. 62.3 Micrograph of a small bronchiole leading into a terminal bronchiole, respiratory bronchiole and alveolar ducts and sacs. Boxes show mucosal protrusions caused by contraction of underlying smooth muscle. (By permission from Kierszenbaum AL 2002 Histology and Cell Biology. St Louis: Mosby.)

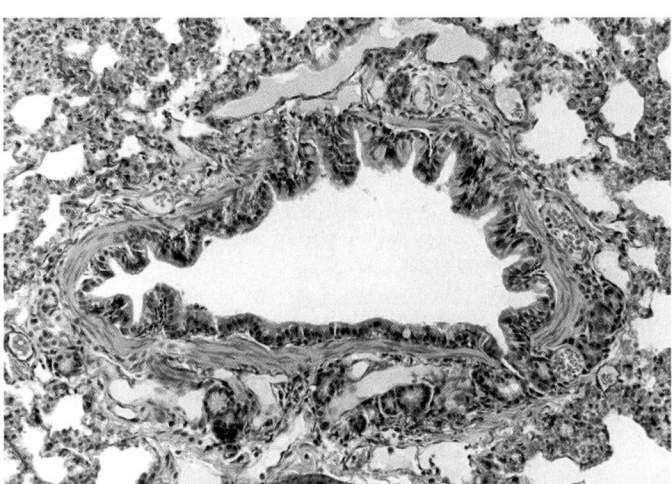

Fig. 62.4 Larger bronchiole stained for elastin, showing smooth muscle in the bronchiolar wall and a few small seromucous glands (below).

of the interalveolar septa (see below). This elastic framework is a vital mechanical element of the lung, and is responsible for elastic recoil during expiration.

In the trachea and extrapulmonary bronchi, the smooth muscle is mainly confined to the posterior, non-cartilaginous part of the tracheal tube. Along the entire intrapulmonary bronchial tree, smooth muscle forms two opposed helical tracts which become thinner and finally disappear at the level of the alveoli. The tone of these muscle fibres is under nervous and hormonal control: groups of muscle cells are coupled by gap junctions to spread excitation within fascicles.

Muscle cell contraction narrows the airway, while relaxation permits bronchodilation. Some tone normally exists in the muscular bands, which relax slightly during inspiration and contract during expiration, thereby assisting the tidal flow of air. Abnormal contraction may be caused by circulating smooth muscle stimulants or by local release of excitants such as serotonin, histamine and leukotrienes, which produces bronchospasm. Numerous mast cells are present in the connective tissue of the respiratory tree, especially towards the bronchioles.

CARTILAGINOUS SUPPORT

The trachea and extrapulmonary bronchi contain a framework of incomplete rings of hyaline cartilage (**Figs 63.12, 62.5**) which are united by fibrous tissue and smooth muscle. Intrapulmonary bronchi contain discontinuous plates or islands of hyaline cartilage in their walls.

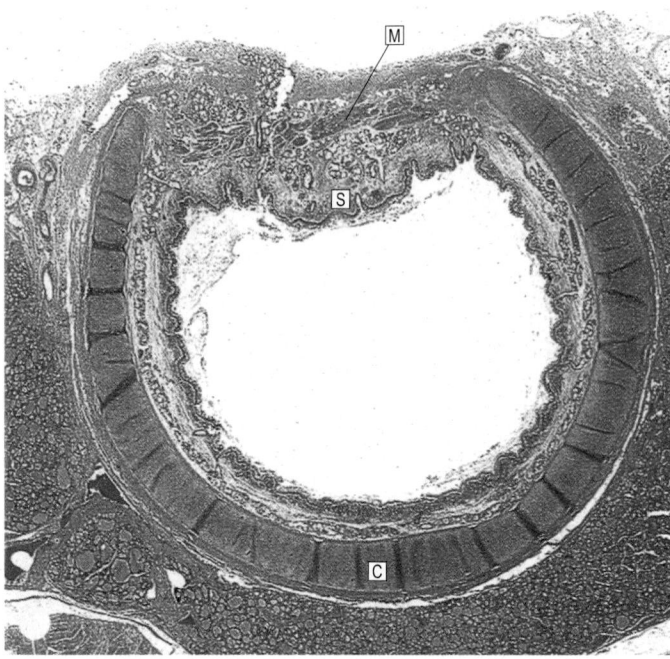

Fig. 62.5 Micrograph of the trachea of a child, sectioned transversely, showing an incomplete cartilage ring (C), joined posteriorly by muscular tissue (M). Seromucous submucosal glands (S) are concentrated in this region and between adjacent cartilages. (By permission from Stevens A, Lowe JS 1996 Human Histology, 2nd edn. London: Mosby.)

Tracheal cartilages – Tracheal cartilages vary from 16 to 20 in number. Anteriorly, each cartilage takes the form of an incomplete ring which surrounds approximately two-thirds of the tracheal circumference (p. 1075). Posteriorly, where the cartilages are deficient, the tube is flat and is completed by fibroelastic tissue and smooth muscle. The cartilages are horizontally stacked and separated by narrow intervals. They are c.4 mm vertically, and c.1 mm thick. Their external surfaces are vertically flat, and their internal surfaces are convex. Two or more cartilages often unite, partially or completely, and sometimes bifurcate at their ends. They may become calcified in the elderly. The cartilages are shorter, narrower and less regular in extrapulmonary bronchi, but they are generally similar in shape and arrangement.

The first and last tracheal cartilages differ from the rest (**Fig. 63.12**). The first cartilage is the broadest. It often bifurcates at one end and is connected by the cricotracheal ligament to the inferior border of the cricoid cartilage, with which it may blend. It may also blend with the second cartilage. The last cartilage is centrally thick and broad and its lower border, the carina, is a triangular hook-shaped process, which curves down and backwards between the bronchi. It forms an incomplete ring on each side, and encloses the start of a principal bronchus.

Bronchial cartilages – The irregularity of the cartilaginous plates in the extrapulmonary bronchi increases as they are traced distally. As the major bronchi approach their lungs and lobes, the plates surround their dorsal aspects. In intrapulmonary bronchi, discontinuous plates of cartilage progressively form less and less of the bronchial wall, and they are not present in the bronchioles (**Fig. 62.2**).

SEROSA

The serosa is formed by the visceral pleura (p. 1067) which is a transparent single sheet of mesothelium covering a thin lamina propria of connective tissue, and is closely attached to the various structures of the lung, except at the hilum. Beneath the serosa, loose connective tissue covers the entire pulmonary surface: it extends from the hilum along the conducting tubes and blood vessels within the substance of the lung. The connective tissue partitions the lung into numerous small lung lobules. These are small polyhedral tissue masses which each receives a lobular bronchiole and the terminal branches of arterioles, venules, lymphatics and nerves. Lobules vary in size, the superficial ones are the largest, and are visible as polygonal areas c.5–15 mm across.

RESPIRATORY SURFACES

Thin-walled respiratory surfaces (alveoli) are distributed as isolated patches within the walls of respiratory bronchi, and as tube-like alveolar ducts and balloon-like alveolar sacs which contain groups of adjacent alveoli (**Fig. 62.3**).

ALVEOLAR AREA

Normal adult human alveoli have a mean total surface area of 143 m^2: an adult respiratory system contains c.300 million alveoli. Their inflated diameter (c.250 μm) varies with lung position, and is greater in the upper regions than in the lower, because of the increased gravitational pressure at the lung base. These values vary considerably between normal young individuals, and the differences become even more marked with age as a result of degenerative changes.

ALVEOLAR STRUCTURE (Figs 62.1, 62.6, 62.7, 62.8, 62.9)

The alveoli are thin-walled pouches which provide the respiratory surface for gaseous exchange. Their walls contain two types of epithelial cell (pneumocytes), which cover a delicate connective tissue within which a network of capillaries ramify. Since the walls are extremely thin, they present a minimal barrier to gaseous exchange between the atmosphere and the blood in the capillaries. Adjacent alveoli are frequently in close contact and then the intervening connective tissue forms the central part of an interalveolar septum. Alveolar macrophages are present within the alveolar lumen, and migrate over the epithelial surface.

Interalveolar septum – The alveolar lining epithelium varies in thickness, but extensive areas of it are as little as 0.05 μm thick (see below). The epithelium lies on a basal lamina, which, in the thin portions of a septum, is fused with the basal lamina surrounding the adjacent capillaries. The total barrier to diffusion between air and blood in these thin portions may be as little as 0.2 μm. The thick portions of a septum contain connective tissue elements, including elastic fibres, collagen type III fibres, resident and migratory cells (**Fig. 62.6**).

Alveolar epithelial cells (pneumocytes) – The alveolar epithelium is a mosaic of Types I and II pneumocytes. Type I pneumocytes form over 90% of the alveolar area and share a fused basal lamina with that of the adjacent capillary endothelium to form the thin portions of interalveolar septa. They are simple squamous epithelial cells with a thin cytoplasm (0.05–0.2 μm) which extends from a thicker perinuclear region, and facilitates gaseous diffusion between the lumen of the alveolus and its capillaries. The edges of adjacent cells overlap, and they are joined by tight junctions which create a strict diffusion barrier between the alveolar surface and underlying tissues. Together with a similar endothelial barrier, this arrangement limits the movement of fluid from blood and interstitial spaces into the alveolar lumen (the blood–air barrier). If damaged, type I cells, which do not divide, are replaced by the proliferation of type II cells which are able to differentiate into type I pneumocytes.

The smaller type II cells are often more numerous than type I cells, but they contribute less than 10% of the surface area. They are rounded cells which protrude from the alveolar surface, particularly at the angles between alveolar profiles. In the human lung they are often associated with interalveolar pores of Köhn. Their cytoplasm contains numerous characteristic secretory lamellar bodies (**Fig. 62.9**), which they can recycle. Ultrastructurally, the lamellar bodies are comprised of concentric whorls of phospholipid-rich membrane, the precursors of alveolar surfactant.

Interalveolar pores (of Köhn) – These are small pores lined by epithelium (usually type II alveolar cells), which cross interalveolar septa to link adjacent alveolar air spaces. Humans have up to seven pores per alveolus, ranging in size from 2 to 13 μm. These small passages may sustain the flow of air, in the event of blockage of one of the alveolar ducts. They are also routes of migration for alveolar macrophages.

Alveolar macrophages – Like macrophages in other sites in the body (p. 80), alveolar macrophages are derived from circulating monocyte precursors. They originate in haemopoietic tissue in the bone marrow, migrate into the alveolar lumen from adjacent blood vessels and connective tissue, and wander about on the epithelial surfaces. Alveolar macrophages clear the respiratory spaces of inhaled particles which

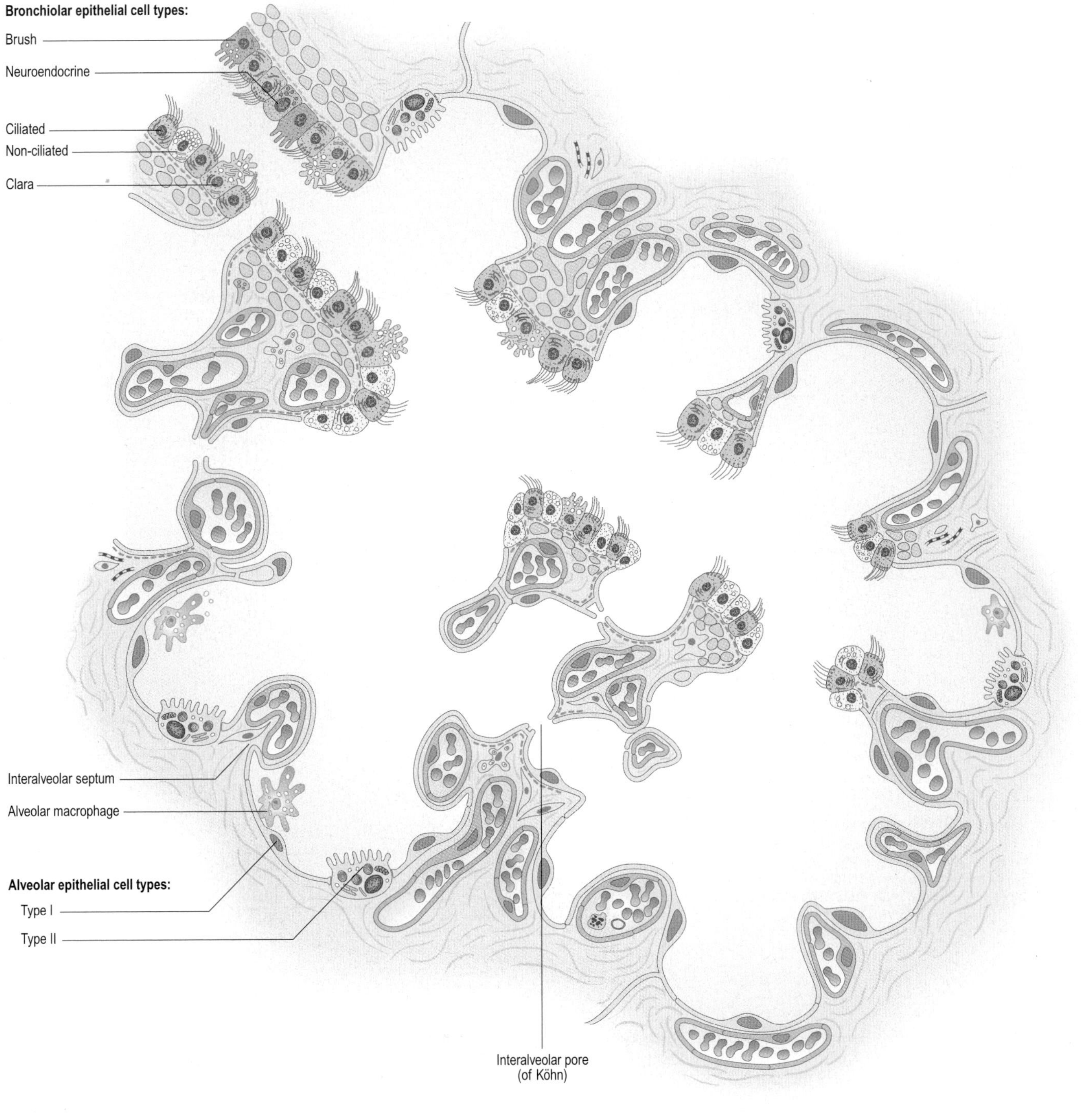

Bronchiolar epithelial cell types:

Brush

Neuroendocrine

Ciliated

Non-ciliated

Clara

Interalveolar septum

Alveolar macrophage

Alveolar epithelial cell types:

Type I

Type II

Interalveolar pore
(of Köhn)

Fig. 62.6 The respiratory portion of the lung and its cell types.

are small enough to reach the alveoli, hence their alternative name of dust cells. Most of them migrate with their phagocytosed load to the bronchioles where they are swept into the mucociliary rejection current and removed from the lung. Others migrate through the epithelium of the alveoli into the lymphatics which drain the lung connective tissue, and thence into lymphoid tissue around the pulmonary lobules. Under normal conditions these cells have a granular cytoplasm because they contain phagocytosed particles: in smokers the latter have a characteristic appearance, and are called tar bodies.

Alveolar macrophages can be recovered from sputum, and are of diagnostic importance if they appear abnormal, for instance, whenever erythrocytes leak from pulmonary capillaries, macrophages which engulf red cells become brick red, and are detectable in 'rusty' sputum. They are typical of congestive heart failure, and therefore often termed heart-failure cells. Macrophages which have migrated back into the connective tissue of the lung settle in patches which are visible beneath

the visceral pleura, e.g. carbon-filled cells give the lungs a mottled appearance. However, if the inhaled particles are abrasive or chemically active, they may elude macrophage removal, and instead damage the respiratory surface, which produces fibrosis and a concomitant reduction in the respiratory area. This occurs in many industrial diseases, e.g. pneumoconiosis, which is due to coal dust, or asbestosis, where the long thin fibres of asbestos can cause considerable damage and may trigger fatal mesothelioma in the pleural lining. When actively phagocytic, macrophages release proteases: if antiproteases (e.g. α_1 antitrypsin), which are normally present in the alveolar lining, are deficient, then macrophage activity may damage the lung. Alveolar macrophages are also involved in the turnover of surfactant.

In pathological conditions other cells, e.g. neutrophil leukocytes and lymphocytes, may enter the alveoli and other parts of the respiratory tree, and their presence imparts a characteristic yellow appearance to the sputum.

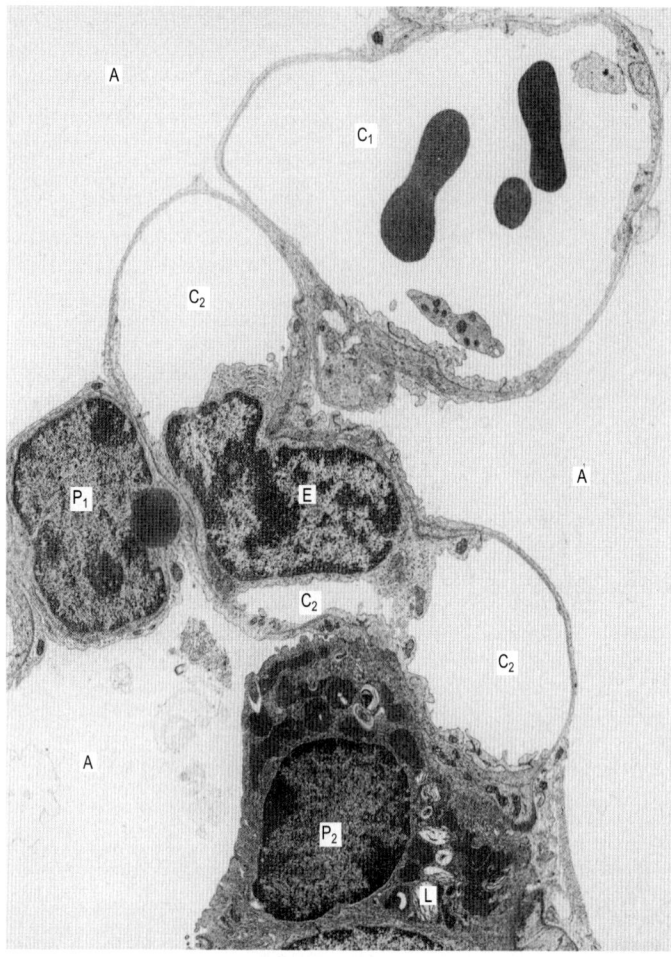

Fig. 62.7 Electron micrograph showing the alveolar septum between three adjacent alveoli (A). The septum contains two capillaries (C_1 and C_2) in section; the lower one is cut obliquely through the nucleus of one of its endothelial lining cells and its lumen in three places. Type I pneumocytes (P_1) line the alveolar air spaces except where a type II pneumocyte ((P_2) bottom centre), with cytoplasmic lamellar bodies, is located. (By permission from Young B, Heath JW 2000 Wheater's Functional Histology. Edinburgh: Churchill Livingstone.)

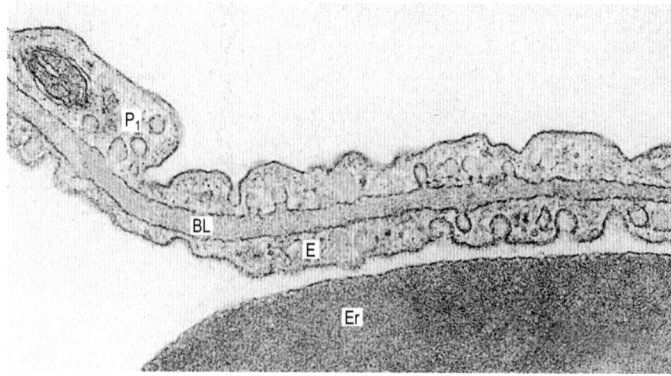

Fig. 62.8 Electron micrograph of the thin portion of an interalveolar septum. Part of an erythrocyte (Er) is shown in the capillary lumen (bottom), which is lined by endothelium (E). The alveolar air space (top) is lined by a type I pneumocyte (P_1). Between the attenuated cytoplasm of the two cells is a shared basal lamina (BL). (By permission from Young B, Heath JW 2000 Wheater's Functional Histology. Edinburgh: Churchill Livingstone.)

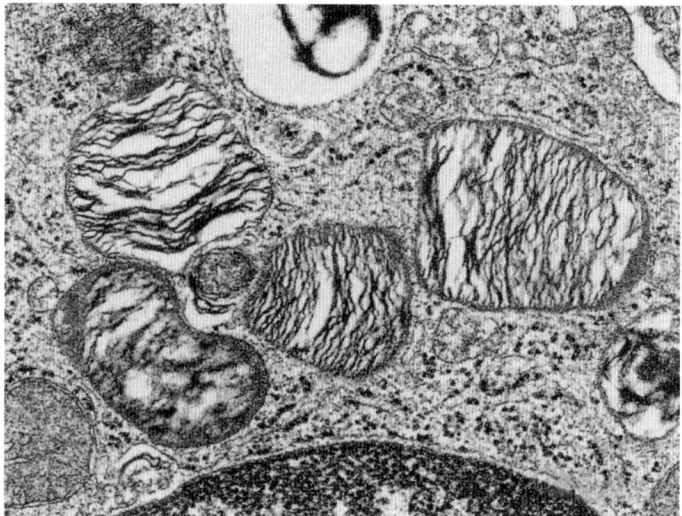

Fig. 62.9 Electron micrograph of cytoplasmic lamellar bodies in a Type II pneumocyte. They are composed mainly of phospholipids which are released by exocytosis and contribute to the surfactant secreted by these pneumocytes and Clara cells of the respiratory bronchioles. (By permission from Young B, Heath JW 2000 Wheater's Functional Histology. Edinburgh: Churchill Livingstone.)

ALVEOLAR SURFACTANT

The alveolar surface is normally covered by a film of pulmonary surfactant, which is a complex mixture, mainly of phospholipids (particularly dipalmitoylphosphatidylcholine and phosphatidylglycerol), with some protein and neutral lipid (Devendra & Spragg 2002). Surfactant is stored in lamellar bodies and secreted in the form of tubular myelin (unrelated to myelin of the nervous system) by type II pneumocytes. It is recycled by type II pneumocytes, or cleared (phagocytosed) by alveolar macrophages. Clara cells of the bronchiolar epithelium are believed to secrete surfactant of a different composition.

Surface tension at the alveolar surface is very high, because the alveoli are minute. This opposes expansion during inspiration, and tends to collapse the alveoli in expiration. The detergent-like properties of pulmonary surfactant greatly reduce the surface tension, and make ventilation of the alveoli much more efficient.

REFERENCES

Devendra G, Spragg RG 2002 Lung surfactant in subacute pulmonary disease. Respir Res 3: 19–22.

Jeffrey PK 2003 Microscopic structure of the lung. In: Gibson GJ, Geddes DM, Costabel V, Stok PJ, Corrin B (eds), Respiratory Medicine, 3rd edn. London: Elsevier Science: 34–50.

Pleura, lungs, trachea and bronchi

The lungs are the essential organs of respiration and are responsible for the uptake of oxygen into the blood and the removal of carbon dioxide. The functional design of the thorax facilitates this complex process. The muscles of respiration and the diaphragm act together to increase the intrathoracic volume: this creates a negative pressure within the pleural space surrounding the lung and causes expansion of the lung. The resultant reduction in the intra-alveolar pressure prompts the conduction of air through the upper respiratory tract into the trachea and airways and thence into the alveoli where gas exchange occurs. The process of breathing exposes the lung to noxious agents including gases, dust particles, bacteria and viruses. The mucous barrier, mucociliary escalator, branching pattern of the airways and the cough reflex are all anatomical defences against these insults. Anatomical defects may compromise respiratory function: for example, chest wall abnormalities may cause restrictive lung disease. Similarly, ultrastructural abnormalities such as ciliary dysfunction (as seen in Kartagener's syndrome) lead to recurrent respiratory infections and airway damage.

PLEURA (Figs 63.1, 63.2, 63.3, 63.4)

Each lung is covered by pleura, a serous membrane arranged as a closed invaginated sac. The visceral or pulmonary pleura adheres closely to the pulmonary surface and its interlobar fissures. Its continuation, the parietal pleura, lines the corresponding half of the thoracic wall and covers much of the diaphragm and structures occupying the middle region of the thorax. The visceral and parietal pleurae are continuous with each other around the hilar structures, and they remain in close, though sliding, contact at all phases of respiration. The potential space between them is the pleural cavity, which is maintained at a negative pressure by the inward elastic recoil of the lung and the outward pull of the chest wall. Any breach of the chest wall and parietal pleura or visceral pleura consequently leads to the accumulation of air within the pleural cavity (pneumothorax). Fluid (hydrothorax), blood (haemothorax) and rarely lymph (chylothorax) can also accumulate in this space. Pneumothoraces may occur spontaneously or following trauma (e.g. rib fractures, penetrating injuries from sharp instruments, iatrogenic injury). Significant air in the pleural space is visible on a chest radiograph: there is separation of the parietal and visceral pleurae and an absence of pulmonary vascular markings in the corresponding area. Occasionally a ball valve-like effect occurs so that air enters the pleural space during inspiration but cannot escape in expiration. This tension pneumothorax can be life threatening and should be suspected whenever there are unilateral decreased breath sounds and hyperresonance on percussion, hypotension, jugular venous distension and contralateral tracheal deviation. A tension pneumothorax requires immediate decompression by the insertion of an intercostal drain or wide bore catheter. Fluid collection in the pleural space may be due to congestive cardiac failure, hypoalbuminaemia, inflammatory, infective, or neoplastic conditions. A pleural effusion causes obliteration of the costophrenic angle and the diaphragm, and a lateral meniscus is visible on a frontal chest radiograph. Drainage of the fluid and subsequent analysis is required for diagnostic purposes. Where there is a collection of pus (empyema) or blood, pleural drainage is essential for therapeutic purposes. Ultrasonography is useful in assessing the size and characteristics of an effusion such as the presence of loculation and debris. It may even demonstrate underlying consolidated lung. Computed tomography is utilized to assess the underlying hidden lung parenchyma and mediastinal glands. For further review of the radiology of the pleurae and lungs, see Armstrong (2000).

The right and left pleural sacs form separate compartments and touch only behind the upper half of the sternal body (**Figs 63.2, 63.3**), although they are also close to each other behind the oesophagus at the midthoracic level. The region between them is the mediastinum (interpleural space). The left pleural cavity is the smaller of the two because the heart extends further to the left. The upper and lower limits of the pleurae are about the same on the two sides, but the left sometimes descends lower in the midaxillary line.

The interlobar fissures (p. 1068) and posterior azygo-oesophageal and retrosternal pleural reflections are the only aspects of the normal pleura that can be visualized on a chest radiograph or CT scan (**Figs 63.8, 63.9**). Demonstration of significant pleural shadowing in any other region usually implies pathological abnormalities of the pleura. Thoracoscopy allows the direct inspection of both the parietal and visceral surfaces. The parietal pleura is translucent and at thoracoscopy the underlying muscles and blood vessels are visible. The visceral pleura is also translucent and has a grey variegated appearance due to the underlying lung and the vascular network in the subpleural layer.

PARIETAL PLEURA

Different regions of parietal pleura are customarily distinguished by name: costovertebral (lines the internal surface of the thoracic wall and the vertebral bodies); diaphragmatic (lies on the thoracic surface of the diaphragm); cervical (lies over the pulmonary apices, and is therefore also called the dome of the pleura); mediastinal (applied to the structures between the lungs).

Costovertebral pleura – Costovertebral pleura lines the sternum, ribs, transversus thoracis and intercostal muscles and the sides of the vertebral bodies, and is easily separated from them. External to the pleura is a thin layer of loose connective tissue, the endothoracic fascia, which corresponds to the transversalis fascia of the abdominal wall. In front, the costal pleura begins behind the sternum where it is continuous with the mediastinal pleura, along a junction extending from behind the sternoclavicular joint down and medially to the midline behind the sternal angle. From here, the right and left costal pleurae descend in contact with each other to the level of the fourth costal cartilages and then diverge. On the right side, the line descends to the back of the xiphisternal joint, while on the left the line diverges laterally and descends at a distance of 2–25 mm from the sternal margin to the sixth costal cartilage, forming the cardiac notch. On each side the costal pleura sweeps laterally, lining the internal surfaces of the costal cartilages, ribs, transversus thoracis and intercostal muscles. Posteriorly it passes over the sympathetic trunk and its branches to reach the sides of the vertebral bodies, where it is again continuous with the mediastinal pleura. The costovertebral pleura is continuous with the cervical pleura at the inner margin of the first rib and below it becomes continuous with the diaphragmatic pleura along a line which differs slightly on the two sides. On the right, this line of costodiaphragmatic reflection begins behind the xiphoid process, passes behind the seventh costal cartilage to reach the eighth rib in the midclavicular line, the tenth rib in the midaxillary line, and then ascends slightly to cross the twelfth rib level with the upper border of the twelfth thoracic spine (**Figs 63.2, 63.3, 63.4**). On the left, the line initially follows the ascending part of the sixth costal cartilage, but then follows a course similar to that on the right, although it may be slightly lower.

Diaphragmatic pleura – The diaphragmatic pleura is a thin, tightly adherent layer which covers most of the upper surface of the diaphragm.

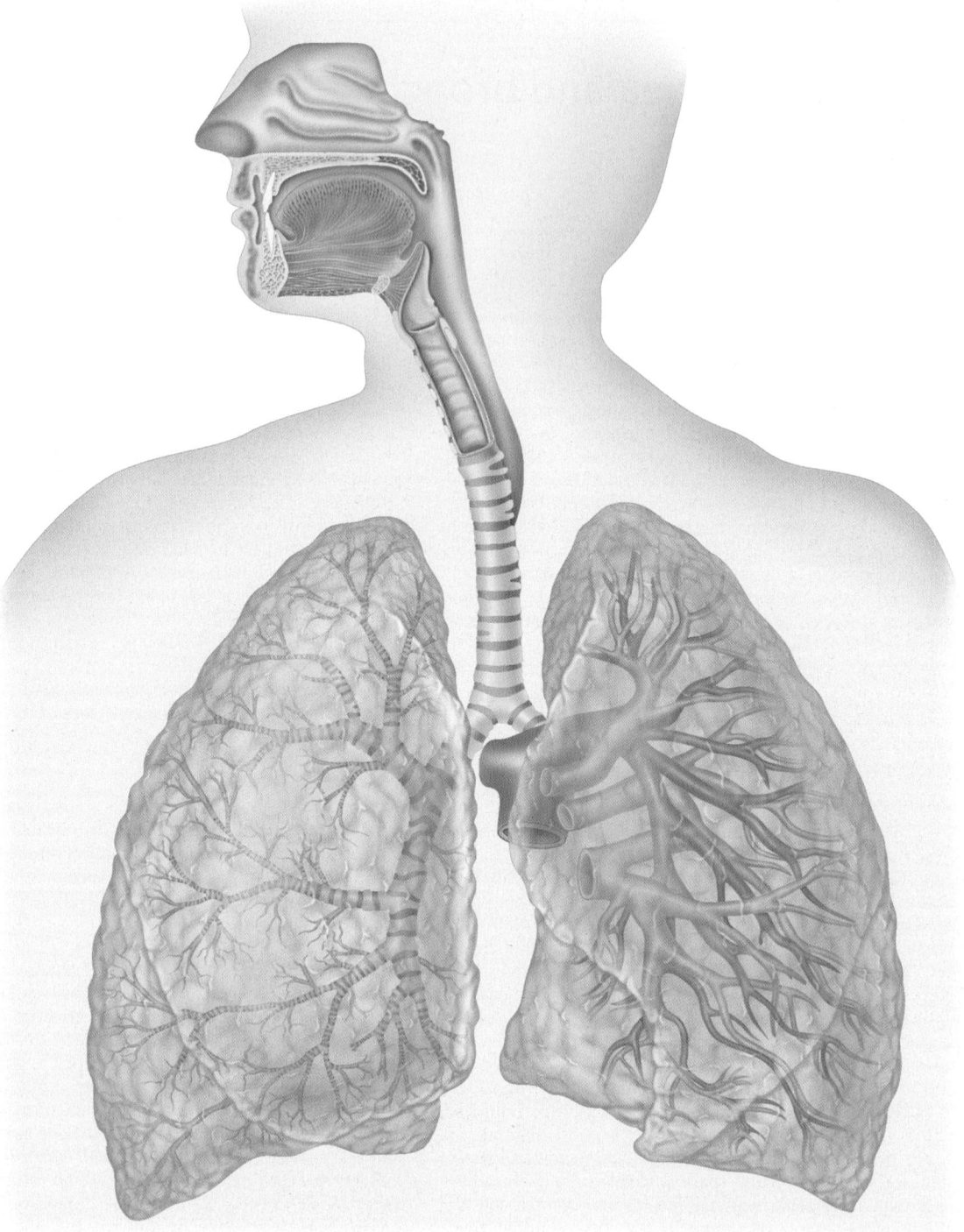

Fig. 63.1 The respiratory tract. Those parts of the tract in the head and upper neck are shown in sagittal section, in the lower neck turned anteriorly and, in the remainder of the tract, from the anterior aspect. The right lung shows the bronchial tree in detail whereas the left lung shows the pulmonary vasculature.

It is continuous with the costal pleura and on its medial aspect is continuous with the mediastinal pleura along the line of attachment of the pericardium to the diaphragm.

Cervical pleura – The cervical pleura is a continuation of the costo-vertebral pleura over the pulmonary apex (**Fig. 63.5**). It ascends medially from the internal border of the first rib to the apex of the lung, as high as the lower edge of the neck of the first rib, and then descends lateral to the trachea to become the mediastinal pleura. As a result of the obliquity of the first rib, the cervical pleura extends 3–4 cm above the first costal cartilage, but not above the neck of the first rib. The cervical pleura is strengthened by a fascial suprapleural membrane, which is attached in front to the internal border of the first rib, and behind to the

anterior border of the transverse process of the seventh cervical vertebra. It contains a few muscular fibres, which spread from the scaleni. Scalenus minimus extends from the anterior border of the transverse process of the seventh cervical vertebra to the inner border of the first rib behind its subclavian groove, and also spreads into the pleural dome, which it therefore tenses: it has been suggested that the suprapleural membrane is the tendon of scalenus medius. The cervical pleura (like the pulmonary apex) reaches the level of the seventh cervical spine 2.5 cm from the midline. Its projection is a curved line from the sternoclavicular joint to the junction of the medial and middle thirds of the clavicle, its summit being 2.5 cm above it. The subclavian artery ascends laterally in a furrow below the summit of the cervical pleura (p. 1068, **Fig. 63.5**).

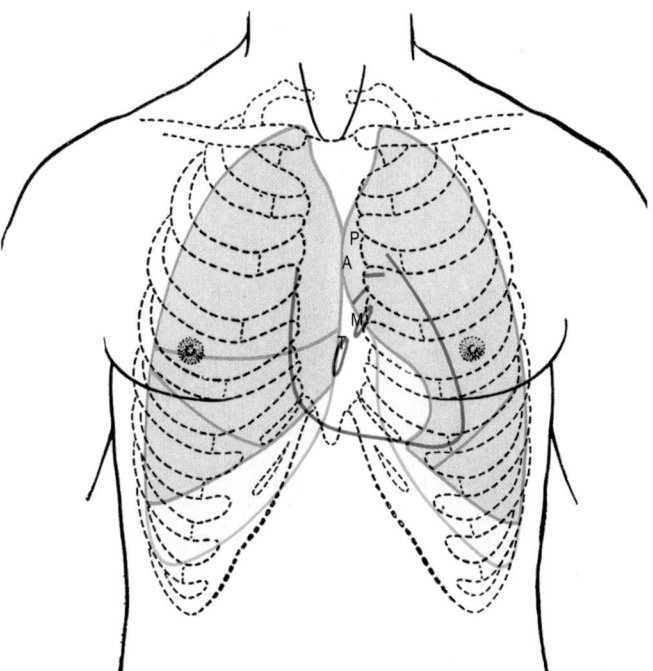

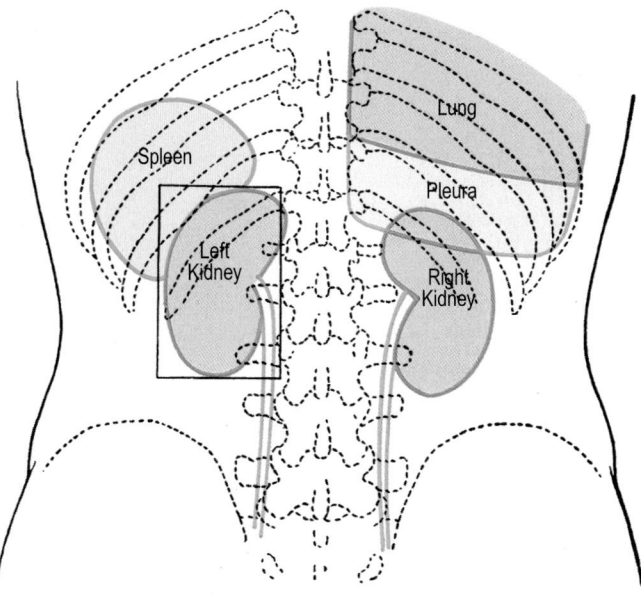

Fig. 63.4 The lower limits of the lung and pleura: posterior view. The lower portions of the lung and pleura are shown on the right side.

Fig. 63.2 Ventral aspect of the thorax, showing surface projections: purple, pulmonary; blue, pleural; red outline, cardiac. **A**, orifice of aorta; **M**, left atrioventricular (mitral) orifice; **P**, orifice of pulmonary trunk; T, right atrioventricular (tricuspid) orifice. Skeletal structures are indicated by broken lines.

Mediastinal pleura – The mediastinal pleura is the lateral boundary of the mediastinum and forms a continuous surface above the hilum of the lung from sternum to vertebral column. On the right it covers the right brachiocephalic vein, the upper part of the superior vena cava, the terminal part of the azygos vein, the right phrenic and vagus nerves, the trachea and oesophagus. On the left it covers the aortic arch, left phrenic and vagus nerves, left brachiocephalic and superior intercostal veins, left common carotid and subclavian arteries, thoracic duct and oesophagus. At the hilum of the lung it turns laterally to form a tube that encloses the hilar structures and is continuous with the pulmonary pleura.

VISCERAL PLEURA
The pulmonary pleura is inseparably adherent to the lung over all its surfaces including those in the fissures, except at the root or hilum of the lung and along a line descending from this, which marks the attachment of the pulmonary ligament (**Figs 63.6, 63.7**).

INFERIOR PULMONARY LIGAMENTS
Below the hilum the mediastinal pleura extends as a double layer, the pulmonary ligament, from the lateral surface of the oesophagus to the mediastinal surface of the lung, where it is continuous with the parietal pleura (**Figs 63.6, 63.7**). It is continuous above with the pleura around the hilar structures and below it ends in a free sickle-shaped border.

PLEURAL RECESSES
The pleura extends considerably beyond the inferior border of the lung, but not as far as the attachment of the diaphragm, which means that the diaphragm is in contact with the costal cartilages and intercostal muscles below the line of pleural reflection from the thoracic wall to the diaphragm. In quiet inspiration the inferior margin of the lung does not reach this reflection, and the costal and diaphragmatic pleurae are separated merely by a narrow slit, the costodiaphragmatic recess. In quiet inspiration the lower limit of the lung is c.5 cm above the lower pleural limit. A similar costomediastinal recess exists behind the sternum and the costal cartilages, where the thin anterior margin of the lung falls short of the line of pleural reflection (**Fig. 60.4**). The extent of this recess, the anterior costomediastinal line of pleural reflection, and the position of the anterior margin of the lung all exhibit individual variation.

The inferior border of the right costodiaphragmatic recess is an important consideration in the surgical posterior approach to the kidney. Usually the pleura crosses the twelfth rib at the lateral border of erector spinae, so that the medial region of the kidney is above the pleural reflection (**Fig. 63.4**). If this rib does not project beyond this

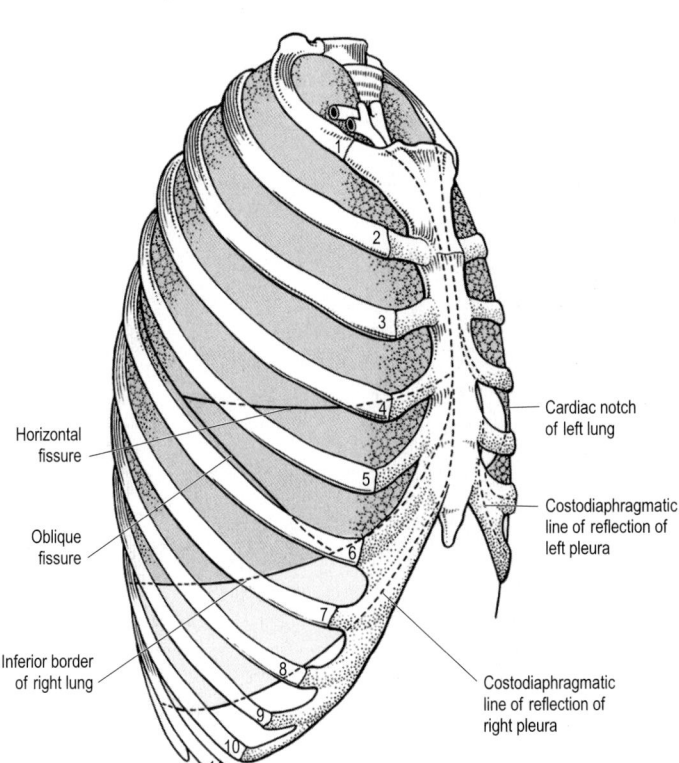

Horizontal fissure

Oblique fissure

Inferior border of right lung

Cardiac notch of left lung

Costodiaphragmatic line of reflection of left pleura

Costodiaphragmatic line of reflection of right pleura

Fig. 63.3 The relations of the pleurae and lungs to the chest wall: right lateral aspect. Purple, lungs, covered with the pleural sacs; blue, pleural sac, with no underlying lung.

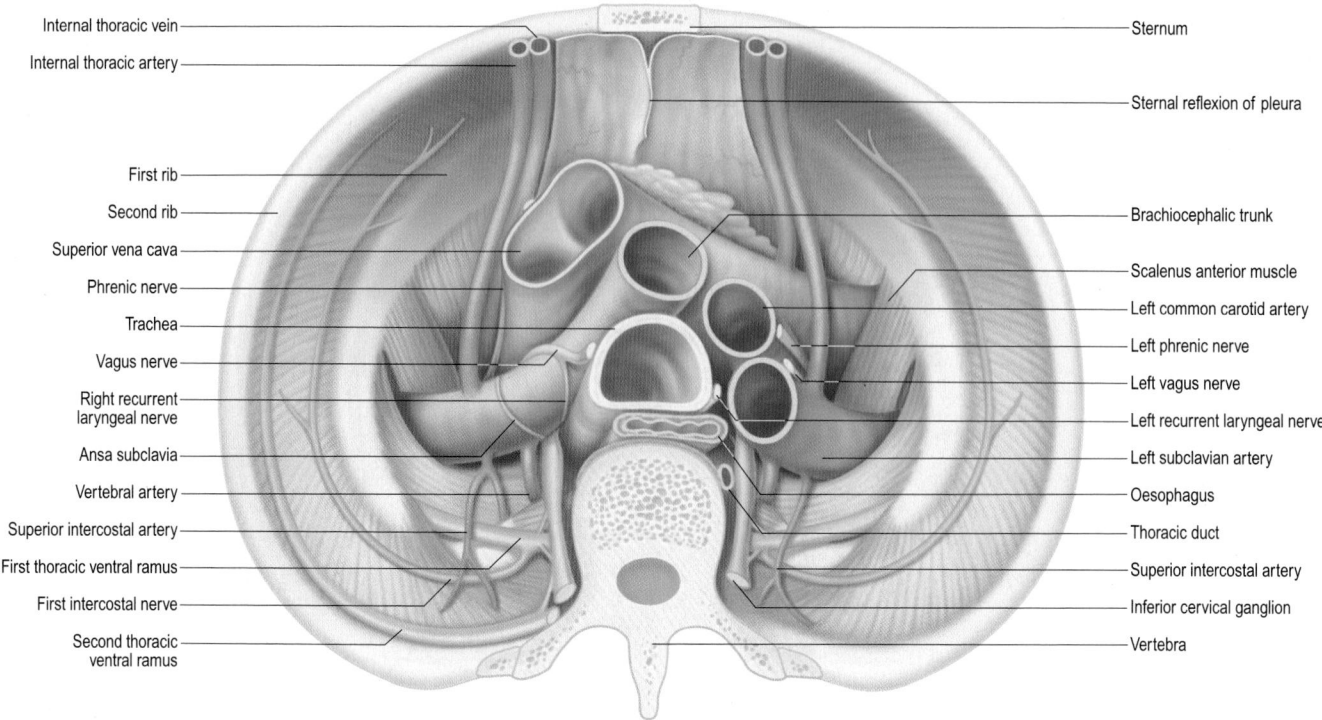

Fig. 63.5 Structures related to the right cervical pleura and left cervical pleura as seen from below.

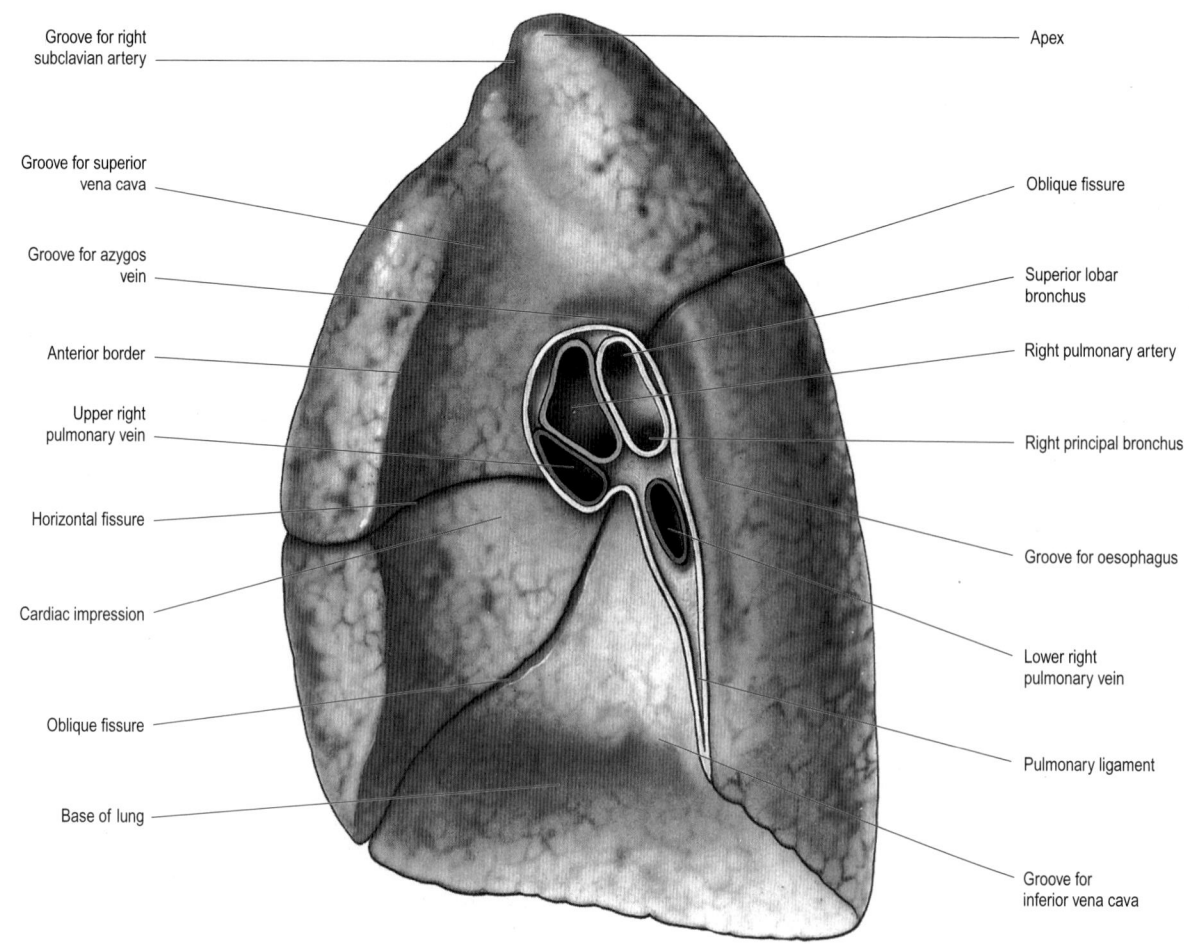

Fig. 63.6 The medial surface of the right lung.

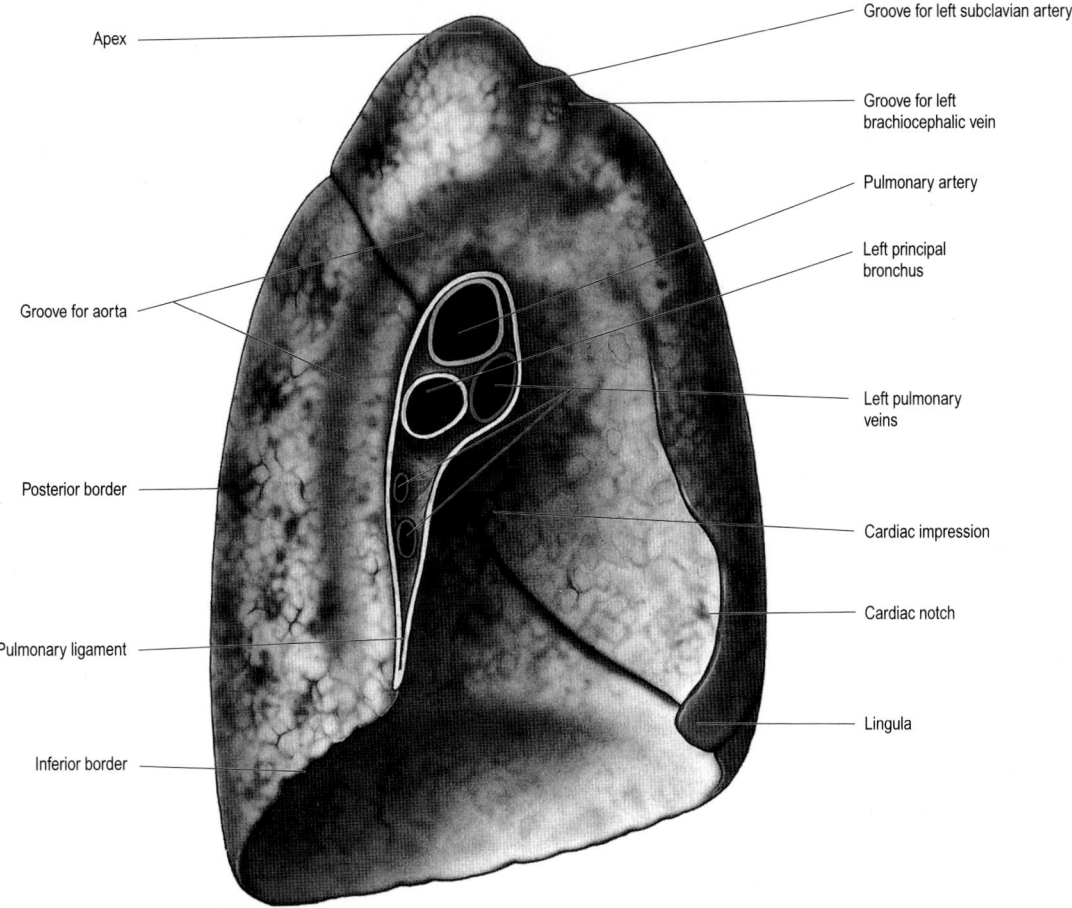

Fig. 63.7 The medial surface of the left lung.

muscle, the eleventh may be mistaken for the twelfth in palpation, and an incision prolonged to this level will damage the pleura. Whether the lowest palpable rib is the eleventh or twelfth can be ascertained by counting from the second rib (identified at its junction with the sternal angle).

VASCULAR SUPPLY AND LYMPHATIC DRAINAGE
The parietal and visceral pleurae are developed from somatopleural and splanchnopleural layers of the lateral plate mesoderm respectively. The parietal pleura is therefore supplied by arteries from somatic sources. The costovertebral pleura is supplied by branches of intercostal and internal thoracic arteries; the mediastinal pleura is supplied by branches from bronchial arteries, upper diaphragmatic arteries, internal thoracic and mediastinal arteries; the cervical pleura is supplied by branches from the subclavian artery; and the diaphragmatic pleura is supplied by the superficial part of the microcirculation of the diaphragmatic muscle. The veins join systemic veins in the thoracic wall which drain into the superior vena cava. Lymph from the costovertebral parietal pleura drains into the internal thoracic chain anteriorly and intercostal chains posteriorly, while that from the diaphragmatic pleura drains into the mediastinal, retrosternal and coeliac axis nodes.

The visceral pleura forms an integral part of the lung and accordingly its arterial supply and venous drainage are provided by the bronchial vessels. The bronchial arteries at the hilum form an annulus that surrounds the main bronchus, and pleural branches from this annulus supply the visceral pleura which faces the mediastinum, interlobar surfaces, apical surface and part of the diaphragmatic surface. The visceral pleura is drained by pulmonary veins, apart from an area around the hilum that drains into bronchial veins. The lymphatic drainage of the visceral pleura is to the deep pulmonary plexus within the interlobar and peribronchial spaces.

INNERVATION
The costal and peripheral diaphragmatic parietal pleurae are innervated by intercostal nerves, and the mediastinal and central diaphragmatic

parietal pleurae are innervated by the phrenic nerve. Irritation of the former results in pain referred along intercostal nerves to the thoracic or abdominal wall, whereas irritation of the diaphragmatic pleurae causes pain that is referred to the lower neck and shoulder tip, i.e. to the C3, 4 dermatomes. The visceral pleura is innervated by visceral afferents that reach it by travelling along the bronchial vessels.

MICROSTRUCTURE
The pleural surface is smooth and moistened by serous fluid. It consists of a single layer of flat mesothelial cells separated by a basal lamina from an underlying lamina propria of loose connective tissue. Ultrastructurally, pleural mesothelial cells are like those of the peritoneum in that they have highly folded basal plasma membranes, their adjacent cell surfaces interdigitate and are joined by desmosomes, and their luminal surfaces bear numerous microvilli and some cilia. Pinocytotic vesicles are common in their cytoplasm.

The deeper layers of the lamina propria are continuous with the tissue surrounding the pulmonary lobules (p. 1070). Blood and lymph vessels and nerves all travel within the pleura.

LUNGS

The lungs are the essential organs of respiration. They are situated on either side of the heart and other mediastinal contents (**Figs 63.1, 63.6, 63.7, 63.9, 63.10, 63.11**). Each lung is free in its pleural cavity, except for its attachment to the heart and trachea at the hilum and pulmonary ligament respectively. When removed from the thorax, a fresh lung is spongy, can float in water, and crepitates when handled, because of the air within its alveoli. It is also highly elastic and so it retracts on removal from the thorax. Its surface is smooth and shiny and is separated by fine, dark lines into numerous small polyhedral domains, each crossed by numerous finer lines, indicating the areas of contact between its most peripheral lobules and the pleural surface.

At birth the lungs are pink, but in adults they are dark grey and patchily mottled. As age advances this maculation becomes black, as granules of inhaled carbonaceous material are deposited in the loose connective tissue near the lung surface. Darkening is often more marked in men than women, and in those who have dwelt in industrial areas or in smokers. The posterior pulmonary border is usually darker than the anterior. In the upper, less movable parts of the lung, this surface pigmentation tends to be concentrated opposite the intercostal spaces. Lungs from fetuses or stillborn infants who have not respired differ from those of infants who have taken a breath, in that they are firm, non-crepitant and do not float in water.

The adult right lung usually weighs c.625 g, and the left 565 g, but they vary greatly. Their weight also depends on the amount of blood or serous fluid contained within them. In proportion to body stature, the lungs are heavier in men than in women.

PULMONARY SURFACE FEATURES

Each lung has an apex, base, three borders and two surfaces (**Figs 63.6, 63.7, 63.11**). In shape each lung approximates to half a cone.

Apex

The apex, the rounded upper extremity, protrudes above the thoracic inlet where it contacts the cervical pleura, and is covered in turn by the suprapleural membrane. Owing to the obliquity of the inlet, the apex rises 3–4 cm above the level of the first costal cartilage although it is level posteriorly with the neck of the first rib. Its summit is c.2.5 cm above the medial third of the clavicle. The apex is therefore in the root of the neck (**Figs 63.1, 63.2, 63.3**). It has been asserted that, because the apex does not rise above the neck of the first rib, it is really intrathoracic, and that it is the anterior surface which ascends highest in inspiration, but this requires confirmation. The subclavian artery arches up and laterally over the suprapleural membrane, grooves the anterior surface of the apex near its summit and separates it from scalenus anterior. Posterior to the apex are the cervicothoracic (stellate) sympathetic ganglion, the ventral ramus of the first thoracic spinal nerve and the superior intercostal artery (**Fig. 63.5**). Scalenus medius is lateral, and the brachiocephalic artery, right brachiocephalic vein and trachea are on the right, while the left subclavian artery and left brachiocephalic vein are on the left.

Base

The basal surface is semilunar and concave, and rests upon the superior surface of the diaphragm, which separates the right lung from the right lobe of the liver and the left lung from the left lobe of the liver, the gastric fundus and spleen. Since the diaphragm extends higher on the right than on the left, the concavity is deeper on the base of the right lung. Posterolaterally, the base has a sharp margin that projects a little into the costodiaphragmatic recess (p. 1065).

The costal surface

The costal surface of the lung is smooth and convex, and its shape is adapted to that of the thoracic wall, which is vertically deeper posteriorly. It is in contact with the costal pleura and exhibits, in specimens preserved *in situ*, grooves that correspond with the overlying ribs.

The medial surface

The medial surface has a posterior vertebral and anterior mediastinal part. The vertebral part lies in contact with the sides of the thoracic vertebrae and intervertebral discs, the posterior intercostal vessels and the splanchnic nerves. The mediastinal area is deeply concave, because it is adapted to the heart at the cardiac impression, which is much larger and deeper on the left lung where the heart projects more to the left of the median plane. Posterosuperior to this concavity is the somewhat triangular hilum, where various structures enter or leave the lung, collectively surrounded by a sleeve of pleura which also extends below the hilum and behind the cardiac impression as the pulmonary ligament (p. 1070).

Other impressions of the lung surface

In addition to these pulmonary features, preserved lungs show a number of other impressions that indicate their relations with surrounding structures (**Figs 59.2, 63.6, 63.7**). On the right lung the cardiac impression is related to the anterior surface of the right auricle, the anterolateral surface of the right atrium and partially to the anterior surface of the right ventricle. The impression ascends anterior to the hilum as a wide groove for the superior vena cava and the end of the

right brachiocephalic vein (**Fig. 63.6**). Posteriorly this groove is joined by a deep sulcus which arches forwards above the hilum and is occupied by the azygos vein. The right side of the oesophagus makes a shallow vertical groove behind the hilum and the pulmonary ligament. Towards the diaphragm it inclines left and leaves the right lung, and therefore does not reach the lower limit of this surface. Posteroinferiorly the cardiac impression is confluent with a short wide groove adapted to the inferior vena cava. Between the apex and the groove for the azygos, the trachea and right vagus are close to the lung, but do not mark it.

On the left lung (**Fig. 63.7**) the cardiac impression is related to the anterior and lateral surfaces of the left ventricle and auricle. The anterior infundibular surface and adjoining part of the right ventricle is also related to the lung as it ascends in front of the hilum to accommodate the pulmonary trunk. A large groove arches over the hilum, and descends behind it and the pulmonary ligament, corresponding to the aortic arch and descending aorta. From its summit a narrower groove ascends to the apex for the left subclavian artery. Behind this, above the aortic groove, the lung is in contact with the thoracic duct and oesophagus. In front of the subclavian groove there is a faint linear depression for the left brachiocephalic vein. Inferiorly, the oesophagus may mould the surface in front of the lower end of the pulmonary ligament.

Pulmonary borders

The inferior border is thin and sharp where it separates the base from the costal surface and extends into the costodiaphragmatic recess. It is more rounded medially where it divides the base from the mediastinal surface. It corresponds, in quiet respiration, to a line drawn from the lowest point of the anterior border which passes to the sixth rib at about the midclavicular line, then to the eighth rib in the midaxillary line (c.10 cm above the costal margin), and then continues posteriorly, medially and slightly upwards to a point 2 cm lateral to the tenth thoracic spine (**Figs 63.2, 63.3, 63.4**). The posterior border separates the costal surface from the mediastinal, and corresponds to the heads of the ribs. It has no recognizable markings and is really a rounded junction of costal and vertebral (medial) surfaces. The thin, sharp, anterior border overlaps the pericardium. On the right it corresponds closely to the costomediastinal line of pleural reflection, and is almost vertical. On the left it approaches the same line above; however, below the fourth costal cartilage it shows a variable cardiac notch, the edge of which passes laterally for c.3.5 cm before curving down and medially to the sixth costal cartilage c.4 cm from the midline. It thus does not reach the line of pleural reflection here (**Figs 63.1, 63.2, 63.3**) and so the pericardium is covered only by a double layer of pleura (area of superficial cardiac dullness, p. ???). However, surgical experience suggests that the line of pleural reflection, the anterior pulmonary margin and the costomediastinal pleural recess are all variable.

PULMONARY FISSURES AND LOBES

Right lung

The right lung is divided into superior, middle and inferior lobes by an oblique and a horizontal fissure (**Fig. 63.6**). The upper, oblique fissure separates the inferior from the middle and upper lobes, and corresponds closely to the left oblique fissure, although it is less vertical, and crosses the inferior border of the lung c.7.5 cm behind its anterior end. On the posterior border it is either level with the spine of the fourth thoracic vertebra or slightly lower. It descends across the fifth intercostal space and follows the sixth rib to the sixth costochondral junction (p. 947). The short horizontal fissure separates the superior and middle lobes. It passes from the oblique fissure, near the midaxillary line, horizontally forwards to the anterior border of the lung, level with the sternal end of the fourth costal cartilage, then passes backwards to the hilum on the mediastinal surface (p. 947). On a frontal chest radiograph (**Fig. 63.8A**) the horizontal fissure is visible in c.60% of the population. The oblique fissure is usually visible on a lateral radiograph (**Fig. 63.8B**) and on a high resolution CT as a curvilinear band from the lateral aspect to the hilum (**Fig. 63.9**).

The small middle lobe is thus cuneiform and includes some of the costal surface, the lower part of the anterior border and the anterior part of the base of the lung. Sometimes the medial part of the upper lobe is partially separated by a fissure of variable depth which contains the terminal part of the azygos vein, enclosed in the free margin of a mesentery derived from the mediastinal pleura, thereby forming the 'lobe of the azygos vein'. This varies in size, and sometimes includes

A

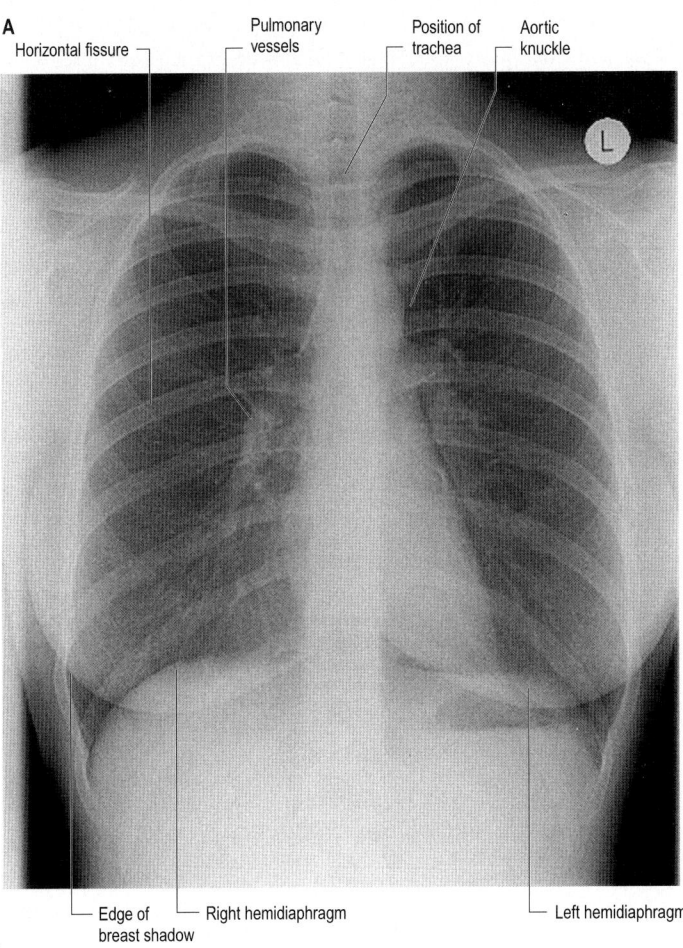

Horizontal fissure — Pulmonary vessels — Position of trachea — Aortic knuckle

Edge of breast shadow — Right hemidiaphragm — Left hemidiaphragm

B

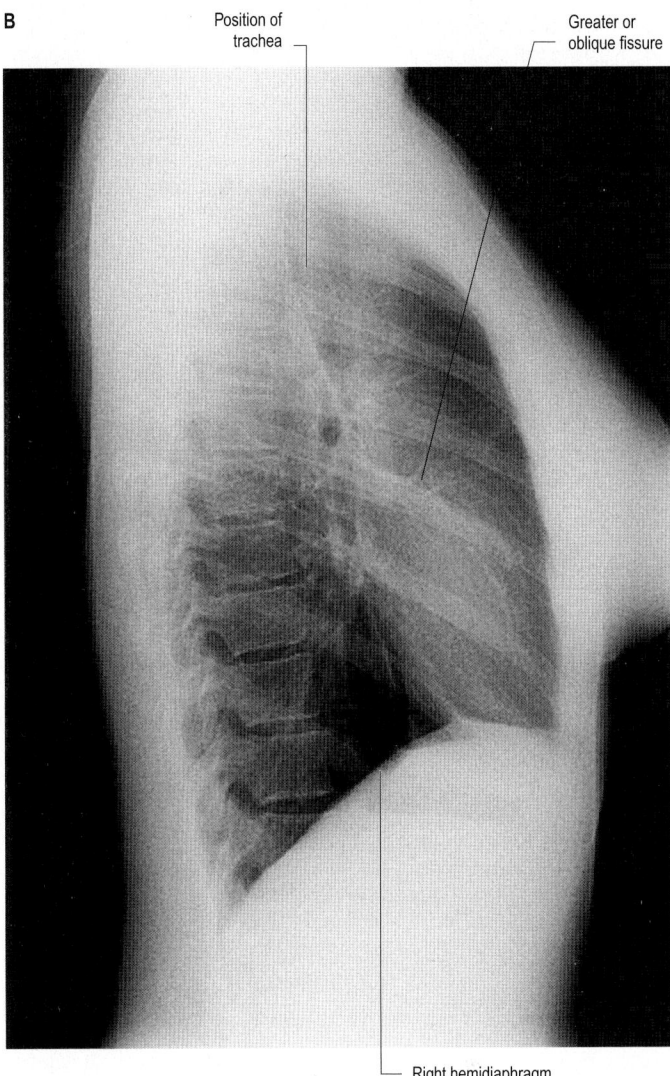

Position of trachea — Greater or oblique fissure

Right hemidiaphragm

Fig. 63.8 Radiograph of chest: **A**, posteroanterior view of adult female and **B**, lateral view.

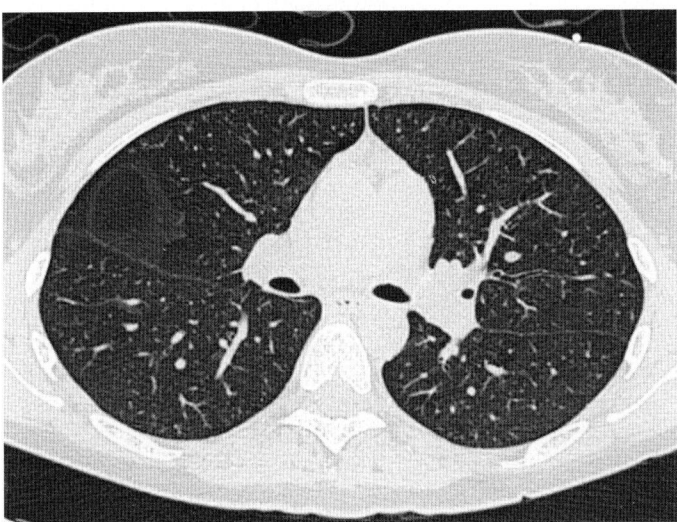

Fig. 63.9 A section of a high resolution computed tomogram of the thorax demonstrating the lung parenchyma and oblique fissures.

the apex of the lung. It is always supplied by one or more branches of the apical bronchus. Radiographically, a pleural effusion may be limited to the azygos fissure. Less common variations are the presence of an inferior accessory fissure, which separates the medial basal segment

from the remainder of the lower lobe, and a superior accessory fissure, which separates the apical segment of the lower lobe from the basal segments.

Left lung

The left lung is divided into a superior and an inferior lobe by an oblique fissure (**Fig. 63.7**) which extends from the costal to the medial surfaces of the lung both above and below the hilum. Superficially this fissure begins on the medial surface at the posterosuperior part of the hilum. It ascends obliquely backwards to cross the posterior border of the lung c.6 cm below the apex, then descends forwards across the costal surface, to reach the lower border almost at its anterior end. It finally ascends on the medial surface to the lower part of the hilum. At the posterior border of the lung the fissure usually lies opposite a surface point 2 cm to the side of the midline between the spines of the third and fourth thoracic vertebrae, but it may be above or below this level. Traced around the chest, the fissure reaches the fifth intercostal space (at or near the midaxillary line) and follows this to intersect the inferior border of the lung close to, or just below, the sixth costochondral junction (7.5 cm from the midline). The left oblique fissure is usually more vertical than the right, and is indicated approximately by the medial border of the scapula when the arm is fully abducted above the shoulder (p. 947). A left horizontal fissure is a normal variant found in c.10% of patients.

The superior lobe, which lies anterosuperior to the oblique fissure, includes the apex, anterior border, much of the costal and most of the medial surfaces of the lung. At the lower end of the cardiac notch a small process, the lingula, is usually present. The larger inferior lobe lies behind and below the fissure, and contributes almost the whole of the base, much of the costal surface and most of the posterior border of the lung.

The diaphragm rises higher on the right to accommodate the liver, and so the right lung is vertically shorter (by 2.5 cm) than the left. However, cardiac asymmetry means that the right lung is broader, and has a greater capacity and weight than the left.

The identification of the completeness of the fissures is important prior to lobectomy, because individuals with incomplete fissures are more prone to develop postoperative air leaks, and may require further procedures such as stapling and pericardial sleeves (see Venuta et al 1998).

Bronchopulmonary segments

Each of the principal bronchi divides into lobar bronchi. Primary branches of the right and left lobar bronchi are termed segmental bronchi because each ramifies in a structurally separate, functionally independent, unit of lung tissue called a bronchopulmonary segment (pp. 1076, 1076, 1077; **Figs 63.10, 63.11, 63.12**).

The main segments are named and numbered as follows:

Right lung	
Superior lobe:	1, apical; 2, posterior; 3, anterior
Middle lobe:	4, lateral; 5, medial
Inferior lobe:	6, superior (apical); 7, medial basal; 8, anterior basal; 9, lateral basal; 10, posterior basal

Left lung	
Superior lobe:	1, apical; 2, posterior; 3, anterior; 4, superior lingular; 5, inferior lingular
Inferior lobe:	6, superior (apical); 8, anterior basal; 9, lateral basal; 10, posterior basal

Each segment is surrounded by connective tissue that is continuous with the visceral pleura, and is a separate respiratory unit. The vascular and lymphatic arrangements of the segments are described on page 1077.

PULMONARY HILA

The pulmonary root (**Figs 59.2, 63.6, 63.7**) connects the medial surface of the lung to the heart and trachea and is formed by a group of structures that enter or leave the hilum. These are the principal bronchus, pulmonary artery, two pulmonary veins, bronchial vessels, a pulmonary autonomic plexus, lymph vessels, bronchopulmonary lymph nodes and loose connective tissue, which are all enveloped by pleura. The pulmonary roots, or pedicles, lie opposite the bodies of the fifth to seventh thoracic vertebrae. Common anterior relations of both hila are the phrenic nerve, pericardiacophrenic artery and vein, and anterior pulmonary plexus. Common posterior relations are the vagus nerve and posterior pulmonary plexus. The pulmonary ligament is inferior. The major structures in both roots are similarly arranged, so that the upper of the two pulmonary veins is in front, the pulmonary artery and principal bronchus are behind, and the bronchial vessels are most posterior. The arrangement of bronchopulmonary segments (p. 1070) and the pulmonary hila permit the resection of localized lesions caused by lung cancer, and abscesses.

Right hilum

The right root is situated behind the superior vena cava and right atrium and below the terminal part of the azygos vein. The sequence from above downwards is superior lobar bronchus, pulmonary artery, principal bronchus, and lower pulmonary vein (Fig. 63.6). In right-sided pulmonary resections the main pulmonary artery is first localized at the angle of the superior vena cava and the azygos vein and the superior pulmonary vein and then the inferior pulmonary vein are dissected out before the appropriate bronchus.

Left hilum

The left root lies below the aortic arch and in front of the descending thoracic aorta. The vertical sequence at the left hilum is pulmonary artery, principal bronchus, and lower pulmonary vein (Fig. 63.7). The

pulmonary artery is longer on the left side: each of its branches from the hilum to the oblique fissure must be identified for pulmonary resections.

SECONDARY PULMONARY LOBULES

Each segmental bronchus supplies a bronchopulmonary segment. Progressive subdivisions of the bronchus occur within each segment and the bronchi become increasingly narrow. All intrapulmonary bronchi are kept patent by cartilaginous plates, which decline in size and number and finally disappear when the tubes are less than 1 mm in diameter (bronchioles). The terminal bronchiole is the most peripheral bronchiole not to have alveoli in its wall. Distal to each terminal bronchiole is an acinus, which consists of three to four orders of respiratory bronchioles, leading to three to eight orders of alveolar ducts. The walls of these ducts consist of alveolar sacs or the mouths of alveoli. The primary lobule is the lung distal to the respiratory bronchiole. The secondary lobule is the smallest subsection of the peripheral lung bounded by connective tissue septa and consists of approximately six terminal bronchioles. The connective tissue septa are uneven in both size and shape.

VASCULAR SUPPLY AND LYMPHATIC DRAINAGE

The lungs have two functionally distinct circulatory pathways. These are the pulmonary vessels, which convey deoxygenated blood to the alveolar walls and drain oxygenated blood back to the left side of the heart, and the much smaller bronchial vessels, which are derived from the systemic circulation and provide oxygenated blood to lung tissues which do not have close access to atmospheric oxygen, e.g. those of the bronchi and larger bronchioles (p. 1077).

The pulmonary artery bifurcates into right and left pulmonary arteries, which pass to the hila of the lungs. On entering the lung tissue, both arteries divide into branches that accompany segmental and sub-segmental bronchi and lie mostly dorsolateral to them. The pulmonary capillaries form plexuses immediately outside the epithelium in the walls and septa of alveoli and alveolar sacs. The plexus forms a single layer in the interalveolar septa; it has meshes smaller than the capillaries, and exceedingly thin walls. Pulmonary veins, two from each lung, drain the pulmonary capillaries. Their radicles coalesce into larger branches which traverse the lung independently of the pulmonary arteries and bronchi. Communicating freely, they form large vessels that ultimately accompany the arteries and bronchial tubes to the pulmonary hilum, where the bronchi often separate the dorsolateral artery and the ventro-medial vein. The pulmonary veins open into the left atrium and convey oxygenated blood for systemic distribution by the left ventricle.

At the hilum, the pulmonary vessels accompany the main bronchial divisions, but this is not the case in the bronchopulmonary segments (p. 1077), where a segmental bronchus, its branches and associated arteries, occupy a central position in each segment, and many tributaries of the pulmonary veins run between segments, serving adjacent segments which drain into more than one vein. Some veins also lie beneath the visceral pleura, including that in the interlobar fissures. Thus a broncho-pulmonary segment is not a complete vascular unit with an individual bronchus, artery and vein. During resection of segments it is obvious that the planes between them are not avascular but are crossed by pulmonary veins and sometimes by branches of arteries. This pattern of bronchi, arteries and veins exhibits considerable variation: veins are the most variable, and arteries are more variable than bronchi.

Pulmonary lymphatic vessels originate in a superficial subpleural plexus. A deep plexus accompanies the branches of the pulmonary vessels and bronchi. Superficial efferents turn round lung borders and the margins of fissures to converge in the bronchopulmonary nodes. There is little anastomosis between the superficial and deep lymphatics, except in the hilar regions. In peripheral parts of the lungs small channels connect superficial and deep lymphatic vessels, and are capable of dilatation to direct lymph from the deep to the superficial channels when outflow from deep vessels is obstructed by pulmonary disease. Deep in the fissures, lymphatic vessels of adjoining lobes connect. Consequently, although there is a tendency for vessels from the upper lobes to pass to the superior tracheobronchial nodes, and those from lower lobes to the inferior tracheobronchial group, these connections are not exclusive. At the level of pulmonary lobation the arrangement of lymphatic vessels follows the central artery of a lobule and its peripheral veins. There are also lymphoid aggregations, non-follicular in appearance, in peribronchial sites and in 'placoid' formations adjoining pulmonary pleura.

A

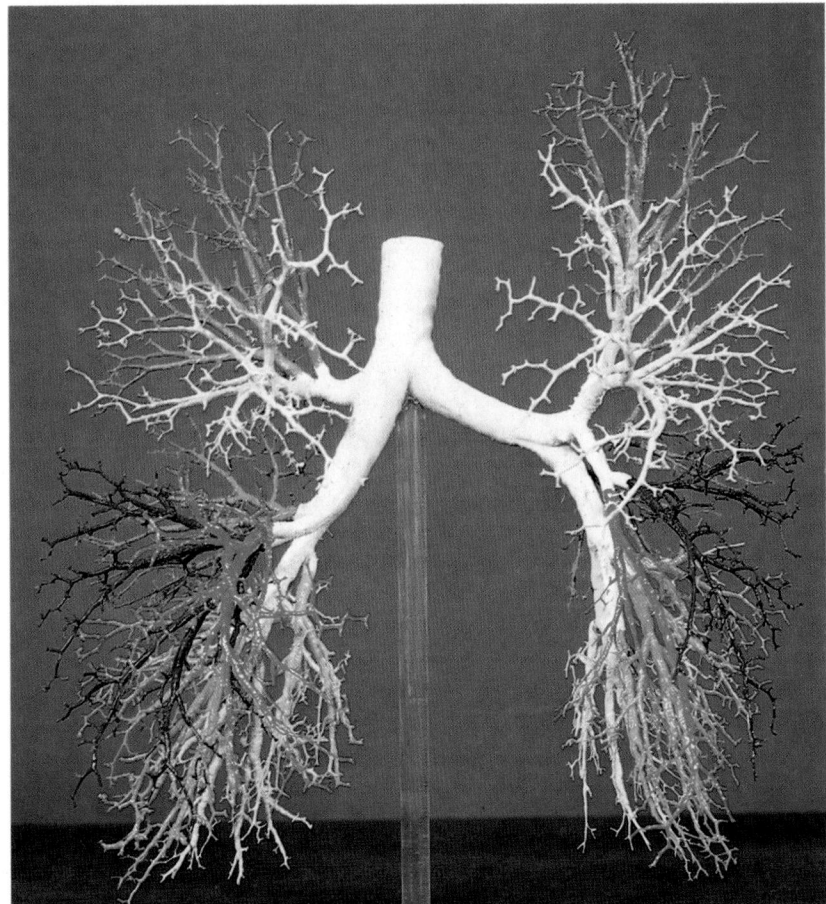

Fig. 63.10 A, A resin corrosion cast of the adult human lower trachea and bronchial tree photographed from the anterior aspect. The segmental bronchi and their main branches have been coloured brown = apical; grey/blue = posterior; pink = anterior; dark blue = lateral (middle lobe) and superior lingular; red = medial (middle lobe) and inferior lingular; dark green = superior (apical) of inferior lobe; yellow = medial basal; orange = anterior basal; blue = lateral basal; light green = posterior basal. **B**, Corrosion cast of the bronchial tree of the right lung, colour coded as in **A** to indicate the territories supplied by different segmental bronchi. **C**, Corrosion cast of the bronchial tree of the left lung, colour coded as in A. Note that in this and other preparations shown in 63.10 many of the finer bronchial branches have been trimmed away to reveal the larger bronchi. (Specimens prepared by MCE Hutchinson; photograph by Kevin Fitzpatrick on behalf of GKT School of Medicine, London.)

B

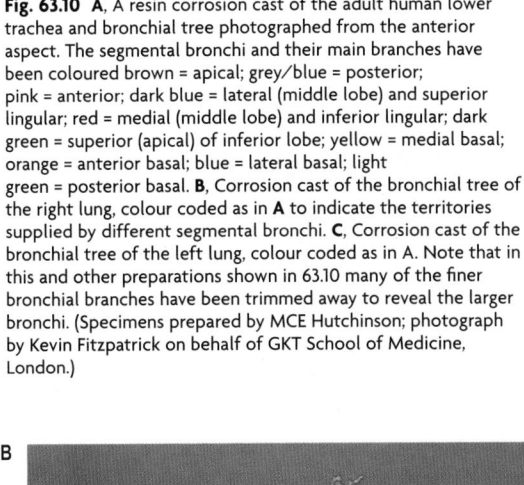

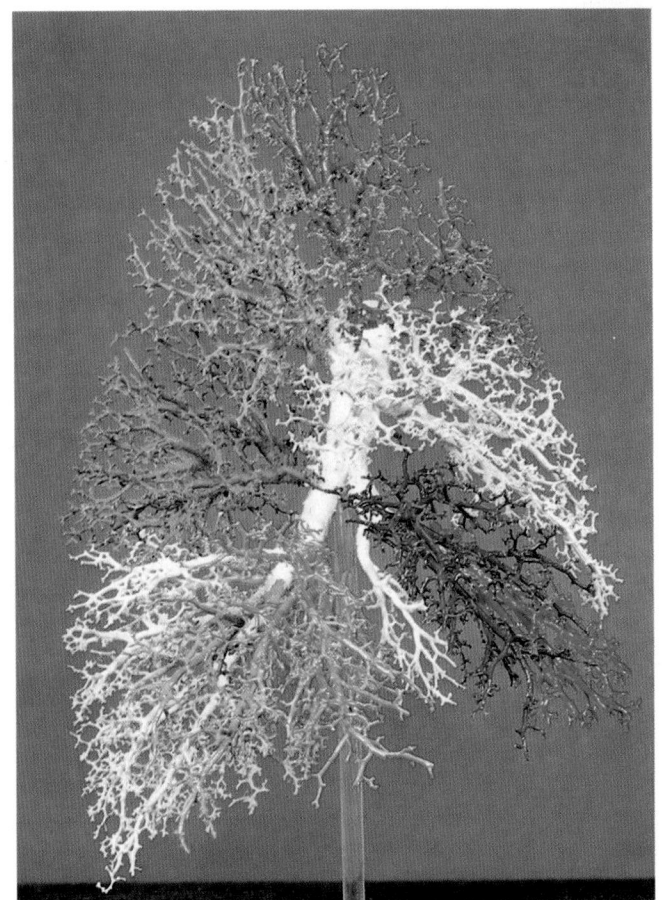

C

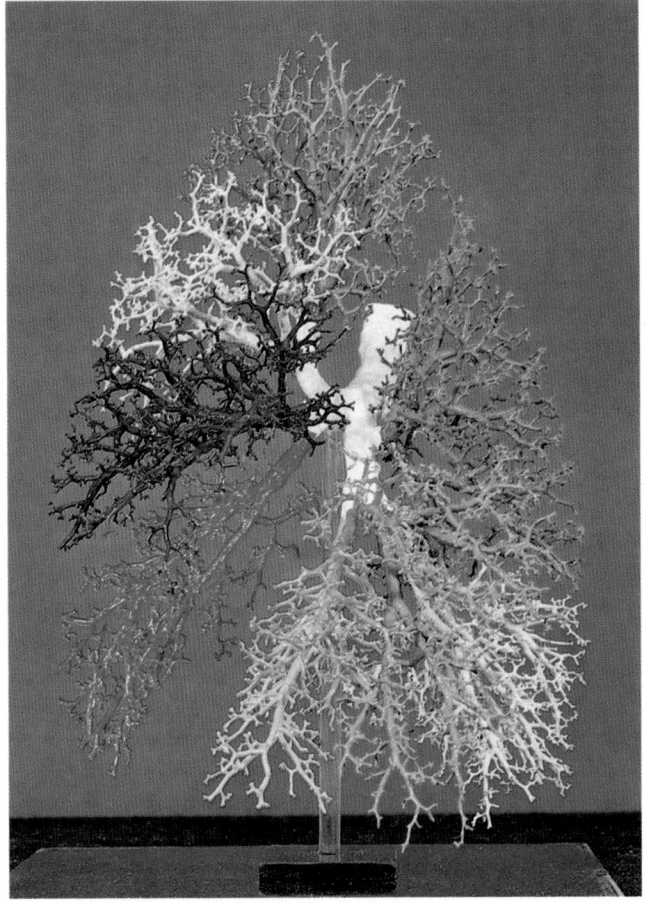

A Anterior view

B Posterior view

C Lateral (costal) aspect

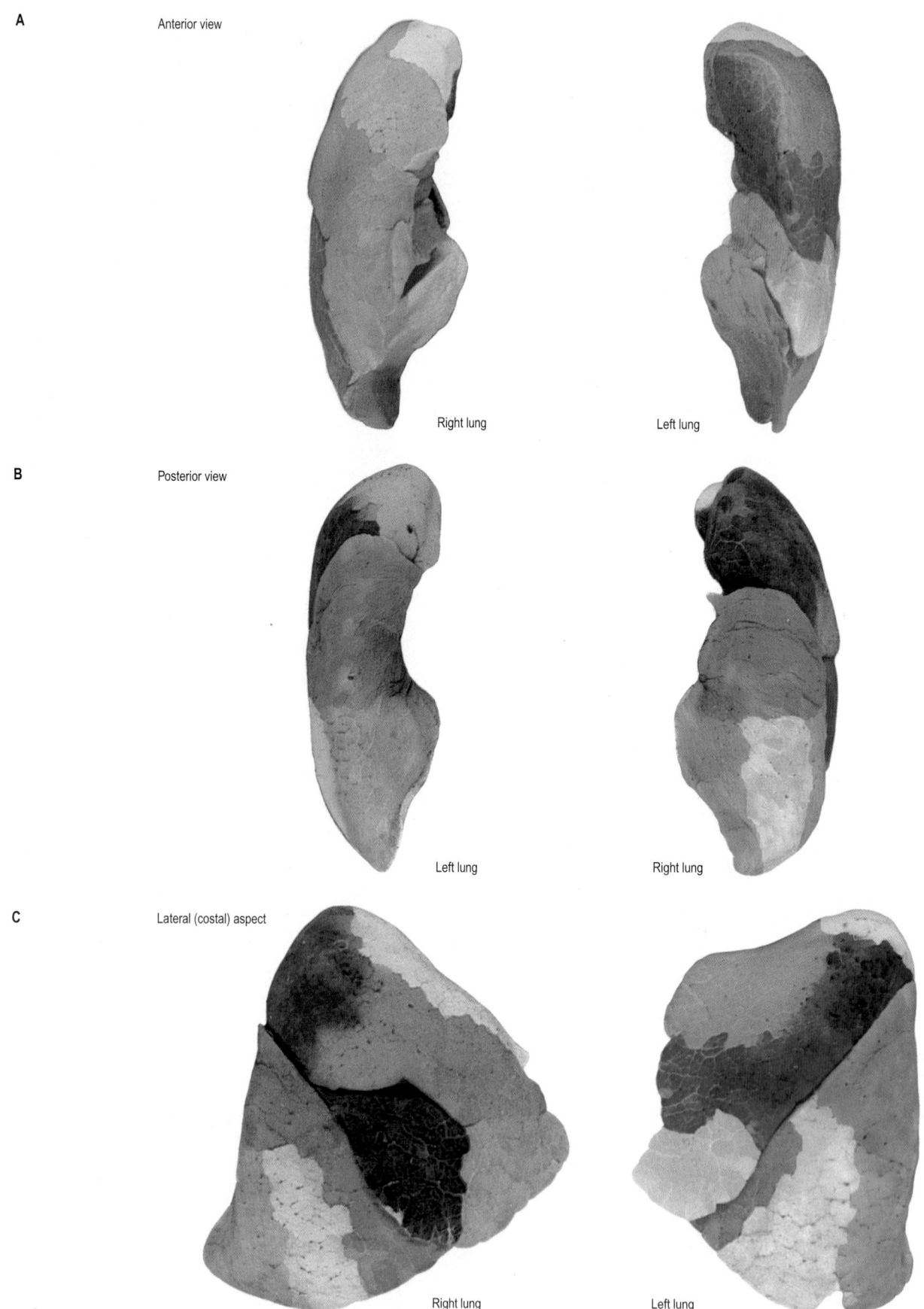

Right lung

Left lung

Left lung

Right lung

Right lung

Left lung

Fig. 63.11 Bronchopulmonary segments of the right and left lungs, coloured to indicate the different territories as in **Fig. 63.10**, except that in the right lung the medial view shows a subsuperior segment which is painted white. The lungs are side by side (right and left). **A**, As seen from anterior aspect; **B**, as seen from posterior aspect; **C**, as seen from lateral aspect. (Prepared by MCE Hutchinson, GKT School of Medicine, London; photograph by Sarah-Jane Smith.)

D Medial hilar aspect

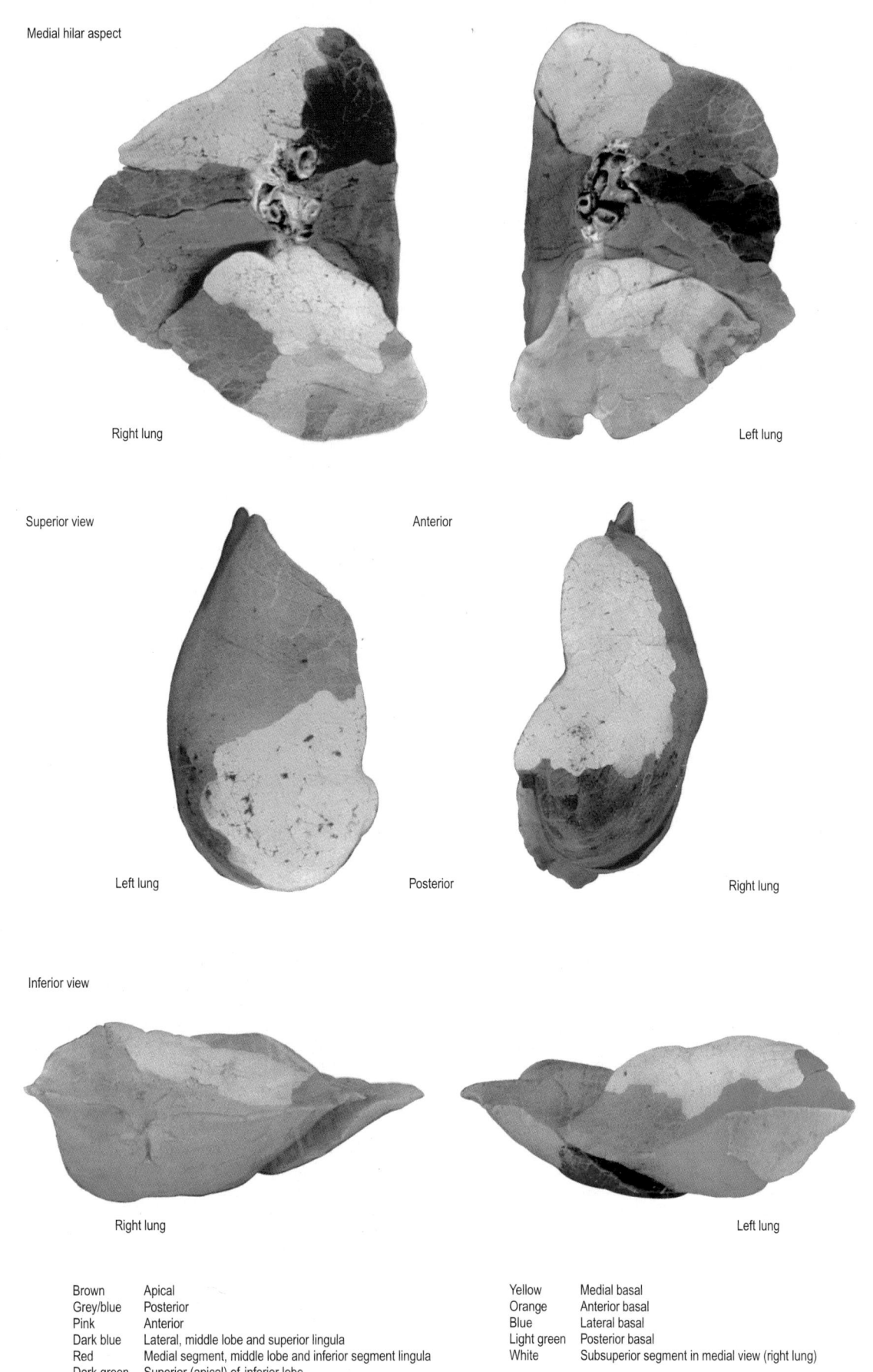

Right lung   Left lung

Superior view   Anterior

Left lung   Posterior   Right lung

E Inferior view

Right lung   Left lung

Brown	Apical
Grey/blue	Posterior
Pink	Anterior
Dark blue	Lateral, middle lobe and superior lingula
Red	Medial segment, middle lobe and inferior segment lingula
Dark green	Superior (apical) of inferior lobe

Yellow	Medial basal
Orange	Anterior basal
Blue	Lateral basal
Light green	Posterior basal
White	Subsuperior segment in medial view (right lung)

Fig. 63.11 (*Cont'd*) **D**, both lungs seen from medial (hilar) aspect; **E**, from inferior view.

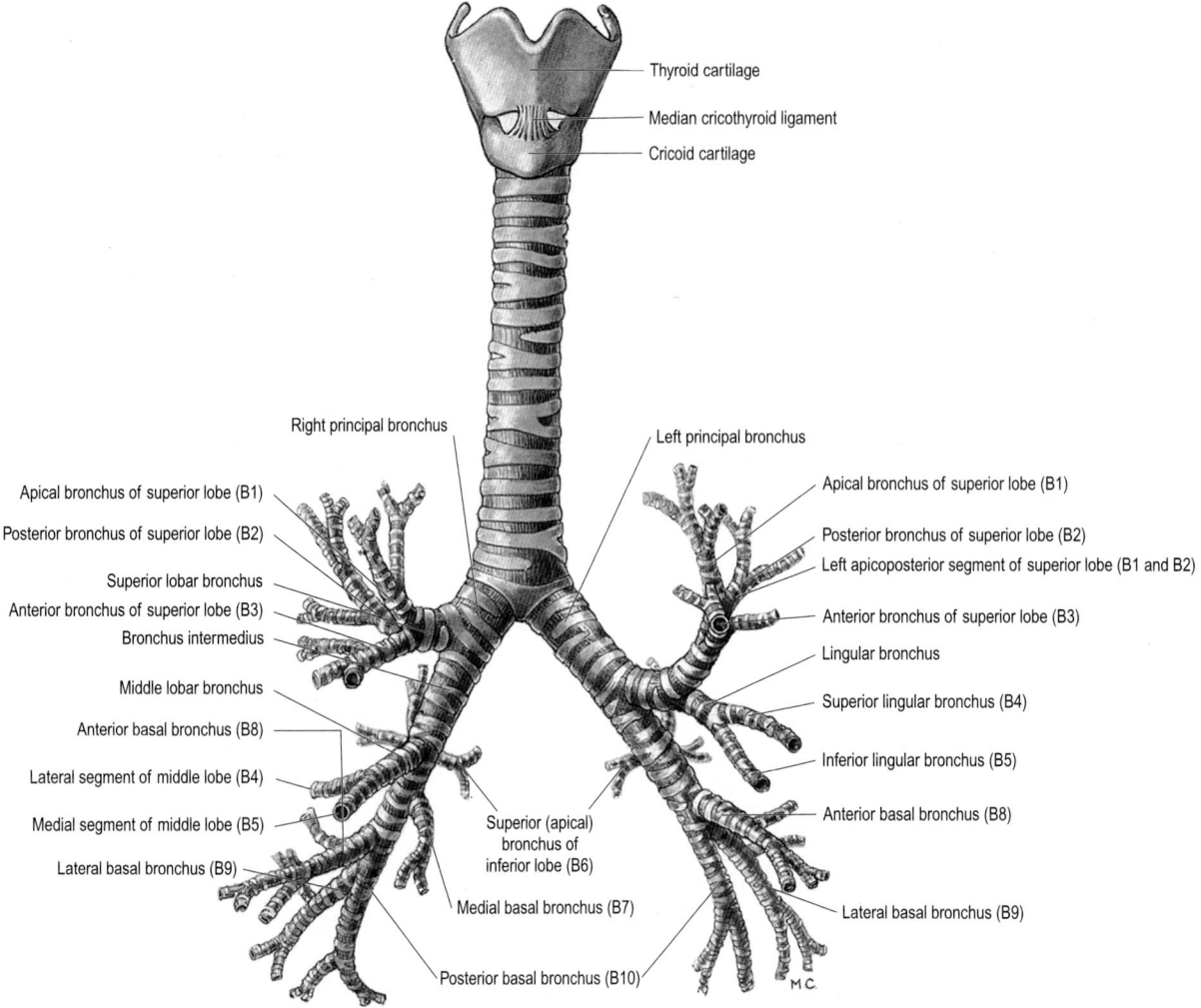

Thyroid cartilage

Median cricothyroid ligament

Cricoid cartilage

Right principal bronchus

Left principal bronchus

Apical bronchus of superior lobe (B1)

Posterior bronchus of superior lobe (B2)

Superior lobar bronchus

Anterior bronchus of superior lobe (B3)

Bronchus intermedius

Middle lobar bronchus

Anterior basal bronchus (B8)

Lateral segment of middle lobe (B4)

Medial segment of middle lobe (B5)

Lateral basal bronchus (B9)

Superior (apical) bronchus of inferior lobe (B6)

Medial basal bronchus (B7)

Posterior basal bronchus (B10)

Apical bronchus of superior lobe (B1)

Posterior bronchus of superior lobe (B2)

Left apicoposterior segment of superior lobe (B1 and B2)

Anterior bronchus of superior lobe (B3)

Lingular bronchus

Superior lingular bronchus (B4)

Inferior lingular bronchus (B5)

Anterior basal bronchus (B8)

Lateral basal bronchus (B9)

M.C.

Fig. 63.12 The cartilages of the larynx, trachea and bronchi: anterior aspect. The bronchopulmonary segments are shown in brackets. (Drawn from a metal cast made by the late Lord Russell Brock, GKT School of Medicine, London.)

Right lung

In the hilum, the union of apical, anterior and posterior veins (draining the upper lobe) with a middle lobar vein (formed by lateral and medial tributaries, **Fig. 63.13**) forms the superior right pulmonary vein. The inferior right pulmonary vein is formed by the hilar union of superior (apical) and common basal veins from the lower lobe. The union of superior and inferior basal tributaries forms the common basal vein.

The right pulmonary artery divides into two large branches as it emerges behind the superior vena cava (**Fig. 63.13**). A lymph node usually occupies the bifurcation. The superior branch, which is the smaller of the two, goes to the superior lobe and usually divides into two further branches, which supply the majority of that lobe. The inferior branch descends anterior to the intermediate bronchus and immediately posterior to the superior pulmonary vein. It provides a small recurrent branch to the superior lobe, then at the point where the horizontal fissure meets the oblique fissure, it gives off the branch to the middle lobe anteriorly, and the branch to the superior segment of the inferior lobe posteriorly. It then continues a short distance before dividing to supply the rest of the inferior lobe segments.

Left lung

In the hilum the superior left pulmonary vein, which drains the upper lobe, is formed by the union of apicoposterior (draining the apical and posterior segments), anterior and lingular veins (**Fig. 63.13**). The inferior left pulmonary vein, which drains the lower lobe, is formed by the hilar union of two veins, superior (apical) and common basal, the latter formed by the union of a superior and an inferior basal vein. All the main tributaries of the pulmonary veins receive smaller tributaries, some intrasegmental and others intersegmental.

The left pulmonary artery emerges from within the concavity of the aortic arch and descends anterior to the descending aorta to enter the oblique fissure (**Fig. 63.13**). The branches of the left pulmonary artery are extremely variable. Usually its first and largest branch is to the anterior segment of the left superior lobe. Prior to reaching the fissure it gives off a variable number of other branches to the superior lobe. As it enters the fissure it usually supplies a large branch to the superior segment of the inferior lobe. Lingular branches arise within the fissure, and the rest of the lower lobe is supplied by many varied branching patterns. It was a surgical aphorism of the late Lord Brock that when performing a left upper lobectomy 'there was always one more branch of the pulmonary artery than you thought!'.

Pulmonary sequestration

When a portion of lung exists without the appropriate bronchovascular connections, it is usually supplied by the systemic vasculature. Pulmonary sequestration segments may be extralobar, in which case they are covered by visceral pleura and usually found below the left lower lobe. Intralobar abnormalities are usually embedded in normal lung, classically the posterior basal segment of the left lower lobe. Extralobar pulmonary sequestration *per se* is asymptomatic, but is often associated with other congenital abnormalities.

Pulmonary arteriography and embolization

A thrombus that forms in the legs or pelvic veins may embolize and travel in the right side of the circulation through the right atrium and right ventricle and then lodge in the pulmonary vasculature. The clinical abnormalities observed depend on the size of the embolus. Large emboli may lodge in the main pulmonary artery branches and cause

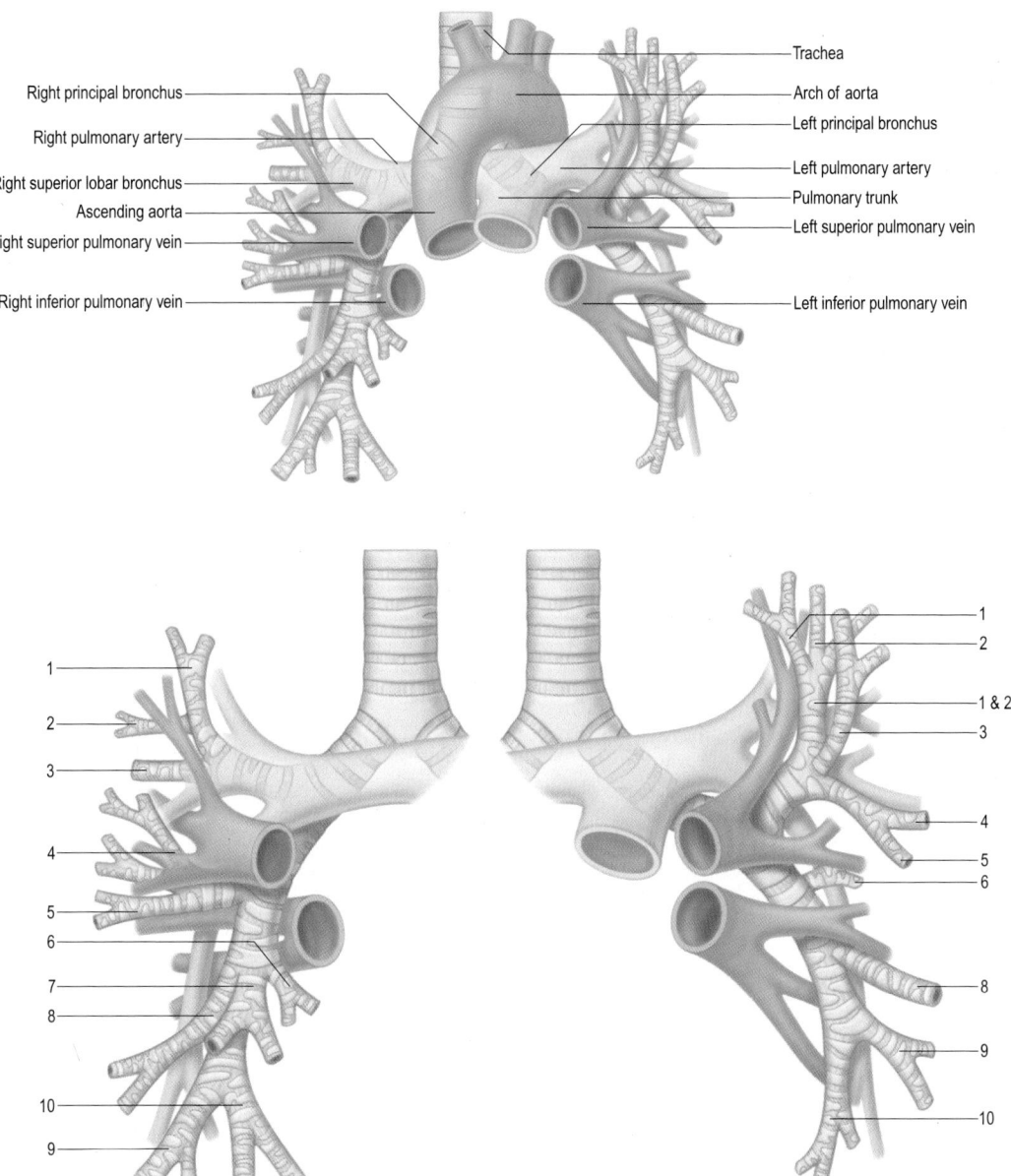

Trachea
Arch of aorta
Left principal bronchus
Left pulmonary artery
Pulmonary trunk
Left superior pulmonary vein
Left inferior pulmonary vein

Right principal bronchus
Right pulmonary artery
Right superior lobar bronchus
Ascending aorta
Right superior pulmonary vein
Right inferior pulmonary vein

Fig. 63.13 The relationship of the central airways with the pulmonary arteries and pulmonary veins.

right ventricular dysfunction and hypoxia. Smaller emboli may lodge in segmental pulmonary arteries and cause pleuritic chest pain, shortness of breath and haemoptysis. Pulmonary emboli cause a ventilation/perfusion mismatch that can have serious physiological implications leading to a significant reduction in the oxygenation of blood. Ventilation/perfusion scans with radiolabelled xenon and technetium usually demonstrate segmental abnormalities in perfusion with normal ventilation in the corresponding regions. Pulmonary emboli may also be evaluated by contrast enhanced spiral CT or pulmonary angiograms and appear as filling defects.

INNERVATION
The lungs are innervated by vagal and sympathetic fibres. The vagal fibres supply the bronchial muscles and glands and are bronchoconstrictor and secretomotor. The efferent sympathetic fibres are inhibitory. They relax the bronchial smooth muscle and also have vasoconstrictor effects.

Pulmonary plexuses
The pulmonary plexuses are anterior and posterior to the other hilar structures of the lungs. The anterior plexus is much smaller and is formed by rami from vagal and cervical sympathetic cardiac nerves as well as direct branches from both sources. The posterior pulmonary

plexus is formed by the rami of vagal cardiac branches from the second to fifth or sixth thoracic sympathetic ganglia. The left plexus also receives branches from the left recurrent laryngeal nerve.

TRACHEA AND BRONCHI

The trachea is a tube formed of cartilage and fibromuscular membrane, lined internally by mucosa (p. 1059). The anterolateral portion is made up of incomplete rings of cartilage, and the posterior aspect by a flat muscular wall. It is c.10–11 cm long, and descends from the larynx (**Fig. 63.12**) from the level of the sixth cervical vertebra to the upper border of the fifth thoracic vertebra, where it divides into right and left principal (pulmonary) bronchi. It lies approximately in the sagittal plane, but its point of bifurcation is usually a little to the right. The trachea is mobile and can rapidly alter in length: thus, during deep inspiration, the bifurcation may descend to the level of the sixth thoracic vertebra (p. 947). Its external transverse diameter is c.2 cm in adult males, and 1.5 cm in adult females. In children it is smaller, more deeply placed and more mobile. The lumen in live adults is c.12 mm in transverse diameter, although this increases after death as the smooth muscle making up its posterior aspect relaxes. In the first postnatal year, the tracheal diameter does not exceed 4 mm, while during later childhood its diameter in millimetres is approximately equal to age in years. The transverse shape of the lumen is variable, especially in the later decades of life, and may be round, lunate or flattened. At bronchoscopy the posterior wall of the trachea bulges into the lumen and this is exaggerated in expiration and coughing. The distal end of the trachea is visible as a concave spur. A tracheal bronchus may occasionally arise from the lateral wall of the trachea, more frequently from the right side: it may be supernumerary or it may represent a displaced upper lobe airway.

TRACHEAL RELATIONS

Cervical part of the trachea

Anterior relations – The cervical trachea is crossed anteriorly by skin and by the superficial and deep cervical fasciae. It is also crossed by the jugular arch and overlapped by sternohyoid and sternothyroid. The second to fourth tracheal cartilages are crossed by the isthmus of the thyroid gland, above which an anastomotic artery connects the bilateral superior thyroid arteries; below this and in front are the pretracheal fascia, inferior thyroid veins, thymic remnants and the thyroid ima artery (when it exists). In children the brachiocephalic artery crosses obliquely in front of the trachea at, or a little above, the upper border of the manubrium; the left brachiocephalic vein may also rise a little above this level.

Posterior relations – Behind the cervical trachea is the oesophagus, which runs between the trachea and the vertebral column. The recurrent laryngeal nerves ascend on each side, in or near the grooves between the sides of the trachea and oesophagus.

Lateral relations – The lateral relations of the trachea are the paired lobes of the thyroid gland, which descend to the fifth or sixth tracheal cartilage, and the common carotid and inferior thyroid arteries.

Thoracic part of the trachea (Figs 63.12, 63.14)

Anterior relations – As it descends through the superior mediastinum, the thoracic trachea lies behind the manubrium of sternum, the attachments of sternohyoid and sternothyroid, the thymic remnants and the inferior thyroid vein. The brachiocephalic and left common carotid arteries come to lie on the right and left respectively of the trachea as they diverge upwards into the neck. At a lower level the aortic arch, the brachiocephalic and left common carotid arteries, left brachiocephalic veins, deep cardiac plexus and some lymph nodes are all anterior to the trachea.

Posterior relations – The oesophagus is posterior to the trachea and separates it from the vertebral column.

Lateral relations – Laterally and on the right are the right lung and pleura, right brachiocephalic vein, superior vena cava, right vagus nerve and azygos vein. On the left are the arch of the aorta, left common carotid and left subclavian arteries. The left recurrent laryngeal nerve is at first situated between the trachea and aortic arch, and then lies in, or just in front of, the groove between the trachea and the oesophagus.

RIGHT MAIN BRONCHUS

The right principal bronchus (**Figs 60.4, 63.12, 63.14**) is wider, shorter and more vertical than the left, being c.2.5 cm long: this explains why inhaled foreign bodies enter it more often than the left. These events are more common in children and they may present with breathlessness, unilateral wheeze or recurrent aspirations. A chest radiograph may show air trapping in the affected lobe. The right main bronchus gives rise to its first branch, the superior lobar bronchus, then enters the right lung opposite the fifth thoracic vertebra. The azygos vein arches over it and the right pulmonary artery lies at first inferior, then anterior, to it. After giving off the superior lobar bronchus, which arises posterosuperior to the right pulmonary artery, the right main bronchus crosses the posterior aspect of the artery, enters the pulmonary hilum posteroinferior to it, and divides into a middle and an inferior lobar bronchus. Normal variants in the bronchial anatomy are occasionally seen and consist of either displaced or supernumerary airways (*see* Ghaye et al 2001). Abnormalities include a common origin of right upper lobe and

right middle lobe; an accessory cardiac bronchus; and a right lower lobe bronchus that may arise from the left main stem bronchus. These anatomic variants are largely asymptomatic, but occasionally may cause haemoptysis, recurrent infection and development of bronchiectasis of the airway.

Right superior lobar bronchus

The right superior lobar bronchus arises from the lateral aspect of the parent bronchus and runs superolaterally to enter the hilum; c.1 cm from its origin it divides into three segmental bronchi.

Segmental anatomy – The apical segmental bronchus continues superolaterally towards the apex of the lung, which it supplies, and divides near its origin into apical and anterior branches. The posterior segmental bronchus serves the posteroinferior part of the superior lobe, passes posterolaterally and slightly superiorly and soon divides into a lateral and a posterior branch. The anterior segmental bronchus runs anteroinferiorly to supply the rest of the superior lobe, and divides near its origin into a lateral and an anterior branch of equal size (p. 1070; **Figs 63.10, 63.11**).

Right middle lobar bronchus

The right middle lobar bronchus starts c.2 cm below the superior lobar bronchus, from the front of right bronchus intermedius and descends anterolaterally.

Segmental anatomy – The right middle lobar bronchus soon divides into a lateral and a medial segmental bronchus: these pass to the lateral and medial parts of the middle lobe, respectively (p. 1070; **Figs 63.10, 63.11**).

Right inferior lobar bronchus

The right inferior lobar bronchus is the continuation of the principal bronchus beyond the origin of the middle lobar bronchus.

Segmental anatomy – At or a little below its origin from the principal bronchus, the right inferior lobar bronchus gives off a large superior (apical) segmental bronchus posteriorly. This runs posteriorly to the upper part of the inferior lobe, and then divides into medial, superior and lateral branches: the first two usually arise from a common stem. After giving off the superior segmental branch, the right inferior lobar bronchus descends posterolaterally. The medial basal segmental bronchus branches from its anteromedial aspect, and runs inferomedially to serve a small region below the hilum. The inferior lobar bronchus continues downwards and then divides into an anterior basal segmental bronchus, which descends anteriorly, and a trunk that soon divides into a lateral basal segmental bronchus, which descends laterally, and a posterior basal segmental bronchus, which descends posteriorly. In more than half of all right lungs a subsuperior (subapical) segmental bronchus arises posteriorly from the right inferior lobar bronchus 1–3 cm below the superior segmental bronchus, and is distributed to the region of lung between the superior and posterior basal segments (p. 1070; **Figs 63.10, 63.11**).

LEFT MAIN BRONCHUS

The left principal bronchus, which is narrower and less vertical than the right, is c.5 cm long, and enters the hilum of the left lung at the level of the sixth thoracic vertebra. Passing to the left inferior to the aortic arch, it crosses anterior to the oesophagus, thoracic duct and descending aorta. The left pulmonary artery is at first anterior and then superior to it. After it enters the hilum, it divides into a superior and an inferior lobar bronchus.

Left superior lobar bronchus

The left superior lobar bronchus arises from the anterolateral aspect of its parent stem, curves laterally and soon divides into two bronchi which correspond to the branches of the right principal bronchus as it supplies the right superior and middle lobes. However, on the left side both are distributed to the left superior lobe because there is no separate middle lobe.

Segmental anatomy – The superior division of the left superior lobar bronchus ascends c.1 cm, gives off an anterior segmental bronchus, continues a further 1 cm as the apicoposterior segmental bronchus and

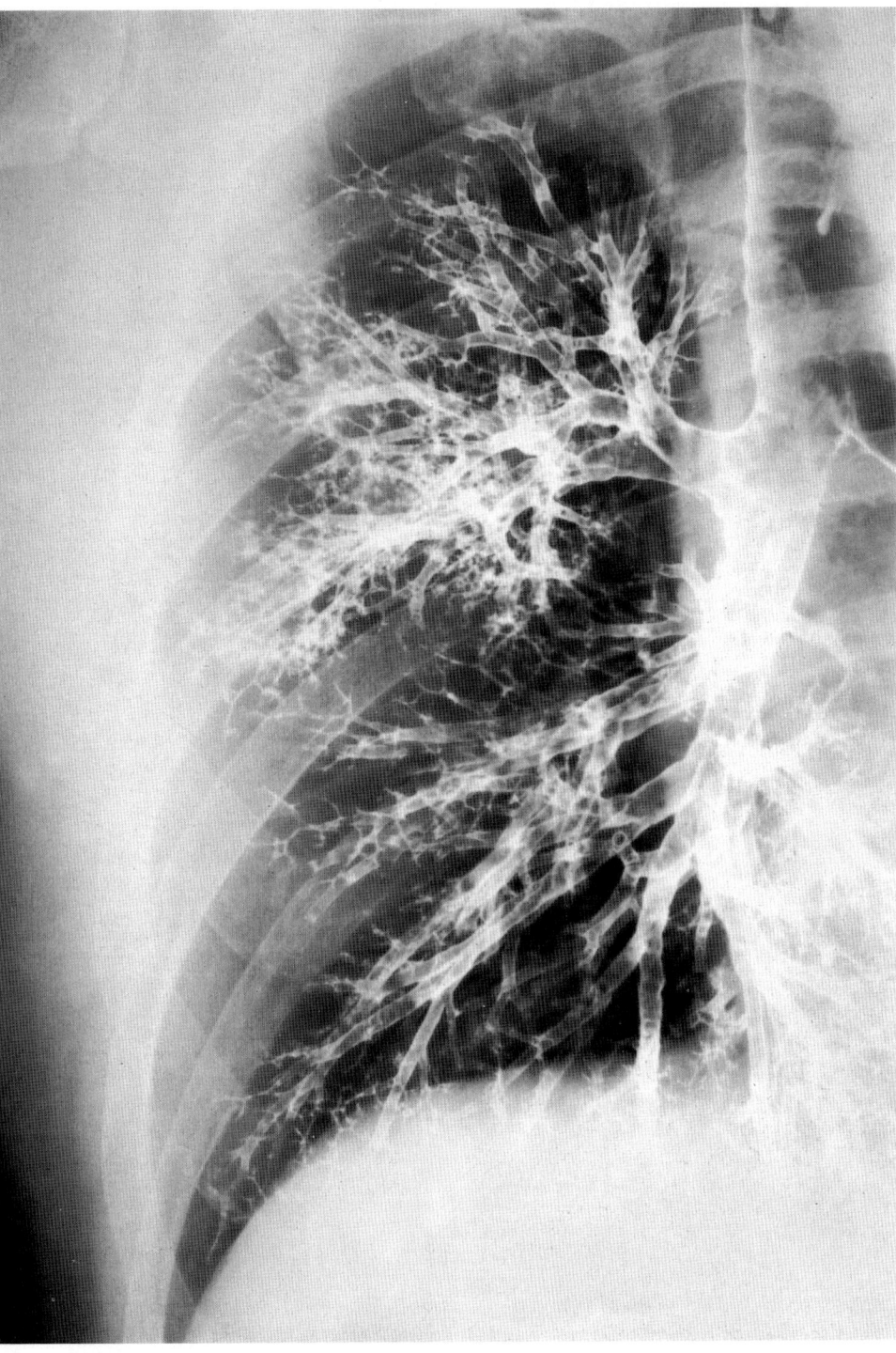

Fig. 63.14 Bronchogram showing the branching pattern of the trachea and bronchi of the right lung, in a slightly oblique anteroposterior view. In this procedure, a radiopaque contrast medium has been introduced into the respiratory tract to coat the walls of the respiratory passages. For identification of the major branches, compare with **Fig. 63.10A**.

then divides into apical and posterior branches. The apical, posterior and anterior segmental bronchi are largely distributed as they are in the right superior lobe. The inferior division descends anterolaterally to the anteroinferior part of the left superior lobe (the lingula) and forms the lingular bronchus, which divides into superior and inferior lingular segmental bronchi. This is different from the pattern in the right middle lobe, where the corresponding distribution is lateral and medial (p. 1070; **Figs 63.10, 63.11**).

Left inferior lobar bronchus
The left inferior bronchus descends posterolaterally and divides to supply territories of the lung that are distributed in essentially the same manner as they are in the right lung.

Segmental anatomy – The superior (apical) segmental bronchus arises from the inferior lobar bronchus posteriorly c.1 cm from its origin. After a further 1–2 cm, the inferior lobar bronchus divides into an antero-medial and a posterolateral stem. The latter divides into lateral and

posterior basal segmental bronchi. The anterior basal segmental bronchus is an independent branch of the inferior lobar bronchus in c.10% of lungs. A subsuperior (subapical) segmental bronchus arises posteriorly from the left inferior lobar bronchus in 30% of lungs (p. 1070; **Figs 63.10, 63.11**).

VASCULAR SUPPLY AND LYMPHATIC DRAINAGE
The trachea is supplied with blood mainly by branches of the inferior thyroid arteries. The bronchial arteries, whose branches ascend to anastomose with the tracheal branches of the inferior thyroid arteries, also supply its thoracic portion. Veins draining the trachea end in the inferior thyroid venous plexus. The lymph vessels pass to the pretracheal and paratracheal lymph nodes.

Bronchial arteries
The bronchial arteries supply oxygenated blood to maintain the pulmonary tissues. They are derived from the descending thoracic aorta either directly or indirectly (Baile 1996). The right bronchial artery is

usually a branch of the third posterior intercostal artery, whilst there are normally two left bronchial arteries (upper and lower) that branch separately from the thoracic aorta. The bronchial arteries accompany the bronchial tree and supply bronchial glands, the walls of the bronchial tubes and larger pulmonary vessels. The bronchial branches form a capillary plexus in the muscular tunic of the air passages, and this supports a second, mucosal plexus, which communicates with branches of the pulmonary artery and drains into the pulmonary veins. Other arterial branches ramify in interlobular loose connective tissue and end partly in deep, and partly in superficial bronchial veins. Some also ramify on the surface of the lung, and form subpleural capillary plexuses. Bronchial arteries supply the bronchial wall as far as the respiratory bronchioles, and anastomose with branches of the pulmonary arteries in the walls of the smaller bronchi and in the visceral pleura. These bronchopulmonary anastomoses may be more numerous in the newborn and are subsequently obliterated to a marked degree. In addition to the main bronchial arteries, smaller bronchial branches arise from the descending thoracic aorta: one of these may lie in the pulmonary ligament and may cause bleeding during inferior lobectomy.

Bronchial veins

The bronchial veins form two distinct systems. Deep bronchial veins commence as intrapulmonary bronchiolar plexuses that communicate freely with the pulmonary veins and eventually join a single trunk that ends in a main pulmonary vein or in the left atrium. Superficial bronchial veins drain extrapulmonary bronchi, visceral pleura and the hilar lymph nodes. They also communicate with the pulmonary veins and end in the azygos vein on the right and in the left superior intercostal or the accessory hemiazygos veins on the left. Bronchial veins do not receive all the blood conveyed by bronchial arteries: some enters the pulmonary veins. The main bronchial arteries and veins run on the dorsal aspect of the extrapulmonary bronchi.

Lymphatic drainage

The deep lymphatic plexus reaches the hilum by travelling along the pulmonary vessels and bronchi. In larger bronchi the deep plexus has submucosal and peribronchial parts, but in smaller bronchi there is only a single plexus that extends to the bronchioles. The walls of the alveoli have no lymphatic vessels.

INNERVATION

The anterior and posterior pulmonary plexuses innervate the trachea and the bronchi (p. 1075). The two plexuses are interconnected. The nerves enter the lung as networks that travel along branches of the bronchi and pulmonary and bronchial vessels as far as the visceral pleura. The trachea is innervated by branches of the vagi, recurrent laryngeal nerves and sympathetic trunks, distributed to the tracheal smooth muscle, mucosal glands and blood vessels. Efferent vagal preganglionic axons synapse on small ganglia within the walls of the tracheobronchial tree: these may act as sites of integration and/or modulation of the input from extrinsic nerves, or permit some local control of aspects of airway function by local reflex mechanisms.

BRONCHOSCOPY

Bronchoscopy allows the direct visualization of the vocal cords, trachea and major airways as far as the first division of the subsegmental airway (Fig. 63.15). Occasionally bronchoscopy can also provide some information about structures adjacent to the airways; for example, significant subcarinal lymphadenopathy may cause splaying or widening of the carina. Bronchoscopy enables the acquisition of samples (e.g. bronchial lavage, bronchial brushings, bronchial and transbronchial biopsies), provides information about staging in lung cancer, and facilitates therapeutic procedures (e.g. foreign body removal, ablation of tumours and insertion of airway stents). The information obtained by continuous (spiral) volume CT scanning can be reconstructed to provide three-dimensional images. These can be used to create endobronchial views (virtual bronchoscopy, Fig 63.15D) or to demonstrate the pulmonary arteries.

PULMONARY DEFENSIVE MECHANISMS

The respiratory tract presents a huge surface area that is vulnerable to desiccation, microbial invasion and the mechanical and chemical effects

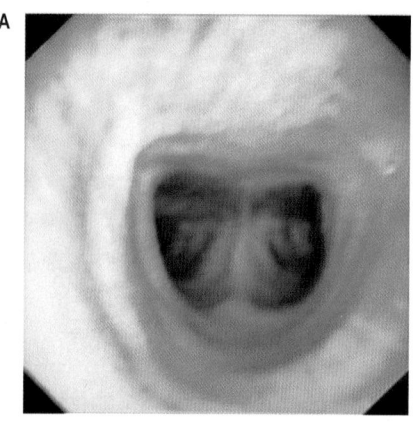
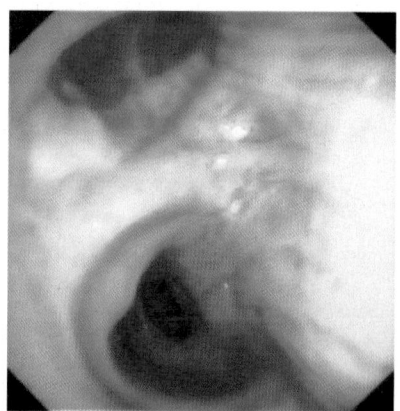
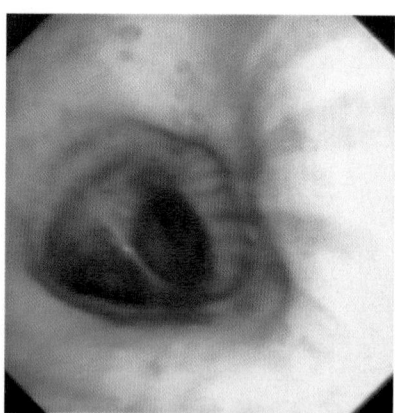

Fig. 63.15 Bronchoscopic view of **A**, distal trachea and carina; **B**, right bronchus intermedius; **C**, left main bronchus. **D**, Virtual CT bronchoscopy with image at carina obtained by planar reconstruction of spiral CT. (By kind permission from GE Medical Systems.)

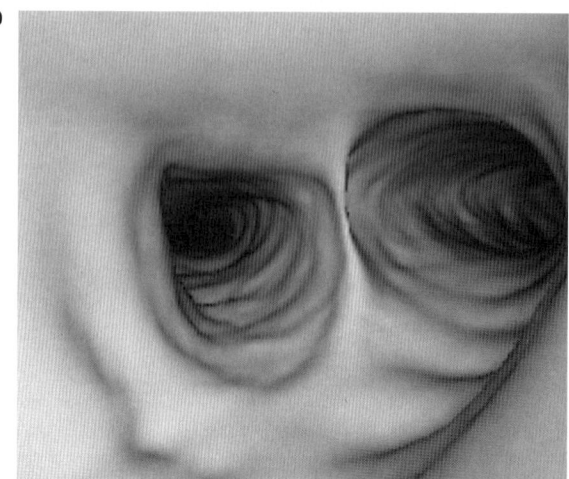

of inhaled particles. Inhaled air is humidified chiefly in the upper respiratory tract where it passes, with some turbulence, over the nasal and buccopharyngeal mucosae. Secretions of the various glands of the bronchial tree also help to prevent desiccation. Goblet cells secrete sulphated acid mucosubstances, and cells in mucous glands beneath the epithelial surface contain mainly carboxylated mucosubstances, particularly those associated with sialic acid, although sulphated groups also occur. In contrast, cells of serous glands contain neutral mucosubstances. Goblet cells respond mainly to local irritation, while tubular glands, both mucous and serous, are mainly under neural and hormonal control. Excessive or altered secretions may obstruct the flow of air. In addition to mucosubstances secreted by bronchial glands, antibacterial and antiviral substances, e.g. lysozyme, antibodies of the IgA type and possibly interferon, also appear in the secreted fluid.

Inhaled particles may be removed via the ciliary rejection current. Cilia sweep the fluid overlying the surfaces of bronchioles, bronchi and trachea upwards at c.1 cm/minute, and much inhaled matter trapped in the viscous fluid may be removed in this way. Particles small enough to reach the alveoli may be removed by alveolar phagocytes (p. 1060). Alveolar epithelium has limited powers of regeneration but normally is continually replaced. The lifespan of alveolar squamous cells is c.3 weeks, that of alveolar phagocytes c.4 days. Inhaled particles may also be cleared by the cough reflex.

Numerous lymphoid nodules (p. 1057) occur in the bronchial lining: they provide foci for the production of lymphocytes and give local immunological protection against infection by cell mediated (T-cell) activities and by the production of immunoglobulins (mainly IgA) from B cells which are passed on to gland cells for secretion to the epithelial surface.

ANATOMY OF COUGHING

Initiation of muscular responses to irritation involves stimulation of sensory endings by mechanical or chemical stimuli. The identity of these afferent terminals is still somewhat uncertain, other than at the laryngeal aditus, where epithelial receptors similar to taste buds are considered responsible. However, at least some of the 'brush cells' of the respiratory epithelium appear to have neural contacts and they may represent sensory cells with basal synaptic outputs (Widdicombe 2002). Other than the larynx, the primary carina and branching points of the tracheobronchial tree appear to be the most sensitive areas of the epithelium lining the airways. Vagal afferents stimulate the cough centre in the brain stem.

Initially there is a deep inspiration, which is followed by forceful contraction of the expiratory muscle and diaphragm against a closed glottis. This leads to an abrupt rise in pleural pressure (6.5 to 13 kPa) and intra-alveolar pressure. Subsequent glottal opening causes a rapid peak expiratory flow of air, followed by some collapse of the trachea and central airways, which is responsible for the post peak plateau in flow.

REFERENCES

Armstrong P 2000 The normal chest. In: Armstrong P, Wilson AG, Dee P, Hansell DM (eds) Images of the Diseases of the Chest. London: Mosby: 21–62.

Baile EM 1996 The anatomy and physiology of the bronchial circulation. J Aerosol Med 9: 1–6.

Ghaye B, Szapiro D, Fanchamps JM, Dondelinger RF 2001 Congenital bronchial abnormalities revisited. Radiographics 21: 105–19.

Jeffrey PK 2003 Microscopic structure of the lung. In: Gibson GJ, Geddes DM, Cosatbel U, Sterk PJ, Corrin B (eds) Respiratory Medicine, 3rd edn. London: Elsevier Science: 34–50.

Venuta F, Rendina EA, De Giacoma T, Flaishman I, Guarino E, Ciccone AM, Ricci C 1998 Technique to reduce air leaks after pulmonary lobectomy. Eur J Cardiothorac Surg 13: 361–4.

Widdicombe J 2002 Neuroregulation of cough: implications for drug therapy. Curr Opin Pharmacol 2: 256–63.

Diaphragm and phrenic nerve

The diaphragm (**Figs 64.1**, **64.2**) is a curved musculofibrous sheet that separates the thoracic from the abdominal cavity. Its mainly convex upper surface faces the thorax, and its concave inferior surface is directed towards the abdomen. The positions of the domes or cupolae of the diaphragm are extremely variable as they depend on body build and the phase of ventilation. Thus the diaphragm will be higher in short, fat people than in tall, thin people, and overinflation of the lung, as occurs for example in emphysema, causes marked depression of the diaphragm. Usually, after forced expiration the right cupola is level anteriorly with the fourth costal cartilage and therefore the right nipple, whereas the left cupola lies approximately one rib lower. With maximal inspiration, the cupola will descend as much as 10 cm, and on a plain chest radiograph the dome coincides with the tip of the sixth rib. In the supine position, the diaphragm will be higher than in the erect position, and when the body is lying on one side, the dependent diaphragm will be considerably higher than the uppermost one.

ATTACHMENTS, ORIGINS, COMPONENTS

The muscle fibres of the diaphragm arise from the highly oblique circumference of the thoracic outlet: the attachments are low posteriorly and laterally, but high anteriorly. Although it is a continuous sheet, the muscle can be considered in three parts, sternal, costal and lumbar, which are based on the regions of peripheral attachment. The sternal part arises by two fleshy slips from the back of the xiphoid process, and is not always present. The costal part arises from the internal surfaces of the lower six costal cartilages and their adjoining ribs on each side, and interdigitates with transversus abdominis (**Fig. 57.17**). The lumbar part arises from two aponeurotic arches, the medial and lateral arcuate ligaments (sometimes termed lumbocostal arches) and from the lumbar vertebrae by two pillars or crura.

The lateral arcuate ligament is a thickened band in the fascia that covers quadratus lumborum, and it arches across the upper part of that

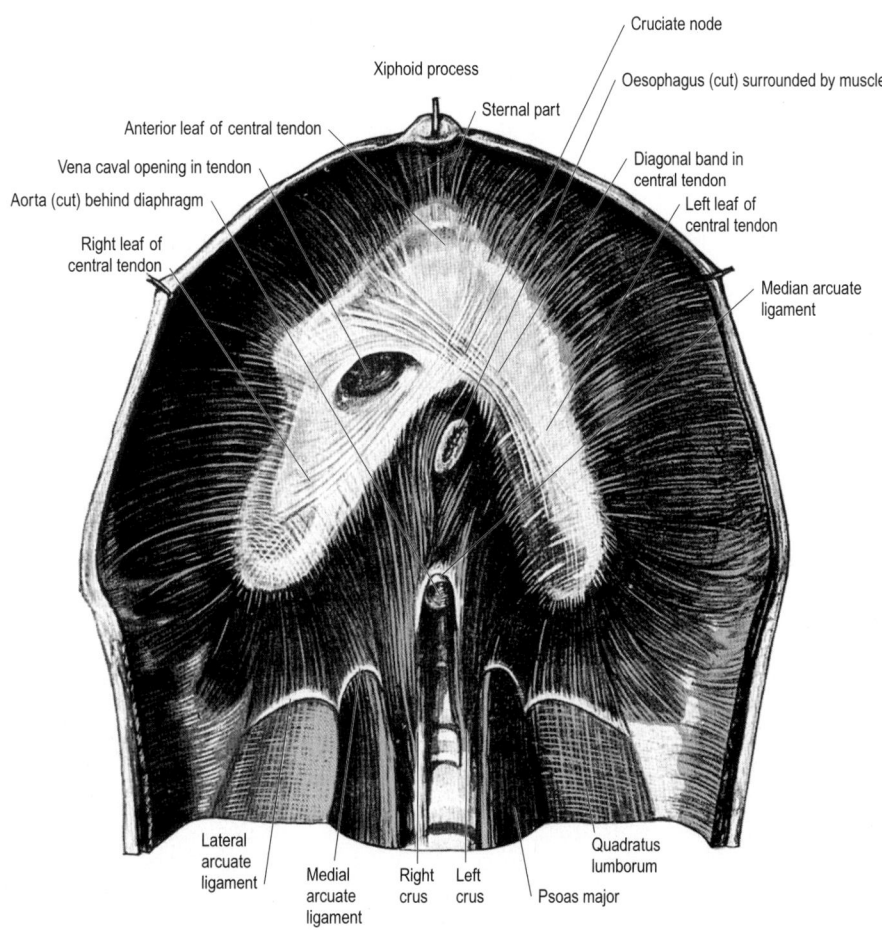

Fig. 64.1 Abdominal aspect of the diaphragm. Note that the fibres descend from their relatively 'high' anterior sternocostal attachments steeply and obliquely to their complex 'low' posterior attachments.

muscle. It is attached medially to the front of the transverse process of the first lumbar vertebra, and laterally to the lower margin of the twelfth rib near its midpoint. The medial arcuate ligament is a tendinous arch in the fascia that covers the upper part of psoas major. Medially, it is continuous with the lateral tendinous margin of the corresponding crus, and is thus attached to the side of the body of the first or second lumbar vertebra. Laterally, it is fixed to the front of the transverse process of the first lumbar vertebra.

The crura are tendinous at their attachments, and blend with the anterior longitudinal ligament of the vertebral column. The right crus is broader and longer than the left, and arises from the anterolateral surfaces of the bodies and intervertebral discs of the upper three lumbar vertebrae. The left crus arises from the corresponding parts of the upper two lumbar vertebrae. The medial tendinous margins of the crura meet in the midline to form an arch, the median arcuate ligament, crossing the front of the aorta at the level of the thoracolumbar disc; it is often poorly defined.

From these circumferential attachments, the fibres of the diaphragm converge into a central tendon. Fibres from the xiphoid process are short, run almost horizontally and are occasionally aponeurotic. Fibres from the medial and lateral arcuate ligaments, and more especially those from the ribs and their cartilages, are longer. They rise almost vertically at first and then curve towards their central attachment. Fibres from the crura diverge, and the most lateral become more lateral as they ascend to the central tendon. Medial fibres of the right crus embrace the oesophagus where it passes through the diaphragm, the more superficial fibres ascend on the left, and deeper fibres cover the right margin (p. 1082). Sometimes, a fleshy fasciculus from the medial side of the left crus crosses the aorta and runs obliquely through the fibres of the right crus towards the vena caval opening, but this fasciculus does not continue upwards around the oesophageal passage on the right side.

The central tendon of the diaphragm is a thin but strong aponeurosis of closely interwoven fibres situated near the centre of the muscle, but closer to the front of the thorax, so that the posterior muscular fibres are longer. In the centre it lies immediately below the pericardium, with which it is partially blended. Its shape is trifoliate. The middle, or anterior, leaf has the form of an equilateral triangle with the apex directed towards the xiphoid process. The right and left folia are tongue-shaped and curve laterally and backwards, the left being a little narrower. The central area of the tendon consists of four well-marked diagonal bands fanning out from a thick central node where compressed tendinous strands decussate in front of the oesophagus and to the left of the vena cava.

SHAPE AND RELATIONSHIPS

The upper surface of the diaphragm lies in relation to three serous membranes. On each side, the pleura separates it from the base of the corresponding lung, and over the middle folium of the central tendon the pericardium is interposed between it and the heart. The latter area, which is almost flat, is referred to as the cardiac plateau. It extends more to the left than the right. In anteroposterior view, the superior profile of the diaphragm rises on either side of the cardiac plateau to a smooth convex dome or cupola, the cupola on the right being higher and slightly broader than that on the left. Most of the inferior surface is covered by peritoneum. The right side is accurately moulded over the convex surface of the right lobe of the liver, the right kidney and right suprarenal (adrenal) gland. The left side conforms to the left lobe of the liver, the fundus of the stomach, the spleen, the left kidney and the left suprarenal gland. In view of these differences in the profile and anatomical relationships of the right and left diaphragm, the side should always be specified in clinical descriptions. At full inspiration, the right hemidiaphragm is found at the anterior sixth rib on a posteroanterior chest radiograph (**Fig. 63.8**). The left hemidiaphragm is c.1.5–2.5 cm lower than the right. Unilateral paralysis may be seen as a raised hemidiaphragm on a chest radiograph.

APERTURES

A number of structures pass between the thorax and abdomen through apertures in the diaphragm. There are three large openings, for the aorta, oesophagus and inferior vena cava (**Fig. 64.2**), and a number of smaller ones.

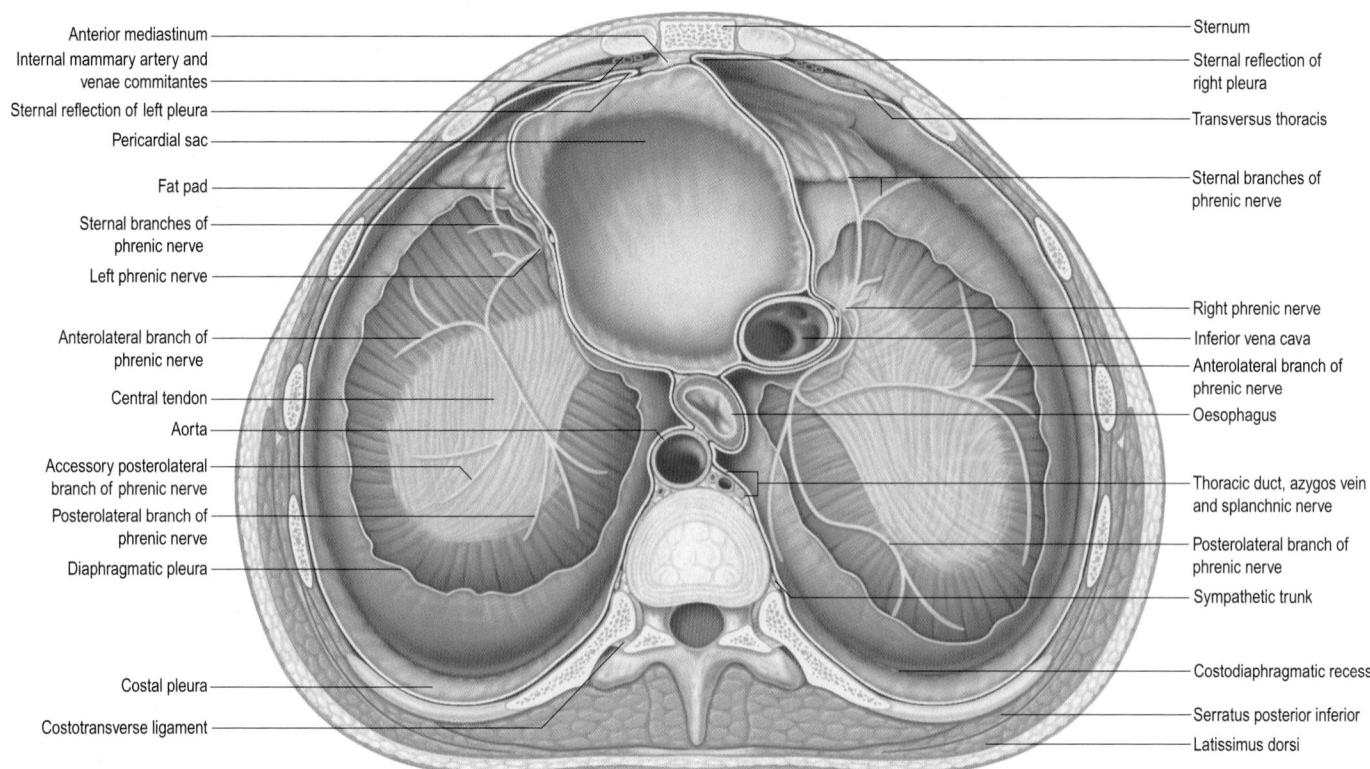

Anterior mediastinum
Internal mammary artery and venae commitantes
Sternal reflection of left pleura
Pericardial sac
Fat pad
Sternal branches of phrenic nerve
Left phrenic nerve
Anterolateral branch of phrenic nerve
Central tendon
Aorta
Accessory posterolateral branch of phrenic nerve
Posterolateral branch of phrenic nerve
Diaphragmatic pleura
Costal pleura
Costotransverse ligament

Sternum
Sternal reflection of right pleura
Transversus thoracis
Sternal branches of phrenic nerve
Right phrenic nerve
Inferior vena cava
Anterolateral branch of phrenic nerve
Oesophagus
Thoracic duct, azygos vein and splanchnic nerve
Posterolateral branch of phrenic nerve
Sympathetic trunk
Costodiaphragmatic recess
Serratus posterior inferior
Latissimus dorsi

Fig. 64.2 Thoracic aspect of the diaphragm. Note that the fibres descend from their relatively 'high' anterior sternocostal attachments steeply and obliquely to their complex 'low' posterior attachments. The phrenic nerves are demonstrated on the diaphragmatic surfaces.

The aortic aperture is the lowest and most posterior of the large openings. It is at the level of the lower border of the twelfth thoracic vertebra and the thoracolumbar intervertebral disc, slightly to the left of the midline. It is an osseo-aponeurotic opening defined by the diaphragmatic crura laterally, the vertebral column posteriorly and the diaphragm anteriorly. Strictly speaking, it lies behind the diaphragm and its median arcuate ligament (when present). Occasionally, some tendinous fibres from the medial parts of the crura also pass behind the aorta, converting the opening into a fibrous ring. The aortic opening transmits the aorta, thoracic duct, lymphatic trunks from the lower posterior thoracic wall and, sometimes, the azygos and hemiazygos veins (p. 1026).

The oesophageal aperture is located at the level of the tenth thoracic vertebra, above, in front of and a little to the left of, the aortic opening. It transmits the oesophagus, gastric nerves, oesophageal branches of the left gastric vessels and some lymphatic vessels. The elliptical opening has a slightly oblique long axis, and is bounded by muscle fibres that originate in the medial part of the right crus and cross the midline. These fibres form a chimney c.2.5 cm long, which accommodates the terminal portions of the oesophagus. The outermost fibres run in a craniocaudal direction, and the innermost fibres are arranged circumferentially. There is no direct continuity between the oesophageal wall and the muscle around the oesophageal opening. The fascia on the inferior surface of the diaphragm, which is continuous with the transversalis fascia (p. 1104) and is rich in elastic fibres, extends upwards into the opening as a flattened cone to blend with the wall of the oesophagus 2–3 cm above the oesophago–gastric (squamocolumnar) junction. Some of its elastic fibres penetrate to the submucosa of the oesophagus. This peri-oesophageal areolar tissue is referred to as the phreno-oesophageal ligament. It connects the oesophagus flexibly to the diaphragm, permitting some freedom of movement during swallowing and ventilation and at the same time limiting upward displacement of the oesophagus.

The vena caval aperture, the highest of the three large openings, lies at about the level of the disc between the eighth and ninth thoracic vertebrae. It is quadrilateral, and located at the junction of the right leaf with the central area of the tendon, so its margins are aponeurotic. It is traversed by the inferior vena cava, which adheres to the margin of the opening, and by some branches of the right phrenic nerve.

There are two lesser apertures in each crus: one transmits the greater and the other the lesser, splanchnic nerve. The ganglionated sympathetic trunks usually enter the abdominal cavity behind the diaphragm, deep to the medial arcuate ligament. Openings for minute veins frequently occur in the central tendon.

On each side of the diaphragm there are small areas where the muscle fibres are replaced by areolar tissue. One, between the sternal and costal parts, contains the superior epigastric branch of the internal thoracic artery and some lymph vessels from the abdominal wall and convex surface of the liver. The other, between the costal part and the fibres that spring from the lateral arcuate ligament, is less constant. When it is present, the posterosuperior surface of the kidney is separated from the pleura only by areolar tissue.

OESOPHAGEAL REFLUX

Reflux of gastric contents into the oesophagus, with risk of inhalation into the lungs is normally prevented by a physiological antireflux barrier located at the gastro–oesophageal junction. The major components of this barrier are the specialized smooth muscle of the wall of the lower oesophagus and the encircling fibres of the crural diaphragm. See also Chapter 71.

HIATUS HERNIA

The diaphragm lends additional power to all expulsive efforts. Thus sneezing, coughing, laughing, crying, urinating, defaecating and expelling the fetus from the uterus, are all preceded by a deep inspiration. A deep inspiration, followed by closure of the glottis, is a common preliminary to powerful recruitment of the trunk muscles, e.g. in lifting heavy weights; the increased intra-abdominal pressure provides pneumatic bracing of the vertebral column. Repeated stress may eventually compromise the integrity of the hiatus, so that the muscular hiatal tunnel widens. There is also laxity of the phreno-oesophageal membrane, which allows the gastro–oesophageal junction to slide into the thorax; this is usually termed a sliding, or type I, hiatus hernia (Kahrilas 2001). Sliding hernias are usually acquired, and they commonly occur in the fifth decade of life. They are found in more than 50% of patients with gastro–oesophageal reflux. This condition induces tonic contraction of the longitudinal oesophageal muscle, which further exacerbates the hiatus hernia. When the stomach herniates into the thorax alongside the oesophagus, it is termed a para-oesophageal, or type II, hiatus hernia.

CONGENITAL HERNIAS/EVENTRATION

Abdominal organs, usually the stomach, may herniate through the diaphragm into the thorax. There are three sites at which such hernias can occur: posterolateral (Bochdalek), subcostosternal (Morgagni) and oesophageal (p. 1093).

The most common is a posterolateral (Bochdalek) hernia, which occurs as a result of a defect in the posterior diaphragm in the region of the tenth or eleventh ribs. It is more common on the left, and presents with abdominal contents in the left hemithorax at birth; clinically significant cases develop hypoxaemia and respiratory failure at birth. A chest radiograph demonstrates mediastinal shift to the contralateral side and the presence of the gastrointestinal contents in the thorax; the diagnosis should be made at routine prenatal ultrasound. Treatment involves decompression of the gastrointestinal contents and cardiopulmonary stabilization. Surgical repair is performed when the patients are stable, but prognosis is determined by the degree of accompanying pulmonary hypoplasia, severity of pulmonary vascular abnormalities and any associated congenital heart defects.

Subcostosternal hernia, first described by Morgagni, is uncommon and occurs through a defect in the anterior diaphragm just lateral to the xiphoid process. It is frequently asymptomatic.

Oesophageal hernia occurs as a result of a defect in the oesophageal aperture, so that part of the stomach herniates into the thorax. It is rarely congenital in origin, usually develops later in life, and is believed to be acquired (p. 1083).

DIAPHRAGMATIC TRAUMA

Closed and penetrating thoracoabdominal injuries may result in rupture or laceration of the diaphragm. With closed injuries and diaphragmatic rupture, there may be subsequent herniation of the abdominal contents into the thorax. Spiral computed tomography with planar reformation should be the primary investigation (Shanmuganathan et al 2000). Magnetic resonance imaging is usually performed when other imaging modalities have produced equivocal findings. Early operative repair is recommended in diaphragmatic trauma, because untreated cases are at risk of developing gastrointestinal obstruction or perforation. Patients with penetrating injuries may require additional assessment by thoracoscopy (Lowdermilk & Naunheim 2000).

VASCULAR SUPPLY AND LYMPHATIC DRAINAGE

The lower five intercostal and subcostal arteries supply the costal margins of the diaphragm while the phrenic arteries supply the main central portion of the diaphragm.

PHRENIC ARTERIES

Two small phrenic vessels help to supply the diaphragm via the abdominal surface (Fig. 91.1). They may arise separately from the aorta, just above its coeliac trunk, by a common aortic stem, or from the coeliac trunk. Occasionally, one is from the aorta, the other from a renal artery. Each artery ascends laterally anterior to a crus of the diaphragm, near the medial border of the suprarenal gland. The left passes behind the oesophagus and forwards on the left side of its diaphragmatic opening. The right phrenic artery passes posterior to the inferior vena cava, and then along the right side of its opening. Each phrenic artery divides into medial and lateral branches near the posterior border of the central tendon. The medial branch curves forwards to anastomose with its fellow in front of the central tendon and with the musculophrenic and pericardiacophrenic arteries. The lateral branch approaches the thoracic wall, and anastomoses with the lower posterior intercostal and musculophrenic arteries. The lateral branch of the right artery supplies the inferior vena cava, whereas the left sends ascending branches to the oesophagus. Invariably there is a communicating artery between the left gastric and inferior phrenic arteries.

PHRENIC VEINS

The phrenic veins follow the corresponding arteries on the inferior diaphragmatic surface. The right phrenic vein ends in the inferior vena cava. The left phrenic vein is often double: one branch ends in the left renal or suprarenal vein, the other passes anterior to the oesophageal opening to join the inferior vena cava.

INNERVATION

The diaphragm receives its motor supply via the phrenic nerves. Sensory fibres are distributed to the peripheral part of the muscle by the lower six or seven intercostal nerves. The right crus of the diaphragm, the fibres of which divide to the right and left of the oesophageal opening, is innervated by both right and left phrenic nerves. There is some evidence that the crural fibres contract slightly before the costal part, and this may be functionally significant.

PHRENIC NERVE

The phrenic nerve is a mixed nerve that provides the sole motor supply to the diaphragm. It arises chiefly from the fourth cervical ramus, but also receives contributions from the third and fifth cervical rami (**Fig. 31.2**). The course of the cervical part of the phrenic nerve is described on page 554. Within the thorax, the phrenic nerve descends anterior to the pulmonary hilum, between the fibrous pericardium and mediastinal pleura, to the diaphragm, accompanied by the pericardio-phrenic vessels. In its thoracic course, each phrenic nerve supplies sensory branches to the mediastinal pleura, fibrous pericardium and parietal serous pericardium. The right and left phrenic nerves differ in their intrathoracic relationships (Rajanna 1947).

Right phrenic nerve

The right phrenic nerve is shorter and more vertical than the left, and is separated at the root of the neck from the second part of the right subclavian artery by scalenus anterior. It is then lateral to the right brachiocephalic vein, the superior vena cava and the fibrous pericardium that covers the right surface of the right atrium and inferior vena cava. The right phrenic nerve divides just above or at the level of the diaphragm.

Left phrenic nerve

At the root of the neck, the left phrenic nerve is commonly stated to leave the medial edge of scalenus anterior and to pass anterior to the first part of the left subclavian artery and behind the thoracic duct. However, sometimes the right and left nerves are symmetric in their cervical course, and so the left phrenic nerve may cross anterior to the second part of the left subclavian artery, separated from it by scalenus anterior at the level of the thoracic inlet. Thereafter, the left phrenic nerve crosses anterior to the left internal thoracic artery, descending across the medial aspect of the apex of the left lung and its pleura to the first part of the subclavian artery, which it crosses obliquely to reach a groove between the left common carotid and subclavian arteries. It passes anteromedially, superficial to the left vagus nerve just above the aortic arch and behind the left brachiocephalic vein, and then passes superficial to the aortic arch and the left superior intercostal vein, anterior to the left pulmonary hilum, to lie between the fibrous pericardium covering the surface of the left ventricle and the mediastinal pleura (**Fig. 63.5**).

Diaphragmatic relationships

The right phrenic nerve traverses the central tendon of the diaphragm, either by the caval aperture or just lateral to it. The left phrenic nerve traverses the muscular part of the diaphragm anterior to the central tendon, just lateral to the left cardiac surface and more anterior than the right phrenic nerve. At the diaphragm or slightly above it, each phrenic nerve supplies fine branches to the parietal pleura above, and the parietal peritoneum below, the central diaphragm. The trunk of each nerve then divides into three branches as it traverses the diaphragm. These are commonly arranged as follows (with some variation): an anterior (sternal) branch, which runs anteromedially towards the sternum and connects with its fellow; an anterolateral branch, which runs laterally anterior to the lateral leaf of the central tendon; a short posterior branch, which divides into a posterolateral ramus coursing behind the lateral leaf and a posterior (crural) ramus supplying the crural fibres. Posterolateral and crural branches may arise separately from the phrenic nerve.

These main branches are often submerged in diaphragmatic muscle or below it. They supply motor fibres to the muscle and sensory fibres to the peritoneum and pleura related to the central part of the diaphragm. They also contain proprioceptive fibres from the musculature. Location of the main branches is of importance in avoiding surgical damage. Radial incisions in the diaphragm from the costal margin to the oesophageal hiatus lead to diaphragmatic paralysis. Thoraco-abdominal incisions in a circumferential manner in the periphery of the diaphragm do not involve any significant branches of the phrenic nerves and preserve diaphragmatic function. Similarly, incisions of the central tendon are safe. The right crus splits to enclose the oesophagus: the right phrenic nerve supplies the part of it to the right of the oesophagus, and the left phrenic nerve supplies the left crus and the part of the right crus that lies on the left of the oesophagus. Phrenic rami connect with branches of the coeliac plexuses on the inferior surface of the diaphragm, and there is a small phrenic ganglion on the right, at the junction of the plexuses. Rami from the plexuses supply the suprarenal glands and, on the right, the hepatic falciform and coronary ligaments, the inferior vena cava and, possibly (via connections with coeliac and hepatic plexuses), the gallbladder (p. 1229).

Lesions of the phrenic nerve

Division of the phrenic nerve in the neck completely paralyses the corresponding half of the diaphragm, which atrophies. If an accessory phrenic nerve exists, section or crushing of the main nerve as it lies on scalenus anterior will not produce complete paralysis. The phrenic nerve may be involved with traumatic lesions of the upper brachial plexus. Historically, it was deliberately injured in order to collapse – and hence rest – the lung in patients with pulmonary tuberculosis. Cardiac surgery is one of the most common causes of phrenic nerve injury, especially as a result of the instillation of saline slush for myocardial preservation. Other causes include thoracic surgery, tumours of the lung or mediastinum, and infections such as typhoid and polio.

Phrenic nerve damage leads to paradoxical movement of the diaphragm that is best observed fluoroscopically, with the patient first in the upright position (diaphragm unloaded), and then supine with a small weight on the abdomen (diaphragm loaded). Diaphragmatic paralysis can also be assessed by ultrasound examination with sniff and cough manoeuvres. Electrical stimulation of the diaphragm, by 'pacing' of one or both phrenic nerves, has been used with some success in infants with central alveolar hypoventilatory syndrome ('Ondine's curse') and in patients with high cervical lesions of the spinal cord, in whom the diaphragm is paralysed, but the lower motor neurones are intact. Electrodes are placed adjacent to the nerves, sometimes in the neck but more usually in the chest, and a ventilatory rhythm is established by trains of stimuli delivered by an implanted device. Because this is an unphysiological way of recruiting the muscle, the fibres must be 'conditioned' during the initial period of stimulation, so that they acquire the necessary resistance to fatigue.

ACCESSORY PHRENIC NERVE

The accessory phrenic nerve is described in Chapter 31.

REFERRED PAIN

Diaphragmatic pain is frequently felt at the tip of the shoulder, reflecting common nerve root origins in the neck. It usually occurs when there is inflammation of the diaphragmatic pleura, e.g. in basal pneumonia, pleural effusions or malignant disease.

ANATOMY OF BREATHING

Breathing is a highly coordinated abdominal and thoracic process. The diaphragm is the major muscle of inspiration, responsible for some 67% of the vital capacity. The external intercostal muscles are most active in inspiration, and the internal intercostals, which are not as strong, are most active in expiration. Increasing the vertical, transverse and anteroposterior dimensions of the chest increases the volume of the pleural space, and the resulting decrease in intrapleural pressure draws air into the lungs. During expiration, the diaphragm relaxes and moves superiorly. Air is expelled from the lungs and the elastic recoil of the lung creates a subatmospheric pressure that returns the lateral and anteroposterior dimensions of the thorax to normal (De Troyer & Estenne 1988, Celli 1998).

During inspiration, the lowest ribs are fixed, and contraction of the diaphragm draws the central tendon downwards. In this movement, the curvature of the diaphragm is scarcely altered. The cupolae move downwards and a little forwards almost parallel to their original positions. The associated downward displacement of the abdominal viscera is permitted by the extensibility of the abdominal wall, but the limit of this extensibility is soon reached. The central tendon, its motion arrested by the abdominal viscera, then becomes a fixed point from which the fibres of the diaphragm continue to contract. This causes the second to tenth ribs to be elevated and the inferior portions of the ribs are turned outwards. The medial aspect of the rib is elevated and this increases the transverse dimension of the chest in the same manner as a bucket handle swinging outwards (**Fig. 64.3A**). This effect is most evident in the lower ribs (seventh to tenth ribs). Movements at the costovertebral joints cause elevation of the anterior ends of the ribs that push the body of the sternum and the upper ribs forwards. This 'pump handle' movement is most evident in the superior ribs (second to sixth ribs) and increases the anteroposterior dimension of the thorax (**Fig. 64.3B**). The right cupola of the diaphragm, which lies on the liver, has a greater resistance to overcome than the left, which lies over the stomach, and so the right crus and the fibres of the right side are more substantial than those of the left. The balance between descent of the diaphragm, protrusion of the abdominal wall ('abdominal' breathing), and elevation of the ribs ('thoracic' breathing), varies in different individuals and with the depth of ventilation. The thoracic element is usually more marked in females, but increases in both sexes during deep inspiration.

Diaphragmatic excursion is c.1.5 cm in quiet breathing. During deep ventilation, the maximum movement ranges from 6 to 10 cm. After a forced inspiration, e.g. when breathing is partially obstructed, the right cupola of the diaphragm can descend to about the level of the eleventh thoracic vertebra, while the left cupola may reach the level of the body of the twelfth. After a forced expiration, the right cupola of the diaphragm is level anteriorly with the fourth costal cartilage, laterally with the fifth, sixth and seventh ribs, and posteriorly with the eighth, and the left cupola is a little lower.

The level of the diaphragm is affected, not only by the phase and depth of ventilation, but also by the degree of distension of the stomach and intestines and the size of the liver. Radiographs show that the height of the diaphragm within the thorax also varies considerably with posture. It is highest when the body is supine, and in this position it performs the greatest ventilatory excursions with normal breathing. When the body is erect the diaphragm is lower, and its ventilatory movements become smaller. The diaphragmatic profile is still lower in the sitting posture, and ventilatory excursions are smallest under these conditions. When the body is horizontal and on one side, the two halves of the diaphragm do not behave in the same way. The uppermost half sinks to a lower level even than in sitting, and moves little with ventilation. The lower half rises higher in the thorax than it does even in the supine position, and its ventilatory excursions are considerably greater. Changes in the level of the diaphragm with alterations in posture explain why patients with severe dyspnoea are most comfortable, and least short of breath, when sitting up.

The primary role of the intercostal muscles is to stiffen the chest wall, preventing paradoxical motion during descent of the diaphragm in inspiration. This becomes most obvious immediately after high spinal injury, when there is flaccid paralysis of the entire trunk and only the diaphragm is left functioning. In a healthy adult with a vital capacity of 4.5 litres, some 3 litres is accounted for by diaphragmatic excursion. Immediately after high spinal injury, the vital capacity decreases to about 300 ml, even though the diaphragm is moving maximally, because some 2.7 litres is lost by paradoxical incursion of the flaccid chest wall as the diaphragm descends. With time (usually several weeks) the paralysis becomes spastic, stiffening the chest wall, and the vital capacity increases towards its phrenic limit of about 3 litres.

In the same way, high spinal injury reveals the role of the abdomen in inspiration and expiration. The abdomen is the major muscle of active expiration in man. During the flaccid stage of high spinal paralysis, the only mechanisms available for returning the relaxed diaphragm into the thorax on expiration are passive recoil of the lungs and chest wall, and the weight of the abdominal viscera. The latter is the most important, and operates only when patients are lying down. If they are sat up or raised upright, they are unable to breathe out. Trussing the abdomen with an elastic binder can help such patients. Conversely, when paralysis becomes spastic, the stiff abdominal wall opposes inspiration.

The role of the abdomen in breathing is often underestimated. If, for example, the anterolateral wall were made of steel, linking the pelvic rim rigidly to the costal margins, inspiration would be impossible. The diaphragm could not descend (because the abdominal contents are incompressible), and the ribs could not rise (because the links to the pelvis would be inextensible). During normal breathing, the abdomen relaxes as the diaphragm contracts. It is possible to oppose this motion by tensing the abdomen, as in the 'beach posture' adopted to exaggerate the size of the chest. In this case, the abdominal contents fix the central tendon of the diaphragm, so that it raises the rib cage as it contracts, but it is a condition of that manoeuvre that the gap between the ribs and the pelvic rim widens.

The ventilatory muscles must also work during sleep, when the pharyngeal muscles relax and upper airway resistance increases. It is now appreciated that in some people, particularly the obese, this relaxation can lead to periodic apnoea and marked hypoxia during sleep. This implies that the pharyngeal muscles have an important ventilatory role in waking life. It is also clear that, although ventilatory

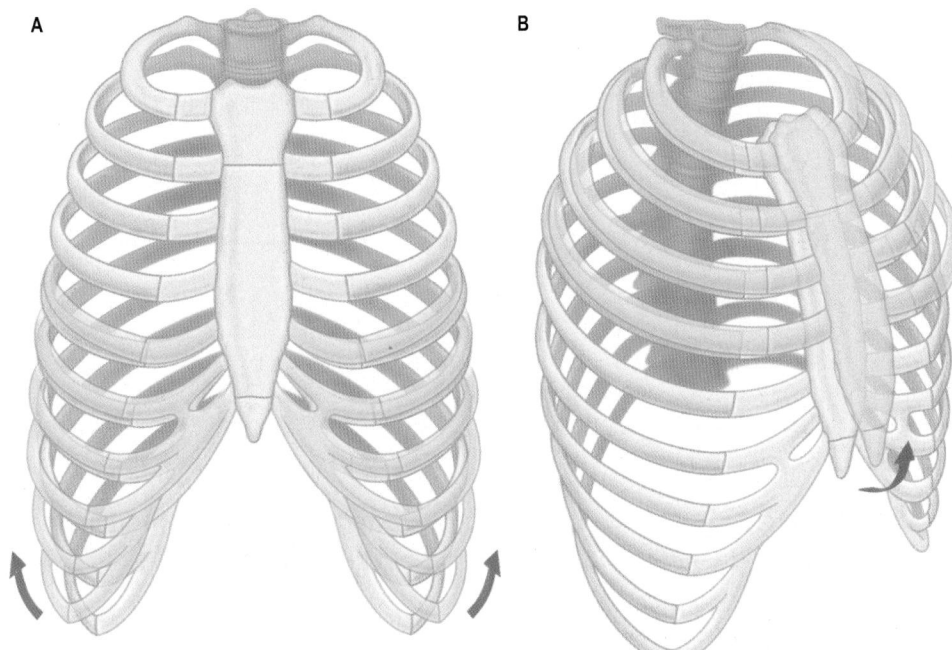

A   B

Fig. 64.3 Movements of the ribs during breathing (**A**) increase the transverse diameter of the chest by the 'bucket handle' movement and (**B**) increase the anteroposterior dimension of the thorax by the 'pump handle' movement.

muscles rarely tire in normal life, they do fatigue when placed under abnormal loads, e.g. in chronic obstructive pulmonary disease.

The different pulmonary regions do not all move equally in ventilation. In quiet ventilation, the juxtahilar part of the lung scarcely moves and the middle region moves only slightly. The superficial parts of the lung expand the most, and the mediastinal surface, posterior border and apex move less, as they are related to less movable structures. The diaphragmatic and costomediastinal regions expand most of all. Most of the volumetric change during ventilation occurs in the alveoli.

REFERENCES

Bohn D 2002 Congenital diaphragmatic hernia. Am J Respir Crit Care Med 166: 911–15.
Reviews the epidemiology, diagnosis and treatment of congenital diaphragmatic hernia.

Celli B 1998 The diaphragm and respiratory muscles. Chest Surg Clin N Am 8: 207–24.

De Troyer A, Estenne M 1988 Functional anatomy of the respiratory muscles. Clin Chest Med 9: 175–93.

Kahrilas PJ 2001 Supraeosophageal complications of reflux disease and hiatal hernia. Am J Med 111(suppl 8A): 51–5.
Reviews gastro–oesophageal reflux and type I sliding hiatus hernia.

Lowdermilk GA, Naunheim KS 2000. Thoracoscopic evaluation and treatment of thoracic trauma. Surg Clin North Am 80: 1535–42.
Discusses the additional benefit and role of video-assisted thoracoscopy in thoracic trauma.

Paterson WG 2001 The normal antireflux mechanism. Chest Surg Clin N Am 11: 473–83.
Describes how the normal anatomy of the distal oesophagus, proximal stomach and the diaphragm serves as an antireflux barrier.

Rajanna MJ 1947 Anatomical and surgical considerations of the phrenic and accessory phrenic nerves. J Inter Coll Surg 60: 42–52.
Describes the anatomical course of the phrenic nerve in 203 cadaveric dissections.

Shanmuganathan K, Killeen K, Mirvis SE, White CS 2000 Imaging of diaphragmatic injuries. J Thorac Imaging 15: 104–11.
Reviews the radiological techniques available in the assessment of the diaphragm after trauma, and the extent and anatomical sites of coexisting thoracoabdominal injuries.

Development of the trachea, lungs and diaphragm

The development of the respiratory system can first be seen at stage 12 (approximately 26 days), when there is a sharp onset of epithelial proliferation within the foregut at regions of the endoderm tube destined to become the lungs, stomach, liver and dorsal pancreas. The future respiratory epithelium bulges ventrally into the investing splanchnopleuric mesenchyme, then grows caudally as a bulb-shaped tube (**Fig. 65.1**). By stage 13, the caudal end of the tube has divided asymmetrically forming the future primary bronchi: with growth the right primary

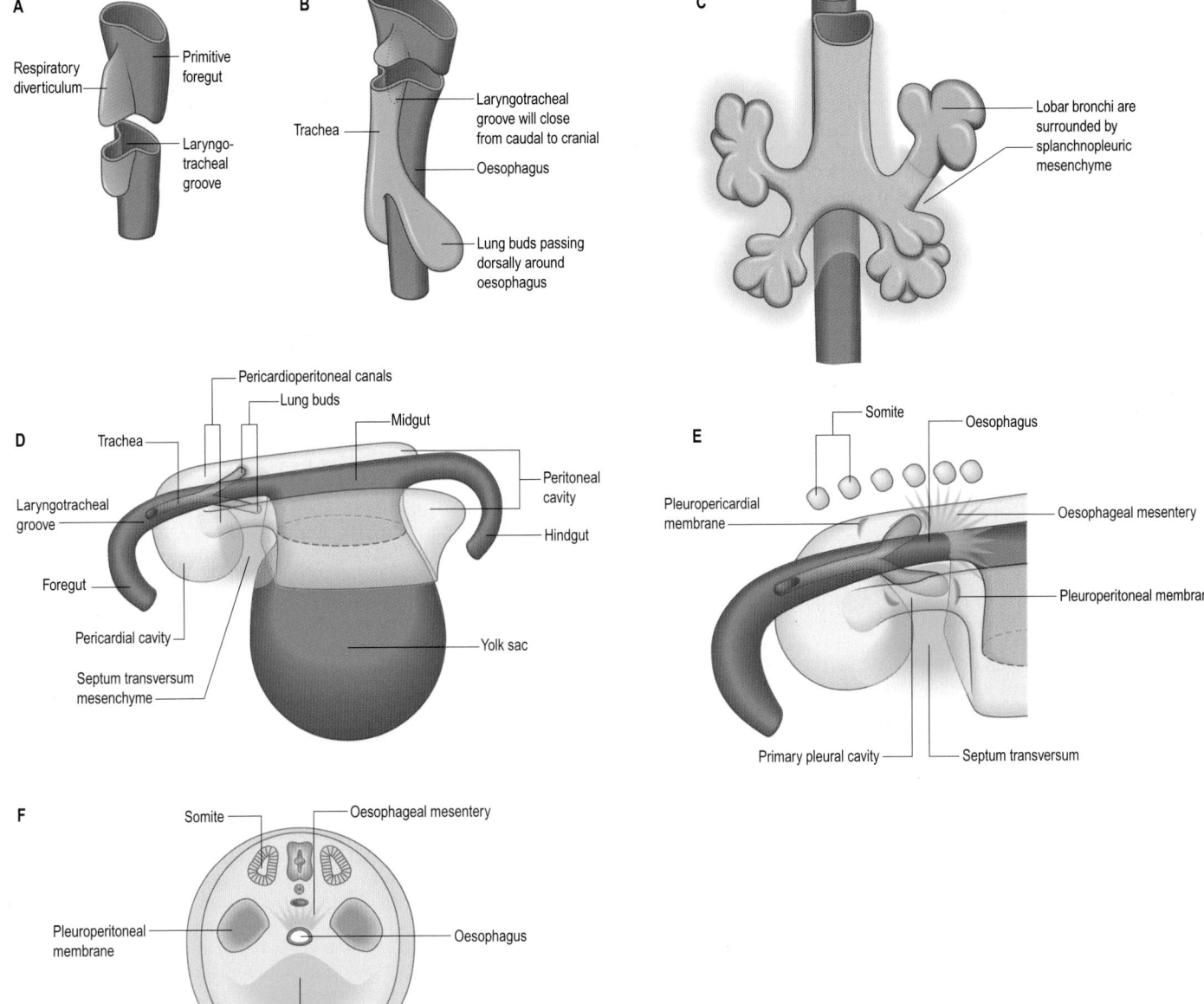

Fig. 65.1 Development of the respiratory tree and diaphragm. **A–C**, Development of the endodermal respiratory tree. **D**, Major epithelial populations in the early embryo from a left dorsolateral view. The lung buds are bulging into the laterally placed pericardioperitoneal canals. **E, F**, Formation of the diaphragm: **E** shows the diaphragmatic components from a left dorsolateral view, and **F** shows the diaphragmatic components viewed from above.

bronchus becomes orientated more caudally whereas the left extends more transversely. The trachea is clearly recognizable at stage 14. From this time the origin of the trachea remains close to its site of evagination from the future oesophagus, however, longitudinal growth of the trachea causes the region of the future carina to descend.

FORMATION OF THE TRACHEA

The trachea starts to develop at stage 12, as a ventral outgrowth from the endodermal foregut into the mesenchyme surrounding the sinus venosus and inflow tract of the heart (**Fig. 90.2**). The point at which the original respiratory diverticulum buds from the foregut, the laryngotracheal groove, remains at a constant level during the embryonic period, and the trachea lengthens distally as the bifurcation point descends. The respiratory diverticulum generally becomes surrounded by angiogenic mesenchyme that connects to the developing sixth aortic arch artery. By stage 17, the mesenchyme around the trachea is beginning to condense to form cartilage.

Initially, the tracheal mesenchyme is continuous with that surrounding the ventral wall of the oesophagus, but progressive lengthening and continued division of the tracheal bud, together with deviation of the lung buds dorsally, isolates the oesophagus and trachea within tissue-specific mesenchyme. This facilitates regional differentiation, not only between trachea and lungs, but also within the lungs themselves, i.e. the number of lobes, or the degree of growth and maturity of a particular lung. The control of the branching pattern of the respiratory tree resides with the splanchnopleuric mesenchyme. Experimental recombination of tracheal mesenchyme with bronchial respiratory endoderm results in inhibition of bronchial branching, whereas recombination of bronchial mesenchyme with tracheal epithelium will induce bronchial outgrowths from the trachea.

In the normal neonate, the trachea is relatively small in relation to the larynx (**Fig. 11.4**). The walls of the trachea are relatively thick and the tracheal cartilages are relatively closer together than in the adult. The trachea commences at the upper border of the sixth cervical vertebra, a relationship that is conserved with growth, and it bifurcates at the level of the third or fourth thoracic vertebra.

ENDOTRACHEAL INTUBATION IN THE NEONATE

The insertion of an endotracheal tube is a procedure that may be required for resuscitation of the newborn at birth and subsequently to enable artificial ventilation. The tube is introduced into either the nose or the mouth and guided through the vocal cords with the help of a laryngoscope. The tip of the tube should be in the midtrachea, well above the carina.

The required length of the tube can be estimated according to birth weight, as in **Table 65.1**, or, in an emergency, by measuring the distance from the tragus of the ear to the tip of the chin; the distance from the lips to the mid-trachea gives approximately the same measurement. Alternatively, a commonly used formula for the estimation of 'tip to lip' tube length is the '1-2-3 = 7-8-9 guideline'. This is based on the observation that, for a baby weighing 1 kg at birth, the distance from the lip to mid-trachea is 7 cm; for a 2-kg baby it is 8 cm and for a 3-kg baby it is 9 cm. For nasotracheal tubes, the formula takes into account the nasopharyngeal length needed and becomes '1-2-3 = 8-10-12'. These figures are also achieved by using the 7-8-9 figures plus the birth weight in kilograms.

Confirmation of correct positioning of the endotracheal tube is obtained radiologically, either from a chest X-ray or, in order to minimize exposure of the baby to radiation, from a 'coned view' of the trachea. The anatomical reference points used for the X-ray to assess the position of the endotracheal tube are the clavicles, the bodies of the vertebrae and the carina (although the last of these is not always visible on X-ray). Previously, it was advised that the tip of the endotracheal tube should be placed just below the clavicles, at the level of the first rib or 1–2 cm above the carina. Recently, this has been revised because positioning of the clavicles can vary according to angulation and placement of the baby, and the carina cannot always be identified. It is now suggested that the body of the first thoracic vertebra (T1) is a more stable reference point as the target for the tip of the endotracheal tube. The length of the trachea in the neonate can be as short as 3.1 cm in premature infants, and the T1-to-carina distance ranges from 1.4 cm in babies weighing 500–1000 g, to 1.8 cm in those weighing 3001–3500 g. Relevant anatomical reference points are given in **Table 65.2**.

Table 65.1 Guidelines for endotracheal tube length

Birth weight (kg)	Nose to midtrachea (cm)	Lips to midtrachea (cm)
0.5	—	6.2
0.75	—	6.5
1.0	8	6.8
1.5	9	7.3
2.0	10	7.9
2.5	11	8.5
3.0	12	9.1
3.5	13	9.7

(By permission from Hodson WA, Truog WE 1987 Special techniques in managing respiratory problems. In: Avery GB (ed) Neonatology: Pathophysiology and Management in the Newborn, 3rd edn. Philadelphia: Lippincott.)

Table 65.2 Key anatomical points relevant to endotracheal tube positioning in the neonate

Structure	Vertebral level
Vocal cords	C1–2
Thoracic inlet	T1
Carina	T3–4, or T4

(Data from Blayney MP, Logan DR 1994 First thoracic vertebral body as reference for endotracheal tube placement. Arch Dis Child 71:F32–35.)

POSTNATAL TRACHEAL DEVELOPMENT

The postnatal development of the trachea and bronchi is described in Chapter 63 (p. 1075).

FORMATION OF THE LUNGS

The lung buds grow dorsally, passing each side of the relatively smaller oesophagus and bulge into the medial walls of the laterally situated pericardioperitoneal canals (**Figs 65.1, 65.2**). The investing splanchnopleuric mesenchyme surrounding the lung buds contains a mixed population of cells, some destined to pattern endodermal epithelium and others to produce the endothelial network that will surround the future airsacs. Further mesenchymal cells will differentiate as the smooth muscle cells that surround both the respiratory tubes and the blood vessels. In stage 13 embryos, proliferation of the adjacent splanchnopleuric coelomic epithelium (of the primary pleural cavities) is especially evident. The proliferative activity decreases in stage 14, and the mesenchyme becomes arranged in zones around the developing endoderm. At stage 15, angiogenetic mesenchyme is apparent around the primary bronchi. It forms an extensive capillary network around each lung bud, receiving blood from the developing sixth aortic arch artery and draining it into an anastomosis connected to the dorsal surface of the left atrium. After this stage, the coelomic epithelium at the perimeter of the lung surface follows a differentiation pathway to form the visceral pleura.

The lung buds on each side of the oesophagus project dorsally into the pericardioperitoneal canals at stage 15; lobar or secondary bronchi can be seen at stage 16; and the bronchopulmonary segments are present at stage 17. Later stages of respiratory development involve the repeated division of the bronchial tree to form the subsegmental bronchi.

Stage 17 correlates to approximately 7 weeks, when the embryo has achieved a crown–rump length of c.12 mm.

The development of the lungs now moves into the fetal period (stage 23) and continues into the neonatal and postnatal periods.

STAGES OF LUNG DEVELOPMENT

On the basis of histology, lung development progresses through pseudoglandular, canalicular, saccular and alveolar stages.

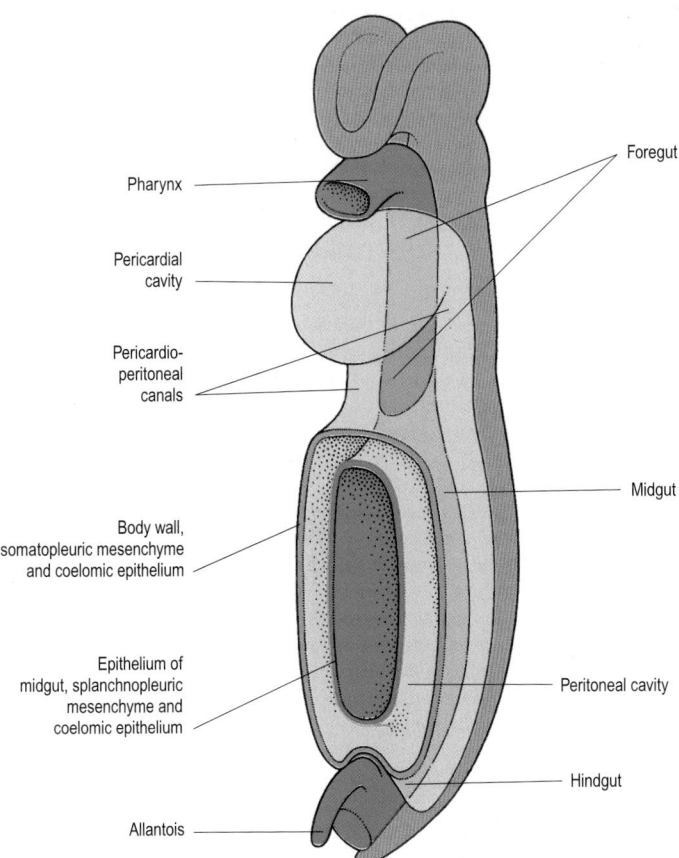

Fig. 65.2 Major epithelial populations within the early embryo. The early gut tube is close to the notochord and neural tube dorsally. The splanchnopleuric layer of the intraembryonic coelomic epithelium is in contact with the foregut ventrally and laterally, with the midgut laterally, and with the hindgut ventrally and laterally.

Labels on figure:
Pharynx
Pericardial cavity
Pericardio-peritoneal canals
Body wall, somatopleuric mesenchyme and coelomic epithelium
Epithelium of midgut, splanchnopleuric mesenchyme and coelomic epithelium
Allantois
Foregut
Midgut
Peritoneal cavity
Hindgut

Pseudoglandular stage (7–17 weeks)

The pseudoglandular stage covers the development of the lower conducting airways and the appearance of the acinar structures. The growth and branching of the endoderm epithelium is controlled by the local investing splanchnopleuric mesenchyme. The airways begin to differentiate during this stage. They are lined proximally by high columnar epithelium and distally by cuboidal epithelium: the upper airways subsequently become lined with pseudostratified epithelium. Mucous glands develop by the twelfth week and enlarge in the submucosa. Secretory activity has been identified in the trachea at 14 weeks. The splanchnopleuric mesenchyme condenses around the epithelium and differentiates into smooth muscle and connective tissue cell types. Cartilage differentiation in the airways is poorly described, and it is not clear if cartilage is synthesized in the pseudoglandular stage.

Canalicular stage (17–26 weeks)

During the canalicular phase, about three generations of branching take place, after which the amount of mesenchyme around the branching tips of the dividing respiratory tree decreases and the distal airspaces widen. At 23 weeks, longitudinal sections of the future distal regions show a sawtooth margin, which may indicate the site of further acini. Peripheral growth is accompanied by an increase in the capillary network around the distal airspaces. In many places, the capillaries are in close contact with the respiratory cuboidal epithelium, and here the respiratory epithelial cells decrease in height and begin to differentiate as type I pneumocytes. The cells that remain cuboidal are type II pneumocytes, which are believed to be the stem cells of the alveolar epithelium: they develop an increasing number of lamellar bodies which store surfactant from 6 months of gestation. Apposition of the capillary networks to the thin pneumocytes and reduction of the interstitial tissue of the lung are prerequisites for future effective gas exchange.

Saccular stage (24 weeks to birth)

At the saccular stage, thin walled terminal saccules are apparent. The saccules will become alveolar ducts as development proceeds. The expansion of the prospective respiratory airspaces that occurs during this period leads to a further decrease in the amount of interstitial tissue. The capillary networks become closely opposed as the airspaces get closer together. Invaginations termed secondary crests develop from the saccule walls. As a crest protrudes into a saccule, part of the capillary network becomes drawn into it. After the later expansion of the saccules on each side of the crest, a double capillary layer becomes annexed between what are now alveolar walls. During the saccular stage, elastin is deposited beneath the epithelium, which is an important step for future alveolar formation. In addition, surfactant production matures, and this increases the chances of survival of a preterm neonate.

Alveolar stage (28 weeks to 8 years)

Exactly when the saccular structure of the lung can be termed alveolar is not yet clear: opinions range from 28 to 32 weeks. The distal airspaces expand during late gestation and continue to do so after birth. This process is accompanied by fusion of adjacent capillary nets, so that shortly after birth there is an extensive double capillary net. Fusion of these layers is apparent at 28 days postnatally and extensive at 1.5 years; it is probably complete by 5 years. The alveolar stage continues into childhood, perhaps up to 8 years of age, although the time at which alveolar formation is complete has not yet been established.

INTERACTIONS OF EARLY LUNG DEVELOPMENT

Each lung develops by a process of dichotomous branching. For branching to occur, a cleft must develop in the tip (or side) of the epithelial tube. The epithelium then evaginates each side of the cleft, forming new branches that lengthen, and the process is then repeated. Differences have been noted between mesenchyme closely associated with the endoderm epithelium and that some distance away. At the tips of the developing epithelial buds, the mesenchyme is flattened and densely packed. In contrast, along the side of the bud and in the clefts, the mesenchyme forms an ordered row of cuboidal cells. Cells in both arrangements send processes towards the epithelial basal lamina, which is thicker in the clefts, but so attenuated as to be almost indistinguishable on the tips of the buds where the epithelium and mesenchymal cells form intimate contacts. Tenascin, an extracellular matrix molecule (also known as hexabrachion or cytotactin), is present in the budding and distal tip regions, but absent in the clefts. Conversely, fibronectin, an extracellular matrix molecule found commonly in basal laminae, is found in the clefts and along the sides of the developing bronchi, but not on the budding and distal tips.

Some authors have disputed whether the pseudoglandular stage covers the development of the complete bronchial tree, and suggest that lung development can be divided into causally distinct bronchial and respiratory systems, both of which proceed in the canalicular, saccular and alveolar stages (Merkus et al 1996). This proposal is supported by the fact that the epithelium of the developing bronchial system is columnar, whereas in the respiratory system it is cuboidal and composed of precursors of type II pneumocytes, which exhibit early stages of multilamellar bodies. The sharp demarcation between alveolar epithelium and bronchial epithelium that persists throughout development has led to the proposal that the bronchial and respiratory systems each originate from a different portion of the primordial respiratory diverticulum. The type II pneumocyte is the key cell in pulmonary acinus formation, because it is the stem cell that produces type I pneumocytes, and which ultimately matures into a surfactant-producing cell. The cells at the distal end of the bronchial system are non-ciliated Clara cells, which develop slowly prenatally.

The pattern of lung development resides within the local splanchnopleuric mesenchyme, which may be destined to become interstitial connective tissue of the lung, smooth muscle cells that surround either the airways or the blood vessels, endothelial networks (both blood vascular and lymphatic) or blood cells of the pulmonary and bronchial circulations.

Lung fibroblasts influence the rate of cytodifferentiation and maturity of the lung epithelium. Those from the pseudoglandular stage stimulate epithelial cell proliferation, whereas fibroblasts from the saccular stage promote differentiation. The latter secrete an oligopeptide, fibroblast-pneumocyte factor, which stimulates neighbouring type II pneumocytes in the developing alveolar walls to produce the surfactant phospholipid, saturated phosphatidylcholine, contained in multilamellar bodies. In recent years, premature babies and those who needed to be delivered preterm have been given cortisol, which binds to specific receptors in lung mesenchyme and causes release of fibroblast-pneumocyte factor, thus accelerating lung maturity.

There is a sexual dimorphism in lung development. Androgens delay fetal lung maturation while stimulating fetal lung growth; male type II cells are less mature than their female counterparts, perhaps because androgens block the effects of cortisol on fibroblast-pneumocyte factor concentrations.

The development of lung smooth muscle has been demonstrated immunohistochemically using antibodies against cytoskeletal and contractile proteins. The local lung mesenchyme is initially immuno-positive for vimentin. In cells that are destined to become smooth muscle, vimentin is replaced by desmin; the expression of both desmin and smooth muscle myosin indicates that the cell is terminally differentiated. However, cells containing α-smooth muscle actin, which form a thick coat around the primitive airways, have a more extensive distribution than the cells containing either desmin or smooth muscle myosin, and occur in regions of epithelial cleft formation, which suggests that they may be associated with branching morphogenesis.

Endothelial development is seen in the pseudoglandular stage when capillary networks form around the developing lung buds. These will become the capillary anastomoses around the future alveoli. The mesenchyme produces both the endothelium of the vessel tunica intima and the smooth muscle cells of the tunica media. Vimentin occurs in the cells around developing vessels in the pseudoglandular stage, but is replaced by desmin in the saccular stage.

MATURATION OF THE LUNGS

There are three prerequisites for normal lung development, namely sufficient intrathoracic space, normal fetal breathing movements and sufficient amniotic fluid.

Whereas many fetal organs are able to grow to normal proportions even if they are in abnormal locations, this is not the case for the lungs. Lung growth becomes impaired by restricted expansion, and it is suggested that distension of the developing lung may provide a major stimulus to growth during normal development. Absence or impairment of fetal breathing movements, and defects affecting diaphragmatic activity, are all associated with pulmonary hypoplasia. It is believed that normal fetal breathing movements increase the lung volume and stimulate growth of the distal airspaces. Fetal breathing movements involve rhythmic activation of the diaphragm and muscles of the upper respiratory tract; movements are very small compared with those seen after birth, because the airways are filled with lung fluid.

During development, the mucous glands of the trachea and bronchi secrete a lung fluid, which usually passes up the respiratory tract to mix with the amniotic fluid. The relationship between lung fluid and amniotic fluid is far more complex than was previously believed. Pulmonary hypoplasia at birth is often associated with severe congenital urinary obstruction and oligohydramnios, e.g. Potter's syndrome. In renal agenesis, reduced bronchial branching occurs as early as 12–14 weeks of gestation (i.e. at a time before amniotic fluid is produced by the kidneys), which suggests that a direct renal factor supports lung development. Later, the presence of amniotic fluid is necessary for normal fetal lung development. The fetal lung is a net fluid secretor. Most of the fluid produced remains within the lungs as a mechanical effect of the amniotic fluid pressure, and normally only a small amount of this fluid contributes to the amniotic fluid. The normal functioning of the kidneys regulates the volume and pressure of the lung airway fluid and may in turn provide the pressure needed for expansion and enlargement of the bronchial and pulmonary systems. Interestingly, prolonged experimental lung drainage accelerates the maturity of the alveolar cells, possibly because of an inappropriate signal that birth is imminent.

Normal postnatal pulmonary arterial development

Immediately after birth, dramatic remodelling of the pulmonary vasculature occurs to effect an abrupt reduction of pulmonary vascular resistance. This process continues at a rapid rate throughout the first 1–2 months, while the lungs adapt to extrauterine life, and then more slowly throughout childhood. Failure to remodel in the presence of an anatomically normal heart leads to persistent pulmonary hypertension. Normal postnatal pulmonary arterial development in the full-term neonate can be divided into three stages:

Stage one – lasts from birth to about postnatal day 4, and concerns the immediate adaptation to extrauterine life. At birth, the endothelial cells of the precapillary arteries are squat and have narrow bases on the sub-endothelium, a low surface:volume ratio and many surface projections. Five minutes after birth, the endothelial cells are thinner and gradually show less cell overlap, the surface:volume ratio increases, few cell projections are seen, the vessel wall becomes thinner and the lumen diameter increases (**Fig. 65.3**). The smooth muscle cells show a significant reduction in diameter during this time.

Stage two – lasts from around day 4 to 3–4 weeks, and is the time when the cells deposit matrix around themselves to fix their new positions. At birth, the internal elastic lamina of the small muscular arteries consists only of amorphous elastin in a basal lamina-like matrix. By 3 weeks of age, a definitive elastic lamina is evident, although it is heavily fenestrated, permitting contact between the endothelial cells and the smooth muscle cells.

Stage three – continues into adulthood. The intrapulmonary arteries increase in size and their walls increase in thickness. However, from birth all the pulmonary vascular smooth muscle cells from the hilum to the precapillary bed are immature and maturation is not advanced until 2 years. As the distal airspaces expand, there is a process of fusion of the capillary nets from one alveolus to another, forming, for a period, an extensive double capillary net. Fusion of these layers can be seen from postnatal day 28. It becomes more extensive by 1.5 years and it is believed to be complete by 5 years.

The lungs at birth

The amount and type of connective tissue in the lung changes after birth. The neonatal lung has abundant type III and type IV collagen, but little type I collagen, which is seen in mature lungs. The former collagen types are not so strong, suggesting that the neonatal lung is more plastic – a phenotype that would facilitate the changes in cell shape and orientation that characterize adaptation to extrauterine life. The rapid

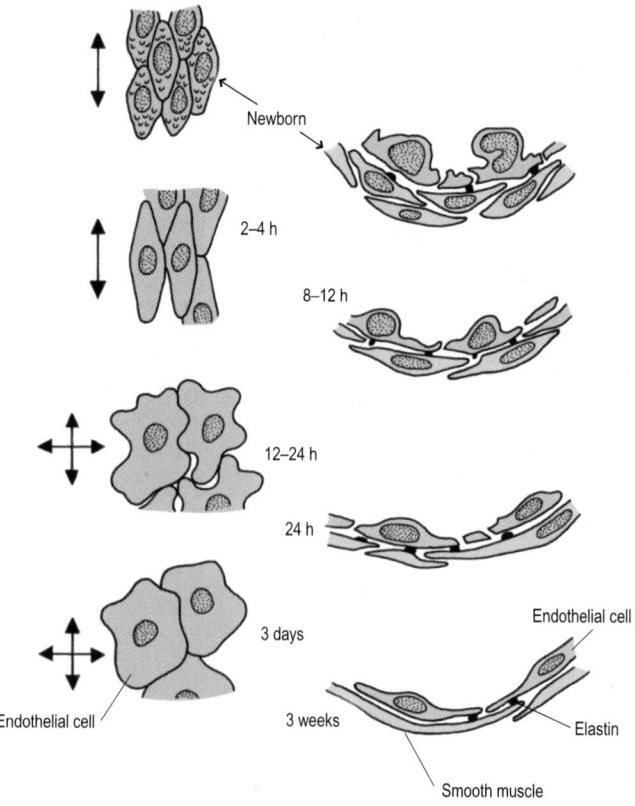

Fig. 65.3 En face views (left) and transverse sections (right) showing the changes in the endothelial and smooth muscle cells of small muscular pulmonary arteries accompanying terminal bronchi from the neonatal period to 3 weeks after birth. (From Haworth SG 1992 Pathophysiological and metabolic manifestations of pulmonary vascular disease in children. Herz 17(4): 254–261. By permission of Urban and Vogel.)

deposition of type I collagen postnatally gives structural stiffness to the blood vessel walls.

In the neonate, the lungs are relatively shorter and broader than those in the adult (Figs 65.4, 11.4). The respiratory rate in a full-term infant is 40–44 breaths/min (normal resting rate in an adult male is 12 breaths/min). Lung development continues from the alveolar stage at birth through the neonatal period and into childhood, perhaps up to 8 years of age, although the time at which this stage is complete has not yet been established.

CONGENITAL MALFORMATIONS OF THE TRACHEA, BRONCHI AND LUNGS

Tracheomalacia and bronchomalacia

Abnormalities in cartilage development lead to the development of excessive laxity in the affected airways: these abnormalities are termed tracheomalacia when the trachea is affected, and bronchomalacia when the bronchi are involved. The abnormality may involve a small localized area, or may be more generalized (e.g. Williams–Campbell syndrome, in which there is diffuse bronchomalacia from the second to the seventh generation of bronchi). Tracheobronchomalcia leads to collapse and obstruction of the airways. It usually presents in early infancy with cough, tachypnoea, stridor and wheeze. Patients with significant obstruction and apnoea may be treated by aortopexy, the aorta being lifted off the trachea by means of suturing in the adventitia of the aorta to the sternum. Some patients have associated congenital heart anomalies (14%), tracheo-oesophageal fistula (10%) and other syndromes (8%) (Masters et al 2002).

Tracheo-oesophageal fistulae

Tracheo-oesophageal fistulae are the most common abnormalities of the lower respiratory tract: they occur in c.1 in 3000 births. They present in the newborn with recurrent cough, choking spells and regurgitation of feeds, primarily as a result of the accumulation of secretions and saliva in the mouth and aspiration of gastric acid into the lungs.

The separation of the respiratory and enteric tubes normally occurs at about stage 15, during weeks 4–5. Failure of separation at this time leads to the development of a tracheo-oesophageal fistula. The anomaly may be compounded by a failure of growth of the proximal oesophagus.

Normally, the oesophagus lengthens with the rapid elongation of the embryo up to 7 weeks. The rapid proliferation of the oesophageal lumen partially obliterates the lumen and recanalization is not complete until 8 weeks. The cellular processes that lead to separation of the trachea and oesophagus occasionally produce oesophageal atresia. Tracheo-oesophageal atresia is rare, with an incidence of c. 1 in 3000 to 1 in 4500 births, depending on the population. Five types of tracheo-oesophageal fistulae may be recognized (Fig. 65.5). In almost all cases, the oesophagus ends blindly and the stomach is connected to the lower end of the trachea. Because of this connection, the abdomen becomes rapidly distended with air once the baby is delivered and starts breathing. Prenatally, polyhydramnios may be a clinical feature, but may not be apparent until the third trimester. In two of the five types of tracheo-oesophageal fistulae there is no communication between the stomach and the upper gut. Such cases are identifiable on ultrasound, as the stomach should always be visible at a 20-week examination, and its absence on ultrasound should prompt further evaluation at 24–26 weeks.

Tracheo-oesophageal fistula is commonly associated with other congenital anomalies, including cardiovascular defects (30%), anorectal (15%) and genitourinary anomalies (15%). These defects may be combined in the VATER syndrome, which involves vertebral, anorectal, cardiac and oesophageal anomalies, together with radial aplasia and the presence of a single umbilical artery.

Agenesis and aplasia of the lungs

Agenesis/aplasia of the lungs are extremely rare congenital abnormalities, in which there may be unilateral or bilateral absence of the lung. In agenesis, the airway stump is absent – i.e. there is absence of the trachea in bilateral disease, or of the primary bronchus in unilateral disease. In aplasia, there is a rudimentary airway stump, but absence of any distal lung. Tracheal agenesis or aplasia is often associated with other ipsilateral congenital malformations. The contralateral lung is enlarged, with a greater number of alveoli, but has a normal bronchial pattern. Individuals with aplasia may present with recurrent infection, dyspnoea and reduced exercise capacity, and there may be pooling of bronchial secretions, with secondary infection and overspill of infected secretions into the contralateral normal lung.

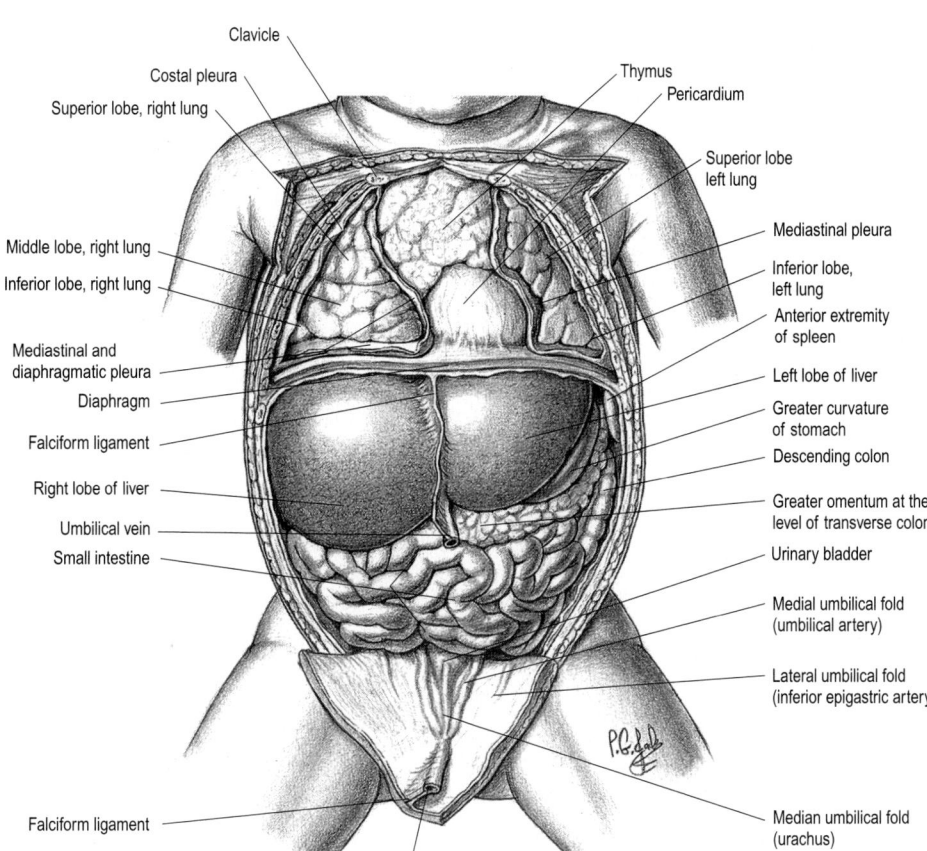

Clavicle
Costal pleura
Superior lobe, right lung
Thymus
Pericardium
Superior lobe left lung
Mediastinal pleura
Middle lobe, right lung
Inferior lobe, right lung
Inferior lobe, left lung
Anterior extremity of spleen
Mediastinal and diaphragmatic pleura
Left lobe of liver
Diaphragm
Greater curvature of stomach
Falciform ligament
Descending colon
Right lobe of liver
Greater omentum at the level of transverse colon
Umbilical vein
Urinary bladder
Small intestine
Medial umbilical fold (umbilical artery)
Lateral umbilical fold (inferior epigastric artery)
Falciform ligament
Median umbilical fold (urachus)
Umbilical vein

Fig. 65.4 Abdominal and thoracic viscera *in situ* in a full-term neonate. The anterior thoracic and abdominal wall has been removed. The lower abdominal wall has been deflected downwards.

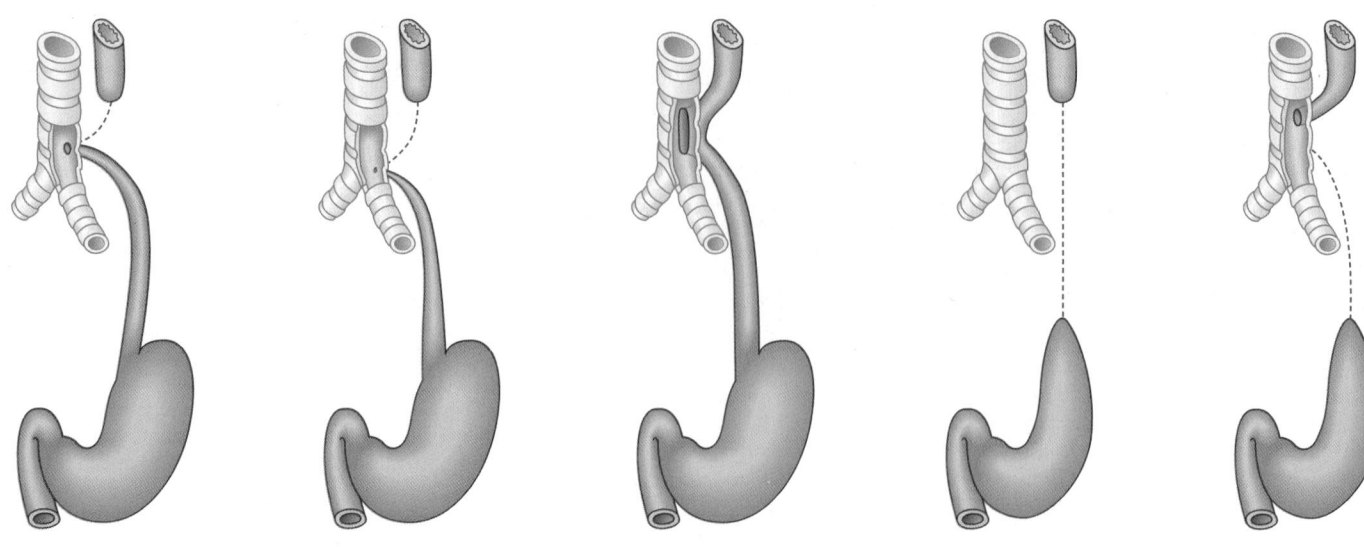

Fig. 65.5 Examples of tracheo-oesophageal fistulae and oesophageal atresia.

Bronchogenic cysts

Bronchogenic cysts are formed during development when an area of bronchial tissue becomes separated from the developing bronchus and forms a thin walled cyst lined by respiratory epithelium. By order of frequency, they may be found in the carinal (51%), right para-tracheal (19%), para-oesophageal (14%), hilar (9%) and, occasionally (7%), in pericardial, retrosternal and para-vertebral regions.

Bronchial atresia

Bronchial atresia is a congenital condition in which a major bronchus or segmental airway ends blindly or with a thin membrane. Pulmonary development normally occurs distally, and over time this tissue becomes distended with debris and mucus (bronchocoele), with adjacent over-inflated lung tissue. It characteristically affects the left upper lobe (64% of cases) and the chest radiographic findings are of a perihilar ovoid density with strands projecting into a localized area of hyperlucent lung. The left lower lobe is affected in 14% of cases and the right lower and right middle lobe in 8% of cases. The majority of cases are asymptomatic and are revealed as incidental findings on chest radiographs.

THORACIC WALL AND PLEURAL CAVITIES

For the lungs to function, they must be surrounded by a complete pleural cavity slightly larger than the capacity of the lungs. The synchronous development of the thoracic cage, diaphragm and the pleural cavities is therefore of vital importance for the normal development of the lungs and postnatal functioning of the respiratory system.

In stage 14 embryos, the heart is at the level of the upper cervical somites and above the upper limb buds. The thoracic somites are opposite the midgut. The putative thoracic region contains the pericardial cavity ventrally and the pericardioperitoneal canals posteriorly, on each side of the foregut. The future pleural cavities are as yet undefined regions of the pericardioperitoneal canals. Below the heart, septum transversum mesenchyme (p. 209) that has arisen from the caudal pericardial wall is being invaginated by endodermal epithelial cells from the foregut hepatic primordium.

Whereas the lung buds are invested by splanchnopleuric mesenchyme derived from the medial walls of the pericardioperitoneal canals, the lateral walls produce somatopleuric mesenchyme, which contributes to the body wall. This latter mesenchyme is penetrated by the developing ribs that arise from the thoracic sclerotomes. In the midline, the somatopleuric mesenchyme gives rise to the sternum and costal cartilages. The bony and cartilaginous cage provides insertions for the intercostal muscles, which arise from the ventrolateral edge of the epithelial plate of the somites. The somatopleuric coelomic epithelium, after its proliferative phase, gives rise to the parietal layer of pleura.

As the lung buds project into the pericardioperitoneal canals, they subdivide them into primary pleural coeloms around the lung buds cranially, and paired peritoneal coeloms caudally, that are continuous with the wider peritoneal coelom around the mid- and hindguts. The communications with the pericardial and peritoneal coeloms become the pleuropericardial and pleuroperitoneal canals, respectively (**Fig. 65.1**). When separation between these fluid-filled major coelomic regions is advancing towards completion, they are named the pericardial, pleural and peritoneal cavities. In early embryos, the cavities retain substantial volumes of fluid and their walls are separate. They provide the route for a primitive type of circulation until superceded by the blood vascular system. In later fetal and postnatal life, cavity walls are coapted, so that a mere microscopic film of serous fluid intervenes between them.

A curved elevation of tissue, the pulmonary ridge, develops on the lateral wall of the pleural coelom and partly encircles the pleuro-pericardial canal. The ridge is continuous with the dorsolateral edge of the septum transversum. The developing lung bud abuts on the ridge, which as a result divides into two diverging membranes meeting at the septum transversum. One is cranially placed and termed the pleuro-pericardial membrane. Embedded within it are the common cardinal vein and phrenic nerve, which reach the septum transversum by this route. The other membrane, caudally placed, is termed the pleuroperitoneal membrane. As the apical part of the lung forms it invades and splits the body wall and extends cranially on the lateral aspect of the common cardinal vein, preceded by an extension from the primary pleural coelom to form part of the secondary, definitive, pleural sac. In this way the common cardinal vein and the phrenic nerve come to lie medially in the mediastinum. The pleuropericardial canal, which lies medial to the vein, is gradually narrowed to a slit, which is soon obliterated by the apposition and fusion of its margins (**Fig. 65.1**). Closure occurs early and is mainly effected by the growth and expansion of the surrounding viscera (heart and great vessels, lungs, trachea and oesophagus), and not by active growth of the pleuropericardial membrane across the opening to the root of the lung.

In addition to its extension in a cranial direction, the lung and its associated visceral and parietal pleurae also enlarge ventromedially and caudodorsally. With the ventromedial extension, the lungs and pleurae therefore excavate and split the somatopleuric mesenchyme over the pericardium, separating the latter from the ventral and lateral thoracic walls (**Fig. 65.6**). Thus the ventrolateral fibrous pericardium, parietal serous pericardium and mediastinal parietal pleura, although topographically deep, are somatopleuric in origin.

NEONATAL THORAX

The neonatal thorax has a rounded circumference rather than the dorsoventrally flattened profile of the adult. The chest wall in the neonate is relatively soft and flexible, which makes it subject to collapse during negative pressure generation.

At all ages, there is a reduction, if not loss, of tonic intercostal activity during rapid eye movement (REM) sleep. The mechanism is believed to be related to a descending spinal inhibition of the muscle spindle

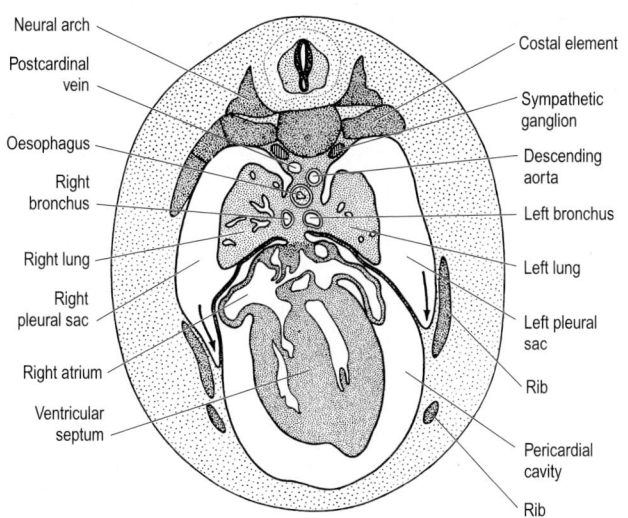

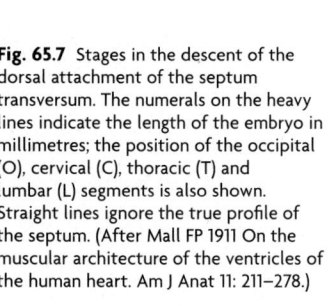

Fig. 65.7 Stages in the descent of the dorsal attachment of the septum transversum. The numerals on the heavy lines indicate the length of the embryo in millimetres; the position of the occipital (O), cervical (C), thoracic (T) and lumbar (L) segments is also shown. Straight lines ignore the true profile of the septum. (After Mall FP 1911 On the muscular architecture of the ventricles of the human heart. Am J Anat 11: 211–278.)

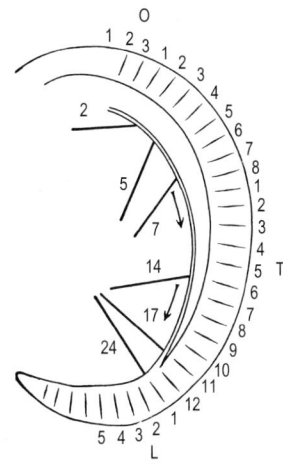

Fig. 65.6 Transverse section of a 2-mm human embryo, showing how the pleural sacs extend ventrally on each side of the pericardium and split the body wall. The arrows indicate the directions of growth of the two secondary pleural sacs.

system. In addition, although during REM sleep the diaphragm descends further, this inspiratory effort is dissipated in sucking in the ribs and enlarging the abdomen, thus the rib cage and abdominal ventilatory movements become out of phase. The neonate is at particular risk in this respect, firstly because the chest wall is flexible, and secondly because much of the infant sleep activity is of the REM type.

FORMATION OF THE DIAPHRAGM

The separation of the pleural and peritoneal cavities is effected by development of the diaphragm (**Fig. 65.1**). This forms from a portion of the septum transversum mesenchyme above the developing liver. The septum transversum is a population of mesenchymal cells that arises from the coelomic wall of the caudal part of the pericardial cavity. As the population proliferates, it forms a condensation of mesenchyme, caudal to the pericardial cavity and extending from the ventral and lateral regions of the body wall to the foregut. Dorsal to it on each side is the relatively narrow pleuroperitoneal canal. The endodermal hepatic bud grows into the caudal part of the septum transversum, whereas the cranial portion will form the diaphragm.

Medial to the pleuroperitoneal canals are the oesophagus and stomach with their dorsal mesentery and, at the root of the latter, the dorsal aorta. Dorsolateral to the canals are the pleuroperitoneal membranes, which remain small. Dorsally are the mesonephric ridges, suprarenal (adrenal) glands and gonads. Just as the enlargement of the pleural cavity cranially and ventrally is effected by a process of burrowing into the body wall, so its caudodorsal enlargement is effected in the same way. The expanding pleural cavities extend into the mesenchyme dorsal to the suprarenal glands, the gonads and (degenerating) mesonephric ridges. Thus somatopleuric mesenchyme is peeled off the dorsal body wall to form a substantial portion of the dorsolumbar part of the diaphragm. The pleuroperitoneal canal is closed by the fusion of its edges, which are carried together from posterolaterally to anteromedially by growth of the organs surrounding it and in particular that of the suprarenal gland. The right pleuroperitoneal canal closes earlier than the left, which presumably explains why an abnormal communication persisting between the pleural and peritoneal cavities is more frequently encountered on the left.

While these changes occur, the septum transversum undergoes a progressive alteration in relative position. In a 2-mm human embryo,

the dorsal border of the septum transversum lies opposite the second cervical segment but, as the embryo grows and the heart enlarges, it migrates caudally. At first the ventral border moves more rapidly than the dorsal, but after the embryo has attained a length of 5 mm, the dorsal border migrates more rapidly (**Fig. 65.7**). When the dorsal border of the septum transversum lies opposite the fourth cervical segment, the phrenic nerve (C3, 4 and 5) and portions of the corresponding myotomes grow into it and accompany it in its later migrations (**Fig. 65.1**). It is not until the end of the second month that the dorsal border of the septum transversum is opposite the last thoracic and first lumbar segments, the final position occupied by some of the dorsal attachments of the diaphragm. However, the main derivatives of the central part of the diaphragm lie at considerably more cranial levels.

The components of the diaphragm are therefore the oesophageal mesentery and paired pleuroperitoneal membranes (posteriorly); septum transversum mesenchyme (ventrally); and excavated body wall (laterally).

Neonatal diaphragm

The diaphragm is relatively flat at birth, and gains its dome shape with growth of the thorax and abdominal viscera. The neonatal diaphragm exhibits an exaggerated asymmetric movement, in which the posterior portion shows a considerably greater excursion than the anterior portion. The flatter configuration means that it is potentially less effective in compressing the abdominal contents and expanding the lower thorax during ventilation.

Diaphragmatic herniae

Diaphragmatic herniae may result from failure of fusion of the component parts or from a primary defect. Posterolateral defects (Bochdalek's hernia) are the most common (85–90%) and may be bilateral (5%) or unilateral. Of the unilateral defects, the left side is more commonly affected (80%). These hernias have been attributed to failure of fusion of the pleuroperitoneal membrane; however, this view has been challenged recently. Hernias between the costal and sternal origins (Morgagni hernia) are rare (1–2%). Midline defects in the central tendon arise from septum transversum defects. The incidence of congenital diaphragmatic hernias is about 1:3000 to 1:5000 in neonates, with a prenatal incidence of 1:2000. There is a high association of diphragmatic hernias with other anomalies.

Diaphragmatic hernias can be diagnosed by ultrasound examination. The presence of bowel in the thorax and mediastinal shift may be seen. The main causes of death in babies with diaphragmatic hernias are pulmonary hypoplasia and hypertension, which occur as a result of the limited expansion of the lung during development.

REFERENCES

Harding R, Hoope SB 1999 Lung development and maturation. In: Rodeck CH, Whittle MJ (eds) Fetal Medicine: Basic Science and Clinical Practice, Ch 16. Edinburgh: Churchill Livingstone: 181–96.

Johnson P 1999 Thoracic malformations. In: Rodeck CH, Whittle MJ (eds) Fetal Medicine: Basic Science and Clinical Practice, Ch 52. Edinburgh: Churchill Livingstone: 651–63.
Presents the aetiology, diagnosis and treatment of the main thoracic malformations seen in neonates.

Masters IB, Chang AB, Patterson L et al 2002 Series of laryngomalacia, tracheomalacia, and bronchomalacia disorders and their associations with other conditions in children. Pediatr Pulmonol 34: 189–95.
A detailed prospective study of 299 cases of bronchomalacia.

Merkus PJ, ten Have-Opbroek AA, Quanjer PH 1996 Human lung growth: a review. Pediatr Pulmonol 21: 383–97.

ABDOMEN AND PELVIS

Editors:

Jeremiah C Healy *(Lead Editor)*
Neil R Borley *(Editor, chapters 66–89, 108)*
Thomas Ind *(Editor, chapters 103–107)*
Jonathan Glass *(Editor, chapters 91–101)*
Anthony Mundy *(Editor, chapters 91–101, 108)*
Patricia Collins *(Embryology, Growth and Development)*
Caroline Wigley *(Microstructure)*

With specialist contributions on clinical and functional anatomy by

Clive Bartram *(chapter 84),* **Gina Brown** *(83),* **Helen Cox** *(70),*
Gregory P Sadler *(87, 89),* **Giles Toogood** *(85, 86)*

Critical reviewers:

John Bidmead *(chapters 102–108),* **Paul Cartwright** *(66),*
Stuart Stanton *(102–108)*

Surface anatomy of the abdomen and pelvis

ABDOMINAL PLANES AND REGIONS

For descriptive purposes, the abdomen can be divided by a number of imaginary horizontal and vertical lines drawn using the skeletal landmarks of the thorax and abdomen (**Fig. 66.1**). Projection of these lines into the sagittal or transverse planes can then be used to define certain abdominal 'planes'. Apart from dividing the abdomen into different regions for descriptive purposes, these planes are also of value in defining approximate vertebral levels and the positions of some relatively fixed intra-abdominal structures.

VERTICAL PLANES

In addition to the midline, which passes through the xiphisternal process and the pubic symphysis, there are two paramedian planes which are projected from the midclavicular line (also sometimes called the lateral or the mammary line). This line passes through the midpoint of the clavicle, crosses the costal margin just lateral to the tip of the ninth costal cartilage, and passes through a point mid way between the anterior superior iliac spine and the symphysis pubis. It approximates to, but does not exactly correspond to, the lateral border of rectus abdominis.

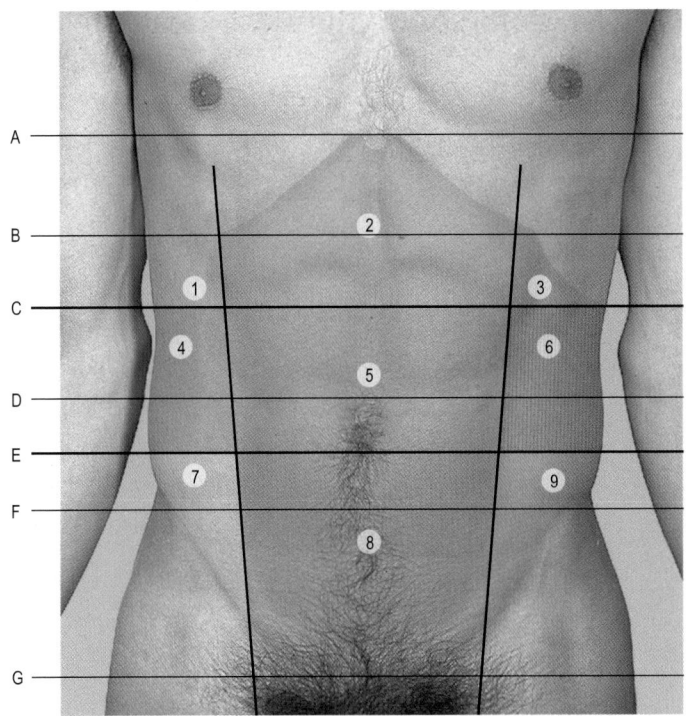

Fig. 66.1 Planes and regions of the abdomen. (Photograph by permission from Lumley JSP 2002 Surface Anatomy, 3rd edn. Edinburgh: Churchill Livingstone.)

Key for planes:
A. Xiphisternal plane. **B.** Transpyloric plane. **C.** Subcostal plane. **D.** Supracristal plane.
E. Transtubercular plane. **F.** Interspinous plane. **G.** Pubic crest plane.

Key for nine regions of the abdomen:
1. Right hypochondrium. **2.** Epigastric. **3.** Left hypochondrium. **4.** Right lumbar.
5. Central/umbilical. **6.** Left lumbar. **7.** Right iliac fossa. **8.** Suprapubic/hypogastrium.
9. Left iliac fossa.

HORIZONTAL PLANES

Several horizontal planes have been defined, but only the subcostal and transtubercular planes are in common clinical use.

The xiphisternal plane runs horizontally through the xiphoid processes at the level of the ninth thoracic vertebra. It demarcates the level of the cardiac plateau on the central part of the upper border of the liver.

The transpyloric plane lies midway between the suprasternal notch of the manubrium and the upper border of the pubic symphysis. It usually lies at the level of the body of the first lumbar vertebra near its lower border and meets the costal margins at the tips of the ninth costal cartilages, where a distinct 'step' may be felt at the costal margin. The linea semilunaris crosses the costal margin on the transpyloric plane. The hilum of both kidneys, the origin of the superior mesenteric artery, the termination of the spinal cord, the neck, adjacent body and head of the pancreas, and the confluence of the superior mesenteric and splenic veins as they form the hepatic portal vein may all lie in this plane. The pylorus may be found in the transpyloric plane, but is not a constant feature.

The subcostal plane is a line joining the lowest point of the costal margins, formed by the tenth costal cartilage on each side. It usually lies at the level of the body of the third lumbar vertebra, the origin of the inferior mesenteric artery from the aorta, and the third part of the duodenum, although this varies with posture.

The supracristal plane joins the highest point of the iliac crest on each side. It usually lies at the level of the body of the fourth lumbar vertebra, and marks the level of bifurcation of the abdominal aorta. On the posterior abdominal surface, it is a common level for the identification of the fourth lumbar vertebra, and is used to perform lumbar puncture at the L4–5 or L5–S1 intervertebral level, which is safely below the termination of the spinal cord.

The transtubercular plane joins the tubercles of the iliac crests and usually lies at the level of the body of the fifth lumbar vertebra near its upper border. It indicates, or is just above, the confluence of the common iliac veins and marks the origin of the inferior vena cava.

The interspinous plane joins the centres of the anterior superior spines of the iliac crests. It passes through either the lumbosacral disc, or the sacral promontory, or just below them, depending on the degree of lumbar lordosis, sacral inclination and curvature.

The plane of the pubic crest lies at the level of the inferior end of the sacrum or part of the coccyx, depending on the degree of lumbar lordosis, sacral inclination and curvature.

ABDOMINAL REGIONS

The abdomen can be divided into nine arbitrary regions by the subcostal and transtubercular planes and the two midclavicular planes projected onto the surface of the body. These regions are used in practice for descriptive localization of the position of a mass or the localization of a patient's pain. They may also be used in the description of the location of the abdominal viscera. The nine regions thus formed are: epigastrium; right and left hypochondrium; central or umbilical; right and left lumbar; hypogastrium or suprapubic; right and left iliac fossa.

ANTERIOR ABDOMINAL WALL (Fig. 66.2)

SKELETAL LANDMARKS

The superior boundary of the anterior abdominal wall is formed by several clear landmarks. In the midline superiorly lies the xiphoid

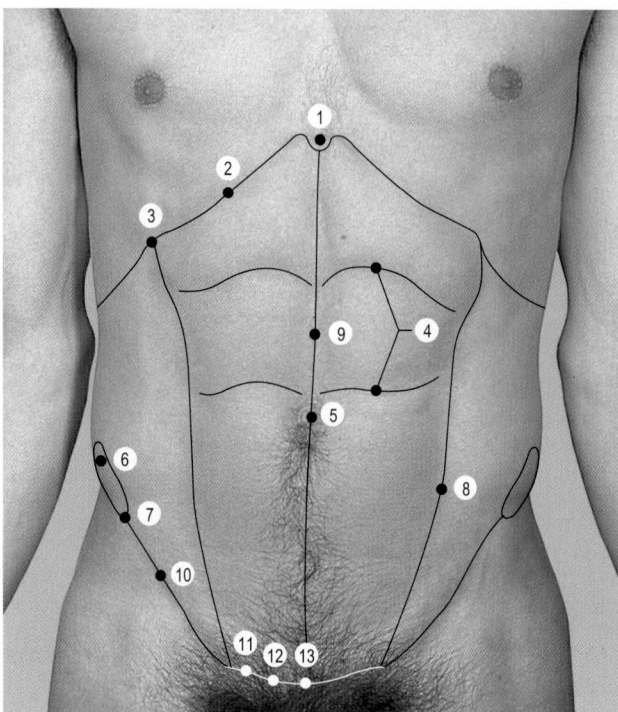

1. Xiphoid process. 2. Costal margin. 3. Tip of the ninth costal cartilage.
4. Tendinous intersections. 5. Umbilicus. 6. Iliac crest. 7. Anterior superior iliac spine.
8. Linea semilunaris. 9. Linea alba. 10. Inguinal ligament. 11. Pubic tubercule.
12. Pubic crest. 13. Pubic symphysis.

Fig. 66.2 Anterior abdominal wall landmarks. (Photograph by permission from Lumley JSP 2002 Surface Anatomy, 3rd edn. Edinburgh: Churchill Livingstone.)

process. From this the costal margins extend to either side from the seventh costal cartilage at the xiphisternal joint to the tip of the twelfth rib; the latter is often difficult to feel in the obese or if it is short. The lowest part of the costal margin lies in the midaxillary line and is formed by the inferior margin of the tenth costal cartilage. The tip of the lower border of the ninth costal cartilage can usually be defined as a distinct 'step' along the costal margin.

The inferior boundary of the anterior abdominal wall is formed, in order, by: the iliac crest, which descends from the tubercle to the anterior superior iliac spine; the inguinal ligament, which runs downwards and forwards to the pubic tubercle; and the pubic crest, which runs from the pubic tubercle laterally to the pubic symphysis in the midline. The pubic tubercle can be identified by direct palpation in thin individuals and can be detected, even in the obese, by palpation of the tendon of adductor longus, which runs up to its attachment on the pubis directly below the pubic tubercle. The tendon is best felt in tension with the hip flexed, abducted and externally rotated.

The posterolateral boundary is defined by the midaxillary line.

SOFT TISSUE LANDMARKS

Umbilicus

The umbilicus is an obvious but very inconstant landmark. In the supine adult, it usually lies at the level of the disc between the third and fourth lumbar vertebrae. The bifurcation of the abdominal aorta then lies c.2 cm caudal to the umbilicus. In the erect position, in children and in the obese, or individuals with a pendulous abdomen, the umbilicus may lie at a lower level.

Rectus abdominis

In a thin and muscular individual, the tendinous intersections of rectus abdominis (p. 1106) may be visible when it is tensed by lifting the head against resistance or by sitting up. These intersections are usually situated at the level of the umbilicus, the level of the xiphoid process and midway between these two points.

Linea alba

The linea alba (p. 1106) is usually only visible in thin muscular individuals. It is wide and obvious above the umbilicus, but is almost linear and invisible below this level.

Linea semilunaris

The linea semilunaris (p. 1106) lies along the lateral margin of the rectus sheath and is visible as a shallow curved groove in muscular individuals when the abdominal muscles are tensed, e.g. by sitting up from the lying position.

Inguinal region

The two commonly described surface markings in the inguinal region (p. 1106) are the mid-inguinal point and the midpoint of the inguinal ligament.

Mid-inguinal point

The mid-inguinal point lies at the midpoint of the line between the symphysis pubis and the anterior superior iliac spine. It is superior to the point of palpation of the pulse of the femoral artery as it emerges from beneath the inguinal ligament. The approximate surface marking of the deep inguinal ring lies immediately above the mid-inguinal point, and is a useful landmark for palpation of the origin of an indirect inguinal herniae sac.

Midpoint of the inguinal ligament

The midpoint of the inguinal ligament lies halfway between the pubic tubercle and the anterior superior iliac spine. It lies directly lateral to the origin of the inferior epigastric vessels as they lie on the posterior wall of the inguinal canal.

INTRA-ABDOMINAL VISCERA (Fig. 66.3)

The surface markings of the intra-abdominal viscera are variable and depend on age, body habitus, nutritional state, phase of ventilation and body position. The use of radiological imaging of the abdominal viscera means that the location of the viscera by surface markings is almost

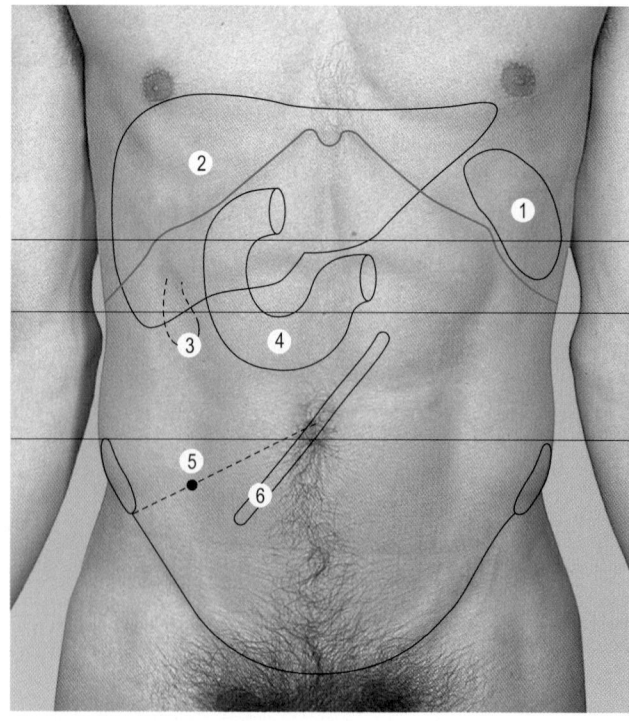

1. Spleen. 2. Liver. 3. Gallbladder. 4. Duodenum. 5. Appendix.
6. Root of small bowel mesentery.

Fig. 66.3 Intra-abdominal visceral landmarks. (Photograph by permission from Lumley JSP 2002 Surface Anatomy, 3rd edn. Edinburgh: Churchill Livingstone.)

obsolete in modern clinical practice. The following descriptions are at best regarded as the most common or approximate markings in a healthy supine individual.

STOMACH

The stomach lies in a curve within the left hypochondrium and epigastrium although, when distended and pendulous, it may lie as far down as the central or hypogastric regions. The epigastrium is the usual place to auscultate for a 'succussion splash' caused by chronic gastric stasis in upper intestinal obstruction.

DUODENUM

The first part of the duodenum sometimes lies just above the transpyloric plane, depending on its mobility and length. The second part usually lies in the transpyloric plane just to the right of the midline, and the third part usually lies in the subcostal plane across the midline. The fourth part often lies in the transpyloric plane to the left of the midline, although its position varies according to the length of its mesentery.

SMALL BOWEL AND ITS MESENTERY

The small bowel is usually referred to as lying in the central umbilical region, but often occupies part of both iliac fossae, both lumbar regions and the hypogastrium. The small bowel mesentery runs obliquely in a line from a point 2 cm to the left of the body of the second lumbar vertebra above the subcostal plane, to a point just anterior to the right sacroiliac joint just below the interspinous plane.

APPENDIX

The appendix is highly variable both in its length and in its position. Its base is commonly referred to as lying beneath a point marked two-thirds of the way along a line joining the umbilicus to the anterior superior iliac spine.

LIVER

The inferior border of the liver extends along a line that passes from the right tenth costal cartilage to the left fifth rib in the midclavicular line. The upper border of the liver follows a line that passes from the fifth rib in the midclavicular line on the right to the equivalent point on the left. This upper border curves slightly downwards at its centre and crosses the midline behind the xiphoid. The right border of the liver is curved to the right and joins the upper and lower right limits. The outline of the liver may be defined by the dull note it gives on percussion when compared with the resonance of the lungs above and the hollow abdominal viscera below.

The lower edge of a normal liver cannot usually be palpated, even in women and children, in whom the liver is at a slightly lower level. What is often mistaken for the liver in abdominal palpation is the bulge of rectus abdominis above its upper tendinous intersection.

GALLBLADDER

The fundus of the gallbladder is very variable in location. It is commonly identified with the tip of the ninth costal cartilage (in the transpyloric plane), near the junction of the linea semilunaris with the costal margin.

SPLEEN

The spleen lies beneath the ninth, tenth and eleventh ribs on the left side. Its surface markings can be delineated on the lower posterior thoracic wall by defining its axis, which extends from a point 5 cm to the left of the midline at the level of the tenth thoracic spine, and passes laterally along the line of the tenth rib to the midaxillary line.

RETROPERITONEAL VISCERA (Fig. 66.4)

PANCREAS

The surface projection of the head of the pancreas lies within the duodenal curve. The neck lies in the transpyloric plane, behind the pylorus in the midline. The body passes obliquely up and left for c.10 cm, its left part lying a little above the transpyloric plane. The tail lies a little above and to the left of the intersection of the transpyloric and left lateral planes.

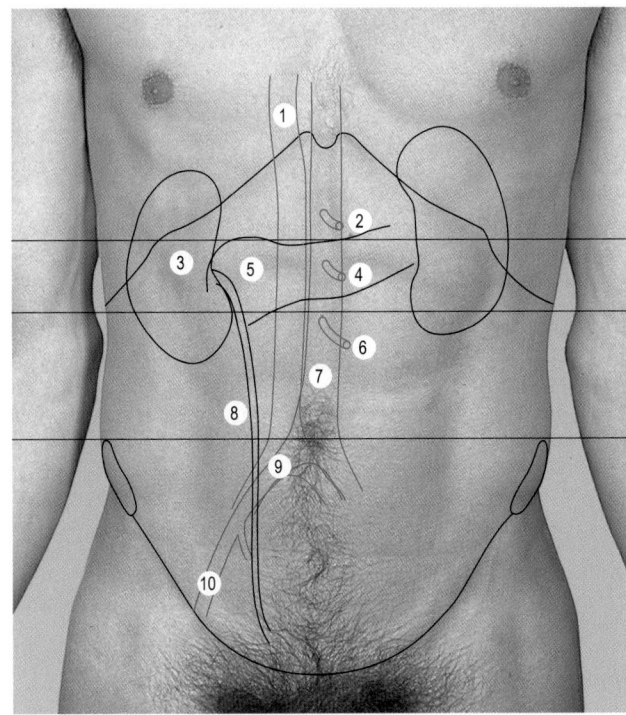

1. Inferior vena cava. 2. Coeliac artery. 3. Right kidney. 4. Superior mesenteric artery. 5. Head of pancreas. 6. Inferior mesenteric artery. 7. Aorta. 8. Right ureter. 9. Common iliac artery. 10. External iliac artery.

Fig. 66.4 Retroperitoneal visceral landmarks. (Photograph by permission from Lumley JSP 2002 Surface Anatomy, 3rd edn. Edinburgh: Churchill Livingstone.)

KIDNEY

The anterior and posterior surface projections of the kidneys are related to anterior and posterior abdominal wall landmarks. The right kidney lies c.1.25 cm lower than the left. On the anterior surface, the centre of the hilum lies in the transpyloric plane c.5 cm from the midline and slightly medial to the tip of the ninth costal cartilage. From the hilum, the outline of the anterior surface can be drawn c.11 cm long and 4.5 cm broad, the upper pole being c.2.5 cm and the lower 7.5 cm from the midline. As the transverse axis is oblique, the width thus shown is 1.5 cm less than the actual width of the kidney. On the posterior surface, the centre of the hilum lies opposite the lower border of the spinous process of the first lumbar vertebra and c.5 cm from the midline. The outline of the posterior surface can be traced similarly to the anterior surface. The lower pole is c.2.5 cm above the summit of the iliac crest. The kidneys are c.2.5 cm lower in the standing than in the supine individual; they ascend and descend a little with respiration, which is of particular importance in endoscopic renal surgery. The lower pole of the normal right kidney may occasionally be felt in the thin individual, especially the female, by bimanual palpation on full inspiration.

URETER

The ureter starts on either side approximately at the transpyloric plane (the left higher than the right), c.5 cm from the midline. Each passes downwards and somewhat medially to enter the bladder at a point marked superficially by the position of the pubic tubercle.

ABDOMINAL AORTA

The abdominal aorta starts just to the left of the midline, at the level of the body of the twelfth thoracic vertebra. It continues downwards for 10 cm as a band 2 cm wide, and bifurcates at the level of the fourth lumbar vertebra (which is marked by the transtubercular plane), 1.5 cm below and to the left of the umbilicus. The pulsations of the aorta can be felt in a thin individual in the supine position by pressing firmly in the midline backwards onto the vertebral column. An easily palpable aorta in an obese person should raise the suspicion of an aneurysm, to be checked by radiological imaging.

Visceral arteries

The coeliac trunk arises from the aorta immediately after it enters the abdomen at the level of the twelfth thoracic vertebra. The origin of the superior mesenteric artery usually lies above the transpyloric plane, and that of the inferior mesenteric artery lies at the level of the body of the third lumbar vertebra, in the subcostal plane.

Renal arteries

The renal arteries can be projected as broad lines running laterally for 4 cm from the aorta just inferior to the transpyloric plane; the left inclines across the plane.

Iliac arteries

The surface projection of the common iliac artery corresponds to the superior one-third of a broad line, which is laterally slightly convex, from the aortic bifurcation to a point mid way between the anterior superior iliac spine and the pubic symphysis. The external iliac artery corresponds to the inferior two-thirds of this line.

Superior gluteal artery

The surface marking of the exit of the superior gluteal artery from the pelvis corresponds to the junction of the upper and middle thirds of a line joining the posterior superior iliac spine to the apex of the greater trochanter.

Inferior gluteal artery

The surface marking of the exit of the inferior gluteal artery from the pelvis lies near the midpoint of a line joining the posterior superior iliac spine and the ischial tuberosity.

INFERIOR VENA CAVA

The inferior vena cava starts at the level of the body of the fifth lumbar vertebra, usually in the transtubercular plane (2.5 cm below the supracristal plane). From this level it can be represented by a band, running vertically, 2.5 cm to the right of the midline. The inferior vena cava leaves the abdomen by traversing the diaphragm at the level of the eighth thoracic vertebra, directly behind the sternal extremity of the right sixth costal cartilage.

CLINICAL PROCEDURES

PNEUMOPERITONEUM FOR LAPAROSCOPY

The establishment of a pneumoperitoneum is frequently performed by accessing the peritoneal cavity at the level of the umbilicus. Most commonly done just below the umbilicus, the incision through the linea alba allows access to the peritoneum at a point where there is relatively little extraperitoneal fat present and where the linea alba is relatively wide.

SURGICAL INCISIONS

Most surgical incisions are performed according to surgical imperatives rather than anatomical constraints. The paramedian incision has been used to decrease the risk of incisional hernia. The skin and anterior fascial incision is made over the belly of the rectus muscle at the level required. Rectus abdominis is then displaced laterally, in order not to interfere with its neurovascular supply (which enters laterally). The posterior rectus sheath is then incised in the paramedian plane. This approach allows rectus abdominis to lie between the two fascial incisions once the wound is closed.

INTESTINAL STOMAS (ILEOSTOMY, COLOSTOMY, CAECOSTOMY)

Where possible, intestinal stomas are usually formed through transrectus incisions. A cruciate incision is made in the anterior rectus sheath and the muscle fibres parted until the posterior sheath is reached. The latter is then incised without injury to the epigastric vessels (inferior or superior, depending on the level). This incision offers the advantage that fibres of rectus abdominis act to support the stoma: they provide a dynamic, contractile surround that tends to reduce the risk of herniation occurring around the stoma.

SUPRAPUBIC CATHETERIZATION

The urinary bladder is commonly accessed for short- or long-term catheterization through the anterior abdominal wall. As the bladder fills, the upper part of the dome comes to lie in the preperitoneal space in the suprapubic region. It can be relatively easily accessed via transcutaneous puncture in the midline, because there are no major neurovascular structures at this level and the linea alba is relatively thin.

Anterior abdominal wall

The anterior abdominal wall extends from the costal margins and xiphoid process superiorly to the iliac crests, pubis and pubic symphysis inferiorly. It overlaps and is connected to both the posterior abdominal wall and paravertebral tissues. It forms a continuous but flexible sheet of tissue across the anterior and lateral aspects of the abdomen. The anterior abdominal wall is composed of the integument, muscles and connective tissue lining the peritoneal cavity. It has an important role in maintaining the form of the abdomen and is involved in many physiological activities. Anterior abdominal wall tissues form the inguinal canal that connects the abdominal cavity to the scrotum in men or labia majora in women, and also form the umbilicus; both of these sites are of considerable clinical importance.

SKIN AND SOFT TISSUE

The integument of the anterior abdominal wall comprises skin, soft tissues, lymphatic and vascular structures, and segmental nerves. The outer layer is formed from the skin and subcutaneous fat. The skin is non-specialized and variably hirsute, depending on the sex and race. All individuals have some extension of the pubic hair onto the anterior abdominal wall skin, although this is commonly most pronounced in males, in whom the hair may extend almost up to the umbilicus in a triangular pattern. The subcutaneous fat of the abdominal wall is highly variable in thickness and is one of the areas where excess fat is stored during periods of obesity, particularly in males.

VASCULAR SUPPLY AND LYMPHATIC DRAINAGE

The anterior abdominal wall receives its blood supply from paired superior and inferior epigastric arteries running vertically through the tissues, and from paired posterior intercostal, subcostal and lumbar vessels running obliquely around the anterolateral aspects of the abdomen.

Superior epigastric artery and veins (Fig. 67.1)

The superior epigastric artery is a terminal branch of the internal thoracic artery. It descends between the costal and xiphoid slips of the diaphragm, accompanied by two or more veins. The vessels pass anterior to the lower fibres of transversus thoracis and the upper fibres of transversus abdominis. The artery enters the rectus sheath behind rectus abdominis and runs down to anastomose with the inferior epigastric artery at the level of the umbilicus. Branches supply rectus abdominis and perforate the sheath to supply the abdominal skin. A branch given off in the upper rectus sheath passes anterior to the xiphoid process of the sternum and anastomoses with the same contralateral branch. This vessel may give rise to troublesome bleeding during surgical incisions that extend up to and alongside the xiphoid process. The superior epigastric artery supplies small branches to the anterior part of the diaphragm. On the right, small branches reach the falciform ligament, where they anastomose with the hepatic artery.

Inferior epigastric artery and veins (Fig. 67.2)

The inferior epigastric artery originates from the external iliac artery posterior to the inguinal ligament. Its accompanying veins, usually two, drain into the external iliac vein. It curves forwards in the anterior extraperitoneal tissue and ascends obliquely along the medial margin of the deep inguinal ring. It lies posterior to the spermatic cord, but is separated from it by the transversalis fascia. It pierces the transversalis fascia and the attenuated part of the posterior rectus sheath, where it ascends between rectus abdominis and the posterior lamina of the sheath. In this part of its course, it raises the parietal peritoneum of the anterior

abdominal wall as the lateral umbilical fold. It divides into numerous branches, which anastomose with those of the superior epigastric and lower six posterior intercostal arteries. The artery is an important inferomedial relation of the deep inguinal ring, and may be damaged during extensive medial dissection of the deep ring during hernia repair, particularly when this is performed in the preperitoneal plane. The vas deferens in the male, or round ligament in the female, wind laterally round it. It has the following branches: the cremasteric artery, a pubic branch, and muscular and cutaneous branches.

The cremasteric artery accompanies the spermatic cord in males and supplies the cremaster and other coverings of the cord. It anastomoses with the testicular artery. In females it is small and accompanies the round ligament. A pubic branch, near the femoral ring, descends posterior to the pubis and anastomoses with the pubic branch of the obturator artery. Occasionally, the pubic branch of the inferior epigastric is larger than the main obturator artery and supplies the majority of flow into the vessel as it enters the thigh. It is then referred to as the aberrant obturator artery. It lies close to the medial border of the femoral ring and may be damaged in medial dissection of the ring during femoral hernia repair. Muscular branches supply the abdominal muscles and peritoneum, and anastomose with the circumflex iliac and lumbar arteries. Cutaneous branches perforate the aponeurosis of external oblique, supply the skin and anastomose with branches of the superficial epigastric artery.

Sometimes the inferior epigastric artery arises from the femoral artery. It then ascends anterior to the femoral vein, into the abdomen to follow its course as above. It occasionally arises from the external iliac artery, in common with an aberrant obturator artery and, rarely, from the obturator artery.

The superior and inferior epigastric arteries are an important source for a potential collateral circulation between the internal thoracic artery and the external iliac artery in situations in which flow in the thoracic or abdominal aorta is compromised. Small tributaries of the inferior epigastric vein drain the skin around the umbilicus and anastomose with the terminal branches of the umbilical vein, draining the inner surface of the umbilicus via the falciform ligament (p. 1127). These anastomoses may open widely in cases of portal hypertension, with portal venous blood draining into the systemic circulation via the inferior epigastric vessels. The radiating dilated veins seen under the umbilical skin are referred to as the 'caput medusae'.

Posterior intercostal, subcostal and lumbar arteries

The tenth and eleventh posterior intercostal arteries and the subcostal artery emerge from under the subcostal groove of their respective ribs and pass into the tissues of the anterior abdominal wall. They run through the aponeurosis of transversus abdominis and lie deep to the fibres of internal oblique. The lumbar arteries (p. 1119) also cross the aponeurosis of transversus abdominis and lie deep to internal oblique. The arteries on either side run forward, giving off muscular branches to the overlying internal and external oblique, before anastomosing with the lateral branches of the superior and inferior epigastric arteries at the lateral border of the rectus sheath. Perforating cutaneous vessels run vertically through the muscles to supply the overlying skin and subcutaneous tissue. A small contribution to the supply of the lower abdominal muscles comes from branches of the deep circumflex iliac arteries.

Lymphatic drainage

The lymphatic vessels of the anterior abdominal wall lie both superficial and deep to the deep fascia.

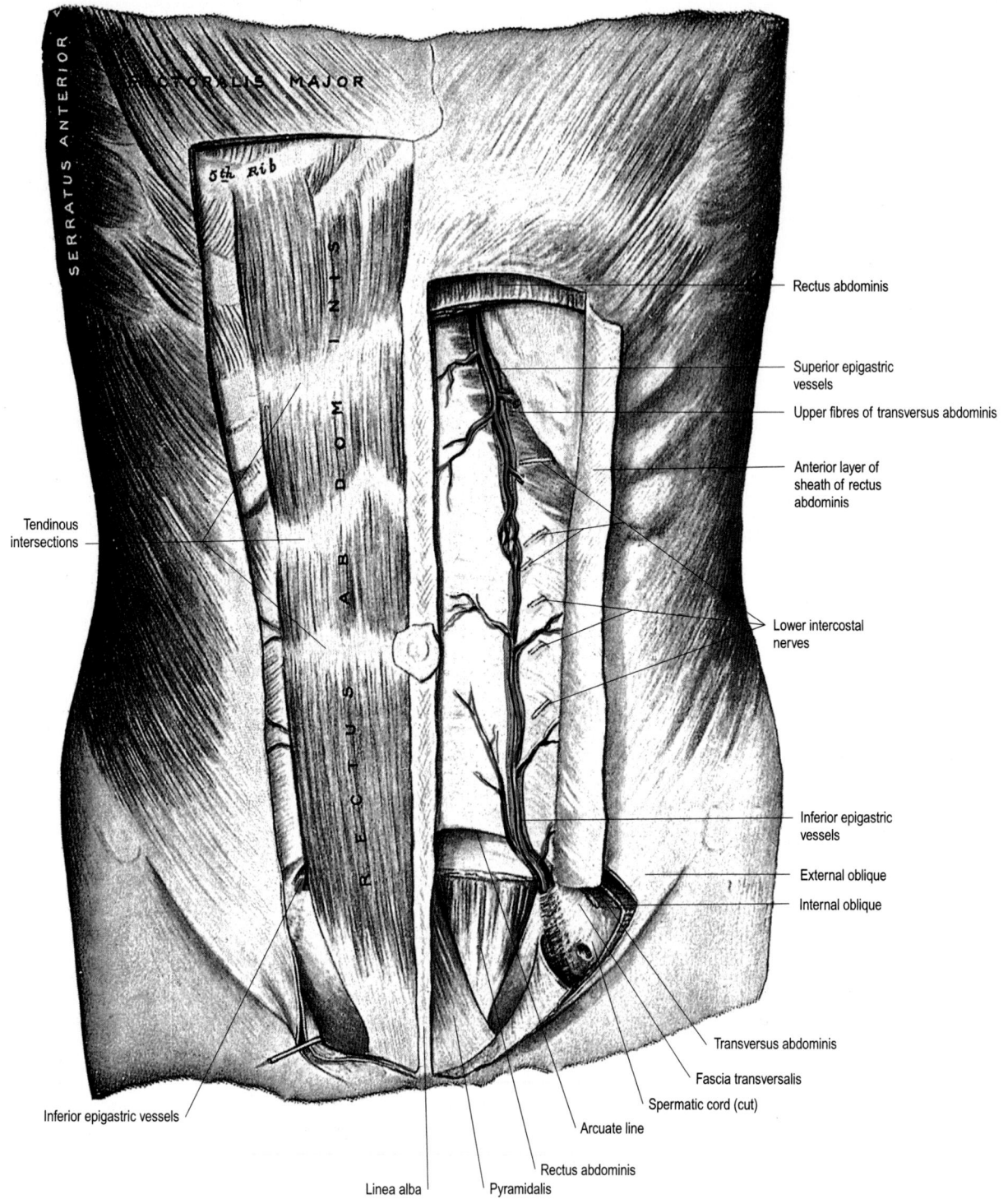

Rectus abdominis

Superior epigastric vessels

Upper fibres of transversus abdominis

Anterior layer of sheath of rectus abdominis

Lower intercostal nerves

Inferior epigastric vessels

External oblique

Internal oblique

Transversus abdominis

Fascia transversalis

Spermatic cord (cut)

Arcuate line

Rectus abdominis

Pyramidalis

Linea alba

Inferior epigastric vessels

Tendinous intersections

SERRATUS ANTERIOR

PECTORALIS MAJOR

5th Rib

RECTUS ABDOMINIS SIN

Fig. 67.1 Right rectus abdominis and left pyramidalis. The greater part of left rectus abdominis has been removed to show the superior and inferior epigastric vessels.

Superficial vessels

The superficial lymphatic vessels accompany the subcutaneous blood vessels. Vessels from the lumbar and gluteal regions run with the superficial circumflex iliac vessels. Those from the infra-umbilical skin run with the superficial epigastric vessels. Both drain into the superficial inguinal nodes. The supra-umbilical region is drained by vessels running obliquely up to the pectoral and subscapular axillary nodes, and there is some drainage to the parasternal nodes.

Deep vessels

The deep lymphatic vessels accompany the deep arteries. The vessels from the posterior portion of the abdominal wall pass with the lumbar arteries to drain into the lateral aortic and retro-aortic nodes. Vessels

from the upper anterior abdominal wall run with the superior epigastric vessels to the parasternal nodes. Vessels of the lower abdominal wall drain into the circumflex iliac, inferior epigastric and external iliac nodes.

SEGMENTAL NERVES

The seventh to the twelfth lower thoracic ventral rami continue anteriorly from the intercostal spaces into the abdominal wall (**Fig. 67.3**). Approaching the anterior ends of their respective spaces, the seventh and eighth nerves curve superomedially across the deep surface of the costal cartilages between the digitations of transverse abdominis. They reach the deep aspect of the posterior layer of the aponeurosis of internal oblique. Both the seventh and eighth nerves then run through

rotation of the trunk against resistance is provided by unilateral contraction of the oblique muscles.

RECTUS ABDOMINIS

Rectus abdominis is a long, strap-like muscle that extends along the entire length of the anterior abdominal wall. It is widest in the upper abdomen and lies just to the side of the midline. The paired recti are separated in the midline by the linea alba (p. 1106) (**Fig. 67.1**).

The muscle fibres of rectus abdominis are interrupted by three fibrous bands or tendinous intersections. One is usually situated at the level of the umbilicus, another opposite the free end of the xiphoid process and a third about midway between the other two. These intersections pass transversely or obliquely across the muscle in a zigzag manner. They are rarely full-thickness and may extend only half-way through the body of the muscle. They usually fuse with the fibres of the anterior lamina of the sheath of the muscle. Sometimes, one or two incomplete intersections are present below the umbilicus. The intersections may occur during development or may represent the myosepta delineating the myotomes that form the muscle.

The medial border of rectus abdominis is closely related to the linea alba. Its lateral border may be visible on the surface of the anterior abdominal wall as a curved groove, the linea semilunaris, which extends from the tip of the ninth costal cartilage to the pubic tubercle. In a muscular individual it is readily visible, even when the muscle is not actively contracting, but in many normal and obese individuals it may be completely obscured.

Attachments – Rectus abdominis arises by two tendons. The larger, lateral tendon is attached to the crest of the pubis and may extend beyond the pubic tubercle to the pectineal line. The medial tendon interlaces with the contralateral muscle and blends with the ligamentous fibres covering the front of the symphysis pubis. Additional fibres may arise from the lower part of the linea alba. Superiorly, rectus abdominis is attached by three slips of muscle to the fifth, sixth and seventh costal cartilages. The most lateral fibres are usually attached to the anterior end of the fifth rib. Sometimes this slip is absent, and occasionally it may extend to the fourth and third ribs. The most medial fibres are occasionally connected to the costoxiphoid ligaments and the side of the xiphoid process. In males, the pubic attachment of rectus abdominis may run over the anterior surface of the symphysis pubis and become continuous with the attachment of the gracilis and the fascia lata to the pubis.

Vascular supply – Rectus abdominis is supplied principally by the superior and inferior epigastric arteries. The inferior epigastric artery tends to be larger in calibre than the superior. Small terminal branches from the lower three posterior intercostal arteries, the subcostal artery, the posterior lumbar arteries and the deep circumflex artery may provide some contribution, particularly to the lateral edges and the lower attachments, and they form small anastomoses with the lateral branches of the epigastric arteries. Rectus abdominis provides an excellent myocutaneous flap, either pedicled or free, because of the excellent vascularity provided by the epigastric vessels and because the muscle belly is separated from surrounding tissue within the rectus sheath. The upper half of the muscle may be used for breast reconstruction or augmentation of tissue loss on the anterior thorax. The lower half may be used in the region of the thigh and may be rotated on its lower attachments, passed through the pelvis and delivered into the perineum for reconstruction after radical pelvic and perineal resections.

Innervation – Rectus abdominis is innervated by the terminal branches of the ventral rami of the lower six or seven thoracic spinal nerves via the lower intercostal and subcostal nerves.

Actions – The recti contribute to the flexion of the trunk (p. 1104). They also contribute to the maintenance of abdominal wall tone required during straining.

Rectus sheath

Rectus abdominis on each side is enclosed by a fibrous sheath. The anterior portion of this sheath extends the entire length of the muscle and fuses with the periosteum of the muscle attachments. Posteriorly, the sheath is complete in the upper two-thirds of the muscle. In the lower one-third, the posterior layer of the sheath stops approximately midway between the umbilicus and the pubis. In most individuals this is a clearly defined line, although the transition may not always be clear-cut in others. The lower border of the posterior sheath is called the arcuate line. Below this level, rectus abdominis is enclosed posteriorly by the transversalis fascia and extraperitoneal connective tissue (**Figs 67.4, 67.5**). The rectus sheath is formed from decussating fibres from all three lateral abdominal muscles. External oblique, internal oblique and transversus abdominis each forms a bilaminar aponeurosis at their medial borders. The fibres from all three anterior leaves run obliquely upwards, whereas the posterior leaves run obliquely downwards at right angles to the anterior leaves.

The anterior rectus sheath is composed of both leaves of the aponeurosis of external oblique and the anterior leaf of the aponeurosis of internal oblique fused together. The posterior rectus sheath is composed of the posterior leaf of the aponeurosis of internal oblique and both leaves of the aponeurosis transversus abdominis (**Fig. 67.6**). Because of this arrangement, both the anterior and posterior layers of the rectus sheath consist of three layers of fibres with the middle layer running obliquely at right angles to the other two. At the midline, the anterior and posterior layers are closely approximated. Fibres of each layer decussate to the opposite side of the sheath, forming a continuous aponeurosis with the contralateral muscles (**Fig. 67.7**). Fibres also decussate anteroposteriorly, crossing from anterior sheath to posterior sheath. The dense fibrous line caused by this decussation is called

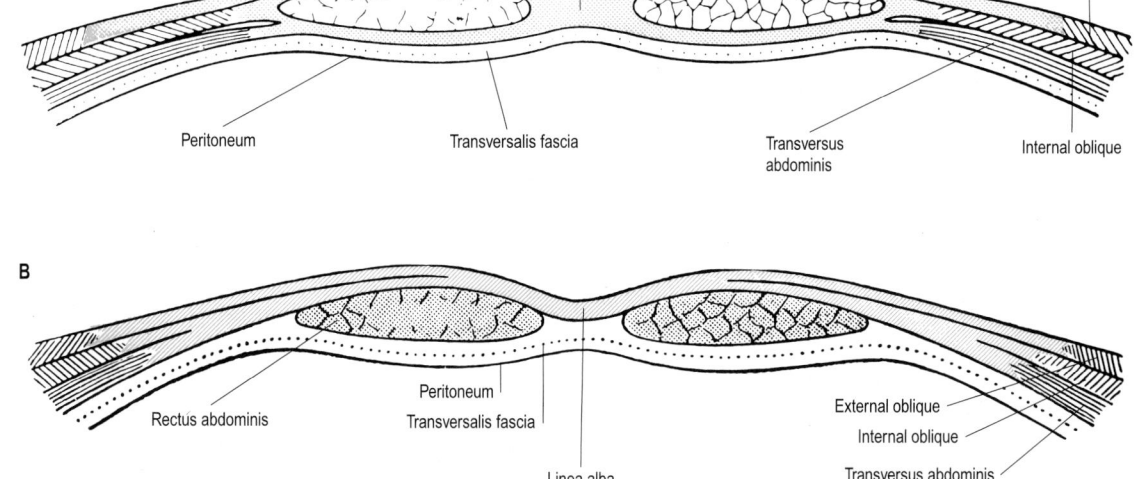

A

Rectus abdominis   Linea alba   External oblique

Fig. 67.4 Transverse sections through the anterior abdominal wall: **A**, immediately above the umbilicus; **B**, below the arcuate line. The bilaminar nature of each muscular aponeurosis is difficult to illustrate in cross-section. The fibres appear to fuse into a single sheet during formation of the rectus sheath. Note that, below the arcuate line, rectus is supported directly by the transversalis fascia.

Peritoneum   Transversalis fascia   Transversus abdominis   Internal oblique

B

Rectus abdominis   Peritoneum   External oblique
Transversalis fascia   Internal oblique
Linea alba   Transversus abdominis

A

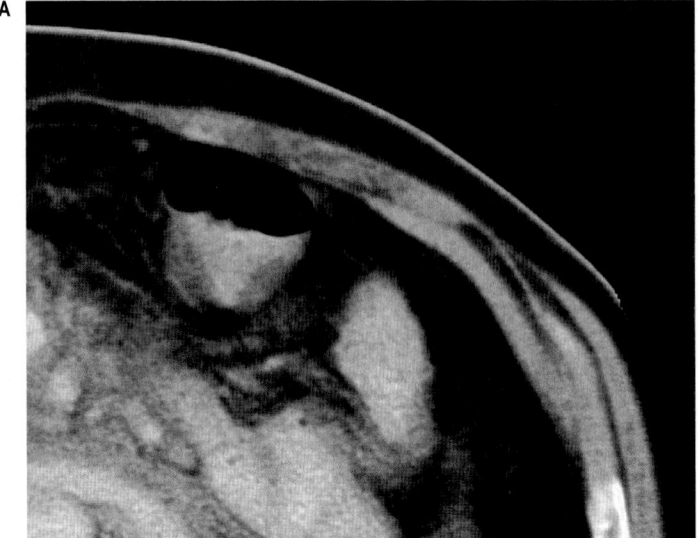

B

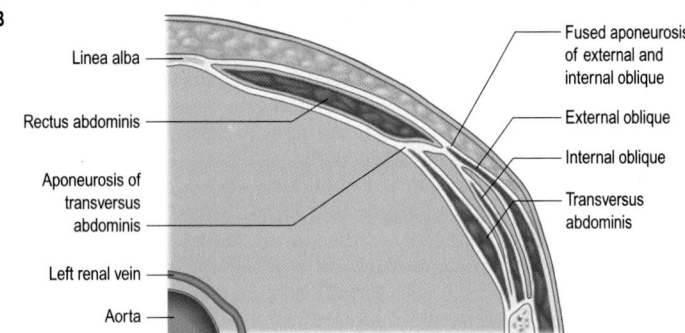

Linea alba

Rectus abdominis

Aponeurosis of transversus abdominis

Left renal vein

Aorta

Fused aponeurosis of external and internal oblique

External oblique

Internal oblique

Transversus abdominis

Fig. 67.5 Rectus sheath. Computed tomography scan (**A**) and diagram (**B**) of the anterior abdominal wall, demonstrating the formation of the rectus sheath above the umbilicus. The anterior rectus sheath is composed of both leaves of the aponeurosis of external oblique and the anterior leaf of the aponeurosis of internal oblique, fused together. The posterior rectus sheath is composed of the posterior leaf of the aponeurosis of internal oblique and both leaves of the aponeurosis of transversus abdominis.

A

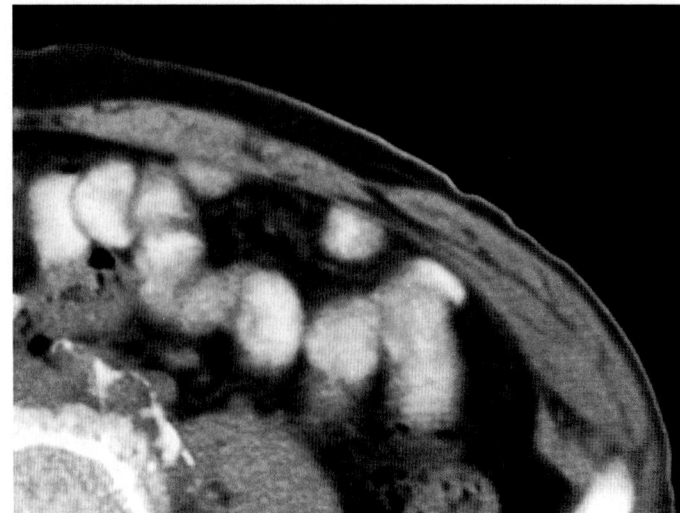

B

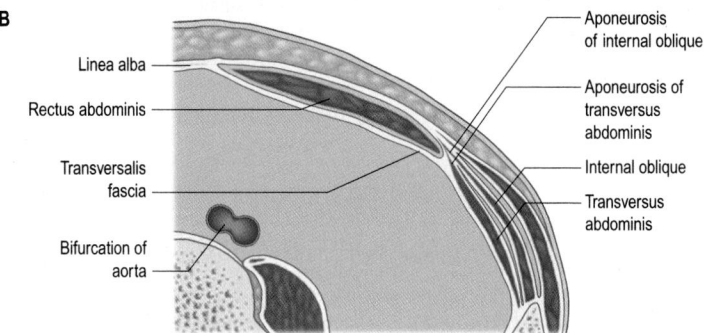

Linea alba

Rectus abdominis

Transversalis fascia

Bifurcation of aorta

Aponeurosis of internal oblique

Aponeurosis of transversus abdominis

Internal oblique

Transversus abdominis

Fig. 67.6 Rectus sheath. Computed tomography scan (**A**) and diagram (**B**) of the anterior abdominal wall, demonstrating the formation of the rectus sheath below the umbilicus. Below the umbilicus, the posterior rectus sheath is formed by the transversalis fascia and extraperitoneal connective tissue.

the linea alba. The external oblique, internal oblique and transversus abdominis muscles can thus be regarded as paired, digastric muscles with a central tendon in the form of the linea alba. These decussating fibres maybe used to identify the midline during surgical incisions, since they can be seen as oblique fibres crossing at right angles. Below the level of the arcuate line, the fibres forming the posterior rectus sheath rapidly cease running behind the rectus and all leaves pass into the anterior rectus sheath.

Linea alba

The linea alba is a tendinous raphe extending from the xiphoid process to the symphysis pubis and pubic crest. It lies between the two recti and is formed by the interlacing and decussating aponeurotic fibres of external oblique, internal oblique and transversus abdominis. It is visible only in the lean and muscular, as a slight groove in the anterior abdominal wall. A fibrous cicatrix, the umbilicus, lies a little below the midpoint of the linea alba, and is covered by an adherent area of skin. Below the umbilicus, the linea alba narrows progressively as the rectus muscles lie closer together. Above the umbilicus, the rectus muscles diverge from one other and the linea alba is correspondingly broader. The linea alba has two attachments at its lower end: its superficial fibres are attached to the symphysis pubis, and its deeper fibres form a triangular lamella that is attached behind rectus abdominis to the posterior surface of the pubic crest on each side. This posterior attachment of linea alba is named the 'adminiculum lineae albae'. The linea alba is crossed from side to side by a few minute vessels.

In the fetus, the umbilicus transmits the umbilical vessels, urachus and, up to the third month, the vitelline or yolk stalk. It closes a few

days after birth, but the vestiges of the vessels and urachus remain attached to its deep surface. The remnant of the fetal left umbilical vein forms the round ligamentum of the liver. The obliterated umbilical arteries form the medial umbilical ligaments, enclosed in peritoneal folds of the same name. The partially obliterated remains of the urachus persist as the median umbilical ligament.

Divarication of the recti

Thinning and widening of the upper linea alba may occur, most commonly as a result of obesity or chronic straining. This process disrupts the arrangement of the fibres of the bilaminar aponeurosis. Contraction of the anterolateral abdominal muscles fails to be transmitted across the midline through the linea alba and increased intra-abdominal pressure causes the abdominal viscera to protrude beneath the thinned tissue as a broad midline bulge. The recti become widely separated or divaricated. This is not true herniation, as all the layers of the abdominal wall in that region are intact.

Umbilical hernia

There are three varieties of umbilical hernia. In true congenital herniation, a defect is present from birth. This is usually simply the result of failure of closure of the umbilicus after retraction of the umbilical gut loop. Less commonly, the gut loop does not retract and remains, in part, outside the abdominal cavity. An infantile umbilical hernia is caused by stretching of the umbilical scar tissue, associated with increased intra-abdominal pressure. An acquired umbilical or paraumbilical hernia actually occurs through small areas of weakness in the linea alba, above or below the umbilical scar.

PYRAMIDALIS

Attachments – Pyramidalis is a triangular muscle that lies in front of the lower part of rectus abdominis within the rectus sheath. It is attached

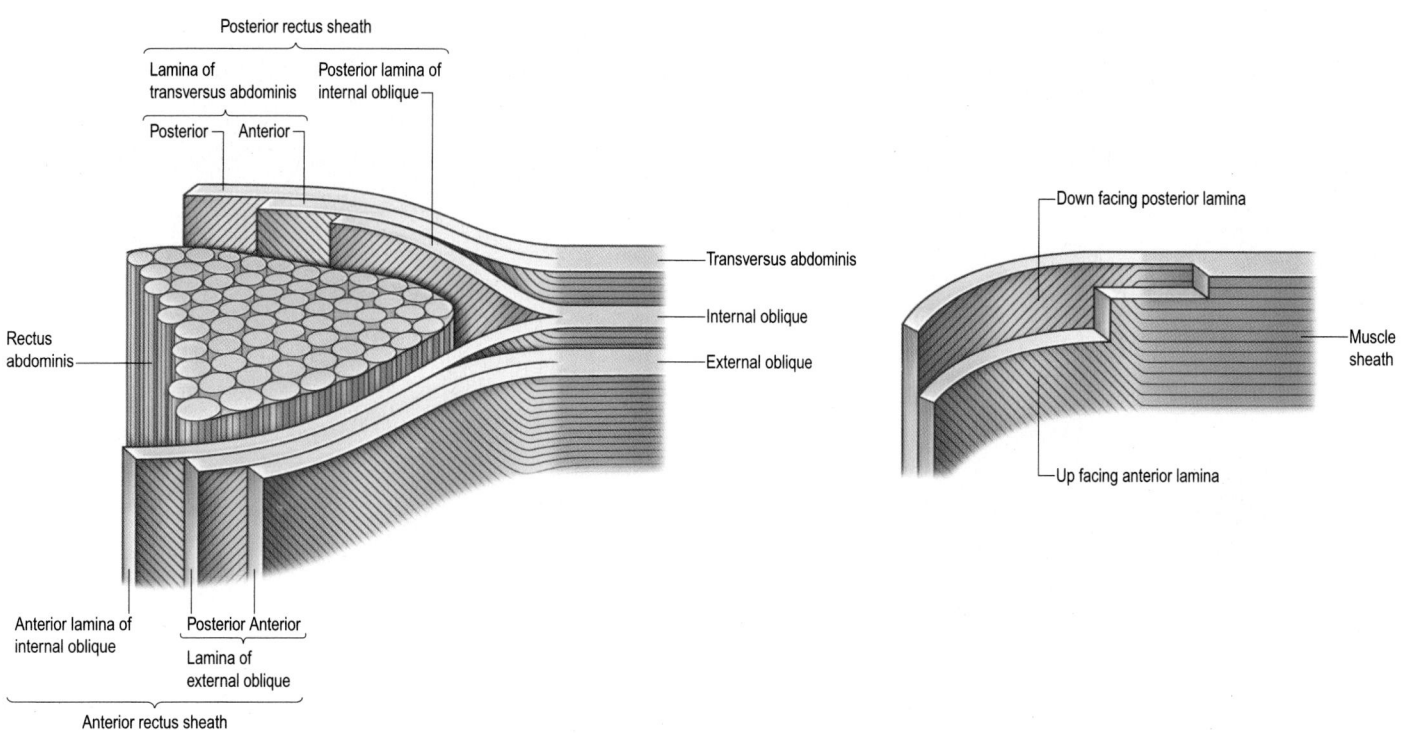

Fig. 67.7 The concept of bilaminar aponeuroses of the external oblique muscles. Note that the fibres of the superficial and deep layers are approximately at right angles; decussations occur as part of the linea alba. (Modified from Rizk NN 1980 A new description of the anterior abdominal wall in man and mammals. J Anat 131: 373–385. By permission Blackwell Publishing.)

by tendinous fibres to the front of the pubis and to the ligamentous fibres in front of the symphysis. The muscle diminishes in size as it runs upwards, and ends in a pointed apex that is attached medially to the linea alba. This attachment usually lies midway between the umbilicus and pubis, but may occur higher. The muscle varies considerably in size. It may be larger on one side than on the other, absent on one or both sides, or even doubled.

Vascular supply – Pyramidalis is supplied by branches of the inferior epigastric artery, with some contribution from the deep circumflex iliac artery. A small artery frequently crosses the midline posterior to the belly of the muscle to anastomose with the contralateral vessel. This may cause troublesome bleeding during surgical incisions that run down as far as the lower rectus sheath above the symphysis pubis.

Innervation – Pyramidalis is supplied by the terminal branches of the subcostal nerve, which is the ventral ramus of the twelfth thoracic spinal nerve.

Actions – Pyramidalis contributes to tensing the lower linea alba, but is of doubtful physiological significance.

EXTERNAL OBLIQUE (Fig. 67.8)

Attachments – External oblique is the largest and the most superficial of the three lateral abdominal muscles. It curves around the lateral and anterior parts of the abdomen and is attached to the external surfaces and inferior borders of the lower eight ribs. The attachments rapidly become muscular and interdigitate with the lower attachment of serratus anterior and latissimus dorsi along an oblique line that extends downwards and backwards. The upper attachments are close to the cartilages of the corresponding ribs, the middle ones arise from the ribs at some distance from their cartilages and the lowest are close to the apex of the cartilage of the twelfth rib. The fibres of external oblique diverge as they pass to their lower attachments. Those from the lower two ribs pass nearly vertically downwards and are attached to the anterior half or more of the outer lip of the anterior segment of the iliac crest. The middle and upper fibres pass downwards and forwards and end in the anterior aponeurosis, along a line drawn vertically from the ninth costal cartilage to a little below the level of the umbilicus. The

muscle fibres rarely descend beyond a line from the anterior superior iliac spine to the umbilicus. The posterior border of the muscle is free (**Fig. 67.10**).

The inguinal ligament is formed by the margin of the aponeurosis of external oblique extending between the anterior superior iliac spine and the pubic tubercle (p. 1107). The deep fibres of the aponeurosis of external oblique are not initially parallel to the long axis of the inguinal ligament: they approach the ligament obliquely at an angle of 10–20°. On reaching the ligament, fibres turns medially, and most run along the ligament to reach the pubic tubercle. The deepest fibres of the aponeurosis spread out posteromedially to insert into the pectineal line.

The upper and lower rib attachments of the muscle may be absent. Digitations or even the entire muscle may be reduplicated. The upper attachments of the muscle are sometimes continuous with pectoralis major or serratus anterior.

Vascular supply – External oblique is supplied by branches from the lower posterior intercostal and subcostal arteries, the superior and inferior epigastric arteries, the superficial and deep circumflex arteries and the posterior lumbar arteries.

Innervation – External oblique is innervated by the terminal branches of the lower five intercostal nerves and the subcostal nerve from the ventral rami of the lower six thoracic spinal nerves.

Actions – External oblique contributes to the maintenance of abdominal tone (p. 1104), increasing intra-abdominal pressure and lateral flexion of the trunk against resistance.

Inguinal ligament

The inguinal ligament is the thick, inrolled lower border of the aponeurosis of external oblique and stretches from the anterior superior iliac spine to the pubic tubercle. Its grooved abdominal surface forms the 'floor' of the inguinal canal. The ligament is not linear and has an inferior and an anterior convexity. At its lower border, it is continuous with the fascia lata. The lateral half is rounded and lies more obliquely than the medial half. The latter gradually widens towards its attachment to the pubis, where it becomes more horizontal and supports the spermatic cord. At the medial end, some fibres do not attach to the pubic tubercle but extend in two directions. Some expand posteriorly

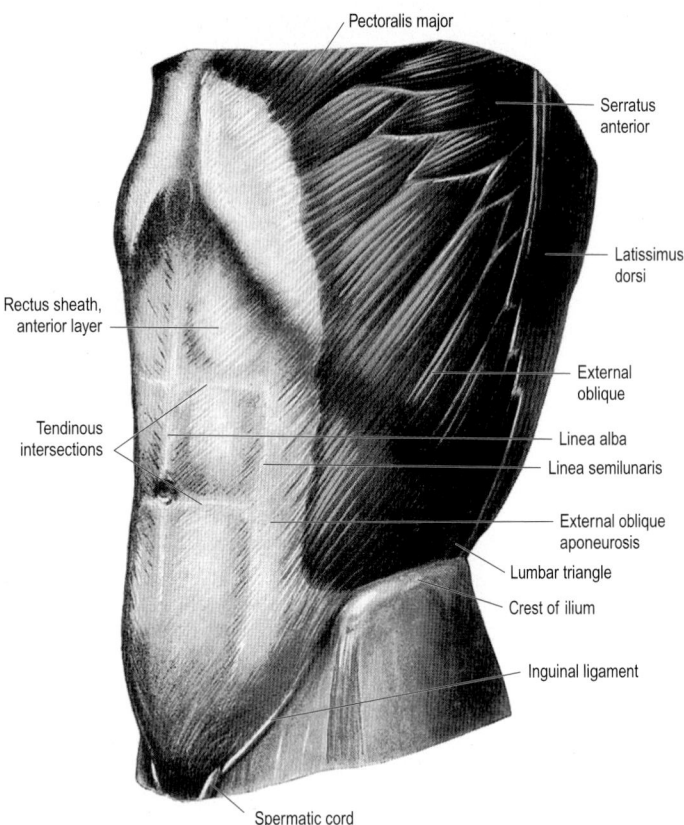

Fig. 67.8 The left anterolateral abdominal wall muscles, showing the external oblique and rectus sheath, together with the aponeurosis of external oblique.

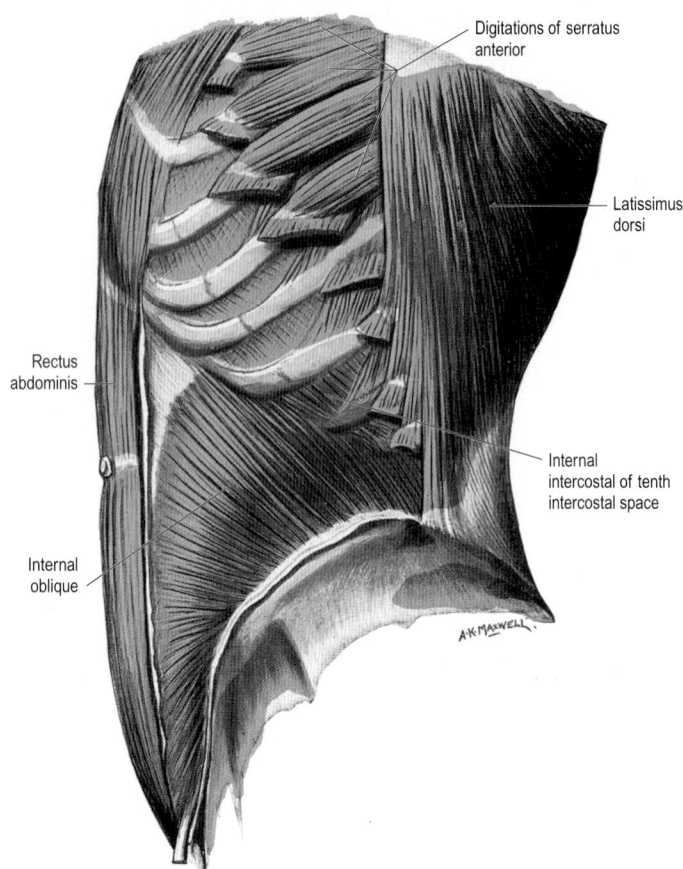

Fig. 67.9 Muscles of the left side of the trunk. External oblique has been removed to show internal oblique, but its digitations from the ribs have been preserved. The sheath of rectus abdominis has been opened and its anterior lamina removed.

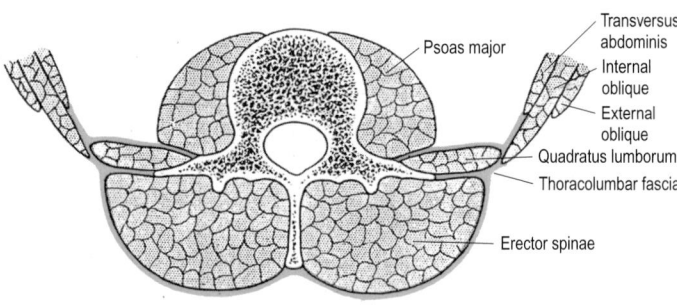

Fig. 67.10 Transverse section through the posterior abdominal wall, showing the posterior attachment of the anterolateral abdominal wall muscles. All other connective tissue strata have been omitted.

and laterally to attach to the pectineal line, forming the lacunar ligament complex. Other fibres pass upwards and medially behind the superficial inguinal ring and external oblique to join the rectus sheath and the linea alba. These constitute the reflected part of the inguinal ligament. Fibres from either side decussate in the linea alba, similarly to the aponeurosis of the abdominal muscles (p. 1105).

INTERNAL OBLIQUE (Fig. 67.9)

Attachments – Internal oblique lies deep to external oblique for the majority of its course. It is thinner and less bulky than external oblique. Its fibres arise from the lateral two-thirds of the grooved upper surface of the inguinal ligament, where they form a common attachment with the iliac fascia to the inguinal ligament. Laterally, internal oblique is also attached to the anterior two-thirds of the intermediate line of the anterior segment of the iliac crest, and posteriorly some fibres are attached to the thoracolumbar fascia (**Fig. 67.10**). The fibres originating from the posterior end of the iliac attachment pass upwards and laterally and are attached to the inferior borders and tips of the lower three or four ribs and their cartilages. Here, the attachments merge with those of the internal intercostals. The uppermost of these fibres form a short, free superior border. The fibres attached to the anterior iliac crest diverge and end in the anterior aponeurosis, which gradually broadens from below upwards. The uppermost part of the aponeurosis is attached to the cartilages of the seventh, eighth and ninth ribs. The fibres that originate from the inguinal ligament arch downwards and medially across the spermatic cord in the male and the round ligament of the uterus in the female. They become tendinous, fuse with the corresponding part of the aponeurosis of transversus abdominis, and attach to the crest and medial part of the pectineal line, forming the conjoint tendon.

Vascular supply – Internal oblique is supplied by branches from the lower posterior intercostal and subcostal arteries, the superior and inferior epigastric arteries, the superficial and deep circumflex arteries and the posterior lumbar arteries.

Innervation – Internal oblique is innervated by the terminal branches of the lower five intercostal nerves and the subcostal nerve from the ventral rami of the lower six thoracic spinal nerves, in addition to a small contribution from the iliohypogastric and ilioinguinal nerves from the ventral ramus of the first lumbar spinal nerve.

Actions – Internal oblique contributes to the maintenance of abdominal tone (p. 1104), increasing intra-abdominal pressure, and enables lateral flexion of the trunk against resistance.

CREMASTER

Attachments – Cremaster consists of loosely arranged muscle fasciculi lying along the spermatic cord. It is variable in thickness and is thickest in young men. It may form an incomplete coating around the cord, known as the cremasteric fascia, which extends around the testis but lies within the external spermatic fascia. The attachment of the muscle arises mainly from the inferomedial border of internal oblique and transversus abdominis. A separate tendinous attachment may also occur to the middle of the inguinal ligament, extending as far as the anterior superior iliac spine. The medial portion is attached to the pubic tubercle and lateral pubic crest. The fibres spread out over the lateral aspect of the spermatic cord as it approaches the superficial inguinal ring. The shortest and most superior fasciculi turn inwards in front of the cord to join the medial part. The longer, lateral fasciculi blend with the fascia over the cord and upper part of the tunica vaginalis. In the female, a few fibres descending on the round ligament of the uterus represent the lateral part of cremaster. The medial part of the muscle is variably developed, and may be absent. It is attached to the pubic tubercle and the lateral pubic crest, the conjoint tendon and lower border of transversus abdominis. These fasciculi loop on the posteromedial aspect of the cord, interlacing with those of the lateral part. The entire muscle appears to form continuous loops that pass from the middle of the inguinal ligament as far as the tunica vaginalis, and then return to attach to the pubic tubercle.

Vascular supply – Cremaster is supplied by the cremasteric artery, a branch of the inferior epigastric artery.

Innervation – Cremaster is innervated by the genital branch of the genitofemoral nerve, derived from the first and second lumbar spinal nerves.

Actions – Cremaster pulls the testis up towards the superficial inguinal ring. Although its fibres are striated, it is not usually under voluntary control. Stroking the skin of the medial side of the thigh evokes a reflex contraction of the muscle, the cremasteric reflex, which is most pronounced in children. It may represent a protective reflex, and the cremaster may also have a role in testicular thermoregulation.

TRANSVERSUS ABDOMINIS (Fig. 67.11)

Attachments – Transversus abdominis is the deepest of the lateral abdominal muscles. It is attached to the lateral one-third of the inguinal ligament and the associated iliac fascia, the anterior two-thirds of the inner lip of the anterior segment of the iliac crest, the thoracolumbar fascia between the iliac crest and the twelfth rib, and the internal aspects of the lower six costal cartilages. The costal attachments interdigitate with the attachment of the diaphragm. The muscle ends in an anterior aponeurosis. The lower fibres curve downwards and medially, together with those of the aponeurosis of internal oblique, and insert into the pubic crest and pectineal line to form the conjoint tendon. A band of fibres, sometimes muscular, may run from the lower border of the muscle to the inguinal ligament and is called the interfoveolar ligament. The remainder of the aponeurosis passes medially and the fibres decussate at, and blend with, the linea alba. The upper costal and anterior iliac fibres of transversus abdominis are short. The lower costal and posterior iliac fibres are longer, and the thoracolumbar fibres are longest. Near the xiphoid process, the aponeurosis is formed only 2–3 cm from the linea alba, so the muscular part of transversus abdominis extends behind rectus into the posterior layer of the rectus sheath. The medial edge of the muscle, at the start of the aponeurosis, curves first downwards and laterally, and is furthest from the lateral edge of the rectus sheath at the level of the umbilicus. It then curves downwards and medially towards the middle of the superior crus of the superficial inguinal ring.

Occasional defects filled with fascia may occur in the lower muscular and aponeurotic parts of both internal oblique and transversus abdominis. The two muscles are sometimes fused and, rarely, transversus abdominis may be absent.

Vascular supply – Transversus abdominis is supplied by branches from the lower posterior intercostal and subcostal arteries, the superior and inferior epigastric arteries, the superficial and deep circumflex arteries and the posterior lumbar arteries.

Innervation – Transversus abdominis is innervated by the terminal branches of the lower five intercostal nerves, the subcostal nerve and the iliohypogastric and ilioinguinal nerves. These arise from the ventral rami of the lower six thoracic and first lumbar spinal nerves.

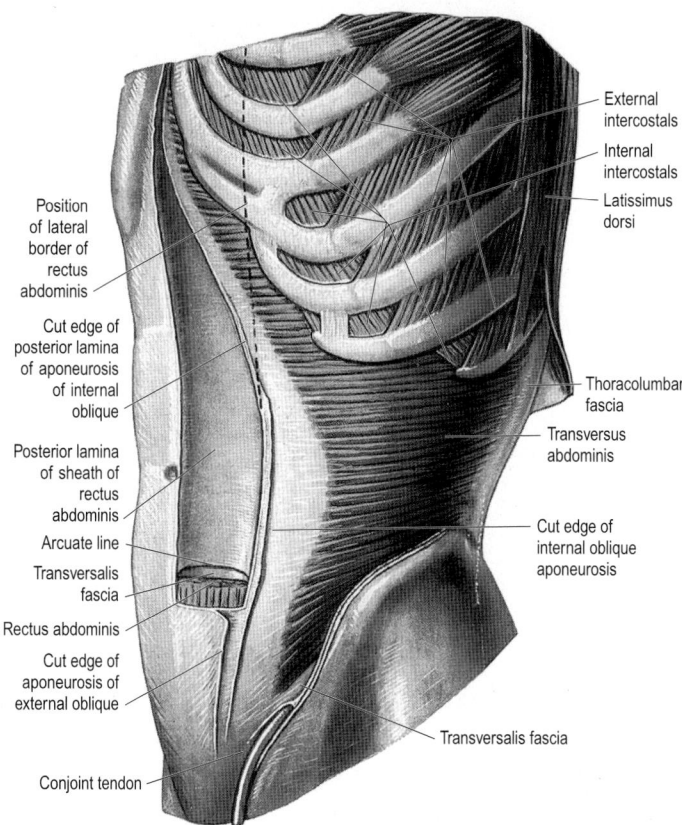

Position of lateral border of rectus abdominis

Cut edge of posterior lamina of aponeurosis of internal oblique

Posterior lamina of sheath of rectus abdominis

Arcuate line

Transversalis fascia

Rectus abdominis

Cut edge of aponeurosis of external oblique

Conjoint tendon

External intercostals

Internal intercostals

Latissimus dorsi

Thoracolumbar fascia

Transversus abdominis

Cut edge of internal oblique aponeurosis

Transversalis fascia

Fig. 67.11 Left transversus abdominis. The aponeurosis of transverses abdominis fuses into the posterior layer of the rectus sheath above the arcuate line.

Actions – Transversus abdominis contributes mainly to the maintenance of abdominal tone and increasing intra-abdominal pressure (p. 1104).

CONJOINT TENDON

The conjoint tendon is formed from the lower fibres of internal oblique and the lower part of the aponeurosis of transversus abdominis. It is attached to the pubic crest and pectineal line. It descends behind the superficial inguinal ring and acts to strengthen the medial portion of the posterior wall of the inguinal canal. The attachment to the pectineal line is frequently absent. Medially, the upper fibres of the tendon fuse with the anterior wall of the rectus sheath, and laterally some fibres may blend with the interfoveolar ligament.

INGUINAL CANAL (Figs 67.12, 67.13, 67.14, 67.15)

The inguinal canal is a natural hiatus in the tissues of the anterior abdominal wall, and is formed from the various layers of the wall in the region of the groin. Its size and form vary with age, and although it is present in both sexes it is most well developed in the male. The canal is an oblique tunnel, with deep and superficial openings or rings. It contains the spermatic cord in males, the round ligament of the uterus in females, and the ilioinguinal nerve in both sexes.

Superficial inguinal ring

The superficial inguinal ring is a hiatus in the aponeurosis of external oblique, just above and lateral to the crest of the pubis. The ring is actually triangular, and its apex points along the line of the deep fibres of the aponeurosis. Although it varies in size, it does not usually extend laterally beyond the medial one-third of the inguinal ligament. The base lies along the crest of the pubis and its sides are the crura of the opening in the aponeurosis. The lateral crus is the stronger and is reinforced by fibres of the inguinal ligament inserted into the pubic tubercle. The medial crus is thin. The fibres attach to the front of the symphysis pubis and interlace with fibres from the opposite side. In the external layer of the investing fascia of external oblique, some fibres arch above the apex of the superficial inguinal ring as intercrural fibres. In the male, the lateral crus is curved to form a groove, in which the spermatic cord rests.

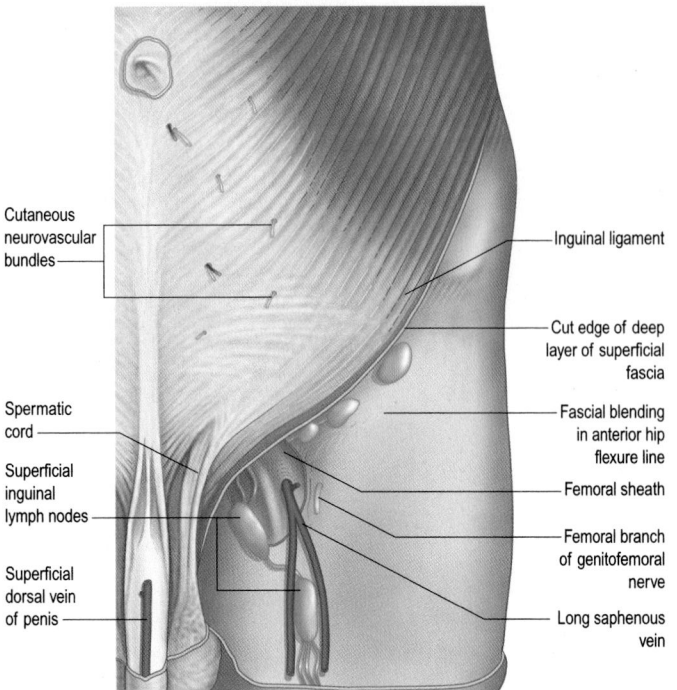

Fig. 67.12 Superficial structures of the inguinal region and lower part of the anterior abdominal wall on the left side.

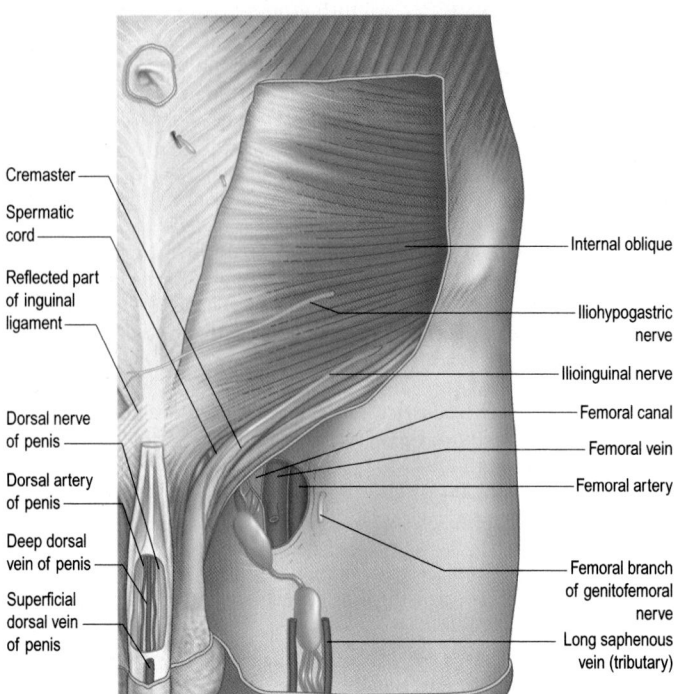

Fig. 67.14 Dissection of the regions shown in **Fig. 67.12**, with part of external oblique removed.

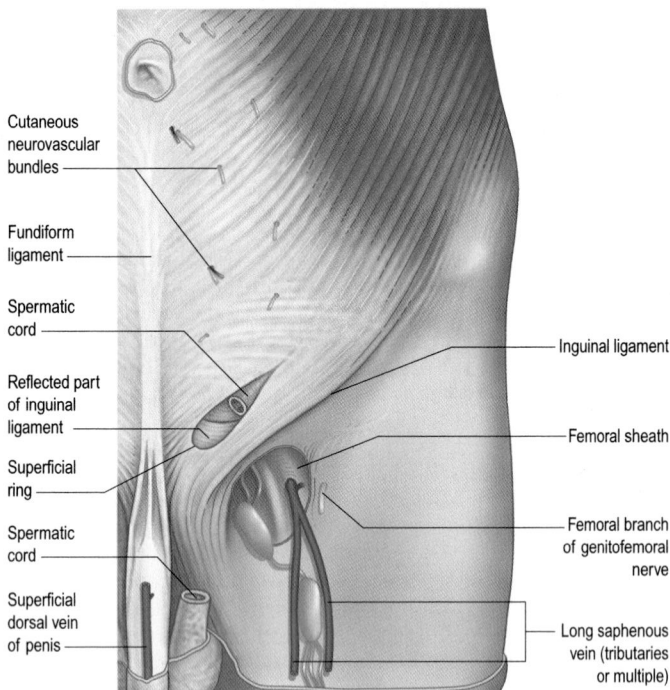

Fig. 67.13 Superficial structures of the inguinal region and lower part of the anterior abdominal wall on the left side, with the superficial aponeurotic layer removed.

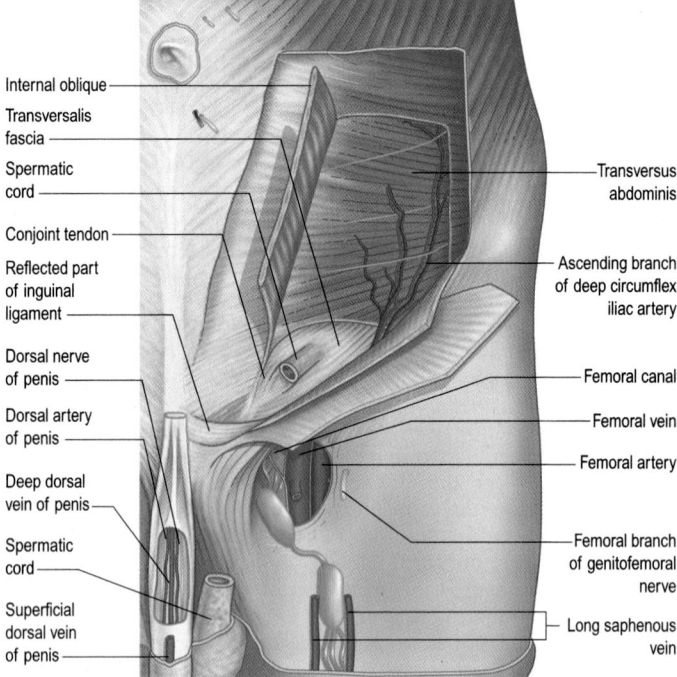

Fig. 67.15 Dissection of the regions shown in **Fig. 67.13**, with parts of external and internal oblique muscles removed.

Fibres from the aponeurosis of external oblique and overlying fascia continue downwards from the crura of the ring, and form a delicate tubular prolongation of fibrous tissue around the spermatic cord and testis. This is the external spermatic fascia and constitutes the outermost covering of the cord. The superficial inguinal ring is only a distinct aperture when the continuity of this fascia with the aponeurosis is interrupted. The ring is smaller in the female.

Deep inguinal ring

The deep inguinal ring is situated in the transversalis fascia, midway between the anterior superior iliac spine and the symphysis pubis c.1.25 cm above the inguinal ligament. It is oval, with an almost vertical long axis. Its size varies between individuals, and it is always much larger in the male. It is related above to the arched lower margin of transversus abdominis, and medially to the inferior epigastric vessels and the interfoveolar ligament, when that is present. Traction on the fascial ring exerted by internal oblique may constitute a valve-like safety mechanism when intra-abdominal pressure is increased.

Boundaries

The inguinal canal is a virtual space lying between the various layers formed from the lower tissues of the anterior abdominal wall. It lies obliquely and slants downwards and medially, parallel with and a little above the inguinal ligament. It extends from the deep to the superficial inguinal rings. Its length depends on the age of the individual, but in the adult is between 3 and 5 cm long. It is bounded anteriorly by the skin, superficial fascia and aponeurosis of external oblique. In its lateral one-third, the anterior wall is reinforced by the muscular fibres of the internal oblique just above their origin from the inguinal ligament. Posterior to the canal lie the reflected inguinal ligament, the conjoint tendon and the transversalis fascia, which separate it from extraperitoneal connective tissue and peritoneum. Superiorly lie the arched fibres of internal oblique and transversus abdominis forming the conjoint tendon. Inferior to the canal is the union of the transversalis fascia with the inguinal ligament and, at the medial end, the lacunar ligament.

In the newborn, the deep and superficial rings are nearly super-imposed and the canal is extremely short. This creates an approximately oval defect in the abdominal wall. As the child grows, the anterior abdominal wall muscles grow rapidly, causing the positions of the rings to separate and the canal to lengthen. The defect thus becomes pro-gressively more oblique until, in adulthood, the presence of separate anterior and posterior canal walls forms a 'flap valve' effect. Increases in intra-abdominal pressure transmitted through the posterior wall and the deep ring are supported by the presence of the thickest part of the overlying anterior wall. At the superficial ring and medial end of the anterior wall, where it is weakest, the posterior wall is strengthened by the conjoint tendon and the reflected inguinal ligament. The fibres of internal oblique and transversus abdominis, which form the conjoint tendon, are constantly active in standing; this activity increases during episodes of increased intra-abdominal pressure.

Relations (Fig. 67.16)

The inferior epigastric vessels are important posterior relations of the medial end of the canal. They lie on the transversalis fascia as they ascend obliquely behind the conjoint tendon into the posterior portion of the rectus sheath.

The inguinal triangle lies in the posterior wall of the canal. It is bounded inferiorly by the medial half of the inguinal ligament, medially by the lower lateral border of rectus abdominis and laterally by the inferior epigastric artery. It overlies the medial inguinal fossa and, in part, the supravesical fossa.

Lacunar ligament

The lacunar ligament is a thick triangular band of tissue lying mainly posterior to the medial end of the inguinal ligament. It measures c.2 cm from base to apex and is a little larger in the male. It is formed from fibres of the medial end of the inguinal ligament and fibres from the fascia lata of the thigh, which join the medial end of the inguinal liga-ment from below. The inguinal fibres run posteriorly and laterally to the medial end of the pectineal line and are continuous with the pectineal fascia. They form a near horizontal, triangular sheet with a curved medial border. This edge forms the lateral border of the femoral canal. The apex of the triangle is attached to the pubic tubercle. A strong fibrous band, the pectineal ligament of Astley Cooper, extends laterally along the pectineal line from the pectineal attachment. The fibres from the fascia lata join the inferior/posterior border of the inguinal liga-ment, which, in combination with fibres from the transversalis fascia, fuses with the pectineal fascia as it joins the thickened periosteum of the pectineal line. This portion of the lacunar ligament forms the lower extension of the medial border of the femoral canal and femoral sheath.

HERNIAS OF THE ANTERIOR ABDOMINAL WALL

INGUINAL HERNIA

An inguinal hernia involves the protrusion of a viscus through the tissues of the inguinal region of the abdominal wall. Although the inguinal canal is arranged such that the weaknesses in the anterior abdominal wall caused by the deep and superficial inguinal rings are supported, the region remains a potential cause of herniation.

Indirect inguinal hernia

An indirect hernia is defined as arising lateral to the inferior epigastric vessels. Many indirect hernias are related to the congenital abnormal persistence of the vaginal process. Other indirect hernias are acquired as a result of progressive weakening of the lateral and posterior walls of the canal. The hernia may pass through the deep ring or may expand the deep ring such that it is no longer a clear entity. Small indirect hernias tend to lie below and lateral to the fibres of the conjoint tendon, but larger hernias often distort and thin the tendon superiorly. Small hernias, which do not protrude beyond the inguinal canal, are covered by the same inner layers as the spermatic cord, including the internal spermatic fascia and cremaster. If the hernia extends through the superficial inguinal ring it is, in addition, covered by external spermatic fascia.

In hernias related to a persistent fully patent vaginal process, the hernia contents descend in front of the testis into the tunica vaginalis (complete congenital hernia) and the vaginal process and tunica form part of the hernial sac. Where the vaginal process is sealed off from the tunica vaginalis, the hernia contents descend to the top of the testis (incomplete congenital hernia). Although both types are related to a congenital abnormality, actual herniation into the potential sac may not occur until adult life, as a consequence of increased intra-abdominal pressure or sudden muscular strain.

Direct inguinal hernia

A direct inguinal hernia is defined as arising medial to the inferior epigastric vessels. Direct hernias are always caused by an acquired weak-ness of the inguinal triangle in the medial posterior wall of the canal, and frequently extend through the anterior wall of the canal or super-ficial ring. The hernia may protrude through the transversalis fascia, between the conjoint tendon and the inferior epigastric vessels, and enter the inguinal canal. It may closely resemble an indirect hernia, in that the coverings are similar. Its clinical presentation can also mimic an indirect inguinal hernia. Other direct hernias arise either between the fibres of the conjoint tendon or by eventration of the tendon such that it forms a thin covering to the hernia. In either case, a hernia enters the lower end of the canal, protruding through the superficial ring medial to the cord, and is covered by external spermatic fascia.

Clinical features of inguinal hernias

Indirect hernias often descend from lateral to medial in the same oblique angle as the canal, because of their origin in the lateral end of the inguinal canal. This is particularly true for congenital hernias. Direct hernias arise from the medial end of the canal and tend to protrude more directly anteriorly. With the patient in the supine position and the hernia reduced, pressure applied over the region of the deep inguinal ring may prevent appearance of an indirect hernia on standing or straining. This method of determining the type of hernia is fraught with

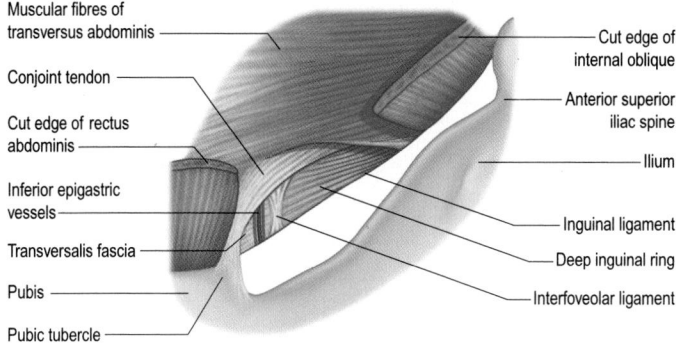

Muscular fibres of
transversus abdominis

Conjoint tendon

Cut edge of rectus
abdominis

Inferior epigastric
vessels

Transversalis fascia

Pubis

Pubic tubercle

Cut edge of
internal oblique

Anterior superior
iliac spine

Ilium

Inguinal ligament

Deep inguinal ring

Interfoveolar ligament

Fig. 67.16 Deep structures of the inguinal canal. The aponeurosis of external oblique has been removed. The fibres of internal oblique and rectus abdominis have been divided for clarity. The structures passing posteroinferiorly to the inguinal ligament have also been excluded for clarity.

difficulties. Indirect hernias may have a wide neck, and occlusion of the deep ring may not be possible with simple digital pressure. An acquired indirect hernia may arise medial to the deep ring. The angle of the descent of the hernia is also an unreliable guide, as it depends on the size of the defect in the posterior wall of the canal, the length of the canal and whether the hernia protrudes through the anterior wall. Direct hernias are more likely to have a wide-necked origin, making strangulation less likely.

Femoral hernia

A femoral hernia protrudes through the femoral ring. The femoral ring is normally closed by a femoral septum of modified extraperitoneal tissue, and is therefore a weak spot. In females, the ring is relatively large and subject to profound changes during pregnancy, explaining why femoral hernias are more common in women. When a section of intestine bulges through the ring, it pushes out a hernial sac of peritoneum. It is covered by extraperitoneal tissue (the femoral septum) and descends along the femoral canal to the saphenous opening. It is prevented from descending further along the femoral sheath by the narrow saphenous opening, by the vessels and by the close attachment of the superficial fascia and sheath to the lower part of the rim of the saphenous opening. The hernia hence turns forwards, distending the cribriform fascia and curving upwards over the inguinal ligament and the lower part of the aponeurosis of external oblique. While in the canal the hernia is usually small, because of the resistance of its surrounds, but enlarges as it escape into the inguinal loose connective tissue. Thus a femoral hernia first descends and then ascends forwards. Hence pressure to reduce it should be directed in the reverse order, with the thighs passively flexed for greatest relaxation.

The coverings of a femoral hernia are, from within outwards: the peritoneum, femoral septum, femoral sheath, cribriform fascia, superficial fascia and skin. A fibrous covering, the fascia propria, may lie outside the peritoneal sac and is frequently separated from it by adipose tissue. It represents a femoral septum thickened to form a membranous sheet by hernial pressure. The fascia propria may easily be mistaken for the sac, and its contained extraperitoneal fat for omentum; the fat may resemble a lipoma, but dissection will reveal the true hernial sac in its centre. The intestine reaches only to the saphenous opening in incomplete femoral hernia, in contradistinction to complete hernia, in which it passes through the opening. The small size of an incomplete hernia renders it difficult to detect and therefore dangerous, especially in the corpulent. The site of strangulation varies: it may be at the neck of the hernial sac; more often it is at the junction of the falciform margin of the saphenous opening with the free edge of the pectineal part of the inguinal ligament; or it may be at the saphenous opening. The site of narrowing should be divided superomedially for a distance of 4–6 mm to avoid all normally positioned vessels and other important structures. However, occasionally the obturator artery is replaced by an enlarged pubic branch of the inferior epigastric artery descending almost vertically to the obturator foramen. This vessel sometimes curves along the edge of the lacunar part of the inguinal ligament, encircling the neck of a hernial sac, and may be inadvertently cut during enlargement of the femoral ring in reducing a femoral hernia.

The pubic tubercle is an important landmark in distinguishing inguinal from femoral hernias; the neck of the hernia is superomedial to it in inguinal hernia, but inferolateral in the femoral form.

LESIONS OF THE INTERCOSTAL NERVES

Lesions of individual intercostal nerves do not produce any appreciable clinical effects. Innervation of the anterolateral muscles is from several different nerves, and it requires several lesions to produce a significant reduction in the tone of any muscle. Because of the overlap between sequential dermatomes, significant cutaneous anaesthesia is felt only after sectioning of at least two or more sequential nerves.

REFERENCES

Cormack GC, George B, Lamberty H 1994 The Arterial Anatomy of Skin Flaps, 2nd edn. London, Edinburgh: Churchill Livingstone: 168–72.
Lytle WJ 1979 Inguinal anatomy. J Anat 128: 581–94.

Rizk NN 1980 A new description of the anterior abdominal wall in man and mammals. J Anat 131: 373–85.
Shafik A 1977 The cremasteric muscle. In: Johnson AD, Gomes WR (eds) The Testis. Academic Press: New York.

Posterior abdominal wall and retroperitoneum

The posterior abdominal wall consists of fasciae, muscles and their vessels and spinal nerves. The overlying skin is continuous with that of the back. It is not easily defined, and is best described as that part of the abdominal wall lying between the two mid-dorsal lines, below the posterior attachments of the diaphragm and above the pelvis. It is continuous laterally with the anterolateral abdominal wall, superiorly with the posterior wall of the thorax behind the attachments of the diaphragm and inferiorly with the structures of the pelvis. The spinal column forms part of its structure and the muscles and fasciae of the back are closely related to it, especially posterolaterally.

The major vessels and lymphatic channels, in addition to the peripheral autonomic nervous systems of the abdomen, pelvis and lower limbs lie on the posterior abdominal wall. These structures, together with several viscera (including the kidneys [Ch. 91], suprarenal (adrenal) glands [Ch. 89], pancreas [Ch. 87], ureters [Ch. 92] and parts of the gut tube [Chs 73, 76–82]), lie beneath the posterior parietal peritoneum. These tissues and their surrounding connective and fascial planes are collectively referred to as the retroperitoneum.

It has been suggested that the retroperitoneum can be divided into several spaces according to their relationships to the fascial layers that surround the kidneys and ureters. In this description, the layers of the perirenal fascia (p. 1114) enclose a perirenal space containing the kidney, suprarenal gland, upper ureter and their neurovascular supply. The anterior layer of the perirenal fascia is continuous across the midline anterior to the main neurovascular structures of the retroperitoneum, and the right and left perirenal spaces communicate, although this channel is limited and contains many of the midline neurovascular structures of the retroperitoneum. Behind the posterior layer of the perirenal fascia lies the posterior pararenal space. Anterior to the anterior layer of the perirenal fascia lies the anterior pararenal space, in which lie several retroperitoneal parts of the gut tube, including the duodenum and pancreas. The anterior pararenal spaces are also continuous across the midline and are limited posteriorly by the anterior communicating layer of the perirenal fascia and anteriorly by the parietal peritoneum. This description helps to explain why moderate amounts of fluid, blood or pus collecting in the retroperitoneum tend to remain constrained within the space in which they are formed although, for pathological processes such as tumour invasion, the fascial planes provide a weak barrier to local spread.

Several structures, such as the pancreas, are referred to as being retroperitoneal. However although they are derived embryologically from the gut tube, they are not readily separated from the other retroperitoneal structures. Several other structures, such as the descending colon, are also referred to as being retroperitoneal, but they remain separated from the other retroperitoneal structures by a clearly defined fascial plane, which corresponds with the plane of fusion of their mesentery during development. This is of relevance during surgical exposure of the retroperitoneal organs and in some pathological processes: those defined by clear fascial planes may be mobilized with little or no risk of bleeding, whereas mobilization of the pancreas, for example, is difficult and often very vascular.

SKIN AND SOFT TISSUES

The skin of the back in the region of the posterior abdominal wall is similar to that of the rest of the trunk. It is supplied by vessels from the musculocutaneous branches of the lumbar arteries and veins, and receives its innervation from the dorsal rami of the lumbar spinal and lower thoracic nerves.

The soft tissues of the posterior abdominal wall and retroperitoneum (p. 743) are composed of several distinct layers of fascia, which divide them into anatomically distinct compartments.

THORACOLUMBAR FASCIA (Figs 67.10, 68.1, 68.2)

The thoracolumbar fascia in the lumbar region is in three layers. The posterior layer is attached to the spines of the lumbar and sacral vertebrae and to the supraspinous ligaments. The middle layer is attached medially to the tips of the transverse processes of the lumbar vertebrae and the intertransverse ligaments, inferiorly to the iliac crest, and superiorly to the lower border of the twelfth rib and the lumbocostal ligament. The

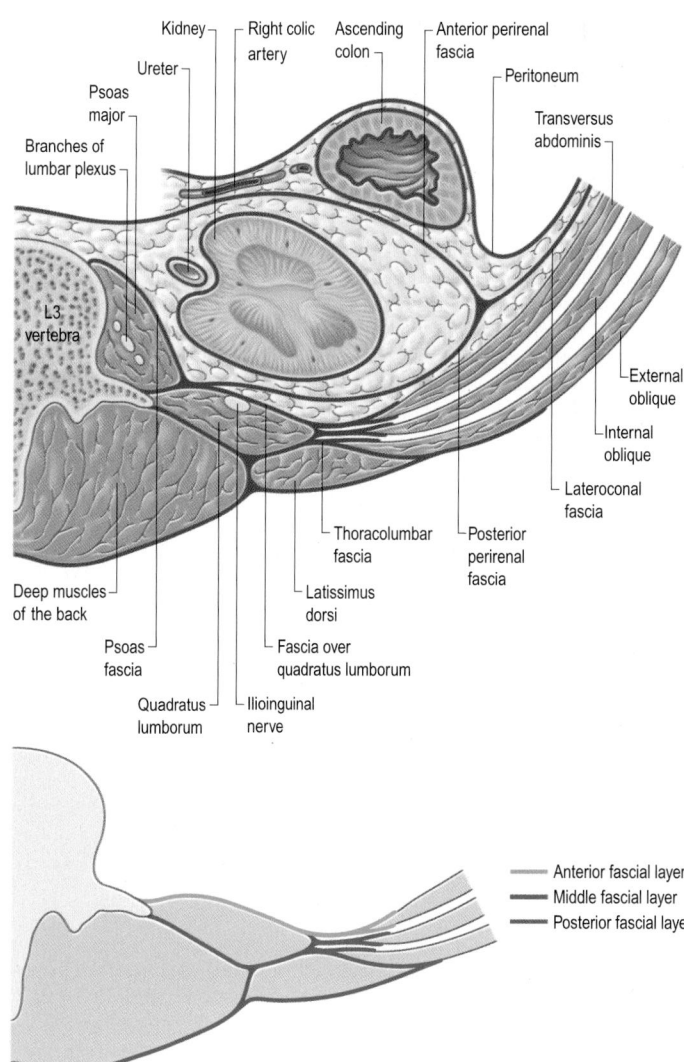

Fig. 68.1 Fascial layers of the upper posterior abdominal wall. **A,** Transverse section just below the level of the hilum of the kidney. For clarity, the deep muscles of the back have not been identified separately. **B,** The separate layers of the thoracolumbar fascia.

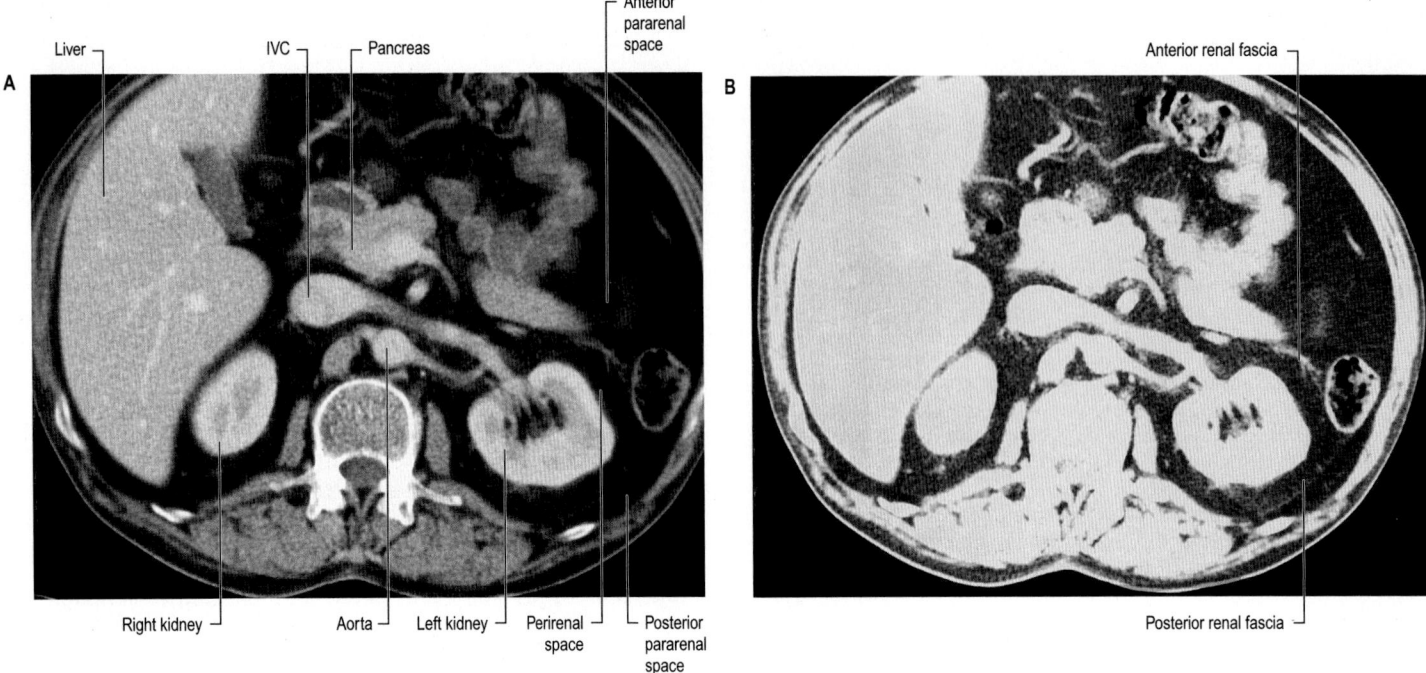

Fig. 68.2 Axial CT scan of the upper abdomen. **A**, On soft-tissue windows, to demonstrate retroperitoneal anatomy. IVC, inferior vena cava. **B**, On narrower window widths, to show the anterior and posterior renal fascia.

anterior layer covers quadratus lumborum and is attached medially to the anterior surfaces of the transverse processes of the lumbar vertebrae behind the lateral part of psoas major. Inferiorly, it is attached to the iliolumbar ligament and the adjoining part of the iliac crest. Superiorly, it is attached to the apex and inferior border of the twelfth rib and then extends to the transverse process of the first lumbar vertebra, to form the lateral arcuate ligament of the diaphragm. The posterior and middle layers of the thoracolumbar fascia unite at the lateral margin of erector spinae. At the lateral border of quadratus lumborum they are joined by the anterior layer, to form the aponeurotic origin of transversus abdominis (p. 1109).

OTHER FASCIAL LAYERS (Fig. 68.3)

Psoas fascia
Psoas major is enclosed within a layer of fascia over its anterior surface. The medial border is continuous with the attachments of the muscle to the transverse processes of the lumbar vertebrae, the bodies of the lumbar vertebrae and the tendinous arches. Superiorly, the fascia forms part of the medial arcuate ligament. Laterally, the fascia blends with the fascia over quadratus lumborum in the upper part of the muscle and is continuous with the iliac fascia lower down. It separates the anterior mass of psoas major from the retroperitoneal structures lying on it. The fascia extends down into the thigh. Inflammatory collections arising from the paraspinal tissues or the retroperitoneal tissues that penetrate through the fascia tend to be confined by it, and they may track down the length of the muscle, to appear in the groin where the fascia is thinnest.

Iliac fascia
The iliac fascia is continuous with and indistinguishable from the psoas fascia. The fascia blends with the anterior layer of the thoracolumbar fascia over quadratus lumborum in the upper retroperitoneum. Lower down, it is attached firmly to the inner aspect of the iliac crest and medially to the periosteum of the ilium at the pelvic brim. It is also attached in the abdomen to the iliopectineal eminence.

Perirenal fascia ‹X ref 7.20.2.1›
The perirenal fascia (p. 1270) is a multilaminated fascial layer that surrounds the kidney, suprarenal glands, upper ureter and associated fat, which all lie in the perirenal space. Although described as having anterior

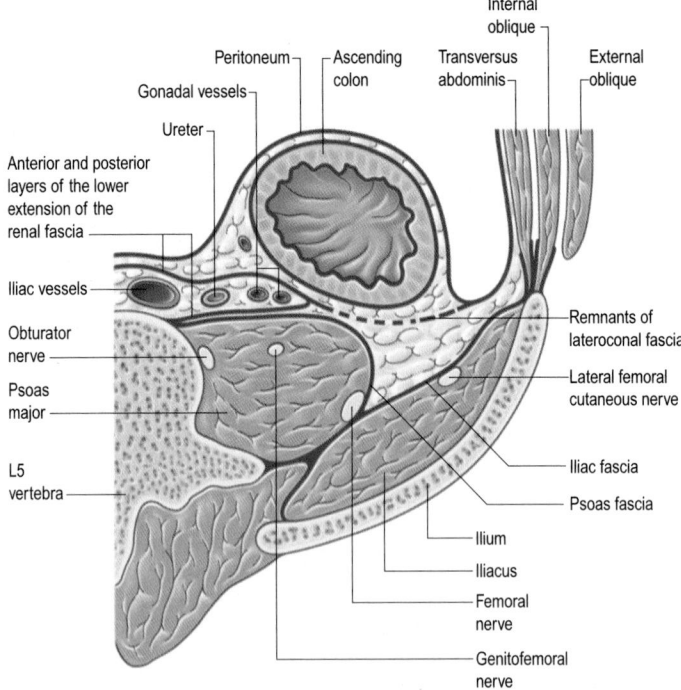

Fig. 68.3 Fascial layers of the lower posterior abdominal wall. Transverse section at the level of the fifth lumbar vertebra.

and posterior layers, these are continuous with each other laterally. The posterior layer of the renal fascia is adherent to the fascia over psoas major, the iliac fascia and the anterior layers of the thoracolumbar fascia. In the obese, there may be some loose adipose tissue between these layers, but it is rarely thick. The anterior part of the renal fascia separates the kidney and the perirenal space from the overlying anterior pararenal space and its associated viscera (on the right the duodenum, ascending colon and right colonic mesentery and on the left the duodenum, descending colon and left colonic mesentery). Inferiorly, the perirenal fascia continues down and encloses the ureter. It becomes progressively thinner towards the brim of the pelvis, where it is no longer distinguishable from the loose general connective tissue of the retroperitoneum.

Lateroconal fascia

The lateroconal fascia is formed from the lateral aspect of the perirenal fascia and extends anterolaterally to fuse with the fascia over transversus abdominis. It divides the anterior and posterior pararenal spaces from each other, but is thinnest in the inferior part of the retroperitoneum.

POSTERIOR EXTRAPERITONEAL CONNECTIVE TISSUE

The retroperitoneum usually contains loose connective tissue between the fascial layers. This is particularly true around the renal fascia and anterior to the psoas and iliac fascia. In all but the thinnest individuals, there is some adipose tissue present in these areas, and in the obese it may be markedly thickened. The retroperitoneal arteries and veins lie within this tissue, but the branches of the lumbar plexus of nerves lie deep to it, beneath the iliac and psoas fascia.

BONES

The posterior abdominal wall is supported by the bony structures of the vertebral column and bony pelvis. These include the lower two ribs (p. 957), the twelfth thoracic and five lumbar vertebrae, and the sacrum and ilium (p. 1425), in addition to their interconnecting ligaments.

MUSCLES (Figs 68.4, 68.5)

The majority of the muscles of the posterior abdominal wall are functionally part of the lower limb or vertebral column. They provide the surface against which the neurovascular structures of the retroperitoneum lie, and they are supported and separated from the majority of the retroperitoneal structures by fascial layers.

QUADRATUS LUMBORUM

Quadratus lumborum is an irregularly shaped quadrilateral muscle, which is broader at its inferior attachment than superiorly.

Attachments – Quadratus lumborum is attached below by aponeurotic fibres to the iliolumbar ligament and the adjacent portion of the iliac crest for c.5 cm. The superior attachment is to the medial half of the lower border of the twelfth rib, and by four small tendons to the apices of the transverse processes of the upper four lumbar vertebrae. Sometimes it is also attached to the transverse process or body of the twelfth thoracic vertebra. Occasionally, a second layer of this muscle is found in front of the first. This duplicated layer is attached to the upper borders of the transverse processes of the lower three or four lumbar vertebrae and to the lower margin and the lower part of the anterior surface of the twelfth rib.

Relations – Anterior to quadratus lumborum are the colon (ascending on the right, descending on the left), kidney, psoas major and minor, and diaphragm. The subcostal, iliohypogastric and ilioinguinal nerves lie on the fascia anterior to the muscle, but are bound down to it by the medial continuation of the transversalis fascia.

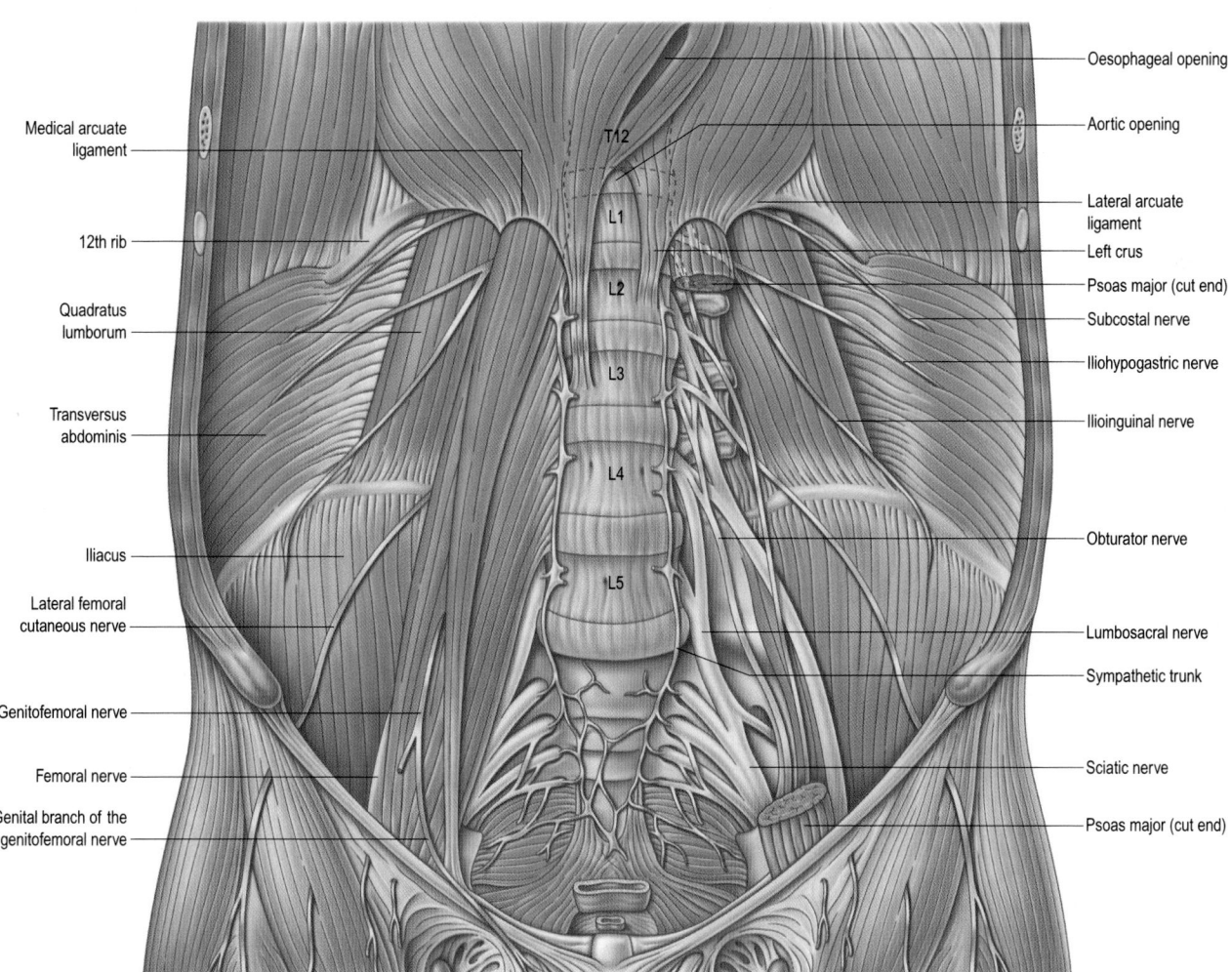

Fig. 68.4 Muscles and nerves of the posterior abdominal wall. The left psoas major has been removed to expose the origins of the lumbar plexus and quadratus lumborum.

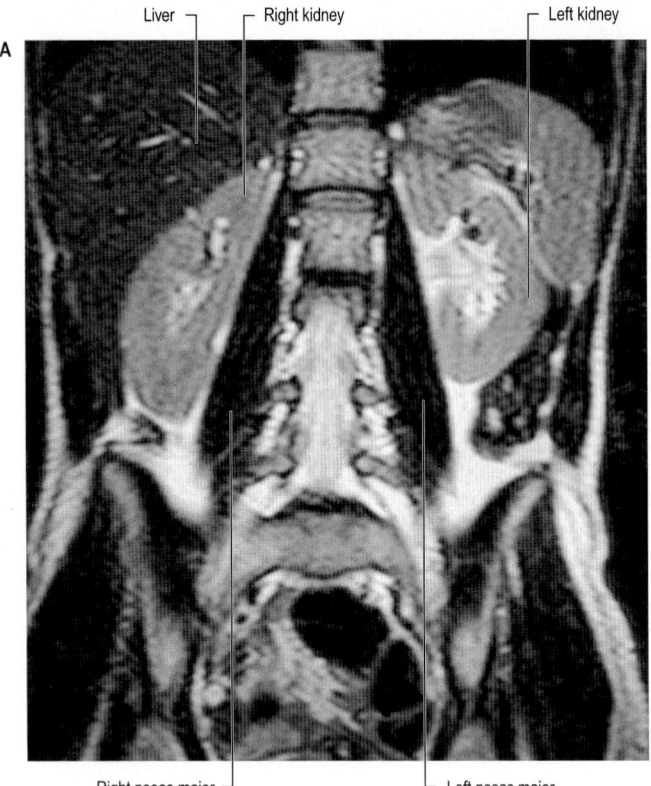

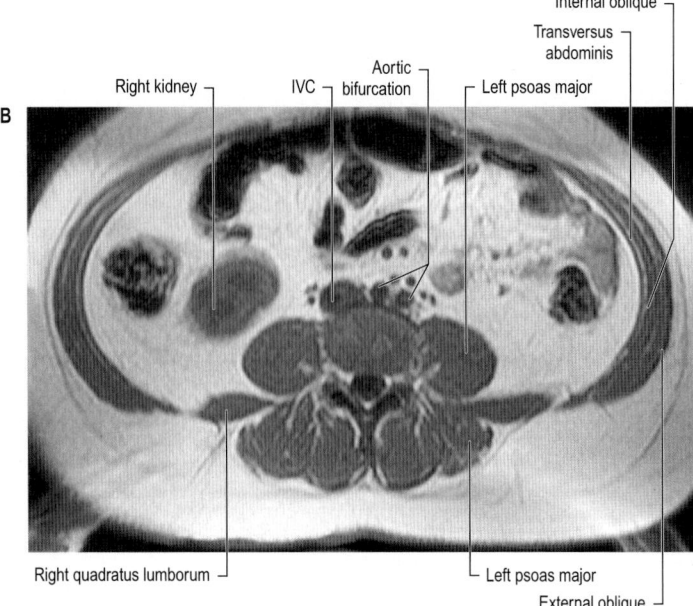

Fig. 68.5 Muscles of the posterior abdominal wall demonstrated on magnetic resonance imaging. **A**, Coronal T2-weighted MR image. **B**, Axial T1-weighted MR image. IVC, inferior vena cava.

Vascular supply – Quadratus lumborum is supplied by branches of the lumbar arteries, the arteria lumbalis ima, the lumbar branch of the iliolumbar artery and branches of the subcostal artery.

Innervation – Quadratus lumborum is innervated by the ventral rami of the twelfth thoracic and upper three or four lumbar spinal nerves.

Actions – Quadratus lumborum fixes the last rib, and acts as a muscle of inspiration by helping to stabilize the lower attachments of the diaphragm. It has been suggested that this action might also provide a fixed base for controlled relaxation of the diaphragm in the precise adjustment of expiration needed for speech and singing. With the pelvis fixed, quadratus acts upon the vertebral column, flexing it to the same side. When both muscles contract, they probably help to extend the lumbar part of the vertebral column.

PSOAS MAJOR
Psoas major has several sites of abdominal attachment. Posteriorly, the attachments are to the anterior surfaces and lower borders of the transverse processes of all the lumbar vertebrae. The muscle arising from these attachments is referred to as the posterior mass. The muscle also has an anterior mass. It consists of two different sets of attachments. The first part is five slips of muscle attached to the bodies of two adjoining vertebrae and their intervertebral disc (from the twelfth thoracic vertebra and the thoracolumbar disc to the lumbosacral disc and the first sacral segment). The second part is a series of tendinous arches extending across the narrow parts of the bodies of the five lumbar vertebrae between these slips. The upper four lumbar intervertebral foramina bear important relations to these attachments of the muscle. The foramina lie anterior to the transverse processes (the posterior attachments) and posterior to the vertebral bodies, discs and tendinous arches (anterior attachments). The roots of the lumbar plexus therefore enter the muscle directly between the two masses and the plexus is lodged within it. The branches then emerge from the borders and surfaces of psoas major.

PSOAS MINOR
Psoas minor (p. 1444) is often absent but, when present, lies anterior to psoas major. It arises from the sides of the bodies of the twelfth thoracic and first lumbar vertebrae and from the disc between them. It

ends in a long, flat tendon, which is attached to the pectineal line and iliopectineal eminence and, laterally, to the iliac fascia.

ERECTOR SPINAE
Erector spinae (p. 764) do not form part of the posterior abdominal wall itself, but are closely associated with the fascial layers of the posterior wall.

ILIACUS
Iliacus (p. 1446) is a triangular sheet of muscle that arises from the superior two-thirds of the concavity of the iliac fossa, the inner lip of the iliac crest, the ventral sacroiliac and iliolumbar ligaments and the upper surface of the lateral part of the sacrum. In front, it reaches as far as the anterior superior and anterior inferior iliac spines, and receives a few fibres from the upper part of the capsule of the hip joint. Most of its fibres converge into the lateral side of the strong tendon of psoas major. It lines the posterior wall of the lesser pelvis formed by the ilium.

POSTERIOR ABDOMINAL WALL HERNIAS
Herniation through the posterior abdominal wall is extremely rare. The fascial layers usually provide an excellent protection against protrusion of the posterior abdominal viscera, which are relatively immobile. However, the posterior free border of external oblique and the inferior free border of latissimus dorsi do give rise to an area of potential weakness, referred to as the lumbar triangle. Spontaneous hernias through this tissue are very rare in the absence of previous surgical access such as a nephrectomy.

VASCULAR SUPPLY AND LYMPHATIC DRAINGE

ABDOMINAL AORTA (Figs 68.6, 68.7)
The abdominal aorta begins at the median, aortic hiatus of the diaphragm, anterior to the inferior border of the twelfth thoracic vertebra and the thoracolumbar intervertebral disc. It descends anterior to the lumbar vertebrae to end at the lower border of the fourth lumbar vertebra, a little to the left of the midline, by dividing into two common iliac arteries. It diminishes rapidly in calibre from above downward, because its branches are large; however, the diameter of the vessel at any

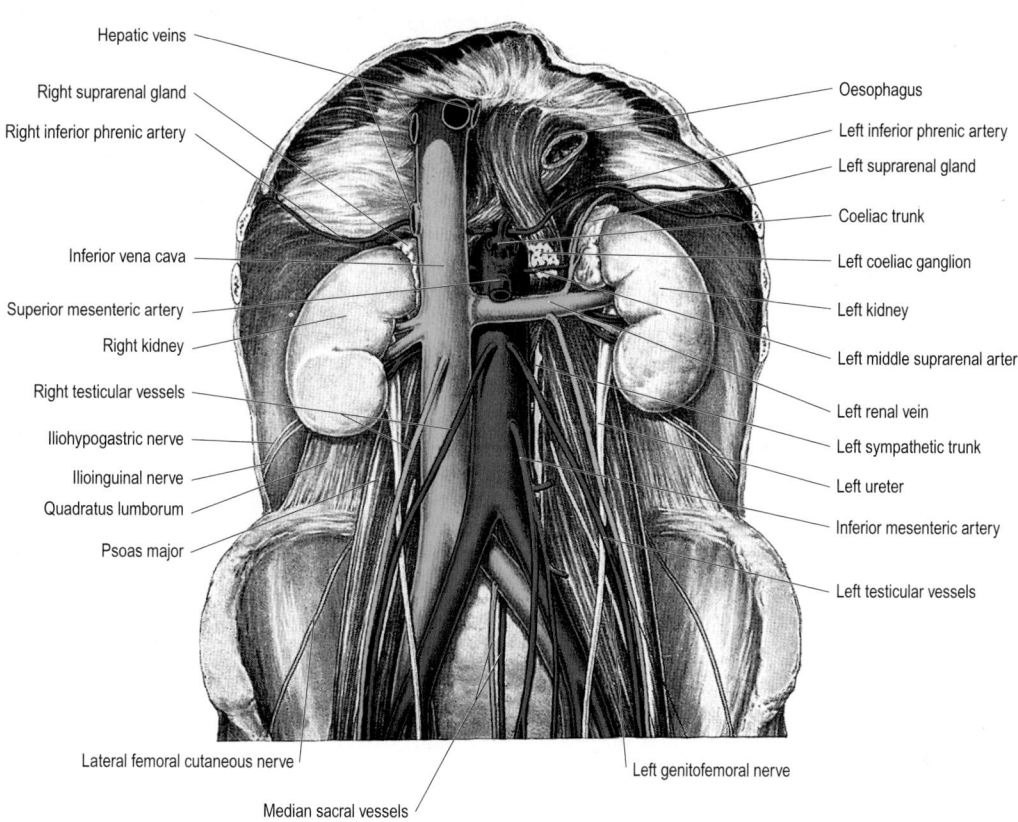

Hepatic veins
Right suprarenal gland
Right inferior phrenic artery
Inferior vena cava
Superior mesenteric artery
Right kidney
Right testicular vessels
Iliohypogastric nerve
Ilioinguinal nerve
Quadratus lumborum
Psoas major

Oesophagus
Left inferior phrenic artery
Left suprarenal gland
Coeliac trunk
Left coeliac ganglion
Left kidney
Left middle suprarenal artery
Left renal vein
Left sympathetic trunk
Left ureter
Inferior mesenteric artery
Left testicular vessels

Lateral femoral cutaneous nerve
Left genitofemoral nerve
Median sacral vessels

Fig. 68.6 The abdominal aorta, inferior vena cava and their branches in the male. The fascia, lymphatics and connective tissue have been removed for clarity.

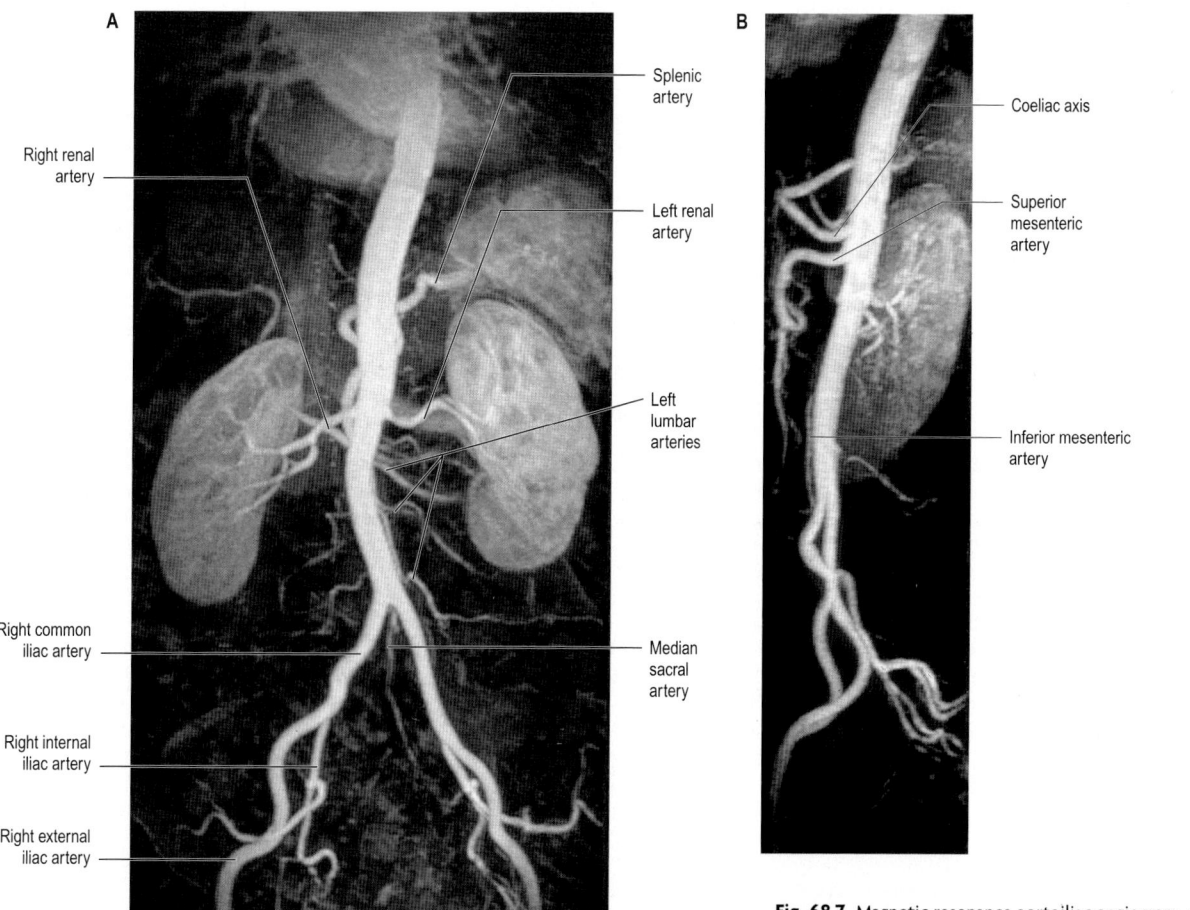

A
B

Right renal artery
Splenic artery
Left renal artery
Coeliac axis
Superior mesenteric artery
Left lumbar arteries
Right common iliac artery
Median sacral artery
Inferior mesenteric artery
Right internal iliac artery
Right external iliac artery

Fig. 68.7 Magnetic resonance aortoiliac angiogram. **A**, Coronal reformat. **B**, Sagittal reformat.

1117

given height tends to increase slightly with age. The cadaveric superior and inferior calibres are between c.9 and 14 mm and 8 and 12 mm, respectively, with little difference between the sexes. The angle of aortic bifurcation varies widely, particularly in the elderly. It has been suggested that the relationship between aortic size and shape is a possible causative factor in the development of abdominal aortic aneurysm (Newman et al 1971). This may be caused by the reflection of transmitted pressure waves, which occurs at junctions between vessels. At the aortic bifurcation, pressure oscillations and possibly turbulence may be set up as a result of differences in the luminal diameters of the common iliac arteries, and so give rise to reflected waves that may injure the intima of the distal abdominal aorta. The role of the relative calibres of the iliac arteries remains uncertain (Shah et al 1978).

Relations

The upper abdominal aorta is related anteriorly to the coeliac trunk and its branches. The coeliac plexus and the lesser sac lie between it and the left lobe of the liver and lesser omentum. Below this, the superior mesenteric artery leaves the aorta, crossing anterior to the left renal vein. The body of the pancreas, with the splenic vein on its posterior surface, extends obliquely up and to the left across the abdominal aorta, separated from it by the superior mesenteric artery and left renal vein. Below the pancreas, the proximal parts of the gonadal arteries, and the third part of the duodenum, lie anteriorly. In its lowest part it is covered by the posterior parietal peritoneum and crossed obliquely by the origin of the small intestinal mesentery.

The thoracolumbar intervertebral discs, the upper four lumbar vertebrae, intervening intervertebral discs and the anterior longitudinal ligament are all posterior to the abdominal aorta. Lumbar arteries arise from its dorsal aspect and cross posterior to it. The third and fourth (and sometimes second) left lumbar veins also cross behind it to reach the inferior vena cava. The aorta may overlap the anterior border of the left psoas major.

On the right, the aorta is related above to the cisterna chyli and thoracic duct, the azygos vein and the right crus of the diaphragm, which overlaps and separates it from the inferior vena cava and right coeliac ganglion. Below the second lumbar vertebra, it is closely applied to the left side of the inferior vena cava. This close relationship occasionally allows the formation of an aorto–caval fistula, particularly after aneurysmal disease surgery or trauma to the aorta.

On the left, the aorta is related above to the left crus of the diaphragm and left coeliac ganglion. Level with the second lumbar vertebra, it is related to the duodenojejunal flexure and the left sympathetic trunk, the fourth part of the duodenum and the inferior mesenteric vessels.

Branches (Fig. 68.8)

The branches of the aorta are described as anterior, lateral and dorsal. The anterior and lateral branches are distributed to the viscera. The dorsal branches supply the body wall, vertebral column, vertebral canal and its contents. The aorta terminates by dividing into the right and left common iliac arteries.

Anterior group (Fig. 68.9)

Coeliac trunk (coeliac axis) – The coeliac trunk is the first anterior branch and arises just below the aortic hiatus at the level of T12/L1 vertebral bodies. It is c.1.5–2 cm long and passes almost horizontally forwards and slightly right above the pancreas and splenic vein. It divides into the left gastric, common hepatic and splenic arteries. The coeliac trunk may also give off one or both of the inferior phrenic arteries. The superior mesenteric artery may arise with the coeliac trunk as a common origin. One or more of the superior mesenteric branches may arise from the coeliac trunk. Anterior to the coeliac trunk lies the lesser sac. The coeliac plexus surrounds the trunk, sending extensions along its branches. On the right lie the right coeliac ganglion, right crus of the diaphragm and the caudate lobe of the liver. To the left lie the left coeliac ganglion, left crus of the diaphragm and the cardiac end of the stomach. The right crus may compress the origin of the coeliac trunk, giving the appearance of a stricture. The head of the pancreas and the splenic vein are inferior to the coeliac trunk.

Superior mesenteric artery – The superior mesenteric artery (p. 1169) originates from the aorta c.1 cm below the coeliac trunk, at the level of the L1–2 intervertebral disc. It lies posterior to the splenic vein and the

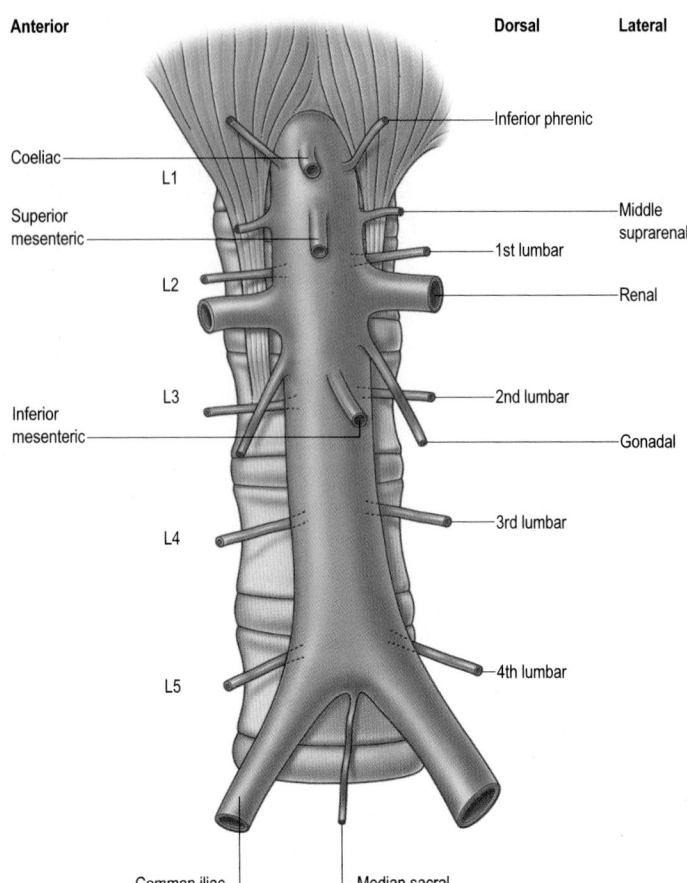

Fig. 68.8 The branches of the abdominal aorta.

body of the pancreas. The left renal vein separates it from the aorta. It runs inferiorly and anteriorly, anterior to the uncinate process of the pancreas and the third part of the duodenum.

Inferior mesenteric artery – The inferior mesenteric artery is usually smaller in calibre than the superior mesenteric artery. It arises from the anterior or left anterolateral aspect of the aorta at about the level of the third lumbar vertebra, 3 or 4 cm above the aortic bifurcation and posterior to the horizontal part of the duodenum.

Lateral group

Suprarenal artery – The middle suprarenal artery arises from the lateral aspect of the abdominal aorta, level with the superior mesenteric artery. It ascends slightly, and runs over the crura of the diaphragm to the suprarenal glands, where it anastomoses with the suprarenal branches of the phrenic and renal arteries. The right middle suprarenal artery passes behind the inferior vena cava and near the right coeliac ganglion. The left middle suprarenal artery passes close to the left coeliac ganglion, splenic artery and the superior border of the pancreas.

Renal artery – The renal arteries are two of the largest branches of the abdominal aorta and arise laterally from the vessel just below the origin of the superior mesenteric artery. The right is longer and usually arises slightly higher than the left. It passes posterior to the inferior vena cava, right renal vein, head of the pancreas and second part of the duodenum. The left renal artery arises a little lower down and passes behind the left renal vein, the body of the pancreas and the splenic vein.

Gonadal artery – The gonadal arteries (p. 1118) are two long, slender vessels that arise from the aorta a little inferior to the renal arteries. Each passes inferolaterally under the parietal peritoneum on psoas major.

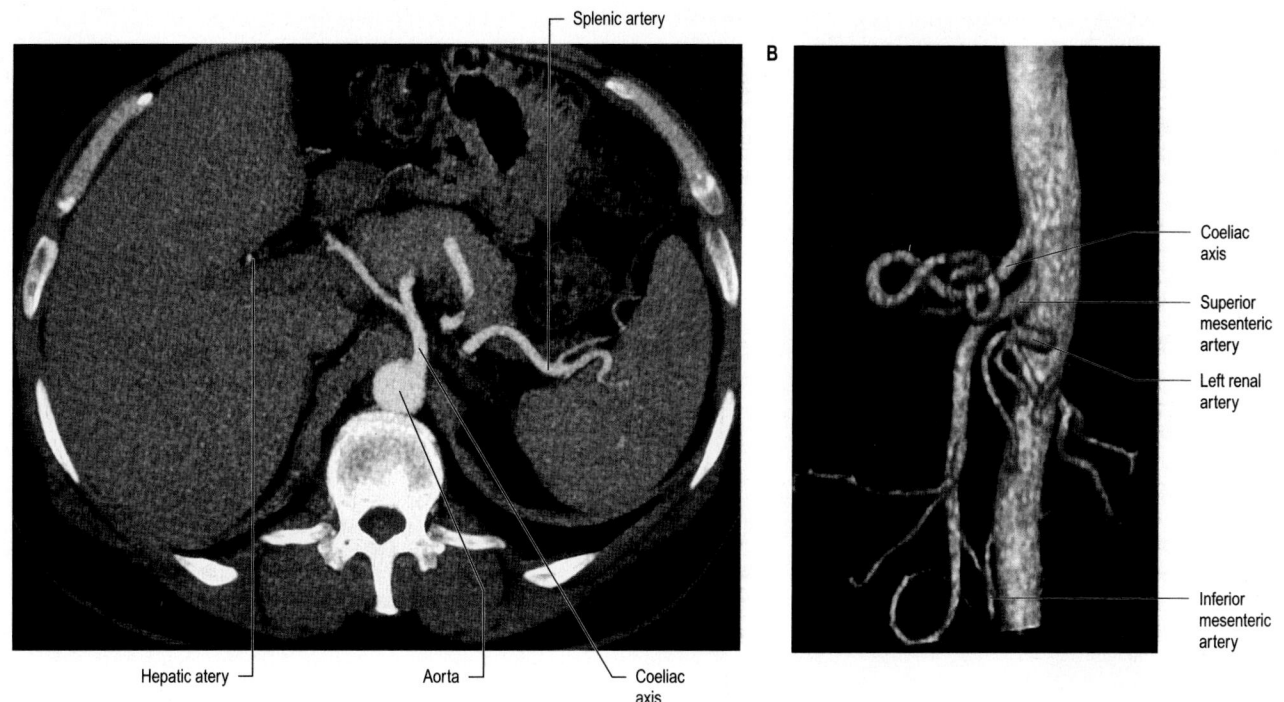

Splenic artery

A

B

Coeliac
axis

Superior
mesenteric
artery

Left renal
artery

Inferior
mesenteric
artery

Hepatic atery

Aorta

Coeliac
axis

Fig. 68.9 Multislice computed tomography angiogram of the abdominal aorta. **A**, Single axial slice from the volume data set at the level of the coeliac axis. **B**, Three-dimensional surface-shaded reformat of the volume dataset acquired on axial multislice CT through the entire abdomen to produce a midline sagittal view of the anterior branches of the aorta.

Dorsal group

Inferior phrenic arteries – The inferior phrenic arteries usually arise from the aorta, just above the level of the coeliac trunk. Occasionally they arise from a common aortic origin with the coeliac trunk, from the coeliac trunk itself or from the renal artery. They contribute to the arterial supply of the diaphragm. Each artery ascends and runs laterally anterior to the crus of the diaphragm, near the medial border of the suprarenal gland. The left passes behind the oesophagus and forwards on the left side of its diaphragmatic opening. The right passes posterior to the inferior vena cava and then along the right of the diaphragmatic opening for the inferior vena cava. Near the posterior border of the central tendon of the diaphragm, each divides into medial and lateral branches. The medial branch curves forwards to anastomose with its fellow in front of the central tendon and with the musculophrenic and pericardiacophrenic arteries. The lateral branch approaches the thoracic wall, and anastomoses with the lower posterior intercostal and musculophrenic arteries. The lateral branch of the right artery provides the arterial supply to the wall of the inferior vena cava, whereas the left sends ascending branches to the serosal surface of the abdominal oesophagus. Each inferior phrenic artery has two or three small suprarenal branches. The capsule of the liver and spleen may also receive a small supply from the arteries.

Lumbar arteries – The lumbar arteries arise in series with the posterior intercostal arteries. There are usually four on each side. They arise from the posterolateral aspect of the aorta, opposite the lumbar vertebrae. A fifth, smaller, pair occasionally arise from the median sacral artery, but lumbar branches of the iliolumbar arteries usually take their place. The lumbar arteries run posterolaterally on the first to the fourth lumbar vertebral bodies, behind the sympathetic trunks, to intervals between the lumbar transverse processes. From here they continue into the muscles of the posterior abdominal wall. The right arteries pass posterior to the inferior vena cava. The upper two on the right side and first left lumbar arteries lie posterior to the corresponding crus of the diaphragm. Arteries of both sides pass under tendinous arches, which span the lateral concavities of the vertebral bodies, which form the attachment of psoas major. They run posterior to the muscle and the lumbar plexus. They then cross the anterior surface of quadratus lumborum, the upper three posterior, and the last usually anterior to it. At the lateral border

of quadratus lumborum they pierce the posterior aponeurosis of transversus abdominis, running forward between it and internal oblique. They anastomose with one another and the lower posterior intercostal, subcostal, iliolumbar, deep circumflex iliac and inferior epigastric arteries.

Dorsal branches – Each lumbar artery has a dorsal branch, which passes backwards between the adjacent transverse vertebral processes to supply the dorsal muscles of the back, the joints and skin of the back. This branch also has a spinal branch which enters the vertebral canal to supply its contents and adjacent vertebra, anastomosing with the arteries above and below it and across the midline. The spinal branch of the first lumbar artery supplies the terminal spinal cord itself; the remainder supply the cauda equina, meninges and vertebral canal. Occlusion of all or most of these arteries by dissection or aneurysm of the abdominal aorta may cause ischaemia of the cauda equina, producing the so-called 'cauda equina syndrome'. This is rare, however, even after infrarenal aortic graft surgery, because of the relatively good collateral circulation of the spinal cord arteries from the descending thoracic aorta. Branches of the lumbar arteries and their dorsal branches supply the adjacent muscles, fasciae, bones, red marrow, ligaments and joints of the vertebral column.

Median sacral artery

The median sacral artery is a small branch that arises from the posterior aspect of the aorta a little above its bifurcation. It descends in the midline, anterior to the fourth and fifth lumbar vertebrae, sacrum and coccyx, and ends in the coccygeal body. At the level of the fifth lumbar vertebra, it is crossed by the left common iliac vein and often gives off a small lumbar artery (arteria lumbalis ima), small branches of which reach the anorectum via the anococcygeal ligament. Anterior to the fifth lumbar vertebra the median sacral artery anastomoses with a lumbar branch of the iliolumbar artery. Anterior to the sacrum it anastomoses with the lateral sacral arteries and sends branches into the anterior sacral foramina.

Aortic surgery and prostheses

Open surgical approaches to the abdominal aorta maybe associated with several potential complications. Injury to the large lymphatic trunks in the upper abdomen may lead to chylous ascites (p. 1122). Disruption of the intermesenteric and inferior mesenteric plexuses rarely causes clinically significant disturbances of autonomic function.

INFERIOR VENA CAVA (Fig. 68.10)

The inferior vena cava conveys blood to the right atrium from all structures below the diaphragm. The majority of its course is within the abdomen, but a small section lies within the fibrous pericardium in the thorax. It is formed by the junction of the common iliac veins anterior to the fifth lumbar vertebral body, a little to its right. It ascends anterior to the vertebral column, to the right of the aorta. It is contained in a deep groove on the posterior surface of the liver, or sometimes in a tunnel completed by a band of liver tissue. It crosses the tendinous part of the diaphragm between its median and right 'leaves' and inclines slightly anteromedially. Passing through the fibrous pericardium and through a posterior inflexion of the serous pericardium, it opens into the inferoposterior part of the right atrium. The abdominal portion of the inferior vena cava is devoid of valves.

Relations of the abdominal part of the inferior vena cava

Anteriorly, the inferior vena cava is related to the right common iliac artery at its origin. It is crossed obliquely by the root of the mesentery and its contained vessels and nerves, and by the right gonadal artery. It lies behind the peritoneum of the posterior abdominal wall and the third part of the duodenum. It ascends behind the head of the pancreas and then the first part of the duodenum, separated from them by the common bile duct and portal vein. Above the duodenum it is again covered by the peritoneum of the posterior abdominal wall, which forms the posterior wall of the epiploic foramen. This separates it from the right free border of the lesser omentum and its contents. Above this it is intimately related to the liver anteriorly.

The lower three lumbar vertebral bodies, their intervertebral discs and the anterior longitudinal ligament and right psoas major, sympathetic trunk and third and fourth lumbar arteries are all posterior to the inferior vena cava. Superior to these structures, the inferior vena cava is related posteriorly to the right crus of the diaphragm, the medial part of the right suprarenal gland, the right coeliac ganglion and the right renal, middle suprarenal and inferior phrenic arteries.

The right ureter, the second part of the duodenum, medial border of the right kidney and the right lobe of the liver are all lateral to the right side of the inferior vena cava. The aorta, the right crus of the diaphragm and the caudate lobe of the liver are all lateral to the left side.

Numerous anomalies may occur in the anatomy of the inferior vena cava, mostly related to its complex formation (p. 1047). It is sometimes replaced, below the level of the renal veins, by two more or less symmetric vessels (**Fig. 68.11**), often associated with the failure of interconnection between the common iliac veins, and as a result of persistence on the left of a longitudinal channel (usually the supra-cardinal or subcardinal vein) that normally disappears in early fetal life. In complete visceral transposition, the inferior vena cava lies to the left of the aorta.

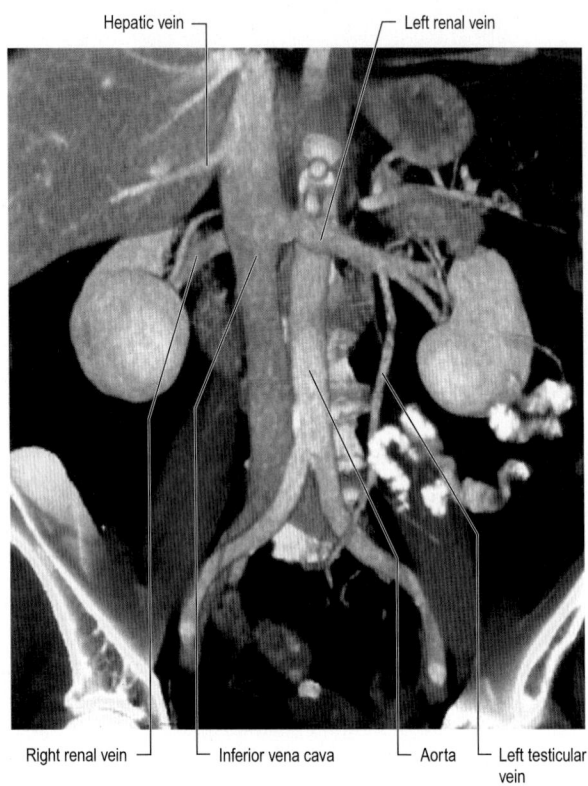

Fig. 68.10 Multislice computed tomography three-dimensional surface-shaded angiogram of the abdominal aorta and inferior vena cavogram.

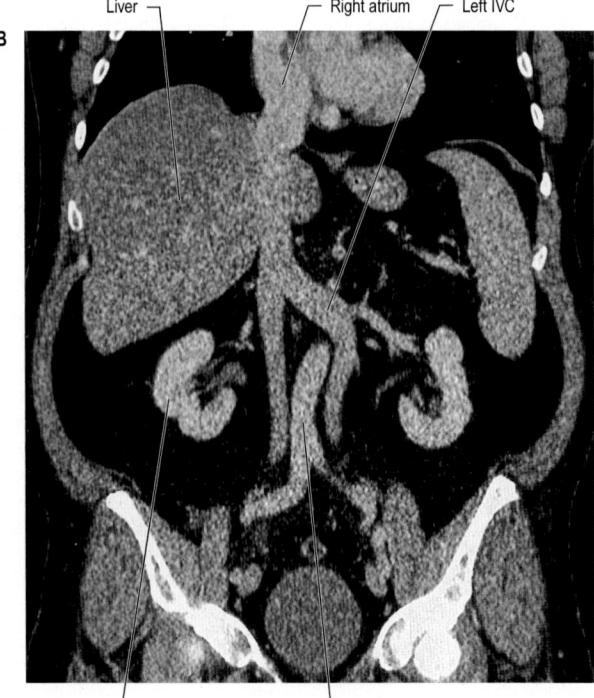

Fig. 68.11 Multislice computed tomography demonstrating a double inferior vena cava (IVC). **A,** Axial CT at the level of the renal hilum, showing an IVC on either side of the aorta. **B,** Coronal reformat showing bilateral IVC joining above the level of the renal veins.

Tributaries (Fig. 68.12)

The abdominal inferior vena cava usually receives the common iliac veins at its origin and the lumbar, right gonadal, renal, right suprarenal, inferior phrenic and hepatic veins during its course.

Lumbar veins

Four pairs of lumbar veins collect blood by dorsal tributaries from the lumbar muscles and skin. These branches anastomose with tributaries of the lumbar origin of the azygos and hemiazygos veins (p. 987). The abdominal tributaries to the lumbar veins drain blood from the posterior, lateral and anterior abdominal walls, including the parietal peritoneum. Anteriorly, the abdominal tributaries anastomose with branches of the inferior and superior epigastric veins. These anastomoses provide routes of continued venous drainage from the pelvis and lower limb to the heart in the event of inferior vena caval obstruction. The abdominal tributaries drain into the superior epigastric veins and hence via the internal thoracic veins to the superior vena cava, whereas the dorsal tributaries carry blood into the azygos and hemiazygos system and hence into the superior vena cava. Near the vertebral column, the lumbar veins drain the vertebral plexuses and are connected by the ascending lumbar vein, which is a vessel running longitudinally anterior to the roots of the transverse processes of the lumbar vertebrae. The third and fourth lumbar veins are fairly consistent in their course and pass forward on the sides of the corresponding vertebral bodies to enter the posterior aspect of the inferior vena cava. The left lumbar veins pass behind the abdominal aorta and are therefore longer. First and second lumbar veins are much more variable and may drain into the inferior vena cava, ascending lumbar vein, or lumbar azygos veins. They are often connected to each other, and the first lumbar vein does not usually enter the inferior vena cava directly, but turns down to join the second.

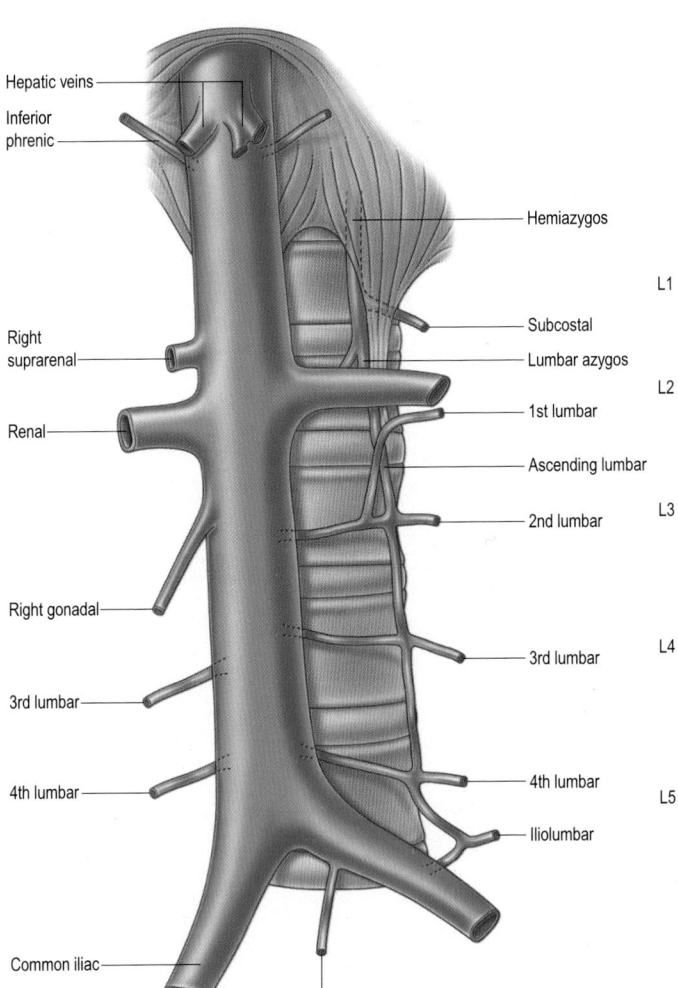

Fig. 68.12 Tributaries of the inferior vena cava and lumbar veins. Only the left lumbar venous system is shown, for clarity.

Alternatively, the first lumbar vein may drain directly into the ascending lumbar vein or pass forward over the first lumbar vertebral body to the lumbar azygos vein. The second lumbar vein may join the inferior vena cava at or near the level of the renal veins. Sometimes it joins the third lumbar vein, or it may drain into the ascending lumbar vein.

Ascending lumbar vein – The ascending lumbar vein connects the common iliac, iliolumbar and lumbar veins. It lies between psoas major and the roots of the lumbar transverse processes. There is considerable variability in the course of this vein and the related lumbar azygos and first lumbar veins. Superiorly, it commonly joins the subcostal vein to form the azygos vein on the right and the hemiazygos on the left. These veins run forward over the twelfth thoracic vertebral body, and pass deep to the crura of the diaphragm and into the thorax. The ascending lumbar vein is usually joined by a small vessel from the back of the inferior vena cava or left renal vein on the left. This little vein represents the azygos line (p. 1047) and is referred to as the lumbar azygos vein. Sometimes the ascending lumbar vein ends in the first lumbar vein, which then skirts the first lumbar vertebra with the first lumbar artery, to join the lumbar azygos vein. In this circumstance the subcostal veins join the azygos vein on the right and the hemiazygos vein on the left.

Gonadal veins

Only the left gonadal vein (pp. 1323, 1306) joins the inferior vena cava directly. It opens into its right anterolateral aspect at an acute angle just inferior to the level of the left renal vein. It is often double all the way to the level of entry into the inferior vena cava.

Renal veins

The renal veins (p. 1247) are large calibre vessels, which lie anterior to the renal arteries and open into the inferior vena cava almost at right angles. The left is three times longer than the right in length (7.5 cm and 2.5 cm, respectively). The left vein lies on the posterior abdominal wall posterior to the splenic vein and body of the pancreas. Close to its opening into the inferior vena cava, it lies anterior to the aorta with the superior mesenteric artery just above it. The right renal vein lies posterior to the second part of the duodenum and sometimes the lateral part of the head of the pancreas.

Suprarenal vein

The right suprarenal vein drains directly into the inferior vena cava at the level of the twelfth thoracic vertebra.

Inferior phrenic veins

The inferior phrenic veins run on the inferior surface of the central tendon of the diaphragm. They drain into the posterolateral aspect of the inferior vena cava around the level of the tenth thoracic vertebra. The left vein tends to drain at a slightly higher level than the right, and runs above the level of the oesophageal opening in the diaphragm. It may be double, with a branch draining into the left renal or suprarenal vein.

Collaterals in inferior vena caval occlusion

Occlusion of the inferior vena cava may follow thrombosis resulting from hypercoagulable conditions, or embolism from lower limb or pelvic thromboses. The increased pressure within the lower body circulation leads to oedema of the legs and back, without ascites. Collateral venous circulation is established through a wide range of anastomoses between branches that drain ultimately to the superior vena cava. The lumbar veins connect to branches of the superior epigastric, circumflex iliac, lateral thoracic and posterior intercostal veins. They also anastomose with tributaries of the azygos, hemiazygos and lumbar azygos veins. The interconnecting vertebral venous plexuses provide an additional route of collateral circulation between the vena cavae.

Inferior vena caval filters

Recurrent embolization of clot from the pelvic or lower limbs veins may be a serious threat to life. In an effort to prevent life-threatening pulmonary embolism, a fenestrated filter may be placed within the inferior vena cava in an effort to trap the clot. These are most commonly inserted by radiological guidance via the internal jugular vein and superior vena cava and placed at a level below the origin of the renal veins. Progressive occlusion of the filter by clot may lead to symptoms of vena caval obstruction. Rarely, damage to the medial wall of the vena cava from the retaining hooks of the filter may lead to the development of an aorto–caval fistula as a result of the close proximity of the aorta at this level.

LYMPHATIC DRAINAGE (Figs 68.13, 68.14, 68.15)

The lymphatic drainage of the muscles, deep tissues and integument of the posterior abdominal wall is broadly divided into four regions. The small upper left and upper right regions drain to the lateral aortic nodes and the ipsilateral axillary lymph nodes. The larger lower left and lower right portions drain to the lateral and retro-aortic lymph nodes, although some drainage also occurs to the left and right superficial inguinal nodes.

The lymphatic drainage of the abdominal viscera occurs almost exclusively through the cisterna chyli and the thoracic duct. Some lymphatic drainage may occur across the diaphragm from the bare area of the liver and the uppermost retroperitoneal tissues, but this is probably of little clinical consequence other than during obstruction of the thoracic duct. The lymph nodes of the retroperitoneum lie around the abdominal aorta and form pre-aortic, lateral aortic and retro-aortic groups. Collectively, they are referred to as the para-aortic lymph nodes and clinically it is difficult to distinguish between them, either at operation or on cross-sectional imaging.

Cisterna chyli and abdominal lymph trunks

The abdominal origin of the thoracic duct lies to the right of the midline at the level of the lower border of the twelfth thoracic vertebral body or the thoracolumbar intervertebral disc. It receives all the lymph delivered by the four main abdominal lymph trunks, which converge to an elongated arrangement of channels, referred to as the abdominal confluence of lymph trunks. This may be a simple duct-like structure

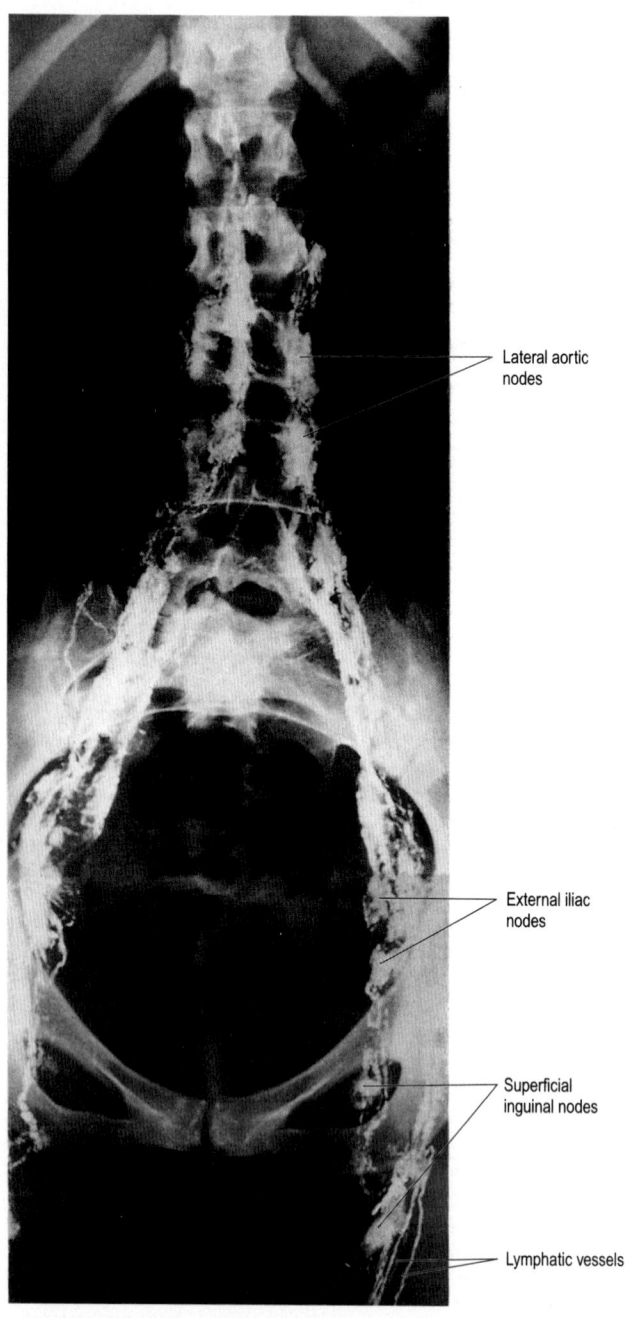

Lateral aortic nodes

External iliac nodes

Superficial inguinal nodes

Lymphatic vessels

Fig. 68.13 Lymphangiogram showing the lateral aortic and proximal iliac lymphatics. The radiograph was taken approximately 3 hours after the injection of contrast medium into the lymphatics of the dorsum of the foot. (Provided by GI Verney, Addenbrooke's Hospital, Cambridge; photographs prepared by Sarah-Jane Smith and Kevin Fitzpatrick on behalf of GKT School of Medicine, London.)

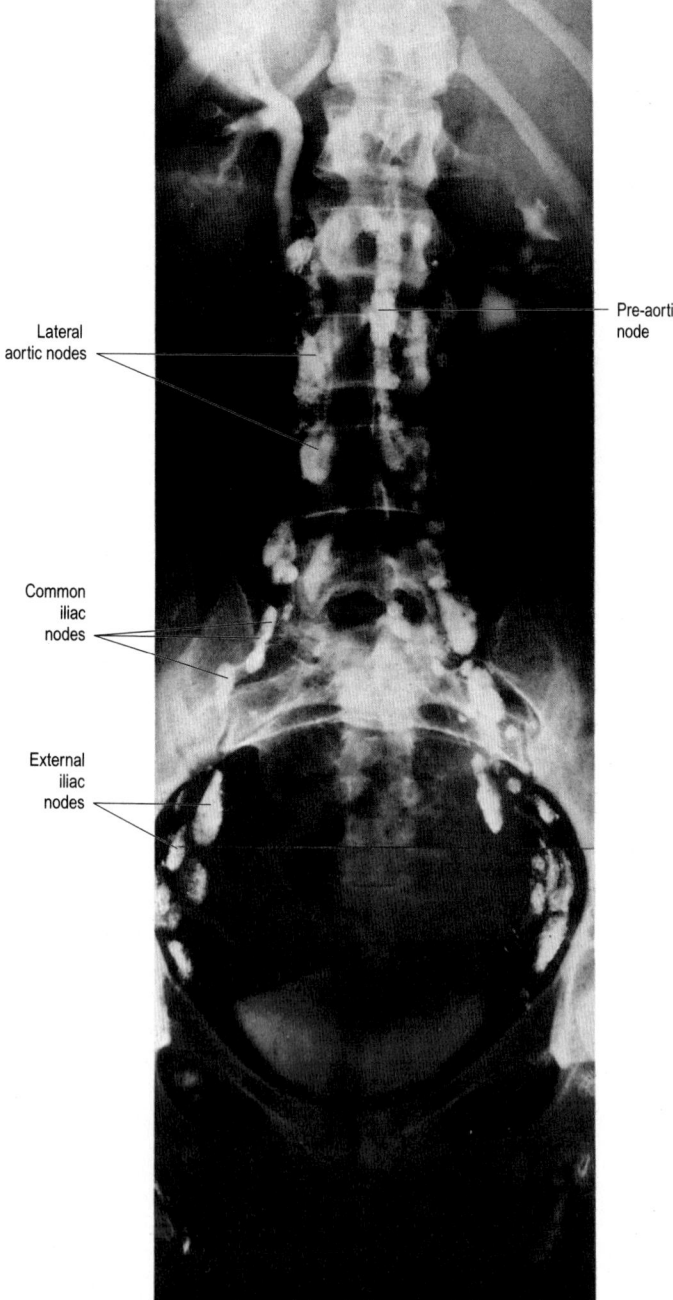

Lateral aortic nodes

Pre-aortic node

Common iliac nodes

External iliac nodes

Fig. 68.14 Lymphangiogram showing the lateral aortic and proximal iliac lymph nodes. The radiograph was taken approximately 24 hours after the injection of contrast medium into the lymphatics of the dorsum of the foot. Intravenous contrast opacifies the renal collecting system. (Provided by JB Kinmonth.)

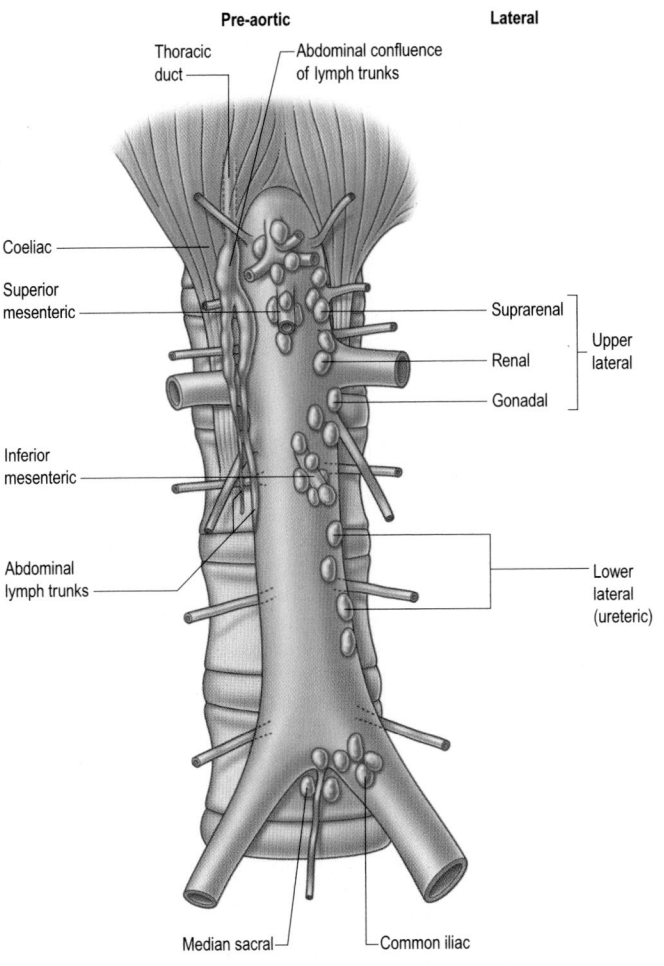

Fig. 68.15 Abdominal lymph node groups. The main pre-aortic groups are shown. Only the left-sided lateral nodes are shown, for clarity.

surgery, particularly dissections carried out around the aorta above the level of the coeliac axis. The large calibre of the trunks, coupled with the volume of lymph flowing through them, means that they do not readily self-seal after injury, and this lead to problematic recurrent chylous (lymphatic) ascites.

The thoracic duct leaves the superior end of the cisterna chyli or the abdominal confluence and immediately passes through the aortic aperture of the diaphragm posterolateral to the aorta.

Pre-aortic group

The pre-aortic groups tend to lie around the origins of the anterior (visceral) arteries and receive lymph from the gastrointestinal tract and its accessory structures (liver, spleen and pancreas) from the abdominal oesophagus to the level of the anus. They give rise to lymphatic vessels, which drain upwards to form the intestinal trunks that enter the abdominal confluence of lymph trunks. They are divisible into coeliac, superior mesenteric and inferior mesenteric groups, being near the origins of these arteries.

Coeliac nodes

The coeliac nodes lie anterior to the abdominal aorta around the origin of the coeliac artery. They are a terminal group and receive lymph draining from the regional lymph nodes around the branches of the coeliac artery (left gastric, hepatic and pancreaticosplenic nodes). They also receive lymph from the lower pre-aortic groups (the superior mesenteric and inferior mesenteric). The coeliac nodes give rise to right and left intestinal lymph trunks.

Gastric – There are a great number of gastric lymph node groups. They drain the stomach, upper duodenum, abdominal oesophagus and the greater omentum. They drain to the coeliac group.

Hepatic – The hepatic nodes extend in the lesser omentum along the hepatic arteries and bile duct. They vary in number and site, but almost always occur at the junction of the cystic and common hepatic ducts (the cystic node), alongside the upper common bile duct and in the anterior border of the epiploic foramen. Hepatic nodes drain the majority of the liver, gallbladder and bile ducts, but also receive drainage from some parts of the stomach, duodenum and pancreas. They drain to the coeliac nodes and thence to the intestinal trunks.

Pancreaticosplenic – The pancreaticosplenic nodes drain the spleen, pancreas and part of the stomach. Their afferents join the coeliac nodes.

Superior mesenteric and inferior mesenteric nodes

The superior and inferior mesenteric nodes lie anterior to the aorta near the origins of their respective arteries. The superior and inferior mesenteric nodes are preterminal groups for the alimentary canal from the duodenojejunal flexure to the upper anal canal. They collect from outlying groups, including the mesenteric, ileocolic, colonic and para-rectal nodes and drain into the coeliac nodes.

Lateral aortic group

The lateral aortic nodes lie on either side of the abdominal aorta anterior to the medial margins of psoas major, diaphragmatic crura and sympathetic trunks. On the right, some nodes lie lateral and anterior to the inferior vena cava near the end of the right renal vein. Nodes rarely lie between the aorta and inferior vena cava where they are closely related. The lateral aortic nodes drain the viscera and other structures supplied by the lateral and dorsal aortic branches. The upper lateral groups receive the lymph drainage directly from the suprarenal glands, kidneys, ureters, gonads, uterine tubes and upper uterus. They also receive lymph directly from the deeper tissues of the posterior abdominal wall. Lymphatics from the pelvis, most of the pelvic viscera, the perineum and the anterolateral abdominal wall pass first to regional nodes largely related to the iliac arteries and their branches. These include the common iliac, external iliac, internal iliac and circumflex iliac nodes, in addition to the inferior epigastric and sacral nodes. Lymph from the lower limbs passes through the pelvic lymph nodes via the iliac groups.

The lateral aortic group drains into the two lumbar lymph trunks, one on each side, which terminate in the confluence of lymph trunks. A few vessels may pass to the pre-aortic and retro-aortic nodes and others cross the midline to flow into the contralateral nodes, forming a loose plexus.

or be duplicated, triplicated or plexiform. When it is wider than the thoracic duct its interior is sometimes irregular and bilocular or trilocular, and may surround intercalated lymph nodes. It is only occasionally a simple, fusiform, saccular dilatation, and the widely used name 'cisterna chyli' best describes these forms.

The abdominal confluence of lymph trunks extends from the beginning of the thoracic duct, vertically downwards for 5–7 cm, and lies anterolateral to the right of the first and second lumbar vertebral bodies and their intervening discs. It lies immediately to the right of the abdominal aorta. Along its length it lies between the territories containing the upper right lateral aortic lymph nodes and right-sided members of the coeliac and superior mesenteric pre-aortic groups, branches from which may drain directly into the various trunks. The upper two right lumbar arteries and the right lumbar azygos vein are between the confluence and the vertebral column. The medial edge of the right crus of the diaphragm lies anterior to the abdominal confluence of lymph trunks. The confluence receives the right and left lumbar and intestinal lymph trunks, although rarely these may drain directly into the thoracic duct.

The lumbar lymph trunks are formed by vessels draining from the lateral aortic nodes. Thus, either directly or after traversing intermediary groups, they carry lymph from: the lower limbs, the full thickness of the pelvic, perineal and infra-umbilical abdominal walls, the deep tissues of most of the supra-umbilical abdominal walls, most of the pelvic viscera, gonads, kidneys and suprarenal glands. The intestinal lymph trunks receive vessels draining from coeliac nodes and, via these nodes, the superior and inferior mesenteric nodes, which are collectively the pre-aortic nodes. Either directly or via intermediary groups, they drain the entire abdominal gastrointestinal tract down to the anus.

The intimate relationship of the cisterna chyli and abdominal lymph trunks to the abdominal aorta may lead to problems after aortic

Retro-aortic group

The retro-aortic group is the smallest of all the para-aortic lymph nodes. They have no particular areas of drainage, although they may receive some lymph directly from the paraspinal posterior abdominal wall. They effectively provide peripheral nodes of the lateral aortic groups and interconnect between surrounding groups.

INNERVATION

The posterior abdominal wall contains the origin of the lumbar plexus and numerous autonomic plexuses and ganglia, which lie close to the abdominal aorta and its branches.

Lumbar ventral rami increase in size from first to last and are joined, near their origins, by grey rami communicantes from the four lumbar sympathetic ganglia. These rami, long and slender, accompany the lumbar arteries round the sides of the vertebral bodies, behind psoas major. Their arrangement is irregular: one ganglion may give rami to two lumbar nerves, one lumbar nerve may receive rami from two ganglia; rami often leave the sympathetic trunk between ganglia. The first and second, and sometimes the third, lumbar ventral rami are each connected with the lumbar sympathetic trunk by a white ramus communicans. The lumbar ventral rami descend laterally into psoas major. The first three and most of the fourth form the lumbar plexus; the smaller moiety of the fourth joins the fifth as a lumbosacral trunk, which joins the sacral plexus. The fourth is often termed the nervus furcalis, being divided between the two plexuses; but the third is occasionally the nervus furcalis; or both third and fourth may be furcal nerves, in which case the plexus is termed prefixed. More frequently, the fifth nerve is furcal, the plexus then being termed postfixed. These variations modify the sacral plexus.

LUMBAR PLEXUS (Fig. 68.16)

The lumbar plexus lies within the substance of the posterior part of psoas major, anterior to the transverse processes of the lumbar vertebrae. It is formed by the first three, and most of the fourth, lumbar ventral rami. The first lumbar ramus receives a branch from the last thoracic ventral ramus. The paravertebral part of psoas major consists of posterior and anterior masses, which arise from different attachments. The lumbar plexus lies between these masses and hence is in 'line' with the intervertebral foramina. Although there may be minor variations, the most common arrangement of the plexus is described here.

The first lumbar ventral ramus, joined by a branch from the twelfth thoracic ventral ramus, bifurcates, and the upper and larger part divides again into the iliohypogastric and ilioinguinal nerves. The smaller lower part unites with a branch from the second lumbar ventral ramus to form the genitofemoral nerve. The remainder of the second, third, and part of the fourth lumbar ventral rami join the plexus and divide into ventral and dorsal branches. Ventral branches of the second to fourth rami join to form the obturator nerve. The main dorsal branches of the second to fourth rami join to form the femoral nerve. Small branches from the dorsal branches of the second and third rami join to form the lateral femoral cutaneous nerve. The accessory obturator nerve, when it exists, arises from the third and fourth ventral branches. The lumbar plexus is supplied by branches from the lumbar vessels which supply psoas major.

The branches of the lumbar plexus are:

Muscular	T12, L1–4
Iliohypogastric	L1
Ilioinguinal	L1
Genitofemoral	L1, L2
Lateral femoral cutaneous	L2, L3
Femoral	L2–4 dorsal divisions
Obturator	L2–4 ventral divisions
Accessory obturator	L2, L3

Division of constituent ventral rami into ventral and dorsal branches is not as clear in the lumbar and lumbosacral plexuses as it is in the brachial plexus. Anatomically, the obturator and tibial nerves (via the sciatic) arise from ventral divisions, and the femoral and peroneal nerves (via the sciatic) from dorsal divisions. Lateral branches of the twelfth thoracic and first lumbar ventral rami are drawn into the gluteal skin,

but otherwise these nerves are typical. The second lumbar ramus is difficult to interpret. It not only contributes substantially to the femoral and obturator nerves, but also has an anterior terminal branch (the genital branch of the genitofemoral) and a lateral cutaneous branch (lateral femoral cutaneous nerve and the femoral branch of the genitofemoral). Anterior terminal branches of the third to fifth lumbar and first sacral rami are suppressed, but the corresponding parts of the second and third sacral rami supply the skin, etc. of the perineum.

Inflammatory processes may occur in the posterior abdominal wall in the tissues anterior to psoas major, such as retrocaecal appendicitis on the right and diverticular abscess on the left. This may cause irritation of one or more of the branches of the lumbar plexus and lead to presenting symptoms of pain or dysaesthesia in the distribution of the affected nerves such as in the thigh, hip or buttock skin.

Muscular branches

Small branches from all five lumbar roots.

Iliohypogastric nerve

Distribution – The iliohypogastric nerve originates from the L1 ventral ramus. It emerges from the upper lateral border of psoas major, crosses obliquely behind the lower renal pole and in front of quadratus lumborum. Above the iliac crest, it enters the posterior part of transversus abdominis. Between transversus abdominis and internal oblique, it divides into lateral and anterior cutaneous branches, and also supplies both muscles. The lateral cutaneous branch runs through internal and external oblique above the iliac crest, a little behind the iliac branch of the twelfth thoracic nerve, and is distributed to the posterolateral gluteal skin. The anterior cutaneous branch runs between and supplies internal oblique and transversus abdominis. It runs through internal oblique c.2 cm medial to the anterior superior iliac spine, and through the external oblique aponeurosis c.3 cm above the superficial inguinal ring, and is then distributed to the suprapubic skin. The iliohypogastric nerve connects with the subcostal and ilioinguinal nerves (**Fig. 67.3**). It is occasionally injured during an oblique surgical approach to the appendix. However, because the suprapubic skin is innervated from several sources, there is rarely any detectable sensory loss. Division of the iliohypogastric nerve above the anterior superior iliac spine may weaken the posterior wall of the inguinal canal and predispose to direct formation of a direct hernia.

Motor – The iliohypogastric nerve supplies a small motor contribution to transversus abdominis and internal oblique, including the conjoint tendon.

Sensory – The iliohypogastric nerve supplies sensory fibres to transversus abdominis, internal oblique and external oblique, and innervates the posterolateral gluteal and suprapubic skin.

Ilioinguinal nerve

Distribution – The ilioinguinal nerve originates from the L1 ventral ramus. It is smaller than the iliohypogastric nerve and arises with it from the first lumbar ventral ramus, to emerge from the lateral border of psoas major, with or just inferior to the iliohypogastric nerve. It passes obliquely across quadratus lumborum and the upper part of iliacus and enters transversus abdominis near the anterior end of the iliac crest. It sometimes connects with the iliohypogastric nerve at this point. It pierces internal oblique and supplies it and then traverses the inguinal canal below the spermatic cord. It emerges with the cord from the superficial inguinal ring to supply the proximal medial skin of the thigh and the skin over the root of the penis and upper part of the scrotum in males, or the skin covering the mons pubis and the adjoining labium majus in females. The ilioinguinal and iliohypogastric nerves are reciprocal in size. The ilioinguinal is occasionally very small and ends by joining the iliohypogastric, a branch of which then takes its place. Occasionally, the ilioinguinal nerve is completely absent when the iliohypogastric nerve supplies its territory. The nerve may be injured during inguinal surgery, particularly for hernia, which produces paraesthesia over the skin of the genitalia. Entrapment of the nerve during surgery may cause troublesome recurrent pain in this distribution.

Motor – The ilioinguinal nerve supplies motor nerves to transversus abdominis and internal oblique.

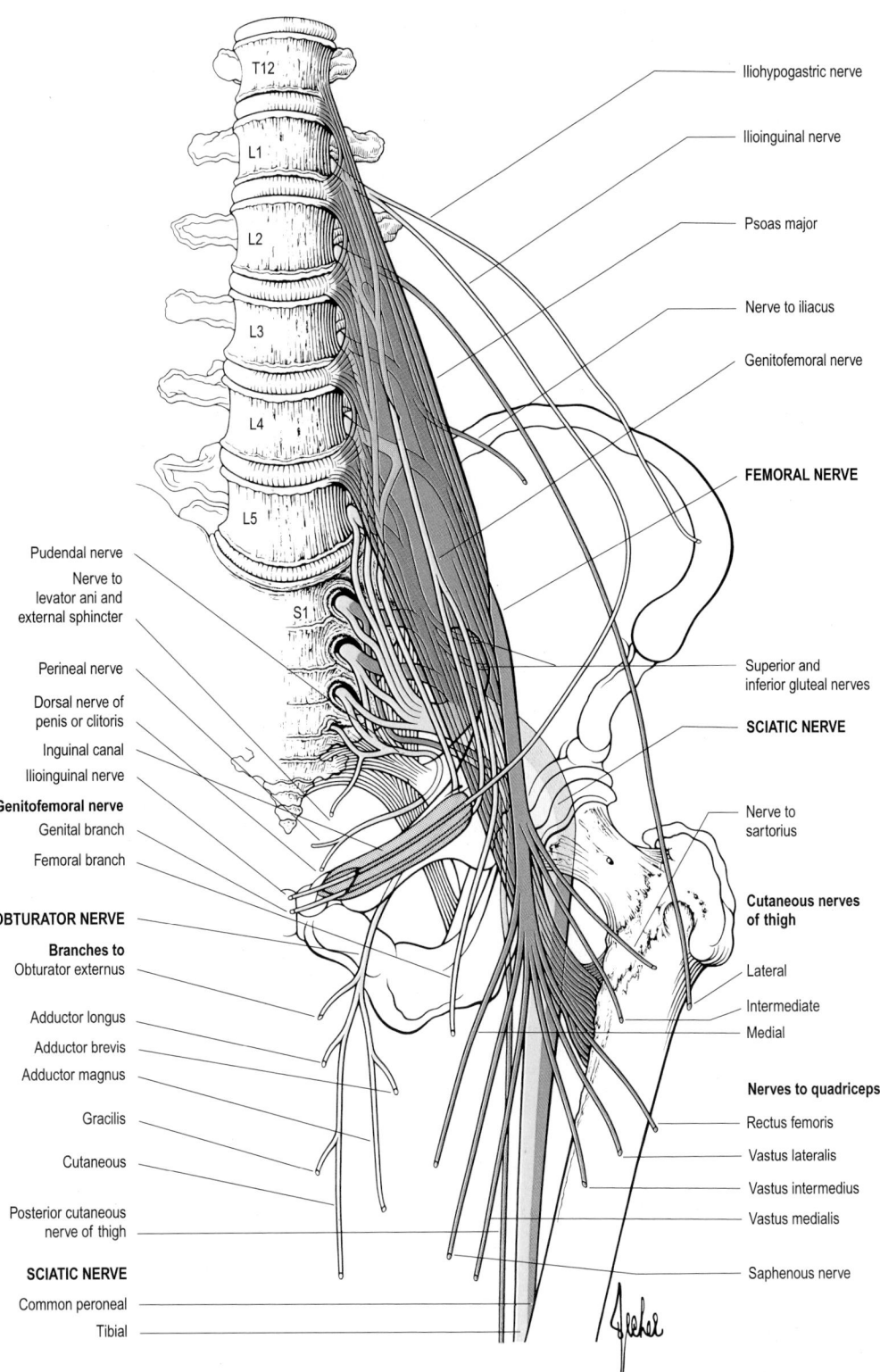

Fig. 68.16 The lumbar plexus, its branches and the muscles which they supply. The ventral branches of the ventral rami are coloured yellow and the dorsal branches orange.

Sensory – The ilioinguinal nerve supplies sensory fibres to transversus abdominis and internal oblique. It innervates the medial skin of the thigh and the skin over the root of the penis and upper part of the scrotum in males or the skin covering the mons pubis and the adjoining labium majus in females.

Genitofemoral nerve

Distribution – The genitofemoral nerve originates from the L1 and L2 ventral rami. It is formed within the substance of psoas major and

descends obliquely forwards through the muscle to emerge on its abdominal surface near the medial border, opposite the third or fourth lumbar vertebra. It descends beneath the peritoneum on psoas major, crosses obliquely behind the ureter and divides above the inguinal ligament into genital and femoral branches. It often divides close to its origin; its branches then emerge separately from psoas major. The genital branch crosses the lower part of the external iliac artery, enters the inguinal canal by the deep ring and supplies cremaster and the skin of the scrotum in males. In females, it accompanies the round ligament and ends in the skin of the mons pubis and labium majus. The femoral branch descends lateral to the external iliac artery, and sends a few fila-ments round it. It then crosses the deep circumflex iliac artery, passes behind the inguinal ligament and enters the femoral sheath lateral to the femoral artery. It pierces the anterior layer of the femoral sheath and fascia lata and supplies the skin anterior to the upper part of the femoral triangle. It connects with the femoral intermediate cutaneous nerve and supplies the femoral artery. The genital branch may be injured during inguinal surgery, in the same way as the ilioinguinal nerve.

Motor – The genitofemoral nerve innervates cremaster via the genital branch.

Cutaneous – The genitofemoral nerve innervates the skin of the scrotum in males or mons pubis and labium majus in females via the genital branch, and the anteromedial skin of the thigh via the femoral branch.

Femoral nerve
The femoral nerve (p. 1455) descends through psoas major and emerges low on its lateral border. It passes between psoas major and iliacus deep to the iliac fascia and runs posterior to the inguinal ligament into the thigh. It gives off branches, which supply iliacus and pectineus and sensory fibres to the femoral artery. Posterior to the inguinal ligament, it lies lateral to the femoral artery and is separated from it by a part of psoas major.

Lateral femoral cutaneous nerve of the thigh
The lateral femoral cutaneous nerve of the thigh (p. 1454) emerges from the lateral border of psoas major and crosses iliacus obliquely towards the anterior superior iliac spine. It supplies sensory fibres to the parietal peritoneum in the iliac fossa. The right nerve passes postero-lateral to the caecum, separated from it by the iliac fascia and peritoneum. The left nerve passes behind the lower part of the descending colon. Both pass behind or through the inguinal ligament c.1 cm medial to the anterior superior iliac spine and anterior to, or through, sartorius into the thigh.

Obturator nerve
The obturator nerve (p. 1455) descends within the substance of psoas major to emerge from its medial border at the level of the pelvic brim. It passes posterior to the common iliac vessels and lateral to the internal iliac vessels. It then descends on the lateral wall of the pelvis attached to the fascia over obturator internus. Here it lies anterosuperior to the obturator vessels before running into the obturator foramen to enter the thigh. It gives no branches in the abdomen or pelvis.

Accessory obturator nerve
When present, the accessory obturator nerve (p. 1456) emerges from the medial border of psoas major and runs along this border over the posterior surface of the superior pubic ramus posterior to pectineus. It gives off branches here to supply pectineus and the hip joint, and it may join with the main obturator nerve.

LUMBOSACRAL PLEXUS
The lumbosacral plexus (p. 1456) provides the nerve supply to the pelvis and lower limb, in addition to part of the autonomic supply to the pelvic viscera. It gives origin to the sciatic, inferior gluteal, superior gluteal and pudendal nerves (p. 1364), in addition to the nerves to quadratus femoris, obturator internus and the posterior cutaneous nerve of the thigh.

LUMBAR SYMPATHETIC SYSTEM
The lumbar part of each sympathetic trunk usually contains four interconnected ganglia. It runs in the extraperitoneal connective tissue anterior to the vertebral column and along the medial margin of psoas major. Superiorly, it is continuous with the thoracic trunk posterior to the medial arcuate ligament. Inferiorly, it passes posterior to the common iliac artery and is continuous with the pelvic sympathetic trunk. On the right side, it lies posterior to inferior vena cava, and on the left it is posterior to the lateral aortic lymph nodes. It is anterior to most of the lumbar vessels, but may pass behind some lumbar veins.

The first, second and sometimes third lumbar ventral spinal rami send white rami communicantes to the corresponding ganglia. Grey rami communicantes pass from all four lumbar ganglia to the lumbar spinal nerves. They are long, and accompany the lumbar arteries round the sides of the vertebral bodies, medial to the fibrous arches to which psoas major is attached. Four lumbar splanchnic nerves pass from the ganglia to join the coeliac, inferior mesenteric (or occasionally abdominal aortic) and superior hypogastric plexuses. The first lumbar splanchnic nerve, from the first ganglion, gives branches to the coeliac, renal and inferior mesenteric plexuses. The second nerve joins the inferior part of the intermesenteric or inferior mesenteric plexus. The third nerve arises from the third or fourth ganglion and passes anterior to the common iliac vessels to join the superior hypogastric plexus. The fourth lumbar splanchnic nerve from the lowest ganglion passes above the common iliac vessels to join the lower part of the superior hypo-gastric plexus, or the inferior hypogastric 'nerve'.

Vascular branches from all lumbar ganglia join the abdominal aortic plexus. Fibres of the lower lumbar splanchnic nerves pass to the common iliac arteries and form a plexus, which continues along the internal and external iliac arteries as far as the proximal part of the femoral artery. Many postganglionic fibres travel in the muscular, cutaneous and saphenous branches of the femoral nerve, supplying vasoconstrictor nerves to the femoral artery and its branches in the thigh. Other post-ganglionic fibres travel via the obturator nerve to the obturator artery. Considerable uncertainty persists regarding the exact path of the sym-pathetic nerve supply to the lower limb (Pick 1970).

Segmental sympathetic supply to abdominal viscera
For information on the plexuses, please see the appropriate chapters: coeliac plexus, superior mesenteric plexus, abdominal aortic plexus (intermesenteric plexus), inferior mesenteric plexus, superior hypo-gastric plexus, inferior hypogastric plexuses.

LUMBAR PARASYMPATHETIC SYSTEM
The parasympathetic supply to the abdominal viscera is provided by the vagus nerve to the coeliac and superior mesenteric plexuses, and from the pelvic splanchnic nerves to the inferior mesenteric, superior hypogastric and inferior hypogastric plexuses.

PARA-AORTIC BODIES
The para-aortic bodies are condensations of chromaffin tissue that are found in close relation to the aortic autonomic plexuses and lumbar sympathetic chains. They are largest in the fetus, become relatively smaller in childhood and have largely disappeared by adulthood. They are most commonly found as a pair of bodies lying anterolateral to the aorta in the region of the intermesenteric, inferior mesenteric and superior hypogastric plexuses. They may lie as high as the coeliac plexus, as low as the inferior hypogastric plexus in the pelvis, or may be closely applied to the sympathetic ganglia of the lumbar chain. Scattered cells that persist into adulthood may, rarely, be the sites of development of tumours of the chromaffin tissue (phaeochromo-cytoma), although these are much more commonly found arising from the cells of the suprarenal medulla. The wide variation in site of persistent para-aortic body tissue accounts for the range of locations of such tumours.

REFERENCES
Burkhill GJC, Healy JC 2000 Anatomy of the retroperitoneum. Imaging 12: 10–20.
Newman DL, Gosling RG, Bowden R 1971 Changes in aortic distensibility and area ratio with the development of atherosclerosis. Atherosclerosis 14: 231–40.
Pick J 1970 The Autonomic Nervous System. Philadelphia: Lippincott.

Shah PM, Scarton HA, Tsapogas MJ 1978 Geometric anatomy of the aorto–common iliac bifurcation. J Anat 126: 451–8.
Both this and the Newman reference describe the anatomical factors that may affect the development of aortoiliac atherosclerosis.

Peritoneum and peritoneal cavity

Chapter

69

PERITONEUM AND PERITONEAL REFLECTIONS

STRUCTURE OF THE PERITONEUM

The peritoneum is the largest serous membrane in the body, and its arrangements are often complex. In males it forms a closed sac, but in females it is open at the lateral ends of the uterine tubes.

It consists of a single layer of flat mesothelial cells lying on a layer of loose connective tissue. The mesothelium usually forms a continuous surface, but in some areas may be fenestrated. Neighbouring cells are joined by junctional complexes, but probably permit the passage of macrophages. The submesothelial connective tissue may also contain macrophages, lymphocytes and adipocytes (in some regions). Mesothelial cells may transform into fibroblasts, which may play an important role in the formation of peritoneal adhesions after surgery or inflammation of the peritoneum.

The peritoneal cavity is a potential space between the parietal peritoneum, which lines the abdominal wall, and infoldings of visceral peritoneum, which suspend the abdominal viscera within the cavity. It contains a small amount of serous fluid, but is otherwise empty. The fluid lubricates the visceral peritoneum and allows the mobile viscera to glide freely on the abdominal wall and each other within the limits dictated by their attachments. It contains water, proteins, electrolytes and solutes derived from interstitial fluid in the adjacent tissues and from the plasma in the local blood vessels. It normally contains a few cells, including desquamated mesothelium, nomadic peritoneal macrophages, mast cells, fibroblasts, lymphocytes and other leukocytes. Some cells, particularly macrophages, migrate freely between the peritoneal cavity and the surrounding connective tissue. Lymphocytes provide both cellular and humoral immunological defence mechanisms within the peritoneal cavity. The intraperitoneal fluid is directed by gravity to dependent sites within the peritoneal cavity, and also flows in a cephalad direction as a consequence of the negative upper intra-abdominal pressures which are generated by respiration.

The peritoneal cavity never contains gas in normal circumstances, although the amount of fluid may be increased in inflammatory conditions of the viscera. In females blood or fluid may occasionally escape from the uterine tubes into the pelvic peritoneal cavity during menstruation.

Extraperitoneal connective tissue separates the parietal peritoneum from the muscular layers of the abdominal walls. The parietal peritoneum covering the anterior abdominal wall and pelvic walls is generally attached only loosely by this tissue, an arrangement which allows for considerable alteration in the size of the bladder and rectum. The extraperitoneal tissue on the inferior surface of the diaphragm and behind the linea alba is denser and more firmly adherent. The extraperitoneal tissue frequently contains large amounts of fat over the posterior abdominal wall, especially in obese males. The visceral peritoneum is firmly adherent to the underlying tissues and cannot be easily detached. Its connective tissue layer is often continuous with the fibrous matrix of the wall of the underlying viscera and rarely contains much loose connective or adipose tissue. The visceral peritoneum is often considered as part of the underlying viscus for clinical and pathological purposes such as the staging of carcinoma.

GENERAL ARRANGEMENT OF THE PERITONEUM (Fig. 69.1)

In utero, the alimentary tract develops as a single tube suspended in the coelomic cavity by ventral and dorsal mesenteries (p. 1254). Ultimately, the ventral mesentery is largely resorbed, although some parts persist in the upper abdomen and form structures such as the falciform ligament. The mesenteries of the intestines in the adult are the remnants of the dorsal mesentery. The migration and subsequent fixation of parts of the gastrointestinal tract produce the so-called 'retroperitoneal' segments of bowel (duodenum, ascending colon, descending colon, and rectum), and four separate intraperitoneal bowel loops suspended by mesenteries of variable lengths. These are all covered by visceral peritoneum which is continuous with the parietal peritoneum covering the posterior abdominal wall. The first intraperitoneal loop is formed by the intraperitoneal oesophagus, the stomach and first part of the duodenum. The second loop is made up of the duodenojejunal junction, jejunum, ileum and occasionally the caecum and proximal ascending colon. The third loop contains the transverse colon and the final loop contains the sigmoid colon and occasionally the distal descending colon.

Where the visceral peritoneum encloses or suspends organs within the peritoneal cavity, the peritoneum and related connective tissues are known as the peritoneal ligaments, omenta or mesenteries. All but the greater omentum are composed of two layers of visceral peritoneum separated by variable amounts of connective tissue. The greater omentum is folded back on itself and is therefore made up of four layers of closely applied visceral peritoneum, which are separated by variable amounts of adipose tissue. The mesenteries attach their respective viscera to the posterior abdominal wall: the attachment is referred to as the mesenteric root, and the peritoneum of the mesentery is continuous with that of the posterior abdominal wall in this area.

Although they are described as intraperitoneal, strictly speaking the suspended organs do not lie within the peritoneal cavity, because they are covered by visceral peritoneum. They are continuous with the extraperitoneal tissues, including the retroperitoneum, via subperitoneal tissue lying between the folds of visceral peritoneum. The loose areolar connective tissues of the extraperitoneal and subperitoneal tissues are sometimes conceptualized as 'spaces' because fluid or blood collects relatively easily within them. The subperitoneal tissues contain the neurovascular bundles and lymphatic channels which supply the suspended organs. In obese individuals, extensive adipose tissue within the mesenteries and omenta may obscure the neurovascular bundles. In contrast, in the very young, the elderly or the malnourished, the mesentery may contain very little adipose tissue and the neurovascular bundles are usually obvious.

Peritoneum of the upper abdomen (Figs 69.2, 69.3, 69.4)

The abdominal oesophagus, stomach, liver and spleen all lie within a double fold of visceral peritoneum which runs from the posterior to the anterior abdominal wall. This fold has no recognized name, but has been referred to as the mesogastrium by Coakley and Hricak 1999 because it is derived from the fetal mesogastrium (p. 1254). It has a complex attachment to the wall of the abdominal cavity and gives rise to the falciform ligament, coronary ligaments, lesser omentum (gastrohepatic and hepatoduodenal ligaments), greater omentum (including gastrocolic ligament), gastrosplenic ligament, splenorenal ligament, and phrenicocolic ligament.

The falciform ligament

The falciform ligament is a thin anteroposterior peritoneal fold which connects the liver to the posterior aspect of the anterior abdominal wall just to the right of the midline. It extends inferiorly to the level of the umbilicus, and is widest between the liver and umbilicus. The ligament narrows superiorly as the distance between the liver and anterior abdominal wall reduces and narrows to just a centimetre or so in height over the superior surface of the liver. Its two peritoneal layers divide to

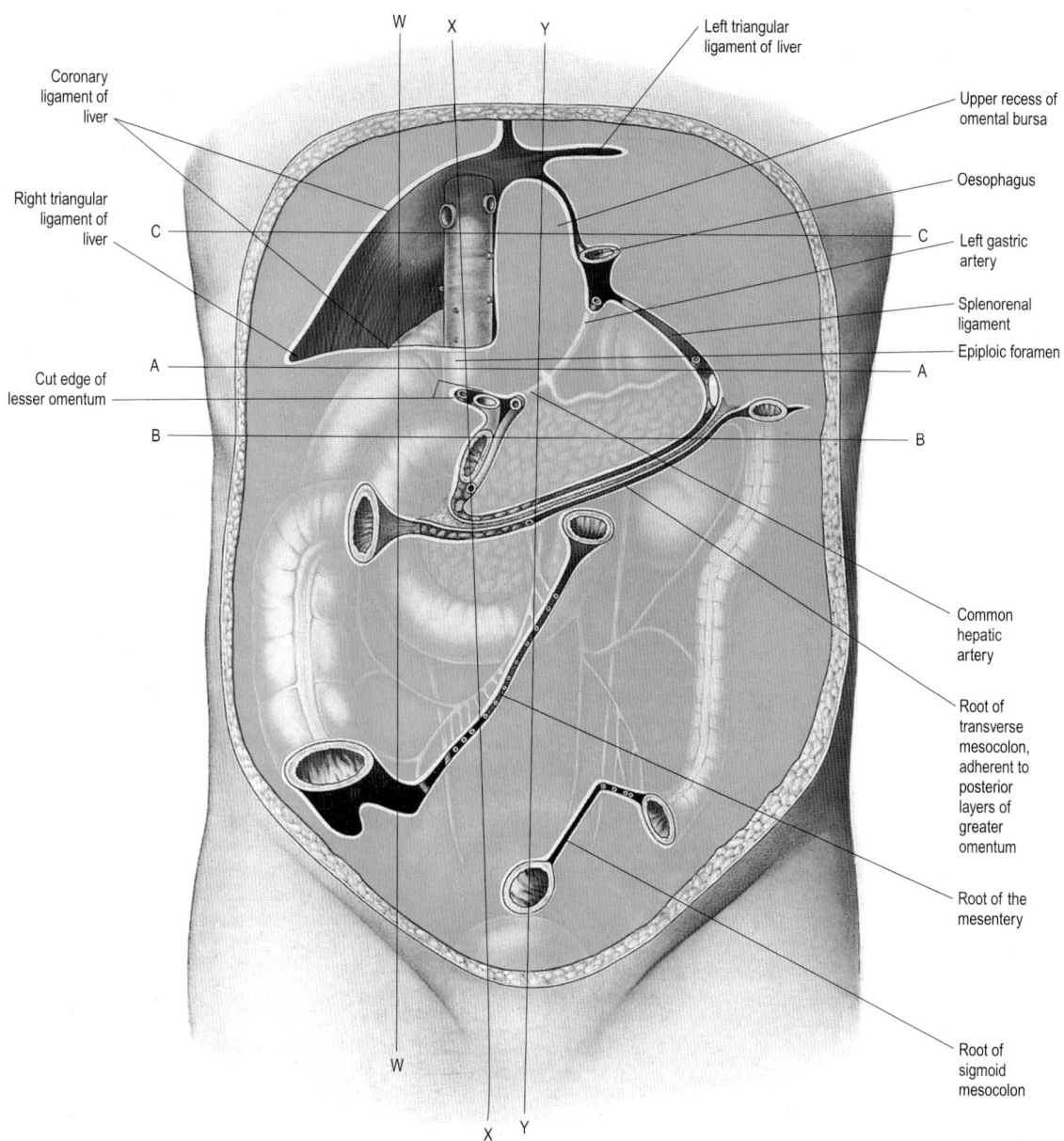

Fig. 69.1 The posterior abdominal wall, showing the lines of peritoneal reflexion, after removal of the liver, spleen, stomach, jejunum, ileum, caecum, transverse colon and sigmoid colon. The various sessile (retroperitoneal) organs are seen shining through the posterior parietal peritoneum. Note: the ascending and descending colon, duodenum, kidneys, suprarenals, pancreas and inferior vena cava. Line WW represents the plane of **Fig. 69.2**. Line YY represents the plane of **Fig. 69.4**. Line XX represents the plane of **Fig. 69.3**. Line AA represents the plane of **Fig. 69.5**. Line BB represents the plane of **Fig. 69.6**. Line CC represents the plane of **Fig. 69.7**.

enclose the liver and are continuous with the visceral peritoneum adherent to the surface of the liver. Superiorly, they are reflected onto the inferior surface of the diaphragm and are continuous with the parietal peritoneum over the right dome. At the posterior limit, or apex, of the falciform ligament, the two layers are also reflected vertically left and right, and are continuous with the anterior layers of the left triangular ligament and the superior layer of the coronary ligament of the liver. The inferior aspect of the falciform ligament forms a free border where the two peritoneal layers become continuous with each other as they fold over to enclose the ligamentum teres (p. 1213). Because the peritoneum of the falciform ligament is continuous with that covering the posterior abdominal wall and the periumbilical anterior abdominal wall, blood arising from retroperitoneal haemorrhage (commonly acute haemorrhagic pancreatitis) may track between the folds of peritoneum and appear as haemorrhagic discolouration around the umbilicus (Cullen's sign). Spread of inflammatory change from the pancreas runs through the gastrohepatic ligament (lesser omentum) and then via the falciform ligament to the umbilicus.

The peritoneal connections of the liver (Figs 69.5, 69.6, 69.7)

The liver is almost completely covered in visceral peritoneum, only the 'bare area' is in direct contact with the right dome of the diaphragm. Peritoneal folds, the ligaments of the liver, run from the liver to the surrounding viscera and to the abdominal wall and diaphragm. They are described in detail in Chapter 85 (p. 1213).

The coronary ligament is formed by the reflection of the peritoneum from the diaphragm onto the posterior surfaces of the right lobe of the liver. Between the two layers of this ligament, a large area of liver, the bare area, is devoid of peritoneal covering. At this point the liver is attached to the diaphragm by areolar tissue and is in continuity inferiorly with the uppermost part of the anterior pararenal space. The layers of the coronary ligament are continuous on the right with the right triangular ligament.

The upper layer of the coronary ligament is continuous superiorly with the peritoneum over the inferior surface of the diaphragm and inferiorly with the peritoneum over the right and superior surfaces of the liver. At the lower margin of the bare area, the lower layer of the

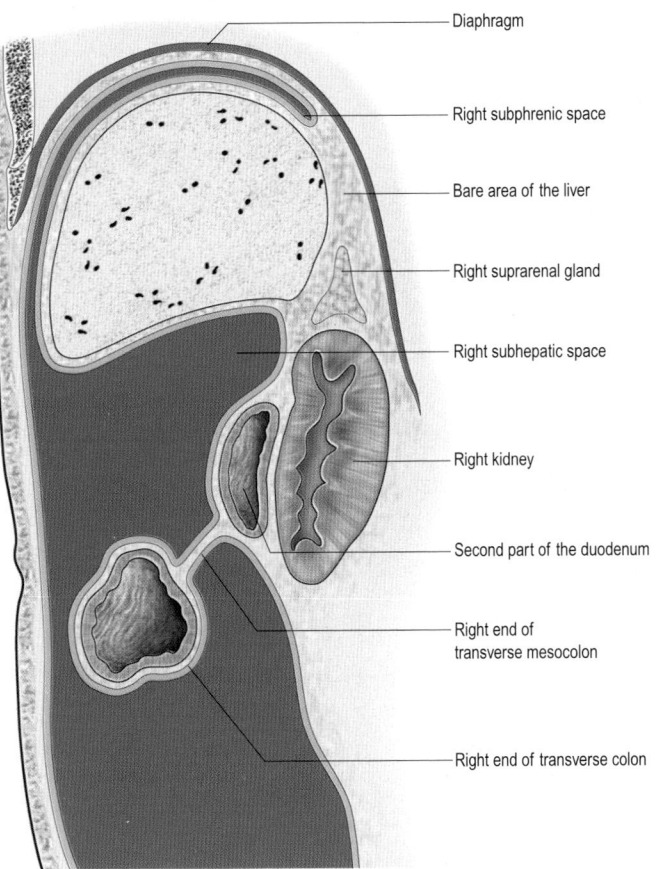

Fig. 69.2 Sagittal section through the abdomen to the right of the epiploic foramen along one line of WW in **Fig. 69.1**.

coronary ligament is continuous inferiorly with the peritoneum of the posterior abdominal wall over the right suprarenal gland and upper pole of the right kidney, and superiorly with the peritoneum over the inferior surface of the liver.

The left triangular ligament is a double layer of peritoneum which extends over the superior border of the left lobe of the liver to a variable length. Medially, its anterior leaf is continuous with the left layer of the falciform ligament. The posterior layer is continuous with the left layer of the lesser omentum. The left triangular ligament lies in front of the abdominal part of the oesophagus, the upper end of the lesser omentum and part of the fundus of the stomach. Intraoperative division of the left triangular ligament permits mobilization of the left lobe of the liver in order to expose the abdominal oesophagus and crura of the diaphragm.

The right triangular ligament is a short V-shaped fold formed by the approximation of the two layers of the coronary ligament at its right lateral end, and is continuous with the peritoneum of the right postero-lateral abdominal wall. The coronary ligament is reflected inferiorly and is directly continuous with the peritoneum over the upper pole of the right kidney. This fold is sometimes referred to as the hepatorenal ligament. The recess formed between the peritoneum of the inferior surface of the liver, the hepatorenal ligament and the peritoneum over the right kidney is known as the hepatorenal pouch (of Morison). In the supine position this is the most dependent part of the peritoneal cavity in the upper abdomen, and is a common site of pathological fluid accumulation.

The peritoneum is reflected inferolaterally from the posterior layer of the left triangular ligament onto the posterior abdominal wall above the oesophageal opening of the diaphragm. It lines the inferior surface of the left dome of the diaphragm and continues backwards onto the posterior abdominal wall. Inferiorly, it is reflected behind the spleen onto the most lateral part of the mesentery of the transverse colon and the splenic flexure. It continues down lateral to the descending colon into the pelvis, and forms the left paracolic 'gutter' (p. 1136). Medially, the peritoneum covering the left upper posterior abdominal wall is reflected anteriorly to form the left layer of the upper end of the lesser omentum, the peritoneum over the left aspect of the abdominal oesophagus and the left layer of the splenorenal ligament.

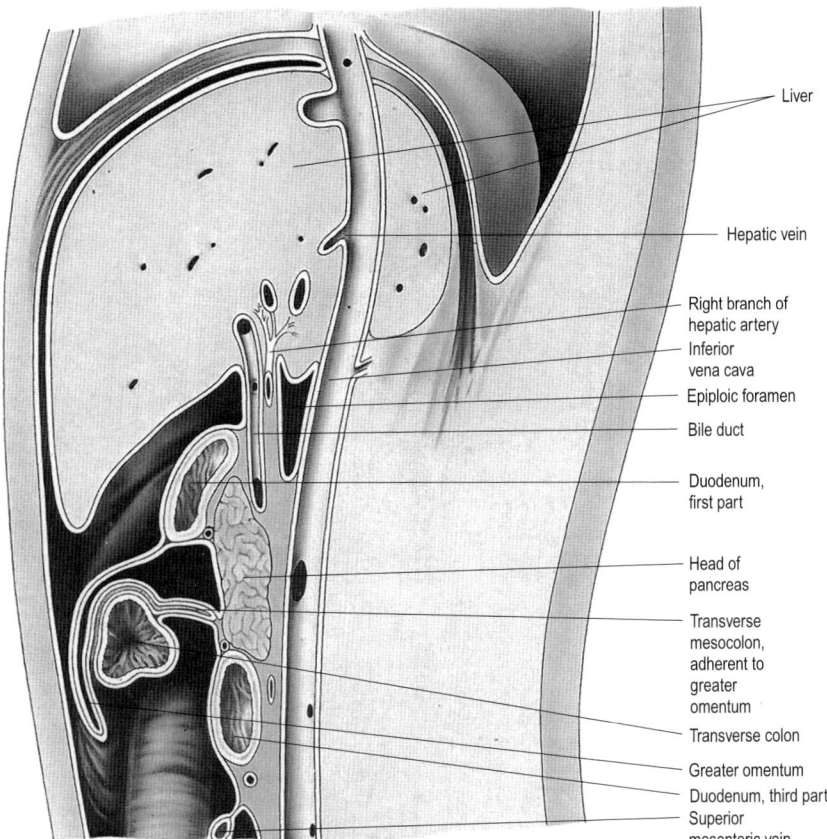

Fig. 69.3 Section through the upper part of the abdominal cavity, along the line XX in **Fig. 69.1**. The boundaries of the epiploic foramen are shown and a small recess of the lesser sac is displayed in front of the head of the pancreas. Note that the transverse colon and its mesocolon are adherent to the posterior two layers of the greater omentum.

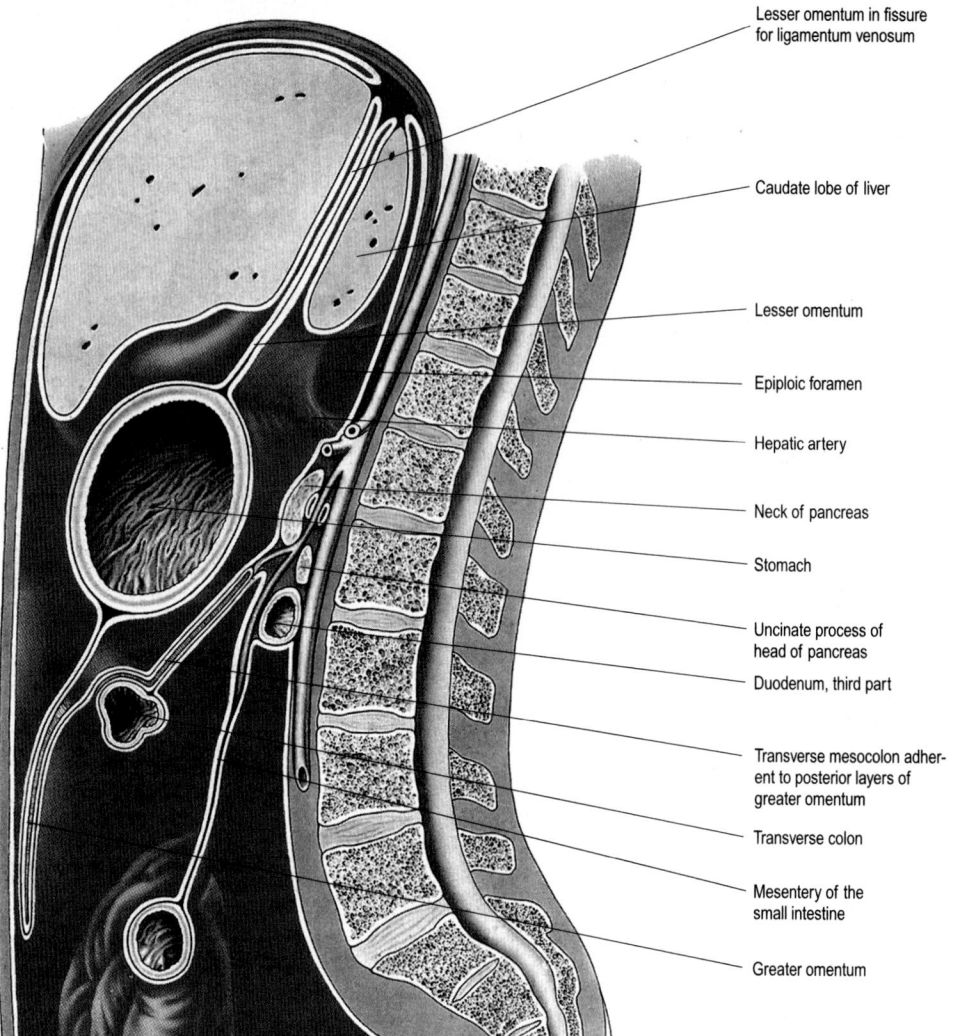

Lesser omentum in fissure for ligamentum venosum

Caudate lobe of liver

Lesser omentum

Epiploic foramen

Hepatic artery

Neck of pancreas

Stomach

Uncinate process of head of pancreas

Duodenum, third part

Transverse mesocolon adherent to posterior layers of greater omentum

Transverse colon

Mesentery of the small intestine

Greater omentum

Fig. 69.4 Sagittal section through the abdomen, approximately in the median plane. Compare with **Fig. 69.1**. The section cuts the posterior abdominal wall along the line YY in **Fig. 69.1**. The peritoneum is shown in blue except along its cut edges, which are left white.

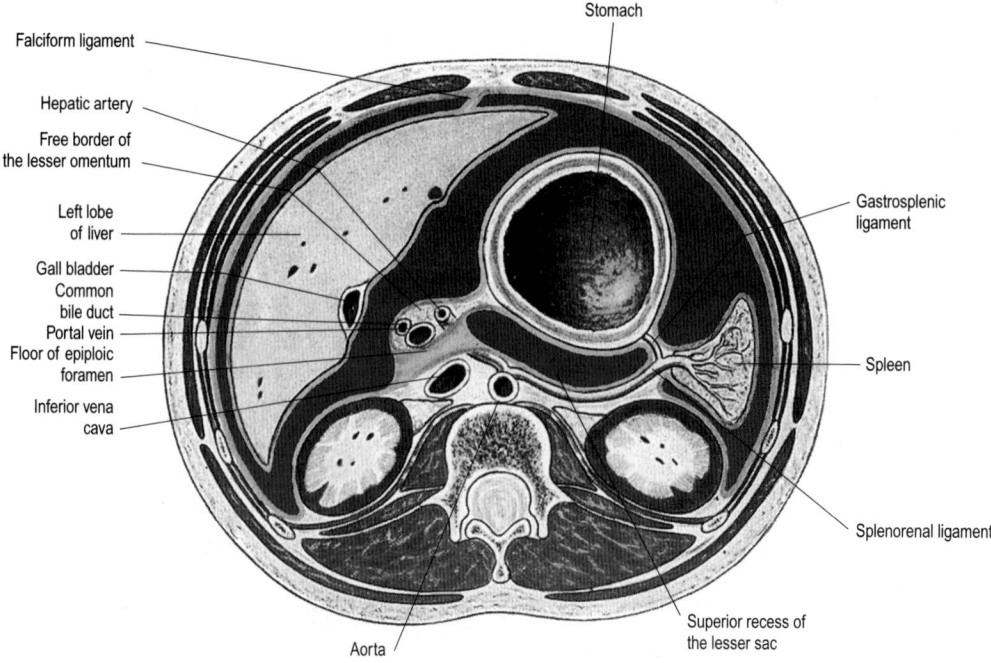

Stomach

Falciform ligament

Hepatic artery

Free border of the lesser omentum

Left lobe of liver

Gall bladder

Common bile duct

Portal vein

Floor of epiploic foramen

Inferior vena cava

Gastrosplenic ligament

Spleen

Splenorenal ligament

Superior recess of the lesser sac

Aorta

Fig. 69.5 Transverse section through the abdomen, at the level of line AA in **Fig. 69.1**, viewed from above. The peritoneal cavity is shown in dark blue; the peritoneum and its cut edges in lighter blue.

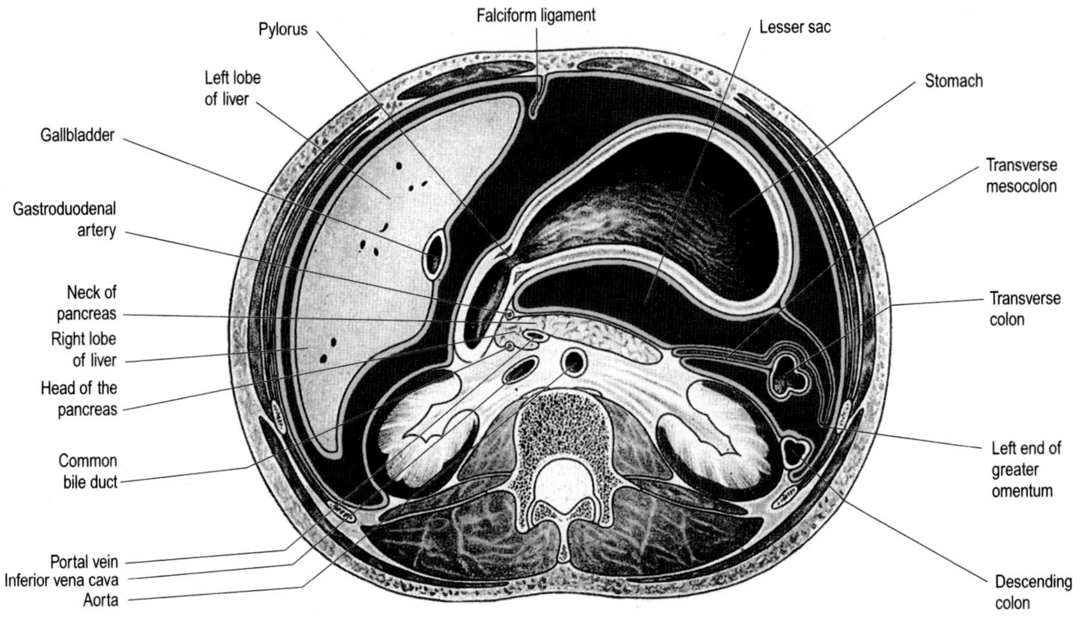

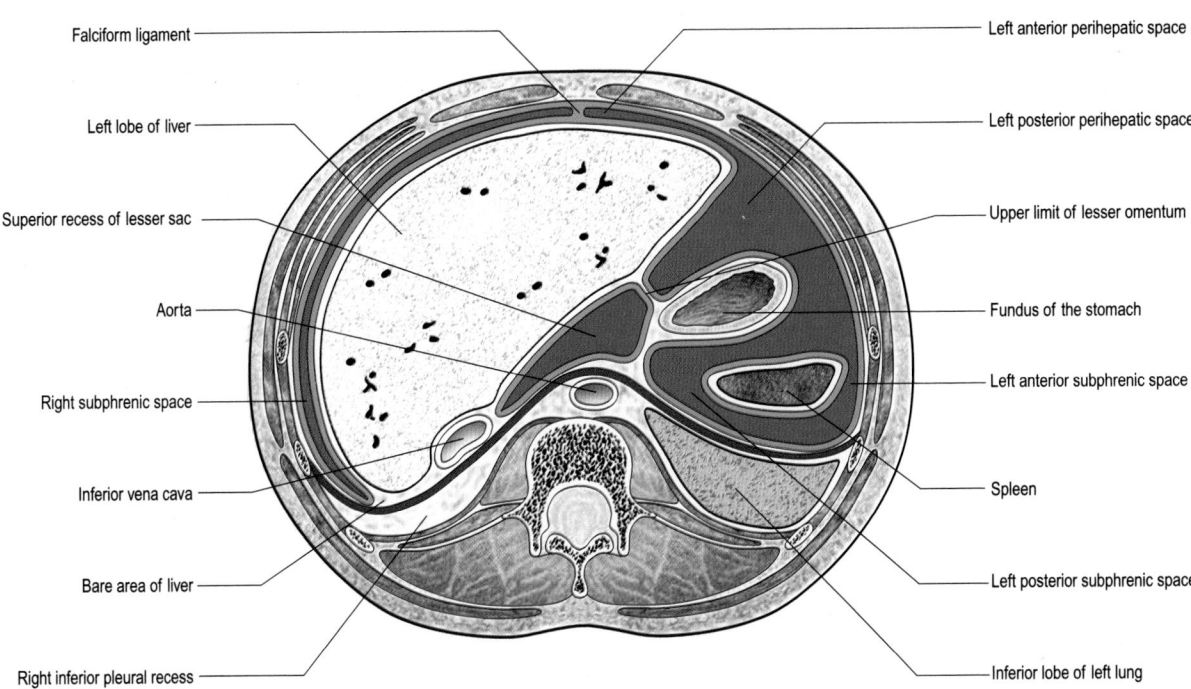

Fig. 69.6 Transverse section through the abdomen at the level of the line BB in **Fig. 69.1**, viewed from above. Colours as in **Fig. 69.5**.

Labels (Fig. 69.6): Pylorus · Falciform ligament · Lesser sac · Left lobe of liver · Stomach · Gallbladder · Transverse mesocolon · Gastroduodenal artery · Transverse colon · Neck of pancreas · Right lobe of liver · Head of the pancreas · Left end of greater omentum · Common bile duct · Portal vein · Inferior vena cava · Aorta · Descending colon

Fig. 69.7 Transverse section through the abdomen at the level of the line CC in **Fig. 69.1**. The line passes through the bare area of the liver at the superior end of the lesser omentum. The parts of the left subphrenic space are clearly seen although they are continuous with each other.

Labels (Fig. 69.7): Falciform ligament · Left anterior perihepatic space · Left lobe of liver · Left posterior perihepatic space · Superior recess of lesser sac · Upper limit of lesser omentum · Aorta · Fundus of the stomach · Right subphrenic space · Left anterior subphrenic space · Inferior vena cava · Spleen · Bare area of liver · Left posterior subphrenic space · Right inferior pleural recess · Inferior lobe of left lung

From the inferior layer of the coronary ligament the peritoneum descends over the anterior surface of the right kidney to the front of the first part of the duodenum and hepatic flexure of the colon. Medially it passes in front of a short segment of the inferior vena cava between the duodenum and liver. At this point the peritoneum forms the posterior wall of the epiploic foramen. It forms a narrow strip, which broadens out as it continues across the midline onto the posterior wall of the lesser sac. It lines the posterior abdominal wall over the diaphragmatic crura, the upper abdominal aorta, the coeliac axis, nodes and plexus and the upper border of the pancreas. Inferiorly, below the liver, the peritoneum continues down on the posterior abdominal wall to the right of the ascending colon, forming the right paracolic 'gutter' between the anterolateral abdominal wall and colon.

The lesser omentum

The lesser omentum is formed of two layers of peritoneum separated by a variable amount of connective tissue and is derived from the ventral mesogastrium. It runs from the inferior visceral surface of the liver to the abdominal oesophagus, stomach, pylorus and first part of the duodenum. Superiorly, its attachment to the inferior surface of the liver forms an L-shape. The vertical component of the L is formed by the fissure for the ligamentum venosum. Inferiorly, the attachment turns and runs horizontally to complete the L in the portal fissure. The vertical and horizontal components of the lesser omentum run between the liver and the stomach and duodenum and are known as the gastrohepatic and hepatoduodenal ligaments, respectively. At the lesser curvature of the stomach, the layers of the lesser omentum split to enclose

1131

the stomach and are continuous with the visceral peritoneum covering the anterior and posterior surfaces of the stomach. The anterior layer of the lesser omentum descends from the fissure for the ligamentum venosum onto the anterior surface of the abdominal oesophagus, stomach and duodenum. The posterior layer descends from the posterior part of the fissure for the ligamentum venosum and runs onto the posterior surface of the stomach and pylorus. The lesser omentum forms the anterior surface of the lesser sac. The gastrohepatic ligament contains the right and left gastric vessels, branches of the vagus nerves, and gastrohepatic lymph nodes between its two layers near their attachment to the stomach. The right lateral border of the lesser omentum is thickened and extends from the junction between the first and second parts of the duodenum to the porta hepatis. This border is free and forms the anterior wall of the epiploic foramen. It contains the portal vein, common bile duct, hepatic artery, portocaval lymph nodes and lymphatics and the hepatic plexus of nerves ensheathed in a perivascular fibrous capsule. Occasionally the free margin extends to the right of the epiploic foramen, runs to the gallbladder and is referred to as the cystoduodenal ligament.

The left border of the lesser omentum is short and runs over the inferior surface of the diaphragm between the liver and medial aspect of the abdominal oesophagus. The lesser omentum is thinner on the left and may be fenestrated or incomplete. The variations in thickness are dependent upon the amount of connective tissue, especially fat.

The greater omentum

The greater omentum is the largest peritoneal fold and hangs inferiorly from the greater curvature of the stomach. It is a double sheet: each sheet consists of two layers of peritoneum separated by a scant amount of connective tissue. The two sheets are folded back on themselves and are firmly adherent to each other. The anterior sheet descends from the greater curvature of the stomach and first part of the duodenum. The most anterior layer is continuous with the visceral peritoneum over the anterior surface of the stomach and duodenum and the posterior layer is continuous with the peritoneum over the posterior wall of the stomach and pylorus. The anterior sheet descends a variable distance into the peritoneal cavity and then turns sharply on itself to ascend as the posterior sheet. The posterior sheet passes anterior to the transverse colon and transverse mesocolon. It is attached to the posterior abdominal wall above the origin of the small intestinal mesentery and anterior to the head and body of the pancreas. The anterior layer of the posterior sheet is continuous with the peritoneum of the posterior wall of the lesser sac. The posterior layer is reflected sharply inferiorly and is continuous with the anterior layer of the transverse mesocolon. The posterior sheet is adherent to the transverse mesocolon at its root and is often known as the gastrocolic ligament, which is the supracolic part of the greater omentum. In early foetal life the greater omentum and transverse mesocolon are separate structures, and this arrangement sometimes persists. During surgical mobilization of the transverse colon, the plane between the transverse mesocolon and greater omentum can be entered opposite the taenia omentalis, and the greater omentum can be separated entirely from the transverse colon and mesocolon if required. Access into the lesser sac can be obtained via this approach if the upper part of the posterior sheet of the greater omentum is then divided. This gives a relatively bloodless plane of entry for surgical access to the posterior wall of the stomach and to the anterior surface of the pancreas. The greater omentum is continuous with the gastrosplenic ligament on the left, and on the right it extends to the start of the duodenum. A fold of peritoneum, the hepatocolic ligament, may run from either the inferior surface of the right lobe of the liver or the first part of the duodenum to the right side of the greater omentum or hepatic flexure of the colon.

The right border of the greater omentum is occasionally adherent to the anterior surface of the ascending colon down as far as the caecum: its peritoneal layers are not continuous with the peritoneum over this part of the colon. A thin sheet of peritoneum referred to as Jackson's membrane may run from the front of the ascending colon and caecum to the posterolateral abdominal wall and may merge with the greater omentum. It often contains several small blood vessels. Occasionally, a band passes from the right side of the ascending colon to the lateral abdominal wall near the level of the iliac crest. It has been called the 'sustentaculum hepatis' but plays no role in the support of the liver. Other folds between the ascending colon and posterolateral abdominal wall may divide the right lateral paracolic gutter into several small recesses. Less commonly the greater omentum is adherent to the anterior

surface of the left colon; very occasionally it extends to the level of the sigmoid colon.

When the undisturbed abdomen is opened, the greater omentum is frequently wrapped around the upper abdominal organs. Only rarely is it evenly dependent anterior to the coils of the small intestine, although this is the disposition which is frequently illustrated. It is usually thin and cribriform, but it always contains some adipose tissue and is a common site for storage of fat in obese individuals, particularly males.

Between the two layers of the anterior fold of the greater omentum, close to the greater curvature of the stomach, the right and left gastroepiploic vessels form a wide anastomotic arc. Numerous vessels are given off from the arc and extend the full length of the omentum. This supply appears to exceed the metabolic requirements of the omentum, and perhaps reflect the role the greater omentum may play in peritoneal disease processes. The greater omentum is highly mobile and frequently becomes adherent to inflamed viscera within the abdominal cavity. This action may help to limit the spread of infection and the omentum may provide a source of well-vascularized tissue to take part in the early reparative process. It contains numerous fixed macrophages, which are easily mobilized. These may accumulate into dense, oval or round visible 'milky-spots'.

The peritoneal connections of the spleen

The peritoneal connections of the spleen include the gastrosplenic, splenorenal and phrenicocolic ligaments, which suspend the spleen in the left upper quadrant of the abdomen. The gastrosplenic ligament runs between the greater curvature of the stomach and the hilum of the spleen and is in continuity with the left side of the greater omentum. The layers of the gastrosplenic ligament separate to enclose the spleen and then rejoin to form the splenorenal ligament and phrenicocolic ligaments. The splenorenal ligament extends from the spleen to the posterior abdominal wall and the phrenicocolic ligament extends to the anterolateral abdominal wall.

The splenorenal ligament is formed from two layers of peritoneum. The anterior layer is continuous medially with the peritoneum of the posterior wall of the lesser sac over the left kidney and runs up to the splenic hilum where it is continuous with the posterior layer of the gastrosplenic ligament. The posterior layer of the splenorenal ligament is continuous laterally with the peritoneum over the inferior surface of the diaphragm and runs onto the splenic surface over the renal impression. The splenic vessels lie between the layers of the splenorenal ligament: the tail of the pancreas is usually present in its lower portion. The gastrosplenic ligament also has two layers. The posterior layer is continuous with the peritoneum of the splenic hilum and the peritoneum over the posterior surface of the stomach. The anterior layer is formed from the peritoneum reflected off the gastric impression of the spleen and is continuous with the peritoneum over the anterior surface of the stomach. The short gastric and left gastroepiploic branches of the splenic artery pass between the layers of the gastrosplenic ligament. The phrenicocolic ligament extends from the splenic flexure of the colon to the diaphragm at the level of the eleventh rib. It extends inferiorly and laterally and is continuous with the peritoneum of the lateral end of the transverse mesocolon at the lateral margin of the pancreatic tail, and the splenorenal ligament at the hilum of the spleen.

A fan-shaped presplenic fold frequently extends from the anterior aspect of the gastrosplenic ligament near the greater curvature of the stomach below the inferolateral pole of the spleen. It blends with the phrenicocolic ligament.

If the peritoneal attachments of the spleen are not recognized during surgery, the splenic capsule is at risk of injury and there may be subsequent serious bleeding. Downward traction on the phrenicocolic ligament during handling of the descending colon, especially during mobilization of the splenic flexure, may cause rupture of the splenic capsule. This is less likely if traction on the phrenicocolic ligament is made laterally or medially. The superior border and anterior diaphragmatic surface of the splenic capsule are often adherent to the peritoneum of the greater omentum. Medial traction on the omentum during surgery may cause splenic capsular injury: such injury is less likely, if any limited traction required is applied inferiorly.

Peritoneum of the lower abdomen

The posterior surface of the lower anterior abdominal wall is lined by parietal peritoneum which extends from the linea alba centrally to the lateral border of quadratus lumborum. Here it is continuous with the peritoneum of the lateral paracolic gutter and is reflected over the sides and front of the ascending colon on the right and the descending colon on the left. Occasionally the ascending and descending colon are suspended by a short mesentery from the posterior abdominal wall. Between the ascending and descending colon, the peritoneum lines the posterior abdominal wall other than the oblique area, where it is reflected anteriorly to form the right and left layers of the small intestinal mesentery. Over the posterior abdominal wall it covers the left and right psoas major, inferior vena cava, duodenum, vertebral column and right and left ureters. At the upper extent of the posterior abdominal wall the peritoneum is reflected anteriorly and is continuous with the peritoneum of the posterior layer of the transverse mesocolon.

Transverse mesocolon

The mesentery of the transverse colon is a broad fold of visceral peritoneum reflected anteriorly from the posterior abdominal wall and suspends the transverse colon in the peritoneal cavity. The root of the transverse mesocolon lies along an oblique line passing from the anterior aspect of the second part of the duodenum, over the head and neck of the pancreas, above the duodenojejunal junction and over the upper pole of the left kidney to the splenic flexure. It varies considerably in length but is shortest at either end. It contains the middle colic vessels and their branches together with branches of the superior mesenteric plexus, lymphatics and regional lymph nodes. Its two layers pass to the posterior surface of the transverse colon where they separate to cover the colon. The upper layer of peritoneum is reflected from the posterior abdominal wall immediately anteriorly and inferiorly and becomes continuous with the posterior layer of the greater omentum to which it is adherent. The lower layer of peritoneum of the transverse mesocolon is continuous with the peritoneum of the posterior abdominal wall. Lateral extensions of the transverse mesocolon produce two shelf-like folds on the right and left sides of the abdominal cavity. On the right the duodenocolic ligament extends from the transverse mesocolon at the hepatic flexure to the second part of the duodenum. On the left the phrenicocolic ligament extends from the transverse mesocolon at the splenic flexure to the diaphragm at the level of the eleventh rib. Near the uncinate process of the pancreas, the root of the transverse mesocolon is closely related to the upper limit of the root of the small intestinal mesentery.

Mesentery of the small intestine

The mesentery of the small intestine is arranged as a complex fan formed from two layers of peritoneum (anterosuperior and posteroinferior) separated by connective tissue and vessels. The root of the mesentery lies along a line running diagonally from the duodenojejunal flexure on the left side of the second lumbar vertebral body to the right sacroiliac joint. The root crosses over the third part of the duodenum, aorta, inferior vena cava, right ureter and right psoas major. The length of the root of the mesentery is c.15 cm long in adults while the mesentery along its intestinal attachment is the same length as the small intestine (c.5 m), and consequently the mesentery is usually thrown into multiple folds along its intestinal border. The average depth of the mesentery from the root to the intestinal border is c.20 cm, but this varies along the length of the small intestine: it is shortest at the jejunum and terminal ileum and longest in the region of the mid ileum. Its two peritoneal layers contain the jejunum, ileum, jejunal and ileal branches of the superior mesenteric vessels, branches of the superior mesenteric plexus, lacteals and regional lymph nodes. Because of the length and mobility of the mesentery, identification of the proximal and distal ends of a loop of small intestine may be difficult through small surgical incisions. Tracing the continuity of the right peritoneal layer of the mesentery onto the posterior abdominal wall above the root towards the ascending colon, and the continuity of the left layer towards the descending and sigmoid colon, may be useful in helping to orientate an individual loop of ileum. The mesentery of the small intestine is sometimes joined to the transverse mesocolon at the duodenojejunal junction by a peritoneal band. Occasionally the fourth part of the duodenum possesses a very short mesentery which is continuous with the upper end of the root of the small bowel mesentery. Pronounced bands of peritoneum may extend to the posterior abdominal wall at the terminal ileum. The root of the mesentery of the small intestine is continuous with the peritoneum surrounding the appendix and caecum in the right iliac fossa.

Mesoappendix

The mesentery of the appendix is a triangular fold of peritoneum around the vermiform appendix. It is attached to the posterior surface of the lower end of the mesentery of the small intestine close to the ileocaecal junction. It usually reaches the tip of the appendix but sometimes fails to reach the distal third, in which case a vestigial low peritoneal ridge containing fat is present over the distal third. It encloses the blood vessels, nerves and lymph vessels of the vermiform appendix, and usually contains a lymph node.

Sigmoid mesocolon

The sigmoid mesocolon shows individual variation in length and depth. The root of the sigmoid colon forms a shallow inverted V with an apex near the division of the left common iliac artery but may vary from a very short straight line at the pelvic brim to a long curved attachment. The upper, left end of the attachment runs medially over the left psoas major. The lower, right end passes into the pelvis towards the midline at the level of the third sacral vertebra. The root extends for a variable distance over the brim of the pelvis and the lower posterior abdominal wall. The anteromedial peritoneal layer of the mesentery of the sigmoid colon is continuous with the peritoneum of the lower left posterior abdominal wall and its posterolateral layer is continuous with the peritoneum of the pelvis and lateral abdominal wall. The proximal and distal ends of the sigmoid colon are occasionally joined together by a fibrous band which is usually associated with a narrow based sigmoid mesentery and may predispose the sigmoid colon to volvulus. Pronounced bands of peritoneum may also be found running from the proximal sigmoid colon to the posterior abdominal wall. The sigmoid and superior rectal vessels run between its layers and the left ureter descends into the pelvis behind its apex.

Peritoneum of the lower anterior abdominal wall (Fig. 69.8)

The peritoneum of the lower anterior abdominal wall is raised into five ridges which diverge as they descend from the umbilicus. These are the median and right and left lateral and medial umbilical folds. The median umbilical fold extends from the umbilicus to the apex of the bladder and contains the urachus or its remnant (p. 1259). The obliterated umbilical artery lies under the medial umbilical fold which ascends from the pelvis to the umbilicus. The supravesical fossa lies between the medial and median umbilical folds on either side of the midline. The lateral umbilical fold covers the inferior epigastric artery below its entry into the rectus sheath, and is separated from the medial umbilical fold by the medial inguinal fossa. The lateral inguinal fossa lies lateral to the lateral umbilical fold, and covers the deep inguinal ring. The femoral fossa lies inferomedial to the lateral inguinal fossa, from which it is separated by the medial end of the inguinal ligament. It overlies the femoral ring (Chapter 67).

Peritoneum of the pelvis

The parietal peritoneum of the posterior surface of the anterior abdominal wall and that lining the posterior abdominal wall continue into the pelvis as the pelvic peritoneum. The pelvic peritoneum then follows the surfaces of the true pelvic viscera and pelvic side walls although there are important differences between the sexes.

Peritoneum of the male pelvis (Fig. 69.9)

In males, the peritoneum of the left lower abdominal wall is reflected from the junction of the sigmoid colon and anterolateral surface of the rectum to line the brim and upper inner surface of the true pelvis. The peritoneum passes down into the true pelvis, lying over the anterior surface of the rectum, which then becomes an extraperitoneal organ. Laterally, the peritoneum is reflected to the pelvic side walls to form the right and left pararectal fossae: these vary in size according to the degree of distension of the rectum. The peritoneum is reflected anteriorly from the anterior surface of the rectum over the upper poles of the seminal vesicles and onto the posterior surface of the bladder, producing the rectovesical pouch. Anteriorly the rectovesical pouch is limited laterally by peritoneal folds, the sacrogenital folds, which extend from the sides of the bladder posteriorly to the anterior aspect of the sacrum. The peritoneum covers the superior surface of the bladder, and forms a paravesical fossa on each side limited laterally by a ridge of peritoneum which contains the ductus deferens. The size of the paravesical fossae depends on the volume of urine in the bladder. When the bladder is empty, a variable transverse vesical fold divides each fossa into two. The

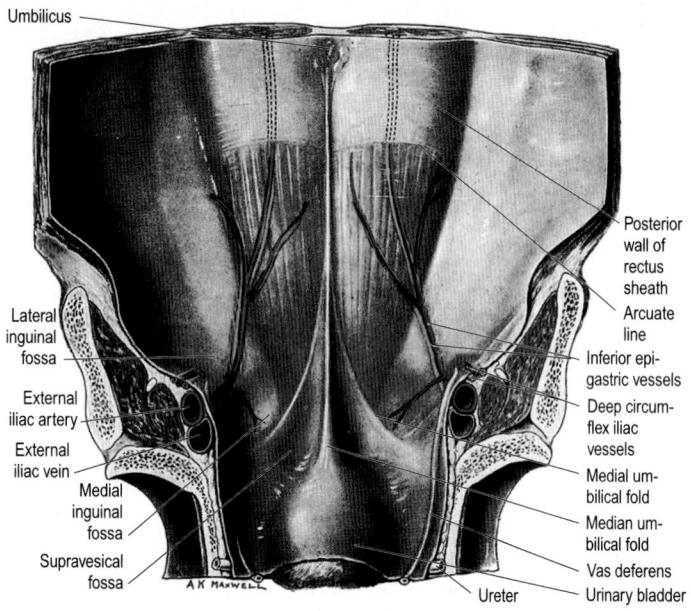

Umbilicus

Lateral
inguinal
fossa

External
iliac artery

External
iliac vein

Medial
inguinal
fossa

Supravesical
fossa

A.K. MAXWELL

Posterior
wall of
rectus
sheath

Arcuate
line

Inferior epi-
gastric vessels

Deep circum-
flex iliac
vessels

Medial umbi-
lical fold

Median um-
bilical fold

Vas deferens

Urinary bladder

Ureter

Fig. 69.8 The infra-umbilical part of the anterior abdominal wall of a male subject: posterior surface, with the peritoneum in situ. Note the pelvic bones flanking the wide greater pelvis (middle) and narrower lesser pelvis (below) containing the bladder.

posterior surface of the lower anterior abdominal wall to the umbilicus (p. 1132). When the bladder distends, the peritoneum is lifted from the lower anterior abdominal wall so that part of the anterior surface of the bladder is in direct contact with the posterior surface of the lower median area of the anterior abdominal wall. This relationship means that a well-distended bladder can be entered by direct puncture through the lower anterior abdominal wall without entering the peritoneal cavity (suprapubic puncture).

Peritoneum of the female pelvis

In females the peritoneum covers the upper rectum as it does in the male, but it descends further over the anterior surface of the rectum. The lateral limit of the pararectal and paravesical fossae is the peritoneum covering the round ligament of the uterus (p. 1133). The rectovesical pouch is occupied by the uterus and vagina. The peritoneum from the rectum is thus reflected anteriorly onto the posterior surface of the posterior fornix of the vagina and the uterus producing the recto-uterine pouch (of Douglas). The peritoneum covers the fundus of the uterus to its anterior (vesical) surface as far as the junction of the body and cervix, from which it is reflected forwards to the upper surface of the bladder, forming a shallow vesico-uterine pouch. Peritoneum is reflected from the bladder to the posterior surface of the anterior abdominal wall as it is in males. Marginal recto-uterine folds correspond to the sacrogenital folds in males and pass back to the sacrum from the sides of the cervix, lateral to the rectum. Peritoneum is reflected from the anterior and posterior uterine surfaces to the lateral pelvic walls as the broad ligament of the uterus. This consists of anteroinferior and posterosuperior layers which are continuous at the upper border of the ligament (p. 1332). The broad ligament extends from the sides of the uterus to the lateral pelvic walls, and contains the uterine tubes in its free superior margins and the ovaries attached to its posterior layer. Below, it is continuous with the lateral pelvic parietal peritoneum. Between the ridges formed by the obliterated umbilical arteries and the ureter, the peritoneum forms a shallow depression on the lateral pelvic wall, the ovarian fossa, which lies behind the lateral attachment of the broad ligament. The ovary usually rests in the fossa in nulliparous females.

anterior ends of the sacrogenital folds may sometimes be joined by a ridge separating a middle fossa from the main rectovesical pouch. Between the paravesical and pararectal fossae the ureters and internal iliac vessels may cause slight elevations in the peritoneum. From the apex of the bladder the peritoneum extends superiorly along the

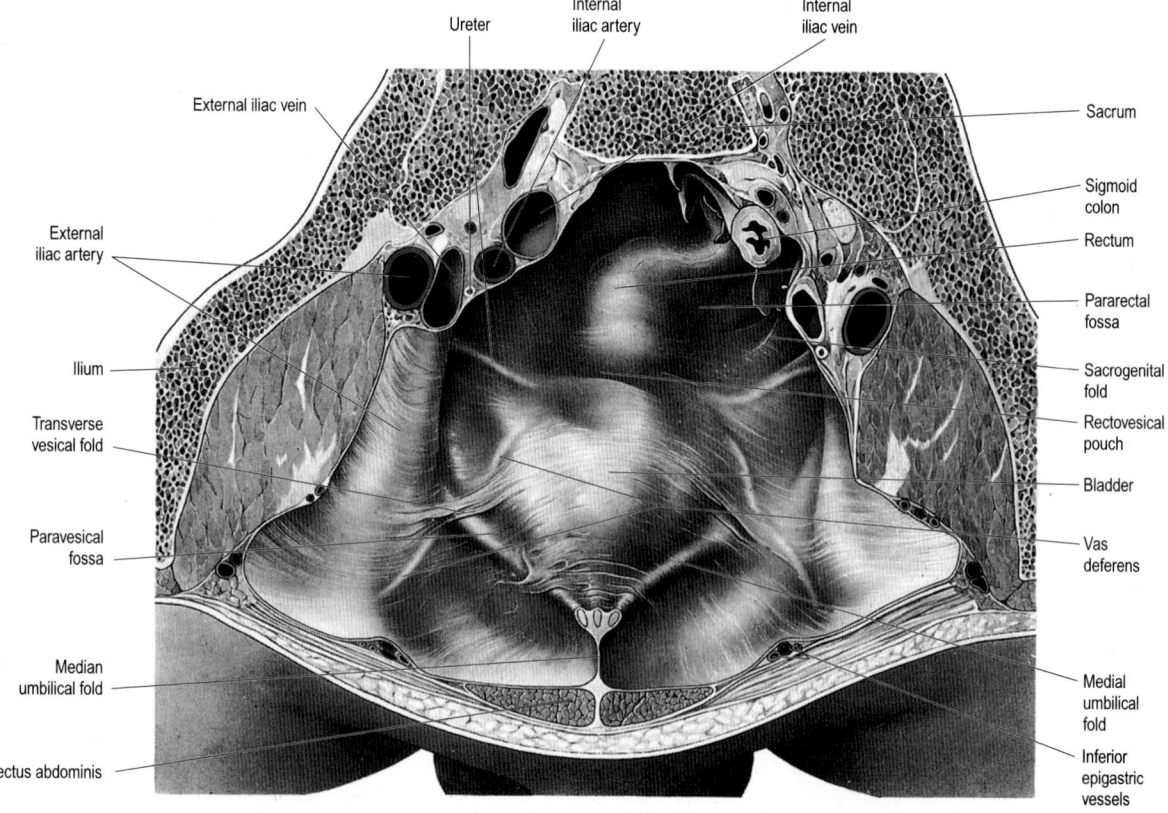

Ureter

Internal
iliac artery

Internal
iliac vein

External iliac vein

External
iliac artery

Ilium

Transverse
vesical fold

Paravesical
fossa

Median
umbilical fold

Rectus abdominis

Sacrum

Sigmoid
colon

Rectum

Pararectal
fossa

Sacrogenital
fold

Rectovesical
pouch

Bladder

Vas
deferens

Medial
umbilical
fold

Inferior
epigastric
vessels

Fig. 69.9 The peritoneum of the male pelvis: anterosuperior view. The median umbilical fold contains both the unpaired median and the paired medial umbilical ligaments in the plane of section in this subject.

PERITONEAL CAVITY

GENERAL ARRANGEMENT OF THE PERITONEAL CAVITY

The peritoneal cavity is a single continuous space between the parietal peritoneum lining the abdominal wall and the visceral peritoneum enveloping the abdominal organs. It consists of a main region, termed the greater sac, which is equivalent to the main abdominal cavity surrounding the majority of the abdominal and pelvic viscera. The lesser sac, or omental bursa, is a small diverticulum lined with peritoneum, which is situated behind the stomach and lesser omentum and in front of the pancreas and retroperitoneum (p. 1135). These two areas communicate via the epiploic foramen.

For clinical purposes the peritoneal cavity can be divided into several spaces because pathological processes are often contained within these spaces and their anatomy may influence diagnosis and treatment. It is useful to divide the peritoneal cavity into two main compartments, supramesocolic and inframesocolic, which are partially separated by the transverse colon and its mesentery (the latter connects the transverse colon to the posterior abdominal wall). The pelvic peritoneal spaces are described above (p. 1133).

Supramesocolic compartment

The supramesocolic space lies above the transverse mesocolon between the diaphragm and the transverse colon. It can be arbitrarily divided into right and left supramesocolic spaces. These regions can be further subdivided into a number of subspaces, which are normally in communication, but are frequently subdivided by inflammatory adhesions in disease. The right supramesocolic space can be divided into three subspaces; the right subphrenic space, the right subhepatic space, and the lesser sac. The left supramesocolic space can be divided into two subspaces; the left subphrenic space and the left perihepatic space.

Right subphrenic space

The right subphrenic space lies between the diaphragm and the anterior, superior and right lateral surfaces of the right lobe of the liver. It is bounded on the left side by the falciform ligament and behind by the upper layer of the coronary ligament. It is a relatively common site for collections of fluid after right sided abdominal inflammation.

Right subhepatic space (hepatorenal recess)

The right subhepatic space lies between the right lobe of the liver and the right kidney. It is bounded superiorly by the inferior layer of the coronary ligament, laterally by the right lateral abdominal wall, posteriorly by the anterior surface of the upper pole of the right kidney and medially by the second part of the duodenum, hepatic flexure, transverse mesocolon and part of the head of the pancreas. In the supine position the posterior right subhepatic space is more dependent than the right paracolic gutter: postoperative infected fluid collections are common in this location.

Lesser sac (omental bursa)

The lesser sac is a cavity lined with peritoneum and connected to the larger general peritoneal cavity (greater sac) by the epiploic foramen. It is considered part of the right supramesocolic space because embryologically the liver grows into the right peritoneal space and stretches the dorsal mesentery to form the lesser sac behind the stomach. The sac varies in size according to the size of the viscera making up its walls. It has posterior and anterior walls as well as superior, inferior, right and left borders.

The anterior wall is made up of the posterior peritoneal layer of the lesser omentum, the peritoneum over the posterior wall of the stomach and first part of the duodenum, and the uppermost part of the anterior layer of the greater omentum. At its right border, the anterior wall is mostly formed by the lesser omentum but moving towards the left, the lesser omentum becomes progressively shorter and more of the anterior wall is formed by the posterior aspect of the stomach and greater omentum.

The posterior wall is formed mainly by the peritoneum covering the posterior abdominal wall in this area. In the lower part, the posterior wall is made up of the anterior layer of the posterior sheet of the greater omentum as it lies on the transverse mesocolon. The posterior wall covers, from below upwards, a small part of the head and the whole neck and body of the pancreas, the medial part of the anterior aspect of the left kidney, most of the left suprarenal (adrenal) gland, the commencement of the abdominal aorta and coeliac artery and part of the diaphragm. The inferior phrenic, splenic, left gastric and hepatic arteries lie partly behind the bursa. Many of these structures form the 'bed' of the stomach and are separated from it only by the linings of the lesser sac.

The superior border of the lesser sac is narrow and lies between the right side of the oesophagus and the upper end of the fissure for the ligamentum venosum. Here peritoneum of the posterior wall of the lesser sac is reflected anteriorly from the diaphragm to join the posterior layer of the lesser omentum.

The inferior border of the lesser sac runs along the line of the fusion of the layers of the greater omentum. This runs from the gastrosplenic ligament to the peritoneal fold behind the first part of the duodenum. In cases where the layers are not completely adherent to each other, the lesser sac may extend as far as the bottom of the two sheets of the greater omentum. In adults, even in these circumstances of separation of the layers, the lowest extent of the inferior border is rarely below the level of the transverse colon.

The right border of the lesser sac is formed by the reflection of the peritoneum from the pancreatic neck and head onto the inferior aspect of the first part of the duodenum. The line of this reflection ascends to the left, along the medial side of the gastroduodenal artery. Near the upper duodenal margin the right border joins the floor of the epiploic foramen round the hepatic artery proper. The epiploic foramen thus forms a break in the right border. Above the epiploic foramen the right border is formed by the reflection of peritoneum from the diaphragm to the right margin of the caudate lobe of the liver and along the left side of the inferior vena cava, enclosing the hepatic recess.

The left border of the lesser sac runs from the left end of the root of the transverse mesocolon and is mostly formed by the inner layer of peritoneum of the splenorenal and gastrosplenic ligaments. The part of the lesser sac lying between the splenorenal and gastrosplenic ligaments is referred to as the splenic recess. Above the level of the spleen, the two ligaments are merged as the short gastrophrenic ligament, which passes forwards from the diaphragm to the posterior aspect of the fundus of the stomach and forms part of the upper left border of the lesser sac. The two layers of the gastrophrenic ligament diverge near the abdominal oesophagus, leaving part of the posterior gastric surface devoid of peritoneum. The left gastric artery runs forwards here into the lesser omentum.

The lesser sac is narrowed by two crescentic peritoneal folds produced by the hepatic and left gastric arteries. The left gastropancreatic fold overlies the left gastric artery as it runs from the posterior abdominal wall to the lesser curvature of the stomach. The right gastropancreatic fold overlies the hepatic artery as it runs from the posterior abdominal wall to the lesser omentum. The folds vary in size. When prominent, they divide the lesser sac into a smaller superior and a larger inferior recess. The superior recess lies posterior to the lesser omentum and liver, and encloses the caudate lobe of the liver, which is covered by peritoneum on both its anterior and posterior surfaces. It extends superiorly into the fissure for the ligamentum venosum and lies adjacent to the right crus of the diaphragm posteriorly. The inferior recess of the lesser sac lies between the stomach and pancreas and is contained in the double sheet of the greater omentum.

Epiploic foramen (of Winslow) – The epiploic foramen (foramen of Winslow, aditus to the lesser sac), is a short, vertical slit, c.3 cm height in adults, in the upper part of the right border of the lesser sac. It leads into the greater sac. The hepatoduodenal ligament, which is formed by the thickened right edge of the lesser omentum extending from the flexure between the first and second parts of the duodenum, forms the anterior margin of the foramen. The anterior border contains the common bile duct (on the right), portal vein (posteriorly) and hepatic artery (on the left) between its two layers. Superiorly the peritoneum of the posterior layer of the hepatoduodenal ligament runs over the caudate lobe of the liver which forms the roof of the epiploic foramen. This layer of peritoneum is then reflected onto the inferior vena cava which forms the posterior margin of the epiploic foramen. At the upper border of the first part of the duodenum the peritoneum runs forwards from the inferior vena cava, above the head of the pancreas, and is continuous with the posterior layer of the lesser omentum, forming the floor of the epiploic foramen. A narrow passage, the vestibule of the lesser sac, may be found to the left of the foramen between the caudate process and the first part of the duodenum. To the right, the rim of the foramen is continuous with the peritoneum of the greater sac. The roof is continuous with the peritoneum on the inferior surface of the right hepatic lobe. The anterior and posterior walls of the foramen are normally apposed.

Left subphrenic space

The left subphrenic space lies between the diaphragm, the anterior and superior surfaces of the left lobe of the liver, the anterosuperior surface of the stomach and the diaphragmatic surface of the spleen. It is bounded to the right by the falciform ligament and behind by the anterior layer of the left triangular ligament. It is much enlarged in the absence of the spleen and is a common site for fluid collection particularly after splenectomy. The left subphrenic space is substantially larger than the right and is sometimes described as being divided into anterior and posterior parts, although no obvious demarcation exists in the absence of disease. The left posterior subphrenic space is small and lies between the fundus of the stomach and the diaphragm above the origin of the splenorenal ligament. The left anterior subphrenic space is large and lies between the superior and anterolateral surfaces of the spleen and the left dome of the diaphragm. Inferiorly and medially, this space is bounded by the splenorenal, gastrosplenic, and phrenicocolic ligaments which produces a partial barrier to the left paracolic gutter. This may explain why left subphrenic collections are less frequent than right subphrenic collections following lower abdominal and pelvic surgery, but the left subphrenic space is the commonest site of fluid collection after upper abdominal, particularly splenic, surgery.

Left perihepatic space

The left perihepatic space is sometimes subdivided into anterior and posterior spaces. The posterior perihepatic space is also known as the left subhepatic space or gastrohepatic recess. The left anterior perihepatic space lies between the anterosuperior surface of the left lobe of the liver and diaphragm. The left posterior perihepatic space lies inferior to the left lobe of the liver, and extends into the fissure for the ligamentum venosum on the right, anterior to the main portal vein. Posteriorly, the lesser omentum separates this space from the superior recess of the lesser sac. On the left, the space is bounded by the lesser curvature of the stomach.

Inframesocolic compartment

The inframesocolic compartment lies below the transverse mesocolon and transverse colon are far as the true pelvis. It is divided in two unequal spaces by the root of the mesentery of the small intestine. It contains the right and left paracolic gutters lateral to the ascending and descending colon. As a consequence of the mobility of the transverse mesocolon and mesentery of the small intestine, disease processes are rarely well contained within these spaces, and fluid within the infracolic space tends to descend into the pelvis or the paracolic gutters.

Right infracolic space

The right infracolic space is a triangular space. It is smaller than its counterpart on the left, and lies posterior and inferior to the transverse colon and mesocolon and to the right of the small intestinal mesentery. The space is narrowest inferiorly because the attachment of the root of the mesentery of the small intestine lies well to the right of the midline. The vermiform appendix often lies in the lower part of the right infracolic space.

Left infracolic space

The left infracolic space is larger than its counterpart on the right and is in free communication with the pelvis to the right of the midline. It lies posterior and inferior to the transverse colon and mesocolon and to the left of the mesentery of the small intestine. The sigmoid colon and its mesentery may partially restrict the flow of fluid or blood into the pelvis to the left of the midline.

Paracolic gutters

The right and left paracolic gutters are peritoneal recesses on the posterior abdominal wall lying alongside the ascending and descending colon. The main paracolic gutter lies lateral to the colon on each side. A less obvious medial paracolic gutter may be formed, especially on the right side, if the colon possesses a short mesentery for part of its length. The right (lateral) paracolic gutter runs from the superolateral aspect of the hepatic flexure of the colon, down the lateral aspect of the ascending colon, and around the caecum. It is continuous with the peritoneum as

it descends into the pelvis over the pelvic brim. Superiorly, it is continuous with the peritoneum which lines the hepatorenal pouch and, through the epiploic foramen, the lesser sac. Bile, pus or blood released from viscera anywhere along its length may run along the gutter and collect in sites quite remote from the organ of origin. In supine patients, infected fluid from the right iliac fossa may ascend in the gutter to enter the lesser sac. In patients nursed in a sitting position, fluid from the stomach, duodenum or gallbladder may run down the gutter to collect in the right iliac fossa or pelvis and may mimic acute appendicitis or form a pelvic abscess. The right paracolic gutter is larger than the left, which together with the partial barrier provided by the phrenicocolic ligament, may explain why right subphrenic collections are more common than left subphrenic collections.

Extraperitoneal subphrenic spaces

There are two potential 'spaces' which actually lie outside the peritoneal coverings of the abdomen but are of clinical relevance because of the possibility that fluid collections will accumulate in them. The right extraperitoneal space is bounded by the two layers of the coronary ligament, the bare area of the liver and the inferior surface of the right dome of the diaphragm. The left extraperitoneal space lies anterior to the left suprarenal gland and upper pole of the left kidney. It contains extraperitoneal connective tissue.

Clinical management of fluid collections in the peritoneal cavity

Fluid collections frequently occur within the peritoneal cavity as a result of a wide range of pathological processes. In the absence of any inflammation, peritoneal adhesions or previous surgery, serous fluid is almost always distributed freely between the peritoneal spaces and is not confined to any particular area. Simple ascites, for example, can therefore be drained freely from any convenient dependent part of the peritoneal cavity. This is most commonly performed by blind or ultrasound guided insertion of a catheter into the lower left or right paracolic gutters. These spaces usually readily fill with fluid and although the colon and some loops of small bowel may be present, their relatively mobility results in very little risk of injury to them.

Fluid collections caused by inflammatory processes are often much more viscid because they contain pus, fibrin or blood and are usually associated with peritoneal inflammation which results in, at least transient, peritoneal adhesions. These factors mean that collections may become localized if the flow of fluid is restricted by the, partial compartmentalization of the peritoneum. Once collected in one 'space', this fluid often becomes further confined by ongoing inflammation and may even form a truly walled-off cavity over time. Any of the spaces of the peritoneum may develop a collection but the subphrenic, subhepatic and pelvic spaces are the commonest since they are most well defined by the fixed peritoneal folds and organs forming their boundaries. These spaces are also the most dependent spaces within the peritoneum in the supine position and consequently any initially free fluid tends to gravitate to them.

Surgical access to the peritoneal spaces is rarely necessary today because of the great advances which have been made in radiologically guided drainage. When necessary, lateral subcostal or intercostal incisions may give adequate access to the subphrenic spaces and the anterior wall of the rectum is also a useful route to access the rectouterine or rectovesical space. Computerized tomography or ultrasound guided drainage offers a much more reliable and versatile method of accessing even difficult spaces such as subhepatic, perihepatic, paracolic or even intermesenteric collections. Posterolateral translumbar or trans-sciatic approaches can be used to access these more difficult areas.

Peritoneal dialysis

The mesothelium resembles vascular endothelium in being a dialysing membrane which fluids and small molecules may traverse. Numerous endocytic vesicles occur near the cell surfaces, the remaining cytoplasm being poor in organelles, indicating low metabolic activity. Normally the volumes of fluid transmitted by peritoneal surfaces are small, but large volumes may be administered via the intraperitoneal route. Conversely, substances such as urea can be dialysed from blood into fluid circulated through the peritoneal cavity.

Ventriculoperitoneal shunts

The absorptive capabilities of the peritoneum can be used to absorb excess transitional fluids from several sites in the body. The commonest of these is the absorption of cerebrospinal fluid drained from the intra-cerebral ventricles or the intrathecal space via a fine calibre catheter. The catheter can be placed within the peritoneum with a one way valve preventing reflux of peritoneal fluid into the cerebrospinal fluid. The fluid is then continuously absorbed maintaining a low pressure within the intrathecal or intraventricular space.

RECESSES OF THE PERITONEAL CAVITY

Peritoneal folds may create fossae or recesses within the peritoneal cavity. These are of clinical interest because a length of intestine may enter one and be constricted by the fold at the entrance to the recess: it may subsequently become a site of internal herniation. The contents of the peritoneal fold may be important if surgical incision is required to reduce such a hernia. Although internal herniation may occur into the lesser sac via the epiploic foramen, the sac is not usually considered to be a peritoneal recess.

Duodenal recesses (Fig. 69.10)

Several folds of peritoneum may exist around the fourth part of the duodenum and the duodenojejunal junction forming several recesses.

Superior duodenal recess

The superior duodenal recess is occasionally present, usually in association with an inferior duodenal recess. It lies to the left of the end of the fourth part of the duodenum, opposite the second lumbar vertebra, and behind a crescentic superior duodenal fold (duodenojejunal fold). The fold has a semilunar free lower edge which merges to the left with the peritoneum anterior to the left kidney. The inferior mesenteric vein is directly behind the junction of the left (lateral) end of this fold and the posterior parietal peritoneum. The recess varies in size but is commonly is c.2 cm deep, admitting a fingertip. It opens downwards, its orifice being in the angle formed by the left renal vein as it passes across the abdominal aorta.

Inferior duodenal recess

The inferior duodenal recess is usually present often associated with a superior recess with which it may share an orifice. It lies to the left of the fourth part of the duodenum, opposite the third lumbar vertebra. It sits behind a non-vascular, triangular inferior duodenal fold (duo-denomesocolic fold), which has a sharp upper edge. It is usually c.3 cm deep, admits one or two fingers and opens upwards towards the superior duodenal recess. It sometimes extends behind the fourth part of the duodenum and to the left, in front of the ascending branch of the left colic artery and the inferior mesenteric vein.

Paraduodenal recess (Fig. 69.11)

The paraduodenal recess may occur in conjunction with superior and inferior duodenal recesses. It is rare in adults but is more commonly seen in newborn children. It lies a little to the left and slightly behind of the fourth part of the duodenum, behind a falciform paraduodenal fold. The free right edge of the fold contains the inferior mesenteric vein and ascending branch of the left colic artery, and represents part of the upper left colic mesentery. Its free edge lies in front of the wide orifice of the recess, which faces right.

Retroduodenal recess

The retroduodenal recess is the largest of the duodenal recesses, but is rarely present. It lies behind the third and fourth parts of the duodenum in front of the abdominal aorta. It ascends nearly to the duodenojejunal junction, is 8–10 cm deep, and bounded on both sides by duodeno-parietal folds. It has a wide orifice which faces down and to the left.

Duodenojejunal recess

The duodenojejunal or mesocolica recess occurs in c.20% of adults. When present, it is almost never associated with any other duodenal recesses. It is c.3 cm deep and lies to the left of the abdominal aorta, between the duodenojejunal junction and the root of the transverse mesocolon. It is bounded above by the pancreas, on the left by the kidney, and below by the left renal vein. It has a circular opening between two peritoneal folds, and faces down and to the right.

Mesentericoparietal recess

The mesentericoparietal recess is only rarely present in adults. It lies just below the third part of the duodenum and invaginates into the upper

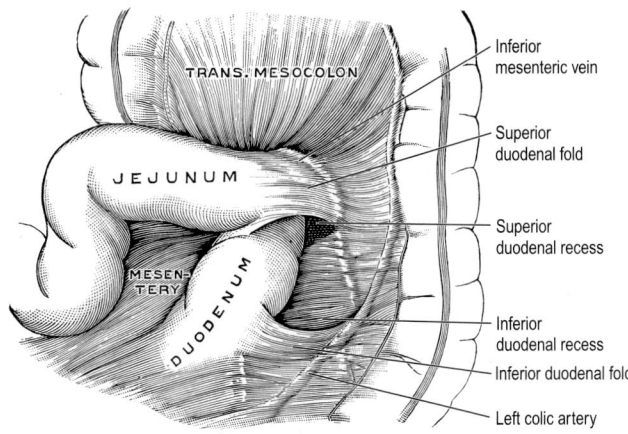

Fig. 69.10 The superior and inferior duodenal recesses. The transverse colon and jejunum have been displaced. (After Jonnesco, from Poirier P, Charpy A 1901 Traite d'Anatomie Humaine. Paris: Masson et Cie.)

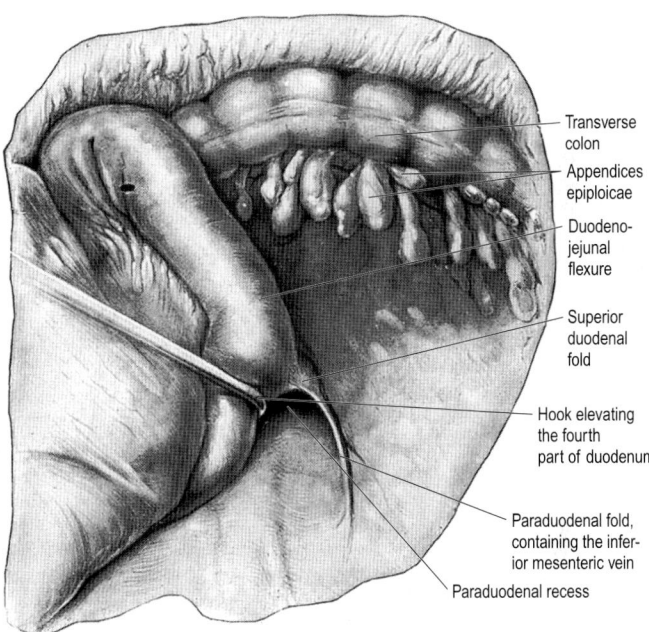

Fig. 69.11 The paraduodenal recess.

part of the mesentery towards the right. Its orifice is large and faces left behind a fold of mesentery raised by the superior mesenteric artery.

Caecal recesses (Fig. 69.12)

Several folds of peritoneum may exist around the caecum and form recesses. Paracaecal recesses are common sites for abscess formation following acute appendicitis.

Superior ileocaecal recess

The superior ileocaecal recess is usually present and best developed in children. It is often reduced and absent in the aged, especially the obese. It is formed by the vascular fold of the caecum, which arches over the anterior caecal artery, supplying the anterior part of the ileocaecal junction, and its accompanying vein. It is a narrow slit bounded in front by the vascular fold, behind by the ileal mesentery, below by the terminal ileum and on the right by the ileocaecal junction. Its orifice opens downwards to the left.

Inferior ileocaecal recess

The inferior ileocaecal recess is well marked in youth but frequently obliterated by fat in adults. It is formed by the ileocaecal fold, which extends from the anteroinferior aspect of the terminal ileum to the

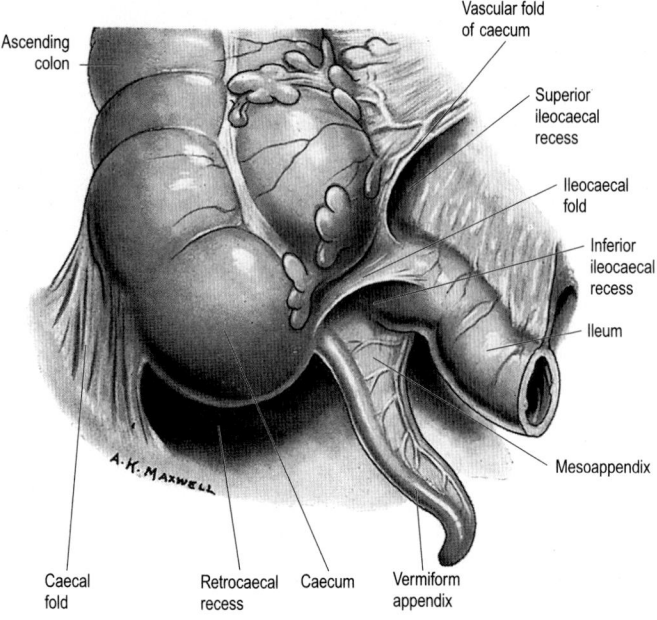

Ascending colon

Vascular fold of caecum

Superior ileocaecal recess

Ileocaecal fold

Inferior ileocaecal recess

Ileum

Mesoappendix

A.K. MAXWELL

Caecal fold

Retrocaecal recess

Caecum

Vermiform appendix

Fig. 69.12 The peritoneal folds and recesses in the caecal region.

front of the mesoappendix (or to the appendix or caecum). It is also known as the 'bloodless fold of Treves', although it sometimes contains blood vessels and will often bleed if divided during surgery. If inflamed, especially when the appendix and its mesentery are retrocaecal, it may be mistaken for the mesoappendix. The recess is bounded in front by the ileocaecal fold, above by the posterior ileal surface and its mesentery, to the right by the caecum, and behind by the upper mesoappendix. Its orifice opens downwards to the left.

Retrocaecal recess

The retrocaecal recess lies behind the caecum. It varies in size and extent and ascends behind the ascending colon, often being large enough to admit an entire finger. It is bounded in front by the caecum (and sometimes the lower ascending colon), behind by the parietal peritoneum and on each side by caecal folds (parietocolic folds) passing from the caecum to the posterior abdominal wall. The vermiform appendix frequently occupies this recess when in the retrocaecal position.

Intersigmoid recess

The intersigmoid recess is constant in fetal life and infancy, but may disappear during later development. It lies behind the apex of the V-shaped parietal attachment of the sigmoid mesocolon and is funnel shaped. It is directed upwards and opens downwards. It varies in size from a slight depression to a shallow fossa. Its posterior wall is formed by the parietal peritoneum of the posterior abdominal wall which covers the left ureter as it crosses the bifurcation of the left common iliac artery. Occasionally the recess is within the layers of the sigmoid mesocolon, and is nearer the bowel wall than the mesenteric root. It is probably produced by an imperfect blending of the mesocolon with the posterior parietal peritoneum.

VASCULAR SUPPLY AND LYMPHATIC DRAINAGE

Parietal and visceral peritoneum develop from the somatopleural and splanchnopleural layers respectively of lateral plate mesoderm (Chapter 108). Parietal peritoneum is therefore supplied by somatic blood vessels of the abdominal and pelvic walls. Its lymphatics join those in the body wall and drain to parietal lymph nodes. Visceral peritoneum is best considered as an integral part of the viscera which it overlies. It derives its blood supply from the viscera, and its lymphatics join the visceral vessels to drain to the regional lymph nodes.

INNERVATION

The parietal peritoneum is innervated by branches from nerves which supply the muscles and skin of the overlying body wall and thus has a similar spinal level of origin. The visceral peritoneum is innervated by branches of visceral afferent nerves which travel with the autonomic supply to the underlying viscera. The different sensations arising from pathologies which affect either the parietal or visceral peritoneum reflect these differences in patterns of innervation. Well-localized pain is elicited by mechanical, thermal or chemical stimulation of the nocioceptors of the parietal peritoneum. The sensation is usually confined to one or two dermatomes for each area of peritoneum stimulated and is both lateralized and well-localized. Somatic nerves of the parietal peritoneum also supply the corresponding segmental areas of skin and muscles and, when the parietal peritoneum is irritated, muscles tend to contract by reflex, causing localized hypercontractility (guarding) or even rigidity of the abdominal wall. The parietal peritoneum on the underside of the diaphragm is supplied with afferent fibres from the phrenic nerves and peripherally by the lower six intercostal nerves and subcostal nerve. Peripheral irritation of the diaphragm may result in pain, tenderness and muscular rigidity in the distribution of the lower thoracic spinal nerves, while central irritation may result in pain in the cutaneous distribution of cervical spinal nerves III–V, i.e. the shoulder region.

The visceral peritoneum and viscera are not affected by these stimuli since the visceral afferent innervation provides a much more limited sensation of discomfort. When stimulated, the sensation of pain is of a less severe nature and referred to the area of abdominal wall according to the region of the intestinal tract affected. Discomfort from foregut structures is felt in the region of the epigastrium, midgut structures in the region of the umbilicus, and hindgut structures in the suprapubic region: none of these sensations shows significant lateralization. However, stretch of the visceral peritoneum is a potent cause of certain sensations and responses. Various neural elements in the visceral walls, mesenteries and overlying peritoneum mediate poorly localized sensations of discomfort when stimulated by stretch, and may also elicit profound reflex autonomic reactions involving vasomotor and cardiac changes. This is of considerable clinical relevance. The effects of division of the parietal peritoneum may be rendered painless by local or regional local anaesthesia. In marked contrast, the direct central connections of the visceral afferents, particularly via the vagus, mean that stretching the visceral peritoneum may have profound effects, and may produce acute haemodynamic instability despite high spinal anaesthesia. Ischaemia of the underlying viscera causes poorly localized abdominal pain, probably due to the spasms of visceral smooth muscle.

REFERENCES

Healy JC, Reznek RH 1999 The anterior abdominal wall and peritoneum. In Butler P, Mitchell A, Ellis H (eds) Applied Radiological Anatomy. Cambridge: Cambridge University Press: 189–200.
Demonstrates the imaging anatomy of the peritoneal spaces and reflections using cross-sectional imaging.

Meyers M 1994 Dynamic Radiology of the Abdomen. Normal and Pathologic Anatomy. New York: Springer.
Provides a systematic application of anatomic and dynamic principles to the understanding and diagnosis of intraabdominal disease.

Coakley FV, Hricak H 1999 Imaging of peritoneal and mesenteric disease: key concepts for the clinical radiologist. Clin Radiol 54: 563–574
Explains the complex anatomy of the upper abdominal peritoneal fold suspending the stomach, liver and spleen.

General microstructure of the gut wall

The gut wall displays a common structural plan which is modified regionally (p. 41) to take account of local functional differences. The general microstructure is best appreciated by reference to the development of the gut (Chapter 90). Much of the alimentary canal originates as a tube of endoderm enclosed in splanchnopleuric mesoderm. Its external surface faces the embryonic coelom, and the endodermal lining forms the epithelium of the canal and also the secretory and ductal cells of various glands which secrete into the lumen, including the pancreas and liver. The splanchnopleuric mesoderm forms the connective tissue, muscle layers, blood vessels and lymphatics of the wall, and its external surface becomes the visceral mesothelium or serosa (p. 41). There is no serosa surrounding the cervical and thoracic portions of the gut, or where the hindgut traverses the pelvic floor: in these sites the gut tube is surrounded by a connective tissue adventitia. Neural elements invade the gut from neural crest tissue (Chapter 14). The smooth muscle of the muscularis externa layers of the alimentary canal is supplemented with striated muscle both cranially (from the branchial arches) and caudally. An outline of the general microstructural organization of the gut wall is shown in **Fig. 70.1**.

MATURE GUT WALL

The gut wall has four main layers, namely mucosa, submucosa, muscularis externa and serosa (p. 41). The mucosa (mucous membrane) is the innermost layer and is subdivided into a lining epithelium, an underlying lamina propria (a layer of loose connective tissue, where many of the glands are also found) and a thin layer of smooth muscle, the muscularis mucosae. The submucosa is a strong and highly vascularized layer of connective tissue. The muscularis externa consists of inner circular and outer longitudinal layers which are present throughout the gut wall: a partial oblique layer is present only in the stomach. The external surface is bounded by a serosa or adventitia, depending on its position within the body.

MUCOSA

Epithelium
The epithelium is a protective barrier and the site of secretion and absorption. Its protective function (against mechanical, thermal and chemical injury) is particularly evident in the oesophagus and in the terminal part of the rectum, where it is thick, stratified, and covered in mucus, which serves as a protective lubricant. Other than in these sites, the epithelium lining the gut wall is single-layered, and either cuboidal (in glands) or columnar. It contains cells modified for absorption as well as various types of secretory cell.

The barrier function and selectivity of absorption depend on tight junctions (p. 7) over the entire epithelium. The surface area of the lumen available for secretion or absorption is increased by the presence of mucosal folds, pits, crypts, villi and glands. Microvilli on the surfaces of individual absorptive cells amplify the area of apical plasma membrane in contact with the contents of the gut. Some glands lie in the lamina propria, some in the submucosa, and others (the liver and pancreas) are totally external to the wall of the gut. All of these glands drain into the lumen of the gut through individual ducts. The epithelium also contains scattered neuroendocrine (enteroendocrine) cells.

Lamina propria
The lamina propria consists of compact connective tissue, often rich in elastin fibres, which supports the surface epithelium and provides nutrient vessels and lymphatics. Lymphoid follicles are present in many regions of the gut, most notably in Peyer's patches. Cells within the lamina propria are the source of growth factors which regulate cell turnover, differentiation and repair in the overlying epithelium.

Muscularis mucosae
The muscularis mucosae is well developed in the oesophagus and in the large intestine, especially in the terminal part of the rectum. In addition, single muscle cells originating from the muscularis mucosae are found inside the villi or between the tubular glands of the stomach and large intestine. By its contraction, the muscularis mucosae can alter the surface configuration of the mucosa locally, allowing it to adapt to the shapes and mechanical forces imposed by the contents of the lumen, and in the intestinal villi, promoting vascular exchange and lymphatic drainage.

SUBMUCOSA
The submucosa contains large bundles of collagen and is the strongest layer of the gut wall. However, it is also pliable and deformable and can therefore adjust to changes in the length and diameter of the gut. It contains the largest arterial network of the wall, which supplies both the mucosa and the muscle coat. The submucosa invades the folds which project into the lumen of the oesophagus and rectum, the rugae of the gastric wall, and the plicae circulares of the small intestine, but does not enter the villi.

MUSCULARIS EXTERNA
The muscularis externa usually consists of distinct inner circular and outer longitudinal layers whose antagonistic activities create waves of peristalsis responsible for the movement of ingested material through the lumen of the gut. In the stomach, where movements are more complex, there is a partial oblique layer, internal to the other two layers. The layer of circular muscle is invariably thicker than the longitudinal muscle, except in the colon, where the longitudinal muscle is gathered into three cords (taenia coli).

The muscularis externa is composed almost exclusively of smooth muscle, except in the upper oesophagus, where smooth muscle blends with striated muscle. Although the oesophageal musculature resembles that of the pharynx, it is entirely under involuntary control. For most of its length, the smooth muscle of the gut wall consists of ill-defined bundles of cells, typically visceral in type, and somewhat larger than vascular smooth muscle cells. They are c.500 μm long, regardless of body size, and are electrically and mechanically coupled. Their fasciculi lack a perimysium, but have sharp boundaries.

The arrangement of the musculature means that a segment of gut can change extensively in diameter (to virtual occlusion of the lumen) and also in length, although elongation is limited by the presence of mesenteries. The co-ordinated activity of the two muscle layers produces a characteristic motor behaviour which is mainly propulsive and directed anally (peristalsis), combined with a non-propulsive motor activity which either mixes the luminal contents, as occurs in the stomach, or partitions them, as occurs at the pyloric sphincter. The muscle maintains constant volume, so that shortening of a segment of the gut wall is accompanied by an increase in muscle layer circumference.

Intestinal smooth muscle exhibits variable and changing degrees of contraction on which rhythmic (or phasic) contractions are superimposed. Slow waves of rhythmic electrical activity, driven by changes in membrane potential in pacemaker cells (interstitial cells), spread throughout the thickness of the circular and longitudinal smooth muscle coats. After spreading circumferentially, slow waves can move in either oral or anal directions, causing segmental contraction. The distances of

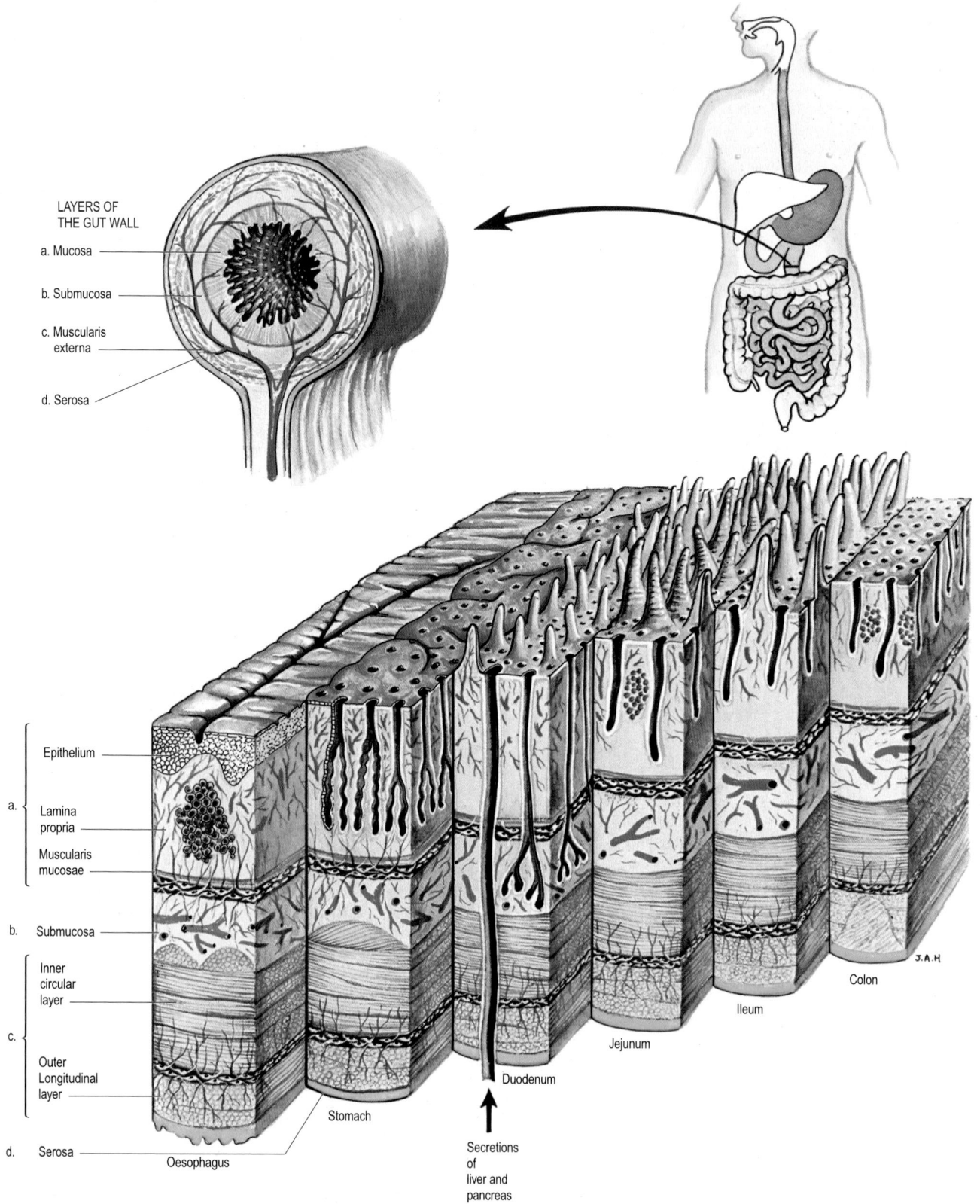

LAYERS OF
THE GUT WALL

a. Mucosa

b. Submucosa

c. Muscularis
externa

d. Serosa

Epithelium

a. Lamina
propria

Muscularis
mucosae

b. Submucosa

Inner
circular
layer

c.

Outer
Longitudinal
layer

d. Serosa

Oesophagus

Stomach

Duodenum

Secretions
of
liver and
pancreas

Jejunum

Ileum

Colon

J.A.H

Fig. 70.1 The general arrangement of the alimentary canal to show the layers of the gut wall at the levels indicated (highly diagrammatic). The transverse colon (above right) has been displaced downwards to reveal the duodenum.

propagation and the patterns of this spontaneous activity vary between areas of the intestine. Neural regulation of slow and phasic contractions involves excitatory and inhibitory transmitters which are released from the myenteric plexus. This motor control is closely co-ordinated with mucosal absorption and secretion and is mediated via intrinsic nerves in the submucous plexus. The peristaltic reflex occurs during passage of luminal contents down the intestine. It involves ascending contraction and descending relaxation: the sensory limb is mediated by sensory neurones that respond to either mucosal stimulation (intrinsic primary afferents) or muscle stretch (extrinsic afferents).

Interstitial cells

Interstitial cells (of Cajal) are thought to act as pacemakers for the myogenic contraction of muscularis externa, establishing the rhythm of bowel contractions through their influence on electrical slow wave activity. They receive modulatory inputs from the enteric nervous system and from the extrinsic innervation of the gut.

Interstitial cells are thin, flat, and branched. They resemble smooth muscle cells because they contain actin and myosin filaments, and are linked by gap junctions to typical smooth muscle cells. However, they are phenotypically distinct from muscle cells because their intermediate filaments are vimentin rather than desmin, (which is typical of muscle cells). They lie in close apposition to varicose nerve endings of at least two types; one contains small, round clear vesicles (50 nm diameter), the other contains flat, discoidal vesicles (70 nm diameter).

The positions of the interstitial cell layers vary regionally. In general, they lie in the same layers as the enteric plexuses. They are scattered among the cells of the circular muscle layer in the oesophagus and stomach, lie between the inner and outer layers of circular smooth muscle in the small intestine, and colocalize with the myenteric plexus and the single layer of the submucosal plexus on the luminal side of the circular component of the muscularis externa, in the large intestine.

SEROSA AND ADVENTITIA

There is a layer of connective tissue external to the muscularis externa. It is of variable thickness and in many places contains adipose tissue. Where the gut is covered by visceral peritoneum, the external layer is a serosa, which consists of a thin connective tissue layer and an external coat of mesothelium. Elsewhere the connective tissue blends with that of the surrounding fasciae and is referred to as an adventitia. Where the alimentary tract is retroperitoneal, the surface facing the abdominal cavity is covered by serosa, and the other parts are covered by adventitia.

VASCULAR PLEXUSES

Vascular plexuses are present at various levels of the wall, especially in the submucosa and mucosa: they connect with plexuses of vessels which supply the surrounding tissues or those entering through the mesentery, and accompany the ducts of outlying glands.

INNERVATION

The gut is densely innervated by the autonomic and enteric nervous systems, and is under extrinsic and intrinsic neuronal control. Neuronal cell bodies of the enteric nervous system lie between the circular and longitudinal components of the muscularis externa (myenteric plexus) and within the submucosa (submucosal plexus). They provide the intrinsic sensory and motor supply of the gut wall and connect with extrinsic sensory, motor and sensorimotor nerves of cranial or spinal origin.

Extrinsic innervation

The extrinsic innervation is derived from neurones outside the gut, and contains functional components from the sympathetic, parasympathetic and visceral sensory divisions of the peripheral nervous system. Visceral sensory endings (p. 59) respond to excessive muscular contraction or distension: their cell bodies are situated in the nodose ganglion of the vagus nerve and in thoracic and lumbar spinal or dorsal root ganglia. The cell bodies of parasympathetic efferent axons lie in the vagal dorsal motor nucleus in the medulla oblongata. Sympathetic efferent fibres arise from the thoracic and lumbar spinal cord and relay in prevertebral sympathetic ganglia (coeliac, mesenteric and pelvic).

A subserosal plexus, which sometimes contains neuronal cell bodies, connects the extrinsic nerve fibres with the myenteric plexus and is particularly prominent near the mesentery. Fibres from this plexus run through the longitudinal muscle layer to reach the myenteric plexus.

Intrinsic innervation (Fig. 70.2)

The intrinsic innervation of the gut wall is derived from neurones which are located entirely within the wall in intramural ganglionated plexuses (for more details see pp. 59, 238). The myenteric (Auerbach's) plexus is a network of fine bundles of axons and small ganglia which lies within the muscularis externa, between the circular and longitudinal layers. It is often associated with secondary and tertiary plexuses of nerve fibres which sometimes contain isolated neuronal cell bodies. There are two or more submucosal plexuses, the most superficial of which is Meissner's plexus.

Non-ganglionated nerve plexuses lie at various levels in the wall, notably in the lamina propria (mucosal plexus); at the interface between the submucosa and muscularis externa; between the circular and longitudinal muscles (the non-ganglionated part of the myenteric plexus); and within the serosa. An additional non-ganglionated plexus lies between the internal and external components of the circular muscle of the small intestine. All parts of the myenteric plexus are continuous not only with each other, but also with the nerve fibre bundles in the circular muscle. The latter are connected to the ganglionated and non-ganglionated plexuses of the submucosa, and these in turn are connected with the mucosal plexus by fibres which pass through the muscularis mucosa.

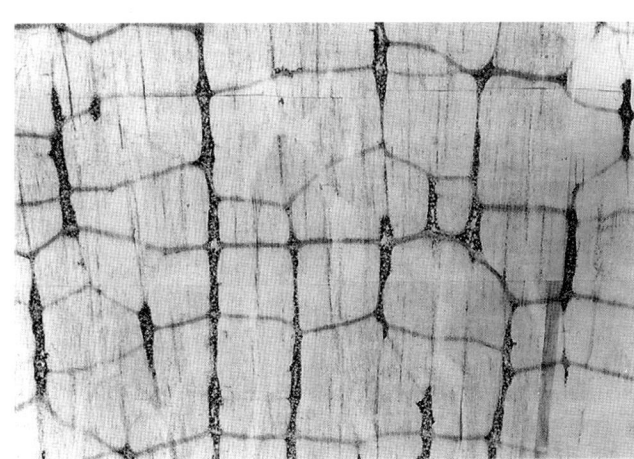

Fig. 70.2 Wall of the small intestine with the mesh-like appearance of the myenteric plexus highlighted by selective neuronal staining. The ganglia are the elongated structures running vertically, comprised of ganglion neurones, joined by connecting strands of nerve fibres. The circular musculature, virtually unstained, runs vertically and the unstained longitudinal musculature runs transversely. (Courtesy of Professor G Gabella, University College, London.) (By kind permission from G Gabella, Department of Anatomy and Embryology, University College, London.)

Stomach and abdominal oesophagus

The stomach is the widest part of the alimentary tract and lies between the oesophagus and the duodenum. It is situated in the upper abdomen, extending from the left upper quadrant downwards, forwards and to the right, lying in the left hypochondriac, epigastric and umbilical areas. It occupies a recess beneath the diaphragm and anterior abdominal wall that is bounded by the upper abdominal viscera on either side. Its mean capacity increases from c.30 ml at birth, to 1000 ml at puberty, to c.1500 ml in adults. The peritoneal surface of the stomach is interrupted by the attachments of the greater and lesser omenta, which define the greater and lesser curvatures separating two surfaces (**Figs 71.1, 71.6**).

PARTS OF THE STOMACH

The stomach is divided for descriptive purposes into the fundus, body, pyloric antrum and pylorus, by arbitrary lines drawn on its external surface. The internal appearance and microstructure of these regions varies to some degree. The fundus is dome shaped and projects above and to the left of the cardiac orifice to lie in contact with the left dome of the diaphragm. It lies above a line drawn horizontally from the incisura cardiaca to the greater curvature. The body extends from the fundus to the incisura angularis, which is a constant external notch at the lower end of the lesser curvature. A line drawn from the incisura angularis to an indentation on the greater curvature defines the lower boundary of the body. The pyloric antrum extends from this line to the sulcus intermedius. At this point, the stomach narrows to become the pyloric canal, which is usually only 1–2 cm in length and terminates at the pyloric orifice.

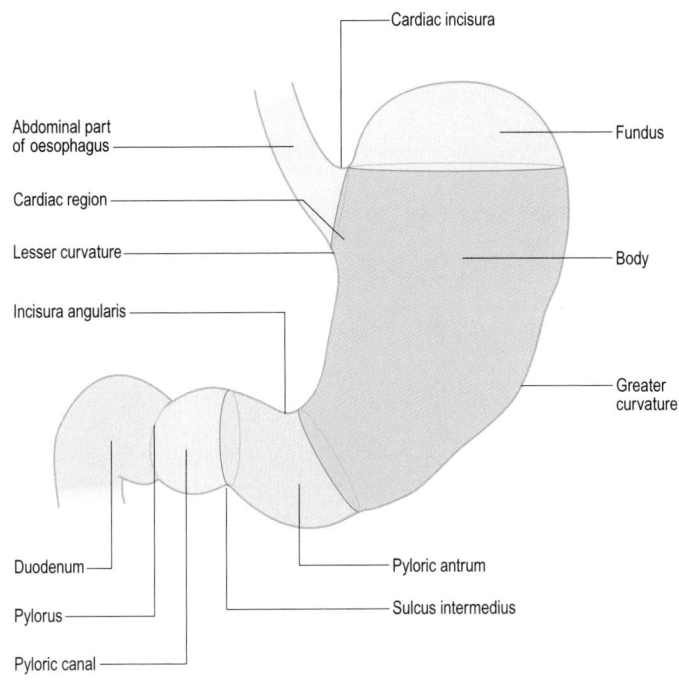

Fig. 71.1 The parts of the stomach.

GASTRIC RELATIONS

GASTRIC CURVATURES

Lesser curvature

The lesser curvature extends between the cardiac and pyloric orifices and forms the medial (posterior and superior) border of the stomach. It descends from the medial side of the oesophagus in front of the decussating fibres of the right crus of the diaphragm. It curves downwards and to the right and lies anterior to the superior border of the pancreas. It ends at the pylorus just to the right of the midline. In the most dependent part there is typically a notch, the incisura angularis, whose position and appearance vary with gastric distension. The lesser omentum is attached to the lesser curvature and contains the right and left gastric vessels.

Greater curvature

The greater curvature is four or five times longer than the lesser. It starts from the incisura cardiaca formed between the lateral border of the abdominal oesophagus and the fundus of the stomach. It arches upwards, posterolaterally and to the left. Its highest convexity, the apex of the fundus, is approximately level with the left fifth intercostal space just below the left nipple in males, but varies with respiration. From this level it sweeps inferiorly and anteriorly, slightly convex to the left, almost as far as the tenth costal cartilage in the supine position, where it turns medially to end at the pylorus. There is frequently a groove, termed the sulcus intermedius, in the curvature close to the pyloric constriction. The start of the greater curvature is covered by peritoneum, which continues over the anterior surface of the stomach. Laterally the greater curvature gives attachment to the gastrosplenic ligament and beyond this to the greater omentum, which contains the gastroepiploic vessels. The gastrosplenic ligament and the greater omentum, together with the gastrophrenic and splenorenal ligaments, are continuous parts of the original dorsal mesogastrium. The names merely indicate regions of the same continuous sheet of peritoneum and associated connective tissue.

Gastric volvulus

Volvulus of the stomach is much less common than volvulus of either the sigmoid colon or caecum. Two types of gastric volvulus may occur. The first, organoaxial volvulus, occurs about a line of rotation running from below the cardiac orifice to the pylorus. The antrum, body and fundus rotate upwards, with the greater curvature coming to lie above the lesser curvature as the volvulus progresses. The second, mesenteroaxial volvulus, occurs about a line drawn 'across' the body of the stomach, usually just above the incisura angularis. This type of volvulus is perpendicular to the line of organoaxial volvulus. The distal body and antrum rotate anteriorly, superiorly and laterally whilst the upper body and fundus rotate posteriorly, medially and inferiorly. Although relatively mobile within the upper abdomen, the stomach is normally tethered to the oesophagus at the gastro-oesophageal junction, to the duodenum at the pylorus, to the spleen by the gastrosplenic omentum, and to the liver by the lesser omentum. The attachment to the transverse colon via the gastrocolic omentum also restrains the stomach but is the most mobile of all. For either type of gastric volvulus to occur, it is necessary for some or all of these points of tethering to be loosened either by previous surgical division or by chronic lengthening and loosening of their connective tissue. Organoaxial volvulus is most common because the lesser omentum, gastrosplenic ligament and gastrocolic omentum are more likely to undergo chronic lengthening by traction than the other attachments of the stomach. Mesenteroaxial volvulus requires the gastro-oesophageal junction and pylorus to be sufficiently mobile as to come into close approximation. These structures are firmly tethered and consequently this form of gastric volvulus is much less common. Despite the profuse gastric arterial supply, either type of volvulus may compromise the vascularity of the stomach.

GASTRIC SURFACES

When the stomach is empty and contracted, the two surfaces tend to lie facing almost superiorly and inferiorly, but with increasing degrees of distension they come to face progressively more anteriorly and posteriorly.

Anterior (superior) surface

The lateral part of the anterior surface is posterior to the left costal margin and in contact with the diaphragm, which separates it from the left pleura, the base of the left lung, the pericardium and the left sixth to ninth ribs (**Fig. 71.2**). It lies posterior to the costal attachments of the upper fibres of transversus abdominis, which separate it from the seventh to ninth costal cartilages. The upper and left part of this surface curves posterolaterally and is in contact with the gastric surface of the spleen. The right half of the anterior surface is related to the left and quadrate lobes of the liver and the anterior abdominal wall. When the stomach is empty, the transverse colon may lie adjacent to the anterior surface. The entire anterior (superior) surface is covered by peritoneum.

Posterior (inferior) surface

The posterior surface lies anterior to the left crus and lower fibres of the diaphragm, the left inferior phrenic vessels, the left suprarenal gland, the superior pole of the left kidney, the splenic artery, the anterior pancreatic surface, the splenic flexure of the colon and the upper layer of the transverse mesocolon (**Fig. 71.3**). Together these form the shallow stomach bed: they are separated from the stomach by the lesser sac (over which the stomach slides as it distends). The upper left part of the surface curves anterolaterally and lies in contact with the gastric surface of the spleen. The greater omentum and the transverse mesocolon separate the stomach from the duodenojejunal flexure and ileum. The posterior surface is covered by peritoneum, except near the cardiac orifice, where a small, triangular area contacts the left diaphragmatic

crus and sometimes the left suprarenal gland. The left gastric vessels reach the lesser curvature at the right extremity of this bare area in the left gastropancreatic fold. The gastrophrenic ligament passes from the lateral aspect of this bare area to the inferior surface of the diaphragm.

GASTRIC ORIFICES

CARDIAC ORIFICE AND GASTRO–OESOPHAGEAL JUNCTION

The opening from the oesophagus into the stomach is the cardiac orifice (**Fig. 71.4**). It is typically situated to the left of the midline behind the seventh costal cartilage at the level of the eleventh thoracic vertebra. It is c.10 cm from the anterior abdominal wall and 40 cm from the incisor teeth. The short abdominal part of the oesophagus curves sharply to the left as it descends and is continuous with the cardiac orifice. The right side of the oesophagus is continuous with the lesser curvature, the left side with the greater curvature. There is no specific anatomical cardiac sphincter related to the orifice.

Internally, the transition between oesophagus and stomach is difficult to define because mucosa of gastric fundal pattern extends a variable distance up into the abdominal oesophagus. It usually forms a 'zig-zag' squamo-columnar epithelial junction with the oesophageal epithelium above this Z line (p. 1152). This is often referred to as the gastro-oesophageal junction, for histological and endoscopic purposes. A sling of longitudinal gastric muscle forms a loop on the superior, left, side of the gastro-oesophageal junction between the oesophagus and the lesser curvature, and this is taken as the external boundary of this junction.

GASTRO-OESOPHAGEAL REFLUX

Reflux of gastric contents into the abdominal and lower thoracic oesophagus as a result of transient relaxation of the lower oesophageal sphincter occurs as a normal event in most individuals for a small percentage of their daily life. It also occurs as a result of a weak lower oesophageal sphincter, or of hiatus hernia which disrupts the normal anatomical barriers (p. 1083). Several anatomical and physiological factors normally prevent gastro-oesophageal reflux. The folds of gastric mucosa present in the gastro-oesophageal junction, the mucosal rosette, contribute to the formation of a fluid- and gas-tight seal. They also help

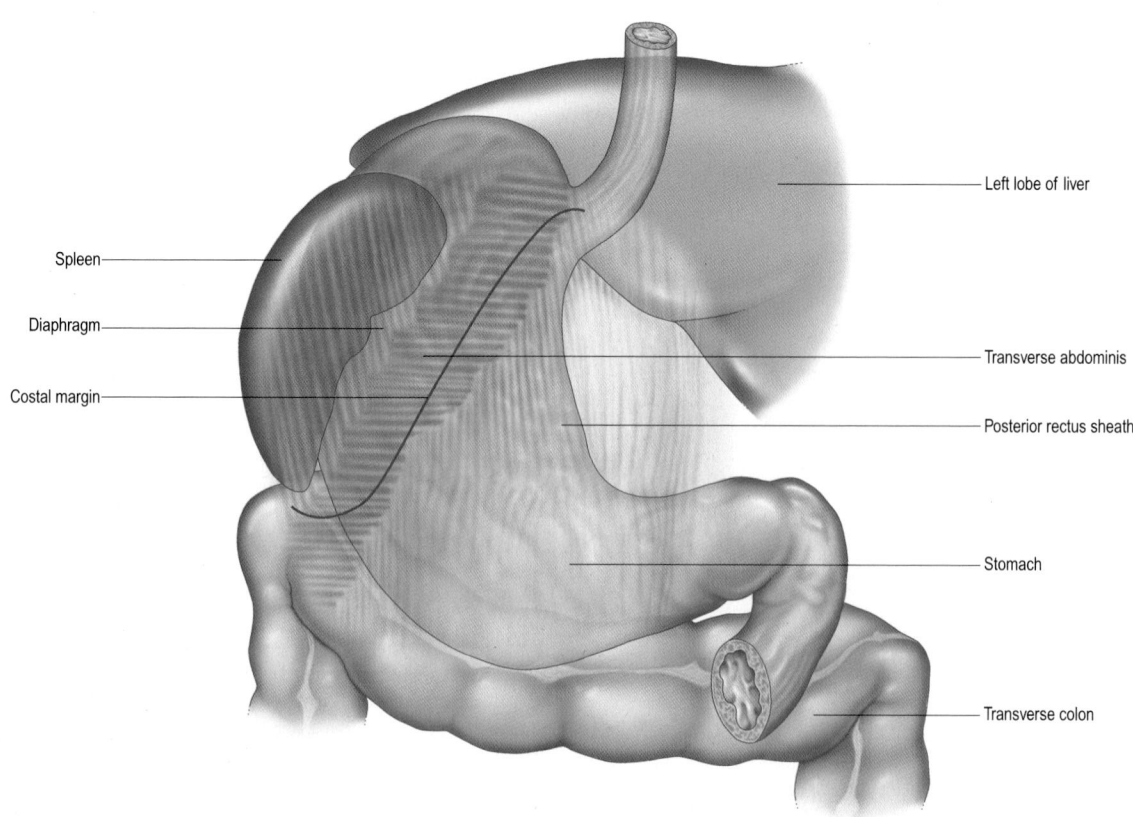

Fig. 71.2 Anterior relations of the stomach, viewed from behind.

Spleen

Diaphragm

Costal margin

Left lobe of liver

Transverse abdominis

Posterior rectus sheath

Stomach

Transverse colon

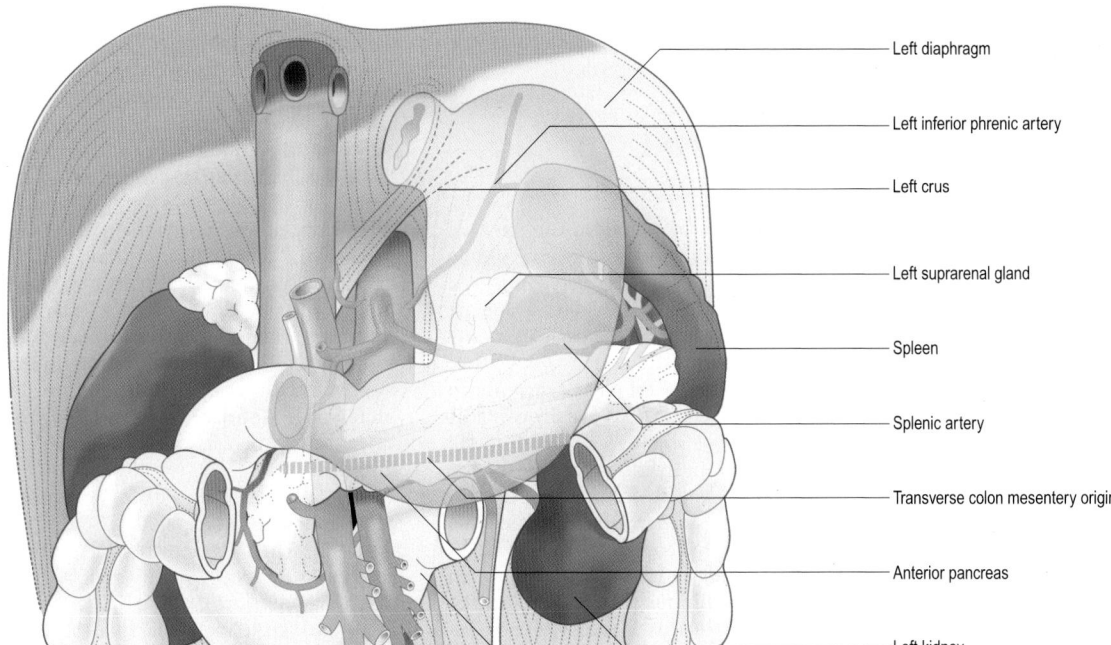

Fig. 71.3 Posterior relations of the stomach.

Left diaphragm

Left inferior phrenic artery

Left crus

Left suprarenal gland

Spleen

Splenic artery

Transverse colon mesentery origin

Anterior pancreas

Left kidney

Duodenojejunal flexure

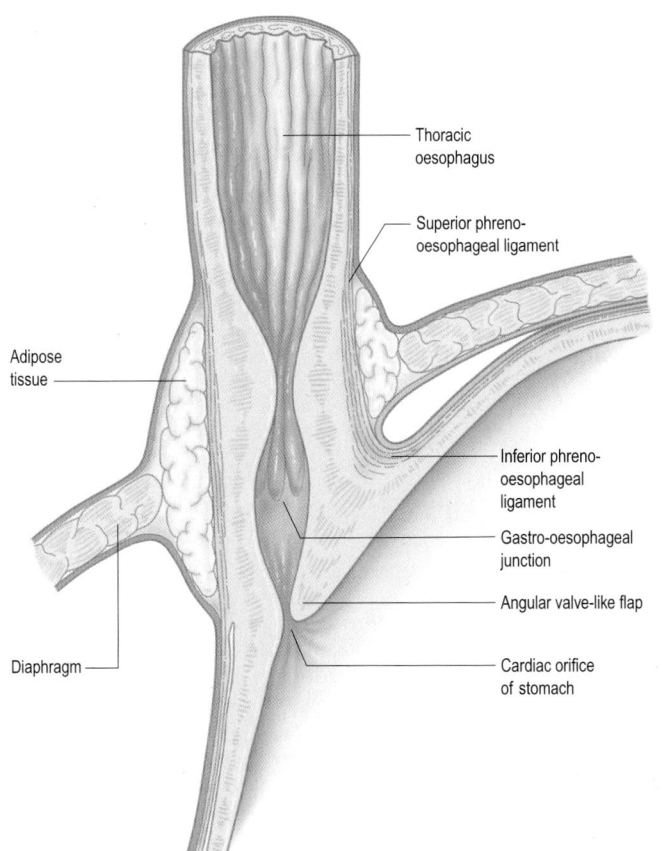

Thoracic oesophagus

Superior phreno-oesophageal ligament

Inferior phreno-oesophageal ligament

Gastro-oesophageal junction

Angular valve-like flap

Cardiac orifice of stomach

Adipose tissue

Diaphragm

Fig. 71.4 The valve-like structure formed by the angle of the wall at the cardiac orifice. (Provided by Donald E Low, Department of Surgery, Virginia Mason, Seattle, USA.)

tonic contractions of the lower oesophageal musculature, which forms an effective high pressure zone (HPZ) (p. 986). The specialized smooth muscle of the wall of the lower oesophagus and the encircling fibres of the crural diaphragm exert a radial pressure that can be measured by a sensing device as it is withdrawn from the stomach into the oesophagus (Paterson 2001). If reflux is to be prevented, this pressure must always exceed the difference between the pressures on either side of the junction, i.e. the difference between intra-abdominal pressure (transferred to the stomach, and augmented by any contraction of the stomach wall itself), and intrathoracic pressure (transferred to the oesophagus).

During expiration, pressure exerted by tonic contraction of the smooth muscle of the lower oesophagus is normally sufficient to oppose the gastro-oesophageal pressure gradient. During inspiration, intra-abdominal pressure rises and intrathoracic pressure becomes more negative, increasing the risk of reflux. This tendency is opposed by additional pressure exerted by contraction of the crural fibres of the diaphragm. (Activation of the crural diaphragm slightly before the costal diaphragm would ensure that contraction of peri-oesophageal fibres preceded the increase in gastro-oesophageal pressure gradient.) The anti-reflux barrier must of course be lowered for swallowing and vomiting. Swallowing is followed immediately by expiration, which relaxes the crural fibres and allows the oesophageal contents to be transferred to the stomach by peristaltic movement. Vomiting is produced by bursts of activity involving co-contraction of the diaphragm, intercostal and abdominal muscles in a pattern distinct from that of respiration: this activity is coordinated with relaxation of the crural fibres around the oesophagus (Miller, 1990).

Barrett's oesophagus
The squamous epithelium lining the lower oesophagus may be pathologically replaced by a columnar, gastric type epithelium. This may occur as islands, strips, or circumferentially, and may extend for a variable length up the lower oesophagus. This process is most likely to be the result of the chronic reflux of gastric contents, acid or alkali, into the oesophagus with a resultant change in mucosal cell type. The abnormal columnar type epithelium present in the anatomical oesophagus is referred to as Barrett's epithelium.

PYLORIC ORIFICE
The pyloric orifice is the opening into the duodenum. The circular pyloric constriction on the surface of the stomach usually indicates the location of the pyloric sphincter and is often marked by a prepyloric vein crossing the anterior surface vertically downwards. The pyloric orifice typically lies 1–2 cm to the right of the midline in the transpyloric plane

to ensure that even low levels of tone within the lower oesophageal wall muscles may occlude the lumen of the junction against low pressures of gastric gas. The angle of the cardiac orifice may help to form a type of 'flap valve' and the length of abdominal oesophagus is buttressed externally by pads of adipose connective tissue at and below the level of the diaphragmatic hiatus. However, the major anti-reflux mechanism is the

with the body supine and the stomach empty. The pyloric sphincter is a muscular ring formed by a marked thickening of the circular gastric muscle interlaced with some longitudinal fibres.

GASTRIC FORM AND INTERNAL APPEARANCES

It is clear from contrast radiographic studies that the form and position of the stomach are extremely variable depending on posture, the volume of its contents, and the surrounding viscera. They are also influenced by the tone of the abdominal wall and gastric musculature and by the build of the individual. The empty stomach is most commonly J-shaped and, in the erect posture, the pylorus descends to the level of the second or the third lumbar vertebra. The lowest part of the antrum often lies below the level of the umbilicus. The fundus usually contains gas. The overall axis of the organ is, therefore, slightly inclined from the vertical (**Figs 71.5, 71.6**). In short, obese individuals the axis of the stomach lies more towards the horizontal as a 'steer-horn' shape.

Variation caused by the contents of the stomach mainly affects the body because the pyloric part usually remains contracted during digestion. As the stomach fills, it expands forwards and downwards but, when the colon or small bowel is distended, the fundus enlarges towards the liver and diaphragm. As stomach capacity increases, the pylorus is displaced to the right and the axis of the whole organ lies in a more oblique direction (**Figs 71.5, 71.6**). In this position the anterior and posterior surfaces tend to face forwards and backwards and the lowest part is the pyloric antrum, which extends below the umbilicus. When intestinal distension interferes with downward expansion of the body, the stomach retains a horizontal position.

INTERNAL APPEARANCES

During endoscopic examination (**Fig. 71.7**), the stomach is typically at least partially distended by air. The cardiac orifice and the lowest portion of the abdominal oesophagus viewed from above are typically closed at rest by tonic contraction of the lower oesophageal musculature. The gastric mucosa lining the orifice is puckered into ridges. It is present for a short but variable distance into the abdominal oesophagus and the transition between columnar and squamous epithelium is usually clearly visible. The presence of abnormal columnar epithelium within the anatomical oesophagus is referred to as Barrett's oesophagus but the precise definition of this condition is difficult. From within the distended stomach, the cardiac orifice appears in the medial wall of the fundus and is asymmetrical. The medial edge of the cardiac orifice is continuous with the medial wall of the body of the stomach. The mucosa is slightly thickened at this point with a raised profile, forming part of the 'mucosal rosette' that lines the orifice. The 'rosette' aids closure of the cardiac orifice and helps prevent reflux of stomach contents into the oesophagus. The medial edge of the orifice is

more clearly visible than the lateral edge as it forms a more acute angle with the mucosal lining of the abdominal oesophagus.

In the partly distended stomach, the mucosa of the fundus is thrown into gentle folds with no particular pattern. As the stomach fills towards capacity, however, these folds rapidly become less pronounced, and the wall is nearly smooth when the stomach is over-inflated. The body of the stomach has the most pronounced mucosal folds. Even in moderate distension, they appear as long, broad mucosal ridges running in sinuous strips from fundus to pyloric antrum (**Fig. 71.6**). They are seen on all mucosal surfaces of the body but are most obvious on the anterolateral, lateral and posterolateral parts (which correspond to the inner surface of the anterior and posterior external surfaces and to the greater curvature). Here they are occasionally called the *magenstrasse*, a reference to their possible role in directing liquid entering the stomach immediately down into the pyloric antrum. These folds are least prominent on the medial surface (corresponding to the inner surface of the lesser curvature), which is much smoother, particularly when the stomach distends.

The areae gastricae within the antrum are small nodular elevations of the mucosal surface that are readily seen on double contrast barium meal (**Fig. 71.6**). The few folds present in the antrum when the stomach is relaxed disappear with distension. The antrum adjacent to the pyloric canal, the prepyloric antrum, has a smooth mucosal surface culminating in a slight puckering of the mucosa at the pyloric orifice caused by the contraction of the pyloric sphincter.

GASTROSTOMY

Since the lower body and antrum of the stomach is related to the posterior aspect of the left anterior abdominal wall, it may usefully be accessed to form a gastrostomy. Its mobility enables the anterior surface of the stomach to be readily approximated to the parietal peritoneum on the posterior surface of the abdominal wall and a communication to be established between the lumen of the stomach and the surface of the skin. Although this may be performed as a direct open surgical procedure under general anaesthetic it is much more commonly performed using a percutaneous puncture guided by either endoscopic visualization of the stomach or radiological imaging. The procedure is made easier by the fact that the anterior surface of the stomach lies most nearly in the vertical plane when the stomach is distended. One of the main hazards of the procedure results from the occasional interposition of the transverse colon between the stomach and anterior abdominal wall. This may lead to inadvertent transfixion of the colon by the needle puncture system. The variable length of the transverse colonic mesentery means that it may sometimes lie adjacent to the anterior gastric surface when a subject is recumbent. These risks may be reduced by radiological guidance.

VASCULAR SUPPLY AND LYMPHATIC DRAINAGE

ARTERIES

The arterial supply to the stomach comes predominantly from the coeliac axis although intramural anastomoses exist with vessels of other origins at the two ends of the stomach (**Figs 71.8, 71.9**). The left gastric artery arises directly from the coeliac axis. The splenic artery gives origin to the short gastric arteries as well as the left gastroepiploic artery and may occasionally give origin to a posterior gastric artery. The hepatic artery gives origin to the right gastric artery and the gastroduodenal artery, which in turn gives origin to the right gastroepiploic artery.

Left gastric artery

The left gastric artery is the smallest branch of the coeliac axis. It ascends to the left of the midline and crosses the left crus of the diaphragm beneath the peritoneum of the upper posterior wall of the lesser sac. Here it lies adjacent to the left inferior phrenic artery and medial or anterior to the left suprarenal gland. It runs forwards into the superior portion of the lesser omentum adjacent to the superior end of the lesser curvature. It turns anteroinferiorly to run along the lesser curvature between the two peritoneal leaves of the lesser omentum. At the highest point of its course, it gives off an oesophageal branch. In its course along the lesser curvature, it gives off multiple branches that run onto the anterior and posterior surfaces of the stomach and anastomose with the right gastric artery in the region of the incisura angularis.

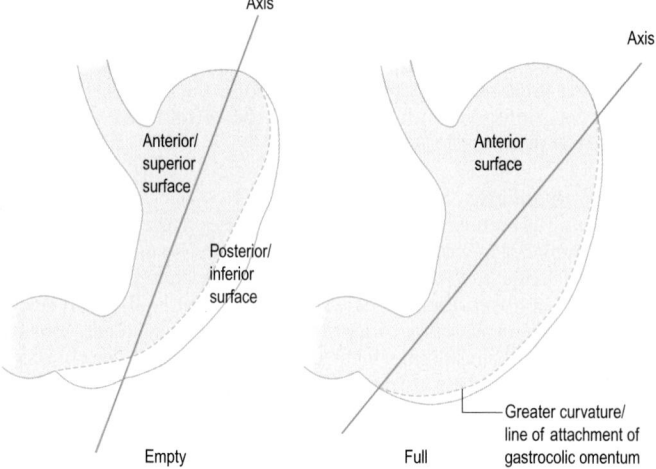

Fig. 71.5 Axes of the empty and full stomach. As the stomach distends, the greater curvature 'rolls' downwards and the anterosuperior surface comes to lie almost completely vertical as the anterior surface.

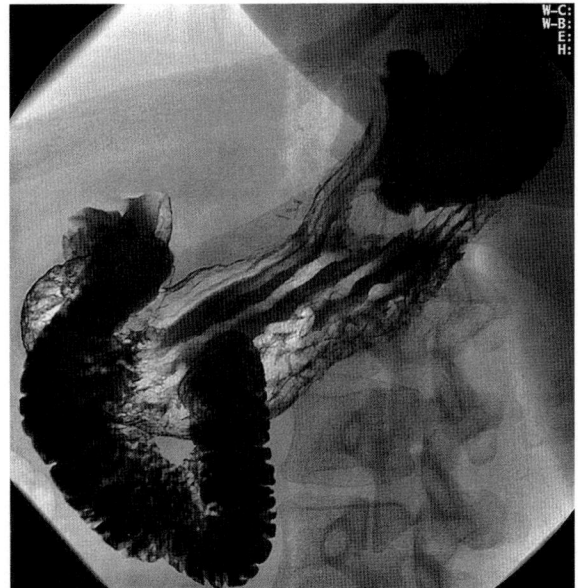

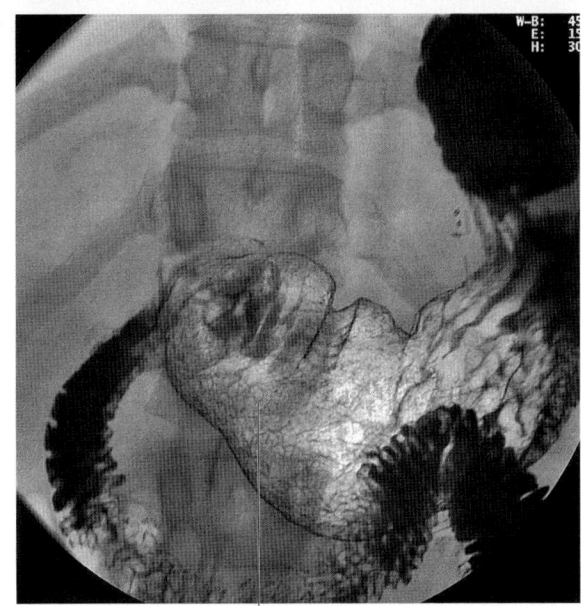

Area gastricae

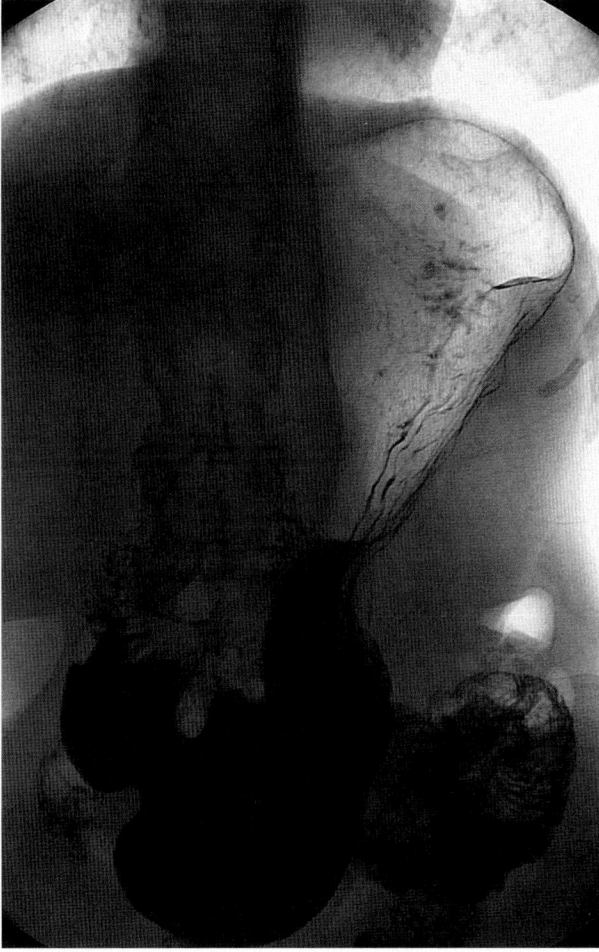

Fig. 71.6 Double contrast barium meal. **A**, Initial stomach filling demonstrates a horizontally lying stomach with prominent gastric rugal folds. **B**, The area gastricae within the antrum are clearly identified on distension of the stomach. **C**, In the erect position the stomach has a more 'J'-shaped configuration.

The left gastric artery may arise from the common hepatic artery or its branches. The most common variant is an origin from the left hepatic artery, when the left gastric artery passes between the peritoneal layers of the superior lesser omentum to reach the lesser curvature of the stomach. Other variants include a common origin with the common hepatic artery. An aberrant left hepatic artery can occasionally arise from the left gastric artery: identification of an aberrant origin may be of importance during surgical mobilization of the upper stomach.

Short gastric arteries
The short gastric arteries are variable in number, commonly between five and seven, and arise from the splenic artery, its divisions, or from the proximal left gastroepiploic artery. They pass between layers of the gastrosplenic ligament to supply the cardiac orifice and gastric fundus, and anastomose with branches of the left gastric and left gastroepiploic arteries. An accessory left gastric artery may arise with these vessels from the distal splenic artery.

Left gastroepiploic artery
The left gastroepiploic artery arises from the splenic artery as its largest branch near the splenic hilum. It runs anteroinferiorly between the layers of the gastrosplenic ligament and into the upper gastrocolic omentum. It lies between the layers of peritoneum close to the greater curvature, running inferiorly to anastomose with the right gastro-

epiploic artery. It gives off gastric branches to the fundus of the stomach through the gastrosplenic ligament and to the body of the stomach through the gastrocolic omentum. These are necessarily longer than the gastric branches of the right gastroepiploic artery and may be 8–10 cm long. Epiploic (omental) branches arise along the course of the vessel and descend between the layers of the gastrocolic omentum into the greater omentum. A particularly large epiploic branch commonly originates close to the origin of the left gastroepiploic artery, descends in the lateral portion of the greater omentum and provides a large arterial supply to the lateral half of the omentum.

Posterior gastric artery
Variant: A distinct posterior gastric artery may occur. When present, it arises from the splenic artery in its middle section posterior to the body of the stomach. It ascends behind the peritoneum of the lesser sac towards the fundus. It reaches the posterior surface of the stomach in the gastrophrenic fold.

Right gastric artery
The right gastric artery arises from the hepatic artery as it passes forwards from the posterior wall of the lesser sac into the lower border of the lesser omentum above the first part of the duodenum. The right gastric artery then runs between the peritoneal layers of the lesser omentum just above the medial end of the lesser curvature. It passes superiorly along the lesser curvature, giving off multiple branches onto

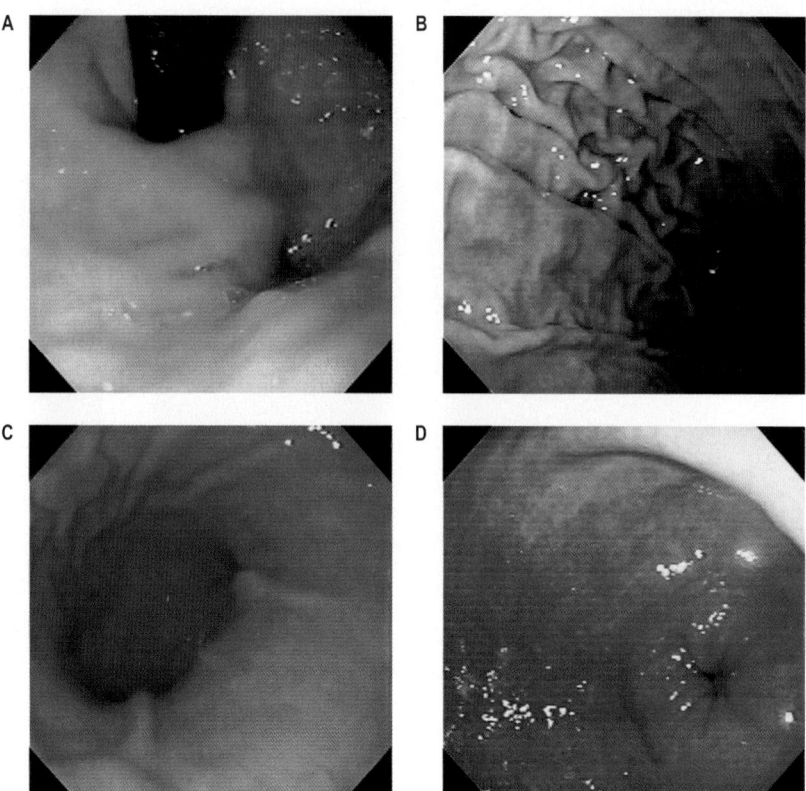

Fig. 71.7 Endoscopic appearance of the stomach: **A**, cardiac orifice from below; **B**, body greater curvature; **C**, body lesser curvature; **D**, pylorus.

the anterior and posterior surfaces of the stomach, and anastomoses with the left gastric artery.

The origin of the right gastric artery is often variant. The most common alternative origins are from the common hepatic, left hepatic, gastroduodenal or supraduodenal arteries.

Gastroduodenal artery

The gastroduodenal artery arises from the common hepatic artery posterior and superior to the first part of the duodenum. It gives origin to the right gastroepiploic and superior pancreaticoduodenal arteries at the lower border of the first part of the duodenum.

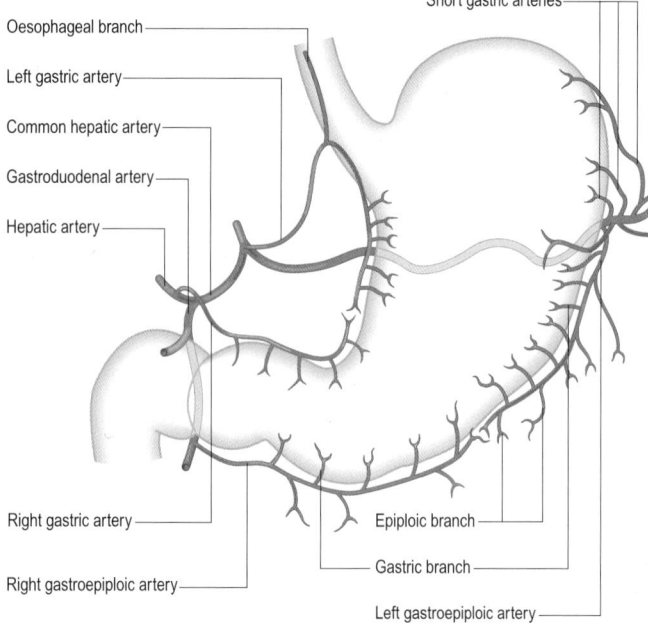

Fig. 71.8 Arterial supply of the stomach.

Right gastroepiploic artery

The right gastroepiploic artery originates from the gastroduodenal artery behind the first part of the duodenum, anterior to the head of the pancreas. It passes inferiorly towards the midline between the layers of the gastrocolic omentum. It lies inferior to the pylorus and then runs laterally along the greater curvature. It ends by anastomosing with the left gastroepiploic artery. It is adjacent to the pylorus but, more distally, lies c.2 cm from the greater curvature of the stomach. Gastric branches ascend onto the anterior and posterior surfaces of the antrum and lower body of the stomach while epiploic branches descend into the greater omentum. It also contributes to the supply of the inferior aspect of the first part of the duodenum.

Arterial anastomoses of the stomach

There is an anastomosis between the oesophageal arteries originating from the thoracic aorta and the vessels supplying the fundus in the region of the cardiac orifice. At the pyloric orifice the extensive network of vessels supplying the duodenum allows for some anastomosis between vessels of superior mesenteric artery origin and the pyloric vessels. The major named vessels supplying the stomach form extensive arterial anastomoses both on the serosal surface and around the curvatures. The right and left gastroepiploic arteries and the left and right gastric arteries anastomose freely with each other along the greater and lesser curvatures respectively. Anastomoses also form between the short gastric and left gastric arteries in the region of the fundus, and between the right gastric and right gastroepiploic arteries in the region of the antrum. In addition to the extensive serosal anastomoses, networks form within the stomach wall at intramuscular, submucosal and mucosal levels. A true plexus of small arteries and arterioles is present within the submucosa: it supplies the mucosa and shows considerable regional variation both in the gastric wall and in the proximal duodenum. The rich arterial supply to the stomach ensures that the high mucosal blood flow required for physiological functioning is maintained even if one or more vessels become occluded. As a consequence, the stomach exhibits considerable resistance to ischaemia even when multiple arterial supplies are lost.

The pyloric arteries are rami of the right gastric and right gastroepiploic arteries and pierce the duodenum distal to the sphincter around its entire circumference. They pass through the muscular layer to the submucosa where they divide into two or three rami, which turn back into the pyloric canal beneath the mucosa and run to the end of the pyloric antrum (**Fig. 71.10**). They supply the entire mucosa of the pyloric

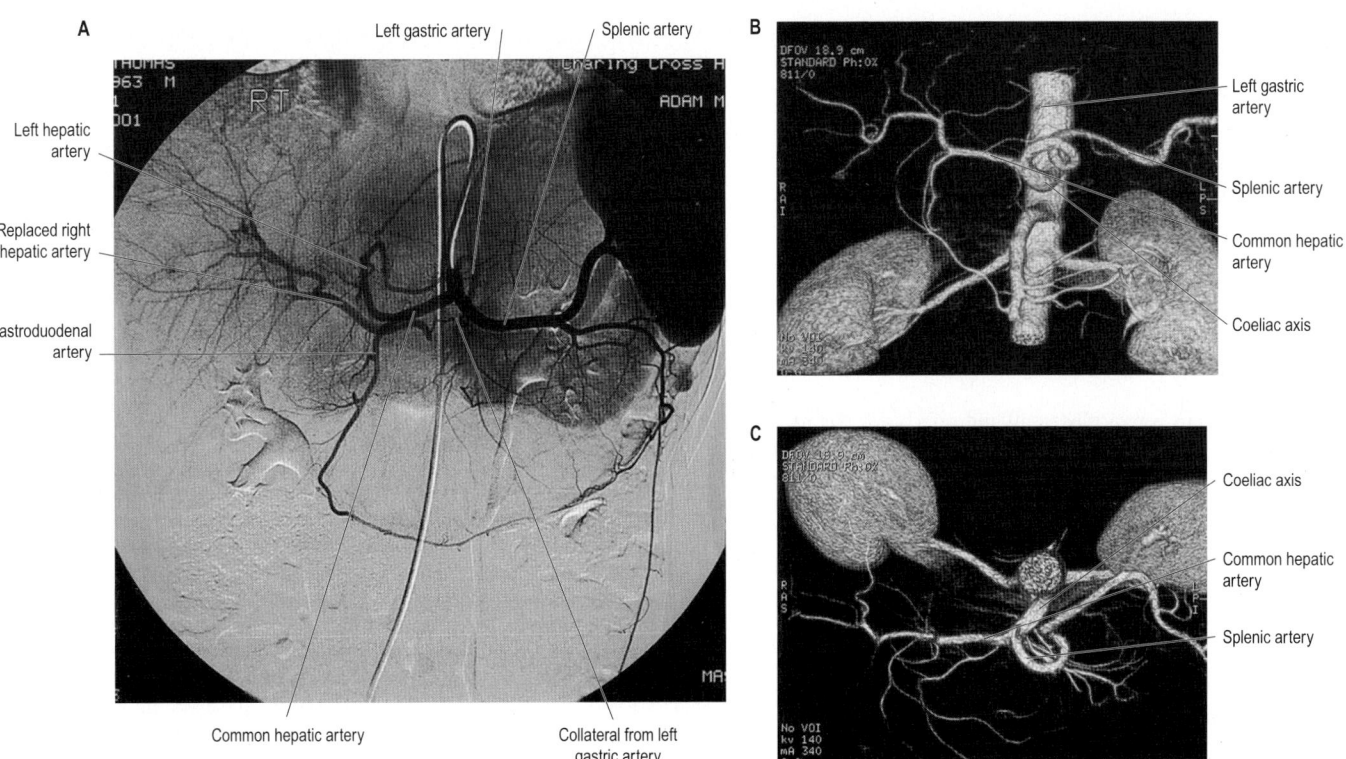

Fig. 71.9 The coeliac axis and its branches demonstrated on: **A**, digital subtraction angiogram demonstrating a replaced right hepatic artery arising from the origin of the superior mesenteric artery and being filled by a collateral from the left gastric artery. (**A**, by kind permission from Dr Adam Mitchell, Charing Cross Hospital London; **B** and **C**, by kind permission from GE Worldwide Medical Systems.)

canal. Branches of these pyloric submucosal arteries may anastomose close to their origin with the duodenal submucosal arteries. Their terminal rami also anastomose with gastric arteries from the prepyloric antrum. The pyloric sphincter is supplied by the gastric and pyloric arteries via rami that leave their parent vessels in the subserosal and submucosal levels to penetrate the sphincter.

Dieu la Foy lesions

Abnormalities of the intramural vascularity of the stomach are a rare cause of bleeding from the upper gastrointestinal tract. So-called 'Dieu la Foy' lesions commonly occur in the proximal body or fundus. When not actively bleeding, they appear as small, raised, red dots marking the mucosal surface of the proximal body or fundus. They were originally thought to be small arteriovenous malformations of the submucosal plexus. It is now considered that such lesions are caused by a larger than normal penetrating arterial vessel running through the muscular coat of the stomach into the submucosa before branching into the submucosal plexus. Although not a pathological abnormality, the vessel has a greater than normal calibre for arteries at this level. The pulsatile flow, combined with its proximity to the overlying mucosa, may then lead to focal ulceration and rupture of the vessel following minor trauma, leading to profuse intraluminal bleeding.

VEINS

The stomach veins drain ultimately into the portal vein. A rich submucosal and intramural network of veins gives rise to veins that usually accompany the corresponding named arteries. They drain either into the splenic or superior mesenteric veins although some pass directly into the portal vein.

Short gastric veins

Four or five short gastric veins drain the gastric fundus and the upper part of the greater curvature. They drain into the splenic vein or one of its large tributaries.

Left gastroepiploic vein

The left gastroepiploic vein drains both anterior and posterior gastric surfaces and the adjacent greater omentum. It runs superolaterally along

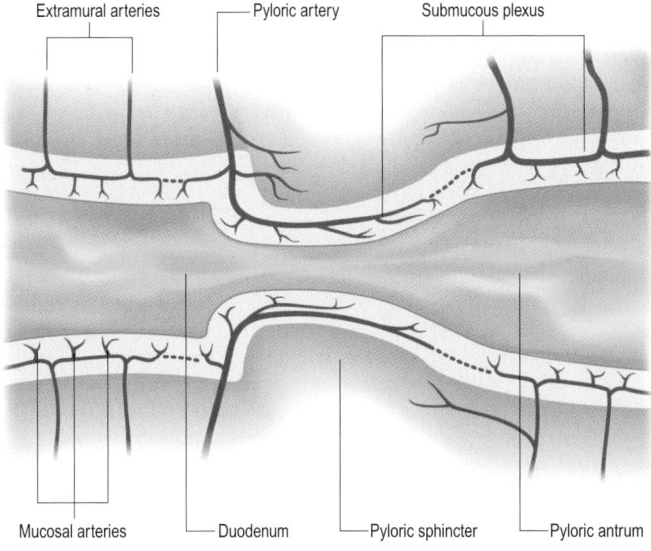

Fig. 71.10 Blood supply of the stomach and the proximal duodenum. A scheme of arterial arrangements at the gastroduodenal junction. Dotted lines indicate sites where the submucous plexus may be non-continuous. Shaded areas represent the muscular layer of the visceral wall. (Redrawn courtesy of C Piasecki, Department of Anatomy, Royal Free Hospital School of Medicine, London and the Journal of Anatomy.)

the greater curvature, between the layers of the gastrocolic omentum. It receives multiple tributaries from the anterior and posterior surfaces of the body of the stomach and the greater omentum, and drains into the splenic vein within the gastrosplenic ligament.

Right gastroepiploic vein

The right gastroepiploic vein drains the greater omentum, distal body and antrum of the stomach. It passes medially, inferior to the greater curvature, in the upper portion of the gastrocolic omentum. Just proximal to the pyloric constriction it passes posteriorly to drain into the superior mesenteric vein below the neck of the pancreas. It may receive the superior pancreaticoduodenal vein close to its entry into the superior mesenteric vein.

Left gastric vein
The left gastric vein drains the upper body and fundus of the stomach. It ascends along the lesser curvature to the oesophageal opening where it receives several lower oesophageal veins. It then curves posteriorly and medially behind the posterior peritoneal surface of the lesser sac. It drains into the portal vein directly at the level of the upper border of the first part of the duodenum.

Right gastric vein
The right gastric vein is typically small and runs along the medial end of the lesser curvature. It passes under the peritoneum as it is reflected from the posterior aspect of the pylorus and first part of the duodenum onto the posterior wall of the lesser sac. It drains directly into the portal vein at the level of the first part of the duodenum. It receives the prepyloric vein as it ascends anterior to the pylorus at the level of the pyloric opening.

Posterior gastric veins
Distinct posterior gastric veins may occur. When present, they accompany the posterior gastric artery from the middle of the posterior surface of the stomach. They drain into the splenic vein and may occur as multiple small vessels.

Gastric varices
Variceal dilatation of the submucosal veins of the stomach may occur in the presence of portal hypertension. The anastomosis between portal and systemic venous circulations occurs around the lower oesophagus and upper stomach. Submucosal veins close to the cardiac orifice may become involved in the pathological flow of blood from the stomach and other upper abdominal viscera into the oesophageal veins. Gastric varices present less commonly in clinical practice than oesophageal varices. Occasionally gastric varices exist without the presence of oesophageal varices. In these circumstances, it may be that the effective 'point of meeting' between portal and systemic venous systems is lower than usual and occurs in the upper stomach rather than the lower oesophagus.

LYMPHATIC DRAINAGE
The stomach has a rich network of lymphatics that connect with lymphatics draining the other visceral organs of the upper abdomen. At the gastro-oesophageal junction the lymphatics are continuous with those draining the lower oesophagus. In the region of the pylorus they are continuous with those draining the duodenum. In the main, they follow the course of the arteries supplying the stomach, however many separate node groups are now recognized (**Fig. 71.11**). The relationship of separate node groups to the regions of the stomach and the vascular territories supplied is of great importance during resection of the stomach, particularly for malignancy. Pancreatic and hepatic lymphatics play a considerable role in draining areas of the stomach during disease.

INNERVATION

The stomach is innervated by sympathetic and parasympathetic fibres. The sympathetic supply originates from the fifth to twelfth thoracic spinal segments and is mainly distributed to the stomach via the greater and lesser splanchnic nerves and the coeliac plexus. Periarterial plexuses form along the arteries and supply the stomach from the coeliac axis. Additional innervation comes from fibres of the hepatic plexus, which pass to the upper body and fundus via the upper limit of the lesser omentum. Some innervation is also provided via direct branches from the greater splanchnic nerves.

The parasympathetic supply is from the vagus nerves (**Fig. 71.12**). Usually one or two rami branch on the anterior and posterior aspects of the gastro-oesophageal junction. The anterior nerves are mostly from the left vagus and the posterior from the right vagus, both emerging from the oesophageal plexus.

The anterior nerves supply filaments to the cardiac orifice and divide near the oesophageal end of the lesser curvature into gastric, pyloric and hepatic branches. Gastric branches (between four and ten) radiate on the anterior surface of the body and fundus. The greater anterior gastric nerve is the major gastric branch and lies in the lesser omentum near the lesser curvature. Pyloric branches (generally two) originate below the cardiac orifice. The smaller of the two nerves runs between the peritoneal layers of the lesser omentum almost horizontally towards its free edge and turns down on the left side of the hepatic artery to reach the pylorus. The larger nerve usually arises from the greater anterior gastric nerve during its course over the anterior surface of the stomach and runs inferomedially to the pyloric antrum. Hepatic branches (one or two) originate from the pyloric branches and run superiorly to contribute to the hepatic plexus.

The posterior nerves produce two main groups of branches, gastric and coeliac. Gastric branches originate behind the cardiac orifice and upper body of the stomach. They radiate over the posterior surface of the body and fundus and extend to the antrum but do not reach the pyloric sphincter. The largest is termed the greater posterior gastric nerve and runs posteriorly along the lesser curvature, giving branches to the coeliac plexus. Coeliac branches are often larger than the gastric branches. They run beneath the peritoneum, deep to the posterior wall of the lesser sac, at the upper limit of the lesser omentum to reach the coeliac plexus. Hepatic branches (one or two) are often small and originate from the coeliac branches. No true plexus occurs on either the anterior or posterior gastric surfaces, but plexuses are present in the submucosa and between the layers of the muscularis externa.

The gastric sympathetic nerves are vasoconstrictor to the gastric vasculature and inhibitory to gastric musculature. The sympathetic supply to the pylorus is motor, and brings about pyloric constriction. The sympathetic supply also conducts afferent impulses that mediate sensations, including pain. The parasympathetic gastric supply is secretomotor to the gastric mucosa and motor to the gastric musculature. It is also responsible for coordinated relaxation of the pyloric sphincter during gastric emptying.

Coeliac plexus
The coeliac plexus is the largest major autonomic plexus, sited at the level of the twelfth thoracic and first lumbar vertebrae. It is a dense network uniting two large coeliac ganglia and surrounds the coeliac artery and the root of the superior mesenteric artery (**Fig. 71.13**). It is posterior to the stomach and lesser sac, anterior to the crura of the diaphragm and the commencement of the abdominal aorta, and lies between the suprarenal glands. The plexus and ganglia are joined by greater and lesser splanchnic nerves and branches from the vagus and phrenic nerves. The plexus extends as numerous secondary plexuses along adjacent arteries.

The coeliac ganglia are irregular masses on each side of the coeliac trunk adjacent to the suprarenal glands. They lie anterior to the crura of the diaphragm. The right ganglion is posterior to the inferior vena cava, the left ganglion posterior to the origin of the splenic artery. The ipsilateral greater splanchnic nerve joins the upper part of each ganglion. The lower part of each ganglion forms a distinct subdivision usually termed the aorticorenal ganglion. This receives the ipsilateral lesser splanchnic nerve and gives origin to the majority of the renal plexus. It most commonly lies anterior to the origin of the renal artery. The coeliac plexus is connected to or gives rise to the phrenic, splenic, hepatic, superior mesenteric, suprarenal, renal and gonadal plexuses.

Phrenic plexus
The phrenic plexus lies around the inferior phrenic arteries on the crura of the diaphragm. It arises as a superior extension of the coeliac ganglion and often receives one or two sensory branches from the phrenic nerve. The left phrenic plexus is usually larger than the right. On the left it supplies branches to the left suprarenal gland and the cardiac orifice of the stomach. The right phrenic plexus joins the phrenic nerve, forming a small phrenic ganglion. This distributes branches to the inferior vena cava, suprarenal gland and hepatic plexus.

REFERRED PAIN
The majority of the sensation of pain arising from the stomach is poorly localized. In common with other structures of foregut origin, it is referred to the central epigastrium. Pain arising from the region of the

A

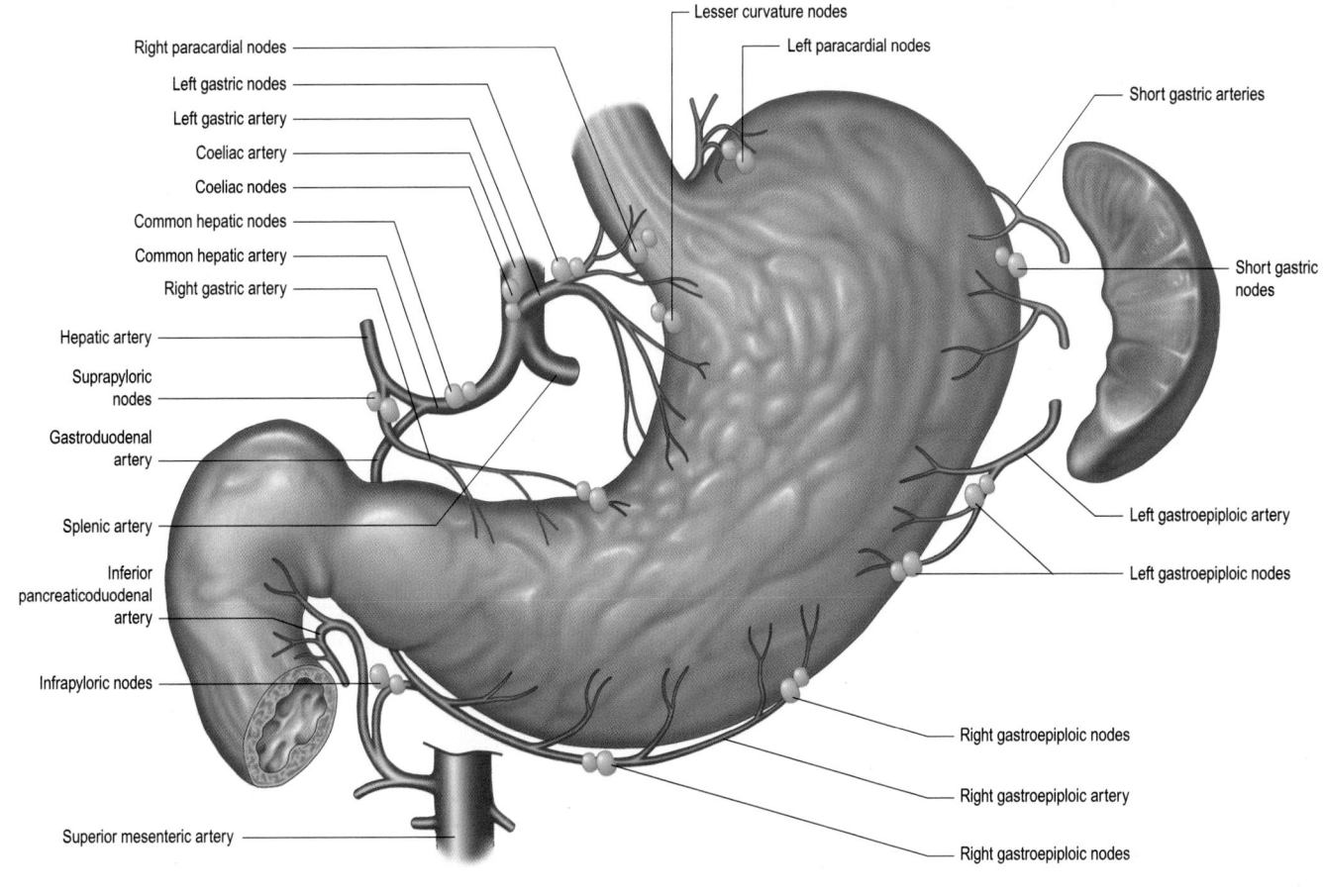

Right paracardial nodes

Left gastric nodes

Left gastric artery

Coeliac artery

Coeliac nodes

Common hepatic nodes

Common hepatic artery

Right gastric artery

Hepatic artery

Suprapyloric nodes

Gastroduodenal artery

Splenic artery

Inferior pancreaticoduodenal artery

Infrapyloric nodes

Superior mesenteric artery

Lesser curvature nodes

Left paracardial nodes

Short gastric arteries

Short gastric nodes

Left gastroepiploic artery

Left gastroepiploic nodes

Right gastroepiploic nodes

Right gastroepiploic artery

Right gastroepiploic nodes

B

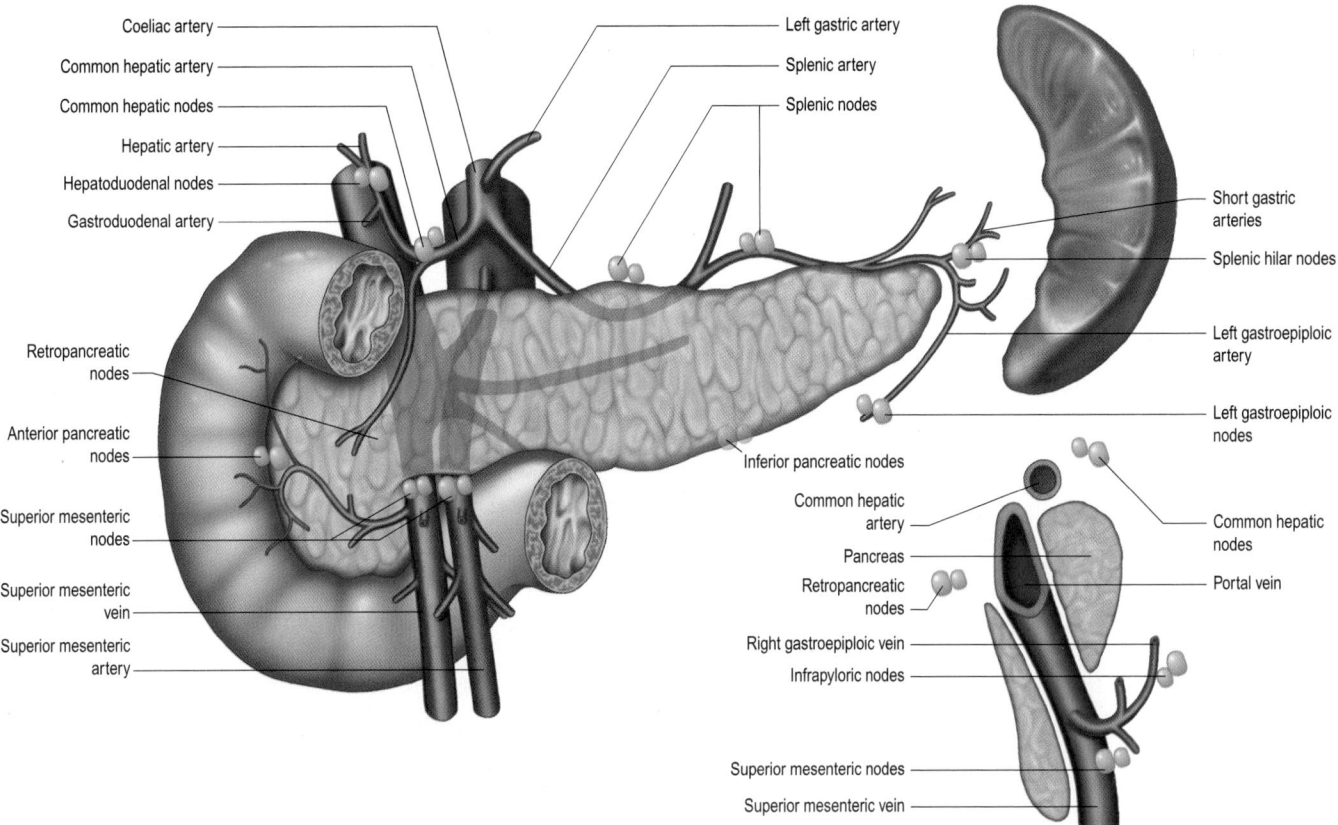

Coeliac artery

Common hepatic artery

Common hepatic nodes

Hepatic artery

Hepatoduodenal nodes

Gastroduodenal artery

Retropancreatic nodes

Anterior pancreatic nodes

Superior mesenteric nodes

Superior mesenteric vein

Superior mesenteric artery

Left gastric artery

Splenic artery

Splenic nodes

Short gastric arteries

Splenic hilar nodes

Left gastroepiploic artery

Left gastroepiploic nodes

Inferior pancreatic nodes

Common hepatic artery

Pancreas

Retropancreatic nodes

Right gastroepiploic vein

Infrapyloric nodes

Common hepatic nodes

Portal vein

Superior mesenteric nodes

Superior mesenteric vein

Fig. 71.11 Lymph node stations of **A**, the stomach and **B**, upper abdominal viscera.

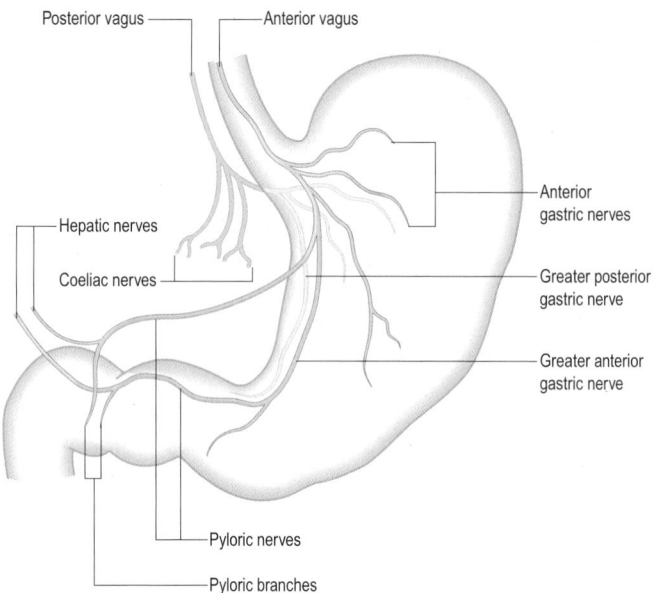

Fig. 71.12 Distribution of the vagal nerves to the stomach.

gastro-oesophageal junction may involve innervation from the oesophagus and is commonly referred to the lower retrosternal and subxiphoid areas.

MICROSTRUCTURE

The gastric wall consists of the major layers found elsewhere in the gut, i.e. mucosa, submucosa, muscularis externa and serosa, together with gastric vessels and nerves (**Figs 71.14, 71.15**). The microstructure reflects the functions of the stomach as an expandable muscular sac lined by secretory epithelium, although there are local structural and functional variations in this pattern.

Mucosa

The mucosa is a thick layer with a soft, smooth surface that is mostly reddish brown in life but pink in the pyloric region. In the contracted stomach the mucosa is folded into numerous folds or rugae, most of

which are longitudinal. They are most marked towards the pyloric end and along the greater curvature (**Fig. 71.7**). The rugae represent large folds in the submucosal connective tissue (see below) rather than variations in the thickness of the mucosa covering them, and they are obliterated when the stomach is distended. As elsewhere in the gut, the mucosa is composed of a surface epithelium, lamina propria and muscularis mucosae.

EPITHELIUM

When viewed microscopically at low magnification, the internal surface of the stomach wall (**Fig. 71.15**) appears honeycombed by small, irregular gastric pits c.0.2 mm in diameter. The base of each gastric pit receives several long, tubular gastric glands that extend deep into the lamina propria as far as the muscularis mucosae. Simple columnar mucus-secreting epithelium covers the entire luminal surface including the gastric pits, and is composed of a continuous layer of surface mucous cells which release gastric mucus from their apical surfaces to form a thick protective, lubricant layer over the gastric lining. This epithelium commences abruptly at the cardiac orifice, where there is a sudden transition from oesophageal stratified epithelium.

Gastric glands

Although all gastric glands are tubular, they vary in form and cellular composition in different parts of the stomach. They can be divided into three groups – the cardiac, principal (in the body and fundus) and pyloric glands. The most highly specialized are the principal glands.

Principal gastric glands

The principal glands are found in the body and fundus, three to seven opening into each gastric pit (**Figs 71.14, 71.15, 71.16**). Their junction with the base of the pit is termed the isthmus of the gland and immediately basal to this is the neck, the remainder being the base. In the walls of the gland are at least five distinct cell types: chief, parietal, mucous neck, stem and neuroendocrine.

The chief (peptic) cells (**Figs 71.14, 71.16**) are the source of the digestive enzymes pepsin and lipase. They are usually basal in position, their shape is cuboidal and their nuclei rounded and euchromatic. They contain secretory zymogen granules and because of the abundant cytoplasmic RNA they are strongly basophilic. The parietal (oxyntic) cells are the source of gastric acid and of intrinsic factor, a glycoprotein necessary for the absorption of vitamin B_{12}. They are large, oval and strongly eosinophilic, with centrally placed nuclei. They are mainly situated in the more apical half of the gland, reaching as far as the isthmus. They occur only at intervals along the walls, and bulge laterally into the surrounding connective tissue. Parietal cells have a unique ultra-structure related to their ability to secrete hydrochloric acid. The luminal side of the cell is deeply invaginated to form a series of blind-ended

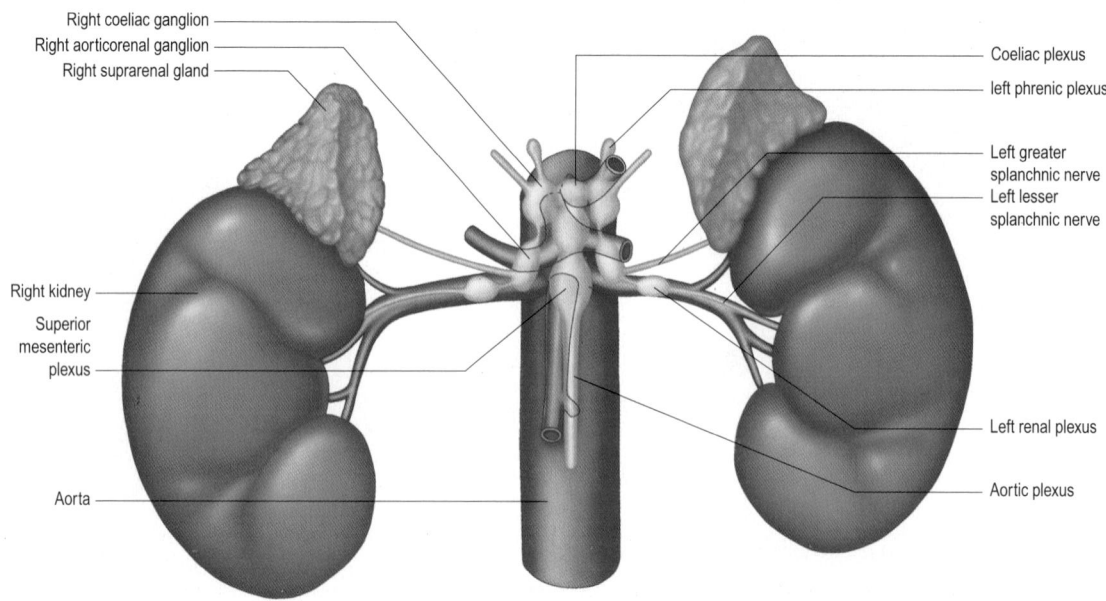

Fig. 71.13 Distribution of the upper abdominal autonomic plexuses.

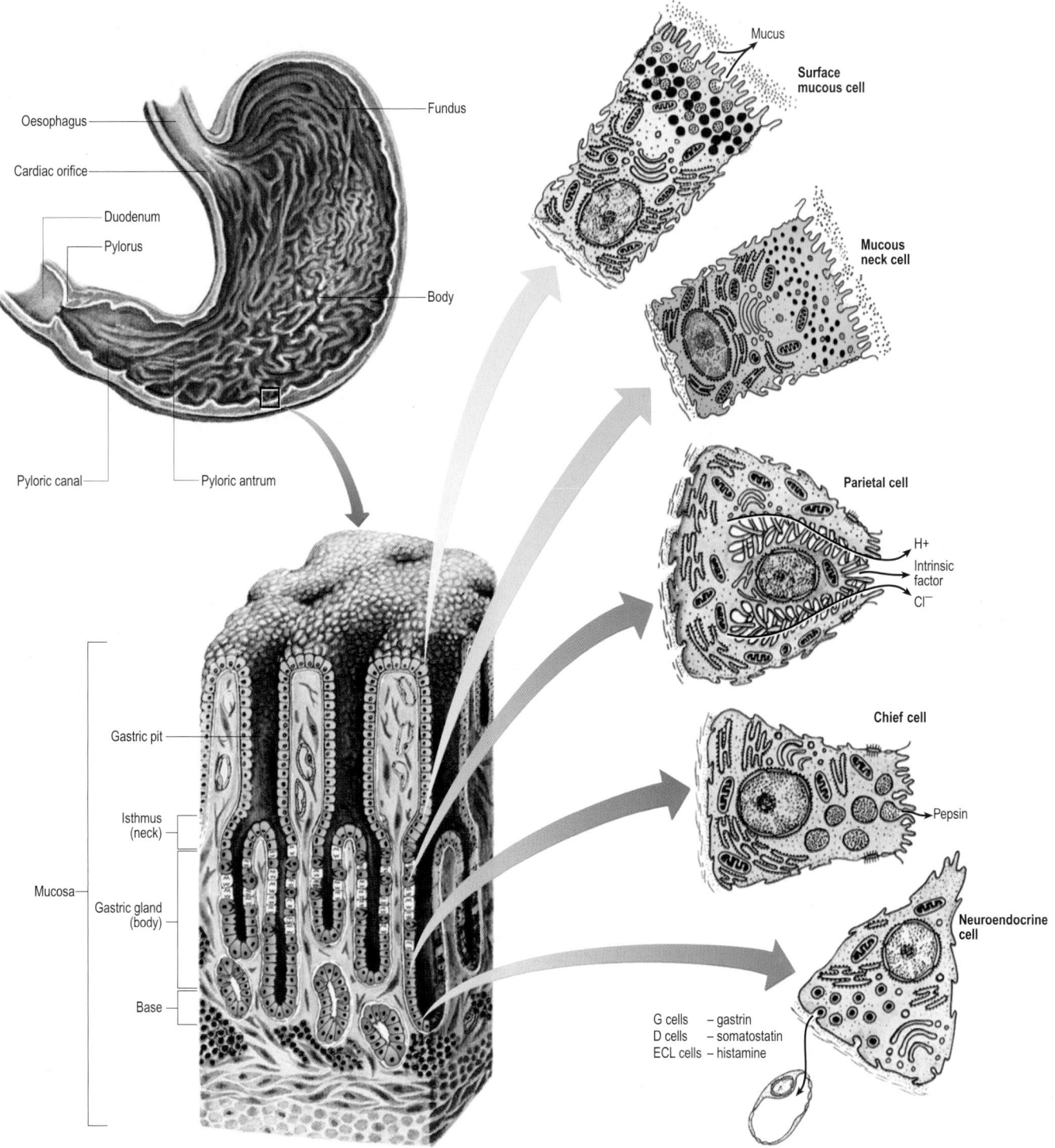

Fig. 71.14 Diagram showing the principal regions of the interior of the stomach and the microstructure of tissues and cells within its wall. Undifferentiated, dividing cells are shown in white.

channels (canaliculi) bearing numerous irregular microvilli. Within the cytoplasm facing these channels are numerous fine membranous tubules (the tubulo-vesicular system) directed towards the canalicular surface. Abundant mitochondria are interspersed among these organelles. The plasma membrane covering the microvilli has a high concentration of H^+/K^+ ATPase antiporter channels that actively secrete hydrogen ions into the lumen, chloride ions following along the electrochemical gradient. The precise structure of the cell varies with its secretory phase: when stimulated, the numbers and surface areas of the microvilli increase up to five-fold, thought to be by the rapid fusion of the tubulo-vesicular system with the plasma membrane. At the end of stimulated secretion, this process is reversed, the excess membrane retreats back into the tubulo-alveolar system and microvilli are lost.

Mucous neck cells are numerous at the necks of the glands and are scattered along the walls of the more basal regions. They are typical mucus-secreting cells, with apical secretory vesicles containing mucins, and basally displaced nuclei. However, their products are distinct histochemically from those of the superficial mucous cells.

Stem cells are relatively undifferentiated mitotic cells from which the other types of gland cell are derived. They are relatively few in number, and are situated in the isthmus region of the gland and bases of the gastric pits. These cells are columnar, with a few short apical microvilli. They periodically undergo mitosis, the cells they produce migrating apically to differentiate into new surface mucous cells, or basally to form mucous neck, parietal and chief cells, and also the neuroendocrine cells. All of these cells have a limited lifespan, especially

1153

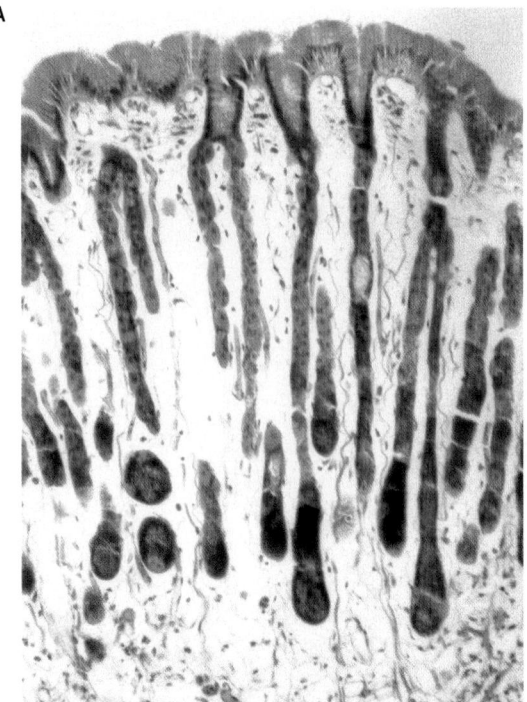

A

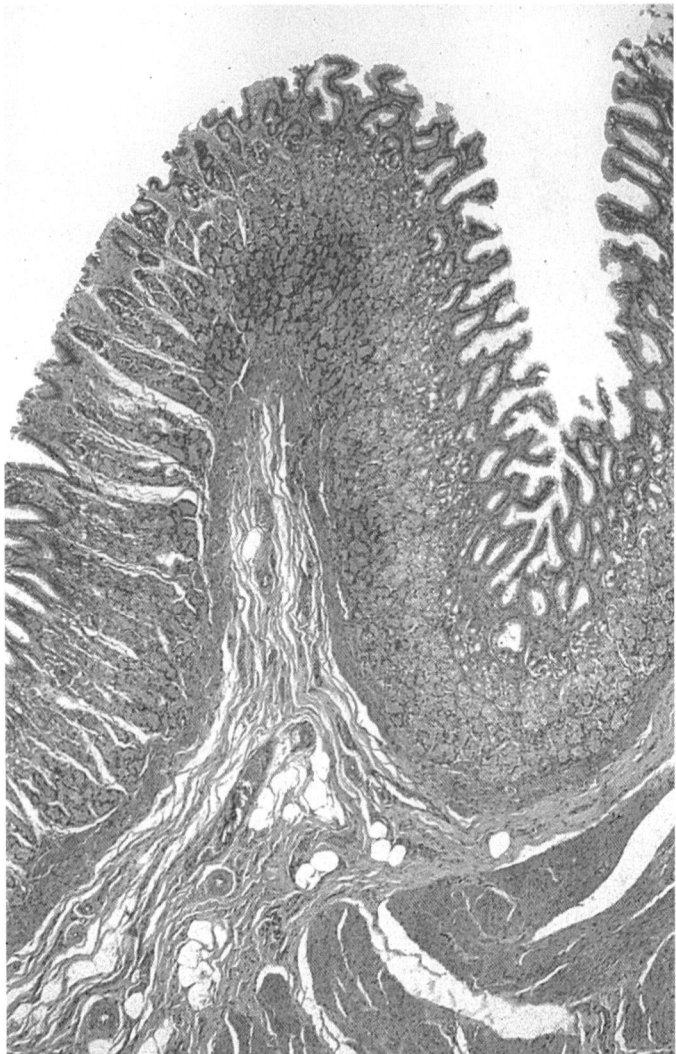

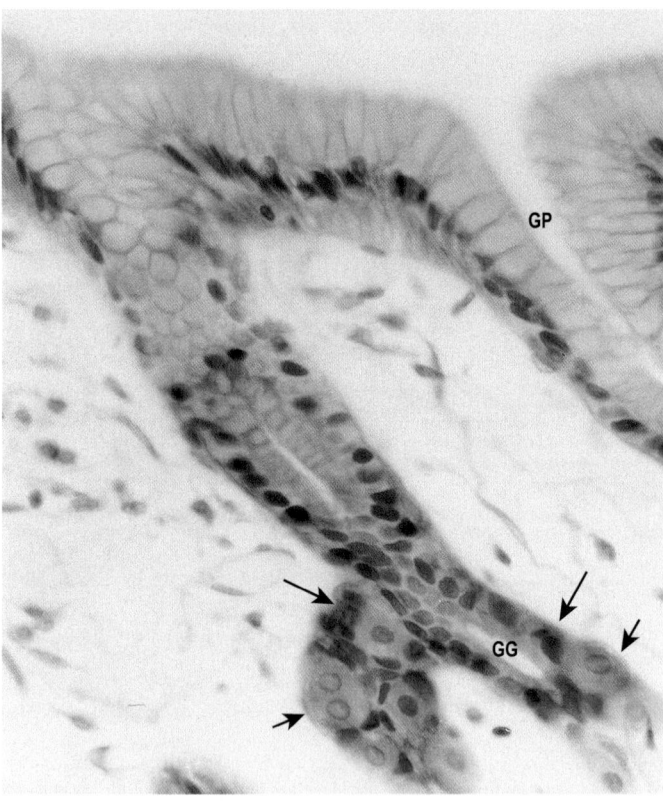

B

Fig. 71.15 Low power micrograph showing the stomach wall, in the region of a longitudinal fold or ruga, visible macroscopically. The surface epithelium is infolded microscopically to form gastric pits, into the bases of which open gastric glands extending through the thickness of the mucosal lamina propria. A muscularis mucosae layer and submucosa follow the contours of the ruga and part of the external muscularis layers is seen below. (By permission from Kierszenbaum AL 2002 Histology and Cell Biology. St Louis: Mosby.)

the mucus-secreting types, and are constantly replaced. The replacement period for surface mucous cells is c.3 days; mucous neck cells are replaced after c.1 week. Other cell types appear to live much longer.

Neuroendocrine (enteroendocrine) cells occur in all types of gastric gland but more frequently in the body and fundus. They are situated mainly in the deeper parts of the glands, among the chief cells. They are basally situated, pleomorphic cells with irregular nuclei surrounded by granular cytoplasm containing clusters of large (0.3 μm) secretory granules. These cells synthesize a number of biogenic amines and polypeptides important in the control of motility and glandular secretion. In the stomach they include cells designated as G cells secreting gastrin, D cells (somatostatin), and ECL (enterochromaffin-like) cells (histamine). They form part of the system of dispersed neuroendocrine cells.

Cardiac glands
Cardiac glands are confined to a small area near the cardiac orifice (**Fig. 71.17**); some are simple tubular glands, others are compound branched tubular. Mucus-secreting cells predominate and parietal and chief cells, although present, are few.

Pyloric glands
Pyloric glands enter as groups of two or three short convoluted tubes into the bases of the deep gastric pits of the pyloric antrum: the pits

Fig. 71.16 A, Micrograph showing gastric glands in the fundic region, opening into the bases of gastric pits lined by mucous cells similar to those covering the epithelial surface. Eosinophilic parietal cells and basophilic chief cells line the glands, shown at higher magnification in **B** (photograph by Sarah-Jane Smith). **B**, Higher power micrograph showing eosinophilic parietal cells (short arrows) and basophilic chief cells (long arrows) lining the gastric glands (GG); these open into gastric pits (GP), which are invaginations of the mucus-secreting surface epithelium.

occupy about two-thirds of the mucosal depth (**Fig. 71.18**). Pyloric glands are mostly populated with mucus-secreting cells, parietal cells are few and chief cells scarce. In contrast, neuroendocrine cells are numerous, especially G cells, which secrete gastrin when activated by appropriate mechanical stimulation (causing increased gastric motility and secretion of gastric juices). Although parietal cells are infrequent in

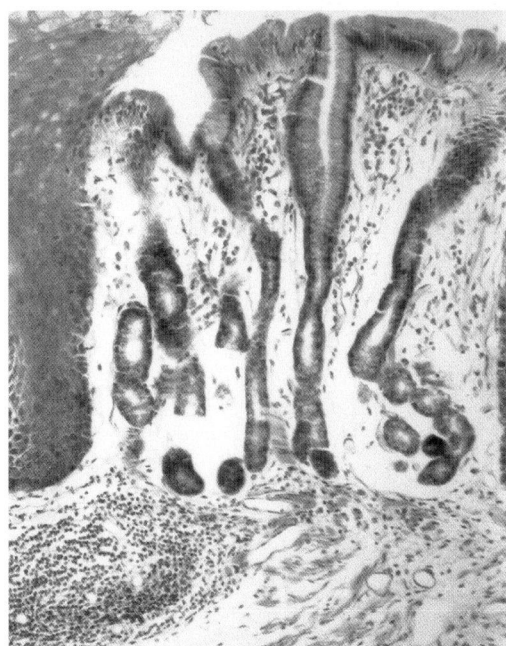

Fig. 71.17 Micrograph showing the junction between the stratified squamous non-keratinizing epithelium of the oesophagus (left) and the stomach, with cardiac glands. A lymphoid follicle (an example of MALT) is seen in the submucosa of the junction zone (bottom left). (Photograph by Sarah-Jane Smith.)

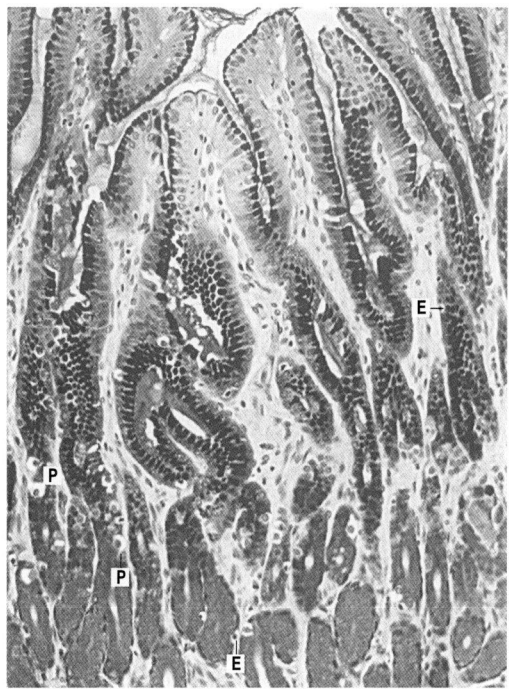

Fig. 71.18 Micrograph showing the pyloric region of the stomach with pyloric glands, stained with the periodic acid-Schiff (PAS) technique to show mucin (magenta) in the gastric pits and glands. Pale staining cells are the larger parietal cells (P) and smaller enteroendocrine cells (E). (By permission from Dr JB Kerr, Monash University, from Kerr JB 1999 Atlas of Functional Histology. London: Mosby.)

pyloric glands, they are always present in fetal and postnatal tissue. In adults they may appear in the duodenal mucosa proximally near the pylorus.

LAMINA PROPRIA

The lamina propria forms a connective tissue framework between the glands and contains lymphoid tissue that collects in small masses, gastric lymphatic follicles, which resemble solitary intestinal follicles (especially in early life). The lamina propria also contains a complex periglandular vascular plexus, which is thought to be important in the maintenance of the mucosal environment, including the removal of bicarbonate produced in the tissues as a counterpart to acid secretion. Neural plexuses are present and contain sensory and motor terminals.

MUSCULARIS MUCOSAE

The muscularis mucosae is a thin layer of smooth muscle fibres lying external to the layer of glands. Its fibres are arranged as inner circular and outer longitudinal layers, and there is also a discontinuous external circular layer. The inner layer sends strands of smooth muscle cells between the glands, and their contraction probably assists in emptying into the gastric pits.

Submucosa

The submucosa is a variable layer of loose connective tissue containing thick collagen bundles, numerous elastin fibres, blood vessels and nervous plexuses, including the ganglionated submucosal (Meissner's) plexus of the stomach.

Muscularis externa

The muscularis externa is a thick muscle coat immediately under the serosa, with which it is closely connected by subserous loose connective tissue. From innermost outwards it has oblique, circular and longitudinal layers of smooth muscle fibres, although the separation between layers may be indistinct in places. The circular layer is poorly developed in the oesophageal region but is thickened at the distal pyloric antrum to form the annular pyloric sphincter. The outer longitudinal layer is most pronounced in the upper two-thirds of the stomach and the inner oblique layer in the lower half.

The actions of the muscularis externa of the stomach produce a churning movement that mixes food with the gastric secretions. When the muscles contract, they reduce the volume of the stomach and throw the mucosa into longitudinal folds or rugae (see above). These flatten as the stomach distends with food and the musculature relaxes and thins. Muscle activity is controlled by a network of unmyelinated autonomic nerve fibres and their ganglia, lying between the muscle layers in the myenteric (Auerbach's) plexus.

Serosa or visceral peritoneum

The serosa is an extension of the visceral peritoneum and covers the entire surface except along the greater and lesser curvatures at the attachment of the greater and lesser omenta, where the peritoneal layers leave space for vessels and nerves. It is also absent from a small posteroinferior area near the cardiac orifice where the stomach contacts the diaphragm at the reflections of the gastrophrenic and left gastropancreatic folds.

REFERENCES

DiDio LJ, Anderson MC 1968 The 'Sphincters' of the Digestive System. Baltimore: Williams and Wilkins.

Japanese Research Society for Gastric Cancer 1998 Japanese Classification of Gastric Carcinoma. Tokyo: Kanehara & Co Ltd and Gastric Cancer 1: 10–24, 25–30.
A detailed, widely accepted, description of the lymph node fields of the upper abdominal viscera, particularly in relation to malignancy.

Silverstein FE, Tytgat GNJ 1991 Atlas of Gastrointestinal Endoscopy. 2nd edition. New York: Gower Medical Publishing.

Microstructure of the small intestine

The intestinal wall is composed of mucosa, submucosa, muscularis externa and serosa or adventitia (**Figs 70.1, 72.1 to 72.7**). The mucosa is thick and very vascular in the proximal small intestine, but thinner and less vascular distally. In places it is ridged by the underlying submucosa to form circular folds, and mucosal finger- or leaf-like intestinal villi cover the whole surface. There are numerous simple tubular intestinal glands or crypts between the bases of the villi, and additional submucosal glands in the duodenum.

CIRCULAR FOLDS

Large, crescentic folds of mucosa (**Figs 72.2, 72.3**) project into the intestinal lumen transversely or slightly obliquely to the long axis. Unlike gastric folds they are not obliterated by distension of the intestine. Most extend round half or two-thirds of the luminal circumference: some are complete circles; some bifurcate and join adjacent folds; some are spiral but extend only once (occasionally two or three times) round the lumen. Larger folds are c.8 mm deep at their broadest, but most are smaller than this, and larger folds often alternate with smaller ones. Folds begin to appear c.2.5–5 cm beyond the pylorus. Distal to the major duodenal papilla they are large and close together, as they also are in the proximal half of the jejunum. From here to midway along the ileum they diminish, and they disappear almost completely in the distal ileum, which accounts for the thinness of this part of the intestinal wall. The circular folds slow the passage of the intestinal contents and increase the absorptive surface. They are visible in radiographs after a barium meal.

INTESTINAL VILLI (Figs 70.1, 72.4, 72.5)

Intestinal villi are highly vascular projections of the mucosal surface, just visible to the naked eye. They cover the entire intestinal mucosa, increase the surface area of the lumen about eight-fold, and give it a velvety texture. Villi are large and numerous in the duodenum and

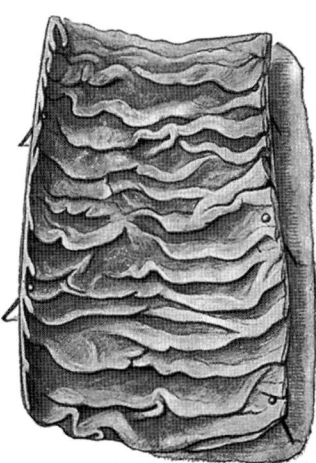

Fig. 72.2 Internal aspect of a representative sample of the proximal jejunum, showing circular folds.

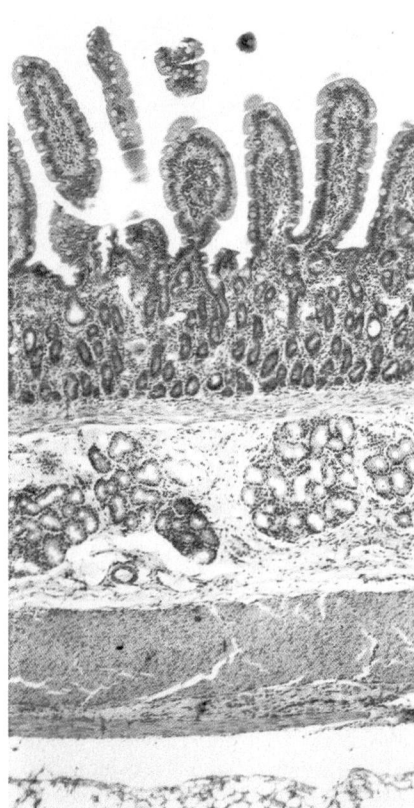

Fig. 72.1 Low-power micrograph showing the wall of the duodenum, with villi projecting into the lumen; intestinal crypts (of Lieberkühn) in the mucosa, seen mainly in transverse section; well-defined muscularis mucosae; submucosal seromucous (Brunner's) glands and muscularis externa. (Photograph by Sarah-Jane Smith.)

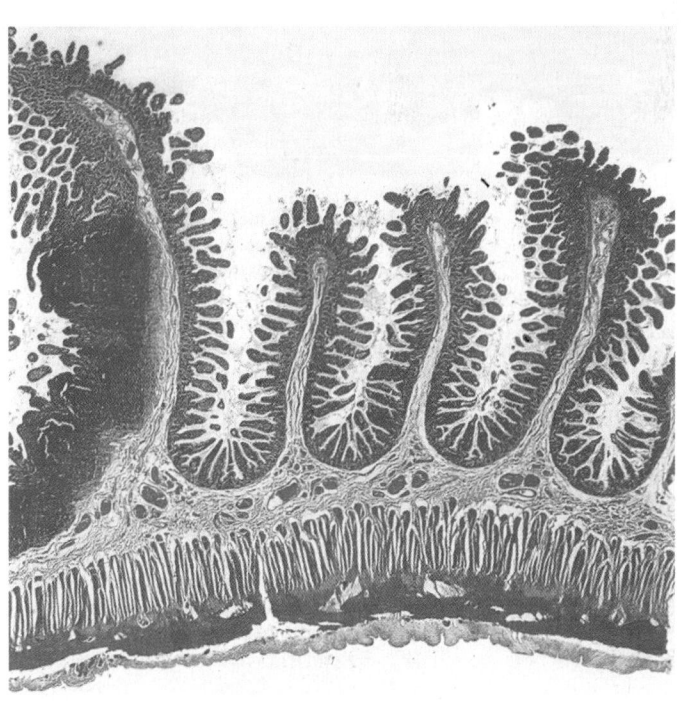

Fig. 72.3 Low-power micrograph showing several circular folds in the wall of the ileum. The folds are covered with villi projecting into the lumen and the submucosa extends into the core of each fold. Circular (innermost) and longitudinal smooth muscle layers form the underlying muscularis externa. Large masses of lymphoid tissue (Peyer's patches) occupy the mucosa at the left of the field. (By permission from Young B, Heath JW 2000 Wheater's Functional Histology. Edinburgh: Churchill Livingstone.)

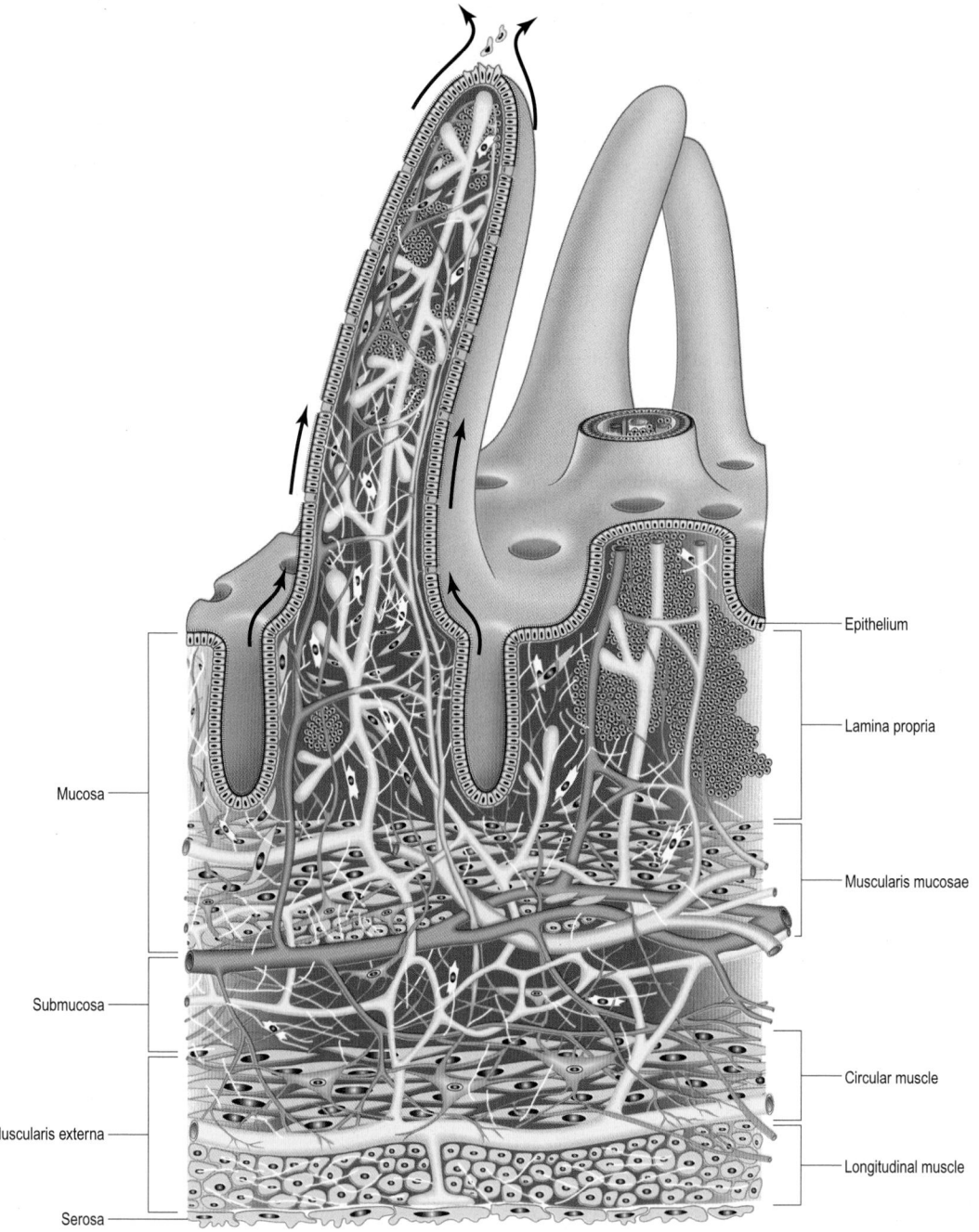

Fig. 72.4 A three-dimensional reconstruction of the architecture of an intestinal villus, indicating the underlying layers of the intestinal wall. Also shown are arteries and arterioles (red), veins and venules (blue), central lacteals and other lymphatic channels (yellow), lymphoid follicles (purple), neural elements (green), smooth muscle fibres (pink), and fibroblasts (white). Note the orifices of the intestinal crypts (of Lieberkühn). Types of cells in the epithelium include absorptive cells, goblet cells and neuroendocrine cells. Arrows indicate the direction of cell migration. The various layers are not drawn to scale.

jejunum, and smaller and fewer in the ileum. In the first part of the duodenum they appear as broad ridges, become tall and foliate in the distal duodenum and proximal jejunum, and then gradually shorten to a finger-like form in the distal jejunum and ileum. Villi vary in density from 10 to 40 per square millimetre and from c.0.5 to 1.0 mm in height.

MUCOSA

The mucosa (**Figs 70.1, 72.5**) consists of epithelium, lamina propria and muscularis mucosae.

EPITHELIUM (Fig. 72.5)

A single-layered epithelium covers the intestinal villi (**Fig. 72.5**), and also lines the intestinal glands (crypts) that open between the bases of

villi. Two types of cell, enterocytes and goblet cells, cover the surfaces of the villi. Microfold cells (M cells) are restricted to the dome epithelium covering localized accumulations of lymphoid tissues. These cell types are all in contact basally with a basal lamina to which they adhere, and all derive from a common stem cell in the intestinal crypts.

Enterocytes

Enterocytes are columnar absorptive cells, c.20 μm tall (**Fig. 72.7**). They are the most numerous type of cell in the intestinal lining, and are responsible for nutrient absorption. Their surfaces bear up to 3000 microvilli, which greatly increase the surface area for absorption. Collectively, microvilli are visible by light microscopy as a brush (striated) border c.1 μm thick: individual microvilli can be resolved only by electron microscopy. Enterocyte nuclei are elongated vertically, mainly euchromatic and located just below the centre of the cell. The

Epithelium

Lamina propria

Muscularis mucosae

Circular muscle

Longitudinal muscle

Mucosa

Submucosa

Muscularis externa

Serosa

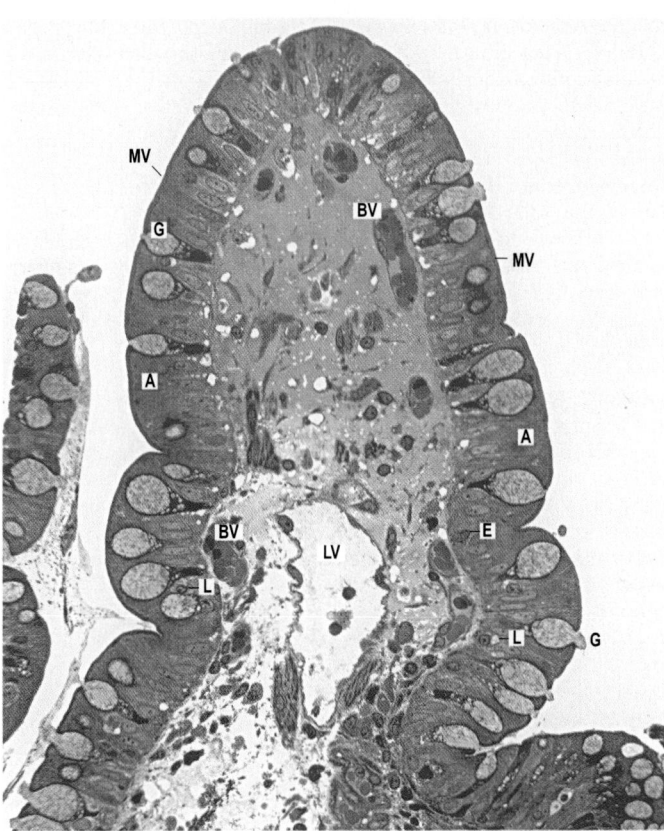

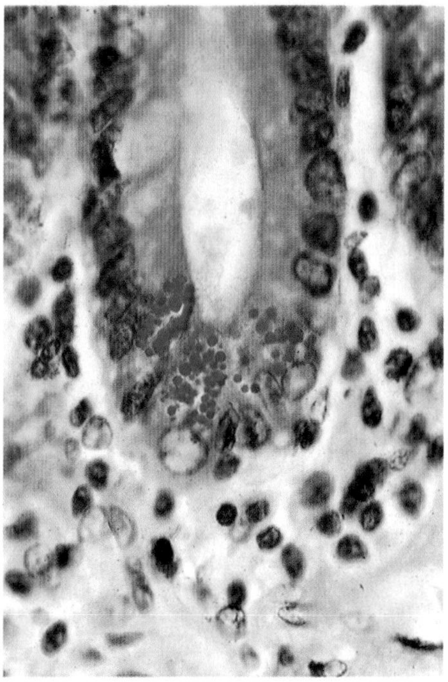

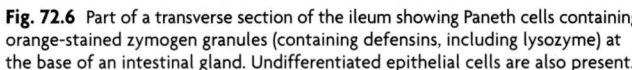

Fig. 72.6 Part of a transverse section of the ileum showing Paneth cells containing orange-stained zymogen granules (containing defensins, including lysozyme) at the base of an intestinal gland. Undifferentiated epithelial cells are also present.

Fig. 72.5 High-power micrograph of an intestinal villus (toluidine blue-stained resin section) showing absorptive enterocytes (A), bearing microvilli (MV) covering its surface, interspersed with goblet cells (G) filled with pale mucinogen granules. Enteroendocrine cells (E) and intraepithelial lymphocytes (L) are also seen. The central core is lamina propria containing blood vessels (BV), a large lacteal lymphatic vessel (LV) and other connective tissue elements; smooth muscle cells are also present. (By permission from Dr JB Kerr, Monash University, from Kerr JB 1999 Atlas of Functional Histology. London: Mosby.)

Goblet cells

Goblet cells are most numerous in the distal small intestine, increasing in number from the duodenum to their highest density in the terminal ileum. They have elongated, basal nuclei, an apical region containing many membrane-bound mucinogen granules (**Fig. 72.7**), and apical surfaces that bear a few short microvilli. Goblet cell mucins contribute to protection against microorganisms and toxins in the gut lumen, and also provide lubrication and mechanical protection from the intestinal contents.

Microfold (M) cells

Microfold cells are present where the epithelium covers lymphoid aggregates (MALT; p. 77) in the intestinal wall. They are cuboidal or flattened in shape and have long, widely spaced microfolds rather than microvilli on their apical surfaces. They sample luminal antigens by endocytosis and transport antigen to lymphocytes that occupy intercellular pockets formed by deep invaginations of the M-cell basolateral plasma membranes. See page 80 for details of antigen processing and presentation.

Lymphocytes

Intraepithelial lymphocytes are found in close association with M cells and also between the basolateral regions of enterocytes and goblet cells. They are migratory cells derived from the underlying lymphoid tissue and constitute an important means of immune defence.

Intestinal glands or crypts

Intestinal glands or crypts (of Lieberkühn) are tubular pits that open into the lumen throughout the intestinal mucosa via small circular apertures between the bases of the villi (**Figs 70.1, 72.1, 72.4**). Their thin walls are composed of columnar enterocytes supplemented by mucous cells, Paneth cells, stem cells and neuroendocrine cells. They are separated by a basement membrane from a rich capillary plexus within the lamina propria.

cells have a lifespan after differentiation of about 5 days, and their position on the villus wall reflects their stage in the life cycle: at the tips of intestinal villi they undergo programmed, apoptotic, cell death and are shed from the epithelium. They are replaced at the base of the villus by stem cell mitosis.

The apical cell surface is resistant to protease attack because microvilli possess a specialized glycoprotein-rich surface coat (glycocalyx) which, with an overlying layer of mucus, protects the epithelium against pancreatic enzymes in the intestinal lumen. The cell coat also contains a number of digestive enzymes as integral membrane proteins. These include enzymes that degrade disaccharides and oligopeptides prior to absorption. Further details of the structure of microvilli are given on page 20.

The luminal surface is an important barrier to diffusion. Nutrients generally have to pass through enterocytes (transcellular absorption) before they reach the underlying lamina propria and its blood vessels and lymphatics (lacteals). Classical epithelial junctional complexes (p. 7) encircle the apical plasma membranes of adjacent enterocytes, and their tight junctions form an effective barrier to non-selective diffusion between the gut lumen and the body as a whole. The lateral plasma membranes of enterocytes are highly folded, interdigitating with each other to form complex intercellular boundaries, anchored periodically by desmosomes, and making contact at gap junctions. The lateral intercellular space expands during active absorption and is an additional conduit (supplementing transport across the basal cell surface) for the passage of fluids, nutrients and other solutes to the vessels of the lamina propria.

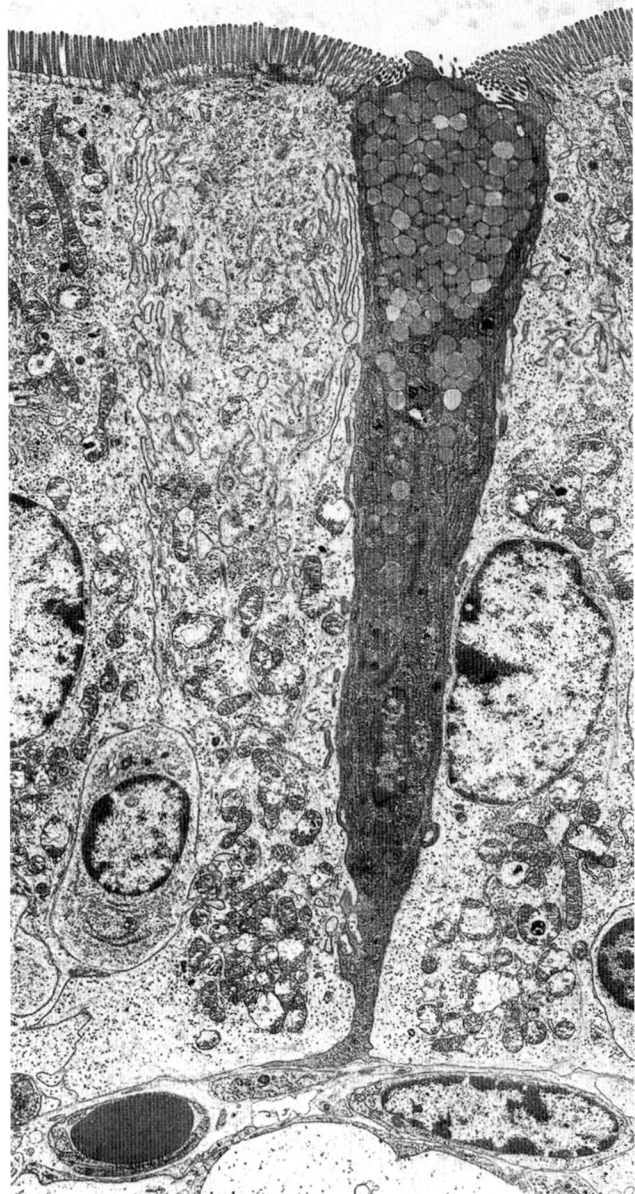

Fig. 72.7 Electron micrograph of columnar enterocytes covering a villus in the small intestine, each with an apical brush border of microvilli. A single goblet cell containing mucinogen granules is also present. The small cell towards the left between two enterocytes is an intraepithelial lymphocyte. A capillary and other connective tissue elements of the lamina propria lie beneath the basal lamina.

Enterocytes – Enterocytes in the crypts secrete ions and alkaline fluid to dilute chyme and aid absorption by structurally similar cells covering the villi.

Mucous cells – The mucous cells in the crypts are similar to the goblet cells of the villi.

Paneth cells – Paneth cells are numerous in the deeper parts of the intestinal crypts, particularly in the duodenum. They are rich in zinc and contain large acidophilic granules (**Fig. 72.6**) that stain strongly with eosin or phosphotungstic haematoxylin. Paneth cells secrete lysozyme, a highly specific antibacterial enzyme, and other defensive proteins (defensins) such as tumour necrosis factor alpha (TNF-α), which protect the intestinal luminal surface.

Stem cells – Stem cells occur in a zone just above the basal region of the crypts and are the source of most of the cell types of the intestinal epithelium. Their progeny, transit (transient) amplifying cells, have one of the most rapid proliferation rates in the body. They migrate out of

the intestinal crypts along the sides of the villi, where they differentiate mainly into the short-lived columnar enterocytes or goblet cells (which are thus continually replaced). When not dividing, their apical surfaces have fewer and more irregular microvilli than the differentiated enterocytes.

Neuroendocrine cells – Several types of neuroendocrine cell are scattered among the walls of the intestinal crypts, and less commonly over the villi. They secrete bioactive peptides, such as gastrin, cholecystokinin and secretin, basally into the surrounding lamina propria. Crypt neuroendocrine cells are derived from stem cells, which also give rise to enterocytes and other epithelial elements. For further details of the dispersed neuroendocrine system see page 180.

LAMINA PROPRIA

The lamina propria is composed of connective tissue and provides mechanical support for the epithelium. It has a rich vascular plexus, receives nutrients absorbed by the enterocytes, and forms the cores of the villi. It also contains lymphoid tissue, fibroblasts and connective tissue extracellular matrix fibres, smooth muscle cells, eosinophils, macrophages, mast cells, capillaries, lymphatic vessels and unmyelinated nerve fibres. Plasma cells are numerous and lymphocytes in many regions are clustered in solitary and aggregated lymphatic follicles, Peyer's patches, some of which extend through the muscularis mucosae into the submucosa.

Core of the villus – Each villus has a core of delicate connective tissue that contains a large blind-ending lymphatic vessel or lacteal (so called because of its content of suspended chylomicrons, the droplets of apoprotein–lipid complex elaborated by enterocytes from absorbed dietary fats). The core also contains blood vessels, nerves and smooth muscle cells derived from fine extensions of the muscularis mucosae. Each lacteal, usually single but occasionally double, starts in a closed dilated extremity near the tip of a villus, and extends through the core to the base of the villus, where it joins a narrower lymphatic plexus in the deeper lamina propria. Its wall is a single layer of endothelial cells. Smooth muscle cells surround the lacteal throughout the villus and their contraction propels its contents into the underlying lymphatic plexus. Capillaries within the core are lined by fenestrated endothelium to facilitate the rapid intake of nutrients diffusing from the covering absorptive epithelium.

Mucosa-associated lymphoid tissue – Mucosa-associated lymphoid tissue (MALT) is found mainly in the lamina propria, but sometimes expands into the submucosa. It is the source of B and T lymphocytes and other related cells for the immune defence of the gut wall (p. 77). MALT consists of lymphoid follicles covered by intestinal epithelium that includes a few M cells.

Solitary lymphoid follicles are scattered along the length of the intestinal mucosa, and are most numerous in the distal ileum. Aggregated follicles, Peyer's patches, are largest and most numerous in the ileum, whilst in the distal jejunum they are small, circular and few; they are only occasionally found in the duodenum. They are usually situated in the intestinal wall opposite the mesenteric attachment. Aggregated lymphoid follicles are circular or oval masses containing 10–260 follicles, varying in length from 2 to 10 cm and visible macroscopically as dome-like elevations. Villi are small or absent over the larger follicular groups.

Like other masses of MALT (except lymph nodes), solitary and aggregated lymphoid follicles are most prominent around the age of puberty, after which they diminish in number and size, although many persist into old age. For further details of intestinal MALT, including Peyer's patches, see the review by Kraehenbuhl and Neutra (1992).

MUSCULARIS MUCOSAE

The muscularis mucosae forms the base of the mucosa, and has external longitudinal and internal circular layers of smooth muscle cells. It follows the surface profiles of the circular folds and sends fine fascicles of smooth muscle cells into the cores of the villi.

SUBMUCOSA

The submucosa is composed of loose connective tissue carrying blood vessels, lymphatics and nerves. Its ridged elevations form the cores of the circular folds. The geometry of its collagen and elastin fibres permits the considerable changes in transverse and longitudinal dimensions that accompany peristalsis, whilst still providing adequate support, elasticity and strength.

SUBMUCOSAL GLANDS

Submucosal glands are limited to the submucosa of the duodenum (**Figs 70.1, 72.1**). Their ducts traverse the muscularis mucosae to enter the bases of the mucosal crypts. They are largest and most numerous near the pylorus, and form an almost complete layer in the proximal half of the descending duodenum. Thereafter they gradually diminish in number and disappear at the duodenojejunal junction. They are small, branched tubuloacinar glands (p. 34): each has several secretory acini lined by low columnar epithelial cells that produce an alkaline (c.pH 9) mucoid secretion which effectively neutralizes acidic chyme from the stomach. Many neuroendocrine cells are present among the acinar cells.

MUSCULARIS EXTERNA

The muscularis externa consists of a thin external longitudinal layer and a thick internal circular layer of smooth muscle cells. It is thicker in the proximal small intestine. For details, see Gabella (1988).

SEROSA

Serosa is visceral peritoneum. It consists of a subserous stratum of loose connective tissue covered by mesothelium. The retroperitoneal portion of the duodenum is mainly covered by a connective tissue adventitia rather than by serosa.

REFERENCES

Gabella G 1988 Structure of intestinal musculature. In: Handbook of Physiology; The Gastrointestinal System I. New York: American Physiological Society and Oxford University Press: 103–39.

Kraehenbuhl JP, Neutra MR 1992 Molecular and cellular basis of immune protection of mucosal surfaces. Physiol Rev 72: 853–79.

Duodenum

The adult duodenum is c.20–25 cm long and is the shortest, widest and most predictably placed part of the small intestine. It is only partially covered by peritoneum although the extent of the peritoneal covering varies along its length: the proximal 2.5 cm is intraperitoneal; the remainder is retroperitoneal. The duodenum forms an elongated 'C' that lies between the level of the first and third lumbar vertebrae in the supine position. The lower 'limb' of the C extends further to the left of the midline than the upper limb. The head and uncinate process of the pancreas lie within the concavity of the C. The duodenum lies entirely above the level of the umbilicus and is described as having four parts (**Figs 73.1, 73.2**).

FIRST (SUPERIOR) PART

The first part of the duodenum is c.5 cm long and starts as a continuation of the duodenal end of the pylorus. It is the most mobile portion of the duodenum. Close to the pylorus, peritoneum covers the anterior, superior and upper part of the posterior aspect where the duodenum forms part of the anterior wall of the epiploic foramen. Here the lesser omentum is attached to its upper border and the greater omentum to its lower border. The first 2 or 3 cm have a bland internal mucosal appearance and readily distend on insufflation during endoscopy. This part is frequently referred to as the duodenal 'cap': it has a triangular, homogeneous appearance during contrast radiology and shows the same pattern of rugae as the pylorus. It is often visible on plain radiographs of the abdomen as an isolated triangular gas shadow to the right of the first or second lumbar vertebra. The first part then passes superiorly, posteriorly and laterally for c.5 cm before curving sharply inferiorly into the superior duodenal flexure, which marks the end of the first part. Through this course it rapidly becomes more retroperitoneal and is covered by peritoneum only on its anterior aspect. From the end of the duodenal cap, the internal appearance is characterized by extensive, deep mucosal folds that involve up to half of the circumference of the lumen. Even during endoscopic insufflation, these folds are pronounced (**Fig. 73.3**) and they are readily seen on contrast radiographs (**Fig. 73.2**). The section from the duodenal cap to the superior duodenal flexure lies posterior and inferior to the quadrate lobe of the liver. At the junction with the second part of the duodenum it lies posterior to the neck of the gallbladder. The first part of the duodenum lies anterior to the gastroduodenal artery, common bile duct and portal vein and antero-superior to the head and neck of the pancreas. The gastroduodenal artery lies immediately posterior to the outer muscular layers of the posterior wall of the first part. Peptic ulceration is commonly found on the posterior wall in this region and penetration of the wall with erosion of the gastroduodenal artery may lead to dramatic haemorrhage. The common hepatic and hepatoduodenal lymph nodes also lie close to the first part of the duodenum and can be visualized using endoscopic ultrasound. This may be important in the staging of gastric, pancreatic or bile duct tumours. The proximity of the common bile duct to the first part of the duodenum allows endoscopic ultrasound examination of the distal common bile duct and the formation of a surgical anastomosis between bile duct and duodenum (choledochoduodenostomy) when required. Penetrating peptic ulceration in the anterior wall may lead to free perforation into the peritoneal cavity because the anterior surface of the first part is covered only by peritoneum.

SECOND (DESCENDING) PART

The second part of the duodenum is c.8–10 cm long. It starts at the superior duodenal flexure and runs inferiorly in a gentle curve, which is convex to the right side of the vertebral column, extending to the lower border of the third lumbar vertebral body. It then turns sharply medially into the inferior duodenal flexure which marks its junction with the third part. It is covered by peritoneum only on its upper anterior surface, lies posterior to the neck of the gallbladder and the right lobe of the liver at its start, and is crossed anteriorly by the transverse colon. The origin of the transverse mesocolon is attached to the anterior surface of the duodenum by loose connective tissue. Below the attachment of the transverse mesocolon, the connective tissue and vessels forming the mesentery of the upper ascending colon and hepatic flexure are loosely attached to the anterior surface of the duodenum. This section of duodenum is at risk of injury during surgical mobilization of the ascending colon. The second part lies anterior to the hilum of the right kidney, the right renal vessels, the edge of the inferior vena cava and the right psoas major. The head of the pancreas and the common bile duct are medial and the hepatic flexure is above and lateral. A small part of the pancreatic head is sometimes embedded in the medial duodenal wall, and pancreatic rests in the duodenal wall produce small filling defects on double contrast barium meal. The internal appearance is similar to that of the distal portion of the first part of the duodenum, with pronounced mucosal folds (**Fig. 73.3**). The common bile duct and pancreatic duct enter the medial wall obliquely and unite to form the hepatopancreatic ampulla (p. 1228). The narrow, distal, end opens on the summit of the major duodenal papilla (ampulla of Vater), situated on the postero-medial wall of the second part c.8–10 cm distal to the pylorus (**Fig. 73.3**). An accessory pancreatic duct may open c.2 cm above the major papilla on a minor duodenal papilla (p. 1233). Peptic ulceration of the second part is less common than that of the first part, but tends to occur on the anterior or lateral wall.

Duodenal diverticula

The duodenum is the most common site for a diverticulum in the small intestine. Diverticula are congenital and usually solitary. They almost always arise in the medial wall of the second part of the duodenum, where they are intimately related to the head of the pancreas. This relationship means that diverticula are frequently related to the major duodenal papilla (ampulla of Vater), and the latter may be found either on the mucosal fold at the mouth of a diverticulum or arising from the mucosa within the body of a diverticulum, particularly on the supero-medial wall. This may complicate interpretation of contrast radiographs of the duodenum or biliary system and may cause difficulties during attempted endoscopic cannulation of the papilla because the diverticulum may restrict access. If the papilla is located on or close to the anterior wall of a diverticulum, the procedure of opening the ampulla with an electrocautery current during attempted cannulation (sphincterotomy) is made more hazardous because the wall is thin at this point and so there is a risk of free perforation into the peritoneal cavity.

THIRD (HORIZONTAL) PART

The third part of the duodenum starts at the inferior duodenal flexure and is c.10 cm long. It runs from the right side of the lower border of the third lumbar vertebra, angled slightly superiorly, across to the left, anterior to the inferior vena cava, and ends in continuity with the fourth part in front of the abdominal aorta. It lies posterior to the transverse mesocolon, the origin of the small bowel mesentery and the superior mesenteric vessels. Peritoneum covers the lower portion of the anterior aspect and is reflected anteriorly to form the posterior layer of the origin of the small bowel mesentery. The anterior surface of the left lateral end, close to the junction with the fourth part, is also covered with peritoneum. The third part is anterior to the right ureter, right psoas

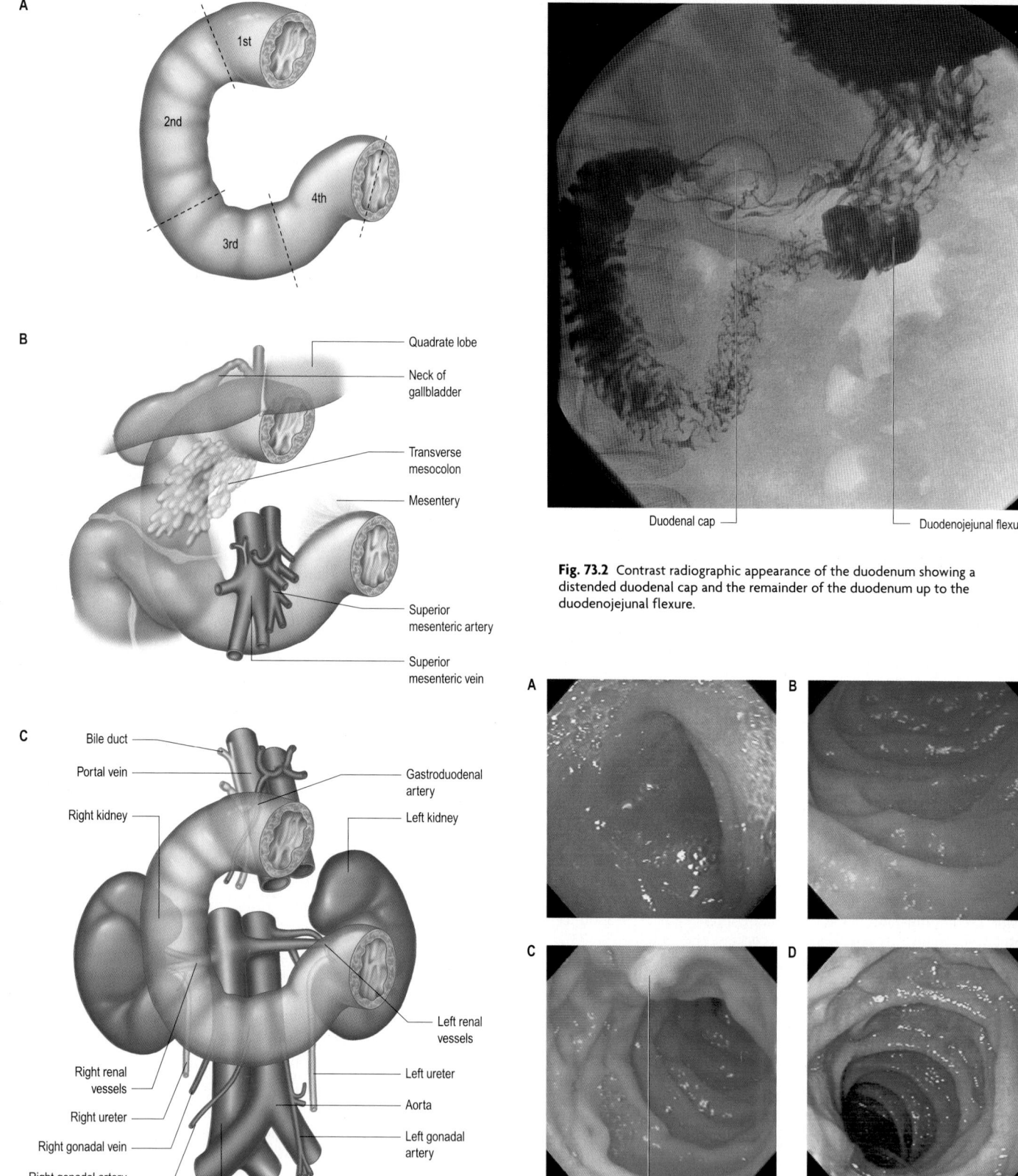

A

1st

2nd

4th

3rd

B

Quadrate lobe

Neck of
gallbladder

Transverse
mesocolon

Mesentery

Superior
mesenteric artery

Superior
mesenteric vein

C

Bile duct

Portal vein

Right kidney

Right renal
vessels

Right ureter

Right gonadal vein

Right gonadal artery

Inferior vena cava

Gastroduodenal
artery

Left kidney

Left renal
vessels

Left ureter

Aorta

Left gonadal
artery

Fig. 73.1 **A**, The four parts of the duodenum. **B**, **C** The relations of the duodenum: **B**, anterior surface; **C**, posterior surface.

Duodenal cap

Duodenojejunal flexure

Fig. 73.2 Contrast radiographic appearance of the duodenum showing a distended duodenal cap and the remainder of the duodenum up to the duodenojejunal flexure.

A

B

C

D

Major duodenal papilla

Fig. 73.3 The endoscopic appearances of the duodenum: **A**, duodenal cap; **B**, distal first part; **C**, second part showing the major duodenal papilla; **D**, third part.

major, right gonadal vessels, inferior vena cava and abdominal aorta (at the origin of the inferior mesenteric artery), and inferior to the head of the pancreas. Anteroinferiorly, loops of jejunum lie in the right and left infracolic compartments. In the mid portion, the third part is potentially 'pinched' between the superior mesenteric vessels just below their origin anteriorly, and the abdominal aorta posteriorly: this arrangement very occasionally gives rise to intermittent obstruction of the duodenum at this point.

FOURTH (ASCENDING) PART

The fourth part of the duodenum is c.2.5 cm long. It starts just to the left of the aorta and runs superiorly and laterally to the level of the upper border of the second lumbar vertebra. It then turns antero-inferiorly at the duodenojejunal flexure and is continuous with the jejunum. The aorta, left sympathetic trunk, left psoas major, left renal and left gonadal vessels are all posterior, and the left kidney and left ureter are posterolateral. The main trunk of the inferior mesenteric vein lies either posterior to the duodenojejunal flexure or beneath the adjacent peritoneal fold. (The duodenojejunal flexure is a useful landmark to locate the vein radiologically or surgically.) Anteriorly are the upper part of the root of the small bowel mesentery, the left lateral transverse mesocolon and transverse colon, which separate it from the stomach. The peritoneum of the root of the small bowel mesentery continues over the anterior surface. The lower border of the body of the pancreas is superior. At its left lateral end, the fourth part becomes progressively covered in peritoneum on its superior and inferior surfaces, such that it is suspended from the retroperitoneum by a double fold of peritoneum, the ligament of Treitz, at the start of the duodenojejunal flexure. The ligament of Treitz is not a mesentery because the vascular supply to the fourth part of the duodenum continues to enter its wall from the posteromedial aspect. It may contain a small slip of muscle called the suspensory muscle of the duodenum. When present, the suspensory muscle contains skeletal muscle fibres that run from the left crus of the diaphragm to connective tissue around the coeliac axis, and smooth muscle fibres that run from the coeliac axis: its function is unknown. The ligament of Treitz is an important landmark in the radiological diagnosis of incomplete rotation and malrotation of the small intestine (p. 1257).

VASCULAR SUPPLY AND LYMPHATIC DRAINAGE

ARTERIES

The main vessels supplying the duodenum are the superior and inferior pancreaticoduodenal arteries. The first and second parts also receive contributions from several sources including the right gastric artery, the supraduodenal artery, the right gastroepiploic artery, the hepatic artery and the gastroduodenal artery. Branches of the superior pancreaticoduodenal artery may contribute to the supply of the pyloric canal, with some anastomosis in the muscular layer across the pyloroduodenal junction.

Gastroduodenal artery

The gastroduodenal artery arises from the common hepatic artery behind, or sometimes above, the first part of the duodenum. It is of moderately large calibre and descends between the first part of the duodenum and the neck of the pancreas, immediately to the right of the peritoneal reflection from the posterior surface of the first part. It usually lies to the left of the common bile duct but is occasionally anterior. At the lower border of the first part of the duodenum it divides into the right gastroepiploic and superior pancreaticoduodenal arteries. Before its division the lowest part of the artery gives rise to small branches that supply the pyloric end of the stomach and the pancreas, and retroduodenal branches that supply the first part and the proximal portion of the second part of the duodenum directly. The supraduodenal artery often arises from the gastroduodenal artery behind the upper border of the first part of the duodenum and supplies the superior aspect of the first part. Although the gastroduodenal artery usually branches from the common hepatic artery it may also arise as a trifurcation with the right and left hepatic arteries. Occasionally the origin is from the superior mesenteric artery or the left hepatic artery, and rarely it may arise from the coeliac axis and right hepatic artery. The

supraduodenal artery occasionally arises from the common hepatic artery or right gastric artery.

Superior pancreaticoduodenal arteries

The superior pancreaticoduodenal artery is usually double. The anterior artery is a terminal branch of the gastroduodenal artery and descends in the anterior groove between the second part of the duodenum and the head of the pancreas. It supplies branches to the first and second parts of the duodenum and to the head of the pancreas, and anastomoses with the anterior division of the inferior pancreaticoduodenal artery. The posterior artery is usually a separate branch of the gastroduodenal artery and is given off at the upper border of the first part of the duodenum. It descends to the right, anterior to the portal vein and common bile duct as the latter lies behind the first part of the duodenum. It then runs behind the head of the pancreas, crosses posterior to the common bile duct (which is embedded in the head of the pancreas), enters the duodenal wall and anastomoses with the posterior division of the inferior pancreaticoduodenal artery. The posterior artery supplies branches to the head of the pancreas, the first and second parts of the duodenum, and several branches to the lowest part of the common bile duct.

Inferior pancreaticoduodenal artery

The inferior pancreaticoduodenal artery arises from the superior mesenteric artery or its first jejunal branch, near the superior border of the third part of the duodenum. It usually divides directly into anterior and posterior branches. The anterior branch passes to the right, anterior to the lower border of the head of the pancreas, and runs superiorly to anastomose with the anterior superior pancreaticoduodenal artery. The posterior branch runs posteriorly and superiorly to the right, lying posterior to the lower border of the head of the pancreas, and anastomoses with the posterior superior pancreaticoduodenal artery. Both branches supply the pancreatic head, its uncinate process and the second and third parts of the duodenum.

Jejunal artery branches

The first jejunal branch of the superior mesenteric artery has branches that supply the fourth part of the duodenum. They frequently form an anastomosis with the terminal branch of the anterior inferior pancreaticoduodenal artery, which means that the fourth part of the duodenum has a potential collateral supply from the coeliac axis and superior mesenteric artery and so is not commonly affected by ischaemia.

VEINS

The duodenal veins drain ultimately into the portal vein. Submucosal and intramural veins give rise to pancreaticoduodenal veins that usually accompany the corresponding named arteries. The superior pancreaticoduodenal vein is formed medial to the mid point of the second part of the duodenum. It runs superomedially on the posterior surface of the head of the pancreas, passes posterior to the distal common bile duct and drains into the portal vein behind the neck of the pancreas. The inferior pancreaticoduodenal vein runs from the anteromedial aspect of the second part of the duodenum inferiorly in the groove between the second and third parts and the head of the pancreas. It usually drains into the superior mesenteric vein but may drain into the right gastroepiploic vein. Small veins from the first and upper second part of the duodenum may drain into the prepyloric vein whilst veins from the third and fourth parts may drain directly into the superior mesenteric vein.

LYMPHATICS

Duodenal lymphatics run to anterior and posterior pancreatic nodes that lie in the anterior and posterior grooves between the pancreatic head and the duodenum. These drain widely into the suprapyloric, infrapyloric, hepatoduodenal, common hepatic and superior mesenteric nodes.

INNERVATION

The duodenum is innervated by the parasympathetic and sympathetic systems. Preganglionic sympathetic fibres originate from neurones in the fifth to the twelfth thoracic spinal segments and travel via the greater and lesser splanchnic nerves to the coeliac plexus where they synapse on neurones in the coeliac ganglion: postganglionic axons are distributed via periarterial plexuses on the branches of the coeliac axis and superior mesenteric artery. The parasympathetic supply is from the vagus nerve via branches from the coeliac plexus.

REFERRED PAIN

In common with other structures derived from the foregut, the visceral sensation of pain arising from the duodenum is poorly localized and referred to the central epigastrium.

REFERENCE

Jackson JE 1999 Vascular anatomy of the gastrointestinal tract. In: Butler P, Mitchell AWM, Ellis H (eds) Applied Radiological Anatomy. Cambridge, UK: Cambridge University Press.
Provides details and illustrations of common vascular variants.

Jejunum and ileum

The small intestine consists of the duodenum, jejunum and ileum and extends from the pylorus to the ileocaecal valve. In the living adult it has a total length of c.5 metres, but this can range widely from less than 3 metres to more than 7 metres. The proximal two-fifths is referred to as the jejunum and the distal three-fifths as the ileum, although there is no clear distinction between the two parts. There is, however, a gradual change in morphology from the proximal to distal ends of the small bowel. The distal 30 cm or so of the ileum is often referred to as the terminal ileum, which has some specialized physiological functions. The jejunum and ileum occupy the central and lower parts of the abdominal cavity and usually lie within the boundary formed by the abdominal colon. They are attached to the posterior abdominal wall by a mesentery and this allows considerable mobility of the loops of small bowel. In the supine position, loops of jejunum may be found anterior to the transverse colon, stomach and even lesser omentum. When upright, loops of ileum may descend into the pelvis anterior to the rectum and, in women, may fill the rectouterine pouch. The majority of the jejunum and ileum is covered anteriorly by the greater omentum (p. 1132). The jejunum and ileum are covered by peritoneum on all but their mesenteric borders where the adipose connective tissue of the mesentery abuts the muscular wall. The peritoneum continues over these tissues to enclose the mesentery (p. 1133). Mesenteric fat covers c.20% of the circumference wall of the ileum and somewhat less of the jejunum.

The mucosa of the jejunum and ileum is thrown into numerous circular folds, plicae circulares, which protrude into the lumen. The submucosa of the small bowel contains aggregates of lymphoid tissue, which are more numerous in the ileum.

JEJUNUM

The jejunum has a median external diameter of c.4 cm and an internal diameter of 2.5 cm. It has a thicker wall than the ileum, and possesses a profuse arterial blood supply so that it appears redder than the ileum. The plicae circulares are most pronounced in the proximal jejunum, where they are more numerous and deeper than elsewhere in the small bowel. They frequently 'branch' around the lumen and may appear to be ranged one on top of another, giving the jejunum a characteristic appearance during single contrast radiography (**Fig. 74.1**). Lymphoid aggregates are almost absent from the proximal jejunum; they are present distally but are still fewer in number and smaller than in the ileum. They are usually discoid in shape and impalpable. In the supine position the jejunum usually occupies the upper left infracolic compartment extending down to the umbilical region. The first loop or two often occupies a recess between the left part of the transverse mesocolon and the left kidney. On supine radiological examination, the jejunal loops are characteristically situated in the upper abdomen, to the left of the midline, whereas the ileal loops tend to lie in the lower right part of the abdomen and pelvis. This distribution can be reversed during ileus or small bowel obstruction due to rotation around the mesenteric attachment following bowel distension.

JEJUNAL FEEDING

In situations where the stomach and duodenum are either unsuitable or unavailable for receiving oral nutrition, delivery of prepared feed to the jejunum is possible. This can be performed either using a surgically created jejunostomy or by insertion of a feeding tube. Because the jejunum is highly mobile, it is possible to bring the first or second loop of jejunum into contact with the abdominal wall to create a surgical jejunostomy. Insertion of a fine-bore feeding tube via the nose as far as the jejunum is also possible. The end of the feeding tube must lie beyond the duodenojejunal flexure to prevent reflux of the feed into the duodenum and stomach; this is usually confirmed by radiological monitoring of the progress of the tube through the duodenum.

ILEUM

The ileum has a median external diameter of 3.5 cm and an internal diameter of 2 cm; it tends to have a thinner wall than the jejunum. The plicae circulares become progressively less obvious in the distal mucosa in the ileum: they tend to be single and flatter with less pronounced crests (**Figs 74.1, 74.2**). The mucosa of the terminal ileum immediately proximal to the ileocaecal valve may appear almost flat. Lymphoid aggregates are larger and more numerous than in the jejunum and may be easily palpable in the terminal ileum. They are most prominent in early childhood, become less so prior to puberty, and are of the adult type by late teenage years. In the supine position, the ileum lies mainly in the hypogastric region and right iliac fossa. The terminal ileum frequently lies in the pelvis, from which it ascends over the right psoas major and right iliac vessels to end in the right iliac fossa, where it opens into the ileocaecal valve.

MECKEL'S DIVERTICULUM

The ileal diverticulum (of Meckel) exists in c.3% of adults: it represents the remnant of the proximal part of the intestino-vitelline duct. It projects from the antimesenteric border of the terminal ileum and is commonly located between 50 and 100 cm from the ileocaecal valve. It has a median length of c.5 cm and often possesses a short 'mesentery' of adipose tissue that extends from the ileal mesentery up to the base. The lumen of the diverticulum is usually wide, with a calibre similar to that of the ileum. The tip is usually free but occasionally may be connected to the anterior abdominal wall near the umbilicus by a fibrous band. The mucosa is ileal in type but small areas may be lined by gastric body type epithelium, which occasionally gives rise to bleeding in the adjacent normal ileal mucosa. Heterotopic areas of pancreatic, colonic or other tissues may occur in its wall. Inflammation may mimic acute appendicitis: Meckel's diverticulum is derived from midgut structures, and so pain is referred to the periumbilical region as it is in early appendicitis.

VASCULAR SUPPLY AND LYMPHATIC DRAINAGE

ARTERIES

The arterial supply to the jejunum and ileum arises from the superior mesenteric artery. Branches divide as they approach the mesenteric border and extend between the serosal and muscular layers. From these, numerous branches traverse the muscle, supplying it and forming an intricate submucosal plexus from which minute vessels pass to the glands and villi. Although there is a profuse anastomotic network of arteries within the mesentery, anastomoses between the terminal branches close to the intestinal wall are few, and alternate vessels are often distributed to opposite sides of the jejunum/ileum (**Fig. 74.3**).

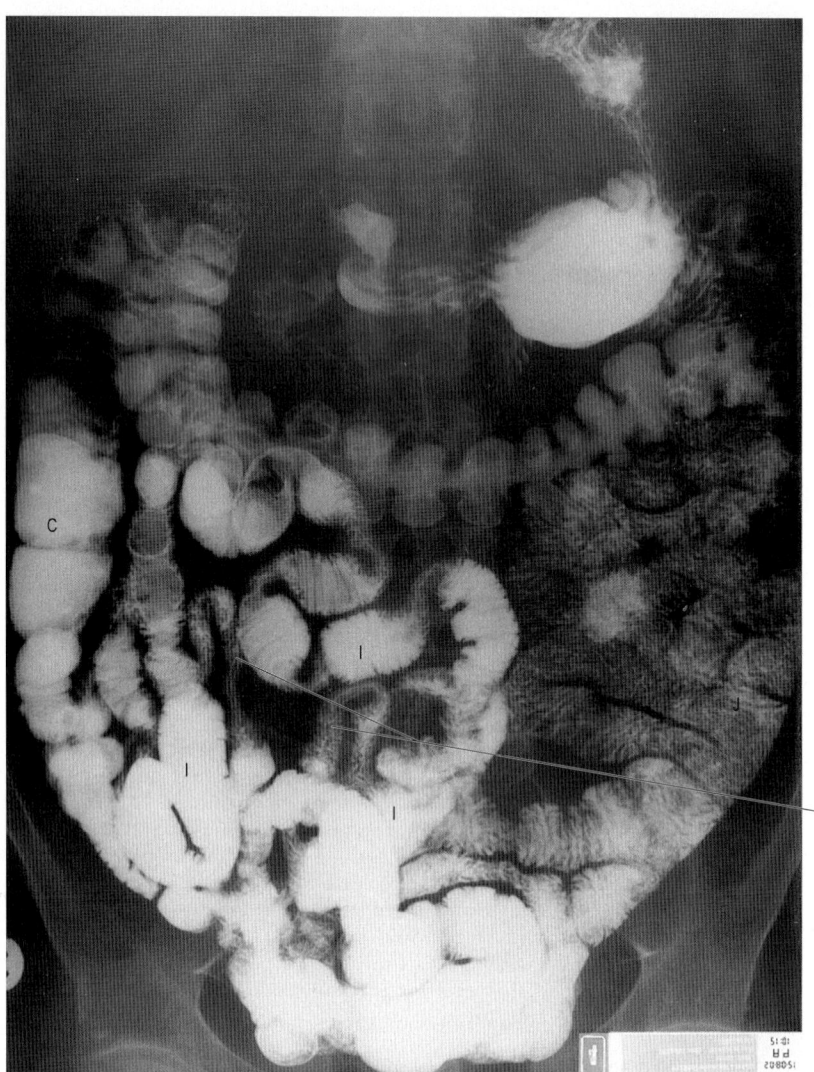

A

Fig. 74.1 Barium studies of the jejunum and ileum. **A**, Barium follow-through. The feathery appearance of the small intestine is due to the plicae circulares, this is most prominent in the jejunum. The constrictions are the result of peristalsis. **B**, Small bowel enema (enteroclysis). The plicae circulares are clearly demonstrated by this technique. C, caecum; I, ileum; J, jejunum; PC, plicae circulares; TI, terminal part of ileum.

Peristalsis

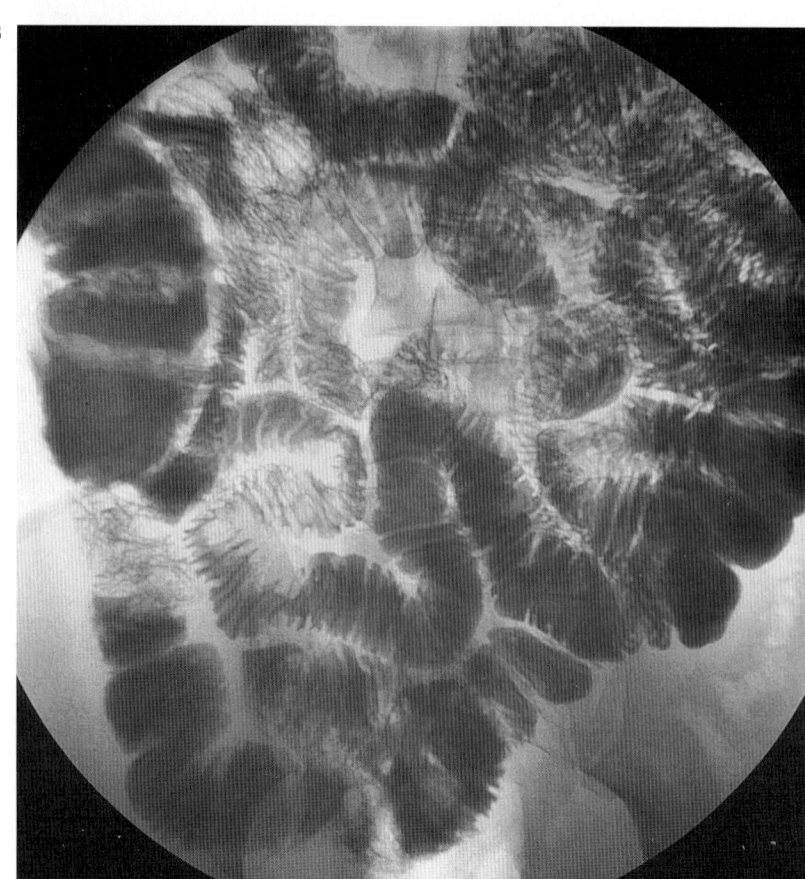

B

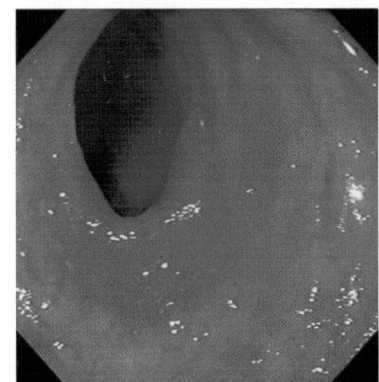

Fig. 74.2 Endoscopic appearance of the terminal ileum.

SUPERIOR MESENTERIC ARTERY

The superior mesenteric artery (**Figs 74.4, 74.5**) originates from the aorta c.1 cm below the coeliac trunk, at the level of the intervertebral disk between the first and second lumbar vertebrae. It runs inferiorly and anteriorly, anterior to the uncinate process of the pancreas and the third part of the duodenum, and posterior to the splenic vein and the body of the pancreas. The left renal vein lies behind it and separates it from the aorta (**Fig. 74.6**).

As it descends in the root of the small bowel mesentery, the artery crosses anterior to the inferior vena cava, right ureter and right psoas major. The calibre of the vessel steadily decreases as successive branches are given off to the loops of jejunum and ileum: it ends in a terminal branch which anastomoses with the ileocolic artery. The superior mesenteric artery gives off the middle colic (p. 1193), right colic (p. 1203), ileocolic, jejunal and ileal branches. A fibrous strand from the region of the last ileal branch may be present in the mesentery and represents the vestige of the embryonic artery that originally connected it to the yolk sac. The superior mesenteric artery may be the source of the common hepatic, gastroduodenal, accessory right hepatic, accessory pancreatic or splenic arteries. It may arise from a common coeliac–mesenteric trunk.

Jejunal branches – Jejunal branches arise from the left side of the upper portion of the superior mesenteric artery (**Figs 74.4, 74.5**). They are usually five to ten in number and are distributed to the jejunum as a series of short arcades. These form a single or occasionally double tier of anastomotic arcs before giving rise to multiple straight vessels that run directly towards the jejunal wall (**Fig. 74.3**). These vessels run almost parallel in the mesentery and are distributed alternately to opposite aspects of its wall. Small twigs supply regional lymph nodes and other structures in the mesentery.

Ileal branches – Ileal branches arise from the left and anterior aspects of the superior mesenteric artery. They are more numerous than the jejunal branches but smaller in calibre. The length of the mesentery is greater in the ileum and the branches form three, four or sometimes five tiers of arcs within the mesentery before giving rise to multiple straight vessels that run directly towards the ileal wall. As with the jejunal branches, these run parallel in the mesentery and are distributed to alternate aspects of the ileum. They are longer and smaller than similar jejunal vessels, particularly in the distal ileum. In the terminal ileum, the arcades receive a contribution from the ileal branch of the ileocolic artery and are often larger in calibre than the mid-ileal vessels.

VEINS

Superior mesenteric vein

The superior mesenteric vein drains the small intestine, caecum, ascending and transverse parts of the colon (**Figs 74.5B, 74.7**). It is formed in the right lower mesentery of the small bowel by the union of tributaries from the terminal ileum, caecum and vermiform appendix. It ascends in the mesentery to the right of the superior mesenteric artery. It passes anterior to the right ureter, inferior vena cava, third part of the duodenum and uncinate process of the pancreas, and joins the splenic vein behind the neck of the pancreas to form the portal vein.

A

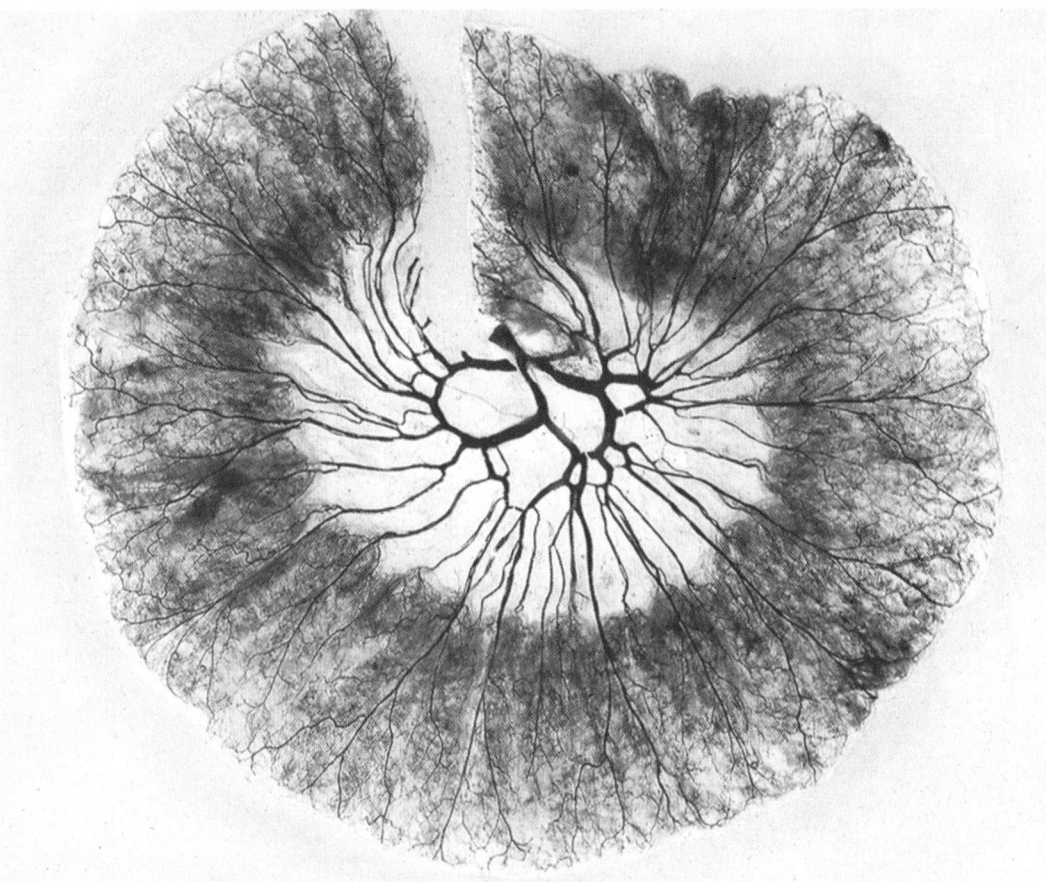

Fig. 74.3 Specimens of the jejunum (**A**) and ileum (**B**) (overleaf) from a subject in whom the superior mesenteric artery was injected with a red coloured mass of gelatin before fixation. Subsequently the specimens were dehydrated and then cleared in benzene followed by methyl salicylate. The largest vessels present are the jejunal and ileal branches of the superior mesenteric artery and these are succeeded by anastomotic arterial arcades, which are relatively few in number (1–3) in the jejunum, becoming more numerous (5–6) in the ileum. From the arcades, straight arteries pass towards the gut wall; frequently, successive straight arteries are distributed to opposite sides of the gut. Note the denser vascularity of the jejunal wall. (Specimens prepared by MCE Hutchinson; photographs by Kevin Fitzpatrick on behalf of GKT School of Medicine, London.)

B

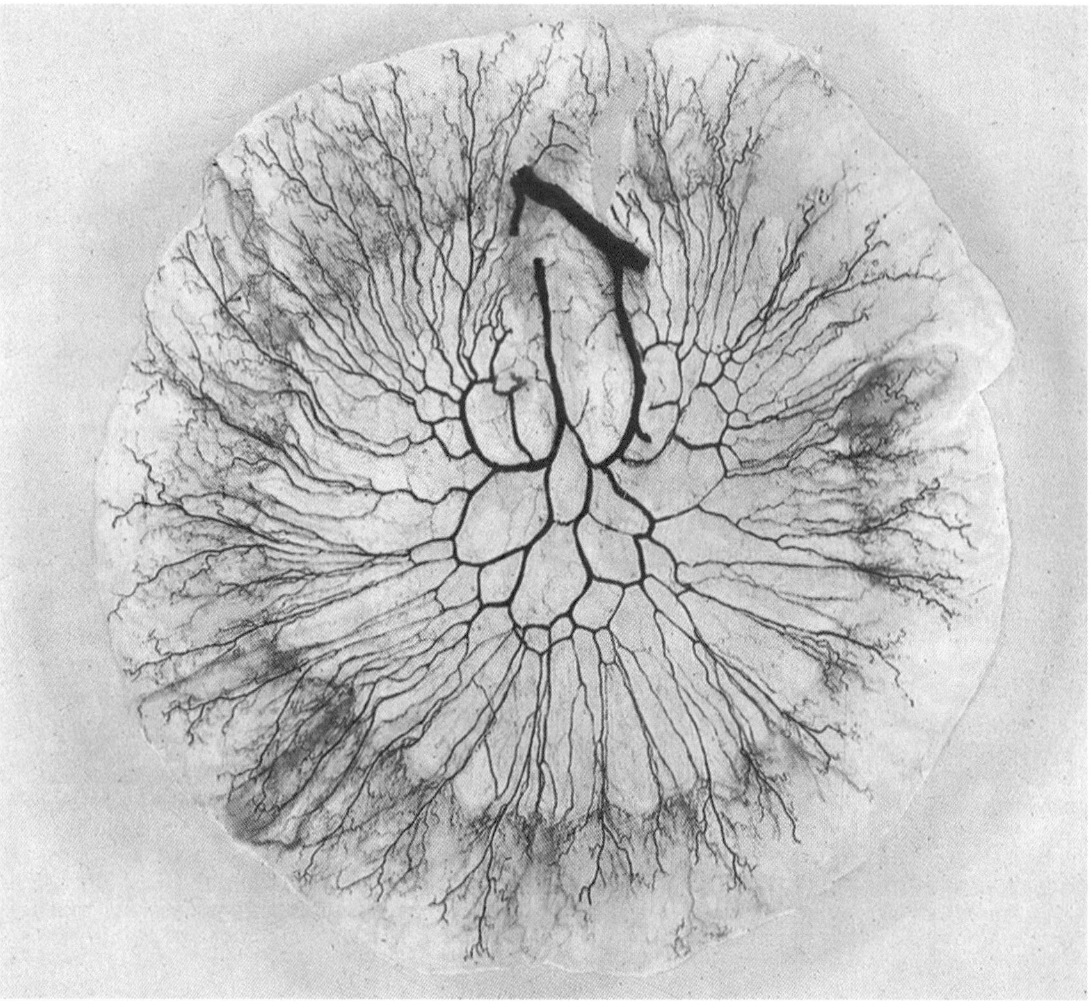

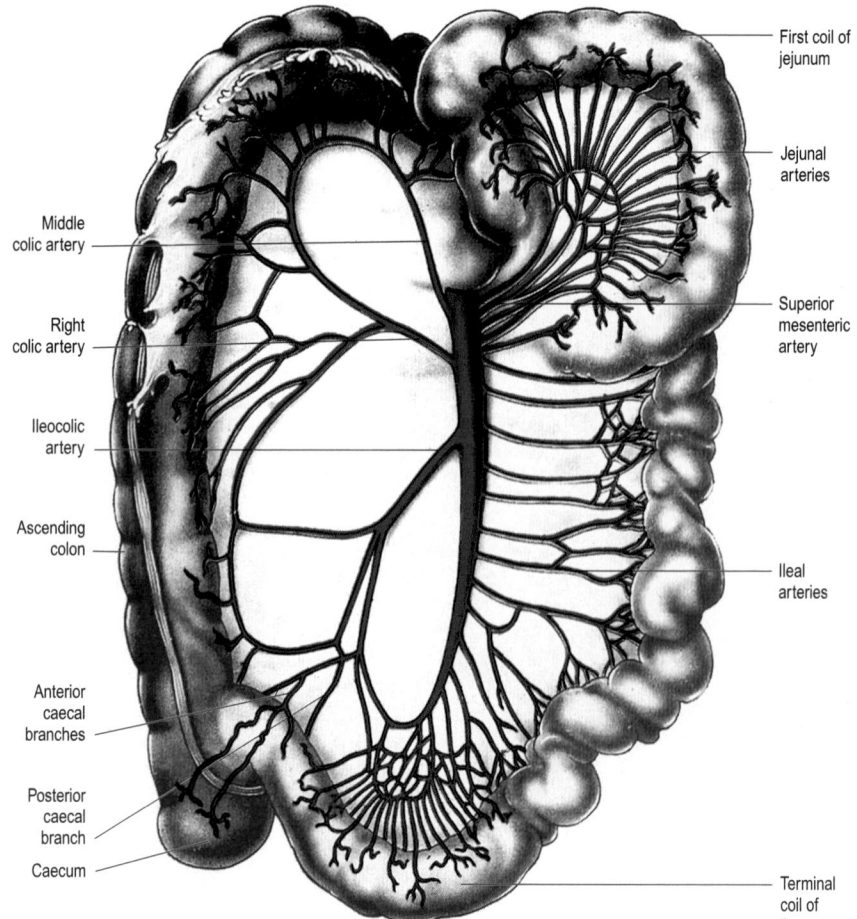

Fig. 74.3 (Cont'd).

First coil of
jejunum

Jejunal
arteries

Middle
colic artery

Right
colic artery

Superior
mesenteric
artery

Ileocolic
artery

Ascending
colon

Ileal
arteries

Anterior
caecal
branches

Posterior
caecal
branch

Caecum

Terminal
coil of
ileum

Fig. 74.4 The superior mesenteric artery and its branches.
The first loop of the jejunum and the terminal loop of the
ileum have been spread out to show the arrangement of
their arteries.

A

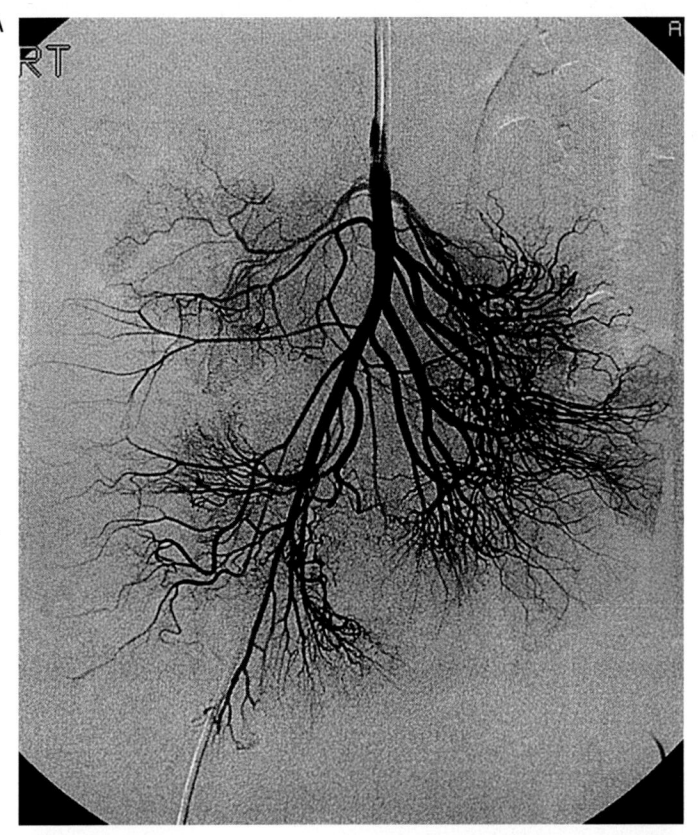

B

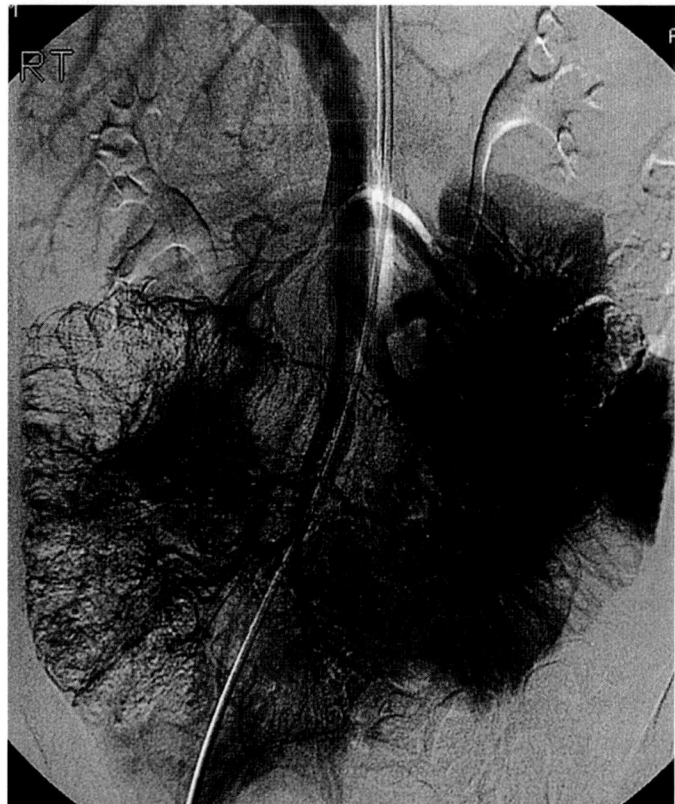

C

Fig. 74.5 The superior mesenteric artery and its branches: digital subtraction angiogram of the superior mesenteric artery (**A**) and vein (**B**); **C**, sagittal reformat of multislice CT superior mesenteric angiogram. (**A**, by kind permission from Dr Adam Mitchell, Charing Cross Hospital, London.) (**B**, by kind permission from Dr Adam Mitchell, Charing Cross Hospital, London; **C**, by kind permission from GE Worldwide Medical Systems.)

Tributaries – The superior mesenteric vein receives jejunal, ileal, ileocolic, right colic (p. 1191), middle colic (p. 1193), right gastroepiploic (p. 1149) and pancreaticoduodenal (p. 1165) veins in a similar distribution to the corresponding arteries.

LYMPHATICS

Lymph vessels, called lacteals, are arranged at two levels within the wall of the small bowel. The first is mucosal and the second in the muscular coat. Lymph vessels from the villi arise from an intricate plexus in the mucosa and submucosa and are joined by vessels from lymph spaces at the bases of solitary lymphoid follicles. They drain to larger vessels at the mesenteric aspect of the gut. The lymph vessels of the muscular tunic form a close plexus that runs mostly between the two muscle layers. They communicate freely with mucosal vessels and also open into vessels at the mesenteric border. Mesenteric lacteals pass between the layers of the mesentery. They drain into a series of mesenteric lymph nodes arranged in tiers within the mesentery which follow the same distribution as the regional arterial supply and which may form a 'chain' along the major arteries. Elsewhere in the ileal and jejunal mesentery they form an extensive network that affords a relatively wide field of lymph node drainage. This arrangement makes radical surgical resection of lymph nodes difficult if the vessels to the remaining unaffected small bowel are to be preserved. The mesenteric nodes drain into superior mesenteric nodes around the root of the superior mesenteric artery.

INNERVATION

SUPERIOR MESENTERIC PLEXUS

The superior mesenteric plexus, an inferior continuation of the coeliac plexus, lies in the preaortic connective tissue around the origin of the superior mesenteric artery, posterior to the pancreas. It receives preganglionic parasympathetic elements via the right vagus nerve. Preganglionic sympathetic fibres originate from neurones in the mid-thoracic spinal segments and travel in the greater and lesser splanchnic nerves to the coeliac and superior mesenteric ganglia where they synapse. The superior mesenteric ganglion lies superiorly in the plexus, usually above the origin of the superior mesenteric artery. Postganglionic axons accompany the superior mesenteric artery into the mesentery and are distributed along branches of the artery.

REFERRED PAIN

In common with other structures derived from the midgut, the visceral sensation of pain arising from the jejunum or ileum is poorly localized. It is commonly referred to the periumbilical region or central epigastrium.

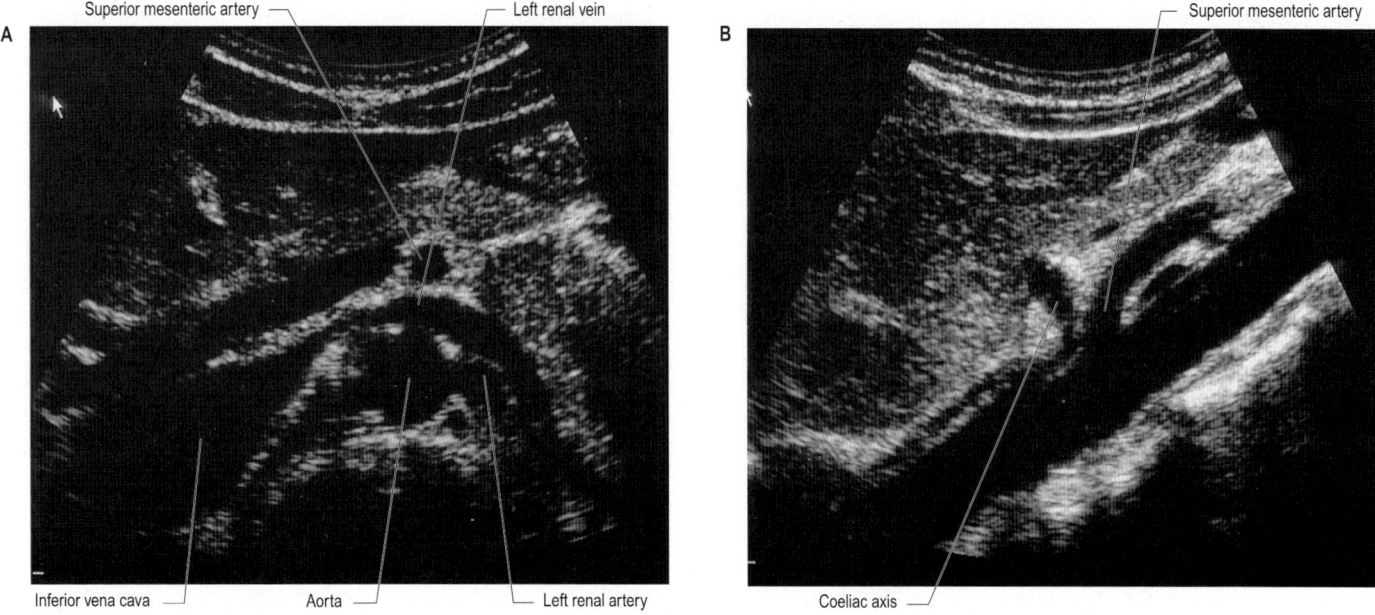

A

Superior mesenteric artery ⎯⎯⎯ | ⎯⎯⎯ Left renal vein

Inferior vena cava ⎯⎯⎯ | Aorta ⎯⎯⎯ | ⎯⎯⎯ Left renal artery

B

⎯⎯⎯ Superior mesenteric artery

Coeliac axis ⎯⎯⎯

Fig. 74.6 Ultrasound images taken through the origin of the superior mesenteric artery demonstrated in the axial (**A**) and sagittal (**B**) planes.

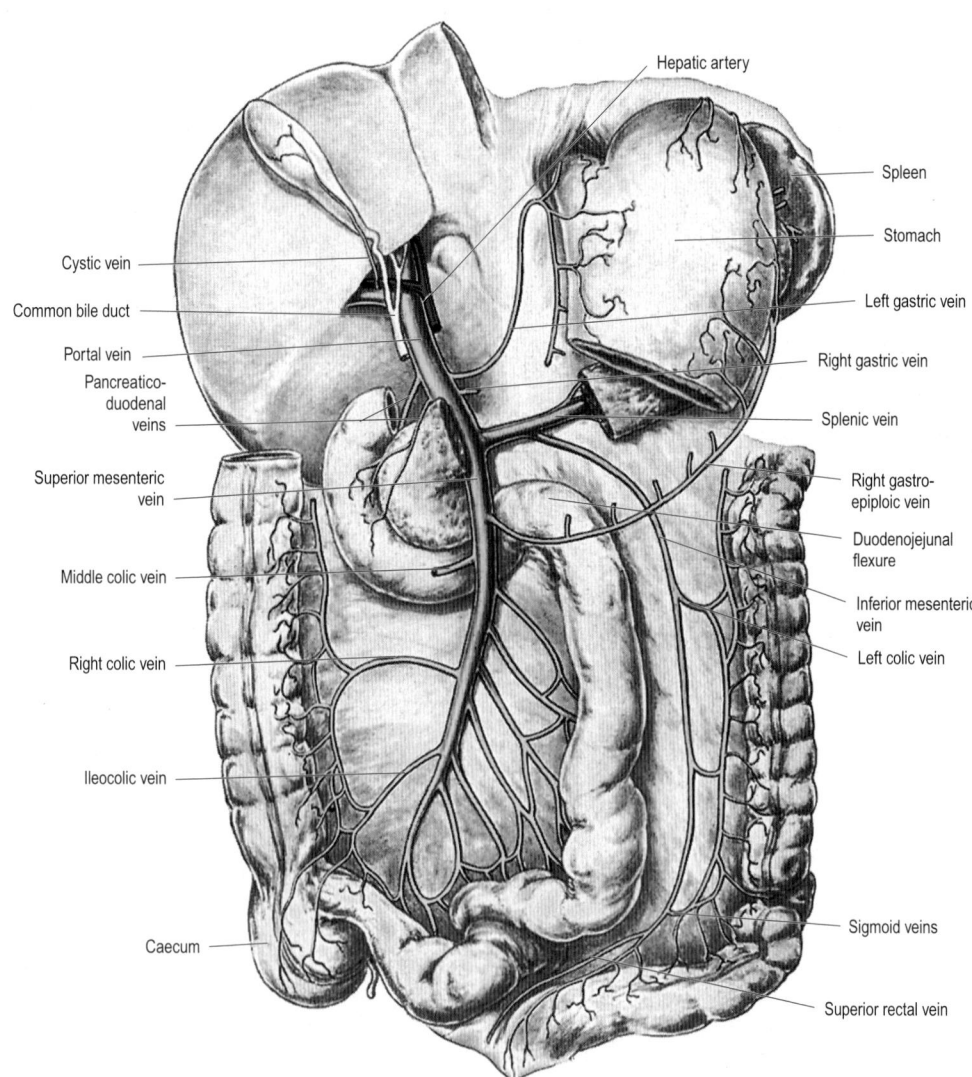

Hepatic artery

Spleen

Stomach

Cystic vein

Common bile duct

Portal vein

Pancreatico-
duodenal
veins

Superior mesenteric
vein

Middle colic vein

Right colic vein

Ileocolic vein

Left gastric vein

Right gastric vein

Splenic vein

Right gastro-
epiploic vein

Duodenojejunal
flexure

Inferior mesenteric
vein

Left colic vein

Sigmoid veins

Caecum

Superior rectal vein

Fig. 74.7 The portal vein and its tributaries (semi-diagrammatic). Portions of the stomach, pancreas and left lobe of the liver and the transverse colon have been removed.

REFERENCES

Kadir S 1991 Atlas of Normal and Variant Angiographic Anatomy. Philadelphia: WB Saunders.

Underhill BML 1955 Intestinal length in man. Br Med J 2: 1243–6.

Microstructure of the large intestine

The layers of tissue in the large intestinal wall (**Figs 70.1, 75.1**) resemble those in the small intestine (Ch. 72), except that villi and circular folds are absent and the glands (crypts) are longer.

MUCOSA

The mucosa is pale, smooth, and, in the colon, raised into numerous crescent-shaped folds between the sacculi. In the rectum it is thicker, darker, more vascular, and more loosely attached to the submucosa.

EPITHELIUM OF THE CAECUM, APPENDIX, COLON AND UPPER
RECTUM (Figs 75.1, 75.2, 75.3)
The luminal surface is lined by columnar cells, mucous (goblet) cells, and occasional microfold (M) cells (p. 1158) that are restricted to the epithelium overlying lymphoid follicles. Columnar and mucous cells are also present in the intestinal glands (crypts) which additionally contain stem cells and neuroendocrine cells. The glands generally lack Paneth cells, but these may be present in the caecum.

Columnar (absorptive) cells – Columnar (absorptive) cells are the most numerous of the epithelial cell types. They are responsible for ion exchange and other transepithelial transport functions including water resorption, particularly in the colon. Although there is some variation in their structure, they all bear apical microvilli, which are shorter and less regular than those on enterocytes in the small intestine. All cells have typical junctional complexes around their apices, and these limit extracellular diffusion from the lumen across the intestine wall.

Mucous (goblet) cells – Mucous cells have a similar structure to those of the small intestine, but are more numerous. They are outnumbered by absorptive cells for most of the length of the colon, but they are equally frequent towards the rectum, where their numbers increase further.

Microfold (M) cells – Microfold cells are similar to those of the small intestine: they are flattened or cuboidal cells with long, blunt micro-folds rather than typical microvilli, and they are restricted to epithelium overlying lymphoid follicles.

Stem cells – Stem cells are the source of the other epithelial cell types in the large intestine. They are located at or near the bases of the intestinal glands, where they divide by mitosis. They provide cells that migrate towards the luminal surface of the intestine: their progeny differentiate, undergo apoptosis and are shed after approximately 5 days.

Neuroendocrine cells – Neuroendocrine cells are situated mainly at the bases of the glands, and secrete basally into the lamina propria.

INTESTINAL GLANDS (CRYPTS) OF THE LARGE INTESTINE
The crypts are narrow perpendicular tubular glands which are longer, more numerous and closer together than those of the small intestine. Their openings give a cribriform appearance to the mucosa in surface view (**Fig. 75.2**). The glands are lined by low columnar epithelial cells, mainly goblet cells (**Figs 75.1, 75.3**), between which are columnar absorptive cells and neuroendocrine cells. Epithelial stem cells at their bases give rise to all three cell types.

LAMINA PROPRIA
The lamina propria is composed of connective tissue that supports the epithelium. It forms a specialized pericryptal fibroblast sheath around each intestinal gland. Solitary lymphoid follicles within the lamina propria are most abundant in the caecum, appendix and rectum, but are also present scattered along the rest of the large intestine. They are similar to those of the small intestine (Ch. 72) and efferent lymphatic vessels originate within them. Lymphatic vessels are absent from the lamina propria core between crypts.

MUSCULARIS MUCOSAE
The muscularis mucosae of the large intestine is essentially similar to that of the small intestine: it has prominent longitudinal and circular layers.

SUBMUCOSA

The submucosa of the large intestine is similar to that of the small intestine.

MUSCULARIS EXTERNA

The muscularis externa has outer longitudinal and inner circular layers of smooth muscle. The longitudinal fibres form a continuous layer but, with the exception of the uniform outer muscle layer of most of the appendix, macroscopically these are aggregated as longitudinal bands or taeniae coli (**Fig. 76.10**). Between the taeniae coli the longitudinal layer is much thinner, less than half the circular layer in thickness. The circular fibres form a thin layer over the caecum and colon, and are aggregated particularly in the intervals between the sacculi. In the rectum they form a thick layer and in the anal canal they form the internal anal sphincter. There is an interchange of fascicles between circular and longitudinal layers, especially near the taeniae coli. Deviation of longitudinal fibres from the taeniae to the circular layer may, in some instances, explain the haustration of the colon.

SEROSA

The serosa or visceral peritoneum is variable in extent. Along the colon the peritoneum forms small fat-filled appendices epiploicae (**Fig. 76.10**) which are most numerous on the sigmoid and transverse colon but generally absent from the rectum. Subserous loose connective tissue attaches the peritoneum to the muscularis externa.

MICROSTRUCTURE OF THE APPENDIX

The layers of the wall of the appendix are essentially those of the rest of the large intestine but some features are notably different and are described here. The serosa forms a complete covering, except along the mesenteric attachment. The longitudinal muscular fibres form a complete layer of uniform thickness, except over a few small areas where both muscular layers are deficient, leaving the serosa and submucosa in contact. At the base of the appendix, the longitudinal muscle thickens to form rudimentary taeniae that are continuous with those of the caecum and colon.

The submucosa typically contains many large lymphoid aggregates that extend from the mucosa and obscure the muscularis mucosae layer: consequently this becomes discontinuous. These aggregates also cause the mucosa to bulge into the lumen of the appendix, so that it narrows irregularly (**Fig. 75.4**). They are absent at birth but accumulate over the first 10 years of life to become a prominent feature. The mucosa is covered by a columnar epithelium as it is elsewhere in the large

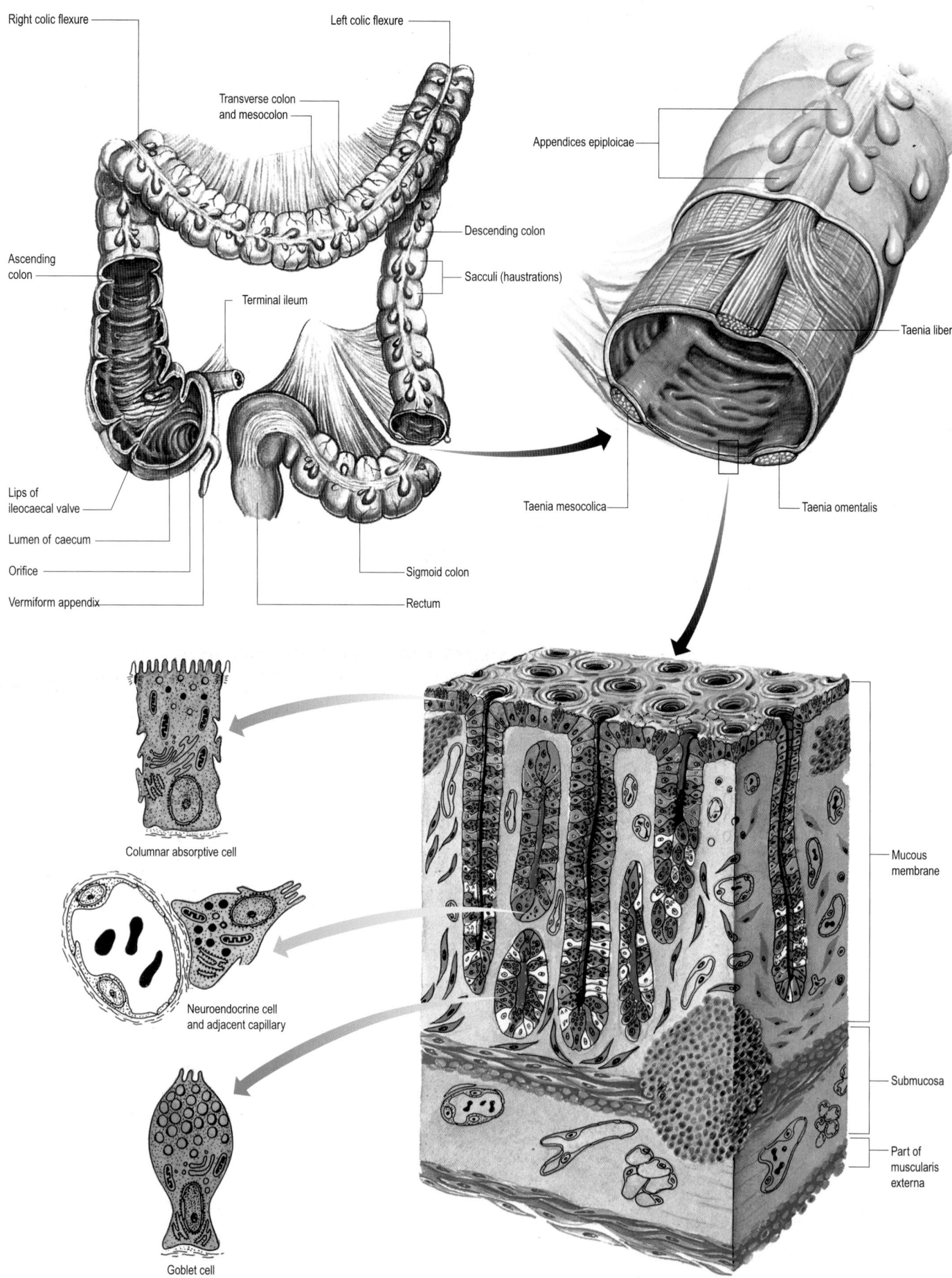

Fig. 75.1 Diagrams showing the major regions of the large intestine, the microstructure of the colonic wall and its epithelial cells. Note the aggregations of lymphocytes (yellow) and undifferentiated epithelial cells (white).

intestine, and M cells are present in the epithelium that overlies the mucosal lymphoid tissue. Glands (crypts) are similar to those of the colon but are fewer in number and thus less densely packed. They penetrate deep into the lymphoid tissue of the mucosal lamina propria (**Fig. 75.4**). The submucosal lymphoid tissue frequently exhibits germinal centres within its follicles (p. 77), indicative of B-cell activation, as it is in secondary lymphoid tissue elsewhere (p. 74). In adults, the normal layered structure of the appendix is lost and the lymphoid follicles atrophy and are replaced by collagenous tissue. In the elderly, the appendix may be filled with fibrous scar tissue.

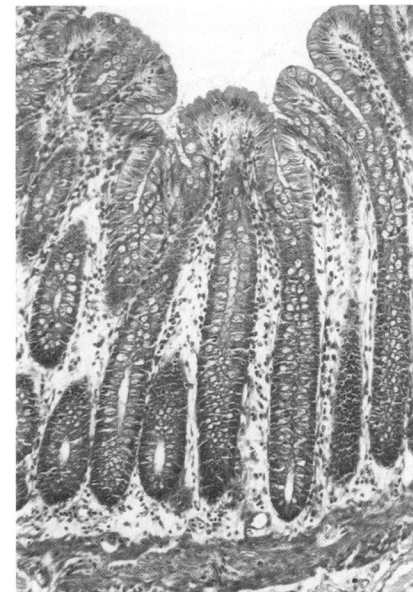

Fig. 75.3 Micrograph showing the colonic mucosa with mucus-secreting surface epithelium and glands (crypts). The smooth muscle of the muscularis mucosae is seen at the bottom of the field. (Photograph by Sarah-Jane Smith.)

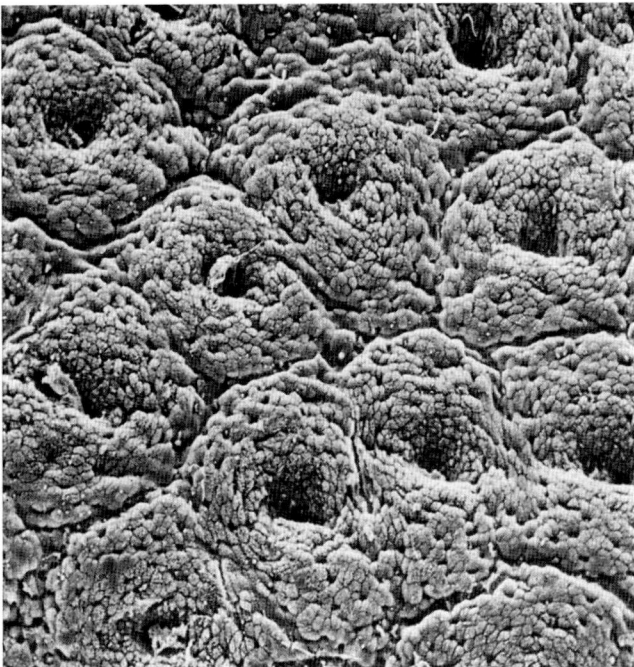

Fig. 75.2 Scanning electron micrograph of the luminal surface of human rectal mucosa. The outlines of absorptive epithelial cells bearing microvilli and the openings of rectal crypts can be seen. (Material provided by DS Rampton; prepared and photographed by Michael Crowder.)

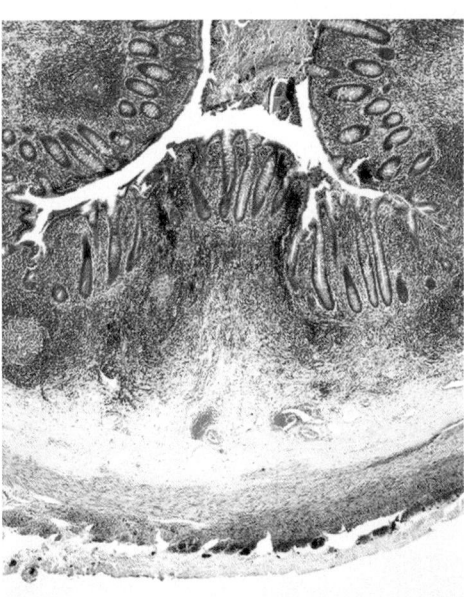

Fig. 75.4 Low-power micrograph of the appendix in transverse section, showing part of its circumference and a faecal pellet lodged in its lumen. Lymphoid tissue (basophilic staining) occupies much of the mucosa between crypts, and part of the submucosa. The muscularis externa and outermost serosa layer are seen at the bottom of the field. (Photograph by Sarah-Jane Smith.)

Overview of the large intestine

The large intestine extends from the distal end of the ileum to the anus, and is c.1.5 m long, although there is considerable variation in its length. Its calibre is greatest near the caecum and gradually diminishes to the level of mid rectum. It enlarges in the lower third of the rectum to form the rectal ampulla above the anal canal. The large intestine differs from the small intestine in that it has a greater calibre; it is for the most part more fixed in position; its longitudinal muscle, though a complete layer, is concentrated into three longitudinal bands, taeniae coli, in all but the distal sigmoid colon and rectum; small adipose projections, appendices epiploicae, are scattered over the free surface of the whole colon (they tend to be absent from the caecum, vermiform appendix and rectum). Moreover, the colonic wall is puckered into sacculations (haustrations), which may, in part, be due to the presence of the taeniae coli, and which may be demonstrated on plain radiographs as incomplete septations arising from the bowel wall. The function of the large intestine is chiefly absorption of fluid and solutes.

Broadly speaking, the large intestine lies in a curve which extends from the right iliac fossa, ascends in the right flank, crosses the mid upper abdomen in a variable course, descends in the left flank, passes through the left iliac fossa and thence posteroinferiorly into the pelvis. (**Fig. 76.1**). It tends to form a border to the loops of the small intestine which are located centrally within the abdomen. The colon commences in the right iliac fossa as the caecum, from which the vermiform

appendix arises. The caecum proceeds directly into the ascending colon which ascends in the right lumbar and hypochondriac regions to the inferior aspect of the liver where it bends to the left forming the hepatic flexure (right colic flexure). The large intestine then loops across the abdomen with an anteroinferior convexity as the transverse colon, and on reaching the left hypochondriac region it curves inferiorly to form the splenic flexure (left colic flexure). The descending colon proceeds through the left lumbar and iliac regions and becomes the sigmoid colon in the left iliac fossa. The sigmoid colon descends deep into the pelvis as the rectum and ends in the anal canal below the level of the pelvic floor.

The large intestine develops as a fully mesenteric organ (p. 1259). However, after the rotation of the gut tube *in utero*, large portions of it come to lie adherent to the retroperitoneum, which means that some parts of the colon are fixed within the retroperitoneum, and other parts are suspended by a mesentery within the peritoneal cavity. Those portions of the colon within the retroperitoneum are separated from other retroperitoneal structures by a thin layer of connective tissue which forms an avascular field during surgical dissection, but which offers little or no barrier to the spread of disease within the retroperitoneum.

The caecum may be within the retroperitoneum, but more frequently is suspended by a short mesentery. The ascending colon is usually a retroperitoneal structure although the hepatic flexure may be suspended

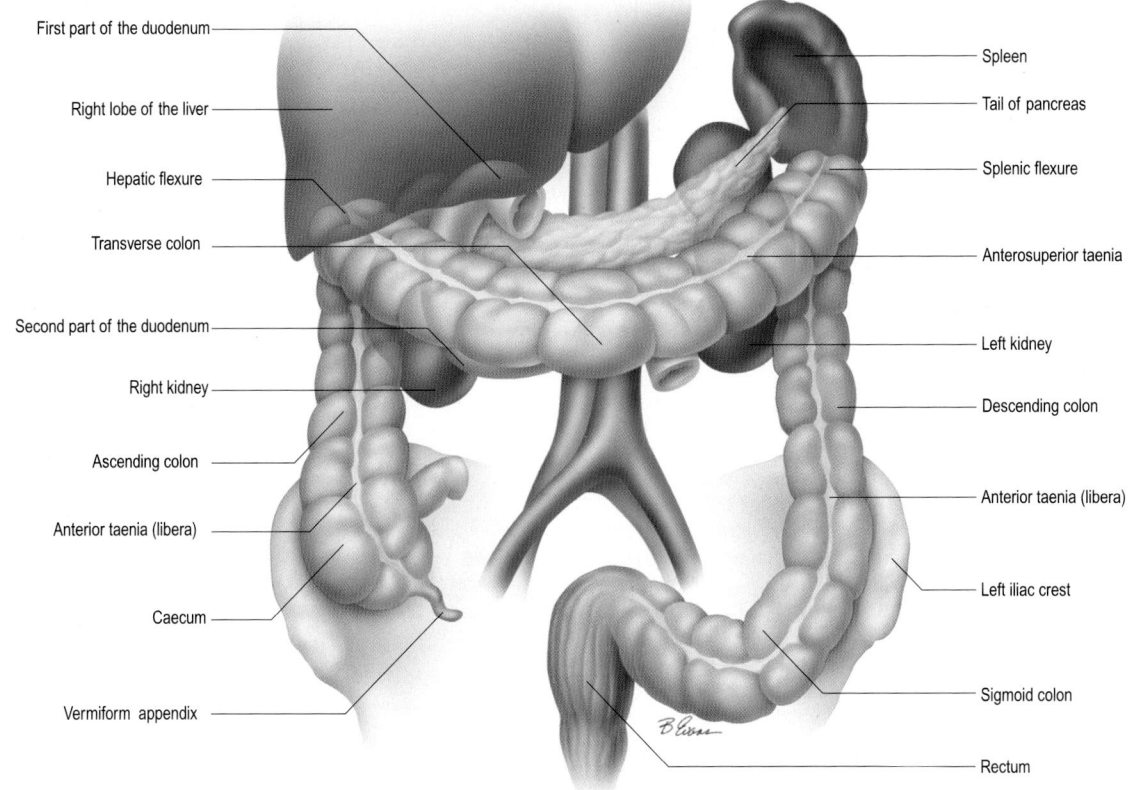

Fig. 76.1 Overview of the abdominal colon and its relations.

by a mesentery. The transverse colon emerges from the retroperitoneum on a rapidly elongating mesentery and lies, often freely mobile, in the upper abdomen. The transverse mesocolon shortens to the left of the upper abdomen and may become retroperitoneal at the splenic flexure. Occasionally the splenic flexure is suspended by a short mesentery. The descending colon is retroperitoneal usually to the level of the left iliac crest. As the colon enters the pelvis it becomes increasingly more mesenteric again at the origin of the sigmoid colon, although the overall length of the sigmoid mesentery is highly variable. The distal sigmoid colon lies on a rapidly shortening mesentery as it approaches the pelvis and by the level of the rectosigmoid junction the mesentery has all but disappeared, so that the rectum enters the pelvis as a retroperitoneal structure. In the neonate and infant, the caecum and proximal ascending colon are often more mobile on a longer mesentery than in the adult.

The mesenteries of the colon consist of visceral peritoneum enclosing connective and adipose tissues which envelop the vessels, nerves and lymphatics as they course from the retroperitoneum. There is a direct communication from the retroperitoneum to the suspended colon within the mesenteries via the so-called subperitoneal space.

EXTERNAL APPEARANCE

The haustrations of the colon are often absent in the caecum proximal to the origin of the ascending colon and are often relatively sparse in the ascending and proximal transverse colon. In these regions the taeniae coli are usually thin and occupy only a small percentage of the circumference of the colon. There are few if any appendices epiploicae on the serosal surface of the caecum, and only a limited number on the surface of the ascending colon. The haustrations become more pronounced from the middle of the transverse colon to the distal portion of the descending colon: the sigmoid colon is often characterized by marked sacculation. The width of the taeniae coli remains fairly constant throughout the length of colon but the number of appendices usually increases, becoming most numerous in the sigmoid colon where they can be fairly large in the obese individual. The taeniae are located in fairly constant positions beneath the serosal surface of the colon except in the transverse colon. They are oriented anteriorly, opposite the midline of the mesenteric attachment on the anti-mesenteric aspect of the colon (taenia libera), posterolaterally (taenia omentalis) and posteromedially (taenia mesocolica) midway between the taenia libera and the mesentery. In the caecum and descending colon, which are partly retroperitoneal structures, the posterolateral taenia is often obscured from view by the peritoneal reflection onto the colonic wall. In the transverse colon, the taeniae are rotated through 90° – anterior being inferior, posteromedial being posterior and posterolateral being superior – as a consequence of the mobility and dependent position of this part of the colon. The taeniae coli broaden to occupy more of the circumference of the sigmoid colon in its distal portion and by the level of the rectosigmoid junction have widened to form distinct anterior and posterior bands, which unite to form a complete longitudinal muscle covering for the rectum. The rectum therefore has no external sacculation and no serosal appendices epiploicae.

INTERNAL APPEARANCE

Throughout its length, the internal aspect of the colon is characterized by the presence of haustrations. These infoldings of the wall consist of mucosa and submucosa, and may partially span the lumen, but they never form a complete, circumferential ring. The pattern of the haustrations and appearance of the colonic mucosa help the clinician appreciate the level reached during flexible endoscopic examinations of the colon. In the portion of the caecum where haustrations occur, the three longitudinal taeniae coli converge to form a characteristic 'trefoil' pattern on the caecal wall (**Fig. 76.2**). Elsewhere, the wall of the lower pole of the caecum is usually devoid of haustrations, although a spiral mucosal pattern is often seen in the region of the appendix orifice (**Fig. 78.3**). The upper caecum and ascending colon possess shallow but long haustrations which may extend across one-third of the lumen (**Fig. 76.3**). This pattern is most pronounced in the transverse colon where the long haustrations often confer a triangular cross section on the lumen (**Fig. 76.4**). The wall of the colon is thinnest in this region and is most at risk of perforation during therapeutic endoscopic procedures. The haustrations of the descending and sigmoid colon tend to be thicker and shorter than those of the transverse colon, which gives a more circular cross-section to the lumen. The overall luminal diameter

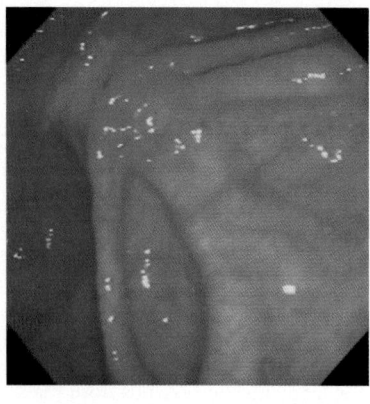

Fig. 76.2 Endoscopic appearance of the caecum. The characteristic trefoil appearance of the confluence of the three taeniae is usually obvious.

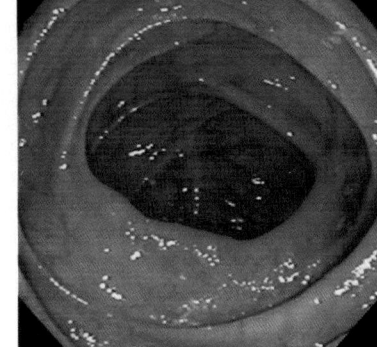

Fig. 76.3 Endoscopic appearance of the ascending colon.

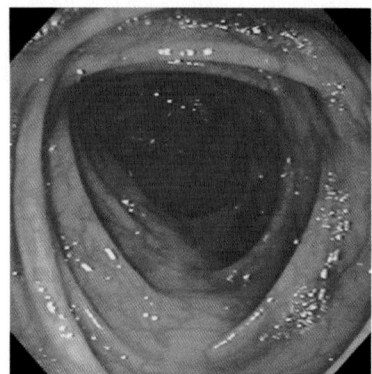

Fig. 76.4 Endoscopic appearance of the transverse colon. The characteristic triangular appearance of the haustrations when viewed collectively is obvious.

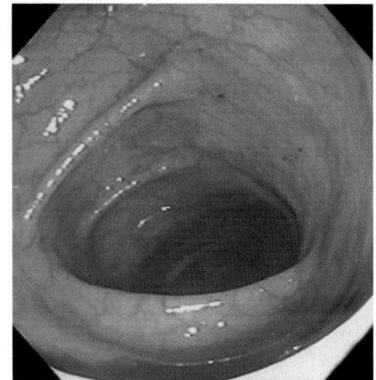

Fig. 76.5 Endoscopic appearance of the descending colon.

is often smallest in the descending colon (**Fig. 76.5**). During endoscopy the pattern of the submucosal vessels becomes more conspicuous in the sigmoid colon (**Fig. 76.6**). (The mobility of the sigmoid colon on its mesentery means that shorter lengths of colon tend to be visible during endoscopy than anywhere else in the colon.) The haustrations of the rectum tend to form consistent and recognizable folds: the

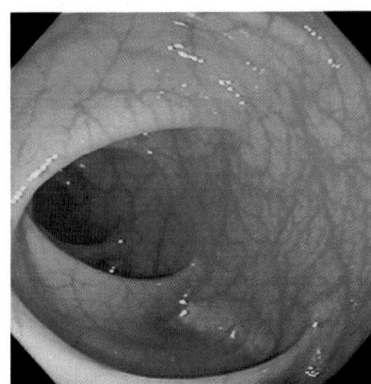

Fig. 76.6 Endoscopic appearance of the sigmoid colon.

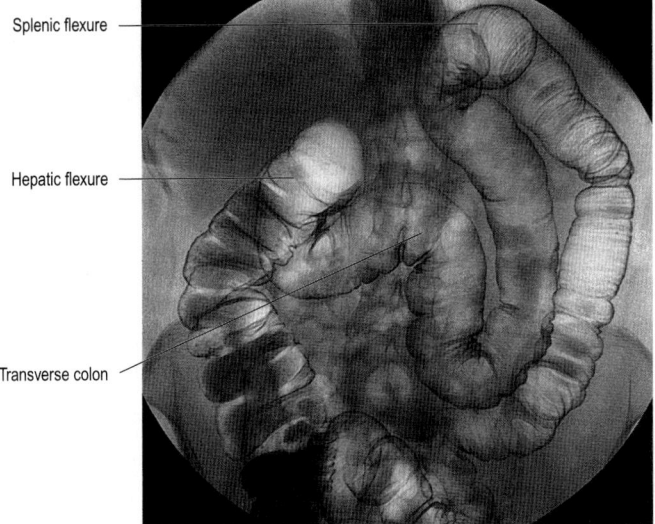

Splenic flexure

Hepatic flexure

Transverse colon

Fig. 76.7 Appearance of the abdominal colon on double contrast barium enema examination demonstrating the transverse colon, hepatic and splenic flexures.

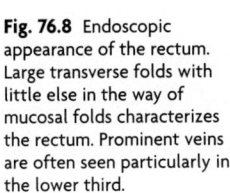
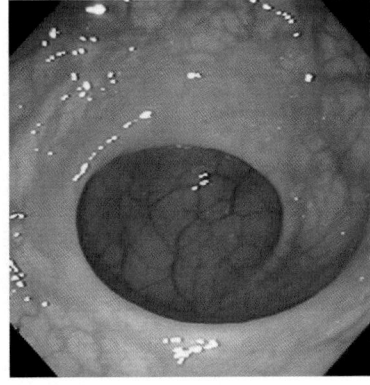

Fig. 76.8 Endoscopic appearance of the rectum. Large transverse folds with little else in the way of mucosal folds characterizes the rectum. Prominent veins are often seen particularly in the lower third.

pattern of the submucosal vessels is more pronounced than anywhere else in the colon (**Fig. 76.8**). Distinct veins are usually visible during endoscopy, and they are most marked above the anorectal junction.

CROSS-SECTIONAL APPEARANCE

Cross-sectional imaging of the colon can be performed with computerized tomography (CT) and magnetic resonance imaging (MRI) permitting visualization of the bowel wall. On axial imaging the colon may be filled with particulate faeces and air (**Fig. 76.9**). The wall in normal individuals is imperceptibly thin. Diverticular disease is very common in adults, and air-filled diverticula are frequently identified as outpouchings of the colonic wall, especially in the sigmoid colon. The air

content and position of the colon facilitate its identification throughout the retroperitoneum and peritoneum suspended by its mesenteries. The caecum and ascending colon often contain faecal residue and are easily identified in the right retroperitoneum. The transverse colon may contain faeces or gas, but lies in a variable position suspended by its mesentery. The descending colon in the left retroperitoneum is frequently collapsed and contains little faecal residue.

The volume data sets produced by modern multislice CT can now produce virtual colonoscopic mucosal images in the distended and cleaned colon, and surface-rendered images of the external surface of the bowel. In addition post-processing allows interrogation of the bowel mucosa in stretched out segments of bowel that can be opened up like a surgical specimen (**Fig. 76.9**). In addition, both CT and MR abdominal angiography are possible following an intravenous injection of contrast: these techniques are less invasive than conventional angiography, which is increasingly being reserved for patients who need interventional procedures performed under imaging guidance.

VASCULAR SUPPLY AND LYMPHATIC DRAINAGE

ARTERIES

The arterial supply of the large intestine is derived from both the superior and inferior mesenteric arteries. Those parts derived from the midgut (caecum, appendix, ascending colon and right two-thirds of the transverse colon) are supplied from colic branches of the superior mesenteric artery; whilst hindgut derivatives (left part of the transverse, descending and sigmoid colon, rectum and upper anal canal) are supplied predominantly from the inferior mesenteric artery, with small contributions from branches of the internal iliac artery. The larger unnamed branches of these vessels ramify between the muscular layers of the colon which they supply. They subdivide into smaller submucosal rami and enter the mucosa. The terminal branches divide into vasa brevia and vasa longa which either enter the colonic wall directly or run through the subserosa for a short distance before crossing the circular smooth muscle to give off branches to the appendices epiploicae (**Fig. 76.10**).

Superior mesenteric artery

The superior mesenteric artery supplies the caecum, appendix, ascending colon and right two-thirds of the transverse colon via the ileocolic, right colic and middle colic branches (**Figs 76.11, 76.12**). The ileocolic artery is formed as the distal continuation of the superior mesenteric artery in the root of the small bowel mesentery after the origin of the last ileal artery. Although it has many variations in its terminal distribution, it usually divides into a superior branch, which anastomoses with the right colic artery, and an inferior branch, which anastomoses with the distal superior mesenteric artery.

The right colic artery usually arises as a common trunk with the middle colic artery. Occasionally it arises separately from the right side of the superior mesenteric artery and is absent rarely. Sometimes it arises from the ileocolic when it is named the accessory right colic artery.

The middle colic artery is one of the first branches of the superior mesenteric artery and usually originates on its anterolateral aspect as a common trunk with the right colic artery. It arises just inferior to the uncinate process of the pancreas, anterior to the third part of the duodenum and ascends in the root of the transverse colon mesentery, just to the right of the midline dividing into terminal branches.

Occasionally the middle colic artery arises separately from the right colic artery. It may arise from the dorsal pancreatic artery and rarely may arise from an accessory or replaced hepatic artery arising from the superior mesenteric artery. The artery may end in left and right main branches but frequently divides into three or more main branches within the mesentery.

A large branch may be present, which runs parallel and posterior to the middle colic artery in the transverse mesocolon. This provides a direct communication between the superior and inferior mesenteric arteries and is known as the arc of Riolan.

Inferior mesenteric artery

The inferior mesenteric artery is usually smaller in calibre than the superior mesenteric artery, and arises from the anterior or left

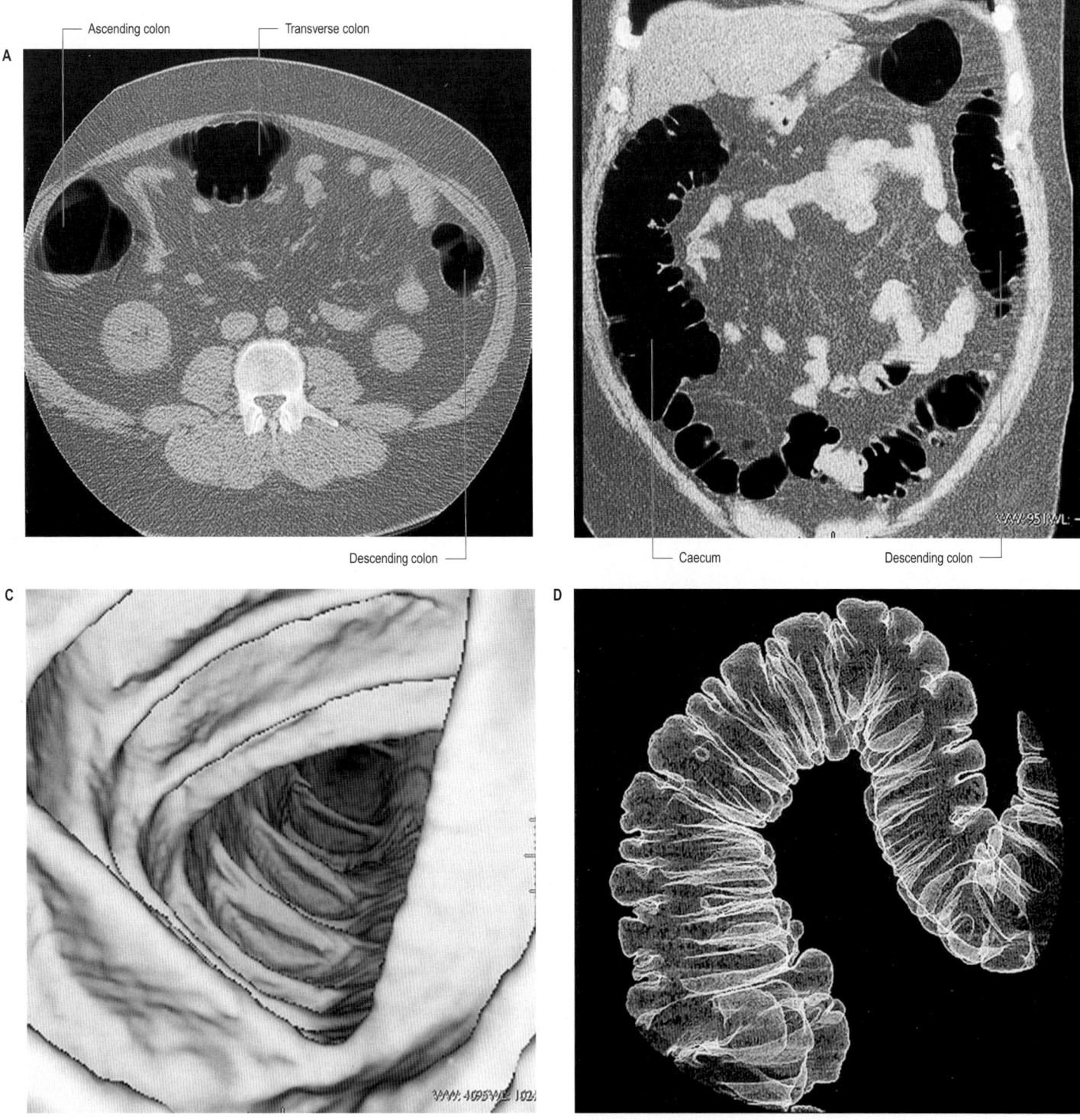

Fig. 76.9 Appearance of the colon on multislice computerized tomographic examination. The data acquired in the axial plane can be presented in a number of ways using multiplanar and volume rendered reformatting as demonstrated below. **A**, Axial CT showing air within the ascending, transverse and descending colon. **B**, Coronal reformat from axial data set showing the caecum, ascending and descending colon. **C**, Volume-rendering of the colonic wall using the axial data set to produce virtual colonoscopic views to show the triangular lumen of the transverse colon. **D**, Volume-rendering of the air-filled colon using the axial data set to give an image similar to a double contrast barium enema. (Images provided by kind permission from GE Worldwide Medical Systems.)

anterolateral aspect of the aorta at about the level of the third lumbar vertebra, 3 or 4 cm above the aortic bifurcation and posterior to the horizontal part of the duodenum. It descends deep to the peritoneum, initially anterior and then to the left of the aorta. It crosses the origin of the left common iliac artery medial to the left ureter and then enters, and continues in, the root of the sigmoid mesocolon as the superior rectal artery. Distally the inferior mesenteric vein is lateral to it. The principal branches are the left colic, sigmoid (of which there may be several) and superior rectal arteries (**Figs 76.11, 76.13**).

MARGINAL ARTERY OF THE COLON (Fig. 76.12)

The marginal artery (marginal artery of Drummond) of the colon is the vessel which lies closest to and parallels the bowel wall. It is formed by the main trunks, and the arcades arising from, the ileocolic and right, middle and left colic arteries. Anastomoses form between the main terminal branches which run parallel to the colon within the mesentery and give rise to vasa recta and vasa brevia to supply the colon. In the region of the splenic flexure the marginal artery receives contributions from the left branch of the middle colic artery – a branch of the

E

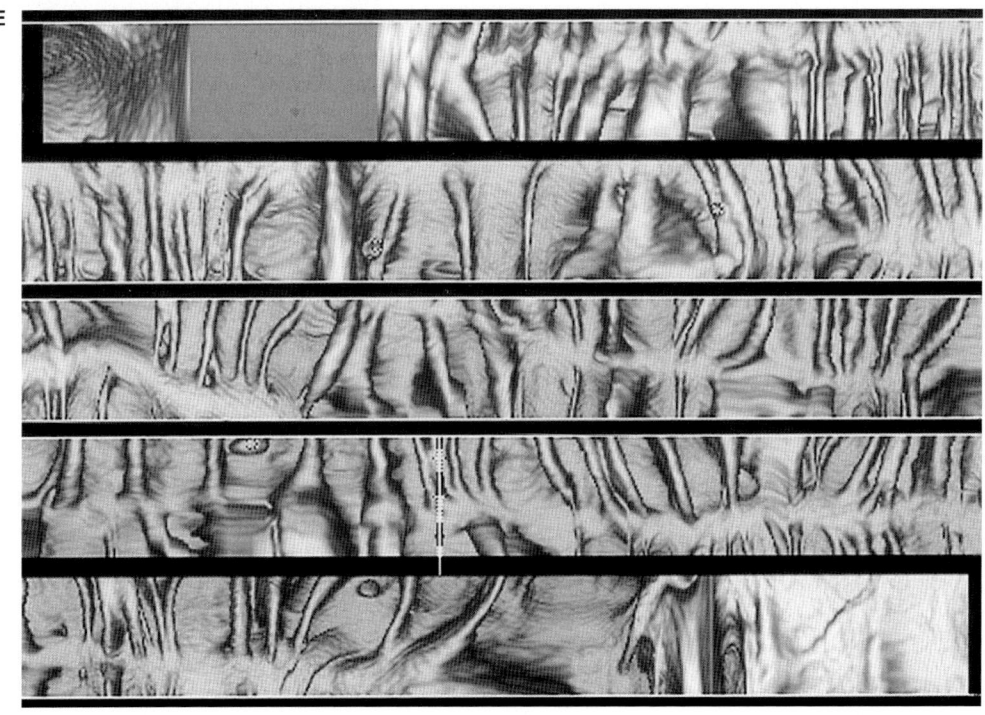

Fig. 76.9 (*Cont'd*) **E**, Volume-rendering of the axial data set to produce a virtual dissection of the transverse colon.

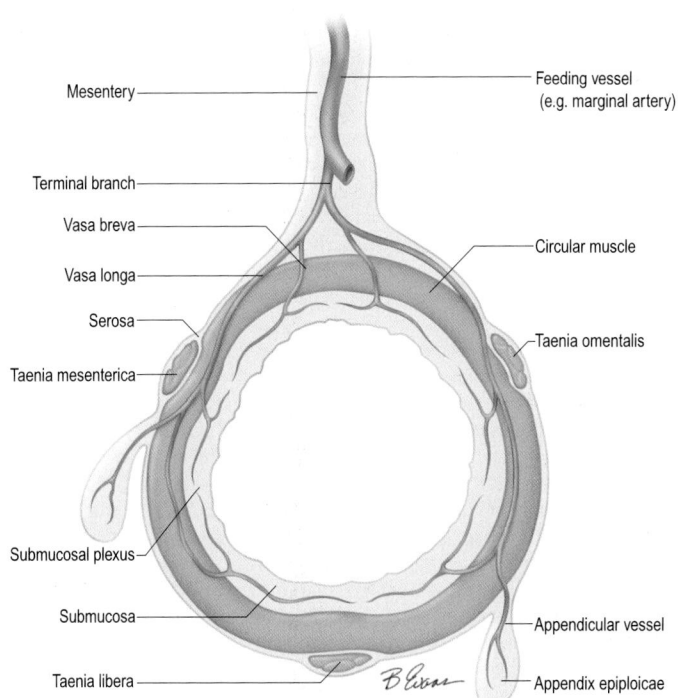

Mesentery

Feeding vessel
(e.g. marginal artery)

Terminal branch

Vasa breva

Circular muscle

Vasa longa

Serosa

Taenia omentalis

Taenia mesenterica

Submucosal plexus

Submucosa

Appendicular vessel

Taenia libera

Appendix epiploicae

Fig. 76.10 Typical pericolic arrangement of arterial vasculature.

superior mesenteric artery – which ramifies and anastomoses with an ascending branch of the left colic artery to supply the upper descending colon. The descending branch of the left colic artery ramifies and anastomoses with upper branches of the highest sigmoid artery to supply the descending colon. The origin of the primary arterial supply for the splenic flexure and distal third of the transverse colon is usually via the left colic artery but may be from the left branch of the middle colic artery. The marginal artery in the region of the splenic flexure may be absent or of such small calibre as to be of little clinical relevance. It may hypertrophy significantly when one of the main visceral arteries is compromised, e.g. following stenosis or occlusion of the inferior mesenteric artery, and it then provides a vessel of collateral supply.

Colonic vascular occlusion

The marginal artery of the colon may become massively dilated when there is chronic, progressive occlusion of the superior mesenteric artery, because under these conditions it is required to supply the majority of the midgut (except the proximal portion which is supplied by collateral vessels from the coeliac artery). Occlusion of the aorta or common iliac arteries may also result in dilatation of the marginal and inferior mesenteric arteries, which become an important collateral supply to the legs via dilated middle rectal vessels arising from the internal iliac artery.

Occlusion of the inferior mesenteric artery does not always result in irreversible ischaemia of the descending and sigmoid colon, because the marginal artery of the colon usually receives an adequate supply from the left branch of the middle colic artery. Moreover, the sigmoid arteries may be supplied by the superior rectal artery, which anastomoses with the middle and inferior rectal arteries. When ischaemia does occur, it is usually maximal in the proximal descending colon because this region is furthest from the collateral arterial supplies.

Vascular ligation in colonic resections

During resection of the descending and sigmoid colon, ligation of the inferior mesenteric artery close to its origin preserves the bifurcation of the left colic artery. This allows continued flow in the left colic artery to the proximal descending colon supplied by flow from the middle colic artery via the marginal artery. Less radical resection, involving ligation of the left colic artery close to its bifurcation, may interfere with or obliterate this supply and render the descending colon more likely to become ischaemic. The same is true for ligation of the left colic vein. If the inferior mesenteric vein is ligated, then the bifurcation of the vein forms the route of venous drainage for the descending colon to the middle colic vein territory. Ligation of the branches separately will impair the venous drainage.

VEINS

The venous drainage of the large intestine is primarily into the hepatic portal vein via the superior mesenteric and inferior mesenteric veins, although a small amount of drainage from the rectum occurs via middle rectal veins into the internal iliac vein and via inferior rectal veins into the pudendal vein. Those parts of the colon derived from the midgut (caecum, appendix, ascending colon and right two-thirds of the transverse colon) drain into colic branches of the superior mesenteric vein, whilst hindgut derivatives (left part of the transverse, descending and sigmoid colon, rectum and upper anal canal) drain into the inferior mesenteric vein.

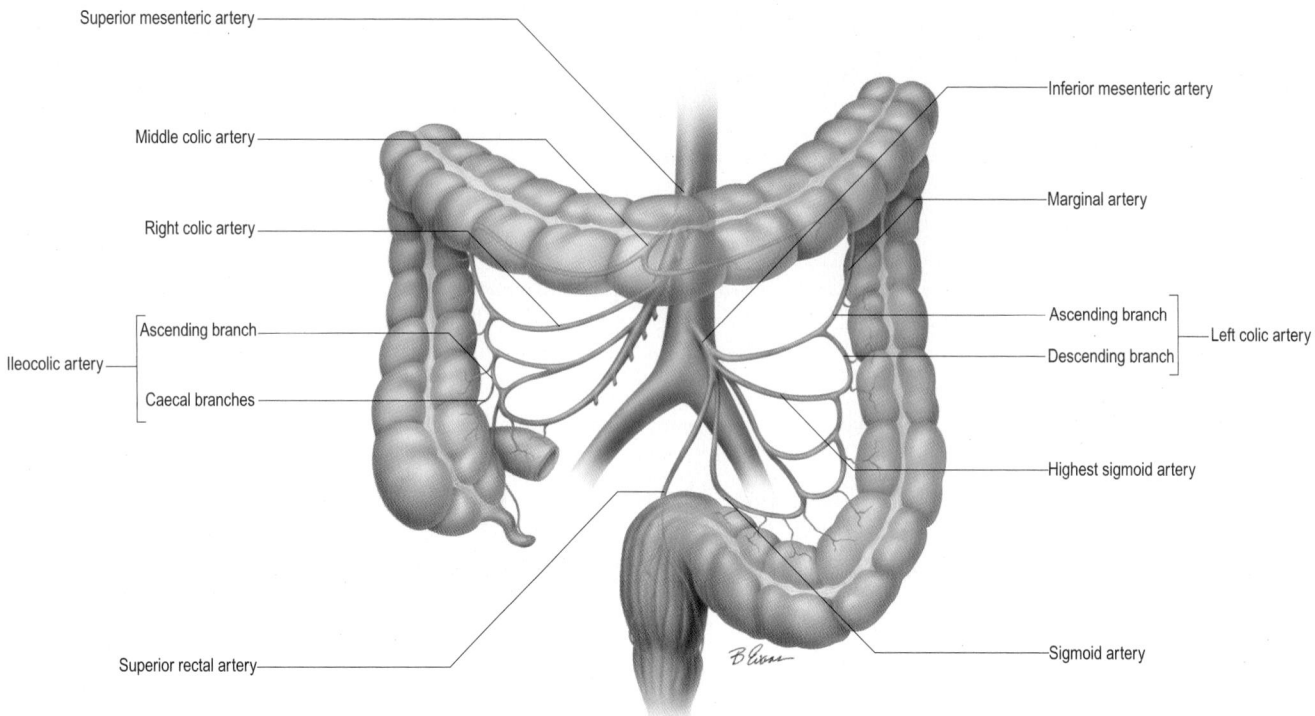

Superior mesenteric artery

Middle colic artery

Right colic artery

Ascending branch

Ileocolic artery

Caecal branches

Inferior mesenteric artery

Marginal artery

Ascending branch

Descending branch

Left colic artery

Highest sigmoid artery

Sigmoid artery

Superior rectal artery

Fig. 76.11 Relations and main branches of the superior and inferior mesenteric arteries.

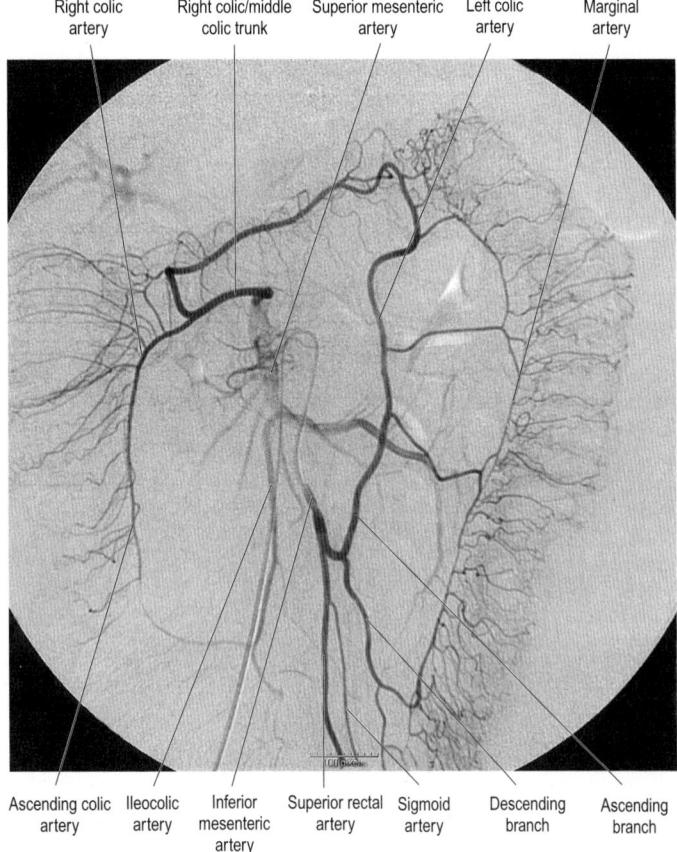

Right colic artery

Right colic/middle colic trunk

Superior mesenteric artery

Left colic artery

Marginal artery

Ascending colic artery

Ileocolic artery

Inferior mesenteric artery

Superior rectal artery

Sigmoid artery

Descending branch

Ascending branch

Fig. 76.12 Digital subtraction arteriogram of the marginal artery running parallel to the colon and anastomosing with the branches of the superior mesenteric artery supplying the right side of the colon. (By kind permission from Dr J Jackson, Hammersmith Hospital, London.)

Superior mesenteric vein

The superior mesenteric vein receives middle colic, right colic and ileocolic veins. Venous blood from the wall of the caecum, appendix, ascending colon and right two-thirds of the transverse colon drains into mesenteric arcades and subsequently into segmental veins, which accompany their respective arteries. The segmental veins drain into the superior mesenteric vein, which lies to the right of the mesenteric artery. The veins tend to follow variations in arterial drainage.

Inferior mesenteric vein

The inferior mesenteric vein drains the rectum, sigmoid, descending and distal transverse colon (**Figs 76.13, 76.14**). It begins as the superior rectal vein, from the rectal plexus, through which it connects with middle and inferior rectal veins. The superior rectal vein leaves the pelvis and crosses the left common iliac vessels medial to the left ureter with the superior rectal artery, and continues upwards as the inferior mesenteric vein. The inferior mesenteric vein lies to left of the inferior mesenteric artery, ascending deep to the peritoneum and anterior to the left psoas major. It may cross the testicular or ovarian vessels or ascend medial to them, and then passes above, or behind, the duodenojejunal flexure. It usually drains into the splenic vein, but occasionally drains into the confluence of the splenic and superior mesenteric veins or directly into the superior mesenteric vein. If a duodenal or paraduodenal fossa exists, the vein is usually in its anterior wall. The inferior mesenteric vein receives tributaries from several sigmoid veins, the middle and the left colic veins.

LYMPHATICS

Lymphatic vessels of the caecum, ascending and proximal transverse colon drain ultimately into lymph nodes related to the superior mesenteric artery, while those of the distal transverse colon, descending colon, sigmoid colon and rectum drain into nodes following the course of the inferior mesenteric artery (**Fig. 76.15**). In cases where the distal transverse colon or splenic flexure is predominantly supplied by vessels from the middle colic artery, the lymphatic drainage of this area may be predominantly to superior mesenteric nodes.

Colic nodes

Lymph nodes related to the colon form four groups, namely epicolic, paracolic, intermediate colic and preterminal colic nodes. Epicolic nodes are minute nodules on the serosal surface of the colon, sometimes in

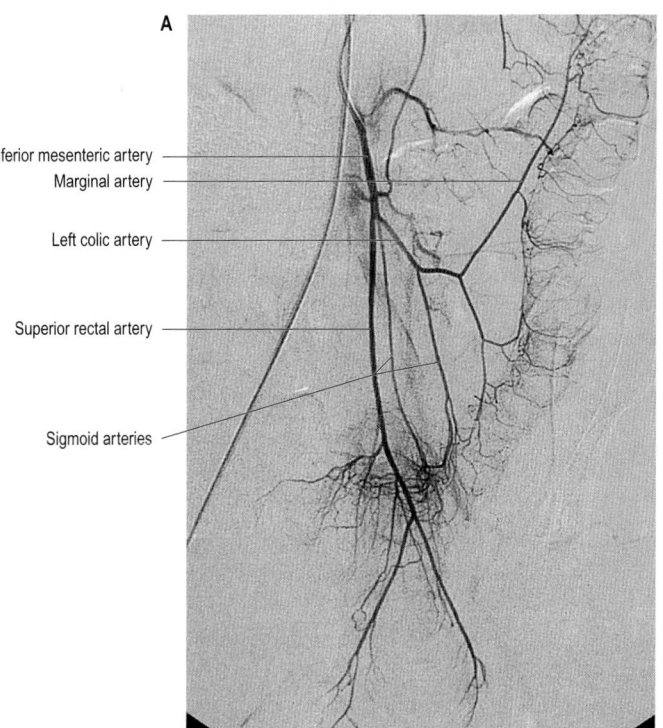

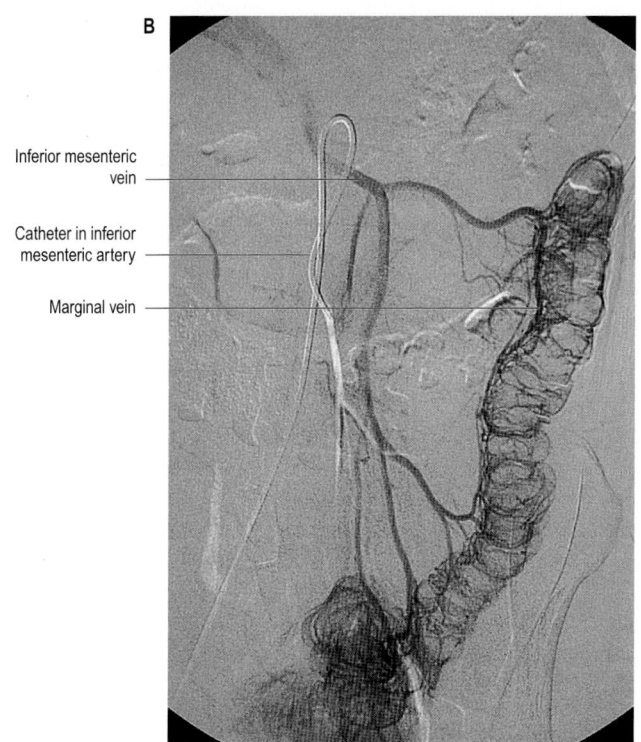

A
Inferior mesenteric artery
Marginal artery
Left colic artery
Superior rectal artery
Sigmoid arteries

B
Inferior mesenteric vein
Catheter in inferior mesenteric artery
Marginal vein

Fig. 76.13 Digital subtraction arteriogram showing **A**, the inferior mesenteric artery and its branches and **B**, the inferior mesenteric vein and its tributaries. (By kind permission from Dr Adam Mitchell, Charing Cross Hospital, London.)

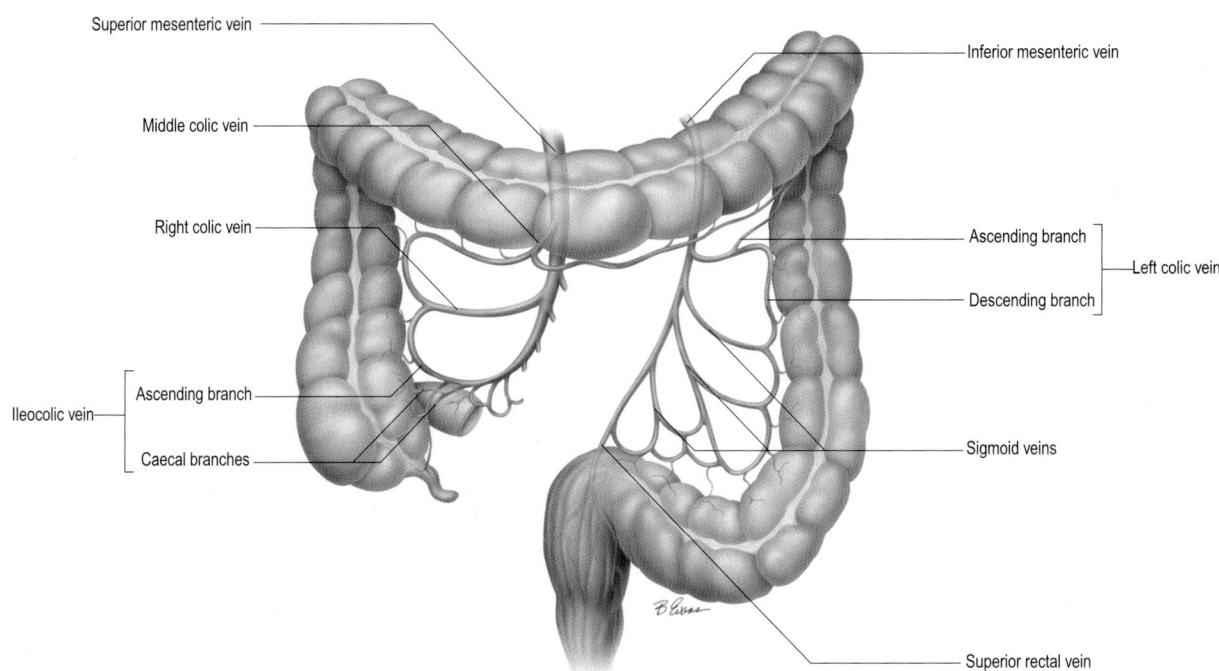

Superior mesenteric vein
Middle colic vein
Right colic vein
Ileocolic vein
  Ascending branch
  Caecal branches
Inferior mesenteric vein
Ascending branch
Descending branch
Left colic vein
Sigmoid veins
Superior rectal vein

Fig. 76.14 Relations and main branches of the superior and inferior mesenteric veins.

the appendices epiploicae. Paracolic nodes lie along the medial borders of the ascending and descending colon and along the mesenteric borders of the transverse and sigmoid colon. Intermediate colic nodes lie along the named colic vessels (the ileocolic, right colic, middle colic, left colic, sigmoid and superior rectal arteries). Preterminal colic nodes lie along the main trunks of the superior and inferior mesenteric arteries and drain into para-aortic nodes at the origin of these vessels. These are commonly referred to as the highest nodes of the territory which they drain.

Lymph node clearance in colorectal cancer resections

Radical lymphadenectomy during resection for colorectal cancer requires removal of the highest possible lymph node draining the area of colon in which the tumour is located. In cases of cancer involving the rectum and sigmoid colon, this usually involves resection of the pre-terminal colic nodes of the inferior mesenteric artery and thus ligation of the inferior mesenteric artery at its root or just below the origin of the left colic artery. A detailed description of the classification of the lymph nodes with regard to the site of the primary tumour within the colon

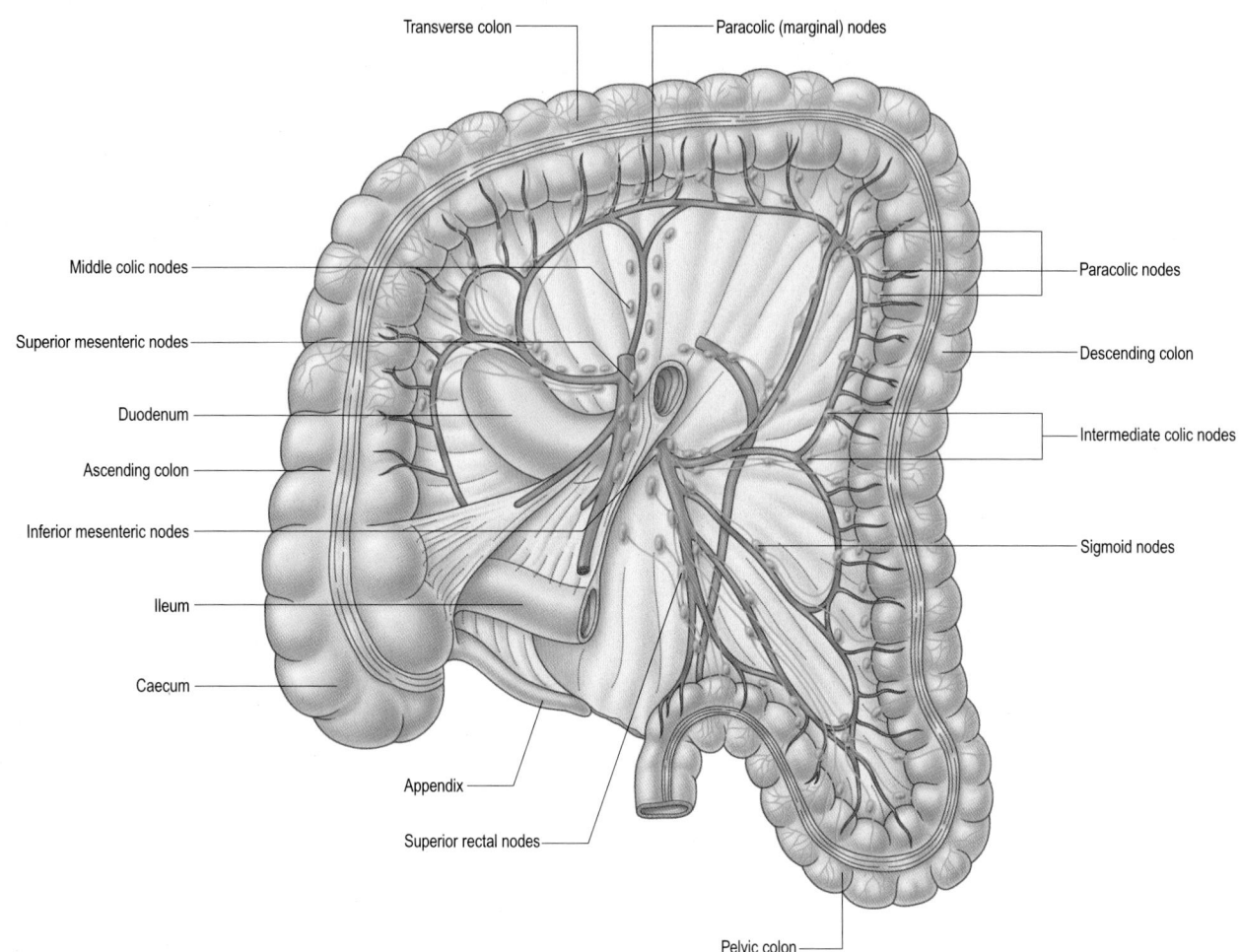

Fig. 76.15 The lymph vessels and nodes of the transverse, descending and sigmoid colon. (After Jamieson JK, Dobson JF 1908 The lymphatics of the colon. Proc R Soc Med 2: 149–174, by permission from the Royal Society of Medicine.)

has been suggested by the Japanese Society for the Cancer of the Colon and Rectum.

INNERVATION

The colon and rectum are innervated by the sympathetic and parasympathetic systems (**Figs 76.16, 76.17**).

The sympathetic supply to the caecum, appendix, ascending colon and right two-thirds of the transverse colon (derivatives of the midgut) originates in the fifth to the twelfth thoracic spinal segments. The preganglionic sympathetic axons which arise from these segments, and which are destined to influence the gut wall, do not synapse locally in the sympathetic chain, but instead are conveyed to the coeliac plexus via the greater and lesser splanchnic nerves, and synapse on ganglionic neurones in the coeliac and superior mesenteric plexuses. Postganglionic axons derived from neurones in these plexuses travel along branches of the superior mesenteric artery, and are distributed to the walls of the colon from periarterial plexuses. The parasympathetic supply is derived from the vagus nerve via the coeliac and superior mesenteric plexuses.

The sympathetic supply of the left third of the transverse colon, the descending and sigmoid colon, rectum and upper anal canal – derivatives of the hindgut – originates in the lumbar and upper sacral spinal segments. The fibres are distributed via the lumbar splanchnic nerves through the abdominal aortic and the inferior mesenteric plexuses and via the sacral splanchnic nerves through the superior and inferior hypogastric plexuses. Postganglionic axons reach the gut wall via periarterial plexuses on branches of the inferior mesenteric artery. The parasympathetic supply travels via the pelvic splanchnic nerves (nervi erigentes) from cell bodies in the second to the fourth sacral spinal segments. Those distributed to the rectum and upper anal canal run through the inferior and superior hypogastric plexuses to branches of the inferior mesenteric artery. Some of those distributed to the

descending and sigmoid colon run via these plexuses; however, a large number of fibres pass directly through the retroperitoneal tissues to the splenic flexure, descending and sigmoid colon independently of the inferior mesenteric artery.

The ultimate distribution within the wall of the large intestine is similar to the small intestine. The colic sympathetic nerves are motor to the ileocaecal valve musculature and inhibitory to mural muscle in the colon and rectum. Some fibres are vasoconstrictor to the colic vasculature. Parasympathetic nerves are motor to the colic and rectal musculature and inhibitory to the internal anal sphincter. Afferent impulses mediating sensations of distension are carried by visceral afferent fibres which travel with the parasympathetic nerves; pain impulses pass in visceral afferents travelling with the sympathetic and parasympathetic nerves supplying the rectum and the upper part of the anal canal.

SUPERIOR MESENTERIC PLEXUS

The superior mesenteric plexus lies in the preaortic connective tissue around the origin of the superior mesenteric artery posterior to the pancreas. It is an inferior continuation of the coeliac plexus, and includes branches from the right vagus nerve and the coeliac plexus. Its branches accompany the superior mesenteric artery into the mesentery, and it divides into secondary plexuses which are distributed along the branches of the artery. The superior mesenteric ganglion lies superiorly in the plexus, usually above the origin of the superior mesenteric artery.

ABDOMINAL AORTIC PLEXUS (INTERMESENTERIC PLEXUS)

The abdominal aortic plexus lies on the sides and front of the aorta, between the origins of the superior and inferior mesenteric arteries. It consists of 4–12 intermesenteric nerves, which are connected by oblique branches. It is continuous above with the coeliac plexus and below with the superior hypogastric plexus. It is formed by parasympathetic and

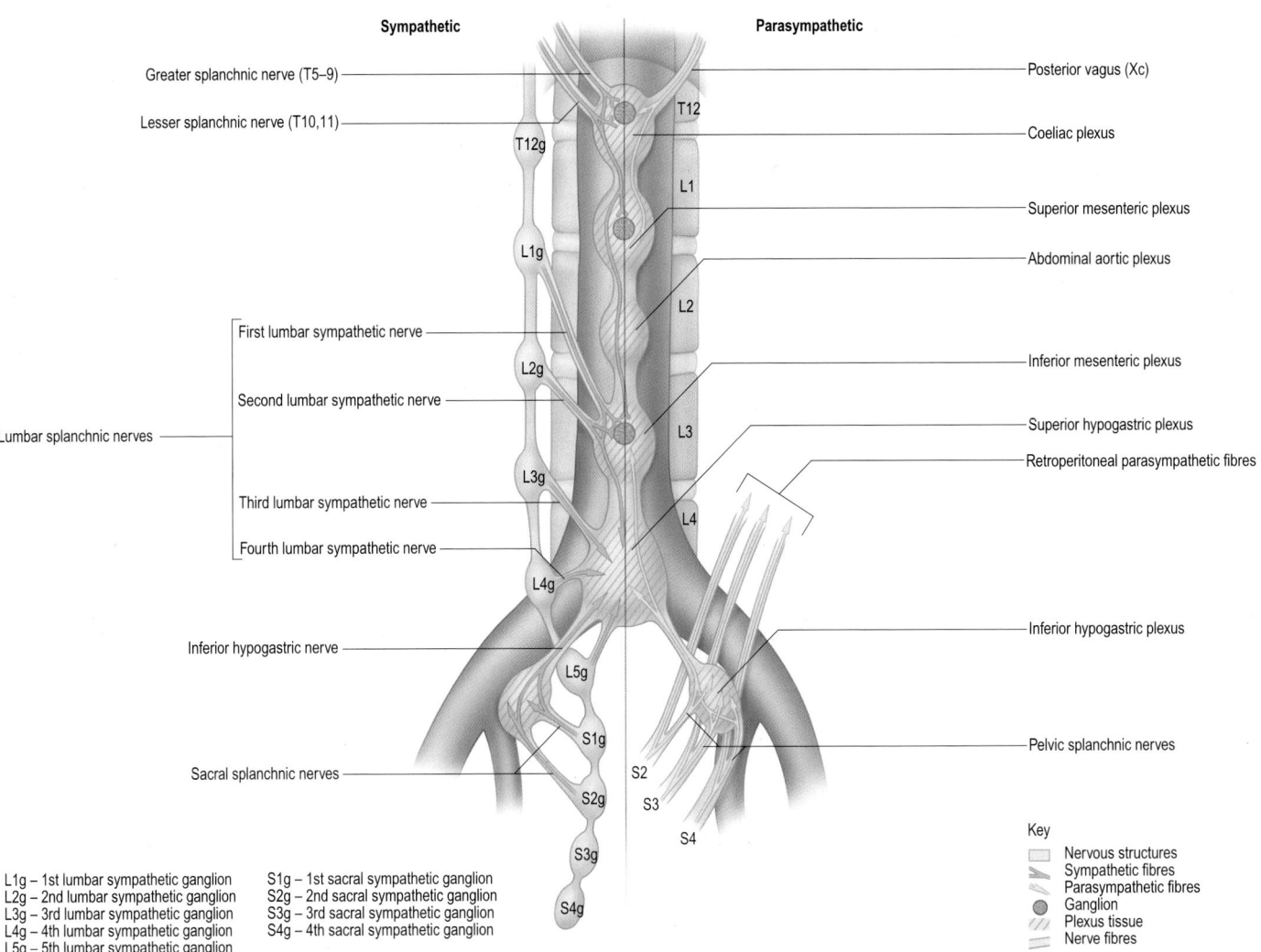

Sympathetic

Greater splanchnic nerve (T5–9)

Lesser splanchnic nerve (T10,11)

T12g

L1g

First lumbar sympathetic nerve

L2g

Second lumbar sympathetic nerve

Lumbar splanchnic nerves

Third lumbar sympathetic nerve

L3g

Fourth lumbar sympathetic nerve

L4g

Inferior hypogastric nerve

L5g

S1g

Sacral splanchnic nerves

S2g

S3g

S4g

Parasympathetic

Posterior vagus (Xc)

T12

Coeliac plexus

L1

Superior mesenteric plexus

Abdominal aortic plexus

L2

Inferior mesenteric plexus

Superior hypogastric plexus

L3

Retroperitoneal parasympathetic fibres

L4

Inferior hypogastric plexus

Pelvic splanchnic nerves

S2

S3

S4

L1g – 1st lumbar sympathetic ganglion
L2g – 2nd lumbar sympathetic ganglion
L3g – 3rd lumbar sympathetic ganglion
L4g – 4th lumbar sympathetic ganglion
L5g – 5th lumbar sympathetic ganglion

S1g – 1st sacral sympathetic ganglion
S2g – 2nd sacral sympathetic ganglion
S3g – 3rd sacral sympathetic ganglion
S4g – 4th sacral sympathetic ganglion

Key
Nervous structures
Sympathetic fibres
Parasympathetic fibres
Ganglion
Plexus tissue
Nerve fibres

Fig. 76.16 Schematic diagram of the autonomic plexuses of the colon and rectum.

sympathetic branches from the coeliac plexus and receives rami from the first and second lumbar splanchnic nerves which contain sympathetic fibres. It is connected with the testicular, inferior mesenteric, iliac and superior hypogastric plexuses.

INFERIOR MESENTERIC PLEXUS

The inferior mesenteric plexus lies around the origin of the inferior mesenteric artery and is distributed along its branches. It is formed predominantly from the aortic plexus and the first and second lumbar splanchnic nerves (sympathetic fibres), but it also receives connections from the superior hypogastric plexus (sympathetic and parasympathetic fibres).

SUPERIOR HYPOGASTRIC PLEXUS

The superior hypogastric plexus lies anterior to the aortic bifurcation, the left common iliac vein, medial sacral vessels, fifth lumbar vertebral body and sacral promontory and between the common iliac arteries. It is often termed the presacral nerve, but is seldom a single nerve and it is prelumbar rather than presacral. Most frequently found to the left side of the midline, it lies in extraperitoneal connective tissue from which the parietal peritoneum can easily be stripped. The breadth and condensation of its constituent nerves vary. The attachment of the sigmoid mesocolon, containing the superior rectal vessels, is anterior and to the left of the lower part of the plexus. The superior hypogastric plexus is formed by branches from the aortic plexus and the third and fourth lumbar splanchnic nerves (which are mainly sympathetic). It may also contain parasympathetic fibres from the pelvic splanchnic nerves – which ascend from the two inferior hypogastric plexuses – via a series of filaments sometimes identified as the right and left hypo-

gastric 'nerves'. The latter lie in loose connective tissue just posterolateral to the start of the mesorectum and pass over the pelvic brim medial to the internal iliac vessels. The superior hypogastric plexus supplies fibres to the inferior mesenteric plexus and to the ureteric, testicular, ovarian and common iliac plexuses.

Preganglionic sympathetic axons originate in the lower three thoracic and upper two lumbar spinal segments; they synapse in the ganglia associated with the lumbar and sacral sympathetic trunk, or in the lower part of the aortic, superior or inferior hypogastric plexuses. Preganglionic parasympathetic axons originate from neurones in the second to fourth sacral spinal segments.

INFERIOR HYPOGASTRIC (PELVIC) PLEXUSES

The inferior hypogastric plexus lies in the thin extraperitoneal connective tissue lateral to the mesorectum. Laterally lie the internal iliac vessels, and attachments of levator ani, coccygeus and obturator internus; superiorly lie the superior vesical and obliterated umbilical arteries; posteriorly lie the sacral and coccygeal plexuses. In males the inferior hypogastric plexus lies posterolaterally on either side of the seminal vesicles, prostate and the posterior part of the urinary bladder. In females each plexus lies lateral to the uterine cervix, vaginal fornix and the posterior part of the urinary bladder, and often extends into the broad ligaments of the uterus.

The inferior hypogastric plexus is formed from the right and left hypogastric 'nerves' – which are mainly sympathetic – and long branches of the parasympathetic pelvic splanchnic nerves (S2, 3, 4). Branches from the lowest lumbar splanchnic nerve and sacral splanchnic nerves may also join the plexus via the hypogastric 'nerves'. In males the plexus supplies the vas deferens, seminal vesicles, prostate, accessory glands and penis. In females it supplies the ovary, fallopian tubes, uterus,

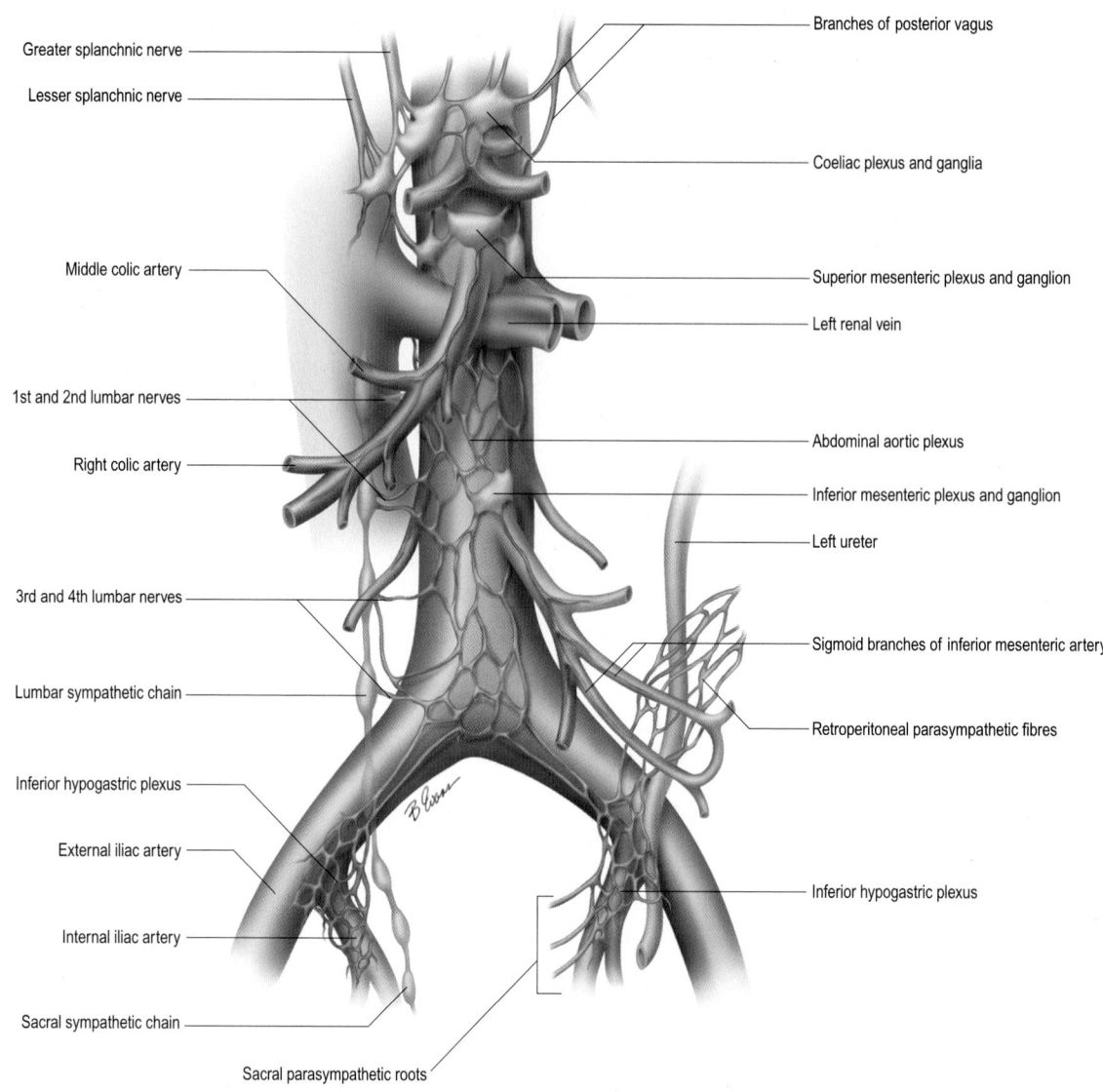

Greater splanchnic nerve

Lesser splanchnic nerve

Middle colic artery

1st and 2nd lumbar nerves

Right colic artery

3rd and 4th lumbar nerves

Lumbar sympathetic chain

Inferior hypogastric plexus

External iliac artery

Internal iliac artery

Sacral sympathetic chain

Sacral parasympathetic roots

Branches of posterior vagus

Coeliac plexus and ganglia

Superior mesenteric plexus and ganglion

Left renal vein

Abdominal aortic plexus

Inferior mesenteric plexus and ganglion

Left ureter

Sigmoid branches of inferior mesenteric artery

Retroperitoneal parasympathetic fibres

Inferior hypogastric plexus

Fig. 76.17 Anatomic illustration of the autonomic plexuses of the colon and rectum.

uterine cervix and vagina. It supplies the urinary bladder and distal ureter in both sexes.

Preganglionic sympathetic axons originate in the lower thoracic and upper two lumbar spinal segments; they synapse in the ganglia associated with the lumbar and sacral sympathetic trunk, or in the lower part of the aortic, superior or inferior hypogastric plexuses. Preganglionic parasympathetic axons originate from neurones in the second to fourth sacral spinal segments.

REFERENCES

Fenlon HM 2002 Virtual colonoscopy. Br J Surg 89(1): 1–3.
Describes and reviews the use of multislice CT to image the colon.
Fisher DF Jr, Fry WJ 1987 Collateral mesenteric circulation. Surg Gynecol Obstet 164(5): 487–92.
Reviews collateral mesenteric circulations that develop during disease processes.
Jackson JE 1999 Vascular anatomy of the gastrointestinal tract. In: Butler P, Mitchell AWM, Ellis H (eds) Applied Radiological Anatomy. Cambridge: Cambridge University Press.

Japanese Society for the Cancer of the Colon and Rectum 1997. Japanese Classification of Colorectal Carcinoma. Tokyo: Kanehara & Co Ltd.
Describes the topography of colonic mesenteric lymph nodes with particular reference to radical excision of carcinoma.
Oliphant M, Berne AS, Meyers MA 1996 The subperitoneal space of the abdomen and pelvis: planes of continuity. Am J Roentgenol 167(6): 1433–9.
Silverstein FE, Tytgat GNJ 1991 Atlas of Gastrointestinal Endoscopy, 2nd edn. London: Gower Medical Publishing.

Caecum

The caecum is a large blind pouch of large intestine lying in the right iliac fossa below the ileocaecal valve and continuing distally as the ascending colon. The blind-ending vermiform appendix usually arises on its medial side at the level of the ileal opening. Its average axial length is c.6 cm and its breadth c.7.5 cm. It rests posteriorly on the right iliacus and psoas major, with the lateral cutaneous nerve of the thigh interposed. Posteriorly lies the retrocaecal recess which frequently contains the vermiform appendix. The anterior abdominal wall is immediately anterior to the caecum except when it is empty, when the greater omentum and some loops of the small intestine may be interposed. Usually the caecum is entirely covered by peritoneum, but occasionally this is incomplete posterosuperiorly where it lies attached to the iliac fascia by loose connective tissue. In early fetal life the caecum is usually short, conical and broad at the base, with an apex turned superomedially towards the ileocaecal junction. As the fetus grows, the caecum increases in length more than in breadth, to form a longer tube with a narrower base but retaining the same inclination. Distal growth later ceases, but the proximal part continues to grow in breadth, so that at birth a narrow vermiform appendix extends from the apex of a conical caecum. This infantile form persists throughout life in only a very small percentage of individuals. Occasionally the conical caecum takes on a quadrate shape as a result of the outgrowth of a saccule on each side of the anterior taenia: the saccules are of equal size and the appendix arises from the depression between them instead of from the apex of a cone. In the normal adult form, the right saccule grows more rapidly than the left, forming a new 'apex'. The original apex, with the appendix attached, is pushed towards the ileocaecal junction.

The caecum commences the process of fluid and electrolyte reabsorption, which occurs to a large extent in the ascending and transverse colon. The distensible nature and 'sac-like' morphology of the caecum are adaptations for the storage of larger volumes of semi-liquid chyme entering from the small bowel via the ileocaecal valve.

ILEOCAECAL VALVE

The ileum opens into the posteromedial aspect of the large intestine at the junction of the caecum and colon. The ileocaecal orifice has a so-called 'valve', consisting of two flaps which project into the lumen of the large intestine (**Figs 77.1, 77.2**). The precise shape and form of the valve varies but in the distended, fixed, caecum the flaps are often semilunar. The upper flap, approximately horizontal, is attached to the junction of the ileum and colon; the lower flap is longer and more concave, and is attached to the junction of the ileum and caecum. At their ends the flaps fuse, continuing as narrow membranous ridges, the frenula of the valve. The orifice may appear in many different shapes depending on the state of contraction or distension of the caecum: it is commonly either a slit or an oval. The margin of the ileocaecal valve is a reduplication of the intestinal mucosa and circular muscle. Longitudinal muscle fibres are partly reduplicated as they enter the valve, but the more superficial fibres and the peritoneum continue from the small to the large intestine without interruption. The valve may prevent reflux of chyme from the caecum to the ileum, and may slow the passage of ileal contents into the caecum when the circular muscle of the valve is contracted by sympathetic stimulation. Although circular and longitudinal muscle layers of the terminal ileum continue into the valve, there is little evidence that it constitutes a true functional sphincter.

The ileal valvular surfaces are covered with villi and have the structure of the small intestinal mucosa, whereas their caecal surfaces have no villi but display numerous orifices of tubular glands peculiar to the colonic mucosa.

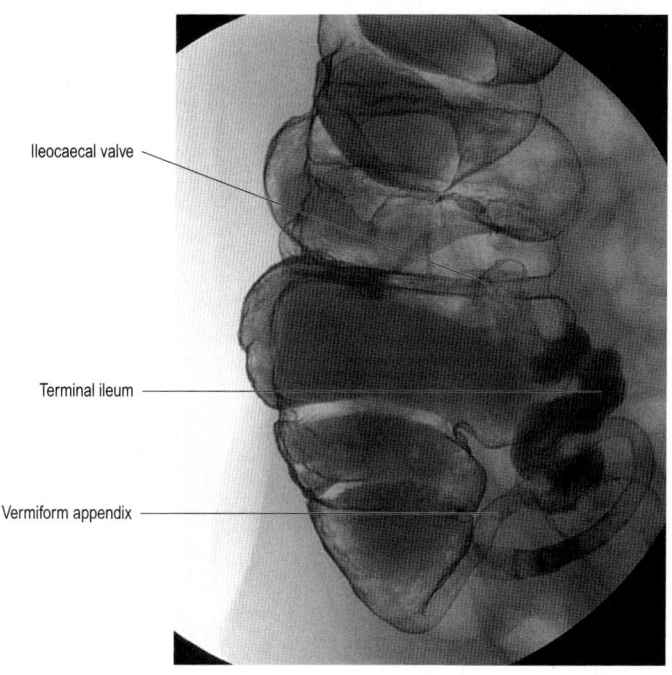

Fig. 77.1 Double contrast barium enema appearance of the caecum and ileocaecal valve.

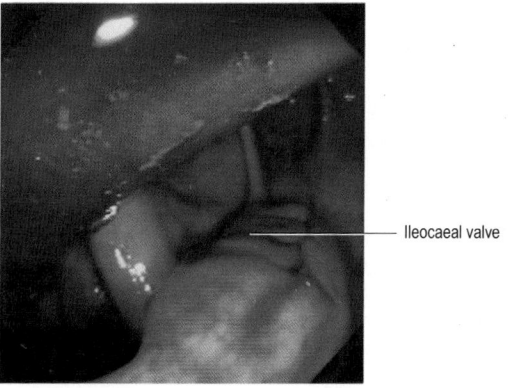

Fig. 77.2 Endoscopic appearance of the ileocaecal valve.

VASCULAR SUPPLY AND LYMPHATIC DRAINAGE

ILEOCOLIC ARTERY

The caecum is supplied principally from the ileocolic artery, which is the last branch from the right side of the superior mesenteric artery (**Fig. 77.3**). It descends to the right beneath the parietal peritoneum

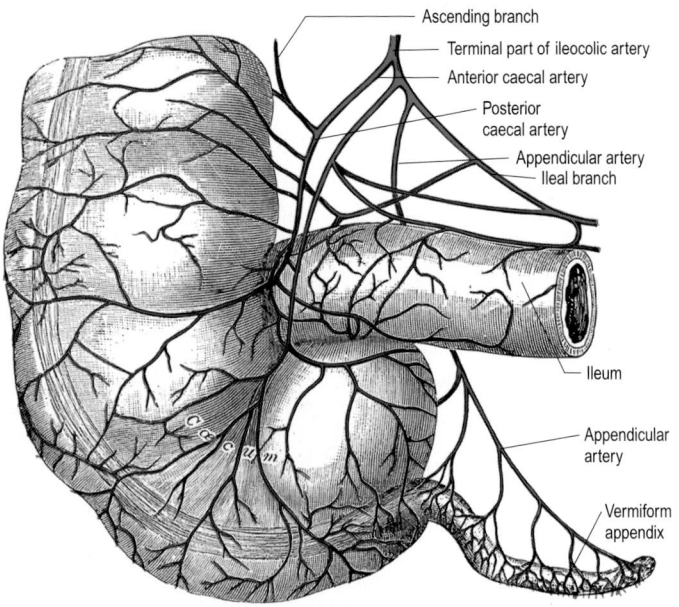

Fig. 77.3 The arteries of the caecum and vermiform appendix.

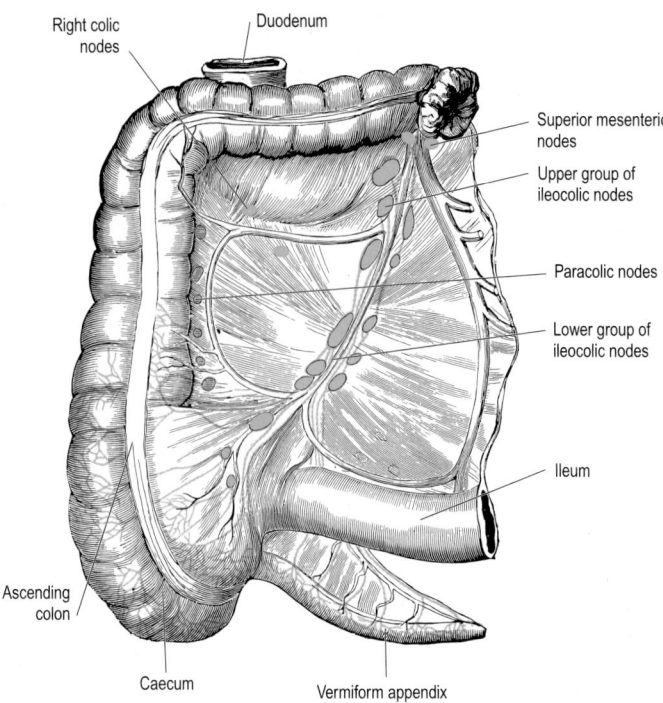

Fig. 77.4 The lymph vessels and nodes of the caecum and vermiform appendix: anterior aspect. (Modified with permission from Elsevier: The Lancet, 1907, 1, 1061–1066.)

into the right iliac fossa, where it divides into two branches: the superior branch anastomoses with the right colic artery, and the inferior branch anastomoses with the end of the superior mesenteric artery. The ileocolic artery crosses anterior to the right ureter, testicular or ovarian vessels, and psoas major.

The inferior branch approaches the superior border of the ileocolic junction. It has the following named branches: ascending (colic) artery (which passes up on the ascending colon); anterior and posterior caecal arteries; appendicular artery (which descends behind the terminal ileum to enter the mesoappendix and gives off a recurrent branch which anastomoses with a branch of the posterior caecal artery); ileal artery (which ascends to the left on the lower ileum, supplies it and anastomoses with the terminal ileal arcade arteries).

ILEAL ARTERIES
The terminal arcades of the ileal arteries provide a collateral supply to the caecum via anastomoses with the ileal branch of the ileocolic artery.

ILEOCOLIC VEIN
The ileocolic vein is formed from superior and inferior tributaries and ascends alongside the ileocolic artery beneath the peritoneum of the ileocaecal mesentery to drain into the superior mesenteric vein. The inferior tributary receives appendicular, anterior and posterior caecal and ileal veins and the superior tributary drains the ascending colic veins.

LYMPHATIC DRAINAGE
Anterior lymphatic vessels pass in front of the caecum and drain to the anterior ileocolic nodes and nodes of the ileocolic chain; posterior vessels ascend behind the caecum to the posterior and inferior ileocolic nodes. Lymph drains from the nodes in the ileocolic chain into the superior mesenteric nodes in the root of the small bowel mesentery (**Fig. 77.4**).

INNERVATION

The caecum is innervated by sympathetic and parasympathetic nerves via the superior mesenteric plexus.

CAECAL VOLVULUS

Because the caecum and ascending colon may possess a mesentery to a variable degree, it is possible for the caecum (and lower portion of the ascending colon) to rotate about their mesenteric attachment (mesentero-axial volvulus) such that the lower pole of the caecum comes to lie in the left or right upper quadrant of the abdomen. The fixed apex of this rotation is formed by the attachment of the caecal mesentery to the retroperitoneum. Volvulus is extremely unlikely in individuals where the caecum and ascending colon possess a short broadly attached mesentery. Volvulus occurs most commonly in those individuals where a large portion of the ascending colon lies on a mesentery and the common origin of the caecal and ascending colic mesentery is narrow. True isolated volvulus of the caecum is extremely rare.

Vermiform appendix

The vermiform appendix is a narrow, vermian (worm-shaped) tube which arises from the posteromedial caecal wall, c.2 cm below the end of the ileum. It may occupy one of several positions (**Fig. 78.1**). Thus it may be retrocaecal, retrocolic (behind the caecum or lower ascending colon respectively), pelvic or descending (when it hangs dependently over the pelvic brim, in close relation to the right uterine tube and ovary in females). These are the commonest positions seen in clinical practice. Other positions are occasionally seen especially when there is a long appendix mesentery allowing greater mobility. These include subcaecal (below the caecum); preilial (anterior to the terminal ileum); postileal (behind the terminal ileum).

The three taeniae coli on the ascending colon and caecum converge on the base of the appendix, and merge into its longitudinal muscle. The anterior caecal taenia is usually distinct and can be traced to the appendix, which affords a guide to its location in clinical practice. The appendix varies from 2 to 20 cm in length: it is often relatively longer in children and may atrophy and shorten after mid-adult life. It is connected by a short mesoappendix to the lower part of the ileal mesentery. This fold is usually triangular, extending almost to the appendicular tip along the whole viscus.

The lumen of the appendix is small and opens into the caecum by an orifice lying below and slightly posterior to the ileocaecal opening. The orifice is sometimes guarded by a semilunar mucosal fold forming a valve (**Fig. 78.2**). The lumen may be widely patent in early childhood and is often partially or wholly obliterated in the later decades of life. The appendix usually contains numerous patches of lymphoid tissue although these tend to decrease in size from early adulthood.

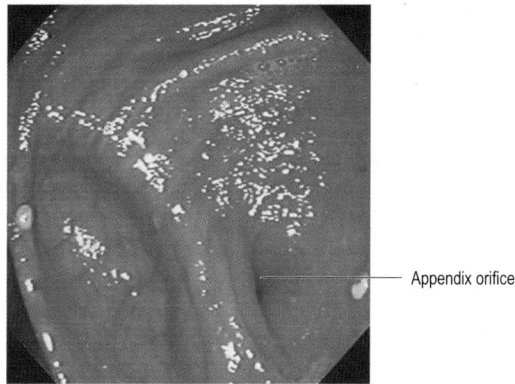

Appendix orifice

Fig. 78.2 Endoscopic appearance of the appendix orifice. The orifice varies from a small depression to an obvious lumenal structure.

VASCULAR SUPPLY AND LYMPHATIC DRAINAGE

APPENDICULAR ARTERY

The main appendicular artery, a branch from the lower division of the ileocolic artery, runs behind the terminal ileum and enters the mesoappendix a short distance from the appendicular base. Here it gives off a recurrent branch, which anastomoses at the base of the appendix with a branch of the posterior caecal artery: the anastomosis is sometimes extensive. The main appendicular artery approaches the tip of the organ, at first near to, and then in the edge of, the mesoappendix. The terminal part of the artery lies on the wall of the appendix and may be thrombosed in appendicitis, which results in distal gangrene or necrosis. Accessory arteries are common, and many individuals possess two or more arteries of supply.

APPENDICULAR VEINS

The appendix is drained via one or more appendicular veins into the posterior caecal or ileocolic vein and thence into the superior mesenteric vein.

LYMPHATICS

Lymphatic vessels in the appendix are numerous: there is abundant lymphoid tissue in its walls. From the body and apex of the appendix 8–15 vessels ascend in the mesoappendix, and are occasionally interrupted by one or more nodes. They unite to form three or four larger vessels which run into the lymphatic vessels draining the ascending colon, and end in the inferior and superior nodes of the ileocolic chain.

INNERVATION

The appendix and overlying visceral peritoneum are innervated by sympathetic and parasympathetic nerves from the superior mesenteric plexus. Visceral afferent fibres carrying sensations of distension and pressure mediate the symptoms of 'pain' felt during the initial stages of appendicular inflammation. In keeping with other structures derived

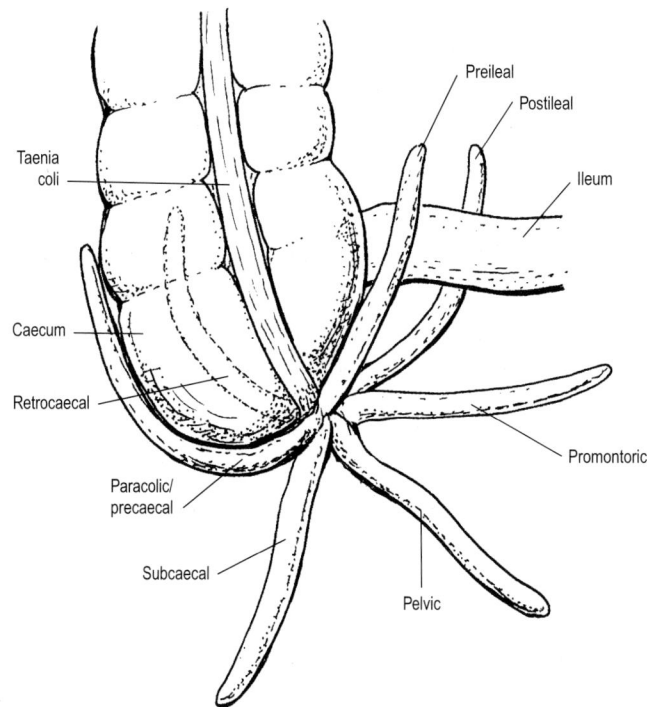

Preileal

Postileal

Ileum

Taenia coli

Caecum

Retrocaecal

Promontoric

Paracolic/ precaecal

Subcaecal

Pelvic

Fig. 78.1 Diagram illustrating the major positions of the appendix encountered at surgery or postmortem.

from the midgut, these sensations are poorly localized initially, and referred to the central (periumbilical) region of the abdomen. It is not until parietal tissues adjacent to the appendix become involved in any inflammatory process that somatic nociceptors are stimulated, and there is an associated change in the nature and localization of pain.

ACUTE APPENDICITIS

The genesis of acute appendicitis varies between individuals. It may follow obstruction of the lumen, when it is a consequence of increased intraluminal pressure and retention of (infected) contents which allows acute suppuration to occur. The size of the orifice of the appendix in some individuals may contribute to the risk that this will happen.

Appendicoliths may be visible on plain radiographs in 7–15% of the normal population: in those patients with acute abdominal pain, their presence indicates a high risk of appendicitis being present. The increased size of the orifice and lumen at the extremes of life may be a reason why acute appendicitis is relatively uncommon in these age groups. Acute appendicitis may also present as a primary suppuration of the tissues of the appendix itself: the reduction in appendicular lymphoid tissue that occurs in later life may be another reason why the disease is infrequent in the elderly. Although the appendix is well supplied by arterial anastomoses at its base, the appendicular artery is an end artery from the midpoint upwards and its close proximity to the wall makes it susceptible to thrombosis during episodes of acute inflammation. This may render the distal appendix ischaemic and explains the frequency of gangrenous perforation seen in the disease.

REFERENCE

Buschard K, Kjaeldgaard A 1973 Investigations and analysis of the positions, fixation, length and embryology of the vermiform appendix. Acta Chir Scand 139: 293–8.

Ascending colon

The ascending colon is c.15 cm long and narrower than the caecum. It ascends to the inferior surface of the right lobe of the liver, on which it makes a shallow depression, and then turns abruptly forwards and to the left, at the hepatic flexure. It is a retroperitoneal structure covered anteriorly and on both sides by peritoneum. Its posterior surface is connected by loose connective tissue to the iliac fascia, the iliolumbar ligament, the quadratus lumborum muscles, the aponeurosis of transversus abdominis, and the anterior peri-renal fascia inferolateral to the right kidney. The lateral femoral cutaneous nerve, usually the fourth lumbar artery, and sometimes the ilioinguinal and iliohypogastric nerves, lie posteriorly as they cross the quadratus lumborum muscles. Laterally the peritoneum forms the paracolic gutter. The ascending colon possesses a narrow mesocolon for part of its course in up to one-third of cases. Anteriorly it is in contact with loops of ileum, the greater omentum and the anterior abdominal wall.

HEPATIC FLEXURE

The hepatic flexure forms the junction of the ascending and transverse colon as the latter turns down, forwards and to the left. It is variable in position and usually has a less acute angle than the splenic flexure. The anterior surface of the lower pole of the right kidney is posterior and the right lobe of the liver is superior and anterolateral. The descending (second) part of the duodenum is medial and the fundus of the gallbladder is anteromedial. The posterior aspect of the hepatic flexure is not covered by peritoneum and is in direct contact with renal fascia.

VASCULAR SUPPLY AND LYMPHATIC DRAINAGE

ARTERIES

Ileocolic artery – ascending branch
The ascending branch of the ileocolic artery supplies the lower half of the ascending colon and anastomoses freely with the right colic artery.

Right colic artery
The right colic artery is a small vessel and may be absent. When present, it arises near the middle of the superior mesenteric artery, or in common with the middle colic artery. It passes towards the ascending colon, deep to the parietal peritoneum and anterior to the right gonadal vessels, right ureter and psoas major. Sometimes it arises more superiorly and crosses the descending duodenum and inferior pole of the right kidney. Near the colon it divides into a descending branch, which anastomoses with the ileocolic artery, and an ascending branch which anastomoses with the middle colic arteries. These form arches from which vessels are distributed to the upper two-thirds of the ascending colon, and to the hepatic flexure.

VEINS
Ascending tributaries of the ileocolic and right colic veins accompany their respective arteries into the root of the mesentery and drain via the ileocolic vein into the superior mesenteric vein. Although the right colic vein usually drains into the superior mesenteric vein, it is occasionally

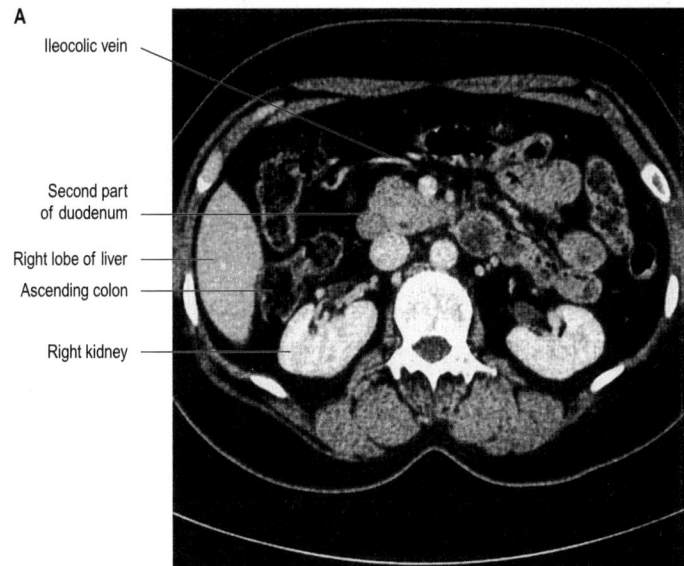

A

Ileocolic vein

Second part of duodenum

Right lobe of liver

Ascending colon

Right kidney

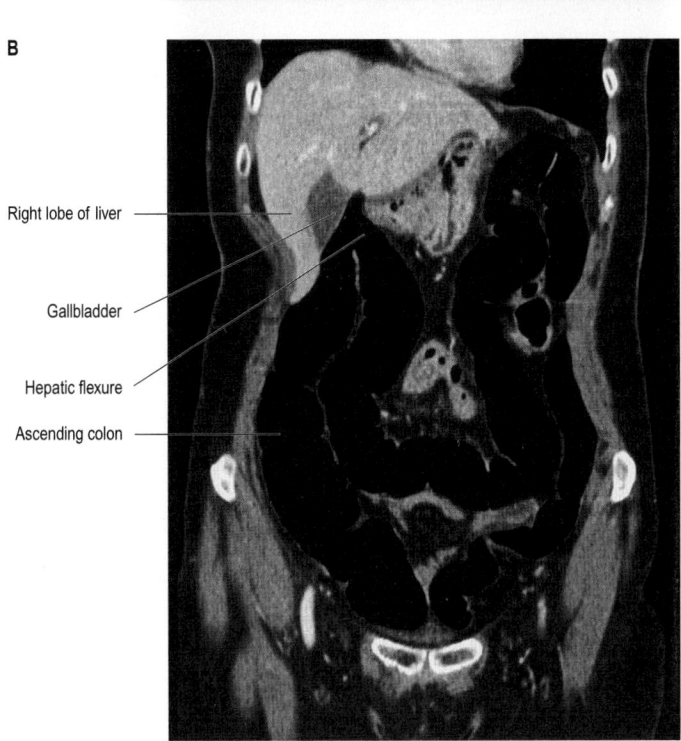

B

Right lobe of liver

Gallbladder

Hepatic flexure

Ascending colon

Fig. 79.1 The relationship of the ascending colon and hepatic flexure to right lobe of liver, kidneys, second part of duodenum, and gallbladder in **A** axial and **B** coronal reformat CT images. (By kind permission from Dr Louise Moore, Chelsea and Westminster Hospital, London.)

absent or may join the right gastroepiploic or inferior pancreaticoduodenal vein to form a 'gastrocolic trunk' which drains into the superior mesenteric vein.

LYMPHATICS

Lymphatic vessels originate from both anterior and posterior aspects of the colon and drain into nodes located along the ascending branch of the ileocolic and the right colic arteries. Lymphatic drainage from the distal ascending colon and hepatic flexure may be predominantly to the nodes of the right colic artery. The lymphatic anastomoses are rich and the preterminal nodes for both routes of drainage are the ileocolic nodes which are located close to the superior mesenteric artery.

INNERVATION

The ascending colon is innervated by sympathetic and parasympathetic nerves via the superior mesenteric plexus.

REFERENCE

Yamaguchi S, Kuroyanagi H, Milson JW, Sim R, Shimada H 2002 Venous anatomy of the right colon: precise structure of the major veins and gastrocolic trunk in 58 cadavers. Dis Colon Rectum 45: 1337–40.

Transverse colon

The transverse colon is c.50 cm long, and extends from the hepatic flexure in the right lumbar region across into the left hypochondriac region, where it curves posteroinferiorly below the spleen as the splenic flexure. It is highly variable in length and position, as may be confirmed by radiological assessment, but it often describes an inverted arch, with its concavity directed posteriorly and superiorly. Near the splenic flexure an abrupt U-shaped curve may descend lower than the main arch. The posterior surface at the hepatic flexure is devoid of peritoneum and is attached by loose connective tissue to the front of the descending part of the duodenum and the head of the pancreas. The transverse colon from here to the splenic flexure is almost completely invested by peritoneum, and is suspended from the anterior border of the body of the pancreas by the transverse mesocolon. The latter is attached from the inferior part of the right kidney, across the second part of the duodenum and pancreas, to the inferior pole of the left kidney. The transverse colon hangs down between the flexures to a variable extent, and sometimes reaches the pelvis. Above it are the liver and gallbladder, the greater curvature of the stomach and the body of the spleen. The transverse colon is usually attached to the greater curvature of the stomach by the gastrocolic ligament, which is in continuity with the greater omentum, lying anteriorly and extending inferiorly (p. 1127). Behind and below the transverse colon lie the descending part of the duodenum, the head of the pancreas, the upper end of the small bowel mesentery, the duodenojejunal flexure and loops of the jejunum and ileum.

The transverse mesocolon permits considerable mobility of the transverse colon: occasionally the colon may be interposed between the liver and the diaphragm (Chilaiditi syndrome), and may be mistaken for free intraperitoneal gas.

SPLENIC FLEXURE

The splenic flexure forms the junction of the transverse and descending colon, and lies in the left hypochondriac region anteroinferior to the lower part of the spleen and anterior to the pancreatic tail. The left kidney lies behind and lateral to it (**Fig. 80.1**). The splenic flexure often adopts a very acute angle such that the end of the transverse colon overlaps the beginning of the descending colon. It lies more superiorly and posteriorly than the right hepatic flexure, and is attached to the diaphragm at the level of the tenth and eleventh ribs by the phrenicocolic ligament (p. 1127) which lies below the anterolateral pole of the spleen.

VASCULAR SUPPLY AND LYMPHATIC DRAINAGE

ARTERIES

The proximal two-thirds of the transverse colon is supplied by the superior mesenteric artery via the middle colic artery. The distal third is usually supplied by the ascending branch of the left colic artery via the marginal artery of the colon, although this is somewhat variable.

Middle colic artery

The middle colic artery leaves the superior mesenteric artery just inferior to the pancreas and anterior to the third part of the duodenum. Initially it passes inferiorly, then turns to run anteriorly and superiorly within the transverse mesocolon, where it usually divides into a right and left branch. The right branch anastomoses with the right colic artery, and the left branch anastomoses with the left colic artery. The arterial arches thus formed lie 3 or 4 cm from the transverse colon, which they supply.

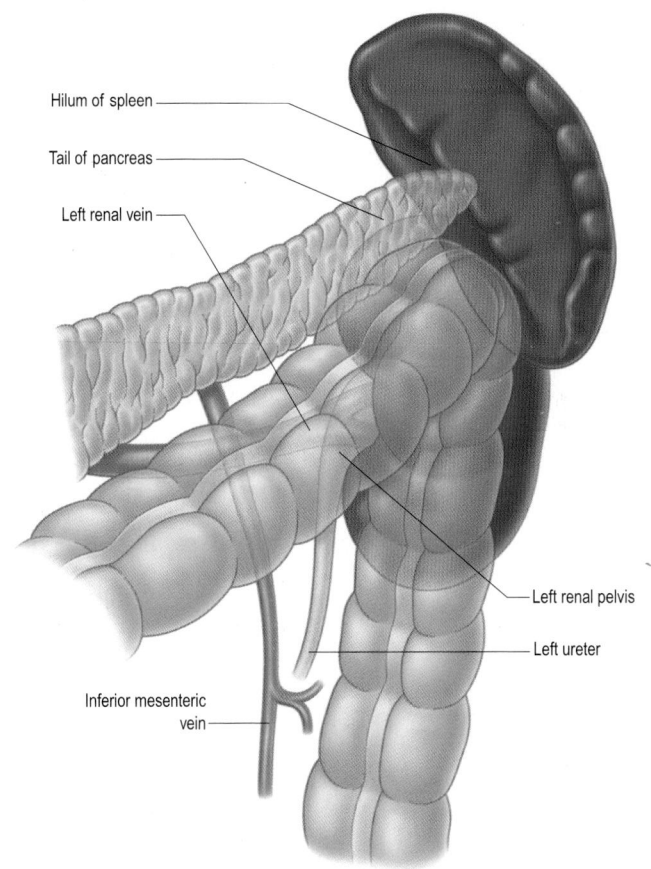

Hilum of spleen

Tail of pancreas

Left renal vein

Left renal pelvis

Left ureter

Inferior mesenteric vein

Fig. 80.1 Relations of the splenic flexure.

Sometimes the middle colic artery divides into three or more branches within the transverse mesocolon, in which case the most lateral branches form the arterial anastomoses.

VEINS

Several tributaries drain into one or more middle colic veins. The middle colic veins drain either into the superior mesenteric vein, just before its junction with the splenic vein, or directly into the hepatic portal vein.

LYMPHATICS

Lymph vessels drain into nodes along the middle colic arteries and then into the superior mesenteric nodes. The predominant lymphatic drainage of the splenic flexure is usually via nodes along the left colic artery which drain into the inferior mesenteric nodes: this arrangement is dependent on the arterial supply to the distal third of the transverse colon.

INNERVATION

The proximal two-thirds of the transverse colon is innervated by sympathetic and parasympathetic nerves via the superior mesenteric plexus. The distal third usually receives a sympathetic supply from the inferior mesenteric plexus and a parasympathetic supply from this plexus and from retroperitoneal fibres which travel in the pelvic splanchnic nerves from neurones in the second, third and fourth sacral segments (p. 1178).

REFERENCE

Murphy JM, Maibaum A, Alexander G, Dixon AK 2000 Chilaiditi's syndrome and obesity. Clin Anat 13(3): 181–4.

Descending colon

The descending colon is c.25 cm long. It descends through the left hypochondriac and lumbar regions, initially following the lateral border of the lower pole of the left kidney, and then descending in the angle between psoas major and quadratus lumborum to the iliac crest. It then curves inferomedially, lying anterior to iliacus and psoas major, to become the sigmoid colon at the inlet of the lesser pelvis. It is a retroperitoneal structure covered anteriorly and on both sides by peritoneum. Its posterior surface is separated by loose connective tissue from the anterior peri-renal fascia inferolateral to the left kidney, the aponeurosis of transversus abdominis, quadratus lumborum, iliacus and psoas major. The subcostal vessels and nerves, iliohypogastric and ilioinguinal nerves, fourth lumbar artery (usually), the lateral femoral cutaneous, femoral and genitofemoral nerves, the gonadal vessels and the external iliac artery all pass behind the descending colon. Loops of jejunum lie anteriorly: if the anterior abdominal walls are relaxed, the most inferior part of the descending colon may be directly palpated transabdominally. The descending colon is smaller in calibre, more deeply placed, and more frequently covered posteriorly by peritoneum, than the ascending colon.

VASCULAR SUPPLY AND LYMPHATIC DRAINAGE

ARTERIES

The arterial supply of the descending colon is from the inferior mesenteric artery via its left colic branch, which also anastomoses with the marginal artery of the colon (in the region of the splenic flexure), and the sigmoid arteries (in the region of the junction with the sigmoid colon).

Left colic artery

The left colic artery ascends anterior to the left psoas major, and divides into ascending and descending branches: this division can occur soon after its origin. The trunk and its branches cross the left ureter and gonadal vessels. The ascending branch passes anterior to the left kidney in the upper left retroperitoneum and anastomoses with the left branch of the middle colic artery in the subperitoneal space within the transverse mesocolon. The descending branch passes laterally in the retroperitoneum approaching the descending colon where it forms part of the marginal artery and anastomoses with the highest sigmoid artery. The arterial arches thus formed supply the distal third of the transverse and the descending colon.

VEINS

The left colic vein is formed from several tributaries including ascending and descending branches which correspond to the equivalent arteries. These tributaries may not form a discrete vein until they drain into the inferior mesenteric vein, and occasionally there may be two distinct veins which both run into the inferior mesenteric vein. The left colic vein usually lies superior to its equivalent artery and has a shorter course because it ascends more steeply to drain into the inferior mesenteric vein.

LYMPHATICS

Lymph vessels drain into nodes along the left colic artery and subsequently into the inferior mesenteric nodes.

INNERVATION

The descending colon receives a sympathetic supply from the inferior mesenteric plexus and a parasympathetic supply from this plexus and from retroperitoneal fibres which travel in the pelvic splanchnic nerves from neurones in the second, third and fourth sacral segments (p. 1178).

B

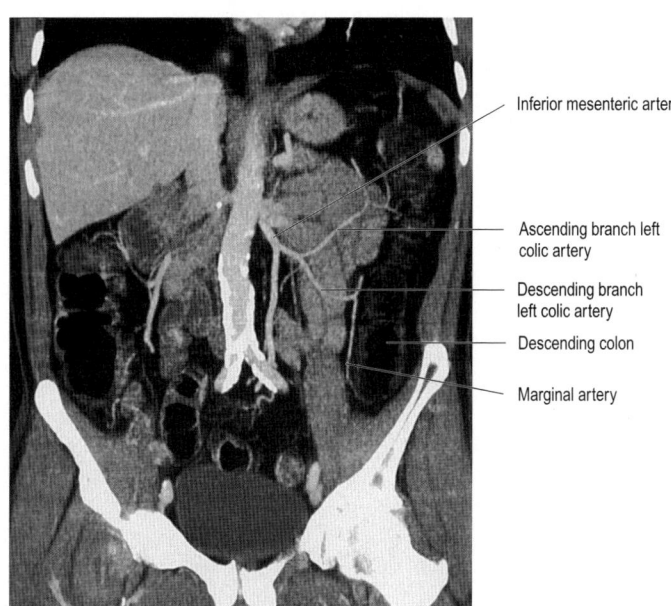

Inferior mesenteric artery

Ascending branch left colic artery

Descending branch left colic artery

Descending colon

Marginal artery

A

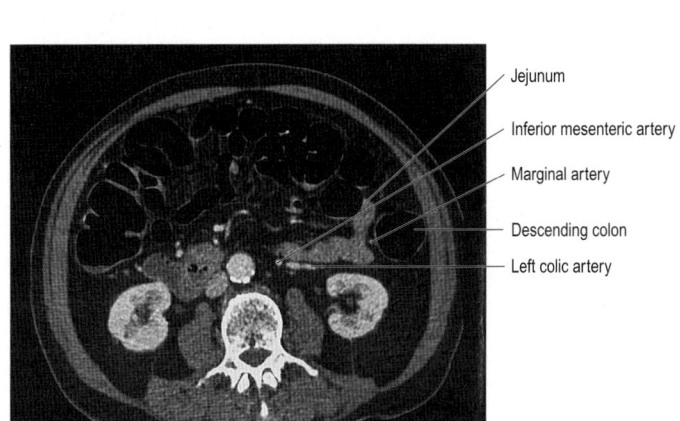

Jejunum

Inferior mesenteric artery

Marginal artery

Descending colon

Left colic artery

Fig. 81.1 The vascular supply of descending colon from the inferior mesenteric artery via left colic artery with ascending and descending branches **A** axial and **B** coronal. CT reformat. (By kind permission from Dr Louise Moore, Chelsea and Westminster Hospital, London.)

Sigmoid colon

The sigmoid colon begins at the pelvic inlet and ends at the rectum. Characteristically it forms a mobile loop which normally lies in the lesser pelvis. It is completely invested in peritoneum and is attached to the posterior pelvic wall and lower posterior abdominal walls by the fan-shaped sigmoid mesocolon. The root of the sigmoid mesocolon has an inverted 'V' attachment to the posterior abdominal wall. The sigmoid colon initially descends adjacent the left pelvic wall, but then comes to lie in an extremely variable position. It may remain folded principally in contact with the peritoneum overlying iliacus, or it may cross the pelvic cavity between the rectum and bladder in males, or the rectum and uterus in females, and it may even reach the right pelvic wall. If long, the sigmoid loop may rise out of the pelvis into the abdominal cavity and lie in contact with loops of ileum. The sigmoid loop ends in a relatively constant position lying just to the left of the midline at the level of the third sacral body, where it bends inferiorly and is continuous with the rectum. The sigmoid loop is fixed at its junctions with the descending colon and rectum but quite mobile between them. Its relations are therefore variable (**Fig. 82.1**). Laterally it is related to the left external iliac vessels, the obturator nerve, ovary or vas deferens and the lateral pelvic wall. Posteriorly lie the left internal iliac vessels, gonadal vessels, ureter, piriformis and sacral plexus. Inferiorly are the bladder in males, or uterus and bladder in females, and superiorly and to the right the sigmoid colon is in contact with loops of the ileum. The gonadal vessels and ureter lie in a distinct fascial plane which is separate from the thin fascial coverings of the mesosigmoid. The fascial plane surrounding the sigmoid can be recognized during dissection of the mesentery of the sigmoid colon

because it does not contain the numerous small vessels which are often present in the loose connective tissue surrounding the ureter and gonadal vessels.

The position and shape of the sigmoid colon vary greatly, depending on its length; the length and mobility of its mesocolon; the degree of distension (when distended it rises into the abdominal cavity, and sinks again into the lesser pelvis when empty); and the condition of the rectum, bladder and uterus (the sigmoid colon tends to rise when these are distended, and to fall when they are empty). The length and diameter of the sigmoid colon also vary in different races.

SIGMOID VOLVULUS

Rotation or volvulus around the mesenteric attachment of the sigmoid colon, similar to the rotation of the caecum around its mesentery, may occur. Only the sigmoid colon is affected, because the descending colon rarely possesses sufficient mesentery to become involved in the rotation. Rotation usually involves at least 270°.

Volvulus is more common as the length of the sigmoid colon increases, producing a 'fan-like' mesentery with a short retroperitoneal attachment. Volvulus does not occur in individuals where the sigmoid colon is short or where the mesentery is short and its attachment runs over the brim of the pelvis. The combination of anatomical features predisposing to sigmoid volvulus is most commonly found in sub-Saharan Africans and chronically institutionalized patients.

DIVERTICULAR DISEASE

The development of acquired diverticula occurs commonly in the sigmoid colon, particularly in white Caucasian populations. The aetiopathogenesis is probably multifactorial and includes dietary factors; however, the location of the diverticula would seem to be related to the underlying anatomy of the wall of the colon. Diverticula commonly occur midway between the antimesenteric and lateral taeniae, i.e. where the wall is potentially weak, not only because the circular muscle lacks the support of the longitudinal muscle, but also because it is traversed here by arteries as they access the submucosal vascular plexus. The predilection of the diverticula for the sigmoid colon probably relates to causative factors rather than intrinsic differences in the structure of its walls. In marked contrast, congenital diverticula may occur anywhere throughout the colon, and are often found adjacent to the mesenteric attachment of the colon.

VASCULAR SUPPLY AND LYMPHATIC DRAINAGE

ARTERIES

Sigmoid (inferior left colic) arteries

There are between two and five sigmoid arteries, which are branches of the inferior mesenteric artery. They descend from the retroperitoneum obliquely within the subperitoneal space anterior to the left psoas major, ureter and gonadal vessels. Branches supply the lower descending colon and sigmoid colon, and anastomose superiorly with the left colic artery and inferiorly with the superior rectal artery (**Fig. 82.2**). Unlike the small intestine, arterial arcades do not form until the arteries are close to the colon wall. At this point small branches arise and anastomose with each other to form a marginal artery along the mesenteric border of the sigmoid colon. A significant space often exists in the mesentery between the highest sigmoid artery and the descending branch of the left colic artery.

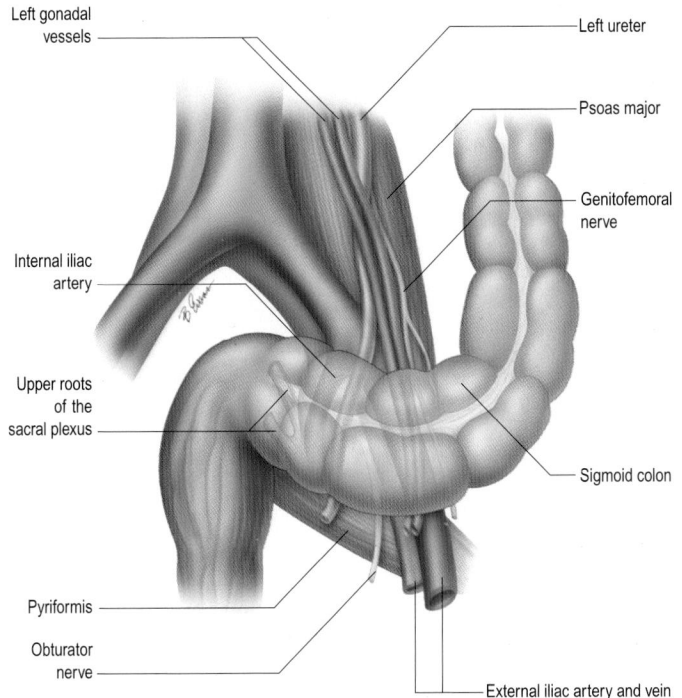

Left gonadal vessels

Internal iliac artery

Upper roots of the sacral plexus

Pyriformis

Obturator nerve

Left ureter

Psoas major

Genitofemoral nerve

Sigmoid colon

External iliac artery and vein

Fig. 82.1 Relations of the sigmoid colon.

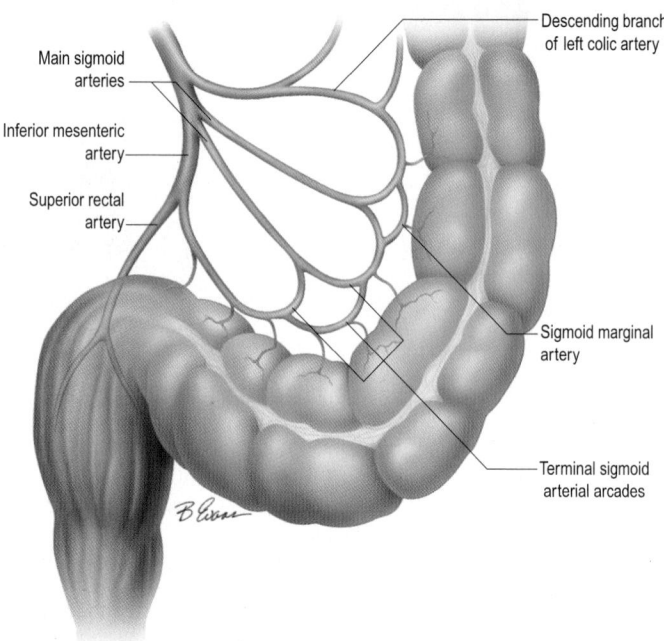

Fig. 82.2 Details of sigmoid colon arterial supply.

Labels in figure:
Main sigmoid arteries
Inferior mesenteric artery
Superior rectal artery
Descending branch of left colic artery
Sigmoid marginal artery
Terminal sigmoid arterial arcades

VEINS

Several sigmoid veins drain the sigmoid colon and run superiorly alongside their respective arteries to drain into the inferior mesenteric vein.

LYMPHATICS

Lymphatic vessels drain into sigmoid nodes in the sigmoid mesocolon and join with superior rectal and left colic vessels to drain into the inferior mesenteric nodes.

INNERVATION

The sigmoid colon receives a sympathetic supply from the inferior mesenteric plexus and a parasympathetic supply from this plexus and from retroperitoneal fibres which travel in the pelvic splanchnic nerves from neurones in the second, third and fourth sacral segments (p. 1178).

Rectum

Although the rectum is continuous with the sigmoid colon, it has several features which distinguish it functionally from the rest of the colon. These features suit its specialized role in defaecation and continence in combination with the anal canal.

The rectum is continuous with the sigmoid colon at the level of the third sacral vertebra and terminates at the upper end of the anal canal. It descends along the sacrococcygeal concavity as the sacral flexure of the rectum, initially inferoposteriorly and then inferoanteriorly to join the anal canal by passing through the pelvic diaphragm. The anorectal junction is 2–3 cm in front of and slightly below the tip of the coccyx, which is opposite the apex of the prostate in males. From this level the anal canal passes inferiorly and posteriorly from the lower end of the rectum. The posterior bend is termed the perineal flexure of the rectum and the angle it forms with the upper anal canal is termed the anorectal angle. The rectum also deviates in three lateral curves. The upper is convex to the right, the middle (the most prominent) bulges to the left, and the lower is convex to the right. Both ends of the rectum are in the median plane (**Fig. 83.1**).

Although variable in absolute length, a common landmark used in clinical practice to define the rectum is a length of 15 cm above the external anal margin. It commences with a similar diameter to the sigmoid colon, more inferiorly it is dilated as the rectal ampulla. The rectum differs from the sigmoid colon in having no sacculations, appendices epiploicae, or mesentery. The taeniae blend c.5 cm above the rectosigmoid junction, forming two wide muscular bands which descend anteriorly and posteriorly in the rectal wall. These then fuse to form an encircling layer of longitudinal muscle, which invests the entire length of the rectum. At the rectal ampulla a few strands of the anterior longitudinal fibres pass forwards to the perineal body, as the musculus recto-urethralis. In addition, two fasciculi of smooth muscle may pass anteroinferiorly from the front of the second and third coccygeal vertebrae to blend with the longitudinal muscle fibres on the posterior wall of the anal canal, forming the rectococcygeal muscles.

The upper third of the rectum is covered by peritoneum on its anterior and lateral aspects. It is related anteriorly to the sigmoid colon or loops of ileum if these lie in the pelvis, otherwise it is related to the urinary bladder in males or cervix and body of the uterus in females. The middle third of the rectum is covered by peritoneum only on the anterior aspect. The peritoneum is reflected superiorly onto the urinary bladder in males, to form the rectovesical pouch, or onto the posterior vaginal wall in females to form the recto-uterine pouch (pouch of Douglas). The level of this reflection is higher in males with the rectovesical pouch is c.7.5 cm (about the length of the index finger) from the anus. In females the recto-uterine pouch is c.5.5 cm from the anus. In the male neonate, peritoneum extends on to the front of the rectum as far as the lower limit of the prostate. Superiorly the peritoneum is firmly attached to the muscle layer of the sigmoid colon by fibrous connective tissue, but as it descends onto the rectum it is more loosely attached by fatty connective tissue, allowing for considerable expansion of the upper half of the rectum (**Figs 83.2, 83.3**).

There are no haustra in the rectum. When empty the mucosa forms a number of longitudinal folds in its lower part which become effaced during distension. In addition the rectum commonly has three (although the number can vary) permanent semilunar transverse or horizontal folds, most marked in rectal distension (**Fig. 76.8**). Two forms of horizontal fold have been recognized. One consists of the mucosa, a circular muscle layer and part of the longitudinal muscle, and is marked externally by an indentation. The other is devoid of longitudinal muscle and has no external marking. The most superior fold at the beginning of the rectum may be either on the left or right and occasionally encircles the rectal lumen. The middle fold is largest and most constant. It lies immediately above the rectal ampulla, projecting from the anterior and right wall just below the level of the anterior peritoneal reflection. The circular muscle is more marked in this fold than in the others. The most inferior and variable fold is found on the left c.2.5 cm below the middle fold. Sometimes a fourth fold is found on the left c.2.5 cm above the middle fold.

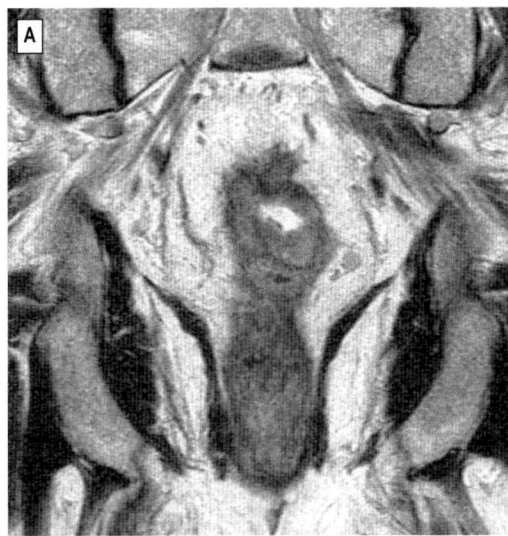

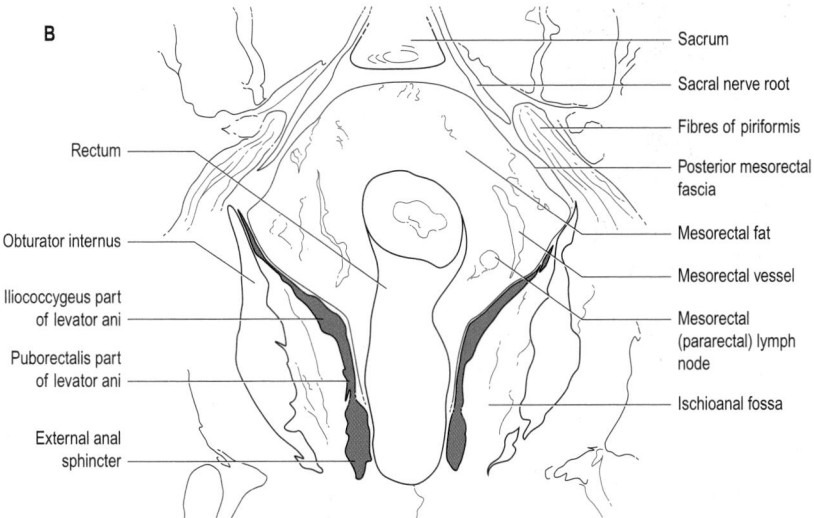

Sacrum

Sacral nerve root

Fibres of piriformis

Posterior mesorectal fascia

Mesorectal fat

Mesorectal vessel

Mesorectal (pararectal) lymph node

Ischioanal fossa

Rectum

Obturator internus

Iliococcygeus part of levator ani

Puborectalis part of levator ani

External anal sphincter

Fig. 83.1 Coronal T2-weighted MRI of the rectum.

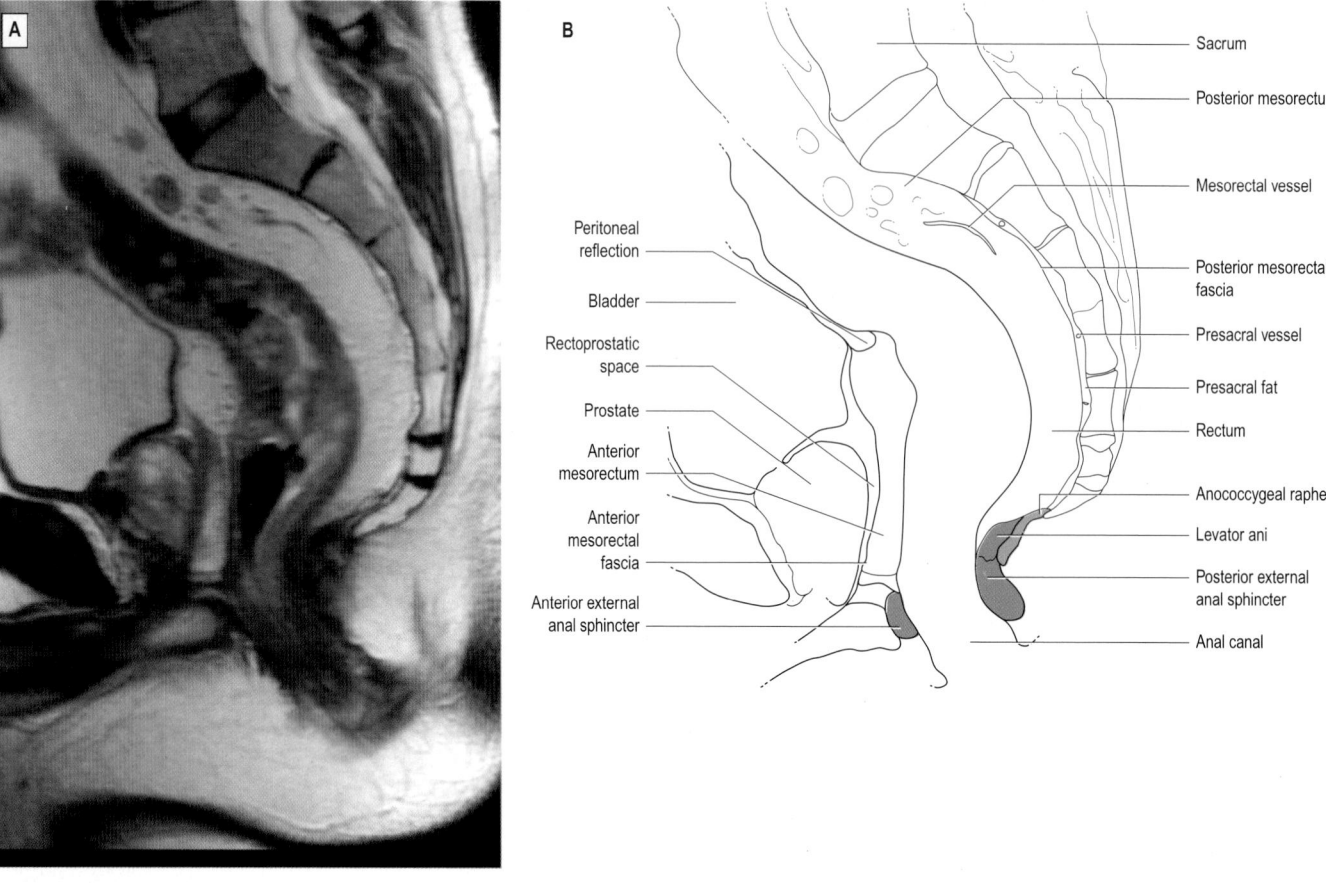

Fig. 83.2 Sagittal T2-weighted MRI of the rectum in the male.

Labels (Fig. 83.2B):
- Sacrum
- Posterior mesorectum
- Mesorectal vessel
- Posterior mesorectal fascia
- Presacral vessel
- Presacral fat
- Rectum
- Anococcygeal raphe
- Levator ani
- Posterior external anal sphincter
- Anal canal
- Peritoneal reflection
- Bladder
- Rectoprostatic space
- Prostate
- Anterior mesorectum
- Anterior mesorectal fascia
- Anterior external anal sphincter

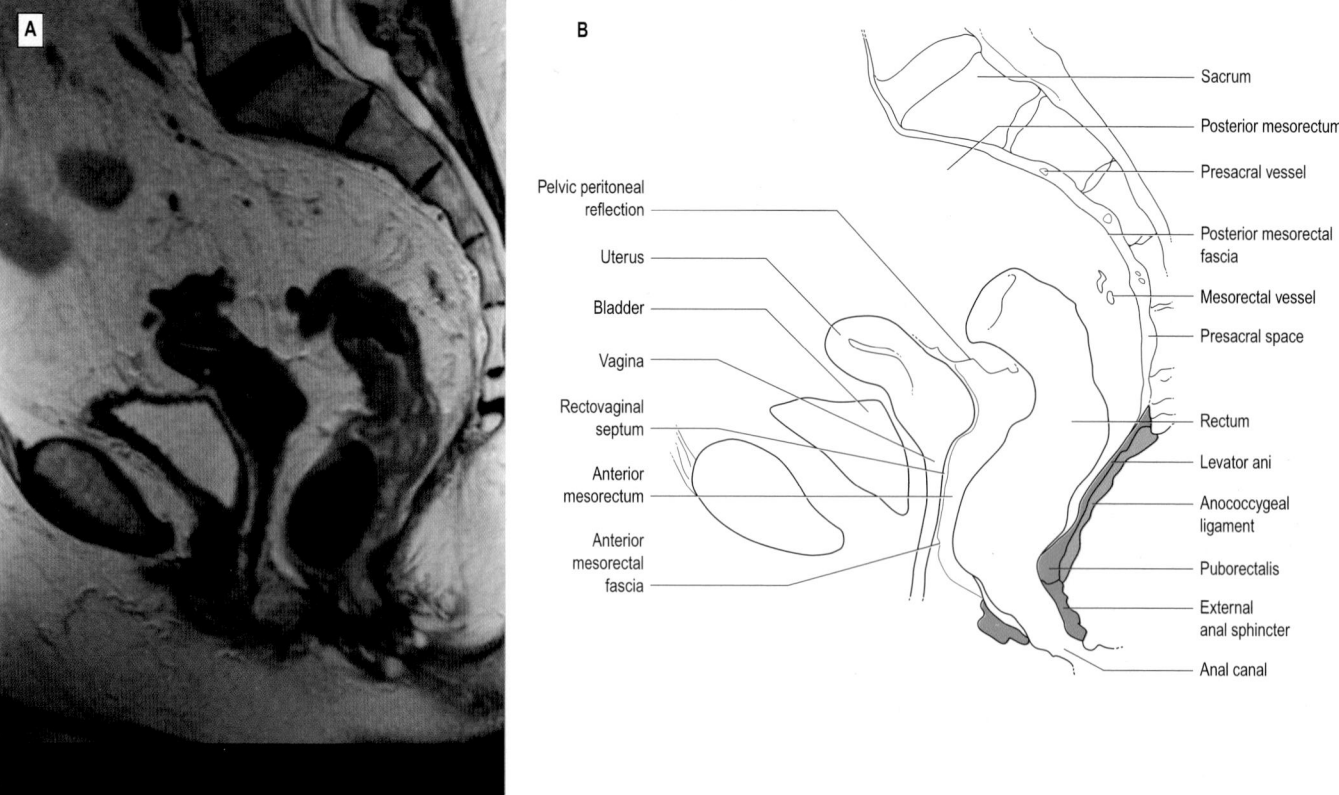

Fig. 83.3 Sagittal T2-weighted MRI of the rectum in the female.

Labels (Fig. 83.3B):
- Sacrum
- Posterior mesorectum
- Presacral vessel
- Posterior mesorectal fascia
- Mesorectal vessel
- Presacral space
- Rectum
- Levator ani
- Anococcygeal ligament
- Puborectalis
- External anal sphincter
- Anal canal
- Pelvic peritoneal reflection
- Uterus
- Bladder
- Vagina
- Rectovaginal septum
- Anterior mesorectum
- Anterior mesorectal fascia

MESORECTUM, RECTAL FASCIAE AND 'SPACES'

The mesorectum (mesentery of the rectum) and its contents are intimately related to the rectum down to the level of levator ani (**Figs 83.4, 83.5, 83.6**).

The mesorectum is a distinct compartment that derives from the embryological hindgut. It contains the superior rectal artery and its branches, the superior rectal vein and tributaries, the lymphatic vessels and nodes along the superior rectal artery, and branches from the inferior mesenteric plexus which descend to innervate the rectum and loose adipose connective tissue.

The mesorectum is enclosed by the mesorectal fascia which is a distinct covering derived from the visceral peritoneum. It is also known

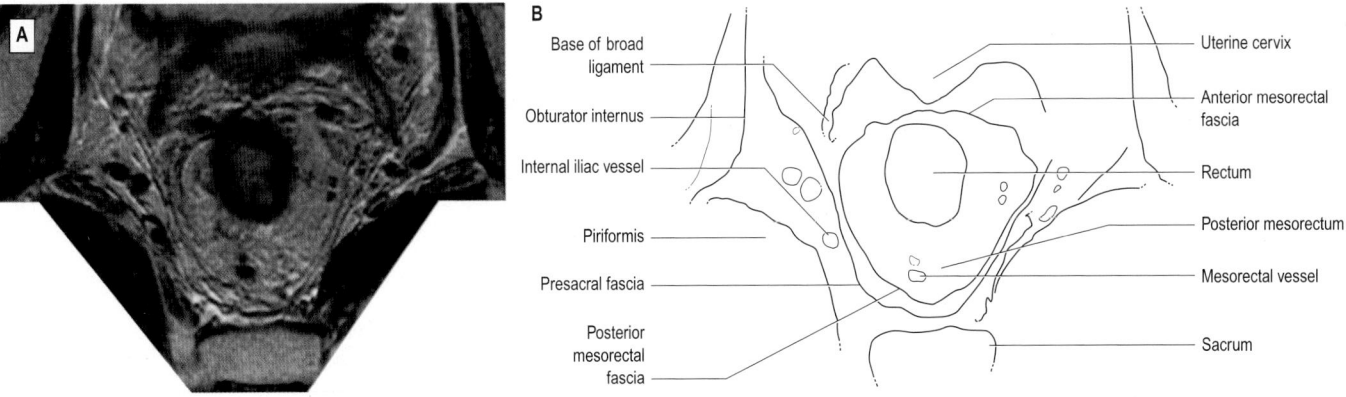

Fig. 83.4 Axial T2-weighted MRI of the upper rectum in the female.

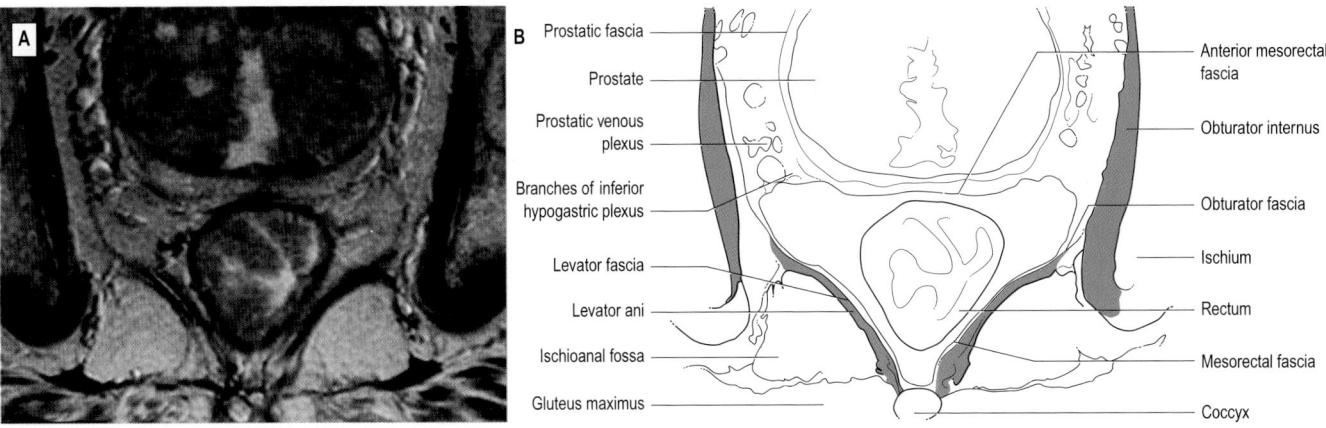

Fig. 83.5 Axial T2-weighted MRI of the mid rectum below the peritoneal reflection in a male.

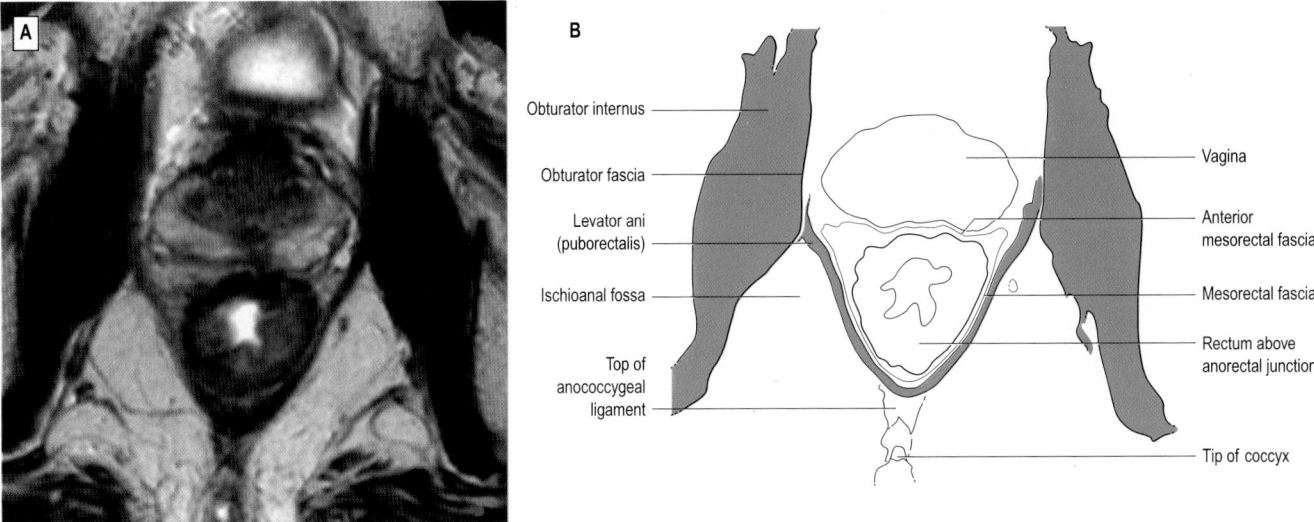

Fig. 83.6 Axial T2-weighted MRI of the low rectum below the peritoneal reflection in a female.

as the visceral fascia of the mesorectum, fascia propria of the rectum or the presacral wing of the hypogastric sheath. The fascia bounds the mesorectum posteriorly and thus lies anterior to the retrorectal space and the presacral fascia. The mesorectum and its fascia are surrounded by loose areolar tissue which separates them from the posterior and lateral walls of the true pelvis. Superiorly, the mesorectal fascia blends with the connective tissue bounding the sigmoid mesentery. Laterally, the mesorectal fascia extends around the rectum and becomes continuous with a denser condensation of fascia anteriorly. In males this anterior fascia is known as the rectovesical fascia of Denonvilliers. In females it forms the fascia of the rectovaginal septum.

On MRI scanning, the mesorectum is seen as a fat-containing envelope in which vessels are depicted as low signal due to signal void produced by blood flow. Lymph nodes appear as high signal ovoid structures. Small nerves within the mesorectum are not visualized, but interlacing connective tissue within the mesorectum can be seen as low signal intensity strands. The mesorectal fascia is demonstrated on axial views as a low signal layer surrounding the mesorectum, which corresponds to the distinct condensation of fascia seen on histological sections containing the mesorectum (Brown et al 1999) (Fig. 83.4). Identification of the involvement of this layer by malignant tumours of the rectum on MRI scanning may help plan preoperative radiotherapy, and predict the chance of successful surgical resection.

Anterolaterally, branches of the inferior hypogastric plexus and branches of the middle rectal artery and veins run into the mesorectum. They are ensheathed by fascia and together are referred to as the 'lateral rectal ligaments'. The number and calibre of the middle rectal vessels are highly variable. They may be very small or even absent (Sato & Sato 1991). The 'lateral ligaments' are not seen on MRI or CT scanning, and only appear as an identifiable structure with surgical traction on the rectum. The fascia of the 'ligaments' is flimsy and they probably play very little role in support of the rectum.

The parietal fascia that covers the levator and pelvic side-wall muscles forms a denser condensation of fascial tissue overlying the sacrum (Fig. 83.7).

RELATIONS OF THE RECTUM

Posterior to the rectum and mesorectum, and separated from them by the presacral fascia in the median plane are the lower three sacral vertebrae, coccyx, median sacral vessels, and the lowest portion of the sacral sympathetic chain. Laterally, the upper part of the rectum is related to the pararectal fossa and its contents (sigmoid colon or terminal ileum), while below the peritoneal reflection lie piriformis, the anterior rami of the lower three sacral and coccygeal nerves, sympathetic trunk, lower lateral sacral vessels, the coccygei and levatores ani muscles. Anteriorly above the level of the peritoneal reflection lie loops of

sigmoid colon or terminal ileum – if these lie in the pelvis – otherwise the rectum is related to the upper parts of the base of the bladder in males, or cervix/body of the uterus and upper vagina in females. The lower parts of the base of the bladder, the seminal vesicles, vas deferens, terminal parts of the ureters, and the prostate in males (Figs 83.5, 83.6), or the lower part of the vagina in females lie below the reflection. In females, the rectovaginal septum is composed of a condensation of connective tissue which is continuous with the connective tissue of the outer layers of the rectal and vaginal walls. In postmenopausal females, and following childbirth, the connective tissue of the rectovaginal septum may atrophy or be thinned, reducing the support for the anterior rectal and posterior vaginal wall.

RECTAL PROLAPSE

Prolapse of the rectum involving all layers of the rectal wall may occur. The precise aetiology is not known. During prolapse, the mid and upper rectum descends towards the pelvic floor on straining. This descent tends to occur within the lumen of the rectum as a form of intussusception, and may be a consequence of the large diameter of the lower rectal ampulla and relative fixation of the anorectal junction and anal canal. The upper mesorectum is formed by relatively loose adipose connective tissue, and so relatively little tissue actually fixes the mid and upper rectum in position within the pelvis. The 'lateral ligaments' are composed mainly of vascular structures and offer only limited support against rectal descent. Chronic enlargement of the anorectal space bound by levatores ani commonly occurs in patients suffering rectal prolapse, but it is thought to be a consequence rather than a cause of the prolapse. During prolapse, the recto-uterine pouch in females also descends with the anterior rectal wall, and in extreme cases may become everted through the anus between the layers of rectal wall. This rarely happens to the rectovesical pouch in males.

RECTOCOELE

When the rectovaginal septum is grossly effaced, especially in postmenopausal females, the pressure of defaecation transmitted forward along the sacral flexure of the rectum can eventually cause bulging of the rectal wall into the posterior vagina, and, in extreme cases, through the vaginal introitus. Failure of support of the rectum and perineum by the puborectalis and pubovaginalis muscles contributes to this prolapse by allowing descent of the posterior perineum during straining.

MESORECTAL EXCISION IN RECTAL CANCER

An important concept in the oncological treatment of adenocarcinoma of the rectum is the integrity of the rectum and its mesorectal tissue. The epirectal and pararectal lymphatic tissues are located throughout the

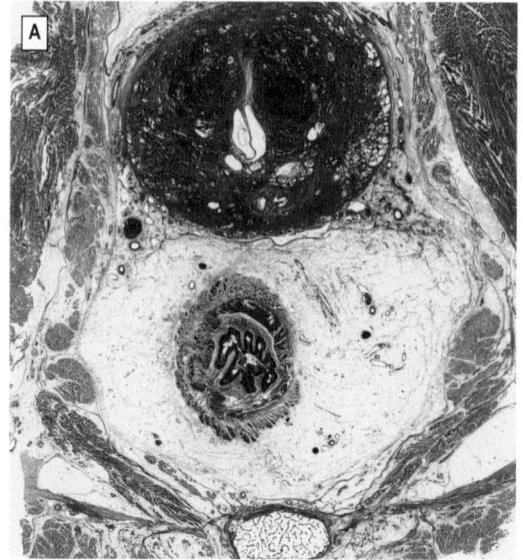

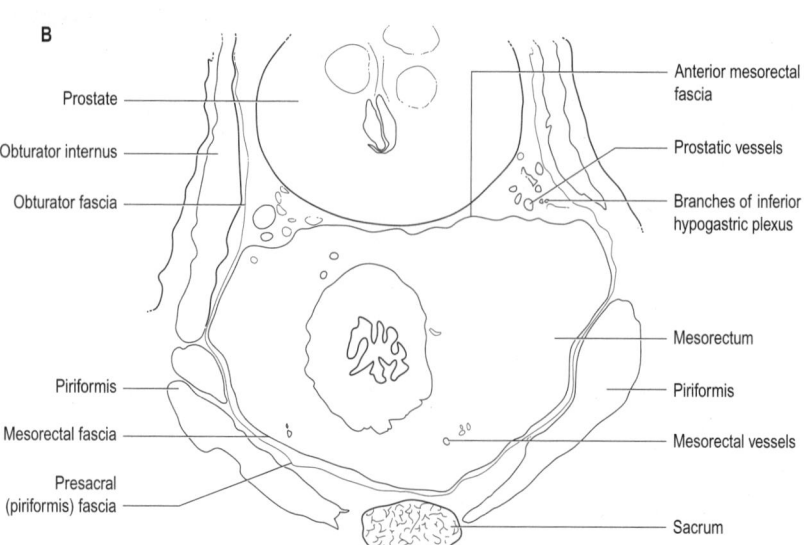

Fig. 83.7 Wholemount cadaveric specimen of the mid rectum in a male.

mesorectum. If the mesorectum is divided or disrupted during surgical excision of rectal carcinoma, involved nodes may be left in situ, which may predispose to local recurrence of tumour (Heald et al 1982). Oncological excision of the rectum involves mobilization of the rectum in the plane formed by the mesorectal fascia posterolaterally around the mesorectum. This plane allows the rectum and mesorectum to be removed as a whole without disruption of the presacral fascia and its underlying venous plexus. It is continuous with the plane between the mesentery surrounding the origin of the superior rectal artery and the presacral fascia over the sacral promontory, which is opened during mobilization of the inferior mesenteric artery origin prior to ligation. The mesorectal plane extends laterally and anteriorly, disrupted only by small branches of the middle rectal vessels, and is continuous with the rectovesical or rectovaginal fascia, which provides a similar oncological plane of dissection. Since the inferior hypogastric nerves are closely related to the plane of the mesorectal fascia in its upper third, dissection must spare the nerves if bladder dysfunction (and erectile dysfunction in males) is to be avoided following surgery. Complete excision of the rectum – total mesorectal excision – involves mobilization of this plane to the level of levatores ani. During the excision it is important to follow the sacral curve of the rectum to prevent entry into the presacral fascia or anococcygeal ligament.

LOCAL EXCISION OF THE RECTUM

Full thickness excision of lesions of the rectal wall is possible in those parts of the rectum lying below the peritoneal reflections in the extra-peritoneal compartment. The mesorectal adipose tissue contains any leakage of contents and provides support to the closure of the defect in the rectal wall. Since only the lower third of the rectum is wholly extraperitoneal, full thickness local excisions of the rectum should be avoided on the anterior wall of the middle third and anterolateral walls of the upper third of the rectum. The height to which such excision can be performed anteriorly in females is lower than in males, because of the lower level of the peritoneal reflection which makes entry into the peritoneal cavity more likely.

VASCULAR SUPPLY AND LYMPHATIC DRAINAGE

ARTERIES

The principal arterial supply to the upper two-thirds of the rectum is the superior rectal artery. Branches of the middle rectal artery provide some additional supply to the middle third, and ascending branches of the inferior rectal artery supply the distal third. A small contribution also comes from the median sacral artery, which is the terminal midline branch of the aorta and enters the posterior wall of the anorectal junction on the sacrorectal fascia (**Fig. 83.8**).

Superior rectal artery – The superior rectal artery is the principal continuation of the inferior mesenteric artery. It descends into the pelvis in the sigmoid mesocolon, crosses the left common iliac vessels and passes over the sacral promontory usually just to the left of the midline. It is straddled by the inferior hypogastric nerves on either side. It lies anterior to the upper sacral vertebrae and passes into the upper mesorectum. It descends, initially in the midline, and divides into two branches at the level of the third sacral vertebra. These lie initially posterolateral, then lateral, to the rectal wall as they descend one on each side of the rectum. Terminal branches pierce the muscle wall from the level of the upper mesorectum to enter the rectal submucosa, where they anastomose with ascending branches of the inferior rectal arteries.

Middle rectal arteries – The middle rectal arteries arise from the anterior division of the internal iliac artery and enter the mesorectum antero-laterally in the 'lateral rectal ligaments'. They are frequently absent (Sato & Sato 1991). When present they provide an arterial supply to the muscle of the mid and lower rectum, but form only poor anastomoses with the superior and inferior rectal arteries.

Inferior rectal arteries – The inferior rectal arteries are terminal branches of the internal pudendal arteries. They enter the upper anal canal laterally and supply the internal and external sphincters, the anal canal below its valves, and the perianal skin. They also provide ascending branches in

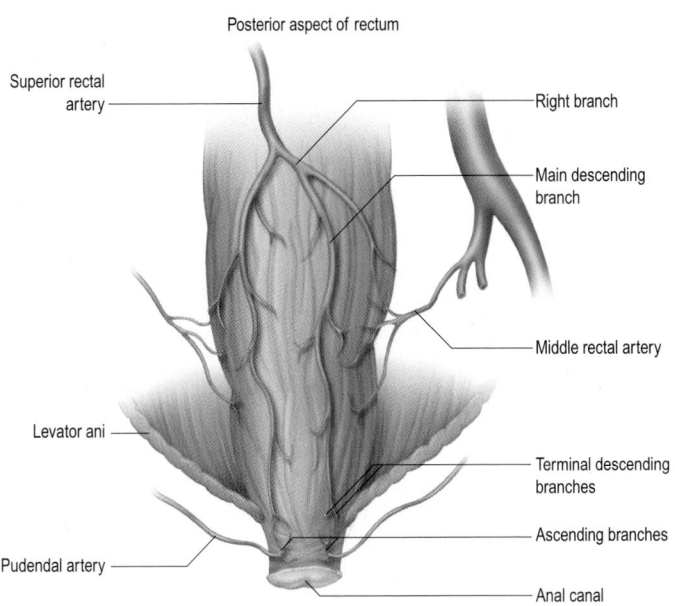

Posterior aspect of rectum

Superior rectal
artery

Right branch

Main descending
branch

Middle rectal artery

Levator ani

Terminal descending
branches

Ascending branches

Pudendal artery

Anal canal

Fig. 83.8 Details of the arterial supply of the rectum (viewed from behind).

the submucosa, which anastomose with the terminal branches of the superior rectal artery.

VEINS

Rectal venous plexus – The rectal venous plexus surrounds the rectum, and connects anteriorly with the vesical plexus in males or the utero-vaginal plexus in females. It consists of an internal part, beneath the rectal and anal epithelium, and an external part outside the muscular wall. In the anal canal the internal plexus displays longitudinal dilatations, connected by transverse branches in circles immediately above the anal valves. The dilatations are most prominent in the left lateral, right anterolateral and right posterolateral sectors. The internal plexus drains mainly to the superior rectal vein but connects widely with the external plexus. The inferior portion of the external plexus is drained by the inferior rectal vein into the internal pudendal vein, the middle portion by a middle rectal vein into the internal iliac vein, and its superior part by the superior rectal vein, which is the start of the inferior mesenteric vein. Communication between portal and systemic venous systems is thus established in the rectal plexus.

Superior rectal veins – The superior rectal veins are formed from the internal rectal plexus. The tributaries of the superior rectal vein ascend in the rectal submucosa as about six vessels of considerable size which pierce the rectal wall c.7.5 cm above the anus. The branches unite to form the superior rectal vein, which runs along the superior rectal artery in the root of the mesorectum and mesosigmoid, passes to the left of the midline and continues as the inferior mesenteric vein.

Middle rectal veins – The middle rectal veins pass alongside the middle rectal arteries to drain into the anterior division of the internal iliac vein on the lateral wall of the pelvis.

LYMPHATICS

Lymphatics draining the rectum and the upper anal canal above the level of the dentate line pass superiorly, initially through the rectal wall, and then as a fine network over the surface of the rectum, before draining into epirectal nodes in the mesorectum. They usually lie very close to the outer fibres of the rectal longitudinal muscle. The pararectal nodes lie within the mesorectum, a variable distance from the rectal wall. The overall direction of drainage is upwards along the branches of the superior rectal artery. The nodes lie within the loose adipose connective tissue of the mesorectum. Drainage to intermediate groups occurs up to the nodes near the origin of the inferior mesenteric artery (**Fig. 83.9**).

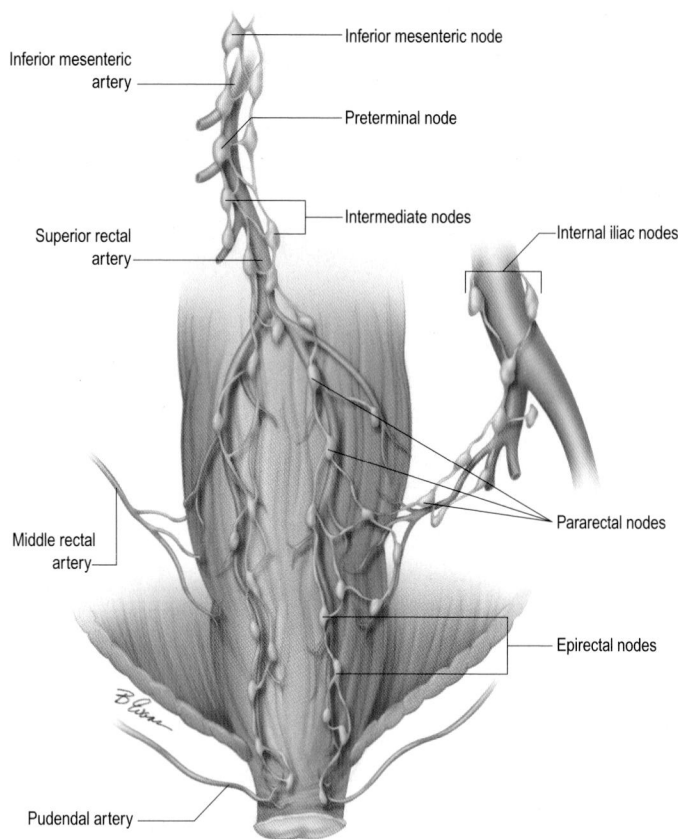

Inferior mesenteric node

Inferior mesenteric artery

Preterminal node

Intermediate nodes

Internal iliac nodes

Superior rectal artery

Pararectal nodes

Middle rectal artery

Epirectal nodes

Pudendal artery

Fig. 83.9 Lymph nodes of the rectum and upper anal canal (viewed from behind).

INNERVATION

The rectum is innervated primarily via the inferior mesenteric plexus. Both sympathetic and parasympathetic fibres (p. 1185) form a plexus along branches of the superior rectal artery. A small contribution is also made by fibres of the middle rectal plexus along the branches of the middle rectal artery. These are derived from the inferior hypogastric plexus (p. 1185). The role of rectal innervation in continence and its relation to anal innervation is dealt with on page 1210.

REFERENCES

Broden B, Snellman B 1968 Procidentia of the rectum studied with cineradiography. A contribution to the discussion of causative mechanisms. Dis Colon Rectum 11: 330–47.

Brown G, Richards CJ, Newcombe RG et al 1999 Rectal carcinoma: thin-section MR imaging for staging in 28 patients. Radiology 211(1): 215–22.

Heald RJ, Husband EM, Ryall RDH 1982 The mesorectum in rectal cancer surgery: the clue to pelvic recurrence? Br J Surg 69: 613–16.
Original description of the mesorectal plane and its relevance to the surgical excision of rectal tumours.

Sato K, Sato T 1991 The vascular and neuronal composition of the lateral ligament of the rectum and the rectosacral fascia. Surg Radiol Anat 13(1): 17–22.

Anal canal

The anal canal begins at the anorectal junction and ends at the anal verge (**Figs 84.1, 84.2, 84.3, 84.4**). It is angulated in relation to the rectum because the pull of the sling-like puborectalis produces the anorectal angle. It lies 2–3 cm in front of and slightly below the tip of the coccyx, which is opposite the apex of the prostate in males. The anal verge is marked by a sharp turn where the squamous epithelium which lines the lower anal canal becomes continuous with the skin of the perineum. The pigmentation of skin around the anal verge demarcates the extent of the external sphincter. Identification of the anal verge may be difficult, particularly in males in whom the perineum may 'funnel' upwards into the lower anal canal. However, the characteristic puckering of the external epithelium caused by the penetrating fibres of the conjoint longitudinal layer (p. 1208) makes a useful landmark. The functional anal canal is represented by a zone of high pressure which roughly equates to the anatomical canal. The anal canal consists of an inner epithelial lining, a vascular subepithelium, the internal and external anal sphincters and fibromuscular supporting tissue. It is between 2.5 and 5 cm long in adults although the anterior wall is slightly shorter than the posterior. It is usually shorter in females. At rest it forms an oval slit in the anteroposterior plane rather than a circular canal due to the arrangement of the external anal sphincter.

The anal canal is attached posteriorly to the coccyx by the anococcygeal ligament, a midline fibroelastic structure which may possess some skeletal muscle elements, and which runs between the posterior aspect of the external sphincter and the coccyx. Just above this is the raphe of the levator plate, the fusion of the two halves of the iliococcygeus, which merges anteriorly with puborectalis. Between these two structures is a potential 'postanal' space.

The anus is surrounded laterally and posteriorly by loose adipose tissue within the ischioanal fossae, a potential pathway for the spread of perianal sepsis from one side to the other (p. 1366). The ischial spines may be palpated laterally. The pudendal nerves pass over the ischial spines at this point (p. 1126) and pudendal nerve motor terminal latency may be measured digitally using a modified electrode worn on the examining glove.

Anteriorly the perineal body separates the anal canal from the membranous urethra and penile bulb in males or from the lower vagina in females.

LINING OF THE ANAL CANAL

The upper portion of the anal canal is lined by columnar epithelium similar to that of the rectum. It contains secretory and absorptive cells with numerous tubular glands or crypts. The subepithelial tissues are mobile and relatively distensible and possess profuse submucosal arterial and venous plexuses. Terminal branches of the superior rectal vessels pass downwards towards the anal columns. The submucosal veins drain into the submucosal rectal venous plexus and also through the fibres of the upper internal anal sphincter into an intermuscular venous plexus.

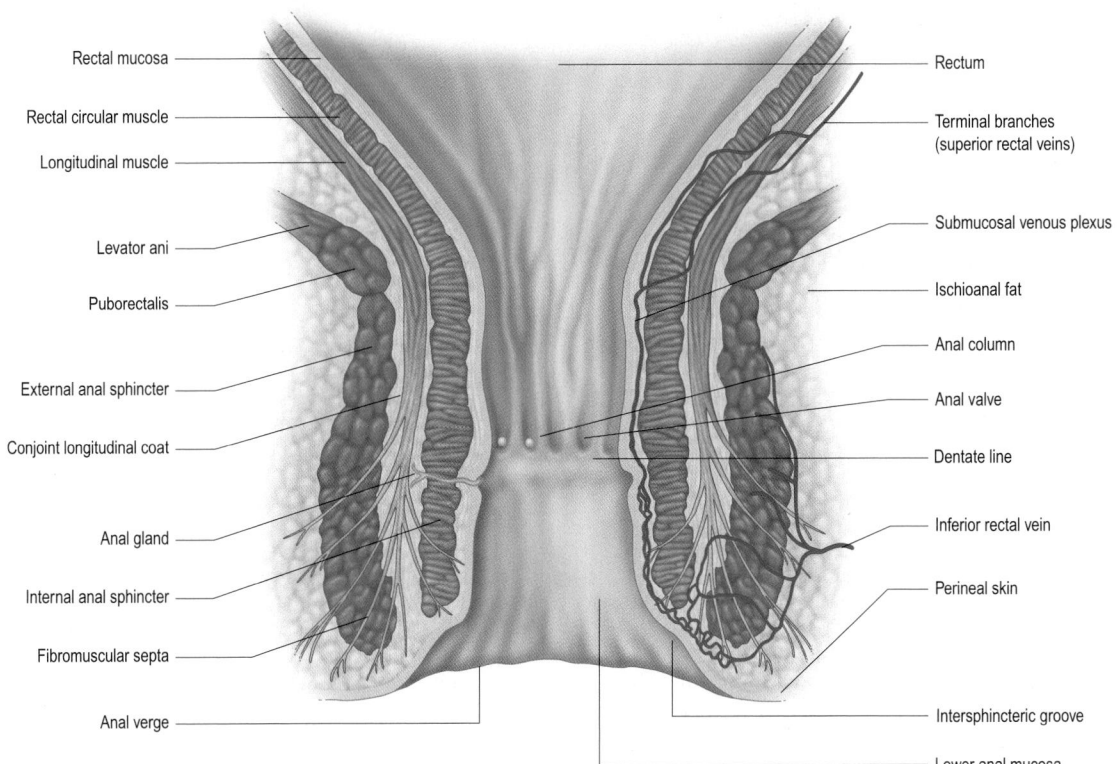

Fig. 84.1 Coronal section through the anal canal. Glandular and vascular structures are only shown unilaterally for clarity.

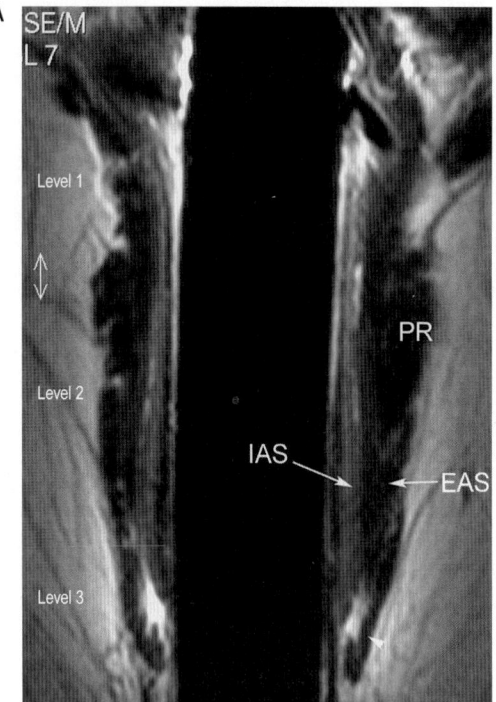

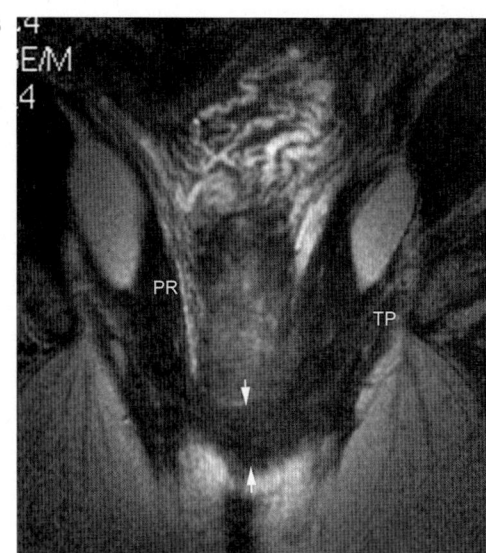

Fig. 84.2 **A**, Mid-coronal MRI endocoil image of the anal canal. **B**, Anterior coronal MRI endocoil section in a woman showing the transverse perineii (TP) joining the external anal sphincter anteriorly (between arrows). EAS, external anal sphincter; IAS, internal anal sphincter; PR, puborectalis.

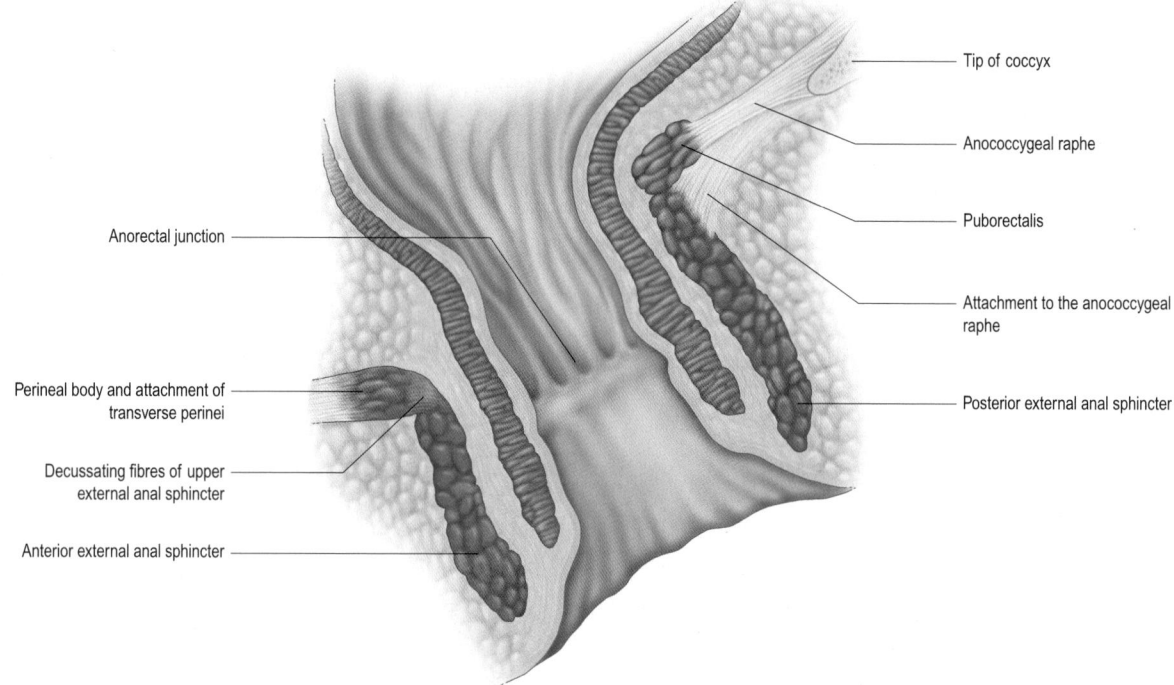

Fig. 84.3 Sagittal section through the anal canal. The anal canal is angled posteriorly with the anterior sphincteric structures appearing to be lower than posterior structures. The glandular, vascular and fibromuscular structures and the conjoint longitudinal coat have been omitted for clarity. EAS, external anal sphincter.

There are 6–10 vertical folds, the anal columns, in the mid anal canal. They tend to be obvious in children but less well-defined in adults. Each column contains a terminal radicle of the superior rectal artery and vein: the vessels are largest in the left-lateral, right-posterior and right-anterior quadrants of the wall of the canal where the subepithelial tissues expand into three 'anal cushions'. The cushions seal the anal canal, helping to maintain continence to flatus and fluid. They are also important in the pathogenesis of haemorrhoids. The lower ends of the columns may form small crescentic folds called the anal valves, between which lie small recesses referred to as anal sinuses. The anal valves and sinuses together form the dentate (or pectinate) line. About six anal glands open into small depressions in the anal valves, the anal crypts.

The glands, which are branched, are lined by stratified columnar epithelium. Cystic dilatations may be seen in the glands, which may extend through the internal sphincter and even into the external sphincter (Seow-Cheon Ho 1994).

The mucosa below the dentate line is smooth, and termed the pectin. It is non-keratinized stratified squamous epithelium which lacks sweat and sebaceous glands and hair follicles, but contains numerous somatic nerve endings. It extends down to the intersphincteric groove, a depression at the lower border of the internal sphincter. The canal below the intersphincteric groove is lined by hair-bearing, keratinizing, stratified epithelium which is continuous with the perianal skin. The submucosa in this region contains profuse arterial and venous plexuses

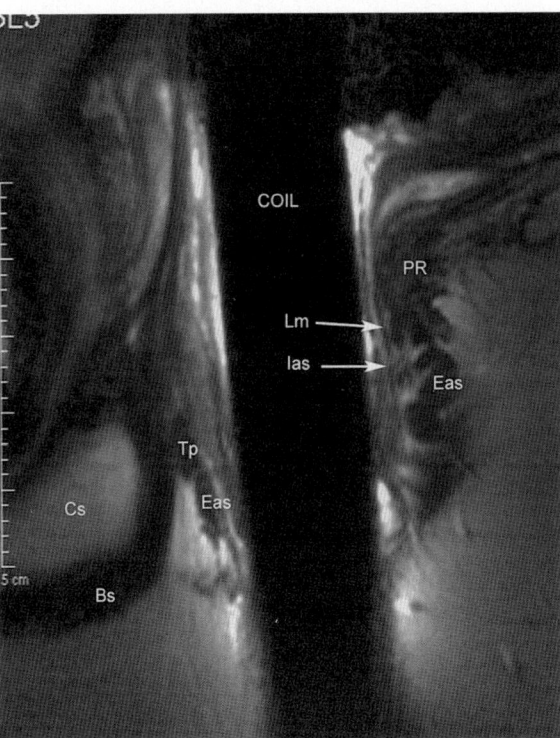

Fig. 84.4 MRI endocoil mid sagittal view of the anal canal in a man. Cs, corpus spongiosus; Tp, transverse perineii; Eas, external anal sphincter; Lm, longitudinal muscle; Ias, internal anal sphincter; PR, puborectalis; Bs, bulbospongiosus.

and has more connective tissue than the upper canal. It may be tethered to fibres of the conjoint longitudinal layer in the region of the intersphincteric groove.

The junction between the columnar and squamous epithelia is referred to as the anal transition zone (ATZ), which is variable in height and position, and often contains islands of squamous epithelium extending up into the columnar mucosa. Nerve endings including thermoreceptors exist in the submucosa around the upper ATZ. They probably play a role in continence by providing a highly specialized 'sampling' mechanism by which the contents of the lower rectum are identified during periods when the upper anal canal relaxes to allow rectal contents to come into contact with the upper anal canal epithelium (Duthie & Gairns 1960).

The well-defined muscularis mucosae of the rectum continues into the upper canal. Fibres from the longitudinal muscle pass through the internal sphincter and surround the submucosal venous plexus, before turning upwards to merge with the muscularis mucosae to form the musculus submucosae ani.

Referred pain
Pain in the anus is usually felt with a high degree of acuity and is well localized to the perineum and anal canal itself.

Haemorrhoids
Haemorrhoids represent abnormal enlargement of the anal cushions. The partial drainage of the venous plexus into the intermuscular plane may play a role in this chronic engorgement as a result of obstruction of the venous flow during prolonged straining and defaecation. Since the subepithelial vascular cushions of the upper, mid and lower anal canal form a continuous plexus, the differentiation of haemorrhoids into internal and external is somewhat arbitrary. The laxity of the upper anal canal submucosa is probably responsible for the fact that internal haemorrhoids may form more easily, although engorgement of the plexus deep to the lower anal epithelium may also occur. Since the epithelium in the lower canal is well supplied with sensory nerve endings, acute distension or invasive treatment to haemorrhoids in this area causes profound discomfort, whereas invasive or destructive therapy with relatively few symptoms is possible in the upper canal because the latter is lined with insensate columnar mucosa.

Anal fissures
Vertical breaks in the anal epithelium are not uncommon in human beings. The development of chronic, non-healing fissures is less common. They are more likely to develop in the anterior, and particularly the posterior, midline of the anus, possibly because stress within the anal canal is concentrated in these regions by the arrangement of the external sphincter fibres. The relative paucity of the arterial supply in these regions probably contributes to poor healing. Persistent hypertonicity of the anal sphincter is a primary pathogenic factor, possibly developing as a consequence of disordered local reflex mechanisms between the lower rectum and internal anal sphincter.

Cryptoglandular sepsis and fistula in ano
Infection of the anal glands is the main cause of anal sepsis and cryptogenic fistula formation (Parks et al 1976). Because many of these glands extend into the intersphincteric plane, so-called cryptoglandular sepsis may readily spread into this tissue plane. The commonest route of drainage of this sepsis is downwards between the internal and external anal sphincters to appear beneath the skin at the anal verge. Rupture or drainage of the sepsis at this point will form a fistula in ano in the intersphincteric plane. Less commonly, the infection drains outwards from the intersphincteric plane. It passes through the fibres of the external anal sphincter, possibly along the spreading septa of the conjoint longitudinal coat to appear in the perianal skin outside the external anal sphincter as a transphincteric fistula. If the sepsis does not originate in the intersphincteric plane, drainage is likely to be beneath the anal mucosa alone with the formation of a submucous fistula.

Sepsis within the ischioanal fossa surrounding the lower anal canal can spread with relative ease since the connective tissue is mostly loose adipose tissue. Pus may spread posteriorly, behind the lower anal canal, into the contralateral ischioanal fossa due to the absence of any septa or ligamentous attachments of the lower anal canal (Parkes 1961).

MUSCLES OF THE ANAL CANAL
The anal canal is encircled by the internal and external anal sphincters, separated by the longitudinal layer, and has connections superiorly to puborectalis and the transverse perineii (p. 1358) (**Figs 84.5, 84.6**).

Internal anal sphincter

Attachments – The internal anal sphincter is a well-defined ring of obliquely orientated smooth muscle fibres continuous with the circular muscle of the rectum, terminating at the junction of the superficial and subcutaneous components of the external sphincter. Its thickness varies between 1.5 and 3.5 mm, depending upon the height within the anal canal and whether the canal is distended. It is usually thinner in females and becomes thicker with age. It may also be thickened in disease processes such as rectal prolapse and chronic constipation. The lower portion of the sphincter is crossed by fibres from the conjoint longitudinal coat which pass into the submucosa of the lower canal.

Vascular supply – The internal anal sphincter is supplied from the terminal branches of the superior rectal vessels and branches of the inferior rectal vessels.

Innervation – The internal anal sphincter is innervated by the sympathetic and parasympathetic systems from fibres extending down from the lower rectum. Sympathetic fibres originate in the lower two lumbar segments, are distributed to the sphincter via the inferior hypogastric plexus, and cause contraction of the sphincter. Parasympathetic fibres originate in the second to fourth sacral spinal segments, are distributed through the inferior hypogastric plexus, and cause relaxation of the sphincter. The internal anal sphincter relaxes following stimulation of the rectum suggesting that local reflex pathways exist between the lower rectal sensory fibres and sphincteric motor fibres. This relaxation also occurs on stimulation of somatic sensory nerves present in the pelvic floor indicating that an additional reflex pathway exists via the sacral spinal segments.

EXTERNAL ANAL SPHINCTER
The external anal sphincter is an oval tube-shaped complex of striated muscle, composed mainly of type 1 (slow twitch) skeletal muscle fibres, which are well suited to prolonged contraction.

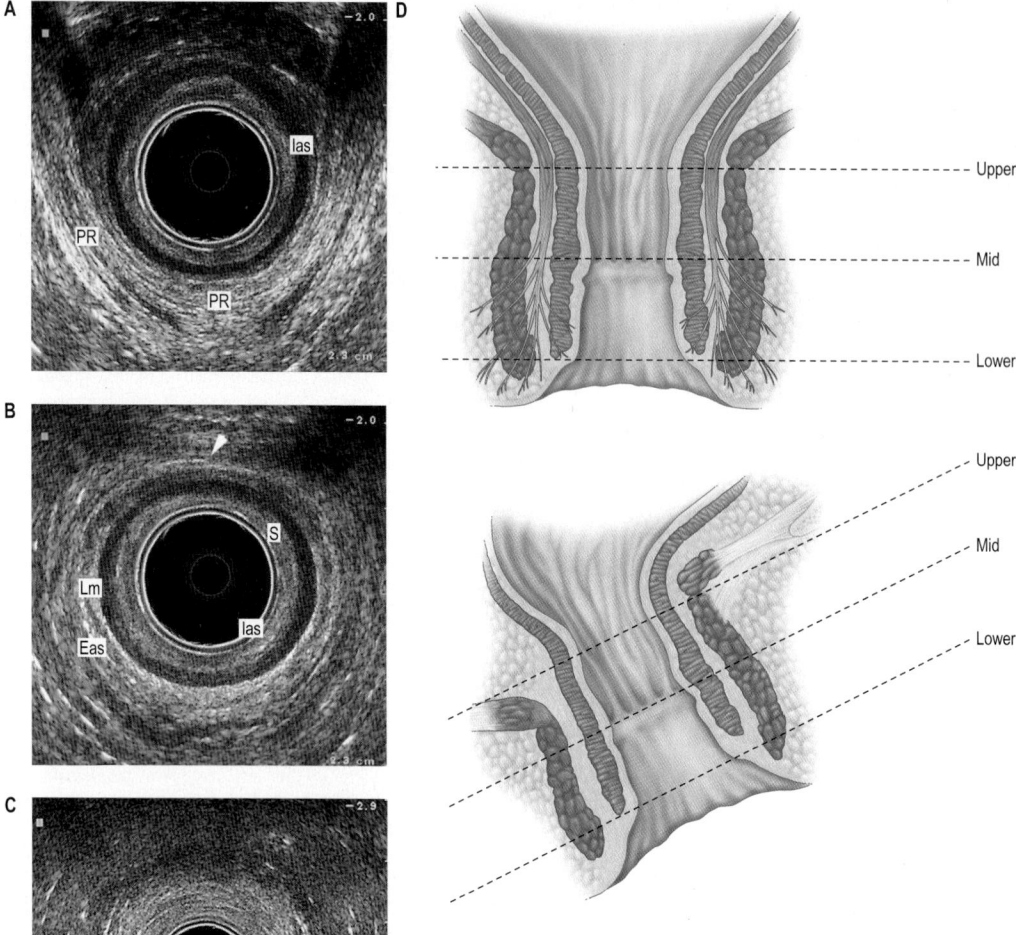

Fig. 84.5 A–C, Axial views of the anal canal at three levels on endoanal ultrasound in a woman. The endoanal ultrasound probe is the black structure centrally. **A**, Upper anal canal. The 'U' shape of the puborectalis (PR) is visible. Ias, internal anal sphincter. **B**, Middle anal canal. The external anal sphincter (Eas) is now a complete ring anteriorly (arrowhead). Lm, longitudinal muscle; S, subepithelial tissues **C**, Lower anal canal. Below the termination of the internal anal sphincter, the longitudinal layer extends through the subcutaneous external anal sphincter (between arrowheads). **D**, Key for levels of the anal canal.

Although previously described as consisting of deep, superficial and subcutaneous parts, the external anal sphincter forms a single functional and anatomical entity. Endoanal ultrasound and magnetic resonance imaging reveal that the uppermost fibres blend with the lowest fibres of puborectalis. Anteriorly some of these upper fibres decussate into the superficial transverse perineal muscles and posteriorly, some fibres are attached to the anococcygeal raphe. The majority of the middle fibres of the external anal sphincter surround the lower part of the internal sphincter. This portion is attached anteriorly to the perineal body and posteriorly to the coccyx via the anococcygeal ligament. Some fibres from each side of the sphincter decussate in these areas to form a commissure in the anterior and posterior midline. The lower fibres lie below the level of the internal anal sphincter and are separated from the lowest anal epithelium by submucosa.

The length and thickness of the external anal sphincter varies between the sexes: in females, the anterior portion tends to be shorter, the wall may be slightly thinner, and the tube may take the form of an asymmetrical cone (Rociu et al 2000). In women the transverse perineii and bulbospongiosus fuse with the external sphincter in the lower part of the perineum. In men the annular external sphincter is separate from the central point of the perineum into which the transverse perineii and bulbospongiosus fuse, so that there is a surgical plane of cleavage between the external sphincter and perineum (**Fig. 84.7**).

Vascular supply – The external anal sphincter is supplied from the terminal branches of the inferior rectal vessels with a small contribution from the median sacral artery.

Innervation – The external anal sphincter is innervated by the inferior rectal branch of the pudendal nerve originating in the anterior divisions of the second to fourth sacral nerve roots.

FIBROMUSCULAR STRUCTURES OF THE ANAL CANAL

The longitudinal layer and conjoint longitudinal coat

The longitudinal layer is situated between the internal and external sphincters and contains a fibromuscular layer, the conjoint longitudinal coat, and the intersphincteric space with its connective tissue components (Lunniss & Phillips 1992). The longitudinal layer has a muscular and fibroelastic component. The muscle part is formed by fusion of striated muscle fibres from puboanalis, the innermost part of puborectalis, with smooth muscle from the longitudinal muscle of the rectum. Endoanal ultrasound and magnetic resonance imaging demonstrate either muscle bundles or incomplete sheets of muscle extending down between the sphincters in the upper canal in both sexes: in men these often end just above the lower border of the internal sphincter. The layer then becomes completely fibroelastic, and splits into septa running between bundles of the subcutaneous external sphincter to terminate in the perianal skin. The area bounded by these septa is generally referred to as the perianal space. The most peripheral of the septa extend between the fibres of the external sphincter into the ischioanal fat. The most central septa pass through the fibres of the internal sphincter to reach the anal lining and may help to form the intersphincteric groove.

The conjoint longitudinal coat is innervated by autonomic fibres from the same origin as those supplying the internal sphincter.

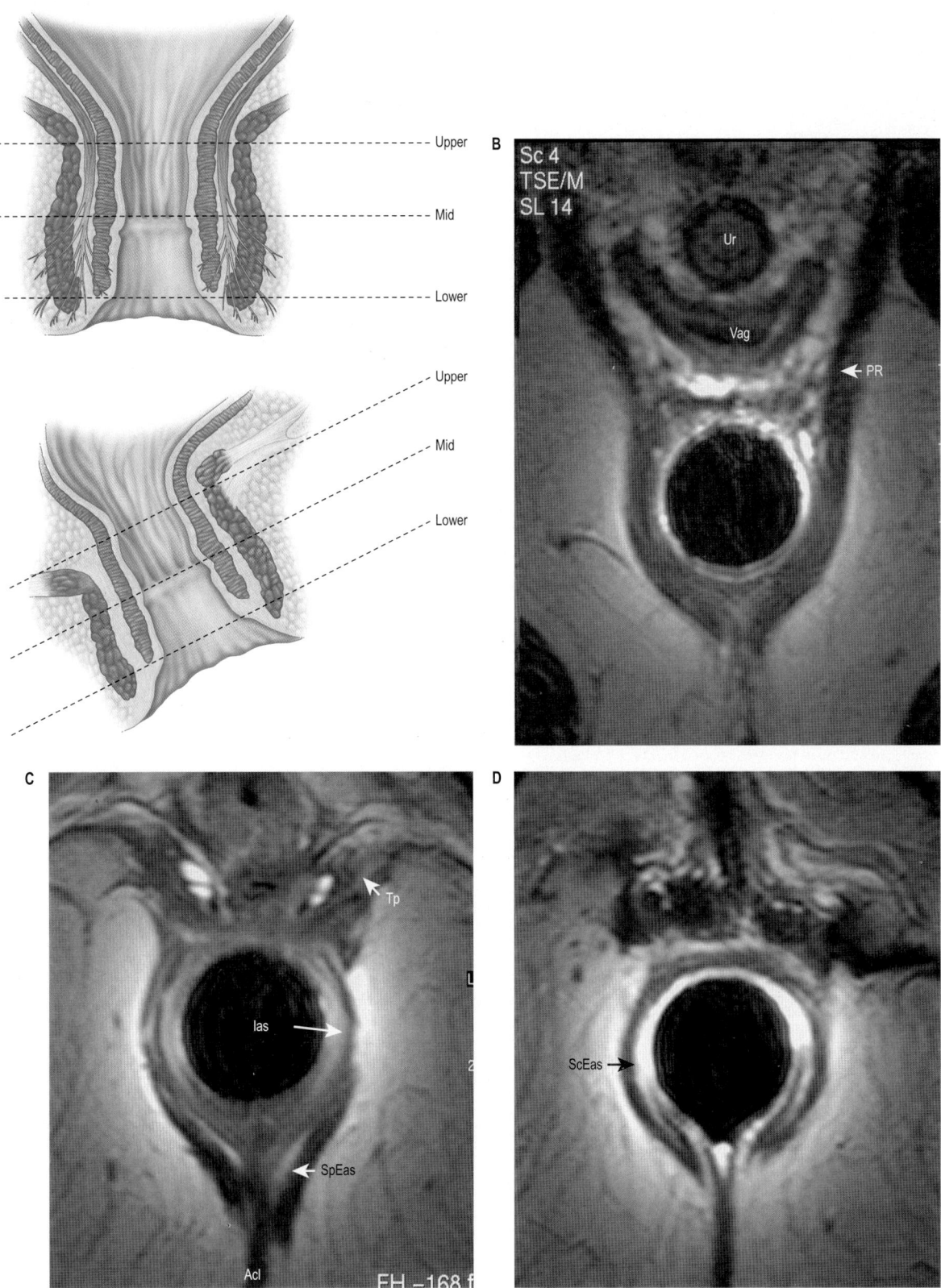

Fig. 84.6 MRI scan images of the anal canal. **A**, Key for levels of the anal canal. **B**, Upper anal canal. High in the canal with the sling of puborectalis (PR) extending anteriorly to the pubic bones. Vag, vagina; Ur, urethra. **C**, Mid anal canal. Mid canal level shows the transverse perineii (Tp) fusing into the external anal sphincter anteriorly. The superficial (middle) external anal sphincter (SpEas) is attached either side of the anococcygeal ligament (Acl). Ias, internal anal sphincter. **D**, Low anal canal. Low canal level, below the internal anal sphincter. ScEas, subcutaneous (lower) part of the external anal sphincter.

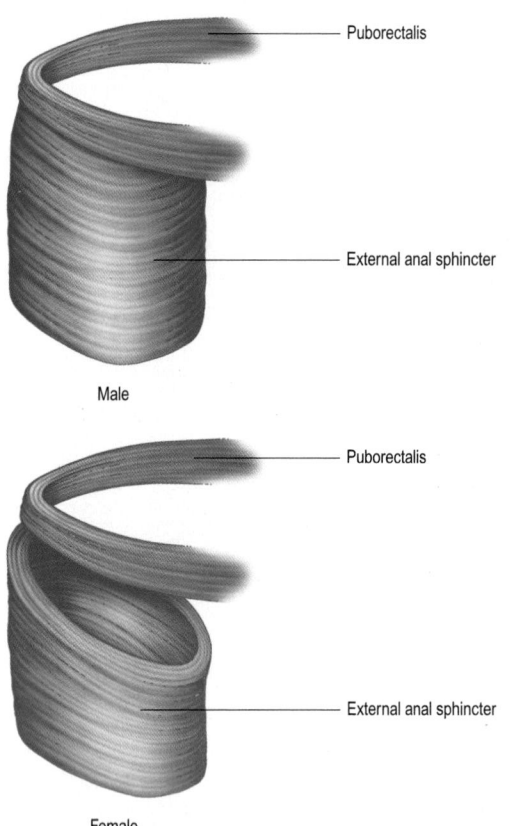

Male

Female

Fig. 84.7 Typical male and female external anal sphincter anatomy. The puborectalis is shown in isolation with the external anal sphincter viewed from superolateral. The anterior portion of the external anal sphincter is typically shorter and thinner in females.

Other fibromuscular structures

A layer of smooth muscle, yellow elastic fibres, and collagenous connective tissue is found in the anal submucosa, inferior to the anal sinuses. It is derived mainly from strands of the conjoint longitudinal coat, which descend inwards between the fibres of the internal sphincter. Some of the strands end by turning outwards around the lower edge of the internal sphincter to rejoin the main longitudinal layer. Most continue obliquely downwards and insert into the dermis below the intersphincteric groove. These attachments may help to form the corrugations seen in the perianal skin. The septa end in a honeycomb-like arrangement of fibres, which prevents easy distension of the lowest anal lining. This may explain the severe pain produced by pus or blood which collects here, since small volumes of fluid rapidly produce high pressure within the subepithelium.

VASCULAR SUPPLY AND LYMPHATIC DRAINAGE

ARTERIES

The arterial supply to the anal canal is derived from terminal branches of the superior rectal artery, the inferior rectal branch of the pudendal artery and branches of the median sacral artery. The supply to the anal canal lining is not distributed uniformly. The anterior and, more particularly, the posterior, midline epithelia have a relatively poorer arterial supply than that lining the lateral portions of the canal (Klosterhalfen et al 1989). This is of relevance in the perpetuation of chronic anal fissures (p. 1207).

VEINS

The venous drainage of the upper anal canal mucosa, internal anal sphincter and conjoint longitudinal coat passes via the terminal branches of the superior rectal veins into the inferior mesenteric vein. The lower anal canal and external sphincter drain via the inferior rectal branch of the pudenal vein into the internal iliac vein.

LYMPHATICS

Lymphatics from the upper anal mucosa, internal anal sphincter and conjoint longitudinal coat drain upwards into the submucosal and intramural lymphatics of the rectum. The lower anal canal epithelium and external anal sphincter lymphatics drain downwards via perianal plexuses into vessels which drain into the external inguinal lymph nodes. The lymphatics of puborectalis drain into the internal iliac lymph nodes. This arrangement has considerable importance for tumours of the lower rectum and upper anal canal. If the tumour is confined to the tissue of origin, malignant spread is confined to the mesorectal lymph nodes. However, if the tumour involves puborectalis or tissues associated with the external anal sphincter, the possibility of lymph node spread to these other groups may require radical excision and much more extensive surgery.

ANORECTAL CONTINENCE

To keep the anal canal closed the pressure within the anal canal has to be higher than in the rectum. The resting pressure in the canal is maintained mainly by tonic activity of the internal sphincter, with sudden increases of intrarectal pressure, as with coughing or exertion, compensated for by rapid contraction of the external sphincter and puborectalis. Angulation of the anorectal junction and the 'flap valve' theory is no longer considered important in continence. The internal sphincter does not close the canal completely, and the (c.7 mm) gap is sealed by the vascular subepithelial tissues.

DEFECATION

Defecation is a conscious physiological act in response to feeling the need to pass stool in the rectum, requiring coordinated relaxation of the pelvic floor muscles and anal sphincter. The dynamics have been studied using pressure measurements in the colon, rectum and anus (Herbst et al 1997) and by various imaging techniques including fluoroscopy, ultrasonography and magnetic resonance imaging (Kruyt et al 1991).

The process is initiated by mass colonic contractions driving faeces into the rectum. Rectal distension lowers internal sphincter tone in preparation for defecation. Defecation may be deferred by conscious contraction of the external anal sphincter until contractions cease and retrograde rectal peristalsis moves stool out of the distal rectum, so that the sensation to defecate passes off. Initiation of defecation involves relaxation of the pelvic floor muscles and external sphincter, so that the pelvic floor descends and the anal canal opens. Abdominal contraction will aid expulsion from the rectum, but continuing mass colonic contractions push more faeces down into the rectum, so that the entire left colon may be emptied.

Integrating the sensory input from the anal canal in order to control the activity of the anal musculature occurs at many levels in the nervous system, including the spinal cord, brain stem, thalamus and cortex. Neural activity monitors and regulates defecation, and other more subtle behaviours within the rectum and anal canal, such as the separation of faeces from rectal gas; local adjustments to faecal consistency and quantities; self-cleansing movements in the rectum and anal canal; and coordination with other actions of the perineal and abdominal muscles.

ANAL INCONTINENCE

Anal incontinence is common and may occur for a variety of reasons. Abnormal high rectal pressures, as in severe diarrhoea, may overcome a normal sphincter, and autonomic disorders may produce abnormal motor activity or loss of normal sensation, so that there is no awareness of stool. There may also be damage to the anal sphincter, mostly from vaginal delivery, or atrophy of the external sphincter from pudendal damage, also of obstetric origin, except in the elderly. A damaged sphincter will not be able to overcome normal fluctuations of intrarectal pressures, or there may be a combination of damage and rectal dysfunction resulting in anal incontinence.

REFERENCES

Duthie HL, Gairns FW 1960 Sensory nerve-endings and sensation in the anal region of man. Br J Surg 47: 585–95.

Herbst F, Kamm MA, Morris GP, Britton K, Woloszko J, Nicholls RJ 1997 Gastrointestinal transit and prolonged ambulatory colonic motility in health and faecal incontinence. Gut 41: 381–9.

Klosterhalfen B, Vogel P, Rixen H, Mittermayer C 1989 Topography of the inferior rectal artery: a possible cause of chronic primary anal fissure. Dis Colon Rectum 32: 43–52.
A detailed postmortem angiographic study demonstrating the arrangement of anal arterial supply

Kruyt RH, Delemarre JB, Doornbos J, Vogel HJ 1991 Normal anorectum: dynamic MR imaging anatomy. Radiology 179(1): 159–63.
Describes the MR anatomy of the anorectum in relation to surrounding structures and the anorectal angle at rest, during perineal contraction, and during straining, in asymptomatic subjects

Lunniss PJ, Phillips RK 1992 Anatomy and function of the anal longitudinal muscle. Br J Surg 79: 882–4.

Parkes AG 1961 The pathogenesis and treatment of fistula in ano. Br Med J 1: 463–9.
An early, full description of the relationship between the anatomy of anal glands and cryptoglandular sepsis

Parks AG, Gordon PH, Hardcastle JD 1976 A classification of fistula-in-ano. Br J Surg 63(1): 1–12.
A classification of anal fistulas based on the pathogenesis of the disease and the normal muscular anatomy of the pelvic floor

Rociu E, Stoker J, Eijkemans MJ, Lameris JS 2000 Normal anal sphincter anatomy and age- and sex-related variations at high-spatial-resolution endoanal MR imaging. Radiology 217: 395–401.

Seow-Choen F, Ho JM 1994 Histoanatomy of anal glands. Dis Colon Rectum 37: 1215–18.

SECTION **7** Chapter **84**

Liver

The liver is the largest of the abdominal viscera, occupying a substantial portion of the upper abdominal cavity. It performs a wide range of metabolic activities necessary for homeostasis, nutrition and immune defence. It is composed largely of epithelial cells (hepatocytes), which are bathed in blood derived from the hepatic portal veins and hepatic arteries. There is continuous chemical exchange between the cells and the blood. Hepatocytes are also associated with an extensive system of minute canals, which form the biliary system into which products are secreted. The liver is important in the removal and breakdown of toxic, or potentially toxic, materials from the blood. It regulates blood glucose and lipids, and plays a role in the storage of certain vitamins, iron, and other micronutrients as well as breaking down or modifying amino acids. It is involved in a plethora of other biochemical reactions. Since the majority of these processes are exothermic, a substantial part of the thermal energy production of the body, especially at rest, is provided by the liver. The liver is populated by phagocytic macrophages, which form part of the mononuclear phagocyte system of the body, and are important in the removal of particulates from the blood stream. In fetal life the liver is an important site of haemopoiesis.

The liver lies in the upper right part of the abdominal cavity. It occupies most of the right hypochondrium and epigastrium, although it frequently extends into the left hypochondrium as far as the left lateral line. In adults the liver weighs c.2% of body mass. The liver has an overall wedge shape, which is in part determined by the form of the upper abdominal cavity into which it grows. The narrow end of the wedge lies towards the left hypochondrium, with the anterior edge pointing anteriorly and inferiorly. The superior and right lateral aspects are shaped by the anterolateral abdominal and chest wall as well as the diaphragm. The inferior aspect is shaped by the adjacent viscera. In life it is reddish brown in colour and although firm and pliant its weight and texture depend in part on the volume of venous blood it contains. The liver capsule plays an important part in maintaining the integrity of its shape. Once the capsule is lacerated, the liver tissue is easily parted and provides only limited support for surgical sutures. These features, in combination with its exceptional vascular supply, make the liver prone to potentially lethal injuries if it is split open.

The liver is probably supported in its position in the upper abdomen by several factors. Tone in the anterolateral abdominal muscles is important in holding many viscera, including the liver, in place. Ligamentous attachments of the liver capsule to the diaphragm and anterior abdominal wall (p. 1213) provide some support, and prevent rotation of the liver about its vascular attachments at the porta hepatis (p. 1215) and hepatic veins (p. 1220). The liver is also attached to the relatively fixed retroperitoneal inferior vena cava by the hepatic and caudate veins. The relative importance of these attachments can be seen after orthotopic liver transplantation where, despite the absence of ligamentous structures, the liver remains within the right upper quadrant although it is more prone to torsion and rotation.

EXTERNAL FEATURES

Hepatic attachments

The liver is attached to the anterior abdominal wall, diaphragm and other viscera by several ligaments, which are formed from condensations of the peritoneum as described on page 1127.

Falciform ligament

The liver is attached in front to the anterior abdominal wall by the falciform ligament. The two layers of this ligament descend from the posterior surface of the anterior abdominal wall and diaphragm and turn onto the anterior and superior surfaces of the liver. On the dome of the superior surface, the right leaf runs laterally and is continuous with the upper layer of the coronary ligament. The left layer of the falciform ligament turns medially and is continuous with the anterior layer of the left triangular ligament. The ligamentum teres – which represents the obliterated left umbilical vein – (p. 1215) runs in the lower free border of the falciform ligament and continues into a fissure on the inferior surface of the liver.

Coronary ligament

The coronary ligament is formed by the reflection of the peritoneum from the diaphragm onto the posterior surfaces of the right lobe of the liver. Between the two layers of this ligament there is a large triangular area of liver devoid of peritoneal covering called the 'bare area' of the liver. Here the liver is attached to the diaphragm by areolar tissue and is in continuity inferiorly with the anterior pararenal space. The coronary ligament is continuous on the right with the right triangular ligament. On the left, it becomes closely applied, and forms the left triangular ligament. The upper layer of the coronary ligament is reflected superiorly onto the inferior surface of the diaphragm and inferiorly onto the right and superior surface of the liver. The lower layer of the coronary ligament reflects inferiorly over the right suprarenal gland and right kidney, and superiorly onto the inferior surface of the liver. Surgical division of the right triangular and coronary ligaments allows the right lobe of the liver to be brought forward, and exposes the lateral aspect of the inferior vena cava behind the liver.

Triangular ligaments

The left triangular ligament is a double layer of peritoneum which extends to a variable length over the superior border of the left lobe of the liver. Medially the anterior leaf is continuous with the left layer of the falciform ligament. The posterior layer is continuous with the left layer of the lesser omentum. The left triangular ligament lies in front of the abdominal part of the oesophagus, the upper end of the lesser omentum and part of the fundus of the stomach. Division of the left triangular ligament allows the left lobe of the liver to be mobilized for exposure of the abdominal oesophagus and crura of the diaphragm.

The right triangular ligament is a short structure which lies at the apex of the 'bare area' of the liver and is continuous with the layers of the coronary ligament.

Lesser omentum

The lesser omentum is a fold of peritoneum which extends from the lesser curve of the stomach and proximal duodenum to the inferior surface of the liver. The attachment to the inferior surface of the liver is L-shaped. The vertical component follows the line of the fissure for the ligamentum venosum – the fibrous remnant of the ductus venosus. More inferiorly the attachment runs horizontally to complete the L in the porta hepatis. At its upper end, the superior layer of lesser omentum is continuous on the left with the posterior layer of the left triangular ligament, and the inferior layer is continuous on the right with the coronary ligament as it encloses the inferior vena cava. At its lower end, the two layers diverge to surround the structures of the porta hepatis. A thin fibrous condensation of fascia usually runs from the medial end of the porta hepatis into the fissure in the inferior surface which contains the ligamentum teres. This fascia is continuous with the lower border of the falciform ligament when the ligamentum teres re-emerges at the inferior border of the liver. Care should be taken when dividing the lesser omentum, since an aberrant left hepatic artery may run in the medial end.

Hepatic surfaces (Fig. 85.1)

The liver is usually described as having superior, anterior, right, posterior and inferior surfaces, and has a distinct inferior border. However, superior, anterior and right surfaces are continuous and no definable borders separate them. It would be more appropriate to group them as the diaphragmatic surface, which is mostly separated from the inferior, or visceral surface, by a narrow inferior border. The border is rounded between the right and inferior surfaces, but becomes angled much more sharply between the anterior and inferior surfaces. This part of the inferior border is notched by the ligamentum teres, just to the right of the midline. The inferior border follows the right costal margin lateral to the fundus of the gallbladder, which usually corresponds to a second notch, 4–5 cm to the right of the midline. To the left of the ligamentum teres, the inferior border ascends below the medial end of the right costal margin. It crosses the infrasternal angle to pass behind the medial end of the left costal margin near the tip of the eighth costal cartilage. At the infrasternal angle the inferior border is related to the anterior abdominal wall and is accessible to examination by percussion, but is not usually palpable. In the midline, the inferior border of the liver is near the transpyloric plane, about a hand's breadth below the xiphisternal joint. In women and children the border often projects a little below the right costal margin.

Superior surface

The superior surface is the largest surface and lies immediately below the diaphragm, separated from it by peritoneum except for a small triangular area where the two layers of the falciform ligament diverge. The majority of the superior surface lies beneath the right dome; however, centrally there is a shallow cardiac impression corresponding to the position of the heart above the central tendon of the diaphragm. The left side of the superior surface lies beneath part of the left dome of the diaphragm. The superior surface blends imperceptibly with the anterior, right and posterior surfaces over the 'dome' of the liver. It is related to the right diaphragmatic pleura and base of the right lung, to the pericardium and ventricular part of the heart, and to part of the left diaphragmatic pleura and base of the left lung.

Anterior surface

The anterior surface, which is approximately triangular and convex, is covered by peritoneum except at the attachment of the falciform ligament. Much of it is in contact with the anterior attachment of the diaphragm. On the right the diaphragm separates it from the pleura and sixth to tenth ribs and cartilages, and on the left from the seventh and eighth costal cartilages. The thin margins of the base of the lungs are thus quite close to the upper part of this surface, more extensively so on the right. The median area of the anterior surface lies behind the xiphoid process and the anterior abdominal wall in the infracostal angle.

Right surface

The right surface is covered by peritoneum and lies adjacent to the right dome of the diaphragm which separates it from the right lung and pleura and the seventh to eleventh ribs. Above and lateral to its upper third, lie both the right lung and basal pleura between the diaphragm and the seventh and eighth ribs. The diaphragm, the costodiaphragmatic recess lined by pleura, and the ninth and tenth ribs all lie lateral to the middle third of the right surface. Lateral to the lower third, the diaphragm and thoracic wall are in direct contact. Rarely, the hepatic flexure and proximal transverse colon may lie on a long mesentery over the right and superior surfaces of the liver, referred to as Chilaiditi syndrome.

Liver biopsy – The liver lies conveniently close to the abdominal wall on its right and lateral anterior surfaces. Under normal circumstances, no other structures lie between the liver parenchyma and the diaphragm overlying the intercostal spaces of the ninth and tenth ribs. During deep inspiration the lung may descend to fill the pleura-lined costodiaphragmatic recess as far down as the tenth rib, but on forced expiration it also shrinks, and the eight or even seventh intercostal space may come into direct contact with the diaphragm overlying the liver. Blind percutaneous needle biopsy of the liver can be achieved through these intercostal spaces provided the patient can 'fix' the position of the liver by holding a forced expiration, and so ensure that the lung is not interposed between the body wall and the diaphragm. More commonly, biopsy is performed under ultrasound guidance. This

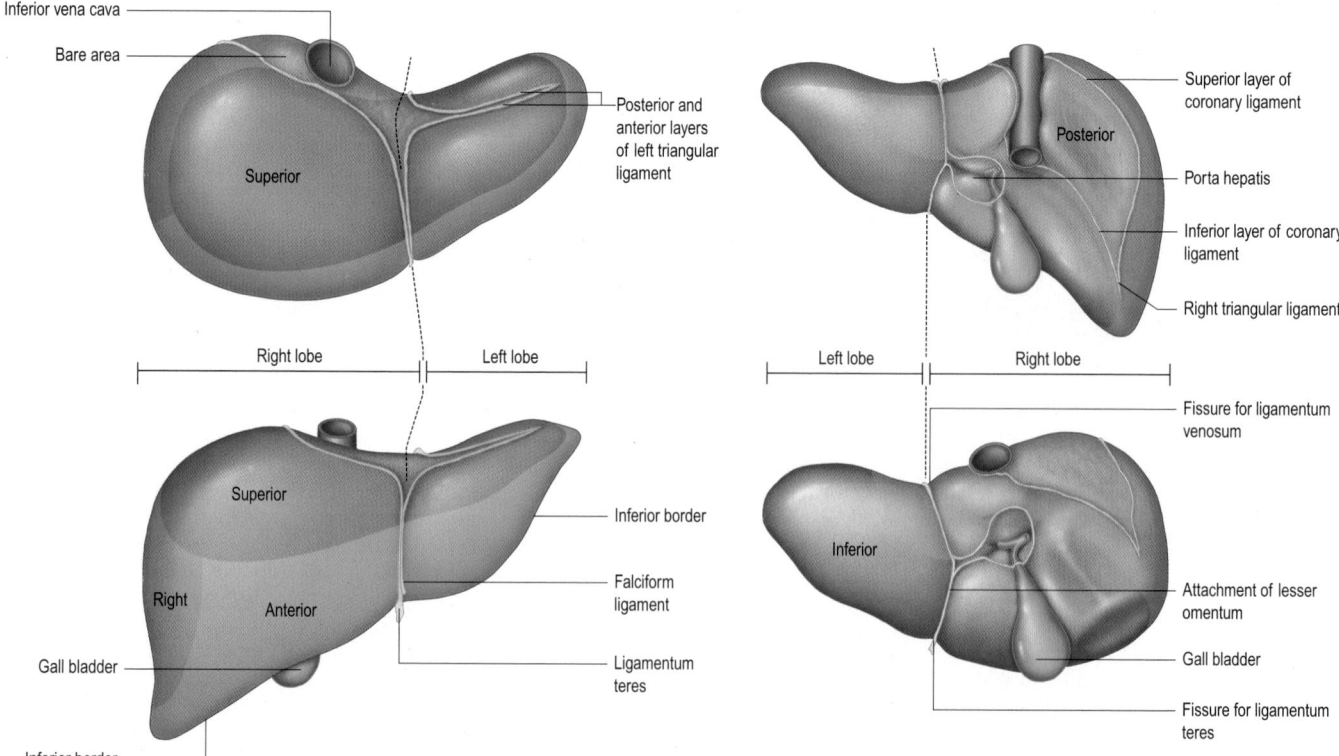

Fig. 85.1 The surfaces and external features of the liver. Top left, superior view; top right, posterior view; bottom left, anterior view; bottom right, inferior view.

not only ensures the lung is not liable to injury, but that the biopsy is directed to specific lesions within the parenchyma.

Posterior surface

The posterior surface is convex, wide on the right, but narrow on the left. A deep median concavity corresponds to the forward convexity of the vertebral column close to the attachment of the ligamentum venosum. Much of the posterior surface is attached to the diaphragm by loose connective tissue, which forms the so-called 'bare area'. The 'bare area' is triangular in shape. It is bounded above and below by the layers of the coronary ligament and its apex is directed down to the right, running into the right triangular ligament. Lateral to its lower end, the 'bare area' is an anterior relation of the upper pole of the left suprarenal gland. The inferior vena cava lies in a groove or tunnel in the medial end of the 'bare area'. To the left of the caval groove the posterior surface of the liver is formed by the caudate lobe, which is covered by a layer of peritoneum. This peritoneum is continuous with that of the inferior layer of the coronary ligament and the layers of the lesser omentum. The potential space between these three peritoneal layers is often referred to as the superior omental recess. The caudate lobe is related to the diaphragmatic crura above the aortic opening and the right inferior phrenic artery. It is separated by these structures from the descending thoracic aorta.

The fissure for the ligamentum venosum separates the posterior aspect of the caudate from the main part of the left lobe. The fissure cuts deeply in front of the caudate lobe and contains the two layers of the lesser omentum. Below, it curves laterally to the left end of the porta hepatis. The ligamentum venosum is attached below to the posterior aspect of the left branch of the portal vein. It ascends in the floor of the fissure and passes laterally. At the upper end of the caudate lobe it joins the left hepatic vein near its entry into the inferior vena cava, or sometimes the vena cava itself.

The posterior surface over the left lobe bears a shallow oesophageal impression near the upper end of the fissure for the ligamentum venosum caused by the abdominal part of the oesophagus. The posterior surface of the left lobe to the left of this impression is related to part of the fundus of the stomach (**Fig. 85.2**)

Inferior surface

The inferior surface is bounded by the inferior edge of the liver. It blends with the posterior surface in the region of the origin of the lesser omentum, the porta hepatis and the lower layer of the coronary ligament. It is marked near the midline by a sharp fissure which contains the ligamentum teres – the obliterated fetal left umbilical vein. Occasionally this fissure is bridged by liver tissue to form a tunnel. Posteriorly the inferior surface is related to the ligamentum venosum and the gallbladder. The latter usually lies in a shallow fossa but may vary from having a short mesentery, to being completely intrahepatic when it lies within a cleft in the liver parenchyma (p. 1227). Between the fissure for the ligamentum teres and the gallbladder lies the quadrate lobe.

The inferior surface of the left lobe is related inferiorly to the fundus of the stomach and the upper lesser omentum. The quadrate lobe lies adjacent to the pylorus, first part of the duodenum and the lower part of the lesser omentum. Occasionally the transverse colon lies between the duodenum and the quadrate lobe. To the right of the gallbladder, the inferior surface is related to the hepatic flexure of the colon, the right suprarenal gland and right kidney, and the first part of the duodenum.

The inferior surface may demonstrate a pronounced 'mound' of liver tissue close to the left border of the fissure for the ligamentum teres. This is referred to as the tuber omentale.

The porta hepatis (Figs 85.3, 85.4) – The porta hepatis is the area of the inferior surface through which all the neurovascular and biliary structures, except the hepatic veins, enter and leave the liver. It is situated between the quadrate lobe in front and the caudate process behind. The porta hepatis is actually a deep fissure into which the portal vein, hepatic artery and hepatic nervous plexus ascend into the parenchyma of the liver. The right and left hepatic bile ducts and some lymph vessels emerge from it. At the porta hepatis, the hepatic ducts lie anterior to the portal vein and its branches, and the hepatic artery with its branches lies between the two. All these structures are enveloped in the perivascular fibrous capsule – hepatobiliary capsule of Glisson – a sheath of loose connective tissue which surrounds the vessels as they course through the portal canals in the liver. It is also continuous with the fibrous

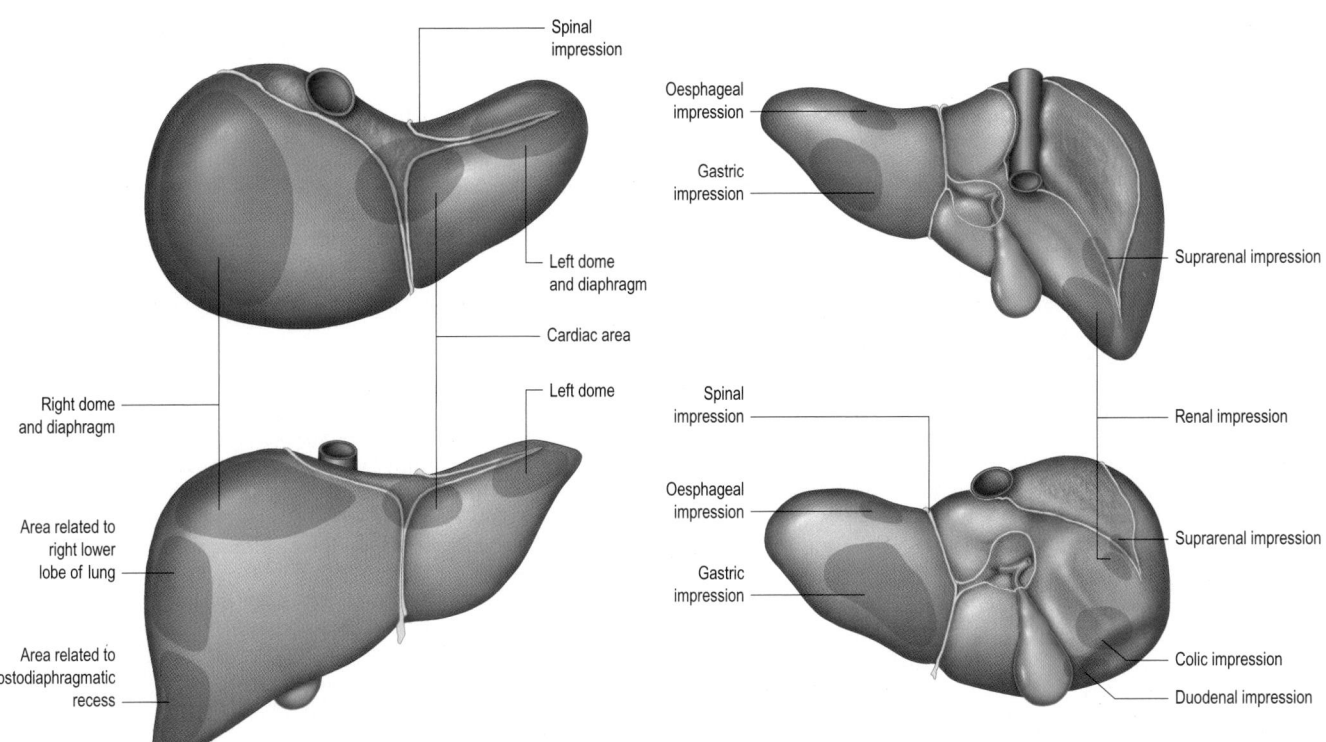

Fig. 85.2 Relations of the liver. Top left, superior view; top right, posterior view; bottom left, anterior view; bottom right, inferior view.

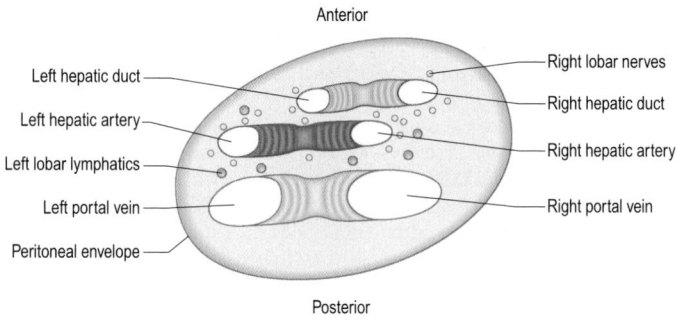

Anterior

Left hepatic duct

Left hepatic artery

Left lobar lymphatics

Left portal vein

Peritoneal envelope

Right lobar nerves

Right hepatic duct

Right hepatic artery

Right portal vein

Posterior

Fig. 85.3 Cross-section of the structures at the porta hepatis.

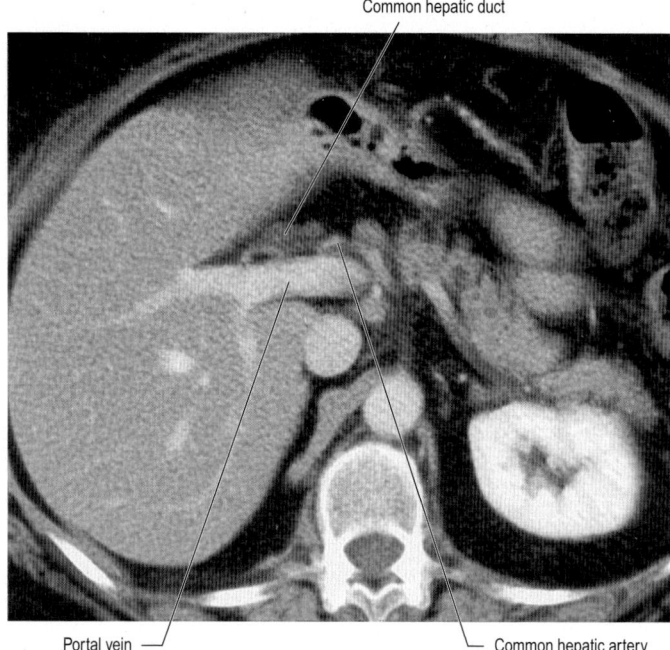

Common hepatic duct

Portal vein

Common hepatic artery

Fig. 85.4 Axial CT of the porta hepatis. The hepatic ducts lie anteriorly, the portal vein posteriorly, and hepatic artery between the two.

hepatic capsule. The dense aggregation of vessels, supporting connective tissue, and liver parenchyma just above the porta hepatis is often referred to as the 'hilar plate' of the liver. It may be dissected surgically to gain access to the intrahepatic branches of the bile ducts and vessels. The left hepatic duct remains extrahepatic as it runs down to the bifurcation along the base of segment IV – the quadrate lobe. This extrahepatic length of duct is particularly useful when performing high biliary duct reconstructions where a length of jejunum is anastomosed to form a biliary enteric bypass, for strictures of the common hepatic duct.

LOBATION AND SEGMENTATION

The liver has four lobes or eight segments, depending on whether it is defined by its gross anatomical appearance or by its internal architecture. Classification of the liver by internal architecture divides it into lobes, segments or sectors. The biliary, hepatic arterial and portal venous supply of the liver tend to follow very similar distributions used to define the hepatic segments. The hepatic venous anatomy follows a markedly different pattern. At the edge of segments, there is considerable overlap between vascular and biliary structures and segments are not identifiable by either gross external or internal examination of the liver. The value of the segmental classification, according to vascular

and biliary supply, is that surgical resection of a segment, multiple segments or a whole lobe, may be planned and performed to encounter the fewest possible major vascular structures. The surface of the liver is often marked by indentations or accessory fissures which do not relate directly to the lobes or segments. They occur most often over the superior, right, and anterior surfaces.

Gross anatomical lobes

Historically the gross anatomical appearance of the liver has been divided into right, left, caudate and quadrate lobes by the surface peritoneal and ligamentous attachments. The falciform ligament superiorly and the ligamentum venosum (p. 1219) inferiorly, mark the division between right and left lobes. On the inferior surface, to the right of the groove formed by the ligamentum venosum, there are two prominences separated by the porta hepatis. The quadrate lobe lies anteriorly, the caudate lobe posteriorly. The gallbladder usually lies in a shallow fossa to the right of the quadrate lobe.

Right lobe

The right lobe is the largest in volume and contributes to all surfaces. It is demarcated by the line of attachment of the falciform ligament superiorly. Inferiorly the fissure for the ligamentum teres, the groove for the ligamentum venosum, and the attachment of the lesser omentum, mark its border.

The inferior border of the right lobe, to the right of the gallbladder, often demonstrates a bulge of tissue, which when pronounced, is referred to as Riedel's lobe. Although the right inferior border of the liver is not usually palpable, the presence of a Riedel's lobe may be clinically detectable and may give rise to confusion as an apparent pathological right upper quadrant mass.

Quadrate lobe

The quadrate lobe is only visible from the inferior surface. It is bounded by the gallbladder fossa to the right, a short portion of the inferior border anteriorly, the fissure for the ligamentum teres to the left, and the porta hepatis posteriorly. In gross anatomical descriptions it is said to be a lobe arising from the right lobe; however, it is functionally related to the left lobe.

Caudate lobe

The caudate lobe is visible on the posterior surface. It is bounded on the left by the fissure for the ligamentum venosum, below by the porta hepatis, and on the right by the groove for the inferior vena cava. Above, it continues into the superior surface on the right of the upper end of the fissure for the ligamentum venosum. Below and to the right, it is connected to the right lobe by a narrow caudate process, which is immediately behind the porta hepatis and above the epiploic foramen. Depending on the depth of the fissure for the ligamentum venosum, the caudate lobe often has an anterior surface, which forms the posterior wall of the fissure and is in contact with the hepatic part of the lesser omentum. In gross anatomical descriptions this lobe is said to arise from the right lobe, but it is functionally separate.

Left lobe

The left lobe is the smaller of the two 'main' lobes. It lies to the left of the falciform ligament, has no subdivisions, and ends in a thin apex pointing into the left upper quadrant. Since it is substantially thinner than the right lobe it is more flexible. It is nearly as large as the right lobe in young children, possibly due to a more even distribution in portal and hepatic arterial supply, which may progressively come to favour growth of the right lobe during development of the body cavity. A fibrous band may be present at the left end of the adult left lobe: it represents an atrophied remnant of the more extensive left lobe found in children. If present, it contains atrophied bile ducts called the hepatic vasa aberrantia. Similar remnants may occur in the inferior border of the lobe and near the inferior vena cava.

Couinaud segments (Figs 85.5, 85.6)

Although a variety of definitions have been used to describe the anatomy of the liver segments, the most widely accepted clinical nomenclature is that described by Couinaud (1957), and Healey and Schroy (1953).

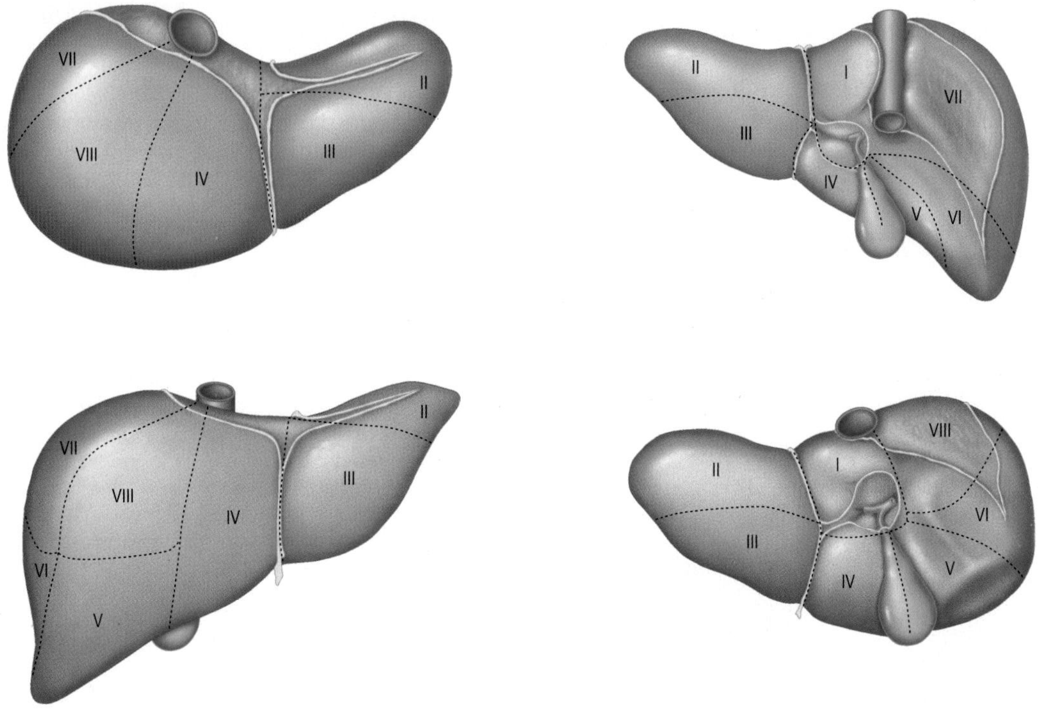

Fig. 85.5 Segmentation of the liver – Couinaud. Top left, superior view; top right, posterior view; bottom left, anterior view; bottom right, inferior view. The segments are sometimes referred to by name – I, caudate (sometimes subdivided into left and right parts); II, lateral superior; III, lateral inferior; IV, medial (sometimes subdivided into superior and inferior parts); V, anterior inferior; VI, posterior inferior; VII, posterior superior; VIII, anterior superior.

The internal architecture of the liver is divided into segments, commonly referred to as Couinaud's segments. Couinaud based his work on the distribution of the portal and hepatic veins whilst Healey and Schroy studied the arterial and biliary anatomy.

The liver is divided by the 'principal plane' into two halves of approximately equal size. The principal plane is defined by an imaginary parasagittal line from the gallbladder anteriorly to the inferior vena cava posteriorly. The usual functional division of the liver into right and left lobes lies along this plane. The liver is further subdivided into segments, each supplied by a principal branch of the hepatic artery, portal vein and bile duct. Segments I, II, III and IV make up the functional left lobe, and segments V, VI, VII and VIII make up the functional right lobe. The right lobe can be further divided into a posterior and anterior section or sector. The right posterior section is made up of segments VI and VII, and the right anterior section is made up of segments V and VIII. The left lobe can also be divided into sections: segment IV is referred to as the left medial section, and segments II and III as the left lateral section. The hepatic veins lie in liver parenchyma between the sections. Segment I corresponds to the gross anatomical caudate lobe and segment IV to the quadrate lobe.

The delineation of the internal liver architecture has been confirmed by cross-sectional imaging techniques as well as hepatic portography and arteriography. On axial CT and MRI, segment I is situated posterior and to the right of the inferior vena cava; segments VII, VIII, IV and II run in a clockwise fashion above the portal vein; and segments VI, V, IV and III are situated in a similar manner below the portal vein.

The value of the identification of the liver segments and sections according to vascular and biliary supply is that surgical resection of a segment, section, multiple segments, a lobe or greater volume of tissue may be performed whilst encountering the least number of possible major vascular structures.

Liver resection
Surgical resection of the liver for primary and secondary neoplasia is now routine, and there is very low morbidity and mortality. Knowledge of the internal anatomy of the liver is essential. As much as 80% of the liver mass can be removed safely. The liver has the unique capacity of regeneration, and will regrow to its original size some 6–12 months after resection.

The identification of the hepatic arterial and portal venous segmentation means that lesions seen on cross-sectional imaging can be placed within segments, so that the feasibility of resection can be assessed. Although detailed arterial and portal venous imaging is usually required to allow definitive surgical planning, understanding the segmental anatomy of the liver has allowed considerable advances to be made. Since the hepatic venous anatomy differs widely from the portal and arterial anatomy, resections rarely lie within wholly convenient vascular planes. Currently, the main limitation to liver resection is not the difficulty of segmental anatomy but the involvement of vital structures such as the inferior vena cava, or the need to preserve an adequate volume of functioning liver tissue after resection.

Resection of the liver can be described as either non-anatomical or anatomical. Non-anatomical resections are usually minor and the lines of resection are not related to Couinaud's segments. Major resections usually follow the planes between the segments and are anatomical. The nomenclature of liver resections has been historically confusing. Recently, Strasberg (1997) has attempted to simplify this by describing the removal of segments V to VIII as a right hemihepatectomy. The resection of liver has otherwise been described with respect to sections and segments. For example, removal of segments IV to VIII is a right trisectionectomy, involving the removal of the right posterior, right anterior and left medial sections. Major anatomical liver resections involve control of the appropriate inflow and outflow to the part of liver to be resected. Once the inflow has been stopped a line of ischaemic demarcation appears which then guides the surgeon along a plane of resection.

Liver transplantation
Liver transplantation is an established form of treatment for patients with end stage liver disease. Orthotopic transplantation involves a standard hepatectomy including the hepatic inferior vena cava. The implant of the graft then requires a superior and inferior caval anastomosis, followed by anastomosis of the portal vein. In adults, most surgeons use venovenous bypass during the anhepatic phase of the transplant. This allows splanchnic and systemic venous blood to return to the heart via the internal jugular vein. The transplant is completed by performing the arterial and biliary anastomoses.

For children, a cadaveric liver may be split into two along the lines of segmentation such that a single liver can be used for two transplants, usually an adult and a child or two small adults. Live donor liver transplants may be performed since the left lateral section and sometimes a right hemiliver (segments V to VIII) can be removed from a healthy donor and then transplanted.

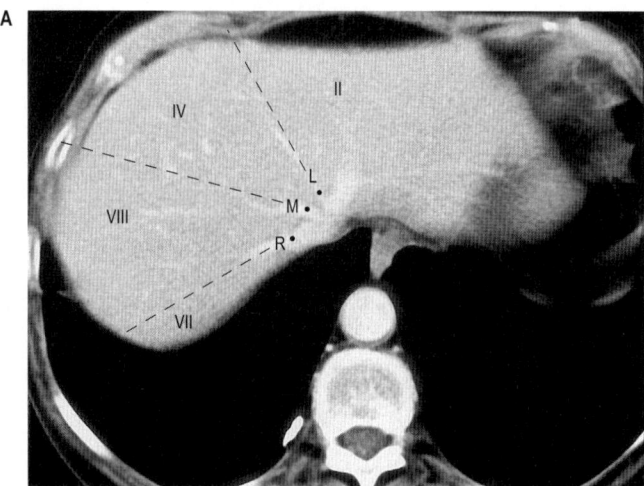

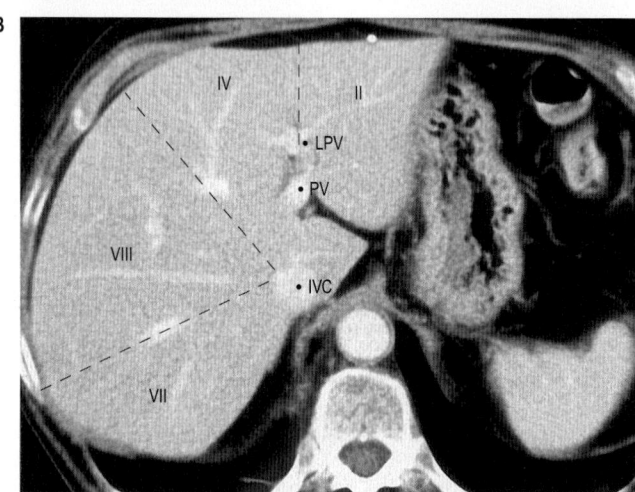

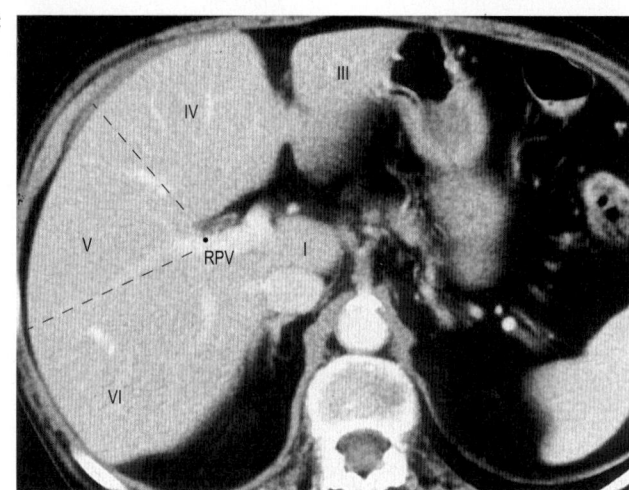

Fig. 85.6 Couinaud segments of the liver seen on axial CT scan. **A**, Contrast enhanced CT shows the left (L), middle (M), and right (R) hepatic veins at the superior aspect of the liver. **B**, Inferior to this the caudate lobe (segment I) lies between the inferior vena cava (IVC) and the main portal vein (PV). The left portal vein (LPV) separates segment II superiorly from segment III inferiorly. **C**, The right portal vein (RPV) divides segments V and VI inferiorly (C) from segments VII and VIII superiorly (B).

VASCULAR SUPPLY AND LYMPHATIC DRAINAGE

The vessels connected with the liver are the portal vein, hepatic artery and hepatic veins. The portal vein and hepatic artery ascend in the lesser omentum to the porta hepatis, where each bifurcates. The hepatic bile duct and lymphatic vessels descend from the porta hepatis in the same omentum (**Figs 85.3, 85.4**). The hepatic veins leave the liver via the posterior surface and run directly into the inferior vena cava.

HEPATIC ARTERY (Figs 85.7, 85.8)

In adults the hepatic artery is intermediate in size between the left gastric and splenic arteries. In fetal and early postnatal life it is the largest branch of the coeliac axis. After its origin from the coeliac axis, it passes anteriorly and laterally below the epiploic foramen to the upper aspect of the superior part of the duodenum. The artery may be subdivided into the common hepatic artery – from the coeliac trunk to the origin of the gastroduodenal artery – and the hepatic artery 'proper' – from that point to its bifurcation. It passes anterior to the portal vein and ascends between the layers of the lesser omentum. It lies anterior to the epiploic foramen and passes in the free border of the lesser omentum medial to the common bile duct and anterior to the portal vein. At the porta hepatis it divides into right and left branches before these run into the parenchyma of the liver. The right hepatic artery usually crosses posterior (occasionally anterior) to the common hepatic duct. It almost always divides into an anterior branch supplying segments V and VIII, and a posterior branch supplying segments VI and VII. The anterior division often supplies a branch to segment I and the gallbladder. The segmental arteries are macroscopically end arteries although some collateral circulation occurs between segments via fine terminal branches.

There are a small number of normal variants, which are important to demonstrate angiographically because they may influence surgical and interventional radiological procedures. A vessel which supplies a lobe in addition to its normal vessel is defined as an accessory artery. A replaced hepatic artery is a vessel that does not originate from an orthodox position and is the sole supply to that lobe. Rarely a replaced common hepatic artery arises from the superior mesenteric artery. More commonly a replaced right hepatic artery or an accessory right hepatic artery arises from the superior mesenteric artery (**Fig. 85.8B**). In this

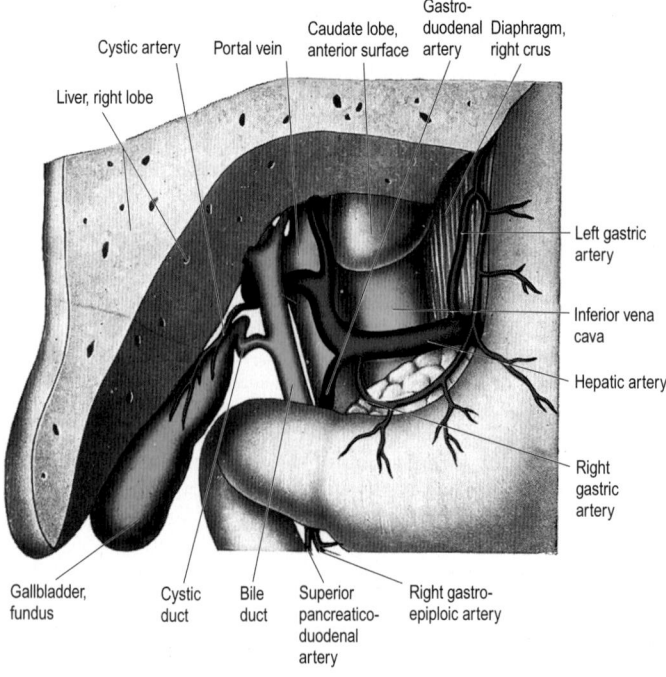

Fig. 85.7 Dissection to show the relations of the hepatic artery, bile duct and portal vein to each other in the lesser omentum: anterior aspect.

A

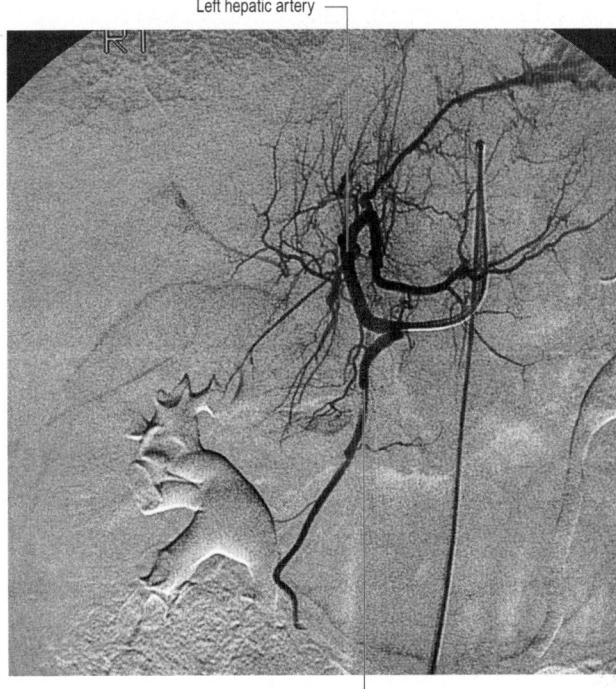

Left hepatic artery

Gastroduodenal artery

B

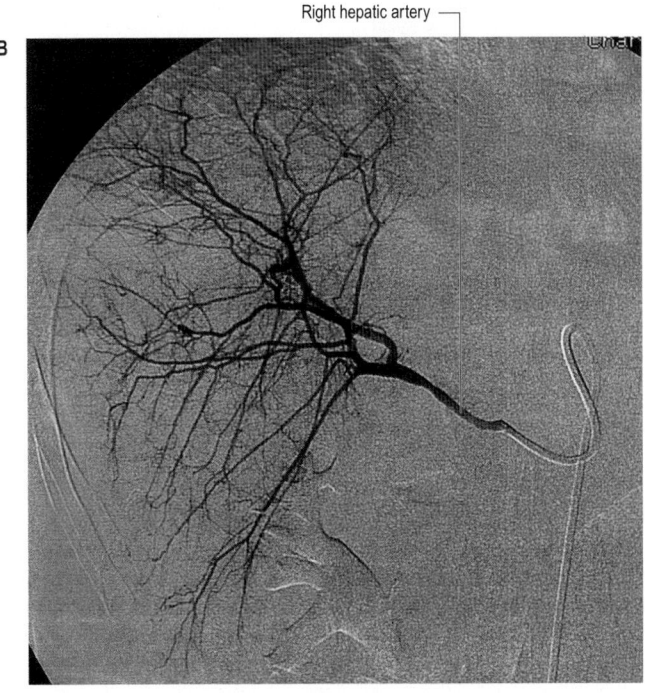

Right hepatic artery

Fig. 85.8 Hepatic arteriogram. **A**, A selective hepatic arteriogram shows normal left hepatic artery branches and small right hepatic artery branches. **B**, The right hepatic artery is arising from the origin of the superior mesenteric artery.

case they run behind the portal vein and bile duct in the lesser omentum. Occasionally, a replaced left hepatic artery or an accessory branch arises from the left gastric artery. This provides a source of collateral arterial circulation in cases of occlusion of the vessels in the porta hepatis and may be injured during mobilization of the stomach as it lies in the upper portion of the lesser omentum. Rarely, accessory left or right hepatic arteries may also arise from the gastroduodenal artery or aorta.

The hepatic artery gives off right gastric, gastroduodenal and cystic branches as well as direct branches to the bile duct from the right hepatic and sometimes the supraduodenal artery.

VEINS

The liver has two venous systems. The portal system conveys venous blood from the majority of the gastrointestinal tract and its associated organs to the liver. The hepatic venous system drains blood from the liver parenchyma into the inferior vena cava.

Portal venous system

The portal system includes all the veins draining the abdominal part of the digestive tube with the exception of the lower anal canal, but including the abdominal part of the oesophagus. It also drains the spleen, pancreas and gallbladder. The portal vein conveys the blood from these viscera to the liver, where it ramifies like an artery, and ends in the sinusoids from which vessels again converge to reach the inferior vena cava via the hepatic veins (p. 1222). The blood running through the portal system therefore passes through two sets of 'exchange' vessels, namely the capillaries of the gut, spleen, pancreas or gallbladder, and the hepatic sinusoids.

In adults, the portal vein and its tributaries have no valves. In fetal life and for a short postnatal period valves are demonstrable in its tributaries, but they usually atrophy. Rarely some persist in an atrophic form into adulthood.

Portal vein (Figs 88.3, 85.9, 85.10)

The portal vein begins at the level of the second lumbar vertebra and is formed from the convergence of the superior mesenteric and splenic veins. It is c.8 cm long and lies anterior to the inferior vena cava and posterior to the neck of the pancreas. It lies obliquely to the right and ascends behind the first part of the duodenum, the common bile duct and gastroduodenal artery. At this point it is directly anterior to the inferior vena cava. It enters the right border of the lesser omentum, and ascends anterior to the epiploic foramen to reach the right end of the porta hepatis. It then divides into right and left main branches which accompany the corresponding branches of the hepatic artery into the liver. In the lesser omentum it lies posterior to both the common bile duct and hepatic artery. It is surrounded by the hepatic nerve plexus and accompanied by many lymph vessels and some lymph nodes. The right branch usually receives the cystic vein and then enters the right lobe. In common with the hepatic artery, it usually forms an anterior division supplying segments V and VIII and a posterior division supplying segments VI and VII. The anterior division may give a branch to segment I. The left branch has a longer extraparenchymal course and tends to lie slightly more horizontal than the right branch but is often of smaller calibre. It gives off branches to segments I (caudate), II, III and IV (quadrate). As it enters the left lobe it is joined by para-umbilical veins and the ligamentum teres, which contains the functionless and partly obliterated left umbilical vein. It is connected to the inferior vena cava by the ligamentum venosum, a vestige of the obliterated ductus venosus. The small extrahepatic section of the left branch, from which the branches to segments II, III and IV arise, is a persistent part of the left umbilical vein.

The portal vein receives many branches including the splenic, superior mesenteric, left gastric, right gastric, para-umbilical and cystic veins. Portal venous blood is one route through which hepatic metastases from gastrointestinal primary malignancies may spread. Blood within the portal vein flows at such a rate that streaming may occur so that the blood from the splenic vein tends to remain on the left side of the portal blood stream and drain preferentially to the left main branch. The clinical evidence to support this is very limited since colorectal cancer metastases commonly occur in the right lobe.

The portal vein supplies the liver with c.5% of its resting oxygen consumption but significantly more of its metabolic nutrition. Progressive occlusion of the hepatic artery rarely results in complete necrosis of the liver, which is due principally to the blood supply derived from the portal vein.

Porto-systemic shunts

Increase in the pressure within the portal venous system may occur for a wide range of reasons. Chronic hypertension of the portal system results in dilatation of the portal vein and its tributaries in response to the raised postcapillary pressure. Tiny venous channels not normally visible may dilate and become engorged. In those areas where these veins form anastomoses with veins draining into the systemic venous circulation, a reversal of flow may occur due to the pressure difference within the two systems. Portal venous blood then flows into the

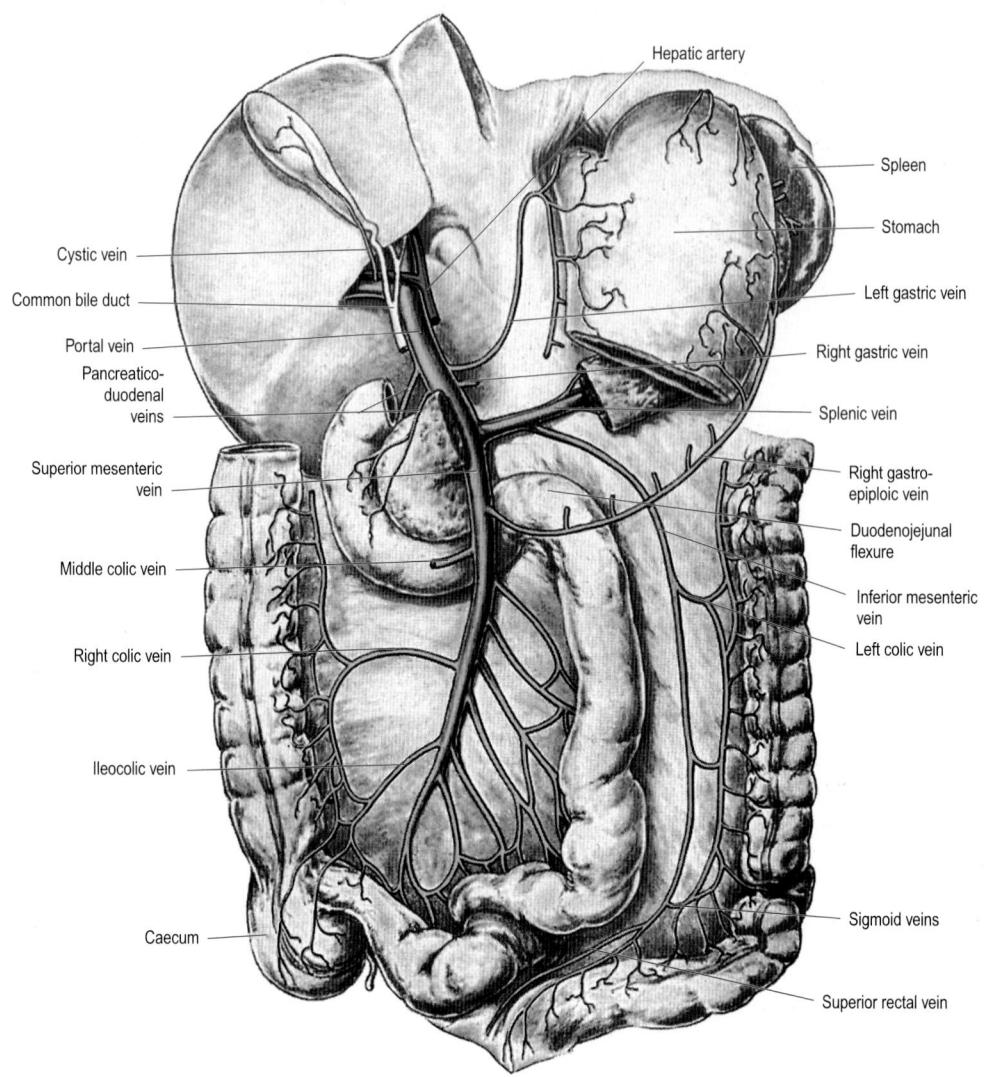

Hepatic artery

Spleen

Stomach

Cystic vein

Left gastric vein

Common bile duct

Right gastric vein

Portal vein

Pancreatico-
duodenal
veins

Splenic vein

Superior mesenteric
vein

Right gastro-
epiploic vein

Duodenojejunal
flexure

Middle colic vein

Inferior mesenteric
vein

Right colic vein

Left colic vein

Ileocolic vein

Sigmoid veins

Caecum

Superior rectal vein

Fig. 85.9 The portal vein and its tributaries (semi-diagrammatic). Portions of the stomach, pancreas and left lobe of the liver and the transverse colon have been removed.

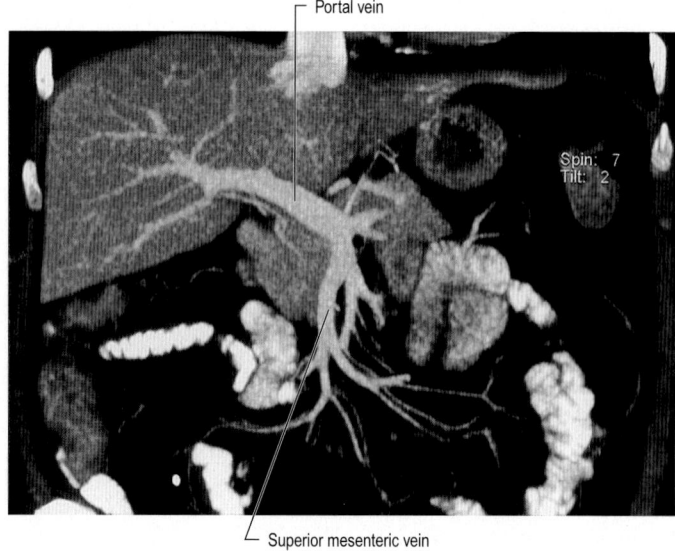

Portal vein

Spin: 7
Tilt: 2

Superior mesenteric vein

Fig. 85.10 Coronal CT of the portal vein and superior mesenteric vein.

systemic circulation without having been processed by the liver tissue. The following are common sites of porto-systemic shunts.

- Between the left gastric and lower oesophageal veins (portal) and the lower branches of the oesophageal veins draining into the azygos and accessory hemiazygos veins (systemic). Enlargement of these anastomoses may result in the formation of varices, either oesophageal or gastric. These may give rise to potentially fatal torrential bleeding.
- Between the superior rectal veins (portal) and the middle and inferior rectal veins draining into the internal iliac and pudendal veins (systemic). The dilated veins may be seen on the rectal wall, but rarely give rise to troublesome bleeding and are not a cause for internal haemorrhoids.
- Between persistent tributaries of the left branch of the portal vein running in the ligamentum teres and the peri-umbilical branches of the superior and inferior epigastric veins (systemic), forming the so-called 'caput medusae'.
- Between intraparenchymal branches of the right branch of the portal vein lying in liver tissue exposed in the 'bare area' and retroperitoneal veins draining into the lumbar, azygos and hemiazygos veins.
- Between omental and colonic veins (portal) and retroperitoneal veins (systemic) in the region of the hepatic and splenic flexure.
- Rarely, between a patent ductus venosus connected to the left branch of the portal vein and the inferior vena cava.

Hepatic veins (Figs 85.6A, 85.11, 85.12)

The hepatic veins convey blood from the liver to the inferior vena cava. The tributaries arise within the parenchyma of the liver and have a thin

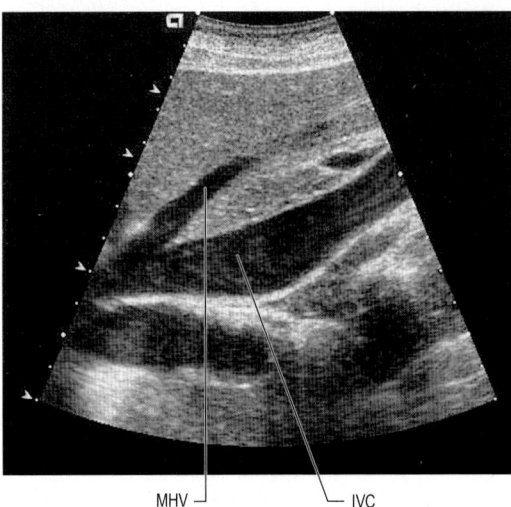

Fig. 85.11 Sagittal ultrasound of the middle hepatic vein. Middle hepatic vein (MHV) draining into the inferior vena cava (IVC).

tunica adventitia which binds them to the walls of their canals within the liver. They are a major source of bleeding following open liver injury since they are less able to collapse sufficiently to allow haemostasis to occur. The veins commence as intralobular veins, which drain the sinusoids and lead to sublobular veins, which eventually unite into hepatic veins. These emerge from the posterior hepatic surface to open directly into the inferior vena cava in its groove on the posterior hepatic surface. Hepatic veins are arranged in upper and lower groups. The upper group are usually large veins and commonly referred to as the right, middle and left hepatic veins. The right hepatic vein drains segments V, VI, VII and VIII. The middle hepatic vein lies between segments IV and VIII and drains both these segments and segment V. The left hepatic vein drains segments II and III with some drainage from segment IV. The lower group vary in number and extent of distribution. They are small veins draining directly into the inferior vena cava from segment I and occasionally from segments VII and VIII. The hepatic veins have no valves. The caudate lobe often has small veins draining

directly into the inferior vena cava and therefore may hypertrophy in conditions involving thrombosis of the large hepatic veins, e.g. Budd–Chiari syndrome.

Transjugular intraparenchymal porto-systemic shunt (TIPS) procedure for portal hypertension

In situations where severe, possibly life-threatening, complications due to chronic portal hypertension exist, the formation of a large calibre anastomosis between portal and systemic circulations may be used to reduce the intraportal pressure. The safest way to perform this is to use the proximity of the hepatic veins and dilated portal branches within the liver parenchyma. Balloon catheters introduced via the internal jugular vein can be passed down the superior and inferior vena cava into the hepatic veins. Under radiological guidance, puncture across an appropriate strip of liver tissue can be achieved into a dilated portal branch. Balloon rupture and dilatation of this tissue 'window' can then be performed with relative safety, since the surrounding liver tissue provides some degree of support to the damaged tissue.

LYMPHATICS

Lymph from the liver has abundant protein content. Lymphatic drainage from the liver is wide and may pass to nodes both above and below the diaphragm. This can be seen since obstruction of the hepatic venous drainage increases the flow of lymph in the thoracic duct. Hepatic collecting vessels are divided into superficial and deep systems.

Superficial hepatic vessels

The superficial vessels run in subserosal areolar tissue over the whole surface of the liver and drain in four directions.

Lymph vessels from the majority of the posterior surface, the surface of the caudate lobe, and the posterior part of the inferior surface of the right lobe, accompany the inferior vena cava and drain into pericaval nodes. Vessels in the coronary and right triangular ligaments may directly enter the thoracic duct without any intervening node.

Vessels from the majority of the inferior surface, anterior surface and most of the superior surface all converge on the porta hepatis to drain into the hepatic nodes.

A few lymph vessels from the posterior surface of the lateral end of the left lobe pass towards the oesophageal opening to drain into the paracardiac nodes.

One or two lymph trunks from the right surface and right end of the superior surface accompany the inferior phrenic artery across the right crus to drain into the coeliac nodes.

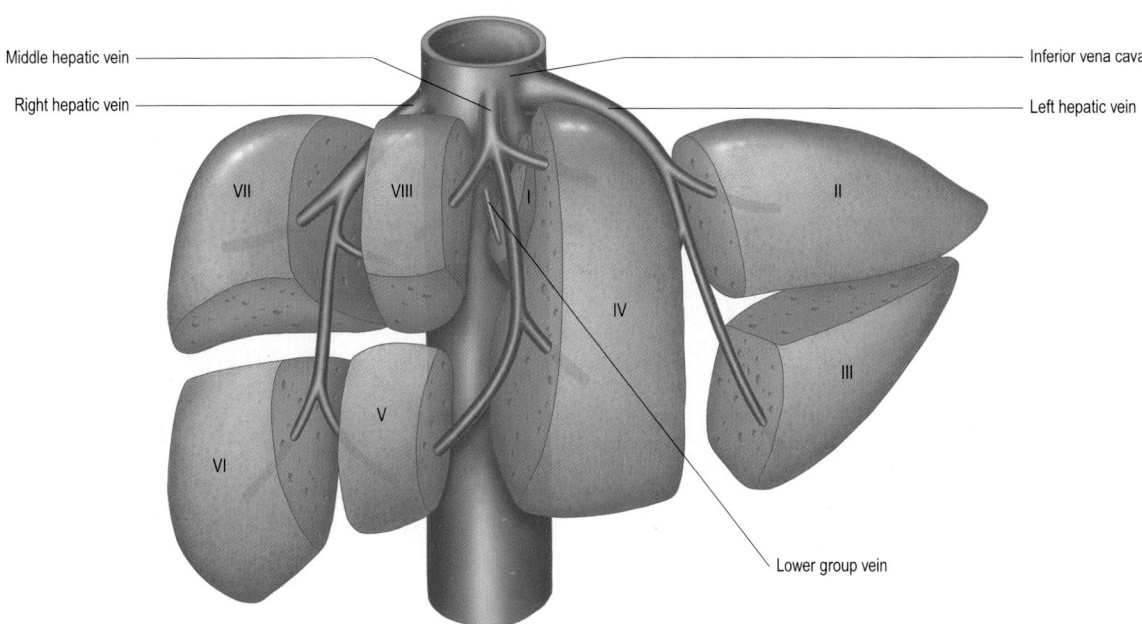

Fig. 85.12 Arrangement of the hepatic venous territories. Multiple lower group veins may be present. Individual segments may drain into more than one hepatic venous territory.

Deep hepatic lymphatics

The great majority of the liver parenchyma is drained by lymphatic vessels within the substance of the liver. The fine lymphatic vessels merge to form larger vessels. Some run superiorly through the parenchyma to form the ascending trunks. They accompany the hepatic veins and pass through the caval opening in the diaphragm to drain into nodes round the end of the inferior vena cava. Vessels from the lower portion of the liver form descending trunks which emerge from the porta hepatis to drain into the hepatic nodes.

INNERVATION

The liver has a dual innervation. The parenchyma is supplied by hepatic nerves, which arise from the hepatic plexus and contain sympathetic and parasympathetic (vagal) fibres (p. 1150). They enter the liver at the porta hepatis and largely accompany the hepatic arteries and bile ducts. A very few may run directly within the liver parenchyma. The capsule is supplied by some fine branches of the lower intercostal nerves, which also supply the parietal peritoneum, particularly in the area of the 'bare area' and superior surface. This is seen clinically when distension or disruption of the liver capsule causes quite well localized sharp pain.

HEPATIC PLEXUS

The hepatic plexus is the largest derivative of the coeliac plexus. It also receives branches from the anterior and posterior vagi. It accompanies the hepatic artery and portal vein and their branches into the liver, where its fibres run close to the branches of the vessels. These branches not only supply vasomotor fibres to the hepatic vessels and biliary tree, but also innervate the hepatocytes directly and are involved in the control of some homeostatic mechanisms. Branches to the gallbladder form a delicate cystic plexus. Multiple fine branches from the plexus supply the common and hepatic bile ducts directly. The vagal fibres are motor to the musculature of the gallbladder and bile ducts and inhibitory to the sphincter of the bile duct.

Nerves run from the hepatic plexus with the branches of the common hepatic artery to supply, or contribute to the supply of, foregut derivatives. Branches may run inferiorly from the plexus to accompany the right gastric artery and contribute to the supply of the pylorus; with the gastroduodenal artery and branches to reach the pylorus and the first part of the duodenum; with the right gastroepiploic artery to provide a small contribution to the supply the right side of the stomach and the greater curvature. The superior pancreaticoduodenal extension supplies the descending part of the duodenum, the pancreatic head, and the intrapancreatic part of the common bile duct.

REFERRED PAIN

Pain arising from the parenchyma of the liver is poorly localized. In common with other structures of foregut origin, pain is referred to the central epigastrium. Stretch of or involvement of the liver capsule by inflammatory or neoplastic processes rapidly produces well-localized pain of a 'somatic' nature.

MICROSTRUCTURE

The liver is essentially an epithelial-mesenchymal outgrowth of the caudal part of the foregut, with which it retains its connection via the biliary tree. The surface of the liver facing the peritoneal cavity is covered by a typical serosa, the visceral peritoneum. Beneath this, and enclosing the whole structure, is a thin (50–100 μm) layer of connective tissue from which extensions pass into the liver as connective tissue septa and trabeculae. Branches of the hepatic artery and hepatic portal vein, together with bile ductules and ducts, run within these connective tissue trabeculae which are termed portal tracts (portal canals). The combination of the two types of vessel and a bile duct is termed a portal triad; these structures are usually accompanied by one or more lymphatic vessels.

The liver parenchyma consists of a complex network of epithelial cells, supported by connective tissue, and perfused by a rich blood supply from the hepatic portal vein and hepatic artery. The epithelial cells, hepatocytes, carry out the major metabolic activities of this organ, but additional cell types possess storage, phagocytic and mechanically supportive functions. In the mature liver, hepatocytes are arranged mainly in plates – or cords, as seen in two-dimensional sections – usually only one cell thick. Until about seven years of age, plates are normally two cells thick (p. 1255). Between the plates are venous sinusoids, which anastomose with each other via gaps in the hepatocyte plates.

Bile secreted by the hepatocytes is collected in a network of minute tubes (canaliculi). The hepatocytes can therefore be regarded as exocrine cells, secreting bile to the alimentary tract ultimately via the hepatic ducts and bile duct. However, their other metabolic orientation is towards the blood, with which hepatocytes carry out complex biochemical exchanges. The fetal liver is a major haemopoietic organ; erythrocytes, leukocytes and platelets develop from the mesenchyme covering the sinusoidal endothelium.

LOBULATION OF THE LIVER (Figs 85.13, 85.14)

In humans, the arrangement of hepatic plates into discrete lobules is less clear than in some species, where the classic lobular units of structure are delimited microscopically by distinct connective tissue septa. These lobules are comprised of polygonal (often hexagonal)

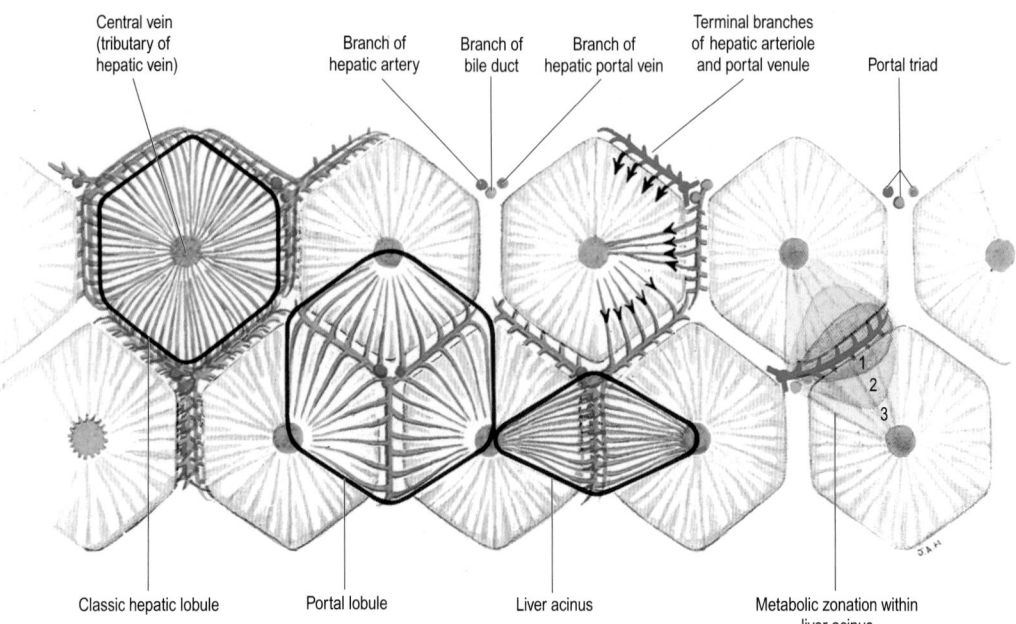

Central vein (tributary of hepatic vein)

Branch of hepatic artery

Branch of bile duct

Branch of hepatic portal vein

Terminal branches of hepatic arteriole and portal venule

Portal triad

Classic hepatic lobule

Portal lobule

Liver acinus

Metabolic zonation within liver acinus

Fig. 85.13 The histological organization of the liver, showing the principal types of subdivisions which have been proposed. For purposes of clarity, the territories of the classic hepatic lobules are shown as regular hexagons, unlike their real appearance which is highly variable. The portal lobule, centred on the portal triad and biliary drainage is also shown. Liver function is emphasized by the territory of the liver acinus, which centres on blood flow to sectors of adjacent hepatic lobules (see text) and reflects gradients of metabolism across its zones.

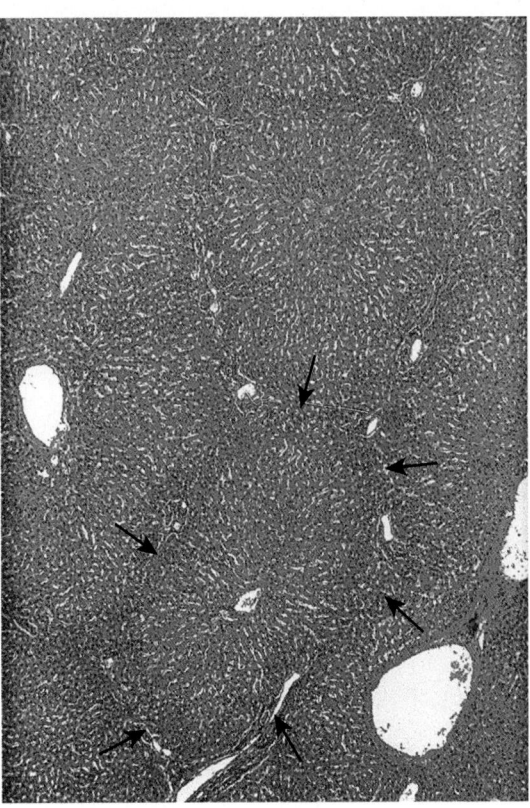

Fig. 85.14 The structural organization of human liver tissue into lobules, bordered by delicate connective tissue septa (arrows) in which run branches of the hepatic portal vein, hepatic artery and bile duct, grouped as portal triads. A central vein drains each lobule. (By permission from Dr JB Kerr, Monash University, from Kerr JB 1999 Atlas of Functional Histology. London: Mosby.)

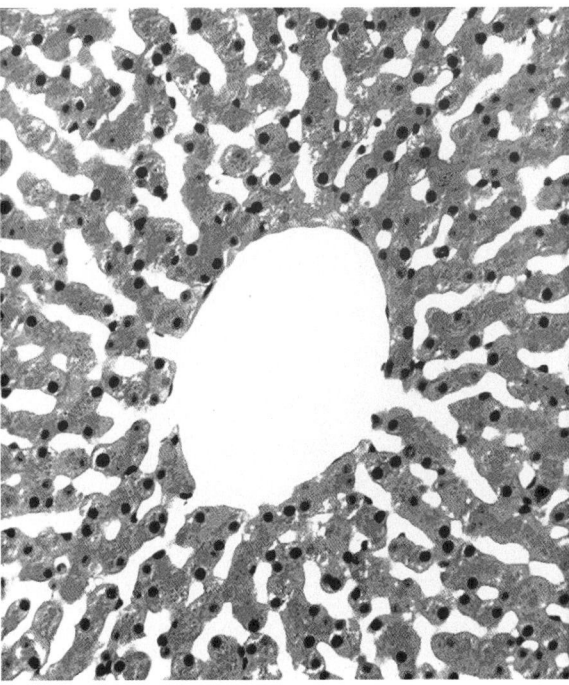

Fig. 85.15 A central vein draining a hepatic lobule. The surrounding liver parenchyma consists of plates (cords) of hepatocytes radiating from the central vein and interposed hepatic sinusoids through which blood flows towards the central vein. (By permission from Dr JB Kerr, Monash University, from Kerr JB 1999 Atlas of Functional Histology. London: Mosby.)

clusters of hepatocytes, about 1 mm in diameter, bounded by loose connective tissue which in humans is scant. Within each lobular unit, hepatic plates with intervening sinusoids radiate around a central vein, a tributary of the hepatic vein draining the tissue. These plates do not pass straight to the periphery of a lobule like the spokes of a wheel but run irregularly, as they anastomose and branch. Detailed studies of human liver, using three-dimensional reconstruction and morphometric analysis, combined with histopathological observations, have revealed a highly orderly arrangement of the human liver into functional units, the liver (portal) acini. They are approximately oval masses of tissue, centred on a terminal branch of a hepatic arteriole and portal venule, and with their long axes defined by the territory between two adjacent central veins. Each acinus includes the hepatic tissue served by these afferent vessels and is bounded by the territories of other acini.

The acinar definition of hepatic micro-organization has clarified important problems of liver histopathology, especially the development of zones of anoxic damage, glycogen deposition and removal, and of toxic trauma, which are all related to the direction of blood flow and thus tend to follow the acinar pattern. There are also real metabolic differences between hepatocytes within the acini and so they are divided into three zones: zone 1 (periportal) nearest to the terminal branches of afferent vessels; zone 2 intermediate zone; and zone 3 around the central venous drainage.

BLOOD SUPPLY

Preterminal hepatic arterioles in the portal canals branch to convey arterial blood to the sinusoids by several routes, mainly via a fine capillary plexus which drains to branches of the portal veins. Some arterial blood passes directly to the hepatic sinusoids, bypassing these capillary plexuses; but they represent only a small part of the total flow. Sinusoids thus contain mixed venous and arterial blood. Central veins from adjacent lobules form interlobular veins, which unite as hepatic veins, draining blood to the inferior vena cava. Hepatic veins draining the tissue run quite separately with respect to the portal triad system, freely crossing the boundaries of triad territories.

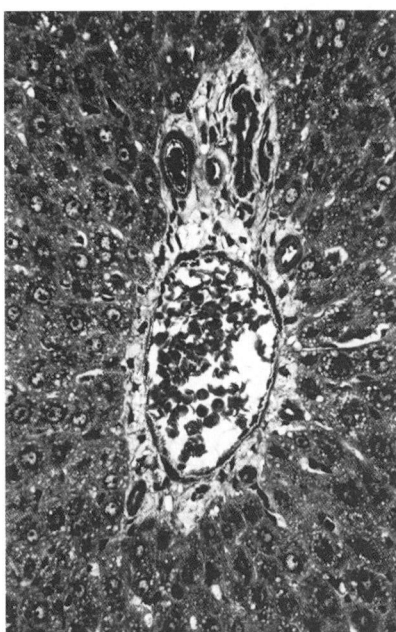

Fig. 85.16 A portal triad in the liver, toluidine blue stained. It contains branches of the hepatic portal vein (centre; generally the largest profile), the hepatic artery (here, a small arteriole, top left profile) and the elongated profile of a bile duct, with typical round epithelial cell nuclei (top right). Other small bile ductule and arteriolar branches are also visible. (Photograph by Sarah-Jane Smith.)

CELLS OF THE LIVER (Figs 85.15, 85.16)

Cells of the liver include hepatocytes, hepatic stellate cells – also known as perisinusoidal lipocytes, or Ito cells – sinusoidal endothelial cells, macrophages (Kupffer cells), the cells of the biliary tree – cuboidal to columnar epithelium – and connective tissue cells of the capsule and portal tracts.

Hepatocytes (Figs 85.17, 85.18, 85.19, 85.20)

About 80% of the liver volume and 60% of its cell number are formed by hepatocytes (parenchymal cells). They are polyhedral, with 5–12 sides and are from 20 to 30 µm across. Their nuclei are round, euchromatic and often tetraploid, polyploid or multiple – two or more in each cell. Their cytoplasm typically contains much rough and smooth endoplasmic reticulum, many mitochondria, lysosomes and

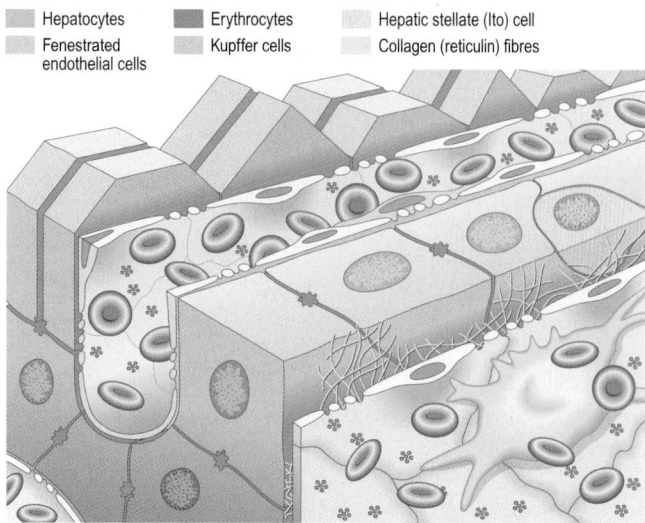

Hepatocytes
Fenestrated endothelial cells
Erythrocytes
Kupffer cells
Hepatic stellate (Ito) cell
Collagen (reticulin) fibres

Fig. 85.17 The chief cellular features of a hepatic cord, showing hepatocytes, grooved by bile canaliculi. A discontinuous fenestrated endothelium lines the sinusoids, shown containing erythrocytes. Also shown are a Kupffer cell and a hepatic stellate cell. Fine collagen fibres occupy the space of Disse.

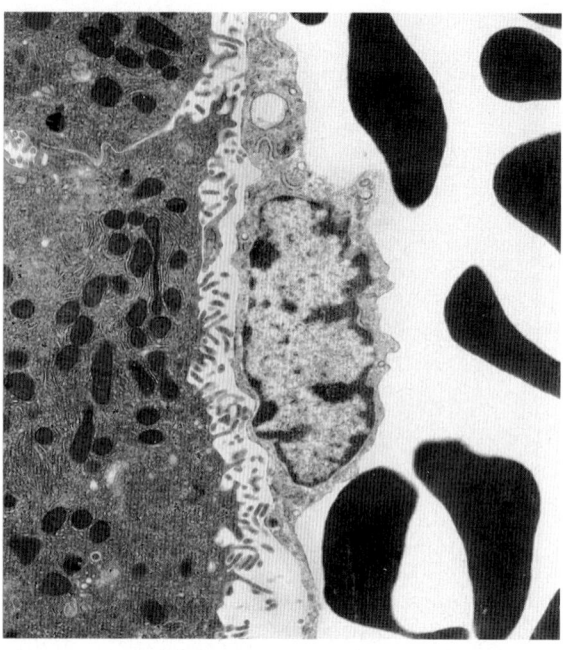

Fig. 85.18 High power electron micrograph of the border of a hepatic sinusoid showing two hepatocytes, with their plasma membranes facing a sinusoid containing erythrocytes. Their lateral membranes enclose a small bile canaliculus (top left). The sinusoid is lined by fenestrated endothelial cells; the nucleus of an endothelial cell is seen in the centre of the field. The endothelium lacks a basal lamina and is separated from hepatocytes by the space of Disse, into which hepatocyte microvilli project. (By permission from Young B, Heath JW 2000 Wheater's Functional Histology. Edinburgh: Churchill Livingstone.)

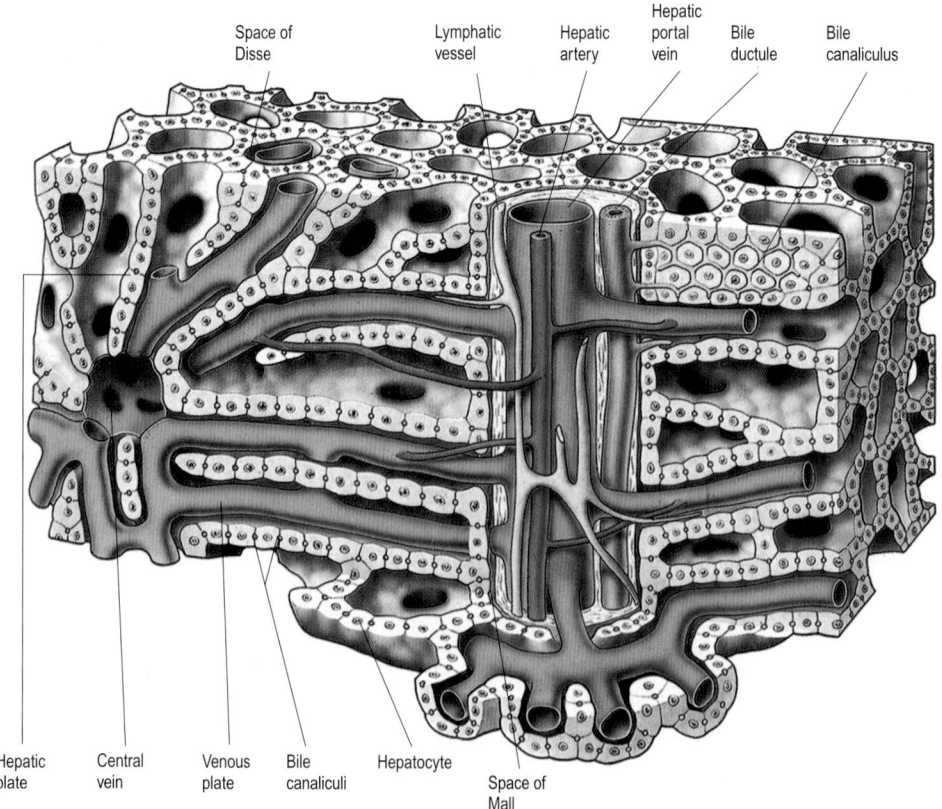

Space of Disse
Lymphatic vessel
Hepatic artery
Hepatic portal vein
Bile ductule
Bile canaliculus

Hepatic plate
Central vein
Venous plate
Bile canaliculi
Hepatocyte
Space of Mall

Fig. 85.19 Diagram of hepatic microstructure. Perisinusoidal endothelial cells and macrophages (Kupffer cells) are not shown. (Modified after H Elias, Department of Anatomy, Chicago Medical School.)

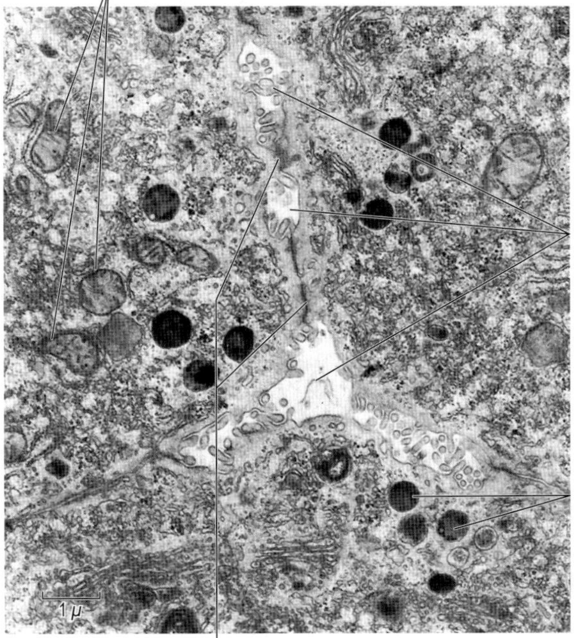

Fig. 85.20 Electron micrograph showing portions of three adjacent hepatocytes and the intervening bile canaliculi, bounded by tight junctions.

well-developed Golgi apparatus, features indicating a high metabolic activity. Glycogen granules and lipid vacuoles are usually prominent. Numerous, large peroxisomes and vacuoles containing enzymes, e.g. urease in distinctive crystalline forms, indicate the complex metabolism of these cells. Their role in iron metabolism is shown by the presence of storage vacuoles containing crystals of ferritin and haemosiderin.

The surfaces of hepatocytes facing the sinusoids exhibit numerous microvilli, c.0.5 µm long, which create a large area of membrane – 70% of the hepatocyte surface – exposed to blood plasma. Elsewhere, hepatocytes are linked by numerous gap junctions and desmosomes. Lateral plasma membranes of adjacent hepatocytes form microscopic channels, the bile canaliculi, which are specialized regions of inter-cellular space formed by apposing grooves in hepatocyte plasma membranes, sealed from extraneous interstitial space by tight junctions. Numerous membrane-bound exocytotic vesicles cluster near the lumen of the canaliculi, since the secretion of bile components is targeted to the canalicular plasma membrane. These canaliculi form the origins of the biliary tree and their tight junctions prevent bile from entering interstitial fluid or blood plasma: this is the blood–bile barrier.

Hepatic stellate cells

Hepatic stellate cells are also known as perisinusoidal lipocytes or Ito cells and are much less numerous than hepatocytes. They are irregular in outline and lie within the hepatic plates, between the bases of hepatocytes. They are thought to be mesenchymal in origin and are characterized by numerous cytoplasmic lipid droplets. These cells secrete most of the intralobular matrix components, including collagen type III (reticular) fibres. They store the fat-soluble vitamin A in their lipid droplets and are a significant source of growth factors active in liver homeostasis and regeneration. Hepatic stellate cells also play a major role in pathological processes. In response to liver damage, they become activated and predominantly myofibroblast-like. They are responsible for the replacement of toxically damaged hepatocytes with collagenous scar tissue – hepatic fibrosis, seen initially in zone 3, around central veins. This can progress to cirrhosis, where the parenchymal architecture and pattern of blood flow are destroyed, with major systemic consequences.

Sinusoidal endothelial cells

Hepatic venous sinusoids are generally wider than blood capillaries and are lined by a thin but highly fenestrated endothelium which lacks a basal lamina (**Fig. 85.18**). The endothelial cells are typically flattened, each with a central nucleus and joined to each other by junctional complexes. The fenestrae are grouped in clusters with a mean diameter of 100 nm, allowing plasma direct access to the basal plasma membranes of hepatocytes. Their cytoplasm contains numerous typical transcytotic vesicles.

Kupffer cells

Kupffer cells are hepatic macrophages derived from circulating blood monocytes. They are long-term hepatic residents, lying within the sinusoidal lumen (**Fig. 85.17**), attached to the endothelial surface. They originate in the bone marrow, and form a major part of the mono-nuclear phagocyte system (p. 81), responsible for removing cellular and microbial debris from the circulation, and secreting cytokines involved in defence. Kupffer cells remove aged and damaged red cells from the hepatic circulation, a function normally shared with the spleen, but fulfilled entirely by the liver after splenectomy. Kupffer cells are irregular in shape, with long processes extending into the sinusoidal lumen.

HEPATIC PLATES (CORDS)

The endothelial linings of the sinusoids are separated from hepatocytes of the hepatic plates by a narrow gap, the perisinusoidal space of Disse which is normally about 0.2–0.5 µm wide, but distends in anoxic conditions. It contains fine collagen fibres – chiefly type III, with some types I and IV – the microvilli of adjacent hepatocytes, and occasional non-myelinated nerve terminals. There is no basal lamina within the space of Disse.

Minute bile canaliculi form nets with polygonal meshes in the hepatic plates. Each polygonal hepatocyte is surrounded by canaliculi except on the surfaces – at least two – facing sinusoids. Hepatic plates thus enclose a network of canaliculi which pass to the lobular periphery, where they join to form narrow intralobular ductules (terminal ductules or the canals of Hering) lined by squamous or cuboidal epithelium. These enter bile ductules in the portal canals, lined by cuboidal or columnar cells. The flow of bile is thus towards the periphery of lobules, in the opposite direction to the blood flow, which is centripetal.

REFERENCES

Couinaud C 1957 Le foie: etudes anatomique et chirurgicules. Masson: Paris.
   The original description of hepatic segmentation by Couinaud
Healey JE, Schroy PC 1953 Anatomy of the biliary ducts within the human liver; analysis of the prevailing pattern of branchings and the major variations of the biliary ducts. Arch Surg 66: 599–616.

Mitchell AWM, Dick R 1999 Liver, gall-bladder, pancreas and spleen. In: Butler P, Mitchell AWM, Ellis H (eds) Applied Radiological Anatomy. Cambridge: Cambridge University Press: 239–58.
Strasberg SM 1997 Terminology of liver anatomy and liver resections: coming to grips with hepatic babel. J Am Coll Surg 184: 413–34.
   A review and suggested system for the clinical nomenclature of liver surgery according to segmental anatomy

Gallbladder and biliary tree

The biliary tree consists of the system of vessels and ducts which collect and deliver bile from the liver parenchyma to the second part of the duodenum. It is conventionally divided into intrahepatic and extra-hepatic biliary ducts. The intrahepatic ducts are formed from the larger bile canaliculi (p. 1222) which come together to form segmental ducts. These fuse close to the porta hepatis into right and left hepatic ducts. The extrahepatic biliary tree consists of the right and left hepatic ducts, the common hepatic duct, the cystic duct and gallbladder and the common bile duct (**Fig. 86.1**).

GALLBLADDER (Fig. 86.2)

The gallbladder is a flask-shaped, blind-ending diverticulum attached to the common bile duct by the cystic duct. In life, it is grey-blue in colour and usually lies attached to the inferior surface of the right lobe of the liver by connective tissue. In the adult the gallbladder is between 7 and 10 cm long with a capacity of up to 50 ml. It usually lies in a shallow fossa in the liver parenchyma covered by peritoneum continued from the liver surface. This attachment can vary widely. At one extreme the gallbladder may be almost completely buried within the liver surface, having no peritoneal covering (intraparenchymal pattern); at the other extreme it may hang from a short mesentery formed by the two layers of peritoneum separated only by connective tissue and a few small vessels (mesenteric pattern). The gallbladder is described as having a fundus, body and neck. The neck lies at the medial end close to the porta hepatis, and almost always has a short peritoneal covered attachment to the liver (mesentery); this mesentery usually contains the cystic artery. The mucosa at the medial end of the neck is obliquely ridged, forming

a spiral groove continuous with the spiral valve of the cystic duct. At its lateral end the neck widens out to form the body of the gallbladder and this widening is often referred to in clinical practice as 'Hartmann's pouch'. The neck lies anterior to the second part of the duodenum.

The body of the gallbladder normally lies in contact with the liver surface. When the neck possesses a mesentery, this rapidly shortens along the length of the body as it comes to lie in the gallbladder fossa. It lies anterior to the second part of the duodenum and the right end of the transverse colon. The fundus lies at the lateral end of the body and usually projects past the inferior border of the liver to a variable length. It often lies in contact with the anterior abdominal wall behind the ninth costal cartilage where the lateral edge of the right rectus abdominis crosses the costal margin. This is the location where enlarge-ment of the gallbladder is best sought on clinical examination. The fundus commonly lies adjacent to the transverse colon.

The gallbladder varies in size and shape. The fundus may be elongated and highly mobile. Rarely the fundus of the gallbladder is folded back upon the body of the gallbladder, the so-called Phrygian cap. On ultrasound this may be wrongly interpreted as an apparent septum within an otherwise normal gallbladder. Rarely, the gallbladder may be bifid or completely duplicated, usually with a duplicated cystic duct.

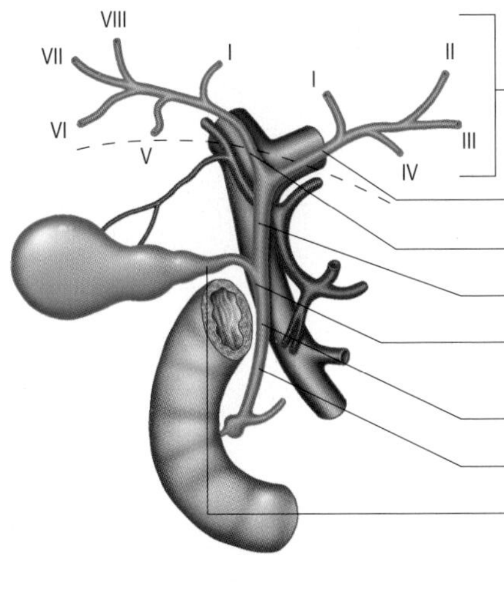

Fig. 86.1 Overall arrangement of the intrahepatic and extrahepatic biliary tree. The biliary tree to the level of the segmental ducts shown in relation to the conventional arterial anatomy. The segmental ducts often branch just before, or are multiple, as they enter the main lobar ducts, but are shown as single ducts for clarity here. Note that segment I usually has drainage to both right and left hepatic ducts. The level of the liver parenchyma at the porta hepatis is shown by the dashed black line. Duodenum, brown; portal veins, blue; hepatic arteries, red.

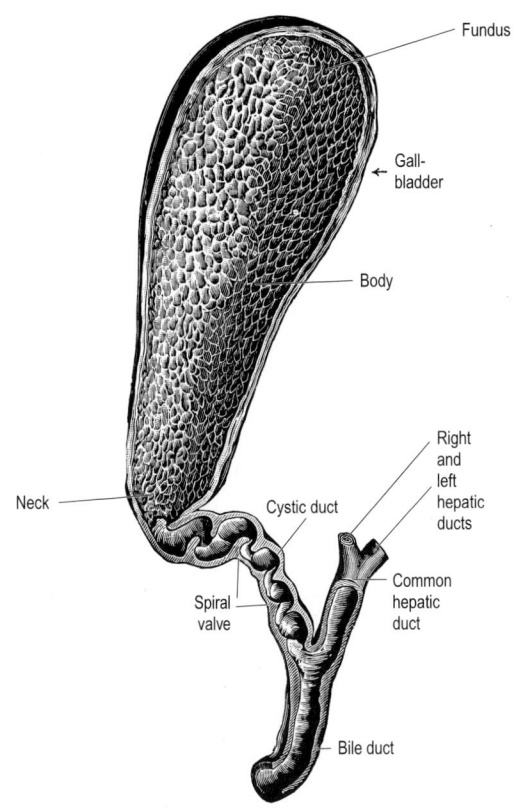

Fig. 86.2 Interior of the gallbladder and bile ducts.

EXTRAHEPATIC BILIARY TREE

CYSTIC DUCT

The cystic duct drains the gallbladder into the common bile duct. It is between 3 and 4 cm long, passes posteriorly to the left from the neck of the gallbladder, and joins the common hepatic duct to form the common bile duct. It almost always runs parallel to, and is adherent to, the common hepatic duct for a short distance before joining it. The junction usually occurs near the porta hepatis but may be lower down in the free edge of the lesser omentum. The cystic duct may have several important variations in its anatomy. Rarely, the cystic duct lies along the right edge of the lesser omentum all the way down to the level of the duodenum before the junction is formed, but in these cases the cystic and common bile ducts are usually closely adherent. The cystic duct occasionally drains into the right hepatic duct in which case it may be elongated, lying anterior or posterior to the common hepatic duct, and joins the right hepatic duct on its left border. Rarely, the duct is double or even absent in which case the gallbladder drains directly into the common bile duct. One or more accessory hepatic ducts occasionally emerge from segment V of the liver and join either the right hepatic duct, the common hepatic duct, the common bile duct, the cystic duct, or the gallbladder directly. These variations in cystic duct anatomy are of considerable importance during surgical excision of the gallbladder. Ligation or clip occlusion of the cystic duct must be performed at an adequate distance from the common bile duct to prevent angulation or damage to it. Accessory ducts must not be confused with the right hepatic or common hepatic ducts.

The mucosa of the cystic duct bears 5–12 crescentic folds, continuous with those in the neck of the gallbladder. They project obliquely in regular succession, appearing to form a spiral valve when the duct is cut in longitudinal section. When the duct is distended, the spaces between the folds dilate and externally it appears twisted like the neck of the gallbladder.

HEPATIC BILE DUCTS

The main right and left hepatic ducts emerge from the liver and unite near the right end of the porta hepatis as the common hepatic duct. This descends about 3 cm before being joined on its right at an acute angle by the cystic duct to form the common bile duct. The common hepatic duct lies to the right of the hepatic artery and anterior to the portal vein in the free edge of the lesser omentum.

COMMON BILE DUCT (Figs 86.3, 86.4)

The common bile duct is formed near the porta hepatis, by the junction of the cystic and common hepatic ducts. It is usually between 6 and 8 cm long. Its diameter tends to increase somewhat with age but is usually around 6 mm in adults. It descends posteriorly and slightly to the left, anterior to the epiploic foramen, in the right border of the lesser omentum. It lies anterior and to the right of the portal vein and to the right of the hepatic artery. It passes behind the first part of the duodenum with the gastroduodenal artery on its left, and then runs in a groove on the superolateral part of the posterior surface of the head of the pancreas (**Fig. 87.1**). It lies anterior to the inferior vena cava and is sometimes embedded in the pancreatic tissue. The duct may lie close to the medial wall of the second part of the duodenum or as much as 2 cm from it. Even when it is embedded in the pancreas, a groove in the gland marking its position can be palpated behind the second part of the duodenum.

Hepatopancreatic ampulla (of Vater)

As it lies medial to the second part of the duodenum, the common bile duct approaches the right end of the pancreatic duct. The ducts enter the duodenal wall together, and usually unite to form the hepatopancreatic ampulla. Rarely the common bile duct and pancreatic duct drain into the duodenum separately. Circular muscle usually surrounds the lower part of the common bile duct (bile duct sphincter) and frequently also surrounds the terminal part of the main pancreatic duct (pancreatic duct sphincter) and the hepatopancreatic ampulla (sphincter of Oddi). When all elements are present, this arrangement may allow for separate control of pancreatic and common bile duct emptying. Division of the upper part of the ampulla and ampullary sphincter (sphincterotomy) may be required to allow access to the common bile duct during endoscopic retrograde cholangiography).

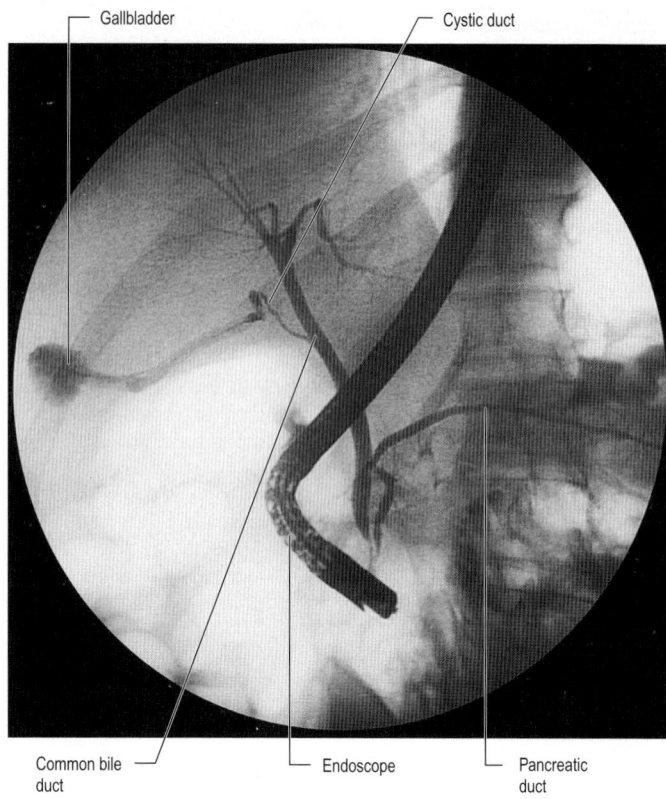

Gallbladder — Cystic duct

Common bile duct — Endoscope — Pancreatic duct

Fig. 86.3 Endoscopic retrograde cholangiopancreatogram.

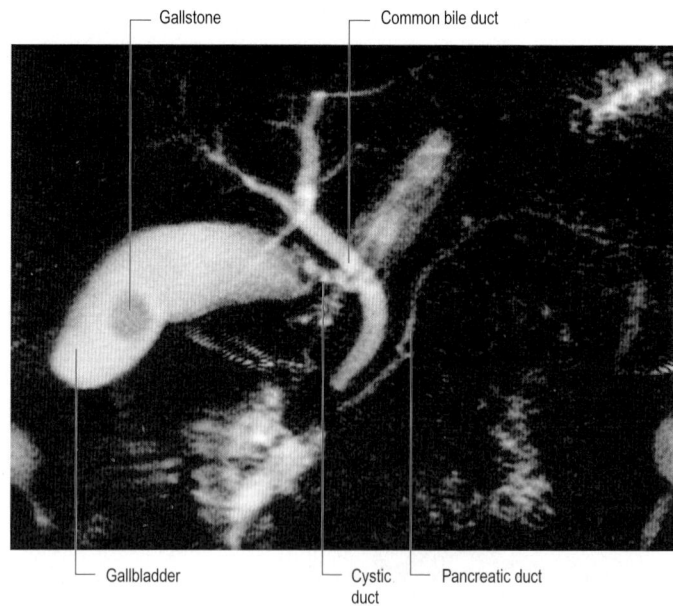

Gallstone — Common bile duct

Gallbladder — Cystic duct — Pancreatic duct

Fig. 86.4 Magnetic resonance cholangiopancreatogram.

Calot's triangle

The near triangular space formed between the cystic duct, the common hepatic duct and the inferior surface of segment V of the liver (Suzuki et al 2000), is commonly referred to as Calot's triangle. It is enclosed by the double layer of peritoneum which forms the short mesentery of the cystic duct. Since the two layers are not closely opposed, there is an appreciable amount of loose connective tissue within the triangle. It is perhaps better described as a pyramidal 'space' with one apex lying at the junction of the cystic duct and fundus of the gallbladder, one at the porta hepatis, and two closer apices at the attachments of the gallbladder to the liver bed. The base of the triangle thus lies on the inferior surface of the liver. This space usually contains the cystic artery as it approaches the gallbladder, the cystic lymph node and lymphatics from the gallbladder, one or two small cystic veins, the autonomic nerves running to the gallbladder and some loose adipose tissue. It may contain any accessory ducts which drain into the gallbladder from the liver. Appreciation of the variations in ductal and arterial anatomy as they relate to the triangle are of considerable importance during excision of the gallbladder in order to avoid mistakenly ligating the common hepatic or common bile duct.

BILIARY STONES

Gallstones usually form in the gallbladder. As the gallbladder empties, gallstones move towards the cystic duct. When small stones enter the cystic duct they may irritate the columnar mucosa which leads to spasm of the smooth muscle in the cystic duct wall. This spasm generates pain known as biliary colic, which is often very severe. The mucosal folds in the neck of the gallbladder and the cystic duct provide a common site of entrapment of gallstones. Stones occluding the neck of the gall-bladder may cause a sterile distension of the gallbladder; providing the gallbladder has not undergone acute inflammation previously it remains non-fibrotic and readily distensible, and an enlarged fundus often becomes palpable below the costal margin. Stones lodged in the distal cystic duct may cause swelling in the tissues around the duct. Due to the close relationship of the distal cystic duct to the common hepatic duct, this swelling may give rise to secondary compression of the common hepatic duct with resultant partial obstruction to the flow of bile and the appearance of mild jaundice; so called 'Mirizzi syndrome'. Once stones have passed through the cystic duct they often become impacted at the junction of the common bile duct and pancreatic duct just proximal to the hepatopancreatic ampulla, producing obstructive jaundice.

ENDOSCOPIC CHOLANGIOGRAPHY

The common bile duct may be accessed endoscopically from the duo-denum for diagnostic cholangiography and therapeutic interventions. Due to the angled relationship of the distal common bile duct and pancreatic duct, direct cannulation of the bile duct may be difficult. When the duct lies in a more vertical position, embedded within the wall of the duodenum, a direct incision in the base of the hepato-pancreatic ampulla and the adjacent wall of the duodenum (pre-cut sphincterotomy) may expose the duct to allow cannulation. This is occasionally associated with haemorrhage due to the duodenal wall vessels. Division of the smooth muscle fibres of the common bile duct sphincter may be necessary for endoscopic access to the bile duct but it often results in uncontrolled reflux of duodenal contents into the distal common bile duct, and this may result in recurrent biliary infections.

BILIARY DRAINAGE

The proximity of the fundus of the gallbladder to the anterior abdominal wall provides a useful route of access for percutaneous drainage of a distended, obstructed gallbladder. It is rarely obscured by liver tissue, can often be accessed below the costal margin, and is most often per-formed under ultrasound guidance. Because of the nature of the cystic duct, drainage of the gallbladder is rarely adequate to decompress the biliary tree if it is blocked, and this must be achieved endoscopically, surgically or by a percutaneous, transhepatic approach. This latter technique requires the identification of dilated intrahepatic bile ducts, usually by ultrasound imaging with direct guided puncture via a right subcostal approach. Percutaneous access is obtained via segment III in the left lobe of the liver and via segments V and VI in the right lobe of the liver.

VASCULAR SUPPLY AND LYMPHATIC DRAINAGE

CYSTIC ARTERY

The cystic artery usually arises from the right hepatic artery. It usually passes posterior to the common hepatic duct and anterior to the cystic duct to reach the superior aspect of the neck of the gallbladder. It divides into superficial and deep branches. The superficial branch ramifies on the inferior aspect of the gallbladder body, the deep branch on the superior aspect. These arteries anastomose over the surface of the body

and fundus. The cystic artery may arise from the common hepatic artery, sometimes from the left hepatic artery, and rarely from the gastroduo-denal or superior mesenteric arteries. In these cases it crosses anterior (or less commonly posterior) to the common bile duct or common hepatic duct to reach the gallbladder. An accessory cystic artery may arise from the common hepatic artery or one of its branches and the cystic artery often bifurcates close to its origin, giving rise to two vessels which approach the gallbladder. Multiple fine arterial branches may arise from the parenchyma of segments IV or V of the liver and con-tribute to the supply of the body, particularly when the gallbladder is substantially intrahepatic. This makes the gallbladder relatively resistant to necrosis during inflammation which otherwise occludes the cystic artery.

The cystic artery gives rise to multiple fine branches which supply the common and lobar hepatic ducts and upper part of the common bile duct. These fine branches form a network which anastomoses with the vessels ascending around the common bile duct and with the vessels from the liver parenchyma which descend with the right and left hepatic ducts.

DUCTAL ARTERIES

The common bile duct and hepatic ducts are supplied by a fine network of vessels, which lie in close proximity to the ducts themselves. This network usually has contributions from several sources. Disruption of the network during surgical exposure of the bile ducts over a long length frequently causes chronic ischaemia and a resultant stenosis of the duct. Approaches which spare the network are necessary to avoid this complication.

Anterior to the common bile duct, two to four ascending vessels arise from the retroduodenal branch of the gastroduodenal artery as it crosses the anterior surface of the duct at the upper border of the duodenum. Three or four descending branches of the right hepatic and cystic arteries arise as these vessels pass close to the lower common hepatic duct. These ascending and descending arteries form long narrow anastomotic channels along the length of the duct, which are approximately disposed into medial and lateral 'trunks' although they may lie more anterolateral and posteromedial.

Posteriorly, a retroportal artery often arises from the coeliac axis, superior mesenteric artery or one of their major branches close to the origin from the aorta. It runs upwards on the posterior surface of the portal vein. It usually ends by joining the retroduodenal artery close to the lower end of the supraduodenal bile duct, but occasionally it passes up behind the bile duct to join the right hepatic artery. When present, the retroportal artery contributes to the arterial network supplying the supraduodenal bile duct system.

CYSTIC VEINS

The venous drainage of the gallbladder is rarely by a single cystic vein. There are usually multiple small veins. Those arising from the superior surface of the body and neck lie in areolar tissue between the gallbladder and liver and enter the liver parenchyma to drain into the segmental portal veins. The remainder form one or two small cystic veins, which enter the liver either directly or after joining the veins draining the hepatic ducts and upper bile duct. Only rarely does a single or double cystic vein drain into the right portal branch.

LYMPHATICS

Numerous lymphatic vessels run from the submucosal and subserosal plexuses on all aspects of the gallbladder and cystic duct. Those on the hepatic aspect of the gallbladder connect with the intrahepatic lymph vessels. The remainder drain into the cystic node, which usually lies above the cystic duct in the tissue of Calot's triangle. This node, and some lymphatic channels which bypass the cystic node, drain into a node lying in the anterior border of the free edge of the lesser omentum. Hepatic nodes lying in the porta hepatis collect lymph from vessels accompanying the hepatic ducts and the upper part of the bile duct. Lymphatics from the lower part of the common bile duct drain into the inferior hepatic and upper pancreaticosplenic nodes.

INNERVATION

The gallbladder and the extrahepatic biliary tree are innervated by branches from the hepatic plexus (p. 1222). The retroduodenal part of the common bile duct also has contributions from the pyloric branches of the vagi, which also innervate the smooth muscle of the hepato-pancreatic ampulla.

REFERRED PAIN

In common with other structures of foregut origin, pain from stretch of the common bile duct or gallbladder is referred to the central epigastrium. Involvement of the overlying somatic peritoneum produces pain which is more localized to the right upper quadrant.

MICROSTRUCTURE

GALLBLADDER (Fig. 86.5)

The fundus of the gallbladder is covered by a serosa (p. 41), but this only covers the inferior surfaces and sides of the body and neck of the gallbladder unless the gallbladder is mesenteric. Beneath it is subserous loose connective and adipose peritoneal tissue. The gallbladder wall microstructure generally resembles that of the small intestine. The mucosa is yellowish-brown and elevated into minute rugae with a honeycomb appearance (**Fig. 86.2**). In section, projections of the mucosa into the gallbladder lumen resemble intestinal villi, but these are not fixed structures and the surface flattens as the gallbladder fills with bile. Its epithelium is a single layer of columnar absorptive cells bearing apical microvilli. Goblet cells are absent. Basally, the spaces between epithelial cells are dilated. Many capillaries lie beneath the basement membrane. The epithelial cells actively absorb water and solutes from the bile to concentrate it, up to ten-fold. The thin fibromuscular layer is composed of fibrous tissue mixed with smooth muscle cells which are arranged loosely in longitudinal, circular and oblique bundles.

BILE DUCTS

The large biliary ducts have external fibrous and internal mucosal layers. The former is fibrous connective tissue which contains a variable amount of longitudinal, oblique and circular smooth muscle cells. The mucosa is continuous with that of the hepatic ducts, gallbladder and

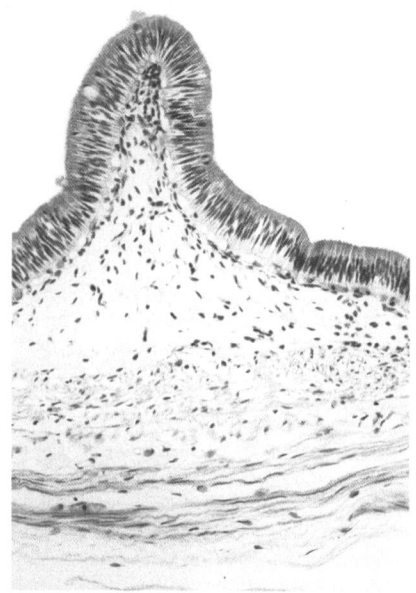

Fig. 86.5 Low power micrograph showing the gallbladder wall, with a mucosal projection which flattens in the full gallbladder, and the thin muscular layer. (Photograph by Sarah-Jane Smith.)

duodenum. The epithelium is columnar. Many tubuloalveolar mucous glands occur in the walls of these ducts.

Expulsion of gallbladder contents is under neuroendocrine control. Fat in the duodenum causes the release of cholecystokinin (CCK), stimulating the gallbladder to contract because muscle cells in its walls have surface receptors for CCK. When the pressure exceeds 100 mm of bile, the sphincter of Oddi relaxes and bile enters the duodenum. The termination of the united bile and pancreatic ducts is packed with villous, valvular folds of mucosa with muscle cells in their connective tissue cores. Contraction is thought to result in retraction and clumping of the folds, preventing reflux of duodenal contents and controlling the exit of bile.

REFERENCES

Suzuki M, Akaishi S, Rikiyama T, Naitoh T, Rahman MM, Matsuno S. 2000. Laparoscopic cholecystectomy, calot's triangle, and variations in cystic arterial supply. Surgical Endoscopy 14: 141–4.

IHPBA Brisbane 2000 Terminology of Liver Anatomy and Restrictions.

Pancreas

The pancreas is the largest of the digestive glands and performs a range of both endocrine and exocrine functions. The major part of the gland is exocrine, secreting a range of enzymes which are involved in the digestion of lipids, carbohydrates and proteins. The endocrine function of the pancreas is derived from cells scattered throughout the substance of the gland. They take part in glucose homeostasis as well as being involved in the control of upper gastrointestinal motility and function.

The pancreas is salmon pink in colour with a firm, lobulated smooth surface. The main portion of the pancreas is divided into four parts – head, neck, body and tail – and it possesses one accessory lobe (the uncinate process) (**Fig. 87.1**). The division into the parts is purely on the basis of anatomical relations and there are only very minor functional or anatomical differences between them. The uncinate process is an anatomically and embryologically distinct portion of the pancreas. In adults the pancreas measures between 12 and 15 cm long and is shaped as a flattened 'tongue' of tissue, thicker at its medial end (head) and thinner towards the lateral end (tail). With age, the amount of exocrine tissue tends to decline, as does the amount of fatty connective tissue within the substance of the gland, and this leads to a progressive thinning atrophy which is particularly noticeable on CT scanning. The pancreas lies within the curve of the first, second and third parts of the duodenum, and extends transversely and slightly upwards across the posterior abdominal wall to the hilum of the spleen, behind the stomach. It does not lie in one plane. It is effectively 'draped' over the other structures in the retroperitoneum and the vertebral column and so forms a distinct shallow curve, the neck and medial body being the most anterior parts. Because of its flattened shape, the parts of the pancreas, particularly the body, are often referred to as having surfaces and borders.

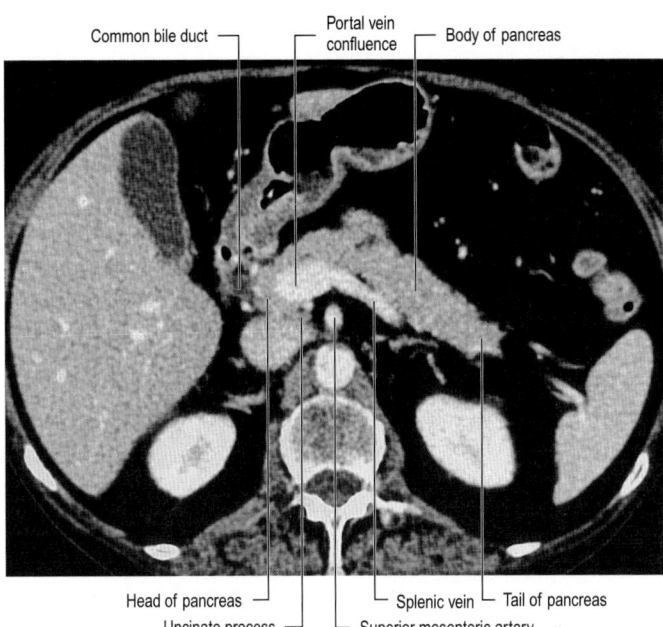

Common bile duct — Portal vein confluence — Body of pancreas

Head of pancreas — Splenic vein — Tail of pancreas
Uncinate process — Superior mesenteric artery

Fig. 87.1 CT scan of pancreas.

HEAD

The head of the pancreas lies to the right of the midline, anterior and to the right side of the vertebral column. It is the thickest and broadest part of the pancreas but is still flattened in the anteroposterior plane. It lies within the curve of the duodenum. Superiorly it lies adjacent to the first part of the duodenum but close to the pylorus the duodenum is on a short mesentery, and here the duodenum lies anterior to the upper part of the head (p. 1163). The duodenal border of the head is flattened and slightly concave, and is firmly adherent to the second part of the duodenum. Occasionally a small part of the head is actually embedded in the wall of the second part of the duodenum. The superior and inferior pancreaticoduodenal arteries lie between the head and the duodenum in this area. The inferior border lies superior to the third part of the duodenum and is continuous with the uncinate process (p. 1233). Close to the midline, the head is continuous with the neck. The boundary between head and neck is often marked anteriorly by a groove for the gastroduodenal artery and posteriorly by a similar but deeper deep groove containing the union of the superior mesenteric and splenic veins to form the portal vein.

Anterior surface (Fig. 87.2) – The anterior surface of the head is covered in peritoneum and is related to the origin of the transverse mesocolon.

Posterior surface – The posterior surface of the head is related to the inferior vena cava, which ascends behind it and covers almost all of this aspect. It is also related to the right renal vein and the right crus of the diaphragm.

NECK

The neck of the pancreas is only c.2 cm wide and links the head and body. It is often the most anterior portion of the gland. It is defined as that portion of the pancreas which lies anterior to the portal vein, and is closely related to the upper posterior surface. The lower part of the neck lies anterior to the superior mesenteric vein just before the formation of the portal vein. This is important during surgery for pancreatic cancer since malignant involvement of these vessels may make resection impossible. The anterior surface of the neck is covered with peritoneum. It lies adjacent to the pylorus just inferior to the epiploic foramen. The gastroduodenal and anterior superior pancreaticoduodenal arteries descend in front of the gland in the region of the junction of the neck and head.

BODY

The body of the pancreas runs from the left side of the neck to the tail. It is the longest portion of the gland and becomes progressively thinner and less broad towards the tail. It is slightly triangular in cross-section and is described as having three surfaces: anterosuperior, posterior and anteroinferior.

Anterosuperior surface – The anterosuperior surface of the pancreas makes up most of the anterior aspect of the gland close to the neck. Laterally, it narrows and lies slightly more superiorly to share the anterior aspect with the anteroinferior surface. It is covered by peritoneum, which runs anteroinferiorly from the surface of the gland to be continuous with the anterior, ascending layer of the greater omentum (p. 1132), (**Fig. 69.4**). It is separated from the stomach by the lesser sac.

Posterior surface (Fig. 87.3) – The posterior surface of the pancreas is devoid of peritoneum. It lies anterior to the aorta and the origin of the

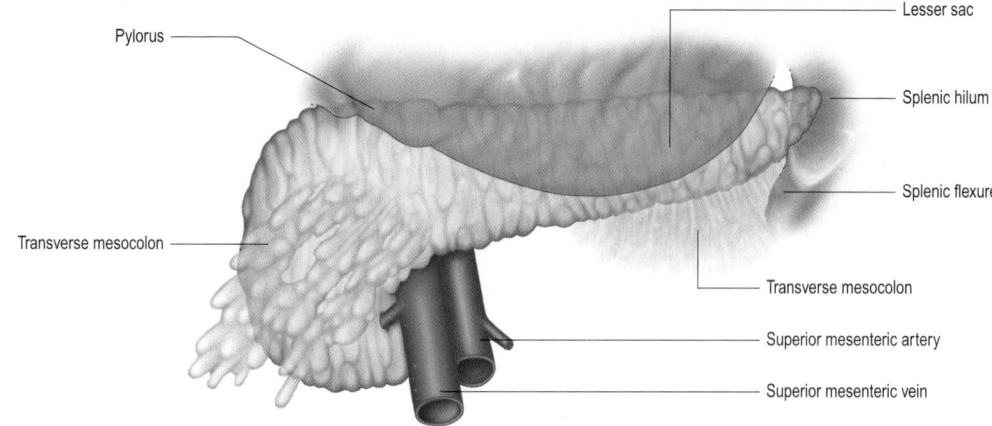

Fig. 87.2 Anterior relations of the pancreas. The extent of the lesser sac varies slightly between individuals. The splenic flexure may lie below or anterior to part of the tail.

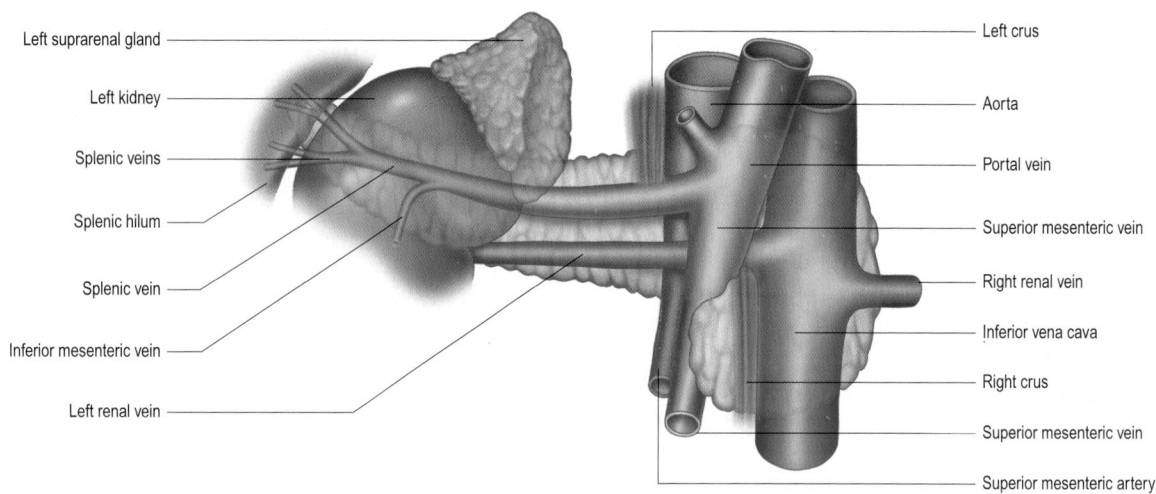

Fig. 87.3 Posterior relations of the pancreas. The posterior surfaces of the pancreas with their relations (viewed from behind).

superior mesenteric artery, the left crus of the diaphragm, left suprarenal gland and the left kidney and renal vessels, particularly the left renal vein. It is closely related to the splenic vein which runs from left to right forming a shallow groove in the gland. The splenic vein lies between the posterior surface and the other posterior relations. The left kidney is also separated from the posterior surface by perirenal fascia and fat.

Anteroinferior surface – The anteroinferior surface of the pancreas begins as a narrow strip just to the left of the neck. As the body runs laterally, it broadens out to form more of the anterior aspect of the body. It is covered by peritoneum which is continuous with that of the posteroinferior layer of the transverse mesocolon. The fourth part of the duodenum, the duodenojejunal flexure and coils of jejunum lie inferiorly. The lateral end of the inferior border often lies superior and posterior to the splenic flexure. The peritoneum of the anterosuperior layer of the transverse mesocolon is reflected onto the upper part of the anteroinferior surface.

Superior border – On the right side the superior border of the pancreas is initially blunt and somewhat flat. As the gland is followed to the left, the surface changes to become narrower and sharper. An omental tuberosity usually projects from the right end of the superior border above the level of the lesser curvature of the stomach, in contact with the posterior surface of the lesser omentum. The superior border is related to the coeliac artery. The common hepatic artery runs to the right just above the gland, the splenic artery runs to the left along the superior border. The course of the artery is often highly tortuous and it tends to rise above the level of the superior border at several points along its course.

Anterior border – The anterior border of the pancreas separates the anterosuperior from the anteroinferior surfaces. The two layers of the transverse mesocolon diverge along this border. One passes up over the anterosuperior surface whilst the other runs downwards and backwards over the anteroinferior surface.

Inferior border – The inferior border of the pancreas separates the posterior from the anteroinferior surfaces. At the medial end of the inferior border, adjacent to the neck of the pancreas, the superior mesenteric vessels emerge from behind the gland. More laterally, the inferior mesenteric vein runs under the border to join the splenic vein on the posterior surface. This is a useful site of identification of the inferior mesenteric vein during left-sided colonic resections and on CT imaging.

TAIL

The tail of the pancreas is the narrowest, most lateral portion of the gland and lies between the layers of the splenorenal ligament (p. 1132). It is continuous medially with the body and is between 1.5 and 3.5 cm long in adults. It may finish at the base of the splenorenal ligament or extend up nearly as far as the splenic hilum, in which case it is prone to injury at splenectomy during ligation of the splenic vessels. Posteriorly it is related to the splenic branches of the splenic artery and the splenic vein and its tributaries. The tip of the tail may lie in contact with the splenic hilum.

UNCINATE PROCESS

The uncinate process of the pancreas extends from the inferior lateral end of the head of the gland. It is embryologically separate from the rest of the gland, and as a consequence of its development it lies posterior to the superior mesenteric vessels. These lie in close contact to its anterior surface as they descend and run forward into the root of the ileal mesentery. Posteriorly it lies in front of the aorta, and inferiorly it lies on the upper surface of the third part of the duodenum. Tumours of the uncinate process do not cause obstruction to the common bile duct but frequently compress the third part of the duodenum as a result of this close relationship.

PANCREATIC DUCTS

The exocrine pancreatic tissue drains into multiple small lobular ducts, which drain into a single main, and usually, a single accessory duct (**Fig. 86.3**).

The main pancreatic duct runs within the substances of the gland from left to right. It tends to lie more towards the posterior than anterior surface. It is formed by the junction of several lobular ducts in the tail. As it runs within the body it increases in calibre as it receives further lobular ducts, which join it almost at right angles to the axis of the main duct to form a 'herringbone pattern'. On ultrasound the duct can often be demonstrated, measuring c.3 mm in diameter in the head, 2 mm in the body, and 1 mm in the tail in adults. As it reaches the neck of the gland it usually turns inferiorly and posteriorly towards the bile duct, which lies on its right side. The two ducts enter the wall of the descending part of the duodenum obliquely and unite in a short dilated hepatopancreatic ampulla (p. 1163).

A separate accessory pancreatic duct usually drains the lower part of the head and uncinate process. It is much smaller in calibre than the main duct and forms within the substance of the head from several lobular ducts. It ascends anterior to the main duct and usually communicates with it through several small branches. The accessory duct occasionally opens onto a small rounded minor duodenal papilla, which lies about 2 cm anterosuperior to the major papilla. If the duodenal end of the accessory duct fails to develop, the duct drains along the connecting channels into the main duct.

The main and accessory pancreatic ducts demonstrate some variability in their anatomy (**Fig. 87.4**). Occasionally the accessory duct is absent and the main duct drains the uncinate process directly. The main duct may drain directly into the duodenum and the uncinate process drains via an accessory duct. Rarely the two ducts are conjoined.

VASCULAR SUPPLY AND LYMPHATIC DRAINAGE

ARTERIES (Fig. 87.5)

The pancreas has a rich arterial supply derived from the coeliac axis and superior mesenteric arteries via both named vessels and multiple small un-named vessels.

Inferior pancreaticoduodenal artery

The inferior pancreaticoduodenal artery arises from the superior mesenteric artery or its first jejunal branch, near the superior border of the third part of the duodenum. It usually divides directly into anterior and posterior branches. The anterior branch passes to the right, anterior to the lower border of the head of the pancreas, and runs superiorly to anastomose with the anterior superior pancreaticoduodenal artery. The posterior branch runs posteriorly and superiorly to the right, lying posterior to the lower border of the head of the pancreas and anastomoses with the posterior superior pancreaticoduodenal artery. Both branches supply the pancreatic head, its uncinate process and the second and third parts of the duodenum.

Superior pancreaticoduodenal artery

The superior pancreaticoduodenal artery is usually double. The anterior artery is a terminal branch of the gastroduodenal artery and descends in the anterior groove between the second part of the duodenum and head of the pancreas. It supplies branches to the head of the pancreas. It anastomoses with the anterior division of the inferior pancreaticoduodenal artery. The posterior artery is usually a separate branch of

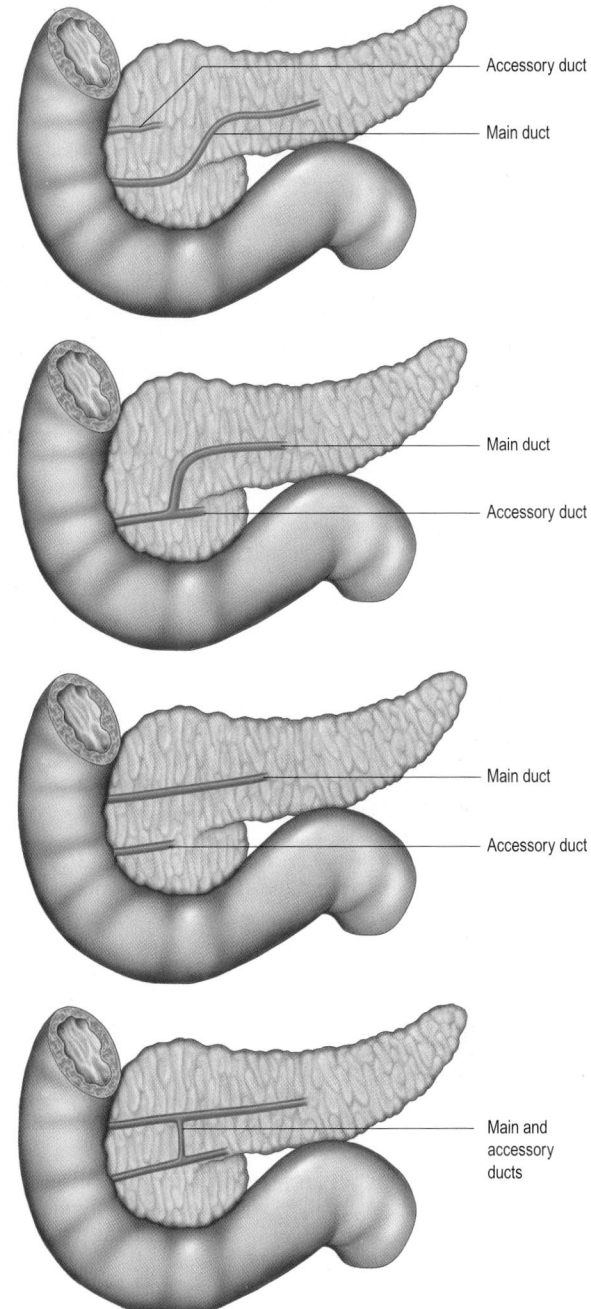

Fig. 87.4 Variations in the ductal anatomy of the pancreas.

the gastroduodenal artery arising at the upper border of the first part of the duodenum. It descends to the right, anterior to the portal vein and common bile duct, where the duct passes behind the first part of the duodenum. The artery runs posterior to the head of the pancreas and then crosses posterior to the common bile duct embedded in the head of the pancreas. It enters the duodenal wall and anastomoses with the posterior division of the inferior pancreaticoduodenal artery. The posterior superior artery supplies branches to the head of the pancreas and the first and second parts of the duodenum.

Pancreatic branches

The pancreas is supplied by numerous small arterial branches which usually run into the gland directly from their arteries of origin. These are particularly numerous in the region of the neck, body and tail. Most originate from the splenic artery as it runs along the superior border of the gland and supply the left part of the body and tail. A dorsal branch descends posterior to the pancreas, dividing into right and left branches. It sometimes arises from the superior mesenteric, middle colic, hepatic or rarely, the coeliac artery. The right branch is often double and runs

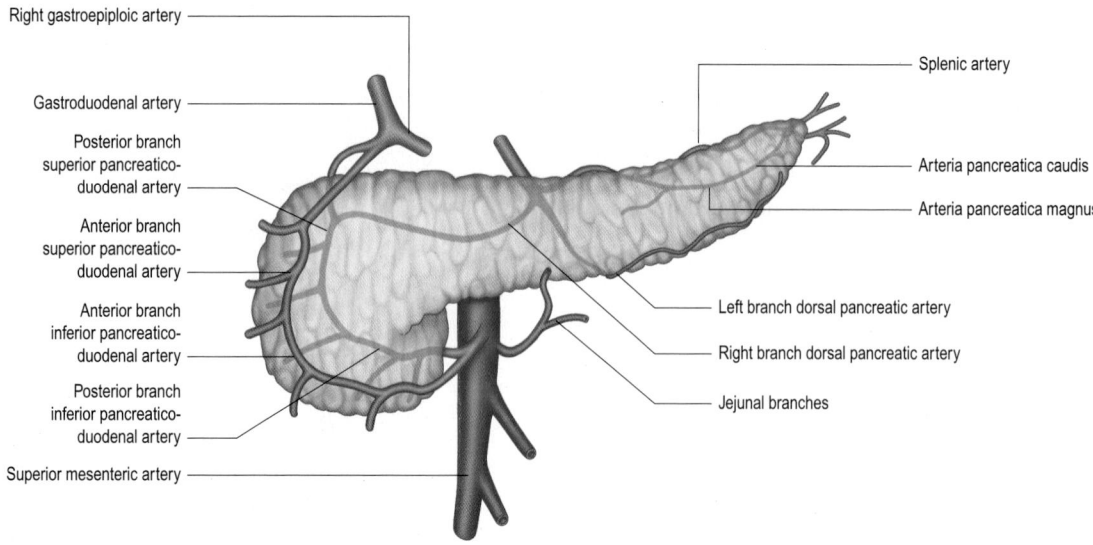

Right gastroepiploic artery

Gastroduodenal artery

Posterior branch
superior pancreatico-
duodenal artery

Anterior branch
superior pancreatico-
duodenal artery

Anterior branch
inferior pancreatico-
duodenal artery

Posterior branch
inferior pancreatico-
duodenal artery

Superior mesenteric artery

Splenic artery

Arteria pancreatica caudis

Arteria pancreatica magnus

Left branch dorsal pancreatic artery

Right branch dorsal pancreatic artery

Jejunal branches

Fig. 87.5 Arterial supply of the pancreas.

between the neck and uncinate process to form a prepancreatic arterial arch as it anastomoses with a branch from the anterior superior pancreaticoduodenal artery. The left branch runs along the inferior border to the pancreatic tail where it anastomoses with the greater pancreatic artery (arteria pancreatica magna) and the artery to tail of the pancreas (arteria caudae pancreatis).

Small un-named branches also arise from the first jejunal arcade of the superior mesenteric artery and the arterial branches of the retro-peritoneal vessels.

Small arteries characteristically run along the inferior and superior borders of the gland, either lying in a deep groove or within the tissue of the gland. They supply branches, which penetrate the substance of the gland at right angles to the vessel and receive contributions from the arteries supplying the gland but mainly from the inferior and superior pancreaticoduodenal arteries. They may bleed profusely on cutting the parenchyma of the gland during resection and usually require ligation.

VEINS

The venous drainage of the pancreas is primarily into the portal system. The head and neck drain primarily via superior and inferior pancreatico-duodenal veins (p. 1165). The body and tail drain mostly via small veins running directly into the splenic vein along the posterior aspect of the gland or occasionally directly into the portal vein. Small venous channels exist between the gland and the retroperitoneal veins, draining into the lumbar veins and these may hypertrophy and become clinically significant in cases of portal hypertension.

LYMPHATICS

Lymph capillaries commence around the pancreatic acini. The larger lymph vessels follow the arterial supply and drain into the lymph nodes around the pancreas and adjacent node groups. The tail and body lymphatics drain mostly into the pancreaticosplenic nodes although some drain directly to pre-aortic nodes. Lymphatics from the neck and head drain more widely into nodes along the pancreaticoduodenal, superior mesenteric and hepatic arteries. Drainage also occurs to the pre-aortic nodes and coeliac axis nodes. There are no lymphatics in the pancreatic islets.

INNERVATION OF THE EXOCRINE PANCREAS

The exocrine lobules of the pancreas are innervated by a fine network of sympathetic and parasympathetic fibres. The sympathetic supply originates from the sixth to tenth thoracic spinal segments and is mainly distributed to the pancreas via the sympathetic contribution to the coeliac ganglia. The postganglionic fibres are distributed to the gland via the arterial supply as periarterial plexuses. The parasympathetic

supply is from the posterior vagus nerve and the parasympathetic com-ponent of the coeliac plexus. The supply to the gland is both vasomotor (sympathetic) and parenchymal (sympathetic and parasympathetic) in distribution. The exocrine lobules are innervated by a fine network of parasympathetic and sympathetic fibres. Sensory fibres running from the gland run in both the sympathetic and parasympathetic systems. These mediate the sensation of pain arising from the gland and may also carry other sensory information. In chronic inflammation or inoperable tumours of the gland, thermal or chemical ablation of the coeliac plexus may be required to control chronic pain mediated by these fibres.

REFERRED PAIN

Pain arising in the pancreas is poorly localized. In common with other foregut structures, the majority of pain arising from the pancreas is referred to the epigastrium. Inflammatory or infiltrative processes arising from the gland rapidly involve the tissues of the retro-peritoneum and their supply from somatic nerves, and this is referred to the posterior paravertebral region around the lower thoracic spine.

PANCREATITIS AND PSEUDOCYST

Pancreatitis is one of the major pathological processes affecting the pancreas. Gallstones lying within the common bile duct are associated with pancreatitis. The presence of a common drainage for the common bile duct and the pancreatic duct may allow reflux of bile or pancreatic enzymes into the pancreatic duct during the passage of a gallstone through the ampulla. This may also occur due to oedema of the common bile duct wall even when the gallstones have not entered the common ampulla.

Inflammation in the pancreas may cause a range of secondary pathologies. The course of the superior mesenteric artery and vein behind the neck and between the inferior border and uncinate process makes these vessels vulnerable to compression and secondary inflam-mation, which may result in an inflammatory aneurysm of the superior mesenteric artery or thrombosis of the superior mesenteric vein. Inflammatory aneurysms may rupture producing major haemorrhage. Thrombosis of the superior mesenteric vein may cause potentially lethal venous ischaemia of the small intestine. Thrombosis of smaller arterial branches such as the origin of the middle colic artery may also occur, causing ischaemia of individual organs such as the transverse colon.

The profuse arterial and venous supply to the gland makes it particularly prone to haemorrhage. The extravasated blood collects in the retroperitoneal tissues as the neck and body of the gland lie largely in the loose connective tissue of the retroperitoneum. The pancreas lies

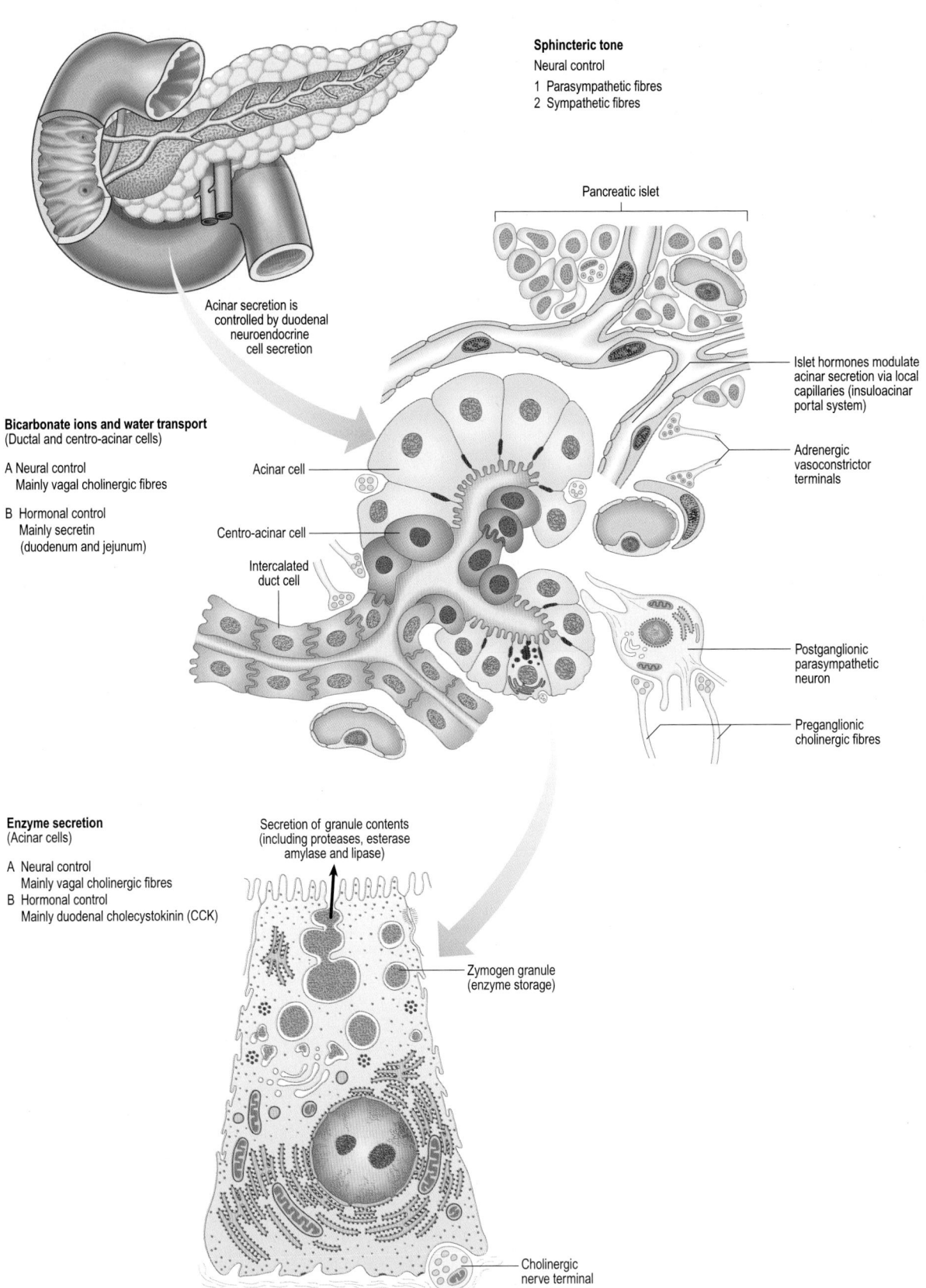

Sphincteric tone
Neural control
1 Parasympathetic fibres
2 Sympathetic fibres

Acinar secretion is controlled by duodenal neuroendocrine cell secretion

Bicarbonate ions and water transport
(Ductal and centro-acinar cells)

A Neural control
  Mainly vagal cholinergic fibres

B Hormonal control
  Mainly secretin
  (duodenum and jejunum)

Pancreatic islet

Islet hormones modulate acinar secretion via local capillaries (insuloacinar portal system)

Acinar cell

Adrenergic vasoconstrictor terminals

Centro-acinar cell

Intercalated duct cell

Postganglionic parasympathetic neuron

Preganglionic cholinergic fibres

Enzyme secretion
(Acinar cells)

A Neural control
  Mainly vagal cholinergic fibres
B Hormonal control
  Mainly duodenal cholecystokinin (CCK)

Secretion of granule contents (including proteases, esterase amylase and lipase)

Zymogen granule (enzyme storage)

Cholinergic nerve terminal

Fig. 87.6 Microstructure of the exocrine pancreas and the mechanisms by which its secretion is controlled.

anterior to the thoracolumbar and perirenal fasciae and the blood can track freely in the retroperitoneal tissues to appear either in the flanks – so-called Grey–Turner's sign – in the groins, or above the iliac crest where the iliac fascia is attached. Blood tracking laterally from the head of the pancreas may enter the lesser omentum and 'bare area' of the liver, from where it may run forward into the falciform ligament and appear around the skin of the umbilicus – so-called Cullen's sign.

During acute episodes of inflammation, the close anterior relationship of the stomach may contribute to gastric stasis and vomiting. The origin of the superior mesenteric plexus also lies close to the pancreas and secondary inflammation in the tissues around the pancreas may affect the autonomic supply to the midgut and contribute to the paralytic ileus which frequently develops.

In severe cases, pancreatic inflammation may cause the collection of fluid within and around the pancreatic tissue. Intrapancreatic collections frequently resolve spontaneously over time but coalescence of the fluid may occur anterior to the pancreas beneath the layer of peritoneum covering its anterior surfaces, although this actually lies beneath the posterior wall of the lesser sac. If this collection persists and grows, the peritoneum anterior and superior to the pancreas is stretched and comes to lie in contact with the anterior wall of the lesser sac. This collection is referred to as a pseudocyst. The anterior wall of the pseudocyst is formed of the twin layers of peritoneum lying adjacent to the posterior wall of the stomach, the lesser omentum and, occasionally, the gastrosplenic ligament. The lateral wall of the pseudocyst includes the splenorenal ligament. The posterior wall is a mixture of fibrous tissue resulting from previous inflammation, the anterior surface of the pancreas and the retroperitoneal tissues. Treatment of the pseudocyst usually involves drainage of the contents into the lumen of the stomach. This may be established endoscopically by placement of a drain through the posterior stomach wall and the two thickened layers of peritoneum into the cyst. Alternatively, the drain may be placed using radiological guidance, via the anterior abdominal wall and the anterior stomach wall.

PANCREATIC RESECTION

Resection of the pancreas is complicated by several factors. The extensive vascular supply requires careful haemostasis. Spleen-preserving resections may be undertaken if the underlying pathology does not involve the splenic vein as it lies in the groove on the posterior surface of the gland, although the multiple small pancreatic veins draining into it may cause troublesome bleeding. Resection of the head and neck is possible provided the plane between the neck and the portal vein has not been involved by disease. Occasional small venous branches may enter the portal vein directly and may also cause bleeding during this mobilization. Resection of the head and neck are always accompanied by resection of the distal first and second parts of the duodenum because of the dense adherence between the two and the common arterial supply. Resection without removal of the proximal part of the first part of the duodenum and pylorus – pylorus preserving pancreatectomy – may be possible provided the arterial supply to the pylorus from the stomach, and directly from the pre-pyloric vessels, is adequate.

MICROSTRUCTURE (Figs 87.6, 87.7, 87.8)

The pancreas is composed of two different types of glandular tissue. The main tissue mass is exocrine (p. 34), in which are embedded pancreatic islets of endocrine cells (p. 34).

EXOCRINE PANCREAS

The exocrine pancreas is a branched acinar gland, surrounded and incompletely lobulated by delicate loose connective tissue. It is formed of pyramidal, secretory cells arranged mainly as spherical clusters, or

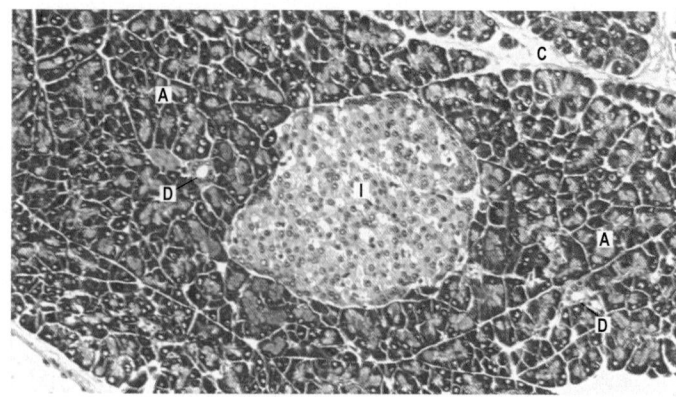

Fig. 87.7 Pancreatic tissue. Exocrine acinar cells (A) are deeply stained basally, indicating the high ribosomal concentration. Small ducts (D) are shown. An endocrine islet (of Langerhans) (I) is shown centrally, with pale-staining cells surrounded by a network of capillaries, seen as clear spaces. Connective tissue septa (C) separate lobules. (By permission from Dr JB Kerr, Monash University, from Kerr JB 1999 Atlas of Functional Histology. London: Mosby.)

acini. A narrow intercalated, intralobular duct originates within each secretory acinus, lined initially by flattened or cuboidal centro-acinar cells. These small ductules form branching links which run within and between adjacent acini, explaining why structurally distinct intralobular pancreatic ducts are infrequent (*see* Kerr 1999, for details). More distally, these are replaced by taller cuboidal and eventually columnar epithelium in the larger interlobular ducts. The latter are surrounded by loose connective tissue of the septa, containing smooth muscle and autonomic nerve fibres. Neuroendocrine cells are present amongst the columnar ductal cells and mast cells are numerous in the surrounding connective tissue.

Acinar cells

Acinar cells of the exocrine pancreas have a basal nucleus and, in their basal cytoplasmic domain, abundant rough endoplasmic reticulum which results in their basophilic staining characteristics. Dense secretory zymogen granules stain deeply with eosin in the apical region. A prominent supranuclear Golgi complex is surrounded by large, membrane-bound granules containing the proteinaceous constituents of pancreatic secretion, including enzymes which are only active after release. Ganglionic neurones and cords of undifferentiated epithelial cells are also found within the acini. The structure of the exocrine pancreas and its functional regulation are summarized in **Fig. 87.6**.

ENDOCRINE PANCREAS (Fig. 87.8)

The endocrine pancreas consists of pancreatic islets of Langerhans, composed of spherical or ellipsoid clusters of cells embedded in the exocrine tissue. The human pancreas may contain more than a million islets, usually most numerous in the tail. An islet is a mass of polyhedral cells, each in close proximity to fenestrated capillaries and a rich autonomic innervation. Specialized staining procedures or immunohistochemical techniques are necessary to distinguish the three major types of cell, designated alpha, beta and delta. Their general organization is shown in **Fig. 87.8**.

The most numerous cells, types alpha and beta, secrete glucagon and insulin respectively. Alpha cells tend to be concentrated at the periphery of islets, and beta cells more centrally. A third type, the delta cell, secretes somatostatin and gastrin, and like alpha cells, is peripherally placed within the islets. A minor cell type, the F cell, secretes pancreatic

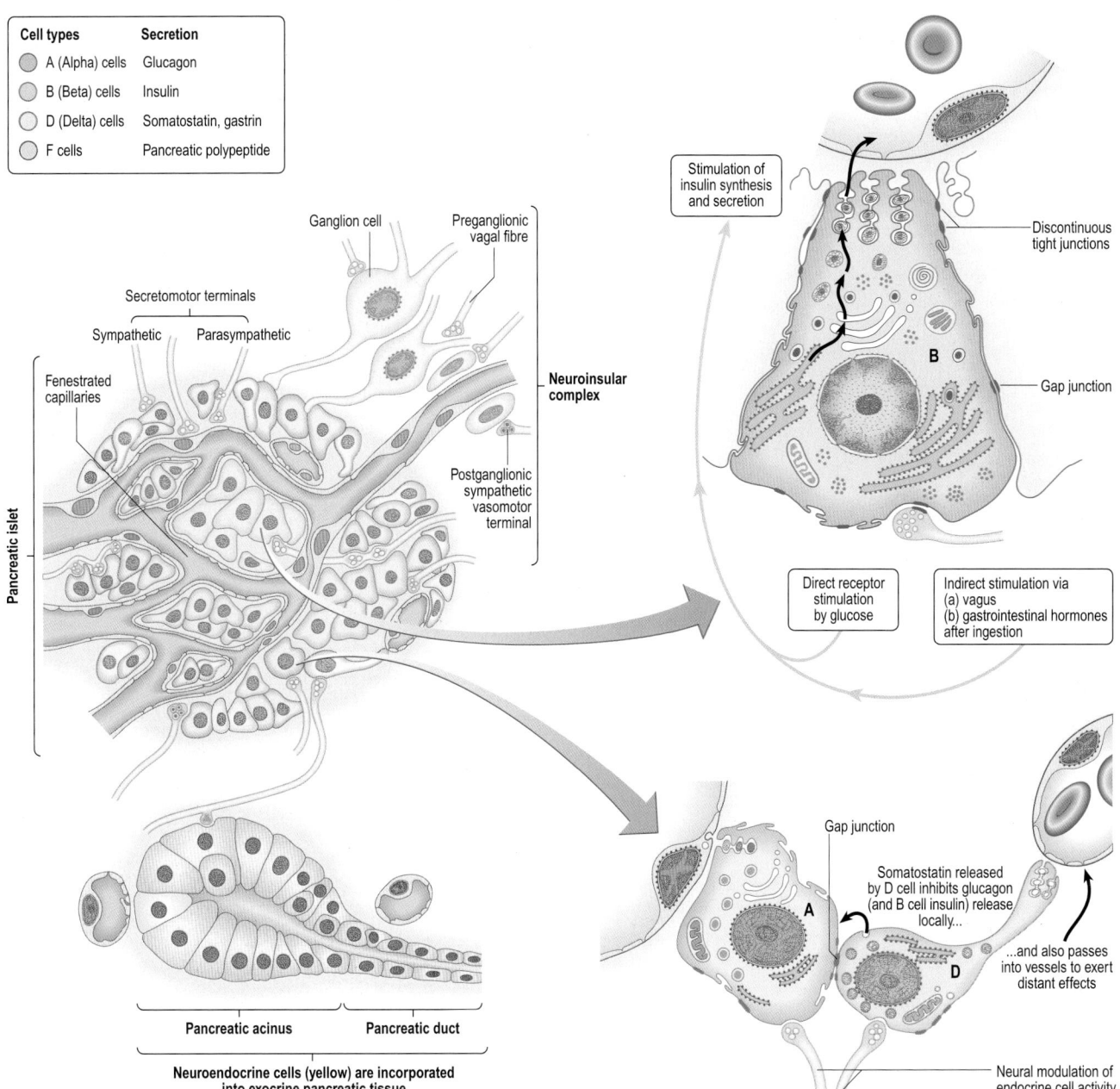

Cell types	Secretion
A (Alpha) cells	Glucagon
B (Beta) cells	Insulin
D (Delta) cells	Somatostatin, gastrin
F cells	Pancreatic polypeptide

Fig. 87.8 Microstructure and control of function of the endocrine pancreas.

polypeptide (PP), which is stored in smaller secretory granules. The autonomic transmitters acetylcholine (ACh) and noradrenalin affect islet cell secretion. ACh augments insulin and glucagon release, noradrenalin inhibits glucose-induced insulin release and they may also affect somatostatin and PP secretion.

Innervation of endocrine pancreas

The innervation of the endocrine islets is almost exclusively from the parasympathetic system. Fine branches ramify among the cells and form plexuses around the islets. Fibres frequently synapse with acinar cells before innervating the islets, suggesting a close linkage between neural control of exocrine and endocrine components. Many fibres enter the islets with the arterioles. Parasympathetic ganglia lie in the connective tissue within and between lobules, and in the former case are frequently associated with islet cells, forming neuroinsular complexes. Both alpha and beta cells are involved in these neuroinsular complexes. Three types of nerve terminal are seen in islets. Cholinergic terminals have agranular vesicles with a diameter of 30–50 nm, adrenergic terminals have dense-cored vesicles with a diameter of 30–50 nm and a third, uncharacterized, type have dense-cored vesicles with a diameter of 60–200 nm (Smith & Porte 1976).

No selective link with any one type of insular cell has been found. Sometimes more than one type of terminal contacts a single cell and some of the chemical synapses between axon terminals and islet cells show narrow areas in the synaptic clefts suggesting an electrical synapse or gap junction. Such junctions also occur between islet cells, and electrical coupling of nerve supply to a functional network of islet cells may occur (Orci 1974).

REFERENCES

Kerr JB 1999 Atlas of Functional Histology, Chapter 14. London: Mosby.
Orci L 1974 A portrait of a pancreatic B-cell. Diabetologia 10: 163–87.

Smith PH, Porte D Jr 1976 Neuropharmacology of the pancreatic islets. Annu Rev Pharmacol Toxicol 16: 269–85.

Spleen (Fig. 88.1)

The spleen consists of a large encapsulated mass of vascular and lymphoid tissue situated in the upper left quadrant of the abdominal cavity between the fundus of the stomach and the diaphragm. Its shape varies from a slightly curved wedge to a 'domed' tetrahedron. The shape is mostly determined by its relations to neighbouring structures during development. The superolateral aspect is shaped by the left dome of the diaphragm with the inferomedial aspect being influenced mostly by the neighbouring splenic flexure of the colon, the right kidney and stomach. Its long axis lies approximately in the plane of the tenth rib. Its posterior border is c.4 cm from the mid-dorsal line at the level of the tenth thoracic vertebral spine. Its anterior border usually reaches the mid-axillary line.

The size and weight of the spleen vary with age and between the sexes. It can also vary slightly in the same individual under different conditions. In the adult it is usually c.12 cm long, 7 cm broad and between 3 and 4 cm wide. It is comparatively largest in the young child, and although its weight increases during puberty, by adulthood it is relatively smaller in comparison to the neighbouring organs. It tends to diminish in size and weight in senescence. Its average adult weight is about 150 g although the normal range is wide, between 80 g and 300 g, in part reflecting the amount of blood it contains.

Additional collections of fully functional splenic tissue may exist near the spleen, especially within the gastrosplenic ligament and greater omentum. These accessory spleens, or spleniculi, are usually isolated but can be connected to the spleen by thin bands of similar tissue. They may be numerous and widely scattered in the abdomen. The spleen may retain its fetal lobulated form or show deep notches on its diaphragmatic surface and inferior border in addition to those usually present on the superior border.

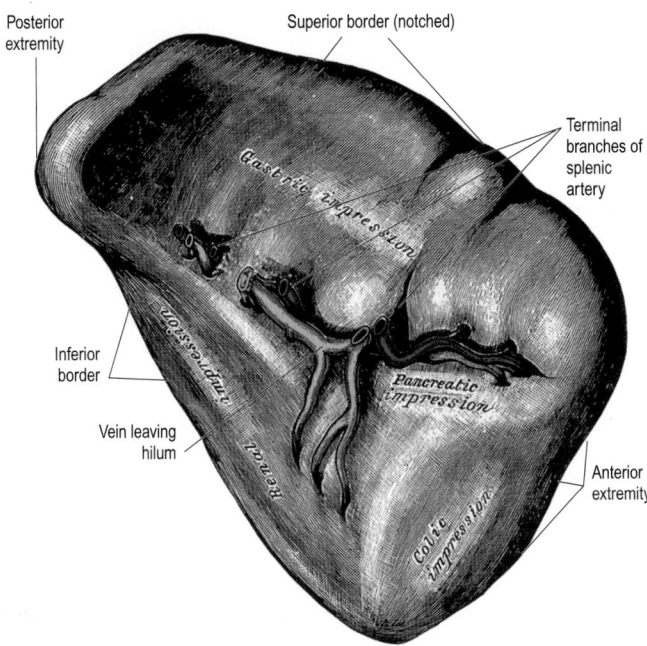

Fig. 88.1 The visceral surface of the spleen.

RELATIONS

The spleen has a superolateral diaphragmatic and an inferomedial visceral surface. There are superior and inferior borders and anterior and posterior extremities or poles. The diaphragmatic surface is convex and smooth and faces mostly superiorly and laterally although the posterior part may face posteriorly and almost medially as it approaches the inferior border. The diaphragmatic surface is related to the abdominal surface of the left dome of the diaphragm which separates it from the basal pleura, the lower lobe of the left lung and the ninth to eleventh left ribs. The pleural costodiaphragmatic recess extends down as far as its inferior border. The visceral surface faces inferomedially towards the abdominal cavity and is irregular. It is marked by gastric, renal, pancreatic and colic impressions. The gastric impression faces anteromedially and is broad and concave where the spleen lies adjacent to the posterior aspect of the fundus, upper body and upper greater curvature of the stomach. It is separated from the stomach by a peritoneal recess, which is limited by the gastrosplenic ligament. The renal impression is slightly concave and lies on the lowest part of the visceral surface. It is separated from the gastric impression above by a raised strip of splenic tissue and the splenic hilum. It faces inferomedially and slightly backwards, being related to the upper and lateral area of the anterior surface of the left kidney and sometimes to the superior pole of the left suprarenal gland. The colic impression lies at the inferior pole of the spleen and is usually flat. It is related to the splenic flexure of the colon and the phrenicocolic ligament. The pancreatic impression is often small when present and lies between the colic impression and the lateral part of the hilum. It is related to the tail of the pancreas which lies in the splenorenal ligament. The hilum of the spleen lies in the visceral surface closer to the inferior border and anterior extremity. It is a long fissure pierced by several irregular apertures through which the branches of the splenic artery and vein as well as nerves and lymphatics enter and leave the spleen.

The superior border separates the diaphragmatic surface from the gastric impression and is usually convex. Near the anterior extremity there may be one or two notches persisting from the lobulated form of the spleen in early fetal life. These notches are often absent and are not a reliable guide to the identification of the spleen during clinical examination. The inferior border separates the renal impression from the diaphragmatic surface and lies between the diaphragm and the upper part of the lateral border of the left kidney. It is more blunt and rounded than the superior border and corresponds in position to the eleventh rib's lower margin. The posterior extremity, or superior pole, usually faces the rounded vertebral column. The anterior extremity, or inferior pole, is larger and less angulated than the posterior extremity and connects the lateral ends of the superior and inferior borders. It is related to the colic impression and may lie adjacent to the splenic flexure and the phrenicocolic ligament.

PERITONEAL CONNECTIONS OF THE SPLEEN (Fig. 88.2)

The spleen is almost entirely covered by peritoneum, which is firmly adherent to its capsule. Recesses of the greater sac separate it from the stomach and left kidney. It develops in the upper dorsal mesogastrium (p. 1254), (**Figs 90.6, 90.7, 90.8**) and remains connected to the posterior abdominal wall, anterolateral abdominal wall and stomach by three folds of peritoneum. The posterior connection is the splenorenal ligament, the anterolateral connection is the phrenicocolic ligament, and the anterior connection is the gastrosplenic ligament. The splenorenal ligament is formed from two layers of peritoneum. The anterior layer is continuous with the peritoneum of the posterior wall of the lesser sac over the left kidney and is continuous with peritoneum

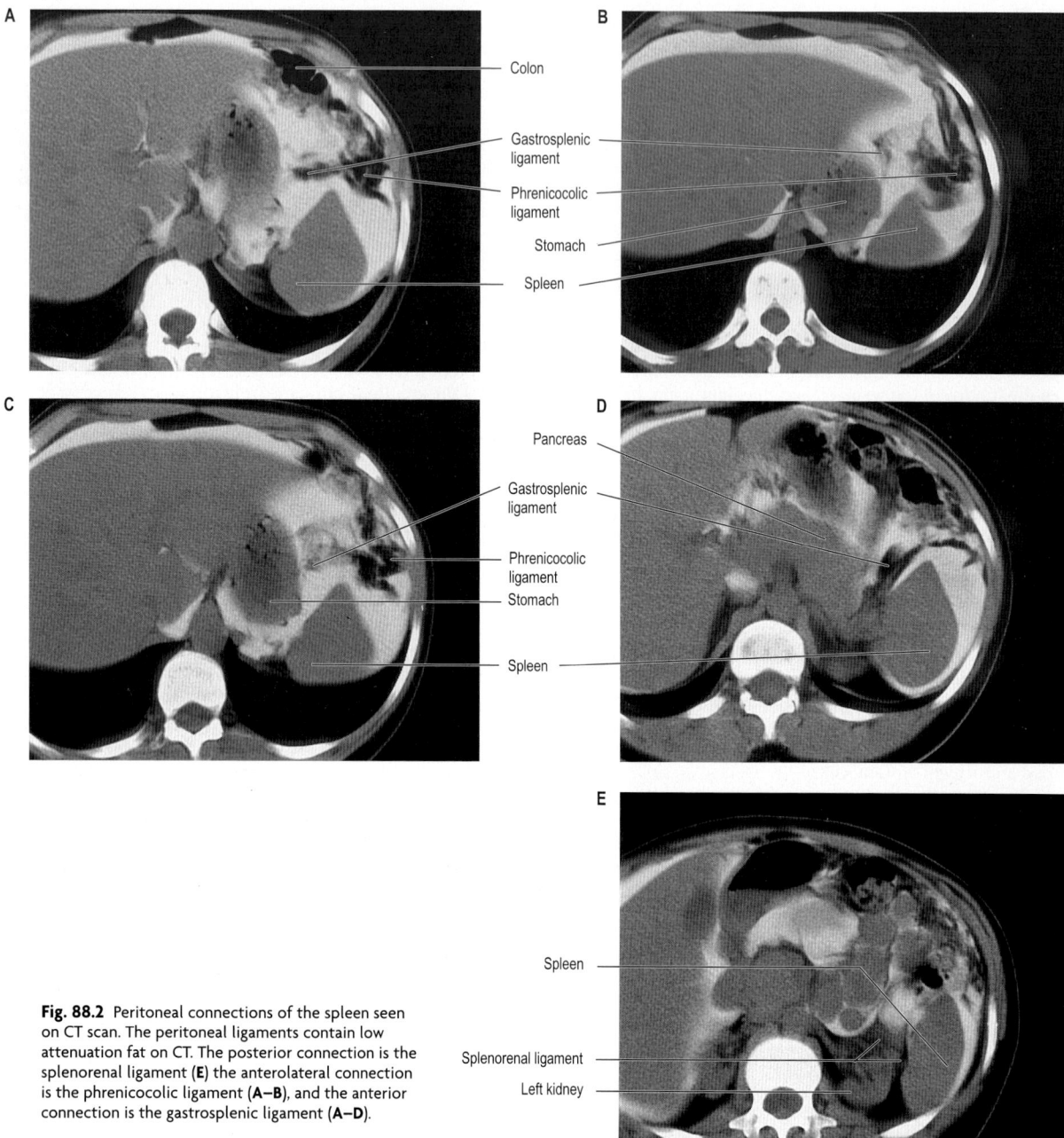

Fig. 88.2 Peritoneal connections of the spleen seen on CT scan. The peritoneal ligaments contain low attenuation fat on CT. The posterior connection is the splenorenal ligament (**E**) the anterolateral connection is the phrenicocolic ligament (**A–B**), and the anterior connection is the gastrosplenic ligament (**A–D**).

of the splenic hilum where it runs into the posterior layer of the gastrosplenic ligament. The posterior layer of the splenorenal ligament is continuous with the peritoneum over the inferior surface of the diaphragm and runs onto the splenic surface over the renal impression. The splenic vessels lie between the layers of the splenorenal ligament and the tail of the pancreas is usually present in its lower portion (**Fig. 69.5**). The length of the splenorenal ligament may vary. Longer ligaments tend to make the spleen more mobile and may predispose the spleen to injury due to rotational shear forces during trauma but also make the mobilization of the spleen easier during surgery. The presence of the pancreatic tail within the splenorenal ligament must be remembered as it can be injured during ligation of the splenic vessels causing pancreatitis or a pancreatic duct fistula to form.

The gastrosplenic ligament also has two layers. The posterior is continuous with the peritoneum of the splenic hilum and that over the posterior aspect of the stomach. The anterior layer is formed from the peritoneum reflected off the gastric impression and reaches the greater curvature of the stomach anteriorly. The short gastric and left gastroepiploic branches of the splenic artery pass between its layers. Division of the gastrosplenic ligament during surgery may be hazardous if the ligament is short since ligation of the short gastric vessels may risk injury to the greater curvature of the stomach.

The phrenicocolic ligament extends from the splenic flexure of the colon to the diaphragm at the level of the eleventh rib. It extends inferiorly and laterally and is continuous with the peritoneum of the lateral end of the transverse mesocolon at the lateral margin of the pancreatic tail, and the splenorenal ligament at the hilum of the spleen.

If the peritoneal attachments of the spleen are not recognized surgery may risk injury to the splenic capsule and subsequent serious bleeding. Downward traction on the phrenicocolic ligament during handling of the descending colon, especially during mobilization of the splenic flexure, may cause rupture of the splenic capsule. This is less likely if traction on the phrenicocolic ligament is made laterally or medially. The superior border and anterior diaphragmatic surface are often adherent to the peritoneum of the greater omentum. Medial traction on the omentum during surgery may cause capsular injury which is less likely if any limited traction required is applied inferiorly. The diaphragmatic surface of the spleen is occasionally adherent to the peritoneum over the inferior surface of the diaphragm. These adhesions often occur after inflammation in the spleen but may also be present congenitally.

SPLENOMEGALY

Any massive immune response may be accompanied by splenic enlargement. This also occurs in many other systemic inflammatory and degenerative conditions. In splenomegaly, the anterior border, anterior diaphragmatic surface and notched superior border may become clearly palpable below the left costal margin; the notches are often exaggerated and may be clearly palpable. The transverse colon and splenic flexure are displaced downward.

SPLENIC TRAUMA

Because of its relatively mobile peritoneal connections, the spleen is particularly prone to rotational injury during rapid deceleration or compressions. This may lead to tearing injuries to the splenic vessels at the hilum or burst injuries of the splenic pulp. Fractures of the overlying lower left ribs may cause sharp penetrating injuries to the splenic capsule and pulp. The spleen may also be injured during surgical procedures by tearing of its capsule through peritoneal adhesions and connections. Minor capsular tears may be treated by application of various haemostatic substances to the exposed pulp. Direct sutured repair of more extensive tears of the spleen is rarely successful because of the fragile nature of the splenic pulp. Moderately severe injuries may be treated by compression of the splenic tissue until haemostasis occurs but extensive burst injuries or major injuries to the hilar vessels usually require splenectomy.

SPLENECTOMY

Partial splenectomy is followed by rapid regeneration of lost tissue and there is no significant loss in any of the functions of the spleen. Total splenectomy has few haematological consequences since the functions of the spleen are largely assumed by the liver. There is, however, a loss in immune function, particularly in the antibody response to systemic infections with encapsulated bacteria. This is referred to as 'overwhelming post-splenectomy sepsis syndrome'. It is particularly a problem when the spleen is lost in early childhood, but is still a significant risk even if the spleen is lost in late adult life. Splenectomy in adults is usually followed by an increased white blood cell count with increased lymphocytic, neutrophil, eosinophil and platelet counts in the peripheral blood. These effects fade and disappear within a few weeks.

VASCULAR SUPPLY AND LYMPHATIC DRAINAGE

SPLENIC ARTERY

The spleen is supplied exclusively from the splenic artery. This is the largest branch of the coeliac axis and its course is among the most tortuous in the body (**Fig. 87.5**). From its origin the artery runs a little way inferiorly, then turns rapidly to the left to run initially horizontally above the level of the neck of the pancreas, before ascending as it passes more laterally. It is less steeply inclined than the body and tail of the pancreas and so comes to lie posterior to the superior border of the gland. It lies in multiple loops or even coils which appear above the superior border of the pancreas and descend to lie behind the gland. The splenic artery lies anterior to the left kidney and left suprarenal gland. It runs in the splenorenal ligament posterior to the tail of the pancreas and divides into two or three main branches before entering the hilum of the spleen. As these branches enter the hilum they divide further into four or five segmental arteries. These vessels each supply a segment of the splenic tissue. There is relatively little arterial collateral circulation between the segments which means that occlusion of a segmental vessel often leads to infarction of part of the spleen. There is, however, considerable venous collateral circulation between the segments, which makes segmental resection of the spleen practically impossible. The splenic artery gives off various branches to the pancreas in its course (p. 1233) and gives off short gastric arteries to the stomach just prior to dividing or from its terminal branches (p. 1147).

SPLENIC VEIN (Fig. 88.3)

The splenic vein is formed by five or six tributaries emerging from the hilum of the spleen. It is actually formed within the splenorenal ligament close to the tip of the tail of the pancreas. The splenic vein tributaries are thin walled and often spread over several centimetres as the hilum is long and thin (**Fig. 88.1**). This is important during surgical removal of the spleen since the venous tributaries must be divided close to the hilum to avoid injury to the pancreatic tail. They should be ligated in several groups to prevent the risk of avulsion of the veins from the splenic hilum and profuse bleeding, before the resection is complete.

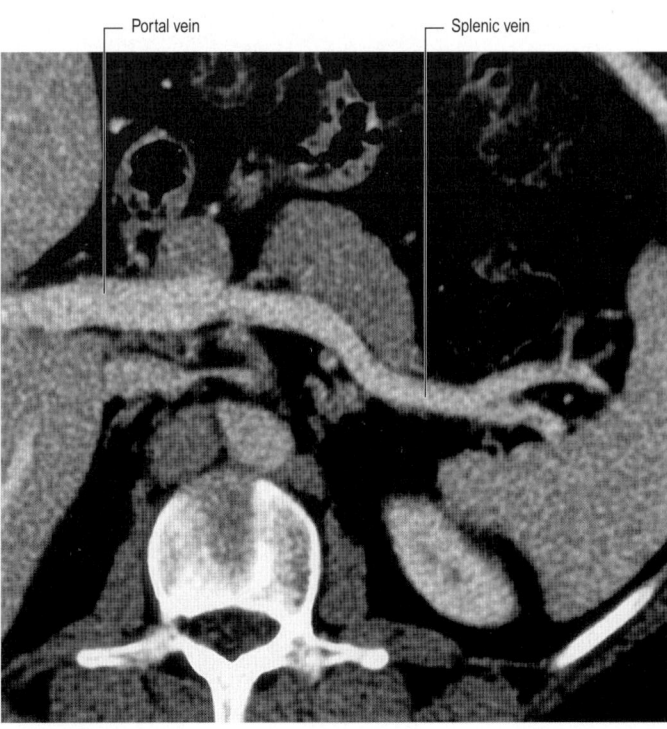

Fig. 88.3 Axial oblique CT slice of the portal vein and splenic vein.

The splenic vein runs in the splenorenal ligament below the splenic artery and posterior to the tail of the pancreas. It descends to the right, and crosses the posterior abdominal wall inferior to the splenic artery and posterior to the body of the pancreas. It receives numerous short tributaries from the gland. It crosses anterior to the left kidney and renal hilum. It is separated from the left sympathetic trunk and left crus of the diaphragm by the left renal vessels, and from the abdominal aorta by the superior mesenteric artery and left renal vein. It ends behind the neck of the pancreas, where it joins the superior mesenteric vein to form the portal vein. The short gastric and left gastro-epiploic veins drain into the splenic vein through the folds of the gastrosplenic ligament near its origin (p. 1149).

LYMPHATICS

Lymphatic vessels drain along the splenic trabeculae to pass out of the hilum into the lymphatic vessels accompanying the splenic artery and vein. The vessels run posterior to pancreas close to the splenic artery and drain into nodes at the hilum, along the splenic artery and into the coeliac nodes.

INNERVATION

The spleen is innervated by the splenic plexus. This is formed by branches of the coeliac plexus, left coeliac ganglion, and right vagus. It accompanies the splenic artery. The fibres are mainly sympathetic and terminate in blood vessels and non-striated muscle of the splenic capsule and trabeculae. These fibres appear to be mainly noradrenergic vasomotor, concerned with the regulation of blood flow through the spleen. Adrenergic agonists inhibit the concentration of red cells in the splenic blood (so called 'plasma skimming') indicating that sympathetic activity causes an increase in the 'fast' circulation of the spleen as opposed to slow filtration (p. 1244) (Reilly 1985).

REFERRED PAIN

The majority of the sensation of pain arising from the pulp of the spleen is poorly localized. In common with other structures of foregut origin, it is referred to the central epigastrium. Distension of the splenic capsule stretches the parietal layers of the peritoneum and produces pain localized to the posterior left upper quadrant.

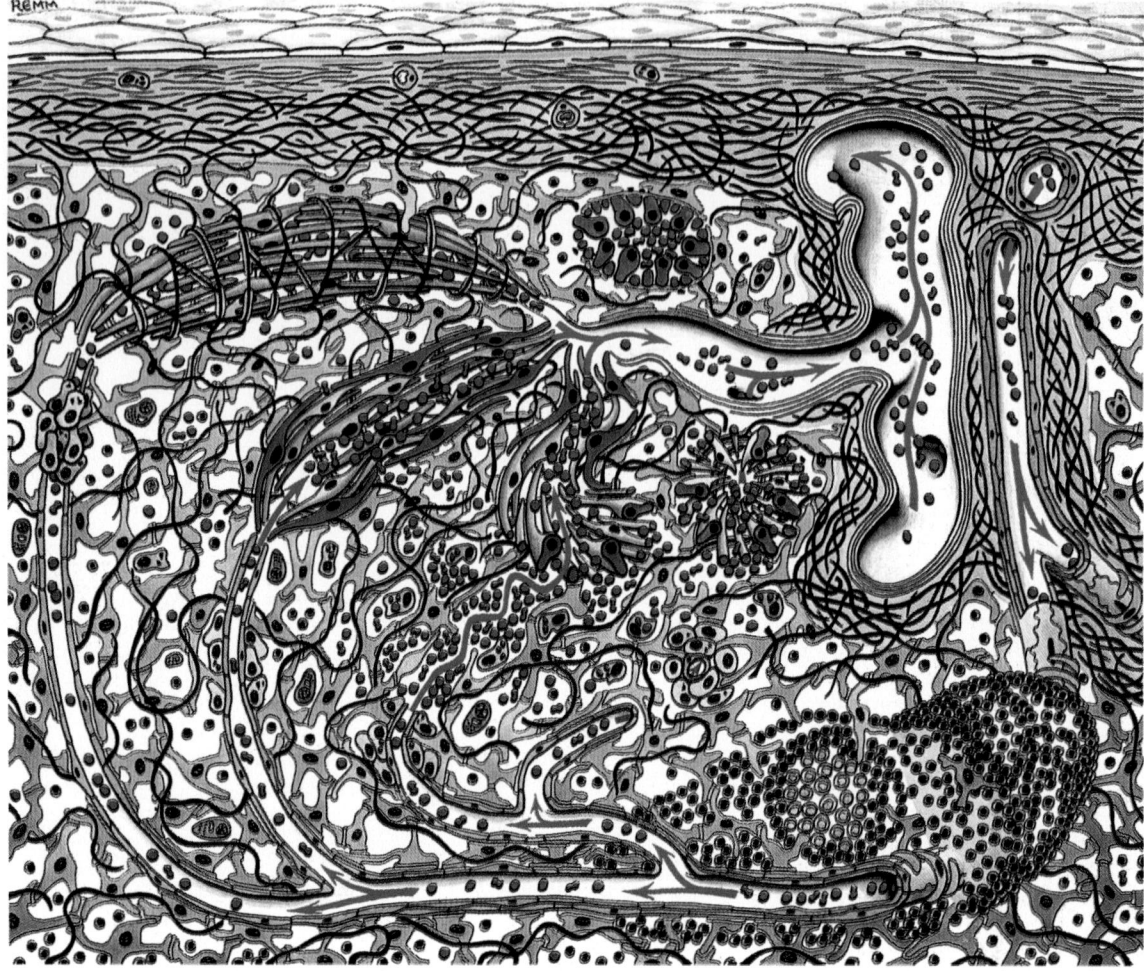

Fig. 88.4 The main features of splenic structure, not to scale. Shown are the capsule, trabeculae, reticular fibres and cells, the perivascular lymphoid sheaths and follicles (white pulp), and the cellular cords and venous sinusoids of the red pulp. The 'open' and 'closed' theories of splenic circulation are illustrated, although it is likely that most of the circulation is of the open form. The venous sinusoids are lined by specialized 'stave' cells (blue) with their intercellular gaps over-emphasized for clarity.

MICROSTRUCTURE (Figs 88.4, 88.5, 88.6, 88.7)

The spleen is essentially concerned with phagocytosis and immune responses. In the fetus it is also an important site of haemopoiesis. Postnatally it may become haemopoietic in certain pathological conditions. Although important to the defence of the body it is not absolutely essential since many of its functions can be assumed by the liver and by other lymphoid tissues if the spleen is removed.

Microscopically, the parenchymal tissue of the spleen consists of two major components, known as white pulp and red pulp, from their appearance when a fresh spleen is transected. The white pulp is composed of lymphoid tissue (p. 74) in which B and T lymphocytes mature and proliferate under antigenic stimulation. The red pulp is a unique

Fig. 88.5 A section through the spleen. White pulp is present as ovoid areas of basophilic tissue, many with germinal centres (GC) due to the high density of lymphocytes surrounding splenic arterioles (periarteriolar lymphoid sheaths, PALS). Arterioles derive from trabecular arteries (TA). Paler areas within the white pulp are germinal centres. Red pulp (RP) lies between white pulp tissue and consists of splenic sinusoids and intervening cellular cords. Part of the capsule is seen top right. (By permission from Dr JB Kerr, Monash University, from Kerr JB 1999 Atlas of Functional Histology. London: Mosby.)

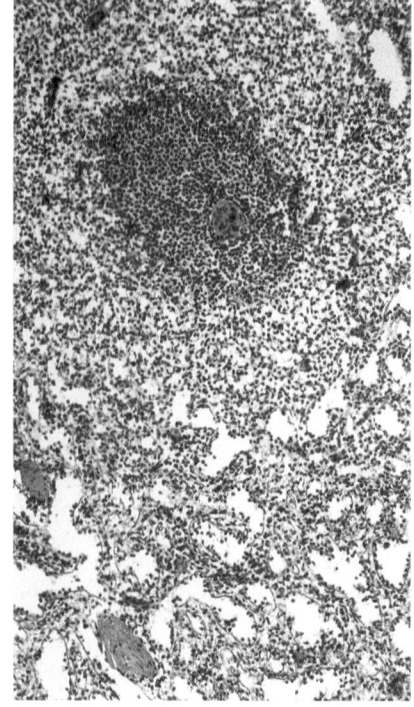

Fig. 88.6 Medium power view of the junctional zone between the densely packed lymphocytes of white pulp (top), surrounding a small eccentrically placed penicillar arteriole, and the open sinusoids and cellular cords of red pulp, below. A section of fibromuscular trabecular tissue (pink) is seen at the bottom left of the field. (Photograph by Sarah-Jane Smith.)

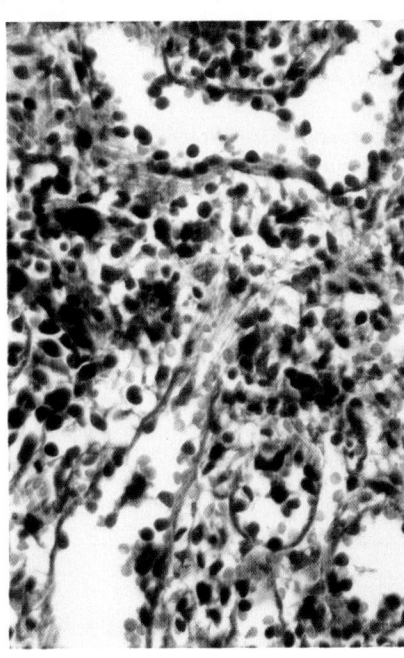

Fig. 88.7 High power micrograph of spleen, trichrome-stained, showing splenic sinusoids (open spaces) in red pulp and cellular cords in between. One sinusoid is sectioned tangentially through its wall to show, centre field, the fine parallel strap-like endothelial stave cells. The nuclei of stave cells lining transversely sectioned sinusoids bulge into the lumen, which also contains migratory lymphocytes and erythrocytes re-entering the circulation. Numerous orange erythrocytes are also seen outside the circulation, within the splenic cords, which are populated by macrophages. (Photograph by Sarah-Jane Smith.)

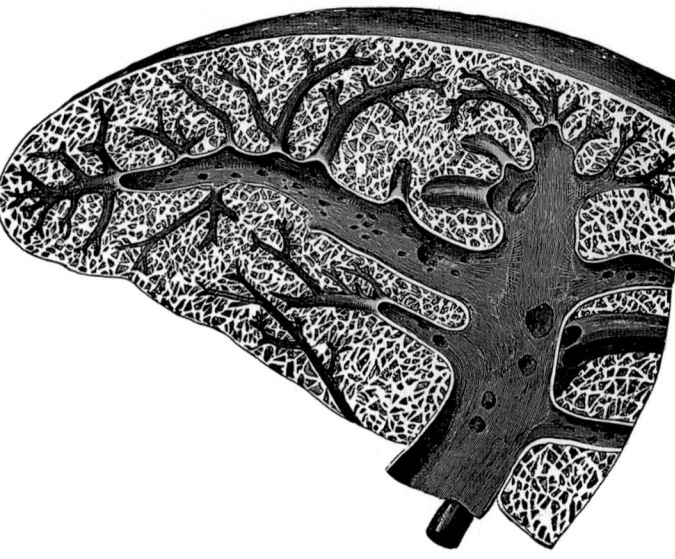

Fig. 88.8 Transverse section through the spleen, showing the trabecular tissue and the splenic vein and its tributaries (from the first edition of Gray's Anatomy, 1858). (From the first edition of Gray's Anatomy, 1858.)

filtration device with which the spleen clears particulate material from the blood as it perfuses the spleen. Red pulp is composed of a complex system of interconnected spaces populated by large numbers of phagocytic macrophages (p. 80). These cells remove effete red blood cells, microorganisms, cellular debris and other particulate matter from the circulation.

FIBROUS FRAMEWORK OF THE SPLEEN

The serosa of the peritoneum covers the entire organ except at its hilum and along the lines of reflexion of the splenorenal and gastrosplenic ligaments. Deep to this layer is the connective tissue capsule, a continuous layer c.1.5 mm thick, containing abundant collagen (type I) but also some elastin fibres. The capsule has an outer and an inner lamina in which the directions of collagen fibres differ, increasing its strength. Numerous trabeculae extend from the capsule into the substance of the spleen, branching within it to form a supportive framework. The largest trabeculae enter at the hilum and provide a conduit for the splenic vessels and nerves, dividing into branches in the splenic pulp (**Figs 88.4, 88.8**). Within the spleen, branching trabeculae are continuous with a delicate network of fine collagen (type III, reticular) fibres pervading both the white and red pulp, which is laid down by numerous fibroblasts present in its meshes.

WHITE PULP (Fig. 88.6)

In the spleen parenchyma, branches of the splenic artery radiate out from the hilum within trabeculae, ramifying and narrowing to arterioles. In their terminal few millimetres, their connective tissue adventitia is replaced by a sheath of T-lymphocytes, the periarteriolar lymphatic sheath (PALS). This sheath is enlarged in places by lymphoid follicles (p. 74), which are aggregations of B lymphocytes visible to the naked eye on the freshly cut spleen surface as white semi-opaque dots, 0.25–1 mm in diameter, which contrast with the surrounding deep reddish-purple of the red pulp. Follicles are usually situated near the terminal branches of arterioles and typically protrude to one side of the vessel, which therefore appears eccentrically placed within the follicle. Arterioles branch laterally within follicles to form a series of parallel terminal arterioles – called penicilli, or penicillar arterioles, from their resemblance to the penicillium mould.

Like the periarteriolar sheaths, follicles are centres of lymphocyte proliferation as well as aggregation, and when antigenically stimulated, the white pulp increases in size as lymphocytes proliferate. The primary follicles become intensely active in B-cell proliferation, and they develop germinal centres, as are found in lymph nodes (p. 75). The presentation of antigen by follicular dendritic cells (p. 81) is involved in this process. The germinal centres regress when the infection subsides. Follicles generally atrophy with increasing age and may be absent in the very elderly.

RED PULP (Figs 88.4, 88.7)

The red pulp constitutes the majority (75%) of the total splenic volume. Within it lie large numbers of venous sinusoids which drain into tributaries of the major splenic veins. The sinusoids are separated from each other by a fibrocellular network, the reticulum, formed by numerous reticular fibroblasts, and small bundles of delicate collagen type III fibres, in the meshes of which lie splenic macrophages. Seen in two-dimensional sections, these intersinusoidal regions appear as strips of tissue, the splenic cords, which alternate with splenic sinuses (**Figs 88.4, 88.7**). In reality they form a three-dimensional continuum around the venous spaces.

Venous sinusoids

Venous sinusoids are elongated ovoid vessels c.50 µm in diameter, lined by a characteristic, 'incomplete' endothelium unique to the spleen. The endothelial cells are long and narrow, aligned with the long axis of the sinusoid – for this reason they are often called stave cells, reminiscent of planks in a barrel (**Figs 88.4, 88.7**). They are attached at intervals along their length to their neighbours by short stretches of intercellular junctions which alternate with intercellular slits through which blood can pass. A perforated, discontinuous basal lamina is present on the aspect of the sinus facing away from the lumen. The presence of slits between the endothelial cells allows blood cells to squeeze into the lumen of the sinusoid from the surrounding splenic cords. The sinusoids are supported externally by circumferential and longitudinal reticular fibres which are connected to the fibrous reticulum around them.

Reticular tissue of the splenic cords

A population of large, stellate fibroblasts, the reticular cells, lie around the sinusoids, amongst the network of collagen fibres. The flattened extensions of these cells help to divide the reticular space into a series of defined compartments containing macrophages. Reticular cells synthesize the matrix components of the reticulum, including collagen and proteoglycans. Blood is released into the reticular space from the ends of capillaries which originate from penicillar arterioles. As it percolates through the spaces within cords, macrophages are able to remove particulate material, including ageing and damaged erythrocytes, from the blood. Under conditions where there are many damaged erythrocytes in the circulation to be removed by splenic macrophages, the reticular cells proliferate and increase the size of the red pulp considerably, thus causing enlargement of the whole spleen, and in extreme cases, splenomegaly.

MARGINAL ZONE

The marginal zone lies at the interface between the white and red pulp. It is a region of great importance to the function of the spleen. Here the lymphocytes are more loosely arranged than in the white pulp, and are held in a dense network of reticular fibres and cells. The arterioles leaving the white pulp are surrounded by a small aggregation of macrophages, the periarteriolar macrophage sheath. The marginal zone is a region where blood is delivered into the red pulp, and also where many lymphocytes leave the circulation to migrate into their respective T- and B-lymphocyte areas of the white pulp.

SPLENIC MICROCIRCULATION (Fig. 88.4)

The segmental splenic arteries enter the hilum and ramify in the trabeculae throughout the organ. The splenic vein forms in the ligament from an equal number of tributaries emerging from the hilum. Small arteries tapering to arterioles pass through the white pulp then turn abruptly to form penicillar branches which, after a course of c.0.5 mm, pass out of the white pulp into the marginal zone and red pulp. The passage of blood through the vascular compartments between the arterioles and splenic veins is referred to collectively as the intermediate circulation of the spleen. Ultimately, blood is passed to the venous sinusoids from which it enters venules leading to small veins – running within trabeculae – and thence into larger veins draining the spleen at its hilum.

Open and closed splenic circulations

Views on the intermediate circulation of the spleen differ on whether blood passes from the arterioles (or their terminal capillaries) directly into the venous sinuses (a closed circulation), or is instead discharged into a network of spaces in the splenic cords before entering the sinuses through the minute slits in their walls (an open circulation). In humans, evidence favours the presence of an anatomically and physiologically open circulation, in which blood percolates slowly through the reticular tissue of the splenic cords and filters through slits in the sinus walls before joining the majority of the blood flow. There is thought to be an additional closed vascular route but this is likely to provide only a minor contribution to splenic circulation; however, this has not been determined conclusively.

REFERENCE ‹H7.18.7›

Reilly FD 1985 Innervation and vascular pharmacodynamics of the mammalian spleen. Experientia 41: 187–92.

Suprarenal (adrenal) gland (Figs 89.1, 89.2)

The suprarenal (adrenal) glands lie immediately superior and slightly anterior to the upper pole of either kidney. Golden yellow in colour, each gland possesses two functionally and structurally distinct areas: an outer cortex and an inner medulla. The glands are surrounded by connective tissue containing perinephric fat and they are enclosed within the renal fascia. They are separated from the kidneys by a small amount of fibrous tissue. In the adult the glands measure c.50 mm vertically, 30 mm transversely and 10 mm anteroposteriorly. They each weigh c.5 g (the medulla being about one-tenth of the total weight). The dimensions of the suprarenal glands *in vivo* have been defined by Vincent and colleagues (1994) using computed tomography (CT). The mean dimensions of the body of the suprarenal gland are 0.61 cm (right) and 0.79 cm (left). The mean dimensions of suprarenal limbs are 0.28 cm (right) and 0.33 cm (left). No individual suprarenal limb should measure more than 6.5 mm across.

The glands are macroscopically slightly different in external appearance (**Fig. 89.1**). The right gland is pyramidal in shape and has two well-developed lower projections (limbs) giving a cross-sectional appearance similar to a broad-headed arrow. The left gland has a more semilunar form and is flattened in the anteroposterior plane. The left gland is marginally larger than the right. The bulk of the right suprarenal sits on the apex of the right kidney and usually lies slightly higher than the left gland, which sits on the anteromedial aspect of the upper pole of the left kidney.

At birth the glands are comparatively larger and are approximately one-third the size of the ipsilateral kidney. The cortex of each gland reduces in size immediately after birth and the medulla grows comparatively little. By the end of the second month the weight of the suprarenal has reduced by 50%. The glands begin to grow by the end of the second year and regain their weight at birth by puberty. There is little further weight increase in adult life.

Small accessory suprarenal glands composed mainly of cortical tissue may occur in the areolar tissue near the main suprarenal glands. Accessory glands, cortical bodies, may also occur in the spermatic cord, epididymis and broad ligament of the uterus.

A. Anterior aspect

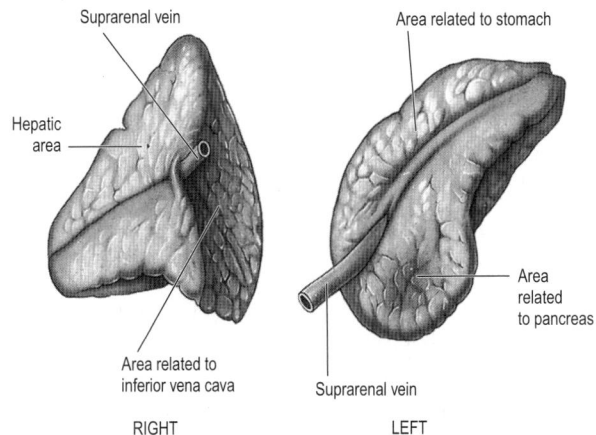

B. Posterior aspect

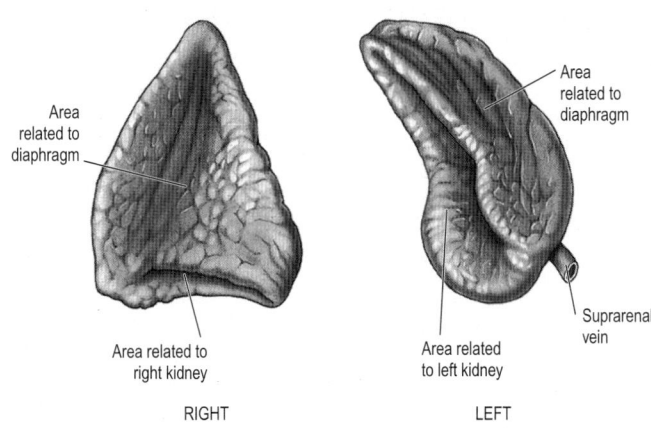

Fig. 89.1 Suprarenal glands: anterior (**A**) and posterior (**B**) aspects.

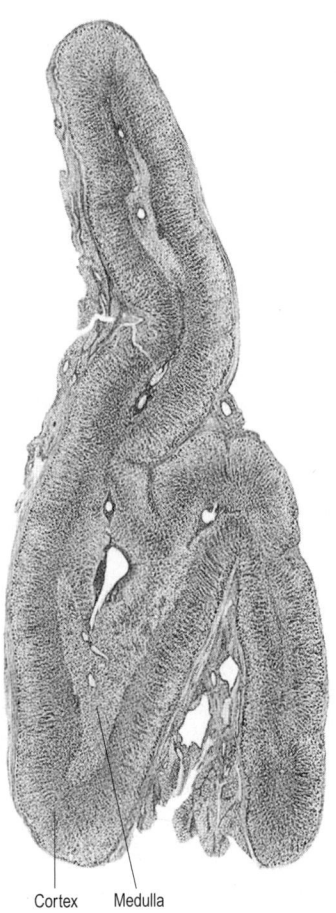

Fig. 89.2 Vertical section through a whole adult human suprarenal gland.

1245

RIGHT SUPRARENAL GLAND (Fig. 89.3)

The right suprarenal gland lies posterior to the inferior vena cava from which it is only separated by a thin layer of fascia and connective tissue. It is posterior to the right lobe of the liver and lies anterior to the right crus of the diaphragm and superior pole of the right kidney (**Fig. 89.3**). Its inferior surface is referred to as the base and adjoins the anterosuperior aspect of the superior pole of the right kidney. It often overlaps the apex of the upper pole of the right kidney as the two lower projections (limbs) straddle the renal tissue. The anterior surface faces slightly laterally and possesses two distinct facets. The medial facet is somewhat narrow, runs vertically and lies posterior to the inferior vena cava. The lateral facet is triangular and lies in contact with the bare area of the liver. The lowest part of the anterior surface may be covered by peritoneum, reflected onto it from the inferior layer of the coronary ligament. At this point it may lie posterior to the lateral border of the second part of the duodenum. Below the apex, near the anterior border of the gland, the hilum lies in a short sulcus from which the right suprarenal vein emerges to join the inferior vena cava. This vein is particularly short and makes surgical resection of the gland potentially hazardous, because ligation may be difficult. The vein may be avulsed from the inferior vena cava during surgery or occasionally by high-energy deceleration injuries. The posterior surface is divided into upper and lower areas by a curved transverse ridge. The large upper area is slightly convex and rests on the diaphragm. The small lower area is concave and lies in contact with the superior aspect of the upper pole of the right kidney. The medial border of the gland is thin and lies lateral to the right coeliac ganglion and the right inferior phrenic artery as the artery runs over the right crus of the diaphragm.

LEFT SUPRARENAL GLAND

The left suprarenal gland lies closely applied to the left crus of the diaphragm and is separated from it only by a thin layer of fascia and connective tissue (**Fig. 89.3**). The medial aspect is convex whilst the lateral aspect is concave since it is shaped by the medial side of the superior pole of the left kidney. The superior border is sharply defined while the inferior surface is more rounded. The anterior surface has a large superior area covered by peritoneum on the posterior wall of the lesser sac, which separates it from the cardia of the stomach and sometimes from the posterior aspect of the spleen. The smaller inferior area is not covered by peritoneum and lies in contact with the pancreas and splenic artery. The hilum faces inferiorly from the medial aspect and is near the lower part of the anterior surface. The left suprarenal vein emerges from the hilum and runs inferomedially to join the left renal vein. The posterior surface is divided by a ridge into a lateral area adjoining the kidney and a smaller medial area which lies in contact with the left crus of the diaphragm. The convex medial border lies lateral to the left coeliac ganglion and the left inferior phrenic and left gastric arteries, which ascend on the left crus of the diaphragm.

SUPRARENAL GLAND EXCISION

Removal of one or both suprarenal glands may be performed either through 'open surgery' or via a laparoscopic approach. There are essentially three 'open surgical' methods for removing the suprarenal glands. The posterior and lateral approaches involve removal of either the eleventh or twelfth ribs. The surgeon remains in the retroperitoneal plane and accesses the gland via the perirenal fat. This approach can be performed laparoscopically, but is difficult: landmarks are not easily identified because of the surrounding fat and the 'workspace' is frequently small. Not surprisingly, few surgeons employ this approach.

During laparoscopic surgery the anterior, transperitoneal approach is most commonly used. The patient is placed in the lateral decubitus position. On the left side, the splenic flexure is mobilized inferiorly revealing the kidney. The lateral phrenicocolic ligament is then fully divided allowing the spleen to be mobilized medially and exposing the splenorenal ligament. Division of the splenorenal ligament with the patient in the lateral decubitus position allows the spleen to 'drop' medially exposing the plane between the splenic hilum and medial border of the left kidney. Here the pancreatic tail is identified as it runs to the hilum of the spleen. The renal fascia is divided to expose the suprarenal gland lying over the superomedial aspect of the upper pole of the kidney. On the right side, the right triangular ligament of the liver is divided. This allows the liver to be retracted caudally. In most individuals the inferior vena cava is easily identified behind the peritoneum lateral to the second part of the duodenum. The peritoneal reflection on the inferior border of the liver is divided from the inferior vena cava to the lateral border of the liver. This exposes the suprarenal gland in the angle between the inferior vena cava and liver. The peritoneal reflection along the lateral aspect of the inferior vena cava is divided and the gland is then mobilized laterally exposing the suprarenal vein, which often emerges from the posterior aspect of the inferior vena cava. Once the suprarenal vein is divided the small middle suprarenal arteries running from the aorta behind the cava to the gland are easily identified. The gland is then usually mobilized very easily in a lateral direction. However, the gland can lie either behind the inferior vena cava or under the liver, in which case dissection at the junction of the liver and inferior vena cava often becomes very difficult.

In obese (or Cushingoid) patients, identification of a relatively normal size suprarenal gland can be extremely difficult and time consuming. The suprarenal vein emerges from the lower medial border of the gland and it is often a very substantial structure. In contrast, the supplying arteries tend to be rather smaller in size and individual arteries are often difficult to identify during surgery.

The anterior open approach follows the procedure as described above through either a subcostal or a midline incision.

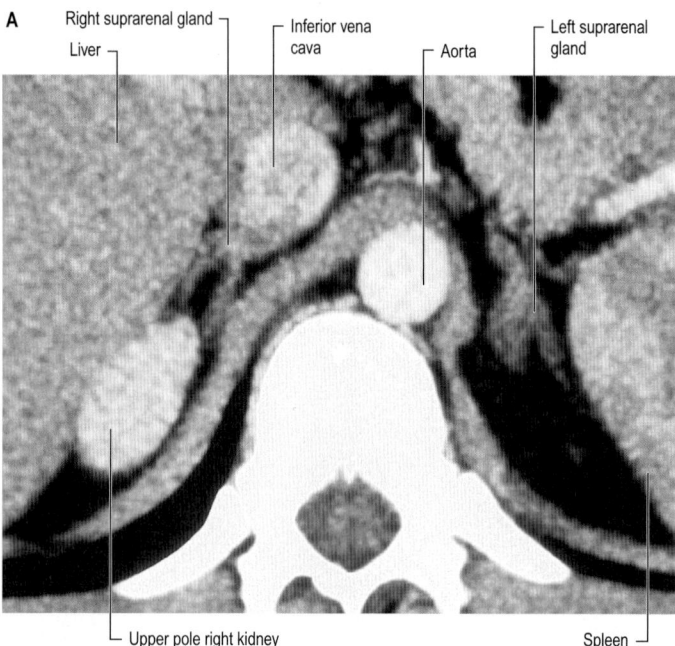

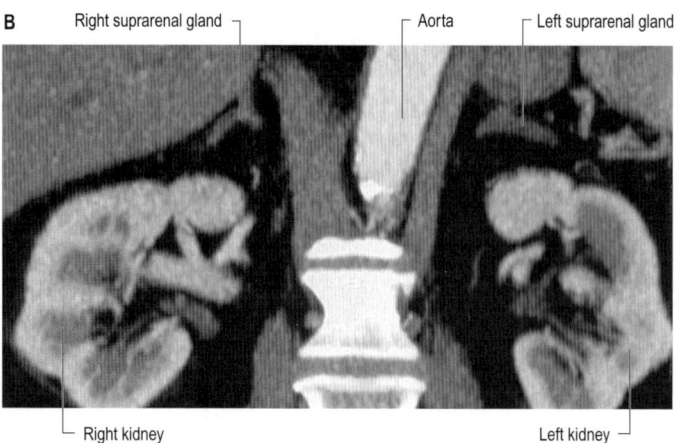

Fig. 89.3 **A**, Axial and **B**, coronal multislice CT scans of the right and left suprarenal glands.

VASCULAR SUPPLY AND LYMPHATIC DRAINAGE

ARTERIES

The suprarenal glands are very vascular. Each gland is supplied by superior, middle and inferior suprarenal arteries, whose main branches may be duplicated or even multiple. They ramify over the capsule before entering the gland to form a subcapsular plexus, from which fenestrated sinusoids pass around clustered glomerulosal cells and between columns in the zona fasciculata to a deep plexus in the zona reticularis. From this plexus venules pass between medullary chromaffin cells to medullary veins, which they enter between prominent bundles of smooth muscle fibres. Some relatively large arteries bypass this indirect route and pass directly to the medulla (see **Fig. 89.5**).

Superior suprarenal arteries

The superior suprarenal artery arises from the inferior phrenic artery, which is a branch of the abdominal aorta (p. 1119). It is often small and may be absent.

Middle suprarenal arteries (See also p. 1247)

The middle suprarenal artery arises from the lateral aspect of the abdominal aorta, at the level of the superior mesenteric artery. It ascends slightly and runs over the crura of the diaphragm to the suprarenal glands, where it anastomoses with the suprarenal branches of the inferior phrenic and renal arteries. The right middle suprarenal artery passes behind the inferior vena cava and near the right coeliac ganglion. It is frequently multiple. The left middle suprarenal artery passes close to the left coeliac ganglion, splenic artery and the superior border of the pancreas.

Inferior suprarenal arteries

The inferior suprarenal arteries arise from the renal arteries (p. 1118), usually from the main renal artery but occasionally from its upper pole branches.

VEINS

Medullary veins emerge from the hilum to form a suprarenal vein, which is usually single. The right vein is very short, passing directly and horizontally into the posterior aspect of the inferior vena cava. An accessory vein is occasionally present and runs from the hilum superomedially to join the inferior vena cava above the right suprarenal vein. The left suprarenal vein descends medially, anterior and lateral to the left coeliac ganglion. It passes posterior to the pancreatic body and drains into the left renal vein. Since the venous drainage from each gland is usually via a single vein, damage to a suprarenal vein is more likely to cause infarction of that gland than damage to one of the suprarenal arteries.

LYMPHATIC DRAINAGE

Small lymphatic channels from both cortex and medulla drain to the hilum where larger calibre lymphatics emerge to drain directly into the lateral groups of para-aortic nodes (p. 1123).

INNERVATION

SUPRARENAL PLEXUS

The suprarenal gland, relative to its size, has a larger autonomic supply than any other organ. The suprarenal plexus on each side lies between the medial aspect of the glands and the coeliac and aorticorenal ganglia. It contains mostly preganglionic sympathetic fibres which originate in the lower thoracic spinal segments and which reach the plexus via branches from the coeliac ganglion and plexus, and via the greater splanchnic nerve. These fibres synapse, often in deep invaginations, with large medullary chromaffin cells, which may thus be considered as homologous with postganglionic sympathetic neurones. A preponderance of non-myelinated axons has been described in the human suprarenal plexus.

Both cortex and medulla also contain acetylcholinesterase (AChE)-positive fibres which presumably reach the gland from the coeliac plexus: some synapse with ganglion cells in the zonae fasciculata and reticularis.

MICROSTRUCTURE

In section, the suprarenal gland has an outer cortex, which is yellowish in colour and forms the main mass, and a thin medulla, forming about one-tenth of the gland, which is dark red or greyish, depending on its content of blood (**Fig. 89.2**). The medulla is completely enclosed by cortex, except at the hilum. The gland has a thick collagenous capsule, which extends deep trabeculae into the cortex. The capsule contains a rich arterial plexus which supplies branches to the gland.

SUPRARENAL CORTEX (Figs 89.4, 89.5)

The suprarenal cortex consists of the zona glomerulosa, zona fasciculata and zona reticularis (**Figs 89.4, 89.5**). The outer subcapsular zona glomerulosa consists of a narrow region of small polyhedral cells in rounded clusters. The cells have deeply staining nuclei and a basophilic cytoplasm containing a few lipid droplets. Ultrastructurally, the cytoplasm displays abundant smooth endoplasmic reticulum, which is typical of cells which synthesize steroids. Deep to this, the broader zona fasciculata consists of large polyhedral basophilic cells arranged in straight columns, two cells wide, with parallel fenestrated venous sinusoids between them. The cells contain many lipid droplets and large amounts of smooth endoplasmic reticulum. The innermost part of the cortex, the zona reticularis, consists of branching interconnected columns of rounded cells whose cytoplasm also contains smooth endoplasmic reticulum, many lysosomes and aggregates of brown lipofuscin pigment which accumulate with age.

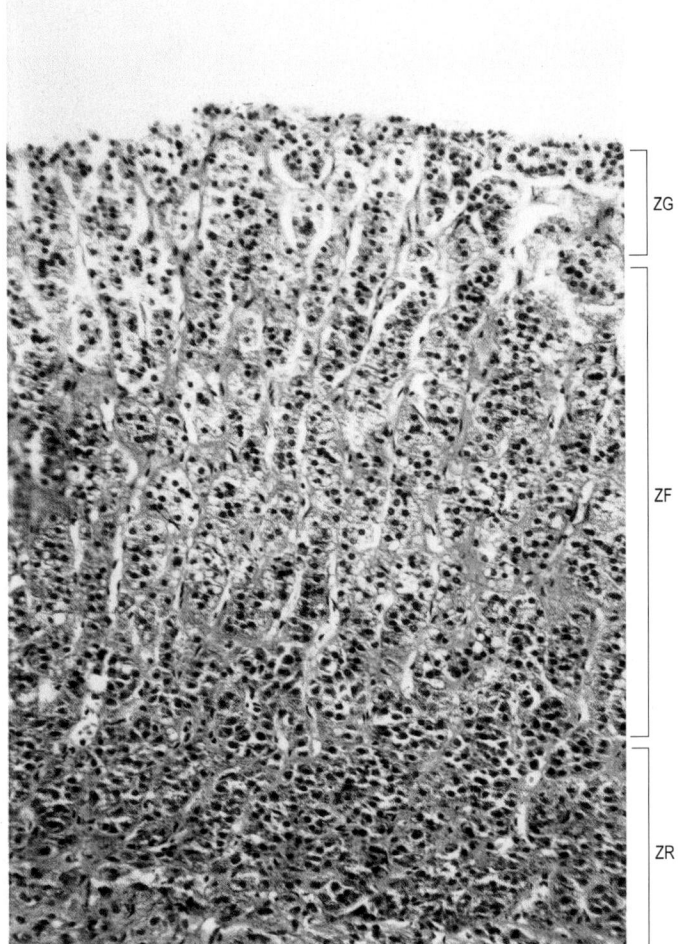

Fig. 89.4 Cortex of the suprarenal gland. Beneath the capsule (top, absent from this specimen) is the thin zona glomerulosa (ZG), then the zona fasciculata (ZF) which occupies much of the cortex, and innermost, the zona reticularis (ZR). Sinusoids (clear spaces) and a delicate connective tissue (green) surround groups of endocrine cells, defining the organization of cells in the three functional zones. (Photograph by Sarah-Jane Smith.)

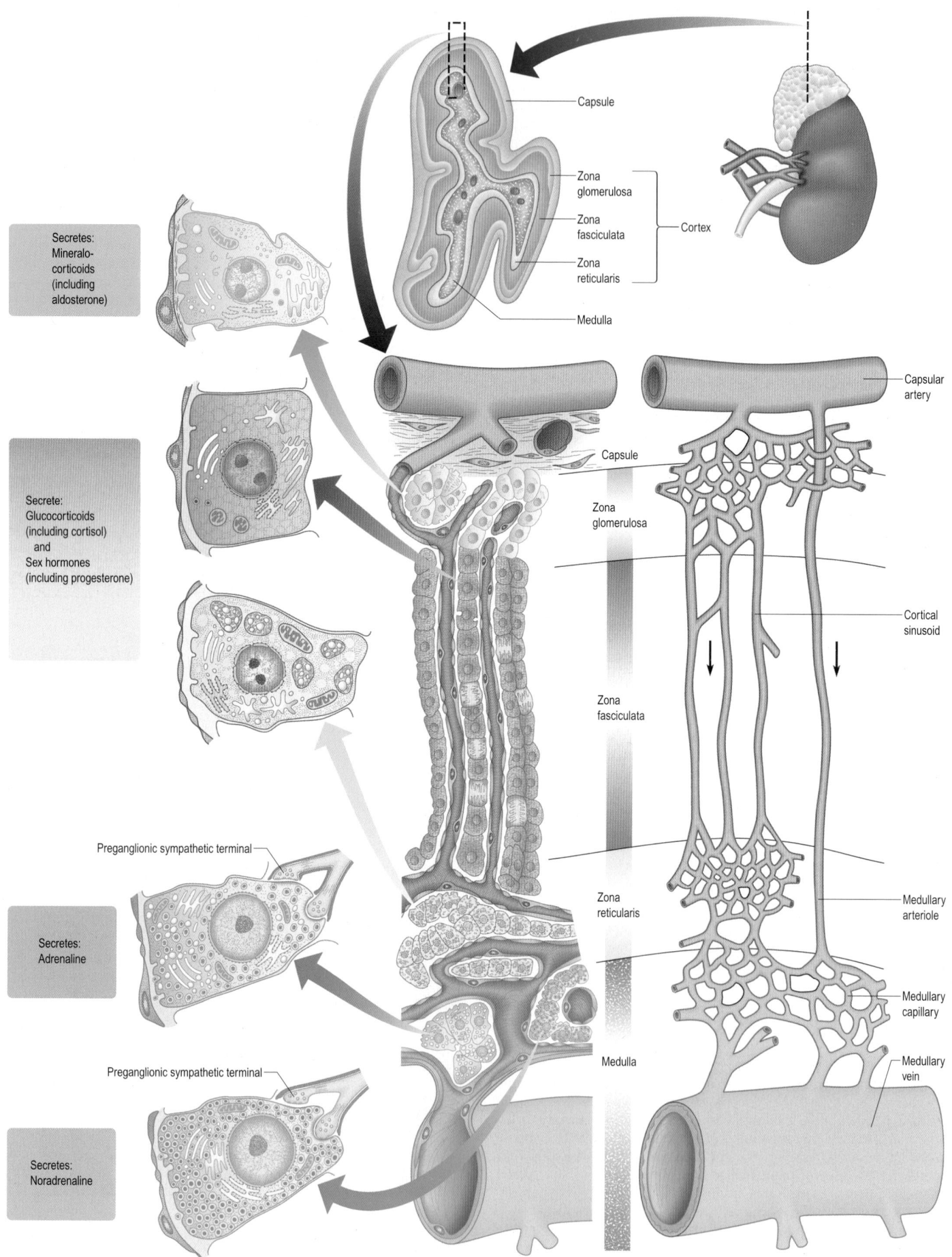

Fig. 89.5 The gross sectional appearance, microstructure, vasculature and ultrastructure of the suprarenal gland. Brief functional summaries are appended.

Cortical cells produce several hormones and the cells of the zonae fasciculata and reticularis are also rich in ascorbic acid. Cells in the zona glomerulosa produce mineralocorticoids, e.g. aldosterone, which regulates electrolyte and water balance; cells in the zona fasciculata produce hormones maintaining carbohydrate balance (glucocorticoids) e.g. cortisol (hydrocortisone); cells in the zona reticularis produce sex hormones (progesterone, oestrogens and androgens). The cortex is essential to life; complete removal is lethal without replacement therapy. It exerts considerable control over lymphocytes and lymphoid tissue: increase in secretion of corticosteroids can result in a marked reduction in lymphocyte numbers.

The deeper part of the zona fasciculata widens in pregnancy and in women of childbearing age in summer. Cortical atrophy in elderly males is greatest in the same region.

SUPRARENAL MEDULLA (Fig. 89.6)

The suprarenal medulla is composed of groups and columns of chromaffin cells (phaeochromocytes) separated by wide venous sinusoids and supported by a network of reticular fibres. Chromaffin cells, so-called from their colour reaction to dichromate fixatives, form part of the neuroendocrine system (p. 180) and are functionally equivalent to postganglionic sympathetic neurones. They are neural crest derivatives (p. 244) and synthesize, store (as granules), and release the catecholamines noradrenaline (norepinephrine) and adrenaline (epinephrine) into the venous sinusoids. Release is under preganglionic sympathetic control; single or small groups of sympathetic neurons are found in the medulla.

The majority of chromaffin cells synthesize adrenaline and store it in small granules with a dense core. Less numerous noradrenaline-secreting cells have larger granules with a dense eccentric core. Some cells synthesize both hormones. Chromogranin proteins package catecholamines within the granules, which also contain enkephalins, opiate-like proteins that may have endogenous analgesic effects in some circumstances. All of the cells are large, with large nuclei and

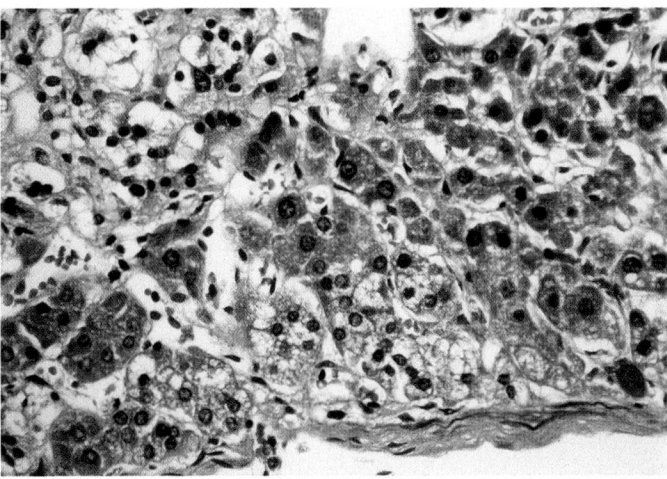

Fig. 89.6 Section through the medulla of the suprarenal gland (trichrome-stained), showing large deeply staining chromaffin cells and a nerve fibre bundle (stained green, below). (Photograph by Sarah-Jane Smith.)

basophilic, faintly granular cytoplasm. They form single rows along the venous sinusoids. Sympathetic axon terminals synapse with the chromaffin cells on their surfaces which face away from the sinusoids (**Fig. 89.5**).

The sinusoids, which are lined by fenestrated endothelium, drain to the central medullary vein and hilar suprarenal vein. Normally, little adrenaline or noradrenaline is released but in response to fear, anger or stress, secretion is increased. Unlike the cortex, the suprarenal medulla is not essential to life.

REFERENCE

Vincent JM, Morrison ID, Armstrong P, Reznek RH 1994 The size of normal adrenal glands on computed tomography. Clin Radiol 49: 453–55.

Development of the peritoneal cavity, the gastrointestinal tract and its adnexae

Chapter

90

POSTPHARYNGEAL FOREGUT

The postdiaphragmatic gut is subdivided into three embryological portions: fore- mid- and hindgut, but there are no corresponding fundamental morphological and cytological distinctions between the three parts (**Fig. 90.1**). Thus the foregut produces a portion of the duodenum as does the midgut, and the midgut similarly produces large intestine, as does the hindgut. The differences between portions of the gut develop as a result of interactions between the three embryonic tissue layers which give rise to the gut, namely the endodermal inner epithelium, the thick layer of splanchnopleuric mesenchyme, and the outer layer of proliferating splanchnopleuric coelomic epithelium.

The epithelial layer of the mucosa and connected ducts and glands are derived from the endodermal epithelium. The lamina propria and muscularis mucosa, the connective tissue of the submucosa, the muscularis externa and the external connective tissue are all derived from the splanchnopleuric mesenchyme. The outer peritoneal epithelium is derived from the splanchnopleuric coelomic epithelium.

Throughout the gut, blood vessels, lymphatics and lymph nodes develop from local populations of angiogenic mesenchyme. The nerves, which are distributed within the enteric and autonomic systems, are derived from the neural crest (p. 254). There is a craniocaudal develop-

mental gradient along the gut in that the stomach and small intestine develop in advance of the colon.

Fig. 90.2A,B shows the gut in a stage 12 embryo in relation to the other developing viscera, especially the heart and liver. **Fig. 90.3** shows the overall development of the gut from stages 13–17. These diagrams should be compared. **Fig. 90.1** shows the fundamental relationship of the intraembryonic coelom to the developing gut.

All regions of the gut develop from epithelial/mesenchymal interactions which are dependent on the sequential expression of a range of basic and specific genes; on the regulation of the developmental clock, seen in all areas of development; on endogenous regulatory mechanisms and local environmental influences (Lebenthal 1989). Although all these factors pertain to the whole range of developing tissues, local differences in any one of these factors along the length of the developing gut promotes the differentiation of, for example, the gastric mucosa and hepatocytes; the rotation of the midgut; and the final disposition of the sessile portions of the fully formed gastrointestinal tract. The gut is functional prior to birth and able to interact with the extrauterine environment in preterm infants.

OESOPHAGUS

The oesophagus can be distinguished from the stomach at stage 13 (embryo 5 mm). It elongates during successive stages and its absolute length increases more rapidly than the embryo as a whole. Cranially it is invested by splanchnopleuric mesenchyme posterior to the developing trachea, and more caudally between the developing lungs and pericardio-peritoneal canals posterior to the pericardium (for details of tracheo-oesophageal fistulae see p. 1091). Caudal to the pericardium, the terminal, pregastric segment of the oesophagus has a short thick dorsal meso-oesophagus (from splanchnopleuric mesenchyme), while ventrally it is enclosed in the cranial stratum of the septum transversum mesenchyme. Each of the above are continuous caudally with their respective primitive dorsal and ventral mesogastria (p. 1254). Thus the oesophagus has only limited areas related to a primary coelomic epithelium. However, note the subsequent development of the para-oesophageal right and left pneumatoenteric recesses (see **Fig. 90.7**), the relation of the ventral aspect of the middle third of the oesophagus to the oblique sinus of the pericardium, and the relation of its lateral walls in the lower thorax to the mediastinal pleura. All the foregoing are secondary extensions from the primary coelom.

The oesophageal mucosa consists of two layers of cells by stage 15 (week 5), but the proliferation of the mucosa does not occlude the lumen at any time. The mucosa becomes ciliated at 10 weeks, and stratified squamous epithelium is present at the end of the 5th month: occasionally patches of ciliated epithelium may be present at birth. Circular muscle can be seen at stage 15 but longitudinal muscle has not been identified until stage 21. Neuroblasts can be demonstrated in the early stages; the myenteric plexuses have cholinesterase activity by 9.5 weeks and ganglion cells are differentiated by 13 weeks. It has been suggested that the oesophagus is capable of peristalsis in the first trimester. Oesophageal atresia is one of the more common obstructive conditions of the alimentary tract: fetuses swallow amniotic fluid, and so the condition may be indicated by polyhydramnios.

Oesophagus at birth

At birth the oesophagus extends 8–10 cm from the cricoid cartilage to the gastric cardiac orifice. It starts and ends 1–2 vertebrae higher than in the adult, extending from between the fourth to the sixth cervical vertebra to the level of the ninth thoracic vertebra (**Fig. 11.5**). Its average diameter is 5 mm and it possesses the constrictions seen in the

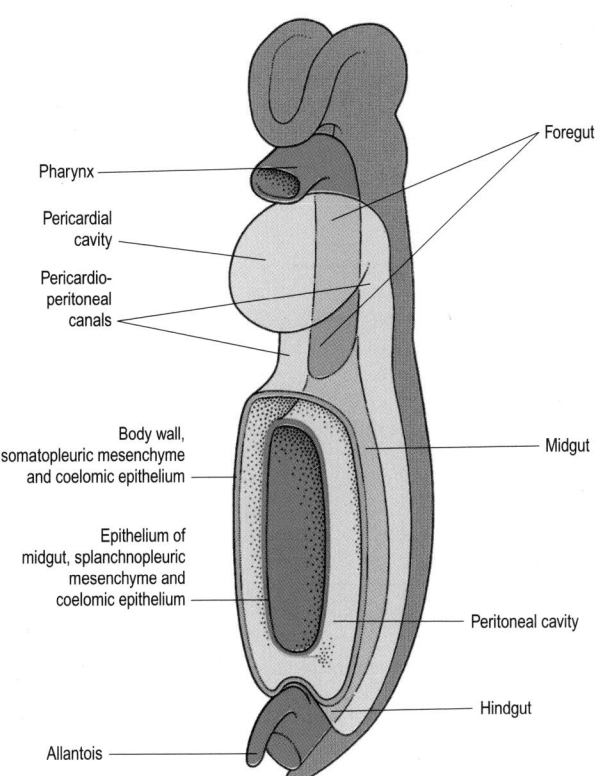

Fig. 90.1 Major epithelial populations within the early embryo. The early gut tube is close to the notochord and neural tube dorsally. The splanchnopleuric layer of the intraembryonic coelomic epithelium is in contact with the foregut ventrally and laterally, with the midgut laterally and with the hindgut ventrally and laterally.

Pharynx

Pericardial cavity

Pericardio-peritoneal canals

Body wall, somatopleuric mesenchyme and coelomic epithelium

Epithelium of midgut, splanchnopleuric mesenchyme and coelomic epithelium

Allantois

Foregut

Midgut

Peritoneal cavity

Hindgut

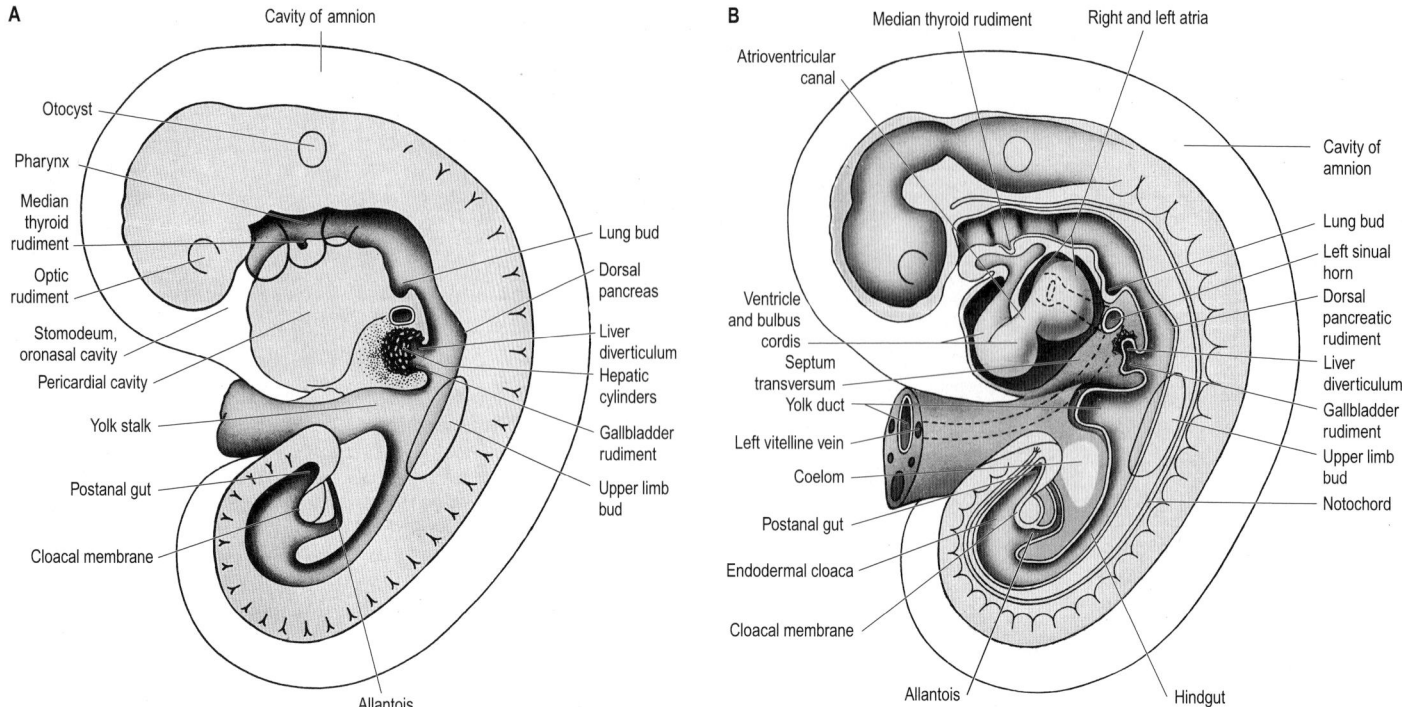

Fig. 90.2 A, The digestive tube of a human embryo at stage 12, with 29 paired somites, a CR length of 3.4 mm and an estimated age of 27 days. Note pharyngeal development. **B**, Reconstruction of a human embryo at the end of the fourth week. The alimentary canal and its outgrowths are shown in median section. The brain is shown in outline, but the spinal cord is omitted. The heart is shown in perspective, the left horn of the sinus venosus having been divided. The somites are indicated in outline. (Modified with permission from Streeter GL 1942 Developmental horizons in human embryos. Contrib Embryol Carnegie Inst Washington 30: 211–245.)

adult. The narrowest constriction is at its junction with the pharynx, where the inferior pharyngeal constrictor muscle functions to constrict the lumen: this region may be easily traumatized with instruments or catheters. In the neonate the mucosa may contain scattered areas of ciliated columnar epithelium, but these disappear soon after birth. Peristalsis along the oesophagus and at the lower oesophageal sphincter is immature at birth and results in frequent regurgitation of food in the newborn period. The pressure at the lower oesophageal sphincter approaches that of the adult at 3–6 weeks of age.

STOMACH

At the end of the fourth and beginning of the fifth week the stomach can be recognized as a fusiform dilation cranial to the wide opening of the midgut into the yolk sac (**Figs 90.2, 90.3**). By the fifth week this opening has narrowed into a tubular vitelline intestinal duct, which soon loses its connection with the digestive tube. At this stage the stomach is median in position and separated cranially from the pericardium by the septum transversum (see **Fig. 90.5**), which extends caudally on to the cranial side of the vitelline intestinal duct and ventrally to the somatopleure. Dorsally, the stomach is related to the aorta and, reflecting the presence of the pleuroperitoneal canals on each side, is connected to the body wall by a short dorsal mesentery, the dorsal mesogastrium (see **Fig. 90.7**). The latter is directly continuous with the dorsal mesentery (mesenteron) of almost all of the remainder of the intestine (except its caudal short segment).

In human embryos of 10 mm (stage 15–16), the characteristic gastric curvatures are already recognizable. Growth is more active along the dorsal border of the viscus: its convexity markedly increases and the rudimentary fundus appears. Because of more rapid growth along the dorsal border, the pyloric end of the stomach turns ventrally and the concave lesser curvature becomes apparent (**Figs 90.3, 90.6**). The stomach is now displaced to the left of the median plane and apparently becomes physically rotated, which means that its original right surface becomes dorsal and its left surface becomes ventral. Accordingly the right vagus is distributed mainly to the dorsal, and the left vagus mainly to the ventral, surfaces of the stomach. The dorsal mesogastrium increases in depth and becomes folded on itself. The ventral mesogastrium becomes more coronal than sagittal. The pancreaticoenteric recess (see **Fig. 90.7**), hitherto usually described as a simple depression on the right

side of the dorsal mesogastrium, becomes dorsal to the stomach and excavates downwards and to the left between the folded layers. It may now be termed the inferior recess of the bursa omentalis. Put simply, the stomach has undergone two 'rotations'. The first is 90° clockwise, viewed from the cranial end, the second is 90° clockwise, about an anteroposterior axis. The displacement, morphological changes and apparent 'rotation' of the stomach have been attributed variously to its own and surrounding differential growth changes, extension of the pancreaticoenteric recess with changes in its mesenchymal walls, and pressure, particularly that exerted by the rapidly growing liver.

Mucosa

Mucosal and submucosal development can be seen in the 8th to 9th weeks. No villi form in the stomach, unlike other regions of the gut; instead glandular pits can be seen in the body and fundus. These develop in the pylorus and cardia by weeks 10 and 11 when parietal cells can be demonstrated. Although acid secretion has not been demonstrated in the fetal stomach before 32 weeks' gestation, preterm infants from 26 weeks' gestation onwards are able to secrete acid soon after birth. Intrinsic factor has been detected after 11 weeks. This increases from the 14th to 25th week, at which time the pylorus, which contains more parietal cells than it does in the adult, also contains a relatively larger quantity of intrinsic factor. The significance of the early production of intrinsic factor and the late production of acid by the parietal cells is not known. Chief cells can be identified after weeks 12–13, although they cannot be demonstrated to contain pepsinogen until term. Mucous neck cells actively produce mucus from week 16. Gastrin-producing cells have been demonstrated in the antrum between 19 and 20 weeks and gastrin levels have been measured in cord blood and in the plasma at term. Cord serum contains gastrin levels 2–3 times higher than those in maternal serum.

Muscularis

The stomach muscularis externa develops its circular layer at 8–9 weeks, when neural plexuses are developing in the body and fundus. The longitudinal muscle develops slightly later. The pyloric musculature is thicker than the rest of the stomach: in general, the thickness of the total musculature of the stomach at term is reduced compared to the adult.

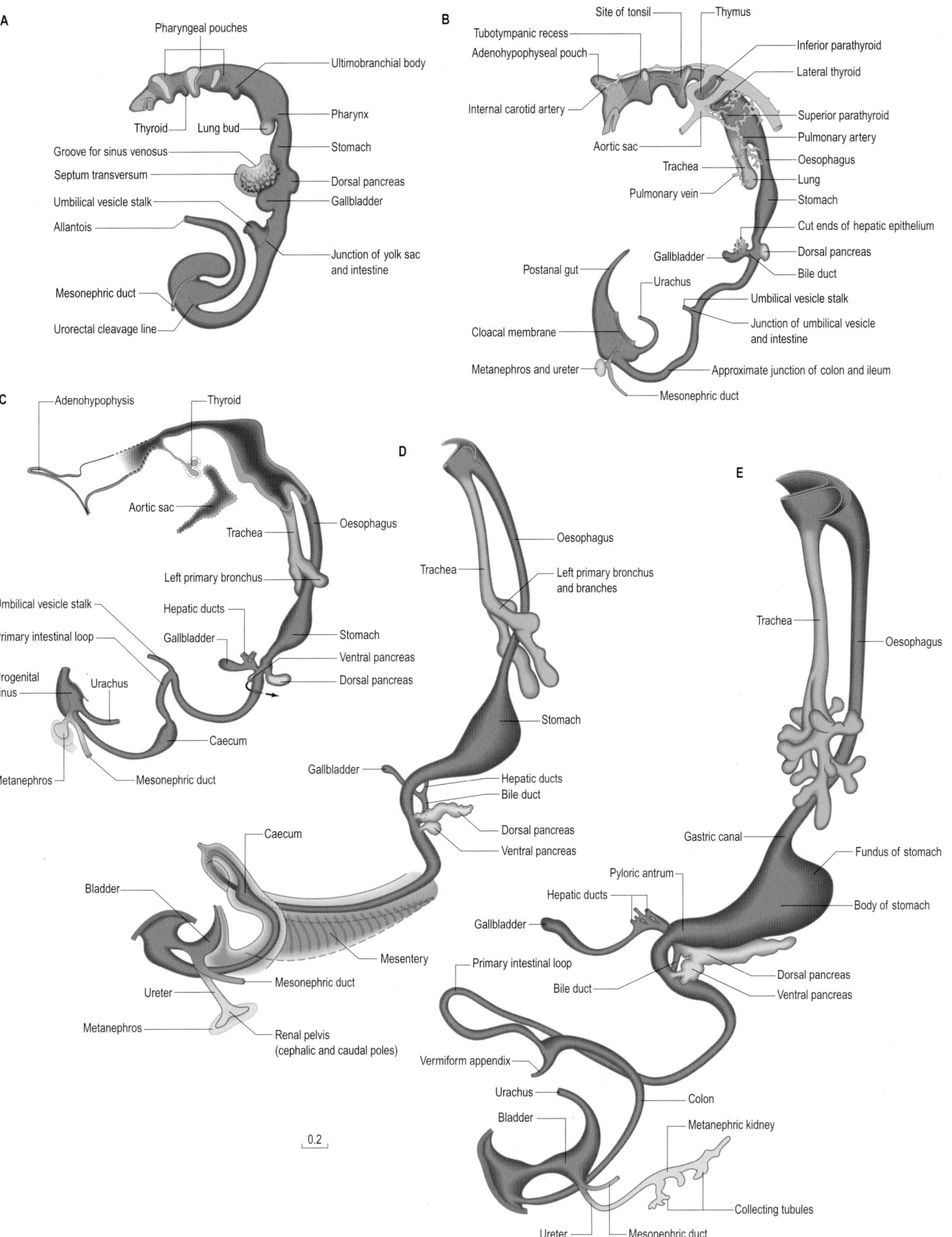

Fig. 90.3 The shape of the endodermal epithelium of the gut at succeeding stages. The scale is constant illustrating the enormous growth of the gut over a 13-day period. **A**, stage 13; **B**, stage 14; **C**, stage 15; **D**, stage 16 and **E**, stage 17. Note the separation of the respiratory diverticulum, the elongation of the foregut and expansion of the stomach, the formation of the hepatic and pancreatic diverticula, the lengthening of the midgut loop which protrudes into the umbilical cord, and the separation of the cloaca into enteric and allantoic portions. (Modified from O'Rahilly and Muller. Developmental Stages in Human Embryos 1987 Carnegie Institution of Washington. Pub 637.)

Serosa

The serosa of the stomach is derived from the splanchnopleuric coelomic epithelium. No part of this serosa undergoes absorption. The original left side of the gastric serosa faces the greater sac, the right side faces the lesser sac.

Stomach at birth

The stomach exhibits fetal characteristics until just after birth when the initiation of pulmonary ventilation, the reflexes of coughing and swallowing, and crying, cause the ingestion of large amounts of air and liquid. Once postnatal swallowing has started the stomach distends to four or five times its contracted state, and shifts its position in relation to the state of expansion and contraction of the other abdominal viscera, and to the position of the body. In the neonate, the anterior surface of the stomach is generally covered by the left lobe of the liver, which extends nearly as far as the spleen (**Figs 11.4, 65.5**). Only a small portion of the greater curvature of the stomach is visible anteriorly. The capacity of the stomach is 30–35 ml in the full-term neonate, rising to 75 ml in the second week and 100 ml by the fourth week (adult capacity is on average 1000 ml). The mucosa and submucosa are relatively thicker than in the adult, however, the muscularis is only moderately developed and peristalsis is not coordinated. At birth gastric acid secretion is low, which means that gastric pH is high for the first 12 postnatal hours. It falls rapidly with the onset of gastric acid secretion, usually after the first feed. Acid secretion usually remains low for the first 10 days postnatally. Gastric emptying and transit times are delayed in the neonate.

DUODENUM

The duodenum develops from the caudal part of the foregut and the cranial part of the midgut. A ventral mesoduodenum, which is continuous cranially with the ventral mesogastrium, is attached only to the foregut portion. Posteriorly the duodenum has a thick dorsal mesoduodenum which is continuous with the dorsal mesogastrium cranially and the dorsal mesentery of the midgut caudally. Anteriorly the extreme caudal edge of the ventral mesentery of the foregut extends onto the short initial segment of the duodenum. The liver arises as a diverticulum from the ventral surface of the duodenum at the foregut–midgut junction, i.e. where the midgut is continuous with the yolk sac wall (the cranial intestinal portal). The ventral pancreatic bud also arises from this diverticulum. The dorsal pancreatic bud evaginates posteriorly into the dorsal mesoduodenum slightly more cranially than the hepatic diverticulum. The rotation, differential growth, and cavitations related to the developing stomach and omenta cause corresponding movements in the duodenum, which forms a loop directed to the right, with its original right side now adjacent to the posterior abdominal wall. This shift is compounded by the migration of the bile duct and ventral pancreatic duct around the duodenal wall. Their origin shifts until it reaches the medial wall of the second part of the fully formed duodenum: the bile duct passes posteriorly to the duodenum and travels in the free edge of the ventral duodenum and ventral mesogastrium. Local adherence and subsequent absorption of part of the duodenal serosa and the parietal peritoneum results in almost the whole of the duodenum, other than a short initial segment, becoming retroperitoneal (sessile).

Duodenal atresia is a developmental defect found in 1 in 5000 live births (Whittle 1999). It may be associated with an annular pancreas which may compress the duodenum externally (20% of duodenal atresia), or with abnormalities of the bile duct. In 40–60% of cases the atresia is complete and pancreatic tissue fills the lumen. The condition can be diagnosed on ultrasound examination, which reveals a typical double bubble appearance caused by fluid enlarging the stomach and the proximal duodenum. Polyhydramnios is invariably present and often the indication for the scan. Duodenal atresia commonly occurs with other developmental defects, e.g. cardiac and skeletal anomalies and in Down's syndrome.

DORSAL AND VENTRAL MESENTERIES OF THE FOREGUT

The epithelium of the stomach and duodenum does not rotate relative to its investing mesenchyme. The rotation includes the coelomic epithelial walls of the pericardioperitoneal canals, which are on each side of the stomach and duodenum and form its serosa, and the elongating dorsal mesogastrium or the much shorter dorsal mesoduodenum. A ventral mesogastrium can be seen when the distance between the stomach and liver increases. Whereas the dorsal mesogastrium takes origin from the posterior body wall in the midline, its connection to the greater

curvature of the stomach, which lengthens as the stomach grows, becomes directed to the left as the stomach undergoes its first rotation. With the second rotation a portion of the dorsal mesogastrium now faces caudally. The ventral mesogastrium remains as a double layer of coelomic epithelium which encloses mesenchyme and forms the lesser omentum (see **Figs 90.7, 90.8B**).

Movement of the stomach is associated with an extensive lengthening of the dorsal mesogastrium, which becomes the greater omentum, and which now, from its posterior origin, droops caudally over the small intestine, then folds back anteriorly and ascends to the greater curvature of the stomach. The greater omentum is therefore composed of a fold containing, technically, four layers of peritoneum. The dorsal mesoduodenum, or suspensory ligament of the duodenum, is a much thicker structure, and it fixes the position of the duodenum when the rest of the midgut and its dorsal mesentery elongate and pass into the umbilical cord. For a more detailed account of this process see page 1256.

SPECIAL GLANDS OF THE POSTPHARYNGEAL FOREGUT

Pancreas

The pancreas develops from two evaginations of the foregut which fuse to form a single organ. A dorsal pancreatic bud can be seen in stage 13 embryos as a thickening of the endodermal tube which proliferates into the dorsal mesogastrium (**Figs 90.3, 90.4**). A ventral pancreatic bud

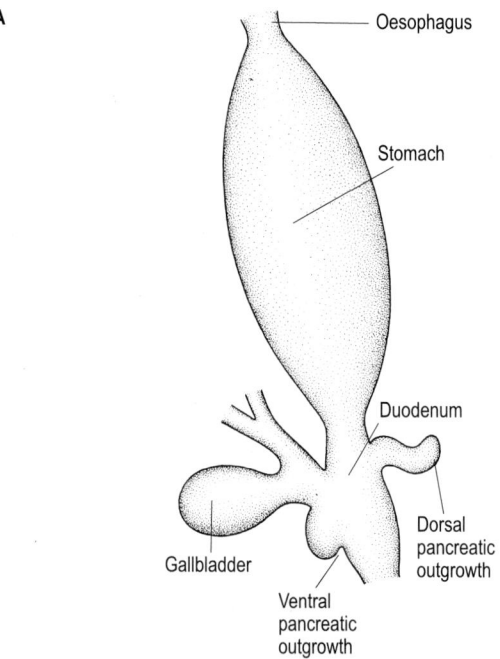

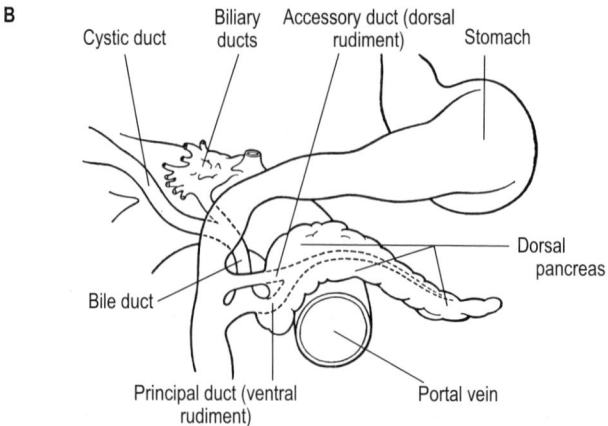

Fig. 90.4 Development of the pancreas in a human embryo. **A**, An early stage, 7.5 mm embryo; lateral view. **B**, A later stage, 14.5 mm embryo; ventral view. (Modified with permission from Streeter GL 1942 Developmental horizons in human embryos. Contrib Embryol Carnegie Inst Washington 30: 211–245.)

evaginates in close proximity to the liver primordium but cannot be clearly identified until stage 14 when it appears as an evagination of the bile duct itself. At stage 16 (5 weeks) differential growth of the wall of the duodenum results in movement of the ventral pancreatic bud and the bile duct to the right side and ultimately to a dorsal position. It is not clear whether there is a corresponding shift of mesenchyme during this rotation. However, the ventral pancreatic bud and the bile duct rotate from a position within the ventral mesogastrium (ventral meso-duodenum) to one in the dorsal mesogastrium (dorsal mesoduodenum) which is destined to become fixed onto the posterior abdominal wall. By stage 17 the ventral and dorsal pancreatic buds have fused, although the origin of the ventral bud from the bile duct is still obvious. Three-dimensional reconstruction of the ventral and dorsal pancreatic buds have confirmed that the dorsal pancreatic bud forms the anterior part of the head, the body and the tail of the pancreas and the ventral pancreatic bud forms the posterior part of the head and the posterior part of the uncinate process. The ventral pancreatic bud does not form all of the uncinate process (Collins 2002).

The developing pancreatic ducts usually fuse in such a way that most of the dorsal duct drains into the proximal part of the ventral duct (**Figs 90.3, 90.4**). The proximal portion of the dorsal duct usually persists as an accessory duct. The fusion of the ducts takes place late in development or in the postnatal period: 85% of infants have patent accessory ducts as compared to 40% of adults. Fusion may not occur in 10% of individuals, in which case separate drainage into the duodenum is maintained, so-called pancreatic divisum. Failure of the ventral pancreatic diverticulum to migrate will result in an annular pancreas which may constrict the duodenum locally.

The ventral pancreas does not always extend anterior to the superior mesenteric vein but remains related to its right lateral surface. Initially the body of the pancreas extends into the dorsal mesoduodenum and then cranially into the dorsal mesogastrium. As the stomach rotates, this portion of the dorsal mesogastrium is directed to the left forming the posterior wall of the lesser sac. The posterior layer of this portion of dorsal mesogastrium fuses with the parietal layer of the coelom wall (peritoneum) and the pancreas becomes mainly retroperitoneal. The region of fusion of the dorsal mesogastrium does not extend so far left as to include the tail of the pancreas which passes into the spleno-renal (lienorenal) ligament. The anterior border of the pancreas later provides the main line of attachment for the posterior leaves of the greater omentum.

Cellular development of the pancreas

The early specification of pancreatic endoderm involves the proximity of the notochord to the dorsal endoderm, which locally represses the expression of Shh transcription factor. Endoderm caudal to the pancreatic region does not respond to notochordal signals. The ventral pancreatic endoderm does not seem to undergo the same induction. Pancreatic mesenchyme is derived from two regions. The mesenchyme which surrounds the dorsal pancreatic bud proliferates from the splanchnopleuric coelomic epithelium of the medial walls of the pericardioperitoneal canals, whereas the ventral pancreatic bud is invested by septum transversum mesenchyme and by mesenchyme derived from the lower ventral walls of the pericardioperitoneal canals.

The primitive endodermal ductal epithelium provides the stem cell population for all the secretory cells of the pancreas. Initially these endocrine cells are located in the duct walls or in buds developing from them, and later they accumulate in pancreatic islets. The remaining primitive duct cells will differentiate into definitive ductal cells. In the fetus they develop microvilli and cilia but lack the lateral interdigitations seen in the adult. Branches of the main duct become interlobular ductules which terminate as blind ending acini or as tubular, acinar elements.

The ductal branching pattern and acinar structure of the pancreas is determined by the pancreatic mesenchyme. This mesenchyme gives rise to connective tissue between the ducts which, in the fetus, appears to be important in stimulating pancreatic proliferation and maintaining the relative proportions of acinar, α and β cells during development. It also provides cell lines for smooth muscle within the pancreas. Angiogenic mesenchyme invades the developing gland to produce blood and lymphatic vessels.

The process of islet differentiation is divided into two phases (Collins 2002). Phase I, characterized by proliferation of polyhormonal cells, occurs from weeks 9–15. Phase II, characterized by differentiation of

monohormonal cells, is seen from week 16 onwards. The β cells, producing insulin and amylin, differentiate first, followed by α-cells which produce glucagon. The δ cells which produce somatostatin are seen after 30 weeks. The dorsal bud gives rise mostly to α cells, and the ventral bud to most of the pancreatic polypeptide producing cells. The β cells develop from the duct epithelium throughout development and into the neonatal period. Later, in weeks 10–15, some of the primitive ducts differentiate into acinar cells in which zymogen granules or acinar cell markers can be detected at 12–16 weeks.

The pancreas in the neonate has all of the normal subdivisions of the adult. The head is proportionately large in the newborn and there is a smooth continuation between the body and the tail. The inferior border of the head of the pancreas is found at the level of the second lumbar vertebra. The body and tail pass cranially and to the left, and the tail is in contact with the spleen (**Fig. 11.4**).

Liver

The liver is one of the most precocious embryonic organs and is the main centre for haemopoiesis in the fetus. It develops from an endodermal evagination of the foregut and from septum transversum mesenchyme which is derived from the proliferating coelomic epithelium in the proto-cardiac region. The development of the liver is intimately related to the development of the heart. The vitelline veins, succeeded by the umbilical veins passing to the sinus venosus are disrupted by the enlarging septum transversum to form a hepatic plexus, the forerunner of the hepatic sinusoids (p. 1046). (See Collins 2002 for a detailed account of hepatic development.)

Early liver development

As the head fold and early intraembryonic coelom form, the ventral parietal wall of the pericardial cavity gives rise to populations of cells termed precardiac or cardiac mesenchyme. Hepatic endoderm is induced to proliferate by this mesenchyme, although all portions of the early heart tube, truncus arteriosus, atria, ventricle, both endocardium and myocardium, have hepatic induction potency which is tissue-specific, but not species-specific. As the heart and foregut become separated by the accumulation of the cardiac mesenchyme, the mesenchyme itself is renamed septum transversum. It is seen as a ventral mass, caudal to the heart which passes dorsally on each side of the developing gut to join the mesenchyme proliferating from the walls of the pericardioperitoneal canals. The majority of the cells within the septum transversum are destined to become hepatic mesenchyme.

In the stage 11 embryo the location of the hepatic endoderm has been identified at the superior boundary of the rostral intestinal portal. By stage 12, the hepatic endodermal primordium is directed ventrally and begins to proliferate as a diverticulum. There are two parts: a caudal part, which will produce the cystic duct and gallbladder, and a cranial part which forms the liver biliary system (**Figs 90.3, 90.5**). The cells start to express liver-specific molecular markers and glycogen storage.

Around the cranial portion of the hepatic diverticulum the basal lamina is progressively disrupted and individual epithelial cells migrate into the surrounding septum transversum mesenchyme. The previously smooth contour of the diverticulum merges into columnar extensions of endoderm, the epithelial trabeculae, which stimulate the hepatic mesenchymal cells to form blood islands and endothelium. The advance of the endodermal epithelial cells promotes the conversion of progressively more hepatic mesenchyme into endothelium and blood cells, and only a little remains to form the scanty liver capsule and interlobular connective tissue. This invasion by the hepatic epithelium is completed in stage 13, when it approaches the caudal surface of the pericardial cavity, and is separated from it only by a thin lamina of mesenchyme which will give rise to part of the diaphragm.

During this early phase of development the liver is far more highly vascularized than the rest of the gut. The hepatic capillary plexus is connected bilaterally with the right and left vitelline veins. Dorso-laterally they empty by multiple channels into enlarged hepatocardiac channels, which lead to the right and left horns of the sinus venosus; usually the channel on the right side is most developed. Both left and right channels bulge into the pericardioperitoneal canals, forming sites for the exchange of fluid from the coelom into the vascular channels. The growth of the hepatic tissue in these regions is sometimes referred to as the left and right horns of the liver.

The liver remains proportionately large during its development and constitutes a sizeable organ dorsal to the heart at stage 14 (**Fig. 90.8B,C**),

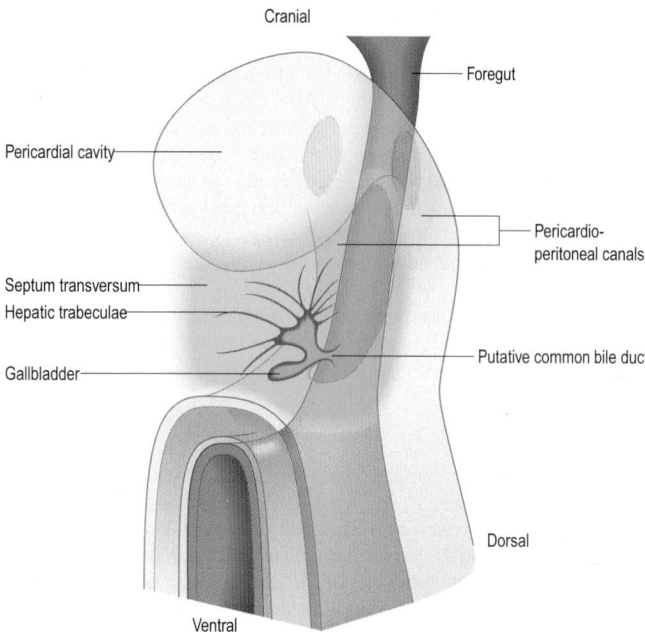

Cranial

Foregut

Pericardial cavity

Pericardio-
peritoneal canals

Septum transversum
Hepatic trabeculae

Putative common bile duct

Gallbladder

Dorsal

Ventral

Fig. 90.5 The hepatic endodermal primordium proliferates ventrally into the septum transversum mesenchyme. The endodermal cells forming the hepatic trabeculae will become hepatocytes; the septum transversum mesenchymal cells will become the endothelium of the liver sinusoids and early blood cells. (Modified with permission from Collins P 2002 Embryology of the liver and bile ducts. In: Howard, ER, Stringer MD, Clombani PM (eds) Surgery of the Liver, Bile Ducts and Pancreas in Children, Chapter 7, Part 3. London: Arnold.)

then more caudally placed by stage 16. By this stage hepatic ducts can be seen separating the hepatic epithelium from the extrahepatic biliary system, but even at stage 17 the ducts do not penetrate far into the liver.

Maturation of the liver
At 3 months' gestation, the liver almost fills the abdominal cavity and its left lobe is nearly as large as its right. When the haematopoietic activity of the liver is assumed by the spleen and bone marrow the left lobe undergoes some degeneration and becomes smaller than the right. The liver remains relatively larger than in the adult throughout the remainder of gestation. In the neonate it constitutes 4% of the body weight, compared to 2.5–3.5% in adults. It is in contact with the greater part of the diaphragm and extends below the costal margin anteriorly, and in some cases to within 1 cm of the iliac crest posteriorly. The left lobe covers much of the anterior surface of the stomach and constitutes nearly one-third of the liver (**Figs 11.4, 65.5**). Although its haemopoietic functions cease before birth its enzymatic and synthetic functions are not completely mature at birth.

Development of intrahepatic biliary ducts
The development of the intrahepatic biliary ducts follows the branching pattern of the portal vein radicles (Collins 2002). The cranial hepatic diverticulum gives rise to the liver hepatocytes, the intrahepatic large bile ducts (right and left hepatic ducts, segmental ducts, area ducts and their first branches) and the small bile ducts (septal bile ducts, interlobular ducts and bile ductules). The portal and hepatic veins arise together from the vitelline veins. Early in development the accumulation of mesenchyme around these veins is similar, whereas later mesenchyme increases around the portal veins. This is a prerequisite for bile duct development. Primitive hepatocytes surround the portal vein branches and associated mesenchyme and form a sleeve of cells termed the ductal plate. Portions of the ductal plate divide to produce lines of epithelial cells which migrate close to a portal vein branch where they differentiate into bile ducts. As the bile ducts develop, angiogenic mesenchymal cells form blood vessels which connect to the hepatic artery from 10 weeks. Thus the portal triads are patterned by the portal vein radicles which initially induce bile duct formation and then artery formation. The development of the biliary system extends from the hilum to the periphery. Abnormalities of the biliary tree are associated with abnormalities of the branching pattern of the portal vein. The

developing bile ducts remain patent throughout development; the solid stage of ductal development previously promulgated has been refuted. Atresia of the extrahepatic bile ducts has been noted, often in assocition with extrahepatic atresia. The cause of this condition is not clear; inflammatory process may be involved, although some cases have features of ductal plate malformation (Howard 2002).

Development of extrahepatic biliary ducts
The caudal part of the hepatic endodermal diverticulum forms the extrahepatic biliary system, the common hepatic duct, gallbladder, cystic duct and common bile duct.

The bile duct, which originated from the ventral wall of the foregut (now duodenum), migrates with the ventral pancreatic bud first to the right and then dorsomedially into the dorsal mesoduodenum. The right and left hepatic ducts arise from the cranial end of the common hepatic duct from 12 weeks' gestation.

Atresia of the extrahepatic bile ducts in neonates occurs alone or in conjunction with a range of other anomalies, including situs inversus, malrotation, polysplenia and cardiac defects. In such cases the intrahepatic bile ducts have a mature tubular shape but also show features of ductal plate malformation.

In the neonate the gallbladder has a smaller peritoneal surface than in the adult, and its fundus often does not extend to the liver margin. It is generally embedded in the liver and in some cases may be covered by bands of liver. After the second year the gallbladder assumes the relative size it has in the adult.

MIDGUT

The midgut forms the third and fourth parts of the duodenum, jejunum, ileum and two-thirds of the way along the transverse colon: its development produces most of the small and a portion of the large intestine. In embryos of stages 10 and 11 it extends from the cranial to the caudal intestinal portals and communicates directly with the yolk sac over its entire length. Although it has a dorsal wall, at these stages the lateral walls have not yet formed. By stage 12 the connection with the yolk sac has narrowed such that the midgut has ventral walls cranially and caudally. This connection is reduced to a yolk stalk containing the vitellointestinal duct during stage 13, at which time the yolk sac appears as a sphere in front of the embryo. Posterior to the midgut the splanchnopleuric coelomic epithelia converge forming the dorsal mesentery. Ventrolaterally the intraembryonic coelom is in wide communication with the extraembryonic coelom. At stage 14 the midgut has increased in length more than the axial length of the embryonic body and, with elongation of the dorsal mesentery, it bulges ventrally, deviating from the median plane. For all these stages consult **Fig. 90.3**.

PRIMARY INTESTINAL (OR MIDGUT) LOOP
The midgut loop can first be seen at stage 15 when a bulge, the caecal bud, can be discerned on the lower limb of the loop, caudal to the yolk stalk (which arises from the apex or summit of the loop) (**Figs 90.3, 90.6**). Later, the original proximal limb of the loop moves to the right and the distal limb to the left. The longest portion of the dorsal mesentery is at the level of the yolk stalk: there is less relative lengthening near the caudal end of the duodenum or the cranial half of the colon. The midgut extends into the umbilical coelom having already rotated through an angle of 90° (anticlockwise viewed from the ventral aspect). This relative position is approximately maintained so long as the protrusion persists, during which time the proximal limb which forms the small intestine elongates greatly. It becomes coiled, and its adjacent mesentery adopts a pleated appearance. The origin of the root of the mesentery is initially both median and vertical, while at its intestinal attachment it is elongated like a ruffle and folded along a horizontal zone. The mesenteric sheet and its contained vessels has spiralled through 90°. The distal, colic, part of the loop elongates less rapidly and has no tendency to become coiled. By the time the fetus has attained a length of 40 mm (10 weeks), the peritoneal cavity has enlarged and the relative size of the liver and mesonephros is much less. The re-entry of the gut occurs rapidly and in a particular sequence during which it continues the process of rotation. The proximal loop returns first, with the jejunum mainly on the left and the ileum mainly on the right of the subhepatic abdominal cavity. As they re-enter the abdominal cavity the coils of jejunum and ileum slide inwards over the right aspect of the descending mesocolon, and so displace the descending colon to the

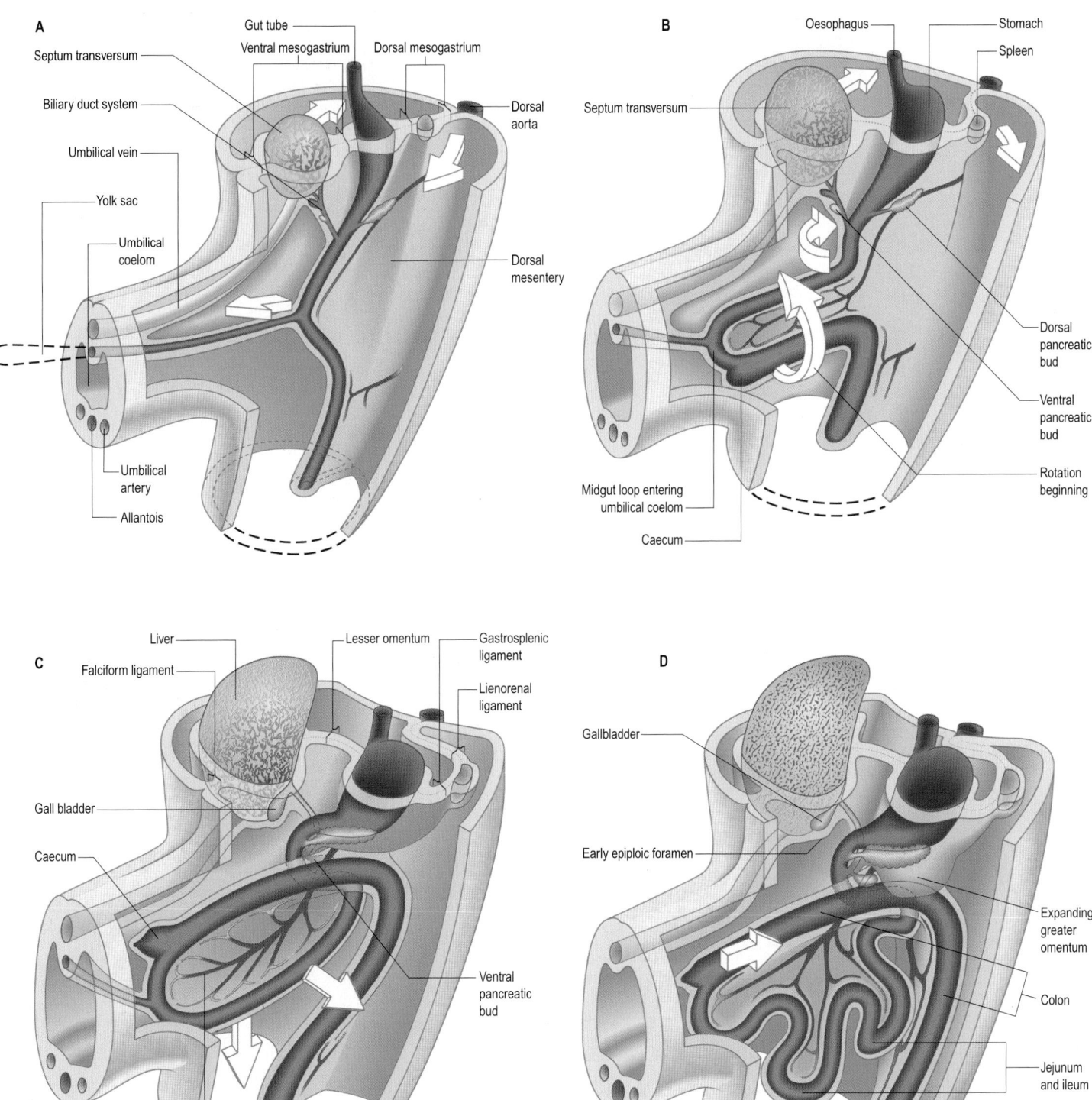

A

Septum transversum

Biliary duct system

Umbilical vein

Yolk sac

Umbilical coelom

Gut tube

Ventral mesogastrium

Dorsal mesogastrium

Dorsal aorta

Dorsal mesentery

Umbilical artery

Allantois

B

Oesophagus

Stomach

Spleen

Septum transversum

Dorsal pancreatic bud

Ventral pancreatic bud

Rotation beginning

Midgut loop entering umbilical coelom

Caecum

C

Liver

Falciform ligament

Lesser omentum

Gastrosplenic ligament

Lienorenal ligament

Gall bladder

Caecum

Ventral pancreatic bud

Superior mesenteric artery (axis of midgut rotation)

D

Gallbladder

Early epiploic foramen

Expanding greater omentum

Colon

Jejunum and ileum

Fig. 90.6 Three-dimensional schematization of the major developmental sequences of the subdiaphragmatic embryonic and fetal gut, together with its associated major glands, peritoneum and mesenteries: left anterolateral aspect. The development sequence **A–F** spans 1.5 months to the perinatal period.

left. The transverse colon passes superiorly to the origin of the root of the mesentery. The caecum is the last to re-enter and at first lies on coils of ileum on the right. Later development of the colon leads to its elongation and to the establishment of the hepatic and splenic flexures.

Anomalies of midgut rotation

If the midgut loop fails to return to the abdominal cavity at the appropriate time a range of ventral defects can result. Failure of obliteration of the vitelline-intestinal duct connecting the midgut to the yolk sac results in Meckel's diverticulum. This may present as a short segment of vitelline duct attached to the original ventral side of the ileum; it may remain attached to the umbilicus as a fistula; or it may remain as a ligamentous attachment to the umbilicus.

An umbilical hernia occurs when loops of gut protrude into a widened umbilical cord at term. The degree of protuberance may increase when the infant cries, which raises the intra-abdominal pressure: these hernias usually resolve without treatment. Exomphalos is a ventral wall defect

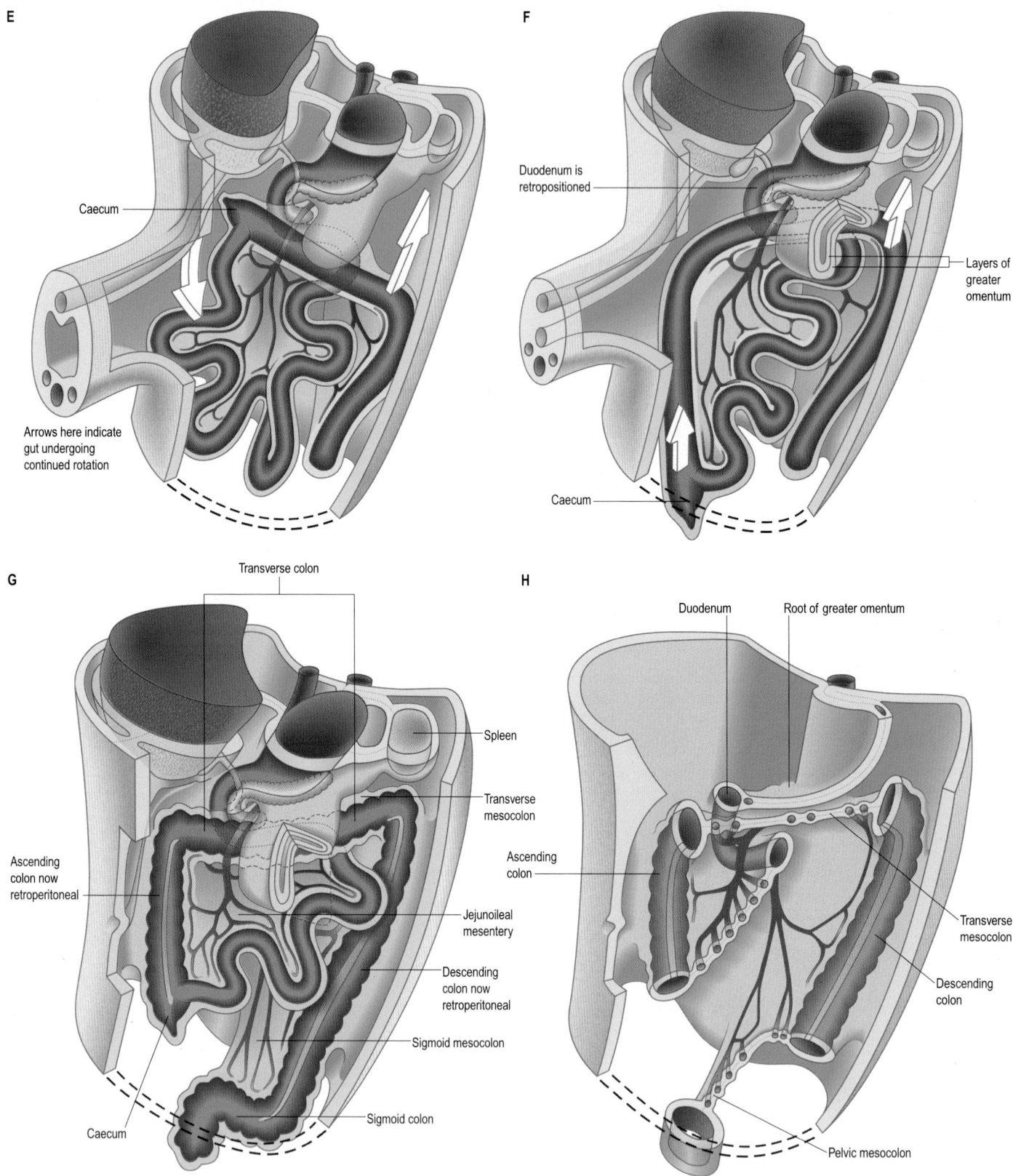

E

Caecum

Arrows here indicate
gut undergoing
continued rotation

F

Duodenum is
retropositioned

Layers of
greater
omentum

Caecum

G

Transverse colon

Ascending
colon now
retroperitoneal

Spleen

Transverse
mesocolon

Jejunoileal
mesentery

Descending
colon now
retroperitoneal

Sigmoid mesocolon

Caecum

Sigmoid colon

H

Duodenum   Root of greater omentum

Ascending
colon

Transverse
mesocolon

Descending
colon

Pelvic mesocolon

Fig. 90.6 (*Cont'd*) Three-dimensional schematization of the major developmental sequences of the subdiaphragmatic embryonic and fetal gut, together with its associated major glands, peritoneum and mesenteries: left anterolateral aspect. The development sequence **A–F** spans 1.5 months to the perinatal period. **H** denotes the general disposition of the remaining viscera, mesenteric roots with their lines of attachment, and principal contained vessels, which approximate to the adult state for comparison.

with midline herniation of the intra-abdominal contents into the base of the umbilical cord. Herniated viscera are covered by the peritoneum internally and amnion externally. The omphalocoele so formed ranges in size from a large umbilical hernia to a very large mass containing most of the visceral organs. Even after the exomphalos has been repaired these babies will still have a deficient anterior abdominal wall.

Gastroschisis is a para-umbilical defect of the anterior abdominal wall associated with evisceration of the abdominal organs. The organs are not enclosed in membranes, thus gastroschisis can be detected by prenatal ultrasonography and differentiated from exomphalos. Gastroschisis is thought to result from periumbilical ischaemia caused by vascular compromise of either the umbilical vein or arteries. The incidence of this condition appears to be increasing, especially in babies born to young women less than 20 years old (Whittle 1999).

Congenital volvulus arises if the midgut loop does not rotate appropriately. A number of types of this condition are identified. Left-sided colon occurs if the midgut loop has not rotated at all; mixed rotation results in the caecum lying inferior to the pylorus; failure of attachment of the peritoneum appropriately may result in the small intestine being attached at only two points on the posterior abdominal wall. All of these arrangements lead to a risk of volvulus which may result in necrosis of the gut.

The position and configuration of the duodenal loop are of particular importance in children. The normal duodenal loop has a U-shaped configuration. The suspensory ligament of the duodenum (ligament of Treitz) is usually found to the left of the body of the first or second lumbar vertebral body after normal gut rotation: any other position of this ligament may indicate some degree of gut malrotation. On barium studies the duodenojejunal flexure should thus lie to the left of the upper lumbar spine at the level of the pylorus.

If the caecum has remained in the right upper quadrant it may become fixed in that position by peritoneal attachments passing to the right, so called Ladd's bands. These may compress the underlying duodenum and give rise to duodenal stenosis. The high positioning of the caecum close to the duodenal jejunal flexure, in some cases in the midline, is associated with later development of volvulus.

The identification of intestinal malrotation can be made by X-ray investigation, however, ultrasonography has the advantage of showing the position of the superior mesenteric vein and artery. The vein should lie to the right of the artery. Most cases of volvulus will show inversion of this normal relationship, but malrotation can occur with apparently normally related vessels, particularly in malrotation with bowel obstruction due to Ladd's bands and not volvulus.

UMBILICAL CORD (See also p. 1341)

During the period when the midgut loop protrudes into the umbilical coelom, the edges of the ventral body wall are becoming relatively closer, forming a more discrete root for the umbilical cord. Somatic mesenchyme, which will form the ventral body wall musculature, migrates into the somatopleuric mesenchyme and passes ventrally toward the midline. The umbilical cord forms all of the ventral body wall between the pericardial bulge and the developing external genitalia. It encloses a portion of the extraembryonic coelom, the umbilical coelom, into which midgut loop protrudes. When the midgut loop is abruptly returned to the abdominal cavity the more recognizable umbilical cord forms. The vitellointestinal duct and vessels involute. The cranial end of the allantois becomes thinned and its lumen partially obliterated, and it forms the urachus. The mesenchymal core of the umbilical cord is derived by coalescence from somatopleuric amniotic mesenchyme, splanchnopleuric vitellointestinal (yolk sac) mesenchyme, and splanchnopleuric allantoic (connecting stalk) mesenchyme. These various layers become fused and are gradually transformed into the viscid, mucoid connective tissue (Wharton's jelly) which characterizes the more mature cord. The changes in the circulatory system result in a large cranially oriented left umbilical vein (the right umbilical vein regresses), and two spirally disposed umbilical arteries.

MATURATION OF THE SMALL INTESTINE

Mucosa

The exact timing of the cellular morphogenesis of the gut is difficult to establish, especially as it undergoes a proximodistal gradient in maturation. Developmental differences between parts of the small intestine or colon have not yet been correlated with age. The endodermal cells of the small intestine proliferate and form a layer some three to four cells thick with mitotic figures throughout. From 7 weeks, blunt projections of the endoderm have begun to form in the duodenum and proximal jejunum; these are the developing villi which increase in length until in the duodenum the lumen becomes difficult to discern. The concept of occlusion of the lumen and recanalization which is described in many accounts of development does not match the cytodifferentiation which occurs in the gut epithelia. Thus it is no longer thought that there is secondary recanalization of the gut lumen. By 9 weeks the duodenum, jejunum and proximal ileum have villi and the remaining distal portion of ileum develops villi by 11 weeks. The villi are covered by a simple epithelium. Primitive crypts, epithelial downgrowths into the mesen-

chyme between the villi, appear between 10 and 12 weeks similarly along a craniocaudal progression. Brunner's glands are present in the duodenum from 15 weeks and the muscularis mucosa can be seen in the small intestine from 18 weeks.

Whereas mitotic figures are initially seen throughout the endodermal layer of the small intestine prior to villus formation, by 10–12 weeks they are limited to the intervillous regions and the developing crypts. It is believed that an 'adult' turnover of cells may exist when rounded-up cells can be observed at the villus tips, in position for exfoliation. The absorptive enterocytes have microvilli at their apical borders before 9 weeks. An apical tubular system appears at this time composed of deep invaginations of the apical plasma membrane and membrane-bound vesicles and tubules; many lysosomal elements (meconium corpuscles) appear in the apical cytoplasm. These latter features are more developed in the ileum than jejunum, are most prominent at 16 weeks, and diminish by 21 weeks. There are abundant deposits of glycogen in the fetal epithelial cells, and it has been suggested that prior to the appearance of hepatic glycogen the intestinal epithelium serves as a major glycogen store. Goblet cells are present in small numbers by 8 weeks, Paneth's cells differentiate at the base of the crypts in weeks 11 and 12, and enteroendocrine cells appear between weeks 9 and 11. M cells (membrane or microfold cells) are present from 14 weeks.

Meconium can be detected in the lumen of the intestine by the 16th week. It is derived from swallowed amniotic fluid which contains vernix and cellular debris, salivary, biliary, pancreatic and intestinal secretions, and sloughed enterocytes. As the mixture passes along the gut, water and solutes are removed and cellular debris and proteins concentrated. Meconium contains enzymes from the pancreas and proximal intestine in higher concentrations in preterm than full-term babies.

Muscularis layer

The muscularis layer is derived from the splanchnopleuric mesenchyme as it is in other parts of the gut. Longitudinal muscle can be seen from 12 weeks. At 26–30 weeks the gut shows contractions without regular periodicity; from 30–33 weeks repetitive groups of regular contractions have been seen in preterm neonates.

Serosa

The small intestine possesses only a dorsal mesentery. The movement of the root of this dorsal mesentery, and the massive lengthening of its enteric border in order to match the longitudinal growth of the gut tube, reflect the spiralizing of the midgut loop in the umbilical coelom. The specific regions of adherence of the serosa and parietal peritoneum of the small intestine in the peritoneal cavity are given on page 1261.

Small intestine at birth

In the neonate the small intestine forms an oval-shaped mass with its greater diameter transversely orientated in the abdomen, rather than vertically as in the adult (**Fig. 65.5**). The mass of the small intestine inferior to the umbilicus is compressed by the urinary bladder which is anterior at this point. The small intestine is 300–350 cm long at birth and its width when empty is 1–1.5 cm. The ratio between the length of the small and large intestine at birth is similar to the adult ratio. The mucosa and submucosa are fairly well developed and villi are present throughout the small intestine, however, some epithelial differentiation is incomplete. The muscularis is very thin, particularly the longitudinal layer, and there is little elastic tissue in the wall. There are few or no circular folds in the small intestine, and the jejunum and ileum have little fat in their mesentery.

PRIMITIVE HINDGUT

Just as the foregut has an extensive, ventral endodermal diverticulum which contributes to a system separate from the gut, so too the hindgut has a ventral diverticulum, the allantois, destined for a different system. However, unlike the respiratory diverticulum of the foregut the allantois is formed very early in development, prior even to formation of the embryonic endoderm and tail folding. With the reorganization of the caudal region of the embryo at stage 10, part of the allantois is drawn into the body cavity. The early embryonic hindgut thus consists of a dorsal tubular region extending from the caudal intestinal portal to the cloacal membrane, and a ventral blind-ending allantois extending from the cloacal region into the connecting stalk. The slightly dilated cavity, lined by endoderm, that cranially receives the enteric hindgut proper and the root of the allantoenteric diverticulum is termed the endodermal cloaca. It is closed ventrally by the cloacal membrane (endoderm opposed to proctodeal ectoderm), and it also has, transiently, a small recess of endoderm in the root of the tail, the postanal gut. As elsewhere, the hindgut, allantois and endodermal cloaca are encased in splanchnopleuric mesenchyme. Proliferation of the mesenchyme and endoderm in the angle of the junction of hindgut and allantois produces a urorectal septum (**Fig. 109.4**). Continued proliferation of the urorectal septum and elongation of the endodermal structures thrusts the endodermal epithelium towards the cloacal membrane with which it fuses centrally, separating the presumptive rectum and upper anal canal (dorsally) from the presumptive urinary bladder and urogenital sinus (ventrally) (**Figs 109.4, 109.7**). The cloacal membrane is thus divided into anal (dorsal) and urogenital (ventral) membranes. The nodal centre of division is the site of the future perineal body, the functional centre of the perineum. Details of the development of the allantoic hindgut are given on page 1391.

ENTERIC HINDGUT

The development of the large intestine, whether derived from mid- or hindgut, seems to be similar. The proximal end of the colon can be first identified at stage 15 when an enlargement of a local portion of gut on the caudal limb of the midgut loop defines the developing caecum. An evagination of the distal portion of the caecum forms the vermiform appendix at stage 17 (**Fig. 90.3**). Apart from the embryonic studies of Streeter (1942) there is little information about the development of the large intestine in humans. The early endodermal lining of the colon appears stratified, and mitoses occur throughout the layers. A series of longitudinal folds arise initially at the rectum and caecum and later in the regions of colon between these two points. The folds segment into villi with new villi forming between. The developing mucosa invaginates into the underlying mesenchyme between the villi to form glands which increase in number by splitting longitudinally from the base upwards. The villi gradually diminish in size and are absent by the time of birth.

MATURATION OF THE LARGE INTESTINE

The similarity of development of the small and large intestines is further mirrored in their cytological differentiation. Fetal gut from 11 weeks shows dipeptidase activity in the colon as well as in the small intestine. Throughout preterm development meconium corpuscles are seen in the colon and in the small intestine: they are believed to be the phagocytosed remains of neighbouring cells which have died as a result of programmed cell death.

There is little direct evidence of colonic function in the human fetus and neonate. However, the specific results of mammalian studies are being correlated to human studies where possible. A number of distinct and important differences between the function of adult and fetal colon have been reported.

Mucosa

The absorption of glucose and amino acids does not take place through the colonic mucosa in adult life, but there is evidence of direct absorption of these nutrients during development. At birth the normal cycle of bile acids is not mature. In the adult, bile is secreted by the liver, stored in the gallbladder and then secreted into the intestine where it is absorbed by the jejunum and ileum. In the fetus and neonate, the transport of bile acids by an active process from the ileum does not occur, and so bile salts pass on into the colon. In the adult the presence of bile salts in the colon stimulates the secretion of water and electrolytes which results in diarrhoeal syndrome; however, the fetal and neonatal colon seems protected from this effect. The colon is not considered a site of significant nutrient absorption in the adult, and yet neonates are unable to assimilate the full lactose load of a normal breast feed from the small intestine and a large proportion of it may be absorbed from the colon. Thus it appears that the colon fulfills a slightly different role in the preterm and neonatal period, conserving nutrient absorption and minimizing fluid loss until the neonate has adjusted to extrauterine life, oral feeding, and the establishment of the symbiotic bacterial flora.

Muscularis

The muscularis is present and functioning by the 8th week, when peristaltic waves have been observed. The specific orientation of the

longitudinal muscle layer into taeniae coli occurs in the 11th to 12th weeks when haustra appear. The enteric nerves are present in Meissner's and Auerbach's plexuses at 8 and 12 weeks respectively: there is a craniocaudal migration of neurones into the gut wall. A normal distribution of ganglion cells has been noted in preterm babies of 24 weeks, although there is a region devoid of ganglia just above the anal valves. Abnormal migration of neural crest cells to the gut may give rise to Hirschsprung's disease (p. 1261). Puborectalis appears in 20–30 mm embryos, following opening of the anal membrane.

Serosa

The development of the serosa of the intestine is considered with the development of the peritoneal cavity (p. 1261).

Colon at birth

In the neonate the colon is c.66 cm long and averages 1 cm in width. The caecum is relatively smaller than in the adult; it tapers into the vermiform appendix. The ascending colon is shorter in the neonate, reflecting the shorter lumbar region. The transverse colon is relatively long, whereas the descending colon is short, but twice the length of the ascending colon (**Figs 11.4, 65.5**). The sigmoid colon may be as long as the transverse colon; it often touches the inferior part of the anterior body wall on the left and, in c.50% of neonates, part of the sigmoid colon lies in the right iliac fossa. The muscularis, including the taeniae coli, is poorly developed in the colon as it is in the small intestine. Appendices, epiploicae and haustra are not present, which gives a smooth external appearance to the colon. Haustra appear within the first 6 months. The rectum is relatively long; its junction with the anal canal forms at nearly a right angle.

ANAL CANAL

Mesenchymal proliferation occurs around the rim of the ectodermal aspect of the anal membrane which thus comes to lie at the bottom of a depression, the proctodeum (**Fig. 109.4**). With the absorption and disappearance of the anal membrane the anorectum communicates with the exterior. The lower part of the anal canal is formed from the proctodeal ectoderm and underlying mesenchyme, but its upper part is lined by endoderm. The line of union corresponds with the edges of the anal valves in the adult. The dual origin of the anal canal is reflected in its innervation: the endodermal portion is innervated by autonomic nerves, and the ectodermal proctodeum is innervated by spinal nerves.

In the fourth and fifth weeks a small part of the hindgut, the postanal gut, projects caudally beyond the anal membrane towards the region of the tail; it usually disappears before the end of the fifth week.

Imperforate anus is a term used to describe many different anorectal malformations. The most common is anal agenesis which is found in c.45% of all cases of imperforate anus. The condition is usually associated with a fistula which opens into the vulva (females) or into the urethra (males). It is more rare for the anal membrane to fail to perforate. The condition cannot reliably be diagnosed prenatally by ultrasound diagnosis, and it may be confused with Hirschsprung's disease and colonic atresia. The prognosis is good for low lesions of the anal canal. The principal concern in all cases is the degree of bowel control, urinary control and in some cases sexual function, which is compromised by the condition. Anorectal malformations may be indicators of other abnormalities, for example those forming the 'VATER' syndrome (Vertebral, Anal, Tracheo-Oesophageal and Renal abnormalities).

DEVELOPMENT OF GUT-ASSOCIATED LYMPHOID TISSUE AND ENTERIC NERVOUS SYSTEM

DEVELOPMENT OF GUT-ASSOCIATED LYMPHOID TISSUE

The neonatal gut becomes colonized by a range of bacterial flora, some of which exist in a symbiotic relationship with their host, some of which may be considered pathogenic. The gut plays a significant role in the defence of the body. Individual lymphocytes appear in the lamina propria of the gut from approximately week 12 of development, and lymphoid aggregates, Peyer's patches, have been noted between 15 and 20 weeks: it is not clear whether these cells migrate in from distant sources or differentiate from the investing mesenchyme. The endodermal epithelium overlying the lymphoid aggregates is often distorted into a dome shape. The cells within the dome are a mixed population of enterocytes, endocrine cells, goblet cells and M cells. M cells are specialized to provide a mechanism for the transport of micro-organisms and intact macromolecules across the epithelium to the intraepithelial space and lamina propria. They have been observed in the fetus by 17 weeks; it is believed that they are formed by a specialized epithelial/mesenchymal interaction of the endoderm and underlying lymphoid type mesenchyme.

There are similarly specialized epithelial cells between the enterocytes. Intraepithelial leukocytes account for c.15% of the epithelial cells of the gut in the adult. They have been observed at 11 weeks, with a distribution of c.3 intraepithelial leukocytes/100 gut epithelial cells. Both T and B lymphocytes have been described in the developing gut wall. For an account of the development of the immune cells of the gut consult Butzner & Befus (1989).

DEVELOPMENT OF THE ENTERIC NERVOUS SYSTEM

Enteric neurones are derived from trunk neural crest cells at somite levels 1–7 and from 28 onwards (**Fig. 14.11** and p. 254). After neurulation the crest cells begin their ventral migration and invade the gut via the dorsal mesentery. Glial cells associated with the gut have been identified as arising from similar levels. The local splanchnopleuric mesenchyme patterns the crest cells such that those which enter the gut layers attain an enteric fate, whereas those that remain outside the gut become committed as parasympathetic postganglionic neurones. The enteric neurones also migrate to the glands of the gut, e.g. the pancreas.

Hirschsprung's disease

Hirschsprung's disease is usually characterized by an aganglionic portion of gut which does not display peristalsis, and a dilated segment of colon proximal to this site. Histologically there is either an absence or a reduction in the number of ganglia and postganglionic neurones in the myenteric plexus; postganglionic innervation of the muscle layers is also often defective. It is believed that the condition is caused by a failure of neural crest cells to colonize the gut wall appropriately. An over-abundance of basal laminal components, perhaps at the mesothelial/mesenchyme interface, may prevent the early migrating neural crest cells from penetrating the gut wall; their new position outside the gut does not confer on them the environmental stimuli for enteric nerve differentiation and so non-enteric development occurs in local ganglia adjacent to the gut (Gershon 1987). A variable length of large intestine may be affected: the lower and midrectum are the most common sites, but in severe cases the rectum, sigmoid, descending and even proximal colon can be aganglionic. The chronic dilatation of the colon or rectum proximal to the affected segment gives rise to the common name, megacolon. It occurs as a consequence of functional obstruction due to the failure of peristalsis within the affected segment, and the dilated colon is structurally normal. Occasionally aganglionosis affects only a very short length of rectum proximal to the anorectal junction and the degree of functional obstruction is minimal: in these cases of 'ultrashort segment Hirschsprung's disease', clinical abnormalities arise later in life. Infants with Hirschsprung's disease show delay in the passage of meconium, constipation, vomiting and abdominal distension.

FUNCTIONAL MATURITY OF THE GUT AT BIRTH

After birth the first passage of stool of the newborn is termed meconium. This is a dark, sticky, viscid substance formed from the passage of amniotic fluid, sloughed cells, digestive enzymes and bile salts along the fetal gut. Meconium becomes increasingly solid as gestation advances but does not usually pass out of the fetal body while *in utero*. Fetal distress produced by anoxia may induce the premature defecation of meconium into the amniotic fluid, with the risk of its inhalation. At birth the colon contains 60–200 g of meconium. The majority of neonates defaecate within the first 24 hours after birth. Delayed passage of stool beyond this time is associated with Hirschsprung's disease (p. 1261) or imperforate anus (p. 1261). The normal passage of meconium continues for the first 2 or 3 days after birth, and is followed by a transition to faecal stools by day 7.

DEVELOPMENT OF THE PERITONEAL CAVITY

The early development of the intraembryonic coelom which gives rise to the peritoneal cavity is described on pages 198 and 207. **Fig. 10.23** show the shape of the early peritoneal cavity and indicate the mesenchymal populations derived from its epithelial walls. Initially the peritoneal cavity associated with the lower end of the foregut has separate right and left components, the pleuroperioneal canals (**Fig. 90.1**). At the level of the midgut, the pleuroperitoneal canals join a confluent cavity surrounding the developing gut, which transitorily is in communication with the extraembryonic coelom.

The description of the development of the peritoneal cavity which follows pertains to changes which occur as a consequence of the differential growth of the gut.

PERITONEUM

Peritoneum develops from a specific portion of the intraembryonic coelomic walls (pp. 198, 207). Initially the intraembryonic coelomic epithelium is a pseudostratified germinal layer from which cellular progeny with different fates arise in specific sites and at specific developmental times. The portion which will give rise to the peritoneum is derived from the lower portion of the pericardioperitoneal canals and the somatopleure and splanchnopleure associated with the lower foregut, midgut and upper portions of the hind gut (**Figs 10.24, 90.1**).

The proliferative splanchnopleuric epithelium produces cell populations for the mucosa and muscularis of the gut and also the lamina propria and epithelium of the visceral peritoneum, (the serosa of the gut wall). The somatopleuric epithelium gives rise to the lamina propria and epithelium of the parietal peritoneum. The visceral and parietal peritoneal layers constitute a mesothelium, which denotes their origin from the intraembryonic mesoderm of the coelomic wall.

As the gut grows, splanchnic mesenchyme accumulates around the endodermal epithelium and the whole unit generally moves ventrally. There is a concomitant enlargement of the caudal ends of the developing pericardioperitoneal (pleuroperitoneal) canals and developing peritoneal cavity. The medial walls of the intraembryonic coelom move closer and there is a relative decrease in the mesenchyme between them. The regions where the medial portions of the intraembryonic coelom come together are termed mesenteries. They are composed of two layers of peritoneum with intervening mesenchyme and contain the neurovascular structures which pass to and from the gut. At the caudal ends of the pleuroperitoneal canals the gut has both ventral and dorsal mesenteries, whereas caudal to this there is only a dorsal mesentery.

The mesenteries attached to the gut tube lengthen to permit large movements or rotations of the gut tube. Later, when part or the whole of the mesentery lies against the parietal peritoneum, their apposed surfaces fuse and are absorbed, i.e. they become sessile. Only those viscera developed in direct apposition to one of the primary coelomic regions, or a secondary extension of the latter, retain a partial or almost complete visceral serous cover. Thus the original line of reflexion of mesenteries becomes altered, or in some cases the organ may become retroperitoneal. These mechanisms are significant throughout the subdiaphragmatic gut, but are predominant in the small and large intestine. All serous membranes may vary their thickness, lines of reflexion, disposition, 'space' enclosed and their channels of communication, by a process of areal and thickness growth on one aspect combined with cavitation (leading to expanding embryonic recess formation) on the other (**Fig. 90.7A**).

Although all of the gut tube and its derived glands are associated with mesenteries formed as described above, the nomenclature for some portions of the gut and glands is different. Thus the mesenteries of the stomach are called omenta and the reflections of peritoneum around the liver, which develop from a confluence of splanchnopleuric, somatopleuric and septum transversum-derived portions, are called ligaments.

The movements of the developing viscera within the peritoneal cavity occur with associated movements of the mesothelia which surround them. The descriptions of peritoneal cavity development which follow are thus describing a sequence of changes which affect a complex space and its boundaries.

Mesenteries of the developing gut

The cervicothoracic oesophagus develops between the pericardioperitoneal canals (**Fig. 90.1**). It is encased in prevertebral, retrotracheal

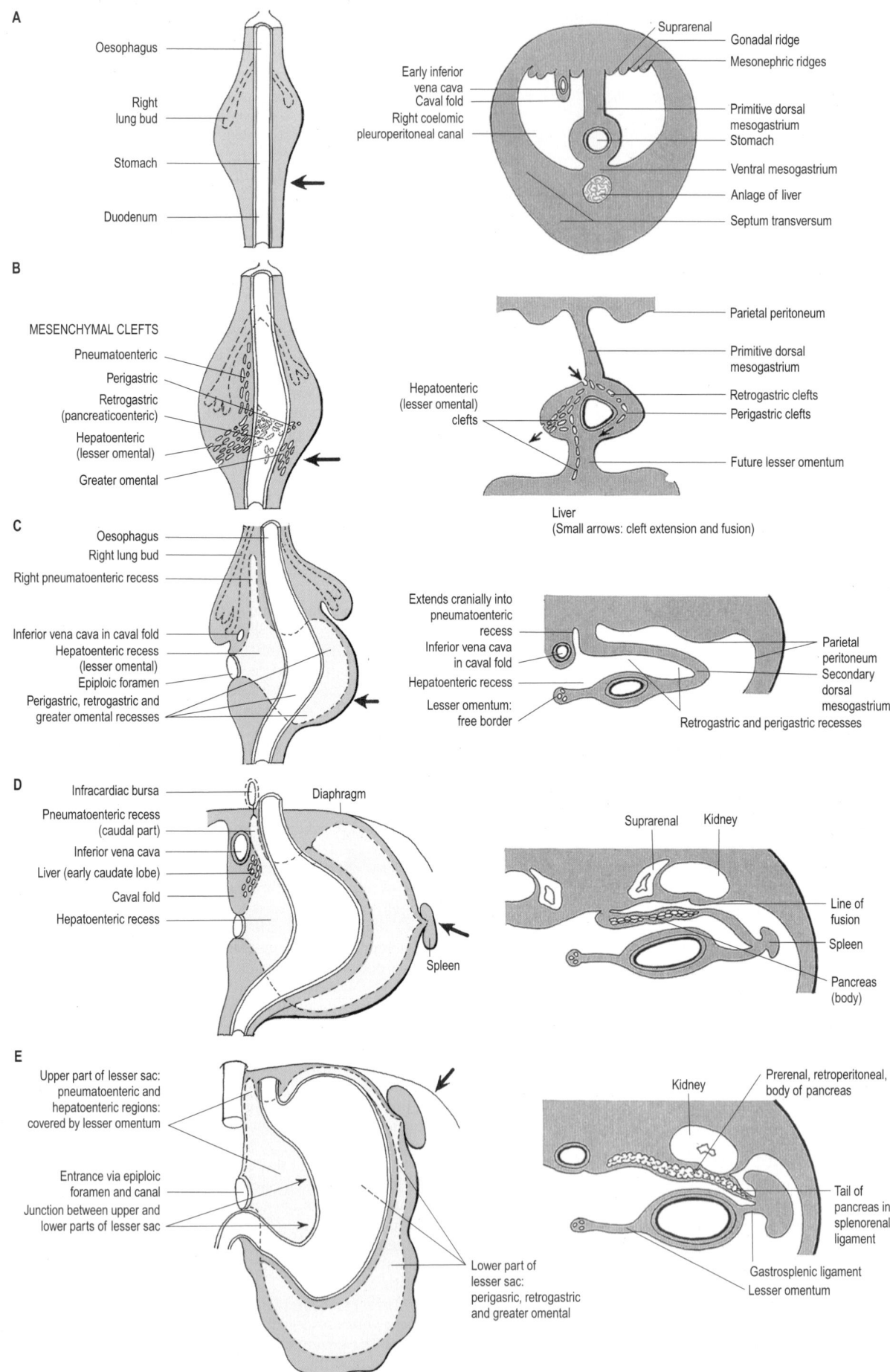

Fig. 90.7 Development of the subdiaphragmatic foregut and the right and left pericardioperitoneal/pleuroperitoneal canals, with particular reference to the terminal oesophagus, stomach, duodenum, spleen, the lesser sac of peritoneum and omenta: seen in semicoronal section (left column) and transverse section at the levels indicated (right column).

and retrocardiac mesenchyme. As the pericardioperitoneal canals expand with the developing lung buds, and the diaphragm forms immediately below them, the oesophagus at this level has no true dorsal or ventral mesentery. At superior and intermediate thoracic levels parts of the lateral aspects of the oesophagus are closely related to the secondary, mediastinal, parietal pleura. In the lower thorax the oesophagus inclines ventrally anterior to the descending thoracic aorta. The dorsocaudally sloping midline diaphragm between oesophageal and aortic orifices may be homologized with part of a dorsal meso-oesophagus, and is used in that context in descriptions of diaphragmatic development. A ventral midline diaphragmatic strip may also be considered to be a derivative of a ventral meso-oesophagus, however, this region is more usually thought of as septum transversum.

The alimentary tube, from the diaphragm to the start of the rectum, initially possesses a sagittal dorsal mesentery. Its line of continuity with the dorsal parietal peritoneum (i.e. its 'root' or 'line of reflexion') is initially also midline.

The abdominal foregut, from the diaphragm to the future hepato-pancreatic duodenal papilla, also has a ventral mesentery. This extends from the ventrolateral margins of the abdominal oesophagus and as yet 'unrotated' primitive stomach and proximal duodenum, cranially to the future diaphragm and anteriorly to the ventral abdominal wall (to the level of the cranial rim of the umbilicus). Caudally, between umbilicus and duodenum, it presents a crescentic free border.

The midgut and hindgut have no ventral mesentery; thus the pleural and supra-umbilical peritoneal cavities are initially, and transiently, bilaterally symmetrical above the umbilicus. Below the umbilicus, the peritoneal cavity is freely continuous across the midline ventral to the gut (**Fig. 90.5**).

Foregut mesenteries

The ventral and dorsal foregut mesenteries are relatively large compared with the slender endodermal tubes they encase: they are composed of mesenchyme sandwiched between two layers of splanchnopleuric coelomic epithelium. (Compare the endodermal profile seen in **Fig. 90.3** with the endoderm and surrounding splanchnopleure in **Fig. 90.8**.) A complex series of recesses develop in the splanchnopleuric mesenchyme and become confluent. As a result of foregut rotation, differential growth of stomach, liver, pancreas and spleen, and completion of the diaphragm, the territories of the greater sac and lesser sac (omental bursa) are delimited, and the mesenteric complexes of these organs (omenta and 'ligaments') are defined (**Figs 90.6, 90.7, 90.8**).

Consequences of rotation of the stomach

A number of processes occur concurrently which conceptually can be visualized as the movement of the right pleuroperitoneal canal to a position posterior to the stomach such that its communication with the remainder of the peritoneal cavity is reduced (p. 1252). These processes include the differential growth of the walls of the stomach, the formation and specific local extension of the omenta (dorsal and ventral meso-gastria), the growth of the liver and particularly of the vessels and ducts which enter and leave the liver. These developments permit stomach expansion both anteriorly and posteriorly when food is ingested and free movement of peristalsis. The right pleuroperitoneal canal forms a discrete region of the peritoneal cavity, the lesser sac, and the remaining left pleuroperitoneal canal and the remainder of the peritoneal cavity form the greater sac. The entrance to the original right pleuroperitoneal canal (lesser sac) becomes reduced in size. It is called the epiploic foramen, foramen of Winslow, or the aditus of the omental bursa (bursa omentalis) (**Fig. 90.8C**).

Early stages of lesser sac development

The lesser sac is first indicated by the appearance of multiple clefts in the para-oesophageal mesenchyme on both left and right aspects of the oesophagus. Although they may become confluent, the left clefts are transitory and soon atrophy. The right clefts merge to form the right pneumatoenteric recess that extends from the oesophageal end of the lesser curvature of the stomach as far as the caudal aspect of the right lung bud. At its gastric end it communicates with the general peritoneal cavity and lies ventrolateral to the gut; more rostrally it lies directly lateral to the oesophagus. It is not, as commonly stated, a simple progressive excavation of the right side of the dorsal mesogastrium. The right pneumatoenteric recess undergoes further extension, subdivision and modification (**Fig. 90.8A**). From its caudal end a second process of cleft

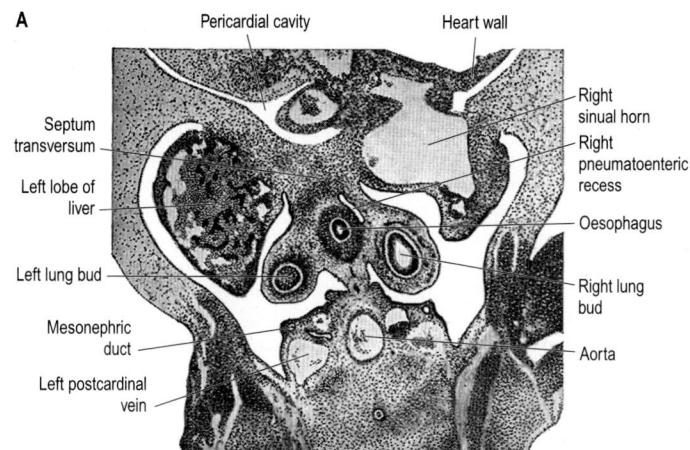

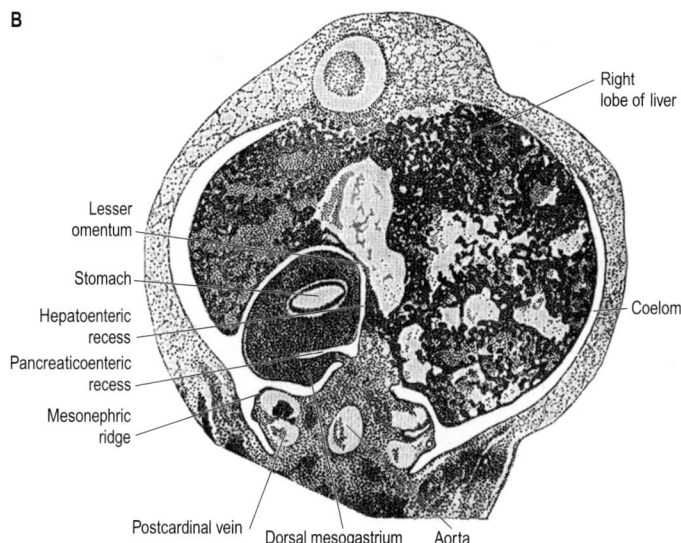

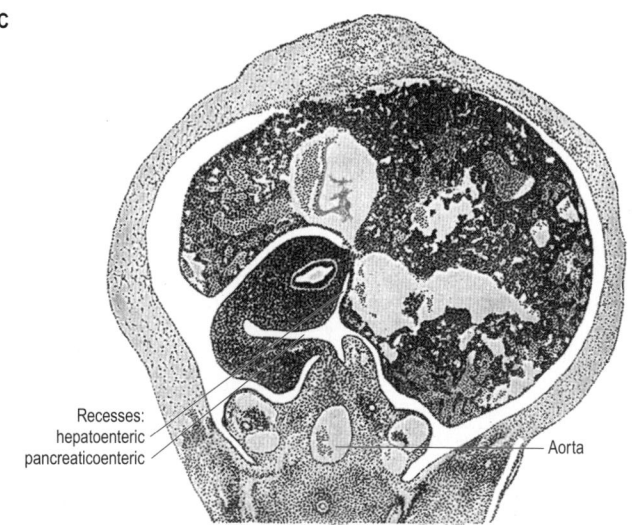

Fig. 90.8 **A**, Transverse section of a human embryo, 8 mm long, showing the right pneumatoenteric recess. **B**, Transverse section through the same embryo as A but 530 mm more caudally. Note that rotation of the stomach has taken place and that the sinusoidal spaces in the liver communicate freely with one another. **C**, Transverse section through the same embryo as B, but 150 mm more caudally. Compare with the preceding figure and observe that the omental bursa (pancreaticoenteric recess) communicates with the general peritoneal cavity at this level.

and cavity formation occurs which produces the hepatoenteric recess. This thins and expands the splanchnopleure between the liver and the stomach and proximal duodenum, and reaches the diaphragm (**Figs 90.7C, 90.8B,C**). The resulting, structurally bilaminar, mesenteric sheet is the lesser omentum. It is derived, cranially to caudally, from the small meso-oesophagus; the much larger ventral mesogastrium and the most caudal free border, is from the ventral mesoduodenum. As differential growth of the duodenum occurs, the biliary duct is repositioned and most of the duodenum becomes sessile. The duodenal attachment of the free border and a continuous neighbouring strip of the lesser omentum become confined to the upper border of a short segment of its superior part. The contrasting growth and positioning of its attached viscera cause the free border to change gradually from the horizontal to the vertical. It carries the bile duct, portal vein and hepatic artery, and its hepatic end is reflected around the porta hepatis. An alternative name for this part of the lesser omentum is the hepatoduodenal ligament: it forms the anterior wall of the epiploic foramen. The floor of the foramen is the initial segment of the superior part of the duodenum, its posterior wall is the peritoneum covering the immediately subhepatic part of the inferior vena cava, and its roof the peritonealized caudate process of the liver. The major part of the lesser omentum from the lesser gastric curvature passes in an approximately coronal plane to reach the floor of the increasingly deep groove for the ductus venosus on the hepatic dorsum: this part is sometimes called the hepatogastric ligament.

Ligaments of the liver

The liver is precociously large during development because of its early role in haematopoiesis. Thus the liver mass projects into the abdominal cavity with equal growth on the two sides of the peritoneal cavity. The ligaments associated with the liver develop from the ventral mesogastrium – which passes from the foregut to the ventral abdominal wall down to the cranial rim of the intestinal portal – and from the reflections of peritoneum from the liver to the diaphragm.

The medial portions of the germinative coelomic epithelial walls containing splanchnopleuric mesenchyme, septum transversum mesenchyme and developing liver constitute the early ventral mesogastrium (**Fig. 90.5**). The mesenchyme between these layers is continuous superiorly with the septum transversum mesenchyme of the diaphragm. The coelomic epithelial layers of the ventral mesogastrium almost touch anterior and posterior to the liver, and are separated by a slender lamina of mesenchyme. They form the falciform ligament and the lesser omentum respectively, and where they are in contact with the liver directly they form visceral peritoneum.

When the diaphragm is formed above the liver (p. 1093), local cavities coalesce and open into the general coelomic cavity as extensions of the greater (and lesser) sacs. In this way almost all the ventrosuperior, visceral and some of the posterior aspects of the liver become peritonealized. The process of extending the greater sac continues over the right lobe and stops when the future superior and inferior layers of the coronary ligament and the right triangular ligament are defined. Those, plus a medial boundary provided by an extension of the lesser sac, enclose the 'bare area' of the liver where loose areolar tissue of septum transversum origin persists. Later in development, when the haematopoietic function of the liver declines, the left lobe becomes relatively smaller than the right, which presumably accounts for the smaller size of the left triangular ligament.

Where the superior layers of the coronary and left triangular ligaments meet they continue as a (bilaminar) ventral mesentery attached to the ventrosuperior aspects of the liver. Its somewhat arched umbilicohepatic free caudal border carries the left umbilical vein. As the ventral body wall develops this falciform ligament, which initially attaches to the early cranial intestinal portal, is drawn to the diminishing cranial rim of the umbilicus. It may be considered the final ventral part of the ventral mesogastrium, although its free border has a ventral mesoduodenal origin. Its passage to the ventral body wall becomes increasingly oblique, curved and falciform (sickle-shaped) as the umbilicus becomes more defined.

In the early embryo the connection between one pericardioperitoneal canal and the other was directly across the ventral surface of the cranial midgut, immediately caudal to the developing primitive ventral mesogastrium. By stage 14 the passage from one side of the falciform ligament to the other necessitates passing below the greatly enlarged liver, or the curved lower edge of the falciform ligament, or the lesser omentum. The position of the falciform ligament is of clinical interest

in the neonate in diagnosing pneumoperitoneum because it is silhouetted by air on abdominal X-rays.

Caval fold

The caval fold is a linear eminence, with divergent cranial and caudal ends, which passes from the upper abdominal to the lower thoracic region and protrudes from the dorsal wall of the pleuroperitoneal canal. Cranially it becomes continuous, lateromedially, with the root of the pulmonary anlage and pleural coelom, the uppermost portion of the septum transversum mesenchyme, and the retrocardiac mediastinal mesenchyme. Caudally it forms an arch with dorsal and ventral horns. The dorsal horn merges with the primitive dorsal mesentery and the mesonephric ridge and associated gonad and suprarenal (adrenal) gland. The ventral horn is confluent with the dorsal surface of the septal mesenchyme.

Thus the caval fold is a zone where intestinal, mesenteric, intermediate, hepatic, pericardial, pulmonary and mediastinal mesenchymes meet and blend. It provides a mesenchymal route for the upper abdominal, transdiaphragmatic and transpericardial parts of the inferior vena cava, and it is also prominent in the development of parts of the liver, lesser sac of peritoneum, and certain mesenteries. The left fold regresses whereas the right fold enlarges rapidly (**Fig. 90.7**).

The pneumatoenteric recess continues to expand to the right into the substance of the caval fold. It stops near the left margin of the hepatic part of the inferior vena cava, which remains extraperitoneal and crosses the base of the now roughly triangular bare area of the liver and this new expanded line of reflexion. With closure of the pleuroperitoneal canals the rostral part of the right pneumatoenteric recess is sequestered by the diaphragm but often persists as a small serous sac in the right pulmonary ligament. The remaining caval fold mesenchyme to the left of the inferior vena cava – which forms the right wall of the upper part of the lesser sac – becomes completely invaded by embryonic hepatic tissue and is transformed into the caudate lobe of the liver. This smooth, vertically elongated mass projects into the cavity of the lesser sac: both its posterior, and much of its anterior, surfaces become peritonealized as a result of the increasing depth of the groove for the ductus venosus and the attachment of the lesser omentum to its floor.

Later stages of lesser sac development

The lower (inferior) part of the lesser sac starts development at c.8–9 mm CR length. At this stage, the early pneumatoenteric and hepatoenteric recesses are well established. Progressive differential gastric growth produces an elliptical transverse sectional profile, with a right-sided lesser curvature, which corresponds to the original ventral border of the gastric tube. The lesser omental gastric part of the ventral mesogastrium remains attached to this border. The greater curvature of the stomach is a new, rapidly expanding, region: its convex profile projects mainly to the left, but also cranially and caudally (**Fig. 90.7**). The original dorsal border of the gastric tube now traverses the dorsal aspect of the expanding rudiment, curving along a line near the lesser curvature. The primitive dorsal mesogastrium is transiently attached to it, and blends with the thick layer of compound gastric mesenchyme clothing the posterior aspect and greater curvature of the miniature stomach. Because of its thickness, the mesenchyme projects cranially, caudally, and particularly to the left, beyond the 'new' greater curvature of the endodermal lining of the stomach.

The processes already described in relation to the ventral mesenteries now supervene. Multiple clefts appear at various loci in the mesenchyme, and there are local mesenchyme to epithelial transitions. The groups of clefts rapidly coalesce to form transiently isolated closed spaces which soon join with each other and with the preformed upper part of the lesser sac; the newly formed epithelia join the coelomic epithelium. In sequence, the initial loci occur in the compound posterior gastric mesenchyme nearer the lesser curvature and along its zone of blending with the primitive dorsal mesogastrium; in the dorsal mesoduodenum; and independently in the caudal rim, where greater curvature mesenchyme and dorsal mesogastrium blend. As these cavities become confluent and their 'reniform' expansion follows, matches and then exceeds that of the gastric greater curvature, there are several major sequelae. The primitive dorsal mesogastrium increases in area by intrinsic growth, and, as cavitation proceeds, by incorporating substantial contributions from the dorsal lamella separated by cleavage of the posterior gastric mesenchyme. It is now called the secondary dorsal mesogastrium (**Fig. 90.7C**). The gastric attachment of the secondary dorsal mesogastrium changes progressively: it may be regarded as a set of somewhat spiral lines, longitudinally disposed, that move with time to the left, from near the lesser curvature, towards and finally reaching, the definitive greater curvature. The parietal mesogastrial and (cleaving) mesoduodenal attachment remains, for a time, in the dorsal midline, but subsequently undergoes profound changes. With the confluence of the cavities that collectively form the lower part of the lesser sac, its communication with the upper part – which corresponds to the lesser gastric curvature and right and left gastropancreatic folds – becomes better defined. Ventral to the lower part of the cavity postcleavage splanchnopleure covers the posteroinferior surface of the stomach and a short proximal segment of the duodenum. This ventral wall is continued beyond the greater curvature and duodenum as the splanchnopleuric strip of visceral attachment of the secondary dorsal mesogastrium and mesoduodenum. The radial width of the strip is relatively short cranially (gastric fundus) and gradually increases along the descending left part of the greater curvature. It is longest throughout the remaining perimeter of the greater curvature as far as the duodenum: this prominent part shows continued marginal (caudoventral and lateral) growth with extended internal cavitation (its walls constitute the expanding greater omentum, **Fig. 90.7E**). The margins of the cavity of the inferior part of the lesser sac are limited by the reflexed edges of the ventrally placed strata derived from the secondary dorsal mesogastrium just described. These converge to form the splanchnopleuric dorsal wall, which is initially 'free' throughout except at its midline dorsal root. At roughly midgastric levels, the pancreatic rudiment grows obliquely encased in this dorsal wall; its tail ultimately reaches the left limit of the lesser sac at the level of the junction between gastric fundus and body.

Greater omentum

The greater omentum continues to grow both laterally, and particularly caudoventrally. It covers and is closely applied to the transverse mesocolon, transverse colon and inframesocolic and infracolic coils of small intestine (**Fig. 90.6D–G**). At this stage the quadrilaminar nature of the dependent part of the greater omentum is most easily appreciated. 'Simple' mesenteries are bilaminar: they possess two mesothelial surfaces derived from splanchnopleuric coelomic epithelium, which enclose a connective tissue core derived from splanchnopleuric mesenchyme. In the greater omentum, the gastric serosa covering its posteroinferior surface (single mesothelium) and the anterosuperior serosa (single mesothelium) converge to meet at the greater curvature and initial segment of the duodenum. The resulting bilaminar mesentery continues caudoventrally as the 'descending' stratum of the omentum. This, on reaching the omental margins, is reflexed and now passes craniodorsally to its parietal root as the 'ascending' posterior bilaminar stratum. The two bilaminar strata are initially in fairly close contact caudally, but separated by a fine, fluid-containing, cleft-like extension of the lower part of the lesser sac. The posterior mesothelium of the posterior stratum makes equally close contact with the anterosuperior surface of the transverse colon, starting at the taenia omentalis, and with its transverse mesocolon.

Maturation of the lesser sac

At this stage, and subsequently, it is convenient to designate the lower part of the lesser sac as consisting of three subregions: retrogastric, perigastric and greater omental (**Fig. 90.7E**). The names are self-explanatory but their confines are all modified by various factors. Two phenomena are particularly prominent: gastric 'descent' relative to the liver, and fusion of peritoneal layers with altered lines of reflexion, adhesion of surfaces and loss of parts of cavities.

After the third month hepatic growth diminishes, particularly of the left lobe, and the whole organ recedes into the upper abdomen. Meanwhile the stomach elongates and some descent occurs, despite its relatively fixed cranial and caudal ends. This produces the angular flexure of the stomach which persists postnatally. The concavity of the lesser curvature is now directed more precisely to the right, the lesser omentum is more exactly coronal and its free border vertical. Ventral to the liver the free border of the falciform ligament passes steeply craniodorsally from umbilicus to liver (see disposition in neonate in **Figs 65.5, 11.4 and 11.5**). The mesenchymal dorsal wall of the lower part of the lesser sac, which is crossed obliquely by the growing pancreas, has hitherto remained free and retained its original dorsal midline root. Substantial areas now fuse with adjacent peritonealized surfaces of retroperitoneal viscera, the parietes, or another mesenteric

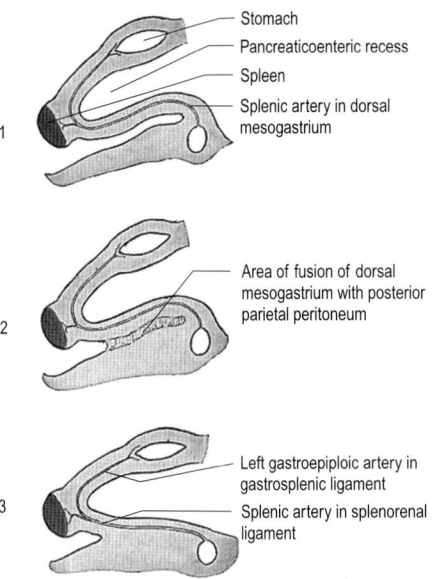

Fig. 90.9 Fusion of the proximal part of the dorsal mesogastrium with the peritoneum on the posterior abdominal wall. Note also the conversion of the dorsal mesogastrium into the gastrosplenic and lienorenal ligaments. 1, Transverse section of an embryo in which the dorsal mesogastrium is still at the stage shown in **Fig. 90.8A**. 2 and 3, Transverse sections of older embryos made at the same level, simplified by retaining the shape and size of the stomach and spleen.

Labels in figure:
- Stomach
- Pancreaticoenteric recess
- Spleen
- Splenic artery in dorsal mesogastrium
- Area of fusion of dorsal mesogastrium with posterior parietal peritoneum
- Left gastroepiploic artery in gastrosplenic ligament
- Splenic artery in splenorenal ligament

sheet or fold. Where sheets fuse there is a variable loss of apposed mesothelia and some continuity of their mesenchymal cores, but they remain surgically separable and no vascular anastomosis develops across the interzone. Above the pancreas the posterior secondary dorsomesogastrial wall of the sac becomes closely applied to the peritoneum covering the posterior abdominal wall and its sessile organs, the diaphragm, much of the left suprarenal gland, the ventromedial part of the upper pole of the left kidney, the initial part of the abdominal aorta, the coeliac trunk and its branches, and other vessels, nerves, and lymphatics (**Figs 90.7D,E, 11.5**). Their peritoneal surfaces fuse. However, albeit with some tissue loss, a single mesothelium remains covering these structures, intercalated as a new secondary dorsal wall for this part of the lesser sac (**Fig. 90.9**).

The pancreas grows from the duodenal loop, penetrating the substance of the dorsal mesoduodenum and secondary dorsal mesogastrium, their mesenchymes and mesothelia initially clothing its whole surface, except where there exist peritoneal lines of reflexion. Its posterior peritoneum becomes closely applied to that covering all the posterior abdominal wall structures it crosses (the inferior vena cava, abdominal aorta, splenic vein, superior mesenteric vessels, inferior mesenteric vein, portal vein, left renal vessels, the caudal pole of the left suprarenal, a broad ventral band on the left kidney and various muscles (**Fig. 11.4**). The intervening peritoneal mesothelia fuse and atrophy, and the mesenchymal cores form fascial sheaths and septa. The pancreas is now sessile. The peritoneum covering the upper left part of its head, neck and the anterosuperior part of its body forms the central part of the dorsal wall of the lesser sac. The pancreatic tail remains peritonealized by a persisting part of the secondary dorsal mesogastrium as it curves from the ventral aspect of the left kidney towards the hilum of the spleen. The infracolic parts of the pancreas are covered with greater sac peritoneum. In the greater omental subregion of the lower part of the lesser sac two contrasting forms of mesenteric adhesion occur. The posterior 'returning' bilaminar stratum of the omentum undergoes partial fusion with the peritoneum of the transverse colon at the taenia omentalis and with its mesocolon. The layers remain surgically separable: no anastomosis occurs between omental and colic vessels.

The original dorsal midline attachment to the parietes of the foregut dorsal mesentery is profoundly altered during the development of the lesser sac and its associated viscera. However, despite the extensive areas of fusion, virtually the whole of the gastric greater curvature (other than a small suboesophageal area) and its topographical continuation (the inferior border of the first 2–3 cm of the duodenum), retain true mesenteric derivatives of the secondary dorsal mesogastrium and its continuation, the dorsal mesoduodenum. Although regional names are used to assist identification and description, it must be emphasized that they are all merely subregions of one continuous sheet.

The upper (oesophagophrenic) part of the lesser omentum arches across the diaphragm. As this bilaminar mesentery approaches the oesophageal hiatus its laminae diverge, skirting the margins of the hiatus. They then descend for a limited distance and with variable inclination, to enclose reciprocally shaped areas on the dorsum of the gastric fundus and diaphragm. The area may be roughly triangular to quadrangular; it contains areolar tissue and constitutes the bare area of the stomach or, when large, the left extraperitoneal space. Its right lower angle is the base of the left gastropancreatic fold, and its left lower angle reconstitutes the bilaminar mesentery. The root of the latter arches downwards and to the left across the diaphragm and suprarenal gland and gives the gastrophrenic ligament to the gastric fundus. It continues to arch across the ventral surface of the upper part of the left kidney, and its layers part to receive the pancreatic tail: they initially extend to the hilum of the spleen as the splenorenal (lienorenal) ligament (**Figs 90.6, 90.9**). The left half of this bilaminar 'ligament' provides an almost complete peritoneal tunic for the spleen. It then reunites with its fellow at the opposite rim of the splenic hilum, and continues to the next part of the gastric greater curvature as the gastrosplenic ligament. The remaining part (perhaps two-thirds) of the gastric greater curvature and its short duodenal extension provide attachment for the anterior, 'descending', bilaminar stratum of the greater omentum. Its returning, posterior, bilaminar stratum continues to its parietal root (which extends from the inferior limit assigned to the splenorenal ligament), and curves caudally and to the right along the anterior border of the body of the pancreas, immediately cranial to the line of attachment of the transverse mesocolon. Crossing the neck of the pancreas, the same curve is followed for a few centimetres on to its head; the omental root then sharply recurves cranially and to the left, to reach the inferior border of the duodenum. Thus it reaches that part of the lesser sac provided by cleavage of the dorsal mesoduodenum from the greater sac. It enters the epiploic foramen, traverses the epiploic canal between the caudate hepatic process and proximal duodenum, then crosses the right gastropancreatic fold, and descends behind the proximal duodenum to enter the right marginal strip enclosed by the greater omentum. The definitive origins of the peritoneum from the posterior abdominal wall are shown in the adult in **Figs 69.1, 69.4** and **69.5**.

Peritoneum associated with the mid- and hindgut

It is convenient to consider the mesenteries of the small and large intestine after rotation and the principal growth patterns have been achieved and the developing pancreas is becoming retroperitoneal.

Small intestine

Most of the duodenal loop encircles the head of the pancreas and is retroperitoneal. The peritoneum principally covers its ventral and convex aspects. Areas not covered are a short initial segment of the superior (first) part, which is more completely peritonealized because it gives attachment to the right margins of the greater and lesser omenta; where the transverse colon is closely apposed to the descending (second) part, or where the latter is crossed by the root of the transverse mesocolon; where the mesentery crosses the transverse (third) part, and descends across the ascending (fourth) part from its upper extremity at the duodenojejunal flexure. These regions are illustrated in the adult in **Fig. 69.1**. In addition, one or more of up to six different duodenal recesses may develop. Their variations in shape and size, their intestinal, mesenteric and vascular relations, and, when adequately recorded, the frequencies and disposition of their orifices, are given on page 1137.

From a mesenteric standpoint, the succeeding small intestine, from the duodenojejunal flexure to the ileocaecal junction, undergoes less modification of its embryonic form than other gut regions. Its early dorsal mesentery is a continuous, single (but structurally bilaminar) sheet, with a midline parietal attachment (line of reflexion, or 'root'). The attachment of the root becomes an oblique narrow band from the left aspect of the second lumbar vertebra to the cranial aspect of the right sacroiliac joint.

Ascending colon

The caecum and vermiform appendix arise as a diverticulum from the antimesenteric border of the caudal limb of the midgut loop, consequently the caecum does not possess a primitive mesocaecum. These regions of the gut undergo long periods of growth, often asymmetrical, and their final positions, dimensions and general topography show considerable variation. The vermiform appendix is almost wholly clothed with visceral peritoneum, derived from the diverging layers of its rather diminutive mesoappendix. The latter should perhaps be regarded as a direct derivative of the primitive dorsal mesentery, and perhaps a similar status for the vascular fold of the caecum should be considered.

The colonic gut retains its primitive dorsal mesentery, the mesocolon, until the differential growth, rotation and circumabdominal displacement of this part of the gut tube nears completion. Its original root is still vertical in the dorsal midline, although the mesocolon diverges from it widely as an incomplete, flattened pyramid, to reach its colonic border at the future taenia mesocolica. During the fourth and fifth months substantial areas of the primitive mesocolon adhere to, then fuse with, the parietal peritoneum. In this way, some colonic segments become sessile while others have a shorter mesocolon with an often profoundly altered parietal line of attachment. The mesocolon of the transverse and sigmoid segments normally persists, while the ascending colon, right (hepatic) flexure and descending colon become sessile: the ascending or descending, or both, colonic segments may also retain a mesocolon which varies from a localized 'fold' to a complete mesocolon. When sessile, the ventral, medial and lateral aspects of the ascending or descending colon are clothed with peritoneum, and the protrusion of the viscus produces medial and lateral peritoneal paracolic gutters on each side. This form of apposition to underlying structures proceeds from the ascending colon to include the right colic (hepatic) flexure, and thence continues anteroinferiorly to the left, so involving the right-sided initial segment of the transverse colon.

Transverse colon

The right extremity of the transverse colon is sessile, and is separated by fibroareolar tissue from the anterior aspect of the descending (second) part of the duodenum and the corresponding aspect of most of the head of the pancreas. The remainder of the transverse colon, up to and including the left (splenic) colic flexure, is almost completely peritonealized by the diverging layers of the transverse mesocolon. The root of the latter reaches the neck and whole extent of the anterior border of the body of the pancreas. The long axis of the definitive pancreas lies obliquely. The splenic colonic flexure is considerably more rostral than the hepatic flexure and consequently the root of the mesocolon curves obliquely upwards as it crosses the upper abdomen from right to left. As it expands, the posteroinferior wall of the greater omental part of the lesser sac gradually covers, and becomes closely applied to, the transverse mesocolon and its contained colon, finally projecting beyond the latter. Craniocaudal adherence now occurs between the omental wall and the pericolonic and mesocolonic layers.

Descending colon

The left colic flexure receives much of its peritoneal covering from the left extremity of the transverse mesocolon. It is also often connected to the parietal peritoneum of the diaphragm over the tenth and eleventh ribs by a phrenicocolic ligament. The latter sometimes blends with a presplenic fold that radiates from the gastrosplenic ligament. The descending colon becomes sessile. The process of fusion and obliteration of both ascending and descending mesocolons starts laterally and progresses medially.

Sigmoid colon

The sigmoid colon is most variable in its length and disposition. It retains its dorsal mesocolon, but the initial midline dorsal attachment of its root is considerably modified in its definitive state.

Rectum

The rectum continues from the ventral aspect of the third sacral vertebra to its anorectal (perineal) flexure anteroinferior to the tip of the coccyx: the distance changes with age. All aspects of the rectum are encased by mesenchyme, and the early dorsally placed mass is named, by some authorities, the dorsal mesorectum. However, the latter does not form a true mesentery: with progressive skeletal development it is reduced to a woven fibroareolar sheet which displays patterned variations in thickness and fibre orientation. The sheet is closely applied to the ventral concavity of the sacrum and coccyx, and encloses numerous fibromuscular and neurovascular elements. The rectum therefore becomes sessile, and visceral peritoneum is restricted to its lateral and ventral surfaces (**Fig. 109.4**).

With the disappearance of the postanal gut by the end of the fifth week, the ventrolateral peritoneum reaches the superior surface of the pelvic floor musculature: this condition persists until late in the fourth month. In the male the ventral rectal peritoneum is reflected over the posterior surface of the prostate, bladder trigone and associated structures. In the female the ventral peritoneum initially receives a reflection which covers almost the whole posterior aspect of the vagina, and is continued over the uterus. Subsequently, the closely apposed walls of these deep peritoneal pouches fuse over much of their caudal extent, their mesothelia are lost, and the viscera are separated by an intervening, bilaminar (surgically separable), fibrous stratum. In the male this becomes the rectovesical fascia and posterior wall of the prostatic sheath. In the female it becomes the rectovaginal septum between the lower part of the vagina and the rectum (**Fig. 11.5**). The proximal third of the rectum is covered by peritoneum ventrolaterally: the lateral extensions of this tunic are triangular and deep proximally, but taper to an acute angle by the middle third of the rectum. The middle third of the rectum is covered by peritoneum only on its ventral surface, where it forms the posterior wall of the shallower rectovesical or rectovagino-uterine pouch. The remaining rectum and anal canal are extraperitoneal.

NEONATAL PERITONEAL CAVITY

The fully formed peritoneal cavity, although complex topographically, remains a single cavity with numerous intercommunicating regions, pouches and recesses (**Fig. 11.5**). The only small peritoneal sacs to separate completely from the main cavity are the infracardiac bursa (**Fig. 90.7D**) and the tunica vaginalis testis (**Fig. 109.17**).

In fetal life the greater omental cavity extends to the internal aspect of the lateral and caudal edges of the omentum. Postnatally a slow but progressive fusion of the internal surfaces occurs with obliteration of the most dependent part of the cavity: this proceeds rostrally and, when mature, the cavity does not usually extend appreciably beyond the transverse colon. Transverse mesocolon–greater omentum fusion begins early while the umbilical hernia of the midgut has not returned. It starts between the right margin of the early greater omentum and near the root of the presumptive mesocolon, and later spreads to the left.

In the neonate the peritoneal cavity is ovoid (**Figs 11.4, 65.5**). It is fairly shallow from anterior to posterior because the bilateral posterior extensions on each side of the vertebral column, which are prominent in the adult, are not present (**Fig. 11.5**). Two factors lead to the protuberance of the anterior abdominal wall in the neonate and infant. The diaphragm is flatter in the newborn, which produces a caudal displacement of the viscera. The pelvic cavity is very small in the neonate, which means that organs which are normally pelvic in the adult, i.e. urinary bladder, ovaries and uterus, all extend superiorly into the abdomen (**Fig. 11.5**). The pelvic cavity is joined to the abdominal cavity at less of an acute angle in the neonate because there is no lumbar vertebral curve and only a slight sacral curve.

The peritoneal attachments are similar to the adult. However, the greater omentum is relatively small: its constituent layers of peritoneum may not be completely fused, and it does not extend much below the level of the umbilicus (**Fig. 11.5**). Generally the length of the mesentery of the small intestine and of the transverse and sigmoid mesocolons are longer than in the adult, whereas the area of attachment of the ascending and descending colons is relatively smaller. The peritoneal mesenteries and omenta contain little fat.

SPLEEN

The spleen appears about the sixth week as a localized thickening of the coelomic epithelium of the dorsal mesogastrium near its cranial end (**Figs 90.6, 90.7, 90.9**). The proliferating cells invade the underlying angiogenetic mesenchyme, which becomes condensed and vascularized. The process occurs simultaneously in several adjoining areas which soon fuse to form a lobulated spleen of dual origin (from coelomic epithelium and from mesenchyme of the dorsal mesogastrium). The enlarging spleen projects to the left, so that its surfaces are covered by the peritoneum of the mesogastrium on its left aspect, which forms a boundary of the general extrabursal (greater) sac. When fusion occurs between the dorsal wall of the lesser sac and the dorsal parietal peritoneum, it does not extend to the left as far as the spleen, which remains

connected to the dorsal abdominal wall by a short splenorenal ligament. Its original connection with the stomach persists as the gastrosplenic ligament. The earlier lobulated character of the spleen disappears, but is indicated by the presence of notches on its upper border in the adult.

The histogenesis of the spleen has attracted relatively little attention. The vascular reticulum is well developed at 8–9 weeks, and contains immature reticulocytes and numerous closely spaced thin-walled vascular loops. Differentiation of blood cells, macrophages, and of arteries, veins, capillaries and sinusoids has occurred by the eleventh to twelfth week. Initially the capsule consists of cuboidal cells bearing cilia and microvilla.

The spleen displays various developmental anomalies, including complete agenesis, multiple spleens or polysplenia, isolated small additional spleniculi and persistent lobulation. Asplenia and polysplenia are associated with other anomalies especially those involving the cardiac and pulmonary systems. Accessory spleens are very common in neonates, located in the greater omentum. At birth the spleen weighs, on average, 13 g (**Fig. 11.4**). It doubles its weight in the first postnatal year and triples it by the end of the third year.

SUPRARENAL GLANDS

The suprarenal (adrenal) cortex is formed during the second month by a proliferation of the coelomic epithelium. Cells pass into the underlying mesenchyme between the root of the dorsal mesogastrium and the mesonephros (**Fig. 14.11**). The proliferating tissue, which extends from the level of the sixth to the twelfth thoracic segments, is soon disorganized dorsomedially by invasion of neural crest cells from somite levels 18–24, which form the medulla, and also by the development of venous sinusoids. The latter are joined by capillaries, which arise from adjacent mesonephric arteries and penetrate the cortex in a radial manner. When proliferation of the coelomic epithelium stops the cortex is enveloped ventrally, and later dorsally, by a mesenchymal capsule which is derived from the mesonephros. The subcapsular nests of cortical cells are the rudiment of the zona glomerulosa: they proliferate cords of cells which pass deeply between the capillaries and sinusoids. The cells in these cords degenerate in an erratic fashion as they pass towards the medulla, becoming granular, eosinophilic and ultimately autolysed. These cords of cells constitute the fetal cortex, which undergoes rapid involution during the first two years after birth. The fascicular and reticular zones of the adult cortex are proliferated from the glomerular zone after birth.

The most common abnormality of suprarenal gland development is congential adrenal hyperplasia, which occurs in 1:5000–1:15 000 births. This condition is caused by a group of autosomal recessive disorders in which there are deficiencies in enzymes required for the synthesis of cortisol. In 90% of cases the cause is deficiency of the enzyme 21-hydroxylase, producing an accumulation of 17-hydroxyprogesterone, which is converted to androgens. The levels of androgens increase by several hundred times, causing female embryos and fetuses to undergo external genital masculinization ranging from clitoral hypertrophy to formation of a phallus and scrotum: masculinization of the brain has also been suggested. In male embryos the levels do not cause any changes in external genitalia. Signs of androgen excess may appear in childhood with precocious masculinization and accelerated growth (Lewis, Yaron & Evans 1999).

SUPRARENAL GLANDS IN THE NEONATE

The suprarenal glands are relatively very large at birth (**Figs 11.4, 109.8**) and constitute 0.2% of the entire body weight, compared with 0.01% in the adult. The left gland is heavier and larger than the right, as it is in the adult. At term each gland weighs c.4 g; the average weight of the two glands is 9 g (average in the adult is 7–12 g). The glands involute rapidly in the neonatal period when each gland loses 25% of its mass; the average weight of both glands is 5 g by the end of the second week, and 4 g by 3 months. Birth weight is not regained until puberty. The cortex of the suprarenal gland is thicker than in the adult and the medulla of the gland is small. Early studies on fetal suprarenal glands described extensive degeneration and necrosis of fetal zone cells; however, it is believed that these studies showed disease processes rather than the normal involution of the gland. With normal involution the fetal zone cells of the postnatal gland become smaller and they assume the appearance and organization typical of zona fasciculata.

REFERENCES

Butzner JD, Befus AD 1989 Interactions among intraepithelial leucocytes and other epithelial cells in intestinal development and function. In: Lebenthal E (ed) Human Gastrointestinal Development, Chapter 37. New York: Raven Press.

Collins P 2002 Embryology of the pancreas. In: Howard ER, Stringer MD, Colombani PM (eds) Surgery of the Liver, Bile Ducts and Pancreas in Children, Part 8. London: Arnold: 479–92.
Covers pancreatic morphogenesis, the timescale of development, the origin of pancreatic cell lines and factors that regulate pancreatic development.

Collins P 2002 Embryology of the liver and bile ducts. In: Howard ER, Stringer MD, Colombani PM (eds) Surgery of the Liver, Bile Ducts and Pancreas in Children, Part 3. London: Arnold: 91–102.
Covers morphogenesis of the liver and early hepatic circulation, the origin of hepatic cell lines and the development of the extra- and intrahepatic biliary systems.

Gershon MD 1987 Phenotypic expression by neural crest-derived precursors of enteric neurons and glia. In: Madreson PFA (ed) Developmental and Evolutionary Aspects of the Neural Crest. New York: John Wiley.
Describes a mouse model of Hirschsprung's disease.

Howard ER 2002 Biliary atresia: etiology, management and complications. In: Howard ER, Stringer MD, Colombani PM (eds) Surgery of the Liver, Bile Ducts and Pancreas in Children, Part 3. London: Arnold: 103–32.
Reviews the aetiology and clinical presentation of biliary atresia, including the congenital, infective and anatomical factors that are related to the condition.

Lebenthal E 1989 Concepts in gastrointestinal development. In: Lebenthal E (ed) Human Gastrointestinal Development, Chapter 1. New York: Raven Press.
This chapter is the first in a volume dedicated to the development of structure and function of the gut, liver and pancreas. Includes the development of the immunological surveillance mechanisms and gastrointestinal flora .

Lewis P, Yaron Y, Evans MI 1999 Fetal endocrine disorders. In: Rodeck CH, Whittle MJ (eds) Fetal Medicine: Basic Sciences and Clinical Practice, Chapter 62. Edinburgh: Churchill Livingstone: 829–34.
Reviews the diagnosis and treatment of common fetal endocrine disorders, particularly of the suprarenal and thyroid glands.

Streeter GL 1942 Developmental horizons in human embryos. Descriptions of age group XI, 13 to 20 somites, and age group XII, 21 to 29 somites. Contrib Embryol Carnegie Inst Washington 30: 211–45.

Whittle MJ 1999 Gastrointestinal abnormalities. In: Rodeck CH, Whittle MJ (eds) Fetal Medicine: Basic Sciences and Clinical Practice, Chapter 54. Edinburgh: Churchill Livingstone: 703–714.
Reviews the diagnosis and treatment of abnormalities of the gastrointestinal tract.

Kidney

The kidneys excrete the end products of metabolism and excess water. Both of these actions are essential to the control of concentrations of various substances in the body fluids, e.g. maintaining electrolyte and water balance approximately constant in the tissue fluids. The kidneys also have endocrine functions producing and releasing erythropoietin which affects red blood cell formation, renin which influences blood pressure, 1,25-hydroxycholecalciferol, which is involved in the control of calcium metabolism and is a derivative of vitamin D, and perhaps modifies the action of the parathyroid hormone, and various other soluble factors with metabolic actions.

The kidneys in the fresh state are reddish-brown. They are situated posteriorly behind the peritoneum on each side of the vertebral column and are surrounded by adipose tissue. Superiorly they are level with the upper border of the twelfth thoracic vertebra, inferiorly with the third lumbar vertebra. The right is usually slightly inferior to the left, probably reflecting its relationship to the liver. The left is a little longer and narrower than the right and lies nearer the median plane (**Fig. 91.1**).

The long axis of each kidney is directed inferolaterally and the transverse axis posteromedially. Hence the anterior and posterior aspects usually described are in fact anterolateral and posteromedial. The transpyloric plane passes through the superior part of the right renal hilum and the inferior part of the left (p. 1099).

Each kidney is c.11 cm in length; 6 cm in breadth and 3 cm in antero-posterior dimension. The left kidney may be 1.5 cm longer than the right; it is rare for the right kidney to be more than 1 cm longer than the left. The average weight is c.150 g in men and 135 g in women. In thin individuals with a lax abdominal wall the lower pole may just be felt in full inspiration by bimanual lumbar examination, but this is unusual.

In the fetus and newborn, the kidney has c.12 lobules (**Fig. 91.2**). These are fused in adults to present a smooth surface although traces of lobulation may remain.

Absent and ectopic kidneys – A single absent kidney is seen in c.1 in 1200 individuals and results from failure of metanephric blastema to

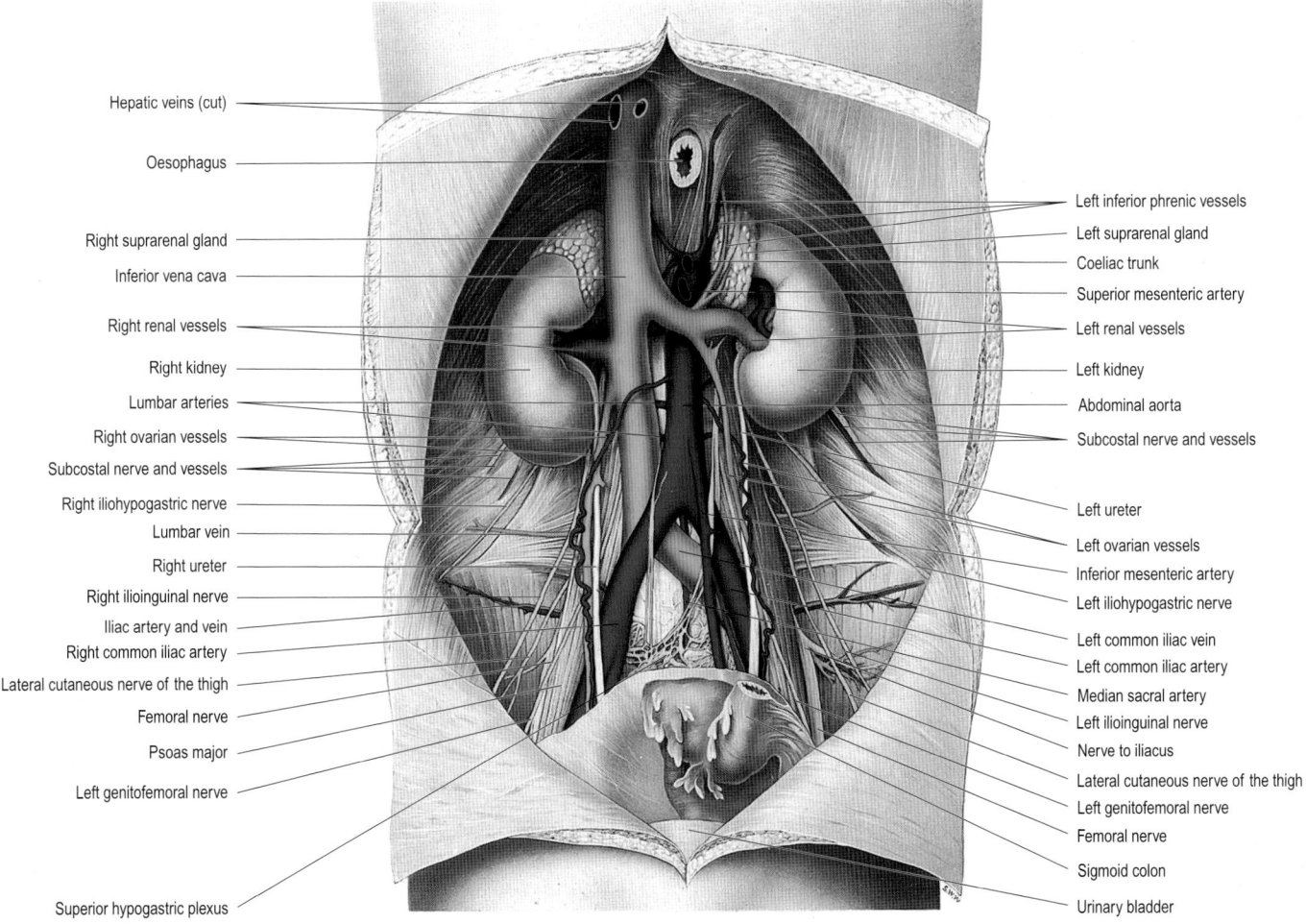

Hepatic veins (cut)	Left inferior phrenic vessels
Oesophagus	Left suprarenal gland
Right suprarenal gland	Coeliac trunk
Inferior vena cava	Superior mesenteric artery
Right renal vessels	Left renal vessels
Right kidney	Left kidney
Lumbar arteries	Abdominal aorta
Right ovarian vessels	Subcostal nerve and vessels
Subcostal nerve and vessels	
Right iliohypogastric nerve	Left ureter
Lumbar vein	Left ovarian vessels
Right ureter	Inferior mesenteric artery
Right ilioinguinal nerve	Left iliohypogastric nerve
Iliac artery and vein	Left common iliac vein
Right common iliac artery	Left common iliac artery
Lateral cutaneous nerve of the thigh	Median sacral artery
Femoral nerve	Left ilioinguinal nerve
Psoas major	Nerve to iliacus
Left genitofemoral nerve	Lateral cutaneous nerve of the thigh
	Left genitofemoral nerve
	Femoral nerve
	Sigmoid colon
Superior hypogastric plexus	Urinary bladder

Fig. 91.1 Dissection to show the relations of structures on the posterior abdominal wall (female subject).

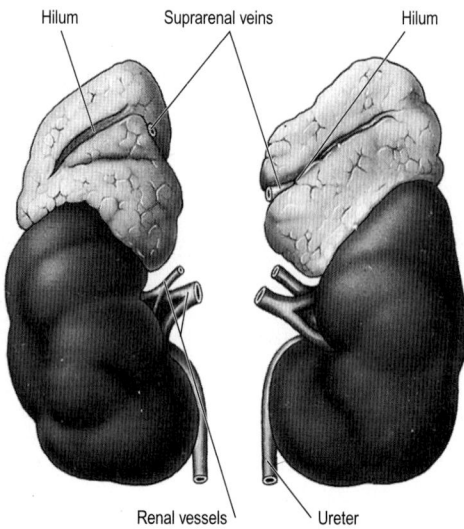

Fig. 91.2 The kidneys and suprarenal glands of a newborn infant: anterior aspect. Note the lobulation of the renal surface and relative size of the organs.

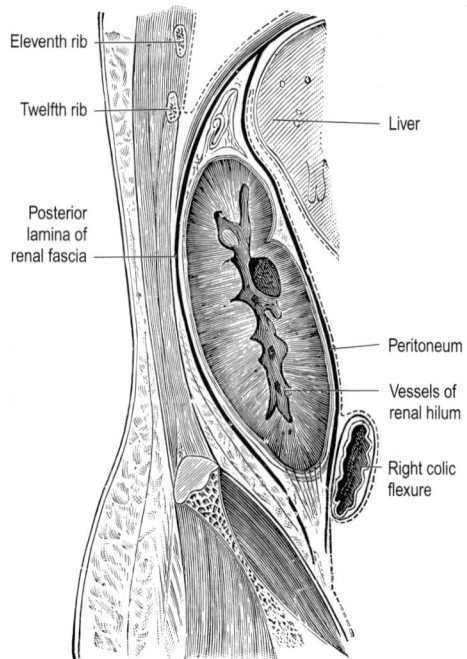

Fig. 91.3 Sagittal section through the posterior abdominal wall showing the relations of the renal fascia of the right kidney.

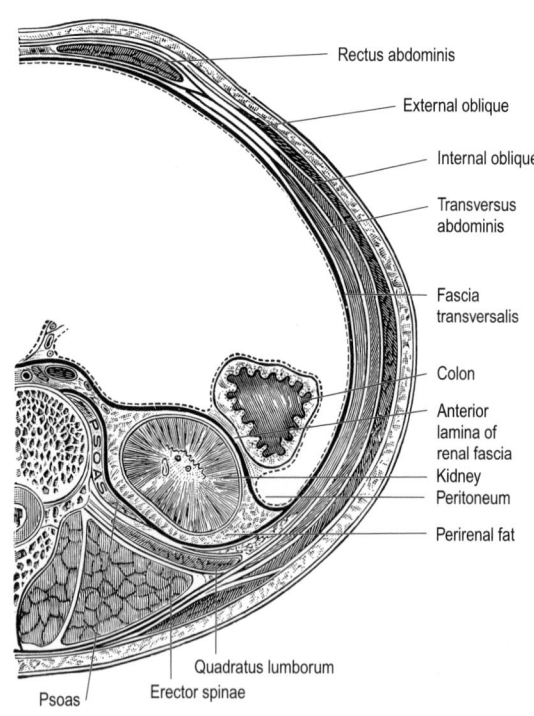

Fig. 91.4 Transverse section, showing the relations of the renal fascia.

join with a ureteric bud on the affected side. It has no clinical sequelae but may frequently be associated with absence of the ipsilateral vas deferens and/or epididymis and may be associated with other congenital anomalies including imperforate anus, cardiac valvular anomalies and oesophageal atresia. A single kidney often shows compensatory hypertrophy. The life expectancy of individuals with a single kidney is the same as those with two kidneys.

Failure of the kidney to ascend *in utero* to the correct position in the renal fossa results in renal ectopia. Most commonly the kidney is found in the pelvis: this occurs in c.1 in 2500 live births. Kidneys so placed often have associated malrotation anomalies, and may have marked fetal lobulation. Pelvic kidneys frequently become hydronephrotic as a result of an anterior placed ureter and an anomalous arterial supply. An associated pelviureteric junction obstruction is often present.

Very rarely and despite the normal location of the ureteric orifices within the bladder, the two renal masses may be on the same side. This is termed crossed renal ectopia and usually the two renal masses are fused in such circumstances. A solitary crossed renal ectopia may be associated with skeletal and other genitourinary anomalies.

Horseshoe kidney – Horseshoe kidneys are found in 1 in 400 individuals. A transverse bridge of renal tissue, the isthmus, which usually but not invariably contains functioning renal substance, connects the two renal masses. The isthmus lies between the inferior poles, most commonly anterior to the great vessels. The ureters curve anterior to the connection and may have a high insertion into the renal pelvis.

The blood supply to horseshoe kidneys is variable. One vessel to each moiety is seen in 30% of horseshoe kidneys. Multiple anomalous vessels are common and the isthmus may be supplied by a vessel directly from the aorta or from branches of the inferior mesenteric, common iliac or external iliac arteries. In view of this variable arterial anatomy, angiography is very helpful when planning renal surgery on horseshoe kidneys.

Horseshoe kidneys can have an associated congenital pelviureteric junction obstruction in up to 30%. Anomalous vessels crossing the ureter and the abnormal course of the ureter as it passes over renal substance may also cause obstruction. Horseshoe kidneys have an increased incidence of stone disease, probably as a consequence of areas of inefficient drainage.

PERIRENAL FASCIA (Figs 91.3, 91.4)

The perirenal fascia is a dense, elastic connective tissue sheath which envelops each kidney and suprarenal gland together with a layer of surrounding perirenal fat. The kidney and its vessels are embedded in perirenal fat, which is thickest at the renal borders and prolonged at the hilum into the renal sinus.

The perirenal fascia was originally described as being made up of two separate entities, the posterior fascia of Zuckerkandl and the anterior fascia of Gerota which fused laterally to form the lateral conal fascia. According to this view, the lateral conal fascia continued anterolaterally behind the colon to blend with the parietal peritoneum.

However, work by Mitchell (1950) showed that the perirenal fascia is not made up of distinct fused fasciae, but is in fact a single multi-laminated structure which is fused posteriomedially with the muscular fasciae of psoas major and quadratus lumborum. It then extends anterolaterally behind the kidney as a bilaminated sheet, which at a variable point divides into a thin lamina which passes around the front of the kidney as the anterior perirenal fascia, and a thicker posterior lamina which continues anterolaterally as the lateral conal fascia (and fuses with the parietal peritoneum.

Classically, the anterior perirenal fascia was thought to blend into the dense mass of connective tissue surrounding the great vessels in the root of the mesentery behind the duodenum and pancreas, thereby preventing communication between perirenal spaces across the midline. However inspection of CT and anatomical sections of cadavers following the injection of small volumes of contrast and coloured latex respectively into the perirenal space revealed that fluid could extend across the midline at the third to fifth lumbar levels through a narrow channel measuring 2–10 mm in AP dimension. In the midline the anterior and posterior renal fasciae fuse superiorly and are attached to the crus of their respective hemidiaphragms. Inferiorly the fasciae separate for a variable craniocaudal distance along most of the length of each kidney. The posterior perirenal fascia fuses with the muscular fascia of psoas major whilst the anterior perirenal fascia extends across the midline in front of the great vessels and so communication between the two sides is permitted. Below this level the two fasciae once again merge and are attached to the great vessels or iliac vessels. The containment of fluid to one side of the perirenal space that is observed in over two thirds of clinical cases is attributed to the presence of fibrous septae.

Above the suprarenal glands the anterior and posterior perirenal fasciae were previously said to fuse with each other and to the diaphragmatic fascia. This description of a closed superior cone is not universally accepted. Cadaveric experiments have shown the superior aspect of the perirenal space to be open and in continuity with the bare area of the liver on the right and the subphrenic extraperitoneal space on the left. The posterior fascial layer blends bilaterally with the fascia of psoas major and quadratus lumborum as well as the inferior phrenic fascia. The anterior fascial layer on the right blends with the right inferior coronary ligament at the level of the upper pole of the kidney and bare area of the liver. On the left the anterior layer fuses with the gastrosplenic ligament at the level of the suprarenal gland.

There is some debate concerning the inferior fusion of the perirenal fascia. Many investigators believe that inferiorly the anterior and posterior leaves of the perirenal fascial fuse to produce an inverted cone which is open to the pelvis at its apex. Laterally the anterior and posterior leaves fuse with the iliac fascia, and medially they fuse with the periureteric connective tissue. The inferior apex of the cone is open anatomically towards the iliac fossa but rapidly becomes sealed in inflammatory disease. An alternative view is based on the dissection of recently deceased cadavers after injections of coloured latex into the perirenal space: these have shown that the anterior and posterior perirenal fasciae merge to form a single multilaminar fascia which contains the ureter in the iliac fossa. Anteriorly this common fascia is loosely connected to the parietal peritoneum, and so denies free communication between the perirenal space and the pelvis, and also denies communication between the perirenal and pararenal spaces.

A simple nephrectomy for benign disease removes the kidney from within perirenal fascia; a radical nephrectomy for cancer removes the entire contents of the perirenal space including the perirenal fascia, in order to give adequate clearance around the tumour.

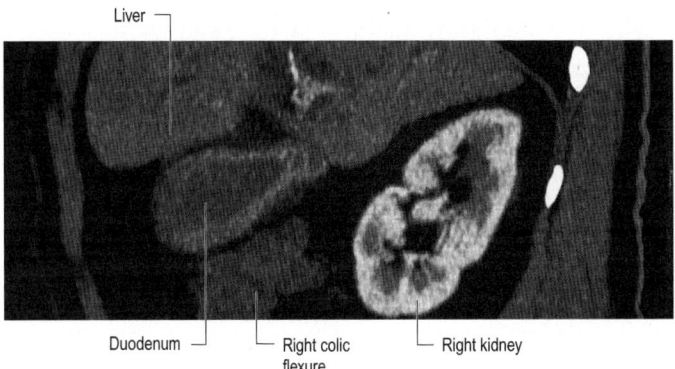

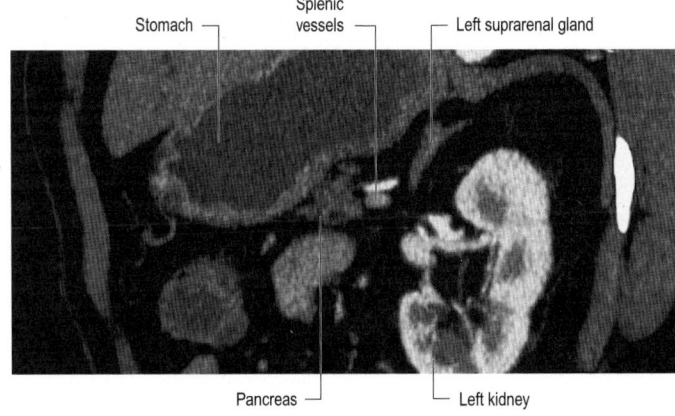

Fig. 91.5 Multislice CT scan of the kidneys. **A**, Coronal oblique reformat showing both kidneys and the suprarenal glands. **B**, Sagittal oblique of the right kidney lying posterior to the right lobe of the liver, duodenum and right colic flexure. **C**, Sagittal oblique of the left kidney lying posterior to the stomach, pancreas and the splenic vessels.

RENAL RELATIONS (Fig. 91.5)

The superior poles of both kidneys are thick and round and each is related to its suprarenal gland. The inferior poles are thinner and extend to within 2.5 cm of the iliac crests. The lateral borders are convex. The left kidney is covered superiorly by peritoneum, which separates it from the spleen, and below this is in contact with the descending colon (**Fig. 91.6A**). The peritoneum of the greater sac separates the lateral border of the right kidney from the right lobe of the liver. The medial borders are convex adjacent to the poles, concave between them and slope inferolaterally. In each a deep vertical fissure opens anteromedially as the hilum, which is bounded by anterior and posterior lips and contains the renal vessels and nerves and the renal pelvis. The relative positions of the main hilar structures are the renal vein anterior, the renal artery intermediate and the pelvis of the kidney posterior. Usually an arterial branch from the main renal artery runs over the superior margin of the renal pelvis to enter the hilum on the posterior aspect of the pelvis, and a renal venous tributary often leaves the hilum in the same plane.

Above the hilum the medial border is related to the suprarenal gland and below to the origin of the ureter.

The convex anterior surface of the kidney actually faces anterolaterally and its relations differ on the right and left. Likewise the posterior surface of the kidneys in reality faces posteromedially. Its relations are similar on both sides of the body.

ANTEROLATERAL SURFACE OF RIGHT KIDNEY (Fig. 91.6A)

A small area of the superior pole is in contact with the right suprarenal gland, indeed the suprarenal gland may overlap the upper part of the medial border of the superior pole. A large area below this (about three-quarters of the anterior surface) is immediately related to the renal impression on the right lobe of the liver. A narrow medial area is related to the descending part of the duodenum. Inferiorly the anterior surface is in contact laterally with the right colic flexure and medially with part of the small intestine. The areas related to the small intestine and in

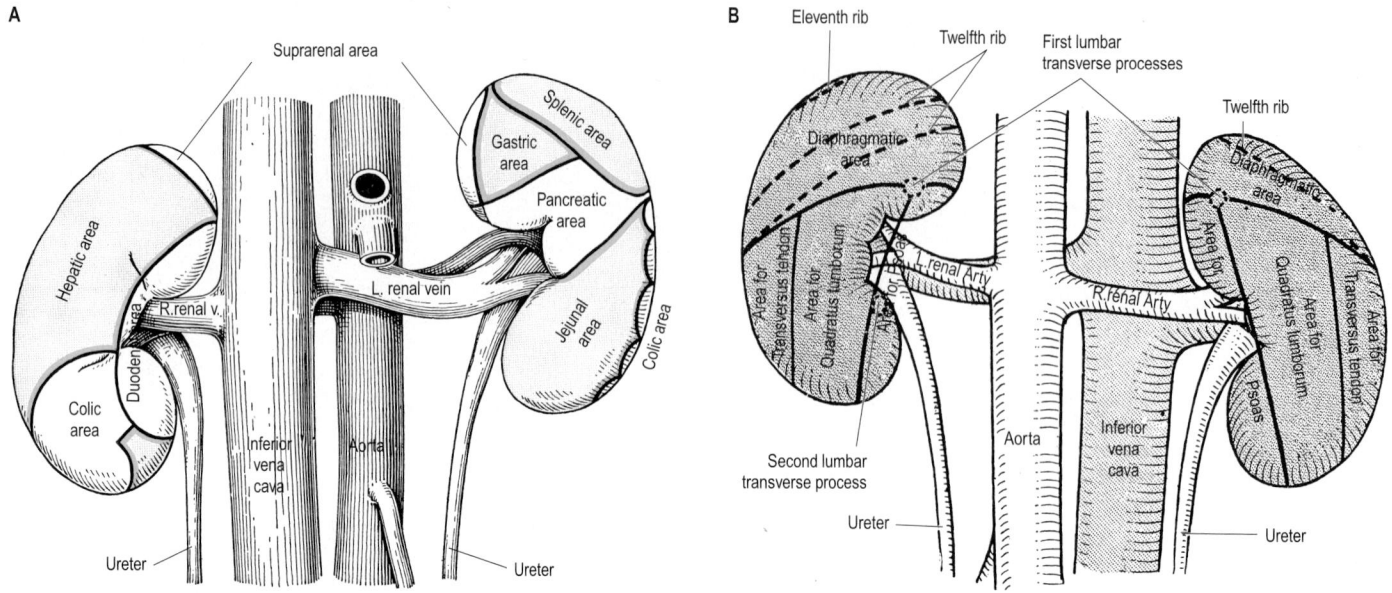

Fig. 91.6 A, The anterior surfaces of the kidneys, showing the areas related to neighbouring viscera. Areas coloured pale blue are separated from adjacent viscera by the peritoneum. **B**, The posterior surfaces of the kidneys, showing the areas of relation to the posterior abdominal wall.

contact with the liver are covered by peritoneum which overlies the renal fascia, whereas the suprarenal, duodenal and colic areas are devoid of peritoneum.

ANTEROLATERAL SURFACE OF LEFT KIDNEY (Fig. 91.6A)
A small medial area of the superior pole is related to the left suprarenal gland. Approximately the upper two-thirds of the lateral half of the anterior surface is related to the spleen. A central quadrilateral area lies in contact with the pancreas and the splenic vessels. Above this a small variable triangular region, between the suprarenal and splenic areas, is in contact with the stomach. Below the pancreatic and splenic areas, a narrow lateral strip which extends to the lateral border of the kidney is related to the left colic flexure and the beginning of the descending colon. An extensive medial area is related to loops of jejunum. The gastric area is covered with the peritoneum of the lesser sac (omental bursa) and the splenic and jejunal areas are covered by the peritoneum

of the greater sac. Behind the peritoneum covering the jejunal area, branches of the left colic vessels are related to the kidney. The suprarenal, pancreatic and colic areas are devoid of peritoneum.

POSTEROMEDIAL SURFACE OF BOTH KIDNEYS (Figs 91.6B, 91.7)
The posteromedial surface of the kidneys is embedded in fat and devoid of peritoneum (**Figs 91.3, 91.4**). It is anterior to the diaphragm, the medial and lateral arcuate ligaments, psoas major, quadratus lumborum and the aponeurotic tendon of transversus abdominis, the subcostal vessels and subcostal, iliohypogastric, and ilioinguinal nerves. The upper pole of the right kidney is level with the twelfth rib, and that of the left with the eleventh and twelfth ribs. The diaphragm separates the kidney from the pleura, which descends to form the costodiaphragmatic recess. Sometimes its muscle is defective or absent in a triangle immediately above the lateral arcuate ligament, and this allows perirenal adipose tissue to contact the diaphragmatic pleura.

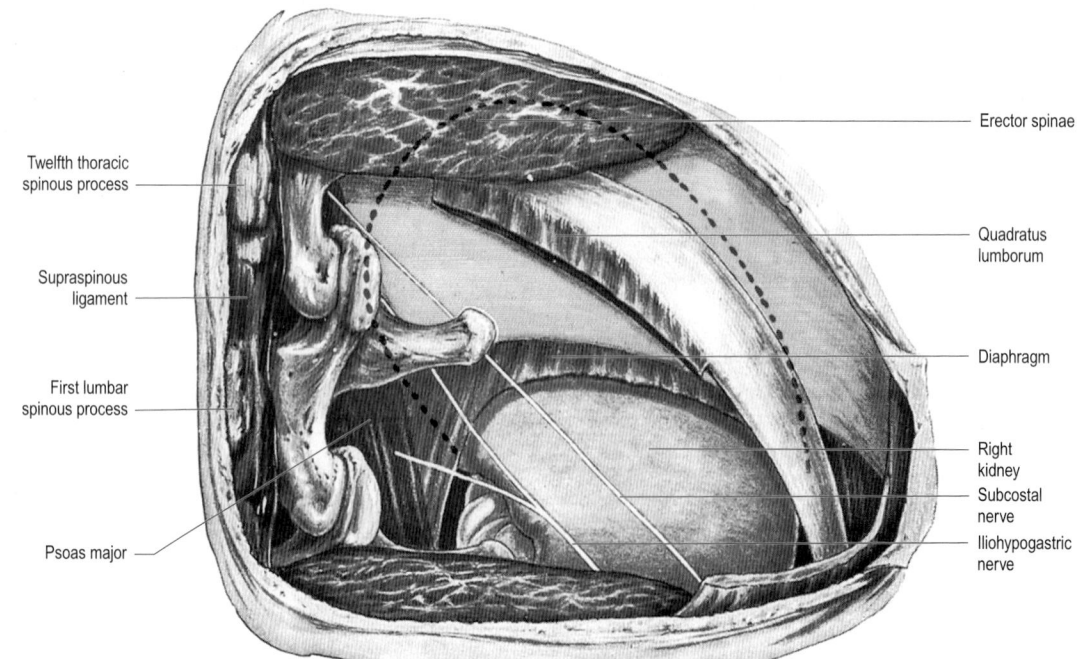

Fig. 91.7 The right kidney (posterior exposure). The blue area represents the pleura, the broken red line the upper part of the kidney. The subcostal nerve has been displaced downwards. Parts of the diaphragm and quadratus lumborum have been resected.

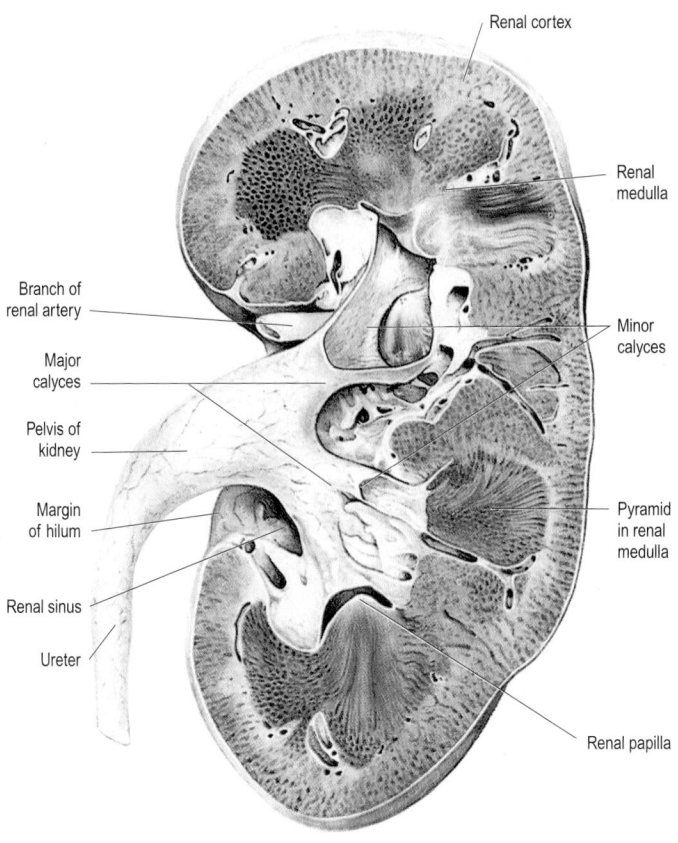

Renal cortex

Renal medulla

Branch of renal artery

Major calyces

Pelvis of kidney

Margin of hilum

Renal sinus

Ureter

Minor calyces

Pyramid in renal medulla

Renal papilla

Fig. 91.8 Longitudinal section through a kidney to show the normal macroscopic appearance: note the pelvis of the ureter and its division into calyces. The pelvis and major calyces have not been opened.

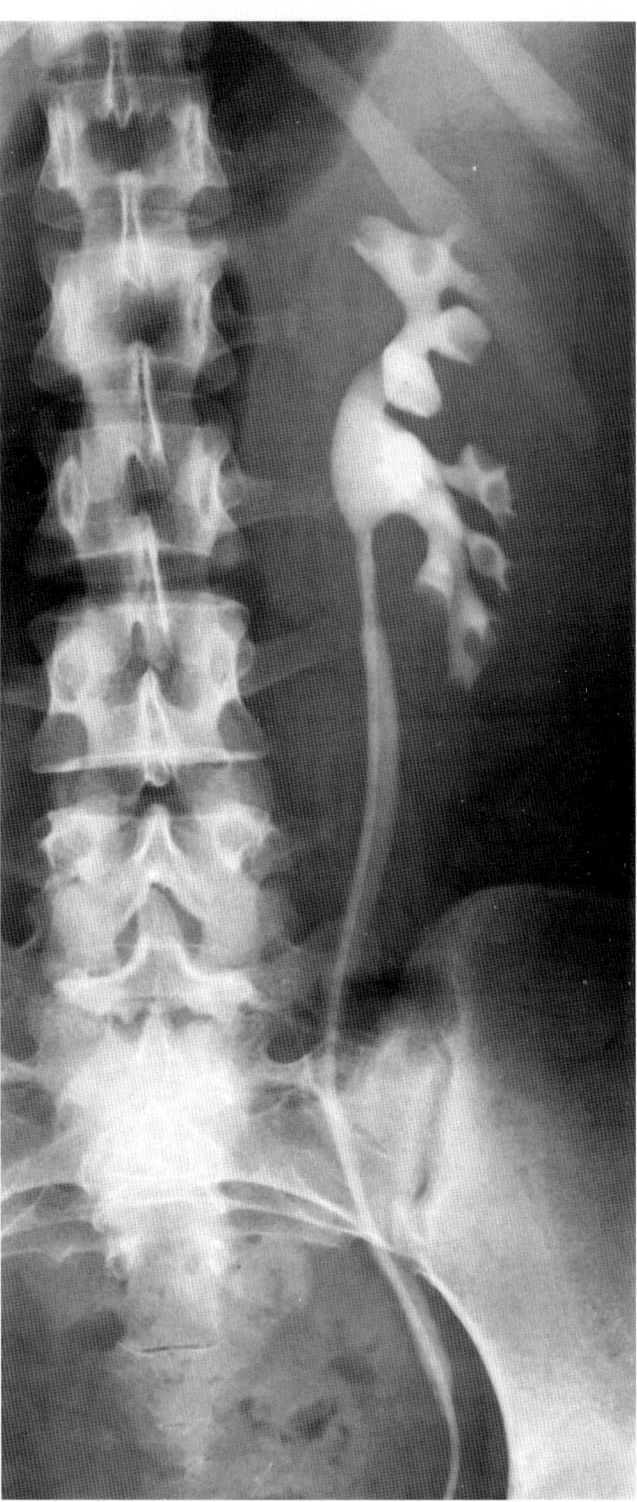

Fig. 91.9 A left retrograde pyelogram. Contrast medium which has been introduced into the calyces, pelvis and upper ureter via a ureteric catheter can be clearly identified. This technique affords considerably better visualization of the calyces than can be achieved by the intravenous method. Note the relation of the ureter to the tips of the lumbar transverse processes and the characteristic 'cupping' or 'champagne glass' profiles of the tips of the lesser calyces where they surround the renal pyramids. 'Calyx' means a cup and such 'cupping' of the minor calyces is the normal appearance. (The major calyces are not cups and are hence inappropriately named.)

GENERAL RENAL STRUCTURE (Fig. 91.8)

The postnatal kidney has a thin capsule, easily removed, composed of collagen-rich tissue with some elastic and smooth muscle fibres. In renal disease it may become adherent. The kidney itself can be divided into an internal medulla and external cortex.

The renal medulla consists of pale, striated, conical renal pyramids, their bases peripheral, their apices converging to the renal sinus. At the renal sinus they project into calyces as papillae.

The renal cortex is subcapsular, arching over the bases of the pyramids and extending between them towards the renal sinus as renal columns. The peripheral regions are cortical arches and are traversed by radial, lighter-coloured medullary rays, separated by darker tissue, the convoluted part. The rays taper towards the renal capsule and are peripheral prolongations from the bases of renal pyramids. The cortex is histologically divisible into outer and inner zones; the inner is demarcated from the medulla by tangential blood vessels (arcuate arteries and veins), which lie at the junction of the two, but a thin layer of cortical tissue (subcortex) appears on the medullary side of this zone. The cortex close to the medulla is sometimes termed juxtamedullary.

RENAL CALYCES AND PELVIS (Fig. 91.9)

The hilum of the kidney leads into a central renal sinus, lined by the renal capsule and almost filled by the renal pelvis and vessels, the remaining space being filled by fat. Within the renal sinus, the collecting tubules of the nephrons of the kidney open onto the summits of the renal papillae to drain into minor calyces, funnel-shaped expansions of the upper urinary tract (**Figs 91.9, 91.15**). The renal capsule covers the external surface of the kidney and continues through the hilum to line the sinus and fuse with the adventitial coverings of the minor calyces. Each minor calyx surrounds either a single papilla or, more rarely, groups of two or three papillae. The minor calyces unite with their neighbours to form two or possibly three larger chambers, the major calyces. The calyces of each kidney are usually arranged in seven pairs (seven ventral and seven dorsal) although there is wide variation. The calyces drain into the infundibula. The renal pelvis is normally formed from the junction of two infundibula, one from the upper and one from the lower pole calyces, but there may be a third, draining the calyces in

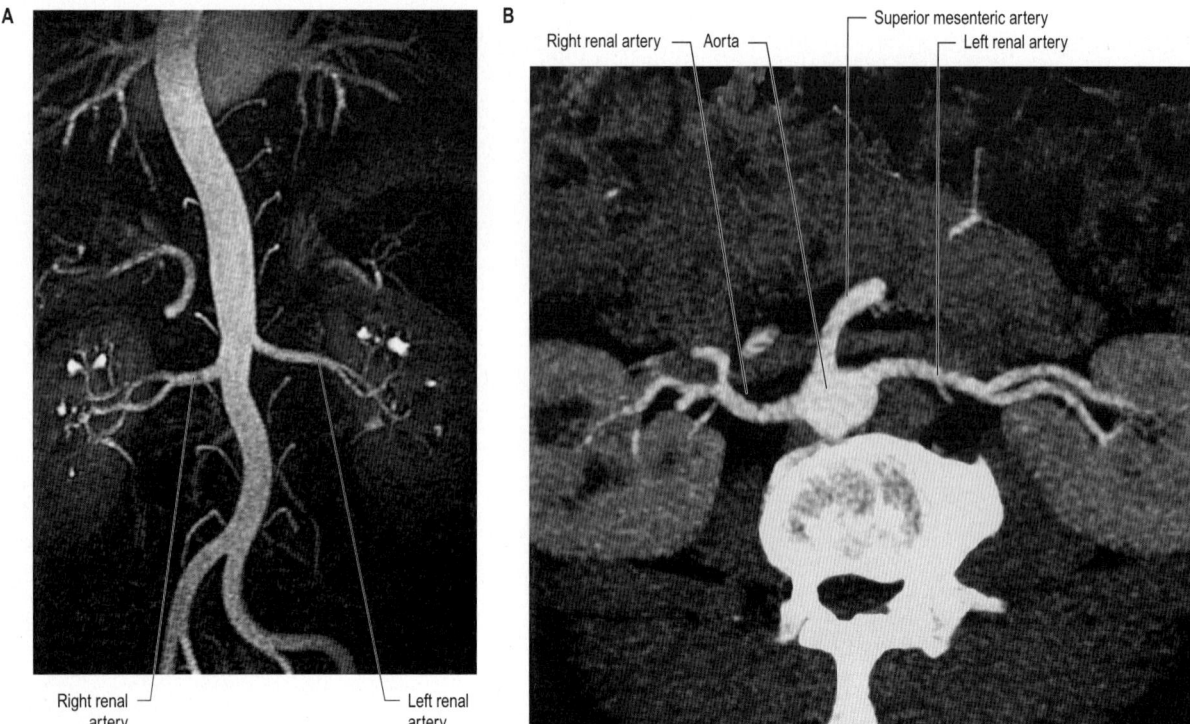

A

Right renal
artery

Left renal
artery

B

Right renal artery — Aorta — Superior mesenteric artery — Left renal artery

Fig. 91.10 Multislice CT renal angiogram. **A**, Coronal reformat. **B**, Axial reformat.

the mid-portion of the kidney. The calyces are usually grouped so that three pairs drain into the upper pole infundibulum and four pairs into the lower pole infundibulum. If there is a middle infundibulum, the distribution is normally three pairs at the upper pole, two in the middle, and two at the lower pole. There is considerable variation in the arrangement of the infundibula and in the extent to which the pelvis is intrarenal or extrarenal. The funnel-shaped renal pelvis tapers as it passes inferomedially, traversing the renal hilum to become continuous with the ureter (**Figs 92.1, 91.8, 91.9, 91.15**). It is rarely possible to determine precisely where the renal pelvis ceases and the ureter begins: the region is usually extrahilar and normally lies adjacent to the lower part of the medial border of the kidney. Rarely, the entire renal pelvis has been found to lie inside the sinus of the kidney so that the pelviureteric region occurs either in the vicinity of the renal hilum or completely within the renal sinus.

The calyces, renal pelvis and ureter are well-demonstrated radiologically following an intravenous injection of radio-opaque contrast which is excreted in the urine (intravenous urography – IVU) (**Fig. 92.1**); or after the introduction of radio-opaque contrast into the ureter by catheterization through a cystoscope (ascending or retrograde pyelography (**Fig. 91.9**). Normal cupping of the minor calyces by projecting renal papillae may be obliterated by conditions that cause hydronephrosis, chronic distension of the ureter and renal pelvis due to upper or lower urinary tract obstruction resulting in elevated intrapelvic pressure.

RENAL CALCULI

An understanding of intrarenal and ureteric anatomy is essential when managing patients with calculi, particularly now that minimal invasive techniques are available to treat this common pathology.

Smaller renal calculi are treated with extracorporeal shock wave lithotripsy. Stones in the lower pole of the kidney clear less well if the angle between the infundibulum of the calyx containing the stone and the ureter is acute, or if there is a particularly long and narrow infundibulum.

Percutaneous stone extraction is most frequently achieved by puncturing a posterior calyx with a needle. Posterior calyces are seen to lie more medially when looking at an intravenous urogram because of the normal rotation of the kidney.

Ureteric calculi tend to be arrested in their descent in either the pelviureteric region, the point where the ureter passes over the pelvic

brim, or the vesicoureteric junction, because these are the three areas where the ureter is narrowest.

VASCULAR SUPPLY AND LYMPHATIC DRAINAGE

ARTERIES (Figs 91.1, 91.10)

The paired renal arteries take c.20% of cardiac output to supply organs that represent less than one-hundredth of total body weight. They supply the kidneys through a number of subdivisions described sequentially as segmental, lobar, interlobar, and arcuate arteries. These are end arteries with no anastomoses. The arcuate arteries further divide into interlobular arteries which give rise to the afferent arteries to the glomeruli.

The renal arteries branch laterally from the aorta just below the origin of the superior mesenteric artery. Both cross the corresponding crus of the diaphragm at right angles to the aorta (**Figs 91.1, 91.11**). The right renal artery is longer and often higher, passing posterior to the inferior vena cava, right renal vein, head of the pancreas and descending part of the duodenum. The left renal artery is a little lower and passes behind the left renal vein, the body of the pancreas and splenic vein. It may be crossed anteriorly by the inferior mesenteric vein.

A single renal artery to each kidney is present in c.70% of individuals. The arteries vary in their level of origin and in their calibre, obliquity and precise relations. In its extrarenal course each renal artery gives off one or more inferior suprarenal arteries, a branch to the ureter and branches which supply perinephric tissue, the renal capsule and the pelvis. Near the renal hilum, each artery divides into an anterior and a posterior division, and these divide into segmental arteries supplying the renal vascular segments. Accessory renal arteries are common (30% of individuals), and usually arise from the aorta above or below the main renal artery and follow it to the renal hilum. They are regarded as persistent embryonic lateral splanchnic arteries. Accessory vessels to the inferior pole cross anterior to the ureter and may, by obstructing the ureter, cause hydronephrosis. Rarely, accessory renal arteries arise from the coeliac or superior mesenteric arteries near the aortic bifurcation or from the common iliac arteries.

Segmental arteries (Fig. 91.12)

The segmental arteries branch successively into lobar, interlobar, arcuate and interlobular arteries, afferent and efferent glomerular arterioles

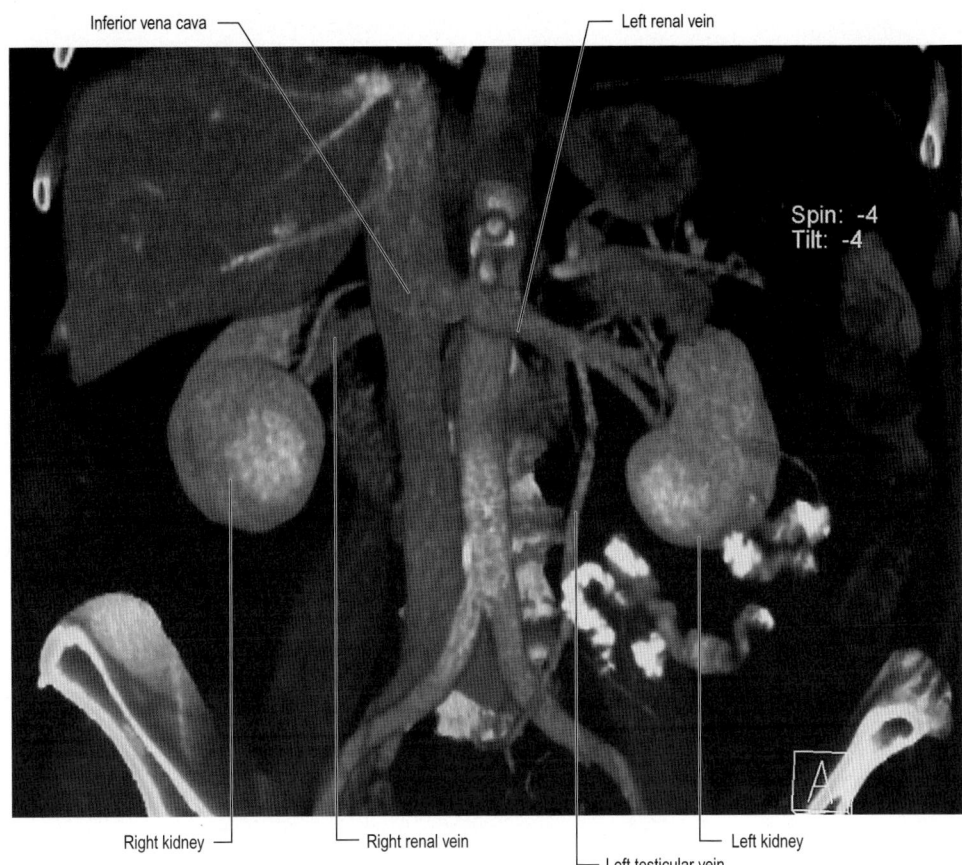

Inferior vena cava

Left renal vein

Spin: -4
Tilt: -4

Right kidney

Right renal vein

Left kidney

Left testicular vein

Fig. 91.11 CT renal venogram. Acquired from a multislice CT examination and reconstructed as a 3D surface shaded reformat.

and cortical intertubular capillary plexuses. The cortical venous radicles drain them and also the vasa recta and associated capillary plexuses of the medulla into the renal vein (**Figs 91.12, 91.15**). Renal vascular segmentation was originally recognized by John Hunter in 1794, but the first detailed account of the primary pattern was produced in the 1950s from casts and radiographs of injected kidneys. Five arterial segments have been identified. The apical segment occupies the anteromedial region of the superior pole. The superior (anterior) segment includes the rest of the superior pole and the central anterosuperior region. The inferior segment encompasses the whole lower pole. The middle (anterior) segment lies between the anterior and inferior segments. The posterior segment includes the whole posterior region between the apical and inferior segments.

This is the pattern most commonly seen and although there can be considerable variation it is the pattern that clinicians most frequently encounter when performing partial nephrectomy. Whatever pattern is present, it must be emphasized that vascular segments are supplied by virtual end arteries. In contrast, larger intrarenal veins have no segmental organization and anastomose freely.

Brödel (1911) described a relatively avascular longitudinal zone (the 'bloodless' line of Brödel) along the convex renal border, which was proposed as the most suitable site for surgical incision. However, many vessels cross this zone, and it is far from 'bloodless': planned radial or intersegmental incisions are preferable. Knowledge of the vascular anatomy of the kidney is important when undertaking partial nephrectomy for renal cell cancers. In this surgery the branches of the renal artery are defined so that the surgeon may safely excise the renal substance containing the tumour whilst not compromising the vascular supply to the remaining renal tissue.

Lobar, interlobar, arcuate and interlobular arteries

Initial branches of segmental arteries are lobar, usually one to each renal pyramid. Before reaching the pyramid they subdivide into two or three interlobar arteries, extending towards the cortex around each pyramid. At the junction of the cortex and medulla, interlobar arteries dichotomize into arcuate arteries which diverge at right angles. As they arch between cortex and medulla, each divides further, ultimately supplying interlobular arteries which diverge radially into the cortex. The terminations of adjacent arcuate arteries do not anastomose but end in

the cortex as additional interlobular arteries. Though most interlobular arteries come from arcuate branches, some arise directly from arcuate or even terminal interlobar arteries (**Fig. 91.15**).

Interlobular arteries ascend towards the superficial cortex or may branch occasionally en route (**Fig. 91.15**). Some are more tortuous and recurve towards the medulla at least once before proceeding towards the renal surface. Others traverse the surface as perforating arteries to anastomose with the capsular plexus (which is also supplied from the inferior suprarenal, renal and gonadal arteries).

Afferent and efferent arterioles

Afferent glomerular arterioles are mainly the lateral rami of interlobular arteries. A few arise from arcuate and interlobar arteries when they vary their direction and angle of origin: deeper ones incline obliquely back towards the medulla, the intermediate pass horizontally, and the more superficial approach the renal surface obliquely before ending in a glomerulus (**Figs 91.13, 91.15**).

From most glomeruli (except those at juxtamedullary and some at intermediate cortical levels) efferent glomerular arterioles soon divide to form a dense peritubular capillary plexus around the proximal and distal convoluted tubules. In the main renal cortical circulation there are thus two sets of capillaries in series, glomerular and peritubular, linked by efferent glomerular arterioles. From the venous ends of the peritubular plexuses fine radicles converge to join interlobular veins, one with each interlobular artery. Many interlobular veins begin beneath the fibrous renal capsule by the convergence of several stellate veins, which drain the most superficial zone of the renal cortex and so are named from their surface appearance. Interlobular veins pass to the corticomedullary junction. They also receive some ascending vasa recta and end in arcuate veins, which accompany arcuate arteries, and anastomose with neighbouring veins. Arcuate veins drain into interlobar veins, which anastomose and form the renal vein.

The vascular supply of the renal medulla is largely from efferent arterioles of juxtamedullary glomeruli, supplemented by some from more superficial glomeruli, and 'aglomerular' arterioles (probably from degenerated glomeruli). Efferent glomerular arterioles passing into the medulla are relatively long, wide vessels, and contribute side branches to neighbouring capillary plexuses before entering the medulla, where each divides into 12–25 descending vasa recta. As their name suggests,

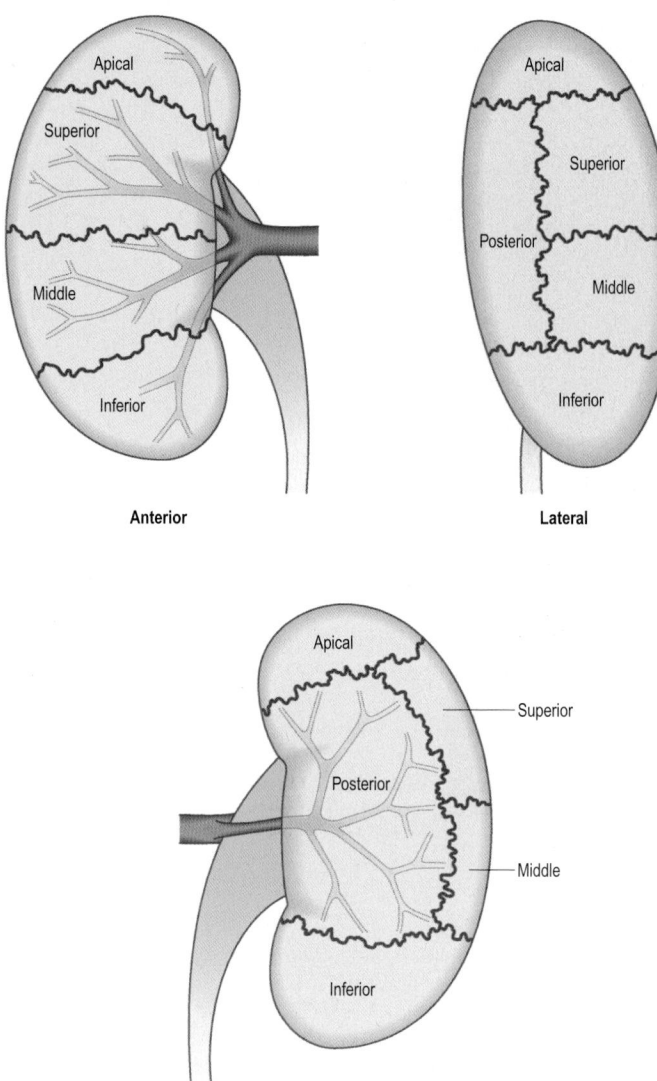

Anterior

Lateral

Posterior

Fig. 91.12 Segmental arterial anatomy of the right kidney. (By permission from Walsh PC, Retik AB, Vaughan ED et al (eds) 2002 Campbell's Urology, 8th edn. Philadelphia: Saunders.)

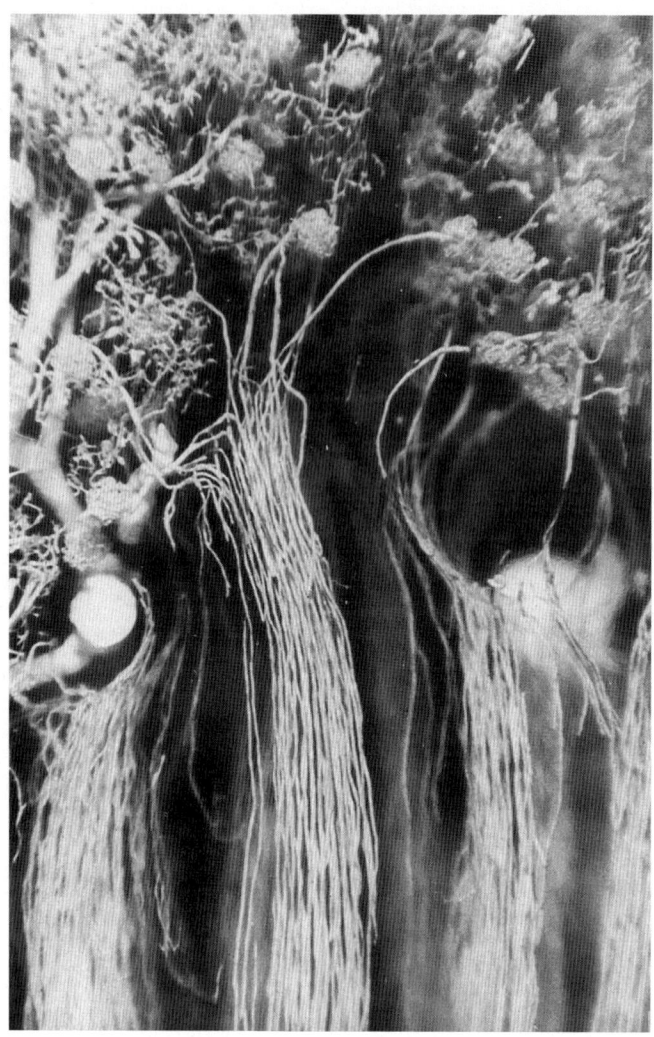

Fig. 91.13 'Microfil' injection of the arterial tree of human kidney, high power micrograph. The juxtamedullary efferent arterioles leave the glomeruli to form medullary vascular bundles (descending vasa recta). (Preparation provided by DB Moffat, Department of Anatomy, University College of Wales, Cardiff.)

these run straight to varying depths in the renal medulla, contributing side branches to a radially elongated capillary plexus (**Fig. 91.15**) applied to the descending and ascending limbs of renal loops and to collecting ducts. The venous ends of capillaries converge to the ascending vasa recta, which drain into arcuate or interlobular veins. An essential feature of the vasa recta (particularly in the outer medulla) is that both ascending and descending vessels are grouped into vascular bundles, within which the external aspects of both types are closely apposed, bringing them close to the limbs of renal loops and collecting ducts. As these bundles converge centrally into the renal medulla they contain fewer vessels: some terminate at successive levels in neighbouring capillary plexuses. This proximity of descending and ascending vessels with each other and adjacent ducts provides the structural basis for the counter-current exchange and multiplier phenomena (**Figs 91.13, 91.15**).

These complex renal vascular patterns show regional specializations which are closely adapted to the spatial organization and functions of renal corpuscles, tubules and ducts (**Figs 91.13, 91.14, 91.15**).

Renal, interlobar and arcuate arteries are typical large muscular arteries and the interlobular vessels resemble small muscular arteries. Afferent glomerular vessels have a typical arteriolar structure with a muscular coat two to three cells thick; this coat and the connective tissue components of the wall diminish near a glomerulus until a point 30–50 μm proximal to it where arteriolar cells begin to show modifications typical of the juxtaglomerular apparatus (p. 1283). The efferent arterioles from most cortical glomeruli have thicker walls and a narrower calibre than corresponding afferents. Although the afferent arteriole

is generally considered to be solely responsible for tubuloglomerular feedback, the role of the efferent arteriole in this process has been reviewed by Davis (1991). The peritubular and medullary capillaries possess a well-defined basal lamina and their endothelial cells have typically fenestrated cytoplasm, as in ascending vasa recta, whereas the descending vasa recta have thicker, continuous endothelium.

VEINS (Fig. 91.11)

The large renal veins lie anterior to the renal arteries and open into the inferior vena cava almost at right angles. The left is three times longer than the right (7.5 cm and 2.5 cm) and for this reason the left kidney is the preferred side for live donor nephrectomy. It runs from its origin in the renal hilum, posterior to the splenic vein and the body of pancreas, and then across the anterior aspect of the aorta, just below the origin of the superior mesenteric artery. The left gonadal vein enters it from below and the left suprarenal vein, usually receiving one of the left inferior phrenic veins, enters it above but nearer the midline. The left renal vein enters the inferior vena cava a little superior and to the right. The right renal vein is behind the descending duodenum and sometimes the lateral part of the head of the pancreas.

The left renal vein may be double, one vein passing posterior, the other anterior, to the aorta before joining the inferior vena cava. This is sometimes referred to as persistence of the 'renal collar'. The anterior vein may be absent so that there is a single retroaortic left renal vein. Because of its close relationship with the aorta, the left renal vein may be ligated during surgery for aortic aneurysm. This seldom results in any harm to the kidney, provided that the ligature is placed to the right

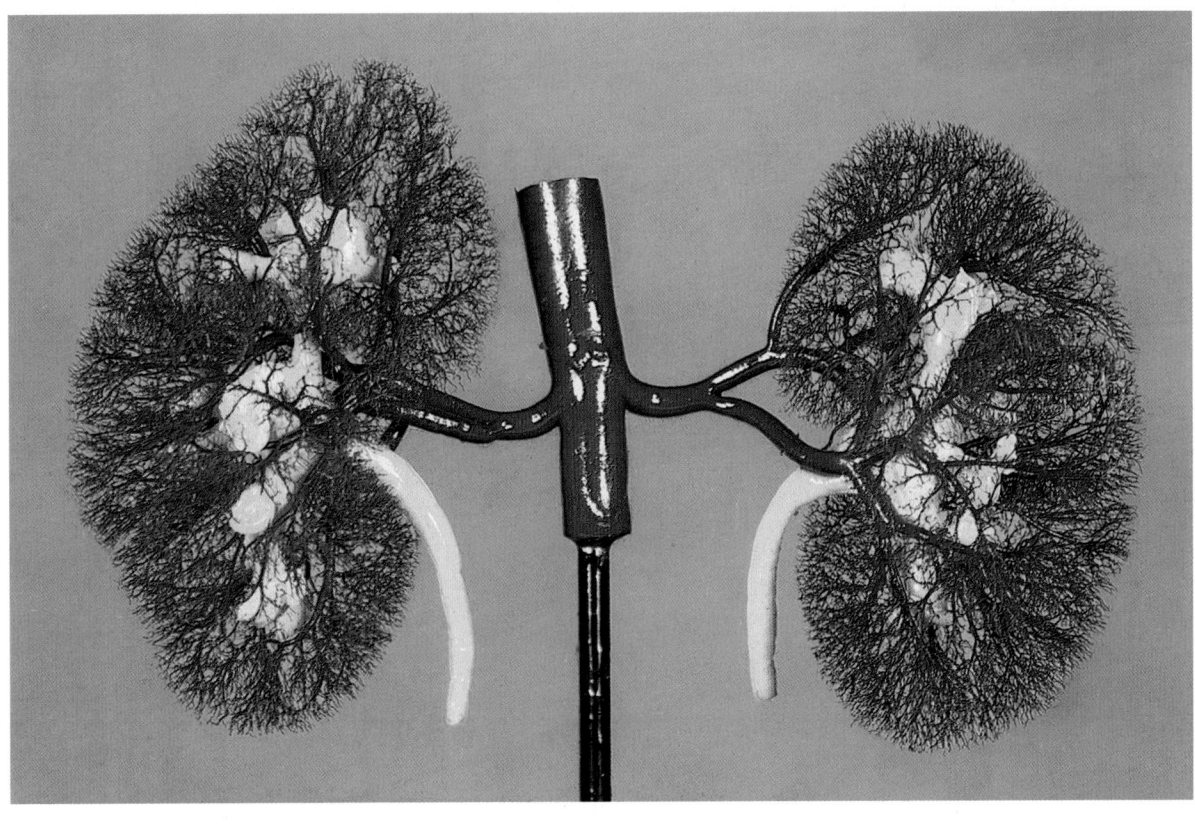

Fig. 91.14 Resin corrosion cast of human kidneys. Ureter, pelvis and calyces are yellow; aorta, renal arteries and their branches are red. Compare with **Figs 91.9, 91.10A**. (Prepared by the late DH Tompsett of the Royal College of Surgeons of England. By permission of the Museums of The Royal College of Surgeons.)

of the draining gonadal and suprarenal veins, because these usually provide adequate collateral venous drainage. The right renal vein has no significant collateral drainage and cannot be ligated with impunity.

LYMPHATIC DRAINAGE

Renal lymphatic vessels begin in three plexuses, around the renal tubules, under the renal capsule, and in the perirenal fat (the latter two connect freely). Collecting vessels from the intrarenal plexus form four or five trunks which follow the renal vein to end in the lateral aortic nodes; as they leave the hilum the subcapsular collecting vessels join them. The perirenal plexus drains directly into the same nodes.

INNERVATION

A dense plexus of autonomic nerves around the renal artery is formed by rami from the coeliac ganglion and plexus, aorticorenal ganglion, lowest thoracic splanchnic nerve, first lumbar splanchnic nerve and aortic plexus. Small ganglia occur in the renal plexus, the largest usually behind the origin of the renal artery. The plexus continues into the kidney around the arterial branches to supply the vessels, renal glomeruli, and tubules, especially the cortical tubules. Axons from plexuses around the arcuate arteries innervate juxtamedullary efferent arterioles and vasa recta, which control the blood flow between the cortex and medulla without affecting the glomerular circulation. Axons from the renal plexus contribute to ureteric and gonadal plexuses. The ureteric plexus receives, in its upper part, branches from the renal and aortic plexuses, in its intermediate part, branches from the superior hypogastric plexus and hypogastric nerve, and in its lower part, branches from the hypogastric nerve and inferior hypogastric plexus. This supply influences the inherent motility of the ureter.

MICROSTRUCTURE (Fig. 91.15)

The kidney is composed of many tortuous, closely packed uriniferous tubules, bounded by a delicate connective tissue in which run blood vessels, lymphatics and nerves. Each tubule consists of two embryologically distinct parts (p. 1373), the nephron, which produces urine, and the collecting duct, which completes the concentration of urine and through which urine passes out of the kidney to the ureter and urinary bladder.

The nephron consists of a renal corpuscle, concerned with filtration from the plasma, and a renal tubule, concerned with selective resorption from the filtrate to form the urine. Collecting ducts carry fluid from several renal tubules to a terminal papillary duct, opening into a minor calyx at the apex of a renal papilla (**Fig. 91.15A**). Papillary surfaces show numerous minute orifices of these ducts and pressure on a fresh kidney expresses urine from them.

RENAL CORPUSCLE (Figs 91.16, 91.17)

Renal corpuscles are small rounded structures averaging c.0.2 mm in diameter, visible in the renal cortex deep to a narrow peripheral cortical zone (**Figs 91.15, 91.16**). There are one to two million renal corpuscles in each kidney, their number decreasing with age. Each has a central glomerulus of vessels and a glomerular (Bowman's) capsule, from which the renal tubule originates.

Glomerulus

A glomerulus is a collection of convoluted capillary blood vessels, united by a delicate mesangial matrix and supplied by an afferent arteriole which enters the capsule opposite the urinary pole, where the filtrate enters the tubule. An efferent arteriole emerges from the same point, the vascular pole of the corpuscle. Glomeruli are simple in form until late prenatal life; some remain so for about 6 months after birth, the majority maturing by 6 years and all by 12 years (p. 1373).

Bowman's capsule (Figs 91.16, 91.18, 91.19, 91.20)

Bowman's capsule is the blind expanded end of a renal tubule, and is deeply invaginated by the glomerulus. It is lined by a simple squamous epithelium on its outer (parietal) wall; its glomerular, juxtacapillary (visceral) wall is composed of specialized epithelial podocytes. Between the two walls of the capsule is a flattened urinary space, continuous with the proximal convoluted tubule (**Figs 91.15B, 91.16**). The basal lamina of the visceral capsular podocytes is shared with that of the glomerular endothelium.

Podocytes surrounding the capillary loops are stellate cells, whose major (primary) foot processes curve around capillaries. These branch to form secondary processes which are applied closely to the basal lamina and they, or tertiary processes, give rise to the terminal pedicels (**Figs 91.18, 91.19, 91.20**). Pedicels of one cell alternate with those of an adjacent cell and interdigitate tightly with each other. Pedicels are separated by narrow (25 nm) gaps, the filtration slits (**Figs 91.18,**

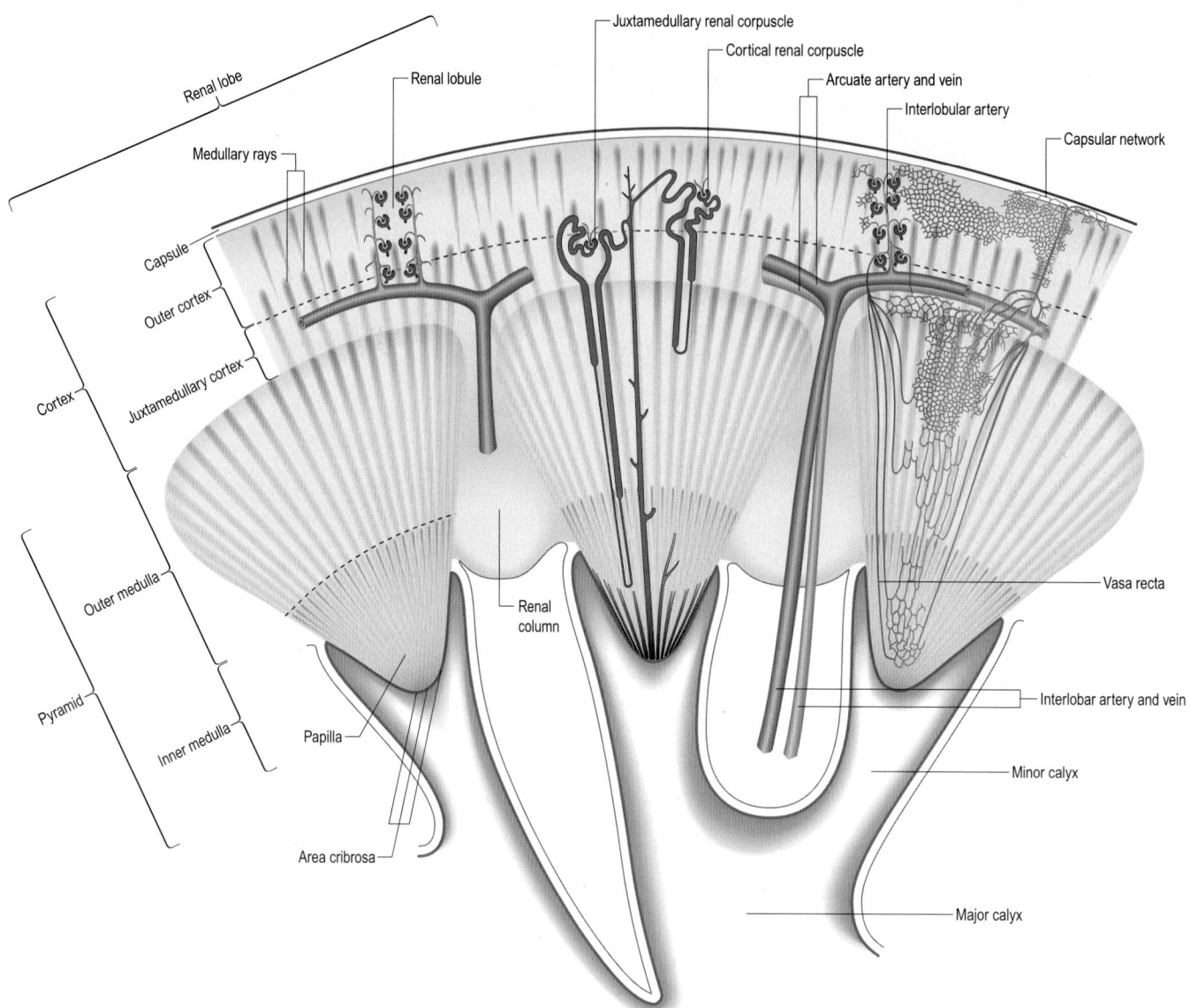

Fig. 91.15 The structural and functional organization of the kidney. The major structures in the kidney cortex and medulla (left), the position of cortical and juxtamedullary nephrons (middle) and the major blood vessels (right).

91.20). The latter are covered by a dense, membranous slit diaphragm, through which filtrate must pass to enter the urinary space.

The glomerular endothelium is finely fenestrated. The principal barrier to the passage of fluid from capillary lumen to urinary space is the shared endothelial and podocyte basal lamina (**Fig. 91.20**). This is c.0.33 μm thick in man, and is produced by the fusion of endothelial and podocyte laminae; it is finely fibrillar and shows three layers. The first layer, towards the endothelial surface, and the third layer are pale-staining (lamina rara interna and lamina rara externa, respectively); the middle layer is dense and fibrous (lamina densa). This arrangement differs from basal laminae elsewhere, and reflects its dual origin. The glomerular basal lamina acts as a selective filter, allowing the passage from blood, under pressure, of water and various small molecules and ions in the circulation. Haemoglobin may cross the filter, but larger molecules and those of similar size with a negative charge, are largely retained. Most protein that does enter the filtrate is selectively resorbed and degraded by cells of the proximal convoluted tubule.

Irregular mesangial cells, with phagocytic and contractile properties, lie within the delicate supportive mesangial matrix (mesangium) of the glomerulus, which they secrete. The mesangium is a specialized connective tissue which binds the loop of glomerular capillaries and fills the spaces between endothelial surfaces that are not invested by podocytes (**Fig. 91.15B**). Mesangial cells are related to vascular pericytes (p. 146) and are concerned with the turnover of glomerular basal lamina. They clear the glomerular filter of, e.g. immune complexes and cellular debris,

and their contractile properties help to regulate blood flow. Similar cells, the extraglomerular mesangial (lacis) cells, lie outside the glomerulus at the vascular pole and form part of the juxtaglomerular apparatus.

RENAL TUBULE

A renal or uriniferous tubule consists of a glomerular capsule leading into a proximal convoluted tubule, connected to the capsule by a short neck which continues into a sinuous or coiled convoluted part (**Fig. 91.15B**). This straightens as it approaches the medulla and becomes the descending thick limb of the loop of Henle which is connected to the ascending limb by an abrupt U-turn. The limbs of the loop of Henle are narrower and thin-walled as they traverse the deeper medullary tissue, forming the descending and ascending thin segments. The ascending thick limb continues into the distal tubule. The tubule wall shows a focal thickening, the macula densa, where it comes close to the vascular pole of its parent glomerulus at the start of the convoluted part of the distal tubule. The nephron finally straightens once more as the connecting tubule, which ends by joining a collecting duct.

Collecting ducts originate in the cortical medullary rays and join others at intervals. They finally open into wider papillary ducts which open on to a papilla; their numerous orifices form a perforated area cribrosa on the surface at its tip (**Fig. 91.15B**).

Renal tubules are lined throughout by a single-layered epithelium (**Figs 91.15B, 91.16, 91.21**). The type of epithelial cell varies according to the functional roles of the different regions, e.g. active transport and

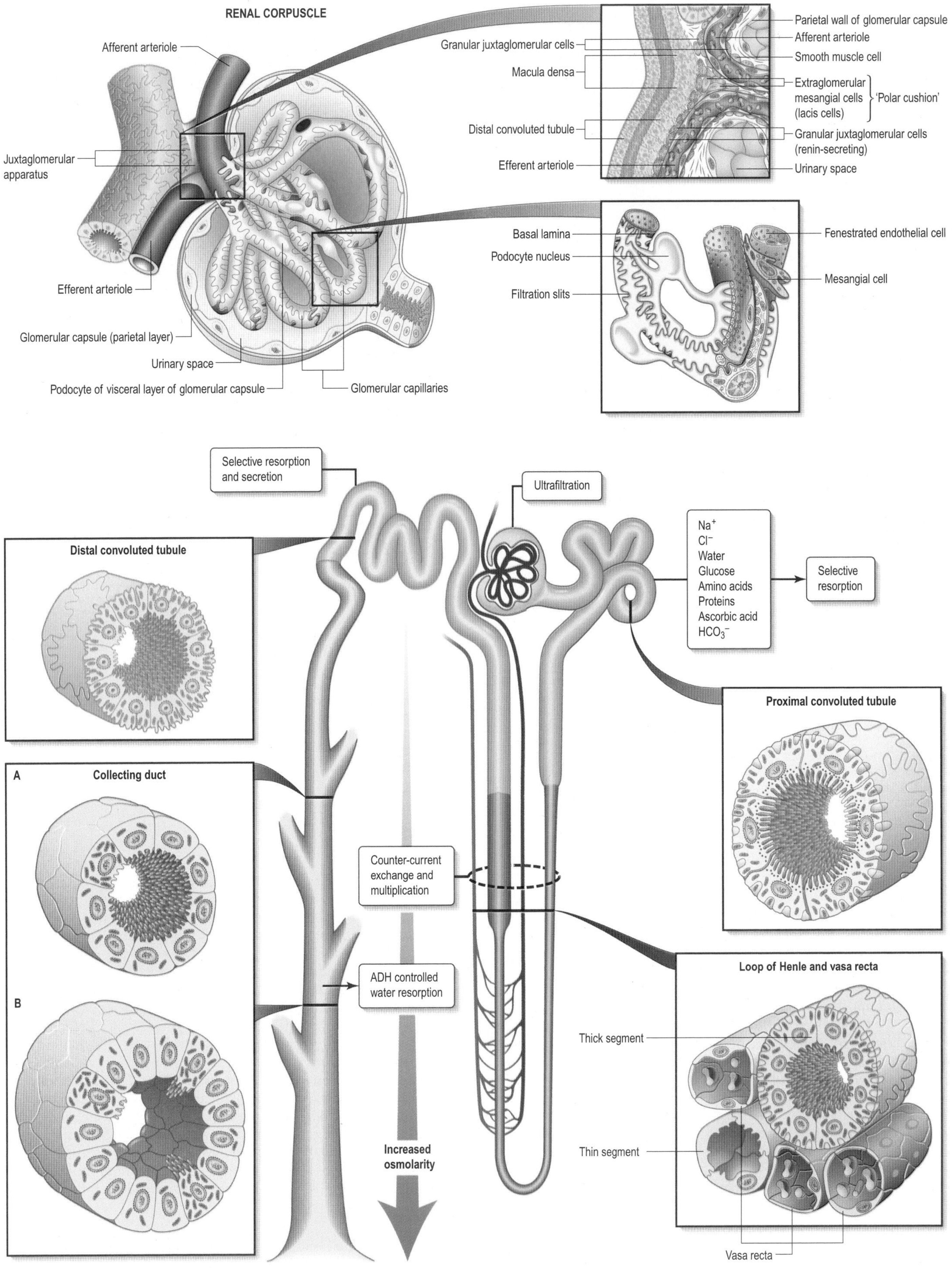

Fig. 91.15 (*Cont'd*) **B**, The regional microstructure and principal activities of a kidney nephron and collecting duct. For clarity, a nephron of the long loop (juxtamedullary) type is shown.

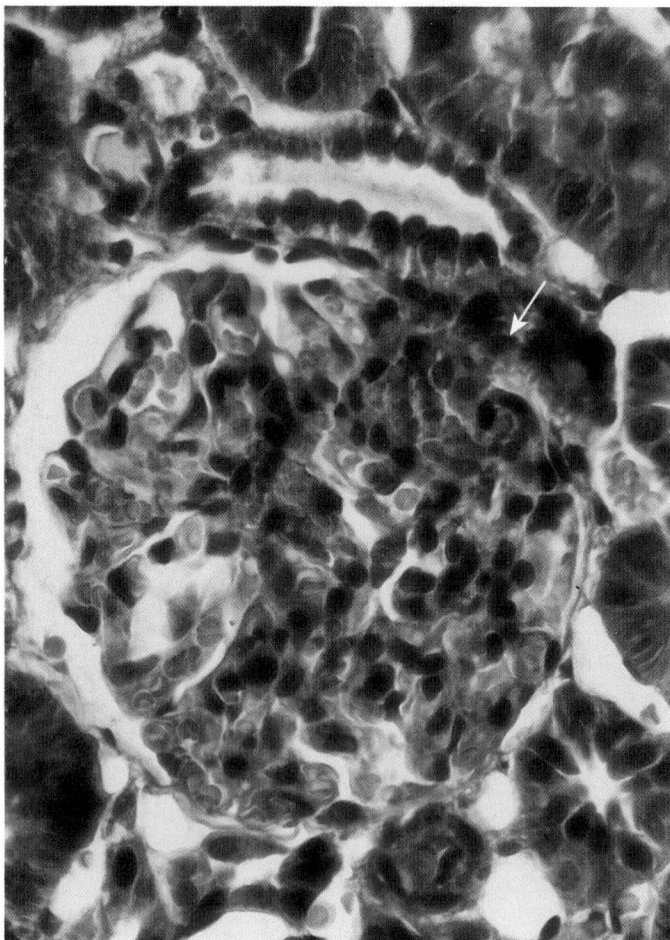

Fig. 91.16 A renal corpuscle in the kidney cortex (trichrome-stained), showing a glomerulus (centre) within its capsule, enclosing the urinary space (left). An arteriole containing erythrocytes is seen at the vascular pole of the capsule (arrow), where it is associated with the macula densa of a distal convoluted tubule (DCT, top). The macula densa comprises a group of more closely packed, taller cells in part of the DCT wall adjacent to the glomerulus. Profiles of proximal convoluted tubules (with brush borders obscuring their lumen) are also visible (e.g. top right). (Photograph by Kevin Fitzpatrick on behalf of GKT School of Medicine, London.)

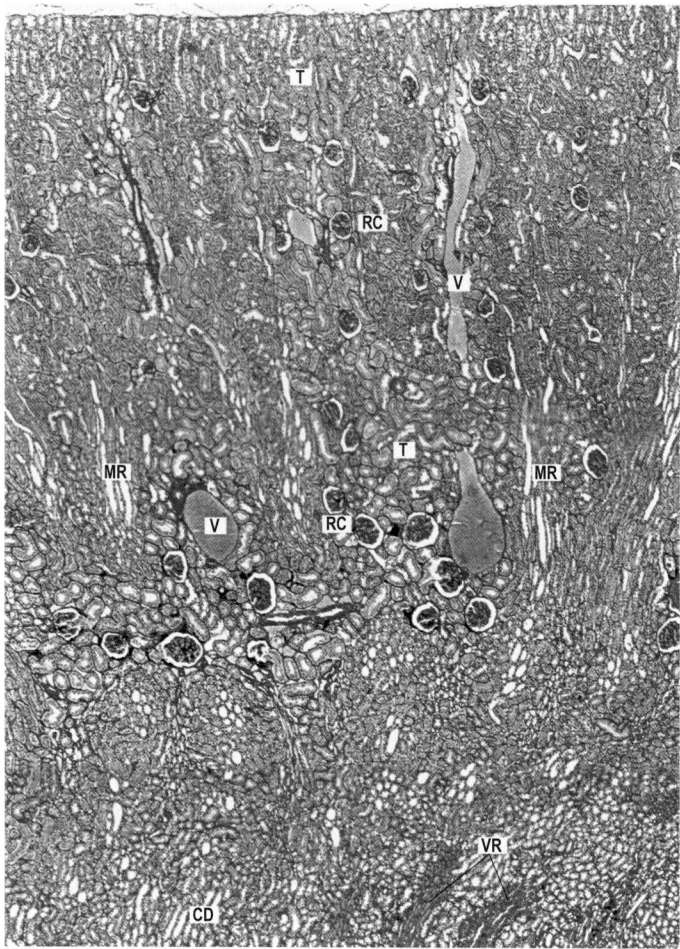

Fig. 91.17 Renal cortex and medulla. The cortex contains renal corpuscles (RC), renal tubules (T), blood vessels (V), and medullary rays (MR). The medulla contains many tubules of the loops of Henle and collecting ducts (CD), sectioned in transverse, oblique and longitudinal planes, and islands of capillaries, the vasa recta (VR). (By permission from Dr JB Kerr, Monash University, from Kerr JB 1999 Atlas of Functional Histology. London: Mosby.)

passive diffusion of various ions and water into and out of the tubules; reabsorption of organic components such as glucose and amino acids; uptake of any proteins which leak through the glomerular filter.

The proximal convoluted tubule is lined by cuboidal or low columnar epithelium and has a brush border of tall microvilli on its luminal surface. The shape of the cells depends on tubular fluid pressure, which in life distends the lumen and flattens the cells; their shape becomes taller when glomerular blood pressure falls postmortem or at biopsy. The cytoplasm of proximal tubular cells is strongly eosinophilic and their nuclei are euchromatic and central. By light microscopy their bases show faint striations, which ultrastructurally are seen to be due to a complex series of infoldings of the basal plasma membrane, between which numerous mitochondria are orientated perpendicularly. The lateral surfaces of adjacent epithelial cells interdigitate to increase the complexity of the basolateral plasma membrane. Taking into account

the microvilli on their luminal surfaces, these cells possess large areas of plasma membrane in contact with tubular fluid and the extratubular space: this arrangement facilitates the transport of ions and small molecules against steep concentration gradients. The abundant mitochondria supply the energy, as ATP, needed for this process. Sodium/potassium adenosine triphosphatase (Na/K ATPase) is located in apical and basal membranes, and the cytoplasm contains numerous other enzymes concerned with ion transport. Water and other solutes pass between cells (paracellular transport) passively along osmotic and electrochemical gradients, probably through leaky apical tight junctions. Pinocytotic vesicles are found near the apical surface, and represent the means by which small proteins and peptides from the filtrate are internalized and degraded by associated lysosomes. Peroxisomes and lipid droplets abound in the cytoplasm.

The loop of Henle consists of a thin segment (c.30 μm in diameter), lined by low cuboidal to squamous cells, and a thick segment (c.60 μm in diameter) composed of cuboidal cells like those in the distal convoluted tubule. The thin segment forms most of the loop in

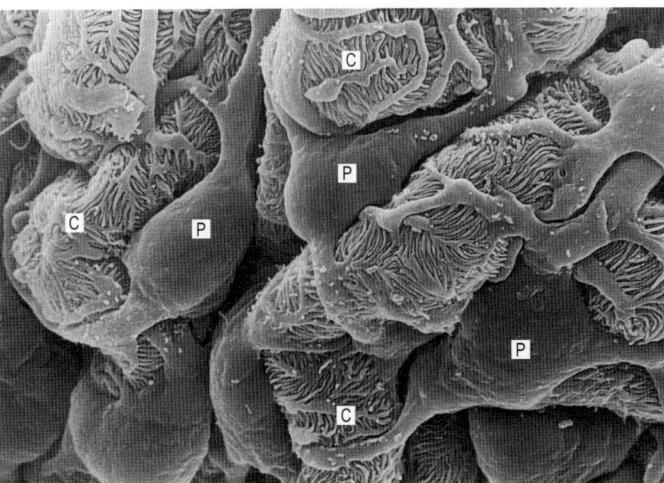

Fig. 91.18 Scanning electron micrograph showing podocytes forming the visceral layer of Bowman's capsule in the renal corpuscle. Podocyte cell bodies (P) send out primary processes which branch several times to end in fine pedicels which wrap tightly around the glomerular capillaries (C), interdigitating with similar pedicels from a neighbouring podocyte. The pedicels and their underlying basal lamina form an important part of the glomerular filtration apparatus. (By permission of Igaku-Shoin, from Fujita T, Tanaka K, Tokunaga J 1981 SEM Atlas of Cells and Tissues, Vol 3.)

Cells of the distal tubule are cuboidal and resemble those in the proximal tubule. They have few microvilli, and so the tubular lumen has a more distinct outline. The basolateral folds containing mitochondria are deep, almost reaching the luminal aspect (**Fig. 91.15B**). Enzymes concerned in active transport of sodium, potassium and other ions are abundant. At the junction of the straight and convoluted regions the distal tubule comes close to the vascular pole of its parent renal corpuscle. Here, tubular cells form a sensory structure, the macula densa, which is concerned with the regulation of blood flow and thus filtration rate. Cells in the terminal part of the distal tubule have fewer basal folds and mitochondria and constitute a connecting duct formed from metanephric mesenchyme during embryogenesis. Collecting ducts are lined by simple cuboidal or columnar epithelium, which increases in height from the cortex, where they receive the contents of distal tubules, to the wide papillary ducts which discharge at the area cribrosa. The pale-staining principal cells have relatively few organelles or lateral interdigitations and only occasional microvilli. A second cell type, intercalated or dark cells (also present in smaller numbers in the distal convoluted tubule), have longer microvilli and more mitochondria. These secrete H⁺ into the filtrate and function in the maintenance of acid–base homeostasis.

PRODUCTION OF URINE (Fig. 91.22)

Glomerular filtration

Glomerular filtration is the passage of water containing dissolved small molecules from the blood plasma to the urinary space in the glomerular capsule. Larger molecules, e.g. plasma proteins above c.70 kilodaltons and those with a net negative charge, polysaccharides and lipids, are largely retained in blood by the selective permeability of the glomerular basal lamina.

Filtration occurs along a steep pressure gradient between the large glomerular capillaries and the urinary space, the principal structure separating the two being the glomerular basal lamina. This gradient far exceeds the colloid osmotic pressure of blood which opposes the outward flow of filtrate. In the peripheral renal cortex the arteriolar pressure gradient is enhanced by the higher calibre of afferent, compared

juxtamedullary nephrons which reach deep into the medulla. Few organelles appear in cells lining the thin segment, indicating that these cells play a passive, rather than an active, role in ion transport. The thick segment is composed of cuboidal epithelium with many mitochondria, deep basolateral folds and short apical microvilli, indicating a more active metabolic role. The thick limb of the loop of Henle is the source of Tamm–Horsfall protein in normal urine.

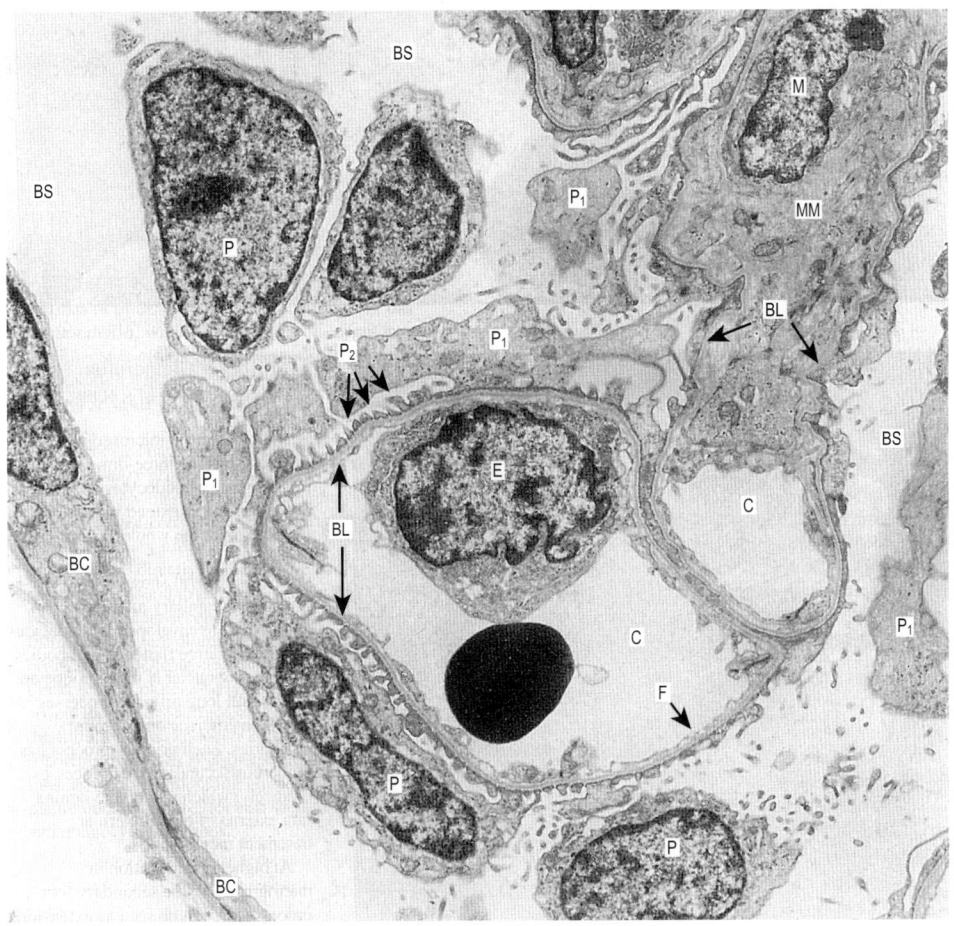

Fig. 91.19 Capillary loops (C) of the renal glomerulus; one profile contains an electron-dense erythrocyte. Capillaries are lined by a fenestrated endothelium (F) and endothelial cell nuclei (E) are seen bulging into the capillary lumina. The nuclei of several epithelial podocytes (P) of the visceral layer of Bowman's capsule can be seen. Their primary processes (P₁) give rise to numerous secondary foot processes (P₂) and these, or tertiary processes, rest on the glomerular basal lamina (BL). A mesangial stalk is shown at the top right, comprising mesangial cells (M) and a dense mesangial matrix (MM), which supports the capillary loops. The mesangium is separated from the capillary lumen only by the endothelial cell cytoplasm, whereas the podocytes and their basal laminae continue around the mesangial stalk and separate it from the urinary (Bowman's) space (BS), which ramifies throughout the glomerulus. Part of the outer parietal layer of Bowman's capsule (BC) is seen to the left. (By permission from Young B, Heath JW 2000 Wheater's Functional Histology. Edinburgh: Churchill Livingstone.)

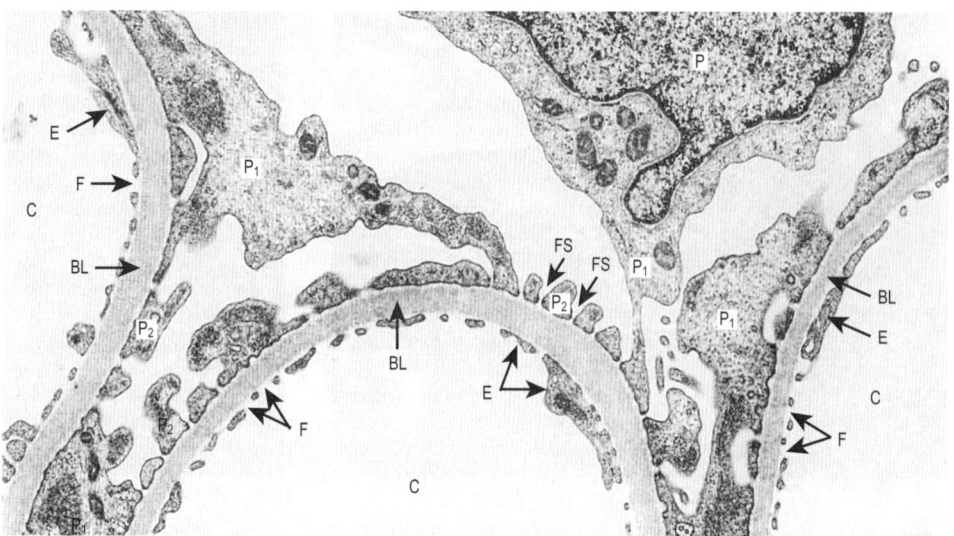

Fig. 91.20 Filtration apparatus of the renal corpuscle, formed by the fenestrated capillary endothelial cells, the filtration slits between podocyte pedicels and their thick, shared basal lamina. BL, basal lamina; C, capillary loops; E, endothelial cell cytoplasm; F, fenestrations; P, podocyte, P_1, primary processes and P_2, secondary foot processes which rest on the glomerular basal lamella. (By permission from Young B, Heath JW 2000 Wheater's Functional Histology. Edinburgh: Churchill Livingstone.)

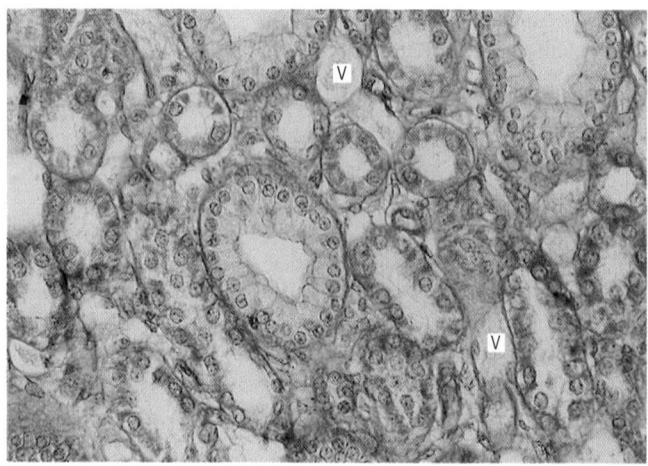

Fig. 91.21 Part of the renal medulla (trichrome stained) in cross-section. Note large collecting ducts and small thin segments of the loop of Henle, interspersed with vasa recta (V).

with efferent, glomerular arterioles. In all glomeruli the rate of filtration can be altered by changes in the tone of the glomerular arterioles. When first formed, the glomerular filtrate is isotonic with glomerular blood and has an identical concentration of ions and small molecules.

Selective resorption

Selective resorption from the filtrate is an active process and occurs mainly in the proximal convoluted tubules, which resorb glucose, amino acids, phosphate, chloride, sodium, calcium and bicarbonate; they also take up small proteins by endocytosis. Cells of the proximal tubules are permeable to water, which passes out of the tubules passively, so that the filtrate remains locally isotonic with blood. The rest of the tubule reabsorbs most of the water (variable, but up to 95%), such that when it reaches the calyces, urine is generally much reduced in volume and hypertonic to blood. This depends on the establishment of high osmolality in the medullary interstitium, which exerts considerable osmotic pressure on water-permeable regions of the tubule (**Fig. 91.22**).

Countercurrent multiplier mechanism

The countercurrent multiplier mechanism is responsible for producing a high osmolality in the extratubular interstitial tissue of the renal medulla. Water passes freely from the tubular lumen into the adjacent medullary interstitium along the descending limb of the loop of Henle. This part of the tubule is less permeable to solutes. In the thick segment of the ascending limb, sodium and chloride ions are actively transported

from the tubule lumen to interstitial spaces, whilst the tubular epithelium remains impermeable to water. The increased interstitial osmolality causes water to be withdrawn from the descending part of the loop, thus concentrating the filtrate. Tubular fluid flows in a countercurrent on its descent into and ascent out of the medulla: it is augmented by new isotonic fluid entering the loop and depleted by hypotonic fluid leaving the loop, as solutes are actively resorbed.

In this way the osmotic gradient within the interstitium is multiplied from the corticomedullary boundary to the medullary pyramids, where it reaches an equilibrium of four to five times the osmolality of plasma. Urea contributes c.50% of the medullary osmotic strength, mainly contributed passively by the medullary part of the collecting ducts. These are generally highly permeable to urea, and permeability is enhanced by antidiuretic hormone (ADH, vasopressin). Although the tonicity of the tubular fluid changes during its passage through the steep osmotic gradient within the medulla, the osmotic gradient between ascending and descending limbs at each level never exceeds 200 mOsm/kg, a force which can be sustained by the cells of the tubular wall.

Countercurrent exchange mechanism (Fig. 91.13B)

Rapid removal of ions from the renal medulla by the circulation of blood is minimized by another looped countercurrent system. This is the countercurrent exchange mechanism, in which arterioles entering the medulla pass for long distances parallel to the venules leaving it, before ending in capillary beds around tubules. This close apposition of oppositely flowing blood allows the direct diffusion of ions from out-flowing to inflowing blood, so that the vasa recta (**Figs 91.13, 91.15A**) conserve the high osmotic pressure in the medulla.

Concentration of urine

Because sodium and chloride ions are selectively resorbed by the cells of the ascending limbs and distal tubules under aldosterone control (p. 1247), the filtrate at the distal end of the convoluted tubules is hypotonic. As it reaches the collecting ducts, fluid descends again through the medulla and thus re-enters a region of high osmotic pressure. The cells lining the collecting ducts are variably permeable to water, under the influence of neurohypophyseal ADH. Water follows an osmotic gradient into the adjacent extratubular spaces, so that the tonicity of the filtrate gradually rises along collecting ducts, until at the tip of the renal pyramids it is above that of blood. As much as 95% of water in the original glomerular filtrate is thus resorbed into blood. This complex system is highly flexible and the balance between the rate of filtration and absorption can be varied to meet current physiological demands.

Control of hydrogen and ammonium ion concentrations is essential to the regulation of acids and bases in the blood; secretion of various ions occurs at several sites. Over 91% of ingested potassium is excreted in urine, largely through secretion by cells of the distal tubule and collecting duct. For further details of renal physiology see Davies et al 2001.

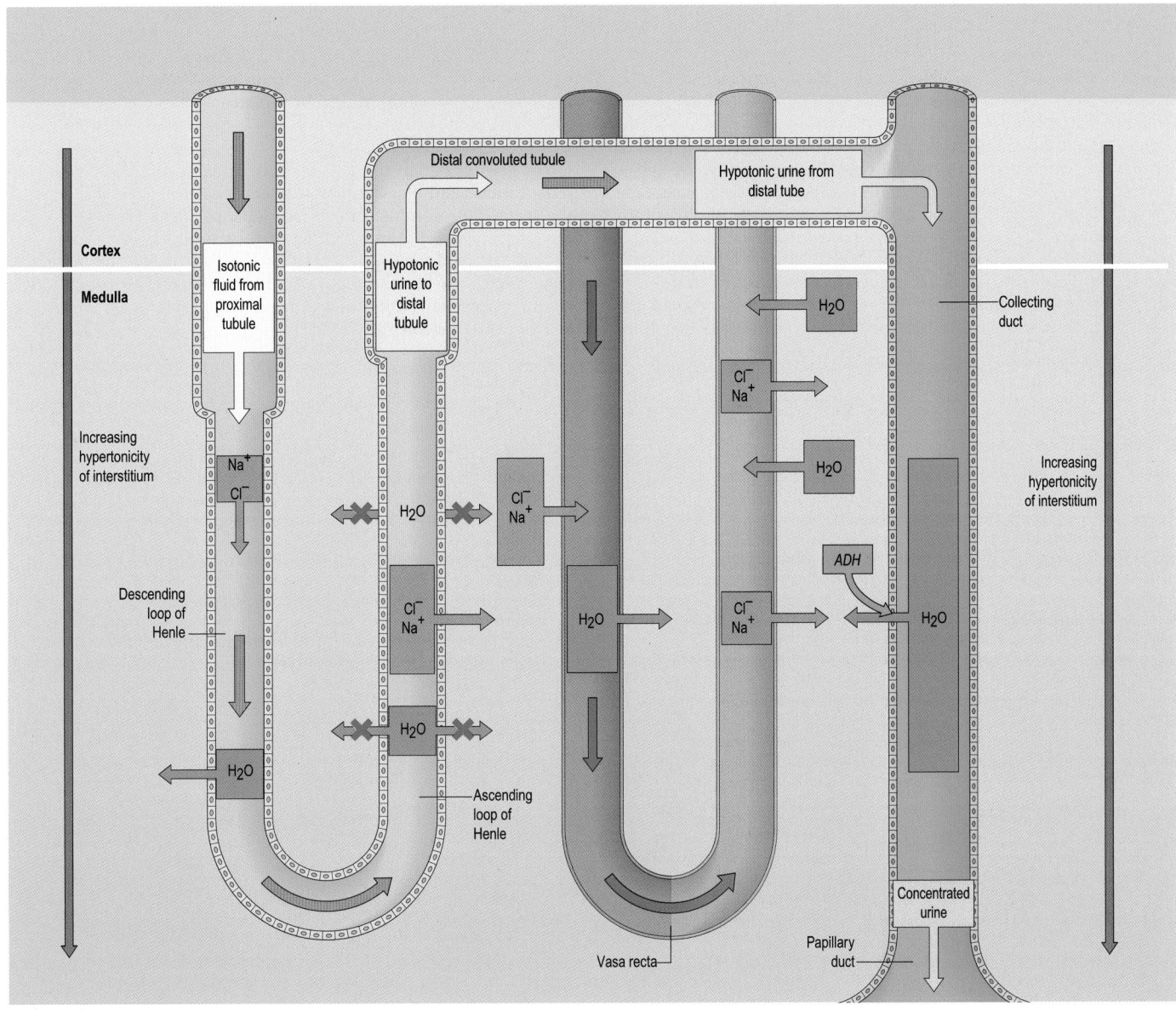

Fig. 91.22 The inter-relationships between the countercurrent multiplier and exchange mechanisms which operate in the renal medulla. The movements of ions and water and the action of antidiuretic hormone (ADH) are indicated. For further details see text. (By permission from Stevens A, Lowe JS 1996 Human Histology, 2nd edn. London: Mosby.)

JUXTAGLOMERULAR APPARATUS

The juxtaglomerular apparatus provides a tubuloglomerular feedback system which maintains systemic arterial blood pressure during a reduction in vascular volume and decrease in filtration rate. The afferent and efferent arterioles at the vascular pole of a glomerulus and the macula densa of the distal tubule of the same nephron lie in close proximity, enclosing a small cone of tissue populated by extraglomerular mesangial (lacis) cells (**Fig. 91.15B**). The cells of the tunica media of the afferent and, to a lesser extent, efferent, arterioles differ from typical smooth muscle cells. They are large, rounded myoepithelioid cells and their cytoplasm contains many mitochondria and dense, renin-containing vesicles, 10–40 nm in diameter. These juxtaglomerular cells form one element of the juxtaglomerular apparatus.

The second element of the juxtaglomerular apparatus is the sensory component, the macula densa of the distal tubule. Up to 40 cells in the tubule wall form a cluster of taller, more tightly packed cells with large, oval nuclei (**Fig. 91.16**). Their mitochondria are concentrated apically. Macula densa cells are osmoreceptors, sensing the NaCl content of the filtrate after its passage through the loop of Henle. When NaCl concentrations in the filtrate change, tubuloglomerular feedback mechanisms operate to maintain the inverse relationship between salt concentration and glomerular filtration rate. Juxtaglomerular cells release renin, an

enzyme which acts on circulating angiotensinogen (a liver protein) to activate the cascade whereby angiotensin II increases blood pressure (and therefore filtration rate), stimulates aldosterone and ADH release and increases sodium ion and water resorption, primarily from the distal tubule, to increase plasma volume. Macula densa cells are thought to respond to high salt concentration in the distal tubule by releasing nitric oxide, which inhibits the tubuloglomerular feedback response and reduces filtration rate. The role of macula densa cells in the stimulation of renin release to increase filtration rate is less well understood.

The third element of the juxtaglomerular apparatus is a population of extraglomerular mesangial cells which form a network (or lace, hence their alternative name of lacis cells) of stellate cells connecting the macula densa sensory cells with the juxtaglomerular effector cells. It is likely that extraglomerular mesangial cells transmit the sensory signal, possibly through gap junctions. They may also signal to contractile glomerular mesangial cells and effect vasoconstriction directly within the glomerulus. Adrenergic nerve fibres occur in small numbers among these cells.

RENAL CALYCES AND PELVIS

The wall of the proximal part of the urinary tract is composed of three layers, an outer connective tissue adventitia, an intermediate layer of smooth muscle and an inner mucosa. The mucosal lining of the renal calyces and pelvis is identical in structure to that of the ureter (p. 1288) and will not be considered further here. The adventitia consists of loose fibroelastic connective tissue which merges with retroperitoneal areolar tissue. Proximally the coat fuses with the fibrous capsule of the kidney lining the renal sinus.

The smooth muscle of the renal calyces and pelvis is composed of two distinct types of smooth muscle cell. One type of muscle cell is identical to that described for the ureter and can be traced proximally through the pelviureteric region and renal pelvis as far as the minor calyces. The other type of cell forms the muscle coat of each minor calyx and continues into the major calyces and pelvis where it forms a distinct inner layer. The cells also form a thin sheet of muscle which covers each minor calyx and extends across the renal parenchyma between the attachments of neighbouring minor calyces, thereby linking each minor calyx to its neighbours. This discrete inner layer of atypical smooth muscle ceases in the pelviureteric region so that the proximal ureter lacks such an inner layer. Pacemaker cells that initiate renal pelvic and ureteric peristalsis are sited within the calyces. These allow coordinated peristalsis of the ureter c.6 times a minute.

OTHER RENAL CELLS

Other cells essential to renal structure and function lie between the renal tubules and blood vessels. Connective tissue is inconspicuous in the cortex but prominent in the medulla, particularly in the papillae. Medullary interstitial cells, which may be modified fibroblasts, form vertical stacks of tangentially orientated cells between the more distal collecting ducts, like the rungs of a ladder. These cells secrete prostaglandins and may contribute, with cortical tubular cells, to the renal source of erythropoietin.

REFERENCES

Brodel M 1911 The intrinsic blood-vessels of the kidney and their significance in nephrotomy. John Hopkins Hosp Bull 12: 10–13.
  Original description of a relatively avascular longitudinal zone within the kidney, proposed as a site for surgical incision.

Burkhill GJC, Healy JC 2000 Anatomy of the peritoneum. Imaging 12: 10–20.
  Review of the imaging literature describing the contentious anatomy of the perirenal fascia.

Davies A, Blakeley AGH, Kidd C 2001 The renal system. In: Human Physiology, Chapter 8. Edinburgh: Churchill Livingstone: 713–97.

Davies JM 1991 The role of the efferent arteriole in tubuloglomerular feedback. Kidney Int (Suppl) 32: S71–3.

Gosling JA, Dixon JS 1974 Species variation in the location of upper urinary tract pacemaker cells. Invest Urol 11: 418.
  Early paper describing the identification of pacemaker cells in various species.

Merklin RJ, Michels NA 1958 The variant renal and suprarenal blood supply with data on the inferior phrenic, ureteral, and gonadal arteries: a statistical analysis based on 185 dissections and a review of the literature. J Int Coll Surg; 29: 41–76.
  A review of renal vascular anatomy in almost 11,000 kidneys.

Mitchell GAG 1950 The renal fascia. Br J Surg 37: 257–66.
  Demonstrating that the perirenal fascia is a multilaminate structure rather than a single fused fascia.

Novick AC 1998 Anatomic approaches in nephron-sparing surgery for renal cell carcinoma. Atlas Urol Clin North Am 6: 39.

Ureter

The ureters are muscular tubes whose peristaltic contractions convey urine from the kidneys to the urinary bladder (**Fig. 92.1**). Each measures 25–30 cm in length and is thick-walled, narrow, and continuous superiorly with the funnel-shaped renal pelvis. Each descends slightly medially anterior to psoas major, and enters the pelvic cavity where it curves laterally, then medially, as it runs down to open into the base of the urinary bladder. Its diameter is c.3 mm but is slightly less at its junction with the renal pelvis, at the brim of the lesser pelvis near the medial border of psoas major, and where it runs within the wall of the urinary bladder, which is its narrowest part. These are the commonest sites for renal stone impaction. The renal pelvis has already been described (p. 1274).

RELATIONS (Fig. 92.2)

In the abdomen the ureter descends posterior to the peritoneum on the medial part of psoas major, which separates it from the tips of he lumbar transverse processes. During surgery on intraperitoneal structures, the ureter can be tented up as the peritoneum is drawn anteriorly, resulting in inadvertent ureteric injury. Anterior to psoas major it crosses in front of the genitofemoral nerve and is obliquely crossed by the gonadal vessels. It enters the lesser pelvis anterior to either the end of the common iliac or the start of the external iliac vessels.

The inferior vena cava is medial to the right ureter while the left ureter is lateral to the aorta. The inferior mesenteric vein has a long retroperitoneal course lying close to the medial aspect of the left ureter.

At its origin the right ureter is usually overlapped by the descending part of the duodenum. It descends lateral to the inferior vena cava, and is crossed anteriorly by the right colic and ileocolic vessels. Near the superior aperture of the lesser pelvis it passes behind the lower part of the mesentery and terminal ileum. The left ureter is crossed by the gonadal and left colic vessels (**Fig. 92.3**). It passes posterior to loops of jejunum and sigmoid colon and its mesentery in the posterior wall of the intersigmoid recess.

In the pelvis the ureter lies in extraperitoneal areolar tissue. At first it descends posterolaterally on the lateral wall of the lesser pelvis along the anterior border of the greater sciatic notch. Opposite the ischial spine it turns anteromedially into fibrous adipose tissue above levator ani to reach the base of the bladder. On the pelvic wall it is anterior to the internal iliac artery and the beginning of its anterior trunk, posterior to which are the internal iliac vein, lumbosacral nerve and sacroiliac joint. Laterally it lies on the fascia of obturator internus. It progressively crosses to become medial to the umbilical, inferior vesical, and middle rectal arteries.

In males (**Fig. 92.2**), the pelvic ureter hooks under the vas deferens (**Fig. 98.1**), then passes in front of and slightly above the upper pole of the seminal vesicle to traverse the bladder wall obliquely before opening at the ipsilateral trigonal angle (**Fig. 98.2**). Its terminal part is surrounded by tributaries of the vesical veins. In females, the pelvic part at first has the same relations as in males, but anterior to the internal iliac artery it is immediately behind the ovary, forming the posterior boundary of the ovarian fossa (p. 1321). In the anteromedial part of its course to the bladder it is related to the uterine artery, uterine cervix and vaginal fornices. It is in extraperitoneal connective tissue in the infero-medial part of the broad ligament of the uterus where it may be damaged during hysterectomy. In the broad ligament, the uterine artery is anterosuperior to the ureter for 2.5 cm and then crosses to its medial side to ascend alongside the uterus. The ureter turns forwards slightly above the lateral vaginal fornix and is generally 2 cm lateral to the supra-vaginal part of the uterine cervix in this location. It then inclines medially to reach the bladder, with a variable relation to the front of the

vagina. As the uterus is commonly deviated to one side, one ureter, usually the left, may be more extensively apposed to the vagina, and may cross the midline.

The distal 1–2 cm of each ureter is surrounded by an incomplete collar of non-striated muscle, which forms a sheath (of Waldeyer). The ureters pierce the posterior aspect of the bladder and run obliquely through its wall for a distance of 1.5–2.0 cm before terminating at the ureteric orifices. This arrangement is believed to assist in the prevention of reflux of urine into the ureter, since the intramural ureters are thought to be occluded during increases in bladder pressure. There is no evidence of a classic ureteral sphincter mechanism in man. The longi-tudinally oriented muscle bundles of the terminal ureter continue into the bladder wall and at the ureteric orifices become continuous with the superficial trigonal muscle. In the distended bladder, in both sexes, the ureteric openings are c.5 cm apart, and c.2.5 cm apart when the bladder is empty.

Duplex ureters – In 1 in 125 individuals, two ureters drain the renal pelvis on one side; this is termed a duplex system. Bilateral duplex ureters occur in c.1 in 800 cases. The duplex ureters derive from two ureteric buds arising from the mesonephric duct. They are contained in a single fascial sheath and may fuse at any point along their course or may be separate until they insert through separate ureteric orifices into the bladder. Care must be taken not to compromise the blood supply of the second ureter when excising or reimplanting a single ureter of a duplex.

The ureter from the upper pole of the kidney (the longer ureter) inserts more medially and caudally in the bladder than the ureter from the lower pole (the shorter ureter). This reflects their embryological development: the ureteric bud which is initially more proximal on the mesonephric duct has a shorter time to be pulled cranially in the bladder and so it inserts more distally in the mature bladder. The ureter from the lower pole has a shorter intramural course than the longer ureter and is prone to reflux.

Ectopic ureters – Single ureters and more commonly the longer ureter of a duplex system can insert more caudally and medially than normal in some individuals. In the male the ureter can insert at the bladder neck or posterior urethra, or rarely into the seminal vesicle, but it always inserts cranial to the external urethral sphincter. In the female, ectopic insertion can be distal to the external urethral sphincter in the urethra, or into the vagina, resulting in persistent childhood incontinence.

Uretoroceles – A ureterocele is a cystic dilatation of the lower end of the ureter: the ureteric orifice is covered by a membrane which expands as it is filled with urine and then deflates as it empties. Uretoroceles can vary in size with resultant obstructive 'back pressure' changes seen in the ureter and pelvicalyceal system proximally. They usually do not cause bladder outflow obstruction except for the rare prolapsing uretorocele. Prolapsing uretoroceles, though small, prolapse from their position around the uretero-vesical junction region in to the urethra, causing intermittent bladder outflow obstruction. They are identified antenatally with ultrasound and can result in obstruction to the ureter. In adults uretoroceles tend to be bilateral and small. They can produce obstruction to the ureter but commonly produce no clinical manifestations.

Retrocaval ureter – A persistence of the posterior cardinal vein, associated with high confluence of the right and left common iliac veins or a double inferior vena cava, may result a retrocaval ureter which passes behind the inferior vena cava before it emerges in front of

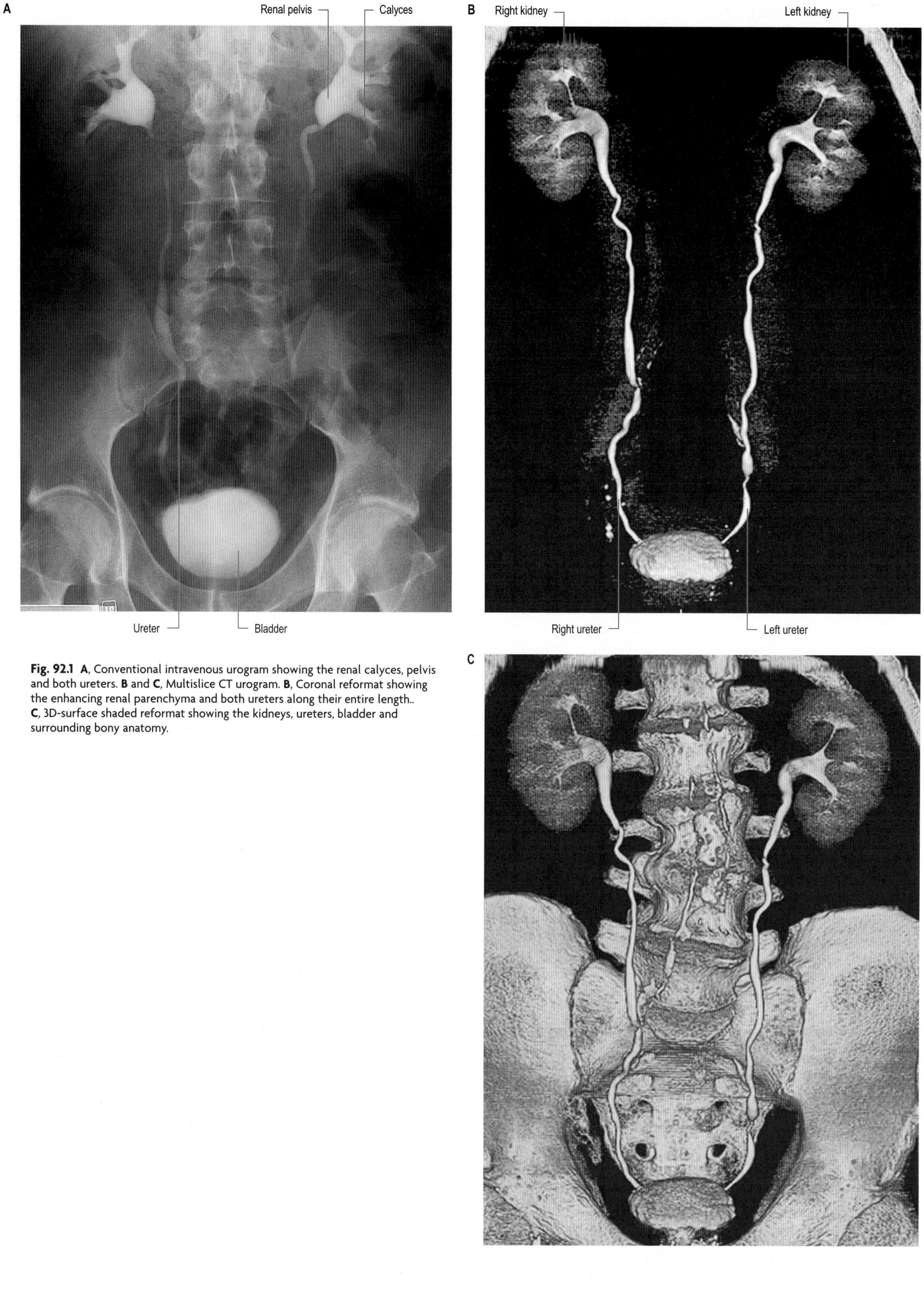

A

Renal pelvis — ⌐ Calyces

Ureter — ⌐ Bladder

B

Right kidney — Left kidney —

Right ureter — Left ureter —

Fig. 92.1 A, Conventional intravenous urogram showing the renal calyces, pelvis and both ureters. **B** and **C**, Multislice CT urogram. **B**, Coronal reformat showing the enhancing renal parenchyma and both ureters along their entire length.. **C**, 3D-surface shaded reformat showing the kidneys, ureters, bladder and surrounding bony anatomy.

C

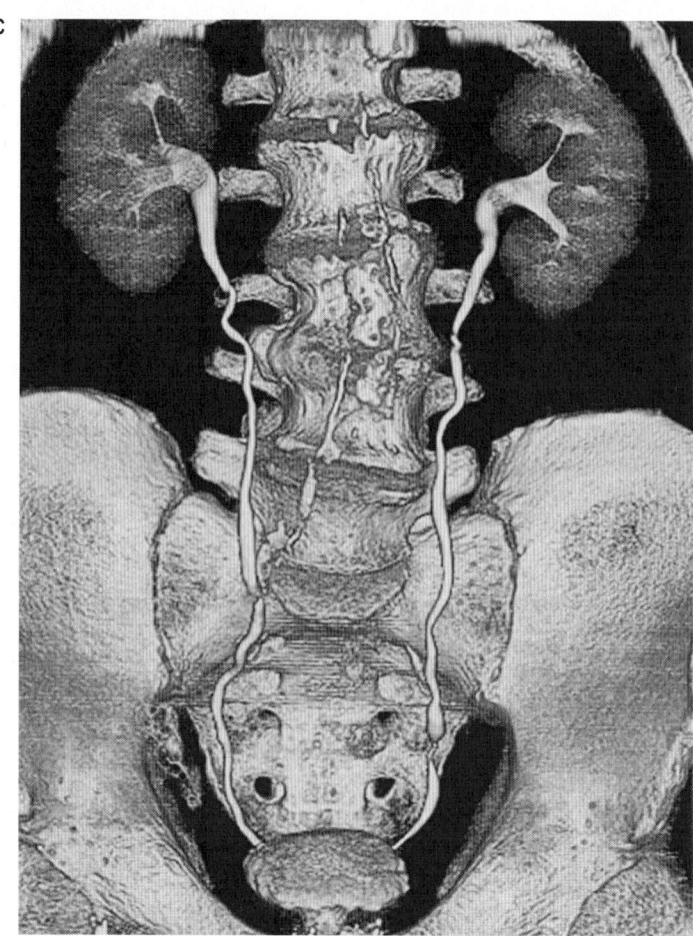

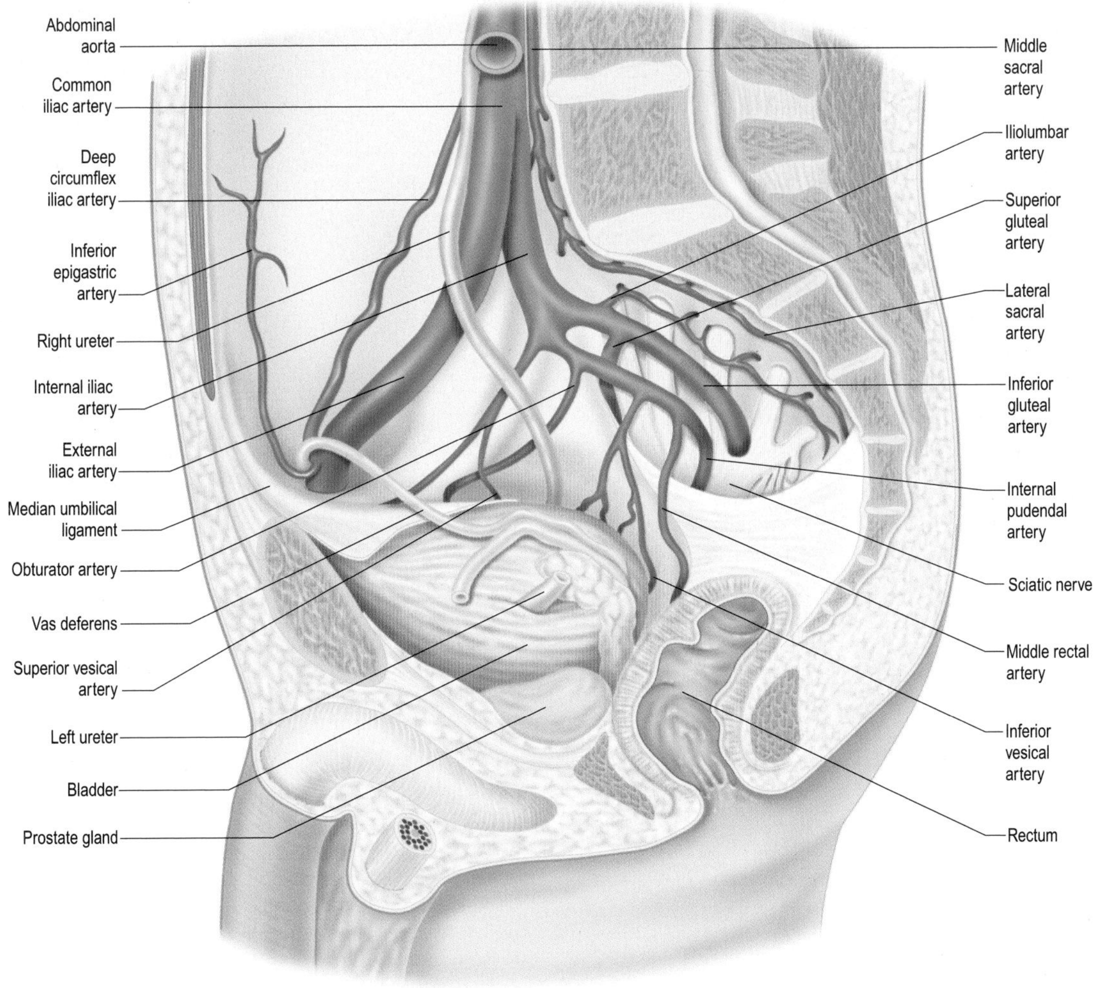

Fig. 92.2 Relations of lower right ureter in male. (By permission from Walsh PC, Retik AB, Vaughan ED et al (eds) 2002 Campbell's Urology, 8th edn. Philadelphia: Saunders.)

it to pass from medial to lateral. Retrocaval ureter occurs in c.1 in 1500 individuals. Most commonly it has no clinical sequelae although it can result in upper ureteric obstruction.

VASCULAR SUPPLY AND LYMPHATIC DRAINAGE

ARTERIES AND VEINS (Fig. 92.3)

The ureter is supplied by branches from the renal, gonadal, common iliac, internal iliac, vesical and uterine arteries and the abdominal aorta. The pattern of distribution is subject to much variation. There is a good longitudinal anastomosis between these branches on the wall of the ureter, which means that the ureter can be safely transected at any level intraoperatively, and a uretero-ureterostomy performed, without compromising its viability. The branches from the inferior vesical artery are constant in their occurrence and supply the lower part of the ureter as well as a large part of the trigone of the bladder. The branch from the renal artery is also constant and is preserved whenever possible in renal transplantation to ensure good vascularity of the ureter. The venous drainage generally follows the arterial supply.

LYMPHATIC DRAINAGE

Lymph vessels begin in submucosal, intramuscular and adventitial plexuses, which all communicate. Collecting vessels from the upper ureter may join the renal collecting vessels or pass directly to the lateral aortic nodes near the origin of the gonadal artery; those from its lower abdominal part go to the common iliac nodes; and those from its pelvic part end in the common, external or internal iliac nodes.

INNERVATION

The ureter is supplied from the lower three thoracic, first lumbar, and the second to fourth sacral segments of the spinal cord by branches from the renal and aortic plexuses, and the superior and inferior hypogastric plexuses. The ureteric nerves consist of relatively large bundles of axons which form an irregular plexus in the adventitia of the ureter. Numerous smaller branches penetrate the ureteric muscle coat. Some of the adventitial nerves accompany the blood vessels and branch with them as they extend into the muscle layer. Others are unrelated to the vascular supply and lie free in the adventitial connective tissue around the circumference of the ureter. There is a gradual increase in innervation from the renal pelvis and upper ureter (which has a sparse distribution of autonomic nerves) to a maximum density in the juxtavesical segment. There are at least three different phenotypes: cholinergic, noradrenergic and peptidergic (substance P). Other neurotransmitters also exist, so the control mechanisms are likely to be complex. The functional significance of these different types of autonomic nerve fibres in relation to ureteric smooth muscle activity is not fully understood, however, it is recognized that nerves are not essential for the initiation and propagation of ureteric contraction waves.

A branching plexus of fine axons occurs within the lamina propria and extends from the inner aspect of the muscle coat towards the base of the urothelium. These axons are cholinergic and, while some form perivascular plexuses, others lie in isolation from the vascular supply. A similar distribution of noradrenergic and peptidergic nerves has been observed throughout the lamina propria. The functional significance of these nerves, which are not related to blood vessels, remains unclear, but it seems probable that at least some of them are sensory in function.

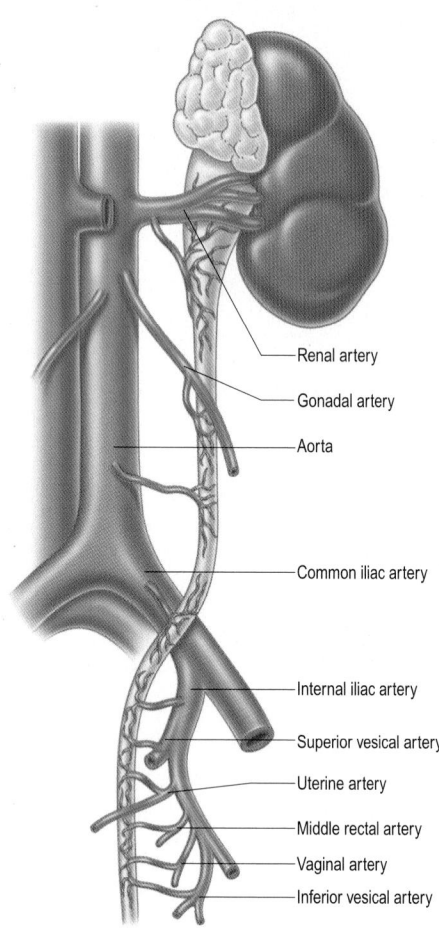

Fig. 92.3 Course of the left ureter, showing how the proximal part takes its blood supply medially, and the distal part is supplied laterally. (By permission from Walsh PC, Retik AB, Vaughan ED et al (eds) 2002 Campbell's Urology, 8th edn. Philadelphia: Saunders.)

REFERRED PAIN

Excessive distension of the ureter or spasm of its muscle may be caused by a stone (calculus) and provokes severe pain (ureteric colic, which is commonly, but mistakenly, called renal colic). The pain, spasmodic and agonizing, particularly if the obstruction is gradually forced down the ureter by the muscle spasm, is referred to cutaneous areas innervated from spinal segments which supply the ureter, mainly T11–L2. It shoots down and forwards from the loin to the groin and scrotum or labium majus and may extend into the proximal anterior aspect of the thigh by projection to the genitofemoral nerve (L1, 2). The cremaster, which has the same innervation, may reflexly retract the testis.

MICROSTRUCTURE

The wall of the ureter is composed of an external adventitia, a smooth muscle layer and an inner mucosal layer (**Fig. 92.4**). The last consists of the urothelium and an underlying connective tissue lamina propria.

The ureteric adventitial blood vessels and connective tissue fibres are orientated parallel to the long axis of the ureter. Throughout its length, the muscle coat of the ureter is fairly uniform in thickness and in cross-section measures c.750–800 μm in width. The muscle bundles which constitute this coat are frequently separated from one another by relatively large amounts of connective tissue. However, branches which interconnect muscle bundles are common and there is frequent interchange of muscle fibres between adjacent bundles. As a consequence of this extensive branching, individual muscle bundles do not spiral around the ureter, but form a complex meshwork of interweaving bundles. In addition, unlike the gut (Chapter 72), the muscle bundles are so

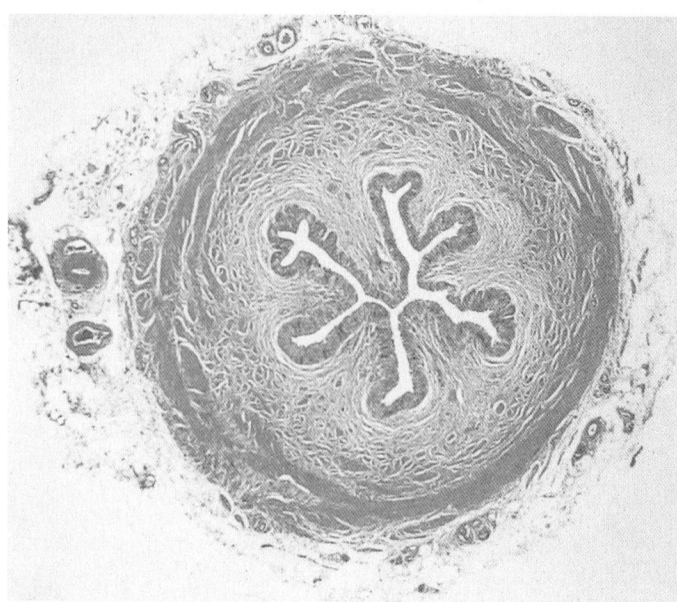

Fig. 92.4 Transverse section of ureter. The walls are muscular and are lined by a specialized urothelium. (By permission from Stevens A, Lowe JS 1996 Human Histology, 2nd edn. London: Mosby.)

arranged that morphologically distinct longitudinal and circular layers cannot be clearly distinguished. In the upper part of the ureter, the inner muscle bundles tend to lie longitudinally while those on the outer aspect have a circular or oblique orientation. In its middle and lower parts, there are additional outer longitudinally orientated fibres. As the ureterovesical junction is approached, the muscle coat consists predominantly of longitudinally orientated muscle bundles.

The mucosa of the ureter consists of an epithelium, the urothelium, on the deep aspect of which is a layer of subepithelial fibroelastic connective tissue lamina propria. The latter varies in thickness from 350–700 μm and is a conduit for small blood vessels and bundles of non-myelinated nerve fibres. Occasional lymphocytes may be present in the lamina propria but their aggregation into definitive lymph nodules is rare. The urothelium is usually extensively folded, giving the ureteric lumen a stellate outline.

URETERIC PERISTALSIS

Under normal conditions contraction waves originate in the proximal part of the upper urinary tract and are propagated in an anterograde direction towards the bladder. Atypical smooth muscle cells in the wall of the minor calyces act individually or collectively as pacemaker sites. A peristaltic wave begins at one (or possibly more) of these sites. Once initiated, the contraction is propagated through the wall of the adjacent major calyx and activates the smooth muscle of the renal pelvis. Contraction waves are propagated away from the kidney, and so undesirable pressure rises are not directed against the renal parenchyma. Since several potential pacemaker sites exist, the initiation of contraction waves is unimpaired by partial nephrectomy: the minor calyces spared by the resection remain *in situ* to continue their pacemaking function.

Experimental evidence indicates that autonomic nerves do not play a major part in the propagation of peristalsis. It seems more likely that they play a modulatory role on the contractile events occurring in the musculature of the upper urinary tract. The most likely mechanism to account for impulse propagation is myogenic conduction as a result of the electrotonic coupling of one muscle cell to its immediate neighbours by means of intercellular 'gap' junctions. There are numerous regions of close approach between ureteric smooth muscle cells and also between both types of muscle cell in the renal pelvis and calyces. It is therefore reasonable to assume that in the upper urinary tract this type of intercellular junction may be responsible for the conduction of excitation from one myocyte to the next.

Bladder

The urinary bladder is a reservoir (**Figs 93.1, 93.2, 98.1**). It varies in size, shape, position and relations, according to its content and the state of neighbouring viscera. When empty, it lies entirely in the lesser pelvis but as it distends it expands anterosuperiorly into the abdominal cavity. When empty, it is somewhat tetrahedral and has a base (fundus), neck, apex, a superior and two inferolateral surfaces.

The base (fundus) of the bladder is triangular and posteroinferior. In females it is closely related to the anterior vaginal wall (**Fig. 102.1**); in males it is related to the rectum although it is separated from it above by the rectovesical pouch and below by the seminal vesicle and vas deferens on each side (**Figs 93.2, 98.1**). In a triangular area between the vasa deferentia, the bladder and rectum are separated only by rectovesical fascia, commonly known as Denonvillier's fascia. The inferior part of this area may be obliterated by approximation of the ampullae of the vas deferens above the prostate.

The neck is the lowest region and is also the most fixed. It is 3–4 cm behind the lower part of the symphysis pubis, which is a little above the plane of the inferior aperture of the lesser pelvis. The bladder neck is the internal urethral orifice and alters little in position with varying conditions of the bladder and rectum. In males the neck rests on, and is in direct continuity with, the base of the prostate; in females it is related to the pelvic fascia, which surrounds the upper urethra.

The vesical apex in both sexes faces towards the upper part of the symphysis pubis. The median umbilical ligament (urachus, **Fig. 109.1**)

ascends behind the anterior abdominal wall from the apex to the umbilicus, covered by peritoneum to form the median umbilical fold.

The triangular superior surface is bounded by lateral borders from the apex to the ureteric entrances and by a posterior border , which joins them. In males the superior surface is completely covered by peritoneum, which extends slightly onto the base and continues posteriorly into the rectovesical pouch and anteriorly into the median umbilical fold (p. 1133). It is in contact with the sigmoid colon and the terminal coils of the ileum. In females the superior surface is largely covered by peritoneum, which is reflected posteriorly onto the uterus at the level of the internal os (i.e. the junction of the uterine body and cervix), to form the vesicouterine pouch. The posterior part of the superior surface, devoid of peritoneum, is separated from the supravaginal cervix by fibroareolar tissue (p. 1133).

In males, each inferolateral surface is separated anteriorly from the pubis and puboprostatic ligaments by the (potential) retropubic space. In females the relations are similar, except that the pubovesical ligaments replace the puboprostatic ligaments. The inferolateral surfaces are not covered by peritoneum.

As the bladder fills it becomes ovoid. In front it displaces the parietal peritoneum from the suprapubic region of the abdominal wall. Its inferolateral surfaces become anterior and rest against the abdominal wall without intervening peritoneum for a distance above the symphysis pubis which varies with the degree of distension, but is commonly

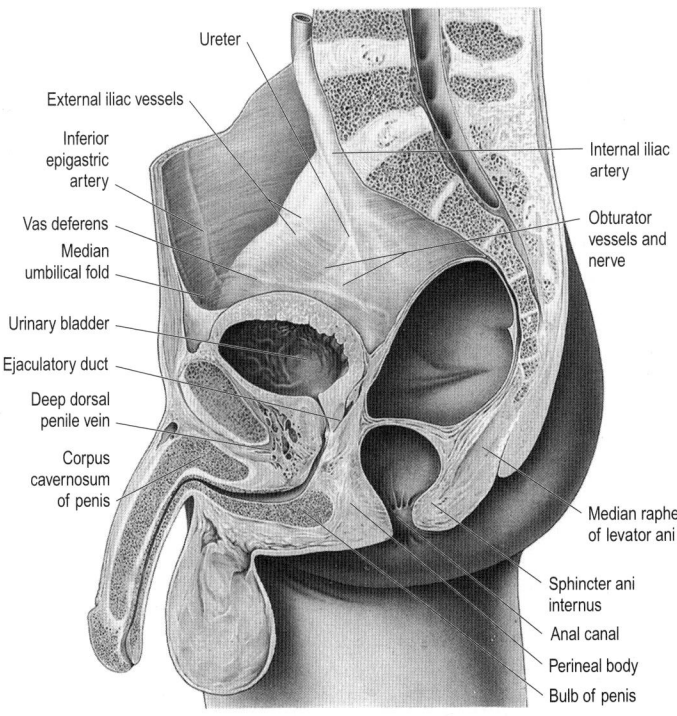

Fig. 93.1 Median sagittal section to show male internal and external genitalia, bladder. A number of structures (e.g. obturator vessels, ureter) are only faintly visible through the overlying peritoneum.

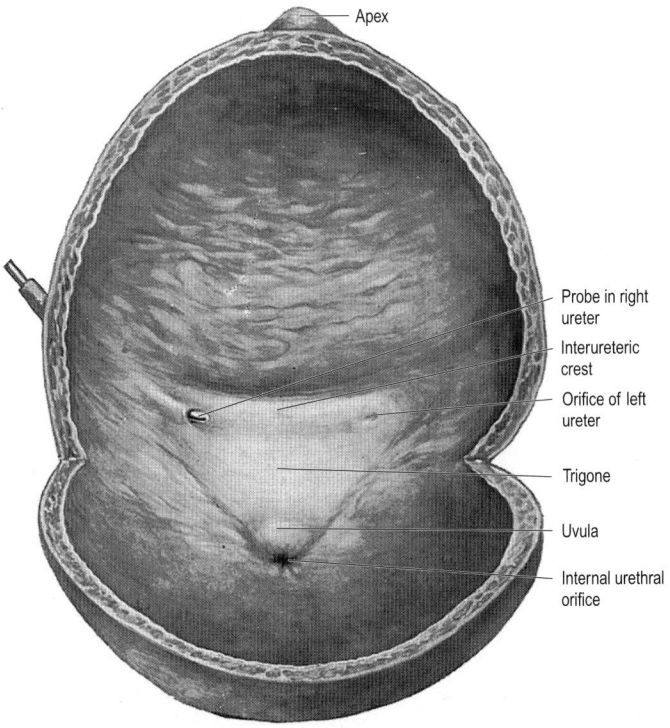

Fig. 93.2 Anterior aspect of the interior of the urinary bladder.

5–7 cm. The distended bladder may be punctured just above the symphysis pubis without traversing the peritoneum (suprapubic cystostomy): surgical access to the bladder through the anterior abdominal wall is usually by this route. The summit of the full bladder points up and forwards above the attachment of the median umbilical ligament, so that the peritoneum forms a supravesical recess of varying depth between the summit and the anterior abdominal wall: this recess often contains coils of small intestine. A distended bladder may be ruptured in lower abdominal or pelvic injuries, either extraperitoneally or, if the superior surface is involved, with tearing of the peritoneum and escape of urine into the peritoneal cavity.

At birth, the bladder is relatively higher than in the adult, and the internal urethral orifice is level with the upper symphyseal border. The bladder is then abdominal rather than pelvic, and extends about two-thirds of the distance towards the umbilicus. Urine samples may therefore be obtained in children by performing suprapubic needle puncture. The bladder progressively descends, and reaches the adult position shortly after puberty.

Congenital abnormalities of the bladder are described on page 1379.

LIGAMENTS OF BLADDER (Fig. 69.9)

The bladder is anchored inferiorly by condensations of pelvic fascia which attach it to the pubis, lateral pelvic side-walls, and rectum.

In both sexes stout bands of fibromuscular tissue extend from the bladder neck to the inferior aspect of the pubic bones. These structures are the pubovesical ligaments. They constitute the superior extensions of the pubourethral ligaments in the female or the puboprostatic ligaments in the male. The pubovesical ligaments lie on each side of the median plane, leaving a midline hiatus through which numerous small veins pass. A number of other so-called ligaments have been described in relation to the base of the urinary bladder. The reflections of the peritoneum from the bladder to the side-walls of the pelvis form the lateral ligaments, and the sacrogenital folds constitute the posterior ligaments: they are not true ligaments, but condensations of connective tissue around the major neurovascular structures. They are described as ligaments in routine clinical use.

The apex of the bladder is connected to the umbilicus by the remains of the urachus, which forms the median umbilical ligament. The lumen of the lower part of the urachus may persist throughout life and communicate with the cavity of the bladder. From the superior surface of the bladder the peritoneum is carried off in a series of folds, the 'false' ligaments of the bladder. Anteriorly there are three folds, the median umbilical fold over the median umbilical ligament and two medial umbilical folds over the obliterated umbilical arteries.

BLADDER INTERIOR

VESICAL MUCOSA (Fig. 93.2)

The vesical mucosa is attached only loosely to subjacent muscle for the most part: it folds when the bladder empties, and the folds are effaced as it fills. Over the trigone, immediately above and behind the internal urethral orifice, it is adherent to the subjacent muscle layer and always smooth (**Fig. 93.2**). The anteroinferior angle of the trigone is formed by the internal urethral orifice, its posterolateral angles by the ureteric orifices. The superior trigonal boundary is a slightly curved interureteric crest, which connects the two ureteric orifices and is produced by the continuation into the vesical wall of the ureteric internal longitudinal muscle. Laterally this ridge extends beyond the ureteric openings as ureteric folds, produced by the terminal parts of the ureters which run obliquely through the bladder wall. At cystoscopy the interureteric crest appears as a pale band and is a guide to the ureteric orifices in catheterization.

TRIGONE

The smooth muscle of the trigone consists of two distinct layers, sometimes termed the superficial and deep trigonal muscles. The latter is composed of muscle cells, indistinguishable from those of the detrusor, and is simply the posteroinferior portion of the detrusor muscle proper. Confusion might be avoided if the term deep trigonal muscle was abandoned in favour of the more accurate term trigonal detrusor muscle. The superficial trigonal muscle represents a morphologically distinct

component of the trigone, which, unlike the detrusor, is composed of relatively small diameter muscle bundles continuous proximally with those of the intramural ureters. The superficial trigonal muscle is relatively thin but is generally described as becoming thickened along its superior border to form the interureteric crest. Similar thickenings occur along the lateral edges of the superficial trigone. In both sexes the superficial trigone muscle becomes continuous with the smooth muscle of the proximal urethra, and extends in the male along the urethral crest as far as the openings of the ejaculatory ducts.

URETERIC ORIFICES

The slit-like ureteric orifices are placed at the posterolateral trigonal angles (**Fig. 93.2**). In empty bladders they are c.2.5 cm apart, and c.2.5 cm from the internal urethral orifice; in distension these measurements may be doubled.

INTERNAL URETHRAL ORIFICE

The internal urethral orifice is sited at the trigonal apex, the lowest part of the bladder, and is usually somewhat crescentic in section. There is often an elevation immediately behind it in adult males (particularly past middle age) which is caused by the median prostatic lobe, sometimes known as the uvula of the bladder.

BLADDER NECK

The smooth muscle of the bladder neck is histologically, histochemically and pharmacologically distinct from the detrusor muscle proper and so the bladder neck should be considered as a separate functional unit. The arrangement of smooth muscle in this region is quite different in males and females, and therefore each sex will be described separately.

FEMALE

The female bladder neck consists of morphologically distinct smooth muscle. The large diameter fasciculi characteristic of the detrusor are replaced in the region of the bladder neck by small diameter fasciculi which extend obliquely or longitudinally into the urethral wall.

In the normal female the bladder neck sits above the pelvic floor supported predominantly by the pubovesical ligaments, the endopelvic fascia of the pelvic floor and levator ani. These support the urethra at rest; with elevated intra-abdominal pressure the levators contract, increasing urethral closure pressure to maintain continence. This anatomical arrangement commonly alters after parturition and with increasing age, such that the bladder neck lies beneath the pelvic floor, particularly when the intra-abdominal pressure rises: the mechanism described above then fails to maintain continence (stress incontinence as a result of urethral hypermobility).

MALE

In the male, the bladder neck is completely surrounded by a circular collar of smooth muscle which extends distally to surround the pre-prostatic portion of the urethra. Because of the location and orientation of its constituent fibres, the term preprostatic sphincter is suitable for this particular component of urinary tract smooth muscle. This is a genital sphincter mechanism with a well-defined adrenergic innervation, which ensures anterograde ejaculation by closing the bladder neck during seminal emission. Distally, this muscle merges with and becomes indistinguishable from the musculature in the stroma and capsule of the prostate gland.

Whether this preprostatic sphincter replaces, or is additional to, the bladder neck muscle pattern seen in the female is unclear, but it is probably additional.

BLADDER OUTFLOW OBSTRUCTION

In progressive chronic obstruction to micturition, e.g. by prostatic enlargement or urethral stricture, bladder muscle hypertrophies. The muscle fasciculi increase in size and, because they interlace in all directions, a thick-walled 'trabeculated bladder' is produced. Mucosa between the fascicles forms 'diverticula'. When outflow is thus obstructed, emptying is not complete: some urine remains and may become infected, and infection may ascend to the kidneys. Back pressure from a chronically distended bladder may gradually dilate the ureters and renal pelves (so-called 'hydronephrosis') and even the renal collecting tubules, which can result in progressive renal impairment.

VASCULAR SUPPLY AND LYMPHATIC DRAINAGE

ARTERIES (Fig. 108.4)

The bladder is supplied principally by the superior and inferior vesical arteries, derived from the anterior trunk of the internal iliac artery, supplemented by the obturator and inferior gluteal arteries. In the female additional branches are derived from the uterine and vaginal arteries.

Superior vesical artery

The superior vesical artery supplies many branches to the fundus of the bladder. The artery to the vas deferens often originates from one of these and accompanies the vas deferens to the testis, where it anastomoses with the testicular artery. Other branches supply the ureter. The beginning of the superior vesical artery is the proximal, patent section of the fetal umbilical artery.

Inferior vesical artery

The inferior vesical artery often arises with the middle rectal artery from the internal iliac artery. It supplies the base of the bladder, prostate, seminal vesicles and lower ureter. Prostatic branches communicate across the midline. The inferior vesical artery may sometimes provide the artery to the vas deferens.

VEINS (Fig. 93.3)

The veins which drain the bladder form a complicated plexus on its inferolateral surfaces and pass backwards in the lateral ligaments of the bladder to end in the internal iliac veins.

LYMPHATIC DRAINAGE (Fig. 108.6)

Lymphatics which drain the bladder begin in mucosal, intermuscular and serosal plexuses. There are three sets of collecting vessels, most of which end in the external iliac nodes. Vessels from the trigone emerge on the exterior of the bladder to run superolaterally. Vessels from the superior surface of the bladder converge to the posterolateral angle and pass superolaterally to the external iliac nodes (one may go to the internal or common iliac group). Vessels from the inferolateral surface of the bladder ascend to join those from the superior surface or run to the lymph nodes in the obturator fossa.

Minute nodules of lymphoid tissue may occur along the vesical lymph vessels.

Innervation

The nerves supplying the bladder arise from the pelvic plexuses, which are a mesh of autonomic nerves and ganglia on the lateral aspects of the rectum, internal genitalia and bladder base. They consist of both sympathetic and parasympathetic components, each of which contains both efferent and afferent fibres. The innervation of the bladder has been reviewed in some detail by Mundy (1999).

EFFERENT FIBRES

Parasympathetic fibres arise from the second to the fourth sacral segments of the spinal cord and enter the pelvic plexuses on the posterolateral aspects of the rectum as the pelvic splanchnic nerves or nervi erigentes. The sympathetic fibres are derived from the lower three thoracic and upper two lumbar segments of the spinal cord. These form the coeliac and mesenteric plexuses around the great vessels in the abdomen from which the hypogastric plexuses descend into the pelvis as fairly discrete nerve bundles within the extraperitoneal connective tissue posterior to the ureter on each side. The anterior part of the pelvic plexus is known as the vesical plexus. Small groups of autonomic neurones occur within the plexus and throughout all regions of the bladder wall. These multipolar intramural neurones are rich in acetylcholinesterase (AChE) and occur in ganglia consisting of up to 20 nerve cell bodies. Numerous preganglionic autonomic fibres form both axosomatic and axodendritic synapses with the ganglionic neurones. The majority of the preganglionic nerve terminals correspond morphologically to presumptive cholinergic fibres. Noradrenergic terminals also relay on cell bodies in the pelvic plexus: it is not known whether similar nerves synapse on intramural bladder ganglia.

The urinary bladder (including the trigonal detrusor muscle) is profusely supplied with nerves which form a dense plexus among the detrusor muscle cells. The majority of these nerves contain AChE and occur in abundance throughout the muscle coat of the bladder. Axonal varicosities adjacent to detrusor muscle cells possess features which are considered to typify cholinergic nerve terminals and contain clusters of small (50 nm diameter) agranular vesicles together with occasional large (80–160 nm diameter) granulated vesicles and small mitochondria. Terminal regions approach to within 20 nm of the surface of the muscle cells and may be partially surrounded by Schwann cell cytoplasm, or more often are naked nerve endings. The human detrusor muscle possesses a sparse supply of sympathetic noradrenergic nerves which generally accompany the vascular supply and only rarely extend among the myocytes. Nonadrenergic, noncholinergic nerves have been identified, and a number of other neurotransmitters or neuromodulators have been detected in intramural ganglia, including the peptide somatostatin. The superficial trigonal muscle is associated with more noradrenergic (sympathetic) fibres than cholinergic (parasympathetic) nerves. This difference supports the view that the superficial trigonal muscle should be regarded as 'ureteric' rather than 'vesical' in origin. However it must be emphasized that the superficial trigonal muscle forms a very minor part of the total muscle mass of the bladder neck and proximal urethra in either sex and is probably of little significance in the physiological mechanisms which control these regions.

The smooth muscle of the bladder neck in males is predominantly orientated obliquely or circularly and is sparsely supplied with cholinergic (parasympathetic) nerves but possesses a rich noradrenergic (sympathetic) innervation. A similar distribution of autonomic nerves also occurs in the smooth muscle of the prostate gland, seminal vesicles and vasa deferentia. Stimulation of sympathetic nerves causes contraction of smooth muscle in the wall of the genital tract resulting in seminal emission. Concomitant sympathetic stimulation of the proximal urethral smooth muscle causes sphincteric closure of the preprostatic sphincter, thereby preventing reflux of ejaculate into the bladder. Although this genital function of the bladder neck of the male is well established, it is not known whether the smooth muscle of this region

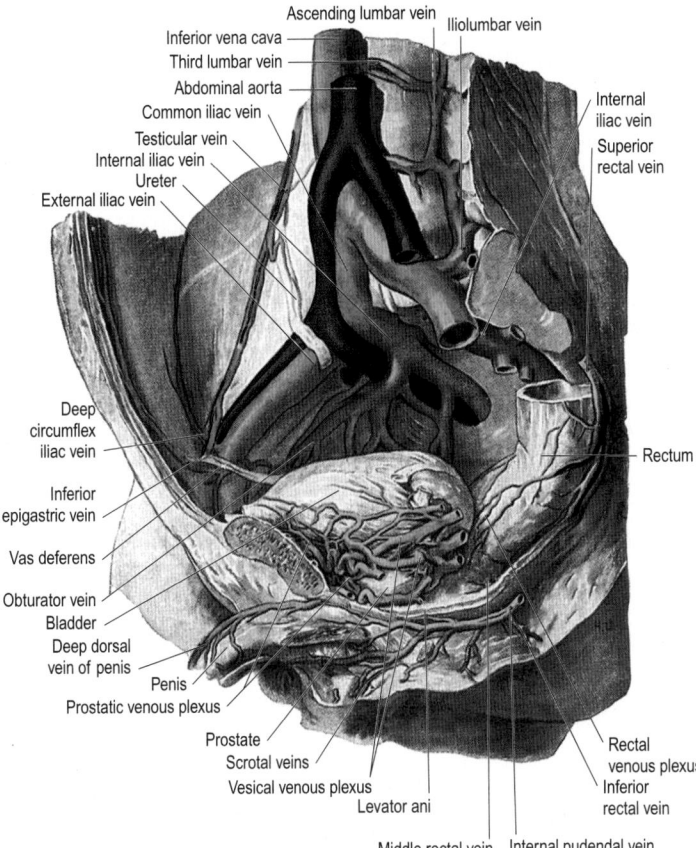

Inferior vena cava
Third lumbar vein
Abdominal aorta
Common iliac vein
Testicular vein
Internal iliac vein
Ureter
External iliac vein

Ascending lumbar vein
Iliolumbar vein

Internal iliac vein
Superior rectal vein

Deep circumflex iliac vein
Inferior epigastric vein
Vas deferens
Obturator vein
Bladder
Deep dorsal vein of penis
Penis
Prostatic venous plexus
Prostate
Scrotal veins
Vesical venous plexus
Levator ani

Rectum

Rectal venous plexus
Inferior rectal vein

Middle rectal vein   Internal pudendal vein

Fig. 93.3 The veins of the right half of the male pelvis. (After Spalteholtz W 1924 Die Arterien der Herzwand. Anatomische Untersuchungen an Menschen and Tieren. Leipzig: Hirzel.)

plays an active role in maintaining urinary continence. In contrast, the smooth muscle of the bladder neck of the female receives relatively few noradrenergic nerves but is richly supplied with presumptive cholinergic fibres. The sparse supply of sympathetic nerves presumably relates to the absence of a functioning 'genital' portion of the wall of the female urethra.

The lamina propria of the fundus and inferolateral walls of the bladder is virtually devoid of autonomic nerve fibres, apart from some noradrenergic and occasional presumptive cholinergic perivascular nerves. However, as the urethral orifice is approached, the density of nerves unrelated to blood vessels increases. At the bladder neck and trigone a nerve plexus extends throughout the lamina propria. The constituent nerves are cholinesterase positive and run through the connective tissue independent of blood vessels. Some of the larger diameter axons are myelinated and others lie adjacent to the basal urothelial cells. As in the ureter, the subepithelial nerve plexus of the bladder is assumed to subserve a sensory function in the absence of any obvious effector target sites.

AFFERENT FIBRES

Vesical nerves are also concerned with pain and awareness of distension and are stimulated by distension or spasm due to a stone, inflammation or malignant disease; they travel in sympathetic and parasympathetic nerves, predominantly the latter. Division of the sympathetic paths (e.g. 'presacral neurectomy'), or of the superior hypogastric plexus, therefore does not materially relieve vesical pain, whereas considerable relief follows bilateral anterolateral cordotomy. Since nerve fibres mediating awareness of distension travel in the posterior columns (fasciculus gracilis), the patient still retains awareness of the need to micturate after anterolateral cordotomy. The nerve endings detecting noxious stimuli are probably of more than one type: a subepithelial plexus of fibres containing dense vesicles, probably afferent endings, has been described.

MECHANISM AND CONTROL OF MICTURITION (Fig. 93.4)

Micturition consists of a storage phase and a voiding phase. During the storage phase the bladder accommodates an increasing volume of urine without any change in intravesical pressure. This is partly because of its viscoelastic properties, and partly because a gateing mechanism in the spinal cord reflexly inhibits preganglionic parasympathetic (efferent) activity, and a similar mechanism in the pelvic ganglia prevents the transmission of preganglionic activity to postganglionic parasympathetic neurones until preganglionic activity reaches a threshold level (giving an all-or-none effect). These properties are augmented by sufficient activity of the distal urethral sphincter to maintain urethral closure. This activity is controlled centrally by a storage centre within the rostral pons (called the L-centre because of its lateral location, p. 349). Mean bladder capacity in male adults varies around 400 ml. Micturition commonly occurs at smaller volumes. Filling to c.500 ml may be tolerated, but beyond this pain is caused by tension in the wall, leading to the urgent desire to micturate. Pain is referred to the cutaneous areas supplied by spinal segments supplying the bladder (T10–L2, S2–4), including the lower anterior abdominal wall, perineum and penis.

With threshold afferent stimulation, efferent impulses from the micturition centre in the rostral pons (also called the M-centre because of its relative medial location) (p. 349). activate descending spinal pathways to the intermediolateral grey column of the second, third and fourth sacral spinal segments where the cell bodies of the preganglionic parasympathetic nerves are located. Their axons run to the pelvic (inferior hypogastric) plexuses as the pelvic splanchnic nerves, and synapse on postganglionic parasympathetic neurones in ganglia within the plexuses and within the wall of the bladder. Postganglionic fibres ramify throughout the thickness of the detrusor smooth muscle coat. The profuse distribution of these motor nerves emphasizes the importance of the parasympathetic nervous system in initiating and sustaining bladder contraction during micturition. Just before the onset of voiding, the distal urethral sphincter is relaxed by central inhibition of its motor neurones (which are also located in the second, third and fourth sacral spinal segments), by the same nerve pathway which activates the preganglionic parasympathetic nerves. Activation of the parasympathetic innervation of the bladder causes the release of acetylcholine. This activates muscarinic receptors in the detrusor layer of the bladder wall and this causes bladder contraction. Relaxation of the urethra is currently believed to be due to the release of nitric oxide from these same parasympathetic nerves in the bladder neck and urethra. The central integration of the nervous control of the bladder and urethra is essential for normal micturition.

MICROSTRUCTURE (Fig. 93.4)

The wall of the urinary bladder consists of three layers, an outer adventitial layer of soft connective tissue (which in some regions possesses a serosal covering of peritoneum), a smooth muscle coat (the detrusor muscle), and an inner mucosal layer which lines the interior of the bladder.

The serous layer is restricted to the superior and, in males, part of the posterior, surfaces of the bladder. It consists of mesothelium and underlying connective tissue as elsewhere in the peritoneum. The detrusor muscular layer is composed of relatively large diameter interlacing bundles of smooth muscle cells arranged as a complex meshwork. Three ill-defined layers are present and arranged in such a way that longitudinally orientated muscle bundles predominate on the inner and outer aspects of a substantial middle circular layer. Posteriorly, some of the outer longitudinal bundles pass over the bladder base and fuse with the capsule of the prostate or with the anterior vaginal wall. Other bundles extend to the anterior aspect of the rectum as the rectovesical muscle. Anteriorly some of the outer longitudinal bundles continue into the pubovesical ligaments and contribute to the muscular component of these structures. As in the muscle coat of the ureter, exchange of fibres between adjacent muscle bundles frequently occurs within the bladder wall. Functionally, therefore, the detrusor acts as a single unit of interlacing smooth muscle.

The mucosa has a structure similar to that of the ureters. The mucosal lamina propria forms a relatively thick layer, varying in depth from 500 μm in the fundus and inferolateral walls to c.100 μm in the trigone. Small bundles of smooth muscle cells form an incomplete and rudimentary muscularis mucosae. An extensive network of blood vessels is present throughout the lamina propria and supplies a plexus of thin-walled fenestrated capillaries which lie in grooves at the base of the urothelium. In addition to the urothelium, the epithelium of the bladder neck and trigone also contains a cell which is characterized by the presence of numerous large membrane-bound vesicles each containing a central dense granule: these cells belong to the dispersed neuroendocrine system (p. 180).

Several morphological variations have been described in the mucosa of the bladder. Since they occur in otherwise normal healthy adults, they are not considered to represent pathological conditions. One of the commonest epithelial variants found in bladder biopsy samples or at postmortem are so-called Von Brunn's nests, proliferations of morphologically normal basal urothelial cells which project into the underlying connective tissue of the lamina propria and are particularly frequent in the trigone. They may undergo central involution which results in areas of oedematous-looking mucosa termed cystitis cystica. Mucus-secreting glands with single or branched ducts are frequently observed in the bladder mucosa, and are particularly numerous near the ureteric and internal urethral orifices. Non-keratinizing squamous metaplasia of the vaginal type frequently occurs in the urinary bladder mucosa, especially over the trigone, commonly in adult females, and rarely in males. It is of no pathological significance when confined to the trigone.

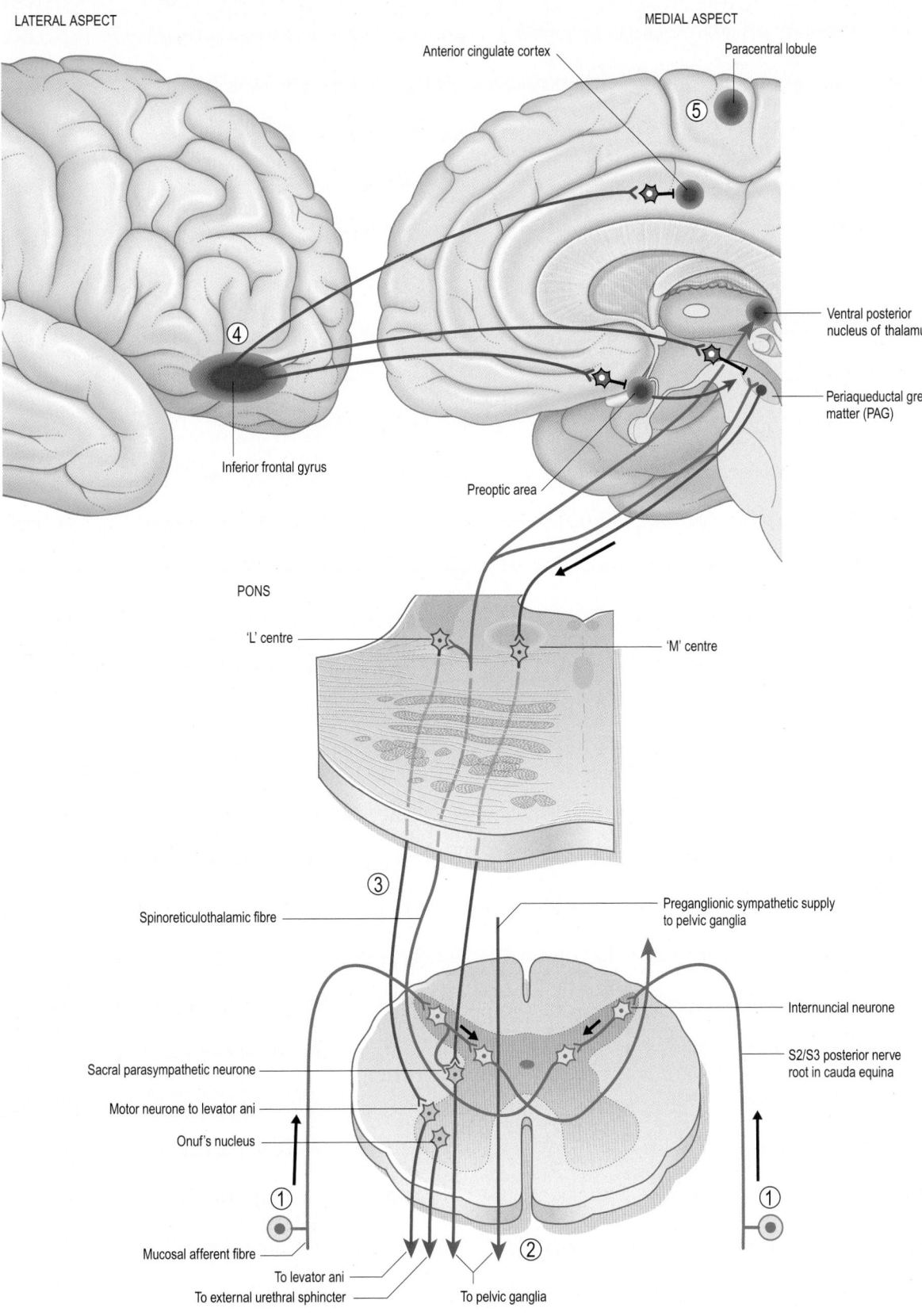

Fig. 93.4 Control of micturition. The micturition control centre is in the paramedian pontine reticular formation on each side. It comprises a medially placed micturition centre, 'M' and laterally placed storage centre, 'L'. Neurones project from the 'M' centre and to the storage centre 'L' to parasympathetic neurones in segments 2–4 of the sacral spinal cord, and to Onuf's nucleus, which is in the same segments, and which innervates the external urethral sphincter. At higher levels, neurones in the right prefrontal and anterior cingulate cortex, right preoptic nucleus and periaqueductal grey matter, are involved in the control of micturition. Vesical afferents from stretch receptors in the detrusor and trigonal mucosa relay the extent of bladder filling to the brain stem and thalamus via spinoreticulothalamic fibres (1). Activity in the sympathetic system that maintains bladder compliance increases (via β_2 receptors detrusor fibres) and parasympathetic activity is inhibited (2). Spinoreticular fibres synapsing in the 'L' nucleus in the pons activate Onuf's nucleus to increase the tone of the external sphincter (3). If micturition is deferred, fibres projecting from the inferior frontal gyrus inhibit the right anterior cingulate gyrus, preoptic area and periaqueductal grey matter) (4). Voluntary contraction of the pelvic floor musculature, controlled by the prefrontal cortex driving the perineal 'area' of the motor cortex (5) cannot be long sustained once filling is complete. (By permission from FitzGerald MJT, Folan-Curren J 2001 Clinical Neuroanatomy, 4th edn. London: Saunders.)

REFERENCES

Klutke CG, Siegel CL 1995 Functional female pelvic anatomy. Urol Clin North Am 22(3): 487–98.

Mundy AR, Fitzpatrick J, Neal D, George N 1999 Structure and function of the lower urinary tract. In: The Scientific Basis of Urology, Chapter 11. Oxford: Isis Medical Media: 217–42.
Explains the neurological components of bladder function from the higher cortical centres to molecular events within the cells of the detrusor muscle.

Male urethra

The male urethra is 18–20 cm long and extends from the internal orifice in the urinary bladder to the external opening, or meatus, at the end of the penis. It may be considered in two parts (**Figs 93.1, 94.1**). The relatively long anterior urethra (c.16 cm long) lies within the perineum (proximally) and the penis (distally) surrounded by the corpus spongiosum and is functionally a conduit. The relatively short posterior urethra (4 cm) lies in the pelvis proximal to the corpus spongiosum and is acted upon by the urogenital sphincter mechanisms and also acts as a conduit.

The anterior urethra is subdivided into a proximal component, the bulbar urethra, which is surrounded by the bulbospongiosus and is entirely within the perineum, and a pendulous or penile component, which continues on to the tip of the penis.

The posterior urethra is divided into preprostatic, prostatic, and membranous segments.

In the flaccid penis, the urethra as a whole presents a double curve (**Fig. 93.1**). Except during the passage of fluid along it, the urethral canal is a mere slit: in transverse section, the slit is transversely arched

in the prostatic part, in the preprostatic and membranous portions it is stellate, in the bulbar and penile portions it is transverse, while at the external orifice it is sagittal.

PREPROSTATIC PART

The preprostatic urethra is c.1–1.5 cm in length, extending almost vertically from the bladder neck to the superior aspect of the verumontanum. In addition to the smooth muscle bundles which run in continuity from the bladder neck down to the prostatic urethra, and distinct from the smooth muscle within the prostate, smooth muscle bundles surround the bladder neck and preprostatic urethra: they are arranged as a distinct circular collar which has its own distinct adrenergic innervation. The bundles which form this 'preprostatic sphincter' are small in size compared with the muscle bundles of the detrusor and are separated by a relatively larger connective tissue component rich in elastic fibres. Unlike the detrusor and the rest of the urethral smooth muscle (common to both sexes), the preprostatic sphincter is almost totally devoid of parasympathetic cholinergic nerves but is richly supplied with sympathetic noradrenergic nerves. Contraction of the preprostatic sphincter serves to prevent the retrograde flow of ejaculate through the proximal urethra into the bladder, and can maintain continence when the external sphincter has been damaged. It is extensively disrupted in the vast majority of men undergoing bladder neck surgery, e.g. transurethral resection of the prostate, which results in retrograde ejaculation.

PROSTATIC PART

The prostatic urethra is c.3–4 cm in length and tunnels through the substance of the prostate closer to the anterior than the posterior surface of the gland. It is continuous above with the preprostatic part and emerges from the prostate slightly anterior to its apex (the most inferior point of the prostate). The urethra turns anteriorly as it passes through the prostate making an angle of c.35°. Throughout most of its length the posterior wall possesses a midline ridge, the urethral crest, which projects into the lumen causing it to appear crescentic in transverse section. On each side of the crest there is a shallow depression, termed the prostatic sinus, the floor of which is perforated by the orifices of c.15–20 prostatic ducts. An elevation, the verumontanum (colliculus seminalis), at about the middle of the length of the urethral crest, contains the slit-like orifice of the prostatic utricle. On both sides of, or just within, this orifice are the two small openings of the ejaculatory ducts. The prostatic utricle is a cul-de-sac c.6 mm long, which runs upwards and backwards in the substance of the prostate behind its median lobe. Its walls are composed of fibrous tissue, muscular fibres and mucous membrane; the latter is pitted by the openings of numerous small glands. The prostatic utricle develops from the paramesonephric ducts or urogenital sinus, and is thought to be homologous with the vagina of the female (p. 1385). It is sometimes called the 'vagina masculina', but the more usual view is that it is a uterine homologue and hence the term 'utricle'.

The lowermost part of the prostatic urethra is fixed by the puboprostatic ligaments and is therefore immobile.

MEMBRANOUS PART

The membranous part of the urethra is the shortest (c.1.5 cm), least dilatable and, with the exception of the external orifice, the narrowest, section of the urethra. It descends with a slight ventral concavity from

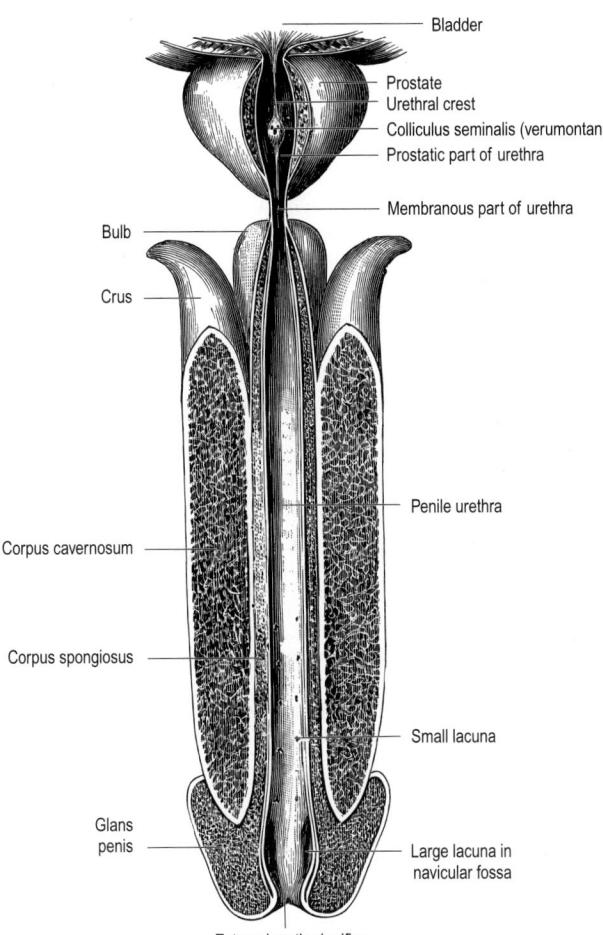

Bladder
Prostate
Urethral crest
Colliculus seminalis (verumontanum)
Prostatic part of urethra
Membranous part of urethra
Bulb
Crus
Corpus cavernosum
Corpus spongiosus
Penile urethra
Small lacuna
Glans penis
Large lacuna in navicular fossa
External urethral orifice

Fig. 94.1 The whole length of the lumen of the male urethra exposed by an incision extending into it from its dorsal aspect. Note openings of prostatic utricle and ejaculatory ducts on the colliculus seminalis (verumontanum).

the prostate to the bulb of the penis (**Fig. 93.1**), passing through the perineal membrane, c.2.5 cm posteroinferior to the pubic symphysis. The wall of the membranous urethra consists of a muscle coat, separated from the epithelial lining by a narrow layer of fibroelastic connective tissue. The muscle coat consists of a relatively thin layer of bundles of smooth muscle, which are continuous proximally with those of the prostatic urethra, and a prominent outer layer of circularly orientated striated muscle fibres, which form the external urethral sphincter, as it is commonly known. The bladder neck is sometimes called the proximal sphincter mechanism, to distinguish it from the distal sphincter mechanism. This latter term has considerable value because it recognizes that the sphincter-active membranous urethra consists of several components, namely, urethral smooth muscle; urethral striated muscle (rhabdosphincter), which is the most important component; and the periurethral part of levator ani, which is important to resist surges of intra-abdominal pressure (e.g. on coughing or exercise). The external sphincter represents the point of highest intraurethral pressure in the normal, contracted state. The intrinsic striated muscle component is devoid of muscle spindles. The striated muscle fibres themselves are unusually small in cross-section (15–20 μm diameter), and are physiologically of the slow twitch type, unlike the pelvic floor musculature, which is a heterogeneous mixture of slow and fast twitch fibres of larger diameter. The slow twitch fibres of the external sphincter are capable of sustained contraction over relatively long periods of time and actively contribute to the tone, which closes the urethra and maintains urinary continence.

The urethral sphincter mechanism is described on page 1367.

ANTERIOR PART

The anterior or spongiose part of the urethra lies within the corpus spongiosum penis (p. 1315). It is c.15 cm long when the penis is flaccid and extends from the end of the membranous urethra to the external urethral orifice on the glans penis. It starts below the perineal membrane at a point anterior to the lowest level of the symphysis. This part of the anterior urethra is surrounded by bulbospongiosus and is called the bulbar urethra. It is the widest part of the urethra. The bulbourethral glands open into this section of the urethra c.2.5 cm below the perineal membrane.

From here, when the penis is flaccid, the urethra curves downwards as the penile urethra. It is a narrow, transverse slit when empty, and has a diameter of c.6 mm when passing urine. It is dilated at its termination within the glans penis where it is known as the navicular fossa. The external urethral orifice is the narrowest part of the urethra, and is a sagittal slit, c.6 mm long, bounded on each side by a small labium.

The epithelium of the urethra, particularly in the bulbar and distal penile segments, presents the orifices of numerous small mucous glands and follicles situated in the submucous tissue and named the urethral glands. It also contains a number of small pit-like recesses, or lacunae, of varying sizes whose orifices are directed forwards. One, larger than the rest, the lacuna magna, is situated on the roof of the navicular fossa.

TRAUMATIC INJURY TO THE URETHRA

The urethra may be ruptured by a fall-astride (or straddle) injury to the bulbar urethra in the perineum, or by an injury related to a pelvic fracture. These injuries usually affect the junction of the membranous with the bulbar segments across the perineal membrane. One complication of such injuries is extravasation of urine. After an injury to the bulbar urethra, urine usually extravasates between the perineal membrane and the membranous layer of the superficial fascia (clinically known as Colles' fascia). As both of these are attached firmly to the ischiopubic rami, extravasated fluid cannot pass posteriorly because the two layers are continuous around the superficial transverse perineal muscles. Laterally, the spread of urine is blocked by the pubic and ischial rami. Urine cannot enter the lesser pelvis through the perineal membrane if this remains intact, so it makes its way anteriorly into the loose connective tissue of the scrotum and penis and thence to the anterior abdominal wall. If the posterior urethra is injured, urine is extravasated into the pelvic extraperitoneal tissue: if the perineal membrane is torn as well extravasation may also occur into the perineum.

CONGENITAL ANOMALIES OF THE URETHRA

Hypospadias, found in c.1 in 300 boys, most often results in the urethra opening in the distal penis; sometimes it opens on the ventral aspect of the penis or more proximally up to the perineum. There is also an associated abnormality of the prepuce, which is longer dorsally and lacking ventrally, and often an associated chordee which causes a ventral curvature of the penis. It is important that this anomaly be identified prior to circumcision, because the abnormal foreskin is sometimes used for surgical correction of the deformity. Posterior urethral valves occur in 1 in 5000 to 8000 males and the most common cause of urinary outflow obstruction in male infants. The commest type (Type I) are believed to occur if the Wolffian ducts open too anteriorly onto the primitive prostatic urethra. This abnormal migration of the ducts leaves behind thick vestigial tissue that forms rigid valve cusps extending caudally from the verumontanum.

Very rarely urethral duplication is seen. When present the two urethrae almost invariably lie on top of each other rather than side by side. It is possible that one of the urethrae, most likely the more dorsal, may be blind ending.

VASCULAR SUPPLY AND LYMPHATIC DRAINAGE

URETHRAL ARTERY

The urethral artery arises from the internal pudendal artery or common penile artery just below the perineal membrane and travels through the corpus spongiosum, to reach the glans penis. It supplies the urethra and erectile tissue around it. In addition, the urethra is supplied by the dorsal penile artery, via its circumflex branches on each side and, retrograde from the glans, by its terminal branches. The blood supply through the corpus spongiosum is so plentiful that the urethra can be divided without compromising its vascular supply.

VEINS

The venous drainage of the anterior urethra is to the dorsal veins of the penis and internal pudendal veins, which drain to the prostatic plexus. The posterior urethra drains into the prostatic and vesical venous plexuses, which drain into the internal iliac veins.

LYMPHATIC DRAINAGE

Vessels from the posterior urethra pass mainly to the internal iliac nodes; a few may end in the external iliac nodes. Vessels from the membranous urethra accompany the internal pudendal artery. Vessels from the anterior urethra accompany those of the glans penis, ending in the deep inguinal nodes. Some may end in superficial nodes; others may traverse the inguinal canal to end in the external iliac nodes.

INNERVATION

The prostatic plexus supplies the smooth muscle of the prostate and prostatic urethra. It is derived from the pelvic plexus on each side and lies on the posterolateral aspect of the seminal vesicle and prostate on each side. Lesser cavernous nerves pierce the bulb of the corpus spongiosum proximally to supply the penile urethra. The greater cavernous nerves carry the sympathetic supply, which causes contraction of the preprostatic sphincter during ejaculation and prevents reflux of ejaculate into the bladder. The parasympathetic preganglionic fibres come from the second to fourth sacral segments. The nerve supply of the intrinsic muscle striated component (or rhabdosphincter) of the distal sphincter mechanism (or external sphincter) is controversial. It is generally believed to be supplied by neurones in Onuf's nucleus and by perineal branches of the pudendal nerve lying on the perineal aspect of the pelvic floor. In both instances the axons arise from neurones in S2, 3 and 4. Fibres from Onuf's nucleus (which is somatic) travel with the pelvic plexus on each side until they branch off and run on the pelvic aspect of the pelvic floor to enter the membranous urethra.

MICROSTRUCTURE

The epithelium lining the preprostatic urethra and the proximal part of the prostatic urethra is a typical urothelium. It is continuous with that lining the bladder, and with the epithelium lining the ducts of the prostate and bulbourethral glands, the seminal vesicles, and the vasa deferentia and ejaculatory ducts. These relationships are important in the spread of urinary tract infections.

Below the openings of the ejaculatory ducts the epithelium changes to a pseudostratified or stratified columnar type, which lines the membranous urethra and the major part of the penile urethra. Mucus-secreting cells are common throughout this epithelium and frequently occur in small clusters in the penile urethra. Branching tubular para-urethral glands secrete protective mucus onto the urethral epithelial lining and are especially numerous on its dorsal aspect. In older men many of the deep recesses of the urethral mucosa contain concretions similar to those found within prostatic glands (p. 1302). Towards the distal end of the penile urethra the epithelium changes once again, becoming stratified squamous in type with well-defined connective tissue papillae. This epithelium also lines the navicular fossa and becomes keratinized at the external meatus. The epithelial cells lining the navicular fossa are glycogen-rich. This may provide a substrate for commensal lactobacilli which, as in the female vagina (p. 1353), provide a defence against pathogenic organisms.

REFERENCE

Chancellor MB, Yoshimura N 2002 Physiology and pharmacology of the bladder and urethra. In: Walsh PC et al (eds) Campbell's Urology Study Guide, 2nd edn. Philadelphia: Saunders: Chapter 23.

Female urethra

The female urethra is c.4 cm long and 6 mm in diameter. It begins at the internal urethral orifice of the bladder, approximately opposite the middle of the symphysis pubis, and runs anteroinferiorly behind the symphysis pubis, embedded in the anterior wall of the vagina. It crosses the perineal membrane and ends at the external urethral orifice as an anteroposterior slit with rather prominent margins situated directly anterior to the opening of the vagina and c.2.5 cm behind the glans clitoridis (**Fig. 108.10**). It sometimes opens into the anterior vaginal wall. Except during the passage of urine, the anterior and posterior walls of the urethra are in apposition and the epithelium is thrown into longitudinal folds, one of which, on the posterior wall of the canal, is termed the urethral crest. Many small mucous urethral glands and minute pit-like recesses or lacunae open into the urethra. On each side, near the lower end of the urethra, a number of these glands are grouped together and open into a duct, named the para-urethral duct: each duct runs down in the submucous tissue and ends in a small aperture on the lateral margin of the external urethral orifice.

VASCULAR SUPPLY, LYMPHATIC DRAINAGE AND INNERVATION

Arteries – The blood supply to the female urethra is derived from the vesical and vaginal arteries, principally the latter.

Veins – The venous plexus around the urethra drains into the vesical venous plexus around the bladder neck, and into the internal pudendal veins. An erectile plexus of veins along the length of the urethra is continuous with the erectile tissue of the vestibular bulb.

Lymphatic drainage – The urethral lymphatics drain into the internal and external iliac nodes.

Innervation – Parasympathetic preganglionic fibres from the second to fourth segments of the sacral spinal cord run in the pelvic splanchnic nerves and synapse in the vesical plexus in or near the bladder wall (p. 1291): postganglionic fibres are distributed to the smooth muscle of the urethral wall. Somatic fibres to the striated muscle are derived from the same sacral segments, and run in the pelvic splanchnic nerves but do not synapse in the vesical plexus. Sensory fibres run in the pelvic splanchnic nerves to the second to fourth segments of the sacral spinal cord. Postganglionic sympathetic fibres arise from the plexus around the vaginal arteries.

MICROSTRUCTURE (Fig. 95.1)

The wall of the female urethra consists of an outer muscle coat and an inner mucosa, which lines the lumen and is continuous with that of the bladder. The muscle coat consists of an outer sheath of striated muscle (external urethral sphincter or distal sphincter mechanism together with an inner coat of smooth muscle fibres. The female external urethral sphincter is anatomically separate from the adjacent periurethral striated muscle of the anterior pelvic floor. The fibres of the sphincter are arranged like a signet ring. They form a sleeve which is thickest anteriorly in the middle one-third of the urethra, and is relatively deficient posteriorly. The striated muscle extends into the anterior wall of both the proximal and distal thirds of the urethra but is deficient posteriorly in these regions. The muscle cells forming the external urethral sphincter are all small diameter, slow twitch, fibres.

The smooth muscle coat extends throughout the length of the urethra and consists of slender muscle bundles, the majority of which are orientated obliquely or longitudinally. A few circularly arranged muscle fibres occur in the outer aspect of the non-striated muscle layer and intermingle with the skeletal muscle fibres forming the inner part of the external urethral sphincter. Proximally the urethral smooth muscle extends as far as the bladder neck where it is replaced by fascicles of detrusor smooth muscle. This region in the female lacks a well-defined circular smooth muscle component comparable with the preprostatic sphincter of the male. Distally, urethral smooth muscle bundles terminate in the subcutaneous adipose tissue surrounding the external urethral meatus.

The smooth muscle of the female urethra receives an extensive presumptive cholinergic parasympathetic nerve supply, but contains relatively few noradrenergic nerves. In the absence of an anatomical sphincter, competence of the female bladder neck and proximal urethra is unlikely to be totally dependent on smooth muscle activity, and is more probably related to the support provided by the ligamentous

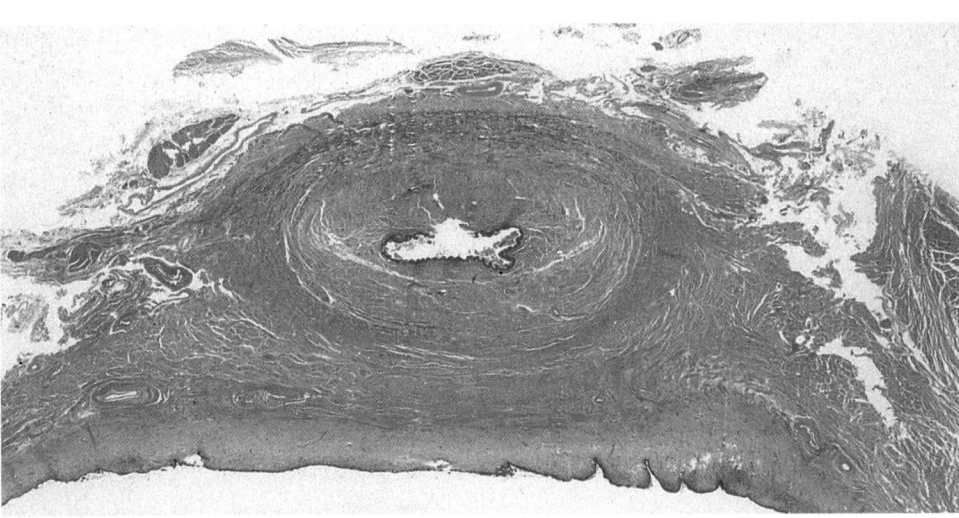

Fig. 95.1 Transverse section through the female urethra. The lumen (centre field) is lined by a stratified squamous non-keratinizing epithelium, continuous with the keratinized epithelium of the genital vestibule (below) into which it opens. The urethral mucosa is surrounded by a circular smooth muscular layer. (By kind permission of Anthony R Mundy.)

structures which surround them. The innervation and longitudinal orientation of most of the muscle fibres suggest that urethral smooth muscle in the female is active during micturition, serving to shorten and widen the urethral lumen.

The mucosa lining the female urethra consists of a stratified epithelium and a supporting lamina propria of loose fibroelastic connective tissue. The latter is bulky and well-vascularized, and contains numerous thin-walled veins. Its abundant elastic fibres are orientated both longi-tudinally and circularly around the urethra. The lamina propria contains a fine nerve plexus, believed to be derived from sensory branches of the pudendal nerves. The proximal part of the urethra is lined by urothelium, identical in appearance to that of the bladder neck. Distally the epithelium changes into a non-keratinizing stratified squamous type which lines the major portion of the female urethra. This epithelium is keratinized at the external urethral meatus where it becomes continuous with the skin of the vestibule.

REFERENCE

Chancellor MB, Yoshimura N 2002 Physiology and pharmacology of the bladder and urethra. In: Walsh PC et al (eds) Campbell's Urology Study Guide, 2nd edn. Philadelphia; Saunders: Chapter 23.

Prostate

The prostate is a pyramidal fibromuscular gland which surrounds the prostatic urethra from the bladder base to the membranous urethra and is itself surrounded by a thin but tough connective tissue capsule (**Figs 94.1, 98.1, 101.1, 96.1, 96.2**). It lies at a low level in the lesser pelvis, behind the inferior border of the symphysis pubis and pubic arch and anterior to the rectal ampulla, through which it may be palpated. Being somewhat pyramidal, it presents a base or vesical aspect superiorly, an apex inferiorly and posterior, anterior and two inferolateral surfaces. The prostatic base measures about 4 cm transversely. The gland is c.2 cm in anteroposterior and 3 cm in its vertical diameters, and weighs c.8 g in youth, but almost invariably enlarges with the development of benign prostatic hyperplasia (BPH), weighing usually c.40 g, but sometimes as much as 150 g or even more after the first five decades of life (p. 1301).

Superiorly the base is largely contiguous with the neck of the bladder. The urethra enters the prostate near its anterior border. The apex is inferior, surrounding the junction of the prostatic and membranous parts of the posterior urethra.

The anterior surface lies in the arch of the pubis, separated from it by a venous plexus (Santorini's plexus) and loose adipose tissue. It is transversely narrow and convex, extending from the apex to the base. Near its superior limit it is connected to the pubic bones by the puboprostatic ligaments. The urethra emerges from this surface antero-superior to the apex of the gland. The anterior part of the prostate is relatively deficient in glandular tissue and is largely composed of fibro-muscular tissue.

The inferolateral surfaces are related to the muscles of the pelvic sidewall: the anterior fibres of levator ani embrace the prostate in the pubourethral sling or pubourethralis. These muscles are separated from the prostate by a thin layer of connective tissue.

The posterior surface is separated from the rectum by the prostatic capsule and by Denonvillier's fascia, a dense condensation of pelvic fascia which develops by obliteration of the rectovesical peritoneal pouch. It is obliterated from below upwards as fetal life progresses so that at birth this fascia separates the prostate, the seminal vesicles and the ampullae of the vasa deferentia from the rectum. The posterior surface is transversely flat and vertically convex. Near its superior (juxtavesical) border is a depression where it is penetrated by the two ejaculatory ducts. Below this is a shallow, median sulcus, usually considered to mark a partial separation into right and left lateral lobes.

The anterior and lateral aspects of the prostate are covered by a layer of fascia derived from the endopelvic fascia on each side. The prostatic venous plexus (**Fig. 93.3**) lies between this extension of the endopelvic fascia and the capsule of the prostate. Anteroinferiorly the fascia and the capsule of the prostate merge and blend with the puboprostatic ligaments.

The prostate is traversed by the urethra and ejaculatory ducts, and contains the prostatic utricle. The urethra usually passes between its anterior and middle thirds. The ejaculatory ducts pass anteroinferiorly through its posterior region to open into the prostatic urethra (p. 1295).

ZONAL ANATOMY OF THE PROSTATE
(Figs 96.1, 96.2)

The prostate gland was initially thought to be divided into five anatomical lobes, but it is now recognized that five lobes can only be distinguished in the fetal gland prior to 20 weeks' gestation. Between then and the onset of BPH, three lobes are recognizable, two lateral and a median lobe. This simplified view of prostatic lobation is retained

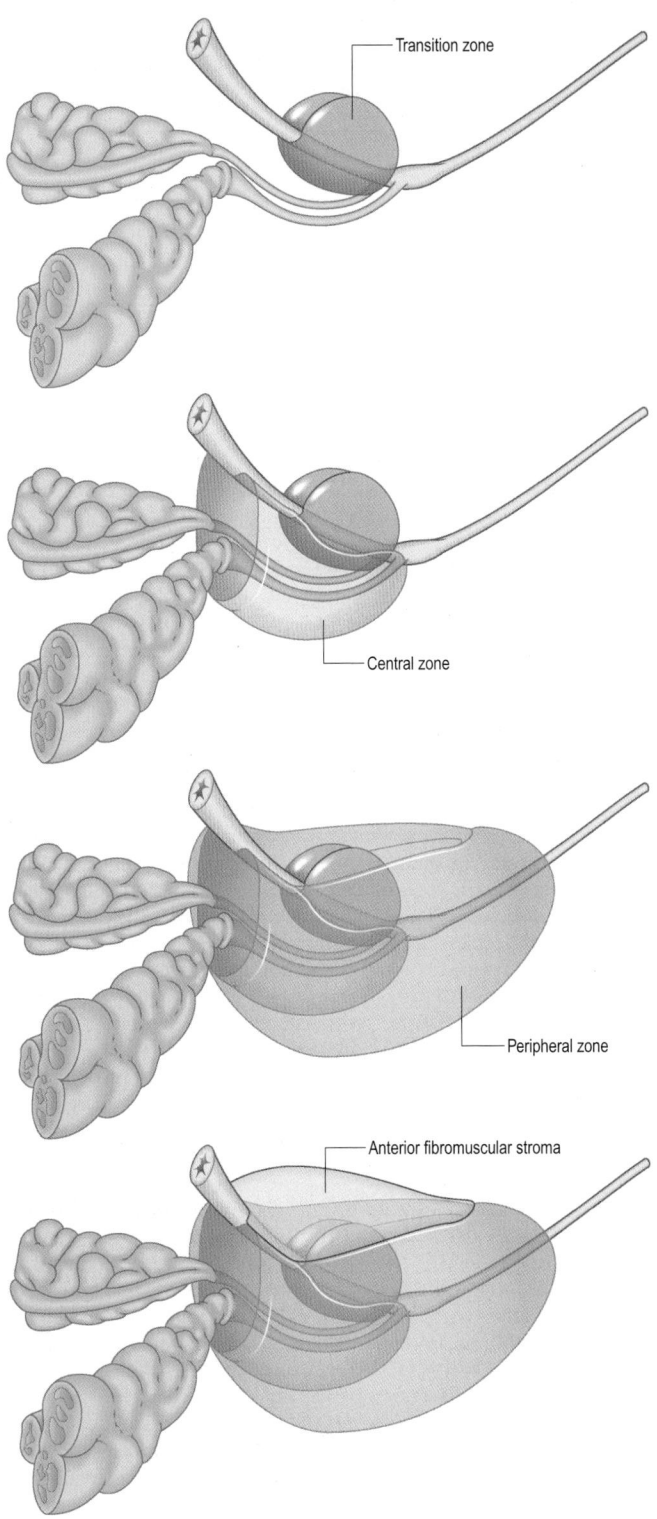

Transition zone

Central zone

Peripheral zone

Anterior fibromuscular stroma

Fig. 96.1 Zonal anatomy of the prostate. (By permission from Walsh PC, Retik AB, Vaughan ED et al (eds) 2002 Campbell's Urology, 8th edn. Philadelphia: Saunders.)

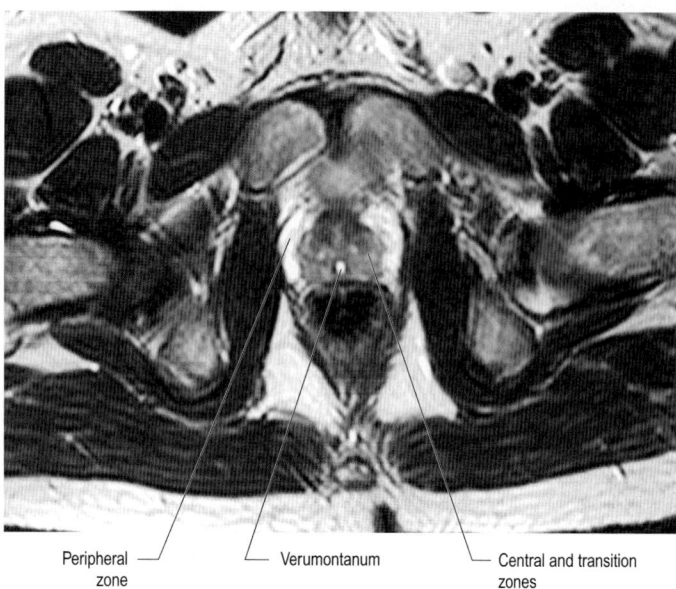

Peripheral zone — Verumontanum — Central and transition zones

Fig. 96.2 T2-weighted axial MRI scan of the prostate in a young man showing the normal high signal of the peripheral zone, intermediate signal central and transitional zones, and verumontanum in the central gland.

because clinicians refer to left and right 'lobes' when describing rectally palpable and endoscopically visible abnormalities in the diseased state when prostatic anatomy is distorted by BPH.

From an anatomical and particularly from a morbid anatomical perspective, the glandular tissue may be subdivided into three distinct zones, peripheral (70% by volume), central (25% by volume), and transition (5% by volume) (**Fig. 96.2**). Non-glandular tissue (fibro-muscular stoma) fills up the space between the peripheral zones anterior to the preprostatic urethra. The central zone surrounds the ejaculatory ducts posterior to the preprostatic urethra and is more or less conical in shape with its apex at the verumontanum. The transition zone lies around the distal part of the preprostatic urethra just proximal to the apex of the central zone and the ejaculatory ducts. Its ducts enter the prostatic urethra just below the preprostatic sphincter and just above the ducts of the peripheral zone. The peripheral zone is cup-shaped and encloses the central transition zone and the preprostatic urethra except anteriorly, where the space is filled by the anterior fibromuscular stoma. Simple mucus-secreting glands lie in the tissue around the preprostatic urethra, above the transition zone and surrounded by the preprostatic sphincter. These simple glands are similar to those in the female urethra and unlike the glands of the prostate.

The zonal anatomy of the prostate is clinically important because most carcinomas arise in the peripheral zone, whereas BPH affects the transition zone, which may grow to form the bulk of the prostate. BPH begins as micronodules in the transition zone; these grow and coalesce to form macronodules around the inferior margin of the preprostatic urethra, just above the verumontanum. Macronodules in turn compress the surrounding normal tissue of the peripheral zone posteroinferiorly thereby creating a 'false capsule' around the hyperplastic tissue, which coincidentally provides a plane of cleavage for surgical enucleation of the hyperplastic tissue. As the transition zone grows, it produces the appearance of 'lobes' on either side of the urethra above. These lobes may, in due course, compress or distort the preprostatic and prostatic parts of the urethra to produce symptoms. The central zone surrounding the ejaculatory ducts is rarely involved in any disease. It shows certain histochemical characteristics which are different from the rest of the prostate and is thought to be derived from the Wolffian duct system (much like the epididymi, vasa deferentia and seminal vesicles), whereas the rest of the prostate is derived from the urogenital sinus (p. 1393).

The zonal anatomy may be distinguished to some extent on radio-logical imaging. On transrectal ultrasonography (TRUS) the central and peripheral zones are generally of uniform low-level echogenicity, although slight differences may be appreciated. The preprostatic urethra is surrounded by a less echogenic area which corresponds to the preprostatic sphincter, periurethral glandular tissue and transition zone. It is often possible to see the ejaculatory ducts coursing to the prostatic urethra on sagittal scans of the gland. The seminal vesicles are hypoechoic/anechoic sacculated structures which lie superoposterior to the gland.

On magnetic resonance (MR) imaging the prostate gland has a zonal anatomy on T2-weighted images (**Fig. 96.2**). The normal peripheral zone has high signal intensity, as does fluid within the seminal vesicles. The central and transition zones have relatively low signal and are often referred to as the 'central gland'. The verumontanum may be seen as high signal within the central gland.

The relationship of the zones of the gland normally changes with age. The central zone atrophies, and the transition zone enlarges secondary to BPH. This often produces a low signal band at the margin of the hypertrophied transition and compressed peripheral zones, the surgical pseudocapsule, which is well seen on T2-weighted MR images. The fluid-containing seminal vesicles appear very high signal on T2-weighted images

VASCULAR SUPPLY AND LYMPHATIC DRAINAGE

ARTERIES (Fig. 108.4)

The prostate is supplied by branches from the inferior vesical, internal pudendal and middle rectal arteries. They perforate the gland along a posterolateral line from the junction of the prostate with the bladder down to the apex of the gland.

VEINS

The veins run into a plexus around the anterolateral aspects of the prostate, posterior to the arcuate pubic ligament and the lower part of symphysis pubis, anterior to the bladder and prostate (**Fig. 93.3**). The chief tributary is the deep dorsal vein of the penis. The plexus also receives anterior vesical and prostatic rami (which connect with the vesical plexus and internal pudendal vein), and drains into vesical and internal iliac veins.

LYMPHATIC DRAINAGE

Collecting vessels from the vas deferens end in the external iliac nodes, while those from the seminal vesicle drain to the internal and external iliac nodes. Prostatic vessels end mainly in internal iliac, sacral and obturator nodes. A vessel from the posterior surface accompanies the vesical vessels to the external iliac nodes and one from the anterior surface reaches the internal iliac group by joining vessels which drain the membranous urethra.

INNERVATION

The prostate has an abundant nerve supply from the inferior hypo-gastric (pelvic) plexus. The prostatic capsule is covered by numerous nerve fibres and ganglia, which form a periprostatic nerve plexus. The greatest density of nerves is found in the preprostatic sphincter, followed by the anterior fibromuscular stroma, and the peripheral zone is the least densely innervated. Nerves containing neuropeptide Y and vaso-intestinal polypeptide (VIP) are localized in the subepithelial connective tissue, in the smooth muscle layers of the gland, and in the walls of its blood vessels. Neurovascular bundles containing nerves which supply the prostate, seminal vesicles, prostatic urethra, ejaculatory ducts, corpora cavernosa, corpus spongiosum, membranous and penile urethra and bulbourethral glands are closely applied to, but separable from, the posterolateral margins of the prostate. These nerves are frequently damaged during radical prostate surgery for organ-confined prostate cancer, producing impotence (p. 1317).

MICROSTRUCTURE (Figs 96.3, 96.4)

The prostate is grey to reddish in colour according to its activity, and is very dense. It is enclosed by a thin, but strong fibrous capsule within a sheath derived from pelvic fascia and containing a venous plexus. The capsule is firmly adherent to the gland and is continuous with a median septum and with numerous fibromuscular septa which divide the glandular tissue into indistinct lobules.

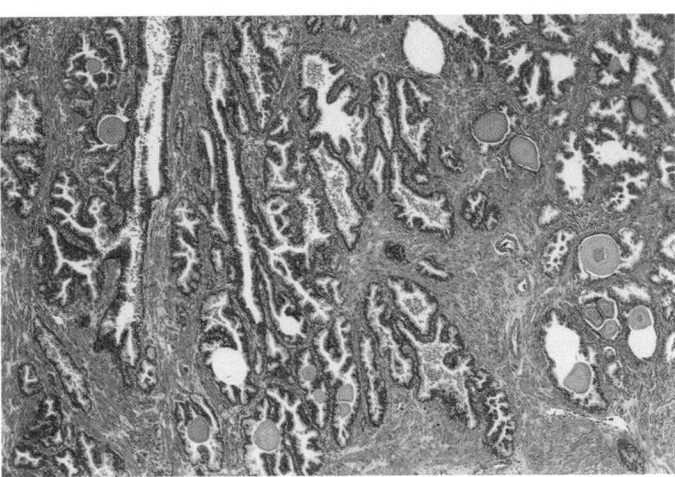

Fig. 96.3 Main prostatic glands with several prostatic concretions (corpora amylacea) as seen centre right. The lining epithelium is typically variable, from cuboidal to pseudostratified columnar, with complex infolded regions. Several ducts are seen, top left. (Photograph by Sarah-Jane Smith.)

The muscular tissue is mainly smooth. Anterior to the urethra a layer of smooth muscle merges with the main mass of muscle in the fibro-muscular septa. Superiorly it blends with vesical smooth muscle. Anterior to this smooth muscle a transversely crescent-shaped mass of skeletal muscle is continuous inferiorly with the sphincter urethrae in the deep perineal pouch. Its fibres pass transversely internal to the capsule, and are attached to it laterally by diffuse collagen bundles; other collagen bundles pass posteromedially, merging with the prostatic fibromuscular

septa and the septum of the urethral crest. This muscle, supplied by the pudendal nerve, probably compresses the urethra but it may pull the urethral crest back and the prostatic sinuses forwards, dilating the urethra. Glandular contents may be expelled simultaneously into the urethra when it has expanded in this way, so that it contains 3–5 ml seminal fluid prior to ejaculation.

The glandular tissue consists of numerous follicles with frequent internal papillae. Follicles open into elongated canals which join to form 12–20 main ducts. The follicles are separated by loose connective tissue, supported by extensions of the fibrous capsule and muscular stroma and enclosed in a delicate capillary plexus. Follicular epithelium is variable but predominantly columnar and either single-layered or pseudostratified. Prostatic ducts open mainly into the prostatic sinuses in the floor of the prostatic urethra. They have a bilayered epithelium, the luminal layer is columnar and the basal layer is populated by small cuboidal cells. Small colloid amyloid bodies are frequent in the follicles (**Fig. 96.3**). Prostatic and seminal vesicular secretions form the bulk of seminal fluid. Prostatic secretions are slightly acid, and contain acid phosphatase, amylase, prostate specific antigen and fibrinolysin as well as zinc. Numerous neuroendocrine cells, containing neurone-specific enolase, chromogranin and serotonin, are present in the glandular epithelium. Their numbers decline after middle age and their function is unknown.

Histological sections just above the level of the verumontanum show two concentric, partially circumurethral, zones of glandular tissue (**Fig. 96.4**). The larger outer zone is the peripheral zone which has long, branched glands, whose ducts open mainly into the prostatic sinuses. The inner zone is the transition zone and consists of glands whose ducts open on the floor of the prostatic sinuses and colliculus seminalis and a group of simple mucosal glands, surrounding the preprostatic urethra. Anteriorly, in the prostatic isthmus, the peripheral zone and submucosal glands are absent. Carcinomas arise almost exclusively in the peripheral zone, whereas the transition zone is prone to BPH.

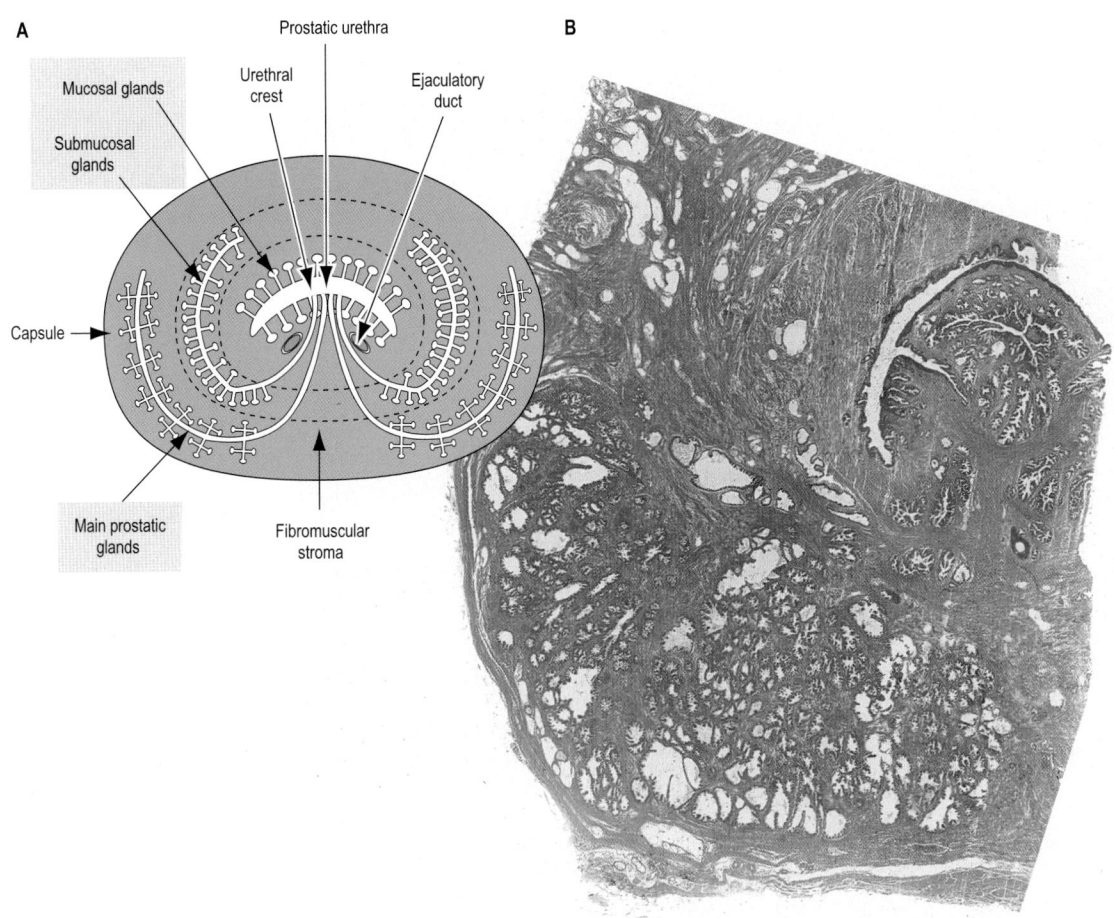

Fig. 96.4 A, Microstructure of the prostate. **B**, The prostate gland is shown in transverse hemisection at the level of the urethral crest. Periurethral submucosal glands are commonly involved in benign prostatic hypertrophy, whereas the peripheral glands are the usual site of origin of carcinoma. (By permission from Kierszenbaum AL 2002 Histology and Cell Biology. St Louis: Mosby.)

AGE CHANGES IN THE PROSTATE

At birth, the prostate has a system of ducts embedded in a stroma which forms a large part of the gland. Follicles are represented by small end-buds on the ducts. Before birth there is hyperplasia and squamous metaplasia of the epithelium of the ducts, colliculus seminalis and prostatic utricle, possibly due to maternal oestrogens in the fetal blood. This subsides after birth and is followed by a period of quiescence lasting for 12–14 years.

At puberty, between the ages of approximately 14 and 18 years, the prostate gland enters a maturation phase: it more than doubles in size during this time. Growth is almost entirely due to follicular development, partly from end-buds on ducts, and partly from modification of the ductal branches. Morphogenesis and differentiation of the epithelial cords starts in an intermediate part of the epithelial anlage and proceeds to the urethral and subcapsular parts of the gland; the latter is reached by the age of 17–18 years. The glandular epithelium is initially multi-layered squamous or cuboidal, and is transformed into a pseudostratified epithelium consisting of basal, exocrine secretory (including mucous) and neuroendocrine cells. The mucous cells are temporary, and are lost as the gland matures. The remaining exocrine secretory cells produce a number of products including acid phosphatase, prostate-specific antigen and β-microseminoprotein. This growth of the secretory component is associated with a condensation of the stroma, which diminishes relative to the glandular tissue. These changes are probably a response to the secretion of testosterone by the testis.

During the third decade the glandular epithelium grows by irregular multiplication of the epithelial infoldings into the lumen of the follicles.

After the third decade the size remains virtually unaltered until 45–50 years, when the epithelial foldings tend to disappear, follicular outlines become more regular, and amyloid bodies increase in number. All these changes are signs of prostatic involution.

After 45–50 years the prostate tends to develop BPH. The nature of BPH has been outlined earlier in this chapter. It is an age-related condition: if a man lives long enough then it is inevitable, although it is not always symptomatic.

REFERENCE

Mundy AR, Fitzpatrick J, Neal D, George N (eds) 1999 The prostate and benign prostatic hyperplasia. In: The Scientific Basis of Urology, Chapter 13. Oxford: Isis Medical Media: 257–76.
Includes a review of prostatic zonal anatomy.

Testes and epididymes

The testes are the primary reproductive organs or gonads in the male. They are ovoid reproductive and endocrine organs responsible for sperm production and are suspended in the scrotum by scrotal tissues including the non-striated dartos muscle and the spermatic cords. Average testicular dimensions are 4–5 cm in length, 2.5 cm in breadth and 3 cm in anteroposterior diameter; their weight varies from 10.5–14 g. The left testis usually lies lower than the right testis. Each testis lies obliquely within the scrotum, its upper pole tilted anterolaterally and the lower posteromedially (**Fig. 97.1**). The anterior aspect is convex, the posterior nearly straight, with the spermatic cord attached to it. Anterior, medial and lateral surfaces and both poles are convex, smooth and covered by the visceral layer of the serosal tunica vaginalis, which separates them from the parietal layer and the scrotal tissues external to this. Between these two layers there is always a very fine film of fluid. This fluid layer can increase on occasions, creating a hydrocele. The posterior aspect is only partly covered by tunica serosa; the epididymis adjoins its lateral part.

TESTIS

The testis is invested by three coats, which are, from outside inwards, the tunica vaginalis, tunica albuginea and tunica vasculosa. Each testis is separated from its fellow by a fibrous median raphe, which is deficient superiorly.

TUNICA VAGINALIS

The tunica vaginalis (**Figs 97.1, 991.**) is the lower end of the peritoneal processus vaginalis, whose formation precedes the descent of the fetal testis from the abdomen to the scrotum (p. 1388). After this migration, the proximal part of the tunica, from the internal inguinal ring almost to the testis, contracts and is obliterated, leaving a closed distal sac into which the testis is invaginated. The tunica is reflected from the testis

onto the internal surface of the scrotum, so forming the visceral and parietal layers of the tunica. The visceral layer covers all aspects of the testis except most of the posterior aspect. Posteromedially it is reflected forwards to the parietal layer. Posterolaterally it passes to the medial aspect of the epididymis and lines the epididymal sinus, and then passes laterally to its posterior border where it is reflected forwards to become continuous with the parietal layer. The visceral and parietal layers are continuous at both poles but at the upper pole the visceral layer surmounts the head of the epididymis before reflexion.

The more extensive parietal layer reaches below the testis and ascends in front of and medial to the spermatic cord. The inner surface of the tunica vaginalis has a smooth, moist mesothelium: the potential space between its visceral and parietal layers is termed the cavity of the tunica vaginalis.

TUNICA ALBUGINEA

The tunica albuginea is a dense, bluish-white covering for the testis. It is composed mainly of interlacing bundles of collagen fibres, and is covered externally by the visceral layer of the tunica vaginalis, except at the epididymal head and tail and the posterior aspect of the testis, where vessels and nerves enter. It covers the tunica vasculosa and, at the posterior border of the testis, projects into the testicular interior as a thick, incomplete, fibrous septum, the mediastinum testis, which extends from the upper to the lower end of the testis (**Fig. 97.2**). Testicular vessels run within the mediastinum testis.

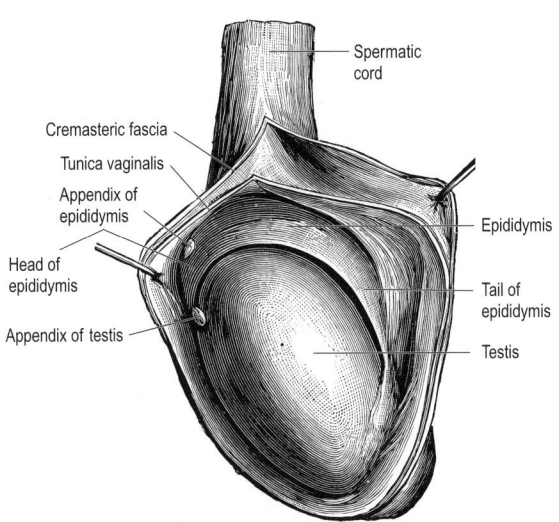

Fig. 97.1 The left testis, exposed by incising and laying open the cremasteric fascia and parietal layer of the tunica vaginalis on the lateral aspect of the testis.

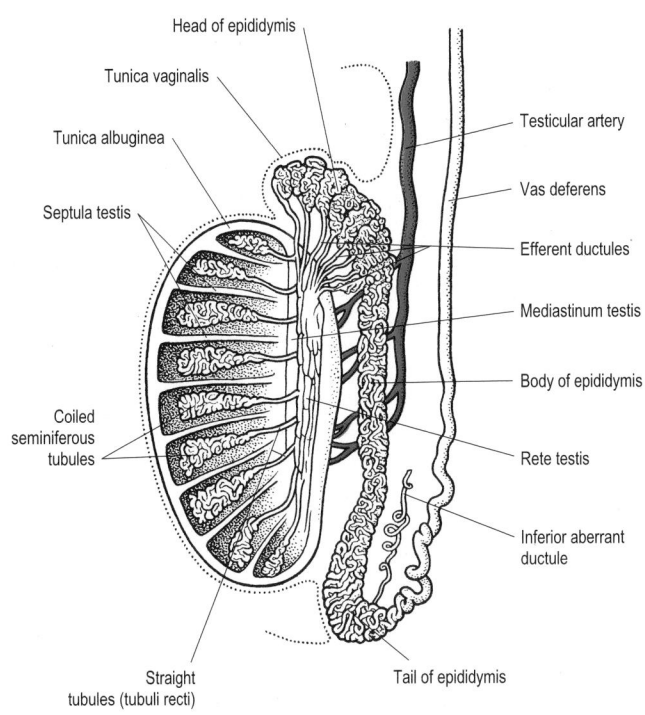

Fig. 97.2 Vertical section through the testis and epididymis, showing the arrangement of the ducts of the testis and the mode of formation of the vas deferens.

TUNICA VASCULOSA

The tunica vasculosa contains a plexus of blood vessels and delicate loose connective tissue, and extends over the internal aspect of the tunica albuginea, covering the septa and therefore all the testicular lobules.

UNDESCENDED TESTIS (See also p. 1306.)

In the early fetal period the testes are located posteriorly in the abdominal cavity. Their descent to the scrotum appears to be under hormonal control (gonadotropins and androgens) (p. 1388). Testicular descent may be arrested at any point along its route into the scrotum and a clinically undescended testis may be in the abdomen, at the deep inguinal ring, in the inguinal canal, or between the superficial inguinal ring and the scrotum.

A unilateral undescended testis is present in 3% of boys at birth and 1% of boys by 3 months of age. Bilateral maldescent is seen in just over 1% of male births. Undescended testes are associated with infertility. There is evidence that surgical correction of an undescended testis at any age may not improve its spermatogenesis, but significant impairment of fertility is probably only seen in men with bilateral undescended testis. Leydig cell function is not usually affected by maldescent, so androgen production usually remains within the normal range and erectile potency function is unaffected. Patients with an undescended testis are at increased risk of testicular tumour, particularly seminoma, and require surgical intervention as early as possible to ensure its correct location. The risk is highest in abdominal testes. Surgery may not reduce the risk of tumour development, but maximizes the chance of early detection of any tumour.

An undescended testis can usually be found by ultrasonography if it is in or close to the inguinal canal. Laparoscopy is more reliable in the pelvis.

Retention in the inguinal canal is often complicated by congenital hernia, because the processus vaginalis remains patent. The testis may traverse the canal but reach an abnormal site.

OBLITERATED PART OF THE PROCESSUS VAGINALIS

The obliterated part of the processus vaginalis is often seen as a fibrous thread in the anterior part of the spermatic cord, extending from the internal end of the inguinal canal – where it is connected to the peritoneum – as far as the tunica vaginalis. Sometimes it disappears within the cord. However, its proximal part may remain patent, so that the peritoneal cavity communicates with the tunica vaginalis, or the proximal processus may persist, although it may be shut off distally from the tunica. Occasionally its cavity may persist at an intermediate level as a cyst. When patent, its cavity may admit a loop of intestine, to form an indirect inguinal hernia (p. 1111). The processus is usually obliterated by 18 months of age.

HYDROCELE, SPERMATOCELE, EPIDIDYMAL CYST

In congenital hydrocele the fluid is in the tunical sac, which communicates with the peritoneal cavity through a non-obliterated processus vaginalis. Infantile hydrocele occurs when the processus is obliterated only at or near the deep inguinal ring. It resembles vaginal hydrocele, but fluid extends up the cord into the inguinal canal. If the processus is obliterated at both the deep inguinal ring and above the epididymis, leaving a central open part, this may distend as an encysted hydrocele of the cord. A spermatocele is a cyst related to the caput epididymis: it may contain spermatozoa and it is probably a retention cyst of one of the seminiferous tubules. Removal is usually unnecessary and may result in epididymal obstruction. The same applies to a simple epididymal cyst, which may have a similar aetiology to a spermatocele but remains free of sperm.

EPIDIDYMIS (Fig. 97.2)

The epididymis lies posteriorly and slightly lateral to the testis, with the vas deferens along its medial side (**Fig. 97.2**), (Ch. 98). It has an expanded head or globus major superiorly, a body (corpus) and a tail (cauda or globus minor). Its overall length is 6–7 cm and it consists of the single convoluted ductus epididymis formed by the union of the efferent ducts of the testis, which attach to the rete testis. From the tail, the vas deferens ascends medially to the deep inguinal ring, within the spermatic cord. The epididymis is invested by tunica vaginalis, some-

what less closely applied than it is to the testis, except at its posterior margin. Laterally there is a deep groove, the sinus epididymis, between the epididymis and the testis.

TESTICULAR AND EPIDIDYMAL APPENDICES

At the upper extremities of the testis and epididymis are two small, stalked bodies, the appendix testis and appendix epididymis. They are developmental remnants of the paramesonephric ducts (Müllerian) duct and the mesonephros, respectively (**Figs 97.1, 99.1**), (p. 1385). They are liable to undergo torsion.

TESTICULAR TORSION

The testis and epididymis are usually fixed to their surrounding tissues. In some patients this fixation may be insufficient, a condition which allows the structures to twist within the tunica vaginalis. This is termed testicular torsion and normally results in severe scrotal pain. This is a surgical emergency. Histopathological changes leading to gangrene occur in the testis if the twist is not reversed within 4–6 hours. The injury results from venous and then arterial occlusion. Fertility may be affected by an episode of torsion. Other structures may also twist within the scrotum, e.g. the testicular appendix (otherwise termed the hydatid of Morgagni) and the appendix epididymis. Torsion of these structures may result in scrotal pain, which is usually far more localized than the pain of testicular torsion.

VASCULAR SUPPLY AND LYMPHATIC DRAINAGE

TESTICULAR ARTERIES

The testicular arteries are two long, slender vessels, which arise anteriorly from the aorta a little inferior to the renal arteries. Each passes infero-laterally under the parietal peritoneum on psoas major. The right testicular artery lies anterior to the inferior vena cava and posterior to the horizontal part of the duodenum, right colic and ileocolic arteries, root of the mesentery and terminal ileum. The left testicular artery lies posterior to the inferior mesenteric vein, left colic artery and lower part of the descending colon. Each artery crosses anterior to the genito-femoral nerve, ureter and the lower part of the external iliac artery and passes to the deep inguinal ring to enter the spermatic cord and travel via the inguinal canal to enter the scrotum. At the posterosuperior aspect of the testis the testicular artery divides into two branches on its medial and lateral surfaces: these pass through the tunica albuginea and ramify in the tunica vasculosa. Terminal branches enter the testis over its surface. Some pass into the mediastinum testis and loop back before reaching their distribution. Capillaries lying next to seminiferous tubules penetrate the layers of interstitial tissue and are of interest as part of the 'blood–testis' barrier. They run either parallel to the tubules or across them but do not enter their walls. They are separated from germinal and supporting cells by a basement membrane and variable amounts of fibrous tissue containing interstitial cells: selective exchange phenomena involving androgens and immune substances occur here.

In the abdomen the testicular artery supplies perirenal fat, the ureter and iliac lymph nodes, and in the inguinal canal it supplies cremaster. Sometimes the right testicular artery passes posterior to the inferior vena cava. The testicular arteries represent persistent lateral splanchnic aortic branches which enter the mesonephros and cross ventral to the supracardinal vein, but dorsal to the subcardinal vein. Normally the lateral splanchnic artery – which persists as the right testicular artery – passes caudal to the suprasubcardinal anastomosis, which forms part of the inferior vena cava. When it passes cranial to the anastomosis, the right testicular artery is behind the inferior vena cava.

The testis also receives blood from the cremasteric branch of the inferior epigastric artery, and from the artery to the vas deferens. Interference with the testicular artery high in the abdomen therefore usually leaves the testis unharmed, whereas interruption in the region of the spermatic cord may interfere with all of these vessels and lead to infarction. Indeed it has been proposed that the correct way of treating varicoceles is to ligate both the testicular artery and vein high up, which also has the advantage of ligating the venae comitantes of the artery.

These small veins anastomose with the internal spermatic veins and can be responsible for recurrence of the varicocele.

TESTICULAR VEINS (Fig. 97.3)

The testicular veins emerge posteriorly from the testis, drain the epididymis and unite to form the pampiniform plexus, which is a major component of the spermatic cord, and ascends anterior to the vas deferens. In the inguinal canal the plexus is drained by three or four veins which run into the abdomen through the deep inguinal ring. Within the abdomen these veins coalesce into two veins, which ascend on each side of the testicular artery, anterior to psoas major and the ureter, and behind the peritoneum. The left veins pass behind the lower descending colon and inferior margin of the pancreas and are crossed by the left colic vessels, and the right veins pass behind the terminal ileum and horizontal part of the duodenum and are crossed by the root of the mesentery, ileocolic and right colic vessels. The veins join to form single right or left testicular veins: the right testicular vein opens into the inferior vena cava at an acute angle just inferior to the level of the renal veins, and the left testicular vein opens into the left renal vein at a right angle. The testicular veins contain valves.

The testicular veins in the scrotum and inguinal canal are frequently varicose. Varicocele formation, which is almost always on the left, is perhaps due to the orthogonal junction of the left testicular and renal veins. There is evidence that the presence of a varicocele raises testicular temperature and impairs fertility. In fact most varicoceles are treated (surgically) for pain rather than infertility. Varicoceles can also be treated by radiological embolization of the left testicular vein via a right femoral vein approach. After ligation of a varicocele, venous return is by the small veins of the vas deferens, cremaster and scrotal tissues.

LYMPHATIC DRAINAGE OF THE TESTIS

Testicular vessels start in a superficial plexus under the tunica vaginalis, and a deep plexus in the substance of the testis and epididymis. Four to eight collecting trunks ascend in the spermatic cord and accompany the testicular vessels on psoas major, ending in the lateral aortic and pre-aortic nodes.

INNERVATION

Testicular nerves accompany the testicular vessels and are derived from the tenth and eleventh thoracic spinal segments via the renal and aortic autonomic plexuses. Catecholaminergic nerve fibres form plexuses around smaller blood vessels and among the interstitial cells in the testis and epididymis.

MICROSTRUCTURE

TESTIS (Figs 97.4, 97.5)

The surface of the testis is covered closely by the visceral tunica vaginalis, a layer of flat mesothelial cells similar to and continuous with the peritoneal lining. It is separated from the parietal tunica vaginalis, the outer layer of the double fold of peritoneum, which accompanies the descending testis (p. 1388), by a potential space containing serous fluid, which acts as a lubricant and allows movement of the testis within the scrotum. The testicular capsule proper, the tunica albuginea, is tough and collagenous and thickened posteriorly as the mediastinum testis. Beneath the tunica albuginea is a thin layer of connective tissue containing the superficial blood vessels. Blood vessels, lymphatics and the genital ducts enter or leave the body of the testis at the mediastinum.

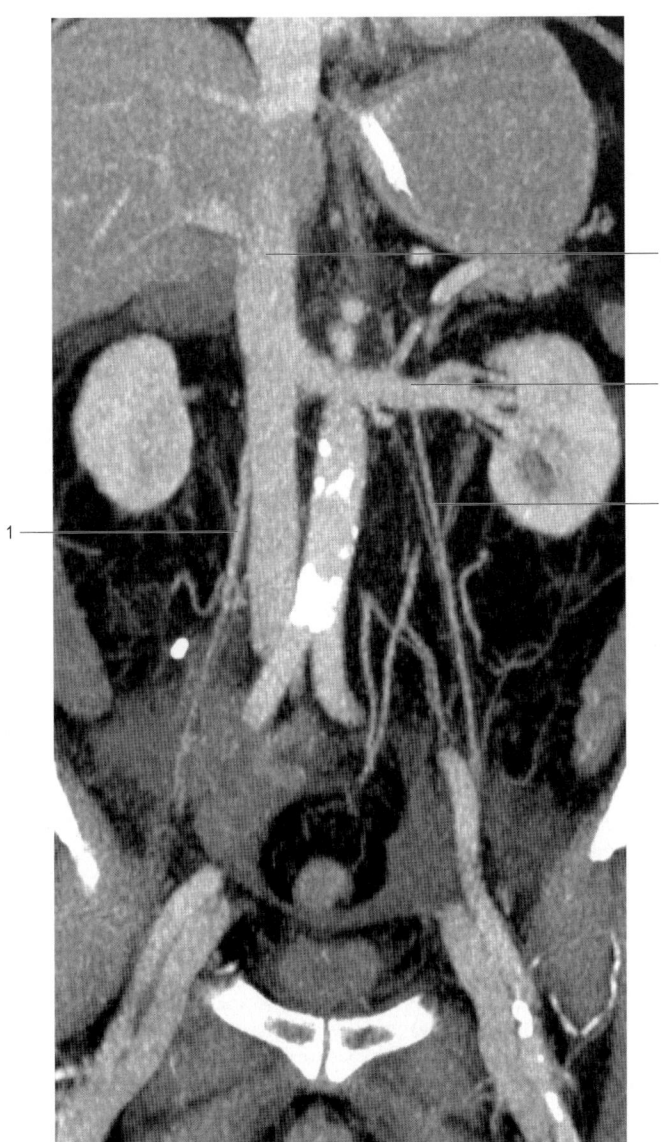

1. Right testicular vein. 2. Inferior vena cava. 3. Left renal vein. 4. Left testicular vein.

Fig. 97.3 Multislice CT of the inferior vena cava showing the left testicular vein draining to the left renal vein and the right testicular vein draining directly to the inferior vena cava.

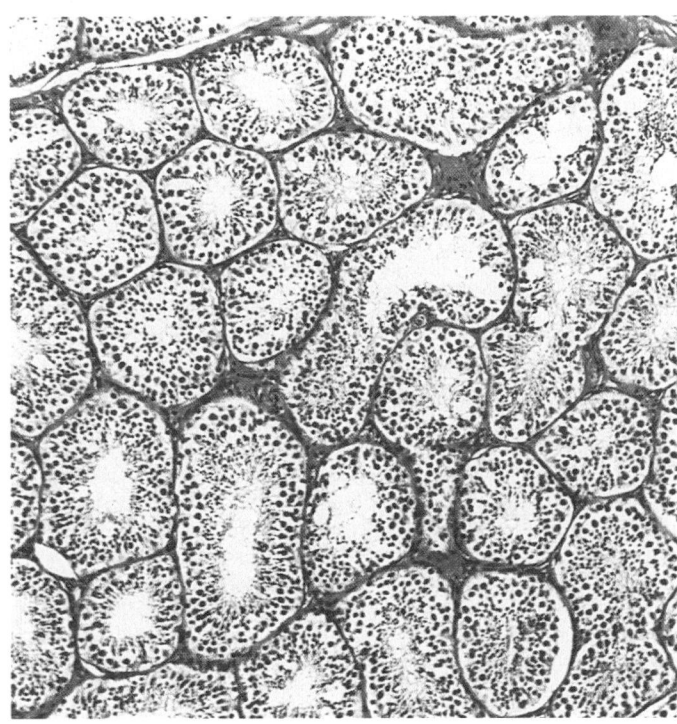

Fig. 97.4 Seminiferous tubules (cut in various planes of section), and the interstitial tissue of the testis. The seminiferous tubules are highly convoluted and lined by a stratified epithelium which consists of cells in various stages of spermatogenesis and spermiogenesis (collectively referred to as the spermatogenic series). Non-spermatogenic cells are the Sertoli cells. (By permission from Young B, Heath JW 2000 Wheater's Functional Histology. Edinburgh: Churchill Livingstone.)

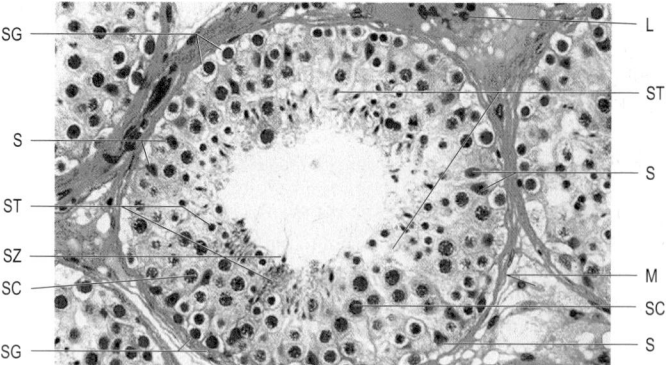

SG — L
S — ST
ST — S
SZ —
SC — M
SG — SC
— S

Fig. 97.5 Human seminiferous tubule showing the differentiation sequence of spermatozoa from basally situated spermatogonia (SG). Large primary spermatocytes (SC) have characteristic threadlike chromatin in various stages of prophase of the first meiotic division. Smaller haploid spermatids (ST) have round nuclei initially, but mature to possess the dense, elongated nuclei and flagellae of spermatozoa (SZ). Sertoli cells (S) are identified from their oval or pear-shaped nuclei orientated perpendicular to the basal lamina, and prominent nucleoli. The tubule is surrounded by peritubular myoid cells (M) and clusters of large endocrine Leydig cells (L) are seen in the interstitial connective tissue. (By permission from Dr JB Kerr, Monash University, from Kerr JB 1999 Atlas of Functional Histology. London: Mosby.)

Septa from the mediastinum extend internally to partition the testis into c.250 lobules (**Fig. 97.2**). These differ in size, and are largest and longest in the centre. Each lobule contains one to four convoluted seminiferous tubules, which are much-coiled loops whose free ends both open into channels (the rete testis) within the mediastinum. The loose connective tissue between seminiferous tubules contains several layers of contractile peritubular myoid cells, and clusters of steroid-producing interstitial (Leydig) cells (**Fig. 97.5**).

There are 400–600 seminiferous tubules in each testis and the length of each is 70–80 cm. Their diameter varies from 0.12–0.3 mm. They are pale in early life, but in old age they contain much fat and are deep yellow. Each tubule is surrounded by a basal lamina, on which rests a complex, stratified seminiferous epithelium containing spermatogenic cells and supportive Sertoli cells. When active, the spermatogenic cells include basally situated spermatogonia and their progeny in the adluminal compartment, spermatocytes, spermatids and mature spermatozoa (**Fig. 97.5**). Among the spermatids may be residual bodies, which are spherical structures derived from surplus spermatid cytoplasm shed during maturation and phagocytosed by Sertoli cells. For a review of the ultrastructural features of the human testis, with emphasis on spermatogenesis and the cytology of the Leydig cells, see Kerr (1991).

Spermatogonia

Spermatogonia, the stem cells for all spermatozoa, are descended from primordial germ cells which migrate into the genital cords of the developing testis (p. 1386). In the fully differentiated testis they are located along the basal laminae of the seminiferous tubules. Several types of spermatogonia are recognized on the basis of cell and nuclear dimensions, distribution of nuclear chromatin (dark, condensed or pale, euchromatic) and histochemical and ultrastructural data. The three basic groups of spermatogonia are dark type A (Ad), pale type A (Ap), and type B. Ad cells divide mitotically to maintain the population of spermatogonia which, before puberty, is small but increases under androgenic stimulation. Some divisions give rise to Ap cells which also divide mitotically but remain linked in clusters by fine cytoplasmic bridges. These are the precursors of type B cells, which are committed to the spermatogenic sequence. At about the time type B cells enter a final round of DNA synthesis, without undergoing cytokinesis, they leave the basal compartment and cross the blood–testis barrier to enter meiotic prophase as primary spermatocytes. These coordinated processes are under the control of Sertoli cells.

Primary and secondary spermatocytes

Primary spermatocytes have a diploid chromosome number but duplicated sister chromatids (DNA content is thus 4N, where N is the DNA content of haploid spermatozoa). They are all at some stage of a long meiotic prophase (p. 24) of c.3 weeks. Primary spermatocytes are characteristically large cells (**Fig. 97.5**) with large round nuclei in which the nuclear chromatin is condensed into dark, threadlike, coiled chromatids at different stages in the process of crossing over and genetic exchange between chromatids of maternal and paternal homologues. These cells give rise to secondary spermatocytes with a haploid chromosome complement (but 2N DNA content), the reduction division is designated as meiosis I. Few secondary spermatocytes are seen in tissue sections because they rapidly undergo the second meiotic (equatorial) division, where sister chromatids separate (DNA content is now N), to form haploid spermatids. Theoretically each primary spermatocyte produces four spermatids, but some degenerate during maturation so that the yield is lower.

Spermatids

Spermatids do not divide again but gradually mature into spermatozoa by a series of nuclear and cytoplasmic changes known as spermiogenesis. All of these maturational changes take place while the spermatids remain closely associated with Sertoli cells and linked by cytoplasmic bridges with each other. The first phase of spermiogenesis is the Golgi phase, during which hydrolytic enzymes accumulate in Golgi vesicles, which coalesce into a single large acrosomal vesicle, close to the nucleus. The pair of centrioles migrates to the opposite posterior pole. The distal centriole begins to generate the axoneme, a circular arrangement of nine microtubule doublets surrounding a central pair. In the cap phase, which follows, the acrosomal vesicle flattens and envelops the anterior half of the nucleus to form an acrosomal cap. This comes to occupy the presumptive anterior pole of the spermatozoon, furthest from the tubule lumen.

During the acrosome phase, nuclear chromatin condenses and the nucleus elongates to a spearhead shape. The anterior cytoplasmic volume reduces considerably, bringing the wall of the acrosomal vesicle into contact with the plasma membrane. A perinuclear sheath of microtubules develops from the posterior edge of the acrosome to form the manchette, extending towards the posterior pole. The axonemal complex continues to extend into the developing tail region, which protrudes into the tubule lumen. Prominent mitochondria migrate through a neck region, which forms at the posterior pole of the nucleus and contains the centrioles, and along the axoneme into the developing middle piece. Here they assemble into a helical sheath of mitochondria which surrounds a ring of nine coarse fibres forming around the axonemal complex along its length in the developing tail.

In the final phase of maturation, excess cytoplasm is detached as a residual body which is phagocytosed and degraded by Sertoli cells. During the formation of residual bodies, spermatids lose their cytoplasmic bridges and separate from each other before being released into their tubule.

Spermatozoa (Fig. 97.6)

As it is released from the wall of the seminiferous tubule into the lumen, the spermatozoon is non-motile but structurally mature (**Fig. 97.6**). Its expanded head contains little cytoplasm and is connected by a short constricted neck to the tail. The tail is a complex flagellum, which greatly exceeds the head region in volume, and is divided into middle, principal and end pieces. The head has a maximum length of c.4 μm and a maximum diameter of 3 μm, and contains the elongated, flattened nucleus with condensed, deeply staining chromatin and the acrosomal cap anteriorly. The latter contains acid phosphatase, hyaluronidase, neuraminidase and proteases necessary for fertilization (p. 185). The neck is c.0.3 μm long. In its centre is a well-formed centriole, corresponding to the proximal centriole of the spermatid from which it differentiated. The axonemal complex is derived from the distal centriole. A small amount of cytoplasm exists in the neck, covered by a plasma membrane continuous with that of the head and tail.

The middle piece of the tail is a long cylinder, c.1 μm in diameter and 7 μm long. It consists of an axial bundle of microtubules, the axoneme, outside which is a cylinder of nine dense outer fibres, surrounded by a helical mitochondrial sheath. At the caudal end of the middle piece is an electron-dense body, the anulus. The principal piece of the tail becomes the motile part of the cell. It is c.40 μm long and 0.5 μm in diameter and forms the majority of the spermatozoon. The axoneme and the surrounding dense fibres are continuous from the neck region through the whole length of the tail except for its terminal 5–7 μm, in which the axoneme alone persists. In this terminal end piece the tail

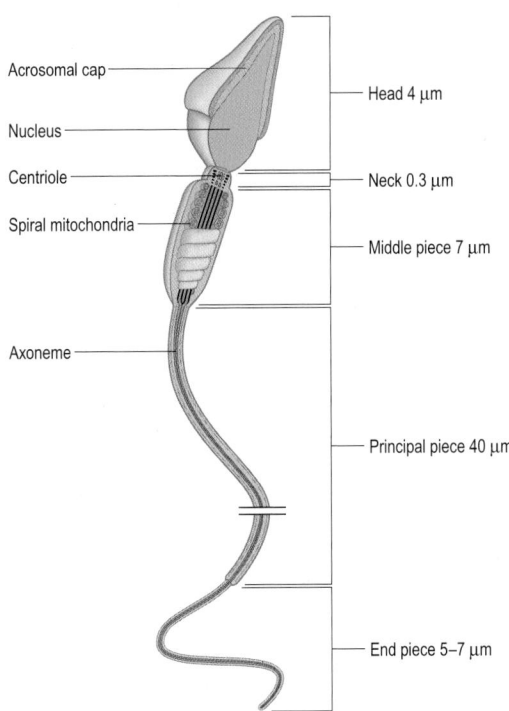

Acrosomal cap

Nucleus

Centriole

Spiral mitochondria

Axoneme

Head 4 μm

Neck 0.3 μm

Middle piece 7 μm

Principal piece 40 μm

End piece 5–7 μm

Fig. 97.6 The main ultrastructural features of a mature spermatozoon.

thus has the typical structure of a flagellum, with a simple nine plus two arrangement of microtubules.

Sertoli cells

Sertoli cells are the supporting, non-spermatogenic cells of the seminiferous tubules and form a major cellular component of the tubule before puberty, and in the elderly. They are variable in overall cell shape, but they all contact the basal lamina and their cytoplasm extends to the tubule lumen. Here, their apical plasma membranes form complex recesses which envelop spermatids and spermatozoa until the latter are mature enough for release. Long cytoplasmic processes also extend between the spermatogonia in the basal compartment and spermatocytes in the adluminal compartment of the tubule. Adjacent Sertoli cell processes are joined at this level by tight junctions, which create a diffusion barrier between the extratubular and intratubular compartments. This is the blood–testis barrier which, if breached by traumatic or inflammatory events, can allow immune responses to develop against sperm antigens, resulting in subfertility. For a general review of the blood–testis barrier see Johnson and Gomes (1977).

The Sertoli cell nucleus is euchromatic and irregular or pear-shaped, and contains one or two prominent nucleoli. It is usually aligned perpendicular to the basal lamina. The cytoplasm contains many lysosomes, consistent with its phagocytic phenotype. Sertoli cells provide trophic support for the surrounding germ cells, secrete androgen-binding protein and play an important role in controlling spermatocyte and spermatid differentiation and maturation. The proteinaceous fluid they secrete into the tubule lumen provides nutrients and facilitates the transport of spermatozoa into the excurrent duct system. Sertoli cells change considerably during the spermatogenic cycle and respond to the hypophyseal hormones, luteinizing hormone (LH) and follicle-stimulating hormone (FSH).

Spermatogenic cycle

At any locus in a seminiferous tubule, generation of germ cells occurs in a cycle, with a periodicity of c.16 days. Stages in the cycle are characterized by the presence of different combinations of cells within the spermatogenic sequence. The generation of a mature spermatozoon from a spermatogonium takes four such cycles, or c.64 days. In cross-section, the seminiferous tubule shows more than one phase of the cycle around its circumference, as waves of progression through a spermatogenic cycle occur in spirals down the length of the tubule.

Testicular interstitial tissue

The tissues between the seminiferous tubules include various connective tissue components, peritubular myoid cells, vessels and nerves. The myoid cells are contractile and their rhythmic activity propels non-motile spermatozoa through the tubule towards the rete testis and excurrent ductal system. Clusters of steroid-secreting interstitial Leydig cells lie between the tubules. Leydig cells are large polyhedral cells with an eccentric nucleus containing one to three nucleoli. Their pale staining cytoplasm contains a considerable amount of smooth endoplasmic reticulum, lipid droplets and unique needle-shaped crystalloid inclusions up to 20 μm long (crystals of Reinke), of unknown function. Leydig cells synthesize and secrete androgens, stimulated by LH and prolactin, which induces expression of the LH receptor. The activity of Leydig cells varies with age: they are active in fetal life in the development of the genital tract but decline in function postpartum until the onset of puberty.

EFFERENT DUCTULES AND EPIDIDYMIS (Fig. 97.7)

The process of spermatogenesis described above occurs in the highly coiled parts of the seminiferous tubules. As the latter reach the apical part of the lobule towards the mediastinum they become much less convoluted. They form the short tubuli recti, lined by cuboidal epithelium lacking spermatogenic cells. Tubuli recti enter the fibrous tissue of the mediastinum testis as a close network of anastomosing tubes, the rete testis, lined by a flat epithelium. At the upper pole of the mediastinum, 12–20 efferent ductules (ductuli efferentes) perforate the tunica albuginea and leave the testis for the epididymis. The efferent ductules are lined by a ciliated columnar epithelium which also contains shorter, actively endocytic, non-ciliated cells. External to the epithelium, the ductules are surrounded by a thin circular coat of smooth muscle.

Initially the ductules are straight. They become enlarged and very convoluted and form the conical lobules of the epididymis, which make up its head (caput). Each lobular duct, 15–20 cm in length, opens into the single duct of the epididymis, whose coils form the epididymal body (corpus) and tail (cauda). When the coils are unravelled, the tube measures more than 6 metres, increasing in thickness as it approaches the epididymal tail, where it becomes the vas deferens. The coils are held together by bands of fibrous connective tissue. In the epididymal duct the muscle is thicker and the epithelium is composed of columnar pseudostratified cells (**Fig. 97.7**). The muscle undergoes peristaltic contractions to propel spermatozoa towards the tail region, where they are stored.

The epithelium contains two main cell types, principal and basal cells, and the less common apical cells and clear cells. Principal cells are tall columnar cells with basally located, elongated, oval nuclei. They bear long (15 μm) regular apical microvilli termed stereocilia, because

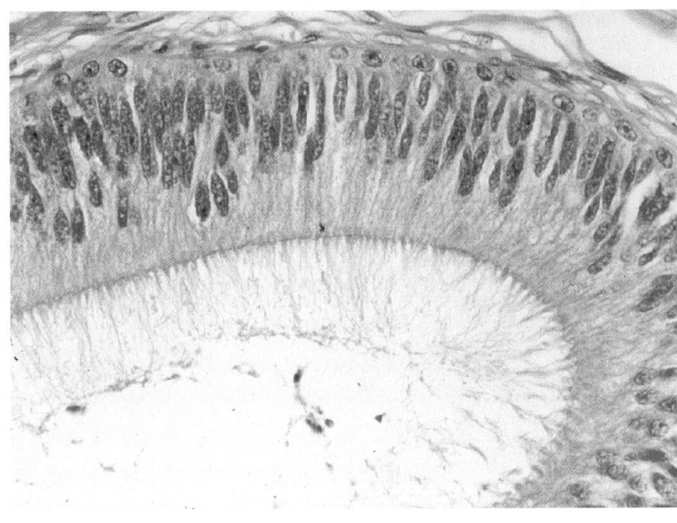

Fig. 97.7 The lining of the epididymis. The pseudostratified epithelium consists of two major cell types, principal cells with long apical stereocilia, and basal cells. (By permission from Kierszenbaum AL 2002 Histology and Cell Biology. St Louis: Mosby.)

they were once thought to be immotile cilia. They function to resorb fluid from the testicular secretions and c.90% of the total is absorbed in the epididymis. These cells also secrete glycoproteins essential for the maturation of spermatozoa and endocytose various other components of the seminal fluid. Basal cells lie between the bases of the principal cells and are thought to be the precursors of principal cells. Apical cells have numerous mitochondria and are most abundant in the head of the epididymis. Clear cells are columnar cells, most numerous in the tail region, with few microvilli but numerous endocytic vesicles and lipid droplets. Their functions are unknown.

MATURATION OF SPERMATOZOA

Functional maturation is a complex process. Spermatozoa show little independent motility while still in the male genital tract, though when removed from the epididymis they may display circular or even forward directional movements if taken from the cauda epididymis near the beginning of the vas deferens. Apart from this immature motility, spermatozoa are largely transported through the genital tract first by ciliary action and then by peristaltic contractions of the duct walls. Human spermatozoa do not undergo any demonstrable structural changes during their passage through the epididymis, but there is evidence of biochemical and functional modifications. Evidence from restorative surgery after vasectomy indicates that at least part of the human epididymis is essential for acquisition of mature motile activity.

Motility of spermatozoa

It is now generally accepted that the tail executes undulatory movements in one plane. It has also been suggested that a helical component is superimposed upon these movements, and that there are perhaps two separable mechanisms to account for sperm motility, one involving flat waves travelling along the tail, the other associated with torsional activity. The latter type of movement has been linked with the unequal size and distribution of the dense fibres, and the asymmetry of the spermatozoan head. It has also been suggested that the central pair of fine fibrils act as axial stiffeners.

As soon as they are ejaculated the spermatozoa display their full pattern of motility. The factors which trigger these movements are not yet clear: the other constituents of semen, which are derived from the epididymis, testis, seminal vesicle and prostate, are generally considered to exert an activating influence. Spermatozoa have been recovered in a motile state in human cervical mucus several days after insemination and will survive in this condition for as long as 7 days when implanted into such secretions *in vitro*. In view of the speed with which spermatozoa reach the infundibulum of the uterine tube, and the brevity of their fertilizing power, these survival periods may be of little significance. Spermatozoa have been shown to reach their tubal destination in a manner of minutes after ejaculation in some mammals; experiments on recently excised human uteri and tubes indicate a time of c.70 minutes. The conclusion must be that factors other than their own motility (1.5–3.0 mm/min) are responsible for the transport of spermatozoa from the site of deposition in the vaginal fornix to the ovarian end of the uterine tube: there is considerable evidence that contraction of the uterine and tubal musculature is responsible.

Capacitation

After ejaculation into the female genital tract, spermatozoa undergo the final step in their maturation, a process known as capacitation. This normally requires exposure to the secretions of the uterine tube: a spermatozoon is unable to penetrate the corona radiata to fertilize an ovum until it has been within the female genital tract for a period of time, usually a few hours.

AGE CHANGES IN THE TESTIS

Functionally, the fetal testis is predominantly an endocrine gland which produces testosterone and a specifically fetal gonadal hormone, the anti-Müllerian hormone. These two hormones play crucial roles in the induction and regulation of male sexual differentiation. The seminiferous tubules do not become canalized until approximately the seventh month of gestation, although this may occur later.

Postnatally the testis gradually changes its role, but retains the ability to manufacture testosterone and other regulatory materials, e.g. the peptide hormone oxytocin, which act in either an endocrine or a paracrine fashion.

At puberty, the testis becomes primarily a source of spermatozoa. The fetal Leydig cells, which are responsible for the androgen-induced differentiation of the male genitalia, degenerate after birth, and are replaced, during puberty, by an adult population of androgen-producing cells which persist throughout adult life. The testes grow slowly until the age of c.10 or 11 years, at which time there is a marked acceleration of growth rate, and spermatogenesis begins.

There is no definite age for the onset of the progressive testicular involution associated with advancing age. Testicular size, sperm quality and quantity, and the numbers of Sertoli cells and Leydig cells, have all been reported to decrease in the elderly. Leydig cell activity is driven by LH: the decrease in Leydig cell function in the elderly, as part of what has been described as the normal ageing process, may be affected by changes in the secretion of LH, which is controlled by the hypothalamus. The volume occupied by the seminiferous tubules decreases, whereas that occupied by interstitial tissue remains approximately constant. The most frequently observed histological change in the ageing testis is variation in spermatogenesis in different seminiferous tubules, so that it is complete, though reduced, in some, but absent in others, when sclerosis may occur. In tubules where spermatogenesis is complete, morphological abnormalities may be observed in the germ cells, including multinucleation. Germ cell loss generally begins with the spermatids, but progressively affects the earlier germ cell types, i.e. the spermatocytes and spermatogonia. Sertoli cells are also affected by ageing, and show a range of morphological changes including dedifferentiation, mitochondrial metaplasia and multinucleation. In the Leydig cells there is a decrease in the quantity of smooth endoplasmic reticulum and mitochondria, while lipid droplets, crystalline inclusions and residual bodies increase and some cells become multinucleate. Tubules in which the entire epithelium has been lost have been observed in testes where other tubules appeared normal. The development of tubular involution with advancing age is similar to that observed after experimental ischaemia, suggesting that vascular lesions may be involved in age-related testicular atrophy. However, there is no abrupt change in testicular function equivalent to the female climacteric.

REFERENCES

Kerr JB 1991 Ultrastructure of the seminiferous epithelium and intertubular tissue of the human testis. J Electron Microsc Tech 19: 215–40.
Reviews the ultrastructural features of the human testis, with emphasis on spermatogenesis and cytology.

Johnson AD, Gomes WR (eds) 1977 The Testis, Vol 4. Advances in Physiology, Biochemistry and Function. New York: Academic Press.
A general review of the blood–testis barrier.

Vas deferens and ejaculatory ducts

VAS DEFERENS (Fig. 98.1)

The vas deferens is a muscular tube, 45 cm long, which conveys sperm to the ejaculatory ducts, and is the distal continuation of the epididymis, starting at the epididymal tail (**Fig. 97.2**). At first it is very tortuous, but it becomes straighter, and ascends along the posterior aspect of the testis, medial to the epididymis. From the superior pole of the testis it ascends in the posterior part of the spermatic cord, and traverses the inguinal canal. At the internal (deep) inguinal ring the vas deferens leaves the cord, curves round the lateral side of the inferior epigastric artery and ascends for c.2.5 cm anterior to the external iliac artery. It then turns back and inclines slightly down and obliquely across the external iliac vessels to enter the lesser pelvis, where, situated retroperitoneally, it continues posteriorly, medial to the obliterated umbilical artery, the obturator nerve and vessels, and the vesical vessels (**Fig. 93.1**). It crosses the ureter (**Fig. 98.1**) and bends acutely to pass anteromedially between the posterior surface of the bladder and the upper pole of the seminal vesicle. It then descends in contact with the seminal vesicle, gradually approaching the opposite duct. Here it lies between the base of the bladder and the rectum, from which it is separated by Denonvillier's fascia. It finally descends to the base of the prostate, where it joins the duct of the seminal vesicle at an acute angle to form the ejaculatory duct (**Fig. 101.1**). It feels cord-like when grasped because of its thick wall and small lumen. Posterior to the bladder the lumen becomes dilated and tortuous and is termed the ampulla; beyond this, where it joins the duct of the seminal vesicle, it is again greatly diminished in calibre (**Fig. 98.1**).

The vasa deferentia may be congenitally absent, most commonly in association with the presence of one or two abnormal gene loci at the cystic fibrosis site. This condition results in azoospermia.

ABERRANT DUCTULES

A narrow, blind, caudal aberrant ductule often occurs, usually connected with the caudal part of the epididymal duct or with the start of the vas deferens. Uncoiled, it varies in length from 5 to 35 cm; it may be dilated near its end, but is otherwise uniform in calibre. In structure it is similar to the vas deferens. Occasionally it is not connected with the epididymis. A rostral aberrant ductule may occur in the epididymal head, connected with the rete testis. Aberrant ductules are derived from mesonephric tubules (p. 1375).

PARADIDYMIS

The paradidymis is a small collection of convoluted tubules, found anteriorly in the spermatic cord above the epididymal head. The tubules are lined by ciliated columnar epithelium and probably represent the remains of the mesonephros (p. 1375).

EJACULATORY DUCTS

The ejaculatory ducts are formed on each side by the union of the duct of the seminal vesicle with the ampulla of the vas (**Figs 93.1, 101.1**). Each is almost 2 cm in length, starts from the base of the prostate, runs anteroinferiorly between its median and right or left lobes, and skirts the prostatic utricle to end on the verumontanum at two slit-like orifices on, or just within, the utricular opening. The ducts diminish and converge towards their ends.

VASCULAR SUPPLY, LYMPHATIC DRAINAGE AND INNERVATION

Each vas deferens has its own artery, usually derived from the superior vesical artery, which anastomoses with the testicular artery to supply the epididymis and testis. Veins drain from the vas deferens and seminal vesicles to the pelvic venous plexus. Lymphatic vessels drain to the external and internal iliac nodes.

The vasa deferentia are innervated by a rich autonomic plexus composed mainly of sympathetic nerve fibres derived from the pelvic plexus.

MICROSTRUCTURE

The wall of the vas deferens has loose connective tissue externally, a thick middle muscular layer and an internal mucosal layer. The muscular layer is composed of smooth muscle fibres arranged in external longitudinal and internal circular sheets. An additional internal longitudinal layer is present at the origin of the duct where it leaves the tail of the epididymis, however all muscle layers intermingle. The mucosa is folded longitudinally and its epithelium is columnar and non-ciliated through most of the duct. Towards its distal end a pseudostratified columnar epithelium appears, the tallest cells of which bear non-motile stereocilia (elongated microvilli), similar to those of the epididymis. The connective tissue of the lamina propria contains elastic fibres.

The walls of the ejaculatory ducts are thin. They contain an outer fibrous layer, which is much reduced beyond their entrance into the prostate, a thin layer of smooth muscle fibres with an outer circular and inner longitudinal orientation, and a mucosa lined by columnar epithelium. The ducts dilate during ejaculation.

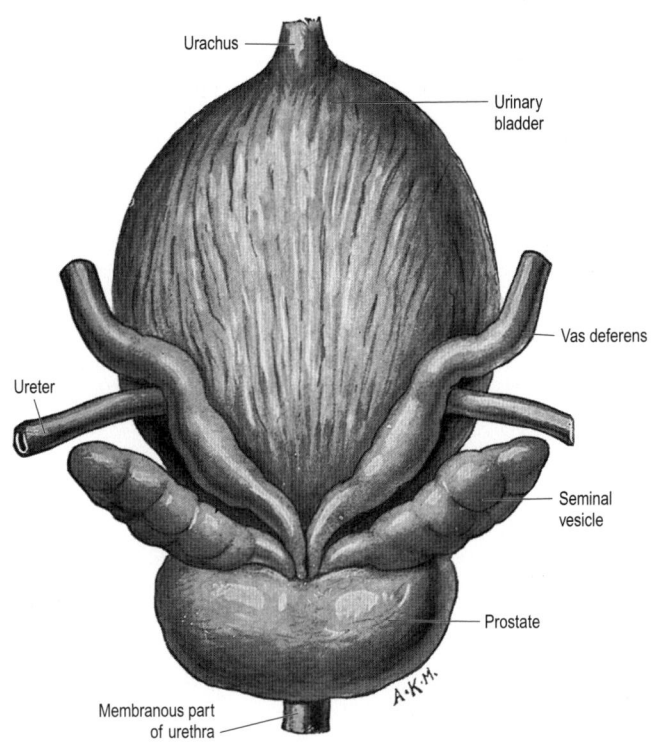

Fig. 98.1 Posterosuperior aspect of the male internal urogenital organs.

Labels: Urachus · Urinary bladder · Vas deferens · Ureter · Seminal vesicle · Prostate · Membranous part of urethra · A·K·M·

Spermatic cord and scrotum

SPERMATIC CORD

As the testis traverses the abdominal wall into the scrotum during early life, it carries its vessels, nerves and vas deferens with it. These meet at the deep inguinal ring to form the spermatic cord, which suspends the testis in the scrotum and extends from the deep inguinal ring to the posterior aspect of the testis. The left cord is a little longer than the right. Between the superficial ring and testis the cord is anterior to the rounded tendon of adductor longus. It is crossed anteriorly by the superficial and posteriorly by the deep external pudendal arteries respectively. The cord traverses the inguinal canal with its walls as relations: the ilioinguinal nerve is inferior. In the canal the cord acquires coverings from the layers of the abdominal wall, which extend into the scrotal wall as the internal spermatic, cremasteric and external spermatic fasciae.

The internal spermatic fascia is a thin, loose layer around the spermatic cord and it is derived from the transversalis fascia. The cremasteric fascia contains fasciculi of skeletal muscle united by loose connective tissue to form the cremaster, which is continuous with internal oblique. The external spermatic fascia, a thin fibrous stratum continuous above with the aponeurosis of external oblique, descends from the crura of the superficial ring.

The spermatic cord contains the vas deferens; testicular artery and veins, cremasteric artery (a branch of the inferior epigastric artery) and artery to the vas deferens (from the superior vesical artery); genital branch of the genitofemoral nerve, cremasteric nerve and sympathetic components of the testicular plexus, which are joined by filaments from the pelvic plexus accompanying the artery to the vas deferens; 4–8 lymph vessels draining the testis. All of these structures are conjoined by loose connective tissue.

SCROTUM (Fig. 99.1)

The scrotum is a cutaneous fibromuscular sac containing the testes and lower parts of the spermatic cords. It hangs below the pubic symphysis between the anteromedial aspects of the thighs. It is divided into right and left halves by a cutaneous raphe, which continues ventrally to the inferior penile surface and dorsally along the midline of the perineum to the anus. The raphe indicates the bilateral origin of the scrotum from the genital swellings. The left side of the scrotum is usually lower because the left spermatic cord is longer.

The external appearance varies. When warm, and in the elderly and debilitated, the scrotum is smooth, elongated and flaccid. When cold, and in the young and robust, it is short, corrugated and closely applied to the testes because of the contraction of the dartos muscle. It consists of skin, dartos muscle and external spermatic, cremasteric and internal spermatic fasciae. The internal spermatic fascia is loosely attached to the parietal layer of the tunica vaginalis (**Fig. 99.1**).

The scrotal skin is thin, pigmented and often rugose. It bears thinly scattered, crisp hairs, whose roots are visible through the skin. It has sebaceous glands, whose secretion has a characteristic odour, and also numerous sweat glands, pigment cells and nerve endings. These nerve endings respond to mechanical stimulation of the hairs and skin and to variations in temperature. There is no subcutaneous adipose tissue.

The dartos muscle is a thin layer of smooth muscle, which is continuous beyond the scrotum with the superficial inguinal and perineal fasciae. It extends into the scrotal septum, which connects the raphe to the inferior surface of the penile radix and divides the scrotum into two cavities. The septum contains all the layers of scrotal wall except skin. The dartos muscle is closely united to the skin, but is connected to subjacent parts by delicate loose connective tissue, giving it marked

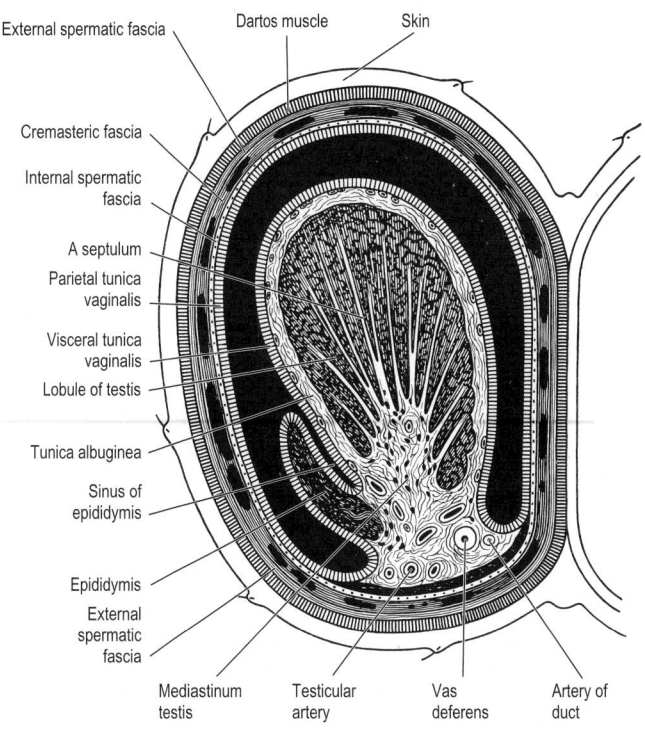

Fig. 99.1 Transverse section through the left half of the scrotum and the left testis. The tunica vaginalis is represented as artificially distended (as would occur in a hydrocoele) to show its visceral and parietal layers.

independence. A fibromuscular 'scrotal ligament' extends from the dartos sheet to the inferior testicular pole, and may play a role in thermoregulation of the testis.

VASCULAR SUPPLY AND LYMPHATIC DRAINAGE OF THE SCROTUM

Arteries supplying the scrotum (Figs 108.4, 100.3) – The arteries supplying the scrotum include the external pudendal branches of the femoral artery, the scrotal branches of the internal pudendal artery, and a cremasteric branch from the inferior epigastric artery. Dense subcutaneous plexuses of scrotal vessels carry a substantial blood flow, which facilitates heat loss. Arteriovenous anastomoses of a simple but large-calibre type are also prominent.

Veins (Fig. 93.3) – The veins follow the corresponding arteries.

Lymphatic drainage – The skin of the scrotum is drained by vessels, which accompany the external pudendal blood vessels to the superficial inguinal nodes.

INNERVATION

The scrotum is innervated by the ilioinguinal nerve, the genital branch of the genitofemoral nerve, the two posterior scrotal branches of the perineal nerve, and the perineal branch of the posterior femoral cutaneous nerve. The anterior third of the scrotum is supplied mainly from the first lumbar spinal segment (by way of the ilioinguinal and genitofemoral nerves), while the posterior two-thirds are innervated principally from the third sacral spinal cord segment (via the perineal and posterior femoral cutaneous nerves). The ventral axial line of the lower limb passes between these areas. A spinal anaesthetic, therefore, must be injected much higher to anaesthetize the anterior region.

Penis

The penis, the male copulatory organ, consists of an attached root (radix) in the perineum and a free, normally pendulous, body (corpus), which is completely enveloped in skin.

SKIN

The penile skin is remarkably thin, dark and loosely connected to the tunica albuginea. At the corona of the penis it is folded to form the prepuce or foreskin, which variably overlaps the glans. The internal preputial layer is confluent at the neck with the thin skin covering and adhering firmly to the glans, and by this with the urethral mucosa at the external urethral orifice. On the urethral aspect of the glans a median fold, the frenulum, passes from the deep surface of the prepuce to the glans immediately proximal to the orifice. Cutaneous sensitivity, which is high over the surface of the glans, is accentuated near the frenulum. The prepuce and glans penis enclose a potential cleft, the preputial sac, and two shallow fossae flank the frenulum.

ROOT (Fig. 100.1)

The root of the penis consists of three masses of erectile tissue in the urogenital triangle, namely the two crura and the bulb, firmly attached to the pubic arch and perineal membrane respectively. The crura are the posterior regions of the corpora, and the bulb is the posterior end of the corpus spongiosum.

Each penile crus (**Fig. 100.1**) starts behind as a blunt, elongate but rounded process, attached firmly to the everted edge of the ischiopubic ramus and covered by ischiocavernosus. Anteriorly it converges towards its fellow and is slightly enlarged posterior to this. Near the inferior symphyseal border the two crura come together and continue as the corpora cavernosa of the body of the penis.

The bulb of the penis (**Fig. 100.1**) lies between the crura and is firmly connected to the inferior aspect of the perineal membrane, from which it receives a fibrous covering. Oval in section, the bulb narrows anteriorly into the corpus spongiosum, down and forwards at this point. Its convex superficial surface is covered by bulbospongiosus. Its flattened deep surface is pierced above its centre by the urethra, which traverses it to reach the corpus spongiosum.

BODY (Fig. 100.2)

The body of the penis contains three elongated erectile masses, capable of considerable enlargement when engorged with blood during erection. When flaccid the penis is cylindrical, but when erect it is triangular with rounded angles. The surface which is posterosuperior during erection, is termed the dorsum of the penis and the opposite aspect is the ventral surface. The erectile masses are the right and left corpora cavernosa, and the median corpus spongiosum, which are continuations of the crura and bulb of the penis respectively.

CORPORA CAVERNOSA

The corpora cavernosa of the penis form most of the body. In close apposition throughout, they share a common fibrous envelope and are separated only by a median fibrous septum. On the urethral surface their combined mass has a wide median groove, adjoining the corpus spongiosum (**Fig. 100.2**); dorsally a similar but narrower groove contains the deep dorsal vein. The corpora end distally in the hollow, proximal aspect of the glans penis in a rounded cone, on which each has a small terminal projection (**Fig. 100.1**). They are enclosed in a strong fibrous tunica albuginea, consisting of superficial and deep strata. The super-

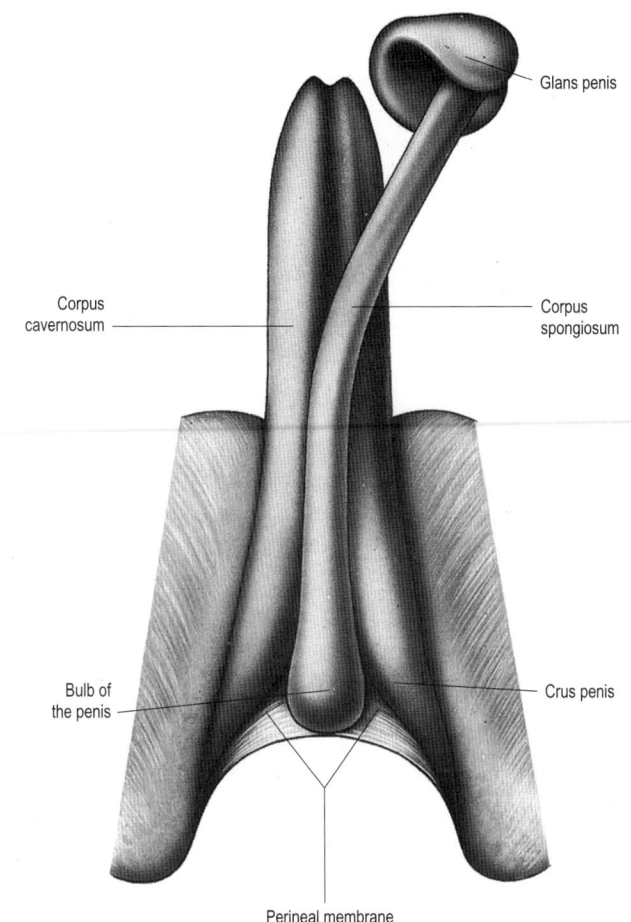

Fig. 100.1 Ventral aspect of the constituent erectile masses of the penis in erect position. The glans penis and the distal part of the corpus spongiosum are shown detached from the corpora cavernosa penis and turned to the left.

ficial fibres are longitudinal, and form a single tube round both corpora. The deep fibres are circularly orientated and surround each corpus separately, joining together as a median septum of the penis. The median septum is thick and complete proximally so that the corporal bodies can be separated proximally for 5–7 cm. Distally it consists of a pectiniform (comb-like) series of bands and is called the pectiniform septum, which is incomplete and allows cross-circulation of blood between the two corpora.

CORPUS SPONGIOSUM

The corpus spongiosum of the penis is traversed by the urethra. It adjoins the median groove on the urethral surface of the conjoined corpora cavernosa. It is cylindrical, tapering slightly distally, and surrounded by a tunica albuginea. Near the end of the penis it expands into a somewhat conical enlargement, the glans penis (**Figs 100.1, 100.2**).

The glans penis projects dorsally over the end of the corpora cavernosa, and has a shallow concave surface to which they are attached. The corona glandis projects from its base, overhanging an obliquely

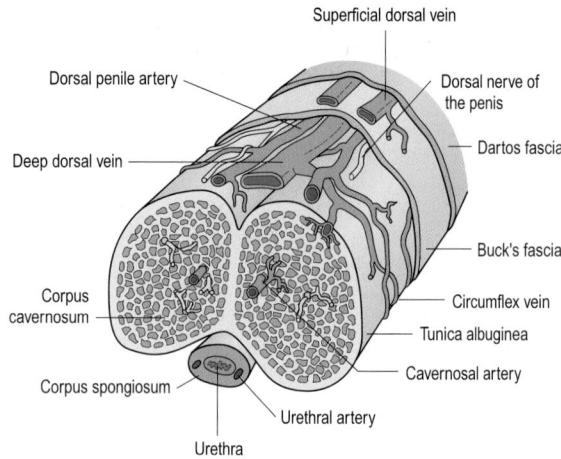

Fig. 100.2 Transverse section of penis. (By permission from Eardley I, Sethia K 1998 Erectile Dysfunction. London: Mosby.)

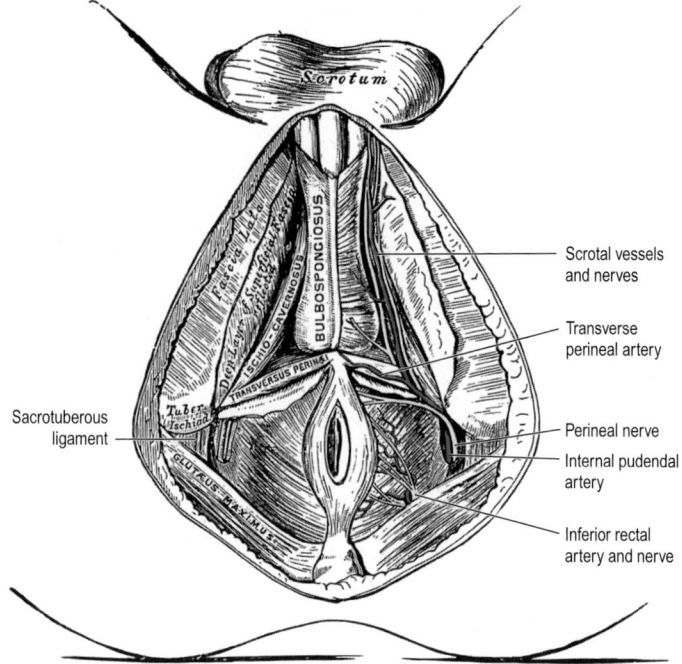

Fig. 100.3 The superficial branches of the internal pudendal artery in the male.

grooved neck of the penis. Numerous small preputial glands on the corona glandis and penile neck secrete sebaceous smegma. The navicular fossa of the urethra is in the glans and opens by a sagittal slit on or near its apex.

SUPERFICIAL PENILE FASCIA

The superficial penile fascia is devoid of fat, and consists of loose connective tissue, invaded by a few fibres of dartos muscle from the scrotum (p. 1313). Indeed, clinically, it is commonly call the dartos layer. As in the suprapubic abdominal wall, the deepest layer is condensed to form a distinct tough fascial sheath known as Buck's fascia. It surrounds both corpora cavernosa and splits to enclose the corpus spongiosum, separating the superficial and deep dorsal veins. At the penile neck it blends with the fibrous covering of all three corpora. Proximally, it is continuous with the dartos muscle and with the fascia covering the urogenital region of the perineum (p. 1367).

SUSPENSORY LIGAMENTS OF PENIS

The body of the penis is supported by two ligaments, the fundiform and triangular ligaments, which are continuous with its fascia and consist largely of elastin fibres. The fundiform ligament, stems from the lowest part of the linea alba, and splits into two lamellae which skirt the penis and unite below with the scrotal septum. The triangular suspensory ligament, deep to the fundiform ligament, is attached above to the front of the pubic symphysis, and blends below, on each side, with the fascia penis.

VASCULAR SUPPLY AND LYMPHATIC DRAINAGE

PERINEAL ARTERY (Fig. 100.3)
The perineal artery leaves the internal pudendal artery (**Fig. 108.4**) near the anterior end of its canal and approaches the scrotum in the superficial perineal region, between bulbospongiosus and ischiocavernosus. Beyond the perineal membrane, and near its base, a small transverse branch passes medially, inferior to the superficial transverse perineal muscle, to anastomose with its contralateral fellow, and with the posterior scrotal and inferior rectal arteries; collectively these vessels supply tissues between the anus and the penile bulb. The posterior scrotal arteries, distributed to the scrotal skin, dartos and perineal muscles, are usually terminal branches of the perineal artery but may also arise from its transverse branch.

ARTERY OF THE BULB OF THE PENIS
The artery of the bulb of the penis is short but wide. It runs medially through the deep transverse perineal muscle to the penile bulb, which it penetrates. It supplies the corpus spongiosum and the bulbourethral gland.

CAVERNOSAL ARTERY (DEEP ARTERY OF THE PENIS)
The cavernosal artery is a terminal branch of the internal pudendal artery. It passes through the perineal membrane to enter the crus penis. It runs the length of the corpus cavernosum and supplies its erectile tissue. Within the corpus the cavernosal arteries divide into branches running in the trabeculae. Some end directly in capillary networks which open into the cavernous spaces, and others become convoluted and somewhat dilated helicine arteries, which then open into the cavernous spaces. Helicine arteries are most abundant in the posterior regions of the corpora cavernosa.

DORSAL ARTERY OF THE PENIS
The dorsal artery of the penis is the other terminal branch of the internal pudendal artery. It runs between the crus penis and pubic symphysis, and then pierces the suspensory ligament of the penis to run along its dorsum to the glans, where it forks into branches to the glans and prepuce. In the penis it lies deep to Buck's fascia between the dorsal nerve and deep dorsal vein, the latter being most medial. It supplies penile skin by branches which run through the dartos layer. It gives off circumflex branches which run around the shaft of the penis deep to and then within Buck's fascia to supply the tunica albuginea of the corpus cavernosum, anastomosing through the tunica with the cavernosal system. These vessels also supply the corpus spongiosum.

DORSAL VEINS OF THE PENIS (Fig. 93.3)
The veins which drain the corpora cavernosa leave the corpora by passing obliquely through the tunica albuginea via a series of small vessels. These small veins run into the circumflex veins which run circumferentially around the shaft of the penis from its ventral aspect, where they receive tributaries from the corpus spongiosum, to its dorsal aspect, where they drain into the deep dorsal vein. The dorsal veins, superficial and deep, are unpaired. The superficial dorsal vein drains the prepuce and penile skin. It runs back in subcutaneous tissue and inclines right or left, before it opens into one of the external pudendal veins. The deep dorsal vein lies deep to Buck's fascia. It receives blood from the glans penis and corpora cavernosa penis, and courses back in the midline between the paired dorsal arteries. Near the root of the penis it passes deep to the suspensory ligament and through a gap between the arcuate pubic ligament and anterior margin of the perineal membrane. It divides into right and left branches which connect below the symphysis pubis with the internal pudendal veins and ultimately enter the prostatic plexus.

LYMPHATIC DRAINAGE OF THE PENIS

The penile skin is drained by vessels, which, with those of the perineal skin, accompany the external pudendal blood vessels to the superficial inguinal nodes. Lymph vessels from the glans pass to the deep inguinal and external iliac nodes. Lymph vessels from the erectile tissue and penile urethra pass to the internal iliac lymph nodes.

INNERVATION

The nerves to the corpora cavernosa form two groups, the lesser and greater cavernous nerves, which arise from the front of the pelvic (inferior hypogastric) plexus and join branches from the pudendal nerve before passing below the pubic arch. Lesser cavernous nerves pierce the fibrous penile sheath proximally to supply the erectile tissue of the corpus spongiosum and penile urethra. Greater cavernous nerves proceed on the dorsum of the penis, where they connect with the dorsal nerve, and supply the erectile tissue: some filaments reach the erectile tissue of the corpus spongiosum. Stimulation of the sympathetic supply to the male genital organs produces vasoconstriction (the parasympathetic is vasodilator), contraction of the seminal vesicles and prostate, and seminal emission. Parasympathetic fibres are vasodilator and come from the second, third and fourth sacral spinal segments via the pudendal nerve and pelvic plexuses. On the glans and bulb of the penis some cutaneous filaments innervate lamellated corpuscles and many terminate in characteristic end bulbs.

MICROSTRUCTURE

The internal surfaces of the fibrous sheaths of the corpora cavernosa and their dividing septum give rise to numerous trabeculae. These cross the corpora cavernosa in all directions and divide them into a series of cavernous spaces, which gives them a spongy appearance (**Fig. 100.2**). The trabeculae are composed of collagen and elastin fibres, and smooth muscle cells. They contain numerous vessels and nerves. The cavernous spaces are filled with blood during erection, but many are empty in the flaccid penis. They are lined by flat non-fenestrated endothelial cells. The fibrous tunica albuginea of the corpus spongiosum is thinner, whiter and more elastic than that of the corpora cavernosa. It is formed partly of smooth muscle cells: a layer of the same tissue surrounds the urethral epithelium and the paraurethral glands.

ERECTION AND EJACULATION

Erection is purely vascular. It occurs in response to parasympathetic stimulation and is independent of compression by the ischiocavernosi and bulbospongiosus, although these may contribute to maximum rigidity. Sexual arousal leads to rapid inflow from the helicine arteries following relaxation of the smooth muscle of the corpora cavernosa, an event which is dependent on the production of nitrous oxide and cyclic GMP. This inflow of blood fills the cavernous spaces leading to tumescence. The resulting distension converts tumescence to erection by pressure on the subtunical veins, which drain the erectile tissue, thereby obstructing them. The pressure within the corpora cavernosa is maintained at 100 mmHg to maintain penile erection. Continuing cutaneous stimulation of the glans and frenulum contributes significantly to maintaining erection and initiating orgasm and ejaculation. Erection is thus dependent on a normal psychogenic response to stimulation, intact parasympathetic nerves, corporal smooth muscle capable of relaxation, patent arteries capable of delivering blood at the required rate, and a normal venous system.

Ejaculation consists of two processes: emission and ejaculation. Emission is the transmission of seminal fluid from the vasa, prostate and seminal vesicles into the prostatic urethra under sympathetic control. Ejaculation is the onward transmission of seminal fluid from the prostatic urethra to the exterior. This has autonomic and somatic components. The first discernible part of the process is contraction of bulbospongiosus, which contracts about six times under somatic control. The way in which seminal fluid crosses the external urethral sphincter into the bulbar urethra is not clear: it is known to be under autonomic control and is timed such that from the second to the final contraction of bulbospongiosus the ejaculate appears from the external meatus, in some younger men in a pulsatile fashion.

Failure to achieve tumescence with adequate stimulation is termed impotence or more recently and politically correctly, erectile dysfunction. The mechanism of erection is complex: failure in any of the previously mentioned components can result in impotence. The commonest causes include psychogenic disturbance with failure to relax cavernous smooth muscle; arterial insufficiency, as a result of atheromatous disease; and damage to the parasympathetic nervous system secondary to diabetes or following pelvic surgery such as radical prostatectomy, radical cystectomy or bowel resection. Pharmacotherapy is predominantly directed at achieving cavernosal smooth muscle relaxation.

Detumescence is effected through the sympathetic pathway. Failure of an erection to detumesce is termed priapism. This can occur spontaneously but is most commonly seen with conditions that impair blood flow by increasing its viscosity such as sickle cell anaemia or leukaemia, or as a consequence of drug treatment when given by injection. These conditions result in ischaemia of the corporal smooth muscle, which causes pain within the penis.

Peyronie's disease produces a bend in the erect penis. This is most commonly a dorsal curvature and results from a localized thickening or plaque of the corpora cavernosa which prevents expansion of a segment during erection.

REFERENCES

Lepor H, Gregerman M, Crosby R, Mostofi FK, Walsh PC 1985 Precise localization of the autonomic nerves of the pelvic plexus to the corpora cavernosa: a detailed anatomical study of the adult male pelvis. J Urol 133: 207–212.

Mundy AR, Fitzpatrick J, Neal D, George N (eds) 1999 Male sexual function. In: The Scientific Basis of Urology, Chapter 12. Isis Medical Media: 243–53.

Accessory glandular structures

SEMINAL VESICLES (Figs 101.1, 101.2)

The two seminal vesicles are sacculated, contorted tubes located between the bladder and rectum (**Figs 98.1, 101.1**). Each vesicle is c.5 cm long, somewhat pyramidal, the base being directed up and posterolaterally. Essentially, the seminal vesicle is a single coiled tube with irregular diverticula (**Fig. 101.1**); the coils and diverticula are connected by fibrous tissue. The diameter of the tube is 3–4 mm and its uncoiled length is 10–15 cm. The upper pole is a cul-de-sac, the lower narrows to a straight duct, which joins the vas deferens to form the ejaculatory duct. The anterior surface contacts the posterior aspect of the bladder, and extends from near the entry of the ureter to the prostatic base. The posterior surface is related to the rectum, from which it is separated by Denonvillier's fascia. The seminal vesicles diverge superiorly. They are related to the vas deferens and the terminations of the ureters, and are partly covered by peritoneum. Each has a dense, fibromuscular sheath. Along the medial margin of each vesicle is the ampulla of the vas deferens. The veins of the prostatic venous plexus, which drain posteriorly to the internal iliac veins, lie laterally.

BULBOURETHRAL GLANDS

The two bulbourethral glands are small round yellow somewhat lobulated masses c.1 cm in diameter (**Fig. 109.19**). They lie lateral to the membranous urethra above the perineal membrane and penile bulb and are enclosed by fibres of the urethral sphincter. The excretory duct of each, almost 3 cm long, passes obliquely forwards external to the mucosa of the membranous urethra and penetrates the perineal membrane. It opens by a minute orifice on the floor of the bulbar urethra c.2.5 cm below the perineal membrane. In later decades the glands generally diminish in size.

VASCULAR SUPPLY AND LYMPHATIC DRAINAGE

The arteries to the seminal vesicles are derived from the inferior vesical and middle rectal arteries. The veins and lymphatics accompany these arteries.

INNERVATION

The innervation of the seminal vesicles and bulbourethral glands is derived from the pelvic plexuses.

MICROSTRUCTURE

SEMINAL VESICLE

The paired seminal vesicles, together with the ampulla of the vas deferens and the ejaculatory ducts, form a functional unit which develops slowly until the onset of puberty. After puberty the vesicles form sac-like structures which contribute up to 85% of the seminal fluid. They are mainly concerned with secretion of seminal coagulating proteins, fructose, prostaglandins and other specific proteins in an alkaline, viscous yellowish fluid.

The wall of the seminal vesicle is composed of an external connective tissue layer, a middle smooth muscle layer – which is thinner than in the vas deferens and arranged in external longitudinal and internal circular layers – and an internal mucosal layer with a highly folded, labyrinthine structure. The cuboidal to pseudostratified columnar epithelium of the mucosa shows features typical of protein-secreting cells. The vesicles are not reservoirs for spermatozoa as their name suggests, because spermatozoa are stored mainly in the epididymis. They contract during ejaculation, and their secretion forms most of the ejaculate.

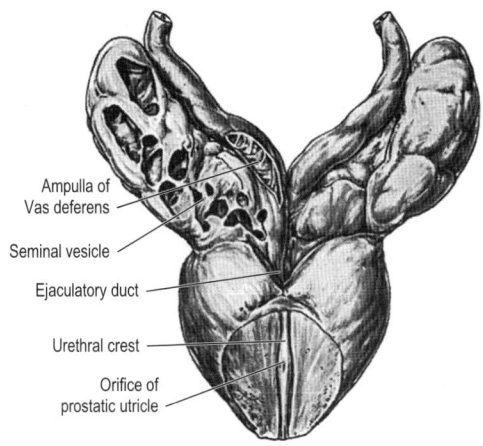

Fig. 101.1 Anterior aspect of the seminal vesicles, terminal parts of the vasa deferentia and the prostate. The lamina of the right seminal vesicle, the ampulla of the right vas deferens and of the prostatic part of the urethra have been exposed by appropriate removal of tissues.

Ampulla of Vas deferens

Seminal vesicle

Ejaculatory duct

Urethral crest

Orifice of prostatic utricle

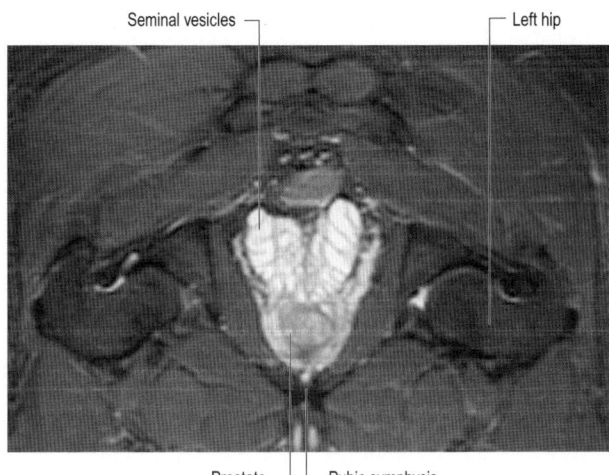

Seminal vesicles — Left hip

Prostate — Pubic symphysis

Fig. 101.2 Axial oblique MRI (STIR sequence) demonstrates normal high signal within prominent seminal vesicles lying above the prostate in a young man.

BULBOURETHRAL GLANDS

Each bulbourethral gland consists of several lobules held together by a fibrous capsule. The secretory units are mainly tubulo-alveolar in form. The glandular epithelium, which is columnar, secretes acid and neutral mucins into the penile (spongiose) urethra prior to ejaculation, and these have a lubricating function. The main secretory duct is lined by a stratified columnar epithelium. Diffuse lymphoid tissue (MALT; p. 77) is associated with the glands.

Ovaries

The ovaries are paired ovoid structures, homologous with the testes, but smaller (**Figs 102.1**, **102.2**, **102.3**, **102.4**, **103.2**). They have an average volume of 11 cm³ in reproductively mature women. The ovaries are dull white in colour and consist of dense fibrous tissue in which ova are embedded. Before regular ovulation begins they have a smooth surface, but thereafter their surfaces are distorted by scarring that follows the degeneration of successive corpus lutea.

In embryonic and early fetal life the ovaries are situated in the lumbar region near the kidneys, and they gradually descend into the lesser pelvis. In the neonate, they are c.1.3 cm long, 0.6 cm wide, and 0.4 cm thick. Prior to the first menstrual period (menarche) the ovaries are about a third of the normal reproductive adult size. They gradually increase in size with body growth. They are mobile structures and may change their position to some extent according to the state of the surrounding organs such as the intestines.

During pregnancy, the ovaries are lifted high in the pelvis and, by 14 weeks of gestation, become partly abdominal structures. By the third trimester they are totally abdominal structures and lie vertically behind and lateral to the parous uterus. The ovaries more than double their size by term. Following childbirth, the ovarian position varies. They are displaced in the first pregnancy and usually never return to their original location. During the early menopause, the average size of the ovary is 2.0 × 1.5 × 0.5 cm and this reduces to 1.5 × 7.5 × 0.5 cm in late menopause.

Accessory ovaries may occur in the mesovarium or in the adjacent part of the broad ligament.

The description that follows refers to the ovarian condition in nulliparous women, except where otherwise stated.

RELATIONS (Fig. 102.4)

The ovaries lie on each side of the uterus close to the lateral pelvic wall (**Fig. 102.4**). They are suspended in the pelvic cavity by a double

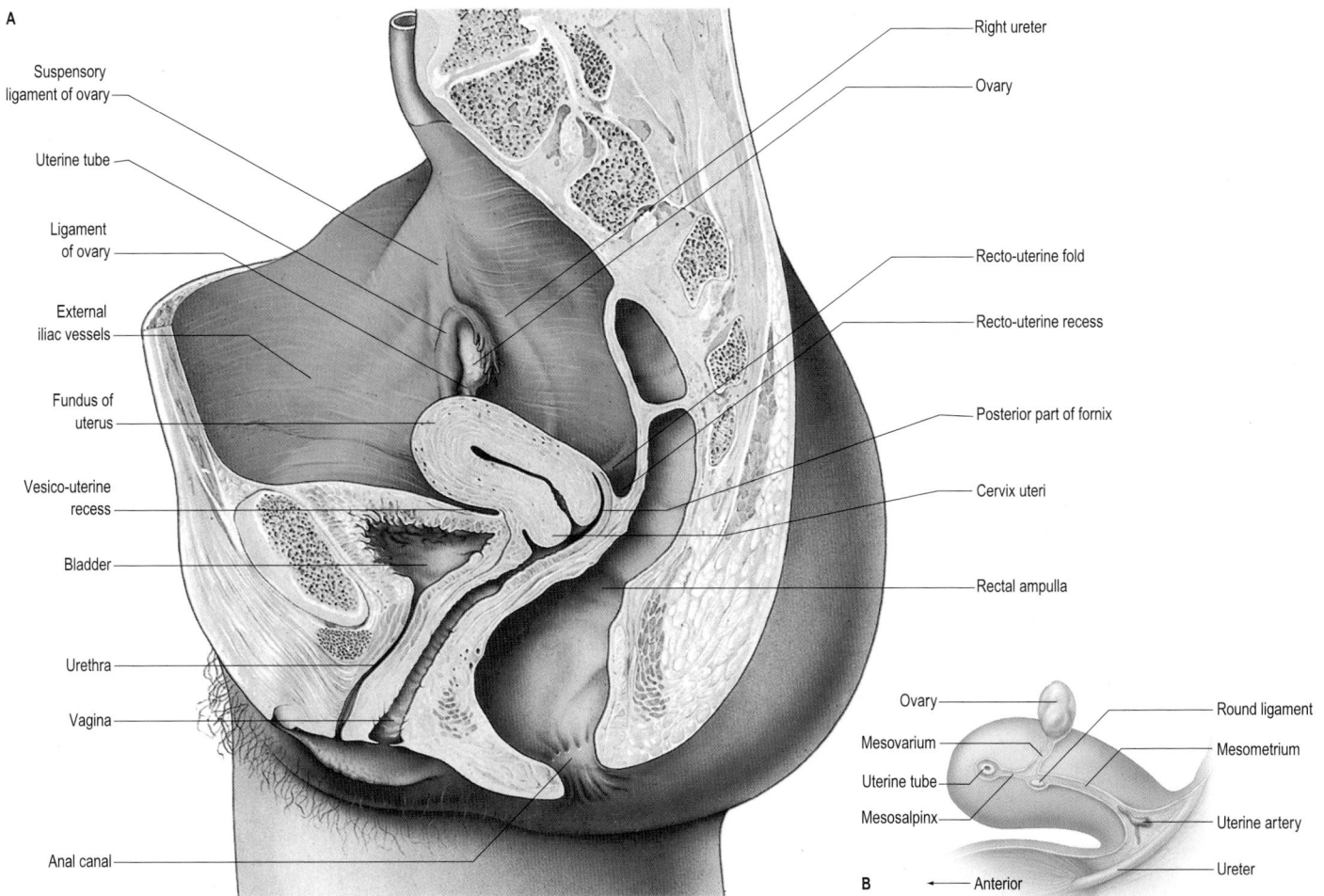

Fig. 102.1 A, Median sagittal section through a human female pelvis. Peritoneum: blue. **B**, Sagittal section showing the peritoneal attachments of the ovary.

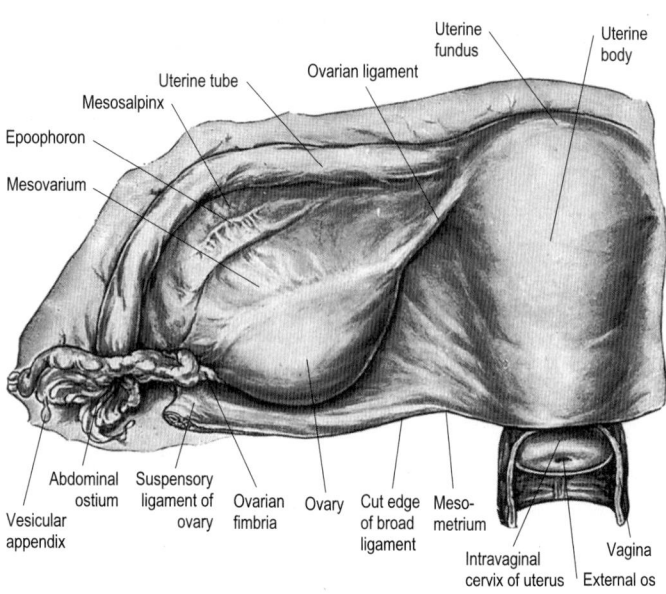

Fig. 102.2 Posterosuperior aspect of the uterus and the left broad ligament. The ligament has been spread out and the ovary is displaced downwards.

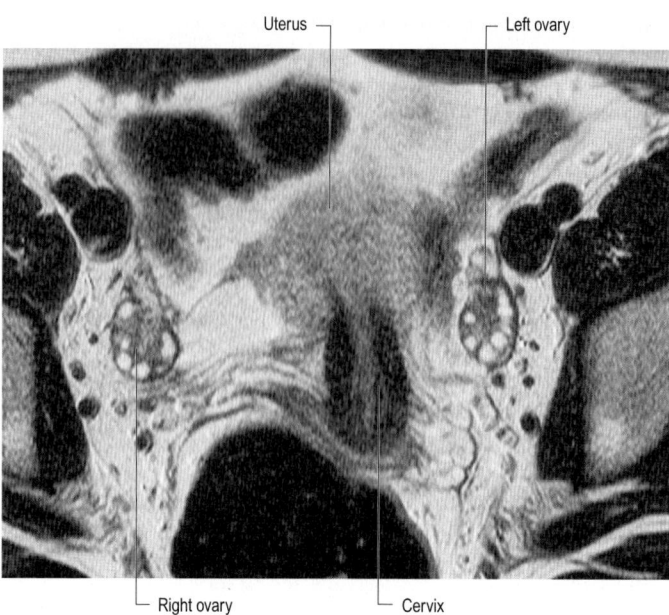

Fig. 102.4 Axial T2-weighted images through the female pelvis showing the anteverted uterus with ovaries on either side close to the pelvic wall. Both ovaries contain multiple small high-signal follicles.

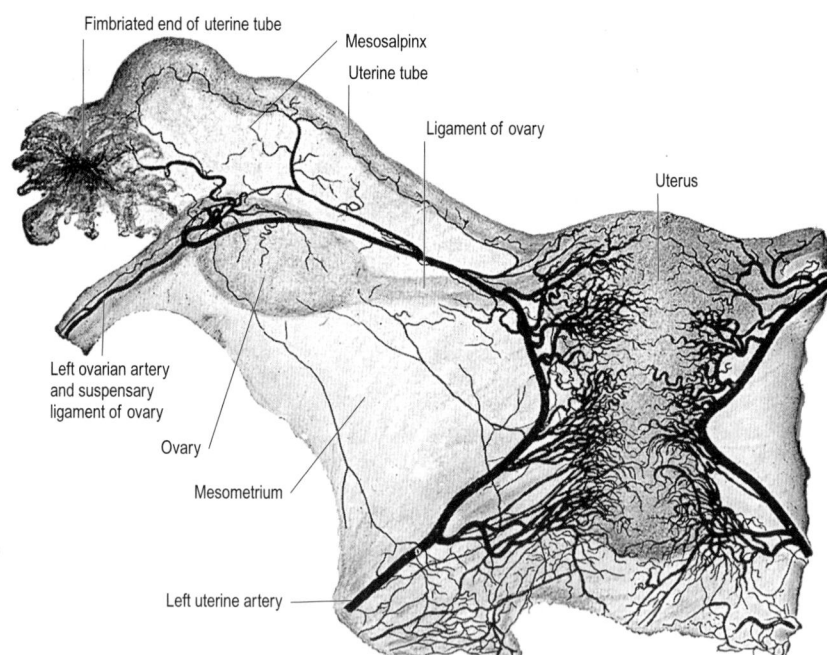

Fig. 102.3 Posterior aspect of a cleared injected specimen to show the distribution of the left uterine and ovarian arteries of a female aged 17 years. (Prepared by Hamilton Drummond.)

fold of peritoneum, the mesovarium, which attaches to the upper limit of the posterior aspect of the broad uterine ligament (**Fig. 102.2**). The long axis of each ovary is vertical in the erect position. During pregnancy they may be horizontal or oblique. Compare **Figs 102.1** and **102.2**.

The ovary has lateral and medial surfaces, superior and inferior extremities, or poles, and anterior and posterior borders. The lateral surface of the ovary contacts parietal peritoneum in the ovarian fossa. Behind the ovarian fossa are extraperitoneal structures, including the ureter, internal iliac vessels, obturator vessels and nerve, and the origin of the uterine artery. The medial surface faces the uterus and uterine vessels in the broad ligament, and the peritoneal recess here is termed the ovarian bursa. Above the superior extremity are the fimbria and distal section of the uterine tube. The inferior extremity points downwards towards the pelvic floor. The anterior border faces the posterior leaf of the broad ligament and contains the mesovarium. The posterior border is free and faces the peritoneum, which overlies the upper part of the internal iliac artery and vein, and the ureter.

On the right side, superior and lateral to the ovary, are the ileocaecal junction, caecum and appendix. On the left side, the sigmoid colon passes over the superior pole of the ovary and joins the rectum, which lies between the medial surfaces of both ovaries.

PERITONEAL ATTACHMENTS (Fig. 102.2)

SUSPENSORY (INFUNDIBULOPELVIC) LIGAMENT

The suspensory (infundibulopelvic) ligament of the ovary is a peritoneal fold, which is attached to the upper part of the lateral surface of the ovary. It contains the ovarian vessels and nerves and passes superiorly over the external iliac vessels, genitofemoral nerve and ureter (**Fig. 102.1**) to join the peritoneum, which covers psoas major. On the right side the suspensory ligament is attached to a fold of peritoneum that is posterior and inferior to the caecum and appendix. On the left side the peritoneal attachment is higher than on the right, and is lateral to the junction of the descending and sigmoid colons.

OVARIAN LIGAMENTS

The ovarian ligament attaches the uterine (inferiomedial) extremity of the ovary to the lateral angle of the uterus, posteroinferior to the uterine tube. It lies in the posterior leaf of the broad ligament and contains some smooth muscle cells. The ovarian ligament is continuous with the medial border of the round ligament (p. 1389), both of which are remnants of the gubernaculum (Ch. 109).

MESOVARIUM

The mesovarium is a short peritoneal fold, which attaches the ovary to the back of the broad ligament. It carries blood vessels and nerves to the ovarian hilum. The uterine tube arches over the ovary, and ascends in relation to its mesovarian border, then curves over its tubal end and passes down on its posterior, free border and medial surface (**Fig. 102.1**).

VASCULAR SUPPLY AND LYMPHATIC DRAINAGE (Fig. 102.3)

ARTERIES

The ovarian arteries are branches of the abdominal aorta and originate below the renal arteries. They correspond to the testicular arteries (**Fig. 91.1**). Each descends behind the peritoneum in the paracolic gutter, and at the brim of the pelvis crosses the external iliac artery and vein to enter the true pelvic cavity. Here the artery turns medially in the ovarian suspensory ligament and continues into the uterine broad ligament, below the uterine tube. At the ovarian level it passes back in the mesovarium and divides into branches that supply the ovary. Branches also supply the uterine tube, and, on each side, a branch passes lateral to the uterus to unite with the uterine artery. Other branches accompany the round ligaments through the inguinal canal to the skin of the labium majus and the inguinal region.

Early in intrauterine life the ovaries flank the vertebral column inferior to the kidneys, and so the ovarian arteries are relatively short – the arteries gradually lengthen as the ovaries descend into the pelvis.

The vessels supplying the ovary dilate during pregnancy as their anastamoses form part of the uterine and tubal circulation (**Fig. 102.3**), and this results in a swollen mesovarium and ovary.

VEINS

The ovarian veins emerge from the ovary as a plexus (pampiniform plexus) in the mesovarium and suspensory ligament. Two veins issue from the plexus and ascend with the ovarian artery. Their further course is similar to that of the testicular veins. They usually merge into a single vessel before entering either the inferior vena cava on the right side, or the renal vein on the left side. They may contain valves. The ovarian veins are much enlarged in pregnancy.

LYMPHATIC DRAINAGE

Lymph drainage is via three main routes. Lymph vessels ascend along the ovarian artery to preaortic and lateral aortic nodes situated near the origin of the renal arteries. Lymph may drain directly to lumboaortic, iliac and obturator nodes, which then drain into para-aortic nodes, or it may drain along the round liagament to the inguinal nodes and across the uterus to the contralateral pelvic nodes.

INNERVATION

The ovarian plexuses consist of postganglionic sympathetic, parasympathetic and visceral afferent fibres. The efferent sympathetic fibres are derived from the tenth and eleventh thoracic spinal segments and are probably vasoconstrictor, whereas the parasympathetic fibres, from the inferior hypogastric plexuses, are probably vasodilator. Little is known of their actual distribution or function. Histochemical studies have demonstrated the presence of cholinergic and adrenergic nerve fibres in both the ovaries and ovarian ligaments.

The nerves accompany the ovarian artery to the ovary and uterine tube. The upper part of the ovarian plexus is formed from branches of the renal and aortic plexuses, and the lower part is reinforced from the superior and inferior hypogastric plexuses. Autonomic fibres do not reach the ovarian follicles and are not required for ovulation.

REFERRED PAIN

Sensory fibres accompany the sympathetic nerves, and so ovarian pain can be periumbilical. It is often perceived in the right or left iliac fossa due to local inflammation. Ovarian pain can also be perceived on the medial side of the thigh in the cutaneous distribution of the obturator nerve, presumably because the ovary lies close to the obturator nerve in the ovarian fossa, and so any inflammation of the ovary or peritoneum in the ovarian fossa may affect the obturator nerve.

MICROSTRUCTURE

In young females the surface of the ovary is covered by a single layer of cuboidal epithelium, which contains some flatter cells. It appears dull white, in contrast to the shiny smooth peritoneal mesothelial covering of the mesovarium, with which it is continuous. A white line around the anterior mesovarian border usually marks the transition between peritoneum and ovarian epithelium. The surface epithelium is also termed the germinal epithelium, but this is a misnomer, because it is not the source of germ cells (p. 1386). In adults, c.85% of ovarian cancers arise from neoplastic changes in the surface epithelium.

Immediately beneath the epithelium there is a tough collagenous coat, the tunica albuginea. The ovarian tissue it surrounds is divisible into a cortex, which contains the ovarian follicles, and a medulla, which receives the ovarian vessels and nerves at the hilum (**Fig. 102.5**).

OVARIAN CORTEX

Before puberty, the cortex forms c.35%, the medulla c.20%, and interstitial cells up to 45%, of the volume of the ovary. After puberty the cortex forms the major part of the ovary, and encloses the medulla except at the hilum. It contains the ovarian follicles at various stages of development, and corpora lutea and their degenerative remnants, depending on age or stage of the menstrual cycle. The follicles and structures derived from them are embedded in a dense stroma composed of a meshwork of thin collagen fibres and fusiform fibroblast-like cells arranged in characteristic whorls. Stromal cells differ from fibroblasts in general connective tissue in that they contain lipid droplets, which accumulate in pregnancy. Stromal cells give rise to the thecal layers of maturing ovarian follicles. The theca interna becomes steroid-secreting in the corpus luteum.

MEDULLA

The medulla is highly vascular, much more so than the cortex. It contains numerous veins and spiral arteries, which enter the hilum from the mesovarium and lie within a loose connective tissue stroma. Small numbers of cells (hilus cells) with characteristics similar to interstitial (Leydig) cells in the testis are found in the medulla at the hilum, and they may be a source of androgens.

OVARIAN FOLLICLES

Primordial follicle

The formation of the female gamete is a complex process. At birth, the ovarian cortex contains a superficial zone of primordial follicles. These consist of primary oocytes c.25 μm in diameter, each surrounded by a single layer of flat follicular cells (**Fig. 102.6**). The oocyte nuclei are slightly eccentric and have a characteristically prominent nucleolus. They contain the diploid number of chromosomes (duplicated as sister chromatids), arrested at the diplotene stage of meiotic prophase since before birth. The prenatal development of primordial follicles is described on page 1386. Many follicles degenerate either during prepubertal (including prenatal) life, or through atresia at some stage after beginning the process of cyclical maturation during the childbearing period. Their remnants are visible as atretic follicles, the remains of which accumulate throughout the period of reproductive life. After puberty, a cohort of up to 20 primordial follicles, (fewer with advancing age) become activated in each menstrual cycle. Their development takes a number of cycles. Of the follicles activated in each cohort, usually only one follicle from one or other ovary becomes dominant, reaches maturity and releases its oocyte at ovulation.

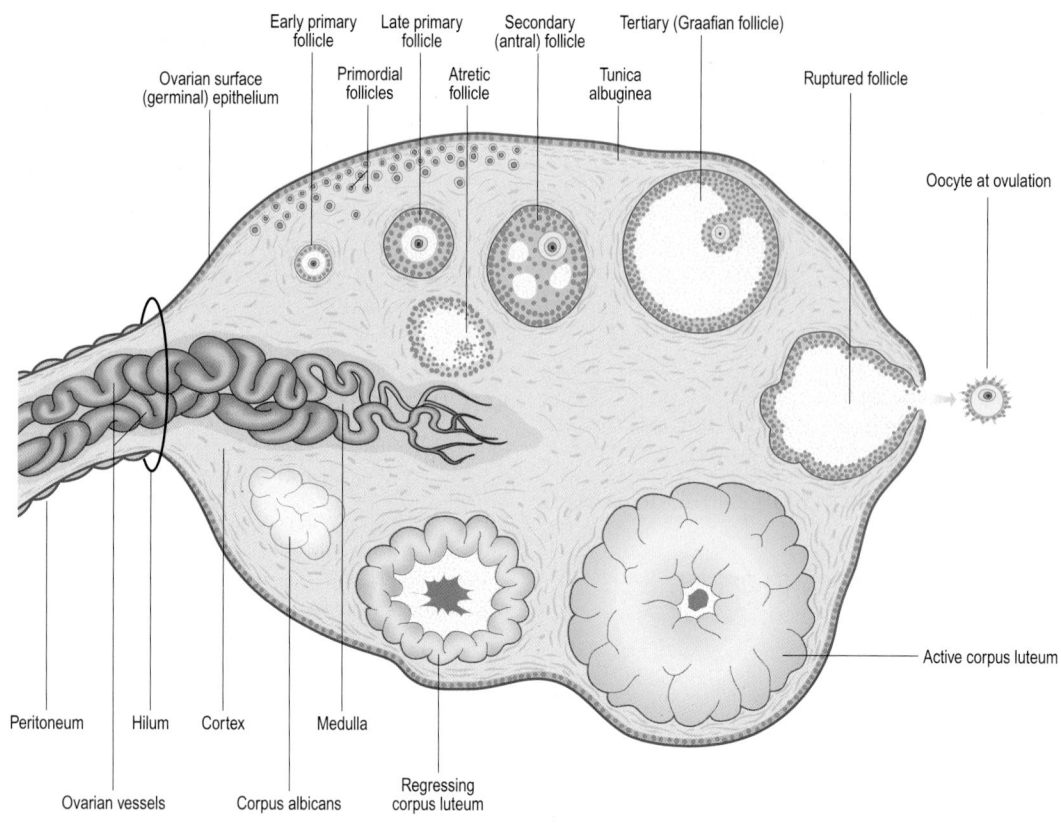

Fig. 102.5 The microstructure of the ovary and follicles at various stages in their cyclical development and the formation of corpora lutea and albicans. Note that in the human ovary, developing follicles are rarely seen.

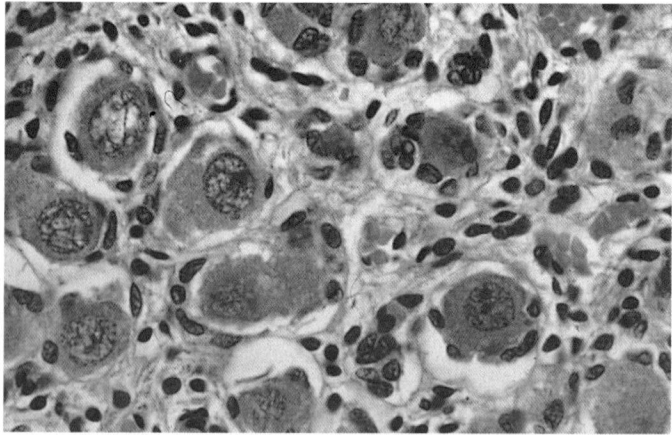

Fig. 102.6 High power micrograph of primordial follicles in the ovarian cortex of a 32-week fetus. A single layer of flattened follicular cells surrounds each large primary oocyte. (By permission from Stevens A, Lowe JS 1996 Human Histology, 2nd edn. London: Mosby.)

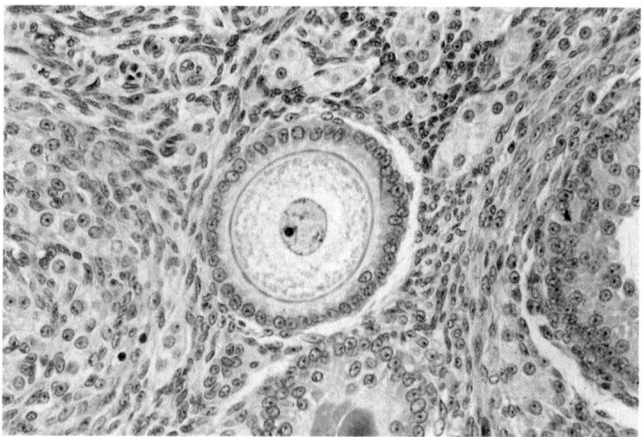

Fig. 102.7 Primary follicle (rat) showing the zona pellucida between the oocyte and a single layer of cuboidal follicular (granulosa) cells.

Primary follicle

The first sign of activation is a change in the follicle cells from flattened to cuboidal. This is followed by their proliferation to give rise to a multilayered follicle consisting of granulosa cells surrounded by a thick basal lamina. Stromal cells immediately surrounding the follicle begin to differentiate into spindle-shaped cells, which constitute the theca folliculi (the presumptive theca interna). They are later accompanied by a more fibrous theca externa. At the same time the oocyte increases in size and secretes a thick layer of extracellular proteoglycan-rich material, the zona pellucida, between its plasma membrane and the surrounding granulosa cells of the early follicle (Fig. 102.7). This is important for the process of fertilization (p. 185). The granulosa cells in contact with the zona pellucida send cytoplasmic processes radially inwards and these

contact oocyte microvilli at gap junctions, indicating communication between them (for a review see Buccione et al 1990). The follicular cells, in particular the granulosa cells, which are in functional contact with each other through gap junctions, continue to proliferate and so the thickness of the late primary follicle wall increases.

Secondary (antral) follicle

As the number of granulosa cells continues to increase, cavities begin to form between them (Fig. 102.8) filled with a clear fluid (liquor folliculi) containing hyaluronate, growth factors, and steroid hormones secreted by the granulosa cells. The follicle is now about 200 μm in diameter and usually lies deep in the cortex. These cavities coalesce to form one large fluid-filled space, the antrum. This is surrounded by a

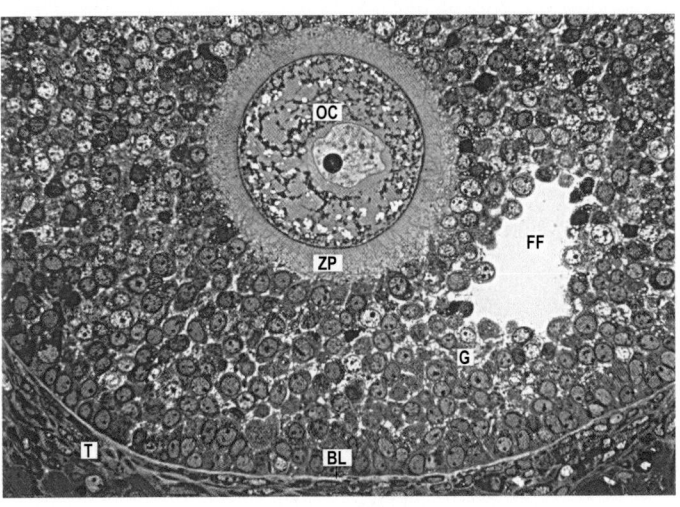

Fig. 102.8 Early antral (secondary) follicle showing the development of a fluid-filled antrum (follicular fluid, FF) within the granulosa cell layer. The oocyte (OC) is separated from the granulosa cells (G) by a pale-staining zona pellucida (ZP). Note the relative size of the oocyte and its nucleus and prominent nucleolus, compared with follicular cells. The follicle is surrounded by a basal lamina (BL) and a thecal cell layer (T). (By permission from Dr JB Kerr, Monash University, from Kerr JB 1999 Atlas of Functional Histology. London: Mosby.)

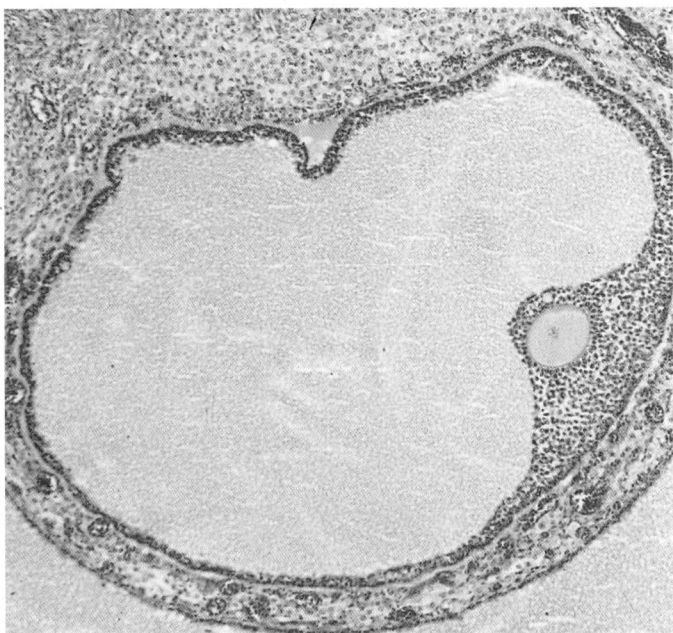

Fig. 102.9 A mature tertiary (Graafian) follicle, with an eccentrically located oocyte surrounded by a cumulus oophorus (of granulosa cells) within the fluid-filled antrum. (By permission from Stevens A, Lowe JS 1996 Human Histology, 2nd edn. London: Mosby.)

thin, uniform layer of granulosa cells, except at one pole of the follicle where a thickened granulosa layer envelopes the eccentrically placed oocyte, to form the cumulus oophorus (**Fig. 102.9**). The oocyte has now reached its maximum size of about 80 µm and the inner and outer thecae are clearly differentiated. As follicles mature, the theca interna becomes more prominent and its cells more rounded and typical of steroid-secreting endocrine cells. These cells produce androstenedione from which the granulosa cells synthesize oestrogens (primarily oestradiol). Follicular development is stimulated by follicle-stimulating hormone (FSH).

Tertiary follicle

Although a number of follicles may progress to the secondary stage by about the first week of a menstrual cycle, usually only one follicle, from either one of the two ovaries, proceeds to the tertiary stage, and the remainder become atretic. The surviving follicle increases in size considerably as the antrum takes up fluid from the surrounding tissues and expands to a diameter of c.2 cm. The cumulus oophorus surrounding the oocyte thins. The term Graafian follicle is often used to describe this mature follicular stage. The oocyte and a surrounding ring of tightly adherent cells, the corona radiata, breaks away from the follicle wall and floats freely in the follicular fluid. The primary oocyte, which has remained in the first meiotic prophase since fetal life, completes its first meiotic division to produce the almost equally large secondary oocyte and a minute first polar body with very little cytoplasm. The secondary haploid oocyte immediately begins its second meiotic division, but when it reaches metaphase, the process is arrested until fertilization has occurred. The follicle moves to the superficial cortex, causing the surface of the ovary to bulge. The tissues at the point of contact (the stigma) with the tough tunica albuginea and ovarian surface epithelium are eroded until the follicle ruptures and its contents are released into the peritoneal cavity for capture by the fimbria of the uterine (Fallopian) tube (p. 1329). The oocyte at ovulation is still surrounded by its zona pellucida and corona radiata of granulosa cells. If fertilization does not occur, it begins to degenerate after 24 to 48 hours.

Corpus luteum

After ovulation, the walls of the empty follicle collapse and fold. The granulosa cells increase in size and synthesize a cytoplasmic carotenoid pigment (lutein) giving them a yellowish colour (hence corpus luteum). These large (30–50 µm) granulosa lutein cells form most of the corpus luteum (**Fig. 102.10**). The basal lamina surrounding the follicle breaks down, and numerous smaller theca lutein cells infiltrate the folds of the cellular mass, accompanied by capillaries and connective tissue. Extravasated blood from thecal capillaries accumulates in the centre as a small clot, but this rapidly resolves and is replaced by connective tissue. Ultrastructurally, all lutein cells have a cytoplasm filled with abundant smooth endoplasmic reticulum, characteristic of steroid synthesizing endocrine cells. Granulosa lutein cells secrete progesterone and oestradiol (from aromatization of androstenedione, which is synthesized by theca lutein cells). The two cell types also respond differently to circulating gonadotropins. Theca lutein cells express receptors for, and respond to, human chorionic gonadotrophin (hCG). If the oocyte is not fertilized, the corpus luteum (of menstruation) functions for c.12 to 14 days after ovulation, then atrophies. The lutein cells undergo fatty degeneration, autolysis, removal by macrophages and gradual replacement with fibrous tissue. Eventually, after c.2 months, a small, whitish scar-like corpus albicans is all that remains.

If fertilization does occur, implantation of the blastocyst into the uterine endometrium usually begins seven days later and the embryonic trophoblast then starts to produce hCG. The chorionic gonadotrophin stimulates the corpus luteum of menstruation to grow, and it becomes a corpus luteum of pregnancy. It normally increases in size from c.10 mm in diameter to 25 mm around 8 weeks of gestation (p. 1323) and can be seen clearly on the ovary on ultrasound. It secretes progesterone, oestrogen and relaxin, and functions throughout pregnancy, although it gradually regresses as its endocrine functions are largely replaced by the placenta after c.8 weeks' gestation. Its diameter is reduced by the end of pregnancy to c.1 cm. In the next few months it degenerates, like the corpus luteum of menstruation, to form a corpus albicans.

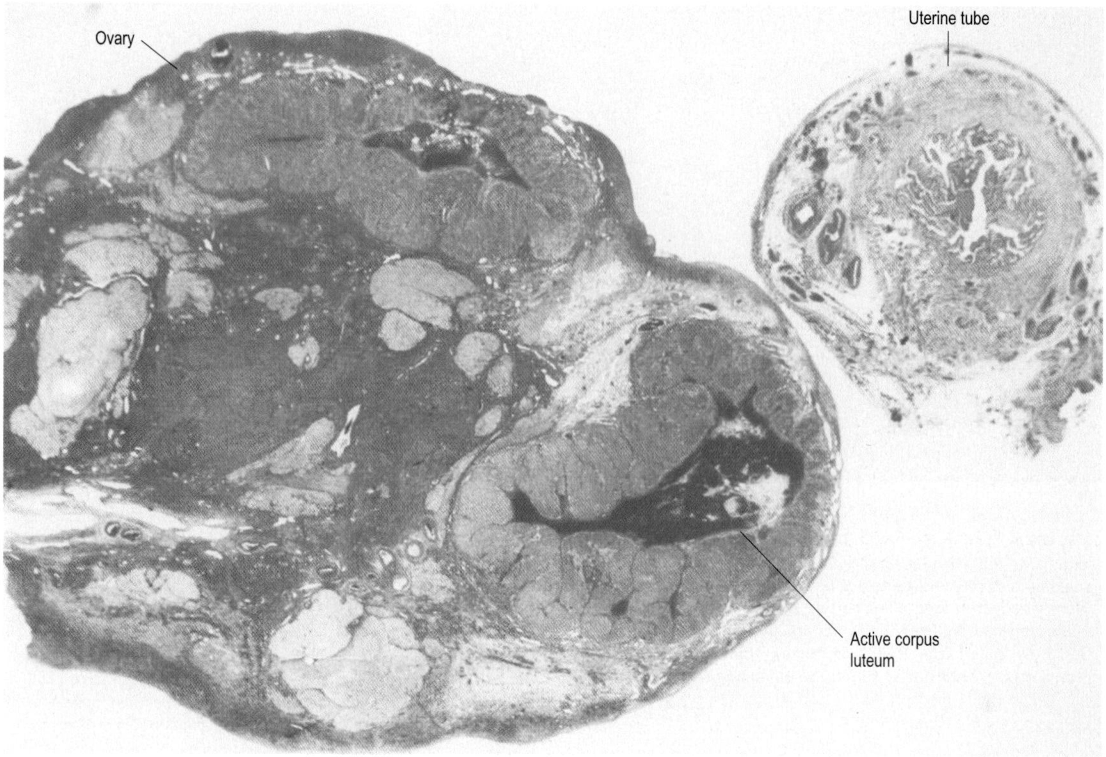

Fig. 102.10 Low-power micrograph showing the human ovary in reproductive maturity. The large structure on the right is an active corpus luteum and several other corpora lutea are at various stages of degeneration and the formation of corpora albicans. The uterine tube is seen in transverse section to the right of the ovary. (By permission from Young B, Heath JW 2000 Wheater's Functional Histology. Edinburgh: Churchill Livingstone.)

OVARY IN THE MENOPAUSE

At the menopause (usually in the 45–55-year-age range), ovulation ceases and various microscopic changes ensue within the ovarian tissues. The stroma becomes denser, the tunica albuginea thickens and the ovarian surface epithelium thins. However, many follicles persist within the cortex. Some lack oocytes, and others contain oocytes, providing the possibility of ovulation if the hormonal changes were to be reversed. Some abnormal follicles may become cystic as age progresses, and this is quite a common feature in later years.

OVARIAN CYSTS

An ovary may contain a functional or pathological cyst. Prior to ovulation a Graafian follicle can be seen on the surface of the ovary and can be as large as 1 cm. After ovulation, the corpus luteum develops, and this can also be visualized on the surface of the ovary. These normal functional cysts can sometimes be confused with ovarian cystic pathology on ultrasound.

A Graafian follicle can fail to rupture and continue to enlarge, reaching sizes of 5 or 6 cm. When rupture eventually occurs the process can cause severe pain. Corpus luteal cysts can also develop into larger than average structures. This is especially so in the first trimester of pregnancy when large cysts can be identified on ultrasound scan and cause concern. They usually regress as pregnancy advances and rarely cause symptoms.

Benign and malignant neoplasms of the ovary can produce fluid (usually a serous, mucinous, or sebaceous fluid) and develop into cysts. Sometimes these cysts become very large and can reach sizes of 30 or 40 cm. When a pathological cyst becomes very large, movement within the pelvis and abdomen can result in torsion around the suspensory ligament. This causes ischaemic pain, and the ovary becomes gangrenous and requires surgical excision.

Polcystic ovaries occur in one in five women and are part of a genetically inherited condition associated with subfertility, irregular periods, androgenic signs, early baldness in the woman's father, insulin resistance, and late-onset diabetes. Structurally, polycystic ovaries are about one and a half times the size of a normal ovary and have a glistening white surface. They consist of 20 to 40 small (2–5 mm diameter) cysts on the surface of the ovary, which encircle a denser than normal stroma. The classic description of this appearance on ultrasound is that of a string of pearls. For an extensive review on this and other aspects of polycystic ovaries see Dunaif and Thomas (2002).

REFERENCES

Buccione R, Schroeder AC, Eppig JJ 1990 Interactions between somatic cells and germ cells throughout mammalian oogenesis. Biol Reprod 43: 543–7.

Dunaif A, Thomas A 2001 Current concepts in the polycystic ovary syndrome. Annu Rev Med 52: 401–19.

Uterine tubes

The two uterine (Fallopian) tubes lie on each side of the uterus in the upper margin of the broad ligament (mesosalpinx) (**Figs 103.1**, **103.2**, **103.3**). They are c.10 cm long and are pinkish red in colour.

The medial opening of the tube (the uterine os) is located at the superior angle of the uterus. The tube passes laterally and superiorly and consists of four main parts: intramural; isthmus; ampulla; and fimbria. The intramural part is c.0.7 mm wide, 1 cm long, and lies within the myometrium. It is continuous laterally with the isthmus, which is 1 to 5 mm wide and 3 cm long, and is rounded, muscular and firm. Its lumen is narrow and exhibits three to five longitudinal major folds with a variable degree of relatively simple secondary folding. The isthmus is continuous laterally with the ampulla, the widest portion of the tube with a maximum luminal diameter of c.1 cm. The ampulla is c.5 cm long and has a thin wall and a tortuously folded luminal surface marked by 4 to 5 major longitudinal ridges on which lie secondary folds, creating an extensive, labyrinthine surface area (see **Fig. 103.5**). Typically, fertilization takes place in its lumen. The ampulla opens into the funnel-shaped infundibulum at the abdominal os. Numerous mucosal finger-like folds, c.1 mm wide, the fimbriae, are attached to the ends of the infundibulum (**Fig. 102.2**). They extend from its inner circumference beyond the muscular wall of the tube. One of these, the ovarian fimbria, is longer and more deeply grooved than the others, and is typically applied to the tubal pole of the ovary. At the time of ovulation the fimbriae swell and extend as a result of engorgement of the vessels in the lamina propria, which aids capture of the released oocyte. All fimbriae are covered, like the mucosal lining throughout the tube, by a ciliated epithelium whose cilia beat towards the ampulla.

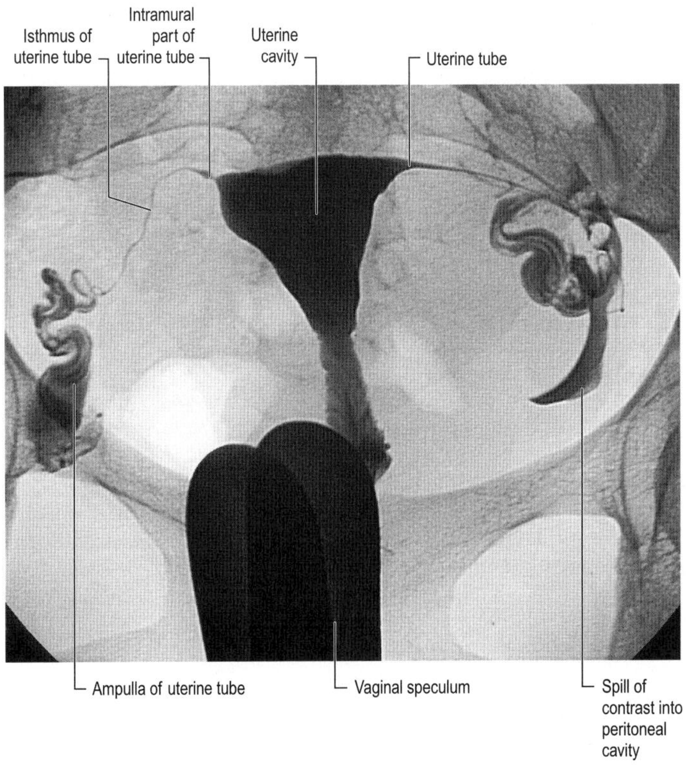

TUBAL PREGNANCY AND BLOCKAGE

After fertilization the segmenting zygote normally enters the uterus. Occasionally it may adhere to and develop in the tube. A tubal pregnancy is the commonest variety of ectopic gestation. Ectopic gestations usually end with extrusion through the abdominal ostium or natural death and resorption. Occasionally they can continue to expand and rupture through the uterine tube causing severe haemorrhage.

Uterine tubes may be blocked intrinsically or extrinsically by scar tissue. The most common causes of tubal blockage include infection, endometriosis, and adhesions from previous surgery. The two most common methods for assessing tubal patency are laparoscopic dye insufflation (LDI) (**Fig. 103.4**) and hysterosalpingography (HSG) (**Fig. 103.1**). LDI involves a general anaesthetic and the insertion of an endoscope (laparoscope) into the abdomen. Blue dye is inserted through the cervical os and is seen to spill from the fimbriated end in a patent uterine tube (**Fig. 103.4**). This technique also allows inspection of any abnormal features that might cause extrinsic blockage of the tube, e.g. endometriosis or adhesions. HSG involves the injection of a radiopaque dye through the cervical os (**Fig. 103.1**) and assessing tubal patency radiologically. It has the advantage of allowing assessment of the cavity of the uterus and uterine tubes.

Isthmus of uterine tube ⌐ Intramural part of uterine tube ⌐ Uterine cavity ⌐ Uterine tube

Ampulla of uterine tube ⌐ Vaginal speculum ⌐ Spill of contrast into peritoneal cavity

Fig. 103.1 Digitally subtracted hysterosalpingogram. Radiopaque contrast is introduced via a catheter inserted through the cervical os. The catheter is introduced using a vaginal speculum. The contrast fills the triangular uterine cavity. The lumina of the narrow intramural and isthmic parts of the uterine tubes may be traced inferolaterally from the superior angles. They expand into the wider ampullae. Some contrast media has escaped into the pelvic cavity from the abdominal ostia. (By kind permission from Dr Julia Hillier, Chelsea and Westminster Hospital, London.)

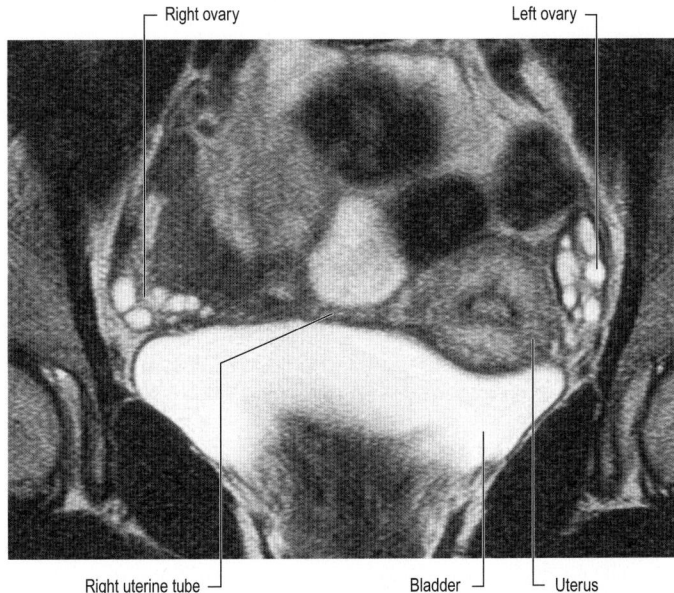

Right ovary ⌐ Left ovary ⌐

Right uterine tube ⌐ Bladder ⌐ Uterus

Fig. 103.2 Coronal T2-weighted MRI in a young female showing the anteverted uterus lying above the bladder. The right ovary is clearly seen at the lateral margin of the right uterine tube. Both ovaries contain high signal follicles.

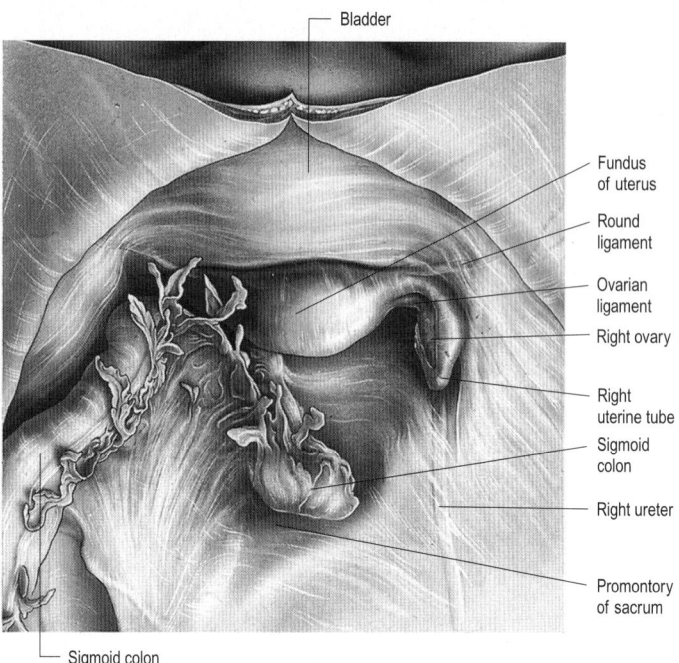

Fig. 103.3 The female pelvis and its contents.

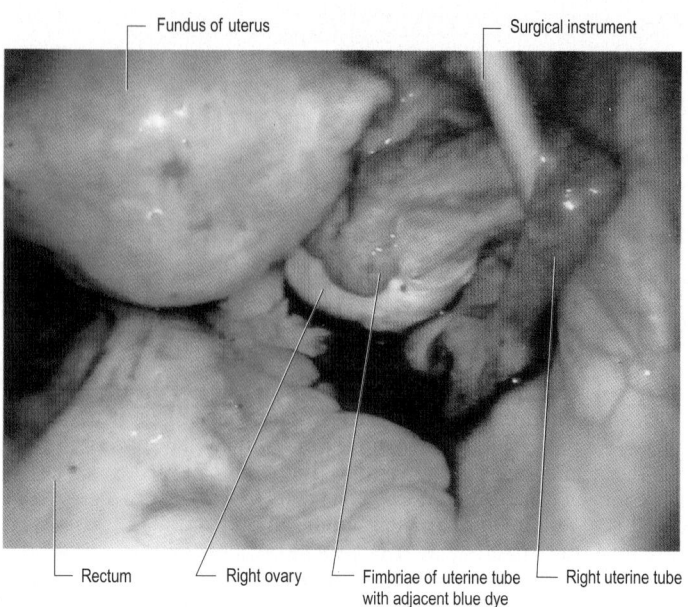

Fig. 103.4 Photograph taken at laparoscopy demonstrating the infundibulum of the uterine tube with its fimbriae. Blue dye has been injected through the cervix and is seen spilling from the infundibulum. This is a test of tubal patency in a woman with infertility.

Tubal inflammation sometimes results in the fimbriated end becoming blocked by adhesions. Pus may collect in the tube causing a pyosalpinx, or fluid may accumulate as a result of mucosal inflammation and this causes a hydrosalpinx. Pelvic peritonitis is said to occur more frequently in females because infection of the vagina, uterus or of the uterine tube may spread directly to the peritoneum via the abdominal ostium.

RELATIONS

The mesosalpinx is inferior, and the ovarian ligament is inferior and medial, to the tube (**Fig. 102.2**). The mesovarium and ovary lie inferiorly at its fimbrial end. The round ligament is anterior to the tube. The superior and posterior surfaces of the tube lie free in the peritoneal cavity (**Figs 102.1, 102.2**).

PERITONEAL ATTACHMENTS

The uterine tube is attached on its inferior surface to a double fold of peritoneum in the broad ligament called the mesosalpinx (p. 1332). The vessels, nerves and lymphatics that supply the uterine tube lie within the mesosalpinx (p. 1328).

VESTIGIAL STRUCTURES

The epoophoron (**Fig. 102.2**) lies in the lateral part of the mesosalpinx between the ovary and uterine tube. It consists of 10 to 15 short, blind-ending transverse ductules, which converge towards the ovary. Their other ends open into a rudimentary longitudinal duct, the duct of the epoophoron (duct of Gartner). This runs medially in the broad ligament, parallel with the lateral part of the uterine tube (p. 1332). There are often one or more small cystic vesicular appendices between the epoophoron and the fimbriated end of the tube. The duct of the epoophoron can occasionally be followed along the uterus nearly to the internal os where it penetrates the muscular wall of the uterus and descends in the wall of the cervix, gradually approaching the mucosa without actually reaching it. It then descends in the lateral wall of the vagina to end near or at the free margin of the hymen. The paroophoron consists of a few rudimentary tubules scattered in the broad ligament between the epoophoron and uterus, and is most easily seen in children. Both the epoophoron and paroophoron are remnants of mesonephric

tubules. The duct of the epoophoron is a persistent part of the mesonephric duct (p. 1375).

VASCULAR SUPPLY AND LYMPHATIC DRAINAGE

ARTERIES

The blood supply to the uterine tubes is derived from ovarian and uterine stems. The lateral third of the tube is supplied by the ovarian artery (p. 1323), which continues in the mesosalpinx to anastomose with branches from the uterine artery (p. 1333). The branches from the uterine artery supply the medial two-thirds of the tube.

VEINS

Venous drainage is similar to the arterial supply. The venous drainage for the lateral two-thirds of the uterine tube is via the pampiniform plexus to the ovarian veins. The latter open into the inferior vena cava on the right side and the renal vein on the left side. The medial two-thirds of the tube drain via the uterine plexus to the internal iliac vein.

LYMPHATIC DRAINAGE

Lymph drainage is via ovarian vessels to the para-aortic nodes (p. 1323) and uterine vessels to the internal iliac chain (p. 1323). It is possible for lymph to reach the inguinal nodes via the round ligament.

INNERVATION

Nerve fibres are distributed largely with the ovarian and uterine arteries. Most of the tube has a dual sympathetic and parasympathetic supply. Preganglionic parasympathetic fibres are derived from the vagus for the lateral half of the tube, and pelvic splanchnic nerves for the medial half. Sympathetic supply is derived from the tenth thoracic to the second lumbar spinal segments. Visceral afferent fibres travel with the sympathetic nerves, and enter the cord through corresponding dorsal roots. They may also accompany parasympathetic fibres. The ampullary submucosa contains modified Pacinian corpuscles.

REFERRED PAIN

Pain from tubal disease is classically described as occurring in the iliac fossa as a result of local peritoneal irritation. As with pain from the ovary (p. 1323), this can sometimes cause discomfort in the distribution of the obturator nerve on the medial aspect of the thigh.

MICROSTRUCTURE

The walls of the uterine tubes show typical visceral mucosal, muscular and serosal layers (pp. 41, 41). The mucosa is thrown into longitudinal folds (**Fig. 103.5**), which are most pronounced distally at the infundibulum and decrease to shallow bulges in the intrauterine (intramural) portion. The mucosa is lined by a single-layered, tall, columnar epithelium, which contains mainly ciliated cells and secretory (peg) cells (so-called because they project into the lumen further than their ciliated neighbours), and occasional intraepithelial lymphocytes. In the tube, ciliated cells predominate distally (**Fig. 103.5**) and secretory cells proximally. Their activities vary with the stage in the menstrual cycle and with age. Secretory cells are most active around the time of ovulation. Their secretions include nutrients for the gametes and aid capacitation of the spermatozoa. Ciliated cells increase in height and develop more cilia in the oestrogenic first half of the menstrual cycle. Their cilia waft the oocyte from the open-ended infundibulum towards the uterus in fluids secreted by the peg cells. The epithelium regresses in height towards the end of the cycle and postmenopausally, when ciliated cells are reduced in number.

The lamina propria provides vascular connective tissue support and abundant lymphatic drainage vessels. The smooth muscle of the muscularis is arranged as an inner circular, or spiral, layer and an outer, thinner, longitudinal layer. Together, their contractile activity produces peristaltic movements of the tube, which assist propulsion of the gametes and the fertilized ovum. The uterine tubes are covered externally by a highly vascular serosa.

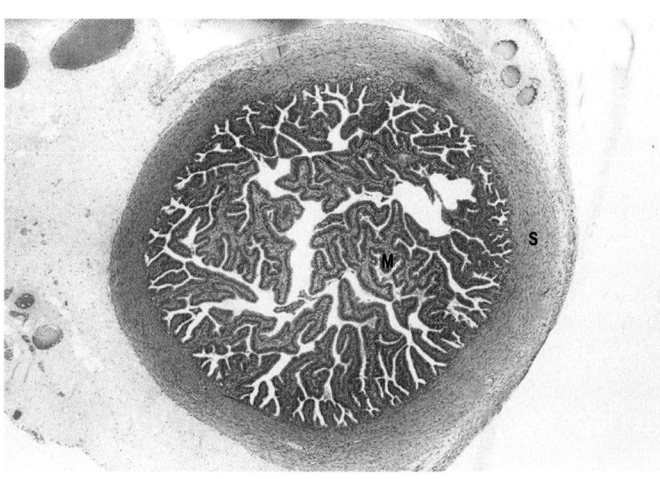

Fig. 103.5 Ampullary region of uterine tube showing the two layers of smooth muscle (S) surrounding the mucosa (M), with its complex folds projecting into the lumen. (By permission from Dr JB Kerr, Monash University, from Kerr JB 1999 Atlas of Functional Histology. London: Mosby.)

Uterus

The uterus is a hollow, thick-walled and muscular organ. It is normally situated in the lesser pelvis between the urinary bladder and the rectum (**Fig. 103.3**).

The uterus is divided into two main regions. The body of the uterus (corpus uteri) forms the upper two-thirds, and the cervix (cervix uteri) forms the lower third (**Figs 102.1, 104.1**). The body of the uterus is pear shaped and contains a lumen that is flat anteroposteriorly. The cervix is narrower and is cylindrical in shape. The uterine tubes are attached to the upper part of the body of the uterus with their ostia opening into the lumen (**Ch. 103**). The lower portion of the cervix continues into the vagina. The adult non-pregnant uterus is c.7.5 cm long, 5.0 cm in breadth, 2.5 cm thick, and weighs between 30 and 40 gm.

UTERINE BODY (CORPUS UTERI) (Figs 104.2, 104.3)

The body of the uterus extends from the fundus at its uppermost part to the cervix inferiorly (**Fig. 104.1**). Near its upper end, the body receives uterine tubes on both sides (**Figs 103.1, 103.2**). The point of fusion between the uterine tube and body is called the uterine cornu. Infero-anterior to the cornu is the round ligament and inferoposterior is the ovarian ligament (**Figs 103.3, 102.1, 102.2**). The fundus is superior to the entry points of the uterine tubes, and the uterine body narrows as it extends towards the cervix.

The dome-like fundus is covered by peritoneum, which is continuous with that of neighbouring surfaces. It is contacted by coils of small intestine and occasionally by distended sigmoid colon. The lateral margins of the body are convex, and on each side their peritoneum is reflected laterally to form the broad ligament, which extends as a flat sheet to the pelvic wall.

The anterior surface of the uterine body is covered by peritoneum, which is reflected onto the bladder at the uterovesical fold. This normally occurs at the level of the internal os, which is the most inferior margin of the body of the uterus. Between the bladder and uterus there is the vesico-uterine pouch, which is obliterated when the bladder is distended. When the bladder is empty, the vesico-uterine pouch is usually empty, but it may be occupied by part of the small intestine.

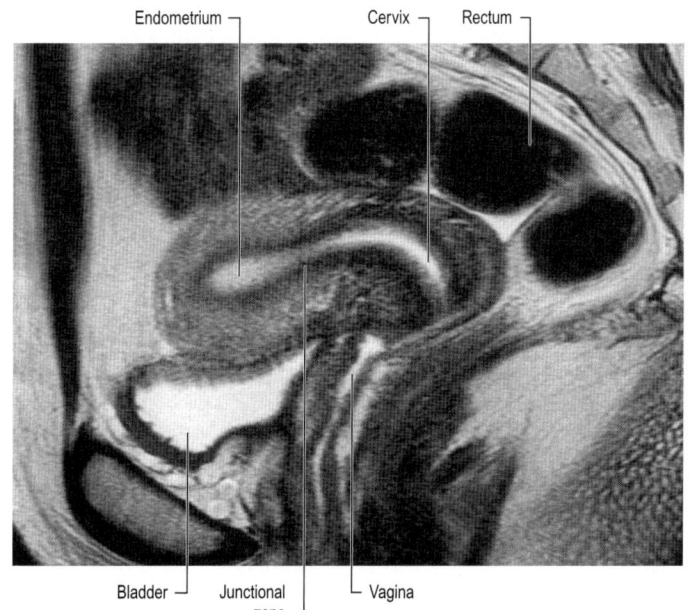

Fig. 104.2 Sagittal MRI in a young female. On T2-weighted MRI the uterus displays a zonal anatomy, with three distinct zones: the endometrium; junctional zone; and myometrium. The endometrium and uterine cavity appear as a high-signal stripe. A band of low signal, the junctional zone, borders the endometrium. This represents the inner myometrium, which blends with the low-signal band of fibrous cervical stroma at the level of the internal os.

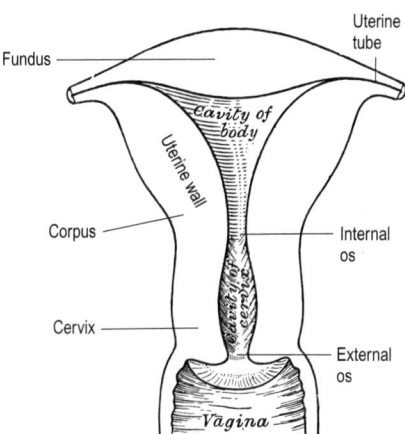

Fig. 104.1 Sectional diagram showing the interior divisions of the uterus and its continuity with the vagina.

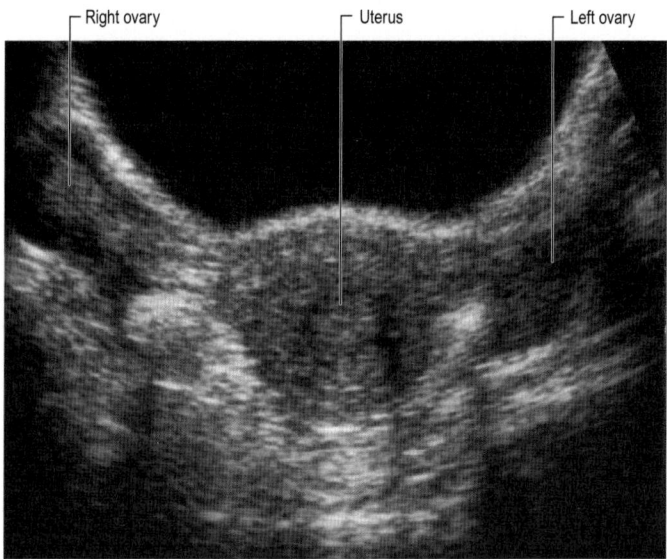

Fig. 104.3 Transabdominal ultrasound of the female pelvis showing the uterus and both ovaries.

The posterior surface of the uterus is convex transversely. Its peritoneal covering continues down to the cervix and upper vagina and is then reflected back to the rectum (**Fig. 102.1**) along the surface of the recto-uterine pouch (of Douglas), which lies posterior to the uterus. The sigmoid colon lies posterior to the uterus, although the terminal ileal coil usually separates the two.

The cavity of the uterine body measures c.6 cm from the external os of the cervix to the wall of the fundus and is flat in its anteroposterior plane (**Figs 103.1, 104.1**). In coronal section (**Fig. 104.1**) it is triangular, broad above where the two uterine tubes join the uterus, and narrow below at the internal os of the cervix.

CERVIX (CERVIX UTERI)

The adult, non-pregnant cervix is c.2.5 cm long. It is narrower and more cylindrical than the corpus, is widest at its midlevel, and round in section. The upper end communicates with the uterine body via the internal os and the lower end opens into the vagina at the external os. In nulliparous women, the external os is usually a circular aperture, whereas after childbirth it is a transverse slit. There are two longitudinal ridges, one each on its anterior and posterior walls, that give off small oblique palmate folds. These ascend laterally like the branches of a tree (arbor vitae uteri). The folds on opposing walls interdigitate to close the canal. The narrower isthmus of the cervix forms the upper third. Although unaffected in the first month of pregnancy, it is gradually taken up into the uterine body during the second month to form the 'lower uterine segment'. In non-pregnant women the isthmus undergoes menstrual changes, although these are less pronounced than those in the uterine body.

The external end of the cervix bulges into the anterior wall of the vagina, which divides it into supravaginal and vaginal regions (**Figs 102.1, 104.4**). The supravaginal part of the cervix is separated in front from the bladder by cellular connective tissue, the parametrium, which also passes to the sides of the cervix and laterally between the two layers of the broad ligaments. The uterine arteries flank the cervix in this tissue and the ureters descend forwards in it c.2 cm from the cervix, curving under the arch formed by the uterine arteries. The relation of the arteries to the ureters is not always symmetrical. Posteriorly the supravaginal cervix is covered by peritoneum, which continues caudally on to the posterior vaginal wall and is then reflected onto the rectum via the recto-uterine recess (**Fig. 102.1**). Posteriorly, it is related to the rectum, from which it may be separated by a terminal ileal coil.

The vaginal part of the cervix projects into the vaginal cavity forming grooves around its perimeter termed vaginal fornices.

VARIATIONS

Sometimes there is failure in fusion of the paramesonephric (Müllerian) ducts. This results in a uterus that is not pear shaped and has a varying degree of septation. The most extreme example is often **associated with a septate vagina, two cervices, and two discrete uteri each** with one uterine tube (**Fig. 109.15**). This is called a didelphine uterus. Sometimes there is just a septum (septate uterus) or partial clefting of the uterus (bicornuate uterus).

RELATIONS AND POSITIONS (Fig. 104.4)

The bladder and uterovesical space are anterior to the uterus. The rectum and the recto-uterine pouch are posterior. The broad ligaments are lateral to the uterus. The long axis usually lies along the axis of the pelvic inlet, but since the uterus is movable, its position varies with distension of the bladder and rectum. Except when displaced by a much distended bladder, the long axis of the uterus is nearly at right angles to that of the vagina; the axis of the vagina corresponds to the axis of the pelvic outlet.

In the adult nulliparous state the uterus normally tilts forward along its long axis (**Fig. 104.4**), a state which is normally described as anteflexed. With the bladder empty the whole uterus leans forwards at an angle to the vagina, and in this position is described as anteverted. In 10 to 15% of women the whole uterus leans backwards at an angle to the vagina and is said to be retroverted. A uterus that angles backwards on the cervix is described as retroflexed.

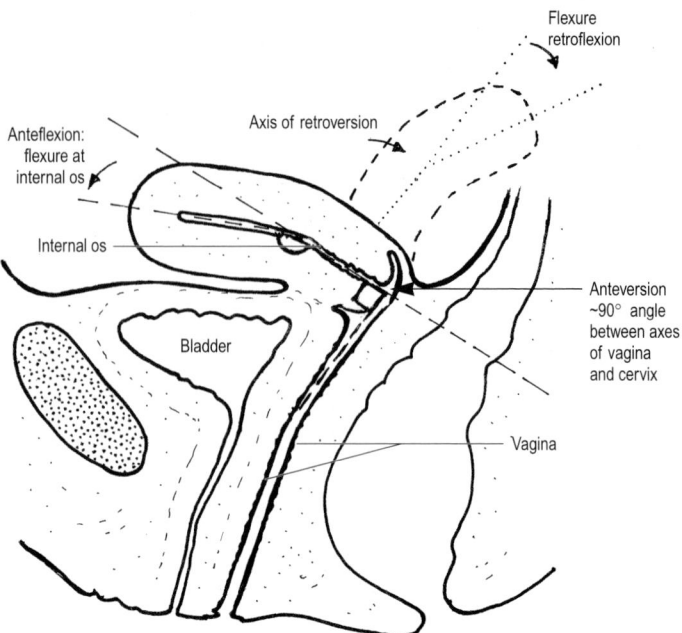

Fig. 104.4 Variations in uterine position.

UTERINE LIGAMENTS

The uterus is continuous with a number of 'ligaments'. Some of these are true ligaments in that they have a fibrous composition and supply support to the uterus. Some ligaments provide no support to the uterus, and others only consist of folds of peritoneum.

PERITONEAL FOLDS
The peritoneal folds are the anterior and posterior ligaments of the uterus, and the broad ligament.

Uterovesical fold
The uterovesical fold or anterior ligament consists of peritoneum reflected onto the bladder from the uterus at the junction of its cervix and body.

Rectovaginal fold
The rectovaginal fold or posterior ligament consists of peritoneum reflected from the posterior vaginal fornix on to the front of the rectum, thereby forming the deep recto-uterine pouch. It is bounded anteriorly by the uterus, supravaginal cervix and posterior vaginal fornix. Posteriorly it is bounded by the rectum. Laterally it is bounded by the uterosacral ligaments (p. 1333).

Broad ligament
The broad ligaments extend, one from each side of the uterus, to the lateral walls of the pelvis, where they become continuous with the peritoneum. The upper border is free. The lower border is continuous with the peritoneum over the bladder, rectum and pelvic sidewall. They are continuous with each other at the free edge via the uterine fundus and diverge below near the superior surfaces of levatores ani. In the free border on either side lies a uterine tube.

The uterus and the broad ligament form a septum across the lesser pelvic cavity, dividing it into an anterior part containing the bladder and a posterior part containing the rectum, terminal ileum and part of the sigmoid colon. With the bladder empty, the uterus and broad ligament are inclined forwards so that the posterior surface faces up and back, and the anterior surface faces down and forwards. As the bladder fills, the plane of the ligament tilts backwards and the free borders become superior so that the layers face anteriorly and posteriorly. The broad ligament is divided into an upper mesosalpinx, a posterior mesovarium and an inferior mesometrium.

Mesosalpinx – The mesosalpinx is attached above to the uterine tube and posteroinferiorly to the mesovarium. Superior and laterally it is attached to the suspensory ligament of the ovary and medially it is attached to the ovarian ligament. The fimbria of the tubal infundibulum projects from its free lateral end. Between the ovary and uterine tube the mesosalpinx contains vascular anastomoses between the uterine and ovarian vessels, the epoophoron, and the paroophoron (p. 1384).

Mesovarium – The mesovarium projects from the posterior aspect of the broad ligament, of which it is the smaller part. It is attached to the hilum of the ovary and carries vessels and nerves to the ovary.

Mesometrium – The mesometrium is the largest part of the broad ligament, and extends from the pelvic floor to the ovarian ligament and uterine body. The uterine artery passes between its two peritoneal layers c.1.5 cm lateral to the cervix. The uterine artery crosses the ureter shortly after its origin from the internal iliac artery and gives off a branch that passes superiorly to the uterine tube, where it anastomoses with the ovarian artery. Between the pyramid formed by the infundibulum of the tube, the upper pole of the ovary, and the lateral pelvic wall, the mesometrium contains ovarian vessels and nerves within a fibrous suspensory ligament of the ovary (infundibulopelvic ligament). This ligament continues laterally over the external iliac vessels as a distinct fold. The mesometrium also encloses the proximal part of the round ligament of the uterus, as well as smooth muscle and loose connective tissue.

LIGAMENTS

These consist of the round, uterosacral, transverse cervical and pubocervical ligaments.

Round ligaments

The round ligaments are narrow somewhat flattened bands 10 to 12 cm long, which pass diagonally down and laterally within the mesometrium from the upper part of the uterus to the pelvic floor. They are attached superiorly to the uterine wall just below and anterior to the lateral cornua. Each ligament continues laterally downwards across the vesical, obturator and external iliac vessels, the obturator nerve, and the obliterated umbilical artery. At the start of the inferior epigastric artery, the round ligament enters the deep inguinal ring. It traverses the inguinal canal and finally splits into strands that merge with surrounding connective tissue terminating in the mons pubis above the labium majus. Near the uterus the round ligament contains much smooth muscle but this gradually diminishes until the terminal part is purely fibrous. It contains blood vessels, nerves and lymphatics. The latter drain the uterine region around the entry of the uterine tube to the superficial inguinal lymph nodes. Uterine neoplasms may spread by this route. In the fetus a projection of the peritoneum (processus vaginalis) is carried with the round ligament for a short distance into the inguinal canal. This is generally obliterated in adults, although it is sometimes patent even in old age. In the canal the ligament receives the same coverings as the spermatic cord, although they are thinner and blend with the ligament itself, which may not reach the mons pubis. The round and ovarian ligaments both develop from the gubernaculum (p. 1389) and are continuous.

Uterosacral ligaments

The uterosacral ligaments are recto-uterine folds and contain fibrous tissue and smooth muscle. They pass back from the cervix and uterine body on both sides of the rectum, and they are attached to the front of the sacrum. The ligaments can be palpated laterally on rectal examination. On vaginal examination they can be felt as thick bands of tissue passing downwards on both sides of the posterior fornix.

Transverse cervical ligaments

The transverse cervical ligaments (cardinal ligaments, ligaments of Mackenrodt) extend from the side of the cervix and lateral fornix of the vagina to attach extensively on the pelvic wall. At the level of the cervix, some fibres interdigitate with fibres of the uterosacral ligaments. They are continuous with the fibrous tissue around the lower parts of the ureters and pelvic blood vessels.

Pubocervical ligament

Fibres of the pubocervical ligament pass forward from the anterior aspect of the cervix and upper vagina to diverge around the urethra. These fibres attach to the posterior aspect of the pubic bones.

UTERINE SUPPORT

While the uterosacral and transverse cervical ligaments may act in varying measure as mechanical supports of the uterus, levatores ani and coccygei, the urogenital diaphragm and the perineal body appear at least as important in this respect. There has been renewed interest in the supporting structures of the pelvis, and the subject has been reviewed in detail by DeLancey (2000).

Occasionally, the muscular and ligamentous support of the uterus fails, which results in prolapse of the uterus through the vagina. In the most extreme example, procidentia, it prolapses all the way through the vagina. Uterine prolapse usually occurs in association with prolapse of other organs such as the vagina and rectum. It is more common in women who have gone through childbirth and is the result of successive weakening of the pelvic floor during parturition. There is also an inherited component to pelvic-floor prolapse.

VASCULAR SUPPLY AND LYMPHATIC DRAINAGE

ARTERIES

The uterine artery arises as a branch of the anterior division of the internal iliac artery and crosses anterior to the ureter to give off two main branches. These pass superiorly and inferiorly along the lateral surface of the uterus. The uterine artery supplies the uterine body, the uterine cervix, the uterine tubes, and the upper part of the vagina.

From its origin, the uterine artery crosses the ureter anteriorly in the broad ligament before branching at the level of the uterus. One major branch ascends the uterus tortuously within the broad ligament until it reaches the region of the ovarian hilum where it anastomoses with branches of the ovarian artery. Another branch descends to supply the cervix and anastomoses with branches of the vaginal artery to form two median longitudinal vessels, the azygos arteries of the vagina, which descend anterior and posterior to the vagina. Although there are anastomoses with the ovarian and vaginal arteries, the dominance of the uterine artery is indicated by its marked hypertrophy during pregnancy.

The tortuosity of the vessels as they ascend in the broad ligaments is repeated in their branches within the uterine wall. Each uterine artery gives off numerous branches. These enter the uterine wall, divide and run circumferentially as groups of anterior and posterior arcuate arteries. They ramify and narrow as they approach the anterior and posterior midline so that no large vessels are present in these regions. However, the left and right arterial trees anastomose across the midline and unilateral ligation can be performed without serious effects. The arcuate arteries supply many tortuous radial branches, which pass centripetally through the deeper myometrial layers, supplying these *en route*, to reach the endometrium.

Terminal branches in the uterine muscle are tortuous and are called helicine arterioles. They provide a series of dense capillary plexuses in the myometrium and endometrium. From the arcuate arteries many helical arteriolar rami pass into the endometrium. Their detailed appearance changes during the menstrual cycle. In the proliferative phase helical arterioles are less prominent, whereas they grow in length and calibre, becoming even more tortuous in the secretory phase.

VEINS

The venous drainage of the uterus is via the uterine veins, which extend laterally in the broad ligaments and drain into the internal iliac veins. The uterine veins run a course adjacent to the arteries in the broad ligament and pass over the ureters. The uterine venous plexus anastomoses with the vaginal and ovarian venous plexuses.

LYMPHATIC DRAINAGE

Uterine lymphatics exist in the superficial (subperitoneal) and deep parts of the uterine wall. Collecting vessels from the cervix pass laterally in the parametrium to the external iliac nodes, posterolaterally to the internal iliac nodes, and posteriorly to the rectal and sacral nodes. Some cervical efferents may reach the obturator or gluteal nodes. Vessels from the lower part of the uterine body pass mostly to the external iliac nodes, with those from the cervix. From the upper part of the body, the fundus and the uterine tubes, vessels accompany those of the ovaries to the lateral aortic and pre-aortic nodes. A few pass to the external iliac nodes. The region surrounding the isthmic part of the uterine tube is drained along the round ligament to the superficial inguinal nodes. Uterine lymph vessels enlarge greatly during pregnancy.

INNERVATION

Uterine nerves arise predominantly from the inferior hypogastric plexus. Some branches descend with the vaginal arteries. Other branches pass directly to the cervix uteri. Some branches ascend with, or near, the uterine arteries in the broad ligament.

Nerves to the cervix form a plexus that contains small paracervical ganglia. Sometimes one ganglion is larger and is termed the uterine cervical ganglion. Nerves accompanying the uterine arteries supply the uterine body and tube, and connect with tubal nerves from the inferior hypogastric plexus and with the ovarian plexus. The uterine nerves ramify in the myometrium and endometrium, and usually accompany the vessels. Efferent preganglionic sympathetic fibres are derived from the last thoracic and first lumbar spinal segments. The sites of their postganglionic neurones are unknown. Preganglionic parasympathetic fibres arise in the second to fourth sacral spinal segments and relay in the paracervical ganglia. Sympathetic activity may produce uterine contraction and vasoconstriction and parasympathetic activity may produce uterine inhibition and vasodilatation, but these activities are complicated by hormonal control of uterine functions.

MICROSTRUCTURE

The uterine wall is composed of three main layers. From its lumen outwards these are the endometrium (mucosa), myometrium (smooth muscle layer) and perimetrium (serosa) or adventitia, depending on region. The myometrium is by far the largest component.

ENDOMETRIUM

The mucosal layer forming the endometrium is continuous below with the vaginal mucosa through the external os, and with the peritoneum through the abdominal os of the uterine tubes. It is formed by a layer of connective tissue, the endometrial stroma, which supports a single-layered columnar epithelium continuous with large numbers of tubular endometrial (uterine) glands running perpendicular to the luminal surface or slightly coiled (**Fig. 104.5**). These glands penetrate as far as the boundary with the myometrium. In the uterine body the surface epithelium is ciliated and cuboidal before puberty but becomes columnar and is usually non-ciliated over large areas in the adult uterus. The endometrial glands are composed largely of columnar cells secreting glycoproteins and glycogen, variably with the stages of the menstrual cycle (p. 1335). The stroma consists of a highly cellular connective tissue between the endometrial glands, and contains blood and lymphatic vessels. The endometrium undergoes a number of changes during the menstrual cycle (p. 1335). For a review of endometrial structure see Spornitz (1992).

Endometriosis

In some women, endometrial tissue can exist outside the uterus, a condition called endometriosis. This can occur anywhere, including the lung and bowel, but is most common on the pelvic peritoneum and ovary. Endometriosis may result in a number of symptoms which correlate with the cyclical hormonal influences that occur on endometrial cells. When endometriosis occurs in the pelvis, women develop painful periods and painful intercourse. When endometriosis occurs on the ovary, a cyst of endometrial tissue, an endometrioma, can occur. These are sometimes called chocolate cysts because they contain old blood from repeated monthly haemorrhage into the cyst. The cause of endometriosis is unknown. However, a number of theories exist, including retrograde menstruation and abnormal cell development.

MYOMETRIUM (Fig. 104.5)

The myometrium is a fibromuscular layer that forms most of the uterine wall. In nulliparous women it is dense and c.1.3 cm thick at the uterine midlevel and fundus but thin at the tubal orifices. It is composed largely of smooth muscle fasciculi mingled with loose connective tissue, blood vessels, lymphatic vessels and nerves.

The body of the uterus is often described as having four more or less distinct muscular layers. The innermost layer (submucosal layer) is composed mostly of longitudinal and some oblique smooth muscle.

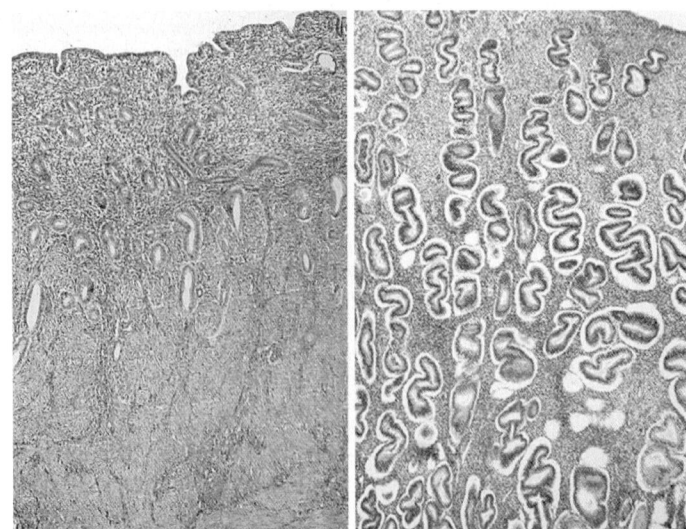

Fig. 104.5 **A**, Low-power micrograph of the uterine wall, including endometrium, glands and myometrium. **B**, Higher-power micrograph of the endometrium, showing the coiled glands typical of the secretory second half of the menstrual cycle. (By permission from Kierszenbaum AL 2002 Histology and Cell Biology. St Louis: Mosby.)

Where the lumen of the uterine tube passes through the uterine wall, this layer forms a circular muscle coat. External to the submucosal layer is the vascular layer, a zone rich in blood vessels as well as longitudinal muscle. Next is a layer of predominantly circular muscle, the supra-vascular layer. The outer, thin, longitudinal muscle layer, the subserosal layer, lies adjacent to the perimetrium.

The fibromuscular fascicles of the outer two layers converge at the lateral angles of the uterus, and continue into the uterine tubes and the round and ovarian ligaments. Some fascicles enter the broad ligaments, others turn back into the uterosacral ligaments. At the junction between the body and the cervix, the smooth muscle merges with dense irregular connective tissue containing both collagen and elastin, and forms the majority of the cervical wall.

Bilateral longitudinal fascicles extend in the lateral submucosal layer from the fundal angle to the cervix. Their muscle fibres differ structurally from those of typical myometrium, and they may provide fast conducting pathways which coordinate the contractile activities of the uterine wall.

During pregnancy the muscle hypertrophies, and the individual fibres are greatly enlarged. Their numbers also increase by proliferative hyperplasia. The numbers of gap junctions coupling adjacent fibres also increase, indicating greater coordination of their contractility. During pregnancy, contractility is inhibited by relaxin, which is secreted by the ovarian corpus luteum and placenta (p. 1325).

Leiomyoma

Benign tumours of myometrial cells are are called leiomyomata (fibroids). The aetiology of these benign tumours is unknown. However, they are more common in women of Afro-Caribbean origin than in Caucasian women. Over a third of women of reproductive age have fibroids. If they project predominantly into the cavity of the uterus they are termed submucous fibroids. Submucous fibroids increase the surface area of the endometrium and can result in heavy menstrual bleeding. Fibroids that are predominantly on the surface of the uterus are called subserous and those that exist predominantly within the myometrium are called intramural. Most women have no symptoms from their fibroids but occasionally they can get pain from a degenerating fibroid as well as excessive menstrual blood loss. Large fibroids can cause particular problems in pregnancy where they are more likely to degenerate and cause pain and can also obstruct labour. Occasionally a fibroid may develop a blood supply from another organ such as the omentum. It then loses its supply from the uterus and becomes a parasytic fibroid.

Adenomyosis

Sometimes areas of endometrial tissue can exist deep within the myometrium. This tissue responds to cyclical changes in oestrogen and progesterone. However, as the endometrial lining cannot be expelled through the cervix, and is in effect trapped, it causes painful periods. This condition is known as adenomyosis and is characterized by ill-defined thickening of the low signal junctional zone and sometimes areas of high signal on MRI scans.

PERIMETRIUM

The perimetrium (serosa) is composed of peritoneum (mesothelium overlying a thin connective tissue lamina propria), which covers the uterine body and supravaginal cervix posteriorly, but anteriorly covers only the body. Over the most inferior quarter of the uterine length the peritoneum is separated posteriorly from the underlying uterus by loose cellular connective tissue and large veins. Beneath the peritoneum there is a subserous layer of loose, more fibrous tissue.

UTERINE CERVIX (Fig. 104.6)

Except for the lower part, the uterine cervix is lined by a single-layered, columnar epithelium with tubular glands, which overlies a fibroelastic connective tissue stroma containing relatively little smooth muscle. The elastic component of the cervical stroma is essential to the stretching capacity of the cervix during childbirth. Its lower region (approximately one-third, but variable), including its vaginal surface, is covered by non-keratinizing stratified squamous epithelium, which contains glycogen. None of the mucosa is shed during menstruation and so, unlike the body of the uterus, it is not divided into functional and basal layers and lacks spiral arteries.

For most of the upper part of the endocervical canal the mucosa is c.3 mm thick. It is lined by a deeply folded surface epithelium of columnar mucous cells continuous with branched tubular cervical glands, which are lined by a similar secretory epithelium (**Fig. 104.6**). Ciliated cells are also present in patches at the surface. The cervical glands extend obliquely upwards and outwards from the canal. They secrete clear, alkaline mucus, which is relatively viscous except at the midpoint of the menstrual cycle, when their more copious, less viscous, secretions favour sperm motility. Not uncommonly, the aperture of a gland becomes blocked and it then fills with mucus to form a Nabothian cyst (or follicle), up to 5 mm or more in diameter.

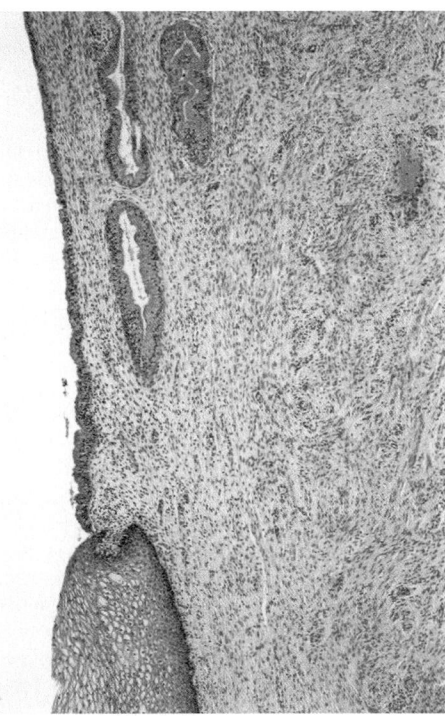

Fig. 104.6 The transformation zone of the uterine cervix. The single-layered columnar epithelium of the endocervical canal (above left) changes abruptly to the stratified squamous non-keratinizing epithelium (below) of the external os and ectocervix. (Photograph by Sarah-Jane Smith.)

The squamocolumnar junction between the columnar secretory epithelium of the endocervical canal and the stratified squamous covering of the ectocervix is abrupt (**Fig. 104.6**). Its precise location varies with age and, to a lesser extent, with the stage in the menstrual cycle. It approximates to the position of the external os, which is its usual prepubertal location. At puberty, the endocervical columnar epithelium responds to oestrogenic stimulation and extends distally on the ectocervix. This area of columnar cells on the ectocervix forms an area that is red and raw in appearance called an ectropion (cervical erosion). It is then exposed to the acidic environment of the vagina (p. 1353) and through a process of squamous metaplasia, a stratified squamous ectocervical epithelium effectively regrows over the exposed area, resulting in a transformation zone. Other hyperoestrogenic states such as pregnancy and the use of oral contraceptive pills can also result in an ectropion. This is important clinically as this area is the most usual site of epithelial abnormalities that may progress to malignancy. In addition, the new stratified epithelium frequently occludes the ducts of endocervical glands in the region and Nabothian cysts develop. In postmenopausal women, the squamocolumnar junction recedes into the endocervical canal.

CYCLICAL CHANGES IN THE UTERUS

Throughout the period of reproductive life (except during pregnancy and lactation), a series of closely interrelated cyclical changes occur in the ovary, uterus and vagina. Each cycle extends over a period of c.28 days. In the ovarian cycle one follicle usually reaches full maturity, ruptures and releases its secondary oocyte. The wall of the follicle is then transformed into an important endocrine gland, the corpus luteum. About 10 days after ovulation the corpus luteum begins to regress, then ceases to function and is replaced by fibrous tissue.

The changes of the uterine cycle (menstrual cycle) chiefly involve the lining endometrium of the body and fundus of the uterus and may be divided into three phases: menstrual; proliferative; and secretory.

MENSTRUAL PHASE (Fig. 104.7)

Prior to menstruation three strata can be recognized in the endometrium (**Fig. 104.7**). These are the stratum compactum, spongiosum and basale. In the stratum compactum, next to the free surface, the necks of the glands are only slightly expanded and the stromal cells show a distinct decidual reaction. In the stratum spongiosum, the uterine glands are tortuous, dilated and ultimately only separated from one another by a small amount of interglandular tissue. The stratum basale, next to the uterine muscle, is thin and contains the tips of the uterine glands embedded in an unaltered stroma.

The upper two strata are often grouped together as the functional layer, stratum functionalis, of the endometrium, and the lower (basal) layer is the stratum basalis. As regression of the corpus luteum occurs, those parts of the stroma showing a decidual reaction together with the glandular epithelium undergo degenerative changes and the endometrium often diminishes in thickness. Blood escapes from the superficial vessels of the endometrium forming small haematomata beneath the surface epithelium. The superficial part of the endometrium, next to the free surface, is shed piecemeal, leaving mainly the basal zone, adjacent to the uterine muscle (**Fig. 104.7**). Approximately two-thirds to three-quarters of the thickness of the endometrium may be shed. Blood and necrotic endometrium then begin to appear in the uterine lumen, and are discharged from the uterus through the vagina. This menstrual flow lasts from 3 to 6 days. The amount of tissue lost is variable, but usually the stratum compactum and most of the spongiosum are desquamated.

PROLIFERATIVE PHASE (Fig. 104.8)

In the early proliferative phase, and even before the menstrual flow ceases, the epithelium from the persisting basal parts of the uterine glands grows luminally over the denuded surface of the endometrium. Re-epithelialization is complete by 5 to 6 days after the start of menstruation. Initially the tissue is only 1–2 mm thick and lined by low cuboidal epithelium. The glands are straight and narrow with short columnar cells. The apical cell surface contains microvilli, and some ciliated cells are present. The stroma is dense and contains small numbers of lymphocytes among the larger population of mesenchymally derived

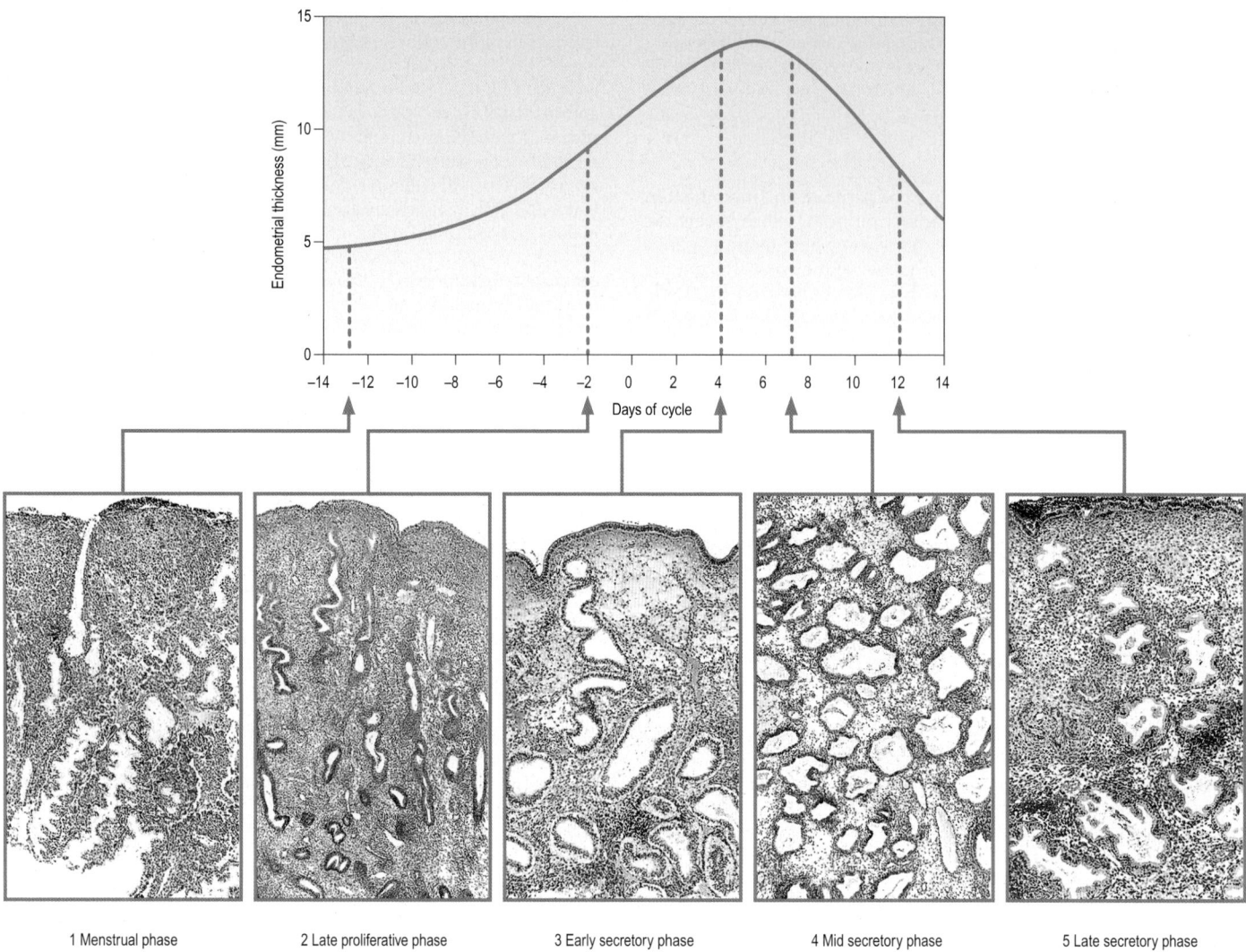

1 Menstrual phase   2 Late proliferative phase   3 Early secretory phase   4 Mid secretory phase   5 Late secretory phase

Fig. 104.7 Stages in the menstrual cycle. The top panel shows the variation in thickness of endometrium during an idealized 28-day cycle in which ovulation occurs at day 0. Measurements were made by transvaginal ultrasound. The five lower panels are histological sections of endometrium at the cycle times indicated. (By permission from Buckley CH, Fox H 1989 Biopsy Pathology of the Endometrium. London: Chapman and Hall Medical.)

cells. During days 10 to 12 of the proliferative phase the endometrium grows in response to the presence in the bloodstream of oestrogen produced by the ovary (**Fig. 104.8**), which acts through receptors present on both the stromal and epithelial cells of the endometrium. Mitoses are seen and the glands become distinctly tortuous. Their lining epithelial cells become tall columnar (**Fig. 104.7**).

SECRETORY PHASE (Fig. 104.9)

The secretory phase coincides with the luteal phase of the ovarian cycle. Ovulation occurs c.14 days before the onset of the next menstrual flow. The changes occurring in the secretory phase depend upon the presence in the bloodstream of progesterone and oestrogens, secreted by the corpus luteum (**Fig. 104.8**). Steroid receptors in the endometrium respond by activating a programme of new gene expression to produce, in the following 7 days, a highly regulated sequence of differentiative events, which are presumably required to prepare the tissue for blastocyst implantation. Part of the response is direct, but there is evidence that some of the effects may be mediated through growth factors. The first morphological effects of progesterone are evident 24 to 36 hours after ovulation. In the early secretory phase, glycogen masses (known incorrectly as 'subnuclear vacuoles') appear in the basal cytoplasm of the epithelial cells lining the glands, where they are often associated with lipid. Nuclei are thus displaced towards the centre of the cells (**Fig. 104.9**). Giant mitochondria appear and are associated with semi-rough endoplasmic reticulum. A prominent nuclear channel system is present. A notable increase in polarization of the gland cells occurs and Golgi apparatus and secretory vesicles accumulate in the supranuclear

cytoplasm. Nascent secretory products may be detected immuno-histochemically within the gland cells. Progestational effects on the stroma are also evident in the early secretory phase. Nuclear enlargement occurs and the packing density of the resident mesenchymal cells increases, due in part to the increase in volume of gland lumens and onset of secretory activity in the epithelial compartment.

By the mid-secretory phase the endometrium may be up to 6 mm deep. The basal epithelial glycogen mass is progressively transferred to the apical cytoplasm, allowing the return of nuclei to the cell base. The Golgi apparatus becomes dilated and products including glycogen, mucin and other glycoproteins are released from the glandular epithelium into the lumen by a combination of apocrine and exocrine mechanisms: this activity reaches a maximum c.6 days after ovulation. These secretory changes are considerably less pronounced in the basal gland cells and the luminal epithelium than in the glandular cell population of the stratum functionalis. There is a notable stromal oedema and a corresponding decrease in the density of collagen fibrils. At the same time the endoplasmic reticulum and Golgi apparatus become more prominent, and there is evidence for the synthesis of collagen as well as its endocytosis and degradation, presumably reflecting matrix remodelling.

In the late secretory phase glandular secretory activity declines. Decidual differentiation occurs in the superficial stromal cells surrounding blood vessels. This transformation includes rounding of the nucleus and an increase in the cytoplasmic volume with a concurrent increase and dilatation of the rough endoplasmic reticulum and Golgi systems and cytoplasmic accumulation of lipid droplets and glycogen.

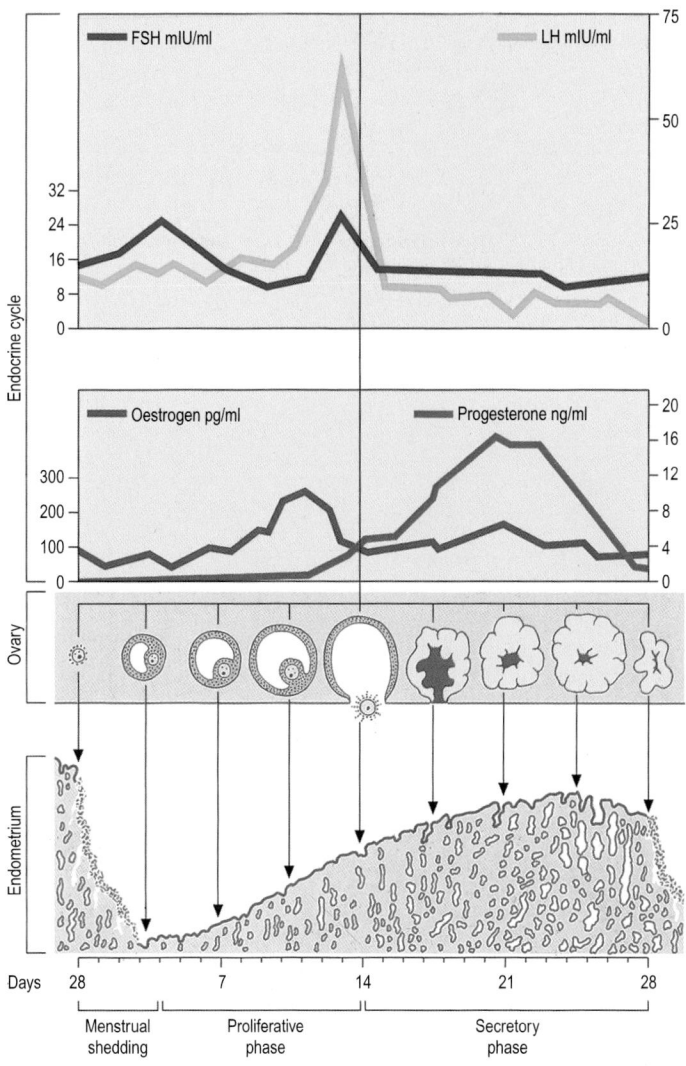

Fig. 104.8 Some salient features of the female reproductive cycle. Note the periodic changes that occur during the non-pregnant state of the ovarian cycle and the concomitant endometrial changes of the menstrual (uterine) cycle, and variations in circulating plasma hormone levels, and the consequences of pregnancy. FSH, follicle stimulating hormone; LH, luteinizing hormone. (Modified from Wendell-Smith CP, Williams PL, Treadgold S 1984 Basic Human Embryology, 3rd edn. Baltimore: Urban and Schwarzenberg.)

The cells begin to produce basal lamina components including laminin and type IV collagen.

VASCULAR CHANGES DURING THE MENSTRUAL CYCLE

The vascular bed of the endometrium undergoes significant changes during the menstrual cycle. The arteries to the endometrium arise from a myometrial plexus and consist of short, straight vessels to the basal portion of the endometrium and more muscular spiral arteries to its superficial two-thirds. The capillary bed consists of an endothelium with a basal lamina that is discontinuous in the proliferative phase, becoming more distinct by the mid-secretory phase. Pericytes are present, some of which resemble smooth muscle cells, and these are sometimes enclosed within the basal lamina. The pericytes make contact with the endothelial cells by means of cytoplasmic extensions that project through the basal lamina. Enlargement of the pericytes starts in the early secretory phase and leads to a conspicuous cuff of cells in the mid- and late-secretory phases. The venous drainage, consisting of narrow perpendicular vessels that anastomose by cross branches, is common to both the superficial and basal layers of the endometrium. The arterial supply to the basal part of the endometrium remains unchanged during the menstrual cycle. However, the spiral arteries to the superficial strata lengthen disproportionately. They become increasingly coiled and their tips approach more closely the uterine epithelium during the secretory phase of the menstrual cycle. This leads to a slowing of the circulation

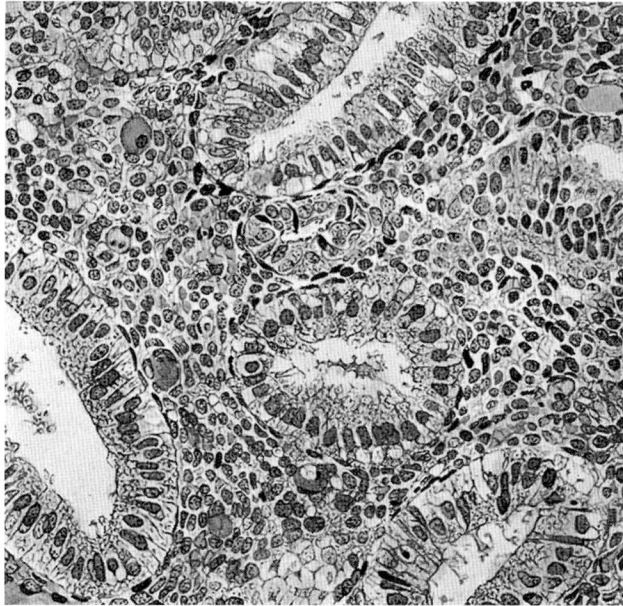

Fig. 104.9 Section of human endometrium at about day 17 of the menstrual cycle (early secretory phase). The accumulation of secretory material in the basal parts of the epithelial cells lining the glands has displaced the nuclei towards the lumen of the gland. (Lent by Gordon Museum, London.)

in the superficial strata with some vasodilation. Immediately before the menstrual flow these vessels begin to constrict intermittently, causing stasis of the blood and anaemia of the superficial strata. During the periods of relaxation of the vessels, blood escapes from the devitalized capillaries and veins, thus causing the menstrual blood loss.

During the proliferative, early, and mid-secretory phases of the cycle, the bone-marrow derived cells present in the endometrium are mainly macrophages and classic T cells, and there are very few B cells. In the late secretory phase, an unusual, large, granular lymphocyte population is recruited to the tissue and is found mainly in the stromal compartment.

If fertilization of the ovum does not occur, the corpus luteum undergoes degeneration. The breakdown of the endometrium that follows this cessation of function is due to the reducing levels of progesterone and oestrogen.

MAGNETIC RESONANCE IMAGING OF THE UTERUS (Fig. 104.2)

On T2-weighted magnetic resonance imaging (MRI) (Fig. 104.2), the uterus displays a zonal anatomy, with three distinct zones: the endometrium; junctional zone; and myometrium. The endometrium and uterine cavity appear as a high-signal stripe the thickness of which varies with the menstrual cycle. In the early proliferative phase it measures up to 5 mm, widening to up to 1 cm in the mid-secretory phase. A band of low signal, the junctional zone, borders the endometrium. This represents the inner myometrium, which blends with the low-signal band of fibrous cervical stroma at the level of the internal os. The junctional zone appears low signal because the cells of the myometrium have a low water content when compared to those of the outer myometrium. The junctional zone is of constant thickness and signal throughout the menstrual cycle, measuring c.5 mm. The outer myometrium is of medium signal intensity in the proliferative phase, becoming of high signal intensity in the mid-secretory phase because of the increased vascularity and prominence of the arcuate vessels.

In prepubertal females, the uterus is smaller (only 4 cm in length) and on T2-weighted images the endometrium is minimal or absent, with an indistinct junctional zone. In postmenopausal women, the corpus decreases in size and the zonal anatomy is indistinct.

On T2-weighted MRI the cervix has an inner low-signal stroma continuous with the junctional zone of the uterus. Often this is surrounded by an outer zone of intermediate signal intensity, which is continuous with the outer myometrium. The appearances do not change with the menstrual cycle or oral contraceptive pill use. The central stripe is very high signal and is a consequence of the secretions produced by the endocervical glands.

REFERENCES

DeLancey JO 2000 Anatomy. In: Stanton SL, Monga A (eds) Clinical Urogynaecology, 2nd edition. London: Churchill Livingstone.
An overview of the support of the pelvic floor in relation to female prolapse and incontinence.

Spornitz UM 1992 The functional morphology of the human endometrium and decidua. Adv Anat Embryol Cell Biol 124: 1–99.

Implantation, placentation, pregnancy and parturition

FERTILIZATION AND IMPLANTATION

Fertilization usually occurs in the lateral or ampullary part of the uterine tube, and is followed c.26–40 hours later by the first cleavage. The dividing preimplantation embryo is conveyed along the tube to the uterine cavity by ciliary action and is aided by muscular tubal contractions. The journey takes c.3 days. The blastocyst adheres to the endometrium after it hatches from the zona pellucida. The outer cells of the blastocyst, the trophoblast or trophectoderm, are flattened polyhedral cells, which possess ultrastructural features typical of a transporting epithelium. The trophoblast covering the inner cell mass is the polar trophoblast and that surrounding the blastocyst cavity is the mural trophoblast.

Implantation involves the initial attachment of polar trophectoderm to endometrial luminal epithelium. The trophectoderm then penetrates the epithelium and underlying basal lamina and implants into the stroma using a combination of motile and locally degradative activities. There are two distinct cell arrangements in the trophoblast: an inner cytotrophoblast of cuboidal cells; and an outer multinucleated mass of cytoplasm, the syncytiotrophoblast. The latter penetrates the uterine luminal epithelium and sends finger-like projections between adjacent epithelial cells towards the underlying basal lamina. The two layers become interlocked by numerous tight junctions. Preimplantation embryos produce proteases (responsible for degrading basal lamina extracellular matrix molecules), which probably mediate penetration of the subepithelial basal lamina by the syncytiotrophoblast. Implantation continues with erosion of maternal vascular endothelium and glandular epithelium, and phagocytosis of secretory products, until the blastocyst occupies an uneven implantation cavity in the stroma (interstitial implantation). In the early postimplantation phase, the maternal surface is resealed by re-epithelialization and the formation of a plug, which may contain fibrin.

The syncytiotrophoblast secretes a hormone, human chorionic gonadotrophin (hCG), which may be detected in the urine from as early as 10 days after fertilization, and forms the basis for tests for early pregnancy. HCG prolongs the life of the corpus luteum, which continues to secrete progesterone and oestrogens during approximately the first two months of pregnancy. Thereafter, these and other hormones are produced by the placenta.

Menstruation ceases on successful implantation. The endometrium, known as the decidua of pregnancy, thickens to form a suitable nidus for the conceptus. Decidualization of the endometrial stroma may occur without an intrauterine pregnancy, e.g. in the presence of an ectopic pregnancy, after prolonged treatment with progesterone, and in the late secretory phase of a non-conception cycle.

Decidual differentiation is not evident in the stroma at the earliest stages of implantation, and it may not be until a week later that fully differentiated cells are present. During decidualization the interglandular tissue increases in quantity. It contains a substantial population of leukocytes (large granular lymphocytes, macrophages and T cells) distributed amongst large decidual cells. Decidual cells are mesenchymally derived stromal cells which contain varying amounts of glycogen, lipid, and vimentin-type intermediate filaments in their cytoplasm. They are generally rounded, but their shape may vary depending on the local packing density. They may contain one, two or sometimes three nuclei and frequently display rows of club-like cytoplasmic protrusions enclosing granules. The cells are associated with a characteristic capsular basal lamina. Decidual cells produce a range of secretory products, including insulin-like growth factor, binding protein 1 (IGF-BP1) and prolactin, which may be taken up by the trophoblast. These secretions probably play a role in the maintenance and growth of the conceptus in the early part of postimplantational development, and can be detected in amniotic fluid in the first trimester of pregnancy.

Extracellular matrix, growth factors and protease inhibitors produced by the decidua all probably modulate the degradative activity of the trophoblast and support placental morphogenesis and placental accession to the maternal blood supply. Formation of the haemochorial placenta requires a developmental progression (where the development proceeds in a specific order over time), which is specified in the trophoblast but is dependent on the maternal environment for its correct expression. Immunological rejection of the semi-allogenec conceptus does not occur because the trophoblast expresses human leukocyte antigen-G (HLA-G) which downregulates the maternal immune response.

Once implantation is complete, distinctive names are applied to different regions of the decidua. The part covering the conceptus is the decidua capsularis; that between the conceptus and the uterine muscular wall is the decidua basalis (where the placenta subsequently develops); that which lines the remainder of the body of the uterus is the decidua parietalis (**Fig. 105.1**). There is no evidence that their respective resident maternal cell populations exhibit site-specific properties.

FETAL MEMBRANES

The implanting conceptus consists of three cavities and surrounding epithelia. The original blastocyst cavity, now termed the extraembryonic

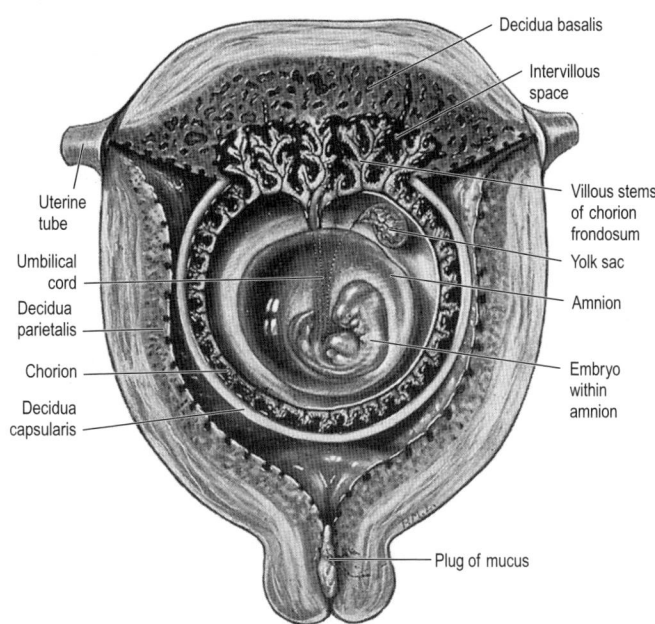

Decidua basalis

Intervillous space

Villous stems of chorion frondosum

Yolk sac

Amnion

Embryo within amnion

Plug of mucus

Uterine tube

Umbilical cord

Decidua parietalis

Chorion

Decidua capsularis

Fig. 105.1 The gravid uterus in the second month. A placental site precisely in the uterine fundus as indicated in the plan is, however, rather unusual. The dorsal, ventral or lateral wall of the corpus uteri is more usual.

coelom or chorionic cavity, is large compared to the embryo within (**Figs 10.9**, **10.10**). The trophoblast becomes lined by a mesothelium derived from cells proliferating close to the inner cell mass. These two layers collectively form the chorion. The part of the chorion overlying the implantation site that will give rise to the placenta is termed the chorion frondosum, reflecting the abundance of proliferating villi. The early villi degenerate as the placenta enlarges, initially at the abembryonic pole, and then later over most of the enlarging chorion, leaving the smooth chorion laeve.

The embryo is formed from upper epiblast and lower hypoblast layers (Ch. 10). A small amniotic cavity develops above the epiblast and a larger yolk sac develops beneath the hypoblast. Both cavities are covered externally by a mesothelium, which is continuous with the inner lining of the trophoblast. The amnion is thus composed of epiblast-derived cells and mesothelium. The yolk sac wall is composed of hypoblast derived cells, extraembryonic mesenchyme and mesothelium.

A fourth cavity, the allantois, develops as a caudal hypoblastic diverticulum that becomes embedded within the extraembryonic mesenchyme, which forms the connecting stalk of the embryo. It does not have a direct mesothelial covering.

In the early stages the amnion and yolk sac are suspended within the chorionic cavity (see **Fig. 105.3**). With embryonic and fetal growth the amniotic cavity expands until it fills the chorionic cavity and abuts against the chorion.

AMNION (CHORIO-AMNION)

Between the tenth and twelfth weeks of pregnancy the amniotic cavity expands and the chorion frondosum regresses to form the chorion laeve, which is in turn apposed to the decidua capsularis. During the same period the amnion and chorion fuse to form the chorio-amnion, and this avascular membrane persists to term.

The original amniotic cells develop from the edges of the epiblast of the embryonic disc and are ultimately connected directly to the skin at the umbilical region. As the fetus grows and the amniotic cavity expands, the amniotic membrane extends along the connecting stalk and forms the outer covering of the umbilical cord. For details of the formation of the umbilical cord see page 1259. After birth, the site of this embryonic/extraembryonic junction is important, because the extraembryonic cell lines will die, causing the umbilical cord to degenerate and detach from the body wall. In cases of anomalous development of the ventral body wall, e.g. gastroschisis and exomphalos, there may be insufficient skin in this region and a large ventral wall defect may result.

The inner surface of the amnion consists of a simple cuboidal epithelium with a microvillous apical surface beneath which is a cortical web of intermediate filaments and microfilaments. There are no tight junctional complexes between adjacent cells and cationic dyes penetrate between the cells as far as the basal lamina. The intercellular clefts present scattered desmosomes, but elsewhere the clefts widen and contain interlacing microvilli. These features are consistent with selective permeability properties. The epithelium synthesizes and deposits extracellular matrix into the compact layer of acellular stroma located beneath the basal lamina, as well as the basal lamina itself.

Human amniotic epithelial cells are thought to be pluripotential because they arise so early from the conceptus. They can be distinguished from the epiblast cells from day 8. Recent studies have shown that amniotic cells lack the major histocompatibility complex antigen. The amnion can therefore be exposed to the maternal immune system without eliciting a maternal immune response. Cultured human amniotic epithelial cells express a range of neural and glial markers, including glial fibrillary acidic protein (GFAP), myelin basic protein, vimentin and neurofilament proteins, suggesting that these cells may supply neurotrophic factors to the amniotic fluid. Amnion is used in the repair of corneas after trauma and as a graft material for reconstructing vaginas in women with cloacal abnormalities.

Towards the end of gestation increasing numbers of amniotic cells undergo apoptosis. Apoptotic cells become detached from the amnion and are found in the amniotic cavity at term. The highest incidence is in weeks 40–41, independent of the onset of labour. Apoptosis may play a role in the fragility and rupture of the fetal membranes at term.

The chorion at term consists of an inner cellular layer containing fibroblasts and a reticular layer of fibroblasts and Hofbauer cells, which resembles the mesenchyme of an intermediate villus. The outer layer consists of cytotrophoblast 3 to 10 cells deep, resting on a pseudobasal lamina, which extends beneath and between the cells. Occasional

obliterated villi within the trophoblast layer are the remnants of villi present in the chorion frondosum of the first trimester. Although the interface between the trophoblast and decidua parietalis is uneven, no trophoblast infiltration of the parietalis occurs.

AMNIOTIC FLUID

The amniotic fluid, or liquor amnii, is derived from multiple sources throughout gestation. These include secretions from amnion epithelium, filtration of fluid from maternal vessels via the parietal decidua and amniochorion, filtration from the fetal vessels via the chorionic plate or the umbilical cord, and fetal urine. In early pregnancy, diffusion from intracorporeal vessels via fetal skin provides another source. Once the gut is formed, fetal swallowing of amniotic fluid is a normal occurrence. The fluid is absorbed into the fetal circulation and passes via the placental barrier into the maternal circulation. There is rapid exchange between the amniotic fluid and maternal and fetal circulations via the placenta and fetal kidneys.

In the early stages amniotic fluid resembles blood plasma in composition and is probably formed largely by transport across the amniotic membrane. As pregnancy advances, it becomes progressively more dilute, partly by the addition of fetal urine. It contains less than 2% of solids, including urea, inorganic salts, a small amount of protein and frequently a trace of sugar. Glycoprotein secretions from amniotic epithelium include fibronectin. There is experimental evidence of a considerable and rapid flux of water across the amniotic membrane.

By the end of the third month the expanding amnion has extensive contact with the chorion laeve, and only these thin membranes separate the amniotic fluid from the decidua parietalis, the tissues and vessels of which provide another route for the exchange of water and dissolved substances. Secretory products of maternal decidua, including prolactin and insulin-like growth factor binding protein 1 (IGF-BP1), are present in the liquor. The amount of amniotic fluid increases in quantity up to the sixth or seventh month and then diminishes slightly. At the end of pregnancy it is usually somewhat less than a litre. It provides a buoyant medium, which supports the delicate tissues of the young embryo and allows free movement of the fetus during the later stages of pregnancy. It also diminishes the risk to the fetus of injury from without.

A volume of amniotic fluid in excess of 2 litres is generally considered to be abnormal and constitutes polyhydramnios. A deficiency is termed oligohydramnios. Both conditions may be associated with fetal abnormalities, e.g. fetuses with agenesis of the kidneys or atresia of the lower urinary tract are often associated with oligohydramnios. Similarly, pulmonary hypoplasia at birth may be caused by severe congenital urinary obstruction because a reduction in the amniotic fluid pressure permits fluid produced in the fetal lungs to escape and this compromises lung expansion. Cases of oesophageal atresia or anencephaly, in which swallowing is impossible or impaired, and open spina bifida, are often associated with polyhydramnios. Impaired swallowing combined with these neural defects is accompanied by direct discharge of cerebrospinal fluid (CSF) into the amniotic liquor. In fetuses with spina bifida and some other neural tube defects the concentration of α-fetoprotein in the amniotic fluid is exceptionally high and is used to diagnose these abnormalities.

YOLK SAC

As the secondary yolk sac forms it delineates a cavity lined with parietal, and perhaps visceral, hypoblast, which is continuous with the developing endoderm from the primitive streak (Ch. 10). The yolk sac becomes coated with extraembryonic mesenchyme, which forms mesenchymal and mesothelial layers. The inner cells of the yolk sac (denoted endoderm in many studies, although this layer is restricted to the embryo itself) are columnar with numerous microvilli and pinocytotic vesicles. They contain abundant rough endoplasmic reticulum, well-developed Golgi apparatus, and numerous mitochondria.

The outer mesothelium also exhibits microvilli, which are covered by a mucus layer. The cells appear less active than the inner yolk sac cells. The mesothelium may provide a protective coat to prevent damage caused by compression or friction of the yolk sac wall against the chorionic cavity lining. The intervening mesenchymal layer is the main site for blood vessel and cell formation in the early embryo.

The yolk sac remains within the extraembryonic coelom (chorionic cavity) throughout gestation. It becomes located between the amnion and chorion as they fuse near the placental attachment of the umbilical cord. It continues to grow slowly and is sometimes found at term in this

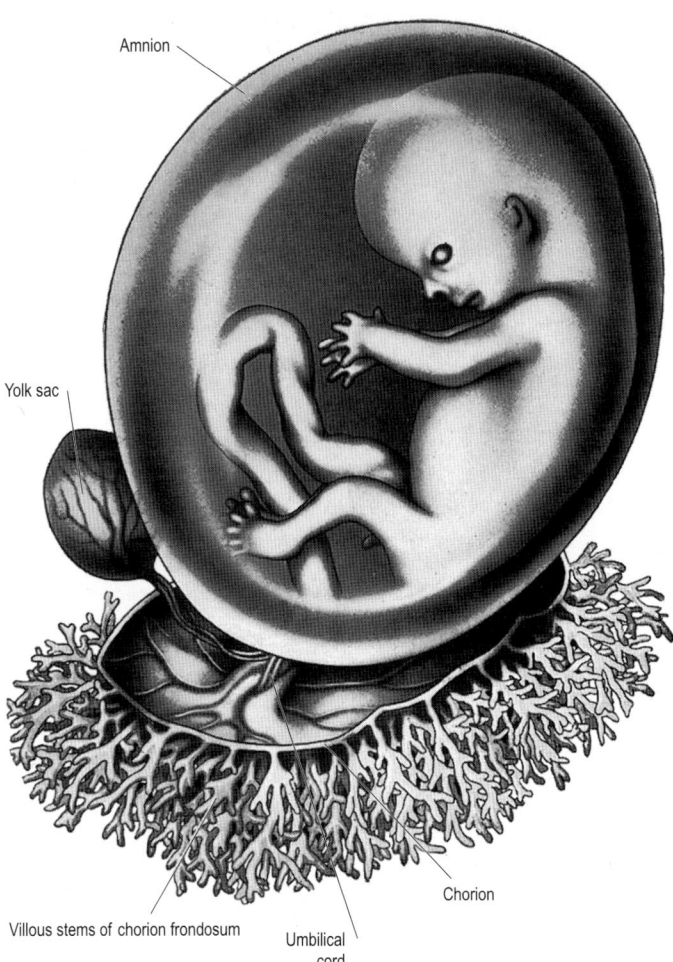

Fig. 105.2 A fetus of c.8 weeks, enclosed in the amnion, magnified c.2.5 diameters. A part of the chorion frondosum with its branching villous stems is shown in the lower part of the figure. The villous stems have been detached from the basal plate, which is not shown here.

Labels on figure: Amnion / Yolk sac / Villous stems of chorion frondosum / Umbilical cord / Chorion

site as a small vesicle, usually less than 5 mm in diameter. The yolk stalk and contained endodermal duct gradually elongate with the growth in length of the umbilical cord (**Fig. 105.2**).

ALLANTOIS

The allantoenteric diverticulum (**Fig. 105.3**) arises early in the third week as a solid, endodermal outgrowth from the dorsocaudal part of the yolk sac into the mesenchyme of the connecting stalk. It soon becomes canalized. When the hindgut is developed, the proximal (enteric) part of the diverticulum is incorporated in its ventral wall. The distal (allantoic) part remains as the allantoic duct and is carried ventrally to open into the ventral aspect of the cloaca or terminal part of the hindgut (**Fig. 105.3**). The allantois is a site of angiogenesis, which gives rise to the umbilical vessels and placental circulation. The extraembryonic mesenchyme around the allantois forms the connecting stalk, which is later incorporated into the umbilical cord.

In the fetus, the allantoic duct, which is confined to the proximal end of the umbilical cord, elongates and thins. However, it may persist as an interrupted series of epithelial strands at term, in which case the proximal strand is often continuous at the umbilicus with the median intra-abdominal urachus, and this in turn continues into the apex of the bladder.

UMBILICAL CORD

The formation of the connecting stalk is described in Chapter 10, and the early formation of the umbilical cord is described on page 1259

(**Fig. 105.3**). The umbilical cord ultimately consists of an outer covering of flattened amniotic epithelial cells and an interior mass of mesenchyme of diverse origins (**Fig. 10.22**), which contains two endodermal tubes, the yolk and allantoic ducts, and their associated vitelline and allantoic (umbilical) blood vessels.

The mesenchymal core is derived from the somatopleuric extra-embryonic mesenchyme covering the amniotic folds, splanchnopleuric extraembryonic mesenchyme of the yolk stalk (which carries the vitelline vessels and clothes the endodermal yolk duct), and similar allantoic mesenchyme of the connecting stalk (which clothes the allantoic duct and initially carries two umbilical arteries and two umbilical veins). These various mesenchymal compartments fuse and are gradually transformed into the loose connective tissue (Wharton's jelly), which characterizes the more mature cord. The tissue consists of widely spaced elongated fibroblasts separated by a delicate three-dimensional meshwork of fine collagen fibres, which contains a variety of hydrated glycosaminoglycans, and is particularly rich in hyaluronic acid.

The yolk stalk and endodermal duct remain within the cord. The allantois extends only into the proximal part of the umbilical cord. It may remain as a series of epithelial strands.

The vitelline and allantoic (umbilical) vessels, which are initially symmetrical, become modified as a result of changes in the circulation. The vitelline vessels involute, whereas most of the allantoic (umbilical) vessels persist. The right umbilical vein disappears but the two umbilical arteries normally remain; occasionally one umbilical artery may disappear. The vessels of the umbilical cord are rarely straight, and are usually twisted into either a right- or left-handed cylindrical helix. The number of turns involved ranges from a few to over 300. This conformation may be produced by unequal growth of the vessels, or by torsional forces imposed by fetal movements. Its functional significance is obscure. Perhaps the pulsations and contractions of the helical vessels assist the venous return to the fetus in the umbilical vein.

Mature umbilical vessels, particularly the arteries, have a strong muscular coat, which contracts readily in response to mechanical stimuli. The outermost bundles pursue an interlacing spiral course, and when they contract they produce shortening of the vessel and thickening of the media, with folding of the interna and considerable narrowing of the lumen. This action may account for the periodic sharp constrictions of contour, the so-called valves of Hoboken, which often characterize these vessels.

The fully developed umbilical cord is on average some 50 cm long and 1–2 cm in diameter. Its length varies from 20–120 cm. Exceptionally short or long cords are associated with fetal problems and complications during labour. The cord usually attaches to the placenta, but in a minority of cases velamentous insertion is observed (i.e. into the membranes) and this may be associated with vulnerability to injury and fetal haemorrhage.

DEVELOPMENT OF THE PLACENTA

The human placenta is initially labyrinthine as the early villous stems are formed, and becomes villous as generations of terminal villi develop. Maternal blood bathes the surfaces of the chorion that bound the intervillous space and the placenta is therefore defined as haemochorial. Different grades of fusion exist between the maternal and fetal tissues in many other mammals (e.g. epitheliochorial, syndesmochorial, endotheliochorial). The chorion is vascularized by the allantoic blood vessels of the body stalk and so the human placenta is also termed chorio-allantoic (whereas in some mammals a choriovitelline placenta either exists alone or supplements the chorio-allantoic variety). In addition, the human placenta is said to be dediduate because maternal tissue is shed with the placenta and membranes at term as part of the afterbirth.

As the blastocyst implants, the syncytiotrophoblast invades and digests the uterine tissues, including the glands and walls of maternal blood vessels (**Figs 10.8, 10.9**). The syncytiotrophoblast increases rapidly in thickness over the embryonic pole. A progressively thinner layer covers the rest of the wall towards the abembryonic pole. Microvillus-lined clefts and lacunar spaces develop in the syncytiotrophoblastic envelope (days 9–11 of pregnancy) and establish communications with one another. Initially, many of these spaces contain maternal blood derived from dilated uterine capillaries and veins, as the walls of the vessels are partially destroyed. As the conceptus grows, the lacunar spaces enlarge, and become confluent to form an intervillous space.

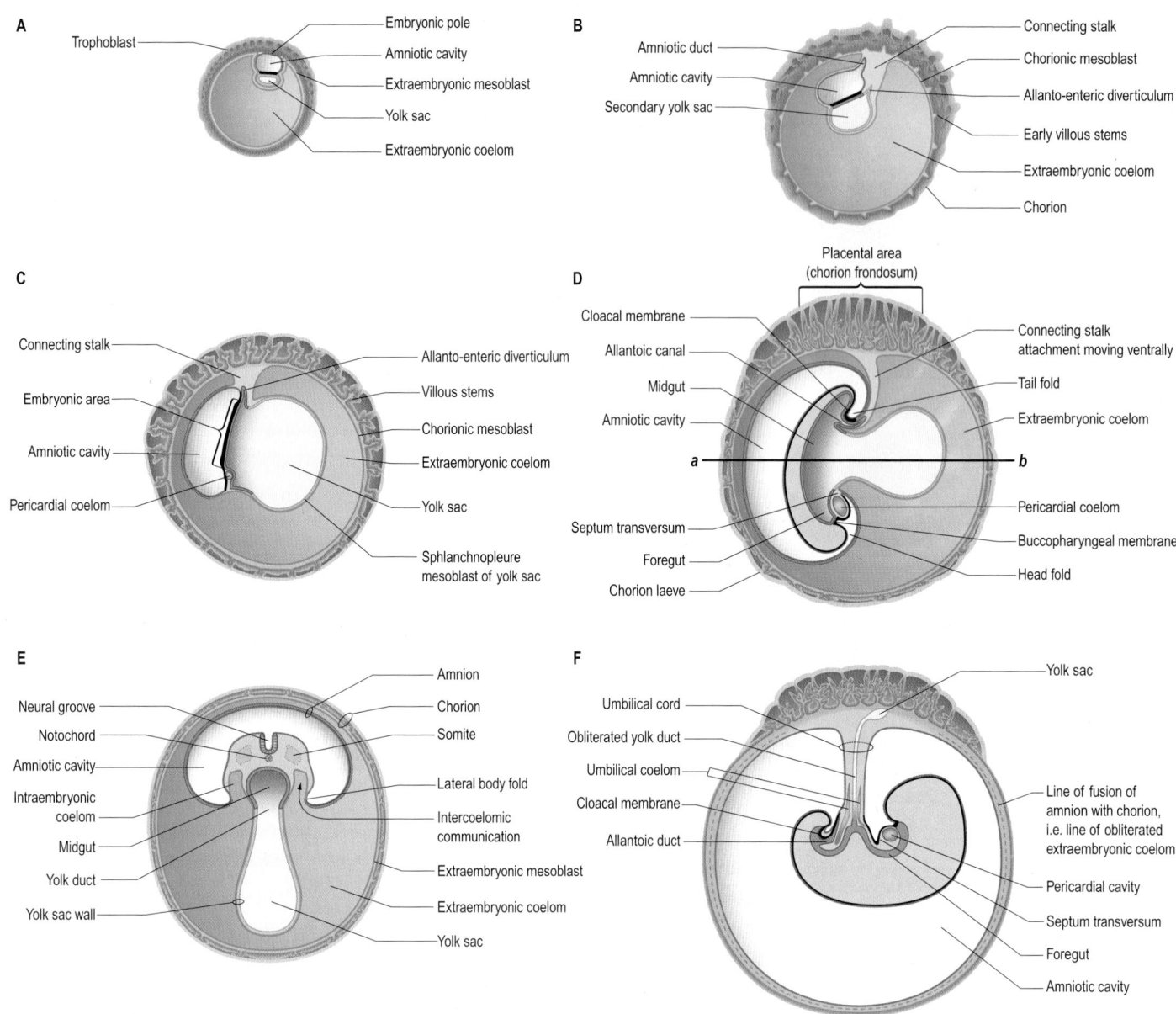

Fig. 105.3 Diagrams showing: **A**, an early stage in development of the human blastocyst; **B**, blastocyst sectioned so the embryo is longitudinally sectioned showing the early formation of the allantois and the connecting stalk; **C**, longitudinal section of embryo at a later stage of development; the pericardial cavity can be see at the most rostral part of the embryonic area; **D**, longitudinal section of embryo at a later stage showing formation of the head and tail folds, the expansion of the amnion and the delimitation of the umbilicus; **E**, a transverse section along the line a–b in **D**. Observe that the intraembryonic coelom communicates freely with the extraembryonic coelom; **F**, longitudinal section of embryo at a later stage showing full expansion of the amniotic cavity and the umbilical cord.

The projections of syncytiotrophoblast into the maternal decidua are called primary villi. They are invaded first with cytotrophoblast and then with mesenchyme (days 13–15) to form secondary placental villi. Fetal capillaries develop in the mesenchymal core of the villi. The cytotrophoblast within the villi continues to grow through the invading syncytiotrophoblast and makes direct contact with the decidua basalis, forming anchoring villi. Further cytotrophoblast proliferation occurs laterally so that neighbouring outgrowths meet to form a spherical cytotrophoblastic shell around the conceptus (**Figs 10.9, 105.4**). Lateral projections from the main stem villus form true and terminal villi (**Fig. 105.4**).

As secondary villi form, single mononuclear cells become detached from the distal cytotrophoblast and infiltrate the maternal decidua. This process occurs in two phases: an initial infiltration of the decidua basalis, when interstitial extravillous trophoblast tends to accumulate in the vicinity of maternal spiral arteries; and a second wave of migration so that extravillous trophoblast reaches the inner one-third of the myometrium. At the same time, cytotrophoblast from the shell penetrates into and migrates along the inner walls of maternal spiral arteries (endovascular extravillous trophoblast) so that by the 18th week it has

reached the inner myometrial segments. The interstitially migrating cells appear to have the capacity to invade arteries from their adventitia, and are presumably involved in the remodelling of the maternal arteries. The latter lose smooth muscle and associated elastic and collagenous matrix, which is replaced with non-resistive fibrinoid, an arrangement that permits an expansion of the vessels and as much as a 20-fold increase in the flow of blood into the intervillous space. Common pregnancy pathologies, including intrauterine growth retardation, pre-eclampsia and spontaneous abortion, are all associated with incomplete vascular remodelling, which probably reflects a failure of penetration by extravillous trophoblast.

With the onset of the embryonic heartbeat, a primitive circulation exists between the yolk sac, the embryo and the chorio-allantoic placenta. The embryonic side of the placenta is termed the chorionic plate and the maternal side the basal plate. Growing free villi permeate the inter-villous space and are spanned by the early villous stems and their branches.

Expansion of the entire conceptus is accompanied by radial growth of the villi and, simultaneously, an integrated tangential growth and expansion of the trophoblastic shell. Eventually each villous stem forms

NUTRITION THROUGHOUT GESTATION

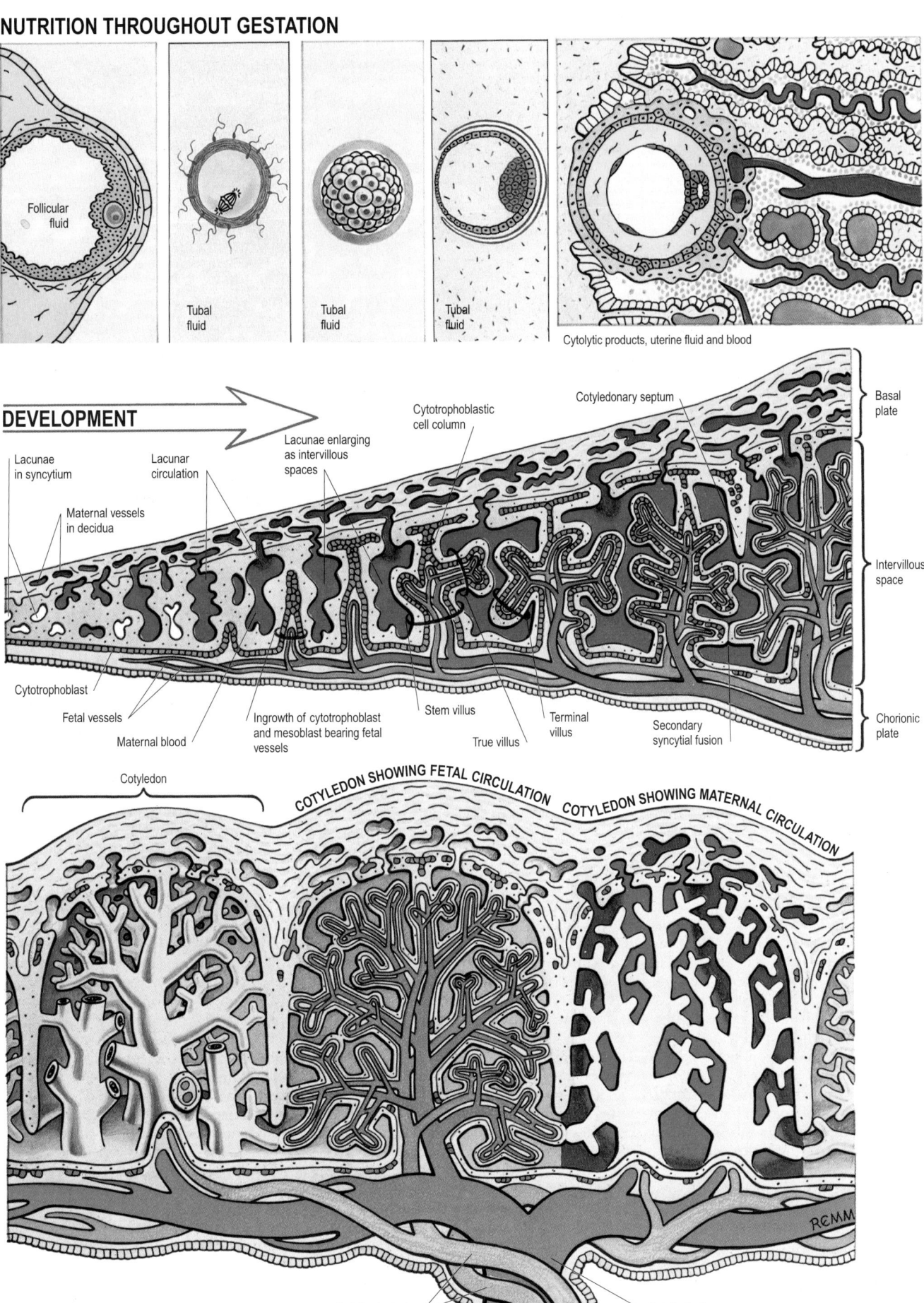

Fig. 105.4 Nutrition of oocyte, zygote, morula, free and implanted blastocyst, embryo and fetus throughout gestation. Embryonic and placental development proceed from left to right. Aspects of mature placental structure and circulation are shown below.

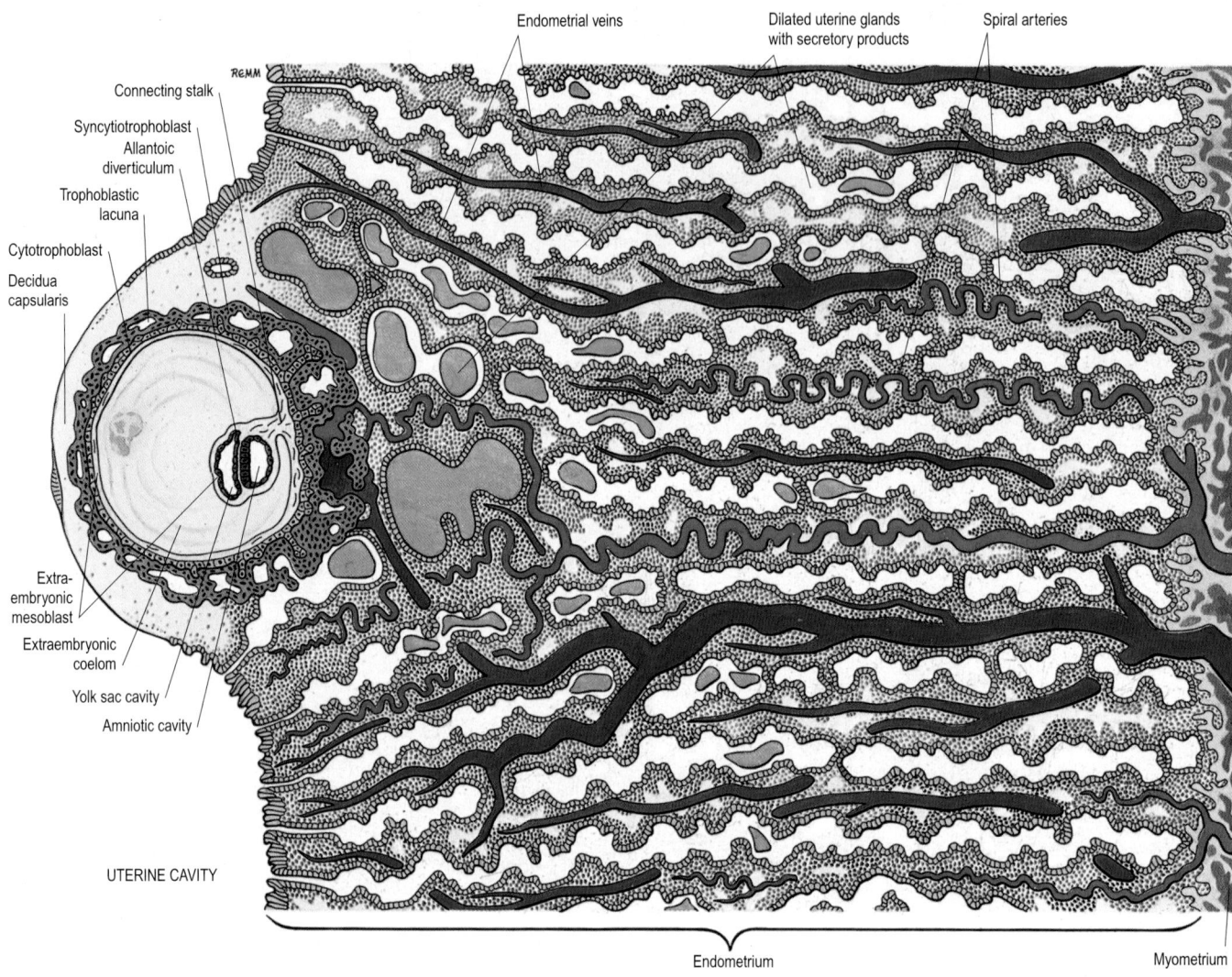

Endometrial veins

Dilated uterine glands
with secretory products

Spiral arteries

Connecting stalk

Syncytiotrophoblast
Allantoic
diverticulum

Trophoblastic
lacuna

Cytotrophoblast

Decidua
capsularis

Extra-
embryonic
mesoblast

Extraembryonic
coelom

Yolk sac cavity

Amniotic cavity

UTERINE CAVITY

Endometrium

Myometrium

Fig. 105.5 The general structure of the implanting blastocyst and its relationship to the tissues of the endometrium on the fifteenth day after fertilization. Note the arrangement and gradation in thickness of the syncytial trophoblast, which has eroded the maternal tissues. Some of the deeper trophoblastic lacunae already contain maternal blood.

a complex consisting of a single trunk attached by its base to the chorion, from which second and third order branches (intermediate and terminal villi) arise distally. Terminal villi are specialized for exchange between fetal and maternal circulations. Each one starts as a syncytial outgrowth and is invaded by cytotrophoblastic cells, which then develop a core of fetal mesenchyme as the villus continues to grow. The core is vascularized by fetal capillaries (i.e. each villus passes through primary, secondary and tertiary grades of histological differentiation). The germinal cytotrophoblast continues to add cells that fuse with the overlying syncytium and so contribute to the expansion of the haemochorial interface. Terminal villi continue to form and branch within the confines of the definitive placenta throughout gestation, projecting in all directions into the intervillous space (**Fig. 105.4**).

From the third week until about the second month of pregnancy, the entire chorion is covered with villous stems. They are thus continuous peripherally with the trophoblastic shell, which is in close apposition with both the decidua capsularis and the decidua basalis. The villi adjacent to the decidua basilis are stouter, longer and show a greater profusion of terminal villi. As the conceptus continues to expand, the decidua capsularis is progressively compressed and thinned, the circulation through it is gradually reduced and adjacent villi slowly atrophy and disappear. This process starts at the abembryonic pole, and by the end of the third month, the abembryonic hemisphere of the conceptus is largely denuded. Eventually the whole chorion apposed to the decidua capsularis is smooth (the chorion laeve). In contrast, the villous stems of the disc-shaped region of chorion apposed to the decidua basalis increase greatly in size and complexity (the chorion frondosum),

and together with the decidua basalis constitutes the definitive placental site.

Coincidentally with the growth of the embryo and the expansion of the amnion, the decidua capsularis is thinned and distended (**Figs 105.5, 105.1**) and the space between it and the decidua parietalis gradually obliterated. By the second month of pregnancy the three endometrial strata recognizable in the premenstrual phase, compactum, spongiosum and basale, are better differentiated and easily distinguished. In the spongiosum the glands are compressed and appear as oblique slit-like fissures lined by low cuboidal cells. By the beginning of the third month of pregnancy the decidua capsularis and decidua parietalis are in contact, while by the fifth month the decidua capsularis is greatly thinned, and during the succeeding months (**Fig. 105.6**) it virtually disappears.

INTERVILLOUS SPACE

The intervillous space, at first spanned by the early villous stems and their branches, is increasingly permeated by growing free villi (**Figs 105.4, 105.7, 105.8**). It contains the circulating maternal blood. On its fetal aspect, it is bounded by a chorionic plate, which consists of syncytial, cytotrophoblastic and mesenchymal layers of the chorion. The latter carry radicles of the umbilical vessels and fuse laterally with the mesenchyme of the expanding amnion. On its maternal aspect it is bounded by a basal plate, which consists of an incomplete peripheral syncytium with an outer cytotrophoblastic shell and columns of cytotrophoblast, which extend deeper into the maternal decidual stroma. The trophoblast and adjacent decidua are enmeshed in layers of fibrinoid

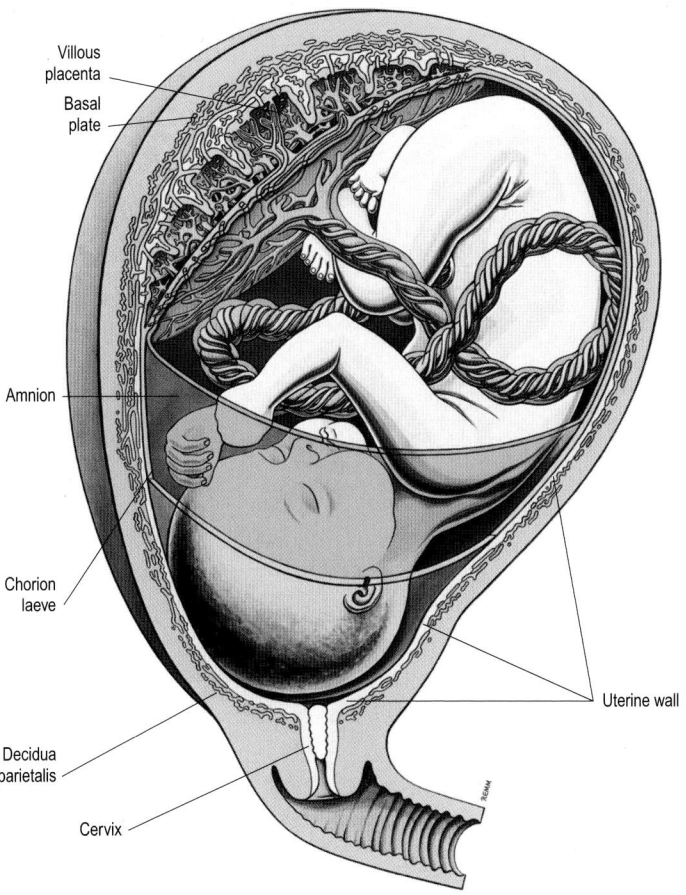

Villous
placenta

Basal
plate

Amnion

Chorion
laeve

Decidua
parietalis

Cervix

Uterine wall

Fig. 105.6 A full-term human fetus *in utero*, including a sectional view of the placenta, the amnion (mauve), chorion (green), uterine wall and cervix (yellow), the cervix with a plug of mucus in the cervical canal, the umbilical cord and its contained vessels, and the rugose vaginal wall. Note the characteristic flexed posture of the fetus and its limbs, and the overall position within the uterus that the fetus commonly occupies. The single umbilical vein carries oxygenated blood, the two umbilical arteries carry deoxygenated blood. These vessels arborize in the chorionic plate (seen through the overlying amnion) and their branches pass into the villous stems. The latter span the intervillous space where they branch into intermediate and terminal villi. Incomplete placental septa project from the basal plate towards the chorionic plate.

and basement membrane-like extracellular matrix to form a complex junctional zone. Where a discrete layer of fibrinoid is present between the trophoblastic shell and decidual stroma it is known as Nitabuch's layer. The intervillous space from chorionic to basal plates contains the main trunks of the villous stems dividing into their intermediate and terminal villi. The trunk and its branches may be regarded as the essential structural, functional and growth unit of the developing placenta.

The maternal blood vessels approach and reach the intervillous space through the various layers of the basal plate. The spiral arteries of the endometrium open through gaps in the cytotrophoblastic shell and peripheral syncytium. They probably do not open directly into the intervillous space until as late as the tenth week. At term, from the inner myometrium to the intervillous space, the walls of most spiral arteries consist of fibrinoid matrix within which cytotrophoblast is embedded. This arrangement allows expansion of the arterial diameter (and so an increased blood flow) independent of the local action of vasocontrictive agents. Endothelial cells, where present, are often hypertrophic.

The veins that drain the blood away from the intervillous space pierce the basal plate and join tributaries of the uterine veins. The presence of a marginal venous sinus, which hitherto has been described as a constant feature occupying the peripheral margin of the placenta and communicating freely with the intervillous space, has not been confirmed.

Experimental studies have shown that radio-opaque material injected into the aorta passes in spurts or jets to the intervillous space and at

sufficient pressure to drive it towards the chorion, thus preventing a short circuit of arterial blood into the venous openings. The openings of the coiled arteries show intermittent activity. Myometrial contractions alter the pressure in the intervillous space and promote placental venous drainage.

CHORIONIC PLATE

The chorionic plate is covered on its fetal aspect by the amniotic epithelium, on the stromal side of which is a connective tissue layer carrying the main branches of the umbilical vessels (**Figs 105.4, 105.7**). Subjacent to this is a diminishing layer of cytotrophoblasts and then the inner syncytial wall of the intervillous space. The connective tissue layer is formed by fusion between the mesenchyme-covered surfaces of amnion and chorion. It is more fibrous and less cellular than Wharton's jelly (of the umbilical cord), except near the larger vessels. The vessels radiate and branch from the cord attachment, with variations in the branching pattern, until they reach the bases of the trunks of the villous stems and then arborize within the intermediate and terminal villi. There are no anastomoses between vascular trees of adjacent stems. The two umbilical arteries are normally joined at, or just before they enter, the chorionic plate, by some form of substantial transverse anastomosis, (Hyrtl's anastomosis).

BASAL PLATE

The basal plate, from fetal to maternal aspect, consists of the outer wall of the intervillous space. In different places, this may contain syncytium, cytotrophoblast or fibrinoid matrix, Rohr's stria of fibrinoid, remnants of the cytotrophoblastic shell, Nitabuch's stria of fibrinoid, and maternal decidua (**Figs 105.4, 105.7**).

Nitabuch's stria and the decidua basilis contain cytotrophoblast and multinucleate trophoblast giant cells derived from the mononuclear cytotrophoblast population, which infiltrates the decidua basilis during the first 18 weeks of pregnancy. These cells penetrate as far as the inner one-third of the myometrium, but can often be observed at or near the decidual–myometrial junction. They are not found in the decidua parietalis or the adjacent myometrium, from which it may be inferred that the placental bed giant cell represents a differentiative end stage in the extravillous trophoblast lineage.

The striae of fibrinoid are irregularly interconnected and variable in prominence. Strands pass from Nitabuch's stria into the adjacent decidua, which contains basal remnants of the endometrial glands and large and small decidual cells scattered in a connective tissue framework. The latter supports an extensive venous plexus.

Throughout the second half of pregnancy the basal plate becomes thinned and progressively modified. There is a relative diminution of the decidual elements, increasing deposition of fibrinoid, and admixture of fetal and maternal derivatives.

STRUCTURE OF A VILLUS

Chorionic villi are the essential structures involved in exchanges between mother and fetus. The villous tissues separating fetal and maternal blood are therefore of crucial functional importance.

From the chorionic plate, progressive branching occurs into the villous tree, as stem villi give way to intermediate and terminal villi. Each villus has a core of connective tissue containing collagen types I, III, V and VI, as well as fibronectin. Cross-banded fibres (30–35 nm) of type I collagen often occur in bundles. Type III collagen is present as thinner (10–15 nm) beaded fibres, which form a meshwork that often encases the larger fibres. Collagens V and VI are present as 6–10 nm fibres closely associated with collagens I and III. Laminin and collagen type IV are present in the stroma associated with basal laminae surrounding fetal vessels and in the trophoblast basal lamina. Overlying this matrix are ensheathing cyto- and syncytial trophoblast cells bathed by the maternal blood in the intervillous space (**Figs 105.4, 105.7, 105.9**). Cohesion between the cells of the cytotrophoblast and also between the cytotrophoblast and the syncytium is provided by numerous desmosomes between the apposed plasma membranes.

In earlier stages, the cytotrophoblast forms an almost continuous layer on the basal lamina. After the fourth month it gradually expends itself producing syncytium, which comes to lie on the basal lamina over an increasingly large area and becomes progressively thinner. A few cytotrophoblastic cells, usually disposed singly, persist until term. In the first and second trimester cytotrophoblastic sprouts, covered in

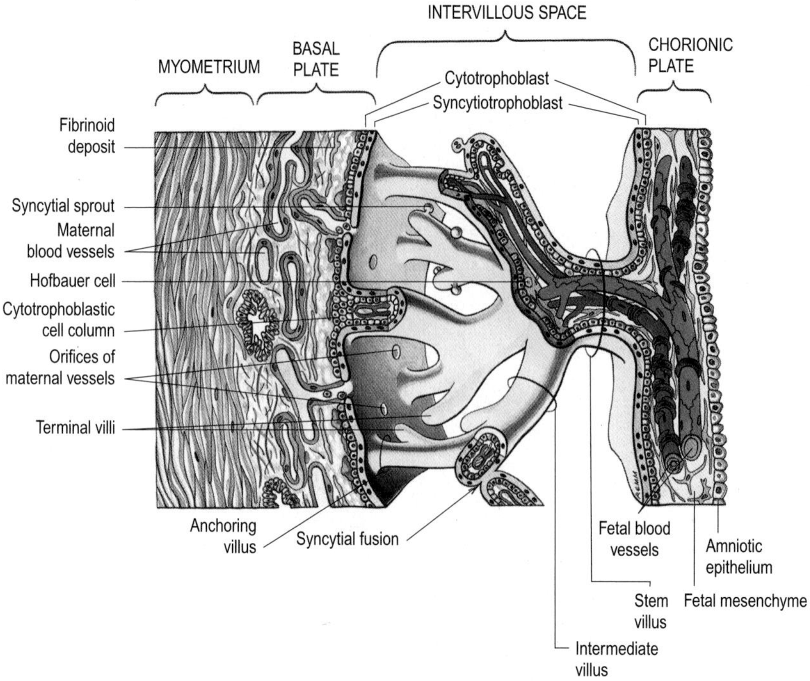

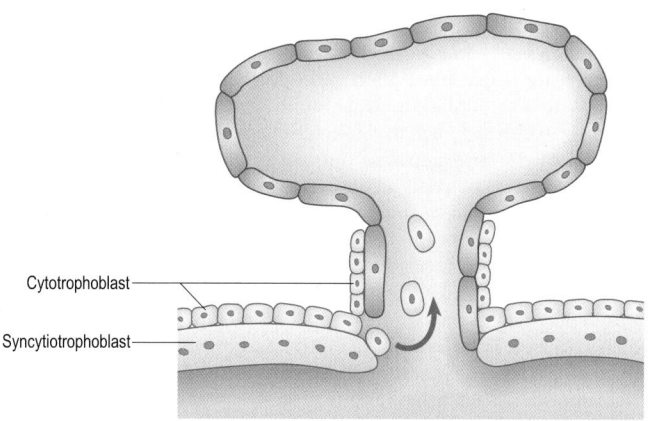

INTERVILLOUS SPACE

MYOMETRIUM   BASAL PLATE   CHORIONIC PLATE

Cytotrophoblast
Syncytiotrophoblast

Fibrinoid deposit

Syncytial sprout

Maternal blood vessels

Hofbauer cell

Cytotrophoblastic cell column

Orifices of maternal vessels

Terminal villi

Anchoring villus   Syncytial fusion

Fetal blood vessels   Amniotic epithelium

Stem villus   Fetal mesenchyme

Intermediate villus

Fig. 105.7 The arrangement of the placental tissues. The intervillous space is spanned by a villous stem and its divisions. The sectioned surfaces show the disposition of the fetal and maternal blood vessels, the amniotic epithelium, the cellular and syncytial layers of trophoblast and the complex junctional zone between the fetal and maternal tissues in the basal plate, which contains deposits of fibrinoid material and isolated masses of peripheral syncytium. Note surface syncytial sprouts and Hofbauer cells (large phagocytic cells) associated with a terminal villus. Syncytial fusion is occurring between the tips of two terminal villi.

Cytotrophoblast

Syncytiotrophoblast

Fig. 105.8 A syncytial sprout.

syncytium, are present; they represent a stage in the development of new villi (**Fig. 105.8**). Cytotrophoblast columns at the tips of anchoring villi extend from the villous basal lamina to the maternal decidual stroma.

The cells of the villous cytotrophoblast (Langhans cells) are pale-staining with a slight basophilia. Ultrastructurally, they have a rather electron-translucent cytoplasm, and relatively few organelles. These cells contain intermediate filaments particularly in association with desmosomes. Between the desmosomes, the membranes of adjacent cells are separated by c.20 nm. Sometimes the intercellular gap widens to accommodate microvillous projections from the cell surfaces, and it occasionally contains patches of fibrinoid.

A smaller population of intermediate cytotrophoblast may also be found in the chorionic villi. This postmitotic population represents a state of partial differentiation between the cytotrophoblast stem cell and the overlying syncytium.

The syncytium is an intensely active tissue layer across which most transplacental transport must occur. It secretes a range of placental hormones into the maternal circulation. Syncytial cytoplasm is more strongly basophilic than that of the Langhans cells and is packed with organelles consistent with its secretory phenotype. Where the plasma membrane adjoins basal lamina it is often infolded into the cytoplasm, whereas the surface bordering the intervillous space is set with numerous long microvilli, which constitute the brush border seen by light microscopy.

Glycogen is thought to be present in both layers of the trophoblast at all stages, although it is not always possible to demonstrate its presence histochemically. Lipid droplets occur in both layers and are free in the core of the villus. In the trophoblast they are found principally within the cytoplasm, but they also occur in the extracellular space between cytotrophoblast and syncytium, and between the individual cells of the cytotrophoblast. The droplets diminish in number with advancing age and may represent fat in transit from mother to fetus, and/or a pool of precursors for steroid synthesis. Membrane-bound granular bodies of moderate electron density occur in the cytoplasm, particularly in the syncytium, some of which are probably secretion granules. Other membrane-bound bodies, lysosomes and phagosomes, are involved in the degradation of materials engulfed from the intervillous space.

In the immature placenta, syncytial sprouts (**Fig. 105.8**) represent the first stages in the development of new terminal villi, which later become invaded by cytotrophoblast and villous mesenchyme. Occasionally, adjacent syncytial sprouts make contact and fuse to form slender syncytial bridges. The sprouts may become detached, forming maternal syncytial emboli, which pass to the lungs. It has been computed that some 100,000 sprouts pass daily into the maternal circulation. In the lungs they provoke little local reaction and apparently disappear by lysis. However, they may occasionally form foci for neoplastic growth. Syncytial sprouts are present in the term placenta, but are usually degenerating.

Syncytial knots are aggregates of degenerating nuclei, which may represent a sequestration phenomenon by which senescent nuclear material is removed from adjacent metabolically active areas of syncytium.

Fibrinoid deposits are frequently found on the villous surface in areas lacking syncytiotrophoblast. They may constitute a repair mechanism in which the fibrinoid forms a wound surface that is subsequently re-epithelialized by trophoblast. The extracellular matrix glycoprotein tenascin has been localized in the stroma adjacent to these sites.

The core of a villus contains small and large reticulum cells, fibroblasts, and large phagocytic Hofbauer cells, which are more numerous in early pregnancy. Early mesenchymal cells probably differentiate into small reticulum cells, which in turn produce fibroblasts or large reticulum cells. The small reticulum cells appear to delimit a collagen-free stromal channel system through which Hofbauer cells migrate. Mesenchymal collagen increases from a network of fine fibres in early mesenchymal villi to a densely fibrous stroma within stem villi in the second and third trimester. After approximately 14 weeks, the stromal channels found in immature intermediate villi are infilled by collagen to give the fibrous stroma characteristic of the stem villus.

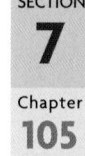

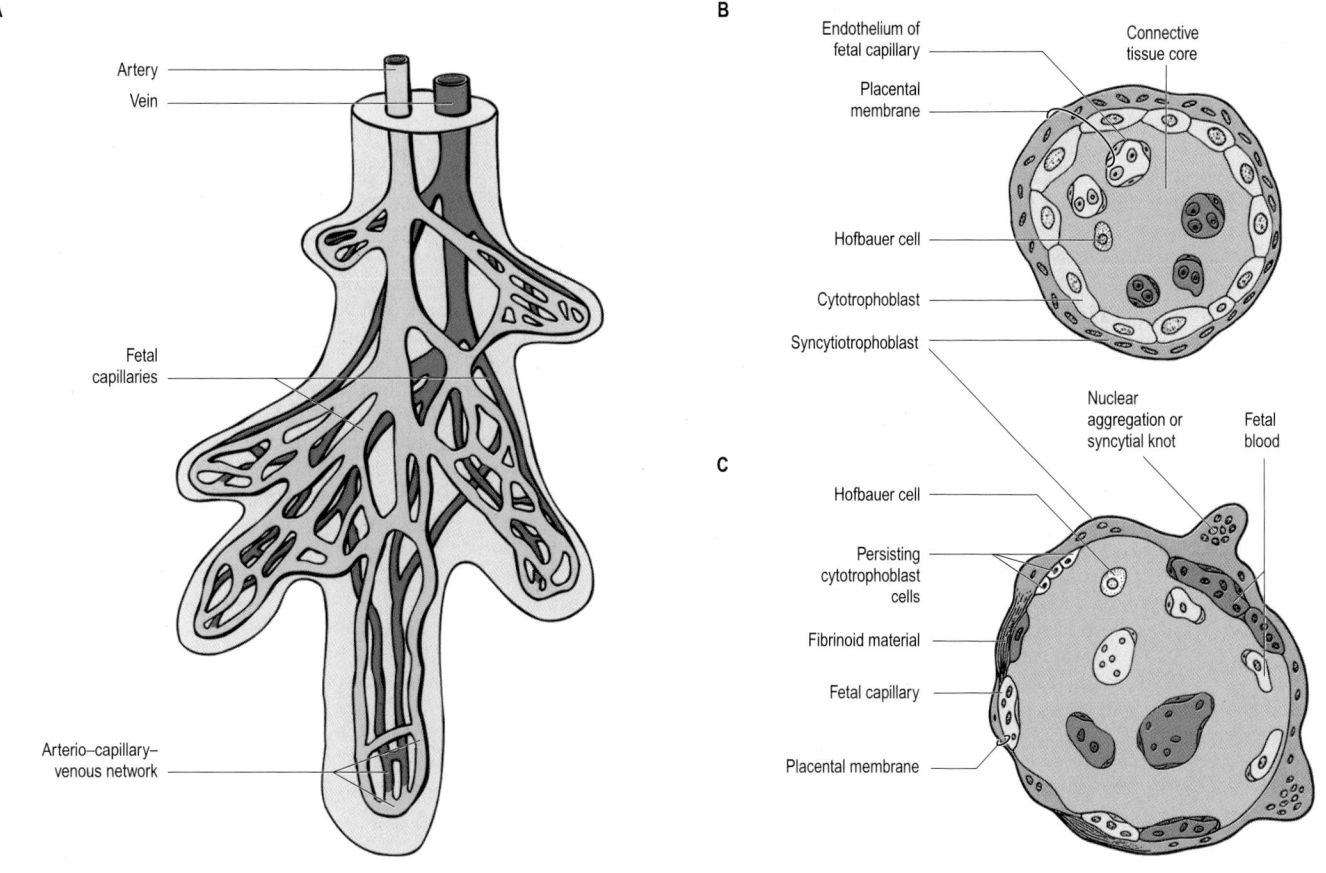

Fig. 105.9 A, Chorionic villus and its arterio–capillary–venous system carrying fetal blood. The artery carries deoxygenated blood and waste products from the fetus, whereas the vein carries oxygenated blood and nutrients to the fetus. Sections through a chorionic villus at 10 weeks, **B**, and at full term, **C**. The villi are bathed externally in maternal blood. The placental membrane, composed of fetal tissues, separates the maternal blood from the fetal blood.

Fetal vessels include arterioles and capillaries. Pericytes may be found in close association with the capillary endothelium. From late first trimester the vessels are surrounded externally by a basal lamina. From the second trimester (and a little later in terminal villi), dilated thin-walled capillaries are found immediately adjacent to the villous trophoblast; their respective basal laminae apparently fuse to produce a vasculo–syncytial interface.

MATURATION AND FUNCTIONS OF THE PLACENTA

In the early stages of placental development the blood in the fetal vessels is separated from the maternal blood in the intervillous space by the fetal vascular endothelial cells, the connective tissue of the villus, the subepithelial basal lamina and its covering of cyto- and syncytial trophoblast. These constitute a placental barrier interposed between the bloodstreams. It is a selectively permeable barrier and allows water, oxygen and other nutritive substances and hormones to pass from mother to fetus, and some of the products of excretion to pass from fetus to mother.

Throughout pregnancy, the placenta increases its surface area and thickness, and there are concomitant increases in the size, length and complexity of branching of the villous stems. At term, the placental diameter varies from 200 to 220 mm, the mean placental weight is 470 g, its mean thickness is 25 mm and the total villous surface area exceeds 10 m^2. The placental barrier becomes reduced in thickness during gestation. After the fourth month the villous syncytium comes into direct apposition with the subepithelial basal lamina over an increasing area (80% at term) and it becomes thinner. The fetal capillaries approach the surface of the terminal villi and become dilated.

The mechanism of transfer of substances across the placental barrier is complex. The volume of maternal blood circulating through the intervillous space has been assessed at 500 ml per minute. Simple diffusion suffices to explain gaseous exchange. Transfer of ions and other water-soluble solutes is by paracellular and transcellular diffusion and transport, although the relative importance of each of these for most individual solutes is unknown, and the paracellular pathway is morphologically undefined. Glucose transfer involves facilitated diffusion, while active transport mechanisms carry calcium and at least some amino acids. The fat-soluble and water-soluble vitamins are likely to pass the placental barrier with different degrees of facility. The water-soluble vitamins B and C pass readily. Water is interchanged between fetus and mother (in both directions) at c.3.5 litres per hour. The transfer of substances of high molecular weight, such as complex sugars, some lipids and hormonal and non-hormonal proteins, varies greatly in rate and degree, and is not so well understood. Energy-dependent selective transport mechanisms including receptor-mediated transcytosis are likely to be involved.

Lipids may be transported unchanged through and between the cells of the trophoblast to the core of the villus. The passage of maternal antibodies (immunoglobulins) across the placental barrier confers some degree of passive immunity on the fetus. In this instance it is widely accepted that transfer is by micropinocytosis. Investigation of trans-placental mechanisms is complicated by the fact that the trophoblast itself is the site of synthesis and storage of certain substances, e.g. glycogen.

The placenta is an important endocrine organ. Some steroid hormones, various oestrogens, β-endorphins, progesterone, hCG and human chorionic somatomammotropin (hCS), which is also known as placental lactogen (hPL), are synthesized and secreted by the syncytium. The trophoblast also contains enzyme systems that are associated with the synthesis of steroid hormones.

It has been suggested that leukocytes may migrate from the maternal blood through the placental barrier into the fetal capillaries. It has also been shown that some fetal and maternal red blood cells may cross the barrier. The former may have important consequences, e.g. in Rhesus incompatibility.

The majority of drugs are small molecules, which are sufficiently lipophilic to pass the barrier. Many are tolerated by the fetus, but some may exert grave teratogenic effects on the developing embryo (e.g. thalidomide). A well-documented association exists between maternal alcohol ingestion and fetal abnormalities. Addiction of the fetus can occur to substances of maternal abuse such as cocaine and heroin.

A wide variety of bacteria, spirochaetes, protozoa and viruses, including human immunodeficiency virus (HIV), are known to pass the placental barrier from mother to fetus, although the mechanism of transfer is uncertain. The presence of maternal rubella in the early months of pregnancy is of especial importance in relation to the production of congenital anomalies.

THE PLACENTA AT TERM

After delivery of the fetus the placenta becomes separated from the uterine wall and, together with the so-called 'membranes', is expelled as the afterbirth. Separation takes place along the plane of the stratum spongiosum and extends beyond the placental area, detaching the villous placenta, with associated fibrinoid matrix and small amounts of decidua basale, and the chorio-amnion, together with a superficial layer of the fused decidua capsularis and decidua parietalis.

The process of separation ruptures many uterine vessels. However, under normal circumstances postpartum haemorrhage is limited after delivery of the placenta and membranes because the firm contraction of the muscular wall of the uterus closes the torn ends of the vessels. When the placenta and membranes have been expelled, a thin layer of stratum spongiosum is left as a lining for the uterus.It soon degenerates and is cast off in the early part of the puerperium. A new epithelial lining for the uterus is regenerated from the remaining stratum basale. The chorio-amnion is continuous with the placenta at its margin and constitutes the 'membranes' familiar in obstetrics.

When ligature of the umbilical cord is delayed, the blood volume of the child is, on average, appreciably greater than it is when the ligature is applied at the earliest possible moment. It appears that in the former case much of the blood in the fetal placental vessels is transferred from the placenta to the fetus.

The expelled placenta is a flattened discoidal mass with an approximately circular or oval outline (**Fig. 105.10**). It has an average volume of 500 ml (range 200–950 ml), an average weight of 470 g (range 200–800 g), an average diameter of 185 mm (range 150–200 mm), an average thickness of 23 mm (range 10–40 mm), and an average surface area of c.30 000 mm². Thickest at its centre (the original embryonic pole), it rapidly thins towards its periphery where it continues as the chorion laeve.

Macroscopically, the fetal or inner surface, covered by amnion, is smooth, shiny and transparent, so that the mottled appearance of the subjacent chorion, to which it is closely applied, can be seen. The umbilical cord is usually attached near the centre of the fetal surface, and branches of the umbilical vessels radiate out under the amnion from this point; the veins being deeper and larger than the arteries. The remains of the yolk sac can sometimes be identified beneath the amnion and close to the attachment of the cord, as a minute vesicle, up to 5 mm in diameter. A fine thread, which is a vestige of the yolk stalk, is attached to it.

The maternal surface of the placenta is finely granular and mapped into some 15–30 lobes by a series of fissures or grooves. The placental lobes correspond in large measure to the major branches of distribution of the umbilical vessels, and this is particularly well seen in specimens which have been X-rayed after intravascular injection of radio-opaque media. The lobes are often somewhat loosely termed cotyledons. The grooves correspond to the bases of incomplete placental septa, which become increasingly prominent from the third month onwards. They extend from the maternal aspect of the intervillous space (the basal plate) towards, but do not quite reach, the chorionic plate. The septa are complex structures composed of components of the cytotrophoblastic shell and residual syncytium, together with maternally derived material including decidual cells, occasional blood vessels and gland remnants, collagenous and fibrinoid extracellular matrix and, in the later months of pregnancy, foci of degeneration. The nature of the maternal surface of the expelled placenta is determined by the tissue plane of separation of the placenta at parturition.

PLACENTAL VARIATIONS

The placenta is usually attached to the posterior wall of the uterus near the fundus, with its centre in or near the median plane. The site of attachment is determined by the point where the blastocyst becomes embedded, but the factors on which this depends are not understood. The placenta may be attached at any point on the uterine wall, offering no complications to a normal labour unless it is so low down that it overlies the internal os, in which case serious antepartum haemorrhage may occur, especially if it is nearly central in position. This occurs in c.1 in 400 pregnancies and is known as placenta praevia. (Extrauterine sites of implantation are described in Ch. 10.)

The umbilical cord, although usually attached near the centre of the placenta, may reach it at any point between its centre and margin; the latter condition is known as a battledore placenta. Occasionally the cord fails to reach the placenta itself and ends in the membranes in its vicinity. When insertion of the cord is so velamentous, the larger branches of the umbilical vessels traverse the membranes before they reach and ramify on the placenta. A small accessory (succenturiate) placental lobe is occasionally present, connected to the main organ by membranes and blood vessels. It may be retained *in utero* after delivery of the main placental mass and prolong postpartum haemorrhage. Occasionally other degrees of division occur (bipartite or tripartite placentae).

Other variations include placenta membranacea, in which villous stems and their branches persist over the whole chorion, and placenta circumvallata, where the placental margin is undercut by a deep groove. Pathological forms of adherence or penetration include: placenta accreta, which displays exceptional adherence to the decidua basalis; placenta increta, in which the myometrium is invaded; and placenta percreta, when the invasion by placental tissue passes completely through the uterine wall.

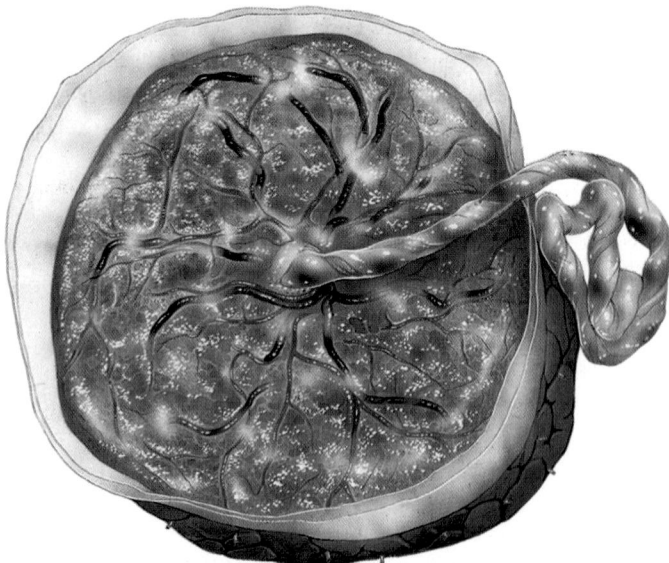

Fig. 105.10 The fetal surface of a recently delivered placenta. The spiral umbilical vessels in the umbilical cord, and their radiating branches shine through the transparent amnion. The maternal surface is exposed in the lower and right corner of the figure. Note the fringes of amnion and chorion, the majority of which have been cut away near the placental margin. (Drawn from a coloured photograph provided by EF Gibberd.)

NUTRITION OF THE EMBRYO

In early development the blastomeres derive their nourishment in part from stores laid down in the cytoplasm of the primary oocyte. These stores are not as extensive as those found in the yolk of most non-mammalian species, and it is assumed that the human embryo also derives nutrition from tubal and uterine secretions. The cleaving embryo uses pyruvate rather than glucose as an energy substrate, but switches to utilizing glucose at the blastocyst stage. New protein production occurs during the preimplantation phase, but ongoing protein breakdown is responsible for a slight net decrease in protein content.

During the process of implantation, breakdown products derived from lysed uterine tissues may provide a source of nutrition. There follows a period of about two weeks during which the embryonic disc is dependent on nutrients obtained from the fluid-filled cavities of the amnion, the coelom and the yolk sac. These fluids contain products arising from extravasated maternal blood absorbed by trophoblasts. However, early in development these sources of supply diminish. After gastrulation the lumen of the neural tube is isolated by closure of the neuropores, the extraembryonic coelom becomes greatly reduced (**Fig. 105.3**) and is later shut off from the intraembryonic coelom, and the yolk sac is separated from the gut by the narrowing of the yolk duct. Absorption of nutrients over the surface of the embryo becomes inadequate as the surface-to-volume ratio decreases. It therefore becomes imperative that some other source of nutrients should be available at an early stage. This involves the maternal circulation coming into close, although indirect, apposition with the developing embryonic circulation.

The differentiating angioblastic mesenchyme in which the embryonic vessels and erythrocytes develop is first formed early in the third week from the extraembryonic mesenchyme beneath the mesothelium that clothes the yolk sac. Slightly later, angioblastic mesenchyme appears around the allantois in the connecting stalk, within the mesenchyme of the chorion, and, later still, within the embryonic area. Spaces form within the angioblastic mesenchyme, and the cells lining these spaces differentiate into typical flattened endothelial cells. Neighbouring spaces join to form capillary plexuses. Meanwhile, small localized groups of mesenchymal cells project into the spaces and become cut off to form blood islands, their cells differentiating into embryonic erythrocytes.

The development of extraembryonic vessels around the chorion (**Fig. 105.4**) and within the early placenta, which form an intimate relationship with the maternal circulation, occurs ahead of embryonic development. Thus chorionic villi and the intervillous space are enlarging when the primitive streak forms. By the time the body plan stage is attained and the heart beats, an early circulation is present.

ANATOMY OF PREGNANCY AND PARTURITION

During pregnancy many morphological changes occur in the female reproductive system and associated abdominal structures. The uterus enlarges to accommodate the developing fetus and placenta, and there are various alterations in the pelvic walls, floor and contents which allow for this expansion, and also anticipate parturition. At the end of this period dramatic changes take place, which facilitate the passage of the baby through the birth canal. These alterations are often neglected by anatomists, but they represent an important aspect of normal reproductive morphology, and have considerable clinical significance.

UTERINE SIZE IN PREGNANCY

The uterus grows dramatically during pregnancy and increases in weight from c.50 g at the beginning of pregnancy to up to 1 kg at term. Most of this gain in weight results from increases in the vascularity and tissue fluid of the uterine wall, together with myometrial growth (Ch. 104). The increased growth of the uterine wall is driven by a combination of mechanical stretching as the conceptus grows, and the stimulus of oestrogen and progesterone. The smooth muscle mass of the myometrium is thought to increase mainly by hypertrophy, although some hyperplasia occurs early on in pregnancy.

As pregnancy proceeds, the uterus expands out of the pelvic basin and is usually palpable just above the pubic symphysis by the twelfth week, unless the uterus is retroverted (Ch. 104), in which case it may not be palpable in the abdomen until a little later. In past obstetric practice, anatomical surface landmarks such as the pubic symphysis, umbilicus and xiphisternum were used to estimate uterine size and therefore gestational age. So, for example, by the twentieth week of pregnancy the uterine fundus has usually risen to the level of the umbilicus, and by 36 weeks the uterine fundus has reached the xiphisternum. However, with the advent of diagnostic ultrasound (which allows both accurate dating of pregnancy and detection of many fetal anomalies), it has become clear that there is great variation in uterine size for a given gestation, and that clinical estimates based on anatomical landmarks are of

limited value. In late pregnancy, fetal size and growth can be assessed by serial measurement of the distance between the pubic symphysis and the uterine fundus. The symphysis–fundus measurements act primarily as a screening method, and more accurate ultrasound assessment of fetal biometry is usually held in reserve (**Fig. 105.11**).

RELATIONS OF THE UTERUS IN PREGNANCY

With uterine expansion, the ovaries and uterine tubes are displaced upwards and laterally. The round ligaments become hypertrophied and their course from the cornual regions of the uterus down to the internal inguinal ring becomes more vertical. The broad ligament tends to open out to accommodate the massive increase in the sizes of the uterine and ovarian vessels. The uterine veins in particular can reach c.1 cm in diameter and, for this reason, they appear to act as a significant reservoir for blood after uterine contraction. Lymphatics and nerves similarly proliferate, although the significance of the increased innervation is not clear, because paraplegic women are able to labour normally, albeit painlessly.

The uterine fundus comes into contact with the anterior abdominal wall at c.16–20 weeks' gestation. Later in pregnancy the increase in intra-abdominal pressure produced by the gravid uterus may produce eversion of the umbilicus. On the skin over the abdomen, a combination of stretching and hormonal changes may produce stretch marks (striae gravidarum). In multiparous patients, separation of right and left rectus abdominis may allow the uterine fundus to fall forwards to some extent.

In the supine position, the pregnant woman in late pregnancy is vulnerable to aortocaval compression, as the enlarged uterus presses on, and reduces blood flow in, the great vessels. Symptoms of nausea and faintness may be obvious, and uteroplacental blood flow may be impaired in some cases.

The jejunum, ileum and transverse colon tend to be displaced upwards by the enlarging uterus, whereas the caecum and appendix are displaced to the right, and the sigmoid colon posteriorly and to the left. Upward and lateral displacement of the appendix in later pregnancy can cause difficulties in the diagnosis of appendicitis. The ureters are pushed laterally by the enlarging uterus and in late pregnancy can be compressed at the level of the pelvic brim, resulting in hydronephrosis and loin pain. However, mild ureteric dilatation is normal in pregnancy, caused by progesterone-induced relaxation of smooth muscle in the ureteric walls. The axis of the uterus is shifted or dextrorotated by the presence of the sigmoid colon and this may lead to inadvertent incision into large uterine vessels at the time of lower segment caesarean section unless the operator is aware of any such rotation.

MATERNAL RESPIRATION, MICTURITION AND COLORECTAL CONTROL

As the uterus grows there is some outward displacement of the chest, with flaring of the ribs. Although vital capacity is unchanged, tidal air is said to increase by 200 ml and residual volume to fall by the same amount. The respiratory rate may increase somewhat even in early pregnancy, possibly due to the effect of progesterone, while in late pregnancy, uterine expansion may limit diaphragmatic excursion. The bladder becomes hyperaemic in early pregnancy, and there is also an increase in the frequency of micturition because of the raised glomerular filtration rate at that time, and later due to pressure from the presenting part on the bladder. Such pressure may also provoke urinary stress incontinence in the third trimester.

Changes in colorectal control are not very significant during pregnancy itself, although some women are troubled by constipation. Rectal sphincter damage can occur during childbirth and may lead to significant faecal incontinence if not recognized and adequately repaired at the time.

PELVIC CHANGES IN PREGNANCY

The presence of a pregnant uterus results in a change in the centre of gravity of the body, especially in late pregnancy (**Fig. 105.12**). In order to compensate for this, the mother tends to straighten her cervical and thoracic spine, and throw her shoulders back, resulting in a compensatory lumbar lordosis. There is also a softening of the pubic symphysis and sacroiliac joints, caused by production of relaxin and other pregnancy hormones. This increased mobility produces a form of pelvic instability so that the pregnant woman tends to walk with a waddling gait. The result of this softening is an increase in pelvic

A

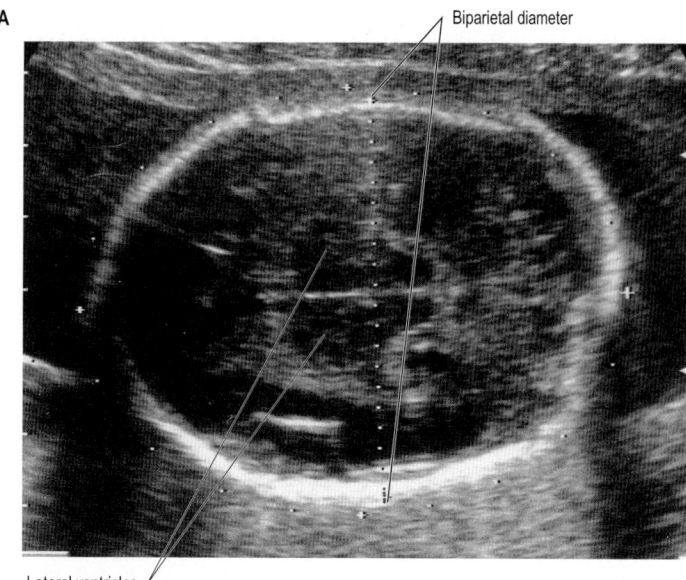

Biparietal diameter

Lateral ventricles

B

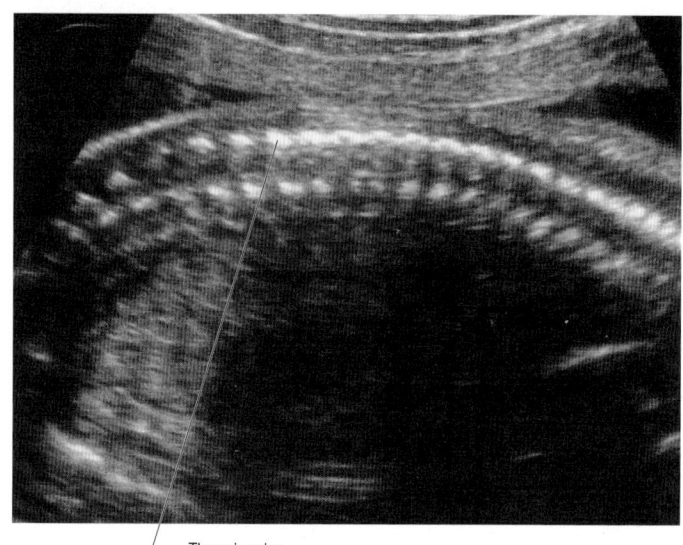

Thoracic spine

C

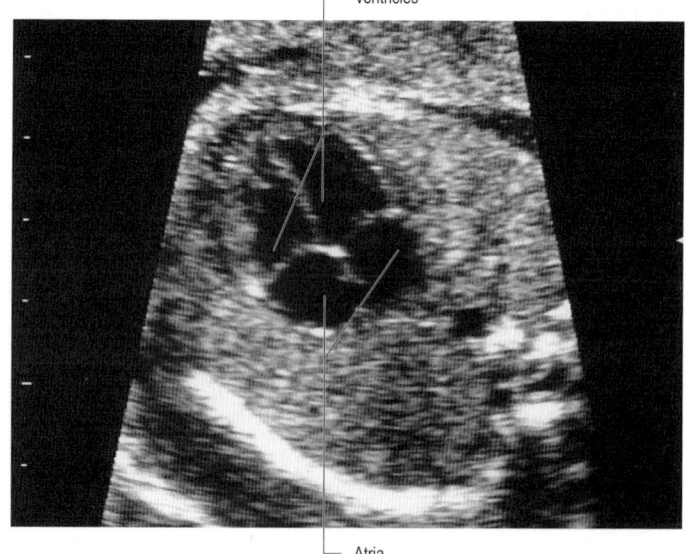

Ventricles

Atria

Fig. 105.11 Transabdominal ultrasound on a 16-week fetus. **A**, Biparietal diameter (an accurate method of dating the pregnancy). **B**, Longitudinal view of the thoracic spine. **C**, Four-chamber view of the heart (used to detect foetal anomalies). (By kind permission from Carien Laubscher, Superintendent in Ultrasound, Chelsea and Westminster Hospital, London.)

Placenta   Fetal leg   Fetal arm

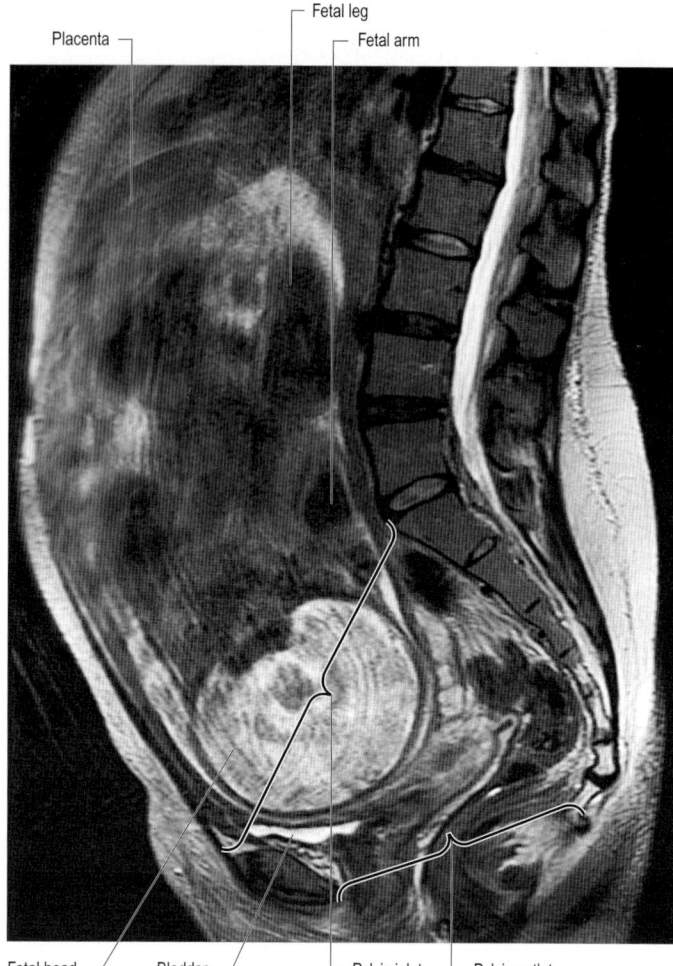

Fetal head   Bladder   Pelvic inlet   Pelvic outlet

Fig. 105.12 Sagittal T2-weighted scan, showing a normal cephalic presentation and the positions of the pelvic inlet and outlet at 30 weeks' pregnancy. (By kind permission from Kelly Wimpey, Superintendent in MRI, Chelsea and Westminster Hospital, London.)

diameter, which is of benefit during the time of labour. Significant joint relaxation can be associated with pain, sometimes called pelvic arthropathy, and in severe cases radiographs show that when a woman stands on one leg the two halves of the symphysis are almost at different levels. Rotation of the sacrum at the sacroiliac joint may increase the diameter of the pelvic outlet.

BIRTH CANAL AND PERINEUM DURING PARTURITION

The uterine cervix is required to serve two functions in relation to pregnancy and parturition. For 9 months the cervix is a relatively rigid fibromuscular structure, which retains the products of conception within the uterus, and yet, within a few hours during active labour, it has to dilate rapidly to allow the fetus to descend through the birth canal. In fact this transition is not as abrupt as might first appear, and there is considerable softening and shortening of the cervix in the weeks before the onset of labour. A corresponding increase in uterine activity is usually apparent during this prelabour period. The rigidity of the cervix appears to be related to the orientation of its collagen fibres within a regular connective tissue matrix. Softening of the cervix prior to and during labour is associated with a loss of this pattern of fibre distribution and a large increase in tissue water.

LABOUR

The onset of labour is defined as the combination of regular and usually painful uterine contractions of sufficient intensity to produce progressive effacement and dilatation of the cervix. It is often difficult to define the exact time of the onset of labour, except retrospectively. The pain of labour contractions is thought to be caused by myometrial ischaemia produced by a reduction in uterine blood flow during the peak of a contraction. Uterine contractions direct the fetus against the cervix and at the same time result in retraction of the upper uterine segment, drawing the fibromuscular cervix upwards past the presenting part. The process of labour is described as having three main stages, as follows.

First stage – The first stage is defined as the period during which the cervix dilates as it is drawn up into the lower portion of the uterus until there is no longer any cervix palpable on vaginal examination, and thus no further impediment to the descent of the fetus through the birth canal.

Second stage – The second stage begins once the cervix is fully dilated, and ends with the delivery of the baby. Uterine contractions produce the descent of the fetal presenting part. Pressure at this stage on the pelvic diaphragm and rectum produces in the mother a reflex desire to 'bear down'. Thus involuntary maternal effort using the diaphragm and abdominal musculature augments uterine activity to help deliver the child.

The head of the baby usually enters the pelvis with the occiput facing laterally. Further descent of the head results in the occiput contacting the gutter-shaped pelvic floor formed by levator ani. This promotes flexion and rotation of the occiput to the anterior position. With further descent the occiput escapes under the symphysis pubis and the head is born by extension. At this point, the baby's head regains its normal relationship with its shoulders, and slight rotation (or restitution) of the head is seen. Further external rotation occurs as the leading shoulder is directed medially by the maternal pelvic floor. The body of the baby is now born by lateral flexion as one shoulder slips underneath the symphysis and the posterior shoulder is drawn over the frenulum.

Third stage – The third stage is defined as the time from delivery of the fetus until delivery of the placenta. This process is usually expedited by the administration of oxytocic drugs in an attempt to limit maternal blood loss.

FACTORS AFFECTING THE PROGRESS OF LABOUR

Many factors affect the progress of labour including the quality of uterine contractions, the size of the maternal bony pelvis, the size and position of the baby's head and the extent to which the skull will mould to the shape of the pelvis (**Fig. 105.12**). The complex nature of these interactions means that it is generally not possible to predict the outcome of labour with any degree of accuracy, and most pregnant women will be offered a trial of labour if there is any doubt, providing the baby is in cephalic presentation. Poor progress during labour is predominantly a problem in the first labour because of the combination of incoordinate uterine action and increased soft tissue resistance at the level of the cervix, pelvic diaphragm and perineum. Treatment of such primigravidae is aimed at improving uterine activity through the combination of artificial rupture of the fetal membranes and administration of an intravenous infusion of oxytocin. Over 80% of cases will respond to such a regime, the remainder usually requiring caesarean delivery. In multiparous women, slow progress in labour may be due to inadequate uterine contractions but is more commonly due to mechanical problems such as a large baby. Use of oxytocin in the context of such genuine mechanical difficulties can lead to uterine rupture.

OBSTETRIC EMERGENCIES

Fetal distress – The unborn baby derives its oxygen from the mother via the placenta and umbilical cord. Fetal hypoxia may occur if the uteroplacental circulation is inadequate, if the placenta separates from the uterine wall or if the cord is compressed. During labour, uterine contractions tend to reduce placental perfusion. In addition, cord compression may occur during contractions, particularly if the amniotic fluid volume is reduced. Indirect evidence of fetal hypoxia can be inferred from certain changes in the fetal heart rate such as reduced variation and decelerations occurring in the rate after uterine contractions. Confirmation of hypoxia can be achieved by obtaining a blood sample from the fetal scalp and measuring the acid–base balance of the specimen. Confirmation of significant hypoxia acidosis during labour (pH < 7.20) is an indication for immediate delivery.

Prolapsed cord – The umbilical cord may prolapse through the cervix into the vagina once the fetal membranes rupture. Conditions that prevent the fetal head from fully occupying the maternal pelvis will predispose to this problem, i.e. pelvic tumours (fibroids), ovarian cysts, placenta praevia and prematurity. Compression of the cord by the presenting part of the fetus, or an umbilical artery spasm will lead to fetal hypoxia and death if untreated. The treatment is either funic replacement (pushing the cord back above the fetal head) or immediate caesarean section, and the risk of perinatal death rises as the interval from diagnosis to delivery increases.

Antepartum haemorrhage – The two most serious causes of antepartum haemorrhage are placenta praevia and placental abruption.

Placenta praevia – In early pregnancy the placental disc occupies a large proportion of the uterine cavity and will often appear to be situated near the internal os, on ultrasonographic or MRI examination (**Fig. 105.13**). In the majority of cases where the placenta appears low in early pregnancy, growth and stretching of the uterus will usually draw the placenta upwards away from the cervix by the end of pregnancy. In c.1% of pregnancies the position of the placenta will remain over, or in close proximity to, the internal cervical os at the end of pregnancy. This condition is called placenta praevia and is associated with vaginal bleeding during pregnancy and labour. The blood loss can be life-threatening for the mother. The diagnosis is confirmed by ultrasound examination and the usual therapeutic goal is to prolong pregnancy with hospitalization and if necessary provide blood transfusion until the fetus is of sufficient maturity to be delivered. Caesarean section is required and the procedure may be very haemorrhagic because of the increased vascularity of the lower uterine segment.

Placental abruption – Placental abruption, i.e. premature separation of the placenta from the uterine wall, is an emergency that may occur in either pregnancy or labour, and remains a significant cause of intra-uterine death. The diagnosis is suggested by the onset of constant and severe abdominal pain, with the uterus appearing rigid and tender on abdominal palpation. Placental separation is usually accompanied by bleeding but the blood may initially be contained within the uterus and not be obvious on external examination. Release of thromboplastin from the damaged placenta into the maternal circulation causes disseminated intravascular coagulation and consumption of clotting factors, which may predispose to further maternal haemorrhage at the time of delivery. Transfusion of blood and clotting factors may be required to resuscitate the mother. If the fetus is showing signs of distress on presentation, caesarean section is usually undertaken.

Postpartum haemorrhage – Prior to separation of the placenta, a large proportion of the mother's cardiac output passes through the uterine circulation. After separation in the third stage of labour, exsanguination is only prevented by marked uterine contraction, with criss-crossing myometrial fibres acting as a tourniquet, restricting blood flow to the area that was the placental site. Therefore, any condition that predisposes to poor uterine contraction, such as retained placental tissue or blood clot within the uterus, will increase the likelihood of haemorrhage immediately after delivery.

The other major cause of postpartum bleeding is that of trauma to the genital tract. Tearing will be found most frequently in the perineum and vagina but on occasion cervical laceration or even uterine rupture may be responsible for bleeding. Primary management of postpartum haemorrhaging is aimed at administering oxytocic drugs and resuscitating the mother with intravenous fluid. If this fails to stem the bleeding, then exploration of the genital tract under anaesthesia is undertaken to exclude retained placental tissue or genital tract trauma.

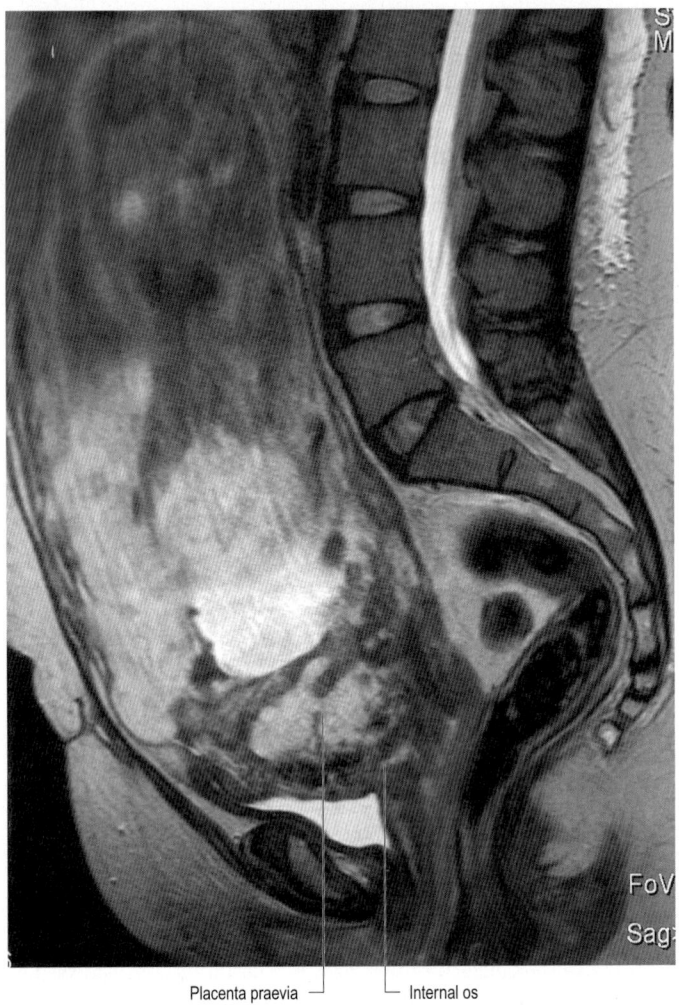

Placenta praevia — | — Internal os

Fig. 105.13 Sagittal T2-weighted scan showing a placenta praevia overlying the internal cervical os at 36 weeks' pregnancy. (By kind permission from Kelly Wimpey, Superintendent in MRI, Chelsea and Westminster Hospital, London.)

Vagina

The vagina is a fibromuscular tube lined by non-keratinized stratified epithelium (**Figs 102.1A,B, 102.2, 104.1, 104.4, 106.3**). It extends from the vestibule (the cleft between the labia minora) to the uterus.

The vagina ascends posteriorly and superiorly at an angle of over 90° to the uterine axis. This angle varies with the contents of the bladder and rectum, and the width increases as it ascends. Above the level of the hymen, the inner surfaces of the anterior and posterior vaginal walls are ordinarily in contact with each other forming a transverse slit. Its anterior wall is 7.5 cm in length and the posterior wall is 9 cm long on average.

The upper end of the vagina surrounds the vaginal projection of the uterine cervix. The vaginal mucosa is attached to the uterine cervix higher on the posterior cervical wall than on the anterior. The annular recess between the cervix and vagina forms four fornices. These are called the anterior, posterior and, two lateral fornices. Although the different parts of this recess are given separate names, the recess is essentially continuous.

Occasionally remnants of the duct of Gartner (p. 1384), Gartner's cysts, can be seen protruding through the lateral fornices or lateral parts of the vagina. These normal embryological remnants can some-times be confused with cancerous lesions and cause clinical concern during a routine cervical screening examination. They are normally asymptomatic.

RELATIONS

The bladder and urethra are anterior to the vagina. The rectum and anal canal are posterior and separated from the upper part by the recto-uterine pouch (p. 1332).

The anterior wall of the vagina is related to the urethra (which is embedded in it) inferiorly, and to the base of the bladder in its middle and upper portions. The posterior wall is covered by peritoneum in its upper quarter. It is separated from the rectum by the recto-uterine pouch superiorly, and by moderately loose connective tissue in its middle half (Denonvillier's fascia). In its lower quarter it is separated from the anal canal by the musculofibrous perineal body. Laterally are levator ani muscles (p. 1358) and pelvic fascia. As the ureters pass anteromedially to reach the fundus of the bladder, they pass close to the lateral fornices. As they enter the bladder the ureters are usually anterior to the vagina (p. 1375). At this point, each ureter is crossed transversely by a uterine artery (p. 1333).

VAGINAL FISTULA

Childbirth can be complicated by cephalopelvic disproportion where the pelvic cavity is too small for the size of the fetal head. This results in obstructed labour, which is treated by Caesarean section. In the developing world, where early recourse to Caesarean section is not available, this can cause a prolonged labour and necrosis of the vagina anteriorly due to pressure of the fetal head. This necrosis can cause a connection between the bladder and vagina (vesicovaginal fistula), which results in urinary incontinence. Other causes of a vesicovaginal fistula include cancer, post-radiation therapy, and trauma. A connection can also occur between the vagina and rectum, resulting in a recto-vaginal fistula.

VASCULAR SUPPLY AND LYMPHATIC DRAINAGE

ARTERIES
Arterial supply is derived from the vaginal, uterine, internal pudendal and middle rectal branches of the internal iliac arteries. The vaginal artery often gives off two or three branches that correspond to the inferior vesical artery in males. They descend on the vagina and supply the mucous membrane. Branches are also sent to the vestibular bulb, vesical fundus, and adjacent part of the rectum.

VEINS
The vaginal veins, one on each side, form from lateral plexuses that connect with uterine, vesical and rectal plexuses and drain to the internal iliac veins. The uterine and vaginal plexuses may provide collateral venous drainage to the lower limb.

LYMPHATIC DRAINAGE
Vaginal lymphatic vessels link with those of the cervix uteri, rectum and vulva. They form three groups but the regions drained are not sharply demarcated. Upper vessels accompany the uterine artery to the internal and external iliac nodes. Intermediate vessels accompany the vaginal artery to the internal iliac nodes. Vaginal vessels below the hymen, and from the vulva and perineal skin, pass to the superficial inguinal nodes.

INNERVATION

Innervation is derived from the vaginal plexuses and pelvic splanchnic nerves (p. 1126). The lower vagina is supplied by the pudendal nerve (p. 1457). Many nerve fibres in the lamina propria and muscle are probably cholinergic. Vaginal nerves from the lower parts of the inferior hypogastric and uterovaginal plexuses follow the vaginal arteries to supply the vaginal walls, the erectile tissue of the vestibular bulbs and clitoris (cavernous nerves of the clitoris), the urethra and the greater vestibular glands. The nerves contain many parasympathetic fibres, which are vasodilatory to the erectile tissue.

SPECULUM EXAMINATION (Figs 106.1, 106.2)

The vagina is examined using either a bivalve or angled (Sim's) speculum. A bivalve speculum (**Fig. 106.1A**) exposes the cervix, vaginal fornices, and lateral walls of the vagina. The angled (Sim's) speculum (**Fig. 106.1B**) is used to assess for uterine and vaginal prolapse.

MICROSTRUCTURE

The vagina has an inner mucosal and an external muscular layer. The lamina propria of the mucosa contains many thin-walled veins.

MUCOSA (Figs 106.2)
The mucosa adheres firmly to the muscular layer. There are two median longitudinal ridges on its epithelial surface, one anterior and the other posterior. Numerous transverse bilateral rugae extend from these vaginal

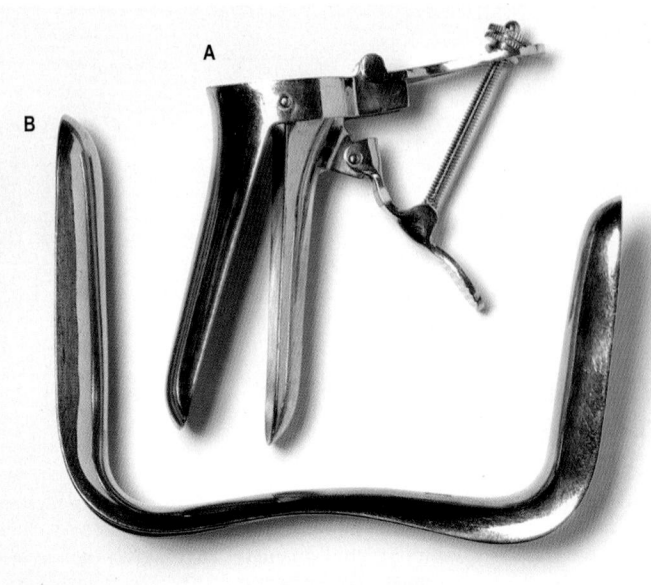

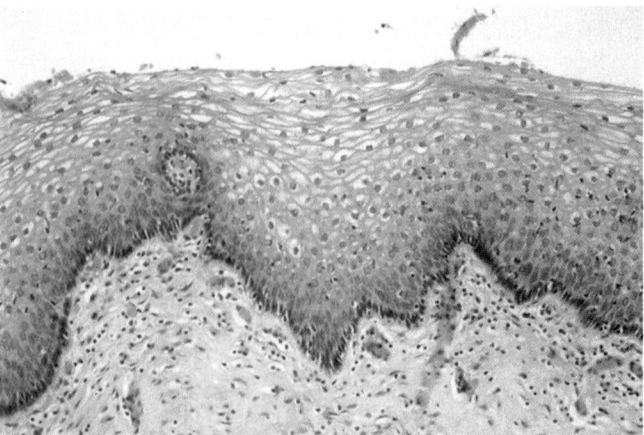

Fig. 106.2 Section through the mucosa of the vagina, showing the non-keratinized stratified squamous epithelium and the lamina propria beneath. Note the papillated interface between the epithelium and underlying connective tissue. Haematoxylin and eosin.

Fig. 106.1 A, bivalve speculum (Cuscos') used for exposing the cervix and lateral vaginal walls during clinical examination. **B,** An angled speculum (Sim's) used for exposing the vaginal walls during clinical examination.

columns. They are divided by sulci of variable depth, giving an appearance of conical papillae, which are most numerous on the posterior wall and near the orifice, and which are especially well developed before parturition. The epithelium is non-keratinized, stratified, squamous similar to, and continuous with, that of the ectocervix (p. 1334). After puberty it thickens and its superficial cells accumulate glycogen, which gives them a clear appearance in histological preparations.

The vaginal epithelium does not change markedly during the menstrual cycle, but its glycogen content increases after ovulation and then diminishes towards the end of the cycle. Natural vaginal bacteria, particularly *Lactobacillus acidophilus*, break down glycogen in the desquamated cellular debris to lactic acid. This produces a highly acidic (pH 3) environment, which inhibits the growth of most other micro-organisms. The amount of glycogen is less before puberty and after the menopause, when vaginal infections are more common. There are no mucous glands, but a fluid transudate from the lamina propria and mucus from the cervical glands lubricate the vagina.

MUSCULAR LAYERS

The muscular layers are composed of smooth muscle and consist of a thick outer longitudinal and an inner circular layer. Longitudinal fibres are continuous with the superficial muscle fibres of the uterus, and the strongest fasciculi are those attached to the rectovesical fascia on each side. The two layers are not distinct but connected by oblique decussating fasciculi. The lower vagina is also surrounded by the skeletal muscle fibres of bulbospongiosus. A layer of loose connective tissue, containing extensive vascular plexuses, surrounds the muscle layers.

Female external genital organs

The female external genitalia (**Figs 107.1**, **107.2**) include the mons pubis, labia majora, labia minora, clitoris, vestibule, vestibular bulb and the greater vestibular glands. The term pudendum, or vulva, includes all these parts.

SKIN

MONS PUBIS

The mons pubis is the rounded eminence that is anterior to the pubic symphysis. It is formed by a mass of subcutaneous adipose connective tissue. In adults, the mons is covered by coarse hair. This hair is usually limited above by a horizontal boundary. (In males there is a continuation of pubic hair to the umbilicus.)

LABIA MAJORA (Fig. 107.1)

The labia majora are two prominent, longitudinal, cutaneous folds extending back from the mons pubis to the perineum. They form the lateral boundaries of the pudendal cleft, into which the vagina and urethra open. Each labium has an external, pigmented surface, covered with crisp hairs and a pink, smooth, internal surface with large sebaceous follicles. Between these surfaces there is much loose connective and adipose tissue, intermixed with smooth muscle resembling the scrotal

dartos muscle, together with vessels, nerves and glands. The uterine round ligament may end in the adipose tissue and skin in the front part of the labium. A persistent processus vaginalis and congenital inguinal hernia may also reach a labium. The labia are thicker in front, where they join to form the anterior commissure. Posteriorly they do not join but merge into neighbouring skin, ending near and almost parallel to each other. The connecting skin between them posteriorly forms a ridge called the posterior commissure. This overlies the perineal body and is the posterior limit of the vulva. The interval between this and the anus is c.2.5 to 3 cm thick and is termed the 'gynaecological' perineum.

LABIA MINORA (Figs 107.1, 107.2)

The labia minora are two small cutaneous folds, devoid of fat, that lie between the labia majora. They extend from the clitoris obliquely down, laterally and back for c.4 cm, flanking the vaginal orifice. In virgins their posterior ends may be joined by the cutaneous frenulum of the labia minora. Anteriorly, each labium minus bifurcates. The upper layer passes above the clitoris to form with its fellow a fold, the prepuce, which overhangs the glans of the clitoris. The lower layer passes below the clitoris to form with its fellow the frenulum of the clitoris. Sebaceous follicles are numerous on the apposed labial surfaces. Sometimes an extra labial fold (labium tertium) is found on one or both sides between the labia minora and majora.

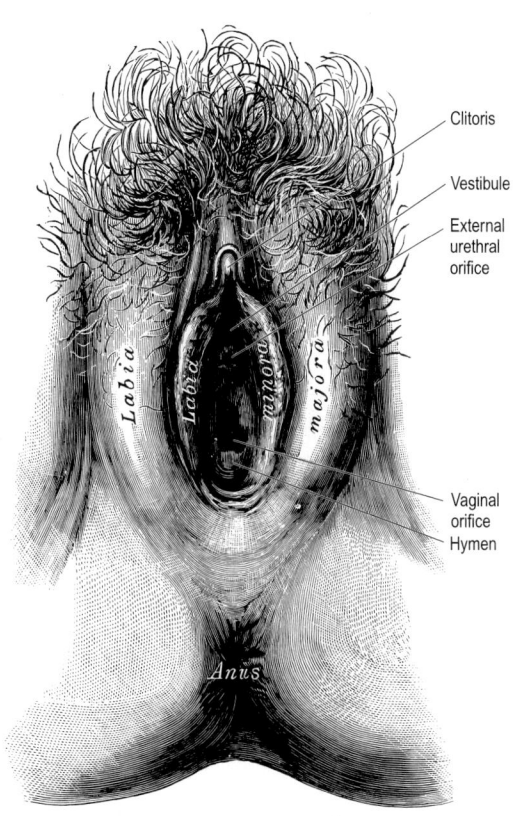

Fig. 107.1 The female external genitalia.

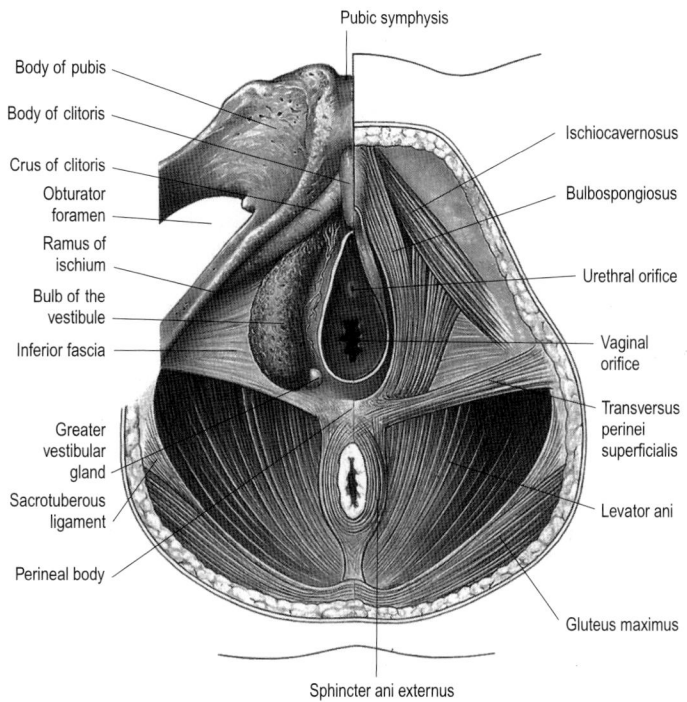

Fig. 107.2 The female perineum. On the right side the bulb of the vestibule and greater vestibular gland are shown. On the left side the muscles superficial to these structures are shown.

VESTIBULE (Fig. 107.2)

The vestibule is the cavity that lies between the labia minora. It contains the vaginal and external urethral orifices and the openings of the two greater vestibular glands and those of numerous, mucous, lesser vestibular glands. There is a shallow vestibular fossa between the vaginal orifice and the frenulum of the labia minora.

CLITORIS (Fig. 107.2)

The clitoris is an erectile structure, homologous with the penis, which lies posteroinferior to the anterior commissure. It is partially enclosed by the anterior bifurcated ends of the labia minora. The corpus clitoridis has two corpora cavernosa, which are composed of erectile tissue and enclosed in dense fibrous tissue separated medially by an incomplete fibrous pectiniform septum. Each corpus cavernosum is connected to its ischiopubic ramus by a crus.

The glans of the clitoris is a small round tubercle of spongy erectile tissue. Its epithelium has high cutaneous sensitivity, which is important in sexual responses. The clitoris, like the penis, has a 'suspensory' ligament and two small muscles, ischiocavernosi, attached to its crura (p. 1316). In many anatomical details it is a small version of the penis, but differs from it in being separate from the urethra.

VAGINAL ORIFICE (INTROITUS) (Fig. 107.2)

The introitus is usually a sagittal slit positioned posteroinferior to the urethral meatus. Its size varies. It is capable of great distension during parturition and to a lesser degree during coitus.

HYMEN VAGINAE

The hymen is a thin fold of mucous membrane situated just within the vaginal orifice. The internal surfaces of the folds are normally in contact each other and the vaginal orifice appears as a cleft between them.

The hymen varies greatly in shape and area. When stretched, it is annular and widest posteriorly. Sometimes it is semilunar, concave towards the mons pubis. Occasionally it is cribriform or fringed. It may be absent or form a complete, imperforate hymen. When it is ruptured, small round carunculae hymenales (also known as carunculae myrtiformis) are its remnants. It has no established function.

EXTERNAL URETHRAL ORIFICE (URINARY MEATUS) (Fig. 107.2)

The urethra opens into the vestibule c.2.5 cm inferiorly to the clitoris and anterior to the vaginal orifice. The meatus is usually a short, sagittal cleft with slightly raised margins and is very distensible. It varies in shape, and the aperture may exhibit either rounded, slit-like, crescentic or stellate forms.

BULBS OF THE VESTIBULE (Fig. 107.2)

The bulbs of the vestibule are homologues of the single penile bulb and corpus spongiosum. They are two elongate erectile masses, flanking the vaginal orifice and united in front of it by a narrow commissura bulborum (pars intermedia). Each lateral mass is c.3 cm in length. Their posterior ends are expanded and are in contact with the greater vestibular glands. Their anterior ends are tapered and joined to one another by a commissure, and to the clitoris by two slender bands of erectile tissue. Their deep surfaces contact the inferior aspect of the urogenital diaphragm. Superficially each is covered by the bulbospongiosus posteriorly. Thus the female corpus spongiosum is split into bilateral masses, except in its most anterior region, by the vestibule and the vaginal and urethral orifices.

GREATER VESTIBULAR GLANDS (GLANDS OF BARTHOLIN) (Fig. 107.2)

The greater vestibular glands (glands of Bartholin)are homologues of the male bulbourethral glands. They consist of two small, round or oval reddish-yellow bodies, flanking the vaginal orifice, in contact with, and often overlapped by, the posterior end of the vestibular bulb. Each opens into the vestibule, by a duct of c.2 cm, in the groove between the hymen and a labium minus.

The glands are composed of tubulo-acinar tissue. The secretory cells are columnar and secrete a clear or whitish mucus with lubricant properties. They are stimulated by sexual arousal.

Ducts connecting the greater vestibular glands with the vagina may become blocked with proteinaceous material. This can cause the secretion from the gland to accumulate within it forming a cyst (Bartholin's cyst), which can appear as a pea- to grape-sized swelling bulging unilaterally from the lower part of the vulvovaginal margin. Occasionally a cyst becomes infected, forming an abscess. Treatment is surgical, by excision or marsupialization.

VASCULAR SUPPLY AND LYMPHATIC DRAINAGE

ARTERIES

The arterial blood supply of the female external genitalia resembles that of homologous structures in males. Thus it is derived from the superficial and deep external pudendal branches of the femoral artery and the internal pudendal artery on each side. The blood supply is substantial and consequently haemorrhage from vulval injuries may be severe.

VEINS

Venous drainage of the vulval skin is via external pudendal veins to the long saphenous vein. Venous drainage of the clitoris mirrors that of the penis and is via deep dorsal veins to the internal pudendal vein and superficial dorsal veins to the external pudendal and long saphenous veins (p. 1203).

LYMPHATIC DRAINAGE

Lymphatic drainage of the vulva is via a meshwork of connecting vessels that emerge into three or four collecting trunks around the mons pubis. They drain to superficial inguinal nodes, then deep femoral nodes and eventually to pelvic nodes. The last of the deep femoral nodes lies under the inguinal ligament and is often called Cloquet's node. Lymph vessels in the perineum and lower part of the labia majora drain to the rectal lymphatic plexus (p. 1203). Lymph vessels from the clitoris and labia minora drain to deep inguinal nodes and direct clitoral efferents may pass to the internal iliac nodes.

INNERVATION

The sensory innervation of the anterior and posterior parts of the labium majus differ, as they do in the scrotum. The anterior third of the labium majus is supplied by the ilioinguinal nerve (L1). The posterior two-thirds are supplied by the labial branches of the perineal nerve (S3). The lateral aspect of the labium majus also receives nervous innervation from the perineal branch of the posterior cutaneous nerve of the thigh (S2).

AGE-RELATED CHANGES

Before adolescence, the mons pubis is relatively flat and the labia minora are poorly formed. The hymenal ring is normally narrow and well formed. During adolescence, coarse hair forms over the mons and labia majora. The labia minora also become more prominent and flap like. The hymenal ring normally ruptures after first sexual intercourse but can rupture earlier due to other non-sexual physical activity. After the menopause, pubic hair thins and labial tissue atrophies slightly.

True pelvis, pelvic floor and perineum

TRUE PELVIS AND PELVIC FLOOR

The true pelvis is a bowl-shaped structure formed from the sacrum, pubis, ilium, ischium, the ligaments which interconnect these bones and the muscles which line their inner surfaces. The true pelvis is considered to start at the level of the plane passing through the promontory of the sacrum, the arcuate line on the ilium, the iliopectineal line and the posterior surface of the pubic crest. This plane, or 'inlet' lies at an angle of between 35 and 50° up from the horizontal and above this the bony structures are sometimes referred to as the false pelvis. They form part of the walls of the lower abdomen. The floor or 'outlet' of the true pelvis is formed by the muscles of levator ani. Although the floor is gutter shaped, it generally lies in a plane between 5 and 15° up from the horizontal. This difference between the planes of the inlet and outlet is the reason why the true pelvis is said to have an axis (lying perpendicular to the plane of both inlet and outlet) which progressively changes through the pelvis from above downwards. The details of the topography of the bony and ligamentous pelvis is considered fully on page 1428.

Muscles and fasciae of the pelvis

PELVIC MUSCLES (Figs 108.1, 108.2)

The muscles arising within the pelvis form two groups. Piriformis and obturator internus, although forming part of the walls of the pelvis, are considered as primarily muscles of the lower limb. Levator ani and coccygeus form the pelvic diaphragm and delineate the lower limit of the true pelvis. The fasciae investing the muscles are continuous with visceral pelvic fascia above, perineal fascia below and obturator fascia laterally.

PIRIFORMIS (See also p. 1357.)

Piriformis forms part of the posterolateral wall of the true pelvis. It is attached to the anterior surface of the sacrum, the gluteal surface of the ilium near the posterior inferior iliac spine, the capsule of the adjacent sacroiliac joint and sometimes to the upper part of the pelvic surface of the sacrotuberous ligament. It passes out of the pelvis through the greater sciatic foramen. Within the pelvis, the anterior surface of piriformis is related to the rectum (especially on the left), the sacral plexus of nerves and branches of the internal iliac vessels. The posterior surface lies against the sacrum.

OBTURATOR INTERNUS (See also p. 1357.)

Obturator internus and the fascia over its upper inner (pelvic) surface form part of the anterolateral wall of the true pelvis. It is attached to the structures surrounding the obturator foramen; the inferior ramus of the pubis, the ischial ramus, the pelvic surface of the hip bone below and behind the pelvic brim, and the upper part of the greater sciatic foramen. It also attaches to the medial part of the pelvic surface of the obturator

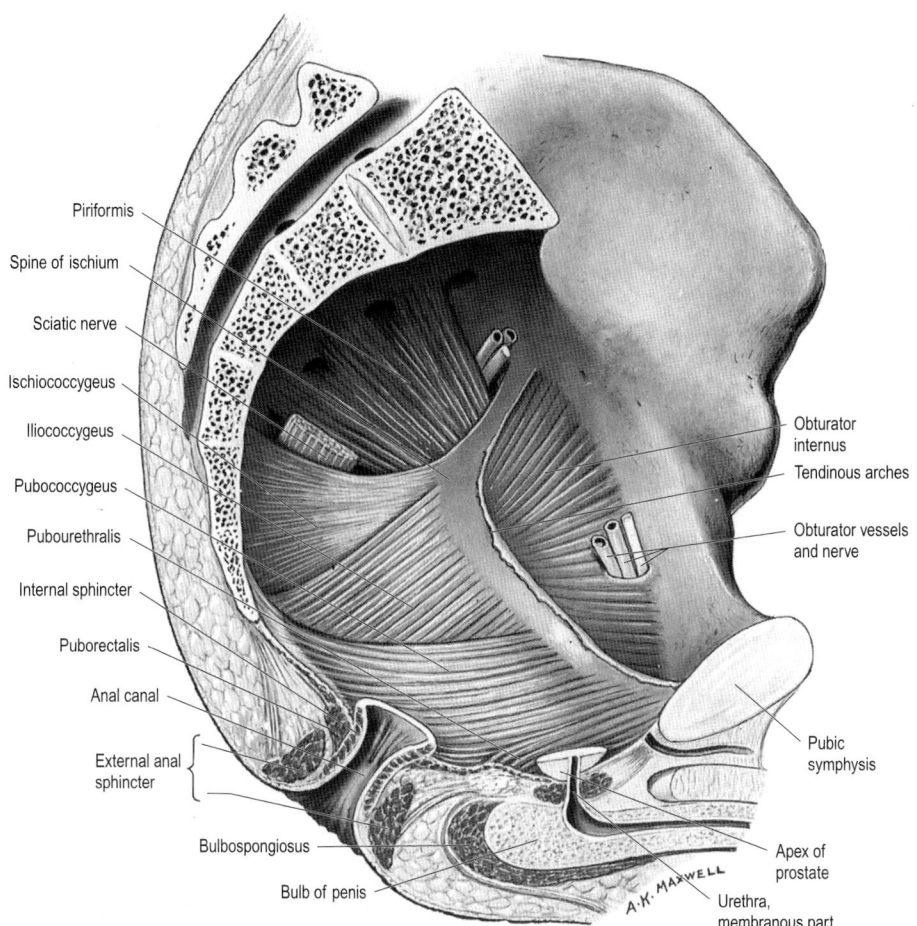

Fig. 108.1 Muscles of the male pelvis – lateral view. The superior gluteal and obturator vessels and nerves have been divided close to their exit from the pelvis. The rectum, bladder and upper prostate have been omitted for clarity.

Piriformis

Spine of ischium

Sciatic nerve

Ischiococcygeus

Iliococcygeus

Pubococcygeus

Pubourethralis

Internal sphincter

Puborectalis

Anal canal

External anal sphincter

Bulbospongiosus

Bulb of penis

Obturator internus

Tendinous arches

Obturator vessels and nerve

Pubic symphysis

Apex of prostate

Urethra, membranous part

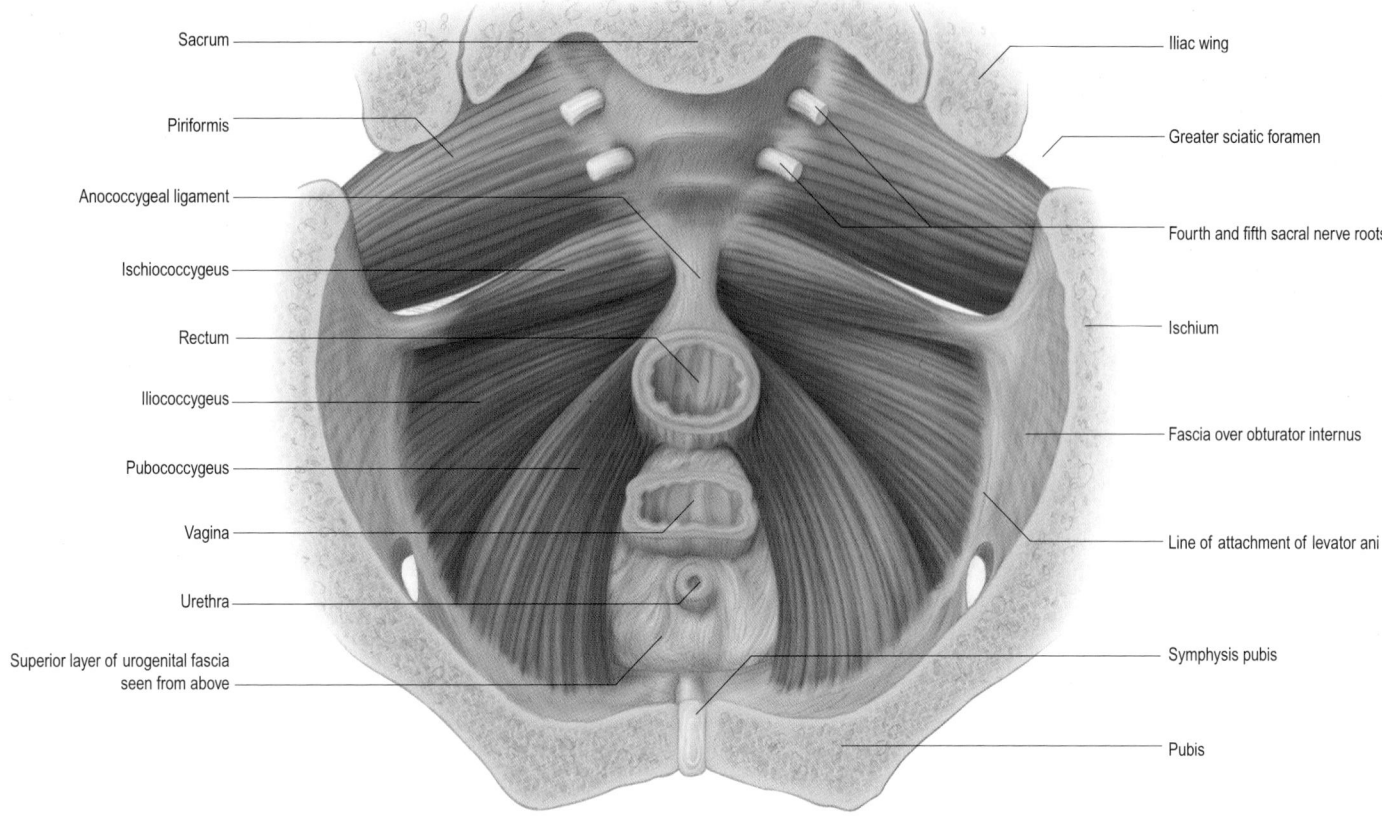

Sacrum

Piriformis

Anococcygeal ligament

Ischiococcygeus

Rectum

Iliococcygeus

Pubococcygeus

Vagina

Urethra

Superior layer of urogenital fascia
seen from above

Iliac wing

Greater sciatic foramen

Fourth and fifth sacral nerve roots

Ischium

Fascia over obturator internus

Line of attachment of levator ani

Symphysis pubis

Pubis

Fig. 108.2 Muscles of the female pelvis viewed from above. The sacral nerve roots have been divided close to the sacral foramina. The anorectal junction, vagina and urethra have been divided at the level of the pelvic floor.

membrane. The muscle is covered by a thick fascial layer and the fibres themselves cannot be seen directly from within the pelvis. This fascia gives attachment to some of the fibres of levator ani and thus only the upper portion of the muscle lies lateral to the contents of the true pelvis, whilst the lower portion forms part of the boundaries of the ischioanal fossa. In the male, the upper portion lies lateral to the bladder, the obturator and vesical vessels, and the obturator nerve. In the female, the attachments of the broad ligament of the uterus, the fallopian end of the uterine tubes, and the uterine vessels, also lie medial to obturator internus and its fascia.

LEVATOR ANI (ISCHIOCOCCYGEUS, ILIOCOCCYGEUS, PUBOCOCCYGEUS)

Levator ani is a broad muscular sheet of variable thickness attached to the internal surface of the true pelvis and forms a large portion of the pelvic floor. The muscle is subdivided into named portions according to their attachments and the pelvic viscera to which they are related. These parts are often referred to as separate muscles, but the boundaries between each part cannot be easily distinguished and they perform many similar physiological functions. The separate parts are referred to as ischiococcygeus, iliococcygeus and pubococcygeus. Pubococcygeus is often subdivided into separate parts according to the pelvic viscera to which they relate, i.e. pubourethralis and puborectalis in the male, pubovaginalis and puborectalis in the female. Levator ani arises from each side of the walls of the pelvis. Fibres from ischiococcygeus attach to the sacrum and coccyx but the remaining parts of the muscle converge in the midline. The fibres of iliococcygeus join by a partly fibrous inter-section and form a raphe posterior to the anorectal junction. Closer to the anorectal junction and elsewhere in the pelvic floor, the fibres are more nearly continuous with those of the opposite side and the muscle forms a sling (puborectalis and pubovaginalis or pubourethralis).

Attachments

Ischiococcygeus – The ischiococcygeal part may be referred to as a separate muscle, sometimes named coccygeus. It lies as the most posterosuperior portion of levator ani and arises as a triangular

musculotendinous sheet with its apex attached to the pelvic surface and tip of the ischial spine. The base of the muscle is attached to the lateral margins of the coccyx and the fifth sacral segment. Ischiococcygeus is rarely absent, but may be nearly completely tendinous rather than muscular. It lies on the pelvic aspect of the sacrospinous ligament and may be fused with it, particularly if mostly tendinous. The sacrospinous ligament may represent a degenerate part or an aponeurosis of the muscle since the muscle and ligament are coextensive.

Iliococcygeus – The iliococcygeal part is attached to the inner surface of the ischial spine below and anterior to the attachment of ischio-coccygeus and to the obturator fascia as far forward as the obturator canal (**Fig. 108.1**). The most posterior fibres are attached to the tip of the sacrum and coccyx but most join with fibres from the opposite side to form a raphe. This raphe is effectively continuous with the fibro-elastic anococcygeal ligament, which is closely applied to its inferior surface and some muscle fibres may attach into the ligament. The raphe provides a strong attachment for the pelvic floor posteriorly and must be divided to allow wide excisions of the anorectal canal during abdomino-perineal excisions for malignancy. An accessory slip may arise from the most posterior part and is sometimes referred to as iliosacralis.

Pubococcygeus – The pubococcygeal part is attached to the back of the body of the pubis and passes back almost horizontally. The most medial fibres run directly lateral to the urethra and its sphincter as it passes through the pelvic floor. In males these fibres therefore lie lateral and inferior to the prostate and are referred to as pubourethralis. They form part of the urethral sphincter complex together with the intrinsic striated and smooth musculature of the urethra and fibres decussate across the midline directly behind the urethra. In females the fibres of this part of the muscle run further back to from a sling around the posterior wall of the vagina and are referred to as pubovaginalis. In both sexes fibres from this part of pubococcygeus attach to the perineal body and a few elements also attach to the anorectal junction. Some of these fibres, sometimes called puboanalis, decussate and blend with the longitudinal rectal muscle and fascial elements to contribute to the conjoint longitudinal coat of the anal canal. Behind the rectum

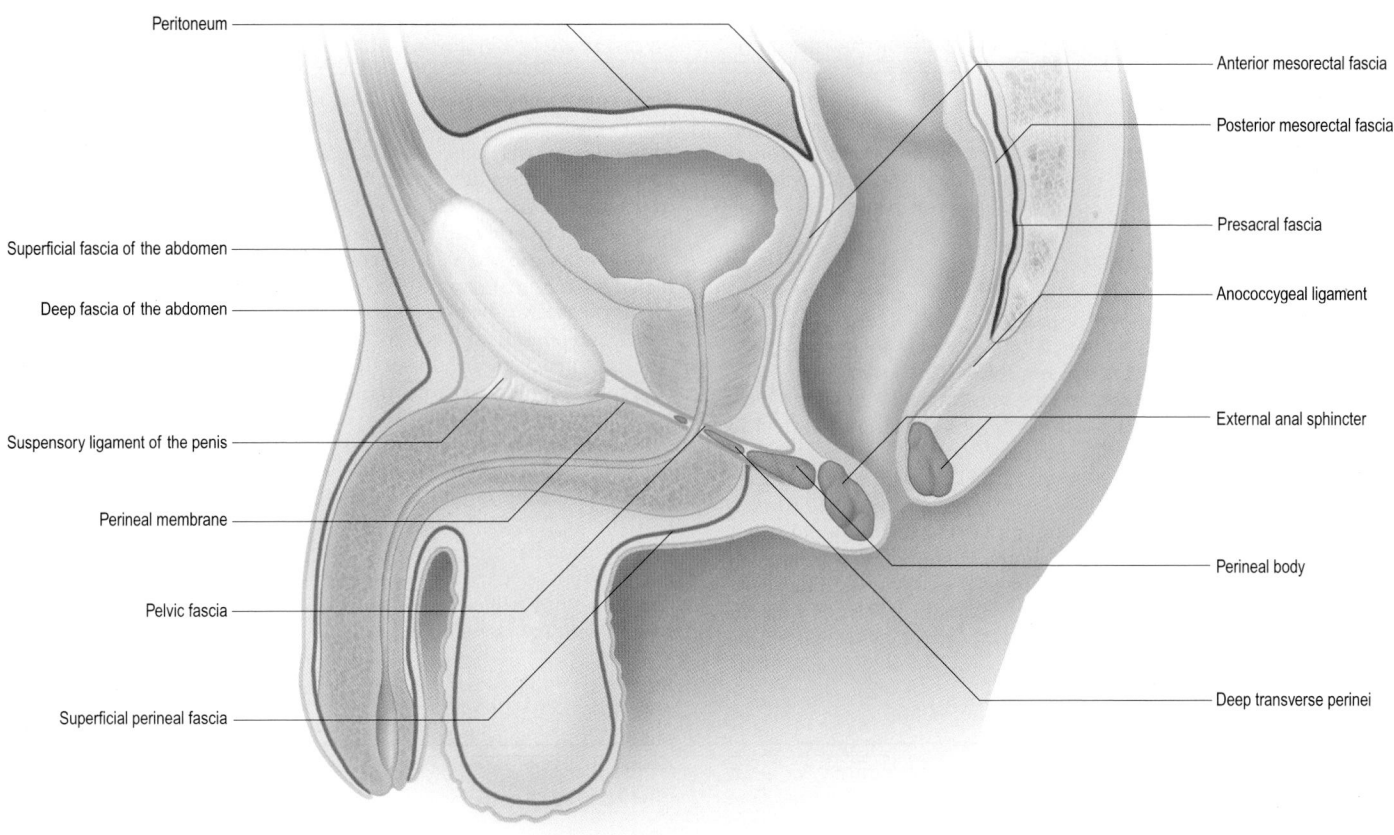

Fig. 108.3 Fasciae of the pelvis and perineum. Median sagittal section in the male. The deep fascia of the abdominal wall, the layers of the urogenital fascia and the mesorectal fascia are in green, the peritoneum in blue, the superficial fascia of the abdominal wall and perineum in red. Muscles are shown in brown.

Labels (top to bottom, left):
Peritoneum
Superficial fascia of the abdomen
Deep fascia of the abdomen
Suspensory ligament of the penis
Perineal membrane
Pelvic fascia
Superficial perineal fascia

Labels (top to bottom, right):
Anterior mesorectal fascia
Posterior mesorectal fascia
Presacral fascia
Anococcygeal ligament
External anal sphincter
Perineal body
Deep transverse perinei

some fibres of pubococcygeus form a tendinous intersection as part of the levator raphe but a thick muscular sling, puborectalis, wraps around the anorectal junction. Some fibres blend with those of the external anal sphincter.

Relations
The superior, pelvic surface of levator ani is separated only by fascia (superior pelvic diaphragmatic, visceral and extraperitoneal (p. 1359) from the urinary bladder, prostate or uterus and vagina, rectum and peritoneum. Its inferior, perineal, surface forms the medial wall of the ischioanal fossa and the superior wall of the anterior recess of the fossa, both being covered by inferior pelvic diaphragmatic fascia. The posterior border is separated from the coccyx by areolar tissue. The medial borders of the two levator muscles are separated by the visceral outlet, through which pass the urethra, vagina, and anorectum.

Vascular supply
Levator ani is supplied by branches of the inferior gluteal artery, the inferior vesical artery and the pudendal artery.

Innervation
Fibres originating mainly in the second, third and fourth sacral spinal segments reach levator ani from below and above by a variety of routes (Wendell-Smith & Wilson 1991). Most commonly pubococcygeus (puborectalis and pubovaginalis or pubourethralis) is supplied by second and third sacral spinal segments via the pudendal nerve, and ischiococcygeus and iliococcygeus by direct branches of the sacral plexus from third and fourth sacral spinal segments.

Actions
Pubococcygeus is a lateral compressor of the various visceral canals which cross the pelvic floor. The puborectalis part also reinforces the external anal sphincter and helps to create the anorectal angle. It also reduces the anteroposterior dimension of the ano–urogenital hiatus.

Iliococcygeus and, to a lesser extent, the less muscular ischiococcygeus, assist puborectalis in contributing to anorectal and urinary continence. It is well recognized that levator ani must relax appropriately to permit expulsion of urine and particularly faeces. Levator ani also forms much of the basin-shaped muscular pelvic diaphragm, which supports the pelvic viscera and it contracts with abdominal muscles and the abdominothoracic diaphragm to raise intra-abdominal pressure. Like the abdominothoracic diaphragm, but unlike abdominal muscles, levator ani is also active in the inspiratory phase of quiet respiration. In the pregnant female, the shape of the pelvic floor may help to direct the fetal head into the anteroposterior diameter of the pelvic outlet.

PELVIC FASCIAE (Fig. 108.3)

The pelvic fasciae may be conveniently divided into the parietal pelvic fascia, which mainly forms the coverings of the pelvic muscles, and the visceral pelvic fascia, which forms the coverings of the pelvic viscera, their supplying vessels and nerves. The visceral pelvic fascia is described with the pelvic viscera.

PARIETAL PELVIC FASCIA
The parietal pelvic fascia on the pelvic surface of obturator internus is well differentiated as the obturator fascia. Above, it is connected to the posterior part of the arcuate line of the ilium, and is continuous with iliac fascia. Anterior to this, as it follows the line of origin of obturator internus, it is gradually separated from the attachment of the iliac fascia and a portion of the periosteum of the ilium and pubis spans between them. It arches below the obturator vessels and nerve, investing the obturator canal, and is attached anteriorly to the back of the pubis. Behind the obturator canal the fascia is markedly aponeurotic and gives a firm attachment to levator ani. Below the attachment of levator ani it is thin and forms part of the lateral wall of the ischioanal fossa in the perineum. It is continuous with the pelvic periosteum and thus the fascia over piriformis.

FASCIA OVER PIRIFORMIS

The fascia of piriformis is very thin, and fuses with the periosteum on the front of the sacrum at the margins of the anterior sacral foramina. It ensheathes the sacral anterior primary rami which emerges from these foramina, and the nerves are often described as lying behind the fascia. The internal iliac vessels lie in front of the fascia over piriformis and their branches draw out sheaths of the fascia and extraperitoneal tissue into the gluteal region, above and below piriformis.

FASCIA OF THE PELVIC DIAPHRAGM

The fascia of the pelvic diaphragm covers both of the surfaces of the pelvic diaphragm. On the lower surface is the thin inferior fascia of the pelvic diaphragm, which is continuous with the obturator fascia laterally. It covers the medial wall of the ischioanal fossa and blends below with fasciae on the urethral sphincter and the external anal sphincter. On the upper surface is the superior fascia of the pelvic diaphragm which is generally known clinically as the endopelvic fascia.

It is attached anteriorly to the back of the body of the pubis, c.2 cm above its lower border, and extends laterally across the superior ramus of the pubis, blending with the obturator fascia and continuing along an irregular line to the spine of the ischium. It is continuous posteriorly with the fascia over piriformis and the anterior sacrococcygeal ligament. Medially, the superior fascia of the pelvic diaphragm blends with the visceral pelvic fascia. The fascia over obturator internus above the attachment of levator ani is therefore composed of the obturator fascia itself, the superior and inferior pelvic diaphragmatic fasciae and fibres from levator ani. The thickening where these structures fuse is the tendinous arch of levator ani. Below it, within the superior fascia, is the tendinous arch of the pelvic fascia, a thick white band extending from the lower part of the symphysis pubis to the inferior margin of the spine of the ischium (arcus tendineous fasciae pelvis). This is the attachment of the lateral, 'true' ligament of the urinary bladder. Anteriorly the same fascia forms two thick bands, the paired puboprostatic ligaments in the male, or the pubourethral ligaments in the female.

PRESACRAL FASCIA

The presacral fascia lies between the posterior aspect of the mesorectal fascia and the superior pelvic diaphragmatic fascia. It is a hammock-like sheet extending between the tendinous arches of the pelvic fascia on either side. Below, it extends to the anorectal junction, where it fuses with the posterior aspect of the mesorectal fascia at the level of the anorectal junction. Above, it can be traced to the origin of the superior hypogastric plexus where it becomes progressively thinner over the promontory of the sacrum and becomes continuous with the retroperitoneal tissues. The right and left hypogastric nerves and inferior hypogastric plexuses lie on its surface and the presacral veins lie immediately posterior to it. It forms a distinct layer which can be seen both on magnetic resonance images of the pelvis and during surgery. The fascia provides an important landmark because extension of rectal tumours through it significantly reduces the chance of curative resectional surgery being possible. Dissection in the plane posterior to it may result in bleeding from the presacral veins and, since the adventitia of the veins is partly attached to the posterior surface of the fascia, the haemorrhage may be severe because the veins are unable to contract down properly.

Vascular supply and lymphatic drainage of the pelvis

The true pelvis contains the internal iliac arteries and veins as well as the lymphatics draining the majority of the pelvic viscera. The common and external iliac vessels as well as the lymphatics draining the lower limb lie along the pelvic brim and in the lower retroperitoneum, but are conveniently discussed together with the vessels of the true pelvis.

ARTERIES OF THE PELVIS

COMMON ILIAC ARTERIES

The abdominal aorta bifurcates into the right and left common iliac arteries anterolateral to the left side of the fourth lumbar vertebral body. These arteries diverge as they descend to divide at the level of the sacroiliac joint into external and internal iliac arteries. The external iliac artery is the principal artery of the lower limb and the internal iliac artery provides the principal supply to the pelvic viscera and walls, the perineum and the gluteal region.

Right common iliac artery – The right common iliac artery is approximately 5 cm long and passes obliquely across part of the fourth and the fifth lumbar vertebral bodies. The sympathetic rami to the pelvic plexus and, at its division, the ureter, cross anterior to it. It is covered by the parietal peritoneum, which separates it from the coils of the small intestine. Posteriorly, it is separated from the fourth and fifth lumbar vertebral bodies and their intervening disc by the right sympathetic trunk, the terminal parts of the common iliac veins and the start of the inferior vena cava, the obturator nerve, lumbosacral trunk and iliolumbar artery. Lateral to its upper part are the inferior vena cava and the right common iliac vein and lower down is the right psoas major. The left common iliac vein is medial to the upper part.

Left common iliac artery – The left common iliac artery is shorter than the right and is approximately 4 cm long. Lying anterior to it are the sympathetic rami to the pelvic plexus, the superior rectal artery and, at its terminal bifurcation, the ureter. The sympathetic trunk, the fourth and fifth lumbar vertebral bodies and intervening disc, the obturator nerve, lumbosacral trunk and iliolumbar artery are all posterior to it. The left common iliac vein is posteromedial to the artery while the left psoas major lies lateral to it.

Branches – In addition to the external iliac and internal iliac terminal branches, each common iliac artery gives small branches to the peritoneum, psoas major, ureter, adjacent nerves and surrounding areolar tissue. Occasionally the common iliac artery gives rise to the iliolumbar artery and accessory renal arteries if the kidney is low lying.

INTERNAL ILIAC ARTERIES (Fig. 108.4)

Each internal iliac artery, c.4 cm long, begins at the common iliac bifurcation, level with the lumbosacral intervertebral disc and anterior to the sacroiliac joint. It descends posteriorly to the superior margin of the greater sciatic foramen where it divides into an anterior trunk, which continues in the same line towards the ischial spine, and a posterior trunk, which passes back to the greater sciatic foramen. Anterior to the artery are the ureter and, in females, the ovary and fimbriated end of the uterine tube. The internal iliac vein, lumbosacral trunk and sacroiliac joint are posterior. Lateral is the external iliac vein, between the artery and psoas major and inferior to this is the obturator nerve. The parietal

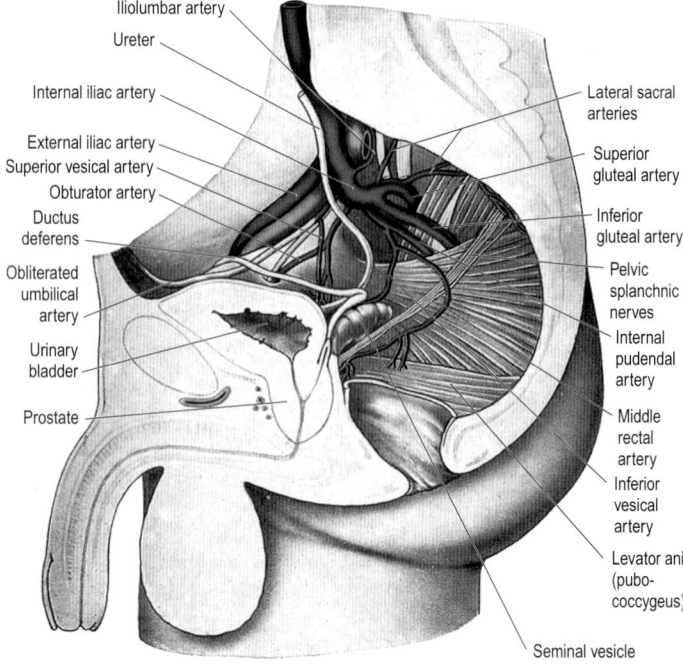

Fig. 108.4 Arteries of the male pelvis. The internal iliac vein and its tributaries and the rectum have been omitted for clarity.

peritoneum is medial, separating it from the terminal ileum on the right and the sigmoid colon on the left. Tributaries of the internal iliac vein are also medial.

In the fetus the internal iliac artery is twice the size of the external and is the direct continuation of the common iliac artery. The main trunk ascends on the anterior abdominal wall to the umbilicus, converging on the contralateral artery. The two arteries run through the umbilicus to enter the umbilical cord as the umbilical arteries. At birth, when placental circulation ceases, only the pelvic segment remains patent as the internal iliac artery and part of the superior vesical artery; the remainder becomes a fibrous medial umbilical ligament. In males, the patent part usually gives off an artery to the vas deferens.

Posterior trunk branches

Iliolumbar artery – The iliolumbar artery is the first branch of the posterior trunk and ascends laterally anterior to the sacroiliac joint and lumbosacral nerve trunk. It lies posterior to the obturator nerve and external iliac vessels and reaches the medial border of psoas major, dividing behind it into the lumbar and iliac branches. The lumbar branch supplies psoas major and quadratus lumborum and anastomoses with the fourth lumbar artery. It sends a small spinal branch through the intervertebral foramen between the fifth lumbar and first sacral vertebrae, to supply the cauda equina. The iliac branch supplies iliacus; between the muscle and bone it anastomoses with the iliac branches of the obturator artery. A large nutrient branch enters an oblique canal in the ilium. Other branches runs around the iliac crest, contribute to the supply of the gluteal and abdominal muscles, and anastomose with the superior gluteal, circumflex iliac and lateral circumflex femoral arteries.

Lateral sacral arteries – The lateral sacral arteries are usually double or if single divide rapidly into superior and inferior branches. The superior and larger artery passes medially into the first or second anterior sacral foramen, supplies the sacral vertebrae and contents of the sacral canal and leaves the sacrum via the corresponding dorsal foramen to supply the skin and muscles dorsal to the sacrum. The inferior or lateral sacral artery crosses obliquely anterior to piriformis and the sacral anterior spinal rami, then descends lateral to the sympathetic trunk to anastomose with its fellow and the median sacral artery anterior to the coccyx. Its branches enter the anterior sacral foramina and are distributed like those of the superior artery.

Superior gluteal artery – The superior gluteal artery is the largest branch of the internal iliac and effectively forms the main continuation of its posterior trunk. It runs posteriorly between the lumbosacral trunk and the first sacral ramus or between the first and second rami, then turns slightly inferiorly leaving the pelvis by the greater sciatic foramen above piriformis and dividing into superficial and deep branches. In the pelvis it supplies piriformis, obturator internus and a nutrient artery to the ilium. The superficial branch enters the deep surface of gluteus maximus. Its numerous branches supply the muscle and anastomose with the inferior gluteal branches while others perforate the tendinous medial attachment of the muscle to supply the skin over the sacrum where they anastomose with the posterior branches of the lateral sacral arteries. The deep branch of the superior gluteal artery passes between gluteus medius and the bone, soon dividing into superior and inferior branches. The superior branch skirts the superior border of gluteus minimus to the anterior superior iliac spine and anastomoses with the deep circumflex iliac artery and the ascending branch of the lateral circumflex femoral artery. The inferior branch runs through gluteus minimus obliquely, supplies it and gluteus medius and anastomoses with the lateral circumflex femoral artery. A branch enters the trochanteric fossa to join the inferior gluteal artery and ascending branch of the medial circumflex femoral artery while other branches run through gluteus minimus to supply the hip joint.

The superior gluteal artery occasionally arises directly from the internal iliac artery with the inferior gluteal artery and sometimes from the internal pudendal artery.

Anterior trunk branches

Superior vesical artery (See also p. 1361.) – The superior vesical artery is the first large branch of the anterior trunk. It lies on the lateral wall of the pelvis just below the brim and runs anteroinferiorly medial to the

periosteum of the posterior surface of the pubis. It supplies the distal end of the ureter, the bladder, the proximal end of the vas deferens and the seminal vesicles. It also gives origin to the umbilical artery in the foetus, which remains as a fibrous cord, the medial umbilical ligament, in the adult. This vessel occasionally remains patent as a small artery supplying the umbilicus.

Inferior vesical artery (See also p. 1361.) – The inferior vesical artery may arise as a common branch with the middle rectal artery. In the female it is often replaced by the vaginal artery. It supplies the bladder, the prostate, the seminal vesicles and the vas deferens.

Middle rectal artery (See also p. 1361.) – The middle rectal artery is often multiple and may be small. It runs into the lateral fascial coverings of the mesorectum. It occasionally arises close to or in common with the origin of the inferior vesical artery in males.

Vaginal artery (See also p. 1361.) – In females the vaginal artery may replace the inferior vesical artery. It may arise from the uterine artery close to its origin.

Obturator artery – The obturator artery runs anteroinferiorly from the anterior trunk on the lateral pelvic wall to the upper part of the obturator foramen. It leaves the pelvis via the obturator canal and divides into anterior and posterior branches. In the pelvis it is related laterally to the fascia over obturator internus and is crossed on its medial aspect by the ureter and, in the male, by the vas deferens. In the nulliparous female the ovary lies medial to it. The obturator nerve is above the artery, the obturator vein below it. In the pelvis the obturator artery provides iliac branches to the iliac fossa. These supply the bone and iliacus and anastomose with the iliolumbar artery. A vesical branch runs medially to the bladder and sometimes replaces the inferior vesical branch of the internal iliac artery. A pubic branch usually arises just before the obturator artery leaves the pelvis, and ascends over the pubis to anastomose with the contralateral artery and the pubic branch of the inferior epigastric artery.

Outside the pelvis the anterior and posterior terminal branches encircle the foramen between obturator externus and the obturator membrane. The anterior branch curves anteriorly on the membrane and then inferiorly along its anterior margin to supply branches to obturator externus, pectineus, the femoral adductors and gracilis. It anastomoses with the posterior branch and the medial circumflex femoral artery. The posterior branch follows the posterior margin of the foramen and turns anteriorly on the ischial part to anastomose with the anterior branch. It supplies the muscles attached to the ischial tuberosity and anastomoses with the inferior gluteal artery. An acetabular branch enters the hip joint at the acetabular notch, ramifies in the fat of the acetabular fossa and sends a branch along the ligament of the femoral head.

Occasionally the obturator artery is replaced by an enlarged pubic branch of the inferior epigastric artery (p. 1101) which descends almost vertically to the obturator foramen. It usually lies near the external iliac vein, lateral to the femoral ring, and is rarely injured during inguinal or femoral hernia surgery. Sometimes it curves along the edge of the lacunar part of the inguinal ligament, partly encircling the neck of a hernial sac, and may be inadvertently cut during enlargement of the femoral ring in reducing a femoral hernia.

Uterine artery (See also p. 1361.) – The uterine artery is an additional branch in females. It is a large branch which arises below the obturator artery on the lateral wall of the pelvis and runs inferomedially into the broad ligament of the uterus.

Internal pudendal artery (in the pelvis) (See also p. 1361.) – The internal pudendal artery arises just below the origin of the obturator artery. It descends laterally to the inferior rim of the greater sciatic foramen, where it leaves the pelvis between piriformis and ischiococcygeus to enter the gluteal region. It then curves around the dorsum of the ischial spine to enter the perineum by the lesser sciatic foramen. This course effectively allows the nerve to wrap around the posterior limit of levator ani at its attachment to the ischial spine and so gain access to the perineum. In the pelvis the internal pudendal artery crosses anterior to piriformis, the sacral plexus and the inferior gluteal artery. Behind the ischial spine it is covered by gluteus maximus, with the pudendal nerve medial and the nerve to obturator internus lateral to it. Several muscular branches leave the pudendal artery in the pelvis and gluteal region to supply the adjacent muscles and nerves.

Inferior gluteal artery – The inferior gluteal artery is the larger terminal branch of the anterior internal iliac trunk and principally supplies the buttock and thigh. It descends posteriorly, anterior to the sacral plexus and piriformis but posterior to the internal pudendal artery. It passes between the first and second or second and third sacral anterior spinal nerve rami, then between piriformis and ischiococcygeus. It runs through the lower part of the greater sciatic foramen to reach the gluteal region. The artery runs inferiorly between the greater trochanter and ischial tuberosity with the sciatic and posterior femoral cutaneous nerves deep to gluteus maximus. It continues down the thigh, supplying the skin and anastomosing with branches of the perforating arteries. The inferior gluteal and internal pudendal arteries often arise as a common stem from the internal iliac, sometimes with the superior gluteal artery. Inside the pelvis the inferior gluteal artery gives branches to piriformis, ischiococcygeus and iliococcygeus. Occasionally it contributes to the middle rectal arterial supply and, in the male, supplies vessels to the seminal vesicles and prostate.

EXTERNAL ILIAC ARTERIES

The external iliac arteries are of larger calibre than the internal iliac artery. Each artery descends laterally along the medial border of psoas major from the common iliac bifurcation to a point midway between the anterior superior iliac spine and the symphysis pubis. It enters the thigh posterior to the inguinal ligament to become the femoral artery.

On the right the artery is separated from the terminal ileum and, usually, the appendix by the parietal peritoneum and extraperitoneal tissue. On the left the artery is separated from the sigmoid colon and coils of the small intestine lie anteromedially. At its origin the artery may be crossed by the ureter. It is also crossed by the gonadal vessels, the genital branch of the genitofemoral nerve, the deep circumflex iliac vein and the vas deferens (male) or round ligament (female). Posterior to the artery the iliac fascia separates it from the medial border of psoas major. The external iliac vein lies partly posterior to its upper part but is more medial to it below. Laterally, it is related to psoas major which is covered by the iliac and psoas fascia. Numerous lymph vessels and nodes lie on its front and sides.

The external iliac artery is principally the artery of the lower limb and as such has few branches in the pelvis. Apart from very small vessels to psoas major and neighbouring lymph nodes, the artery has no branches until it gives off the inferior epigastric and deep circumflex iliac arteries which arise near to its passage under the inguinal ligament.

Deep circumflex iliac artery – The deep circumflex iliac artery branches laterally from the external iliac artery almost opposite the origin of the inferior epigastric artery. It ascends and runs laterally to the anterior superior iliac spine behind the inguinal ligament in a sheath formed by the union of the transversalis and iliac fasciae. There it anastomoses with the ascending branch of the lateral circumflex femoral artery, pierces the transversalis fascia and skirts the internal lip of the iliac crest. About halfway along the iliac crest it runs through transversus abdominis and then between transversus and internal oblique to anastomose with the iliolumbar and superior gluteal arteries. At the anterior superior iliac spine it gives off a large ascending branch, which runs between internal oblique and transversus abdominis. It supplies both muscles and anastomoses with the lumbar and inferior epigastric arteries.

Inferior epigastric artery (See also p. 1362.) – The inferior epigastric artery originates from the external iliac artery posterior to the inguinal ligament. It curves forwards in the anterior extraperitoneal tissue and ascends obliquely along the medial margin of the deep inguinal ring where it continues as an artery of the anterior abdominal wall.

VEINS OF THE PELVIS

The true pelvis contains a large number of veins which drain the wall and most of the viscera contained within the pelvis and carry venous blood from the gluteal region, thigh the hip. The external iliac veins, lying close to the brim of the pelvis, carry the venous drainage of most of the lower limb. There is considerable variation in the venous drainage of the pelvis and although the major veins frequently follow their

named arterial counterparts, the small tributaries exhibit a great deal of variation between individuals.

COMMON ILIAC VEINS (Fig. 108.5)

The common iliac vein is formed by the union of external and internal iliac veins, anterior to the sacroiliac joints. It ascends obliquely to end at the right side of the fifth lumbar vertebra, uniting at an acute angle with the contralateral vessel to form the inferior vena cava. The right common iliac vein is shorter and more nearly vertical, lying posterior then lateral to its artery. The right obturator nerve passes posterior. The left common iliac vein is longer and more oblique and lies first medial, then posterior to its artery. It is crossed anteriorly by the attachment of the sigmoid mesocolon and superior rectal vessels. Each vein receives iliolumbar and sometimes lateral sacral veins. The left common iliac usually drains the median sacral vein. There are no valves in these veins. The left common iliac vein occasionally ascends to the left of the aorta to the level of the kidney where it receives the left renal vein and crosses anterior to the aorta to join the inferior vena cava. This vessel represents the persistent caudal half of the left postcardinal or supracardinal vein.

Median sacral veins – The medial sacral veins accompany the corresponding artery anterior to the sacrum, and unite to form a single vein which usually ends in the left common iliac vein. Sometimes it ends at the common iliac junction.

Internal pudendal veins – The internal pudendal veins are venae comitantes of the internal pudendal artery. They unite as a single vessel ending in the internal iliac vein. They receive veins from the penile bulb and the scrotum (males) or clitoris and labia (females) and the inferior rectal veins.

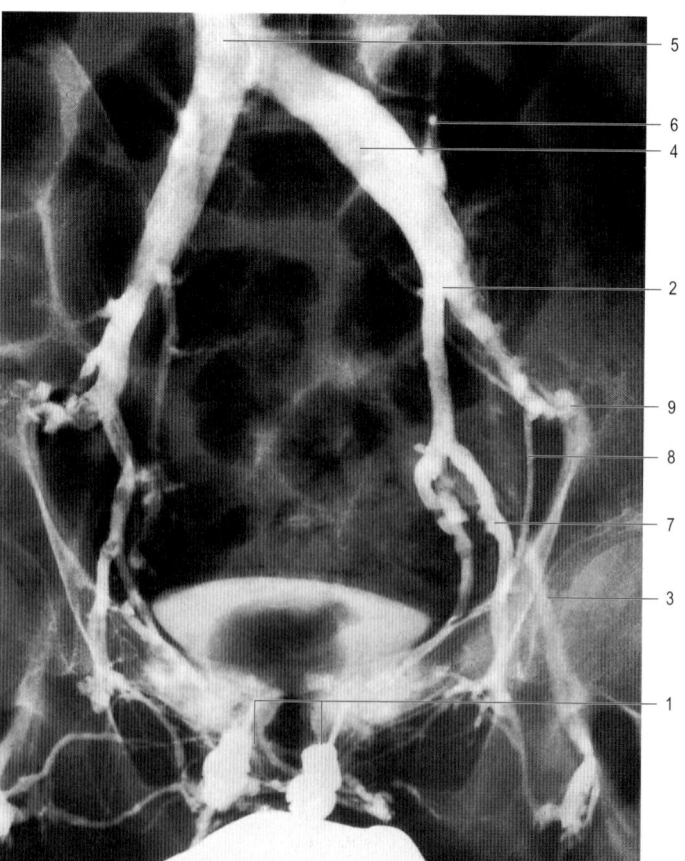

1. Injected contrast medium in pubic bones.   2. Internal iliac vein receiving anterior and posterior tributaries.   3. External iliac vein (faintly outlined).   4. Common iliac vein.   5. Inferior vena cava. 6. Ascending lumbar vein.   7. Obturator vein.   8. Internal pudendal vein.   9. Gluteal vein.

Fig. 108.5 Venogram showing the veins of the pelvis and groin. Contrast medium has been injected into the bodies of the pubic bones. (Provided by M Lea Thomas.)

INTERNAL ILIAC VEIN

The internal iliac vein is formed by the convergence of several veins above the greater sciatic foramen. It does not have the predictable trunks and branches of the internal iliac artery but its branches drain the same territories. It ascends posteromedial to the internal iliac artery to join the external iliac vein, forming the common iliac vein at the pelvic brim, anterior to the lower part of the sacroiliac joint. It is covered antero-medially by parietal peritoneum. Its tributaries are the gluteal, internal pudendal and obturator veins, which originate outside the pelvis; the lateral sacral veins which run from the anterior surface of the sacrum; and the middle rectal, vesical, uterine and vaginal veins which originate in the venous plexuses of the pelvic viscera.

The venous drainage of the leg may be blocked by thrombosis involving the external iliac systems and the inferior vena cava. Under these circumstances, the pelvic veins, particularly the internal iliac tributaries, enlarge and provide a major avenue of venous return from the femoral system. Surgical interference with these veins may seriously compromise venous drainage and precipitate oedema of one or both legs.

Superior gluteal veins – The superior gluteal veins are the venae comitantes of the superior gluteal artery. They receive branches corresponding to branches of the artery and enter the pelvis via the greater sciatic foramen, above piriormis. They join the internal iliac vein, frequently as a single trunk.

Inferior gluteal veins – The inferior gluteal veins are venae comitantes of the inferior gluteal artery. They begin proximally and posterior in the thigh, where they anastomose with the medial circumflex femoral and first perforating veins. They enter the pelvis low in the greater sciatic foramen, joining to form a vessel opening into the distal (lower) part of the internal iliac vein. They connect with the superficial gluteal veins by perforating veins (Doyle 1970) analogous to the sural perforating veins. They probably have a venous 'pumping' role, and provide collaterals between the femoral and internal iliac veins.

Obturator vein – The obturator vein begins in the proximal adductor region and enters the pelvis via the obturator foramen. It runs posteriorly and superiorly on the lateral pelvic wall below the obturator artery and between the ureter and internal iliac artery to end in the internal iliac vein. It is sometimes replaced by an enlarged pubic vein, which joins the external iliac vein.

Lateral sacral veins – The lateral sacral veins accompany the lateral sacral arteries, and are interconnected by a sacral venous plexus.

Middle rectal vein – The middle rectal vein begins in the rectal venous plexus and drains the rectum and mesorectum. It often receives tributaries from the bladder and the prostate and seminal vesicle (males) and the posterior aspect of the vagina (females). It is variable in size and runs laterally on the pelvic surface of levator ani to end in the internal iliac vein.

EXTERNAL ILIAC VEIN

The external iliac vein is the proximal continuation of the femoral vein. It begins posterior to the inguinal ligament, ascends along the pelvic brim and ends anterior to the sacroiliac joint by joining the internal iliac vein to form the common iliac vein. On the right it lies medial to the external iliac artery, gradually inclining behind it as it ascends. On the left it is wholly medial. Disease of the external iliac artery may cause it to adhere closely to the vein at the point where it is in contact, and, particularly on the right side, the walls of the vessels may become fused, making dissection hazardous. Medially the external iliac vein is crossed by the ureter and internal iliac artery. In males it is crossed by the vas deferens, in females by the round ligament and ovarian vessels. Lateral to it lies psoas major, except where the artery intervenes. The vein is usually valveless, but may contain a single valve. It tributaries are the inferior epigastric, deep circumflex iliac and pubic veins.

Inferior epigastric vein– One or two inferior epigastric veins accompany the artery and drain into the external iliac vein a little above the inguinal ligament.

Deep circumflex iliac vein – The deep circumflex vein is formed from venae comitantes of the corresponding artery. It joins the external iliac

vein a little above the inferior epigastric veins after crossing anterior to the external iliac artery.

Pubic vein – The pubic vein connects the external iliac and the obturator vein. It ascends on the pelvic surface of the pubis with the pubic branch of the inferior epigastric artery. It sometimes replaces the normal obturator vein.

LYMPHATIC DRAINAGE OF THE PELVIS

COMMON ILIAC NODES (Fig. 108.6)

The common iliac nodes are grouped around the artery, and one or two lie inferior to the aortic bifurcation and anterior to the fifth lumbar vertebra or sacral promontory. They drain the external and internal iliac nodes and connect to the lateral aortic nodes. They usually lie in medial, lateral and anterior chains around the artery, the lateral being the main route. Since they receive drainage from both internal and external iliac nodes, the common iliac nodes receive the entire lymphatic drainage of the lower limb.

EXTERNAL ILIAC NODES

The external iliac nodes usually form three subgroups, lateral, medial and anterior to the external iliac vessels. The medial nodes are considered the main channel of drainage, collecting lymph from the lower limb via the inguinal nodes, the deeper layers of the infra-umbilical abdominal wall, the adductor region of the thigh, the glans penis or clitoris, the membranous urethra, prostate, fundus of the bladder, uterine cervix and upper vagina. Their efferents pass to the common iliac nodes.

Inferior epigastric and circumflex iliac nodes – The inferior epigastric and circumflex iliac nodes are associated with their vessels and drain the corresponding areas to the external iliac nodes.

INTERNAL ILIAC NODES (Fig. 108.7)

The internal iliac nodes surround the branches of the internal iliac vessels and receive afferents from most of the pelvic viscera (with the exception of the gonads and the rectum), deeper parts of the perineum and the gluteal and posterior femoral muscles. They drain to the common iliac

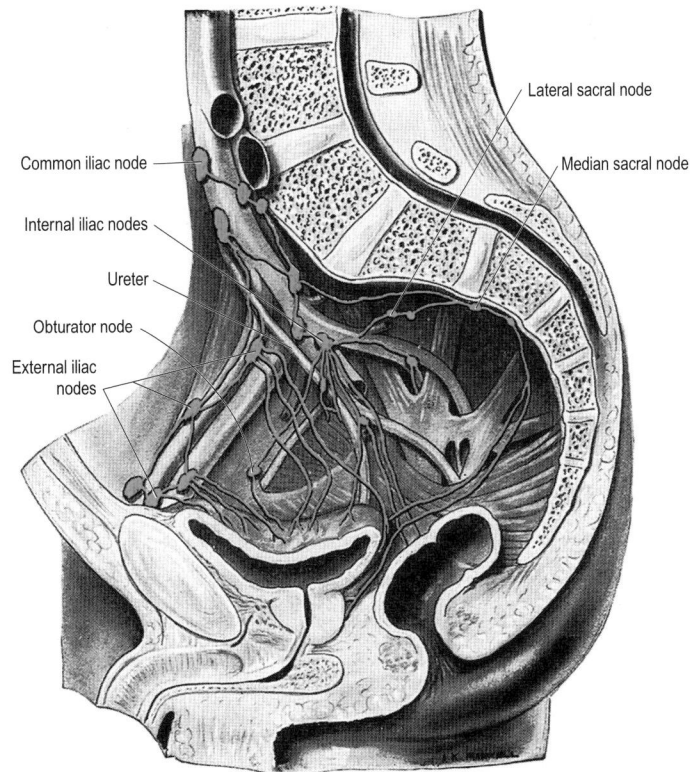

Lateral sacral node

Median sacral node

Common iliac node

Internal iliac nodes

Ureter

Obturator node

External iliac nodes

Fig. 108.6 Lymphatic drainage of the male pelvis and urinary bladder.

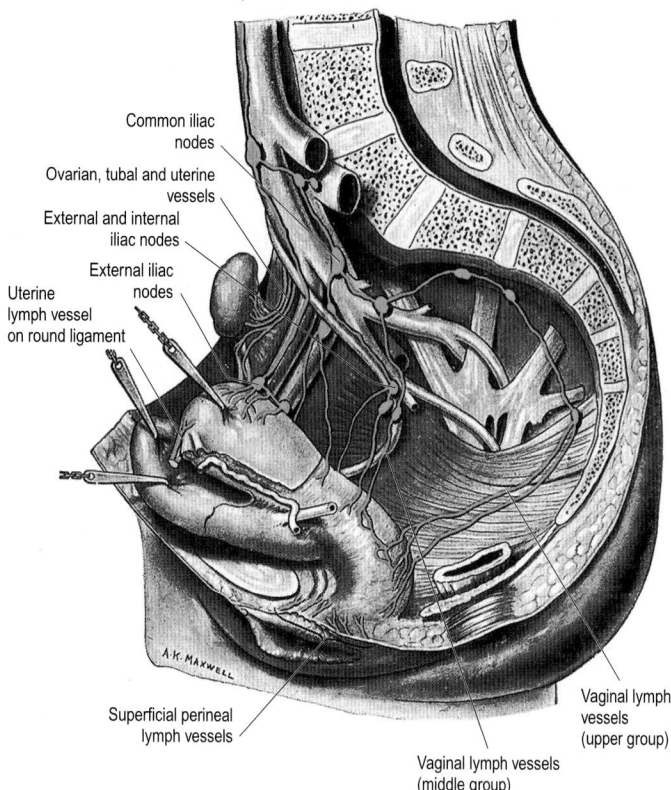

Common iliac
nodes

Ovarian, tubal and uterine
vessels

External and internal
iliac nodes

External iliac
nodes

Uterine
lymph vessel
on round ligament

Superficial perineal
lymph vessels

Vaginal lymph
vessels
(upper group)

Vaginal lymph vessels
(middle group)

A·K·MAXWELL

Fig. 108.7 Lymphatic drainage of the female pelvis. (After Cuneo and Marcille.)

nodes. The individual groups are considered in the description of the viscera. There are frequent connections between the right and left groups particularly when they lie close to the anterior and posterior midlines.

Innervation of the pelvis

The pelvis contains the lumbosacral nerve trunk, the sacral plexus, the coccygeal plexus and the pelvic parts of the sympathetic and parasympathetic systems. These supply the somatic and autonomic innervation to the majority of the pelvic visceral organs, the pelvic floor and perineum, the gluteal region and the lower limb.

The ventral rami of the sacral and coccygeal spinal nerves form the sacral and coccygeal plexuses. The upper four sacral ventral rami enter the pelvis by the anterior sacral foramina, the fifth between the sacrum and coccyx, while that of the coccygeal nerve curves forwards below the rudimentary transverse process of the first coccygeal segment. The first and second sacral ventral rami are large, the third to fifth diminish progressively and the coccygeal is the smallest. Each receives a grey ramus communicans from a corresponding sympathetic ganglion. Visceral efferent rami leave the second to fourth sacral rami as pelvic splanchnic nerves, containing parasympathetic fibres which reach minute ganglia in the walls of the pelvic viscera.

LUMBOSACRAL TRUNK AND SACRAL PLEXUS (Fig. 111.41)

The sacral plexus is formed by the lumbosacral trunk, the first to third sacral ventral rami and part of the fourth, the remainder of the last joining the coccygeal plexus.

The lumbar part of the lumbosacral trunk contains part of the fourth and all the fifth lumbar ventral rami; it appears at the medial margin of psoas major, and descends over the pelvic brim anterior to the sacroiliac joint to join the first sacral ramus. The greater part of the second and third sacral rami converge on the inferomedial aspect of the lumbosacral trunk in the greater sciatic foramen to form the sciatic nerve. The ventral and dorsal divisions of the nerves do not separate physically from each other but the fibres remain separate within the rami, and ventral and dorsal divisions of each contributing root join

within the sciatic nerve. The fibres of the dorsal divisions will go on to form the common peroneal nerve and the ventral division fibres form the tibial nerve. The sciatic nerve occasionally divides into common peroneal and tibial nerves inside the pelvis. In these cases the common peroneal nerve usually runs through piriformis.

The sacral plexus lies against the posterior pelvic wall anterior to piriformis, posterior to the internal iliac vessels and ureter, and behind the sigmoid colon on the left. The superior gluteal vessels run between the lumbosacral trunk and first sacral ventral ramus or between the first and second sacral rami, while the inferior gluteal vessels lie between the first and second or second and third sacral rami (**Fig. 108.8**).

The sacral plexus is not commonly involved in malignant tumours of the pelvis because in lies behind the relatively dense presacral fascia which resists all but locally very advanced malignant infiltration. When it occurs, there is intractable pain in the distribution of the branches of the plexus which may be very difficult to treat. The plexus may also be involved in the reticuloses or be affected by plexiform neuromas.

BRANCHES OF THE SACRAL PLEXUS

The branches of the sacral plexus are:

	Ventral divisions	Dorsal divisions
Nerve to quadratus femoris and gemellus inferior	L4,5, S1	
Nerve to obturator internus and gemellus superior	L5, S1,2	
Nerve to piriformis		S2 (S1)
Superior gluteal nerve		L4,5, S1
Inferior gluteal nerve		L5, S1,2
Posterior femoral cutaneous nerve	S2,3	S1,2
Tibial (sciatic) nerve	L4,5, S1,2,3	
Common peroneal (sciatic) nerve		L4,5, S1,2
Perforating cutaneous nerve		S2,3
Pudendal nerve	S2,3,4	
Nerves to levator ani and external anal sphincter	S4	
Pelvic splanchnic nerves		S2,3 (S4)

The course and distribution of most of the branches of the sacral plexus are covered fully on page 1456.

PUDENDAL NERVE (IN THE PELVIS)

The pudendal nerve arises from the ventral divisions of the second, third and fourth sacral ventral rami and is formed just above the superior border of the sacrotuberous ligament and the upper fibres of ischiococcygeus. It leaves the pelvis via the greater sciatic foramen between piriformis and ischiococcygeus, enters the gluteal region and crosses the sacrospinous ligament close to its attachment to the ischial spine. The nerve lies medial to the internal pudendal vessels on the spine. It accompanies the internal pudendal artery through the lesser sciatic foramen into the pudendal (Alcock's) canal on the lateral wall of the ischioanal fossa. In the posterior part of the canal it gives rise to the inferior rectal nerve, the perineal nerve and the dorsal nerve of the penis or clitoris.

SACRAL VISCERAL BRANCHES

These arise from the second to fourth sacral ventral rami to innervate the pelvic viscera; they are termed pelvic splanchnic nerves.

SACRAL MUSCULAR BRANCHES

Several muscular branches arise from the fourth sacral ventral ramus to supply the superior surface of levator ani and the upper part of the external anal sphincter. The branches to levator ani enter the superior

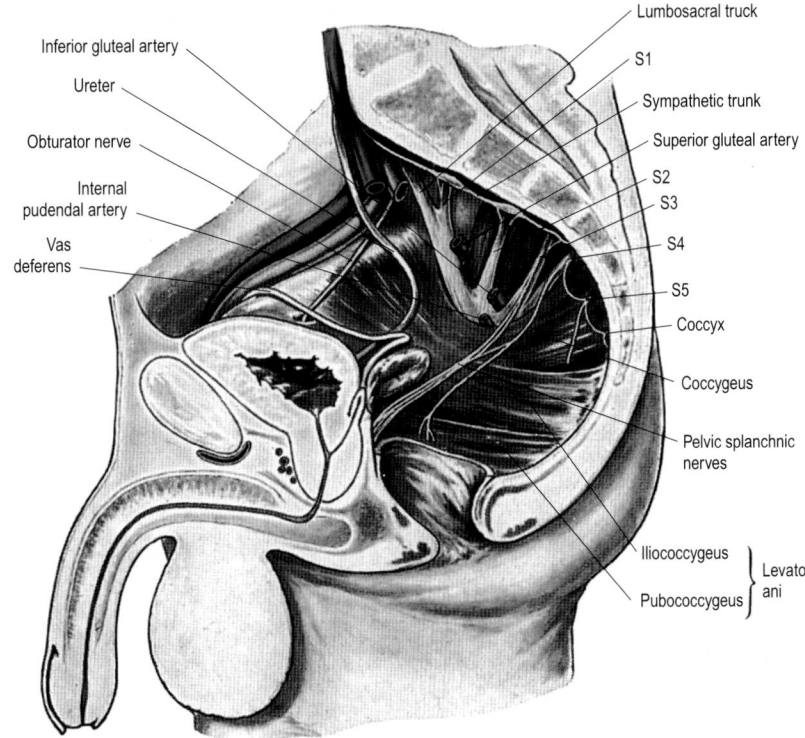

Inferior gluteal artery

Ureter

Obturator nerve

Internal pudendal artery

Vas deferens

Lumbosacral truck

S1

Sympathetic trunk

Superior gluteal artery

S2

S3

S4

S5

Coccyx

Coccygeus

Pelvic splanchnic nerves

Iliococcygeus

Pubococcygeus

Levator ani

Fig. 108.8 The lumbosacral plexus in the pelvis. The pelvic viscera have been omitted for clarity.

(pelvic) surface of the muscle whilst the branch to the external anal sphincter (also referred to as the perineal branch of the fourth sacral nerve) reaches the ischioanal fossa by running through ischiococcygeus or between ischiococcygeus and iliococcygeus. It supplies the skin between the anus and coccyx via its cutaneous branches.

COCCYGEAL PLEXUS

The coccygeal plexus is formed by a small descending branch from the fourth sacral ramus and by the fifth sacral and coccygeal ventral rami. The fifth sacral ventral ramus emerges from the sacral hiatus, curves round the lateral margin of the sacrum below its cornu and pierces ischiococcygeus from below to reach its upper, pelvic surface. Here it is joined by a descending branch of the fourth sacral ventral ramus, and the small trunk so formed descends on the pelvic surface of ischio-coccygeus. They join the minute coccygeal ventral ramus which emerges from the sacral hiatus and curves round the lateral coccygeal margin to pierce coccygeus to reach the pelvis. This small trunk is the coccygeal plexus. Anococcygeal nerves arise from it and form a few fine filaments which pierce the sacrotuberous ligament to supply the adjacent skin.

PELVIC PART OF THE SYMPATHETIC SYSTEM

The pelvic sympathetic trunk lies in the extraperitoneal tissue anterior to the sacrum beneath the presacral fascia. It lies medial or anterior to the anterior sacral foramina and has four or five interconnected ganglia. Above, it is continuous with the lumbar sympathetic trunk. Below the lowest ganglia the two trunks converge to unite in the small ganglion impar anterior to the coccyx. Grey rami communicantes pass from the ganglia to sacral and coccygeal spinal nerves but there are no white rami communicantes. Medial branches connect across the midline and twigs from the first two ganglia join the inferior hypogastric plexus or the hypogastric 'nerve'. Other branches form a plexus on the median sacral artery.

VASCULAR BRANCHES

Postganglionic fibres pass through the grey rami communicantes to the roots of the sacral plexus. Those forming the tibial nerve are conveyed to the popliteal artery and its branches in the leg and foot whilst those in the pudendal and superior and inferior gluteal nerves accompany the same named arteries to the gluteal and perineal tissues. Branches may also supply the pelvic lymph nodes.

Preganglionic fibres for the rest of the lower limb are derived from the lower three thoracic and upper two or three lumbar spinal segments. They reach the lower thoracic and upper lumbar ganglia through white rami communicantes and descend through the sympathetic trunk to synapse in the lumbar ganglia. Postganglionic fibres pass from these ganglia via grey rami communicantes to the femoral nerve which carries them to the distribution of the femoral artery and its branches. Some fibres descend through the lumbar ganglia to synapse in the upper two or three sacral ganglia, from which postganglionic axons join the tibial nerve to supply the popliteal artery and its branches in the leg and foot.

Sympathetic denervation of vessels in the lower limb can be effected by removing or ablating the upper three lumbar ganglia and the intervening parts of the sympathetic trunk, which is rarely useful in treating vascular insufficiency of the lower limb.

PERINEUM
Muscles and fasciae of the perineum

The perineum is an approximately diamond-shaped region which lies below the pelvic floor, between the inner aspects of the thighs and anterior to the sacrum and coccyx. It is usually described as if from the position of an individual lying supine with the hip joints in abduction and partial flexion. The surface projection of the perineum and the form of the skin covering it varies considerably depending on the position of the thighs but the deep tissues themselves occupy relatively fixed positions. The perineum is bounded anteriorly by the pubic symphysis and its arcuate ligament, posteriorly by the coccyx, anterolaterally by the ischiopubic rami and the ischial tuberosities and posterolaterally by the sacrotuberous ligaments. The deep limit of the perineum is the inferior surface of the pelvic diaphragm and its superficial limit is the skin which is continuous with that over the medial aspect of the thighs and the lower abdominal wall. An arbitrary line joining the ischial tuberosities (the interischial line) divides the perineum into an anterior urogenital triangle and a posterior anal triangle. The urogenital triangle faces downwards and forwards, whereas the anal triangle faces downwards and backwards.

The male urogenital triangle contains the bulb and attachments of the penis (**Fig. 108.9**, Chapter 100) and the female urogenital triangle contains the mons pubis, the labia majora, the labia minora, the clitoris and the vaginal and urethral orifices (Chapter 107).

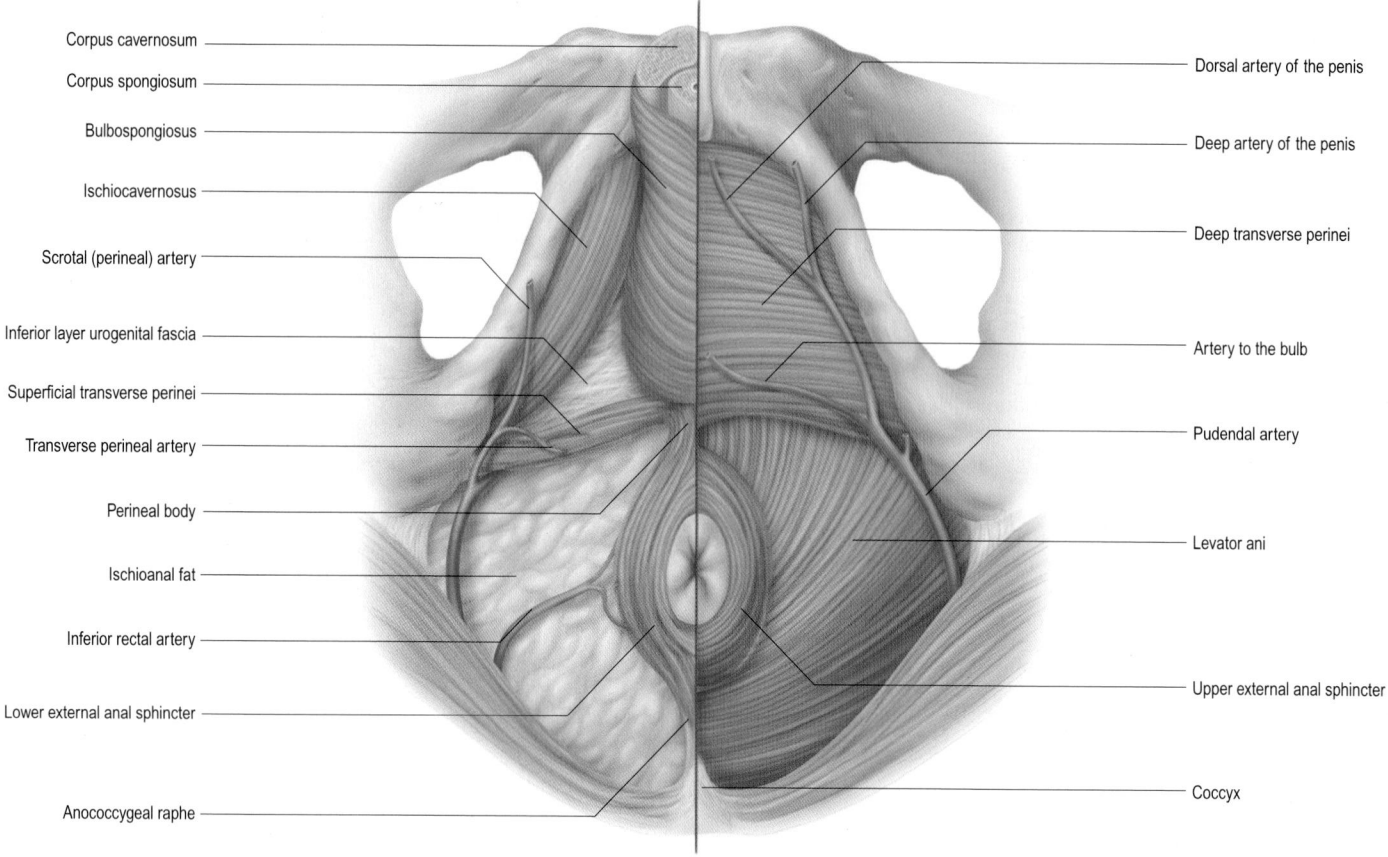

Corpus cavernosum

Corpus spongiosum

Bulbospongiosus

Ischiocavernosus

Scrotal (perineal) artery

Inferior layer urogenital fascia

Superficial transverse perinei

Transverse perineal artery

Perineal body

Ischioanal fat

Inferior rectal artery

Lower external anal sphincter

Anococcygeal raphe

Dorsal artery of the penis

Deep artery of the penis

Deep transverse perinei

Artery to the bulb

Pudendal artery

Levator ani

Upper external anal sphincter

Coccyx

Fig. 108.9 Muscles and fasciae of the male perineum. On the left side the skin and superficial fascia of the perineum only have been removed. The perineal (scrotal) artery has been shown as it runs forward into the scrotal tissues. On the right side, the corpora cavernosa and corpus spongiosum and their associated muscles, the superficial perineal muscles and inferior layer of the urogenital fascia have been removed to reveal the underlying deep muscles and arteries of the perineum. All veins and nerves have been omitted for clarity.

ANAL TRIANGLE

The structure of the anal triangle is similar in males and females. The main difference reflects the wider transverse dimension of the triangle in females as a result of the larger size of the pelvic outlet (p. 1430). The anal triangle contains the anal canal and its sphincters, and the ischioanal fossa and its contained nerves and vessels. It is lined by superficial and deep fascia.

Superficial fascia
The superficial fascia of the region is thin and is continuous with the superficial fascia of the skin of the perineum, thighs and buttocks.

Deep fascia
The deep fascia lines the inferior surface of levator ani and is continuous at its lateral origin with the fascia over obturator internus below the attachment of levator. It lines the deep portion of the ischioanal fossa and its lateral walls.

Ischioanal fossa
The ischioanal fossa is an approximately horse-shoe shaped region filling the majority of the anal triangle. The 'arms' of the horseshoe are triangular in cross section because levator ani slopes downwards towards the anorectal junction (**Fig. 84.1**). Although it is often referred to as a space, it is filled with loose adipose tissue and occasional blood vessels. The anal canal and its sphincters lie in the centre of the horse-shoe. Above them the deep medial limit of the fossa is formed by the deep fascia over levator ani. The outer boundary of the fossa is formed anterolaterally by the deep fascia over obturator internus deeply and the periosteum of the ischial tuberosities more superficially. Posterolaterally the outer boundary is formed by the lower border of gluteus maximus and the sacrotuberous ligament. Anteriorly, the superficial boundary

of the fossa is formed by the posterior aspect of the muscles of the urogenital triangle. Deep to this there is no fascial boundary between the fossa and the tissues deep to the perineal membrane (p. 1367) as far anteriorly as the posterior surface of the pubis below the attachment of levator ani. Posteriorly, the fossa contains the attachment of the external anal sphincter to the tip of the coccyx: above and below this the adipose tissue of the fossa is uninterrupted across the midline. These continuations of the ischioanal fossa mean that infections, tumours and fluid collections within may not only enlarge relatively freely to the side of the anal canal but may also spread with little resistance to the opposite side and deep to the perineal membrane. The internal pudendal vessels and accompanying nerves lie in the lateral wall of the ischioanal fossa, enclosed in fascia to form the pudendal canal. The inferior rectal vessels and nerves cross the fossa from the pudendal canal and often branch within it. The fossa is an important surgical plane during resections of the anal canal and anorectal junction for malignancy. It provides an easy plane of dissection with relatively few vessels encountered, which encompasses all of the muscular structures of the anal canal. It leads to the inferior surface of levator ani through which the dissection is carried.

External anal sphincter (See also p. 1366.)
The external anal sphincter is an oval tube of striated muscle which surrounds the lowest part of the anal canal. The upper most (deepest) fibres blend with the lowest fibres of puborectalis and the two are seen to be continuous on endoanal ultrasound and magnetic resonance imaging. Anteriorly some of these upper fibres decussate into the superficial transverse perineal muscles and posteriorly, some fibres are attached to the anococcygeal raphe. The majority of the middle fibres of the external anal sphincter surround the lower part of the internal sphincter. This portion is attached anteriorly to the perineal body and posteriorly to the coccyx via the anococcygeal ligament. Some fibres

from each side of the sphincter decussate in these areas to form a sort of commissure in the anterior and posterior midline. The anterior and posterior attachments of the external anal sphincter give the muscular tube an oval profile lying anteroposteriorly. The lower fibres lie below the level of the internal anal sphincter and are separated from the lowest anal epithelium only by submucosa.

Anococcygeal ligament

The anococcygeal ligament is a layered musculotendinous structure running between the middle portion of the external anal sphincter and the coccyx. The lowest portion of the presacral fascia lies above the deep part of the ligament and between the two lie the most posterior fibres of the raphe of iliococcygeus. These three structures together are sometimes referred to as the postanal plate. Division of the anococcygeal raphe may cause descent of the anal canal and a lowering of the posterior part of the anal triangle but does not demonstrably interfere with the process of defaecation.

UROGENITAL TRIANGLE

The urogenital triangle is bounded posteriorly by the interischial line which usually overlies the posterior border of the transverse perineal muscles. Anteriorly and laterally it is bounded deeply by the symphysis pubis and ischiopubic rami. In males, the urogenital triangle extends superficially to encompass the scrotum and the root of the penis. In females, it extends to the lower limit of the labia and mons pubis. The urogenital triangle is divided into two parts by a strong perineal membrane. The deep perineal space lies above the membrane and below it is the superficial perineal space.

The female urogenital triangle includes muscles, fasciae and spaces similar to those in the male. There are some differences in size and disposition caused by the presence of the vagina and female external genitalia.

DEEP PERINEAL SPACE

The deep perineal space was long regarded as an anatomical region between the urogenital diaphragm and the perineal membrane which contained the urethra and urethral sphincter. However, the urogenital diaphragm does not exist and the urethral sphincter, previously thought to be the principle content of the deep perineal space where it was described as surrounding the urethra, is now recognized to be contained within the urethra. The deep perineal space is bounded deeply by the endopelvic fascia of the pelvic floor and superficially by the perineal membrane. Between these two fascial layers lie the deep transverse perinei, superficial to the urethral sphincter mechanism and pubourethralis, and in females superficial to the compressor urethrae and sphincter urethrovaginalis. These muscles do not form a true diaphragmatic sheet as such because fibres from several parts extend through the visceral outlet in the pelvic floor into the lower reaches of the pelvic cavity.

Perineal membrane (inferior fascia of the urogenital diaphragm)

The perineal membrane is a triangular membrane which stretches almost horizontally across the urogenital triangle. It is attached laterally to the periosteum of the ischiopubic rami and its apex is attached to the arcuate ligament of the pubis. It is particularly thick in this area and is referred to as the transverse perineal ligament. The posterior border is fused with the deep part of the perineal body and is continuous with the fascia over the deep transverse perinei.

In the male, the perineal membrane is crossed by the urethra, 2–3 cm behind the inferior border of the symphysis pubis; the vessels and nerves to the bulb of the penis; the ducts of the bulbourethral glands, posterolateral to the urethral orifice; the deep dorsal vessels and dorsal nerves of the penis, behind the pubic arch in the midline; and the posterior scrotal vessels and nerves, anterior to the transverse perinei.

In the female the perineal membrane is less well defined than in the male. It is divided almost into two halves by the vagina and urethra such that it forms a triangle on each side of these structures and the pubourethral ligament (the female equivalent of the transverse perineal ligament in males) links the two sides anteriorly behind the pubic arch. It is crossed by the urethra, 2–3 cm behind the inferior border of the symphysis pubis; the vagina, centrally; the ducts of Bartholin's glands, posterolateral to the urethral orifice; the deep dorsal vessels and dorsal

nerves of the clitoris, behind the pubic arch in the midline; the posterior labial vessels and nerves, anterior to the transverse perinei.

Deep transverse perinei

The deep transverse perinei form an incomplete sheet of muscle extending across the urogenital triangle from the medial aspects of the ischiopubic rami. Posteriorly the sheet is attached to the perineal body where its fibres decussate with those of the opposite side. Anteriorly, the muscles are deficient and the visceral structures pass across the endopelvic fascia and the perineal membrane. Some fibres pass to the deep part of external anal sphincter posteriorly and sphincter urethrae anteriorly. Together with the superficial transverse perinei the muscles act to tether the perineal body in the median plane and may help support the visceral canals which pass through them. They are supplied by the perineal branches of the pudendal vessels and nerves.

The urethral sphincter mechanism

The urethral sphincter mechanism consists of the intrinsic striated and smooth muscle of the urethra and the pubourethralis component of levator ani which surrounds the urethra at the point of maximum concentration of those muscles. It surrounds the membranous urethra in the male and the middle and lower thirds of the urethra in the female. In the male, fibres also reach up to the lowest part of the neck of the bladder and, between the two, fibres lie on the surface of the prostate. The bulk of the fibres surround the membranous urethra and some fibres are attached to the inner surface of the ischiopubic ramus. In the female, the sphincter mechanism surrounds more than the middle third of the urethra. It blends above with the smooth muscle of the bladder neck and below with the smooth muscle of the lower urethra and vagina.

Actions – The urethral sphincter mechanism compresses the urethra, particularly when the bladder contains fluid. Its location around the region of highest urethral closing pressure suggests that it plays an important role in the continence of urine. Like bulbospongiosus, it is relaxed during micturition, but it contracts to expel final drops of urine, or of semen in the male, from the bulbar urethra. It may be stimulated via a vaginal tampon electrode as has been used in the treatment of stress incontinence of urine in females.

Innervation – The urethral sphincter mechanism extends from the perineum through the urogenital hiatus into the pelvic cavity. It probably receives innervation via the perineal branch of the pudendal nerve from below and direct branches from the sacral plexus and the pelvic splanchnic nerves from above (Wendell-Smith & Wilson 1991). All these nerves originate in the second, third and fourth sacral spinal segments.

Compressor urethrae

Compressor urethrae exists in females and arises from the ischiopubic rami of each side by a small tendon. Fibres pass anteriorly to meet their contralateral counterparts in a flat band which lies anterior to the urethra, below sphincter urethrae (**Fig. 108.10**). A variable number of fibres from the same origin fan medially to reach the lower walls of the vagina. These fibres may rarely reach as far posteriorly as the perineal body.

Sphincter urethrovaginalis

Sphincter urethrovaginalis exists in females and arises from the perineal body. Its fibres pass forwards on either side of the vagina and urethra to meet their contralateral counterparts in a flat band, anterior to the urethra, below compressor urethrae (**Fig. 108.10**).

Actions – The direction of the fibres of compressor urethrae and sphincter urethrovaginalis suggests that they produce elongation as well as compression of the membranous urethra and thus aid continence in females.

SUPERFICIAL PERINEAL SPACE (Fig. 108.11)

The superficial perineal space lies below the perineal membrane and is limited superficially by the superficial perineal fascia. It contains the corpora cavernosa and corpus spongiosum, ischiocavernosus, bulbospongiosus and the superficial transverse perinei and branches of the pudendal vessels and nerves. In the female it is crossed by the urethra and vagina and contains the clitoris. In the male it contains the urethra which runs in the root of the penis.

A

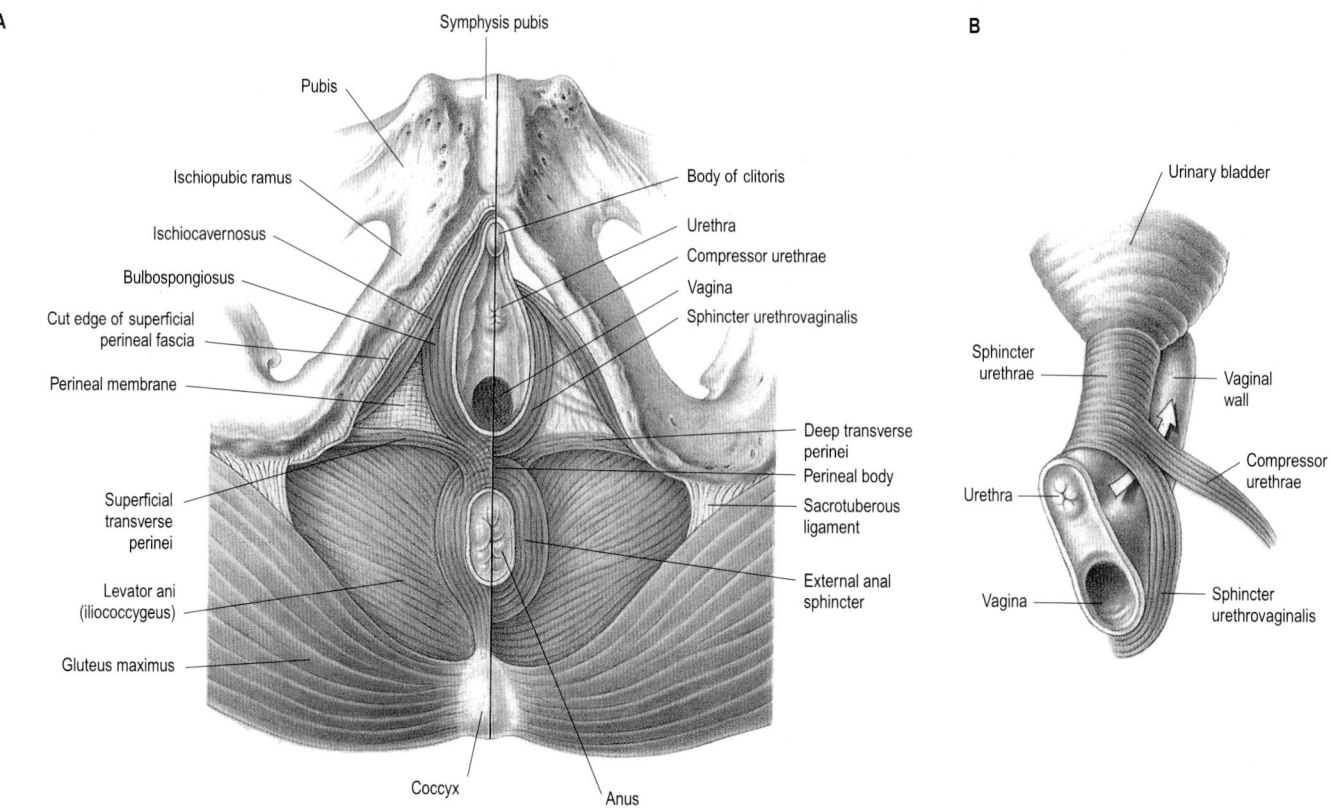

Fig. 108.10 Muscles of the female perineum. On the right side, the membranous layer of superficial fascia has been removed (note the cut edge). On the left side, superficial perineal muscles and overlying fascia have been removed to show the deep perineal muscles. The smaller figure illustrates the continuity of the deep perineal muscles with sphincter urethrae.

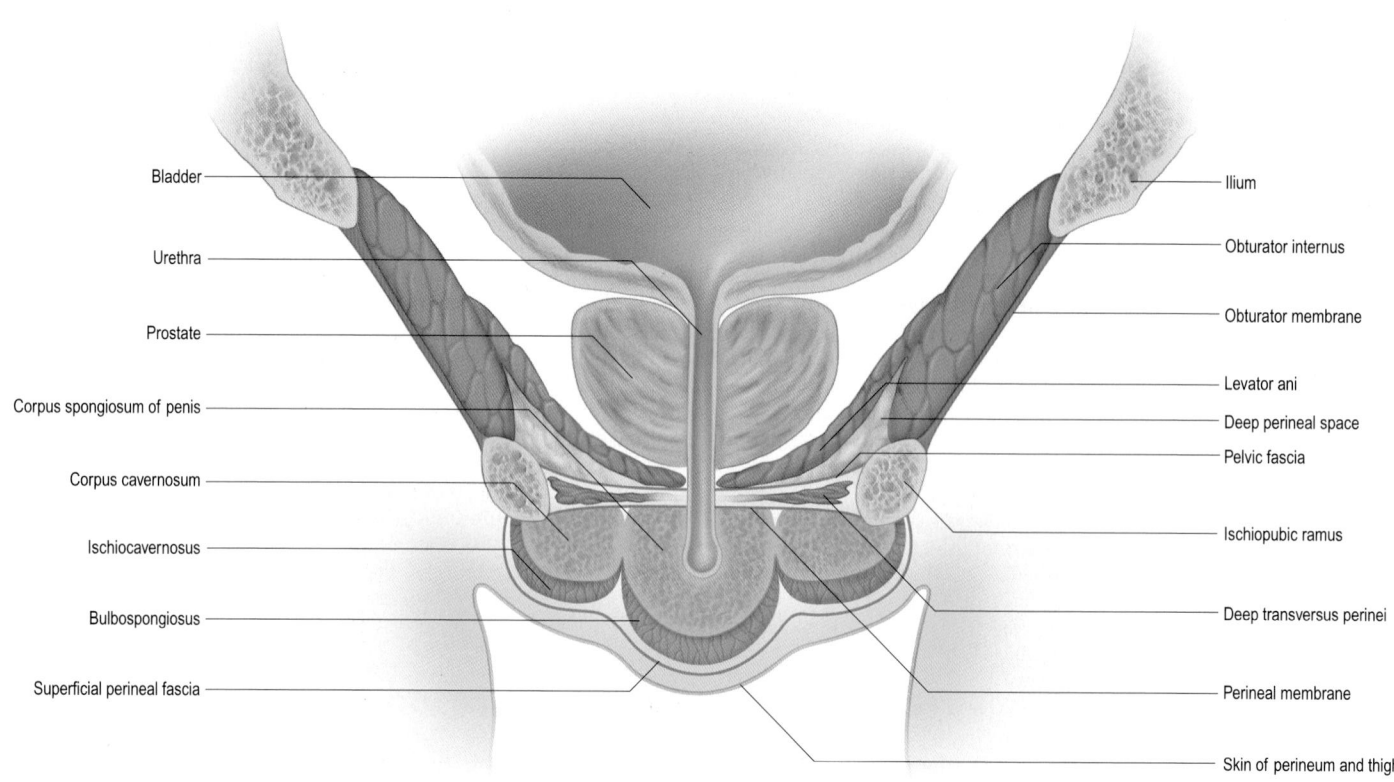

Fig. 108.11 Muscles and fasciae of the male perineum – coronal view. The section passes through the bulb of the penis at the level of the urethra. The deep perineal space is continuous with the ischioanal fossa posteriorly. The layers of the urogenital fascia and the superficial fascia of the perineum are in green and muscles are shown in brown.

Superficial perineal fascia

The superficial fascia of the urogenital triangle (Colles' fascia) forms a clear, surgically recognizable plane beneath the skin of the anterior perineum. It is firmly attached posteriorly to the fascia over the superficial transverse perinei and the posterior limit of the perineal membrane. Laterally, it is attached to the margins of the ischiopubic rami as far back as the ischial tuberosities. From here it runs more superficially to the skin of the urogenital triangle, lining the external genitalia before running anteriorly into the skin of the lower abdominal wall where it is continuous with the membranous fascia (Scarpa's fascia). In the male, the superficial perineal fascia covers the corpora cavernosa from their attachment to the ischiopubic rami and is continuous with the fascia of the penis. It is also continuous with the fascial layer in the skin of the scrotum containing the dartos muscle. In females the fascia follows the same limits but is much less extensive in the labia majora.

Since the superficial perineal fascia is in continuity with the fascia of the anterior abdominal wall but tethered firmly by its posterolateral attachments, fluid, blood or pus may track freely from the lower anterior abdominal wall into the superficial perineal space. Similarly blood, urine or fluid accumulating in the superficial space due to trauma or surgery on the urogenital triangle will spread throughout the tissues of the triangle including the scrotum or labia majora but cannot pass posteriorly into the anal triangle or laterally into the medial thigh.

Deep perineal fascia

The deep perineal fascia is attached to the ischiopubic rami and to the posterior margin of the perineal membrane and perineal body over the membranous layer. In front it fuses with the suspensory ligament of the penis or clitoris and the fasciae of external oblique and the rectus sheath.

Perineal body

The perineal body is a poorly defined aggregation of fibromuscular tissue located in the midline at the junction between the anal and urogenital triangles. It is attached to many structures in both the deep and superficial urogenital spaces. Posteriorly fibres from the middle part of the external anal sphincter and the conjoint longitudinal coat merge with the body. Superiorly it is continuous with the rectoprostatic or rectovaginal septum including fibres from levator ani (puborectalis or pubovaginalis). Anteriorly, the deep transverse perinei, the superficial transverse perinei and bulbospongiosus also attach and contribute fibres to it (**Fig. 108.3**). The perineal body is continuous with the perineal membrane and the superficial perineal fascia. Since the superficial perineal fascia runs forward into the skin of the perineum, the perineal body is tethered to the central perineal skin, which is often puckered over it. In males this is continuous with the perineal raphe in the skin of the scrotum. In females, the perineal body lies directly posterior, and is attached, to the posterior commissure of the labia majora and the introitus of the vagina.

The anus can be surgically detached from the perineal body without any clinical consequences. However, spontaneous lacerations of the body sustained during childbirth are often associated with damage to the anterior fibres of the external anal sphincter. The deliberate division of the perineal body to facilitate delivery (episiotomy) is angled laterally to avoid such injuries. The perineal body is often used for the positioning of radiological markers used to determine the amount of descent the perineum undergoes during straining in order to assess pelvic floor dysfunction.

Superficial transverse perinei

The superficial transverse perinei are narrow strips of muscle which run more or less transversely across the superficial perineal space anterior to the anus. The muscles are occasionally small and rarely absent. On each side the muscle is attached to the medial and anterior aspects of the ischial tuberosity. Medially the fibres mostly run into the perineal body although some may pass into bulbospongiosus or external anal sphincter on the same side.

Bulbospongiosus

Bulbospongiosus differs between the sexes. In the male it lies in the midline, anterior to the perineal body and consists of two symmetrical parts united by a median fibrous raphe. The fibres attach to the perineal body, in which they decussate, and are attached to the transverse superficial perinei and the external anal sphincter. The fibres diverge like the halves of a feather from the median raphe. A thin layer of posterior fibres unites with the posterior portion of the perineal membrane. The majority of the middle fibres encircle the bulb of the penis and adjacent corpus spongiosum and attach to an aponeurosis on the dorsal surfaces. The anterior fibres spread out over the sides of the corpora cavernosa, ending partly in them, anterior to ischiocavernosus, and partly in a tendinous expansion which covers the dorsal vessels of the penis.

Actions – Bulbospongiosus helps to empty the urethra of urine after the bladder has emptied. It may assist in the final stage of erection as the middle fibres compress the erectile tissue of the bulb and the anterior fibres contribute by compressing the deep dorsal vein of the penis. It contracts six or seven times during ejaculation, assisting in the expulsion of semen.

In the female bulbospongiosus also attaches to the perineal body, but the muscle on each side is separate and covers the superficial parts of the vestibular bulbs and greater vestibular glands. They run anteriorly on either side of the vagina to attach to the corpora cavernosa clitoridis. A few fibres cross over the dorsum of the body of the clitoris. The muscle acts to constrict the vaginal orifice and express the secretions of the greater vestibular glands. Anterior fibres contribute to erection of the clitoris by compressing its deep dorsal vein.

Ischiocavernosus (Figs 108.12, 108.13)

In the male ischiocavernosus covers the crus penis and is attached by tendinous and muscular fibres to the medial aspect of the ischial tuberosity behind, and to the ischial ramus on both sides of the crus. The fibres end in an aponeurosis attached to the sides and under surface of the crus penis. In the female, ischiocavernosus is related to a smaller crus clitoris and has a much smaller attachment to the ischiopubic ramus, but is otherwise similar to the corresponding muscle in the male.

Action – Ischiocavernosus compresses the crus penis in males and may help to maintain penile erection. The muscles form a triangle on each side of the midlines with bulbospongiosus medially and the superficial transverse perinei posteriorly attached to the perineal membrane. When contracted, ischiocavernosi act together to stabilize the erect penis. In the female ischiocavernosus may help to promote clitoral erection.

Vascular supply and lymphatic drainage of the perineum (Figs 108.4, 108.5)

ARTERIES OF THE PERINEUM

Internal pudendal artery (in the perineum)

The internal pudendal artery enters the perineum around the posterior aspect of the ischial spine. It runs on the lateral wall of the ischioanal fossa in the pudendal (Alcock's) canal with the pudendal veins and the pudendal nerve. The canal is formed by the connective tissue binding the vessels and nerve to the perineal surface of the obturator internus fascia. The canal lies c.4 cm above the lower limit of the ischial tuberosity. Approaching the margin of the ischial branch, it proceeds above or below the inferior fascia of the urogenital diaphragm along the medial margin of the inferior pubic ramus and ends behind the inferior pubic ligament.

In the male the internal pudendal artery gives a branch to the bulb of the penis before it divides into the cavernosal and dorsal arteries of the penis. The internal pudendal artery distal to its perineal branch has been named the artery of the penis in view of its distribution. The artery to the bulb supplies the corpus spongiosum, the cavernoid artery to the penis supplies the corpus cavernosa on each side and the dorsal artery runs on the dorsal aspect of the penis, supplying circumflex branches to the corpora cavernosa and corpus spongiosum before they end by anastomosing in the coronal sulcus to supply the glans penis and its overlying skin.

In the female the artery to the bulb is distributed to the erectile tissue of the vestibular bulb and vagina. The cavernosal artery is much smaller and supplies the corpora cavernosa of the clitoris and the dorsal artery supplies the glans and prepuce of the clitoris.

Branches of the internal pudendal artery are sometimes derived from an accessory pudendal artery, which is usually a branch of the pudendal before its exit from the pelvis.

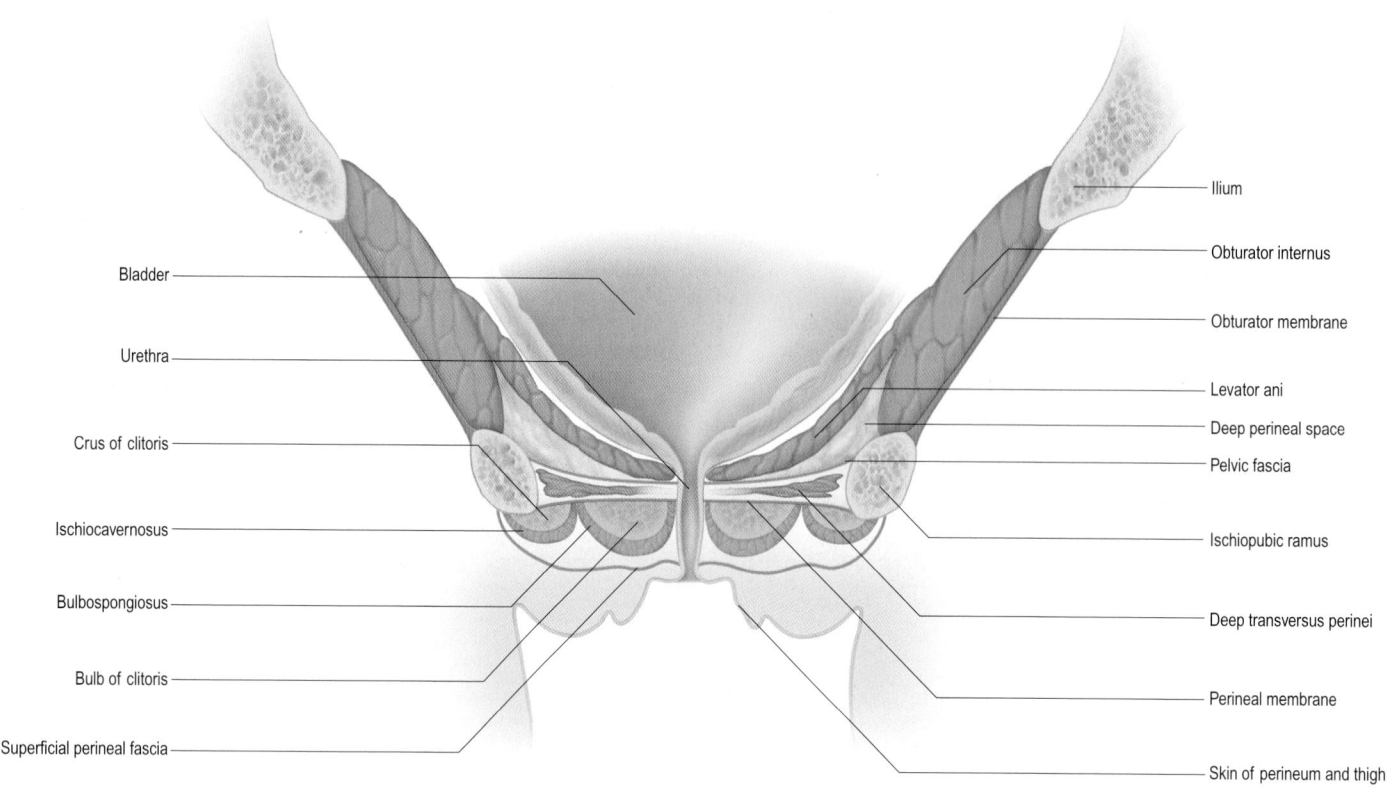

Fig. 108.12 Muscles and fasciae of the female perineum – coronal view. The section passes through the bulb of the clitoris at the level of the urethra. The deep perineal space is continuous with the ischioanal fossa posteriorly. The layers of the perineal fascia and the superficial fascia of the perineum are in green and muscles are shown in brown.

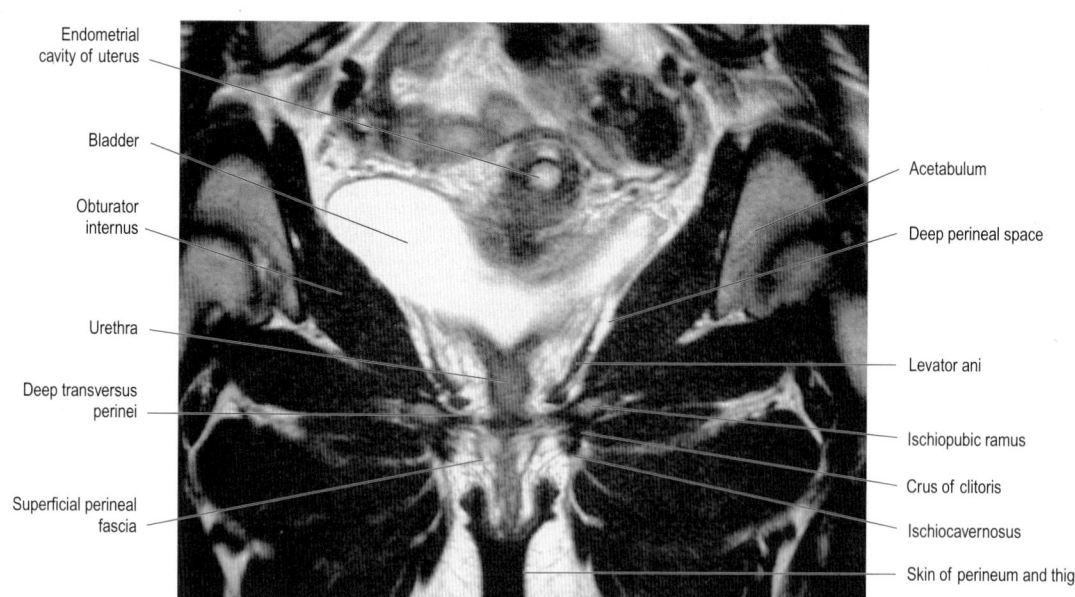

Fig. 108.13 Muscles and fasciae of the female perineum – coronal T2-weighted MRI. (Provided by Dr J Lee and Ms K Wimpey, Chelsea and Westminster Hospital, London.)

Inferior rectal artery (See also p. 1370.)

The inferior rectal artery arises just after the pudendal artery enters the canal on the lateral wall of the ischioanal fossa. It runs antero-medially through the adipose tissue of the ischioanal fossa to reach the deep portion of the external anal sphincter. It often branches before reaching the sphincter. During dissections of the anal canal, particularly during perineal excisions of the anorectum, the inferior rectal vessels are encountered in the ischioanal fossa and must be secured before division or they tend to retract laterally to the canal, where they can cause troublesome bleeding.

Perineal artery

The perineal artery is a branch of the internal pudendal artery near the anterior end of the pudendal canal, and runs through the inferior fascia of the urogenital diaphragm. In the male it approaches the scrotum in the superficial perineal space, between bulbospongiosus and ischio-cavernosus. A small transverse branch passes medially, inferior to the superficial transverse perineal muscle, to anastomose with the contra-lateral artery and with the posterior scrotal and inferior rectal arteries. It supplies the transverse perinei, the perineal body and the posterior attachment of the bulb of the penis. The posterior scrotal arteries are usually terminal branches of the perineal artery but may also arise from its transverse branch. They are distributed to the scrotal skin and dartos muscle in the male and supply the perineal muscles. In the female the perineal artery runs an almost identical course and gives rise to similar branches. The posterior scrotal arteries are replaced by posterior labial arteries.

VEINS OF THE PERINEUM: INTERNAL PUDENDAL VEINS

The internal pudendal veins are venae comitantes of the internal pudendal artery and unite as a single vessel ending in the internal iliac vein. The perineal tributaries receive veins from the penile bulb and the scrotum (males) or clitoris and labia (females) and the inferior rectal veins join towards the posterior end of the pudendal canal.

LYMPHATIC DRAINAGE OF THE PERINEUM

The lymphatics from the skin of the penis and scrotum (male) or skin of the clitoris and labia (female) drain together with lymphatics from the perineal skin to the superficial inguinal nodes and thence to the deep inguinal nodes. The glans, corpora cavernosa and corpus spongiosum of the penis or clitoris drain directly to the deep inguinal nodes.

Innervation of the perineum: pudendal nerve (in the perineum)

The pudendal nerve gives rise to the inferior rectal, perineal and dorsal nerves of the penis or clitoris.

The pudendal nerve is readily found in its very constant position over the ischial spine. It may be 'blocked' by infiltration with a local anaesthetic applied via a needle passed through the lateral wall of the vagina to cause anaesthesia of the perineal and anal skin. It may also be palpated here through the lateral wall of the rectum and motor terminal latencies measured.

INFERIOR RECTAL NERVE

The inferior rectal nerve runs through the medial wall of the pudendal canal with the inferior rectal vessels. It crosses the ischioanal fossa to supply the external anal sphincter, the lining of the lower part of the anal canal, and the circumanal skin. It frequently breaks into terminal branches just before reaching the lateral border of the sphincter. Its cutaneous branches distributed around the anus overlap the perineal branch of the posterior femoral cutaneous nerve and the scrotal or labial nerves. The inferior rectal nerve occasionally arises directly from the sacral plexus and crosses the sacrospinous ligament or reconnects with the pudendal nerve. In females the inferior rectal nerve may supply sensory branches to the lower part of the vagina.

PERINEAL NERVE

The perineal nerve is the inferior and larger terminal branch of the pudendal nerve in the pudendal canal. It runs forwards below the internal pudendal artery and accompanies the perineal artery, dividing into posterior scrotal or labial and muscular branches. The posterior scrotal or labial nerves are usually double and have medial and lateral branches which run over the perineal membrane and pass forwards in the lateral part of the urogenital triangle with the scrotal (or labial) branches of the perineal artery. They supply the skin of the scrotum or labia majora, overlapping the distribution of the perineal branch of the posterior femoral cutaneous and inferior rectal nerve. In females the posterior labial branches also supply sensory fibres to the skin of the lower vagina.

Muscular branches arise directly from the pudendal nerve to supply the superficial transverse perinei, bulbospongiosus, ischiocavernosus, deep transverse perinei, sphincter urethrae and the anterior parts of the external anal sphincter and levator ani. In males a nerve to the bulb of the urethra leaves the nerve to the bulbospongiosus, piercing it to supply the corpus spongiosum penis and ends in the urethral mucosa.

DORSAL NERVE OF THE PENIS OR CLITORIS

The dorsal nerve of the penis or clitoris runs anteriorly above the internal pudendal artery along the ischiopubic ramus deep to the inferior fascia of the urogenital diaphragm. It supplies the corpus cavernosum and accompanies the dorsal artery of the penis or clitoris between the layers of the suspensory ligament. In males it runs on the dorsum of the penis to end in the glans. In females the dorsal nerve of the clitoris is very small.

REFERENCES

Doyle JF 1970 The perforating veins of the gluteus maximus. Ir J Med Sci 3: 285–8.

Wendell-Smith C P, Wilson PM 1991 The vulva, vagina and urethra and the musculature of the pelvic floor. In: Philipp E, Setchell M, Ginsburg J (eds) Scientific Foundations of Obstetrics and Gynaecology. Oxford: Butterworth-Heinemann: 84–100.

Development of the urogenital system

URINARY SYSTEM

The urinary and reproductive systems develop from intermediate mesenchyme and are intimately associated with one another especially in the earlier stages of their development. The urinary system develops ahead of the reproductive or genital systems.

Intermediate mesenchyme is disposed longitudinally in the trunk, subjacent to the somites (in the folded embryo), at the junction between the splanchnopleuric mesenchyme (adjacent to the gut medially) and the somatopleuric mesenchyme (subjacent to the ectoderm laterally) (**Fig. 109.1**). In lower vertebrates, intermediate mesenchyme typically develops serial, segmental epithelial diverticuli termed nephrotomes. Each nephrotome encloses a cavity, the nephrocoele, which communicates with the coelom through a peritoneal funnel, the nephrostome (**Fig. 109.2**). The dorsal wall of a nephrotome evaginates as a nephric tubule. The dorsal tips of the cranial nephric tubules bend caudally and fuse to form a longitudinal primary excretory duct, which grows caudally and curves ventrally to open into the cloaca. The more caudally placed, and therefore chronologically later, tubules open secondarily into this duct or into tubular outgrowths from it. Glomeruli, specific arrangements of capillaries and overlying coelomic epithelium, arise from the ventral wall of the nephrocoele (internal glomeruli) or the roof of the coelom adjacent to the peritoneal funnels (coelomic or external glomeruli), or in both situations (**Fig. 109.2**).

It has been customary to regard the renal excretory system as three organs, the pronephros, mesonephros and metanephros, succeeding

each other in time and space, such that the last to develop is retained as the permanent kidney (**Fig. 109.1, 109.2**). However, it is difficult to provide reliable criteria by which to distinguish these stages or to define their precise limits in embryos.

PRONEPHROS

The intermediate mesenchyme becomes visible in stage 10 embryos and can be distinguished as a nephrogenic cord when 10 somites are present. A pronephros is present in human embryos only as clusters of cells in the most cranial portions of the nephrogenic cord (**Figs 109.1, 109.2**). More caudally, similar groups of cells appear and become vesicular. The dorsal ends of the most caudal of the vesicles join the primary excretory duct. Their central ends are connected with the coelomic epithelium by cellular strands, which probably represent rudimentary peritoneal funnels. Glomeruli do not develop in association with these cranially situated nephric tubules, which ultimately disappear. It is doubtful whether external glomeruli develop in human embryos.

Primary excretory duct

In stage 11 embryos of c.14 somites, the primary excretory duct can be seen as a solid rod of cells in the dorsal part of the nephrogenic cord. Its cranial end is about the level of the ninth somite and its caudal tip merges with the undifferentiated mesenchyme of the cord. It differentiates before any nephric tubules, and when the latter appear it is at first unconnected with them. In older embryos the duct has lengthened

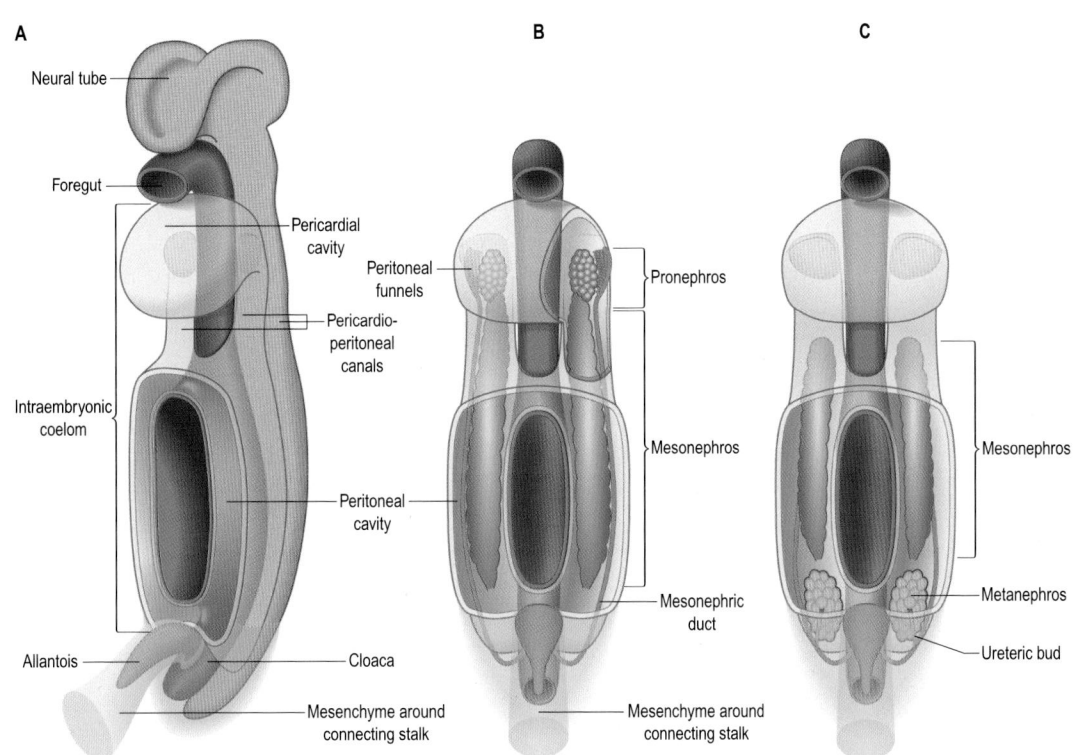

Fig. 109.1 A, Major epithelial populations within a stage 10 embryo, viewed from a ventrolateral position. **B**, Position of pronephros and mesonephros on the posterior thoracic and abdominal wall. **C**, Position of mesonephros and metanephros.

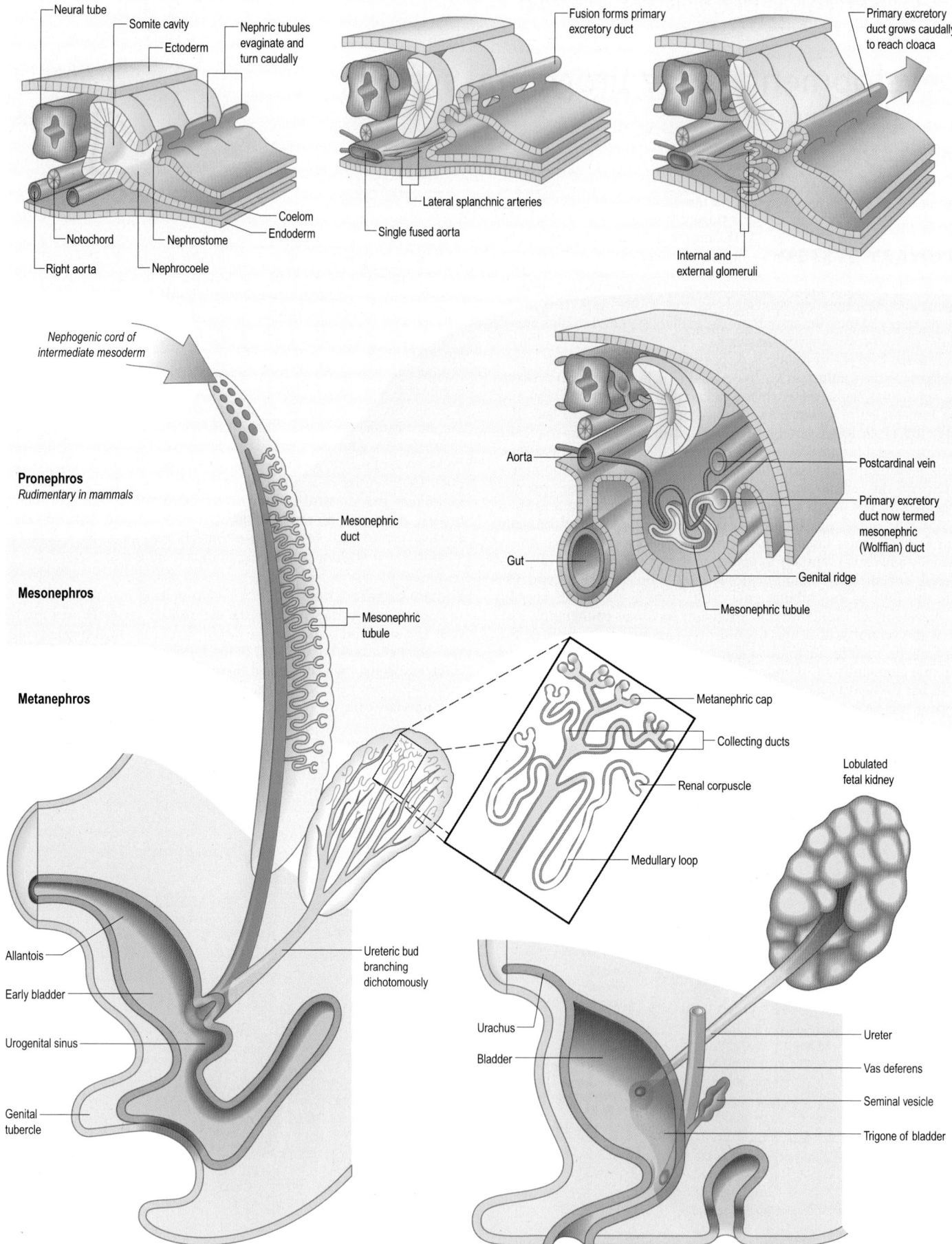

Fig. 109.2 Principal features of the primitive vertebrate nephric system for comparison with the development of the human nephric system. A considerable period of embryonic and fetal life has necessarily been compressed into a single diagram. (Modified from Williams PL, Wendell-Smith CP, Treadgold S 1969 Basic Human Embryology, 2nd edn. Philadelphia: Lippincott.)

and its caudal end becomes detached from the nephrogenic cord to lie immediately beneath the ectoderm. From this level it grows caudally, independent of the nephrogenic mesenchyme, and then curves ventrally to reach the wall of the cloaca. It becomes canalized progressively from its caudal end to form a true duct, which opens into the cloaca in embryos at stage 12 (**Fig. 109.1C**). Clearly, up to this stage the name 'duct' is scarcely appropriate.

MESONEPHROS

From stage 12 mesonephric tubules, which develop from the intermediate mesenchyme between somite levels 8–20, begin to connect to the primary excretory duct, which is now renamed the mesonephric duct. More caudally, a continuous ridge of nephrogenic mesenchyme extends to the level of somite 24. The mesonephric tubules (nephrons) are not metameric – there may be two or more mesonephric tubules opposite each somite.

Within the mesonephros, each tubule first appears as a condensation of mesenchyme cells, which epithelialize and form a vesicle. One end of the vesicle grows towards and opens into the mesonephric duct, while the other dilates and invaginates. The outer stratum forms the glomerular capsule, while the inner cells differentiate into mesonephric podocytes, which clothe the invaginating capillaries to form a glomerulus. The capillaries are supplied with blood through lateral branches of the aorta. It has been estimated that 70–80 mesonephric tubules and a corresponding number of glomeruli develop. However, these tubules are not all present at the same time, it is rare to find more than 30–40 in an individual embryo, because the cranial tubules and glomeruli develop and atrophy before the development of those situated more caudally.

By the end of the sixth week each mesonephros is an elongated, spindle-shaped organ that projects into the coelomic cavity, one on each side of the dorsal mesentery, from the level of the septum transversum to the third lumbar segment. This whole projection is called the mesonephric ridge, mesonephros, or Wolffian body (**Fig. 109.1B, C**). It develops subregions, and a gonad develops on its medial surface (p. 1381). There are striking similarities in structure between the mesonephros and the permanent kidney or metanephros, but the mesonephric nephrons lack a segment that corresponds to the descending limb of the loop of Henle. The mesonephros is believed to produce urine by stage 17. A detailed comparison of the development and function of the mesonephros and metanephros in staged human embryos is not available.

In stage 18 embryos (13–17 mm) the mesonephric ridge extends cranially to about the level of rib 9. In both sexes the cranial end of the mesonephros atrophies, and in embryos 20 mm in length (stage 19) a mesonephros is found only in the first three lumbar segments, although it may still possess as many as 26 tubules. The most cranial one or two tubules persist as rostral aberrant ductules (**Fig. 109.13**); the succeeding five or six tubules develop into either the efferent ductules of the testis and lobules of the head of the epididymis (male), or the tubules of the epoöphoron (female); the caudal tubules form the caudal aberrant ductules and the paradidymis (male), or the paroöphoron (female) (p. 1384).

Mesonephric duct

Once mesonephric nephrons connect to the primary excretory duct it is renamed the mesonephric duct. This runs caudally in the lateral part of the nephric ridge, and at the caudal end of the ridge it projects into the cavity of the coelom in the substance of a mesonephric fold (**Fig. 109.3**). As the mesonephric ducts from each side approach the urogenital sinus the two mesonephric folds fuse, between the bladder ventrally and the rectum dorsally, forming a transverse partition across the cavity of the pelvis, which is somewhat inappropriately called the genital cord (**Fig. 109.3**). In the male the peritoneal fossa between the bladder and the genital cord becomes obliterated, but it persists in the female as the uterovesical pouch. The mesonephric duct itself becomes the canal of the epididymis, vas deferens and ejaculatory duct (p. 1382).

Urogenital sinus

The primitive hindgut ends in a cloacal region. This is connected ventrally with a blind-ending diverticulum, the allantois, which is intimately related to the development of the caudal portion of the urinary system. The enteric and allantoic portions of the hindgut are separated by the proliferation of the urorectal septum, a partition of mesenchyme and

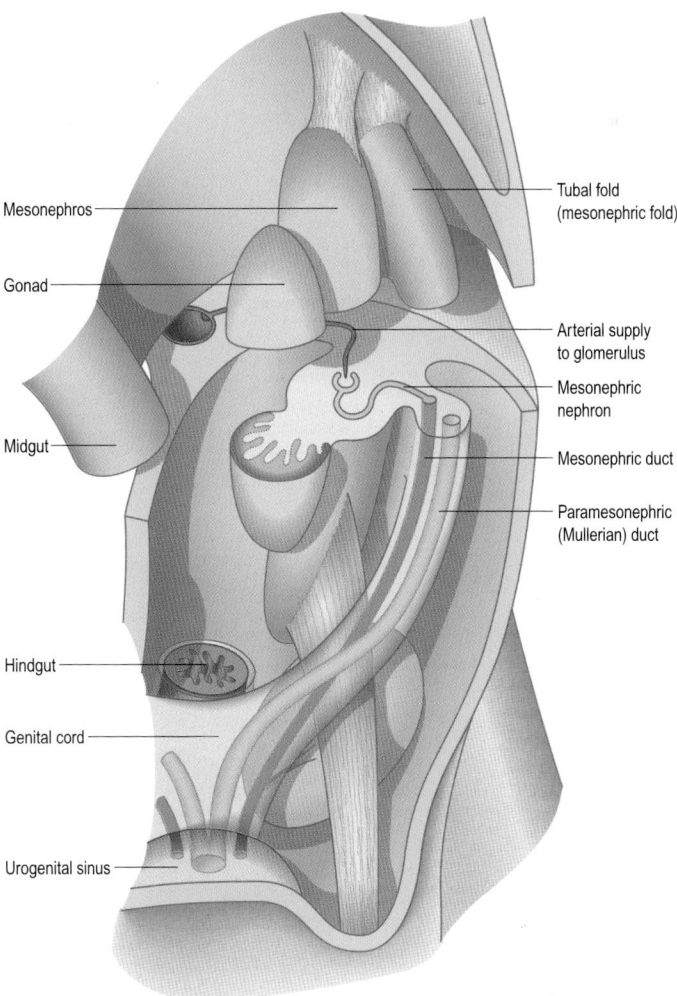

Fig. 109.3 Arrangement of mesonephric duct from mesonephros to urogenital sinus. The duct runs within the tubal fold with the paramesonephric duct. For later development, *see* **Fig. 109.14**. (Redrawn from Tuchmann-Duplessis H, Haegel P 1972 Illustrated Human Embryology, Vol 2 Organogenesis. London: Chapman and Hall.)

endoderm in the angle of the junction of hindgut and allantois (**Fig. 109.4**). The endodermal epithelium beneath the mesenchyme of the urorectal septum approaches and fuses with the cloacal membrane, thereby dividing the membrane into anal (dorsal) and urogenital (ventral) membranes, and the cloacal region into dorsal and ventral portions. The dorsal portion of the cloacal region is the putative rectum. The ventral portion can be further divided into: a cranial vesicourethral canal, continuous above with the allantoic duct; a middle, narrow channel, the pelvic portion; and a caudal, deep, phallic section, which is closed externally by the urogenital membrane. The second and third parts together constitute the urogenital sinus.

METANEPHROS

The pronephros and mesonephros are linear structures. They both contain stacks of tubules distributed along the craniocaudal axis of the embryo, an arrangement that results in the production of hypotonic urine. In marked contrast, the tubules in the metanephric kidney are arranged concentrically, and the loops of Henle are directed towards the renal pelvis. This arrangement allows different concentration gradients to develop within the kidney and results in the production of hypertonic urine. Metanephric nephrons do not join with the existing mesonephric duct but with an evagination of that duct, which branches dichotomously to produce a characteristic pattern of collecting ducts.

The metanephric kidney develops from three sources. An evagination of the mesonephric duct, the ureteric bud, and a local condensation of mesenchyme, the metanephric blastema, form the nephric structure (**Fig. 109.5**). Angiogenic mesenchyme migrates into the metanephric blastema slightly later to produce the glomeruli and vasa recta. It is

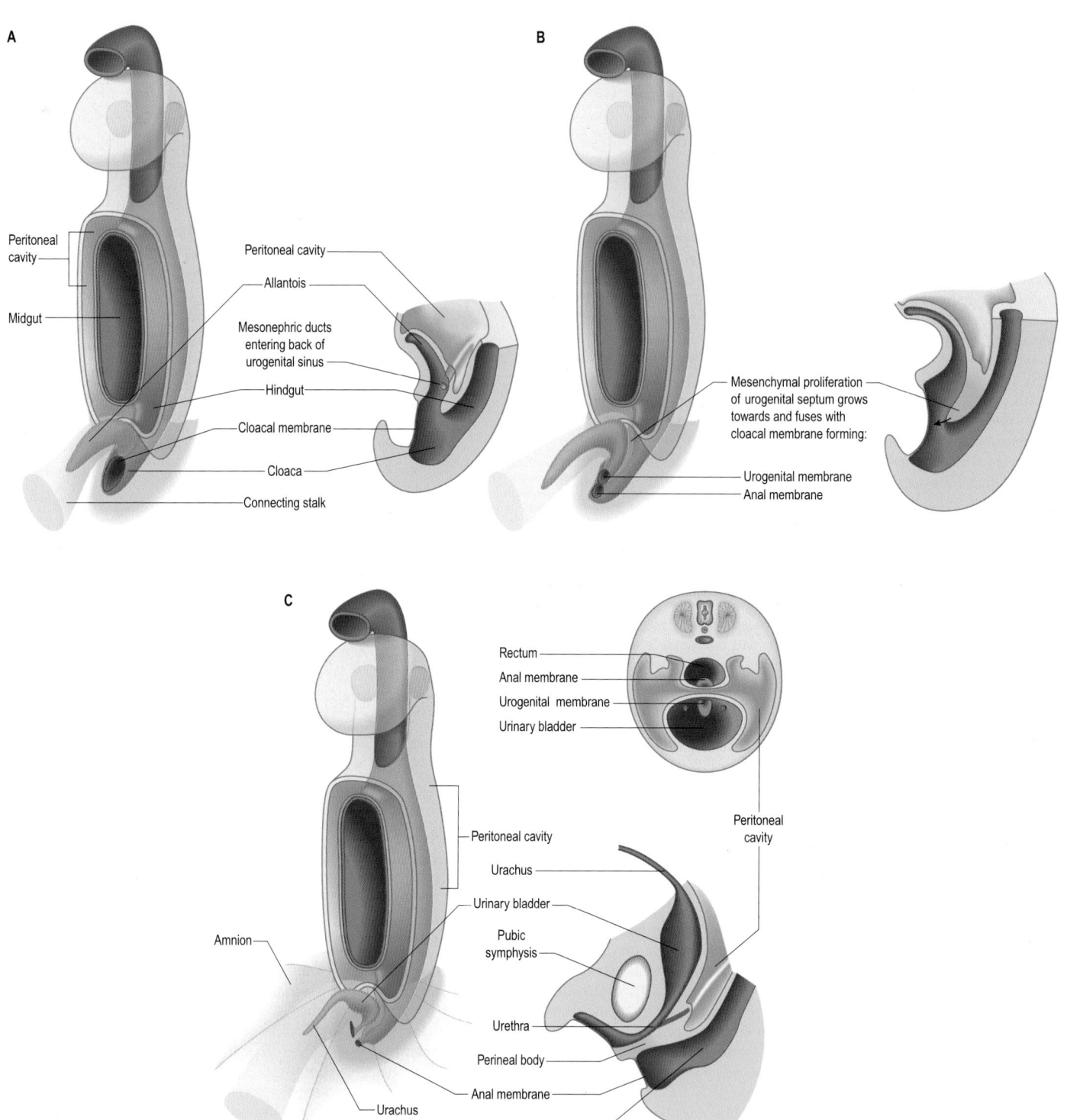

Fig. 109.4 The division of the hindgut into urinary and enteric parts. Left ventrolateral view of the intraembryonic coelom and corresponding midsagittal sections. **A**, Early cloaca. **B**, Proliferation of urorectal septum. **C**, Complete separation of urethra and anal canal, and position of perineal body (also includes a sagittal section which permits a view into the bladder and rectum).

possible that an intact nerve supply is also required for metanephric kidney induction.

An epithelial/mesenchymal interaction between the duct system and the surrounding mesenchyme occurs in both mesonephric and metanephric systems. In the mesonephric kidney, development proceeds in a craniocaudal progression, and cranial nephrons degenerate before caudal ones are produced. In the metanephric kidney a proportion of the mesenchyme remains as stem cells that continue to divide and which enter the nephrogenic pathway later when the individual collecting ducts lengthen. The temporal development of the metanephric kidney is patterned radially, such that the outer cortex is the last part to be formed. The following interactions occur in the development of the

metanephric kidney (**Fig. 109.5**). The ureteric bud undergoes a series of bifurcations within the surrounding metanephric mesenchyme, and forms smaller ureteric ducts. At the same time the metanephric mesenchyme condenses around the dividing ducts to form S-shaped clusters, which transform into epithelia and fuse with the ureteric ducts at their distal ends. Blood vessels invade the proximal ends of the S-shaped clusters to form vascularized glomeruli.

The ureteric bud bifurcates when it comes into contact with the metanephric blastema in response to extracellular matrix molecules synthesized by the mesenchyme. Both chondroitin sulphate proteoglycan synthesis and chondroitin sulphate glycosaminoglycan processing are necessary for the dichotomous branching of the ureteric bud. In

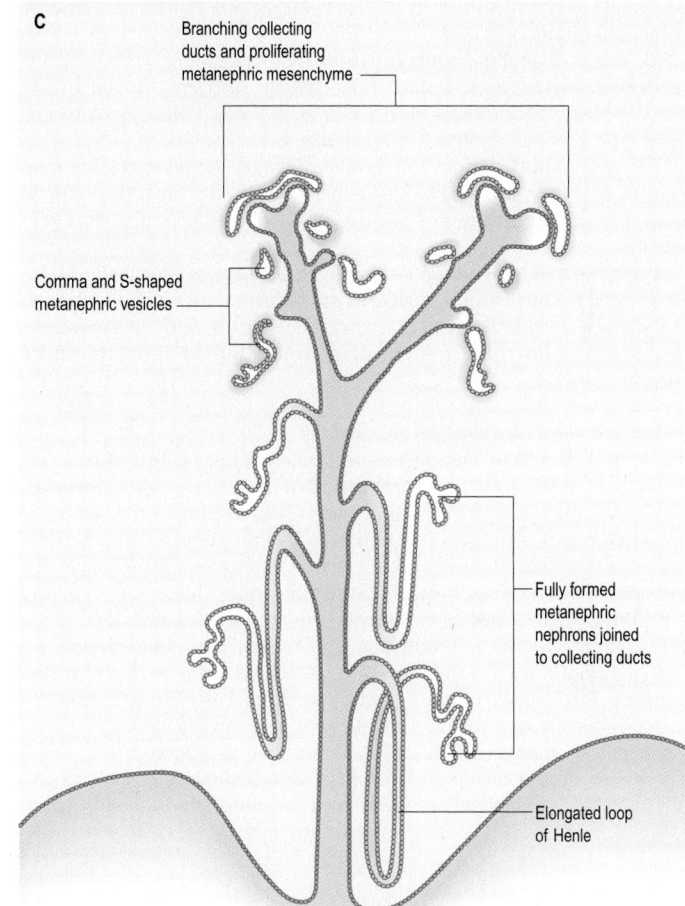

Fig. 109.5 Overview of metanephric kidney development. **A**, The ureteric bud arises from the mesonephric duct. The metanephric mesenchyme proliferates and separates with each subdivision of the ureteric bud. **B**, The metanephric mesenchyme converts to epithelia, forms comma and S-shaped vesicles, which become metanephric nephrons. **C**, All stages of metanephric development are present concurrently. The most recently formed are on the outer aspect of the kidney.

metanephric culture, incubation of fetal kidneys in β-D-xyloside, an inhibitor of chrondroitin sulphate synthesis, dramatically inhibits ureteric bud branching.

Subsequent divisions of the ureteric bud and associated mesenchyme define the gross structure of the kidney and the major and minor calyces, the distal branches of the ureteric ducts that will form the collecting ducts of the kidney. As the collecting ducts elongate the metanephric mesenchyme condenses around them. An adhesion molecule, syndecan, can be detected between the mesenchymal cells in the condensate. The cells switch off expression of N-CAM (cell adhesion molecules), fibronectin and collagen I, and start to synthesize L-CAM (also called E cadherin) and the basal lamina constituents laminin and collagen IV. The mesenchymal clusters are thus converted to small groups of epithelial cells, which undergo complex morphogenetic changes. Each epithelial group elongates, and forms first a comma-shaped, then an

S-shaped, body, which continues to elongate and subsequently fuses with a branch of the ureteric duct at its distal end, while expanding as a dilated sac at its proximal end. The latter involutes, and cells differentiate locally such that the outer cells become the parietal glomerular cells, while the inner ones become visceral epithelial podocytes. The podocytes develop in close proximity to invading capillaries derived from angiogenic mesenchyme outside the nephrogenic mesenchyme. This third source of mesenchyme produces the endothelial and mesangial cells within the glomerulus. The (metanephric-derived) podocytes and the angiogenic mesenchyme produce fibronectin and other components of the glomerular basal lamina. The isoforms of type-IV collagen within this layer follow a specific programme of maturation as the filtration of macromolecules from the plasma becomes restricted.

Platelet derived growth factor (PDGF) β-chain and the PDGF receptor β-subunit (PDGFR β) have been detected in developing human glomeruli between 54 and 109 days' gestation. PDGF β-chain is localized in the differentiating epithelium of the glomerular vesicle during its comma and S-shaped stages, while PDGFR β is expressed in the undifferentiated metanephric blastema, vascular structures and interstitial cells. Both PDGF β-chain and PDGFR β are expressed by mesangial cells, which may promote further mesangial cell proliferation.

Metanephric mesenchyme will develop successfully in vitro, which makes experimental perturbation of kidney development comparatively easy to evaluate. Early experimental studies demonstrated that other mesenchymal populations, and spinal cord, were able to induce ureteric bud division and metanephric development. Nerves enter the developing kidney very early, travelling along the ureter. If developing kidney rudiments are incubated with antisense oligonucleotides, which neutralize nerve growth factor receptor (NGF-R) mRNA, nephrogenesis is completely blocked, suggesting that metanephric mesenchyme induction is a response to innervation. The powerful inductive effect of the spinal cord on metanephric mesenchyme may be a further expression of this phenomenon.

All stages of nephron differentiation are present concurrently in the developing metanephric kidney (**Fig. 109.5**). Antigens for the brush border of the renal tubule appear when the S-shaped body has formed. They appear first in the inner cortical area.

The metanephric kidney is lobulated throughout fetal life, but this condition usually disappears during the first year after birth (**Fig. 109.8**, p. 1378). Varying degrees of lobulation occasionally persist throughout life.

The growth of left and right kidneys is well matched during development. Fetal kidney volume increases most during the second trimester in both sexes. For reasons that are not understood, male fetuses show greater values for renal volume than female fetuses from the third trimester onwards.

Endocrine development of the kidney

The kidney functions not only as an excretory organ, but also as an endocrine organ, secreting hormones that are concerned with renal haemodynamics. Before birth homeostasis is controlled by the placenta. The fetal kidney produces amniotic fluid. The kidneys of premature babies of less than 36 weeks are immature. They contain incompletely differentiated cortical nephrons, which compromise their ability to maintain homeostasis. Problems of immaturity are further compounded by the effects of hypoxia and asphyxia, which modify renal hormones.

Renal hormones include the renin–angiotensin system, renal prostaglandins, the kallikrein–kinin system, and renal dopamine. Renin is found in the smooth muscle cells of arterioles, interlobular arteries and branches of the renal artery, and has also been described in the distal convoluted tubule cells. Kallikrein has been demonstrated in rat fetal kidney, and prostaglandins have been demonstrated in the renal medulla and renal tubule. Renal dopamine is produced (mainly) by the enzymatic conversion of L-dopa to dopamine in the early segments of the proximal convoluted tubule, and is also sourced locally from dopaminergic nerves. Other renal hormones include an antihypertensive lipid, which is produced in the interstitial cells of the renal medulla, and, possibly, histamine and serotonin. Growth factors produced by human embryonic kidney cells include erythropoietin and interleukin β (which stimulate megakaryocyte maturation) and transforming growth factor-β.

Ascent of the kidney

The metanephric kidney is initially sacral. As the ureteric outgrowth lengthens, it becomes positioned more and more cranially. The metanephric pelvis lies on a level with the second lumbar vertebra when the embryo reaches a length of c.13 mm. During this period the ascending kidney receives its blood supply sequentially from arteries in its immediate neighbourhood, i.e. the middle sacral and common iliac arteries. The definitive renal artery is not recognizable until the beginning of the third month. It arises from the most caudal of the three suprarenal arteries, all of which represent persistent mesonephric or lateral splanchnic arteries. Additional renal arteries are relatively common, and may enter at the hilum or at the upper or lower pole of the gland – they also represent persistent mesonephric arteries.

Ureter

The wall of the ureter is initially highly permeable. Its lumen later becomes obliterated and is subsequently recanalized. Both of these processes begin in intermediate portions of the ureter and proceed cranially and caudally. Recanalization is not associated with metanephric function, but perhaps reflects the rapid elongation of the ureter as the embryo grows. Two fusiform enlargements appear at the lumbar and pelvic levels of the ureter at 5 and 9 months, respectively (the pelvic is inconstant). As a result the ureter shows a constriction at its proximal end (pelviureteric region) and another as it crosses the pelvic brim. A third narrowing is always present at its distal end and is related to the growth of the bladder wall.

At first the distal end of the ureter is connected to the dorsomedial aspect of the mesonephric duct, but, as a result of differential growth, this connection comes to lie lateral to the duct.

Urinary bladder

The urinary bladder develops from the cranial vesicourethral canal, which is continuous above with the allantoic duct (**Figs 109.4, 109.6, 109.7**). The mesonephric ducts open into the urogenital sinus early in development. The ureters develop as branches of the mesonephric ducts, which attain their own access to the developing bladder, and their orifices open separately into the bladder on the lateral side of the opening of the mesonephric ducts. Later the two orifices become separated still further and, although the ureter retains its point of entry into the bladder, the mesonephric duct opens into that part of the urogenital sinus that subsequently becomes the prostatic urethra (**Fig. 109.6**). The triangular region of absorption of the mesonephric ducts contributes to the trigone of the bladder and dorsal wall of the proximal half of the prostatic urethra, i.e. as far as the opening of the prostatic utricle and ejaculatory ducts, or its female homologue, the whole female urethral dorsal wall. The remainder of the vesicourethral canal forms the body of the bladder and urethra, and its apex is prolonged to the umbilicus as a narrow canal, the urachus.

The fetal bladder can be identified by ultrasound examination at 9–11 weeks' gestation and the absence of a bladder image is considered abnormal at 13 weeks or later.

NEONATAL URINARY SYSTEM

At birth the two kidneys weigh c.23 g. They function early in development and produce the amniotic fluid that surrounds the fetus. The lobulated appearance of fetal kidneys is still present at birth (**Figs 11.4, 109.8**). Addition of new cortical nephrons continues in the first few months of postnatal life after which general growth of the glomeruli and tubules results in the disappearance of lobulation. The renal blood flow is lower in the neonate – adult values are attained by the end of the first year. The glomerular filtration rate at birth is c.30% of the adult value, which is attained by 3–5 months of age.

The neonatal urinary bladder is egg-shaped and the larger end is directed downwards and backwards (**Figs 11.4, 11.5, 109.9, 109.10**). Although described as an abdominal organ, nearly one half of the neonatal bladder lies below a line drawn from the promontory of the sacrum to the upper edge of the pubic symphysis, i.e. within the cavity of the true pelvis. From the bladder neck, the bladder extends anteriorly and slightly upwards in close contact with the pubis until it reaches the anterior abdominal wall. The apex of the contracted bladder lies at a point midway between the pubis and the umbilicus. When the bladder is filled with urine the apex may extend up to the level of the umbilicus. It is therefore possible to obtain urine by inserting a needle, connected to a syringe, into the bladder through the abdominal wall c.2 cm above the symphysis pubis and aspirating the contents into the sterile syringe. The success rate of the procedure is variable and depends upon the bladder being full. Recently, a much higher success rate has been reported by using an ultrasound scanner to locate the bladder and confirm that it contains urine prior to the insertion of the needle.

There is no true fundus in the fetal bladder as there is in the adult. Although the anterior surface is not covered with peritoneum, peritoneum extends posteriorly as low as the level of the urethral orifice. Because the apex of the bladder is relatively high, pressure on the lower abdominal wall will express urine from an infant bladder. Moreover, because the bladder remains connected to the umbilicus by the obliterated remains of the urachus (**Fig. 65.5**), stimulation of the umbilicus can initiate micturition in babies. The elongated shape of the bladder in neonates means that the ureters are correspondingly reduced in length and they lack a pelvic portion. The bladder does not gain its adult, pelvic, position until about the sixth year. A distinct interureteric fold is present in the contracted neonatal bladder.

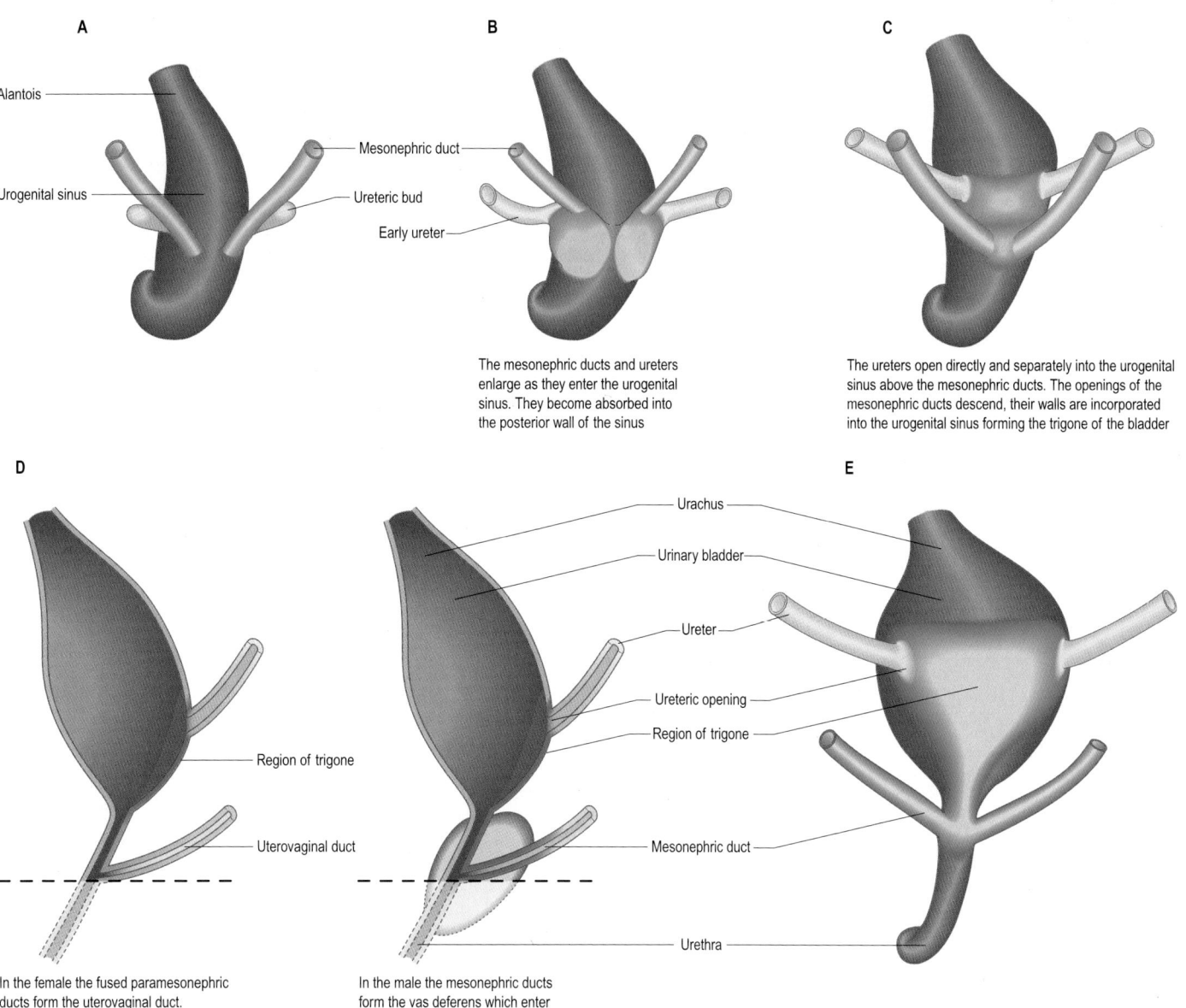

A

Alantois

Urogenital sinus

Mesonephric duct

Ureteric bud

Early ureter

B

The mesonephric ducts and ureters enlarge as they enter the urogenital sinus. They become absorbed into the posterior wall of the sinus

C

The ureters open directly and separately into the urogenital sinus above the mesonephric ducts. The openings of the mesonephric ducts descend, their walls are incorporated into the urogenital sinus forming the trigone of the bladder

D

Region of trigone

Uterovaginal duct

In the female the fused paramesonephric ducts form the uterovaginal duct. The mesonephric ducts degenerate.

In the male the mesonephric ducts form the vas deferens which enter the urethra through the prostate gland.

E

Urachus

Urinary bladder

Ureter

Ureteric opening

Region of trigone

Mesonephric duct

Urethra

Fig. 109.6 Development of the urinary part of the urogenital sinus and formation of the trigone of the bladder. **A–C** and **E**, Posterior views. **D**, Male and female, midsagittal sections. (Redrawn from Tuchmann-Duplessis H, Haegel P 1972 Illustrated Human Embryology, Vol 2 Organogenesis. London: Chapman and Hall.)

ANOMALIES OF THE URINARY SYSTEM

Anomalies of the urinary system are relatively common (3% of live births). Renal agenesis is the absence of one or both kidneys. In unilateral renal agenesis, the remaining kidney exhibits compensatory hypertrophy and produces a nearly normal functional mass of renal tissue. Problems with kidney ascent can result in a pelvic kidney. Alternatively, the kidneys may fuse together at their caudal poles producing a horseshoe kidney, which cannot ascend out of the pelvic cavity because the inferior mesenteric artery prevents further migration.

It was thought that renal cysts arose from clumps of vesicular cells, which persisted when the tips of branches from the ureteric diverticulum failed to fuse with metanephrogenic cap tissue. It is now believed that they are wide dilatations of a part of otherwise continuous nephrons. In most cases, autosomal dominant polycystic kidney disease results from mutations of *PKD1* or *PKD2* genes which are expressed in human embryos from 5–6 weeks of development within the mesonephros and later the metanephros (Chauvet et al 2002). In this condition the cystic dilatation may affect any part of the nephron, from Bowman's capsule to collecting tubules. Less common is infantile cystic renal disease, inherited as a recessive trait, where the proximal and distal tubules are dilated to some degree but the collecting ducts are grossly affected.

Abnormalities of the ventral body wall caudal to the umbilicus, especially with inappropriate siting of the genital tubercle (p. 1393) can result in exstrophy of the bladder (**Fig. 109.11**). In this condition the urorectal septum (internal) is associated with the genital tubercle (external), which means that the urogenital and anal membranes are widely separated. When the urogenital membrane involutes, the posterior surface of the bladder is exposed to the anterior abdominal wall. The lower part of the abdominal wall is therefore occupied by an irregularly oval area, covered with mucous membrane, on which the two ureters open. The periphery of this extroverted area, which is covered by urothelium, becomes continuous with the skin (**Fig. 109.19**).

The routine use of ultrasound as an aid to *in-utero* diagnosis of abnormalities has revealed a prevalence of 1–2 abnormal fetuses per 1000 ultrasound procedures. Of these, 20–30% are anomalies of the genitourinary tract, and can be detected as early as 12–15 weeks' gestation. However, the decision to be made after such a diagnosis is by no means clear. Urinary obstruction is considered an abnormality, yet transient modest obstruction is considered normal during canalization of the urinary tract, and has been reported in 10–20% of fetuses in the third trimester. A delay in canalization, or in the rupture of the cloacal membrane, can produce a dilatation. Similarly, the closure of the urachus at 32 weeks may be associated with high-resistance outflow for the system, which again produces transient obstruction. The degree to which obstruction may cause renal parenchymal damage cannot be assessed in a developing kidney, which may have primary nephrogenic dysgenesis.

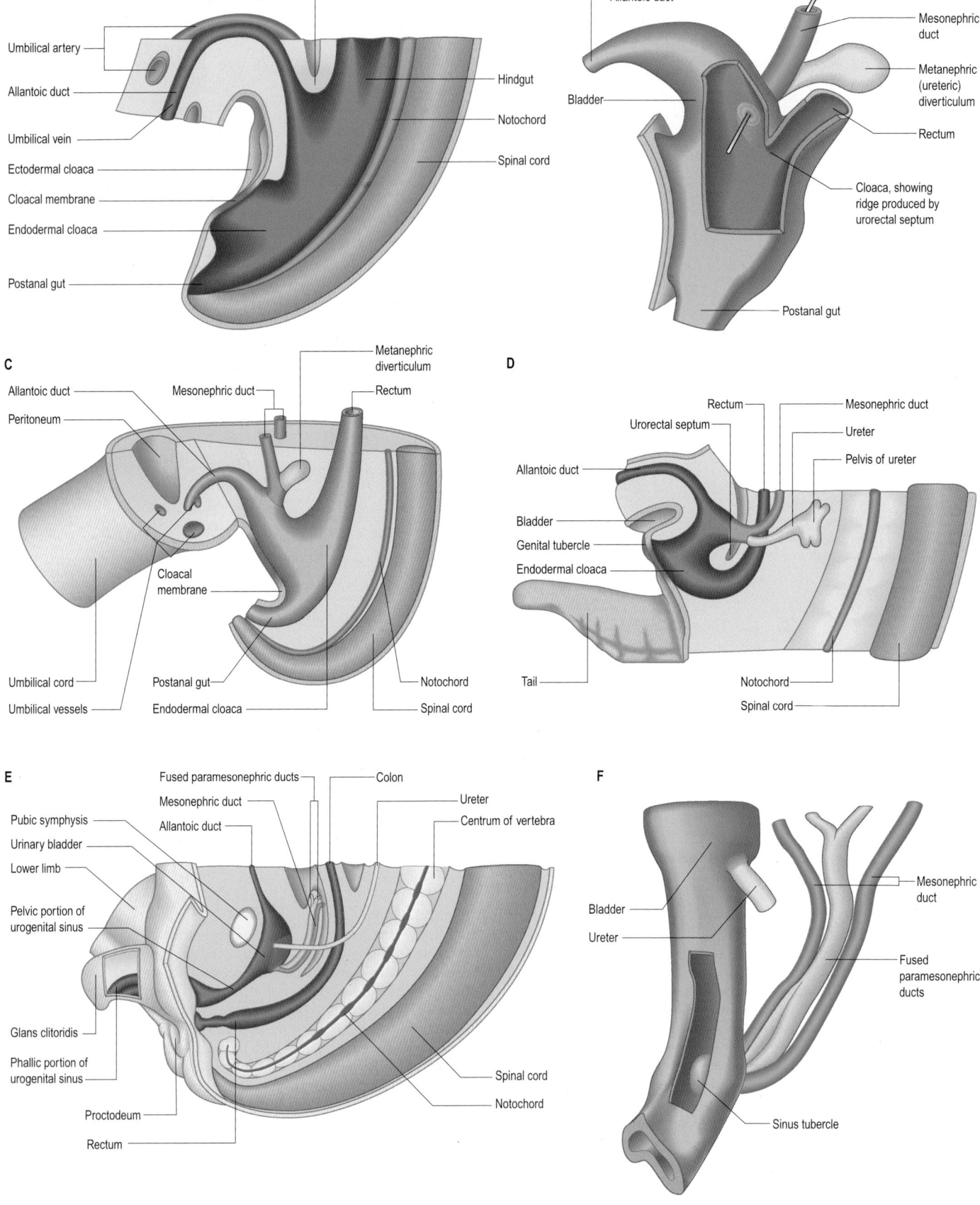

Fig. 109.7 **A**, The caudal end of a human embryo, c.4 weeks, showing the left lateral aspects of the spinal cord, notochord and endodermal cloaca. **B**, The endodermal cloaca of a human embryo, near the end of the fifth week. Part of the left wall of the cloaca, including the left mesonephric duct, has been removed, together with the adjoining portions of the walls of the developing bladder and rectum. A piece of the ectoderm around the cloacal membrane has been left *in situ*. A wire is shown passing along the right mesonephric duct into the cloaca. **C**, The caudal end of a human embryo, c.5 weeks, showing the endodermal cloaca. **D**, The caudal end of a human embryo, c.6 weeks. The cloaca is becoming divided by the urorectal septum. **E**, The caudal end of a female human fetus, $8\frac{1}{2}$–9 weeks, from the left-hand side showing structures in and near the median plane. The cloaca is now completely divided into urogenital and intestinal segments. **F**, Part of the vesicourethral portion of the endodermal cloaca of a female human fetus, $8\frac{1}{2}$–9 weeks. The sinus tubercle is the elevation on the posterior wall of the urogenital sinus, caused by the fusion with the paramesonephric ducts.

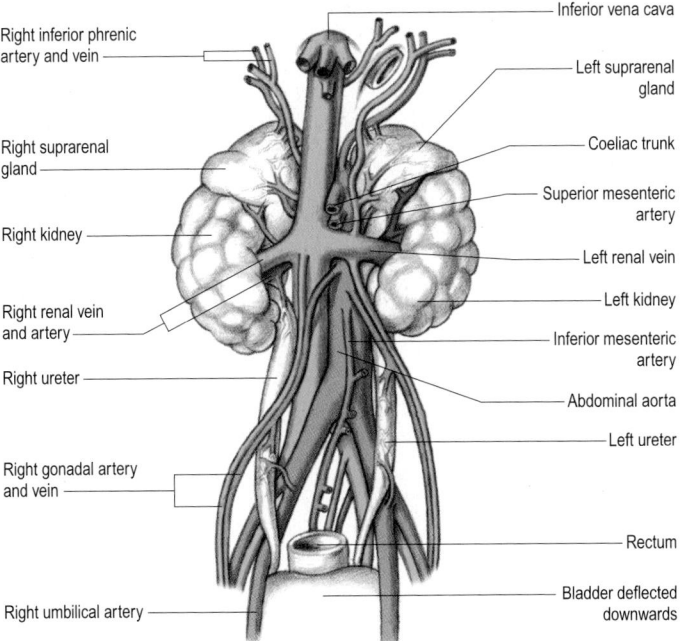

Fig. 109.8 Posterior abdominal wall of a full-term neonate. Note the lobulated kidneys and relatively wide calibre of the ureters. (After Crelin ES 1969 Anatomy of the Newborn. Philadelphia: Lea and Febiger.)

The volume of amniotic fluid is used as an indicator of renal function, but, because other sources produce amniotic fluid in early gestation, amniotic volume does not reflect fetal urinary output until the second trimester. Too little amniotic fluid is termed oligohydramnios, too much, hydramnios. Although variation in the amount of amniotic fluid may suggest abnormalities of either the gut or kidneys, it is not always possible to correlate even severe oligohydramnios with renal dysfunction. There is an important relationship between the volume of amniotic fluid, lung development and maturity, and oligohydramnios has been shown to be associated with pulmonary hypoplasia.

REPRODUCTIVE SYSTEM

Development of the reproductive organs from the intermediate mesenchyme starts from stage 14, c.10 days later than the urinary system. Bilateral paramesonephric (Müllerian) ducts develop alongside the mesonephric ducts, and the midportion of each mesonephros undergoes thickening to form the gonadal ridge. Although the primordial germ cells are delineated very early in development, they are sequestered in the extraembryonic tissues until the gonadal ridge is ready to receive them. It was thought that development to one or other sexual phenotype occurred after migration of the primordial germ cells to the indifferent gonads. However, it is now recognized that the development of male or female gonads, genital ducts and external genitalia is far more complicated, and is the result of a complex interplay between genetic expression, timing of development and the influence of sex hormones. As development proceeds, a significant proportion of early embryonic urinary tissue is incorporated into the reproductive tracts, especially in the male. The earliest stage of reproductive development, prior to the arrival of the primordial germ cells into the gonad, is termed the indifferent or ambisexual stage.

EARLY GONADAL DEVELOPMENT (AMBISEXUAL OR INDIFFERENT STAGE)
Essentially four different cell lineages contribute to the gonads. Cells are derived from: proliferating coelomic epithelium on the medial side of the mesonephros; underlying mesonephric mesenchyme; invading angiogenic mesenchyme already present in the mesonephros; and primordial germ cells that arise from the epiblast very early in development and later migrate from the allantoic wall.

The formation of the gonads is first indicated by the appearance of an area of thickened coelomic epithelium on the medial side of the mesonephric ridge in the fifth week, stage 16 (**Figs 109.12, 109.13, 109.16**). Elsewhere on the surface of the ridge the coelomic epithelium is one or two cells thick, but over this gonadal area it becomes multilayered. Thickening rapidly extends in a longitudinal direction until it

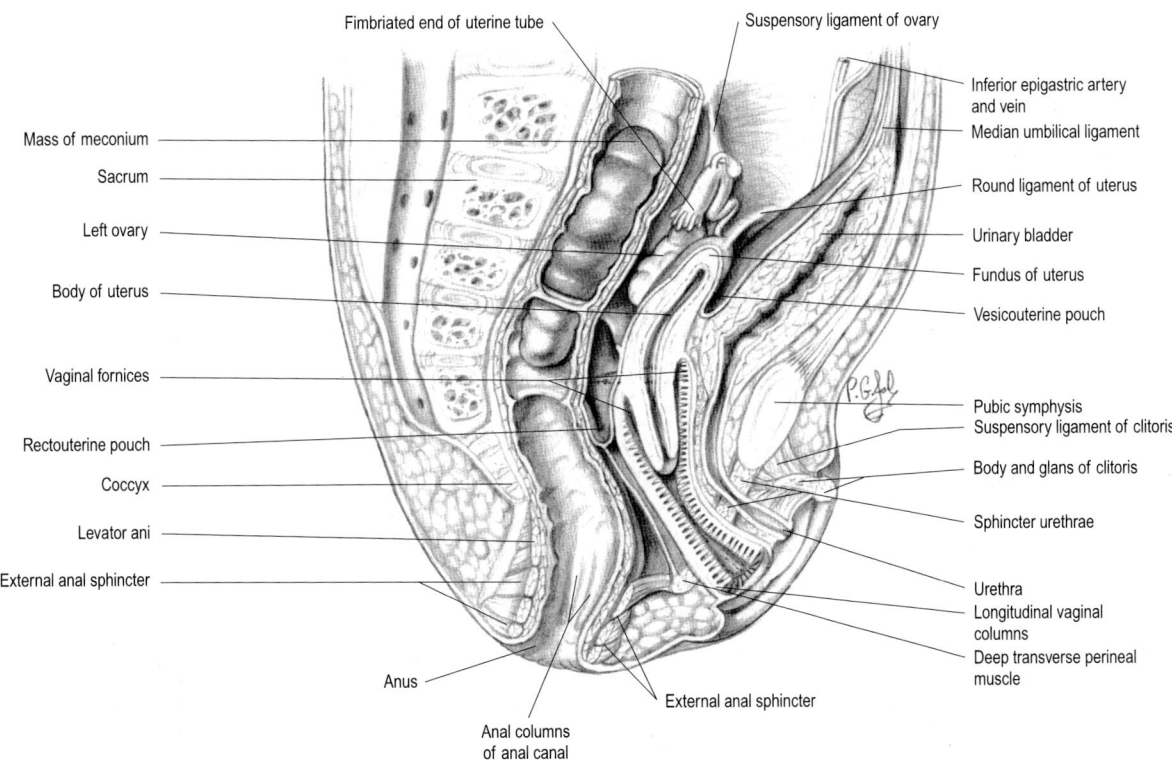

Fig. 109.9 Midsagittal section through the pelvis of a full-term female neonate. Note the abdominal position of the urinary bladder and uterus. (After Crelin ES 1969 Anatomy of the Newborn. Philadelphia: Lea and Febiger.)

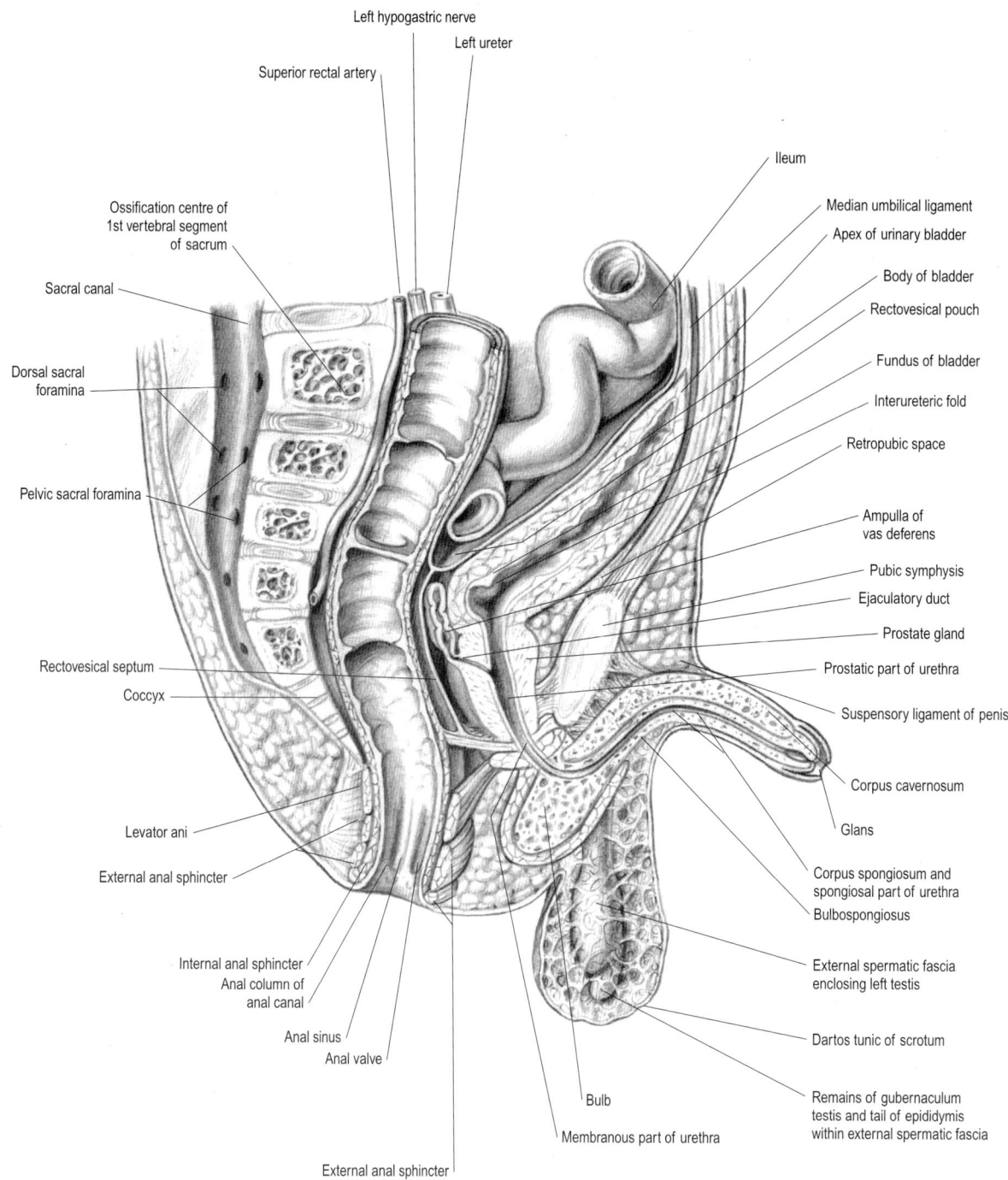

Left hypogastric nerve

Left ureter

Superior rectal artery

Ossification centre of
1st vertebral segment
of sacrum

Ileum

Median umbilical ligament

Apex of urinary bladder

Sacral canal

Body of bladder

Rectovesical pouch

Dorsal sacral
foramina

Fundus of bladder

Interureteric fold

Retropubic space

Pelvic sacral foramina

Ampulla of
vas deferens

Pubic symphysis

Ejaculatory duct

Prostate gland

Rectovesical septum

Prostatic part of urethra

Coccyx

Suspensory ligament of penis

Corpus cavernosum

Levator ani

Glans

External anal sphincter

Corpus spongiosum and
spongiosal part of urethra

Bulbospongiosus

Internal anal sphincter
Anal column of
anal canal

External spermatic fascia
enclosing left testis

Anal sinus

Dartos tunic of scrotum

Anal valve

Bulb

Membranous part of urethra

Remains of gubernaculum
testis and tail of epididymis
within external spermatic fascia

External anal sphincter

Fig. 109.10 Midsagittal section through the pelvis of a full-term male neonate. Note the abdominal position of the urinary bladder. (After Crelin ES 1969 Anatomy of the Newborn. Philadelphia: Lea and Febiger.)

covers nearly the whole of the medial surface of the ridge. The thickened epithelium continues to proliferate, displacing the renal corpuscles of the mesonephros in a dorsolateral direction and forms a projection into the coelomic cavity, the gonadal ridge. Surface depressions form along the limits of the ridge, which is thus connected to the mesonephros by a broad mesentery, the mesogenitale. In this way the mesonephric ridge becomes subdivided into a lateral part, the tubal fold, containing the mesonephric and paramesonephric ducts, and a medial part, the gonadal fold. The tubal fold also contains the nephric tubules and glomeruli at its base (**Fig. 109.3**).

Up to the seventh week the ambisexual gonad possesses no sexually differentiating feature. From stage 16 the proliferating coelomic epithelium forms a number of cellular epithelial cords (sometimes called primary sex cords), separated by mesenchyme. The cords remain at the periphery of the primordium and form a cortex. Proliferation and labyrinthine cellular condensation of the mesonephric mesenchyme,

including angiogenic mesenchyme, produces a central medulla (**Fig. 109.16**).

REPRODUCTIVE DUCTS

The paramesonephric Müllerian ducts develop in embryos of both sexes, but become dominant in the development of the female reproductive system. They are not detectable until the embryo reaches a length of 10–12 mm (early sixth week). Each begins as a linear invagination of the coelomic epithelium, the paramesonephric groove, on the lateral aspect of the mesonephric ridge near its cranial end. The blind caudal end continues to grow caudally into the substance of the ridge as a solid rod of cells, which becomes canalized as it lengthens. Throughout the extent of the mesonephros it is lateral to the mesonephric duct, which acts as a guide for it. The paramesonephric duct reaches the caudal end of the mesonephros in the eighth week. It turns medially and crosses ventral to the mesonephric duct to enter the genital cord, where it bends

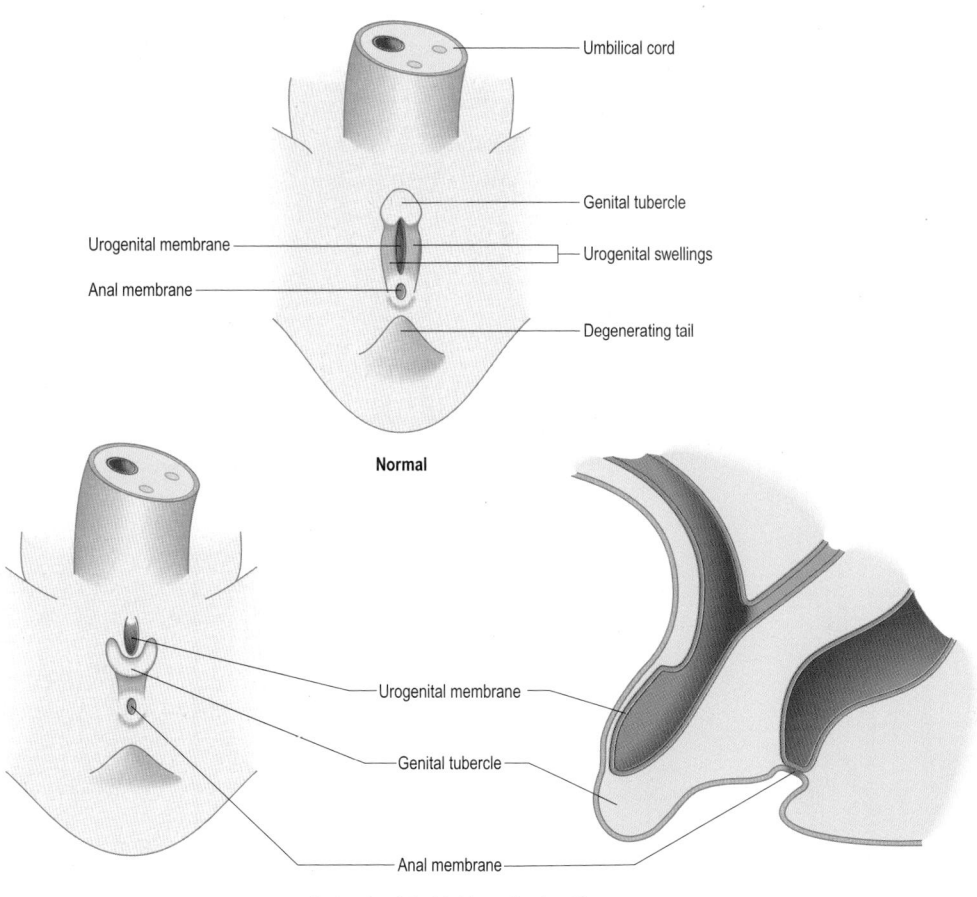

Normal

Exstrophy of the bladder and epispadias

Fig. 109.11 Bladder exstrophy. Misalignment of the genital tubercle and urogenital swellings with the urogenital membrane during early development results in subsequent malposition of the bladder, urethra and associated sphincters. The disappearance of the urogenital membrane exposes the posterior wall of the bladder, and the urethral opening is on the superior side of the penis or clitoris. (Redrawn from Tuchmann-Duplessis H, Haegel P 1972 Illustrated Human Embryology, Vol 2 Organogenesis. London: Chapman and Hall.)

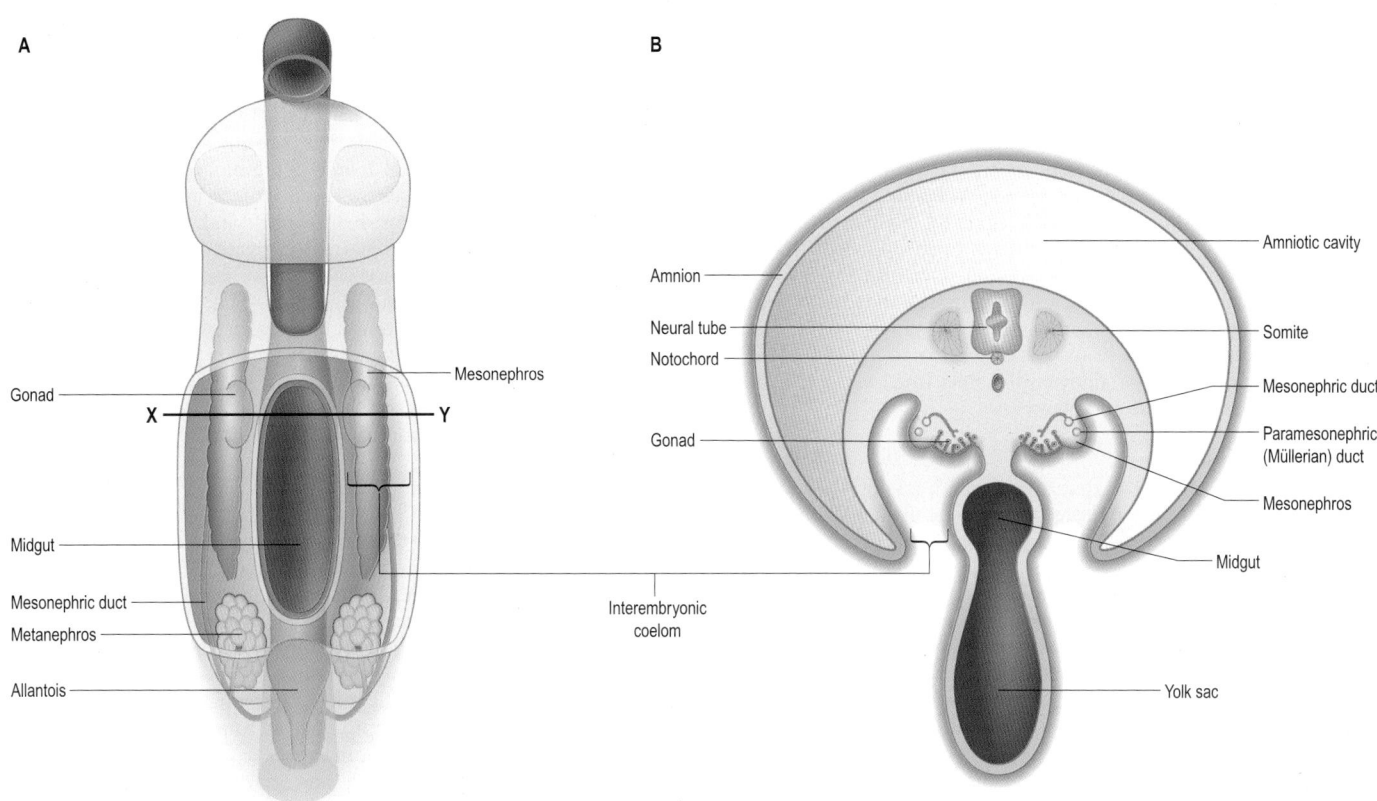

Fig. 109.12 A, Position of the gonads on the posterior abdominal wall, anteromedial to the mesonephros. **B**, Transverse section of figure **A**, through the line X–Y.

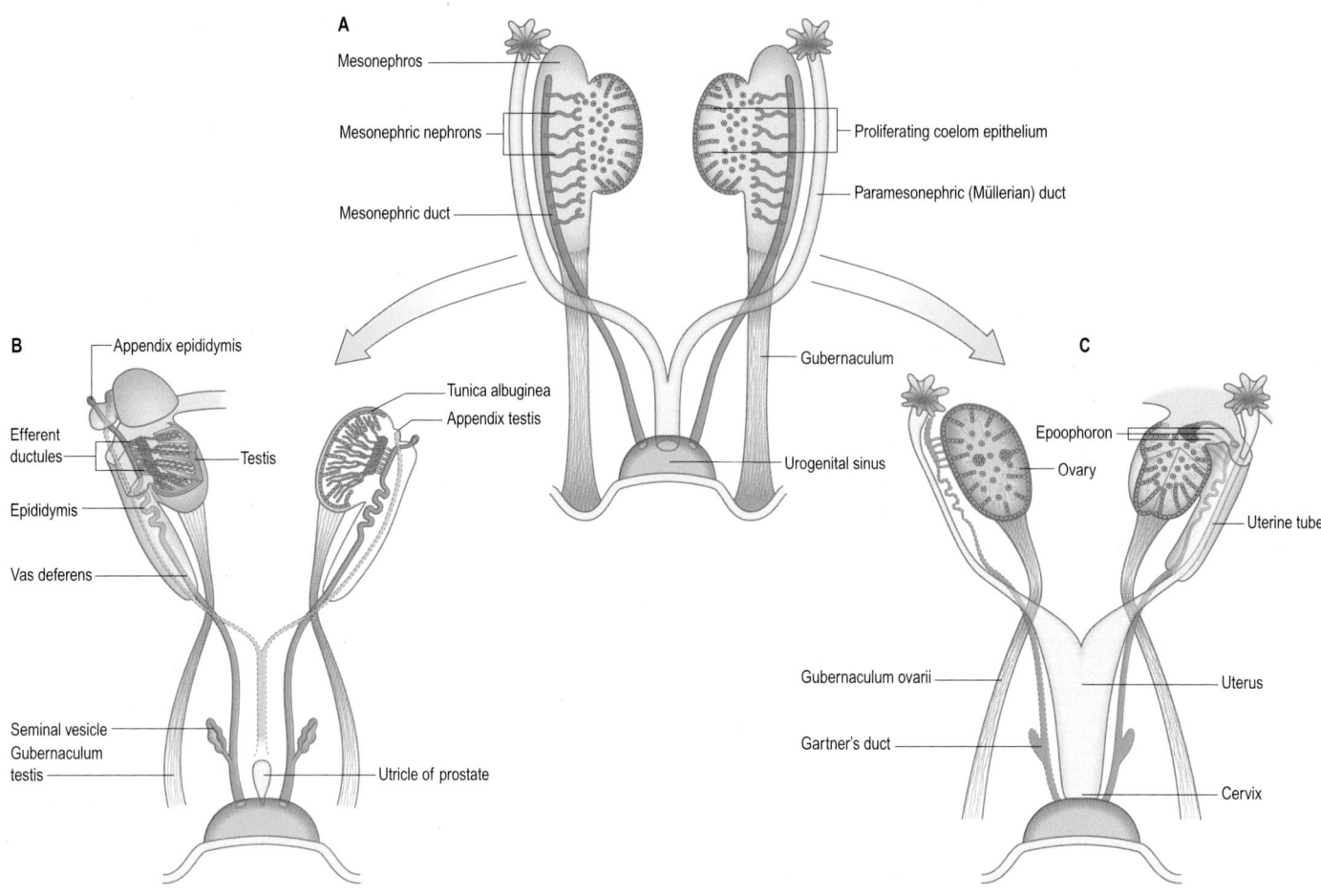

A

Mesonephros

Mesonephric nephrons

Mesonephric duct

Proliferating coelom epithelium

Paramesonephric (Müllerian) duct

B

Appendix epididymis

Efferent ductules

Epididymis

Vas deferens

Seminal vesicle
Gubernaculum testis

Testis

Tunica albuginea

Appendix testis

Utricle of prostate

Gubernaculum

Urogenital sinus

C

Epoophoron

Ovary

Uterine tube

Gubernaculum ovarii

Gartner's duct

Uterus

Cervix

Fig. 109.13 A, Indifferent or ambisexual stage of development. **B**, Male. The mesonephric ducts are retained (left) and the paramesonephric ducts involute (right). **C**, Female. The paramesonephric (Müllerian) ducts are retained (right) and the mesonephric ducts involute (left).

caudally in close apposition with its fellow from the opposite side (**Fig. 109.13**). The two ducts reach the dorsal wall of the urogenital sinus during the third month, and their blind ends produce an elevation called the Müllerian sinus tubercle (**Fig. 109.19**).

At the end of the indifferent stage each paramesonephric duct consists of vertical cranial and caudal parts and an intermediate horizontal region. The mesonephric ducts course caudally, medial to the paramesonephric ducts, and both duct systems open into the urogenital sinus. The genital ducts possess an external serosa on some surfaces derived from coelomic epithelium, a smooth muscle muscularis derived from underlying mesenchyme, and an internal mucosa derived from either the mesonephric duct or from the invaginated tube of coelomic epithelium that forms the paramesonephric duct. The layers are invaded by angiogenic mesenchyme and by nerves.

Uterus and uterine tubes

In the female the mesonephric duct is vestigial. Cranially it becomes the longitudinal duct of the epoöphoron, while caudally it is referred to as Gartner's duct (**Table 109.1**). The cranial part of the paramesonephric ducts forms the uterine tubes, and the original coelomic invagination remains as the pelvic opening of the tube. The fimbriae become defined as the cranial end of the mesonephros degenerates. The caudal vertical parts of the two ducts fuse with each other to form the uterovaginal primordium (**Figs 109.13, 109.14, 109.19**). This gives rise to the lower part of the uterus and, as it enlarges, it takes in the horizontal parts to form the fundus and most of the body of the adult uterus. A constriction between the body of the uterus and the cervix can be found at 9 weeks. The stroma of the endometrium and the uterine musculature develop from the surrounding mesenchyme of the genital cord.

Failure of fusion of the two paramesonephric ducts can lead to a range of anomalies summarized in **Fig. 109.15**. These fusions can also contribute to anomalies of vaginal development.

At birth the uterus is 2.5–5 cm long (average 3.5 cm), 2 cm wide between the uterine tubes, and c.1.3 cm thick (**Figs 11.4, 11.5, 109.9**). The body of the uterus is smaller than the uterine cervix, which forms two-thirds or more of the length. The isthmus between the body and the cervix is absent. The fetal female reproductive tract is affected by maternal hormones and undergoes some enlargement in the fetus. The endocervical glands are active before birth and the cervical canal is usually filled with mucus. The uterus is relatively large at birth, and subsequently involutes to about one-third of its length and more than half of its weight. The neonatal size and weight of the uterus are not regained until puberty. The uterine tubes are relatively short and wide.

The position of the uterus in the pelvic cavity depends to a great extent on the state of the bladder anteriorly and the rectum posteriorly. If the bladder contains only a small amount of urine the uterus may be anteverted but it is often in a direct line with the vagina (**Figs 109.9, 109.19**).

Vagina

At c.60 mm crown rump (CR) length an epithelial proliferation, the sinuvaginal bulb, arises from the dorsal wall of the urogenital sinus in the region of the sinus tubercle. Its origin marks the site of the future hymen. The proliferation gradually extends cranially as a solid anteroposteriorly flattened plate inside the tubular condensation of the uterovaginal primordium, which will eventually become the fibromuscular vaginal wall. The caudal tip of the paramesonephric duct epithelium recedes until, at about the 140 mm stage, its junction with the epithelial proliferation lies in the cervical canal.

Starting from its caudal end, and gradually extending cranially through its whole extent, the solid plate formed by the sinus proliferation enlarges into a cylindrical structure. Thereafter the central cells desquamate to establish the vaginal lumen. The extent to which mesonephric and paramesonephric ducts contribute directly to the formation

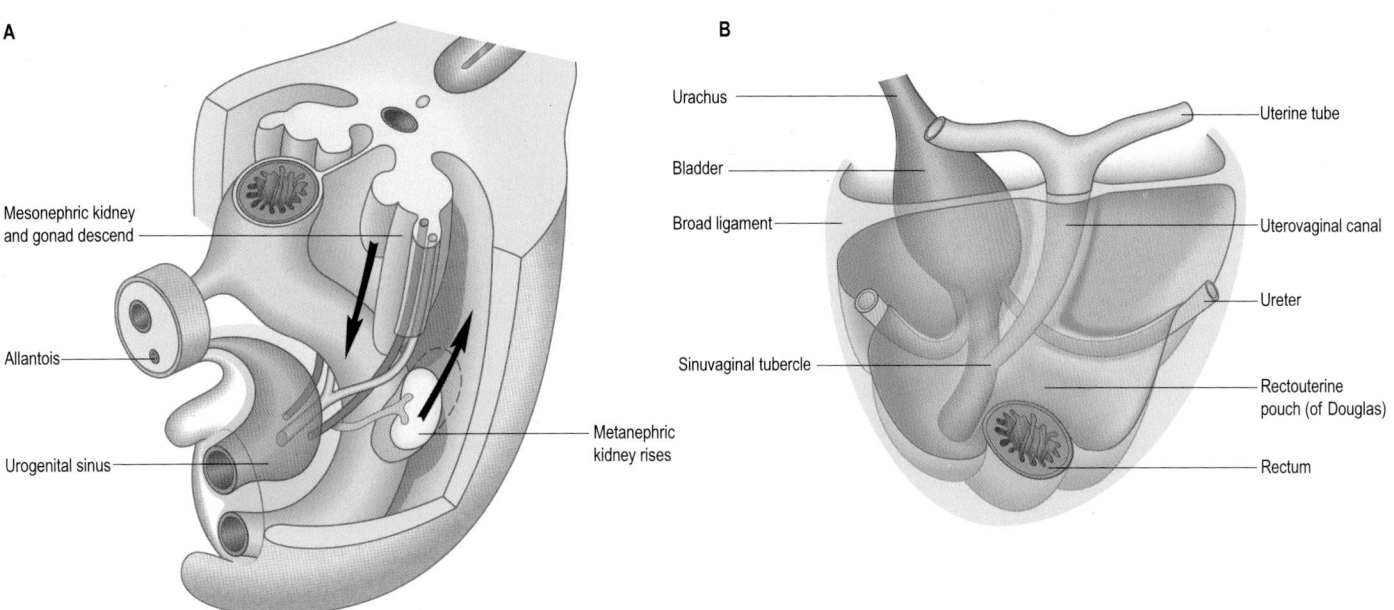

Fig. 109.14 Relative movements of the gonads and associated tubes. **A**, Gonads and mesonephros move caudally, the metanephros ascends. **B**, Posterior view of the mesonephric ducts (ureters) and the fused paramesonephric ducts (uterovaginal canal) in the female. For earlier development, see **Fig. 109.3**. (Redrawn from Tuchmann-Duplessis H, Haegel P 1972 Illustrated Human Embryology, Vol 2 Organogenesis. London: Chapman and Hall.)

of the vagina is controversial. As the upper end of the vaginal plate enlarges it grows up to embrace the cervix, and then is excavated to produce the vaginal fornices. Anomalies of paramesonepric duct fusion can produce related vaginal anomalies (**Fig. 109.15**). The urogenital sinus undergoes relative shortening craniocaudally to form the vestibule, which opens on the surface through the cleft between the genital folds. The lower end of the vaginal plate grows caudally so that in 109 mm embryos the vaginal rudiment approaches the vestibule. In fetuses of 162 mm the vaginal lumen is complete except at the cephalic end where the fornices are still solid; they are hollow by 170 mm. At approximately half way through gestation (180 mm) the genital canal is continuous with the exterior. During the later months of fetal life the vaginal epithelium is greatly hypertrophied, apparently under the influence of maternal hormones, but after birth it assumes the inactive form of childhood.

In the neonate, the vagina is c.2.5–3.5 cm long and 1.5 cm wide at the fornices. The uterine cervix extends into the vagina for c.1 cm. The posterior vaginal wall is longer than the anterior wall, which gives the vagina a distinct curve (**Figs 11.5, 109.9, 109.19**). The cavity is filled with longitudinal columns covered with a thick layer of cornified, stratified squamous epithelium. These cells slough off after birth when the effect exerted by maternal hormones is removed.

The orifice of the vagina is surrounded by a thick elliptical ring of connective tissue, the hymen (**Fig. 109.9**). During childhood the hymen becomes a membranous fold along the posterior margin of the vaginal lumen. Should the fold form a complete diaphragm across the vaginal lumen it is termed an imperforate hymenal membrane.

Reproductive ducts in the male

In the male, the most paramesonephric ducts atrophy (**Fig. 109.13**) under the influence of anti-Müllerian hormone (AMH), which is released locally by the Sertoli cells of the testis. Vestigial structures are therefore most likely to persists cranially and/or caudally, at the limits of the local effects of AMH. A vestige of the cranial end of the duct persists as the appendix testis (**Figs 109.13, 109.19, Table 109.1**). The fused caudal ends of the two ducts are connected to the wall of the urogenital sinus by a solid utricular cord of cells, which soon merges with a proliferation of sinus epithelium, the sinu-utricular cord. The latter is similar to, but less extensive than, the sinus proliferation in the female. The proliferating epithelium is claimed to be an intermingling of the endoderm of the urogenital sinus with the lining epithelia of the mesonephric and paramesonephric ducts, which have extended on to the surface of the sinus tubercle. As the sinu-utricular cord grows, so the utricular cord recedes from the tubercle. In the second half of fetal life the composite

cord acquires a lumen and becomes dilated to form the prostatic utricle, the lining of which consists of hyperplastic stratified squamous epithelium (**Figs 109.13, 109.19**). The sinus tubercle becomes the colliculus seminalis.

The main reproductive ducts in the male are derived from the mesonephric ducts, which are subsumed into the male reproductive system as the metanephric kidney develops (p. 1373). The mesonephric duct gives rise to the canal of the epididymis, vas deferens and ejaculatory duct. The seminal vesicle and the ampulla of the vas deferens appear as a common swelling at the end of the mesonephric duct during the end of the third and into the fourth month. Their appearance coincides with degeneration of the paramesonephric ducts, although no causal relation between the two events has been established. Separation into two rudiments occurs at c.125 mm crown–heel length. The seminal vesicle elongates, its duct is delineated and hollow diverticula bud from its wall. About the sixth month (300 mm crown–heel length) the growth rate of both vesicle and ampulla is greatly increased. **Figure 109.10** shows the position of the ampulla of the vas deferens in the neonate, possibly in response to increased secretion of prolactin by the fetal or maternal hypophysis, or to the effects of placental hormones. The tubules of the prostate show a similar increase of growth rate at this time.

PRIMORDIAL GERM CELLS

The primordial germ cells are formed very early from the epiblast. They are large cells, 12 to 20 μm in diameter, in comparison with most somatic cells. They are characterized by vesicular nuclei with well-defined nuclear membranes and by a tendency to retain yolk inclusions long after these have disappeared from somatic cells. It is not yet clear whether the primordial germ cells are derived from particular blastomeres during cleavage, if they constitute a clonal line from a single blastomere, or if they are the product of a progressive concentration of the nucleus of the fertilized ovum by unequal partition at successive mitoses. Primordial germ cells spend the early stages of development within the extra-embryonic tissues near the end of the primitive streak and in the connecting stalk. In this situation they are away from the inductive influences to which the majority of the somatic cells are subjected during early development.

Primordial germ cells can be identified in human embryos in stage 11 when the number of cells is probably not more than 20–30. When the tail fold has formed they appear within the endoderm and the splanchnopleuric mesenchyme and epithelium of the hindgut as well as in the adjoining region of the wall of the yolk sac. They migrate dorso-cranially in the mesentery, by amoeboid movements and by growth

1 Partial or total failure of fusion of the terminal portion of the paramesonephric (Müllerian) ducts

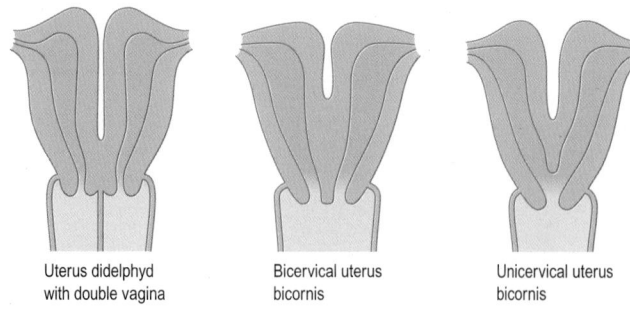

Uterus didelphyd
with double vagina

Bicervical uterus
bicornis

Unicervical uterus
bicornis

2 Partial or total atresia of the terminal portion of one or both paramesonephric (Müllerian) ducts

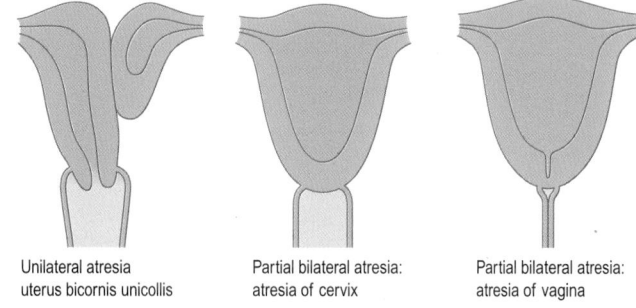

Unilateral atresia
uterus bicornis unicollis

Partial bilateral atresia:
atresia of cervix

Partial bilateral atresia:
atresia of vagina

3 Failure of resorption of the uterovaginal septum after fusion of the paramesonephric (Müllerian) ducts

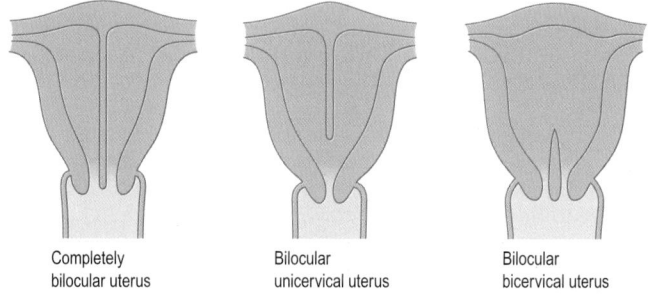

Completely
bilocular uterus

Bilocular
unicervical uterus

Bilocular
bicervical uterus

Fig. 109.15 Uterovaginal malformations. (Redrawn from Tuchmann-Duplessis H, Haegel P 1972 Illustrated Human Embryology, Vol 2 Organogenesis. London: Chapman and Hall.)

displacement, and pass around the dorsal angles of the coelom (medial coelomic bays) to reach the genital ridges from stage 15 (**Fig. 109.16**). It is believed that the genital ridges exert long-range effects on the migrating primordial germ cells, in terms of controlling their direction of migration and supporting the primordial germ-cell population.

Primordial germ cells proliferate both during and after migration to the mesonephric ridges. Cells which do not complete this migration degenerate. After segregation, when they are often termed primary gonocytes, they divide to form secondary gonocytes.

DEVELOPMENT OF THE GONADS

The factors that lead to formation of either testis or ovary are described below and in **Fig. 109.16**. The morphological events which occur in each type of gonadal development are presented first.

Testis

Most studies support the hypothesis that the seminiferous tubules are formed from cords of epithelial cells derived from the proliferating coelomic epithelium (**Figs 109.13, 109.16**). The cords lengthen, partly by addition from the coelomic epithelium, and encroach on the medulla, where they unite with a network of cells derived from the mesonephric mesenchyme destined to become the rete testis. Primordial germ cells are incorporated into the cords, which later become enlarged and canalized to form the seminiferous tubules. The cells derived from the surface of the early gonad form the supporting Sertoli cells. Sertoli cells proliferate throughout development and perhaps into childhood. When they stop dividing they mature and cannot be reactivated. Each Sertoli

cell can only support a fixed number of germ cells during their development into spermatozoa, i.e. the number of Sertoli cells produced at this time determines the maximal limit of sperm output. Because the germ cells make up the bulk of the adult testis, the number of Sertoli cells is a major determinant of the size to which the testes will grow (factors which impair the process of spermatogenesis, resulting in the loss of germ cells, will also affect testicular size). Variation in Sertoli cell number is probably the most important factor in accounting for the enormous variation in sperm counts between individual men, whether fertile or infertile. Indeed, the available data for adult men indicate that Sertoli cell numbers vary across a fifty-fold range. Although some of this variation may result from attrition of Sertoli cell numbers because of ageing, the major differences in Sertoli cell numbers will have been determined by events in fetal and/or childhood life.

The interstitial cells of the testis are derived from mesenchyme and possibly also from coelomic epithelial cells that do not become incorporated into the tubules. Among other cell lines they form the embryonic and fetal cells of Leydig, which secrete testosterone. A later migration of mesenchyme beneath the coelomic epithelium forms the tunica albuginea of the testis.

The cords of the rete testis become connected to the glomerular capsules in the persisting part of the mesonephros. Ultimately they become connected to the mesonephric duct by the five to twelve most cranial persisting mesonephric tubules. These become exceedingly convoluted and form the lobules of the head of the epididymis. The mesonephric duct, which was the primitive 'ureter' of the mesonephros, becomes the canal of the epididymis and the vas deferens of the testis. The seminiferous tubules do not acquire lumina until the seventh month; the tubules of the testicular rete become canalized somewhat earlier.

Disorders of development of the testis and reproductive tract in the male fetus seem to be increasing in incidence. Testicular maldescent (cryptorchidism) and hypospadias appear to have doubled or trebled in incidence in the last 30–50 years, while testicular cancer has increased by an even greater margin and is now the commonest cancer of young men. Although testicular cancer is primarily a disease of young men (95% of cases affect 15- to 45-year-old males) it is now established that this age-incidence reflects activation of premalignant carcinoma-in-situ (CIS) cells, which are present at birth and which almost certainly arise during fetal life. It has been suggested that CIS cells are primordial germ cells that have failed to develop normally. Abnormalities of development of the testis and reproductive tract (e.g. gonadal dysgenesis, cryptorchidism, small testes) are important risk factors for the development of testicular cancer. However, the most dramatic change that appears to have occurred in the relatively recent past is a fall in sperm counts of around 40–50% (1% per year over the last 50 years). Although this dramatic decrease is obviously manifest only in adulthood, as with testicular cancer, it is thought that an explanation for this is impaired testicular development during fetal or childhood life.

Ovary

In its earliest stages, the ovary closely resembles the testis, although it is slower to differentiate its characteristically female features (**Figs 109.13, 109.16**). Few, if any, of the epithelial cords invade the medulla. The majority remain in the cortex, where they may be joined by a second proliferation from the coelomic epithelium overlying the gonad. In histological sections of ovaries from the third and subsequent months, the epithelial cords appear as clusters of cells, which may contain primitive germ cells, separated by fine septa of undifferentiated mesenchyme. An ovarian rete condenses in the medullary mesenchyme and some of its cords may join mesonephric glomeruli. The medulla subsequently regresses, and connective tissue and blood vessels from this region invade the cortex to form the ovarian stroma. During this invasion the clusters of epithelial cortical cells break into individual groups of supporting cells (now identified as granulosa cells), which surround the primordial germ cells (now identified as primary oocytes) that have entered the prophase of the first meiotic division. Primary oocytes are derived from a mitotic division of the primordial germ cells (naked oogonia). Their epithelial capsules consist of flattened pregranulosa cells derived from proliferations of coelomic epithelium. The ovary now has its full complement of primary oocytes. The majority undergo atresia at various stages during their development, but the remainder resume development after puberty, when they complete the first meiotic division shortly before ovulation (p. 1323). The granulosa cells at this

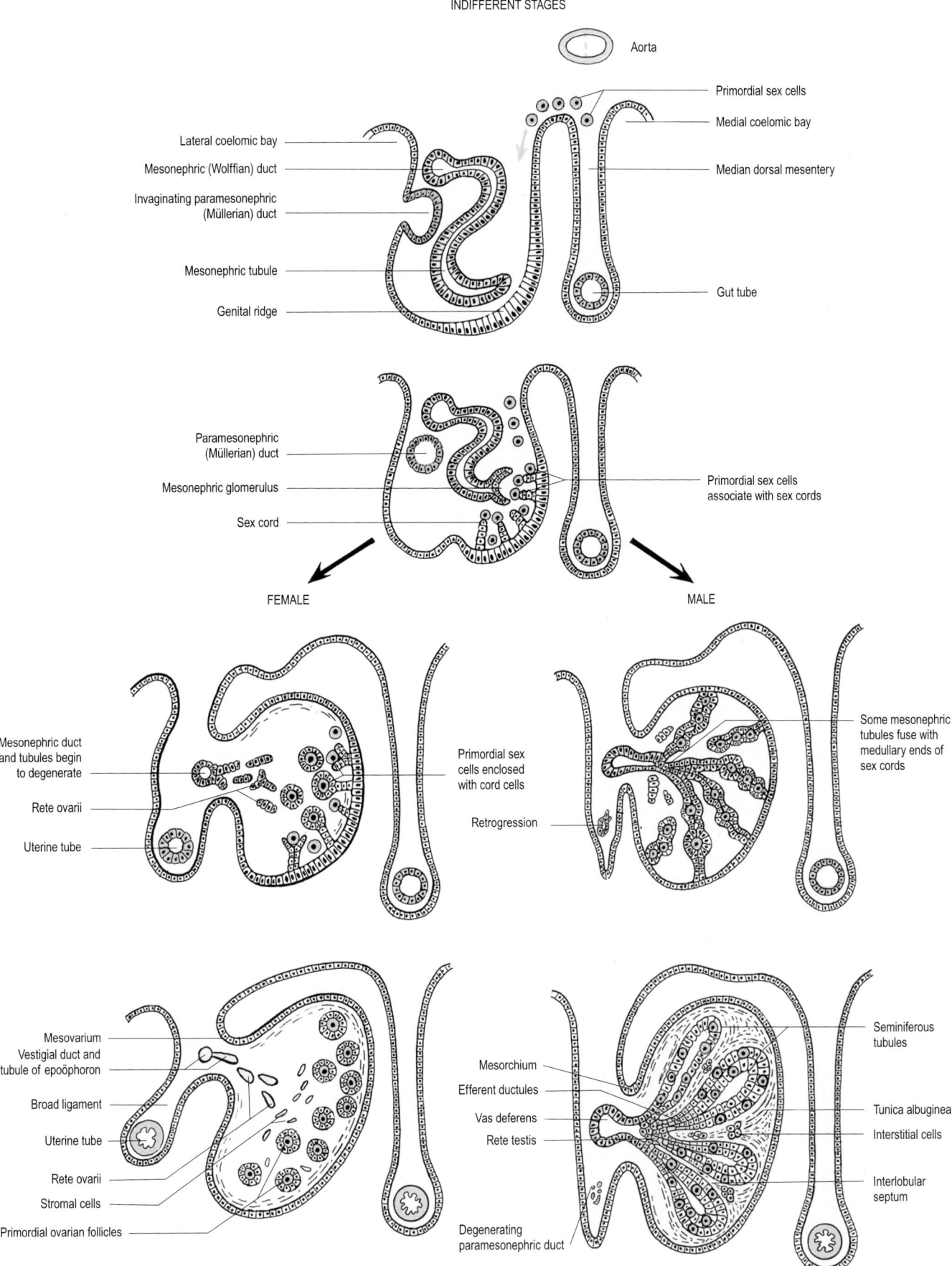

INDIFFERENT STAGES

Aorta

Primordial sex cells

Medial coelomic bay

Lateral coelomic bay

Median dorsal mesentery

Mesonephric (Wolffian) duct

Invaginating paramesonephric
(Müllerian) duct

Mesonephric tubule

Genital ridge

Gut tube

Paramesonephric
(Müllerian) duct

Mesonephric glomerulus

Sex cord

Primordial sex cells
associate with sex cords

FEMALE

MALE

Mesonephric duct
and tubules begin
to degenerate

Rete ovarii

Uterine tube

Primordial sex
cells enclosed
with cord cells

Retrogression

Some mesonephric
tubules fuse with
medullary ends of
sex cords

Mesovarium
Vestigial duct and
tubule of epoöphoron

Broad ligament

Uterine tube

Rete ovarii

Stromal cells

Primordial ovarian follicles

Mesorchium

Efferent ductules

Vas deferens

Rete testis

Degenerating
paramesonephric duct

Seminiferous
tubules

Tunica albuginea

Interstitial cells

Interlobular
septum

Fig. 109.16 Development of the gonads and associated ducts as seen in transverse section to show the fate of the primordial sex cells, mesonephric duct and tubules and paramesonephric duct in the two sexes. (Modified from Williams PL, Wendell-Smith CP, Treadgold S 1969 Basic Human Embryology, 2nd edn, Philadelphia: Lippincott.)

time enlarge and multiply to form the stratum granulosum and, as they do so, they become surrounded by thecal cells, which differentiate from the stroma.

Only the middle part of the gonadal ridge produces the ovary. Its cranial part is sterile and becomes the suspensory ligament of the ovary (infundibulopelvic fold of peritoneum). Its caudal region, also sterile, is incorporated into the ovarian ligament.

Sex determination in the embryo

It was believed that the gonads were indifferent or ambisexual until the arrival of the primordial germ cells in the gonadal ridge, at which point the sex of the embryo was 'turned on' by the presence of the male or female germ cells. It now seems that the germ cells may be essentially irrelevant to testis determination; embryos in which the genital ridges are devoid of germ cells may still have morphologically normal testis development. It is not clear if the germ cells are necessary for ovarian determination. They are required for the proper organization and differentiation of the ovary, and their absence results in the development of 'streak gonads', where only lines of follicular cells can be seen, as in Turner's syndrome.

The processes of sex determination and differentiation involve interacting pathways of gene activity, which lead to the total patterning of the embryo as either male or female.

In one model of sex determination in humans, the female pathway is considered to be the default pathway. According to this model, the Y chromosome of a male embryo diverts development into the testicular pathway, and the resulting changes that convert an indifferent gonad to a testis produce a range of local and widely acting hormones, which collectively generate all the secondary sexual characteristics.

The possession of a Y chromosome is usually associated with a male developmental pathway. The male-determining region of the Y chromosome, which is located near its tip, is termed the testis-determining factor (TDF), and is regarded by some as the 'master switch' that programmes the direction of sexual development. It has been suggested that the TDF acts initially within the epithelial cords of cells derived from the coloemic epithelium of the ambisexual gonad. These cells can potentially differentiate into either Sertoli or granulosa cells (the supporting cells for the germ cells in the testis and ovary respectively). TDF directs their development into Sertoli cells, which then influence the differentiation of the other cell types in the testicular pathway, so that Leydig cells appear later, and the connective tissue becomes organized into a male pattern. The germ cells are also affected by this environment. When they arrive they become enclosed within the Sertoli cells and enter mitotic arrest (which is characteristic of spermatogenesis), instead of entering meiosis and meiotic arrest (which characterizes oogenesis). Thus the development of male characteristics follows the expression of TDF, and female characteristics develop in its absence.

Subsequent development of the male phenotype requires fetal secretion of both testosterone and anti-Müllerian hormone (AMH), (also called Müllerian inhibiting substance or MIS), and the development of the appropriate cytoplasmic testosterone-binding protein. Sertoli cells synthesize AMH, which causes the regression of the Müllerian ducts, and Leydig cells produce testosterone, which promotes the development of the mesonephric ducts, sets into process the development of male external genitalia, and sensitizes other tissues to testosterone (p. 1388). Absence of the testosterone-binding protein results in XY individuals with testes and degenerated Müllerian ducts, but because they cannot respond to the circulating testosterone produced by their testes they develop female secondary sexual characteristics.

Studies on the exact position of the TDF have been based on deletion mapping the Y chromosome in a class of XX males arising from abnormal X:Y interchange at meiosis. In all mammals tested a conserved sequence that mapped to the Y chromosome was found. The sequence formed part of a gene in the sex-determining region of the Y chromosome, and was therefore termed SRY. It is believed to be genetically and functionally equivalent to TDF. This gene is first expressed in cells located centrally in the developing gonad and then later in the cranial and caudal poles in supporting cells, called pre-Sertoli cells, which are derived from the coelomic epithelium. Studies indicate that SRY initiates testis formation from the indifferent gonad by directing the development of supporting-cell precursors as Sertoli rather than granulosa cells (Albrecht & Eicher 2001).

The possession of a Y chromosome expressing SRY and TDF may, therefore, underlie the switch to development of the male phenotype, by initiating Sertoli cell differentiation. An alternative view is that the possession of TDF accelerates the development of the gonads in XY embryos generally, so that testes are larger and more advanced than ovaries of the same age. Male human fetuses are generally bigger than females from 12 weeks' gestation, indeed males are already slightly ahead of females at six weeks' gestation, just prior to testicular differentiation. It has been suggested that this difference in the growth rate is encoded in the sex chromosomes. Once gonadal development has started, the difference in size between testes and ovaries becomes proportionately much greater than the overall size difference between XY and XX fetuses. (Interestingly, the right gonad develops slightly ahead of the left, an observation which may be correlated with the finding that testes are more often on the right side, and ovaries on the left, in hermaphrodites.)

Although a fetus is exposed to maternal hormones, the accelerated development of the testis at early embryological stages ensures arrest of meiosis of the germ cells, and the production of local hormones that masculinize the male embryo before the development of the reproductive tract and ovaries of the female. The range of intersex conditions, of phenotypic sex that is not correlated to genotype, and the effect of multiple X chromosomes in males, suggests that the male developmental pathway involves many testis determining genes, whereas only a single X chromosome determines the female default pathway. Once testicular differentiation and male hormone secretion have begun, other Y-chromosomal genes are required to maintain spermatogenesis and complete spermiogenesis. The impairment of oogenesis by other chromosomal abnormalities is much less severe than the impairment of spermatogenesis.

DESCENT OF THE GONADS

The gonads develop on the posterior abdominal wall bilaterally along the central portion of the mesonephros. This region receives a rich blood supply, which is directed to the gonads as the mesonephros involutes. Both gonads descend, the testis to lie outside the abdominal cavity, and the ovary to the pelvis, however, they retain their early blood supply from the dorsal aorta.

Descent of the testis

Each testis initially lies on the dorsal abdominal wall. As it enlarges, its cranial end degenerates and the remaining organ therefore occupies a more caudal position. It is attached to the mesonephric fold by the mesorchium (the mesogenitale of the undifferentiated gonad), a peritoneal fold that contains the testicular vessels and nerves and a quantity of undifferentiated mesenchyme. It also acquires a secondary attachment to the ventral abdominal wall, which has a considerable influence on its subsequent movements. At the point where the mesonephric fold bends medially to form the genital cord (**Fig. 109.3**), it becomes connected to the lower part of the ventral abdominal wall by an inguinal fold of peritoneum. The mesenchymal cells occupying the core of the inguinal fold condense as another cord, the gubernaculum (**Figs 109.3, 109.13, 109.17**). This extends from the epidermal ectoderm, which will later form the scrotum, through the inguinal fold and the mesorchium to the caudal pole of the testis. It travels through the site of the future inguinal canal, which is formed around it by the differentiating muscles of the abdominal wall. At the end of the second month the caudal part of the ventral abdominal wall is horizontal but, after the return of the intestine to the peritoneal cavity, it grows in length and becomes progressively more vertical. As the umbilical artery runs ventrally from the dorsal to the ventral wall, it pulls up a falciform peritoneal fold, which forms the medial boundary of a peritoneal fossa, the saccus vaginalis or lateral inguinal fossa, into which the testis projects. This lower end of the fossa protrudes down the inguinal canal, along the ventrosuperior aspect of the gubernaculum, as the processus vaginalis (**Figs 109.17, 109.19**).

The mechanism of testicular descent has been variously ascribed to shortening and active contraction of the gubernaculum, increased intra-abdominal pressure, a simple growth process, and the effect on the convex surface of the gland of the active contraction of the lower fibres of internal oblique, which squeeze it through the canal. (For a review of testicular descent in the human see Barteczko & Jacob 2000.) The gubernaculum precedes the testis both spatially and in rate of growth, and forms a tapering column of soft tissue with the diminutive testis at its cranial pole. It continues to grow until the seventh month, by which time its caudal part has filled the future inguinal canal and has begun

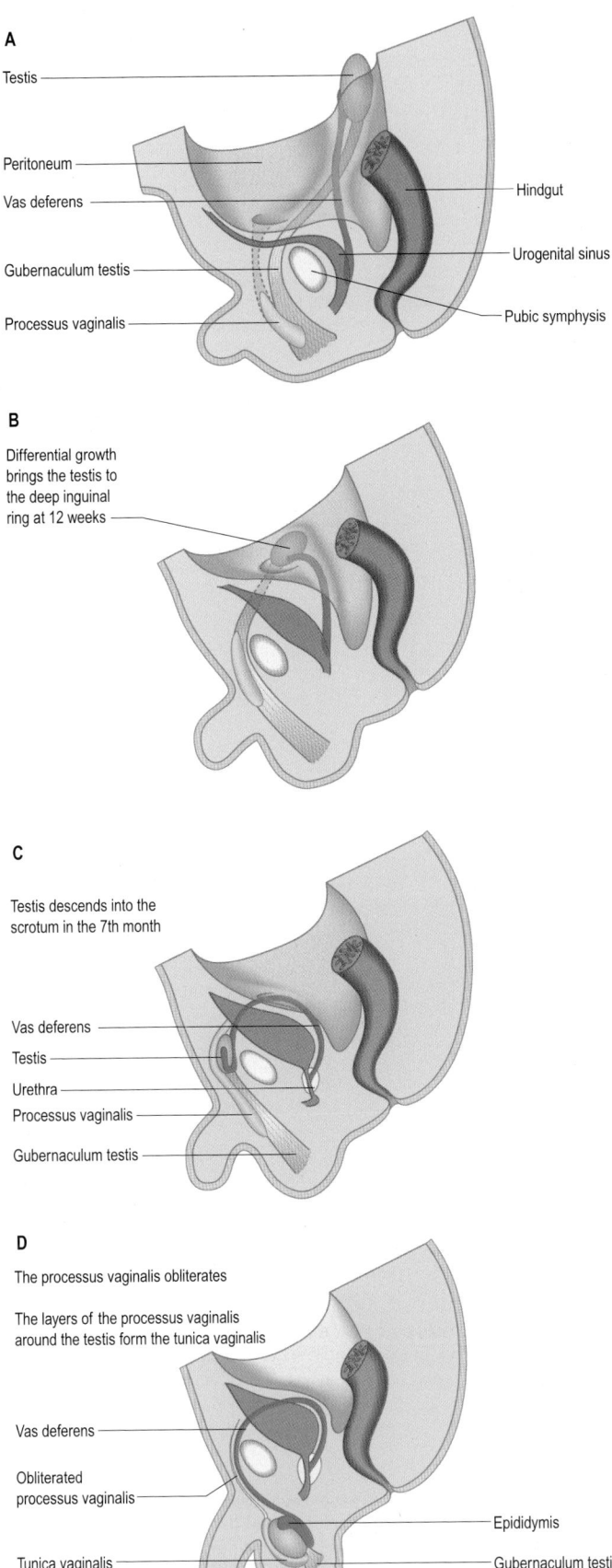

A

Testis

Peritoneum

Vas deferens

Gubernaculum testis

Processus vaginalis

Hindgut

Urogenital sinus

Pubic symphysis

B

Differential growth brings the testis to the deep inguinal ring at 12 weeks

C

Testis descends into the scrotum in the 7th month

Vas deferens

Testis

Urethra

Processus vaginalis

Gubernaculum testis

D

The processus vaginalis obliterates

The layers of the processus vaginalis around the testis form the tunica vaginalis

Vas deferens

Obliterated processus vaginalis

Tunica vaginalis

Epididymis

Gubernaculum testis

Fig. 109.17 Descent of the testis. The testis is always retroperitoneal. (Redrawn from Tuchmann-Duplessis H, Haegel P 1972 Illustrated Human Embryology, Vol 2 Organogenesis. London: Chapman and Hall.)

to expand the developing scrotum. In this it also precedes the processus vaginalis. It does not develop attachments to skin, nor is there any evidence that it produces the radiating extensions into suprapubic, perineal or femoral sites that are often cited to explain the various forms of ectopic testis. By virtue of its soft consistency, gubernacular tissue (which in the early stage is formed mainly of hyaluronic acid) may offer a route of low resistance to the descending testis. It stops growing in the last two months of gestation, and this, coupled with an accelerating rate of growth in the testis and epididymis, may be a factor in testicular descent as far as the inguinal canal.

The mechanism of the final rapid descent of the testis into the scrotum is not yet clear, although endocrine effects are certainly important. Experimentally, division of the genitofemoral nerve prevents both inguinoscrotal testicular descent and differentiation and migration of the gubernaculum. It has been suggested that androgens act on neurones, the axons of which run in the genitofemoral nerve, stimulating release of neurotransmitters, which might act as second messengers for androgens, from the nerve endings. A peptide neurotransmitter, calcitonin gene-related peptide (CGRP), is present in the genitofemoral nerve and its cell bodies in the spinal cord. CGRP causes the gubernacula from newborn male mice to contract rhythmically, whereas CGRP antagonists inhibit this contraction.

The caudal pole of the testis is retained in apposition with the deep inguinal ring by the gubernaculum during the sixth and seventh months. The testes finally descend into the scrotum before birth (**Fig. 11.4**), the left testis usually migrating ahead of the right. In full-term male neonates 90% have descended testes. In premature babies descent may not be complete. As the testis descends it is preceded by the processus vaginalis. The distal end of the processus vaginalis, into which the testis projects, forms the tunica vaginalis testis. The portion associated with the spermatic cord in the scrotum and inguinal canal normally becomes obliterated, and usually leaves a fibrous remnant. At birth the processus vaginalis is collapsed but not necessarily obliterated. It remains patent for up to 14 days in nearly 70% of male infants, but by 20 days after birth it is partially (or completely) obliterated in 80% of male infants, the left side before the right.

In a few cases the original cavity within the processus may persist, in whole or in part, in any location. These variations may form the walls of hernial sacs or encysted fluid sites. When a patent processus retains a connection with the general peritoneal cavity it provides a preformed sac for a potential oblique inguinal hernia. It may be occluded at its upper end and be shut off from the tunica vaginalis and yet remain patent in the intervening section. The patent portion may become distended with fluid, and present as an encysted hydrocoele of the spermatic cord. The spermatic cord is relatively large in the neonate, as are the seminal vesicles and adjacent ampullae of the vas deferens.

In aberrant testicular descent the testis may remain in the abdomen, or it may fail to reach the scrotum and may then lie in the perineum, at the root of the penis, at the superficial inguinal ring, or in the upper part of the thigh.

The testis must follow the processus vaginalis. Should the latter, for any reason, follow a structure other than the scrotal extension of the gubernaculum, malposition of the testis will result. Traditionally, these malpositions have been associated with certain additional extensions of gubernacular tissue. The largest extension normally passes to the scrotum. Lesser extensions have been described as gaining attachment to the perineum, the root of the penis, the pubis, the inguinal ligament, and the neighbourhood of the saphenous opening. However, there is considerable doubt about these lesser expansions (the so-called 'tails of Lockwood'). They may reflect premature and abnormal fibrous partitioning of the gubernacular mesenchyme.

Descent of the ovary

The relative movements of the ovary are less extensive than those of the testis. Like the testis, the ovary ultimately reaches a lower level than it occupies in the early months of fetal life, but it does not leave the pelvis to enter the inguinal canal, except in certain anomalies. The ovary is connected to the medial aspect of the mesonephric fold by the mesovarium (homologous with the mesorchium), and to the ventral abdominal wall by the inguinal fold (**Figs 109.13, 109.18**). A mesenchymatous gubernaculum develops in this fold but, as it traverses the mesonephric fold, it acquires an additional attachment to the lateral margin of the uterus near the entrance of the uterine tube. Its lower part, caudal to this uterine attachment, becomes the round ligament of

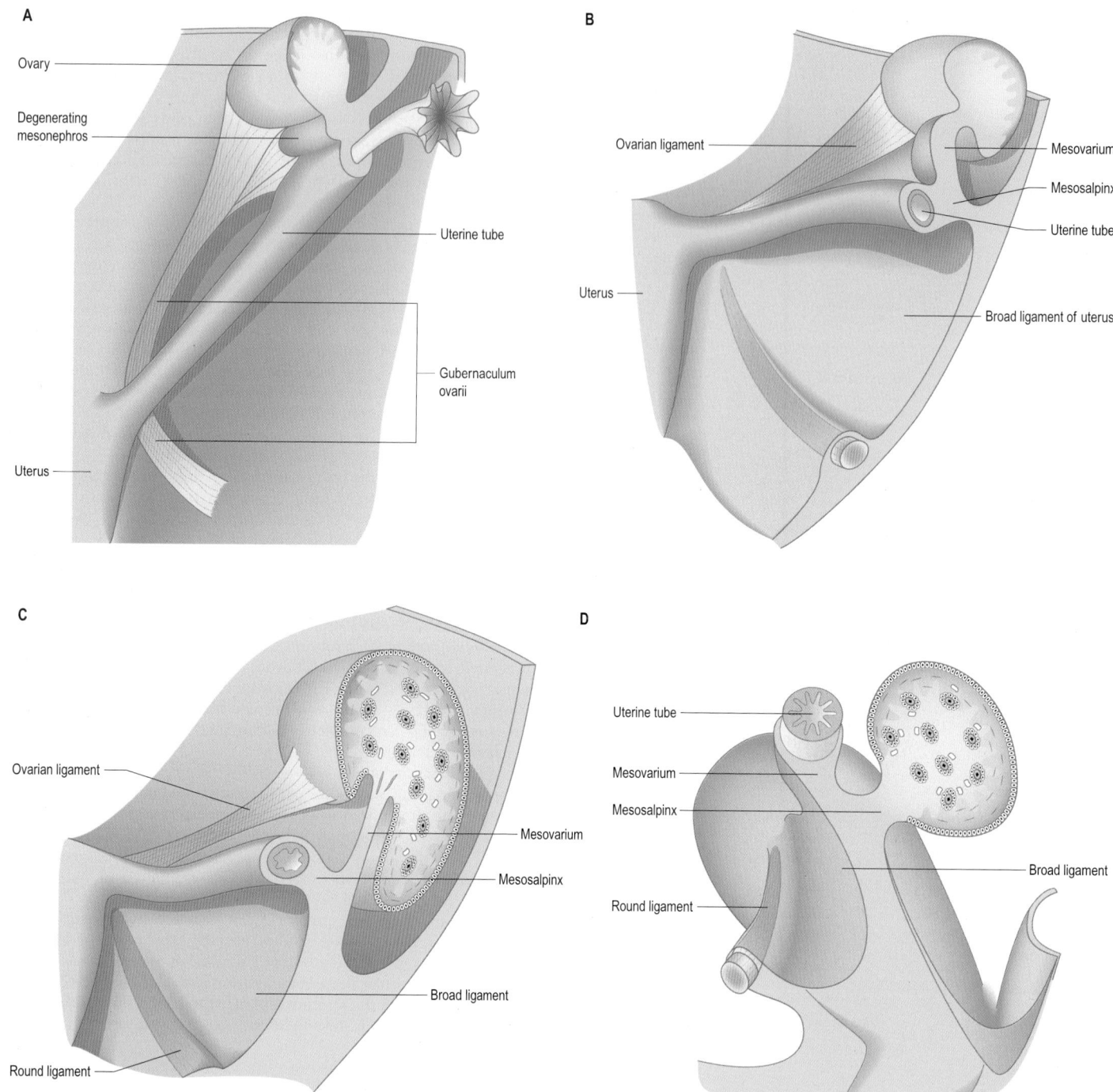

Fig. 109.18 Descent of the ovary. **A**, Early developing left ovary and uterine tube. **B**, Start of posterior movement of ovary. **C**, Left ovary in definitive posterior position. **D**, Parasagittal section of the ligaments associated with the ovary viewed from a left lateral position. (Redrawn from Tuchmann-Duplessis H, Haegel P 1972 Illustrated Human Embryology, Vol 2 Organogenesis. London: Chapman and Hall.)

the uterus and the part cranial to this becomes the ovarian ligament. Collectively these structures are homologous with the gubernaculum testis in the male (**Figs 109.18, 109.19**). This new uterine attachment may be correlated with the restricted ovarian descent. At first the ovary is attached to the medial side of the mesonephric fold but, in accordance with the manner in which the two mesonephric folds form the genital cord (**Figs 109.3, 109.13**), it is finally connected to the posterior layer of the broad ligament of the uterus. The gubernacula thus persist in the female, unlike the male, as bilateral fibrous bands or ligaments. Experimentally, they do not contract in response to application of CGRP (*see* above). They do not extend into the labia majora, as frequently described, but to the connective tissue just external to the external ring of the inguinal canal. The saccus vaginalis is present in the female. Its prolongation into the inguinal canal (sometimes termed the canal of

Nuck) is normally completely obliterated, but may remain patent and form the sac of a potential indirect inguinal hernia.

In the neonate the ovaries lie in the lower part of the iliac fossae. The long axis of the ovary is almost vertical. It becomes temporarily horizontal during descent, but regains the vertical when it reaches the ovarian fossa. The ovaries complete their descent into the ovarian fossae in early childhood. Thus, at birth the ovary and the lateral end of the corresponding uterine tube lie above the pelvic brim. They do not sink into the lesser pelvis until the latter enlarges sufficiently to contain both of them and the other pelvic viscera, including the bladder. The combined weight of the ovaries at birth is c.0.3 g, which is relatively large, and much larger than the combined weight of the testes (**Figs 11.4, 109.9**). The ovaries double in weight during the first 6 postnatal weeks. They bear surface furrows, which disappear during the second and third

INDIFFERENT STAGE

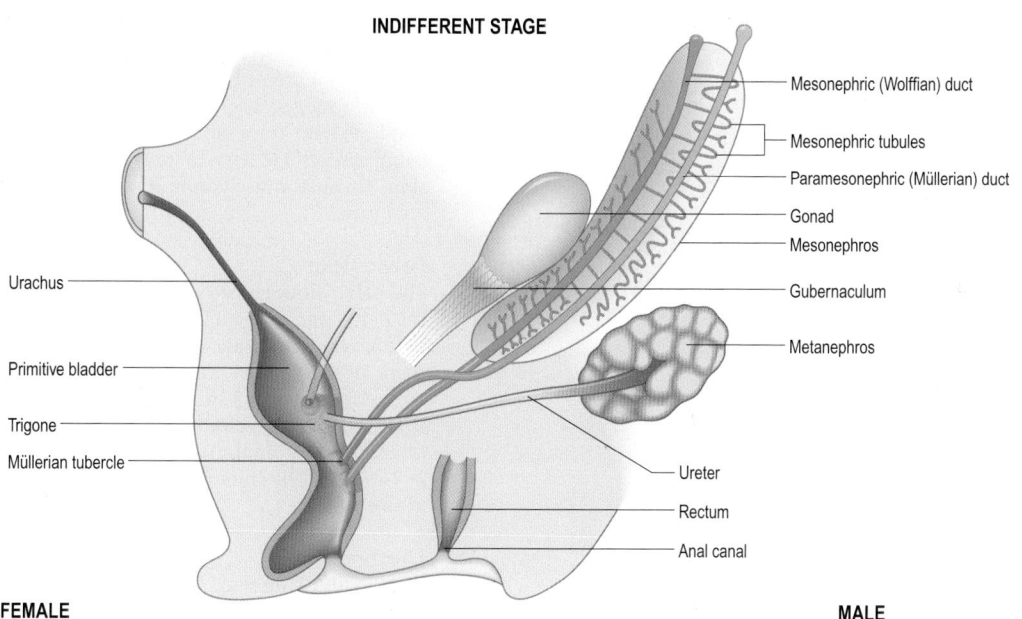

Mesonephric (Wolffian) duct
Mesonephric tubules
Paramesonephric (Müllerian) duct
Gonad
Mesonephros
Gubernaculum
Metanephros
Ureter
Rectum
Anal canal

Urachus
Primitive bladder
Trigone
Müllerian tubercle

FEMALE / MALE

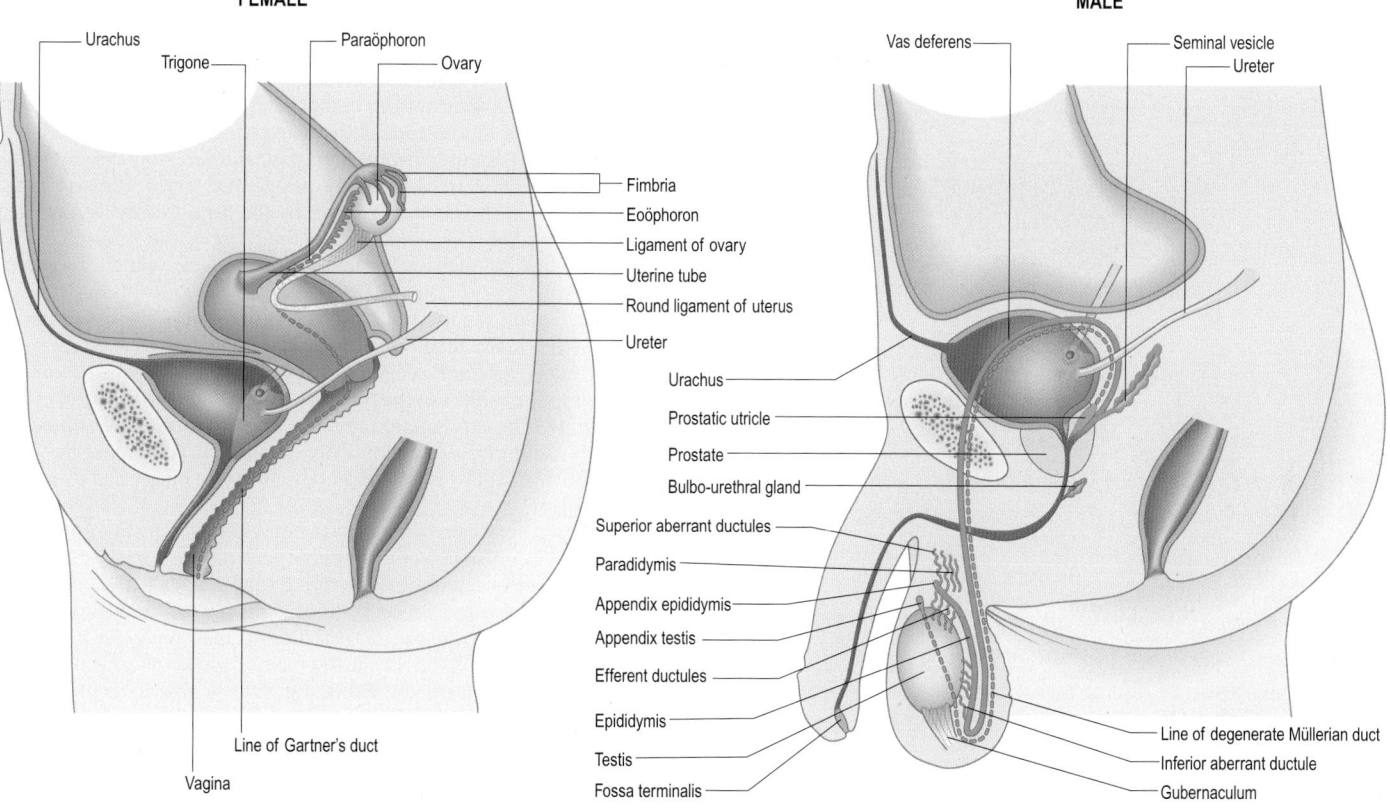

FEMALE

Urachus
Trigone
Paraöphoron
Ovary
Fimbria
Eoöphoron
Ligament of ovary
Uterine tube
Round ligament of uterus
Ureter
Line of Gartner's duct
Vagina

MALE

Vas deferens
Seminal vesicle
Ureter
Urachus
Prostatic utricle
Prostate
Bulbo-urethral gland
Superior aberrant ductules
Paradidymis
Appendix epididymis
Appendix testis
Efferent ductules
Epididymis
Testis
Fossa terminalis
Line of degenerate Müllerian duct
Inferior aberrant ductule
Gubernaculum

Fig. 109.19 The development of the urogenital system from the indifferent stage to the definitive male and female conditions. (Modified from Williams PL, Wendell-Smith CP, Treadgold S 1969 Basic Human Embryology, 2nd edn. Philadelphia: Lippincott.)

postnatal months. All of the primary oocytes for the reproductive life of a female are present in her ovaries by the end of the first trimester of pregnancy. Of the 7,000,000 primary oocytes estimated to be present at the fifth month of gestation, 1,000,000 remain at birth, 40,000 by puberty, and only 400 are ovulated during reproductive life.

CLOACA AND EXTERNAL GENITALIA

The cloaca is that region at the end of the primitive hindgut, which is continuous with the allantois, a ventral diverticulum (**Fig. 109.7**). The allantois passes into the connecting stalk of the early embryo prior to tail folding and is then drawn into the body cavity after stage 10. It retains an extension into the connecting stalk, and later into the umbilicus, throughout embryonic life. The cloaca is a slightly dilated cavity lined with endoderm. It is initially connected cranially to the enteric hindgut, and ventrocaudally is in contact with overlying ectoderm at the cloacal

membrane. Proliferation of mesenchyme at the angle of the junction of the hindgut and allantois produces a urorectal septum, which grows caudally and eventually produces fusion of the endodermal epithelium with the cloacal membrane (**Figs 109.4, 109.7, 109.20**). The cloaca is thus divided into a presumptive rectum and anal canal dorsally, and a presumptive urinary bladder and urogenital sinus ventrally, and the cloacal membrane is divided into anal and urogenital membranes respectively. The nodal centre of division is the site of the future perineal body. The urogenital sinus receives the mesonephric and paramesonephric ducts.

Anomalies of cloacal subdivision may result in a range of defects. In extroversion of the cloaca (ectopia cloacae), the urorectal septum does not develop. The defect is complicated by a failure of mesenchymal migration around the ventral body wall to support the umbilical cord and this results in a large abdominal defect with a central colonic

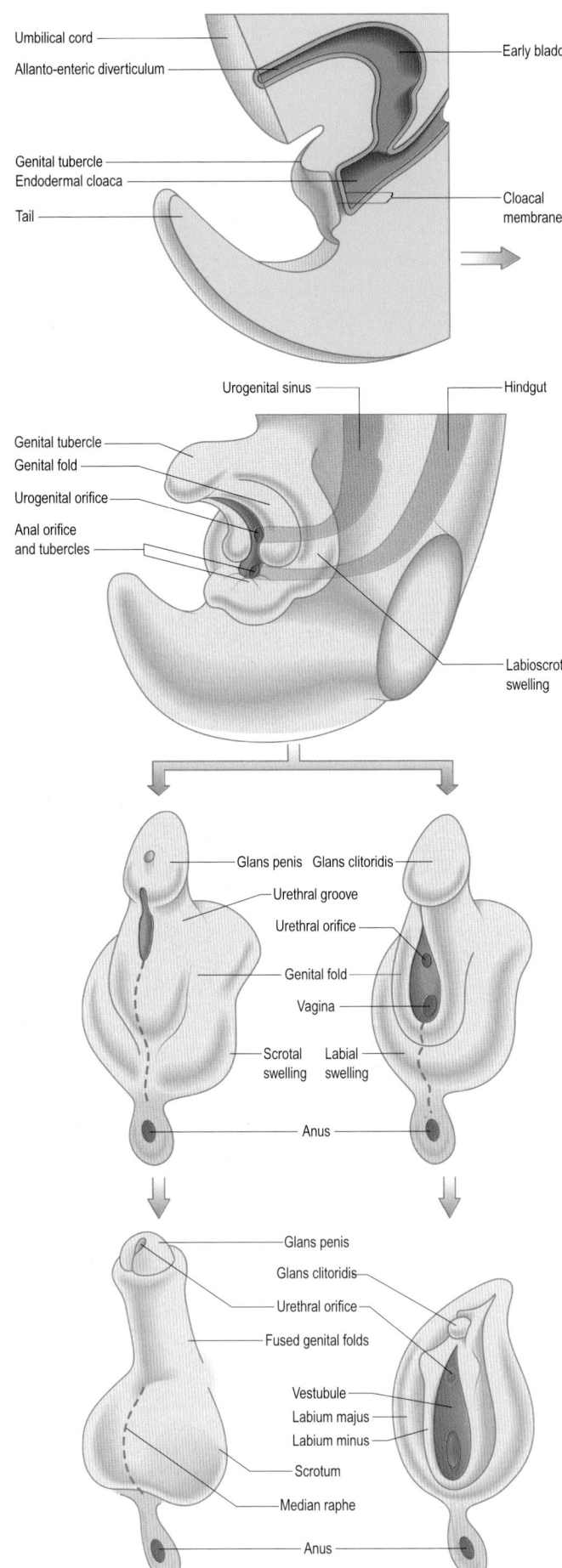

Umbilical cord
Allanto-enteric diverticulum
Genital tubercle
Endodermal cloaca
Tail
Early bladder
Cloacal membrane

Urogenital sinus
Hindgut
Genital tubercle
Genital fold
Urogenital orifice
Anal orifice and tubercles
Labioscrotal swelling

Glans penis Glans clitoridis
Urethral groove
Urethral orifice
Genital fold
Vagina
Scrotal swelling Labial swelling
Anus

Glans penis
Glans clitoridis
Urethral orifice
Fused genital folds
Vestubule
Labium majus
Labium minus
Scrotum
Median raphe
Anus

Fig. 109.20 The development of the external genitalia from the indifferent stage to the definitive male (left) and female (right) conditions.

portion and bilateral bladder components. With only partial development of the urorectal septum, the urogenital sinus may remain with a high confluence of bladder, vagina and rectum. The cloacal membrane may be abnormally elongated and prematurely ruptured throughout its whole extent, prior to the formation of the urorectal septum, or, in some cases, there may be only a small sinus opening externally at the skin. The anal musculature is often present but not associated with the anal canal.

Pelvic floor

The pelvic floor consists of the ligamentous supports of the cervix, and the pelvic and urogenital diaphragms, and constitutes another partition that traverses the body cavity. Little is known about pelvic floor development in the human. The striated muscle is derived from the somatic epithelial plates in a similar manner to the muscles of the ventrolateral body wall. Puborectalis appears in 20–30 mm embryos, following opening of the anal membrane, and striated muscle fibres can be seen at 15 weeks. The smooth muscle of the urethral sphincter is also present at this time.

Urethra

The urethra is derived from endoderm, as are the prostate gland and vagina (both outgrowths of the lower urogenital sinus or urethra), and the other small glandular structures that develop around the caudal body orifices.

In the male, the prostatic urethra proximal to the orifice of the prostatic utricle is derived from the vesicourethral part of the cloaca and the incorporated caudal ends of the mesonephric ducts. The remainder of the prostatic part, the membranous part, and probably the part within the bulb, are all derived from the urogenital sinus. The succeeding section, as far as the glans, is formed by the fusion of the genital folds (**Fig. 109.20**) and so is contained in the shaft of the penis. The short section within the glans is formed from ectoderm, which invaginates into the glans.

In the female, the urethra is derived entirely from the vesicourethral region of the cloaca, including the dorsal region derived from the mesonephric ducts. It is homologous with the part of the prostatic urethra proximal to the orifices of the prostatic utricle and the ejaculatory ducts. The region of the early urethra remains open to form the vestibule into which the definitive urethra and vagina open. It is believed that these regions are invaded by ectoderm because they are innervated by somatic nerves.

Urethral defects caused by arrests of development are not uncommon in the male. In epispadias the urethra opens on the dorsal aspect of the penis at its junction with the anterior abdominal wall. This anomaly is considered to be a less severe form of exstrophy of the bladder. In the simplest form of hypospadias, the urethra may open on the ventral (perineal) aspect of the penis at the base of the glans, and the part of the urethra that is normally within the glans is absent. In more severe cases the genital folds fail to fuse, and the urethra opens on the ventral aspect of a malformed penis just in front of the scrotum. A still greater degree of this malformation is accompanied by failure of the genital swellings to unite with each other. In these cases the scrotum is divided and, since the testes are also frequently undescended, the resemblance to the labia majora is very striking. Male children suffering from this deformity are often mistaken for girls. In such cases it is important to determine at the earliest stage not only the chromosomal sex of the infant but also the internal anatomy and stage of development of the internal genital tract. Sex assignment and rearing will depend on these factors.

The urethral sphincter first forms as a mesenchymal condensation around the urethra in 12–15 mm (stage 18) embryos, after division of the cloaca. The mesenchyme proliferates and becomes defined at the bladder neck in 31 mm embryos, and along the anterior part of the urethra by 69 mm. The muscle fibres differentiate after 15 weeks' gestation, at which time both smooth and striated fibres are present. In females there is continuity between the smooth muscle of the urethral wall and of the bladder. In males the muscle fibres are less abundant because of the local development of the prostate. Striated muscle fibres form around the smooth muscle initially in the anterior wall of the urethra and later encircle the smooth muscle layer. The origin of the striated muscle is not known – it could be derived from the myogenic cells from which puborectalis develops. The smooth and striated components of the urethral sphincter are closely related, but there is no mixing of fibres as occurs in the anorectal sphincter.

Prostate gland

The prostate gland arises during the third month from interactions between the urogenital sinus mesenchyme and the endoderm of the proximal part of the urethra. Early outgrowths, some 14 to 20 in number, arise from the endoderm around the whole circumference of the tube, but mainly on its lateral aspects and excluding the dorsal wall above the utricular plate. They give rise to the outer glandular zone of the prostate (p. 1301). Later outgrowths from the dorsal wall above the mesonephric ducts arise from the epithelium of mixed urogenital, mesonephric and possibly paramesonephric, origin covering the cranial end of the sinus tubercle. They produce the internal zone of glandular tissue. The outgrowths, which are at first solid, branch, become tubular and invade the surrounding mesenchyme. The latter is differentiating into smooth muscle, associated blood and lymphatic vessels and connective tissue and is invaded by autonomic nerves.

Similar outgrowths occur in the female but remain rudimentary. The urethral glands correspond to the mucosal glands around the upper part of the prostatic urethra, and the para-urethral glands correspond to the true prostatic glands of the external zone.

The bulbourethral glands in the male, and the greater vestibular glands in the female, arise as diverticula from the epithelial lining of the urogenital sinus.

External genitalia

Patterning of the external genitalia may be achieved by mechanisms similar to those that pattern the face and limb. In the cranial region neural crest mesenchyme makes an important contribution to the organization of the pharyngeal arches and the regions around the upper sphincters. Neural crest also arises from the tail-bud region, specifically from a population of cells termed the caudoneural hinge, which share the same molecular markers as the primitive node (p. 241). The neural tube at this level is derived from a mesenchymal/epithelial transformation of caudoneural-hinge cells, which form a cylinder. Neural crest cells delaminate from the dorsal surface of the cylinder in a rostrocaudal direction. It is not known whether neuronal neural crest arising from secondary neurulation processes contributes to the caudal interface between endoderm and ectoderm.

The external genitalia, like the gonads, pass through an indifferent state before distinguishing sexual characters appear (**Fig. 109.20**). From stage 13, primordia of the external genitalia, composed of underlying proliferating mesenchyme covered with ectoderm, arise around the cloacal membrane, between the primitive umbilical cord and the tail. During stage 15 the cloacal membrane is divided by the urorectal septum into a cranial urogenital membrane and a caudal anal membrane (**Figs 109.4, 109.14**). Local ectodermal/mesenchymal interactions give rise to the anal sphincter, which will develop without the presence of the urorectal septum or the anal canal. A surface elevation, the genital tubercle, appears at the cranial end of the urogenital membrane and two lateral ridges, the genital or urethral folds, form each side of the membrane (**Fig. 109.20**). The genital tubercle forms a distinct primordium, which will become the glans of either the penis or the clitoris. Elongation of the genital folds and urogenital membrane produces a primitive phallus. As this structure grows it is described as having a cranial surface analogous to the dorsum of the penis, and a caudal surface analogous to the perineal surface of both sexes. The urogenital sinus, contiguous with the internal aspect of the urogenital membrane, becomes attenuated within the elongating phallus forming the primitive urethra. The urogenital membrane breaks down at about stage 19 (20 mm, 6.5 weeks) allowing communication of ectoderm and endoderm at the edges of the disrupted membrane and continuity of the urogenital sinus with the amniotic cavity. Urine can escape from the urinary tract from this time. The endodermal layer of the attenuated distal portion of the urogenital sinus, which is now displayed on the caudal aspect of the phallus, is termed the urethral plate. As mesenchyme proliferates within the genital folds, the urethral plate sinks into the body of the phallus forming a primary urethral groove. The genital folds meet proximally in a transverse ridge immediately ventral to the anal membrane.

While these changes are in progress two labioscrotal (genital) swellings appear, one on each side of the base of the phallus, and extend caudally, separated from the genital folds by distinct grooves (**Figs 109.20, 109.21**).

As a general rule, epithelium, which can be touched easily and has a somatic innervation, is derived from ectoderm. In the buccal cavity and pharynx the ectoderm/endoderm zone is towards the posterior third of the tongue – touch here usually elicits the gag reflex. In the anal canal the outer portion, distal to the anal valves, is derived from ectoderm and has a somatic innervation, whereas the epithelium proximal to the valves is derived from endoderm and has an autonomic innervation.

Homologies of the parts of the urogenital system are shown in Table 109.1.

Male genitalia

The growth of male external characteristics is stimulated by androgens regardless of the genetic sex. The male phallus enlarges to form the penis. The genital swellings meet each other ventral to the anus and unite to form the scrotum (**Fig. 109.20**). The genital folds fuse with each other from behind forwards, enclosing the phallic part of the urogenital sinus behind to form the bulb of the urethra and closing the definitive urethral groove in front to form the greater part of the spongiose urethra. Fusion of the folds results in the formation of a median raphe and occurs in such a way that the lining of the postglandular urethra is mainly, perhaps wholly, endodermal in origin. Thus, as the phallus lengthens, the urogenital orifice is carried onwards until it reaches the base of the glans at the apex of the penis. From the tip of the phallus an ingrowth of surface ectoderm occurs within the glans to meet and fuse with the penile urethra. Subsequent canalization of the ectoderm permits a continuation of the urethra within the glans.

The glans and shaft of the penis are recognizable by the third month. The prepuce also begins to develop in the third month, when the primary external orifice of the urethra is still at the base of the glans. A ridge consisting of a mesenchymal core covered by epithelium appears proximal to the neck of the penis and extends forwards over the glans. A solid lamella of epithelium deep to this ridge extends backwards to the base of the glans. The ventral extremities of the ridge curve backwards to become continuous with the genital folds at the margins of the urethral orifice. As the urethral folds meet to form the terminal part of

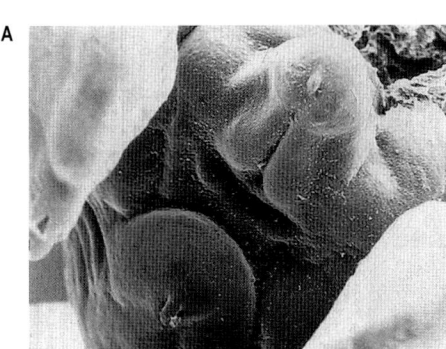 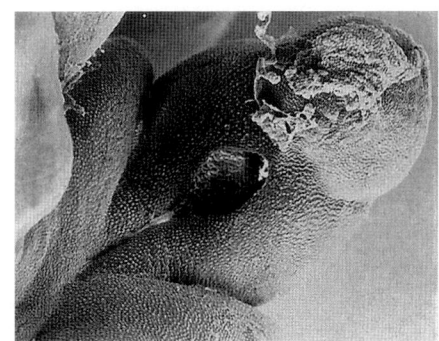 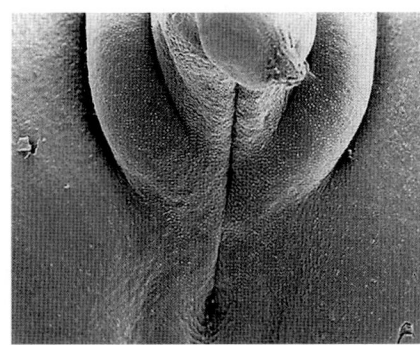

Fig. 109.21 Scanning electron micrographs of early human external genitalia. **A**, Indifferent stage in a human embryo estimated as 42 postovulatory days. **B**, A human female embryo at 12 weeks' development. The genital folds are not fused. **C**, A human male embryo at 12 weeks. Fusion of the genital folds has occurred. (Photographs by P Collins.)

Table 109.1 Homologies of the parts of the urogenital system in male and female

Gonad	Testis	Ovary
Gubernacular cord	Gubernaculum testis	Ovarian and round ligaments
Mesonephros (Wolffian body)	Appendix of epididymis (?) Efferent ductules Lobules of epididymis Paradidymis Aberrant ductules	Appendices vesiculosae (?) Epoöphoron Paroöphoron
Mesonephric duct (Wolffian duct)	Duct of epididymis Vas deferens Ejaculatory duct Part of bladder and prostatic urethra	Duct of epoöphoron (Gartner's duct) Part of bladder and urethra
Paramesonephric (or Müllerian) duct	Appendix of testis Prostatic utricle	Uterine tube Uterus Vagina (?)
Allantoic duct	Urachus	Urachus

Cloaca:
  dorsal part
 	
  ventral part
 	
  urogenital sinus
	
	Rectum and upper part of anal canal
	Most of bladder
	Part of prostatic urethra
	Prostatic urethra distal to utricle
	Bulbo-urethral glands
	Rest of urethra to glans
		
		Rectum and upper part of anal canal
		Most of bladder and the urethra
		
		Greater vestibular glands
		Vestibule

Genital folds	Ventral penis	Labia minora
Genital tubercle	Glans penis Urethra in glans	Clitoris

the urethra, the ventral horns of the ridge fuse to form the frenulum. The epithelial lamella breaks down over the dorsum and sides of the glans to form the preputial sac, and thus free the prepuce from the surface of the glans. Thereafter the prepuce grows as a free fold of skin, which covers the terminal part of the glans. Although the prepuce and glans begin to separate from the fifth month in utero, they may still be joined at birth. The preputial sac may not be complete until 6–12 months or more after birth and, even then, the presence of some connecting strands may still interfere with the retractability of the prepuce.

The mesenchymal core of the phallus is comparatively undifferentiated in the first two months, but the blastemata of the corpora cavernosa become defined during the third month. Nerves are present in the differentiating mesenchyme from the seventh week. Despite containing less smooth muscle and elastic tissue than the adult, the neonatal penis is capable of erection.

The scrotum is formed by proliferation of the genital swellings, which are the anchoring points for the gubernaculum testis. The genital swellings fuse across the midline covering the base of the penis. The testes descend into the scrotum prior to birth. In the neonate the penis and scrotum are relatively large. The scrotum has a broad base which does not narrow until after the first year. Both the septum and the walls of the scrotum are relatively thicker than in adults.

Female genitalia

The female phallus, which exceeds the male in length in the early stages, becomes the clitoris. The genital swellings remain separate as the labia majora and the genital folds also remain separate, forming the labia minora (**Fig. 109.20**). The perineal orifice of the urogenital sinus is retained as the cleft between the labia minora, above which the urethra and vagina open. The prepuce of the clitoris develops in the same way as its male homologue. By the fourth month the female external genitalia can no longer be masculinized by androgens.

At birth neonatal females have relatively enlarged labia minora, clitoris and labia majora. The labia majora are united by a posterior

labial commissure and each contains the distal end of the round ligament of the uterus, the gubernaculum ovarii (**Fig. 109.18**).

There is evidence that in certain tissues, e.g. urogenital sinus and genital swellings, testosterone is converted into 5α-dihydrotestosterone. In XY individuals with a genetic deficiency of the enzyme responsible for this conversion, not only functioning testes but also female external genitalia with an enlarged clitoris and a small vaginal pouch, are present, suggesting that external genital development is under the control of 5α-dihydrotestosterone. Such individuals are usually raised as girls. However, at puberty the external genitalia become responsive to testosterone, which causes masculinization at this stage.

MATURATION OF THE REPRODUCTIVE ORGANS AT PUBERTY

Until the adolescent growth spurt the reproductive organs grow very slowly. Generally the changes occur over a time period termed puberty. The sequence of these events is much less variable than the age at which they take place. The sequence of puberty in girls and boys is shown in **Fig. 109.22**.

In girls the appearance of the breast bud is usually the first sign of puberty. The uterus and vagina develop simultaneously with the breast. Menarche occurs after the peak of the height spurt – onset is more closely related to radiological than to chronological age. It has been suggested that the menarche occurs as a critical weight of c.50 kg is attained, and certainly sports and excessive restriction of diet, which may reduce weight below this level, can cause amenorrhoea in women who were previously menstruating normally. Tall girls reach sexual maturity earlier than short ones, but girls with a late adolescent growth spurt and later puberty are ultimately taller on the average than those who pass through the menarche early, for they have longer to grow. A girl who has begun to menstruate can be predicted to grow a further 7.5 cm at most. Menarche marks a definitive stage of uterine development but does not mean attainment of full reproductive function. Many of the early menstrual cycles may not involve ovulation.

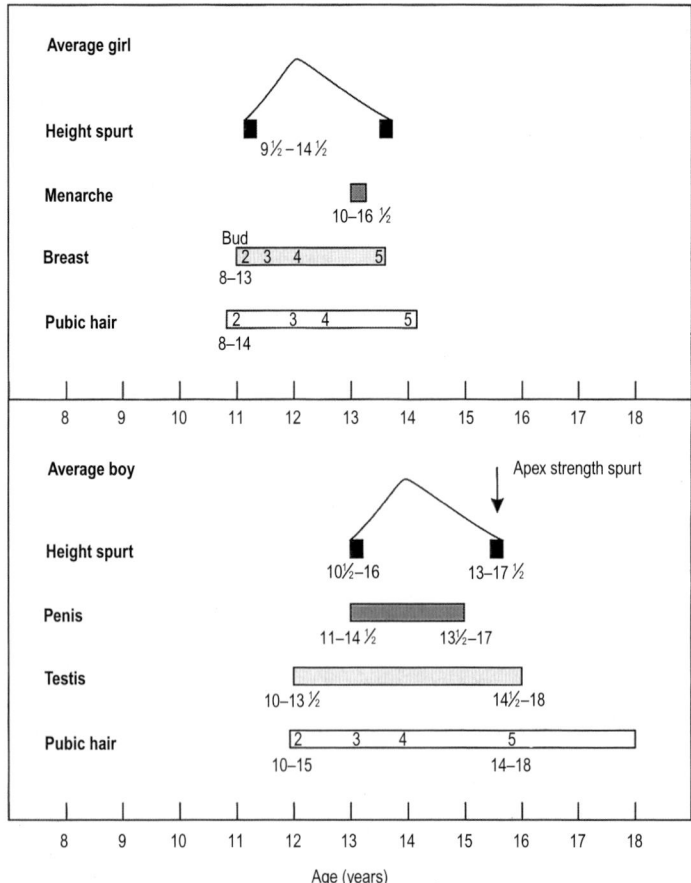

Fig. 109.22 Events which occur at adolescence in average girls and boys. The figures beneath the bars indicate the range of ages within which each event may begin and end. Figures within the bars indicate the developmental stage. (Adapted with permission from Tanner JM 1962 Growth at Adolescence, 2nd edn. Oxford: Blackwell Publishing.)

The earliest sign of puberty in boys is the growth of the testes and scrotum. The volume of the testes may be estimated – the average adult volume is 20 ml – and a volume of 6 ml indicates that puberty has started. Later the penis, prostate and seminal vesicles begin to enlarge. Increased testosterone levels produced by the Leydig cells of the testes promote changes in the larynx, skin and distribution of bodily hair.

REFERENCES

Albrecht KH, Eicher EM 2001 Evidence that SRY is expressed in pre-Sertoli cells and Sertoli and granulosa cells have a common precursor. Dev Biol 240(1): 92–107.

Barteczko KJ, Jacob MI 2000 The testicular descent in human. Origin, development and fate of the gubernaculum Hunteri, processus vaginalis peritonei and gonadal ligaments. Adv Anat Embryol Cell Biol 156: III–X, 1–98. Springer.
Includes scanning electron microscopy images and three-dimensional reconstructions of the human testis from stage 14. The caudal ligaments of the ovary and uterus are also considered.

Chauvet V, Qian F, Boute N et al 2002 Expression of PKD1 and PKD2 transcripts and proteins in human embryo and during normal kidney development. Am J Pathol 160: 973–83.

Sharpe RM, McKinnell C, Kivlin C, Fisher JS 2003 Proliferation and functional maturation of Sertoli cells, and the relevance to disorders of testis function in adulthood. Reproduction 125: 769–84.

PELVIC GIRDLE AND LOWER LIMB

Editors:

Andrew Williams *(Lead Editor)*

Richard LM Newell *(Editor)*

Mark S Davies *(Editor, chapter 115)*

Patricia Collins *(Embryology, Growth and Development)*

Critical reviewers:

Paul Cartwright *(chapter 110)*, **Thomas Ind** *(111)*

General organization and surface anatomy of the lower limb

This chapter is divided into two sections. The first is an overview of the general organization of the lower limb, with particular emphasis on the fascial skeleton, distribution of the major blood vessels and lymphatic channels, and of the branches of the lumbar and sacral plexuses: it is intended to complement the detailed regional anatomy described in Chapters 111 to 115. The second section describes the surface anatomy of the lower limb.

The structure of the lower limb is determined by its adaptations for weightbearing, locomotion and the maintenance of equilibrium (stability). Indeed, the adaptations for weightbearing and for stability, and the differing developmental histories of the limbs account for the major structural and functional differences between the lower limb and the upper limb. There are two important anatomical junctional or transitional zones between the trunk and the lower limb through which longitudinally running nerves and vessels pass in both directions. These zones are the inguinal (pelvicrural) and the gluteal (buttock) regions. The latter includes the junctional zones between the limb and the abdominopelvic cavity (via the greater sciatic foramen) and between the limb and the perineum (via the lesser sciatic foramen).

SKIN, FASCIA AND SOFT TISSUES

In the young adult the skin of the lower limb is generally stronger and thicker than that of the upper limb: weightbearing skin, e.g. of the sole of the foot, is particularly thickened. The skin of the buttocks and posterior thigh bears weight in the sitting position. The skin over the anterior aspect of the lower leg is particularly fragile and vulnerable in the elderly. Body hair is usually well developed in all areas except the sole and posterior ankle.

FASCIAL SKELETON
The well-defined 'fascial skeleton' of the lower limb forms a tough circumferential 'stocking-like' structure that constrains the musculature. Septa pass from this outer fascial sheath to the bones within, confining the functional muscle groups within osteofascial compartments. The tough fascia gives additional areas of attachment to the muscles and ensures that they work to maximal effect. Thickenings in the ensheathing layer may act as additional tendons and form fibrous retinacula where tendons cross joints.

Although these fascial layers and planes are particularly prominent in the embalmed cadaver, they are also very real and significant structures in the living. The pattern of soft-tissue organization directs the physiological action of the muscles and is crucial for efficient venous return from the limb. The fascial planes also control and direct the spread of pathological fluids (blood, pus) within the limb and play an important part in determining the degree and direction of displacement seen in long bone fractures.

Fasciocutaneous system
The fascial septa dictate the pathways of cutaneous arteries, which subsequently perforate and ramify on the fascial 'stocking' before supplying the skin.

OSTEOFASCIAL COMPARTMENTS IN THE LOWER LIMB
There are three functional compartments in the thigh: anterior (extensor), posterior (flexor) and medial (adductor) (p. 1461). Only the anterior and posterior compartments are separated by distinct fascial septa. A very definite fascial separation into anterior (extensor), posterior (flexor) and lateral (evertor) compartments exists in the leg: compartment syndrome is most common in this region (p. 1489). Osteofascial compartments in the foot are described on page 1509.

All osteofascial compartments are traversed by vessels and nerves that also supply the muscles within the compartments (pp. 1461, 1489).

Compartment syndrome – The limiting walls of osteofascial compartments are largely inelastic: any condition that leads to an increase in the volume of the compartmental contents is therefore likely to cause an increase in intracompartmental pressure. Such conditions include muscle swelling caused by trauma or overuse, haemorrhage and local infection. If untreated, this increased pressure will lead to damage to the nerves and vessels traversing the compartment – which will have severe consequences for those parts of the limb distal to the compartment – and produce necrosis of the intracompartmental muscles.

BONES AND JOINTS (Figs 110.1, 110.2)

The bones of the lower limb are: the three fused components of the pelvic girdle; the femur and its associated patella (thigh); the tibia and fibula (leg); the tarsus, metatarsus and phalanges (foot). The innominate bone (especially the ilium and ischium) and the femur, tibia and bones of the hindfoot are strong and their external (cortical) and internal (trabecular) structure are adapted for weightbearing.

The pelvic girdle connects the lower limb to the axial skeleton via the sacroiliac joint, an originally synovial joint in which mobility has been sacrificed for stability and strength for effective weight transmission from the trunk to the lower limb. The anterior joint of the pelvic girdle is the pubic symphysis, a secondary cartilaginous joint that may move slightly during hip and sacroiliac movement and during childbirth. The hip joint, a synovial ball-and-socket joint, exhibits a very effective compromise between mobility and stability, allowing movement in all three orthogonal planes. The more distal joints have gained mobility at the expense of stability. The knee joint anatomically includes the patellofemoral joint, a synovial joint allowing the patella to move over the distal femur. The main component of the knee joint is a bicompartmental synovial joint between femur and tibia allowing flexion, extension and some medial and lateral rotation of the leg. It is not a true hinge joint as its axes of flexion and extension are variable and there is coupled rotation. The tibia and fibula articulate with each other at the superior and inferior tibiofibular joints. The superior joint, a plane synovial joint, allows slight gliding movement only. The inferior joint, a fibrous joint, lies just above the ankle and allows significant rotation of the fibula linked to ankle motion. The ankle (talocrural) joint is formed by the inferior tibia and fibula 'gripping' the talus. It allows dorsiflexion and plantarflexion. There are multiple joints in the foot: these can be simplified by considering the hindfoot, midfoot and forefoot. These joints allow the complex movements of which the foot is capable, making the foot well adapted to provide a platform for standing and for shock absorption and propulsion in gait.

Both knee and ankle are commonly subject to closed injuries: the virtually subcutaneous position of the knee makes it liable to open injury and infection. Although the ankle is a frequently injured weightbearing joint, the prevalence of degenerative arthritis as a clinical presentation is surprisingly low when compared with that found in the hip and knee.

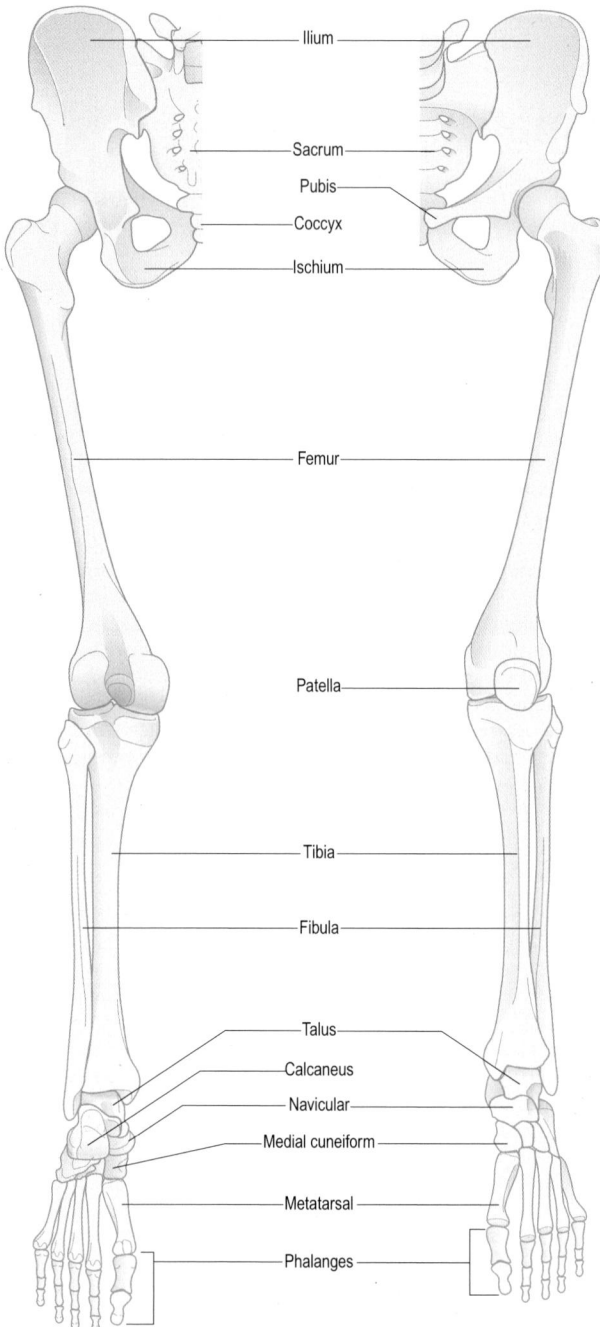

Fig. 110.1 Overview of bones of the lower limb: posterior aspect. (From Aids to the Examination of the Peripheral Nervous System. 2000. 4th edn. London: Saunders. With permission of Guarantors of Brain.)

Fig. 110.2 Overview of bones of the lower limb: anterior aspect. (From Aids to the Examination of the Peripheral Nervous System. 2000. 4th edn. London: Saunders. With permission of Guarantors of Brain.)

MUSCLES

The effects of developmental extension and medial rotation of the limb are most evident in the relative positions of the muscle groups in the thigh and the leg, and in the adult pattern of segmental innervation (dermatomes) (pp. 175). In general terms, the anterior aspect of the adult limb is the extensor aspect, while the flexors lie posteriorly; the reverse is true at the hip. As a result of this rotation, the dermatomes tend to spiral around the limb rather than lie parallel to its long axis.

The role of the muscles of the lower limb in the maintenance of equilibrium during locomotion and while standing has often been overlooked. Many of the muscles act frequently or predominantly from their distal attachments. During both stance and locomotion, it is often

the distal attachment that is fixed and the proximal that is mobile, as in the predominant action of gluteus medius as a pelvic stabilizer rather than as a hip abductor. In contrast, in the upper limb for most of the time the proximal muscle attachments are fixed and the distal attachments are mobile as the hand moves in space. The lower limb contains many muscles that act upon more than one joint: indeed it is unusual for any joint of the lower limb to move in isolation.

Muscles of the lower limb may be subdivided into muscles of the iliac region, gluteal region, thigh, leg and foot. (Note that, according to anatomical convention, 'leg' refers to the part of the lower limb between the knee and ankle.) In both thigh and leg, the functional groups of muscles are contained in osteofascial compartments that are particularly well defined and of major clinical significance in the leg. The muscles acting within these closed osteofascial compartments also assist and maintain drainage of the venous system against gravity.

The main muscles of the iliac region are psoas major and iliacus, a functional unit comprising the major flexors of the hip and running from the lumbar spine and inner surface of the ilium respectively to the lesser trochanter of the femur. The much less important and inconstantly present psoas minor runs from the lumbar spine to the pubis.

The muscles of the gluteal region include the named gluteal muscles and the deeper-lying short lateral rotators of the hip joint. Gluteus maximus lies most superficially, running from the posterior pelvis to the proximal femur and fascia lata. It is a powerful extensor of the hip joint, acting more often to extend the trunk on the femur than to extend the limb on the trunk. Gluteus medius and minimus, attaching proximally to the outer iliac surface and distally to the greater trochanter of the femur, are abductors of the hip whose most important action is to stabilize the pelvis on the femur during locomotion. They are helped in this function by tensor fasciae latae, a more anteriorly placed muscle arising from the anterolateral ilium and inserting into the fascia lata. Two of the short lateral rotators of the hip, piriformis and obturator internus, attach proximally within the pelvis, while the others – obturator externus, the gemelli and quadratus femoris – attach externally. All attach distally to the proximal femur.

The muscles of the thigh lie in three functional compartments: anterior (extensor), medial (adductor) and posterior (flexor). The anterior or extensor compartment includes sartorius and the quadriceps group. Sartorius and rectus femoris attach proximally to the pelvis and can thus act on the hip joint as well as the knee. The remaining components of the quadriceps, the vastus muscles, attach proximally to the femur only, and, acting as a unit, are powerful knee extensors. The medial or adductor compartment contains the named adductor muscles and gracilis; pectineus may also be included. These muscles connect the anterior pelvis and the femur: adductor magnus also attaches proximally to the ischial tuberosity. The posterior ('hamstring') compartment includes semitendinosus, semimembranosus and biceps femoris. These muscles attach proximally to the pelvis (ischial tuberosity) and act both to extend the trunk on the femur and to flex and rotate the knee. Adductor magnus, as reflected by the extent of its proximal attachment and by its dual innervation, shares the first of these functions with the hamstrings. Biceps femoris is the only thigh muscle that attaches distally to the fibula: it has no tibial attachment.

The muscles of the leg also comprise three functional compartments. The anterior or extensor compartment includes the extensors (dorsiflexors) of the ankle and the long extensors of the toes. Tibialis anterior, the main ankle dorsiflexor, also inverts the foot at the subtalar joint, while the smallest muscle of the compartment, peroneus (fibularis) tertius, is a dorsiflexor that everts the foot. The posterior or flexor (plantarflexor) compartment has superficial and deep components. The superficial component contains the gastrocnemius and soleus, powerful plantar flexors of the ankle, and the small and inconsistent plantaris. All attach distally via the calcaneal (Achilles) tendon. Popliteus, a rotator of the knee, lies most proximally in the deep leg. Gastrocnemius, plantaris and popliteus are the only leg muscles attached proximally to the femur and can thus act on the knee as well as the ankle. The remaining leg muscles attach proximally to the tibia, fibula or both, and to the interosseous membrane. The deep flexor compartment proper contains the long flexors of the toes together with tibialis posterior, the main invertor of the foot. The lateral compartment contains the main evertors of the foot, peroneus (fibularis) longus and brevis: both are also plantar flexors at the ankle.

The muscles of the foot are arranged in layers. They facilitate action of the muscles originating from the leg acting via the long tendons passing through the foot and control foot posture during its various functions.

VASCULAR SUPPLY AND LYMPHATIC DRAINAGE

ARTERIAL SUPPLY (Figs 110.3, 110.4)

The main artery of the lower limb distal to the inguinal ligament and the gluteal fold is the continuation of the external iliac artery, which starts as the femoral artery in the anterior compartment of the thigh. It becomes the popliteal artery in the posterior compartment of the thigh and then divides into its terminal branches in the posterior compartment of the leg. The obturator and inferior gluteal vessels also contribute to the supply of the proximal part of the limb. In the embryo the inferior gluteal artery supplied the main axial artery of the limb, which is represented in the adult by the arteria comitans nervi ischiadici (artery to the sciatic nerve, p. 1470).

The bones of the lower limb receive their arterial supply from nutrient vessels, metaphyseal arterial branches of the peri-articular anastomoses, and the arteries supplying the muscles that attach to their periosteum. The pattern of arterial supply is particularly relevant to fracture healing, the spread of infection and malignancy, and the planning of reconstructive surgical procedures. For further details consult Cormack and Lamberty (1994), Taylor and Razaboni (1994) and Crock (1996).

VENOUS DRAINAGE (Figs 110.5, 110.6, 110.7, 110.8)

The veins of the lower limb can be subdivided, like those of the upper limb, into superficial and deep groups. The superficial veins are subcutaneous and lie in the superficial fascia; the deep veins (beneath the deep fascia) accompany the major arteries. Both groups have valves, which are more numerous in the deep veins and also more numerous than in the veins of the upper limb. Venous plexuses occur within and between some of the lower limb muscles.

The principal named superficial veins are the long and short saphenous veins. Their numerous tributaries are mainly unnamed. For details and variations consult Kosinski (1926).

Deep veins of the lower limbs accompany the arteries and their branches. Plantar digital veins arise from plexuses in the plantar regions of the toes, connect with dorsal digital veins and unite into four plantar metatarsal veins. These run in the intermetatarsal spaces and connect by perforating veins with dorsal veins, then continue to form a deep plantar venous arch accompanying the plantar arterial arch. From this arch, medial and lateral plantar veins run near the corresponding arteries: they communicate with the long and short saphenous veins before forming the posterior tibial veins behind the medial malleolus. The posterior tibial veins accompany the posterior tibial artery. They receive veins from the calf muscles, especially the venous plexus in soleus, and connect with superficial veins and with the peroneal veins. The latter, running with their artery, receive branches from soleus and superficial veins.

The anterior tibial veins are continuations of the venae comitantes of the dorsalis pedis artery. They leave the extensor region between the tibia and fibula, pass through the proximal end of the interosseous membrane, and unite with the posterior tibial veins to form the popliteal vein at the distal border of popliteus.

Venous (muscle) pumps

In a standing position, venous return from the lower limb depends largely on muscular activity, especially contraction of the calf and foot muscles, known as the 'muscle pump', whose efficiency is aided by the tight sleeve of deep fascia. 'Perforating' veins connect the long saphenous vein with the deep veins, particularly near the ankle, distal calf and knee. Their valves are arranged so as to prevent flow of blood from the deep to the superficial veins. At rest, pressure in a superficial vein is equal to the height of the column of blood extending from that vein to the heart. When calf muscles contract, blood is pumped proximally in the deep veins and is normally prevented from flowing into the superficial veins by the valves in the perforating veins. During relaxation, blood may be aspirated from the superficial into the deep veins. If the valves in the perforating veins become incompetent, these veins become 'high pressure leaks' during muscular contraction, and the superficial veins become dilated and varicose. Similar perforating connections occur in the antero-lateral region, where varicosities may also occur. Veins connecting the long saphenous vein to the femoral vein in the adductor canal may become varicose (Dodd & Cockett 1976).

Venous plexuses

Venous plexuses may be intramuscular (soleus) or intermuscular (in the foot and gluteal region). The plexuses communicate with the axially running deep veins and are components of the 'muscle pump' mechanism.

LYMPHATIC DRAINAGE (Fig. 110.9)

Most lymph from the lower limb traverses a large intermediary inguinal group of nodes. Peripheral nodes are few and all are deeply sited. Except for an inconsistent node lying proximally on the interosseous membrane near the anterior tibial vessels, they occur only in the popliteal fossa. Enlarged popliteal nodes may be palpated along the line of the popliteal vessels while the passively supported knee is gradually moved from extension to semi-flexion. Inguinal nodes are found superficial and deep to the deep fascia. The deep nodes are few and lie alongside the medial aspect of the femoral vein. The superficial nodes may be divided into a lower vertical group that clothe the proximal part of the long saphenous vein, and an upper group that lie parallel to, but below, the inguinal ligament and which are related to the superficial circumflex iliac and superficial external pudendal vessels. Lymph from the lower limb passes from the inguinal nodes to the external and common iliac nodes, and ultimately drains to the lateral aortic group. Deep gluteal lymph reaches the same group through the internal and common iliac chains.

Lymphatic drainage of superficial tissues

The superficial lymph vessels begin in subcutaneous plexuses. Collecting vessels leave the foot medially, along the long saphenous vein, or laterally with the short saphenous vein. Medial vessels are larger and more numerous. They start on the tibial side of the dorsum of the foot, and ascend anterior or posterior to the medial malleolus. Thereafter both sets converge on the long saphenous vein and accompany it to the distal superficial inguinal nodes. Lateral vessels begin on the fibular side of the dorsum of the foot, and some cross anteriorly in the leg to join the medial vessels and so pass to the distal superficial inguinal lymph nodes. Others accompany the short saphenous vein to the

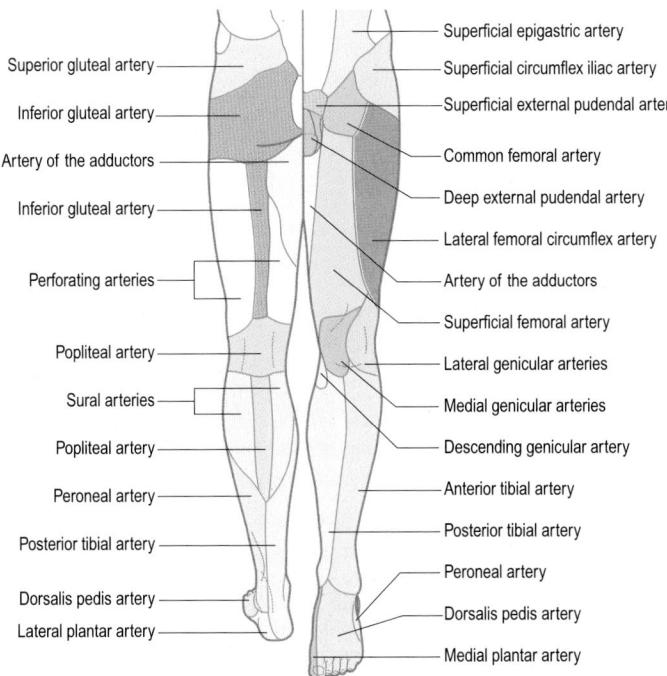

Fig. 110.3 The anatomical territories served by the cutaneous blood supply to the lower limb. (By permission from Cormack GC, Lamberty BGH 1994 The Arterial Anatomy of Skin Flaps, 2nd edn. Edinburgh: Churchill Livingstone.)

Superficial epigastric artery
Superior gluteal artery
Superficial circumflex iliac artery
Inferior gluteal artery
Superficial external pudendal artery
Artery of the adductors
Common femoral artery
Inferior gluteal artery
Deep external pudendal artery
Perforating arteries
Lateral femoral circumflex artery
Artery of the adductors
Superficial femoral artery
Popliteal artery
Lateral genicular arteries
Sural arteries
Medial genicular arteries
Popliteal artery
Descending genicular artery
Peroneal artery
Anterior tibial artery
Posterior tibial artery
Posterior tibial artery
Peroneal artery
Dorsalis pedis artery
Dorsalis pedis artery
Lateral plantar artery
Medial plantar artery

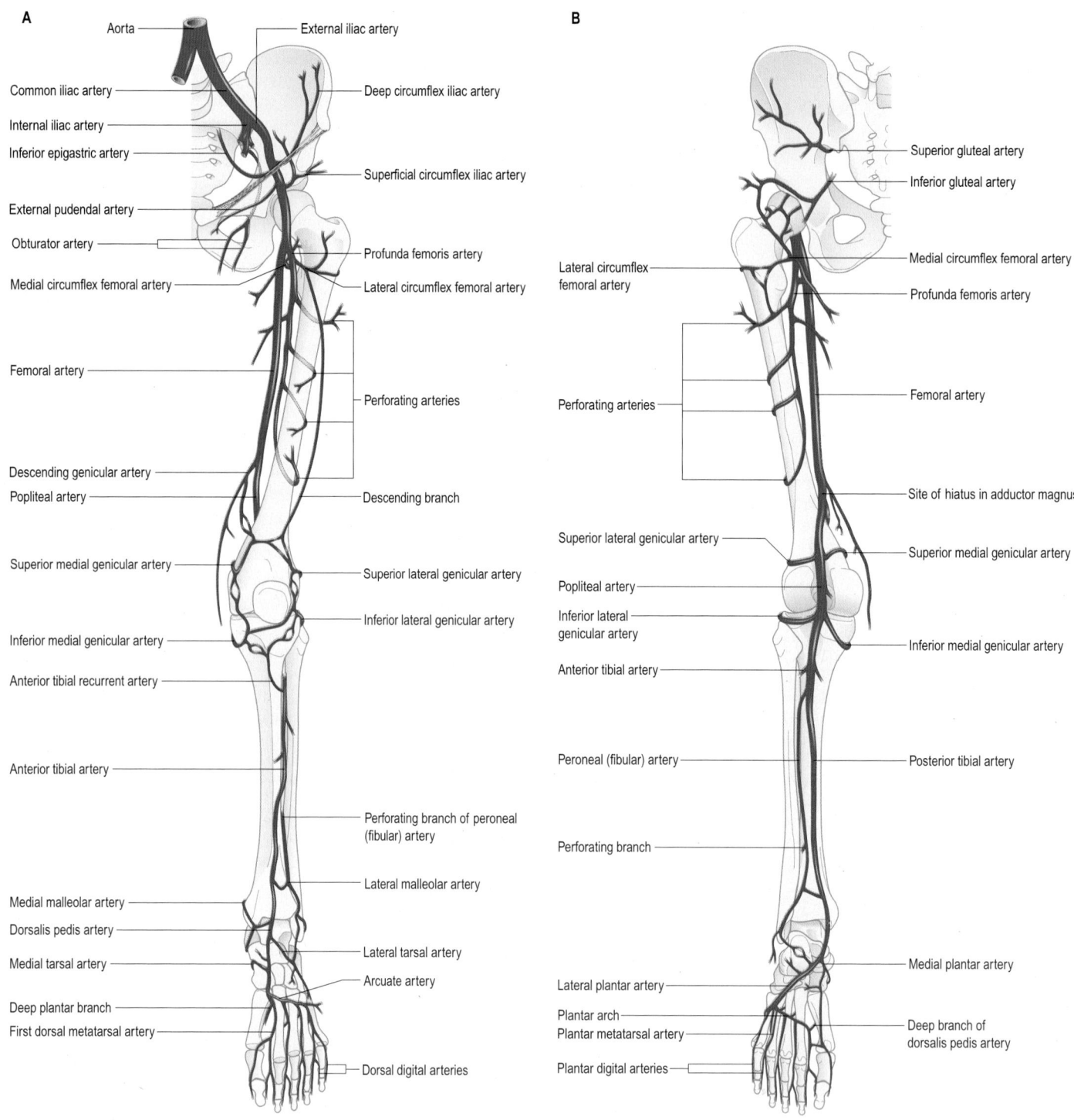

A

Aorta

External iliac artery

Common iliac artery

Deep circumflex iliac artery

Internal iliac artery

Inferior epigastric artery

Superficial circumflex iliac artery

External pudendal artery

Obturator artery

Profunda femoris artery

Medial circumflex femoral artery

Lateral circumflex femoral artery

Femoral artery

Perforating arteries

Descending genicular artery

Popliteal artery

Descending branch

Superior medial genicular artery

Superior lateral genicular artery

Inferior lateral genicular artery

Inferior medial genicular artery

Anterior tibial recurrent artery

Anterior tibial artery

Perforating branch of peroneal (fibular) artery

Lateral malleolar artery

Medial malleolar artery

Dorsalis pedis artery

Medial tarsal artery

Lateral tarsal artery

Arcuate artery

Deep plantar branch

First dorsal metatarsal artery

Dorsal digital arteries

B

Superior gluteal artery

Inferior gluteal artery

Medial circumflex femoral artery

Lateral circumflex femoral artery

Profunda femoris artery

Perforating arteries

Femoral artery

Site of hiatus in adductor magnus

Superior lateral genicular artery

Superior medial genicular artery

Popliteal artery

Inferior lateral genicular artery

Anterior tibial artery

Inferior medial genicular artery

Peroneal (fibular) artery

Posterior tibial artery

Perforating branch

Medial plantar artery

Lateral plantar artery

Plantar arch

Plantar metatarsal artery

Deep branch of dorsalis pedis artery

Plantar digital arteries

Fig. 110.4 Overview of arteries of the lower limb. **A**, Anterior. **B**, Posterior.

popliteal nodes. Superficial lymph vessels from the gluteal region run anteriorly to the proximal superficial inguinal nodes.

Lymphatic drainage of deeper tissues

The deep vessels accompany the anterior and posterior tibial, peroneal, popliteal and femoral vessels. The deep vessels from the foot and leg are interrupted by popliteal nodes; those from the thigh pass to the deep inguinal nodes. The deep lymph vessels of the gluteal and ischial regions follow their corresponding blood vessels. Those accompanying the superior gluteal vessels end in a node near the intrapelvic part of the superior gluteal artery, near the superior border of the greater sciatic foramen, while those which follow the inferior gluteal vessels traverse one or two of the small nodes below piriformis and pass to the internal iliac nodes.

INNERVATION

Overview of the plexuses

The lumbar and sacral plexuses innervate the lower limb. The lumbar plexus lies deep within psoas major, anterior to the transverse processes of the first three lumbar vertebrae. The sacral plexus lies in the pelvis on the anterior surface of piriformis, deep to the pelvic fascia, which separates it from the inferior gluteal and pudendal vessels. The lumbo-sacral trunk (L4 and L5) emerges medial to psoas major and lies on the ala of the sacrum before crossing the pelvic brim to join the anterior primary ramus of S1.

LESIONS OF THE LUMBAR AND SACRAL PLEXUSES

The deep and protected situation of the plexuses means that lesions are not common. The lumbar plexus may be involved in retroperitoneal

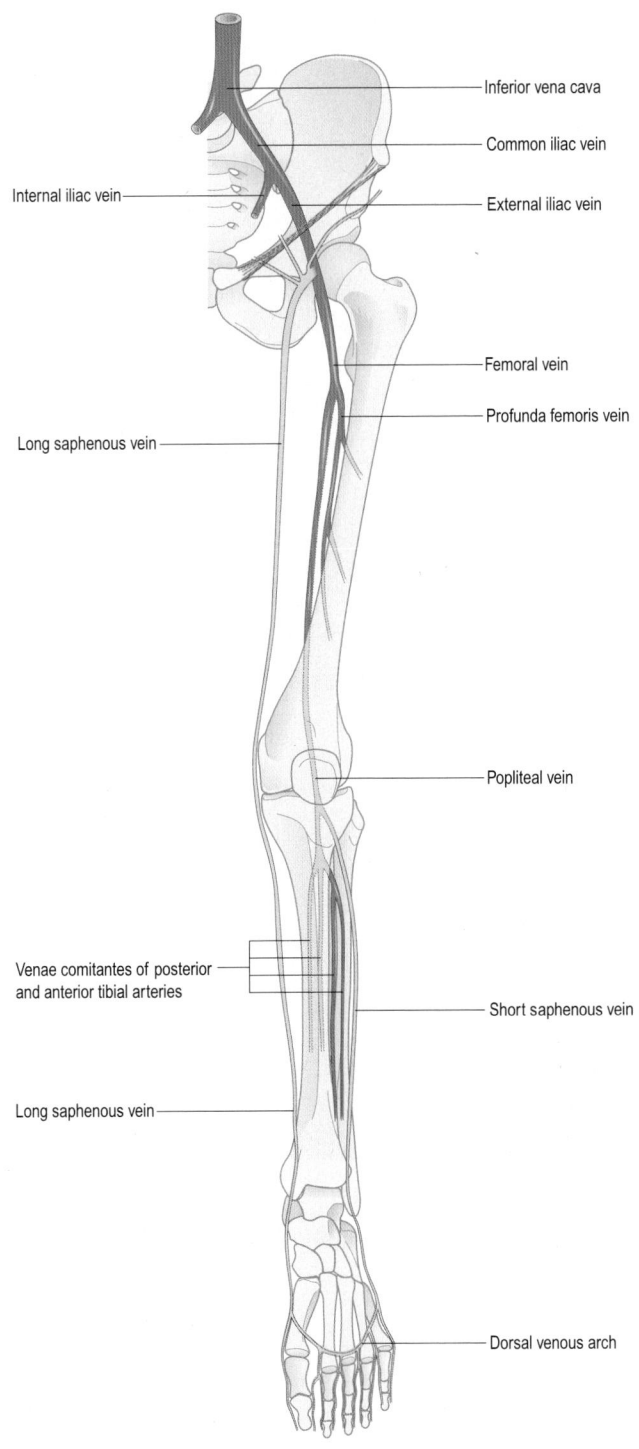

Fig. 110.5 Overview of veins of the lower limb.

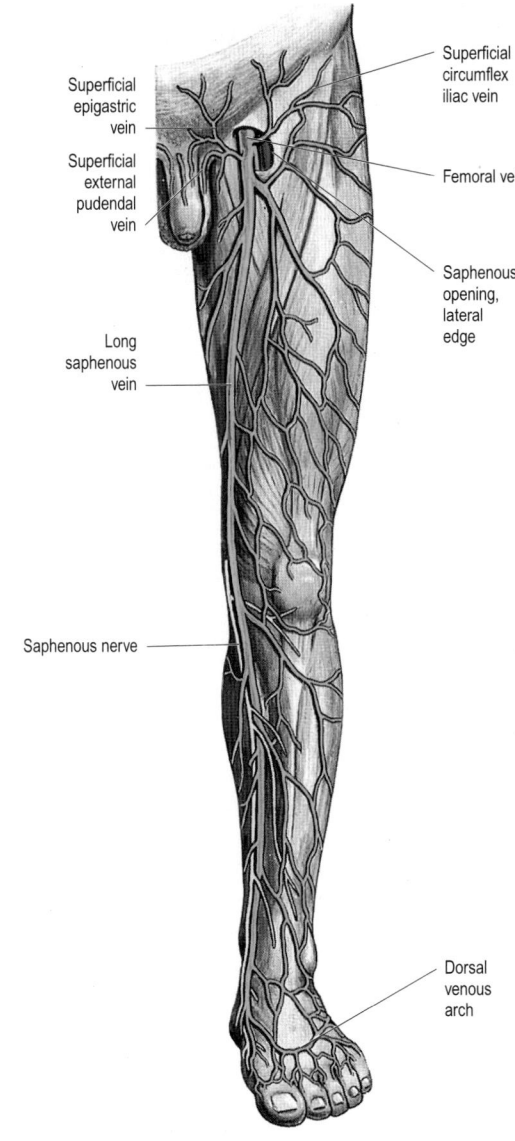

Fig. 110.6 The long saphenous vein and its tributaries.

pathology, and the sacral plexus may be invaded by spreading pelvic malignancy. Both may be involved in the reticuloses, affected by plexiform neuromas, or damaged in fractures of the lumbar spine and pelvis or in other conditions that cause severe retroperitoneal and pelvic haemorrhage. Temporary lesions may occur after pregnancy and childbirth, e.g. after difficult forceps delivery of a large baby. Pain, which may be diffuse, is the most common feature, and there is often clinical involvement of several roots.

OVERVIEW OF THE PRINCIPAL NERVES OF THE LOWER LIMB
(Figs 110.10, 110.11)

Femoral nerve (L2–4)
The femoral nerve is the nerve of the anterior compartment of the thigh. It arises from the posterior divisions of the second to fourth lumbar

ventral rami, descends through psoas major and emerges on its lateral border to pass between psoas and iliacus and enter the thigh behind the inguinal ligament and lateral to the femoral sheath. Its terminal branches form in the femoral triangle c.2 cm distal to the inguinal ligament. In the abdomen the nerve supplies small branches to iliacus and a branch to the proximal part of the femoral artery. It subsequently supplies a large cutaneous area on the anterior and medial thigh, medial leg and foot, and gives articular branches to the hip and knee. The femoral nerve is described in detail on page 1455.

Obturator nerve (L2–4)
The obturator nerve is the nerve of the medial compartment of the thigh. It arises from the anterior divisions of the second to fourth lumbar ventral rami, descends through psoas major and emerges from its medial border at the pelvic brim. It crosses the sacroiliac joint behind the common iliac artery and lateral to the internal iliac vessels, runs along the lateral pelvic wall on obturator internus, and enters the thigh through the upper part of the obturator foramen. Near the foramen it divides into anterior and posterior branches, separated at first by part of obturator externus and more distally by adductor brevis. It gives articular branches to the hip and knee, and may supply skin on the medial thigh and leg. The obturator nerve is described in detail on page 1455.

Sciatic nerve (L4, L5, S1–3)
The sciatic nerve is the nerve of the posterior compartment of the thigh and, via its major branches, of all the compartments of the lower leg

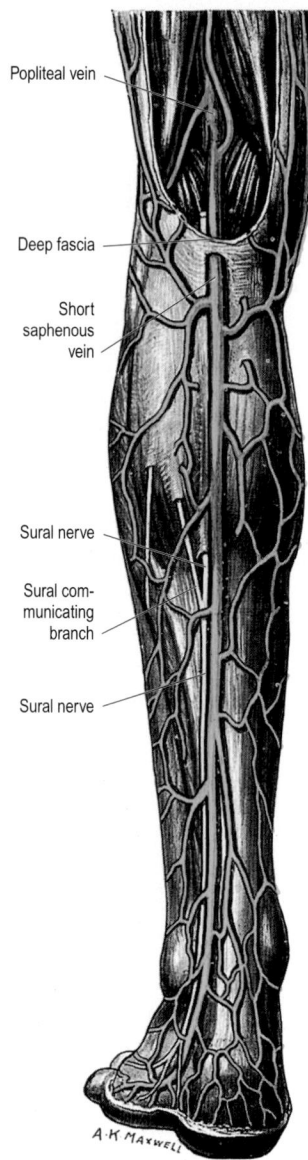

Popliteal vein

Deep fascia

Short saphenous vein

Sural nerve

Sural communicating branch

Sural nerve

A·K·MAXWELL

Fig. 110.7 The short saphenous vein and its tributaries.

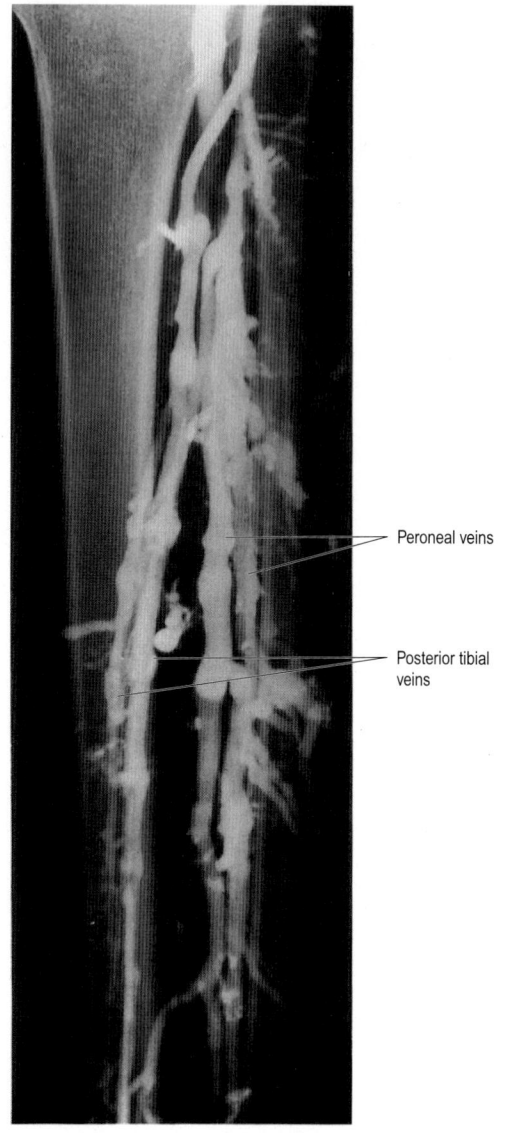

Peroneal veins

Posterior tibial veins

Fig. 110.8 Venogram of the leg to show the deep veins; the valves are clearly demonstrated. (Provided by Sean Gallagher, GKT School of Medicine, London; photograph by Sarah-Jane Smith.)

and foot. Formed in the pelvis from the ventral rami of the fourth lumbar to third sacral spinal nerves, it is 2 cm wide at its origin and is the thickest nerve in the body. It enters the lower limb via the greater sciatic foramen below piriformis and descends between the greater trochanter and ischial tuberosity. The nerve passes along the back of the thigh, where it is crossed by the long head of biceps femoris, and divides into the tibial and common peroneal (fibular) nerves proximal to the knee. The actual level of division is very variable since the tibial and common peroneal nerves are structurally separate and only loosely connected throughout their proximal course. The sciatic gives off articular branches that supply the hip joint through its posterior capsule (these are sometimes derived directly from the sacral plexus) and the knee joint. All the hamstring muscles, including the ischial part of adductor magnus, but not the short head of biceps femoris, are supplied by the medial (tibial) component of the sciatic nerve. The short head of biceps is supplied by the lateral (common peroneal) component. The sciatic nerve is described in detail on page 1456.

Tibial nerve (L4, L5, S1–3)
The tibial nerve arises from the anterior division of the sacral plexus. It descends along the back of the thigh and popliteal fossa to the distal border of popliteus, then passes anterior to the arch of soleus with the popliteal artery and continues into the leg. In the popliteal fossa it lies lateral to the popliteal vessels, becomes superficial to them at the knee and crosses to the medial side of the artery. In the leg it is the nerve of

the posterior compartment and descends with the posterior tibial vessels to lie between the heel and the medial malleolus. It ends beneath the flexor retinaculum by dividing into the medial and lateral plantar nerves. The tibial nerve supplies articular branches to the knee and ankle. Its cutaneous area of supply, including its terminal branches, includes the back of the calf, the whole of the sole, the lateral border of the foot and the medial and lateral sides of the heel. The tibial nerve is described in detail on page 1504.

Common peroneal nerve (L4, L5, S1, S2)
The common peroneal nerve (common fibular nerve) is derived from the posterior division of the sacral plexus. In the leg it is the nerve of the anterior and lateral compartments. It descends obliquely along the lateral side of the popliteal fossa to the fibular head, lying between the tendon of biceps femoris and the lateral head of gastrocnemius. It curves lateral to the neck of the fibula deep to peroneus longus and divides into superficial and deep peroneal (fibular) nerves: the common peroneal nerve is easily injured at the fibular neck. Before it divides, it gives off articular branches to the knee and the superior tibiofibular joints and cutaneous branches. Its cutaneous area of supply, including its terminal branches, includes the anterolateral and lateral surfaces of the leg and most of the dorsum of the foot. The common peroneal nerve is described in detail on page 1504.

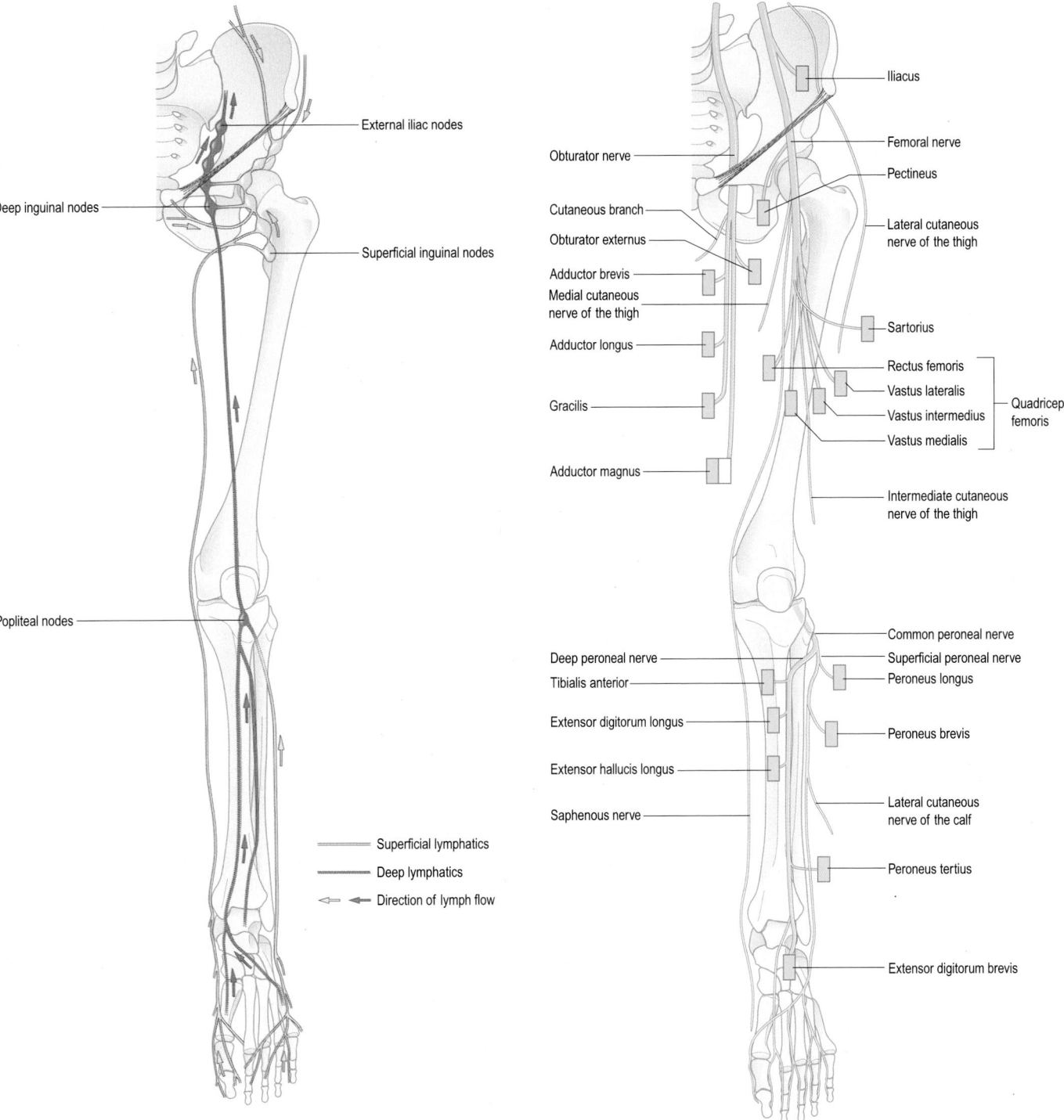

Fig. 110.9 Lymphatics of the lower limb.

Fig. 110.10 Nerves on the anterior aspect of the lower limb, their cutaneous branches, and the muscles they supply. (From Aids to the Examination of the Peripheral Nervous System. 2000. 4th edition. London: Saunders. With permission of Guarantors of Brain.)

Gluteal nerves

The gluteal nerves arise from the posterior division of the sacral plexus. The superior gluteal nerve (L4, L5, S1) leaves the pelvis through the greater sciatic notch above piriformis and supplies gluteus medius, gluteus minimus, tensor fasciae latae and the hip joint. The inferior gluteal nerve (L5, S1, S2) passes through the greater sciatic notch below piriformis and supplies gluteus maximus. The gluteal nerves are described in detail on page 1456.

AUTONOMIC INNERVATION

The autonomic supply to the limbs is exclusively sympathetic. The preganglionic sympathetic inflow to the lower limb is derived from neurones in the lateral horn of the lower thoracic (T10, T11) and upper lumbar (L1, L2) spinal cord segments. Fibres pass in white rami communicantes to the sympathetic chain and synapse in the lumbar and sacral ganglia. Postganglionic fibres pass in grey rami communicantes

to enter the lumbar and sacral plexuses, and many are distributed via the cutaneous branches of the nerves derived from these plexuses. The blood vessels to the lower limb receive their sympathetic supply via adjacent peripheral nerves. Postganglionic fibres accompanying the iliac arteries are destined mainly for the pelvis but may supply vessels in the upper thigh.

Surgical lumbar sympathectomy may be indicated in arterial disease. Surgical or chemical (phenol injection) sympathectomy may be used to treat rest pain or other troublesome sensory symptoms in arterial disease or in causalgia. The segment of the chain including the second and third lumbar ganglia is removed: preservation of the first lumbar ganglion is said to lessen the risk of ejaculatory problems.

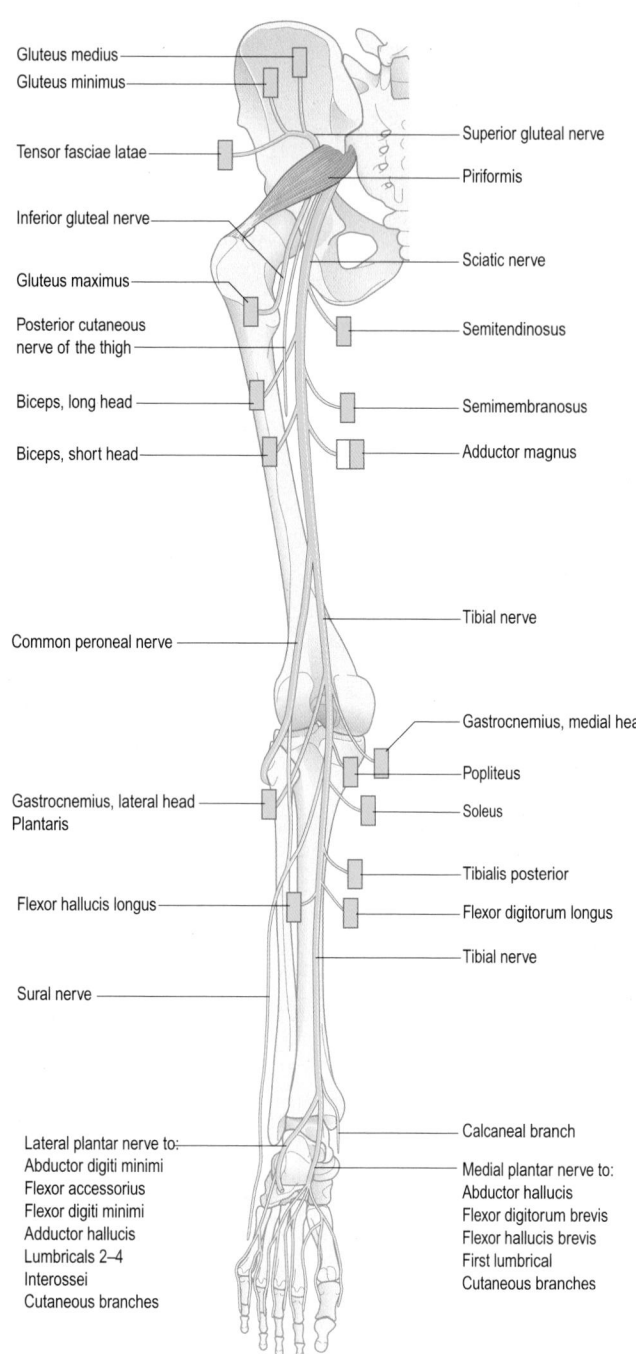

Gluteus medius

Gluteus minimus

Tensor fasciae latae

Inferior gluteal nerve

Gluteus maximus

Posterior cutaneous
nerve of the thigh

Biceps, long head

Biceps, short head

Common peroneal nerve

Gastrocnemius, lateral head
Plantaris

Flexor hallucis longus

Sural nerve

Lateral plantar nerve to:
Abductor digiti minimi
Flexor accessorius
Flexor digiti minimi
Adductor hallucis
Lumbricals 2–4
Interossei
Cutaneous branches

Superior gluteal nerve

Piriformis

Sciatic nerve

Semitendinosus

Semimembranosus

Adductor magnus

Tibial nerve

Gastrocnemius, medial head

Popliteus

Soleus

Tibialis posterior

Flexor digitorum longus

Tibial nerve

Calcaneal branch

Medial plantar nerve to:
Abductor hallucis
Flexor digitorum brevis
Flexor hallucis brevis
First lumbrical
Cutaneous branches

Fig. 110.11 Nerves on the posterior aspect of the lower limb, their cutaneous branches, and the muscles they supply. (From Aids to the Examination of the Peripheral Nervous System. 2000. 4th edn. London: Saunders. With permission of Guarantors of Brain.)

SURFACE ANATOMY

SKELETAL LANDMARKS

Pelvis (Fig. 110.12)

An oblique skin crease, the fold of the groin, marks the junction of the front of the thigh with the anterior abdominal wall, and corresponds fairly accurately to the inguinal ligament. The anterior superior iliac spine lies at the lateral end of the fold and can always be palpated. At its medial end, the fold reaches the pubic tubercle. From the anterior superior iliac spine, the iliac crest is easily palpable along its entire length. It terminates posteriorly as the posterior superior iliac spine, which may be felt in the depression seen just above the buttock. This depression lies at the level of the second sacral segment, at the level of the middle of the sacroiliac joint and the termination of the spinal dural sac. The ischial tuberosity may be palpated in the lower part

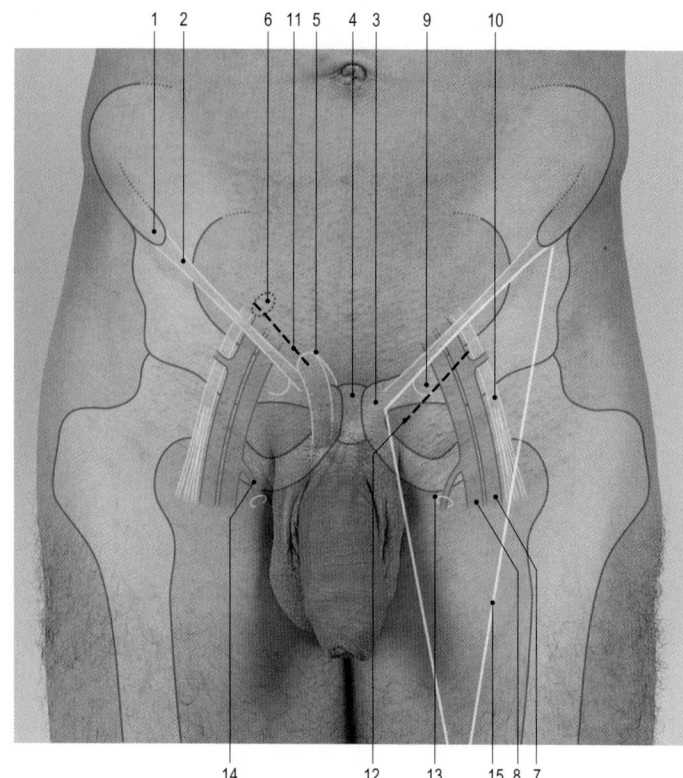

1. Anterior superior iliac spine. 2. Inguinal ligament. 3. Pubic tubercle.
4. Symphysis pubis. 5. Superficial inguinal ring. 6. Deep inguinal ring.
7. Femoral artery. 8. Femoral vein. 9. Femoral canal. 10. Femoral nerve.
11. Inguinal hernia incision. 12. Femoral hernia incision. 13. Saphenous opening.
14. Long saphenous vein. 15. Femoral triangle.

Fig. 110.12 Inguinal region (bones and soft tissues) and femoral triangle (vessels and nerves). (Photograph by Sarah-Jane Smith. Artwork modified from Lumley JSP 2002 Surface Anatomy, 3rd edn. Edinburgh: Churchill Livingstone.)

of the buttock. It is covered by gluteus maximus when the hip joint is extended, but can be identified without difficulty when the hip is flexed, e.g. in the sitting position, when the tuberosity emerges from under cover of the lower border of gluteus maximus and becomes subcutaneous, separated from the skin only by a pad of fat and the ischial bursa. In this position, the weight of the body is supported by the ischial tuberosities.

Femur (Figs 110.13, 110.14, 110.15)

The greater trochanter of the femur, which is the only palpable part of the proximal portion of the femur, lies the breadth of the subject's hand below the midpoint of the iliac crest. It can be both seen and felt as a prominence in front of the hollow on the side of the gluteal region. The lower end of the femur is less deeply placed. When the knee is flexed passively, the medial surface of the medial condyle and the lateral surface of the lateral condyle of the femur may both be palpated, and portions of the femoral articular surface can be examined on each side of the lower part of the patella.

Patella

The patella can be readily identified. When the quadriceps is relaxed in the fully extended knee, the patella can be tilted and moved on the lower end of the femur. The lower limit of the patella lies more than 1–2 cm above the line of the knee joint.

Knee (Figs 110.16, 110.17)

The patella and the medial and lateral condyles of the femur have been described above. The tibial condyles form visible and palpable landmarks at the medial and lateral sides of the patellar tendon. The latter may be traced downwards from the apex of the patella to the tibial tubercle, which is easily seen as well as felt. When the knee is flexed, the anterior margins of the tibial condyles can be felt: each forms the lower boundary of a depression at the side of the patellar tendon. The lateral

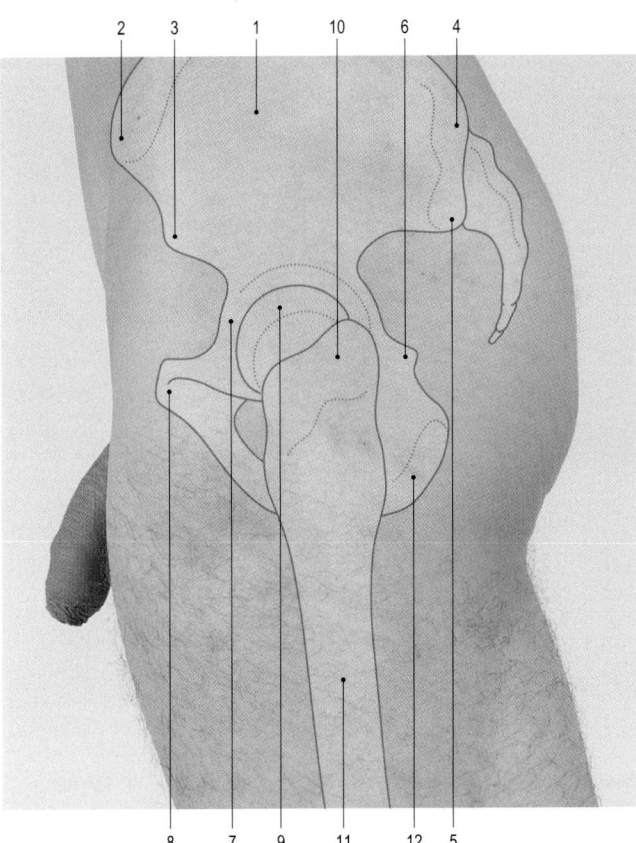

1. Ilium.   2. Anterior superior iliac spine.   3. Anterior inferior spine.
4. Posterior superior iliac spine.   5. Posterior inferior iliac spine.   6. Ischial spine.
7. Iliopubic eminence.   8. Body of pubis.   9. Head of femur.   10. Greater trochanter.
11. Shaft of femur.   12. Ischial tuberosity.

Fig. 110.13 Lateral aspect of the hip joint: bones. (Photograph by Sarah-Jane Smith. Artwork modified from Lumley JSP 2002 Surface Anatomy, 3rd edn. Edinburgh: Churchill Livingstone.)

condyle is the more prominent of the two. The joint line of the tibio-femoral joint corresponds to the upper margins of the tibial condyles and can be represented by a line drawn round the limb at this level. The anterior horns of the menisci lie in the angles between this line and the edges of the patellar tendon. The iliotibial tract is attached to a prominence, Gerdy's tubercle, on the anterior aspect of the lateral condyle, 1 cm below the joint line and c.2 cm lateral to the tibial tubercle.

The head of the fibula forms a slight surface elevation on the upper part of the posterolateral aspect of the leg. It lies vertically below the posterior part of the lateral condyle of the femur, not less than 1 cm below the level of the knee joint.

Leg and ankle (Fig. 110.18)

The subcutaneous medial surface of the tibia corresponds to the flat anteromedial aspect of the leg. Above, this surface merges into the medial condyle of the tibia, and below it is continuous with the visible prominence of the medial malleolus of the tibia. The sinuous anterior border of the tibia can be felt distinctly throughout most of its extent, but inferiorly it is somewhat masked by the tendon of tibialis anterior, which lies to its lateral side. The lateral malleolus of the fibula forms a conspicuous projection on the lateral side of the ankle: it descends to a more distal level than the medial malleolus and is placed on a more posterior plane. The lateral aspect of the lateral malleolus is continuous above with an elongated, subcutaneous, triangular area of the lower shaft of the fibula. The lateral part of the anterior margin of the lower end of the tibia can be detected immediately in front of the base of the lateral malleolus; the line of the ankle joint can be gauged from it.

Foot (Figs 110.19, 110.20)

On the dorsum of the foot, the anterior part of the upper surface of the calcaneus can be identified a little in front of the lateral malleolus. When the foot is passively inverted, the upper and lateral part of the

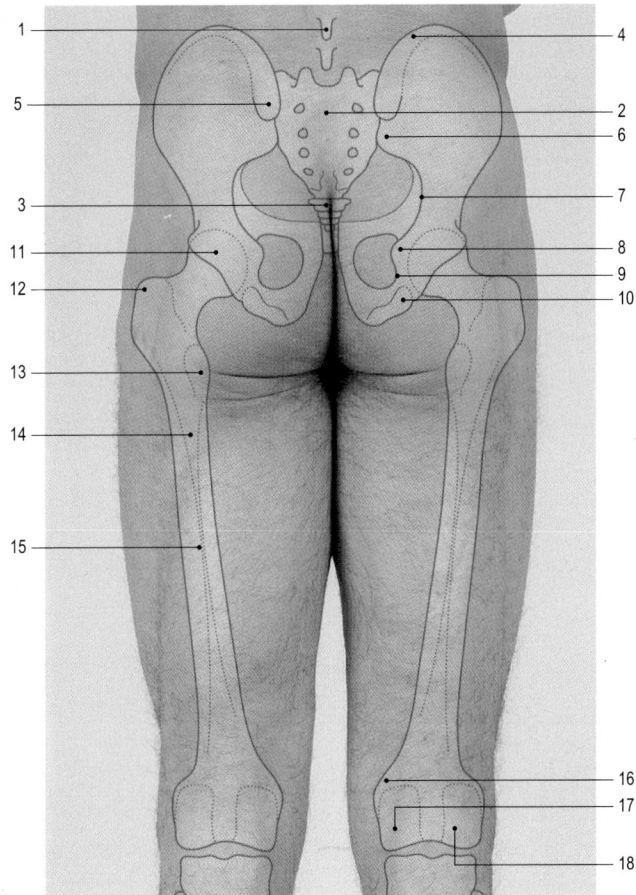

1. Fourth lumbar spine.   2. Sacrum.   3. Coccyx.   4. Iliac crest.
5. Posterior superior iliac spine.   6. Posterior inferior iliac spine.   7. Greater sciatic notch.
8. Ischial spine.   9. Lesser sciatic notch.   10. Ischial tuberosity.   11. Head of femur.
12. Greater trochanter.   13. Lesser trochanter.   14. Gluteal tuberosity.   15. Linea aspera.
16. Adductor tubercle.   17. Medial femoral condyle.   18. Lateral femoral condyle.

Fig. 110.14 Gluteal region and posterior aspect of the thigh: bones. (Photograph by Sarah-Jane Smith. Artwork modified from Lumley JSP 2002 Surface Anatomy, 3rd edn. Edinburgh: Churchill Livingstone.)

head of the talus can be both seen and felt 3 cm anterior to the distal end of the tibia; it is obscured by the extensor tendons when the toes are dorsiflexed.

The dorsal aspects of the bodies of the metatarsal bones can be felt more or less distinctly, although they tend to be obscured by the extensor tendons of the toes. The tuberosity on the base of the fifth metatarsal bone forms a distinct projection, which can be both seen and felt, halfway along the lateral border of the foot.

The flat lateral surface of the calcaneus can be palpated on the lateral aspect of the heel and can be traced forwards below the lateral malleolus, where it is hidden by the tendons of peroneus longus and brevis. The peroneal tubercle, when sufficiently large, can be felt 2 cm below the tip of the lateral malleolus. A palpable depression just anterior to the lateral malleolus leads to the lateral end of the sinus tarsi.

On the medial side of the foot, the sustentaculum tali of the calcaneus can be felt 2 cm vertically below the medial malleolus. The medial aspect of the calcaneus can be felt (indistinctly) below and behind the sustentaculum tali. The most conspicuous bony landmark on the medial side of the foot is the tuberosity of the navicular bone, which is usually visible and can always be felt 2.5 cm anterior to the sustentaculum tali. Anterior to this, the medial cuneiform bone can be identified by tracing the tendon of tibialis anterior into it. The upper and medial parts of the joint between the medial cuneiform and the first metatarsal can be felt as a narrow groove.

When the foot is placed on the ground, it rests on the posterior part of the inferior surface of the calcaneus, the heads of the metatarsal bones and, to a lesser extent, on its lateral border. The instep, which corresponds to the medial longitudinal arch of the foot, is elevated

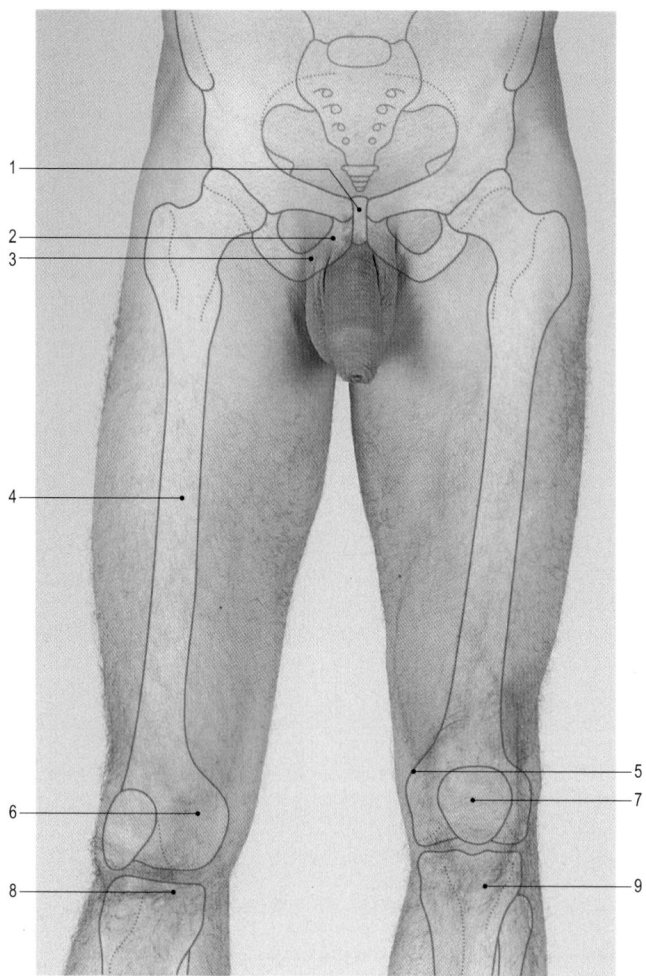

1. Symphysis pubis. **2.** Body of pubis. **3.** Inferior pubic ramus. **4.** Femur. **5.** Adductor tubercle. **6.** Medial femoral condyle. **7.** Patella. **8.** Medial tibial plateau. **9.** Tibial tuberosity.

Fig. 110.15 Anterior and medial aspect of the thigh: bones. (Photograph by Sarah-Jane Smith. Artwork modified from Lumley JSP 2002 Surface Anatomy, 3rd edn. Edinburgh: Churchill Livingstone.)

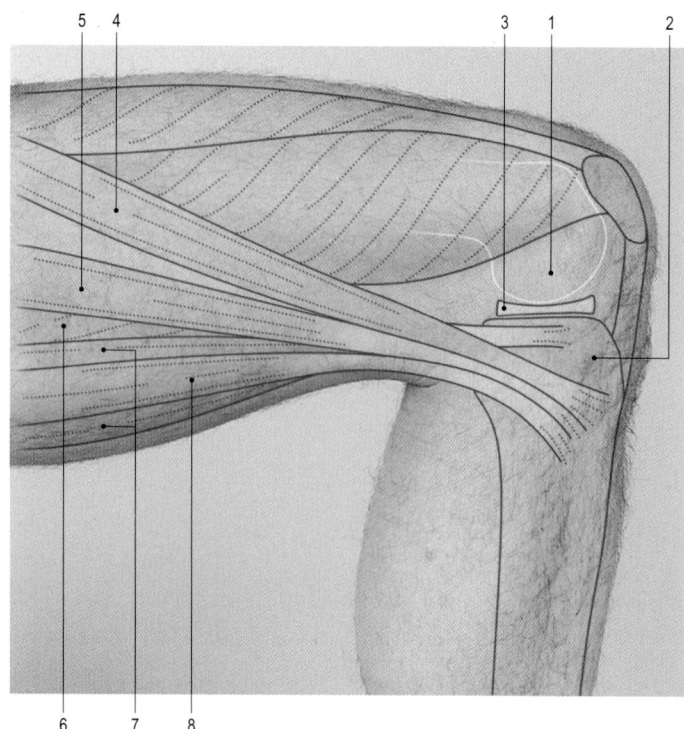

1. Medial femoral condyle. **2.** Medial tibial condyle. **3.** Medial meniscus. **4.** Sartorius. **5.** Gracilis. **6.** Adductor magnus. **7.** Semimembranosus. **8.** Semitendinosus.

Fig. 110.16 Medial aspect of the flexed knee: bone and muscles. (Photograph by Sarah-Jane Smith. Artwork modified from Lumley JSP 2002 Surface Anatomy, rd edn. Edinburgh: Churchill Livingstone.)

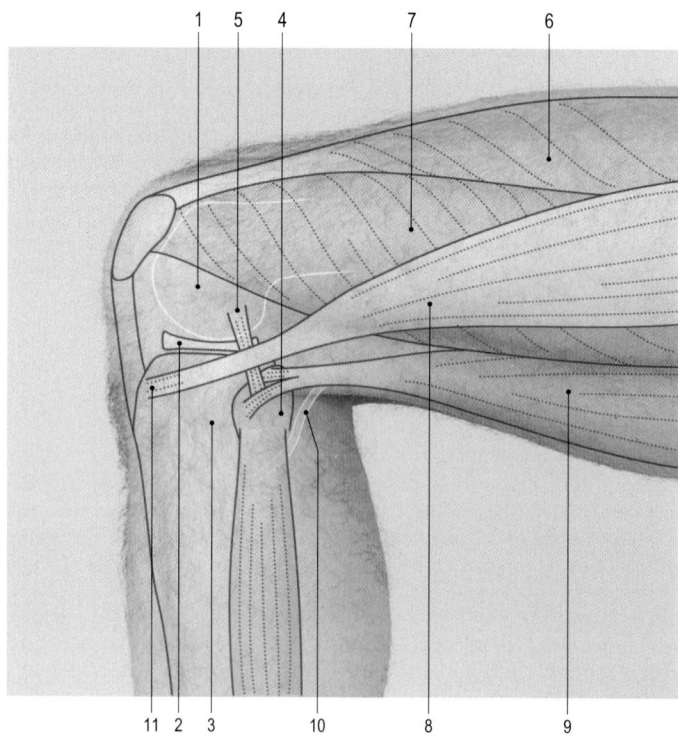

1. Lateral femoral condyle. **2.** Lateral meniscus. **3.** Lateral tibial condyle. **4.** Head of fibula. **5.** Lateral collateral ligament. **6.** Rectus femoris. **7.** Vastus lateralis. **8.** Iliotibial band. **9.** Biceps femoris. **10.** Common peroneal nerve. **11.** Gerdy's tubercle.

Fig. 110.17 Lateral aspect of the flexed knee: bone and soft tissues. (Photograph by Sarah-Jane Smith. Artwork modified from Lumley JSP 2002 Surface Anatomy, 3rd edn. Edinburgh: Churchill Livingstone.)

from the ground. The medial and lateral tubercles of the calcaneus can be identified on the posterior part of the inferior surface of the calcaneus, but they are obscured by the tough fibro-fatty pad that covers them. The heads of the metatarsal bones are similarly covered by a thick pad, which forms the ball of the foot. The foot is at its widest at this level, reflecting the slight splay of the metatarsal bones as they pass anteriorly.

The calcaneocuboid joint lies 2 cm behind the tubercle on the base of the fifth metatarsal bone and is practically in line with the talonavicular joint, whose position may be gauged from the position of the head of the talus. The tarsometatarsal joints lie on a line joining the tubercle of the fifth metatarsal bone to the tarsometatarsal joint of the great toe. When the latter joint cannot be felt on the medial border of the foot, its position may be indicated 2.5 cm in front of the tuberosity of the navicular bone. The joint between the second metatarsal and the intermediate cuneiform lies some 2–3 mm behind the line of the other tarsometatarsal joints. The metatarsophalangeal joints lie 2.5 cm behind the webs of the toes.

MUSCULOTENDINOUS AND LIGAMENTOUS LANDMARKS

Buttock and hip (Figs 110.13, 110.21)

The bulky prominence of the buttock is caused by the forward tilt of the pelvis (which throws the ischium backwards), the size of gluteus maximus, and the large amount of subcutaneous fat.

The horizontal gluteal fold marks the upper limit of the posterior aspect of the thigh. It does not correspond to the lower border of gluteus maximus but is caused by fibrous connections between the skin and the deep fascia. The natal cleft, which separates the buttocks inferiorly, starts above at the third or fourth sacral spine.

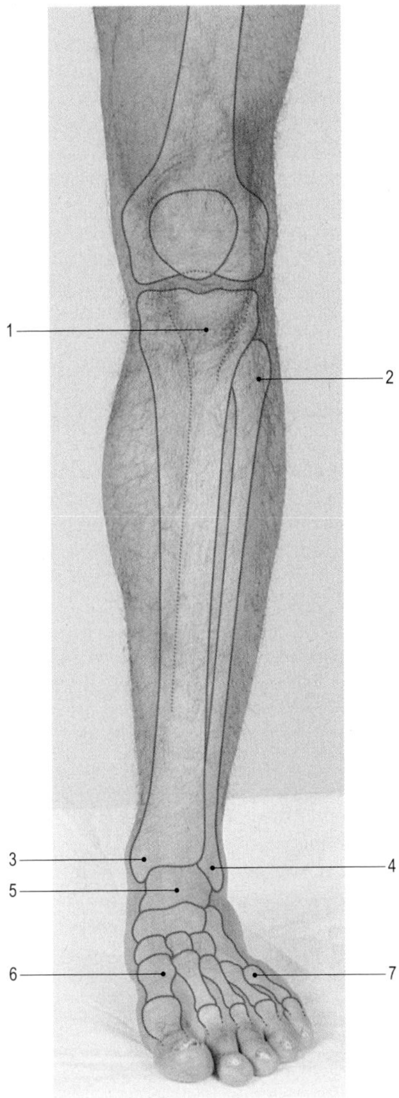

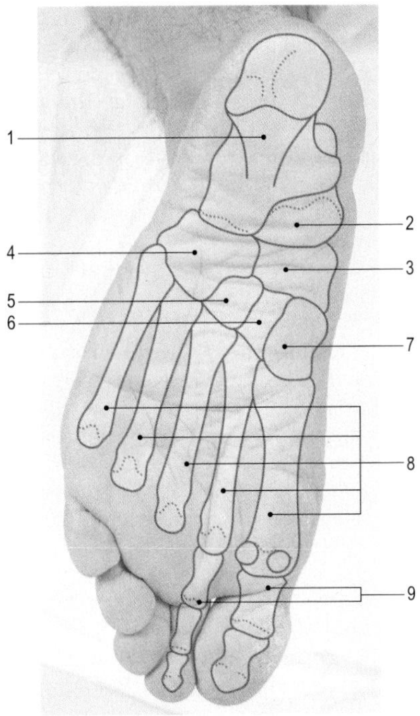

1. Calcaneus.
2. Talus.
3. Navicular.
4. Cuboid.
5. Lateral cuneiform.
6. Intermediate cuneiform.
7. Medial cuneiform.
8. Metatarsals.
9. Phalanges.

Fig. 110.20 Sole of the foot: bones. (Photograph by Sarah-Jane Smith. Artwork modified from Lumley JSP 2002 Surface Anatomy, 3rd edn. Edinburgh: Churchill Livingstone.)

1. Tibia.
2. Fibula.
3. Medial malleolus.
4. Lateral malleolus.
5. Talus.
6. First metatarsal.
7. Fifth metatarsal.

Fig. 110.18 Anterior aspect of the lower leg: bones. (Photograph by Sarah-Jane Smith. Artwork modified from Lumley JSP 2002 Surface Anatomy, 3rd edn. Edinburgh: Churchill Livingstone.)

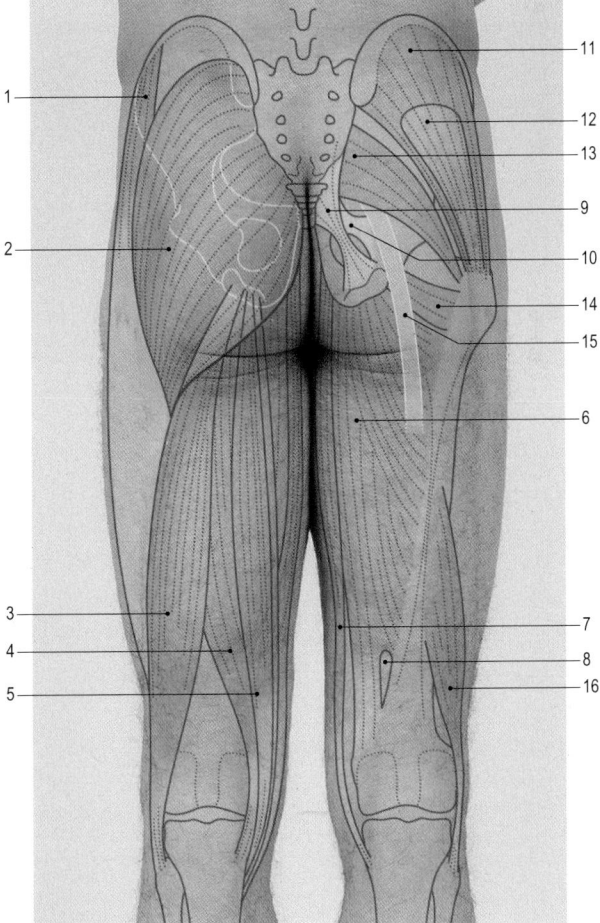

1. Tensor fasciae latae.   2. Gluteus maximus.   3. Long head of biceps femoris.
4. Semitendinosus.   5. Semimembranosus.   6. Adductor magnus.   7. Gracilis.
8. Adductor hiatus.   9. Sacrotuberous ligament.   10. Sacrospinous ligament.
11. Gluteus medius.   12. Gluteus minimus (deep to medius).   13. Piriformis.
14. Quadratus femoris.   15. Sciatic nerve.   16. Short head of biceps femoris.

Fig. 110.21 Gluteal region and posterior aspect of the thigh: superficial (left limb) and deep (right limb) muscles. (Photograph by Sarah-Jane Smith. Artwork modified from Lumley JSP 2002 Surface Anatomy, 3rd edn. Edinburgh: Churchill Livingstone.)

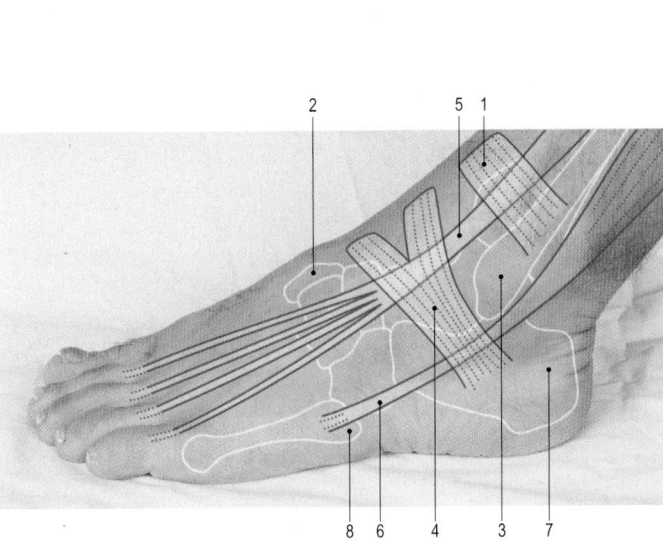

1. Superior extensor retinaculum.   2. Medial cuneiform   3. Lateral malleolus.
4. Inferior extensor retinaculum.   5. Tendon of extensor digitorum.
6. Tendon of peroneus brevis.   7. Calcaneus.   8. Tuberosity of fifth metatarsal.

Fig. 110.19 Left foot and ankle, lateral view. (Photograph by Sarah-Jane Smith.)

The upper border of gluteus maximus begins on the iliac crest c.3 cm lateral to the posterior superior iliac spine and runs downwards and laterally to the apex of the greater trochanter. Its lower border corresponds to a line drawn from the ischial tuberosity, through the midpoint of the gluteal fold, to a point c.9 cm below the greater trochanter. Although gluteus maximus overlaps the ischial tuberosity in the standing position, on sitting it slides superiorly posterior to the tuberosity, leaving it free to bear weight. The muscle can be felt to contract when the hip is extended against resistance.

Gluteus medius completely covers the underlying gluteus minimus. Both muscles lie in a slight depression superolateral to gluteus maximus and inferior to the anterior portion of the iliac crest. They constitute the major abductors of the hip and are demonstrated by asking the subject to stand on one limb. The ipsilateral muscles contract and tilt the pelvis in order to stabilize the centre of gravity, and the contralateral gluteal fold will rise. If the hip abductors are paralysed, e.g. in congenital dislocation of the hip or in a long-standing fracture of the neck of the femur, this mechanism is disturbed and the normal tilting of the pelvis does not occur. Indeed, when the patient stands on the affected hip, the pelvis tilts downwards on the contralateral side (Trendelenburg's sign).

Thigh (Figs 110.12, 110.13, 110.16, 110.17, 110.22)

The inguinal ligament can be felt running between the anterior superior iliac spine and the pubic tubercle when the thigh is abducted and externally rotated. Just distal to the inguinal ligament, but running horizontally, is the hip flexure line (Holden's line), where the deep layer of superficial fascia of the abdominal wall meets the fascia lata of the thigh.

The shallow depression lying immediately below the fold of the groin corresponds to the femoral triangle (p. 1419). It is bounded on its lateral side by the strap-like sartorius. The latter can be both seen and felt in a reasonably thin and muscular subject when the hip is flexed in the sitting position, while keeping the knee extended, especially when the thigh is slightly abducted and rotated laterally. The muscle can be traced downwards and medially from the anterior superior iliac spine to approximately half-way down the medial side of the thigh. Distally, it may be identified as a soft longitudinal ridge passing towards the posterior part of the medial femoral condyle. The adductor group of muscles forms the bulky, fleshy mass at the upper part of the medial side of the thigh. The medial border of adductor longus forms the medial boundary of the femoral triangle and can be felt as a distinct ridge when the thigh is adducted against resistance. At its upper end, its tendon of origin immediately below the pubic tubercle can be identified and felt between the finger and thumb, which is a useful guide to this bony landmark.

The forward convexity of the front of the thigh is caused by the curvature of the femur covered by the fleshy mass of quadriceps femoris. Rectus femoris appears as a ridge passing down the anterior aspect of the thigh when the sitting subject flexes the hip with the knee extended. Vastus medialis constitutes the bulge above and medial to the patella. Vastus lateralis forms the elevation above and lateral to the patella, more proximal and less pronounced than that of vastus medialis. Vastus intermedius is hidden by the other three muscles.

The flattened appearance of the lateral aspect of the thigh is produced by the iliotibial tract, which is a thickened portion of the deep fascia of the thigh (fascia lata). It stands out as a strong, visible ridge on the lateral aspect of the knee when the knee is either extended against gravity or when the opposite limb is lifted from the floor while standing.

Knee (Fig. 110.23)

The large depression that can be seen at the back of the knee when the joint is actively flexed against resistance corresponds to the popliteal

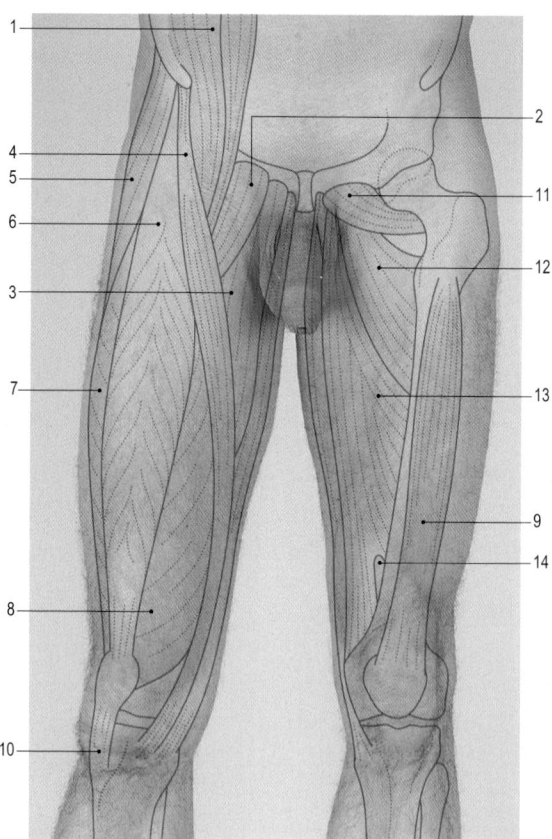

Note: items 6–10 make up the quadriceps muscle.
1. Iliopsoas. **2.** Pectineus. **3.** Adductor longus. **4.** Sartorius. **5.** Tensor fasciae latae. **6.** Rectus femoris. **7.** Vastus lateralis. **8.** Vastus medialis. **9.** Vastus intermedius. **10.** Patellar tendon. **11.** Obturator externus. **12.** Adductor brevis. **13.** Adductor magnus. **14.** Adductor hiatus.

Fig. 110.22 Anterior and medial aspect of the thigh: superficial (right limb) and deep (left limb) muscles. (Photograph by Sarah-Jane Smith. Artwork modified from Lumley JSP 2002 Surface Anatomy, 3rd edn. Edinburgh: Churchill Livingstone.)

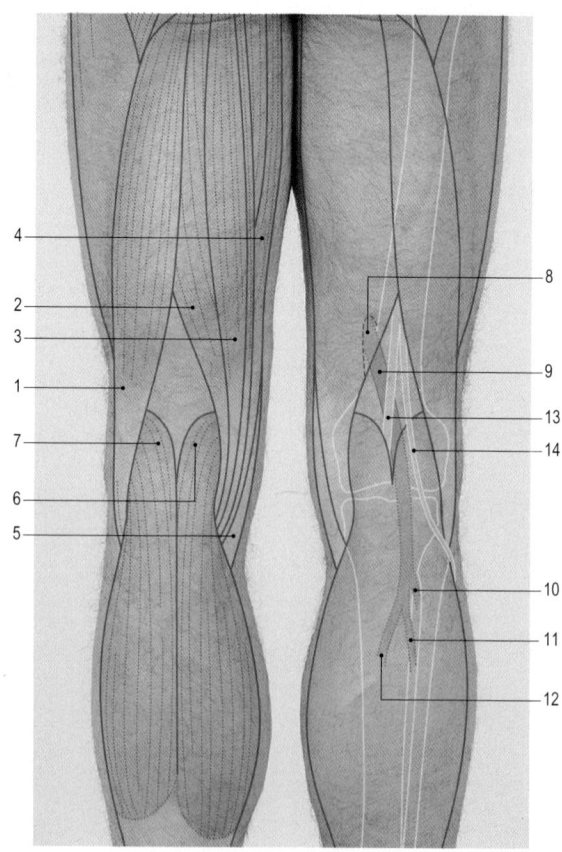

1. Biceps femoris. **2.** Semimembranosus. **3.** Semitedinosus. **4.** Gracilis. **5.** Sartorius. **6.** Gastronemius, medial head. **7.** Gastronemius, lateral head. **8.** Adductor hiatus. **9.** Popliteal artery. **10.** Anterior tibial artery. **11.** Peroneal artery. **12.** Posterior tibial artery. **13.** Tibial nerve. **14.** Common peroneal nerve.

Fig. 110.23 Popliteal fossa: soft tissues. (By permission from Lumley JSP 2002 Surface Anatomy, 3rd edn. Edinburgh: Churchill Livingstone.)

fossa. The transverse skin crease of the popliteal fossa is 2–3 cm above the tibiofemoral joint line. The fossa is bounded on the lateral side by the prominent tendon of biceps femoris, which can be felt between the finger and thumb and can be traced downwards to the head of the fibula. Three tendons can be felt on the medial side of the fossa. Semitendinosus is the most lateral and posterior, and gracilis is the most medial and anterior. These two tendons stand out sharply and can be seen when the knee is flexed against resistance and the limb actively adducted. The third tendon is that of semimembranosus: it is more deeply situated and can be felt in the interval between the tendons of semitendinosus and gracilis. It is much thicker than the other two tendons and broadens rapidly as it is traced upwards. Distally, in thin individuals, the upper border of the pes anserinus can be palpated. The upper borders of the two heads of gastrocnemius form the medial and lateral inferior boundaries of the popliteal fossa.

The lateral collateral ligament may be felt passing from the tip of the fibular head to the lateral epicondyle of the femur when the knee is flexed and laterally directed pressure is applied to the medial side of the knee. The medial patellofemoral ligament may be felt overlying the medial femoral condyle in the flexed knee, running between the midpoint of the medial patella and medial femoral epicondyle.

Leg (Figs 110.16, 110.17, 110.18, 110.24, 110.25, 110.26, 110.27)

The muscles in the anterior osteofascial compartment of the leg form a gentle prominence over the upper two-thirds of its anterolateral aspect: this prominence is accentuated when the foot is actively dorsiflexed. In the lower third of the leg these muscles are replaced by their tendons. The tendon of tibialis anterior can be seen just lateral to the anterior border of the tibia and traced downwards and medially across the front of the ankle. The other tendons cannot be examined satisfactorily above the ankle. Immediately above the medial malleolus and close to the

medial border of the tibia, the tendons of tibialis posterior and flexor digitorum longus can be felt (rather indistinctly) when the foot is actively inverted and plantar flexed.

On the lateral aspect of the leg, peroneus longus can be seen as a narrow ridge during active eversion and plantarflexion of the foot. It covers and hides peroneus brevis. Both muscles cover the lateral aspect of the fibula, which means that the shaft of the fibula can only be

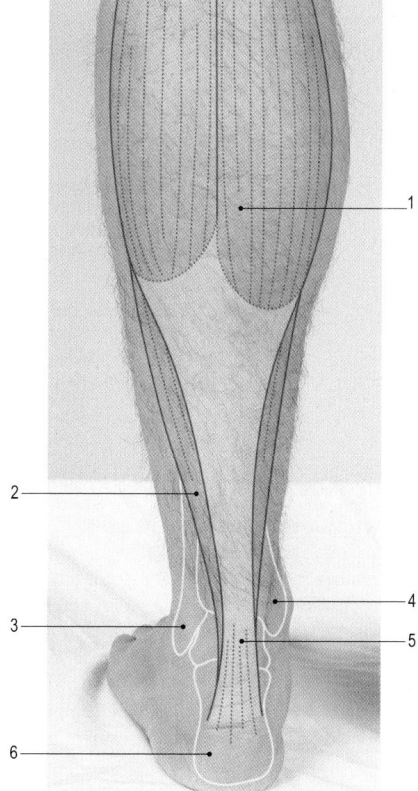

1. Gastrocnemius.
2. Soleus.
3. Medial malleolus.
4. Lateral malleolus.
5. Calcaneus tendon (Achilles tendon).
6. Calcaneus

Fig. 110.25 Left calf and ankle, posterior view with foot plantigrade. (Photograph by Sarah-Jane Smith.)

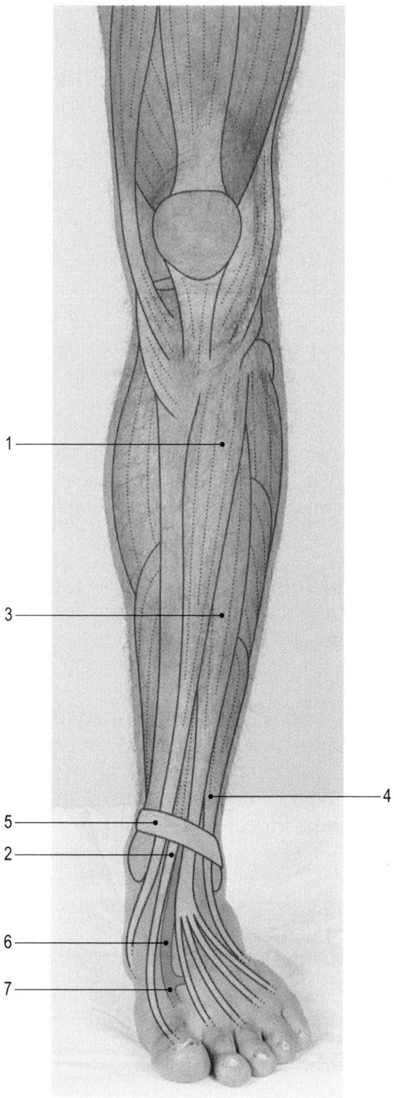

1. Tibialis anterior.
2. Extensor hallucis longus.
3. Extensor digitorum longus.
4. Peroneus tertius.
5. Superior extensor retinaculum.
6. Dorsalis pedis artery.
7. First dorsal metatarsal artery.

Fig. 110.24 Anterior aspect of the lower leg: muscles. (Photograph by Sarah-Jane Smith. Artwork modified from Lumley JSP 2002 Surface Anatomy, 3rd edn. Edinburgh: Churchill Livingstone.)

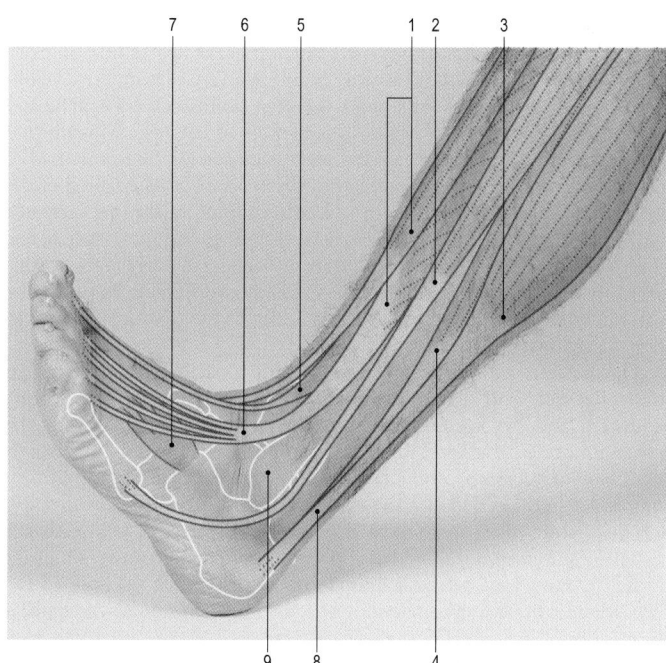

1. Tibialis anterior. 2. Peroneus longus. 3. Gastrocnemius 4. Soleus.
5. Tendon of extensor hallucis longus. 6. Tendons of extensor digitorum longus.
7. Extensor digitorum brevis. 8. Calcaneus tendon (Achilles tendon) 9. Lateral malleolus.

Fig. 110.26 Left leg and foot, lateral view with ankle dorsiflexed. (Photograph by Sarah-Jane Smith.)

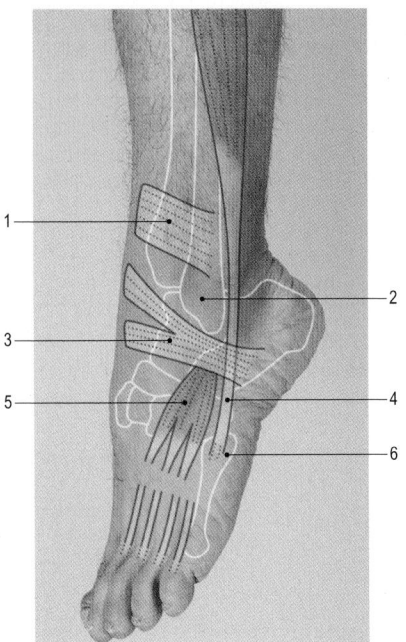

1. Superior extensor retinaculum.
2. Lateral malleolus.
3. Inferior extensor retinaculum.
4. Tendon of peroneus brevis.
5. Extensor digitorum brevis.
6. Tuberosity of fifth metatarsal.

Fig. 110.27 Left leg and foot, ankle plantar flexed, lateral view. (Photograph by Sarah-Jane Smith.)

palpated indistinctly between its neck and its lower subcutaneous triangular area.

The bulky prominence of the calf of the leg is formed by gastrocnemius and soleus, both of which can be identified either when the foot is plantar flexed against resistance, or when the heel is raised from the ground by standing on tiptoes. The two heads of gastrocnemius unite to form the inferior angle of the popliteal fossa. The medial head of gastrocnemius descends to a lower level than its lateral head. Soleus lies deep to gastrocnemius; when tensed, it bulges from under gastrocnemius, particularly on the lateral side, and its fleshy belly extends to a more distal level. Both muscles end below in the conspicuous calcaneal tendon, which can be gripped between the finger and thumb and followed downwards to its insertion into the posterior aspect of the calcaneus.

Foot (Figs 110.19, 110.20, 110.26, 110.27)

When the toes are actively dorsiflexed, the belly of extensor digitorum brevis forms a small elevation on the dorsum of the foot, a little in front of the lateral malleolus. It is the only muscle that arises from the dorsum of the foot. The tendon of tibialis anterior stands out conspicuously on the medial side when active dorsiflexion of the toes is combined with inversion: it can be traced downwards and medially to the medial cuneiform bone. Also in dorsiflexion, the tendon of extensor hallucis longus can be identified lateral to tibialis anterior. Still more laterally, and immediately in front of the lateral part of the inferior end of the tibia, the tendons of extensor digitorum longus and peroneus tertius are crowded together as they pass through the fibrous loop of the inferior extensor retinaculum. More distally, these tendons diverge to their insertions.

The tendon of tibialis posterior winds posterior to the medial malleolus and then curves forwards in the interval between this bony landmark and the sustentaculum tali to reach the tuberosity of the navicular bone. The tendon is thrown into relief when the foot is forcibly plantar flexed and inverted. The tendon of flexor digitorum longus lies midway between the medial margin of the calcaneal tendon and the margin of the medial malleolus. It curves forwards below tibialis posterior and lies on the medial aspect of the sustentaculum tali. From there, it passes forwards and laterally to the centre of the sole of the foot, where it breaks up into tendons for the lateral four toes. The tendon of flexor hallucis longus lies inferior to, and grooves, the sustentaculum tali. As it passes forward to the great toe, it crosses the line of the flexor digitorum longus opposite the interval between the sustentaculum tali and the tuberosity of the navicular bone. Abductor hallucis may be seen in some subjects as a fleshy mass across the instep of the foot, passing from the medial calcaneal tubercle to the ball of the great toe.

The plantar fascia is most easily palpated along its medial border, in the sole of the foot when the toes are maximally dorsiflexed. Its precise origin is difficult to palpate because of the thickness of the heel pad,

but it is easily palpated just distal to the heel pad as far as the ball of the foot.

SURFACE MARKINGS OF VESSELS, PULSES AND NERVES

Arteries

The femoral artery enters the thigh at the fold of the groin, at a point midway between the anterior superior iliac spine and the pubic symphysis, directly anterior to the hip joint. Its course can be represented by the upper two-thirds of a line joining that point to the adductor tubercle when the flexed thigh is abducted slightly and rotated laterally.

The popliteal artery may be represented approximately by a line extending from the junction of the middle and lower thirds of the thigh, 2.5 cm medial to its posterior midline, to the midpoint between the femoral condyles, and continuing inferolaterally to the level of the tibial tuberosity, medial to the fibular neck. The artery bifurcates into the anterior and posterior tibial arteries at the lower border of popliteus.

The anterior tibial artery may be represented by a line that begins 2.5 cm inferior to the medial side of the head of the fibula and runs downwards and slightly medially to the midpoint between the two malleoli.

The posterior tibial artery corresponds to a line drawn from the level of the neck of the fibula to a point midway between the medial malleolus and calcaneal tendon, along the midline of the back of the calf. The same line represents the course of the tibial nerve. At first the nerve lies lateral to the popliteal artery, then gradually crosses the vessel to gain its medial side. The trunk of the medial plantar artery begins midway between the medial malleolus and heel (medial calcaneal tubercle) and extends towards the first interdigital cleft as far as the navicular bone.

Pulses

Femoral artery pulse – At its origin the pulsations of the femoral artery can be felt, and in this situation the vessel can be compressed against the superior ramus of the pubis or the head of the femur. Like the carotid pulse, the femoral pulse is of value in assessing whether there is any significant cardiac output in cases of circulatory collapse. It is a common site for radiological catheter insertion and for arterial puncture for blood gas analysis.

Popliteal artery pulse – The pulse of the popliteal artery is the most difficult of the peripheral pulses to feel because the artery lies deep in the popliteal fossa. It is best examined with the subject lying supine or prone, with the knee flexed, in order to relax the tense popliteal fascia that roofs the popliteal fossa. The popliteal pulse is then felt by deep pressure over the midline of the fossa against the popliteal surface of the femur.

Posterior tibial artery pulse – The pulse of the posterior tibial artery can be felt by gentle palpation behind the medial malleolus as the artery lies between the tendons of flexor hallucis longus and flexor digitorum longus.

Dorsalis pedis arterial pulse – The dorsalis pedis arterial pulse is found by palpation against the underlying tarsal bones immediately lateral to the tendon of extensor hallucis longus.

Veins

The surface marking for the femoral vein is immediately medial to the femoral pulse. The long saphenous vein terminates c.2 cm inferior to the femoral pulse. Its course may be marked out in the thigh by a line passing from this point downwards and backwards to a point the breadth of the subject's hand behind the medial border of the patella.

The long saphenous vein can often be seen as it runs upwards and backwards across the medial surface of the tibia a little above and in front of the medial malleolus: this is a useful site for obtaining surgical venous access or for harvesting vein for cardiac bypass surgery. It is accompanied in this region by the saphenous nerve, which is usually anterolateral, but may be posterior to, the vein. The vein and nerve then run proximally and posteriorly along the medial border of the tibia to reach a point the breadth of the subject's hand posterior to the medial border of the patella. The short saphenous vein may be represented by a line which runs from the posterior surface of the lateral malleolus up the midline of the calf to the popliteal fossa: with the sural nerve it is the key anatomical guide to surgical dissection of the popliteal fossa.

The dorsal venous arch forms a conspicuous feature on the dorsum of the foot and curves, convex forwards, across the metatarsus. The long saphenous vein arises from its medial end and runs upwards and backwards immediately in front of the medial malleolus. The short saphenous vein arises from the lateral end of the arch and passes backwards and inferior to, and then upwards and posterior to, the lateral malleolus.

Femoral venous cannulation

While femoral venous puncture is relatively easy and supplies ready access to the right atrium, the use of this approach is relatively unpopular for long-term cannulation because of a higher incidence of thrombosis and sepsis. It is, however, a useful site for venous sampling in a patient with collapsed veins. For femoral venous cannulation the skin puncture site is approximately 1 cm medial to the femoral artery and just below the inguinal ligament. After skin puncture the needle is advanced with the syringe at an angle of 30° to the skin, aiming cephalad.

Nerves (Fig. 110.28)

The surface marking for the femoral nerve in the inguinal region is immediately lateral to the femoral pulse. The surface marking for the course of the saphenous nerve is described with the course of the long saphenous vein (see above).

The course of the sciatic nerve can be represented by a line that starts at a point midway between the posterior superior iliac spine and ischial tuberosity, curves outwards and downwards through a point midway between the greater trochanter and the ischial tuberosity, and then continues vertically downwards in the midline of the posterior aspect of the thigh to the upper angle of the popliteal fossa, where it divides into the tibial and common peroneal nerves (if it has not already done so at a higher level).

The course of the common peroneal nerve can be indicated by a line that runs from the upper angle of the popliteal fossa, along the medial side of the tendon of biceps femoris and then curves downwards and forwards around the neck of the fibula. The nerve is palpable medial and, more distally to the tendon of biceps and over the neck of the

fibula, although here it is less distinct as it passes deep to the origin of peroneus longus. At the neck of the fibula the nerve is at particular risk of damage either from a tightly applied plaster cast or from a fracture.

The deep peroneal nerve starts on the lateral aspect of the neck of the fibula, passes downwards and medially, and rapidly becomes associated with the anterior tibial artery, which it accompanies to the ankle. The superficial peroneal nerve also begins on the lateral aspect of the neck of the fibula. It descends to a point on the anterior border of peroneus longus, at the junction of the middle and lower thirds of the leg, where it pierces the deep fascia and divides into medial and lateral branches. The latter gradually diverge as they descend to reach the dorsum of the foot and may be seen if the foot is pulled into maximal plantarflexion and adduction.

With one exception, the cutaneous nerves of the foot are not normally visible. The superficial peroneal nerve is usually easily seen and palpated over the dorsolateral aspect of the ankle and midfoot when the ankle is plantar flexed and the fourth toe passively flexed. This is particularly true in individuals with little subcutaneous fat. Whilst the lateral branch is usually seen, the medial branch is rarely visible. These superficial nerves are at risk from surgery in the anterior ankle region (especially during arthroscopy): they can be identified reliably by passive plantarflexion and inversion of the foot whilst running the blunt end of a ballpoint pen across the anterior ankle. An easily palpable click will localize the nerves, even in patients who are not thin.

Dermatomes (Figs 110.29, 110.30, 110.31)

Our knowledge of the extent of individual dermatomes, especially in the limbs, is largely based on clinical evidence. The dermatomes of the lower limb arise from spinal nerves T12 to S3.

The preaxial border starts near the midpoint of the thigh and descends to the knee. It then curves medially, descending to the medial malleolus and the medial side of the foot and hallux. The postaxial border starts in the gluteal region and descends to the centre of the popliteal fossa, then deviates laterally to the lateral malleolus and the lateral side of the

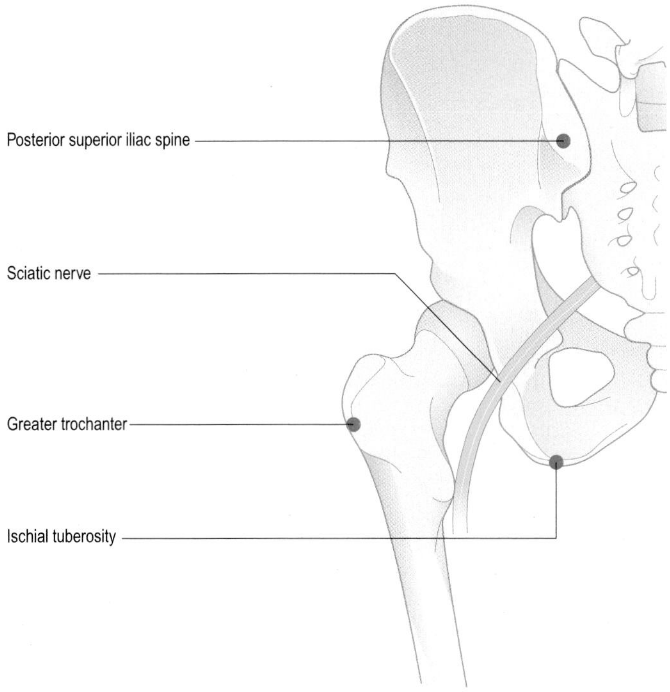

Fig. 110.28 Surface markings of the sciatic nerve. The line of the nerve joins the midpoint between the ischial tuberosity and the posterior superior iliac spine with the midpoint between the ischial tuberosity and the greater trochanter and then continues vertically down the back of the thigh. (From Ellis H, Feldman S 1997 Anatomy for Anaesthetists, 7th edn. Oxford: Blackwell Science. By permission of Blackwell Publishing.)

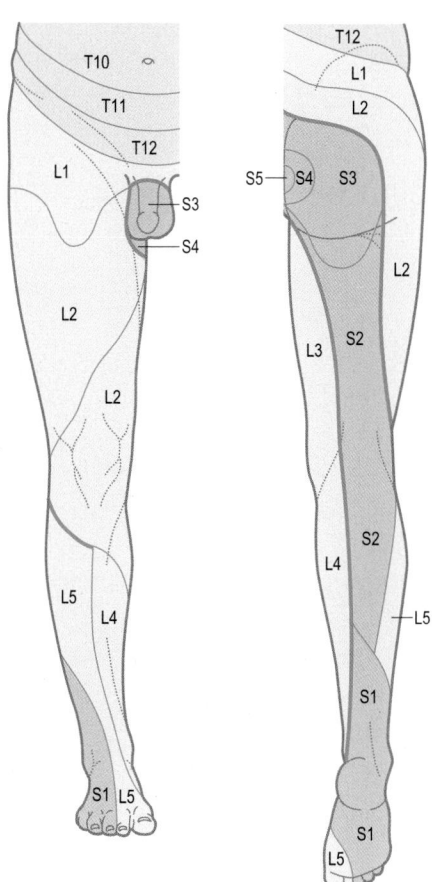

Fig. 110.29 Dermatomes of the lower limb. There is considerable variation and overlap between dermatomes, but the overlap across axial lines (heavy black) is minimal.

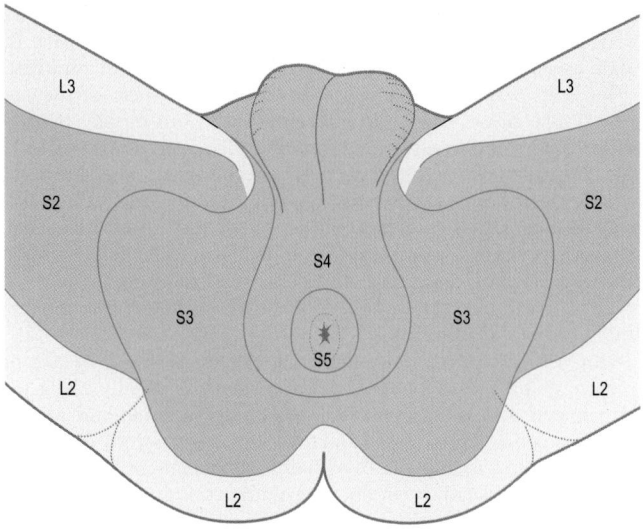

Fig. 110.30 Dermatomes of the perineum.

foot. The ventral and dorsal axial lines exhibit corresponding obliquity. The ventral starts proximally at the medial end of the inguinal ligament and descends along the posteromedial aspect of the thigh and leg to end proximal to the heel. The dorsal axial line begins in the lateral gluteal region and descends posterolaterally in the thigh to the knee; it inclines medially and ends proximal to the ankle. Considerable overlap exists between adjacent dermatomes innervated by nerves derived from consecutive spinal cord segments.

Myotomes
Tables 110.1 to **110.4** summarize the predominant segmental origin of the nerve supply for each of the lower limb muscles and for movements that take place at the joints of the lower limb: damage to these segments or to their motor roots results in maximum paralysis. Data are based chiefly on clinical evidence (Sharrad 1995).

Reflexes
Knee jerk (L2–4) – With the patient supine and the knee supported and partially flexed, the patellar tendon is struck at its midpoint: this should elicit contraction of the quadriceps, which extends the knee.

Ankle jerk (S1, 2) – With the patient supine and the lower limb externally rotated and partially flexed at hip and knee, the foot is passively dorsiflexed to stretch the calcaneal tendon, which is then struck with a percussion hammer. Contraction of the calf muscles plantar flexes the ankle. The reflex can also be examined with the patient kneeling on a chair.

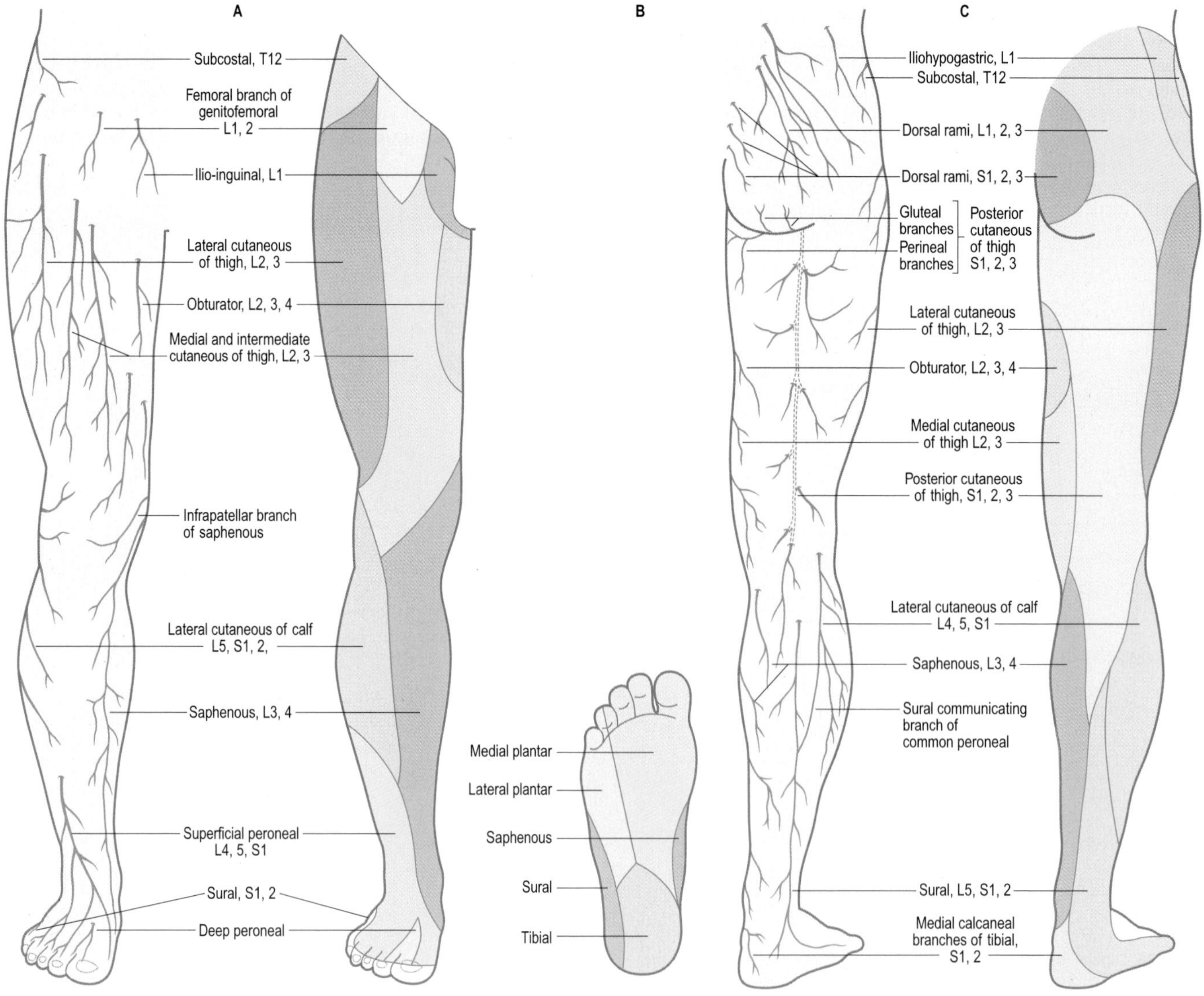

A

Subcostal, T12

Femoral branch of genitofemoral L1, 2

Ilio-inguinal, L1

Lateral cutaneous of thigh, L2, 3

Obturator, L2, 3, 4

Medial and intermediate cutaneous of thigh, L2, 3

Infrapatellar branch of saphenous

Lateral cutaneous of calf L5, S1, 2,

Saphenous, L3, 4

Superficial peroneal L4, 5, S1

Sural, S1, 2

Deep peroneal

B

Medial plantar

Lateral plantar

Saphenous

Sural

Tibial

C

Iliohypogastric, L1
Subcostal, T12

Dorsal rami, L1, 2, 3

Dorsal rami, S1, 2, 3

Gluteal branches — Perineal branches — Posterior cutaneous of thigh S1, 2, 3

Lateral cutaneous of thigh, L2, 3

Obturator, L2, 3, 4

Medial cutaneous of thigh L2, 3

Posterior cutaneous of thigh, S1, 2, 3

Lateral cutaneous of calf L4, 5, S1

Saphenous, L3, 4

Sural communicating branch of common peroneal

Sural, L5, S1, 2

Medial calcaneal branches of tibial, S1, 2

Fig. 110.31 The cutaneous nerves of the right lower limb, their areas of distribution and segmental origins. **A**, Anterior aspect; **B**, sole of foot; **C**, posterior aspect. In **C**, the interrupted line represents the trunk of the posterior cutaneous nerve of the thigh, most of which lies deep to the fascia lata.

Table 110.1 Movements, muscles and segmental innervation in the lower limb

Joint	Movement	Muscle	Innervation	L1	L2	L3	L4	L5	S1	S2	S3
HIP	FLEXION	Psoas major	Spinal nn. L1–3	▩	▩						
		Iliacus	Femoral n.		▩						
		Pectineus	Femoral n.		▩						
		Rectus femoris	Femoral n.			▩	▩				
		Adductor longus	Obturator n.		▩	▩					
		Sartorius	Femoral n.								
	EXTENSION	Gluteus maximus	Inferior gluteal n.					▩	▩		
		Adductor magnus	Obturator & tibial nn.		▩	▩					
		Hamstrings	Mainly tibial nn.						▩		
	MEDIAL ROTATION	Iliacus	Femoral n.		▩						
		Gluteus medius & minimus	Superior gluteal n.					▩	▩		
		Tensor fasciae latae	Superior gluteal n.					▩			
	LATERAL ROTATION	Superior & inferior gemelli	Lumbosacral plexus								
		Quadratus femoris	Lumbosacral plexus								
		Piriformis	Lumbosacral plexus						▩		
		Obturator internus	Lumbosacral plexus						▩		
		Obturator externus	Obturator n.								
		Sartorius	Femoral n.								
	ADDUCTION	Gracilis	Obturator n.								
		Adductor longus	Obturator n.		▩	▩					
		Adductor magnus	Obturator & tibial nn.		▩	▩					
		Adductor brevis	Obturator n.		▩						
		Pectineus	Femoral n.		▩						
	ABDUCTION	Tensor fasciae latae	Superior gluteal n.					▩	▩		
		Gluteus medius & minimus	Superior gluteal n.					▩	▩		
		Piriformis	Lumbosacral plexus						▩		
KNEE	FLEXION	Hamstrings:									
		Semimembranosus	Tibial n.						▩		
		Semitendinosus	Tibial n.						▩		
		Biceps femoris	Tibial & common peroneal nn.						▩		
		Gastrocnemius	Tibial n.								
	EXTENSION	Quadriceps femoris:									
		Rectus femoris	Femoral n.			▩	▩				
		Vastus lateralis	Femoral n.			▩	▩				
		Vastus intermedius	Femoral n.			▩	▩				
		Vastus medialis	Femoral n.			▩	▩				
ANKLE	DORSIFLEXION	Tibialis anterior	Deep peroneal n.					▩			
		Extensor digitorum longus	Deep peroneal n.					▩			
		Extensor hallucis longus	Deep peroneal n.					▩			
		Peroneus tertius	Deep peroneal n.					▩			
	PLANTARFLEXION	Gastrocnemius	Tibial n.						▩		
		Soleus	Tibial n.						▩		
		Flexor digitorum longus	Tibial n.						▩		
		Flexor hallucis longus	Tibial n.						▩		
		Peroneus longus	Superficial peroneal n.								
		Tibialis posterior	Tibial n.								
	INVERSION	Tibialis anterior	Deep peroneal n.					▩			
		Tibialis posterior	Tibial n.								
	EVERSION	Peroneus longus	Superficial peroneal n.								
		Peroneus tertius	Deep peroneal n.								
		Peroneus brevis	Superficial peroneal n.								
TOES	FLEXION	Flexor digitorum longus	Tibial n.						▩		
		Flexor hallucis longus	Tibial n.						▩		
		Flexor hallucis brevis	Medial plantar n.								
		Flexor digitorum brevis	Medial plantar n.								
		Flexor digitorum accessorius	Lateral plantar n.								
		Flexor digiti minimi brevis	Lateral plantar n.								
		Abductor hallucis	Medial plantar n.								
		Abductor digiti minimi	Lateral plantar n.								
		Lumbricals	Medial & lateral plantar nn.								
	EXTENSION	Extensor digitorum longus	Deep peroneal n.					▩			
		Extensor hallucis longus	Deep peroneal n.								
		Extensor digitorum brevis	Deep peroneal n.								
	ABDUCTION	Abductor hallucis	Medial plantar n.								
		Abductor digiti minimi	Lateral plantar n.								
		Dorsal interossei	Lateral plantar n.								
	ADDUCTION	Plantar interossei	Lateral plantar n.								
		Adductor hallucis	Lateral plantar n.								

1415

Table 110.1 complements the mainly topographical description of muscles in Chapters 111–115 by bringing together information about the innervation and functions of the muscles of the lower limb. To achieve this, some simplification has been necessary. **Movements.** At the central nervous level of control, muscles are not recognized as individual actuators but as components of movement. Muscles may contribute to several types of movement, acting variously as prime movers, antagonists, fixators or synergists. A muscle that crosses two joints can produce more than one movement, and one or other of these functions may be emphasized when the proximal and distal attachments are fixed by the action of gravity or other muscles. Even a muscle that acts across one joint can produce a combination of movements, such as flexion with medial rotation, or extension with adduction, and some muscles have therefore been included in more than one place in the table. **Nerve roots.** The spinal roots listed as contributing to the innervation of muscles varies in different texts: this is a reflection of the often unreliable nature of the information available. The most positive identifications have been obtained by stimulating spinal roots electrically, and recording the evoked electromyographic activity in the muscles. However, this is a laborious process, and data of this quality are in limited supply. Much of the information in the table is based on neurological experience gained in examining the effects of lesions, and some of it is far from new. **Major and minor contributions.** Spinal roots have been given the same shading when they innervate a muscle to a similar extent or when differences in their contribution have not been described. Heavy shading has been used to indicate roots from which there is known to be a dominant contribution. From a clinical viewpoint, some of these roots may be regarded as innervating the muscle almost exclusively. Minor contributions have been retained in the table in order to increase its utility in other contexts, such as electromyography and comparative anatomy. **Clinical testing.** For diagnostic purposes, it is neither necessary nor possible to test every muscle, and the experienced neurologist can cover every clinical possibility with a much shorter list. Red has been used to highlight those muscles or movements that have diagnostic value. The emphasis in these tables is on the differentiation of lesions at different root levels. The preferred criteria for including a given muscle on this list are that it is visible and palpable; that its action is isolated or can be isolated by the examiner; that it is innervated by one peripheral nerve or (predominantly) one root; that is has a clinically elicitable reflex; and that it is useful in differentiating between different nerves, roots or levels of lesion.

Table 110.2 Segmental innervation of the muscles of the lower limb

L1	Psoas major, psoas minor
L2	Psoas major, iliacus, sartorius, gracilis, pectineus, adductor longus, adductor brevis
L3	Quadriceps, adductors (magnus, longus, brevis)
L4	Quadriceps, tensor fasciae latae, adductor magnus, obturator externus, tibialis anterior, tibialis posterior
L5	Gluteus medius, gluteus minimus, obturator internus, semimembranosus, semitendinosus, extensor hallucis longus, extensor digitorum longus, peroneus tertius, popliteus
S1	Gluteus maximus, obturator internus, piriformis, biceps femoris, semitendinosus, popliteus, gastrocnemius, soleus, peronei (longus and brevis), extensor digitorum brevis
S2	Piriformis, biceps femoris, gastrocnemius, soleus, flexor digitorum longus, flexor hallucis longus, some intrinsic foot muscles
S3	Some intrinsic foot muscles (except abductor hallucis, flexor hallucis brevis, flexor digitorum brevis, extensor digitorum brevis)

Table 110.3 Segmental innervation of joint movements of the lower limb

Hip	Flexors, adductors, medial rotators	L1–3
	Extensors, abductors, lateral rotators	L5, S1
Knee	Extensors	L3,4
	Flexors	L5, S1
Ankle	Dorsiflexors	L4, 5
	Plantarflexors	S1, 2
Foot	Invertors	L4, 5
	Evertors	L5, S1
	Intrinsic muscles	S2, 3

Table 110.4 The movements and muscles tested to determine the location of a lesion in the lower limb

Movement	Muscle	Upper motor neurone	Root	Reflex	Nerve
Hip flexion	Iliopsoas	++	L1, 2		Femoral
Hip adduction	Adductors		L2, 3	(+)	Obturator
Hip extension	Gluteus maximus		L5, S1		Sciatic
Knee flexion	Hamstrings	+	S1		Sciatic
Knee extension	Quadriceps		L3, 4	++	Femoral
Ankle dorsiflexion	Tibialis anterior	++	L4		Deep peroneal
Ankle eversion	Peronei		L5, S1		Superficial peroneal
Ankle inversion	Tibialis posterior		L4, 5		Tibial
Ankle plantarflexion	Gastrocnemius/soleus		S1, 2	++	Tibial
Big toe extension	Extensor hallucis longus		L5	(Babinski reflex)	Deep peroneal

The muscles listed in the column Upper motor neurone are those which are preferentially affected in upper motor neurone lesions. The root level is the principal supply to a muscle.

Plantar reflex – The plantar reflex is a superficial reflex whose elicitation forms an important part of the clinical examination of the central nervous system. With the foot relaxed and warm, the outer edge of the sole is stroked longitudinally with a hard object (traditionally the examiner's nail or a key). This should elicit flexion of the toes, although the normal adult response varies with the strength of the stimulus. In adults with upper motor neurone lesions, the response includes extension of the great toe (Babinski's sign).

CLINICAL PROCEDURES

NERVE BLOCKS

Nerves can be effectively blocked with local anaesthetic injection for surgical or post-injury pain relief. The useful blocks in the lower limb are around the hip, for thigh and knee pain, and around the ankle, for foot surgery. For the deeper nerves around the hip, the use of a nerve stimulator needle is very helpful to localize the nerve precisely before infiltration of local anaesthetic. For example, to provide pain relief for total knee replacement, blockade of the sciatic nerve in the buttock, femoral nerve in the anterior groin, and obturator nerve in the medial groin, may be undertaken. To allow 'awake foot surgery' the posterior tibial nerve at the posteromedial ankle, the sural nerve at the posterolateral ankle and the superficial peroneal nerves at the anterior ankle, are blocked at the ankle.

DETERMINATION OF LOCATION OF A LESION

The principles of testing muscle innervation in clinical neurological examination are given on page 814. **Table 110.4** gives a list of movements and muscles of the lower limb chosen according to these principles. In practice, these tests would be combined with tests of sensory function.

INJECTION AND ASPIRATION

Intramuscular injection

Intramuscular injections into the buttock should be avoided, to prevent iatrogenic damage to the sciatic nerve. If the buttock is to be used, the safe area is the true upper and outer quadrant, which is identified with the whole buttock exposed. The injection is then given mainly into gluteus medius rather than into gluteus maximus, provided a sufficiently long needle is used: most so-called 'intramuscular' injections given into the buttock are actually given into the fat. A safe alternative is to inject into the lateral aspect of the thigh (vastus lateralis).

Joint injection and aspiration

Careful aseptic technique is essential for all joint aspirations and injections.

Hip joint – With the patient lying supine, and after the positions of the femoral artery and the anterior superior iliac spine have been marked out, the needle is introduced anteriorly c.5 cm distal to the anterior superior iliac spine and c.4 cm lateral to the femoral pulse, and passed posteriorly, a little proximally (cephalad), and medially.

Knee joint – The lateral retropatellar approach is used. With the patient supine and the knee extended, the needle is introduced at the level of the superior border of the patella and guided towards the suprapatellar pouch.

Ankle joint – The anterior approach entails introducing the needle between the tendons of tibialis anterior and extensor hallucis longus with the ankle partially plantar flexed, keeping the needle tangential to the curve of the talus.

ARTHROSCOPY PORTALS

The placement of portals for arthroscopy is critical, partly to maximize surgical access for visualization and for surgical instruments, but to also avoid damage to structures such as nerves and blood vessels. The knee is the joint most frequently examined in this way.

Knee

For the knee, the standard portals are anterior. When the knee is flexed at a right angle, 'soft triangles' bordered by the patellar tendon, the femoral condyles and the tibia and anterior horns of the menisci are palpable on either side of the superior third of the patellar tendon. Small 'stab' incisions can be made in the apices of these triangular areas at about the level of the inferior pole of the patella for the anterolateral portal, and slightly lower for the anteromedial portal. These portals will allow passage of an arthroscope and instruments, with good access to most of the joint. The fat pad is close by: passage through it will hamper the view and subsequent surgery. The patellar tendon and the infrapatellar branch of the saphenous nerve are at risk from the incisions. The nerve is less vulnerable than the tendon: its position is variable but it usually lies below the appropriate portal sites. However, in the days of open meniscal surgery, the nerve was usually divided and painful neuroma formation was not uncommon.

Posteromedial and posterolateral portals are useful when better access to the posterior knee is required. The saphenous and common peroneal nerves respectively are at risk with these approaches, and anatomical knowledge is vital to safe portal placement. Laterally the incision should be anterior to the tendon of biceps, which can easily be palpated. Medially the situation is more difficult because the saphenous nerve and vein run over the medial epicondylar region of the knee the breadth of the subject's hand posterior to the medial border of the patella. It is essential that sharp incision includes the skin only, and that dissection down to the joint capsule is undertaken bluntly. If the medial meniscus is sutured, the capsule must be exposed before tying off sutures to avoid ensnaring the nerve. In lateral meniscal repair a useful guide to avoid injury to the common peroneal nerve is never to allow needles or sutures to pass medial to the tendon of popliteus whilst viewing arthroscopically.

Hip

Hip arthroscopy is not yet a common procedure but is increasingly being used. There are a number of portals. The anterolateral portal is sited on the skin c.4 cm lateral to the femoral pulse and 4 cm inferior to the inguinal ligament. A needle traversing the skin 30–45° cephalad is passed under X-ray control into the joint. Once the synovial cavity is entered the 'vacuum' is lost and the joint can be distracted. Other more lateral portals can be used: the lateral cutaneous nerve of the thigh and the sciatic nerve are potentially at risk.

Ankle

The use of ankle arthroscopy is well established, especially in treating sports-related injuries. Anterior portals are standard. The anteromedial can be placed to pass just medial to the tendon of tibialis anterior, in the palpable soft spot. However, this comes close to the long saphenous vein and nerve: limiting the sharp incision to the skin, followed by blunt deeper dissection reduces the risk. Alternatively the anteromedial portal can be chosen to pass between the lateral edge of tibialis anterior and extensor hallucis longus. The anterolateral portal is placed with the help of the arthroscope in the joint to check the position of a preliminary needle passed into the joint. The portal should pass lateral to peroneus tertius and extensor digitorum longus. The intermediate dorsal cutaneous branch of the superficial peroneal nerve is at risk as it crosses the ankle anterior to the lateral malleolus, and therefore it is wise to ink in the nerves and blood vessels before making any incision. The nerves can be felt at the front of the ankle even in obese patients. They are often seen if the ankle is maximally pulled into plantarflexion and are seen to flick as the barrel of a pen is pulled across the front of the ankle. Posterior ankle arthroscopy is controversial: there is a view that the proximity of the neurovascular bundle (medially) and the sural nerve (laterally) renders it too hazardous. Keeping lateral to the tendon of flexor hallucis will safeguard the medial neurovascular bundle.

SURGICAL INCISIONS

Hip

Hip joint surgery is usually undertaken for paediatric problems, trauma, or arthroplasty in arthritis. Anterior and anterolateral approaches, often used in children, put the lateral cutaneous nerve of the thigh at considerable risk. Even in more lateral approaches, the lateral cutaneous nerve of the thigh and the femoral and sciatic nerves are all at risk through traction. A popular anterolateral approach to the hip joint involves splitting and separating forwards the anterior part of gluteus medius and vastus lateralis as a single sheet of tissue for subsequent reattachment to the greater trochanter. This technique relies on the anatomical continuity of the tissue. If the splitting of gluteus medius is more than a few centimetres superior to the tip of the greater trochanter then the superior gluteal nerve and vessels are at risk, and weakness of hip abduction and a limp may result.

Knee

Most open knee surgery can be undertaken through an anterior midline longitudinal incision, which gives good access and means that any future surgery can usually be undertaken via the same wound. New incisions run the risk of skin necrosis and poor wound healing as a consequence of interfering with the cutaneous blood supply. Inevitable interruption of the cutaneous nerves, including the infrapatellar branch of the saphenous nerve, means that there is always numbness lateral to a longitudinal incision.

The extensile approach to the posterior knee is extensive. The key is to expose the sural nerve and short saphenous vein and to trace them proximally. This will lead the surgeon into the popliteal fossa and, after opening the deep fascia, safely to the neurovascular bundle. The wound crosses a flexure crease. A scar perpendicular to the crease might induce a fixed flexion contracture of the joint and therefore, as at the anterior elbow, an S-shaped incision is employed where the transverse segment runs in the line of the flexure crease.

Foot and ankle

Incisions around the foot and ankle frequently put cutaneous nerves at risk: such an injury can cause a distressing painful neuroma. The sural nerve at the ankle has a notorious tendency to form neuromas, often after repair of a ruptured calcaneal tendon. Bunion surgery is also problematic and can be undertaken through an internervous plane with a dorsomedial incision over the first metatarsophalangeal joint, rather than the traditional dorsal approach.

REFERENCES

Cormack GC, Lamberty BGH 1994 See Bibliography.

Crock HV 1996 Atlas of Vascular Anatomy of the Skeleton and Spinal Cord. London: Martin Dunitz.

Dodd H, Cockett FB 1976 The Pathology and Surgery of the Veins of the Lower Limb, 2nd edn. Edinburgh: Churchill Livingstone.

Kosinski C 1926 Observations on the superficial venous system of the lower extremity. J Anat 60: 131–42.

Sharrard WJW 1955 The distribution of the permanent paralysis in the lower limb in poliomyelitis; a clinical and pathological study. J Bone Joint Surg Br 37-B(4): 540–58.

Taylor GI, Razaboni RM (eds) 1994 Michel Salmon: Anatomic Studies, Book 1. Arteries of the Muscles of the Extremities and Trunk. St. Louis: Quality Medical Publishing.

Pelvic girdle, gluteal region and hip joint

The term pelvic girdle is usually taken to be synonymous with a single 'innominate bone', though a girdle in other contexts is a complete ring. This implies that the human pelvis includes two pelvic girdles. Functionally it is more rational to consider a single pelvic 'girdle', which consists of the two innominate bones and the sacrum (strictly a part of the vertebral column). This strong pelvic girdle is virtually incapable of independent movement except during parturition in the female. It provides a weightbearing and protective structure, an attachment for trunk and limb muscles, and the skeletal framework of the birth canal. It is also best considered as a complete ring in the assessment of bony injuries.

The gluteal region or buttock is an area encompassed by the gluteal fold inferiorly, a line joining the greater trochanter and the anterior superior iliac spine laterally, the iliac crest superiorly and the midline medially. It consists of a large bulk of skeletal muscle covering large and vulnerable neurovascular structures, and incorporates junctional (transitional) zones between the limb, pelvis and perineum at the sciatic foramina. Direct and indirect musculoskeletal injuries may entail damage to the sciatic nerve and gluteal vessels.

The mobile yet very stable hip joint is deeply placed and well protected, but has important anatomical relations, especially anteriorly and posteriorly, which should be borne in mind during the management of trauma and degenerative arthritis, which commonly affect this joint. Its posterior relations lie in the gluteal region; anteriorly lies the junctional zone between pelvis and limb. This pelvicrural 'foramen', which lies between the inguinal ligament anteriorly and the pubis and ilium posteriorly, transmits numerous structures between the anterior thigh and pelvis.

SKIN

See also page 1399.

VASCULAR SUPPLY AND LYMPHATIC DRAINAGE
Most of the skin of the buttock is supplied by musculocutaneous perforating vessels from the superior and inferior gluteal arteries. There are also small peripheral contributions from similar branches of the internal pudendal, iliolumbar, sacral, and first (profunda) perforating arteries. The arterial supply of the skin of the upper thigh is described on page 1461. For further detail consult Cormack and Lamberty (1994).

Cutaneous veins are tributaries of vessels that correspond to the named arteries. Cutaneous lymphatic drainage is to the superficial inguinal nodes.

INNERVATION/DERMATOMES
See page 1399.

SOFT TISSUE

FASCIA

Superficial fascia
The superficial fascia of the buttock is continuous superiorly with that over the low back, and contains a considerable quantity of coarse fat. The superficial fascia of the thigh consists, as elsewhere in the limbs, of loose areolar tissue containing a variable amount of fat. In some regions, particularly near the inguinal ligament, it splits into recognizable layers, between which may be found the branches of superficial vessels and nerves. It is thick in the inguinal region, where its two layers enclose

the superficial inguinal lymph nodes, long saphenous vein and other smaller vessels. Here the superficial layer is continuous with the abdominal superficial layer. The deep layer, a thin fibroelastic stratum, is most marked medial to the long saphenous vein and inferior to the inguinal ligament, and extends between the subcutaneous vessels and nerves and the deep fascia, with which it fuses a little below the ligament. (The line of fusion lies in the floor of the ventral flexure line of Holden or 'groove associated with the hip joint'.) This membranous fascia completes the saphenous opening, blending with its circumference and with the femoral sheath. Over the opening it is perforated by the long saphenous vein, by the superficial branches of the femoral artery except the superficial circumflex iliac (which perforates the fascia lata separately), and lymphatic vessels, hence the term cribriform fascia (Latin *cribrum* = a sieve).

Deep fascia
The deep fascia covering the gluteal muscles varies in thickness. Over maximus it is thin, but over the anterior two-thirds of medius it forms the thick, strong gluteal aponeurosis. This is attached to the lateral border of the iliac crest superiorly, and splits anteriorly to enclose tensor fasciae latae and posteriorly to enclose gluteus maximus (p. 1444).

Fascia lata
The fascia lata, the wide deep fascia of the thigh, is thicker in the proximal and lateral parts of the thigh where tensor fasciae latae and an expansion from gluteus maximus are attached to it. It is thin posteriorly and over the adductor muscles, but thicker around the knee, where it is strengthened by expansions from the tendon of biceps femoris laterally, sartorius medially, and quadriceps femoris anteriorly. The fascia lata is attached superiorly and posteriorly to the back of the sacrum and coccyx, laterally to the iliac crest, anteriorly to the inguinal ligament and superior ramus of the pubis, and medially to the inferior ramus of the pubis, the ramus and tuberosity of the ischium, and the lower border of the sacrotuberous ligament. From the iliac crest it descends as a dense layer over gluteus medius to the upper border of gluteus maximus, where it splits into two layers, one passing superficial and the other deep to the muscle, to reunite at its lower border.

Iliotibial tract
Over the flattened lateral surface of the thigh, the fascia lata thickens to form a strong band, the iliotibial tract. The upper end of the tract splits into two layers, where it encloses and anchors tensor fasciae latae and receives, posteriorly, most of the tendon of gluteus maximus. The superficial layer ascends lateral to tensor fasciae latae to the iliac crest; the deeper layer passes up and medially, deep to the muscle, and blends with the lateral part of the capsule of the hip joint. Distally, the iliotibial tract is attached to a smooth, triangular, anterolateral facet on the lateral condyle of the tibia (Gerdy's tubercle) where it is superficial to and blends with an aponeurotic expansion from vastus lateralis. When the leg is extended it stands out as a strong, visible ridge on the anterolateral aspect of the knee.

Distally, the fascia lata is attached to all exposed bony points around the knee joint, such as the condyles of the femur and tibia, and the head of the fibula. On each side of the patella the deep fascia is reinforced by transverse fibres, which attach the vasti to it. The stronger lateral fibres are continuous with the iliotibial tract.

Intermuscular septa
The fascia lata is continuous with two intermuscular septa, which are attached to the whole of the linea aspera and its prolongations above

and below. The lateral, stronger septum, which extends from the attachment of gluteus maximus to the lateral condyle, lies between vastus lateralis in front and the short head of biceps femoris behind and provides partial attachment for them. The medial, weaker septum lies between vastus medialis and the adductors and pectineus. Numerous smaller septa, such as that separating the thigh adductors and flexors, pass between the individual muscles, ensheathing them and sometimes providing partial attachment for their fibres.

SAPHENOUS OPENING (Fig. 111.1)

The saphenous opening is an aperture in the deep fascia, lateral and a little distal to the medial part of the inguinal ligament, which allows passage to the long saphenous vein and other smaller vessels. The cribriform fascia, which is pierced by these structures, fills in the aperture and must be removed to reveal it. Adjacent subsidiary openings may exist to transmit venous tributaries, but these openings are more usually in the floor of the fossa. In the adult the approximate centre of the opening is c.3 cm inferior and 3 cm lateral to the pubic tubercle. It varies considerably in size, with a height of 1.5–9 cm and a width of 1–4 cm. The fascia lata in this part of the thigh displays superficial and deep strata (not to be confused with the superficial and deep layers of the superficial fascia described above). They lie respectively anterior and posterior to the femoral sheath; the somewhat spiral circumference of the saphenous opening is formed where the two are in continuity.

The superficial stratum, lateral and superior to the saphenous opening, is attached to the crest and anterior superior spine of the ilium, to the whole length of the inguinal ligament, and to the pecten pubis together with the lacunar ligament. It is reflected inferolaterally from the pubic tubercle as the arched falciform margin, which forms the superior, lateral and inferior boundaries of the saphenous opening: this margin adheres to the anterior layer of the femoral sheath, and the cribriform fascia is attached to it. The falciform margin is considered to have superior and inferior cornua. The inferior cornu is well defined, and is continuous behind the long saphenous vein with the deep stratum of the fascia lata.

The deep stratum is medial to the saphenous opening and is continuous with the superficial stratum at its lower margin. Traced upwards, it covers pectineus, adductor longus and gracilis, passes behind the femoral sheath, to which it is closely united, and continues to the pecten pubis.

FEMORAL SHEATH (Fig. 111.2)

The femoral sheath is formed by distal prolongations of the transversalis fascia anterior to the femoral vessels, and of the iliac fascia posteriorly, together forming a short funnel, wider proximally, its distal end fusing

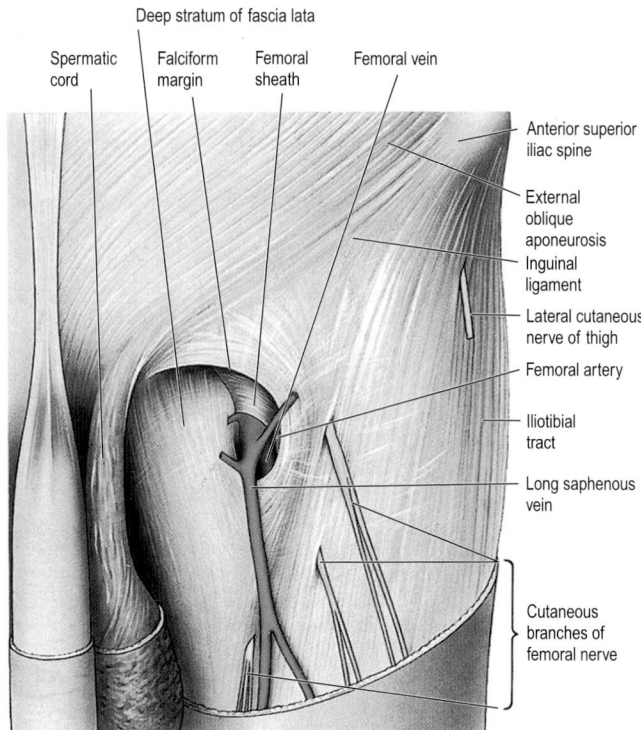

Fig. 111.1 The left saphenous opening, after removal of the cribriform fascia.

with the vascular fascia 3 or 4 cm distal to the ligament. At birth the sheath is shorter; it elongates when extension at the hips becomes habitual. The femoral branch of the genitofemoral nerve perforates its vertical lateral wall. The medial wall slopes laterally and is pierced by the long (great) saphenous vein and lymphatic vessels. Like the carotid sheath, the femoral sheath encloses a mass of connective tissue in which the vessels are embedded. Three compartments are described: a lateral one containing the femoral artery, an intermediate one for the femoral vein, and most medial and smallest, the femoral canal, which contains the lymph vessels and a lymph node embedded in areolar tissue. The presence of this canal allows the femoral vein to distend. The

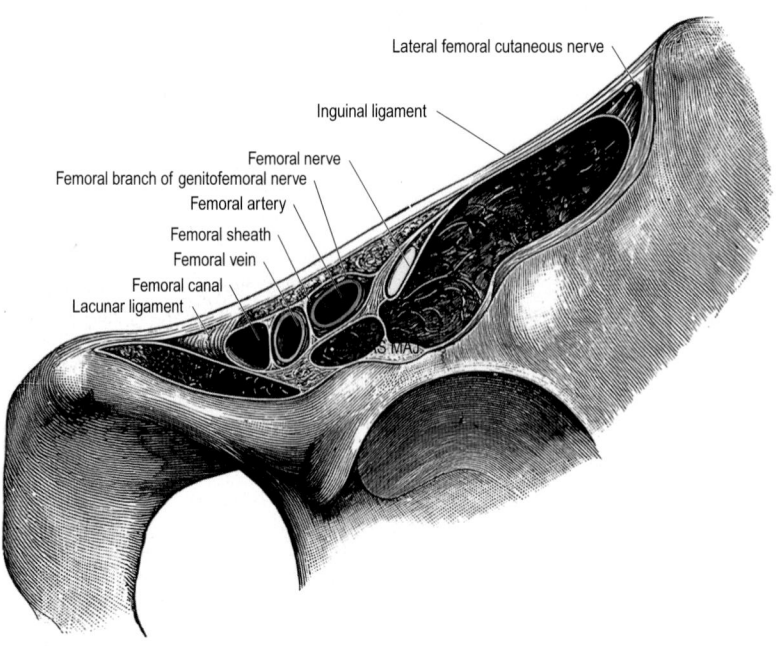

Fig. 111.2 Structures passing beneath the left inguinal ligament.

canal is conical, c.1.25 cm in length. Its proximal end is the outer femoral ring, bounded in front by the inguinal ligament, behind by pectineus and its fascia, medially by the crescentic edge of the lacunar ligament and laterally by the femoral vein. The spermatic cord, or the round ligament, is just above its anterior margin, while the inferior epigastric vessels are near its anterolateral rim. It is larger in women than in men: this is due partly to the greater breadth of the pelvis and partly to the smaller size of the femoral vessels in women. The ring is filled by condensed extraperitoneal tissue, the femoral septum, covered by the parietal peritoneum. The femoral septum is traversed by numerous lymph vessels that connect the deep inguinal to the external iliac lymph nodes.

Femoral hernia
Femoral hernia is described with other groin hernias on page 1111.

FEMORAL TRIANGLE
The femoral triangle is a depressed area of the thigh lying distal to the inguinal fold. Its apex is distal, its limits are the medial margin of sartorius laterally, the medial margin of adductor longus medially and the inguinal ligament proximally (the base). Its floor is provided laterally by iliacus and psoas major, medially by pectineus and adductor longus. The femoral vessels, passing from midbase to apex, are in the deepest part of the triangle. Lateral to the artery the femoral nerve divides. The triangle also contains fat and lymph nodes.

BURSAE RELATED TO GLUTEUS MAXIMUS
There are three bursae deep to gluteus maximus: the trochanteric, over the greater trochanter; the gluteofemoral, between the tendon of gluteus maximus and that of vastus lateralis; and the ischiofemoral, over the gluteal tuberosity, which is less commonly present.

OBTURATOR MEMBRANE (Fig. 111.3)
The obturator membrane is a thin aponeurosis that closes (obturates) most of the obturator foramen, leaving a superolateral aperture, the obturator canal, through which the obturator vessels and nerve leave the pelvis and enter the thigh. The membrane is attached to the sharp margin of the obturator foramen except at its inferolateral angle, where it is fixed to the pelvic surface of the ischial ramus, i.e. internal to the foramen. Its fibres are arranged mainly transversely in interlacing bundles;

the uppermost bundle, which is attached to the obturator tubercles, completes the obturator canal. The two surfaces of the obturator membrane provide attachment for the two obturator muscles, internus and externus, and some fibres of the pubofemoral ligament of the hip joint are attached to the external surface.

BONE

INNOMINATE BONE (Figs 111.4, 111.5)

Topography
The innominate or hip bone is large, irregular, constricted centrally and expanded above and below. Its lateral surface has a deep, cup-shaped acetabulum, articulating with the femoral head, anteroinferior to which is the large, oval or triangular obturator foramen. Above the acetabulum the bone widens into a plate with a sinuously curved iliac crest.

The bone articulates in front with its fellow to form the pelvic girdle. Each has three parts, ilium, ischium and pubis, connected by cartilage in youth but united as one bone in adults. The principal union is in the acetabulum. The ilium includes the upper acetabulum and expanded area above it; the ischium includes the lower acetabulum and bone posteroinferior to it; the pubis forms the anterior acetabulum, separating the ilium from ischium, and the anterior median region where the pubes meet.

Acetabulum (Fig. 111.6)
The acetabulum is an approximately hemispherical cavity central on the lateral aspect of the innominate bone, facing anteroinferiorly and surrounded by an irregular margin deficient inferiorly at the acetabular notch. The acetabular fossa forms the central floor and is rough and non-articular. The articular lunate surface is widest above (the 'dome'), where weight is transmitted to the femur. Fractures through this region therefore often lead to poor outcomes. All three innominate elements contribute to the acetabulum, but unequally. The pubis forms the antero-superior fifth of the articular surface, the ischium forms the floor of the fossa and rather more than the posteroinferior two-fifths of the articular surface, and the ilium forms the remainder. A linear defect may cross the acetabular surface from the superior border to the acetabular fossa, but does not follow any junction between the main morphological parts of the innominate bone.

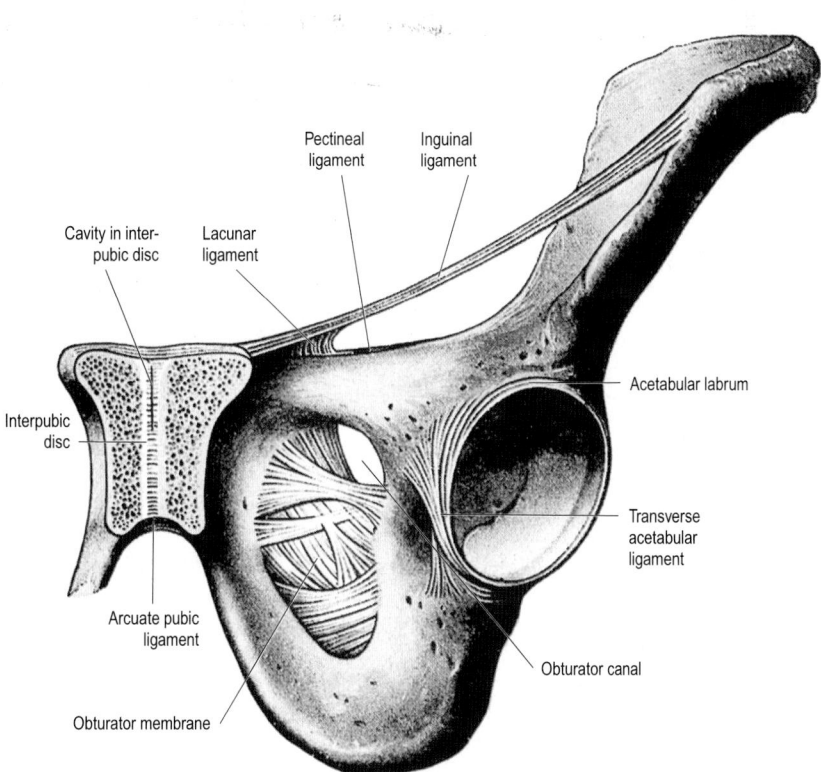

Fig. 111.3 Oblique coronal section showing the left obturator membrane.

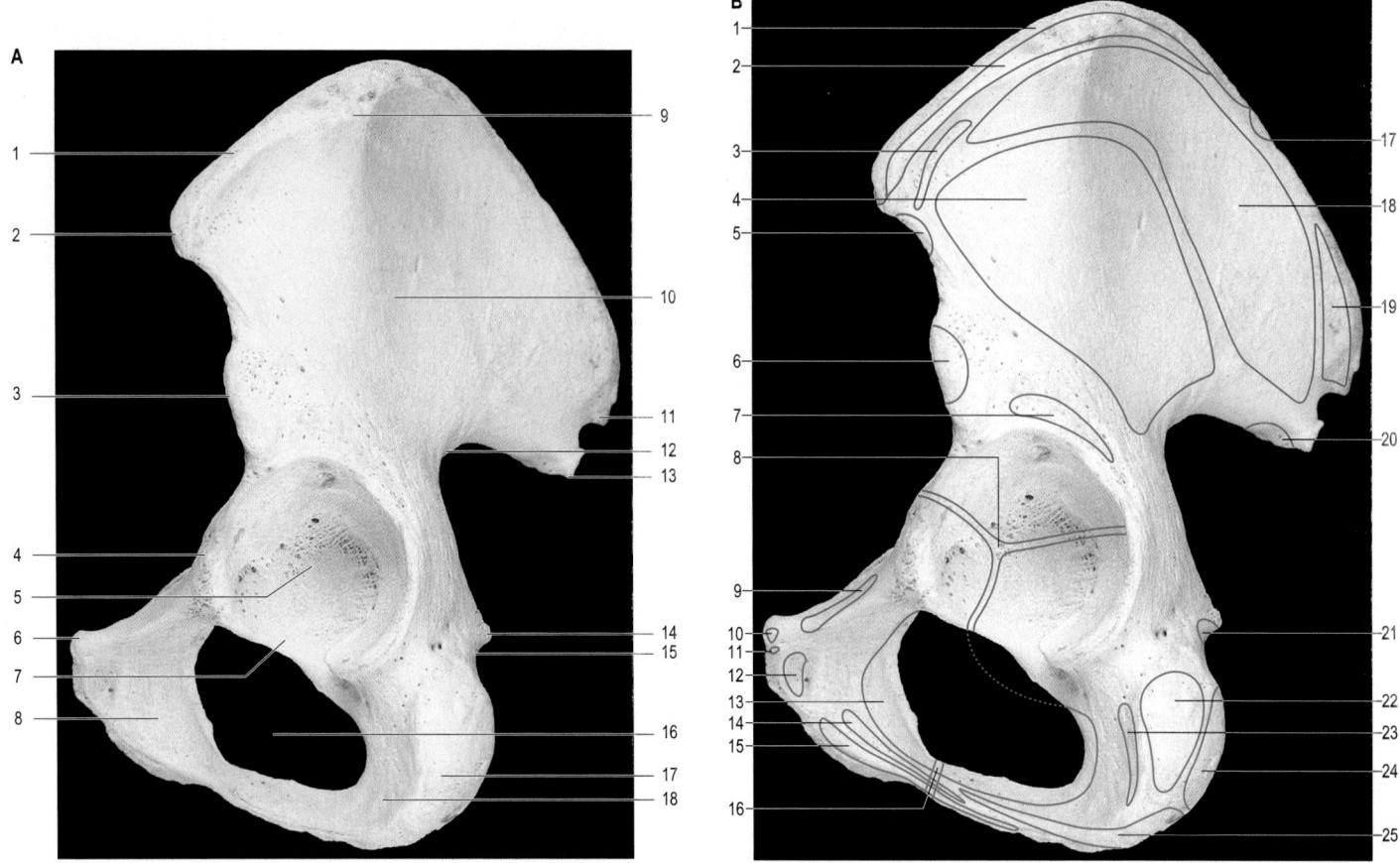

Part A: **1.** Iliac crest. **2.** Anterior superior iliac spine. **3.** Anterior inferior iliac spine. **4.** Iliopubic (iliopectineal) eminence. **5.** Acetabulum. **6.** Pubic tubercle. **7.** Acetabular notch. **8.** Pubis. **9.** Tubercle of iliac crest. **10.** Ilium. **11.** Posterior superior iliac spine. **12.** Greater sciatic notch. **13.** Posterior inferior iliac spine. **14.** Ischial spine. **15.** Lesser sciatic notch. **16.** Obturator foramen. **17.** Ischial tuberosity. **18.** Ischium.

Part B: **1.** Internal oblique. **2.** External oblique. **3.** Tensor fasciae latae. **4.** Gluteus minimus. **5.** Sartorius. **6.** Rectus femoris, straight head. **7.** Rectus femoris, reflected head. **8.** Junction between ilium, pubis and ischium. **9.** Pectineus. **10.** Rectus abdominis, lateral head. **11.** Pyramidalis. **12.** Adductor longus. **13.** Obturator externus. **14.** Adductor brevis. **15.** Gracilis. **16.** Junction between pubis and ischium. **17.** Latissimus dorsi. **18.** Gluteus medius. **19.** Gluteus maximus. **20.** Piriformis. **21.** Gemellus superior. **22.** Semimembranosus. **23.** Quadratus femoris. **24.** Biceps femoris and semitendinosus. **25.** Adductor magnus.

Fig. 111.4 Left innominate bone, external aspect. **B,** The muscle attachments. (Photographs by Sarah-Jane Smith.)

Obturator foramen

The obturator foramen lies below and slightly anterior to the acetabulum, between the pubis and ischium. It is bordered above by the grooved obturator surface of the superior pubic ramus, medially by the pubic body and its inferior ramus, below by the ischial ramus, and laterally by the anterior border of the ischial body, including the margin of the acetabular notch. The foramen is almost closed by the obturator membrane (p. 1421), which is attached to its margins, except above, where a communication remains between the pelvis and thigh. This free edge is attached to an anterior obturator tubercle at the anterior end of the inferior border of the superior pubic ramus, and a posterior obturator tubercle on the anterior border of the acetabular notch; these tubercles are sometimes indistinct. Since the tubercles lie in different planes and the obturator groove crosses the upper border of the foramen, the acetabular rim is in fact a spiral. The foramen is large and oval in males, but smaller and nearly triangular in females.

Structure

The thicker parts of the innominate bone are trabecular, encased by two layers of compact bone, while the thinner parts, as in the acetabulum and central iliac fossa, are often translucent and consist of one lamina of compact bone. In the upper acetabulum and along the arcuate line, i.e. the route of weight transmission from the sacrum to the femur, the amount of compact bone is increased and the subjacent trabecular bone displays two sets of pressure lamellae. These start together near the upper auricular surface and diverge to impinge on two strong buttresses of compact bone, from which two similar sets of lamellar arches start and converge on the acetabulum. The anterior iliac crest has been much studied as regards distribution of cortical and trabecular bone.

Whitehouse (1977) has surveyed these studies: his own observations, by scanning electron micrography, indicate that the cortical bone is very porous, being only 75% bone, decreasing to 35% near the anterior superior iliac spine. Denser cortical bone starts at the margins of the crest and thickens rapidly below it on both aspects of the iliac blade.

Studies of the internal stresses within the innominate have revealed a systemic pattern of trabeculae that corresponds well with the expected patterns of theoretical stress trajectories (Holm 1980), though the patterns are much more complicated than in any other major bone. Stresses are higher in the acetabular than in the iliac region. In the ilium, stresses on the pelvic surface are much less than those on the gluteal surface.

Muscle attachments

See individual bones.

Vascular supply

In the infant, nutrient arteries are clearly demonstrable for each component of the innominate bone. Each nutrient artery branches in fan-like fashion within its bone of supply (Crock 1996). Later, a periosteal arterial network develops, with contributions from numerous local arteries (see under individual bones).

Innervation

A periosteal network receives contributions from local nerves which supply muscles attaching to the periosteum and the joints in which the innominate bone is involved. Autonomic nerves accompany nutrient arteries and branch within the bone.

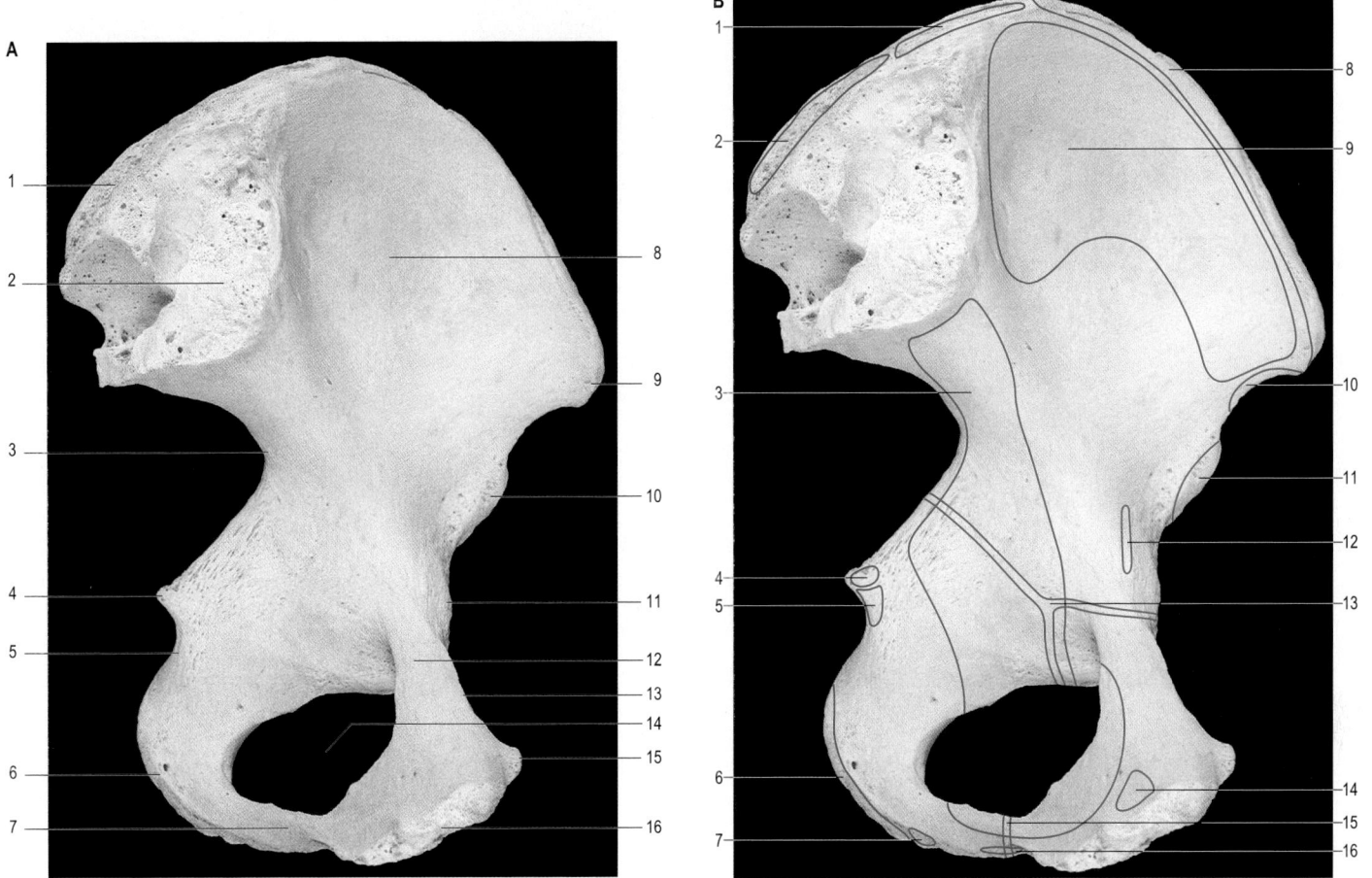

Part A: **1.** Iliac tuberosity. **2.** Auricular surface. **3.** Greater sciatic notch. **4.** Ischial spine. **5.** Lesser sciatic notch. **6.** Ischial tuberosity. **7.** Ischiopubic (inferior pubic) ramus. **8.** Iliac fossa. **9.** Anterior superior iliac spine. **10.** Anterior inferior iliac spine. **11.** Iliopubic (iliopectineal) eminence. **12.** Superior pubic ramus. **13.** Pecten pubis. **14.** Obturator foramen. **15.** Pubic tubercle. **16.** Symphyseal surface.

Part B: **1.** Quadratus lumborum. **2.** Erector spinae. **3.** Obturator internus. **4.** Coccygeus. **5.** Levator ani. **6.** Sacrotuberous ligament. **7.** Transversus perinei superficialis. **8.** Transversus abdominis. **9.** Iliacus. **10.** Sartorius. **11.** Rectus femoris. **12.** Psoas minor. **13.** Junction between ilium, ischium and pubis (triradiate cartilage). **14.** Levator ani. **15.** Junction between ischium and pubis. **16.** Sphincter urethrae.

Fig. 111.5 Left innominate bone, internal (pelvic) aspect. **B**, The muscle attachments. (Photographs by Sarah-Jane Smith.)

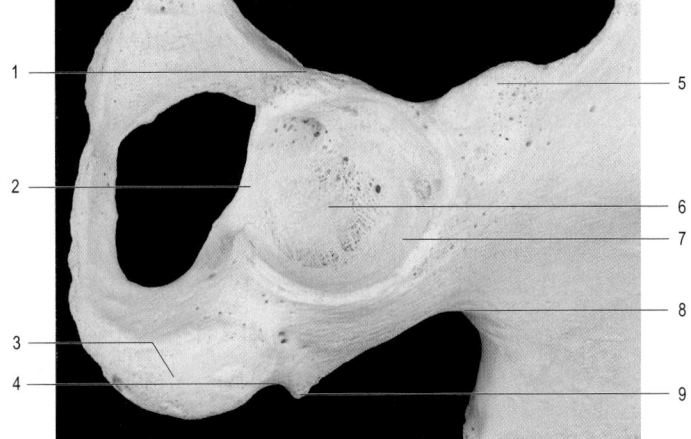

1. Iliopubic eminence. **2.** Acetabular notch. **3.** Ischial tuberosity. **4.** Lesser sciatic notch. **5.** Anterior inferior iliac spine. **6.** Acetabular fossa. **7.** Lunate (articular) surface. **8.** Greater sciatic notch. **9.** Ischial spine.

Fig. 111.6 Left acetabulum. (Photograph by Sarah-Jane Smith.)

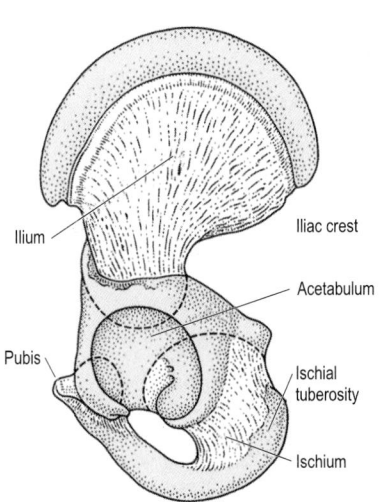

Fig. 111.7 The innominate bone at birth. Blue = unossified (cartilaginous) regions.

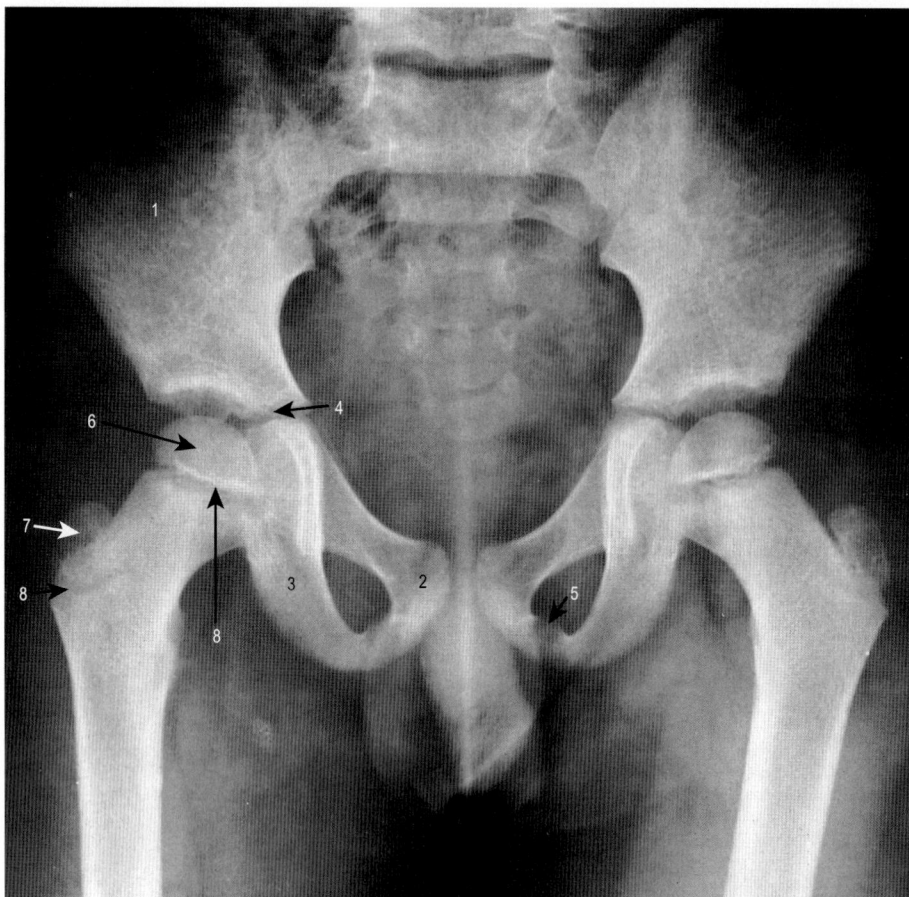

1. Ilium.
2. Pubis.
3. Ischium.
4. Part of triradiate growth cartilage.
5. Cartilage between pubic and ischial rami.
6. Superior femoral epiphysis.
7. Ossifying greater trochanter.
8. Cartilaginous growth plates.

Fig. 111.8 Anteroposterior radiograph of the pelvis of a boy aged 7.

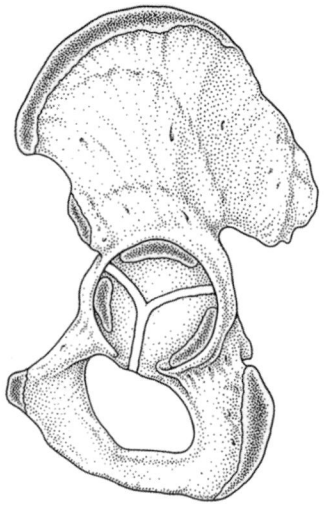

Fig. 111.9 The adolescent innominate bone. More heavily stippled areas indicate the secondary centres of ossification. Blue = unossified (cartilaginous) regions.

Ossification (Figs 111.7, 111.8, 111.9)

Ossification is by three primary centres, one each for the ilium, ischium and pubis. The iliac centre appears above the greater sciatic notch prenatally at about the ninth week, the ischial centre in its body in the fourth month, and the pubic centre in its superior ramus between the fourth and fifth months. At birth the whole iliac crest, the acetabular floor and inferior margin are still cartilaginous. The acetabulum is still a cartilaginous cup with a triradiate stem extending medially to the pelvic surface as a Y-shaped epiphyseal plate between the ilium, ischium and pubis, and including the anterior inferior iliac spine. Cartilage along the inferior margin also covers the ischial tuberosity, forms con-

joined ischial and pubic rami, and continues to the pubic symphyseal surface and along the pubic crest to its tubercle.

The ossifying ischium and pubis fuse to form a continuous body ramus at the seventh or eighth year. Secondary centres, other than for the acetabulum, appear about puberty and fuse between the fifteenth and twenty-fifth years. There are usually two for the iliac crest (which rapidly fuse), and single centres for the ischial tuberosity (in cartilage close to the inferior acetabular margin and spreading forwards), anterior inferior iliac spine (although it may ossify from the triradiate cartilage), and symphyseal surface of the pubis (the pubic tubercle and crest may have separate centres). Progression of the ossification of the iliac crest in girls is a useful guide to skeletal maturity and helps the timing of surgery for spinal deformity.

Between the ages of 8 and 9 years three major centres of ossification appear in the acetabular cartilage. The largest appears in the anterior wall of the acetabulum and fuses with the pubis, the second in the iliac acetabular cartilage superiorly, fusing with the ilium, and the third in the ischial acetabular cartilage posteriorly, fusing with the ischium. At puberty these epiphyses expand towards the periphery of the acetabulum and contribute to its depth (Ponseti 1978). Fusion between the three bones within the acetabulum occurs between the sixteenth and eighteenth years. Delaere et al (1992) have suggested that ossification of the ilium is similar to that of a long bone, possessing three cartilaginous epiphyses and one cartilaginous process, although it tends to undergo osteoclastic resorption comparable with that of cranial bones. During development the acetabulum increases in breadth at a faster rate than it does in depth.

Avulsion fractures of pelvic apophyses may occur from excessive pull on tendons, usually in athletic adolescents. The most frequent injuries are to the ischial tuberosity (hamstrings) and anterior inferior iliac spine (rectus femoris).

PUBIS (Figs 111.4, 111.5)

Topography

The pubis is the ventral part of the innominate bone and forms a median cartilaginous pubic symphysis with its fellow. From its anteromedial body a superior ramus passes up and back to the acetabulum and an inferior ramus passes back, down and laterally to join the ischial ramus inferomedial to the obturator foramen.

The body, anteroposteriorly compressed, has anterior, posterior and symphyseal (medial) surfaces and an upper border, the pubic crest. The anterior surface also faces inferolaterally; it is rough superomedially and smooth elsewhere, giving attachment to medial femoral muscles. The smooth posterior surface faces upwards and backwards as the oblique anterior wall of the lesser pelvis and is related to the urinary bladder. The symphyseal surface is elongated and oval, united by cartilage to its fellow at the pubic symphysis. Denuded of cartilage it has an irregular surface of small ridges and furrows or nodular elevations, varying considerably with age, features which are of forensic value. The pubic crest is the rounded upper border of the body which overhangs the anterior surface; its lateral end is the rounded pubic tubercle. Both crest and tubercle are palpable, the latter partly obscured in males by the spermatic cord that crosses above it from the scrotum to the abdomen. The pubic rami diverge posterolaterally from the lateral corners of the body.

The anterior surface of the pubic body faces the femoral adductor region. The anterior pubic ligament attaches to its medial part and to a rough strip, which is wider in females. The posterior surface is separated from the urinary bladder by retropubic fat. The puboprostatic ligaments are attached medial to levator ani.

Superior pubic ramus

The superior pubic ramus passes upwards, backwards and laterally from the body, superolateral to the obturator foramen, to reach the acetabulum. It is triangular in section and has three surfaces and borders. Its anterior, pectineal surface, tilted slightly up, is triangular in outline and extends from the pubic tubercle to the iliopubic eminence. It is bounded in front by the rounded obturator crest and behind by the sharp pecten pubis (pectineal line) which, with the crest, is the pubic part of the linea terminalis (i.e. anterior part of the pelvic brim). The posterosuperior, pelvic surface, medially inclined, is smooth and narrows into the posterior surface of the body, which is bounded above by the pecten pubis and below by a sharp inferior border. The obturator surface, directed down and back, is crossed by the obturator groove sloping down and forwards. Its anterior limit is the obturator crest and its posterior limit is the inferior border.

Inferior pubic ramus

The inferior pubic ramus, an inferolateral process of the body, descends inferolaterally to join the ischial ramus medial to, and below, the obturator foramen. The union may be locally thickened, but not obviously so in adults. The ramus has two surfaces and borders. The anteroexternal surface, continuous above with that of the pubic body, faces the thigh and is marked by muscles. It is limited laterally by the margin of the obturator foramen and, medially, by the rough anterior border. The posterointernal surface is continuous above with that of the body and is transversely convex: its medial part is often everted in males and connected to the crus of the penis. This surface faces the perineum medially, its smooth lateral part tilted up towards the pelvic cavity.

The internal surface is indistinctly divided into medial, intermediate and lateral areas. The medial area faces inferomedially in direct contact with the crus of the penis or clitoris and is limited above and behind by an indistinct ridge for attachment of the fascia overlying the superficial perineal muscles. The medial margin of the ramus, strongly everted in males, provides attachment for the fascia lata and the membranous layer of the superficial perineal fascia.

Pubic tubercle

The pubic tubercle provides a medial attachment for the inguinal ligament in the floor of the superficial inguinal ring and is crossed by the spermatic cord.

Pecten pubis

The pecten pubis is the sharp, superior edge of the pectineal surface. The conjoint tendon and lacunar ligament are attached at its medial end. A strong fibrous pectineal ligament is attached along the rest of its surface. The smooth pelvic surface is separated from parietal peritoneum only by areolar tissue, in which the lateral umbilical ligament descends forwards across the ramus and, laterally, the vas deferens passes backwards. The obturator groove, converted to a canal by the upper borders

of the obturator membrane and obturator muscles, transmits the obturator vessels and nerve from the pelvis to the thigh. Some fibres of the pubofemoral ligament are attached to the lateral end of the obturator crest.

Muscle attachments

The tendon of adductor longus is attached on the anterior surface of the body, in the angle between its upper end and the pubic crest. Below adductor longus, gracilis attaches to a line near the medial border extending down to the inferior ramus. Lateral to gracilis, adductor brevis is attached to the body and inferior ramus. Obturator externus is attached laterally to the anterior surface, spreading onto both rami.

Anterior fibres of levator ani are attached on the posterior surface of the body near its centre. More laterally, obturator internus is attached, extending onto both rami.

Pectineus is attached to the pectineal surface of the superior ramus along its upper part.

Gracilis, adductor brevis and obturator externus are attached in mediolateral order to the external surface of the inferior ramus. Adductor magnus usually extends from the ischial ramus on to the lower part of the inferior pubic ramus between adductor brevis and obturator externus. Some inner fibres of sphincter urethrae may be attached to the intermediate area of the internal surface, related to the dorsal nerve of the penis or clitoris, internal pudendal vessels and their fascial sheath. Fibres of obturator internus are attached to the lateral area.

Ascending loops of cremaster are attached to the pubic tubercle. Lateral to the tubercle, on the pubic crest, the lateral part of rectus abdominis and, below it, pyramidalis are attached. Medially the crest is crossed by the medial part of rectus abdominis, ascending from ligamentous fibres interlacing in front of the pubic symphysis.

Psoas minor, when present, is attached near the centre of the pecten pubis.

Vascular supply

The pubis is supplied by a periosteal anastomosis of branches from the obturator, inferior epigastric and medial circumflex femoral arteries. The superficial and deep external pudendal arteries may also contribute. Multiple vascular foramina are present, mainly at the lateral (acetabular) end of the bone, but there is no consistently placed nutrient foramen.

Innervation

The periosteum of the pubis is innervated by branches of nerves which supply muscles attached to the bone, the hip joint and the symphysis pubis.

Ossification

Ossification of the pubis is described on page 1421.

ILIUM (Figs 111.4, 111.5)

Topography

The ilium has upper and lower parts and three surfaces. The smaller, lower part forms a little less than the upper two-fifths of the acetabulum. The upper part is much expanded, and has gluteal, sacropelvic and iliac (internal) surfaces. The posterolateral gluteal surface is an extensive rough area; the anteromedial iliac fossa is smooth and concave; the sacropelvic surface is medial and posteroinferior to the fossa, from which it is separated by the medial border.

Iliac crest

The iliac crest is the superior border of the ilium, convex upwards but sinuously curved, internally concave in front, and convex behind. Its ends project as anterior and posterior superior iliac spines. The anterior superior iliac spine is palpable at the lateral end of the inguinal fold. The posterior superior iliac spine is not palpable but is often indicated by a dimple c.4 cm lateral to the second sacral spine above the medial gluteal region (buttock).

The lateral end of the inguinal ligament is attached to the anterior superior iliac spine.

The crest has ventral and dorsal segments: the ventral is slightly more than the anterior two-thirds of the crest and its prominence is associated with changes in iliac form as a result of the emergence of the upright posture; the dorsal segment, which occupies approximately the posterior third in man, exists in all land vertebrates. The ventral segment of the crest has internal and external lips; the rough intermediate zone is narrowest centrally. The tubercle of the crest projects onto the outer lip c.5 cm posterosuperior to the anterior superior spine. The dorsal segment has two sloping surfaces separated by a longitudinal ridge ending at the posterior superior spine. The summit of the crest, a little behind its midpoint, is level with the interval between the third and fourth lumbar spines. The interosseous and posterior sacroiliac ligaments arise from the medial margin of the dorsal segment.

Anterior border

The anterior border descends to the acetabulum from the anterior superior spine. Superiorly it is concave forwards. Inferiorly is a rough anterior inferior iliac spine, immediately above the acetabulum, which is divided indistinctly into an upper area for the straight part of rectus femoris and a lower area extending laterally along the upper acetabular margin to form a triangular impression for the iliofemoral ligament.

Posterior border

The posterior border is irregularly curved and descends from the posterior superior spine, at first forwards, with a posterior concavity forming a small notch. At the lower end of the notch is a wide, low projection, the posterior inferior iliac spine. Here the border turns almost horizontally forwards for c.3 cm then down and back to join the posterior ischial border. Together these borders form a deep greater sciatic notch, bounded above by the ilium and below by the ilium and ischium.

The upper fibres of the sacrotuberous ligament are attached to the upper part of the posterior border. The superior rim of the notch is related to the superior gluteal vessels and nerve. The lower part of the border (i.e. the lower margin of the greater sciatic notch) is covered by piriformis and related to the sciatic nerve, which, however, largely adjoins the ischium.

Medial border

The medial border separates the iliac fossa and the sacropelvic surface. It is indistinct near the crest, rough in its upper part, then sharp where it bounds an articular surface for the sacrum, and finally rounded. The latter part is the arcuate line, which inferiorly reaches the posterior part of the iliopubic (iliopectineal) eminence, marking the union of the ilium and pubis.

Gluteal surface

The gluteal surface, facing inferiorly in its posterior part and laterally and slightly downwards in front, is bounded above by the iliac crest, below by the upper acetabular border and by the anterior and posterior borders. It is rough and curved, convex in front, concave behind, and marked by three gluteal lines. The posterior gluteal line is shortest, descending from the external lip of the crest c.5 cm in front of its posterior limit and ending in front of the posterior inferior iliac spine. Above, it is usually distinct, but inferiorly it is ill-defined and frequently absent. The anterior gluteal line, the longest, begins near the midpoint of the superior margin of the greater sciatic notch and ascends forwards into the outer lip of the crest, a little anterior to its tubercle. The inferior gluteal line, rarely well-marked, begins posterosuperior to the anterior inferior iliac spine, curving posteroinferiorly to end near the apex of the greater sciatic notch. Between the inferior gluteal line and the acetabular margin is a rough, shallow groove. Behind the acetabulum the lower gluteal surface is continuous with the posterior ischial surface, the unions marked by a low elevation.

The articular capsule is attached to an area adjoining the acetabular rim, most of which is covered by gluteus minimus. Posteroinferiorly, near the union of the ilium and ischium, the bone is related to piriformis.

Iliac fossa

The iliac fossa, the internal concavity of the ilium, faces antero-superiorly. It is limited above by the iliac crest, in front by the anterior border and behind by the medial border, separating it from the sacropelvic surface. It forms the smooth and gently concave posterolateral wall of the greater pelvis. Below it is continuous with a wide shallow groove which is bounded laterally by the anterior inferior iliac spine and medially by the iliopubic eminence.

The wide groove between the anterior inferior iliac spine and iliopubic eminence is occupied by the converging fibres of iliacus laterally and the tendon of psoas major medially: the tendon is separated from bone by a bursa. The right iliac fossa contains the caecum, and often the vermiform appendix and terminal ileum. The left iliac fossa houses the end of the descending colon.

Sacropelvic surface

The sacropelvic surface, the posteroinferior part of the medial iliac surface, is bounded posteroinferiorly by the posterior border, antero-superiorly by the medial border, posterosuperiorly by the iliac crest and anteroinferiorly by the line of fusion of the ilium and ischium. It is divided into iliac tuberosity, auricular and pelvic surfaces. The iliac tuberosity, a large, rough area below the dorsal segment of the iliac crest, shows cranial and caudal areas separated by an oblique ridge and connected to the sacrum by the interosseous sacroiliac ligament. The sacropelvic surface gives attachment to the posterior sacroiliac ligaments and, behind the auricular surface, to the interosseous sacroiliac ligament. The iliolumbar ligament is attached to its anterior part. The auricular surface, immediately anteroinferior to the tuberosity, articulates with the lateral sacral mass. Shaped like an ear, its widest part is anterosuperior, its 'lobule' posteroinferior and on the medial aspect of the posterior inferior spine. Its edges are well defined, but the surface, though articular, is rough and irregular. It articulates with the sacrum and is reciprocally shaped. The anterior sacroiliac ligament is attached to its sharp anterior and inferior borders. The narrow part of the pelvic surface, between the auricular surface and the upper rim of the greater sciatic notch, often shows a rough preauricular sulcus for the lower fibres of the anterior sacroiliac ligament, more apparent in females. For the reliability of this feature as a sex discriminant see Finnegan (1978) and Brothwell and Pollard (2001). The pelvic surface is anteroinferior to the acutely recurved part of the auricular surface, contributing to the lateral wall of the lesser pelvis. Its upper part, facing down, is between the auricular surface and the upper limb of the greater sciatic notch. Its lower part faces medially and is separated from the iliac fossa by the arcuate line. Anteroinferiorly it extends to the line of union of the ilium and ischium. This is usually obliterated, but passes from the depth of the acetabulum to approximately the middle of the inferior limb of the greater sciatic notch.

Muscle attachments

The attachment of sartorius extends down the anterior border below the anterior superior spine.

The iliac crest gives attachment to lateral abdominal and dorsal muscles, and to fasciae and muscles of the lower limb. The fascia lata and iliotibial tract are attached to the outer lip and tubercle of its ventral segment. Tensor fasciae latae is attached anterior to the tubercle. The lower fibres of external oblique and, just behind the summit of the crest, the lowest fibres of latissimus dorsi are attached to its anterior two-thirds. A variable interval exists between the most posterior attachment of external oblique and the most anterior attachment of latissimus dorsi, and here the crest is the base of the lumbar triangle. Internal oblique is attached to the intermediate area of the crest. Transversus abdominis is attached to the anterior two-thirds of the inner lip of the crest, and behind this to the thoracolumbar fascia and quadratus lumborum. The highest fibres of gluteus maximus are attached to the dorsal segment of the crest on its lateral slope. Erector spinae arises from the medial slope of the dorsal segment. The straight part of rectus femoris is attached to the upper area of the anterior inferior spine. Some fibres of piriformis are attached in front of the posterior inferior spine on the upper border of the greater sciatic notch.

The gluteal surface is divided by three gluteal lines into four areas. Behind the posterior line, the upper rough part is for the attachment of the upper fibres of gluteus maximus and the lower, smooth region for part of the sacrotuberous ligament and iliac head of piriformis. Gluteus medius is attached between the posterior and anterior lines, below the iliac crest, and gluteus minimus is attached between the anterior and inferior lines. The fourth area, below the inferior line, contains vascular foramina.

The reflected head of rectus femoris attaches to a curved groove above the acetabulum.

Iliacus is attached to the upper two-thirds of the iliac fossa and is related to its lower third.

The medial part of quadratus lumborum is attached to the anterior part of the sacropelvic surface, above the iliolumbar ligament. Piriformis is sometimes partly attached lateral to the preauricular sulcus, and part of obturator internus is attached to the more extensive remainder of the pelvic surface.

Vascular supply
Branches of the iliolumbar artery run between iliacus and bone; one or more enter large nutrient foramina lying posteroinferiorly in the iliac fossa. The superior gluteal, obturator and superficial circumflex iliac arteries contribute to the periosteal supply. The obturator artery may supply a nutrient branch. Vascular foramina on the iliac gluteal aspect may lead into large vascular canals in the bone.

Innervation
The periosteum is innervated by branches of nerves which supply muscles attached to the bone, the hip joint and the sacroiliac joint.

Ossification
Ossification of the ilium is described on page 1421.

ISCHIUM (Figs 111.4, 111.5, 111.10)

Topography
The ischium, the inferoposterior part of the innominate bone, has a body and ramus. The body has upper and lower ends and femoral, posterior and pelvic surfaces. Above, it forms the inferoposterior part of the acetabulum; below, its ramus ascends anteromedially at an acute angle to meet the descending pubic ramus and complete the obturator foramen. The ischiofemoral ligament is attached to the lateral border below the acetabulum.

The femoral surface faces downwards, forwards and laterally towards the thigh. It is bounded in front by the margin of the obturator foramen. The lateral border, indistinct above but well defined below, forms the lateral limit of the ischial tuberosity. At a higher level the femoral surface is covered by piriformis, from which it is partially separated by the sciatic nerve and the nerve to quadratus femoris. The posterior surface, facing superolaterally, is continuous above with the iliac gluteal surface, and here a low convexity follows the acetabular curvature. Inferiorly, this surface forms the upper part of the ischial tuberosity, above which is a wide, shallow groove on its lateral and medial aspects. Above the ischial tuberosity the posterior surface is crossed by the tendon of obturator internus and the gemelli. The nerve to quadratus femoris lies between these structures and the bone. The ischial tuberosity

is a large, rough area on the lower posterior surface and inferior extremity of the ischium. Though obscured by gluteus maximus in hip extension, it is palpable in flexion. It is 5 cm from the midline and about the same distance above the gluteal fold. It is elongated, widest above, and tapers inferiorly. The ischial posterior aspect lies between the lateral and posterior borders. The posterior border blends above with that of the ilium, helping to complete the inferior rim of the greater sciatic notch, the posterior end of which has a conspicuous ischial spine. Below this, the rounded border forms the floor of the lesser sciatic notch, between the ischial spine and tuberosity. The pelvic surface is smooth and faces the pelvic cavity; inferiorly it forms part of the lateral wall of the ischiorectal fossa.

Ischial ramus
The ischial ramus has anteroinferior and posterior surfaces continuous with those of the inferior pubic ramus: the anteroinferior surface is roughened by the attachment of the medial femoral muscles. The smooth posterior surface is partly divided into perineal and pelvic areas, like the inferior pubic ramus. The upper border completes the obturator foramen; the rough lower border, together with the medial border of the inferior pubic ramus, bounds the subpubic angle and pubic arch.

The fascia overlying the superficial perineal muscles is attached below the ridge between the perineal and pelvic areas of the posterior surface of the ischial ramus. Above the ridge are areas for the attachment of the crus of the penis or clitoris and sphincter urethrae. The lower border of the ramus is an attachment for the fascia lata and a membranous layer of the superficial perineal fascia.

Ischial tuberosity
The ischial tuberosity is divided nearly transversely into upper and lower areas. The upper area is subdivided by an oblique line into a superolateral and an inferomedial part. The lower area, narrowing as it curves onto the inferior ischial aspect, is subdivided by an irregular vertical ridge into lateral and medial areas. The medial is covered by fibroadipose tissue, usually containing the ischial bursa of gluteus maximus, which supports the body in sitting. Medially the tuberosity is limited by a curved ridge passing on to the ramus, to which the sacrotuberous ligament and its falciform process are attached.

Ischial spine (Fig. 111.11)
The ischial spine projects downwards and a little medially. The sacrospinous ligament (p. 1439) is attached to its margins, separating the greater from the lesser sciatic foramen. The ligament is crossed posteriorly by the internal pudendal vessels and the nerve to obturator internus.

Muscle attachments
Part of obturator externus is attached to the lower femoral surface of the ischial body.

The anterior surface of the ischial ramus faces the adductor region. Obturator externus above, anterior fibres of adductor magnus and near the lower border, gracilis, are all attached here. Between adductor magnus and gracilis the attachment of adductor brevis may descend from the inferior pubic ramus. The posterior surface is divided into pelvic and perineal areas. The pelvic area, facing back, has part of obturator internus attached to it. The perineal area faces medially: its upper part is related to the crus of the penis or clitoris, and sphincter urethrae, ischiocavernosus and the transverse superficial perineal muscle are attached below this.

The ischial tuberosity gives attachment to the posterior femoral muscles. Quadratus femoris is attached along the upper part of its lateral border. The upper area of the tuberosity is subdivided by an oblique line into a superolateral part for semimembranosus and an inferomedial part for the long head of biceps femoris and semitendinosus. The lower area is subdivided by an irregular vertical ridge into lateral and medial areas. The larger lateral area is for part of adductor magnus.

Superomedial to the tuberosity the posterior surface has a wide, shallow groove, usually covered by hyaline cartilage, with a bursa between it and the tendon of obturator internus. Gemellus inferior is attached to the lower margin of the groove, near the tuberosity. Gemellus superior is attached to the upper margin, near the ischial spine.

The pelvic surface of the ischial spine gives attachment to coccygeus (coextensive with the sacrospinous ligament) and to the most posterior fibres of levator ani.

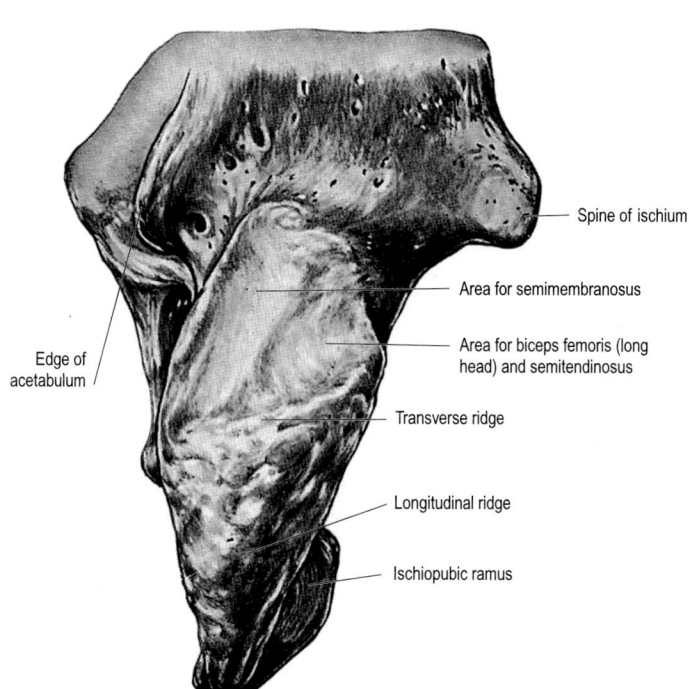

Spine of ischium

Area for semimembranosus

Area for biceps femoris (long head) and semitendinosus

Edge of acetabulum

Transverse ridge

Longitudinal ridge

Ischiopubic ramus

Fig. 111.10 The left ischial tuberosity: posterior aspect.

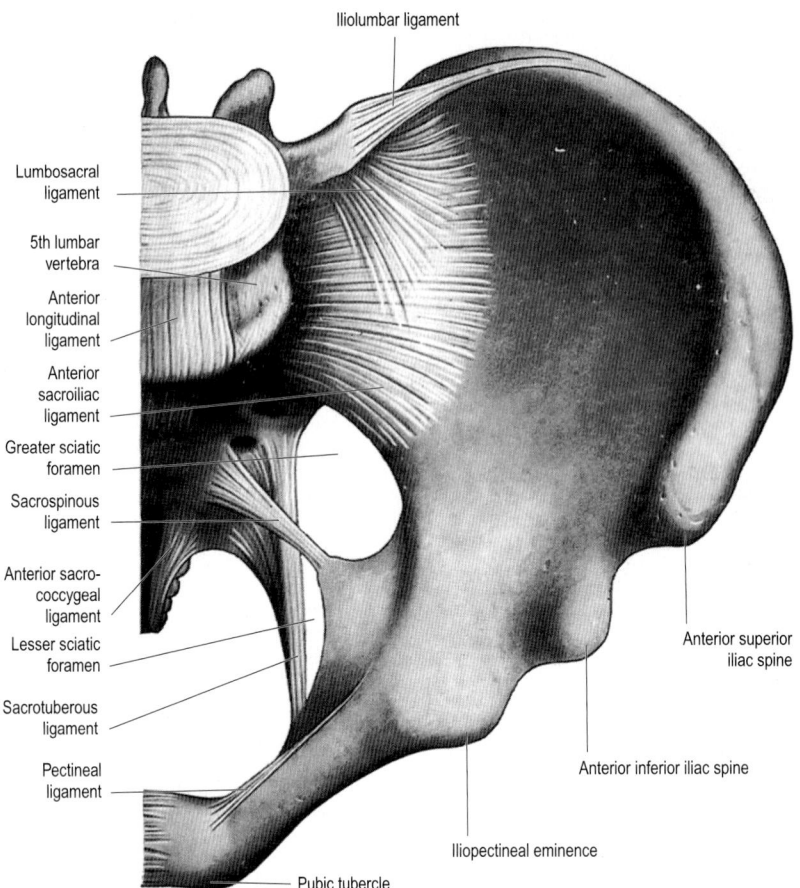

Iliolumbar ligament

Lumbosacral ligament

5th lumbar vertebra

Anterior longitudinal ligament

Anterior sacroiliac ligament

Greater sciatic foramen

Sacrospinous ligament

Anterior sacro-coccygeal ligament

Lesser sciatic foramen

Sacrotuberous ligament

Pectineal ligament

Pubic tubercle

Anterior superior iliac spine

Anterior inferior iliac spine

Iliopectineal eminence

Fig. 111.11 Joints and ligaments of the left half of the pelvis: anterior aspect.

Obturator internus is attached to the upper part of the smooth pelvic ischial surface, converging on the lesser sciatic notch (foramen) and covering the rest of this surface except the pelvic aspect of the ischial spine. The muscle and its fascia separate the bone from the ischiorectal fossa.

Vascular supply
There are multiple vascular foramina at the acetabular margins, and a few are usually present on the pelvic surface. The bone is supplied by branches of the obturator, medial circumflex femoral and inferior gluteal arteries.

Innervation
The periosteum is innervated by branches of nerves that supply the hip joint and muscles attached to the bone.

Ossification
Ossification of the ischium is described on page 1421.

SACRUM
See page 749.

COCCYX
See page 754.

THE SKELETAL PELVIS AS A WHOLE (Fig. 111.12)
The term pelvis ('basin') is applied vaguely to the skeletal ring formed by the innominate bones and the sacrum, the cavity therein, and even the entire region where the trunk and lower limbs meet. It is used here in the skeletal sense, to describe the irregular osseous girdle between the femoral heads and fifth lumbar vertebra. It is large because its primary function is to withstand the forces of body weight and musculature. In this section, its obstetric, forensic and anthropological significance will be considered.

The pelvis can be regarded as having greater and lesser segments, the true and false pelves. The segments are arbitrarily divided by an oblique plane passing through the sacral promontory posteriorly and the lineae terminales elsewhere. Each linea terminalis includes the iliac arcuate line, iliopectineal line (pecten), and pubic crest. The segments are continuous, and the parts of the body cavity that they enclose are also continuous through the pelvic inlet (superior pelvic aperture).

The greater pelvis
The greater pelvis consists of iliac blades above the lineae terminales and the sacral base. This junctional zone is structurally massive and forms powerful arches from the acetabular fossae to the vertebral column around the visceral cavity, which is part of the abdomen. It has little anterior wall because of the pelvic inclination.

The pelvic inlet (superior pelvic aperture)
The pelvic inlet may be round or oval, and is indented posteriorly by the sacral promontory. Its boundary, the pelvic brim, is obstetrically important and has also long been measured for anthropological reasons, as has the pelvic cavity.

By convention, the pelvic inlet is described in three dimensions. The anteroposterior diameter (true conjugate) is measured between the midpoints of the sacral promontory and upper border of the symphysis pubis and is c.10 cm in the adult male and 11.2 cm in the adult female. The transverse diameter is the maximum distance between similar points (assessed by eye) on opposite sides of the pelvic brim and is c.12.5 cm in the male and 13.1 cm in the adult female. The oblique diameter is measured from the iliopubic eminence to the opposite sacroiliac joint and is c.12 cm in the adult male compared to 12.5 cm in the adult female. These measurements differ between racial groups.

The articulated bony pelvis
The lesser pelvis encloses a true basin when soft tissues of the pelvic floor are in place. Skeletally it is a narrower continuation of the greater pelvis, with irregular but more complete walls around its cavity. Of obstetric importance, it has a curved median axis, and superior and inferior openings. The superior opening is occupied by viscera. The pelvic floor and its sphincters largely close the inferior opening.

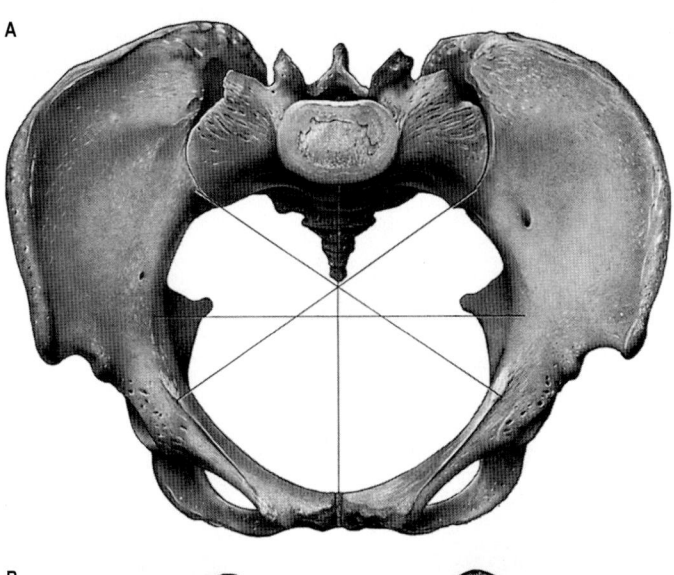

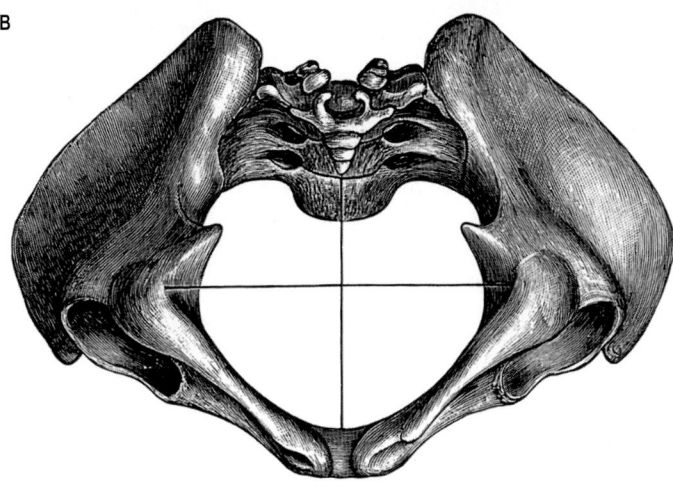

Fig. 111.12 The diameters of the female lesser pelvis: **A**, pelvic inlet (superior aperture); **B**, pelvic outlet (inferior aperture) – oblique diameter not shown.

Cavity of the lesser pelvis

The cavity of the lesser pelvis is short, curved, and markedly longer in its posterior wall. Anteroinferiorly it is bounded by pubic bones, their rami and symphysis. Posteriorly it is bounded by the concave anterior sacral surface and coccyx. Laterally on each side its margins are the smooth quadrangular pelvic aspect of the fused ilium and ischium. The region so enclosed is the pelvic cavity proper, through which pass the rectum, bladder and parts of the reproductive organs. The cavity in females must also permit passage of the fetal head.

The pelvic cavity diameters are measured at approximately the mid level and also vary with different racial groups. The anteroposterior diameter is measured between the midpoints of the third sacral segment and posterior surface of the symphysis pubis and is c.10.5 cm in the male and 13 cm in the adult female. The transverse diameter is the widest transverse distance between the side walls of the cavity, and often the greatest transverse dimension in the whole cavity. It measures c.12 cm in the adult male and 12.5 cm in the adult female. The oblique diameter is the distance from the lowest point of one sacroiliac joint to the mid-point of the contralateral obturator membrane and measures c.11 cm in the male and 13.1 cm in the adult female.

The pelvic outlet (inferior pelvic aperture)

Less regular in outline than the pelvic inlet, the pelvic outlet is indented behind by the coccyx and sacrum and bilaterally by the ischial tuberosities. Its perimeter thus consists of three wide arcs. Anteriorly is the pubic arch, between the converging ischiopubic rami. Posteriorly and laterally on both sides are the sciatic notches between the sacrum and ischial tuberosities. These are divided by the sacrotuberous and sacrospinous ligaments into greater and lesser sciatic foramina.

With ligaments included, the pelvic outlet is rhomboidal. Its anterior limbs are the ischiopubic rami (joined by the inferior pubic ligament) and its posterior margins are the sacrotuberous ligaments, with the coccyx in the midline. The outlet is thus not rigid in its posterior half, being limited by ligaments and the coccyx, all slightly yielding. Even with the sacrum taken as the posterior midline limit (more reliable for measurement), there may be slight mobility at the sacroiliac joints. Note also that a plane of the pelvic outlet is merely conceptual. The anterior, ischiopubic part has a plane which is inclined down and back to a transverse line between the lower limits of the ischial tuberosities, and the posterior half has a plane approximating to the sacrotuberous ligaments, sloping down and forwards to the same line.

Three measurements are made for the pelvic outlet. The antero-posterior diameter is usually measured from the coccygeal apex to the midpoint of the lower rim of the symphysis. The lowest sacral point may also be used (male 8 cm, female 12.5 cm). The transverse (bituberous) diameter is measured between the ischial tuberosities at the lower borders of their medial surfaces (male 8.5 cm, female 11.8 cm). The oblique diameter extends from the midpoint of the sacrotuberous ligament on one side to the contralateral ischiopubic junction (male 10 cm, female 11.8 cm).

Other measurements

Apart from these main measurements, by consensus the basis of pelvic osteometry, other planes and measurements are used in obstetric practice. The plane of greatest pelvic dimensions is an obstetric concept. It represents the most capacious pelvic level, between the pelvic brim and midlevel plane, and corresponds with the latter anteriorly at the middle part of the symphysis pubis and posteriorly at the level of the second and third sacral segments.

The plane of least dimensions is said to be at about midpelvic level. Its transverse diameter is between the apices of the ischial spines. This measurement is c.9.5 cm in an adult female and is just wide enough to allow passage of the biparietal diameter of a fetal head (c.9 cm). Not surprisingly, most difficulty in parturition occurs here.

The above measurements are sometimes made in clinical practice using X-ray or MRI pelvimetry. Measurement is not possible without radiological techniques, and even these do not take into account the soft tissues. Anatomical measurements have been made in the past and were performed at physical and vaginal examination. However, these manual measurements have proven to be of little clinical value and are now obsolete.

Morphological classification of pelves

Interest in the dimensions described above is primarily obstetric and, less frequently, forensic. All pelvic measurements display individual variation and the values quoted are means from limited surveys. Sexual and racial differences also occur. These measurements have been analysed by many anatomists, anthropologists, obstetricians and radiologists in attempts to classify human pelves, especially female. The four most common terms used today are gynaecoid, anthropoid, platypelloid and android. The gynaecoid pelvis is the traditional Western female pelvis with a heart-shaped brim and the measurements described above. An anthropoid pelvis has a larger midcavity and a wide anteroposterior inlet which is oval in shape. An anthropoid pelvis is more common in women of African origin and may be associated with a 'high assimilation' pelvis where there is an additional lumbar vertebra. A platypelloid pelvis is flat and oval from side to side at the brim. It is a contracted pelvis that is rarely seen nowadays, having previously been associated with rickets. An android pelvis has a triangular brim and is the shape of a male pelvis.

Pelvic axes and inclination (Fig. 111.13)

The axis of the superior pelvic aperture traverses its centre at right angles to its plane, directed down and backwards. When prolonged (projected) it passes through the umbilicus and midcoccyx. An axis is similarly established for the inferior aperture: projected upwards it impinges on the sacral promontory. Axes can likewise be constructed for any plane, and one for the whole cavity is a concatenation of an infinite series of such lines. It follows the curvature of the cavity, indicated by the profile of the sacrum and coccyx in lateral views. The form of this pelvic axis and the disparity in depth between the anterior and posterior contours of the cavity are prime factors in the mechanism of fetal transit in the pelvic canal.

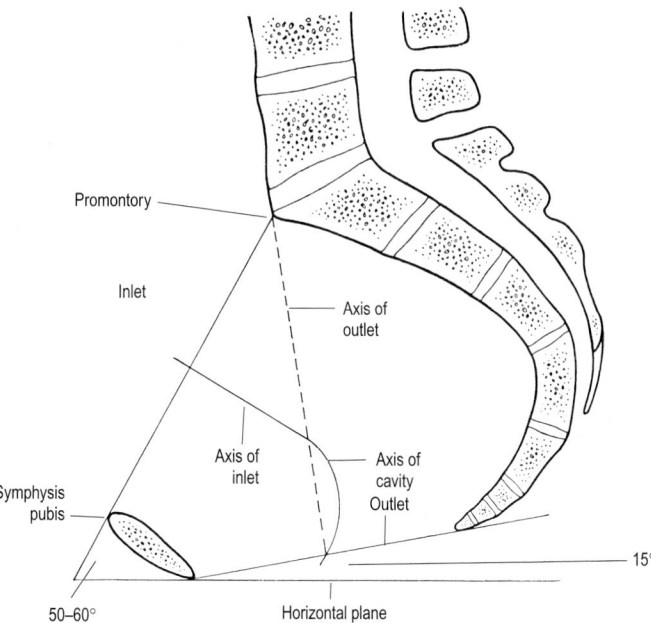

Fig. 111.13 Median sagittal section through the female pelvis, showing the planes of the inlet and outlet and the axis of the pelvic cavity.

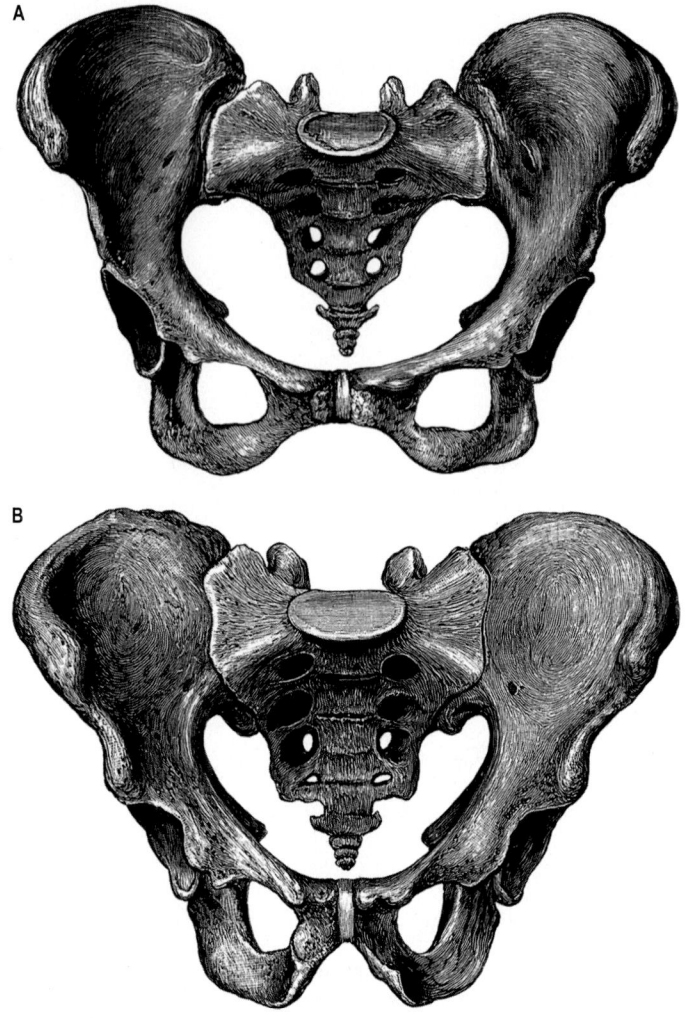

Fig. 111.14 The anterior aspect of the pelvis: **A**, female; **B**, male.

In the standing position the pelvic canal curves obliquely backwards relative to the trunk and abdominal cavity. The whole pelvis is tilted forwards, the plane of the pelvic brim making an angle of 50–60° with the horizontal. The plane of the pelvic outlet is tilted to c.15°. Therefore, the posterior parts of both planes are above the anterior. Strictly, the pelvic outlet has two planes, an anterior passing backwards from the pubic symphysis and a posterior passing forwards from the coccyx, both descending to meet at the intertuberous line. In standing, the pelvic aspect of the symphysis pubis faces as much upwards as backwards and the sacral concavity is directed anteroinferiorly. The front of the symphysis and anterior superior iliac spines are in the same vertical plane. In sitting, body weight is transmitted through inferomedial parts of the ischial tuberosities, with variable soft tissues intervening. The anterior superior iliac spines are in a vertical plane through the acetabular centres, and the whole pelvis is tilted back with the lumbosacral angle somewhat diminished at the sacral promontory.

Pelvic mechanism

The skeletal pelvis supports and protects the contained viscera, but is primarily part of the lower limbs, affording wide attachment for leg and trunk muscles. It constitutes the major mechanism for transmitting the weight of the head, trunk and upper limbs to the lower limbs. It may be considered as two arches divided by a vertical transacetabular plane. The posterior arch, chiefly concerned in transmitting weight, consists of the upper three sacral vertebrae and strong pillars of bone from the sacroiliac joints to the acetabular fossae. The anterior arch, formed by the pubic bones and their superior rami, connects these lateral pillars as a tie beam to prevent separation; it also acts as a compression strut against medial femoral thrust. The sacrum, as the summit of the posterior arch, is loaded at the lumbosacral joint. Theoretically this force has two components, one thrusting the sacrum downwards and backwards between the iliac bones, the other thrusting its upper end downwards and forwards. Sacral movements are regulated by osseous shape and massive ligaments. The first component therefore acts against the wedge, its tendency to separate iliac bones resisted by the sacroiliac and iliolumbar ligaments and symphysis pubis.

Vertical coronal sections through the sacroiliac joints suggest division of the (synovial) articular region of the sacrum into three segments. In the anterosuperior segment, involving the first sacral vertebra, the articular surfaces are slightly sinuous and almost parallel. In the middle segment the posterior width between the articular markings is greater than the anterior, and centrally a sacral concavity fits a corresponding iliac convexity, an interlocking mechanism relieving the strain on the

ligaments produced by body weight. In the posteroinferior segment the anterior sacral width is greater than the posterior and here its sacral surfaces are slightly concave. Anteroinferior sacral dislocation by the second component (of force) is prevented, therefore, mainly by the middle segment, owing to its cuneiform shape and interlocking mechanism. However, some rotation occurs, in which the anterosuperior segment tilts down and the posteroinferior segment up. 'Superior' segmental movement is limited to a small degree by wedging but primarily by tension in the sacrotuberous and sacrospinous ligaments. In all movements the sacroiliac and iliolumbar ligaments and symphysis pubis resist separation of the iliac bones.

SEXUAL DIFFERENCES IN THE PELVIS (Fig. 111.14)

The pelvis provides the most marked skeletal differences between male and female. Distinction can be made even during fetal life, particularly in the subpubic arch. In infancy, dimensions of the whole pelvis are greater in males than in females, but the size of the pelvic cavity is usually greater in females. This distinction prevails in childhood, but the difference is maximal at c.22 months. Sexual differences in adults are divisible into metrical and non-metrical features: the range of most features overlaps between the sexes.

Differences are inevitably linked to function. While the primary pelvic function in both sexes is locomotor, the pelvis, particularly the lesser pelvis, is adapted to parturition in females, and these changes variably affect the proportions and dimensions of the greater pelvis. Since males are distinctly more muscular and therefore more heavily built, overall pelvic dimensions, such as the intercristal measurement (distance between the iliac crests), are greater, markings for muscles and ligaments more pronounced, and general architecture heavier. The male iliac crest is more rugged and more medially inclined at its anterior end; in females the crests are less curved in all parts. The iliac blades are more vertical in females, but do not ascend so far; the iliac fossae are therefore shallower and each iliopectineal line more vertical. These iliac peculiarities probably account for the greater prominence of female hips.

The male is relatively and absolutely more heavily built above the pelvis, with consequent differences at the lumbosacral and hip joints. The sacral basal articular facet for the fifth lumbar vertebra and intervening disc is more than a third of the total sacral basal width in males but less than a third in females, in whom the sacrum is also relatively broader, accentuating this difference. The female has relatively broader sacral alae. The male acetabulum is absolutely larger, and its diameter is approximately equal to the distance between its anterior rim and symphysis pubis. In females, acetabular diameter is usually less than this distance, not only because it is absolutely smaller but also because the anterolateral wall of the cavity is comparatively and often absolutely wider. The height of the female symphysis and adjoining parts of the pubis and ischium, which form the anterior pelvic wall, are also absolutely less, producing a somewhat triangular obturator foramen, which is more ovoid in males. Differing pubic growth is also expressed in the subpubic arch below the symphysis and between the inferior pubic rami. It is more angular in males, being 50–60°; in females it is rounded, less easy to measure and usually 80–85°. A greater separation of the pubic tubercles in females contributes to the pubic width. The ischiopubic rami are also much more lightly built and narrowed near the symphysis; in males they bear a distinctly rough, everted area for attachment of the penile crura, the corresponding attachment for the clitoris being poorly developed. Ischial spines are closer in males and are more inturned. The greater sciatic notch is usually wider in females: mean values for males and females are 50.4° and 74.4°, respectively. The greater female values for angle and width are associated with increased backward sacral tilt and greater anteroposterior pelvic diameter, especially at lower levels.

The sacrum also displays metrical sexual differences. Female sacra are less curved, the curvature being most marked between the first and second segments and the third and fifth, with an intervening flatter region. Male sacra are more evenly curved, relatively long and narrow and more often exceeding five segments (by addition of a lumbar or coccygeal vertebra). The sacral index compares sacral breadth (between the most anterior points on the auricular surfaces) with length (between midpoints on the anterior margins of the promontory and apex): average values for males and females are 105% and 115%. Auricular surfaces are relatively smaller and more oblique in females, but extend onto the upper three sacral vertebrae in both sexes. The dorsal auricular border is more concave in females. Many differences may be summarized in the generalization that the pelvic cavity is longer and more conical in males, shorter and more cylindrical in females; the axis is curved in both. Differences are greater at the inferior aperture than the brim, where in absolute measurements males are not as different from females as sometimes stated. The superior aperture is more likely to be anthropoid or android in males and gynaecoid or android in females, but there is overlap between the sexes.

In forensic practice, identification of human skeletal remains (which are sometimes fragmentary) usually involves diagnosis of sex, and this is most certainly established from the pelvis. Even parts of the pelvis may be useful. Several studies of metrical characteristics in various pelvic regions have been made, leading to the production of various indices. The ilium has received particular attention, e.g. one index compares the pelvic and sacroiliac parts of the bone. A line is extended back from the iliopectineal eminence to the nearest point on the anterior auricular margin and thence to the iliac crest. The auricular point divides this chilotic line into anterior (pelvic) and posterior (sacral) segments, each expressed as a percentage of the other. Chilotic indices display reciprocal values in the sexes: the pelvic part of the chilotic line is predominant in females, and the sacral part in males. Detailed metrical studies of the ilium have indicated its limited reliability in 'sexing' pelves. However, the higher incidence and definition of the female preauricular sulcus is recognized. The desirability of correlating all available metrical data is to be emphasized; when a range of pelvic data can be combined, especially if they are metrical, 95% accuracy should be achieved. Complete accuracy has been claimed when the rest of the skeleton is available. Assessment of sex from isolated and often incomplete human remains is less reliable.

For details, consult Mays (1998) and Brothwell and Pollard (2001).

FEMUR

Topography (Figs 111.15, 111.16)

The femur is the longest and strongest bone in the human body. Its length is associated with a striding gait, its strength with weight and muscular forces. Its shaft, almost cylindrical in most of its length and bowed forward, has a proximal round, articular head projecting mainly medially on its short neck, which is a medial curvature of the proximal shaft. The distal extremity is more massive and is a double 'knuckle' (condyle) that articulates with the tibia. In standing, the femoral shafts are oblique and their heads are separated by the pelvic width. The shafts converge downwards and medially to the knees and almost touch: they lie below the hip joints. Since the tibia and fibula descend vertically from the knees, the ankles are also in the line of body weight in standing or walking. Femoral obliquity varies but is greater in women, reflecting the relatively greater pelvic breadth and shorter femora. Proximally the femur consists of a head, neck, and greater and lesser trochanters.

Femoral head (Fig. 111.17)

The femoral head faces anterosuperomedially to articulate with the acetabulum. The head, often described as rather more than half a 'sphere', is not part of a true sphere but is spheroidal and is part of the surface of an ovoid. Its smoothness is interrupted posteroinferior to its centre by a small, rough fovea.

The head is intracapsular, encircled distal to its equator by the acetabular labrum. Its periphery is distinct, except anteriorly, where the articular surface extends to the neck. The ligamentum teres attaches to the fovea. The anterior surface of the head is separated inferomedially from the femoral artery by the tendon of psoas major, the psoas bursa, and the articular capsule.

Femoral neck (Fig. 111.17)

The femoral neck is c.5 cm long, narrowest in its mid part and widest laterally, and connects the head to the shaft at an angle of c.125° (angle of inclination; neck–shaft angle): this facilitates movement at the hip joint, enabling the limb to swing clear of the pelvis. The neck also provides a lever for the action of the muscles acting about the hip joint, which are attached to the proximal femur. The neck–shaft angle is widest at birth and diminishes until adolescence; it is smaller in females. The neck is laterally rotated with respect to the shaft (angle of anteversion) some 10–15°, although values of this angle vary between individuals and between populations (Eckhoff et al 1994). The contours of the neck are rounded: the upper surface is almost horizontal and slightly concave, the lower is straighter but oblique, directed inferolaterally and backwards to the shaft near the lesser trochanter. On all aspects the neck expands as it approaches the articular surface of the head. The anterior surface of the neck is flat and marked at the junction with the shaft by a rough intertrochanteric line. The posterior surface, facing posteriorly and superiorly, is transversely convex, and concave in its long axis; its junction with the shaft is marked by a rounded intertrochanteric crest. There are numerous vascular foramina, especially anteriorly and posterosuperiorly.

The anterior surface is intracapsular, the capsule attaching laterally to the intertrochanteric line. Facets, often covered by extensions of articular cartilage, and various imprints frequently occur here. These facets may sometimes be associated with squatting. One such feature, the cervical fossa, may be a racial characteristic. On the posterior surface the capsule does not reach the intertrochanteric crest; little more than the medial half of the neck is intracapsular. The anterior surface adjoining the head and covered by cartilage is related to the iliofemoral ligament. A groove, produced by the tendon of obturator externus as it approaches the trochanteric fossa, spirals across the posterior surface of the neck in a proximolateral direction.

Greater trochanter (Fig. 111.17)

The greater trochanter is large and quadrangular, projecting up from the junction of the neck and shaft. Its posterosuperior region projects superomedially to overhang the adjacent posterior surface of the neck and here its medial surface presents the rough trochanteric fossa. The proximal border of the trochanter lies the breadth of the subject's hand below the iliac tubercle, level with the centre of the femoral head. It has an anterior rough impression. Its lateral surface is divided by an oblique, flat strip, wider above, which crosses it down and forwards. This surface

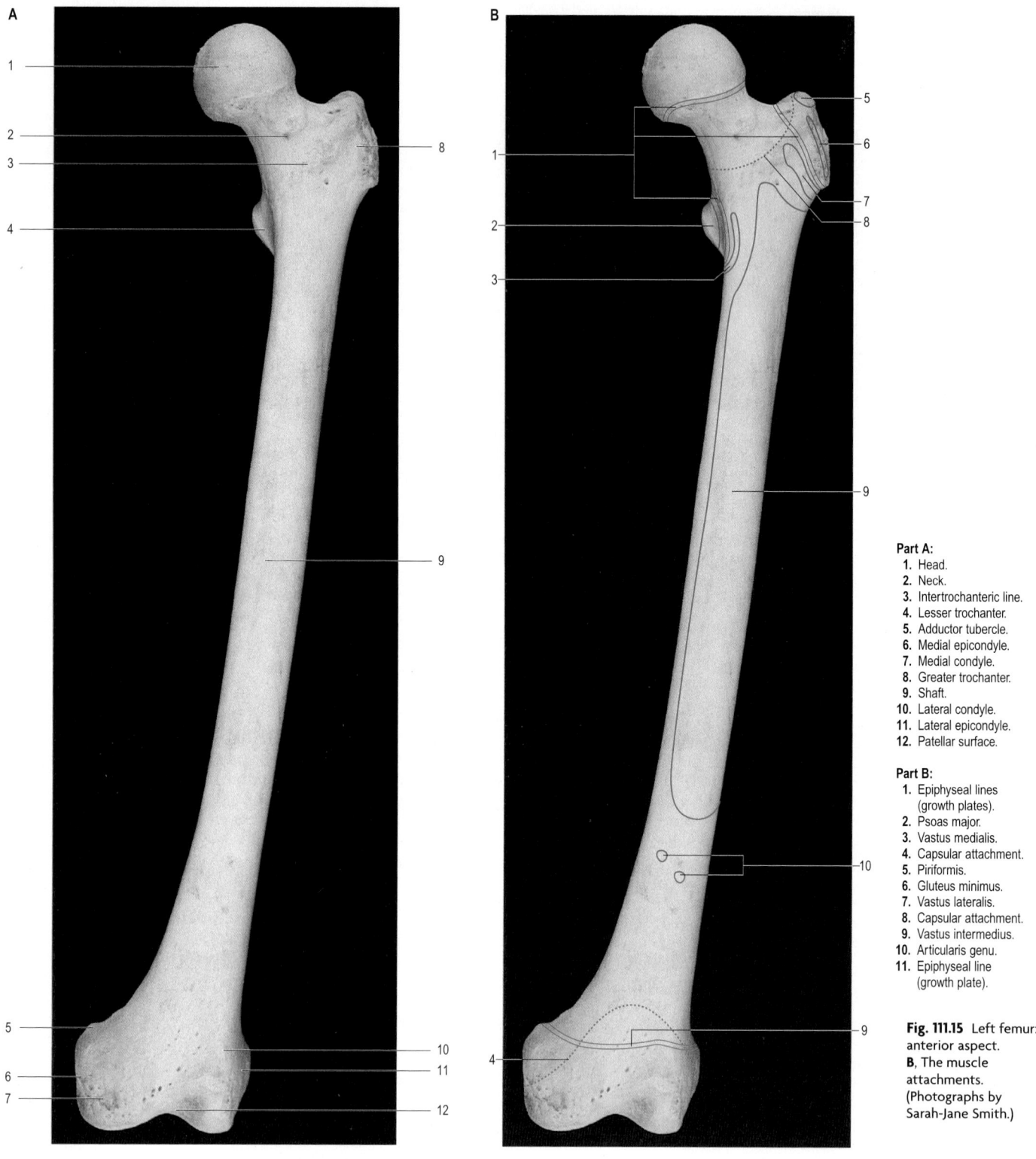

Part A:
1. Head.
2. Neck.
3. Intertrochanteric line.
4. Lesser trochanter.
5. Adductor tubercle.
6. Medial epicondyle.
7. Medial condyle.
8. Greater trochanter.
9. Shaft.
10. Lateral condyle.
11. Lateral epicondyle.
12. Patellar surface.

Part B:
1. Epiphyseal lines (growth plates).
2. Psoas major.
3. Vastus medialis.
4. Capsular attachment.
5. Piriformis.
6. Gluteus minimus.
7. Vastus lateralis.
8. Capsular attachment.
9. Vastus intermedius.
10. Articularis genu.
11. Epiphyseal line (growth plate).

Fig. 111.15 Left femur: anterior aspect. **B,** The muscle attachments. (Photographs by Sarah-Jane Smith.)

is palpable, especially when the muscles are relaxed. The trochanteric fossa occasionally presents a tubercle or exostosis.

Lesser trochanter

The lesser trochanter is a conical posteromedial projection of the shaft at the posteroinferior aspect of its junction with the neck. Its summit and anterior surface are rough, but its posterior surface, at the distal end of the intertrochanteric crest, is smooth. It is not palpable.

Intertrochanteric line

The intertrochanteric line, a prominent ridge at the junction of the anterior surfaces of the neck and shaft, descends medially from a superomedial tubercle on the anterior aspect of the greater trochanter

to a point on the lower border of the neck, anterior to the lesser trochanter, where there may also be a tubercle. This line is the lateral limit of the hip joint capsule anteriorly. The upper and lower bands of the iliofemoral ligament are attached to its proximal and distal ends and tubercles. Distally it is continuous with the spiral line.

Intertrochanteric crest

The intertrochanteric crest, a smooth ridge at the junction of the posterior surface of the neck with the shaft, descends from the postero-superior angle of the greater trochanter medially down to the lesser trochanter. A little above its centre is a low, rounded quadrate tubercle. Above the tubercle it is covered by gluteus maximus, from which it is separated distally by quadratus femoris and the upper border of adductor magnus.

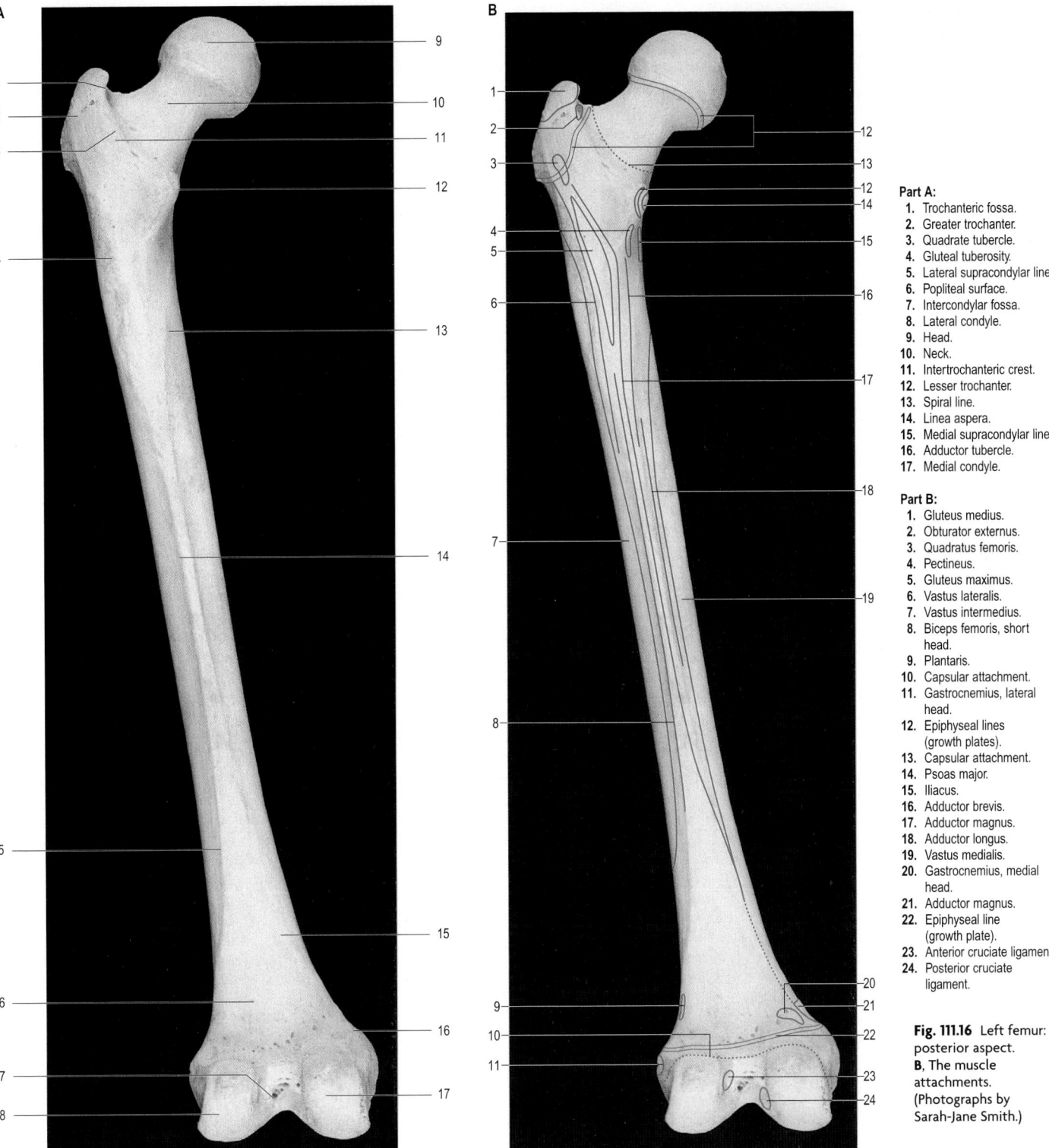

A
1
2
3
4
5
6
7
8

9
10
11
12
13
14
15
16
17

B
1
2
3
4
5
6
7
8
9
10
11

12
13
12
14
15
16
17
18
19
20
21
22
23
24

Part A:
1. Trochanteric fossa.
2. Greater trochanter.
3. Quadrate tubercle.
4. Gluteal tuberosity.
5. Lateral supracondylar line.
6. Popliteal surface.
7. Intercondylar fossa.
8. Lateral condyle.
9. Head.
10. Neck.
11. Intertrochanteric crest.
12. Lesser trochanter.
13. Spiral line.
14. Linea aspera.
15. Medial supracondylar line.
16. Adductor tubercle.
17. Medial condyle.

Part B:
1. Gluteus medius.
2. Obturator externus.
3. Quadratus femoris.
4. Pectineus.
5. Gluteus maximus.
6. Vastus lateralis.
7. Vastus intermedius.
8. Biceps femoris, short head.
9. Plantaris.
10. Capsular attachment.
11. Gastrocnemius, lateral head.
12. Epiphyseal lines (growth plates).
13. Capsular attachment.
14. Psoas major.
15. Iliacus.
16. Adductor brevis.
17. Adductor magnus.
18. Adductor longus.
19. Vastus medialis.
20. Gastrocnemius, medial head.
21. Adductor magnus.
22. Epiphyseal line (growth plate).
23. Anterior cruciate ligament.
24. Posterior cruciate ligament.

Fig. 111.16 Left femur: posterior aspect. **B**, The muscle attachments. (Photographs by Sarah-Jane Smith.)

Gluteal tuberosity

The gluteal tuberosity may be an elongated depression or a ridge. It may in part be prominent enough to be called a third trochanter.

Shaft (Figs 111.15, 111.16)

The shaft is surrounded by muscles and is impalpable. The distal anterior surface, for 5–6 cm above the patellar articular surface, is covered by a suprapatellar bursa, between bone and muscle. The distal lateral surface is covered by vastus intermedius. The medial surface, devoid of attachments, is covered by vastus medialis.

The shaft is narrowest centrally, expanding a little proximally, particularly towards its distal end. Its long axis makes an angle of c.10° with the vertical, and diverges c.5–7° from the long axis of the tibia. Its middle third has three surfaces and borders. The extensive anterior surface, smooth and gently convex, is between the lateral and medial borders, which are both round and indistinct. The posterolateral surface is bounded posteriorly by the broad, rough linea aspera, usually a crest with lateral and medial edges. Its subjacent compact bone is augmented to withstand compressive forces, which are concentrated here by the anterior curvature of the shaft. The linea aspera receives adductor longus, intermuscular septa and the short head of biceps femoris, inseparably blended at their attachment. Perforating arteries cross the linea laterally under tendinous arches in adductor magnus and biceps. Nutrient foramina, directed proximally, appear in the linea aspera, varying in number and site, one usually near its proximal end, a second usually near its distal end. The medial surface is posteromedial, smooth like the others, bounded in front by the indistinct medial border and behind by the linea aspera. In its proximal third the shaft has a fourth, posterior

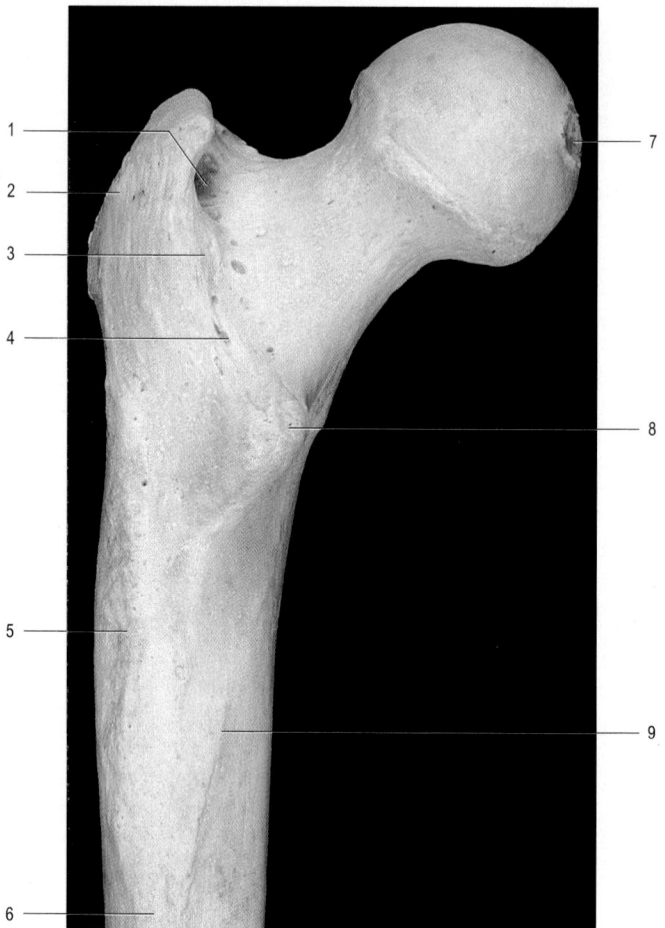

1. Trochanteric fossa. 2. Greater trochanter. 3. Quadrate tubercle. 4. Intertrochanteric crest.
5. Gluteal tuberosity. 6. Linea aspera. 7. Fovea for ligamentum teres attachment.
8. Lesser trochanter. 9. Spiral line.

Fig. 111.17 Proximal end of left femur: posterior aspect. (Photograph by Sarah-Jane Smith.)

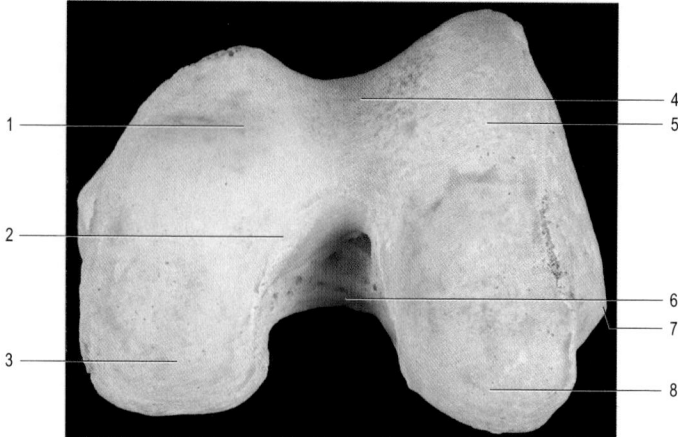

1. Medial oblique groove. 2. Semilunar area. 3. Medial condyle. 4. Patellar surface.
5. Lateral oblique groove. 6. Intercondylar notch. 7. Lateral epicondyle. 8. Lateral condyle.

Fig. 111.18 Distal end of left femur: articular surface. (Photograph by Sarah-Jane Smith.)

surface, bounded medially by a narrow, rough spiral line that is continuous proximally with the intertrochanteric line and distally with the medial edge of linea aspera. Laterally this surface is limited by the broad, rough, gluteal tuberosity, ascending a little laterally to the greater trochanter and descending to the lateral edge of the linea aspera. In its distal third the shaft also has a fourth, posterior surface, between the medial and lateral supracondylar lines, which is continuous above with the corresponding edges of the linea aspera. The lateral line is most distinct in its proximal two-thirds, where the short head of biceps femoris and lateral intermuscular septum are attached. Its distal third has a small rough area for the attachment of plantaris, often encroaching on the popliteal surface. The medial line is indistinct in its proximal two-thirds, where vastus medialis is attached. Proximally, the shaft is crossed by femoral vessels entering the popliteal fossa from the adductor canal. It is often sharp for 3 or 4 cm proximal to the adductor tubercle.

The popliteal surface is also triangular. In its distal medial part it is rough and slightly elevated. Forming the proximal floor of the popliteal fossa, it is covered by variable amounts of fat that separate the popliteal artery from bone. The superior medial genicular artery, a branch of the popliteal artery, arches medially above the medial condyle. It is separated from bone by the medial head of gastrocnemius. The latter is attached a little above the condyle; further distally there may be a smooth facet underlying a bursa for the medial head of gastrocnemius. More medially, there is often an imprint proximal to the articular surface: in flexion this is close to a rough tubercle on the medial tibial condyle for the attachment of semimembranosus. The superior lateral genicular artery arches up laterally proximal to the lateral condyle but is separated from bone by the attachment of plantaris to the distal part of the lateral supracondylar line.

Distal end (Fig. 111.18)

The distal end of the femur is widely expanded as a bearing surface for transmission of weight to the tibia. It has two massive condyles, which are partly articular. Anteriorly the condyles unite and continue into the shaft; posteriorly they are separated by a deep intercondylar fossa and project beyond the plane of the popliteal surface. The articular surface is a broad area, like an inverted U, for the patella and the tibia. The patellar surface extends anteriorly on both condyles, especially the lateral. It is transversely concave, vertically convex and grooved for the posterior patellar surface. The tibial surface is divided by the intercondylar fossa but is anteriorly continuous with the patellar surface. Its medial part is a broad strip on the convex inferoposterior surface of the medial condyle, and is gently curved with a medial convexity. Its lateral part covers similar aspects of the lateral condyle but is broader and passes straight back. The tibial surfaces are transversely convex in all directions. The anteroposterior curvature of both surfaces is not uniform. The exact pattern is controversial. One view is that in both tibial portions of the femoral condyles the sagittal radius of curvature is ever decreasing (a 'closing helix'). More recently it has been suggested that the medial articular surface describes arcs of two circles. The more posterior has a smaller radius. Laterally there may only be one arc of fixed curvature with a radius similar to that of the posterior arc of the medial femoral articular surface. These differences are important determinants of knee joint motion.

Patellar surface (trochlear groove) – The patellar surface extends more proximally on the lateral side. Its proximal border is therefore oblique and runs distally and medially, separated from the tibial surfaces by two faint grooves that cross the condyles obliquely. The lateral groove is the more distinct. It runs laterally and slightly forwards from the front of the intercondylar fossa and expands to form a faint triangular depression, resting on the anterior edge of the lateral meniscus with the knee fully extended. The medial groove is restricted to the medial part of the medial condyle and rests on the anterior edge of the medial meniscus in full extension. Where it ceases, the patellar surface continues back to the lateral part of the medial condyle as a semilunar area adjoining the anterior region of the intercondylar fossa. This area articulates with the medial vertical facet of the patella in full flexion; it is not distinct in outline in most femora. In habitual squatters articular cartilage may extend to the lateral aspect of the lateral condyle under vastus lateralis.

The trochlear groove helps to stabilize the patella. An abnormally shallow groove predisposes to instability.

Intercondylar fossa – The intercondylar fossa separates the two condyles distally and behind. In front it is limited by the distal border of the patellar surface, and behind by an intercondylar line, separating it from the popliteal surface. It is intracapsular but largely extrasynovial. Its lateral wall, the medial surface of the lateral condyle, bears a flat posterosuperior impression which spreads to the floor of the fossa near the intercondylar line for the proximal attachment of the anterior cruciate ligament. The medial wall of the fossa, i.e. the lateral surface of the medial condyle, bears a similar larger area, but far more anteriorly, for the proximal attachment of the posterior cruciate ligament. Both impressions are smooth and largely devoid of vascular foramina, whereas the rest of the fossa is rough and pitted by vascular foramina. A bursal recess between the ligaments may ascend to the fossa. The capsular ligament and, laterally, the oblique popliteal ligament, are attached to the intercondylar line. The ligamentum mucosum (infrapatellar synovial fold or plica) is attached to the anterior border of the fossa.

Lateral condyle (Figs 111.18, 111.19) – The lateral condyle is larger anteroposteriorly than the medial. Its most prominent point is the lateral epicondyle to which the lateral collateral ligament is attached. A short groove, deeper in front, separates the lateral epicondyle inferiorly from the articular margin. This groove allows the tendon of popliteus to run deep to the lateral collateral ligament and insert inferior and anterior to the ligament insertion. Adjoining the joint margin is a strip of condyle, 1 cm broad. It is intracapsular and covered by synovial membrane except for the attachment of popliteus.

The medial surface is the lateral wall of the intercondylar fossa. Its lateral surface projects beyond the shaft. Part of the lateral head of gastrocnemius is attached to an impression posterosuperior to the lateral epicondyle.

Medial condyle – The medial condyle has a bulging convex medial aspect, which is easily palpable. Proximally its adductor tubercle, which may only be a facet rather than a projection, receives the tendon of adductor magnus. The medial prominence of the condyle, the medial epicondyle, is anteroinferior to the tubercle. The lateral surface of the condyle is the medial wall of the intercondylar fossa. The condyle projects distally so that, despite the obliquity of the shaft, the profile of the distal end is almost horizontal. A curved strip, c.1 cm wide, adjoining the medial articular margin, is covered by synovial membrane and is inside the joint capsule. Proximal to this, the medial epicondyle receives the medial collateral ligament.

Structure (Fig. 111.20)
The femoral shaft is a cylinder of compact bone with a large medullary cavity. The wall is thick in its middle third, where the femur is narrowest and the medullary cavity most capacious. Proximally and distally the compact wall becomes progressively thinner, and the cavity gradually fills with trabecular bone. The extremities, especially where articular, consist of trabecular bone within a thin shell of compact bone, their trabeculae being disposed along lines of greatest stress. At the proximal end the main trabeculae form a series of plates orthogonal to the articular surface, converging to a central dense wedge, which is supported by strong trabeculae passing to the sides of the neck, especially along its upper and lower profiles. Force applied to the femoral head is therefore transmitted to the wedge and thence to the junction of the neck and shaft. This junction is strengthened by dense trabeculae extending laterally from the lesser trochanter to the end of the superior aspect of the neck, thus resisting tensile or shearing forces applied to the neck through the head. Tensile and compressive tests indicate that axial trabeculae of the femoral head withstand much greater stresses than peripheral trabeculae. A smaller bar across the junction of the greater trochanter with the neck and shaft resists shearing produced by muscles attached to it. These two bars are proximal layers of arches between the sides of the shaft and transmit to it forces applied to the proximal end. A thin vertical plate, the calcar femorale, ascends from the compact wall near the linea aspera into the trabeculae of the neck. Medially it joins the posterior wall of the neck; laterally it continues into the greater trochanter, where it disperses into general trabecular bone. It is thus in a plane anterior to the trochanteric crest and base of the lesser trochanter. Newell (1997), in a review of the calcar femorale, has described its three-dimensional anatomy in terms of the work of Dixon (1910), who was the first to recognize the deficiencies of the classic two-dimensional description of the architecture of the proximal femur. Dixon suggested that the trabecular framework of the proximal femur was spiral, and that the 'arches' were simplified sectional profiles of this spiral. At the distal end of the femur, trabeculae spring from the entire internal surface of compact bone, descending perpendicular to the articular surface. Proximal to the condyles these are strongest and most

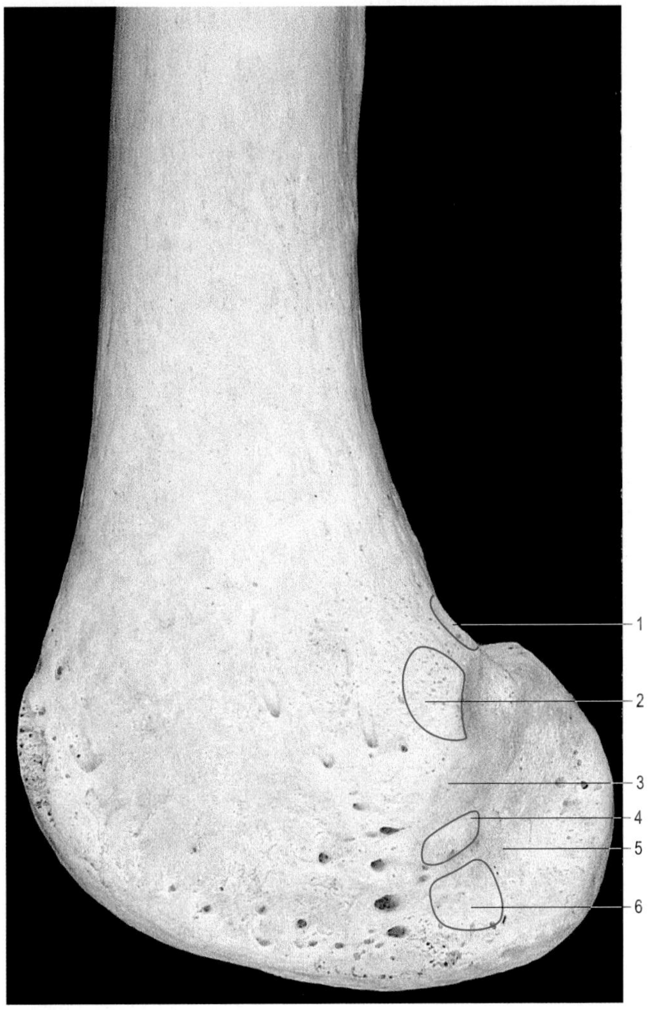

1. Attachment of plantaris.   2. Attachment of lateral head of gastrocnemius.
3. Lateral epicondyle.   4. Attachment of lateral collateral ligament.
5. Groove for popliteus in full flexion.   6. Attachment of popliteus.

Fig. 111.19 Distal end of left femur: lateral aspect. (Photograph by Sarah-Jane Smith.)

accurately perpendicular. Horizontal planes of trabecular bone, arranged like crossed girders, form a series of cubical compartments.

Muscle attachments
The greater trochanter provides attachment for the smaller gluteal muscles. Gluteus minimus is attached to its rough anterior impression and gluteus medius to its lateral oblique strip. The bone is separated from the tendon of gluteus medius by a bursa. The area behind is covered by deep fibres of gluteus maximus, with part of its trochanteric bursa interposed. The tendon of piriformis is attached to the upper border of the trochanter and the common tendon of obturator internus and the gemelli are attached to its medial surface. The trochanteric fossa receives the tendon of obturator externus.

Psoas major is attached to the summit and anteromedial surface of the lesser trochanter. Iliacus is attached to the medial or anterior surface of its base, descending a little behind the spiral line as its tendon fuses with that of psoas. Adductor magnus (upper part) passes over its posterior surface, sometimes separated by an interposed bursa.

The most proximal fibres of vastus lateralis are attached to the proximal end of the intertrochanteric line, and those of vastus medialis are attached distally. Quadratus femoris is attached to the quadrate tubercle and the immediately distal bone. Vastus intermedius is attached to the anterior and lateral surfaces of the shaft in their proximal three-quarters. Slips of articularis genu are attached distal to this.

The gluteal tuberosity receives the deeper fibres of the distal half of gluteus maximus and, at its medial edge, pubic fibres of adductor magnus. Distal to this, adductor magnus is attached to the linea aspera

A

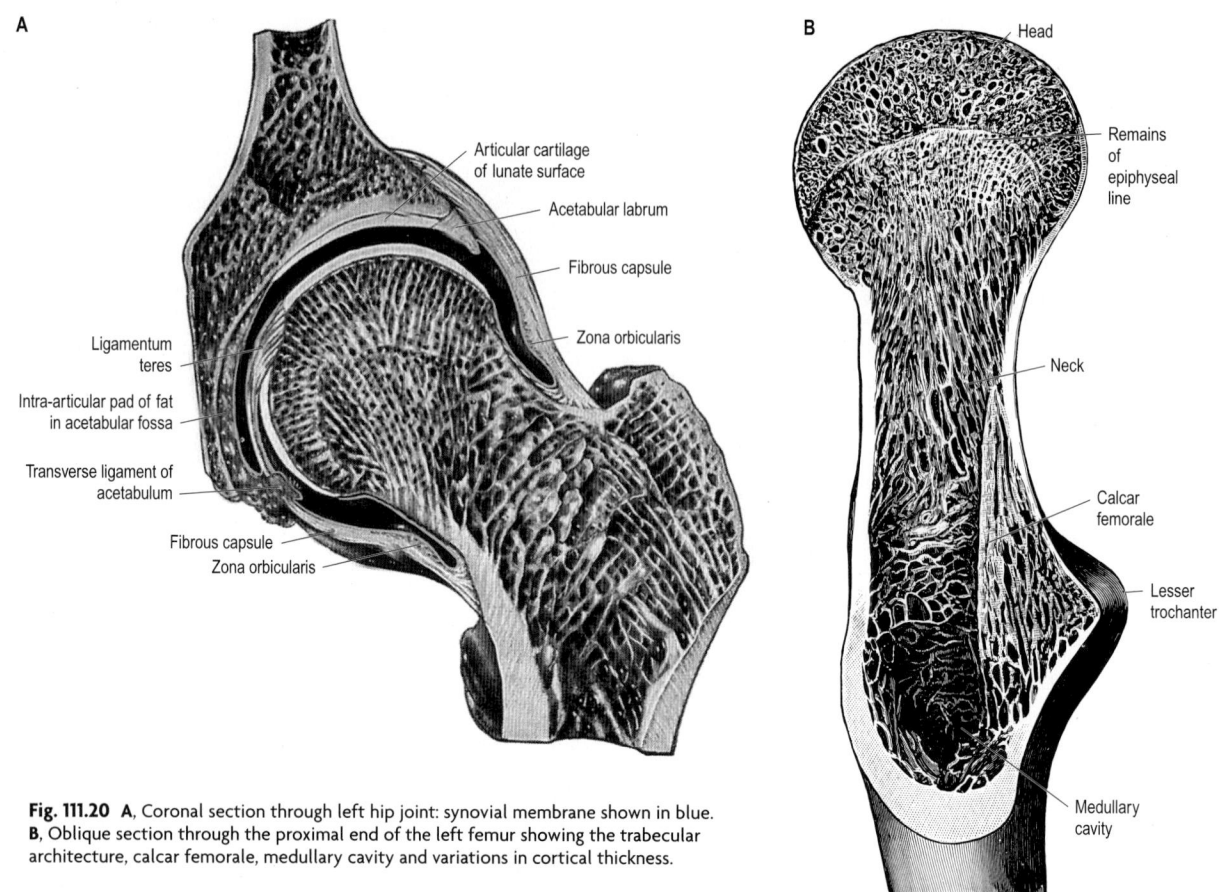

Articular cartilage
of lunate surface

Acetabular labrum

Fibrous capsule

Zona orbicularis

Ligamentum
teres

Intra-articular pad of fat
in acetabular fossa

Transverse ligament of
acetabulum

Fibrous capsule

Zona orbicularis

B

Head

Remains
of
epiphyseal
line

Neck

Calcar
femorale

Lesser
trochanter

Medullary
cavity

Fig. 111.20 A, Coronal section through left hip joint: synovial membrane shown in blue.
B, Oblique section through the proximal end of the left femur showing the trabecular
architecture, calcar femorale, medullary cavity and variations in cortical thickness.

and aponeurotically to the proximal part of the medial supracondylar ridge. Its remaining fibres form a large tendon attached to the adductor tubercle, with an aponeurotic expansion to the distal part of the medial supracondylar ridge.

Pectineus and adductor brevis are attached to the posterior femoral surface between the gluteal tuberosity and spiral line. The pectineal attachment is a line, sometimes slightly rough, from the base of the lesser trochanter to the linea aspera. Adductor brevis is attached lateral to pectineus and beyond this to the proximal part of the linea aspera, medial to adductor magnus.

Adductor longus, intermuscular septa and the short head of biceps femoris are attached to the linea aspera.

Vastus lateralis has a linear attachment from the anterior surface of the base of the greater trochanter to the proximal end of the gluteal tuberosity, and along the lateral margin of the latter to the proximal half of the lateral edge of the linea aspera. Vastus medialis is attached from the distal end of the intertrochanteric line along the spiral line to the medial edge of the linea aspera and thence to the medial supracondylar line, which also receives many fibres from the aponeurotic attachments of adductor magnus.

The medial head of gastrocnemius is attached to the posterior surface a little above the medial condyle.

The short head of biceps femoris is attached to the proximal two-thirds of the lateral supracondylar line. Plantaris attaches to the line distally. There is an attachment of vastus medialis to the proximal two-thirds of the medial supracondylar line.

Part of the lateral head of gastrocnemius is attached postero-superiorly to the lateral epicondyle. Popliteus is attached anteriorly in the groove on the outer aspect of the lateral epicondyle. Its tendon passes deep to the lateral collateral ligament (**Fig. 111.19**). The tendon lies in the groove in full knee flexion; in extension it crosses the articular margin and may form an impression on it.

Vascular supply (Fig. 111.21)

For details consult Crock (1980, 1996).

The blood supply of the femoral head is derived from an arterial ring around the neck, just outside the attachment of the fibrous capsule, constituted by the medial and lateral circumflex arteries with minor con-

tributions from the superior and inferior gluteal vessels (see trochanteric anastomosis, p. 1453). From this ring, ascending cervical branches pierce the capsule (under its zona orbicularis, p. 1440) to ascend the neck beneath the reflected synovial membrane. These vessels become the retinacular arteries and form a subsynovial intra-articular ring. Here the vessels are at risk with a displaced fracture of the femoral neck. Interruption of blood supply in this way can lead to avascular necrosis of the femoral head. If the fracture is intra-articular then not only is the intraosseous blood supply damaged but the retinacular vessels can also be vulnerable. If the fracture is extracapsular, the retinacular vessels will remain intact and avascular necrosis of the femoral head does not occur. The ascending cervical vessels give off metaphyseal branches that enter the neck, while the intra-articular ring gives off lateral and inferior epiphyseal branches. A small medial epiphyseal supply, of importance in early childhood, reaches the head along the ligamentum teres (p. 1441) by the acetabular branches of the obturator and medial circumflex femoral arteries, which anastomose with the other epiphyseal vessels. During growth, the epiphyseal plate separates the territories of the metaphyseal and epiphyseal vessels; after osseous union of the head and neck, they anastomose freely. Observations on developmental patterns of this supply in late fetal and early postnatal periods have revealed that although medial and lateral circumflex arteries at first contribute equally, two major branches of the medial provide the final supply, both posterior to the neck. The supply from the lateral circumflex diminishes and the arterial ring is interrupted. As the femoral neck elongates, the extracapsular circle becomes more distant from the epiphyseal part of the head.

The trochanteric regions and subtrochanteric shaft are supplied by the trochanteric and cruciate arterial anastomoses (p. 1453). More distally in the shaft, nutrient foramina, directed proximally, are found in the linea aspera, varying in number and site: one is usually near its proximal end and a second usually near its distal end. The main nutrient artery is usually derived from the second perforating artery (see profunda femoris, p. 1451). If two nutrient arteries occur, they may branch from the first and third perforators. Periosteal vessels arise from the perforators and from the profunda, and run circumferentially rather than longitudinally. The distal metaphysis has many vascular foramina. Arterial supply here is from the genicular anastomosis (p. 1486).

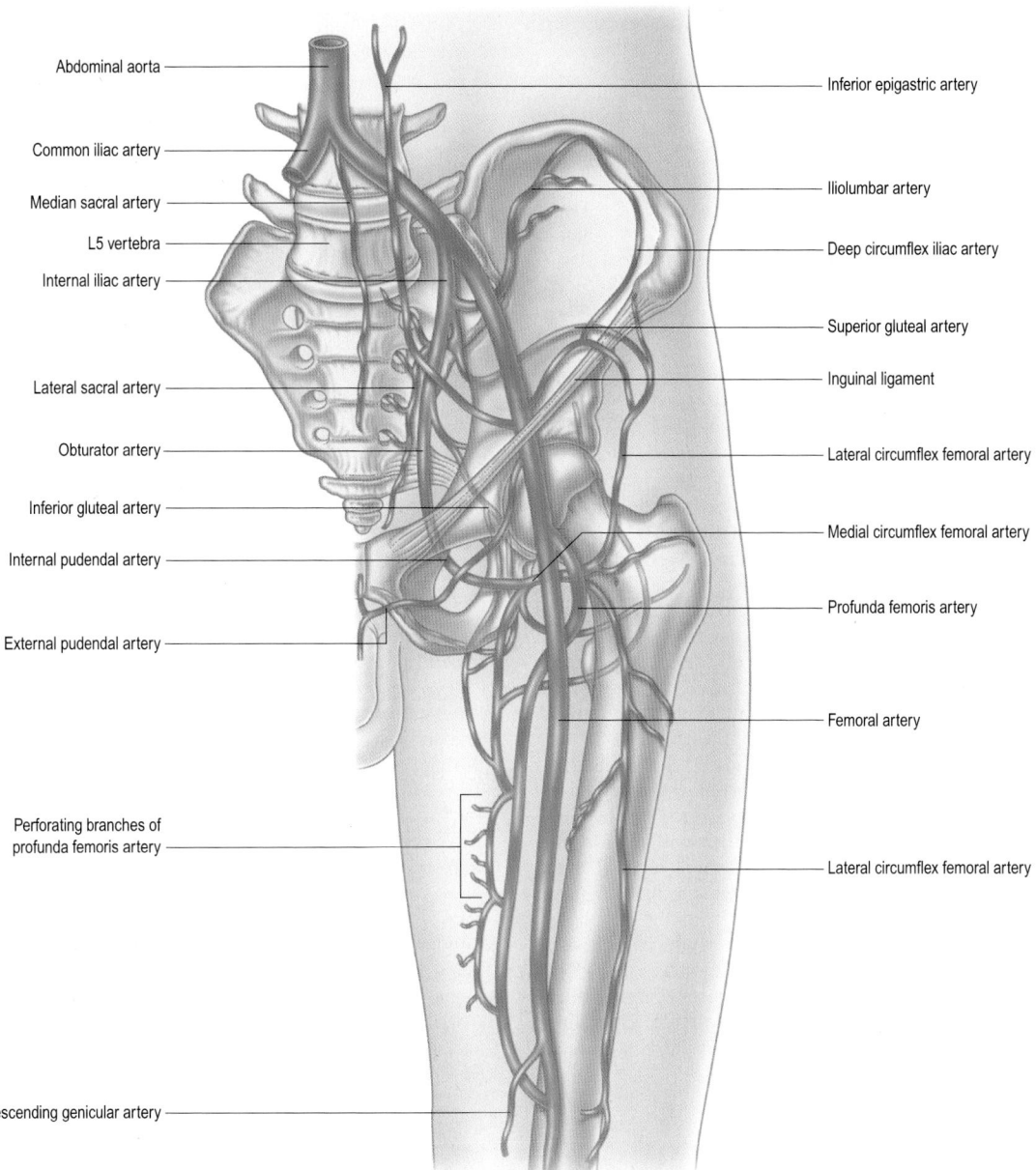

Abdominal aorta

Common iliac artery

Median sacral artery

L5 vertebra

Internal iliac artery

Lateral sacral artery

Obturator artery

Inferior gluteal artery

Internal pudendal artery

External pudendal artery

Perforating branches of
profunda femoris artery

Descending genicular artery

Inferior epigastric artery

Iliolumbar artery

Deep circumflex iliac artery

Superior gluteal artery

Inguinal ligament

Lateral circumflex femoral artery

Medial circumflex femoral artery

Profunda femoris artery

Femoral artery

Lateral circumflex femoral artery

Fig. 111.21 Collateral circulation around the hip and upper thigh.

The pattern of venous drainage of the head and neck corresponds in general to that of the arteries, though there may be a single large cervical vein posteroinferiorly.

Innervation

The periosteal innervation is derived proximally from nerves that supply the hip joint (p. 1440), distally from those supplying the knee (p. 1482), and in all areas from nerves that innervate muscles attached to the bone.

Ossification (Figs 111.15, 111.16, 111.22)

The femur ossifies from five centres: in the shaft, head, greater and lesser trochanters and the distal end. Other than the clavicle, it is the first long bone to ossify. The process starts in the midshaft in the seventh prenatal week and extends to produce a miniature shaft that is largely ossified at birth. Secondary centres appear in the distal end (from which the condyles and epicondyles are formed) during the ninth month, in the head during the first six months after birth, in the greater trochanter during the fourth year and in the lesser between the twelfth and fourteenth year. The centre in the cartilaginous head is restricted to it until the tenth year, so that the epiphyseal line (**Fig. 111.8**) is horizontal and the inferomedial part of the articular surface is on the neck. The medial epiphyseal margin later grows over this part of the articular surface. Thus, the mature epiphysis is a hollow cup on the summit of

the neck. The epiphyseal line follows the articular margin except where it is separated superiorly from the articular surface by a non-articular area where blood vessels enter the head (Trueta 1957). The epiphyses fuse independently: the lesser trochanter soon after puberty, then the greater, the head in the fourteenth year in females, seventeenth in males, and the distal end in the sixteenth year in females, eighteenth in males. The distal epiphyseal plate traverses the adductor tubercle.

Growth plate considerations

Trauma to any epiphyseal plate can lead to bony union between epiphysis and metaphysis, and so cause premature cessation of growth. Any surgery in the hip region in children can injure the growth plate, resulting in abnormal proximal femoral development. In the case of fractures involving the epiphysis, restoration of normal bony alignment as soon as possible is essential to minimize the risk of subsequent abnormal growth.

The growth plate represents a line of weakness and predisposes to fracture from injury. Such injuries affecting the capital epiphysis are uncommon.

As well as acute injury, a more chronic fracture through the capital epiphysis occurs in 'slipped upper femoral epiphysis'. The condition affects pubescent adolescents, especially males. Endocrinological abnormality may be related. The femoral head epiphysis displaces posteriorly

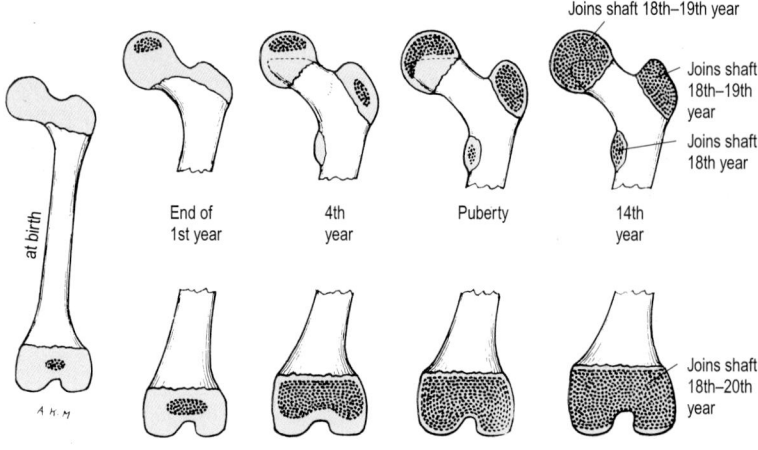

Joins shaft 18th–19th year

Joins shaft 18th–19th year

Joins shaft 18th year

at birth

End of 1st year

4th year

Puberty

14th year

Joins shaft 18th–20th year

Fig. 111.22 Stages in ossification of the femur (not to scale). Blue = unossified (cartilaginous) regions.

off the femoral neck. If it heals in this position, lower limb deformity and restricted hip movement occur. A classic hallmark is obligatory external rotation of the femur as the hip is flexed. Treatment varies according to the time taken for the 'slip' to occur. Normal anatomical restoration is rarely possible in 'acute' cases. The position of the femoral head may be accepted as it is and fixed with screws in this position to stop further displacement. This treatment will deliberately cause premature growth plate fusion and so prevent future 'slippage'. Since the distal femoral growth plate produces the vast majority of femoral length, an acceptable limb length difference usually results.

Infection of bone in neonates and young children tends to arise via bacteria in the blood stream which usually 'seed' in the metaphyseal region, probably as a consequence of the vascular 'arcade' arrangement of arteries in this part of the bone. The proximal femoral growth plate is intra-articular. As a result infection in the proximal femoral metaphysis can spread into the joint and result in a septic arthritis that can destroy the hip joint permanently.

The distal end of the femur is the only epiphysis in which ossification consistently starts just before birth, a most reliable indicator that a dead newborn child was viable. Since the epiphyseal plate is level with the adductor tubercle, the epiphysis is partly extra-articular. Operations here may damage the distal epiphyseal cartilage in children and result in subsequent shortening of the leg.

JOINTS

PUBIC SYMPHYSIS
The pubic bones meet in the midline at the pubic symphysis, a secondary cartilaginous joint (**Fig. 111.3**).

Articulating surfaces
The articulating surfaces are the medial (symphyseal) surfaces of the pubic bones, each covered by a thin layer of tightly adherent hyaline cartilage (surface growth cartilage in the young). The junction is not flat but marked by reciprocal crests and papillae. Theoretically this would resist shearing. The surfaces of hyaline cartilage are connected by fibrocartilage, varying in thickness and constituting the interpubic disc. The symphysis often contains a cavity, probably due to absorption. It rarely appears before the tenth year and is non-synovial. The cavity, which is better developed in females, is usually posterosuperior but may reach the front or even occupy most of the cartilage.

Ligaments
The interpubic disc is strengthened anteriorly by several interlacing collagenous fibrous layers, passing obliquely from bone to bone, decussating and interweaving with fibres of the external oblique aponeuroses and the medial tendons of the recti abdominis. These layers constitute the anterior pubic ligament. There are also less well-developed posterior fibres, sometimes named the posterior pubic ligament. The main ligaments of the joint are the superior and arcuate pubic ligaments. The superior pubic ligament connects the bones above, extending to the pubic tubercles. The arcuate pubic ligament, a thick arch of fibres, connects the lower borders of the symphyseal pubic surfaces bounding the pubic arch. Superiorly it blends with the interpubic disc

and extends laterally attached to the inferior pubic rami. Its inferior edge is separated from the anterior border of the perineal membrane by an opening for the deep dorsal vein of the penis or clitoris.

Vascular supply
The pubic symphysis is supplied by pubic branches of the obturator, superficial external pudendal and inferior epigastric arteries.

Innervation
The pubic symphysis is innervated by branches from the iliohypogastric, ilioinguinal and pudendal nerves.

Factors maintaining stability
The interpubic disc and the superior and arcuate ligaments are the main stabilizing factors of the pubic symphysis.

Movements
Angulation, rotation and displacement are possible but slight and are likely during movement at the sacroiliac and hip joints. Excessive movement may occur as a sports injury. Some separation occurs late in gestation and during childbirth: on occasion this is considerable.

Relations and 'at risk' structures
Anteriorly the pubic symphysis is related to superficial fascia and skin. Because of the obliquity of the joint, the proximal shafts of the penis and clitoris also lie anterior to its lower half. Inferiorly the urethra lies c.2.5 cm away in the male, and somewhat closer in the female, as it passes through the perineal membrane. Closer to the joint, the deep dorsal vein of the penis or clitoris passes between the arcuate ligament and the anterior border of the perineal membrane. Posteriorly the upper part of the joint is separated from the inferolateral surfaces of the bladder by the retropubic fat pad. Inferiorly in the male the prostatic venous plexus separates the prostate from the lower part of the joint. The region is sometimes termed the retropubic space. Because of these relations traumatic disruption of the anterior bony pelvis may be associated with serious urogenital injury.

SACROILIAC JOINT (Fig. 111.23)
The sacroiliac joint is a synovial articulation between the sacral and iliac auricular surfaces. Fibrous adhesions and gradual obliteration occur in both sexes, earlier in males, and after the menopause in females. Radiological evidence of obliteration in normal subjects is occasionally seen before 50 years, but is not uncommon thereafter. In old age the joint may be completely fibrosed and occasionally even ossified.

Articulating surfaces
The surfaces are nearly flat only in infants; in adults they are irregular, often markedly so, and sometimes sinuous. The curvatures and irregularities, greater in males, are reciprocal: they restrict movements and contribute to the considerable strength of the joint in transmitting weight from the vertebral column to the lower limbs. The sacral surface is covered by hyaline cartilage, which is thicker anteriorly than posteriorly in adults. The thinner cartilage on the iliac surface, earlier thought to be fibrocartilage, is also hyaline as confirmed by the presence of type II collagen.

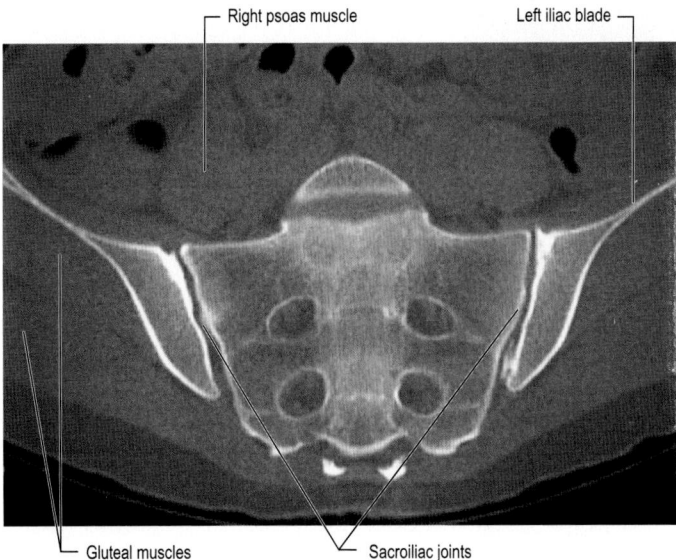

Right psoas muscle · Left iliac blade

Gluteal muscles · Sacroiliac joints

Fig. 111.23 Multislice CT of the sacroiliac joints in an adult female, reformatted in the coronal plane. (By kind permission from Dr Justin Lee, Chelsea and Westminster Hospital, London.)

Fibrous capsule

The capsule is attached close to both articular margins.

Ligaments

Anterior sacroiliac ligament (Fig. 111.11) – The anterior sacroiliac ligament, an anteroinferior capsular thickening, is particularly well-developed near the arcuate line and the posterior inferior iliac spine, where it connects the third sacral segment to the lateral side of the preauricular sulcus. It is thin elsewhere.

Interosseous sacroiliac ligament – The interosseous sacroiliac ligament is the major bond between the bones, filling the irregular space postero-superior to the joint. It is covered superficially by the posterior sacroiliac ligament. Its deeper part has superior and inferior bands passing from depressions posterior to the sacral auricular surface to those on the iliac tuberosity. These bands are covered by, and blend with, a more super-ficial fibrous sheet connecting the posterosuperior margin of a rough area posterior to the sacral auricular surface to the corresponding margins of the iliac tuberosity. This sheet is often partially divided into superior and inferior parts, the former uniting the superior articular process and lateral crest on the first two sacral segments to the neigh-bouring ilium as a short posterior iliac ligament (**Fig. 45.49**).

The posterior sacroiliac ligament (Fig. 45.59) – The posterior sacroiliac ligament lies over the interosseous ligament: the dorsal rami of the sacral spinal nerves and vessels intervene. It consists of several weak fasciculi connecting the intermediate and lateral sacral crests to the posterior superior iliac spine and posterior end of the internal lip of the iliac crest. Inferior fibres, from the third and fourth sacral segments, ascend to the posterior superior iliac spine and posterior end of the internal lip of the iliac crest: they may form a separate long posterior sacroiliac ligament. This ligament is continuous laterally with part of the sacrotuberous ligament and medially with the posterior lamina of the thoracolumbar fascia.

Iliolumbar ligament – See page 761.

Sacrotuberous ligament (Figs 111.11, 45.59) – The sacrotuberous ligament is broadly attached by its base to the posterior superior iliac spine. It is partly blended with the posterior sacroiliac ligaments to the lower trans-verse sacral tubercles and the lateral margins of the lower sacrum and upper coccyx. Its oblique fibres descend laterally, converging to form a thick, narrow band that widens again below and is attached to the medial margin of the ischial tuberosity. It then spreads along the ischial ramus as the falciform process, whose concave edge blends with the fascial sheath of the internal pudendal vessels and pudendal nerve. The

lowest fibres of gluteus maximus are attached to the posterior surface of the ligament; superficial fibres of the lower part of the ligament continue into the tendon of biceps femoris. The ligament is pierced by the coc-cygeal branches of the inferior gluteal artery, the perforating cutaneous nerve and filaments of the coccygeal plexus.

Sacrospinous ligament (Fig. 111.11) – The thin, triangular sacrospinous ligament extends from the ischial spine to the lateral margins of the sacrum and coccyx anterior to the sacrotuberous ligament, with which it blends. Its anterior surface is coccygeus: muscle and ligament are coextensive and are the anterior and posterior aspects of the same structure. The sacrospinous ligament is often regarded as a degenerate part of coccygeus.

Sciatic foramina (Fig. 111.11) – The sacrotuberous and sacrospinous liga-ments convert the sciatic notches into foramina.

Greater sciatic foramen – The greater sciatic foramen is bounded antero-superiorly by the greater sciatic notch, posteriorly by the sacrotuberous ligament and inferiorly by the sacrospinous ligament and ischial spine. It is partly filled by the emerging piriformis, above which the superior gluteal vessels and nerve leave the pelvis. Below it, the inferior gluteal vessels and nerve, internal pudendal vessels and pudendal nerve, sciatic and posterior femoral cutaneous nerves and the nerves to obturator internus and quadratus femoris all leave the pelvis.

Lesser sciatic foramen – The lesser sciatic foramen is bounded anteriorly by the ischial body, superiorly by its spine and sacrospinous ligament, and posteriorly by the sacrotuberous ligament. It transmits the tendon of obturator internus, the nerve to obturator internus, and the internal pudendal vessels and pudendal nerve.

Vascular supply

The arterial supply is derived from the iliolumbar, superior gluteal and superior lateral sacral arteries, with corresponding venous drainage. Lymphatic drainage follows the arteries, reaching the iliac and lumbar nodes.

Innervation

The innervation of the sacroiliac joint is controversial and not generally agreed. Results of reported studies vary. It probably receives branches from the anterior and posterior primary rami of the first two sacral spinal nerves, and from the superior gluteal nerve. The obturator nerve and the lumbosacral trunk may also contribute. It is difficult to apply Hilton's law (p. 110) to this joint.

Factors maintaining stability

The sacroiliac joint is one of the most stable joints in the body, and supports the weight of the trunk. The reciprocal irregularity of the joint surfaces allows very little movement. The tendency of the sacrum to be forced downwards by the trunk is resisted by the extremely strong posterior ligaments, while the iliolumbar ligaments help to resist dis-placement of the fifth lumbar vertebra over the sacrum. The sacrotuberous and sacrospinous ligaments oppose upward tilting of the lower part of the sacrum under downward thrust at its upper end.

Movements

Primary movement of the sacroiliac joint is minimal: all muscles that cross the joint act on the lumbar spine or on the hip. Such movements as do occur are mainly imposed on the joint as the pelvis moves. Data from living subjects are technically difficult to obtain, and those based on plain radiographs are unreliable. Studies using implanted tantalum spheres and biplanar radiography have shown mean rotational ranges of less than 2°. Even when there is recordable movement, the direction of movement is irregular. Biplanar radiography has also shown that the axes of movement of the sacroiliac joint during hip movement are oblique, and that the axes differ in flexion and extension.

During pregnancy the pelvic joints and ligaments loosen under the influence of the hormone relaxin. Movements in the joints increase. Relaxation renders the sacroiliac locking mechanism less effective, permitting greater rotation and perhaps allowing alterations in pelvic diameters at childbirth, although the effect is probably small. The impaired locking mechanism diverts the strain of weightbearing to the ligaments, with frequent sacroiliac strain after pregnancy.

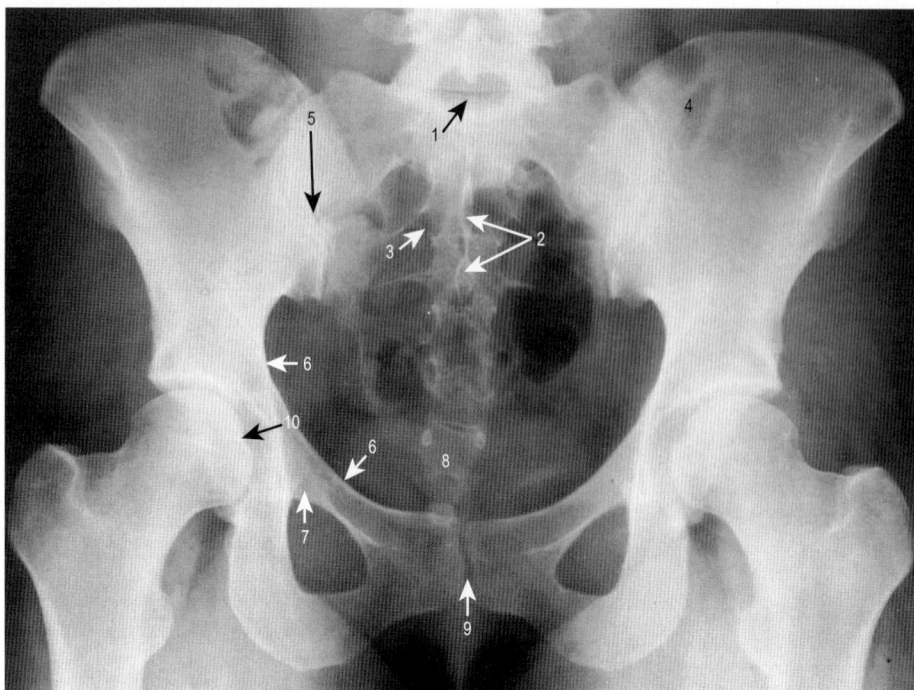

1. Sacral promontory.
2. Sacral spines.
3. Margin of anterior sacral foramen.
4. Gas in pelvic colon.
5. Sacroiliac joint.
6. Pelvic brim.
7. Obturator groove.
8. Coccyx.
9. Symphysis pubis.
10. Fovea of femoral head.

Fig. 111.24 Anteroposterior radiograph of adult female pelvis.

Relations and 'at risk' structures

The sacroiliac joints have many important anterior relations. The internal and external iliac veins join to form the common iliac veins immediately anteriorly, separating the joints from the bifurcations of the common iliac arteries and, more anteriorly, the ureters. The lumbosacral trunk and the obturator nerve cross the anterior aspect of the joint behind the vessels. Piriformis partly attaches to the anterior capsule, separating the joint from the upper part of the sacral plexus.

Variants

Accessory sacroiliac articulations are not uncommon. They develop behind the articular surface between the lateral sacral crest and posterior superior iliac spine and iliac tuberosity, and are acquired fibrocartilaginous joints resulting from the stresses of weightbearing. They have a joint capsule, are saddle-shaped, and may be single, double, unilateral or bilateral (Weisl 1954).

HIP JOINT (Figs 111.24, 111.25, 111.26)

The hip joint is a multiaxial synovial joint of ball-and-socket (spheroidal, cotyloid) type.

Articular surfaces (Figs 111.3, 111.17, 111.25)

The femoral head articulates with the cup-shaped (cotyloid) acetabulum, its centre lying a little below the middle third of the inguinal ligament. (The profile of the anterior margin of the joint is parallel to the middle third of the inguinal ligament.) The articular surfaces are reciprocally curved but neither coextensive nor completely congruent. The close-packed position is in full extension, with slight abduction and medial rotation. As in the shoulder joint, the surfaces are considered ovoid or spheroid rather than spherical, but this is controversial. Evidence favours spheroid and slightly ovoid surfaces, which become almost spherical with advancing age. The femoral head is covered by articular cartilage, except for a rough pit for the ligamentum teres. In front the cartilage extends laterally over a small area on the adjoining neck; it is thickest centrally. Cartilage thickness is maximal anterosuperiorly in the acetabulum and anterolaterally on the femoral head. The acetabular articular surface is an incomplete ring, the lunate surface, broadest above where the pressure of body weight falls in the erect posture, and narrowest in its pubic region. It is deficient inferiorly opposite the acetabular notch and covered by articular cartilage, which is thickest where the surface is broadest. The acetabular fossa within it is devoid of cartilage but contains fibroelastic fat largely covered by synovial membrane. Acetabular depth is increased by the acetabular labrum, a fibrocartilaginous rim attached to the acetabular margin. This deepens the cup and bridges the acetabular notch as the transverse acetabular ligament. The

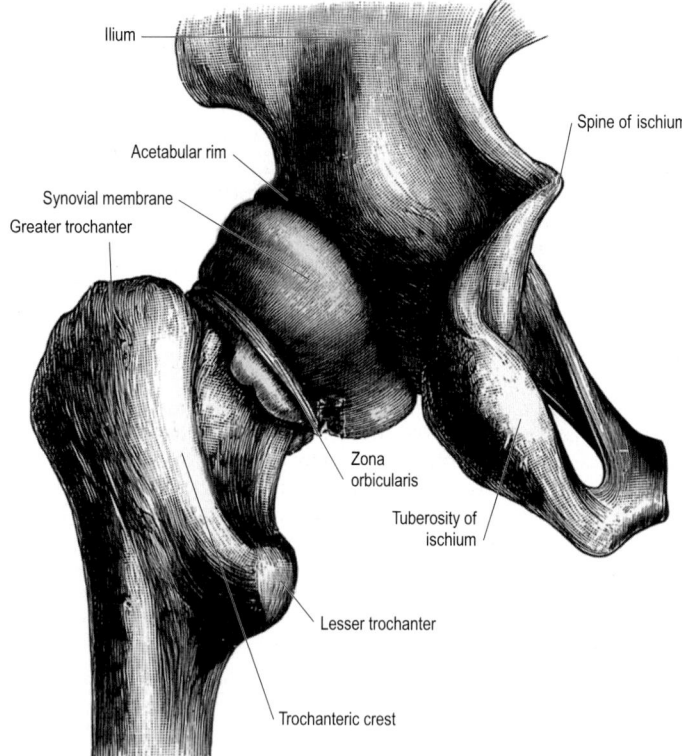

Fig. 111.25 Synovial cavity of left hip joint (distended): posterior aspect.

labrum is triangular in section, attaching by the base of the triangle to the acetabular rim while the apex is its free margin. The diameter of the acetabular cavity is constricted by the labral rim, which embraces the femoral head, maintaining joint stability both as a static restraint and by providing proprioceptive information.

Fibrous capsule

The capsule is strong and dense, and is attached above to the acetabular margin 5–6 mm beyond its labrum, in front to the outer labral aspect and, near the acetabular notch, to the transverse acetabular ligament

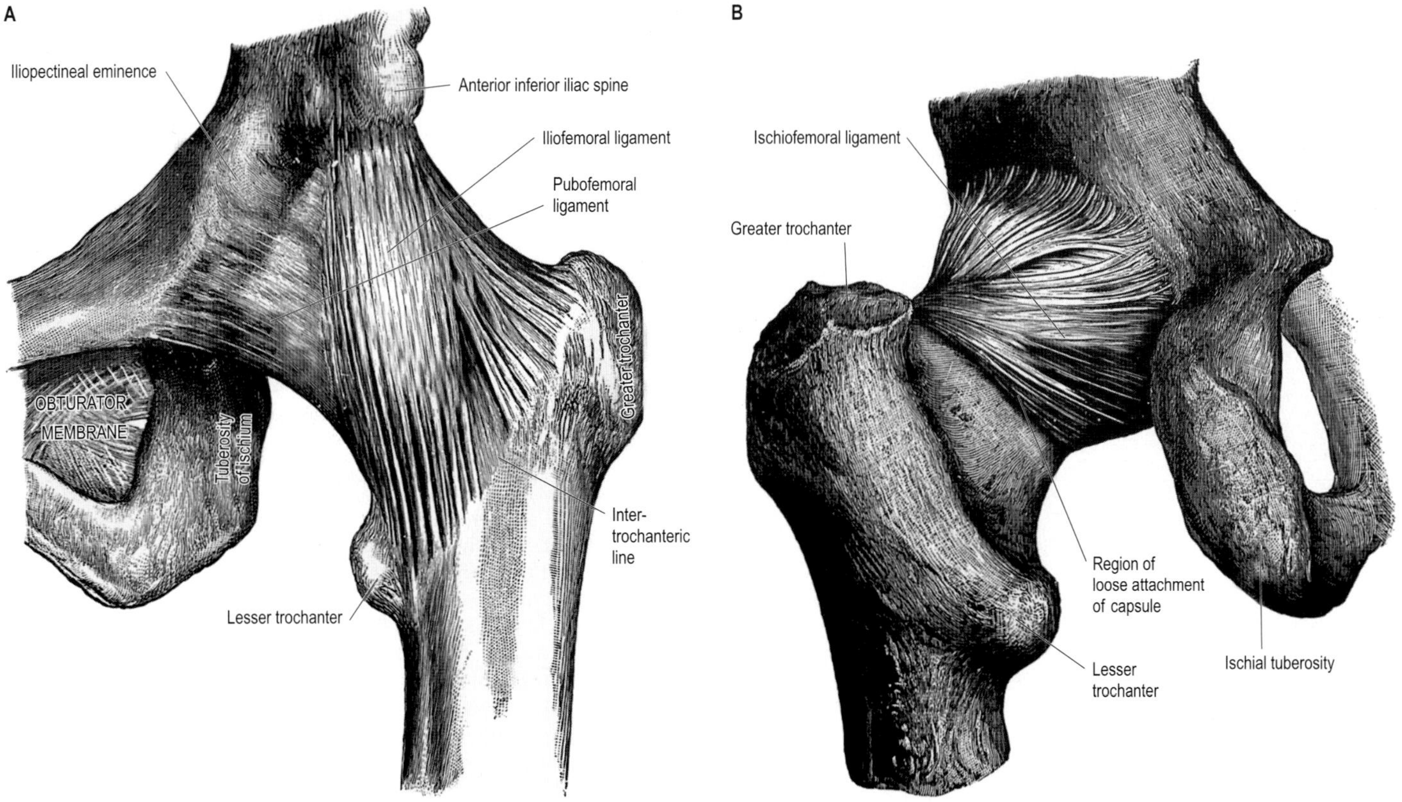

A

B

Fig. 111.26 The left hip joint: **A**, anterior aspect; **B**, posterior aspect.

and the adjacent rim of the obturator foramen. It surrounds the femoral neck and is attached anteriorly to the intertrochanteric line, superiorly to the base of the femoral neck, posteriorly c.1 cm above the intertrochanteric crest, and inferiorly to the femoral neck near the lesser trochanter. Anteriorly many fibres ascend along the neck as longitudinal retinacula, containing blood vessels for both the femoral head and neck. The capsule is thicker anterosuperiorly, where maximal stress occurs, particularly in standing; posteroinferiorly it is thin and loosely attached. It has two sets of fibres, circular and longitudinal. The circular fibres (zona orbicularis) are internal and form a collar round the femoral neck. Though partly blended with the pubofemoral and ischiofemoral ligaments, these fibres are not directly attached to bone. Externally, longitudinal fibres are most numerous in the anterosuperior region, reinforced by the iliofemoral ligament. The capsule is also strengthened by the pubofemoral and ischiofemoral ligaments; externally it is rough, covered by muscles and separated from psoas major and iliacus by a bursa. The capsular attachment to the femur lies well distal to the growth plate of the femoral head both anterior and posteriorly, making the upper femoral epiphysis entirely intracapsular. The capsular attachment also intersects the growth plate of the greater trochanter on the upper surface of the base of the neck (**Figs 111.15, 111.16**).

Ligaments (Fig. 111.26)

The ligaments of the hip joint are the iliofemoral, pubofemoral, ischiofemoral, transverse acetabular and the ligamentum teres. As the hip moves so the capsular ligaments, as capsular thickenings, wind and unwind, tightening around the hip, affecting stability, excursion and joint capacity. As a result of the last point, a hip containing fluid is most comfortable held a little flexed as this provides the largest volume for joint distension. See Fuss and Bacher (1991) for details.

Iliofemoral ligament

The iliofemoral ligament is very strong and shaped like an inverted Y, lying anteriorly and intimately blended with the capsule. Its apex is attached between the anterior inferior iliac spine and acetabular rim, its base to the intertrochanteric line. Fuss and Bacher distinguish a weaker central section, referred to as the greater iliofemoral ligament, with thicker, more dense margins – the lateral and medial iliofemoral ligaments. The oblique lateral ligament attaches to a tubercle at the supero-

lateral end of the intertrochanteric line; the vertical medial ligament reaches the inferomedial end.

Pubofemoral ligament – The pubofemoral ligament is triangular, its base attaching to the iliopubic eminence, superior pubic ramus, obturator crest and obturator membrane. It blends distally with the capsule and deep surface of the medial iliofemoral ligament. Fuss and Bacher consider this ligament to consist of four crura.

Ischiofemoral ligament – The ischiofemoral ligament thickens the back of the capsule and consists of three distinct parts. The central part, the superior ischiofemoral ligament, spirals superolaterally from the ischium, where it is attached posteroinferior to the acetabulum, behind the femoral neck to attach to the greater trochanter deep to the iliofemoral ligament. Some fibres blend with the zona orbicularis. Lateral and medial inferior ischiofemoral ligaments embrace the posterior circumference of the femoral neck.

Transverse acetabular ligament (Fig. 111.3) – The transverse acetabular ligament is part of the labrum but has no cartilage cells. Its strong, flat fibres cross the acetabular notch forming a foramen through which vessels and nerves enter the joint.

Ligamentum teres (ligament of the head of the femur) (Fig. 111.27) – The ligamentum teres is a triangular somewhat flattened band, its apex attached anterosuperiorly in the fovea on the femoral head. Its base is principally attached on both sides of the acetabular notch, between which it blends with the transverse ligament. It also receives weaker contributions from the margins of the acetabular fossa. Ensheathed by synovial membrane, it varies in strength. Occasionally its synovial sheath exists alone, without a core; rarely both ligament and sheath are absent. The ligament appears to tense when the thigh is semi-flexed and adducted, and to relax in abduction.

Synovial membrane

Starting from the femoral articular margin, the synovial membrane covers the intracapsular part of the femoral neck, then passes to the internal surface of the capsule to cover the acetabular labrum, ligamentum teres and fat in the acetabular fossa. It is thin on the deep

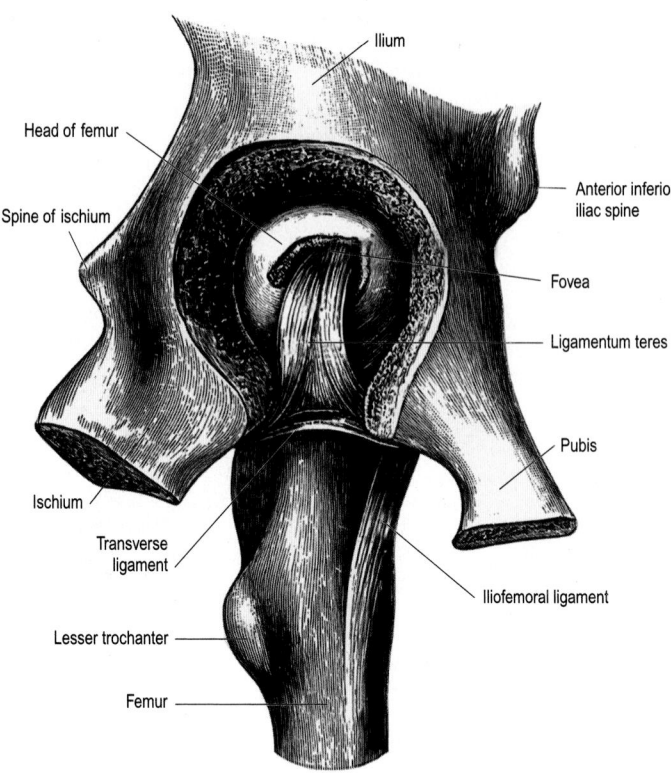

Fig. 111.27 Left hip joint, opened by removal of the acetabular floor from within the pelvis.

surface of the iliofemoral ligament where it is compressed against the femoral head and sometimes is even absent here.

Bursae

The hip joint may communicate with the subtendinous iliac (psoas) bursa by a circular aperture between the pubofemoral ligament and the vertical band of the iliofemoral ligament. More distant bursae are associated with the tendons of attachment of glutei medius and minimus at the greater trochanter, and between gluteus maximus and vastus lateralis.

Vascular supply and lymphatic drainage

Articular arteries are branches from the obturator, medial circumflex femoral, and superior and inferior gluteal arteries, with corresponding venous drainage. They form the cruciate and trochanteric anastomoses (p. 1453). Lymphatics from the front of the hip joint drain to the deep inguinal nodes, while those from the medial and posterior aspects run with the obturator and gluteal arteries respectively to reach the internal iliac nodes.

Innervation

The nerve supply to the hip is from the femoral nerve or its muscular branches, the obturator and accessory obturator nerves, the nerve to quadratus femoris and the superior gluteal nerves.

Factors maintaining stability

The femoral head is closely fitted to the acetabulum in an area exceeding half a sphere, and is embraced closely by its labrum, which restrains it in the socket. In addition a 'vacuum effect' is present. The thick capsule is reinforced by the three major ligaments, of which the iliofemoral is the strongest, and is progressively tightened when the femur extends to the line of the trunk. The pubofemoral and ischiofemoral ligaments also tighten and, as the joint approaches close packing, resistance to an extending torque rapidly increases. In addition, the transverse ligament and the ligament of the head contribute to stability. The hip joint is thus very stable. Traumatic dislocation usually requires extreme violence, and only slight separation can be achieved by strong traction on the intact joint. To aid insertion of an arthroscope, a needle is first inserted

into the joint to release the suction effect. With traction the joint will then open sufficiently.

Movements and muscles

Movements

Movements of the hip joint can be categorized as flexion–extension, adduction–abduction, medial and lateral rotation, and circumduction, conveniently considered as rotations around three orthogonal axes. When femoral movements are considered in relation to the articular surfaces, the length and angulation of the neck in relation to the shaft must be remembered. When the thigh is flexed or extended, the femoral head 'spins' in the acetabulum on an approximately transverse axis. Conversely, the acetabula rotate around similar axes in flexion and extension of the trunk on stationary femoral heads.

With the foot stationary on the ground, medial and lateral femoral rotation have a vertical axis through the centre of the femoral head and medial condyle. Such axial medial rotation is the inevitable conjunct rotation accompanying terminal extension of the knee and is often referred to as 'screw-home'. The reverse occurs in initial flexion at the knee joint. The 'screw-home' phenomenon allows achievement of a 'closed packed position' for the tibiofemoral joint, so aiding stability in the extended knee. Because of the relation of this axis to the whole femur (with its angulated neck and oblique shaft), during medial rotation the medial condyle moves very little on the medial tibial condyle, while the lateral condyle moves forwards on its tibial surface, and the greater trochanter moves simultaneously in a forward arc: converse movements occur during lateral rotation. With the foot in loose contact or free, medial and lateral adjunct rotation of the whole lower limb occur around variable axes, all passing through the femoral head and any part of the foot. Conversely, with one foot stationary and the other free, the whole trunk may rotate on one femoral head, as in cross-kicking. Abduction and adduction are around an anteroposterior axis through the femoral head, but since this is not truly spherical no axis is satisfactory. Some kinesiologists refer to a mechanical axis coincident with the topographical long axis of the femoral neck, impinging on the approximate centre of the articular surface of the head, making extension and flexion of the thigh relatively pure 'spins' at the hip joint and most effective in tightening or relaxing the capsular ligaments. All other movements are regarded as pure or impure swings. While this permits analysis closer to actual articular function than a cardinal triaxial system, related arbitrarily to the 'anatomical' position, the mechanical axis is itself (incorrectly) regarded by some as dynamic because forms of apparent dynamic 'spin' may occur in many positions. This view stems from an imprecise definition of the varieties of axes employed in arthrokinematics. The mechanical axis is not dynamic relative to the femur. It is stationary during pure spins, and moves relative to its coarticular surface in chordal or arcuate paths during pure or impure swings respectively.

Simple flexion is possible to 110–120° from the vertical; extension beyond the vertical is limited (perhaps 10–20°). Both movements are augmented by adjustments of the spinal column and pelvis, flexion of the knee and concomitant medial or lateral hip rotation. For example, knee flexion (lessening tension in the posterior femoral muscles) increases hip flexion to 120°; the thigh can be drawn passively to the trunk, though with some spinal flexion. Extension in walking and running is increased by forward inclination of the body, pelvic tilting and rotation and lateral hip rotation (Joseph 1975). Abduction and adduction can be similarly increased.

Muscles producing movements

Flexion is produced by psoas major and iliacus, assisted by pectineus, rectus femoris and sartorius. The adductors, particularly adductor longus, also assist, especially in early flexion from full extension.

Extension is produced by gluteus maximus and the hamstring (posterior femoral) muscles. In the fully erect posture with pendent arms a vertical line through the centre of gravity of the body passes behind a line joining the centres of the femoral heads. Consequently, the body tends to incline backwards but is counterbalanced by ligamentous tension and congruence and compression of the articular surfaces with the hip joints in the close-packed position. Under increased loading of the trunk or leaning backwards, these resistive but passive factors are assisted by active contraction of the hip flexors. In swaying forwards at the ankles, or when the arms are stretched forward, and also in forward bending at the hip, the line of body weight moves in front of the transverse axis. The posture adopted, or the rate of change of posture, is largely controlled by the hamstrings which, although powerful flexors of the knee, are equally strong extensors of the hip. Gluteus maximus only becomes active when the thigh is extended against resistance, as in rising from a bending position or climbing.

Abduction is produced by gluteus medius and minimus, assisted by tensor fasciae latae and sartorius. Abduction is limited by adductor tension, the pubofemoral ligament and the medial band of the ilio-femoral ligament. These muscles are consistently involved in walking or running, contracting periodically at precise phases of the walking or running cycle.

Adduction is produced by adductors longus, brevis and magnus, assisted by pectineus and gracilis. Adduction is limited by contact with the opposite limb but its range is wider with the thigh flexed, when it is limited by the abductor muscles, the lateral band of the iliofemoral ligament and ligament of the femoral head.

Medial rotation is produced by tensor fasciae latae and the anterior fibres of gluteus minimus and medius. It is relatively weak and is limited by the lateral rotators, ischiofemoral ligament and the posterior part of the capsule. Electromyographic data suggest that the adductors usually assist in medial rather than lateral rotation, but this is, of course, dependent on the primary position.

Lateral rotation is produced by the obturator muscles, the gemelli and quadratus femoris, assisted by piriformis, gluteus maximus and sartorius. It is a powerful action and limited by tension in the medial rotators and the lateral band of the iliofemoral ligament.

Relations and 'at risk' structures

The joint capsule is surrounded by muscles (**Fig. 111.28**). Anteriorly, lateral fibres of pectineus separate its most medial part from the femoral vein. Lateral to this the tendon of psoas major, with iliacus lateral to it, descends across it, partly separated by a bursa. The femoral artery is anterior to the tendon, with the femoral nerve deep in a groove between the tendon and iliacus. More laterally the straight head of rectus femoris crosses the joint with a deep layer of the fascial iliotibial tract, which blends with the capsule under the lateral border of the muscle. Superiorly, the reflected head of rectus femoris contacts the capsule medially, while gluteus minimus covers it laterally, being closely adherent. Inferiorly, lateral fibres of pectineus adjoin the capsule and, more posteriorly, obturator externus spirals obliquely to its posterior aspect. Posteriorly, the lower capsule is covered by the tendon of obturator externus, separating it from quadratus femoris and accompanied by an ascending branch of the medial circumflex femoral artery. Above this the tendon of obturator internus and the gemelli contact the joint, separating it from the sciatic nerve. The nerve to quadratus femoris is deep to the

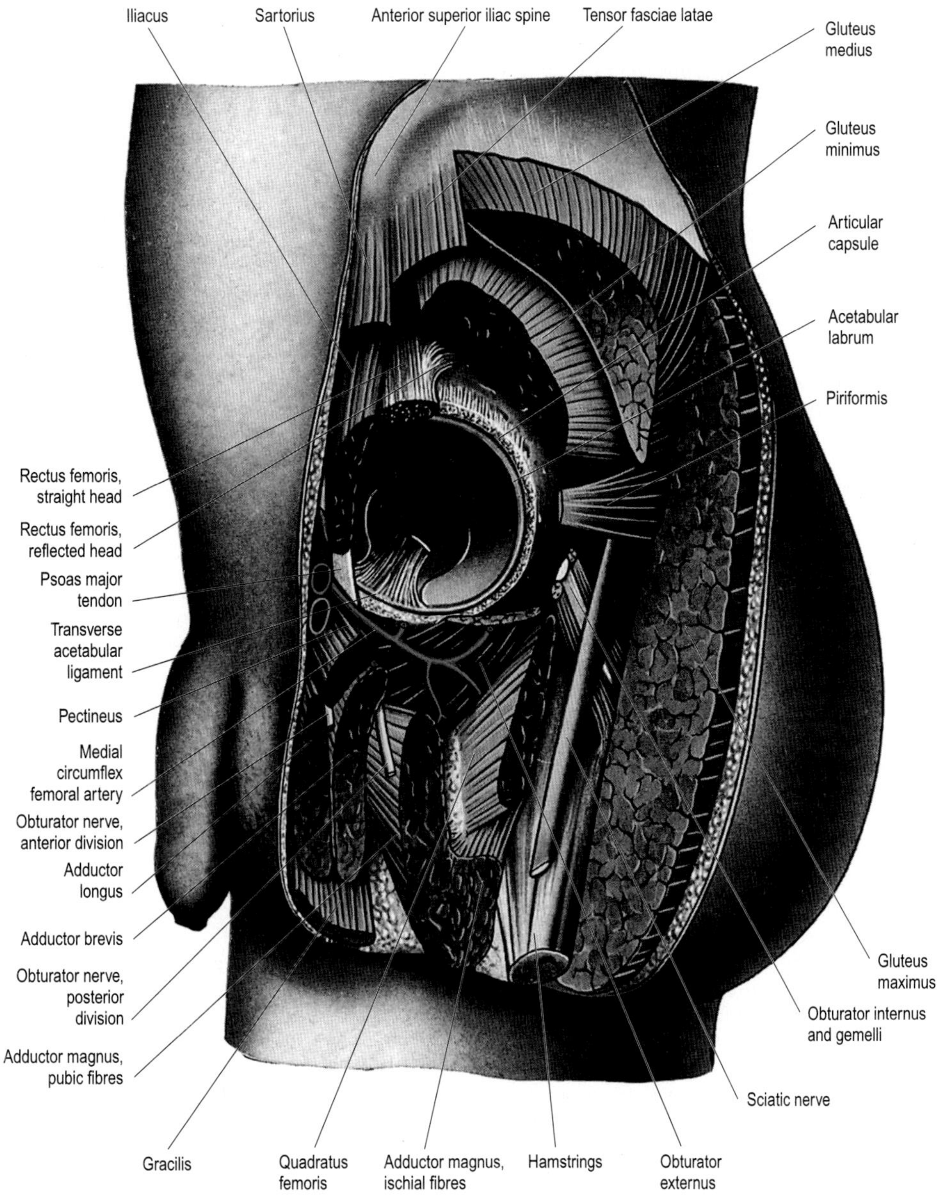

Fig. 111.28 Dissection to display the structures surrounding the left hip joint. The femoral head has been disarticulated and removed.

obturator internus tendon, and descends most medially on the capsule. Above this, the posterior surface of the joint is crossed by piriformis.

Hip and groin pain

There are a number of possible causes for the painful hip and groin. True hip joint pain is usually felt deep in the crease of the groin. A patient with pain over the lateral aspect of the hip usually has a local problem such as trochanteric bursitis. Pain in the buttock is only occasionally from the hip joint: most frequently it is referred from the lumbosacral spine. Vascular claudication is another cause of buttock pain. Groin pain may be due to inguinal or femoral hernias. In the younger age group groin pain afflicts those engaged in sport, especially running ball sports. Here the pain is sometimes from a hernia but more commonly related to adductor tendinitis secondary to acute or chronic overload of the adductor longus tendon. Another common problem is attritional chronic overload of the anterior abdominal wall at its attachments to the pubis and inguinal ligament, or of external oblique at the external inguinal ring. Rarely problems at the symphysis pubis occur. Great care is required to localize the causative problem.

MUSCLES

MUSCLES OF THE ILIAC REGION

Although there is no 'iliac region' as such, this heading conveniently describes a group of three muscles that originate from the lumbar vertebral column (psoas major and minor) and the ilium (iliacus). Two (psoas major and iliacus) are attached together on the femur as flexors and are often considered as a functional unit, iliopsoas. Psoas minor only reaches the pubis, and acts on the spine and sacroiliac joint.

Iliac fascia

The iliac fascia covers psoas and iliacus. It is thin above, but thickens progressively towards the inguinal ligament. The part covering psoas is thickened above as the medial arcuate ligament. Medially, the fascia over psoas is attached by a series of fibrous arches to the intervertebral discs, the margins of vertebral bodies, and the upper part of the sacrum. Laterally, it blends with the fascia anterior to quadratus lumborum above the iliac crest, and with the fascia covering iliacus below the crest.

The iliac part is connected laterally to the whole of the inner lip of the iliac crest and medially to the pelvic brim, where it blends with the periosteum. It is attached to the iliopectineal eminence, where it receives a slip from the tendon of psoas minor, when that muscle is present. The external iliac vessels are anterior to the fascia but the branches of the lumbar plexus are posterior. The fascia is separated from the peritoneum by loose extraperitoneal tissue. Lateral to the femoral vessels, the iliac fascia is continuous with the posterior margin of the inguinal ligament and the transversalis fascia. Medially it passes behind the femoral vessels to become the pectineal fascia, attached to the pecten pubis. At the junction of its lateral and medial parts it is attached to the iliopectineal eminence and the capsule of the hip joint. It thus forms a septum between the inguinal ligament and the hip bone, dividing the space here into a lateral part, the lacuna musculorum, containing psoas major, iliacus and the femoral nerve, and a medial part, the lacuna vasorum, transmitting the femoral vessels (**Fig. 111.2**). The iliac fascia continues downward to form the posterior wall of the femoral sheath.

PSOAS MAJOR (Fig. 111.29)

Attachments – Psoas major is a long muscle that lies on either side of the lumbar vertebral column and the pelvic brim. Its proximal attachments are complex. They include the anterior surfaces and lower borders of the transverse processes of all the lumbar vertebrae. There are five digitations, each from the bodies of two adjoining vertebrae and their intervertebral disc. The highest of these arises from the lower margin of the body of the twelfth thoracic vertebra, the upper margin of the body of the first lumbar vertebra and the interposed thoracolumbar disc. The lowest arises from the adjacent margins of the bodies of the fourth and fifth lumbar vertebrae and the interposed disc. A series of tendinous arches extend across the narrow parts of the bodies of the lumbar vertebrae between the digitations already described. The lumbar arteries and veins, and filaments from the sympathetic trunk, pass medial to these arches.

The upper four lumbar intervertebral foramina bear important relations to these attachments of the muscle. The foramina lie anterior

to the transverse processes and posterior to the attachments to vertebral bodies, discs and tendinous arches. Thus, the roots of the lumbar plexus enter the muscle directly, the plexus is lodged within it, and its branches emerge from its borders and surfaces.

The muscle descends along the pelvic brim, continues posterior to the inguinal ligament and anterior to the capsule of the hip joint, and converges to a tendon which, having received on its lateral side nearly all the fibres of iliacus, becomes attached to the lesser trochanter of the femur. The large subtendinous iliac bursa, which occasionally communicates with the cavity of the hip joint, separates the tendon from the pubis and the capsule of the joint.

The complex vertebral attachments of psoas major sometimes display minor numerical variations.

Relations – The upper limit of psoas major is posterior to the diaphragm in the lowest part of the posterior mediastinum. It may be in contact with the posterior extremity of the pleural sac. In the abdomen its anterolateral surface is related to the medial arcuate ligament (an arched thickening in the general psoas fascia), extraperitoneal tissue and peritoneum, the kidney, psoas minor, renal vessels, ureter, testicular or ovarian vessels and genitofemoral nerve. Anteriorly, the right psoas is overlapped by the inferior vena cava and crossed by the end of the ileum; the left psoas is crossed by the colon. Its posterior surface is related to the transverse processes of the lumbar vertebrae and the medial edge of quadratus lumborum. The lumbar plexus is embedded posteriorly in the substance of psoas major. Medially the muscle is related to the bodies of the lumbar vertebrae and lumbar vessels. Along its anteromedial margin it is in contact with the sympathetic trunk, aortic lymph nodes and, along the pelvic brim, with the external iliac artery. This margin is covered by the inferior vena cava on the right side, and lies posterior and lateral to the abdominal aorta on the left side. In the thigh, psoas is related anteriorly to the fascia lata and the femoral artery, and posteriorly to the capsule of the hip joint from which it is separated by a bursa. At its medial border, it is related to pectineus and the medial circumflex femoral artery, and to the femoral vein, which may overlap it slightly. At its lateral border it is related to the femoral nerve and iliacus. The femoral nerve descends at first through the fibres of psoas major, and then in the furrow between it and iliacus.

Branches of the lumbar plexus diverge from the abdominal part of psoas. Emerging from the lateral border, from above downwards, are the iliohypogastric, ilioinguinal and lateral femoral cutaneous and femoral nerves. From the anterolateral surface the genitofemoral nerve emerges, and the obturator and accessory obturator nerves and the upper root of the lumbosacral trunk all emerge from the medial border.

Vascular supply – Psoas major is supplied by a rich network of arteries derived from the lumbar, iliolumbar, obturator, external iliac and femoral arteries. In general terms, the upper part of the muscle is supplied by the lumbar arteries, the mid part by the anterior branch of the iliolumbar artery (the main artery to the muscle) with contributions from the deep circumflex and external iliac arteries, and the distal part by the femoral artery and its branches. The psoas sheath has an arterial supply independent from that of the muscle, though the same vessels contribute.

Innervation – Psoas major is innervated by the ventral rami of the lumbar spinal nerves, mainly L1 and 2 with some contribution from L3.

Actions – Psoas major acts together with iliacus; the combination is referred to as iliopsoas. See below with iliacus.

Clinical anatomy: testing – See below after iliacus.

PSOAS MINOR (Fig. 111.29)

Attachments – Psoas minor is absent in c.40% of subjects. When present, it lies anterior to psoas major, entirely within the abdomen. It arises from the sides of the bodies of the twelfth thoracic and first lumbar vertebrae and from the disc between them. It ends in a long, flat tendon which is attached to the pecten pubis and iliopectineal eminence and, laterally, to the iliac fascia.

Relations – Psoas minor lies on psoas major, and its proximal anterior relations are those of the anterior or anteromedial surface of that muscle.

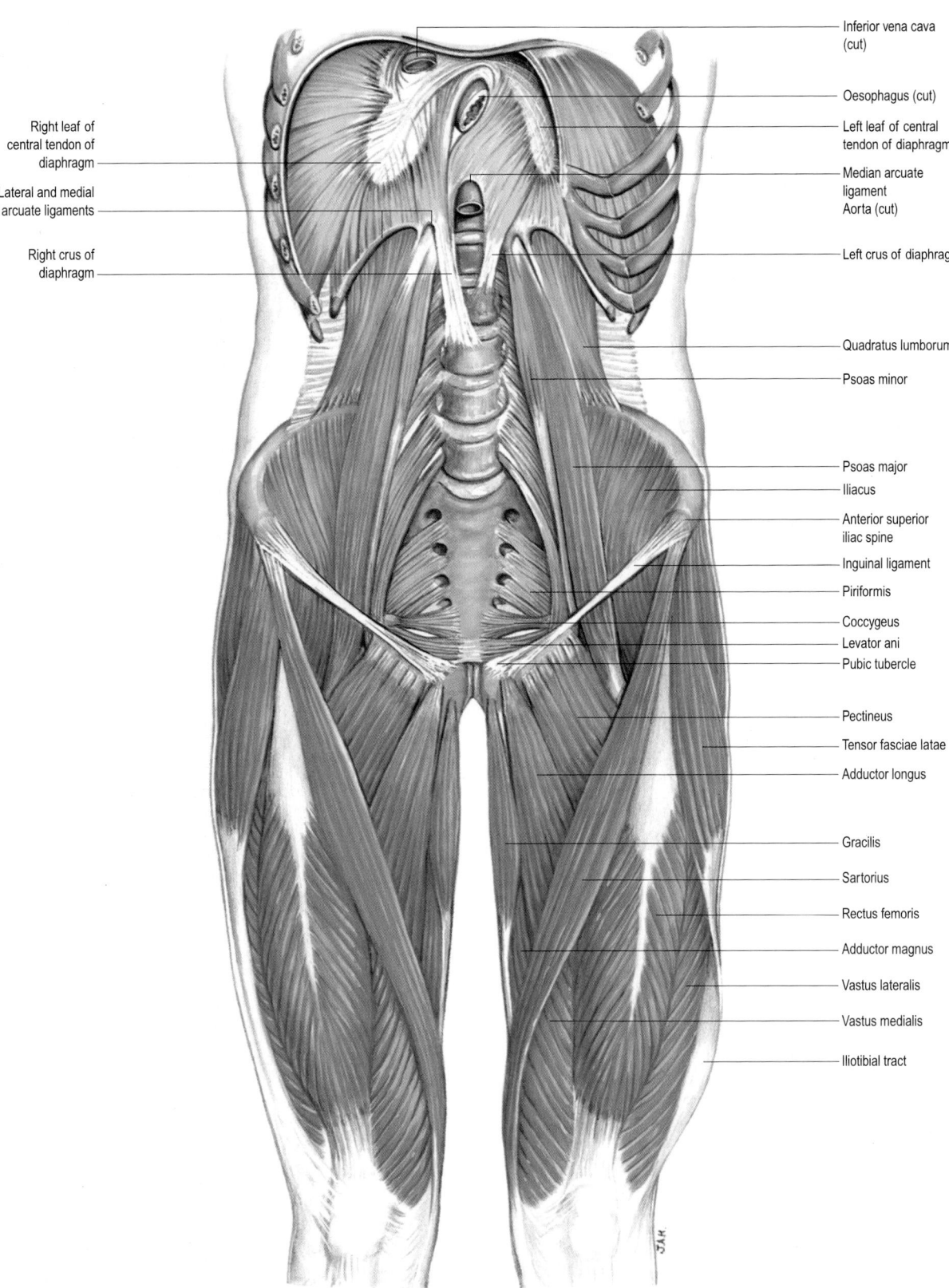

Inferior vena cava (cut)

Oesophagus (cut)

Left leaf of central tendon of diaphragm

Median arcuate ligament
Aorta (cut)

Left crus of diaphragm

Quadratus lumborum

Psoas minor

Psoas major

Iliacus

Anterior superior iliac spine

Inguinal ligament

Piriformis

Coccygeus

Levator ani

Pubic tubercle

Pectineus

Tensor fasciae latae

Adductor longus

Gracilis

Sartorius

Rectus femoris

Adductor magnus

Vastus lateralis

Vastus medialis

Iliotibial tract

Right leaf of central tendon of diaphragm

Lateral and medial arcuate ligaments

Right crus of diaphragm

Fig. 111.29 View of the abdomen, pelvis and thighs, showing abdominal aspect of the diaphragm, hip flexors and superficial muscles of the thigh.

Vascular supply – The main arterial supply to psoas minor is from the lumbar arteries, though there may be minor contributions from other vessels of the network that supplies psoas major (p. 1449).

Innervation – Psoas minor is innervated by a branch from L1.

Action – Psoas minor is probably a weak flexor of the trunk.

Testing – Psoas minor cannot be tested clinically.

ILIACUS (Fig. 111.29)

Attachments – Iliacus is a triangular sheet of muscle that arises from the superior two-thirds of the concavity of the iliac fossa, the inner lip of the iliac crest, the ventral sacroiliac and iliolumbar ligaments, and the upper surface of the lateral part of the sacrum (**Fig. 45.31**). In front, it reaches as far as the anterior superior and anterior inferior iliac spines, and receives a few fibres from the upper part of the capsule of the hip joint. Most of its fibres converge into the lateral side of the strong tendon of psoas major, and the muscles then insert together into the lesser trochanter, but some fibres are attached directly to the femur for c.2.5 cm below and in front of the lesser trochanter.

Relations – In the abdomen, the anterior surface of iliacus is related to its fascia (which separates the muscle from extraperitoneal tissue and peritoneum), the lateral femoral cutaneous nerve, the caecum (on the right) and the iliac part of the descending colon (on the left). On its posterior surface is the iliac fossa, at its medial border, psoas major and the femoral nerve. In the thigh, its anterior surface is in contact with the fascia lata, rectus femoris, sartorius and profunda femoris artery, and its posterior surface is in contact with the capsule of the hip joint, from which it is separated by a bursa it shares with psoas major.

Vascular supply – Iliacus is supplied by the same arterial network as psoas major (p. 1449), and there is mutual overlap of the arterial territories of each muscle. The main supply is from the iliac branches of the anterior iliolumbar artery, with contributions from the deep circumflex iliac, obturator and femoral systems.

Innervation – Iliacus is innervated by branches of the femoral nerve, L2 and 3.

Actions of iliopsoas – Psoas major, acting from above together with iliacus, flexes the thigh upon the pelvis. Electromyographic studies do not support the common view that psoas major acts as a medial rotator of the hip joint, but activity has been described in lateral rotation, particularly in the young. When psoas major and iliacus of both sides act from below, they contract powerfully to bend the trunk and pelvis forwards against resistance, as in raising the trunk from the recumbent to the sitting posture when undertaking a 'sit-up' exercise.

Electromyography does not support the anatomical prediction that unilateral action of psoas causes lateral and forward flexion of the trunk to that side.

In symmetrical standing, iliopsoas has some action from below to maintain the vertebral column upright. Psoas major is active in balancing the trunk while sitting.

Clinical anatomy: testing – Both psoas and iliacus may be the sites of pathological collections of fluid. An abscess (typically tuberculous) of vertebral origin may track down through psoas and present as a mass in the thigh. Haematoma or infection within the iliacus fascia may present as a mass or as a flexion deformity of the hip.

Iliopsoas may be tested clinically by actively flexing the hip against resistance, in the supine position with hip and knee flexed.

PIRIFORMIS (Fig. 111.30)

Attachments – Piriformis occupies a central position in the buttock, where it lies in the same plane as gluteus medius. It arises from the anterior surface of the sacrum by three digitations, which are attached to the portions of bone between the pelvic sacral foramina, and to the grooves leading from the foramina (**Fig. 45.31**). It also arises from the gluteal surface of the ilium near the posterior inferior iliac spine, from the capsule of the adjacent sacroiliac joint, and sometimes from the upper part of the pelvic surface of the sacrotuberous ligament. The

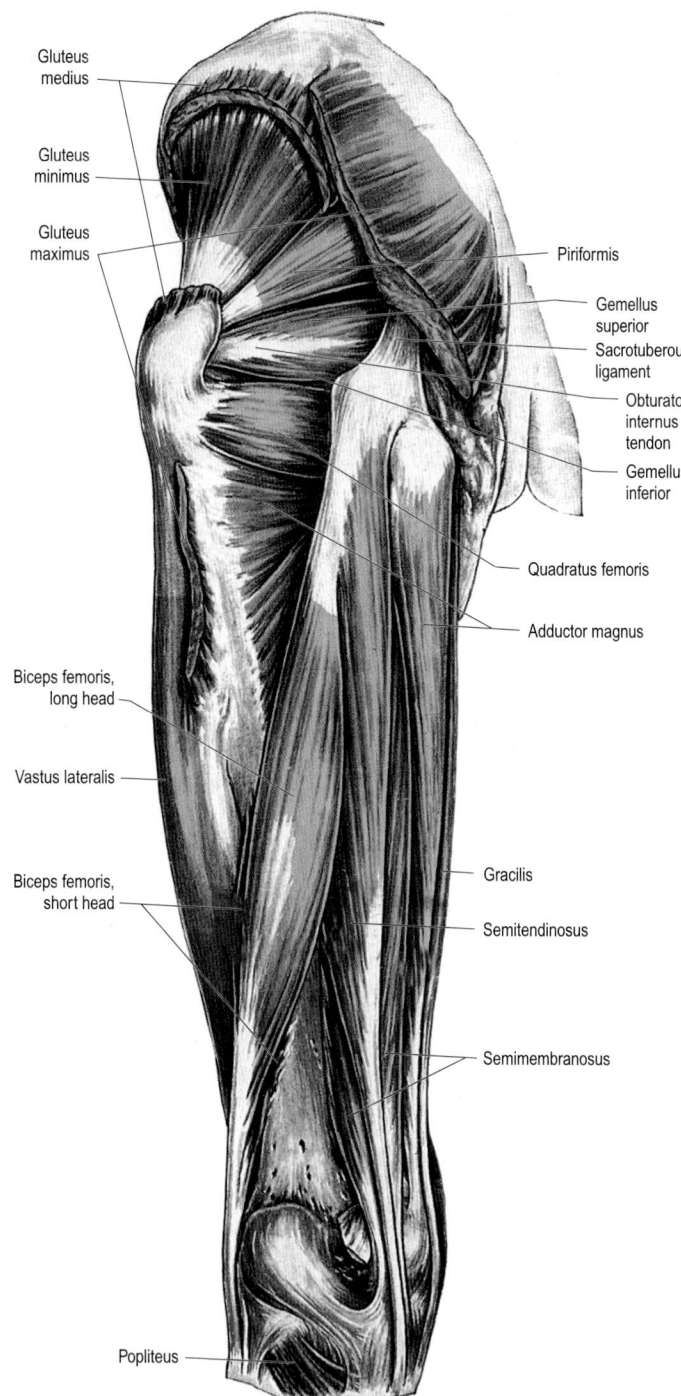

Gluteus medius

Gluteus minimus

Gluteus maximus

Piriformis

Gemellus superior

Sacrotuberous ligament

Obturator internus tendon

Gemellus inferior

Quadratus femoris

Adductor magnus

Biceps femoris, long head

Vastus lateralis

Biceps femoris, short head

Gracilis

Semitendinosus

Semimembranosus

Popliteus

Fig. 111.30 Muscles of the left gluteal region and posterior thigh.

muscle passes out of the pelvis through the greater sciatic foramen, which it substantially fills. Here it constitutes an important surgical landmark for structures that emerge above and below it. It inserts into the medial side of the upper border of the greater trochanter of the femur via a rounded tendon that lies behind and above, but is often partially blended with, the common tendon of obturator internus and the gemelli. The muscle itself may be fused with gluteus medius.

Relations – Within the pelvis, the anterior surface of piriformis is related to the rectum (especially on the left), the sacral plexus of nerves and branches of the internal iliac vessels. The posterior surface lies against the sacrum. Outside the pelvis, its anterior surface is in contact with the posterior surface of the ischium and capsule of the hip joint and its posterior surface with gluteus maximus. Its upper border is in contact with gluteus medius and the superior gluteal vessels and nerve, its lower border with coccygeus and gemellus superior. The inferior gluteal and internal pudendal vessels, the sciatic, posterior femoral cutaneous and pudendal nerves, and muscular branches from the sacral plexus appear in the buttock in the interval between piriformis and gemellus superior. The relationship between piriformis and the sciatic nerve is variable. The undivided nerve may emerge above the muscle (usual) or through the muscle. The major divisions of the nerve may lie either side of the muscle, or (the most common variant) one division passes between the heads of a divided muscle and one division either above or below.

Piriformis can occasionally cause entrapment of the sciatic nerve in the buttock, giving rise to the so-called 'piriformis syndrome'.

Vascular supply – In the buttock, piriformis is supplied mainly from the superior gluteal artery, with contributions from the gemellar branches of the internal pudendal. There may be a separate branch from the inferior gluteal artery. In the pelvis the main supply is from the lateral sacral artery, with contributions from both gluteal vessels.

Innervation – Piriformis is innervated by branches from L5, S1 and 2.

Actions – Piriformis rotates the extended thigh laterally, but abducts the flexed thigh.

Clinical anatomy: testing – Clinically it is not possible to test piriformis alone; however, for suspected injury to piriformis the best provocative test is to ask the seated subject to abduct the thighs. Buttock pain suggests piriformis injury.

OBTURATOR INTERNUS (Fig. 111.31)

Attachments – Obturator internus is situated partly within the true pelvis and partly posterior to the hip joint. It arises from the internal surface of the anterolateral wall of the lesser pelvic cavity. Its attachments, which almost surround the obturator foramen, are to the inferior ramus of the pubis, the ischial ramus, and the pelvic surface of the hip bone below and behind the pelvic brim, to the upper part of the greater sciatic foramen above and behind, to the obturator foramen below and in front (**Fig. 111.5B**). It also arises from the medial part of the pelvic surface of the obturator membrane, from the tendinous arch that completes the obturator canal, and, to a small extent, from the obturator fascia that covers the muscle. The fibres converge rapidly towards the lesser sciatic foramen and end in four or five tendinous bands on the deep surface of the muscle. These bands make a lateral right-angled turn around the grooved surface of the ischium between its spine and

tuberosity. The grooved surface is covered with a smooth layer of hyaline cartilage and is separated from the tendon by a bursa: ridges on the surface correspond to furrows between the tendinous bands. These bands leave the pelvis through the lesser sciatic foramen and unite to form a single flattened tendon that passes horizontally across the capsule of the hip joint. The gemelli fuse with this tendon before it inserts into an anterior impression on the medial surface of the greater trochanter anterosuperior to the trochanteric fossa. A long, narrow bursa is usually interposed between the tendon and the capsule of the hip joint, and occasionally communicates with the bursa between the tendon and the ischium.

Relations – Within the pelvis, the anterolateral surface of the muscle is in contact with the obturator membrane and inner surface of the lateral wall of the pelvis. Its posteromedial surface is related to the obturator fascia, the origin of levator ani, and the sheath that surrounds the internal pudendal vessels and pudendal nerve, and forms the lateral wall of the ischiorectal fossa. Outside the pelvis, the muscle is covered by gluteus maximus, is crossed posteriorly by the sciatic nerve and passes behind the hip joint. As the tendon of obturator internus emerges from the lesser sciatic foramen it is overlapped both above and below by the two gemelli, which form a muscular canal for it. Near its termination the gemelli pass anterior to the tendon and form a groove in which it lies.

Vascular supply – The main arterial supply of the extrapelvic part of obturator internus is from the gemellar branches of the internal pudendal artery. The intrapelvic part is supplied by the obturator artery, which gives branches to both surfaces of the muscle: it is also supplied by small branches from the internal pudendal artery.

Innervation – Obturator internus is innervated by the nerve to obturator internus, L5 and S1.

Actions – See below, with obturator externus.

OBTURATOR EXTERNUS (Fig. 111.32)

Attachments – Obturator externus is a flat, triangular muscle covering the external surface of the anterior pelvic wall. It arises from the medial two-thirds of the external surface of the obturator membrane, and from the adjacent bone of the pubic and ischial rami, extending for a short distance onto their pelvic surfaces between the margin of the obturator foramen and the obturator membrane. The whole muscle, and the

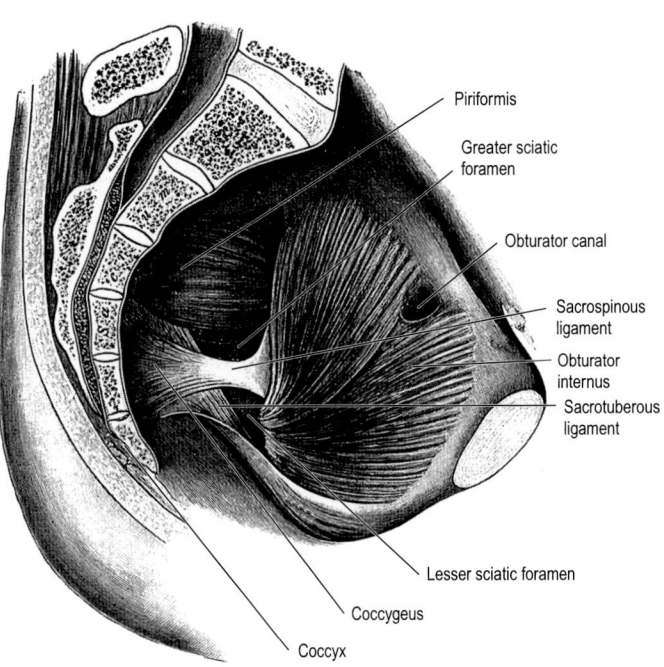

Fig. 111.31 The left obturator internus: pelvic aspect.

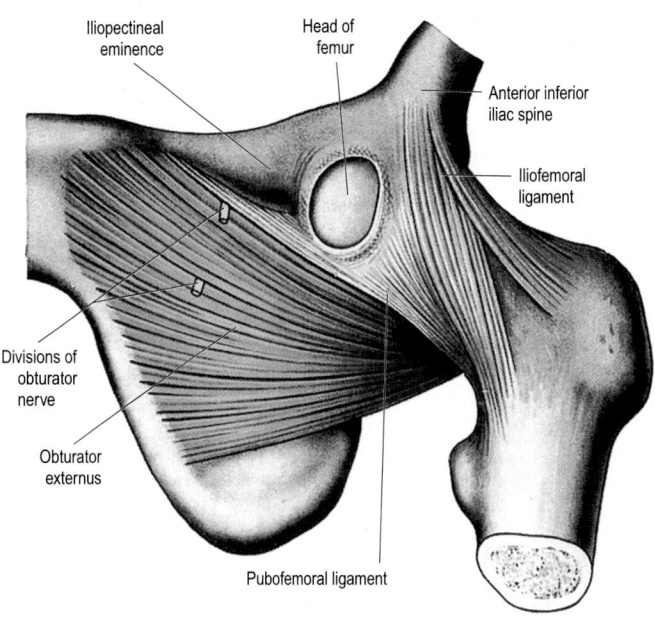

Fig. 111.32 The left obturator externus: anteroinferior aspect. The bursa of the psoas major tendon, which in this specimen communicated with the synovial cavity of the hip joint, has been opened to expose the head of the femur.

tendon into which its fibres converge, spirals backwards, laterally and upwards, and crosses the back of the neck of the femur and lower part of the capsule of the hip joint to end in the trochanteric fossa of the femur.

Relations – A bursa, which communicates with the hip joint, may be interposed between the tendon and the hip joint capsule and femoral neck. The obturator vessels lie between the muscle and the obturator membrane. The anterior branch of the obturator nerve reaches the thigh by passing in front of the muscle, and the posterior branch by piercing it.

Vascular supply – Obturator externus receives a variable pattern of supply from the obturator and medial circumflex femoral arteries.

Innervation – Obturator externus is innervated by the posterior branch of the obturator nerve, L3 and 4.

Actions – It has been suggested that the short muscles around the hip joint, pectineus, piriformis, obturators, gemelli and quadratus femoris, are more important as postural muscles than as prime movers, acting as adjustable ligaments to maintain the stability and integrity of the hip. However, these muscles are largely inaccessible to direct observation, and because of the hazards presented by their close relationship to important neurovascular structures there is a total lack of electromyographic data in man. In both bipedal walking and vertical climbing obturator externus is recruited during the early part of swing phase: in climbing it effects lateral rotation of the thigh, and in walking it probably counteracts the tendency to medial rotation produced by the anterior adductor muscles at this stage of the cycle. Obturator internus differs from externus in its pattern of use but its role in bipedal walking remains unclear. Its attachments suggest that it, like the gemelli, is a lateral rotator of the extended thigh and an abductor of the flexed thigh. These actions may be used to antagonize unwanted components of movement produced by the primary locomotor muscles.

Testing – The short rotators cannot be tested individually, but external rotation of the extended hip and abduction of the flexed hip against resistance tests them as a group.

GEMELLUS INFERIOR AND GEMELLUS SUPERIOR (Fig. 111.30)

Attachments – Gemellus inferior arises from the upper part of the ischial tuberosity, immediately below the groove for the tendon of obturator internus. It blends with the lower border of this tendon, and inserts with it into the medial surface of the greater trochanter.

Gemellus superior, the smaller of the two gemelli, arises from the dorsal surface of the ischial spine, blends with the upper border of the tendon of obturator internus, and inserts with it into the medial surface of the greater trochanter. It is sometimes absent.

The two gemelli can be regarded as accessory to obturator internus.

Relations – The relations of the gemelli are as for the extrapelvic part of obturator internus.

Vascular supply – The superior gemellus is supplied by the internal pudendal artery and its gemellar branches, by the inferior and sometimes also by the superior gluteal artery. The inferior gemellus is supplied mainly by the medial circumflex femoral artery.

Innervation – Gemellus superior is innervated by the nerve to obturator internus, L5 and S1. Gemellus inferior is innervated by the nerve to quadratus femoris, L5 and S1.

Actions – The gemelli rotate the extended thigh laterally and abduct the flexed thigh.

Testing – See testing of obturator externus above.

QUADRATUS FEMORIS (Fig. 111.30)

Attachments – Quadratus femoris is a flat, quadrilateral muscle lying between gemellus inferior and the upper margin of adductor magnus, from which it is separated by the transverse branch of the medial circumflex femoral artery. It arises from the upper part of the external aspect of the ischial tuberosity and inserts into a small tubercle a little

above the middle of the trochanteric crest of the femur and into the bone for a short distance below. It may be absent.

Relations – The muscle passes behind the hip joint and the neck of the femur, separated from them by the tendon of obturator externus and the ascending branch of the medial circumflex femoral artery (which may cause troublesome bleeding if injured during the posterior approach to the hip). The sciatic nerve crosses the muscle posteriorly. A bursa is often present between the muscle and the lesser trochanter.

Vascular supply – Branches pass to the superficial surface of the muscle from the inferior gluteal artery and from the medial circumflex femoral artery. The latter vessel also supplies the deep surface.

Innervation – Quadratus femoris is innervated by the nerve to quadratus femoris, L5 and S1.

Action – Quadratus femoris produces lateral rotation of the thigh.

Testing – See testing of obturator externus.

TENSOR FASCIAE LATAE (Fig. 111.29)

Attachments – Tensor fasciae latae arises from the anterior 5 cm of the outer lip of the iliac crest, from the lateral surface of the anterior superior iliac spine and part of the border of the notch below it between gluteus medius and sartorius, and from the deep surface of the fascia lata. Proximal attachments may extend to the aponeurotic fascia superficial to gluteus medius. It descends between, and is attached to, the two layers of the iliotibial tract of the fascia lata and usually ends approximately one-third of the way down the thigh, although it may reach as far as the lateral femoral condyle.

Vascular supply – The muscle itself is supplied mainly by a large ascending branch of the lateral circumflex femoral artery. The tensor fasciae latae musculocutaneous flap is raised on this pedicle. The superior part of the muscle receives branches from the superior gluteal artery. The fascia surrounding the muscle is supplied superficially by the superficial circumflex iliac artery and on its deep surface by the lateral circumflex femoral artery.

Innervation – Tensor fasciae latae is innervated by the superior gluteal nerve, L4, 5 and S1.

Actions – Tensor fasciae latae, acting through the iliotibial tract, extends the knee with lateral rotation of the leg; it may also assist in abduction and medial rotation of the thigh, though its role as an abductor is controversial. The muscle helps to maintain upright posture whilst minimizing energy expenditure on muscle activity: when the subject is standing it acts from below to steady the pelvis on the head of the femur and, through the iliotibial tract, to steady the condyles of the femur on the tibial condyles whilst the knee extensors are relaxed. Some authors consider the iliotibial tract to be more important in steadying the pelvis than tensor fasciae latae. The muscle aids gluteus medius in postural abduction at the hip. Postural control is its main function.

In the last 20° or so of extension the pull of the iliotibial tract is anterior to the flexion axis of the knee and so the tensor fasciae latae is a weak extensor. Flexion beyond 20° leads to the iliotibial tract passing posterior to the flexion axis so that the muscle becomes a weak flexor.

Testing – When the thigh is flexed against gravity and the knee is extended, an angular depression appears immediately below the anterior superior iliac spine: its lateral boundary is tensor fasciae latae. If the thigh is then abducted against resistance, the muscle can be seen to act.

GLUTEUS MAXIMUS (Fig. 111.33)

Attachments – Gluteus maximus is the largest and most superficial muscle in the gluteal region. It is a broad, thick quadrilateral mass, which, with its overlying adipose fascia, forms the familiar prominence of the buttock. Gluteus maximus is thicker and more extensive in man than in any non-human primate, developments that are associated with the evolutionary transition to bipedality and a permanently upright posture. The muscle has a coarse fascicular architecture, with large bundles of fibres separated by fibrous septa. It arises from the posterior

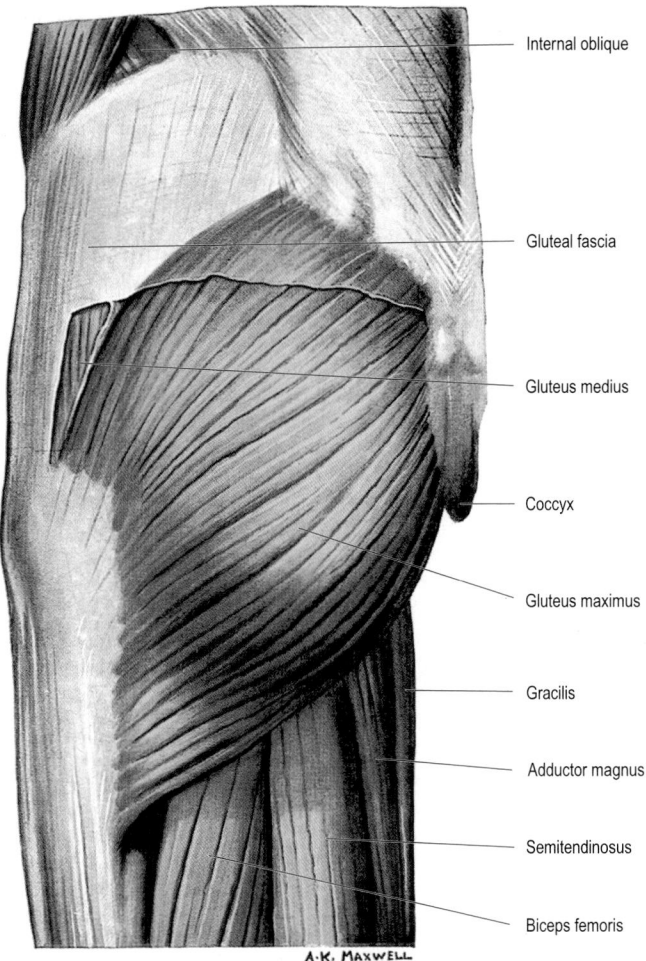

Internal oblique

Gluteal fascia

Gluteus medius

Coccyx

Gluteus maximus

Gracilis

Adductor magnus

Semitendinosus

Biceps femoris

A·K· MAXWELL

Fig. 111.33 The left gluteus maximus, posterior view. A triangular piece of gluteal fascia has been removed to expose part of gluteus medius.

gluteal line of the ilium, and the rough area of bone, including the crest, immediately above and behind it; from the aponeurosis of erector spinae; the dorsal surface of the lower part of the sacrum and the side of the coccyx; the sacrotuberous ligament; and the fascia (gluteal aponeurosis) which covers gluteus medius. There may be additional slips from the lumbar aponeurosis or ischial tuberosity. The muscle may also be bilaminar. The fibres descend laterally; the upper part of the muscle, together with the superficial fibres of the lower part, ends in a thick tendinous lamina which passes lateral to the greater trochanter and is attached to the iliotibial tract of the fascia lata. The deeper fibres of the lower part of the muscle are attached to the gluteal tuberosity between vastus lateralis and adductor magnus.

Relations – A thin fascia separates the superficial surface of gluteus maximus from the overlying thick adipose subcutaneous tissue. Its deep surface is related to the ilium, sacrum, coccyx, and sacrotuberous ligament, part of gluteus medius, piriformis, the gemelli, obturator internus, quadratus femoris, the ischial tuberosity, greater trochanter, and the attachments of biceps femoris, semitendinosus, semimembranosus and adductor magnus. Bursae related to gluteus maximus are described on page 1421. The superficial division of the superior gluteal artery reaches the deep surface of the muscle between piriformis and gluteus medius. The inferior gluteal and internal pudendal vessels, the sciatic, pudendal and posterior femoral cutaneous nerves, muscular branches from the sacral femoral cutaneous nerves, and muscular branches from the sacral plexus all leave the pelvis below piriformis. The first perforating artery and the terminal branches of the medial circumflex femoral artery are also deep to the lower part of gluteus maximus. Its upper border is thin and overlies gluteus medius. Its prominent lower border is free and slopes downwards and laterally. It is crossed by the horizontal gluteal fold (the posterior flexure line of the hip joint), which marks the upper limit of the back of the thigh on the surface.

Vascular supply – The dominant vascular pedicle is usually that of the inferior gluteal artery, which supplies approximately two-thirds of the muscle. The remainder is supplied mainly by the superior gluteal artery, though this may sometimes be the dominant vessel. The lateral and distal borders of the muscle receive a supply from the first profunda perforator and from the medial circumflex femoral artery. Minor branches may be derived from the lateral circumflex femoral, lateral sacral and internal pudendal arteries.

Gluteus maximus muscle and musculocutaneous flaps may be based on either of the gluteal vessels or on the first profunda perforator, depending on the site and size of the defect requiring coverage.

Innervation – Gluteus maximus is innervated by the inferior gluteal nerve, L5 and S1 and 2.

Actions – Acting from the pelvis, gluteus maximus can extend the flexed thigh and bring it into line with the trunk. Acting from its distal attachment, it may prevent the forward momentum of the trunk from producing flexion at the supporting hip during bipedal gait. The muscle is inactive during standing, swaying forwards at the ankle joints, or bending forwards at the hip joints to touch the toes. However, it acts with the hamstrings in raising the trunk after stooping, by rotating the pelvis backwards on the head of the femur. It is intermittently active in the walking cycle and in climbing stairs, and continuously active in strong lateral rotation of the thigh. Its upper fibres are active in powerful abduction of the thigh. It is a tensor of the fascia lata, and through the iliotibial tract it stabilizes the femur on the tibia when the knee extensor muscles are relaxed.

Testing – Extension of the hip against resistance, in the supine or prone position.

GLUTEUS MEDIUS (Figs 111.30, 111.33)

Attachments – Gluteus medius is a broad, thick muscle. It arises from the outer surface of the ilium between the iliac crest and posterior gluteal line above and the anterior gluteal line below, and also from the strong fascia superficial to its upper part. The fibres converge to a flat tendon that attaches to a ridge that slants downwards and forwards on the lateral surface of the greater trochanter.

A deep slip of the muscle may be attached to the upper border of the trochanter. The posterior edge of gluteus medius sometimes blends with piriformis.

Relations – The posterior third of gluteus medius is covered by gluteus maximus, but it is superficial in its anterior two-thirds, where it is covered only by a strong layer of deep fascia. Its deep surface is related to gluteus minimus. Branches of the deep divisions of the superior gluteal nerve and artery run between the muscles and are vulnerable during anterolateral approaches to the hip that involve splitting gluteus medius (**Fig. 111.34**). Where the tendon glides on the anterosuperior part of the lateral surface of the trochanter, a bursa (trochanteric bursa of gluteus medius) separates it from the bone.

Vascular supply – The main supply to gluteus medius is from the deep branch of the superior gluteal artery. The distal part of the muscle is supplied from the trochanteric anastomosis (p. 1453).

Innervation – Gluteus medius is innervated by the superior gluteal nerve, L4, 5 and S1.

Actions – Considered below with gluteus minimus.

Clinical anatomy: testing – Considered below with gluteus minimus.

GLUTEUS MINIMUS (Fig. 111.30)

Attachments – Gluteus minimus lies deep to gluteus medius, which it resembles. The fan-shaped muscle arises from the outer surface of the ilium between the anterior and inferior gluteal lines and, behind, from the margin of the greater sciatic notch. The fibres converge below to the deep surface of an aponeurosis that ends in a tendon which is attached to an anterolateral ridge on the greater trochanter and contributes an expansion to the capsule of the hip joint.

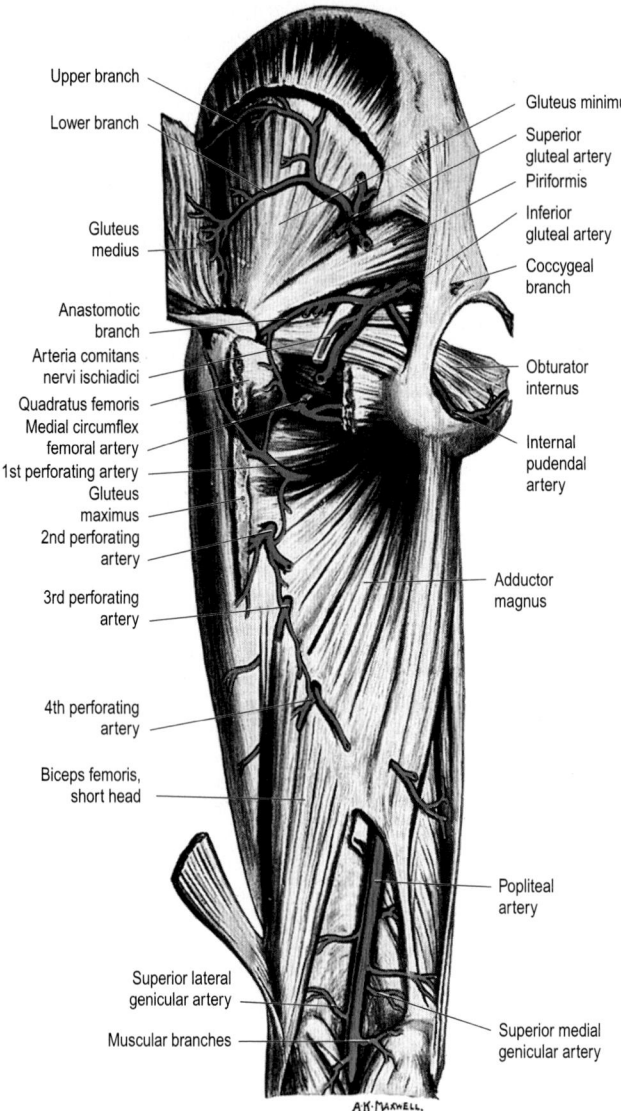

Upper branch

Lower branch

Gluteus
medius

Anastomotic
branch

Arteria comitans
nervi ischiadici

Quadratus femoris

Medial circumflex
femoral artery

1st perforating artery

Gluteus
maximus

2nd perforating
artery

3rd perforating
artery

4th perforating
artery

Biceps femoris,
short head

Superior lateral
genicular artery

Muscular branches

Gluteus minimus

Superior
gluteal artery

Piriformis

Inferior
gluteal artery

Coccygeal
branch

Obturator
internus

Internal
pudendal
artery

Adductor
magnus

Popliteal
artery

Superior medial
genicular artery

A.K.MAXWELL.

Fig. 111.34 The arteries of the left gluteal and posterior femoral regions.

The muscle may divide into anterior and posterior parts. Separate slips may pass to piriformis, gemellus superior, or vastus lateralis.

Relations – Branches of the deep division of the superior gluteal artery and nerve run on the superficial surface of the muscle. The reflected tendon of rectus femoris and the capsule of the hip joint are deep to gluteus minimus. A bursa (trochanteric bursa of gluteus minimus) separates the tendon from the medial part of the anterior surface of the greater trochanter.

Vascular supply – Gluteus minimus is supplied from both its surfaces, from the main trunk and the deep branch of the superior gluteal artery, with a contribution at its femoral attachment from the trochanteric anastomosis (p. 1453).

Innervation – Gluteus minimus is innervated by the superior gluteal nerve, L4, 5 and S1.

Actions of gluteus medius and minimus – Both gluteus medius and minimus, acting from the pelvis, abduct the thigh, and their anterior fibres rotate it medially. Acting from the femur, they play an essential part in maintaining the trunk upright when the foot of the opposite side is raised from the ground in walking and running. In this phase the body weight tends to make the pelvis sag downwards on the unsupported side. This is counteracted by the gluteus medius and minimus of the supporting side, which, acting from below, exert such powerful traction on the hip bone that the pelvis is actually raised a little on the unsupported side. In symmetrical standing with the feet somewhat separated, the abductor muscles are usually electrically 'silent', but with the feet placed parallel and close together they are active.

Clinical anatomy: testing – The supportive effect of the glutei (medius and minimus) on the pelvis when the contralateral foot is raised depends on the following conditions. The two muscles, and their innervation, must be functioning normally. The components of the hip joint, which forms the fulcrum, must be in their usual relation. The neck of the femur must be intact, with its normal angulation to the shaft.

When any one of these conditions is not fulfilled, e.g. in paralysis of the glutei, congenital dislocation of the hip, or coxa vara, the supporting mechanism is upset and the pelvis sinks on the unsupported side when the patient tries to stand on the affected limb. This is known clinically as Trendelenburg's sign. Sufferers from paralysis of gluteus medius and minimus have a characteristic lurching gait. Provided that these muscles are intact, paralysis of other muscles acting on the hip joint produces remarkably little deficit in walking, or even in running.

Gluteus medius and minimus may be tested together by medial (internal) rotation of the thigh against resistance, in the supine position with hip and knee flexed. Both muscles may be tested together with tensor fasciae latae by abduction of the lower limb against resistance, in the supine position with the knee extended.

VASCULAR SUPPLY

ILIAC VESSELS

See page 1362.

EXTERNAL ILIAC ARTERIES
See page 1362.

EXTERNAL ILIAC VEINS
See page 1362.

FEMORAL VESSELS

FEMORAL ARTERY (Figs 111.2, 111.35, 111.36, 111.37, 112.1, 112.2)

The femoral artery is a continuation of the external iliac. It begins behind the inguinal ligament, midway between the anterior superior iliac spine and the pubic symphysis, descends along the anteromedial part of the thigh in the femoral triangle, enters and passes through the adductor (subsartorial) canal, and becomes the popliteal artery as it passes through an opening in adductor magnus near the junction of the middle and distal thirds of the thigh. Its first three or four centimetres are enclosed, with its vein, in the femoral sheath. The part of the artery proximal to the origin of profunda femoris is often clinically termed the common femoral, while that distal to the profunda origin is termed the superficial femoral artery.

Rarely, the femoral artery divides, distal to the origin of the profunda femoris artery, into two trunks that reunite near the adductor opening. It may be replaced by the inferior gluteal artery, accompanying the sciatic nerve to the popliteal fossa and representing a proximal persistence of the original axial artery. The external iliac artery is then small, ending as the profunda femoris artery.

Femoral sheath
See page 1419.

Femoral triangle
See page 1419.

Relations of the femoral artery in the femoral triangle

Anterior to the artery are the skin, superficial fascia, superficial inguinal lymph nodes, fascia lata, femoral sheath, superficial circumflex iliac vein (crossing in the superficial fascia) and the femoral branch of the genitofemoral nerve (which is at first lateral then anterior). Near the apex of the triangle, the medial femoral cutaneous nerve crosses the artery from the lateral to the medial side. Posteriorly lie the femoral sheath and the tendons of psoas, pectineus and adductor longus. The artery is separated from the hip joint by the tendon of psoas major, from pectineus by the femoral vein and profunda vessels, and from adductor longus by the femoral vein. Proximally, the nerve to pectineus passes

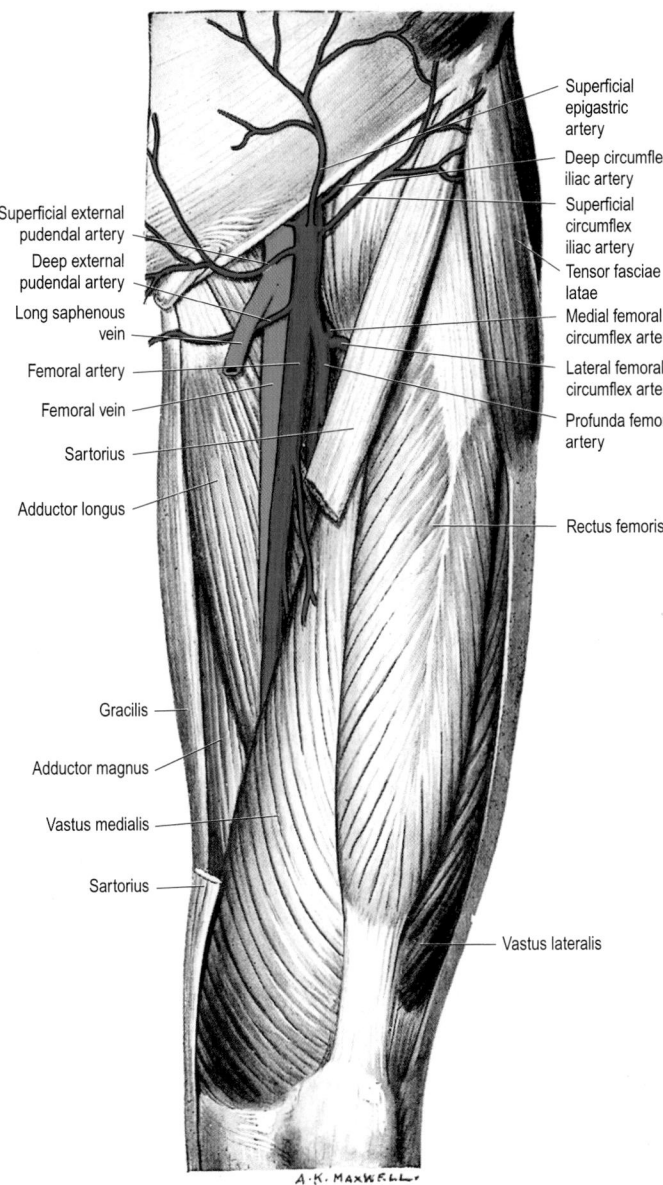

Superficial
epigastric
artery

Deep circumflex
iliac artery

Superficial
circumflex
iliac artery

Tensor fasciae
latae

Medial femoral
circumflex artery

Lateral femoral
circumflex artery

Profunda femoris
artery

Rectus femoris

Superficial external
pudendal artery

Deep external
pudendal artery

Long saphenous
vein

Femoral artery

Femoral vein

Sartorius

Adductor longus

Gracilis

Adductor magnus

Vastus medialis

Sartorius

Vastus lateralis

A·K·MAXWELL·

Fig. 111.35 The left femoral vessels.

medially behind the artery. The femoral nerve lies lateral to the artery. The femoral vein is medial to the artery in the proximal part of the triangle and becomes posterior distally at the apex.

Adductor (subsartorial) canal

See page 1461.

Relations of the femoral artery in the adductor canal

See page 1469.

Clinical anatomy

Compression of the femoral artery is most effective just distal to the inguinal ligament, where it is superficial and separated from the bone (iliopubic eminence) only by the psoas tendon. For this reason arterial injury proximal to the inguinal ligament, such as laceration by a knife cannot be controlled simply by compression. Gaining proximal control of bleeding involves major exposure of the more proximal arteries as a life-saving manoeuvre.

Minor branches in the proximal thigh (Fig. 111.35)

Superficial epigastric artery

The superficial epigastric artery arises anteriorly from the femoral artery c.1 cm distal to the inguinal ligament. It traverses the cribriform fascia to ascend anterior to the ligament and run in the abdominal superficial fascia almost to the umbilicus. It supplies the superficial inguinal lymph

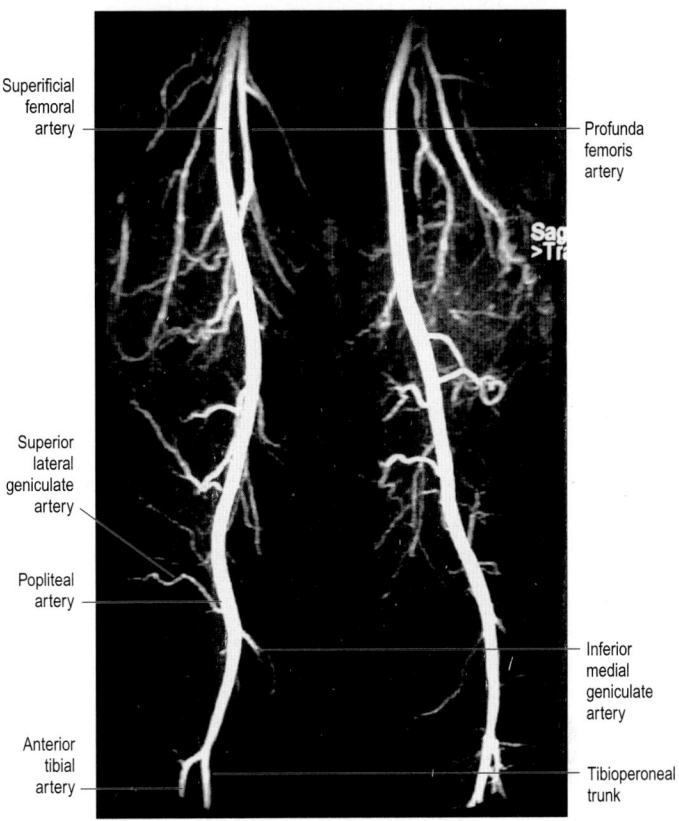

Superficial
femoral
artery

Profunda
femoris
artery

Superior
lateral
geniculate
artery

Popliteal
artery

Inferior
medial
geniculate
artery

Anterior
tibial
artery

Tibioperoneal
trunk

Fig. 111.36 Magnetic resonance angiogram (MRA) of the femoral and popliteal arteries. (By kind permission from Dr Justin Lee, Chelsea and Westminster Hospital, London.)

nodes and superficial fascia and skin, anastomosing with branches of the inferior epigastric and its contralateral fellow.

Superficial circumflex iliac artery

The superficial circumflex iliac artery is the smallest superficial branch of the femoral artery and arises near or with the superficial epigastric artery. It usually emerges through the fascia lata, lateral to the saphenous opening, and turns laterally distal to the inguinal ligament towards the anterior superior iliac spine. It supplies the skin, superficial fascia and superficial inguinal lymph nodes, anastomosing with the deep circumflex iliac, superior gluteal and lateral circumflex femoral arteries.

The superficial circumflex iliac artery is the basis for the important axial-pattern pedicled groin skin flap. Free flaps based on the vessel may also be raised.

Superficial external pudendal artery

The superficial external pudendal artery arises medially from the femoral artery, close to the preceding branches. Emerging from the cribriform fascia, it passes medially, usually deep to the long saphenous vein, across the spermatic cord (or round ligament) to supply the lower abdominal, penile, scrotal or labial skin, anastomosing with branches of the internal pudendal artery.

Deep external pudendal artery

The deep external pudendal artery passes medially across pectineus and anterior or posterior to adductor longus, covered by fascia lata which it pierces to supply the skin of the perineum and scrotum or labium majus. Its branches anastomose with the posterior scrotal or labial branches of the internal pudendal artery.

Muscular branches

These branches supply sartorius, vastus medialis and the adductors.

Profunda femoris artery (Figs 111.35, 111.36, 111.37, 112.2)

The profunda femoris artery (deep femoral artery) is a large branch that arises laterally from the femoral artery c.3.5 cm distal to the inguinal ligament. At first lateral to the femoral artery, it spirals posterior to this

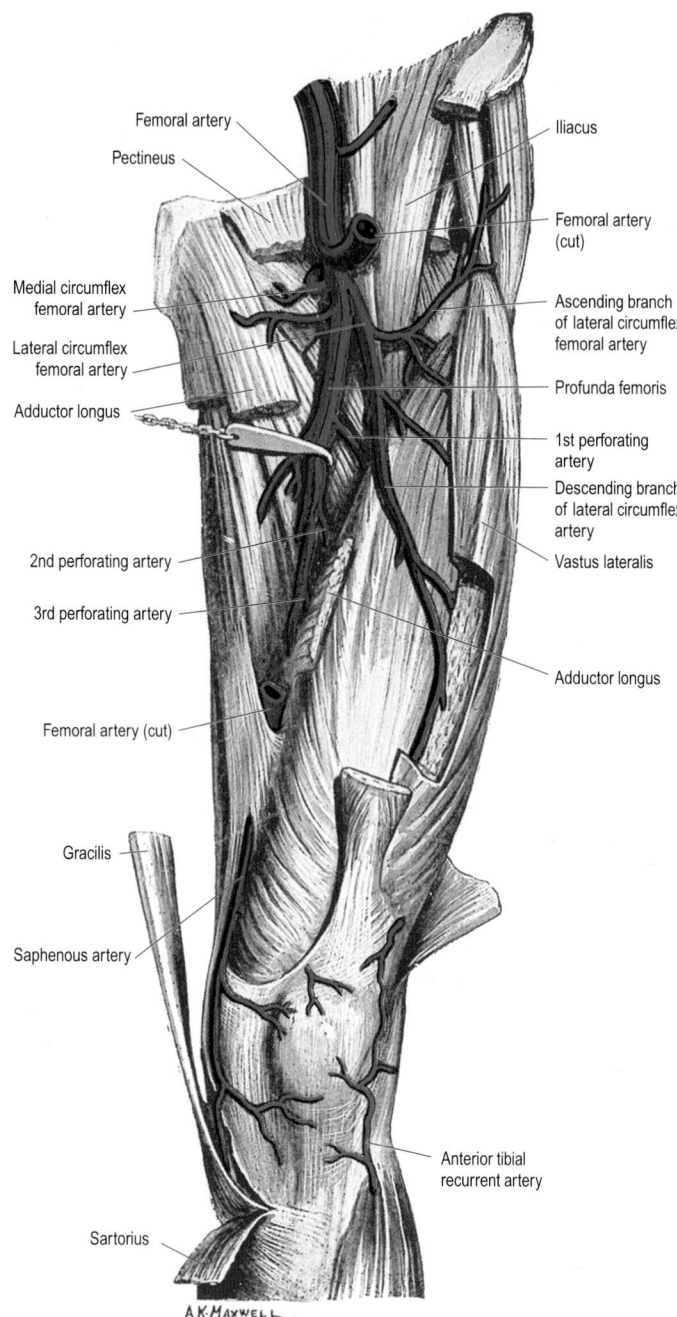

Fig. 111.37 The left profunda femoris artery and its branches.

and the femoral vein to reach the medial side of the femur. It passes between pectineus and adductor longus, then between the latter and adductor brevis, before it descends between adductor longus and adductor magnus. It pierces adductor magnus and anastomoses with the upper muscular branches of the popliteal artery. This terminal part is sometimes named the fourth perforating artery.

The profunda is the main supply to the adductor, extensor and flexor muscles; it also anastomoses with the internal and external iliac arteries above and the popliteal artery below.

The origin of the profunda femoris is sometimes medial, or rarely posterior on the femoral artery; if the former, it may cross anterior to the femoral vein and then pass backwards around its medial side.

Relations
Posteriorly, in proximodistal order, lie iliacus, pectineus, adductor brevis and adductor magnus. Anteriorly are the femoral and profunda veins and distally adductor longus, which separate the profunda from the main femoral artery. Laterally vastus medialis separates the proximal part of the artery from the femur.

Branches of profunda femoris in the proximal thigh

Lateral circumflex femoral artery (Fig. 111.37) – The lateral circumflex femoral artery is a laterally running branch given off near the root of the profunda. It passes between divisions of the femoral nerve, posterior to sartorius and rectus femoris and divides into ascending, transverse and descending branches. It may arise from the femoral artery. The ascending branch ascends along the intertrochanteric line, under tensor fasciae latae, lateral to the hip joint. It anastomoses with the superior gluteal and deep circumflex iliac arteries, supplying the greater trochanter, and, with branches of the medial circumflex femoral, forms an anastomotic ring round the femoral neck, from which ring the femoral neck and head are supplied. The descending branch, sometimes direct from the profunda or the femoral, descends posterior to rectus femoris, along the anterior border of vastus lateralis, which it supplies: a long branch descends in vastus lateralis to the knee, anastomosing with the lateral superior genicular branch of the popliteal, accompanied by the nerve to vastus lateralis. The transverse branch, the smallest, passes laterally anterior to vastus intermedius and pierces vastus lateralis to wind round the femur, just distal to the greater trochanter. It anastomoses with the medial circumflex, inferior gluteal and first perforating arteries (cruciate anastomosis, p. 1453). The ascending branch forms the pedicle of the tensor fasciae latae musculocutaneous flap (p. 1448). The descending branch supplies the anterolateral thigh fasciocutaneous flap, which is based on the fasciocutaneous perforators that arise from the descending branch.

Medial circumflex femoral artery (Fig. 111.37) – The medial circumflex femoral artery usually originates from the posteromedial aspect of the profunda, but often originates from the femoral artery itself. It supplies the adductor muscles and curves medially round the femur between pectineus and psoas major and then obturator externus and adductor brevis, finally appearing between quadratus femoris and the upper border of adductor magnus, dividing into transverse and ascending branches. The transverse branch takes part in the cruciate anastomosis. The ascending branch ascends on the tendon of obturator externus, anterior to quadratus femoris, to the trochanteric fossa, where it anastomoses with branches of the gluteal and lateral circumflex femoral arteries. An acetabular branch at the proximal edge of adductor brevis enters the hip joint under the transverse acetabular ligament with one from the obturator artery. It supplies the fat in the fossa, and reaches the femoral head along its ligament. For details of the blood supply of the proximal end of the femur consult Crock (1996).

Perforating arteries and distal branches – See page 1469.

FEMORAL VEIN (Figs 111.2, 111.35)
The femoral vein accompanies its artery, beginning at the adductor opening as the continuation of the popliteal vein, and ending posterior to the inguinal ligament as the external iliac vein. In the distal adductor canal, it is posterolateral to the femoral artery; more proximally in the canal, and in the distal femoral triangle (i.e. its apex), it is posterior to it; proximally, at the base of the triangle, it is medial. The vein occupies the middle compartment of the femoral sheath, between the femoral artery and canal, fat in the latter allowing expansion of the vein. It has many muscular tributaries: c.4–12 cm distal to the inguinal ligament the profunda femoris vein (deep femoral vein) joins it posteriorly and then the long saphenous vein (see below), which enters anteriorly. Veins accompanying the superficial epigastric, superficial circumflex iliac and external pudendal arteries join the long saphenous vein before it enters the saphenous opening. Lateral and medial circumflex femoral veins are usually tributaries of the femoral. There are usually four or five valves in the femoral vein: the two most constant are just distal to the entry of the profunda femoris and near the inguinal ligament.

Profunda femoris vein
The profunda femoris vein lies anterior to its artery, and has tributaries corresponding to the branches of the artery. Through these tributaries it connects distally with the popliteal and proximally with the inferior gluteal veins. It sometimes drains medial and lateral circumflex femoral veins. It has a valve just before it terminates.

Long saphenous vein (Fig. 110.6)
The long saphenous vein (great saphenous vein), the longest vein in the body, starts distally as a continuation of the medial marginal vein of the

foot, and ends in the femoral vein a short distance distal to the inguinal ligament. It ascends c.2.5–3 cm anterior to the tibial malleolus, crosses the distal third of the medial surface of the tibia obliquely to its medial border, then ascends a little behind the border to the knee. Proximally it is posteromedial to the medial tibial and femoral condyles (lying the breadth of the subject's hand posterior to the medial edge of the patella), and then ascends the medial aspect of the thigh. It passes through the saphenous opening and finally opens into the femoral vein. The 'centre' of the opening is often said to be 2.5–3.5 cm inferolateral to the pubic tubercle, and the vein is then represented by a line drawn from this point to the femoral adductor tubercle. However, the saphenous opening varies greatly in size and disposition so that this 'centre' is not a reliable surface marking for the saphenofemoral junction.

In its course through the thigh the long saphenous vein is accompanied by branches of the medial femoral cutaneous nerve. At the knee the saphenous branch of the descending genicular artery (the saphenous artery) and, in the leg and foot, the saphenous nerve, are anterior to it. The vein is often duplicated, especially distal to the knee. It has from 10 to 20 valves, which are more numerous in the leg than the thigh. One is present just before it pierces the cribriform fascia, another at its junction with the femoral vein. In almost its entire extent the vein lies in superficial fascia, but it has many connections with the deep veins, especially in the leg.

Tributaries

At the ankle the long saphenous vein drains the sole by medial marginal veins. In the leg it often connects with the short saphenous vein and with deep veins via perforating veins. Just distal to the knee it usually receives three large tributaries: from the front of the leg, from the tibial malleolar region (connecting with some of the 'perforating' veins) and from the calf (communicating with the short saphenous vein). The tributary draining the tibial malleolar region is formed distally from a fine network or 'corona' of delicate veins over the medial malleolus, and then ascends the medial aspect of the calf as the posterior arch vein (Dodd and Cockett 1976). This vein was first illustrated by Leonardo da Vinci, whose name is sometimes given to it. It connects with posterior tibial venae comitantes by a series of perforating (communicating) veins. There are usually three, equally spaced between the medial malleolus and the midcalf. More than three such perforators are uncommon, and an arch vein perforator above midcalf is only very rarely found.

Above the posterior crural arch vein, perforating veins join the long saphenous vein or one of its main tributaries at two main sites. The first is at a level in the upper calf indicated by its name, the tibial tubercle perforator; the second is in the lower/intermediate third of the thigh where it perforates the deep fascial roof of the subsartorial canal to join the femoral vein.

In the thigh the long saphenous vein receives many tributaries. Some open independently, whilst others converge to form large named channels that frequently pass towards the basal half of the femoral triangle before joining the long saphenous near its termination. These may be grouped as follows: one or more large posteromedial tributaries, one or more large anterolateral tributaries, four or more peri-inguinal veins. The posteromedial vein of the thigh, large and sometimes double, drains a large superficial region indicated by its name: it has (as have the other tributaries) radiological and surgical significance. One of its lower radicles is often continuous with the short saphenous vein. The posteromedial vein is sometimes named the accessory saphenous vein, though some restrict the term accessory to a lower (more distal) postero-medial tributary when two (or more) are present. Another large vessel, the anterolateral vein of the thigh (anterior femoral cutaneous vein), usually commences from an anterior network of veins in the distal thigh and crosses the apex and distal half of the femoral triangle to reach the long saphenous vein. As the latter traverses the saphenous opening, it is joined by the superficial epigastric, superficial circumflex iliac and superficial external pudendal veins. Their mode of union varies. Superficial epigastric and circumflex iliac veins drain the inferior abdominal wall, the latter also receiving tributaries from the proximo-lateral region of the thigh. The superficial epigastric or the femoral vein may connect with the lateral thoracic veins by means of a thoraco-epigastric vein running superficially on the anterolateral aspect of the trunk. This vein connects the inferior and superior caval areas of drainage and may be dilated and visible in cases of inferior caval obstruction. Superficial external pudendal veins drain part of the scrotum/labia; one is joined by the superficial dorsal vein of the penis/clitoris. The deep external pudendal veins join the long saphenous vein at the saphenous opening.

The long saphenous vein is often harvested for grafts used both in peripheral and coronary arterial surgery.

GLUTEAL VESSELS

See pages 1453 and 1362.

ARTERIAL ANASTOMOSES OF THE HIP (Fig. 111.21)

TROCHANTERIC ANASTOMOSIS

The trochanteric anastomosis lies near the trochanteric fossa of the femur. It is an anastomosis between the ascending branch of the medial circumflex femoral artery and descending branches of the superior and inferior gluteal arteries. The lateral circumflex femoral artery and the first perforating artery from the profunda may also contribute, creating an extracapsular 'arterial ring of the femoral neck' (Crock 1996). Branches from this ring, the retinacular vessels, pierce the capsule and ascend along the femoral neck to give the main blood supply to the head of the femur.

CRUCIATE ANASTOMOSIS

The cruciate anastomosis lies at the level of the lesser trochanter, near the lower edge of the femoral attachment of quadratus femoris. It is an anastomosis between the transverse branches of the medial and lateral circumflex femoral arteries, a descending branch of the inferior gluteal artery and an ascending branch from the first perforating artery.

These anastomoses are the proximal elements of an anastomotic chain of arteries on the back of the thigh that forms a route of collateral circulation when the femoral artery is blocked proximal to the profunda origin (see p. 1469 for details).

LYMPHATIC NODES AND LYMPH DRAINAGE

SUPERFICIAL INGUINAL NODES (Fig. 111.38)

The superficial inguinal nodes form proximal and distal groups. The proximal group usually consists of five or six nodes just distal to the inguinal ligament. Its lateral members receive afferent vessels from the gluteal region and the adjoining infra-umbilical anterior abdominal wall. Medial members receive superficial vessels from the external genitalia (including the inferior vagina), inferior anal canal and perianal region, adjoining abdominal wall, umbilicus and uterine vessels accompanying the round ligament. The distal group usually consists of four or five nodes along the termination of the long saphenous vein. They receive all the superficial vessels of the lower limb, except those from the posterolateral calf. All superficial inguinal nodes drain to the external iliac nodes, some via the femoral canal and others anterior or lateral to the femoral vessels. Numerous vessels interconnect individual nodes.

Superficial inguinal nodes are frequently enlarged in disease or injury in their region of drainage. Thus the proximal inguinal nodes are almost invariably affected in malignant or infective disease of the prepuce, penis, labia majora, scrotum, perineum, anus and lower vagina, or in diseases affecting the skin and superficial structures in these regions, in the infra-umbilical part of the abdominal wall or in the gluteal region. The distal group is implicated only in disease or injury of the limb.

DEEP INGUINAL NODES (Fig. 111.39)

The deep inguinal nodes vary from one to three, and are situated medial to the femoral vein. One lies just distal to the saphenofemoral junction, another in the femoral canal, and the most proximal node lies laterally in the femoral ring. The middle node is the most inconstant and the proximal node is often absent. All receive deep lymphatics accompanying the femoral vessels, lymph vessels from the glans penis or clitoris and a few efferents from the superficial inguinal nodes. Their own efferents traverse the femoral canal to the external iliac nodes.

INNERVATION

LUMBAR PLEXUS AND BRANCHES

See pages 1124 and 1402.

A

Superficial inguinal nodes
(proximal group)

Superficial inguinal nodes
(distal group)

Long saphenous
vein

B

Popliteal nodes

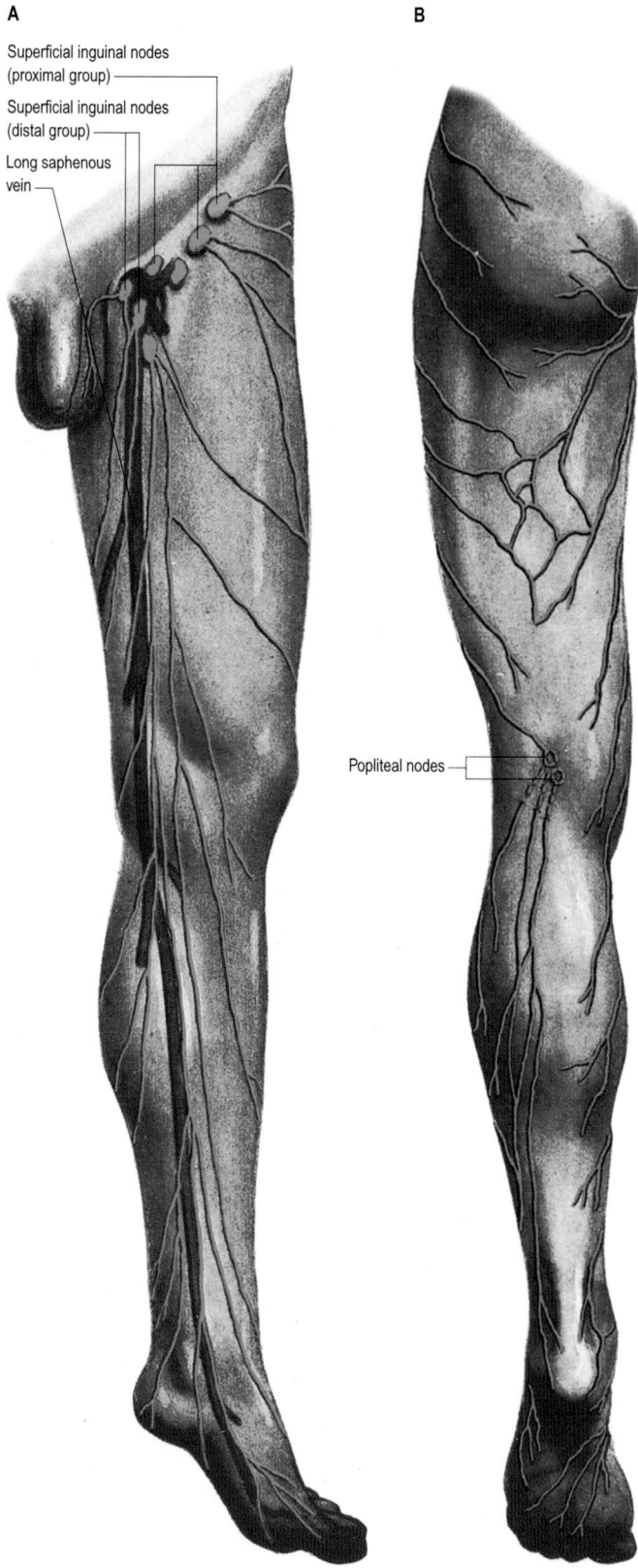

Fig. 111.38 The lymphatic drainage of the superficial tissues of the lower limb (semi-diagrammatic): **A**, anteromedial aspect; **B**, posterior aspect.

Iliohypogastric nerve (L1)
See page 1124.

Ilioinguinal nerve (L1)
See page 1124.

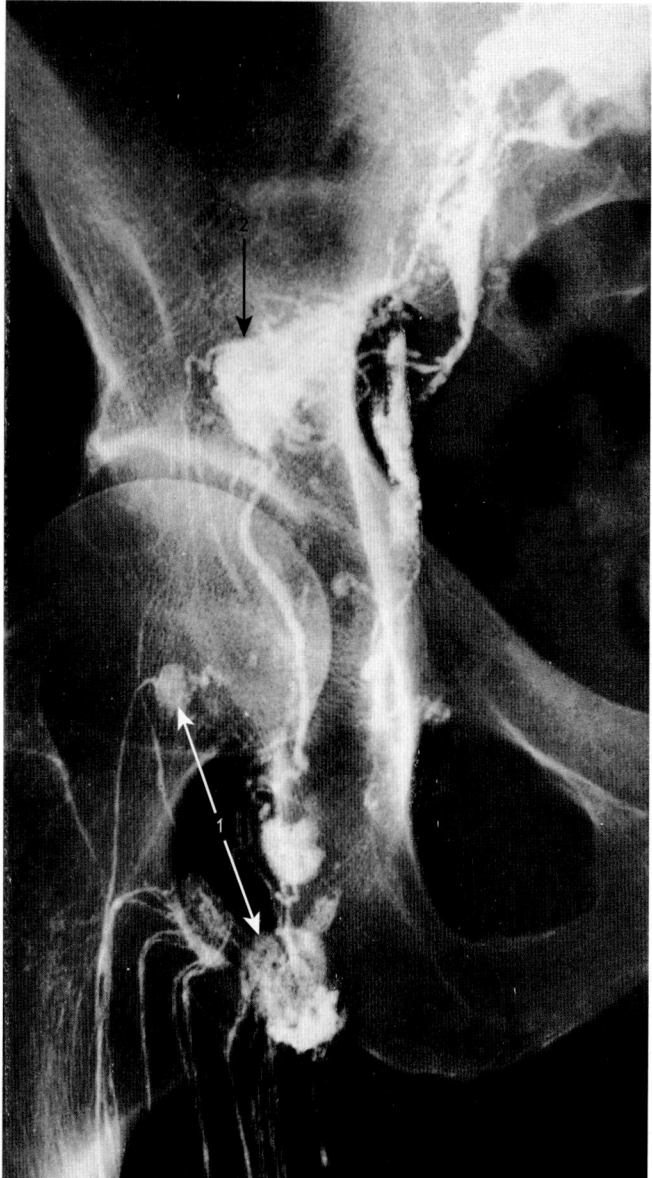

1. Inguinal nodes. 2. External iliac node.

Fig. 111.39 Lymphangiogram showing the inguinal lymph vessels and nodes. (Provided by JB Kinmonth.)

Genitofemoral nerve
See page 1125.

Lateral cutaneous nerve of the thigh

The lateral cutaneous nerve of the thigh arises from the dorsal branches of the second and third lumbar ventral rami and emerges from the lateral border of psoas major, crossing the iliacus obliquely towards the anterior superior iliac spine. It supplies the parietal peritoneum in the iliac fossa. The right nerve passes posterolateral to the caecum, separated from it by the fascia iliaca and peritoneum; the left passes behind the lower part of the descending colon. Both pass behind or through the inguinal ligament, variably medial to the anterior superior iliac spine (commonly c.1 cm) and anterior to or through sartorius into the thigh, where they divide into anterior and posterior branches. The anterior branch becomes superficial c.10 cm distal to the anterior superior iliac spine and supplies the skin of the anterior and lateral thigh as far as the knee. It connects terminally with the cutaneous branches of the anterior division of the femoral nerve and the infrapatellar branch of the saphenous nerve, forming the peripatellar plexus. The posterior branch pierces the fascia lata higher than the anterior, and divides to supply the skin on the lateral surface from the greater trochanter to about midthigh. It may also supply the gluteal skin.

Lesions of the lateral cutaneous nerve of the thigh

The nerve may become entrapped as it passes through or deep to the inguinal ligament just medial to the anterior superior iliac spine. This can produce an area of impaired sensation, often with pain and paraesthesia on the anterolateral aspect of the thigh (meralgia paraesthetica) in the distal cutaneous distribution of the nerve. This area does not extend across the midline anteriorly, it does not extend below the knee and it does not extend behind the hamstring tendons laterally. Exceptionally the posterior branch of the lateral cutaneous nerve of the thigh may be affected separately: this supplies a thin strip from the greater trochanter of the femur down about two-thirds of the way to the knee. This branch leaves the main trunk of the nerve, usually distal to the inguinal ligament, and it then turns laterally to pierce tensor fasciae latae, where it may become entrapped.

Femoral nerve (Fig. 111.40)

The femoral nerve, the largest branch of the lumbar plexus, arises from the dorsal branches (posterior divisions) of the second to fourth lumbar ventral rami. It descends through psoas major, emerging low on its lateral border, and then passes between psoas and iliacus, deep to the iliac fascia. Passing behind the inguinal ligament into the thigh, it splits into anterior and posterior divisions. Behind the inguinal ligament it is separated from the femoral artery by part of psoas major. In the abdomen the nerve supplies small branches to iliacus and pectineus and a branch to the proximal part of the femoral artery; the latter branch sometimes arises in the thigh.

Nerve to pectineus

The nerve to pectineus branches from the medial side of the femoral nerve near the inguinal ligament. It passes behind the femoral sheath and enters the anterior aspect of the muscle.

Anterior division of the femoral nerve

The anterior division of the femoral nerve supplies intermediate and medial cutaneous nerves of the thigh and branches to sartorius.

Intermediate cutaneous nerve of the thigh – See page 1470.

Medial cutaneous nerve of the thigh – See page 1470.

Nerve to sartorius – See page 1470.

Posterior division of the femoral nerve

The branches of the posterior division of the femoral nerve are the saphenous nerve and branches to quadriceps femoris and the knee joint.

Saphenous nerve – See page 1487.

Muscular branches – The muscular branches of the posterior division of the femoral nerve supply quadriceps femoris. A branch to rectus femoris enters its proximal posterior surface and also supplies the hip joint. A larger branch to vastus lateralis forms a neurovascular bundle with the descending branch of the lateral circumflex femoral artery in its distal part and also supplies the knee joint. A branch to vastus medialis descends through the proximal part of the adductor canal, lateral to the saphenous nerve and femoral vessels. It enters the muscle at about its midpoint, sending a long articular filament distally along the muscle to the knee. Two or three branches to vastus intermedius enter its anterior surface about midthigh: a small branch from one of these descends through the muscle to supply articularis genu and the knee joint.

Vascular branches

Vascular branches of the femoral nerve supply the femoral artery and its branches.

Lesions of the femoral nerve

The main trunk of the femoral nerve is not subject to an entrapment neuropathy, but may be compressed by retroperitoneal tumours or retroperitoneal haemorrhage in patients on anticoagulants or with a bleeding diathesis. A localized lesion of the femoral nerve may occur in diabetes mellitus (one of the forms of diabetic amyotrophy). The striking feature of femoral neuropathy is wasting and weakness of quadriceps femoris: this results in considerable difficulty in walking, with a tendency

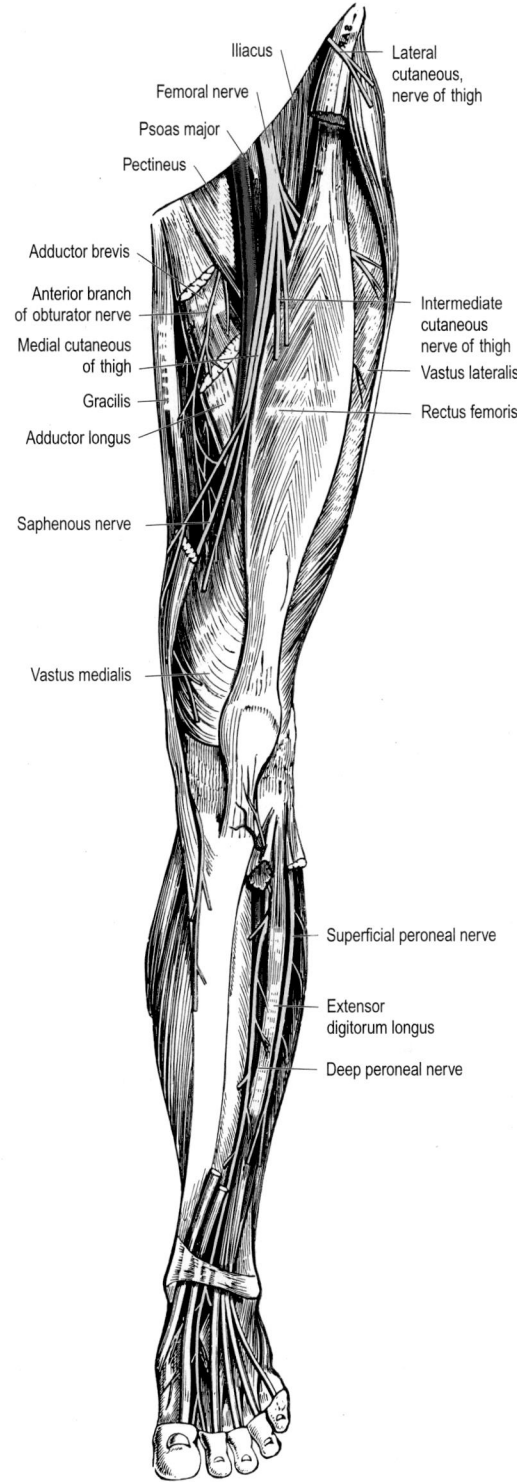

Fig. 111.40 The nerves of the left lower limb: anterior aspect.

Labels on figure:
Iliacus
Femoral nerve
Psoas major
Pectineus
Adductor brevis
Anterior branch of obturator nerve
Medial cutaneous of thigh
Gracilis
Adductor longus
Saphenous nerve
Vastus medialis
Lateral cutaneous, nerve of thigh
Intermediate cutaneous nerve of thigh
Vastus lateralis
Rectus femoris
Superficial peroneal nerve
Extensor digitorum longus
Deep peroneal nerve

for the leg to collapse. Pain and paraesthesia may occur on the anterior and medial aspect of the thigh, extending down the medial aspect of the leg in the distribution of the saphenous branch of the femoral nerve.

Obturator nerve

The obturator nerve arises from the ventral branches of the second to fourth lumbar ventral rami. The branch from the third is the largest while that from the second is often very small. The nerve descends in psoas major, emerging from its medial border at the pelvic brim to pass behind the common iliac vessels and lateral to the internal iliac vessels. It then descends forwards along the lateral wall of the lesser pelvis on obturator internus, anterosuperior to the obturator vessels, to the obturator foramen, entering the thigh by its upper part. Near the foramen it divides into anterior and posterior branches, separated at first by part of obturator externus and lower down by adductor brevis.

Anterior branch (Fig. 111.40)

The anterior branch leaves the pelvis anterior to obturator externus, descending in front of adductor brevis, behind pectineus and adductor longus. At the lower border of adductor longus it communicates with the medial cutaneous and saphenous branches of the femoral nerve, forming a subsartorial plexus (p. 1470) that supplies the skin on the medial side of the thigh. It descends on the femoral artery, which its termination supplies. Near the obturator foramen the anterior branch supplies the hip joint. Behind pectineus it supplies adductor longus, gracilis, usually adductor brevis and often pectineus, and connects with the accessory obturator nerve when it is present. Occasionally the communicating branch to the femoral medial cutaneous and saphenous branches continues as a cutaneous branch to the thigh and leg, emerging from behind the distal border of adductor longus to descend along the posterior margin of sartorius to the knee, where it pierces the deep fascia, connects with the saphenous nerve and supplies the skin halfway down the medial side of the leg.

Posterior branch

The posterior branch pierces obturator externus anteriorly, supplies it and passes behind adductor brevis to the front of adductor magnus, dividing into branches to this and adductor brevis when the latter is not supplied by the anterior division. It usually sends an articular filament to the knee joint which perforates adductor magnus distally or traverses its opening with the femoral artery to enter the popliteal fossa. Here it descends on the popliteal artery to the back of the knee, pierces its oblique posterior ligament and supplies the articular capsule. It gives filaments to the popliteal artery.

Lesions of the obturator nerve

Isolated lesions of the obturator nerve are extremely rare, but may occasionally occur as a result of direct trauma (sometimes during parturition) or in anterior dislocations of the hip. The nerve may also be damaged by a rare obturator hernia, or involved together with the femoral nerve in retroperitoneal lesions close to their origins from the lumbar plexus. A nerve entrapment syndrome causing chronic medial thigh pain is described in athletes with large adductor muscles.

Accessory obturator nerve

Occasionally present (10%), the accessory obturator nerve is small and arises from the ventral branches of the third and fourth lumbar ventral rami. It descends along the medial border of psoas major, crosses the superior pubic ramus behind pectineus and divides into branches, one entering the deep surface of pectineus, another supplying the hip joint and a third connecting with the anterior branch of the obturator nerve. Sometimes the accessory obturator nerve is very small and supplies only pectineus. Any branch may be absent and others may occur, one sometimes supplying adductor longus.

SACRAL PLEXUS AND BRANCHES (Fig. 111.41)

The branches of the sacral plexus are:

	Ventral divisions	Dorsal divisions
To quadratus femoris and gemellus inferior	L4, 5, S1	
To obturator internus and gemellus superior	L5, S1, 2	
To piriformis		S(1), 2
Superior gluteal		L4, 5, S1
Inferior gluteal		L5, S1, 2
Posterior femoral cutaneous	S2, 3	S1, 2
Tibial (sciatic)	L4, 5, S1, 2, 3	
Common peroneal (sciatic)		L4, 5, S1, 2
Perforating cutaneous		S2, 3
Pudendal	S2, 3, 4	
To levator ani, coccygeus and sphincter ani externus	S4	
Pelvic splanchnic	S2, 3, (4)	

Sciatic nerve (Fig. 111.42)

The sciatic nerve is 2 cm wide at its origin and is the thickest nerve in the body. It leaves the pelvis via the greater sciatic foramen below piriformis and descends between the greater trochanter and ischial tuberosity, along the back of the thigh, dividing into the tibial and common peroneal (fibular) nerves at a varying level proximal to the knee. Superiorly it lies deep to gluteus maximus, resting first on the posterior ischial surface with the nerve to quadratus femoris between them. It then crosses posterior to obturator internus, the gemelli and quadratus femoris, separated by the latter from obturator externus and the hip joint. It is accompanied medially by the posterior femoral cutaneous nerve and the inferior gluteal artery. More distally it lies behind adductor magnus and is crossed posteriorly by the long head of biceps femoris. It corresponds to a line drawn from just medial to the midpoint between the ischial tuberosity and greater trochanter to the apex of the popliteal fossa (see p. 1410).

Articular branches arise proximally to supply the hip joint through its posterior capsule: these are sometimes derived directly from the sacral plexus. Muscular branches are distributed to biceps femoris, semitendinosus, semimembranosus and the ischial part of adductor magnus.

The point of division of the sciatic nerve into its major components (tibial and common peroneal) is very variable. The common site is at the junction of the middle and lower thirds of the thigh, near the apex of the popliteal fossa. The division may occur at any level above this, though rarely below it. It is not uncommon for the major components to leave the sacral plexus separately, in which case the common peroneal component usually passes through piriformis at the greater sciatic notch while the tibial component passes below the muscle.

Lesions of the sciatic nerve

The sciatic nerve supplies the knee flexors and all the muscles below the knee, so that a complete palsy of the sciatic nerve results in a flail foot and severe difficulty in walking. This is rare and usually related to trauma. The nerve is vulnerable in posterior dislocation of the hip. As it leaves the pelvis it passes either behind piriformis or sometimes through the muscle and at that point it may become entrapped (the piriformis syndrome: this is a common anatomical variant but an extremely rare entrapment neuropathy, see p. 1446). External compression over the buttock (e.g. in patients who lie immobile on a hard surface for a considerable length of time) can injure the nerve. Sadly the most common cause of serious sciatic nerve injury (and consequent major medicolegal claims) is iatrogenic. It may be damaged in misplaced therapeutic injections into gluteus maximus. The safe zone for deep intramuscular injections here is the upper outer quadrant of the buttock. Perhaps safer still is to inject into the quadriceps, though this can produce problems of its own, e.g. haemorrhage, leading to contracture of the muscle, which limits knee motion. Sciatic nerve palsy occurs after total hip replacement or similar surgery in c.1% of cases. This can be due to sharp injury, burning from bone cement, traction from instruments, manipulation of the hip, inadvertent lengthening of the femur, or haematoma surrounding the nerve or within its soft tissue coverings. Haematoma is characterized by the development of severe pain in the immediate postoperative period. Early surgical exploration and evacuation of haematoma can reverse the nerve lesion. Unfortunately the other causes may not be influenced. The majority are temporary. Complete sciatic nerve palsy is very rare. For some reason, possibly anatomical, the common peroneal part is more usually affected alone. The patient has a foot drop and a high stepping gait.

Inferior gluteal nerve

The inferior gluteal nerve arises from the dorsal branches of the fifth lumbar and first and second sacral ventral rami. It leaves the pelvis via the greater sciatic foramen below piriformis, and divides into branches that enter the deep surface of gluteus maximus.

Superior gluteal nerve

The superior gluteal nerve arises from the dorsal branches of the fourth and fifth lumbar and first sacral ventral rami. It leaves the pelvis via the greater sciatic foramen above piriformis with the superior gluteal vessels, and divides into superior and inferior branches. The superior branch accompanies the upper branch of the deep division of the superior gluteal artery to supply gluteus medius and occasionally gluteus minimus. The inferior branch runs with the lower ramus of the deep division of

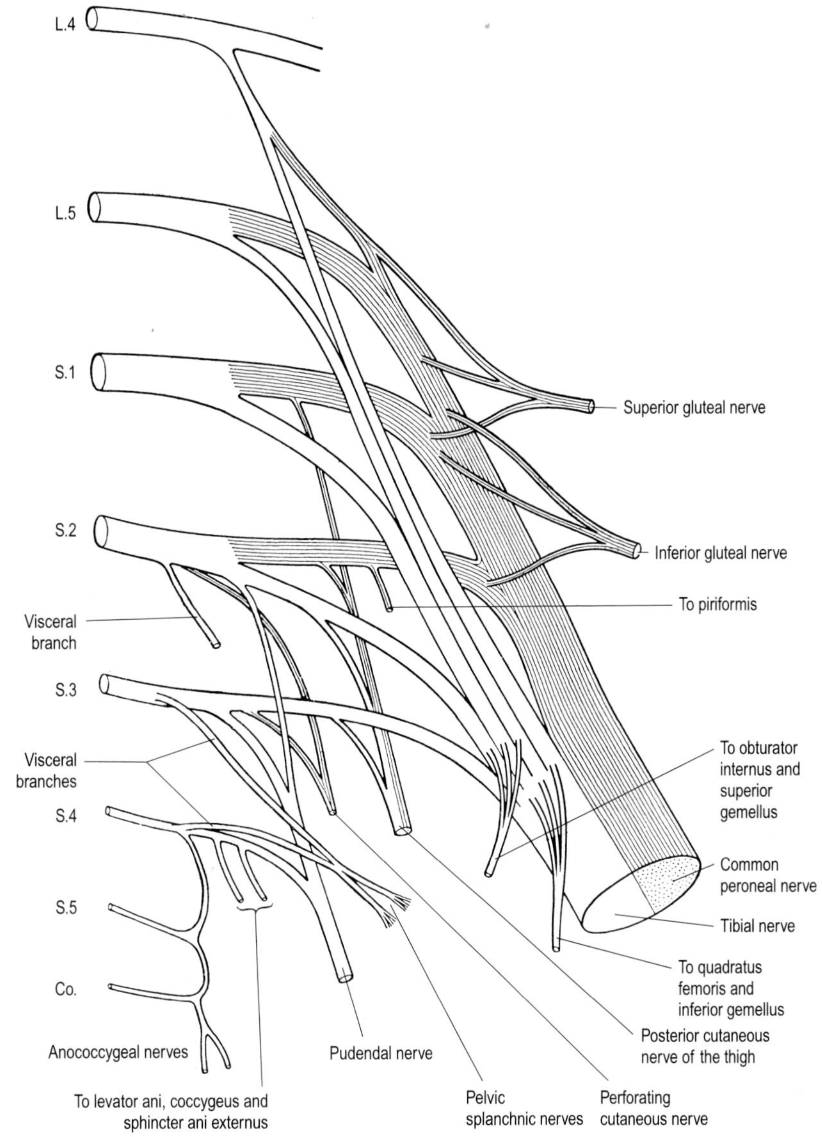

Fig. 111.41 The sacral and coccygeal plexuses. The dorsal rami are not shown. Ventral (anterior) divisions are not shaded. The contribution from S2 to the pelvic splanchnic nerves has been cut before it joins those from S3 and S4.

the superior gluteal artery across gluteus minimus, supplying the glutei medius and minimus and ending in tensor fasciae latae.

Pudendal nerve
See pages 1126 and 1364.

Perforating cutaneous nerve
The perforating cutaneous nerve usually arises from the posterior aspects of the second and third sacral ventral spinal rami. It pierces the sacrotuberous ligament, curves round the inferior border of gluteus maximus and supplies the skin over the inferomedial aspect of this muscle. The nerve may arise from the pudendal nerve or, if absent, may be replaced either by a branch from the posterior femoral cutaneous nerve or from the third and fourth, or fourth and fifth, sacral ventral rami.

Nerve to quadratus femoris and gemellus inferior
The nerve to quadratus femoris and gemellus inferior arises from the ventral branches of the fourth lumbar to the first sacral ventral rami. It leaves the pelvis via the greater sciatic foramen below piriformis, descends on the ischium deep to the sciatic nerve, gemelli and the tendon of obturator internus and supplies gemellus inferior, quadratus femoris and the hip joint.

Nerve to obturator internus and gemellus superior
The nerve to obturator internus and gemellus superior arises from the ventral branches of the fifth lumbar and first and second sacral ventral

rami. It leaves the pelvis like the nerve to quadratus femoris and gemellus inferior, supplies a branch to the upper posterior surface of gemellus superior, crosses the ischial spine lateral to the internal pudendal vessels, re-enters the pelvis via the lesser sciatic foramen and enters the pelvic surface of obturator internus.

Posterior cutaneous nerve of the thigh
The posterior cutaneous nerve of the thigh arises from the dorsal branches of the first and second and the ventral branches of the second and third sacral rami. It leaves the pelvis via the greater sciatic foramen below piriformis and descends under gluteus maximus with the inferior gluteal vessels, lying posterior or medial to the sciatic nerve. It descends in the back of the thigh superficial to the long head of biceps femoris, deep to the fascia lata. Behind the knee it pierces the deep fascia and accompanies the short saphenous vein to midcalf, its terminal twigs connecting with the sural nerve. Its branches are all cutaneous and are distributed to the gluteal region, perineum and the flexor aspect of the thigh and leg. Three or four gluteal branches curl round the lower border of gluteus maximus to supply the skin over its inferolateral area. The perineal branch supplies the superomedial skin in the thigh, curves forwards across the hamstrings below the ischial tuberosity, pierces the fascia lata and runs in the superficial perineal fascia to the scrotal or labial skin, communicating with the inferior rectal and posterior scrotal branches of the perineal nerve. It gives numerous branches to the skin of the back and medial side of the thigh, the popliteal fossa and the proximal part of the back of the leg.

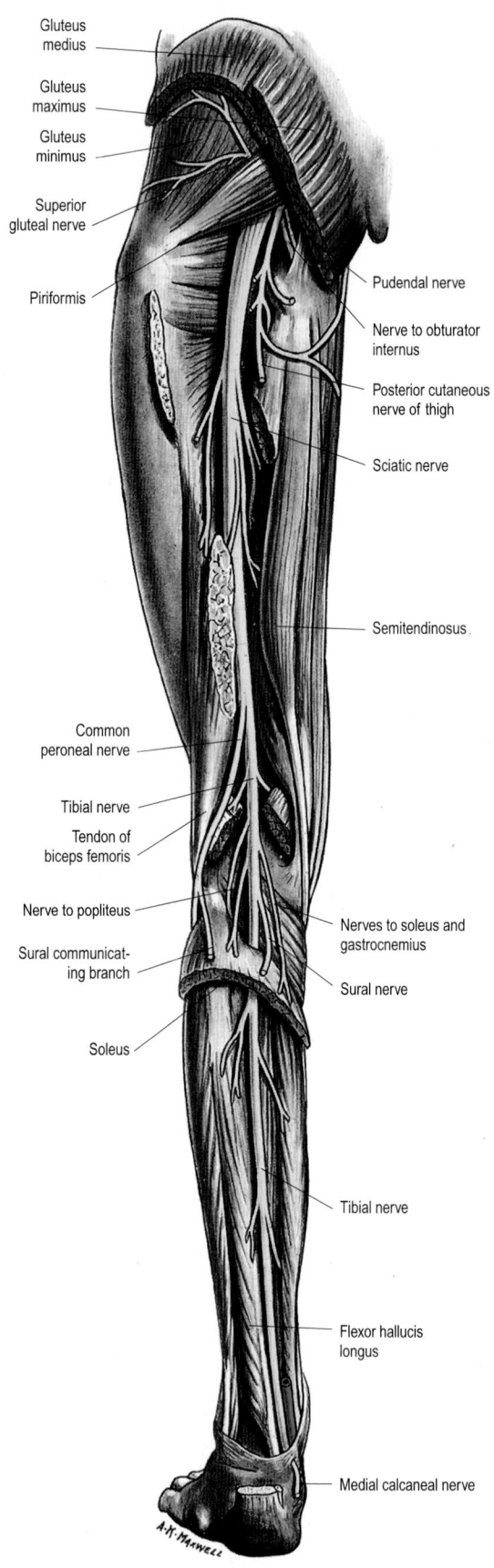

Gluteus
medius

Gluteus
maximus

Gluteus
minimus

Superior
gluteal nerve

Piriformis

Pudendal nerve

Nerve to obturator
internus

Posterior cutaneous
nerve of thigh

Sciatic nerve

Semitendinosus

Common
peroneal nerve

Tibial nerve

Tendon of
biceps femoris

Nerve to popliteus

Sural communicat-
ing branch

Soleus

Nerves to soleus and
gastrocnemius

Sural nerve

Tibial nerve

Flexor hallucis
longus

Medial calcaneal nerve

Fig. 111.42 The nerves of the left lower limb: posterior aspect.

Nerve to piriformis

The nerve to piriformis usually arises from the dorsal branches of the first and second sacral ventral rami (sometimes only the second) and enters the anterior surface of piriformis.

Visceral branches of sacral plexus

See pages 1126 and 1364.

Pelvic muscular branches of sacral plexus

See page 1364.

REFERENCES

Bogduk N 1997 Clinical Anatomy of the Lumbar Spine and Sacrum, 3rd edn. Edinburgh: Churchill Livingstone.

Brothwell DR, Pollard AM (eds) 2001 Handbook of Archaeological Sciences. Chichester: Wiley.

Cormack GC, Lamberty BGH 1994 See Bibliography.

Crock HV 1980 An atlas of the arterial supply of the head and neck of the femur in man. Clin Orthop 152: 17–25.

Crock HV 1996 Atlas of Vascular Anatomy of the Skeletal and Spinal Cord. London: Martin Dunitz.

Delaere O, Kok V, Nyssen-Behets C, Dhem A 1992 Ossification of the human fetal ilium. Acta Anat 143: 330–4.

Dixon AF 1910 The architecture of the cancellous tissue forming the upper end of the femur. J Anat Physiol 44: 223–30.
A neglected and original work with far-reaching implications for the understanding of femoral structure.

Dodd H, Cockett FB 1976 The Pathology and Surgery of the Veins of the Lower Limb, 2nd edn. Edinburgh: Churchill Livingstone.

Eckhoff DG, Kramer RC, Watkins JJ, Alongi CA, van Gerven DP 1994 Variation in femoral anteversion. Clin Anat 7: 72–5.

Finnegan M 1978 Non-metric variation of the infracranial skeleton. J Anat 125: 33–7.
A reference text for forensic and osteo-archaeological work.

Fuss FK, Bacher A 1991 New aspects of the morphology and function of the human hip joint ligaments. Am J Anat 192: 1–13.

Holm NJ 1980 The internal stress pattern of the os coxae. Acta Orthop Scand 51: 421–8.
Biomechanical information, relevant to the function of the hip and pelvis.

Joseph J 1975 Movements at the hip joint. Ann R Coll Surg Eng 56: 192–201.

Mays S 1998 The Archaeology of Human Bones. London: Routledge.

Newell RLM 1997 The calcar femorale: a tale of historical neglect. Clin Anat 10: 27–33.

Ponseti IV 1978 Growth and development of the acetabulum in the normal child. J Bone Joint Surg 60A: 575–85.

Trueta J 1957 The normal vascular anatomy of the femoral head during growth. J Bone Joint Surg 39B: 353–8.

Weisl H 1954 The articular surfaces of the sacro-iliac joint and their relation to the movements of the sacrum. Acta Anat 22: 1–14.

Whitehouse WJ 1977 Cancellous bone in the anterior part of the iliac crest. Calcif Tissue Res 23: 67–76.
Detailed information on the internal structure of a site that is commonly used for marrow biopsy.

Thigh

The thigh consists of a cylinder of compact bone, the femoral shaft, which is completely enclosed by muscle groups through which important neurovascular pathways run. The muscle is limited circumferentially by a tough fascial tube, the fascia lata, and its functional groups are contained within osteofascial compartments defined by fascial septa which join the bone with the enclosing fascia (p. 1461). The femoral artery gives off its major branch, the profunda femoris, in the anterior compartment, and the sciatic nerve usually divides into its main branches, the tibial and common peroneal, as it passes through the posterior compartment. The femoral nerve divides soon after entering the anterior compartment beneath the inguinal ligament. The obturator nerve enters the region proximally and medially from the pelvis and divides into its main branches which run anterior and posterior to adductor longus. The presence and position of the femoral neck cause the femoral shaft to lie obliquely, which means that the anterior (extensor) muscle group, the quadriceps, runs obliquely distally and medially and so applies a pull to the patella which is both laterally and proximally directed. The adductor muscles occupy the region between the quadriceps and the medial margin of the thigh. They are attached distally to the posterior surface of the femur and lie more posteriorly than the quadriceps. The posterior (flexor) muscle group, the hamstrings, lie behind the adductors. The attachments of these muscles determine the displacement of femoral shaft fractures. Knowledge of the anatomy of the thigh is important in the assessment and management of arterial disease.

SKIN

CUTANEOUS VASCULAR SUPPLY AND LYMPHATIC DRAINAGE

The skin of the thigh distal to the inguinal ligament and gluteal fold is supplied mainly by branches of the femoral and profunda femoris arteries. There is some contribution from the obturator, inferior gluteal and popliteal arteries and from direct cutaneous, musculocutaneous and fasciocutaneous vessels. For further details consult Cormack and Lamberty (1994).

Cutaneous veins are tributaries of vessels that correspond to the named arteries. Cutaneous lymphatic drainage is to the superficial inguinal nodes, mainly via collecting trunks accompanying the long saphenous vein.

CUTANEOUS INNERVATION
See page 1399.

SOFT TISSUE

FEMORAL SHEATH AND FEMORAL TRIANGLE
The femoral sheath and femoral triangle are described on page 1419.

FASCIAL COMPARTMENTS (Figs 112.1, 112.2)
There are three functional muscle compartments in the thigh, namely, anterior (extensor), posterior (flexor) and medial (adductor). The anterior and posterior are true osteofascial compartments, limited peripherally by the fascia lata and separated from each other by the femur and the medial and lateral intermuscular septa. The adductor compartment only exists in the proximal part of the thigh and is not a true anatomical compartment, in that it is not limited by fascial planes. The muscles in the three compartments are described on page 1461. Adductor magnus, adductor longus and pectineus could each be considered to be constituents of two compartments, i.e. adductor magnus

in the posterior and the medial compartments, and adductor longus and pectineus in the anterior and the medial compartments.

The nerve supply to the compartments of the thigh mainly follows the 'one compartment – one nerve' principle. Thus the femoral nerve supplies the anterior compartment muscles, the obturator nerve supplies the medial compartment muscles, and the sciatic nerve supplies those in the posterior compartment. The dual functional and compartmental attribution of adductor magnus and pectineus are reflected by their dual nerve supplies.

The arterial supply to the compartmental muscle groups cannot be expressed so simply. All receive a supply from the femoral system, particularly from the profunda femoris and its branches. The adductors receive a contribution from the obturator artery, and the hamstrings receive a proximal supply from the inferior gluteal artery. Further details are given in the descriptions of the individual muscles.

ADDUCTOR CANAL (Figs 112.1, 112.2)
The adductor canal (Hunter's canal; subsartorial canal) is an aponeurotic tunnel in the middle third of the thigh. It runs from the apex of the femoral triangle to an opening in adductor magnus through which the femoral vessels reach the popliteal fossa. It is triangular in section, and bounded anterolaterally by vastus medialis, posteriorly by adductor longus, distally by adductor magnus and anteromedially by a strong aponeurosis that extends between the adductors across the vessels to vastus medialis. Sartorius is anterior. The canal contains the femoral artery and vein, the descending genicular and muscular branches of the femoral artery and their corresponding venous tributaries, the saphenous nerve, and the nerve to vastus medialis (until it enters its muscle).

FEMUR

The shaft of the femur is described on page 1431.

MUSCLES

ANTERIOR COMPARTMENT (Figs 111.29, 112.1, 112.2)
The muscles of the anterior compartment include tensor fasciae latae (see p. 1448), sartorius and rectus femoris, which can act at both hip and knee joints, and vasti medialis, lateralis, and intermedius, which act only at the knee. Articularis genu, a derivative of vastus intermedius, completes the group: it retracts the synovial capsule of the knee joint. Rectus femoris and the vasti extend the knee joint through a common tendon and hence are considered as one muscle called quadriceps femoris. Adductor longus and pectineus are sometimes considered to be part of both the anterior and the adductor compartment.

Sartorius

Attachments (Fig. 112.3) – Sartorius is a narrow strap muscle, and is the longest muscle in the body. It arises by tendinous fibres from the anterior superior iliac spine and the upper half of the notch below it. It crosses the thigh obliquely over to the medial side, then descends more vertically to the medial side of the knee. The muscle fibres terminate at this point and a thin, flattened tendon curves obliquely forwards and expands into a broad aponeurosis. The aponeurosis is attached to the proximal medial surface of the tibia in front of gracilis and semitendinosus, together forming the 'pes anserinus'. A slip from its upper margin blends with the capsule of the knee joint, and another from its lower margin merges with the superficial layer of the

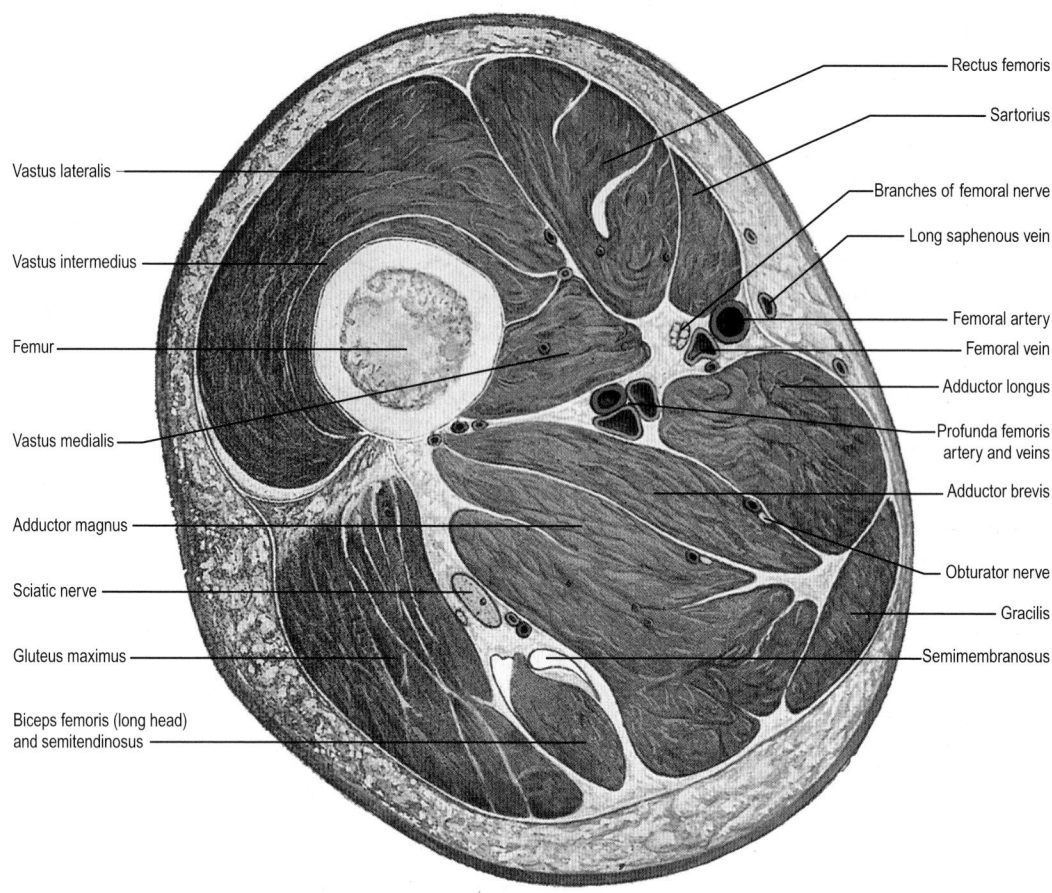

Vastus lateralis

Vastus intermedius

Femur

Vastus medialis

Adductor magnus

Sciatic nerve

Gluteus maximus

Biceps femoris (long head)
and semitendinosus

Rectus femoris

Sartorius

Branches of femoral nerve

Long saphenous vein

Femoral artery

Femoral vein

Adductor longus

Profunda femoris
artery and veins

Adductor brevis

Obturator nerve

Gracilis

Semimembranosus

Fig. 112.1 Transverse (axial) section through the left thigh at the level of the apex of the femoral triangle.

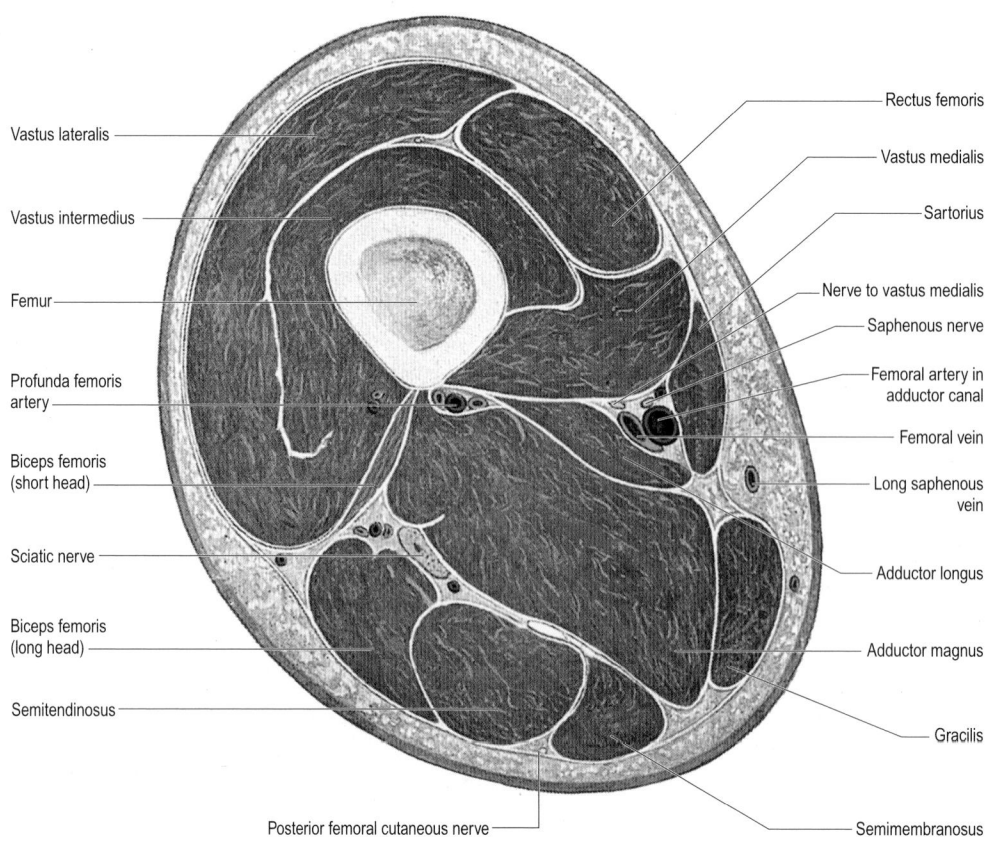

Vastus lateralis

Vastus intermedius

Femur

Profunda femoris
artery

Biceps femoris
(short head)

Sciatic nerve

Biceps femoris
(long head)

Semitendinosus

Posterior femoral cutaneous nerve

Rectus femoris

Vastus medialis

Sartorius

Nerve to vastus medialis

Saphenous nerve

Femoral artery in
adductor canal

Femoral vein

Long saphenous
vein

Adductor longus

Adductor magnus

Gracilis

Semimembranosus

Fig. 112.2 Transverse (axial) section through the middle of the left thigh.

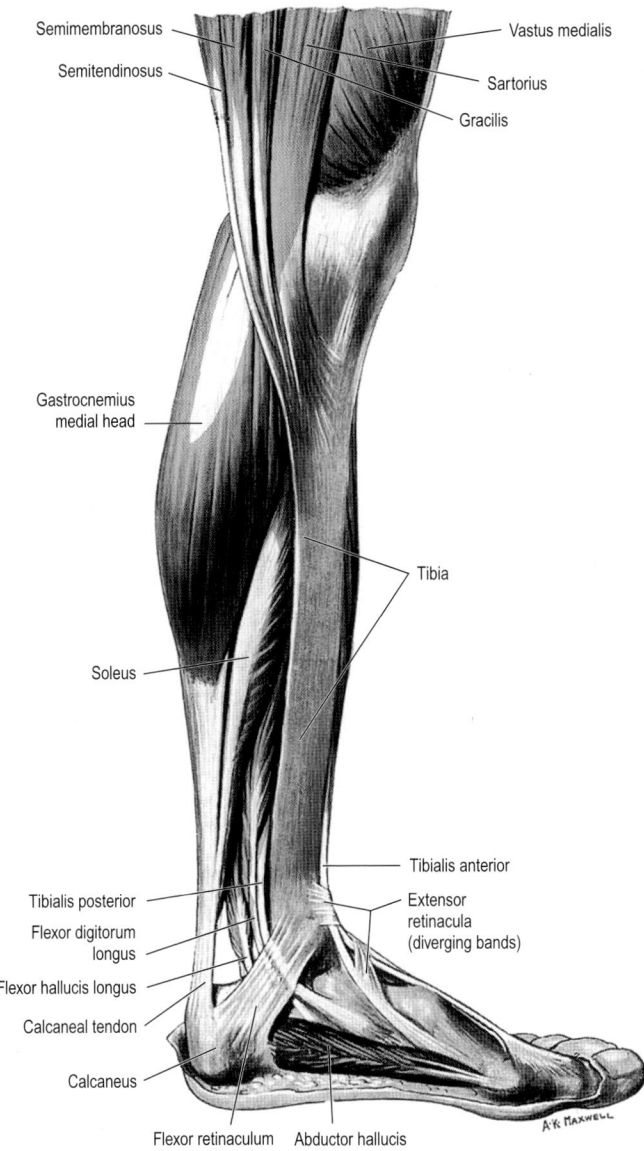

Semimembranosus

Semitendinosus

Gastrocnemius
medial head

Soleus

Tibialis posterior

Flexor digitorum
longus

Flexor hallucis longus

Calcaneal tendon

Calcaneus

Vastus medialis

Sartorius

Gracilis

Tibia

Tibialis anterior

Extensor
retinacula
(diverging bands)

Flexor retinaculum   Abductor hallucis

A·K·MAXWELL

Fig. 112.3 Muscles of the left leg: medial aspect.

deep fascia on the medial side of the leg. This sheet of tissue passes inferiorly to lie superficial to and over the distal insertions of gracilis and semitendinosus. It has to be split by sharp dissection to reveal these two tendons if they need to be harvested, e.g. in cruciate ligament surgery.

In some cases sartorius is absent, while in others it is doubled: when this occurs, the extra head is attached to the pectineal line or to the femoral sheath. Variations in the insertion of sartorius in relation to the knee axis have been described.

Relations – The femoral triangle, in the upper third of the thigh, is formed by the medial border of sartorius (lateral side), the medial border of adductor longus (medial side), and the inguinal ligament (base). The femoral artery descends through this triangle from the middle of the base to the apex. In the middle third of the thigh, the femoral artery and vein, the saphenous nerve and the nerve to vastus medialis are all contained in the adductor canal, which is covered anteriorly by a strong stratum of deep fascia and by sartorius. The fascia bridges the interval between the adductors and quadriceps: it must be incised to expose the vessels.

Vascular supply – The main arterial supply to sartorius is derived from the femoral system, and enters the medial half of the muscle from its deep surface. The superior group may arise from the common femoral, the main trunk of the profunda, the artery of the quadriceps, the super-

ficial femoral or the lateral circumflex femoral artery. There may be an additional proximal supply from the superficial circumflex iliac artery. The middle group arises from the superficial femoral artery. The distal group arises from the superficial femoral within the adductor canal and from the descending genicular artery.

Innervation – Sartorius is innervated by the femoral nerve, L2 and 3.

Actions – Sartorius assists in flexing the leg at the knee, and the thigh on the pelvis, particularly when these two movements are combined. It also helps to abduct the thigh and to rotate it laterally. (Together with inversion of the foot, these movements bring the sole of the foot into direct view.) The fact that sartorius represents only 1% of the physiological cross-sectional area of all muscles which cross the hip or knee joint suggests that its role in walking is a minor one. In a subject ascending steps, electromyographic activity of sartorius increases during lateral rotation of the thigh at the end of the swing phase immediately preceding heel strike, which presumably decelerates the limb. Sartorius may therefore have a substantial involvement in climbing.

Testing – When it contracts against gravity, as it usually does, sartorius can be both seen and felt in the living subject.

Adductor longus
See page 1465.

Iliacus
See page 1446.

Psoas major and minor
See page 1444.

Pectineus
See page 1444.

Quadriceps femoris (Fig. 111.29, 112.1, 112.2)
Quadriceps femoris, the great extensor muscle of the leg, covers almost all of the front and sides of the femur. It can be divided into four parts, each named individually. One, rectus femoris, arises from the ilium and travels straight down the middle of the thigh, its shape and path determining its name. The other three arise from the shaft of the femur and surround it (apart from the linea aspera) from the trochanters to the condyles: vastus lateralis is lateral to the femur, vastus medialis is medial to it, and vastus intermedius lies in front of the femur. Rectus femoris crosses both hip and knee joints, while the three vasti only cross the knee joint.

The tendons of the four components of quadriceps unite in the lower part of the thigh to form a single strong tendon attached to the base of the patella, and some fibres continue over it to blend with the patellar tendon. The patella is a sesamoid bone in the quadriceps tendon, and the patellar tendon, which extends from the patellar apex to the tubercle of the tibia, is the continuation of the main tendon. The medial and lateral patellar retinacula are expansions from its borders. The suprapatellar bursa (a synovial extension of the knee joint) lies between the femur and the suprapatellar part of the quadriceps tendon. The deep infrapatellar bursa lies between the patellar tendon and the proximal end of the tibia.

The arterial supply to the quadriceps group has been traditionally ascribed to a single branch of either the profunda femoris or of the lateral circumflex femoral, the 'artery of the quadriceps'. This vessel, which may be large, occasionally arises directly from the femoral artery. However, according to Taylor and Razaboni (1994) this artery does not supply all four components of the quadriceps: vastus medialis is supplied directly from the (superficial) femoral artery. The supply of the individual muscle components is described below: their sheaths may have an additional and variable supply.

Quadriceps as a group shows little anatomical variation.

Rectus femoris

Attachments – Rectus femoris is fusiform. Its superficial fibres are bipennate, the deep fibres parallel. It has a double origin on the ilium: a straight tendon arises from the anterior inferior iliac spine, and a thinner, flatter reflected tendon from a groove above the acetabulum and from the fibrous capsule of the hip joint. The two unite at an acute angle and spread into an aponeurosis that is prolonged downwards on the anterior surface of the muscle: the muscular fibres arise from this aponeurosis. The fibres end in a broad, thick aponeurosis that forms over the lower two-thirds of its posterior surface and gradually narrows into the thick, flat tendon by which it is attached to the base of the patella. This constitutes the superficial central part of the quadriceps tendon.

Rectus femoris may arise from the anterior superior iliac spine, and its reflected head may be absent.

Relations – Proximally the muscle is covered by tensor fasciae latae, iliacus and sartorius. The reflected head lies beneath gluteus minimus. The capsule of the hip, vastus intermedius, the anterior borders of vasti lateralis and medius, the lateral circumflex femoral artery and branches of the femoral nerve all lie deep to rectus femoris.

Vascular supply – There are two main pedicles, a superior and an inferior. The superior enters rectus femoris at the junction of its upper and middle thirds and arises from the 'artery of the quadriceps'. The inferior and larger branch arises from the 'artery of the quadriceps' at about midthigh level and enters the muscle a few centimetres more distally. There are additional contributions from the lateral circumflex femoral and, less often, the superficial circumflex iliac arteries.

Vastus medialis and vastus medialis obliquus

Attachments – Vastus medialis arises from the lower part of the intertrochanteric line, spiral line, medial lip of the linea aspera, proximal part of the medial supracondylar line, the tendons of adductor longus and magnus, and the medial intermuscular septum. Its fibres pass downwards and forwards at an angle of c.15° to the long axis of the femur, most of them into an aponeurosis on the deep surface of the muscle which is attached to the medial border of the patella and quadriceps tendon. An expansion from this aponeurosis reinforces the capsule of the knee joint and is attached below to the medial condyle of the tibia.

The lowest fibres are much more horizontal and form a bulge in the living subject, medial to the upper half of the patella. Some authors distinguish this part of the muscle as the vastus medialis obliquus, with fibres that originate largely from the tendon of adductor magnus and insert into the medial border of the patella. It plays an important role in the function of patellofemoral joint.

Relations – Vastus medialis is partly covered by rectus femoris and sartorius. In the central part of the thigh it forms the lateral wall of the adductor (Hunter's) canal.

Vascular supply – Vastus medialis is supplied by three branches of the (superficial) femoral artery. The superior and middle branches arise, sometimes from a common trunk, proximal to the adductor canal, while the inferior arises within the canal. There may also be minor branches from the profunda and descending genicular arteries.

Vastus lateralis

Attachments – Vastus lateralis is the largest component of quadriceps femoris. It arises by a broad aponeurosis from the upper part of the intertrochanteric line, the anterior and inferior borders of the greater trochanter, the lateral lip of the gluteal tuberosity, and the proximal half of the lateral lip of the linea aspera. This aponeurosis covers the proximal three-quarters of the muscle; many additional fibres arise from its deep surface. A few fibres also arise from the tendon of gluteus maximus and the lateral intermuscular septum between vastus lateralis and the short head of biceps femoris. The muscular mass thus formed is attached to a strong aponeurosis on the deep surface of the lower part of the muscle. This narrows to a flat tendon, which is attached to the base and lateral border of the patella and blends into the compound quadriceps femoris tendon. It contributes an expansion to the capsule of the knee joint which descends to the lateral condyle of the tibia and blends with the iliotibial tract.

Relations – Vastus lateralis is covered laterally by the fascia lata and the aponeurotic insertions of tensor fasciae latae and gluteus maximus. It is separated from vastus intermedius by branches of the femoral nerve

and the lateral circumflex femoral artery. Posteriorly it is separated from biceps femoris by the lateral intermuscular septum.

Vascular supply – There are three main arteries of supply: the superior medial artery arises directly from the lateral circumflex femoral, the inferior medial (the largest of the three) from the 'artery of the quadriceps', and the lateral from the first perforating branch of the profunda femoris artery.

Vastus intermedius

Attachments – Vastus intermedius arises from the anterior and lateral surfaces of the upper two-thirds of the femoral shaft, and from the lower part of the lateral intermuscular septum. Its fibres end on the anterior surface of the muscle in an aponeurosis which forms the deep part of the quadriceps tendon and is attached to the lateral border of the patella and the lateral condyle of the tibia.

Vastus intermedius appears to be inseparable from vastus medialis. However, when rectus femoris is reflected a narrow cleft can be seen extending upwards from the medial border of the patella between the two muscles, sometimes as far as the lower part of the intertrochanteric line, beyond which the two muscles are frequently fused.

Relations – Vastus intermedius is almost completely covered by the other quadriceps components, except laterally where a small part becomes superficial behind vastus lateralis.

Vascular supply – Vastus intermedius receives a lateral artery of supply, which arises from the 'artery of the quadriceps', and a medial artery that arises directly from the profunda. Arteries to the other quadriceps components may also contribute. There is an anastomotic network deep to the muscle: this supplies the suprapatellar pouch and articularis genu and may form a collateral pathway when the (superficial) femoral artery is blocked.

Articularis genu
Articularis genu is a small muscle, usually distinct from vastus intermedius but occasionally blending with it. It consists of several muscular bundles that arise from the anterior surface of the lower part of the femoral shaft and are attached to a proximal reflection of the synovial membrane of the knee joint. It is visible during knee arthroscopy when viewed looking superiorly from within the suprapatellar pouch (**Fig. 112.4**).

Innervation of quadriceps group
Quadriceps femoris and articularis genu are supplied by the femoral nerve, L2, 3 and 4.

Actions of quadriceps group
Quadriceps femoris extends the knee. Rectus femoris helps to flex the thigh on the pelvis; if the thigh is fixed, it helps to flex the pelvis on the thigh. Rectus can flex the hip and extend the knee simultaneously. Electromyographic studies indicate that the three vasti are not equally active in different phases of extension or rotation. There is little or no activity in quadriceps during standing. Rectus femoris pulls the patella along the line of the mechanical axis of the lower limb (i.e. the line connecting the centres of the hip, knee, and ankle) because its attachment is anterior to the hip joint. The remaining quadriceps are attached to the shaft of the femur and so the pull is lateral as well as proximal. An extremely important dynamic function of vastus medialis obliquus is to counter this lateral vector on the patella during knee motion. Other static factors that help are the depth of the femoral trochlear groove, the buttressing effect of the lateral femoral condyle in the groove, and the restraining action of the medial patellofemoral ligament. Inadequacy of vastus medialis obliquus is a factor in producing patellar instability and pain. Strengthening of this muscle to improve patellar 'tracking' on the femur and stability is a cornerstone in physiotherapy regimens for patellofemoral problems.

Articularis genu retracts the synovial suprapatellar bursa proximally during extension of the leg, presumably to prevent interposition of redundant synovial folds between patella and femur.

Testing
The quadriceps group is tested by extending the knee against resistance, in the supine position with the hip flexed.

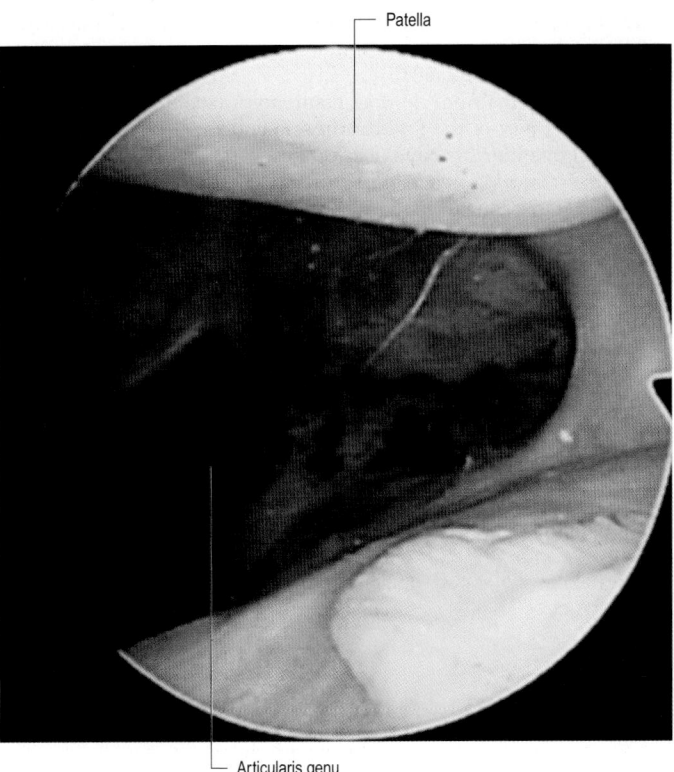

Fig. 112.4 Articularis genu seen from within the suprapatellar pouch at arthroscopy. (By kind permission from Smith and Nephew Endoscopy.)

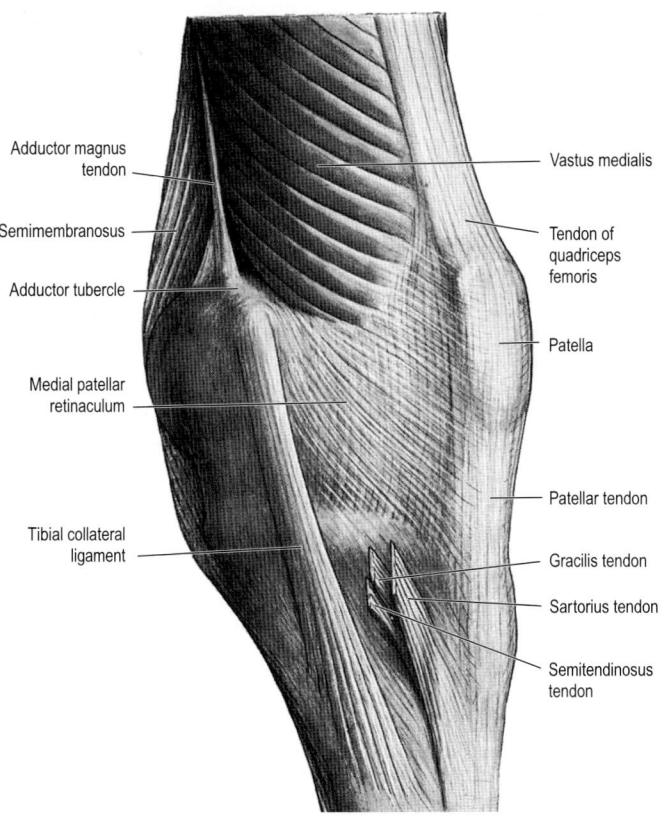

Fig. 112.5 Anteromedial aspect of the left knee joint.

ADDUCTOR COMPARTMENT (Fig. 112.5)

The muscles of the adductor compartment – gracilis, pectineus, adductor longus, adductor brevis, and adductor magnus – have evolved, as their nerve supply suggests, from both flexor and extensor columns. All five muscles cross the hip joint, but only gracilis reaches beyond the knee. They are known collectively as the adductors of the thigh, although their actions are more complex than this, e.g. acting from below they have important roles in balancing the trunk on the lower limb during walking.

Their blood supply is derived from the profunda, medial circumflex femoral, (superficial) femoral and obturator arteries. The profunda (or sometimes the first perforator) supplies a large branch, the 'artery of the adductor muscles'.

Gracilis (Figs 111.29, 112.1, 112.2)

Attachments – Gracilis is the most superficial of the adductor group. It is thin and flat, broad above, narrow and tapering below. It arises by a thin aponeurosis from the medial margins of the lower half of the body of the pubis, the whole of the inferior pubic ramus, and the adjoining part of the ischial ramus (**Fig. 111.28**). The fibres descend vertically into a rounded tendon, often harvested as a knee ligament graft, which passes across the medial condyle of the femur posterior to the tendon of sartorius. It then curves around the medial condyle of the tibia, where it fans out and is attached to the upper part of the medial surface of the tibia, just below the condyle. A few fibres from the lower part of the tendon continue into the deep fascia of the lower leg. Often there is a slip that blends with the tendon of the medial head of gastrocnemius. Unless divided this can lead to problems during surgical harvesting of the gracilis tendon.

Relations – The muscle is covered medially by the fascia lata throughout most of its length. Deep to gracilis lie adductor brevis and adductor magnus. The tibial attachment is immediately proximal to that of semitendinosus, and its upper edge is overlapped by the tendon of sartorius, with which it is partly blended. It is separated from the medial collateral ligament of the knee joint by the tibial intertendinous bursa.

Vascular supply – The arterial supply to gracilis enters via its lateral surface. The main pedicle arises from the 'artery to the adductors' of the profunda and enters at the junction of the upper and middle thirds of the muscle. The gracilis musculocutaneous flap is based on this pedicle. A less important artery enters the distal third of the muscle from the femoral artery. There is a minor proximal supply from the medial circumflex femoral.

Innervation – Gracilis is innervated by the obturator nerve, L2 and 3.

Actions – Gracilis flexes the leg and rotates it medially. It may also act as an adductor of the thigh. When the foot is fixed, gracilis rotates the femur and pelvis laterally on the tibia, and helps balance the trunk during walking.

Testing – While palpating over the tendon posteromedially at the flexed knee, the knee is actively further flexed and the leg actively medially rotated. Gracilis can also be tested with the other adductors of the hip.

Adductor longus (Figs 112.1, 112.2, 112.6)

Attachments – Adductor longus, the most anterior of the three adductors, is a large, fan-shaped muscle that lies in the same plane as pectineus. It arises by a narrow tendon with a flattened (sometimes C-shaped) cross-section, which is attached to the front of the pubis in the angle between the crest and the symphysis. It expands into a broad fleshy belly which descends posterolaterally and inserts by an aponeurosis into the linea aspera in the middle third of the femur, between vastus medialis and adductors magnus and brevis, usually blending with all of them. Its proximal attachment is vulnerable to overload from sporting activity: this is one cause of sport-related groin pain.

Adductor longus is occasionally double.

Relations – Anterior to adductor longus are the spermatic cord, fascia lata (which separates it from the long saphenous vein) and, near its attachment, the femoral artery and vein and sartorius. Posterior to it are adductor brevis and adductor magnus, the anterior branch of the obturator nerve and, near its attachment, the profunda femoris vessels. Lateral is pectineus, and gracilis is medial.

1465

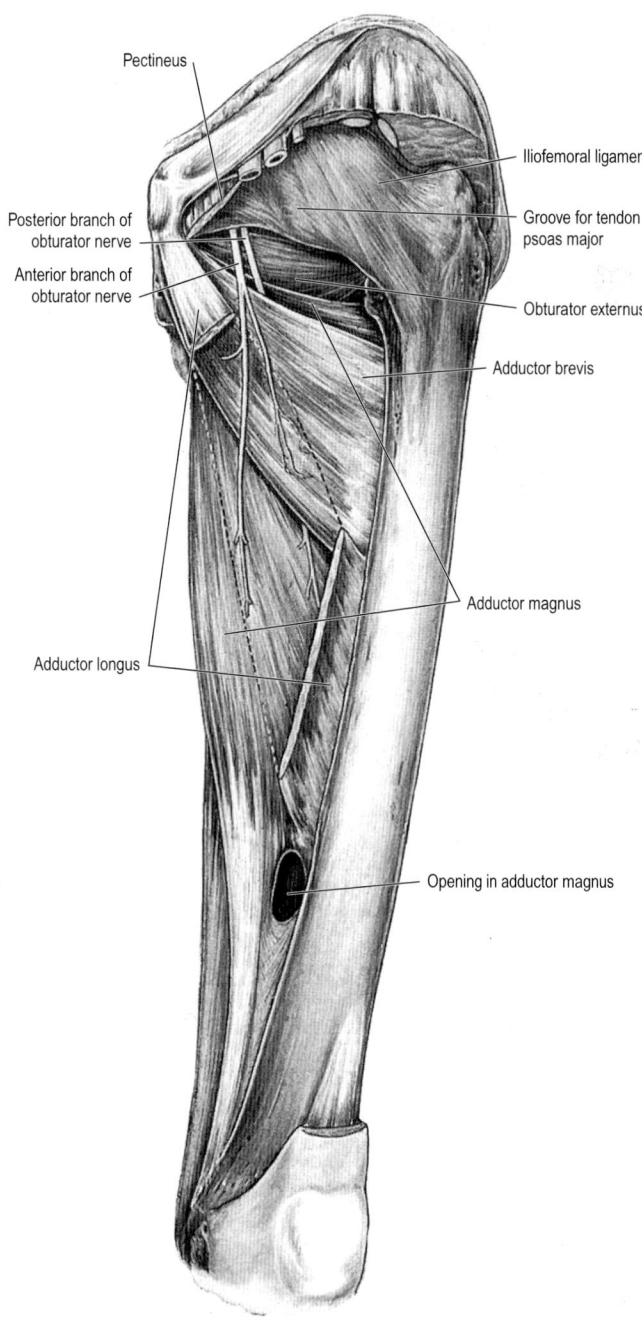

Pectineus

Iliofemoral ligament

Posterior branch of
obturator nerve

Groove for tendon of
psoas major

Anterior branch of
obturator nerve

Obturator externus

Adductor brevis

Adductor magnus

Adductor longus

Opening in adductor magnus

Fig. 112.6 Adductor muscles of the left thigh: anterior aspect. Most of adductor longus has been excised; its borders are indicated by interrupted lines.

Vascular supply – The main supply to adductor longus is to the central part of the muscle from the 'artery to the adductors' of the profunda. There is an additional proximal supply from the medial circumflex femoral artery, and a more distal supply from the femoral artery and sometimes the descending genicular artery.

Innervation – Adductor longus is innervated by the anterior division of the obturator nerve, L2, 3 and 4.

Actions – The actions of the named adductors as a group are discussed below, after each muscle has been described.

Testing – The adductors are tested as a group by adduction of the thigh against resistance, in the supine position and with the knee extended.

Adductor brevis (Figs 112.1, 112.6)

Attachments – Adductor brevis lies posterior to pectineus and adductor longus. It arises by a narrow attachment from the external aspect of the

body and inferior ramus of the pubis, between gracilis and obturator externus. Like adductor longus it is somewhat triangular, and expands as it descends posterolaterally to insert via an aponeurosis into the femur, along a line from the lesser trochanter to the linea aspera, and on the upper part of the linea immediately behind pectineus and the upper part of adductor longus.

Adductor brevis often has two or three separate parts, or may be integrated into adductor magnus.

Relations – Anteriorly lie pectineus, adductor longus, the profunda femoris artery, and the anterior branch of the obturator nerve; posteriorly are adductor magnus and the posterior branch of the obturator nerve. The upper border of adductor brevis is related to the medial circumflex femoral artery, obturator externus, and the conjoined tendon of psoas major and iliacus. Its lower border is related to gracilis and adductor magnus. The second, or first and second perforating arteries pierce it near its femoral attachment.

Vascular supply – The vascular supply to adductor brevis is variable. Usually the main supply is directly from the profunda femoris distally and from the 'artery to the adductors' more proximally. There is an additional proximal supply from the medial circumflex femoral artery. The deep surface receives branches from the obturator artery.

Innervation – Adductor brevis is innervated by the obturator nerve, L2 and 3.

Actions – The actions of the named adductors as a group are discussed below, after each muscle has been described.

Testing – Adductor brevis is tested in the same way as adductor longus.

Adductor magnus (Figs 111.30, 112.1, 112.2, 112.6)

Attachments– Adductor magnus, a massive triangular muscle, arises from a small part of the inferior ramus of the pubis, from the conjoined ischial ramus, and from the inferolateral aspect of the ischial tuberosity. The short, horizontal fibres from the pubic ramus are inserted into the medial margin of the gluteal tuberosity of the femur, medial to gluteus maximus; this part of the muscle, in a plane anterior to the rest, is sometimes called adductor minimus. The fibres from the ischial ramus fan out downwards and laterally, to insert via a broad aponeurosis into the linea aspera and the proximal part of the medial supracondylar line. The medial part of the muscle, composed mainly of fibres from the ischial tuberosity, is a thick mass which descends almost vertically, and ends in the lower third of the thigh in a rounded tendon, which can be palpated proximal to its attachment to the adductor tubercle on the medial condyle of the femur. The tendon is connected by a fibrous expansion to the medial supracondylar line.

The long, linear attachment of the muscle is interrupted by a series of osseo-aponeurotic openings, bridged by tendinous arches attached to the bone. The upper four are small and transmit the perforating branches and the termination of the profunda femoris artery. The lowest is large and allows the femoral vessels to cross to the popliteal fossa.

The vertical, ischiocondylar part of the muscle varies in its degree of separation from the rest. The upper border of adductor magnus may fuse with quadratus femoris.

Relations – Anteriorly lie pectineus, adductor brevis and adductor longus, the femoral and profunda vessels, and the posterior branch of the obturator nerve. A bursa separates the proximal part of the muscle from the lesser trochanter of the femur. Posteriorly are the sciatic nerve, gluteus maximus, biceps femoris, semitendinosus and semi-membranosus. The superior border is parallel with quadratus femoris, and the transverse branch of the medial circumflex femoral artery passes between the muscles. The medial border is related to gracilis, sartorius and the fascia lata.

Vascular supply – As expected from its position, adductor magnus is supplied from both its anterior and posterior aspects. The contribution from the anterior compartment is the more important. Here the obturator, profunda femoris and (superficial) femoral arteries contribute; the main supply is directly from the distal part of the profunda. Distally there may be contributions from the femoral and descending genicular arteries.

Posteriorly there are branches from the medial circumflex femoral, the first and second perforating and the popliteal vessels.

Innervation – Adductor magnus is composite and is doubly innervated by the obturator nerve and the tibial division of the sciatic nerve (L2, 3 and 4); the latter supplies the ischiocondylar part. Both nerves are derived from anterior divisions in the lumbosacral plexus, indicating a primitive flexor origin for both parts of the muscle.

Actions of the named adductors – Extensive or forcible adduction of the femur is not often required. Although the adductors can act in this way, they more commonly act as synergists in the complex patterns of gait activity, and to some degree as controllers of posture. They are active during flexion and extension of the knee. Magnus and longus are probably medial rotators of the thigh. The adductors are inactive during adduction of the abducted thigh in the erect posture (when gravity assists), but active in other postures, such as the supine position, or during adduction of the flexed thigh when standing. They are also active during flexion (longus) and extension (magnus) of the thigh at the hip joint. In symmetrical easy standing their activity is minimal.

Testing – The adductors are usually tested as a group by adduction of the thigh against resistance, in the supine position with the knee extended. The tendon of adductor magnus can be felt just proximal to the adductor tubercle on the medial condyle of the femur. Clinical testing of the other actions mentioned above is not feasible for the individual muscles.

Pectineus (Fig. 111.29)

Attachments – Pectineus is a flat, quadrangular muscle in the femoral triangle. It may also be considered as part of the anterior compartment of the thigh. It arises from the pecten pubis, from the bone in front of it between the iliopectineal eminence and the pubic tubercle, and from the fascia on its own anterior surface. The fibres descend posterolaterally and are attached along a line from the lesser trochanter to the linea aspera.

Pectineus may be bilaminar, in which case the two layers receive separate nerve supplies. Proximally it may be partially or wholly attached to the capsule of the hip joint.

Relations – Pectineus is related anteriorly to the fascia lata, which separates it from the femoral vessels and long saphenous vein; posteriorly to the capsule of the hip joint, adductor brevis, obturator externus and the anterior branch of the obturator nerve; laterally to psoas major and the medial circumflex femoral vessels; and medially to the lateral margin of adductor longus.

Vascular supply – The main arterial supply to pectineus is derived from the medial circumflex femoral artery, which enters the superficial surface of the muscle. There may be a branch from the (common) femoral more proximally, and a deep supply from the obturator artery.

Innervation – Pectineus is innervated by the femoral nerve, L2 and 3, and accessory obturator nerve, L3, when present. Occasionally it receives a branch from the obturator nerve. The muscle may be incompletely divided into dorsal and ventral strata, which are supplied respectively by the obturator and femoral (or rarely accessory obturator) nerves.

Actions – Pectineus adducts the thigh and flexes it on the pelvis.

Testing – The action of pectineus cannot be tested clinically in isolation.

POSTERIOR COMPARTMENT (Fig. 111.30)

The posterior femoral muscles, biceps femoris, semitendinosus, and semimembranosus, are colloquially termed the 'hamstrings'. They cross both hip and knee joints, and integrate extension at the hip with flexion at the knee. As the muscles span the back of the knee, they form the proximal lateral and medial margins of the popliteal fossa (p. 1471). The actions of these muscles and their clinical anatomy will be considered as a group after they have been described individually.

The muscles of the posterior compartment receive their blood supply from the perforating branches of the profunda femoris, most importantly through the first perforator. This vessel has important anastomoses with the inferior gluteal artery (on or within semitendinosus) and with the

medial circumflex femoral artery, while the third perforator anastomoses with the medial superior genicular artery within the short head of biceps. This anastomotic chain forms an important collateral arterial pathway when the femoral artery is blocked (p. 1470).

Semitendinosus (Figs 111.30, 112.2)

Attachments – Semitendinosus, notable for the length of its tendon, is posteromedial in the thigh. It arises from an inferomedial impression on the upper area of the ischial tuberosity (**Fig. 111.4**), by a tendon it shares with the long head of biceps femoris, and from an aponeurosis connecting the adjacent surfaces of the two muscles for c.7.5 cm from their origin. The belly is fusiform and ends a little below midthigh in a long, rounded tendon that runs on the surface of semimembranosus. The tendon curves around the medial condyle of the tibia, passes over the medial collateral ligament of the knee joint (from which it is separated by a bursa, the 'pes bursa'), and inserts into the upper part of the medial surface of the tibia behind the attachment of sartorius and distal to that of gracilis (**Fig. 112.3**). At its termination it is united with the tendon of gracilis and gives off a prolongation to the deep fascia of the leg and to the medial head of gastrocnemius. A tendinous interruption is usually present near the midpoint of the muscle, which may also receive a muscular slip from the long head of biceps femoris. These connections with the medial head of gastrocnemius and biceps can cause difficulty when harvesting the tendon surgically for a graft.

Relations – Semitendinosus lies on semimembranosus throughout its length. The relations of the distal part of the muscle are described above and with the pes anserinus (p. 1478).

Vascular supply – The two main arteries of supply to semitendinosus are superior and inferior. The superior is derived from either the medial circumflex femoral artery or from the first perforating artery. The inferior and larger branch arises from the first perforator distal to the origin of the superior branch. There is an accessory supply at the attachments of the muscle: at the ischial attachment this is derived from the inferior gluteal artery, and at the tibial attachment from the medial inferior genicular artery.

Innervation – Semitendinosus is innervated by the sciatic nerve, L5, S1 and 2, through its tibial division.

Semimembranosus (Figs 111.30, 112.2, 112.7, 112.8)

Attachments – Semimembranosus, so named because of the flattened form of its upper attachment, is posteromedial in the thigh. It arises by a long, flat tendon from a superolateral impression on the ischial

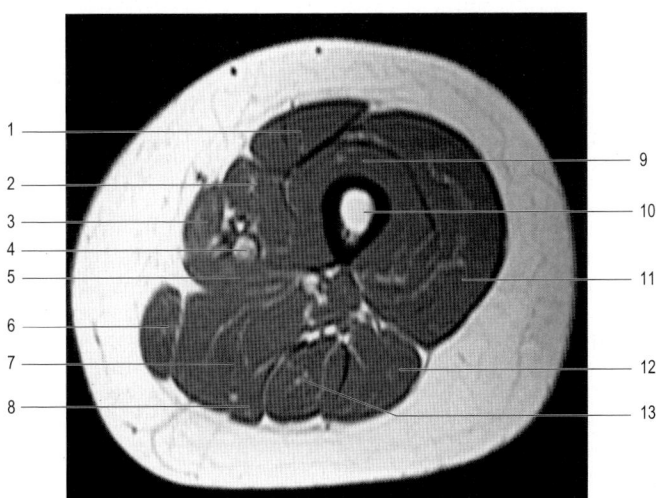

1. Rectus femoris.   2. Vastus medialis.   3. Sartorius.   4. Femoral vein.   5. Adductor longus.
6. Gracilis.   7. Adductor magnus.   8. Semimembranosus.   9. Vastus intermedius.   10. Femur.
11. Vastus lateralis.   12. Long head of biceps femoris.   13. Semitendinosus.

Fig. 112.7 Axial T1-weighted magnetic resonance image of the thigh of an adult female at a level approximately that of the section illustrated in **Fig. 112.8**. (By kind permission from Dr Justin Lee, Chelsea and Westminster Hospital, London.)

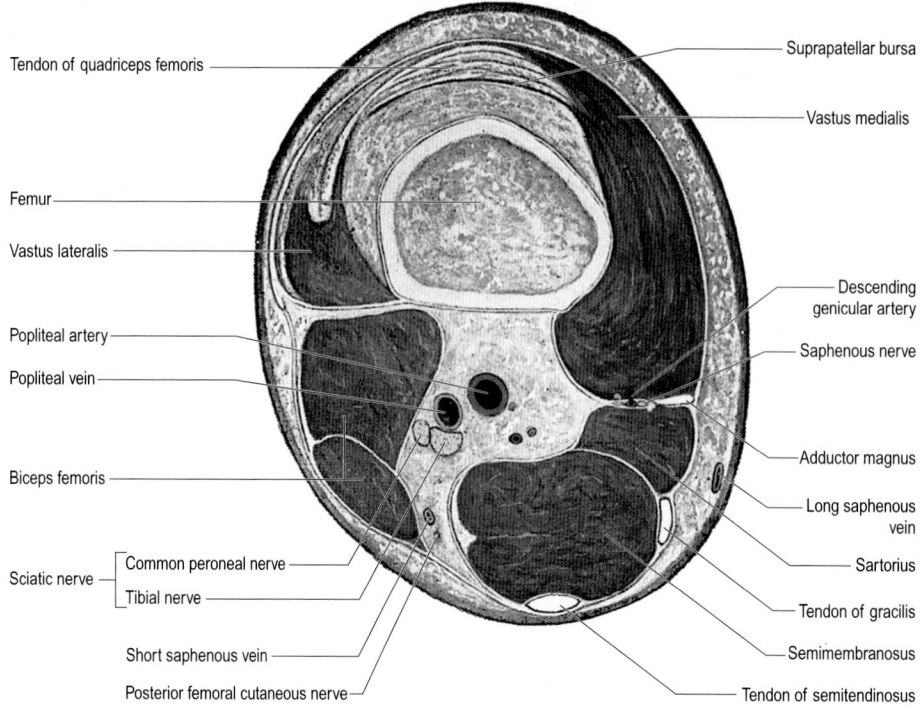

Tendon of quadriceps femoris

Femur

Vastus lateralis

Popliteal artery

Popliteal vein

Biceps femoris

Sciatic nerve — Common peroneal nerve — Tibial nerve

Short saphenous vein

Posterior femoral cutaneous nerve

Suprapatellar bursa

Vastus medialis

Descending genicular artery

Saphenous nerve

Adductor magnus

Long saphenous vein

Sartorius

Tendon of gracilis

Semimembranosus

Tendon of semitendinosus

Fig. 112.8 Transverse (axial) section through the thigh, c.4 cm proximal to the adductor tubercle of the femur.

tuberosity (**Fig. 111.4**). Inferomedially the tendinous fibres intermingle to some extent with those of biceps femoris and semitendinosus. The tendon receives, from the ischial tuberosity and ramus, two fibrous expansions that flank adductor magnus. It then broadens and descends deep to semitendinosus and the long head of biceps femoris. Muscle fibres arise from the tendon at about midthigh and converge to a second aponeurosis on the posterior aspect of the lower part of the muscle, which tapers to the heavy, rounded tendon of the distal attachment. The tendon divides at the level of the knee into five components. The main one is attached to a tubercle (sometimes called the tuberculum tendinis) on the posterior aspect of the medial tibial condyle. The others are: a series of slips to the medial margin of the tibia, immediately behind the medial collateral ligament; a thin fibrous expansion to the fascia over popliteus; a cord-like tendon to the inferior lip and adjacent part of the groove on the back of the medial tibial condyle, deep to the medial collateral ligament; and a strong expansion which passes obliquely upwards to the femoral intercondylar line and lateral femoral condyle and forms much of the oblique popliteal ligament of the knee joint.

Semimembranosus varies considerably in size, and may be absent. It may be double, arising mainly from the sacrotuberous ligament. Slips to the femur or to adductor magnus may occur.

Relations – Semimembranosus overlaps the popliteal vessels and is itself partly overlapped by semitendinosus throughout its extent (**Fig. 111.30**). Its deep surface lies on adductor magnus. The sciatic nerve lies laterally and surprisingly close to the surface. The distal end of the muscle partially overlies the medial head of gastrocnemius before passing anteromedially to it. An important bursa lies between the semi-membranosus tendon and gastrocnemius, and often communicates with the knee joint and with a smaller bursa between the tendon and the posterior tibial margin.

Vascular supply – Semimembranosus is supplied from the perforating arteries, usually from all, though predominantly from the first. Some-times the predominant artery arises from the fourth perforator. A branch of the femoral or popliteal artery supplies the distal part of the muscle, and there may be a contribution from the inferior gluteal artery at the proximal attachment.

Innervation – Semimembranosus is innervated by the sciatic nerve, L5, S1 and 2, through its tibial division.

Biceps femoris (Figs 111.30, 112.1, 112.2, 112.7, 112.8)

Attachments – Biceps femoris occupies a posterolateral position in the thigh. It has two proximal attachments. One, the long head, arises from an inferomedial impression on the upper area of the ischial tuberosity (**Fig. 111.4**), via a tendon which it shares with semitendinosus, and from the lower part of the sacrotuberous ligament. The other, the short head, arises from the lateral lip of the linea aspera, between adductor magnus and vastus lateralis. This attachment extends proximally almost to gluteus maximus and distally along the lateral supracondylar line to within 5 cm of the lateral femoral condyle, and from the lateral inter-muscular septum. The long head forms a fusiform belly that descends laterally across the sciatic nerve. The fibres end in an aponeurosis which covers the posterior surface of the muscle. This aponeurosis receives on its deep surface the fibres of the short head, and gradually narrows to a tendon (the lateral hamstring). The main part of the tendon splits round the fibular collateral ligament and is attached to the head of the fibula. The remainder splits into three laminae. The intermediate lamina fuses with the fibular collateral ligament, while the others pass superficial and deep to the ligament to attach to the lateral condyle of the tibia.

The short head may be absent. Additional slips may arise from the ischial tuberosity, linea aspera, or medial supracondylar line.

Relations – Proximally biceps femoris is covered by gluteus maximus, but elsewhere it lies superficially. Deep to it lie semimembranosus proximally, and the sciatic nerve, adductor magnus and the lateral head of gastrocnemius more distally. Semitendinosus and semimembranosus lie medially. The common peroneal nerve descends along the medial border of the tendon and separates it distally from the lateral head of gastrocnemius. As a guide during surgery, it is safest to find a nerve proximally and dissect it free distally. The common peroneal nerve is found emerging posterior to the biceps tendon, which is thus a useful landmark to find the nerve and also to avoid injury to the nerve. For example, when the lateral meniscus is sutured arthroscopically, care must be taken that all needle passages are anterior to biceps. The nerve is adherent to the biceps tendon: if part of the fibular head or the biceps attachment, usually with the insertion of the lateral collateral ligament, is avulsed, then the tendon will retract the nerve proximally. This may contribute to the cause of common peroneal nerve traction injury. It also means that at surgical exploration the nerve lies in an abnormal position and will be more prone to inadvertent injury. If there is a fibular fracture then the nerve may actually lie within the fracture gap. A bursa may lie between the tendon and the fibular collateral ligament.

Vascular supply – The long head of biceps femoris is supplied by the first and second perforating arteries, with accessory supplies at the ischial attachment from the inferior gluteal and medial circumflex femoral arteries and in the distal quarter from the lateral superior genicular artery. The short head is supplied superiorly by the second or third perforating artery and inferiorly by the lateral superior genicular artery.

Innervation – Biceps femoris is innervated by the sciatic nerve, L5, S1 and 2; the long head through the tibial division and the short head through the common peroneal division, which reflects the composite derivation from flexor and extensor musculature.

Actions of posterior femoral muscles – Acting from above, the posterior femoral muscles flex the knee. Acting from below, they extend the hip joint, pulling the trunk upright from a stooping posture against the influence of gravity, biceps being the main agent. When the knee is semi-flexed, biceps femoris can act as a lateral rotator and semimembranosus and semitendinosus as medial rotators of the lower leg on the thigh at the knee. When the hip is extended, biceps is a lateral rotator and semi-membranosus and semitendinosus are medial rotators of the thigh. As is the case with quadriceps femoris, the adductors and gluteus maximus, the hamstrings are quiescent in easy symmetrical standing. However, any action that takes the centre of gravity in front of a transverse axis through the hip joints, e.g. forward reaching, forward sway at the ankle joints, or forward bending at the hips, is immediately accompanied by strong contraction of the hamstrings. (This is in marked contrast to gluteus maximus, which contracts only when there is a call for powerful extension at the hip joint.)

When the knee is flexed against resistance, the tendon of biceps can be felt lateral to the popliteal fossa. Medial to the fossa, the tendons of gracilis (which is the more medial) and semitendinosus stand out sharply. The semimembranosus tendon is just palpable in the interval between them (and also by deep pressure from a 'pincer' grip beyond their margins). There is some evidence that semimembranosus, semi-tendinosus and biceps femoris, although they cross both hip and knee joints, may produce movement at one of these joints without resisting antagonists at the other. Usually, however, each of these muscles contracts as a whole, and whether or not movement takes place at hip or knee is determined by other muscles which act as fixators of these joints.

Testing – The posterior femoral muscles are tested clinically by active knee flexion against resistance in the supine or prone position. In the prone position the individual hamstring tendons can be identified more easily.

When relaxed, these muscles show considerable variation in length: in some individuals the muscles are so short that they impose a serious limitation on flexion of the trunk at the hip joints when the knees are kept extended. Movements such as stooping must then be accomplished by flexing the vertebral column or squatting. Perhaps the need for more stress on the lumbar spine accounts for the occurrence of hamstring tightness in adolescents who develop spondylolysis. These muscles are prone to tearing, which may be related to the relative complexity of muscles that cross two joints, or to the fact that they are subject to large forces including eccentric contractions.

VASCULAR SUPPLY AND LYMPHATIC DRAINAGE

FEMORAL ARTERY AND VEIN DISTAL TO THE FEMORAL TRIANGLE

Adductor (subsartorial) canal
See page 1461.

Relations of the femoral artery in the adductor canal
(Figs 111.35, 111.36, 112.2)
Anterior to the artery are the skin, superficial and deep fasciae, sartorius and the fibrous roof of the canal. The saphenous nerve is first lateral,

then anterior and finally medial. Posterior are adductor longus and adductor magnus; the femoral vein is also posterior proximally, but becomes lateral distally. Anterolateral are vastus medialis and its nerve.

Descending genicular artery (Fig. 113.1)
The descending genicular artery, the distal branch of the femoral artery, arises just proximal to the adductor opening and immediately supplies a saphenous branch. It then descends in vastus medialis, anterior to the tendon of adductor magnus, to the medial side of the knee, where it anastomoses with the medial superior genicular artery. Muscular branches supply vastus medialis and adductor magnus and give off articular branches that anastomose round the knee joint. One articular branch crosses above the femoral patellar surface, forming an arch with the lateral superior genicular artery and supplying the knee joint. The saphenous branch (saphenous artery) emerges distally through the roof of the adductor canal to accompany the saphenous nerve to the medial side of the knee. It passes between sartorius and gracilis and supplies the skin of the proximomedial area of the leg, anastomosing with the medial inferior genicular artery.

Femoral vein in the thigh
See page 1450.

DISTAL BRANCHES OF PROFUNDA FEMORIS
See page 1451 for a description of the main trunk and proximal branches of profunda femoris.

Perforating arteries (Fig. 111.34)
The perforating arteries perforate the attachment of adductor magnus to reach the flexor aspect of the thigh. There are three perforating branches, and the profunda itself becomes the fourth perforator. They pass close to the linea aspera under small tendinous arches and give off muscular, cutaneous and anastomotic branches. Diminished, they pass deep to the short head of biceps femoris (the first usually through the attach-ment of gluteus maximus), traverse the lateral intermuscular septum and enter vastus lateralis. The first arises proximal to adductor brevis, the second anterior and the third distal to the muscle. The first perforating artery passes back between pectineus and adductor brevis (sometimes through the latter), pierces adductor magnus near the linea aspera to supply adductor brevis, adductor magnus, biceps femoris and gluteus maximus, and anastomoses with the inferior gluteal, medial and lateral circumflex femoral and second perforating arteries. The larger second perforating artery, often arising with the first, pierces the attachments of adductor brevis and magnus, divides into the ascending and descend-ing branches supplying the posterior femoral muscles and anastomoses with the first and third perforating arteries. The femoral nutrient artery usually arises from it. When two nutrient arteries exist they usually arise from the first and third perforators. The third perforating artery starts distal to adductor brevis, pierces the attachment of adductor magnus and divides into branches to the posterior femoral muscles. It anastomoses proximally with the perforating arteries, and distally with the end of the profunda and muscular branches of the popliteal. The femoral nutrient artery may arise from it. Side branches of the diaphyseal nutrient and other branches of the profunda provide subsidiary cortical arteries.

The perforating arteries form a double chain of anastomoses, first in the adductor muscles and subsequently near the linea aspera.

Muscular branches
Numerous muscular branches arise from the profunda femoris artery. Some end in the adductors, and others pierce adductor magnus, supply the flexors and anastomose with the medial circumflex femoral artery and superior muscular branches of the popliteal artery. The profunda is thus the main supply to the femoral muscles.

Anastomoses on the back of the thigh
See also page 1453 and **Figure 111.21**.
An important chain of anastomoses extends on the back of the thigh from the gluteal region to the popliteal fossa. It is formed in proximo-distal order by anastomoses between the gluteal arteries and terminals of the medial circumflex femoral artery; the circumflex femoral arteries and the first perforating artery; the perforating arteries themselves; and between the fourth perforating artery and the superior muscular branches of the popliteal artery.

Collateral circulation in proximal femoral occlusion

After occlusion of the femoral artery proximal to the origin of the profunda femoris artery, five main anastomotic channels are available. These are between: branches of the superior and inferior gluteal arteries, the medial and lateral circumflex femoral arteries and the first perforating branch of the profunda femoris artery; the obturator branch of the internal iliac artery and the medial circumflex femoral artery; the internal pudendal branch of the internal iliac artery and the superficial and deep external pudendal branches of the femoral artery; a deep circumflex iliac branch of the external iliac artery, the lateral circumflex femoral branch of the profunda femoris artery and the superficial circumflex iliac branch of the femoral artery; the inferior gluteal branch of the internal iliac artery and perforating branches of the profunda femoris artery.

ARTERIA COMITANS NERVI ISCHIADICI (ARTERY TO SCIATIC NERVE)

The arteria comitans nervi ischiadici is usually a very small vessel. It is a branch of the internal iliac artery, and runs on the surface of, or within, the sciatic nerve. It represents the primitive axial artery of the lower limb, and occasionally remains as a large vessel, in which case the femoral artery is usually much reduced in size. The artery may participate in collateral circulatory pathways.

LONG SAPHENOUS VEIN

The long saphenous vein is described in detail on page 1452.

INGUINAL LYMPH NODES

See page 1453.

INNERVATION

FEMORAL NERVE

The femoral nerve is described in detail on page 1455.

MEDIAL CUTANEOUS NERVE OF THE THIGH

The medial cutaneous nerve of the thigh is at first lateral to the femoral artery. It crosses anterior to the artery at the apex of the femoral triangle, and divides into anterior and posterior branches. Before doing so, it sends a few rami through the fascia lata to supply the skin of the medial side of the thigh, near the long saphenous vein: one ramus emerges via the saphenous opening, another becomes subcutaneous about mid-thigh. The anterior branch descends on sartorius, perforates the fascia lata beyond midthigh, and divides into a branch which supplies the skin as low as the medial side of the knee, and another which crosses to the lateral side of the patella and connects with the infrapatellar branch of the saphenous nerve. The posterior branch descends along the posterior border of sartorius to the knee, pierces the fascia lata, connects with the saphenous nerve, and gives off several cutaneous rami, some as far as the medial side of the leg. The nerve contributes to the sub-sartorial plexus (p. 1470).

INTERMEDIATE CUTANEOUS NERVE OF THE THIGH

The intermediate cutaneous nerve of the thigh pierces the fascia lata c.8 cm below the inguinal ligament, either as two branches or as one trunk that quickly divides into two. These descend on the front of the thigh, supplying the skin as far as the knee and ending in the peripatellar plexus (p. 1471). The lateral branch of the intermediate cutaneous nerve communicates with the femoral branch of the genitofemoral nerve, frequently piercing sartorius and sometimes supplying it.

NERVE TO SARTORIUS

The main nerve to sartorius arises from the femoral nerve in common with the intermediate cutaneous nerve of the thigh.

LATERAL CUTANEOUS NERVE OF THE THIGH

See page 1457.

SUBSARTORIAL NERVE PLEXUS

The medial cutaneous nerve of the thigh forms a subsartorial plexus with branches of the saphenous and obturator nerves, deep to the fascia lata, at the lower border of adductor longus. When the communicating branch of the obturator nerve is large and reaches the leg, the posterior branch of the medial cutaneous nerve is small, and ends in the plexus from which it gives rise to a few cutaneous filaments.

POSTERIOR CUTANEOUS NERVE OF THE THIGH

See page 1457.

SAPHENOUS NERVE

See page 1487.

OBTURATOR NERVE

See page 1455.

SCIATIC NERVE

See page 1467.

REFERENCES

Cormack GC, Lamberty BGH 1994 See Bibliography.

Taylor GI, Razaboni RM (eds) 1994 Michael Salmon: Anatomic Studies. Book 1, Arteries of the Muscles of the Extremities and the Trunk. St Louis: Quality Medical Publishing.

A translated, updated and edited version of a classic French text, first published in 1933. Now a major source-book in plastic surgery.

Knee

The knee is the largest synovial joint in the body. It consists of three distinct and partially separated compartments, which form a complex 'hinge' joint. This arrangement offers a fulcrum for propulsive muscles, and allows the limb to be folded away in confined spaces and to get closer to ground. The price of its mobility is a tendency to instability. To counter this tendency a complex ligament arrangement, vulnerable to injury, has evolved. The understanding of knee anatomy has improved considerably in recent years, driven in large measure by the advances in surgery in this region.

SKIN

CUTANEOUS VASCULAR SUPPLY AND LYMPHATIC DRAINAGE
(Fig. 113.1)

The arterial supply of the skin covering the knee is derived from genicular branches of the popliteal artery, the descending genicular branch of the femoral artery, and the anterior recurrent branch of the anterior tibial artery, with small contributions from the arteries to vastus medialis and the hamstrings. For further details consult Cormack and Lamberty (1994).

Cutaneous veins are tributaries of the vessels that correspond to the named arteries. Cutaneous lymphatic drainage is to the superficial inguinal nodes, and possibly also to the popliteal nodes and thence to the deep inguinal group.

CUTANEOUS INNERVATION

Infrapatellar branch of saphenous nerve

See Tennant et al (1998).

The infrapatellar branch of the saphenous nerve crosses the anterior aspect of the knee from the medial side. It is invariably divided in most anterior approaches to the knee: this accounts for the numbness that inevitably occurs lateral to a longitudinal anterior knee scar. A painful neuroma may form if the nerve is partially divided, e.g. by the incision for an arthroscopy portal or a small medial arthrotomy. Unfortunately the position of the nerve relative to the line of the joint is variable. In most cases it crosses just below the joint line, passing over the patellar tendon at its insertion into the tibia.

Peripatellar plexus

Proximal to the knee, the infrapatellar branch of the saphenous nerve connects with branches of the medial and intermediate femoral cutaneous nerves. Distal to the knee it connects with other branches of the saphenous nerve, and laterally with the lateral cutaneous femoral nerve, forming a peripatellar plexus.

SOFT TISSUE

POPLITEAL FOSSA (Figs 111.42, 113.2, 113.3, 113.4)

The popliteal fossa is a rhomboidal region posterior to the knee joint, which is more apparent when disturbed by dissection. Biceps femoris (proximal) and plantaris and the lateral head of gastrocnemius (distal) form the lateral borders; semitendinosus and semimembranosus (proximal) and the medial head of the gastrocnemius (distal) form the medial borders; and anteriorly, the femoral popliteal surface, oblique popliteal ligament, posterior aspect of the proximal tibia and the fascia covering the popliteus collectively form the floor. The fossa is covered posteriorly by the popliteal fascia, which is perforated by the short saphenous vein and sural nerve. The two latter structures are the key to the direct posterior approach to the knee. They should be identified and

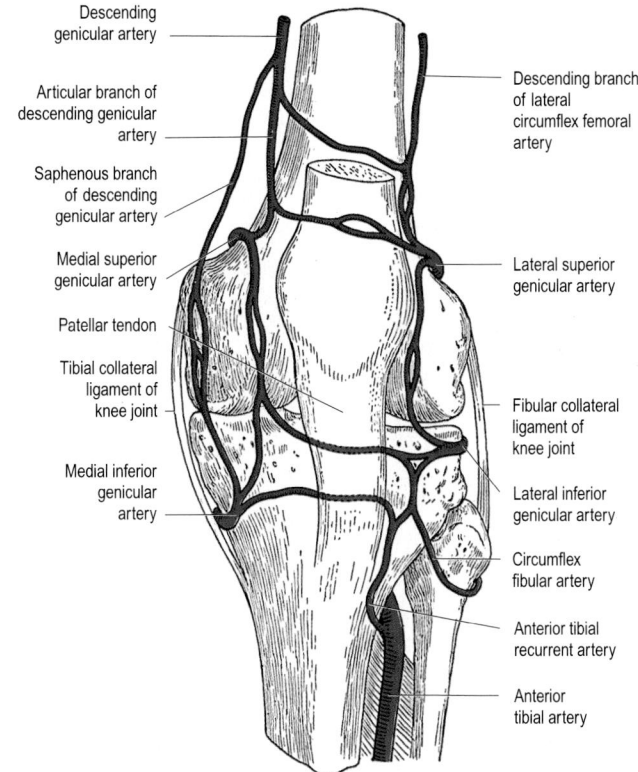

Fig. 113.1 The arterial anastomoses around the left knee joint (schematic).

Descending genicular artery

Articular branch of descending genicular artery

Saphenous branch of descending genicular artery

Medial superior genicular artery

Patellar tendon

Tibial collateral ligament of knee joint

Medial inferior genicular artery

Descending branch of lateral circumflex femoral artery

Lateral superior genicular artery

Fibular collateral ligament of knee joint

Lateral inferior genicular artery

Circumflex fibular artery

Anterior tibial recurrent artery

Anterior tibial artery

'followed' into the popliteal fossa by incision of the deep fascia, which they perforate. (Note that 'popliteal fascia' refers to part of the general investing layer of deep fascia that forms a 'roof' for the fossa. This must be carefully distinguished from the 'fascia of popliteus', which forms part of the floor.)

Contents

Until disturbed, the popliteal fossa is c.2.5 cm wide. Its contents are largely hidden, especially in its distal part, where the heads of gastrocnemius are in contact. When its boundaries are separated, its contents are revealed as the popliteal vessels, tibial and common peroneal nerves, short saphenous vein, sural nerve, posterior femoral cutaneous nerve, an articular branch from the obturator nerve, lymph nodes and fat. The tibial nerve descends centrally immediately anterior to the popliteal fascia, crossing the vessels posteriorly from lateral to medial. The common peroneal nerve descends laterally near the tendon of biceps femoris. Popliteal vessels are deep and united by dense areolar tissue. They lie on the floor of the fossa, the vein superficial to the artery. Proximally, the thick-walled vein lies lateral to the artery, crossing to its medial side distally; sometimes it is double, when the artery lies between the veins, which are usually interconnected. An articular branch from the obturator nerve descends on the artery to the knee. Six or seven popliteal lymph nodes are embedded in the fat, one under the popliteal fascia near the end of the short saphenous vein, one between the popliteal artery and knee joint, the others around the popliteal vessels.

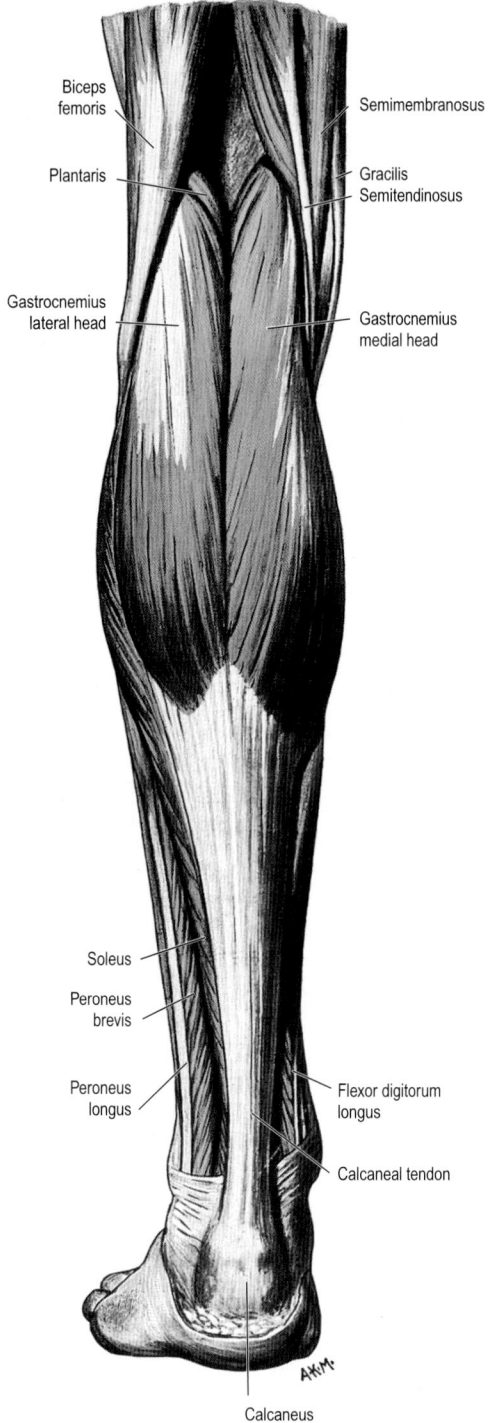

Fig. 113.2 Muscles of the left calf: superficial group. (From Schaefer EA, Symington J, Bryce TH (eds) 1915 Quain's Anatomy, 11th edn. London: Longmans, Green, with permission from Pearson Education.)

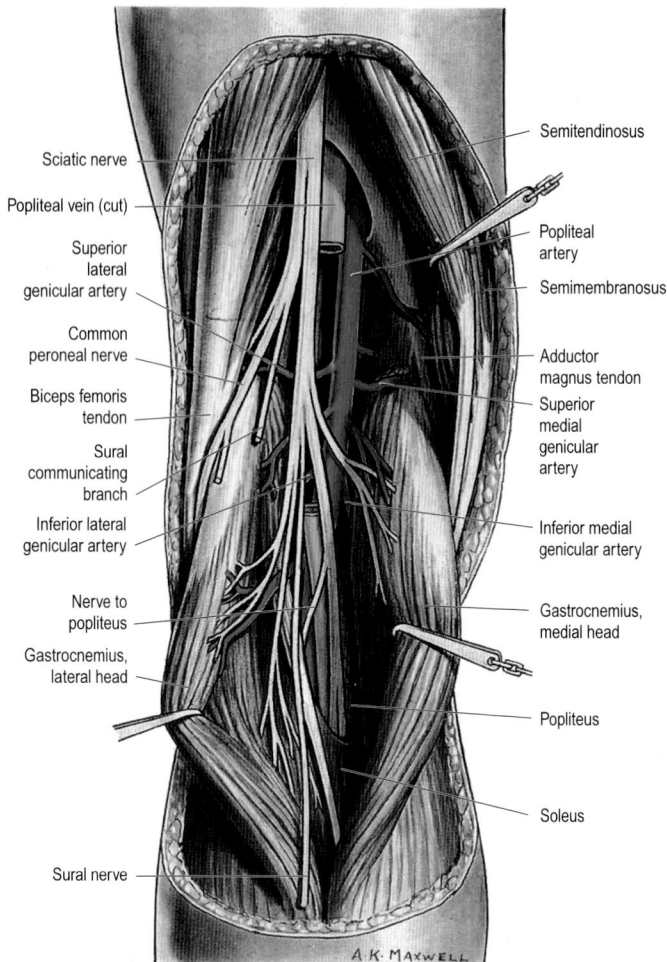

Fig. 113.3 Left popliteal fossa: the heads of gastrocnemius and medial hamstrings have been retracted.

BONE

PATELLA (Figs 113.5, 113.6, 113.7, 113.8)

Topography

The patella is the largest sesamoid bone. It is embedded in the tendon of quadriceps femoris, anterior to the knee joint. The patella is flat, distally triangular, proximally curved, and has anterior and posterior surfaces, three borders and an apex. In the living, its distal apex is a little proximal to the line of the knee joint when standing.

The subcutaneous, convex anterior surface is perforated by nutrient vessels. It is longitudinally striated, separated from skin by a prepatellar bursa, and covered by an expansion from the tendon of quadriceps femoris, which blends distally with superficial fibres of the patellar tendon (patellar ligament), the continued tendon of quadriceps. The posterior surface has a proximal smooth, oval articular area, crossed by a smooth vertical ridge, which fits the groove on the femoral patellar surface and divides the patellar articular area into medial and lateral facets; the lateral is usually larger. Each facet is divided by faint horizontal lines into equal thirds. A seventh 'odd' facet is present as a narrow strip, which is proximally broader, along the extreme medial border of the patella: it contacts the medial femoral condyle in deep flexion. Distal to the articular surface the apex is roughened by the attachment of the patellar tendon. Proximal to this, the area between the roughened apex and the articular surface is covered by an infrapatellar pad of fat. The articular cartilage is the thickest in the body, reflecting the magnitude of the stresses to which it is subjected.

The thick superior border (surface) slopes down and forwards. The medial and lateral borders are thinner and converge distally: the expansions of the tendons of vastus medialis and lateralis (medial and lateral patellar retinacula respectively) are attached to them. The lateral retinaculum receives contributions from the iliotibial tract. Ossification occasionally extends from its lateral margin into the tendon of vastus lateralis.

The shape of the patella can vary: certain configurations are associated with patellar instability. Not infrequently a bipartite patella is seen on radiographs. The bone seems to be in two parts, usually with a smaller superolateral fragment. This has long been attributed to the presence of a separate ossification centre, but in some cases could represent an ununited stress fracture.

Structure

The patella consists of almost uniformly dense trabecular bone, covered by a thin compact lamina. Trabeculae beneath the anterior surface are parallel with the surface; elsewhere they radiate from the articular surface into the substance of the bone.

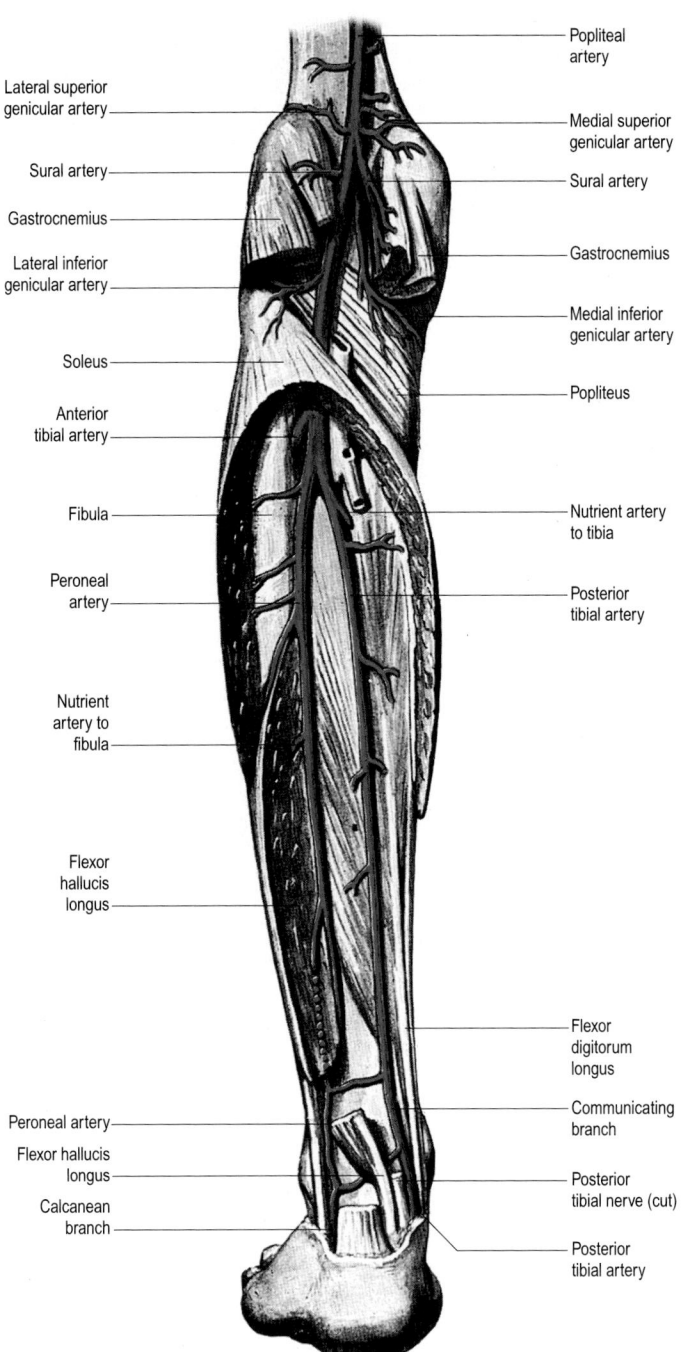

Fig. 113.4 Left popliteal, posterior tibial and peroneal arteries: posterior aspect.

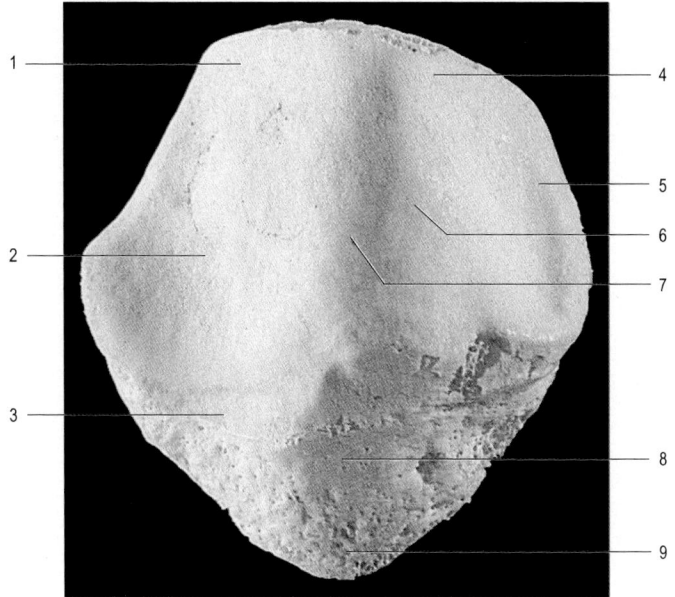

1. Upper lateral facet: in contact with femur in flexion.
2. Lower lateral facet: in contact with femur in extension.
3. Area overlain by edge of circumferential fat pad.
4. Upper medial facet: in contact with femur in flexion.
5. Medial vertical ('odd') facet: in contact with femur in extreme flexion.
6. Lower medial facet: in contact with femur in extension.
7. Ridge.
8. Area covered by infrapatellar fat pad.
9. Area for attachment of patellar tendon.

Fig. 113.5 Left patella: articular (posterior) surface. (Photograph by Sarah-Jane Smith.)

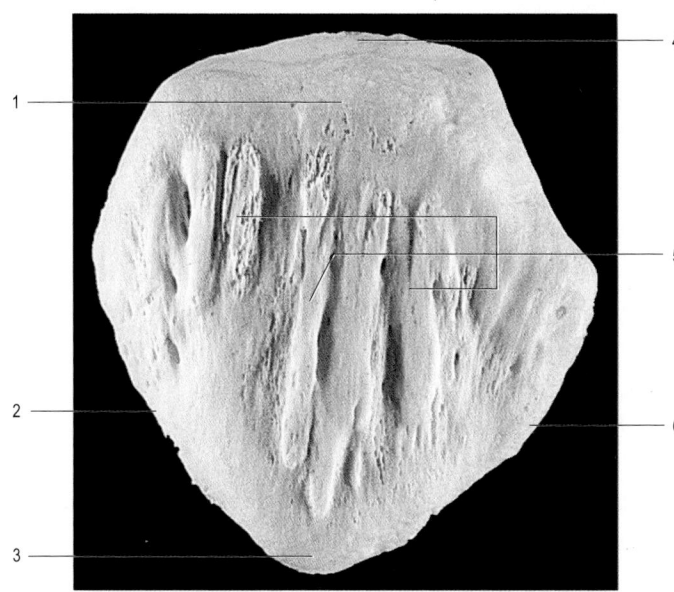

1. Area of attachment of rectus femoris.
2. Medial border: attachment of medial retinaculum (expansion).
3. Apex.
4. Area of attachment of vastus intermedius.
5. Markings of attachment of quadriceps tendon.
6. Lateral border: attachment of lateral retinaculum (expansion).

Fig. 113.6 Left patella: anterior aspect. (Photograph by Sarah-Jane Smith.)

Muscle attachments

Quadriceps femoris is attached on the superior surface, except near its posterior margin; the attachment extends down and forwards onto the anterior surface. The attachment for rectus femoris lies anteroinferior to that for vastus intermedius. Rough markings can be traced in continuity around the periphery of the bone from the anterosuperior surface to the deep surface of the apex. They represent the attachments of the lateral and medial vasti and the patellar tendon respectively.

Vascular supply

The arterial supply of the patella is derived from the genicular anastomosis (p. 1486), particularly from the superior and inferior genicular arteries and from the anterior tibial recurrent artery. There is a prepatellar arterial plexus.

Ossification

Several centres appear during the third to sixth years and quickly coalesce. Accessory marginal centres appear later and fuse with the central mass.

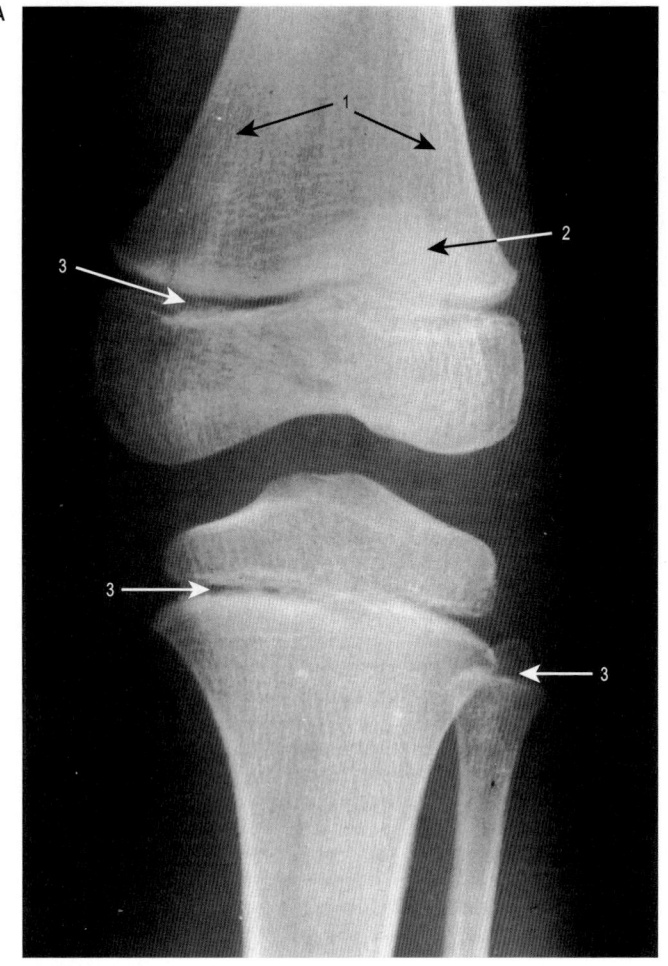

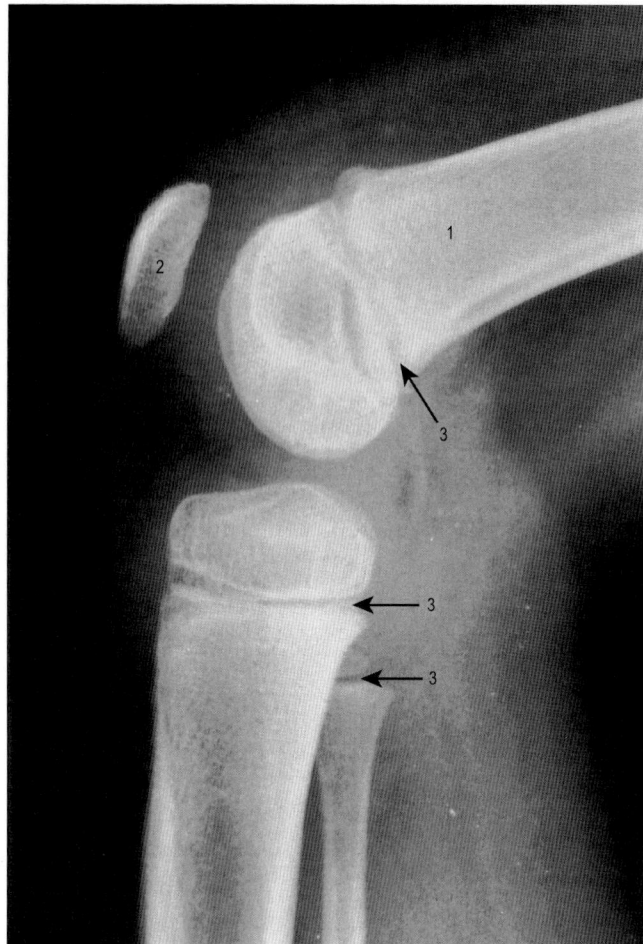

1. Femoral metaphysis. 2. Patella. 3. Cartilaginous growth plates.

Fig. 113.7 Anteroposterior (**A**) and lateral (**B**) radiographs of the knee in a girl aged 6.

FEMUR
See page 1431.

TIBIA
See page 1490.

FIBULA
See page 1493.

JOINTS

PATELLOFEMORAL JOINT
The patellofemoral joint, which is part of the knee joint, is a synovial joint.

Articulating surfaces (Figs 113.9, 113.10)
The articular surface of the patella is adapted to that of the femur (pp. 111–116), which extends onto the anterior surfaces of both condyles like an inverted U. Since the whole area is concave transversely and convex in the sagittal plane, it is an asymmetrical sellar surface. The 'odd' facet contacts the lateral anterior end of the medial femoral condyle in full flexion, when the highest lateral patellar facet contacts the anterior part of the lateral condyle. As the knee extends, the middle patellar facets contact the lower half of the femoral surface; in full extension only the lowest patellar facets are in contact with the femur. In summary, on flexion the patellofemoral contact point moves proximally. The contact area also broadens to cope with the increasing stress that accompanies rising flexion.

Patellar tendon sheath and patellar tendon (Fig. 112.5)
The patellar tendon (patellar ligament) is the central band of the tendon of quadriceps femoris, and is continued distally from the patella to the tibial tuberosity. It is strong, flat and c.8 m in length. Proximally it is attached to the apex and adjoining margins, and to roughened areas on the anterior surface and on a depression on the distal posterior patellar surface. Distally it is attached to the superior smooth area of the tibial tuberosity. This insertion is oblique, and is more distal laterally. Its superficial fibres are continuous over the patella with the tendon of quadriceps femoris, the medial and lateral parts of which descend, flanking the patella, to the sides of the tibial tuberosity, where they merge into the fibrous capsule as the medial and lateral patellar retinacula. The patellar tendon is separated from the synovial membrane by a large infrapatellar fat pad and from the tibia by a bursa (p. 1482). It lies within its own well-defined sheath.

When undertaking a tibial osteotomy, the tibia may be cut from lateral to medial just above the patellar tendon insertion. Failure to appreciate the obliquity of the tendon's tibial attachment may lead to inadvertent division of the tendon, with disastrous results.

All other aspects of the patellofemoral joint are described with the tibiofemoral joint.

TIBIOFEMORAL JOINT
The tibiofemoral joint is a complex synovial joint.

Articulating surfaces

Tibial surface (Figs 113.11, 113.12, 113.13)
The proximal tibial surface slopes posteriorly and downwards relative to the long axis of the shaft. The tilt, which is maximal at birth, decreases with age, and is more marked in habitual squatters. The posterior

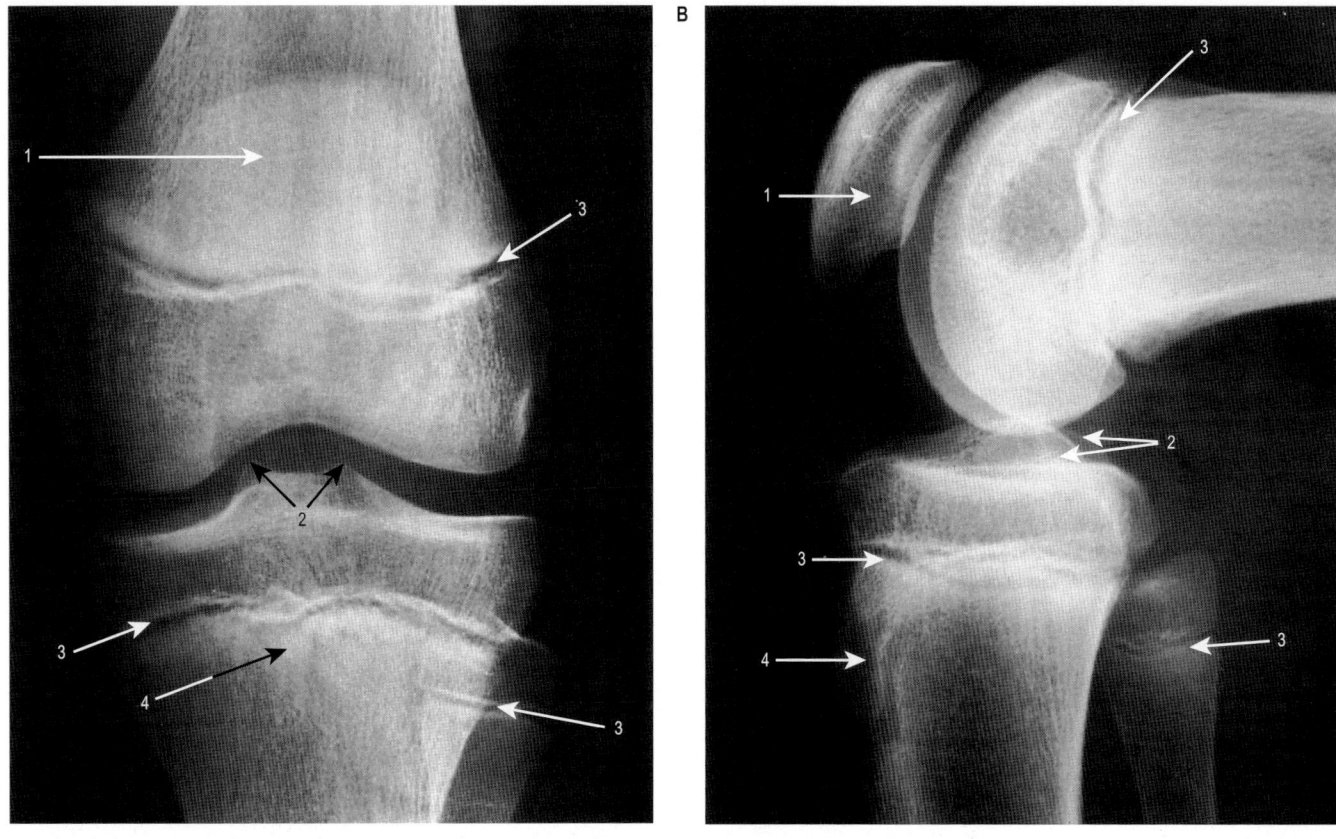

A   B

1. Patella.   2. Intercondylar eminence.   3. Cartilaginous growth plates.   4. Prolongation of proximal tibial epiphysis and growth plate forming the tibial tuberosity.

Fig. 113.8 Anteroposterior (**A**) and lateral (**B**) radiographs of the knee in a boy aged 14.

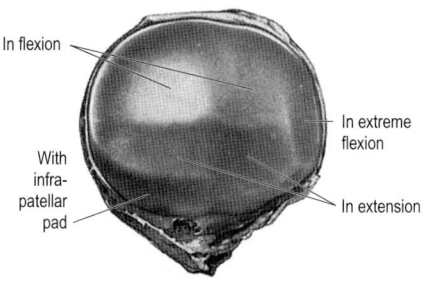

In flexion

In extreme
flexion

With
infra-
patellar
pad

In extension

Fig. 113.9 The articular surface of the left patella showing areas of contact with the femur and infrapatellar fat pad in different positions of the knee.

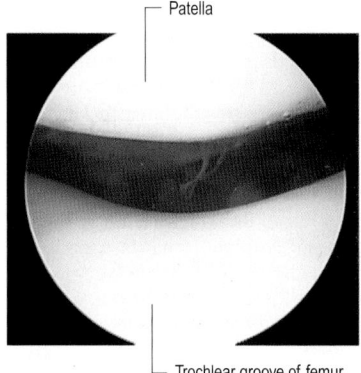

Patella

Trochlear groove of femur

Fig. 113.10 The left patellofemoral joint at arthroscopy. (By kind permission from Smith and Nephew Endoscopy.)

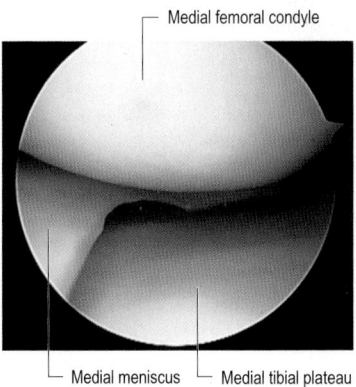

Medial femoral condyle

Medial meniscus   Medial tibial plateau

Fig. 113.11 The medial compartment of the left knee joint at arthroscopy, showing articular surfaces and the medial meniscus. (By kind permission from Smith and Nephew Endoscopy.)

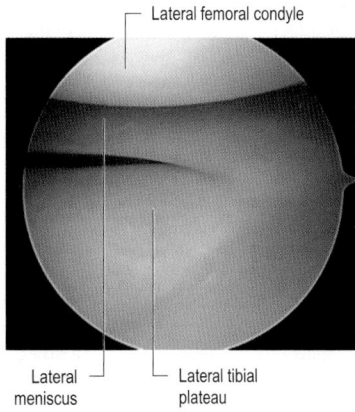

Lateral femoral condyle

Lateral
meniscus   Lateral tibial
plateau

Fig. 113.12 The lateral compartment of the left knee joint at arthroscopy, showing articular surfaces and the lateral meniscus. (By kind permission from Smith and Nephew Endoscopy.)

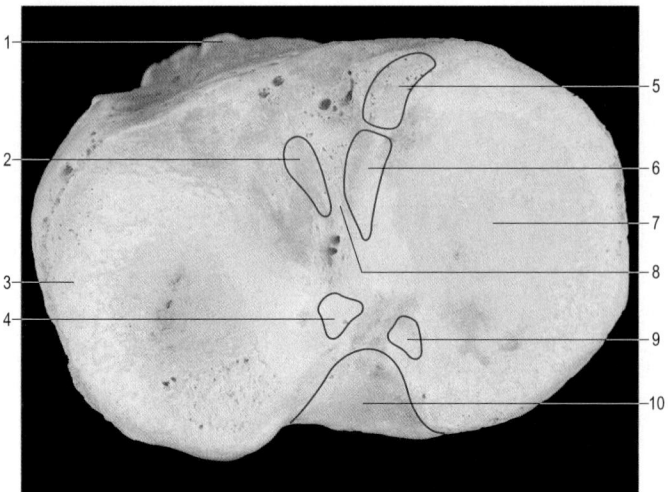

1. Tibial tuberosity.   2. Attachment of anterior horn, lateral meniscus.   3. Lateral condyle.
4. Attachment of posterior horn, lateral meniscus.   5. Attachment of anterior horn, medial meniscus.
6. Attachment of anterior cruciate ligament.   7. Medial condyle.   8. Intercondylar eminence.
9. Attachment of posterior horn, medial meniscus.   10. Attachment of posterior cruciate ligament.

Fig. 113.13 The left tibial plateau. (Photograph by Sarah-Jane Smith.)

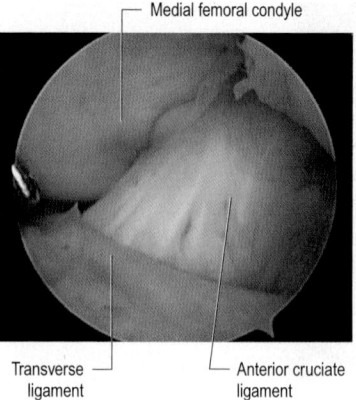

Fig. 113.14 The intercondylar notch at arthroscopy, showing the anterior cruciate and intermeniscal ligaments. (By kind permission from Smith and Nephew Endoscopy.)

surface, distal to the articular margin, displays a horizontal, rough groove to which the capsular and posterior parts of the medial collateral ligaments are attached. The anteromedial surface of the tibia is a rough strip, separated from the medial surface of the shaft by an inconspicuous ridge. The medial patellar retinaculum is attached to the medial and anterior condylar surfaces, which are marked by vascular foramina.

The medial articular surface is oval (long axis anteroposterior) and longer than the lateral tibial condyle. Around its anterior, medial, and posterior margins, it is related to the medial meniscus, and the meniscal imprint, wider behind, narrower anteromedially, is often discernible. The surface is flat in the posterior half with the more anterior surface sloping upwards c.10°. Much of the posterior surface is covered by the meniscus, so that overall a concave surface is presented to the medial femoral condyle. Its lateral margin is raised as it reaches the intercondylar region.

The lateral condyle overhangs the shaft posterolaterally above a small circular facet for articulation with the fibula. The articular surface is more circular and coapted to its meniscus. In the sagittal plane the articular surface is fairly flat centrally; anteriorly and posteriorly the articular surfaces fall away inferiorly. Overall this creates a rather convex surface, so that, with the lateral femoral condyle in contact, there are anterior and posterior recesses (of triangular section), which are occupied by the anterior and posterior meniscal horns. Elsewhere the surface has a raised medial margin that spreads to the lateral intercondylar tubercle. Its articular margins are sharp, except posterolaterally, where the edge is round and smooth: here the tendon of popliteus is in contact with bone.

Intercondylar area (intercondylar eminence) (Fig. 113.14)
The rough-surfaced area between the condylar articular surfaces is narrowest centrally where there is an intercondylar eminence, the edges of which project slightly proximally as the lateral and medial intercondylar tubercles. The intercondylar area widens behind and in front of the eminence as the articular surfaces diverge.

The anterior intercondylar area is widest anteriorly. Anteromedially, anterior to the medial articular surface, is a depression in which the anterior horn of the medial meniscus is attached. Behind this a smooth area receives the anterior cruciate ligament. The anterior horn of the lateral meniscus is attached anterior to the intercondylar eminence, lateral to the anterior cruciate ligament. The eminence, with medial and lateral tubercles, is the narrow central part of the area. The raised tubercles provide some stabilizing influence on the femur.

The posterior horn of the lateral meniscus is attached to the posterior slope of the intercondylar area. The posterior intercondylar area inclines down and backwards behind the posterior horn of the lateral meniscus. A depression behind the base of the medial intercondylar tubercle is

for the posterior horn of the medial meniscus. The rest of the area is smooth and provides attachment for the posterior cruciate ligament, spreading back to a ridge for the capsular ligament.

Femoral surface
The femoral condyles, bearing articular cartilage, are almost wholly convex. The shapes of their sagittal profiles are somewhat controversial. One view is that they are spiral with a curvature increasing posteriorly ('a closing helix'), that of the lateral condyle more rapidly. An alternative view is that the articular surface for contact with the tibia on the medial femoral condyle describes the arcs of two circles. According to this view, the anterior arc makes contact with the tibia near extension and is part of a virtual circle of larger radius than the more posterior arc, which makes contact during flexion. Laterally there may only be a single radius of curvature of a single arc.

Tibiofemoral congruence is improved by the menisci, which are shaped to produce concavity of the surfaces presented to the femur: the combined lateral tibiomeniscal surface is deeper. The lateral femoral condyle has a faint groove anteriorly which rests on the peripheral edge of the lateral meniscus in full extension. A similar groove appears on the medial condyle, but does not reach its lateral border, where a narrow strip contacts the medial patellar articular surface in full flexion. These grooves demarcate the femoral patellar and condylar surfaces. The differences between the shapes of the articulating surfaces correlate with the movements of the joint.

Menisci (Figs 113.11, 113.12, 113.15, 113.16)
The menisci (semilunar cartilages) are crescentic laminae deepening the articulation of the tibial surfaces that receive the femur. Their peripheral attached borders are thick and convex, their free borders thin and

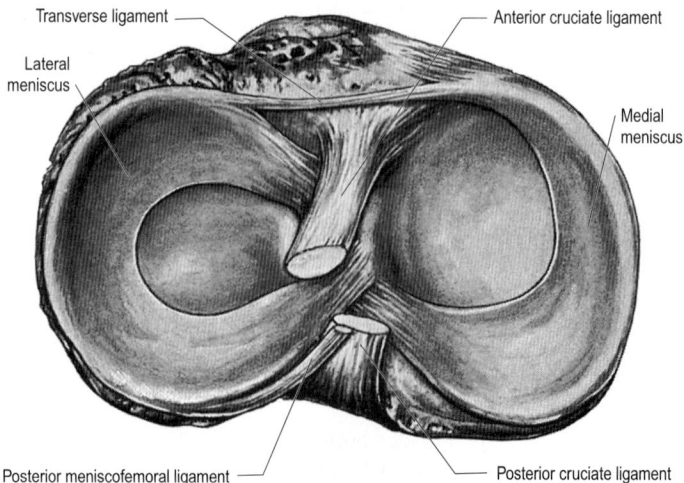

Fig. 113.15 Superior aspect of the left tibia, showing the menisci and the attachments of the cruciate ligaments.

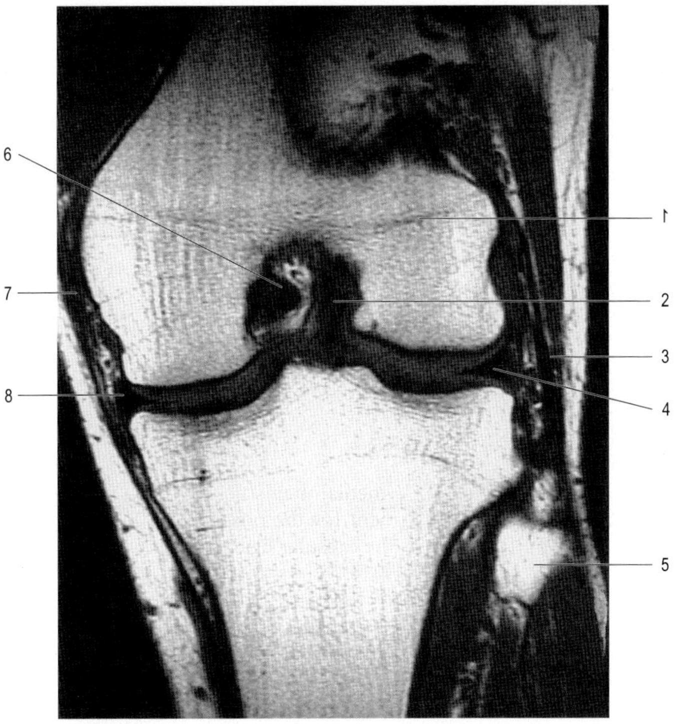

1. Epiphyseal line. 2. Anterior cruciate ligament. 3. Lateral collateral ligament.
4. Lateral meniscus. 5. Head of fibula. 6. Posterior cruciate ligament.
7. Medial collateral ligament. 8. Medial meniscus.

Fig. 113.16 Coronal T1-weighted magnetic resonance image (MRI) of the knee in an adult male. (By kind permission from Dr Justin Lee, Chelsea and Westminster Hospital, London.)

concave. Their peripheral zone is vascularized by capillary loops from the fibrous capsule and synovial membrane, while their inner regions are avascular. Tears of the menisci are common. Most are in the avascular zones and, if treatment is needed, are best resected. Peripheral tears in the vascular zone have the capacity to heal which makes repair a possibility. The meniscal horns are richly innervated compared with the remainder of the meniscus. The central thirds are devoid of innervation (Gronblad et al 1985). The proximal surfaces are smooth and concave and in contact with the articular cartilage on the femoral condyles. The distal surfaces are smooth and flat, resting on the tibial articular cartilage. Each covers approximately two-thirds of its tibial articular surface. Canal-like structures open onto the surface of menisci in infants and young children and may transport nutrients to deeper avascular areas.

Two structurally different regions of the menisci have been identified. The central two-thirds consists of radially organized collagen bundles, and the peripheral third consists of larger circumferentially arranged bundles (Ghadially et al 1983). The articular surfaces of the central part are lined by thinner collagen bundles parallel to the surface, while the outer portion is covered by synovium. This structural arrangement suggests specific biomechanical functions, principally compression centrally and tension peripherally. Compositional changes occur with ageing and degeneration within the menisci: these reduce the ability to resist tensional forces. Outward displacement of the menisci by the femoral condyles is resisted by firm anchorage of the peripheral circumferential fibres to the intercondylar bone at the meniscal horns.

Menisci spread load by increasing the congruity of the articulation, give stability by their physical presence and as providers of proprioceptive feedback, probably assist lubrication, and may cushion extremes of flexion and extension.

Medial meniscus (Figs 113.11, 113.16)
The medial meniscus, broader posteriorly, is almost a semicircle in shape. It is attached by its anterior horn to the anterior tibial intercondylar area in front of the anterior cruciate ligament; the posterior fibres of the anterior horn are continuous with the transverse ligament. The anterior horn is in the floor of a depression medial to the upper part of the patellar tendon. The posterior horn is fixed to the posterior tibial intercondylar area, between the attachments of the lateral meniscus

and posterior cruciate ligament. Its peripheral border is attached to the fibrous capsule and the deep surface of the medial collateral ligament. The tibial attachment is known as the 'coronary ligament'. Collectively these attachments ensure that the medial meniscus is relatively fixed and moves much less than the lateral meniscus.

Lateral meniscus (Fig. 113.12)
The lateral meniscus forms approximately four-fifths of a circle, and covers a larger area than the medial meniscus. Its breadth, except that of the short tapering horns, is uniform. It is grooved posterolaterally by the popliteal tendon, which separates it from the fibular collateral ligament. Its anterior horn is attached in front of the intercondylar eminence, posterolateral to the anterior cruciate ligament, with which it partly blends. Its posterior horn is attached behind this eminence, in front of the posterior horn of the medial meniscus. Its anterior attachment is twisted: the free margin faces posterosuperiorly, and the anterior horn rests on the anterior slope of the lateral intercondylar tubercle. Near its posterior attachment it commonly sends a posterior meniscofemoral ligament superomedially behind the posterior cruciate ligament to the medial femoral condyle. An anterior meniscofemoral ligament may also connect the posterior horn to the medial femoral condyle anterior to the posterior cruciate ligament. The meniscofemoral ligaments are often the sole attachments of the posterior horn of the lateral meniscus. More medially, part of the tendon of popliteus is attached to the lateral meniscus, and so mobility of its posterior horn may be controlled by the meniscofemoral ligaments and popliteus. A meniscofibular ligament occurs in c.80% of knee joints. There is a tibial attachment via a coronary ligament, but the meniscus has no peripheral attachment in the region of popliteus, the popliteus hiatus.

Discoid lateral meniscus – A discoid lateral meniscus occurs in 2–5% of the population, often bilaterally. The distinguishing features of a discoid lateral meniscus are its shape and posterior ligamentous attachments. The following classification of the abnormality is based on Watanabe et al (1979). In its mildest form, the partial discoid meniscus is simply a wider form of the normal lateral meniscus. The tapered free margin is interposed between femoral and tibial condyles, but it does not completely cover the tibial plateau. A complete discoid meniscus appears as a biconcave disc with a rolled medial edge and totally covers the lateral tibial plateau. The Wrisberg type of meniscus has the same shape as a complete discoid meniscus, but its only peripheral posterior attachment is by the meniscofemoral ligaments. The normal tibial attachment of the posterior horn of the lateral meniscus is lacking, but the posterior meniscofemoral ligament persists. As a result, this type of meniscus is attached anteriorly to the tibia and posteriorly to the femur, which renders the posterior horn unstable. Under these circumstances, the meniscus is liable to get caught between the femur and tibia: this accounts for the classic presenting symptom of the 'clunking knee' in some patients. The aetiology of discoid meniscus is not clear. Most are asymptomatic, and are often found by chance at arthroscopy. They may cause difficulty in gaining access to the lateral compartment at arthroscopy.

Discoid medial meniscus is extremely rare.

Transverse [intermeniscal] ligament (Figs 113.14, 113.15)
The transverse ligament connects the anterior convex margin of the lateral meniscus to the anterior horn of the medial meniscus. It varies in thickness and is often absent. Its exact role is not established, but presumably it augments the anterior meniscal attachments and helps resist tension created in the longitudinal circumferential fibres of the menisci when loaded. A posterior meniscomeniscal ligament is sometimes present.

Meniscofemoral ligaments (Figs 113.17, 113.18)
The two meniscofemoral ligaments (MFLs) connect the posterior horn of the lateral meniscus to the inner (lateral) aspect of the medial femoral condyle. The anterior MFL (aMFL; ligament of Humphry) passes anterior to the posterior cruciate ligament. The posterior MFL (pMFL; ligament of Wrisberg) passes behind the posterior cruciate and attaches proximal to the margin of attachment of the posterior cruciate.

Anatomical studies found that at least one meniscofemoral ligament was present in 92% of cadaveric knees examined, whilst both coexisted in 32% (Gupte et al 2003). Biomechanical studies have revealed the cross-sectional area and strength of the meniscofemoral ligaments to

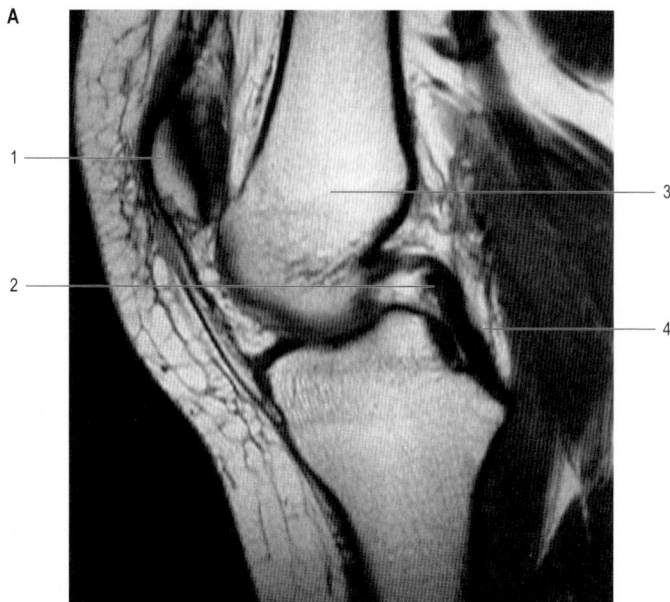

1. Patella.   2. Anterior meniscofemoral ligament of Humphry.   3. Epiphyseal line.
4. Posterior cruciate ligament.

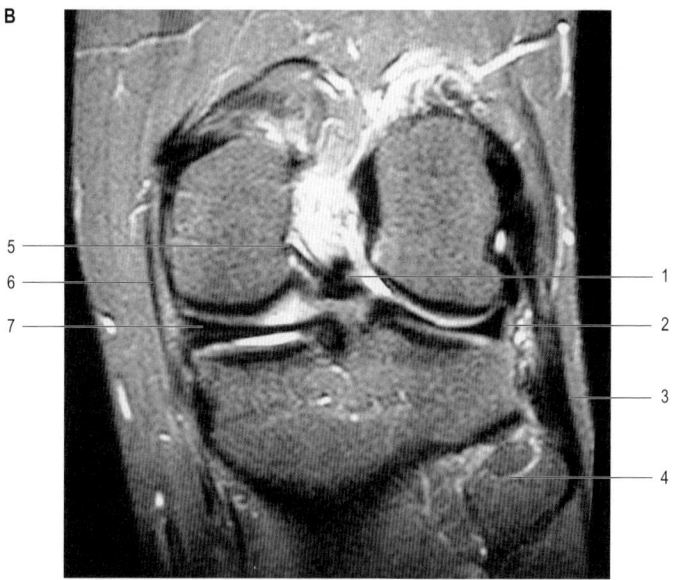

1. Posterior cruciate ligament.   2. Lateral meniscus.   3. Lateral collateral ligament.
4. Head of fibula.   5. Anterior meniscofemoral ligament of Humphry.
6. Medial collateral ligament.   7. Medial meniscus.

Fig. 113.17 A, Sagittal T1-weighted and **B**, coronal STIR magnetic resonance images (MRI) of the knee in an adult male showing the anterior meniscofemoral ligament. (By kind permission from Dr Justin Lee, Chelsea and Westminster Hospital, London.)

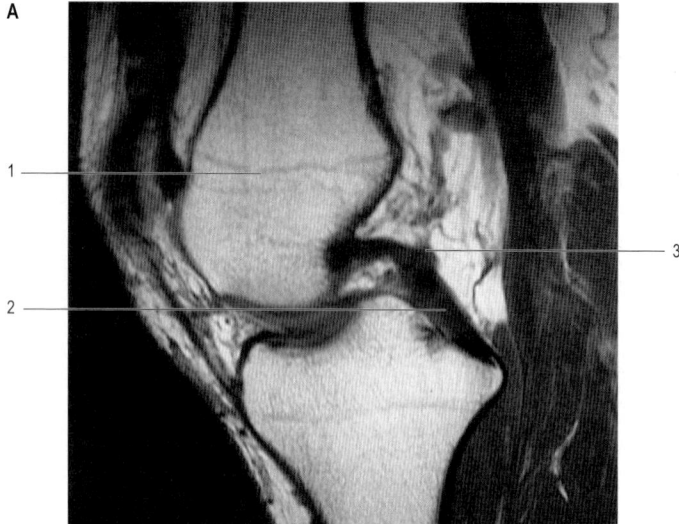

1. Epiphyseal line.   2. Posterior cruciate ligament.
3. Posterior meniscofemoral ligament of Wrisberg.

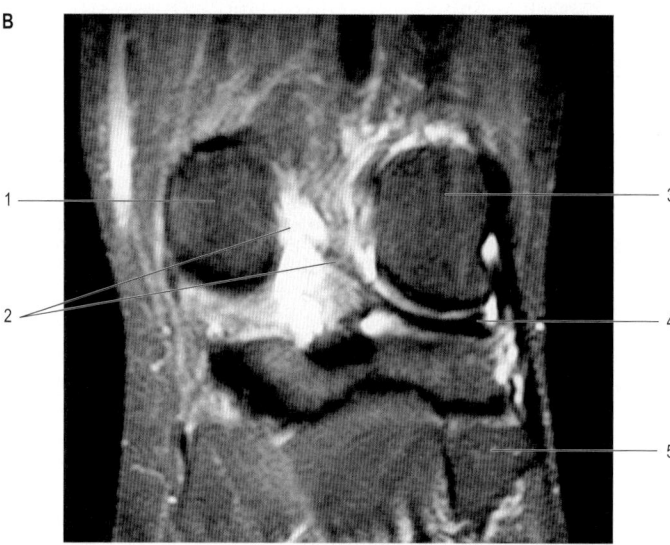

1. Medial femoral condyle.   2. Posterior meniscofemoral ligament of Wrisberg.
3. Lateral femoral condyle.   4. Lateral meniscus.   5. Head of fibula.

Fig. 113.18 A, Sagittal T1-weighted and **B**, coronal STIR magnetic resonance images (MRI) of the knee in an adult male showing the posterior meniscofemoral ligament. (By kind permission from Dr Justin Lee, Chelsea and Westminster Hospital, London.)

be comparable to those of the posterior fibre bundle of the posterior cruciate ligament.

The meniscofemoral ligaments may act as secondary restraints to the posterior cruciate ligament in reducing displacement due to posteriorly directed forces on the tibia. These ligaments are also involved in controlling the motion of the lateral meniscus in conjunction with the tendon of popliteus during flexion.

Soft tissues

Recent advances in knee ligament surgery have contributed to a better understanding of the anatomy of the medial and lateral soft tissues of the knee.

Capsule and retinacula

The capsule is a fibrous membrane of variable thickness. The individual thickenings are referred to as discrete ligaments. Anteriorly it is replaced by the patellar tendon and does not pass proximal to the patella or over the patellar area. Elsewhere it lies deep to expansions from vasti medialis and lateralis, separated from them by a plane of loose connective tissue containing blood vessels. The expansions are attached to the patellar margins and patellar tendon, extending back to the corresponding collateral ligaments and distally to the tibial condyles. They form medial and lateral patellar retinacula, the lateral being augmented by the iliotibial tract.

Posteriorly the capsule contains vertical fibres that arise from the articular margins of the femoral condyles and intercondylar notch and from the proximal tibia. The fibres mainly pass down and medially. The oblique popliteal ligament is a well-defined thickening across the posteromedial capsule, and includes a contribution from the extensive insertion of semimembranosus.

Medial soft tissues (Figs 112.5, 113.19)

The medial soft tissues are arranged in three layers (Warren and Marshall 1979). Layer 1 is the most superficial and is the deep fascia that invests sartorius. The saphenous nerve and its infrapatellar branch are superficial to the fascia. Sartorius inserts into the fascia rather than having a distinct tendon. The pes anserinus is not a site of three distinct tendons

collateral ligament it is thick and has vertically orientated fibres that make up the deep medial collateral ligament. Fibres from it connect to the medial meniscus. Anteriorly the separation of the superficial and deep parts of the medial collateral ligament is distinct. Posteriorly 'layers 2 and 3' blend to form a conjoined posteromedial capsule.

Lateral soft tissues (Figs 113.20, 113.21)

The lateral soft tissues are also arranged in three layers (Seebacher et al 1982). Most superficial is the lateral patellar retinaculum. The middle layer consists of the lateral collateral ligament, popliteofibular ligament, fabellofibular ligament and arcuate ligament. The deep layer is the lateral capsule.

The lateral retinaculum consists of superficial oblique and deep transverse portions. The former runs from the iliotibial band to the patella. The latter is thicker and subdivided into three parts: the lateral patellofemoral ligament, running from the lateral patellar border to the lateral epicondyle of the femur; the transverse retinaculum, running from the iliotibial band to the mid patella; and the patellotibial band, running from the patella to the lateral tibia.

The fascia lata and the iliotibial band lie posterior to the lateral retinaculum. They come together distally to insert into the tibia at Gerdy's tubercle on the anterolateral proximal tibia. Some fibres continue to the tibial tuberosity. Proximally the fascia lata merges with the lateral intermuscular septum. Posteriorly it blends with the biceps fascia. Here, as it emerges from behind the biceps tendon, the common peroneal nerve lies in a thin layer of fat bound by the fascia.

The lateral collateral ligament arises from the lateral epicondyle of the femur posterior to the popliteus insertion and just proximal to the popliteus groove. It is a cord-like structure that passes distally, superficial to the popliteus tendon and deep to the lateral retinaculum, to the fibula, where it blends with the biceps tendon just anterior to the apex of the fibular head. It is separated from the capsule by a thin layer of fat and the inferior lateral genicular vessels.

The single most important stabilizer of the posterolateral knee is the popliteofibular ligament. It passes from the popliteus tendon at a level just below the joint line, posteriorly, laterally and inferiorly, to the fibular head. It is probably what was previously described as the short

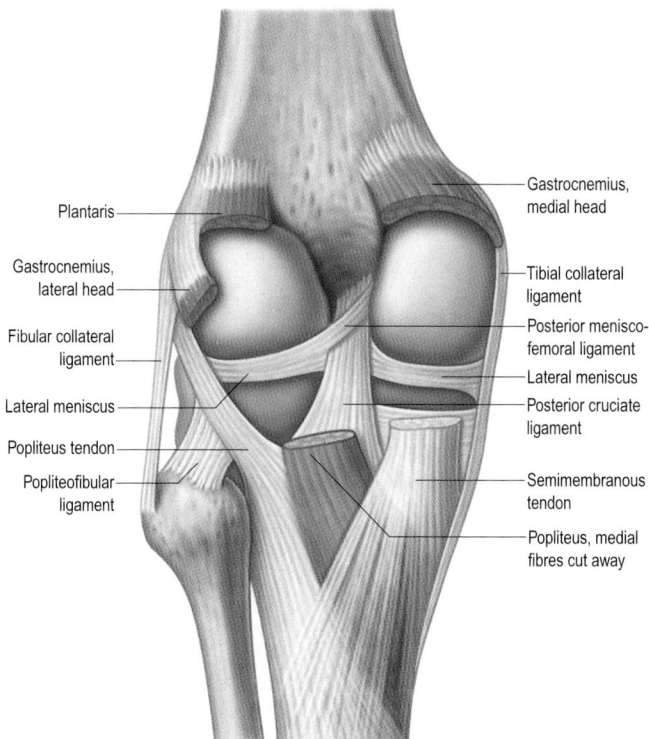

Fig. 113.19 Posterior dissection of the left knee. The fibrous capsule has been removed, exposing the unopened synovial membrane (blue). The synovial cavity has been partially distended by injection.

and their insertions as often described. The 'layer 1' fascia spreads inferiorly and anteriorly to lie superficial to the very distinct tendons of gracilis and semitendinosus and their insertions. The latter two tendons are commonly harvested for ligament reconstruction surgery. To gain access to them the upper edge of sartorius can be identified. The sartorius (layer 1) fascia is then incised to reveal the tendons. Deep to them is the pes bursa, which overlies the superficial medial collateral ligament. This can become inflamed, especially in running athletes.

Posteriorly, 'layer 1' overlies the tendons of gastrocnemius and the structures of the popliteal fossa. Anteriorly, 'layer 1' blends with the anterior limit of 'layer 2' and the medial patellar retinaculum. More inferiorly, 'layer 1' blends with periosteum.

From the medial border of the patella a condensation of tissue passes to the medial epicondyle of the femur (the medial patellofemoral ligament), the anterior horn of the medial meniscus (the meniscopatellar ligament), and the medial tibia (the patellotibial ligament).

'Layer 2' is the plane of the superficial medial collateral ligament. The tendons of gracilis and semitendinosus lie between layers 1 and 2. The superficial medial collateral ligament has parallel and oblique portions. The former contains vertically orientated fibres that pass from the medial epicondyle of the femur to a large insertion on the medial tibia. It extends an average 5 cm distal to the joint line. Its anterior edge is rolled and easily seen just posterior to the insertions of gracilis and semitendinosus once 'layer 1' has been opened. The posterior oblique fibres run posteroinferiorly from the medial epicondyle of the femur to blend with the underlying 'layer 3' (capsule), effectively to insert on the posteromedial tibial articular margin and posterior horn of the medial meniscus. This area is reinforced by a part of the insertion of semimembranosus. There is a vertical split in 'layer 2' anterior to the superficial medial collateral ligament. The fibres anterior to the split pass superiorly to blend with vastus medialis fascia and 'layer 1' in the medial patellar retinaculum. The fibres posterior to the split pass superiorly to the medial epicondyle and thence anteriorly as the medial patellofemoral ligament.

'Layer 3' is the capsule of the knee joint and can be separated from 'layer 2' everywhere except anteriorly close to the patella, where it blends with the more superficial layers. Deep to the superficial medial

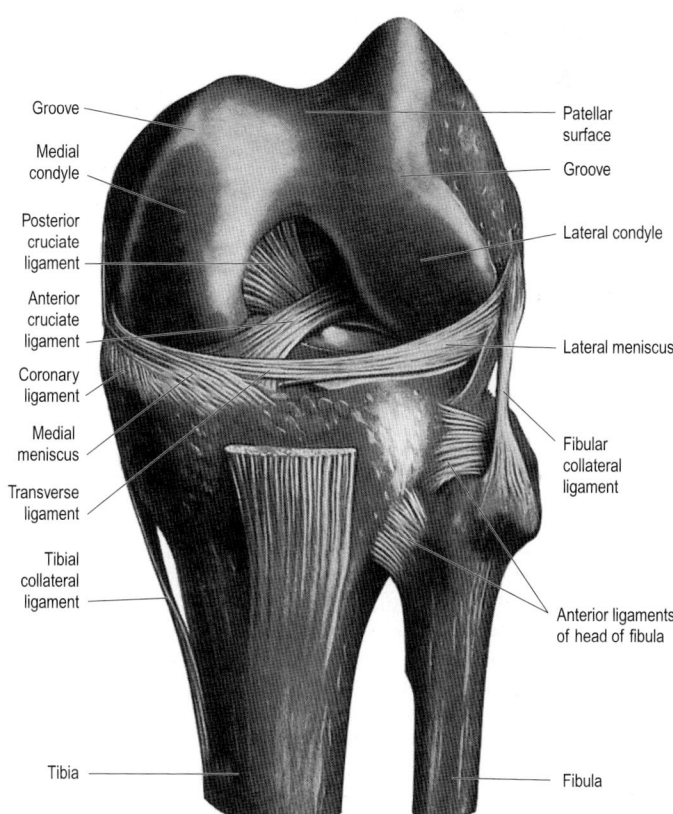

Fig. 113.20 The left knee joint in full flexion: dissection from anterior aspect.

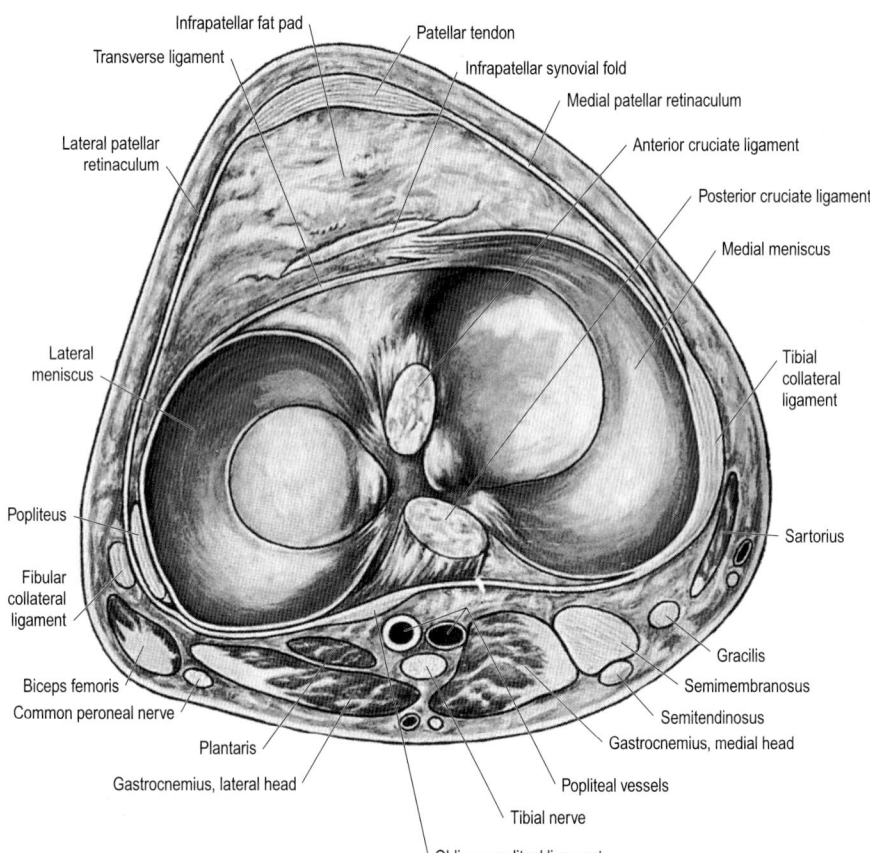

Infrapatellar fat pad

Transverse ligament

Patellar tendon

Infrapatellar synovial fold

Medial patellar retinaculum

Anterior cruciate ligament

Posterior cruciate ligament

Medial meniscus

Lateral patellar retinaculum

Lateral meniscus

Tibial collateral ligament

Popliteus

Sartorius

Fibular collateral ligament

Biceps femoris

Common peroneal nerve

Gracilis

Semimembranosus

Semitendinosus

Gastrocnemius, medial head

Plantaris

Gastrocnemius, lateral head

Popliteal vessels

Tibial nerve

Oblique popliteal ligament

Fig. 113.21 Transverse (axial) section of the left knee joint to show the relations of the joint.

lateral genual ligament. As a passive 'tether' combined with the popliteus tendon proximal to it, it resists external rotation of the tibia. Its connection to the popliteus tendon also allows 'dynamic' tensioning.

The fabellofibular ligament is a condensation of fibres running from the fabella, or if absent, the lateral head of gastrocnemius, to the fibular styloid. The arcuate ligament is a condensation of fibres passing from the fibular styloid, posteromedially over the emerging popliteus tendon below the level of the tibial joint surface to insert into the tibial intercondylar area. The lateral joint capsule is thin and blends posteriorly with the arcuate ligament. Anteriorly it forms the weak lax coronary ligament, which attaches the inferior border of the meniscus to the lateral tibia.

Ligaments

Cruciate ligaments

The cruciate ligaments are very strong and are located a little posterior to the articular centre. They are termed cruciate because they cross: anterior and posterior refer to their tibial attachments. Synovial membrane almost surrounds the ligaments but is reflected posteriorly from the posterior cruciate to adjoining parts of the capsule. The intercondylar part of the posterior region of the fibrous capsule therefore has no synovial covering.

Anterior cruciate ligament (Figs 113.14, 113.15) – The anterior cruciate ligament is attached to the anterior intercondylar area of the tibia, just anterior and slightly lateral to the medial tibial eminence, partly blending with the anterior horn of the lateral meniscus. It ascends posterolaterally, twisting on itself and fanning out to attach high on the posteromedial aspect of the lateral femoral condyle (Girgis et al 1975). Its average length is 38 mm, and average width is 11 mm. It is formed of two, or possibly three, functional bundles. These are not distinct visually but can be identified by dissection. They are named anteromedial, intermediate, and posterolateral, according to their tibial attachments (Amis and Dawkins 1991).

Absent anterior cruciate ligament – Congenital absence of the anterior cruciate ligament is rare and is usually seen in association with lower limb dysplasia (Thomas et al 1985). Knee instability can result. It can

be extremely troublesome and difficult to treat when precipitated by limb-lengthening surgery for the dysplasia-induced short limb.

Posterior cruciate ligament (Figs 113.15, 113.20, 113.22) – The posterior cruciate ligament is thicker and stronger than the anterior cruciate ligament. This is perhaps surprising because its rupture is usually better tolerated than that of the anterior cruciate. Its average length is 38 mm and average width is 13 mm.

The posterior cruciate ligament is attached to the lateral surface of the medial femoral condyle and extends up onto the anterior part of

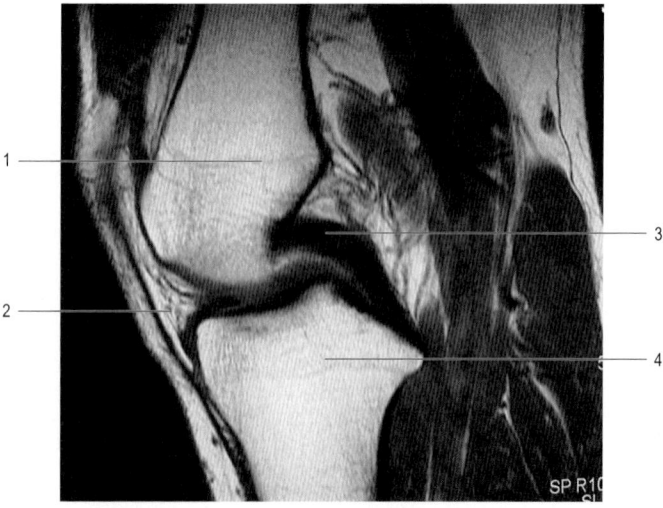

1. Femoral epiphyseal line. 2. Infrapatellar fat pad. 3. Posterior cruciate ligament. 4. Tibial epiphyseal line.

Fig. 113.22 Sagittal T1-weighted magnetic resonance image (MRI) of the knee in an adult male showing the posterior cruciate ligament. (By kind permission from Dr Justin Lee, Chelsea and Westminster Hospital, London.)

the roof of the intercondylar notch, where its attachment is extensive in the anteroposterior direction. Its fibres are adjacent to the articular surface. They pass distally and posteriorly to a fairly compact attachment posteriorly in the intercondylar region and in a depression on the adjacent posterior tibia. This gives a fan-like structure in which fibre orientation is variable. Anterolateral and posteromedial bundles have been defined: they are named (against convention) according to their femoral attachments. The anterolateral bundle tightens in flexion whilst the posteromedial is tight in extension of the knee. Each bundle slackens as the other tightens. Unlike the anterior cruciate ligament, it is not isometric during knee motion, i.e. the distance between attachments varies with knee position.

Synovial membrane, plicae and fat pads

The synovial membrane of the knee is the most extensive and complex in the body. It forms a large suprapatellar bursa between quadriceps femoris and the lower femoral shaft at the proximal patellar border (**Figs 113.23, 113.24**). The bursa is an extension of the joint cavity and is sustained by articularis genu, which is attached to it. Alongside the patella the membrane extends beneath the aponeuroses of the vasti, especially under vastus medialis. It extends the breadth of the subject's hand above the superior pole of the patella. Distal to the patella, the synovial membrane is separated from the patellar tendon by an infrapatellar fat pad. As it covers the fat pad, the membrane projects into the joint as two fringes, alar folds, which bear villi. The folds converge posteriorly to form a single infrapatellar fold or plica (ligamentum mucosum), which curves posteriorly to its attachment in the femoral intercondylar fossa (**Fig. 113.25**). This fold may be a vestige of the inferior boundary of an originally separate femoropatellar joint. The extent of the infrapatellar plica ranges from a thin cord to a complete sheet that can cause obstruction to instrument passage in knee arthroscopy. When substantial, it has been mistaken for the anterior cruciate ligament, which is directly posterior to it. The medial plica extends in the midline anteriorly from the medial alar fold medially to the suprapatellar

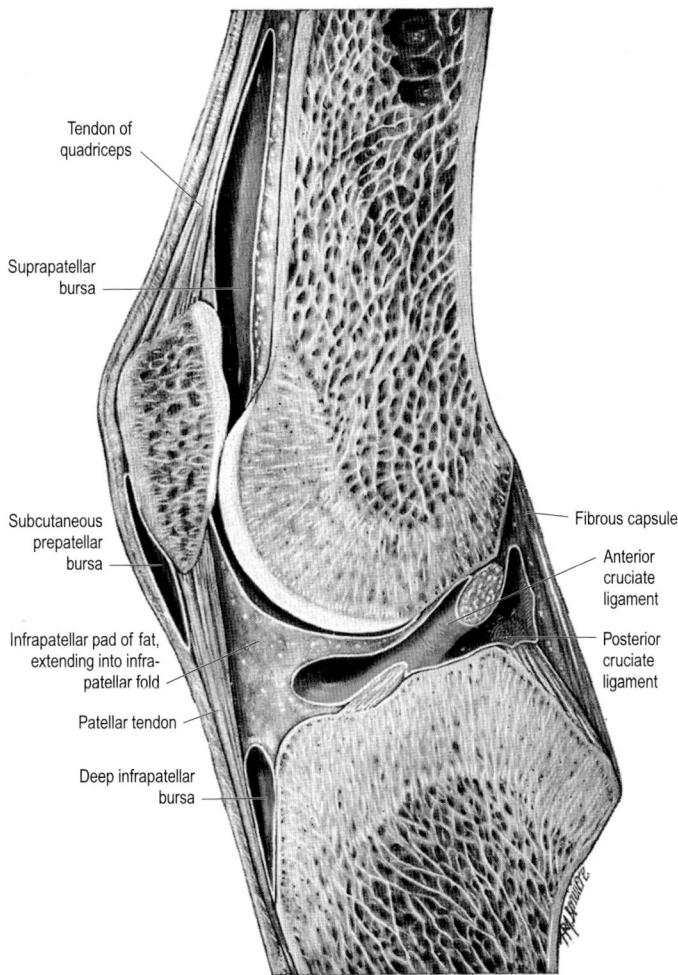

Fig. 113.24 Sagittal section through the left knee joint: lateral aspect. The synovial membrane is coloured blue.

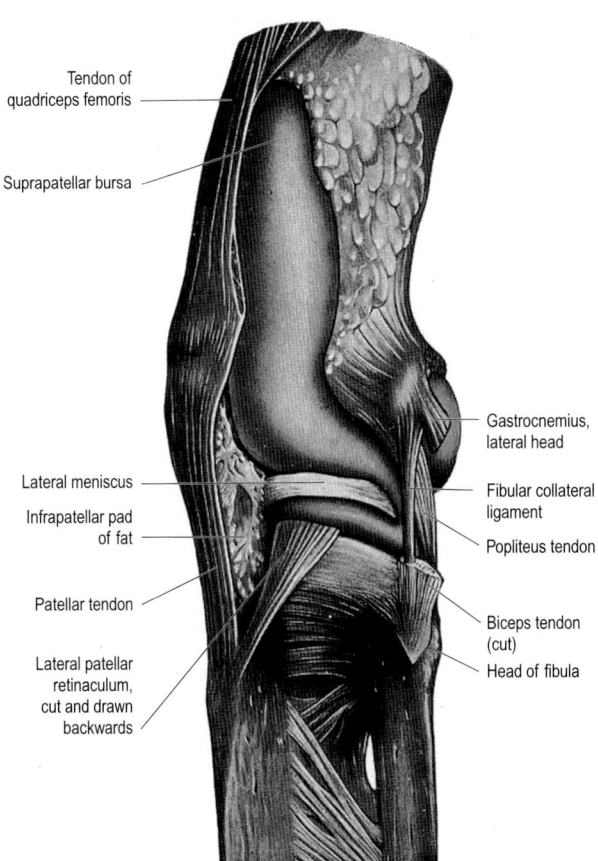

Fig. 113.23 Dissection of the left knee joint: lateral aspect. The synovial cavity has been distended by injection and the synovial membrane is coloured blue.

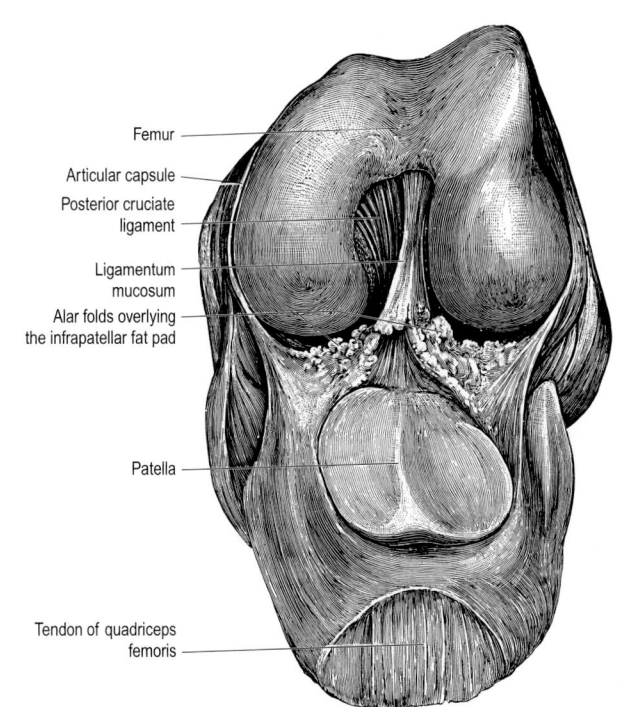

Fig. 113.25 Left knee joint in full flexion: the quadriceps tendon has been sectioned and the patellar flap retracted distally.

pouch. Occasionally it can be thickened and inflamed, usually following acute or chronic trauma.

The suprapatellar plicae are remnants of an embryonic septum that completely separates the suprapatellar pouch from the knee joint. Very occasionally a septum persists, either in its entirety, or perforated by a small peripheral opening. Loose bodies can lie hidden above this septum.

The infrapatellar fat pad is the largest part of a circumferential fatty ring, covered with synovium, which extends around the patellar margins (Newell 1991).

At the sides of the joint the synovial membrane descends from the femur and lines the capsule as far as the menisci, whose surfaces have no synovial covering. Posterior to the lateral meniscus the membrane forms a subpopliteal recess between a groove on the meniscal surface and the tendon of popliteus (**Fig. 113.19**): this may connect with the superior tibiofibular joint (p. 1483). The relation of the synovial membrane to the cruciate ligaments is described on page 1480.

Bursae
There are numerous bursae associated with the knee.

Anterior to the knee there is a large subcutaneous prepatellar bursa between the lower patella and skin; a small deep infrapatellar bursa between the tibia and patellar tendon; a subcutaneous infrapatellar bursa between the distal part of the tibial tuberosity and skin; and a large suprapatellar bursa which is the superior extension of the knee joint cavity (**Fig. 113.24**). Lateral to the knee there are bursae between: the lateral head of gastrocnemius and the joint capsule (which is sometimes continuous with the joint); the fibular collateral ligament and the tendon of biceps femoris; the fibular collateral ligament and the tendon of popliteus; the tendon of popliteus and the lateral femoral condyle, which is usually an extension from the joint. The last two bursae may communicate.

The arrangement of bursae medial to the knee is complex. The bursa between the medial head of gastrocnemius and the fibrous capsule is prolonged between the medial tendon of gastrocnemius and the tendon of semimembranosus (the semimembranosus bursa) and usually communicates with the joint. The bursa between the tendon of semimembranosus and the medial tibial condyle and the medial head of gastrocnemius may communicate with this bursa. There is a bursa between the medial collateral ligament and the tendons of sartorius, gracilis and semitendinosus (the 'pes bursa'). Bursae variable in both number and position lie deep to the medial collateral ligament between the capsule, femur, medial meniscus, tibia or tendon of semimembranosus. Occasionally there may be a bursa between the tendons of semimembranosus and semitendinosus.

Posteriorly, bursae are variable.

The clinically important bursae are the anterior group, the pes bursa, and the semimembranosus bursa. The subcutaneous prepatellar bursa and infrapatellar bursa can be inflamed as 'housemaid's knee' and 'clergyman's knee'. The pes bursa can be inflamed in athletes. In adults inflammation producing a popliteal fossa swelling commonly occurs secondary to degeneration within the knee joint. Regardless of size and position it almost always arises from the plane between semimembranosus and the medial tendon of gastrocnemius.

Vascular supply and lymphatic drainage of knee joint
There is an intricate arterial anastomosis around the patella and femoral and tibial condyles. A superficial network spreads between the fascia and skin around the patella and in the fat deep to the patellar tendon. A deep network lies on the femur and tibia near the adjoining articular surfaces, and supplies the bone and marrow, the articular capsule, synovial membrane and the cruciate ligaments (**Fig. 113.1**). The vessels involved are the superior, middle and inferior genicular branches of the popliteal artery, descending genicular branches of the femoral artery, the descending branch of the lateral circumflex femoral artery, the circumflex fibular artery and the anterior and posterior tibial recurrent arteries. For details consult Scapinelli (1968).

The venous drainage corresponds in name to the arterial supply and runs with it; the named smaller veins drain into the popliteal and femoral veins.

Lymphatic drainage is to the popliteal nodes. Most of the lymph vessels accompany the genicular arteries; some vessels from the joint drain directly into a node between the popliteal artery and the posterior capsule. The popliteal nodes drain mainly into the deep inguinal group.

Innervation of knee joint
The knee joint is innervated by branches from the obturator, femoral, tibial and common peroneal nerves (Freeman & Wyke 1967). The genicular branch of the obturator nerve is the terminal branch of its posterior division. Muscular branches of the femoral nerve, especially to vastus medialis, supply terminal branches to the joint. Genicular branches from the tibial and common peroneal nerves accompany the genicular arteries: those from the tibial nerve run with the medial and middle genicular arteries, while those from the common peroneal nerve run with the lateral genicular and anterior tibial recurrent arteries.

Movements and muscles

Movements
Movements at the knee are customarily described as flexion, extension, internal (medial) and external (lateral) rotation. Flexion and extension differ from true hingeing in that (a) the articular surface profiles of the femoral and tibial articular surfaces produce a variably placed axis of rotation during the flexion arc, and (b) when the foot is fixed, flexion entails corresponding conjunct (coupled) external (lateral) rotation. These conjunct rotations are a product of the geometry of the articular surfaces and, to an extent, the disposition of the associated ligaments. There is differential motion in the medial and lateral tibiofemoral compartments. Laterally there is considerable displacement of the femur on the tibia, with rolling as well as sliding at the joint surface, whereas medially for most of the flexion arc there is minimal relative motion of the femur and tibia, with the motion being almost exclusively one joint surface sliding on the other. In full flexion the lateral femoral condyle is close to subluxation off the posterior lateral tibia. Medially there is only significant posterior femoral displacement beyond 120° by passive means. The menisci move with the femoral condyles, the anterior horns more than the posterior, and the lateral far more than the medial.

The axial rotations have a smaller range than the arc of flexion and extension. These rotations are conjunct, and integral with flexion and extension, i.e. they are obligatory. They can also be adjunct and independent, i.e. voluntary, and are best demonstrated with the knee semi-flexed. Therefore the degree of axial rotation varies with flexion and extension.

The range of extension is c.5–10° beyond straight. Active flexion is c.120° with the hip extended, 140° when it is flexed, and 160° when aided by a passive element, e.g. sitting on the heels. Voluntary rotation is c.60–70°, but conjunct rotation only c.20°.

Conjunct medial rotation of the femur on the tibia in the later stages of extension is part of a 'locking' mechanism, so-called 'screw-home', which is an asset when the fully extended knees are subjected to strain. Full extension is the close-packed position, with maximal spiralization and tightening of the ligaments. The roles of the articular surfaces, musculature and ligaments in generating conjunct rotations remain controversial (Girgis et al 1975, Rajendran 1985), but the following points can be made. The lateral combined meniscotibial 'receiving surface' is smaller, more circular and more deeply concave. Since the articular surface is virtually convex in sagittal section the depth of the receiving surface is largely due to the presence of the lateral meniscus. The lateral femoral articular surface is also smaller. Consequently, the lateral femoral condyle approaches full congruence with the opposed surface c.30° before full extension (well before the medial condyle). Simple extension cannot continue, but medial rotation of the femur occurs on a vertical axis through its head and medial condyle: the medial femoral condyle moves very little in the sagittal plane and is stabilized by the upslope of the anterior half of the medial tibia, while rotation of the lateral femoral condyle and meniscus brings the anterior horn of the latter onto the anterior downslope of the lateral tibial condyle. Rotation and extension follow simultaneously and smoothly until final close packing of both condyles coincides. At the beginning of flexion from full extension (with the foot fixed) lateral femoral rotation occurs, which 'unlocks' the joint. While joint surfaces and many ligaments are involved, electromyographic evidence reveals that contraction of popliteus is important, and that it pulls down and backwards on the lateral femoral condyle, lateral to the axis of femoral rotation. It also retracts the posterior horn during lateral rotation and continuing flexion, via its attachment to the lateral meniscus, and so prevents traumatic compression.

Any position of extension adopted is a balance between forces (torque) extending the joint and passive mechanisms resisting them. The range near to close packing is functionally important. In symmetrical standing, the line of body weight is anterior to the transverse axes of the knee joints, but the passive mechanisms noted above preserve posture with minimal muscular effort (Joseph 1960). Active contraction of the extensors and a close-packed position only occur in asymmetrical postures, e.g. in leaning forward, heavy loading, or when powerful thrust is needed.

In extension, parts of both cruciate ligaments, the tibial and fibular collateral ligaments, the posterior capsular region, the oblique posterior ligament, skin and fasciae are all taut. Passive and sometimes active tension exists in the hamstrings and gastrocnemius, and the anterior part of the medial meniscus is compressed between the femoral and tibial condyles. During extension the patellar tendon is tightened by quadriceps femoris but is relaxed in the erect attitude. When the knee flexes, the fibular collateral ligament and the posterior part of the medial collateral ligament relax but the cruciate ligaments and the anterior part of the medial collateral ligament remain taut: the posterior parts of the menisci are compressed between the femoral and tibial condyles. Flexion is checked by quadriceps femoris, anterior parts of the capsule, posterior cruciate ligament and compression of soft tissues behind the knee. In extreme passive flexion, contact of the calf with the thigh may be the limiting factor and parts of both cruciate ligaments are also tense. In addition to conjunct rotation with terminal extension or initial flexion, relaxed collateral ligaments also allow independent medial and lateral rotation (adjunct rotation) when the joint is flexed.

Accessory movements – Wider rotation can be obtained by passive movements when the knee is semi-flexed. To a limited extent, the tibia can also be translated back and forwards on the femur. Abduction and adduction are prevented in full extension by the collateral ligaments and secondary restraints such as the cruciate ligaments. With the knee slightly flexed, limited adduction and abduction are possible, both passive and active. Slight separation of the femur and tibia can be produced by strong traction.

Muscles producing the movements
Flexion: biceps femoris, semitendinosus and semimembranosus, assisted by gracilis, sartorius and popliteus. With the foot stationary, gastrocnemius and plantaris also assist.
Extension: quadriceps femoris, assisted by tensor fasciae latae.
Medial rotation of the flexed leg: popliteus, semimembranosus and semitendinosus, assisted by sartorius and gracilis.
Lateral rotation of the flexed leg: biceps femoris.

Relations and 'at risk' structures
Anteriorly are the tendon of quadriceps femoris (which encloses and is attached to the non-articular surfaces of the patella), the patellar tendon, tendinous expansions from vastus medialis and lateralis (which extend over the anteromedial and anterolateral aspects of the capsule respectively), and the patellar retinacula. Posteromedial is sartorius, and the tendon of gracilis which lies along its posterior border, both descending across the joint. Posterolaterally the biceps tendon and the common peroneal nerve which lies medial to it are in contact with the capsule, separating it from popliteus (**Fig. 113.21**). Posteriorly the popliteal artery and associated lymph nodes lie on the oblique popliteal ligament: the popliteal vein is posteromedial or medial, and the tibial nerve is posterior to both. The nerve and vessels are overlapped by both heads of gastrocnemius and laterally by plantaris. Gastrocnemius contacts the capsules either side of the vessels. Semimembranosus lies between the capsule and semitendinosus, medial to the medial head of gastrocnemius.

Factors maintaining stability
The control of the stability of the knee is of considerable importance.

Patellofemoral joint
The alignment of the femoral and tibial shafts is such that the pull of the quadriceps on the patella imparts a force on the patella that is directed both superiorly and laterally. The static bony factors that counter this tendency to move laterally are the congruity of the patellofemoral joint and the buttressing effect of the larger lateral part of the trochlear groove. If the patella is small, or resides too high above the trochlea, or if the trochlear groove is too shallow, then instability may result. The static ligamentous factors are the medial patellofemoral ligament and medial retinaculum.

Dynamic muscular control is important. The most distal part of vastus medialis, vastus medialis obliquus, contains transverse fibres: these pull the patella medially, which counters the tendency to lateral movement. It is this muscle that is preferentially strengthened in a physiotherapy programme aimed at treating patellofemoral problems.

Tibiofemoral joint
The tibiofemoral joint surfaces are inherently unstable, especially laterally. Medially some stability is afforded by the relatively concave tibial surface and the relatively fixed posterior horn of the medial meniscus. Both medially and laterally the menisci are helpful, particularly as they move with the femoral condyles. Ligaments play a major role in providing stability: their function is partly static, in that they bind the bones in positions of extreme stress, but they also provide proprioceptive feedback which aids coordination of stabilizing muscle activity. Taking a somewhat 'two-dimensional' view, the medial and lateral collateral ligaments may be considered as resistors of valgus and varus force on the knee respectively, and the anterior and posterior cruciate ligaments as resistors of anterior and posterior tibial translation respectively. However in reality the situation is more complex than this. The stresses are rarely applied in orthogonal planes and so a combination of forces, especially rotational, is involved. Moreover, many structures other than the collateral and cruciate ligaments are involved in stabilizing the joint. The 'posterolateral corner', which resists tibial external rotation, consists of the popliteofibular, fabellofibular, arcuate, and lateral collateral ligaments and iliotibial band, together with popliteus, the lateral head of gastrocnemius and biceps femoris. The 'posteromedial corner', which resists tibial rotation, consists of the posterior oblique portion of the superficial medial collateral ligament, the capsule (including the oblique popliteal ligament) and semimembranosus. Since stresses are often a combination of force plus rotation, structures usually operate together rather than in isolation.

Loading at the knee
During level walking, the force across the tibiofemoral joint for most of the cycle is between two and four times body weight, and can be more. In contrast, the force across the patellofemoral joint is no more than 50% body weight. Peak force transmission across the joint increases sequentially as the menisci, articular cartilage and subchondral bone are damaged or removed. Walking up or down stairs has little influence on tibiofemoral forces, but significantly increases patellofemoral forces to two (walking up) or three (walking down) times body weight, reflecting the changed angle of the quadriceps tendon and patellar tendon during flexion. There are two mechanisms for ameliorating forces transmitted across the patella: the extensor lever arm is lengthened as the axis of rotation moves posteriorly during flexion, and the contact area between the patella and femur almost triples between 30° and 90°. To cope with the potential large forces from activities such as running, the patella has the thickest articular cartilage in the body.

SUPERIOR TIBIOFIBULAR JOINT (Fig. 113.26)
The superior (proximal) tibiofibular joint is an almost plane synovial joint between the lateral tibial condyle and fibular head.

Articulating surfaces
The articulating surfaces vary in size, form and inclination. The joint line may be transverse or oblique. The fibular facet is usually elliptical or circular, almost flat or slightly grooved. The surfaces are covered with hyaline cartilage.

Fibrous capsule
The capsule is attached to the margins of the rims of facets on the tibia and fibula and is thickened anteriorly and posteriorly.

Ligaments
The ligaments of the superior tibiofibular joint are not entirely separate from the capsule. The anterior ligament is made up of two or three flat bands which pass obliquely up from the fibular head to the front of the lateral tibial condyle: it is closely related to the tendon of biceps. The posterior ligament is a thick band that ascends obliquely between the posterior aspect of the fibular head and the lateral tibial condyle: it is covered by the popliteal tendon.

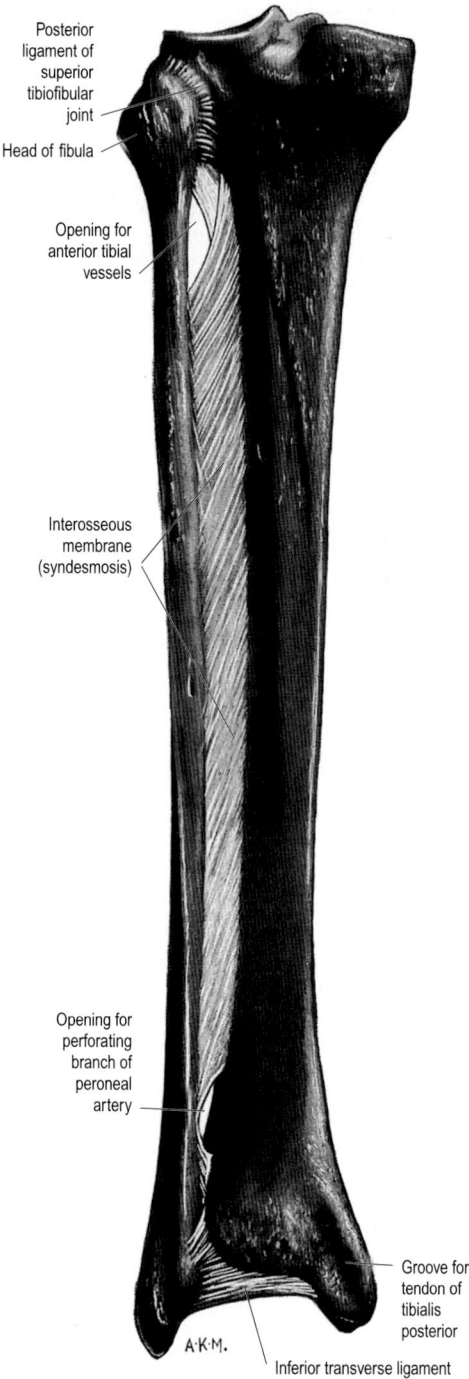

Posterior
ligament of
superior
tibiofibular
joint

Head of fibula

Opening for
anterior tibial
vessels

Interosseous
membrane
(syndesmosis)

Opening for
perforating
branch of
peroneal
artery

A·K·M.

Groove for
tendon of
tibialis
posterior

Inferior transverse ligament

Fig. 113.26 Posterior aspect of the interosseous membrane. Note the contrasting direction of the fibre bundles around the vascular openings.

Synovial membrane

The synovial membrane of the superior tibiofibular joint is sometimes (c.10%) continuous with that of the knee joint via the subpopliteal recess.

Vascular supply and lymphatic drainage

The superior tibiofibular joint receives an arterial supply from the anterior and posterior tibial recurrent branches of the anterior tibial artery. Lymphatics follow the arteries and drain to the popliteal nodes.

Innervation

The superior tibiofibular joint is innervated by branches from the common peroneal nerve and from the nerve to popliteus.

Factors maintaining stability

Stability of the superior tibiofibular joint is maintained by the fibrous capsule and the anterior and posterior ligaments, assisted by the biceps tendon and the interosseous membrane.

Movements

Very little movement other than limited gliding takes place at the superior tibiofibular joint. Some movement must occur in conjunction with movement occurring at the inferior tibiofibular joint (p. 1515); however, fusion of the superior tibiofibular joint seems to have no effect on the ankle.

Relations and 'at risk' structures

The common peroneal nerve runs posterior to the fibular head, medial to the tendon of biceps, which is closely associated with the anterior capsule. The anterior and posterior tibial branches of the popliteal artery, and the peroneal artery, are all vulnerable inferomedial to the joint.

MUSCLES

QUADRICEPS FEMORIS
See page 1463.

ARTICULARIS GENU
See page 1464.

MEDIAL AND LATERAL HEADS OF GASTROCNEMIUS
See page 1499.

SOLEUS
See page 1500.

POPLITEUS (Figs 113.27, 113.28, 113.29)

Attachments

Popliteus is a flat muscle that forms the floor of the lower part of the popliteal fossa. It arises within the capsule of the knee joint by a strong

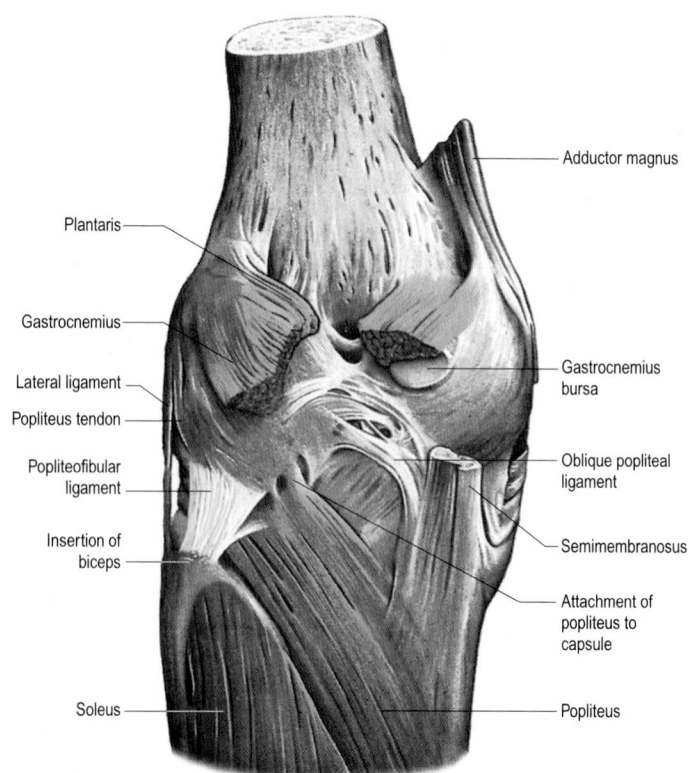

Plantaris

Gastrocnemius

Lateral ligament

Popliteus tendon

Popliteofibular
ligament

Insertion of
biceps

Soleus

Adductor magnus

Gastrocnemius
bursa

Oblique popliteal
ligament

Semimembranosus

Attachment of
popliteus to
capsule

Popliteus

Fig. 113.27 Posterior aspect of the left knee.

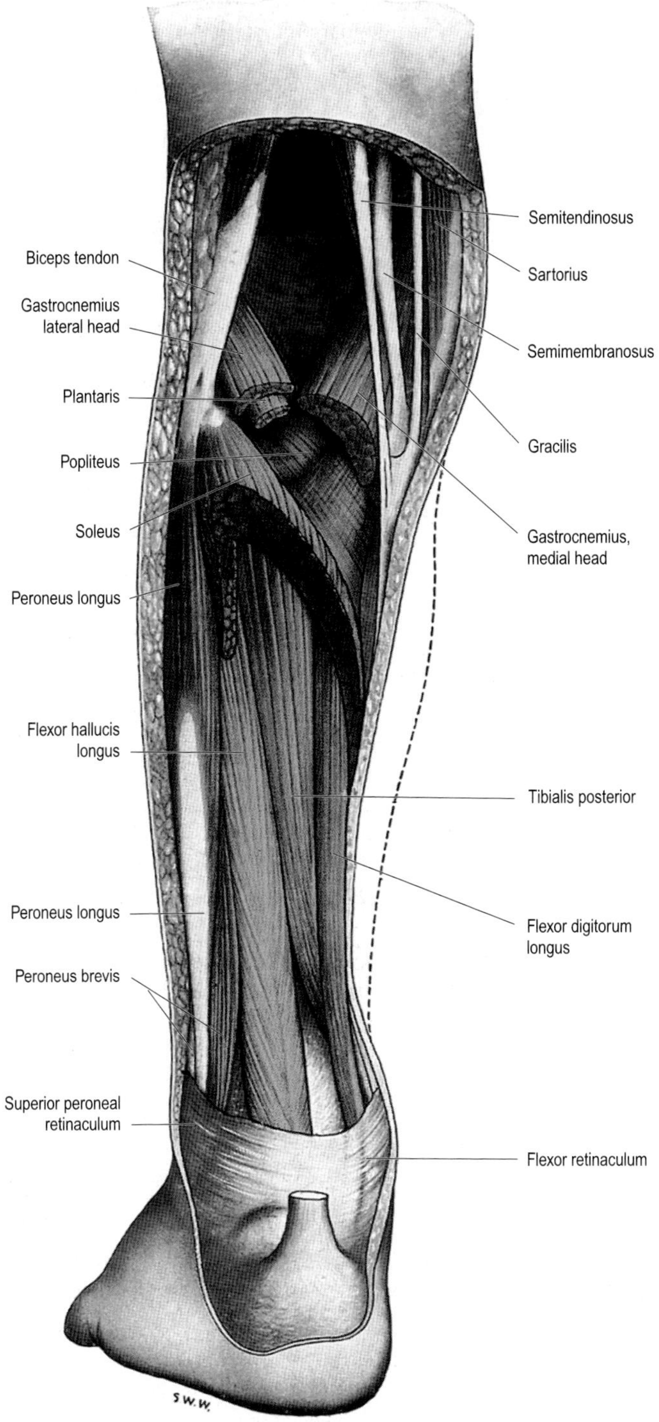

Fig. 113.28

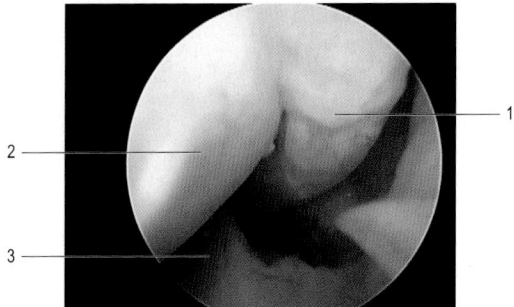

1. Intra-articular part of popliteus tendon.   **2.** Lateral femoral condyle.   **3.** Lateral meniscus.

Fig. 113.29 Intra-articular popliteus tendon at arthroscopy. (By kind permission from Smith and Nephew Endoscopy.)

Biceps tendon

Gastrocnemius lateral head

Plantaris

Popliteus

Soleus

Peroneus longus

Flexor hallucis longus

Peroneus longus

Peroneus brevis

Superior peroneal retinaculum

Semitendinosus

Sartorius

Semimembranosus

Gracilis

Gastrocnemius, medial head

Tibialis posterior

Flexor digitorum longus

Flexor retinaculum

S W. W.

Fig. 113.28 Deep muscles of the left calf in a child aged 8.

tendon, c.2.5 cm long, which is attached to a depression at the anterior end of the groove on the lateral aspect of the lateral condyle of the femur (**Fig. 111.19**). Medially this tendon is joined by collagenous fibres from the arcuate popliteal ligament, from the fibrous capsule adjacent to the lateral meniscus, and from the outer margin of the meniscus.

Popliteus is attached to the medial aspect of the fibular head by the popliteofibular ligament, which passes laterally and inferiorly from the popliteus tendon in a sheet of tissue c.2 cm². This ligament is the single most important stabilizer of the posterolateral region of the knee and resists external rotation of the tibia on the femur. Failure to recognize and reconstruct damage to this ligament and to the related ligamentous structures is the most common reason for a poor result from technically well-performed reconstructive cruciate ligament surgery.

Fleshy fibres expand from the inferior limit of the tendon to form a somewhat triangular muscle that descends medially to be inserted into the medial two-thirds of the triangular area above the soleal line on the posterior surface of the tibia, and into the tendinous expansion that covers its surface.

An additional head may arise from the sesamoid in the lateral head of gastrocnemius. Very rarely, two other muscles may be found deeply behind the knee. Popliteus minor runs from the posterior surface of the lateral condyle, medial to plantaris, to the oblique popliteal ligament. Peroneotibialis runs deep to popliteus from the medial side of the fibular head to the upper end of the soleal line.

Relations

Popliteus is covered posteriorly by a tight aponeurotic expansion, which is largely derived from the tendon of semimembranosus. Gastrocnemius, plantaris, the popliteal vessels and the tibial nerve all lie on the expansion. The popliteal tendon is intracapsular and is deep to the fibular collateral ligament of the knee and the tendon of biceps femoris (**Fig. 113.21**). It is invested on its deep surface by synovial membrane, and grooves the posterior border of the lateral meniscus and the adjoining part of the tibia before it emerges inferior to the posterior band of the arcuate ligament (**Fig. 113.27**). In this region, the 'popliteus hiatus', the lateral meniscus has no peripheral attachment, and is rather mobile.

Vascular supply

The arterial supply of popliteus is derived mainly from the medial and lateral inferior genicular arteries. The latter may cross superficial or deep to the muscle. There are additional contributions from the nutrient artery to the tibia, the proximal part of the tibial artery and from the posterior tibial recurrent artery.

Innervation

Popliteus is innervated by the tibial nerve, L4 and 5 and S1.

Actions

Popliteus rotates the tibia medially on the femur or, when the tibia is fixed, rotates the femur laterally on the tibia. It is usually regarded as the muscle that 'unlocks' the joint at the beginning of flexion of the fully extended knee: electromyography supports this view. Its connection with the arcuate popliteal ligament, fibrous capsule and lateral meniscus has led to the suggestion that popliteus may retract the posterior horn of the lateral meniscus during lateral rotation of the femur and flexion of the knee joint, so protecting the meniscus from being crushed between the femur and the tibia during these movements. The muscle is markedly active in crouching, perhaps to provide stability as the tibia internally rotates during flexion of the knee. However, the main function is likely to be provision of dynamic stability to the posterolateral part of the knee by preventing excessive external rotation of the tibia, partly by its direct action, but especially by tensing the popliteofibular ligament.

Testing

Popliteus plays a part in medially rotating the leg with the non-weightbearing knee flexed, but its individual action cannot be isolated clinically. Damage to the popliteus complex of ligament and tendon as a static 'tether' is manifest by excessive external rotation of the tibia on the femur at 90° and especially at 30° of knee flexion.

BICEPS FEMORIS
See page 1468.

PLANTARIS
See page 1499.

SEMIMEMBRANOSUS
See page 1467.

VASCULAR SUPPLY AND LYMPHATIC DRAINAGE

ARTERIES

Popliteal artery (Figs 112.8, 113.4, 113.30)

The popliteal artery, which is the continuation of the femoral artery, crosses the popliteal fossa. From the opening in adductor magnus it descends laterally to the intercondylar fossa, inclining obliquely to the distal border of popliteus, where it divides into the anterior and posterior tibial arteries. This division usually occurs at the proximal end of the asymmetrical crural interosseous space between the wide tibial metaphysis and the slender fibular metaphysis. The artery is relatively tethered at the adductor magnus hiatus and again distally by the fascia related to soleus. It is therefore vulnerable to traction during knee injuries, e.g. dislocation.

The artery may divide into its terminal branches proximal to popliteus, in which case the anterior tibial artery sometimes descends anterior to the muscle. There may be a true 'trifurcation' into anterior and posterior tibial and peroneal branches. Either the anterior tibial or the posterior tibial artery may be reduced or increased in size. The size of the peroneal artery is usually inversely related to the size of the anterior and posterior tibial arteries, either of whose function the peroneal artery may assume.

The popliteal artery may pass medially beneath the medial head of gastrocnemius, or may pass beneath an aberrant band of muscle in the popliteal fossa: in either case, contraction of the muscles may occlude the artery. This condition, popliteal arterial entrapment, may present with claudication on exercise in a young male patient.

Relations

Anteriorly, from proximal to distal, are fat covering the femoral popliteal surface, the capsule of the knee joint, and the fascia of popliteus. Posteriorly are semimembranosus (proximally) and gastrocnemius and plantaris (distally). In between, the artery is separated from the skin and fasciae by fat and crossed from its lateral to its medial side by the tibial nerve and popliteal vein: the vein lies between the nerve and artery and is adherent to the latter. Laterally are biceps femoris, the tibial nerve, popliteal vein and lateral femoral condyle (all proximal), and plantaris and the lateral head of gastrocnemius (distal). Medially are semimembranosus and the medial femoral condyle (proximal), and the tibial nerve, popliteal vein and medial head of gastrocnemius (distally). The relations of the popliteal lymph nodes are described on page 1487.

Branches (other than terminal)

Genicular anastomosis (Figs 113.1, 113.4) – There is an intricate arterial anastomosis around the patella and femoral and tibial condyles. A superficial network spreads between the fascia and skin around the patella and in the fat deep to the patellar tendon. A deep network lies on the femur and tibia near the adjoining articular surfaces, and supplies the bone and marrow, articular capsule and synovial membrane. The vessels involved are the medial and lateral superior genicular, the medial and lateral inferior genicular, the descending genicular, the descending branch of the lateral circumflex femoral, the circumflex fibular and the anterior and posterior tibial recurrent arteries.

Superior genicular arteries – The superior genicular arteries branch from the popliteal artery, curving round proximal to both femoral condyles to reach the anterior aspect of the knee. The medial superior genicular artery lies under semimembranosus and semitendinosus, proximal to the medial head of gastrocnemius and deep to the tendon of adductor magnus. It divides into a branch to vastus medialis that anastomoses with the descending genicular and medial inferior genicular arteries, and a branch that ramifies on the femur and anastomoses with the lateral superior genicular artery. Its size varies inversely with that of the descending genicular artery. The lateral superior genicular artery passes under the tendon of biceps femoris and divides into superficial and deep branches. The superficial branch supplies vastus lateralis and anastomoses with the descending branch of the lateral circumflex femoral and lateral inferior genicular arteries, while the deep branch anastomoses with the medial superior genicular artery, forming an anterior arch across the femur with the descending genicular artery. The superficial branch is vulnerable if the lateral patellar retinaculum is divided surgically.

Middle genicular artery – The middle genicular artery is small. It arises from the popliteal artery near the posterior centre of the knee joint. It pierces the oblique popliteal ligament to supply the cruciate ligaments and synovial membrane.

Inferior genicular arteries – The medial and lateral inferior genicular arteries arise from the popliteal artery deep to gastrocnemius. The medial is deep to the medial head of gastrocnemius. It descends along the proximal margin of popliteus, which it supplies, passes inferior to the medial tibial condyle, under the medial collateral ligament, and then ascends anteromedial to the joint at the anterior border of the medial collateral ligament. It supplies the joint and the tibia, and anastomoses with the lateral inferior and medial superior genicular arteries and with the anterior tibial recurrent artery and saphenous branch of the descending genicular artery. The lateral inferior genicular artery runs laterally across popliteus and forwards over the fibular head to the front of the knee joint, passing under the lateral head of gastrocnemius, the fibular collateral ligament and the tendon of biceps femoris. Its branches anastomose with the medial inferior and lateral superior genicular, anterior and posterior tibial recurrent and circumflex fibular arteries.

Cutaneous branches: the superficial sural arteries – The superficial sural arteries are three vessels which leave the popliteal artery, or its side branches, descend between the heads of gastrocnemius and perforate

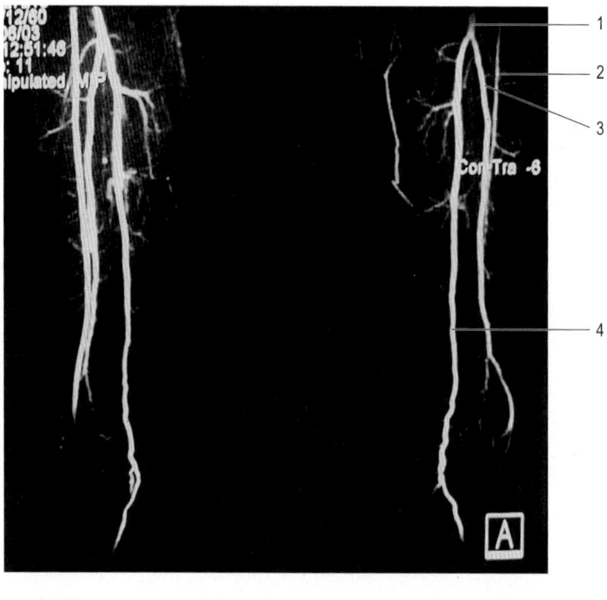

1. Tibioperoneal trunk. 2. Anterior tibial artery. 3. Peroneal artery. 4. Posterior tibial artery.

Fig. 113.30 Magnetic resonance angiogram (MRA) of major branches of the popliteal artery. (By kind permission from Dr Justin Lee, Chelsea and Westminster Hospital, London.)

the deep fascia to supply the skin on the back of the leg. The central or median vessel is usually larger than the medial and lateral, and usually accompanies the sural nerve.

Fasciocutaneous free and pedicled flaps may be raised on the superficial sural arteries.

Superior muscular branches – The superior muscular branches are two or three vessels that arise proximally and pass to adductor magnus and the knee flexors. They anastomose with the termination of the profunda femoris artery.

Sural arteries – The two sural arteries are large and arise behind the knee joint to supply gastrocnemius, soleus and plantaris. They are used in gastrocnemius musculocutaneous flaps (p. 1499).

VEINS

Popliteal vein (Fig. 110.7)
The popliteal vein ascends through the popliteal fossa to the opening in adductor magnus where it becomes the femoral vein. Its relationship to the popliteal artery changes as the vein ascends. Distally it is medial to the artery, between the heads of gastrocnemius it is superficial (posterior) to it, and proximal to the knee joint it is posterolateral to the artery. Its tributaries are the short saphenous vein, veins corresponding to branches of the popliteal artery, and muscular veins, including a large branch from each head of gastrocnemius. There are usually four valves in the popliteal vein.

Long saphenous vein
See page 1452.

Short saphenous vein (Fig. 110.7)
The short saphenous vein (small saphenous vein) begins posterior to the lateral malleolus as a continuation of the lateral marginal vein. In the lower third of the calf it ascends lateral to the calcaneal tendon, lying on the deep fascia and covered only by superficial fascia and skin. Inclining medially to reach the midline of the calf, it penetrates the deep fascia, within which it ascends on gastrocnemius, only emerging between the deep fascia and gastrocnemius gradually at about the junction of the intermediate and proximal thirds of the calf (usually well below the lower limit of the popliteal fossa). Continuing its ascent, it passes between the heads of gastrocnemius then proceeds to its termination in the popliteal vein in the popliteal fossa, 3–7.5 cm above the knee joint.

Tributaries
The short saphenous vein connects with deep veins on the dorsum of the foot, receives many cutaneous tributaries in the leg, and sends several communicating branches proximally and medially to join the long saphenous vein. Sometimes a communicating branch ascends medially to the accessory saphenous vein (see p. 1452): this may be the main continuation of the short saphenous vein. In the leg the short saphenous vein lies near the sural nerve. It has 7–13 valves, one near its termination. Its mode of ending is variable: it may join the long saphenous vein in the proximal thigh or it may bifurcate, one branch joining the long saphenous, the other the popliteal or deep posterior femoral veins. Sometimes it ends distal to the knee in the long saphenous or deep sural muscular veins.

POPLITEAL LYMPH NODES (Fig. 111.38)
There are usually approximately six small lymph nodes embedded in the fat of the popliteal fossa. One, near the end of the short saphenous vein, drains the superficial region served by the vein. Another lies between the popliteal artery and the posterior aspect of the knee joint, receiving direct vessels from the knee joint and from those accompanying the genicular arteries. The remainder flank the popliteal vessels, receiving trunks that accompany the anterior and posterior tibial vessels. Popliteal efferents ascend close to the femoral vessels to reach the deep inguinal nodes; some may accompany the long saphenous vein to the superficial inguinal nodes.

Inflammation of the popliteal nodes is often caused by lateral lesions of the heel.

INNERVATION

SAPHENOUS NERVE (Fig. 111.40)
The saphenous nerve is the largest cutaneous branch of the femoral nerve. It descends lateral to the femoral artery into the adductor canal (p. 1461), where it crosses anteriorly to become medial to the artery. At the distal end of the canal it leaves the artery and emerges through the aponeurotic covering with the saphenous branch of the descending genicular artery. As it leaves the adductor canal it gives off an infrapatellar branch that contributes to the peripatellar plexus and then pierces the fascia lata between the tendons of sartorius and gracilis, becoming subcutaneous to supply the prepatellar skin. It descends along the medial tibial border with the long saphenous vein and divides distally into a branch which continues along the tibia to the ankle and a branch which passes anterior to the ankle to supply the skin on the medial side of the foot, often as far as the first metatarsophalangeal joint. The saphenous nerve connects with the medial branch of the superficial peroneal nerve. Near midthigh, it gives a branch to the subsartorial plexus (p. 1470). The nerve may be subject to an entrapment neuropathy as it leaves the adductor canal.

Infrapatellar branch of saphenous nerve
See page 1471.

PERIPATELLAR PLEXUS
See page 1471.

OBTURATOR NERVE
See page 1455.

SCIATIC NERVE
See page 1458.

TIBIAL NERVE
See page 1504.

COMMON PERONEAL NERVE
See page 1504.

SURAL NERVE
See page 1505.

REFERENCES

Amis AA, Dawkins GP 1991 Functional anatomy of the anterior cruciate ligament. Fibre bundle actions related to ligament replacements and injuries. J Bone Joint Surg 73B: 260–7.

Cormack GC, Lamberty BGH 1994 See Bibliography.

Freeman MAR, Wyke B 1967 The innervation of the knee joint. J Anat 101: 505–32.

Ghadially FN, Lalonde J-M A, Wedge JH 1983 Ultrastructure of normal and torn menisci of the human knee joint. J Anat 136: 773–91.

Girgis FG, Marshall JL, Al Monajem ARS 1975 The cruciate ligaments of the knee joint. Clin Orthop 106: 216–31.

Gronblad M, Korkala O, Leisi P, Karaharju E 1985 Innervation of synovial membrane and meniscus. Acta Orthop Scand 56: 484–6.

Gupte CM, Bull AMJ, Thomas RD, Amis AA 2003 A review of the function and biomechanics of the meniscofemoral ligaments. Arthroscopy 19: 161–71.
A comprehensive review of the properties of these hitherto poorly understood ligaments.

Joseph J 1960 Man's Posture: Electromyographic Studies. Springfield, Illinois: Thomas.

Newell RLM 1991 A complete intra-articular fat pad around the human patella. J Anat 179: 232.
Shows that the infrapatellar and suprapatellar fat pads are not isolated and separate structures.

Rajendran K 1985 Mechanism of locking at the knee joint. J Anat 143: 189–94.

Scapinelli R 1968 Studies on the vasculature of the human knee joint. Acta Anat 70: 305–31.

Primary source of detail, complementing the work of Crock (q.v.) on the vasculature of the bones of the lower limb.

Seebacher JR, Inglis AE, Marshall JL, Warren RF 1982 The structure of the postero-lateral aspect of the knee. J Bone Joint Surg 64A: 536–41.

Work that established the current interpretation of the anatomy of the soft tissues of the knee.

Tennant TD, Birch NC, Holmes MJ, Birch R, Goddard NJ 1998 Knee pain and the infrapatellar branch of the saphenous nerve. J Roy Soc Med 91: 573–5.

Recognizes the clinical significance of this small but important nerve branch.

Thomas P, Jackson AM, Aichroth PM 1985 Congenital absence of the anterior cruciate ligament. J Bone Joint Surg 67B: 572–5.

A rare but important congenital anomaly.

Warren LF, Marshall JL 1979 The supporting structures and layers on the medial side of the knee: an anatomical analysis. J Bone Joint Surg 61A: 56–62.

Watanabe M, Takeda S, Ikeuchi H 1979 Atlas of Arthroscopy. Berlin: Springer-Verlag.

Leg

This chapter describes the shafts of the tibia and fibula, the interosseous membrane between them, and the soft tissues that surround them. The tibiofibular joints are described on pages 1483 and 1525.

The region is commonly injured and is often the site of vascular problems. The anatomy of the deep and superficial veins and their connections has great clinical relevance, as does that of the anterior and posterior tibial and peroneal arteries. The fascial skeleton (p. 1399) determines the function of the leg muscles in their osteofascial compartments, the pathways of neurovascular structures, and the spread and confinement of pathological fluids (which is especially relevant to compartment syndrome). The patterns of attachment of muscles and fasciae to bone also determine the directions of displacement of fractures. The main branches of the sciatic nerve run through the region, each in a different osteofascial compartment.

SKIN

VASCULAR SUPPLY AND LYMPHATIC DRAINAGE

The arterial supply mainly involves branches of the popliteal, anterior tibial, posterior tibial and peroneal vessels (**Fig. 110.3**). There are multiple fasciocutaneous perforators from each vessel, passing along intermuscular septa to reach the skin, as well as musculocutaneous perforators from the surface of gastrocnemius. These are useful in providing local plastic surgical flaps. In some areas there is also a direct cutaneous supply from vessels accompanying cutaneous nerves, e.g. the descending genicular (saphenous branch) and sural arteries. Fasciocutaneous and direct cutaneous branches have a longitudinal orientation in the skin, whereas the musculocutaneous branches are more radially oriented. For further details consult Cormack and Lamberty (1994).

Cutaneous veins are tributaries of vessels that correspond to the named arteries. Medial cutaneous lymphatic collecting vessels accompany the long saphenous veins to the superficial inguinal nodes, and those from the lateral and posterior sides of the leg accompany the short saphenous vein and pierce the deep fascia to drain into the popliteal nodes.

INNERVATION

See page 1399.

SOFT TISSUE

DEEP FASCIA

The deep fascia of the leg, the fascia cruris, is continuous with the fascia lata and is attached around the knee to the patella, the patellar tendon, the tuberosity and condyles of the tibia, and the head of the fibula. Posteriorly, where it forms the popliteal fascia, which covers the popliteal fossa, it is strengthened by transverse fibres and perforated by the short saphenous vein and sural nerve. It receives lateral expansions from the tendon of biceps femoris and multiple medial expansions from the tendons of sartorius, gracilis, semitendinosus and semimembranosus. It blends with the periosteum on the subcutaneous surface of the tibia and the head and malleolus of the fibula, and is continuous below with the extensor and flexor retinacula (p. 1507). It is thick and dense in the proximal and anterior part of the leg, and fibres of tibialis anterior and extensor digitorum longus are attached to its deep surface. It is thinner posteriorly where it covers gastrocnemius and soleus. On the lateral side it is continuous with the intermuscular septa of the lower leg, the anterior and posterior crural intermuscular septa, which are attached to the anterior and posterior borders of the fibula respectively. Several slender fascial extensions enclose individual muscles (see osteofascial compartments below). A broad transverse intermuscular septum, the deep transverse fascia of the leg, passes between the superficial and deep muscles in the calf.

DEEP TRANSVERSE FASCIA

The deep transverse fascia of the leg is a fibrous stratum between the superficial and deep muscles of the calf. It extends transversely from the medial margin of the tibia to the posterior border of the fibula. Proximally, where it is thick and dense, it is attached to the soleal ridge of the tibia and to the fibula, inferomedial to the attachment of soleus. Between these bony attachments it is continuous with fascia covering popliteus and receives an expansion from the tendon of semimembranosus. At intermediate levels it is thin, but distally, where it covers the tendons behind the malleoli, it is again thick and continuous with the flexor and superior peroneal retinacula (p. 1508).

INTEROSSEOUS MEMBRANE (Fig. 113.26)

The interosseous membrane connects the interosseous borders of the tibia and fibula, and separates the anterior and posterior muscles in the leg, some of which are attached to it. The anterior tibial artery passes forwards through a large oval opening near the proximal end of the membrane; distally the perforating branch of the peroneal artery pierces it. Its fibres are predominantly oblique, and most descend laterally. Those which descend medially include a bundle at the proximal border of the proximal opening. The membrane is continuous distally with the interosseous ligament of the distal tibiofibular joint. Tibialis anterior, extensors digitorum longus and hallucis longus, peroneus tertius, the anterior tibial vessels and deep peroneal nerve are all anterior to it, and tibialis posterior and flexor hallucis longus are posterior.

RETINACULA

See page 1507.

OSTEOFASCIAL COMPARTMENTS

The compartments of the leg are particularly well defined and are the commonest sites of osteofascial compartment syndrome (p. 1399). There are three main compartments, anterior (extensor), lateral (peroneal) and posterior (flexor). They are enclosed peripherally by the unyielding deep fascia and separated from each other by the bones and interosseous membrane and by the anterior and posterior intermuscular septa that pass from the deep fascia to the fibula. The anterior compartment, the least expansile of the three, is surrounded by the deep fascia, the tibia, the interosseous membrane and the anterior intermuscular septum. The lateral compartment lies between the intermuscular septa, bordered laterally by the deep fascia and medially by the fibula. The posterior compartment is bounded by the deep fascia, the posterior intermuscular septum, both bones and the interosseous membrane. Its relatively expansile superficial component is separated from the more tense deep component by the deep transverse fascia, reinforced by the deep aponeurosis of soleus.

The nerve supply of the muscles in the compartments follows the 'one compartment – one nerve' principle. The nerve of the anterior compartment is the deep peroneal, that of the lateral compartment the superficial peroneal, and that of the posterior compartment the tibial nerve. Most of the muscles in the anterior compartment are supplied by the anterior tibial artery, with an additional contribution from the peroneal artery to extensor hallucis longus. Muscles in the posterior compartment are supplied by the popliteal, posterior tibial and peroneal arteries. Muscles in the lateral compartment are supplied by the anterior

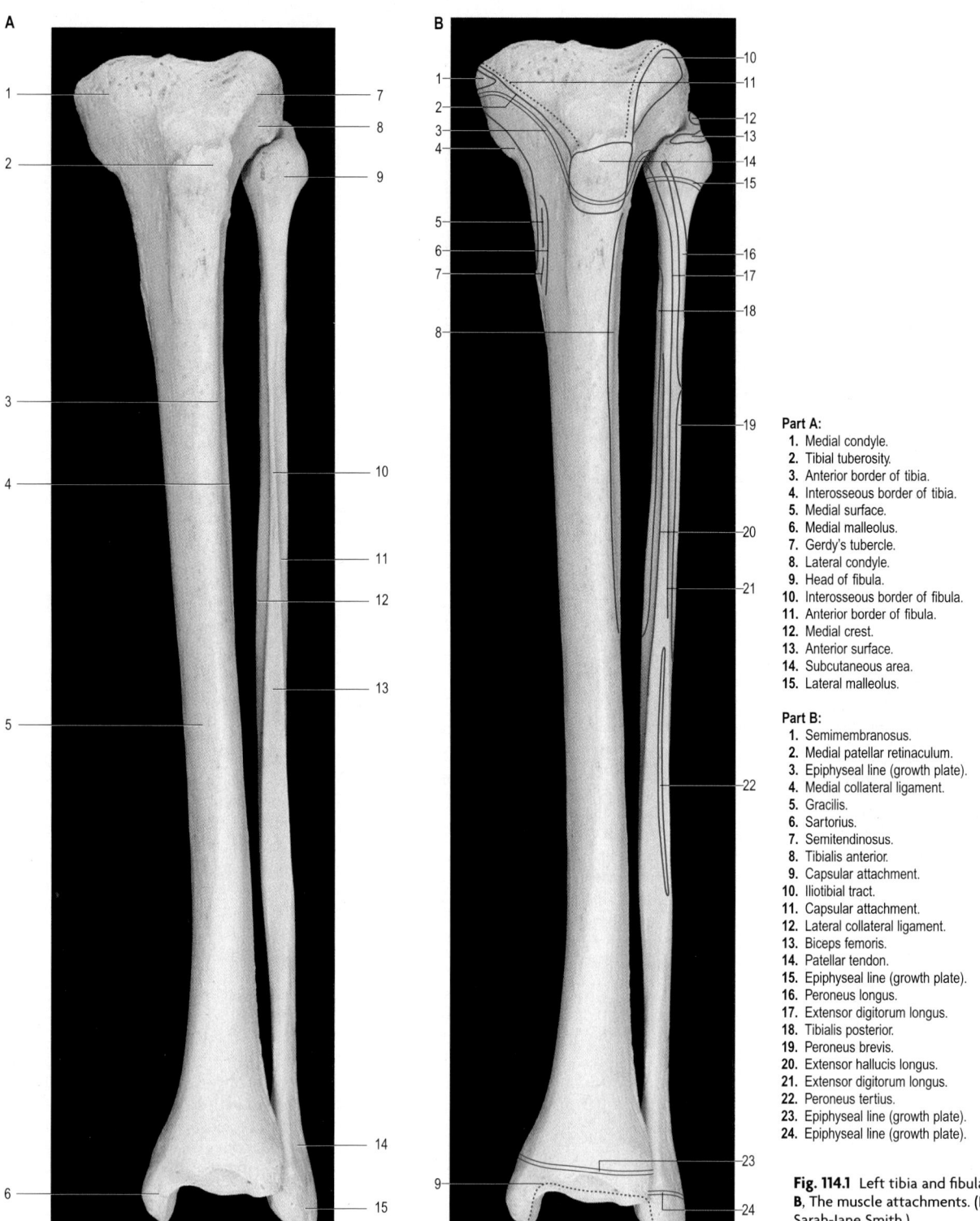

Part A:
1. Medial condyle.
2. Tibial tuberosity.
3. Anterior border of tibia.
4. Interosseous border of tibia.
5. Medial surface.
6. Medial malleolus.
7. Gerdy's tubercle.
8. Lateral condyle.
9. Head of fibula.
10. Interosseous border of fibula.
11. Anterior border of fibula.
12. Medial crest.
13. Anterior surface.
14. Subcutaneous area.
15. Lateral malleolus.

Part B:
1. Semimembranosus.
2. Medial patellar retinaculum.
3. Epiphyseal line (growth plate).
4. Medial collateral ligament.
5. Gracilis.
6. Sartorius.
7. Semitendinosus.
8. Tibialis anterior.
9. Capsular attachment.
10. Iliotibial tract.
11. Capsular attachment.
12. Lateral collateral ligament.
13. Biceps femoris.
14. Patellar tendon.
15. Epiphyseal line (growth plate).
16. Peroneus longus.
17. Extensor digitorum longus.
18. Tibialis posterior.
19. Peroneus brevis.
20. Extensor hallucis longus.
21. Extensor digitorum longus.
22. Peroneus tertius.
23. Epiphyseal line (growth plate).
24. Epiphyseal line (growth plate).

Fig. 114.1 Left tibia and fibula: anterior aspect. B, The muscle attachments. (Photographs by Sarah-Jane Smith.)

tibial and peroneal arteries, and to a small extent proximally by a branch from the popliteal system. The details of supply for each muscle are described on page 1495.

TRAUMA

The leg is especially vulnerable to trauma. The soft tissues of the shin are thin and the subcutaneous position of the medial tibia means that even trivial soft tissue injury can lead to serious problems such as ulceration and osteomyelitis. In the elderly these soft tissues are often especially thin and unhealthy, reflecting the effects of ageing and venous stasis. In the young, tibial fractures are common and, partly due to poor soft tissue coverage, may be open injuries. Reduction of blood supply to the bone, caused by stripping of attached soft tissues, and the risk of contamination add greatly to the risk of non-union and infection of the

fracture. At the junction of the middle and lower thirds of the tibia the blood supply to the bone is relatively poor. Fractures here are less likely to unite.

BONE

TIBIA (Figs 114.1, 114.2)

The tibia lies medial to the fibula and is exceeded in length only by the femur. Its shaft is triangular in section and has expanded ends: a strong medial malleolus projects distally from the smaller distal end. The anterior border is sharp and curves medially towards the medial malleolus. Together with the medial and lateral borders it defines the three surfaces of the bone. The exact shape and orientation of these

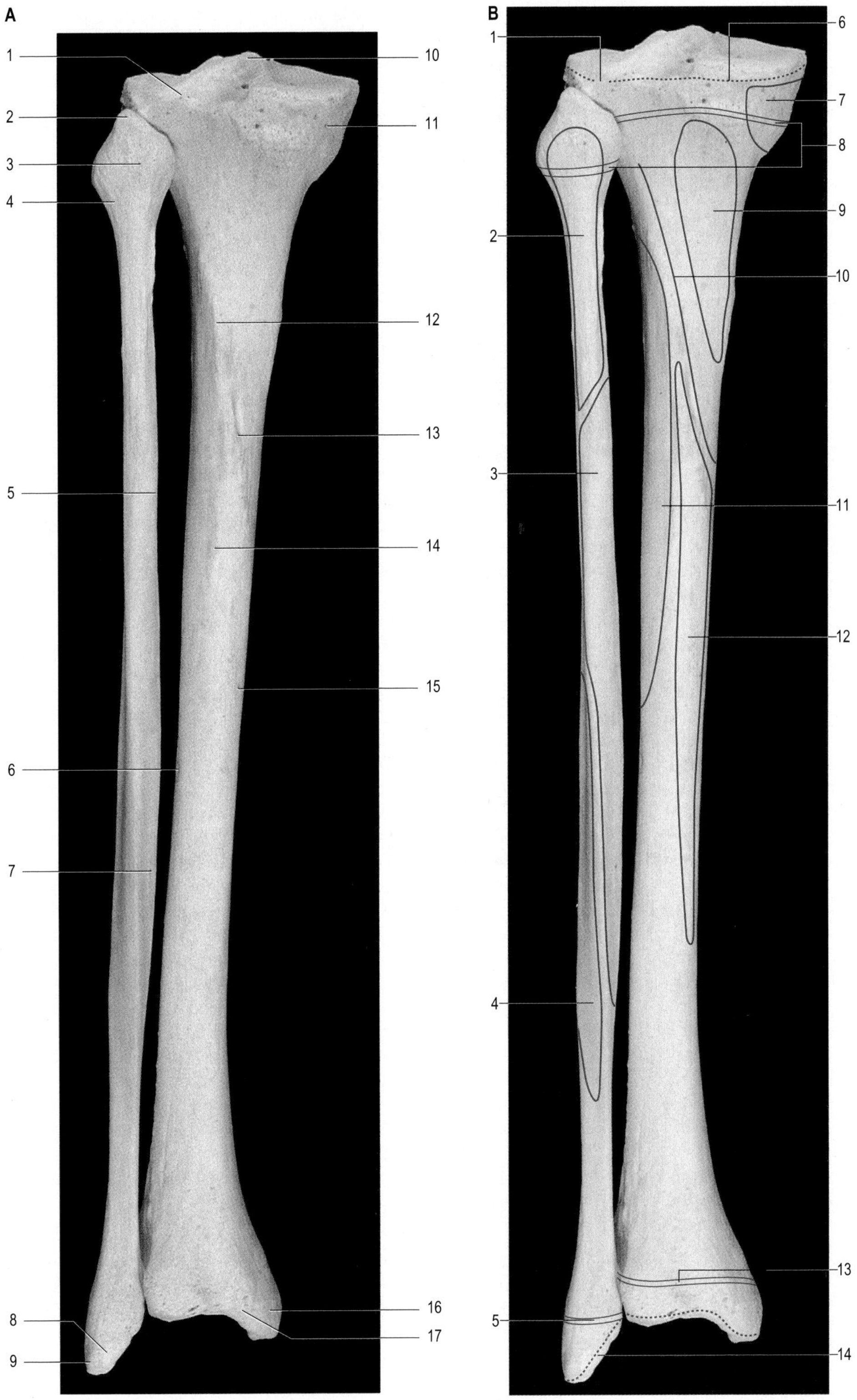

A

1
2
3
4
5
6
7
8
9

10
11
12
13
14
15
16
17

B

1
2
3
4
5

6
7
8
9
10
11
12
13
14

Part A:
1. Groove for tendon of popliteus.
2. Styloid process (apex) of fibula.
3. Head of fibula.
4. Neck of fibula.
5. Medial crest.
6. Interosseous border of tibia.
7. Posterior border.
8. Groove for peroneal tendons.
9. Lateral malleolus.
10. Intercondylar eminence.
11. Groove for semimembranosus attachment.
12. Soleal line.
13. Nutrient foramen.
14. Vertical line.
15. Medial border of tibia.
16. Medial malleolus.
17. Groove for tibialis posterior tendon.

Part B:
1. Gap in capsule for popliteus tendon.
2. Soleus.
3. Flexor hallucis longus.
4. Peroneus brevis.
5. Epiphyseal line (growth plate).
6. Capsular attachment.
7. Semimembranosus.
8. Epiphyseal lines (growth plates).
9. Popliteus.
10. Soleus.
11. Tibialis posterior.
12. Flexor digitorum longus.
13. Epiphyseal line (growth plate).
14. Capsular attachment.

Fig. 114.2 Left tibia and fibula: posterior aspect.
B, The muscle attachments. (Photographs by Sarah-Jane Smith.)

surfaces show individual and racial variations, some of which may be related to function.

Proximal end
The expanded proximal end is a bearing surface for body weight, which is transmitted through the femur. It has massive medial and lateral condyles, an intercondylar area and a tibial tuberosity.

Condyles – The tibial condyles overhang the proximal posterior surface of the shaft. Both have proximal articular surfaces separated by an irregular intercondylar area. The condyles are visible and palpable at the sides of the patellar tendon: the lateral is more prominent. In the passively flexed knee the anterior margins of the condyles are palpable in fossae flanking the patellar tendon.

The fibular facet on the lateral condyle faces distally and posterolaterally. The angle of inclination of the superior tibiofibular joint varies but may be horizontal or oblique. Superomedial to it the condyle is grooved posteriorly by the tendon of popliteus, with a synovial recess between the tendon and bone. The anterolateral aspect of the condyle is separated from the lateral surface of the shaft by a sharp margin for the attachment of deep fascia. The distal attachment of the iliotibial tract makes a flat but definite marking (which is triangular and facet-like) on its anterior aspect. This is Gerdy's tubercle and is usually palpable.

The anterior condylar surfaces are continuous with a large triangular area where the apex is distal and formed by the tibial tuberosity, and the lateral edge is a sharp ridge between the lateral condyle and lateral surface of the shaft.

The condyles, their articular surfaces and the intercondylar area are described in more detail on page 1474.

Tibial tuberosity – The tibial tuberosity is the truncated apex of a triangular area where the anterior condylar surfaces merge. It projects only a little, and is divided into a distal rough and a proximal smooth region. The distal region is palpable and is separated from skin by the subcutaneous infrapatellar bursa. A line across the tibial tuberosity marks the distal limit of the proximal tibial growth plate (**Fig. 114.1**). The patellar tendon is attached to the smooth bone proximal to this, its superficial fibres reaching a rough area distal to the line. The deep infrapatellar bursa and fibroadipose tissue intervene between the bone and tendon proximal to its site of attachment. The latter may be marked distally by a slight oblique ridge, to which the more lateral fibres insert more distally than the medial fibres. This knowledge is vital to avoid damaging the tendon when sawing the tibia transversely just above the tibial tuberosity in a lateral to medial direction, e.g. in performing an osteotomy. In habitual squatters a vertical groove on the anterior surface of the lateral condyle is occupied by the lateral edge of the patellar tendon in full flexion of the knee.

Shaft

The shaft is triangular in section and has (antero)medial, lateral and posterior surfaces separated by anterior, lateral (interosseous) and medial borders. It is thinnest at the junction of the middle and distal thirds, expanding towards both ends.

The anterior border descends from the tuberosity to the anterior margin of the medial malleolus and is subcutaneous throughout. Except in its distal fourth, where it is indistinct, it is a sharp crest. It is slightly sinuous, and turns medially in the distal fourth. The interosseous border begins distal and anterior to the fibular facet and descends to the anterior border of the fibular notch; it is indistinct proximally. The interosseous membrane is attached to most of its length, connecting tibia to fibula. The medial border descends from the anterior end of the groove on the medial condyle to the posterior margin of the medial malleolus. Its proximal and distal fourths are ill defined but its central region is sharp.

The anteromedial surface, between the anterior and medial borders, is broad, smooth and almost entirely subcutaneous. The lateral surface, between the anterior and interosseous borders, is also broad and smooth. It faces laterally in its proximal three-fourths and is transversely concave. Its distal fourth swerves anteriorly, because of the medial deviation of the anterior and distal interosseous borders. This part of the surface is somewhat convex. The posterior surface, between the interosseous and medial borders, is widest above, where it is crossed distally and medially by an oblique, rough soleal line. A faint vertical line descends from the centre of the soleal line, but soon fades. A large vascular groove adjoins the end of the line and descends distally into a nutrient foramen: it may be lateral or medial to the vertical line. Deep fascia and, proximal to the medial malleolus, the medial end of the superior extensor retinaculum, are attached to the anterior border. Posterior fibres of the medial collateral ligament and slips of semimembranosus and the popliteal fascia are attached to the medial border proximal to the soleal line, and some fibres of soleus and the fascia covering the deep calf muscles are attached distal to the line. The distal medial border merges into the medial lip of a groove for the tendon of tibialis posterior. The interosseous membrane is attached to the lateral border, except at its extremes. It is proximally indistinct where a large gap in the membrane transmits the anterior tibial vessels. Distally the border is the anterior boundary of the fibular notch, to which the anterior tibiofibular ligament is attached.

Proximally the medial surface bears, near the medial border, an area c.5 cm long and 1 cm wide for the attachment of the anterior part of the medial collateral ligament. The remaining surface is subcutaneous but crossed obliquely by the long saphenous vein.

The proximal two-thirds of the lateral surface gives attachment to tibialis anterior. Its distal third, devoid of attachments, is crossed in mediolateral order by the tendons of tibialis anterior (lying just lateral to the anterior border) and extensor hallucis longus, the anterior tibial vessels and deep peroneal nerve, extensor digitorum longus and peroneus tertius.

On the posterior surface, popliteus is attached in a triangular area proximal to the soleal line, except near the fibular facet. The popliteal aponeurosis, soleus and its fascia, and the deep transverse fascia are attached to the soleal line. Proximally the line does not reach the interosseous border, and it bears a tubercle for the medial end of the tendinous soleal arch. Lateral to the tubercle, the posterior tibial vessels and tibial nerve descend on tibialis posterior. Distal to the soleal line, a vertical line separates the attachments of flexor digitorum longus and tibialis posterior. Nothing is attached to the distal quarter of this surface, but it is crossed medially by the tendon of tibialis posterior travelling to a posterior groove on the medial malleolus. Flexor digitorum longus crosses obliquely behind tibialis posterior; the posterior tibial vessels and nerve and flexor hallucis longus contact only the lateral part of the distal posterior surface.

Distal end

The slightly expanded distal end of the tibia has anterior, medial, posterior, lateral and distal surfaces. It projects inferomedially as the medial malleolus. The distal end of the tibia, when compared to the proximal end, is laterally rotated (tibial torsion). The torsion starts *in utero* and progresses throughout childhood and adolescence to skeletal maturity. Tibial torsion is c.30° in Caucasian and Asian populations, but is significantly greater in people of African origin (Eckhoff et al 1994). In women it is not uncommon to see some persistence of the femoral neck anteversion that is seen in the newborn. This causes the femoral shaft and knee to be internally rotated. To prevent the feet turning inwards, the tibia can develop a compensatory external torsion.

The smooth anterior surface bulges beyond the distal surface, from which it is separated by a narrow groove, continuing the lateral surface of the shaft. The capsule of the ankle joint is attached to an anterior groove near the articular surface. The medial surface is smooth and continuous above and below with the medial surfaces of the shaft and malleolus: it is subcutaneous and visible. The posterior surface is crossed near its medial end by a nearly vertical but slightly oblique groove, which is usually conspicuous and extends to the posterior surface of the malleolus. Elsewhere it is smooth and continuous with the posterior surface of the shaft. The posterior groove is adapted to the tendon of tibialis posterior, which usually separates that of flexor digitorum longus from the bone. More laterally, the posterior tibial vessels and nerve and flexor hallucis longus contact this surface. The lateral surface is the triangular fibular notch: its anterior and posterior edges project and converge proximally to the interosseous border. The floor of the notch is roughened proximally by a substantial interosseous ligament but is smooth distally and sometimes covered by articular cartilage. The anterior and posterior tibiofibular ligaments are attached to the edges of the notch. The distal surface, articulating with the talus, is wider in front, concave sagittally and transversely slightly convex, i.e. saddle-shaped. Medially it continues into the malleolar articular surface. This articular surface may extend into the groove that separates it from the anterior surface of the shaft. Such extensions, medial or lateral or both, are squatting facets, and they articulate with reciprocal talar facets in extreme dorsiflexion. These features have been used in the evaluation of the racial origins of skeletal material.

Medial malleolus – The short thick medial malleolus has a smooth lateral surface with a crescentic facet that articulates with the medial talar surface. Its anterior aspect is rough and its posterior aspect continues the groove from the posterior surface of the shaft for the tendon of tibialis posterior. The distal border is pointed anteriorly, posteriorly depressed, and gives attachment to the deltoid ligament. The medial malleolus ends proximal to the lateral malleolus, which is also more posterior. The capsule of the ankle joint is attached to its anterior surface, and the flexor retinaculum to its prominent medial border.

Muscle attachments

The patellar tendon is attached to the tibial tuberosity.

Semimembranosus is attached to the distal edge of the groove on the posterior surface of the medial condyle. A tubercle at the lateral end of the groove is the main attachment of the tendon of this muscle.

Slips from the tendon of biceps femoris are attached anteroproximal to the fibular facet on the lateral condyle. Distal to the facet, proximal fibres of extensor digitorum longus and (occasionally) peroneus longus are attached.

Slips of semimembranosus are attached to the medial border of the shaft posteriorly, proximal to the soleal line. Some fibres of soleus attach to the posteromedial surface distal to the line.

Semimembranosus is attached to the medial surface proximally, near the medial border, behind the attachment of the anterior part of the medial collateral ligament. Anterior to this (from anterior to posterior), are the linear attachments of the tendons of sartorius, gracilis and semitendinosus: these rarely mark the bone.

Tibialis anterior is attached to the proximal two-thirds of the lateral surface.

Popliteus is attached to the posterior surface in a triangular area proximal to the soleal line, except near the fibular facet. Soleus and its associated fascia are attached to the soleal line itself.

Flexor digitorum longus and tibialis posterior are attached to the posterior surface distal to the soleal line, medial and lateral respectively to the vertical line.

Vascular supply

The proximal end of the tibia is supplied by metaphyseal vessels from the genicular arterial anastomosis (p. 1486).

The nutrient foramen usually lies near the soleal line and transmits a branch of the posterior tibial artery. However, this nutrient vessel may arise at the level of the popliteal bifurcation or branch from the anterior tibial artery. On entering the bone it divides to give more ascending than descending branches. The periosteal supply to the shaft arises from the anterior tibial artery and from muscular branches.

The distal metaphysis is supplied by branches from the anastomosis around the ankle (p. 1524).

Innervation

The proximal and distal ends of the tibia are innervated by branches from the nerves that supply the knee joint (p. 1482) and ankle joint (p. 1524) respectively. The periosteum of the shaft is supplied by branches from the nerves that innervate the muscles attached to the tibia.

Ossification (Figs 113.7, 113.8, 114.1, 114.2, 114.3)

The tibia ossifies from three centres, one in the shaft and one in each epiphysis. Ossification begins in midshaft at about the seventh intrauterine week. The proximal epiphyseal centre is usually present at birth: at c.10 years a thin anterior process from the centre descends to form the smooth part of the tibial tuberosity. A separate centre for the tuberosity may appear at about the twelfth year and soon fuses with the epiphysis. Distal strata of the epiphyseal plate are composed of dense collagenous tissue in which the fibres are aligned with the patellar tendon. Concentration of traction stress may account for Osgood–Schlatter disease, in which fragmentation of the epiphysis of the tuberosity occurs during adolescence. It produces a painful swelling in the region of the tuberosity. Healing occurs once the growth plate fuses, leaving a bony protrusion. Prolonged periods of traction with the knee extended, in both children and adolescents, can lead to growth arrest of the anterior part of the

proximal epiphysis, which results in bowing of the proximal tibia as the posterior tibia continues to grow. The proximal epiphysis fuses in the sixteenth year in females and the eighteenth in males.

The distal epiphyseal centre appears early in the first year and joins the shaft in about the fifteenth year in females and the seventeenth in males. The medial malleolus is an extension from the distal epiphysis and starts to ossify in the seventh year: it may have its own separate centre.

FIBULA (Figs 114.1, 114.2)

The fibula is much more slender than the tibia and is not directly involved in transmission of weight. It has a proximal head, a narrow neck, a long shaft and a distal lateral malleolus. The shaft varies in form, being variably moulded by attached muscles: these variations may be confusing.

Head

The head of the fibula projects in front, behind and laterally. A round facet on its proximomedial aspect articulates with a facet on the inferolateral surface of the lateral tibial condyle. It faces proximally and anteromedially at an angle which is roughly horizontal or at c. 45°. A blunt apex (styloid process) projects proximally from the posterolateral aspect of the head and is palpable c.2 cm distal to the knee joint. The fibular collateral ligament is attached in front of the apex, embraced by the main attachments of biceps femoris. The tibiofibular capsular ligament is attached to the margins of the articular facet.

The common peroneal nerve crosses posterolateral to the neck and can be rolled against bone there.

Shaft (Fig. 114.4)

The shaft has three borders and surfaces, each associated with a particular group of muscles. The anterior border ascends proximally from the apex of an elongated triangular area that is continuous with the lateral malleolar surface to the anterior aspect of the fibular head. The posterior border, continuous with the medial margin of the posterior groove on the lateral malleolus, is usually distinct distally but often rounded in its proximal half. The interosseous border is medial to the anterior border and usually more posterior; in the proximal two-thirds of the bone they approximate, the 'surface' being narrowed to 1 mm or less.

The lateral surface, between the anterior and posterior borders and associated with the peroneal muscles, faces laterally in its proximal three-fourths. The distal quarter spirals to become continuous with the posterior groove of the lateral malleolus. The anteromedial (sometimes simply termed anterior, or medial) surface, between the anterior and interosseous borders, usually faces anteromedially but often directly anteriorly. It is associated with the extensor muscles. Though wide

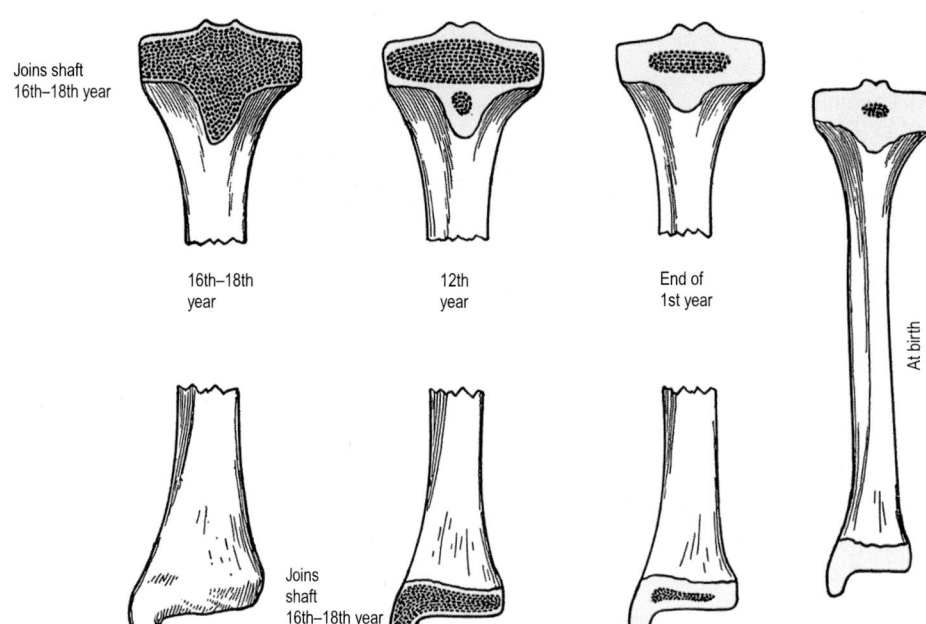

Joins shaft
16th–18th year

16th–18th year

12th year

End of 1st year

At birth

Joins shaft
16th–18th year

Fig. 114.3 Stages in the ossification of the tibia (not to scale). Blue = unossified (cartilaginous) regions.

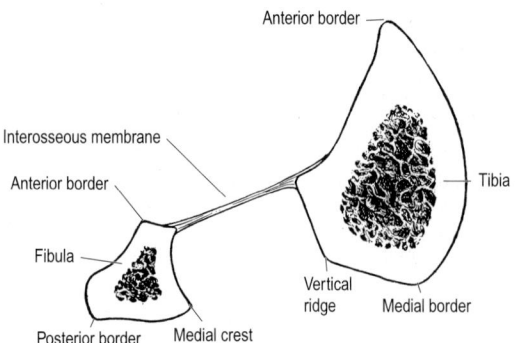

Fig. 114.4 Transverse (axial) section through the left tibia and fibula, showing the attachment of the interosseous membrane.

distally, it narrows in its proximal half and may become merely a ridge. The posterior surface, between the interosseous and posterior borders, is the largest and is associated with the flexor muscles. Its proximal two-thirds is divided by a longitudinal medial crest, separated from the interosseous border by a grooved surface that is directed medially. The remaining surface faces posteriorly in its proximal half; its distal half curves onto the medial aspect. Distally this area occupies the fibular notch of the tibia, which is roughened by the attachment of the principal interosseous tibiofibular ligament. The triangular area proximal to the lateral surface of the lateral malleolus is subcutaneous; muscles cover the rest of the shaft.

The anterior border is divided distally into two ridges that enclose a triangular subcutaneous surface. The anterior intermuscular septum is attached to its proximal three-fourths. The lateral end of the superior extensor retinaculum is attached distally on the anterior border of the triangular area. The lateral end of the superior peroneal retinaculum is attached distally on the posterior margin of the triangular area. The interosseous border ends at the proximal limit of the rough area for the interosseous ligament. The interosseous membrane attached to this border does not reach the fibular head, leaving space for the anterior tibial vessels. The posterior border is proximally indistinct, and the posterior intermuscular septum is attached to all but its distal end. The medial crest is related to the peroneal artery. Attached to the medial crest is a layer of deep fascia, which separates the tendon of tibialis posterior from flexor hallucis longus and flexor digitorum longus.

Lateral malleolus (Fig. 114.5)

The distal end forms the lateral malleolus, which projects distally and posteriorly. Its lateral aspect is subcutaneous while its posterior aspect has a broad groove with a prominent lateral border. Its anterior aspect is rough, round and continuous with the tibial inferior border. The medial surface has a triangular articular facet, vertically convex, its apex distal, which articulates with the lateral talar surface. Behind this facet is a rough malleolar fossa pitted by vascular foramina. The posterior tibiofibular ligament and, more distally, the posterior talofibular ligament, are attached posteriorly in the fossa. The anterior talofibular ligament is attached to the anterior surface of the lateral malleolus; the calcaneofibular ligament is attached to the notch anterior to its apex. The tendons of peroneus brevis and longus groove its posterior aspect: the latter is superficial and covered by the superior peroneal retinaculum (p. 1508).

Muscle attachments

The main attachments of biceps femoris embrace the fibular collateral ligament in front of the apex (styloid process) of the fibular head. Extensor digitorum longus is attached to the head anteriorly, peroneus longus anterolaterally, and soleus posteriorly.

Extensor digitorum longus, extensor hallucis longus and peroneus tertius are attached to the anteromedial (extensor) surface.

Peroneus longus is attached to the whole width of the lateral (peroneal) surface in its proximal third, but in its middle third only to its posterior part, behind peroneus brevis. The latter continues its attachment almost to the distal end of the shaft.

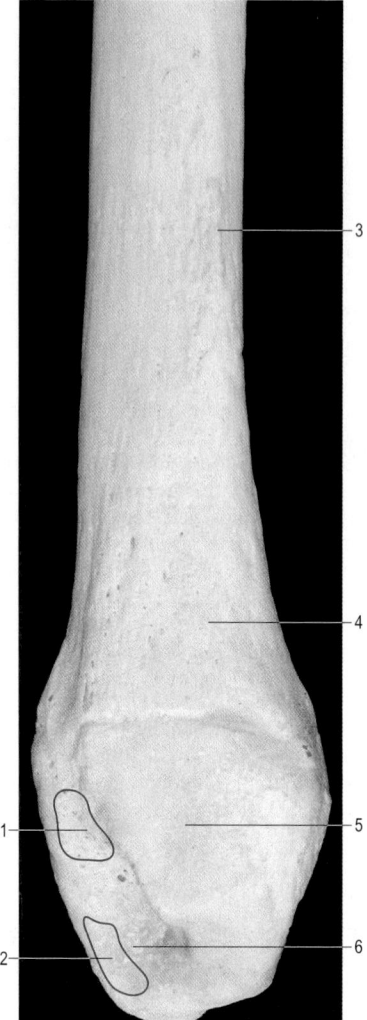

1. Attachment of posterior tibiofibular ligament.
2. Attachment of posterior talofibular ligament.
3. Area for attachments of interosseous ligament.
5. Articular facet for talus.
6. Malleolar fossa.

Fig. 114.5 Distal end of left fibula: medial aspect. (Photograph by Sarah-Jane Smith.)

Muscle attachments to the posterior surface, which is divided longitudinally by the medial crest, are complex. Between the crest and interosseous border the posterior surface is concave. Tibialis posterior is attached throughout most (the proximal three-fourths) of this area; an intramuscular tendon may ridge the bone obliquely. Soleus is attached between the crest and the posterior border on the proximal fourth of the posterior surface; its tendinous arch is attached to the surface proximally. Flexor hallucis longus is attached distal to soleus on the posterior surface and almost reaches the distal end of the shaft.

Vascular supply

A little proximal to the midpoint of the posterior surface (c.14–19 cm from the styloid process), the fibular shaft is pierced by a nutrient foramen, directed distally, which receives a branch of the peroneal artery (p. 1503). The detailed anatomy of the peroneal artery in relation to the fibula is the key to raising osteofasciocutaneous free flaps incorporating segments of the bone. Free vascularized diaphysis grafts may also be taken on a peroneal arterial pedicle. The proximal and distal ends receive metaphyseal vessels from the genicular (p. 1486) and ankle (p. 1524) arterial anastomoses respectively.

Innervation

The proximal and distal ends of the bone are supplied by branches of nerves that innervate the knee and superior tibiofibular joint and the ankle and inferior tibiofibular joints respectively. The periosteum of the shaft is supplied by branches from the nerves that innervate the muscles attached to the fibula.

Ossification (Figs 114.6, 114.7)

The fibula ossifies from three centres, one each for the shaft and the extremities. The process begins in the shaft at about the eighth intrauterine week, in the distal end in the first year, and in the proximal end

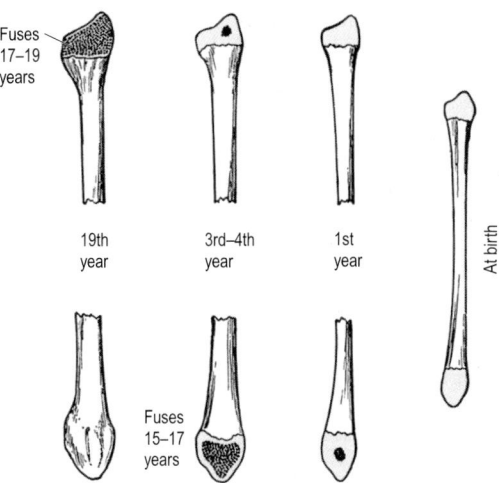

Fuses
17–19
years

19th
year

3rd–4th
year

1st
year

At birth

Fuses
15–17
years

Fig. 114.6 Stages in the ossification of the fibula (not to scale). Blue = unossified (cartilaginous) regions.

at about the third year in females and the fourth in males. The distal epiphysis unites with the shaft at about the fifteenth year in females and the seventeenth in males, whereas the proximal epiphysis does not unite until about the seventeenth year in females and the nineteenth in males, despite having appeared earlier. In this respect the fibula reverses the usual pattern of ossification in long bones.

MUSCLES

The muscles of the leg consist of an anterior group of extensor muscles, which produce dorsiflexion (extension) of the ankle; a posterior group of flexor muscles, which produce plantar flexion (flexion); and a lateral group of muscles derived from the extensors, the peronei. The greater bulk of the muscles in the calf is consistent with the powerful propulsive role of the plantar flexors in walking and running.

ANTERIOR OR EXTENSOR COMPARTMENT (Figs 114.8, 114.9, 114.10, 114.11) The anterior compartment contains muscles that dorsiflex the ankle when acting from above, and act from below to pull the body forward on the fixed foot during walking. Two of the muscles, the common digital extensor and extensor hallucis longus, also extend the toes, and two muscles, tibialis anterior and peroneus tertius, have the additional actions of inversion and eversion respectively.

Tibialis anterior

Attachments – Tibialis anterior is a superficial muscle and is therefore readily palpable lateral to the tibia. It arises from the lateral condyle and proximal half to two-thirds of the lateral surface of the tibial shaft; the adjoining anterior surface of the interosseous membrane; the deep surface of the deep fascia; and the intermuscular septum between itself and extensor digitorum longus. The muscle descends vertically and ends in a tendon on its anterior surface in the lower third of the leg. The tendon passes through the medial compartments of the superior and inferior retinacula (p. 1507), inclines medially, and is inserted into the medial and inferior surfaces of the medial cuneiform and the adjoining part of the base of the first metatarsal bone.

Attachments to the talus, first metatarsal head, base of the proximal phalanx of the hallux, and extensor retinaculum have been recorded.

Relations – Tibialis anterior overlaps the anterior tibial vessels and deep peroneal nerve in the upper part of the leg. It lies on the tibia and interosseous membrane. Extensor digitorum longus and extensor hallucis longus lie laterally.

Vascular supply – The main body of tibialis anterior is supplied by a series of medial and anterior branches of the anterior tibial artery: the branches may occur in two columns. There is a proximal accessory supply from the anterior tibial recurrent artery. The tendon is supplied

A

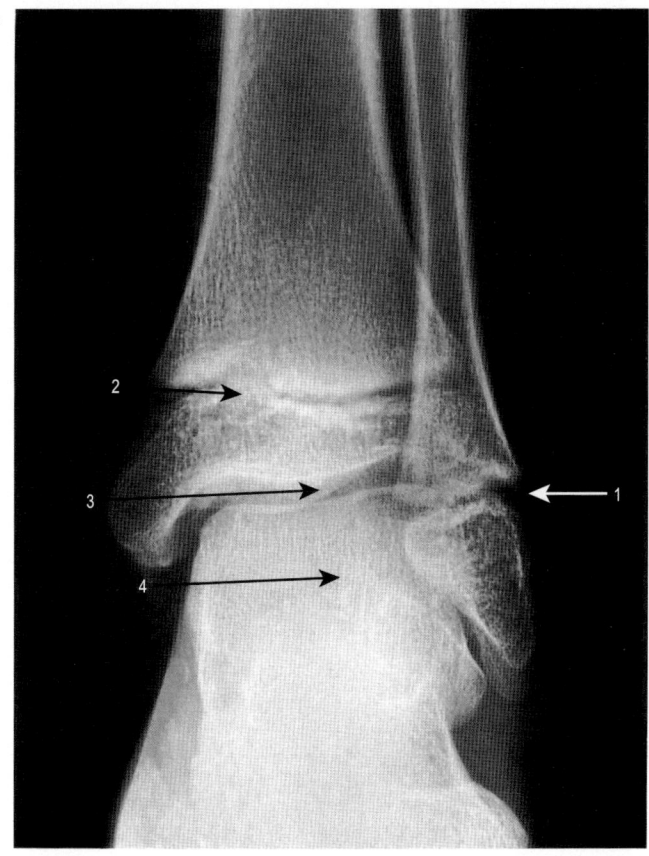

1. Inferior growth plate of fibula.   2. Inferior growth plate of tibia.   3. Ankle joint.   4. Talus.

B

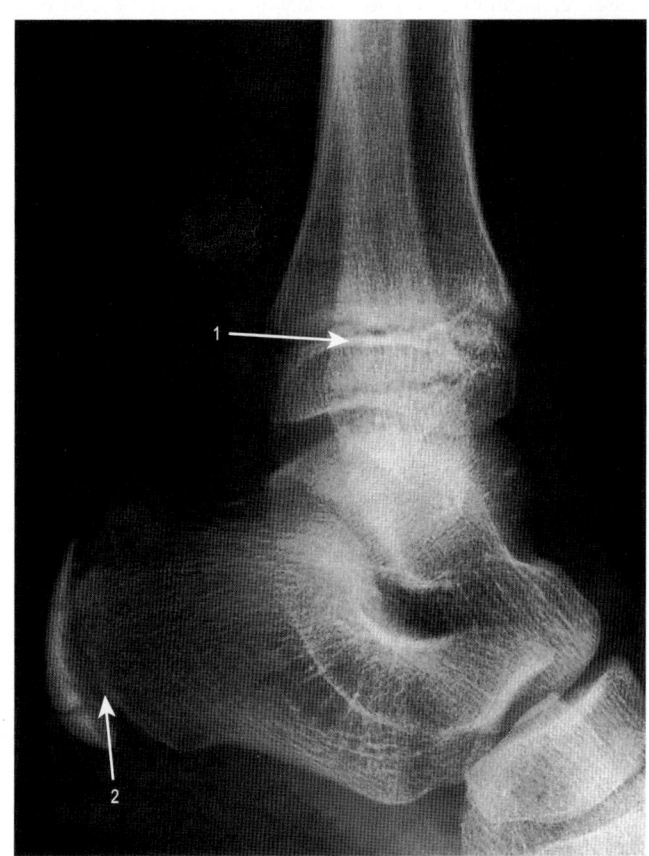

1. Tibial growth plate.   2. Posterior growth plate of calcaneus.

Fig. 114.7 Radiograph of ankle of child of 10 in plantar flexion. **A**, Oblique anteroposterior view. Note that the fibular growth plate is approximately at the level of the ankle joint. **B**, Lateral view. Note the trabecular pattern in the calcaneus.

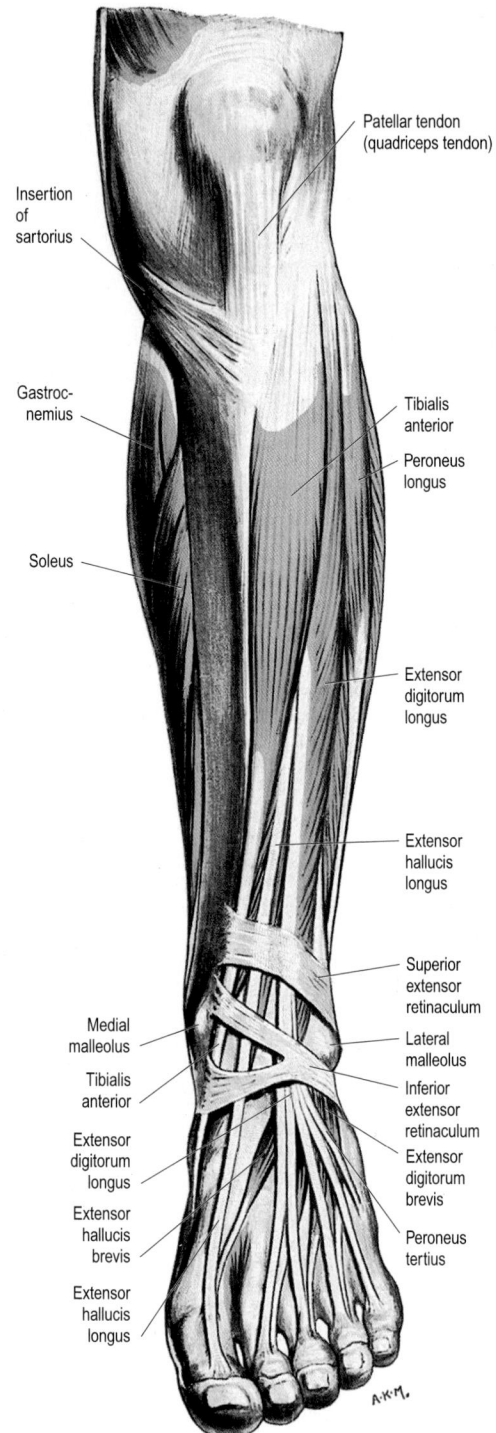

Insertion of sartorius

Gastroc-nemius

Soleus

Medial malleolus

Tibialis anterior

Extensor digitorum longus

Extensor hallucis brevis

Extensor hallucis longus

Patellar tendon (quadriceps tendon)

Tibialis anterior

Peroneus longus

Extensor digitorum longus

Extensor hallucis longus

Superior extensor retinaculum

Lateral malleolus

Inferior extensor retinaculum

Extensor digitorum brevis

Peroneus tertius

Fig. 114.8 Muscles of the left leg: anterior aspect. (From Schaefer EA, Symington J, Bryce TH (eds) 1915 Quain's Anatomy, 11th edn. London: Longmans, Green, with permission from Pearson Education.)

by the anterior medial malleolar artery and network, dorsalis pedis artery, medial tarsal arteries, and medial malleolar and calcaneal branches of the posterior tibial artery.

Innervation – Tibialis anterior is innervated by the deep peroneal nerve, L4 and 5.

Actions – Tibialis anterior is a dorsiflexor of the ankle joint and invertor of the foot. It is most active when both movements are combined, as in walking. Its tendon can be seen through the skin lateral to the anterior border of the tibia and can be traced downwards and medially across the front of the ankle to the medial side of the foot. It elevates the first metatarsal base and medial cuneiform and rotates their dorsal aspects laterally.

The muscle is usually quiescent in a standing subject, since the weight of the body acts through a vertical line that passes anterior to the ankle joints. Acting from below, it helps to counteract any tendency to overbalance backwards by flexing the leg forwards at the ankle. It has a role in supporting the medial longitudinal arch of the foot: although electromyographic activity is minimal during standing, it is manifest during any movement that increases the arch, such as toe-off in walking and running.

Testing – Tibialis anterior can be seen to act when the foot is dorsiflexed against resistance.

Extensor hallucis longus

Attachments – Extensor hallucis longus lies between, and partly deep to, tibialis anterior and extensor digitorum longus. It arises from the middle half of the medial surface of the fibula, medial to extensor digitorum longus, and to a similar extent from the adjacent anterior surface of the interosseous membrane. Its fibres run distally and end in a tendon that forms on the anterior border of the muscle. The tendon passes deep to the superior extensor retinaculum and through the inferior extensor retinaculum (p. 1507), crosses to the medial side of the anterior tibial vessels near the ankle, and is inserted into the dorsal aspect of the base of the distal phalanx of the hallux. At the metatarsophalangeal joint a thin prolongation from each side of the tendon covers the dorsal surface of the joint. An expansion from the medial side of the tendon to the base of the proximal phalanx is usually present.

Extensor hallucis longus is sometimes united with extensor digitorum longus. It may send a slip into the second toe.

Relations – The anterior tibial vessels and deep peroneal nerve lie between extensor hallucis longus and tibialis anterior. Extensor hallucis longus lies lateral to the artery proximally, crosses it in the lower third of the leg, and is medial to it on the foot.

Vascular supply – Extensor hallucis longus is supplied by the anterior tibial artery via obliquely running branches, with a variable contribution from the perforating branch of the peroneal artery. More distally, the tendon is supplied via the anterior medial malleolar artery and network, the dorsalis pedis artery, and the arteries of the first ray with perforating branches from the medial sole.

Innervation – Extensor hallucis longus is innervated by the deep peroneal nerve, L5.

Actions – Extensor hallucis longus extends the phalanges of the hallux and dorsiflexes the foot. When the hallux is actively extended, relatively little external force is required to overcome the extension of the distal phalanx, whereas considerable force is needed to overcome the extension of the proximal phalanx.

Testing – When the hallux is extended (dorsiflexed) against resistance, the tendon of extensor hallucis longus can be seen and felt on the lateral side of the tendon of tibialis anterior. This is a useful and very specific test of the integrity of the L5 spinal nerve.

Extensor digitorum longus

Attachments – Extensor digitorum longus arises from the lateral condyle of the tibia, proximal three-quarters of the medial surface of the fibula, adjacent anterior surface of the interosseous membrane, deep surface of the deep fascia, anterior crural intermuscular septum, and the septum between itself and tibialis anterior. These origins form the walls of an osseo-aponeurotic tunnel. Extensor digitorum longus becomes tendinous at about the same level as tibialis anterior, and the tendon passes behind the superior extensor retinaculum and within a loop of the inferior extensor retinaculum (p. 1507) with peroneus tertius (**Figs 115.2, 115.3**). It divides into four slips, which run forward on the dorsum of the foot and are attached in the same way as the tendons of extensor digitorum in the hand. At the metatarsophalangeal joints the tendons to the second, third and fourth toes are each joined on the lateral side by a tendon of extensor digitorum brevis. The dorsal digital expansion thus formed on the dorsal aspect of the proximal phalanx, like that on the fingers, receives contributions from the lumbrical and interosseous muscles. The expansion narrows as it approaches a

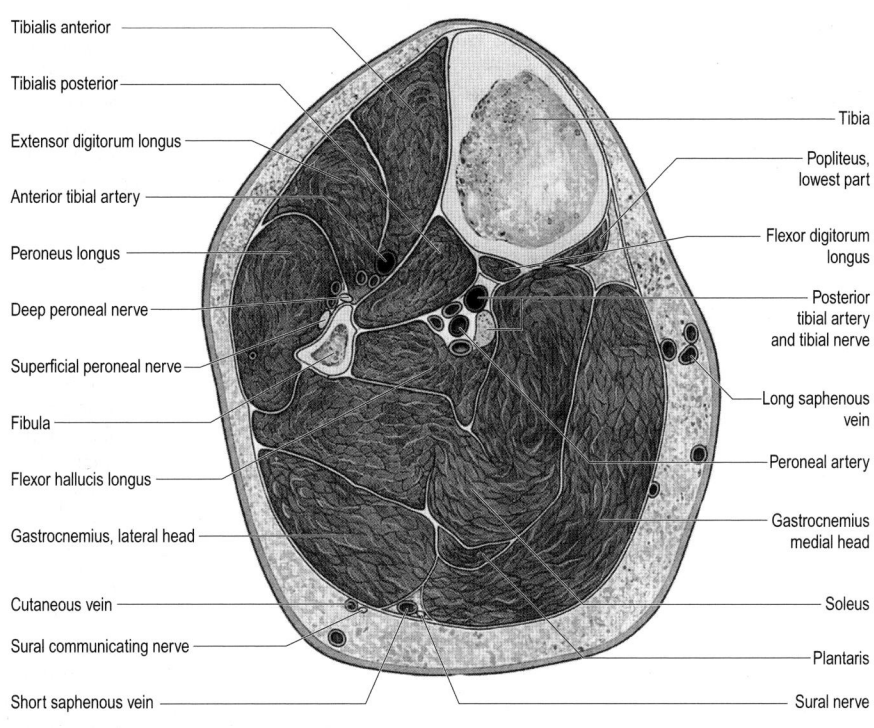

Tibialis anterior

Tibialis posterior

Extensor digitorum longus

Anterior tibial artery

Peroneus longus

Deep peroneal nerve

Superficial peroneal nerve

Fibula

Flexor hallucis longus

Gastrocnemius, lateral head

Cutaneous vein

Sural communicating nerve

Short saphenous vein

Tibia

Popliteus,
lowest part

Flexor digitorum
longus

Posterior
tibial artery
and tibial nerve

Long saphenous
vein

Peroneal artery

Gastrocnemius
medial head

Soleus

Plantaris

Sural nerve

Fig. 114.9 Transverse (axial) section through the left leg, c.10 cm distal to the knee joint.

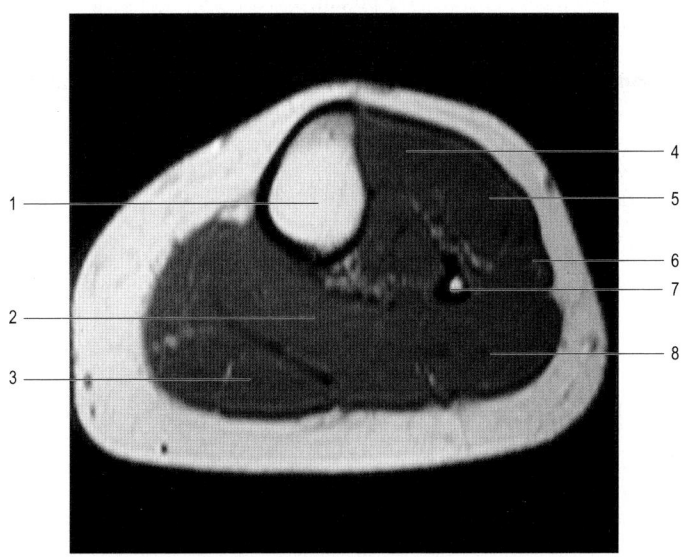

1. Tibia.   2. Soleus.   3. Medial head of gastrocnemius.   4. Tibialis anteroir.
5. Extensor digitorum longus.   6. Peroneus longus.   7. Fibula.   8. Lateral head of gastrocnemius.

Fig. 114.10 Axial T1-weighted magnetic resonance image (MRI) of the leg at a level similar to that of **Fig. 114.9**. (By kind permission from Dr Justin Lee, Chelsea and Westminster Hospital, London.)

proximal interphalangeal joint, and divides into three slips. These are an intermediate slip, attached to the base of the middle phalanx, and two collateral slips, which reunite on the dorsum of the middle phalanx and are attached to the base of the distal phalanx.

The tendons to the second and fifth toes are sometimes doubled, and accessory slips may be attached to metatarsals or to the hallux.

Relations – Extensor digitorum longus lies on the lateral tibial condyle, fibula, lower end of the tibia, ankle joint and extensor brevis. Tibialis anterior and extensor hallucis longus lie medially in the leg, and the peroneal muscles lie laterally. In the upper part of the leg the anterior

tibial vessels and deep peroneal nerve lie between extensor digitorum longus and tibialis anterior; the nerve runs obliquely medially beneath its upper part.

Vascular supply – The main blood supply to extensor digitorum longus is derived from anteriorly and laterally placed branches of the anterior tibial artery, supplemented distally from the perforating branch of the peroneal artery. Proximally there may also be a supply from the lateral inferior genicular, popliteal or anterior tibial recurrent arteries. At the ankle and in the foot, the tendons are supplied by the anterior lateral malleolar artery and network, and by lateral tarsal, metatarsal plantar and digital arteries.

Innervation – Extensor digitorum longus is innervated by the deep peroneal nerve, L5, S1.

Actions – Extensor digitorum longus extends the toes, and it dorsiflexes the ankle synergistically with tibialis anterior and extensor hallucis longus. Acting with the latter it tightens the plantar aponeurosis.

Testing – The tendons of extensor digitorum longus can be seen when the toes are extended (dorsiflexed) against resistance.

Peroneus tertius

Attachments – Peroneus tertius (fibularis tertius) is a uniquely human muscle. It often appears to be part of extensor digitorum longus, and might be described as its 'fifth tendon'. The muscle fibres operating on this tendon arise from the distal third or more of the medial surface of the fibula, the adjoining anterior surface of the interosseous membrane, and the anterior crural intermuscular septum. The tendon passes behind the superior extensor retinaculum and within the loop of the inferior extensor retinaculum it shares with extensor digitorum longus (p. 1507 and **Figs 115.2, 115.3**). It is inserted into the medial part of the dorsal surface of the base of the fifth metatarsal bone, and a thin expansion usually extends forwards along the medial border of the shaft of the bone.

Peroneus tertius is highly variable in its form and muscle bulk but is rarely completely absent. It may be attached to the fourth metatarsal rather than the fifth.

Relations – Peroneus tertius lies lateral to extensor digitorum longus.

1497

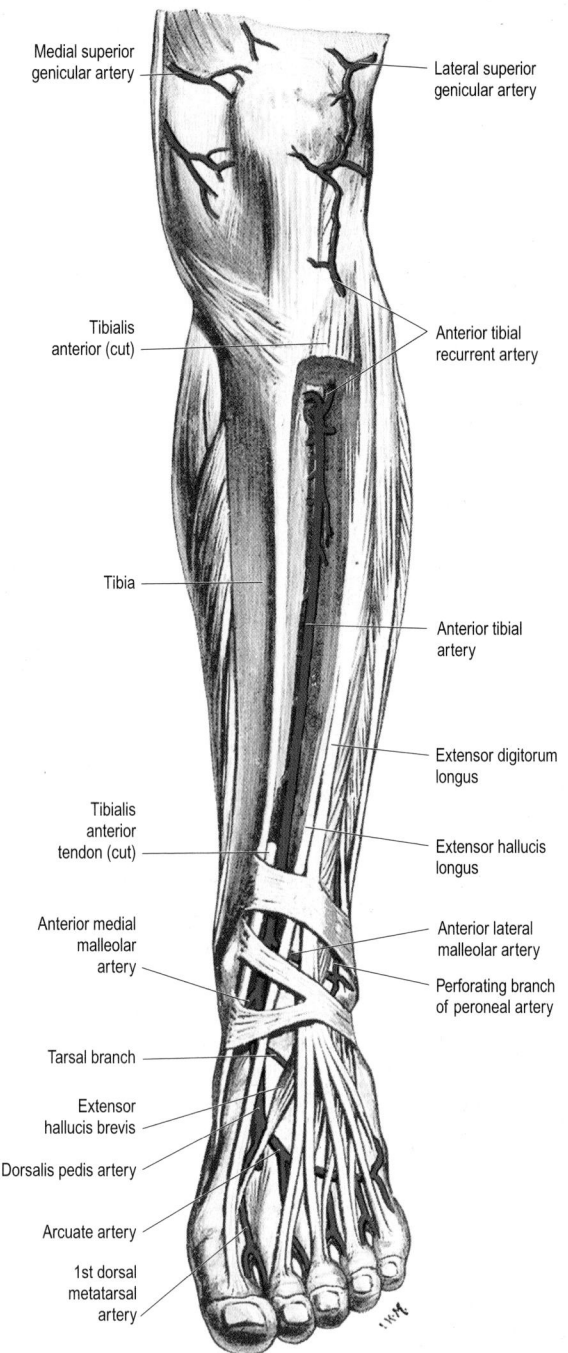

Medial superior
genical artery

Lateral superior
genicular artery

Tibialis
anterior (cut)

Anterior tibial
recurrent artery

Tibia

Anterior tibial
artery

Extensor digitorum
longus

Tibialis
anterior
tendon (cut)

Extensor hallucis
longus

Anterior medial
malleolar
artery

Anterior lateral
malleolar artery

Perforating branch
of peroneal artery

Tarsal branch

Extensor
hallucis brevis

Dorsalis pedis artery

Arcuate artery

1st dorsal
metatarsal
artery

Fig. 114.11 The left anterior tibial and dorsalis pedis arteries. To expose the anterior tibial artery a large part of tibialis anterior has been excised and extensor hallucis longus is retracted laterally.

Vascular supply – Peroneus tertius is supplied by the same vessels as extensor digitorum longus. In the foot it receives an additional supply from the termination of the arcuate artery and the fourth dorsal metacarpal artery.

Innervation – Peroneus tertius is innervated by the deep peroneal nerve, L5, S1.

Actions – During the swing phase of gait (**Fig. 115.38**) electromyographic studies show that peroneus tertius acts with extensor digitorum longus and tibialis anterior to produce dorsiflexion and eversion of the foot (Jungers et al 1993). This levels the foot and helps the toes to clear the ground, an action that improves the economy of bipedal walking. Peroneus tertius is not active during stance phase, a finding that contradicts suggestions that it acts primarily to support the

lateral longitudinal arch or to transfer the centre of pressure of the foot medially.

Testing – Peroneus tertius cannot be tested in isolation, but its tendon can sometimes be seen when the foot is dorsiflexed against resistance.

LATERAL (PERONEAL OR FIBULAR) COMPARTMENT (Figs 113.2, 113.28, 114.8, 114.9, 114.10)

The lateral compartment contains peroneus (fibularis) longus and peroneus (fibularis) brevis. Both evert the foot and are plantar flexors of the ankle, and both probably play a part in balancing the leg on the foot in standing and walking.

Peroneus longus

Attachments – Peroneus longus is the more superficial of the two lateral compartment muscles. It arises from the head and proximal two-thirds of the lateral surface of the fibula, the deep surface of the deep fascia, the anterior and posterior crural intermuscular septa, and occasionally by a few fibres from the lateral condyle of the tibia. The muscle belly ends in a long tendon that runs distally behind the lateral malleolus in a groove it shares with the tendon of peroneus brevis. The groove is converted into a canal by the superior peroneal retinaculum, so that the tendon of peroneus longus, and that of peroneus brevis which lies behind it, are contained in a common synovial sheath. If the peroneal retinaculum is ruptured by injury and fails to heal, the tendons can dislocate from the groove. The peroneus longus tendon runs obliquely forwards across the lateral side of the calcaneus, below the peroneal trochlea and the tendon of peroneus brevis, and beneath the inferior peroneal retinaculum. It crosses the lateral side of the cuboid and then runs under the cuboid in a groove that is converted into a canal by the long plantar ligament (**Fig. 115.35**). It crosses the sole of the foot obliquely and is attached by two slips to the lateral side of the base of the first metatarsal bone and the medial cuneiform; occasionally a third slip is extended to the base of the second metatarsal bone. The tendon changes direction below the lateral malleolus and on the cuboid bone. At both sites it is thickened and at the second a sesamoid fibrocartilage (sometimes a bone, the os peroneum) usually develops within it. A second synovial sheath invests the tendon as it crosses the sole of the foot.

Relations – Proximally peroneus longus lies posterior to extensor digitorum longus and anterior to soleus and flexor hallucis longus. Distally in the leg it lies posterior to peroneus brevis. Between its attachments to the head and shaft of the fibula there is a gap through which the common peroneal nerve passes.

Vascular supply of lateral compartment – Usually the predominant supply of the lateral compartment muscles is derived from superior and inferior branches of the anterior tibial artery; the superior is commonly much the larger. There is also a lesser, variable, contribution from the peroneal artery in the distal part of the leg. A peroneal branch may replace the inferior anterior tibial branch; less often the peroneal artery provides the main supply to the whole compartment. The upper part of peroneus longus is also supplied by the circumflex fibular artery, which is usually a branch of the anterior tibial artery but sometimes arises more proximally. The companion artery to the common peroneal nerve, a branch of the popliteal artery, provides a minor contribution proximally. Distally the tendons are supplied by the peroneal perforating, anterior lateral malleolar, lateral calcaneal, lateral tarsal, arcuate, lateral and medial plantar arteries (**Fig. 115.16**).

Innervation – Peroneus longus is innervated by the superficial peroneal nerve, L5, S1.

Actions – There is little doubt that peroneus longus can evert the foot and plantar flex the ankle, and possibly act on the leg from its distal attachments. The oblique direction of its tendon across the sole would also enable it to support the longitudinal and transverse arches of the foot. With the foot off the ground, eversion is visually and palpably associated with increased prominence of both tendon and muscle. It is not clear to what extent this helps to maintain plantigrade contact of the foot in normal standing, but electromyographic records show little or no peroneal activity under these conditions. Peroneal activity is necessary to stand plantigrade with the legs crossed. Peroneus longus and brevis come strongly into action to maintain the concavity of the foot during toe-off and tip-toeing. If the subject deliberately sways to one side, the peronei contract on that side, but their involvement in postural activity between the foot and leg remains uncertain.

Testing – Peroneus longus and brevis are tested together by eversion of the foot against resistance: the tendons can be identified laterally at the ankle and in the foot.

Peroneus brevis

Attachments – Peroneus brevis arises from the distal two-thirds of the lateral surface of the fibula, anterior to peroneus longus, and from the anterior and posterior crural intermuscular septa. It passes vertically downwards and ends in a tendon that passes behind the lateral malleolus together with, but anterior to, that of peroneus longus. The two tendons run deep to the superior peroneal retinaculum in a common synovial sheath. The tendon of peroneus brevis then runs forwards on the lateral side of the calcaneus above the peroneal trochlea and the tendon of peroneus longus, and is inserted into a tubercle on the base of the fifth metatarsal bone, on its lateral side.

Relations – Anteriorly lie extensor digitorum longus and peroneus tertius. Peroneus longus and flexor hallucis longus are posterior. On the lateral surface of the calcaneus the tendons of peronei longus and brevis occupy separate osseo-aponeurotic canals formed by the calcaneus and the inferior peroneal retinaculum; each tendon is enveloped in a separate forward prolongation of the common synovial sheath (**Fig. 115.2**).

Vascular supply – See under peroneus longus.

Innervation – Peroneus brevis is innervated by the superficial peroneal nerve, L5, S1.

Actions – Peroneus brevis may limit inversion of the foot and so relieve strain on the ligaments that are tightened by this movement (lateral part of interosseous talocalcaneal, lateral talocalcaneal and calcaneofibular), see page 1524. It participates in eversion of the foot and may help to steady the leg on the foot.
See also under peroneus longus.

Testing – See under peroneus longus.

Variants of peroneal muscles – Tendinous slips from peroneus longus may extend to the base of the third, fourth or fifth metatarsal bone, or to adductor hallucis. Fusion of peroneus longus and brevis can occur but is rare. Two other peroneal muscles are described arising from the fibula between peronei longus and brevis. These are peroneus accessorius, whose tendon joins that of peroneus longus in the sole, and peroneus quartus, which arises posteriorly and inserts into the calcaneus or into the cuboid. For variants of peroneus tertius, see page 1497.

POSTERIOR (FLEXOR) COMPARTMENT
The muscles in the posterior compartment of the lower leg form superficial and deep groups, separated by the deep transverse fascia (p. 1489).

For detail of the extramuscular and intramuscular patterns of arterial supply to these muscles consult Taylor and Razaboni (1994). Brief descriptions of the extramuscular vessels are given below.

Superficial flexor group (Figs 112.3, 113.2, 114.9, 114.10)
The superficial flexors gastrocnemius, plantaris and soleus form the bulk of the calf. Gastrocnemius and soleus – the triceps surae – constitute a powerful muscular mass whose main function is plantar flexion of the foot, although soleus in particular has an important postural role (see below). Their large size is one of the most characteristic features of the musculature of man, being related directly to his upright stance and mode of progression. Gastrocnemius and plantaris act on both knee and ankle joints, soleus on the latter alone.

Gastrocnemius

Attachments – Gastrocnemius is the most superficial muscle of the group and forms the 'belly' of the calf. It arises by two heads, connected

to the condyles of the femur by strong, flat tendons. The medial, larger, head is attached to a depression at the upper and posterior part of the medial condyle behind the adductor tubercle, and to a slightly raised area on the popliteal surface of the femur just above the medial condyle. The lateral head is attached to a recognizable area on the lateral surface of the lateral condyle and to the lower part of the corresponding supracondylar line. Both heads also arise from subjacent areas of the capsule of the knee joint. The tendinous attachments expand to cover the posterior surface of each head with an aponeurosis, from the anterior surface of which the muscle fibres arise. The fleshy part of the muscle extends to about midcalf. The muscle fibres of the larger medial head extend lower than those of the lateral head. As the muscle descends, the muscle fibres begin to insert into a broad aponeurosis that develops on its anterior surface; up to this point the muscular masses of the two heads remain separate. The aponeurosis gradually contracts and receives the tendon of soleus on its deep surface to form the calcaneal or Achilles tendon.

On occasion the lateral head, or the whole muscle, is absent. A more frequent variation is a third head, which arises from the popliteal surface of the femur.

Relations – Proximally, the two heads of gastrocnemius form the lower boundaries of the popliteal fossa. The lateral head is partially overlaid by the tendon of biceps femoris, the medial head by semimembranosus. Over the rest of its length the muscle is superficial, and the two heads can easily be seen in the living subject. The superficial surface of the muscle is separated by the deep fascia from the short saphenous vein and the peroneal communicating and sural nerves. The common peroneal nerve crosses the lateral head of the muscle, partly under cover of biceps femoris. The deep surface lies posterior to the oblique popliteal ligament, popliteus, soleus, plantaris, popliteal vessels and the tibial nerve. A bursa, which communicates with the knee joint, is located anterior to the tendon of the medial head. If the bursa expands into the popliteal fossa it does so in the plane between the medial head of gastrocnemius and semimembranosus. The tendon of the lateral head frequently contains a fibrocartilaginous or bony sesamoid, the fabella, where it moves over the lateral femoral condyle. A sesamoid may occasionally occur in the tendon of the medial head. These can be seen on radiographs and may be mistaken for loose bodies in the knee joint.

Vascular supply – Each head of gastrocnemius is supplied by its own sural artery. These arteries are branches of the popliteal artery. They arise variably, usually at the level of the tibiofemoral joint line. The medial sural artery almost always arises more proximally than the lateral: the medial may arise proximal to the joint line, the lateral sometimes distal to the line. Each sural artery enters the muscle head with its nerve of supply, the pedicle entering the muscle near its axial border at the level of the middle of the popliteal fossa. Medial or lateral gastrocnemius musculocutaneous flaps may be raised, each utilizing one of the heads of the muscle based on its own sural artery. Minor accessory sural arteries arise from the popliteal or from the superior genicular vessels.

The blood supply to the calcaneal tendon is poor: the predominant artery is a recurrent branch of the posterior tibial artery and this mainly supplies peritendinous tissues (Taylor & Razaboni 1994).

Innervation – Gastrocnemius is innervated by the tibial nerve, S1 and 2.

Actions – The action of gastrocnemius is considered with soleus.

Testing – Gastrocnemius is tested by plantar flexion of the foot against resistance, in the supine position and with the knee extended.

Plantaris

Attachments – Plantaris arises from the lower part of the lateral supracondylar line and the oblique popliteal ligament. Its small fusiform belly is 7–10 cm long and ends in a long slender tendon which crosses obliquely between gastrocnemius and soleus, runs distally along the medial border of the calcaneal tendon, and fuses or inserts with it.

The muscle is sometimes double, and is absent in c.10% of cases. Occasionally, its tendon merges with the flexor retinaculum or with the fascia of the leg.

Vascular supply – Plantaris is supplied superficially by the lateral sural and popliteal arteries, and deeply by the lateral superior genicular artery. The distal tendon shares a blood supply with the calcaneal tendon.

Innervation – Plantaris is innervated by the tibial nerve, often from the ramus that supplies the lateral head of gastrocnemius, S1 and 2.

Actions – Plantaris is the lower limb equivalent of palmaris longus, and in many mammals it is well developed and inserts directly or indirectly into the plantar aponeurosis. In man the muscle is almost vestigial and is normally inserted well short of the plantar aponeurosis, usually into the calcaneus. It is therefore presumed to act with gastrocnemius.

Soleus

Attachments – Soleus is a broad flat muscle situated immediately deep (anterior) to gastrocnemius. It arises from the posterior surface of the head and proximal quarter of the shaft of the fibula; the soleal line and the middle third of the medial border of the tibia; and from a fibrous band between the tibia and fibula that arches over the popliteal vessels and tibial nerve. This origin is aponeurotic: most of the muscular fibres arise from its posterior surface and pass obliquely to the tendon of insertion on the posterior surface of the muscle. Other muscle fibres arise from the anterior surface of the aponeurosis. They are short, oblique and bipennate in arrangement, and converge on a narrow, central intramuscular tendon that merges distally with the principal tendon. The latter gradually becomes thicker and narrower, and joins the tendon of gastrocnemius to form the calcaneal tendon. The muscle is covered proximally by gastrocnemius, but below midcalf it is broader than the tendon of gastrocnemius and is accessible on both sides of the tendon.

An accessory part of the muscle is sometimes present distally and medially. It may be inserted into the calcaneal tendon, the calcaneus or the flexor retinaculum.

Relations – The superficial surface of soleus is in contact with gastrocnemius and plantaris. Its deep surface is related to flexor digitorum longus, flexor hallucis longus, tibialis posterior and the posterior tibial vessels and tibial nerve, from all of which it is separated by the deep transverse fascia of the leg (p. 1489).

Vascular supply – There are two main arteries of supply to soleus: the superior arises from the popliteal artery at about the level of the soleal arch, and the inferior from the proximal part of the peroneal artery or sometimes from the posterior tibial artery. A secondary supply comes from the lateral sural, peroneal or posterior tibial vessels.

There is a venous plexus within the muscle belly that is important physiologically as part of the muscle pump complex (p. 1401). Pathologically, it is the usual site of deep vein thrombosis.

Innervation – Soleus is innervated by two branches from the tibial nerve, S1 and 2.

Actions – See under triceps surae.

Testing – Soleus is tested by plantar flexion of the foot against resistance in the supine position, with hip and knee flexed: the muscle belly can be palpated separately from those of gastrocnemius.

Actions of triceps surae – The two heads of gastrocnemius, together with soleus, form a tripartite muscular mass sharing the calcaneal tendon and are sometimes termed the triceps surae. These muscles are the chief plantar flexors of the foot. Gastrocnemius is also a flexor of the knee. They are usually large and correspondingly powerful.

Gastrocnemius provides force for propulsion in walking, running and leaping. Soleus, acting from below, is said to be more concerned with steadying the leg on the foot in standing. This postural role is also suggested by its high content of slow, fatigue-resistant (type 1) muscle fibres. In many adult mammals the proportion of this type of fibre in soleus approaches 100%. However, such a rigid separation of functional roles seems unlikely in man: soleus probably participates in locomotion, and gastrocnemius in posture. Nevertheless, the ankle joint is loose-packed in the erect posture, and since the weight of the body acts through a vertical line that passes anterior to the joint, a strong brace is required behind the joint to maintain stability. Electromyography shows that these forces are supplied mainly by soleus: during symmetrical standing, soleus is continuously active, whereas gastrocnemius is recruited only intermittently. The relative contributions of soleus and gastrocnemius to phasic activity of the triceps surae in walking have yet to be satisfactorily analysed.

Deep flexor group (Figs 112.3, 113.28, 114.9)

The deep flexor group, lying beneath (anterior to) the deep transverse fascia, includes one muscle, popliteus, that acts on the knee joint; the others – flexor digitorum longus, flexor hallucis longus and tibialis posterior – are all plantar flexors of the ankle in addition to their specific actions on joints of the foot and digits.

Popliteus

See page 1484.

Flexor digitorum longus

Attachments – Flexor digitorum longus is thin and pointed proximally and gradually widens as it descends. It arises from the posterior surface of the tibia medial to tibialis posterior from just below the soleal line to within 7 or 8 cm of the distal end of the bone; it also arises from the fascia covering tibialis posterior. The muscle ends in a tendon that extends along almost the whole of its posterior surface. The tendon gradually crosses tibialis posterior and passes behind the medial malleolus where it shares a groove with tibialis posterior, from which it is separated by a fibrous septum. Each tendon thus occupies its own compartment lined by a synovial sheath. It then curves obliquely forwards and laterally, in contact with the medial side of the sustentaculum tali, passes deep to the flexor retinaculum, and enters the sole of the foot (**Fig. 115.43**). Here it crosses superficial to the tendon of flexor hallucis longus and receives a strong slip from it. It continues across the sole to form the whole of the long flexor tendon of the fifth toe and contributes to those of the second, third and fourth toes. It may also send a slip to the tendon of flexor hallucis longus. The tendons of flexor accessorius insert into the long flexor tendons of the second, third and fourth digits. Flexor hallucis longus makes a variable contribution through the connecting slip mentioned above. The long flexor tendons of the lateral four digits are attached to the plantar surfaces of the bases of their distal phalanges: each passes between the slips of the corresponding tendon of flexor digitorum brevis at the base of the proximal phalanx.

A supplementary head of the muscle, flexor accessorius longus, with its own tendon, may arise from the fibula, tibia or deep fascia and insert into the main tendon or into flexor accessorius in the foot. There may be communicating slips to tibialis anterior or to flexor hallucis longus.

Relations – Flexor digitorum longus lies medial to flexor hallucis longus. In the leg its superficial surface is in contact with the deep transverse fascia, which separates it from soleus, and distally from the posterior tibial vessels and tibial nerve. Its deep surface is related to the tibia and to tibialis posterior. In the foot it is covered by abductor hallucis and flexor digitorum brevis and crosses superficial to flexor hallucis longus.

Vascular supply – A series of transversely running branches of the posterior tibial artery enters the lateral border of flexor digitorum longus. There may be a secondary supply from peroneal branches to flexor hallucis longus. The tendons are supplied by the vessels of the ankle and sole.

Innervation – Flexor digitorum longus is innervated by branches of the tibial nerve, L5, S1 and S2.

Actions – See under flexor hallucis longus.

Testing – Flexor digitorum longus is tested by flexing the toes against resistance.

Flexor hallucis longus

Attachments – Flexor hallucis longus arises from the distal two-thirds of the posterior surface of the fibula except for the lowest 2.5 cm; the adjacent interosseous membrane and the posterior crural intermuscular septum; and from the fascia covering tibialis posterior, which it overlaps to a considerable extent. Its fibres pass obliquely down to a tendon that occupies nearly the whole length of the posterior aspect of the muscle. This tendon grooves the posterior surface of the lower end of the tibia, then, successively, the posterior surface of the talus and the inferior surface of the sustentaculum tali of the calcaneus (**Fig. 115.3**). Fibrous bands convert the grooves on the talus and calcaneus into a canal lined by a synovial sheath. In dancers, overuse causes thickening of the tendon in this region, and pain and even 'triggering' can occur (hallux saltans). In the sole of the foot, the tendon crosses flexor digitorum longus from lateral to medial, curving obliquely superior to it. At the crossing point the long digital flexor receives a fibrous slip from the tendon of flexor hallucis longus. The tendon then crosses the lateral part of flexor hallucis brevis to reach the interval between the sesamoid bones under the head of the first metatarsal. It continues on the plantar aspect of the hallux, and runs in an osseo-aponeurotic tunnel to be attached to the plantar aspect of the base of the distal phalanx. The tendon is retained in position over the lateral part of flexor hallucis brevis by the diverging stems of the distal band of the medial intermuscular septum.

The distal extent of the muscle belly is a striking characteristic: in the posterior surgical approach to the ankle, flexor hallucis is unmistakeable since its muscle fibres insert almost to calcaneal level. In athletes the muscle fibres may be present so far inferiorly into the tendon that they cause impingement when pulled into the tunnel at the talus.

The connecting slip to flexor digitorum longus varies in size: it usually continues into the tendons for the second and third toes but is sometimes restricted to the second and occasionally extends to the fourth.

Relations – Superficial are soleus and the calcaneal tendon, from which flexor hallucis longus is separated by the deep transverse fascia. Deep are the fibula, tibialis posterior, peroneal vessels, distal part of the interosseous membrane and the tibiotalar joint. Laterally lie the peronei; medially are tibialis posterior, posterior tibial vessels and the tibial nerve. Flexor hallucis longus is an important surgical landmark at the ankle: staying lateral to it prevents injury to the neurovascular bundle.

Vascular supply – Flexor hallucis longus is supplied by numerous branches of the peroneal artery. The tendon is supplied by arteries of the ankle and foot.

Innervation – Flexor hallucis longus is innervated by branches of the tibial nerve, L5, S1 and 2 (mainly S1).

Testing – Flexor hallucis longus is tested by flexion of the hallux against resistance.

Actions of deep digital flexors – Both flexor hallucis longus and flexor digitorum longus can act as plantar flexors but this action is weak compared with gastrocnemius and soleus. When the foot is off the ground, both muscles flex the phalanges of the toes, acting primarily on the distal phalanges. When the foot is on the ground and under load, they act synergistically with the small muscles of the foot and, especially in the case of flexor digitorum longus, with the lumbricals and interossei to maintain the pads of the toes in firm contact with the ground, enlarging the weightbearing area and helping to stabilize the heads of the metatarsal bones, which form the fulcrum on which the body is propelled forwards. Activity in the long digital flexors is minimal during quiet standing, so they apparently contribute little to the static maintenance of the longitudinal arch, but they become very active during toe-off and tip-toe movements.

Tibialis posterior

Attachments – Tibialis posterior is the most deeply placed muscle of the flexor group. At its origin it lies between flexor hallucis longus and flexor digitorum longus, and is overlapped by both, but especially by the former. Its proximal attachment consists of two pointed processes, separated by an angular interval that is traversed by the anterior tibial vessels. The medial process arises from the posterior surface of the interosseous membrane, except at its most distal part, and from a lateral area on the posterior surface of the tibia between the soleal line above and the junction of the middle and lower thirds of the shaft below. The lateral part arises from a medial strip of the posterior fibular surface in

its upper two-thirds. The muscle also arises from the deep transverse fascia, and from the intermuscular septa that separate it from adjacent muscles. In the distal quarter of the leg its tendon passes deep to that of flexor digitorum longus, with which it shares a groove behind the medial malleolus, each enclosed in a separate synovial sheath. It then passes deep to the flexor retinaculum and superficial to the deltoid ligament (p. 1524) to enter the foot. In the foot it is at first inferior to the plantar calcaneonavicular ligament, where it contains a sesamoid fibrocartilage. The tendon then divides into two. The more superficial and larger division, which is a direct continuation of the tendon, is attached to the tuberosity of the navicular, from which fibres continue to the inferior surface of the medial cuneiform. A tendinous band also passes laterally and a little proximally to the tip and distal margin of the sustentaculum tali. The deeper lateral division gives rise to the tendon of origin of the medial limb of flexor hallucis brevis, and then continues between this muscle and the navicular and medial cuneiform to end on the intermediate cuneiform and the bases of the second, third and fourth metatarsals; the slip to the fourth metatarsal is the strongest.

The slips to the metatarsals vary in number. Slips to the cuboid and lateral cuneiform may also occur. An additional muscle, the tibialis secundus, has been described running from the back of the tibia to the capsule of the ankle joint.

Relations – The superficial surface of tibialis posterior is separated from soleus by the deep transverse fascia, and is related to flexor digitorum longus, flexor hallucis longus, the posterior tibial vessels, the tibial nerve and the peroneal vessels. The deep surface is in contact with the interosseous membrane, tibia, fibula and tibiotalar joint.

Vascular supply – Tibialis posterior is supplied by numerous branches of small calibre arising from the posterior tibial and peroneal arteries. The tendon is supplied by arteries of the medial malleolar network and by the medial plantar artery.

Innervation – Tibialis posterior is innervated by the tibial nerve, L4 and 5.

Actions – Tibialis posterior is the principal invertor of the foot, although it may assist in vigorous plantar flexion. By reason of its insertions into the cuneiform bones and the bases of the metatarsals, it has long been thought to assist in elevating the longitudinal arch of the foot, although electromyography shows that it is actually quiescent in standing. It is phasically active in walking, during which it probably acts with the intrinsic foot musculature and the lateral calf muscles to control the degree of pronation of the foot and the distribution of weight through the metatarsal heads. It is said that when the body is supported on one leg, the invertor action of tibialis posterior, exerted from below, helps to maintain balance by resisting any tendency to sway laterally. However, any act of balancing demands the cooperation of many muscles, including groups acting on the hip joints and vertebral column. However, it is undeniable that devastating collapse of the medial longitudinal arch can accompany tibialis posterior rupture.

Testing – Tibialis posterior is tested by inversion of the foot against resistance: the tendon can be seen and felt just proximal to the medial malleolus. The muscle may also be tested by standing on one leg and raising the heel from the ground.

VASCULAR SUPPLY

ANTERIOR TIBIAL ARTERY (Figs 113.4, 113.30, 113.1, 114.11, 114.12, 115.16)
The anterior tibial artery is the terminal branch of the popliteal artery and arises at the distal border of popliteus. At first in the flexor compartment, it passes between the heads of tibialis posterior and through the oval aperture in the proximal part of the interosseous membrane to reach the extensor region, passing medial to the fibular neck. It is vulnerable here during tibial osteotomy. Descending anteriorly on the membrane it approaches the tibia and, distally, lies anterior to it. At the ankle it is midway between the malleoli, and continues on the dorsum of the foot as the dorsalis pedis artery.

The anterior tibial artery may be small but is rarely absent. Its function may be replaced by perforating branches from the posterior

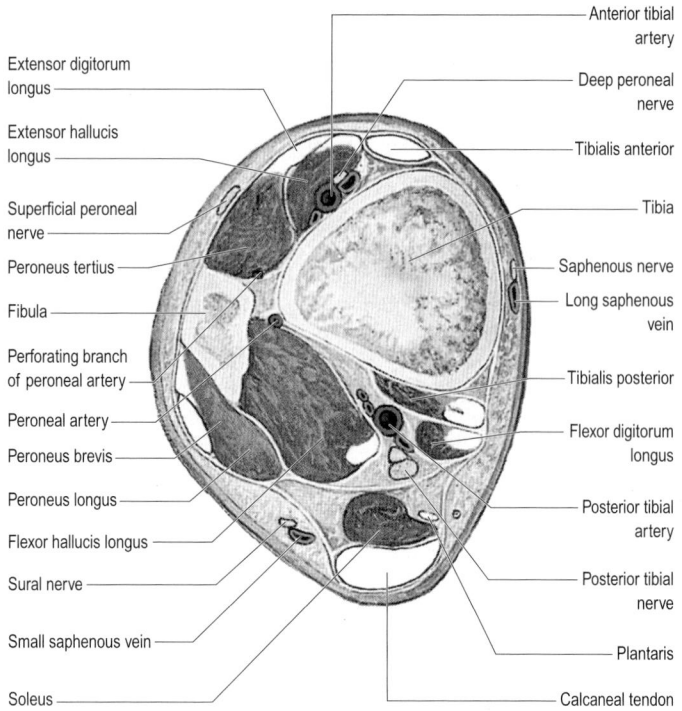

Extensor digitorum longus

Extensor hallucis longus

Superficial peroneal nerve

Peroneus tertius

Fibula

Perforating branch of peroneal artery

Peroneal artery

Peroneus brevis

Peroneus longus

Flexor hallucis longus

Sural nerve

Small saphenous vein

Soleus

Anterior tibial artery

Deep peroneal nerve

Tibialis anterior

Tibia

Saphenous nerve

Long saphenous vein

Tibialis posterior

Flexor digitorum longus

Posterior tibial artery

Posterior tibial nerve

Plantaris

Calcaneal tendon

Fig. 114.12 Transverse section through the left leg, c.6 cm proximal to the tip of the medial malleolus.

tibial artery or by the perforating branch of the peroneal artery. It occasionally deviates laterally, regaining its usual position at the ankle. It may also be larger than normal, in which case its territory of supply in the foot may be increased to include the plantar surface.

Relations

In its proximal two-thirds the anterior tibial artery lies on the interosseous membrane, and in its distal third it is anterior to the tibia and ankle joint. Proximally it lies between tibialis anterior and extensor digitorum longus, then between tibialis anterior and extensor hallucis longus. At the ankle it is crossed superficially from the lateral side by the tendon of extensor hallucis longus and then lies between this tendon and the first tendon of extensor digitorum longus. Its proximal two-thirds are covered by adjoining muscles and deep fascia, its distal third by the skin, fasciae and extensor retinacula. It is accompanied by venae comitantes. The deep peroneal nerve, curling laterally round the fibular neck, reaches the lateral side of the artery where it enters the extensor region, is anterior to the artery in the middle third of the leg, and becomes lateral again distally.

Branches

The named branches of the anterior tibial artery are the posterior and anterior recurrent tibial, muscular, perforating, and anterior medial and lateral malleolar arteries.

Posterior tibial recurrent artery

The posterior tibial recurrent artery is an inconstant branch that arises before the anterior tibial reaches the extensor compartment. It ascends anterior to popliteus with the recurrent nerve to that muscle, anastomosing with the inferior genicular branches of the popliteal artery. It supplies the superior tibiofibular joint.

Anterior tibial recurrent artery

The anterior tibial recurrent artery arises near the posterior tibial recurrent artery. It ascends in tibialis anterior, ramifies on the front and sides of the knee joint and joins the patellar network, anastomosing with the genicular branches of the popliteal and circumflex fibular arteries.

Numerous branches supply the adjacent muscles. Some then pierce the deep fascia to supply the skin, while others traverse the interosseous membrane to anastomose with branches of the posterior tibial and peroneal arteries.

Perforating branches

Most of the fasciocutaneous perforators pass along the anterior peroneal fascial septum behind extensor digitorum longus before penetrating the deep fascia to supply the skin.

Anterior medial malleolar artery

The anterior medial malleolar artery arises c.5 cm proximal to the ankle. It passes posterior to the tendons of extensor hallucis longus and tibialis anterior medial to the joint, where it joins branches of the posterior tibial and medial plantar arteries.

Anterior lateral malleolar artery

The anterior lateral malleolar artery runs posterior to the tendons of extensor digitorum longus and peroneus tertius to the lateral side of the ankle and anastomoses with the perforating branch of the peroneal artery and ascending branches of the lateral tarsal artery.

POSTERIOR TIBIAL ARTERY (Figs 113.4, 113.30, 113.1)

The posterior tibial artery begins at the distal border of popliteus, between the tibia and fibula. It descends medially in the flexor compartment and divides under abductor hallucis, midway between the medial malleolus and the medial tubercle of the calcaneus, into the medial and lateral plantar arteries. The artery may be much reduced in length or in calibre: the peroneal artery then takes over its distal territory of supply and may consequently be increased in size.

Relations

The posterior tibial artery is successively posterior to tibialis posterior, flexor digitorum longus, the tibia and the ankle joint. Proximally, gastrocnemius, soleus and the deep transverse fascia of the leg are superficial to the artery, and distally it is covered only by skin and fascia. It is parallel with and c.2.5 cm anterior to the medial border of the calcaneal tendon; terminally it is deep to the flexor retinaculum and abductor hallucis. The artery is accompanied by two veins and the tibial nerve. The nerve is at first medial to the artery but soon crosses behind it and subsequently becomes largely posterolateral.

Branches

The named branches of the posterior tibial artery are the circumflex fibular, nutrient, muscular, perforating, communicating, medial malleolar, calcaneal, lateral and medial plantar, and peroneal arteries.

Circumflex fibular artery

The circumflex fibular artery, which sometimes arises from the anterior tibial artery, passes laterally round the neck of the fibula through the soleus to anastomose with the lateral inferior genicular, medial genicular and anterior tibial recurrent arteries. It supplies bone and articular structures.

Nutrient artery of the tibia

The nutrient artery of the tibia arises from the posterior tibial near its origin. After giving off a few muscular branches it descends into the bone immediately distal to the soleal line. It is one of the largest of the nutrient arteries.

Muscular branches

Muscular branches are distributed to the soleus and deep flexors of the leg.

Perforating branches

Approximately five fasciocutaneous perforators emerge between flexor digitorum longus and soleus and pass through the deep fascia, often accompanying the perforating veins that connect the deep and superficial venous systems. The arterial perforators then divide into anterior and posterior branches to supply periosteum and skin. These vessels are utilized in raising medial fasciocutaneous perforator flaps in the leg.

Communicating branch
The communicating branch runs posteriorly across the tibia c.5 cm above its distal end, deep to flexor hallucis longus, to join a communicating branch of the peroneal artery.

Medial malleolar branches
The medial malleolar branches pass round the tibial malleolus to the medial malleolar network, which supplies the skin.

Calcaneal branches
Calcaneal branches arise just proximal to the terminal division of the posterior tibial artery. They pierce the flexor retinaculum to supply fat and skin behind the calcaneal tendon and in the heel, and muscles on the tibial side of the sole. They anastomose with medial malleolar arteries and calcaneal branches of the peroneal artery.

Medial plantar artery (Fig. 115.42)
The medial plantar artery is the smaller terminal branch of the posterior tibial artery and passes distally along the medial side of the foot, medial to the medial plantar nerve. At first deep to abductor hallucis, it runs distally between this muscle and flexor digitorum brevis, and supplies both. Near the first metatarsal base, its size, already diminished by muscular branches, is further reduced by a superficial stem that divides to form three superficial digital branches. These accompany the digital branches of the medial plantar nerve and join the first to third plantar metatarsal arteries. The main trunk of the medial plantar artery then runs on to reach the medial border of the hallux where it anastomoses with a branch of the first plantar metatarsal artery.

Lateral plantar artery (Fig. 115.42)
The lateral plantar artery is the larger terminal branch of the posterior tibial artery. It passes distally and laterally to the fifth metatarsal base, lateral to the lateral plantar nerve. (The medial and lateral plantar nerves lie between the corresponding plantar arteries.) Turning medially, with the deep branch of the lateral plantar nerve, it reaches the interval between the first and second metatarsal bases, and unites with the dorsalis pedis artery to complete the plantar arch. As it passes laterally, it is first between the calcaneus and abductor hallucis, then between flexor digitorum brevis and flexor accessorius. Running distally to the fifth metatarsal base, it passes between flexor digitorum brevis and abductor digiti minimi and is covered by the plantar aponeurosis, superficial fascia and skin.

Branches – Muscular branches supply the adjoining muscles. Superficial branches emerge along the lateral intermuscular septum to supply the skin and subcutaneous tissue lateral in the sole. Anastomotic branches run to the lateral border of the foot, joining branches of the lateral tarsal and arcuate arteries. Sometimes a calcaneal branch pierces abductor hallucis to supply the skin of the heel.

PERONEAL ARTERY (Figs 113.4, 113.30, 114.11, 114.12)
The peroneal artery arises from the posterior tibial artery c. 2.5 cm distal to popliteus and passes obliquely to the fibula, descending along its medial crest either in a fibrous canal between tibialis posterior and flexor hallucis longus or within flexor hallucis longus. Reaching the inferior tibiofibular syndesmosis, it divides into calcaneal branches that ramify on the lateral and posterior surfaces of the calcaneus. Proximally it is covered by soleus and the deep transverse fascia between soleus and the deep muscles. Distally it is overlapped by flexor hallucis longus.

The peroneal artery may branch high from the posterior tibial artery or may even branch from the popliteal artery separately, giving a true 'trifurcation'. It may also branch more distally from the posterior tibial artery, sometimes 7 or 8 cm distal to popliteus. Its size tends to be inversely related to the size of the other arteries of the leg. It may be reduced in size but is more often enlarged, when it may join, reinforce or replace the posterior tibial artery in the distal leg and foot. An enlarged perforating branch may replace the dorsalis pedis artery: the dorsalis pedis pulse will then be absent.

Branches
The peroneal artery has muscular, nutrient, perforating, communicating and calcaneal branches.

Muscular branches
Multiple short branches supply soleus, tibialis posterior, flexor hallucis longus and the peroneal muscles.

Nutrient artery
The nutrient artery branches from the main trunk c.7 cm from its origin and enters the fibula 14–19 cm from the styloid process.

Perforating branches
The main perforating branch traverses the interosseous membrane c.5 cm proximal to the lateral malleolus to enter the extensor compartment, where it anastomoses with the anterior lateral malleolar artery. Descending anterior to the inferior tibiofibular syndesmosis, it supplies the tarsus and anastomoses with the lateral tarsal artery. This branch is sometimes enlarged and may replace the dorsalis pedis artery.

Fasciocutaneous perforators from the lateral muscular branches pass along the posterior peroneal fascial septum to penetrate the deep fascia and reach the skin. These vessels are utilized in raising fasciocutaneous posterolateral leg flaps.

Communicating branch
The communicating branch connects to a communicating branch of the posterior tibial artery c.5 cm proximal to the ankle.

Calcaneal branches
Calcaneal (terminal) branches anastomose with the anterior lateral malleolar and calcaneal branches of the posterior tibial artery.

DEEP AND SUPERFICIAL VENOUS SYSTEM (Fig. 110.8)
See also page 1401.

Posterior tibial veins
The posterior tibial veins accompany the posterior tibial artery. They receive tributaries from the calf muscles (especially from the venous plexus in the soleus) and connections from superficial veins and the peroneal veins.

Peroneal veins
The peroneal veins, running with their artery, receive tributaries from soleus and from superficial veins.

Anterior tibial veins
The anterior tibial veins, continuations of the venae comitantes of the dorsalis pedis artery, leave the anterior compartment between the tibia and fibula and pass through the proximal end of the interosseous membrane. They unite with the posterior tibial veins to form the popliteal vein at the distal border of popliteus.

Long saphenous vein
See page 1452.

Short saphenous vein
See page 1487.

Venous disease
Chronic venous disease is common. If the superficial veins of the lower limb are overdistended then they may develop short dilated segments or varicosities. Varicose veins can occur as a consequence of venous valve failure. This can be at the proximal end of the long saphenous vein at the saphenofemoral junction, or in the perforating veins that pass from the superficial system to the high-pressure deep veins. Varicose veins have thin walls and 'leak' red blood cells into adjacent soft tissues. As these cells are broken down haemosiderin is deposited in the soft tissues causing a brown pigmentation. This phenomenon, together with the fact that venous stasis produces oedema, renders the soft tissues of the leg unhealthy and prone to ulceration, particularly after minor trauma.

Acute venous disease occurs most commonly in the leg. The deep veins in the calf may have relatively slow blood flow at times and thrombi can be generated. The deep vein thrombosis can detach and cause life-threatening pulmonary embolism. Blockage of the normal venous system may contribute to an increased local venous pressure and oedema.

INNERVATION

TIBIAL NERVE

The tibial nerve, the larger sciatic component, is derived from the ventral branches (anterior division) of the fourth and fifth lumbar and first to third sacral ventral rami. It descends along the back of the thigh and popliteal fossa to the distal border of popliteus. It then passes anterior to the arch of soleus with the popliteal artery and continues into the leg. In the thigh it is overlapped proximally by the hamstring muscles but it becomes more superficial in the popliteal fossa, where it is lateral to the popliteal vessels. At the level of the knee the tibial nerve becomes superficial to the popliteal vessels and crosses to the medial side of the artery. In the distal popliteal fossa it is overlapped by the junction of the two heads of gastrocnemius.

In the leg the tibial nerve descends with the posterior tibial vessels to lie between the heel and the medial malleolus. Proximally it is deep to soleus and gastrocnemius, but in its distal third is covered only by skin and fasciae, overlapped sometimes by flexor hallucis longus. At first medial to the posterior tibial vessels, it crosses behind them and descends lateral to them until it bifurcates. It lies on tibialis posterior for most of its course except distally, where it adjoins the posterior surface of the tibia. The tibial nerve ends under the flexor retinaculum by dividing into the medial and lateral plantar nerves.

Branches

The branches of the tibial nerve are articular, muscular, sural, medial calcaneal and medial and lateral plantar. The sural nerve is described on page 1505 and the distal branches on page 1544.

Articular branches

Articular branches accompany the superior, inferior medial and middle genicular arteries to the knee joint. They form a plexus with a branch from the obturator nerve and supply the oblique posterior ligament. The branches accompanying the superior and inferior genicular arteries also supply the medial part of the capsule. Just before the tibial nerve bifurcates it supplies the ankle joint.

Muscular branches

Proximal muscular branches arise between the heads of gastrocnemius and supply gastrocnemius, plantaris, soleus and popliteus. The nerve to soleus enters its superficial aspect. The branch to popliteus descends obliquely across the popliteal vessels, curling round the distal border of the muscle to its anterior surface. It also supplies tibialis posterior, the proximal tibiofibular joint and the tibia, and gives off an interosseous branch that descends near the fibula to reach the distal tibiofibular joint.

Muscular branches in the leg, either independently or by a common trunk, supply soleus (on its deep surface), tibialis posterior, flexor digitorum longus and flexor hallucis longus. The branch to flexor hallucis longus accompanies the peroneal vessels.

Lesions of the tibial nerve

The tibial nerve is vulnerable to direct injury in the popliteal fossa, where it lies superficial to the vessels at the level of the knee. It may be damaged in compartment syndrome affecting the deep flexor compartment of the calf. The nerve may be entrapped beneath the flexor retinaculum at the ankle, resulting in tarsal tunnel syndrome.

COMMON PERONEAL NERVE

The common peroneal nerve (common fibular nerve) is approximately half the size of the tibial nerve and is derived from the dorsal branches of the fourth and fifth lumbar and first and second sacral ventral rami. It descends obliquely along the lateral side of the popliteal fossa to the fibular head, medial to biceps femoris. It lies between the bicipital tendon, to which it is bound by fascia, and the lateral head of gastrocnemius. The nerve then passes into the anterolateral muscle compartment through a tight opening in the thick fascia overlying tibialis anterior. It curves lateral to the fibular neck, deep to peroneus longus, and divides into superficial and deep peroneal nerves.

The course of the common peroneal nerve can be indicated by a line from the apex of the popliteal fossa, passing distally, medial to the biceps tendon, to the back of the head of the fibula, where the nerve can be rolled against the bone.

Branches

The common peroneal nerve has articular and cutaneous branches. It terminates as the superficial and deep peroneal nerves.

Articular branches

There are three articular branches. Two accompany the superior and inferior lateral genicular arteries, and may arise in common. The third, the recurrent articular nerve, arises near the termination of the common peroneal nerve. It ascends with the anterior recurrent tibial artery through tibialis anterior and supplies the anterolateral part of the knee joint capsule and the proximal tibiofibular joint.

Cutaneous branches

The two cutaneous branches, often from a common trunk, are the lateral sural and sural communicating nerves. The lateral sural nerve (lateral cutaneous nerve of the calf) supplies the skin on the anterior, posterior and lateral surfaces of the proximal leg. The sural communicating nerve arises near the head of the fibula and crosses the lateral head of gastrocnemius to join the sural nerve (p. 1505). It may descend separately as far as the heel.

Lesions of the common peroneal nerve

The common peroneal nerve is relatively unprotected as it traverses the lateral aspect of the neck of the fibula and is easily compressed at this site, e.g. by plaster casts or ganglia. The nerve may also become entrapped between the attachments of peroneus longus to the head and shaft of the fibula. Traction lesions can accompany dislocations of the lateral compartment of the knee, and are most likely to occur if the distal attachments of biceps and the ligaments that insert into the fibular head are avulsed, possibly with a small part of the fibular head. Because it is tethered to the bicipital tendon by dense fascia, the nerve is pulled proximally. Patients with such injury present with foot drop, which is usually painless. Examination reveals weakness of ankle dorsiflexion, extensor hallucis longus and eversion of the foot, but inversion and plantar flexion are normal and the ankle reflex is preserved. Since the nerve divides at the fibular neck into the superficial peroneal and the deep peroneal nerves, all lesions damaging the nerve at this level may damage the main trunk of the nerve or either of its branches. A lesion of the superficial branch causes weakness of foot eversion with sensory loss on the lateral aspect of the leg, which extends onto the dorsum of the foot.

SUPERFICIAL PERONEAL NERVE

The superficial peroneal nerve (superficial fibular nerve) begins at the common peroneal bifurcation. It is at first deep to peroneus longus, and passes anteroinferiorly between the peronei and extensor digitorum longus to pierce the deep fascia in the distal third of the leg, where it divides into medial and lateral branches. Between the muscles it supplies peroneus longus, peroneus brevis and the skin of the lower leg.

Branches

The medial branch passes anterior to the ankle and divides into two dorsal digital nerves: one supplies the medial side of the great toe, and the other supplies the adjacent sides of the second and third toes. The medial branch communicates with the saphenous and deep peroneal nerves. The smaller lateral branch traverses the dorsum of the foot laterally. It divides into dorsal digital branches that supply the contiguous sides of the third to fifth toes and the skin of the lateral aspect of the ankle, where it connects with the sural nerve. Both branches, especially the lateral, are at risk during the placement of portal incisions for arthroscopy.

Branches of the superficial peroneal nerve supply the dorsal skin of all the toes except that of the lateral side of the fifth toe (supplied by the sural nerve) and the adjoining sides of the great and second toes (supplied by the medial terminal branch of the deep peroneal nerve). Some of the lateral branches of the superficial peroneal nerve are frequently absent and are replaced by sural branches.

Lesions of the superficial peroneal nerve

The superficial peroneal nerve can be subject to entrapment as it penetrates the deep fascia of the leg. It may also be involved in compartment syndrome affecting the lateral compartment.

DEEP PERONEAL NERVE

The deep peroneal nerve (deep fibular nerve) begins at the common peroneal bifurcation, between the fibula and the proximal part of peroneus longus. It passes obliquely forwards deep to extensor digitorum longus to the front of the interosseous membrane and reaches the anterior tibial artery in the proximal third of the leg. It descends with the artery to the ankle, dividing there into lateral and medial terminal branches. It is first lateral to the artery, then anterior, and again lateral at the ankle.

Branches

The deep peroneal nerve supplies muscular branches to tibialis anterior, extensor hallucis longus, extensor digitorum longus and peroneus tertius, and an articular branch to the ankle joint.

The lateral terminal branch crosses the ankle deep to extensor digitorum brevis, enlarges as a pseudoganglion and supplies extensor digitorum brevis. From the enlargement three minute interosseous branches supply the tarsal and metatarsophalangeal joints of the middle three toes; the first branch also supplies the second dorsal interosseous.

The medial terminal branch runs distally on the dorsum of the foot lateral to the dorsalis pedis artery, and connects with the medial branch of the superficial peroneal nerve in the first interosseous space. It divides into two dorsal digital nerves, which supply adjacent sides of the great and second toes. Before dividing, it gives off an interosseous branch which supplies the first metatarsophalangeal joint and the first dorsal interosseous. The deep peroneal nerve may end as three terminal branches.

Lesions of the deep peroneal nerve

The deep peroneal nerve supplies the muscles of the anterior tibial compartment. Consequently damage to this nerve, as in compartment syndrome affecting the anterior compartment, results in weakness of ankle dorsiflexion and extension of all toes. Sensory impairment is confined to the first interdigital cleft.

SAPHENOUS NERVE

See page 1487.

SURAL NERVE

The sural nerve descends between the heads of gastrocnemius, pierces the deep fascia proximally in the leg, and is joined at a variable level by the sural communicating branch of the common peroneal nerve. Some authors term this branch the lateral sural cutaneous nerve, and the main trunk (from the tibial nerve) the medial sural cutaneous nerve. The sural nerve descends lateral to the calcaneal tendon, near the short saphenous vein, to the region between the lateral malleolus and the calcaneus and supplies the posterior and lateral skin of the distal third of the leg. It then passes distal to the lateral malleolus along the lateral side of the foot and little toe, supplying the overlying skin. It connects with the posterior femoral cutaneous nerve in the leg and with the superficial peroneal nerve on the dorsum of the foot.

The surface marking at the ankle is a line parallel to the calcaneal tendon half-way between the tendon and the lateral malleolus. However, its position is variable and it is at risk from any surgery in this region. Rather like the radial nerve at the wrist, the sural nerve has a tendency to form painful neuromas. The nerve is harvested for grafting on occasion because it is sensory only, superficial, and easily identified.

REFERENCES

Cormack GC, Lamberty BGH 1994 See Bibliography.

Eckhoff DG, Kramer RC, Watkins JJ, Burke BJ, Alongi CA, Stamm ER, van Gerven DP 1994 Variation in tibial torsion. Clin Anat 7: 76–9.

Jungers WL, Meldrum DJ, Stern JT Jr 1993 The functional and evolutionary significance of the human peroneus tertius muscle. J Hum Evol 25: 377–86.

Taylor GI, Razaboni RM (eds) 1994 Michael Salmon: Anatomic Studies. Book 1, Arteries of the Muscles of the Extremities and the Trunk. St Louis: Quality Medical Publishing.
A translated, unpaid and edited version of a classic French text, first published in 1933. Now a major source-book in plastic surgery.

Foot and ankle

The human foot is a complex structure adapted to allow orthograde bipedal stance and locomotion. It is the only part of the body which is in regular contact with the ground. There are 28 major bones in the human foot, including the sesamoid bones of the first metatarso-phalangeal joint and 31 major joints, including the ankle joint. For a comprehensive account of the anatomy of the foot and ankle, consult Sarrafian 1993.

SKIN

CUTANEOUS VASCULAR SUPPLY AND LYMPHATIC DRAINAGE

The arterial supply to the skin of the foot is rich and is derived from branches of the three major arteries that supply the foot, namely the dorsalis pedis, posterior tibial and peroneal. The dorsal skin is supplied by the dorsalis pedis and a continuation of this artery, the first dorsal metatarsal artery, with smaller contributions from the anterior peroneal artery and the marginal anastomotic arteries on the medial and lateral borders of the foot. The plantar skin is supplied by perforating branches of the medial and lateral plantar arteries. In the forefoot, the supply is from cutaneous branches of the common digital arteries. The main blood supply to the medial aspect of the heel arises from the medial calcaneal branches of the lateral plantar artery passing through the flexor retinaculum. The lateral heel skin is supplied by the posterior peroneal artery and the lateral tarsal artery. Cutaneous venous drainage is via dorsal and plantar venous arches, which drain into medial and lateral marginal veins. On the dorsum there are two superficial and one deep venous networks, separated by the deep and superficial dorsal fasciae. On the plantar aspect there is a very superficial network forming an intradermal and subdermal mesh that drains to the medial and lateral marginal veins. The deep venous network has branches that accompany the medial and lateral plantar arteries. Uniquely within the lower limb, venous flow is bidirectional and, when valves are present, flow is from the plantar to the superficial dorsal system. From here, blood leaves the foot in the superficial and deep veins of the lower limb.

Superficial lymphatic drainage is via vessels that accompany the long saphenous vein medially and the short saphenous vein laterally and drain via the inguinal lymph nodes. Deep lymphatic vessels accompany the dorsalis pedis, posterior tibial and peroneal arteries and pass via the popliteal lymph nodes.

CUTANEOUS INNERVATION (Fig. 115.1)

The fourth and fifth lumbar and first sacral spinal nerve roots supply sensation to the foot. Dorsal sensation is provided medially by the saphenous nerve, centrally by the superficial peroneal nerve and laterally by the sural nerve; the deep peroneal nerve supplies the dorsum of the first web space. The plantar aspect of the foot is supplied by the medial and lateral plantar nerves, which arise as terminal branches of the tibial nerve. The medial plantar nerve supplies sensation to the plantar aspect of the hallux, the second, the third and the medial half of the fourth toes. The lateral plantar nerve supplies the remaining lateral aspect of the fourth and the entire fifth toe. The heel is innervated by calcaneal branches of the tibial nerve. Injury to any of these nerves can lead to painful neuromata and loss of protective sensation. The sural nerve is especially prone to neuroma formation.

SOFT TISSUES

RETINACULA OF THE ANKLE JOINT

In the vicinity of the tibiotalar joint, the tendons of the muscles of the leg are bound down by localized thickenings of the deep fascia, forming

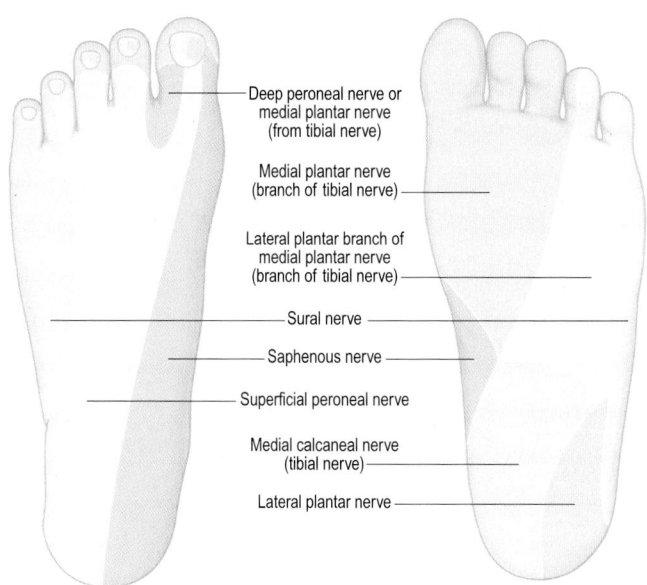

Fig. 115.1 Cutaneous innervation of the foot. **A**, Dorsum. **B**, Plantar aspect.

Deep peroneal nerve or medial plantar nerve (from tibial nerve)

Medial plantar nerve (branch of tibial nerve)

Lateral plantar branch of medial plantar nerve (branch of tibial nerve)

Sural nerve

Saphenous nerve

Superficial peroneal nerve

Medial calcaneal nerve (tibial nerve)

Lateral plantar nerve

retinacular bands that prevent bowstringing of the tendons. There are superior and inferior extensor, flexor and peroneal retinacula.

Extensor retinacula

Superior extensor retinaculum

The superior extensor retinaculum (**Figs 114.8, 115.2**) binds down the tendons of tibialis anterior, extensor hallucis longus, extensor digitorum longus and peroneus tertius immediately above the anterior aspect of the tibiotalar joint. The anterior tibial vessels and deep peroneal nerve pass deep to the retinaculum. The superficial peroneal nerve passes superficially. The retinaculum is attached laterally to the distal end of the anterior border of the fibula and medially to the anterior border of the tibia. Its proximal border is continuous with the fascia cruris, and dense connective tissue connects its distal border to the inferior extensor retinaculum. Only the tendon of tibialis anterior has a synovial sheath here.

Inferior extensor retinaculum

The inferior extensor retinaculum (**Figs 114.8, 115.2**) is a Y-shaped band lying anterior to the tibiotalar joint. The stem of the Y is at the lateral end, where it is attached to the upper surface of the calcaneus, in front of the sulcus calcanei. The band passes medially, forming a strong loop around the tendons of peroneus tertius and extensor digitorum longus (**Fig. 115.3**). From the deep surface of the loop, a band passes laterally behind the interosseous talocalcaneal ligament and the cervical ligament and is attached to the sulcus calcanei. At the medial end of the loop, the Y is completed by two diverging bands, which continue further medially. The more proximal band has two layers. The deep layer passes deep to the tendons of extensor hallucis longus and tibialis anterior, but superficial to the anterior tibial vessels and deep peroneal nerve, to reach the medial malleolus. The superficial layer crosses superficial to

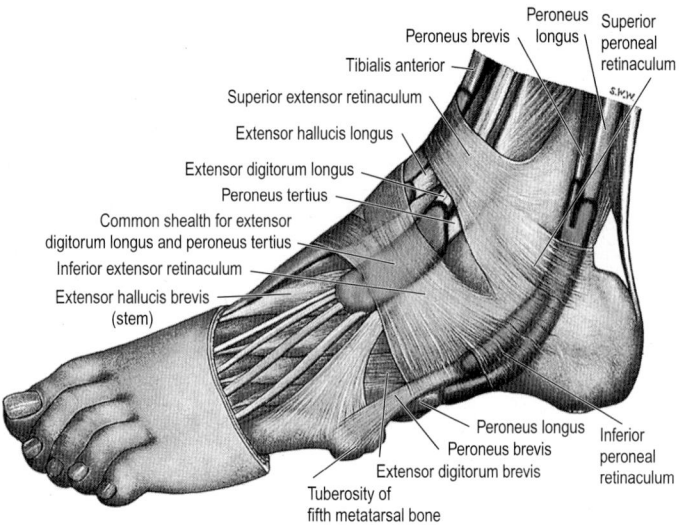

Fig. 115.2 The synovial sheaths of the tendons of the left ankle: lateral aspect.

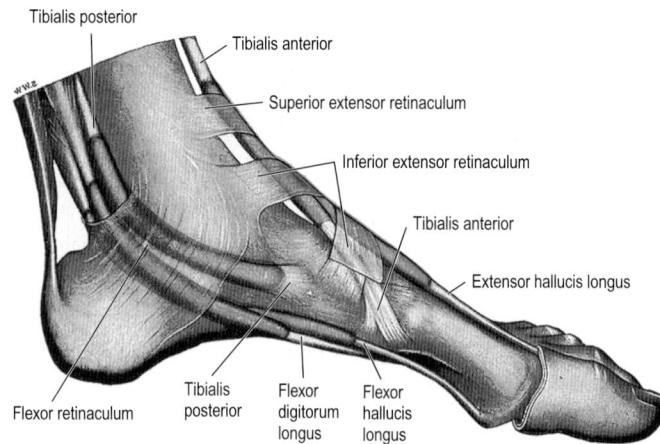

Fig. 115.4 The synovial sheaths of the tendons of the left ankle: medial aspect.

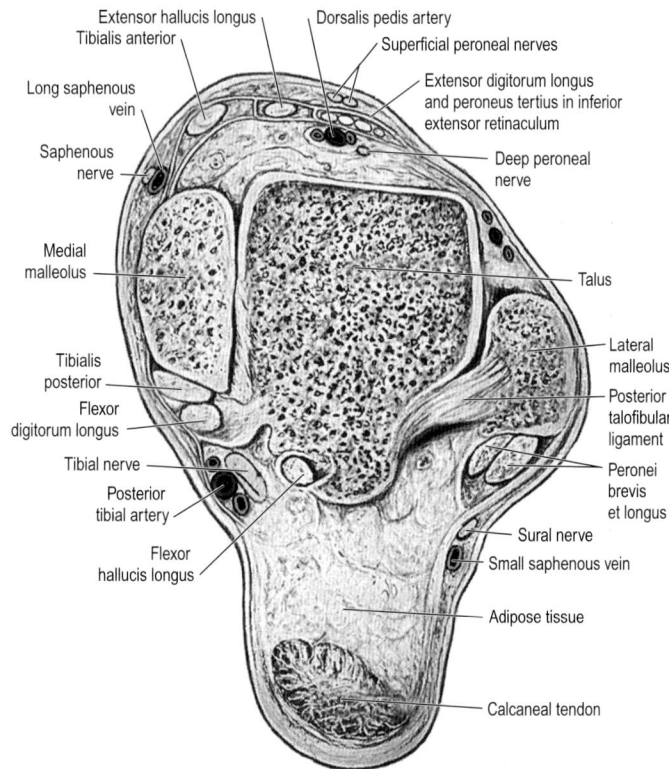

Fig. 115.3 Horizontal section through the inferior part of the left talocrural joint: inferior (distal) aspect.

the tendon of extensor hallucis longus and then adheres firmly to the deep one; in some cases it continues superficial to the tendon of tibialis anterior to reach the tibia. The more distal band extends downwards and medially and is attached to the plantar aponeurosis. It is superficial to the tendons of extensor hallucis longus and tibialis anterior, the dorsalis pedis artery and the terminal branches of the deep peroneal nerve.

Flexor retinaculum

The flexor retinaculum (**Fig. 115.4**) is attached anteriorly to the tip of the medial malleolus, distal to which it is continuous with the deep fascia on the dorsum of the foot; it continues posteriorly to the medial process of the calcaneus and the plantar aponeurosis. Proximally, there

is no clear demarcation between its border and the deep fascia of the lower leg, especially the deep transverse layer of the deep fascia. Distally, its border is continuous with the plantar aponeurosis, and many fibres of abductor hallucis are attached to it. The flexor retinaculum converts grooves on the tibia and calcaneus into canals for the tendons, and bridges over the posterior tibial vessels and tibial nerve. As these structures enter the sole they are, from medial to lateral, the tendons of tibialis posterior and flexor digitorum longus, the posterior tibial vessels, the tibial nerve and the tendon of flexor hallucis longus (**Fig. 115.3**).

Peroneal retinacula

The peroneal retinacula (**Figs 113.28, 115.2**) are fibrous bands that retain the tendons of peroneus longus and brevis in position as they curve round the lateral side of the ankle.

Superior peroneal retinaculum

The superior peroneal retinaculum extends from the back of the lateral malleolus to the deep transverse fascia of the lower leg and the lateral surface of the calcaneus. Damage to the retinaculum can lead to instability of the peroneal tendons.

Inferior peroneal retinaculum

The inferior peroneal retinaculum is continuous in front with the inferior extensor retinaculum, and is attached posteriorly to the lateral surface of the calcaneus. Some of its fibres are fused with the periosteum on the peroneal trochlea (tubercle) of the calcaneus, forming a septum between the tendons of peroneus longus and brevis.

SYNOVIAL SHEATHS IN THE ANKLE REGION

The tendons that cross the ankle joint are all deflected to some degree from a straight course, and must therefore be held down by retinacula and enclosed in synovial sheaths.

Anterior to the ankle, the sheath for tibialis anterior extends from the proximal margin of the superior extensor retinaculum to the interval between the diverging limbs of the inferior retinaculum (**Fig. 115.4**). A common sheath encloses the tendons of extensor digitorum longus and peroneus tertius, starting just above the level of the malleoli, and reaching to the level of the base of the fifth metatarsal bone (**Fig. 115.2**). The sheath for extensor hallucis longus starts just below that for extensor digitorum longus and reaches to the base of the first metatarsal bone (**Fig. 115.2**).

Medial to the ankle, the sheath for tibialis posterior starts c.4 cm above the malleolus and ends just proximal to the attachment of the tendon to the tuberosity of the navicular. The sheath for flexor hallucis longus reaches the level of the malleolus proximally, and the base of the first metatarsal bone distally. A fibrous nodule can form in the tendon, just proximal to the tendon sheath, as a result of overuse, especially in dancers, and catch in the sheath causing 'triggering' of the great toe, 'hallux saltans'. Surgical opening of the sheath may be required. In athletes, the muscle belly of flexor hallucis longus may be abnormally large and extend more distally than usual. It too can catch at the opening of the sheath. The sheath for flexor digitorum longus starts slightly above the malleolus and ends at the navicular.

Lateral to the ankle, the tendons of peroneus longus and brevis are enclosed in a sheath that is single proximally but double distally (**Fig. 115.2**). From the tip of the lateral malleolus it extends for about 4 cm both proximally and distally.

PLANTAR FASCIA

The plantar fascia (**Fig. 115.5**) or aponeurosis is composed of densely compacted collagen fibres orientated mainly longitudinally, but also transversely. Its medial and lateral parts overlie the intrinsic muscles of the hallux and fifth toe; its dense central part overlies the long and short digital flexors.

The central part is the strongest and thickest. It is narrow posteriorly, where it is attached to the medial process of the calcaneal tuberosity proximal to flexor digitorum brevis. It becomes broader and somewhat thinner as it diverges towards the metatarsal heads. Just proximal to these it divides into five bands, one for each toe. As these five bands diverge below the metatarsal shafts, they are united by transverse fibres. Proximal, plantar and a little distal to the metatarsal heads and the metatarsophalangeal joints, the superficial stratum of each band is connected to the dermis by skin ligaments (retinacula cutis). These skin ligaments reach the skin of the ball of the foot proximal to, and in the floors of, the furrows that separate the toes from the sole (**Fig. 115.6A**).

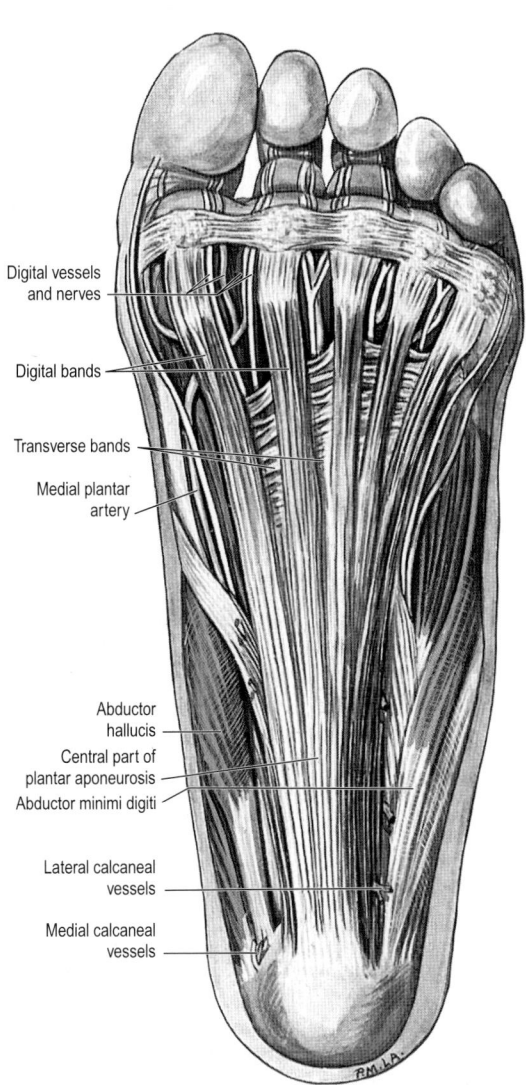

Digital vessels and nerves

Digital bands

Transverse bands

Medial plantar artery

Abductor hallucis

Central part of plantar aponeurosis

Abductor minimi digiti

Lateral calcaneal vessels

Medial calcaneal vessels

Fig. 115.5 The plantar aponeurosis of the left foot.

These cutaneous retinacula condense proximally to form a sagittal septum, but diverge distally into numerous bundles and lamellae that pass at right-angles through bundles of the plantar interdigital ligament. The deep stratum of each digital band of the aponeurosis divides into two septa that flank the digital flexor tendons, separating them from the lumbrical muscles and the digital vessels and nerves. These septa pass deeply to fuse with the interosseous fascia, the deep transverse metatarsal ligaments, the plantar ligaments of the metatarsophalangeal joints, and the periosteum and fibrous flexor sheaths at the base of each proximal phalanx. Pads of fat develop in the webs between the metatarsal heads and the bases of the proximal phalanges; they cushion the digital nerves and vessels from adjoining tendinous structures and extraneous plantar pressures. Vertical strands of collagen from the digital fibrous flexor sheaths tie these four fat pads to the superficial stratum of the plantar aponeurosis and, through this, to the skin (**Fig. 115.6B**). Just distal to the metatarsal heads, a plantar interdigital ligament (superficial transverse metatarsal ligament) blends progressively with the deep aspect of the superficial stratum of the plantar aponeurosis where it enters the toes (**Fig. 115.6A,B**). The central part of the plantar aponeurosis thus provides an intermediary structure between the skin and the osteoligamentous framework of the foot, via numerous cutaneous retinacula and deep septa extending to the metatarsals and phalanges. It is also continuous with the medial and lateral parts, and at the junctions two intermuscular septa, medial and lateral, extend in oblique vertical planes between the medial, intermediate and lateral groups of plantar muscles to reach bone. Thinner horizontal intermuscular septa, passing between muscle layers, are derived from the vertical intermuscular septa.

The lateral part of the plantar aponeurosis, which covers abductor digiti minimi, is thin distally and thick proximally, where it forms a strong band, sometimes containing muscle fibres, between the lateral process of the calcaneal tuberosity and the base of the fifth metatarsal bone. It is continuous medially with the central part of the aponeurosis, and with the fascia on the dorsum of the foot around its lateral border.

The medial part of the plantar aponeurosis, which covers abductor hallucis, is thin. It is continuous proximally with the flexor retinaculum, medially with the fascia dorsalis pedis, and laterally with the central part of the plantar aponeurosis.

FASCIAL COMPARTMENTS OF THE FOOT

There are four main compartments of the plantar aspect of the foot (Jones 1949) (**Fig. 115.7**). The medial compartment contains abductor hallucis and flexor hallucis brevis. It is bounded medially and inferiorly by the extension of the plantar aponeurosis, laterally by an intermuscular septum, and dorsally by the first metatarsal. The central compartment contains flexor digitorum brevis, the lumbricals, flexor accessorius and adductor hallucis. It is bounded by the plantar aponeurosis inferiorly, the osseofascial tarsometatarsal structures dorsally and intermuscular septa medially and laterally. The lateral compartment contains abductor digiti minimi and flexor digiti minimi brevis. Its boundaries are the fifth metatarsal dorsally, the plantar aponeurosis inferiorly and laterally, and an intermuscular septum medially. The interosseous compartment contains the seven interossei and its boundaries are the interosseous fascia and the metatarsals. (Of relevance in calcaneal fractures is a fifth deep central compartment within the central compartment, which contains flexor accessorius alone.)

A compartment syndrome results from an increase in intracompartmental pressure such that venous drainage is impaired. As blood enters at arterial pressure, the compartment pressure increases further and this prevents inflow of arterial blood, leading to muscle and nerve ischaemia. Failure to release the compartment surgically results in necrosis. The five compartments in the foot of clinical significance are the medial, central, lateral, interosseous and calcaneal compartments, and they may all need release. The most common cause of compartment syndrome in the foot is trauma, which is usually high-energy. Crush injuries, calcaneal fractures and disruption of the tarsometatarsal joints are the usual injury patterns associated with compartment syndrome of the foot.

Although there are several fascial layers on the dorsum of the foot, effectively there is one dorsal compartment.

Deep dorsal fascia

The deep fascia on the dorsum of the foot (fascia dorsalis pedis) is a thin layer, continuous above with the inferior extensor retinaculum; it covers the dorsal extensor tendons.

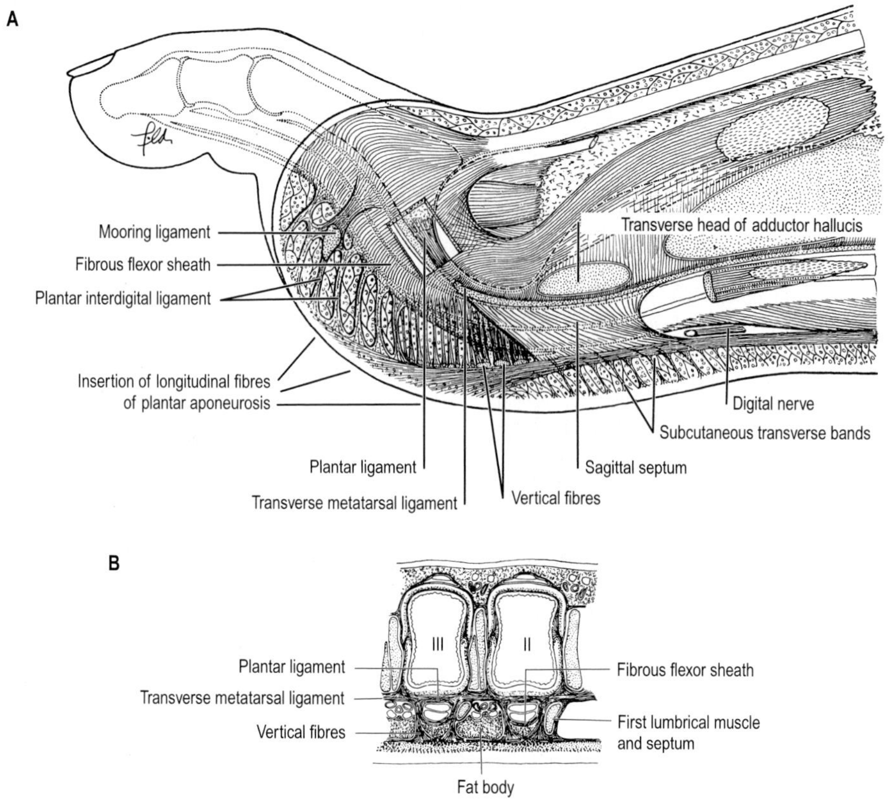

A

Mooring ligament

Fibrous flexor sheath

Plantar interdigital ligament

Transverse head of adductor hallucis

Insertion of longitudinal fibres
of plantar aponeurosis

Digital nerve

Subcutaneous transverse bands

Plantar ligament

Sagittal septum

Transverse metatarsal ligament

Vertical fibres

Fig. 115.6 Details of the tendinous and fibrous architecture of various regions on the plantar aspect of the right foot. **A**, Sagittal section through the second interosseous cleft, showing the internal architecture of the three major areas of the ball of the foot. The sagittal septum is attached to the proximal phalanx via the transverse metatarsal ligament and the plantar ligament of the joint. The vertical fibres and the lamellae of the plantar interdigital ligament are attached to the proximal phalanx via the fibrous flexor sheath. **B**, Transverse section through the heads of the second (II) and third (III) metatarsal bones, showing the course of the collagen fibre bundles in the submetatarsal cushions and around the joints. Fat covers the fibrous flexor sheath inside the cushion; the digital nerves and vessels are lodged between the cushions. (**A**, from Bojsen-Møller and Flagstad 1976, J Anat 121: 599–611. By permission from Blackwell Publishing Ltd.)

B

Plantar ligament

Transverse metatarsal ligament

Vertical fibres

Fibrous flexor sheath

First lumbrical muscle and septum

Fat body

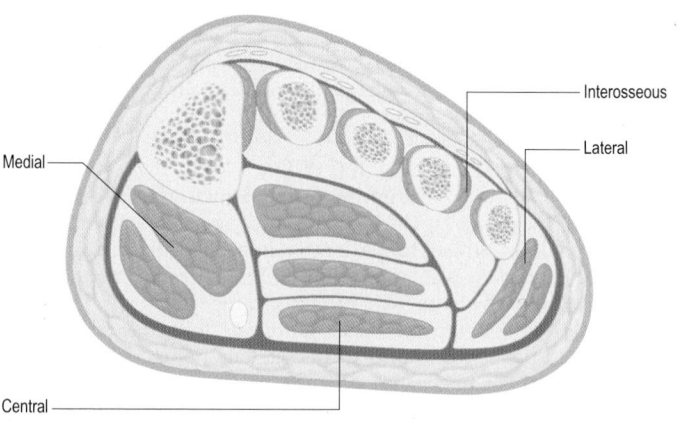

Medial

Central

Interosseous

Lateral

Fig. 115.7 Transverse section through the midfoot, showing the main fascial compartments.

Lateral intermuscular septum

The lateral intermuscular septum is incomplete, especially at its proximal end. Distally, its deep attachments are to the fibrous sheath of peroneus longus and to the fifth metatarsal bone.

Medial intermuscular septum

The medial intermuscular septum is incomplete and divides into three bands, proximal, intermediate and distal, each of which displays lateral and medial divisions as it approaches its deep attachment. The proximal band is attached laterally to the cuboid and blends medially with the tendon of tibialis posterior. The middle band is attached laterally to the cuboid and the long plantar ligament and medially to the medial cuneiform bone. The distal band divides to enclose the tendon of flexor hallucis longus and is attached to the fascia over flexor hallucis brevis.

SPECIALIZED ADIPOSE TISSUE (HEEL AND METATARSAL PAD)

The heel pad is subject to repeated high impacts and is anatomically adapted to withstand these pressures. The average heel pad is 18 mm thick and the mean epidermal thickness is 0.64 mm (dorsal epidermal thickness averages 0.069 mm). The heel pad contains elastic adipose tissue organised as spiral fibrous septa anchored to each other, to the calcaneus and to the skin. The septa are U-shaped fat-filled columns designed to resist compressive loads and are reinforced internally with elastic diagonal and transverse fibres, which separate the fat into compartments.

In the forefoot, the subcutaneous tissue consists of fibrous lamellae arranged in a complex whorl containing adipose tissue attached via vertical fibres to the dermis superficially and the plantar aponeurosis deeply. The fat is particularly thick in the region of the metatarsophalangeal joints, which cushions the foot during the toe-off phase of gait. Like the heel pad, the metatarsal fat pad is designed to withstand compressive and shearing forces. Atrophy of either is a cause of persistent pain.

BONE

Functionally, the skeleton of the foot may be divided into tarsus, metatarsus and phalanges. Here the terms 'plantar' and 'dorsal' are used, rather than anterior and posterior, which are less appropriate. The terms 'proximal' and 'distal' are used with the same significance as in limbs generally. Rotation that occurs in the early stages of the development of the limbs produces a lateral thumb in the hand, and a medial great toe in the foot.

DISTAL TIBIA

The distal end of the tibia has anterior, medial, posterior, lateral and distal surfaces, and projects inferomedially as the medial malleolus. It is laterally rotated relative to the proximal tibia (tibial torsion). The smooth anterior surface bulges slightly and ends distal to the distal surface. The medial surface is smooth and subcutaneous. It is continuous with the shaft proximally and the medial malleolus distally. The posterior surface is smooth and is separated from the medial surface by a prominent ridge that passes inferomedially to the posterior aspect of the medial malleolus. The lateral surface is the triangular fibular notch, which is roughened proximally but smooth distally, where it is sometimes covered by articular cartilage. The distal surface articulates with the talus and is wider anteriorly than posteriorly. It is concave sagittally and slightly convex transversely and continues medially into

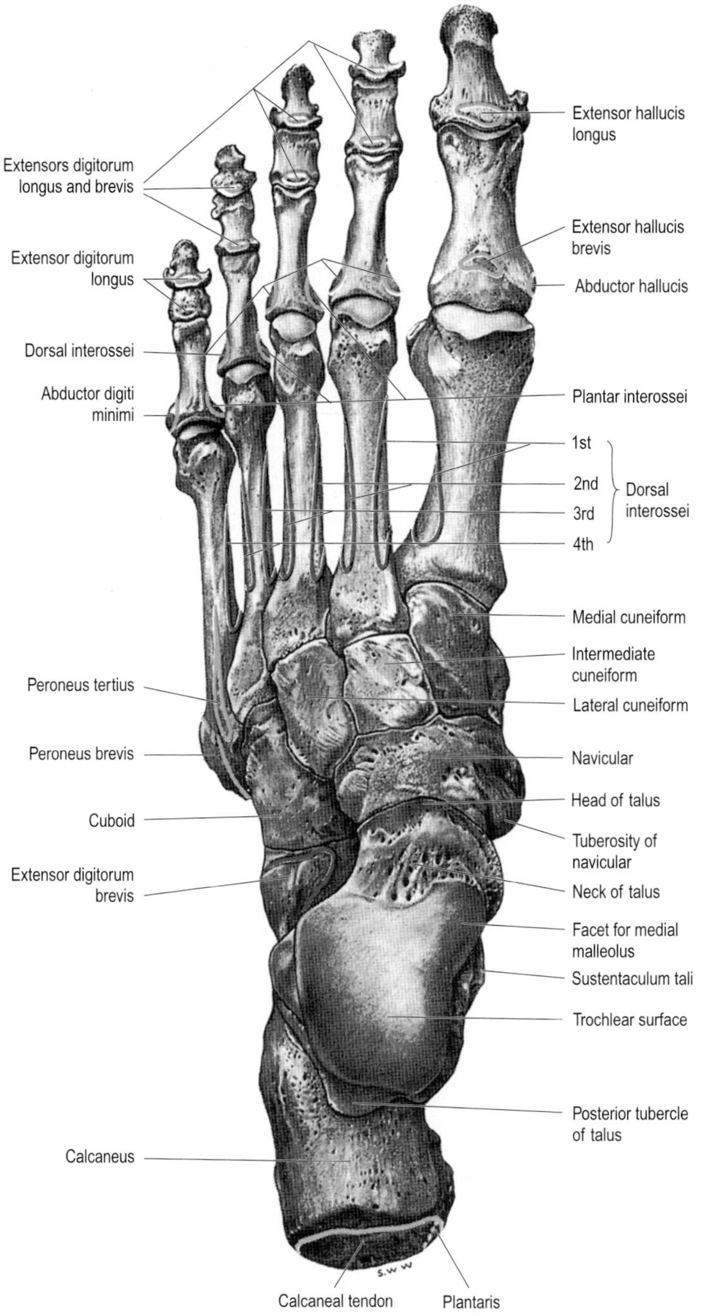

Fig. 115.8 (Dorsal aspect labels)

Extensors digitorum longus and brevis

Extensor digitorum longus

Dorsal interossei

Abductor digiti minimi

Peroneus tertius

Peroneus brevis

Cuboid

Extensor digitorum brevis

Calcaneus

Extensor hallucis longus

Extensor hallucis brevis

Abductor hallucis

Plantar interossei

1st
2nd } Dorsal
3rd interossei
4th

Medial cuneiform

Intermediate cuneiform

Lateral cuneiform

Navicular

Head of talus

Tuberosity of navicular

Neck of talus

Facet for medial malleolus

Sustentaculum tali

Trochlear surface

Posterior tubercle of talus

Calcaneal tendon   Plantaris

Fig. 115.8 Dorsal aspect of the skeleton of the left foot.

Fig. 115.9 (Plantar aspect labels)

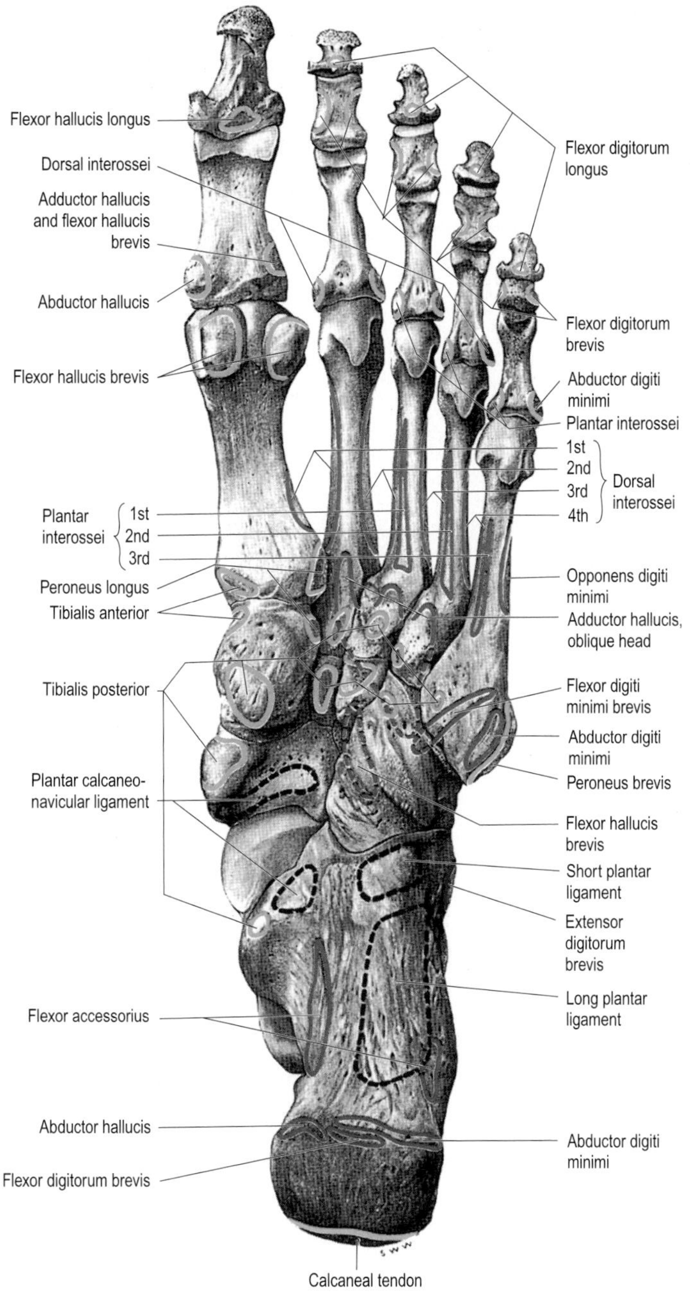

Flexor hallucis longus

Dorsal interossei

Adductor hallucis and flexor hallucis brevis

Abductor hallucis

Flexor hallucis brevis

Plantar interossei { 1st
2nd
3rd }

Peroneus longus

Tibialis anterior

Tibialis posterior

Plantar calcaneo-navicular ligament

Flexor accessorius

Abductor hallucis

Flexor digitorum brevis

Flexor digitorum longus

Flexor digitorum brevis

Abductor digiti minimi

Plantar interossei

1st
2nd } Dorsal
3rd interossei
4th

Opponens digiti minimi

Adductor hallucis, oblique head

Flexor digiti minimi brevis

Abductor digiti minimi

Peroneus brevis

Flexor hallucis brevis

Short plantar ligament

Extensor digitorum brevis

Long plantar ligament

Abductor digiti minimi

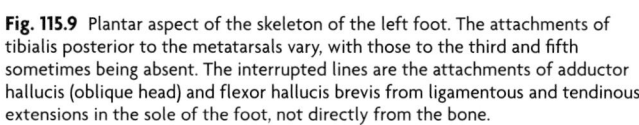

Calcaneal tendon

Fig. 115.9 Plantar aspect of the skeleton of the left foot. The attachments of tibialis posterior to the metatarsals vary, with those to the third and fifth sometimes being absent. The interrupted lines are the attachments of adductor hallucis (oblique head) and flexor hallucis brevis from ligamentous and tendinous extensions in the sole of the foot, not directly from the bone.

the malleolar articular surface. The medial malleolus is short and thick and has a smooth lateral surface with a crescentic facet that articulates with the medial surface of the talar body.

Muscle attachments – The interosseous membrane, the deltoid, and the anterior and posterior tibiofibular ligaments are attached to the distal tibia. No muscles are attached to the bone in this region.

Vascular supply – The distal tibia is supplied by an arterial network formed by branches of the dorsalis pedis, posterior tibial and peroneal arteries.

Innervation – The distal tibia is innervated by branches from the deep peroneal, posterior tibial, saphenous and sural nerves.

Ossification – The distal epiphyseal centre appears early in the first year of life and fuses at 15 years in females and 17 years in males. In 47% of females and 17% of males, an accessory ossification centre appears at

the tip of the medial malleolus. This fuses during the eighth year in females and the ninth in males, and fusion occurs during the eleventh year. It should not be confused with an os subtibiale, which is a rare accessory bone found on the posterior aspect of the medial malleolus.

DISTAL FIBULA

The distal end of the fibula or lateral malleolus projects distally and posteriorly relative to the medial malleolus. Its lateral aspect is subcutaneous, the posterior surface has a broad groove with a prominent lateral border, and the anterior surface is rough and round and articulates with the anteroinferior aspect of the tibia. The medial surface has a triangular articular facet, vertically convex and its apex distal, which articulates with the lateral talar surface. Behind the facet is a rough malleolar fossa.

Muscle attachments – There are no muscles attached to the distal fibula below the level of the interosseous ligament. The ligamentous attachments are those of the lateral ligament complex, i.e. the anterior talofibular, the calcaneofibular and the posterior talofibular ligaments. The interosseous ligament is attached on its medial surface.

The medial surface of the fibula gives rise to the extensor hallucis longus, extensor digitorum longus and the peroneus tertius muscles. The lateral surface has the origin of the peroneus longus and brevis muscles. The posterior surface gives origin to the flexor hallucis longus and soleus muscles lateral to the medial crest of the fibula; medial to it arises the tibialis posterior muscle.

Vascular supply – The distal fibula is supplied by an arterial network made up of branches of the dorsalis pedis, posterior tibial and peroneal arteries.

Innervation – The distal fibula is innervated by the deep peroneal, tibial, saphenous and sural nerves.

Ossification – The distal fibular ossification centre appears in the first year of life and fuses at 17 years. An os subfibulare is a separate entity and lies posterior to the tip of the fibula, whereas the distal fibular apophysis lies anterior. An os retinaculi is rarely encountered: If present, it overlies the bursa of the distal fibula within the peroneal retinaculum.

TARSUS

The seven tarsal bones occupy the proximal half of the foot (**Figs 115.8, 115.9, 115.10**). The tarsus and carpus are homologous, but the tarsal elements are larger, to support and distribute weight. As in the carpus, tarsal bones are arranged in proximal and distal rows, but medially there is an additional single intermediate tarsal element. The proximal row is made up of the talus and calcaneus; the long axis of the talus is inclined anteromedially and down, its distal head is medial to the calcaneus and at a higher level. The distal row contains, from medial to lateral, the medial, intermediate and lateral cuneiforms and the cuboid; they are roughly in parallel and form a transverse arch that is dorsally convex. Medially, the navicular is interposed between the talus and cuneiforms. Laterally, the calcaneus articulates with the cuboid.

The tarsus and metatarsus are arranged to form intersecting longitudinal and transverse arches. Hence thrust and weight are not transmitted from the tibia to the ground (or *vice versa*) directly through the tarsus, but are distributed through the tarsal and metatarsals to the ends of the longitudinal arches. For the purposes of description, each tarsal bone is arbitrarily considered to be cuboidal in form, with six surfaces. The ossification sites and dates are summarised in **Fig. 115.11**.

TALUS

The talus is the link between the foot and leg, through the ankle joint (**Fig. 115.12**)

Head – Directed distally and somewhat inferomedially, the head has a distal surface, oval and convex; its long axis is also inclined inferomedially to articulate with the proximal navicular surface. The plantar surface of the head has three articular areas, separated by smooth ridges. The most posterior and largest is oval, slightly convex and rests on a shelf-like medial calcaneal projection, the sustentaculum tali. Anterolateral to this and usually continuous with it, a flat articular facet rests on the anteromedial part of the dorsal (proximal) calcaneal surface; distally it continues into the navicular surface. Medial to these two calcaneal facets, a part of the talar head is covered with articular cartilage, continuous with the calcaneal and navicular areas (**Fig. 115.12B**) and in contact with the plantar calcaneonavicular ligament, which is covered here, superiorly, by fibrocartilage. When the foot is inverted passively, the dorsolateral aspect of the head is visible and palpable c.3 cm distal to the tibia; it is hidden by extensor tendons when the toes are dorsiflexed.

Neck – The neck is the narrow, medially inclined region between the head and body. Its rough surfaces are for ligaments. The medial plantar surface has a deep sulcus tali which, when the talus and calcaneus are articulated, forms a roof to the sinus tarsi, which is occupied by interosseous talocalcaneal and cervical ligaments.

The long axis of the neck, inclined downwards, distally and medially, makes an angle of c.150° with that of the body; it is smaller (130–140°) at birth, accounting in part for the inverted foot in young children. The dorsal talonavicular ligament and ankle articular capsule are attached distally to its dorsal surface, leaving its proximal part intracapsular. The medial articular facet and part of the trochlear surface may extend onto the neck. The anterior talofibular ligament is attached laterally on the neck, spreading along the adjacent anterior border of the lateral surface. The interosseous talocalcaneal and cervical ligaments are attached to the inferior surface of the neck. A dorsolateral squatting facet commonly occurs on the neck in those who habitually adopt this position. It articulates with the anterior tibial margin in extreme dorsiflexion; the facet may be double.

Body – The body is cuboidal, covered dorsally by a trochlear surface articulating with the distal end of the tibia. It is anteroposteriorly convex, gently concave transversely, widest anteriorly and, therefore, sellar. The triangular lateral surface is smooth and vertically concave for articulation with the lateral malleolus. Superiorly, it is continuous with the trochlear surface; inferiorly its apex is a lateral process. Proximally, the medial surface is (posterosuperiorly) covered by a comma-shaped facet, which is deeper in front and articulates with the medial malleolus. Distally, this surface is rough and contains numerous vascular foramina. The small posterior surface is a rough projecting posterior process, and is marked by an oblique groove between two tubercles that contains the tendon of flexor hallucis longus. The lateral tubercle is usually larger; the medial is less prominent and immediately behind the sustentaculum tali (**Fig. 115.18**). The plantar surface articulates with the middle one-third of the dorsal calcaneal surface by an oval concave facet, its long axis directed distolaterally at an angle of c.45° with the median plane.

The medial edge of the trochlear surface is straight, but its lateral edge inclines medially in its posterior part and is often broadened into a small elongated triangular area, which is in contact with the posterior tibiofibular ligament in dorsiflexion.

The posterior talofibular ligament is attached to the posterior process. It extends up to the groove, or depression, between the process and posterior trochlear border. The posterior talocalcaneal ligament is attached to its plantar border. The groove between the tubercles of the process contains the tendon of flexor hallucis longus, continuing distally into the groove on the plantar aspect of the sustentaculum tali. The medial talocalcaneal ligament is attached below to the medial tubercle, whereas above the tubercle the most posterior superficial fibres of the deltoid ligament are attached. The deep fibres of the deltoid ligament are attached still higher to the rough area immediately below the comma-shaped articular facet on the medial surface (**Fig. 115.12C**).

Muscle attachments – No muscles are attached to the talus. However, many ligaments are attached to it, because it is involved in ankle, subtalar and talocalcaneonavicular joints (**Figs 115.13, 115.14, 115.15**).

Vascular supply – The talar blood supply is rather tenuous because of the lack of muscle attachments. The first comprehensive understanding of its blood supply was provided by Wildenauer in 1950. The extraosseous blood supply to the talus is via the posterior tibial, dorsalis pedis and peroneal arteries (**Fig. 115.16**). The artery of the tarsal canal arises from the posterior tibial artery 1 cm proximal to the origin of the medial and lateral plantar arteries (**Fig. 115.17**). It passes anteriorly between the sheath of flexor digitorum longus and flexor hallucis longus to enter the tarsal canal, in which it lies anteriorly, close to the talus. Branches from the arterial network in the tarsal canal enter the talus. The artery continues through the tarsal canal into the tarsal sinus, where it anastomoses with the artery of the tarsal sinus, forming a vascular sling under the talar neck. A branch of the artery of the tarsal canal known as the deltoid branch passes deep to the deltoid ligament and supplies part of the medial talar body. Sometimes it arises from the posterior tibial artery; rarely, it arises from the medial plantar artery. In talar fractures it may be the only remaining arterial supply to the talus to maintain the viability of the talar body. The dorsalis pedis artery supplies superior neck branches to the talar neck and also gives off the artery of the tarsal sinus. This large vessel is always present and anastomoses with the artery of the tarsal canal. The artery of the tarsal sinus receives a contribution from the perforating peroneal artery and supplies direct branches into the talus. The peroneal artery provides small branches which form a plexus of vessels posteriorly with branches

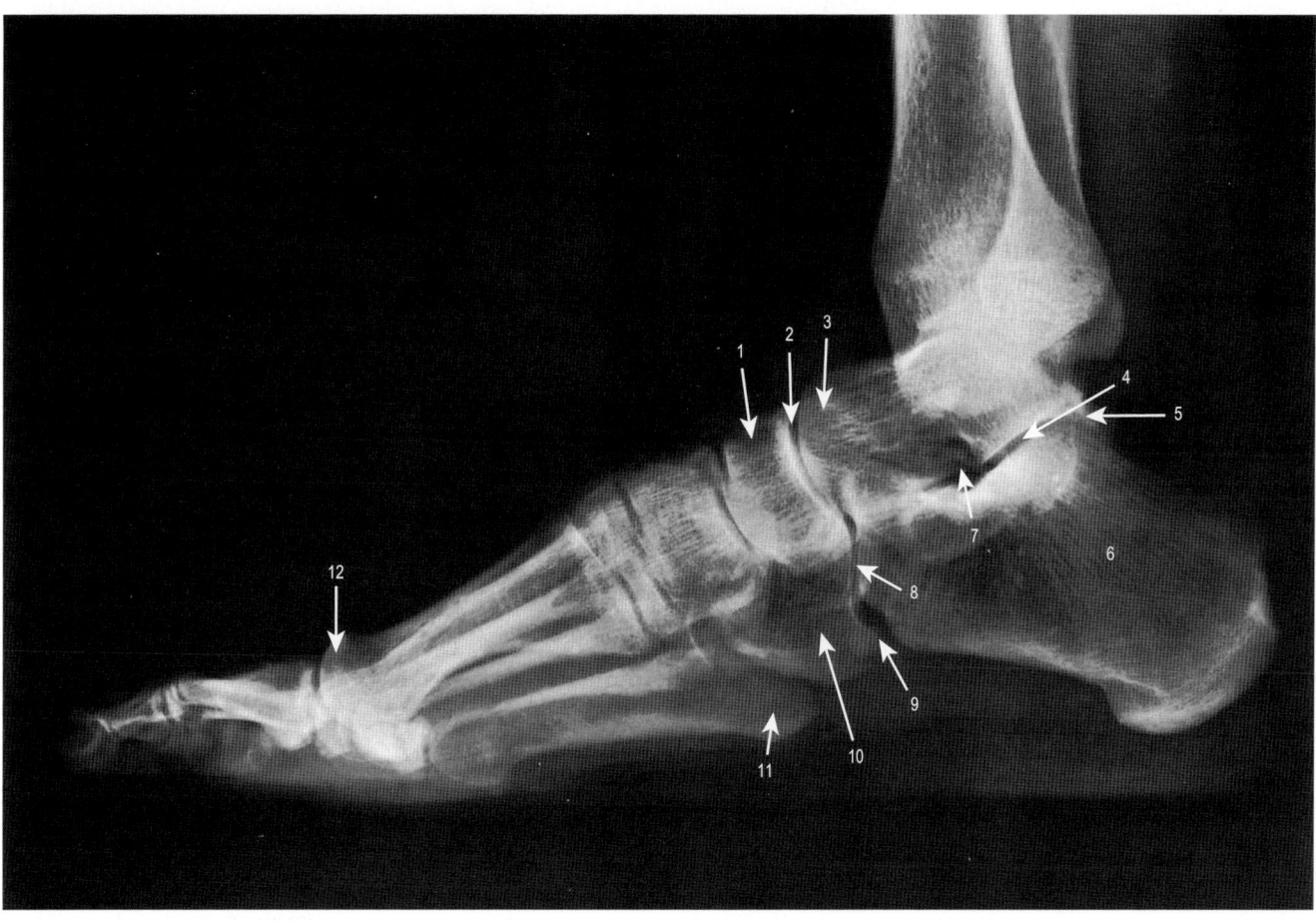

1. Navicular.   2. Talonavicular joint.   3. Head of talus.   4. Subtalar joint.   5. Os trigonum.   6. Calcaneus (note trabecular pattern).   7. Sinus tarsi.   8. Calcaneocuboid joint.
9. Sesamoid in tendon of peroneus longus.   10. Cuboid.   11. Tuberosity on base of fifth metatarsal.   12. Head of first metatarsal.

Fig. 115.10   Lateral radiograph of ankle and foot in full plantigrade contact with the ground, during symmetrical standing, in a man aged 44 years.

of the posterior tibial artery. The contribution of the peroneal artery to the talar blood supply is not considered important.

The intraosseous blood supply of the talar head comes medially from branches of the dorsalis pedis and laterally from branches from the anastomosis between the artery of the tarsal canal and the tarsal sinus. The middle one-third of the talar body, except for the most extreme superior aspect, and the lateral one-third, except for the posterior aspect, are supplied mainly by the anastomotic artery in the tarsal canal. The medial one-third is supplied by the deltoid artery.

Innervation – The talus is innervated by branches from the deep peroneal, posterior tibial, saphenous and sural nerves.

Ossification – A single ossific centre appears prenatally at 6 months (**Fig. 115.11**). The posterior process (Steida) is a separate bone in c.5% of individuals and arises from a separate ossification centre, which appears between 8 and 11 years. In athletes and dancers, it can cause impingement against the posterior tibia, producing pain and sometimes requiring surgical removal. Another more rare accessory bone is the os supratalare, which lies on the dorsal aspect of the talus; it rarely measures more than 4 mm in length.

Talar fractures

The fact that the talus has no muscular attachments and that 70% of its surfaces are covered by articular cartilage means that displaced talar neck fractures, with interruption of the blood supply to the talar body, can result in avascular necrosis and non-union. In general, in undisplaced fractures, these complications do not occur. If, at 8 weeks after fracture of the talar neck, a subchondral lucency is seen in the talar dome on radiographs (Hawkin's sign), it may be assumed that vascularity to the talar body is intact and that the fracture will proceed to unite.

CALCANEUS

The calcaneus (**Fig. 115.18**), the largest tarsal bone, projects posterior to the tibia and fibula as a short lever for muscles of the calf attached to its posterior surface. It is irregularly cuboidal, its long axis inclined distally upwards and laterally. The superior or proximal surface is divisible into three. The posterior one-third is rough and concavo-convex; the convexity is transverse and supports fibroadipose tissue (Kager's fat pad) between the calcaneal tendon and ankle joint. The middle one-third carries the posterior talar facet, which is oval and convex anteroposteriorly. The anterior one-third is partly articular; distal (anterior) to the posterior articular facet, a rough depression narrows into a groove on the medial side, the sulcus calcanei, which completes the sinus tarsi with the talus. (The sinus tarsi is a conical hollow bounded by the talus medially, superiorly and laterally, with the superior surface of the calcaneus below. It is continuous with the tarsal canal.) Distal and medial to this groove, an elongated articular area covers the sustentaculum tali, and extends distolaterally on the body of the bone. This facet is often divided by a non-articular interval at the anterior limit of the sustentaculum tali, forming middle and anterior talar facets, the incidence of which varies with sex and race. Rarely, all three facets on the upper surface of the calcaneus are fused into one irregular area. A detailed analysis of patterns of anterior talar articular facets in a series of 401 Indian calcanei revealed four types. Type I (67%) showed one continuous facet on the sustentaculum extending to the distomedial calcaneal corner; type II (26%) presented two facets, one sustentacular and one distal calcaneal; type III (5%) possessed only a single sustentacular facet; and type IV (2%) showed all anterior and posterior facets confluent.

The anterior surface is the smallest, and is an obliquely set concavo-convex articular facet for the cuboid.

The posterior surface is divided into three regions. These are a smooth proximal (superior) area separated from the calcaneal tendon

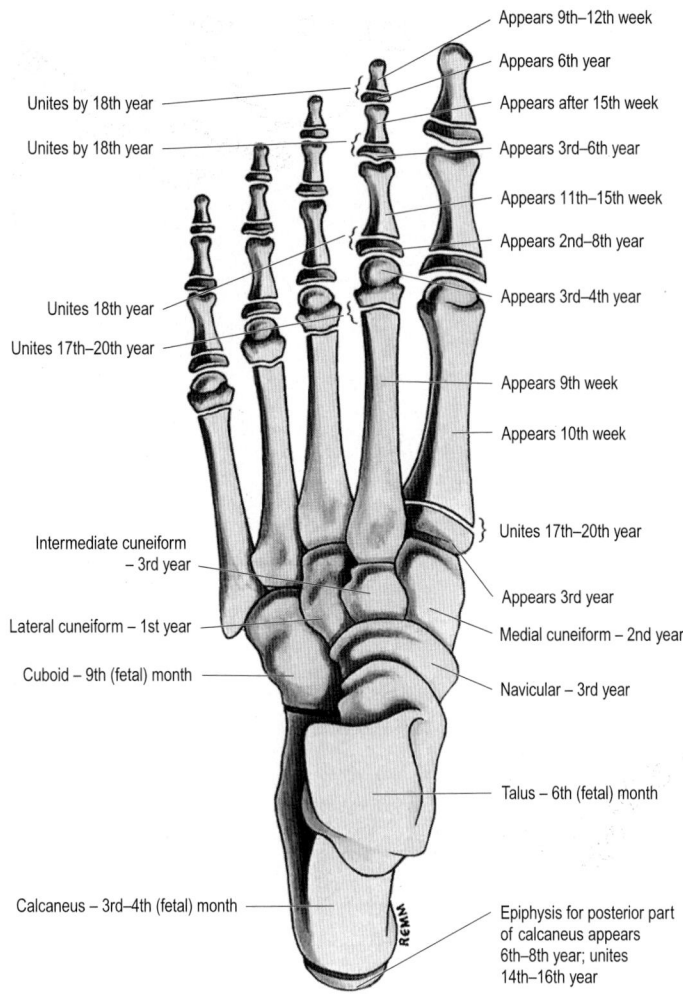

Appears 9th–12th week

Appears 6th year

Unites by 18th year

Appears after 15th week

Unites by 18th year

Appears 3rd–6th year

Appears 11th–15th week

Appears 2nd–8th year

Unites 18th year

Appears 3rd–4th year

Unites 17th–20th year

Appears 9th week

Appears 10th week

Intermediate cuneiform – 3rd year

Unites 17th–20th year

Lateral cuneiform – 1st year

Appears 3rd year

Medial cuneiform – 2nd year

Cuboid – 9th (fetal) month

Navicular – 3rd year

Talus – 6th (fetal) month

Calcaneus – 3rd–4th (fetal) month

Epiphysis for posterior part of calcaneus appears 6th–8th year; unites 14th–16th year

Fig. 115.11 Ossification of the bones of the foot.

by a bursa and adipose tissue, a middle area, the largest, limited above by a groove and below by a rough ridge for the calcaneal tendon, and a distal (inferior) area inclined downwards and forwards, vertically striated, which is the subcutaneous weight-bearing surface.

The plantar surface is rough, especially proximally as the calcaneal tuberosity, the lateral and medial processes of which extend distally, separated by a notch. The medial is longer and broader (**Fig. 115.18B**). Further distally, an anterior tubercle marks the distal limit of the attachment of the long plantar ligament.

The lateral surface is almost flat. It is proximally deeper and palpable on the lateral aspect of the heel distal to the lateral malleolus. Distally, it presents the peroneal tubercle (**Fig. 115.18C**), which is exceedingly variable in size and, when well developed, palpable 2 cm distal to the lateral malleolus. It has an oblique groove for the tendon of peroneus longus and a shallower proximal one for the tendon of peroneus brevis. About 1 cm or more behind and above the peroneal tubercle, a second elevation may exist for attachment of the calcaneofibular part of the lateral ligament.

The medial surface is vertically concave, and its concavity is accentuated by the sustentaculum tali, which projects medially from the distal part of its upper border (**Fig. 115.18D**). Superiorly, the process bears the middle talar facets and inferiorly a groove continuous with that on the talar posterior surface for the tendon of flexor hallucis longus (**Fig. 115.18B**). The medial aspect of the sustentaculum tali can be felt immediately distal to the tip of the medial malleolus; occasionally it is also grooved by the tendon of flexor digitorum longus.

Muscle (and ligament) attachments – The interosseous talocalcaneal and cervical ligaments and the medial root of the inferior extensor retinaculum are attached in the calcaneal sulcus. The non-articular area distal to the posterior talar facet is the site of attachment of extensor

digitorum brevis (in part), the principal band of the inferior extensor retinaculum and the stem of the bifurcated ligament.

Abductor hallucis and the superficial part of the flexor retinaculum and, distally, the plantar aponeurosis and flexor digitorum brevis, are all attached to the medial process of the calcaneal tuberosity at its prominent medial margin. Abductor digiti minimi is attached to the lateral process, extending medially to the medial process. The long plantar ligament is attached to the rough region between the process proximally, and extends to the anterior tubercle distally. The short plantar ligament is attached to the tubercle and the area distal to it. The lateral tendinous head of flexor accessorius is attached distal to the lateral process near the lateral margin of the long plantar ligament. Plantaris is attached to the posterior surface, which is wider below, and near the medial side of the calcaneal tendon. The anterior part of the lateral surface is crossed by the peroneal tendons, but is largely subcutaneous. The calcaneofibular ligament is attached c.1–2 cm proximal to the peroneal tubercle, usually to a low, rounded elevation.

The sustentaculum tali is dorsally part of the talocalcaneonavicular joint; its plantar surface is grooved by the tendon of flexor hallucis longus and margins of the groove give attachment to the deep part of the flexor retinaculum. The plantar calcaneonavicular ligament is attached distally to the medial margin of the sustentaculum, which is narrow, rough and convex. A slip from the tendon of tibialis posterior, and superficial fibres of the deltoid and medial talocalcaneal ligaments, are attached proximally. Distal to the attachment of the deltoid ligament, the tendon of flexor digitorum longus is related to the margin of the sustentaculum and may groove it. The large medial head of flexor accessorius is attached distal to the groove for flexor hallucis longus.

Vascular supply – The calcaneus receives its arterial supply from the medial and lateral calcaneal arteries (arising from the posterior tibial and peroneal arteries, respectively), peroneal artery, posterior calcaneal anastomosis (formed from the posterior tibial and peroneal arteries), medial and lateral plantar arteries, artery of tarsal sinus and tarsal canal, branches of the proximal lateral tarsal artery and perforating peroneal arteries.

Innervation – The calcaneus is innervated by branches of the tibial, sural and the deep peroneal nerves.

Ossification – The calcaneus is the only tarsal bone that always has two ossification centres (**Fig. 115.11**). In addition to the main ossific centre, there is a scale-like posterior apophysis that covers most of the posterior, and part of the plantar, surfaces. The main centre appears prenatally in the third month, whereas the posterior apophysis appears in the sixth year in females and the eighth in males, fusing in the fourteenth and sixteenth years, respectively.

In 2% of individuals, an os calcaneus secondarius is encountered, which is an accessory bone rather than a secondary ossific centre. If present, it is located on the dorsal beak or anterior process of the calcaneus in an interval between the anteromedial aspect of the calcaneus, the proximal end of the cuboid and navicular, and the head of the talus. Other rare accessory bones of the os calcis include the calcaneus accessorius in the region of the peroneal tubercle, the os sustentaculi on the posterior aspect of the sustentaculum, the os subcalcis on the plantar aspect of the calcaneus slightly posterior to the origin of the plantar aponeurosis, and the os aponeurosis plantaris, which lies within the plantar aponeurosis in close proximity to the medial tuberosity of the calcaneus.

NAVICULAR

The navicular (**Fig. 115.19**) articulates between the talar head proximally and cuneiform bones distally. Its distal surface is transversely convex and divided into three facets (the medial being the largest) for articulation with the cuneiforms. The proximal surface, oval and concave, articulates with the talar head. The dorsal surface is rough and convex; the medial, also rough, continues into a prominent tuberosity, palpable c.2.5 cm distal and plantar to the medial malleolus. The plantar surface, rough and concave, is separated from the tuberosity medially by a groove. The lateral surface is rough, irregular and often bears a facet for articulation with the cuboid.

The facet for the medial cuneiform is roughly triangular, its rounded apex is medial and its 'base' often markedly curved; those for the intermediate and lateral cuneiforms are also triangular, with plantar apices.

A

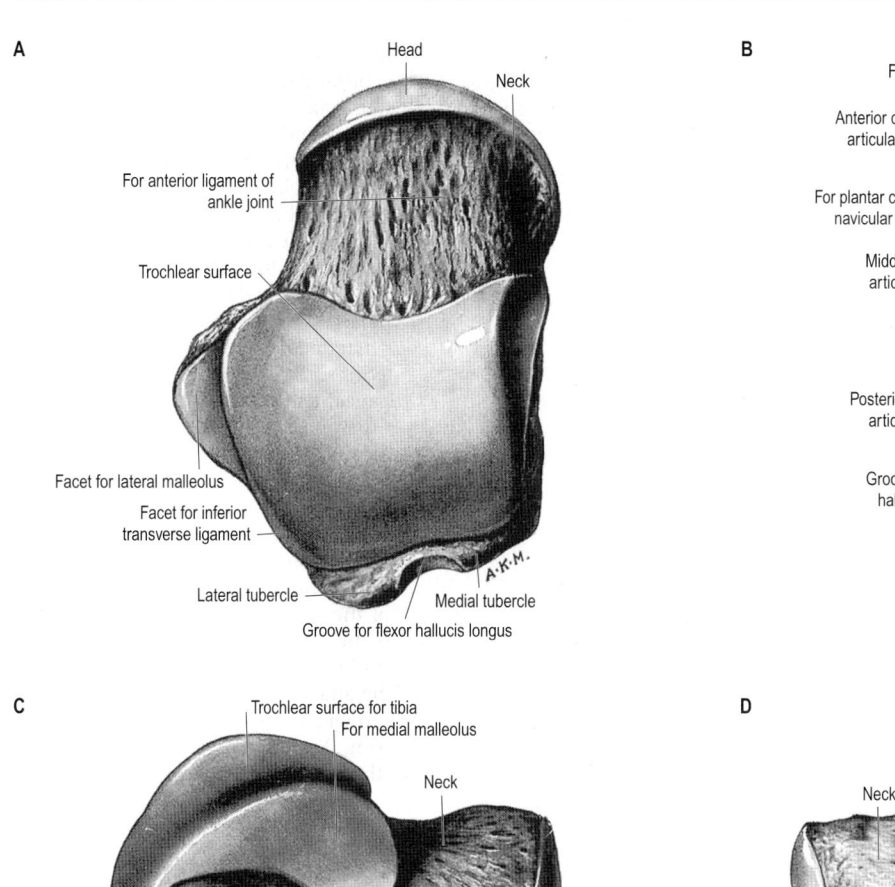

Head

Neck

For anterior ligament of
ankle joint

Trochlear surface

Facet for lateral malleolus

Facet for inferior
transverse ligament

Lateral tubercle

Medial tubercle

Groove for flexor hallucis longus

B

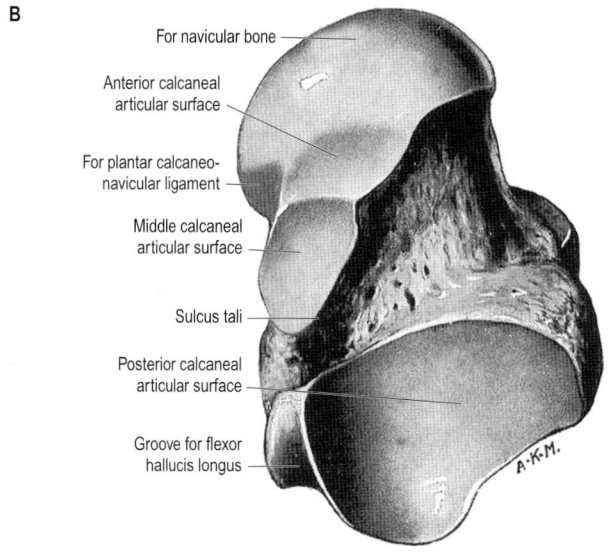

For navicular bone

Anterior calcaneal
articular surface

For plantar calcaneo-
navicular ligament

Middle calcaneal
articular surface

Sulcus tali

Posterior calcaneal
articular surface

Groove for flexor
hallucis longus

C

Trochlear surface for tibia

For medial malleolus

Neck

For navicular

Lateral
tubercle

Medial
tubercle

For deltoid
ligament

Groove for flexor
hallucis longus

For plantar calcaneonavicular
ligament

D

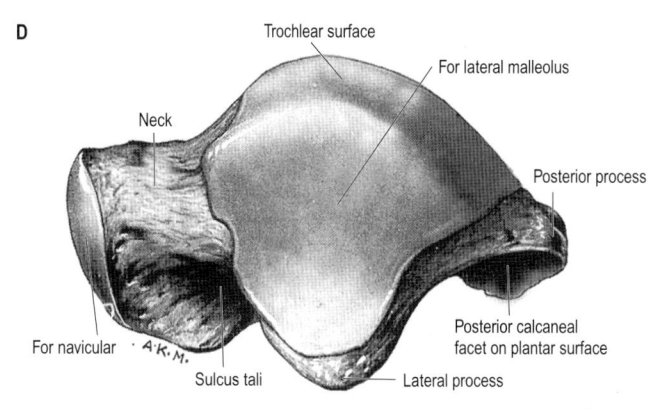

Trochlear surface

For lateral malleolus

Neck

Posterior process

For navicular

Sulcus tali

Posterior calcaneal
facet on plantar surface

Lateral process

Fig. 115.12 The left talus. **A**, Dorsal (superior) aspect; **B**, plantar (inferior) aspect; **C**, medial aspect; **D**, lateral aspect.

The facet for the lateral cuneiform may approach a wide crescent or a semicircle rather than a triangle (**Fig. 115.19A**). Dorsal talonavicular, cuneonavicular and cubonavicular ligaments are attached to the dorsal navicular surface.

Muscle (and ligament) attachments – The tuberosity is the main attachment of tibialis posterior and a groove lateral to it transmits part of the tendon distally to the cuneiforms and middle three metatarsal bases. The plantar calcaneonavicular ligament is attached to a slight projection lateral to the groove and adjacent to the proximal surface. The calcaneonavicular part of the bifurcated ligament is attached to the rough part of the lateral surface.

Vascular supply – The dorsal aspect of the navicular is supplied either from a branch of, or directly from, the dorsalis pedis artery. Its plantar aspect is supplied from the medial plantar artery, and the tuberosity is supplied by an anastomosis from the dorsalis pedis and medial plantar arteries.

Innervation – The navicular is innervated by the deep peroneal and medial plantar nerves.

Ossification – The navicular ossic centre appears during the third year (**Fig. 115.11**) and is sometimes affected by avascular necrosis between the ages of 4 and 7 years (Köhler's disease). An accessory navicular bone is found in c.5% of individuals. It arises from a separate ossification

centre in the navicular tuberosity region. There are three distinct types. Type 1 is a small accessory bone without attachment to the body of the navicular, and probably represents a sesamoid bone within the plantar aspect of the tibialis posterior tendon at the level of the inferior calcaneonavicular ligament. A type 2 accessory navicular is a definite part of the body of the navicular, but the tuberosity is separated by a fibrocartilaginous plate (synchondrosis). A type 3 accessory navicular is united by a bony ridge, producing a cornuate navicular. Only type 2 variants tend to produce symptoms.

Rarely, the navicular is bipartite and it arises from two distinct centres of ossification. This can lead to premature degeneration within the talonavicular joint (Muller–Weiss disease). On occasion, a small bone is found within the talonavicular joint on its dorsal aspect. Referred to as an os talonaviculare dorsale, it represents either a separate accessory bone or a fractured osteophyte of the proximal dorsal aspect of the navicular.

CUBOID

The cuboid, most lateral in the distal tarsal row, is between the calcaneus proximally and the fourth and fifth metatarsals distally (**Fig. 115.20**). Its dorsolateral surface is rough, for the attachment of ligaments. The plantar surface is crossed distally by an oblique groove for the tendon of peroneus longus and bounded proximally by a ridge that ends laterally in the tuberosity of the cuboid, the lateral aspect of which is faceted for a sesamoid bone or cartilage frequently found in the peroneus longus tendon. Proximal to its ridge, the rough plantar surface extends

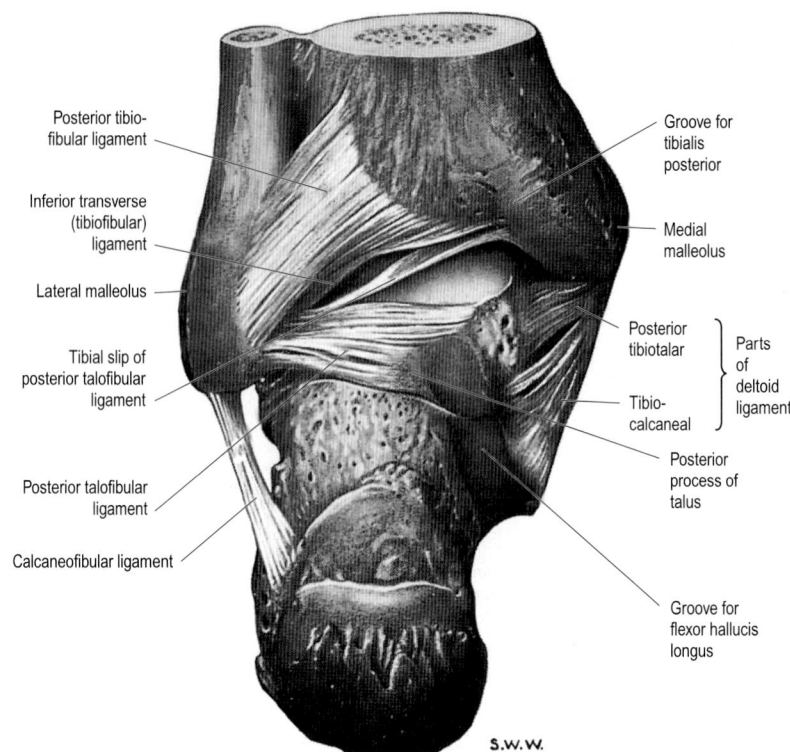

Fig. 115.13 Posterior aspect of the left ankle joint. (Drawn from a specimen in the Museum of the Royal College of Surgeons of England, with permission from the Council.)

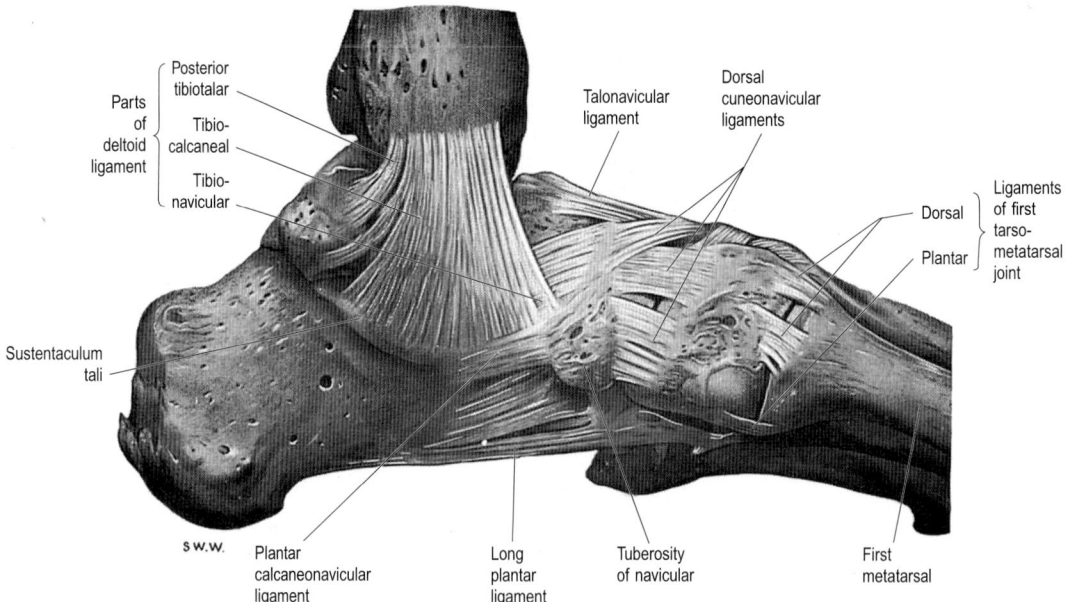

Fig. 115.14 Medial aspect of the left ankle and tarsal joints. (Drawn from a specimen in the Museum of the Royal College of Surgeons of England, with permission from the Council.)

proximally and medially because of the obliquity of the calcaneocuboid joint, making its medial border much longer than the lateral. The lateral surface is rough; the groove for peroneus longus extends from a deep notch on its plantar edge. The medial surface, which is much more extensive and partly non-articular, bears an oval facet for the lateral cuneiform, and proximal to this another (sometimes absent) for the navicular: the two form a continuous surface separated by a smooth vertical ridge. The distal surface is divided vertically into a medial quadrilateral articular area for the fourth metatarsal base and a lateral triangular area, its apex lateral, for the fifth metatarsal base. The proximal surface, triangular and concavo-convex, articulates with the distal calcaneal surface; its medial plantar angle projects proximally and inferior to the distal end of the calcaneus.

Muscle (and ligament) attachments – The dorsal calcaneocuboid, cubonavicular, cuneocuboid and cubometatarsal ligaments are attached to the dorsal surface. Deep fibres of the long plantar ligament are attached to the proximal edge of the plantar ridge. Slips from the tendons of tibialis posterior and flexor hallucis brevis are attached to the projecting proximomedial part of the plantar surface. Interosseous, cuneocuboid and cubonavicular ligaments are attached to the rough part of the medial cuboidal surface. Proximally, the medial calcaneocuboid ligament, which is the lateral limb of the bifurcated ligament, is also attached to this surface.

Vascular supply – The cuboid is supplied by deep branches of the medial and lateral plantar arteries. There is also a small dorsal supply from the dorsal arterial network.

Innervation – The cuboid is innervated by branches from the lateral plantar, sural and deep peroneal nerves.

Ossification – The cuboid frequently begins to ossify before birth, but has generally appeared 6 months after birth (**Fig. 115.11**). An os cuboides secundarium, an accessory bone, is rarely found in close proximity to the cuboid on its plantar aspect.

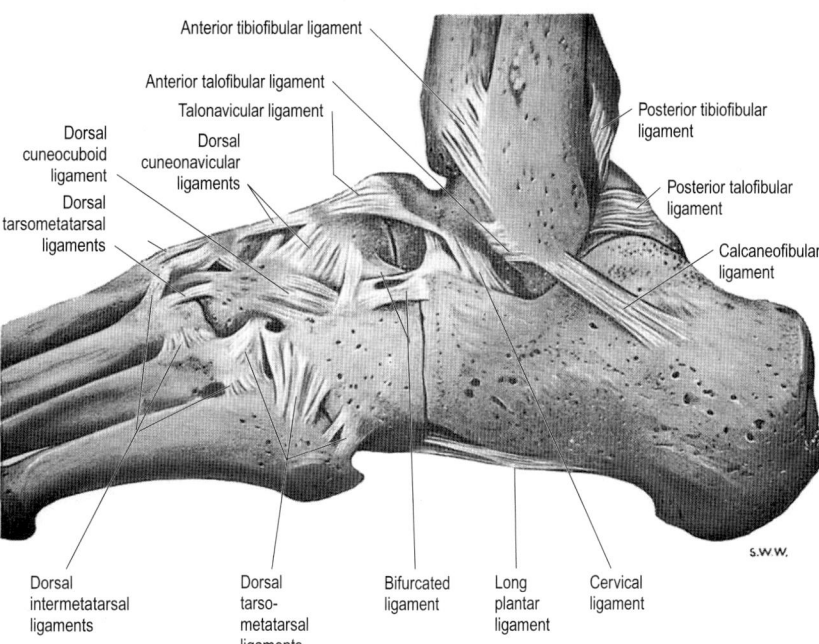

Fig. 115.15 Lateral aspect of the left ankle and tarsal joints. (Drawn from a specimen in the Museum of the Royal College of Surgeons of England, with permission from the Council.)

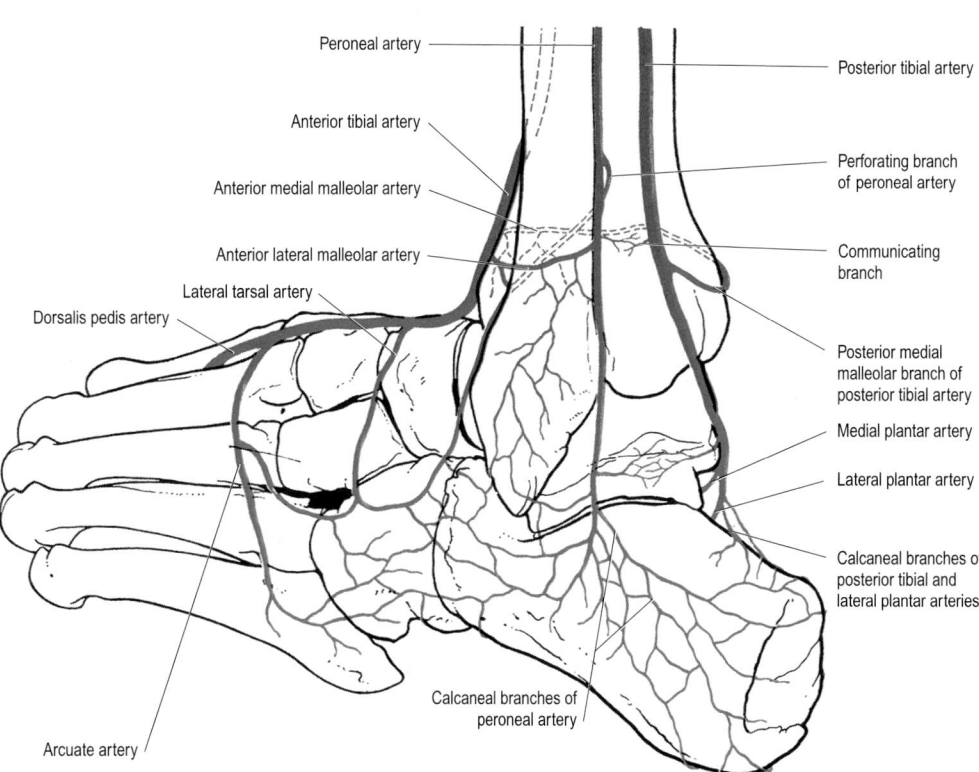

Fig. 115.16 The arterial anastomoses of the ankle, tarsus and metatarsus.

CUNEIFORMS

The wedge-like cuneiform bones articulate with the navicular proximally and the bases of the first to third metatarsals distally; the medial is the largest, the intermediate the smallest. The dorsal surfaces of the intermediate and lateral cuneiforms form the base of the wedge. The wedge is reversed in the medial cuneiform, which is a prime factor in shaping the transverse arch. The proximal surfaces of all three form a concavity for the navicular. The medial and lateral cuneiforms project distally beyond the intermediate cuneiform and so form a recess for the second metatarsal base.

Medial cuneiform

The medial cuneiform (**Fig. 115.21**) articulates with the navicular and first metatarsal base. It has a rough, narrow dorsal surface. The distal surface is a reniform facet for the first metatarsal base, its 'hilum' being lateral. The proximal surface bears a piriform facet for the navicular, which is concave vertically and dorsally narrowed. The medial surface,

rough and subcutaneous, is vertically convex; its distal plantar angle carries a large impression for most of the tendon of tibialis anterior (**Fig. 115.21A**). The lateral surface is partly non-articular; along its proximal and dorsal margins there is a smooth right-angled strip for the intermediate cuneiform. Its distal dorsal area is separated by a vertical ridge from a small, almost square facet for the dorsal part of the medial surface of the second metatarsal base. Plantar to this, the medial cuneiform is attached to the medial side of the second metatarsal base by a strong ligament. Proximally, an interosseous intercuneiform ligament connects this surface to the intermediate cuneiform. The distal and plantar area of the surface is roughened by attachment of part of the peroneus longus tendon (**Fig. 115.21B**).

Muscle attachments – The plantar surface receives a slip from the tendon of tibialis posterior, in addition to part of the insertion of the peroneus longus tendon. The medial surface receives the attachment of most of the tibialis anterior tendon.

1517

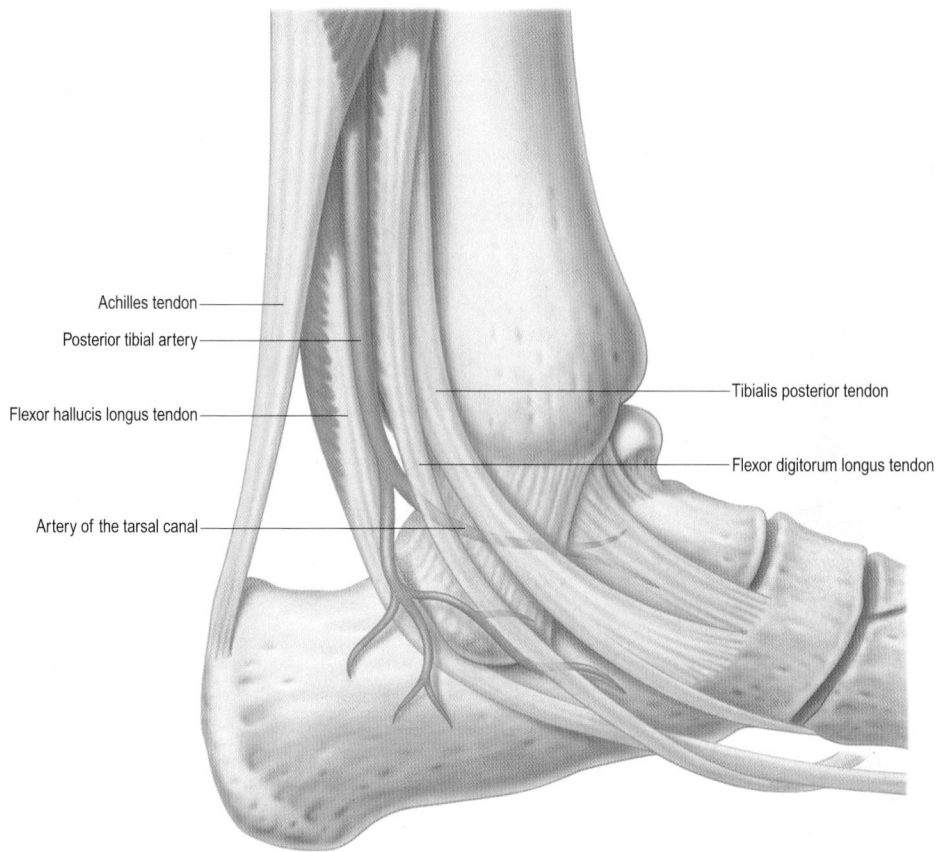

Fig. 115.17 Posteromedial view of ankle demonstrating branches of the posterior tibial artery.

Vascular supply – The medial cuneiform is supplied via its dorsal, medial and lateral surfaces, mainly from the dorsal arterial network.

Innervation – The medial cuneiform is supplied by the deep peroneal and medial plantar nerves.

Ossification – The medial cuneiform may have two separate ossification centres, which appear during the second year of life (**Fig. 115.11**). In 0.5% of individuals, a bipartite medial cuneiform exists, with a horizontal cleavage plane between the two bones.

The os cuneo-1 metatarsale-I plantare is a rare accessory bone that occurs on the plantar aspect of the foot at the base of the first metatarsal and articulates with the plantar base of the first metatarsal and the medial cuneiform.

Intermediate cuneiform

The intermediate cuneiform (**Fig. 115.22**) articulates with the navicular and distally with the second metatarsal base. It has a narrow, plantar surface that receives a slip from the tendon of tibialis posterior. The distal and proximal surfaces, both triangular articular facets, articulate with the second metatarsal base and navicular, respectively. The medial surface is partly articular: along its proximal and dorsal margins a smooth, angled strip, occasionally double, articulates with the medial cuneiform. The lateral surface is also partly articular: along its proximal margin a vertical strip, usually indented, abuts with the lateral cuneiform. Strong interosseous ligaments connect non-articular parts of both surfaces to adjacent cuneiforms.

Muscle attachments – The only muscle that has an attachment to the intermediate cuneiform is part of the tibialis posterior tendon.

Vascular supply – The intermediate cuneiform is supplied via its dorsal, medial and lateral surfaces, mainly from the dorsal arterial network.

Innervation – The intermediate cuneiform is innervated by the deep peroneal and medial plantar nerves.

Ossification – The ossification centre appears during the third year of life (**Fig. 115.11**). The os cuneo-1 metatarsal-II dorsale lies on the dorsal aspect of the joint between the intermediate cuneiform and the second metatarsal, is wedge-shape with its base orientated dorsally, and is rare.

Lateral cuneiform

The lateral cuneiform (**Fig. 115.23**) is between the intermediate cuneiform and cuboid, and also articulates with the navicular and, distally, the third metatarsal base. Like the intermediate cuneiform, its dorsal surface, rough and almost rectangular, is the base of a wedge. The plantar surface is narrow and receives a slip from tibialis posterior and sometimes part of flexor hallucis brevis. The distal surface is a triangular articular facet for the third metatarsal base. The proximal surface is rough on its plantar aspect, but its dorsal two-thirds articulate with the navicular by a triangular facet. The medial surface, partly non-articular, has on its proximal margin a vertical strip, indented for the intermediate cuneiform; on its distal margin, a narrower strip (often two small facets) articulates with the lateral side of the second metatarsal base. The lateral surface, also partly non-articular, bears a triangular or oval proximal facet for the cuboid; a semilunar facet on its dorsal and distal margin articulates with the dorsal part of the medial side of the fourth metatarsal base. Non-articular areas of the medial and lateral surfaces receive intercuneiform and cuneocuboid ligaments, which are important in maintenance of the transverse arch.

Muscle attachments – The plantar surface of the lateral cuneiform receives a slip of the tibialis posterior tendon and, on occasion, part of flexor hallucis brevis.

Vascular supply – The lateral cuneiform is supplied via its dorsal, medial and lateral surfaces, mainly from the dorsal arterial network.

Innervation – The lateral cuneiform is innervated by branches of the deep peroneal and lateral plantar nerves.

Ossification – The lateral cuneiform ossifies during the first year of life (**Fig. 115.11**).

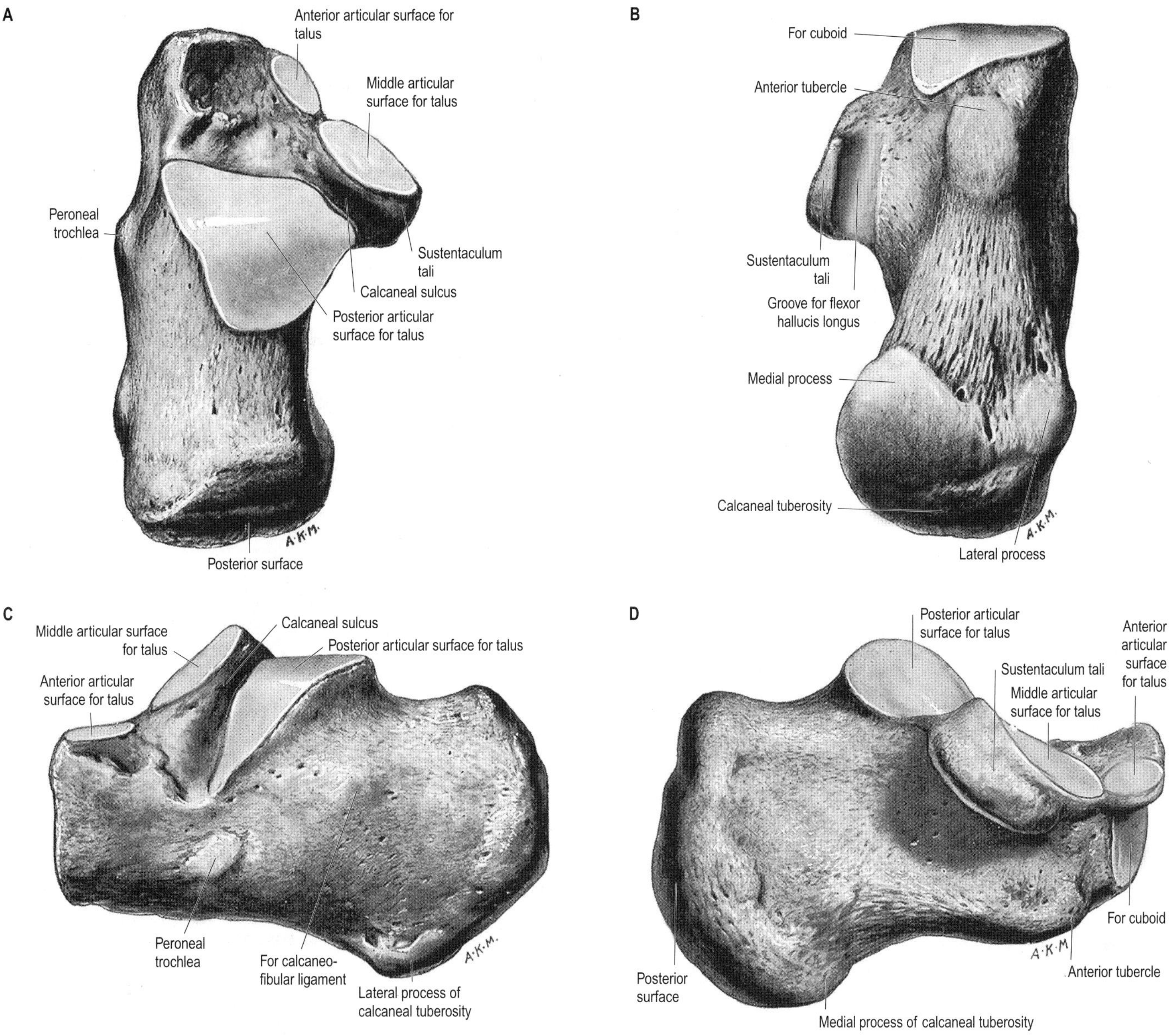

A

Anterior articular surface for talus

Middle articular surface for talus

Peroneal trochlea

Sustentaculum tali

Calcaneal sulcus

Posterior articular surface for talus

Posterior surface

B

For cuboid

Anterior tubercle

Sustentaculum tali

Groove for flexor hallucis longus

Medial process

Calcaneal tuberosity

Lateral process

C

Middle articular surface for talus

Calcaneal sulcus

Posterior articular surface for talus

Anterior articular surface for talus

Peroneal trochlea

For calcaneo-fibular ligament

Lateral process of calcaneal tuberosity

D

Posterior articular surface for talus

Sustentaculum tali

Middle articular surface for talus

Anterior articular surface for talus

Posterior surface

For cuboid

Anterior tubercle

Medial process of calcaneal tuberosity

Fig. 115.18 The left calcaneus. **A**, Dorsal aspect; **B**, plantar aspect; **C**, lateral aspect; **D**, medial aspect.

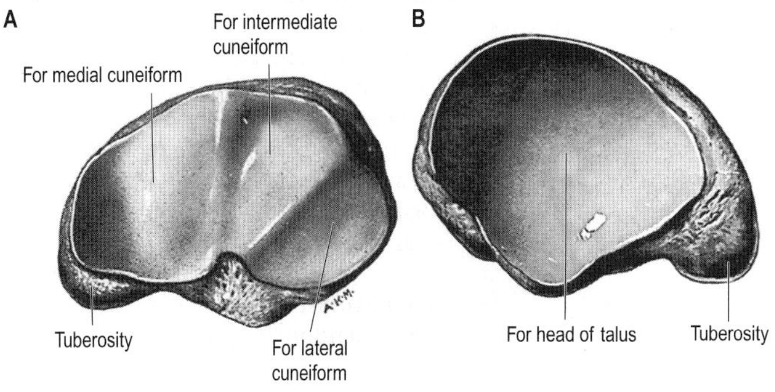

A

For intermediate cuneiform

For medial cuneiform

Tuberosity

For lateral cuneiform

B

For head of talus

Tuberosity

Fig. 115.19 The left navicular. **A**, Distal aspect; **B**, proximal aspect.

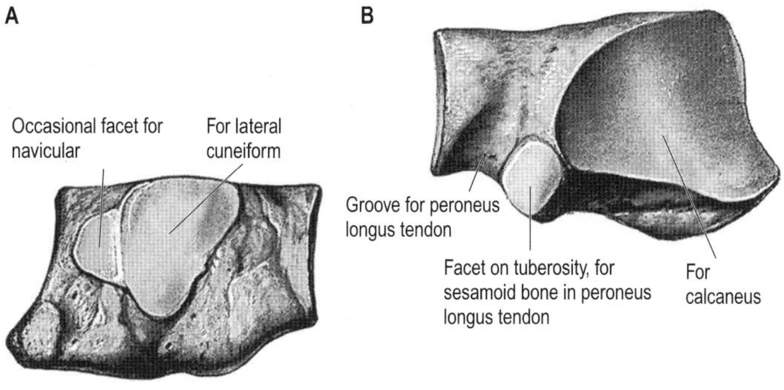

A

Occasional facet for navicular

For lateral cuneiform

B

Groove for peroneus longus tendon

Facet on tuberosity, for sesamoid bone in peroneus longus tendon

For calcaneus

Fig. 115.20 The left cuboid. **A**, Medial aspect; **B**, proximal and lateral aspect.

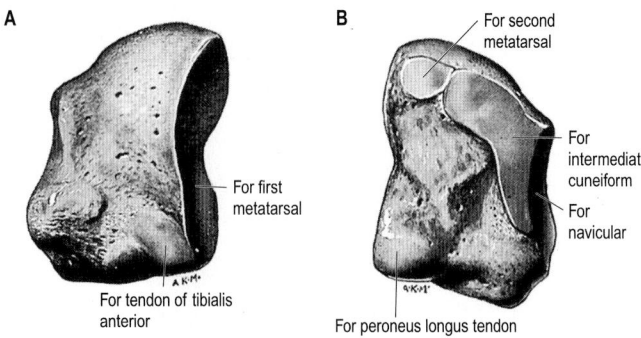

Fig. 115.21 The left medial cuneiform. **A**, Medial aspect; **B**, lateral aspect.

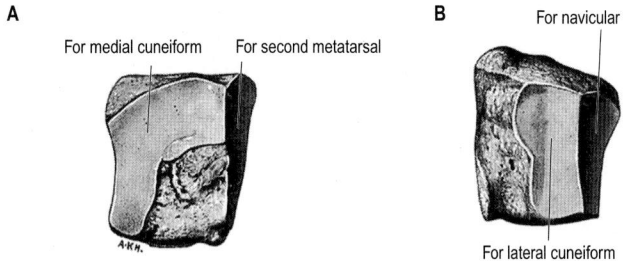

Fig. 115.22 The left intermediate cuneiform. **A**, Distal and medial aspect; **B**, proximal and lateral aspect.

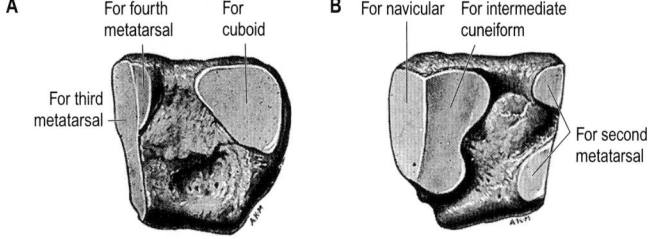

Fig. 115.23 The left lateral cuneiform. **A**, Distal and lateral aspect; **B**, proximal and medial aspect.

TARSAL COALITIONS

Tarsal coalition is a hereditary condition in which there is a fibrous, cartilaginous or osseous union of two or more tarsal bones. Harris and Beath (1948), were the first to understand the association between tarsal coalitions and 'peroneal spastic flat foot'. The condition is believed to arise as a result of a failure of segmentation by primitive mesenchyme. The two most common examples are talocalcaneal and calcaneonavicular coalitions, which usually present with symptoms early in the second decade of life. They are often, but not invariably, associated with flat feet. A talonavicular coalition is rare, but when present is often associated with a 'ball and socket' ankle joint. Resection of a coalition can eradicate pain but rarely increases motion.

METATARSALS

The five metatarsal bones lie distal in the foot and connect the tarsus and phalanges. Like metacarpals, they are miniature long bones, with a shaft, proximal base and distal head. Except for the first and fifth, the shafts are long and slender, longitudinally convex dorsally, and concave on the plantar aspects. Prismatic in section, they taper distally. Their bases articulate with the distal tarsal row and with each other. The line of each tarsometatarsal joint, except the first, inclines proximally and

laterally, metatarsal bases being oblique relative to their shafts. The heads articulate with the proximal phalanges, each by a convex surface that passes farther on to its plantar aspect, where it ends on the summits of two eminences. The sides of the heads are flat, with a depression surmounted by a dorsal tubercle for a collateral ligament of the metatarsophalangeal joint.

On occasion, an os intermetatarseum is encountered between the medial cuneiform and the bases of the first and second metatarsal bones and represents a rare accessory bone in this region.

Individual metatarsals

First metatarsal

The first metatarsal (**Fig. 115.24**) is the shortest and thickest, and has a strong shaft, of marked prismatic form. The base sometimes has a lateral facet or ill-defined smooth area as a result of contact with the second metatarsal. Its large proximal surface, usually indented on the medial and lateral margins, articulates with the medial cuneiform. Its circumference is grooved for tarsometatarsal ligaments and, medially, part of the tendon of tibialis anterior is attached; its plantar angle has a rough, oval, lateral prominence for the tendon of peroneus longus. The medial head of the first dorsal interosseous is attached to the flat lateral surface of the shaft. The large head has a plantar elevation, the crista, which separates two grooved facets (of which the medial is larger), on which sesamoid bones glide.

Muscle attachments – The first metatarsal receives attachments from the tibialis anterior tendon medially, and the peroneus longus tendon on its plantar aspect. It gives origin to the medial head of the first dorsal interosseus muscle on the proximal aspect of the lateral surface.

Vascular supply – The first metatarsal is supplied by the first dorsal and first plantar metatarsal arteries and a superficial branch of the medial plantar artery, which together form a periosteal network. A nutrient artery enters on the lateral surface of the mid-diaphysis. The head receives a medial, lateral and plantar supply from these arteries.

Innervation – The first metatarsal is innervated by the deep peroneal and medial plantar nerves.

Ossification – The first metatarsal has two centres of ossification, one in the shaft, the other in the base (unlike the other metatarsals, in which the secondary ossific centre is distal). They appear during the tenth week of prenatal life and the third year of life, respectively (**Fig. 115.11**).

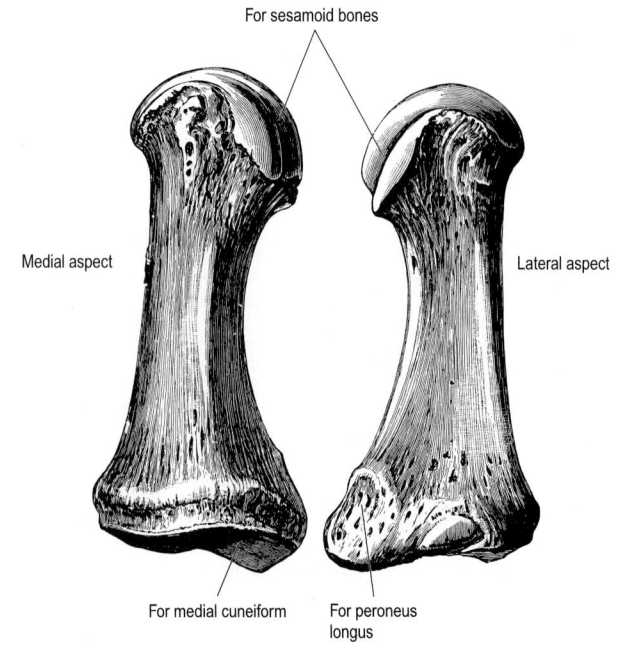

Fig. 115.24 Medial and lateral aspects of the left first metatarsal.

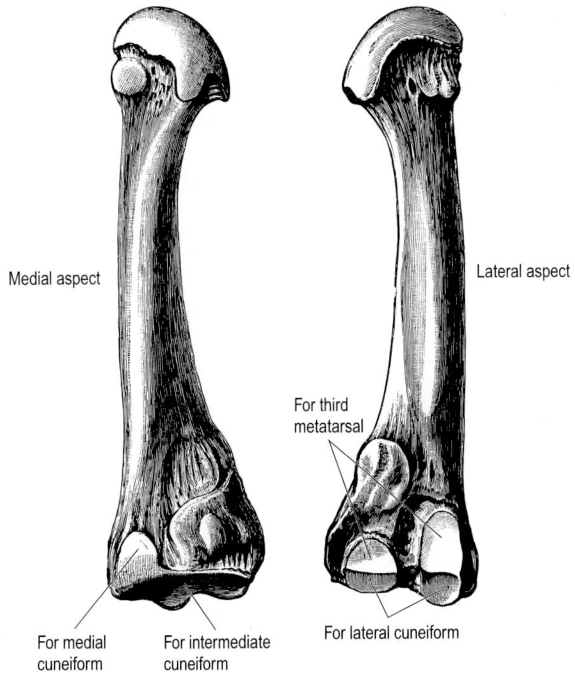

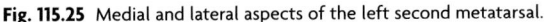

Medial aspect

Lateral aspect

For third
metatarsal

For medial
cuneiform

For intermediate
cuneiform

For lateral cuneiform

Fig. 115.25 Medial and lateral aspects of the left second metatarsal.

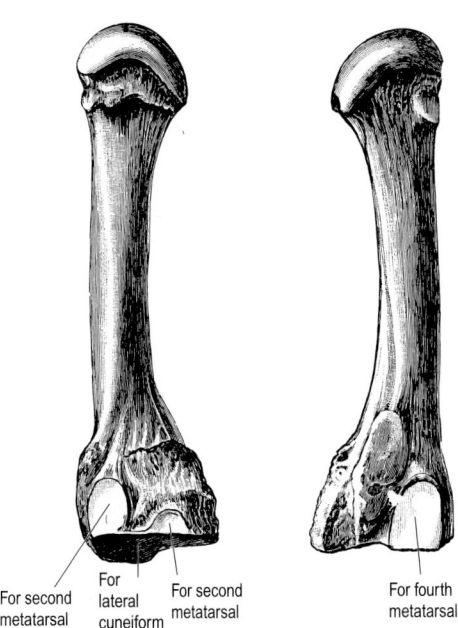

For second
metatarsal

For
lateral
cuneiform

For second
metatarsal

For fourth
metatarsal

Fig. 115.26 Medial and lateral aspects of the left third metatarsal.

The two centres fuse between the seventeenth and twentieth years. Sometimes there is a third centre in the first metatarsal head.

Second metatarsal

The second metatarsal (**Fig. 115.25**) is the longest. Its cuneiform base bears four articular facets. The proximal one, concave and triangular, is for the intermediate cuneiform. The dorsomedial one, for the medial cuneiform, is variable in size and usually continuous with that for the intermediate cuneiform. Two lateral facets, dorsal and plantar, are separated by non-articular bone, each divided by a ridge into distal demifacets, which articulate with the third metatarsal base, and a proximal pair (sometimes continuous) for the lateral cuneiform. The areas of these facets vary, particularly the plantar facet, which may be absent. An oval pressure facet, caused by contact with the first metatarsal, may appear on the medial side of the base, plantar to that for the medial cuneiform. Because of its length, its steep inclination, and the position of its base recessed in the tarsometatarsal joint, it is at risk of stress overload. Perhaps this is why it is a common site for stress fractures in athletes and an avascular phenomenon in its head: Freiberg's infraction.

Muscle attachments – The lateral head of the first dorsal interosseous and the medial head of the second, are attached to the medial and lateral surfaces of the shaft, respectively.

Vascular supply – The blood supply of the second, third and fourth metatarsals follows the same pattern: they are all supplied by branches of the dorsal and plantar metatarsal arteries. The nutrient artery enters the diaphysis on its lateral side near the metatarsal base. A constant plantar vessel supplies the head.

Innervation – The second metatarsal is innervated by branches of the deep peroneal and branches of medial plantar nerve.

Ossification – There are two centres of ossification, one in the shaft and one distally in the metatarsal head (**Fig. 115.11**). Ossification of the shaft starts during the ninth prenatal week and ossification of the metatarsal head starts between the third and fourth years. Fusion occurs between the seventeenth and twentieth years.

Third metatarsal

The third metatarsal (**Fig. 115.26**) has a flat triangular base, articulating proximally with the lateral cuneiform, medially with the second metatarsal, via dorsal and plantar facets, and laterally, via a single facet,

with the dorsal angle of the fourth metatarsal. The medial plantar facet is frequently absent. The third tarsometatarsal joint is relatively stiff and predisposes the third metatarsal to stress fracture.

Muscle attachments – The lateral head of the second dorsal interosseous and first plantar are attached to the medial surface of the shaft. The medial head of the third dorsal interosseous is attached to its lateral surface.

Vascular supply – The blood supply of the third metatarsal is the same as that of the second metatarsal, described above.

Innervation – The third metatarsal is innervated by the deep peroneal and lateral plantar nerves.

Ossification – There are two centres of ossification, one in the shaft and one distally in the metatarsal head (**Fig. 115.11**). Ossification of the shaft starts during the ninth prenatal week and ossification of the metatarsal head starts between the third and fourth years. Fusion occurs between the seventeenth and twentieth years.

Fourth metatarsal

The fourth metatarsal (**Fig. 115.27**) is smaller than the third. Its base has: proximally, an oblique quadrilateral facet for articulation with the cuboid; laterally, a single facet for the fifth metatarsal; medially, an oval facet for the third, sometimes divided by a ridge, the proximal part then articulating with the lateral cuneiform.

Muscle attachments – The lateral head of the third dorsal and second plantar interossei are attached to the medial surface. The medial head of the fourth dorsal interosseous is attached to the lateral surface.

Vascular supply – The blood supply of the fourth metatarsal is the same as that of the second metatarsal, described above.

Innervation – The fourth metatarsal is innervated by the deep peroneal and lateral plantar nerves.

Ossification – There are two centres of ossification, one in the shaft and one distally in the metatarsal head (**Fig. 115.11**). Ossification of the shaft starts during the ninth prenatal week and ossification of the metatarsal head commences between the third and fourth years. Fusion occurs between the seventeenth and twentieth years.

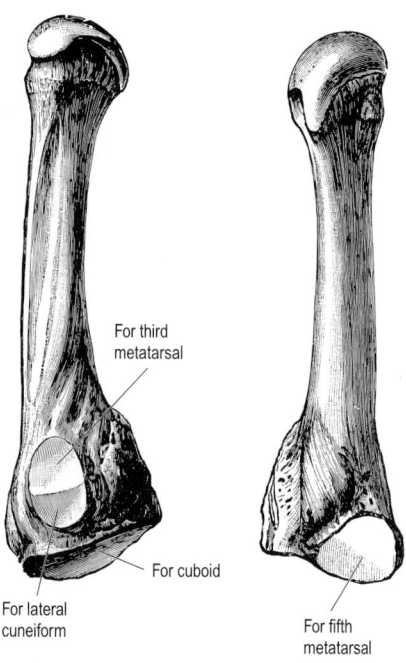

Fig. 115.27 Medial and lateral aspects of the left fourth metatarsal.

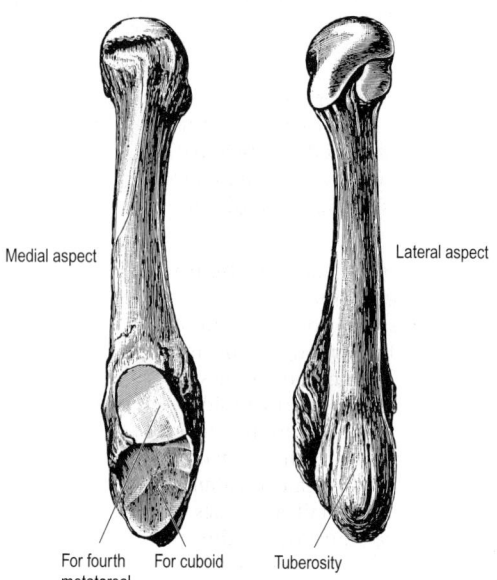

Fig. 115.28 Medial and lateral aspects of the left fifth metatarsal.

Fifth metatarsal

The fifth metatarsal (**Fig. 115.28**) has a tuberosity (styloid process) on the lateral side of its base. The base articulates proximally with the cuboid by a triangular, oblique surface, and medially with the fourth metatarsal. The tuberosity can be seen and felt midway along the lateral border of the foot; in acute inversion it may be fractured. There, injuries are almost always uneventful. However the metaphyseal–diaphyseal junction of the fifth metatarsal base is prone to traumatic or stress fractures, and these have a tendency to delayed and non-union, and often require surgical fixation. It is believed that, because these fractures occur at the level of the nutrient artery foramen and the extraosseous plexus, fracture site avascularity occurs.

Muscle attachments – The tendon of peroneus tertius is attached to the medial part of the dorsal surface and medial border of the shaft, and that of peroneus brevis to the dorsal surface of the tuberosity. A strong band of the plantar aponeurosis, sometimes containing muscle, connects the apex of the tuberosity to the lateral process of the calcaneal tuberosity. It is this attachment, and not that of peroneus brevis, which is responsible for avulsion fractures of the tuberosity. The plantar surface of the base is grooved by the tendon of abductor digiti minimi, and flexor digiti minimi brevis is attached here. The lateral head of the fourth dorsal and the third plantar interossei are attached to the medial side of the shaft.

Vascular supply – The fifth metatarsal is supplied by dorsal and plantar metatarsal arteries and an inconsistent fibular marginal artery. The nutrient artery enters the diaphysis proximally and medially.

Innervation – The fifth metatarsal is innervated by branches from the sural, superficial peroneal and lateral plantar nerves.

Ossification – There are three centres of ossification, one at the base in the region of the tuberosity (an apophysis), one in the shaft and one distally in the metatarsal head. Ossification of the shaft starts during the tenth prenatal week and ossification of the metatarsal head starts between the third and fourth years (**Fig. 115.11**). Fusion of the distal and shaft centres occurs between the seventeenth and twentieth years; the proximal apophysis fuses earlier. An os vesalianum is a rare variant that should not be confused with the basal apophysis.

PHALANGES OF THE FOOT

The phalanges in general resemble those in the hand: there are two in the hallux, and three in each of the other toes (**Figs 115.8, 115.9**). On occasion there are only two phalanges in the little toe and, rarely, this is the case with the other lesser toes. The phalanges of the toes are much shorter than their counterparts in the hand and their shafts, especially those of the proximal set, are compressed from side to side. In proximal phalanges, the compressed shaft is convex dorsally, with a plantar concavity. The base is concave for articulation with a metatarsal head and the head is a trochlea for a middle phalanx. Middle phalanges are small and short, but broader than the proximal. Distal phalanges resemble those in the fingers, but are smaller and flatter. Each has a broad base for articulating with a middle phalanx and an expanded distal. A rough tuberosity on the plantar aspect of the latter is an attachment for the pulp, and a wider area for weight-bearing.

Muscle attachments – Tendons of the long digital flexor and extensors are attached to the plantar and dorsal aspects of the bases of the lateral four distal phalanges. In the hallux, flexor hallucis longus and extensor hallucis longus are similarly attached. The bases of the middle phalanges receive the tendons of flexor digitorum brevis and extensor digitorum brevis. The second, third and fourth proximal phalanges each receives a lumbrical on the medial side and an interosseous on both sides. For further details of muscular, capsular and ligamentous arrangements in the toes refer to **Figs 115.8** and **115.9**. The terminal phalanx of the hallux normally shows a small degree of valgus (lateral) deviation, as may the proximal, even in those who have never worn shoes. The deviation has also been observed in fetal specimens.

Vascular supply – The proximal phalanges receive most of their blood supply from the dorsal digital arteries. The middle phalanges are supplied by plantar and dorsal digital arteries. Distal phalanges receive their supply mainly from plantar digital arteries.

Innervation – The phalanges are innervated by the plantar and dorsal digital nerves.

Ossification – Phalanges are ossified from a primary centre for the shaft and a basal epiphysis (**Fig. 115.11**). Primary centres for the distal phalanges appear between the ninth and twelfth prenatal weeks, and even later in the fifth digit. Primary centres for the proximal phalanges appear between the eleventh and fifteenth weeks, and later for intermediate phalanges, but there is wide variation. Basal centres appear between the second and eighth years (usually second or third in the hallux), uniting by the eighteenth year. Considerable variation probably exists.

SESAMOIDS

Galen is reputed to have first used the term 'sesamoid' because of the resemblance of these bones to sesame seeds. Most sesamoid bones are only a few millimetres in diameter and vary in shape. The location of some sesamoids is constant, but many other sesamoids exist with variable frequency and sites (**Fig. 115.29**). Most sesamoid bones are embedded in tendons in close proximity to joints; however, their precise role is not understood. It is believed that they alter the direction of muscle pull, decrease friction and modify pressure. Some sesamoids ossify, whereas others remain cartilaginous.

Medial and lateral sesamoids of the first metatarsophalangeal joint

The two constant sesamoid bones within the foot are those of the first metatarsophalangeal articulation. The medial sesamoid is generally larger than the lateral sesamoid and lies slightly more distally. During dorsiflexion of the hallux, the sesamoids lie below the first metatarsal head, thus offering protection to the otherwise exposed plantar aspect of the first metatarsal head. The medial (tibial) sesamoid is c.10 mm wide and 14 mm long. The lateral (fibular) sesamoid is c.8 mm wide and 10 mm long. Their overall size varies considerably.

The sesamoids are embedded within the double tendon of flexor hallucis brevis and articulate on their dorsal surface with the plantar facets of the first metatarsal head. The two sesamoids are separated by the crista or intersesamoidal ridge, which provides stability to the sesamoid complex. This ridge can be eroded to the point of obliteration in severe cases of hallux valgus. The sesamoids are connected to the plantar base of the proximal phalanx through the plantar plate, which is an extension of the flexor hallucis brevis tendon. The plantar surface of each sesamoid is covered by a thin layer of the flexor hallucis brevis tendon, whereas the dorsal or superior surface is covered by hyaline cartilage. The sesamoids are suspended by a sling-like mechanism made up of the collateral ligaments of the first metatarsophalangeal joint and the sesamoid ligaments on either side of the joint. The plantar aponeurosis also has an attachment to the sesamoids.

Approximately 30% of sesamoid bones are bipartite. The medial is much more commonly affected. In such cases the condition may be bilateral. The medial sesamoid may have two, three or four parts, but the fibular sesamoid rarely has more than two. The sesamoids may be absent congenitally.

Muscle attachments – The medial sesamoid receives an attachment from abductor hallucis, which has a medial stabilising influence on the sesamoid complex. The lateral sesamoid receives some fibres of the adductor hallucis tendon, which provides lateral stabilisation. The medial and lateral sesamoids are interconnected by the intersesamoid ligament, which forms the floor of the tendinous canal for the flexor hallucis longus tendon.

Vascular supply – There are three patterns of blood supply to the sesamoid bones. In c.50% of cases the arterial supply is derived from the medial plantar artery and the plantar arch, in 25% of cases it is predominantly from the plantar arch and in 25% of cases it is from the medial plantar artery alone. The major arterial blood supply to the sesamoids enters from the proximal and plantar aspects, with only a minor contribution entering through the distal pole. The pattern of vascular supply determines the vulnerability of a sesamoid to avascular necrosis after injury to the bone.

Innervation – The medial and lateral sesamoids are innervated by the plantar digital nerves.

Ossification – The ossific centres of the sesamoids can be multiple or single.

Other sesamoid and accessory bones

Accessory or inconstant sesamoid bones may occur under any weight-bearing surface of the foot, but are most common under the second to fifth metatarsal heads. They are extremely variable in size and their incidence is difficult to determine.

A true sesamoid of the tibialis posterior tendon occurs in c.10% of individuals. It lies on the plantar aspect of the navicular tuberosity within the tibialis posterior tendon at the level of the inferior border of the

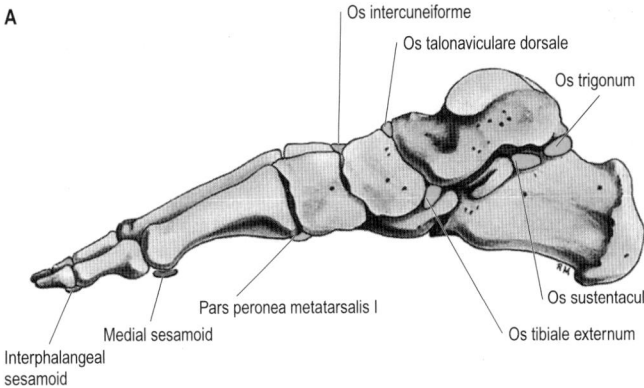

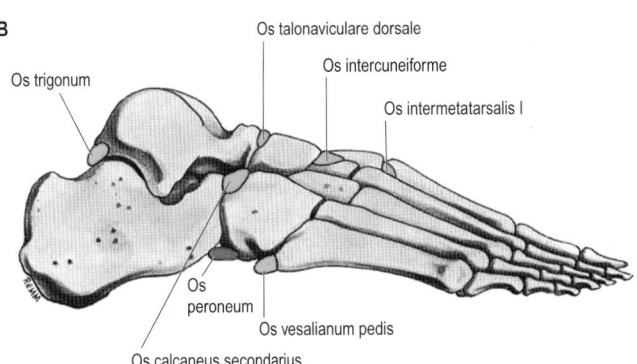

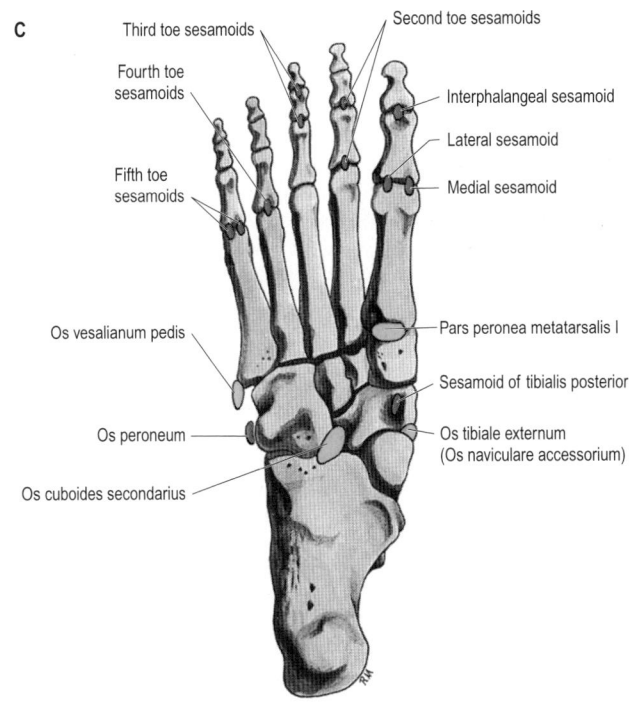

Fig. 115.29 Sites of sesamoid bones (red) and accessory bones (blue) found in the right foot. **A**, Medial aspect; **B**, lateral aspect; **C**, plantar aspect.

calcaneonavicular ligament. Very rarely, a sesamoid is found within the tibialis anterior tendon near its insertion at the level of the anteroinferior corner of the medial cuneiform, where there is an articular facet. An os peroneum is a sesamoid bone within the tendon of peroneus longus that articulates with the lateral wall of the calcaneum, the calcaneocuboid joint or, more frequently, the plantar aspect of the cuboid where there is an articular facet. The os peroneum is situated where the tendon of peroneus longus angles around the plantar aspect of the cuboid on the plantar lateral aspect of the foot. The precise incidence is not known, but it is probably present in 95% of cases; only 20% are ossified, the remainder are cartilaginous.

JOINTS

ANKLE (TALOCRURAL) JOINT

The talocrural joint is approximately a uniaxial hinge. The lower end of the tibia and its medial malleolus, together with the lateral malleolus of the fibula and inferior transverse tibiofibular ligament, form a deep recess ('mortise') for the body of the talus. Although it appears to be a simple hinge, its axis of rotation is dynamic, shifting during dorsi- and plantar flexion. Dorsiflexion is to c.10° with the knee straight, and to c.30° with knee flexion (because of relaxation of the calcaneal tendon). Plantar flexion is to c.30°. Dorsiflexion is the 'close-packed' position, with maximal congruence and ligamentous tension; from this position, all major thrusting movements are exerted, in walking, running and jumping. The malleoli embrace the talus, and even in relaxation no appreciable lateral movement can occur without stretch of the inferior tibiofibular syndesmosis and slight bending of the fibula. The superior talar surface is broader in front, and in dorsiflexion the malleolar gap is increased by slight lateral rotation of the fibula by 'give' at the inferior tibiofibular syndesmosis and gliding at the superior tibiofibular joint.

Articulating surfaces – Articular surfaces are covered by hyaline cartilage. The talar trochlear surface, which is convex parasagittally and gently concave transversely, is wider in front; the distal tibial articular surface is reciprocally curved. The talar articular surface for the medial malleolus is a proximal area on the medial talar surface, and is fairly flat, comma-shaped and deeper anteriorly. The larger lateral talar articular surface is triangular and vertically concave, while the articular surface on the lateral malleolus is reciprocally curved. Posteriorly, the edge between the trochlear and fibular articular surfaces of the talus is bevelled to a narrow, flat triangular area that articulates with the inferior transverse tibiofibular ligament (**Fig. 115.13**); all surfaces are continuous. The bones are connected by a fibrous capsule, medial (deltoid), anterior and posterior talofibular and calcaneofibular ligaments.

Fibrous capsule – Around the joint, the fibrous capsule is thin in front and behind. It is attached proximally to the borders of the tibial and malleolar articular surfaces, and distally to the talus near the margins of its trochlear surface, except in front where it reaches the dorsum of the talar neck. The capsule is strengthened by strong collateral ligaments. Its posterior part is mainly of transverse fibres. It blends with the inferior transverse ligament and is thickened laterally where it reaches the fibular malleolar fossa.

Ligaments – The medial ligament (deltoid collateral) is a strong, triangular band, attached to the apex and the anterior and posterior borders of the medial malleolus (**Fig. 115.14**). Of its superficial fibres, the anterior (tibionavicular) pass forwards to the navicular tuberosity and, behind this, blend with the medial margin of the plantar calcaneo-navicular ligament; intermediate (tibiocalcaneal) fibres descend almost vertically to the entire length of the sustentaculum tali; posterior fibres (posterior tibiotalar) pass posterolaterally to the medial side of the talus and its medial tubercle. The deep fibres (anterior tibiotalar) pass from the tip of the medial malleolus to the non-articular part of the medial talar surface. The ligament is crossed by the tendons of tibialis posterior and flexor digitorum longus. This ligament is rarely injured alone, and is most commonly torn with an associated fracture of the distal fibula. Chronic instability is rare.

The lateral ligament has discrete parts. The anterior talofibular ligament extends anteromedially from the anterior margin of the fibular malleolus to the talus, attached in front of its lateral articular facet and to the lateral aspect of its neck (**Fig. 115.15**). The posterior talofibular ligament runs almost horizontally from the distal part of the lateral malleolar fossa to the lateral tubercle of the posterior talar process (**Fig. 115.13**). A 'tibial slip' of fibres connects it to the medial malleolus. The calcaneofibular ligament, a long cord, runs from a depression anterior to the apex of the fibular malleolus to a tubercle on the lateral calcaneal surface and is crossed by the tendons of peroneus longus and brevis (**Fig. 115.15**). The lateral ligament complex is commonly injured with inversion sprains, often during sport; the posterior talofibular ligament is almost always spared. Although the resulting increased laxity is tolerated in most cases, some require surgical reconstruction.

Synovial membrane – The joint is lined by synovial membrane which projects into the distal tibiofibular joint.

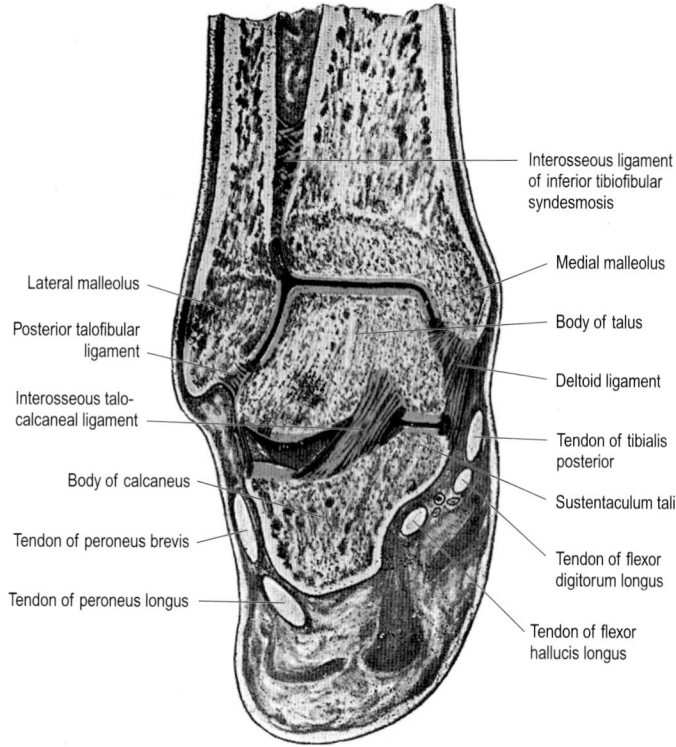

Fig. 115.30 Coronal section through the left ankle and talocalcaneal joints.

Labels (clockwise from top right):
Interosseous ligament of inferior tibiofibular syndesmosis
Medial malleolus
Body of talus
Deltoid ligament
Tendon of tibialis posterior
Sustentaculum tali
Tendon of flexor digitorum longus
Tendon of flexor hallucis longus
Tendon of peroneus longus
Tendon of peroneus brevis
Body of calcaneus
Interosseous talo-calcaneal ligament
Posterior talofibular ligament
Lateral malleolus

Vascular supply and lymphatic drainage – The talocrural joint is supplied by malleolar rami of the anterior and posterior tibial and peroneal arteries. Lymphatic drainage is via vessels accompanying the arteries and via the long and short saphenous veins superficially.

Innervation – The talocrural joint is innervated by branches from the deep peroneal, saphenous, sural and tibial nerves (or medial and lateral plantar nerves, depending on the level of division of the tibial nerve). Occasionally, the superficial peroneal nerve also supplies the ankle joint.

For a comprehensive account of the innervation of the ankle joint (and other foot joints) see Gardner and Gray (1968).

Relations – Anteriorly, from the medial side, are tibialis anterior, extensor hallucis longus, the anterior tibial vessels, deep peroneal nerve, extensor digitorum longus and peroneus tertius; posteriorly from the medial side, are tibialis posterior, flexor digitorum longus, the posterior tibial vessels, tibial nerve, flexor hallucis longus; in the groove behind the lateral malleolus are the tendons of peroneus longus and brevis. The peroneus brevis tendon lies anterior to the longus tendon at this level (**Fig. 115.31**). The long saphenous vein and saphenous nerve cross the ankle joint medial to the tibialis anterior tendon and anterior to the medial malleolus, the nerve lying posterior to the vein.

All the above structures are at risk during surgery on the ankle: the main structures at risk are the neurovascular structures anteriorly and posteromedially. Branches of the superficial peroneal nerve are at risk on the anterolateral aspect of the ankle, particularly during ankle arthroscopy.

Factors maintaining stability – Passive stability is conferred upon the ankle mainly by the medial and lateral ligament complexes, the distal tibiofibular ligaments, the crossing and attached tendon tunnels, the bony contours and the capsular attachments. Dynamic stability is conferred by gravity, muscle action and ground reaction forces. Stability requires the continuous action of soleus, and increases (often involving gastrocnemius) with leaning forward, and *vice versa*. If backward sway takes the projection of the centre of gravity ('weight line') posterior to the transverse axes of the ankle joints, the plantar flexors relax and the dorsiflexors contract.

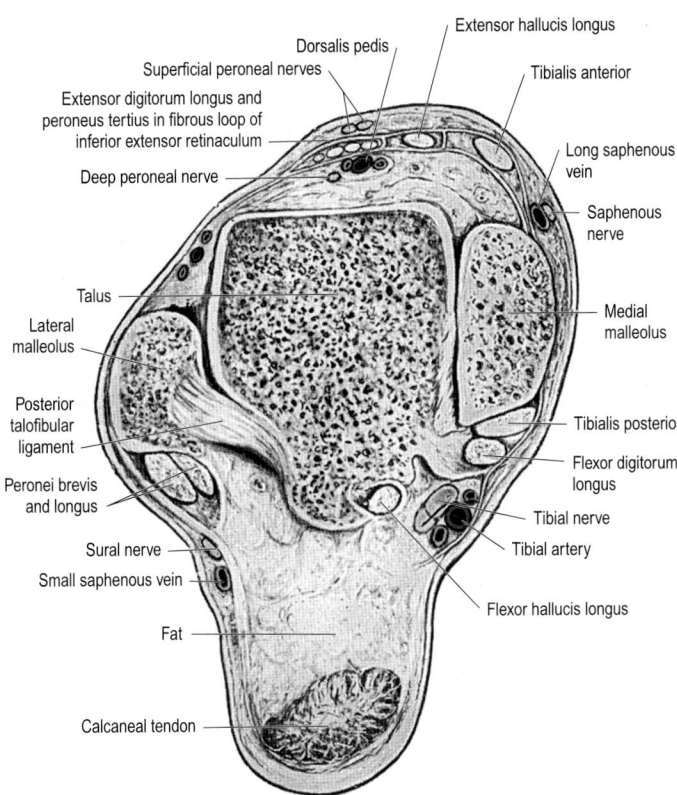

Extensor hallucis longus

Dorsalis pedis

Superficial peroneal nerves

Tibialis anterior

Extensor digitorum longus and
peroneus tertius in fibrous loop of
inferior extensor retinaculum

Long saphenous
vein

Deep peroneal nerve

Saphenous
nerve

Talus

Lateral
malleolus

Medial
malleolus

Posterior
talofibular
ligament

Tibialis posterior

Flexor digitorum
longus

Peronei brevis
and longus

Tibial nerve

Sural nerve

Tibial artery

Small saphenous vein

Fat

Flexor hallucis longus

Calcaneal tendon

Fig. 115.31 Transverse section through the lower part of the left ankle joint: superior aspect.

Failure of the peronei can lead progressively to varus instability, whereas long-standing failure of the tibialis posterior tendon, which is relatively common in the elderly female, can result in valgus instability of the ankle and particularly a planovalgus foot deformity.

Muscles producing movement – Dorsiflexion is produced by tibialis anterior, assisted by extensors digitorum longus and hallucis longus, and peroneus tertius. Plantar flexion is produced by gastrocnemius and soleus, assisted by plantaris, tibialis posterior, flexors hallucis longus and digitorum longus.

Ankle fractures

Ankle fractures are common and of importance because, apart from virtually undisplaced fractures, subsequent morbidity is usual, if anatomical alignment is not restored. Apart from the most simple ankle fractures, most ankle fractures are also associated with a ligamentous injury. Depending on the forces applied, the fracture pattern and concomitant ligament injury can be predicted. The Lauge–Hansen classification, although slightly cumbersome, classifies injuries according to two components: the position of the foot at the time of injury and the direction of the force applied. In a supination/adduction type injury, the foot is supinated and an adduction force is applied, resulting in a transverse fracture of the distal fibula (stage 1), followed by an oblique fracture of the medial malleolus (stage 2). In a supination/external rotation type injury, the first structure to rupture is the anterior inferior tibiofibular ligament, followed in order by a spiral fibular fracture, a posterior malleolar fracture and then a medial malleolar fracture (or deltoid ligament rupture). In pronation/abduction injuries, a transverse medial malleolar fracture is followed by rupture of the anterior and posterior inferior tibiofibular ligaments and interosseous ligament, and then by an oblique fibular fracture. Pronation/external rotation injuries commence with a medial malleolar fracture (or deltoid ligament rupture), followed in turn by rupture of the anterior inferior tibiofibular ligament, the interosseous ligament, the interosseous membrane, a high fibular fracture and fracture of the posterior tibial plafond ('posterior malleolus').

DISTAL TIBIOFIBULAR JOINT

The distal tibiofibular joint is usually considered a syndesmosis; it consists of the anterior and posterior tibiofibular ligaments and the interosseous ligament.

Articulating surfaces – The distal tibiofibular joint is between the rough, medial convex surface on the distal end of the fibula and the rough concave surface of the fibular notch of the tibia. These surfaces are separated distally for c.4 mm by a synovial prolongation from the ankle joint, and may be covered by articular cartilage in their lowest parts.

Fibrous capsule – The distal tibiofibular joint does not have a capsule.

Ligaments – The anterior tibiofibular ligament (**Fig. 115.15**) is a flat band that descends laterally between the adjacent margins of the tibia and fibula, anterior to the syndesmosis. A variant is called Bassett's ligament, which represents a low lying slip of the ligament inserting so far distally on the fibula that it causes irritation of the lateral dome of the talus. It is amenable to arthroscopic removal. The posterior tibiofibular ligament (**Fig. 115.13**) is stronger and is disposed similarly on the posterior aspect of the syndesmosis. Its distal, deep part is the inferior transverse ligament, a thick band of yellow fibres crossing from the proximal end of the lateral malleolar fossa to the posterior border of the tibial articular surface almost to the medial malleolus. The ligament projects distal to the bones, in contact with the talus. Its colour reflects its content of yellow elastic fibres. The interosseous ligament is continuous with the interosseous membrane, it contains many short bands between the rough adjacent tibial and fibular surfaces and is the strongest bond between the bones.

Synovial membrane – The only synovial membrane is a projection of the ankle joint in the lowest 4 mm or so of the inferior tibiofibular joint.

Vascular supply and lymphatic drainage – The tibiofibular joint is supplied by the peroneal perforating branch and medial malleolar rami of the anterior and posterior tibial arteries. Lymphatic drainage is via vessels corresponding to the arteries, and via vessels that accompany the superficial saphenous veins.

Innervation – The distal tibiofibular joint is innervated by branches from the deep peroneal and sural nerves.

Relations – No significant structures pass anterior to the anterior aspect of the distal tibiofibular joint, but the superficial peroneal nerve is at risk during surgery to this area. Posteriorly, the posterior peroneal artery passes over the posterior tibiofibular ligament and is at risk in the posterolateral approach to the fibula.

Factors maintaining stability – Stability is maintained in part by the bone contours, but mainly by the dense anterior and posterior tibiofibular and the interosseous ligaments.

Muscles producing movement – No muscles act on the distal tibiofibular joint, which moves only slightly. Because of the varying slope of the talar lateral malleolar surface, the fibula rotates laterally a little during dorsiflexion at the ankle, the bones being also slightly separated. Testing for a significant disruption of this joint is usually carried out with the patient under anaesthetic and involves applying an external rotation and abduction force, looking for widening of the syndesmosis. Excessive anterior/posterior glide of the fibula relative to the tibia also indicates a disruption of the joint.

TALOCALCANEAL JOINT

Anterior and posterior articulations between the calcaneus and talus form a functional unit often termed the 'subtalar joint'. The posterior articulation is referred to as the talocalcaneal joint and the anterior articulation is regarded as part of the talocalcaneonavicular joint.

The talocalcaneal joint is modified multiaxial and its permitted movements are considered together with those at other tarsal joints. The bones are connected by a fibrous capsule, and by lateral, medial, interosseous talocalcaneal and cervical ligaments.

Articulating surfaces – The subtalar joint proper involves the concave posterior calcaneal facet on the posterior part of the inferior surface of the talus and the convex posterior facet on the superior surface of the calcaneus (**Fig. 115.32**).

Fibrous capsule – The fibrous capsule envelops the joint, its fibres being short and attached to its articular margins; it is split into slips, between which it is thin.

Ligaments

Lateral talocalcaneal ligament – The lateral talocalcaneal ligament is a short flat fasciculus that descends obliquely back from the lateral talar process to the lateral calcaneal surface. It is attached anterosuperior to the calcaneofibular ligament.

Medial talocalcaneal ligament – The medial talocalcaneal ligament connects the medial talar tubercle to the back of the sustentaculum tali and adjacent medial surface of the calcaneus. Its fibres blend with the medial (deltoid) ligament, the most posterior fibres lining the groove for flexor hallucis longus between the talus and calcaneus.

Interosseous talocalcaneal ligament – The interosseous talocalcaneal ligament (**Figs 115.30, 115.32**) is a broad, flat, bilaminar transverse band in the sinus tarsi. It descends obliquely and laterally from the sulcus tali to the calcaneal sulcus. The posterior lamina of the ligament is associated with the talocalcaneal joint, its anterior lamina with the talocalcaneonavicular joint. Its medial fibres are taut in eversion.

Cervical ligament – The cervical ligament (**Fig. 115.15**) is just lateral to the tarsal sinus and attached to the superior calcaneal surface. It is medial to the attachment of extensor digitorum brevis, from where it ascends medially to an inferolateral tubercle on the talar neck (Barclay-Smith 1896). It is considered to be taut in inversion.

Synovial membrane – The synovial membrane of the talocalcaneal joint is separate from other tarsal joints, although direct communication with the ankle joint can occur.

Innervation – The talocalcaneal joint is innervated by branches of the posterior tibial, medial plantar and sural nerves.

Relations – Posteromedially, in the region of the posterior aspect of the talocalcaneal joint lie (from anterior to posterior) the veins on either side of the posterior tibial artery, the tibial nerve and the tendon of flexor hallucis longus. In posteromedial approaches to the ankle and talocalcaneal joints, the neurovascular structures are at risk. On the lateral side, peroneus brevis lies anterior to the longus tendon, passing in close proximity to the talocalcaneal joint, and then passes inferior to the joint, anterior to the tip of the fibula. The sural nerve lies just posterior to the peroneal tendons and is at risk during lateral exposure of the joint.

Factors maintaining stability – Stability is conferred by the bone contours of the hindfoot plus the above mentioned ligaments, although which ligaments provide the most stability is not known. An additional ligamentous restraint is provided by the calcaneofibular component of the lateral ligament complex. The tendons crossing the articulation aid stability.

Muscles producing movement – Heel inversion is controlled by tibialis anterior, tibialis posterior and the gastrocnemius–soleus complex via the calcaneal tendon; the flexors of the long toe also contribute. Heel eversion results from the pull of peroneus longus, brevis and tertius, in addition to the extensors of the long toe.

TALOCALCANEONAVICULAR JOINT

An eloquent account of the talocalcaneonavicular joint was provided by Barclay-Smith in 1896. In clinical practice it is regarded as two joints, i.e. the anterior part of the 'subtalar' joint and the talonavicular joint. It is a compound, multiaxial articulation.

Articulating surfaces – The ovoid talar head is continuous with the triple-faceted anterior area of its inferior surface. The whole fits the concavity formed by the posterior surface of the navicular, the middle and anterior talar facets of the calcaneus, and the superior fibrocartilaginous surface of the plantar calcaneonavicular ligament. The bones are connected by a fibrous capsule and three ligaments: talonavicular, plantar calcaneonavicular, and the calcaneonavicular part of the bifurcated ligaments.

Fibrous capsule – The fibrous capsule is poorly developed, except posteriorly, where it is thick and forms the anterior part of the interosseous ligament filling the tarsal sinus.

Ligaments – The talonavicular ligament (**Figs 115.14, 115.15**) is a broad, thin band; it connects the dorsal surfaces of the neck of the talus and the navicular, and is covered by extensor tendons. The plantar calcaneonavicular ligament and the calcaneonavicular part of the

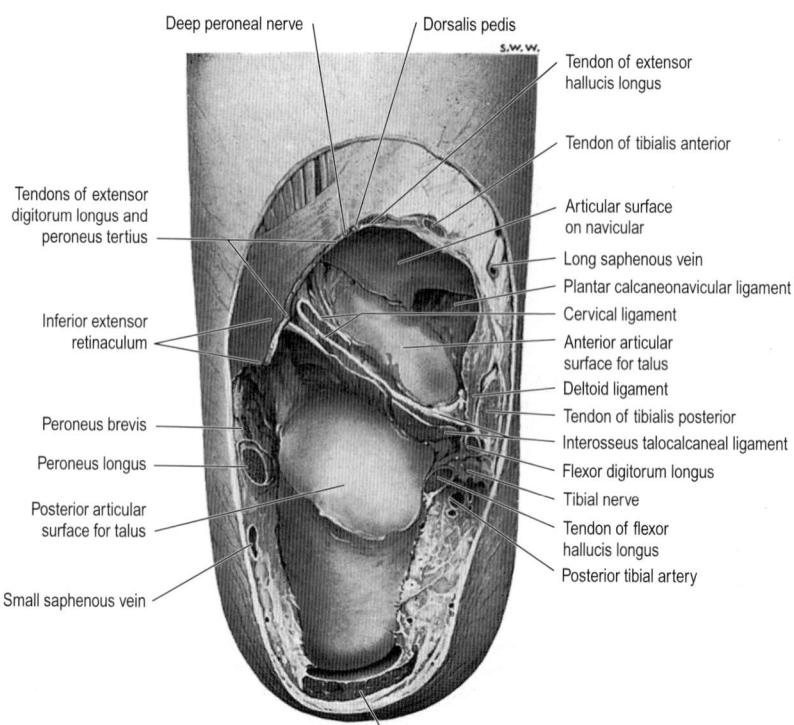

Deep peroneal nerve
Dorsalis pedis
s.w.w.
Tendon of extensor hallucis longus
Tendon of tibialis anterior
Tendons of extensor digitorum longus and peroneus tertius
Articular surface on navicular
Long saphenous vein
Plantar calcaneonavicular ligament
Cervical ligament
Inferior extensor retinaculum
Anterior articular surface for talus
Deltoid ligament
Tendon of tibialis posterior
Peroneus brevis
Interosseus talocalcaneal ligament
Peroneus longus
Flexor digitorum longus
Tibial nerve
Posterior articular surface for talus
Tendon of flexor hallucis longus
Posterior tibial artery
Small saphenous vein
Calcaneal tendon

Fig. 115.32 Left talocalcaneal and talocalcaneonavicular joints, exposed from above by removal of the talus.

bifurcated ligament (**Fig. 115.15**) are the plantar and lateral ligaments of the joint, respectively. Although the calcaneus and navicular do not articulate directly, they are connected by calcaneonavicular and plantar calcaneonavicular ligaments.

The plantar calcaneonavicular (spring) ligament (**Figs 115.14, 115.32, 115.33**) is a broad, thick band connecting the anterior margin of the sustentaculum tali to the plantar surface of the navicular. It ties the calcaneus to the navicular below the head of the talus as part of its articular cavity; it sustains the medial longitudinal arch of the foot. The dorsal surface of the ligament has a triangular fibrocartilaginous facet on which part of the talar head rests (**Fig. 115.32**). Its plantar surface is supported medially by the tendon of tibialis posterior and laterally by the tendons of flexors hallucis longus and digitorum longus; its medial border is blended with the anterior superficial fibres of the medial (deltoid) ligament. The calcaneonavicular ligament is described below as the medial band of the bifurcated ligament.

Synovial membrane – The talocalcaneonavicular joint is synovial and communicates with the talonavicular and talocalcaneal joints.

Innervation – The talocalcaneonavicular joint is innervated by the deep peroneal and medial plantar nerves.

Relations – On the medial side from dorsal to plantar lie the tendon of tibialis posterior and the tendon of flexor digitorum longus above the sustentaculum tali, and the flexor hallucis longus tendon below. At this point, the flexor hallucis longus lies deep to the medial and lateral plantar branches of the posterior tibial artery and nerve. The latter structures are at risk during medial approaches to the joint, e.g. resection of talocalcaneal coalition. Dorsally from medial to lateral lie the tendons of tibialis anterior and extensor hallucis longus, the deep peroneal nerve and the dorsalis pedis artery, the muscle belly of extensor hallucis brevis passing medially and deep to the tendons of extensor digitorum longus

Cuneonavicular and cuboideonavicular ligaments

Fibrous slips from tibialis posterior

Tendon of tibialis posterior

Plantar calcaneonavicular ligament

Groove for flexor hallucis longus

Plantar metatarsal ligaments

Groove for peroneus longus

Long plantar ligament (deep fibres)

Short plantar ligament

S.W.W

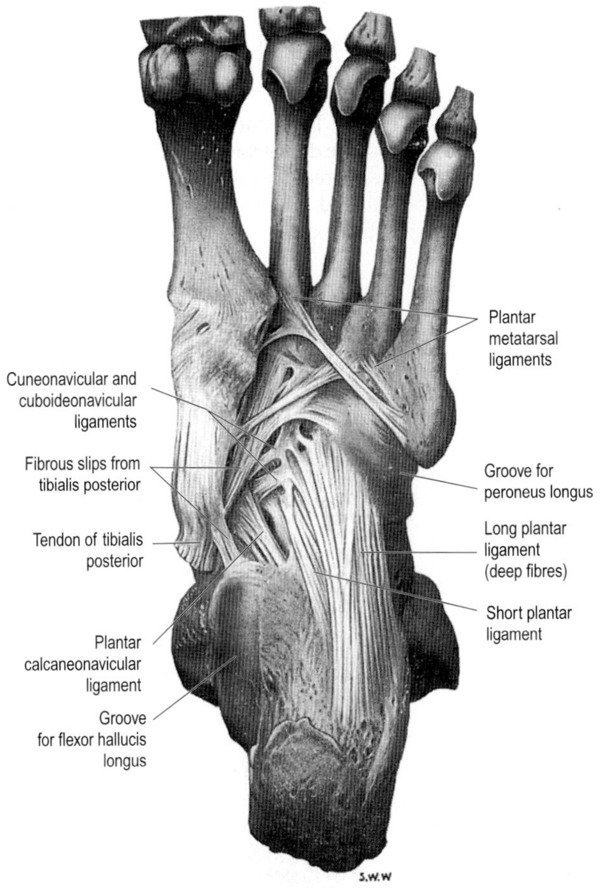

Fig. 115.33 Ligaments on the plantar surface of the left foot. The superficial fibres of the long plantar ligament have been removed. (Drawn from a specimen in the Museum of the Royal College of Surgeons of England, with permission from the Council.)

and peroneus tertius. Structures at risk during the dorsal approach to the talonavicular joint include the branches of the superficial peroneal nerve superficially and the dorsalis pedis artery and deep peroneal nerve deep to the inferior extensor retinaculum.

Factors maintaining stability – Stability is provided as a result of the bone contours, the strong plantar calcaneonavicular (spring) ligament, and the calcaneonavicular component of the bifurcated ligament.

Muscles producing movement – The muscles producing movement are as described above for the talocalcaneal joint.

CALCANEOCUBOID JOINT

The calcaneocuboid joint is at the same level as the talonavicular joint and, together, they represent the transverse tarsal joint. It is a saddle (sellar) or biaxial joint with concavo-convex surfaces.

Articulating surfaces – The articular surfaces of the calcaneocuboid joint, which is 2 cm proximal to the tubercle on the fifth metatarsal base, are between the anterior surface of the calcaneus and the posterior surface of the cuboid.

Fibrous capsule – The fibrous capsule is thickened dorsally as the dorsal calcaneocuboid ligament. The synovial membrane is distinct from other tarsal articulations (**Fig. 115.34**).

Ligaments

Bifurcated ligament – The bifurcated ligament (**Fig. 115.15**) is a strong Y-shaped band. It is attached by its stem proximally to the anterior part of the upper calcaneal surface, and distally it divides into calcaneocuboid and calcaneonavicular parts. The (medial) calcaneocuboid ligament extends to the dorsomedial aspect of the cuboid, forming a main bond between the two rows of tarsal bones; the (lateral) calcaneonavicular ligament is attached to the dorsolateral aspect of the navicular.

Long plantar ligament – The long plantar ligament (**Figs 115.15, 115.33, 115.35**) is the longest ligament associated with the tarsus. It extends from the plantar surface of the calcaneus (anterior to the processes of its tuberosity) and from its anterior tubercle, to the ridge and tuberosity on the plantar surface of the cuboid. Deep fibres are attached to the cuboid and more superficial fibres continue to the bases of the second to fourth, and sometimes fifth, metatarsals. This ligament, with the groove on the plantar surface of the cuboid, makes a tunnel for the tendon of peroneus longus. It is a most powerful factor limiting depression of the lateral longitudinal arch.

Plantar calcaneocuboid ligament – This short plantar ligament (**Fig. 115.33**) is deeper than the long plantar ligament, from which it is separated by areolar tissue. It is a short, wide band of great strength, stretching from the anterior calcaneal tubercle and the depression anterior to it, to the adjoining part of the plantar surface of the cuboid; it also sustains the lateral longitudinal arch.

Synovial membrane – A synovial membrane lines the calcaneocuboid joint.

Innervation – The calcaneocuboid joint is innervated on its plantar aspect by the lateral plantar nerve, and dorsally by the sural and deep peroneal nerves.

Relations – Peroneus longus and abductor digiti minimi pass in close proximity to the joint, with the lateral plantar nerve passing medially. The extensor digitorum brevis overlies the lateral aspect of the joint. The sural nerve and the tendon of peroneus longus itself are at risk during approaches to an os peroneum.

Factors maintaining stability – The calcaneocuboid joint only allows small amounts of movement, and is very stable as a result of the bony contours and the strong ligaments described above.

Muscles producing movement – Movements between the calcaneus and cuboid are gliding, with conjunct rotation upon each other during inversion and eversion of the entire foot. The movements are brought about by the same muscles that act on the talocalcaneal joint and talocalcaneonavicular joint.

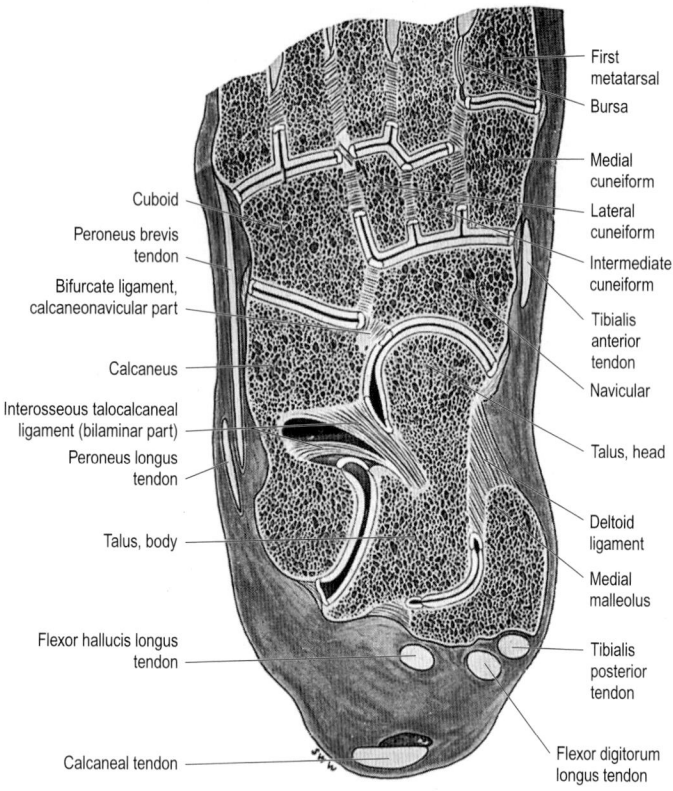

Cuboid

Peroneus brevis tendon

Bifurcate ligament, calcaneonavicular part

Calcaneus

Interosseous talocalcaneal ligament (bilaminar part)

Peroneus longus tendon

Talus, body

Flexor hallucis longus tendon

Calcaneal tendon

First metatarsal

Bursa

Medial cuneiform

Lateral cuneiform

Intermediate cuneiform

Tibialis anterior tendon

Navicular

Talus, head

Deltoid ligament

Medial malleolus

Tibialis posterior tendon

Flexor digitorum longus tendon

Fig. 115.34 Oblique section that descends mediolaterally through the left foot, showing the synovial cavities of the intertarsal and tarsometatarsal joints and the medial malleolar part of the ankle joint: superior aspect. The section passed below the joint between the medial cuneiform and the base of the second metatarsal; no synovial joint was present between the navicular and cuboid. The laminae of the interosseous talocalcaneal ligament form accessory ligaments to the fibrous capsules of the talocalcaneonavicular and subtalar (posterior talocalcaneal) joints. The apparently uniform thickness of the articular cartilages obscures the variations in thickness and curvature that occur in life.

NAVICULOCUNEIFORM JOINTS

The naviculocuneiform joint is a compound joint, often described as plane.

Articulating surfaces – The navicular articulates distally with the cuneiform bones where the distal navicular surface is transversely convex and divided into three facets by low ridges, adapted to the proximal, slightly curved cuneiform surfaces.

Fibrous capsule – The fibrous capsule is continuous with those of the intercuneiform and cuneocuboid joints and it is also connected to the second and third cuneometatarsal joints and intermetatarsal joints between the second to fourth metatarsal bones.

Ligaments

Dorsal and plantar ligaments – The dorsal and plantar ligaments connect the navicular to each cuneiform; of the three dorsal ligaments, one is attached to each cuneiform. The fasciculus from the navicular to the medial cuneiform is continued as the capsule of the joint around its medial aspect, and then blends medially with the plantar ligament. Plantar ligaments have similar attachments and receive slips from the tendon of tibialis posterior.

Synovial membrane – The synovial membrane lines the fibrous capsule in the manner outlined above.

Innervation – The naviculocuneiform joint is innervated dorsally from the deep peroneal nerve. The medial and intermediate naviculocuneiform joints receive a plantar innervation from the medial plantar nerve, and the lateral naviculocuneiform joint is innervated from the lateral plantar nerve.

Relations – The tibialis posterior tendon sends fibres to the medial cuneiform and crosses the joint on its medial side; it is vulnerable to injury when a medial surgical approach is used, as are the dorsal venous arch and the saphenous nerve. The tibialis anterior tendon passes over the dorsomedial aspect of the joint and the extensor hallucis longus tendon is lateral. Over the intermediate cuneiform pass, from medial to lateral, the deep peroneal nerve, the dorsalis pedis artery and the muscle belly of extensor hallucis brevis, all of which are vulnerable during dorsal exposure of the joint. On the lateral aspect of the joint, the superficial structures at risk are the superficial peroneal nerve and the dorsal venous arch.

Muscles producing movement – Movements at the naviculocuneiform, cuboideonavicular, intercuneiform and cuneocuboid joints are merely slight gliding and rotation during pronation or supination of the foot: when alterations occur in a loaded foot in contact with the ground, they increase suppleness when the forefoot is stressed, as in the initial thrust of running and jumping. The muscles responsible for these slight movements are tibialis anterior, tibialis posterior, the peronei and the long toe flexors and extensors.

CUBOIDEONAVICULAR JOINT

The cuboideonavicular joint is usually a fibrous joint, the bones being connected by dorsal, plantar and interosseous ligaments. This syndesmosis is often replaced by a synovial joint, almost plane; its articular capsule and synovial lining are continuous with that of the naviculocuneiform joint. The dorsal ligament extends distolaterally, the plantar nearly transversely from the cuboid to the navicular. The interosseous ligament, made of strong transverse fibres, connects non-articular parts of adjacent surfaces to the two bones (**Fig. 115.34**).

INTERCUNEIFORM AND CUNEOCUBOID JOINTS

The intercuneiform and cuneocuboid joints are all synovial and approximately plane or slightly curved. Their articular capsules and synovial linings are continuous with the naviculocuneiform joints. The bones are connected by dorsal, plantar and interosseous ligaments (**Figs 115.14, 115.15**).

Ligaments

Dorsal and plantar ligaments – The dorsal and plantar ligaments each has three transverse bands, between the medial and intermediate cuneiform, the intermediate and lateral cuneiform, and the lateral cuneiform and cuboid. The plantar ligaments receive slips from the tendon of tibialis posterior.

Interosseous ligaments – The interosseous ligaments connect non-articular areas of adjacent surfaces and are strong agents in maintaining the transverse arch.

Innervation – The intercuneiform and cuneocuboid joints are innervated dorsally via the deep peroneal nerve. The plantar aspect of the medial two joints is innervated from the medial plantar nerve, and the plantar aspect of the lateral joints is innervated from the lateral plantar nerve.

Muscles producing movement – The muscles producing movement are as described above for the naviculocuneiform joint.

TARSOMETATARSAL ARTICULATIONS

Tarsometatarsal articulations are approximately plane synovial joints.

Articulating surfaces – The first metatarsal articulates with the medial cuneiform; the second is recessed between the medial and lateral, articulating with the intermediate cuneiform; the third articulates with lateral cuneiform; the fourth articulates with the lateral cuneiform and cuboid; the fifth articulates with the cuboid. The joints are approximately on a line from the tubercle of the fifth metatarsal to the tarsometatarsal joint of the hallux, except for that between the second metatarsal and intermediate cuneiform, which is 2–3 mm proximal (**Fig. 115.34**).

Fibrous capsule – The hallucal joint has its own capsule; articular capsules and cavities of the second and third are continuous with intercuneiform and naviculocuneiform joints, but separated from the fourth and fifth joints by an interosseous ligament between the lateral cuneiform and fourth metatarsal base.

Ligaments – The bones are connected by dorsal and plantar tarsometatarsal and interosseous cuneometatarsal ligaments.

Dorsal ligaments – The dorsal ligaments are strong and flat. The first metatarsal is joined to the medial cuneiform by an articular capsule; the other tarsometatarsal capsules blend with the dorsal and plantar ligaments. The second metatarsal receives a band from each cuneiform, the third from the lateral cuneiform, the fourth from the lateral cuneiform and cuboid, the fifth from the cuboid alone.

Plantar ligaments – The plantar ligaments are longitudinal and oblique bands, less regular than the dorsal. Those for the first and second metatarsals are strongest; the second and third metatarsals are joined by oblique bands to the medial cuneiform, the fourth and fifth by a few fibres to the cuboid.

Interosseous cuneometatarsal ligaments – There are three interosseous cuneometatarsal ligaments. One (the strongest) passes from the lateral surface of the medial cuneiform to the adjacent angle of the second metatarsal (**Fig. 115.35**). Known as Lisfranc's ligament, it is critical to the stability of the tarsometatarsal joint complex. Disruption of this ligament can lead to instability and deformity and, later, to degenerative changes. A second ligament connects the lateral cuneiform to the adjacent angle of the second metatarsal; it does not divide the joint between the second metatarsal and lateral cuneiform and is inconstant. A third ligament connects the lateral angle of the lateral cuneiform to the adjacent fourth metatarsal base.

Synovial membrane – The first tarsometatarsal joint has its own capsule, with a synovial lining. The other joints are similarly arranged, but there

is a communication between the second and third and between the fourth and fifth tarsometatarsal joints.

Innervation – The interosseous cuneometatarsal ligaments are innervated dorsally via the deep peroneal nerve. The plantar aspect of the medial two joints is innervated from the medial plantar nerve, and the plantar aspects of the lateral joints are innervated from the lateral plantar nerve.

Relations – From medial to lateral, the following structures cross the tarsometatarsal joints across the dorsal aspect: the saphenous nerve, the dorsal venous arch, extensor hallucis longus tendon, the deep peroneal nerve, the dorsalis pedis artery, extensor hallucis brevis, the extensor digitorum longus tendon with the corresponding extensor digitorum brevis to the lateral side, peroneus tertius and peroneus brevis. Branches of the superficial peroneal nerve are variable in location on the dorsum. The sural nerve lies just inferior to the peroneus brevis tendon in the subcutaneous tissues. Surgery of the tarsometatarsal joints is performed through a dorsal approach, and all these structures are potentially at risk.

Factors maintaining stability – The major stabilisers are the ligaments. Although they are dense, this joint complex is vulnerable to injury because of the lack of ligamentous connection between the first and second metatarsal bases. The medial interosseous ligament or Lisfranc's ligament is responsible for the tell-tale avulsion fracture of the second metatarsal base, which may be the only radiographic indication of abnormality after injury to this part of the foot. It is a highly significant injury that is often missed. Failure to recognise and treat this injury by surgical reduction and fixation can lead to long-term disability.

Muscles producing movement – Movements between the tarsal and metatarsal bones are limited to flexion and extension, except in the first tarsometatarsal joint, where some abduction and rotation also occur. Muscles producing this motion are tibialis anterior and peroneus longus. Flexion and extension are brought about by the long and short toe flexors and extensors. Movement between the medial cuneiform and first metatarsal and between the fourth and fifth metatarsals and the cuboid is moderate, to allow the foot to adapt to an uneven surface, whereas movement between the second and third metatarsals and their respective cuneiforms is very limited.

INTERMETATARSAL JOINTS

The intermetatarsal interosseous ligaments are very strong and are present between all the lateral four metatarsals, but are absent between the first and second metatarsals. The base of the second metatarsal is joined to the first tarsometatarsal joint by the medial interosseous ligament (Lisfranc's ligament), connecting the plantar aspect of the second metatarsal to the medial cuneiform.

Ligaments

Dorsal and plantar intermetatarsal ligaments – As with their dorsal counterparts, the plantar intermetatarsal ligaments are longitudinal, oblique or transverse and vary considerably in number and organisation. The plantar ligaments are significantly stronger than the corresponding dorsal ligaments. The strongest is the second oblique plantar ligament, which connects the medial cuneiform to the second and third bases (**Figs 115.33, 115.35**).

Other ligaments – All metatarsal heads are connected indirectly by deep transverse metatarsal ligaments. Dorsal and plantar ligaments pass transversely between adjacent bases. Interosseous ligaments are strong transverse bands connecting non-articular parts of the adjacent surfaces (**Fig. 115.34**).

METATARSOPHALANGEAL ARTICULATIONS

Metatarsophalangeal articulations are ovoid or ellipsoid joints between the rounded metatarsal heads and shallow cavities on the proximal phalangeal bases. They are 2.5 cm proximal to the webs of the toes.

Articulating surfaces – Articular surfaces cover the distal and plantar aspects of the metatarsal heads, but not the dorsal. The plantar aspect of the first metatarsal head has two longitudinal grooves separated by a ridge (the crista). Each articulates with a sesamoid bone embedded in

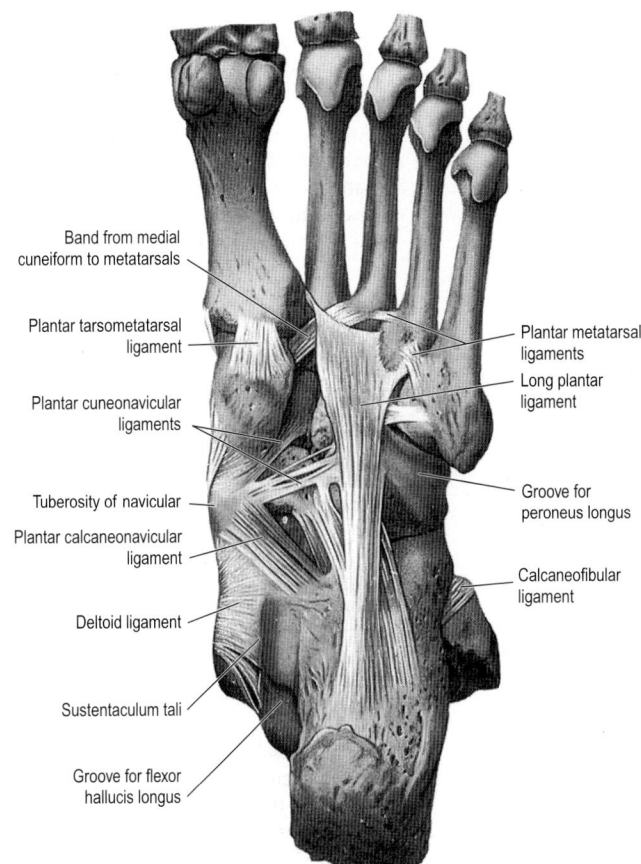

Band from medial
cuneiform to metatarsals

Plantar tarsometatarsal
ligament

Plantar cuneonavicular
ligaments

Tuberosity of navicular

Plantar calcaneonavicular
ligament

Deltoid ligament

Sustentaculum tali

Groove for flexor
hallucis longus

Plantar metatarsal
ligaments

Long plantar
ligament

Groove for
peroneus longus

Calcaneofibular
ligament

S.W.W.

Fig. 115.35 Ligaments of the plantar surface of the left foot. Some of the fibres of the long plantar ligament, which arise in front of the medial tubercle of the calcaneus, have been removed. (Drawn from a specimen in the Museum of the Royal College of Surgeons of England, with permission from the Council.)

the capsule of the joint, formed here by the two tendons of flexor hallucis brevis. The sesamoids are connected to each other by the intersesamoid ligament, which forms the floor of the tendinous canal for the flexor hallucis longus tendon. The medial sesamoid receives an attachment from abductor hallucis and the lateral from adductor hallucis.

Articular areas on the proximal phalangeal bases are concave. Ligaments are capsular, plantar, deep transverse metatarsal and collateral.

Fibrous capsules – Fibrous capsules are attached to their articular margins. They are thin dorsally, and may be separated from the long extensor tendons by small bursae, or they may be replaced by the tendons; they are inseparable from the plantar and collateral ligaments. The plantar aponeurosis blends with the plantar capsule to form the so-called 'plantar plate'. The latter inserts distally via medial and lateral bundles, which insert into the base of the proximal phalanx. The plate is attached to the metatarsal head via a thin synovial fold. Proximally, the plantar plate receives the insertion of the plantar aponeurosis. It also receives an attachment from the accessory collateral ligament.

Ligaments

Plantar ligaments – The plantar ligaments are thick and dense. They are between and blend with the collateral ligaments; their attachment to the metatarsals is loose, but that to the phalangeal bases is firm. Their margins blend with the deep transverse metatarsal ligaments. Their plantar surfaces are grooved for the flexor tendons, the fibrous sheaths of which connect with the edges of the grooves, and their deep surfaces extend the articular areas for metatarsal heads.

Deep transverse metatarsal ligaments – The deep transverse metatarsal ligaments are four short, wide, flat bands uniting the plantar ligaments of adjoining metatarsophalangeal joints. The interossei are dorsal and the lumbricals and digital vessels and nerves are plantar. They resemble the deep transverse metacarpal ligaments, but connect with the plantar ligament of the hallucal metatarsophalangeal joint.

Collateral ligaments – The collateral ligaments are strong cords flanking each joint. They are attached to the dorsal tubercles on the metatarsal heads and the corresponding side of the phalangeal bases and slope downwards and forwards. The first metatarsophalangeal joint also contains metatarso-sesamoid ligaments. On either side, the ligaments arise from the metatarsal head with a narrow origin and fan out to insert on the border of the proximal phalanx and the plantar plate.

Each collateral ligament consists of the phalangeal collateral, which inserts into the base of the proximal phalanx and the accessory collateral ligament, which inserts into the plantar plate.

Synovial membrane – Each metatarsophalangeal joint is a separate synovial joint.

Innervation – The main nerve supply of the metatarsophalangeal joints is from the plantar interdigital nerves, which supply the first, second, third and medial half of the fourth metatarsophalangeal joint on the plantar aspect. Digital branches of the lateral plantar nerve supply the lateral aspect of the fourth and all of the fifth joint on the plantar side. The dorsomedial side of the hallucal metatarsophalangeal joint is supplied by the medial dorsal cutaneous branch of the superficial peroneal nerve. The deep peroneal supplies the lateral side and the medial side of the second toe joint.

Relations – Dorsally, the extensor hallucis longus tendon lies medial to the extensor hallucis brevis tendon. The same arrangement occurs in the lesser toes with the tendons of extensor digitorum longus and brevis. The interossei are plantarmedial and plantarlateral, dorsal to the intermetatarsal ligament, whereas the lumbrical tendons and the digital artery and nerve are plantar to the intermetatarsal ligament. The long and short flexors lie on the plantar aspect of the joint in the midline. If approaching the metatarsophalangeal joint surgically from the plantar surface, it is important not to stray from the midline.

Factors maintaining stability – The first metatarsophalangeal joint owes its stability to its capsuloligamentous structures, and to flexor and extensor hallucis brevis, with a small contribution from flexor and extensor hallucis longus or the bone contours. The lesser toe metatarso-

phalangeal joints are stabilised principally by the collateral ligaments and plantar plates. Rupture of the plantar plate leads to hammer toe deformity.

Muscles producing movement – Movements are like those at the corresponding joints in the hand, but differ in range. Unlike the hand, the range of active extension (50–60°) is greater than that of flexion (30–40°). This is an adaptation to the needs of walking, and is most marked in the hallucal joint, where flexion is a few degrees whereas extension may reach 90°. When the foot is on the ground, metatarsophalangeal joints are already extended to at least 25°, because the metatarsals slope up in the longitudinal arches of the foot (**Fig. 115.36**). The ranges of passive movements in these joints are 90° (extension) and 45° (flexion), according to Kapandji (1974). The following muscles produce movement of the metatarsophalangeal joints:

Flexion – Flexor digitorum brevis, the lumbricals and interossei, assisted by flexors digitorum longus and accessorius. In the fifth toe, flexor digiti minimi brevis assists; in the hallux, flexors hallucis longus and brevis are the only flexors.

Extension – Extensors digitorum longus and brevis, extensor hallucis longus.

Adduction – Adductor hallucis; in the third to fifth toes, the first, second and third plantar interossei, respectively.

Abduction – Abductor hallucis; in the second toe, first and second dorsal interossei; in the third and fourth toes, corresponding dorsal interossei; in the fifth toe, abductor digiti minimi.

Note: The line of reference for adduction and abduction is along the second digit, which has the least mobile metatarsal. This is hence 'abducted' medially or laterally by both its interossei.

Hallux valgus

Hallux valgus is very common, occurring mainly in individuals who have a genetic predisposition. Footwear is implicated in the condition, which presumably accounts for the greater incidence in females. Metatarsus primus varus, an adduction deformity of the first metatarsal, is commonly associated with hallux valgus.

The more round a first metatarsal head, the more prone it is to be unstable. Conversely, a flat metatarsal head is less likely to be associated with hallux valgus. No muscle inserts into the first metatarsal head, and

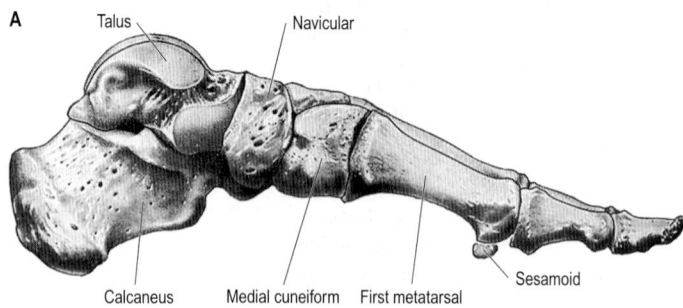

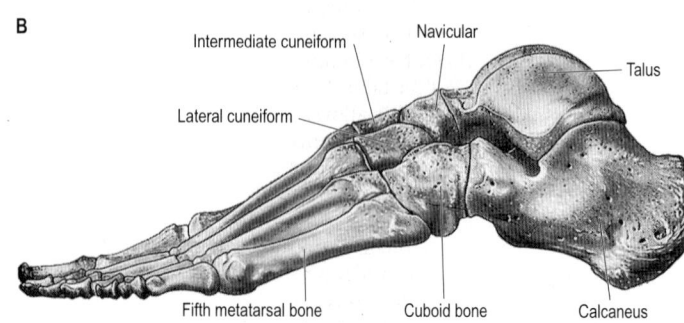

Fig. 115.36 Medial (**A**) and lateral (**B**) aspects of the skeleton of the left foot. Note the height and number of bones in both the medial and lateral longitudinal arches.

therefore its position is determined by the position of the proximal phalanx. As the proximal phalanx moves laterally on the metatarsal head, it pushes the head medially. This leads to attenuation of the medial soft tissue structures and contracture of the lateral ones. The sesamoid sling, which is anchored laterally by adductor hallucis, remains in place as the head moves medially, thus displacing the sesamoids from under the metatarsal head. As this happens, the weakest point of the medial capsule fails, resulting in abductor hallucis slipping under the metatarsal head. This leads to failure of the intrinsic muscles to stabilise the joint, and the pull of abductor hallucis leads to spinning of the proximal phalanx, which results in a pronation deformity. Failure to intervene surgically inevitably results in a progressive deformity.

INTERPHALANGEAL ARTICULATIONS

Interphalangeal articulations are almost pure hinge joints, in which the trochlear surfaces on the phalangeal heads articulate with reciprocally curved surfaces on adjacent phalangeal bases. Each has an articular capsule and two collateral ligaments, as in the metatarsophalangeal joints. The plantar surface of the capsule is a thickened fibrous plate, like the plantar metatarsophalangeal ligaments, and is often termed the plantar ligament.

Movements are flexion and extension, which are greater in amplitude between the proximal and middle phalanges than between the middle and distal. Flexion is marked, but extension is limited by tension of the flexor muscles and plantar ligaments. Abduction, adduction and rotation occur to a minor extent.

Innervation – The interphalangeal articulations are innervated by branches from the plantar interdigital nerves. The medial dorsal cutaneous branch of the superficial peroneal nerve also supplies the hallucal interphalangeal joint. Branches of the deep peroneal, intermediate dorsal cutaneous and sural nerves sometimes supply the joints of the lesser toes.

Muscles producing movement

Flexion – Flexors digitorum longus, brevis and accessorius, flexor hallucis longus.

Extension – Extensors digitorum longus and brevis, extensor hallucis longus.

ARCHES OF THE FOOT

Three main arches are recognised in the foot. They are the medial longitudinal, the lateral longitudinal and the transverse.

MEDIAL LONGITUDINAL ARCH

The medial margin of the foot arches up between the heel and the first metatarsophalangeal joint to form a visible arch (**Fig. 115.36A**). It is made up of the calcaneus, talus, navicular, the three cuneiforms and their three metatarsals. The pillars are the posterior aspect of the calcaneus and the three metatarsal heads. The bones themselves contribute little to the stability of the arch, whereas the ligaments contribute significantly. The most important ligamentous structure is the plantar aponeurosis, which acts as a tie beam between the supporting pillars (Hicks 1953). Dorsiflexion, especially of the hallux, draws the two pillars together, thus heightening the arch. This so-called 'windlass' mechanism was extensively studied by Hicks. Next in importance is the spring ligament, which supports the head of the talus. If this ligament fails, the navicular and calcaneus separate, and this allows the highest point of the arch, the talar head, to lower. The talocalcaneal ligaments and the anterior fibres of the deltoid ligament, from the tibia to the navicular, also contribute.

Muscles also have a role in the maintenance of the medial longitudinal arch. Flexor hallucis longus is important in this regard, and acts as a bowstring. Flexor digitorum longus, abductor hallucis and the medial half of flexor digitorum brevis also contribute, but to a lesser extent. Tibialis posterior and anterior are important in the maintenance of the arch by inverting and adducting the foot, and so help to raise its medial border. The importance of tibialis posterior is manifest by the collapse of the medial longitudinal arch that accompanies failure of the tibialis tendon.

LATERAL LONGITUDINAL ARCH

The bones making up the longitudinal arch are the calcaneus, the cuboid and the fourth and fifth metatarsals (**Fig. 115.36B**). The pillars are the calcaneus and the lateral two metatarsal heads. The bones contribute little to the arch in terms of stability, and ligaments have a more important role. The most significant ligaments are the lateral part of the plantar aponeurosis and the long and short plantar ligaments. The most important contribution to the maintenance of the lateral arch is made by the peroneus longus tendon. The lateral two tendons of flexor digitorum longus (and flexor accessorius) and the muscles of the first layer (lateral half of flexor digitorum brevis and abductor digiti minimi) also assist by preventing separation of the pillars of the arch.

TRANSVERSE ARCH

The bones involved in the transverse arch (**Fig. 115.37**) are the bases of the five metatarsals, the cuboid and the cuneiforms. The intermediate and lateral cuneiforms are wedge-shaped and thus adapted to maintenance of the transverse arch. The stability of the arch is mainly provided by the ligaments, which bind the cuneiforms and the metatarsal bases, and also by the peroneus longus tendon, the pull of which tends to approximate the medial and lateral borders of the foot. A shallow arch is maintained at the metatarsal heads by the deep transverse ligaments, transverse fibres that bind together the digital slips of the plantar aponeurosis, and, to a lesser extent, by the transverse head of adductor hallucis.

BIOMECHANICS OF STANDING, WALKING AND RUNNING

PLANES OF MOTION

Much confusion surrounds the descriptive terms for movement in the foot and ankle. Plantar flexion and dorsiflexion refer to movement in the sagittal plane and occur principally, but not exclusively, at the ankle, metatarsophalangeal and interphalangeal joints. Inversion is tilting of the plantar surface of the foot towards the midline, and eversion is tilting away from the midline. This is motion in the coronal plane and takes place principally in the talocalcaneal and transverse tarsal joints. Adduction is movement of the foot towards the midline in the transverse plane; abduction is movement away from the midline. This movement occurs at the transverse tarsal joints and, to a limited degree, the first tarsometatarsal joint and the metatarsophalangeal joints.

Supination describes a three-dimensional movement and is a combination of adduction, inversion and plantar flexion. Pronation is the opposite motion, i.e. a combination of abduction, eversion and dorsiflexion. Pronation and supination are usually better terms than eversion and inversion, as the latter rarely occur in isolation and the former describe the 'compound' motion that usually occurs.

Active movements occur at the ankle, talocalcaneonavicular and subtalar joints. Movements at the ankle joint are almost entirely restricted to dorsi- and plantar flexion, but slight rotation may occur in

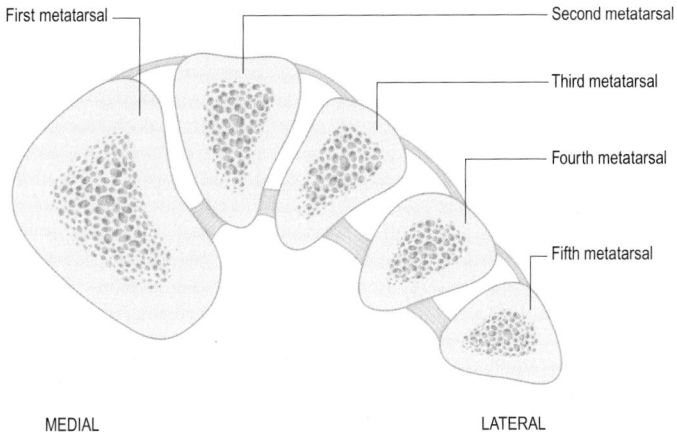

First metatarsal — — Second metatarsal

— Third metatarsal

— Fourth metatarsal

— Fifth metatarsal

MEDIAL   LATERAL

Fig. 115.37 Transverse arch of foot, at the level of the first metatarsal base.

plantar flexion. The ranges of movement at the talocalcaneonavicular and subtalar joint are greater: inversion and eversion mainly occur here.

STANDING

Humans are bipedal: we stand and walk with an erect trunk and knees which are almost straight. Moreover, we are plantigrade, i.e. we set the whole length of the foot down on the ground, whereas most medium to large mammals are digitigrade, i.e. they stand and walk on their toes, and ungulates stand on hooves on the tips of their toes.

When we stand motionless, the ground exerts a force on the feet called the 'ground reaction force', which is equal and opposite to body weight. The latter acts at the 'centre of gravity', a point a little above the hip joints and anterior to the vertebral column. The force on the ground is centred vertically below it, at the centre of pressure. When we stand comfortably, the centre of pressure is usually midway between the insteps of our two feet. We do not remain absolutely still, but sway slightly. As we age, our postural control deteriorates, which is a factor in the development of unsteadiness and risk of falling.

When considering the distribution of load in the lower limb, a knowledge of limb alignment is important. The 'anatomic axis' is produced by lines passing along the shafts of the femur and tibia, and is therefore angled at the knee by 5° to 7°. The 'mechanical axis' is a straight line connecting the centres of the femoral head and ankle. Exactly where the line passes through the knee has yet to be defined: for convenience it is usually taken to pass through the centre, but may well lie more medially. For the tibia, the lines of the mechanical and anatomic axes coincide. Whilst the weight of the body acts in a vertical line from the centre of gravity to the ground, the line of the mechanical axis of the lower limbs is inclined 3° to this in normal stance, with the ankles closer than hips.

In the sagittal plane, body weight acts along a line which passes a few centimetres anterior to the tibiotalar joint, exerting a moment that must be balanced by the plantar flexor muscles. Some electromyographic investigations of standing have found activity mainly in soleus, but others have found moderate activity in gastrocnemius as well. In either case it seems likely that the activity is mainly in type I (slow oxidative) fibres, which can maintain tension more economically than faster fibres could do under the same conditions. Soleus contains c.80% of type I fibres, and gastrocnemius c.50%.

In normal standing, the weight of the body above the knee joint acts slightly anteriorly to the axes of the knees: it exerts a moment that is balanced passively by tension in the ligaments and posterior capsule which prevent hyperextension. If the knees are kept straight, there is little or no electrical activity in the hamstrings and only moderate levels in the quadriceps. Generally, the combined weight of the trunk, arms and head seems to act slightly behind the hip joints, exerting a small moment that is balanced largely by iliopsoas. Thus a relaxed stance, with trunk erect and knees straight, requires very little activity in thigh muscles. This demands low energy consumption and permits long periods of standing. In single leg stance the weight of the upper parts of the body exerts a moment about the supporting hip which must be balanced by abductor muscles, especially tensor fasciae latae and glutei medius and minimus. Damage to the glutei or anterior nerve supply, e.g. during hip surgery, is a potent cause of a limp.

PROPULSION

The contraction of tibialis posterior, gastrocnemius and soleus is the chief factor responsible for propulsion in walking, running and jumping. The propulsive action of these calf muscles is enhanced by arching of the foot and flexion of the toes. In walking, the weight of the foot is taken successively on the heel, lateral border and the ball of the foot. The last part of the foot to leave the ground is the anterior pillar of the medial longitudinal arch and the medial three toes. In the act of running, the heel does not touch the ground, but the point of take-off is still the anterior pillar of the medial longitudinal arch. As the heel leaves the ground, the toes gradually extend. Extension of the hallux particularly, tightens the plantar aponeurosis and thus heightens the arch. At the same time, flexor hallucis longus and flexor digitorum longus elongate, which increases their subsequent contraction. The long and short toe flexors increase the force of take-off by exerting pressure on the ground. The most important muscle in this respect is flexor hallucis longus, which is strongly assisted by the short toe flexors. The lumbricals provide a balancing action to the long toe flexors and prevent buckling of the toes during the toe-off phase of gait.

WALKING

In walking, each foot is on the ground (stance phase) for c.60% of the stride, and off (swing phase) for c.40% (**Fig. 115.38**). Thus single-support phases (one foot on the ground) alternate with double-support phases (two feet). The knee is straight at heel strike and remains nearly straight (10–30°) for most of the stance phase of that leg, bending more only immediately before toe-off. During the swing phase the knee flexes to a maximum of c. 60° at mid-swing.

Stance phase starts with 'heel strike'. With the foot still planted in front of the body, 'foot flat' is reached, and becomes 'mid-stance' when the body comes to be directly above the planted foot. The heel then rises as the contralateral foot makes contact with the ground (the 'double stance' phase). The last event of stance is 'toe off' when the 'swing phase' starts. Early in the stance phase, while it is 'foot flat' in front of the trunk, the foot pushes downwards and forwards on the ground, decelerating the body as well as supporting it. Later, when the foot is behind the trunk, it pushes downwards and backwards, re-accelerating the body (**Fig. 115.38**). The speed, and therefore the kinetic energy, of the body passes through a maximum in each double-support phase, and a minimum in each single-support phase.

The height of the centre of gravity, and so the potential energy of the body, also fluctuates. This is inevitable if the knee is kept nearly straight, making the hip move in a near-circular arc about the ankle of the supporting foot. The vertical component of the total force exerted by both feet on the ground in the double-support phase is greater than body weight, giving the body an upward acceleration. The vertical component of the ground force during the single-support phase is less than body weight, giving the body a downward acceleration. The force fluctuations have to be larger at higher speeds, to give the same vertical movement in less time.

During walking, the potential energy of the body is high when its kinetic energy is low, and vice versa. Energy can thus be swapped back and forth between the two forms, as in a swinging pendulum. A friction-less pendulum would continue swinging forever with no fresh input of energy. In walking, the exchange of potential and kinetic energy is less perfect, and the leg muscles have to do work to replace the energy which is lost at each impact of a foot with the ground. Even so, much less work is needed because of the pendulum principle. A second pendulum effect can be seen in the forward swing of the legs. If the leg were a rigid rod swinging from a fixed pivot, it would swing forward too slowly for normal walking: because it is free to bend at the knee, and because the hip from which it swings rises and falls, the leg swings forward faster with very little need for muscular work.

These pendulum effects ensure that relatively little work is needed to drive the fluctuations of kinetic and potential energy which occur in walking. The additional work needed to overcome air resistance and joint friction is very small, because we travel slowly and have well-lubricated joints. Human walking is economical of energy. Measurements of oxygen consumption show that 70-kg men use only c.230 joules of metabolic energy for every metre they walk at their most economical speed, (c.1.3 metres per second), which is c.140 J/m more than they would use if they stood still. Running uses c.260 J/m more than standing. Walking is economical only near the optimum speed, and the energy cost of fast walking overtakes that of running at c.2 m/s, at which speed adults usually break into a run. Children, with their shorter legs, start running at lower speeds: the theoretical expectation is that the critical speed should be proportional to the square root of leg length.

The function of arm swinging in walking is not fully understood but aids postural stability. For further discussion of standing and walking see Alexander (1992).

Development of walking

The average child sits at 6 months, crawls at 9 months, walks with support at 12 months, and without support at 18 months. The characteristic early gait matures rapidly and is similar to that of the adult by 3 years. Some minor changes occur up to 7 years which are largely a reflection of neurological development, but are also related to stature. Early gait is jerky, unsteady, and wide-based. The arms are held abducted at the shoulder and initially flexed at the elbows. Initial ground contact varies, and heel-toe, whole foot, and toe-heel are all possible. Generally a plantarflexed posture is adopted which contrasts with the adult pattern. In adults, heel strike is accompanied by a straight knee which then flexes. A child strikes the ground with a flexed knee which is then extended in response to weight-bearing, and a short time is spent in single leg stance

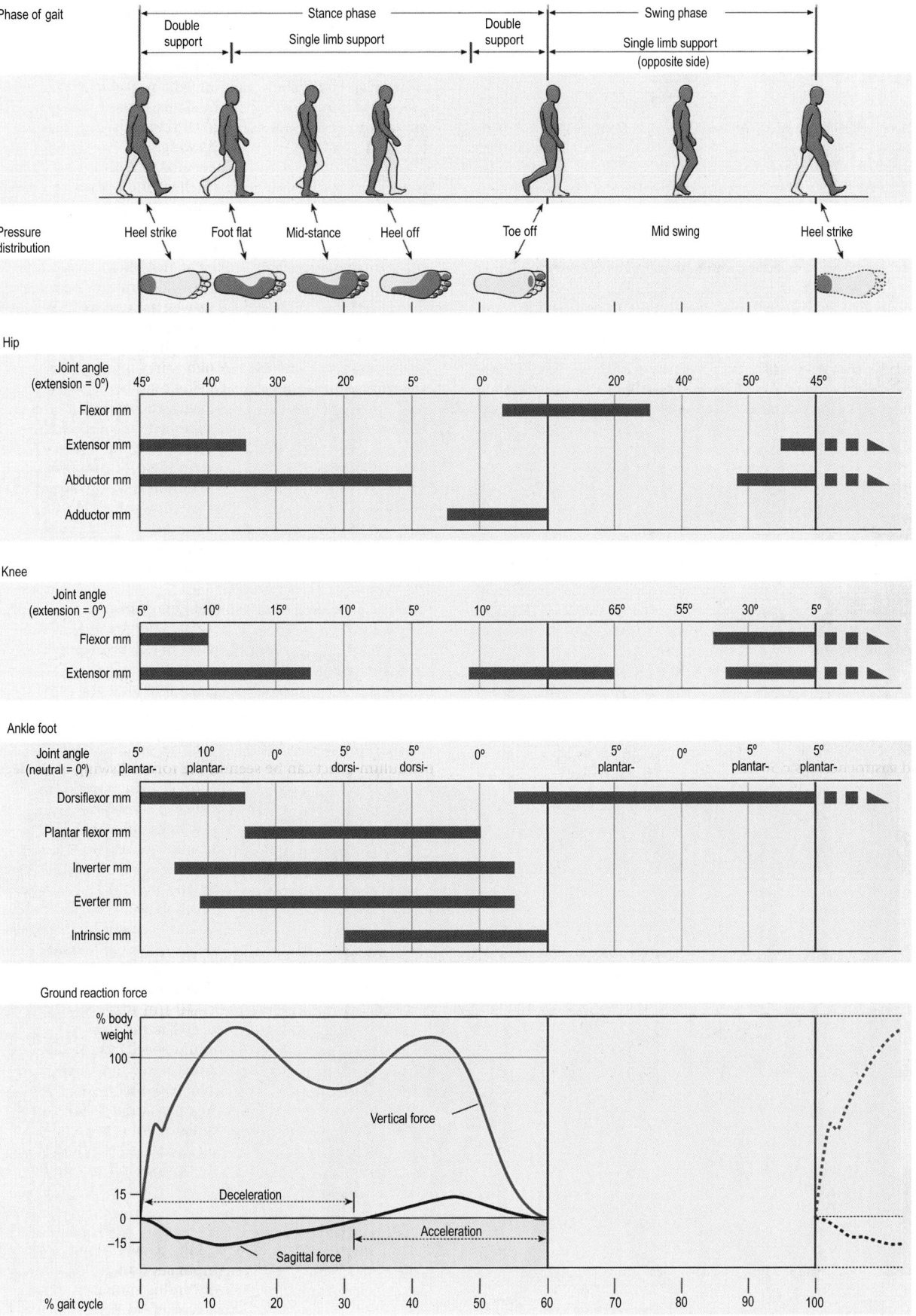

Fig. 115.38 The events that occur during the different phases of a normal gait cycle. Depicted are: distribution of pressure on the plantar surface of the foot; changes in the angles of hip, knee and ankle joints, together with activity in the corresponding muscle groups; and vertical and horizontal (sagittal plane) components of the ground reaction force during stance phase. (Chart collated from various sources by Michael Gunther, Department of Human Anatomy and Cell Biology, University of Liverpool.)

(Fig. 115.39). Maturation is associated with diminution of base width, and increase in step length and velocity. The earliest changes are development of heel-strike, knee flexion during stance, and reciprocal upper limb swing. The period of single leg stance increases.

RUNNING

Walking involves dual-support phases, but in running each foot is on the ground for 40% (jogging) to 27% (sprinting) of the stride, so there is an aerial phase, the 'double float' phase, when neither foot is on the ground. The faster the subject runs, the shorter the stance phase: world-class sprinters spend c.22% of the gait cycle in stance. During each aerial phase the body rises and then falls under gravity, which means that its height and potential energy are maximal in the middle of this phase and minimal at mid-stance, when, in marked contrast to walking, the knee of the supporting leg bends. Walking has been described as 'controlled falling', as the centre of gravity falls from a peak in mid-stance to a low during double support. The analogy that is used for running is an individual on a 'pogo stick'. The runner propels himself from a low point in mid-stance to a peak during double float. During walking, efficiency is maintained by the interchange of potential and kinetic energy. During running, when potential and kinetic energies are in phase, efficiency is maintained in two ways: storage and release of potential energy in the elastic structure of tendons, and transfer of energy between limb segments via muscles which cross two joints (e.g. rectus femoris and hamstrings). The changes in muscle belly lengths are relatively slight during running. The muscles are acting as tensioners of the tendons, indeed, most of the change of length is produced by the stretch and recoil of the tendons. It has been estimated that, of the kinetic and potential energy which is lost and regained in each stance phase, 35% is stored temporarily as elastic strain energy in the Achilles tendon, and 17% in the ligaments of the arch of the foot. Together these springs approximately halve the work required from the muscles.

A tendon is capable of withstanding stresses (force per unit cross-sectional area) of at least 100 N/mm² (10 kg force/mm²). It stretches

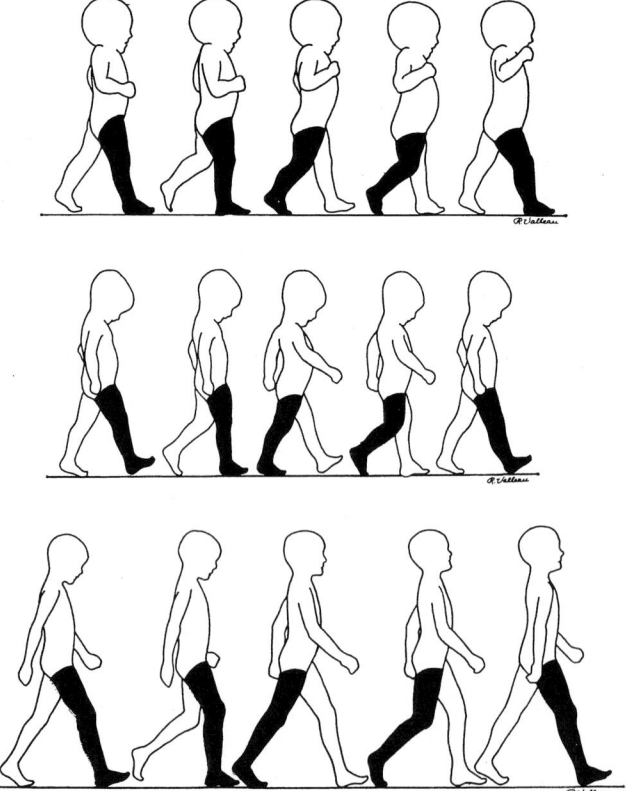

Fig. 115.39 Development of a mature gait. Top: 1-year-old. Note the flexed elbows and lack of arm swing. The foot is plantar flexed at contact. Middle: 3-year-old. Arm swing is now present as is heel strike. Bottom: 6-year-old. There is now an adult-type gait. (By permission from Benson MKD, Fixsen JA, MacNicol MF (eds) 2001 Development of a mature gait. In: Children's Orthopaedics and Fractures, 2nd edn. Edinburgh: Churchill Livingstone.)

elastically by c.8% before breaking, and its recoil returns 93% of the energy used to stretch it. This high energy return is important, not only because it reduces the work required from the muscles, but also because the lost mechanical energy becomes heat: leg tendons with poor energy return would overheat in running, and be damaged. The Achilles tendon is the most important 'spring' in the leg. Most runners strike the ground first with the heel, and the centre of pressure moves rapidly forward to the distal heads of the metatarsals, where it remains for most of the stance phase. A large force is then required in the Achilles tendon to balance the moments about the tibiotalar joint. For a 70-kg man running at middle-distance speed, the peak force in the tendon is c.5000 N (0.5 tonne force), which is enough to stretch it by c.6%. The parts of the tendon which run alongside the muscle bellies of gastrocnemius and soleus must be stretched, as well as the free distal part.

The mean vertical force on the ground during a complete stride cycle of any gait must equal body weight. If the foot is on the ground for only a small fraction of the stride, the forces must then be high. Peak vertical forces on one foot are c.1.0 times body weight in walking, 2.5 times in jogging, and 3.5 times in sprinting. Leg muscles have to exert much larger forces in running than in walking because the ground reaction forces are higher and also because, for a given ground force, flexion of the knee increases the moments about it. The main sources of power are the gastrocnemius–soleus complex at push-off; quadriceps after 'stance-phase reversal' (when the lower limb muscles change from a decelerating role to one of generating power, the generation phase); the hip extensors during late swing and early stance; and the hip abductors just after stance-phase reversal.

As in walking, the ground force acts more or less in line with the leg, so the body is decelerated and reaccelerated during each stance phase. The stance-phase starts with deceleration and absorption of energy. Power is generated after stance-phase reversal as the limb pushes up with the knee extending and foot plantarflexed, and this continues in the swing phase as the limb is accelerated forward. Once the limb is ahead of the trunk, the final phase of swing-phase absorption is initiated, during which the limb is decelerated.

The ground force acts upward on the metatarsal heads, and the Achilles tendon pulls upwards on the calcaneus. The necessary balancing reaction occurs at the ankle, where the tibia presses downwards on the talus. Together these three forces flatten the longitudinal arch of the foot, forcing the ankle 10 mm nearer to the ground than it would be if the foot were rigid. Mechanical tests on amputated feet have shown that the foot is a reasonably good spring, giving an energy return of c.78%. The plantar aponeurosis, long and short plantar ligaments and the plantar calcaneonavicular ligament are all involved in the spring action: they are predominantly collagenous, and presumably have elastic properties similar to those of tendon.

A runner's foot is still moving, typically at about 1.5 m/s, when the heel hits the ground. The impact is cushioned by the subcalcaneal foot pad, supplemented (when shoes are worn) by the compliance of the heel of the shoe. On contact the foot is supinated, which 'locks' the foot as a rigid structure, and is ideal for shock absorption. Immediately after heel strike the trunk progresses over the foot: passive pronation is initiated which makes the foot more flexible and therefore able to adapt to the running surface. As the foot approaches push-off, it becomes supinated again and as a consequence stiffens, which provides an excellent lever. These changes in foot posture cause rotational changes in the leg, and these in turn impact on the knee.

Eighty per cent of runners heel strike, and 20% have a mid-foot strike. In sprinting the forefoot makes contact first to provide the greatest leverage. The knees never fully extend during running: at first contact, the knee is c.25° flexed, increasing to a maximum during stance of c.45° at stance-phase reversal, and decreasing to 20° at toe-off. In running, the swing phase knee flexion increases to c.90° at the end of swing-phase generation (up to c.125° in sprinting), then decreases until contact with the ground again.

MOVEMENTS OF THE FOOT

With the foot on the ground, body weight causes some supination and flattening of the longitudinal arches; about one-third of the weight borne by the forefoot is taken by the head of the first metatarsal. When a resting position becomes active, as occurs on starting to walk, the foot is pronated by muscular effort, and the first metatarsal is depressed (the second less so), which accentuates the longitudinal arch to its maximum height (Hicks 1953). Similar changes can be imposed on a weightbearing foot by active lateral femoral rotation, which is transmitted through the tibia to the talus and entails passive supination of the foot. Medial femoral rotation has an opposite effect. When the foot is grounded and immobile, muscles which move it when it is freely suspended may exert effects on the leg, e.g. the dorsiflexors can then pull the leg forwards at the ankle joint.

The foot has two major functions: to support the body in standing and progression, and to lever it forwards and absorb shock in walking, running and jumping. To fulfil the first function, the pedal platform must be able to spread the stresses of standing and moving and be pliable enough to accommodate walking or running over uneven and sloping surfaces. To fulfil the second function, the foot must be transformable into a strong adjustable lever in order to resist inertia and powerful thrust: a segmented lever can best meet such stresses if it is arched.

In infants and young children, fatty, connective tissue on the plantar aspect may give the foot a flat appearance, indeed, soft tissues modify its appearance to varying degrees at all ages. However, the skeleton of the human foot is normally arched, and the sole of the foot is usually visibly concave. This curvature is customarily analysed into longitudinal and transverse arches. These arches vary individually in height, especially the longitudinal in its medial part. Since they are dynamic, their heights also differ in different phases of activity.

The medial longitudinal arch contains the calcaneus, talus, navicular, cuneiform and medial three metatarsal bones. Its summit, at the superior talar articular surface, takes the full thrust from the tibia and passes it backwards to the calcaneus, and forwards through the navicular and cuneiforms to the metatarsals. When the foot is grounded, these forces are transmitted through the three metatarsal heads and calcaneus (especially its tuberosity). The medial arch is higher, and more mobile and resilient than the lateral arch; its flattening progressively tightens the plantar calcaneonavicular ligament and plantar fascia. The lateral arch is adapted to transmit weight and thrust rather than to absorb such forces: the long plantar and plantar calcaneocuboid ligaments tighten as it flattens.

The lateral arch makes contact with the ground more extensively than the medial arch. As the foot flattens, an increasing fraction of load traverses soft tissues which are inferior to the entire arch. The whole lateral border usually touches the ground, whereas the medial border does not. However the medial border is visibly concave, usually even in standing, which explains the familiar outline of human footprints (though this varies with the position of the feet (**Fig. 115.40**), the development of associated soft tissues, and the nature of the surface). In any activity, as soon as the heel rises, the toes are extended and muscular structures (including the plantar aponeurosis) tighten up in the sole, accentuating the longitudinal arches. It has been suggested that tension diminishes in the deeper plantar ligaments in this phase.

The sole is transversely concave, both in skeletal form and usually in external appearance, and serial transverse arches are most developed inferior to the metatarsus and adjoining tarsus. Transmission of force occurs at the metatarsal heads, to some degree along the lateral border of the foot, and through subjacent soft tissues.

In standing, with only body weight to support, both the intrinsic and extrinsic muscles appear to relax. If the longitudinal arches are allowed to sink as a result of muscular relaxation, the plantar ligaments tie the bones into an arched form. The medial arch is more elevated when the feet are together than when they are apart, i.e. inversion with supination increases as the feet are separated. This medial sag can be countered by voluntary contraction of muscles such as tibialis anterior. Pronation and supination ensure that in standing, whatever the position of the feet, a maximal weight-bearing area is grounded, from the metatarsal heads along the lateral border of the foot to the calcaneus. The twist imparted by pronation (which is partly undone in supination) prompts the likening of the foot to a twisted but resilient plate (**Fig. 115.40**), where adequate ground contact was ensured whatever the angle between the foot and leg, and adaptable resilience was imparted in standing and progression.

PES PLANUS AND PES CAVUS

Pes planus is an excessively flat foot. There is no precise degree of flatness that defines pes planus, but it is either physiological or pathological. Physiological flat feet are flexible and rarely problematic, whereas pathological pes planus is often associated with stiffness and pain. The

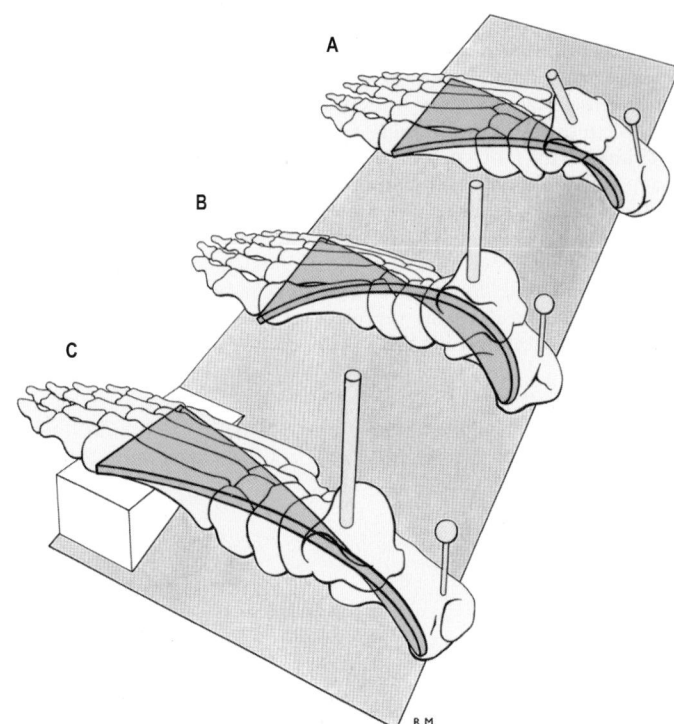

Fig. 115.40 The concept of the foot skeleton as a twisted plate which may be untwisted (supination) or further twisted (pronation) during the maintenance of a plantigrade stance in various positions of the foot. (Based upon MacConaill 1945, 1950.) **A**, The foot skeleton in supination, as in standing with the feet widely separated. Note the marked medial tilting of the talus and, to a lesser degree, of the calcaneus and the depression of the medial longitudinal arch. **B**, Relative pronation of the foot, as in standing with the feet close together. **C**, Supination of the foot when standing on an inclined surface; if the position of the wedge had been reversed, the foot skeleton would, of course, approach maximal pronation.

windlass (or Jack's great toe) test involves passively dorsiflexing the hallux at the metatarsophalangeal joint. This tightens the plantar aponeurosis and, in flexible pes planus, results in accentuation of the medial longitudinal arch. In pathological pes planus, no accentuation of the arch is seen. This test can also be carried out by asking the individual to stand on tiptoe and viewing the hindfoot from behind. In flexible flat feet, the calcaneus swings into a varus position; in pathological pes planus it does not. Causes include tarsal coalition, tibialis posterior tendon disruption, spring ligament rupture, tarsometatarsal arthritis (and subsequent collapse) and hindfoot (talocalcaneal or subtalar joint) degenerative or inflammatory arthritis.

Pes cavus is an excessively high-arched foot. The majority of cases arise as a result of a neurological disorder (e.g., Charcot–Marie–Tooth disease, diastematomyelia, poliomyelitis). Depending on the anatomical location of the deformity, the pes cavus is referred to as hindfoot, midfoot or forefoot cavus. When it involves all three parts of the foot it is called 'global' cavus.

In Charcot–Marie–Tooth disease, an overactive peroneus longus leads to hyperplantar flexion of the first metatarsal. To keep the forefoot in contact with the ground, the affected individual secondarily develops hindfoot varus to compensate. If ignored, the hindfoot varus, which is initially flexible, becomes fixed. The Coleman block test involves standing with the lateral part of the forefoot on a wooden block (Coleman and Chesnut 1977). This effectively balances the forefoot supination and the hindfoot deformity spontaneously corrects if the hindfoot varus is flexible. If the hindfoot is still flexible, surgery only need address the forefoot supination. If fixed, however, the hindfoot deformity also needs to be surgically corrected.

MUSCLES

The intrinsic muscles, i.e. those contained entirely within the foot, follow the primitive limb pattern of dorsal extensors and plantar flexors. The tendons of the extrinsic muscles, which have already been considered, are associated with them topographically and functionally. The intrinsic extensor musculature is limited and, as in the hand, some intrinsic flexor muscles are involved in extensor activities. The tendons of the extrinsic muscles cross the ankle, so moving and stabilising this joint, and those in the foot when they pass more distally. The muscles can be grouped according to their arrangement in the leg. The extensors arise in the anterior compartment of the leg and their tendons pass anterior to the ankle, being bound down by the extensor retinacula. The lateral group, i.e. the peronei, arise from the small lateral compartment of the leg attached to the fibula. Their tendons pass posterior to the lateral malleolus, bound down by the peroneal retinaculum. The posterior group are those comprising the muscles of the calf.

ANTERIOR GROUP

Tibialis anterior, extensor hallucis longus, extensor digitorum longus and peroneus tertius are described in Chapter 114 (pp. 1495–1497).

LATERAL GROUP

Peroneus longus and peroneus brevis are described in Chapter 114 (pp. 1498 and 1499).

POSTERIOR GROUP

Superficial group

Gastrocnemius and soleus are described in Chapter 114 (pp. 1499 and 1500).

Calcaneal tendon (tendocalcaneus, Achilles tendon)

Attachment – The calcaneal tendon (**Figs 112.3, 113.2**) is the thickest and strongest tendon in the human body. It is c.15 cm long, and begins near the middle of the calf, although its anterior surface receives muscle fibres from soleus almost to its lower end. It gradually becomes more rounded to c.4 cm above the calcaneus; below this it expands and becomes attached to the posterior surface of the calcaneus at its mid level. The fibres of the calcaneal tendon are not vertical; rather, they rotate to a variable degree in a spiral manner (Cummins et al 1946).

Vascular supply – The vascular supplies of gastrocnemius and soleus are described in Chapter 114 (pp. 1499 and 1500).

The blood supply to the calcaneal tendon comes distally from the calcaneus and proximally from intramuscular arterial branches. It is believed that there is an area of relatively poor vascularity in the mid-substance of the tendon, although some blood enters the tendon at this point from its anterior surface. During surgery, the paratenon is therefore best left intact in this region.

Innervation – The innervation of gastrocnemius and soleus are described in Chapter 114 (pp. 1499 and 1500).

Relations – The calcaneal tendon is subcutaneous. The sural nerve crosses its lateral border c.10 cm above its insertion. and here it is especially vulnerable to surgical injury. Distally, there are bursae superficial and deep to the tendon. The muscle belly of flexor hallucis longus lies deep to the deep fascia on the anterior surface of the tendon. The neurovascular bundle lies medial to the muscle.

Action – Plantar flexion of the ankle joint. The tendon fibres spiral laterally through 90° as they descend, so that the fibres associated with gastrocnemius come to insert on the bone more laterally, and those associated with soleus more medially.

Heel bursae – There are three locations about the heel where bursae occur. The most common is the retrocalcaneal bursa, which lies between the calcaneal tendon and the superior tuberosity of the calcaneus. An almost constant finding, it has an anterior bursal wall composed of fibrocartilage and a thin posterior wall continuous with the thin epitenon of the calcaneal tendon. Dorsiflexion of the ankle increases pressure within the bursa.

Less common are an adventitious bursa superficial to the calcaneal tendon, and a subcalcaneal bursa between the inferior surface of the calcaneus and the origin of the plantar aponeurosis.

Clinical anatomy – The calcaneal tendon is not the only plantar flexor of the ankle, which is one of the reasons ruptures of the calcaneal tendon can be overlooked. However, it is a frequent site of pathology because of its susceptibility to rupture, undergo degeneration (tendinosis) and become inflamed (paratendonitis). The area of relative avascularity in the mid-substance of the tendon is where the majority of problems occur.

A prominent superolateral calcaneal tuberosity may impinge on the deep aspect of the calcaneal tendon where it inserts onto the calcaneus; this is known as Haglund's disease. It is often associated with a retrocalcaneal bursa, and symptoms are exacerbated by dorsiflexion of the ankle, as this increases the pressure within the bursa and the impingement of calcaneus against the tendon insertion.

Plantaris

The plantaris is described in Chapter 114 (p. 1499).

Deep group

The deep flexors of the calf (**Figs 112.3, 113.28**) include popliteus, which acts on the knee joint. The others, flexor hallucis longus, flexor digitorum longus and tibialis posterior, act on the ankle joint and joints of the foot.

Deep transverse fascia

The deep transverse fascia of the leg is a fibrous stratum between the superficial and deep muscles of the calf, which extends transversely from the medial margin of the tibia to the posterior border of the fibula. Proximally, where it is thick and dense, it is attached to the soleal ridge of the tibia and to the fibula, inferomedial to the attachment of soleus. Between these bony attachments it is continuous with fascia covering popliteus and receives an expansion from the tendon of semimembranosus. At intermediate levels it is thin, but distally, where it covers the tendons behind the malleoli, it is again thick and continuous with the flexor and superior peroneal retinacula.

Flexor hallucis longus

Flexor hallucis longus is described in Chapter 114 (p. 1500).

Flexor digitorum longus

Flexor digitorum longus is described in Chapter 114 (p. 1500).

Tibialis posterior

Tibialis posterior is described in Chapter 114 (p. 1501).

SHORT EXTENSOR TENDONS

Extensor digitorum brevis and extensor hallucis brevis

Attachments – Extensor digitorum brevis (**Figs 114.8, 115.2**) is a thin muscle, arising from the anterior superolateral surface of the calcaneus, in front of the shallow lateral groove for peroneus brevis, from the interosseous talocalcaneal ligament, and from the stem of the inferior extensor retinaculum. It slants distally and medially across the dorsum of the foot, and ends in four tendons. The medial part of the muscle is usually a more or less distinct slip, ending in a tendon that crosses the dorsalis pedis artery superficially to insert into the dorsal aspect of the base of the proximal phalanx of the hallux; this slip is sometimes termed extensor hallucis brevis. The other three tendons attach to the lateral sides of the tendons of extensor digitorum longus for the second, third and fourth toes. The muscle is subject to much variation. There may be accessory slips from the talus and navicular, an extra tendon to the fifth digit, or a lack of one or more tendons. The muscle may be connected to the adjacent dorsal interosseous muscles.

Relations – The most medial tendon, that of extensor hallucis brevis, courses dorsomedially and passes superficial to the dorsalis pedis artery and the deep peroneal nerve. The remaining three tendons pass oblique and deep to the tendons of extensor digitorum longus.

Vascular supply – Extensor digitorum brevis is supplied by a perforating branch of the peroneal artery, the anterior lateral malleolar artery, lateral tarsal arteries, dorsalis pedis arteries, arcuate artery, the first, second and third dorsal metatarsal arteries, proximal and distal perforating arteries, and the dorsal digital arteries to the medial four toes (including the hallux).

Innervation – Extensor digitorum brevis is supplied by the lateral terminal branch of the deep peroneal nerve, L5, S1.

Actions – The muscle assists in extending the phalanges of the middle three toes via the tendons of extensor digitorum longus; in the hallux, it acts only on the proximal phalanx.

Clinical anatomy – Laceration of extensor digitorum brevis leads to little in the way of functional impairment, because the long extensors can compensate for their loss. The proximal part of the muscle can be used as interposition material to prevent bone fusion after resection of a calcaneonavicular bar (a common tarsal coalition). The muscle belly and tendon of extensor hallucis brevis serve as guides to the location of the dorsalis pedis artery and deep peroneal nerve. The distal tendon of extensor hallucis brevis can be used as a local graft.

MUSCLES OF THE SOLE OF THE FOOT

The plantar muscles in the foot can be divided into medial, lateral and intermediate groups. The medial and lateral groups consist of the intrinsic muscles of the hallux and minimus, and the central or inter-mediate group includes the lumbricals, interossei and short digital flexors. It is customary to group them in four layers, as this is the order in which they are encountered during dissection. However, these 'layers' can be overemphasised, and in functional terms the former grouping will often be found more useful.

Plantar muscles of the foot: first layer

This superficial layer (**Fig. 115.41**) includes abductor hallucis, abductor digiti minimi and flexor digitorum brevis. All three extend from the calcaneal tuberosity to the toes, and make up a functional group that assists in maintaining the concavity of the foot.

Abductor hallucis

Attachments – Abductor hallucis arises principally from the flexor retinaculum, but also from the medial process of the calcaneal tuberosity, the plantar aponeurosis, and the intermuscular septum between this muscle and flexor digitorum brevis. The muscle fibres end in a tendon that is attached, together with the medial tendon of flexor hallucis brevis, to the medial side of the base of the proximal phalanx of the hallux. Some fibres are attached more proximally to the medial sesamoid bone of this toe. The muscle may also derive some fibres from the dermis along the medial border of the foot.

Relations – Abductor hallucis (**Fig. 115.41**) lies along the medial border of the foot and covers the origins of the plantar vessels and nerves.

Vascular supply – Abductor hallucis is supplied by the medial malleolar network and its tributaries, medial calcaneal branches of the lateral plantar artery (**Fig. 115.16**), the medial plantar artery (directly and via superficial and deep branches), the first plantar metatarsal artery and perforators and the end of plantar arch.

Innervation – Abductor hallucis is innervated by the medial plantar nerve, S1 and S2. Contraction of the muscle confirms an intact medial plantar nerve when the integrity of this nerve is in question.

Action – Abductor hallucis produces abduction of the hallux, which is a redundant action in the shod population, and is tested by applying a lateral force to the medial aspect of the proximal phalanx and asking the patient to resist.

Clinical anatomy – The deep fascia has been implicated in chronic heel pain, because it can cause entrapment of the first branch of the lateral plantar nerve that lies immediately deep to it. The abductor hallucis fascia is strong and can be used in soft tissue augmentation after hallux valgus correction. Rarely, the muscle can be tight, leading to varus deformity of the foot and a requirement for it to be released. An abductor hallucis flap is sometimes used in soft tissue coverage procedures.

Flexor digitorum brevis

Attachments – Flexor digitorum brevis arises by a narrow tendon from the medial process of the calcaneal tuberosity, from the central part of

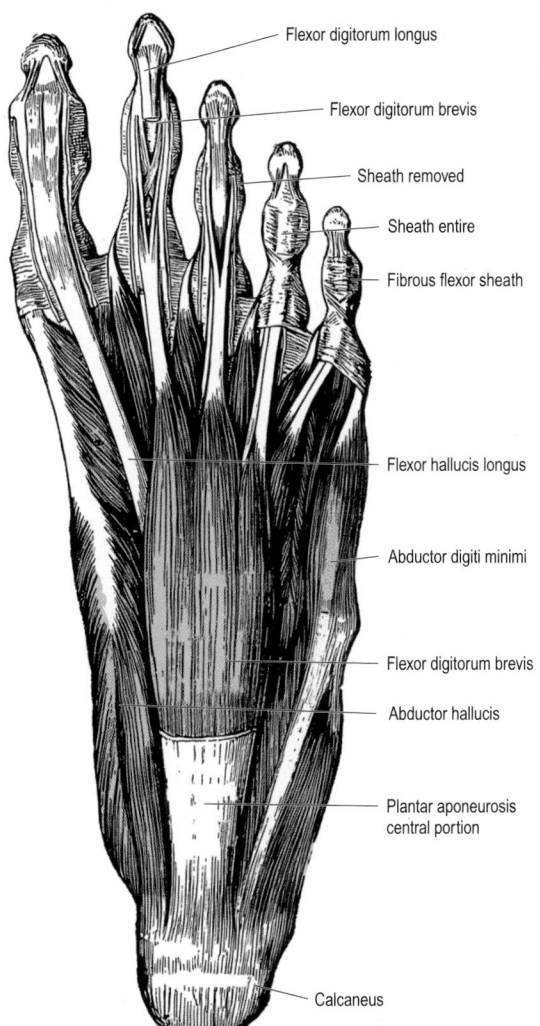

Flexor digitorum longus

Flexor digitorum brevis

Sheath removed

Sheath entire

Fibrous flexor sheath

Flexor hallucis longus

Abductor digiti minimi

Flexor digitorum brevis

Abductor hallucis

Plantar aponeurosis central portion

Calcaneus

Fig. 115.41 The superficial plantar muscles of the left foot.

the plantar aponeurosis, and from the intermuscular septa between it and adjacent muscles. It divides into four tendons, which pass to the lateral four toes; they enter digital tendon sheaths accompanied by the tendons of flexor digitorum longus, which lie deep to them. At the bases of the proximal phalanges, each tendon divides around the corre-sponding tendon of flexor digitorum longus; the two slips then reunite and partially decussate, forming a tunnel through which the tendon of flexor digitorum longus passes to the distal phalanx. The short flexor tendon divides again and attaches to both sides of the shaft of the middle phalanx. The way in which the tendons of flexor digitorum brevis divide and attach to the phalanges is identical to that of the tendons of flexor digitorum superficialis in the hand. The slip to a given toe may be joined by a second, supernumerary slip, be absent, or be replaced by a small muscular slip from the long flexor tendon or from flexor accessorius.

Relations – Flexor digitorum brevis lies immediately deep to the central part of the plantar aponeurosis (**Fig. 115.41**). Its deep surface is separated from the lateral plantar vessels and nerves by a thin layer of fascia.

Vascular supply – Flexor digitorum brevis is supplied by the lateral and medial plantar arteries, the plantar metatarsal arteries and the plantar digital arteries to the lateral four toes.

Nerve supply – Flexor digitorum brevis is innervated by the medial plantar nerve, S1 and S2.

Actions – Flexor digitorum brevis flexes the lesser toes at the proximal interphalangeal joint, with equal effect in any position of the ankle joint.

Clinical anatomy/testing – To test the action of flexor digitorum brevis, the examiner passively extends the distal interphalangeal joint and asks the individual to flex the toes at the proximal interphalangeal joint. Contracture of the flexor tendon can lead to toe deformities, and release or lengthening procedures may be required. The muscle belly is sometimes required for coverage of a soft tissue defect.

Abductor digiti minimi

Attachments – Abductor digiti minimi arises from both processes of the calcaneal tuberosity, from the plantar surface of the bone between them, from the plantar aponeurosis and from the intermuscular septum between the muscle and flexor digitorum brevis. Its tendon glides in a smooth groove on the plantar surface of the base of the fifth metatarsal and is attached, with flexor digiti minimi brevis, to the lateral side of the base of the proximal phalanx of the fifth toe; hence it is more a flexor than an abductor. Some of the fibres arising from the lateral calcaneal process usually reach the tip of the tuberosity of the fifth metatarsal (**Fig. 115.28**) and may form a separate muscle, abductor ossis metatarsi digiti quinti. An accessory slip from the base of the fifth metatarsal is not infrequent.

Relations – Abductor digiti minimi lies along the lateral border of the foot, and its medial margin is related to the lateral plantar vessels and nerve (**Fig. 115.41**).

Vascular supply – Abductor digiti minimi is supplied by the medial and lateral plantar arteries (**Fig. 115.42A**), the plantar digital artery to the lateral side of minimus from the beginning of the plantar arch, the fourth plantar metatarsal artery and end twigs of the arcuate and lateral tarsal arteries (**Fig. 115.16**).

Innervation – Abductor digiti minimi is innervated by the lateral plantar nerve, S1, S2 and S3.

Action – Despite its name, abductor digiti minimi is more a flexor of the little toe metatarsophalangeal joint than an abductor.

Clinical anatomy – Apart from having a role in soft tissue coverage, abductor digiti minimi has little clinical significance.

Plantar muscles of the foot: second layer
Beneath the first muscle layer is a second group of intrinsic muscles, which consists of flexor digitorum accessorius and four lumbrical muscles. The preterminal tendons of flexor hallucis longus and flexor digitorum longus are intimately associated with them.

Flexor hallucis longus

Attachments – Flexor hallucis longus inserts into the base of the hallucal proximal phalanx.

Relations – The flexor hallucis longus tendon passes forward in the second layer like a bowstring. Posteriorly, it lies in a groove beneath the sustentaculum tali. Further forward, it is crossed by the tendon of flexor digitorum longus (knot of Henry). At this point it gives off two strong slips to the medial two divisions of the flexor digitorum tendons. It then passes between the two sesamoids of the first metatarsophalangeal joint, to insert into the base of the proximal phalanx of the hallux. Throughout its length, it is invested in a synovial sheath.

Vascular supply, innervation and action – The vascular supply, innervation and action of flexor hallucis longus are described in Chapter 114 (p. 1500).

Clinical anatomy – Flexor hallucis longus is the plantar flexor of the hallux and is tested by flexion of the interphalangeal joint against resistance. It is involved in posterior ankle impingement syndromes, is prone to tenosynovitis and is occasionally used in tendon transfer

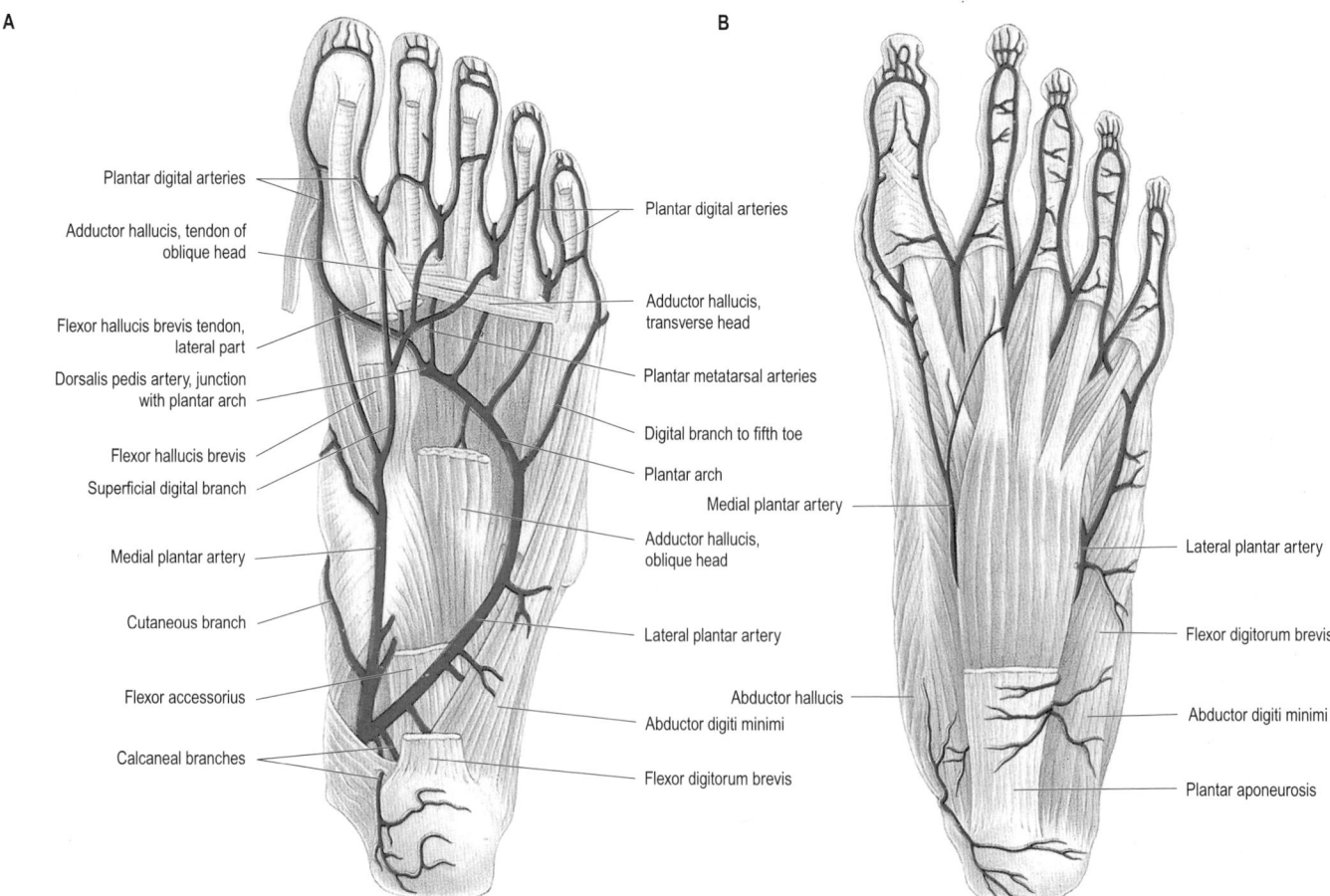

A

Plantar digital arteries
Adductor hallucis, tendon of oblique head
Flexor hallucis brevis tendon, lateral part
Dorsalis pedis artery, junction with plantar arch
Flexor hallucis brevis
Superficial digital branch
Medial plantar artery
Cutaneous branch
Flexor accessorius
Calcaneal branches

Plantar digital arteries
Adductor hallucis, transverse head
Plantar metatarsal arteries
Digital branch to fifth toe
Plantar arch
Medial plantar artery
Adductor hallucis, oblique head
Lateral plantar artery
Abductor hallucis
Abductor digiti minimi
Flexor digitorum brevis

B

Medial plantar artery
Lateral plantar artery
Flexor digitorum brevis
Abductor digiti minimi
Plantar aponeurosis

Fig. 115.42 A, Superficial dissection of the plantar arteries of the left foot. **B**, Deep dissection of the plantar arteries of the left foot.

procedures, e.g. in delayed reconstruction of a rupture of the calcaneal tendon with a large defect between the tendon ends.

Flexor digitorum longus

Attachments – The attachments of flexor digitorum longus are described in Chapter 114 (p. 1500).

Relations – The tendon of flexor digitorum longus enters the sole of the foot on the medial side of the flexor hallucis longus tendon. It receives the insertion of flexor accessorius and passes forward as four separate tendons, deep to the tendons of flexor digitorum brevis. After giving off the lumbricals, it passes through the fibrous sheaths of the lateral four toes.

Vascular supply, innervation and action – The vascular supply, innervation and action of flexor digitorum longus are described in Chapter 114 (p. 1500).

Clinical anatomy – Flexor digitorum longus is rarely affected by pathology, but is implicated in lesser toe deformities such as hammer, claw and mallet toes. It is used in tendon transfer for the surgical treatment of tibialis posterior tendon dysfunction.

Flexor tendon sheaths

The terminations of the tendons of the long and short flexor muscles are contained in osseo-aponeurotic canals similar to those which occur in the fingers. These canals are bounded above by the phalanges, and below by fibrous bands, the digital fibrous sheaths, which arch across the tendons and attach on each side to the margins of the phalanges (**Fig. 115.41**). Along the proximal and intermediate phalanges, the fibrous bands are strong, and the fibres are transverse (annular part); opposite the joints they are much thinner and the fibres decussate (cruciform part). Each osseo-aponeurotic canal has a synovial lining, which is reflected around its tendon; within this sheath, vincula tendinum are arranged as in the fingers.

Flexor digitorum accessorius

Attachments – Flexor digitorum accessorius (**Fig. 115.43**), also known as quadratus plantae, arises by two heads separated by the long plantar ligament. The medial head is larger and more fleshy. It is attached to the medial concave surface of the calcaneus, below the groove for the tendon of flexor hallucis longus. The lateral head is flat and tendinous and is attached to the calcaneus distal to the lateral process of the tuberosity, and to the long plantar ligament. The muscle belly inserts into the tendon of flexor digitorum longus at the point where it is bound by a fibrous slip to the tendon of flexor hallucis longus and where it divides into its four tendons.

The muscle is sometimes absent altogether. It may vary in the number of digits that it supplies: the slip to the fourth is often absent, and a slip to the fifth is sometimes present.

Relations – The medial plantar nerve passes medial to and the lateral plantar nerve passes superficial to flexor accessorius.

Vascular supply – Flexor digitorum accessorius is supplied by the stem of the medial plantar artery (to the medial 'head'), the lateral plantar artery and the plantar arch.

Innervation – Flexor digitorum accessorius is innervated by the lateral plantar nerve, S1, S2 and S3.

Action – By pulling on the tendons of flexor digitorum longus, flexor digitorum accessorius provides a means of flexing the lateral four toes in any position of the ankle joint.

Lumbrical muscles

Attachments – The lumbrical muscles (**Fig. 115.43**) are four small muscles (numbered from the medial side of the foot) which are accessory to the tendons of flexor digitorum longus. They arise from these tendons as far back as their angles of separation, each springing from the sides of two adjacent tendons, except for the first, which arises only from the medial border of the first tendon. The muscles end in tendons that pass

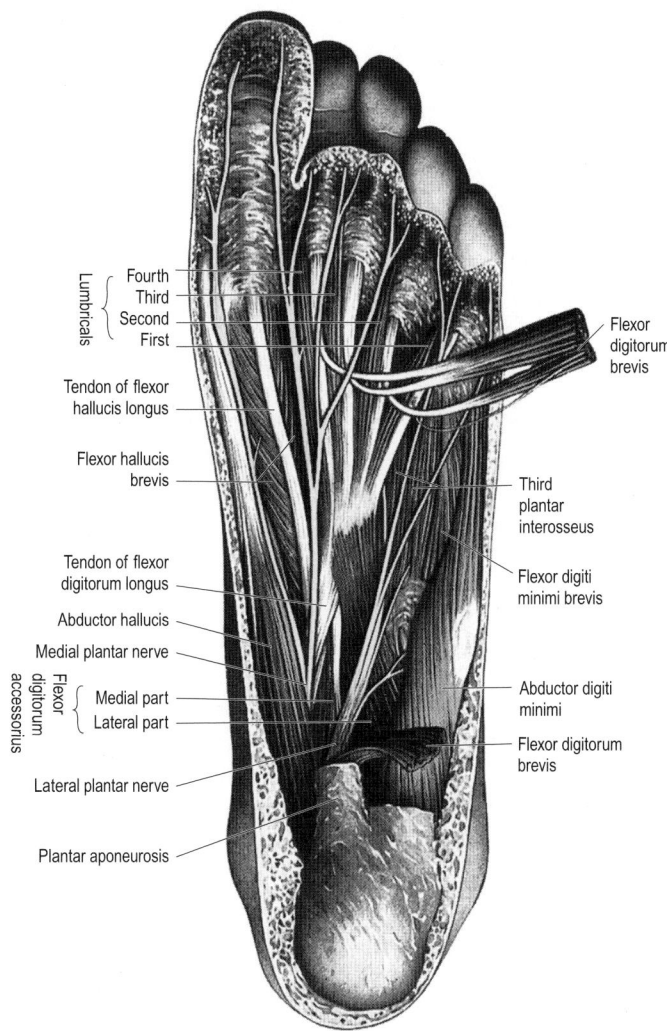

Fig. 115.43 The plantar muscles of the left foot: first and second layers.

distally on the medial sides of the four lesser toes, to be attached to the dorsal digital expansions on their proximal phalanges.

Relations – The lumbricals are intimately related to the flexor digitorum longus tendons before they pass on the plantar surfaces of the deep transverse metatarsal ligaments.

Vascular supply – The lumbricals are supplied by the lateral plantar artery and plantar arch, and by four plantar metatarsal arteries (four distal perforating joined by three proximal perforating arteries). Their tendons are supplied by twigs from the dorsal digital arteries (and their dorsal metatarsal origins) to the lateral four toes.

Innervation – The first lumbrical is supplied by the medial plantar nerve, and the rest are supplied by the deep branch of the lateral plantar nerve, S2 and S3.

Action – The lumbricals maintain extension of the interphalangeal joints of the toes.

Clinical anatomy – In injuries of the tibial nerve, and in conditions such as the hereditary motor–sensory neuropathies (e.g. Charcot–Marie–Tooth disease), lumbrical dysfunction contributes to clawing of the toes.

Plantar muscles of the foot: third layer

The third layer of the foot contains the shorter intrinsic muscles of the hallux and minimus, i.e. flexor hallucis brevis, adductor hallucis and flexor digiti minimi brevis (**Figs 115.44, 115.45**). These are the most deeply situated muscles in the sole, other than the interossei, which are superior to them.

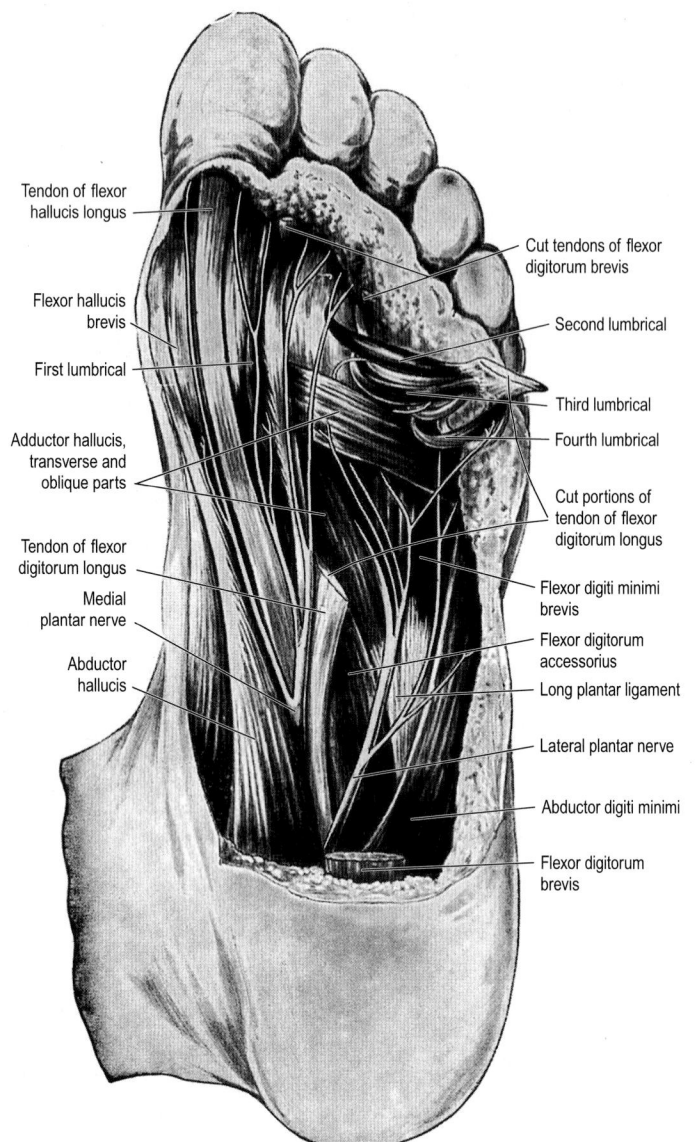

Fig. 115.44 The plantar muscles of the left foot and their nerve supply. Most of flexor digitorum brevis has been removed. The tendon of flexor digitorum longus has been divided, and its distal end has been turned forwards, together with the second, third and fourth lumbricals.

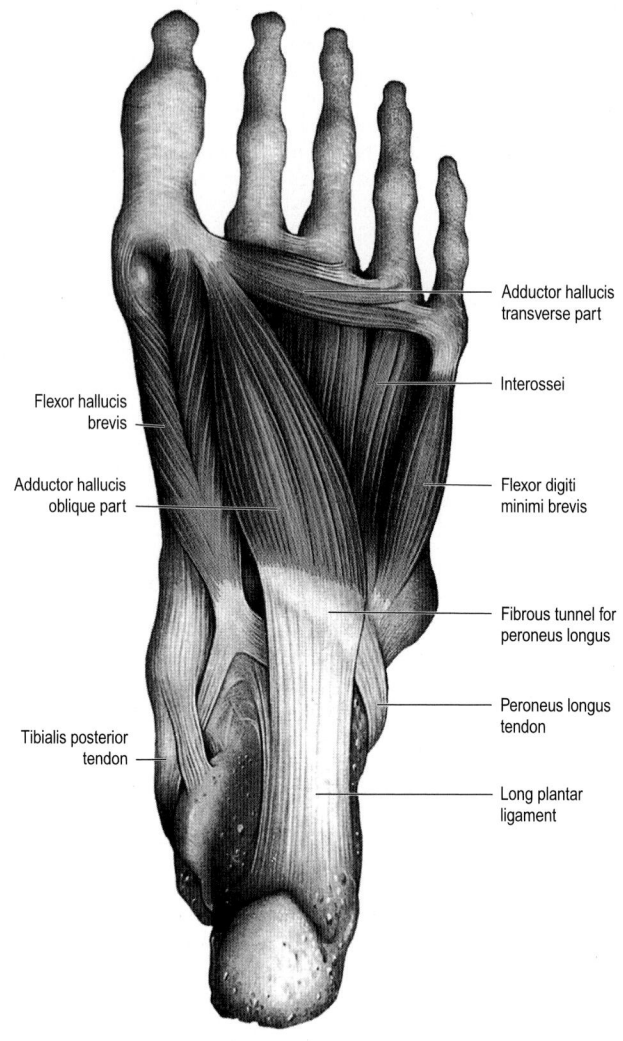

Fig. 115.45 The plantar muscles of the left foot: third layer.

Flexor hallucis brevis

Attachments – Flexor hallucis brevis (**Figs 115.43, 115.45**) has a bifurcate tendon of origin. The lateral limb arises from the medial part of the plantar surface of the cuboid, posterior to the groove for the peroneus longus tendon, and from the adjacent part of the lateral cuneiform. The medial limb has a deep attachment directly continuous with the lateral division of the tendon of tibialis posterior, and a more superficial attachment to the middle band of the medial intermuscular septum. The belly of the muscle divides into medial and lateral parts, the twin tendons of which are attached to the sides of the base of the proximal phalanx of the hallux. A sesamoid bone usually occurs in each tendon near its attachment. The medial part blends with abductor hallucis, and the lateral with adductor hallucis, as they reach their terminations.

Accessory slips may arise proximally from the calcaneus or long plantar ligament. A tendinous slip may extend to the proximal phalanx of the second toe.

Relations – Flexor hallucis brevis lies on the underside of the first metatarsal shaft. Abductor hallucis lies medially. The medial digital nerve to the hallux and the tendon of flexor hallucis longus pass to the

hallux on its plantar surface. On its lateral side, lying more superficially, is the medial plantar nerve.

Vascular supply – Flexor hallucis brevis is supplied by branches of the medial plantar artery, the first plantar metatarsal artery, the lateral plantar artery and the plantar arch.

Innervation – Flexor hallucis brevis is supplied by the medial plantar nerve, S1 and S2.

Action – Flexor hallucis brevis flexes the proximal phalanx of the hallux.

Clinical anatomy/testing – Clinical problems with flexor hallucis brevis relate to sesamoid problems. Excision of both sesamoids leads to disruption of both tendons and a subsequent extension deformity at the first metatarsophalangeal joint, and therefore should not be performed. Testing the tendon is done by asking the individual to flex the first metatarsophalangeal joint with the interphalangeal joint extended, thereby eliminating the action of flexor hallucis longus.

Adductor hallucis

Attachments – Adductor hallucis (**Figs 115.43, 115.45**) arises by oblique and transverse heads. The oblique head springs from the bases of the second, third and fourth metatarsal bones, and from the fibrous sheath of the tendon of peroneus longus. The transverse head, a narrow, flat fasciculus, arises from the plantar metatarsophalangeal ligaments of the third, fourth and fifth toes (sometimes only from the third and fourth), and from the deep transverse metatarsal ligaments between them. The oblique head has medial and lateral parts. The medial part blends with the lateral part of flexor hallucis brevis and is attached to the lateral sesamoid bone of the hallux. The lateral part joins the transverse head and is also attached to the lateral sesamoid bone and directly to the base of the first phalanx of the hallux. There is no phalangeal attachment for the transverse part of the muscle; fibres that fail to reach the lateral sesamoid bone are attached with the oblique part.

In the study by Cralley et al (1975), the transverse part of adductor hallucis was absent in 6% of feet examined. Part of the muscle may be attached to the first metatarsal, constituting an opponens hallucis. A slip may also extend to the proximal phalanx of the second toe.

Relations – Flexor hallucis brevis is proximal and medial. Adductor hallucis lies plantar to the metatarsal shafts and interossei. The long and short toe flexors, and the medial and lateral plantar arteries and nerves, lie superficial to it.

Vascular supply – Adductor hallucis is supplied by branches of the medial plantar artery, the lateral plantar artery, the plantar arch and the first to fourth plantar metatarsal arteries.

Innervation – Adductor hallucis is innervated by the deep branch of the lateral plantar nerve, S2 and S3.

Action – Adductor hallucis partly flexes the proximal phalanx of the hallux, but also stabilises the metatarsal heads.

Clinical anatomy – Adductor hallucis is one of the deforming forces in hallux valgus and needs to be released during a distal soft tissue release when there is a fixed deformity.

Flexor digiti minimi brevis

Attachments – Flexor digiti minimi brevis (**Figs 115.43, 115.45**) arises from the medial part of the plantar surface of the base of the fifth metatarsal bone, and from the sheath of peroneus longus. It has a distal tendon that inserts into the lateral side of the base of the proximal phalanx of the minimus; this tendon usually blends laterally with that of abductor digiti minimi. Occasionally, some of its deeper fibres extend to the lateral part of the distal half of the fifth metatarsal bone, constituting what may be described as a distinct muscle, opponens digiti minimi.

Relations – The fifth metatarsal shaft lies on the deep surface of flexor digiti minimi brevis, the interossei lie medially and the abductor digiti minimi is lateral. The most lateral branch of the lateral plantar nerve lies superficially and just medial to flexor digiti minimi brevis.

Vascular supply – Flexor digiti minimi brevis is supplied by end twigs of the arcuate and lateral tarsal arteries, and the lateral plantar artery and its digital (plantar) branch to the lateral side of minimus.

Innervation – Flexor digiti minimi brevis is innervated by the superficial branch of the lateral plantar nerve, S2 and S3.

Action – Flexor digiti minimi brevis flexes the metatarsophalangeal joint of the little toe.

Plantar muscles of the foot: fourth layer
The fourth muscle layer of the foot consists of the plantar and dorsal interossei. They resemble their counterparts in the hand, but they are arranged relative to an axis through the second and not the third digit, as occurs in the hand, as the second is the least mobile of the metatarsal bones. The tendons of tibialis posterior and peroneus longus are also considered part of the fourth layer.

Dorsal interossei

Attachments – The dorsal interossei (**Fig. 115.46A**) are situated between the metatarsal bones. They consist of four bipennate muscles, each arising by two heads from the sides of the adjacent metatarsal bones. Their tendons are attached to the bases of the proximal phalanges and to the dorsal digital expansions. The first inserts into the medial side of the second toe; the other three pass to the lateral sides of the second, third and fourth toes.

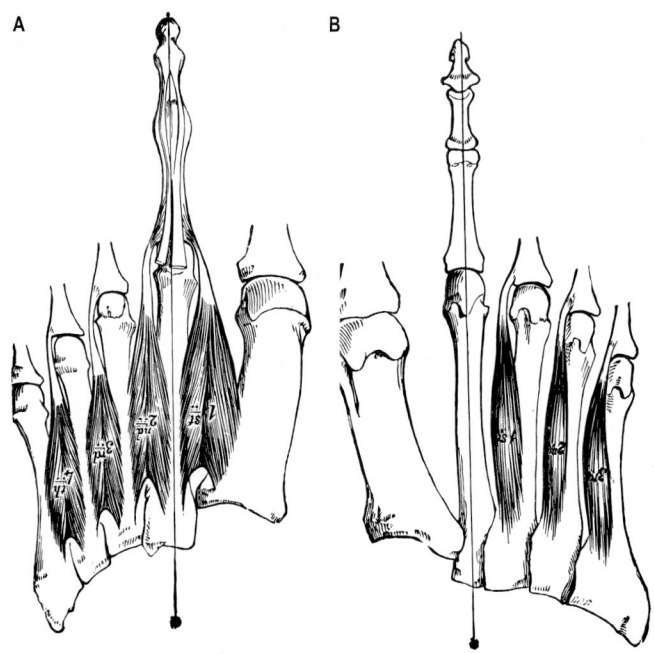

Fig. 115.46 The interossei of the left foot. **A**, Dorsal interossei viewed from the dorsal aspect. **B**, Plantar interossei viewed from the plantar aspect. The axis to which the movements of abduction and adduction are referred is indicated.

Relations – Between the heads of each of the three lateral muscles, there is an angular space through which a perforating artery passes to the dorsum of the foot. Between the heads of the first muscle, the same space transmits the terminal part of the dorsalis pedis artery to the sole.

Vascular supply – Dorsal interossei are supplied by the arcuate artery, lateral and medial tarsal arteries, the first to fourth plantar arteries and the first to fourth dorsal metatarsal arteries (receiving proximal and distal perforating arteries), and by the dorsal digital arteries of the lateral four toes.

Innervation – Dorsal interossei are supplied by the deep branch of the lateral plantar nerve (S2 and S3), except those in the fourth interosseous space, which are supplied by the superficial branch of the lateral plantar nerve. The first dorsal interosseus frequently receives an extra filament from the medial branch of the deep peroneal nerve on the dorsum of the foot, and the second receives a twig from the lateral branch of the deep peroneal nerve.

Action – Dorsal interossei abduct the toes about a longitudinal axis through the second metatarsal. They also flex the metatarsophalangeal joints and extend the interphalangeal joints of the lesser toes. The hallux and little toe have their own abductors.

Clinical anatomy – Denervation of the interossei leads to claw-toe deformities. Development of claw toes should raise the possibility of a neuropathic process (e.g. Charcot–Marie–Tooth disease, diastematomyelia).

Plantar interossei
There are three plantar interossei (**Fig. 115.46B**). They lie below, rather than between, the metatarsal bones, and each is connected to one metatarsal bone only. They arise from the bases and medial sides of the third, fourth and fifth metatarsal bones, and insert into the medial sides of the bases of the proximal phalanges of the same toes, and into their dorsal digital expansions.

Relations – The plantar interossei lie plantar to the dorsal interossei and deep to the muscles of the third layer.

Vascular supply – Plantar interossei are supplied by the lateral plantar artery, the plantar arch, the second to fourth plantar metatarsal arteries and the dorsal digital arteries of the lateral three toes.

Innervation – Plantar interossei are supplied by the deep branch of the lateral plantar nerve (S2 and S3), except those in the fourth interosseous space, which are supplied by the superficial branch of the lateral plantar nerve.

Action – Plantar interossei adduct the third fourth and fifth toes, flex the metatarsophalangeal joints and extend the interphalangeal joints.

Clinical anatomy – The clinical anatomy of the plantar interossei is the same as that of the dorsal interossei.

Tibialis posterior

Tibialis posterior muscles are described in Chapter 114 (p. 1501).

Clinical anatomy – Tibialis posterior is tested by asking an individual to perform a single heel rise and by maximally plantar flexing and inverting the foot against resistance. Tibialis posterior is a powerful muscle which has an excursion of only 1–2 cm. It initiates a heel rise and is responsible for the hindfoot varus that occurs during a single heel rise. It is also very important in the maintenance of the medial longitudinal arch. In overweight individuals with pes planus, unaccustomed activity can lead to inflammation and degeneration of the tendon from the medial malleolar level to its insertion. This leads to elongation of the tendon, attenuation of the spring ligament and progressive collapse of the medial longitudinal arch. As the excursion is so short, the muscle cannot compensate for the tendon lengthening, which results in tibialis posterior tendon dysfunction.

Peroneus longus

Peroneus longus muscles are described in Chapter 114 (p. 1498).

Clinical anatomy – Peroneus longus is tested by asking the individual to evert the foot against resistance. Peroneus longus lies below the peroneal tubercle, and peroneus brevis lies above. Active plantar flexion of the first metatarsal indicates a functioning peroneus longus.

VASCULAR SUPPLY AND LYMPHATIC DRAINAGE

DORSALIS PEDIS ARTERY

The dorsalis pedis artery is the dorsal artery of the foot (**Figs 115.45, 115.47**), and is the continuation of the anterior tibial artery distal to the ankle. It passes to the proximal end of the first intermetatarsal space, where it turns into the sole between the heads of the first dorsal interosseous to complete the plantar arch, and provides the first plantar metatarsal artery.

The artery may be larger, to compensate for a small lateral plantar artery, or replaced by a large perforating branch of the peroneal. It often diverges laterally from its usual route.

Relations – The dorsalis pedis artery successively crosses the talocrural articular capsule, talus, navicular and intermediate cuneiform and their ligaments; superficial to it are the skin, fasciae, inferior extensor retinaculum and, near its termination, extensor hallucis brevis. Medial is the tendon of extensor hallucis longus and lateral are the medial tendon of extensor digitorum longus and medial terminal branch of the deep peroneal nerve. The tendons provide useful landmarks to safe surgical approaches.

Surface anatomy – The pulsation of the dorsal artery of the foot is palpable from the midpoint between the malleoli to the proximal end of the first intermetatarsal space.

Branches

The dorsalis pedis artery gives off the tarsal, arcuate and first dorsal metatarsal arteries.

Tarsal arteries

There are two tarsal arteries, lateral and medial (**Fig. 115.47**). They arise as the dorsalis pedis artery crosses the navicular. The lateral runs laterally under extensor digitorum brevis; it supplies this and the tarsal articulations, and anastomoses with branches of the arcuate, anterior

lateral malleolar and lateral plantar arteries, and the perforating branch of the peroneal artery. Two or three medial tarsal arteries ramify on the medial border of the foot and join the medial malleolar network.

Arcuate artery

The arcuate artery (**Fig. 115.47**) arises near the medial cuneiform, passes laterally over the metatarsal bases, deep to the tendons of the digital extensors, and anastomoses with the lateral tarsal and plantar arteries. It supplies the second to fourth dorsal metatarsal arteries, running distally superficial to the corresponding dorsal interossei, and divides into two dorsal digital branches for the adjoining toes in the interdigital clefts. Proximally, in the interosseous spaces these branches receive proximal perforating branches from the plantar arch. Distally, they are joined by distal perforating branches from the plantar metatarsal arteries. The fourth dorsal metatarsal artery sends a branch to the lateral side of the fifth toe.

First dorsal metatarsal artery

The first dorsal metatarsal artery (**Fig. 115.47**) arises just before the dorsalis pedis artery enters the sole. It runs distally on the first dorsal interosseous and divides at the cleft between the first and second toes. One branch passes under the tendon of extensor hallucis longus and supplies the medial side of the hallux; the other bifurcates to supply the adjoining sides of the hallux and the second toe.

Cutaneous vessels from the dorsalis pedis artery

The dorsalis pedis artery and its first dorsal metatarsal branch give rise to small direct cutaneous branches supplying the dorsal foot skin between the extensor retinaculum and the first web space. This vessel provides the basis of the anatomical rationale for surgically raising a flap of skin over the dorsum of the foot, which can then be used to resurface other areas of the body.

PLANTAR ARCH

The plantar arch (**Fig. 115.42B**) is deeply situated, extending from the fifth metatarsal base to the proximal end of the first interosseous space. Convex distally, it is plantar to the bases of the second to fourth metatarsal bones and corresponding interossei, but dorsal to the oblique part of adductor hallucis.

Branches

The plantar arch gives off three perforating and four plantar metatarsal branches, and numerous branches that supply the skin, fasciae and muscles in the sole. Three perforating branches ascend through the proximal ends of the second to fourth intermetatarsal spaces, between the heads of dorsal interossei, and anastomose with the dorsal metatarsal arteries. Four plantar metatarsal arteries extend distally between the metatarsal bones in contact with the interossei (**Fig. 115.42B**). Each divides into two plantar digital arteries, supplying the adjacent digital aspects. Near its division, each plantar metatarsal sends a distal perforating branch dorsally to join a dorsal metatarsal artery. The first plantar metatarsal artery springs from the junction between the lateral plantar and dorsalis pedis arteries, and sends a digital branch to the medial side of the hallux. The lateral digital branch for the fifth toe arises directly from the lateral plantar artery near the fifth metatarsal base.

Surface anatomy – The lateral plantar artery begins between the heel and medial malleolus, and crosses obliquely to a point 2.5 cm medial to the tuberosity of the fifth metatarsal. With a slight distal convexity, it reaches the proximal end of the first intermetatarsal space.

Clinical anatomy – Haemorrhage from the plantar arch is difficult to stem, because of the depth of the vessel and its important close relations. It must be treated like the palmar arches.

POSTERIOR TIBIAL ARTERY

Before the posterior tibial artery divides into its two main terminal branches, it gives off a communicating branch that runs posteriorly across the tibia c.5 cm above its distal end, deep to flexor hallucis longus, and joins a communicating branch of the peroneal and calcaneal branches, which arise just proximal to the terminal division. They pierce the flexor retinaculum to supply the skin and fat behind the calcaneal tendon. The posterior tibial artery also gives off the artery of

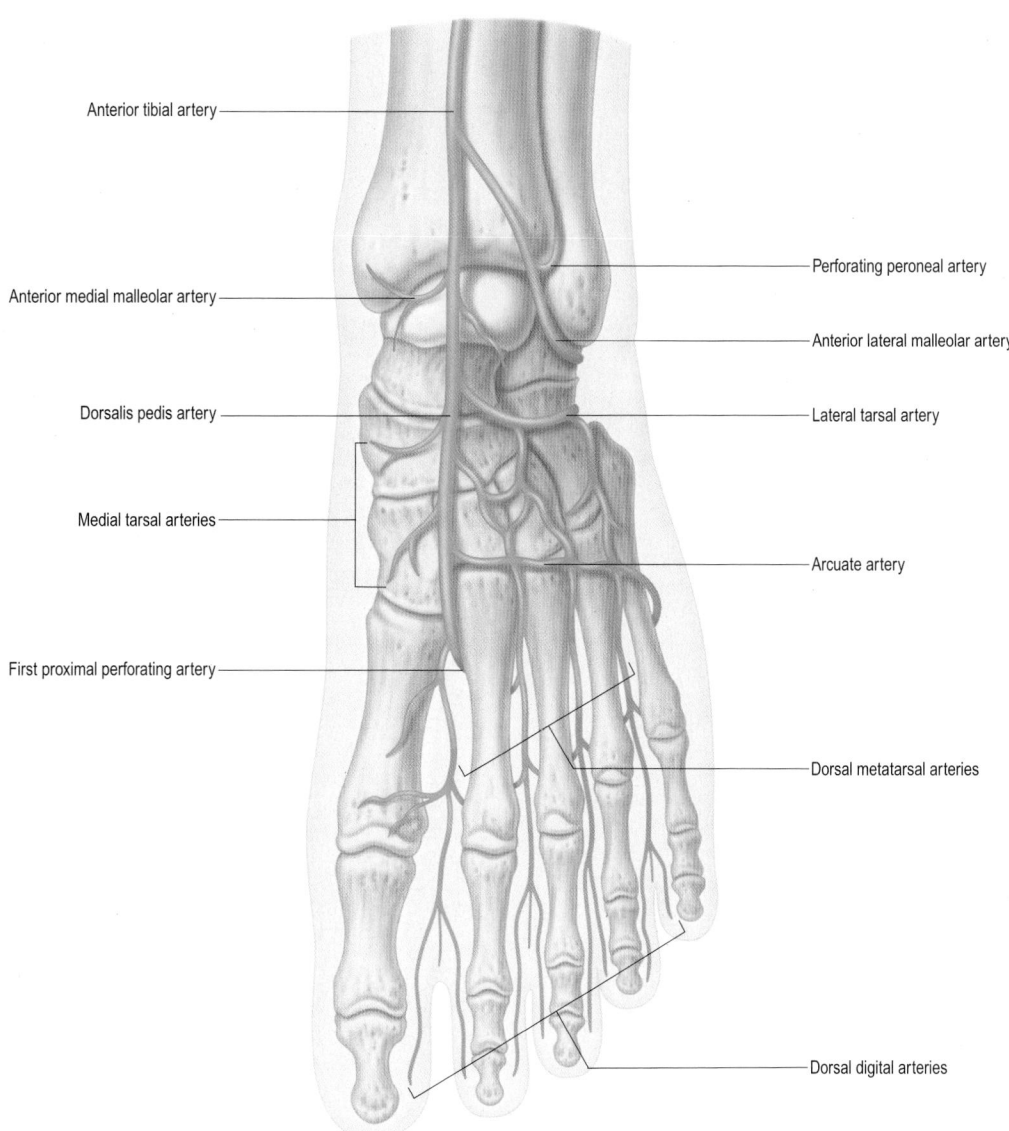

Anterior tibial artery

Anterior medial malleolar artery

Dorsalis pedis artery

Medial tarsal arteries

First proximal perforating artery

Perforating peroneal artery

Anterior lateral malleolar artery

Lateral tarsal artery

Arcuate artery

Dorsal metatarsal arteries

Dorsal digital arteries

Fig. 115.47 Dorsal arteries of the foot.

the tarsal canal. The terminal branches of the posterior tibial artery are the medial and lateral plantar arteries.

Branches

Medial plantar artery

The medial plantar artery (**Fig. 115.42**) is the smaller terminal branch of the posterior tibial. It arises midway between the medial malleolus and the medial calcaneal tubercle and passes distally along the medial side of the foot, with the medial plantar nerve lateral to it. At first deep to abductor hallucis, it runs distally between abductor hallucis and flexor digitorum brevis, supplying both. Near the first metatarsal base, when its calibre is already diminished as a result of supplying numerous muscular branches, it is further diminished by a superficial stem. It passes to the medial border of the hallux, where it anastomoses with a branch of the first plantar metatarsal artery. Its superficial stem then trifurcates and supplies three superficial digital branches that accompany the digital branches of the medial plantar nerve and join the first to third plantar metatarsal arteries.

Lateral plantar artery

The lateral plantar artery (**Fig. 115.42**) is the larger terminal branch of the posterior tibial. It passes distally and laterally to the fifth metatarsal base, the lateral plantar nerve is medial to it. The plantar nerves lie between the plantar arteries. Turning medially, with the deep branch of the nerve, it gains the interval between the first and second metatarsal bases, and unites with the dorsalis pedis artery to complete the plantar

arch. As it passes laterally, it is first between the calcaneus and abductor hallucis, then between flexor digitorum brevis and flexor accessorius. Running distally to the fifth metatarsal base, it passes between flexor digitorum brevis and abductor digiti minimi and is covered by the plantar aponeurosis, superficial fascia and skin.

Muscular branches supply the adjoining muscles. Superficial branches emerge along the intermuscular septum to supply the skin and subcutaneous tissue lateral in the sole. Anastomotic branches run to the lateral border, and join branches of the lateral tarsal and arcuate arteries. Sometimes, a calcaneal branch pierces abductor hallucis to supply the skin of the heel.

DEEP AND SUPERFICIAL VENOUS SYSTEMS IN THE FOOT

Plantar digital veins arise from plexuses in the plantar regions of the toes, connecting with dorsal digital veins and uniting into four plantar metatarsal veins. The latter run in the intermetatarsal spaces and connect by perforating veins with dorsal veins, then continue to form the deep plantar venous arch that accompanies the plantar arterial arch. From this venous arch, medial and lateral plantar veins run near the corresponding arteries and, after communicating with the great and small saphenous veins, form the posterior tibial veins behind the medial malleolus.

The principal named superficial veins are the great and small saphenous. Their numerous tributaries are mostly (but not wholly) unnamed; named vessels will be noted (**Figs 110.6, 110.7**). As in the upper limb, the vessels will be described centripetally from peripheral to major drainage channels.

Dorsal digital veins receive rami from the plantar digital veins in the clefts between the toes and then join to form dorsal metatarsal veins, which are united across the proximal parts of the metatarsal bones in a dorsal venous arch. Proximal to this arch, an irregular dorsal venous network receives tributaries from deep veins and is continuous proximally with a venous network in the leg. At each side of the foot, this network connects with medial and lateral marginal veins, which are both formed mainly by veins from more superficial parts of the sole. In the sole, superficial veins form a plantar cutaneous arch across the roots of the toes and also drain into the medial and lateral marginal veins. Proximal to the plantar arch there is a plantar cutaneous venous plexus, especially dense in the fat of the heel. It connects with the plantar cutaneous venous arch and other deep veins, but drains mainly into the marginal veins. The veins of the sole are an important part of the lower limb 'venous pump' system aiding return of blood up the limb. Intermittent foot compression devices are available to enhance this flow and so reduce the risk of deep vein thrombosis during periods of increased risk, e.g. after surgery.

INNERVATION OF THE FOOT

SUPERFICIAL PERONEAL NERVE
The superficial peroneal nerve is described in Chapter 114 (p. 1504).

DEEP PERONEAL NERVE
The deep peroneal nerve is described in Chapter 114 (p. 1505).

TIBIAL NERVE
The branches of the tibial nerve are articular, muscular, sural, medial calcaneal and the medial and lateral plantar nerves. The course and distribution of the tibial nerve in the calf are described in Chapter 114 (p. 1504).

MEDIAL CALCANEAL NERVE

The medial calcaneal nerve arises from the tibial nerve and perforates the flexor retinaculum to supply the skin of the heel and medial side of the sole.

MEDIAL PLANTAR NERVE

The medial plantar nerve (**Fig. 115.48**) is the larger terminal division of the tibial nerve, and lies lateral to the medial plantar artery. From its origin under the flexor retinaculum, it passes deep to abductor hallucis, then appears between it and flexor digitorum brevis, gives off a medial proper digital nerve to the hallux, and divides near the metatarsal bases into three common plantar digital nerves.

Cutaneous branches pierce the plantar aponeurosis between abductor hallucis and flexor digitorum brevis to supply the skin of the sole of the foot. Muscular branches supply abductor hallucis, flexor digitorum brevis, flexor hallucis brevis and the first lumbrical. The first two arise near the origin of the nerve and enter the deep surfaces of the muscles. The branch to flexor hallucis brevis is from the hallucal medial digital nerve, and that to the first lumbrical from the first common plantar digital nerve. Articular branches supply the joints of the tarsus and metatarsus.

Three common plantar digital nerves pass between the slips of the plantar aponeurosis, each dividing into two proper digital branches. The first supplies adjacent sides of the hallux and second toe and the second supplies adjacent sides of the second and third toes; the third supplies adjacent sides of the third and fourth toes, and also connects with the lateral plantar nerve. The first gives a branch to the first lumbrical. Each proper digital nerve has cutaneous and articular branches: near the distal phalanges a dorsal branch supplies structures around the nail, and the termination of each nerve supplies the ball of the toe. The common digital branches of the medial plantar nerve are distributed in a manner similar to those of the median nerve, as are the motor branches of the two nerves. In the hand, the median nerve supplies abductor and flexor pollicis brevis, opponens pollicis and the first and second lumbricals. An opponens is absent in the foot, but abductor hallucis, flexor hallucis brevis and the first lumbrical are all supplied by the medial plantar nerve. As flexor digitorum brevis and flexor digitorum

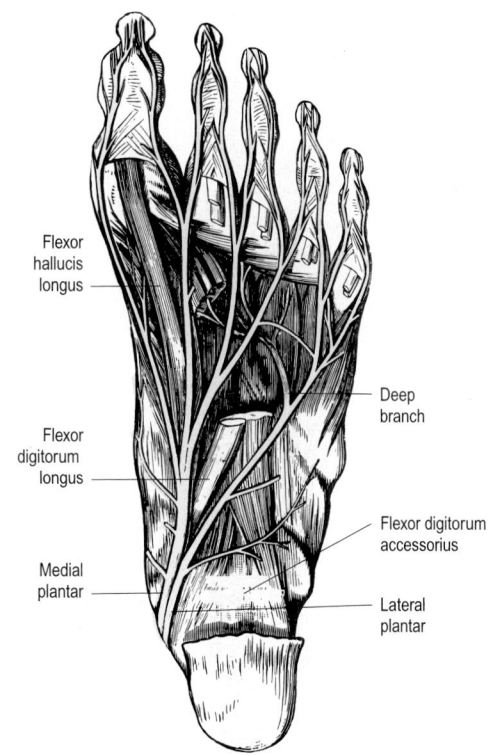

Fig. 115.48 The plantar nerves of the left foot.

superficialis (median nerve) correspond, only the innervation of the second lumbrical differs.

LATERAL PLANTAR NERVE

The lateral plantar nerve (**Fig. 115.48**) supplies the skin of the fifth toe, the lateral half of the fourth toe, and most of the deep muscles of the foot. Its distribution therefore closely resembles that of the ulnar nerve in the hand. It passes laterally forwards medial to the lateral plantar artery, towards the tubercle of the fifth metatarsal. It next passes between flexores digitorum brevis and accessorius, and ends between brevis and abductor digiti minimi by dividing into superficial and deep branches. Before division, it supplies flexor digitorum accessorius and abductor digiti minimi and gives rise to small branches that pierce the plantar fascia to supply the skin of the lateral part of the sole (**Fig. 115.1**). The superficial branch splits into two common plantar digital nerves: the lateral supplies the lateral side of the fifth toe, flexor digiti minimi brevis and the two interossei in the fourth intermetatarsal space; the medial connects with the third common plantar digital branch of the medial plantar nerve and divides into two to supply the adjoining sides of the fourth and fifth toes. The deep branch accompanies the lateral plantar artery deep to the flexor tendons and adductor hallucis and supplies the second to fourth lumbricals, adductor hallucis and all interossei (except those of the fourth intermetatarsal space). Branches to the second and third lumbricals pass distally deep to the transverse head of adductor hallucis, and curl round its distal border to reach them (**Fig. 115.49**).

NERVE ENTRAPMENT SYNDROMES IN THE FOOT
Any nerve of the foot can be affected by entrapment, leading classically to a burning sensation in the distribution of that nerve. Tarsal tunnel syndrome is much less common than carpal tunnel syndrome. The flexor retinaculum can compress the tibial nerve or either of its branches (medial and lateral plantar nerves), but is most commonly compressed by a space-occupying lesion, e.g. ganglion, a leash of vessels or the deep fascia associated with abductor hallucis. Compression of the first branch of the lateral plantar nerve by the deep fascia of abductor hallucis can lead to heel pain. The medial plantar nerve can be irritated at the master knot of Henry: this is usually related to jogging. The master knot of Henry is the anatomical landmark where the tendon of flexor hallucis longus crosses deep to the tendon of flexor digitorum longus, to reach its medial side in the sole of the foot. The superficial peroneal nerve can

be damaged in severe inversion injuries of the ankle, and the deep peroneal nerve is sometimes compressed by osteophytes in the region of the second tarsometatarsal joint. Sural nerve entrapment does not occur from compression by fascial elements; rather, it follows trauma and subsequent scar formation around the nerve. Entrapment of the common digital nerve as it passes under the intermetatarsal ligament of the third (or less commonly the second) webspace can result in a Morton's neuroma, which is probably the most common form of nerve entrapment in the foot.

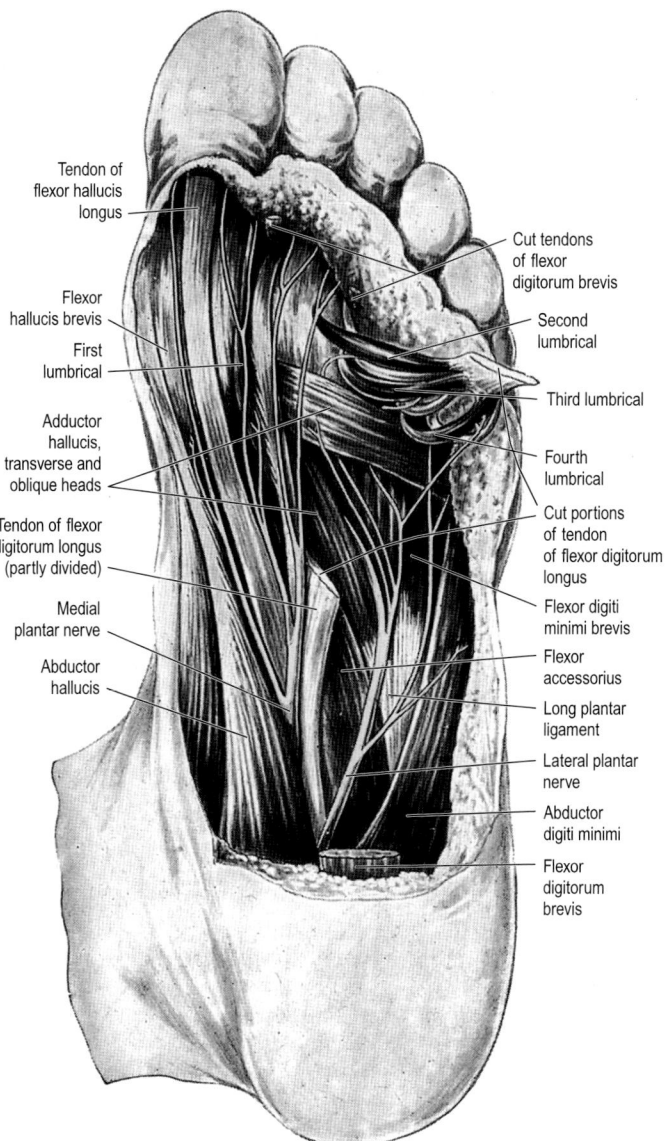

Fig. 115.49 Dissection of the lateral and medial plantar nerves of the left foot. Most of flexor digitorum brevis has been removed. Flexor digitorum longus has been partially divided and its distal end has been displaced, together with the second, third and fourth lumbricals.

Labels on figure:
- Tendon of flexor hallucis longus
- Flexor hallucis brevis
- First lumbrical
- Adductor hallucis, transverse and oblique heads
- Tendon of flexor digitorum longus (partly divided)
- Medial plantar nerve
- Abductor hallucis
- Cut tendons of flexor digitorum brevis
- Second lumbrical
- Third lumbrical
- Fourth lumbrical
- Cut portions of tendon of flexor digitorum longus
- Flexor digiti minimi brevis
- Flexor accessorius
- Long plantar ligament
- Lateral plantar nerve
- Abductor digiti minimi
- Flexor digitorum brevis

REFERENCES

Alexander R McN 1992 The Human Machine. Natural History Museum Publications: London

Barclay-Smith E 1896 The astragalo-calcaneo-navicular joint. J Anat Physiol 30: 390–412.
This paper gave the first description of the astragalo-calcaneo-navicular joint and explained the importance of the joint complex in terms of hindfoot motion.

Coleman S, Chesnut W 1977 A simple test for hindfoot flexibility in the cavovarus foot. Clin Orthop 123: 60–2.

Cralley J, Fitch K, McGonagle W 1975 Lumbrical muscles and contracted toes. Anat Anz 138: 348–53.

Cummins JE, Anson JB, Carr WB, Wright RR, Hauser DWE 1946 The structure of the calcaneal tendon (of Achilles) in relation to orthopedic surgery with additional observations on the plantaris muscle. Surg Gynecol Obstet 83: 107–16.

Gardner E, Gray DJ 1968 The innervation of the joints of the foot. Anat Rec 161: 141–8.

Harris RI, Beath T 1948 Etiology of peroneal spastic flat foot. J Bone Joint Surg [Br] 30: 624–34.

Hicks JH 1953 The mechanics of the foot II. The plantar aponeurosis and the arch. J Anat 88: 25–30.

Jones FW 1949 Structure and Function as Seen in the Foot, 2nd edn. London: Ballière, Tindall and Cox: 63–5. *One of the classic texts on the foot*

Kapandji I A 1970–1974 The Physiology of the Joints. Annotated Diagrams of the Mechanics of the Human Joints, 2nd edn (3 vols translated by L H Honoré: Vol 1 Upper Limb. Vol 2 Lower Limb. Vol 3 The Trunk and the Vertebral Column.) Churchill Livingstone: Edinburgh

Sarrafian SK 1993 Anatomy of the Foot and Ankle, Descriptive, Topographic, Functional, 2nd edn. Philadelphia: Lippincott.

Wildenauer F 1950 Die Blutversorgung des Talus. Z Anat Entwicklungsgesch 115: 32–6.
The first comprehensive account of talar blood supply and the identification of the important artery of the tarsal canal.

Development of the pelvic girdle and lower limb

STAGES OF LOWER LIMB DEVELOPMENT

The lower limb is first recognizable as a laterally projecting ridge at stage 13. By stage 14 the lower limb is closely associated with the wide umbilical cord. During stages 15–17 the limb projects laterally: preaxial growth is only slightly greater than postaxial growth.

By stage 17 the lower limb still has a flattened foot plate. Although a hip region can be identified, there is no true knee as yet. In stage 18 the lower limb appears to be flexed and abducted at the hip with the knee bent, giving the appearance that the knee is facing laterally. Very little skin of the thigh is visible. The soles of the feet face the umbilical cord, and the foot plate has digit rays. During stages 20–23 the digit rays separate, and toes are clearly defined by stage 23. The feet can finally touch at stage 21, when the umbilical cord becomes proportionally smaller and the embryo larger.

The pelvis forms from two hemipelves each of which develops from one cartilaginous focus. Ossification of the pelvis starts with the ilium, which undergoes endochondral ossification at 9.5 weeks. The femur and tibia form in cartilage and the sciatic nerve extends distally to the tibia by stage 18. Cavitation of the hip joint has been reported at 7–8 weeks. The sacroiliac joint can be recognized from 7 weeks: its development is slightly different from that of other synovial joints in that the development of the ilium is ahead of that of the sacrum.

VESSELS IN THE LOWER LIMB (Fig. 116.1)

The axial artery of the lower limb arises from the dorsal root of the umbilical artery and courses along the dorsal surface of the thigh, knee and leg. Below the knee it lies between the tibia and popliteus, and in the leg it lies between the crural interosseous membrane and tibialis posterior. It gives off a perforating artery that traverses the sinal tarsus to form a dorsal network and ends distally in a plantar network. The femoral artery passes along the ventral surface of the thigh, opening a new channel to the lower limb. It arises from a capillary plexus that is connected proximally with the femoral branches of the external iliac artery and distally with the axis artery. At the proximal border of popliteus the axis artery splits into primitive posterior tibial and peroneal branches: these run distally on the dorsal surface of popliteus and tibialis posterior to gain the sole of the foot. At the distal border of popliteus the axis artery gives off a perforating branch that passes ventrally between the tibia and the fibula and then courses to the dorsum of the foot, forming the anterior tibial artery and dorsalis pedis artery. The primitive peroneal artery communicates with the axis artery at the distal border of popliteus and in its course in the leg.

The femoral artery gradually increases in size. Coincidentally, most of the axis artery disappears; however, proximal to its communication with the femoral artery, the root of the axis artery persists as the inferior gluteal artery and the arteria comitans nervi ischiadici.

The proximal parts of the primitive posterior tibial and peroneal arteries fuse: they remain separate distally. Ultimately, much of the primitive peroneal artery disappears; however, a part of the axis artery is incorporated in the permanent peroneal artery. The same considerations apply to anomalies and variations as were described for the developing forelimb.

In the lower limb the preaxial vein becomes the long saphenous vein, which drains into the femoral vein at the saphenous opening. The postaxial vein becomes the short saphenous vein, which passes deep and joins the popliteal vein.

NEONATAL LOWER LIMB

In the neonate the pelvis is cone shaped. The transverse diameter of the true pelvis is 2.2 cm, its anteroposterior diameter 2.8 cm, and the length between the inlet and outlet is 2 cm. The sacrum is proportionately larger than in the adult and the sacral promontory is higher. When walking begins, the sacrum descends between the ilia and the promontory develops. The ilia, ischia and pubic bones are variably ossified at birth (pp. 1424, 1425 and 1427). They meet at the acetabulum, which in the neonate is cartilaginous, relatively large and shallow.

The lower limbs are underdeveloped in the neonate when compared to the upper limbs. They are retained in a flexed position and the leg is proportionately shorter than the thigh. Although the legs appear to be bowed, the tibia and fibula are straight: the illusion of bow legs is caused by the shape of the soft tissues and the slightly more advanced development of the lateral head of gastrocnemius compared to its medial head. The femoral neck is much shorter and forms an acute angle with the shaft. The latter is quite straight, because the adult curvature is acquired with walking. The head of the femur is larger than the acetabular fossa and nearly one-third remains external, which means that the ligamentum teres is relatively very long. Dislocation of the hip joint is relatively easy: the femoral head can be removed from the acetabular fossa laterally, but not posteriorly. The calcaneus and the talus have an ossification centre at birth, and a centre is present in the cuboid in 50% of neonates.

The muscles of the lower limb are much less developed than those in the upper limb. The fetal position often assumed by postnatal babies keeps the thighs in continuous abduction, stretching the adductors. The muscles that will be used for walking are weak; the lack of gluteal development in particular gives the typically diminutive buttocks of the neonate.

In neonates, the feet are usually inverted. They have a greater degree of dorsiflexion caused by the relatively greater area of the trochlea of the talus. Plantar flexion is limited, in part reflecting the shortness of the extensor muscles of the foot. At birth the footprint outlines the whole plantar surface. This is a consequence of the deposition of subcutaneous fat beneath the longitudinal and transverse arches, and so most babies appear flat-footed.

LOWER LIMB ANOMALIES

The categories of limb defects described by Swanson (1976) are given in page 941. Although devised for the upper limb, they apply in the same manner to the lower limb.

Developmental dysplasia of the hip is a term that covers an alteration in hip development before and after birth. The term is now preferred to 'congenital dislocation of the hip'. In the most extreme cases, the femoral head is completely dislocated out of the acetabulum. This condition occurs in c.1 in 100 live births; the ratio of females to males is 6:1. The aetiology is considered to be multifactorial and is associated with first pregnancies, suggesting that both maternal and uterine musculature restrict fetal movement and put postural strain on the fetal hips. Developmental dysplasia of the hip is seen more frequently in breech delivery, especially if the child's knees are extended. The left hip is more frequently affected than the right. This may be because in breech presentation the fetus lies with the right shoulder anterior and the left thigh closest to the maternal sacrum. The physiological effects that cause the maternal ligaments to become temporarily lax prior to delivery are also considered to affect the fetus and to contribute to laxity of the hip capsule.

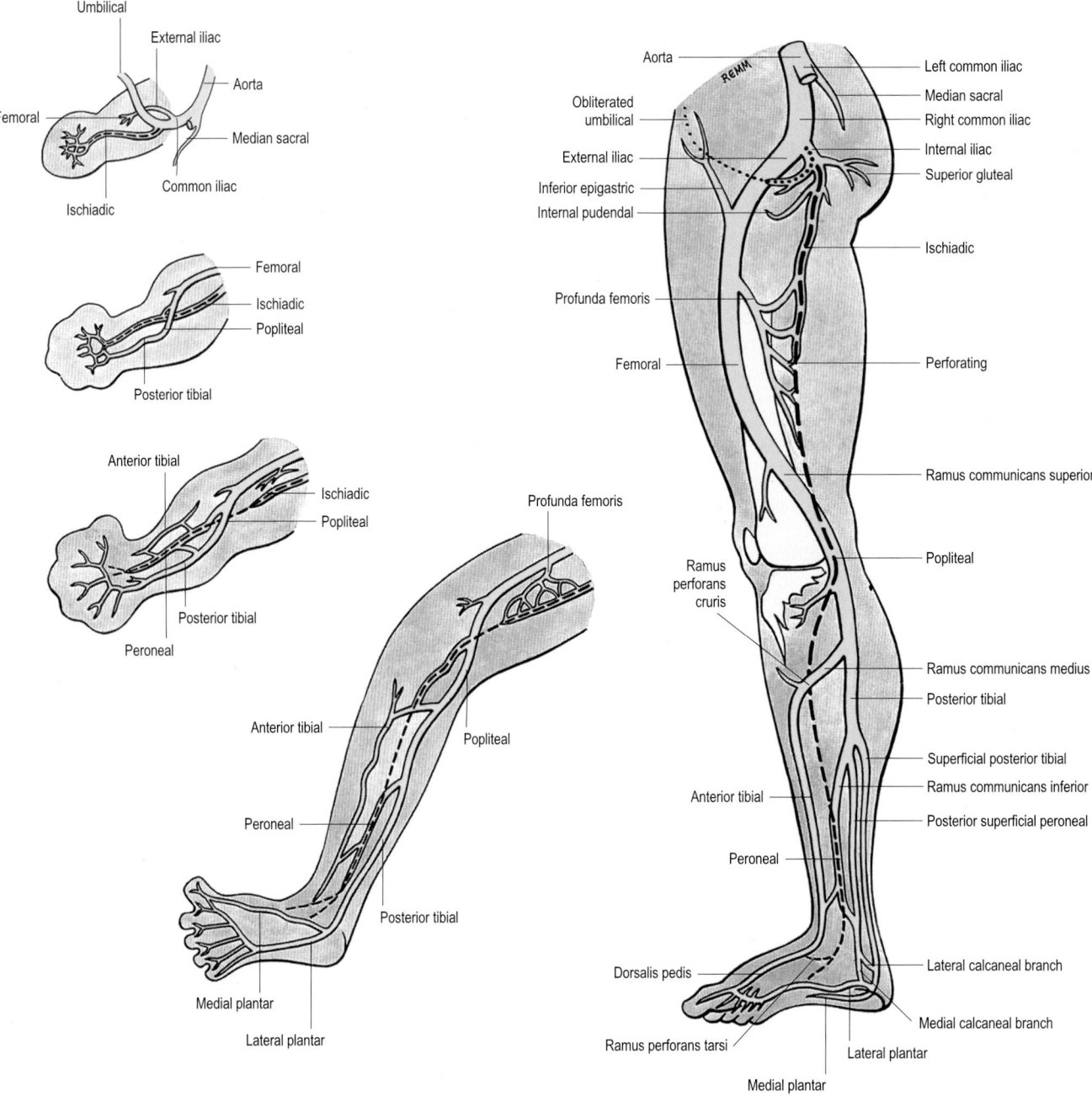

Fig. 116.1 Stages in the development of the arteries of the leg. The original path of the axis artery is indicated by a dashed line. (After Senior, by permission from John Wiley.)

Congenital talipes equinovarus, or club foot, derives its name from a combination of *talus* and *pes*, together with terms describing an elevated heel resembling that of a horse (*equino*), which is also turned inwards (*varus*). It is a common neonatal anomaly and occurs in c.1 per 1000 live births, with males affected twice as often as females. There is some degree of inheritance, so it is not entirely an effect of intrauterine positioning or of oligohydramnios (abnormally little amniotic fluid). Both bones and soft tissues are affected and it is difficult to tell which causes the primary or secondary effect. A number of theories have been proposed to explain the underlying pathogenetic mechanism(s), including abnormal tendon and ligament attachments and delayed muscle maturation. The most widely held theory is that the talus undergoes defective development and that all the other deformities arise as a consequence of this initial defect. The talus is decreased in size by up to 25%. It has a foreshortened neck and decreased body/neck angle, and the subtalar facets are medially rotated. The navicular is small and medially deviated relative to the talus. The calcaneus is also

small and shows varus displacement and equinus tilt: the anterior facets correspond to those of the talus (Barlow & Clarke 1994). The entire affected foot and calf are smaller than their normal counterparts. The foot is inverted and supinated and the forefoot is adducted. The heel is small, rotated inwards and elevated. The calcaneus is inverted beneath the talus. Treatment varies between splintage and repeated complex surgery, which reflects the highly variable severity of the condition and individual response to therapy.

'Flat feet' are common in childhood. The majority are 'flexible' and simply related to posture, whereas 'rigid' flat feet are caused by structural abnormalities. The description of 'rocker bottom' foot is associated with many congenital syndromes. The foot is flat and rigid. The plantar surface appears curved with the apex of the curve at the midtarsal joint. The condition shows an equinus position of the hindfoot. The talus may be vertical and palpable on the plantar surface. A majority of infants with this condition have neurological abnormalities.

REFERENCES

Barlow I, Clarke NMP 1994 Congenital talipes equinovarus. Surgery 12: 211–5.

Swanson AB 1976 A classification for congenital limb malformations. J Hand Surg 1: 8–22.

Eponyms

Achilles tendon: the calcaneal tendon. Achilles in Greek Mythology was slain by a wound in his vulnerable heel inflicted by Paris in the Trojan War.

Adamkiewicz's artery: the largest anterior medullary feeder artery to the anterior spinal artery. It varies in level, arising from the lower (T9–11) posterior intercostal, the subcostal, or less frequently the upper, lumbar (L1–2) arteries. Most often occurs on the left side.
Albert Adamkiewicz (1850–1921), Professor of Pathology, University of Cracow, Poland.

Allen's test: test of sufficiency of the blood supply to the hand by compression and release of the ulnar and radial arteries and observation of the colour change of the hand.
E V Allen (1901–1961), Professor of Medicine, Mayo Clinic, Rochester, Minnesota, USA.

Ammon's horn: the hippocampus.
Friedrich August Von Ammon (1799–1861), Professor of Pathology and Materia Medica, Dresden, Germany.

Andresen lines: structural lines within dentine, representing incremental lines that run more or less perpendicular to the direction of the tubules. They represent an incremental period of about 1 week and are best visualized when longitudinal ground sections are viewed between crossed polars.
Viggo Andresen (1870–1950), orthodontist, Norway.

Arantius' nodules: small nodules in the free border of the aortic valves.
Julio Caesar Aranzio (Arantius) (1530–1589), pupil of Vesalius. Professor of Medicine and Surgery, Bologna, Italy.

Argyll Robertson pupil: pupil reacts to accommodation but not light. Occurs in neurosyphilis.
Douglas Argyll Robertson (1837–1909), ophthalmic surgeon, Edinburgh, UK.

Arnold–Chiari malformation: congenital brain stem and cerebellar herniation through the foramen magnum.
Julius Arnold (1835–1915), Professor of Pathology, Heidelberg, Germany. Hans Chiari (1851–1916), gynaecologist, Austria. Professor of Obstetrics first in Prague, then in Vienna.

Auerbach's plexus: autonomic nervous plexus between circular and longitudinal layers of muscle of the intestine.
Leopold Auerbach (1828–1897), Professor of Neuropathology, Breslau, Poland.

Babinski's sign: upgoing plantar response in pyramidal tract disturbances.
Joseph Babinski (1857–1922), pupil of Charcot, neurologist, Pitié Hôpital, Paris, France.

Baillarger's bands, lines, striae: visible striations seen in sections of the cerebral cortex.
Jules Baillarger (1809–1890), alienist, Charenton Asylum, Paris, France.

Bankart's lesion: detachment of the anteroinferior glenoid labrum and damage to the humeral head, leading to recurrent dislocation of the shoulder.
A S Bankart (1879–1951), surgeon, Royal National Orthopaedic Hospital, London, UK.

Barr body: inactive x chromatin mass in the nucleus of female cells.
Murray Barr (1908–1995), Professor of Anatomy, University of Western Ontario, Canada.

Barret's oesophagus: abnormal columnar ('gastric') cell lining of the lower oesophagus, with risk of development of adenocarcinoma.
Norman Rupert Barrett (1903–1979), surgeon. St Thomas' Hospital and Brompton Hospital, London, UK.

Bartholin's: ducts and gland – the sublingual salivary gland and its ducts;
glands – the greater vestibular glands on either side of the vaginal orifice.
Casper Bartholin (1655–1738), Professor of Medicine, Anatomy and Physics, Copenhagen, Denmark.

Batson's vertebral venous plexus: the valveless vertebral venous veins that communicate with the prostatic venous plexus and explain the readiness with which carcinoma of the prostate spreads to the pelvic bones and vertebrae.
Oscar Batson (1894–1979), Professor of Anatomy, University of Philadelphia, USA.

Battle's sign: bruising over the mastoid process developing two or three days after fracture of the posterior cranial fossa.
William Battle (1855–1936), surgeon, St Thomas' Hospital, London, UK.

Bellini, ducts of: orifices of the renal tubules.
Lorenzo Bellini (1643–1704), Professor of Anatomy, Pisa, Italy.

Bell's palsy: viral infections of the facial nerve.
Sir Charles Bell (1774–1842), surgeon, Middlesex Hospital, London, UK.

Bergmann cells: glial cells of the cerebellum.
Gottlieb Heinrich Bergmann (?–1861), Medical Director of the Hildersheim Asylum, Germany.

Bernouilli effect: fluid flowing through a tube of varying diameter travels fastest and exerts the largest lateral pressure at its narrowest point.
J Bernouilli (1654–1705), mathematician, Switzerland. Shares with Isaac Newton the invention of calculus.

Betz cells: large pyramidal cells of cerebral cortex.
Vladimir Aleksandrovich Betz (1834–1894), Professor of Anatomy, Kiev, Russia.

Bezold's abscess: subperiosteal temporal bone abscess.
Freiderich Bezold (1842–1908), otologist, Munich, Germany.

Bichat's buccal fat pad: the buccal pad of fat – corpus adiposum.
Marie Bichat (1771–1802), Professor of Anatomy and physician, Hôtel Dieu Paris, France. Pioneer in study of tissues.

Billroth's cords: tissue between sinusoids in splenic red pulp.
Christian Albert Theodore Billroth (1829–1894), Professor of Surgery successively at Zurich and Vienna, Austria.

Birbeck granules: small cross-striated granules first reported in the Langerhans cells of the epidermis.
Michael S Birbeck (b.1925), cancer researcher, Institute of Cancer Research, London, UK.

Blaschko lines: pattern adopted by many skin lesions.
Alfred Blaschko (1858–1892), dermatologist, Berlin, Germany.

Bowman's: anterior limiting lamina – anterior elastic membrane of the cornea;
capsule – sheath surrounding the renal glomerulus;
glands – glands in the olfactory mucosa.

1551

Sir William Bowman (1816–1892), surgeon at Birmingham General Hospital then Professor of Anatomy and Physiology, King's College Hospital, London, UK.

Broca's: diagonal band – a fibre tract in the basal forebrain;
area – speech area of cerebral cortex.
Pierre Paul Broca (1824–1880), Professor of Clinical Surgery, Paris, France.

Brödel, bloodless line of: the line of division between the areas of kidney supplied by the anterior and posterior branches of the renal artery.
Max Brödel (1870–1941), medical artist, first at Leipzig then Director of Institute of Art as Applied to Medicine, Baltimore, USA.

Brodmann's area 17, area 18: primary visual cortex.
Korbinian Brodmann (1868–1918), Professor of Anatomy, Tubingen, Germany.

Bruch's choroidal basal lamina: basal membrane of the choroid.
Karl Wilhelm Ludwig Bruch (1819–1884), Professor of Anatomy at Basle, Switzerland, and then Giessen.

Brunner's glands: duodenal glands lying deep to the muscularis mucosae.
Johann Konrad Brunner (1653–1727), Professor of Anatomy successively at Heidelberg and Strasbourg.

Buck's fascia: the penile fascial sheath.
Gordon Buck (1807–1877), surgeon, New York, USA.

Cajal, interstitial cells of: nerve cells of the superficial layer of the cerebral cortex.
Santiago Ramon y Cajal (1852–1934), Professor of Anatomy, Valencia, then Barcelona, then Professor of Histology and Morbid Anatomy, Madrid, Spain.

Calot's triangle: triangle bound by the liver, common hepatic duct and cystic duct.
Jean François Calot (1861–1914), surgeon, Rothschild Hospital, France, where he specialised in the treatment of surgical tuberculosis in children.

Carpenter's syndrome: mental retardation, acrocephaly and syndactyly related to, but genetically distinct from, Alpert's syndrome.
George Carpenter (1859–1910), physician, UK.

Carabelli's cusp or tubercle: an occasional fifth tubercle lingual to the antero-medial cusp of the first upper molar tooth.
Edler Carabelli (1787–1842), Professor of Dental Surgery, Vienna, Austria.

Charcot's artery of cerebral haemorrhage: lenticulostriate branch of middle cerebral artery.
Jean Martin Charcot (1825–1893), neurologist and physician, Salpetrière, Paris, France.

Chassaignac's carotid tubercle: the prominent anterior tubercle of the transverse process of the sixth cervical vertebra against which the carotid artery can be compressed.
Charles Marie Edouard Chassaignac (1805–1879), surgeon, Paris, France.

Clara cells: bronchiolar cells secreting surfactant.
Max Clara (1899–1966) Professor of Anatomy, Leipzig, Germany.

Clarke's column: basal nucleus in posterior horn of spinal grey matter.
Jacob Augustus Lockhart Clarke (1817–1880), neurologist, Hospital for Epilepsy and Paralysis, London, UK.

Claudius, supporting cells of: supporting cells on the floor of the cochlear canal of the inner ear.
Friedrich Matthias Claudius (1822–1869), Professor of Anatomy successively in Kiel and Marburg, Germany.

Cleland's ligament (transverse retrovascular ligament): thin fibres passing from the lateral surfaces of the interphalangeal joints to the skin of the fingers.
John Cleland (1835–1925), Professor of Anatomy, Glasgow, UK.

Cloquet's node (gland): lymph node in the femoral canal.
Jules Germain Cloquet (1790–1883), Professor of Anatomy and Surgery, Paris.

Colles': fascia – continuation of Scarpa's layer of abdominal fascia;
fracture – fracture of the lower end of the radius with dorsal displacement.
Abraham Colles (1773–1843), Professor of Anatomy and Surgery, Royal College of Surgeons of Ireland, Dublin, Ireland.

Cooper's pectineal ligament: thickened periosteum on the penten.
Sir Astley Pastor Cooper (1768–1841), surgeon, Guy's Hospital, London, UK.

Corti, organ of, or rods of: auditory hair cells of the cochlea.
Alfonso Corti (1822–1888), histologist. Held no academic post but worked in Vienna, Berlin, Utrecht and Turin.

Couinard's segments: the segments of the liver.
Claude Couinard (contemporary), Professor of Anatomy and surgeon, Paris, France.

Cowper's glands: the bulbourethral glands.
William Cowper (1666–1709), surgeon, London, UK.

Crouzon's syndrome: craniofacial dysostosis. Premature closures of cranial vault sutures, maxillary hypoplasia and ocular and aural anomalies.
Octave Crouzon (1874–1938), neurologist, Salpêtrière, Paris, France.

Cullen's sign: bluish discolouration at the umbilicus from extravasated blood in ruptured ectopic pregnancy and pancreatitis – an uncommon physical sign.
Thomas Cullen (1869–1953), Professor of Gynaecology, Johns Hopkins Hospital, Baltimore, USA.

Cushingoid syndrome: the syndrome produced by glucocorticosteroid excess.
Harvey Cushing (1869–1939), Professor of Surgery, Harvard, neurosurgeon, Peter Bent Brigham Hospital, Boston, USA.

Cuvier's duct: termination of the cardinal vein in the fetus.
Baron Georges Cuvier (1760–1832), zoologist and palaeontologist, Paris, France.

Darkschewitsch, nucleus of: posterior commissural nucleus.
Liverij Osipovich Darkschewitsch (1858–1925), neuroanatomist, University of Moscow.

Deiters': phalangeal supporting cells – outer hair cells in the organ of Corti;
nucleus – lateral vestibular nucleus of the vestibulocochlear nerve.
Otto Deiters (1834–1863), Professor of Anatomy and Histology, Bonn, Germany.

Denonvillier's fascia: fascia separating the prostate from the rectum.
Charles Pierre Denonvilliers (1808–1872), Professor of Anatomy, Paris, France.

De Quervain's disease: stenosing tenovaginitis of the tendon sheath of abductor pollicis longus and extensor pollicis brevis.
Fritz de Quervain (1868–1940), Professor of Surgery, Berne, Switzerland.

Descemet's posterior limiting lamina: posterior membrane of the cornea.
Jean Descemet (1732–1810), Professor of Anatomy and Surgery, Paris.

Dissé, perisinusoidal space of: space between the venous sinusoid and the hepatic cells.
Josef Disśe (1852–1912), anatomist, Germany

Douglas, pouch of: rectouterine peritoneal pouch.
James Douglas (1675–1742), anatomist and obstetrician, London, UK.

Drummond, marginal artery (or arch) of: the anastomoses between the ileo-colic, right colic, middle colic, left colic and sigmoid arteries (the arch of Roilan is the part of this arch between the middle and left colic artery).
Hamilton Drummond (1882–1925), surgeon, Newcastle Upon Tyne, UK.

Dupuytren's contracture: contraction and fibrosis of the palmar (and occasionally the plantar) fascia.
Baron Guillaume Dupuytren (1777–1835), surgeon, Hôtel Dieu, Paris, France.

(von) Ebner's: glands – serous glands in relation to the circumvallate papillae on the dorsum of the tongue;
lines –incremental lines of dentine.

Victor Ritter Von Rosenstein Ebner (1842–1925), Professor of Histology and Embryology, Innsbruck, Austria.

Edinger–Westphal nucleus: midbrain nucleus containing preganglionic neurons destined to synapse in the ciliary ganglion; it lies close to the nucleus of the oculomotor nerve.
Ludwig Edinger (1855–1918), Professor of Anatomy, Frankfurt-am-Main, Germany.
Karl Westphal (1833–1890), Professor of Psychiatry, Berlin, Germany.

Erb–Duchenne paralysis: the result of injury to the C5 and C6 roots of the brachial plexus.
Wilhelm Erb (1840–1921), Professor of Neurology, Heidelberg, Germany.
G B A Duchenne (1806–1875), neurologist, Paris, France.

Eustachian: tube – the pharyngotympanic tube;
valve – inferior vena caval valve in right atrium.
Bartolomeo Eustachi (1513?–1574), Professor of Anatomy, Rome, Italy, and physician to the Pope.

Fallopian: aqueduct or canal – canal for facial nerve in the temporal bone;
tube – the uterine tube.
Gabrielle Fallopio (1523–1562), Professor of Anatomy, Padua, Italy; a pupil of Vesalius.

Fallot's tetralogy: congenital heart disease comprising pulmonary stenosis, right ventricular hypertrophy, ventricular septal defect and over-riding of the aorta.
Etienne Fallot (1850–1911), Professor of Medicine, Marseilles, France.

Fordyce's spots: small mucosal cysts of cheeks, lips and tongue.
J Fordyce (1858–1925), dermatologist, New York, USA.

Forel's fields (decussation): ventral tegmental decussation between the red nuclei.
August Forel (1848–1931), anatomist and neurologist, Zurich, Switzerland.

Frey's syndrome: sweating in distribution of auriculotemporal nerve triggered by eating ('auriculo-gustatory sweating') after injury to the facial nerve.
Luiji Frey (1889–1944), neurologist, Warsaw, Poland.

Froehse, arcade of: arcade between the two layers of supinator; it transmits the posterior interosseous nerve.
Fritz Froehse, anatomist, Germany.

Froriep's ganglion: inconstant ganglion on posterior aspect of hypoglossal nerve.
August Froriep (1849–1917), physiologist, Tübingen, Germany.

Galen's: nerve (ansa galeni) – branch of the superior laryngeal nerve to the recurrent laryngeal nerve;
(deep galenic venous system) vein – the great cerebral vein.
Claudius Galen (130–200 AD), born Pergamum, Asia Minor, studied there and in Smyrna, Corinth and Alexandria. Physician to Marcus Aurelius and taught Anatomy and Medicine in Rome. Author of numerous texts on anatomy, surgery and medicine.

Gartner's duct: paravaginal duct; mesonephric duct remnant.
Hermann Treschow Gärtner (1785–1827), surgeon in Norwegian and then Danish army.

Gennari's, stria (white line) of: characteristic line in occipital visual cortex.
Francesco Gennari (1750–1795), physician, Parma, Italy.

Gerdy's tubercle: the attachment of the ilio-tibial tract to the proximal tibia.
Pierre Nicolas Gerdy (1797–1856), surgeon and pathologist, Paris, France.

Gerota's fascia: the renal fascia; encapsulates the perinephric fat.
Dumitru Gerota (1867–1939), Professor of Surgery, Bucharest, Romania.

Giacomini's band: band on surface of the uncus.
Carlo Giacomini (1840–1898), Professor of Anatomy, Turin, Italy.

Glisson's capsule: the fibrous capsule of the liver.
Francis Glisson (1597–1677), Regius Professor of Medicine, Cambridge. Described rickets in 1671.

Goethe, ossicle of: the incus (an auditory ossicle).
Johann Wolfgang Goethe (1749–1832), poet, philosopher and scientist, Germany.

Golgi: complexes or apparatus or bodies – membranous cellular organelles;
cells or neurones – GABA-ergic cerebellar interneurones;
corpuscles – tactile end organs in skin and muscle.
Camillo Golgi (1844–1926), Professor of Histology and Anatomy successively in Padua and then Sienna, Italy.

Graafian follicle: the mature ovarian follicle.
Regnier de Graaf (1641–1673), anatomist and physician, Delft, Holland.

Grayson's ligament: fascial fibres which pass from the lateral sides of the phalanges volar to the neurovascular bundle.
J Grayson, Professor of Anatomy, Manchester, UK.

Grey Turner's sign: bluish discoloration in the left loin caused by extravasated blood in acute pancreatitis – an uncommon physical sign.
George Grey Turner (1877–1951), Surgeon at Royal Victoria Infirmary, Newcastle Upon Tyne and the Professor of Surgery, Royal Postgraduate Medical School, Hammersmith, London, UK.

Guerin's fracture: a LeFort I level fracture of the maxilla (see below).
Alphonse Guerin (1816–1895), surgeon, Paris, France.

Guyon's canal: canal for the ulnar nerve and vessels; defined medially by the pisiform, and posteriorly by the flexor retinaculum.
Jean Casimir Guyon (1831–1920), surgeon, Paris, France.

Haller's cells: infraorbital ethmoid cells (synonym: orbitoethmoidal cells) which may be specified as either anterior or posterior ethmoid. They may lie lateral to the infundibulum and then open in to the middle meatus. They grow into the bony orbital floor and may obstruct the ostia of either the ethmoid infundibulum or the maxillary sinus during endonasal procedures.
Albrecht von Haller (1708–1777), Professor of Anatomy, Physiology, Surgery and Botany, University of Göttingen, Germany.

Harris's growth lines: transverse juxta-epiphyseal lines of long bones seen on X-ray and representing temporary growth arrest.
Henry Harris (1886–1951), Professor of Anatomy, Cambridge, UK.

Hartmann's pouch: dilatation above the neck of the gallbladder – a pathological entity produced by a contained gallstone.
Henri Hartmann (1860–1952), Professor of Surgery, Faculty of Medicine, Paris, France.

Haversian: systems – cylindrical units of tissue (osteons) in compact bone;
canals – central vascular channels in Haversian systems.
Clopton Havers (1817–1894), physician practising first in London, then in Isle of Wight, UK.

Henle's: layer – outer layer of cells in the root sheath of a hair;
loop – the looped portion of the renal tubule.
Friedrich Gustav Henle (1808–1885), Professor of Anatomy successively in Zurich, Heidelberg and Göttingen, Germany.

Hensen: node of – thickening at the site of the first formation of the primitive streak;
supporting cells of – in the organ of Corti (see above) to the outer side of the cells of Deiters (see above).
Viktor Hensen (1834–1924), Professor of Physiology, Kiel, Germany.

Hering–Brewer reflex: lung stretch reflex mediated by the vagus.
Carl Ewald Hering (1834–1918), physiologist, Vienna and then Leipzig.

Josef Brewer (1842–1925), psychiatrist and physiologist, Vienna, where he collaborated with Hering.

Hering's canal: fine terminal ductules lined by cuboidal epithelium, linking the intralobular bile canaliculi with bile ducts in the portal canals.
Carl Ewald Hering (1834–1918), physiologist, Vienna and Leipzig

Heschl's transverse temporal gyri: gyri on temporal lobe of brain.
Richard Heschl (1824–1881), Professor of Pathology, Cracow, and then of Clinical Medicine, Graz, Austria.

Heuser's membrane: the parietal hypoblast layer.
Chester Heuser (1885–1965), embryologist, USA.

Hilton's law: nerves crossing a joint supply the joint, the muscles acting on the joint and the skin overlying the joint.
John Hilton (1805–1878), surgeon, Guy's Hospital, London, UK.

1553

Hirschsprung's disease: megacolon resulting from congenital absence of autonomic ganglion cells in distal contracted segment.
Harald Hirschsprung (1830–1916), physician, Queen Louise Children's Hospital, Copenhagen, Denmark.

His: bundle of – the atrioventricular bundle of the heart;
furcula of – an inverted U which appears in the central wall of the developing pharynx.
Wilhelm His (Junior) (1863–1934), Professor of Anatomy successively at Leipzig, Basle, Göttingen and Berlin. Son of Wilhelm His Senior.

His, septum intermedium of: part of the primitive atrial septum.
Wilhelm His (Senior) (1831–1904), Professor of Anatomy and Physiology first in Basle then Leipzig.

Hoboken's valves: valve-like projections in the vessels of the umbilical cord.
Nicolas Von Hoboken (1632–1678), Professor of Anatomy, Harderwyk, then Professor of Medicine and Mathematics in Steinfurt, The Netherlands.

Hofbauer cells: ellipsoid cells in chorionic villi.
Isrid Isidore Hofbauer (1878–1961), gynaecologist, USA.

Holden's line: transverse skin crease at the groin caused by flexion of the hip.
Luther Holden (1815–1905), surgeon, St Bartholomew's Hospital, London, UK.

Horner's syndrome: ptosis and pupillary constriction following interruption of the sympathetic supply to the eyelid and pupil, respectively.
Johann Horner (1831–1886), Professor of Ophthalmology, Zurich, Switzerland.

Howship's lacunae: absorption spaces in bone.
John Howship (1781–1841), surgeon, St George's and Charing Cross Hospitals, London, UK. Suffered himself from osteomyelitis of the tibia and made special study of bone pathology.

Humphrey's ligament: meniscofemoral ligament – Humphrey described this ligament as running from the lateral meniscus to the posterior cruciate ligament.
George Murray Humphrey (1820–1896), Professor of Anatomy and then of Surgery, Cambridge, UK. Founder of Journal of Anatomy.

Hunter's canal: the subsartorial canal.
John Hunter (1728–1793), surgeon, St George's Hospital, London, UK. Described ligation of the femoral artery in the subsartorial canal for popliteal aneurysm.

Huschke, foramen of: deficiency in the floor of the bony part of the external auditory meatus, which usually closes by the fifth year, but may persist throughout life.
Emil Huschke (1797–1858), Professor of Anatomy, Jena, Germany.

Huxley's layer: the inner layer of cells of the root sheath of a hair.
Thomas Henry Huxley (1825–1895), lecturer in Natural History, Royal School of Mines, UK. An early supporter of Darwinism.

Hyrtl's anastomosis (loop): occasional anastomosis between right and left hypoglossal nerves.
Joseph Hyrtl (1811–1894), anatomist, Austria.

Ito, cells of: hepatic stellate cells.
Hayozo Ito (1865–?), Professor of Surgery, Kyoto, Japan.

Jackson's membrane: peritoneal fold between caecum or ascending colon and lateral abdominal wall.
Jabez North Jackson (1868–1935), Professor of Anatomy and Surgery, Kansas City, USA.

Jacobson's organ: the vomeronasal organ.
Ludwig Levin Jacobson (1783–1843), anatomist, Copenhagen, Denmark; later physician in French army.

Kartagener's syndrome: transposition of the viscera associated with abnormal cilia which results in bronchiectasis.
Manes Kartagener (1887–1975), physician, Switzerland.

Kent, bundle of: the atrioventricular bundle (also known as bundle of His, see above).
Albert Kent (1863–1958), Professor of Physiology, Bristol, UK.

Kerckring's valve: valvulae conniventes – the circular folds of the small intestine (already completely described by Fallopio, see above)
Theodor Kerckring (1640–1693), physician and anatomist, Amsterdam, The Netherlands.

Kiesselbach's plexus: site of haemorrhage on nasal septum.
Wilhelm Kiesselbach (1839–1902), ear nose and throat surgeon, Erlangen, Germany.

Killian's dehiscence: gap between the attachments of the inferior constrictor of the pharynx to the cricoid and thyroid cartilages – site of origin of a pharyngeal pouch.
Gustav Killian (1860–1921), Professor of Laryngorhinology successively in Freiburg and Berlin, Germany.

Klippel–Feil syndrome: congenital fusion or reduction in number of cervical vertebrae.
Maurice Klippel (1858–1942), neurologist at Salpetrière, Paris.
André Feil (1884–?), neurologist, France.

Klumpke's paralysis: injury to lowest root of brachial plexus (T1).
Augusta Dejerine-Klumpke (1859–1927), neurologist, Paris, France. Married to another neurologist, Joseph Dejerine.

Klüver–Bucy syndrome: experimental syndrome in rhesus monkey produced by ablation of the temporal limbic system.
Heinrich Klüver (1897–1974), German-born neurologist, USA.
Paul Clancy Bucy (1904–1992), neurologist, USA.

Koch's triangle: triangular area in the wall of the right atrium which marks the site of the atrioventricular node.
Walter Koch (1880–?), physician and pathologist, Berlin and Freiburg, France.

Kohn, interalveolar pores of: pores that link adjacent alveolar air spaces of the lung.
Hans Kohn (1866–?), pathologist, Berlin, Germany.

Kölliker, nucleus of: substantia intermedia centralis in spinal cord.
Rudolf Albert Von Kölliker (1817–1905), anatomist, Switzerland.

Kraissl's lines: lines of greatest tension in the skin.
Cornelius Kraissl (d. 1999), plastic surgeon, New Jersey, USA

Kulchitsky cells: neuroendocrine cells in lung and gut.
Nicholas Kulchitsky (1856–1925), Professor of Histology, Kharkov, Russia. After the Russian revolution he came to London to continue his work in neuropathology at University College.

Kupffer cells: liver macrophages.
Karl Wilhelm Von Kupffer (1829–1902), Professor of Anatomy successively at Kiel, Köningsberg and Munich, Germany.

Labbé's inferior anastomotic vein: connects superficial middle cerebral vein to the transverse sinus.
Leon Labbé (1832–1916), surgeon, France.

Ladd's bands: congenital bands across the duodenum in volvulus neonatorum.
William Edward Ladd (1880–1967), surgeon, Boston Children's Hospital, USA.

Landsmeer's ligament: transverse and oblique retinacular ligaments of the fingers.
Johan Landsmeer (1919–1999), Professor of Anatomy, Leiden, The Netherlands.

Langer's lines: cleavage or crease lines in the skin produced by the arrangement of the subcutaneous fibrous tissues.
Karl Ritter von Edenberg Langer (1819–1887), Professor of Anatomy, Hungary, and then Vienna, Austria

Langerhans: cells – dendritic antigen-presenting cells of skin and other mucosal epithelia;
islets of – clumps of insulin- and other hormone-secreting cells of the pancreas.
Paul Langerhans (1847–1888), Professor of Pathology, Freiburg, Germany. Described the islet cells in his doctorate thesis in 1869, at the age of 22.

Langhans: cells – cytotrophoblastic cells of a chorionic villus lying deep to the syncytiotrophoblast.
Theodore Langhans (1839–1915), pathologist, Berne, Switzerland.

Le Fort: classification of maxillary fractures.
René Le Fort (1829–1893), surgeon, Paris, France.

Leydig cells: the interstitial testosterone-secreting cells of the testis.
Franz Von Leydig (1821–1908), Professor of Histology successively at Würzburg, Tübingen and Bonn, Germany.

Lieberkuhn, crypts of: tubular glands of the small intestine.
Johann Nathaniel Lieberkuhn (1711–1756), physician and anatomist, Berlin, Germany. These glands were described by Malphighi (see below) in 1688.

Lisfranc's ligament: interosseous ligament between the second metatarsal and first cuneiform bone of the foot.
Jaques de St. Martin Lisfranc (1790–1847), Professor of Surgery, Paris, France.

Lissauer, tract of: ascending tract in the spinal cord.
Heinrich Lissauer (1861–1891), neurologist, Breslau.

Lister's tubercle: a prominence on the posterior surface of the distal radius, ulnar to the groove for the tendon of extensor pollicis longus.
Joseph (Lord) Lister (1827–1912), successively Professor of Surgery at Glasgow, Edinburgh and King's College, London, UK.

Littré's glands: submucosal glands of the male urethra.
Alexis Littré (1658–1726), anatomist and surgeon, Paris, France.

Little's area: site of haemorrhage on the nasal septum.
James Laurence Little (1836–1885), Professor of Surgery, University of Vermont, USA.

Lockwood's tails: hypothetical bands interfering with downgrowth of the processus vaginalis, resulting in ectopia testis.
Charles Barrett Lockwood (1856–1914), surgeon, St. Bartholomew's Hospital, London, UK.

Luschka: bursa of – accessory pharyngeal recess in front of the anterior arch of the atlas;
foramen of – lateral aperture in the roof of the fourth cerebral ventricle;
uncovertebral joints of – small synovial joints on either side of the intervertebral cartilaginous joint in cervical vertebrae C3–7 (between the uncinate process of the inferior vertebral body and the bevelled lateral border of the superior body at each level).
Hubert Luschka (1820–1875), Professor of Anatomy, Tübingen, Germany.

Mackenrodt's ligament: the transverse cervical (or cardinal) ligament of the uterus.
Alwin Mackenrodt (1859–1925), Professor of Gynaecology, Berlin, Germany.

Magendie, foramen of: the median aperture in the roof of the fourth ventricle.
François Magendie (1783–1855), physician to the Hôtel Dieu, Paris, France.

Malpighian: corpuscle – splenic corpuscles;
layer – deep layer of the epidermis.
Marcello Malpighi (1628–1694), Professor of Medicine successively in Bologna, Pisa and Messina, Italy. Finally physician to the Papal Court, Rome. Regarded as the founder of microscopic anatomy.

Meckel's: cartilage – the cartilage of the first branchial arch;
diverticulum – the remains of the vitello-intestinal duct.
Johann Meckel (1781–1833), Professor of Anatomy, Halle. His grandfather was Professor of Anatomy in Berlin and described the pterygopalatine ganglion and the dural sac which contains the ganglion of the trigeminal nerve. His father was also Professor of Anatomy in Halle.

Meibomian tarsal glands: the tarsal glands of the eyelid. If blocked they become distended into meibomian cysts.
Heinrich Meibom (1638–1700), Professor of Medicine, History and Poetry, Helmstadt, Germany.

Meissner's: corpuscles – tactile nerve endings in skin;
plexus – submucosal autonomic plexus of the intestine.
George Meissner (1829–1905), Professor of Anatomy and Physiology, Basle, of Zoology and Physiology at Freiburg, and Physiology at Göttingen, Germany.

Merkel cells (or corpuscles): sensory nerve endings in the skin.
Friedrich Sigmund Merkel (1845–1919), Professor of Anatomy successively at Rostock, then Göttingen, Germany.

Meyer's loop: portion of the geniculocalcarine radiation.
Adolf Meyer (1866–1950), neurologist, USA.

Meynert, basal nucleus of: part of the 'substantia innominata' of the basal forebrain: contains large cholinergic neurones that project to the cerebral cortex, amygdala and thalamus.
Theodore Herman Meynert (1833–1892), Professor of Neurology, Vienna, Austria.

Moll's glands: the ciliary glands.
Jacob Antonius Moll (1832–1914), ophthalmologist, The Hague, The Netherlands.

Monro, foramen of: the foramen between the lateral and third ventricles of the brain.
Alexander Monro (1733–1817), Professor of Anatomy, Edinburgh, UK. The chair was also held by his father and his son – all named Alexander.

Montgomery, glands or tubercles of: sebaceous glands situated in the areola of the breast.
William Montgomery (1797–1859), Professor of Midwifery, Dublin, Ireland.
(previously described by Morgagni, see below).

Morgagni: columns of – the columns of the anal canal;
hernia – congenital diaphragmatic hernia between the sternal and costal attachments of the diaphragm.
Giovanni Battista Morgagni (1682–1771), Professor of Anatomy, Padua, Italy, for 59 years. Founder of modern morbid anatomy.

Morison's pouch: the right subhepatic space.
James Rutherford Morison (1853–1939), Professor of Surgery, Durham, UK.

Müller's: cells – neuroglial cells in the retina;
muscle – radial fibres of the ciliary muscles.
Heinrich Müller (1820–1864), Professor of Anatomy, Würzburg, Germany.

Müllerian duct: the paramesonephric duct of the fetus.
Johannes Müller (1801–1858), Professor of Anatomy, Berlin, Germany.

Nabothian cyst: retention cyst of uterine cervix.
Martin Naboth (1675–1721), Professor of Medicine, Leipzig, Germany.

Nissl: granules – basophil granules in cytoplasm of neuronal somata;
stain – specific stain for these granules.
Franz Nissl (1860–1919), neurologist successively of Frankfurt, Heidelberg and Munich, Germany.

Nitabuch's layer or stria: layer in the intervillous spaces of the placenta.
Raissa Nitabuch (19th Century), physician, Germany.

Nuel's spaces: space between outer rods of Corti and hair cells.
Jean Pierre Nuel (1847–1920), Professor of Otology, Louvain and later Liege, Belgium.

Oddi, sphincter of: the sphincter at the termination of the common bile duct.
Ruggero Oddi (1845–1906), surgeon, Rome, Italy. The sphincter had already been described by Glisson (see above) in the 17th century.

Pacchionian bodies: arachnoid granulations.
Antoine Pacchion (1665–1726), physician and anatomist, Rome, Italy.

Pacinian corpuscles: end organs of sensory nerves.
Filippo Pacini (1812–1883), Professor of Anatomy and Physiology successively at Pisa and then Florence, Italy.

Pancoast tumour: apical carcinoma of the lung involving C8 and T1 nerves, the cervical sympathetic chain and upper ribs.
Henry Pancoast (1875–1939), Professor of Radiology, University of Pennsylvania, Philadelphia, USA.

Paneth cells: bacteriocidal lysozyme-secreting cells.
Joseph Paneth (1857–1890), Professor of Physiology first in Breslau, then Vienna, Austria.

Papez circuit: a neuroanatomical circuit mediating emotion, involving the hippocampal formation, mammillary body, anterior nuclei of the thalamus and cingulate gyrus.
James Wenceslas Papez (1883–1958), neurologist, USA.

Passavant's: muscle – upper fibres of palatopharyngeus;
ridge (bar) – projecting ridge, or bar, on posterior wall of pharynx which appears during swallowing.
Phillip Gustav Passavant (1815–1893), surgeon, Frankfurt, Germany.

Petit, canal of: the space between the zonule of Zinn (see below) and the vitreous humour.
François Pourfois de Petit (1664–1741), ophthalmologist, Paris, France.

Peyer's patches: lymphoid aggregates in the ileum.
Johann Conrad Peyer (1653–1712), Professor of Logic, Rhetoric and Medicine in Schaffhausen, Switzerland.

Purkinje: cells – large neurones forming a single eponymous layer in cerebellar cortex;
fibres – subendocardial muscle fibres.
Johannes Purkinje (1787–1869), Professor of Physiology, Breslau and then Prague, Poland.

Ramsay Hunt syndrome: herpes zoster involvement of the geniculate ganglion associated with facial paresis, hyperacusis, unilateral loss of taste, decrease in lacrimation and salivation and otalgia.
James Ramsay Hunt (1874–1937), Professor of Neurology, Columbia University, New York, USA.

Rathke's pouch: diverticulum of roof of stomodaeum which forms the anterior pituitary gland.
Martin Heinrich Rathke (1793–1860), Professor of Zoology and Anatomy, Königsberg, Germany.

Reidel's lobe: supernumerary lobe projecting from right lobe of the liver.
Bernhard Reidel (1846–1916), Professor of Surgery, Jena, Germany.

Reinke's: crystals – rod-shaped crystals in the interstitial cells of the testis and hilus cells of the ovary;
space – chronic laryngitis with swelling of the membranous part of the vocal cords.
Friedrich Berthold Reinke (1862–1919), anatomist, France.

Reissner's membrane: the vestibular membrane of the cochlea.
Ernst Reissner (1824–1878), Professor of Anatomy in Dorpat and then Breslau.

Renshaw's cells: inhibitory interneurones modulating the response of anterior horn cells.
Birdsy Renshaw (1911–1948), neurologist, USA.

Retzius' lines (or striae): brown lines in the dental enamel.
Gustav Magnus Retzius (1842–1919), Professor of Anatomy, Carolinska Institute, Stockholm, Sweden. (Son of Andreas Adolf Retzius 1796–1860, who described the cave of Retzius – the retropubic space – also Professor of Anatomy, Carolinska.)

Rexed's lamina: subdivisions of cells of spinal cord grey matter.
Bror Rexed (1914–?), neuroanatomist, Sweden.

Riolan, arc of: the anastomosis between the middle and left colic arteries.
Jean Riolan (secundus) 1577–1657, Professor of Anatomy and Botany, Paris, France. A great teacher, but rejected the doctrines of William Harvey. Son of Jean Riolan (primus) of Paris.

Rohr's stria: layer of placenta.
Karl Rohr (1863–?), embryologist and gynaecologist, Berne, Switzerland.

Rosenmüller, fossa of: the pharyngeal recess.
Johann Christian Rosenmüller (1779–1820), Professor of Anatomy and Surgery, Leipzig, Germany.

Rosenthal's canal: spiral canal of the cochlea.
Friedrich Christian Rosenthal (1779–1829), Professor of Anatomy, Greifswald, Germany.

Rotter's node: lymph node between pectoralis major and minor.
Josef Rotter (1857–1924), surgeon, Germany.

Ruffini endings (bodies, corpuscles): sensory nerve endings, originally described in skin of fingers.
Angelo Ruffini (1887–1929), Professor of Histology, Bologna, Italy.

Santorini: duct of – the accessory pancreatic duct;
fissures of – two fissures in the anterior cartilaginous wall of the external acoustic meatus;
plexus of – retropubic venous plexus giving rise to pudendal vein.
Giovanni Domenico Santorini (1681–1737), Professor of Medicine and Anatomy, Venice, Italy.

Scarpa's: fascia – the fibrous layer of the superficial fascia of the lower abdomen;
ganglion – the vestibular ganglion.
Antonio Scarpa (1747–1832), Professor of Anatomy, Padua, Italy.

Schlemm, canal of: canal at junction of the cornea and sclera.
Freidrich Schlemm (1795–1858), Professor of Anatomy, Berlin, Germany.

Schmidt–Lanterman incisure or cleft: helical inclusion of glial cytoplasm within the myelin sheath of central and peripheral nerves
Henry Schmidt (1823–1888), pathologist, Charity Hospital, New Orleans, USA.
A J Lanterman (19th Century), anatomist, Strasbourg, France.

Schwann cells: the major glial cell of the peripheral nervous system.
Theodor Schwann (1810–1882), Professor of Anatomy first in Louvain and then Liege, Belgium. One of the instigators of the cell theory.

Schutz's fasciculus: the dorsal longitudinal fasciculus.
Hugo Shutz, neurologist, Leipzig, Germany

Scoog's fibres: transverse fibres of the palmar aponeurosis of the hand.
Tord Skoog (1915–1977), Foundation Professor of Plastic Surgery, University of Uppsala, Sweden.

Sertoli cells: supporting cells of the testicular tubules.
Enrico Sertoli (1842–1910), Professor of Experimental Physiology, Milan, Italy.

Sharpey's fibres: connective tissue joining periosteum to bone.
William Sharpey (1802–1880), Professor of Anatomy successively in Edinburgh and University College, London, UK.

Stahl's deformity: congenital deformity of the ear – broad helix, fossa of the antihelix and upper scaphoid fossa are both absent.
Friedrich Stahl (1811–1879), Physician, Germany.

Stensen's duct: the parotid duct.
Niels Stensen (1638–1686), Professor of Anatomy, Copenhagen, Denmark. Demonstrated the parotid duct at the age of 23.

Struther, ligament of: fibrous band (occasionally ossified) running between medial epicondyle and shaft of the humerus.
Sir John Struthers (1823–1899), Professor of Anatomy, Aberdeen, UK. An authority on the anatomy of whales.

Sylvian: aqueduct – midbrain channel connecting the third and fourth cerebral ventricles;
fissure – the lateral cerebral fissure.
François de la Boe Sylvius (1614–1672), Professor of Medicine, Leyden, The Netherlands.

Tenon's capsule: fascial sheath of the eyeball.
Jaques René Tenon (1724–1816), Professor of Pathology, Academy of Sciences, Paris, France. Chief Surgeon, Salpetrière, Paris. Specialized in ophthalmology.

Testut's ligament: radio-scaphoid-lunate connection.
Leo Testut (1849–1925), Professor of Anatomy, Lyons, France.

Thebesian: valve – valve at orifice of coronary sinus;
veins – venae cordis minimae of heart.
Adam Christian Thebesius (1686–1732), anatomist and pathologist, Leyden, The Netherlands.

Todaro, tendon of: a variable tendinous strand attached to the valvular fold at the termination of the inferior vena cava. It forms the superior border of the triangle of Koch.
Francesco Todaro (1839–1918), Professor of Anatomy at Messina and then Rome, Italy.

Towne's projection: positioning of the head in the radiological examination of the foramen magnum and posterior cranial fossa.
Edward Towne (1883–1957), neurosurgeon, Stanford Medical School, USA.

Treitz, ligament of: 'suspensory' ligament of peritoneum passing from the right crus of the diaphragm to the fourth part of the duodenum.
Wenzel Treitz (1819–1872), Professor of Pathology successively at Cracow and Prague, Czechoslovakia.

Trendelenburg's sign: dipping gait due to hip abductor dysfunction, e.g. in congenital dislocation of the hip or paralysis of gluteus medius and minimus.
Freidrich Trendelenburg (1844–1924), Professor of Surgery successively at Rostock, Bonn and Leipzig, Germany.

Treves, bloodless fold of: peritoneal fold adjacent to mesoappendix.
Sir Frederick Treves (1853–1923), surgeon, London Hospital, UK. Drained the appendix abscess of King Edward VII in 1902.

Valsalva, aortic sinuses of: the aortic sinuses.
Antonio Maria Valsalva (1666–1723), Professor of Anatomy, Bologna, Italy.

Vater, ampulla of: ampulla at junction of common hepatic and pancreatic ducts.
Abraham Vater (1684–1751), Professor of Anatomy, Botany, Pathology and Therapeutics, Wittenburg, Germany.

Vesalius sphenoidal emissary foramen: small foramen for emissary vein immediately anterior and medial to the foramen ovale in the sphenoid bone.
Andreas Vesalius (1514–1564), Professor of Anatomy, Padua, Italy. In 1543 published De Humani Corporis Fabrica, the most famous text of anatomy.

Vidian nerve: nerve of the pterygoid canal.
Guido Guidi Vidius (1500–1561), Professor of Medicine, Pisa, Italy.

Vieussens, anulus of: ansa subclavia of sympathetic nerves.
Raymond de Vieussens (1641–1715), physician and anatomist, Montpellier, France.

Virchow–Robin space: perivascular space in the central nervous system.
Rudolf Ludwig Virchow (1821–1902), Professor of Pathological Anatomy, Würzburg and then Berlin, Germany.
Charles Filippe Robin (1821–1885), Professor of Histology, Paris, France.

Voigt lines: the hair tracts
Christian August Voigt (1809–1890), Professor of Anatomy, Vienna, Austria.

Voit's nerve: branch of the vestibulocochlear nerve that supplies the saccule.
Max Voit (1876–1920), Professor of Anatomy, Göttingen, Germany.

Volkmann's canals: osseous canals carrying blood vessels from the periosteum.
Alfred Wilhelm Volkmann (1800–1877), Professor of Anatomy and Physiology first at Dorpat and later Halle.

Von Brunn's nests: ectopic (subepithelial) urothelial masses in the urinary tract.
Albert Von Brunn (1849–1872), Professor of Anatomy, Göttingen, Germany.

Waldeyer's: sheath – adventitia of distal segments of the ureter; **ring** – a ring of lymphoid tissue which includes the palatine, pharyngeal, tubal and lingual tonsils.
Heinrich Wilhelm Waldeyer (1836–1921), Professor of Pathology at Breslau and then Berlin, Germany.

Wallenberg's syndrome: lesion of the lateral medullary region of the brain stem.
Adolf Wallenberg (1862–1949), physician, Germany.

Wernicke's speech area: motor speech area in superior temporal lobe of cerebral cortex.
Karl Wernicke (1848–1904), Psychiatrist at Breslau and then Halle, Germany.

Wharton's: duct – duct of the submandibular salivary gland; **jelly** – the gelatinous connective tissue of the umbilical cord.
Thomas Wharton (1616 ? –1673), Physician, St Thomas' Hospital, London, UK. Remained on duty there during the Great Plague of 1665.

Whitnall's tubercle: tubercle on the orbital surface of the zygomatic bone.
Samuel Ernest Whitnall (1876–1950), Professor of Anatomy successively at McGill University, Montreal, Canada, and Bristol, UK.

Wiebel–Palade bodies: rod-shaped storage granules in endothelial cells.
Euald Wiebel (contemporary), physician, Switzerland.
George Emil Palade (contemporary), born in Romania, cytologist, Rockefeller Institute, New York, USA, Nobel Prize for Medicine, 1974.

Willis, circle of: the arterial anastomosis at the base of the brain.
Thomas Willis (1621–1675), physician to King James II, practised first in Oxford, then London, UK.

Winslow, foramen of: the epiploic foramen leading to the lesser sac.
Jacob Winslow (1669–1760), Professor of Anatomy and Surgery, Paris, France.

Wrisberg's ligament: band attached to posterior cruciate ligament of the knee.
Heinrich August Wrisberg (1739–1808), Professor of Anatomy, Göttingen, Germany.

Wolffian: body – the mesonephros; **duct** – the mesonephric duct.
Caspar Wolff (1733–1794), born in Berlin, Professor of Anatomy, St Petersburg, Russia, one of the pioneers of embryology.

Zinn, circle (or zonula) of: hyaloid membrane adjacent to the margin of the lens.
Johann Gottfried Zinn (1727–1759), Professor of Medicine and Director of Botanical Gardens, Göttingen, Germany.

Zuckerkandl's fascia: the retrorenal fascia.
Emil Zuckerkandl (1849–1910), Professor of Anatomy at Graz and then Vienna, Austria.

Many of the eponyms listed above are described in more detail in Firkin BG, Whitworth JA 2001 Dictionary of Medical Eponyms. London: Parthenon.

Subject Index

stratum (strata) (*Cont'd*)
corneum 171
of skin 32, 157, 160
deep, of fascia lata 1420
endometrial 1344
granulosum 1388
of skin 157, 160, 160f
lacunosum 407, 407f, 408
lemnisci 346
lucidum 407, 407f
of skin 157, 159f, 160
moleculare 407, 407f, 408
oriens 407, 407f
pyramidalis 407, 407f
radiatum 407, 407f
spinosum, of skin 157, 160
spongiosum, of uterus 1335
superficial, of fascia lata 1420
of tympanic membrane 654–655
zonale 369
see also layer(s); zone(s)
streak, primitive 241, 1340
epithelial–mesenchyme transition 203
formation 192, 193–194
ingression 194, 194f, 206
'streak gonads' 1388
stria(e)
albae 174
fibrinoid 1345
of Gennari 393, 403
gravidarum 174, 1349
longitudinal 266f, 267
medullaris 291, 328, 335f, 339, 384
Nitabuch's 1345
olfactory 432
of olfactory tract 264
rubrae 174
terminalis 287, 288, 369, 379, 421
vascularis, of cochlear duct 671
striation, cross, teeth 596, 597f
striatopallidal system, ventral, projections from amygdala 410
striatum 410f, 419, 420f, **423–427**
afferents and terminals of 423, 424
amygdaloid projections to 410
connections 423–424, 424f
development 264, 423
dorsal 421, 423
afferents to 423–424
connections 423, 425f
efferents 424, 426f
efferents 423, 424, 424f, 425f, 426
neurones 423
ventral 410, 421, 423
afferents to 424–425, 425f, 426f
aminergic inputs 425
connections 423
continuity with dorsal striatum 424, 425
efferents 426, 426f, 427f
see also nucleus (nuclei – nervous), accumbens; tubercle(s), olfactory
see also nucleus, caudate; putamen
stridor, ventilatory 984
striola
of saccule 669
of utricle 668
strip
dorsal, of metacarpals 899, 900
palmar, of metacarpals 899, 900
stripe
aortopulmonary 979
Hensen's 673
para-tracheal 979
posterior tracheal 980

stroke 232, 303, 321–322
stroma
of bone marrow 78
of breast 970
ciliary 707–708
of cornea 703–704
endometrial 1334
of ovary 1386
strut, pterygomaxillary 525
subcortex, connections, somatosensory cortex 399
subglottis 639
infant 640
in speech 644
subiculum 407–408
juxtallocortex 405
projections 408, 408f, 410
subluxation, vertebral ligaments 756
submucosa 41, 1139
anal 1210
of appendix 1173
of hard palate 583
of large intestine 1173
of oesophagus 989
oral 582
of small intestine **1160–1161**
of stomach 1155
subnucleus
caudalis 336
interpolaris 336
oralis 336
rectus 345
substance, perforated
anterior 264, 422f
posterior 342, 375
substance P (SP) 50, 590
globus pallidus 427
striatum 423
substantia
gelatinosa 307, 309, 319–320
nigra 49, 342f, 343f, 344, 427–428
development 260, 262
organization 425f
pars compacta 424, 424f, 425f, 427–428
connections 425f
degeneration in Parkinson's disease 428
pars lateralis 427
pars reticulata 419–420, 425f, 427
efferents 428
striatal efferents to 424, 424f, 425f, 426, 426f
propria (cornea) 703–704, 704f
subthalamus 231, **383–384**, 383f
development 262
sucking, in neonate 269–270
difficulties 270
suckling, oral cavity spaces 611
sulcus (sulci) 87–88
antihelicis transversus 650
calcanei 1513
carotid 465
of cerebellum 353
of cerebral hemispheres 231, **387–389**, 387f, 388f
anterior parolfactory 388
calcarine 388–389, 403
development 266
callosal 388
central 387, 388, 399, 416
development 266
neonates 269
cingulate 388
collateral 387f, 389
development 265f, 266
inferior polar 403

inferior temporal 400
insular 401
intraparietal 399
lateral occipital 403
lunate 403
medial frontal 388
neonatal 269
occipitotemporal 387f, 389
olfactory 389
orbital 389
paracentral 388
parieto-occipital 266, 388, 399
postcentral 399
development 266
posterior parolfactory 388
precentral 396
development 266
rhinal 389
superior polar 403
superior temporal 263f, 400
transverse occipital 403
chiasmatis 462, 465
coronary 946
cruciform 343
fimbriodentate 406
gingival 582, 595
hippocampal 406
development 264
hypothalamic 260, 261f, 288, 369
infraorbital 690
interligamentous 904
intermedius (stomach) 1143
intertuberous 823
labiogingival 611
limitans 291
development 244, 252f, 255
linguogingival 611, 613
malleolar 470
of medulla oblongata
posterolateral 328
ventrolateral 328
nasolabial 497, 507f
olfactory 431
optic 721
paramedian, of cerebellum 353
preauricular, of ilium 1426, 1431
sagittal 461
superior 464
for sagittal sinus 472
sclerae 702
sigmoid 463, 468
of spinal cord
median, posterior 775
posterolateral 775–776
ventral median 307
spiral
external 671
internal 671
terminalis 288f, 421, 584, 614, 999, 1000
transverse 463, 464
tubae 466
tympanic 470, 651, 654
see also groove(s)
summation
spatial 228
temporal 228
summit
of articular eminence 526
of trapezium 896
sunburn 160
'superficial' 3
superficial musculo-aponeurotic system (SMAS) 499
'superior' 3
supination (movement) 882, 902
muscles involved 902
supraglottis 637–638
infant 640
in speech 645

surface(s)
articular
movement **130**, 131, 132f
ovoid 127
shape of **127–128**, 127f, 128f
of synovial joints **108–109**
basal, epithelium 29
of bladder 1289
buccal 590
cellular 5
of heart 996f, 997, **999**, 999f, 1000f
of humerus 823–824, 823f, 824f
of ilium 1426
labial 590
lingual 590
of liver 1214–1216, 1214f
respiratory *see* alveolus (alveoli)
of scapula 819f, 820
of spleen 1239
stellar 127
of stomach 1144, 1144f, 1145f
temporal, of frontal bone 472
volar, of nail 168
surface anatomy *see specific anatomical structures*
surfactant 1062
composition 1062
production
Clara cells 1057, 1062
development 1089
storage 1062
surgical procedures and approaches
access to peritoneal spaces 1136
adenoidectomy 621
ankle arthroscopy 1417
ankle aspiration 1417
ankle injection 1417
aortic 1119–1120, 1122
of appendix, iliohypogastric nerve injury 1124
arthroscopy 1417
axillary abscess incision 817
axillary lymph node dissection 971
axillary lymph node sampling 971
bleeding from superior epigastric vessels 1101
breast conservation 972
breast reconstruction 973
caecostomy 1100
calcaneonavicular bar resection 1537
cannulation
bile duct 1229
femoral vein 1413
internal jugular vein 948
subclavian vein 948
upper arm arteries 812
cardiac, phrenic nerve injury 1084
caroticocavernous sinus fistula 280
chest drain insertion 949
choledochoduodenostomy 1163
cisternal puncture 730–731
colonic resection, vascular ligation 1181
colostomy 1100
commissurotomy 414, 415
cordotomy, dorsolateral 316
coronary angiography 1018
coronary revascularization 1018
corpus callosum division 414, 415, 416f
craniofacial 497
craniotomy, frontotemporal 491
cricothyroid puncture 444
deltoid-splitting, posterior 848
distraction osteogenesis 487
ear surgery
endaural approach 652
inner ear 678
permeatal approach 651